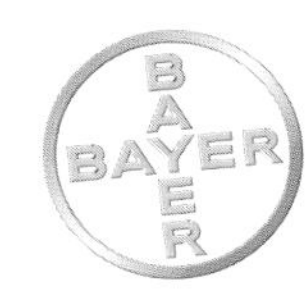

Bayer HealthCare
Animal Health Division

Bayer HealthCare LLC
Animal Health Division
P.O. Box 390
Shawnee Mission
KS 66201-0390

Phone: 913 268 2000
Fax: 913 268 2803

www.bayerDVM.com

Dear Veterinary Student,

What a worthwhile decision you've made to dedicate your talent and energy to the health of animals. At Bayer, we believe the potential for the profession to grow is unlimited, especially when we all work together to keep it alive and well.

With that goal in mind, we'd like to welcome you to the profession by providing you with this complimentary seventh edition of the Compendium of Veterinary Products. The CVP is a valuable in-clinic tool, providing pharmacologic data and label references for products prescribed by veterinarians. As a sponsor for all seven editions, we have been told it is one of the most useful references for veterinary students and professionals alike.

Now, you can also access the CVP online at BayerDVM.com for quick reference, new product information and label updates. Simply select the Resources button from the main menu for the latest product references.

At Bayer, we have not only made it a tradition to keep the veterinary profession strong—we have made it a commitment that extends well into the future with ongoing contributions to veterinary organizations, research, leadership and education.

Most of all, we share your goal of improving the lives of animals and people. And our very best wishes go out to you as you continue your journey.

Sincerely,

Cary Christensen

Cary Christensen, DVM
Director, Veterinary Services

The Compendium of Veterinary Products is produced, printed and published by **North American Compendiums, Ltd.** for distribution by **North American Compendiums, Inc.**

ISBN1-889750-48-4

Printed in Canada

Library of Congress Card Number: 97-643262

Bayer HealthCare
Animal Health Division

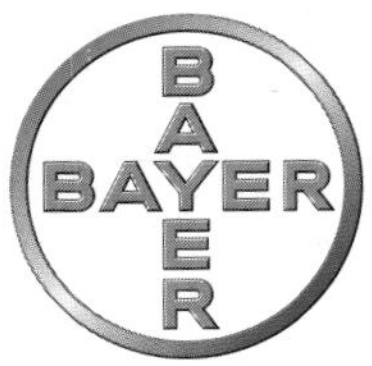

Bayer HealthCare LLC
Animal Health Division
P.O. Box 390
Shawnee Mission
KS 66201-0390

Phone: 913 268 2000
Fax: 913 268 2803

www.bayerDVM.com

Dear Doctor,

The outlook for veterinary medicine is exciting. New technologies and medical options make our food supply safer and help pets live longer, healthier lives. The potential for the veterinary profession to grow is unlimited, especially when we all make a dedicated commitment.

This 7th edition of the *Compendium of Veterinary Products* marks Bayer's 14th year as a sponsor of *CVP*. There was no question about our continued support. We've sponsored all seven editions and we still believe the *CVP* is one of the most useful references for veterinary professionals and students alike.

At Bayer, we're committed to keeping the veterinary profession strong by helping to educate animal owners about the benefits of regular visits with their veterinarians. Bayer's ongoing support for the profession extends to conventions, continuing education seminars, leadership programs, educational symposia, veterinary schools and students. We are dedicated to keeping the veterinary associations healthy, as well, with contributions for the companion animal, equine, livestock and poultry fields.

Most of all, we at Bayer share your commitment to improving the lives of animals and their owners. Our thanks go out to you, not only for your support of Bayer products, but for the differences you make for animals and people.

Sincerely,

John B. Payne

John B. Payne
President & General Manager, North America

Table of Contents

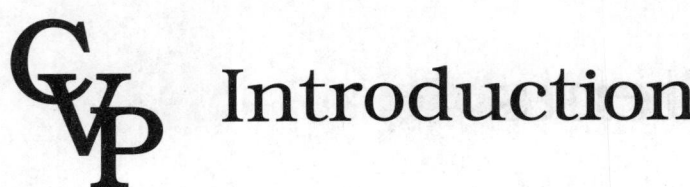

Introduction

FOREWORD

This, the seventh edition of the Compendium of Veterinary Products (CVP), is published in the interest of better communications within the American animal health industry.

COPYRIGHT © 2003

UPDATES ON THE WEB

It's easy to keep up to date with the latest product information.

Visit www.naccvp.com and click on "USA CVP Update".

You will have access to new and changed products, as well as notation of those products discontinued by the manufacturer since November 2002. This is a free service.

DISCLAIMER

Every effort has been made to ensure the accuracy of the information published. However, it remains the responsibility of the readers to familiarize themselves with the product information contained on the product label or package insert.

Inclusion or omission of products does not imply endorsement or criticism by the Publisher or anyone involved in the publication. Inclusion does not imply product availability and/or product registration. Inclusion of editorial articles does not imply endorsement by the organizations who have supplied the material. The Publisher, Editorial Team and all those involved in the production of the Compendium of Veterinary Products cannot be held responsible for publication errors or any consequence that could result from the use of published information.

CD ROM SUBSCRIPTIONS

Products appearing in this seventh edition of the Compendium of Veterinary Products are available on CD ROM for $95.00 plus $8.50 postage and handling.

BOOK SUBSCRIPTIONS

Copies of the CVP are available for $95.00 plus $8.50 postage and handling.

Send check to:

North American Compendiums, Inc.
942 Military Street
Port Huron, MI 48060

Telephone: 810-985-5028
Fax: 810-985-5190
Order Desk: 800-350-0627

or visit our e-commerce site at www.naccvp.com to view all of our products and services.

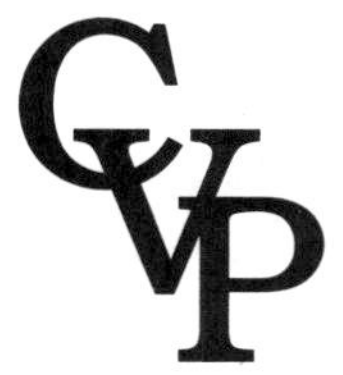

Publisher's Message

We are pleased to present the Seventh Edition of the Compendium of Veterinary Products.

Once again we have worked closely with the manufacturers of pharmaceuticals, biologicals, pesticides and feed additives to bring to our subscribers the most complete set of product data available.

We do not charge for publishing this information. This ensures that we include all products, not just those with major promotional budgets.

Our editorial staff headed by Shirley Inglis, RVT, Dawn Stahle, BBA and Jessie-Lee Schwartz have done a remarkable job in assembling the information. My thanks to them, also our Production Manager Michael Woodley and our printers.

More than ever we believe this reference book will be valuable to all practicing veterinarians, particularly those working with food animals.

We will continue to offer updates at no charge. Please visit our web site at www.naccvp.com and click on "USA CVP Updates". This is a list of changes made since we went to press (November 2002).

Product label information is available on CD ROM and will be accessible in the spring of 2003 on the Internet. Please contact us for more information.

We ask you to mail the subscription registration form found on the last page of this book so that we may contact you with any substantial changes. This edition contains over 4,700 products and numerous indexes.

We welcome any suggestions and criticisms. Please address them to my attention at adrian@naccvp.com .

Adrian J. Bayley, Publisher

North American Compendiums, Inc.
942 Military Street
Port Huron, MI 48060

Telephone:	810-985-5028	Canadian Office:	519-263-3000
Fax:	810-985-5190		519-263-2936

e-mail adrian@naccvp.com

General Considerations

Product Protocol

We have attempted to present as complete a list of animal health products as possible. It should be understood that the protocol for product inclusion was designed as follows:

There is no charge for product listings.

In order to be included, a product must fall under one or more of the following criteria:

1. Pharmaceutical products approved by FDA which have a New Animal Drug Application (NADA) Number, or an Abbreviated New Animal Drug Application (ANADA) Number.
2. Biological and diagnostic products approved by the United States Department of Agriculture (USDA) and manufactured by a licensed establishment.
3. Pesticides and disinfectants approved by the Environmental Protection Agency (EPA) which have an EPA registration number and are used by the veterinary profession.
4. Feed additives or premixes that hold the original NADA or ANADA number.
5. Products that fall within the above criteria which are either sold to veterinarians and/or over the counter (OTC).
6. Products sold exclusively to veterinarians.
7. Products that are sold under private labels and fit the above criteria.

The data updating process

In order to ensure complete and accurate product listings, we are in contact with industry manufacturers and distributors on a continuing basis. To make sure we have included new product lines, we network at industry conferences and trade shows, review government publications, industry journals and web sites. Manufacturers supply product labels and inserts for entry into our database. Label information is captured in a standard format facilitating easy reading by the user.

Disclaimer

Every effort has been made to ensure the accuracy of the information published. However, it remains the responsibility of the readers to familiarize themselves with the product information contained on the product label or package insert.

Inclusion or omission of products does not imply endorsement or criticism by the Publisher or anyone involved in the publication. Inclusion does not imply product availability and/or product registration. Inclusion of editorial articles does not imply endorsement by the organizations who have supplied the material. The Publisher, Editorial Team and all those involved in the production of this publication, cannot be held responsible for publication errors or any consequence that could result from the use of published information.

Missing Products

We will continue to update the contents of this publication. Readers are invited and encouraged to notify the Publisher about products and manufacturers that they feel should be included in the next edition.

Visit www.naccvp.com and click on USA CVP Update.
The site has product label information for new and changed products, and lists products that have been discontinued since publication, November 2002.

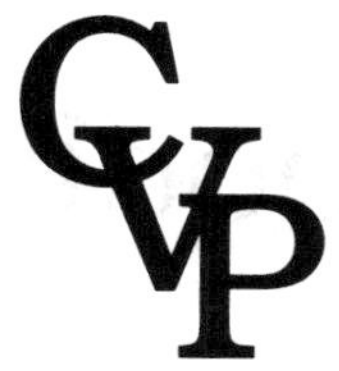

Editorial Message

Welcome to the Seventh Edition of the Compendium of Veterinary Products (CVP). This edition is full of all the new and updated product information that you've come to expect of our first class publication.

Once again, improvements to various sections have been instituted. The Withdrawal Time Charts have been shortened to now include only "Notes" that contain actual withdrawal statements. Also, please refer to our Product Category Index, formerly the Therapeutic Index. This section has been re-organized to reflect in a more straightforward and useful manner, the various categories of products available. Label reference numbers have been included on many of the monographs to aid the updating process.

Would you like to see other product categories added to the CVP? For instance, would nutraceuticals and other alternative medicines exclusively sold by veterinarians have a place in the book? Do you have other product category suggestions for us? Don't hesitate to let us know your suggestions plus any feedback about this edition. Please write to us at the address listed below, or email us at adrian@naccvp.com.

Again we offer our Internet Update Service. Please visit www.nacccvp.com and click on the "USA CVP Update" to read about updates, deletions, additions and erratum since this book went to print (November 2002).

If you would find viewing product label information on your computer helpful, we have subscriptions available to the CVP on CD. See our Introduction on page 6 for more details.

Those responsible for the successful outcome of this edition include: Mike Woodley (Production and Database Manager); Dawn Stahle, BBA (Editorial Assistant); Jessie-Lee Schwartz (Editorial Assistant); Shirley Inglis, RVT (Associate Editor); Douglas White, BA, MA (IT Manager); Pam Ross (Administrative Coordinator); and our Publisher, Adrian Bayley.

North American Compendiums, Inc.
942 Military Street
Port Huron, MI 48060
800-350-0627

What is in the book

The page opposite has been designed so that it may easily be photocopied. We invite you to complete the questionnaire, thereby using every section of the book. We believe this very useful exercise will enable you to fully understand the effectiveness of our various indexes.

and how to use it

1. Name a pharmaceutical that you use on a regular basis. Trade Name ______________________________ (preferably an antibiotic).

2. Go to the Product Index (pages 2415 to 2448 at the back of the book) and find the product.
   The product monograph appears on page # ______
   Manufacturer ______________________________

3. Go to the Manufacturer/Distributor Index (pages 35 to 84 at the front of the book) and find another product that they make.
   Trade Name ______________________________
   The product monograph appears on page # ______

4. Go back to question 2, look up the product in the main section of the book (pages 1001 to 2414).
   What is the general classification (on the right, opposite the Manufacturer's name) of the product?
   ____

5. Find one ingredient in the product. ______________________________

6. Go to the green section and find that ingredient (in bold type). Are there any other products with the same ingredient(s)? ______________________________

7. At the beginning of the pink pages you will find a summary of the Product Category Index. Using your answer to question 4, find the most suitable heading, and the page on which it appears. Page # ______

8. Look for the heading in the Product Category Index, find the product you have chosen in question 1.
   Name another product in the same group. Trade name ______________________________

9. If the product you have chosen is for use in large animals, it may have a withdrawal time. Please look in the yellow pages and find the product you have chosen.
   What is its route of administration? ______________________________

10. Name a vaccine you use on a regular basis. Trade Name ______________________________

11. Go to the main text (pages 1001 to 2414) and find the product. The product appears on page # ______

12. What is the general classification of the vaccine? (on the right, opposite the Manufacturer's name) ________
    In which species is it used? ______________________________

13. Turn to the blue pages and find the species in which the product is used (page heading).
    Page # ______

14. Find the corresponding antigens in the Biological Chart. Follow those columns downwards until you find an 'M' or a 'K' in them. Now follow the line directly to the left and you will find the product you have chosen. Other products with the same antigens will be found above or below the chosen product.

    Name another biological that contains the same antigens ______________________________

American Veterinary Distributors Association (AVDA)

Members

Established in 1976, the American Veterinary Distributors Association (AVDA) is the national trade organization for businesses engaged in the distribution of animal health products.

Active membership is open to firms whose primary business is the wholesale distribution of animal health products. Associate membership is open to manufacturers of animal health products.

There are 26 Active Members (distributors) and 28 Associate Members (manufacturers) and 2 Affiliate Members (distributor buying groups). Active members currently service and sell to over 20,000 veterinary clinics and 40,000 practicing veterinarians on a regular basis, handling many thousands of product lines, and representing more than 500 manufacturers.

Objectives

Some of the objectives of the Association are:

- To further sound business principles in all phases of veterinary product distribution
- To acquire and disseminate business information of value to the veterinary product distribution industry
- To promote and encourage the use of wholesale distributors by veterinarians and veterinary product manufacturers
- To enhance the relationship between veterinary manufacturers, distributors and veterinarians in order to create better communications within the animal health industry
- To assist its members and the veterinary product distribution industry through research and education, in the process of continually improving the distribution of animal health products

Annual Conference

AVDA conducts an annual conference each year featuring speakers, panels and workshops on topics related to the veterinary distribution industry and the management of distributor businesses. National authorities from the industry, government and the academic world take part.

National Association of Wholesalers/Distributors

AVDA is actively affiliated with the National Association of Wholesalers/Distributors (NAW), an organization of more than 120 national wholesaler/distributor trade associations, which collectively represent more than 45,000 wholesaler/distributor firms.

Government Affairs

AVDA serves as a source of information for its member companies on federal and state regulatory and legislative matters that may have impact on their businesses, and from time to time, presents the animal health distribution industry's point of view to legislative and regulatory bodies.

AVDA Members

Bradley Caldwell, Inc.
200 Kiwanis Blvd.
Hazleton, PA 18202

Burns Veterinary Supply
1900 Diplomat Drive
Farmers Branch, TX 75234

The Butler Company
5600 Blazer Parkway
Dublin, OH 43017

Columbus Serum Company
2025 South High Street
Columbus, OH 43207

Great Western Animal Health Supply, Inc.
8433 Washington Place
Albuquerque, NM 87113

Henry Schein Inc.
135 Duryea Rd.
Melville, NY 11747

Lextron, Inc.
PO Box 1240
620 "O" Street
Greeley, CO 80632

Merritt Veterinary Supplies, Inc.
1520 Pineview Road
Columbia, SC 29209

MWI Veterinary Supply Co.
2201 N 20th Street
P.O. Box 47
Nampa, ID 83687

Micro Beef Technologies, Ltd.
P.O. Box 9262
Amarillo, TX 79105

Midwest Veterinary Supply
11965 Larc Industrial Blvd.
Burnsville, MN 55337

Milburn Distributors, Inc.
P.O. Box 42810
Phoenix, AZ 85080

Miller Veterinary Supply Co., Inc.
P.O. Box 470
Fort Worth, TX 76101-0470

Nelson Laboratories
4001 N. Lewis Ave.
Sioux Falls, SD 57104

NLS Animal Health
11407 Cronhill Drive
Owings Mills, MD 21117

Northland Veterinary Supply, Inc.
151 Deposition Dr.
Clear Lake, WI 54005

Northwest Vet Supply, Inc.
P.O. Box 1841
Enid, OK 73702

PCI Animal Health
120 Apollo Street
Brooklyn, NY 11222

R & S Pharma
701 Columbia Ave.
Glasgow, KY 412141

Robert J. Matthews Co.
2850 Nave Road, SE
Massillon, OH 44646-9610

Vet Direct
P.O. Box 1217
Caldwell, ID 83605

Vet Pharm, Inc.
392 15th St. N.E.
Sioux Center, IA 51250

Vetpo Distributors
184 W. 64th Street
Holland, MI 49423

Walco International
P.O. Box 307
East Highway 60
Friona, TX 79035

Webster Veterinary Supply
86 Leonminister Road
Sterling, MA 01564

AVDA Associate Members

ABAXIS
Abbott Laboratories
Addison Biological Laboratory, Inc.
Bayer Animal Health Division
Biocor Animal Health
Boehringer Ingelheim Vetmedica, Inc.
Colorado Serum
DermaPet, Inc.
DVM Pharmaceuticals
Elanco Animal Health
Fort Dodge Animal Health
Innovative Veterinary Diets
Intervet Inc.
Jorgensen Laboratories, Inc.
Kane Enterprises, Inc.
King Animal Health
MAI/Genesis
Merial
Neogen Corporation
Nestlé Purina Petcare
Pharmacia Animal Health
PRN Pharmacal
Schering-Plough Animal Health
Synbiotics Corp.
Tyco Healthcare-Kendall
Veterinary Product Laboratories (VPL)
Virbac
Welch Allyn, Inc.

AVDA Affiliate Members

AgriLabs
Phoenix Pharmaceutical, Inc.

American Veterinary Distributors Association

2105 Laurel Bush Road,
Suite 200
Bel Air, MD 21015

Telelephone: 443-640-1040
Fax: 443-640-1031
www.avda.net

Animal Health Institute (AHI)

The animal health industry continues to demonstrate an ability to adapt and innovate to meet the challenges of the day. During the past year the industry, through the Animal Health Institute, has undertaken a number of initiatives to meet the regulatory and marketplace challenges it faces.

The New World Order

The tragic events of September 11 have altered our way of thinking and doing business. Events that once were inconceivable are now possible eventualities that require planning and preparation.

The impact on the animal health industry is as great as that on any industry. While the focus of the industry has been on working with our customers to prevent the accidental introduction and spread of animal disease, we are now faced with the challenge of working with our customers to think through ways of preventing the intentional introduction of disease.

This new reality also requires increased awareness and willingness to work with law enforcement. For example, increased security in the production of important vaccines to prevent animal health and economic disasters, such as anthrax and foot and mouth disease, must be carefully monitored so that the master cultures used to create these biologicals cannot be used for terrorist activities. Moreover, it is now commonplace, in instances when an outbreak of a new or unusual animal disease is encountered, for law enforcement authorities to ask questions as to the possibility that the outbreak did not occur naturally.

Product Availability

Recognizing the tremendous need for more approved animal medicines to treat sick animals and enhance food production, AHI has made availability of new drugs and vaccines a top priority. A severe backlog in new product reviews at the Center for Veterinary Medicine (CVM) has been a major impediment to our efforts to supply veterinarians and livestock and poultry producers with the steady supply of new and innovative products they rely upon.

Following enactment of the Animal Drug Availability Act in 1996, there was temporary improvement in the review process at CVM. In recent years, however, progress has been reversed, and a severe backlog has developed. Contributing to the problem has been CVM's 1999 announcement of a new framework for evaluating the potential for antibiotic resistance during the approval process. The uncertainty raised by the proposed framework has contributed to an unnavigable maze in the review process.

The current situation with respect to product approval is similar to that faced by the human pharmaceutical industry more than 10 years ago. At that time, the human pharmaceutical industry developed a proposal to provide additional resources to the Food and Drug Administration through user fees in exchange for performance standards that are imposed on the agency. By all measures, the proposal, called the Prescription Drug User Fee Act (PDUFA) has worked well to improve the pace of review of new drug applications. One testament to the success of the program is that Congress has reauthorized it for the second time.

Building on the success of PDUFA, the animal health industry and the Center for Veterinary Medicine have discussed a similar package of performance standards and user fees for animal drugs. A more efficient and predictable review process would create additional incentives for companies to invest research and development dollars on new and innovative products.

Ensuring Continued, Safe Use of Antibiotics

The long-running debate about the use of antibiotics in food animals and the potential for antibiotic resistance has intensified lately. The CVM's proposed withdrawal of fluoroquinolones from use in chickens and turkeys and the organization of consumer groups have elevated the debate.

Antibiotic resistance is an important public health issue. Indeed, there have been numerous reports of growing drug resistance in hospital settings, and among various hospital- and community-acquired infections - none of which are related in any way to animal use of antibiotics.

The debate as it relates to animal use is over the extent to which antibiotic resistant food borne infections arise due to animal administration of antibiotics. In response to the attention and debate over the past several decades, the animal health industry has adopted and cooperated in a number of activities to monitor the potential for antibiotic resistance to arise and implement steps to reduce the potential. Data from a variety of sources indicates these steps are working.

- Since 1996, the federal government, through the National Antimicrobial Resistance Monitoring System (NARMS), has been tracking the trends of resistant bacteria in both humans and animals. This monitoring was implemented as an early warning system against increases in resistance levels that required a management response. Since this surveillance began, the trends in antibiotic resistance in bacteria in humans have generally declined, demonstrating there is not a public health crisis for resistant food borne pathogens. Salmonella resistance to one or more antimicrobials decreased by 30 percent between 1996 and 2000 and Campylobacter resistance decreased by 17 percent between 1997 and 2000.
- The USDA Food Safety Inspection Service data reveal a significant decline in the incidence of Salmonella on carcasses and ground meats since 1996. Reducing bacteria on meat reduced the chance of the transfer of antibiotic resistant bacteria to humans.
- Recent data from the U.S. Centers for Disease Control and Prevention (CDC) show a 23 percent decline in food borne illnesses since 1996. This is consistent with the reductions of bacteria on meat.

Given the lack of public health crisis and the uncertainties about the contribution of animal antibiotic use to the overall antibiotic resistance problem, surveillance and prevention measures have never been more important. A reasonable approach to managing antibiotic resistance as it relates to food borne transmission includes the following steps:

- Prudent use of antimicrobials. General and species-specific judicious-use guidelines already exist and are being implemented on a routine basis. These were developed by the American Veterinary Medical Association with the assistance of the American Association of Swine Veterinarians, American Association of Avian Pathologists, American Association of Bovine Practitioners, American Association of Equine Practitioners, the American Association of Feline Practitioners and the American Animal Hospital Association. The guidelines are posted at http://www.avma.org/scienact/jtua/default.asp. The CDC and the Food and Drug Administration participated in writing the guidelines, and FDA has also posted them at http://www.fda.gov/cvm/fsi/JudUse.htm.
- NARMS was initiated in 1996-97 for surveillance of the incidence of resistant food-borne pathogens in animals and humans. This program can be improved and made more robust with more resources and better coordination among the program participants - CDC, FDA and USDA. In addition, while there is widespread agreement in the medical community that community- and hospital-acquired infections pose a more significant resistance threat compared to food-borne pathogens, there is no systematic surveillance of resistance among these infections.

- The use of risk assessment is vital to identifying public health threats and yielding important information about how to manage those threats. The American Medical Association recognizes that risk assessments should be conducted before decisions are made to remove uses of antimicrobials.
- A useful roadmap for managing antibiotic resistance has been drawn already. The Federal Interagency Public Health Action Plan to Combat Antimicrobial Resistance is a comprehensive, cohesive plan that addresses all aspects of the issue. The task force, comprised of 10 federal agencies and departments, was formed in 1999 and released the plan in early 2001, calling for surveillance, prevention and control, research, and product development. An effective response to antibiotic resistance includes the kind of broad perspective contained in that plan.

AHI Member Companies

Alpharma Inc. Animal Health Division
Bayer, Animal Health Division
Benchmark Biolabs, Inc.
Biotechnical Services, Inc.
Boehringer Ingelheim Vetmedica, Inc.
Colorado Serum Company
Dow AgroSciences
Elanco Animal Health
Fort Dodge Animal Health, Division of Wyeth
ICON Clinical Research, Inc.
Intervet, Inc.
Intrasphere Technologies, Inc.
Merial
Monsanto Company
MVP Laboratories, Inc.
Nestlé Purina PetCare Company
Novartis Animal Health US, Inc.
Nutramax Laboratories, Inc.
Pfizer Animal Health
Pharmacia Animal Health
Phibro Animal Health
Ricerca, Inc.
Schering-Plough Animal Health Corporation
SCIREX Corporation
Texas Vet Lab, Inc.
Virbac Corporation
Woodson-Tenent Laboratories, Inc.

For more information contact:

Animal Health Institute
1325 G Street, NW
Suite 700
Washington, DC 20005-3104

Phone: 202-637-2440
Fax: 202-393-1667
Internet: www.ahi.org

American Animal Hospital Association (AAHA)

Preface

The American Animal Hospital Association is an international organization of more than 27,000 veterinary care providers who treat companion animals. AAHA reminds pet owners that they can help pets live healthier and longer lives by taking their pets to the veterinarian for annual physical exams, vaccinations, and dental care as well as providing pets with fresh water, a balanced diet and exercise. Established in 1933, the association is well known among veterinarians for its high standards for hospitals and pet health care.

Purpose

To provide quality medical care and promote responsible pet ownership and preventative medical care.

The mission of the American Animal Hospital Association is to enhance the abilities of veterinarians to provide quality medical care to companion animals, to enable them to maintain their clinics with high standards of excellence, and to assist them in meeting the needs of their clientele.

Membership Profile

A veterinary hospital seeking AAHA accreditation in the United States and Canada must meet strict standards of excellence in every aspect of operation. In all, there are 12 specific areas in which established AAHA standards must be met, and the Association regularly evaluates each member clinic to assure continued compliance with these standards. The following areas are some of those addressed by the AAHA standards:

- Accurate and thorough record keeping;
- Provide or have access to a 24-hour emergency hospital service;
- Surgery and treatment areas maintained in optimal sterile/sanitary conditions;
- Complete diagnostic facilities must be provided, including examination rooms, radiology, an equipped laboratory, and a library of reference and textbooks;
- Staff that provide nursing care for companion animals must be adequately skilled.

All AAHA hospital members voluntarily meet or exceed the association's standards for facilities, equipment, and quality procedures. They are regularly evaluated by an AAHA consultant to assure continuing compliance.

In addition, every AAHA veterinarian is encouraged to keep up-to-date on major developments in veterinary medicine. The association offers its 27,000 members a wide variety of continuing education opportunities - self-study courses, seminars, lectures, workshops, annual and regional meetings, and publications.

AAHA accredited hospitals are truly distinctive in providing the highest quality care for pets.

For more information about AAHA or a referral to an AAHA-accredited hospital near you, please call 800-883-6301 or contact:

American Animal Hospital Association
P.O. Box 150899
Denver, Colorado
USA 80215-0899

www.aahanet.org

Tel. (303) 986-2800
Fax (303) 986-1700

Academy of Veterinary Consultants (AVC)

AVC MISSION STATEMENT

The Academy of Veterinary Consultants (AVC) is an association of veterinarians involved in beef cattle medicine, herd health programs and consultation. Our mission is to provide continuing education, member support and leadership among various entities of the beef cattle industry. The AVC goal strives for optimum productivity of a safe, high-quality product.

OBJECTIVES OF THE ACADEMY

- To provide education and support to members.
- To maintain a leadership role in the profession and industry, that is not provided by other veterinary organizations.
- To serve as a liaison among the cattle industry, other related professions, the pharmaceutical industry, regulatory agencies and consumers.
- To act as an integrator of production management techniques which meet the need of beef cattle producers

ACTIVITIES

The Academy serves as a representative and liaison of beef cattle veterinarians for interaction with related cattle industry groups. Our association is a direct liaison with the National Cattlemen's Association for their health and beef safety committees. We provide key representation to food animal practitioner groups with direct communication to the USDA. Furthermore, we monitor other organizations such as AHI, CVM, and FSIS whose activities affect the cattle industry.

Established in 1970, the Academy holds three continuing education meetings annually at various sites. These one to two day seminars serve to provide high quality continuing education for consultants and practitioners. Speakers selected from throughout North America provide presentations in their field of expertise to our membership.

The primary educational orientation is directed toward beef cattle with special emphasis on factors that influence feedlot/herd health and performance management.

Regular Academy seminars are taped and a proceedings booklet is published and provided to all current members. Past topics include pathology, physiology, immmunology, parasitology, stress, computers, nutrition, regulatory issues and consultation practice management.

One meeting each year is a "member only" open forum discussion of individual cases, specific medical problems and current issues of concern to our profession and industry. Furthermore, AVC meetings are frequently held in conjunction with regional and national veterinary conferences to provide an even broader scope of continuing education.

MEMBERSHIP

AVC Membership consists of veterinarians from throughout the United States and Canada including feedlot consultants, general practitioners, and veterinarians from industry, universities and diagnostic laboratories.

For membership details, please contact the following address:

Academy of Veterinary Consultants
6610 Amarillo Blvd. West
Amarillo, Texas 79106

Telephone: (806) 353-7478 or (806) 354-2888
Fax: (806) 359-0636

National Association of Veterinary Technicians in America (NAVTA)

Whether you are a highly experienced veterinary technician or a newcomer to the profession, NAVTA has something to offer. NAVTA is committed to the growth and advancement of the veterinary technician profession. Our goal is to help to:

- Influence the future of the profession.
- Be part of the decision-making process that affects veterinary technicians.
- Foster high standards of veterinary care.

How can NAVTA help you grow?

- As an organization, recognized by the AVMA, NAVTA offers strength in numbers which provides a national voice to help protect and promote the veterinary technician profession.
- NAVTA puts its members in touch with leading-edge medical and practice management information through access to continuing education at regional and national meetings.
- NAVTA provides a nationwide network with other veterinary technician professionals to share knowledge, skills, and problem solving strategies.
- Membership offers the opportunity to participate in the election of NAVTA officers, be a candidate for office, and join committees where an active role in the decision making process can be taken.
- The NAVTA journal features continuing education articles and editorials on current issues that affect its members.
- NAVTA's public relations program promotes the veterinary technician profession to help others understand the function, importance and impact of the job and establish a professional image for the veterinary technician.
- NAVTA provides guidance for the development of Veterinary Technician Specialties that will advance the skills, knowledge and recognition of Veterinary Technicians.
- NAVTA promotes a nationwide campaign for National Veterinary Technician Week to educate the public and increase recognition of veterinary technicians as a critical member of the veterinary medical team.

Who is eligible to become a member of NAVTA?

Active Membership

A veterinary technician who is a graduate of an AVMA accredited program and/or is certified, registered or licensed as a veterinary technician is eligible to become an active member.

Associate Membership

If you are not eligible to become an active member but are interested in the Association's goals, you may become an associate member.

Associate members may serve on committees and enjoy other membership benefits, but may not vote or hold office.

For more information please contact:

NAVTA
P.O. Box 224
Battle Ground, IN 47920
www.navta.net

The above information has been taken from the NAVTA membership brochure.

American College of Veterinary Clinical Pharmacology (ACVCP)

The American College of Veterinary Clinical Pharmacology (ACVCP) (www.acvcp.org) is a specialty board recognized by the American Veterinary Medical Association. The primary objectives of the College are to advance the discipline of veterinary clinical pharmacology as a clinical specialty and assure the competence of those who practice in this field by:

- Establishing requirements for veterinary postdoctoral education and experience for certification in the specialty of veterinary clinical pharmacology.
- Examining and certifying veterinarians as having met the requirements to be a specialist in veterinary clinical pharmacology.
- Encouraging veterinary clinical pharmacologists to pursue a program of continuing education for professional advancement throughout their careers.
- Supporting and promoting education and research and other contributions to knowledge relating to veterinary clinical pharmacology.
- Enhancing the exchange of new knowledge in veterinary clinical pharmacology.
- Organizing committees of experts to research and make recommendations to the profession on current problems in veterinary therapeutics.

Prerequisites for Certification

To qualify for Diplomate status, persons must:

- Be legally qualified to practice veterinary medicine in some state, province, or territory or possession of the United States, Canada, or other country.
- Have completed 2 phases of training. A standard training program is one that is conducted under the supervision of a Diplomate of the American College of Veterinary Clinical Pharmacology. The training program must include: (1) *advanced course work,* not in fulfillment of requirements for the Doctor of Veterinary Medicine or equivalent degree; (2) clinical experience, which includes one year of primary patient care, or two years of clinical consultation; and (3) *research* that addresses problems or hypotheses pertinent to veterinary clinical pharmacology. Provision is made for alternate training programs supervised by diplomates of other American veterinary specialty colleges of a clinical discipline or an advisor who has experience consistent with eligibility requirements *for Charter* Diplomates. The alternate program will require mentorship, even if from a distant site, of an ACVCP diplomate. Training programs should be submitted to the ACVCP for review as the program is begun.

  During the first phase of training, it is expected that the applicant will acquire the requisite knowledge to provide the foundation for the practice of the specialty. This includes but is not limited to a thorough understanding of pharmacodynamics, comparative pharmacology, analytical methods, pharmacokinetics, clinical therapeutic trial design, biostatistics, and pathophysiological processes and mechanisms of disease in all important veterinary species. Satisfactory completion of the initial phase of training will be evaluated by acceptable performance on the Phase I objective-type comprehensive examination. The second phase of training should be designed to provide the applicant with the opportunity to apply the basic tools of clinical pharmacology within a clinical milieu. This may include, but is not restricted to the implementation and evaluation of a therapeutic clinical trial, extensive management or consultative support of complex therapeutic problems in at least two important veterinary species, identification of adverse drug reactions, therapeutic drug monitoring, development of rational therapeutic protocols for extra-label drug use in food animals, the determination of appropriate withdrawal times, and individualization of drug dosage. Certification as a Diplomate of the College will be determined on the basis of satisfactory performance on the Phase II written certification examination and submission of two manuscripts based on veterinary clinical pharmacology. Both manuscripts must be non-review articles, published in peer review journals.

For more information contact:

Dawn M. Boothe, DVM, PhD, Dip. ACVCP, ACVIM
Secretary-Treasurer, ACVCP
Department of Physiology & Pharmacology, College of Veterinary Medicine
Texas A&M University, College Station, TX 77843-4466
Tel: (979) 845-9368 Fax: (979) 862-3672
email: dboothe@cvm.tamu.edu

ASPCA

Animal Poison Control Center (APCC)

1-888-4ANI-HELP **1-900-443-0000**

What is the ASPCA Animal Poison Control Center?

The ASPCA Animal Poison Control Center, an operating division of the American Society for the Prevention of Cruelty to Animals (ASPCA) and an allied agency of the University of Illinois College of Veterinary Medicine, is the first and only national, animal-oriented non-profit poison control center in North America. It is a unique emergency hotline providing animal owners and veterinarians with 24-hour-a-day, 7-day-a-week telephone assistance. The center is staffed by 22 veterinarians, of whom four are board certified in toxicology, plus ten certified veterinary technicians.

What makes the ASPCA APCC different from other poison control centers?

The professional veterinary staff of the ASPCA APCC are familiar with how different species respond to poisons and how to properly manage these poisonings. At their fingertips, they have a wide range of information specific to animal poisoning. They also have an extensive collection of individual cases - more than 600,000 - involving pesticide, drug, plant, metal, and other exposures in food-producing and companion animals. This specialized information lets the experienced ASPCA APCC staff make specific diagnostic and treatment recommendations.

What is the cost of this service?

The charge is $45 per case. The charge can be billed to the caller's VISA, MasterCard, Discover, or American Express, or on our 900 line, the charge is billed directly to the caller's phone bill. The ASPCA APCC will do as many follow-up calls as necessary in critical cases, and at an owner's request, will consult with their veterinarian. There is not a charge when the call involves a corporate partner's product. Currently, there are several animal health and agrochemical companies that subscribe to this service, known as the ASPCA Animal Product Safety Service.

What is the Animal Product Safety Service?

The ASPCA Animal Product Safety Service supports corporate product stewardship initiatives by providing an extensive animal product safety and adverse event reporting program. The APSS program provides its subscribers with a toll-free animal product safety number which can be printed on product labels and literature. The APSS program also manages case records, compiles quarterly or monthly reports, and consults with the manufacturer's professional staff to improve product safety. Their reports are in full compliance with EPA and FDA reporting guidelines. Additional services are available to tailor an animal product safety program to meet each manufacturer's needs.

Are there any special services for Veterinary Clinics?

The ASPCA APCC offers the Veterinary Lifeline Partner program for veterinarians using our service. This program makes access to the ASPCA APCC during poison emergencies quicker, easier and more efficient by securely maintaining your clinic's address and credit card information to ensure efficient service in the event of an animal emergency. Your card will not be billed until you call and request our expert poison control services. Enrollment in the program is free, and offers participating members special benefits.

What should be done if an animal is poisoned?

Immediately call the ASPCA APCC. (**888-426-4435**; a $45 consultation fee may apply, **OR 900-443-0000**; $45 consultation fee charged to your telephone bill). Be ready to provide:

- Your name, address, and phone number;
- Information concerning the exposure (the amount of agent, the time since exposure, etc.)
- The species, breed, age, sex, weight, and number of animals involved.
- The agent your animal(s) has been exposed to, if known.
- The problems your animal(s) is experiencing.

If you are unable to access the 900 number, call your telephone company for assistance c the 888 number. When the 888 number is used, your credit card number will likely be requ addition to the above information. [If the agent is part of the Animal Product Safety Serv consultation is at no cost to you.]

How can I receive additional information?

For more information about the center's various services, please contact:

ASPCA Animal Poison Control Center
1717 South Philo Road, Suite #36
Urbana, IL 61802
dfarbman@apcc.aspca.org

1-217-337-5030 (voice)
1-217-337-0599 (fax)
www.apcc.aspca.org

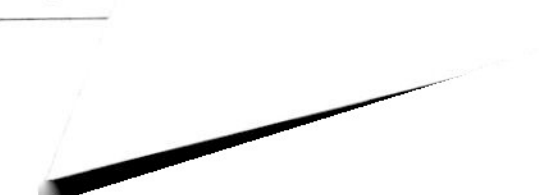

American Veterinary Medical Association (AVMA)

The AVMA is the national organization that represents and serves the interests of the veterinary profession in the United States. The Association's committment is "to advance the science and art of veterinary medicine, including its relationship to public health, biological science, and agriculture".

Established in 1863, the AVMA is a federation of state, territorial, and allied veterinary medical groups. Association policies are established by a House of Delegates comprising delegates from each of these constituent organizations. The House meets once a year.

The AVMA meets the needs of the veterinary profession and the public through many programs. Although most activities directly serve the membership, these same activities benefit the public by promoting animal health care, food safety, and public health and by providing educational materials.

The AVMA publishes two veterinary journals, the Journal of the American Veterinary Medical Association (bi-monthly) and the American Journal of Veterinary Research (monthly). The AVMA supports continuing education efforts through its journals and annual convention. The AVMA also participates in international veterinary activities, and is a member of the World Veterinary Association.

The AVMA provides a variety of services and benefits to its members. Its broader mission is to enhance the profession's image and to ensure that the profession's positions on medical, scientific, political, trade and other matters are presented to industry, government, and the public.

The AVMA is not responsible for and does not endorse the material contained in the Compendium of Veterinary Products, CVP.

Additional information on the AVMA can be obtained by contacting the AVMA at:

American Veterinary Medical Association
'931 North Meacham Road
uite 100
'haumburg, Illinois 60173-4360

. 847-925-8070
847-925-1329

.avma.org

The AVMA Group Health and Life Insurance Trust

For AVMA Members and their Families

This program has been in operation since 1957 under the supervision of nine AVMA member Trustees. The plans are underwritten by New York Life Insurance Company (New York, NY 10010).

The following is a summary of the plans for which U.S. resident members are eligible to apply.

- **Basic Protection Package** - *Protection for your income and family.*
  Long-Term Disability Income
  Decreasing Term Life Insurance
  Accidental Death and Dismemberment
  Rabies Prophylaxis Benefit
- **Major Medical Plan** - *Protection for your health.*
  Medical Coverage of up to $1.5 Million for Eligible Medical Expenses
  "Stop-Loss" feature with choice of deductible
  Preferred Provider Organization Benefits
  Optional Hospital Indemnity Daily Benefit
  Prescription Drug Discount Service
- **Disability Income Plan** - *Protection for your income.*
  Long-Term Disability Benefit up to $7,500 Monthly
  Optional Short-Term Disability Benefits
  Future Purchase Option
- **Professional Overhead Expense** - *Protection for your practice.*
  Up to $10,000 Monthly Benefit
  Paid in addition to any Disability Benefits
  Helps cover office rent, salaries, utilities, and more.
- **Group Term Life/AD&D** - *Protection for your family.*
  Up to $600,000 Member Life Insurance
  Up to $300,000 Spouse Life Insurance
  Discount for non-smokers
  Up to $200,000 Accidental Death and Dismemberment Benefit.

A national network of agents has been appointed by the Trustees to present the Group Health and Life Insurance coverage to AVMA members. Some authorized agents are designated as campus representatives for all U.S. veterinary colleges. They are available to counsel student members regarding special advantages offered to them, especially at graduation, through the AVMA endorsed program.

Call toll-free for information and a listing of authorized representatives.

For more information contact:

The AVMA Group Health and Life Insurance Trust Office
300 South Wacker Drive, 7th Floor
Chicago, Illinois 60606

Tel. 800-621-6360

The AVMA-PLIT

The AVMA-PLIT was established by the American Veterinary Medical Association in 1962 to provide professional liability insurance to AVMA members. The Trust functions independently under an agreement with the AVMA Executive Board which also appoints the Trustees, all of whom are AVMA-member veterinarians.

During its 35-year history, the PLIT has expanded its insurance services to AVMA members to provide a full range of business-related and personal casualty insurance coverages. The Trust's name was changed to AVMA-PLIT in 1997 to reflect the broader scope and reduce the Trust's identity with solely professional liability coverages. The PLIT contracts with insurance companies to provide and underwrite the coverages that are offered by the Trust.

Nearly 70% of AVMA members participate in one or more of the insurance plans offered by the AVMA-PLIT which include: professional liability coverage, extension coverage for loss of or injury to animals in the veterinarian's custody, workers compensation, and business coverages that include: general liability, employment practices liability, business automobile coverage, loss or damage to buildings or equipment, and loss of pharmaceuticals or biologics due to temperature change.

Insurance sales and claims are processed and managed by an insurance broker and administrator, Mack and Parker, Inc. that functions under contract with the AVMA-PLIT and reports directly to the Trustees. Members who desire more information may write or call the AVMA-PLIT at:

AVMA-PLIT
P.O. Box 1629
Chicago, IL 60690-1629

Phone: 800-228-7548 (PLIT)
Fax: 888-754-8329 (PLIT-FAX)
E-mail: avmaplit@mack-parker.com

The AVMA Web Site

http://www.avma.org

What is the AVMA Web site?

The AVMA Web site (www.avma.org) is the online "home" of the American Veterinary Medical Association, an organization representing over 68,000 member veterinarians. Here you will find invaluable public and professional resources reflecting the full scope of veterinary medicine. Whatever your specific interest in the veterinary profession, the AVMA is here to help you get the answers you need.

Veterinary Career Resources

The online **AVMA Veterinary Career Center** brings employers and job seekers the best searching and matching experience available, open to all positions in the veterinary field. Browse as often as you like; or let our electronic Search Agents do it for you, rapidly notifying you by email of matches to your search criteria.

For those wanting to learn about veterinary careers, "About Veterinarians" -- in the Care for Animals area, offers valuable information about the many roles of veterinarians in our society, how to become a veterinarian, and more.

Professional Information Resources

The AVMA's highly regarded journals -- the Journal of the AVMA and the American Journal of Veterinary Research -- are now fully online, in a user-friendly searchable format that also offers printer-friendly versions of the articles for maximum convenience. AVMA Web site visitors can get a head start with these JAVMA resources that are posted online ten to fourteen days in advance of print publication:

- JAVMA News
- Classified Ads
- Meetings & CE
- Educational Opportunities

Other Professional Resources

The AVMA Member Center is the private area of the AVMA Web site and provides quick and convenient access to AVMA services, resources, AVMA policies and guidelines, AVMA Membership Roster, members of the AVMA's volunteer leadership, and other important member information and services.

NOAH® - AMVA's Network of Animal Health

This moderated peer discussion area for veterinarians is available free of charge to all AVMA members. Join your colleagues in these lively discussions to share questions and experiences related to veterinary medicine.

Other resources available in the NOAH area are:

- Compendium of Veterinary Products (sponsored by Bayer, Animal Health Division)
- Material Safety Data Sheets
- Zoonosis Updates

For more information about the AVMA Web site, please contact:

The American Veterinary Medical Association
Center for Information Management
1931 North Meacham Road Phone: (800) 248-2882, ext. 6611
Schaumburg, IL 60173 e-mail: noahelp@avma.org

Visit the AVMA Web site at http://www.avma.org

AVMA Guidelines for Veterinary Prescription Drugs

(Approved by the AVMA House of Delegates, 1998;
Amended by the Executive Board, April 1999)

Key Points

- Veterinary prescription drugs are labeled for use only by or on the order of a licensed veterinarian.
- Veterinary prescription drugs are to be used or prescribed only within the context of a valid veterinarian/client/patient relationship (VCPR).
- Veterinary prescription drugs must be properly labeled before being dispensed.
- Appropriate dispensing and treatment records must be maintained, and veterinary prescription drugs should be dispensed only in quantities required for the treatment of the animal(s) for which the drugs are dispensed.
- Any drug used in a manner not in accordance with its labeling (extra-label use) should be subjected to the same supervisory precautions that apply to veterinary prescription drugs.

The AVMA has prepared the following guidelines as a resource regarding the use and distribution of veterinary prescription drugs. Veterinarians making treatment decisions must use sound clinical judgement and current medical information and must be in compliance with federal, state, and local laws and regulations.

Veterinary Prescription Drugs

Veterinary prescription drugs are those drugs restricted by federal law to use by or on the order of a licensed veterinarian [Section 503(f)Food, Drug, and Cosmetic Act]. The law requires that such drugs be labeled with the statement: "Caution: Federal law restricts this drug to use by or on the order of a licensed veterinarian."

Veterinarian/Client/Patient Relationship

A VCPR exists when all of the following conditions have been met:

- The veterinarian has assumed the responsibility for making clinical judgments regarding the health of the animal(s) and the need for medical treatment, and the client has agreed to follow the veterinarian's instructions.
- The veterinarian has sufficient knowledge of the animal(s) to initiate at least a general or preliminary diagnosis of the medical condition of the animal(s). This means that the veterinarian has recently seen and is personally acquainted with the keeping and care of the animal(s) by virtue of an examination of the animal(s) or by medically appropriate and timely visits to the premises where the animal(s) are kept.
- The veterinarian is readily available for follow-up evaluation, or has arranged for emergency coverage, in the event of adverse reactions or failure of the treatment regimen.

Veterinary Prescription Orders

- Orders issued by licensed veterinarians authorize drug distributors to deliver veterinary prescription drugs to a specific client, or authorize pharmacists to dispense such drugs to a specific client.
- Veterinarians should check with their State Board of Pharmacy and State Veterinary Practice Act to be sure that they are in compliance with state laws.

Labeling & Record Keeping

- Adequate treatment records must be maintained by the veterinarian for at least two years (or as otherwise mandated by law), for all animals treated, to show that the drugs were supplied to clients with whom a valid VCPR has existed. Such records must include the information set forth under Basic Information for Records, Prescriptions, and Labels.
- Food animal owners must also keep treatment records. Owner treatment records have been developed by several producer organizations and are available in conjunction with quality assurance programs.
- All veterinary prescription drugs must be properly labeled when dispensed. A complete label should include the information set forth under Basic Information for Records, Prescriptions, and Labels. If that information is included in the manufacturer's drug label, it is unnecessary to repeat it in the veterinarian's label. If there is inadequate space on the label for complete instructions, the veterinarian must provide additional information to accompany the drug dispensed or prescribed. The veterinarian's additional instructions must be kept in the owner's drug storage area.
- When veterinary prescription drugs are dispensed to companion animal owners, the AVMA recommends that such drugs be placed in child-resistant containers. Such containers are mandated by law in certain states.

Basic Information for Records (R), Prescriptions (P), and Labels (L)

- Name, address, and telephone number of veterinarian (RPL)
- Name (L), address, and telephone number of client (RP)
- Identification of animal(s) treated, species and numbers of animals treated, when possible (RPL)
- Date of treatment, prescribing, or dispensing of drug (RPL)
- Name and quantity of the drug (or drug preparation) to be prescribed or dispensed (RPL)
- Dosage and duration directions for use (RPL)
- Number of refills authorized (RP)

- Cautionary statements, as needed (RPL)
- Expiration date (L)
- Slaughter withdrawal and/or milk withholding times, if applicable (RPL)
- Signature or equivalent (P)

Handling and Storage

The veterinarian should inform clients to whom prescription drugs are delivered or dispensed about appropriate drug handling and storage.

In the clinic, veterinary prescription drugs should be stored separately from over-the-counter drugs, and be easily distinguishable by the professional and paraprofessional staff. Drugs should be stored under conditions recommended by the manufacturer. All drugs should be examined periodically to ensure cleanliness and current dating.

Food animal clients should be advised that veterinary prescription drugs should be securely stored, with access limited to key personnel.

Animal Medicinal Drug Use Clarification Act (AMDUCA) Compliance in Drug Use

The therapeutic administration of any approved dosage form drug in a manner that is not in accordance with the drug's labeling requires additional management. AMDUCA regulations are in force for all approved therapeutic dosage form drugs if administered in a manner not in accordance with the drug's labeling. For such usage, the FDA specifies that the following criteria must be met:

- Make a careful diagnosis and evaluation of the conditions for which the drug is to be used.
- There is no approved animal drug that is labeled for such use, or that contains the same active ingredient in the required dosage form and concentration. Alternatively, an approved animal drug exists, but a veterinarian finds, within the context of a valid veterinarian/client/patient relationship, that the approved drug is clinically ineffective for its intended use.
- Assure that the identity of the treated animal(s) is carefully maintained.
- Establish a substantially extended withdrawal period supported by appropriate scientific information prior to marketing milk, meat, eggs, or other edible products from the treated animal(s).

The use of certain drugs is prohibited in food animals. This list may be amended by the Food and Drug Administration, thus the following list is accurate as of the publication date of this document.

- Prohibited therapy in food animals: chloramphenicol, clenbuterol, diethylstilbestrol, dimetridazole, ipronidazole, other nitroimidazoles, furazolidone, nitrofurazone, other nitrofurans, glycopeptides.
- Prohibited therapy in food animals except approved uses: fluoroquinolone class of antibiotics.
- Prohibited therapy in lactating dairy cows: any sulfonamide except for those specifically approved (sulfadimethoxine, sulfabromethazine and sulfaethoxypyridazine).

In addition to the items set forth under Basic Information for Records, Prescriptions and Labels, AMDUCA regulations specifically add "condition treated" to the record keeping requirement.

AMDUCA does not permit extra -label use of drugs in feed.

Compounding

Compounding is defined as any manipulation to produce a dosage form drug other than that manipulation that is provided for in the directions for use on the labeling of the approved drug product. A few examples include combining drug agents for anesthesia, incorporating a pill into reduced dosage liquid or capsule forms, or creating certain antidotes.

Guidance is found in FDA-CVM Compliance Policy Guide 608.400 "Compounding of Drugs for Use in Animals" issued July 1996.

Food Animal Residue Avoidance Databank (FARAD)

The Food Animal Residue Avoidance Databank (FARAD) is a national food safety project of the US Department of Agriculture Cooperative State Research, Education, and Extension Service in cooperation with University of California-Davis, North Carolina State University, and University of Florida.

FARAD's mission is to provide free expert-mediated consultation to assist in the prevention of chemical residues in foods of animal origin. Since 1982 FARAD has been working with producers, veterinarians, extension specialists and agents who have residue questions. In addition to drug withholding times, FARAD frequently assists practitioners and regulatory agencies in dealing with cases of environmental contaminants including pesticides, herbicides, fungicides and heavy metals.

FARAD has exported its technology to several other countries including the United Kingdom, France, Spain and Canada. Utilizing FARAD's database and software, FARAD centers in those nations provide assistance for questions originating in those countries. FARAD has also been designated a "Center of Excellence" by the United Nations' Food and Agriculture Organization.

FARAD maintains an up-to-date computerized compilation of:

- Current label information, including withdrawal times on all drugs approved for use in food animals in the United States and on hundreds of products used in Canada, Europe, and Australia;
- Official tolerances for drugs and pesticides in tissues, eggs and milk;
- Descriptions and sensitivities of rapid screening tests for detecting residues in tissues, eggs and milk;
- Data on the fate of chemicals in food animals.

How to use FARAD

Information on approved animal health products is available at the FARAD web site http://www.farad.org. Questions can also be emailed to farad@NCSU.edu. FARAD experts can be accessed directly by calling toll-free 1-888-US-FARAD (1-888-873-2723). Most questions can be answered immediately; however, complex responses may require a several days.

Reference Charts

Latin Abbreviations

Abbreviation	Latin	Meaning
ad lib.	*ad libitum*	as much as desired
b.i.d.	*bis in die*	twice daily
q.i.d.	*quarter in die*	four times daily
q.s., or q.s. ad	*quantum sufficit*	quantity sufficient to make
t.i.d.	*ter in die*	three times daily
o.d.	*omnie die*	every day
s.i.d.	*semel in die*	once a day
Rx	*recipe*	take
S., or Sig.	*signa*	Indicates directions to be given on the label of a prescription
a.c.	*ante cibum*	before meals
ad	*ad*	up to; so as to make
ad.	*adde*	add; let there be added
aq.	*aqua*	water
PO	*per os*	orally
p.r.n.	*pro re nata*	when required
gt.	*guttae*	drop

Body Temperature Conversion Chart

°C	°F	°C	°F
36.0	96.8	39.8	103.6
36.5	97.7	40.0	104.0
37.0	98.6	40.2	104.4
37.5	99.5	40.4	104.7
38.0	100.4	40.6	105.1
38.2	100.8	40.8	105.4
38.4	101.1	41.0	105.8
38.6	101.5	41.2	106.2
38.8	101.8	41.4	106.5
39.0	102.2	41.6	106.9
39.2	102.6	41.8	107.2
39.4	102.9	42.0	107.6
39.6	103.3		

Calculations based on the modified formulas: °C = (°F - 32) x (0.5555) and °F = (°C) x (1.8) + 32
Note: 0.5555 substitutes 5/9 and 1.8 substitutes 9/5 in original formulas. Results rounded to one decimal place.

Weights and Measures

Weight Equivalents

Household Measures

1 gt = 0.06 mL
15 gtt = 1 mL
1 tsp = 5 mL
3 tsp = 1 tbsp
1 tbsp = 15 mL
1 jigger = 45 mL
1 teacup = 180 mL
1 glass = 240 mL
1 measuring cup = 240 mL

Abbreviations:

gt = drop
gtt = drops
mL = milliliter
tsp = teaspoon(s)
tbsp = tablespoon

Metric measures

1 metric ton = 1,000 kg
1 metric ton = 2,203 lb (av.)
1 kg = 1,000 g
1 kg = 2.203 lb (av.)
1 g = 1,000 mg
1 g = 0.035 oz (av.)
1 mg = 1,000 µg
1 µg = 0.001 mg (or 1 x 10^{-3} mg)
1 ng = 0.000001 mg (or 1 x 10^{-6} mg)

Abbreviations:

av. = avoirdupois
g = gram(s)
kg = kilogram(s)
lb = pound(s)
mg = milligram(s)
µg = micrograms (it is also abbreviated as mcg)
ng = nanogram
oz = ounce(s)

Avoirdupois* measures

1 lb = 16 oz
1 ton = 2,000 lb
1 oz = 28.35 g
1 lb = 454 g
1 lb = 0.454 kg
1 ton = 907.2 kg
1 ton = 0.907 metric tons

* Avoirdupois is the common system of measuring in USA.

Abbreviations:

g = gram(s)
kg = kilogram(s)
lb = pound(s)
oz = ounce(s)
ton (2000 lb) is also called short ton.

Some apothecary* measures

1 gr = 1/20 scr (or 0.05 scr)
1 gr = 65.8 mg
1 scr = 20 gr
1 scr = 1.3 g
1 dr = 3 scr
1 dr = 3.9 g
1 mg = 0.015 gr
1 g = 15.43 gr
1 oz = 8 dr

* The apothecary measure system has been traditionally used by druggists and pharmacists.

Abbreviations:

dr = dram(s)
g = gram
gr = grain(s)
scr = scruple(s), also represented as ∋

Dosage conversion factors

To convert mg/lb to mg/kg:
mg/kg = mg/lb x 2.2

To convert mg/kg to mg/lb:
mg/lb = mg/kg x 0.454

1 ppm = 1 µg/g or 1 mg/kg

Capacity or Volume Equivalents

Metric

1 L = 1,000 mL
1 mL = 1 cc
30 mL ≅ fl. oz. (av.)
250 mL ≅ 8 fl. oz. (av.)
500 mL ≅ 16 fl. oz. (av.)
0.5 L ≅ 1 pt (av.)
1,000 mL ≅ 32 fl. oz . (av.)
1 L ≅ 1 qt (av.)
100 L = 26.5 gal. (av.)

Abbreviations:

av. = avoirdupois
cc = cubic centimeter
fl oz = fluid ounce(s)
gal = gallon
L = liter
mL = milliliter
pt = pint
qt = quart

Avoirdupois*

1 fl oz = 29.57 mL
1 pt = 16 fl. oz.
1 pt = 473.2 mL
1 qt = 2 pt
1 qt = 0.946 L
1 gal = 4 qt
1 gal = 3.785 L

* Avoirdupois is the common system of measuring in USA.

Abbreviations:

av. = avoirdupois
fl oz = fluid ounce(s), also fl. oz. (av.)
gal = gallon (s), also gal. (av.)
pt = pint(s), also pt (av.)
qt = quart(s), also qt (av.)

Imperial*

1 fl. oz. = 28.4 mL
1 pt = 20 fl oz
1 pt = 568 mL
1 qt = 2 pt
1 qt = 1.136 L
1 gal. = 4 qt
1 gal = 4.55 L
1 bushel = 36.36 L

* The Imperial system conforms to the legal standards of weights and measures of the United Kingdom. It is common in Canada for measuring capacity.

Notice that an *Imperial* fluid ounce equals 28.4 mL, whereas an *avoirdupois* fluid ounce equals 29.57 mL.

Abbreviations:

fl oz = fluid ounce(s), also fl. oz. (imp.)
gal = gallon(s), also gal. (imp.)
imp = Imperial
pt = pint(s), also pt (imp.)
qt = quart(s), also qt (imp.)

Apothecary*

1 min = 1/60 fl dr (0.17 fl dr)
1 min = 0.06 mL
1 fl dr = 60 min
1 fl dr = 3.7 mL
1 fl oz (av.) = 480 min
1 fl oz (av.) = 8 fl dr
1 fl oz (av.) = 29.57 mL

* The apothecary measure system has been traditionally used by druggists and pharmacists.

Abbreviations:

av. = avoirdupois
min = minim (a minim equals one drop - 0.06 mL)
fl dr = fluid dram
fl oz = fluid ounce (avoirdupois)

Notes on measure systems:

- The preceding tables list three measure systems for weight: Metric, Avoirdupois, and Apothecary.
- Listed are four measure systems for capacity or volume: Metric, Avoirdupois (USA), Imperial (UK and Canada) and Apothecary.
- Whenever possible, the Metric System should be used.
- When using the Avoirdupois or Imperial systems for export products, it is recommended to indicate the measuring system being referred to.
- There are other measure systems, e.g. the troy weight system used by jewelers (US and UK), where an ounce equals 31.1 grams.

Weight to Body Surface Area Conversion Chart - Dogs

kg	m^2	kg	m^2	kg	m^2
0.5	0.64	17.0	0.668	34.0	1.060
1.0	0.101	18.0	0.694	35.0	1.081
2.0	0.160	19.0	0.719	36.0	1.101
3.0	0.210	20.0	0.744	37.0	1.121
4.0	0.255	21.0	0.769	38.0	1.142
5.0	0.295	22.0	0.785	39.0	1.162
6.0	0.333	23.0	0.817	40.0	1.181
7.0	0.370	24.0	0.840	41.0	1.201
8.0	0.404	25.0	0.864	42.0	1.220
9.0	0.437	26.0	0.886	43.0	1.240
10.0	0.469	27.0	0.909	44.0	1.259
11.0	0.500	28.0	0.931	45.0	1.278
12.0	0.529	29.0	0.953	46.0	1.297
13.0	0.553	30.0	0.975	47.0	1.302
14.0	0.581	31.0	0.997	48.0	1.334
15.0	0.608	32.0	1.018	49.0	1.352
16.0	0.641	33.0	1.029	50.0	1.371

Calculations based on the modified formula: $\text{BSA in } m^2 = \frac{K\,W^{0.666666666}}{10^4}$

Where BSA = body surface area; m2 = square meters; W = weight in grams; K = 10.1 and 0.666666666 substitutes 2/3 from the original formula1.

Results rounded to the closest millesimal fraction.

[1] Source of original formula: Rosenthal, R.C.: Chemotherapy. *Textbook of Veterinary Internal Medicine,* 4th Ed. (S.J. Ettinger; E.C. Feldman, eds.). W.B. Saunders, Philadelphia, Pa., 1995. Page 478.

Weight to Body Surface Area Conversion Chart - Cats

kg	m2	kg	m2	kg	m2
0.1	0.022	3.0	0.208	6.8	0.360
0.2	0.034	3.2	0.217	7.0	0.366
0.3	0.045	3.4	0.226	7.2	0.373
0.4	0.054	3.6	0.235	7.4	0.380
0.5	0.063	3.8	0.244	7.6	0.387
0.6	0.071	4.0	0.252	7.8	0.393
0.7	0.079	4.2	0.260	8.0	0.400
0.8	0.086	4.4	0.269	8.2	0.407
0.9	0.093	4.6	0.277	8.4	0.413
1.0	0.100	4.8	0.285	8.6	0.420
1.2	0.113	5.0	0.292	8.8	0.426
1.4	0.125	5.2	0.300	9.0	0.433
1.6	0.137	5.4	0.307	9.2	0.439
1.8	0.148	5.6	0.315	9.4	0.445
2.0	0.159	5.8	0.323	9.6	0.452
2.2	0.169	6.0	0.330	9.8	0.458
2.4	0.179	6.2	0.337	10.0	0.464
2.6	0.189	6.4	0.345		
2.8	0.199	6.6	0.352		

Calculations based on the modified formula: $\text{BSA in } m^2 = \frac{W^{0.666666666}}{10^3}$

Where BSA = body surface area; m^2 = square meters; W = weight in grams; and 0.666666666 substitutes 2/3 from the original formula[1].

10^4 has been reduced to 10^3 in order to eliminate the factor K = 10.

Results rounded to the closest millesimal fraction.

[1] Source of original formula: Rosenthal, R.C.: Chemotherapy. *Textbook of Veterinary Internal Medicine,* 4th Ed. (S.J. Ettinger; E.C. Feldman, eds.). W.B. Saunders, Philadelphia, Pa., 1995. Page 478.

Index
Manufacturers/Distributors and their Products

Where possible we have listed the name and address of the manufacturer or distributor responsible for the product in the American market. Page numbers indicate the location of the product monograph.

The information presented has been supplied by the manufacturers and/or distributors. Inclusion or omission of products does not imply endorsement or otherwise, by the publisher or anyone involved in the publication. It must be pointed out that the information is presented as a reference, and it remains the responsibility of the readers to familiarize themselves with the information contained on the label or package insert accompanying each product. Reference to names is not intended as a violation of any trademarks or patents. The Publisher, Editorial Team and all those involved in the production of this publication cannot be held responsible for errors or any consequence that could result from the use of published information.

AGRI LABORATORIES LTD.

20927 STATE ROUTE K
P.O. BOX 3103 (64503)
ST. JOSEPH, MO 64505

Telephone: 816-233-9533
Order Desk: 800-542-8916
Fax: 816-233-9546
Website: www.agrilabs.com

AGRIPHARM/DEALER DISTRIBUTION OF AMERICA

4869 EAST RAINES ROAD
MEMPHIS, TN 38175
Telephone: 901-366-4442

AHC PRODUCTS & PACKAGING, LLC

114C WEST BROADWAY
WINCHESTER, KY 40391
Telephone: 859-737-3441
Fax: 859-737-1143
Website: www.animedproducts.com
Email: ahc@meginc.com

AIRE-MATE, INC.

17335 US 31 NORTH
P.O. BOX 406
WESTFIELD, IN 46074
Telephone: 317-896-2531
Order Desk: 800-544-8990
Fax: 317-896-3788
Website: www.airemate.com
Email: service@airemate.com

AIREX LABORATORIES
Division of The Bullen Companies, Inc.

1640 DELMAR DRIVE
FOLCROFT, PA 19032
Telephone: 610-534-8900
Order Desk: 800-444-8900
Outside USA: 215-724-8100
Fax: 610-534-8912
Website: www.bullenairx.com
Email: bullenairx@bullenairx.com

AIR-TITE PRODUCTS CO., INC.

565 CENTRAL DRIVE
VIRGINIA BEACH, VA 23454
Telephone: 757-340-2501
Order Desk: 800-231-7762
Fax: 757-340-2912
Website: www.air-tite.com
Email: atinfo@air-tite.com

ALCIDE CORPORATION

8561 154TH AVENUE, N.E.
REDMOND, WA 98052
Telephone: 425-882-2555
Order Desk: 800-543-2133
Fax: 425-861-0173
Website: www.alcide.com
Email: info@alcide.com

ALEX C. FERGUSSON INC.

SPRING MILL DRIVE
FRAZER, PA 19355
Telephone: 800-345-1329
Fax: 610-644-8240
Website: www.afco.net
Email: sourcethree@afco.net

ALLIED MONITOR

P.O. BOX 71
201 GOLDEN DRIVE
FAYETTE, MO 65248
Telephone: 660-248-2823
Order Desk: 800-248-9330
Fax: 660-248-1334
Website: www.alliedmonitor.com
Email: allied@coin.org

ALPHARMA INC.
Animal Health Division

ONE EXECUTIVE DRIVE
FORT LEE, NJ 07024
Order Desk: 800-221-5398
Fax: 201-947-3879
Switchboard: 201-947-7774
Technical Information: 201-228-5074
Website: www.alpharma.com
Email: sandy.flick@alpharma.com

ALPHA TECH PET, INC.

789 MASSACHUSETTS AVENUE
LEXINGTON, MA 02420
Telephone: 781-861-7179
Order Desk: 800-222-5537
Fax: 781-863-8505
Website: www.alphatechpet.com

AMERICAN ANIMAL HEALTH, INC.

1401 JOEL EAST ROAD
FORT WORTH, TX 76140
Telephone: 817-293-6363
Order Desk: 800-272-8338
Fax: 817-293-7711
Website: www.aahinc.com

AMERICAN SCIENTIFIC LABORATORIES, INC.

1095 MORRIS AVE.
UNION, NJ 07083
Telephone: 908-629-3490
Order Desk: 800-648-2118
Fax: 908-629-3306

ANIMAL BLOOD BANK

P.O. BOX 1118
DIXON, CA 95620
Telephone: 800-2HELPK9 (800-243-5759)
Fax: 707-678-7357
Website: www.animalbloodbank.com
Email: redcell@aol.com

ANTHONY PRODUCTS CO.
Pacific Animal Health Division

5600 PECK ROAD
ARCADIA, CA 91006
Telephone: 626-357-8711
Order Desk: 800-423-7153
Fax: 626-359-6948

AQUA HEALTH LTD.
A division of Novartis Animal Vaccines, Inc.

37 MCCARVILLE ST.
WEST ROYALTY INDUSTRIAL PARK
CHARLOTTETOWN, PE, CANADA C1E 2A7
Telephone: 208-543-5369
877-544-4966
902-566-4966
Fax: 208-543-5369
902-566-3573
Email: tanya.knudson@ah.novartis.com

ARC LABORATORIES

4280 NORTHEAST EXPRESSWAY
ATLANTA, GA 30340
Telephone: 770-454-3200
Order Desk: 800-755-7056
Fax: 770-454-3214
Fax - Toll-Free: 800-745-0544
Email: pets@gimborn.com

ARGENT CHEMICAL LABORATORIES

8702-152ND AVENUE N.E.
REDMOND, WA 98052
Telephone: 425-885-3777
Order Desk: 800-426-6258
Fax: 425-885-2112
Website: www.argent-labs.com
Email: email@argent-labs.com

ARKO LABORATORIES, LTD.

P.O. BOX 400
HIGHWAY 69 NORTH
JEWELL, IA 50130
Telephone: 515-827-5648
Toll-Free: 800-714-2756
Fax: 515-827-5648

ASPEN VETERINARY RESOURCES, LTD.

3701-A N.E. KIMBALL DRIVE
KANSAS CITY, MO 64161
Telephone: 816-413-1444
Fax: 816-413-1445

BALCHEM CORPORATION

P.O. BOX 175
SLATE HILL, NY 10973
Telephone: 845-355-5300
Fax: 845-355-6314
Website: www.balchem.com
Email: BCP@Balchem.com

BAYER
Animal Health Division

P.O. BOX 390
SHAWNEE MISSION, KS 66201-0390
Customer Service Tel.: 800-633-3796
Customer Service Fax: 800-344-4219
Website: www.bayer-ah.com

BENEPET® PET CARE PRODUCTS

P.O. BOX 8111
ST. JOSEPH, MO 64508-8111
Telephone: 816-279-3449
Toll-Free: 800-825-0341
Fax: 816-279-4725
Email: bsasales@butlersalesassociates.com

BIMEDA, INC.
Div. Cross Vetpharm Group, Ltd.

460 N.W. PARKWAY
RIVERSIDE, MO 64150
Telephone: 816-746-9368
Fax: 816-746-9369
Toll-Free Customer Service: 888-5-BIMEDA or 888-677-6762
Toll-Free Fax: 877-888-7035
Website: www.bimeda.com
Email: sales@bimedaus.com

BIOCOR ANIMAL HEALTH INC.

2720 NORTH 84TH STREET
OMAHA, NE 68134

Telephone:	402-393-7440
Fax:	402-393-4712
Customer Service Tel.:	800-441-7480
Customer Service Fax:	402-393-3455
Website:	www.biocorah.com
Email:	info@biocorah.com

BIOMETALLICS, INC.
Veterinary Science Division

P.O. BOX 2251
PRINCETON, NJ 08543

Telephone:	609-275-0133
Order Desk:	800-999-1961
Fax:	609-275-9485
Email:	Progest1@aol.com

BIOMUNE CO.

8906 ROSEHILL ROAD
LENEXA, KS 66215

Telephone:	913-894-0230
Fax:	913-894-0236

BIONICHE ANIMAL HEALTH USA, INC. (formerly Vetrepharm Research Inc.)

1551 JENNINGS MILL RD.
SUITE 300A
BOGARD, GA 30622

Telephone:	706-549-4503
Order Desk:	888-549-4503
Fax:	706-548-0659
Website:	www.bioniche.com

BIOPURE CORPORATION

11 HURLEY STREET
CAMBRIDGE, MA 02141

Telephone:	617-234-6500
Technical Service:	888-400-0030
Customer Service:	888-337-0929
Fax:	617-234-6850
Website:	www.biopure.com

BIO-TEK INDUSTRIES, INC.

1380 WEST MARIETTA STREET N.W.
P.O. BOX 93746
ATLANTA, GA 30318

Telephone:	404-799-2050
Fax:	404-799-2056
Website:	www.bio-tekusa.com

BIOZYME INCORPORATED

6010 STOCKYARDS EXPRESSWAY
P.O. BOX 4428
ST. JOSEPH, MO 64504

Telephone:	816-238-3326
Toll-Free:	800-821-3070
Fax:	816-238-7549
Website:	www.biozymeinc.com
Email:	support@biozymeinc.com

THE BLOOD BANK OF PROFESSIONAL VETERINARY RESEARCH

1328 WEST COMMERCE STREET
BROWNSTOWN, IN 47220

Telephone:	812-358-9078
Order Desk:	812-358-9078
Fax:	812-358-5600
Email:	profvetr@hsonline.net

BOEHRINGER INGELHEIM VETMEDICA, INC.

2621 NORTH BELT HIGHWAY
ST. JOSEPH, MO 64506-2002

Telephone (main switchboard):	800-821-7467
	816-233-1385
	816-233-2804
Fax:	816-236-2789
Sales Services:	800-325-9167
Technical Information:	800-325-9167
Website:	www.bi-vetmedica.com
	www.productionvalues.us
Email:	info@productionvalues.us

BOU-MATIC
The Dairy Equipment Division of DEC International, Inc.

P.O. BOX 8050
1919 SOUTH STOUGHTON RD.
MADISON, WI 53708

Telephone:	608-222-3484
Order Desk:	608-222-3484
Fax:	608-222-9314
Technical Services:	608-225-3832 Ext. 107
Emergency Response No.:	800-424-9300
Website:	www.boumatic.com

BRINTON LABORATORIES INC.

P.O. BOX 266
208 SOUTH EAST LAKELAND DRIVE
WILLMAR, MN 56201

Telephone:	320-235-8611
Order Desk:	800-533-1899
Fax:	320-235-8629
Website:	www.brintonvet.com
Email:	info@brintonvet.com

THE BUTLER COMPANY

5600 BLAZER PARKWAY
DUBLIN, OH 43017
Telephone: 614-761-9095
Switchboard/Corp. Office
Order Desk: 800-551-3861
Fax: 614-761-1045
Website: www.AccessButler.com

CENTAUR, INC.

P.O. BOX 25667
OVERLAND PARK, KS 66225-5667

Telephone: 913-390-6184
Order Desk: 800-236-6180
Fax: 913-390-5907
Email: centaurunavet@aol.com

CHARITON VET SUPPLY, INC.

P.O. BOX 81
HUNTSVILLE, MO 65259

Telephone: 660-263-8898
Order Desk: 800-748-7837
Fax: 660-263-8860
Website: www.charitonvet.com
Email: cvs@mcmsys.com

CHEMETRICS, INC.

RTE. 28
CALVERTON, VA 20138

Telephone: 540-788-9026
Order Desk: 800-356-3072
Fax: 540-788-1816
Technical Service: 540-788-9026
Website: www.chemetrics.com

CHR. HANSEN BIOSYSTEMS

9015 WEST MAPLE STREET
MILWAUKEE, WI 53215

Telephone: 414-607-5700
Order Desk: 800-543-4422
Fax: 414-607-5701
Technical Information: 800-247-6782
Website: www.chbiosystems.com
Email: las@chr-hansen-us.com

CHURCH & DWIGHT CO., INC.

469 NORTH HARRISON STREET
PRINCETON, NJ 08543

Telephone: 800-221-0453
Customer Service (Orders): 800-631-5591
Customer Service Fax: 800-335-8861
Fax: 609-497-7176
Website: www.ahdairy.com

COLORADO SERUM COMPANY

4950 YORK STREET
P.O. BOX 16428
DENVER, CO 80216-0428

Telephone: 303-295-7527
Order Desk: 800-525-2065
Fax: 303-295-1923
Website: www.colorado-serum.com
Email: colorado-serum@colorado-serum.com or edlehigh@colorado-serum.com

COMBE, INC.

1101 WESTCHESTER AVENUE
WHITE PLAINS, NY 10604-3597
Telephone: 914-694-5454
Order Desk: 914-694-5454
Fax: 914-694-6855
Technical Information: 914-694-5454
Website: www.combe.com
Email: combe@combe.com

CONKLIN COMPANY INC.
Animal Products Division

551 VALLEY PARK DRIVE
P.O. BOX 155
SHAKOPEE, MN 55379
Telephone: 952-445-6010
Order Desk: 800-888-8838
Technical Information: 800-888-8838
Fax: 952-496-4285
Website: www.fastrackmicrobials.com
Email: marketing@conklin.com

CONTEMPORARY PRODUCTS, INC.

P.O. BOX 6067
3788 ELM SPRINGS RD.
SPRINGDALE, AR 72766
Telephone: 479-756-9801
Fax: 479-872-0538

COOK VETERINARY PRODUCTS INC.

1100 W. MORGAN ST.
SPENCER, IN 47460
Telephone: 812-829-4891
Order Desk: 800-826-2380
Fax: 800-837-4130
Website: www.cookgroup.com
Email: cookvetusa@aol.com

CREATIVE SCIENCE™

P.O. BOX 8098
ST. JOSEPH, MO 64508-8098
Telephone: 816-279-3449
Toll-Free: 800-825-0341
Fax: 816-279-4725
Email: bsasales@butlersalesassociates.com

DAIRY ASSOCIATION CO., INC.

P.O. BOX 145
LYNDONVILLE, VT 05851
Telephone: 802-626-3610
Order Desk: 800-232-3610
Fax: 802-626-3433
Website: www.bagbalm.com
Email: info@bagbalm.com

DAVIS MANUFACTURING & PACKAGING, INC.

541 PROCTOR AVENUE
SCOTTDALE (ATLANTA), GA 30079
Telephone: 404-292-2424
Order Desk: 800-292-2424
Fax: 404-292-3049
Website: www.davismfg.com
Email: mail@davismfginc.com

DELMARVA LABORATORIES INC.

1500 HUGUENOT RD.
SUITE 106
MIDLOTHIAN, VA 23113

Telephone: 804-794-7064
Fax: 804-794-7835

DELMONT LABORATORIES, INC.

715 HARVARD AVENUE
P.O. BOX 269
SWARTHMORE, PA 19081-0269

Telephone: 610-543-2747
Order Desk: 800-562-5541
Fax: 610-543-6298
Product Literature: 800-562-5541
Dermatology Information: Dr. Patrick Breen
888-417-9379
Website: www.delmont.com
Email: splvet@delmont.com

DERMAPET

P.O. BOX 59713
POTOMAC, MD 20859

Telephone: 301-983-8387
Order Desk: 800-755-4738
Fax: 301-365-0191
Website: www.dermapet.com
Email: dermapet@aol.com

DIAGNOSTIC PRODUCTS CORPORATION

5700 WEST 96TH STREET
LOS ANGELES, CA 90045-5597

Telephone: 310-645-8200
Sales Services: 310-642-5180
Technical Services: 800-372-1782
Toll-Free: 800-372-1782
Fax: 310-645-9999
Website: www.dpcweb.com
Email: info@dpconline.com

DMS LABORATORIES, INC.

2 DARTS MILL ROAD
FLEMINGTON, NJ 08822

Telephone: 908-782-3353
Order Desk: 800-567-4367
Fax: 908-782-0832
Website: www.rapidvet.com
Email: dmslabs@aol.com

DOMINION VETERINARY LABORATORIES LTD.

1199 SANFORD STREET
WINNIPEG, MB, CANADA R3E 3A1

Telephone: 204-589-7361
Fax: 204-943-9612
Website: www.domvet.com

DUBOIS
Industrial Division of JohnsonDiversey

200 CROWN POINTE PLACE
SHARONVILLE, OH 45241-5412

Telephone: 513-326-8872
Customer Support Center: 800-438-2647
Fax: 513-326-8339
Website: www.duboischemicals.com

DURVET, INC.

P.O. BOX 279
100 S.E. MAGELLAN DRIVE
BLUE SPRINGS, MO 64014

Telephone: 816-229-9101
Order Desk: 800-821-5570
Fax: 816-224-3080
Website: www.durvet.com
Email: info@durvet.com

DVM FORMULA™
a division of Vets Plus, Inc.

102 THIRD AVENUE EAST
KNAPP, WI 54749
Telephone: 715-665-2118
Order Desk: 800-468-3877
Fax: 715-665-2401
Website: www.dvmformula.com
Email: custsvc@vets-plus.com

DVM PHARMACEUTICALS, INC.

50 NORTHWEST 176 STREET
MIAMI, FL 33169
Telephone: 305-575-6200
Order Desk: 800-367-4902
Fax: 305-575-6960
Website: www.DVMPharmaceuticals.com

ECOLAB FOOD AND BEVERAGE DIVISION

370 WABASHA STREET N.
ST. PAUL, MN 55102
Telephone: 888-367-2499
Technical Assistance: 651-293-2818
Fax: 651-293-2260
Website: www.ecolab.com
Email: steve.pasek@ecolab.com

ECOLAB PROFESSIONAL PRODUCTS DIVISION

370 WABASHA STREET N.
N/12
ST. PAUL, MN 55102

Telephone: 800-332-6522
Fax: 651-293-2959
Technical Information: 800-451-7191
Website: www.ecolab.com

ELANCO ANIMAL HEALTH
A Division of Eli Lilly & Co.

4 PARKWOOD SUITE 125
500 EAST 96TH STREET
INDIANAPOLIS, IN 46240-3733

Main Switchboard: 317-433-4800
Customer Service: 317-276-1262
Technical Services: 800-428-4441
Fax: 317-276-4471
Website: www.elanco.com
Email: elanco@elanco.com

EMBREX, INC.

P.O. BOX 13989
RESEARCH TRIANGLE PARK, NC 27709-3989

Telephone: 919-941-5185
Fax: 919-941-5186
Website: www.embrex.com

EQUI AID PRODUCTS, INC.

1517 WEST KNUDSEN DRIVE
PHOENIX, AZ 85027

Telephone: 623-492-9190
Order Desk: 800-735-3399
Fax: 623-492-9385
Website: www.equiaid.com

EQUICARE PRODUCTS
A Division of Farnam Companies, Inc.

301 WEST OSBORN ROAD
PHOENIX, AZ 85013-3928

Telephone: 602-285-1660
Toll-Free: 800-234-2269
Fax: 602-285-1803
Website: www.farnam.com

EUDAEMONIC CORPORATION
An ABS Affiliate

7031 NORTH 16TH STREET
P.O. BOX 594
OMAHA, NE 68101

Telephone: 402-453-6970
Order Desk: 800-553-4550
Fax: 402-453-1052
Website: www.eudaemonic.net
Email: marketing@eudaemonic.net

EVSCO PHARMACEUTICALS
Division of Vétoquinol, USA

P.O. BOX 685
101 LINCOLN AVE., BUENA, NJ 08310

Telephone: 856-697-5115
Customer Service: 800-267-5707
Fax: 856-697-7465

FARNAM COMPANIES, INC.

301 WEST OSBORN ROAD
PHOENIX, AZ 85013-3928

Telephone: 602-285-1660
Toll-Free: 800-234-2269
Fax: 602-285-1803
Website: www.farnam.com

FARNAM COMPANIES, INC., Livestock Division

301 WEST OSBORN ROAD
PHOENIX, AZ 85013-3928

Telephone: 602-285-1660
Toll-Free: 800-234-2269
Fax: 602-285-1803
Website: www.farnam.com

FIEBING COMPANY, INC.

516 S. 2ND ST., P.O. BOX 04125
MILWAUKEE, WI 53204

Telephone: 414-271-5011
Fax: 414-271-3769

FIRST PRIORITY INC.

1585 TODD FARM DRIVE
ELGIN, IL 60123

Telephone: 847-289-1600
Order Desk: 800-650-4899
Fax: 847-289-1223
Website: www.prioritycare.com
Email: custsvc@prioritycare.com

FLEMING LABORATORIES, INC.

P.O. BOX 34384
CHARLOTTE, NC 28234

Telephone: 704-372-5613
Fax: 704-343-9357
Email: flemingg@cetlink.net

FORT DODGE ANIMAL HEALTH Division of Wyeth

800-5TH STREET N.W., P.O. BOX 518
FORT DODGE, IA 50501

Telephone: 515-955-4600
Fax: 515-955-3730
Order Desk Telephone: 800-685-5656
Order Desk Fax: 800-846-8626
Order Desk Email: fdorder@FDAH.com
Professional Services: 800-533-8536
Website: www.wyeth.com/divisions/fort_dodge.asp

G.C. HANFORD MANUFACTURING COMPANY

304 ONEIDA ST.
P.O. BOX 1017
SYRACUSE, NY 13201-1017

Telephone:	315-476-7418
Order Desk:	800-234-4263
Fax:	315-476-7434
Technical Information:	888-23USVET
Website:	www.hanford.com

GLENWOOD, LLC

19 EMPIRE BLVD.
S. HACKENSACK, NJ 07606

Telephone:	201-221-0050
Order Desk:	800-542-0772
Fax:	201-221-0060
Website:	www.glenwood-llc.com
Email:	info@glenwood-llc.com

GOODWINOL PRODUCTS CORP.

41710 WELD COUNTY ROAD 29
PIERCE, CO 80650

Telephone:	970-834-1229
Order Desk:	800-554-1080
Fax:	970-834-0180
Website:	www.goodwinol.com
Email:	Goodwinol@aol.com

GREAT STATES® ANIMAL HEALTH

P.O. BOX 8111
ST. JOSEPH, MO 64508-8111

Telephone:	816-279-3449
Toll-Free:	800-825-0341
Fax:	816-279-4725
Email:	bsasales@butlersalesassociates.com

GREER LABORATORIES, INC.

P.O. BOX 800
639 NUWAY CIRCLE
LENOIR, NC 28645

Telephone:	877-777-1080
Toll-Free Fax:	877-777-1090
Website:	www.greerlabs.com
Email:	salesdept@greerlabs.com

HALOCARBON LABORATORIES
(Division of Halocarbon Products Corp.)

887 KINDERKAMACK ROAD
P.O. BOX 661
RIVER EDGE, NJ 07661
Telephone: 201-262-8899
Order Desk: 800-338-5803
Fax: 201-262-0019
Website: www.halocarbon.com

HAPPY JACK, INCORPORATED

P.O. BOX 475
2122 HIGHWAY 258 SOUTH
SNOW HILL, NC 28580
Telephone: 252-747-2911
Order Desk: 800-326-5225
Fax: 252-747-4111
Website: www.happyjackinc.com
Email: happyjack@happyjackinc.com

HARLMEN CORPORATION

P.O. BOX 451073
OMAHA, NE 68144
Telephone: 402-393-7949
Order Desk: 402-393-7949
Fax: 800-392-0794
Website: www.harlmen.com
Email: info@harlmen.com

THE HARTZ MOUNTAIN CORPORATION

400 PLAZA DRIVE
SECAUCUS, NJ 07094-3688
Telephone: 201-271-4800
Technical Information: 800-275-1414
Fax: 201-271-0357
Website: www.hartz.com

HAWTHORNE PRODUCTS, INC.

16828 NORTH STATE ROAD 167 NORTH
DUNKIRK, IN 47336
Telephone: 765-768-6585
Order Desk: 800-548-5658
Fax: 765-768-7672
Website: www.hawthorne-products.com
Email: don@hawthorne-products.com
OR kim@hawthorne-products.com

HESKA CORPORATION

1613 PROSPECT PARKWAY
FORT COLLINS, CO 80525
Telephone: 970-493-7272
Fax: 970-472-1640
Information/Order Desk: 800-GO-HESKA
Website: www.heska.com
Email: market@heska.com

HORSE HEALTH PRODUCTS
A Division of Farnam Companies, Inc.

301 WEST OSBORN ROAD
PHOENIX, AZ 85013-3928
Telephone: 602-285-1660
Toll-Free: 800-234-2269
Fax: 602-285-1803
Website: www.farnam.com

HORSES PREFER™
a division of Vets Plus, Inc.

102 THIRD AVENUE EAST
KNAPP, WI 54749
Telephone: 715-665-2118
Order Desk: 800-468-3877
Fax: 715-665-2401
Website: www.horsesprefer.com
Email: custsvc@vets-plus.com

H.W. NAYLOR CO. INC.

121 MAIN ST., P.O. BOX 190
MORRIS, NY 13808-0190
Telephone: 607-263-5145
Fax: 607-263-2416

HYGIEIA BIOLOGICAL LABORATORIES

P.O. BOX 8300
1785 E. MAIN STREET, #4
WOODLAND, CA 95776
Lab/Main Office: 530-661-1442 (telephone)
530-661-1633 (fax)
Sales Office: 530-724-3520 (phone & fax)
916-802-1664 (cell phone)
Toll-Free: 888-HYGIEIA
Adverse Reaction Reporting:
530-661-1442 (telephone)
530-661-1633 (fax)
hygieia@compuserve.com (email)
Website: www.hygieialabs.com
Email: info@hygieialabs.com

IDEXX LABORATORIES, INC.

ONE IDEXX DRIVE
WESTBROOK, ME 04092
Telephone: 207-856-0300
Fax: 207-856-0345
Pet Diagnostics/Order Desk: 800-248-2483
Poultry/Livestock Diagnostics: 800-548-9997
Poultry/Livestock Order Desk: 800-943-3999
Website: www.idexx.com
Email: webmaster@idexx.com

IDEXX PHARMACEUTICALS, INC.
A Subsidiary of Idexx Laboratories, Inc.

4249-105 PIEDMONT PARKWAY
GREENSBORO, NC 27410
Telephone: 336-834-6500
Order Desk: 800-374-8006
Fax: 336-834-6502
Website: www.brpharma.com

IMMUCELL CORPORATION

56 EVERGREEN DRIVE
PORTLAND, ME 04103
Telephone: 207-878-2770
Order Desk: 800-444-4614
Fax: 207-878-2117
Website: www.immucell.com

IMMVAC, INC.

6080 BASS LANE
COLUMBIA, MO 65201
Telephone: 573-443-5363
Order Desk: 800-944-7563
Technical Information: 800-944-7563
Fax: 573-874-7108
Website: www.immvac.com
Email: immvac@immvac.com

INTAGRA, INC.

16719 IREDALE PATH
LAKEVILLE, MN 55044
Telephone: 952-898-0422
Order Desk: 800-468-2472
Fax: 952-898-2372
Email: info@intagra.com

INTERCHEM CHEMICAL SPECIALTIES, INC.

3516 NORTH 14TH STREET
ST. LOUIS, MO 63107
Telephone: 314-436-1300
Order Desk: 800-436-9838
Fax: 314-436-1302
Email: INTERCHEM4@AOL.COM

INTERCON CHEMICAL COMPANY

1100 CENTRAL INDUSTRIAL DR.
ST. LOUIS, MO 63110
Telephone: 314-771-6600
Order Desk: 800-325-9218
Fax: 314-771-6608
Website: www.interconchemical.com
Email: inter001@aol.com

INTERVET INC.

405 STATE STREET
P.O. BOX 318
MILLSBORO, DE 19966
Telephone: 800-992-8051
Customer Service: 800-441-8272
Website: www.intervetusa.com
Email: Information.USA@intervet.com

JORGENSEN LABS., INC.

1450 NORTH VAN BUREN AVE.
LOVELAND, CO 80538
Telephone: 970-669-2500
Fax: 970-663-5042
Technical Information: Ask for Vet-Tech
Website: www.jorvet.com
Email: info@jorvet.com

KANE ENTERPRISES, INC.
Ag-Tek Division

P.O. BOX 1043
SIOUX FALLS, SD 57101
Telephone: 605-582-7700
Order Desk: 800-336-8577
Fax: 605-582-7777
Toll-Free Fax: 800-582-7786
Website: www.ag-tek.com
Email: info@ag-tek.com

KENTUCKY PERFORMANCE PRODUCTS

P.O. BOX 1013
VERSAILLES, KY 40383
Telephone: 859-873-2974
Order Desk: 877-230-4565
Fax: 859-879-0770
Website: www.ker.com
Email: orders@ker.com

KENVET
a Division of Loveland Industries, Inc.

P.O. BOX 1289
GREELEY, CO 80632-1289
Telephone: 970-356-8920
Order Desk: 800-356-7202
Toll-Free: 800-356-8920
Fax Orders: 970-356-7964

KING ANIMAL HEALTH

1945 CRAIG ROAD
ST. LOUIS, MO 63146
Telephone: 314-576-6100
Order Desk: 800-738-5464
Fax: 314-469-5749
Technical Information: 800-738-5464
Website: www.soloxine.com
Email: Solox@aol.com

LAKE IMMUNOGENICS, INC.

348 BERG ROAD
ONTARIO, NY 14519
Telephone: 585-265-1973
Order Desk: 800-648-9990
Fax: 585-265-2306
Website: www.lakeimmunogenics.com

LAND O'LAKES, INC.
Animal Milk Products Company

P.O. BOX 64404
MS7405
ST. PAUL, MN 55164-0404
Telephone: 800-618-6455
Order Desk: 800-618-6455
Fax: 651-634-8167
Website: www.lolmilkreplacer.com
Email: animalmilk@landolakes.com

LEGEAR ANIMAL HEALTH PRODUCTS
Division of Goodwinol Products Corp.

41710 WELD COUNTY ROAD 29
PIERCE, CO 80650
Telephone: 970-834-1229
Order Desk: 800-554-1080
Fax: 970-834-0180
Website: www.goodwinol.com
Email: Goodwinol@aol.com

LIFE SCIENCE PRODUCTS®

P.O. BOX 8111
ST. JOSEPH, MO 64508-8111
Telephone: 816-279-3449
Toll-Free: 800-825-0341
Fax: 816-279-4725
Email: bsasales@butlersalesassociates.com

LLOYD LABORATORIES
A Division of LLOYD, Inc.

604 WEST THOMAS AVENUE
P.O. BOX 86
SHENANDOAH, IA 51601
Telephone: 712-246-4000
Order Desk: 800-831-0004
Fax: 712-246-5245
Website: www.lloydinc.com
Email: info@lloydinc.com

LOHMANN ANIMAL HEALTH INTERNATIONAL, MAINE FACILITY

P.O. BOX 255
WATERVILLE, ME 04903-0255
Telephone: 207-873-3989
Domestic Order Desk: 800-655-1342
International Order Desk: 800-639-1581
Fax: 207-873-4975
Website: www.lahinternational.com
Email: info@lahinternational.com

LOHMANN ANIMAL HEALTH INTERNATIONAL, NEW JERSEY FACILITY

2285 EAST LANDIS AVENUE
VINELAND, NJ 08360
Telephone: 856-691-2411
Domestic Order Desk: 800-655-1342
International Order Desk: 800-846-3547
Fax: 856-691-4392
Website: www.lahinternational.com

LOVELAND INDUSTRIES, INC.

P.O. BOX 1289
GREELEY, CO 80632-1289
Telephone: 970-356-8920
Order Desk: 800-356-7202
Toll-Free: 800-356-8920
Fax Orders: 970-356-7964
Website: www.lovelandindustries.com
Email: myron.hillman@loveland.uap.com

LUITPOLD PHARMACEUTICALS, INC. Animal Health Division

ONE LUITPOLD DRIVE
SHIRLEY, NY 11967
Telephone: 631-924-4000
Order Desk: 800-458-0163
Fax: 631-924-1731
Website: www.luitpold.com
Email: jsimpson631@aol.com

MACLEOD PHARMACEUTICALS, INC.

2600 CANTON COURT
SUITE C
FORT COLLINS, CO 80525
Telephone: 970-482-7254
Fax: 970-482-7454
Email: macleod3@verinet.com

MANN LAKE LTD.

501 SOUTH 1ST STREET
HACKENSACK, MN 56452
Order Desk: 800-880-7694
Fax: 218-675-6156
Website: www.mannlakeltd.com
Email: beekeeper@mannlakeltd.com

MED-PHARMEX, INC.

2727 THOMPSON CREEK ROAD
POMONA, CA 91767-1861
Telephone: 909-593-7875
Fax: 909-593-7862
Website: www.med-pharmex.com
Email: medpharmex@aol.com

MEGAN HEALTH, INC.

8620 PENNELL DRIVE
OVERLAND, MO 63114
Telephone: 314-983-9050
Fax: 314-983-9077
Toll-Free: 888-634-2668 ext. 130
Toll-Free Fax: 877-634-2669
Website: www.meganhealth.com
Email: MBoyd@meganhealth.com

MERIAL

3239 SATELLITE BLVD.
BUILDING 500
DULUTH, GA 30096
Telephone: 678-638-3000
Website: www.merial.com

MERIAL SELECT, INC.

P.O. DRAWER 2497
GAINESVILLE, GA 30503
Telephone: 770-536-8787
Order Desk: 770-536-8787
Fax: 770-534-8558

METREX

1717 W. COLLINS AVENUE
ORANGE, CA 92867
Telephone: 800-841-1428
Order Desk: 800-841-1428
Fax: 714-516-7904
Website: www.metrex.com
Email: info@metrex.com

METZ SALES, INC.

522 WEST FIRST STREET
WILLIAMSBURG, PA 16693
Telephone: 814-832-2907
Order Desk: 800-882-8347
Technical Information: 800-882-8347
Fax: 800-882-8347

MG BIOLOGICS

1721 Y AVENUE
AMES, IA 50014
Telephone: 515-769-2340
Fax: 515-769-2390
Website: www.mgbiologics.com
Email: mmeyer@pcpartner.net

MICROBAN SYSTEMS INC.

1135 BRADDOCK AVE.
BRADDOCK, PA 15104
Fax: 412-461-7460
Telephone: 412-351-8686
Fax: 412-351-1394

MID-AMERICAN RESEARCH CHEMICAL CORP.

P.O. BOX 927
COLUMBUS, NE 68602-0927
Telephone: 402-564-7104
Order Desk: 800-228-8508
Technical Information: 800-228-8508
Fax: 402-563-1290
Website: www.marc1.com
Email: marc1@marc1.com

MIDLAND BIOPRODUCTS CORPORATION
Sales and Marketing

800 SNEDDEN DRIVE
P.O. BOX 309
BOONE, IA 50036
Telephone: 515-432-7799
Toll-Free: 800-370-6367
Fax: 515-432-7790
Website: www.midlandbio.com
Email: sales@midlandbio.com

MILK SPECIALTIES CO.

P.O. BOX 278
ILLINOIS & WATER STS.
DUNDEE, IL 60118
Telephone: 800-323-4274
Order Desk: 800-323-5424, Ext. 1162 or Ext. 1143
Fax: 800-423-6455
Website: www.milkspecialties.com
Email: msc@milkspecialties.com

MONSANTO COMPANY
Subsidiary of Pharmacia

800 N. LINDBERGH BOULEVARD
BUILDING B2SC
ST. LOUIS, MO 63167
Telephone: 314-694-1000
Order Desk: 800-233-2999
Website: www.monsanto.com/dairy/

MS BIOSCIENCE, INC.
Division of Milk Specialties Co.

P.O. BOX 278
ILLINOIS AND WATER STREETS
DUNDEE, IL 60118
Sales and Technical Information: 887-772-5825
Fax: 800-423-6455
Website: www.MSBioScience.com

MULTIMIN USA, INC.

31918 COUNTRY CLUB DRIVE
PORTERVILLE, CA 93257-9610
Telephone: 559-791-1000

MVP LABORATORIES, INC.

5404 MILLER AVENUE
RALSTON, NE 68127
Telephone: 402-231-5106
Order Desk: 800-856-4648
Fax: 402-331-8776
Website: www.mvplabs.com
Email: MVPLabs@nfinity.com

NEOGEN CORPORATION

628 WINCHESTER RD.
LEXINGTON, KY 40505
Telephone: 859-254-1221
Order Desk: 800-525-2022
Fax: 859-255-5532
Website: www.neogen.com
Email: inform@neogen.com

NEOTECH, LLC

10061 HWY 22
DRESDEN, TN 38225
Telephone: 731-364-5856
Fax: 731-364-5860
Website: www.neotechvaccines.com
Email: info@neotechvaccines.com

NOVARTIS ANIMAL HEALTH US, INC.

3200 NORTHLINE AVE. SUITE 300
GREENSBORO, NC 27408
Customer Service: 800-332-2761
Professional Services: 800-637-0281
Fax: 336-387-1168
Website: www.ah.novartis.com

NOVARTIS ANIMAL VACCINES, INC.

1447 140TH ST.
LARCHWOOD, IA 51241
Telephone: 712-477-2811
Order Desk: 800-843-3386
Fax: 712-477-2686
Technical Information: 800-454-3424
or 800-843-3386
Website: www.grandlab.com
Email (Product Services):
leann.schulz@ah.novartis.com

ORPHAN MEDICAL, INC.

13911 RIDGEDALE DRIVE
SUITE 250
MINNETONKA, MN 55305
Technical Assistance: 888-867-7426
Order Desk: 800-359-4304

PALA-TECH™ LABORATORIES, INC.

20633 KAFTAN COURT
LAKEVILLE, MN 55044
Telephone: 952-985-0746
Toll-Free: 888-337-2446
Fax: 952-985-7735
Website: www.palatech.com
Email: info@palatech.com

PENNFIELD ANIMAL HEALTH

14040 INDUSTRIAL ROAD
OMAHA, NE 68144

Telephone: 402-330-6000
Order Desk: 800-832-8303
Fax: 402-330-6004
Technical Information: 402-330-6000

PERFORMANCE PRODUCTS, INC.

321 N. 22ND STREET
ST. LOUIS, MO 63103

Telephone: 314-421-0300
Fax: 314-421-3332

PET-AG, INC.

P.O. BOX 396
255 KEYES AVENUE
HAMPSHIRE, IL 60140

Telephone: 847-683-2288
Fax: 847-683-2003
Customer Service: 800-323-6878
Technical Service: 800-323-0877
Website: www.petag.com
Email: domsrvc@petag.com

PFIZER INC.
ANIMAL HEALTH GROUP

235 E. 42ND ST.
NEW YORK, NY 10017

Telephone: 800-877-6250
Fax: 610-363-3280
General: 800-877-6250 or 610-363-3100
Customer Service (Orders): 800-733-5500
Technical Services (USA): 800-366-5288
Technical Services (Canada): 800-461-0917
Website: www.pfizer.com/ah

PHARMACIA ANIMAL HEALTH

7000 PORTAGE ROAD
KALAMAZOO, MI 49001
Telephone: 616-833-4000
Fax: 616-833-4077
Customer Service: 800-793-0596
Website: www.pharmaciaAH.com

PHARMADERM
Veterinary Division of Altana Inc.

60 BAYLIS ROAD
MELVILLE, NY 11747
Telephone: 631-454-7677
Order Desk: 800-432-6673
Fax: 631-454-1572
Website: www.pharmaderm.com
Email: trice@altanainc.com

PHARMX, INC.
Animal Health Technology Division

75 MARKET STREET
SUITE 305
PORTLAND, ME 04101
Telephone: 207-772-2129
Order Desk: 800-787-4276
Technical Information: 800-787-4276
Fax: 207-773-5975
Website: www.phrmx.com
Email: PharmX@Phrmx.com

PHIBRO ANIMAL HEALTH

710 ROUTE 46 EAST - SUITE 401
FAIRFIELD, NJ 07004
Telephone: 973-575-5255
Customer Service: 888-403-0074
Fax: 973-575-4354
Website: www.phibroah.com

PHOENIX PHARMACEUTICAL, INC.

4621 EASTON ROAD
P.O. BOX 8068
ST. JOSEPH, MO 64508
Telephone: 816-364-5777
Order Desk: 800-759-3644
Fax: 816-364-4969
Website: www.phoenixpharmaceutical.com
Email: phoenix@ccp.com

PHOENIX SCIENTIFIC, INC.

3915 S. 48TH ST. TERRACE
P.O. BOX 8039 (64508)
ST. JOSEPH, MO 64503
Telephone: 816-364-3777
Fax: 816-364-3778

PREMIER FARMTECH

3315 NORTH OAK TRAFFICWAY
P.O. BOX 7305, DEPT. 120
KANSAS CITY, MO 64116-0005
Telephone: 877-825-9020
Fax: 816-459-5449

PRN PHARMACAL

8809 ELY ROAD
PENSACOLA, FL 32514
Telephone: 850-476-9462
Order Desk: 800-874-9764
Fax: 850-476-7087
Website: www.prnpharmacal.com
Email: gcushing@prnpharmacal.com

PROFESSIONAL BIOLOGICAL COMPANY

4950 YORK STREET
P.O. BOX 16428
DENVER, CO 80216
Telephone: 303-295-7527
Order Desk: 800-525-2065
Fax: 303-295-1923
Website: www.professionalbiological.com

PROFESSIONAL PHARMACEUTICAL CORPORATION

P.O. BOX 2170
OMAHA, NE 68103
Order Desk: 800-224-4017
Fax: 402-593-2468

PR PHARMACEUTICALS

1512 WEBSTER COURT
P.O. BOX 2126
FORT COLLINS, CO 80524-2126
Telephone: 970-484-5560
Order Desk: 888-484-9249
Fax: 970-484-4941
Website: www.prpharm.com

THE PURDUE FREDERICK COMPANY

ONE STAMFORD FORUM
201 TRESSER BLVD.
STAMFORD, CT 06901-3431
Telephone: 203-588-8000
Fax: 203-588-8850
Website: www.purduepharma.com

Q.A. LABORATORIES

404 ADMIRAL BLVD.
KANSAS CITY, MO 64106
Telephone: 816-421-8081
Fax: 816-421-6572

RECKITT BENCKISER PROFESSIONAL

1655 VALLEY ROAD
WAYNE, NJ 07474
Telephone: 973-633-3600
Order Desk: 800-388-1834
Technical Information: 800-677-9218
Fax: 973-633-3593
Website: www.reckittprofessional.com

RITTER MANUFACTURING, INC.

P.O. BOX 801854
HOUSTON, TX 77280-1854
Telephone: 713-461-4261
Fax: 713-461-5254

ROCHESTER MIDLAND CORP.
Food Safety Division

333 HOLLENBECK STREET
P.O. BOX 31515
ROCHESTER, NY 14603-1515
Telephone: 716-336-2200
Order Desk: 800-RMC-4448
Fax: 716-336-2357
Technical Information: 716-336-2263
Website: www.rochestermidland.com

RX VETERINARY PRODUCTS

4869 EAST RAINES ROAD
MEMPHIS, TN 38175
Telephone: 901-366-4442

SAFE4HOURS

6320 SOUTH SANDHILL ROAD
SUITE 10
LAS VEGAS, NV 89120
Telephone: 702-433-7154
Order Desk: 877-925-6000
Fax: 702-433-7192
Website: www.safe4hours.com
Email: info@safe4hours.com

SCHERING-PLOUGH ANIMAL HEALTH CORPORATION

1095 MORRIS AVE.
UNION, NJ 07083
Telephone: 908-629-3490
Order Desk: 800-648-2118
Fax: 908-629-3306
Customer Service: 800-521-5767
Website: www.sp-animalhealth.com

SERA, INC.

P.O. BOX 15866
SHAWNEE MISSION, KS 66285-5866

Telephone: 913-541-1307
Toll-Free: 800-552-3984
Fax: 913-541-1712
Website: www.seramune.com
Email: cbisera@sound.net

SERGEANT'S PET PRODUCTS INC.

P.O. BOX 18993
MEMPHIS, TN 38181-0993
Telephone: 901-362-1950
Clinical Inquiries:
Manager, Regulatory Affairs: 901-362-1950
Fax: 901-795-9525
Customer Service: 800-224-7387
Fax: 901-795-9525
Website: www.sergeants.com

SKYLABS, LTD.

1000 MACOMB ROAD
RUSHVILLE, IL 62681
Telephone: 217-322-4327
Fax: 217-322-4329

SSI CORPORATION

210 SOUTH CEDAR STREET, P.O. BOX 9
JULESBURG, CO 80737
Telephone: 970-474-0974
Order Desk: 800-654-3668
Fax: 970-474-2186
Email: HOOFSOLUTIONS@CS.com

STEARNS PACKAGING CORPORATION

4200 SYCAMORE AVENUE
P.O. BOX 3216
MADISON, WI 53704
Telephone: 608-246-5150
Order Desk: 800-655-5008
Fax: 608-246-5149
Website: www.stearnspkg.com
Email: stearns@stearnspkg.com

SUNGRO CHEMICALS, INC.

P.O. BOX 24632
LOS ANGELES, CA 90024
Telephone: 213-747-4125
Order Desk: 800-463-9179
Fax: 213-747-0942
Email: lmackson@aol.com

SURENUTRITION
A Division of Farnam Companies, Inc.

301 WEST OSBORN ROAD
PHOENIX, AZ 85013-3928
Telephone: 602-285-1660
Toll-Free: 800-234-2269
Fax: 602-285-1803
Website: www.sure-nutrition.com

SWEETLIX, LLC

1080 WILBANKS ST.
MONTGOMERY, AL 36108
Telephone: 334-834-6510
Toll-Free: 800-325-1486
Fax: 334-264-8673
Website: www.sweetlix.com

SYNBIOTICS CORPORATION

11011 VIA FRONTERA
SAN DIEGO, CA 92127

Customer Service:	800-228-4305
Technical Service:	800-228-4305
Fax:	858-675-2421
Website:	www.synbiotics.com

SYNTROVET INCORPORATED
A division of Schering-Plough Animal Health

P.O. BOX 3182
UNION, NJ 07083

Telephone:	913-888-8876
Order Desk:	800-525-9480
Fax:	913-894-9373

TECHMIX, INC.

740 BOWMAN STREET
STEWART, MN 55385

Telephone:	320-562-2740
Order Desk:	877-466-6455
Fax:	320-562-2125
Website:	www.techmixinc.com
Email:	techmix@hutchtel.net

TECHNIVET

4 INDUSTRY ROAD
BOX 189
BRUNSWICK, ME 04011

Telephone:	207-725-2252
Order Desk:	800-545-2252
Fax:	207-725-2252

TEXAS VET LAB, INC.

1702 NORTH BELL STREET
SAN ANGELO, TX 76903

Telephone:	915-653-4505
Order Desk:	800-284-8403
Fax:	915-653-4501
Website:	www.texasvetlab.com
Email:	txvetlab@wcc.net

THORNELL CORPORATION

160 WHEELOCK RD.
PENFIELD, NY 14526

Telephone:	716-586-5147
Fax:	716-586-1744
Website:	www.thornell.com
Email:	thornco@eznet.net

TOMLYN PRODUCTS
Division of Vétoquinol, USA

P.O. BOX 209
101 LINCOLN AVE., BUENA, NJ 08310
Telephone: 856-697-5115
Customer Service: 800-267-5707
Fax: 856-697-7465
Email: info@tomlyn.com

TRADEWINDS, INC.

20927 STATE ROUTE K
P.O. BOX 3128 (64503)
ST. JOSEPH, MO 64505
Telephone: 877-734-7565
Order Desk: 877-734-7565
Fax: 816-233-9546
Website: www.tradewindsforpets.com

UNITED VACCINES, INC.

P.O. BOX 44220
MADISON, WI 53744-4220
Telephone: 608-277-2030
Order Desk: 800-283-6465
Fax: 608-277-2120

VACCICEL, INC.

101 GREENBRIER STREET
P.O. BOX 847
BELTON, TX 76513
Telephone: 254-939-7778
Fax: 254-939-1955
Email: vaccicel@vvm.com

VEDCO, INC.

5503 CORPORATE DR.
ST. JOSEPH, MO 64507
Telephone: 816-238-8840
Toll-Free: 888-708-3326 (888-70VEDCO)
Fax: 816-238-1837
Website: www.vedco.com/dvmonly/

VET-A-MIX
A Division of LLOYD, Inc.

604 WEST THOMAS AVENUE, P.O. BOX 130
SHENANDOAH, IA 51601

Telephone: 712-246-4000
Order Desk: 800-831-0004
Fax: 712-246-5254
Website: www.lloydinc.com
Email: info@lloydinc.com

VETERINARY DYNAMICS, INC.

1535 TEMPLETON ROAD
TEMPLETON, CA 93465

Telephone: 805-434-0321
Order Desk: 800-654-9743
Fax: 805-434-3840
Website: www.veterinarydynamics.com
Email: vdi@thegrid.net

VETERINARY LABORATORIES, INC.

12340 SANTA FE TRAIL DRIVE
LENEXA, KS 66215

Telephone: 913-888-7500
Order Desk: 800-255-6368
Fax: 913-888-6741

VETERINARY PHARMACEUTICALS COMPANY
Division of Nylos Trading Co. Inc.

P.O. BOX D 3700
POMONA, NY 10970
Telephone: 845-354-8787
Fax: 845-354-8703

VETERINARY PRODUCTS LABORATORIES

301 W. OSBORN
PHOENIX, AZ 85013
Telephone: 800-720-0032
Order Desk: 800-720-0032 Ext 2158, 2283 or 2284
Fax: 800-215-5875
Toll-Free: 888-241-9545
Website: www.vpl.com
Email: info@vpl.com

VETERINARY SPECIALTIES, INC.

28358 WEST VANCE COURT
BARRINGTON, IL 60010
Telephone: 847-304-8708
Order Desk: 888-838-7732
Fax: 847-304-9199

VETLIFE

1001 OFFICE PARK RD.
SUITE 201
WEST DES MOINES, IA 50265
Telephone: 515-224-0788
Order Desk: 888-462-3493
Fax: 515-224-0804
Website: www.vetlife.com
Email: info@vetlife.com

VETREPHARM RESEARCH INC.
(see Bioniche Animal Health USA, Inc.)

VET SOLUTIONS

P.O. BOX 210037
BEDFORD, TX 76095
Telephone: 817-285-8500
Order Desk: 800-285-0508
Fax: 817-285-8100
Website: www.vetsolutions.com

VETS PLUS, INC.
Animal Health & Nutrition

102 THIRD AVENUE EAST
KNAPP, WI 54749
Telephone: 715-665-2118
Order Desk: 800-468-3877
Fax: 715-665-2401
Website: www.vets-plus.com
Email: custsvc@vets-plus.com

VET TEK, INC.

P.O. BOX 279
100 S.E. MAGELLAN DRIVE
BLUE SPRINGS, MO 64014
Telephone: 816-229-9101
Order Desk: 800-821-5570
Fax: 816-224-3080
Website: www.durvet.com
Email: info@durvet.com

VETUS ANIMAL HEALTH
c/o BURNS VETERINARY SUPPLY, INC.

1900 DIPLOMAT DRIVE
FARMERS BRANCH, TX 75234
Telephone: 972-620-9941 or 800-92-BURNS
Order Desk: 800-92-BURNS (National); 877-766-5780 (Baltimore)
Fax: 972-620-1071
Website: www.burnsvet.com
Email: KimA@Dallas.DarbyGroup.com

VIRBAC CORPORATION

P.O. BOX 162059
FORT WORTH, TX 76161
Telephone: 817-831-5030
Order Desk: 800-338-3659
Fax: 817-831-8327
Website: www.virbac.com

VITA-KEY, L.C.

P.O. BOX 823
DECATUR, TX 76234-0823
Telephone: 940-627-3100
Order Desk: 800-539-8482
Fax: 940-627-6810
Website: www.vita-key.com
Email: vita-key@vita-key.com

VORTECH PHARMACEUTICALS, LTD.

6851 CHASE ROAD
DEARBORN, MI 48126
Telephone: 313-584-4088
Order Desk: 800-521-4686
Fax: 313-581-8550
Toll-Free (Inside Michigan): 800-372-2714
Toll-Free (Other States & Canada): 800-521-4686

WEBSTER VETERINARY SUPPLY, INC.

86 LEOMINSTER ROAD
STERLING, MA 01564
Telephone: 978-422-8211
Toll-Free: 800-225-7911
Fax: 978-422-8959
Website: www.webstervet.com
Email: vetsupply@webstervet.com

WELLMARK INTERNATIONAL

1100 E. WOODFIELD ROAD
SUITE 500
SCHAUMBURG, IL 60173
Telephone: 800-766-7661
Fax: 800-426-7473

WEST AGRO, INC.

11100 NORTH CONGRESS AVENUE
KANSAS CITY, MO 64153-1296
Telephone: 816-891-1600
Order Desk: 800-421-1905
Fax: 816-891-6945
Website: www.westagro.com
Email: winston.ingalls@delaval.com

WESTERN CHEMICAL, INC.

1269 LATTIMORE ROAD
FERNDALE, WA 98248
Telephone: 360-384-5898
Order Desk: 800-283-5292
Fax: 360-384-0270
Email: wci@PREMIER1.NET

WESTFALIA•SURGE, INC.

1880 COUNTRY FARM DRIVE
NAPERVILLE, IL 60563
Telephone: 630-369-8100
Order Desk: 800-323-1667
Fax: 630-369-9875
Technical Support: 888-400-5990
Website: www.westfaliasurge.com

W. F. YOUNG, INC.

302 BENTON DRIVE
P.O. BOX 1990
EAST LONGMEADOW, MA 01028-5990
Telephone: 413-526-9999
Order Desk: 800-628-9653
Fax: 413-526-8990
Website: www.absorbine.com
Email: animalhealth@absorbine.com

WILDLIFE PHARMACEUTICALS, INC.

1512 WEBSTER COURT
P.O. BOX 2126
FORT COLLINS, CO 80522-2126
Telephone: 970-484-6267
Fax: 970-482-6184
Website: www.wildpharm.com
Email: info@wildpharm.com

WYSONG CORPORATION

1880 NORTH EASTMAN ROAD
MIDLAND, MI 48642-8896
Telephone: 989-631-0009
Order Desk: 800-748-0188
Fax: 989-631-8801
Website: www.wysong.net
Email: wysong@tm.net

ZINPRO CORPORATION

10400 VIKING DR.
SUITE 240
EDEN PRAIRIE, MN 55344-7298
Telephone: 952-944-2736
Order Desk: 800-445-6145
Fax: 952-944-2749
Website: www.zinpro.com
Email: zinpro@zinpro.com

Brand Name - Ingredient Index

This listing is an alphabetical cross-reference of ingredient and brand names. Names in bold type face are ingredients, and those in regular type face are brand names.

Listings by ingredients are given in the following format:

ingredient(s). Brand Name *(Manufacturer).*

Listings by brand names are given in the following format:

Brand Name *(Manufacturer)*, **ingredient(s).**

Where products have more than one ingredient, the listing will be as follows (example with three ingredients, x, y, and z):

ingredient x, ingredient y, ingredient z. Brand Name *(Manufacturer).*
ingredient y, ingredient z, ingredient x. Brand Name *(Manufacturer).*
ingredient z, ingredient x, ingredient y. Brand Name *(Manufacturer).*
Brand Name *(Manufacturer),* **ingredient x, ingredient y, ingredient z.**

Claims are not made for the therapeutic equivalence of the products listed. Therapeutic efficacy depends upon the amount of drug present in each dose, the pharmaceutical form, the physical nature of the active drug used, the presence of other substances, the method of manufacture, and the exercise of quality control.

Every effort has been made to ensure the accuracy of the information published. However, it remains the responsibility of the readers to familiarize themselves with the product information contained on the product label or package insert. The Publisher, Editorial Team and all those involved in the production of this book, cannot be held responsible for publication errors or any consequence that could result from the use of published information.

#

A

Agri-Cillin™ *(AgriLabs)*, **penicillin G procaine.**

Agri-Mectin™ Equine Paste Dewormer 1.87% *(AgriLabs)*, **ivermectin.**

Agrimycin® 100 *(AgriLabs)*, **oxytetracycline.**

Agrimycin® 200 *(AgriLabs)*, **oxytetracycline.**

Agrimycin®-343 *(AgriLabs)*, **oxytetracycline.**

Agrimycin® Powder *(AgriLabs)*, **oxytetracycline.**

Agri Plus Keto-Nia Drench™ *(Vets Plus)*, **niacin, propylene glycol, vitamins.**

Ag-Tek® Poly-Lube™ *(Kane)*, **lubricating powder.**

Air$_x$® 75 *(Airex)*, **quaternary ammonia.**

Albac® 50 *(Alpharma)*, **bacitracin (zinc).**

Albadry Plus® *(Pharmacia & Upjohn)*, **novobiocin, penicillin G procaine.**

Albamix® Feed Medication *(Pharmacia & Upjohn)*, **novobiocin.**

Albaplex® *(Pharmacia & Upjohn)*, **novobiocin, tetracycline.**

albendazole. Valbazen® Cattle Dewormer Paste *(Pfizer Animal Health)*, Valbazen® Suspension *(Pfizer Animal Health)*.

Albon® Boluses *(Pfizer Animal Health)*, **sulfadimethoxine.**

Albon® Concentrated Solution 12.5% *(Pfizer Animal Health)*, **sulfadimethoxine.**

Albon® Injection 40% *(Pfizer Animal Health)*, **sulfadimethoxine.**

Albon® Oral Suspension 5% *(Pfizer Animal Health)*, **sulfadimethoxine.**

Albon® SR *(Pfizer Animal Health)*, **sulfadimethoxine.**

Albon® Tablets *(Pfizer Animal Health)*, **sulfadimethoxine.**

albuterol sulfate. Torpex™ *(Boehringer Ingelheim)*.

alcohol, butoxypolypropylene glycol, carbomer, chloroxylenol. Swimmer's Ear Astringent *(Vet Solutions)*.

alcohol, camphor, Canada balsam. VetRx™ Small Fur Animal Remedy *(Goodwinol)*.

alcohol, camphor, Canada balsam, corn oil base, oil origanum, oil rosemary. VetRx™ Caged Bird Remedy *(Goodwinol)*, VetRx™ for Cats and Kittens *(Goodwinol)*, VetRx™ for Dogs and Puppies *(Goodwinol)*, VetRx™ Goat & Sheep Remedy *(Goodwinol)*, VetRx™ Pigeon Remedy *(Goodwinol)*, VetRx™ Poultry Remedy *(Goodwinol)*, VetRx™ Rabbit Remedy *(Goodwinol)*.

alcohol, cocamido propyl phosphatidyl, dimonium chloride, propylene glycol. EarMed Cleansing Solution & Wash *(Davis)*.

alcohol, iodide (potassium), iodine, menthol, spearmint oil, witch hazel. Absorbine® RefreshMint® *(W. F. Young)*.

alcohol, quaternary ammonia. Asepti-Wipe™ *(Ecolab Prof. Prod. Div.)*, MetriWipes® *(Metrex)*.

alcohol base, aromatic vegetable oil(s), methyl salicylate, salicylic acid. Bigeloil® *(W. F. Young)*.

alcohol base, glycerine. Corium-20™ *(Virbac)*.

Alfalfa Pellet Horse Wormer *(Farnam)*, **piperazine.**

allantoin, benzalkonium chloride, carbamide. Myosan™ Cream *(Life Science)*, Myosan™ Solution *(Life Science)*.

allantoin, benzocaine, pine tar, propylene glycol, vitamin A, vitamin C (ascorbic acid). A-Plus™ Wound Dressing *(Creative Science)*.

Allercaine™ *(Tomlyn)*, **benzalkonium chloride, denatonium benzoate, lidocaine.**

Allergroom® Shampoo *(Virbac)*, **chitosanide, glycerine, lactic acid, urea.**

Allermyl™ Shampoo *(Virbac)*, **propylene glycol, sodium alkyl ether sulfate, sodium lauryl sulfate.**

Allerpet® C *(V.P.L.)*, **cleaning formulation/spray.**

Allerpet® D *(V.P.L.)*, **cleaning formulation/spray.**

Allerseb-T® Shampoo *(Virbac)*, **coal tar, salicylic acid, sulfur.**

Allerspray™ *(Evsco)*, **benzalkonium chloride, lidocaine.**

All-In-One Calf Bolus *(AgriPharm)*, **fermentation extract(s), microorganisms, vitamins.**

All-In-One Cattle Bolus *(AgriPharm)*, **fermentation extract(s), microorganisms, vitamins.**

All-Pro Biotic™ *(Vets Plus)*, **microorganisms.**

All Purpose Lubricant *(Durvet)*, **aqueous base lubricant(s).**

AloCetic™ Ear Rinse *(DVM)*, **acetic acid, aloe vera.**

aloe, boric acid, acetic acid. EarMed Boracetic® Flush *(Davis)*.

Aloe & Oatmeal Shampoo *(Vet Solutions)*, **aloe vera, oatmeal.**

Aloe & Oatmeal Skin & Coat Conditioner *(Vet Solutions)*, **aloe vera, conditioner formula.**

Aloeclens Otic Cleanser *(Vetus)*, **ear cleanser formula.**

Aloedine® Medicated Shampoo *(Farnam)*, **iodine.**

Aloe Heal™ *(Farnam)*, **aloe vera, vitamin A, vitamin D, vitamin E.**

aloe vera, acetic acid. AloCetic™ Ear Rinse *(DVM)*.

aloe vera, β-[1,4]-linked mannan polymers (Acemannan). CarraVet™ Spray-Gel Wound Dressing *(V.P.L.)*, CarraVet™ Wound Dressing *(V.P.L.)*.

aloe vera, beeswax, emulsifying wax, glycerine, lanolin, petrolatum. Dealer Select Horse Care Hoof Moisturizer *(Durvet)*.

aloe vera, bentonite, boric acid, ferrous sulfate, glycerine, kaolin. Icetight® *(Horse Health)*, Reducine® Poultice *(Equicare)*.

aloe vera, chloroxylenol, humectant(s), vitamins. H-Balm Udder Cream *(Centaur)*.

aloe vera, comfrey. Pad-Tough™ *(Life Science)*.

aloe vera, conditioner formula. Aloe & Oatmeal Skin & Coat Conditioner *(Vet Solutions)*.

aloe vera, emollient(s), ethyl alcohol. Waterless Antibacterial Hand Cleaner *(Davis)*.

aloe vera, emollient(s), peppermint oil. Natural Mint Liniment™ *(Horses Prefer)*.

aloe vera, emollient(s), vitamins. Udder Balm *(Aspen)*, *(First Priority)*.

aloe vera, glycerine, triethanolamine, vitamin E. SoftGuard™ *(Activon)*.

aloe vera, iodide (potassium), isopropyl alcohol, menthol, parachlorometaxylenol, thymol, witch hazel, wormwood oil. Veterinary Liniment *(First Priority)*.

aloe vera, lanolin, moisturizer(s), PABA sun screen, vitamins. Medicated Udder Balm *(First Priority)*.

aloe vera, lanolin, neatsfoot oil, vitamins. Absorbine® Hooflex® Moisturizing Creme *(W. F. Young)*.

aloe vera, lanolin, vitamins. -50 Below *(AgriPharm)*.

aloe vera, moisturizer(s), stain removers, vitamin E. CarraVet™ Multi Purpose Cleansing Foam *(V.P.L.)*.

aloe vera, moisturizer(s), vitamin A, vitamin D, vitamin E. DuraCream *(Durvet)*.

aloe vera, oatmeal. Aloe & Oatmeal Shampoo *(Vet Solutions)*, Oatmeal & Aloe Shampoo *(Davis)*.

aloe vera, oil of lavender, oil of lemongrass, oil of pennyroyal. EarMed Mite Lotion *(Davis)*.

aloe vera, parachlorometaxylenol, propylene glycol. Thrush Treatment *(First Priority)*.

aloe vera, scarlet oil. Scarlet Oil with Aloe Vera *(Life Science)*.

aloe vera, shampoo formula. AlphaLyte® Premium Pet Shampoo *(Alpha Tech Pet)*.

aloe vera, vitamin A, vitamin D, vitamin E. Aloe Heal™ *(Farnam)*.

AlphaLyte® Premium Pet Shampoo *(Alpha Tech Pet)*, **aloe vera, shampoo formula.**

AlphaZyme Plus™ *(Alpha Tech Pet)*, **enzymes.**

Altosid® Cattle Custom Blending Premix *(Wellmark)*, **methoprene.**

Altosid® Premix *(Wellmark)*, **methoprene.**

altrenogest. Regu-Mate® Solution *(Intervet)*.

alum, chloroxylenol. McKillip's Dusting Powder *(Butler)*, *(First Priority)*.

alum, chloroxylenol, ferrous sulfate, tannic acid. Blood Stop Powder *(Aspen)*, *(Durvet)*, *(Vedco)*, Hemostat Powder *(Phoenix Pharmaceutical)*.

alum, copper sulfate, iodoform, tannic acid, activated charcoal. Wonder Dust™ Wound Powder *(Farnam)*.

alum, dimethyl chlorophenol. Equi-Phar™ McKillips Powder *(Vedco)*.

alum, ferric subsulfate, tannic acid, thymol. Blood Stop Powder *(Dominion)*.

alum, ferric sulfate, tannic acid, thymol. Blood Stop Powder *(AgriLabs)*.

aluminum, calcium carbonate, dicalcium phosphate. Neigh-Lox® *(K.P.P.)*.

aluminum chlohydroxy allantoinate, parachlorometaxylenol. Absorbine® Hooflex® Thrush Remedy *(W. F. Young)*.

aluminum chloride, ammonium chloride, bentonite, benzocaine, copper sulfate, diatomaceous earth, ferric subsulfate, iodoform. Clot-It Plus™ *(Evsco)*, Nik Stop® Styptic Powder *(Tomlyn)*.

aluminum chloride, ammonium chloride, bentonite, copper sulfate, diatomite, ferric subsulfate, iodoform. Blood Stop Powder *(Butler)*.

aluminum chloride, ammonium chloride, bentonite, copper sulfate, diatomite, ferrous sulfate, iodine complex (povidone-iodine). Kwik-Stop® Styptic Powder *(ARC)*.

aluminum hydroxide, kaolin, pectin. Anti-Diarrhea Tablets *(ARC)*, Diarrhea Tabs *(Butler)*.

aluminum powder. AluSpray® *(Neogen)*.

aluminum silicate, attapulgite, carob, magnesium trisilicate, pectin. Veda-Sorb Jr Bolus *(Vedco)*.

aluminum silicate, zinc oxide, acetic acid. Ice-O-Poultice® *(Hawthorne)*.

aluminum sulfate, chloroxylenol, collagen, ferric sulfate. Clotisol® Liquid *(BenePet)*.

AluSpray® *(Neogen)*, **aluminum powder.**

A-Lyte Concentrate *(Durvet)*, **amino acids, dextrose, electrolytes.**

A-Lyte Solution *(Durvet)*, **amino acids, dextrose, electrolytes, vitamin B-complex.**

ambicin N. Consept® Barrier Sanitizing Teat Dip *(Westfalia•Surge)*, Consept® Pre+Post Teat Dip *(Westfalia•Surge)*.

Ambi-Pen™ *(Butler)*, **penicillin G benzathine, penicillin G procaine.**

Amcalcilyte Forte *(AgriPharm)*, *(Phoenix Pharmaceutical)*, *(Vedco)*, **amino acids, dextrose, electrolytes.**

Amforol® Suspension *(Fort Dodge)*, **attapulgite, bismuth subcarbonate, kanamycin sulfate, pectin.**

Amforol® Tablets *(Fort Dodge)*, **attapulgite, bismuth subcarbonate, kanamycin sulfate, pectin.**

Amifuse E *(Vetus)*, **amikacin sulfate.**

Amiglyde-V® Injection *(Fort Dodge)*, **amikacin sulfate.**

Amiglyde-V® Intrauterine Solution *(Fort Dodge)*, **amikacin sulfate.**

Amiject D *(Vetus)*, **amikacin sulfate.**

Amikacin C Injection *(Phoenix Pharmaceutical)*, **amikacin sulfate.**

Amikacin E Solution *(Phoenix Pharmaceutical)*, **amikacin sulfate.**

amikacin sulfate. Amifuse E *(Vetus)*, Amiglyde-V® Injection *(Fort Dodge)*, Amiglyde-V® Intrauterine Solution *(Fort Dodge)*, Amiject D *(Vetus)*, Amikacin C Injection *(Phoenix Pharmaceutical)*, Amikacin E Solution *(Phoenix Pharmaceutical)*, Amikacin Sulfate Injection *(Butler)*, *(Vet Tek)*, Amikacin Sulfate Solution *(Vet Tek)*, AmTech AmiMax™ C Injection *(Phoenix Scientific)*, AmTech AmiMax™ E Solution *(Phoenix Scientific)*, CaniGlide™ *(Vedco)*, Equi-Phar EquiGlide™ *(Vedco)*.

Amikacin Sulfate Injection *(Butler)*, *(Vet Tek)*, **amikacin sulfate.**

Amikacin Sulfate Solution *(Vet Tek)*, **amikacin sulfate.**

Amino Acid Bolus *(Vets Plus)*, **amino acids, minerals, vitamins.**

Amino Acid Concentrate *(AgriLabs)*, **amino acids, electrolytes, vitamins.**

Amino Acid Concentrate Oral Solution *(Aspen)*, *(Bimeda)*, **amino acids, dextrose, electrolytes, vitamin B-complex.**

Amino Acid Oral Concentrate *(Phoenix Pharmaceutical)*, **amino acids, dextrose, electrolytes, vitamin B-complex.**

Amino Acid Oral Solution *(Aspen)*, *(Bimeda)*, *(Phoenix Pharmaceutical)*, **amino acids, dextrose, electrolytes, vitamin B-complex.**

amino acids, bicarbonate, microorganisms, minerals, vitamins. Pre-Conditioning/Receiving Formula Gel *(Durvet)*, Ruminant Lactobacillus Gel *(First Priority)*.

amino acids, biotin, vitamins. Dealer Select Horse Care NutriHoof *(Durvet)*.

amino acids, copper. Availa® Cu 100 *(Zinpro)*.

amino acids, copper, iron, vitamin B-complex. NutriVed™ B-Complex Plus Iron Liquid *(Vedco)*.

amino acids, dextrose, electrolytes. A-Lyte Concentrate *(Durvet)*, Amcalcilyte Forte *(AgriPharm)*, *(Phoenix Pharmaceutical)*, *(Vedco)*, Aminocal Plus™ *(Butler)*, AmTech Amcal High Potency Oral Solution *(Phoenix Scientific)*, Glucaminolyte Forte *(AgriPharm)*, *(Vedco)*, Gluco-Amino-Forte Oral Solution *(Phoenix Pharmaceutical)*, Gluco Amino Forte Oral Solution *(Vetus)*, Keto Amino Forte™ *(Butler)*.

amino acids, dextrose, electrolytes, vitamin B-complex. A-Lyte Solution *(Durvet)*, Amino Acid Concentrate Oral Solution *(Aspen)*, *(Bimeda)*, Amino Acid Oral Concentrate *(Phoenix Pharmaceutical)*, Amino Acid Oral Solution *(Aspen)*, *(Bimeda)*, *(Phoenix Pharmaceutical)*, Aminoplex *(Butler)*, Aminoplex Concentrate *(Butler)*, Amino Plus Concentrate *(AgriPharm)*, Amino Plus Solution *(AgriPharm)*, AmTech Amino Acid Oral Concentrate *(Phoenix Scientific)*, AmTech Amino Acid Oral Solution *(Phoenix Scientific)*, Double "A" Concentrate *(Vedco)*, Double "A" Solution *(Vedco)*.

amino acids, dextrose, minerals, vitamins. Tryptophan Plus Gel™ *(Horses Prefer)*.

amino acids, electrolytes. Equi-Phar™ Electramino Paste *(Vedco)*.

amino acids, electrolytes, energy source(s), minerals, vitamins. Energy Drench *(Vedco)*.

amino acids, electrolytes, energy source(s), vitamins. Energy+ *(Butler)*, NRG-Plus™ *(Bimeda)*, Pic-M-Up™ *(AgriPharm)*.

amino acids, electrolytes, fatty acids (essential), minerals. NutriVed™ Chewable Vitamins for Active Dogs *(Vedco)*.

amino acids, electrolytes, glucose. Electramine® *(Life Science)*.

amino acids, electrolytes, minerals, torula yeast. Procal™ Powder *(Butler)*.

amino acids, electrolytes, vitamins. Amino Acid Concentrate *(AgriLabs)*, Amino Acid Solution *(AgriLabs)*, OTC™ Jug *(SureNutrition)*.

amino acids, enzymes, microorganisms, minerals, vitamins, yeast. Vita-Key® Show Cattle Concentrate, Phase II *(Vita-Key)*.

amino acids, enzymes, microorganisms, vitamins, yeast. Vita Boost Paste™ *(AgriLabs)*.

amino acids, fatty acids (essential), minerals, taurine, vitamins. NutriVed™ Chewable Vitamins for Cats *(Vedco)*, NutriVed™ Chewable Vitamins for Kittens *(Vedco)*.

amino acids, fatty acids (essential), minerals, vitamins. NutriVed™ Chewable Vitamins for Dogs *(Vedco)*, NutriVed™ Chewable Vitamins for Puppies *(Vedco)*, NutriVed™ Hypo Allergenic Chewable Tablets *(Vedco)*.

amino acids, fatty acids (omega), vitamins, zinc. Pet Vites O.F.A. Chewable Tablets *(Vetus)*.

amino acids, iron. Availa® Fe 60 *(Zinpro)*.

amino acids, lactic acid producing bacteria, minerals, vitamins. MultiMax™ *(SureNutrition)*.

amino acids, manganese. Availa® Mn 80 *(Zinpro)*.

amino acids, microorganisms, minerals, vitamins. Ruminant LactoBac Gel *(Vedco)*.

amino acids, microorganisms, minerals, vitamins, yeast. Vita-Key® Swine Supplement *(Vita-Key)*.

amino acids, minerals. Availa®-4 *(Zinpro)*, AvailaMin® - Grow/Finish *(Zinpro)*, AvailaMin® - Sow *(Zinpro)*, AvailaMin® - Starter I, II, III *(Zinpro)*, Zinpro+3 *(Zinpro)*.

amino acids, minerals, propylene glycol, vitamins. PRN Hi-Energy Supplement™ *(PRN Pharmacal)*.

amino acids, minerals, selenium, tetrachlorvinphos, vitamins. Vita-Plus® with Equitrol® *(Farnam)*.

amino acids, minerals, taurine, vitamins. Cholodin®-FEL *(MVP)*.

amino acids, minerals, vitamins. Amino Acid Bolus *(Vets Plus)*, Equinime® *(Chariton)*, Maxum® Crumbles *(Horse Health)*, Stam-N-Aid™ *(Neogen)*, Vita Plus® *(Farnam)*.

amino acids, minerals, vitamins, yeast. Vita-Key® Antioxidant Concentrate *(Vita-Key)*, Vita-Key® Equine Supplement *(Vita-Key)*, Vita-Key® Mare & Foal Supplement *(Vita-Key)*.

amino acids, nitrogen, peptides. Arm & Hammer® Bio-Chlor® *(Church & Dwight)*, Arm & Hammer® Fermenten® *(Church & Dwight)*.

amino acids, vitamins. Dealer Select Horse Care Farrier's Select *(Durvet)*.

amino acids, zinc. Availa® Zn 40 *(Zinpro)*, Availa® Zn 100 *(Zinpro)*.

Amino Acid Solution *(AgriLabs)*, **amino acids, electrolytes, vitamins.**

Aminocal Plus™ *(Butler)*, **amino acids, dextrose, electrolytes.**

aminopentamide. Centrine® Injection *(Fort Dodge)*, Centrine® Tablets *(Fort Dodge)*.

Aminoplex *(Butler)*, **amino acids, dextrose, electrolytes, vitamin B-complex.**

Aminoplex Concentrate *(Butler)*, **amino acids, dextrose, electrolytes, vitamin B-complex.**

Amino Plus Concentrate *(AgriPharm)*, **amino acids, dextrose, electrolytes, vitamin B-complex.**

Amino Plus Solution *(AgriPharm)*, **amino acids, dextrose, electrolytes, vitamin B-complex.**

amitraz. Mitaban® *(Pharmacia & Upjohn)*, Preventic® Collar for Dogs *(Virbac)*, Taktic® E.C. *(Intervet)*.

amitraz, pyriproxyfen. Preventic® Plus Tick and Flea IGR Collar for Dogs *(Virbac)*.

Ammonil® Tablets *(King Animal Health)*, **methionine (d-l).**

ammonium bicarbonate, ammonium hydroxide, citric acid, copper carbonate. Cop-R-Sol™ *(Alpharma)*.

ammonium carbonate, camphor, menthol. ZEV *(Dominion)*.

ammonium chloride. Uroeze® *(King Animal Health)*, Uroeze® 200 *(King Animal Health)*.

ammonium chloride, bentonite, benzocaine, copper sulfate, diatomaceous earth, ferric subsulfate, iodoform, aluminum chloride. Clot-It Plus™ *(Evsco)*, Nik Stop® Styptic Powder *(Tomlyn)*.

ammonium chloride, bentonite, copper sulfate, diatomite, ferric subsulfate, iodoform, aluminum chloride. Blood Stop Powder *(Butler)*.

ammonium chloride, bentonite, copper sulfate, diatomite, ferrous sulfate, iodine complex (povidone-iodine), aluminum chloride. Kwik-Stop® Styptic Powder *(ARC)*.

ammonium chloride, benzoic acid, calcium phosphate, sodium bicarbonate, sodium chloride. Expectorant Powder *(First Priority)*.

ammonium chloride, camphor, turpentine. White Liniment *(Butler)*, *(Durvet)*.

ammonium chloride, guaifenesin (glyceryl guaiacolate, guaiacol), phenylephrine hydrochloride, pyrilamine maleate, sodium chloride. Cough Syrup *(Life Science)*.

ammonium chloride, guaifenesin (glyceryl guaiacolate, guaiacol), phenylephrine hydrochloride, pyrilamine maleate, sodium citrate. Anti-Tussive Syrup with Antihistamine *(Vedco)*, ExpectaHist *(Vetus)*.

ammonium chloride, guaifenesin (glyceryl guaiacolate, guaiacol), potassium iodide. AniTuss *(AHC)*, Spec-Tuss™ *(Neogen)*, Tri-Tussin™ Powder *(Creative Science)*.

ammonium chloride, isopropyl alcohol (isopropanol). MetriGuard® *(Metrex)*.

ammonium chloride, methionine (d-l). Fus-Sol™ Drops *(PPI)*.

ammonium hydroxide, citric acid, copper carbonate, ammonium bicarbonate. Cop-R-Sol™ *(Alpharma)*.

amodimethicone, methionine (d-l), minerals, vegetable oil(s), vitamins. Equ-Aid Plus *(Vet-A-Mix)*.

amoxicillin. Amoxi-Drop® *(Pfizer Animal Health)*, Amoxi-Inject® (Cattle) *(Pfizer Animal Health)*, Amoxi-Inject® (Dogs and Cats) *(Pfizer Animal Health)*, Amoxi-Mast® *(Pfizer Animal Health)*, Amoxi-Tabs® (Dogs) *(Pfizer Animal Health)*, Amoxi-Tabs® (Dogs and Cats) *(Pfizer Animal Health)*, Biomox® Oral Suspension *(Delmarva)*, Biomox® Tablets *(Delmarva)*, Robamox®-V Oral Suspension *(Fort Dodge)*, Robamox®-V Tablets *(Fort Dodge)*.

amoxicillin, clavulanic acid. Clavamox® Drops *(Pfizer Animal Health)*, Clavamox® Tablets *(Pfizer Animal Health)*.

Amoxi-Drop® *(Pfizer Animal Health)*, **amoxicillin.**

Amoxi-Inject® (Cattle) *(Pfizer Animal Health)*, **amoxicillin.**

Amoxi-Inject® (Dogs and Cats) *(Pfizer Animal Health)*, **amoxicillin.**

Amoxi-Mast® *(Pfizer Animal Health)*, **amoxicillin.**

Amoxi-Tabs® (Dogs) *(Pfizer Animal Health)*, **amoxicillin.**

Amoxi-Tabs® (Dogs and Cats) *(Pfizer Animal Health)*, **amoxicillin.**

Amphicol® Film-Coated Tablets *(Butler)*, **chloramphenicol.**

Amphyl® Disinfectant Cleaner *(Reckitt Benckiser)*, **phenolic disinfectants.**

ampicillin. Polyflex® *(Fort Dodge)*.

Amprol® 9.6% Oral Solution *(Merial)*, **amprolium.**

Amprol® 25% Type A Medicated Article *(Merial)*, **amprolium.**

Amprol® 128 20% Soluble Powder *(Merial)*, **amprolium.**

amprolium. Amprol® 9.6% Oral Solution *(Merial)*, Amprol® 25% Type A Medicated Article *(Merial)*, Amprol® 128 20% Soluble Powder *(Merial)*, Amprovine® 25% Type A Medicated Article *(Merial)*, Corid® 9.6% Oral Solution *(Merial)*, Corid® 20% Soluble Powder *(Merial)*.

amprolium, ethopabate. Amprol Plus® Type A Medicated Article *(Merial)*.

Amprol Plus® Type A Medicated Article *(Merial)*, **amprolium, ethopabate.**

Amprovine® 25% Type A Medicated Article *(Merial)*, **amprolium.**

AmTech Amcal High Potency Oral Solution *(Phoenix Scientific)*, **amino acids, dextrose, electrolytes.**

AmTech AmiMax™ C Injection *(Phoenix Scientific)*, **amikacin sulfate.**

AmTech AmiMax™ E Solution *(Phoenix Scientific)*, **amikacin sulfate.**

AmTech Amino Acid Oral Concentrate *(Phoenix Scientific)*, **amino acids, dextrose, electrolytes, vitamin B-complex.**

AmTech Amino Acid Oral Solution *(Phoenix Scientific)*, **amino acids, dextrose, electrolytes, vitamin B-complex.**

AmTech Amisol-R Injection *(Phoenix Scientific)*, **magnesium chloride, potassium chloride, sodium acetate, sodium chloride, sodium gluconate.**

AmTech Anthelban V *(Phoenix Scientific)*, **pyrantel pamoate.**

AmTech Aspirin Bolus *(Phoenix Scientific)*, **acetylsalicylic acid.**

AmTech Atropine Sulfate Injection 1/120 Grain *(Phoenix Scientific)*, **atropine sulfate.**

AmTech Calcium Gluconate 23% Solution *(Phoenix Scientific)*, **calcium.**

AmTech Cal-Phos #2 Injection *(Phoenix Scientific)*, **calcium, dextrose, magnesium chloride, sodium hypophosphite.**

AmTech Chlorhexidine Solution *(Phoenix Scientific)*, **chlorhexidine gluconate.**

AmTech Chlortetracycline HCl Soluble Powder *(Phoenix Scientific)*, **chlortetracycline.**

AmTech Clindamycin Hydrochloride Oral Liquid *(Phoenix Scientific)*, **clindamycin hydrochloride.**

AmTech CMPK Injection *(Phoenix Scientific)*, **calcium, magnesium, phosphorus, potassium.**

AmTech Dexamethasone Sodium Phosphate Injection *(Phoenix Scientific)*, **dexamethasone sodium phosphate.**

AmTech Dexamethasone Solution *(Phoenix Scientific)*, **dexamethasone.**

AmTech Dexolyte Solution Injection *(Phoenix Scientific)*, **dextrose, electrolytes.**

AmTech Dextrose Solution 50% *(Phoenix Scientific)*, **dextrose.**

AmTech d-Panthenol Injection *(Phoenix Scientific)*, **dexpanthenol.**

AmTech Epinephrine Injection USP *(Phoenix Scientific)*, **epinephrine.**

AmTech Flunixin Meglumine Injection *(Phoenix Scientific)*, **flunixin meglumine.**

AmTech Furosemide Injection 5% *(Phoenix Scientific)*, **furosemide.**

AmTech GentaMax™ 100 *(Phoenix Scientific)*, **gentamicin.**

AmTech Gentamicin Sulfate Pig Pump Oral Solution *(Phoenix Scientific)*, **gentamicin.**

AmTech GentaPoult™ *(Phoenix Scientific)*, **gentamicin.**

AmTech Guaifenesin Injection *(Phoenix Scientific)*, **guaifenesin (glyceryl guaiacolate, guaiacol).**

AmTech Hypertonic Saline Solution 7.2% *(Phoenix Scientific)*, **sodium chloride.**

AmTech Iron Dextran Injection *(Phoenix Scientific)*, **iron dextran.**

AmTech Iron Dextran Injection-200 *(Phoenix Scientific)*, **iron dextran.**

AmTech Ketamine Hydrochloride Injection, USP *(Phoenix Scientific)*, **ketamine hydrochloride.**

AmTech Lactated Ringers Injection *(Phoenix Scientific)*, **calcium, potassium chloride, sodium chloride, sodium lactate.**

AmTech Levamisole Phosphate Injectable Solution *(Phoenix Scientific)*, **levamisole.**

AmTech Levothyroxine Sodium Tablets *(Phoenix Scientific)*, **levothyroxine.**

AmTech Lidocaine HCl Injectable-2% *(Phoenix Scientific)*, **lidocaine.**

AmTech Mannitol Injection 20% *(Phoenix Scientific)*, **mannitol.**

AmTech Maxim-100 *(Phoenix Scientific)*, **oxytetracycline.**

AmTech Maxim-200® *(Phoenix Scientific)*, **oxytetracycline.**

AmTech Neomycin Oral Solution *(Phoenix Scientific)*, **neomycin.**

AmTech Oxytetracycline HCl Soluble Powder *(Phoenix Scientific)*, **oxytetracycline.**

AmTech Oxytetracycline HCl Soluble Powder-343 *(Phoenix Scientific)*, **oxytetracycline.**

AmTech Oxytocin Injection *(Phoenix Scientific)*, **oxytocin.**

AmTech Phenylbutazone 20% Injection *(Phoenix Scientific)*, **phenylbutazone.**

AmTech Phenylbutazone Tablets, USP 100 mg *(Phoenix Scientific)*, **phenylbutazone.**

AmTech Phenylbutazone Tablets, USP 200 mg *(Phoenix Scientific)*, **phenylbutazone.**

AmTech Phenylbutazone Tablets, USP 1 gram *(Phoenix Scientific)*, **phenylbutazone.**

AmTech Phoenectin® Injection for Cattle and Swine *(Phoenix Scientific)*, **ivermectin.**

AmTech Phoenectin® Liquid for Horses *(Phoenix Scientific)*, **ivermectin.**

AmTech Phoenectin® Paste 1.87% *(Phoenix Scientific)*, **ivermectin.**

AmTech Phoenectin® Pour-On for Cattle *(Phoenix Scientific)*, **ivermectin.**

AmTech ProstaMate® *(Phoenix Scientific)*, **dinoprost (prostaglandin $F_{2\alpha}$).**

AmTech Saline Solution 0.9% *(Phoenix Scientific)*, **sodium chloride.**

AmTech Sodium Iodide 20% Injection *(Phoenix Scientific)*, **sodium iodide.**

AmTech Spectam® Scour-Halt™ *(Phoenix Scientific)*, **spectinomycin.**

AmTech Sterile Water for Injection, USP *(Phoenix Scientific)*, **sterile water.**

AmTech Sulfadimethoxine 12.5% Oral Solution *(Phoenix Scientific)*, **sulfadimethoxine.**

AmTech Sulfadimethoxine Injection - 40% *(Phoenix Scientific)*, **sulfadimethoxine.**

AmTech Sulfadimethoxine Soluble Powder *(Phoenix Scientific)*, **sulfadimethoxine.**

AmTech Tetracycline Hydrochloride Soluble Powder-324 *(Phoenix Scientific)*, **tetracycline.**

AmTech Thiamine Hydrochloride Injection *(Phoenix Scientific)*, **thiamine hydrochloride (B_1).**

AmTech Tripelennamine Hydrochloride Injection *(Phoenix Scientific)*, **tripelennamine hydrochloride.**

AmTech Uterine Bolus *(Phoenix Scientific)*, **urea.**

AmTech Vitamin B Complex *(Phoenix Scientific)*, **vitamin B-complex.**

AmTech Vitamin B Complex Fortified *(Phoenix Scientific)*, **vitamin B-complex.**

AmTech Vitamin B_{12} 1000 mcg *(Phoenix Scientific)*, **vitamin B_{12} (cyanocobalamin).**

AmTech Vitamin B_{12} 3000 mcg *(Phoenix Scientific)*, **vitamin B_{12} (cyanocobalamin).**

AmTech Vitamin B_{12} 5000 mcg *(Phoenix Scientific)*, **vitamin B_{12} (cyanocobalamin).**

AmTech Vitamin C Injectable Solution *(Phoenix Scientific)*, **vitamin C (ascorbic acid).**

AmTech Vitamin K_1 Injection *(Phoenix Scientific)*, **vitamin K_1 (phytonadione).**

AmTech Xylazine HCl Injection 20 mg/mL *(Phoenix Scientific)*, **xylazine hydrochloride.**

AmTech Xylazine HCl Injection 100 mg/mL *(Phoenix Scientific)*, **xylazine hydrochloride.**

amylase, lipase, protease. Pancrezyme® *(King Animal Health)*, Viokase®-V Powder *(Fort Dodge)*, Viokase®-V Tablets *(Fort Dodge)*.

amylase, lipase, protease, vitamin A, vitamin D, vitamin E. PanaKare™ Plus Powder *(Neogen)*, PanaKare™ Plus Tablets *(Neogen)*.

amylase, lipase, protease, vitamins. Pancreatic Plus Powder *(Butler)*, Pancreatic Plus Tablets *(Butler)*, PancreVed Powder *(Vedco)*, PancreVed Tablets *(Vedco)*.

amylase, propylene glycol, protease, surfactant. Enzymatic Detergent *(Vedco)*.

AnaSed® 20 Injection *(Lloyd)*, **xylazine hydrochloride.**

AnaSed® 100 Injectable *(Lloyd)*, **xylazine hydrochloride.**

Anem-X™ 100 *(AgriPharm)*, **iron dextran.**

Anem-X™ 200 *(AgriPharm)*, **iron dextran.**

anhydrous lanolin, citric acid, hyaluronic acid (sodium hyaluronate), sodium citrate, whole blood, adenine. Canine Plasma *(A.B.B.)*, Canine Red Blood Cells *(A.B.B.)*, Canine Whole Blood *(A.B.B.)*, Feline Plasma *(A.B.B.)*, Feline Red Blood Cells *(A.B.B.)*, Feline Whole Blood *(A.B.B.)*.

AniHist *(AHC)*, **guaifenesin (glyceryl guaiacolate, guaiacol), pyrilamine maleate.**

Animal Insecticide *(Durvet)*, **coumaphos.**

Animax® Ointment *(Pharmaderm)*, **neomycin, nystatin, thiostrepton, triamcinolone acetonide.**

AniPrin F *(AHC)*, **acetylsalicylic acid.**

Anipryl® Tablets *(Pfizer Animal Health)*, **selegiline.**

AniPsyll Powder *(AHC)*, **psyllium.**

AniTuss *(AHC)*, **ammonium chloride, guaifenesin (glyceryl guaiacolate, guaiacol), potassium iodide.**

Annihilator™ Insecticide Premise Spray *(Boehringer Ingelheim)*, **deltamethrin.**

Annihilator™ WP Wettable Powder Premise Insecticide *(Boehringer Ingelheim)*, **deltamethrin.**

Antagonil™ *(Wildlife)*, **yohimbine hydrochloride.**

Anthelban V *(Phoenix Pharmaceutical)*, **pyrantel pamoate.**

Anthelcide® EQ Equine Wormer Paste *(Pfizer Animal Health)*, **oxibendazole.**

Anthelcide® EQ Equine Wormer Suspension *(Pfizer Animal Health)*, **oxibendazole.**

Anti-Bacterial Hand Soap *(First Priority)*, **soap formula.**

Anti-Diarrheal Cattle Bolus *(AgriLabs)*, **attapulgite, carob, magnesium trisilicate, pectin.**

Anti-Diarrhea Tablets *(ARC)*, **aluminum hydroxide, kaolin, pectin.**

Antihistamine Granules *(Butler)*, **pseudoephedrine HCl, pyrilamine maleate.**

Anti-Itch Spray *(Vetus)*, **hydrocortisone.**

antioxidants, fatty acids (omega), minerals, soy protein, vitamins. Lickables™ Charge Up!™ *(A.A.H.)*.

antioxidants, fatty acids (omega), minerals, vitamins. Lickables™ Super Charger™ *(A.A.H.)*.

antioxidants, minerals, taurine, vitamins. Lickables™ Hearty Cat™ *(A.A.H.)*.

antioxidants, minerals, vitamins. Lickables™ Hearty Dog™ *(A.A.H.)*.

Antirobe Aquadrops® Liquid *(Pharmacia & Upjohn)*, **clindamycin hydrochloride.**

Antirobe® Capsules *(Pharmacia & Upjohn)*, **clindamycin hydrochloride.**

Antisedan® *(Pfizer Animal Health)*, **atipamezole hydrochloride.**

Antiseptic Iodine Spray *(Dominion)*, **iodine complex (povidone-iodine), isopropyl alcohol (isopropanol).**

Anti-Tussive Syrup with Antihistamine *(Vedco)*, **ammonium chloride, guaifenesin (glyceryl guaiacolate, guaiacol), phenylephrine hydrochloride, pyrilamine maleate, sodium citrate.**

Antivenin *(Fort Dodge)*, **immunoglobulin(s) G.**

Antizol-Vet® *(Orphan Medical)*, **fomepizole.**

A•O•E™, Animal Odor Eliminator *(Thornell)*, **deodorants, neutralizer(s).**

A-Plus™ Wound Dressing *(Creative Science)*, **allantoin, benzocaine, pine tar, propylene glycol, vitamin A, vitamin C (ascorbic acid).**

Apple-Dex® *(Horse Health)*, **electrolytes.**

Apralan® Soluble *(Elanco)*, **apramycin sulfate.**

apramycin sulfate. Apralan® Soluble *(Elanco)*.

Aquacillin™ *(Vedco)*, **penicillin G procaine.**

Aquaject *(Vetus)*, **sterile water.**

aqueous base lubricant(s). All Purpose Lubricant *(Durvet)*, Equi-Phar™ Vedlube O.B. Lubricant *(Vedco)*, Lubri-Nert™ *(Life Science)*, Septi-Lube™ *(Boehringer Ingelheim)*.

arachidonic acid, linoleic acid, linolenic acid, vitamin A, vitamin B_6, vitamin E. Mirra-Coat® for Cats *(Pet-Ag)*.

Arm & Hammer® Bio-Chlor® *(Church & Dwight)*, **amino acids, nitrogen, peptides.**

Arm & Hammer® Fermenten® *(Church & Dwight)*, **amino acids, nitrogen, peptides.**

Armor® *(Westfalia•Surge)*, **iodine.**

arnica, bentonite, boric acid, eucalyptus oil, glycerine, isopropyl alcohol (isopropanol), kaolin, methyl salicylate, peppermint oil, salicylic acid, thymol. Bigeloil® 24-Hour Medicated Poultice *(W. F. Young)*.

aromatic vegetable oil(s), methyl salicylate, salicylic acid, alcohol base. Bigeloil® *(W. F. Young)*.

Arquel® Granules *(Fort Dodge)*, **meclofenamic acid.**

Arquel® Tablets *(Fort Dodge)*, **meclofenamic acid.**

Arrest® Dip/Spray *(Westfalia•Surge)*, **chlorhexidine digluconate.**

arsanilic acid. Pro-Gen® 20% *(Fleming)*, Pro-Gen® 100% *(Fleming)*.

Artec™ Ultra Conditioning Teat Dip *(Ecolab Food & Bev. Div.)*, **heptanoic acid.**

ArthriCare™ Chewable Tablets for Large Dogs *(V.P.L.)*, **acetylsalicylic acid.**

Arthro Ease™ *(Horses Prefer)*, **capsaicin (cayenne pepper extract), emollient(s).**

Asepticare® TB+II *(Ecolab Prof. Prod. Div.)*, **quaternary ammonia.**

Asepti-HB™ *(Ecolab Prof. Prod. Div.)*, **quaternary ammonia.**

Asepti-Wipe™ *(Ecolab Prof. Prod. Div.)*, **alcohol, quaternary ammonia.**

Aspergillus oryzae fermentation extract. Vita Ferm® Pro-Gest *(BioZyme)*, Vita Ferm® Pro-Gest 30 *(BioZyme)*.

Aspergillus oryzae fermentation extract, electrolytes, energy source(s), nutrients, yeast. Vita Charge® Power Drench *(BioZyme)*.

Aspergillus oryzae fermentation extract, minerals, vitamins. K-Zyme® Cat Granules *(BioZyme)*, K-Zyme® Chewable Dog Tablets *(BioZyme)*, K-Zyme® Dog Granules *(BioZyme)*, Vita Charge® 28 Dispersible Powder *(BioZyme)*, Vita Charge® Calf Bolus *(BioZyme)*, Vita Charge® Equine *(BioZyme)*, Vita Charge® Gel Cap *(BioZyme)*, Vita Charge® Paste *(BioZyme)*, Vita Ferm® Breeder Booster+Mag *(BioZyme)*, Vita Ferm® Cattleman's Beefmaker *(BioZyme)*, Vita Ferm® Cattleman's Beefmaker+Mag *(BioZyme)*, Vita Ferm® Concept-Aid *(BioZyme)*, Vita Ferm® Concept-Aid+Mag *(BioZyme)*, Vita Ferm® Concept-Aid A•P *(BioZyme)*, Vita Ferm® Cow Calf 5 *(BioZyme)*, Vita Ferm® Dairy Basemix 12:16 *(BioZyme)*, Vita Ferm® Dairy Basemix 18:6 *(BioZyme)*, Vita Ferm® Dairy Basemix 18:12 *(BioZyme)*, Vita Ferm® Equine *(BioZyme)*, Vita Ferm® Ewe and Lamb *(BioZyme)*, Vita Ferm® Far Out Dry Cow *(BioZyme)*, Vita Ferm® Feedlot Formula *(BioZyme)*, Vita Ferm® Fescue Fiber Buster *(BioZyme)*, Vita Ferm® Fescue Power Keg *(BioZyme)*, Vita Ferm® Formula *(BioZyme)*, Vita Ferm® Grass Enhancer *(BioZyme)*, Vita Ferm® High Mag *(BioZyme)*, Vita Ferm® Natural Protein Pasture Formula (NPPF) *(BioZyme)*, Vita Ferm® Pasture Formula *(BioZyme)*, Vita Ferm® Power Keg *(BioZyme)*, Vita Ferm® Roughage Fortifier *(BioZyme)*, Vita Ferm® Sheep & Goat Keg *(BioZyme)*, Vita Ferm® Sure Champ and Vita Start Pellets *(BioZyme)*, Vita Ferm® Sure Start 2 *(BioZyme)*, Vita Ferm® Sure Start Pac *(BioZyme)*, Vita Ferm® Up Close Dry Cow *(BioZyme)*, Vita Ferm® Vita Grow 32 Natural *(BioZyme)*.

Aspergillus oryzae fermentation extract, minerals, vitamins, yeast. MicroZyme Bolus for Cattle *(Vedco)*.

Aspirin 60 Grain *(Butler)*, **acetylsalicylic acid.**

Aspirin 240 Grain Boluses *(Vedco)*, **acetylsalicylic acid.**

Aspirin 480 Grain Boluses *(Vedco)*, **acetylsalicylic acid.**

Aspirin Bolus *(Aspen)*, *(Durvet)*, **acetylsalicylic acid.**

Aspirin Bolus 240 Grains *(Phoenix Pharmaceutical)*, **acetylsalicylic acid.**

Aspirin Bolus-480 *(AgriLabs)*, **acetylsalicylic acid.**

Aspirin Boluses *(Bimeda)*, *(Butler)*, **acetylsalicylic acid.**

Aspirin Boluses-240 *(AgriLabs)*, **acetylsalicylic acid.**

Aspirin Boluses 240 grains *(AgriPharm)*, **acetylsalicylic acid.**

Aspirin Boluses 240 Grains *(First Priority)*, **acetylsalicylic acid.**

Aspirin Boluses 480 grains *(AgriPharm)*, **acetylsalicylic acid.**

Aspirin Liquid Concentrate *(AgriPharm)*, *(First Priority)*, **acetylsalicylic acid.**

Aspirin Powder *(AgriLabs)*, *(AgriPharm)*, *(Bimeda)*, *(Butler)*, *(First Priority)*, *(Vedco)*, **acetylsalicylic acid.**

Aspirin Powder Molasses-Flavored *(Butler)*, **acetylsalicylic acid.**

Aspirin U.S.P. *(Neogen)*, **acetylsalicylic acid.**

Aspirin U.S.P. Powder *(Neogen)*, **acetylsalicylic acid.**

Asp-Rin Concentrate *(AgriLabs)*, **acetylsalicylic acid.**

Astringent Bolus *(Butler)*, **calcium, copper, iron.**

Atgard® C *(Boehringer Ingelheim)*, **dichlorvos.**

Atgard® Swine Wormer *(Boehringer Ingelheim)*, **dichlorvos.**

atipamezole hydrochloride. Antisedan® *(Pfizer Animal Health)*.

Atroban® 11% EC Insecticide *(Schering-Plough)*, **permethrin.**

Atroban® 42.5% EC *(Schering-Plough)*, **permethrin.**

Atroban® DeLice® Pour-On Insecticide *(Schering-Plough)*, **permethrin.**

Atroban® Extra Insecticide Ear Tags *(Schering-Plough)*, **permethrin, piperonyl butoxide.**

Atroject *(Vetus)*, **atropine sulfate.**

Atropine L.A. *(Butler)*, **atropine sulfate.**

Atropine SA *(Butler)*, **atropine sulfate.**

atropine sulfate. AmTech Atropine Sulfate Injection 1/120 Grain *(Phoenix Scientific)*, Atroject *(Vetus)*, Atropine L.A. *(Butler)*, Atropine SA *(Butler)*, Atropine Sulfate 1/120 *(Neogen)*, *(Vet Tek)*, Atropine Sulfate Injection *(Vedco)*, Atropine Sulfate Injection 1/120 Grain *(Phoenix Pharmaceutical)*, Atropine Sulfate Injection 15 mg/mL L.A. *(RXV)*, Atropine Sulfate L.A. 15 mg/mL *(Neogen)*.

Atropine Sulfate 1/120 *(Neogen)*, *(Vet Tek)*, **atropine sulfate.**

Atropine Sulfate Injection *(Vedco)*, **atropine sulfate.**

Atropine Sulfate Injection 1/120 Grain *(Phoenix Pharmaceutical)*, **atropine sulfate.**

Atropine Sulfate Injection 15 mg/mL L.A. *(RXV)*, **atropine sulfate.**

Atropine Sulfate L.A. 15 mg/mL *(Neogen)*, **atropine sulfate.**

attapulgite. Palapectate™ *(PharmX)*.

attapulgite, activated charcoal. UAA (Universal Animal Antidote) Gel *(Vedco)*.

attapulgite, bismuth subcarbonate, kanamycin sulfate, pectin. Amforol® Suspension *(Fort Dodge)*, Amforol® Tablets *(Fort Dodge)*.

attapulgite, carob, magnesium trisilicate, pectin. Anti-Diarrheal Cattle Bolus *(AgriLabs)*, Gastro-Sorb™ Bolus *(Butler)*, Gastro-Sorb™ Calf Bolus *(Butler)*, Intesti-Sorb Bolus *(AgriPharm)*, Intesti-Sorb Calf Bolus *(AgriPharm)*, Maxi-Sorb Bolus *(Durvet)*, Maxi Sorb Calf Bolus *(Durvet)*, Veda-Sorb Bolus *(Vedco)*.

attapulgite, carob, magnesium trisilicate, pectin, aluminum silicate. Veda-Sorb Jr Bolus *(Vedco)*.

attapulgite, magnesium trisilicate, pectin. Endosorb™ Bolus *(PRN Pharmacal)*, Endosorb™ Suspension *(PRN Pharmacal)*, Endosorb™ Tablets *(PRN Pharmacal)*.

Aureomix® 500 Granular *(Alpharma)*, **chlortetracycline, penicillin G procaine, sulfamethazine.**

Aureomycin® 50 Granular *(Alpharma)*, **chlortetracycline.**

Aureomycin® 90 Granular *(Alpharma)*, **chlortetracycline.**

Aureomycin® 100 Granular *(Alpharma)*, **chlortetracycline.**

Aureomycin® Soluble Powder *(Fort Dodge)*, **chlortetracycline.**

Aureomycin® Soluble Powder Concentrate *(Fort Dodge)*, **chlortetracycline.**

Aureomycin® Sulmet® Soluble Powder *(Fort Dodge)*, **chlortetracycline, sulfamethazine.**

Aureo S 700® Granular 10G *(Alpharma)*, **chlortetracycline, sulfamethazine.**

Aureo S 700® Granular 35G *(Alpharma)*, **chlortetracycline, sulfamethazine.**

AureoZol® 500 Granular *(Alpharma)*, **chlortetracycline, penicillin G procaine, sulfathiazole.**

Aurimite® Insecticide *(Schering-Plough)*, **benzocaine, docusate sodium (dioctyl sodium sulfosuccinate), piperonyl butoxide, pyrethrins.**

Availa®-4 *(Zinpro)*, **amino acids, minerals.**

Availa® Cu 100 *(Zinpro)*, **amino acids, copper.**

Availa® Fe 60 *(Zinpro)*, **amino acids, iron.**

AvailaMin® - Grow/Finish *(Zinpro)*, **amino acids, minerals.**

AvailaMin® - Sow *(Zinpro)*, **amino acids, minerals.**

AvailaMin® - Starter I, II, III *(Zinpro)*, **amino acids, minerals.**

Availa® Mn 80 *(Zinpro)*, **amino acids, manganese.**

Availa® Z/M *(Zinpro)*, **manganese, zinc.**

Availa® Zn 40 *(Zinpro)*, **amino acids, zinc.**

Availa® Zn 100 *(Zinpro)*, **amino acids, zinc.**

Avatec® *(Alpharma)*, **lasalocid sodium.**

Avian Bluelite® *(TechMix)*, **electrolytes, vitamins.**

Avian Vitamins Iodized *(ARC)*, **iodine, vitamins.**

Aviax® *(Phibro)*, **semduramicin sodium.**

Avi-Con *(Vet-A-Mix)*, **vitamins.**

Azium® Powder *(Schering-Plough)*, **dexamethasone.**

Azium® Solution *(Schering-Plough)*, **dexamethasone.**

B

B-1 Powder *(SureNutrition)*, **thiamine hydrochloride (B_1).**

B12-Ject 1000 *(Vetus)*, **vitamin B_{12} (cyanocobalamin).**

B12-Ject 3000 *(Vetus)*, **vitamin B_{12} (cyanocobalamin).**

β-[1,4]-linked mannan polymers (Acemannan). Acemannan Immunostimulant *(V.P.L.)*, CarraSorb™ Freeze-Dried Gel (FDG) *(V.P.L.)*.

β-[1,4]-linked mannan polymers (Acemannan), aloe vera. CarraVet™ Spray-Gel Wound Dressing *(V.P.L.)*, CarraVet™ Wound Dressing *(V.P.L.)*.

Baby Pig Restart™ One-4 *(TechMix)*, **electrolytes, energy source(s), nutrients.**

Bac-Drop Udder Wash *(Ecolab Food & Bev. Div.)*, **phosphoric acid, sulfonic acid.**

Baciferm® Granular 50 *(Alpharma)*, **bacitracin (zinc).**

bacitracin, hydrocortisone acetate, neomycin, polymyxin B. Neobacimyx®-H *(Schering-Plough)*, TriOptic-S® *(Pfizer Animal Health)*, Vetropolycin® HC Ophthalmic Ointment *(Pharmaderm)*.

bacitracin, neomycin, polymyxin B. Mycitracin® Sterile Ointment *(Pharmacia & Upjohn)*, Neobacimyx® *(Schering-Plough)*, TriOptic-P™ *(Pfizer Animal Health)*, Vetro-Biotic® Ointment *(Pharmaderm)*, Vetropolycin® Ophthalmic Ointment *(Pharmaderm)*.

Bicarboject *(Vetus)*, **sodium bicarbonate.**

bicarbonate, dextrose, electrolytes, glycine. Elpak™-G *(Vedco).*

bicarbonate, microorganisms, minerals, vitamins, amino acids. Pre-Conditioning/Receiving Formula Gel *(Durvet)*, Ruminant Lactobacillus Gel *(First Priority).*

Bigeloil® *(W. F. Young)*, **alcohol base, aromatic vegetable oil(s), methyl salicylate, salicylic acid.**

Bigeloil® 24-Hour Medicated Poultice *(W. F. Young)*, **arnica, bentonite, boric acid, eucalyptus oil, glycerine, isopropyl alcohol (isopropanol), kaolin, methyl salicylate, peppermint oil, salicylic acid, thymol.**

Bigeloil® Liquid Gel *(W. F. Young)*, **menthol.**

Big Pine™ *(Intercon)*, **pine oil, quaternary ammonia.**

Bimectin™ Pour-On *(Bimeda)*, **ivermectin.**

Bimesol-R™ Injection *(Bimeda)*, **magnesium chloride, potassium chloride, sodium acetate, sodium chloride, sodium gluconate.**

Biocaine® *(Tomlyn)*, **lidocaine.**

Bio-Cox® 60 Granular *(Alpharma)*, **salinomycin sodium.**

Biodry® *(Pharmacia & Upjohn)*, **novobiocin.**

Bio Guard® Shampoo *(Farnam)*, **shampoo formula.**

Bio-Hoof™ *(Horses Prefer)*, **biotin, methionine, minerals, vitamins.**

Biolyte® *(Pharmacia & Upjohn)*, **dextrose, electrolytes.**

Bio-Meth *(Vet-A-Mix)*, **biotin, methionine (d-l).**

Biomox® Oral Suspension *(Delmarva)*, **amoxicillin.**

Biomox® Tablets *(Delmarva)*, **amoxicillin.**

Bio-Mycin® 200 *(Boehringer Ingelheim)*, **oxytetracycline.**

b-ionone, limonene. MycAseptic® *(Neogen)*, MycAseptic® E *(Neogen).*

Bio-Pine 20 *(Bio-Tek)*, **pine oil.**

Biosol® Liquid *(Pharmacia & Upjohn)*, **neomycin.**

Bio Spot® Flea & Tick Control For Dogs (15 lbs. and Under) *(Farnam)*, **permethrin, pyriproxyfen.**

Bio Spot® Flea & Tick Control For Dogs (Between 15 & 33 lbs.) *(Farnam)*, **permethrin, pyriproxyfen.**

Bio Spot® Flea & Tick Control For Dogs (33 to 66 lbs.) *(Farnam)*, **permethrin, pyriproxyfen.**

Bio Spot® Flea & Tick Control For Dogs (Over 66 lbs.) *(Farnam)*, **permethrin, pyriproxyfen.**

Bio Spot® Stripe-On™ Flea Control For Cats *(Farnam)*, **pyriproxyfen.**

biotin. Biotin-100 *(Vet-A-Mix)*, Biotin™ Gold *(SureNutrition)*, Horse Care Biotin Crumbles *(Durvet)*, Vita•Biotin™ Crumbles *(Horse Health)*, Vita-Min Biotin *(Farnam).*

biotin, linoleic acid, linolenic acid, vitamin A, vitamin B_6, vitamin E. Mirra-Coat® Powder and Liquid *(Pet-Ag).*

biotin, l-lysine, methionine (d-l), vitamin B_6. H.B. 15™ *(Farnam).*

biotin, methionine, minerals, vitamins. Bio-Hoof™ *(Horses Prefer).*

biotin, methionine (d-l). Bio-Meth *(Vet-A-Mix)*, Equi-Phar™ dl-Methionine with Biotin Powder *(Vedco).*

biotin, methionine (d-l), microorganisms, zinc-methionine. Vita-Key® Biotin ZM-80 *(Vita-Key).*

biotin, methionine (d-l), pantothenate. Dealer Select Horse Care Biotin 800 *(Durvet).*

biotin, methionine (d-l), thiamine hydrochloride (B_1), zinc. Hoof Supplement *(First Priority)*, Integrator™ *(Butler).*

biotin, vitamins, amino acids. Dealer Select Horse Care NutriHoof *(Durvet).*

Biotin-100 *(Vet-A-Mix)*, **biotin.**

Biotin™ Gold *(SureNutrition)*, **biotin.**

Biozide® Gel *(PPI)*, **polyvinylpyrrolidone.**

Biozide® Puffer *(PPI)*, **polyvinylpyrrolidone.**

Bird Bene-Bac™ Gel *(Pet-Ag)*, **microorganisms.**

Bird Bene-Bac™ Powder *(Pet-Ag)*, **microorganisms.**

Bi-Sept™ Activator *(Westfalia•Surge)*, **lactic acid.**

Bi-Sept™ Base *(Westfalia•Surge)*, **sodium chlorite.**

BismuKote Paste for Medium & Large Dogs *(Vedco)*, **bismuth subsalicylate.**

BismuKote Paste for Small Dogs *(Vedco)*, **bismuth subsalicylate.**

Bismu-Kote Suspension *(Vedco)*, **bismuth subsalicylate.**

Bismupaste D5 *(Vetus)*, **bismuth subsalicylate.**

Bismupaste D10 *(Vetus)*, **bismuth subsalicylate.**

Bismupaste E20 *(Vetus)*, **bismuth subsalicylate.**

Bismusal *(Bimeda)*, *(Durvet)*, **bismuth subsalicylate.**

Bismusal Suspension *(AgriPharm)*, **bismuth subsalicylate.**

Bismusol *(First Priority)*, **bismuth subsalicylate.**

bismuth subcarbonate, kanamycin sulfate, pectin, attapulgite. Amforol® Suspension *(Fort Dodge)*, Amforol® Tablets *(Fort Dodge).*

bismuth subgallate, bismuth subnitrate, calamine, juniper tar, resorcinol, zinc oxide. Pellitol® Ointment *(Veterinary Specialties).*

bismuth subnitrate, calamine, juniper tar, resorcinol, zinc oxide, bismuth subgallate. Pellitol® Ointment *(Veterinary Specialties).*

bismuth subsalicylate. BismuKote Paste for Medium & Large Dogs *(Vedco)*, BismuKote Paste for Small Dogs *(Vedco)*, Bismu-Kote Suspension *(Vedco)*, Bismupaste D5 *(Vetus)*, Bismupaste D10 *(Vetus)*, Bismupaste E20 *(Vetus)*, Bismusal *(Bimeda)*, *(Durvet)*, Bismusal Suspension *(AgriPharm)*, Bismusol *(First Priority)*, Bismuth Subsalicylate Suspension *(A.A.H.)*, Corrective Suspension *(Phoenix Pharmaceutical)*, Equi-Phar™ BismuKote Paste *(Vedco)*, Gastro-Cote *(Butler)*, PalaBIS™ *(PharmX).*

Bismuth Subsalicylate Suspension *(A.A.H.)*, **bismuth subsalicylate.**

bis-n-tributyltin oxide, quaternary ammonia. Roccal®-D Plus *(Pharmacia & Upjohn).*

Bite Free™ Biting Fly Repellent *(Farnam)*, **butoxypolypropylene glycol, cypermethrin, piperonyl butoxide, pyrethrins.**

Bitter-3™ *(Butler)*, **isopropyl alcohol, oleoresin capsicum, orange peel bitter, propylene glycol, sucrose octyl acetate.**

Bitter Orange™ *(ARC)*, **isopropyl alcohol, oleoresin capsicum, propylene glycol, sucrose octyl acetate.**

Bitter Safe Mist *(Butler)*, **denatonium benzoate, propylene glycol.**

Bizolin®-1 g *(Boehringer Ingelheim)*, **phenylbutazone.**

Bloat Drench™ *(Great States)*, **emulsifiers, vegetable oil(s).**

Bloat Guard® Liquid Type A Medicated Article *(Phibro)*, **poloxalene.**

Bloat Guard® Top Dressing Medicated *(Phibro)*, **poloxalene.**

Bloat Guard® Type A Medicated Article *(Phibro)*, **poloxalene.**

Bloat-Pac® *(Vet-A-Mix)*, **propylene glycol.**

Bloat Release *(AgriLabs)*, **docusate sodium (dioctyl sodium sulfosuccinate).**

Bloat Treatment *(AgriPharm)*, *(Butler)*, *(Durvet)*, **docusate sodium (dioctyl sodium sulfosuccinate).**

Blood Stop Powder *(AgriLabs)*, **alum, ferric sulfate, tannic acid, thymol.**

Blood Stop Powder *(AgriPharm)*, **carboxy methylcellulose, diphenylamine, ferric sulfate.**

Blood Stop Powder *(Aspen)*, **alum, chloroxylenol, ferrous sulfate, tannic acid.**

Blood Stop Powder *(Butler)*, **aluminum chloride, ammonium chloride, bentonite, copper sulfate, diatomite, ferric subsulfate, iodoform.**

Blood Stop Powder *(Centaur)*, **carboxy methylcellulose, diphenylamine, ferric sulfate.**

Blood Stop Powder *(Davis)*, **ferric subsulfate.**

Blood Stop Powder *(Dominion)*, **alum, ferric subsulfate, tannic acid, thymol.**

Blood Stop Powder *(Durvet)*, **alum, chloroxylenol, ferrous sulfate, tannic acid.**

Blood Stop Powder *(First Priority)*, **chloroxylenol, diphenylamine, ferrous sulfate, tannic acid.**

Blood Stop Powder *(Vedco)*, **alum, chloroxylenol, ferrous sulfate, tannic acid.**

Bluelite® C *(TechMix)*, **dextrose, electrolytes.**

Bluelite® Swine Formula *(TechMix)*, **electrolytes, energy source(s).**

Blue Lotion *(AgriLabs)*, **acriflavine, furfural, gentian violet, glycerine, isopropyl alcohol (isopropanol), propylene glycol, sodium propionate, urea.**

Blue Lotion *(Farnam)*, **acriflavine, glycerine, methyl violet, propylene glycol, sodium propionate, urea.**

Blue Lotion Aerosol *(Boehringer Ingelheim)*, **benzyl alcohol, crystal violet, isopropyl alcohol (isopropanol), tannic acid.**

Blue Lotion Topical Antiseptic *(Aspen)*, *(First Priority)*, **benzalkonium chloride, chlorothymol, isopropyl alcohol (isopropanol).**

Blue Snow™ *(Schering-Plough)*, **lanolin, shampoo formula.**

Blu-Gard™ Spray *(Ecolab Food & Bev. Div.)*, **sulfonic acid.**

Blu-Gard™ Teat Dip *(Ecolab Food & Bev. Div.)*, **sulfonic acid.**

Blu-Shield™ Sanitizing Barrier Teat Dip *(Ecolab Food & Bev. Div.)*, **sulfonic acid.**

BMD® 30 *(Alpharma)*, **bacitracin methylene disalicylate.**

BMD® 50 *(Alpharma)*, **bacitracin methylene disalicylate.**

BMD® 60 *(Alpharma)*, **bacitracin methylene disalicylate.**

BMD® Soluble *(Alpharma)*, **bacitracin methylene disalicylate.**

boldenone undecylenate. Equipoise® *(Fort Dodge).*

Boltan III™ *(Butler)*, **carob, kaolin.**

boric acid, acetic acid. DermaPet® MalAcetic™ Conditioner for Dogs and Cats *(DermaPet)*, DermaPet® MalAcetic Otic *(DermaPet)*, DermaPet® MalAcetic™ Shampoo for Dogs and Cats *(DermaPet)*, DermaPet® MalAcetic™ Wet Wipes/Dry Bath *(DermaPet)*, OtoCetic Solution *(Vedco).*

boric acid, acetic acid, aloe. EarMed Boracetic® Flush *(Davis).*

boric acid, camphor, glycerine, zinc sulfate. Eye Rinse *(Butler)*, *(RXV).*

boric acid, camphor, isopropyl alcohol (isopropanol), menthol, salicylic acid, tannic acid. Dry-It *(Q.A. Laboratories).*

boric acid, eucalyptus oil, glycerine, isopropyl alcohol (isopropanol), kaolin, methyl salicylate, peppermint oil, salicylic acid, thymol, arnica, bentonite. Bigeloil® 24-Hour Medicated Poultice *(W. F. Young).*

boric acid, ferrous sulfate, glycerine, kaolin, aloe vera, bentonite. Icetight® *(Horse Health)*, Reducine® Poultice *(Equicare).*

boric acid, glycerine, isopropyl alcohol (isopropanol), lanolin, lidocaine, propylene glycol, salicylic acid, acetic acid. Fresh-Ear *(Q.A. Laboratories).*

boric acid, glycerine, isopropyl alcohol (isopropanol), lidocaine, propylene glycol, salicylic acid, acetic acid. Otic Clear *(Butler).*

C

calcium, magnesium, phosphorus, potassium, vitamins. Mega CMPK Bolus *(AgriPharm)*, Slow Release CMPK Bolus *(PRN Pharmacal)*.
calcium, magnesium, potassium, propylene glycol, vitamin B-complex. Super Calcium Drench *(Vedco)*.
calcium, magnesium, potassium, propylene glycol, vitamins. Calcium Drench Plus Vitamins *(AgriLabs)*, *(Durvet)*.
calcium, magnesium, potassium, vitamins. Calcium Drench *(AgriPharm)*.
calcium, magnesium, selenium, vitamins. Cal-Mag-SV Gel *(Butler)*.
calcium, magnesium chloride, phosphoric acid, potassium chloride, trisodium phosphate. CMPK Gel *(AgriPharm)*.
calcium, magnesium chloride, phosphorus, potassium chloride. C.M.P.K. Gel *(AgriLabs)*, CMPK Gel *(Vedco)*.
calcium, magnesium chloride, potassium chloride, propylene glycol, sodium hypophosphite. 40% CMPK with D_3 Oral Drench *(DVM Formula)*, Oral Calcium Drench *(DVM Formula)*.
calcium, magnesium chloride, potassium chloride, propylene glycol, sodium hypophosphite, vitamin D_3. CMPK D_3 Drench *(Durvet)*.
calcium, magnesium chloride, potassium chloride, tri-calcium phosphate. Oral CMPK Gel *(DVM Formula)*.
calcium, magnesium hydroxide, phosphoric acid, potassium chloride. Cal MPK Gel *(Butler)*.
calcium, magnesium hydroxide, phosphorus, potassium chloride. CMPK Gel *(Durvet)*.
calcium, magnesium sulfate, potassium chloride, sodium chloride. Electrolyte Supplement *(First Priority)*.
calcium, milk protein, nutrients, phosphorus, vitamins. Foal-Lac® Pellets *(Pet-Ag)*.
calcium, phosphorus. Di-Calcium Phosphate *(Neogen)*.
calcium, phosphorus, vitamin A, vitamin D_3. Osteo-Form Powder *(Vet-A-Mix)*, Osteo-Form SA *(Vet-A-Mix)*.
calcium, phosphorus, vitamin D. Calcium Phosphorus Powder *(Pet-Ag)*, Pet-Cal™ *(Pfizer Animal Health)*.
calcium, phosphorus, vitamin D_3. Calcium Phosphorus Tablets *(Pet-Ag)*.
calcium, phosphorus, vitamins. Osteo-Form Tablets *(Vet-A-Mix)*.
calcium, potassium chloride, sodium chloride, sodium lactate. AmTech Lactated Ringers Injection *(Phoenix Scientific)*, Lactated Ringers *(Vet Tek)*, Lactated Ringers Injection *(Phoenix Pharmaceutical)*, Lactated Ringer's Injection *(Vedco)*, Lactated Ringers Injection *(Vetus)*, Lactated Ringers Injection SC *(Butler)*, Lactated Ringer's Injection, USP *(AgriLabs)*, *(Bimeda)*, Lactated Ringer's Solution *(RXV)*.
calcium, potassium chloride, sodium chloride, thiamine hydrochloride (B_1). Happy Jack® Milkade *(Happy Jack)*.
calcium, propylene glycol, tri-calcium phosphate, vitamins. Cal-C-Fresh™ *(Vets Plus)*.
calcium, propylene glycol, vitamin B-complex. Calcium Drench™ *(Vets Plus)*.
calcium, sodium. Cal-Pho-Sol *(Neogen)*.
calcium, tri-calcium phosphate, vitamins. Oral Calcium Gel *(DVM Formula)*.
calcium, vitamin A, vitamin C (ascorbic acid), vitamin D_3. NutriVed™ Calcium Plus Chewable Tablets *(Vedco)*.
calcium, vitamin A, vitamin D. Calcium Gel + Vitamins *(AgriLabs)*.
calcium, vitamin D. Cal Oral Plus™ *(Butler)*.
Calcium 23% Solution *(Vedco)*, **calcium borogluconate.**
calcium borogluconate. Calcium 23% Solution *(Vedco)*.
calcium borogluconate, calcium hypophosphite, dextrose, magnesium borogluconate. Ca-P I.V. Therapy *(RXV)*.
calcium borogluconate, dextrose, magnesium borogluconate, potassium chloride, sodium hypophosphite. CMPK Solution *(Bimeda)*.
calcium carbonate, dicalcium phosphate, aluminum. Neigh-Lox® *(K.P.P.)*.
Calcium Drench *(AgriPharm)*, **calcium, magnesium, potassium, vitamins.**
Calcium Drench™ *(Vets Plus)*, **calcium, propylene glycol, vitamin B-complex.**
Calcium Drench Plus Vitamins *(AgriLabs)*, *(Durvet)*, **calcium, magnesium, potassium, propylene glycol, vitamins.**
Calcium Gel+Selenium *(AgriLabs)*, **calcium, cobalt, magnesium, selenium, vitamins.**
Calcium Gel + Vitamins *(AgriLabs)*, **calcium, vitamin A, vitamin D.**
Calcium Gluconate 23% *(AgriPharm)*, **calcium.**
Calcium Gluconate 23% Solution *(AgriLabs)*, *(Aspen)*, *(Bimeda)*, *(Durvet)*, *(Phoenix Pharmaceutical)*, *(Vet Tek)*, *(Vetus)*, **calcium.**
calcium glycerophosphate, calcium lactate. Calphosan® Solution *(Glenwood)*, Cal-Pho-Sol Solution SA *(Vedco)*.
calcium hydroxide, sodium hydroxide. Dehorning Paste *(AgriPharm)*, D-Horn Paste *(Dominion)*, Dr. Naylor® Dehorning Paste *(H.W. Naylor)*.
calcium hypophosphite, dextrose, magnesium borogluconate, calcium. Norcalciphos™ *(Pfizer Animal Health)*.
calcium hypophosphite, dextrose, magnesium borogluconate, calcium borogluconate. Ca-P I.V. Therapy *(RXV)*.
calcium hypophosphite, dextrose, magnesium borogluconate, potassium chloride, calcium. Cal-MPK 1234™ *(Butler)*.
calcium hypophosphite, dextrose, magnesium chloride, calcium. Cal-MP 1700™ *(Butler)*.
calcium lactate, calcium glycerophosphate. Calphosan® Solution *(Glenwood)*, Cal-Pho-Sol Solution SA *(Vedco)*.
Calcium Oral Gel *(Phoenix Pharmaceutical)*, **calcium, cobalt, magnesium.**
calcium phosphate. PSD Complex II *(PRN Pharmacal)*.
calcium phosphate, magnesium chloride, potassium chloride, calcium. CMPK Gel Plus™ *(Vets Plus)*.
calcium phosphate, sodium bicarbonate, sodium chloride, ammonium chloride, benzoic acid. Expectorant Powder *(First Priority)*.
Calcium Phosphorus Powder *(Pet-Ag)*, **calcium, phosphorus, vitamin D.**
Calcium Phosphorus Tablets *(Pet-Ag)*, **calcium, phosphorus, vitamin D_3.**
Calcium Plus *(First Priority)*, **calcium, cobalt, magnesium.**
Calcium SE *(First Priority)*, **calcium, cobalt, magnesium, selenium, vitamin B-complex.**
Cal Dex #2 *(AgriLabs)*, **calcium, dextrose, magnesium borogluconate, phosphorus.**
Cal-Dex C-M-P-K *(AgriLabs)*, **calcium, dextrose, magnesium borogluconate, potassium chloride, sodium hypophosphite.**
Cal Dex CMPK Injection *(Aspen)*, **calcium, dextrose, magnesium borogluconate, potassium chloride, sodium hypophosphite.**
Cal-Dextro® C *(Fort Dodge)*, **calcium, dextrose.**
Cal-Dextro® K *(Fort Dodge)*, **calcium, dextrose, potassium chloride.**
Cal-Dextro® No. 2 *(Fort Dodge)*, **calcium, dextrose, magnesium borogluconate, phosphorus.**
Cal-Dextro® Special *(Fort Dodge)*, **calcium, dextrose, magnesium borogluconate, phosphorus.**
Calf Quencher *(Vedco)*, **dextrose, electrolytes.**
Calf RD Formula *(TechMix)*, **microorganisms.**
Calf Restart™ One-4 *(TechMix)*, **electrolytes, energy source(s), nutrients.**
Calf Scour Bolus Antibiotic *(Durvet)*, **tetracycline.**
Cal-Gel™ *(Jorgensen)*, **calcium, cobalt, magnesium.**
Cal-Gel 63 *(Durvet)*, **calcium.**
Cal M 64 Plus Se *(Butler)*, **calcium, cobalt, magnesium, selenium.**
Cal-Mag-Co Gel *(Durvet)*, **calcium, cobalt sulfate, magnesium chloride.**
Cal-Mag-SE Gel *(Durvet)*, **calcium, cobalt, magnesium, selenium.**
Cal-Mag-SV Gel *(Butler)*, **calcium, magnesium, selenium, vitamins.**
Cal MP-1000 *(Butler)*, **calcium, dextrose, magnesium chloride, sodium hypophosphite.**
Cal-MP 1700™ *(Butler)*, **calcium, calcium hypophosphite, dextrose, magnesium chloride.**
Cal-MPK™ 1080 Injection *(Butler)*, **calcium, dextrose, magnesium borogluconate, potassium chloride, sodium hypophosphite.**
Cal-MPK 1234™ *(Butler)*, **calcium, calcium hypophosphite, dextrose, magnesium borogluconate, potassium chloride.**
Cal MPK Gel *(Butler)*, **calcium, magnesium hydroxide, phosphoric acid, potassium chloride.**
Cal-Nate 1069™ *(Butler)*, **calcium.**
Cal Oral Plus™ *(Butler)*, **calcium, vitamin D.**
Calox 64 Oral Gel *(Vedco)*, **calcium, cobalt sulfate, magnesium chloride, vitamins.**
Cal Ox 64 Plus SE *(AgriPharm)*, **calcium, cobalt, magnesium, selenium, vitamins.**
CalOx 64 SE Oral Gel *(Vedco)*, **calcium, cobalt, magnesium, selenium, vitamins.**
Cal-Phos #2 *(Vedco)*, **calcium, dextrose, magnesium chloride, sodium hypophosphite.**
Cal-Phos #2 Injection *(AgriLabs)*, **calcium, dextrose, magnesium, phosphorus.**
Cal-Phos #2 Injection *(Phoenix Pharmaceutical)*, **calcium, dextrose, magnesium chloride, sodium hypophosphite.**
Cal-Phos #2 with Potassium Injection *(Phoenix Pharmaceutical)*, **calcium, dextrose, magnesium chloride, potassium chloride, sodium hypophosphite.**
Calphosan® Solution *(Glenwood)*, **calcium glycerophosphate, calcium lactate.**
Cal-Phos Forte *(Bimeda)*, **calcium, dextrose, magnesium, phosphorus.**
Cal-Pho-Sol *(Neogen)*, **calcium, sodium.**
Cal-Pho-Sol Solution SA *(Vedco)*, **calcium glycerophosphate, calcium lactate.**
Calsorb™ *(PRN Pharmacal)*, **calcium.**
Cal Supreme Gel™ *(Bimeda)*, **calcium.**
camphor, Canada balsam, alcohol. VetRx™ Small Fur Animal Remedy *(Goodwinol)*.
camphor, Canada balsam, corn oil base, milk supplement, oil origanum, oil rosemary. VetRx™ Equine Formula *(Goodwinol)*.
camphor, Canada balsam, corn oil base, oil origanum, oil rosemary, alcohol. VetRx™ Caged Bird Remedy *(Goodwinol)*, VetRx™ for Cats and Kittens *(Goodwinol)*, VetRx™ for Dogs and Puppies *(Goodwinol)*, VetRx™ Goat & Sheep Remedy *(Goodwinol)*, VetRx™ Pigeon Remedy *(Goodwinol)*, VetRx™ Poultry Remedy *(Goodwinol)*, VetRx™ Rabbit Remedy *(Goodwinol)*.
camphor, capsicum, menthol. Choate's® Liniment *(Hawthorne)*.
camphor, Churchill's iodine, gum benzoin, rosin, Barbadoes aloes. Shin-Band *(Dominion)*.

camphor, ether, iodine, isopropyl alcohol (isopropanol), turpentine. Harold White's® Leg Paint *(Hawthorne).*
camphor, ether, isopropyl alcohol (isopropanol), menthol. Shin-O-Gel® *(Hawthorne).*
camphor, eucalyptus oil, menthol, phenol, pine oil, scarlet red, thymol. Scarlet Oil Pump Spray *(Dominion).*
camphor, glycerine, zinc sulfate, boric acid. Eye Rinse *(Butler), (RXV).*
camphor, iodide (potassium), iodine, isopropyl alcohol (isopropanol), menthol, thymol. Equi-Phar™ CoolGel *(Vedco).*
camphor, iodide (potassium), iodine, menthol, thymol, benzocaine. Equi-Phar™ BenzaGel *(Vedco).*
camphor, iodine, isopropyl alcohol, menthol, wormwood oil. Dealer Select Horse Care Horse Liniment *(Durvet).*
camphor, iodine, isopropyl alcohol (isopropanol), menthol. Lin-O-Gel® *(Hawthorne).*
camphor, isopropyl alcohol (isopropanol), menthol. Ice-O-Gel® *(Hawthorne).*
camphor, isopropyl alcohol (isopropanol), menthol, salicylic acid, tannic acid, boric acid. Dry-It *(Q.A. Laboratories).*
camphor, isopropyl alcohol (isopropanol), menthol, thymol. Liniment Gel *(First Priority).*
camphor, isopropyl alcohol (isopropanol), menthol, thymol, benzocaine. Liniment Gel with Benzocaine *(First Priority).*
camphor, isopropyl alcohol (isopropanol), menthol, thymol, witch hazel, benzocaine. Benzo-Gel™ *(Butler).*
camphor, menthol, ammonium carbonate. ZEV *(Dominion).*
camphor, methyl salicylate. Vetrolin® Liniment *(Equicare).*
camphor, turpentine, ammonium chloride. White Liniment *(Butler), (Durvet).*
Canada balsam, alcohol, camphor. VetRx™ Small Fur Animal Remedy *(Goodwinol).*
Canada balsam, corn oil base, milk supplement, oil origanum, oil rosemary, camphor. VetRx™ Equine Formula *(Goodwinol).*
Canada balsam, corn oil base, oil origanum, oil rosemary, alcohol, camphor. VetRx™ Caged Bird Remedy *(Goodwinol)*, VetRx™ for Cats and Kittens *(Goodwinol)*, VetRx™ for Dogs and Puppies *(Goodwinol)*, VetRx™ Goat & Sheep Remedy *(Goodwinol)*, VetRx™ Pigeon Remedy *(Goodwinol)*, VetRx™ Poultry Remedy *(Goodwinol)*, VetRx™ Rabbit Remedy *(Goodwinol).*
CaniGlide™ *(Vedco)*, **amikacin sulfate.**
Canine Aspirin Chewable Tablets for Large Dogs *(Pala-Tech)*, **acetylsalicylic acid.**
Canine Aspirin Chewable Tablets For Small and Medium Dogs *(Pala-Tech)*, **acetylsalicylic acid.**
Canine F.A./Plus Chewable Tablets For Large Dogs *(Pala-Tech)*, **fatty acids (omega).**
Canine F.A./Plus Chewable Tablets For Small and Medium Dogs *(Pala-Tech)*, **fatty acids (omega).**
Canine F.A./Plus Granules *(Pala-Tech)*, **fatty acids (omega), minerals, vitamins.**
Canine Fresh Frozen Plasma *(P.V.R.)*, **canine plasma.**
Canine Packed Red Blood Cells *(P.V.R.)*, **RBC's.**
canine pheromone. D.A.P.™ Dog Appeasing Pheromone *(V.P.L.).*
canine plasma. Canine Fresh Frozen Plasma *(P.V.R.).*
Canine Plasma *(A.B.B.)*, **adenine, anhydrous lanolin, citric acid, hyaluronic acid (sodium hyaluronate), sodium citrate, whole blood.**
Canine Red Blood Cells *(A.B.B.)*, **adenine, anhydrous lanolin, citric acid, hyaluronic acid (sodium hyaluronate), sodium citrate, whole blood.**
Canine Thyroid Chewable Tablets *(Pala-Tech)*, **levothyroxine.**
Canine Whole Blood *(A.B.B.)*, **adenine, anhydrous lanolin, citric acid, hyaluronic acid (sodium hyaluronate), sodium citrate, whole blood.**
Canine Whole Blood *(P.V.R.)*, **whole blood.**
Ca-P I.V. Therapy *(RXV)*, **calcium borogluconate, calcium hypophosphite, dextrose, magnesium borogluconate.**
caprine serum fraction. Caprine Serum Fraction, Immunomodulator *(Professional Biological).*
Caprine Serum Fraction, Immunomodulator *(Professional Biological)*, **caprine serum fraction.**
caprylic-capric acid. Bou-Matic Derma-Guard *(Bou-Matic)*, Bou-Matic eXtra-Guard *(Bou-Matic)*, Derma Cide™ *(Westfalia•Surge)*, Derma Sept™ *(Westfalia•Surge).*
capsaicin (cayenne pepper extract). Equine Capsaicin Gel *(Butler)*, Equine Pain Block Gel *(First Priority)*, Sure-Block™ Topical Pain Reliever *(SureNutrition).*
capsaicin (cayenne pepper extract), emollient(s). Arthro Ease™ *(Horses Prefer).*
capsicum, menthol, camphor. Choate's® Liniment *(Hawthorne).*
Capstar® *(Novartis)*, **nitenpyram.**
captan, sulfur. Paraguard™ Shampoo *(First Priority).*
carbadox. Mecadox® 10 *(Phibro)*, MoorMan's® CBX *(ADM).*
carbadox, pyrantel tartrate. MoorMan's® WDC *(ADM).*
carbamide, allantoin, benzalkonium chloride. Myosan™ Cream *(Life Science)*, Myosan™ Solution *(Life Science).*
carbamide (urea) peroxide. Earoxide™ Ear Cleanser *(Tomlyn).*
carbaryl. Adams™ Carbaryl Flea & Tick Shampoo *(Farnam), (V.P.L.)*, Happy Jack® Flea-Tick Powder II *(Happy Jack)*, Mycodex® Pet Shampoo with Carbaryl *(V.P.L.)*, Prozap® Garden & Poultry Dust *(Loveland).*
carbaryl, methoxychlor. Ritter's Tick and Flea Powder *(Ritter).*
carbaryl, n-octyl bicycloheptene dicarboximide, piperonyl butoxide, pyrethrins. Scratchex® Flea & Tick Powder *(Combe).*
carbaryl, piperonyl butoxide, pyrethrins. Adams™ Flea & Tick Dust II *(Farnam), (V.P.L.).*
Carbocaine®-V *(Pharmacia & Upjohn)*, **mepivacaine hydrochloride.**
carbohydrates, minerals, protein(s). Plexamino® Bolus *(Bimeda).*
carbolic acid, eucalyptus oil, menthol, benzocaine. Otisol™ *(Wysong)*, Otisol-O™ *(Wysong).*
carbomer, chloroxylenol, alcohol, butoxypolypropylene glycol. Swimmer's Ear Astringent *(Vet Solutions).*
carboxy methylcellulose. Equi-Phar™ Lubogel-V™ *(Vedco).*
carboxy methylcellulose, diphenylamine, ferric sulfate. Blood Stop Powder *(AgriPharm), (Centaur).*
carboxy methylcellulose, methyl para-hydroxybenzoate, propyl para-hydroxybenzoate, propylene glycol. General Lube *(First Priority).*
carboxy methylcellulose, propylene glycol. Liqui-Lube *(Vetus)*, Lubiseptol *(AgriPharm)*, Lubrivet™ *(Butler)*, Non-Spermicidal - Sterile Lubricating Jelly *(First Priority)*, O B Lube *(AgriLabs), (Centaur)*, Vet Lube *(Phoenix Pharmaceutical).*
carfentanil. Wildnil™ *(Wildlife).*
Carmilax® Bolets® *(Pfizer Animal Health)*, **magnesium hydroxide.**
Carmilax® Powder *(Pfizer Animal Health)*, **magnesium hydroxide.**
carob, kaolin. Boltan III™ *(Butler).*
carob, magnesium trisilicate, pectin, aluminum silicate, attapulgite. Veda-Sorb Jr Bolus *(Vedco).*
carob, magnesium trisilicate, pectin, attapulgite. Anti-Diarrheal Cattle Bolus *(AgriLabs)*, Gastro-Sorb™ Bolus *(Butler)*, Gastro-Sorb™ Calf Bolus *(Butler)*, Intesti-Sorb Bolus *(AgriPharm)*, Intesti-Sorb Calf Bolus *(AgriPharm)*, Maxi-Sorb Bolus *(Durvet)*, Maxi Sorb Calf Bolus *(Durvet)*, Veda-Sorb Bolus *(Vedco).*
carprofen. Rimadyl® Caplets *(Pfizer Animal Health)*, Rimadyl® Chewable Tablets *(Pfizer Animal Health).*
CarraSorb™ Freeze-Dried Gel (FDG) *(V.P.L.)*, **β-[1,4]-linked mannan polymers (Acemannan).**
CarraVet™ Multi Purpose Cleansing Foam *(V.P.L.)*, **aloe vera, moisturizer(s), stain removers, vitamin E.**
CarraVet™ Spray-Gel Wound Dressing *(V.P.L.)*, **β-[1,4]-linked mannan polymers (Acemannan), aloe vera.**
CarraVet™ Wound Dressing *(V.P.L.)*, **β-[1,4]-linked mannan polymers (Acemannan), aloe vera.**
caseinate, skim milk, whey. Vaccine Stabilizer *(Alpharma).*
castor oil, glycerine, petrolatum, zinc oxide, acacia, calamine. Triple Cast™ *(Neogen).*
castor oil, salicylic acid. Wartsoff™ *(Creative Science).*
castor oil, trypsin, balsam peru oil. Granulex® V Aerosol Spray *(Pfizer Animal Health)*, Granulex® V Liquid *(Pfizer Animal Health)*, Trypzyme®-V Aerosol Spray *(V.P.L.)*, Trypzyme®-V Liquid *(V.P.L.).*
Cat Lax® *(Pharmaderm)*, **cod liver oil, petrolatum.**
Cat-Off™ *(Thornell)*, **deodorants, neutralizer(s).**
Cat-Off™ Concentrate *(Thornell)*, **deodorants, neutralizer(s).**
Catron™ IV *(Boehringer Ingelheim)*, **permethrin.**
Cattlyst® 50 *(Alpharma)*, **laidlomycin.**
Caustic Dressing Powder *(Phoenix Pharmaceutical)*, **copper sulfate.**
Caustic Powder *(Butler)*, **copper sulfate.**
Cavicide® *(Metrex)*, **isopropyl alcohol (isopropanol), quaternary ammonia.**
Cefa-Dri® *(Fort Dodge)*, **cephapirin benzathine.**
Cefa-Drops® *(Fort Dodge)*, **cefadroxil.**
cefadroxil. Cefa-Drops® *(Fort Dodge)*, Cefa-Tabs® *(Fort Dodge).*
Cefa-Lak® *(Fort Dodge)*, **cephapirin sodium.**
Cefa-Tabs® *(Fort Dodge)*, **cefadroxil.**
ceftiofur hydrochloride. Excenel® RTU *(Pharmacia & Upjohn).*
ceftiofur sodium. Naxcel® *(Pharmacia & Upjohn).*
Centrine® Injection *(Fort Dodge)*, **aminopentamide.**
Centrine® Tablets *(Fort Dodge)*, **aminopentamide.**
cephapirin benzathine. Cefa-Dri® *(Fort Dodge)*, ToMORROW® *(Fort Dodge).*
cephapirin sodium. Cefa-Lak® *(Fort Dodge)*, ToDAY® *(Fort Dodge).*
Cerulytic™ *(Virbac)*, **benzyl alcohol, hydroxytoluene.**
Cerumene™ *(Evsco)*, **squalane.**
Cerumite 3x *(Evsco)*, **n-octyl bicycloheptene dicarboximide, piperonyl butoxide, pyrethrins.**
Cervizine® Injectable *(Wildlife)*, **xylazine hydrochloride.**
Cestex® *(Pfizer Animal Health)*, **epsiprantel.**
C.E.T.® 0.12% Chlorhexidine Lavage *(Virbac)*, **chlorhexidine gluconate, ethyl alcohol.**
C.E.T.® Chews for Cats *(Virbac)*, **glucose oxidase, lactoperoxidase.**
C.E.T.® Enzymatic Tartar Control Toothpaste *(Virbac)*, **glucose oxidase, lactoperoxidase.**
C.E.T.® Enzymatic Toothpaste *(Virbac)*, **glucose oxidase, lactoperoxidase.**

C.E.T.® FluraFom *(Virbac)*, **fluoride.**

C.E.T.® Oral Hygiene Gel *(Virbac)*, **chlorhexidine gluconate.**

C.E.T.® Oral Hygiene Rinse *(Virbac)*, **chlorhexidine gluconate.**

cetrimide, chlorhexidine gluconate, ethanol. Bou-Matic Kleen & Dri *(Bou-Matic)*.

cetyl alcohol, lanolin, petrolatum, vitamin A, vitamin D, benzethonium chloride. Udder Ointment™ *(LeGear)*.

CGB® Ointment *(PPC)*, **betamethasone, clotrimazole, gentamicin.**

chamomile, conditioners, sunflower oil. Waterless Spray-On Shampoo *(Davis)*.

Champion Protector™ Worm Protector™ 2X *(AgriLabs)*, **pyrantel pamoate.**

Chap-Guard™ Plus *(AgriLabs)*, **emollient(s), vitamins.**

CheckMite+™ *(Mann Lake)*, **coumaphos.**

CheckMite+™ Bee Hive Pest Control Strip *(Bayer)*, **coumaphos.**

Cherryderm™ Grooming Shampoo *(Vetus)*, **coconut oil, shampoo formula.**

Cherry Grooming Shampoo *(Butler)*, **coconut oil, shampoo formula.**

Cherry Grooming Shampoo *(First Priority)*, **shampoo formula.**

chitosanide, docusate sodium (dioctyl sodium sulfosuccinate), lactic acid, propylene glycol, salicylic acid. Epi-Otic® *(Virbac)*.

chitosanide, glycerine, lactic acid, urea. Allergroom® Shampoo *(Virbac)*.

chitosanide, glycerine, oatmeal. Epi-Soothe® Shampoo *(Virbac)*.

chitosanide, lactic acid, benzalkonium chloride. Etiderm® Shampoo *(Virbac)*.

Chlor-A-Clens Cleansing Solution *(Vedco)*, **benzoic acid, chlorhexidine, glycerine, malic acid, propylene glycol, salicylic acid.**

Chlor-A-Clens-L Cleansing Solution *(Vedco)*, **benzoic acid, chlorhexidine, glycerine, lidocaine, malic acid, propylene glycol, zolazepam.**

Chloradine Scrub 4%® *(RXV)*, **chlorhexidine gluconate.**

Chlora-Dip *(First Priority)*, **chlorhexidine gluconate, glycerine.**

chloramphenicol. Amphicol® Film-Coated Tablets *(Butler)*, Bemacol® *(Pfizer Animal Health)*, Chlorbiotic® *(Schering-Plough)*, Duricol™ Chloramphenicol Capsules U.S.P. *(V.P.C.)*, Vetrachloracin® Ophthalmic Ointment *(Pharmaderm)*, Viceton® *(Bimeda)*.

Chlorasan Antiseptic Ointment *(Butler)*, **chlorhexidine.**

Chlorbiotic® *(Schering-Plough)*, **chloramphenicol.**

ChlorhexiDerm™ 2% Shampoo *(DVM)*, **chlorhexidine gluconate.**

ChlorhexiDerm™ Disinfectant *(DVM)*, **chlorhexidine gluconate.**

ChlorhexiDerm™ Flush *(DVM)*, **chlorhexidine gluconate.**

ChlorhexiDerm™ Maximum 4% Shampoo *(DVM)*, **chlorhexidine gluconate.**

ChlorhexiDerm™ Maximum 4% Spray *(DVM)*, **chlorhexidine gluconate.**

ChlorhexiDerm™ Plus Scrub *(DVM)*, **chlorhexidine gluconate.**

ChlorhexiDerm™ S Disinfectant *(DVM)*, **chlorhexidine gluconate.**

chlorhexidine. 4% Maximum Chlorhexidine Shampoo *(Davis)*, Bou-Matic Super Dip *(Bou-Matic)*, Chlorasan Antiseptic Ointment *(Butler)*, Chlorhexidine Ointment 1% *(Phoenix Pharmaceutical)*, ChlorHex Shampoo *(Vedco)*, Clean and Fresh™ *(Butler)*, Fresh Mouth Oral Spray *(Vedco)*, Hexaclens 1 Antiseptic Shampoo *(Vetus)*, Hexaclens 2% Antiseptic Shampoo *(Vetus)*, Hexaseptic Flush *(Vetus)*, Hexoral Rinse *(Vetus)*, Monarch® Prep Udder Wash *(Ecolab Food & Bev. Div.)*, Monarch® Protek® Spray *(Ecolab Food & Bev. Div.)*, Nolvadent® *(Fort Dodge)*, Nolvalube® *(Fort Dodge)*, Nolvasan® Antiseptic Ointment *(Fort Dodge)*, Nolvasan® Cap-Tabs® *(Fort Dodge)*, Nolvasan® S *(Fort Dodge)*, Nolvasan® Shampoo *(Fort Dodge)*, Nolvasan® Skin and Wound Cleanser *(Fort Dodge)*, Nolvasan® Solution *(Fort Dodge)*, Nolvasan® Surgical Scrub *(Fort Dodge)*, Nolvasan® Suspension *(Fort Dodge)*, Nolvasan® Udder Wash Concentrate *(Fort Dodge)*, OralDent *(Phoenix Pharmaceutical)*, Privasan™ Antiseptic Ointment *(First Priority)*.

chlorhexidine, denatonium benzoate, lidocaine. Hexaseptic Flush Plus *(Vetus)*.

chlorhexidine, glycerine. Nolvasan® 5% Teat Dip Concentrate *(Fort Dodge)*, Nolvasan® Teat Dip Concentrate *(Fort Dodge)*.

chlorhexidine, glycerine, lidocaine, malic acid, propylene glycol, zolazepam, benzoic acid. Chlor-A-Clens-L Cleansing Solution *(Vedco)*.

chlorhexidine, glycerine, malic acid, propylene glycol, salicylic acid, benzoic acid. Chlor-A-Clens Cleansing Solution *(Vedco)*.

chlorhexidine, iodine complex (povidone-iodine). Monarch® Protek® Teat Dip *(Ecolab Food & Bev. Div.)*.

chlorhexidine, lidocaine, malic acid, salicylic acid, benzoic acid. Dermachlor™ Plus *(Butler)*.

chlorhexidine, malic acid, propylene glycol, salicylic acid, benzoic acid. Dermachlor™ Rinse *(Butler)*.

chlorhexidine, nicotinamide. Stomadhex™ *(Virbac)*.

chlorhexidine, zinc. Hexoral Zn Rinse *(Vetus)*.

chlorhexidine citrate. ChlorHex Surgical Scrub *(Vedco)*.

chlorhexidine digluconate. Arrest® Dip/Spray *(Westfalia•*Surge), Bactrasan™ Solution *(Aspen)*.

chlorhexidine digluconate, quaternary ammonia. Spectrum™ *(Westfalia•*Surge).

chlorhexidine digluconate, triclosan. Hexadene® Flush *(Virbac)*.

Chlorhexidine Disinfectant Solution *(AgriLabs)*, **chlorhexidine gluconate.**

chlorhexidine gluconate. 2% Chlorhexidine Ointment *(Davis)*, 2% Chlorhexidine Shampoo *(Davis)*, 4% Non-Sting Chlorhexidine Spray *(Davis)*, 20% Chlorhexidine Gluconate Additive *(Davis)*, AmTech Chlorhexidine Solution *(Phoenix Scientific)*, C.E.T.® Oral Hygiene Gel *(Virbac)*, C.E.T.® Oral Hygiene Rinse *(Virbac)*, Chloradine Scrub 4%® *(RXV)*, ChlorhexiDerm™ 2% Shampoo *(DVM)*, ChlorhexiDerm™ Disinfectant *(DVM)*, ChlorhexiDerm™ Flush *(DVM)*, ChlorhexiDerm™ Maximum 4% Shampoo *(DVM)*, ChlorhexiDerm™ Maximum 4% Spray *(DVM)*, ChlorhexiDerm™ Plus Scrub *(DVM)*, ChlorhexiDerm™ S Disinfectant *(DVM)*, Chlorhexidine Disinfectant Solution *(AgriLabs)*, Chlorhexidine Scrub *(A.A.H.)*, Chlorhexidine Scrub 2% *(First Priority)*, Chlorhexidine Scrub 4% *(First Priority)*, Chlorhexidine Solution *(A.A.H.)*, *(Aspen)*, *(Bimeda)*, *(Butler)*, *(Durvet)*, *(First Priority)*, *(Phoenix Pharmaceutical)*, *(Vedco)*, *(Vet Solutions)*, Chlorhexi-Lube *(Durvet)*, *(First Priority)*, Chlor-Scrub 40™ *(Butler)*, Hexadene® Shampoo *(Virbac)*, Hexascrub Medical Scrub 2% *(Vetus)*, Hexascrub Medical Scrub 4% *(Vetus)*, Hexasol Solution *(Vetus)*, Make Your Own Chlorhexidine Shampoo *(Davis)*, Micro Pearls Advantage™ Seba-Hex™ Shampoo *(Evsco)*, ResiChlor™ Leave-on Conditioner *(Virbac)*, TDC/Teat Dip with Chlorhexidine *(Western Chemical)*.

chlorhexidine gluconate, ethanol, cetrimide. Bou-Matic Kleen & Dri *(Bou-Matic)*.

chlorhexidine gluconate, ethyl alcohol. C.E.T.® 0.12% Chlorhexidine Lavage *(Virbac)*.

chlorhexidine gluconate, glycerine. Chlora-Dip *(First Priority)*, Metz Soft-Kote Teat Dip *(Metz)*, Metz Soft-Kote Teat Spray *(Metz)*.

chlorhexidine gluconate, ketoconazole. KetoChlor™ Shampoo *(Virbac)*.

chlorhexidine gluconate, miconazole. Malaseb™ Flush *(DVM)*, Malaseb™ Pledgets *(DVM)*, Malaseb™ Shampoo *(DVM)*, Malaseb™ Spray *(DVM)*.

chlorhexidine gluconate, quaternary ammonia. Bou-Matic Sprayable Supreme *(Bou-Matic)*, Bou-Matic Supreme *(Bou-Matic)*.

chlorhexidine gluconate, zinc. CHX+Zn Oral Mist *(Butler)*.

Chlorhexidine Ointment 1% *(Phoenix Pharmaceutical)*, **chlorhexidine.**

Chlorhexidine Scrub *(A.A.H.)*, **chlorhexidine gluconate.**

Chlorhexidine Scrub 2% *(First Priority)*, **chlorhexidine gluconate.**

Chlorhexidine Scrub 4% *(First Priority)*, **chlorhexidine gluconate.**

Chlorhexidine Solution *(A.A.H.)*, *(Aspen)*, *(Bimeda)*, *(Butler)*, *(Durvet)*, *(First Priority)*, *(Phoenix Pharmaceutical)*, *(Vedco)*, *(Vet Solutions)*, **chlorhexidine gluconate.**

Chlorhexi-Lube *(Durvet)*, *(First Priority)*, **chlorhexidine gluconate.**

ChlorHex Shampoo *(Vedco)*, **chlorhexidine.**

ChlorHex Surgical Scrub *(Vedco)*, **chlorhexidine citrate.**

chlorine dioxide. Ono™ *(PRN Pharmacal)*.

ChlorMax™ 50 *(Alpharma)*, **chlortetracycline.**

chlorothymol, isopropyl alcohol (isopropanol), benzalkonium chloride. Blue Lotion Topical Antiseptic *(Aspen)*, *(First Priority)*.

chloroxylenol. Surgical Scrub and Handwash *(First Priority)*, Surgical Scrub & Handwash *(Vet Solutions)*.

chloroxylenol, alcohol, butoxypolypropylene glycol, carbomer. Swimmer's Ear Astringent *(Vet Solutions)*.

chloroxylenol, alum. McKillip's Dusting Powder *(Butler)*, *(First Priority)*.

chloroxylenol, collagen, ferric sulfate, aluminum sulfate. Clotisol® Liquid *(BenePet)*.

chloroxylenol, copper sulfate. Equi-Phar™ Caustic Powder *(Vedco)*.

chloroxylenol, diphenylamine, ferrous sulfate. Hemostatic Powder *(Butler)*.

chloroxylenol, diphenylamine, ferrous sulfate, tannic acid. Blood Stop Powder *(First Priority)*.

chloroxylenol, ferrous sulfate, tannic acid, alum. Blood Stop Powder *(Aspen)*, *(Durvet)*, *(Vedco)*, Hemostat Powder *(Phoenix Pharmaceutical)*.

chloroxylenol, humectant(s), vitamins, aloe vera. H-Balm Udder Cream *(Centaur)*.

chloroxylenol, salicylic acid, sodium thiosulfate. Equine Medicated Shampoo *(Vet Solutions)*, Universal Medicated Shampoo *(Vet Solutions)*.

chlorpyrifos. Happy Jack® Enduracide® Dip II *(Happy Jack)*, Happy Jack® Paracide II Shampoo *(Happy Jack)*, Pet Care Indoor Premise Spray *(Durvet)*, Scratchex® Flea & Tick Collar for Cats *(Combe)*, Scratchex® Flea & Tick Collar for Dogs *(Combe)*.

Chlor-Scrub 40™ *(Butler)*, **chlorhexidine gluconate.**

chlortetracycline. AmTech Chlortetracycline HCl Soluble Powder *(Phoenix Scientific)*, Aureomycin® 50 Granular *(Alpharma)*, Aureomycin® 90 Granular *(Alpharma)*, Aureomycin® 100 Granular *(Alpharma)*, Aureomycin® Soluble Powder *(Fort Dodge)*, Aureomycin® Soluble Powder Concentrate *(Fort Dodge)*, ChlorMax™ 50 *(Alpharma)*, CLTC® 100 MR *(Phibro)*, CTC 50 *(Durvet)*, CTC Soluble Powder *(AgriLabs)*, CTC Soluble Powder Concentrate *(Durvet)*, Pennchlor 50•G® *(PennField)*, Pennchlor™ 50 Meal *(PennField)*, Pennchlor™ 64 Soluble Powder *(PennField)*, Pennchlor™ 70 Meal *(PennField)*, Pennchlor 90•G® *(PennField)*, Pennchlor 100 Hi-Flo™ Meal *(PennField)*, Pennchlor™ 100-MR *(PennField)*, Pennox 200 Hi-Flo™ Meal *(PennField)*.

chlortetracycline, penicillin G procaine, sulfamethazine. Aureomix® 500 Granular *(Alpharma)*, Pennchlor SP 250® *(PennField)*, Pennchlor SP 500® *(PennField)*.

chlortetracycline, penicillin G procaine, sulfathiazole. AureoZol® 500 Granular *(Alpharma)*.

chlortetracycline, sulfamethazine. Aureomycin® Sulmet® Soluble Powder *(Fort Dodge)*, Aureo S 700® Granular 10G *(Alpharma)*, Aureo S 700® Granular 35G *(Alpharma)*.

Choate's® Liniment *(Hawthorne)*, **camphor, capsicum, menthol.**

choline, fatty acids (essential), methionine (d-l), vitamins. Lipo-Form *(Vet-A-Mix).*
choline, lipids, minerals, vitamins. Geri-Form *(Vet-A-Mix).*
choline, phosphatidylcholine. Cholodin® *(MVP).*
choline bitartrate, inositol, liver, racemethionine, vitamin B-complex. Lipocaps *(Vetus).*
choline chloride. Reashure™ Choline *(Balchem).*
Cholodin® *(MVP),* **choline, phosphatidylcholine.**
Cholodin®-FEL *(MVP),* **amino acids, minerals, taurine, vitamins.**
Chondroprotec® *(Neogen),* **polysulfated glycosaminoglycan.**
chorionic gonadotropin. Chorionic Gonadotropin *(Butler),* Chorulon® *(Intervet).*
Chorionic Gonadotropin *(Butler),* **chorionic gonadotropin.**
chorionic gonadotropin, serum gonadotropin. P.G. 600® Estrus Control *(Intervet).*
Chorulon® *(Intervet),* **chorionic gonadotropin.**
Churchill's iodine, gum benzoin, rosin, Barbadoes aloes, camphor. Shin-Band *(Dominion).*
CHX+Zn Oral Mist *(Butler),* **chlorhexidine gluconate, zinc.**
citric acid. Citric Acid *(AgriLabs), (Alpharma),* Citric Acid Soluble Powder *(AgriPharm).*
Citric Acid *(AgriLabs), (Alpharma),* **citric acid.**
citric acid, copper carbonate, ammonium bicarbonate, ammonium hydroxide. Cop-R-Sol™ *(Alpharma).*
citric acid, copper sulfate. Copper Blue™ *(AgriLabs).*
citric acid, electrolytes, methionine, microorganisms. Greenlyte® *(Bimeda).*
citric acid, hyaluronic acid (sodium hyaluronate), sodium citrate, whole blood, adenine, anhydrous lanolin. Canine Plasma *(A.B.B.),* Canine Red Blood Cells *(A.B.B.),* Canine Whole Blood *(A.B.B.),* Feline Plasma *(A.B.B.),* Feline Red Blood Cells *(A.B.B.),* Feline Whole Blood *(A.B.B.).*
Citric Acid Soluble Powder *(AgriPharm),* **citric acid.**
Clavamox® Drops *(Pfizer Animal Health),* **amoxicillin, clavulanic acid.**
Clavamox® Tablets *(Pfizer Animal Health),* **amoxicillin, clavulanic acid.**
clavulanic acid, amoxicillin. Clavamox® Drops *(Pfizer Animal Health),* Clavamox® Tablets *(Pfizer Animal Health).*
Clean and Fresh™ *(Butler),* **chlorhexidine.**
Clean Crop® Malathion 57EC *(Loveland),* **malathion.**
cleaning formulation/spray. Allerpet® C *(V.P.L.),* Allerpet® D *(V.P.L.).*
ClearCal 50 *(Vedco),* **calcium.**
Clear Eyes *(Farnam),* **sodium chloride, sodium citrate.**
CleaRx® Ear Cleansing Solution *(DVM),* **docusate sodium (dioctyl sodium sulfosuccinate), urea peroxide.**
CleaRx® Ear Drying Solution *(DVM),* **hydrocortisone.**
Cleen Sheen *(Vedco),* **coconut oil, shampoo formula.**
clenbuterol hydrochloride. Ventipulmin® Syrup *(Boehringer Ingelheim).*
Clinacox™ *(Schering-Plough),* **diclazuril.**
Clinafarm® EC *(ASL),* **imazalil.**
Clinafarm® SG *(ASL),* **imazalil.**
Clincaps™ *(Vetus),* **clindamycin hydrochloride.**
ClindaCure™ *(Vedco),* **clindamycin hydrochloride.**
Clinda-Guard™ *(RXV),* **clindamycin hydrochloride.**
clindamycin hydrochloride. AmTech Clindamycin Hydrochloride Oral Liquid *(Phoenix Scientific),* Antirobe Aquadrops® Liquid *(Pharmacia & Upjohn),* Antirobe® Capsules *(Pharmacia & Upjohn),* Clincaps™ *(Vetus),* ClindaCure™ *(Vedco),* Clinda-Guard™ *(RXV),* Clindamycin Hydrochloride Drops *(Phoenix Pharmaceutical),* Clindrops™ *(Vetus).*
Clindamycin Hydrochloride Drops *(Phoenix Pharmaceutical),* **clindamycin hydrochloride.**
Clindrops™ *(Vetus),* **clindamycin hydrochloride.**
CliniCare® Canine Liquid Diet *(Abbott),* **energy source(s), minerals, nutrients, vitamins.**
CliniCare® Feline Liquid Diet *(Abbott),* **energy source(s), minerals, nutrients, vitamins.**
CliniCare® RF Specialized Feline Liquid Diet *(Abbott),* **energy source(s), minerals, nutrients, vitamins.**
Clomicalm® *(Novartis),* **clomipramine hydrochloride.**
clomipramine hydrochloride. Clomicalm® *(Novartis).*
cloprostenol sodium. Estrumate® *(Schering-Plough).*
clorsulon. Curatrem® *(Merial).*
clorsulon, ivermectin. Ivomec® Plus Injection for Cattle *(Merial).*
Clotisol® Liquid *(BenePet),* **aluminum sulfate, chloroxylenol, collagen, ferric sulfate.**
Clot-It Plus™ *(Evsco),* **aluminum chloride, ammonium chloride, bentonite, benzocaine, copper sulfate, diatomaceous earth, ferric subsulfate, iodoform.**
Clot Powder *(Q.A. Laboratories),* **copper sulfate, ferrous sulfate, iodine complex (povidone-iodine).**
clotrimazole. Clotrimazole Solution USP, 1% *(Butler), (Vet Solutions), (Vetus).*
clotrimazole, gentamicin, betamethasone. CGB® Ointment *(PPC),* Genotic B-C™ *(Butler),* MalOtic® Ointment *(Vedco),* Otibiotic Ointment *(Vetus),* Otomax® *(Schering-Plough),* Oto Soothe® Ointment *(RXV),* Tri-Otic® *(Med-Pharmex).*
clotrimazole, gentamicin, mometasone furoate. MometaMax™ Otic Suspension *(Schering-Plough).*
Clotrimazole Solution USP, 1% *(Butler), (Vet Solutions), (Vetus),* **clotrimazole.**
Clout™ All Weather Bait *(Bayer),* **bromethalin.**
Clout™ Place Packs *(Bayer),* **bromethalin.**
Clovite® Conditioner *(Fort Dodge),* **vitamin A, vitamin B_{12} (cyanocobalamin), vitamin D.**
cloxacillin benzathine. Dry-Clox® *(Fort Dodge),* Orbenin®-DC *(Pfizer Animal Health).*
cloxacillin sodium. Dariclox® *(Pfizer Animal Health).*
CLTC® 100 MR *(Phibro),* **chlortetracycline.**
CMPK *(RXV),* **calcium, dextrose, magnesium borogluconate, potassium chloride, sodium hypophosphite.**
CMPK Bolus *(Durvet), (Vets Plus),* **calcium, magnesium, phosphorus, potassium.**
CMPK D_3 Drench *(Durvet),* **calcium, magnesium chloride, potassium chloride, propylene glycol, sodium hypophosphite, vitamin D_3.**
CMPK-Dex *(Vetus),* **calcium, dextrose, magnesium borogluconate, potassium chloride, sodium hypophosphite.**
C.M.P.K. Gel *(AgriLabs),* **calcium, magnesium chloride, phosphorus, potassium chloride.**
CMPK Gel *(AgriPharm),* **calcium, magnesium chloride, phosphoric acid, potassium chloride, trisodium phosphate.**
CMPK Gel *(Durvet),* **calcium, magnesium hydroxide, phosphorus, potassium chloride.**
CMPK Gel *(Vedco),* **calcium, magnesium chloride, phosphorus, potassium chloride.**
CMPK Gel Plus™ *(Vets Plus),* **calcium, calcium phosphate, magnesium chloride, potassium chloride.**
C-M-P-K Injection *(Vet Tek),* **calcium, dextrose, magnesium borogluconate, potassium chloride, sodium hypophosphite.**
CMPK Oral *(AgriPharm),* **calcium, dextrose, magnesium chloride, potassium chloride, sodium phosphate.**
C.M.P.K. Oral Gel *(Phoenix Pharmaceutical),* **calcium, magnesium, phosphorus, potassium.**
CMPK Oral Solution 33% *(Vedco),* **calcium, magnesium, phosphoric acid, potassium.**
CMPK Solution *(Aspen),* **calcium, dextrose, magnesium chloride, potassium chloride, sodium hypophosphite.**
CMPK Solution *(Bimeda),* **calcium borogluconate, dextrose, magnesium borogluconate, potassium chloride, sodium hypophosphite.**
CMPK Solution *(Vedco),* **calcium, dextrose, magnesium chloride, potassium chloride, sodium hypophosphite.**
CMPK with D_3 Drench *(Vets Plus),* **calcium, magnesium, phosphorus, potassium, vitamin D_3.**
coal tar. Hartz® Groomer's Best™ Medicated Shampoo *(Hartz Mountain),* Micro Pearls Advantage™ EVSCO-Tar™ Shampoo *(Evsco),* Nova Pearls™ Coal Tar Spray *(Tomlyn),* Nova Pearls™ Therapeutic Coal Tar Shampoo *(Tomlyn).*
coal tar, menthol, salicylic acid. NuSal-T® Shampoo *(DVM).*
coal tar, salicylic acid, sulfur. Allerseb-T® Shampoo *(Virbac),* LyTar® Shampoo *(DVM),* Sulfur & Tar Medicated Shampoo *(Davis),* T-Lux® Shampoo *(Virbac).*
coal tar, sulfur, triclosan. Sulfodene® Medicated Shampoo & Conditioner for Dogs *(Combe).*
cobalt, magnesium, calcium. Cal "62" Plus Gel *(Aspen),* Calcium Oral Gel *(Phoenix Pharmaceutical),* Calcium Plus *(First Priority),* Cal-Gel™ *(Jorgensen).*
cobalt, magnesium, propionic acid, propylene glycol, vitamins. Keto Oral Gel *(Phoenix Pharmaceutical).*
cobalt, magnesium, propylene glycol, vitamins. Oral Keto Energel *(First Priority).*
cobalt, magnesium, selenium, calcium. Cal M 64 Plus Se *(Butler),* Cal-Mag-SE Gel *(Durvet).*
cobalt, magnesium, selenium, vitamin B-complex, calcium. Calcium SE *(First Priority).*
cobalt, magnesium, selenium, vitamins, calcium. Cal Ox 64 Plus SE *(AgriPharm),* Calcium Gel+Selenium *(AgriLabs),* CalOx 64 SE Oral Gel *(Vedco).*
cobalt glucoheptonate. Copro 25 *(Zinpro).*
cobalt sulfate, copper gluconate, iron. Iron-Plus *(Neogen).*
cobalt sulfate, copper sulfate, hydrochloric acid, manganese sulfate, potassium dichromate. Ema-Sol™ Concentrate *(Alpharma).*
cobalt sulfate, magnesium chloride, calcium. Cal-Mag-Co Gel *(Durvet),* Respond *(Jorgensen),* Super Calcium Gel "62" *(AgriPharm).*
cobalt sulfate, magnesium chloride, vitamins, calcium. Calox 64 Oral Gel *(Vedco).*
cobalt sulfate, magnesium sulfate, polyethelene glycol, propionic acid, silicon dioxide, vitamins. Ketopro Oral Gel *(Vedco).*
Coban® 60 *(Elanco),* **monensin sodium.**
cocamido propyl phosphatidyl, dimonium chloride, propylene glycol, alcohol. EarMed Cleansing Solution & Wash *(Davis).*
Cocoderm Conditioning Shampoo *(Vetus),* **coconut oil, shampoo formula.**
coconut oil, conditioners, shampoo formula. Davis Best Luxury Shampoo *(Davis).*

D

DermaPet® MalAcetic™ Conditioner for Dogs and Cats *(DermaPet)*, **acetic acid, boric acid.**

DermaPet® MalAcetic Otic *(DermaPet)*, **acetic acid, boric acid.**

DermaPet® MalAcetic™ Shampoo for Dogs and Cats *(DermaPet)*, **acetic acid, boric acid.**

DermaPet® MalAcetic™ Wet Wipes/Dry Bath *(DermaPet)*, **acetic acid, boric acid.**

DermaPet® Oatmeal Conditioner *(DermaPet)*, **oatmeal.**

DermaPet® O.F.A. Plus EZ-C Caps (up to 30 lb.) *(DermaPet)*, **fatty acids (omega), vitamin C (ascorbic acid), vitamin E, zinc.**

DermaPet® O.F.A. Plus EZ-C Caps (50-70 lb.) *(DermaPet)*, **fatty acids (omega), vitamin C (ascorbic acid), vitamin E, zinc.**

DermaPet® Seborrheic Shampoo *(DermaPet)*, **salicylic acid, sulfur.**

DermaPet® TrizEDTA™ Aqueous Flush *(DermaPet)*, **EDTA (edetate disodium dihydrate), tromethamine.**

DermaPet® TrizEDTA™ Crystals *(DermaPet)*, **EDTA (edetate disodium dihydrate), tromethamine.**

Derma Sept™ *(Westfalia•Surge)*, **caprylic-capric acid.**

DermaSoothe Oatmeal Leave-On Conditioner *(Davis)*, **conditioners, oatmeal.**

Derma Spray *(Sungro)*, **Melaleuca alternifolia.**

Derma-Vet™ Cream *(Med-Pharmex)*, **neomycin, nystatin, thiostrepton, triamcinolone acetonide.**

Derma-Vet™ Ointment *(Med-Pharmex)*, **neomycin, nystatin, thiostrepton, triamcinolone acetonide.**

Dermazole™ Shampoo *(Virbac)*, **miconazole.**

DermCaps® *(DVM)*, **fatty acids.**

DermCaps® 10 lb. *(DVM)*, **fatty acids.**

DermCaps® 100 lb. *(DVM)*, **fatty acids.**

DermCaps® Economy Size Liquid *(DVM)*, **fatty acids.**

DermCaps® ES *(DVM)*, **fatty acids.**

DermCaps® ES Liquid *(DVM)*, **fatty acids.**

DermCaps® Liquid *(DVM)*, **fatty acids.**

Desicort™ Creme *(Butler)*, **hydrocortisone, zinc oxide.**

deslorelin. Ovuplant™ *(Fort Dodge)*.

desoxicorticosterone pivalate (DOCP). Percorten®-V *(Novartis)*.

detanglers, jojoba oil, keratin, mink oil, d-l-panthenol (vitamin B_5). Lustre Groom Mist™ *(Butler)*.

detergent (enzyme-based). DetergeZyme® *(Metrex)*, EmPower™ *(Metrex)*, MetriSponge® *(Metrex)*, MetriZyme® *(Metrex)*.

detergent mixture. MetriClean2® *(Metrex)*, MetriWash™ *(Metrex)*.

detergent mixture, EDTA (tetrasodium). Lifegard® 900 *(Rochester Midland)*.

detergent mixture, phosphoric acid. Lifegard® 7000 *(Rochester Midland)*, Lifegard® 7500F *(Rochester Midland)*, Lifegard® 7700 *(Rochester Midland)*, Lifegard® 7700ND *(Rochester Midland)*.

detergent mixture, potassium hydroxide, sodium hypochlorite, sodium metasilicate, sodium silicate. Lifegard® 855 Plus *(Rochester Midland)*.

DetergeZyme® *(Metrex)*, **detergent (enzyme-based).**

detomidine hydrochloride. Dormosedan® *(Pfizer Animal Health)*.

Dexaject *(Vetus)*, **dexamethasone.**

Dexalyte *(Butler)*, **electrolytes.**

Dexalyte 8X Powder *(Butler)*, **electrolytes, minerals.**

dexamethasone. AmTech Dexamethasone Solution *(Phoenix Scientific)*, Azium® Powder *(Schering-Plough)*, Azium® Solution *(Schering-Plough)*, Dexaject *(Vetus)*, Dexamethasone 2.0 mg Injection *(Vedco)*, Dexamethasone 2 mg/mL Injection *(RXV)*, Dexamethasone Injection *(AgriLabs)*, *(Vet Tek)*, Dexamethasone Solution *(Aspen)*, *(Butler)*, *(Phoenix Pharmaceutical)*, Dexasone *(RXV)*, Dexazone™ 2 mg *(Bimeda)*.

dexamethasone, neomycin, thiabendazole. Tresaderm® *(Merial)*.

dexamethasone, trichlormethiazide. Naquasone® Bolus *(Schering-Plough)*.

Dexamethasone 2.0 mg Injection *(Vedco)*, **dexamethasone.**

Dexamethasone 2 mg/mL Injection *(RXV)*, **dexamethasone.**

Dexamethasone Injection *(AgriLabs)*, *(Vet Tek)*, **dexamethasone.**

dexamethasone sodium phosphate. AmTech Dexamethasone Sodium Phosphate Injection *(Phoenix Scientific)*, Dexamethasone Sodium Phosphate *(Phoenix Pharmaceutical)*, Dexamethasone Sodium Phosphate Injection *(Butler)*, *(Vedco)*.

Dexamethasone Sodium Phosphate *(Phoenix Pharmaceutical)*, **dexamethasone sodium phosphate.**

Dexamethasone Sodium Phosphate Injection *(Butler)*, *(Vedco)*, **dexamethasone sodium phosphate.**

Dexamethasone Solution *(Aspen)*, *(Butler)*, *(Phoenix Pharmaceutical)*, **dexamethasone.**

Dexasone *(RXV)*, **dexamethasone.**

Dexazone™ 2 mg *(Bimeda)*, **dexamethasone.**

Dexolyte Solution *(Phoenix Pharmaceutical)*, **dextrose, electrolytes.**

dexpanthenol. AmTech d-Panthenol Injection *(Phoenix Scientific)*, D-Panthenol Injectable *(Vedco)*, d-Panthenol Injection *(Butler)*, *(Phoenix Pharmaceutical)*.

Dexsolyte Powder *(Neogen)*, **electrolytes, minerals, sucrose, vitamins.**

dextromethorphan, guaifenesin (glyceryl guaiacolate, guaiacol). Cough Tablets *(Life Science)*.

dextrose. 50% Dextrose Injection, USP *(Bimeda)*, AmTech Dextrose Solution 50% *(Phoenix Scientific)*, Dextrose 50% *(AgriLabs)*, *(AgriPharm)*, *(Durvet)*, Dextrose 50% Solution *(Vedco)*, *(Vetus)*, Dextrose Solution *(Aspen)*, Dextrose Solution 50% *(Butler)*, *(Phoenix Pharmaceutical)*, *(Vet Tek)*, Glucose *(Fort Dodge)*.

dextrose, calcium. Cal-Dextro® C *(Fort Dodge)*.

dextrose, electrolytes. AmTech Dexolyte Solution Injection *(Phoenix Scientific)*, Biolyte® *(Pharmacia & Upjohn)*, Bluelite® C *(TechMix)*, Calf Quencher *(Vedco)*, Deliver® with Dialine™ *(AgriLabs)*, Dexolyte Solution *(Phoenix Pharmaceutical)*, Electrolyte Powder 8X *(Phoenix Pharmaceutical)*, Electrolyte Solution *(AgriLabs)*, *(Vet Tek)*, Electrolyte Solution with Dextrose *(Vedco)*, Electrolyte w/Dextrose Injection *(Aspen)*, Entrolyte® *(Pfizer Animal Health)*, Entrolyte® H.E. *(Pfizer Animal Health)*, Equi-Phar™ Electrolyte with Dextrose *(Vedco)*, Equi-Phar™ Equi-Lyte Powder *(Vedco)*, Hydra-Lyte *(Vet-A-Mix)*, Magna-Lyte *(First Priority)*, Polylites IV *(Butler)*, Sky-Lytes *(Skylabs)*, Vedalyte 8X Powder *(Vedco)*, Vetalyte Plus I.V. Solution *(RXV)*.

dextrose, electrolytes, amino acids. A-Lyte Concentrate *(Durvet)*, Amcalcilyte Forte *(AgriPharm)*, *(Phoenix Pharmaceutical)*, *(Vedco)*, Aminocal Plus™ *(Butler)*, AmTech Amcal High Potency Oral Solution *(Phoenix Scientific)*, Glucaminolyte Forte *(AgriPharm)*, *(Vedco)*, Gluco-Amino-Forte Oral Solution *(Phoenix Pharmaceutical)*, Gluco Amino Forte Oral Solution *(Vetus)*, Keto Amino Forte™ *(Butler)*.

dextrose, electrolytes, glycine. Hy-Sorb™ *(Bimeda)*.

dextrose, electrolytes, glycine, bicarbonate. Elpak™-G *(Vedco)*.

dextrose, electrolytes, glycine, vitamins. Electrolyte HE with Vitamins *(DVM Formula)*.

dextrose, electrolytes, minerals. Stress-Dex® *(Neogen)*.

dextrose, electrolytes, minerals, vitamins. Multi-Electrolytes *(Neogen)*.

dextrose, electrolytes, vitamin B-complex, amino acids. A-Lyte Solution *(Durvet)*, Amino Acid Concentrate Oral Solution *(Aspen)*, *(Bimeda)*, Amino Acid Oral Concentrate *(Phoenix Pharmaceutical)*, Amino Acid Oral Solution *(Aspen)*, *(Bimeda)*, *(Phoenix Pharmaceutical)*, Aminoplex *(Butler)*, Aminoplex Concentrate *(Butler)*, Amino Plus Concentrate *(AgriPharm)*, Amino Plus Solution *(AgriPharm)*, AmTech Amino Acid Oral Concentrate *(Phoenix Scientific)*, AmTech Amino Acid Oral Solution *(Phoenix Scientific)*, Double "A" Concentrate *(Vedco)*, Double "A" Solution *(Vedco)*.

dextrose, electrolytes, vitamins. Ora-Lyte™ Powder *(Butler)*.

dextrose, glycine, minerals. Electrolyte with Thickener *(DVM Formula)*.

dextrose, magnesium, phosphorus, calcium. Cal-Phos #2 Injection *(AgriLabs)*, Cal-Phos Forte *(Bimeda)*.

dextrose, magnesium borogluconate, calcium, calcium hypophosphite. Norcalciphos™ *(Pfizer Animal Health)*.

dextrose, magnesium borogluconate, calcium borogluconate, calcium hypophosphite. Ca-P I.V. Therapy *(RXV)*.

dextrose, magnesium borogluconate, phosphorus, calcium. Cal Dex #2 *(AgriLabs)*, Cal-Dextro® No. 2 *(Fort Dodge)*, Cal-Dextro® Special *(Fort Dodge)*.

dextrose, magnesium borogluconate, potassium chloride, calcium, calcium hypophosphite. Cal-MPK 1234™ *(Butler)*.

dextrose, magnesium borogluconate, potassium chloride, sodium hypophosphite, calcium. Cal Dex CMPK Injection *(Aspen)*, C-M-P-K Injection *(Vet Tek)*, Cal-MPK™ 1080 Injection *(Butler)*, Cal-Dex C-M-P-K *(AgriLabs)*, CMPK-Dex *(Vetus)*, CMPK *(RXV)*.

dextrose, magnesium borogluconate, potassium chloride, sodium hypophosphite, calcium borogluconate. CMPK Solution *(Bimeda)*.

dextrose, magnesium chloride, calcium, calcium hypophosphite. Cal-MP 1700™ *(Butler)*.

dextrose, magnesium chloride, phosphorus, potassium chloride, calcium. Oral Cal MPK *(Durvet)*.

dextrose, magnesium chloride, potassium chloride, sodium hypophosphite, calcium. Cal-Phos #2 with Potassium Injection *(Phoenix Pharmaceutical)*, CMPK Solution *(Vedco)*, *(Aspen)*, M.F.O. Solution *(AgriLabs)*.

dextrose, magnesium chloride, potassium chloride, sodium phosphate, calcium. CMPK Oral *(AgriPharm)*.

dextrose, magnesium chloride, sodium hypophosphite, calcium. AmTech Cal-Phos #2 Injection *(Phoenix Scientific)*, Cal MP-1000 *(Butler)*, Cal-Phos #2 *(Vedco)*, Cal-Phos #2 Injection *(Phoenix Pharmaceutical)*.

dextrose, minerals. Revitilyte™ *(Vets Plus)*, Revitilyte-Gelling™ *(Vets Plus)*.

dextrose, minerals, vitamins, amino acids. Tryptophan Plus Gel™ *(Horses Prefer)*.

dextrose, potassium chloride, calcium. Cal-Dextro® K *(Fort Dodge)*.

Dextrose 50% *(AgriLabs)*, *(AgriPharm)*, *(Durvet)*, **dextrose.**

Dextrose 50% Solution *(Vedco)*, *(Vetus)*, **dextrose.**

Dextrose Solution *(Aspen)*, **dextrose.**

Dextrose Solution 50% *(Butler)*, *(Phoenix Pharmaceutical)*, *(Vet Tek)*, **dextrose.**

D-Horn Paste *(Dominion)*, **calcium hydroxide, sodium hydroxide.**

diatomaceous earth, ferric subsulfate, iodoform, aluminum chloride, ammonium chloride, bentonite, benzocaine, copper sulfate. Clot-It Plus™ *(Evsco)*, Nik Stop® Styptic Powder *(Tomlyn)*.

Diamine Iodide-20 (With Salt) *(First Priority)*, **ethylenediamine dihydroiodide (EDDI).**

Diamine Iodide-40 (With Salt) *(First Priority)*, **ethylenediamine dihydroiodide (EDDI).**

Diamine Iodide (With Sugar) *(First Priority)*, **ethylenediamine dihydroiodide (EDDI).**

Diarrhea Tabs *(Butler)*, **aluminum hydroxide, kaolin, pectin.**

diatomite, ferric subsulfate, iodoform, aluminum chloride, ammonium chloride, bentonite, copper sulfate. Blood Stop Powder *(Butler)*.

diatomite, ferrous sulfate, iodine complex (povidone-iodine), aluminum chloride, ammonium chloride, bentonite, copper sulfate. Kwik-Stop® Styptic Powder *(ARC)*.

diazinon. Patriot™ Insecticide Cattle Ear Tags *(Boehringer Ingelheim)*, Preventef® Flea and Tick Collar for Cats *(Virbac)*, Preventef® Flea and Tick Collar for Dogs *(Virbac)*.

diazinon, coumaphos. Co-Ral® Plus Insecticide Cattle Ear Tag *(Bayer)*.

diazinon, piperonyl butoxide. New Z® Diazinon Insecticide Cattle Ear Tags *(Farnam)*.

diazinon, piperonyl butoxide, pyrethrins. Sunbugger Residual Ant & Roach Spray Aqueous *(Sungro)*.

dibenzoyl peroxide, Melaleuca alternifolia. Equi-Phar™ ThrushGard *(Vedco)*.

Di-Calcium Phosphate *(Neogen)*, **calcium, phosphorus.**

dicalcium phosphate, aluminum, calcium carbonate. Neigh-Lox® *(K.P.P.)*.

dicarboximide, n-octyl bicycloheptene dicarboximide, d-trans allethrin. Hartz® Control Pet Care System® Flea & Tick Conditioning Shampoo for Cats *(Hartz Mountain)*, Hartz® Control Pet Care System® Flea & Tick Conditioning Shampoo for Dogs *(Hartz Mountain)*.

dicarboximide, n-octyl bicycloheptene dicarboximide, piperonyl butoxide, pyrethrins. Hartz® 2 in 1® Flea & Tick Killer for Dogs *(Hartz Mountain)*.

dichloroisocyanurate (sodium). EfferCept® *(Activon)*.

dichloroisocyanurate (sodium), quaternary ammonia, bronopol. ActaCept™ *(Activon)*.

dichlorophene. Happy Jack® Tapeworm Tablets *(Happy Jack)*.

dichlorvos. Atgard® C *(Boehringer Ingelheim)*, Atgard® Swine Wormer *(Boehringer Ingelheim)*, Prozap® Beef & Dairy Spray RTU *(Loveland)*, Prozap® Dairy & Feedlot Insecticide Concentrate *(Loveland)*, Vapona® Concentrate Insecticide *(Boehringer Ingelheim)*.

dichlorvos, n-octyl bicycloheptene dicarboximide, piperonyl butoxide, pyrethrins. Super II Dairy & Farm Spray *(Durvet)*.

dichlorvos, piperonyl butoxide, pyrethrins. Prozap® VIP Insect Spray *(Loveland)*, SK-Surekill® Brand Pyrethrin Plus Fly Spray *(IntAgra)*.

dichlorvos, tetrachlorvinphos. Ravap® E.C. *(Boehringer Ingelheim)*.

diclazuril. Clinacox™ *(Schering-Plough)*.

Dicural® Tablets *(Fort Dodge)*, **difloxacin.**

diethylcarbamazine citrate. Filaribits® *(Pfizer Animal Health)*.

diethylcarbamazine citrate, oxibendazole. Filaribits Plus® *(Pfizer Animal Health)*.

difloxacin. Dicural® Tablets *(Fort Dodge)*.

Digest Aid™ *(Farnam)*, **fermentation extract(s), microorganisms.**

dihydrostreptomycin, penicillin G procaine. Quartermaster® *(Pharmacia & Upjohn)*.

dimethoate. Prozap® Residual Insect Spray 2EC *(Loveland)*.

Di-Methox® 12.5% Oral Solution *(AgriLabs)*, **sulfadimethoxine.**

Di-Methox® Injection-40% *(AgriLabs)*, **sulfadimethoxine.**

Di-Methox® Soluble Powder *(AgriLabs)*, **sulfadimethoxine.**

dimethyl chlorophenol, alum. Equi-Phar™ McKillips Powder *(Vedco)*.

dimethyldodecanamine. Dr. Naylor® Defender® Teat Dip *(H.W. Naylor)*.

dimethyl sulfoxide. Domoso® Gel *(Fort Dodge)*, Domoso® Solution *(Fort Dodge)*.

dimethyl sulfoxide, fluocinolone acetonide. Synotic® Otic Solution *(Fort Dodge)*.

dimonium chloride, propylene glycol, alcohol, cocamido propyl phosphatidyl. EarMed Cleansing Solution & Wash *(Davis)*.

Dineotex *(Stearns)*, **iodine complex (povidone-iodine), phosphoric acid.**

dinoprost (prostaglandin $F_{2\alpha}$). AmTech ProstaMate® *(Phoenix Scientific)*, In-Synch™ *(AgriLabs)*, Lutalyse® Sterile Solution *(Pharmacia & Upjohn)*, ProstaMate™ *(Aspen)*, *(Butler)*, *(RXV)*, *(Vedco)*, *(Vet Tek)*, ProstaMate® *(Phoenix Pharmaceutical)*, *(Vetus)*.

di-n-propyl isocinchomeronate, fenoxycarb, n-octyl bicycloheptene dicarboximide, permethrin, piperonyl butoxide, d-2-allayl-4-hydroxy-3-methyl-2-cyclopenten-1-one. Scratchex® Super Spray™ *(Combe)*.

di-n-propyl isocinchomeronate, n-octyl bicycloheptene dicarboximide, permethrin, piperonyl butoxide, pyrethrins. Adams™ Fly Repellent Concentrate *(V.P.L.)*, Flysect® Super-C *(Equicare)*.

di-n-propyl isocinchomeronate, n-octyl bicycloheptene dicarboximide, permethrin, piperonyl butoxide, pyrethrins, butoxypolypropylene glycol. Adams™ Fly Spray and Repellent *(V.P.L.)*, Flysect® Super-7 *(Equicare)*.

di-n-propyl isocinchomeronate, n-octyl bicycloheptene dicarboximide, permethrin, piperonyl butoxide, pyriproxyfen, d-2-allayl-4-hydroxy-3-methyl-2-cyclopenten-1-one. Sergeant's® PreTect® Flea & Tick Spray for Cats & Kittens *(Sergeant's)*, Sergeant's® PreTect® Flea & Tick Spray for Dogs & Puppies *(Sergeant's)*.

di-n-propyl isocinchomeronate, n-octyl bicycloheptene dicarboximide, piperonyl butoxide, pyrethrins. Adams™ Flea & Tick Mist *(V.P.L.)*, Adams™ Pyrethrin Dip *(Farnam)*, *(V.P.L.)*, EctoKyl™ 3X Flea & Tick Shampoo *(DVM)*, Flea & Tick Mist *(Davis)*, Flysect® Repellent Spray *(Equicare)*, Flysect® Roll-On Fly Repellent Face Lotion *(Equicare)*, Flys-Off® Fly Repellent Ointment *(Farnam)*, Mita-Clear™ *(Pfizer Animal Health)*, Otomite® Plus *(Virbac)*, Performer® Ear Mite Killer *(AgriLabs)*, Pet Care Ear Mite Lotion & Repellent *(Durvet)*, Pet Care Fast Kill Flea & Tick Spray for Dogs & Cats *(Durvet)*, Roll-On™ Fly Repellent *(Farnam)*, Triple Pyrethrins Flea & Tick Shampoo *(Davis)*, Vet-Kem® Triple Action Flea & Tick Shampoo for Dogs, Cats, & Horses *(Wellmark)*, Virbac Pyrethrin Dip™ *(Virbac)*.

di-n-propyl isocinchomeronate, piperonyl butoxide, pyrethrins. Happy Jack® Onex *(Happy Jack)*, Relief! Fly Ointment *(Davis)*, Swat® Fly Repellent Ointment *(Farnam)*, VPL Fly Repellent Ointment *(V.P.L.)*.

di-n-propyl isocinchomeronate, piperonyl butoxide, pyrethrins, butoxypolypropylene glycol. Wipe® Fly Protectant *(Farnam)*.

di-n-propyl isocinchomeronate, piperonyl butoxide, pyrethrins, butoxypolypropylene glycol, cypermethrin. Repel-X® Lotion *(Farnam)*.

Dioctynate *(Butler)*, **docusate sodium (dioctyl sodium sulfosuccinate).**

diphemanil methylsulfate. Bandguard® Cream 2% *(Schering-Plough)*, Bandguard® Spray *(Schering-Plough)*.

diphenhydramine. Histacalm® Shampoo *(Virbac)*, Histacalm® Spray *(Virbac)*, ResiHist® Leave-on Conditioner *(Virbac)*.

diphenylamine, ferric sulfate, carboxy methylcellulose. Blood Stop Powder *(AgriPharm)*, *(Centaur)*.

diphenylamine, ferrous sulfate, chloroxylenol. Hemostatic Powder *(Butler)*.

diphenylamine, ferrous sulfate, tannic acid, chloroxylenol. Blood Stop Powder *(First Priority)*.

Di-Quat 10-S *(Butler)*, **quaternary ammonia.**

Disal® Injection *(Boehringer Ingelheim)*, **furosemide.**

Discourage Taste Deterrent & Training Aid *(Davis)*, **denatonium benzoate, ethyl alcohol.**

Disintegrator® *(Phoenix Pharmaceutical)*, **quaternary ammonia.**

Disposable Enema *(Vedco)*, **docusate sodium (dioctyl sodium sulfosuccinate).**

Dl-Alpha Tocopherol Acetate Injection *(Vedco)*, **vitamin E.**

D'Limonene Dip *(Davis)*, **limonene.**

D'Limonene Shampoo *(Davis)*, **limonene.**

d-l-Methionine Powder™ *(Butler)*, **methionine (d-l).**

DL-Methionine Powder *(First Priority)*, **methionine (d-l).**

d-l-m Tablets *(Butler)*, **methionine (d-l).**

d-l-panthenol (vitamin B_5), detanglers, jojoba oil, keratin, mink oil. Lustre Groom Mist™ *(Butler)*.

docusate sodium (dioctyl sodium sulfosuccinate). Bloat Release *(AgriLabs)*, Bloat Treatment *(AgriPharm)*, *(Butler)*, *(Durvet)*, Dioctynate *(Butler)*, Disposable Enema *(Vedco)*, Enema-DSS *(Butler)*, Enema SA *(Vetus)*.

docusate sodium (dioctyl sodium sulfosuccinate), glycerine. Docu-Soft™ Pet Enema *(Life Science)*.

docusate sodium (dioctyl sodium sulfosuccinate), glycerine, medicinal soap base. Therevac®-SB *(King Animal Health)*.

docusate sodium (dioctyl sodium sulfosuccinate), lactic acid, propylene glycol, salicylic acid, chitosanide. Epi-Otic® *(Virbac)*.

docusate sodium (dioctyl sodium sulfosuccinate), piperonyl butoxide, pyrethrins, benzocaine. Aurimite® Insecticide *(Schering-Plough)*.

docusate sodium (dioctyl sodium sulfosuccinate), propylene glycol. Docusate Solution *(Life Science)*, OtiRinse™ Cleansing/Drying Ear Solution *(DVM)*, Veterinary Surfactant *(Vedco)*, Veterinary Surfactant (D.S.S.) *(First Priority)*.

docusate sodium (dioctyl sodium sulfosuccinate), urea peroxide. ClearR_x® Ear Cleansing Solution *(DVM)*.

Docusate Solution *(Life Science)*, **docusate sodium (dioctyl sodium sulfosuccinate), propylene glycol.**

Docu-Soft™ Pet Enema *(Life Science)*, **docusate sodium (dioctyl sodium sulfosuccinate), glycerine.**

Dog-Off™ *(Thornell)*, **deodorants, neutralizer(s).**

Dolorex® *(Intervet)*, **butorphanol tartrate.**

Dominator® Insecticide Ear Tags *(Schering-Plough)*, **pirimiphos.**

Domitor® *(Pfizer Animal Health)*, **medetomidine hydrochloride.**

Domoso® Gel *(Fort Dodge)*, **dimethyl sulfoxide.**

Domoso® Solution *(Fort Dodge)*, **dimethyl sulfoxide.**

Dopram®-V Injectable *(Fort Dodge)*, **doxapram hydrochloride.**

doramectin. Dectomax® Injectable Solution *(Pfizer Animal Health)*, Dectomax® Pour-On *(Pfizer Animal Health)*.

Dormosedan® *(Pfizer Animal Health)*, **detomidine hydrochloride.**

Double "A" Concentrate *(Vedco)*, **amino acids, dextrose, electrolytes, vitamin B-complex.**

Double "A" Solution *(Vedco)*, **amino acids, dextrose, electrolytes, vitamin B-complex.**

Double Barrel™ VP Insecticide Ear Tags *(Schering-Plough)*, **lambdacyhalothrin, pirimiphos.**

Double Impact™ *(AgriLabs)*, **ivermectin.**

doxapram hydrochloride. Dopram®-V Injectable *(Fort Dodge)*.

Doxirobe™ *(Pharmacia & Upjohn)*, **doxycycline.**

doxycycline. Doxirobe™ *(Pharmacia & Upjohn)*.

D-Panthenol Injectable *(Vedco)*, **dexpanthenol.**

d-Panthenol Injection *(Butler)*, *(Phoenix Pharmaceutical)*, **dexpanthenol.**

Drawing Salve *(Neogen)*, **ichthammol.**

dried colostrum, microorganisms, minerals, vitamins. Colostrum Bolus Forte *(Durvet)*.

dried colostrum, microorganisms, vitamin A, vitamin D, vitamin E. Colostrum Powder *(Vedco)*.

dried colostrum, microorganisms, vitamins. Soluble Colostrum Powder *(Durvet)*.

Dr. Naylor® Blu-Kote® *(H.W. Naylor)*, **acriflavine, gentian violet, sodium propionate.**

Dr. Naylor® Defender® Teat Dip *(H.W. Naylor)*, **dimethyldodecanamine.**

Dr. Naylor® Dehorning Paste *(H.W. Naylor)*, **calcium hydroxide, sodium hydroxide.**

Dr. Naylor® Hoof 'n Heel® *(H.W. Naylor)*, **sodium lauryl sulfate, zinc sulfate.**

Dr. Naylor® Red-Kote® *(H.W. Naylor)*, **isopropyl alcohol (isopropanol), phenol, scarlet red.**

Dr. Naylor® Stop-A-Leak *(H.W. Naylor)*, **ethylacetate, ethylcellulose, iodine, isopropyl alcohol (isopropanol), tannic acid.**

Dr. Naylor® Udder Balm *(H.W. Naylor)*, **8-hydroxyquinolone, lanolin, petrolatum.**

Droncit® (praziquantel) Canine Tablets *(Bayer)*, **praziquantel.**

Droncit® (praziquantel) Feline Tablets *(Bayer)*, **praziquantel.**

Droncit® (praziquantel) Injectable for Dogs and Cats *(Bayer)*, **praziquantel.**

Drontal® (praziquantel/pyrantel pamoate) Tablets *(Bayer)*, **praziquantel, pyrantel pamoate.**

Drontal® Plus (praziquantel/pyrantel pamoate/febantel) Tablets *(Bayer)*, **febantel, praziquantel, pyrantel pamoate.**

Dry-Clox® *(Fort Dodge)*, **cloxacillin benzathine.**

Dry-It *(Q.A. Laboratories)*, **boric acid, camphor, isopropyl alcohol (isopropanol), menthol, salicylic acid, tannic acid.**

d-trans allethrin, dicarboximide, n-octyl bicycloheptene dicarboximide. Hartz® Control Pet Care System® Flea & Tick Conditioning Shampoo for Cats *(Hartz Mountain)*, Hartz® Control Pet Care System® Flea & Tick Conditioning Shampoo for Dogs *(Hartz Mountain)*.

d-trans allethrin, n-octyl bicycloheptene dicarboximide. Hartz® 2 in 1® Rid Flea™ Dog Shampoo with Allethrin *(Hartz Mountain)*.

d-trans allethrin, phenothrin. Duocide® Shampoo *(Virbac)*.

d-trans allethrin, piperonyl butoxide. Mycodex® SensiCare™ Flea & Tick Shampoo *(V.P.L.)*.

D-Trol *(DuBois)*, **quaternary ammonia.**

Duocide® L.A. Spray *(Virbac)*, **n-octyl bicycloheptene dicarboximide, permethrin, pyrethrins.**

Duocide® Shampoo *(Virbac)*, **d-trans allethrin, phenothrin.**

Duo-Pen® *(AgriPharm)*, **penicillin G benzathine, penicillin G procaine.**

DuraCept™ *(Activon)*, **trizinetrione.**

DuraCream *(Durvet)*, **aloe vera, moisturizer(s), vitamin A, vitamin D, vitamin E.**

Duramycin 72-200 *(Durvet)*, **oxytetracycline.**

Duramycin-100 *(Durvet)*, **oxytetracycline.**

Duramycin-324 *(Durvet)*, **tetracycline.**

Duramycin 10 *(Durvet)*, **tetracycline.**

Dura-Pen *(Durvet)*, **penicillin G benzathine, penicillin G procaine.**

Durapen™ *(Vedco)*, **penicillin G benzathine, penicillin G procaine.**

Durasect™ Long-Acting Livestock Pour-On *(Pfizer Animal Health)*, **permethrin.**

Durasect® II Long-Acting Livestock Pour-On *(Pfizer Animal Health)*, **permethrin, piperonyl butoxide, pyrethrins.**

DuraSol™ *(Durvet)*, **acetylsalicylic acid.**

Durazyme Calf Bolus *(Durvet)*, **microorganisms.**

Durazyme Calf Colostrum Supplement *(Durvet)*, **microorganisms, nutrients.**

Durazyme Energy Pack *(Durvet)*, **energy source(s), microorganisms, nutrients.**

Durazyme Paste for Calves *(Durvet)*, **microorganisms, nutrients.**

Duricol™ Chloramphenicol Capsules U.S.P. *(V.P.C.)*, **chloramphenicol.**

Duriron *(Durvet)*, **copper, iron.**

DVMectin™ Liquid for Horses *(DVM)*, **ivermectin.**

DVM Handsoap™ *(DVM)*, **triclosan.**

DVM Tearless™ Shampoo *(DVM)*, **shampoo formula.**

DVM Tearless™ Spray-On Shampoo *(DVM)*, **shampoo formula.**

D-Worm™ 60 Liquid Wormer *(Farnam)*, **pyrantel pamoate.**

D-Worm™ 120 Liquid Wormer *(Farnam)*, **pyrantel pamoate.**

D-Worm™ Dog Wormer Chewable Tablets for Large Dogs *(Farnam)*, **pyrantel pamoate.**

D-Worm™ Dog Wormer Chewable Tablets for Puppies & Small Dogs *(Farnam)*, **pyrantel pamoate.**

D-Worm™ Dog Wormer Tablets for Large Dogs *(Farnam)*, **pyrantel pamoate.**

D-Worm™ Dog Wormer Tablets for Puppies & Small Dogs *(Farnam)*, **pyrantel pamoate.**

D-Worm™ Liquid Wormer for Cats and Dogs *(Farnam)*, **piperazine.**

Dyna-Lode® Equine Supplement *(Harlmen)*, **glycolipids, lecithin, phospholipids, vitamins.**

Dyna-Lode® Supplement for Dogs & Cats *(Harlmen)*, **glycolipids, phospholipids.**

Dyna-Taurine™ *(Harlmen)*, **taurine.**

E

ear cleanser formula. Aloeclens Otic Cleanser *(Vetus)*, Ear Cleansing Solution *(Butler)*, *(Vet Solutions)*, OtiFoam™ Ear Cleanser *(DVM)*, Soothables™ Crystal-Ear *(A.A.H.)*.

Ear Cleansing Solution *(Butler)*, *(Vet Solutions)*, **ear cleanser formula.**

EarMed Boracetic® Flush *(Davis)*, **acetic acid, aloe, boric acid.**

EarMed Cleansing Solution & Wash *(Davis)*, **alcohol, cocamido propyl phosphatidyl, dimonium chloride, propylene glycol.**

EarMed Mite Lotion *(Davis)*, **aloe vera, oil of lavender, oil of lemongrass, oil of pennyroyal.**

EarMed Powder *(Davis)*, **silica.**

Ear Miticide *(Phoenix Pharmaceutical)*, **rotenone.**

Earoxide™ Ear Cleanser *(Tomlyn)*, **carbamide (urea) peroxide.**

EAZI-Breed™ CIDR® Cattle Insert *(Pharmacia & Upjohn)*, **progesterone.**

Ecosect™ Insecticide *(Schering-Plough)*, **potassium salts of fatty acids.**

ECP® Sterile Solution *(Pharmacia & Upjohn)*, **estradiol cypionate.**

Ectiban® D *(Durvet)*, **permethrin.**

Ectiban® DeLice® *(Durvet)*, **permethrin.**

Ectiban® EC *(Durvet)*, **permethrin.**

Ectiban® Synergized DeLice® Pour-On Insecticide *(Durvet)*, **piperonyl butoxide, pyrethrins.**

Ectiban® WP *(Durvet)*, **permethrin.**

Ecto-Foam™ *(Virbac)*, **n-octyl bicycloheptene dicarboximide, piperonyl butoxide, pyrethrins.**

EctoKyl™ 3X Flea & Tick Shampoo *(DVM)*, **di-n-propyl isocinchomeronate, n-octyl bicycloheptene dicarboximide, piperonyl butoxide, pyrethrins.**

EctoKyl® IGR Emulsifiable Concentrate *(DVM)*, **pyriproxyfen.**

EctoKyl™ IGR Pressurized Spray *(DVM)*, **pyriproxyfen, sumethrin, tetramethrin.**

EctoKyl™ IGR Total Release Fogger *(DVM)*, **n-octyl bicycloheptene dicarboximide, permethrin, pyrethrins, pyriproxyfen.**

Ecto-Soothe™ Shampoo *(Virbac)*, **piperonyl butoxide, pyrethrins.**

Ecto-Soothe™ 3X Shampoo *(Virbac)*, **n-octyl bicycloheptene dicarboximide, piperonyl butoxide, pyrethrins.**

EctoZap™ Plus Pour-On Insecticide *(Aspen)*, **permethrin, piperonyl butoxide.**

EctoZap™ Pour-On Insecticide *(Aspen)*, **permethrin.**

Ectrin® Insecticide Cattle Ear Tag *(Boehringer Ingelheim)*, **pyrethrins.**

E.D.D.I. 20 Gr. (Dextrose Base) *(Vedco)*, **ethylenediamine dihydroiodide (EDDI).**

E.D.D.I. 20 Gr. (Organic Iodine Dextrose) *(Phoenix Pharmaceutical)*, **ethylenediamine dihydroiodide (EDDI).**

E.D.D.I. 20 Gr. (Organic Iodine Salt) *(Phoenix Pharmaceutical)*, **ethylenediamine dihydroiodide (EDDI).**

E.D.D.I. 20 Gr. (Salt) *(Vedco)*, **ethylenediamine dihydroiodide (EDDI).**

E.D.D.I. 40 Gr. (Salt) *(Vedco)*, **ethylenediamine dihydroiodide (EDDI).**

EDDI Equine *(Butler)*, **ethylenediamine dihydroiodide (EDDI).**

EDTA (edetate disodium dihydrate), tromethamine. DermaPet® TrizEDTA™ Aqueous Flush *(DermaPet)*, DermaPet® TrizEDTA™ Crystals *(DermaPet)*.

EDTA (tetrasodium), detergent mixture. Lifegard® 900 *(Rochester Midland)*.

EDTA (tetrasodium), lanolin, tromethamine. T8 Solution™ Ear Rinse *(DVM)*.

EfferCept® *(Activon)*, **dichloroisocyanurate (sodium).**

EfferSan™ *(Activon)*, **trizinetrione.**

egg protein. EPIC Daily Feed Supplement for Horses *(Bioniche Animal Health)*, EPIC Neonatal Feed Supplement for Foals *(Bioniche Animal Health)*.

Electramine® *(Life Science)*, **amino acids, electrolytes, glucose.**

Electro Dex® *(Horse Health)*, **electrolytes.**

Electro-Flex™ *(First Priority)*, **free radical scavengers, vitamin C (ascorbic acid), vitamins.**

Electrolyte HE with Vitamins *(DVM Formula)*, **dextrose, electrolytes, glycine, vitamins.**

Electrolyte Pak *(Alpharma)*, **electrolytes.**

Electrolyte Pak Plus Stabilized Vitamin C *(Alpharma)*, **electrolytes, vitamin C (ascorbic acid).**

Electrolyte Powder 8X *(Phoenix Pharmaceutical)*, **dextrose, electrolytes.**

electrolytes. Apple-Dex® *(Horse Health)*, Dexalyte *(Butler)*, Electro Dex® *(Horse Health)*, Electrolyte Pak *(Alpharma)*, Elite™ Electrolyte *(Farnam)*, E-Lyte *(Vedco)*, Endura-Lite™ *(Creative Science)*, Endura-Lyte® *(Life Science)*, Normosol®-R *(Abbott)*, Revitilyte-EQ™ *(Horses Prefer)*, Start To Finish® Sweat Replacer™ *(Milk Specialties)*.

electrolytes, amino acids. Equi-Phar™ Electramino Paste *(Vedco)*.

electrolytes, amino acids, dextrose. A-Lyte Concentrate *(Durvet)*, Amcalcilyte Forte *(AgriPharm)*, *(Phoenix Pharmaceutical)*, *(Vedco)*, Aminocal Plus™ *(Butler)*, AmTech Amcal High Potency Oral Solution *(Phoenix Scientific)*, Glucaminolyte Forte *(AgriPharm)*, *(Vedco)*, Gluco-Amino-Forte Oral Solution *(Phoenix Pharmaceutical)*, Gluco Amino Forte Oral Solution *(Vetus)*, Keto Amino Forte™ *(Butler)*.

electrolytes, dextrose. AmTech Dexolyte Solution Injection *(Phoenix Scientific)*, Biolyte® *(Pharmacia & Upjohn)*, Bluelite® C *(TechMix)*, Calf Quencher *(Vedco)*, Deliver® with Dialine™ *(AgriLabs)*, Dexolyte Solution *(Phoenix Pharmaceutical)*, Electrolyte Powder 8X *(Phoenix Pharmaceutical)*, Electrolyte Solution *(AgriLabs)*, *(Vet Tek)*, Electrolyte Solution with Dextrose *(Vedco)*, Electrolyte w/Dextrose Injection *(Aspen)*, Entrolyte® *(Pfizer Animal Health)*, Entrolyte® H.E. *(Pfizer Animal Health)*, Equi-Phar™ Electrolyte with Dextrose *(Vedco)*, Equi-Phar™ Equi-Lyte Powder *(Vedco)*, Hydra-Lyte *(Vet-A-Mix)*, Magna-Lyte *(First Priority)*, Polylites IV *(Butler)*, Sky-Lytes *(Skylabs)*, Vedalyte 8X Powder *(Vedco)*, Vetalyte Plus I.V. Solution *(RXV)*.

electrolytes, energy source(s). Bluelite® Swine Formula *(TechMix)*.

electrolytes, energy source(s), microorganisms, nutrients. NutriVed™ EnerGel Forte *(Vedco)*.

electrolytes, energy source(s), microorganisms, nutrients, vitamins. Sow & Gilt Restart™ One-4 *(TechMix)*.

electrolytes, energy source(s), minerals, vitamins, amino acids. Energy Drench *(Vedco)*.

electrolytes, energy source(s), nutrients. Baby Pig Restart™ One-4 *(TechMix)*, Calf Restart™ One-4 *(TechMix)*, Vita-Lyte *(Phoenix Pharmaceutical)*.

electrolytes, energy source(s), nutrients, vitamins. Advance™ Arrest® *(Milk Specialties)*, Advance™ Pro-Lyte Plus® *(Milk Specialties)*.

electrolytes, energy source(s), nutrients, yeast, Aspergillus oryzae fermentation extract. Vita Charge® Power Drench *(BioZyme)*.

electrolytes, energy source(s), vitamins. Bovine Bluelite® *(TechMix)*, Equine Bluelite® *(TechMix)*, K-9 Bluelite® *(TechMix)*.

electrolytes, energy source(s), vitamins, amino acids. Energy+ *(Butler)*, NRG-Plus™ *(Bimeda)*, Pic-M-Up™ *(AgriPharm)*.

electrolytes, fatty acids (essential), minerals, amino acids. NutriVed™ Chewable Vitamins for Active Dogs *(Vedco)*.

electrolytes, glucose. Isotone-SA *(Vet-A-Mix)*, Re-Sorb® *(Pfizer Animal Health)*.

electrolytes, glucose, amino acids. Electramine® *(Life Science)*.

electrolytes, glucose, lactic acid producing bacteria. SureLytes™ Plus Carbo Load *(SureNutrition)*.

electrolytes, glucose, microorganisms, nutrients. Ener-Lyte™ *(Aspen)*.

electrolytes, glycine, bicarbonate, dextrose. Elpak™-G *(Vedco)*.

electrolytes, glycine, dextrose. Hy-Sorb™ *(Bimeda)*.

electrolytes, glycine, vitamins, dextrose. Electrolyte HE with Vitamins *(DVM Formula)*.

electrolytes, iron, vitamins. Pig-95 *(Skylabs)*.

electrolytes, methionine, microorganisms, citric acid. Greenlyte® *(Bimeda)*.

electrolytes, microorganisms, organic acidifiers, vitamins. Vit-E-Lyte "Plus" *(Bimeda)*.

electrolytes, microorganisms, vitamins. Revitilyte-Plus™ *(Vets Plus)*.

electrolytes, minerals. Dealer Select Horse Care DurLyte-A *(Durvet)*, Dealer Select Horse Care DurLyte-C *(Durvet)*, Dexalyte 8X Powder *(Butler)*.

electrolytes, minerals, dextrose. Stress-Dex® *(Neogen)*.

electrolytes, minerals, sucrose, vitamins. Dexsolyte Powder *(Neogen)*.

electrolytes, minerals, torula yeast, amino acids. Procal™ Powder *(Butler)*.

electrolytes, minerals, vitamins. Electrolytes-Plus *(Alpharma)*, Vi-tal *(Loveland)*.

electrolytes, minerals, vitamins, dextrose. Multi-Electrolytes *(Neogen)*.

electrolytes, nutrients. Comeback™ *(AgriPharm)*, One Day Response™ *(Farnam, Livestock Div.)*.

electrolytes, oxypolygelatin. RapidVet™ Plasm-ex™ *(DMS Laboratories)*.

electrolytes, vitamin B-complex, amino acids, dextrose. A-Lyte Solution *(Durvet)*, Amino Acid Concentrate Oral Solution *(Aspen)*, *(Bimeda)*, Amino Acid Oral Concentrate *(Phoenix Pharmaceutical)*, Amino Acid Oral Solution *(Aspen)*, *(Bimeda)*, *(Phoenix Pharmaceutical)*, Aminoplex *(Butler)*, Aminoplex Concentrate *(Butler)*, Amino Plus Concentrate *(AgriPharm)*, Amino Plus Solution *(AgriPharm)*, AmTech Amino Acid Oral Concentrate *(Phoenix Scientific)*, AmTech Amino Acid Oral Solution *(Phoenix Scientific)*, Double "A" Concentrate *(Vedco)*, Double "A" Solution *(Vedco)*.

electrolytes, vitamin C (ascorbic acid). Electrolyte Pak Plus Stabilized Vitamin C *(Alpharma)*.

electrolytes, vitamins. Avian Bluelite® *(TechMix)*, Broiler-Pak *(Alpharma)*, Electro R *(Alpharma)*, High Performance Poultry Pak *(Durvet)*, Hog & Cattle Vitamins and Electrolytes *(Fort Dodge)*, Super B-Plex *(Neogen)*, Vitamins and Electrolytes *(Durvet)*, Vitamins and Electrolytes Concentrate *(Alpharma)*, *(Durvet)*, Vitamins & Electrolytes Concentrate *(Fort Dodge)*, Vitamins & Electrolytes "Plus" *(AgriLabs)*, Vitamins & Electrolytes (Soluble) *(Fort Dodge)*, Vita Pak *(Alpharma)*.

electrolytes, vitamins, amino acids. Amino Acid Concentrate *(AgriLabs)*, Amino Acid Solution *(AgriLabs)*, OTC™ Jug *(SureNutrition)*.

electrolytes, vitamins, dextrose. Ora-Lyte™ Powder *(Butler)*.

Electrolyte Solution *(AgriLabs)*, *(Vet Tek)*, **dextrose, electrolytes.**

Electrolyte Solution with Dextrose *(Vedco)*, **dextrose, electrolytes.**

Electrolytes-Plus *(Alpharma)*, **electrolytes, minerals, vitamins.**

Electrolyte Supplement *(First Priority)*, **calcium, magnesium sulfate, potassium chloride, sodium chloride.**

Electrolyte w/Dextrose Injection *(Aspen)*, **dextrose, electrolytes.**

Electrolyte with Thickener *(DVM Formula)*, **dextrose, glycine, minerals.**

Electro R *(Alpharma)*, **electrolytes, vitamins.**

ElectroSol-R *(Phoenix Pharmaceutical)*, **magnesium chloride, potassium chloride, sodium acetate, sodium chloride, sodium gluconate.**

Elimin • Odor® Canine *(Pfizer Animal Health)*, **neutralizer(s).**

Elimin • Odor® Feline *(Pfizer Animal Health)*, **neutralizer(s).**

Elimin • Odor® General Purpose *(Pfizer Animal Health)*, **neutralizer(s).**

Elimin • Odor® Pet Accident *(Pfizer Animal Health)*, **neutralizer(s).**

Elimin • Odor® Pet Stain Eliminator *(Pfizer Animal Health)*, **neutralizer(s), stain removers.**

Elite™ Electrolyte *(Farnam)*, **electrolytes.**

Elpak™-G *(Vedco)*, **bicarbonate, dextrose, electrolytes, glycine.**

E-Lyte *(Vedco)*, **electrolytes.**

Ema-Sol™ Concentrate *(Alpharma)*, **cobalt sulfate, copper sulfate, hydrochloric acid, manganese sulfate, potassium dichromate.**

emollient(s). Protecta-Pad® *(Evsco)*, *(Tomlyn)*.

emollient(s), capsaicin (cayenne pepper extract). Arthro Ease™ *(Horses Prefer)*.

emollient(s), ethyl alcohol, aloe vera. Waterless Antibacterial Hand Cleaner *(Davis)*.

emollient(s), fatty acids. HyLyt*efa® Bath Oil/Coat Conditioner *(DVM)*, HyLyt*efa® Spray-On Shampoo *(DVM)*.

emollient(s), fatty acids, glycerine, hydrolized animal protein, sodium lactate. HyLyt*efa® Hypoallergenic Creme Rinse *(DVM)*.

emollient(s), lanolin, beeswax, comfrey. Equi-Phar™ Miracle Heel *(Vedco)*.

emollient(s), moisturizer(s). Hoof Conditioner *(First Priority)*, Micro Pearls Advantage™ Hydra-Pearls™ Rehydrating Spray *(Evsco)*.

emollient(s), moisturizer(s), PABA sun screen. Frostshield *(Durvet)*.

emollient(s), moisturizer(s), vitamins. Bova Derm® *(Butler)*, Udder Moist *(A.A.H.)*.

emollient(s), peppermint oil, aloe vera. Natural Mint Liniment™ *(Horses Prefer)*.

emollient(s), vitamins. Chap-Guard™ Plus *(AgriLabs)*, Soothables™ Tender Foot *(A.A.H.)*, Udder Balm *(Vedco)*, Udder Comfort Cream *(Phoenix Pharmaceutical)*.

emollient(s), vitamins, aloe vera. Udder Balm *(Aspen)*, *(First Priority)*.

EmPower™ *(Metrex)*, **detergent (enzyme-based).**

emulsifiers, vegetable oil(s). Bloat Drench™ *(Great States)*, Rumen-Eze *(Vet-A-Mix)*.

emulsifying wax, glycerine, lanolin, petrolatum, aloe vera, beeswax. Dealer Select Horse Care Hoof Moisturizer *(Durvet)*.

EmulsiVit E-300 *(Vedco)*, **vitamin E.**

EmulsiVit E/A&D *(Vedco)*, **vitamin A, vitamin D, vitamin E.**

Enacard® Tablets for Dogs *(Merial)*, **enalapril maleate.**

enalapril maleate. Enacard® Tablets for Dogs *(Merial)*.

Encore® *(VetLife)*, **estradiol.**

Endosorb™ Bolus *(PRN Pharmacal)*, **attapulgite, magnesium trisilicate, pectin.**

Endosorb™ Suspension *(PRN Pharmacal)*, **attapulgite, magnesium trisilicate, pectin.**

Endosorb™ Tablets *(PRN Pharmacal)*, **attapulgite, magnesium trisilicate, pectin.**

Endura-Lite™ *(Creative Science)*, **electrolytes.**

Endura-Lyte® *(Life Science)*, **electrolytes.**

Endure™ Sweat-Resistant Fly Spray *(Farnam)*, **butoxypolypropylene glycol, cypermethrin, piperonyl butoxide, pyrethrins.**

Enema-DSS *(Butler)*, **docusate sodium (dioctyl sodium sulfosuccinate).**

Enema SA *(Vetus)*, **docusate sodium (dioctyl sodium sulfosuccinate).**

EnerCal™ *(Vedco)*, **energy source(s), nutrients.**

Energel™ for Cats *(Pet-Ag)*, **minerals, vitamins.**

Energel™ for Dogs *(Pet-Ag)*, **minerals, vitamins.**

Energel™ Powder for Cats *(Pet-Ag)*, **minerals, vitamins.**

Energel™ Powder for Dogs *(Pet-Ag)*, **minerals, vitamins.**

Energy Drench *(Vedco)*, **amino acids, electrolytes, energy source(s), minerals, vitamins.**

Energy+ *(Butler)*, **amino acids, electrolytes, energy source(s), vitamins.**

Energy Plus *(Q.A. Laboratories)*, **energy source(s), vitamins.**

energy source(s), electrolytes. Bluelite® Swine Formula *(TechMix)*.

energy source(s), fatty acids (omega), minerals, vitamins. Nutri-Stat™ *(Tomlyn)*.

energy source(s), microorganisms, nutrients. Durazyme Energy Pack *(Durvet)*.

energy source(s), microorganisms, nutrients, electrolytes. NutriVed™ EnerGel Forte *(Vedco)*.

energy source(s), microorganisms, nutrients, vitamins, electrolytes. Sow & Gilt Restart™ One-4 *(TechMix)*.

energy source(s), minerals, nutrients, vitamins. CliniCare® Canine Liquid Diet *(Abbott)*, CliniCare® Feline Liquid Diet *(Abbott)*, CliniCare® RF Specialized Feline Liquid Diet *(Abbott)*.

energy source(s), minerals, vitamins. High-Cal *(Vet Solutions)*, Nutri-Cal® for Ferrets & Other Small Animals *(Tomlyn)*, Stat *(PRN Pharmacal)*.

energy source(s), minerals, vitamins, amino acids, electrolytes. Energy Drench *(Vedco)*.

energy source(s), nutrients. EnerCal™ *(Vedco)*, Nutri-Cal® *(Evsco)*, Nutri-Cal® for Dogs and Cats *(Tomlyn)*, Nutri-Cal® for Ferrets *(Tomlyn)*.

energy source(s), nutrients, electrolytes. Baby Pig Restart™ One-4 *(TechMix)*, Calf Restart™ One-4 *(TechMix)*, Vita-Lyte *(Phoenix Pharmaceutical)*.

energy source(s), nutrients, vitamins, electrolytes. Advance™ Arrest® *(Milk Specialties)*, Advance™ Pro-Lyte Plus® *(Milk Specialties)*.
energy source(s), nutrients, yeast, Aspergillus oryzae fermentation extract, electrolytes. Vita Charge® Power Drench *(BioZyme)*.
energy source(s), vitamins. Energy Plus *(Q.A. Laboratories)*, Hi-Cal Suspension *(Vedco)*, Liquical™ *(Butler)*, Quick-Start™ *(Vedco)*.
energy source(s), vitamins, amino acids, electrolytes. Energy+ *(Butler)*, NRG-Plus™ *(Bimeda)*, Pic-M-Up™ *(AgriPharm)*.
energy source(s), vitamins, electrolytes. Bovine Bluelite® *(TechMix)*, Equine Bluelite® *(TechMix)*, K-9 Bluelite® *(TechMix)*.
Ener-Lyte™ *(Aspen)*, **electrolytes, glucose, microorganisms, nutrients.**
enrofloxacin. Baytril® (enrofloxacin) 3.23% Concentrate Antimicrobial Solution *(Bayer)*, Baytril® 100 (enrofloxacin) 100 mg/mL Antimicrobial Injectable Solution *(Bayer)*, Baytril® (enrofloxacin) Antibacterial Injectable Solution 2.27% *(Bayer)*, Baytril® (enrofloxacin) Antibacterial Tablets *(Bayer)*, Baytril® (enrofloxacin) Antibacterial Taste Tabs™ *(Bayer)*.
enrofloxacin, silver sulfadiazine. Baytril® Otic (enrofloxacin/silver sulfadiazine) Antibacterial-Antimycotic Emulsion *(Bayer)*.
Entrolyte® *(Pfizer Animal Health)*, **dextrose, electrolytes.**
Entrolyte® H.E. *(Pfizer Animal Health)*, **dextrose, electrolytes.**
Enzymatic Detergent *(Vedco)*, **amylase, propylene glycol, protease, surfactant.**
enzymes. AlphaZyme Plus™ *(Alpha Tech Pet)*, Break-Thru Stain & Odor Remover *(Davis)*, Probios® TC *(Chr. Hansen)*.
enzymes, microorganisms, minerals, vitamins, yeast, amino acids. Vita-Key® Show Cattle Concentrate, Phase II *(Vita-Key)*.
enzymes, microorganisms, vitamins, yeast, amino acids. Vita Boost Paste™ *(AgriLabs)*.
EP-1 3X *(RXV)*, **microorganisms, nutrients.**
EPIC Daily Feed Supplement for Horses *(Bioniche Animal Health)*, **egg protein.**
EPIC Neonatal Feed Supplement for Foals *(Bioniche Animal Health)*, **egg protein.**
epinephrine. AmTech Epinephrine Injection USP *(Phoenix Scientific)*, Epinephrine *(Vedco)*, *(Vet Tek)*, Epinephrine 1:1000 *(AgriPharm)*, *(Durvet)*, *(Neogen)*, Epinephrine Injection *(AgriLabs)*, Epinephrine Injection 1:1000 *(Bimeda)*, Epinephrine Injection 1:1,000 *(Butler)*, Epinephrine Injection USP 1:1000 *(Phoenix Pharmaceutical)*, Epinject *(Vetus)*.
Epinephrine *(Vedco)*, *(Vet Tek)*, **epinephrine.**
Epinephrine 1:1000 *(AgriPharm)*, *(Durvet)*, *(Neogen)*, **epinephrine.**
Epinephrine Injection *(AgriLabs)*, **epinephrine.**
Epinephrine Injection 1:1000 *(Bimeda)*, **epinephrine.**
Epinephrine Injection 1:1,000 *(Butler)*, **epinephrine.**
Epinephrine Injection USP 1:1000 *(Phoenix Pharmaceutical)*, **epinephrine.**
Epinject *(Vetus)*, **epinephrine.**
Epi-Otic® *(Virbac)*, **chitosanide, docusate sodium (dioctyl sodium sulfosuccinate), lactic acid, propylene glycol, salicylic acid.**
Epi-Soothe® Cream Rinse and Conditioner *(Virbac)*, **oatmeal.**
Epi-Soothe® Shampoo *(Virbac)*, **chitosanide, glycerine, oatmeal.**
eprinomectin. Ivomec® Eprinex® Pour-On for Beef and Dairy Cattle *(Merial)*.
epsiprantel. Cestex® *(Pfizer Animal Health)*.
epsom salt, methyl salicylate. Dealer Select Horse Care Epsom Salt Poultice *(Durvet)*.
EqStim® *(Neogen)*, **Propionibacterium acnes.**
Equ-Aid Plus *(Vet-A-Mix)*, **amodimethicone, methionine (d-l), minerals, vegetable oil(s), vitamins.**
Equalizer™ *(Evsco)*, **2-butoxyethanol, isopropyl alcohol.**
Equi Aid CW® *(Equi Aid)*, **pyrantel tartrate.**
Equileve *(Vetus)*, **flunixin meglumine.**
Equimectrin™ Paste 1.87% *(Farnam)*, **ivermectin.**
Equimectrin® Paste 1.87% *(Merial)*, **ivermectin.**
Equimune® I.V. *(Bioniche Animal Health)*, **Mycobacterium cell wall fraction.**
Equine Bene-Bac™ *(Pet-Ag)*, **microorganisms.**
Equine Bluelite® *(TechMix)*, **electrolytes, energy source(s), vitamins.**
Equine Capsaicin Gel *(Butler)*, **capsaicin (cayenne pepper extract).**
Equine Enteric Colloid *(TechMix)*, **fermentation extract(s), microorganisms, psyllium.**
Equine F.A./Plus Granules *(Pala-Tech)*, **fatty acids (omega), minerals, vitamins.**
Equine HoofPro™ Copper Formulation *(SSI Corp.)*, **copper, sulfur.**
Equine HoofPro™ Zinc Formulation *(SSI Corp.)*, **zinc.**
Equine IgG Foalimmune® *(Lake Immunogenics)*, **equine plasma.**
Equine IgG Higamm-Equi™ *(Lake Immunogenics)*, **equine plasma.**
Equine IgG High-Glo *(Mg Biologics)*, **equine plasma.**
Equine Medicated Shampoo *(Vet Solutions)*, **chloroxylenol, salicylic acid, sodium thiosulfate.**
Equine Pain Block Gel *(First Priority)*, **capsaicin (cayenne pepper extract).**
equine plasma. Equine IgG Foalimmune® *(Lake Immunogenics)*, Equine IgG Higamm-Equi™ *(Lake Immunogenics)*, Equine IgG High-Glo *(Mg Biologics)*, Equi-Plas™ *(V.D.I.)*, Immuno-Glo NEP *(Mg Biologics)*, Plasmune J *(Lake Immunogenics)*, Polymune™ *(V.D.I.)*, Polymune™ Plus *(V.D.I.)*.
Equine Psyllium *(First Priority)*, **psyllium.**
equine serum. Normal Equine Serum *(Colorado Serum)*, Normal Serum-Equine *(Professional Biological)*.
Equine Thyroid Supplement *(Pala-Tech)*, **levothyroxine.**
Equinime® *(Chariton)*, **amino acids, minerals, vitamins.**
Equi-Phar™ ArthriBan *(Vedco)*, **acetylsalicylic acid.**
Equi-Phar™ BenzaGel *(Vedco)*, **benzocaine, camphor, iodide (potassium), iodine, menthol, thymol.**
Equi-Phar™ BismuKote Paste *(Vedco)*, **bismuth subsalicylate.**
Equi-Phar™ Caustic Powder *(Vedco)*, **chloroxylenol, copper sulfate.**
Equi-Phar™ CoolGel *(Vedco)*, **camphor, iodide (potassium), iodine, isopropyl alcohol (isopropanol), menthol, thymol.**
Equi-Phar™ dl-Methionine with Biotin Powder *(Vedco)*, **biotin, methionine (d-l).**
Equi-Phar™ Electramino Paste *(Vedco)*, **amino acids, electrolytes.**
Equi-Phar™ Electrolyte with Dextrose *(Vedco)*, **dextrose, electrolytes.**
Equi-Phar™ Equigesic™ *(Vedco)*, **flunixin meglumine.**
Equi-Phar EquiGlide™ *(Vedco)*, **amikacin sulfate.**
Equi-Phar Equi-Hist 1200 Granules *(Vedco)*, **pseudoephedrine HCl, pyrilamine maleate.**
Equi-Phar™ Equi-Lyte Powder *(Vedco)*, **dextrose, electrolytes.**
Equi-Phar™ Equine 7 HSS *(Vedco)*, **sodium chloride.**
Equi-Phar™ Equi-Vita-Phos *(Vedco)*, **microorganisms, minerals, vitamins.**
Equi-Phar™ Folic 20 *(Vedco)*, **folic acid.**
Equi-Phar™ Furosemide Injection 5% *(Vedco)*, **furosemide.**
Equi-Phar™ Horse & Colt Wormer *(Vedco)*, **pyrantel tartrate.**
Equi-Phar™ Ichthammol 20% Ointment *(Vedco)*, **ichthammol.**
Equi-Phar™ LactoBac Gel *(Vedco)*, **microorganisms, vitamins.**
Equi-Phar™ Lubogel-V™ *(Vedco)*, **carboxy methylcellulose.**
Equi-Phar™ McKillips Powder *(Vedco)*, **alum, dimethyl chlorophenol.**
Equi-Phar™ Miracle Heel *(Vedco)*, **beeswax, comfrey, emollient(s), lanolin.**
Equi-Phar™ Nitrofurazone Soluble Dressing *(Vedco)*, **nitrofurazone.**
Equi-Phar™ Phenylbutazone 1 gram Tablets *(Vedco)*, **phenylbutazone.**
Equi-Phar™ Phenylbutazone Injection 20% *(Vedco)*, **phenylbutazone.**
Equi-Phar ProTal™ *(Vedco)*, **pyrantel pamoate.**
Equi-Phar™ Sweet Psyllium *(Vedco)*, **psyllium.**
Equi-Phar™ ThrushGard *(Vedco)*, **dibenzoyl peroxide, Melaleuca alternifolia.**
Equi-Phar™ Vedlube Dry *(Vedco)*, **polyetheline polymer.**
Equi-Phar™ Vedlube O.B. Lubricant *(Vedco)*, **aqueous base lubricant(s).**
Equi-Phar™ Vita Plex Oral Honey *(Vedco)*, **minerals, vitamins.**
EquiPhed *(AHC)*, **pseudoephedrine HCl, pyrilamine maleate.**
Equiphen® Paste *(Luitpold)*, **phenylbutazone.**
Equi-Plas™ *(V.D.I.)*, **equine plasma.**
Equipoise® *(Fort Dodge)*, **boldenone undecylenate.**
Equi-Poultice *(Vetus)*, **magnesium sulfate, methyl salicylate.**
Equi-Prin™ *(First Priority)*, **acetylsalicylic acid.**
Equi-Spot™ Spot-On Fly Control for Horses *(Farnam)*, **permethrin.**
Equitrol® Feed-Thru Fly Control *(Farnam)*, **tetrachlorvinphos.**
Equivim™ *(Butler)*, **minerals, vitamins.**
Equ-SeE *(Vet-A-Mix)*, **selenium, vitamin E.**
Equ-Se5E *(Vet-A-Mix)*, **selenium, vitamin E.**
Eqvalan® Liquid *(Merial)*, **ivermectin.**
Eqvalan® Paste 1.87% *(Merial)*, **ivermectin.**
Eradimite™ *(Fort Dodge)*, **piperonyl butoxide, pyrethrins.**
erythromycin. Gallimycin®-36 *(AgriLabs)*, *(Bimeda)*, Gallimycin®-100 Injection *(Bimeda)*, Gallimycin®-100P *(Bimeda)*, Gallimycin®-200 Injection *(Bimeda)*, Gallimycin®-Dry Cow *(AgriLabs)*, *(Bimeda)*, Gallimycin® PFC *(Bimeda)*.
Esbilac® 2nd Step™ Puppy Weaning Food *(Pet-Ag)*, **weaning formula.**
Esbilac® Liquid *(Pet-Ag)*, **milk replacing formula.**
Esbilac® Powder *(Pet-Ag)*, **milk replacing formula.**
E-SE® *(Schering-Plough)*, **selenium (sodium selenite), vitamin E.**
estradiol. Compudose® *(VetLife)*, Encore® *(VetLife)*.
estradiol, trenbolone acetate. Component® TE-G *(VetLife)*, Component® TE-S *(VetLife)*, Revalor®-200 *(Intervet)*, Revalor®-G *(Intervet)*, Revalor®-H *(Intervet)*, Revalor®-IH *(Intervet)*, Revalor®-IS *(Intervet)*, Revalor®-S *(Intervet)*.
estradiol, trenbolone acetate, tylosin tartrate. Component® TE-G with Tylan® *(VetLife)*, Component® TE-S with Tylan® *(VetLife)*.
estradiol benzoate, progesterone. Component® E-C *(VetLife)*, Component® E-S *(VetLife)*, Synovex® C *(Fort Dodge)*, Synovex® S *(Fort Dodge)*.
estradiol benzoate, progesterone, tylosin tartrate. Component® E-C with Tylan® *(VetLife)*, Component® E-S with Tylan® *(VetLife)*.
estradiol benzoate, testosterone propionate. Component® E-H *(VetLife)*, Synovex® H *(Fort Dodge)*.
estradiol benzoate, testosterone propionate, tylosin tartrate. Component® E-H with Tylan® *(VetLife)*.
estradiol benzoate, trenbolone acetate. Synovex® Plus™ *(Fort Dodge)*.

estradiol cypionate. ECP® Sterile Solution *(Pharmacia & Upjohn).*
Estrumate® *(Schering-Plough),* **cloprostenol sodium.**
ethanol, cetrimide, chlorhexidine gluconate. Bou-Matic Kleen & Dri *(Bou-Matic).*
ethanol, quaternary ammonia. Lysol® Brand II I.C.™ Disinfectant Spray *(Reckitt Benckiser),* Monarch® Super Kabon® *(Ecolab Food & Bev. Div.).*
ether, iodine, isopropyl alcohol (isopropanol), turpentine, camphor. Harold White's® Leg Paint *(Hawthorne).*
ether, isopropyl alcohol (isopropanol), menthol, camphor. Shin-O-Gel® *(Hawthorne).*
ethion. Commando™ Insecticide Cattle Ear Tag *(Boehringer Ingelheim).*
ethopabate, amprolium. Amprol Plus® Type A Medicated Article *(Merial).*
ethylacetate, ethylcellulose, iodine, isopropyl alcohol (isopropanol), tannic acid. Dr. Naylor® Stop-A-Leak *(H.W. Naylor).*
ethyl alcohol, aloe vera, emollient(s). Waterless Antibacterial Hand Cleaner *(Davis).*
ethyl alcohol, chlorhexidine gluconate. C.E.T.® 0.12% Chlorhexidine Lavage *(Virbac).*
ethyl alcohol, denatonium benzoate. Discourage Taste Deterrent & Training Aid *(Davis).*
ethylcellulose, iodine, isopropyl alcohol (isopropanol), tannic acid, ethylacetate. Dr. Naylor® Stop-A-Leak *(H.W. Naylor).*
ethylenediamine dihydroiodide (EDDI). Diamine Iodide-20 (With Salt) *(First Priority),* Diamine Iodide-40 (With Salt) *(First Priority),* Diamine Iodide (With Sugar) *(First Priority),* E.D.D.I. 20 Gr. (Dextrose Base) *(Vedco),* E.D.D.I. 20 Gr. (Organic Iodine Dextrose) *(Phoenix Pharmaceutical),* E.D.D.I. 20 Gr. (Organic Iodine Salt) *(Phoenix Pharmaceutical),* E.D.D.I. 20 Gr. (Salt) *(Vedco),* E.D.D.I. 40 Gr. (Salt) *(Vedco),* EDDI Equine *(Butler),* Hi-Boot® Ethylenediamine Dihydriodide *(WestAgro),* Iodide Powder *(Neogen),* Organic Iodide *(Butler),* Organic Iodide 20 *(Durvet),* Organic Iodide 40 *(Durvet),* Organic Iodide Powder *(Neogen),* Organic Iodine *(AgriLabs), (AgriPharm).*
Etiderm® Shampoo *(Virbac),* **benzalkonium chloride, chitosanide, lactic acid.**
etodolac. EtoGesic® *(Fort Dodge).*
EtoGesic® *(Fort Dodge),* **etodolac.**
eucalyptus oil, glycerine, isopropyl alcohol (isopropanol), kaolin, methyl salicylate, peppermint oil, salicylic acid, thymol, arnica, bentonite, boric acid. Bigeloil® 24-Hour Medicated Poultice *(W. F. Young).*
eucalyptus oil, glycerine, kaolin, methyl salicylate, peppermint oil, salicylic acid. Absorbine® Antiphlogistine® *(W. F. Young).*
eucalyptus oil, isopropyl alcohol (isopropanol), methyl salicylate, parachlorometaxylenol, pine oil, scarlet red, benzyl alcohol. Scarlet Oil *(First Priority).*
eucalyptus oil, malic acid, propylene glycol, salicylic acid, benzoic acid. Euclens Otic Cleanser *(Vetus),* OtiCalm™ Cleansing Solution *(DVM).*
eucalyptus oil, menthol, benzocaine, carbolic acid. Otisol™ *(Wysong),* Otisol-O™ *(Wysong).*
eucalyptus oil, menthol, phenol, pine oil, scarlet red, thymol, camphor. Scarlet Oil Pump Spray *(Dominion).*
eucalyptus oil, methyl salicylate, parachlorometaxylenol, pine oil, scarlet red, benzyl alcohol. Scarlet Oil *(Vedco),* Scarlet Oil Wound Dressing *(AgriPharm).*
eucalyptus oil, methyl salicylate, P-chloro-M-xylenol, pine oil, scarlet red. Scarlex® Scarlet Oil *(Farnam).*
eucalyptus oil, methyl salicylate, pine oil, scarlet red. Scarlet Oil Smear *(First Priority).*
eucalyptus oil, methyl salicylate, pine oil, scarlet red, benzyl alcohol. Scarlet Oil Wound Dressing *(Durvet).*
eucalyptus oil, tea tree oil, denatonium benzoate. Soothables™ Cool Aid *(A.A.H.).*
Euclens Otic Cleanser *(Vetus),* **benzoic acid, eucalyptus oil, malic acid, propylene glycol, salicylic acid.**
Euthasol® *(Delmarva),* **pentobarbital sodium, phenytoin.**
Excalibur® Sheath Cleaner for Horses *(Equicare),* **tea tree oil.**
Excenel® RTU *(Pharmacia & Upjohn),* **ceftiofur hydrochloride.**
Exit™ Insecticide *(AgriPharm),* **permethrin.**
Exit™ II Synergized Formula Insecticide *(AgriPharm),* **permethrin, piperonyl butoxide.**
Exodus™ Paste *(Bimeda),* **pyrantel pamoate.**
Expectade™ Cough Syrup *(PRN Pharmacal),* **guaifenesin (glyceryl guaiacolate, guaiacol), phenylephrine hydrochloride, pyrilamine maleate, sodium citrate.**
ExpectaHist *(Vetus),* **ammonium chloride, guaifenesin (glyceryl guaiacolate, guaiacol), phenylephrine hydrochloride, pyrilamine maleate, sodium citrate.**
Expectorant Powder *(First Priority),* **ammonium chloride, benzoic acid, calcium phosphate, sodium bicarbonate, sodium chloride.**
Eye Rinse *(Butler), (RXV),* **boric acid, camphor, glycerine, zinc sulfate.**
E-Z Copper™ *(SSI Corp.),* **copper sulfate.**

F

F-48 *(Rochester Midland),* **quaternary ammonia.**
Facilitator™ *(Idexx Pharm.),* **hydroxyethylated amylopectin.**
Factrel® *(Fort Dodge),* **gonadorelin.**
famphur. Warbex® Famphur Pour-On for Cattle *(Schering-Plough).*
Farrier's Hoof™ *(Horses Prefer),* **copper, zinc.**
FasCure™ *(KenVet),* **collagen.**
Fast Acting Shampoo *(Davis),* **shampoo formula.**
Fastbreak™ Plus™ *(Boehringer Ingelheim),* **fat product(s), linoleic acid, vitamin A, vitamin D, vitamin E.**
Fastrack® Calf Bolus *(Conklin),* **microorganisms, minerals, nutrients, vitamins, yeast.**
Fastrack® Canine Gel *(Conklin),* **microorganisms, vitamin A, vitamin E, yeast.**
Fastrack® Canine Microbial Supplement *(Conklin),* **microorganisms.**
Fastrack® Equine Gel *(Conklin),* **microorganisms, vitamin A, vitamin E, yeast.**
Fastrack® Kick-Off *(Conklin),* **microorganisms, vitamins, yeast.**
Fastrack® Liquid Dispersible *(Conklin),* **microorganisms, yeast.**
Fastrack® Liquid Dispersible-P *(Conklin),* **microorganisms, yeast.**
Fastrack® Nonruminant Microbial Gel *(Conklin),* **microorganisms, minerals, vitamins, yeast.**
Fastrack® Probiotic Pack *(Conklin),* **microorganisms, yeast.**
Fastrack® Ruminant Bolus *(Conklin),* **microorganisms, minerals, vitamins, yeast.**
Fastrack® Ruminant Microbial Gel *(Conklin),* **microorganisms, minerals, vitamins, yeast.**
Fatal-Plus® Powder *(Vortech),* **pentobarbital sodium.**
Fatal-Plus® Solution *(Vortech),* **pentobarbital sodium.**
fat product(s). Start To Finish® Energy Pak™ 100 *(Milk Specialties).*
fat product(s), lactose, lecithin, minerals, vitamins, whey. Start To Finish® Mare Replacer™ *(Milk Specialties).*
fat product(s), lactose, milk protein, minerals, vitamins, yeast. Start To Finish® Mare & Foal Pellets™ *(Milk Specialties).*
fat product(s), linoleic acid, vitamin A, vitamin D, vitamin E. Fastbreak™ Plus™ *(Boehringer Ingelheim).*
fatty acids. Advance™ Energy Booster 100® *(Milk Specialties),* DermCaps® *(DVM),* DermCaps® 10 lb. *(DVM),* DermCaps® 100 lb. *(DVM),* DermCaps® Economy Size Liquid *(DVM),* DermCaps® ES *(DVM),* DermCaps® ES Liquid *(DVM),* DermCaps® Liquid *(DVM),* Porcine Maximizer™ *(Novartis Animal Vaccines).*
fatty acids, emollient(s). HyLyt*efa® Bath Oil/Coat Conditioner *(DVM),* HyLyt*efa® Spray-On Shampoo *(DVM).*
fatty acids, glycerine, hydrolized animal protein, sodium lactate, emollient(s). HyLyt*efa® Hypoallergenic Creme Rinse *(DVM).*
fatty acids, minerals, vitamins. Super 14™ *(Farnam).*
fatty acids, minerals, vitamins, yeast. Start To Finish® Performance Pellets™ *(Milk Specialties).*
fatty acids, potassium citrate. NutriVed™ Potassium Citrate Granules for Cats and Dogs *(Vedco).*
fatty acids, safflower oil (linoleic acid), vitamin E. Omega EFA™ Capsules *(Butler),* Omega EFA™ Capsules XS *(Butler),* Omega EFA™ Liquid *(Butler),* Omega EFA™ Liquid XS *(Butler).*
fatty acids, selenium, vitamin E. Bovine Maximizer™ *(Novartis Animal Vaccines).*
fatty acids, shampoo formula. D-Basic™ Shampoo *(DVM).*
fatty acids, vitamins, zinc. Happy Jack® Dermaplex™ *(Happy Jack).*
fatty acids (essential). Happy Jack® ToneKote® *(Happy Jack).*
fatty acids (essential), methionine (d-l), vitamins, choline. Lipo-Form *(Vet-A-Mix).*
fatty acids (essential), minerals, amino acids, electrolytes. NutriVed™ Chewable Vitamins for Active Dogs *(Vedco).*
fatty acids (essential), minerals, potassium, taurine, vitamins. Felo-Form *(Vet-A-Mix).*
fatty acids (essential), minerals, taurine, vitamins. NutriVed™ O.F.A. Granules for Cats *(Vedco).*
fatty acids (essential), minerals, taurine, vitamins, amino acids. NutriVed™ Chewable Vitamins for Cats *(Vedco),* NutriVed™ Chewable Vitamins for Kittens *(Vedco).*
fatty acids (essential), minerals, vitamins. Derma-Form Tablets *(Vet-A-Mix),* NutriVed™ O.F.A. Granules for Dogs *(Vedco),* Pet-Tabs®/F.A. Granules *(Pfizer Animal Health),* Sergeant's® Vetscription® Vitamins for Dogs & Puppies *(Sergeant's).*
fatty acids (essential), minerals, vitamins, amino acids. NutriVed™ Chewable Vitamins for Dogs *(Vedco),* NutriVed™ Chewable Vitamins for Puppies *(Vedco),* NutriVed™ Hypo Allergenic Chewable Tablets *(Vedco).*
fatty acids (essential), taurine, vitamins. Sergeant's® Vetscription® Vitamins for Cats & Kittens *(Sergeant's).*
fatty acids (essential), vitamin A, vitamin D, vitamin E, zinc. Pet-F.A. Liquid® *(Pfizer Animal Health).*
fatty acids (essential), vitamin A, vitamin D_3, vitamin E. NutriVed™ O.F.A. Liquid *(Vedco).*
fatty acids (essential), vitamin A, vitamin D_3, vitamin E, zinc. NutriVed™ O.F.A. Chewable Tablets for Large Dogs *(Vedco).*
fatty acids (omega). Canine F.A./Plus Chewable Tablets For Large Dogs *(Pala-Tech),* Canine F.A./Plus Chewable Tablets For Small and Medium Dogs *(Pala-Tech),* DermaPet® EicosaDerm™ *(DermaPet),* Heska® F.A. Granules *(Heska),* NutriVed™ O.F.A. Gel Caps for Large Dogs *(Vedco),* NutriVed™ O.F.A. Gel Caps for Small and Medium Size Dogs *(Vedco).*

fatty acids (omega), minerals, soy protein, vitamins, antioxidants. Lickables™ Charge Up!™ *(A.A.H.)*.

fatty acids (omega), minerals, vitamins. Canine F.A./Plus Granules *(Pala-Tech)*, Derma-Form Granules F.A. *(Vet-A-Mix)*, Equine F.A./Plus Granules *(Pala-Tech)*, Feline F.A./Plus Chewable Tablets *(Pala-Tech)*, Mrs. Allen's Shed-Stop® Granules for Cats *(Farnam)*, Mrs. Allen's Shed-Stop® Granules for Dogs *(Farnam)*.

fatty acids (omega), minerals, vitamins, antioxidants. Lickables™ Super Charger™ *(A.A.H.)*.

fatty acids (omega), minerals, vitamins, energy source(s). Nutri-Stat™ *(Tomlyn)*.

fatty acids (omega), shampoo formula, vitamin E. Omega-Glo E Shampoo *(Vedco)*.

fatty acids (omega), vitamin A, vitamin D, vitamin E. 3V Caps™ for Large & Giant Breeds *(DVM)*, 3V Caps™ for Medium & Large Breeds *(DVM)*, 3V Caps™ for Small & Medium Breeds *(DVM)*, 3V Caps™ Liquid *(DVM)*, Omega-3 Fatty Acid Capsules for Large & Giant Breeds *(Vet Solutions)*, Omega-3 Fatty Acid Capsules for Medium Breeds *(Vet Solutions)*, Omega-3 Fatty Acid Capsules for Small Breeds *(Vet Solutions)*, Omega-3 Fatty Acid Liquid *(Vet Solutions)*.

fatty acids (omega), vitamin A, vitamin D_3, vitamin E, zinc. NutriVed™ O.F.A. Chewable Tablets for Cats *(Vedco)*, NutriVed™ O.F.A. Chewable Tablets for Small and Medium Dogs *(Vedco)*.

fatty acids (omega), vitamin C (ascorbic acid), vitamin E, zinc. DermaPet® O.F.A. Plus EZ-C Caps (up to 30 lb.) *(DermaPet)*, DermaPet® O.F.A. Plus EZ-C Caps (50-70 lb.) *(DermaPet)*.

fatty acids (omega), vitamins, zinc. Palamega™ Complex Chewable Tablets (Liver Flavor) *(Schering-Plough)*.

fatty acids (omega), vitamins, zinc, amino acids. Pet Vites O.F.A. Chewable Tablets *(Vetus)*.

FaVor® *(Pfizer Animal Health)*, **minerals, taurine, vitamins.**

febantel, praziquantel, pyrantel pamoate. Drontal® Plus (praziquantel/pyrantel pamoate/febantel) Tablets *(Bayer)*.

Felaxin® *(Schering-Plough)*, **petrolatum.**

Feline F.A./Plus Chewable Tablets *(Pala-Tech)*, **fatty acids (omega), minerals, vitamins.**

feline pheromones. Feliway® *(Farnam)*, Feliway® Electric Diffuser *(V.P.L.)*, Feliway® Pheromone Spray *(V.P.L.)*.

Feline Plasma *(A.B.B.)*, **adenine, anhydrous lanolin, citric acid, hyaluronic acid (sodium hyaluronate), sodium citrate, whole blood.**

Feline Red Blood Cells *(A.B.B.)*, **adenine, anhydrous lanolin, citric acid, hyaluronic acid (sodium hyaluronate), sodium citrate, whole blood.**

Feline Whole Blood *(A.B.B.)*, **adenine, anhydrous lanolin, citric acid, hyaluronic acid (sodium hyaluronate), sodium citrate, whole blood.**

Feliway® *(Farnam)*, **feline pheromones.**

Feliway® Electric Diffuser *(V.P.L.)*, **feline pheromones.**

Feliway® Pheromone Spray *(V.P.L.)*, **feline pheromones.**

Felo-Form *(Vet-A-Mix)*, **fatty acids (essential), minerals, potassium, taurine, vitamins.**

Felovite®-II with Taurine *(Evsco)*, **minerals, taurine, vitamins.**

Felovite® II with Taurine *(Tomlyn)*, **minerals, taurine, vitamins.**

fenbendazole. MoorMan's® Moorguard® Swine Dewormer *(ADM)*, Panacur® Beef and Dairy Cattle Dewormer *(Intervet)*, Panacur® Cattle Dewormer *(Intervet)*, Panacur® Cattle Dewormer (92 g) *(Intervet)*, Panacur® Granules 22.2% *(Intervet)*, Panacur® Granules 22.2% (Dogs only) *(Intervet)*, Panacur® Granules 22.2% (Horse) *(Intervet)*, Panacur® Horse Dewormer *(Intervet)*, Panacur® Horse Dewormer (25 g) *(Intervet)*, Panacur® Horse Dewormer (57 g) *(Intervet)*, Panacur® Horse Dewormer (92 g) *(Intervet)*, Safe-Guard® 20% Dewormer Type A Medicated Article *(Intervet)*, Safe-Guard® Beef & Dairy Cattle Dewormer *(Intervet)*, Safe-Guard® Beef and Dairy Cattle Dewormer (290 g) *(Intervet)*, Safe-Guard® Cattle Dewormer (92 g) *(Intervet)*, Safe-Guard® Equine Dewormer (25 g) *(Intervet)*, Safe-Guard® Horse Dewormer (92 g) *(Intervet)*, Safe-Guard® Medicated Dewormer for Beef & Dairy Cattle, & Swine *(Intervet)*, Safe-Guard® Medicated Dewormer for Beef & Dairy Cattle (Flaked Meal) *(Intervet)*, Safe-Guard® Medicated Dewormer for Beef & Dairy Cattle (Soft Mini-Pellets) *(Intervet)*, Safe-Guard® Medicated Dewormer for Beef Cattle (20% Protein Block) *(Intervet)*, Safe-Guard® Medicated Dewormer for Beef Cattle (En-Pro-Al® Molasses Block) *(Intervet)*, Safe-Guard® Medicated Dewormer for Swine (EZ Scoop®) *(Intervet)*.

fenbendazole, minerals. Sweetlix® Safe-Guard* Free-Choice Mineral Cattle Dewormer *(Sweetlix)*.

fenbendazole, minerals, protein(s), vitamins. Sweetlix® Safe-Guard® 20% Natural Protein Deworming Block for Beef Cattle *(Sweetlix)*.

fenoxycarb, n-octyl bicycloheptene dicarboximide, permethrin, piperonyl butoxide, d-2-allayl-4-hydroxy-3-methyl-2-cyclopenten-1-one, di-n-propyl isocinchomeronate. Scratchex® Super Spray™ *(Combe)*.

fenvalerate. Fly Guard™ Collar/Brow Band *(Farnam)*.

fermentation extract(s), microorganisms. Digest Aid™ *(Farnam)*.

fermentation extract(s), microorganisms, psyllium. Equine Enteric Colloid *(TechMix)*.

fermentation extract(s), microorganisms, vitamins. All-In-One Calf Bolus *(AgriPharm)*, All-In-One Cattle Bolus *(AgriPharm)*.

Ferret Drops™ *(Tomlyn)*, **iron, liver extract, vitamins.**

Ferret-Off™ *(Thornell)*, **deodorants, neutralizer(s).**

ferric subsulfate. Blood Stop Powder *(Davis)*.

ferric subsulfate, iodoform, aluminum chloride, ammonium chloride, bentonite, benzocaine, copper sulfate, diatomaceous earth. Clot-It Plus™ *(Evsco)*, Nik Stop® Styptic Powder *(Tomlyn)*.

ferric subsulfate, iodoform, aluminum chloride, ammonium chloride, bentonite, copper sulfate, diatomite. Blood Stop Powder *(Butler)*.

ferric subsulfate, tannic acid, thymol, alum. Blood Stop Powder *(Dominion)*.

ferric sulfate, aluminum sulfate, chloroxylenol, collagen. Clotisol® Liquid *(BenePet)*.

ferric sulfate, carboxy methylcellulose, diphenylamine. Blood Stop Powder *(AgriPharm)*, *(Centaur)*.

ferric sulfate, tannic acid, thymol, alum. Blood Stop Powder *(AgriLabs)*.

Ferrodex™ 100 *(AgriLabs)*, **iron dextran.**

Ferrodex™ 200 *(AgriLabs)*, **iron dextran.**

ferrous sulfate, chloroxylenol, diphenylamine. Hemostatic Powder *(Butler)*.

ferrous sulfate, glycerine, kaolin, aloe vera, bentonite, boric acid. Icetight® *(Horse Health)*, Reducine® Poultice *(Equicare)*.

ferrous sulfate, iodine complex (povidone-iodine), aluminum chloride, ammonium chloride, bentonite, copper sulfate, diatomite. Kwik-Stop® Styptic Powder *(ARC)*.

ferrous sulfate, iodine complex (povidone-iodine), copper sulfate. Clot Powder *(Q.A. Laboratories)*.

ferrous sulfate, tannic acid, alum, chloroxylenol. Blood Stop Powder *(Aspen)*, *(Durvet)*, *(Vedco)*, Hemostat Powder *(Phoenix Pharmaceutical)*.

ferrous sulfate, tannic acid, chloroxylenol, diphenylamine. Blood Stop Powder *(First Priority)*.

Fertagyl® *(Intervet)*, **gonadorelin.**

Fiber Forte® Feline *(Life Science)*, **kelp, liver meal, papaya fruit, psyllium.**

Filaribits® *(Pfizer Animal Health)*, **diethylcarbamazine citrate.**

Filaribits Plus® *(Pfizer Animal Health)*, **diethylcarbamazine citrate, oxibendazole.**

Finaplix®-H *(Intervet)*, **trenbolone acetate.**

Finquel® *(Argent)*, **tricaine methanesulfonate.**

fipronil. Frontline® Spray Treatment for Cats & Dogs *(Merial)*, Frontline® Top Spot® for Cats & Kittens *(Merial)*, Frontline® Top Spot® for Dogs & Puppies *(Merial)*.

fipronil, methoprene. Frontline® Plus for Cats & Kittens *(Merial)*, Frontline® Plus for Dogs & Puppies *(Merial)*.

First Companion™ Equi-Spirin *(AgriPharm)*, **acetylsalicylic acid.**

fish oil, iodine, linseed oil, neatsfoot oil, pine tar, turpentine, wheat germ oil. Shur Hoof™ *(Horse Health)*.

fish oil, iodine, linseed oil, pine tar, turpentine, wheat germ oil. Dealer Select Horse Care Hoof Dressing With Brush *(Durvet)*.

Flavomycin® 4 *(Intervet)*, **bambermycins.**

Flavored Aspirin Powder *(First Priority)*, **acetylsalicylic acid.**

Flea & Tick Mist *(Davis)*, **di-n-propyl isocinchomeronate, n-octyl bicycloheptene dicarboximide, piperonyl butoxide, pyrethrins.**

Flea Halt!™ Flea & Tick Repellent Towelettes *(Farnam)*, **n-octyl bicycloheptene dicarboximide, piperonyl butoxide, pyrethrins.**

Flea Halt!™ Flea & Tick Repellent Towelettes for Ferrets *(Farnam)*, **n-octyl bicycloheptene dicarboximide, piperonyl butoxide, pyrethrins.**

Flea, Tick and Lice Shampoo *(Tomlyn)*, **n-octyl bicycloheptene dicarboximide, piperonyl butoxide, pyrethrins.**

florfenicol. Nuflor® Injectable Solution 300 mg/mL *(Schering-Plough)*.

Flucort® Solution *(Fort Dodge)*, **flumethasone.**

FluMeglumine® *(Phoenix Pharmaceutical)*, **flunixin meglumine.**

flumethasone. Flucort® Solution *(Fort Dodge)*.

Flu-Nix™ *(AgriLabs)*, **flunixin meglumine.**

Flunixamine™ *(Fort Dodge)*, **flunixin meglumine.**

flunixin meglumine. AmTech Flunixin Meglumine Injection *(Phoenix Scientific)*, Banamine® Granules *(Schering-Plough)*, Banamine® Injectable Solution *(Schering-Plough)*, Banamine® Paste *(Schering-Plough)*, Equileve *(Vetus)*, Equi-Phar™ Equigesic™ *(Vedco)*, FluMeglumine® *(Phoenix Pharmaceutical)*, Flu-Nix™ *(AgriLabs)*, Flunixamine™ *(Fort Dodge)*, Flunixin Meglumine *(Vet Tek)*, Flunixin Meglumine Injection *(Butler)*, Suppressor® *(RXV)*.

Flunixin Meglumine *(Vet Tek)*, **flunixin meglumine.**

Flunixin Meglumine Injection *(Butler)*, **flunixin meglumine.**

fluocinolone acetonide, dimethyl sulfoxide. Synotic® Otic Solution *(Fort Dodge)*.

fluoride. C.E.T.® FluraFom *(Virbac)*.

Fly Guard™ Collar/Brow Band *(Farnam)*, **fenvalerate.**

FlyPel® Insecticide Spray for Horses *(Virbac)*, **permethrin.**

Fly-Rid Plus *(Durvet)*, **permethrin.**

Flysect® Citronella Spray *(Equicare)*, **butoxypolypropylene glycol, piperonyl butoxide, pyrethrins.**

Flysect® Repellent Spray *(Equicare)*, **di-n-propyl isocinchomeronate, n-octyl bicycloheptene dicarboximide, piperonyl butoxide, pyrethrins.**

Flysect® Roll-On Fly Repellent Face Lotion *(Equicare)*, **di-n-propyl isocinchomeronate, n-octyl bicycloheptene dicarboximide, piperonyl butoxide, pyrethrins.**

Flysect® Super-7 *(Equicare)*, **butoxypolypropylene glycol, di-n-propyl isocinchomeronate, n-octyl bicycloheptene dicarboximide, permethrin, piperonyl butoxide, pyrethrins.**

Flysect® Super-C *(Equicare)*, **di-n-propyl isocinchomeronate, n-octyl bicycloheptene dicarboximide, permethrin, piperonyl butoxide, pyrethrins.**

Flysect® Water-Based Repellent Spray *(Equicare)*, **permethrin, piperonyl butoxide, pyrethrins.**

Flys-Off® Fly Repellent Ointment *(Farnam)*, **di-n-propyl isocinchomeronate, n-octyl bicycloheptene dicarboximide, piperonyl butoxide, pyrethrins.**

Flys-Off® Insect Repellent for Dogs *(Farnam)*, **butoxypolypropylene glycol, piperonyl butoxide, pyrethrins.**

Flys-Off® Lotion Insect Repellent for Dogs *(Farnam)*, **butoxypolypropylene glycol, piperonyl butoxide, pyrethrins.**

Fly-Zap™ Fly Bait *(Aspen)*, **methomyl, tricosene.**

Foal-Lac® Pellets *(Pet-Ag)*, **calcium, milk protein, nutrients, phosphorus, vitamins.**

Foal-Lac® Powder *(Pet-Ag)*, **milk replacing formula.**

Foaming Disinfectant Cleaner *(Davis)*, **quaternary ammonia.**

Foam-Kote 5™ *(Westfalia•Surge)*, **iodine.**

Foam-Kote 10™ *(Westfalia•Surge)*, **iodine.**

Foam Quat *(Vet Solutions)*, **quaternary ammonia.**

folic acid. Equi-Phar™ Folic 20 *(Vedco)*.

folic acid, vitamin E. Folic Acid & Vitamin E Powder *(AHC)*.

Folic Acid & Vitamin E Powder *(AHC)*, **folic acid, vitamin E.**

fomepizole. Antizol-Vet® *(Orphan Medical)*.

Foot Rot & Ringworm Spray *(AgriLabs)*, **benzalkonium chloride.**

formaldehyde. Formaldehyde *(Centaur)*, Formaldehyde Solution *(Vedco)*, Formaldehyde Solution 37% *(Butler)*, *(First Priority)*, *(Phoenix Pharmaceutical)*.

Formaldehyde *(Centaur)*, **formaldehyde.**

formaldehyde, methanol. Paracide-F *(Argent)*, Parasite-S *(Western Chemical)*.

formaldehyde, quaternary ammonia, 2-(hydroxymethyl)-2-nitro-1,3 propanediol. DC&R® Disinfectant *(Loveland)*, Parvosan™ *(KenVet)*.

Formaldehyde Solution *(Vedco)*, **formaldehyde.**

Formaldehyde Solution 37% *(Butler)*, *(First Priority)*, *(Phoenix Pharmaceutical)*, **formaldehyde.**

Formula F-500 *(Aire-Mate)*, **resmethrin.**

Formula V™ Taurine Tablets *(Pet-Ag)*, **taurine.**

Forshner's® Medicated Hoof Packing *(Equicare)*, **petrolatum, pine tar.**

Fortified Vitamin B Complex *(AgriLabs)*, **vitamin B-complex.**

Fortified Vitamin B-Complex *(AgriPharm)*, **vitamin B-complex.**

free radical scavengers, vitamin C (ascorbic acid), vitamins. Electro-Flex™ *(First Priority)*.

Freezex® Freeze *(Hawthorne)*, **menthol.**

Freezex® Hoof Freeze *(Hawthorne)*, **iodide (potassium), iodine, isopropyl alcohol (isopropanol), tannic acid.**

Fresh Cow YMCP Plus *(TechMix)*, **minerals, vitamins, yeast.**

Fresh-Ear *(Q.A. Laboratories)*, **acetic acid, boric acid, glycerine, isopropyl alcohol (isopropanol), lanolin, lidocaine, propylene glycol, salicylic acid.**

Fresh® Iodine Teat Dip (.50%) *(Metz)*, **iodine.**

Fresh® Iodine Teat Dip (1.00%) *(Metz)*, **iodine.**

Fresh Mouth Oral Spray *(Vedco)*, **chlorhexidine.**

Frontline® Plus for Cats & Kittens *(Merial)*, **fipronil, methoprene.**

Frontline® Plus for Dogs & Puppies *(Merial)*, **fipronil, methoprene.**

Frontline® Spray Treatment for Cats & Dogs *(Merial)*, **fipronil.**

Frontline® Top Spot® for Cats & Kittens *(Merial)*, **fipronil.**

Frontline® Top Spot® for Dogs & Puppies *(Merial)*, **fipronil.**

Frostshield *(Durvet)*, **emollient(s), moisturizer(s), PABA sun screen.**

Fulvicin-U/F® Powder *(Schering-Plough)*, **griseofulvin.**

Fulvicin-U/F® Tablets *(Schering-Plough)*, **griseofulvin.**

Fungi-Dry-Ear *(Q.A. Laboratories)*, **acetic acid, isopropyl alcohol (isopropanol), methyl salicylate, propylene glycol, zinc undecylenate.**

Fungisan™ *(Tomlyn)*, **benzalkonium chloride.**

Furall™ (Furazolidone) *(Farnam)*, **furazolidone.**

Fura-Ointment® *(Farnam)*, **nitrofurazone.**

Fura-Septin *(Anthony)*, **nitrofurazone.**

furazolidone. Furall™ (Furazolidone) *(Farnam)*, Furazolidone Aerosol Powder *(V.P.L.)*.

Furazolidone Aerosol Powder *(V.P.L.)*, **furazolidone.**

Fura-Zone *(Neogen)*, **nitrofurazone.**

furfural, gentian violet, glycerine, isopropyl alcohol (isopropanol), propylene glycol, sodium propionate, urea, acriflavine. Blue Lotion *(AgriLabs)*.

Furoject *(Vetus)*, **furosemide.**

furosemide. AmTech Furosemide Injection 5% *(Phoenix Scientific)*, Disal® Injection *(Boehringer Ingelheim)*, Equi-Phar™ Furosemide Injection 5% *(Vedco)*, Furoject *(Vetus)*, Furosemide Injectable 5% *(AgriLabs)*, Furosemide Injection *(AgriLabs)*, Furosemide Injection 5% *(Butler)*, *(Phoenix Pharmaceutical)*, Furosemide Tablets *(Butler)*, *(Vedco)*, Furotabs *(Vetus)*, Salix™ Injection 5% *(Intervet)*, Salix™ Tablets *(Intervet)*.

Furosemide Injectable 5% *(AgriLabs)*, **furosemide.**

Furosemide Injection *(AgriLabs)*, **furosemide.**

Furosemide Injection 5% *(Butler)*, *(Phoenix Pharmaceutical)*, **furosemide.**

Furosemide Tablets *(Butler)*, *(Vedco)*, **furosemide.**

Furotabs *(Vetus)*, **furosemide.**

Fus-Sol™ Drops *(PPI)*, **ammonium chloride, methionine (d-l).**

G

Gainpro®-10 *(Intervet)*, **bambermycins.**

Gallimycin®-36 *(AgriLabs)*, *(Bimeda)*, **erythromycin.**

Gallimycin®-100 Injection *(Bimeda)*, **erythromycin.**

Gallimycin®-100P *(Bimeda)*, **erythromycin.**

Gallimycin®-200 Injection *(Bimeda)*, **erythromycin.**

Gallimycin®-Dry Cow *(AgriLabs)*, *(Bimeda)*, **erythromycin.**

Gallimycin® PFC *(Bimeda)*, **erythromycin.**

Garacin® Piglet Injection *(Schering-Plough)*, **gentamicin.**

Garacin® Pig Pump *(Schering-Plough)*, **gentamicin.**

Garacin® Soluble Powder *(Schering-Plough)*, **gentamicin.**

Garagen™ Ophthalmic Ointment *(PPC)*, **gentamicin.**

Garagen™ Ophthalmic Solution *(PPC)*, **gentamicin.**

Garagen™ Otic Solution *(PPC)*, **betamethasone, gentamicin.**

Garagen™ Topical Spray *(PPC)*, **betamethasone, gentamicin.**

Garasol® Injection (100 mg/mL) *(Schering-Plough)*, **gentamicin.**

Gastro-Cote *(Butler)*, **bismuth subsalicylate.**

GastroGard® *(Merial)*, **omeprazole.**

Gastro-Sorb™ Bolus *(Butler)*, **attapulgite, carob, magnesium trisilicate, pectin.**

Gastro-Sorb™ Calf Bolus *(Butler)*, **attapulgite, carob, magnesium trisilicate, pectin.**

General Lube *(A.A.H.)*, *(Aspen)*, **lubricating jelly.**

General Lube *(First Priority)*, **carboxy methylcellulose, methyl para-hydroxybenzoate, propyl para-hydroxybenzoate, propylene glycol.**

Gen-Gard™ Soluble Powder *(AgriLabs)*, **gentamicin.**

Genotic B-C™ *(Butler)*, **betamethasone, clotrimazole, gentamicin.**

Gentadip *(Med-Pharmex)*, **gentamicin.**

Genta-fuse *(Vetus)*, **gentamicin.**

GentaMax™ 100 *(Phoenix Pharmaceutical)*, **gentamicin.**

gentamicin. AmTech GentaMax™ 100 *(Phoenix Scientific)*, AmTech Gentamicin Sulfate Pig Pump Oral Solution *(Phoenix Scientific)*, AmTech GentaPoult™ *(Phoenix Scientific)*, Garacin® Piglet Injection *(Schering-Plough)*, Garacin® Pig Pump *(Schering-Plough)*, Garacin® Soluble Powder *(Schering-Plough)*, Garagen™ Ophthalmic Ointment *(PPC)*, Garagen™ Ophthalmic Solution *(PPC)*, Garasol® Injection (100 mg/mL) *(Schering-Plough)*, Gen-Gard™ Soluble Powder *(AgriLabs)*, Gentadip *(Med-Pharmex)*, Genta-fuse *(Vetus)*, GentaMax™ 100 *(Phoenix Pharmaceutical)*, Gentamicin Sulfate Solution *(Aspen)*, *(Butler)*, *(RXV)*, *(Vet Tek)*, GentaVed™ 50 *(Vedco)*, GentaVed™ 100 *(Vedco)*, Gentocin® Injection (Cats and Dogs) *(Schering-Plough)*, Gentocin® Ophthalmic Ointment *(Schering-Plough)*, Gentocin® Ophthalmic Solution *(Schering-Plough)*, Gentocin® Pinkeye Spray *(Schering-Plough)*, Gentocin® Solution (Equine) *(Schering-Plough)*, Legacy® *(AgriLabs)*.

gentamicin, betamethasone. Betagen™ Otic Solution *(Med-Pharmex)*, Betagen™ Topical Spray *(Med-Pharmex)*, Garagen™ Otic Solution *(PPC)*, Garagen™ Topical Spray *(PPC)*, Gentamicin Otic Solution *(Butler)*, Gentamicin Topical Spray *(Butler)*, *(RXV)*, Genta-Otic *(Vetus)*, Genta-Spray *(Vetus)*, GentaVed® Otic Solution *(Vedco)*, GentaVed® Topical Spray *(Vedco)*, Gentocin® Durafilm® Solution *(Schering-Plough)*, Gentocin® Otic Solution *(Schering-Plough)*, Gentocin® Topical Spray *(Schering-Plough)*.

gentamicin, betamethasone, clotrimazole. CGB® Ointment *(PPC)*, Genotic B-C™ *(Butler)*, MalOtic® Ointment *(Vedco)*, Otibiotic Ointment *(Vetus)*, Otomax® *(Schering-Plough)*, Oto Soothe® Ointment *(RXV)*, Tri-Otic® *(Med-Pharmex)*.

gentamicin, mometasone furoate, clotrimazole. MometaMax™ Otic Suspension *(Schering-Plough)*.

Gentamicin Otic Solution *(Butler)*, **betamethasone, gentamicin.**

Gentamicin Sulfate Solution *(Aspen)*, *(Butler)*, *(RXV)*, *(Vet Tek)*, **gentamicin.**

Gentamicin Topical Spray *(Butler)*, *(RXV)*, **betamethasone, gentamicin.**

Genta-Otic *(Vetus)*, **betamethasone, gentamicin.**

Genta-Spray *(Vetus)*, **betamethasone, gentamicin.**

GentaVed™ 50 *(Vedco)*, **gentamicin.**

GentaVed™ 100 *(Vedco)*, **gentamicin.**

GentaVed® Otic Solution *(Vedco)*, **betamethasone, gentamicin.**

GentaVed® Topical Spray *(Vedco)*, **betamethasone, gentamicin.**

gentian violet, glycerine, isopropyl alcohol (isopropanol), propylene glycol, sodium propionate, urea, acriflavine, furfural. Blue Lotion *(AgriLabs).*
gentian violet, glycerine, isopropyl alcohol (isopropanol), propylene glycol, urea, acriflavine. Purple Lotion *(Vedco)*, Purple Lotion Wound Dressing *(First Priority).*
gentian violet, isopropyl alcohol (isopropanol), tannic acid, turpentine. Happy Jack® Pad Kote *(Happy Jack).*
gentian violet, sodium propionate, acriflavine. Dr. Naylor® Blu-Kote® *(H.W. Naylor).*
Gent-L-Clens™ *(Schering-Plough)*, **lactic acid, propylene glycol, salicylic acid.**
Gentle Iodine 1% *(Aspen)*, **iodine complex (povidone-iodine), isopropyl alcohol (isopropanol).**
"Gentle" Iodine Wound Spray *(Centaur)*, **iodine complex (povidone-iodine), isopropyl alcohol (isopropanol).**
Gentle Iodine Wound Spray *(First Priority)*, **iodine.**
Gentle Iodine Wound Spray *(Vedco)*, **iodine complex (povidone-iodine), isopropyl alcohol (isopropanol).**
Gentocin® Durafilm® Solution *(Schering-Plough)*, **betamethasone, gentamicin.**
Gentocin® Injection (Cats and Dogs) *(Schering-Plough)*, **gentamicin.**
Gentocin® Ophthalmic Ointment *(Schering-Plough)*, **gentamicin.**
Gentocin® Ophthalmic Solution *(Schering-Plough)*, **gentamicin.**
Gentocin® Otic Solution *(Schering-Plough)*, **betamethasone, gentamicin.**
Gentocin® Pinkeye Spray *(Schering-Plough)*, **gentamicin.**
Gentocin® Solution (Equine) *(Schering-Plough)*, **gentamicin.**
Gentocin® Topical Spray *(Schering-Plough)*, **betamethasone, gentamicin.**
Geri-Form *(Vet-A-Mix)*, **choline, lipids, minerals, vitamins.**
Germicidal Detergent and Deodorant *(Aire-Mate)*, **quaternary ammonia.**
Germicide Solution *(Phoenix Pharmaceutical)*, **quaternary ammonia.**
Glucaminolyte Forte *(AgriPharm)*, *(Vedco)*, **amino acids, dextrose, electrolytes.**
Gluco-Amino-Forte Oral Solution *(Phoenix Pharmaceutical)*, **amino acids, dextrose, electrolytes.**
Gluco Amino Forte Oral Solution *(Vetus)*, **amino acids, dextrose, electrolytes.**
Glucose *(Fort Dodge)*, **dextrose.**
glucose, amino acids, electrolytes. Electramine® *(Life Science).*
glucose, electrolytes. Isotone-SA *(Vet-A-Mix)*, Re-Sorb® *(Pfizer Animal Health).*
glucose, lactic acid producing bacteria, electrolytes. SureLytes™ Plus Carbo Load *(SureNutrition).*
glucose, microorganisms, nutrients, electrolytes. Ener-Lyte™ *(Aspen).*
glucose oxidase, lactoperoxidase. C.E.T.® Chews for Cats *(Virbac)*, C.E.T.® Enzymatic Tartar Control Toothpaste *(Virbac)*, C.E.T.® Enzymatic Toothpaste *(Virbac).*
glutaraldehyde. MetriCide® *(Metrex)*, MetriCide® 28 *(Metrex)*, MetriCide Plus 30® *(Metrex).*
glutaraldehyde, quaternary ammonia. Virocid® *(Merial Select).*
glycerine. Glycerin U.S.P. *(First Priority)*, *(Vedco).*
glycerine, alcohol base. Corium-20™ *(Virbac).*
glycerine, chlorhexidine. Nolvasan® 5% Teat Dip Concentrate *(Fort Dodge)*, Nolvasan® Teat Dip Concentrate *(Fort Dodge).*
glycerine, chlorhexidine gluconate. Chlora-Dip *(First Priority)*, Metz Soft-Kote Teat Dip *(Metz)*, Metz Soft-Kote Teat Spray *(Metz).*
glycerine, docusate sodium (dioctyl sodium sulfosuccinate). Docu-Soft™ Pet Enema *(Life Science).*
glycerine, hydrolized animal protein, sodium lactate, emollient(s), fatty acids. HyLyt*efa® Hypoallergenic Creme Rinse *(DVM).*
glycerine, iodine complex (povidone-iodine). Metz Iodine Teat Dip (0.25%) *(Metz)*, Metz Iodine Teat Dip (0.5%) *(Metz)*, Metz Iodine Teat Dip (1.0%) *(Metz)*, Teat Dip-Lite *(Western Chemical)*, Teat Dip with Glycerin *(Western Chemical)*, Teat-Kote® *(Westfalia•*Surge), Theraderm® 2500 *(Westfalia•*Surge), Theratec™ *(Westfalia•*Surge), Theratec® Plus *(Westfalia•*Surge), West-Vet® Ultradine® *(WestAgro).*
glycerine, isopropyl alcohol (isopropanol), kaolin, methyl salicylate, peppermint oil, salicylic acid, thymol, arnica, bentonite, boric acid, eucalyptus oil. Bigeloil® 24-Hour Medicated Poultice *(W. F. Young).*
glycerine, isopropyl alcohol (isopropanol), lanolin, lidocaine, propylene glycol, salicylic acid, acetic acid, boric acid. Fresh-Ear *(Q.A. Laboratories).*
glycerine, isopropyl alcohol (isopropanol), lanolin, propylene glycol, salicylic acid, acetic acid. OtiClean®-A Ear Cleaning and Deodorant Pads *(ARC).*
glycerine, isopropyl alcohol (isopropanol), lidocaine, propylene glycol, salicylic acid, acetic acid, boric acid. Otic Clear *(Butler).*
glycerine, isopropyl alcohol (isopropanol), methyl violet, propylene glycol, urea, acriflavine. Purple Lotion Wound Dressing *(Durvet).*
glycerine, isopropyl alcohol (isopropanol), propylene glycol, salicylic acid, acetic acid. OtiClean®-A Ear Cleaning Lotion *(ARC).*
glycerine, isopropyl alcohol (isopropanol), propylene glycol, sodium propionate, urea, acriflavine, furfural, gentian violet. Blue Lotion *(AgriLabs).*
glycerine, isopropyl alcohol (isopropanol), propylene glycol, urea, acriflavine, gentian violet. Purple Lotion *(Vedco)*, Purple Lotion Wound Dressing *(First Priority).*
glycerine, kaolin, aloe vera, bentonite, boric acid, ferrous sulfate. Icetight® *(Horse Health)*, Reducine® Poultice *(Equicare).*
glycerine, kaolin, methyl salicylate, peppermint oil, salicylic acid, eucalyptus oil. Absorbine® Antiphlogistine® *(W. F. Young).*
glycerine, lactic acid, propylene glycol, urea, benzalkonium chloride. Humilac® Spray *(Virbac).*
glycerine, lactic acid, urea, chitosanide. Allergroom® Shampoo *(Virbac).*
glycerine, lanolin, petrolatum, aloe vera, beeswax, emulsifying wax. Dealer Select Horse Care Hoof Moisturizer *(Durvet).*
glycerine, lidocaine, malic acid, propylene glycol, zolazepam, benzoic acid, chlorhexidine. Chlor-A-Clens-L Cleansing Solution *(Vedco).*
glycerine, malic acid, propylene glycol, salicylic acid, benzoic acid, chlorhexidine. Chlor-A-Clens Cleansing Solution *(Vedco).*
glycerine, medicinal soap base, docusate sodium (dioctyl sodium sulfosuccinate). Therevac®-SB *(King Animal Health).*
glycerine, menthol, zinc oxide, calamine. Cool-Cast® *(Hawthorne).*
glycerine, methyl violet, propylene glycol, sodium propionate, urea, acriflavine. Blue Lotion *(Farnam).*
glycerine, methyl violet, propylene glycol, urea, acriflavine. Wound-Kote Gentian Violet *(Farnam).*
glycerine, mineral oil, vegetable oil(s). Hairball Solution *(Pet-Ag).*
glycerine, oatmeal, chitosanide. Epi-Soothe® Shampoo *(Virbac).*
glycerine, petrolatum. Hartz® Health measures™ Hairball Remedy *(Hartz Mountain).*
glycerine, petrolatum, zinc oxide, acacia, calamine, castor oil. Triple Cast™ *(Neogen).*
glycerine, pramoxine hydrochloride. Corium-Tx™ *(Virbac).*
glycerine, triethanolamine, vitamin E, aloe vera. SoftGuard™ *(Activon).*
glycerine, zinc sulfate, boric acid, camphor. Eye Rinse *(Butler)*, *(RXV).*
Glycerin U.S.P. *(First Priority)*, *(Vedco)*, **glycerine.**
glyceryl monolaurate. 3M™ Lauricare™ Moisturizing Teat Dip Concentrate *(3M)*, 3M™ Teat Shield™ with Germicide *(3M).*
glycine, bicarbonate, dextrose, electrolytes. Elpak™-G *(Vedco).*
glycine, dextrose, electrolytes. Hy-Sorb™ *(Bimeda).*
glycine, minerals, dextrose. Electrolyte with Thickener *(DVM Formula).*
glycine, vitamins, dextrose, electrolytes. Electrolyte HE with Vitamins *(DVM Formula).*
glycolipids, lecithin, phospholipids, vitamins. Dyna-Lode® Equine Supplement *(Harlmen).*
glycolipids, phospholipids. Dyna-Lode® Supplement for Dogs & Cats *(Harlmen).*
glycopyrrolate. Robinul®-V *(Fort Dodge).*
GME™ Powder and Liquid (Goat's Milk Esbilac®) *(Pet-Ag)*, **goat milk, minerals, vitamins.**
goat milk, minerals, vitamins. GME™ Powder and Liquid (Goat's Milk Esbilac®) *(Pet-Ag).*
Go-Dry™ *(G.C. Hanford)*, **penicillin G procaine.**
Go Max™ Liquid *(Farnam)*, **iron, minerals, selenium, vitamins.**
gonadorelin. Cystorelin® *(Merial)*, Factrel® *(Fort Dodge)*, Fertagyl® *(Intervet).*
Good Start Calf Bolus *(AgriPharm)*, **lactase enzymes, microorganisms, vitamin A, vitamin E.**
Good Start Calf Paste *(AgriPharm)*, **lactase enzymes, microorganisms, vitamin A, vitamin E.**
Goodwinol Ointment *(Goodwinol)*, **benzocaine, lanolin, rotenone.**
Grade A™ *(Intercon)*, **quaternary ammonia.**
Grand Champion® Dri-Kleen™ *(Farnam)*, **shampoo formula.**
Grand Champion® Fly Repellent Formula *(Farnam)*, **piperonyl butoxide, pyrethrins.**
Granulex® V Aerosol Spray *(Pfizer Animal Health)*, **balsam peru oil, castor oil, trypsin.**
Granulex® V Liquid *(Pfizer Animal Health)*, **balsam peru oil, castor oil, trypsin.**
Greenlyte® *(Bimeda)*, **citric acid, electrolytes, methionine, microorganisms.**
Grenade® ER Premise Insecticide *(Schering-Plough)*, **lambdacyhalothrin.**
griseofulvin. Fulvicin-U/F® Powder *(Schering-Plough)*, Fulvicin-U/F® Tablets *(Schering-Plough).*
Groom-Aid® 35x *(Evsco)*, **shampoo formula.**
Groom-Aid® Spray *(Evsco)*, **isopropyl alcohol, lanolin, mineral spirits.**
Grooming Shampoo *(First Priority)*, **coconut oil, shampoo formula.**
Grow Colt® *(Farnam)*, **minerals, vitamins.**
guaifenesin (glyceryl guaiacolate, guaiacol). AmTech Guaifenesin Injection *(Phoenix Scientific)*, Guaifenesin Injection *(Butler)*, *(Phoenix Pharmaceutical)*, Guailaxin® *(Fort Dodge).*
guaifenesin (glyceryl guaiacolate, guaiacol), dextromethorphan. Cough Tablets *(Life Science).*
guaifenesin (glyceryl guaiacolate, guaiacol), phenylephrine hydrochloride, pyrilamine maleate, sodium chloride, ammonium chloride. Cough Syrup *(Life Science).*
guaifenesin (glyceryl guaiacolate, guaiacol), phenylephrine hydrochloride, pyrilamine maleate, sodium citrate. Expectade™ Cough Syrup *(PRN Pharmacal).*
guaifenesin (glyceryl guaiacolate, guaiacol), phenylephrine hydrochloride, pyrilamine maleate, sodium citrate, ammonium chloride. Anti-Tussive Syrup with Antihistamine *(Vedco)*, ExpectaHist *(Vetus).*

guaifenesin (glyceryl guaiacolate, guaiacol), potassium iodide, ammonium chloride. AniTuss *(AHC)*, Spec-Tuss™ *(Neogen)*, Tri-Tussin™ Powder *(Creative Science)*.
guaifenesin (glyceryl guaiacolate, guaiacol), pyrilamine maleate. AniHist *(AHC)*, Hist-EQ Powder *(Butler)*.
Guaifenesin Injection *(Butler)*, *(Phoenix Pharmaceutical)*, **guaifenesin (glyceryl guaiacolate, guaiacol).**
Guailaxin® *(Fort Dodge)*, **guaifenesin (glyceryl guaiacolate, guaiacol).**
gum benzoin, rosin, Barbadoes aloes, camphor, Churchill's iodine. Shin-Band *(Dominion)*.

H

Hairball Preparation *(Vet Solutions)*, **mineral oil, petrolatum.**
Hairball Solution *(Pet-Ag)*, **glycerine, mineral oil, vegetable oil(s).**
hair polish formula. Absorbine® ShowSheen® Hair Polish & Detangler *(W. F. Young)*.
hair spray formula. Dealer Select Horse Care Groom 'N Show *(Durvet)*.
halothane. Halothane, USP *(Halocarbon)*.
Halothane, USP *(Halocarbon)*, **halothane.**
Happy Jack® Cod Liver Oil *(Happy Jack)*, **vitamin A, vitamin D.**
Happy Jack® DD-33™ Flea & Tick Mist *(Happy Jack)*, **permethrin, pyrethrins.**
Happy Jack® Dermaplex™ *(Happy Jack)*, **fatty acids, vitamins, zinc.**
Happy Jack® Ear Canker Powder *(Happy Jack)*, **iodoform, zinc oxide.**
Happy Jack® Enduracide® Dip II *(Happy Jack)*, **chlorpyrifos.**
Happy Jack® Flea Flogger Plus *(Happy Jack)*, **n-octyl bicycloheptene dicarboximide, permethrin, pyrethrins, pyriproxyfen.**
Happy Jack® Flea-Tick Powder II *(Happy Jack)*, **carbaryl.**
Happy Jack® Flea Zinger Plus *(Happy Jack)*, **pyriproxyfen, sumethrin, tetramethrin.**
Happy Jack® Kennel Dip II *(Happy Jack)*, **permethrin, piperonyl butoxide.**
Happy Jack® Kennelspot™ for Dogs (under 33 lbs) *(Happy Jack)*, **permethrin.**
Happy Jack® Kennelspot™ for Dogs (over 33 lbs) *(Happy Jack)*, **permethrin.**
Happy Jack® Liqui-Vict 2X™ *(Happy Jack)*, **pyrantel pamoate.**
Happy Jack® Mange Medicine *(Happy Jack)*, **sulfur.**
Happy Jack® Milkade *(Happy Jack)*, **calcium, potassium chloride, sodium chloride, thiamine hydrochloride (B_1).**
Happy Jack® Mitex™ *(Happy Jack)*, **piperonyl butoxide, pyrethrins.**
Happy Jack® No-Hop Flea-Tick Spray *(Happy Jack)*, **permethrin, pyrethrins.**
Happy Jack® Novation™ Flea & Tick Collar for Dogs *(Happy Jack)*, **deltamethrin.**
Happy Jack® Onex *(Happy Jack)*, **di-n-propyl isocinchomeronate, piperonyl butoxide, pyrethrins.**
Happy Jack® Pad Kote *(Happy Jack)*, **gentian violet, isopropyl alcohol (isopropanol), tannic acid, turpentine.**
Happy Jack® Paracide II Shampoo *(Happy Jack)*, **chlorpyrifos.**
Happy Jack® Sardex II® *(Happy Jack)*, **benzyl benzoate.**
Happy Jack® Skin Balm *(Happy Jack)*, **mercaptobenzothiazole.**
Happy Jack® Tapeworm Tablets *(Happy Jack)*, **dichlorophene.**
Happy Jack® ToneKote® *(Happy Jack)*, **fatty acids (essential).**
Happy Jack® Vita Tabs *(Happy Jack)*, **minerals, vitamins.**
Harold White's® Leg Paint *(Hawthorne)*, **camphor, ether, iodine, isopropyl alcohol (isopropanol), turpentine.**
Hartz® 2 in 1® Flea & Tick Collar for Cats and Kittens *(Hartz Mountain)*, **tetrachlorvinphos.**
Hartz® 2 in 1® Flea & Tick Collar for Dogs and Puppies *(Hartz Mountain)*, **tetrachlorvinphos.**
Hartz® 2 in 1® Flea & Tick Dip for Dogs and Cats *(Hartz Mountain)*, **n-octyl bicycloheptene dicarboximide, piperonyl butoxide, pyrethrins.**
Hartz® 2 in 1® Flea & Tick Killer for Dogs *(Hartz Mountain)*, **dicarboximide, n-octyl bicycloheptene dicarboximide, piperonyl butoxide, pyrethrins.**
Hartz® 2 in 1® Flea & Tick Powder for Cats *(Hartz Mountain)*, **tetrachlorvinphos.**
Hartz® 2 in 1® Flea & Tick Powder for Dogs *(Hartz Mountain)*, **tetrachlorvinphos.**
Hartz® 2 in 1® Flea & Tick Spray for Cats *(Hartz Mountain)*, **tetrachlorvinphos.**
Hartz® 2 in 1® Flea & Tick Spray for Dogs *(Hartz Mountain)*, **tetrachlorvinphos.**
Hartz® 2 in 1® Luster Bath for Cats *(Hartz Mountain)*, **n-octyl bicycloheptene dicarboximide, piperonyl butoxide, pyrethrins.**
Hartz® 2 in 1® Rid Flea™ Dog Shampoo with Allethrin *(Hartz Mountain)*, **d-trans allethrin, n-octyl bicycloheptene dicarboximide.**
Hartz® 2 in 1® Rid Flea™ Dog Shampoo with Pyrethrin *(Hartz Mountain)*, **n-octyl bicycloheptene dicarboximide, piperonyl butoxide, pyrethrins.**
Hartz® Advanced Care™ Brand Flea & Tick Drops Plus+ for Cats and Kittens (10 lbs. & under) *(Hartz Mountain)*, **methoprene, phenothrin.**
Hartz® Advanced Care™ Brand Flea & Tick Drops Plus+ for Cats and Kittens (over 10 lbs.) *(Hartz Mountain)*, **methoprene, phenothrin.**
Hartz® Advanced Care™ Brand Flea & Tick Drops Plus+ for Dogs and Puppies (4 to 15 lbs.) *(Hartz Mountain)*, **methoprene, phenothrin.**
Hartz® Advanced Care™ Brand Flea & Tick Drops Plus+ for Dogs and Puppies (16 to 30 lbs.) *(Hartz Mountain)*, **methoprene, phenothrin.**
Hartz® Advanced Care™ Brand Flea & Tick Drops Plus+ for Dogs and Puppies (31 to 45 lbs.) *(Hartz Mountain)*, **methoprene, phenothrin.**
Hartz® Advanced Care™ Brand Flea & Tick Drops Plus+ for Dogs and Puppies (46 to 60 lbs.) *(Hartz Mountain)*, **methoprene, phenothrin.**
Hartz® Advanced Care™ Brand Flea & Tick Drops Plus+ for Dogs and Puppies (61 to 90 lbs.) *(Hartz Mountain)*, **methoprene, phenothrin.**
Hartz® Advanced Care™ Brand Flea & Tick Drops Plus+ for Dogs and Puppies (Over 90 lbs.) *(Hartz Mountain)*, **methoprene, phenothrin.**
Hartz® Advanced Care® Brand™ Flea Control Capsules™ for Dogs *(Hartz Mountain)*, **methoprene.**
Hartz® Advanced Care™ Brand Once-a-Month™ Flea & Tick Drops for Cats and Kittens (10 lbs. & under) *(Hartz Mountain)*, **phenothrin.**
Hartz® Advanced Care™ Brand Once-a-Month™ Flea & Tick Drops for Cats and Kittens (over 10 lbs.) *(Hartz Mountain)*, **phenothrin.**
Hartz® Advanced Care™ Brand Once-a-Month™ Flea & Tick Drops for Dogs and Puppies (16 to 30 lbs.) *(Hartz Mountain)*, **phenothrin.**
Hartz® Advanced Care™ Brand Once-a-Month™ Flea & Tick Drops for Dogs and Puppies (15 lbs. & under) *(Hartz Mountain)*, **phenothrin.**
Hartz® Advanced Care™ Brand Once-a-Month™ Flea & Tick Drops for Dogs and Puppies (31 to 60 lbs.) *(Hartz Mountain)*, **phenothrin.**
Hartz® Advanced Care™ Brand Once-a-Month™ Flea & Tick Drops for Dogs and Puppies (61 to 90 lbs.) *(Hartz Mountain)*, **phenothrin.**
Hartz® Advanced Care™ Brand Once-a-Month™ Flea & Tick Drops for Dogs and Puppies (over 90 lbs.) *(Hartz Mountain)*, **phenothrin.**
Hartz® Advanced Care® Brand Tick Dabber™ Applicator *(Hartz Mountain)*, **phenothrin.**
Hartz® Control Pet Care System® Flea & Flea Egg Killer for Dogs *(Hartz Mountain)*, **methoprene, tetrachlorvinphos.**
Hartz® Control Pet Care System® Flea & Tick Conditioning Shampoo for Cats *(Hartz Mountain)*, **d-trans allethrin, dicarboximide, n-octyl bicycloheptene dicarboximide.**
Hartz® Control Pet Care System® Flea & Tick Conditioning Shampoo for Dogs *(Hartz Mountain)*, **d-trans allethrin, dicarboximide, n-octyl bicycloheptene dicarboximide.**
Hartz® Control Pet Care System® Flea & Tick Dip for Dogs *(Hartz Mountain)*, **tetrachlorvinphos.**
Hartz® Control Pet Care System® Flea & Tick Repellent for Cats *(Hartz Mountain)*, **tetrachlorvinphos.**
Hartz® Control Pet Care System® Flea & Tick Repellent for Dogs *(Hartz Mountain)*, **tetrachlorvinphos.**
Hartz® Control Pet Care System® Mousse for Cats and Kittens *(Hartz Mountain)*, **methoprene, piperonyl butoxide, pyrethrins.**
Hartz® Control Pet Care System® OneSpot® for Cats and Kittens *(Hartz Mountain)*, **methoprene.**
Hartz® Control Pet Care System® Ultimate Flea Collar® for Cats *(Hartz Mountain)*, **methoprene, tetrachlorvinphos.**
Hartz® Control Pet Care System® Ultimate Flea Collar® for Dogs & Puppies *(Hartz Mountain)*, **methoprene, tetrachlorvinphos.**
Hartz® Easy Wash™ Flea & Tick Shampoo for Dogs *(Hartz Mountain)*, **n-octyl bicycloheptene dicarboximide, piperonyl butoxide, pyrethrins.**
Hartz® Groomer's Best™ Conditioning Shampoo *(Hartz Mountain)*, **shampoo formula.**
Hartz® Groomer's Best™ Medicated Shampoo *(Hartz Mountain)*, **coal tar.**
Hartz® Groomer's Best™ Oatmeal Shampoo *(Hartz Mountain)*, **colloidal oatmeal.**
Hartz® Health measures™ Anti-Itch Hydrocortisone Shampoo *(Hartz Mountain)*, **hydrocortisone.**
Hartz® Health measures™ Anti-Itch Hydrocortisone Spray *(Hartz Mountain)*, **hydrocortisone.**
Hartz® Health measures™ Ear Mite Treatment for Cats *(Hartz Mountain)*, **piperonyl butoxide, pyrethrins.**
Hartz® Health measures™ Ear Mite Treatment for Dogs *(Hartz Mountain)*, **piperonyl butoxide, pyrethrins.**
Hartz® Health measures™ Enteric-Coated Aspirin for Dogs *(Hartz Mountain)*, **acetylsalicylic acid.**
Hartz® Health measures™ Everyday Chewable Vitamins for Cats and Kittens *(Hartz Mountain)*, **minerals, taurine, vitamins.**
Hartz® Health measures™ Everyday Chewable Vitamins for Dogs and Puppies *(Hartz Mountain)*, **minerals, vitamins.**
Hartz® Health measures™ Hairball Remedy *(Hartz Mountain)*, **glycerine, petrolatum.**
Hartz® Health measures™ Hydrocortisone Spot *(Hartz Mountain)*, **hydrocortisone.**
Hartz® Health measures™ Liquid Wormer *(Hartz Mountain)*, **piperazine citrate.**
Hartz® Health measures™ Once-a-month® Wormer for Cats and Kittens *(Hartz Mountain)*, **piperazine adipate.**
Hartz® Health measures™ Once-a-month® Wormer for Dogs *(Hartz Mountain)*, **piperazine adipate.**
Hartz® Health measures™ Once-a-month® Wormer for Large Dogs *(Hartz Mountain)*, **piperazine adipate.**

I

imidacloprid. Advantage® 9 (imidacloprid) Topical Solution for Cats and Kittens (8 Weeks and Older, 9 lbs. and Under) *(Bayer)*, Advantage® 10 (imidacloprid) Topical Solution for Dogs and Puppies (7 Weeks and Older, Under 10 lbs.) *(Bayer)*, Advantage® 18 (imidacloprid) Topical Solution for Cats and Kittens (8 Weeks and Older, Over 9 lbs.) *(Bayer)*, Advantage® 20 (imidacloprid) Topical Solution for Dogs and Puppies (7 Weeks and Older, 11-20 lbs.) *(Bayer)*, Advantage® 55 (imidacloprid) Topical Solution for Dogs and Puppies (7 Weeks and Older, 21-55 lbs.) *(Bayer)*, Advantage® 100 (imidacloprid) Topical Solution for Dogs and Puppies (7 Weeks and Older, Over 55 lbs.) *(Bayer)*.

imidacloprid, permethrin. K9 Advantix™ 10 (imidacloprid/permethrin) For Dogs and Puppies (7 Weeks and Older, 10 lbs. and Under) *(Bayer)*, K9 Advantix™ 20 (imidacloprid/permethrin) For Dogs and Puppies (7 Weeks and Older, 11-20 lbs.) *(Bayer)*, K9 Advantix™ 55 (imidacloprid/permethrin) For Dogs and Puppies (7 Weeks and Older, 21-55 lbs.) *(Bayer)*, K9 Advantix™ 100 (imidacloprid/permethrin) For Dogs and Puppies (7 Weeks and Older, Over 55 lbs.) *(Bayer)*.

imidacloprid, tricosene. QuickBayt™ Fly Bait *(Bayer)*.

imidocarb dipropionate. Imizol® *(Schering-Plough)*.

Imizol® *(Schering-Plough)*, **imidocarb dipropionate.**

Immiticide® *(Merial)*, **melarsomine dihydrochloride.**

Immunoboost® *(Bioniche Animal Health)*, **Mycobacterium cell wall fraction.**

immunoglobulin(s) G. Antivenin *(Fort Dodge)*, Rhodococcus Equi Antibody *(Lake Immunogenics)*.

immunoglobulin(s) G, protein(s). Colostrx® *(Schering-Plough)*.

Immuno-Glo NEP *(Mg Biologics)*, **equine plasma.**

ImmunoRegulin® *(Neogen)*, **Propionibacterium acnes.**

Improved Hoof Dressing *(Fiebing)*, **mineral oil.**

Injectrolyte *(Vetus)*, **magnesium chloride, potassium chloride, sodium acetate, sodium chloride, sodium gluconate.**

Innocugel™ Equine *(Butler)*, **microorganisms, vitamins.**

inositol, liver, racemethionine, vitamin B-complex, choline bitartrate. Lipocaps *(Vetus)*.

InstaMag Bolus *(Vedco)*, **magnesium hydroxide.**

insulin. PZI Vet® *(Idexx Pharm.)*.

In-Synch™ *(AgriLabs)*, **dinoprost (prostaglandin $F_{2}\alpha$).**

Integrator™ *(Butler)*, **biotin, methionine (d-l), thiamine hydrochloride (B_1), zinc.**

Intensive Care Gruel™ (ICG) *(TechMix)*, **nutrients.**

Interceptor® Flavor Tabs® *(Novartis)*, **milbemycin oxime.**

InterSept™ Activator *(Westfalia•Surge)*, **lactic acid.**

InterSept™ Base *(Westfalia•Surge)*, **sodium chlorite.**

Intesti-Sorb Bolus *(AgriPharm)*, **attapulgite, carob, magnesium trisilicate, pectin.**

Intesti-Sorb Calf Bolus *(AgriPharm)*, **attapulgite, carob, magnesium trisilicate, pectin.**

Intrauterine Bolus *(AgriLabs)*, **urea.**

iodide (potassium). Wind-Aid® *(Hawthorne)*.

iodide (potassium), iodine. Lugol's Solution *(Butler)*.

iodide (potassium), iodine, isopropyl alcohol (isopropanol). Iodine 7% Tincture *(AgriLabs)*, Iodine Tincture 7% *(AgriPharm)*, *(Vedco)*, Stronger Iodine Tincture 7% *(Centaur)*, Strong Iodine Tincture *(Butler)*, Strong Iodine Tincture 7% *(Durvet)*, Tincture Iodine 7% *(Bimeda)*.

iodide (potassium), iodine, isopropyl alcohol (isopropanol), menthol, thymol, camphor. Equi-Phar™ CoolGel *(Vedco)*.

iodide (potassium), iodine, isopropyl alcohol (isopropanol), tannic acid. Freezex® Hoof Freeze *(Hawthorne)*.

iodide (potassium), iodine, menthol, spearmint oil, witch hazel, alcohol. Absorbine® RefreshMint® *(W. F. Young)*.

iodide (potassium), iodine, menthol, thymol, benzocaine, camphor. Equi-Phar™ BenzaGel *(Vedco)*.

iodide (potassium), iodine, pine tar. Reducine® Absorbent for Horses *(Equicare)*.

iodide (potassium), iodine, pine tar, ichthammol. Sole Pack™ Hoof Dressing *(Hawthorne)*, Sole Pack™ Hoof Packing *(Hawthorne)*.

iodide (potassium), isopropyl alcohol, menthol, parachlorometaxylenol, thymol, witch hazel, wormwood oil, aloe vera. Veterinary Liniment *(First Priority)*.

Iodide Powder *(Neogen)*, **ethylenediamine dihydroiodide (EDDI).**

iodine. A & L SoftKote *(Bou-Matic)*, Aloedine® Medicated Shampoo *(Farnam)*, Armor® *(Westfalia•Surge)*, Bou-Matic Aloe-Soft *(Bou-Matic)*, Bou-Matic Bovi-Kote *(Bou-Matic)*, Bou-Matic Bovi-Kote 5 *(Bou-Matic)*, Bou-Matic Bovisoft *(Bou-Matic)*, Bou-Matic MaxiSoft *(Bou-Matic)*, Bou-Matic Novablend 10 *(Bou-Matic)*, Bou-Matic Penetrate *(Bou-Matic)*, Bou-Matic Udderdine-5 *(Bou-Matic)*, Bou-Matic Udderdine-10 *(Bou-Matic)*, Bou-Matic Udderdine-12 *(Bou-Matic)*, Bou-Matic Udderdine-502 *(Bou-Matic)*, Derma-Kote™ *(Westfalia•Surge)*, Foam-Kote 5™ *(Westfalia•Surge)*, Foam-Kote 10™ *(Westfalia•Surge)*, Fresh® Iodine Teat Dip (.50%) *(Metz)*, Fresh® Iodine Teat Dip (1.00%) *(Metz)*, Gentle Iodine Wound Spray *(First Priority)*, I-deal™ Barrier Teat Dip *(Ecolab Food & Bev. Div.)*, Iodine Disinfectant *(Durvet)*, IO-Shield® Sanitizing Barrier Teat Dip *(Ecolab Food & Bev. Div.)*, One Step *(Vedco)*, Parvo Guard™ *(First Priority)*, ReFresh® Iodine Teat Dip (1.00%) *(Metz)*, Teat Glo® Sanitizing Teat Dip *(Ecolab Food & Bev. Div.)*, Theratrate™ *(Westfalia•Surge)*, Ultra-Dyne™ *(Westfalia•Surge)*, Xenodine® *(V.P.L.)*, Xenodine® Spray *(V.P.L.)*.

iodine, iodide (potassium). Lugol's Solution *(Butler)*.

iodine, iron, phosphorus, sodium chloride, vitamin A, calcium. Mo' Milk® Feed Mix and Top Dress *(TechMix)*.

iodine, isopropyl alcohol, menthol, wormwood oil, camphor. Dealer Select Horse Care Horse Liniment *(Durvet)*.

iodine, isopropyl alcohol (isopropanol). Iodine Tincture 7% *(Phoenix Pharmaceutical)*, Tincture Iodine 7% *(Aspen)*.

iodine, isopropyl alcohol (isopropanol), iodide (potassium). Iodine 7% Tincture *(AgriLabs)*, Iodine Tincture 7% *(AgriPharm)*, *(Vedco)*, Stronger Iodine Tincture 7% *(Centaur)*, Strong Iodine Tincture *(Butler)*, Strong Iodine Tincture 7% *(Durvet)*, Tincture Iodine 7% *(Bimeda)*.

iodine, isopropyl alcohol (isopropanol), menthol, camphor. Lin-O-Gel® *(Hawthorne)*.

iodine, isopropyl alcohol (isopropanol), menthol, thymol, camphor, iodide (potassium). Equi-Phar™ CoolGel *(Vedco)*.

iodine, isopropyl alcohol (isopropanol), potassium iodide. Iodine Tincture 7% *(First Priority)*.

iodine, isopropyl alcohol (isopropanol), tannic acid, ethylacetate, ethylcellulose. Dr. Naylor® Stop-A-Leak *(H.W. Naylor)*.

iodine, isopropyl alcohol (isopropanol), tannic acid, iodide (potassium). Freezex® Hoof Freeze *(Hawthorne)*.

iodine, isopropyl alcohol (isopropanol), turpentine, camphor, ether. Harold White's® Leg Paint *(Hawthorne)*.

iodine, linseed oil, neatsfoot oil, pine tar, turpentine, wheat germ oil, fish oil. Shur Hoof™ *(Horse Health)*.

iodine, linseed oil, pine tar, turpentine, wheat germ oil, fish oil. Dealer Select Horse Care Hoof Dressing With Brush *(Durvet)*.

iodine, menthol, spearmint oil, witch hazel, alcohol, iodide (potassium). Absorbine® RefreshMint® *(W. F. Young)*.

iodine, menthol, thymol, benzocaine, camphor, iodide (potassium). Equi-Phar™ BenzaGel *(Vedco)*.

iodine, pine tar, ichthammol, iodide (potassium). Sole Pack™ Hoof Dressing *(Hawthorne)*, Sole Pack™ Hoof Packing *(Hawthorne)*.

iodine, pine tar, iodide (potassium). Reducine® Absorbent for Horses *(Equicare)*.

iodine, vitamins. Avian Vitamins Iodized *(ARC)*.

Iodine 7% Tincture *(AgriLabs)*, **iodide (potassium), iodine, isopropyl alcohol (isopropanol).**

I.O. Dine Complex™ Bolus *(PRN Pharmacal)*, **polyvinylpyrrolidone.**

iodine complex (povidone-iodine). Betadine® Solution *(Purdue Frederick)*, Betadine® Surgical Scrub *(Purdue Frederick)*, Bou-Matic Nova Blend VI *(Bou-Matic)*, Controlled Iodine Spray *(Durvet)*, Dairyland Brand Pre-Post 5000 *(Stearns)*, Iodine Scrub *(A.A.H.)*, Iodine Shampoo *(Evsco)*, *(Tomlyn)*, *(Vedco)*, Iodine Topical Solution *(A.A.H.)*, Iofec®-20 Disinfectant *(Loveland)*, "Mild" Iodine Wound Spray *(Centaur)*, Petables™ Clean and Heal Povidone Iodine Bath *(A.A.H.)*, Plexadol™ Shampoo *(Butler)*, Polydine™ Spray *(First Priority)*, Poviderm Medical Scrub *(Vetus)*, Poviderm Medicated Shampoo *(Vetus)*, Poviderm Solution *(Vetus)*, Povidine *(AgriPharm)*, Povidine 0.75% Scrub *(AgriPharm)*, Povidine™ Bolus *(Butler)*, Povidone Iodine Ointment *(First Priority)*, Povidone Iodine Scrub *(First Priority)*, Povidone Iodine Shampoo *(First Priority)*, *(Vedco)*, Povidone Iodine Solution *(First Priority)*, Povidone-Iodine Solution 10% *(Equicare)*, Povidone-Iodine Surgical Scrub 7 1/2% *(Equicare)*, Povidone Scrub *(Butler)*, Povidone Shampoo 5% *(Butler)*, Povidone Solution *(Butler)*, Prodine Ointment *(Phoenix Pharmaceutical)*, Prodine Scrub *(Phoenix Pharmaceutical)*, Prodine Solution *(Phoenix Pharmaceutical)*, PVP Iodine *(Western Chemical)*, PVP Iodine Ointment *(Vedco)*, Response® *(Westfalia•Surge)*, Response II™ *(Westfalia•Surge)*, Rocadyne *(Rochester Midland)*, Teat Guard™ *(Ecolab Food & Bev. Div.)*, Teat Kote 10/III™ *(Westfalia•Surge)*, Vetadine *(Centaur)*, Vetadine Scrub *(Vedco)*, Vetadine Solution *(Vedco)*, Viodine™ Medicated Shampoo *(Equicare)*, V.I.P.-20™ Iodine Shampoo *(Equicare)*, Weladol® Antiseptic Shampoo *(Veterinary Specialties)*, West-Vet® Prepodyne® Scrub *(WestAgro)*, West-Vet® Prepodyne® Solution *(WestAgro)*.

iodine complex (povidone-iodine), aluminum chloride, ammonium chloride, bentonite, copper sulfate, diatomite, ferrous sulfate. Kwik-Stop® Styptic Powder *(ARC)*.

iodine complex (povidone-iodine), chlorhexidine. Monarch® Protek® Teat Dip *(Ecolab Food & Bev. Div.)*.

iodine complex (povidone-iodine), copper sulfate, ferrous sulfate. Clot Powder *(Q.A. Laboratories)*.

iodine complex (povidone-iodine), glycerine. Metz Iodine Teat Dip (0.25%) *(Metz)*, Metz Iodine Teat Dip (0.5%) *(Metz)*, Metz Iodine Teat Dip (1.0%) *(Metz)*, Teat Dip-Lite *(Western Chemical)*, Teat Dip with Glycerin *(Western Chemical)*, Teat-Kote® *(Westfalia•Surge)*, Theraderm® 2500 *(Westfalia•Surge)*, Theratec™ *(Westfalia•Surge)*, Theratec® Plus *(Westfalia•Surge)*, West-Vet® Ultradine® *(WestAgro)*.

iodine complex (povidone-iodine), isopropyl alcohol (isopropanol). Antiseptic Iodine Spray *(Dominion)*, Gentle Iodine 1% *(Aspen)*, "Gentle" Iodine Wound Spray *(Centaur)*, Gentle Iodine Wound Spray *(Vedco)*, Iodine Wound Spray *(AgriLabs)*, Iodine Wound Spray 1.0% *(AgriPharm)*, Iodine Wound Spray 2.44% *(AgriPharm)*.

iodine complex (povidone-iodine), lanolin. Lanodine™ *(Butler)*.

iodine complex (povidone-iodine), lanolin, petrolatum, soybean oil, urea, wheat germ oil, cod liver oil. Vita-Hoof® *(Equicare).*

iodine complex (povidone-iodine), phosphoric acid. Dineotex *(Stearns),* Iosan® *(WestAgro),* K.O. Dyne® *(Westfalia•Surge),* Metz Iodine Detergent *(Metz),* Monarch® Mon-O-Dine *(Ecolab Food & Bev. Div.),* West-Vet® Premise® Disinfectant *(WestAgro).*

iodine complex (povidone-iodine), phosphoric acid, acetic acid. Bou-Matic IO-Wash *(Bou-Matic).*

Iodine Disinfectant *(Durvet),* **iodine.**

Iodine Scrub *(A.A.H.),* **iodine complex (povidone-iodine).**

Iodine Shampoo *(Evsco), (Tomlyn), (Vedco),* **iodine complex (povidone-iodine).**

Iodine Tincture 7% *(AgriPharm),* **iodide (potassium), iodine, isopropyl alcohol (isopropanol).**

Iodine Tincture 7% *(First Priority),* **iodine, isopropyl alcohol (isopropanol), potassium iodide.**

Iodine Tincture 7% *(Phoenix Pharmaceutical),* **iodine, isopropyl alcohol (isopropanol).**

Iodine Tincture 7% *(Vedco),* **iodide (potassium), iodine, isopropyl alcohol (isopropanol).**

Iodine Topical Solution *(A.A.H.),* **iodine complex (povidone-iodine).**

Iodine Wound Spray *(AgriLabs),* **iodine complex (povidone-iodine), isopropyl alcohol (isopropanol).**

Iodine Wound Spray 1.0% *(AgriPharm),* **iodine complex (povidone-iodine), isopropyl alcohol (isopropanol).**

Iodine Wound Spray 2.44% *(AgriPharm),* **iodine complex (povidone-iodine), isopropyl alcohol (isopropanol).**

iodoform, aluminum chloride, ammonium chloride, bentonite, benzocaine, copper sulfate, diatomaceous earth, ferric subsulfate. Clot-It Plus™ *(Evsco),* Nik Stop® Styptic Powder *(Tomlyn).*

iodoform, aluminum chloride, ammonium chloride, bentonite, copper sulfate, diatomite, ferric subsulfate. Blood Stop Powder *(Butler).*

iodoform, tannic acid, activated charcoal, alum, copper sulfate. Wonder Dust™ Wound Powder *(Farnam).*

iodoform, zinc oxide. Happy Jack® Ear Canker Powder *(Happy Jack).*

Iodoject *(Vetus),* **sodium iodide.**

Iofec®-20 Disinfectant *(Loveland),* **iodine complex (povidone-iodine).**

Iosan® *(WestAgro),* **iodine complex (povidone-iodine), phosphoric acid.**

IO-Shield® Sanitizing Barrier Teat Dip *(Ecolab Food & Bev. Div.),* **iodine.**

iron, amino acids. Availa® Fe 60 *(Zinpro).*

iron, calcium, copper. Astringent Bolus *(Butler).*

iron, cobalt sulfate, copper gluconate. Iron-Plus *(Neogen).*

iron, copper. Duriron *(Durvet),* Sav-A-Caf® Finisher Iron *(IntAgra),* Sav-A-Caf® Starter Iron *(IntAgra),* Sav-A-Pig® Oral Iron *(IntAgra).*

iron, liver, minerals, vitamin B_{12}. LIB *(Neogen).*

iron, liver, vitamins. Hi-Vite™ Drops *(Evsco).*

iron, liver extract, vitamins. Ferret Drops™ *(Tomlyn),* Puppy Drops™ *(Tomlyn).*

iron, minerals, selenium, vitamins. Go Max™ Liquid *(Farnam).*

iron, minerals, sorbitol, vitamins. Vi-Sorbin® *(Pfizer Animal Health).*

iron, minerals, vitamins. Red Cell® *(Horse Health).*

iron, petrolatum. Lax'aire® *(Pfizer Animal Health).*

iron, phosphorus, sodium chloride, vitamin A, calcium, iodine. Mo' Milk® Feed Mix and Top Dress *(TechMix).*

iron, vitamin B_{12}. Vitamin B_{12}-Iron Gel™ *(Horses Prefer).*

iron, vitamin B-complex, amino acids, copper. NutriVed™ B-Complex Plus Iron Liquid *(Vedco).*

iron, vitamins. Redglo® *(Equicare),* Vi-Sorbits® *(Pfizer Animal Health).*

iron, vitamins, electrolytes. Pig-95 *(Skylabs).*

iron dextran. AmTech Iron Dextran Injection *(Phoenix Scientific),* AmTech Iron Dextran Injection-200 *(Phoenix Scientific),* Anem-X™ 100 *(AgriPharm),* Anem-X™ 200 *(AgriPharm),* Ferrodex™ 100 *(AgriLabs),* Ferrodex™ 200 *(AgriLabs),* HemaJect 200 *(Vedco),* Iron Dextran-200 *(Durvet),* Iron Dextran Complex *(Premier Farmtech),* Iron Dextran Injection *(Durvet), (Phoenix Pharmaceutical), (Vedco),* Iron Dextran Injection-200 *(Aspen), (Butler), (Phoenix Pharmaceutical),* Iron Hydrogenated Dextran Injection *(Aspen), (V.L.).*

Iron Dextran-200 *(Durvet),* **iron dextran.**

Iron Dextran Complex *(Premier Farmtech),* **iron dextran.**

Iron Dextran Injection *(Durvet), (Phoenix Pharmaceutical), (Vedco),* **iron dextran.**

Iron Dextran Injection-200 *(Aspen), (Butler), (Phoenix Pharmaceutical),* **iron dextran.**

Iron Hydrogenated Dextran Injection *(Aspen), (V.L.),* **iron dextran.**

iron methionine. Meth-Iron 65 *(Zinpro).*

Iron-Plus *(Neogen),* **cobalt sulfate, copper gluconate, iron.**

IsoFlo® *(Abbott),* **isoflurane.**

isoflupredone acetate. Predef® 2X *(Pharmacia & Upjohn).*

isoflupredone acetate, myristyl-gamma-picolinium chloride, neomycin, tetracaine. Neo-Predef® with Tetracaine Powder *(Pharmacia & Upjohn).*

isoflupredone acetate, neomycin, tetracaine. Tritop® *(Pharmacia & Upjohn).*

isoflurane. IsoFlo® *(Abbott),* Isoflurane, USP *(Halocarbon), (Phoenix Pharmaceutical),* Iso-Thesia *(Vetus).*

Isoflurane, USP *(Halocarbon), (Phoenix Pharmaceutical),* **isoflurane.**

isopropyl alcohol. 70% Alcohol Buffered *(Butler).*

isopropyl alcohol, 2-butoxyethanol. Equalizer™ *(Evsco),* See Spot Go!™ *(Tomlyn).*

isopropyl alcohol, lanolin, mineral spirits. Groom-Aid® Spray *(Evsco).*

isopropyl alcohol, menthol, parachlorometaxylenol, thymol, witch hazel, wormwood oil, aloe vera, iodide (potassium). Veterinary Liniment *(First Priority).*

isopropyl alcohol, menthol, wormwood oil, camphor, iodine. Dealer Select Horse Care Horse Liniment *(Durvet).*

isopropyl alcohol, oleoresin capsicum, orange peel bitter, propylene glycol, sucrose octyl acetate. 3-No-Bite Spray *(Vedco),* Bitter-3™ *(Butler).*

isopropyl alcohol, oleoresin capsicum, propylene glycol, sucrose octyl acetate. Bitter Orange™ *(ARC).*

isopropyl alcohol, orange peel bitter, tabasco pepper. Triple-No-Chew *(Q.A. Laboratories),* Triple-No-Chew Spray *(Q.A. Laboratories).*

Isopropyl Alcohol 70% *(AgriLabs), (AgriPharm), (Aspen), (Butler), (Centaur), (Durvet), (First Priority), (Phoenix Pharmaceutical), (Vedco),* **isopropyl alcohol (isopropanol).**

Isopropyl Alcohol 99% *(AgriLabs), (AgriPharm), (Aspen), (Centaur), (First Priority), (Phoenix Pharmaceutical), (Vedco),* **isopropyl alcohol (isopropanol).**

isopropyl alcohol (isopropanol). 70% Isopropyl Alcohol *(Davis),* Isopropyl Alcohol 70% *(AgriLabs), (AgriPharm), (Aspen), (Butler), (Centaur), (Durvet), (First Priority), (Phoenix Pharmaceutical), (Vedco),* Isopropyl Alcohol 99% *(AgriLabs), (AgriPharm), (Aspen), (Centaur), (First Priority), (Phoenix Pharmaceutical), (Vedco),* Isopropyl Rubbing Alcohol U.S.P. *(Dominion).*

isopropyl alcohol (isopropanol), ammonium chloride. MetriGuard® *(Metrex).*

isopropyl alcohol (isopropanol), benzalkonium chloride, chlorothymol. Blue Lotion Topical Antiseptic *(Aspen), (First Priority).*

isopropyl alcohol (isopropanol), benzethonium chloride. V-Tergent® *(Veterinary Specialties).*

isopropyl alcohol (isopropanol), iodide (potassium), iodine. Iodine 7% Tincture *(AgriLabs),* Iodine Tincture 7% *(AgriPharm), (Vedco),* Stronger Iodine Tincture 7% *(Centaur),* Strong Iodine Tincture *(Butler),* Strong Iodine Tincture 7% *(Durvet),* Tincture Iodine 7% *(Bimeda).*

isopropyl alcohol (isopropanol), iodine. Iodine Tincture 7% *(Phoenix Pharmaceutical),* Tincture Iodine 7% *(Aspen).*

isopropyl alcohol (isopropanol), iodine complex (povidone-iodine). Antiseptic Iodine Spray *(Dominion),* Gentle Iodine 1% *(Aspen),* "Gentle" Iodine Wound Spray *(Centaur),* Gentle Iodine Wound Spray *(Vedco),* Iodine Wound Spray *(AgriLabs),* Iodine Wound Spray 1.0% *(AgriPharm),* Iodine Wound Spray 2.44% *(AgriPharm).*

isopropyl alcohol (isopropanol), kaolin, methyl salicylate, peppermint oil, salicylic acid, thymol, arnica, bentonite, boric acid, eucalyptus oil, glycerine. Bigeloil® 24-Hour Medicated Poultice *(W. F. Young).*

isopropyl alcohol (isopropanol), lanolin, lidocaine, propylene glycol, salicylic acid, acetic acid, boric acid, glycerine. Fresh-Ear *(Q.A. Laboratories).*

isopropyl alcohol (isopropanol), lanolin, propylene glycol, salicylic acid, acetic acid, glycerine. OtiClean®-A Ear Cleaning and Deodorant Pads *(ARC).*

isopropyl alcohol (isopropanol), lanolin, propylene glycol, salicylic acid, silicon dioxide, zinc oxide, acetic acid, boric acid. OtiCare®-B Drying Ear Creme *(ARC).*

isopropyl alcohol (isopropanol), lidocaine, propylene glycol, salicylic acid, acetic acid, boric acid, glycerine. Otic Clear *(Butler).*

isopropyl alcohol (isopropanol), menthol, camphor. Ice-O-Gel® *(Hawthorne).*

isopropyl alcohol (isopropanol), menthol, camphor, ether. Shin-O-Gel® *(Hawthorne).*

isopropyl alcohol (isopropanol), menthol, camphor, iodine. Lin-O-Gel® *(Hawthorne).*

isopropyl alcohol (isopropanol), menthol, salicylic acid, tannic acid, boric acid, camphor. Dry-It *(Q.A. Laboratories).*

isopropyl alcohol (isopropanol), menthol, thymol, benzocaine, camphor. Liniment Gel with Benzocaine *(First Priority).*

isopropyl alcohol (isopropanol), menthol, thymol, camphor. Liniment Gel *(First Priority).*

isopropyl alcohol (isopropanol), menthol, thymol, camphor, iodide (potassium), iodine. Equi-Phar™ CoolGel *(Vedco).*

isopropyl alcohol (isopropanol), menthol, thymol, witch hazel, benzocaine, camphor. Benzo-Gel™ *(Butler).*

isopropyl alcohol (isopropanol), mercaptobenzothiazole. Sulfodene® Skin Medication for Dogs *(Combe).*

isopropyl alcohol (isopropanol), methylene blue. Victor Gall Remedy *(Fiebing).*

isopropyl alcohol (isopropanol), methyl salicylate, parachlorometaxylenol, pine oil, scarlet red, benzyl alcohol, eucalyptus oil. Scarlet Oil *(First Priority).*

isopropyl alcohol (isopropanol), methyl salicylate, propylene glycol, zinc undecylenate, acetic acid. Fungi-Dry-Ear *(Q.A. Laboratories).*

isopropyl alcohol (isopropanol), methyl violet, propylene glycol, urea, acriflavine, glycerine. Purple Lotion Wound Dressing *(Durvet).*

isopropyl alcohol (isopropanol), phenol, scarlet red. Dr. Naylor® Red-Kote® *(H.W. Naylor).*

isopropyl alcohol (isopropanol), potassium iodide, iodine. Iodine Tincture 7% *(First Priority).*

isopropyl alcohol (isopropanol), propylene glycol, salicylic acid, acetic acid, glycerine. OtiClean®-A Ear Cleaning Lotion *(ARC)*.

isopropyl alcohol (isopropanol), propylene glycol, sodium propionate, urea, acriflavine, furfural, gentian violet, glycerine. Blue Lotion *(AgriLabs)*.

isopropyl alcohol (isopropanol), propylene glycol, urea, acriflavine, gentian violet, glycerine. Purple Lotion *(Vedco)*, Purple Lotion Wound Dressing *(First Priority)*.

isopropyl alcohol (isopropanol), quaternary ammonia. Cavicide® *(Metrex)*, Kleen-Aseptic® *(Metrex)*.

isopropyl alcohol (isopropanol), tannic acid, benzyl alcohol, crystal violet. Blue Lotion Aerosol *(Boehringer Ingelheim)*.

isopropyl alcohol (isopropanol), tannic acid, ethylacetate, ethylcellulose, iodine. Dr. Naylor® Stop-A-Leak *(H.W. Naylor)*.

isopropyl alcohol (isopropanol), tannic acid, iodide (potassium), iodine. Freezex® Hoof Freeze *(Hawthorne)*.

isopropyl alcohol (isopropanol), tannic acid, turpentine, gentian violet. Happy Jack® Pad Kote *(Happy Jack)*.

isopropyl alcohol (isopropanol), turpentine, camphor, ether, iodine. Harold White's® Leg Paint *(Hawthorne)*.

Isopropyl Rubbing Alcohol U.S.P. *(Dominion)*, **isopropyl alcohol (isopropanol).**

Iso-Thesia *(Vetus)*, **isoflurane.**

Isotone-SA *(Vet-A-Mix)*, **electrolytes, glucose.**

Ivercide™ Equine Paste 1.87% *(Phoenix Pharmaceutical)*, **ivermectin.**

Ivercide™ Injection for Cattle and Swine *(Phoenix Pharmaceutical)*, **ivermectin.**

Ivercide™ Liquid for Horses *(Phoenix Pharmaceutical)*, **ivermectin.**

Ivercide™ Pour-On for Cattle *(Phoenix Pharmaceutical)*, **ivermectin.**

Iverhart™ Plus Flavored Chewables *(Virbac)*, **ivermectin, pyrantel pamoate.**

ivermectin. Acarexx™ *(Idexx Pharm.)*, Agri-Mectin™ Equine Paste Dewormer 1.87% *(AgriLabs)*, AmTech Phoenectin® Injection for Cattle and Swine *(Phoenix Scientific)*, AmTech Phoenectin® Liquid for Horses *(Phoenix Scientific)*, AmTech Phoenectin® Paste 1.87% *(Phoenix Scientific)*, AmTech Phoenectin® Pour-On for Cattle *(Phoenix Scientific)*, Bimectin™ Pour-On *(Bimeda)*, Cooper's® Best Ivermectin Paste 1.87% *(Aspen)*, Double Impact™ *(AgriLabs)*, DVMectin™ Liquid for Horses *(DVM)*, Equimectrin™ Paste 1.87% *(Farnam)*, Equimectrin® Paste 1.87% *(Merial)*, Eqvalan® Liquid *(Merial)*, Eqvalan® Paste 1.87% *(Merial)*, Heartgard® Chewables for Cats *(Merial)*, Heartgard® Chewables for Dogs *(Merial)*, Heartgard® Tablets for Dogs *(Merial)*, Horse Care Ivermectin Paste 1.87% *(Durvet)*, Ivercide™ Equine Paste 1.87% *(Phoenix Pharmaceutical)*, Ivercide™ Injection for Cattle and Swine *(Phoenix Pharmaceutical)*, Ivercide™ Liquid for Horses *(Phoenix Pharmaceutical)*, Ivercide™ Pour-On for Cattle *(Phoenix Pharmaceutical)*, Ivermectin Injection for Cattle and Swine *(Aspen)*, *(Durvet)*, Ivermectin Pour-On *(Aspen)*, *(Durvet)*, Iver-On™ *(Med-Pharmex)*, Iversol *(Med-Pharmex)*, Ivomec® 0.27% Injection for Grower and Feeder Pigs *(Merial)*, Ivomec® 1% Injection for Cattle and Swine *(Merial)*, Ivomec® 1% Injection for Swine *(Merial)*, Ivomec® Pour-On for Cattle *(Merial)*, Ivomec® Premix for Swine Type A Medicated Article *(Merial)*, Ivomec® Sheep Drench *(Merial)*, Ivomec® SR Bolus *(Merial)*, Privermectin™ Drench for Sheep *(First Priority)*, Privermectin™ Equine Oral Liquid *(First Priority)*, Produmec™ Injection for Cattle and Swine *(TradeWinds)*, Produmec™ Pour-On for Cattle *(TradeWinds)*, ProMectin B™ Pour-On For Cattle *(Vedco)*, ProMectin E™ Liquid for Horses *(Vedco)*, ProMectin E™ Paste *(Vedco)*, ProMectin™ Injection for Cattle and Swine *(Vedco)*, Prozap® Ivermectin Pour-On *(Loveland)*, Rotectin™ 1 Paste 1.87% *(Farnam)*, Top Line™ *(AgriLabs)*, UltraMectrin™ Injection *(RXV)*, UltraMectrin™ Pour-On *(RXV)*, Zimecterin® Paste 1.87% *(Farnam)*, *(Merial)*.

ivermectin, clorsulon. Ivomec® Plus Injection for Cattle *(Merial)*.

ivermectin, pyrantel pamoate. Heartgard® Plus Chewables for Dogs *(Merial)*, Iverhart™ Plus Flavored Chewables *(Virbac)*.

Ivermectin Injection for Cattle and Swine *(Aspen)*, *(Durvet)*, **ivermectin.**

Ivermectin Pour-On *(Aspen)*, *(Durvet)*, **ivermectin.**

Iver-On™ *(Med-Pharmex)*, **ivermectin.**

Iversol *(Med-Pharmex)*, **ivermectin.**

Ivomec® 0.27% Injection for Grower and Feeder Pigs *(Merial)*, **ivermectin.**

Ivomec® 1% Injection for Cattle and Swine *(Merial)*, **ivermectin.**

Ivomec® 1% Injection for Swine *(Merial)*, **ivermectin.**

Ivomec® Eprinex® Pour-On for Beef and Dairy Cattle *(Merial)*, **eprinomectin.**

Ivomec® Plus Injection for Cattle *(Merial)*, **clorsulon, ivermectin.**

Ivomec® Pour-On for Cattle *(Merial)*, **ivermectin.**

Ivomec® Premix for Swine Type A Medicated Article *(Merial)*, **ivermectin.**

Ivomec® Sheep Drench *(Merial)*, **ivermectin.**

Ivomec® SR Bolus *(Merial)*, **ivermectin.**

J

jojoba oil, keratin, mink oil, d-l-panthenol (vitamin B_5), detanglers. Lustre Groom Mist™ *(Butler)*.

juniper tar, resorcinol, zinc oxide, bismuth subgallate, bismuth subnitrate, calamine. Pellitol® Ointment *(Veterinary Specialties)*.

Just Born® Milk Replacer for Kittens Powdered Formula *(Farnam)*, **milk replacing formula.**

Just Born® Milk Replacer for Kittens Ready-To-Use Liquid *(Farnam)*, **milk replacing formula.**

Just Born® Milk Replacer for Puppies Powdered Formula *(Farnam)*, **milk replacing formula.**

Just Born® Milk Replacer for Puppies Ready-To-Use Liquid *(Farnam)*, **milk replacing formula.**

K

K9 Advantix™ 10 (imidacloprid/permethrin) For Dogs and Puppies (7 Weeks and Older, 10 lbs. and Under) *(Bayer)*, **imidacloprid, permethrin.**

K9 Advantix™ 20 (imidacloprid/permethrin) For Dogs and Puppies (7 Weeks and Older, 11-20 lbs.) *(Bayer)*, **imidacloprid, permethrin.**

K9 Advantix™ 55 (imidacloprid/permethrin) For Dogs and Puppies (7 Weeks and Older, 21-55 lbs.) *(Bayer)*, **imidacloprid, permethrin.**

K9 Advantix™ 100 (imidacloprid/permethrin) For Dogs and Puppies (7 Weeks and Older, Over 55 lbs.) *(Bayer)*, **imidacloprid, permethrin.**

K-9 Bluelite® *(TechMix)*, **electrolytes, energy source(s), vitamins.**

kanamycin sulfate. Kantrim® *(Fort Dodge)*.

kanamycin sulfate, pectin, attapulgite, bismuth subcarbonate. Amforol® Suspension *(Fort Dodge)*, Amforol® Tablets *(Fort Dodge)*.

Kantrim® *(Fort Dodge)*, **kanamycin sulfate.**

kaolin, activated charcoal. ToxiBan™ Granules *(Vet-A-Mix)*, ToxiBan™ Suspension *(Vet-A-Mix)*.

kaolin, aloe vera, bentonite, boric acid, ferrous sulfate, glycerine. Icetight® *(Horse Health)*, Reducine® Poultice *(Equicare)*.

kaolin, carob. Boltan III™ *(Butler)*.

kaolin, magnesium hydroxide. MVT Powder™ *(Butler)*.

kaolin, methyl salicylate, peppermint oil, salicylic acid, eucalyptus oil, glycerine. Absorbine® Antiphlogistine® *(W. F. Young)*.

kaolin, methyl salicylate, peppermint oil, salicylic acid, thymol, arnica, bentonite, boric acid, eucalyptus oil, glycerine, isopropyl alcohol (isopropanol). Bigeloil® 24-Hour Medicated Poultice *(W. F. Young)*.

kaolin, pectin. Kaolin Pectin *(Bimeda)*, Kaolin-Pectin *(Durvet)*, Kaolin-Pectin Plus *(AgriPharm)*, Kaolin Pectin Suspension *(A.A.H.)*, *(First Priority)*, *(Vedco)*, Kao-Pec *(AgriLabs)*, Kaopectolin *(Aspen)*, Kaopectolin™ *(Butler)*, Kao-Pect+ *(Phoenix Pharmaceutical)*.

kaolin, pectin, aluminum hydroxide. Anti-Diarrhea Tablets *(ARC)*, Diarrhea Tabs *(Butler)*.

kaolin, sorbitol, activated charcoal. ToxiBan™ Suspension with Sorbitol *(Vet-A-Mix)*.

Kaolin Pectin *(Bimeda)*, **kaolin, pectin.**

Kaolin-Pectin *(Durvet)*, **kaolin, pectin.**

Kaolin-Pectin Plus *(AgriPharm)*, **kaolin, pectin.**

Kaolin Pectin Suspension *(A.A.H.)*, *(First Priority)*, *(Vedco)*, **kaolin, pectin.**

Kao-Pec *(AgriLabs)*, **kaolin, pectin.**

Kaopectolin *(Aspen)*, **kaolin, pectin.**

Kaopectolin™ *(Butler)*, **kaolin, pectin.**

Kao-Pect+ *(Phoenix Pharmaceutical)*, **kaolin, pectin.**

Kat-A-Lax* Feline Laxative *(Veterinary Specialties)*, **cod liver oil, petrolatum.**

K-Caps *(Vetus)*, **vitamin K_1 (phytonadione).**

kelp, liver meal, papaya fruit, psyllium. Fiber Forte® Feline *(Life Science)*.

KennelSol™ *(Alpha Tech Pet)*, **quaternary ammonia.**

KenneLSol HC™ *(Alpha Tech Pet)*, **quaternary ammonia.**

KenneLSol-NPV™ *(Alpha Tech Pet)*, **quaternary ammonia.**

KeraSolv® Gel *(DVM)*, **salicylic acid, sodium lactate, urea.**

keratin, mink oil, d-l-panthenol (vitamin B_5), detanglers, jojoba oil. Lustre Groom Mist™ *(Butler)*.

KetaFlo™ *(Abbott)*, **ketamine hydrochloride.**

Ketaject® *(Phoenix Pharmaceutical)*, **ketamine hydrochloride.**

ketamine hydrochloride. AmTech Ketamine Hydrochloride Injection, USP *(Phoenix Scientific)*, KetaFlo™ *(Abbott)*, Ketaject® *(Phoenix Pharmaceutical)*, Ketaset® *(Fort Dodge)*, Keta-Sthetic™ *(RXV)*, Keta-Thesia™ *(Vetus)*, KetaVed™ *(Vedco)*, VetaKet® Injection *(Lloyd)*, Vetalar® *(Fort Dodge)*.

Ketaset® *(Fort Dodge)*, **ketamine hydrochloride.**

Keta-Sthetic™ *(RXV)*, **ketamine hydrochloride.**

Keta-Thesia™ *(Vetus)*, **ketamine hydrochloride.**

KetaVed™ *(Vedco)*, **ketamine hydrochloride.**

Keto Amino Forte™ *(Butler)*, **amino acids, dextrose, electrolytes.**

KetoChlor™ Shampoo *(Virbac)*, **chlorhexidine gluconate, ketoconazole.**

ketoconazole, chlorhexidine gluconate. KetoChlor™ Shampoo *(Virbac)*.

Ketofen® *(Fort Dodge)*, **ketoprofen.**

Keto-Gel™ *(Jorgensen)*, **methionine, propylene glycol, vitamins.**

Keto-Nia-Fresh™ *(Vets Plus)*, **niacin, propylene glycol, vitamin B-complex.**

Keto Oral Gel *(Phoenix Pharmaceutical)*, **cobalt, magnesium, propionic acid, propylene glycol, vitamins.**

Keto Plus Gel™ *(AgriLabs)*, **propylene glycol, vitamins.**

Keto-Plus Gel *(AgriPharm)*, **propylene glycol, vitamins.**
Keto "Plus" Gel *(Durvet)*, **propylene glycol, vitamins.**
Keto Plus Oral Gel *(Butler)*, **propylene glycol, vitamins.**
ketoprofen. Ketofen® *(Fort Dodge)*.
Ketopro Oral Gel *(Vedco)*, **cobalt sulfate, magnesium sulfate, polyethelene glycol, propionic acid, silicon dioxide, vitamins.**
Kiltix® Topical Tick Control *(Bayer)*, **permethrin.**
Kitten Formula *(Vet Solutions)*, **milk replacing formula.**
K-Ject *(Vetus)*, **vitamin K_1 (phytonadione).**
Kleen-Aseptic® *(Metrex)*, **isopropyl alcohol (isopropanol), quaternary ammonia.**
KMR® 2nd Step™ Kitten Weaning Food *(Pet-Ag)*, **weaning formula.**
KMR® Liquid *(Pet-Ag)*, **milk replacing formula.**
KMR® Powder *(Pet-Ag)*, **milk replacing formula.**
K.O. Dyne® *(Westfalia•Surge)*, **iodine complex (povidone-iodine), phosphoric acid.**
K • O • E™, Kennel Odor Eliminator *(Thornell)*, **deodorants, neutralizer(s).**
Kopertox® *(Fort Dodge)*, **copper naphthenate.**
K-Sol *(Alpharma)*, **vitamin K_3 (menadione).**
KV Wound Powder *(KenVet)*, **nitrofurazone.**
Kwik-Stop® Styptic Powder *(ARC)*, **aluminum chloride, ammonium chloride, bentonite, copper sulfate, diatomite, ferrous sulfate, iodine complex (povidone-iodine).**
K-Zyme® Cat Granules *(BioZyme)*, **Aspergillus oryzae fermentation extract, minerals, vitamins.**
K-Zyme® Chewable Dog Tablets *(BioZyme)*, **Aspergillus oryzae fermentation extract, minerals, vitamins.**
K-Zyme® Dog Granules *(BioZyme)*, **Aspergillus oryzae fermentation extract, minerals, vitamins.**

L

lactamide M.E.A., conditioners. Nova Pearls™ Fresh Scent Deodorant Spray for Dogs and Cats *(Tomlyn)*.
lactase enzymes, microorganisms. BP-1 Special Blend *(AgriPharm)*, PP-1 Special Blend *(AgriPharm)*, RXV-PP-1 (Porcine Probiotic Paste) *(AgriPharm)*.
lactase enzymes, microorganisms, vitamin A, vitamin E. Good Start Calf Bolus *(AgriPharm)*, Good Start Calf Paste *(AgriPharm)*.
Lactated Ringers *(Vet Tek)*, **calcium, potassium chloride, sodium chloride, sodium lactate.**
Lactated Ringers Injection *(Phoenix Pharmaceutical)*, **calcium, potassium chloride, sodium chloride, sodium lactate.**
Lactated Ringer's Injection *(Vedco)*, **calcium, potassium chloride, sodium chloride, sodium lactate.**
Lactated Ringers Injection *(Vetus)*, **calcium, potassium chloride, sodium chloride, sodium lactate.**
Lactated Ringers Injection SC *(Butler)*, **calcium, potassium chloride, sodium chloride, sodium lactate.**
Lactated Ringer's Injection, USP *(AgriLabs)*, *(Bimeda)*, **calcium, potassium chloride, sodium chloride, sodium lactate.**
Lactated Ringer's Solution *(RXV)*, **calcium, potassium chloride, sodium chloride, sodium lactate.**
lactic acid. 4XLA® Germicidal Pre- & Post-Milking Teat Dip (Activator) *(Alcide)*, Bi-Sept™ Activator *(Westfalia•Surge)*, InterSept™ Activator *(Westfalia•Surge)*, Uddergold® Germicidal Barrier Teat Dip (Activator) *(Alcide)*.
lactic acid, benzalkonium chloride, chitosanide. Etiderm® Shampoo *(Virbac)*.
lactic acid, propylene glycol, salicylic acid. Gent-L-Clens™ *(Schering-Plough)*.
lactic acid, propylene glycol, salicylic acid, chitosanide, docusate sodium (dioctyl sodium sulfosuccinate). Epi-Otic® *(Virbac)*.
lactic acid, propylene glycol, urea, benzalkonium chloride, glycerine. Humilac® Spray *(Virbac)*.
lactic acid, sodium linear alkylate sulfonate, hydrogen peroxide. Oxy-Gard™ Activated Peroxide Sanitizing Teat Dip *(Ecolab Food & Bev. Div.)*.
lactic acid, urea, chitosanide, glycerine. Allergroom® Shampoo *(Virbac)*.
lactic acid producing bacteria, electrolytes, glucose. SureLytes™ Plus Carbo Load *(SureNutrition)*.
lactic acid producing bacteria, minerals, vitamins, amino acids. MultiMax™ *(SureNutrition)*.
lactic acid producing bacteria, minerals, vitamins, yeast. T.D.N. Mini Rockets *(DVM Formula)*, T.D.N. Mini Rockets™ *(Vets Plus)*, T.D.N. Rockets *(DVM Formula)*, T.D.N. Rockets™ *(Vets Plus)*.
lactoperoxidase, glucose oxidase. C.E.T.® Chews for Cats *(Virbac)*, C.E.T.® Enzymatic Tartar Control Toothpaste *(Virbac)*, C.E.T.® Enzymatic Toothpaste *(Virbac)*.
lactose, lecithin, minerals, vitamins, whey, fat product(s). Start To Finish® Mare Replacer™ *(Milk Specialties)*.
lactose, milk protein, minerals, vitamins. Multi-Milk™ *(Pet-Ag)*.
lactose, milk protein, minerals, vitamins, yeast, fat product(s). Start To Finish® Mare & Foal Pellets™ *(Milk Specialties)*.
laidlomycin. Cattlyst® 50 *(Alpharma)*.
Lamb & Kid Paste *(Durvet)*, **microorganisms.**
lambdacyhalothrin. Grenade® ER Premise Insecticide *(Schering-Plough)*, Saber™ Pour-On Insecticide *(Schering-Plough)*.
lambdacyhalothrin, piperonyl butoxide. Saber™ Extra Insecticide Ear Tags *(Schering-Plough)*.
lambdacyhalothrin, pirimiphos. Double Barrel™ VP Insecticide Ear Tags *(Schering-Plough)*.
Land O Lakes® Instant Amplifier® Max *(Land O'Lakes)*, **neomycin, oxytetracycline, vitamins.**
Land O Lakes® Instant Amplifier® Select *(Land O'Lakes)*, **neomycin, oxytetracycline, vitamins.**
Land O Lakes® Instant Amplifier® Select Plus *(Land O'Lakes)*, **milk replacing formula.**
Land O Lakes® Instant Cow's Match™ *(Land O'Lakes)*, **neomycin, oxytetracycline.**
Land O Lakes® Instant Kid Milk Replacer *(Land O'Lakes)*, **milk replacing formula.**
Land O Lakes® Instant Maxi Care® *(Land O'Lakes)*, **neomycin, oxytetracycline, vitamins.**
Land O Lakes® Instant Nursing Formula *(Land O'Lakes)*, **neomycin, oxytetracycline.**
Land O Lakes® LitterMilk® *(Land O'Lakes)*, **neomycin, oxytetracycline, vitamins.**
Land O Lakes® Mare's Match® *(Land O'Lakes)*, **milk replacing formula.**
Land O Lakes® Mare's Match® Foal Pellets *(Land O'Lakes)*, **milk, whey.**
Land O Lakes® Ultra Fresh® Lamb Milk Replacer *(Land O'Lakes)*, **milk replacing formula.**
Lanodine™ *(Butler)*, **iodine complex (povidone-iodine), lanolin.**
lanolin, beeswax, comfrey, emollient(s). Equi-Phar™ Miracle Heel *(Vedco)*.
lanolin, conditioners. QuikClean™ Waterless Shampoo *(Fort Dodge)*.
lanolin, iodine complex (povidone-iodine). Lanodine™ *(Butler)*.
lanolin, lidocaine, propylene glycol, salicylic acid, acetic acid, boric acid, glycerine, isopropyl alcohol (isopropanol). Fresh-Ear *(Q.A. Laboratories)*.
lanolin, mineral spirits, isopropyl alcohol. Groom-Aid® Spray *(Evsco)*.
lanolin, moisturizer(s), PABA sun screen, vitamins, aloe vera. Medicated Udder Balm *(First Priority)*.
lanolin, neatsfoot oil, petrolatum, pine tar, turpentine. Absorbine® Hooflex® Liquid Conditioner *(W. F. Young)*.
lanolin, neatsfoot oil, pine tar, turpentine. Absorbine® Hooflex® Original Conditioner *(W. F. Young)*.
lanolin, neatsfoot oil, vitamins, aloe vera. Absorbine® Hooflex® Moisturizing Creme *(W. F. Young)*.
lanolin, petrolatum, 8-hydroxyquinolone. Dr. Naylor® Udder Balm *(H.W. Naylor)*.
lanolin, petrolatum, aloe vera, beeswax, emulsifying wax, glycerine. Dealer Select Horse Care Hoof Moisturizer *(Durvet)*.
lanolin, petrolatum, soybean oil, urea, wheat germ oil, cod liver oil, iodine complex (povidone-iodine). Vita-Hoof® *(Equicare)*.
lanolin, petrolatum, vitamin A, vitamin D, benzethonium chloride, cetyl alcohol. Udder Ointment™ *(LeGear)*.
lanolin, propylene glycol, salicylic acid, acetic acid, glycerine, isopropyl alcohol (isopropanol). OtiClean®-A Ear Cleaning and Deodorant Pads *(ARC)*.
lanolin, propylene glycol, salicylic acid, silicon dioxide, zinc oxide, acetic acid, boric acid, isopropyl alcohol (isopropanol). OtiCare®-B Drying Ear Creme *(ARC)*.
lanolin, rotenone, benzocaine. Goodwinol Ointment *(Goodwinol)*.
lanolin, shampoo formula. Blue Snow™ *(Schering-Plough)*.
lanolin, tromethamine, EDTA (tetrasodium). T8 Solution™ Ear Rinse *(DVM)*.
lanolin, vitamins, aloe vera. -50 Below *(AgriPharm)*.
Larvadex® 1% Premix *(Novartis)*, **cyromazine.**
Larvadex® 2SL *(Novartis)*, **cyromazine.**
lasalocid sodium. Advance™ Calvita® Supreme Medicated A.M. Milk Replacer with Bovatec® *(Milk Specialties)*, Avatec® *(Alpharma)*, Bovatec® 68 *(Alpharma)*, Bovatec® 150 FP *(Alpharma)*, Bovatec® Liquid 20 *(Alpharma)*, MoorMan's® Beef Cattle Boost® BT *(ADM)*, MoorMan's® Special Mix Cattle Boost® BT *(ADM)*, Pro-Bac-C *(AgriLabs)*.
Laxade Bolus *(AgriPharm)*, **magnesium hydroxide.**
Laxade Powder *(AgriPharm)*, **magnesium hydroxide.**
Lax'aire® *(Pfizer Animal Health)*, **iron, petrolatum.**
Laxa-Stat™ *(Tomlyn)*, **mineral oil, petrolatum.**
Laxatone® & Tuna Flavor Laxatone® *(Evsco)*, **petrolatum.**
Laxatone® for Cats *(Tomlyn)*, **mineral oil, petrolatum.**
Laxatone® for Ferrets & Other Small Animals *(Tomlyn)*, **mineral oil, petrolatum.**
LD® 1 Udder Wash Base Concentrate *(Alcide)*, **sodium chlorite.**
LD® 2 Udder Wash Activator Concentrate *(Alcide)*, **organic acid.**
LDC-19™ *(Intercon)*, **quaternary ammonia.**
lecithin, minerals, vitamins, whey, fat product(s), lactose. Start To Finish® Mare Replacer™ *(Milk Specialties)*.
lecithin, phospholipids, vitamins, glycolipids. Dyna-Lode® Equine Supplement *(Harlmen)*.
Legacy® *(AgriLabs)*, **gentamicin.**
Legend® (hyaluronate sodium) Injectable Solution (20 mg) *(Bayer)*, **hyaluronic acid (sodium hyaluronate).**

Legend® (hyaluronate sodium) Injectable Solution (40 mg) *(Bayer)*, **hyaluronic acid (sodium hyaluronate).**

levamisole. AmTech Levamisole Phosphate Injectable Solution *(Phoenix Scientific)*, Levamisole Injectable *(AgriLabs)*, Levamisole Phosphate *(Durvet)*, Levamisole Phosphate Injectable Solution, 13.65% *(AgriPharm)*, *(Aspen)*, Levamisole Soluble Pig Wormer *(AgriLabs)*, Levasole® Cattle Wormer Boluses *(Schering-Plough)*, Levasole® Injectable Solution, 13.65% *(Schering-Plough)*, Levasole® Sheep Wormer Boluses *(Schering-Plough)*, Levasole® Soluble Drench Powder *(Schering-Plough)*, Levasole® Soluble Drench Powder (Sheep) *(Schering-Plough)*, Levasole® Soluble Pig Wormer *(Schering-Plough)*, Prohibit® Soluble Drench Powder *(AgriLabs)*, Totalon® Pour-On Dewormer *(Schering-Plough)*.

Levamisole Injectable *(AgriLabs)*, **levamisole.**

Levamisole Phosphate *(Durvet)*, **levamisole.**

Levamisole Phosphate Injectable Solution, 13.65% *(AgriPharm)*, *(Aspen)*, **levamisole.**

Levamisole Soluble Pig Wormer *(AgriLabs)*, **levamisole.**

Levasole® Cattle Wormer Boluses *(Schering-Plough)*, **levamisole.**

Levasole® Injectable Solution, 13.65% *(Schering-Plough)*, **levamisole.**

Levasole® Sheep Wormer Boluses *(Schering-Plough)*, **levamisole.**

Levasole® Soluble Drench Powder *(Schering-Plough)*, **levamisole.**

Levasole® Soluble Drench Powder (Sheep) *(Schering-Plough)*, **levamisole.**

Levasole® Soluble Pig Wormer *(Schering-Plough)*, **levamisole.**

Levo-Powder *(Vetus)*, **levothyroxine.**

Levotabs *(Vetus)*, **levothyroxine.**

levothyroxine. AmTech Levothyroxine Sodium Tablets *(Phoenix Scientific)*, Canine Thyroid Chewable Tablets *(Pala-Tech)*, Equine Thyroid Supplement *(Pala-Tech)*, Levo-Powder *(Vetus)*, Levotabs *(Vetus)*, Levoxine™ Powder *(First Priority)*, NutriVed™ T-4 Chewable Tablets *(Vedco)*, Soloxine® *(King Animal Health)*, T-4 Powder *(Neogen)*, Thyro-L® *(Vet-A-Mix)*, Thyrosyn Tablets *(Vedco)*, Thyro-Tabs® *(Vet-A-Mix)*, Thyroxine-L Powder *(Butler)*, Thyroxine-L Tablets *(Butler)*, Thyrozine *(RXV)*, Thyrozine Powder *(Phoenix Pharmaceutical)*, Thyrozine Tablets *(Phoenix Pharmaceutical)*.

Levoxine™ Powder *(First Priority)*, **levothyroxine.**

LIB *(Neogen)*, **iron, liver, minerals, vitamin B_{12}.**

Lickables™ Charge Up!™ *(A.A.H.)*, **antioxidants, fatty acids (omega), minerals, soy protein, vitamins.**

Lickables™ Hairball Relief *(A.A.H.)*, **petrolatum.**

Lickables™ Hairball Relief Caviar Flavored *(A.A.H.)*, **petrolatum.**

Lickables™ Hearty Cat™ *(A.A.H.)*, **antioxidants, minerals, taurine, vitamins.**

Lickables™ Hearty Dog™ *(A.A.H.)*, **antioxidants, minerals, vitamins.**

Lickables™ Super Charger™ *(A.A.H.)*, **antioxidants, fatty acids (omega), minerals, vitamins.**

lidocaine. AmTech Lidocaine HCl Injectable-2% *(Phoenix Scientific)*, Biocaine® *(Tomlyn)*, DermaCool® with Lidocaine HCl Spray *(Virbac)*, Hexa-Caine *(PRN Pharmacal)*, Lidocaine 2% Injectable *(Bimeda)*, *(Butler)*, Lidocaine HCl 2% *(RXV)*, Lidocaine HCl Injectable 2% *(Aspen)*, Lidocaine Hydrochloride 2% *(Vet Tek)*, Lidocaine Hydrochloride Injectable-2% *(Phoenix Pharmaceutical)*, Lidocaine Hydrochloride Injection 2% *(AgriLabs)*, Lidocaine Injectable 2% *(Vedco)*, Lidoject *(Vetus)*.

lidocaine, benzalkonium chloride. Allerspray™ *(Evsco)*.

lidocaine, benzalkonium chloride, denatonium benzoate. Allercaine™ *(Tomlyn)*.

lidocaine, chlorhexidine, denatonium benzoate. Hexaseptic Flush Plus *(Vetus)*.

lidocaine, malic acid, propylene glycol, zolazepam, benzoic acid, chlorhexidine, glycerine. Chlor-A-Clens-L Cleansing Solution *(Vedco)*.

lidocaine, malic acid, salicylic acid, benzoic acid, chlorhexidine. Dermachlor™ Plus *(Butler)*.

lidocaine, propylene glycol, salicylic acid, acetic acid, boric acid, glycerine, isopropyl alcohol (isopropanol). Otic Clear *(Butler)*.

lidocaine, propylene glycol, salicylic acid, acetic acid, boric acid, glycerine, isopropyl alcohol (isopropanol), lanolin. Fresh-Ear *(Q.A. Laboratories)*.

Lidocaine 2% Injectable *(Bimeda)*, *(Butler)*, **lidocaine.**

Lidocaine HCl 2% *(RXV)*, **lidocaine.**

Lidocaine HCl Injectable 2% *(Aspen)*, **lidocaine.**

Lidocaine Hydrochloride 2% *(Vet Tek)*, **lidocaine.**

Lidocaine Hydrochloride Injectable-2% *(Phoenix Pharmaceutical)*, **lidocaine.**

Lidocaine Hydrochloride Injection 2% *(AgriLabs)*, **lidocaine.**

Lidocaine Injectable 2% *(Vedco)*, **lidocaine.**

Lidoject *(Vetus)*, **lidocaine.**

Lifegard® 256 Plus *(Rochester Midland)*, **quaternary ammonia.**

Lifegard® 800 *(Rochester Midland)*, **polymeric dispersant, potassium hydroxide, sodium metasilicate.**

Lifegard® 855 Plus *(Rochester Midland)*, **detergent mixture, potassium hydroxide, sodium hypochlorite, sodium metasilicate, sodium silicate.**

Lifegard® 900 *(Rochester Midland)*, **detergent mixture, EDTA (tetrasodium).**

Lifegard® 7000 *(Rochester Midland)*, **detergent mixture, phosphoric acid.**

Lifegard® 7500F *(Rochester Midland)*, **detergent mixture, phosphoric acid.**

Lifegard® 7700 *(Rochester Midland)*, **detergent mixture, phosphoric acid.**

Lifegard® 7700ND *(Rochester Midland)*, **detergent mixture, phosphoric acid.**

limonene. Adams™ D-Limonene Flea & Tick Shampoo *(Farnam)*, D'Limonene Dip *(Davis)*, D'Limonene Shampoo *(Davis)*, VIP® Flea Control Shampoo *(V.P.L.)*, VIP® Flea Dip *(V.P.L.)*.

limonene, b-ionone. MycAseptic® *(Neogen)*, MycAseptic® E *(Neogen)*.

linalool, n-octyl bicycloheptene dicarboximide, permethrin, pyriproxyfen. Adams™ Inverted Carpet Spray *(Farnam)*, Sergeant's® PreTect® Household Flea & Tick Spray *(Sergeant's)*.

linalool, permethrin, piperonyl butoxide, pyriproxyfen. Sergeant's® PreTect® Indoor Flea & Tick Fogger *(Sergeant's)*.

linalool, piperonyl butoxide, pyrethrins, pyriproxyfen. Adams™ Carpet Powder *(Farnam)*, Sergeant's® PreTect® Flea & Tick Carpet Powder *(Sergeant's)*.

Lincocin Aquadrops® Liquid *(Pharmacia & Upjohn)*, **lincomycin hydrochloride.**

Lincocin® Injectable *(AgriLabs)*, **lincomycin hydrochloride.**

Lincocin® Sterile Solution *(Durvet)*, **lincomycin hydrochloride.**

Lincocin® Sterile Solution (Dogs and Cats) *(Pharmacia & Upjohn)*, **lincomycin hydrochloride.**

Lincocin® Sterile Solution (Swine) *(Pharmacia & Upjohn)*, **lincomycin hydrochloride.**

Lincocin® Tablets *(Pharmacia & Upjohn)*, **lincomycin hydrochloride.**

Lincomix® 20 Feed Medication *(Pharmacia & Upjohn)*, **lincomycin hydrochloride.**

Lincomix® 50 Feed Medication *(Pharmacia & Upjohn)*, **lincomycin hydrochloride.**

Lincomix® Injectable *(Pharmacia & Upjohn)*, **lincomycin hydrochloride.**

Lincomix® Soluble Powder *(Pharmacia & Upjohn)*, **lincomycin hydrochloride.**

lincomycin hydrochloride. Lincocin Aquadrops® Liquid *(Pharmacia & Upjohn)*, Lincocin® Injectable *(AgriLabs)*, Lincocin® Sterile Solution *(Durvet)*, Lincocin® Sterile Solution (Dogs and Cats) *(Pharmacia & Upjohn)*, Lincocin® Sterile Solution (Swine) *(Pharmacia & Upjohn)*, Lincocin® Tablets *(Pharmacia & Upjohn)*, Lincomix® 20 Feed Medication *(Pharmacia & Upjohn)*, Lincomix® 50 Feed Medication *(Pharmacia & Upjohn)*, Lincomix® Injectable *(Pharmacia & Upjohn)*, Lincomix® Soluble Powder *(Pharmacia & Upjohn)*, Lincomycin Hydrochloride Soluble Powder *(Durvet)*, Lincomycin Soluble *(Alpharma)*, Lincomycin Soluble Powder *(AgriLabs)*, Lincosol Soluble Powder *(Med-Pharmex)*, MoorMan's® LN 10 *(ADM)*.

lincomycin hydrochloride, spectinomycin. Linco-Spectin® Sterile Solution *(Pharmacia & Upjohn)*, L-S 50 Water Soluble® Powder *(Pharmacia & Upjohn)*.

Lincomycin Hydrochloride Soluble Powder *(Durvet)*, **lincomycin hydrochloride.**

Lincomycin Soluble *(Alpharma)*, **lincomycin hydrochloride.**

Lincomycin Soluble Powder *(AgriLabs)*, **lincomycin hydrochloride.**

Lincosol Soluble Powder *(Med-Pharmex)*, **lincomycin hydrochloride.**

Linco-Spectin® Sterile Solution *(Pharmacia & Upjohn)*, **lincomycin hydrochloride, spectinomycin.**

Liniment Gel *(First Priority)*, **camphor, isopropyl alcohol (isopropanol), menthol, thymol.**

Liniment Gel with Benzocaine *(First Priority)*, **benzocaine, camphor, isopropyl alcohol (isopropanol), menthol, thymol.**

Lin-O-Gel® *(Hawthorne)*, **camphor, iodine, isopropyl alcohol (isopropanol), menthol.**

linoleic acid, linolenic acid, vitamin A, vitamin B_6, vitamin E, arachidonic acid. Mirra-Coat® for Cats *(Pet-Ag)*.

linoleic acid, linolenic acid, vitamin A, vitamin B_6, vitamin E, biotin. Mirra-Coat® Powder and Liquid *(Pet-Ag)*.

linoleic acid, vitamin A, vitamin B_6, vitamin E, zinc. Mirra-Coat® (Equine System) *(Pet-Ag)*.

linoleic acid, vitamin A, vitamin D, vitamin E, fat product(s). Fastbreak™ Plus™ *(Boehringer Ingelheim)*.

linolenic acid, minerals, taurine, vitamins. Mrs. Allen's Vita Care® Vitamins for Cats *(Farnam)*, Show Winner!™ Cat Vitamins *(Farnam)*.

linolenic acid, minerals, vitamins. Mrs. Allen's Vita Care® Vitamins for Dogs *(Farnam)*, Nutra-Sure™ Cat Vitamins *(Farnam)*, Pet Vites *(Vetus)*, Show Winner!™ Dog Vitamins *(Farnam)*, Show Winner!™ Kitten Vitamins *(Farnam)*, Show Winner!™ Older Dog Vitamins *(Farnam)*, Show Winner!™ Puppy Vitamins *(Farnam)*.

linolenic acid, vitamin A, vitamin B_6, vitamin E, arachidonic acid, linoleic acid. Mirra-Coat® for Cats *(Pet-Ag)*.

linolenic acid, vitamin A, vitamin B_6, vitamin E, biotin, linoleic acid. Mirra-Coat® Powder and Liquid *(Pet-Ag)*.

linseed oil, neatsfoot oil, pine tar, turpentine, wheat germ oil, fish oil, iodine. Shur Hoof™ *(Horse Health)*.

linseed oil, pine tar, turpentine, wheat germ oil, fish oil, iodine. Dealer Select Horse Care Hoof Dressing With Brush *(Durvet)*.

lipase, protease, amylase. Pancrezyme® *(King Animal Health)*, Viokase®-V Powder *(Fort Dodge)*, Viokase®-V Tablets *(Fort Dodge)*.

lipase, protease, vitamin A, vitamin D, vitamin E, amylase. PanaKare™ Plus Powder *(Neogen)*, PanaKare™ Plus Tablets *(Neogen)*.

lipase, protease, vitamins, amylase. Pancreatic Plus Powder *(Butler)*, Pancreatic Plus Tablets *(Butler)*, PancreVed Powder *(Vedco)*, PancreVed Tablets *(Vedco)*.

lipids, minerals, vitamins, choline. Geri-Form *(Vet-A-Mix)*.

Lipocaps *(Vetus)*, **choline bitartrate, inositol, liver, racemethionine, vitamin B-complex.**

Lipo-Form *(Vet-A-Mix)*, **choline, fatty acids (essential), methionine (d-l), vitamins.**
Lipotinic *(Vet-A-Mix)*, **niacin, vitamin B-complex.**
lipotropics, liver, vitamin B-complex. Methocol™ Capsules *(Life Science).*
Liquamycin® LA-200® *(Pfizer Animal Health)*, **oxytetracycline.**
Liquatone™ *(Westfalia•Surge)*, **quaternary ammonia.**
Liquical™ *(Butler)*, **energy source(s), vitamins.**
Liqui-Char®-Vet *(King Animal Health)*, **activated charcoal.**
Liqui-Char®-Vet with Sorbitol *(King Animal Health)*, **activated charcoal, sorbitol.**
Liquid Asp-Rin™ *(AgriLabs)*, **salicylate (sodium).**
Liquid B Complex *(Alpharma)*, **vitamin B-complex.**
Liquid Vitamin Premix *(Alpharma)*, **vitamins.**
Liqui-Lube *(Vetus)*, **carboxy methylcellulose, propylene glycol.**
Liqui-Prin™ *(AgriPharm), (First Priority)*, **salicylate (sodium).**
liver, minerals, vitamin B$_{12}$, iron. LIB *(Neogen).*
liver, racemethionine, vitamin B-complex, choline bitartrate, inositol. Lipocaps *(Vetus).*
liver, vitamin B-complex, lipotropics. Methocol™ Capsules *(Life Science).*
liver, vitamins, iron. Hi-Vite™ Drops *(Evsco).*
Liver 7 Injection *(Neogen)*, **vitamin B-complex.**
liver extract, vitamins, iron. Ferret Drops™ *(Tomlyn)*, Puppy Drops™ *(Tomlyn).*
liver meal, papaya fruit, psyllium, kelp. Fiber Forte® Feline *(Life Science).*
Lixotinic® *(Pfizer Animal Health)*, **minerals, vitamins.**
l-lysine, methionine (d-l), vitamin B$_6$, biotin. H.B. 15™ *(Farnam).*
Longlife® 90 Day™ Brand Collar for Cats *(Hartz Mountain)*, **tetrachlorvinphos.**
Longlife® 90 Day™ Brand Collar for Dogs *(Hartz Mountain)*, **tetrachlorvinphos.**
Louse Powder with Rabon® *(LeGear)*, **tetrachlorvinphos.**
L-S 50 Water Soluble® Powder *(Pharmacia & Upjohn)*, **lincomycin hydrochloride, spectinomycin.**
Lubiseptol *(AgriPharm)*, **carboxy methylcellulose, propylene glycol.**
lubricating jelly. General Lube *(A.A.H.), (Aspen).*
lubricating powder. Ag-Tek® Poly-Lube™ *(Kane).*
Lubri-Nert™ *(Life Science)*, **aqueous base lubricant(s).**
Lubrivet™ *(Butler)*, **carboxy methylcellulose, propylene glycol.**
lufenuron. Program® 6 Month Injectable for Cats *(Novartis)*, Program® Flavor Tabs® *(Novartis)*, Program® Suspension *(Novartis).*
lufenuron, milbemycin oxime. Sentinel® Flavor Tabs® *(Novartis).*
Lugol's Solution *(Butler)*, **iodide (potassium), iodine.**
Lustre Groom Mist™ *(Butler)*, **d-l-panthenol (vitamin B$_5$), detanglers, jojoba oil, keratin, mink oil.**
Lutalyse® Sterile Solution *(Pharmacia & Upjohn)*, **dinoprost (prostaglandin F$_{2\alpha}$).**
LymDyp™ *(DVM)*, **sulfurated lime.**
Lysol® Brand I.C.™ Quaternary Disinfectant Cleaner *(Reckitt Benckiser)*, **quaternary ammonia.**
Lysol® Brand II I.C.™ Disinfectant Spray *(Reckitt Benckiser)*, **ethanol, quaternary ammonia.**
LyTar® Shampoo *(DVM)*, **coal tar, salicylic acid, sulfur.**

M

Magnalax Bolus *(Phoenix Pharmaceutical)*, **magnesium oxide.**
Magnalax Boluses *(Aspen), (Bimeda), (First Priority)*, **magnesium hydroxide.**
Magnalax Powder *(Bimeda), (Phoenix Pharmaceutical), (Vedco)*, **magnesium hydroxide.**
Magna-Lyte *(First Priority)*, **dextrose, electrolytes.**
Magnapaste™ *(Butler)*, **magnesium sulfate, methyl salicylate.**
Magna-Poultice™ *(First Priority)*, **magnesium sulfate, methyl salicylate.**
magnesium, calcium. Absorbine® ProCMC® *(W. F. Young).*
magnesium, calcium, cobalt. Cal "62" Plus Gel *(Aspen)*, Calcium Oral Gel *(Phoenix Pharmaceutical)*, Calcium Plus *(First Priority)*, Cal-Gel™ *(Jorgensen).*
magnesium, phosphoric acid, potassium, calcium. CMPK Oral Solution 33% *(Vedco).*
magnesium, phosphorus, calcium, dextrose. Cal-Phos #2 Injection *(AgriLabs)*, Cal-Phos Forte *(Bimeda).*
magnesium, phosphorus, potassium, calcium. AmTech CMPK Injection *(Phoenix Scientific)*, CMPK Bolus *(Durvet), (Vets Plus)*, C.M.P.K. Oral Gel *(Phoenix Pharmaceutical)*, Oral CPMK Gel *(First Priority).*
magnesium, phosphorus, potassium, sodium chloride, zinc. Swine Acid-O-Lite™ *(TechMix).*
magnesium, phosphorus, potassium, vitamin D$_3$, calcium. CMPK with D$_3$ Drench *(Vets Plus).*
magnesium, phosphorus, potassium, vitamins, calcium. Mega CMPK Bolus *(AgriPharm)*, Slow Release CMPK Bolus *(PRN Pharmacal).*
magnesium, potassium, propylene glycol, vitamin B-complex, calcium. Super Calcium Drench *(Vedco).*
magnesium, potassium, propylene glycol, vitamins, calcium. Calcium Drench Plus Vitamins *(AgriLabs), (Durvet).*
magnesium, potassium, vitamins, calcium. Calcium Drench *(AgriPharm).*
magnesium, propionic acid, propylene glycol, vitamins, cobalt. Keto Oral Gel *(Phoenix Pharmaceutical).*
magnesium, propylene glycol, vitamins, cobalt. Oral Keto Energel *(First Priority).*
magnesium, selenium, calcium, cobalt. Cal M 64 Plus Se *(Butler)*, Cal-Mag-SE Gel *(Durvet).*
magnesium, selenium, vitamin B-complex, calcium, cobalt. Calcium SE *(First Priority).*
magnesium, selenium, vitamins, calcium. Cal-Mag-SV Gel *(Butler).*
magnesium, selenium, vitamins, calcium, cobalt. Calcium Gel+Selenium *(AgriLabs)*, Cal Ox 64 Plus SE *(AgriPharm)*, CalOx 64 SE Oral Gel *(Vedco).*
magnesium, sulfur. MagSalt™ *(SSI Corp.).*
magnesium borogluconate, calcium, calcium hypophosphite, dextrose. Norcalciphos™ *(Pfizer Animal Health).*
magnesium borogluconate, calcium borogluconate, calcium hypophosphite, dextrose. Ca-P I.V. Therapy *(RXV).*
magnesium borogluconate, phosphorus, calcium, dextrose. Cal Dex #2 *(AgriLabs)*, Cal-Dextro® No. 2 *(Fort Dodge)*, Cal-Dextro® Special *(Fort Dodge).*
magnesium borogluconate, potassium chloride, calcium, calcium hypophosphite, dextrose. Cal-MPK 1234™ *(Butler).*
magnesium borogluconate, potassium chloride, sodium hypophosphite, calcium, dextrose. Cal-Dex C-M-P-K *(AgriLabs)*, Cal Dex CMPK Injection *(Aspen)*, Cal-MPK™ 1080 Injection *(Butler)*, CMPK *(RXV)*, CMPK-Dex *(Vetus)*, C-M-P-K Injection *(Vet Tek).*
magnesium borogluconate, potassium chloride, sodium hypophosphite, calcium borogluconate, dextrose. CMPK Solution *(Bimeda).*
magnesium chloride, calcium, calcium hypophosphite, dextrose. Cal-MP 1700™ *(Butler).*
magnesium chloride, calcium, cobalt sulfate. Cal-Mag-Co Gel *(Durvet)*, Respond *(Jorgensen)*, Super Calcium Gel "62" *(AgriPharm).*
magnesium chloride, phosphoric acid, potassium chloride, trisodium phosphate, calcium. CMPK Gel *(AgriPharm).*
magnesium chloride, phosphorus, potassium chloride, calcium. C.M.P.K. Gel *(AgriLabs)*, CMPK Gel *(Vedco).*
magnesium chloride, phosphorus, potassium chloride, calcium, dextrose. Oral Cal MPK *(Durvet).*
magnesium chloride, potassium chloride, calcium, calcium phosphate. CMPK Gel Plus™ *(Vets Plus).*
magnesium chloride, potassium chloride, propylene glycol, sodium hypophosphite, calcium. 40% CMPK with D$_3$ Oral Drench *(DVM Formula)*, Oral Calcium Drench *(DVM Formula).*
magnesium chloride, potassium chloride, propylene glycol, sodium hypophosphite, vitamin D$_3$, calcium. CMPK D$_3$ Drench *(Durvet).*
magnesium chloride, potassium chloride, sodium acetate, sodium chloride, sodium gluconate. AmTech Amisol-R Injection *(Phoenix Scientific)*, Bimesol-R™ Injection *(Bimeda)*, ElectroSol-R *(Phoenix Pharmaceutical)*, Injectrolyte *(Vetus).*
magnesium chloride, potassium chloride, sodium hypophosphite, calcium, dextrose. Cal-Phos #2 with Potassium Injection *(Phoenix Pharmaceutical)*, CMPK Solution *(Aspen), (Vedco)*, M.F.O. Solution *(AgriLabs).*
magnesium chloride, potassium chloride, sodium phosphate, calcium, dextrose. CMPK Oral *(AgriPharm).*
magnesium chloride, potassium chloride, tri-calcium phosphate, calcium. Oral CMPK Gel *(DVM Formula).*
magnesium chloride, sodium hypophosphite, calcium, dextrose. AmTech Cal-Phos #2 Injection *(Phoenix Scientific)*, Cal MP-1000 *(Butler)*, Cal-Phos #2 *(Vedco)*, Cal-Phos #2 Injection *(Phoenix Pharmaceutical).*
magnesium chloride, vitamins, calcium, cobalt sulfate. Calox 64 Oral Gel *(Vedco).*
magnesium hydroxide. Carmilax® Bolets® *(Pfizer Animal Health)*, Carmilax® Powder *(Pfizer Animal Health)*, InstaMag Bolus *(Vedco)*, Laxade Bolus *(AgriPharm)*, Laxade Powder *(AgriPharm)*, Magnalax Boluses *(Aspen), (Bimeda), (First Priority)*, Magnalax Powder *(Bimeda), (Phoenix Pharmaceutical), (Vedco)*, Milk of Magnesia *(Neogen)*, Polymag™ Bolus *(Butler)*, Polyox® Powder *(Bimeda)*, Polyox® II Bolus *(AgriPharm), (Bimeda)*, Rumalax™ Bolus *(AgriLabs).*
magnesium hydroxide, kaolin. MVT Powder™ *(Butler).*
magnesium hydroxide, phosphoric acid, potassium chloride, calcium. Cal MPK Gel *(Butler).*
magnesium hydroxide, phosphorus, potassium chloride, calcium. CMPK Gel *(Durvet).*
magnesium oxide. Magnalax Bolus *(Phoenix Pharmaceutical)*, MVT™ Bolus Wet Granulation Formula *(Butler)*, Rumen Boluses *(Durvet).*
magnesium oxide, sodium bicarbonate, vitamin B-complex. Buffer Gel™ *(Vets Plus).*
magnesium sulfate, methyl salicylate. Equi-Poultice *(Vetus)*, Magnapaste™ *(Butler)*, Magna-Poultice™ *(First Priority).*
magnesium sulfate, polyethelene glycol, propionic acid, silicon dioxide, vitamins, cobalt sulfate. Ketopro Oral Gel *(Vedco).*
magnesium sulfate, potassium chloride, sodium chloride, calcium. Electrolyte Supplement *(First Priority).*

magnesium trisilicate, pectin, aluminum silicate, attapulgite, carob. Veda-Sorb Jr Bolus *(Vedco)*.

magnesium trisilicate, pectin, attapulgite. Endosorb™ Bolus *(PRN Pharmacal)*, Endosorb™ Suspension *(PRN Pharmacal)*, Endosorb™ Tablets *(PRN Pharmacal)*.

magnesium trisilicate, pectin, attapulgite, carob. Anti-Diarrheal Cattle Bolus *(AgriLabs)*, Gastro-Sorb™ Bolus *(Butler)*, Gastro-Sorb™ Calf Bolus *(Butler)*, Intesti-Sorb Bolus *(AgriPharm)*, Intesti-Sorb Calf Bolus *(AgriPharm)*, Maxi-Sorb Bolus *(Durvet)*, Maxi Sorb Calf Bolus *(Durvet)*, Veda-Sorb Bolus *(Vedco)*.

MagSalt™ *(SSI Corp.)*, **magnesium, sulfur.**

Make Your Own Chlorhexidine Shampoo *(Davis)*, **chlorhexidine gluconate.**

Make Your Own Flea & Tick Shampoo *(Davis)*, **piperonyl butoxide, pyrethrins.**

Malaseb™ Flush *(DVM)*, **chlorhexidine gluconate, miconazole.**

Malaseb™ Pledgets *(DVM)*, **chlorhexidine gluconate, miconazole.**

Malaseb™ Shampoo *(DVM)*, **chlorhexidine gluconate, miconazole.**

Malaseb™ Spray *(DVM)*, **chlorhexidine gluconate, miconazole.**

malathion. Clean Crop® Malathion 57EC *(Loveland)*.

malic acid, propylene glycol, salicylic acid, benzoic acid. Oti-Clens® *(Pfizer Animal Health)*.

malic acid, propylene glycol, salicylic acid, benzoic acid, chlorhexidine. Dermachlor™ Rinse *(Butler)*.

malic acid, propylene glycol, salicylic acid, benzoic acid, chlorhexidine, glycerine. Chlor-A-Clens Cleansing Solution *(Vedco)*.

malic acid, propylene glycol, salicylic acid, benzoic acid, eucalyptus oil. Euclens Otic Cleanser *(Vetus)*, OtiCalm™ Cleansing Solution *(DVM)*.

malic acid, propylene glycol, zolazepam, benzoic acid, chlorhexidine, glycerine, lidocaine. Chlor-A-Clens-L Cleansing Solution *(Vedco)*.

malic acid, salicylic acid, benzoic acid. Derma-Clens® *(Pfizer Animal Health)*.

malic acid, salicylic acid, benzoic acid, chlorhexidine, lidocaine. Dermachlor™ Plus *(Butler)*.

MalOtic® Ointment *(Vedco)*, **betamethasone, clotrimazole, gentamicin.**

mandelic acid. Uddergold® Plus Germicidal Barrier Teat Dip (Activator) *(Alcide)*.

manganese, amino acids. Availa® Mn 80 *(Zinpro)*.

manganese, zinc. Availa® Z/M *(Zinpro)*.

manganese methionine. Manpro 80 *(Zinpro)*, Manpro 160 *(Zinpro)*.

manganese sulfate, potassium dichromate, cobalt sulfate, copper sulfate, hydrochloric acid. Ema-Sol™ Concentrate *(Alpharma)*.

Mange Treatment™ *(LeGear)*, **benzyl benzoate.**

Manniject *(Vetus)*, **mannitol.**

mannitol. AmTech Mannitol Injection 20% *(Phoenix Scientific)*, Manniject *(Vetus)*, Mannitol *(Butler)*, Mannitol Injection *(Vedco)*, Mannitol Injection 20% *(Neogen)*, *(Phoenix Pharmaceutical)*.

Mannitol *(Butler)*, **mannitol.**

Mannitol Injection *(Vedco)*, **mannitol.**

Mannitol Injection 20% *(Neogen)*, *(Phoenix Pharmaceutical)*, **mannitol.**

Man O'War™ Shampoo *(Equicare)*, **shampoo formula.**

Manpro 80 *(Zinpro)*, **manganese methionine.**

Manpro 160 *(Zinpro)*, **manganese methionine.**

MAP®-5 *(Bioniche Animal Health)*, **hyaluronic acid (sodium hyaluronate), sodium chloride, sodium phosphate.**

marbofloxacin. Zeniquin® *(Pfizer Animal Health)*.

Marcicide II *(M.A.R.C.)*, **pine oil, quaternary ammonia.**

Mare-Plus® *(Farnam)*, **minerals, vitamins.**

Marquis™ (15% w/w ponazuril) Antiprotozoal Oral Paste *(Bayer)*, **ponazuril.**

Masti-Clear™ *(G.C. Hanford)*, **penicillin G procaine.**

Maxi-B 1000 *(Durvet)*, **vitamin B-complex.**

Maxiban® 72 *(Elanco)*, **narasin, nicarbazin.**

Maxi/Guard® Oral Cleansing Gel *(Addison)*, **methylcellulose, taurine.**

Maxi/Guard® Zn7™ Derm *(Addison)*, **zinc gluconate.**

Maxi/Guard® Zn7™ Derm Spray *(Addison)*, **zinc gluconate.**

Maxi/Guard® Zn7™ Equine Wound Care Formula *(Addison)*, **zinc gluconate.**

Maxim-200® *(Phoenix Pharmaceutical)*, **oxytetracycline.**

Maxi-Sorb Bolus *(Durvet)*, **attapulgite, carob, magnesium trisilicate, pectin.**

Maxi Sorb Calf Bolus *(Durvet)*, **attapulgite, carob, magnesium trisilicate, pectin.**

Maxum® Crumbles *(Horse Health)*, **amino acids, minerals, vitamins.**

McKillip's Dusting Powder *(Butler)*, *(First Priority)*, **alum, chloroxylenol.**

Mecadox® 10 *(Phibro)*, **carbadox.**

meclofenamic acid. Arquel® Granules *(Fort Dodge)*, Arquel® Tablets *(Fort Dodge)*.

Medalone Cream *(Med-Pharmex)*, **triamcinolone acetonide.**

medetomidine hydrochloride. Domitor® *(Pfizer Animal Health)*.

Medicated Udder Balm *(First Priority)*, **aloe vera, lanolin, moisturizer(s), PABA sun screen, vitamins.**

Medicated Wound Cream *(First Priority)*, **bacitracin (zinc).**

Medicated Wound Powder *(First Priority)*, **bacitracin (zinc), zinc undecylenate.**

medicinal soap base, docusate sodium (dioctyl sodium sulfosuccinate), glycerine. Therevac®-SB *(King Animal Health)*.

Medrol® *(Pharmacia & Upjohn)*, **methylprednisolone.**

Mega CMPK Bolus *(AgriPharm)*, **calcium, magnesium, phosphorus, potassium, vitamins.**

megestrol acetate. Ovaban® Tablets *(Schering-Plough)*.

Melaleuca alternifolia. Derma Spray *(Sungro)*.

Melaleuca alternifolia, dibenzoyl peroxide. Equi-Phar™ ThrushGard *(Vedco)*.

Melaleuca Mist *(Davis)*, **melaleuca oil.**

melaleuca oil. Melaleuca Mist *(Davis)*, Melaleuca Shampoo *(Davis)*.

Melaleuca Shampoo *(Davis)*, **melaleuca oil.**

melarsomine dihydrochloride. Immiticide® *(Merial)*.

melengestrol acetate. MGA® 200 Premix *(Pharmacia & Upjohn)*, MGA® 500 Liquid Premix *(Pharmacia & Upjohn)*.

menthol. Absorbine® Veterinary Liniment *(W. F. Young)*, Absorbine® Veterinary Liniment Gel *(W. F. Young)*, Bigeloil® Liquid Gel *(W. F. Young)*, Freezex® Freeze *(Hawthorne)*, SureTight™ Performance Liniment *(SureNutrition)*.

menthol, ammonium carbonate, camphor. ZEV *(Dominion)*.

menthol, benzocaine, carbolic acid, eucalyptus oil. Otisol™ *(Wysong)*, Otisol-O™ *(Wysong)*.

menthol, camphor, capsicum. Choate's® Liniment *(Hawthorne)*.

menthol, camphor, ether, isopropyl alcohol (isopropanol). Shin-O-Gel® *(Hawthorne)*.

menthol, camphor, iodine, isopropyl alcohol (isopropanol). Lin-O-Gel® *(Hawthorne)*.

menthol, camphor, isopropyl alcohol (isopropanol). Ice-O-Gel® *(Hawthorne)*.

menthol, parachlorometaxylenol, thymol, witch hazel, wormwood oil, aloe vera, iodide (potassium), isopropyl alcohol. Veterinary Liniment *(First Priority)*.

menthol, phenol, pine oil, scarlet red, thymol, camphor, eucalyptus oil. Scarlet Oil Pump Spray *(Dominion)*.

menthol, salicylic acid, coal tar. NuSal-T® Shampoo *(DVM)*.

menthol, salicylic acid, tannic acid, boric acid, camphor, isopropyl alcohol (isopropanol). Dry-It *(Q.A. Laboratories)*.

menthol, spearmint oil, witch hazel, alcohol, iodide (potassium), iodine. Absorbine® RefreshMint® *(W. F. Young)*.

menthol, thymol, benzocaine, camphor, iodide (potassium), iodine. Equi-Phar™ BenzaGel *(Vedco)*.

menthol, thymol, benzocaine, camphor, isopropyl alcohol (isopropanol). Liniment Gel with Benzocaine *(First Priority)*.

menthol, thymol, camphor, iodide (potassium), iodine, isopropyl alcohol (isopropanol). Equi-Phar™ CoolGel *(Vedco)*.

menthol, thymol, camphor, isopropyl alcohol (isopropanol). Liniment Gel *(First Priority)*.

menthol, thymol, witch hazel, benzocaine, camphor, isopropyl alcohol (isopropanol). Benzo-Gel™ *(Butler)*.

menthol, wormwood oil, camphor, iodine, isopropyl alcohol. Dealer Select Horse Care Horse Liniment *(Durvet)*.

menthol, zinc oxide, calamine, glycerine. Cool-Cast® *(Hawthorne)*.

mepivacaine hydrochloride. Carbocaine®-V *(Pharmacia & Upjohn)*.

mercaptobenzothiazole. Happy Jack® Skin Balm *(Happy Jack)*.

mercaptobenzothiazole, isopropyl alcohol (isopropanol). Sulfodene® Skin Medication for Dogs *(Combe)*.

methanol, formaldehyde. Paracide-F *(Argent)*, Parasite-S *(Western Chemical)*.

Methaplex Injection *(PRN Pharmacal)*, **vitamin B-complex.**

Methigel® *(Evsco)*, **methionine (d-l).**

Methio-Form® Chewable Tablets *(Vet-A-Mix)*, **methionine (d-l).**

methionine, microorganisms, citric acid, electrolytes. Greenlyte® *(Bimeda)*.

methionine, minerals, vitamins, biotin. Bio-Hoof™ *(Horses Prefer)*.

methionine, propylene glycol, vitamins. Keto-Gel™ *(Jorgensen)*.

methionine (d-l). Ammonil® Tablets *(King Animal Health)*, d-l-Methionine Powder™ *(Butler)*, DL-Methionine Powder *(First Priority)*, d-l-m Tablets *(Butler)*, Methigel® *(Evsco)*, Methio-Form® Chewable Tablets *(Vet-A-Mix)*, Methio-Tabs® *(Vet-A-Mix)*.

methionine (d-l), ammonium chloride. Fus-Sol™ Drops *(PPI)*.

methionine (d-l), biotin. Bio-Meth *(Vet-A-Mix)*, Equi-Phar™ dl-Methionine with Biotin Powder *(Vedco)*.

methionine (d-l), microorganisms, zinc-methionine, biotin. Vita-Key® Biotin ZM-80 *(Vita-Key)*.

methionine (d-l), minerals, vegetable oil(s), vitamins, amodimethicone. Equ-Aid Plus *(Vet-A-Mix)*.

methionine (d-l), pantothenate, biotin. Dealer Select Horse Care Biotin 800 *(Durvet)*.

methionine (d-l), thiamine hydrochloride (B_1), zinc, biotin. Hoof Supplement *(First Priority)*, Integrator™ *(Butler)*.

methionine (d-l), vitamin B_6, biotin, l-lysine. H.B. 15™ *(Farnam)*.

methionine (d-l), vitamins, choline, fatty acids (essential). Lipo-Form *(Vet-A-Mix)*.

methionine (d-l), zinc sulfate, hydrochloric acid. Zinpro Sulfate & dl-Methionine Liquid *(Alpharma)*.

Methio-Tabs® *(Vet-A-Mix)*, **methionine (d-l).**

Meth-Iron 65 *(Zinpro)*, **iron methionine.**

methocarbamol. Robaxin®-V Injectable *(Fort Dodge)*, Robaxin®-V Tablets *(Fort Dodge)*.

Methocol™ Capsules *(Life Science)*, **lipotropics, liver, vitamin B-complex.**

methomyl, tricosene. Fly-Zap™ Fly Bait *(Aspen)*.

methoprene. Altosid® Cattle Custom Blending Premix *(Wellmark)*, Altosid® Premix *(Wellmark)*, Hartz® Advanced Care® Brand™ Flea Control Capsules™ for Dogs *(Hartz Mountain)*, Hartz® Control Pet Care System® OneSpot® for Cats and Kittens *(Hartz Mountain)*, MoorMan's® Hi-Mag IGR Minerals® *(ADM)*, MoorMan's® IGR Cattle Concentrate *(ADM)*, MoorMan's® IGR Cattle Mix *(ADM)*, MoorMan's® IGR Minerals® *(ADM)*, Vet-Kem® Ovitrol® Spot On® Flea Control for Cats *(Wellmark)*.

methoprene, fipronil. Frontline® Plus for Cats & Kittens *(Merial)*, Frontline® Plus for Dogs & Puppies *(Merial)*.

methoprene, n-octyl bicycloheptene dicarboximide, permethrin, phenothrin, piperonyl butoxide. Vet-Kem® Siphotrol® Plus II Premise Spray *(Wellmark)*.

methoprene, n-octyl bicycloheptene dicarboximide, piperonyl butoxide, pyrethrins. Vet-Kem® Ovitrol® Plus Flea, Tick & Bot Spray *(Wellmark)*.

methoprene, permethrin. Vet-Kem® Ovitrol Plus® Spot On® Flea & Tick Control for Dogs & Puppies (under 30 lbs.) *(Wellmark)*, Vet-Kem® Ovitrol Plus® Spot On® Flea & Tick Control for Dogs & Puppies (over 30 lbs.) *(Wellmark)*, Vet-Kem® Siphotrol® Plus Area Treatment for Homes *(Wellmark)*, Vet-Kem® Siphotrol® Plus Area Treatment Pump Spray for Homes *(Wellmark)*, Vet-Kem® Siphotrol Plus® Fogger *(Wellmark)*.

methoprene, phenothrin. Hartz® Advanced Care™ Brand Flea & Tick Drops Plus+ for Cats and Kittens (10 lbs. & under) *(Hartz Mountain)*, Hartz® Advanced Care™ Brand Flea & Tick Drops Plus+ for Cats and Kittens (over 10 lbs.) *(Hartz Mountain)*, Hartz® Advanced Care™ Brand Flea & Tick Drops Plus+ for Dogs and Puppies (4 to 15 lbs.) *(Hartz Mountain)*, Hartz® Advanced Care™ Brand Flea & Tick Drops Plus+ for Dogs and Puppies (16 to 30 lbs.) *(Hartz Mountain)*, Hartz® Advanced Care™ Brand Flea & Tick Drops Plus+ for Dogs and Puppies (31 to 45 lbs.) *(Hartz Mountain)*, Hartz® Advanced Care™ Brand Flea & Tick Drops Plus+ for Dogs and Puppies (46 to 60 lbs.) *(Hartz Mountain)*, Hartz® Advanced Care™ Brand Flea & Tick Drops Plus+ for Dogs and Puppies (61 to 90 lbs.) *(Hartz Mountain)*, Hartz® Advanced Care™ Brand Flea & Tick Drops Plus+ for Dogs and Puppies (Over 90 lbs.) *(Hartz Mountain)*.

methoprene, piperonyl butoxide, pyrethrins. Hartz® Control Pet Care System® Mousse for Cats and Kittens *(Hartz Mountain)*, Vet-Kem® Ovitrol® Plus Flea & Tick Shampoo for Dogs & Cats *(Wellmark)*.

methoprene, propoxur. Vet-Kem® Breakaway® Plus Flea & Tick Collar for Cats *(Wellmark)*.

methoprene, tetrachlorvinphos. Hartz® Control Pet Care System® Flea & Flea Egg Killer for Dogs *(Hartz Mountain)*, Hartz® Control Pet Care System® Ultimate Flea Collar® for Cats *(Hartz Mountain)*, Hartz® Control Pet Care System® Ultimate Flea Collar® for Dogs & Puppies *(Hartz Mountain)*.

methoxychlor, carbaryl. Ritter's Tick and Flea Powder *(Ritter)*.

methylcarbamate, n-octyl bicycloheptene dicarboximide, phenothrin. Adams™ Dual Action Flea & Tick Collar for Cats *(Farnam)*, Adams™ Dual Action Flea & Tick Collar for Large Dogs *(Farnam)*, Adams™ Dual Action Flea & Tick Collar for Medium Dogs *(Farnam)*.

methylcellulose, taurine. Maxi/Guard® Oral Cleansing Gel *(Addison)*.

methylene blue. Methylene Blue *(Centaur)*.

Methylene Blue *(Centaur)*, **methylene blue.**

methylene blue, isopropyl alcohol (isopropanol). Victor Gall Remedy *(Fiebing)*.

methyl para-hydroxybenzoate, propyl para-hydroxybenzoate, propylene glycol, carboxy methylcellulose. General Lube *(First Priority)*.

methylprednisolone. Medrol® *(Pharmacia & Upjohn)*, Methylprednisolone Tablets *(Boehringer Ingelheim)*, *(Butler)*, *(Vedco)*.

methylprednisolone acetate. Depo-Medrol® *(Pharmacia & Upjohn)*.

Methylprednisolone Tablets *(Boehringer Ingelheim)*, *(Butler)*, *(Vedco)*, **methylprednisolone.**

methyl salicylate, 8-hydroxyquinolone. Bag Salve *(First Priority)*.

methyl salicylate, camphor. Vetrolin® Liniment *(Equicare)*.

methyl salicylate, epsom salt. Dealer Select Horse Care Epsom Salt Poultice *(Durvet)*.

methyl salicylate, magnesium sulfate. Equi-Poultice *(Vetus)*, Magnapaste™ *(Butler)*, Magna-Poultice™ *(First Priority)*.

methyl salicylate, parachlorometaxylenol, pine oil, scarlet red, benzyl alcohol, eucalyptus oil. Scarlet Oil *(Vedco)*, Scarlet Oil Wound Dressing *(AgriPharm)*.

methyl salicylate, parachlorometaxylenol, pine oil, scarlet red, benzyl alcohol, eucalyptus oil, isopropyl alcohol (isopropanol). Scarlet Oil *(First Priority)*.

methyl salicylate, P-chloro-M-xylenol, pine oil, scarlet red, eucalyptus oil. Scarlex® Scarlet Oil *(Farnam)*.

methyl salicylate, peppermint oil, salicylic acid, eucalyptus oil, glycerine, kaolin. Absorbine® Antiphlogistine® *(W. F. Young)*.

methyl salicylate, peppermint oil, salicylic acid, thymol, arnica, bentonite, boric acid, eucalyptus oil, glycerine, isopropyl alcohol (isopropanol), kaolin. Bigeloil® 24-Hour Medicated Poultice *(W. F. Young)*.

methyl salicylate, pine oil, scarlet red, benzyl alcohol, eucalyptus oil. Scarlet Oil Wound Dressing *(Durvet)*.

methyl salicylate, pine oil, scarlet red, eucalyptus oil. Scarlet Oil Smear *(First Priority)*.

methyl salicylate, propylene glycol, zinc undecylenate, acetic acid, isopropyl alcohol (isopropanol). Fungi-Dry-Ear *(Q.A. Laboratories)*.

methyl salicylate, salicylic acid, alcohol base, aromatic vegetable oil(s). Bigeloil® *(W. F. Young)*.

methyl violet. Purple Spray *(AgriPharm)*.

methyl violet, propylene glycol, sodium propionate, urea, acriflavine, glycerine. Blue Lotion *(Farnam)*.

methyl violet, propylene glycol, urea, acriflavine, glycerine. Wound-Kote Gentian Violet *(Farnam)*.

methyl violet, propylene glycol, urea, acriflavine, glycerine, isopropyl alcohol (isopropanol). Purple Lotion Wound Dressing *(Durvet)*.

MetriCide® *(Metrex)*, **glutaraldehyde.**

MetriCide® 28 *(Metrex)*, **glutaraldehyde.**

MetriCide Plus 30® *(Metrex)*, **glutaraldehyde.**

MetriClean2® *(Metrex)*, **detergent mixture.**

MetriGuard® *(Metrex)*, **ammonium chloride, isopropyl alcohol (isopropanol).**

MetriLube® *(Metrex)*, **oil-based lubricant.**

MetriSponge® *(Metrex)*, **detergent (enzyme-based).**

MetriWash™ *(Metrex)*, **detergent mixture.**

MetriWipes® *(Metrex)*, **alcohol, quaternary ammonia.**

MetriZyme® *(Metrex)*, **detergent (enzyme-based).**

Metz Iodine Detergent *(Metz)*, **iodine complex (povidone-iodine), phosphoric acid.**

Metz Iodine Teat Dip (0.25%) *(Metz)*, **glycerine, iodine complex (povidone-iodine).**

Metz Iodine Teat Dip (0.5%) *(Metz)*, **glycerine, iodine complex (povidone-iodine).**

Metz Iodine Teat Dip (1.0%) *(Metz)*, **glycerine, iodine complex (povidone-iodine).**

Metz Soft-Kote Teat Dip *(Metz)*, **chlorhexidine gluconate, glycerine.**

Metz Soft-Kote Teat Spray *(Metz)*, **chlorhexidine gluconate, glycerine.**

M.F.O. Solution *(AgriLabs)*, **calcium, dextrose, magnesium chloride, potassium chloride, sodium hypophosphite.**

MGA® 200 Premix *(Pharmacia & Upjohn)*, **melengestrol acetate.**

MGA® 500 Liquid Premix *(Pharmacia & Upjohn)*, **melengestrol acetate.**

MicaVed® Lotion 1% *(Vedco)*, **miconazole.**

MicaVed® Spray 1% *(Vedco)*, **miconazole.**

Micazole Lotion 1% *(Vetus)*, **miconazole.**

Micazole Spray 1% *(Vetus)*, **miconazole.**

miconazole. Conofite® Cream *(Schering-Plough)*, Conofite® Lotion *(Schering-Plough)*, Conofite® Spray *(Schering-Plough)*, Dermazole™ Shampoo *(Virbac)*, MicaVed® Lotion 1% *(Vedco)*, MicaVed® Spray 1% *(Vedco)*, Micazole Lotion 1% *(Vetus)*, Micazole Spray 1% *(Vetus)*, Miconazole Nitrate Lotion 1% *(Butler)*, Miconazole Nitrate Spray 1% *(Butler)*, Miconosol Lotion 1% *(Med-Pharmex)*, Miconosol Spray 1% *(Med-Pharmex)*, Micro Pearls Advantage™ Miconazole™ Shampoo *(Evsco)*, Micro Pearls Advantage™ Miconazole™ Spray *(Evsco)*, ResiZole™ Leave-on Conditioner *(Virbac)*.

miconazole, chlorhexidine gluconate. Malaseb™ Flush *(DVM)*, Malaseb™ Pledgets *(DVM)*, Malaseb™ Shampoo *(DVM)*, Malaseb™ Spray *(DVM)*.

Miconazole Nitrate Lotion 1% *(Butler)*, **miconazole.**

Miconazole Nitrate Spray 1% *(Butler)*, **miconazole.**

Miconosol Lotion 1% *(Med-Pharmex)*, **miconazole.**

Miconosol Spray 1% *(Med-Pharmex)*, **miconazole.**

Micotil® 300 Injection *(Elanco)*, **tilmicosin.**

Microban® X-580 Institutional Spray Plus *(Microban)*, **n-octyl bicycloheptene dicarboximide, phenol, piperonyl butoxide, pyrethrins, quaternary ammonia.**

Microcillin *(Anthony)*, **penicillin G procaine.**

Micro-D® 500 *(Alpharma)*, **vitamin D_3.**

Micro-D® 1000 *(Alpharma)*, **vitamin D_3.**

MicroMaster® Alert™ Calf Bolus *(Loveland)*, **microorganisms.**

MicroMaster® Avian PAC™ HT *(Loveland)*, **microorganisms.**

MicroMaster® Avian PAC™ Routine *(Loveland)*, **microorganisms.**

MicroMaster® Avian PAC™ Soluble *(Loveland)*, **microorganisms.**

MicroMaster® Avian PAC™ Soluble Plus *(Loveland)*, **microorganisms.**

MicroMaster® Avian Pulse PAC™ *(Loveland)*, **microorganisms.**

MicroMaster® Bovine Paste *(Loveland)*, **microorganisms.**

MicroMaster® Calf PAC™ Soluble *(Loveland)*, **microorganisms.**

MicroMaster® Dairy PAC™ *(Loveland)*, **microorganisms.**

MicroMaster® Equine Gel *(Loveland)*, **microorganisms.**

MicroMaster® Pet Gel *(Loveland)*, **microorganisms.**

MicroMaster® Porcine PAC™ HT *(Loveland)*, **microorganisms.**

MicroMaster® Porcine Paste *(Loveland)*, **microorganisms.**

MicroMaster® Porcine Starter PAC™ *(Loveland)*, **microorganisms.**

MicroMaster® Porcine Starter PAC™ Soluble *(Loveland)*, **microorganisms.**

microorganisms. All-Pro Biotic™ *(Vets Plus)*, Bene-Bac™ Pet Gel *(Pet-Ag)*, Bene-Bac™ Powder *(Pet-Ag)*, Bird Bene-Bac™ Gel *(Pet-Ag)*, Bird Bene-Bac™ Powder *(Pet-Ag)*, BP-1 *(AgriPharm)*, Calf RD Formula *(TechMix)*, Durazyme Calf Bolus *(Durvet)*, Equine Bene-Bac™ *(Pet-Ag)*, Fastrack® Canine Microbial Supplement *(Conklin)*, Lamb & Kid Paste *(Durvet)*, MicroMaster® Alert™ Calf Bolus *(Loveland)*, MicroMaster® Avian PAC™ HT *(Loveland)*, MicroMaster® Avian PAC™ Routine *(Loveland)*, MicroMaster® Avian PAC™ Soluble *(Loveland)*, MicroMaster® Avian PAC™ Soluble Plus *(Loveland)*, MicroMaster® Avian Pulse PAC™ *(Loveland)*, MicroMaster® Bovine Paste *(Loveland)*, MicroMaster® Calf PAC™ Soluble *(Loveland)*, MicroMaster® Dairy PAC™ *(Loveland)*, MicroMaster® Equine Gel *(Loveland)*, MicroMaster® Pet Gel *(Loveland)*, MicroMaster® Porcine PAC™ HT *(Loveland)*, MicroMaster® Porcine Paste *(Loveland)*, MicroMaster® Porcine Starter PAC™ *(Loveland)*, MicroMaster® Porcine Starter PAC™ Soluble *(Loveland)*, Preempt™ *(Milk Specialties)*, *(MS BioScience)*, Probiocin® Oral Gel for Pets *(Chr. Hansen)*, Probios® Bovine One Oral Gel for Ruminants *(Chr. Hansen)*, Probios® Dispersible Powder *(Chr. Hansen)*, Probios® Equine One Oral Gel *(Chr. Hansen)*, Probios® Feed Granules *(Chr. Hansen)*, Probios® Microbial Calf Pac *(Chr. Hansen)*, Probios® Oral Boluses for Ruminants *(Chr. Hansen)*, Probios® Oral Suspension for Swine *(Chr. Hansen)*, Rumen Yeast Caps Plus *(TechMix)*, Zoologic® Bene-Bac™ Large Mammal *(Pet-Ag)*, Zoologic® Bene-Bac™ Powder *(Pet-Ag)*.

microorganisms, citric acid, electrolytes, methionine. Greenlyte® *(Bimeda)*.

microorganisms, fermentation extract(s). Digest Aid™ *(Farnam)*.

microorganisms, lactase enzymes. BP-1 Special Blend *(AgriPharm)*, PP-1 Special Blend *(AgriPharm)*, RXV-PP-1 (Porcine Probiotic Paste) *(AgriPharm)*.

microorganisms, minerals, nutrients, vitamins, yeast. Fastrack® Calf Bolus *(Conklin)*.

microorganisms, minerals, vitamins. Equi-Phar™ Equi-Vita-Phos *(Vedco)*, Power Punch™ *(Vets Plus)*, Vita-Key® Show Cattle Supplement, Phase I *(Vita-Key)*.

microorganisms, minerals, vitamins, amino acids. Ruminant LactoBac Gel *(Vedco)*.

microorganisms, minerals, vitamins, amino acids, bicarbonate. Pre-Conditioning/Receiving Formula Gel *(Durvet)*, Ruminant Lactobacillus Gel *(First Priority)*.

microorganisms, minerals, vitamins, bovine origin glycoproteins. Colostrum-Plus *(Jorgensen)*.

microorganisms, minerals, vitamins, colostrum whey. Oral Probiotic Calf Pak *(AgriPharm)*, Sure-Start Plus *(AgriPharm)*.

microorganisms, minerals, vitamins, dried colostrum. Colostrum Bolus Forte *(Durvet)*.

microorganisms, minerals, vitamins, yeast. Fastrack® Nonruminant Microbial Gel *(Conklin)*, Fastrack® Ruminant Bolus *(Conklin)*, Fastrack® Ruminant Microbial Gel *(Conklin)*.

microorganisms, minerals, vitamins, yeast, amino acids. Vita-Key® Swine Supplement *(Vita-Key)*.

microorganisms, minerals, vitamins, yeast, amino acids, enzymes. Vita-Key® Show Cattle Concentrate, Phase II *(Vita-Key)*.

microorganisms, nutrients. Durazyme Calf Colostrum Supplement *(Durvet)*, Durazyme Paste for Calves *(Durvet)*, EP-1 3X *(RXV)*.

microorganisms, nutrients, electrolytes, energy source(s). NutriVed™ EnerGel Forte *(Vedco)*.

microorganisms, nutrients, electrolytes, glucose. Ener-Lyte™ *(Aspen)*.

microorganisms, nutrients, energy source(s). Durazyme Energy Pack *(Durvet)*.

microorganisms, nutrients, vitamins, electrolytes, energy source(s). Sow & Gilt Restart™ One-4 *(TechMix)*.

microorganisms, organic acidifiers, vitamins, electrolytes. Vit-E-Lyte "Plus" *(Bimeda)*.

microorganisms, potassium, sodium, vitamin E, zinc. Yellow Lite *(AgriPharm)*.

microorganisms, psyllium, fermentation extract(s). Equine Enteric Colloid *(TechMix)*.

microorganisms, vitamin A, vitamin D, vitamin E, dried colostrum. Colostrum Powder *(Vedco)*.

microorganisms, vitamin A, vitamin E, lactase enzymes. Good Start Calf Bolus *(AgriPharm)*, Good Start Calf Paste *(AgriPharm)*.

microorganisms, vitamin A, vitamin E, yeast. Fastrack® Canine Gel *(Conklin)*, Fastrack® Equine Gel *(Conklin)*.

microorganisms, vitamin E. Probios® Plus Natural E Bovine One Oral Gel for Ruminants *(Chr. Hansen)*, Probiotic Plus E for Calves *(Vets Plus)*, Probiotic Plus E for Cattle *(Vets Plus)*.

microorganisms, vitamins. Equi-Phar™ LactoBac Gel *(Vedco)*, Innocugel™ Equine *(Butler)*, Probiotic Power™ *(Vets Plus)*.

microorganisms, vitamins, dried colostrum. Soluble Colostrum Powder *(Durvet)*.

microorganisms, vitamins, electrolytes. Revitilyte-Plus™ *(Vets Plus)*.

microorganisms, vitamins, fermentation extract(s). All-In-One Calf Bolus *(AgriPharm)*, All-In-One Cattle Bolus *(AgriPharm)*.

microorganisms, vitamins, yeast. Fastrack® Kick-Off *(Conklin)*.

microorganisms, vitamins, yeast, amino acids, enzymes. Vita Boost Paste™ *(AgriLabs)*.

microorganisms, yeast. Fastrack® Liquid Dispersible *(Conklin)*, Fastrack® Liquid Dispersible-P *(Conklin)*, Fastrack® Probiotic Pack *(Conklin)*.

microorganisms, zinc-methionine, biotin, methionine (d-l). Vita-Key® Biotin ZM-80 *(Vita-Key)*.

Micro Pearls Advantage™ Benzoyl-Plus *(Evsco)*, **benzoyl peroxide.**

Micro Pearls Advantage™ Dermal-Soothe™ Anti-Itch Cream Rinse *(Evsco)*, **promoxine.**

Micro Pearls Advantage™ Dermal-Soothe™ Anti-Itch Shampoo *(Evsco)*, **promoxine.**

Micro Pearls Advantage™ Dermal-Soothe™ Anti-Itch Spray *(Evsco)*, **moisturizer(s), promoxine.**

Micro Pearls Advantage™ EVSCO-Tar™ Shampoo *(Evsco)*, **coal tar.**

Micro Pearls Advantage™ Hydra-Pearls™ Cream Rinse *(Evsco)*, **moisturizer(s), rinse formula.**

Micro Pearls Advantage™ Hydra-Pearls™ Rehydrating Spray *(Evsco)*, **emollient(s), moisturizer(s).**

Micro Pearls Advantage™ Hydra-Pearls™ Shampoo *(Evsco)*, **moisturizer(s), shampoo formula.**

Micro Pearls Advantage™ Miconazole™ Shampoo *(Evsco)*, **miconazole.**

Micro Pearls Advantage™ Miconazole™ Spray *(Evsco)*, **miconazole.**

Micro Pearls Advantage™ Seba-Hex™ Shampoo *(Evsco)*, **chlorhexidine gluconate.**

Micro Pearls Advantage™ Seba-Moist™ Shampoo *(Evsco)*, **salicylic acid, sulfur.**

Micro-Vet™ Equine Traditional Blend *(Boehringer Ingelheim)*, **minerals, vitamins.**

MicroZyme Bolus for Cattle *(Vedco)*, **Aspergillus oryzae fermentation extract, minerals, vitamins, yeast.**

Milbemite™ Otic Solution *(Novartis)*, **milbemycin oxime.**

milbemycin oxime. Interceptor® Flavor Tabs® *(Novartis)*, Milbemite™ Otic Solution *(Novartis)*.

milbemycin oxime, lufenuron. Sentinel® Flavor Tabs® *(Novartis)*.

"Mild" Iodine Wound Spray *(Centaur)*, **iodine complex (povidone-iodine).**

milk, whey. Land O Lakes® Mare's Match® Foal Pellets *(Land O'Lakes)*.

Milkin Mix *(Skylabs)*, **minerals, vitamins.**

Milk of Magnesia *(Neogen)*, **magnesium hydroxide.**

milk protein, minerals, vitamins, lactose. Multi-Milk™ *(Pet-Ag)*.

milk protein, minerals, vitamins, yeast, fat product(s), lactose. Start To Finish® Mare & Foal Pellets™ *(Milk Specialties)*.

milk protein, nutrients, phosphorus, vitamins, calcium. Foal-Lac® Pellets *(Pet-Ag)*.

milk replacing formula. Esbilac® Liquid *(Pet-Ag)*, Esbilac® Powder *(Pet-Ag)*, Foal-Lac® Powder *(Pet-Ag)*, Just Born® Milk Replacer for Kittens Powdered Formula *(Farnam)*, Just Born® Milk Replacer for Kittens Ready-To-Use Liquid *(Farnam)*, Just Born® Milk Replacer for Puppies Powdered Formula *(Farnam)*, Just Born® Milk Replacer for Puppies Ready-To-Use Liquid *(Farnam)*, Kitten Formula *(Vet Solutions)*, KMR® Liquid *(Pet-Ag)*, KMR® Powder *(Pet-Ag)*, Land O Lakes® Instant Amplifier® Select Plus *(Land O'Lakes)*, Land O Lakes® Instant Kid Milk Replacer *(Land O'Lakes)*, Land O Lakes® Mare's Match® *(Land O'Lakes)*, Land O Lakes® Ultra Fresh® Lamb Milk Replacer *(Land O'Lakes)*, Nurturall®-C for Kittens *(V.P.L.)*, Nurturall®-C for Puppies *(V.P.L.)*, PetLac™ Powder *(Pet-Ag)*, Puppy Formula *(Vet Solutions)*, SPF-Lac® *(Pet-Ag)*, Veta-Lac® Canine *(Vet-A-Mix)*, Veta-Lac® Feline *(Vet-A-Mix)*, Vita Ferm® Milk-N-More Non-Medicated Milk Replacer *(BioZyme)*, Zoologic® Milk Matrix 20/14 *(Pet-Ag)*, Zoologic® Milk Matrix 20/20 *(Pet-Ag)*, Zoologic® Milk Matrix 23/30 *(Pet-Ag)*, Zoologic® Milk Matrix 25/13 *(Pet-Ag)*, Zoologic® Milk Matrix 30/55 *(Pet-Ag)*, Zoologic® Milk Matrix 33/40 *(Pet-Ag)*, Zoologic® Milk Matrix 42/25 *(Pet-Ag)*.

milk supplement, oil origanum, oil rosemary, camphor, Canada balsam, corn oil base. VetRx™ Equine Formula *(Goodwinol)*.

mineral oil. Improved Hoof Dressing *(Fiebing)*, Mineral Oil *(AgriLabs)*, *(AgriPharm)*, *(Aspen)*, *(Dominion)*, *(Durvet)*, *(Vedco)*, Mineral Oil 95 V *(Butler)*, Mineral Oil 95 Viscosity *(First Priority)*, Mineral Oil 150 Viscosity *(First Priority)*, Mineral Oil Light *(Centaur)*, *(Phoenix Pharmaceutical)*.

Mineral Oil *(AgriLabs)*, *(AgriPharm)*, *(Aspen)*, *(Dominion)*, *(Durvet)*, *(Vedco)*, **mineral oil.**

mineral oil, petrolatum. Hairball Preparation *(Vet Solutions)*, Laxa-Stat™ *(Tomlyn)*, Laxatone® for Cats *(Tomlyn)*, Laxatone® for Ferrets & Other Small Animals *(Tomlyn)*.

mineral oil, turpentine. Vita Oil *(Hawthorne)*.

mineral oil, vegetable oil(s), glycerine. Hairball Solution *(Pet-Ag)*.

Mineral Oil 95 V *(Butler)*, **mineral oil.**

Mineral Oil 95 Viscosity *(First Priority)*, **mineral oil.**

Mineral Oil 150 Viscosity *(First Priority)*, **mineral oil.**

Mineral Oil Light *(Centaur)*, *(Phoenix Pharmaceutical)*, **mineral oil.**

minerals. Ab-Sorb™ Bolus *(Bimeda)*, Mineral Vet 5 *(Neogen)*, Multimin™ *(Multimin)*, Vionate® Vitamin Mineral Powder *(ARC)*.

minerals, amino acids. Availa®-4 *(Zinpro)*, AvailaMin® - Grow/Finish *(Zinpro)*, AvailaMin® - Sow *(Zinpro)*, AvailaMin® - Starter I, II, III *(Zinpro)*, Zinpro+3 *(Zinpro)*.

minerals, amino acids, electrolytes, fatty acids (essential). NutriVed™ Chewable Vitamins for Active Dogs *(Vedco)*.

minerals, dextrose. Revitilyte™ *(Vets Plus)*, Revitilyte-Gelling™ *(Vets Plus)*.

minerals, dextrose, electrolytes. Stress-Dex® *(Neogen)*.

minerals, dextrose, glycine. Electrolyte with Thickener *(DVM Formula)*.

minerals, electrolytes. Dealer Select Horse Care DurLyte-A *(Durvet)*, Dealer Select Horse Care DurLyte-C *(Durvet)*, Dexalyte 8X Powder *(Butler)*.

minerals, fenbendazole. Sweetlix® Safe-Guard* Free-Choice Mineral Cattle Dewormer *(Sweetlix)*.

minerals, nutrients, vitamins, energy source(s). CliniCare® Canine Liquid Diet *(Abbott)*, CliniCare® Feline Liquid Diet *(Abbott)*, CliniCare® RF Specialized Feline Liquid Diet *(Abbott)*.

minerals, nutrients, vitamins, yeast, microorganisms. Fastrack® Calf Bolus *(Conklin)*.

minerals, potassium, taurine, vitamins, fatty acids (essential). Felo-Form *(Vet-A-Mix)*.

minerals, propylene glycol, vitamins, amino acids. PRN Hi-Energy Supplement™ *(PRN Pharmacal)*.

minerals, protein(s), carbohydrates. Plexamino® Bolus *(Bimeda)*.

minerals, protein(s), vitamins. Protobolic™ Bolus Improved *(Butler)*.

minerals, protein(s), vitamins, fenbendazole. Sweetlix® Safe-Guard® 20% Natural Protein Deworming Block for Beef Cattle *(Sweetlix)*.

minerals, selenium, tetrachlorvinphos, vitamins, amino acids. Vita-Plus® with Equitrol® *(Farnam)*.

minerals, selenium, vitamins, iron. Go Max™ Liquid *(Farnam)*.

minerals, sorbitol, vitamins, iron. Vi-Sorbin® *(Pfizer Animal Health)*.

minerals, soy protein, vitamins, antioxidants, fatty acids (omega). Lickables™ Charge Up!™ *(A.A.H.)*.

minerals, sucrose, vitamins, electrolytes. Dexsolyte Powder *(Neogen)*.

minerals, taurine, vitamins. FaVor® *(Pfizer Animal Health)*, Felovite®-II with Taurine *(Evsco)*, Felovite® II with Taurine *(Tomlyn)*, Hartz® Health measures™ Everyday Chewable Vitamins for Cats and Kittens *(Hartz Mountain)*, TunaVite™ *(Vedco)*.

minerals, taurine, vitamins, amino acids. Cholodin®-FEL *(MVP)*.

minerals, taurine, vitamins, amino acids, fatty acids (essential). NutriVed™ Chewable Vitamins for Cats *(Vedco)*, NutriVed™ Chewable Vitamins for Kittens *(Vedco)*.

minerals, taurine, vitamins, antioxidants. Lickables™ Hearty Cat™ *(A.A.H.)*.

minerals, taurine, vitamins, fatty acids (essential). NutriVed™ O.F.A. Granules for Cats *(Vedco)*.

minerals, taurine, vitamins, linolenic acid. Mrs. Allen's Vita Care® Vitamins for Cats *(Farnam)*, Show Winner!™ Cat Vitamins *(Farnam)*.

minerals, tetrachlorvinphos, vitamins. Sweetlix® Rabon® Mineral/Vitamin Molasses Block *(Sweetlix)*.

minerals, torula yeast, amino acids, electrolytes. Procal™ Powder *(Butler)*.

minerals, vegetable oil(s), vitamins, amodimethicone, methionine (d-l). Equ-Aid Plus *(Vet-A-Mix)*.

minerals, vitamin B_{12}, iron, liver. LIB *(Neogen)*.

minerals, vitamins. Energel™ for Cats *(Pet-Ag)*, Energel™ for Dogs *(Pet-Ag)*, Energel™ Powder for Cats *(Pet-Ag)*, Energel™ Powder for Dogs *(Pet-Ag)*, Equi-Phar™ Vita Plex Oral Honey *(Vedco)*, Equivim™ *(Butler)*, Grow Colt® *(Farnam)*, Happy Jack® Vita Tabs *(Happy Jack)*, Hartz® Health measures™ Everyday Chewable Vitamins for Dogs and Puppies *(Hartz Mountain)*, Lixotinic® *(Pfizer Animal Health)*, Mare-Plus® *(Farnam)*, Micro-Vet™ Equine Traditional Blend *(Boehringer Ingelheim)*, Milkin Mix *(Skylabs)*, Pet-Form® *(Vet-A-Mix)*, Pet-Tabs® *(Pfizer Animal Health)*, Pet-Tabs® Jr. *(Pfizer Animal Health)*, Pet-Tabs® Plus *(Pfizer Animal Health)*, Pet-Tinic® *(Pfizer Animal Health)*, Poult Pak *(Alpharma)*, Stock Power *(LeGear)*, Superior-Vita-Min Blend™ *(Horses Prefer)*, Unipet Nutritabs® *(Pharmacia & Upjohn)*, Vita-15™ Injection *(Neogen)*, Vita-Key® Brood Mare Supplement *(Vita-Key)*.

minerals, vitamins, amino acids. Amino Acid Bolus *(Vets Plus)*, Equinime® *(Chariton)*, Maxum® Crumbles *(Horse Health)*, Stam-N-Aid™ *(Neogen)*, Vita Plus® *(Farnam)*.

minerals, vitamins, amino acids, bicarbonate, microorganisms. Pre-Conditioning/Receiving Formula Gel *(Durvet)*, Ruminant Lactobacillus Gel *(First Priority)*.

minerals, vitamins, amino acids, dextrose. Tryptophan Plus Gel™ *(Horses Prefer)*.

minerals, vitamins, amino acids, electrolytes, energy source(s). Energy Drench *(Vedco)*.

minerals, vitamins, amino acids, fatty acids (essential). NutriVed™ Chewable Vitamins for Dogs *(Vedco)*, NutriVed™ Chewable Vitamins for Puppies *(Vedco)*, NutriVed™ Hypo Allergenic Chewable Tablets *(Vedco)*.

minerals, vitamins, amino acids, lactic acid producing bacteria. MultiMax™ *(SureNutrition)*.

minerals, vitamins, amino acids, microorganisms. Ruminant LactoBac Gel *(Vedco)*.

minerals, vitamins, antioxidants. Lickables™ Hearty Dog™ *(A.A.H.)*.

minerals, vitamins, antioxidants, fatty acids (omega). Lickables™ Super Charger™ *(A.A.H.)*.

minerals, vitamins, Aspergillus oryzae fermentation extract. K-Zyme® Cat Granules *(BioZyme)*, K-Zyme® Chewable Dog Tablets *(BioZyme)*, K-Zyme® Dog Granules *(BioZyme)*, Vita Charge® 28 Dispersible Powder *(BioZyme)*, Vita Charge® Calf Bolus *(BioZyme)*, Vita Charge® Equine *(BioZyme)*, Vita Charge® Gel Cap *(BioZyme)*, Vita Charge® Paste *(BioZyme)*, Vita Ferm® Breeder Booster+Mag *(BioZyme)*, Vita Ferm® Cattleman's Beefmaker *(BioZyme)*, Vita Ferm® Cattleman's Beefmaker+Mag *(BioZyme)*, Vita Ferm® Concept-Aid *(BioZyme)*, Vita Ferm® Concept-Aid+Mag *(BioZyme)*, Vita Ferm® Concept-Aid A•P *(BioZyme)*, Vita Ferm® Cow Calf 5 *(BioZyme)*, Vita Ferm® Dairy Basemix 12:16 *(BioZyme)*, Vita Ferm® Dairy Basemix 18:6 *(BioZyme)*, Vita Ferm® Dairy Basemix 18:12 *(BioZyme)*, Vita Ferm® Equine *(BioZyme)*, Vita Ferm® Ewe and Lamb *(BioZyme)*, Vita Ferm® Far Out Dry Cow *(BioZyme)*, Vita Ferm® Feedlot Formula *(BioZyme)*, Vita Ferm® Fescue Fiber Buster *(BioZyme)*, Vita Ferm® Fescue Power Keg *(BioZyme)*, Vita Ferm® Formula *(BioZyme)*, Vita Ferm® Grass Enhancer *(BioZyme)*, Vita Ferm® High Mag *(BioZyme)*, Vita Ferm® Natural Protein Pasture Formula (NPPF) *(BioZyme)*, Vita Ferm® Pasture Formula *(BioZyme)*, Vita Ferm® Power Keg *(BioZyme)*, Vita Ferm® Roughage Fortifier *(BioZyme)*, Vita Ferm® Sheep & Goat Keg *(BioZyme)*, Vita Ferm® Sure Champ and Vita Start Pellets *(BioZyme)*, Vita Ferm® Sure Start 2 *(BioZyme)*, Vita Ferm® Sure Start Pac *(BioZyme)*, Vita Ferm® Up Close Dry Cow *(BioZyme)*, Vita Ferm® Vita Grow 32 Natural *(BioZyme)*.

minerals, vitamins, biotin, methionine. Bio-Hoof™ *(Horses Prefer)*.

minerals, vitamins, bovine origin glycoproteins, microorganisms. Colostrum-Plus *(Jorgensen)*.

minerals, vitamins, choline, lipids. Geri-Form *(Vet-A-Mix)*.

minerals, vitamins, colostrum whey, microorganisms. Oral Probiotic Calf Pak *(AgriPharm)*, Sure-Start Plus *(AgriPharm)*.

minerals, vitamins, dextrose, electrolytes. Multi-Electrolytes *(Neogen)*.

minerals, vitamins, dried colostrum, microorganisms. Colostrum Bolus Forte *(Durvet)*.

minerals, vitamins, electrolytes. Electrolytes-Plus *(Alpharma)*, Vi-tal *(Loveland)*.

minerals, vitamins, energy source(s). High-Cal *(Vet Solutions)*, Nutri-Cal® for Ferrets & Other Small Animals *(Tomlyn)*, Stat *(PRN Pharmacal)*.

minerals, vitamins, energy source(s), fatty acids (omega). Nutri-Stat™ *(Tomlyn)*.

minerals, vitamins, fatty acids. Super 14™ *(Farnam)*.

minerals, vitamins, fatty acids (essential). Derma-Form Tablets *(Vet-A-Mix)*, NutriVed™ O.F.A. Granules for Dogs *(Vedco)*, Pet-Tabs®/F.A. Granules *(Pfizer Animal Health)*, Sergeant's® Vetscription® Vitamins for Dogs & Puppies *(Sergeant's)*.

minerals, vitamins, fatty acids (omega). Canine F.A./Plus Granules *(Pala-Tech)*, Derma-Form Granules F.A. *(Vet-A-Mix)*, Equine F.A./Plus Granules *(Pala-Tech)*, Feline F.A./Plus Chewable Tablets *(Pala-Tech)*, Mrs. Allen's Shed-Stop® Granules for Cats *(Farnam)*, Mrs. Allen's Shed-Stop® Granules for Dogs *(Farnam)*.

minerals, vitamins, goat milk. GME™ Powder and Liquid (Goat's Milk Esbilac®) *(Pet-Ag)*.

minerals, vitamins, iron. Red Cell® *(Horse Health)*.

minerals, vitamins, lactose, milk protein. Multi-Milk™ *(Pet-Ag)*.

minerals, vitamins, linolenic acid. Mrs. Allen's Vita Care® Vitamins for Dogs *(Farnam)*, Nutra-Sure™ Cat Vitamins *(Farnam)*, Pet Vites *(Vetus)*, Show Winner!™ Dog Vitamins *(Farnam)*, Show Winner!™ Kitten Vitamins *(Farnam)*, Show Winner!™ Older Dog Vitamins *(Farnam)*, Show Winner!™ Puppy Vitamins *(Farnam)*.

minerals, vitamins, microorganisms. Equi-Phar™ Equi-Vita-Phos *(Vedco)*, Power Punch™ *(Vets Plus)*, Vita-Key® Show Cattle Supplement, Phase I *(Vita-Key)*.

minerals, vitamins, whey, fat product(s), lactose, lecithin. Start To Finish® Mare Replacer™ *(Milk Specialties)*.

minerals, vitamins, yeast. Fresh Cow YMCP Plus *(TechMix)*.

minerals, vitamins, yeast, amino acids. Vita-Key® Antioxidant Concentrate *(Vita-Key)*, Vita-Key® Equine Supplement *(Vita-Key)*, Vita-Key® Mare & Foal Supplement *(Vita-Key)*.

minerals, vitamins, yeast, amino acids, enzymes, microorganisms. Vita-Key® Show Cattle Concentrate, Phase II *(Vita-Key)*.

minerals, vitamins, yeast, amino acids, microorganisms. Vita-Key® Swine Supplement *(Vita-Key)*.

minerals, vitamins, yeast, Aspergillus oryzae fermentation extract. MicroZyme Bolus for Cattle *(Vedco)*.

minerals, vitamins, yeast, fat product(s), lactose, milk protein. Start To Finish® Mare & Foal Pellets™ *(Milk Specialties)*.

minerals, vitamins, yeast, fatty acids. Start To Finish® Performance Pellets™ *(Milk Specialties)*.

minerals, vitamins, yeast, lactic acid producing bacteria. T.D.N. Mini Rockets *(DVM Formula)*, T.D.N. Mini Rockets™ *(Vets Plus)*, T.D.N. Rockets *(DVM Formula)*, T.D.N. Rockets™ *(Vets Plus)*.

minerals, vitamins, yeast, microorganisms. Fastrack® Nonruminant Microbial Gel *(Conklin)*, Fastrack® Ruminant Bolus *(Conklin)*, Fastrack® Ruminant Microbial Gel *(Conklin)*.

minerals, vitamins, zinc. Zinc Plus™ Tablets *(Butler)*.

minerals (complexed). 4-Plex *(Zinpro)*, 4-Plex-C *(Zinpro)*.

mineral spirits, isopropyl alcohol, lanolin. Groom-Aid® Spray *(Evsco)*.

Mineral Vet 5 *(Neogen)*, **minerals.**

mink oil, d-l-panthenol (vitamin B_5), detanglers, jojoba oil, keratin. Lustre Groom Mist™ *(Butler)*.

Mint Disinfectant *(Air-Tite)*, **quaternary ammonia.**

Mirra-Coat® (Equine System) *(Pet-Ag)*, **linoleic acid, vitamin A, vitamin B_6, vitamin E, zinc.**

Mirra-Coat® for Cats *(Pet-Ag)*, **arachidonic acid, linoleic acid, linolenic acid, vitamin A, vitamin B_6, vitamin E.**

Mirra-Coat® Powder and Liquid *(Pet-Ag)*, **biotin, linoleic acid, linolenic acid, vitamin A, vitamin B6, vitamin E.**
Mitaban® *(Pharmacia & Upjohn)*, **amitraz.**
Mita-Clear™ *(Pfizer Animal Health)*, **di-n-propyl isocinchomeronate, n-octyl bicycloheptene dicarboximide, piperonyl butoxide, pyrethrins.**
Mitaplex-P™ *(Tomlyn)*, **piperonyl butoxide, pyrethrins.**
moisturizer(s). Nova Pearls™ Power Moisturizing Spray Mist *(Tomlyn)*, Nova Pearls™ Spray On Moisturizer for Cat Dander Relief *(Tomlyn)*.
moisturizer(s), deodorants. Nova Pearls™ Fresh Scent Deodorant Spray for Ferrets *(Tomlyn)*.
moisturizer(s), emollient(s). Hoof Conditioner *(First Priority)*, Micro Pearls Advantage™ Hydra-Pearls™ Rehydrating Spray *(Evsco)*.
moisturizer(s), PABA sun screen, emollient(s). Frostshield *(Durvet)*.
moisturizer(s), PABA sun screen, vitamins, aloe vera, lanolin. Medicated Udder Balm *(First Priority)*.
moisturizer(s), promoxine. Micro Pearls Advantage™ Dermal-Soothe™ Anti-Itch Spray *(Evsco)*.
moisturizer(s), rinse formula. Micro Pearls Advantage™ Hydra-Pearls™ Cream Rinse *(Evsco)*.
moisturizer(s), shampoo formula. DermaPet® Hypoallergenic Conditioning Shampoo *(DermaPet)*, Micro Pearls Advantage™ Hydra-Pearls™ Shampoo *(Evsco)*, Nova Pearls™ 5 to 1 Concentrate Shampoo *(Tomlyn)*, Nova Pearls™ Sensitive Skin Shampoo *(Tomlyn)*.
moisturizer(s), stain removers, vitamin E, aloe vera. CarraVet™ Multi Purpose Cleansing Foam *(V.P.L.)*.
moisturizer(s), vitamin A, vitamin D, vitamin E, aloe vera. DuraCream *(Durvet)*.
moisturizer(s), vitamins. Teat Elite *(AgriPharm)*.
moisturizer(s), vitamins, emollient(s). Bova Derm® *(Butler)*, Udder Moist *(A.A.H.)*.
MometaMax™ Otic Suspension *(Schering-Plough)*, **clotrimazole, gentamicin, mometasone furoate.**
mometasone furoate, clotrimazole, gentamicin. MometaMax™ Otic Suspension *(Schering-Plough)*.
Mo' Milk® Feed Mix and Top Dress *(TechMix)*, **calcium, iodine, iron, phosphorus, sodium chloride, vitamin A.**
Monarch® Mon-O-Dine *(Ecolab Food & Bev. Div.)*, **iodine complex (povidone-iodine), phosphoric acid.**
Monarch® Prep Udder Wash *(Ecolab Food & Bev. Div.)*, **chlorhexidine.**
Monarch® Protek® Spray *(Ecolab Food & Bev. Div.)*, **chlorhexidine.**
Monarch® Protek® Teat Dip *(Ecolab Food & Bev. Div.)*, **chlorhexidine, iodine complex (povidone-iodine).**
Monarch® Super Kabon® *(Ecolab Food & Bev. Div.)*, **ethanol, quaternary ammonia.**
monensin sodium. Coban® 60 *(Elanco)*, Rumensin® 80 *(Elanco)*.
Monteban® 45 *(Elanco)*, **narasin.**
MoorMan's® Beef Cattle Boost® BT *(ADM)*, **lasalocid sodium.**
MoorMan's® BMD® 30 *(ADM)*, **bacitracin methylene disalicylate.**
MoorMan's® CBX *(ADM)*, **carbadox.**
MoorMan's® Dust with Co-Ral® Insecticide *(ADM)*, **coumaphos.**
MoorMan's® Fly Spray *(ADM)*, **piperonyl butoxide, pyrethrins.**
MoorMan's® Hi-Mag IGR Minerals® *(ADM)*, **methoprene.**
MoorMan's® IGR Cattle Concentrate *(ADM)*, **methoprene.**
MoorMan's® IGR Cattle Mix *(ADM)*, **methoprene.**
MoorMan's® IGR Minerals® *(ADM)*, **methoprene.**
MoorMan's® LN 10 *(ADM)*, **lincomycin hydrochloride.**
MoorMan's® Moorguard® Swine Dewormer *(ADM)*, **fenbendazole.**
MoorMan's® NT 10/10 *(ADM)*, **neomycin, oxytetracycline.**
MoorMan's® Special Mix Cattle Boost® BT *(ADM)*, **lasalocid sodium.**
MoorMan's® TYS 5/5 *(ADM)*, **sulfamethazine, tylosin phosphate.**
MoorMan's® WDC *(ADM)*, **carbadox, pyrantel tartrate.**
morantel tartrate. Rumatel® *(Phibro)*.
moxidectin. Cydectin® Pour-On *(Fort Dodge)*, ProHeart® 6 *(Fort Dodge)*, ProHeart® Tablets *(Fort Dodge)*, Quest® 2% Equine Oral Gel *(Fort Dodge)*.
Mrs. Allen's Shed-Stop® Granules for Cats *(Farnam)*, **fatty acids (omega), minerals, vitamins.**
Mrs. Allen's Shed-Stop® Granules for Dogs *(Farnam)*, **fatty acids (omega), minerals, vitamins.**
Mrs. Allen's Vita Care® Vitamins for Cats *(Farnam)*, **linolenic acid, minerals, taurine, vitamins.**
Mrs. Allen's Vita Care® Vitamins for Dogs *(Farnam)*, **linolenic acid, minerals, vitamins.**
Multi-Electrolytes *(Neogen)*, **dextrose, electrolytes, minerals, vitamins.**
MultiMax™ *(SureNutrition)*, **amino acids, lactic acid producing bacteria, minerals, vitamins.**
Multi-Milk™ *(Pet-Ag)*, **lactose, milk protein, minerals, vitamins.**
Multimin™ *(Multimin)*, **minerals.**
Multi-Pak/256 *(Alpharma)*, **vitamins.**
Multi-Purpose Disinfectant *(LeGear)*, **quaternary ammonia.**
Multi-Quat 128 *(Intercon)*, **quaternary ammonia.**
Multi Quat TB™ *(Intercon)*, **quaternary ammonia.**
mupirocin. Bactoderm® *(Pfizer Animal Health)*.
MU-SE® *(Schering-Plough)*, **selenium (sodium selenite), vitamin E.**
MVT™ Bolus Wet Granulation Formula *(Butler)*, **magnesium oxide.**
MVT Powder™ *(Butler)*, **kaolin, magnesium hydroxide.**
MycAseptic® *(Neogen)*, **b-ionone, limonene.**
MycAseptic® E *(Neogen)*, **b-ionone, limonene.**
Mycitracin® Sterile Ointment *(Pharmacia & Upjohn)*, **bacitracin, neomycin, polymyxin B.**
Mycobacterium cell wall fraction. Equimune® I.V. *(Bioniche Animal Health)*, Immunoboost® *(Bioniche Animal Health)*, Regressin®-V *(Bioniche Animal Health)*.
Mycodex® All-In-One™ Spray *(V.P.L.)*, **n-octyl bicycloheptene dicarboximide, piperonyl butoxide, pyrethrins, pyriproxyfen.**
Mycodex® Environmental Control™ Aerosol Household Spray *(V.P.L.)*, **pyriproxyfen, sumethrin, tetramethrin.**
Mycodex® Environmental Control™ Aerosol Room Fogger *(V.P.L.)*, **n-octyl bicycloheptene dicarboximide, permethrin, pyrethrins, pyriproxyfen.**
Mycodex® Pearlescent Grooming Shampoo *(V.P.L.)*, **shampoo formula.**
Mycodex® Pet Shampoo with 3X Pyrethrins *(V.P.L.)*, **piperonyl butoxide, pyrethrins.**
Mycodex® Pet Shampoo with Carbaryl *(V.P.L.)*, **carbaryl.**
Mycodex® SensiCare™ Flea & Tick Shampoo *(V.P.L.)*, **d-trans allethrin, piperonyl butoxide.**
Mycodex® SensiCare™ Flea & Tick Spray *(V.P.L.)*, **piperonyl butoxide, pyrethrins.**
Myosan™ Cream *(Life Science)*, **allantoin, benzalkonium chloride, carbamide.**
Myosan™ Solution *(Life Science)*, **allantoin, benzalkonium chloride, carbamide.**
myristyl-gamma-picolinium chloride, neomycin, tetracaine, isoflupredone acetate. Neo-Predef® with Tetracaine Powder *(Pharmacia & Upjohn)*.

N

naled. Bansect® Flea & Tick Collar for Cats *(Sergeant's)*, Bansect® Flea & Tick Collar for Dogs *(Sergeant's)*.
naltrexone hydrochloride. Trexonil™ *(Wildlife)*.
Naquasone® Bolus *(Schering-Plough)*, **dexamethasone, trichlormethiazide.**
narasin. Monteban® 45 *(Elanco)*.
narasin, nicarbazin. Maxiban® 72 *(Elanco)*.
Natural Mint Liniment™ *(Horses Prefer)*, **aloe vera, emollient(s), peppermint oil.**
Natural Solvent™ *(Butler)*, **solvent(s).**
Naxcel® *(Pharmacia & Upjohn)*, **ceftiofur sodium.**
neatsfoot oil, petrolatum, pine tar, turpentine, lanolin. Absorbine® Hooflex® Liquid Conditioner *(W. F. Young)*.
neatsfoot oil, pine tar, turpentine, lanolin. Absorbine® Hooflex® Original Conditioner *(W. F. Young)*.
neatsfoot oil, pine tar, turpentine, wheat germ oil, fish oil, iodine, linseed oil. Shur Hoof™ *(Horse Health)*.
neatsfoot oil, vitamins, aloe vera, lanolin. Absorbine® Hooflex® Moisturizing Creme *(W. F. Young)*.
Neigh-Lox® *(K.P.P.)*, **aluminum, calcium carbonate, dicalcium phosphate.**
Nemex™ Tabs *(Pfizer Animal Health)*, **pyrantel pamoate.**
Nemex™-2 Suspension *(Pfizer Animal Health)*, **pyrantel pamoate.**
Neo-325 Soluble Powder *(Bimeda)*, **neomycin.**
Neobacimyx® *(Schering-Plough)*, **bacitracin, neomycin, polymyxin B.**
Neobacimyx®-H *(Schering-Plough)*, **bacitracin, hydrocortisone acetate, neomycin, polymyxin B.**
Neomix® 325 Soluble Powder *(Pharmacia & Upjohn)*, **neomycin.**
Neomix® AG 325 Medicated Premix *(Pharmacia & Upjohn)*, **neomycin.**
Neomix® AG 325 Soluble Powder *(Pharmacia & Upjohn)*, **neomycin.**
neomycin. AmTech Neomycin Oral Solution *(Phoenix Scientific)*, Biosol® Liquid *(Pharmacia & Upjohn)*, Neo-325 Soluble Powder *(Bimeda)*, Neomix® 325 Soluble Powder *(Pharmacia & Upjohn)*, Neomix® AG 325 Medicated Premix *(Pharmacia & Upjohn)*, Neomix® AG 325 Soluble Powder *(Pharmacia & Upjohn)*, Neomycin 200 *(Aspen)*, Neomycin 325 *(AgriLabs)*, *(Durvet)*, Neomycin Oral Solution *(AgriLabs)*, *(Durvet)*, *(Phoenix Pharmaceutical)*, Neo-Sol® 50 *(Alpharma)*, Neosol-Oral *(Med-Pharmex)*, Neosol Soluble Powder *(Med-Pharmex)*, Neoved 200 *(Vedco)*, Neovet 325/100 *(AgriPharm)*, Neovet® Neomycin Oral Solution *(AgriPharm)*.
neomycin, nystatin, thiostrepton, triamcinolone acetonide. Animax® Ointment *(Pharmaderm)*, Dermagen™ Cream *(Butler)*, Dermagen™ Ointment *(Butler)*, Dermalog® Ointment *(RXV)*, Dermalone™ Ointment *(Vedco)*, Derma-Vet™ Cream *(Med-Pharmex)*, Derma-Vet™ Ointment *(Med-Pharmex)*, Panolog® Cream *(Fort Dodge)*, Panolog® Ointment *(Fort Dodge)*, Quadritop™ Cream *(Vetus)*, Quadritop™ Ointment *(Vetus)*.
neomycin, oxytetracycline. Advance™ Calf Medic® Concentrate *(Milk Specialties)*, Advance™ Calvita® Deluxe Medicated Milk Replacer *(Milk Specialties)*, Advance™ Calvita® Supreme Medicated A.M. Milk Replacer with OTC/Neo *(Milk Specialties)*, Land O Lakes® Instant Cow's Match™ *(Land O'Lakes)*, Land O Lakes® Instant Nursing Formula *(Land O'Lakes)*, MoorMan's® NT 10/10 *(ADM)*, Neo-Oxy 10/5 Meal

(PennField), Neo-Oxy 10/10 Meal (PennField), Neo-Oxy 50/50 Meal (PennField), Neo-Oxy 100/50 Meal (PennField), Neo-Oxy 100/50 MR (PennField), Neo-Oxy 100/100 Meal (PennField), Neo-Terramycin® 50/50 (Phibro), Neo-Terramycin® 50/50D (Phibro), Neo-Terramycin® 100/50 (Phibro), Neo-Terramycin® 100/50D (Phibro), Vita Ferm® Milk-N-More Medicated Milk Replacer with Neo/OTC (BioZyme).

neomycin, oxytetracycline, vitamins. Land O Lakes® Instant Amplifier® Max (Land O'Lakes), Land O Lakes® Instant Amplifier® Select (Land O'Lakes), Land O Lakes® Instant Maxi Care® (Land O'Lakes), Land O Lakes® LitterMilk® (Land O'Lakes).

neomycin, polymyxin B, bacitracin. Mycitracin® Sterile Ointment (Pharmacia & Upjohn), Neobacimyx® (Schering-Plough), TriOptic-P™ (Pfizer Animal Health), Vetro-Biotic® Ointment (Pharmaderm), Vetropolycin® Ophthalmic Ointment (Pharmaderm).

neomycin, polymyxin B, bacitracin, hydrocortisone acetate. Neobacimyx®-H (Schering-Plough), TriOptic-S® (Pfizer Animal Health), Vetropolycin® HC Ophthalmic Ointment (Pharmaderm).

neomycin, tetracaine, isoflupredone acetate. Tritop® (Pharmacia & Upjohn).

neomycin, tetracaine, isoflupredone acetate, myristyl-gamma-picolinium chloride. Neo-Predef® with Tetracaine Powder (Pharmacia & Upjohn).

neomycin, thiabendazole, dexamethasone. Tresaderm® (Merial).

Neomycin 200 (Aspen), **neomycin.**

Neomycin 325 (AgriLabs), (Durvet), **neomycin.**

Neomycin Oral Solution (AgriLabs), (Durvet), (Phoenix Pharmaceutical), **neomycin.**

Neo-Oxy 10/5 Meal (PennField), **neomycin, oxytetracycline.**

Neo-Oxy 10/10 Meal (PennField), **neomycin, oxytetracycline.**

Neo-Oxy 50/50 Meal (PennField), **neomycin, oxytetracycline.**

Neo-Oxy 100/50 Meal (PennField), **neomycin, oxytetracycline.**

Neo-Oxy 100/50 MR (PennField), **neomycin, oxytetracycline.**

Neo-Oxy 100/100 Meal (PennField), **neomycin, oxytetracycline.**

Neo-Predef® with Tetracaine Powder (Pharmacia & Upjohn), **isoflupredone acetate, myristyl-gamma-picolinium chloride, neomycin, tetracaine.**

Neo-Sol® 50 (Alpharma), **neomycin.**

Neosol-Oral (Med-Pharmex), **neomycin.**

Neosol Soluble Powder (Med-Pharmex), **neomycin.**

Neo-Terramycin® 50/50 (Phibro), **neomycin, oxytetracycline.**

Neo-Terramycin® 50/50D (Phibro), **neomycin, oxytetracycline.**

Neo-Terramycin® 100/50 (Phibro), **neomycin, oxytetracycline.**

Neo-Terramycin® 100/50D (Phibro), **neomycin, oxytetracycline.**

Neoved 200 (Vedco), **neomycin.**

Neovet 325/100 (AgriPharm), **neomycin.**

Neovet® Neomycin Oral Solution (AgriPharm), **neomycin.**

Neurosyn™ Tablets (Boehringer Ingelheim), **primidone.**

neutralizer(s). Compliance™ Neutralizing Powder (Metrex), Elimin • Odor® Canine (Pfizer Animal Health), Elimin • Odor® Feline (Pfizer Animal Health), Elimin • Odor® General Purpose (Pfizer Animal Health), Elimin • Odor® Pet Accident (Pfizer Animal Health).

neutralizer(s), deodorants. A • O • E™, Animal Odor Eliminator (Thornell), Cat-Off™ (Thornell), Cat-Off™ Concentrate (Thornell), Dog-Off™ (Thornell), Ferret-Off™ (Thornell), K • O • E™, Kennel Odor Eliminator (Thornell), Pleascent® Puppy (Thornell), Skunk-Off® (Thornell).

neutralizer(s), shampoo formula, deodorants. Skunk-Off® Shampoo (Thornell).

neutralizer(s), stain removers. Elimin • Odor® Pet Stain Eliminator (Pfizer Animal Health).

New-Hoof™ Concentrate (Vets Plus), **copper.**

New-Hoof Topical™ (Vets Plus), **copper.**

New Z® Diazinon Insecticide Cattle Ear Tags (Farnam), **diazinon, piperonyl butoxide.**

New Z® Permethrin Insecticide Cattle Ear Tags (Farnam), **permethrin.**

Nexaband® Liquid (Abbott), **cyanoacrylate (formulated).**

Nexaband® S/C (Abbott), **cyanoacrylate (formulated).**

NFZ® Puffer (AgriLabs), (Aspen), (Durvet), (Loveland), **nitrofurazone.**

nfz® puffer (AgriPharm), **nitrofurazone.**

NFZ® Wound Dressing (Loveland), **nitrofurazone.**

Nia-Bol™ (Great States), **niacin.**

niacin. Nia-Bol™ (Great States), Niacin Bolus (Vets Plus), Nu-Keto™ Bolus (Butler).

niacin, propylene glycol, vitamin B_6, vitamin B_{12} (cyanocobalamin). Super Keto Drench (Vedco).

niacin, propylene glycol, vitamin B-complex. Keto-Nia-Fresh™ (Vets Plus).

niacin, propylene glycol, vitamins. Agri Plus Keto-Nia Drench™ (Vets Plus), Niacin-Energy Drench Plus Vitamins (AgriLabs), (Durvet), Oral Keto-Energy Drench (DVM Formula), Oral Keto-Energy Gel (DVM Formula).

niacin, vitamin B-complex. Lipotinic (Vet-A-Mix).

Niacin Bolus (Vets Plus), **niacin.**

Niacin-Energy Drench Plus Vitamins (AgriLabs), (Durvet), **niacin, propylene glycol, vitamins.**

Nicarb® 25% (Phibro), **nicarbazin.**

nicarbazin. Nicarb® 25% (Phibro).

nicarbazin, narasin. Maxiban® 72 (Elanco).

nicotinamide, chlorhexidine. Stomadhex™ (Virbac).

Nik Stop® Styptic Powder (Tomlyn), **aluminum chloride, ammonium chloride, bentonite, benzocaine, copper sulfate, diatomaceous earth, ferric subsulfate, iodoform.**

nisin. Wipe Out® Dairy Wipes (ImmuCell).

nitenpyram. Capstar® (Novartis).

nitrofurazone. Equi-Phar™ Nitrofurazone Soluble Dressing (Vedco), Fura-Ointment® (Farnam), Fura-Septin (Anthony), Fura-Zone (Neogen), KV Wound Powder (KenVet), NFZ® Puffer (AgriLabs), nfz® puffer (AgriPharm), NFZ® Puffer (Aspen), (Durvet), (Loveland), NFZ® Wound Dressing (Loveland), Nitrofurazone (Aspen), Nitrofurazone Dressing (Durvet), Nitrofurazone Dressing 0.2% (AgriLabs), (AgriPharm), Nitrofurazone Ointment (Phoenix Pharmaceutical), Nitrofurazone Soluble Dressing (Butler), (Med-Pharmex), Nitrozone™ Ointment (Bimeda).

Nitrofurazone (Aspen), **nitrofurazone.**

Nitrofurazone Dressing (Durvet), **nitrofurazone.**

Nitrofurazone Dressing 0.2% (AgriLabs), (AgriPharm), **nitrofurazone.**

Nitrofurazone Ointment (Phoenix Pharmaceutical), **nitrofurazone.**

Nitrofurazone Soluble Dressing (Butler), (Med-Pharmex), **nitrofurazone.**

nitrogen, peptides, amino acids. Arm & Hammer® Bio-Chlor® (Church & Dwight), Arm & Hammer® Fermenten® (Church & Dwight).

Nitrozone™ Ointment (Bimeda), **nitrofurazone.**

No Chew Spray (Vetus), **denatonium benzoate.**

n-octyl bicycloheptene dicarboximide, d-trans allethrin. Hartz® 2 in 1® Rid Flea™ Dog Shampoo with Allethrin (Hartz Mountain).

n-octyl bicycloheptene dicarboximide, d-trans allethrin, dicarboximide. Hartz® Control Pet Care System® Flea & Tick Conditioning Shampoo for Cats (Hartz Mountain), Hartz® Control Pet Care System® Flea & Tick Conditioning Shampoo for Dogs (Hartz Mountain).

n-octyl bicycloheptene dicarboximide, permethrin, phenothrin, piperonyl butoxide, methoprene. Vet-Kem® Siphotrol® Plus II Premise Spray (Wellmark).

n-octyl bicycloheptene dicarboximide, permethrin, piperonyl butoxide. War Paint™ Insecticidal Paste (Loveland).

n-octyl bicycloheptene dicarboximide, permethrin, piperonyl butoxide, d-2-allayl-4-hydroxy-3-methyl-2-cyclopenten-1-one, di-n-propyl isocinchomeronate, fenoxycarb. Scratchex® Super Spray™ (Combe).

n-octyl bicycloheptene dicarboximide, permethrin, piperonyl butoxide, pyrethrins, butoxypolypropylene glycol, di-n-propyl isocinchomeronate. Adams™ Fly Spray and Repellent (V.P.L.), Flysect® Super-7 (Equicare).

n-octyl bicycloheptene dicarboximide, permethrin, piperonyl butoxide, pyrethrins, di-n-propyl isocinchomeronate. Adams™ Fly Repellent Concentrate (V.P.L.), Flysect® Super-C (Equicare).

n-octyl bicycloheptene dicarboximide, permethrin, piperonyl butoxide, pyriproxyfen, d-2-allayl-4-hydroxy-3-methyl-2-cyclopenten-1-one, di-n-propyl isocinchomeronate. Sergeant's® PreTect® Flea & Tick Spray for Cats & Kittens (Sergeant's), Sergeant's® PreTect® Flea & Tick Spray for Dogs & Puppies (Sergeant's).

n-octyl bicycloheptene dicarboximide, permethrin, pyrethrins. Duocide® L.A. Spray (Virbac).

n-octyl bicycloheptene dicarboximide, permethrin, pyrethrins, pyriproxyfen. Adams™ Room Fogger with Sykillstop™ (Farnam), (V.P.L.), EctoKyl™ IGR Total Release Fogger (DVM), Happy Jack® Flea Flogger Plus (Happy Jack), IGR House & Area Fogger (Durvet), Mycodex® Environmental Control™ Aerosol Room Fogger (V.P.L.), OmniTrol IGR Fogger (Vedco), Virbac KnockOut® ES Area Treatment (Virbac), Virbac KnockOut® Room and Area Fogger (Virbac).

n-octyl bicycloheptene dicarboximide, permethrin, pyriproxyfen. Sergeant's® Flea-Free Breeze™ (Sergeant's).

n-octyl bicycloheptene dicarboximide, permethrin, pyriproxyfen, linalool. Adams™ Inverted Carpet Spray (Farnam), Sergeant's® PreTect® Household Flea & Tick Spray (Sergeant's).

n-octyl bicycloheptene dicarboximide, phenol, piperonyl butoxide, pyrethrins, quaternary ammonia. Microban® X-580 Institutional Spray Plus (Microban).

n-octyl bicycloheptene dicarboximide, phenothrin, methylcarbamate. Adams™ Dual Action Flea & Tick Collar for Cats (Farnam), Adams™ Dual Action Flea & Tick Collar for Large Dogs (Farnam), Adams™ Dual Action Flea & Tick Collar for Medium Dogs (Farnam).

n-octyl bicycloheptene dicarboximide, piperonyl butoxide, pyrethrins. Adams™ Water Based Flea and Tick Mist (Farnam), (V.P.L.), Cerumite 3x (Evsco), Dairy Bomb-55 (Durvet), Ecto-Foam™ (Virbac), Ecto-Soothe™ 3X Shampoo (Virbac), Flea Halt!™ Flea & Tick Repellent Towelettes (Farnam), Flea Halt!™ Flea & Tick Repellent Towelettes for Ferrets (Farnam), Flea, Tick and Lice Shampoo (Tomlyn), Hartz® 2 in 1® Flea & Tick Dip for Dogs and Cats (Hartz Mountain), Hartz® 2 in 1® Luster Bath for Cats (Hartz Mountain), Hartz® 2 in 1® Rid Flea™ Dog Shampoo with Pyrethrin (Hartz Mountain), Hartz® Easy Wash™ Flea & Tick Shampoo for Dogs (Hartz Mountain), Pyrethrin Plus Shampoo (Vedco), Scratchex® Flea & Tick Shampoo (Combe).

n-octyl bicycloheptene dicarboximide, piperonyl butoxide, pyrethrins, butoxypolypropylene glycol. Pet Guard™ Gel (Virbac).

n-octyl bicycloheptene dicarboximide, piperonyl butoxide, pyrethrins, carbaryl. Scratchex® Flea & Tick Powder *(Combe).*

n-octyl bicycloheptene dicarboximide, piperonyl butoxide, pyrethrins, dicarboximide. Hartz® 2 in 1® Flea & Tick Killer for Dogs *(Hartz Mountain).*

n-octyl bicycloheptene dicarboximide, piperonyl butoxide, pyrethrins, dichlorvos. Super II Dairy & Farm Spray *(Durvet).*

n-octyl bicycloheptene dicarboximide, piperonyl butoxide, pyrethrins, di-n-propyl isocinchomeronate. Adams™ Flea & Tick Mist *(V.P.L.)*, Adams™ Pyrethrin Dip *(Farnam), (V.P.L.)*, EctoKyl™ 3X Flea & Tick Shampoo *(DVM)*, Flea & Tick Mist *(Davis)*, Flysect® Repellent Spray *(Equicare)*, Flysect® Roll-On Fly Repellent Face Lotion *(Equicare)*, Flys-Off® Fly Repellent Ointment *(Farnam)*, Mita-Clear™ *(Pfizer Animal Health)*, Otomite® Plus *(Virbac)*, Performer® Ear Mite Killer *(AgriLabs)*, Pet Care Ear Mite Lotion & Repellent *(Durvet)*, Pet Care Fast Kill Flea & Tick Spray for Dogs & Cats *(Durvet)*, Roll-On™ Fly Repellent *(Farnam)*, Triple Pyrethrins Flea & Tick Shampoo *(Davis)*, Vet-Kem® Triple Action Flea & Tick Shampoo for Dogs, Cats, & Horses *(Wellmark)*, Virbac Pyrethrin Dip™ *(Virbac).*

n-octyl bicycloheptene dicarboximide, piperonyl butoxide, pyrethrins, methoprene. Vet-Kem® Ovitrol® Plus Flea, Tick & Bot Spray *(Wellmark).*

n-octyl bicycloheptene dicarboximide, piperonyl butoxide, pyrethrins, pyriproxyfen. Adams™ Flea & Tick Mist with Sykillstop™ *(Farnam), (V.P.L.)*, Mycodex® All-In-One™ Spray *(V.P.L.)*, Sergeant's® PreTect® Flea & Tick Shampoo for Cats and Kittens *(Sergeant's).*

Nolva-Cleanse™ *(Fort Dodge)*, **propylene glycol.**

Nolvadent® *(Fort Dodge)*, **chlorhexidine.**

Nolvalube® *(Fort Dodge)*, **chlorhexidine.**

Nolvasan® 5% Teat Dip Concentrate *(Fort Dodge)*, **chlorhexidine, glycerine.**

Nolvasan® Antiseptic Ointment *(Fort Dodge)*, **chlorhexidine.**

Nolvasan® Cap-Tabs® *(Fort Dodge)*, **chlorhexidine.**

Nolvasan® Otic *(Fort Dodge)*, **otic solvent, surfactant.**

Nolvasan® S *(Fort Dodge)*, **chlorhexidine.**

Nolvasan® Shampoo *(Fort Dodge)*, **chlorhexidine.**

Nolvasan® Skin and Wound Cleanser *(Fort Dodge)*, **chlorhexidine.**

Nolvasan® Solution *(Fort Dodge)*, **chlorhexidine.**

Nolvasan® Surgical Scrub *(Fort Dodge)*, **chlorhexidine.**

Nolvasan® Suspension *(Fort Dodge)*, **chlorhexidine.**

Nolvasan® Teat Dip Concentrate *(Fort Dodge)*, **chlorhexidine, glycerine.**

Nolvasan® Udder Wash Concentrate *(Fort Dodge)*, **chlorhexidine.**

Non-Spermicidal - Sterile Lubricating Jelly *(First Priority)*, **carboxy methylcellulose, propylene glycol.**

Norcalciphos™ *(Pfizer Animal Health)*, **calcium, calcium hypophosphite, dextrose, magnesium borogluconate.**

Normal Equine Serum *(Colorado Serum)*, **equine serum.**

Normal Serum-Equine *(Professional Biological)*, **equine serum.**

Normosol®-R *(Abbott)*, **electrolytes.**

Nova Pearls™ 5 to 1 Concentrate Shampoo *(Tomlyn)*, **moisturizer(s), shampoo formula.**

Nova Pearls™ Antiseborrheic Shampoo *(Tomlyn)*, **salicylic acid, sulfur.**

Nova Pearls™ Coal Tar Spray *(Tomlyn)*, **coal tar.**

Nova Pearls™ Dry Skin Bath for Dogs *(Tomlyn)*, **salicylic acid, sulfur.**

Nova Pearls™ Fresh Scent Deodorant Spray for Dogs and Cats *(Tomlyn)*, **conditioners, lactamide M.E.A..**

Nova Pearls™ Fresh Scent Deodorant Spray for Ferrets *(Tomlyn)*, **deodorants, moisturizer(s).**

Nova Pearls™ Power Moisturizing Spray Mist *(Tomlyn)*, **moisturizer(s).**

Nova Pearls™ Sensitive Skin Shampoo *(Tomlyn)*, **moisturizer(s), shampoo formula.**

Nova Pearls™ Spray On Moisturizer for Cat Dander Relief *(Tomlyn)*, **moisturizer(s).**

Nova Pearls™ Therapeutic Coal Tar Shampoo *(Tomlyn)*, **coal tar.**

novobiocin. Albamix® Feed Medication *(Pharmacia & Upjohn)*, Biodry® *(Pharmacia & Upjohn).*

novobiocin, penicillin G procaine. Albadry Plus® *(Pharmacia & Upjohn).*

novobiocin, prednisolone, tetracycline. Delta Albaplex® / Delta Albaplex® 3X *(Pharmacia & Upjohn).*

novobiocin, tetracycline. Albaplex® *(Pharmacia & Upjohn).*

NRG-Plus™ *(Bimeda)*, **amino acids, electrolytes, energy source(s), vitamins.**

Nuflor® Injectable Solution 300 mg/mL *(Schering-Plough)*, **florfenicol.**

Nu-Keto™ Bolus *(Butler)*, **niacin.**

Nurturall®-C for Kittens *(V.P.L.)*, **milk replacing formula.**

Nurturall®-C for Puppies *(V.P.L.)*, **milk replacing formula.**

NuSal-T® Shampoo *(DVM)*, **coal tar, menthol, salicylic acid.**

Nutra-Sure™ Cat Vitamins *(Farnam)*, **linolenic acid, minerals, vitamins.**

Nutri-Cal® *(Evsco)*, **energy source(s), nutrients.**

Nutri-Cal® for Dogs and Cats *(Tomlyn)*, **energy source(s), nutrients.**

Nutri-Cal® for Ferrets *(Tomlyn)*, **energy source(s), nutrients.**

Nutri-Cal® for Ferrets & Other Small Animals *(Tomlyn)*, **energy source(s), minerals, vitamins.**

nutrients. Advance™ RuMin 8™ *(Milk Specialties)*, Intensive Care Gruel™ (ICG) *(TechMix)*, Weight Builder™ *(Farnam).*

nutrients, electrolytes. Comeback™ *(AgriPharm)*, One Day Response™ *(Farnam, Livestock Div.).*

nutrients, electrolytes, energy source(s). Baby Pig Restart™ One-4 *(TechMix)*, Calf Restart™ One-4 *(TechMix)*, Vita-Lyte *(Phoenix Pharmaceutical).*

nutrients, electrolytes, energy source(s), microorganisms. NutriVed™ EnerGel Forte *(Vedco).*

nutrients, electrolytes, glucose, microorganisms. Ener-Lyte™ *(Aspen).*

nutrients, energy source(s). EnerCal™ *(Vedco)*, Nutri-Cal® *(Evsco)*, Nutri-Cal® for Dogs and Cats *(Tomlyn)*, Nutri-Cal® for Ferrets *(Tomlyn).*

nutrients, energy source(s), microorganisms. Durazyme Energy Pack *(Durvet).*

nutrients, microorganisms. Durazyme Calf Colostrum Supplement *(Durvet)*, Durazyme Paste for Calves *(Durvet)*, EP-1 3X *(RXV).*

nutrients, phosphorus, vitamins, calcium, milk protein. Foal-Lac® Pellets *(Pet-Ag).*

nutrients, vitamins. PerforMax™ Ration Maximizer *(Equicare).*

nutrients, vitamins, electrolytes, energy source(s). Advance™ Arrest® *(Milk Specialties)*, Advance™ Pro-Lyte Plus® *(Milk Specialties).*

nutrients, vitamins, electrolytes, energy source(s), microorganisms. Sow & Gilt Restart™ One-4 *(TechMix).*

nutrients, vitamins, energy source(s), minerals. CliniCare® Canine Liquid Diet *(Abbott)*, CliniCare® Feline Liquid Diet *(Abbott)*, CliniCare® RF Specialized Feline Liquid Diet *(Abbott).*

nutrients, vitamins, yeast, microorganisms, minerals. Fastrack® Calf Bolus *(Conklin).*

nutrients, yeast, Aspergillus oryzae fermentation extract, electrolytes, energy source(s). Vita Charge® Power Drench *(BioZyme).*

Nutri-Stat™ *(Tomlyn)*, **energy source(s), fatty acids (omega), minerals, vitamins.**

NutriVed™ B-Complex Plus Iron Liquid *(Vedco)*, **amino acids, copper, iron, vitamin B-complex.**

NutriVed™ Calcium Plus Chewable Tablets *(Vedco)*, **calcium, vitamin A, vitamin C (ascorbic acid), vitamin D_3.**

NutriVed™ Chewable Vitamins for Active Dogs *(Vedco)*, **amino acids, electrolytes, fatty acids (essential), minerals.**

NutriVed™ Chewable Vitamins for Cats *(Vedco)*, **amino acids, fatty acids (essential), minerals, taurine, vitamins.**

NutriVed™ Chewable Vitamins for Dogs *(Vedco)*, **amino acids, fatty acids (essential), minerals, vitamins.**

NutriVed™ Chewable Vitamins for Kittens *(Vedco)*, **amino acids, fatty acids (essential), minerals, taurine, vitamins.**

NutriVed™ Chewable Vitamins for Puppies *(Vedco)*, **amino acids, fatty acids (essential), minerals, vitamins.**

NutriVed™ Chewable Zinpro® Tablets *(Vedco)*, **zinc-methionine.**

NutriVed™ EnerGel Forte *(Vedco)*, **electrolytes, energy source(s), microorganisms, nutrients.**

NutriVed™ FlatuEx Chewable Tablets *(Vedco)*, **simethicone.**

NutriVed™ Hypo Allergenic Chewable Tablets *(Vedco)*, **amino acids, fatty acids (essential), minerals, vitamins.**

NutriVed™ Hypo-K Granules *(Vedco)*, **potassium.**

NutriVed™ O.F.A. Chewable Tablets for Cats *(Vedco)*, **fatty acids (omega), vitamin A, vitamin D_3, vitamin E, zinc.**

NutriVed™ O.F.A. Chewable Tablets for Large Dogs *(Vedco)*, **fatty acids (essential), vitamin A, vitamin D_3, vitamin E, zinc.**

NutriVed™ O.F.A. Chewable Tablets for Small and Medium Dogs *(Vedco)*, **fatty acids (omega), vitamin A, vitamin D_3, vitamin E, zinc.**

NutriVed™ O.F.A. Gel Caps for Large Dogs *(Vedco)*, **fatty acids (omega).**

NutriVed™ O.F.A. Gel Caps for Small and Medium Size Dogs *(Vedco)*, **fatty acids (omega).**

NutriVed™ O.F.A. Granules for Cats *(Vedco)*, **fatty acids (essential), minerals, taurine, vitamins.**

NutriVed™ O.F.A. Granules for Dogs *(Vedco)*, **fatty acids (essential), minerals, vitamins.**

NutriVed™ O.F.A. Liquid *(Vedco)*, **fatty acids (essential), vitamin A, vitamin D_3, vitamin E.**

NutriVed™ Potassium Citrate Granules for Cats and Dogs *(Vedco)*, **fatty acids, potassium citrate.**

NutriVed™ T-4 Chewable Tablets *(Vedco)*, **levothyroxine.**

nystatin, thiostrepton, triamcinolone acetonide, neomycin. Animax® Ointment *(Pharmaderm)*, Dermagen™ Cream *(Butler)*, Dermagen™ Ointment *(Butler)*, Dermalog® Ointment *(RXV)*, Dermalone™ Ointment *(Vedco)*, Derma-Vet™ Cream *(Med-Pharmex)*, Derma-Vet™ Ointment *(Med-Pharmex)*, Panolog® Cream *(Fort Dodge)*, Panolog® Ointment *(Fort Dodge)*, Quadritop™ Cream *(Vetus)*, Quadritop™ Ointment *(Vetus).*

O

Oxy-Gard™ Activated Peroxide Sanitizing Teat Dip *(Ecolab Food & Bev. Div.)*, **hydrogen peroxide, lactic acid, sodium linear alkylate sulfonate.**

Oxyglobin® Solution *(Biopure)*, **hemoglobin glutamer-200 (bovine).**

Oxy-Mycin® 100 *(AgriPharm)*, **oxytetracycline.**

Oxy-Mycin® 200 *(AgriPharm)*, **oxytetracycline.**

oxypolygelatin, electrolytes. RapidVet™ Plasm-ex™ *(DMS Laboratories)*.

oxytetracycline. Agrimycin® 100 *(AgriLabs)*, Agrimycin® 200 *(AgriLabs)*, Agrimycin®-343 *(AgriLabs)*, Agrimycin® Powder *(AgriLabs)*, AmTech Maxim-100 *(Phoenix Scientific)*, AmTech Maxim-200® *(Phoenix Scientific)*, AmTech Oxytetracycline HCl Soluble Powder *(Phoenix Scientific)*, AmTech Oxytetracycline HCl Soluble Powder-343 *(Phoenix Scientific)*, Bio-Mycin® 200 *(Boehringer Ingelheim)*, Duramycin 72-200 *(Durvet)*, Duramycin-100 *(Durvet)*, Liquamycin® LA-200® *(Pfizer Animal Health)*, Maxim-200® *(Phoenix Pharmaceutical)*, OT 200 *(Vetus)*, OTC 50 *(Durvet)*, Oxy 500 Calf Bolus *(Boehringer Ingelheim)*, Oxy 1000 Calf Bolus *(Boehringer Ingelheim)*, Oxybiotic™-100 *(Butler)*, Oxybiotic™-200 *(Butler)*, OxyCure™-100 *(Vedco)*, OxyCure™ 200 *(Vedco)*, Oxy-Mycin® 100 *(AgriPharm)*, Oxy-Mycin® 200 *(AgriPharm)*, Oxytetracycline-343 *(Durvet)*, Oxytet Soluble *(Alpharma)*, Pennox™ 50 Meal *(PennField)*, Pennox 100 Hi-Flo™ Meal *(PennField)*, Pennox™ 100-MR *(PennField)*, Pennox™ 200 Injectable *(PennField)*, Pennox™ 343 Soluble Powder *(PennField)*, Promycin™ 100 *(Phoenix Pharmaceutical)*, Terramycin® 10 TM-10® *(Phibro)*, Terramycin® 50 *(Phibro)*, Terramycin® 100 *(Phibro)*, Terramycin® 100 for Fish *(Phibro)*, Terramycin® 200 *(Phibro)*, Terramycin-343® Soluble Powder *(Pfizer Animal Health)*, Terramycin® Scours Tablets *(Pfizer Animal Health)*, Terramycin® Soluble Powder *(Pfizer Animal Health)*, Terra-Vet 100 *(Aspen)*, Terra Vet Soluble Powder *(Aspen)*, Terra-Vet Soluble Powder 343 *(Aspen)*, Tetravet-CA™ *(Alpharma)*, Tetroxy®-100 *(Bimeda)*, Tetroxy® HCA Soluble Powder *(Bimeda)*, Tetroxy® LA *(Bimeda)*, TM-50® *(Phibro)*, TM-50®D *(Phibro)*, TM-100® *(Phibro)*, TM-100®D *(Phibro)*.

oxytetracycline, neomycin. Advance™ Calf Medic® Concentrate *(Milk Specialties)*, Advance™ Calvita® Deluxe Medicated Milk Replacer *(Milk Specialties)*, Advance™ Calvita® Supreme Medicated A.M. Milk Replacer with OTC/Neo *(Milk Specialties)*, Land O Lakes® Instant Cow's Match™ *(Land O'Lakes)*, Land O Lakes® Instant Nursing Formula *(Land O'Lakes)*, MoorMan's® NT 10/10 *(ADM)*, Neo-Oxy 10/5 Meal *(PennField)*, Neo-Oxy 10/10 Meal *(PennField)*, Neo-Oxy 50/50 Meal *(PennField)*, Neo-Oxy 100/50 Meal *(PennField)*, Neo-Oxy 100/50 MR *(PennField)*, Neo-Oxy 100/100 Meal *(PennField)*, Neo-Terramycin® 50/50 *(Phibro)*, Neo-Terramycin® 50/50D *(Phibro)*, Neo-Terramycin® 100/50 *(Phibro)*, Neo-Terramycin® 100/50D *(Phibro)*, Vita Ferm® Milk-N-More Medicated Milk Replacer with Neo/OTC *(BioZyme)*.

oxytetracycline, polymyxin B. Terramycin® Ophthalmic Ointment *(Pfizer Animal Health)*.

oxytetracycline, vitamins, neomycin. Land O Lakes® Instant Amplifier® Max *(Land O'Lakes)*, Land O Lakes® Instant Amplifier® Select *(Land O'Lakes)*, Land O Lakes® Instant Maxi Care® *(Land O'Lakes)*, Land O Lakes® LitterMilk® *(Land O'Lakes)*.

Oxytetracycline-343 *(Durvet)*, **oxytetracycline.**

Oxytet Soluble *(Alpharma)*, **oxytetracycline.**

oxytocin. AmTech Oxytocin Injection *(Phoenix Scientific)*, Oxoject *(Vetus)*, Oxytocin Injection *(AgriLabs)*, *(Aspen)*, *(Bimeda)*, *(Butler)*, *(Phoenix Pharmaceutical)*, *(RXV)*, *(Vedco)*, *(Vet Tek)*.

Oxytocin Injection *(AgriLabs)*, *(Aspen)*, *(Bimeda)*, *(Butler)*, *(Phoenix Pharmaceutical)*, *(RXV)*, *(Vedco)*, *(Vet Tek)*, **oxytocin.**

P

P-128 *(First Priority)*, **quaternary ammonia.**

PABA sun screen, emollient(s), moisturizer(s). Frostshield *(Durvet)*.

PABA sun screen, vitamins, aloe vera, lanolin, moisturizer(s). Medicated Udder Balm *(First Priority)*.

Pad-Tough™ *(Life Science)*, **aloe vera, comfrey.**

PalaBIS™ *(PharmX)*, **bismuth subsalicylate.**

Palamega™ Complex Chewable Tablets (Liver Flavor) *(Schering-Plough)*, **fatty acids (omega), vitamins, zinc.**

Palapectate™ *(PharmX)*, **attapulgite.**

Palaprin® 65 *(PharmX)*, **acetylsalicylic acid.**

Palaprin® 325 *(PharmX)*, **acetylsalicylic acid.**

Panacur® Beef and Dairy Cattle Dewormer *(Intervet)*, **fenbendazole.**

Panacur® Cattle Dewormer *(Intervet)*, **fenbendazole.**

Panacur® Cattle Dewormer (92 g) *(Intervet)*, **fenbendazole.**

Panacur® Granules 22.2% *(Intervet)*, **fenbendazole.**

Panacur® Granules 22.2% (Dogs only) *(Intervet)*, **fenbendazole.**

Panacur® Granules 22.2% (Horse) *(Intervet)*, **fenbendazole.**

Panacur® Horse Dewormer *(Intervet)*, **fenbendazole.**

Panacur® Horse Dewormer (25 g) *(Intervet)*, **fenbendazole.**

Panacur® Horse Dewormer (57 g) *(Intervet)*, **fenbendazole.**

Panacur® Horse Dewormer (92 g) *(Intervet)*, **fenbendazole.**

PanaKare™ Plus Powder *(Neogen)*, **amylase, lipase, protease, vitamin A, vitamin D, vitamin E.**

PanaKare™ Plus Tablets *(Neogen)*, **amylase, lipase, protease, vitamin A, vitamin D, vitamin E.**

Pancreatic Plus Powder *(Butler)*, **amylase, lipase, protease, vitamins.**

Pancreatic Plus Tablets *(Butler)*, **amylase, lipase, protease, vitamins.**

PancreVed Powder *(Vedco)*, **amylase, lipase, protease, vitamins.**

PancreVed Tablets *(Vedco)*, **amylase, lipase, protease, vitamins.**

Pancrezyme® *(King Animal Health)*, **amylase, lipase, protease.**

Panmycin Aquadrops® *(Pharmacia & Upjohn)*, **tetracycline.**

Panolog® Cream *(Fort Dodge)*, **neomycin, nystatin, thiostrepton, triamcinolone acetonide.**

Panolog® Ointment *(Fort Dodge)*, **neomycin, nystatin, thiostrepton, triamcinolone acetonide.**

Pantek® Cleanser *(Loveland)*, **cresol.**

pantothenate, biotin, methionine (d-l). Dealer Select Horse Care Biotin 800 *(Durvet)*.

papaya fruit, psyllium, kelp, liver meal. Fiber Forte® Feline *(Life Science)*.

parachlorometaxylenol, aluminum chlohydroxy allantoinate. Absorbine® Hooflex® Thrush Remedy *(W. F. Young)*.

parachlorometaxylenol, copper sulfate. Proud Flesh Powder *(First Priority)*.

parachlorometaxylenol, pine oil, scarlet red, benzyl alcohol, eucalyptus oil, isopropyl alcohol (isopropanol), methyl salicylate. Scarlet Oil *(First Priority)*.

parachlorometaxylenol, pine oil, scarlet red, benzyl alcohol, eucalyptus oil, methyl salicylate. Scarlet Oil *(Vedco)*, Scarlet Oil Wound Dressing *(AgriPharm)*.

parachlorometaxylenol, propylene glycol, aloe vera. Thrush Treatment *(First Priority)*.

parachlorometaxylenol, thymol, witch hazel, wormwood oil, aloe vera, iodide (potassium), isopropyl alcohol, menthol. Veterinary Liniment *(First Priority)*.

Paracide-F *(Argent)*, **formaldehyde, methanol.**

Paraguard™ Shampoo *(First Priority)*, **captan, sulfur.**

Parasite-S *(Western Chemical)*, **formaldehyde, methanol.**

para-tertiary-amylphenol, ortho-benzyl-para-chlorophenol, orthophenylphenol. PHD 22.5 *(Bio-Tek)*.

Parr Quat *(Butler)*, **quaternary ammonia.**

Parr Quat 4X *(Butler)*, **quaternary ammonia.**

Parvo Guard™ *(First Priority)*, **iodine.**

Parvosan™ *(KenVet)*, **2-(hydroxymethyl)-2-nitro-1,3 propanediol, formaldehyde, quaternary ammonia.**

Parvosol® II RTU *(KenVet)*, **quaternary ammonia.**

Patriot™ Insecticide Cattle Ear Tags *(Boehringer Ingelheim)*, **diazinon.**

Paylean® 9 *(Elanco)*, **ractopamine hydrochloride.**

P-chloro-M-xylenol, pine oil, scarlet red, eucalyptus oil, methyl salicylate. Scarlex® Scarlet Oil *(Farnam)*.

PearLyt™ Shampoo *(DVM)*, **shampoo formula.**

pectin, aluminum hydroxide, kaolin. Anti-Diarrhea Tablets *(ARC)*, Diarrhea Tabs *(Butler)*.

pectin, aluminum silicate, attapulgite, carob, magnesium trisilicate. Veda-Sorb Jr Bolus *(Vedco)*.

pectin, attapulgite, bismuth subcarbonate, kanamycin sulfate. Amforol® Suspension *(Fort Dodge)*, Amforol® Tablets *(Fort Dodge)*.

pectin, attapulgite, carob, magnesium trisilicate. Anti-Diarrheal Cattle Bolus *(AgriLabs)*, Gastro-Sorb™ Bolus *(Butler)*, Gastro-Sorb™ Calf Bolus *(Butler)*, Intesti-Sorb Bolus *(AgriPharm)*, Intesti-Sorb Calf Bolus *(AgriPharm)*, Maxi-Sorb Bolus *(Durvet)*, Maxi Sorb Calf Bolus *(Durvet)*, Veda-Sorb Bolus *(Vedco)*.

pectin, attapulgite, magnesium trisilicate. Endosorb™ Bolus *(PRN Pharmacal)*, Endosorb™ Suspension *(PRN Pharmacal)*, Endosorb™ Tablets *(PRN Pharmacal)*.

pectin, kaolin. Kaolin Pectin *(Bimeda)*, Kaolin-Pectin *(Durvet)*, Kaolin-Pectin Plus *(AgriPharm)*, Kaolin Pectin Suspension *(A.A.H.)*, *(First Priority)*, *(Vedco)*, Kao-Pec *(AgriLabs)*, Kaopectolin *(Aspen)*, Kaopectolin™ *(Butler)*, Kao-Pect+ *(Phoenix Pharmaceutical)*.

Pellitol® Ointment *(Veterinary Specialties)*, **bismuth subgallate, bismuth subnitrate, calamine, juniper tar, resorcinol, zinc oxide.**

Pen-Aqueous *(AgriPharm)*, *(Durvet)*, **penicillin G procaine.**

Pene-Mite™ *(Farnam)*, **piperonyl butoxide, pyrethrins.**

Penicillin 100 *(Alpharma)*, **penicillin G procaine.**

penicillin G benzathine, penicillin G procaine. Ambi-Pen™ *(Butler)*, Combicillin *(Anthony)*, Combicillin-AG *(Anthony)*, Duo-Pen® *(AgriPharm)*, Dura-Pen *(Durvet)*, Durapen™ *(Vedco)*, Sterile Penicillin G Benzathine and Penicillin G Procaine *(Aspen)*, *(G.C. Hanford)*, Twin-Pen™ *(AgriLabs)*.

penicillin G potassium. Penicillin G Potassium *(AgriLabs)*, Penicillin G Potassium, USP *(AgriPharm)*, *(Bimeda)*, *(Durvet)*, Penicillin G Potassium USP *(Fort Dodge)*, R-Pen *(Alpharma)*.

Penicillin G Potassium *(AgriLabs)*, **penicillin G potassium.**

Penicillin G Potassium, USP *(AgriPharm)*, *(Bimeda)*, *(Durvet)*, **penicillin G potassium.**

Penicillin G Potassium USP *(Fort Dodge)*, **penicillin G potassium.**

penicillin G procaine. Agri-Cillin™ *(AgriLabs)*, Aquacillin™ *(Vedco)*, Go-Dry™ *(G.C. Hanford)*, Masti-Clear™ *(G.C. Hanford)*, Microcillin *(Anthony)*, Pen-Aqueous *(AgriPharm)*, *(Durvet)*, Penicillin 100 *(Alpharma)*, Penicillin G Procaine *(G.C. Hanford)*, Penicillin G Procaine 50 *(Alpharma)*, Sterile Penicillin G Procaine *(Aspen)*, Sterile Penicillin G Procaine Aqueous Suspension *(Butler)*.

Penicillin G Procaine *(G.C. Hanford)*, **penicillin G procaine.**

penicillin G procaine, dihydrostreptomycin. Quartermaster® *(Pharmacia & Upjohn)*.

penicillin G procaine, novobiocin. Albadry Plus® *(Pharmacia & Upjohn)*.

penicillin G procaine, penicillin G benzathine. Ambi-Pen™ *(Butler)*, Combicillin *(Anthony)*, Combicillin-AG *(Anthony)*, Duo-Pen® *(AgriPharm)*, Dura-Pen *(Durvet)*, Durapen™ *(Vedco)*, Sterile Penicillin G Benzathine and Penicillin G Procaine *(Aspen)*, *(G.C. Hanford)*, Twin-Pen™ *(AgriLabs)*.

penicillin G procaine, sulfamethazine, chlortetracycline. Aureomix® 500 Granular *(Alpharma)*, Pennchlor SP 250® *(PennField)*, Pennchlor SP 500® *(PennField)*.

penicillin G procaine, sulfathiazole, chlortetracycline. AureoZol® 500 Granular *(Alpharma)*.

Penicillin G Procaine 50 *(Alpharma)*, **penicillin G procaine.**

Pennchlor 50•G® *(PennField)*, **chlortetracycline.**

Pennchlor™ 50 Meal *(PennField)*, **chlortetracycline.**

Pennchlor™ 64 Soluble Powder *(PennField)*, **chlortetracycline.**

Pennchlor™ 70 Meal *(PennField)*, **chlortetracycline.**

Pennchlor 90•G® *(PennField)*, **chlortetracycline.**

Pennchlor 100 Hi-Flo™ Meal *(PennField)*, **chlortetracycline.**

Pennchlor™ 100-MR *(PennField)*, **chlortetracycline.**

Pennchlor SP 250® *(PennField)*, **chlortetracycline, penicillin G procaine, sulfamethazine.**

Pennchlor SP 500® *(PennField)*, **chlortetracycline, penicillin G procaine, sulfamethazine.**

Pennox™ 50 Meal *(PennField)*, **oxytetracycline.**

Pennox 100 Hi-Flo™ Meal *(PennField)*, **oxytetracycline.**

Pennox™ 100-MR *(PennField)*, **oxytetracycline.**

Pennox 200 Hi-Flo™ Meal *(PennField)*, **chlortetracycline.**

Pennox™ 200 Injectable *(PennField)*, **oxytetracycline.**

Pennox™ 343 Soluble Powder *(PennField)*, **oxytetracycline.**

Pentasol® Powder *(Delmarva)*, **pentobarbital sodium.**

pentobarbital sodium. Fatal-Plus® Powder *(Vortech)*, Fatal-Plus® Solution *(Vortech)*, Pentasol® Powder *(Delmarva)*, Sleepaway® *(Fort Dodge)*, Socumb™-6 gr *(Butler)*, Sodium Pentobarbital Injection *(Butler)*, Somlethol *(Webster)*.

pentobarbital sodium, phenytoin. Beuthanasia®-D Special *(Schering-Plough)*, Euthasol® *(Delmarva)*.

Pentothal® Sterile Powder (Veterinary) *(Abbott)*, **thiopental (sodium).**

peppermint oil, aloe vera, emollient(s). Natural Mint Liniment™ *(Horses Prefer)*.

peppermint oil, salicylic acid, eucalyptus oil, glycerine, kaolin, methyl salicylate. Absorbine® Antiphlogistine® *(W. F. Young)*.

peppermint oil, salicylic acid, thymol, arnica, bentonite, boric acid, eucalyptus oil, glycerine, isopropyl alcohol (isopropanol), kaolin, methyl salicylate. Bigeloil® 24-Hour Medicated Poultice *(W. F. Young)*.

peptides, amino acids, nitrogen. Arm & Hammer® Bio-Chlor® *(Church & Dwight)*, Arm & Hammer® Fermenten® *(Church & Dwight)*.

peracetic acid, hydrogen peroxide. Compliance™ *(Metrex)*.

Percorten®-V *(Novartis)*, **desoxicorticosterone pivalate (DOCP).**

PerforMax™ Ration Maximizer *(Equicare)*, **nutrients, vitamins.**

Performer® Ear Mite Killer *(AgriLabs)*, **di-n-propyl isocinchomeronate, n-octyl bicycloheptene dicarboximide, piperonyl butoxide, pyrethrins.**

Permectrin™ II *(Aspen)*, *(Boehringer Ingelheim)*, **permethrin.**

Permectrin™ CDS Pour-On *(Boehringer Ingelheim)*, **permethrin, piperonyl butoxide.**

Permectrin™ Fly & Louse Dust *(Boehringer Ingelheim)*, **permethrin.**

Permectrin™ Pour-On *(Boehringer Ingelheim)*, **permethrin.**

permethrin. 1% Permethrin Pour-On *(Durvet)*, Adams™ Spot-On Flea & Tick Control Large Dogs *(Farnam)*, Adams™ Spot-On Flea & Tick Control Small Dogs *(Farnam)*, Atroban® 11% EC Insecticide *(Schering-Plough)*, Atroban® 42.5% EC *(Schering-Plough)*, Atroban® DeLice® Pour-On Insecticide *(Schering-Plough)*, Back Side® *(AgriLabs)*, Bansect® Squeeze-On Flea & Tick Control for Dogs (under 33 lbs) *(Sergeant's)*, Bansect® Squeeze-On Flea & Tick Control for Dogs (over 33 lbs) *(Sergeant's)*, Boss® Pour-On Insecticide *(Schering-Plough)*, Catron™ IV *(Boehringer Ingelheim)*, Dealer Select Horse Care Permeth 5 Fly Spray *(Durvet)*, Defend® EXspot® Treatment for Dogs *(Schering-Plough)*, Durasect™ Long-Acting Livestock Pour-On *(Pfizer Animal Health)*, Ectiban® D *(Durvet)*, Ectiban® DeLice® *(Durvet)*, Ectiban® EC *(Durvet)*, Ectiban® WP *(Durvet)*, EctoZap™ Pour-On Insecticide *(Aspen)*, Equi-Spot™ Spot-On Fly Control for Horses *(Farnam)*, Exit™ Insecticide *(AgriPharm)*, FlyPel® Insecticide Spray for Horses *(Virbac)*, Fly-Rid Plus *(Durvet)*, Happy Jack® Kennelspot™ for Dogs (under 33 lbs) *(Happy Jack)*, Happy Jack® Kennelspot™ for Dogs (over 33 lbs) *(Happy Jack)*, Horse Lice Duster™ III *(Farnam)*, Kiltix® Topical Tick Control *(Bayer)*, New Z® Permethrin Insecticide Cattle Ear Tags *(Farnam)*, Permectrin™ II *(Aspen)*, *(Boehringer Ingelheim)*, Permectrin™ Fly & Louse Dust *(Boehringer Ingelheim)*, Permectrin™ Pour-On *(Boehringer Ingelheim)*, Permethrin 0.25% Dust *(AgriLabs)*, Permethrin 10% *(Durvet)*, ProTICall® Insecticide for Dogs *(Schering-Plough)*, Prozap® Drycide® *(Loveland)*, Prozap® Insectrin® Dust *(Loveland)*, Prozap® Insectrin® X *(Loveland)*, Scratchex® 30 Day Flea & Tick Treatment (30 lbs. & under) *(Combe)*, Scratchex® 30 Day Flea & Tick Treatment (over 30 lbs.) *(Combe)*, Screwworm Ear Tick Aerosol *(Durvet)*, Sungro Permith *(Sungro)*, UltraSpot™ by Absorbine® *(W. F. Young)*.

permethrin, imidacloprid. K9 Advantix™ 10 (imidacloprid/permethrin) For Dogs and Puppies (7 Weeks and Older, 10 lbs. and Under) *(Bayer)*, K9 Advantix™ 20 (imidacloprid/permethrin) For Dogs and Puppies (7 Weeks and Older, 11-20 lbs.) *(Bayer)*, K9 Advantix™ 55 (imidacloprid/permethrin) For Dogs and Puppies (7 Weeks and Older, 21-55 lbs.) *(Bayer)*, K9 Advantix™ 100 (imidacloprid/permethrin) For Dogs and Puppies (7 Weeks and Older, Over 55 lbs.) *(Bayer)*.

permethrin, methoprene. Vet-Kem® Ovitrol Plus® Spot On® Flea & Tick Control for Dogs & Puppies (under 30 lbs.) *(Wellmark)*, Vet-Kem® Ovitrol Plus® Spot On® Flea & Tick Control for Dogs & Puppies (over 30 lbs.) *(Wellmark)*, Vet-Kem® Siphotrol® Plus Area Treatment for Homes *(Wellmark)*, Vet-Kem® Siphotrol® Plus Area Treatment Pump Spray for Homes *(Wellmark)*, Vet-Kem® Siphotrol Plus® Fogger *(Wellmark)*.

permethrin, phenothrin, piperonyl butoxide, methoprene, n-octyl bicycloheptene dicarboximide. Vet-Kem® Siphotrol® Plus II Premise Spray *(Wellmark)*.

permethrin, piperonyl butoxide. Atroban® Extra Insecticide Ear Tags *(Schering-Plough)*, Back Side™ Plus *(AgriLabs)*, Buzz Off™ Pour-On *(Boehringer Ingelheim)*, EctoZap™ Plus Pour-On Insecticide *(Aspen)*, Exit™ II Synergized Formula Insecticide *(AgriPharm)*, Happy Jack® Kennel Dip II *(Happy Jack)*, Permectrin™ CDS Pour-On *(Boehringer Ingelheim)*, Poridon™ *(Neogen)*, Synergized DeLice® Pour-On Insecticide *(Schering-Plough)*, Ultra Boss® Pour-On Insecticide *(Schering-Plough)*.

permethrin, piperonyl butoxide, d-2-allayl-4-hydroxy-3-methyl-2-cyclopenten-1-one, di-n-propyl isocinchomeronate, fenoxycarb, n-octyl bicycloheptene dicarboximide. Scratchex® Super Spray™ *(Combe)*.

permethrin, piperonyl butoxide, n-octyl bicycloheptene dicarboximide. War Paint™ Insecticidal Paste *(Loveland)*.

permethrin, piperonyl butoxide, pyrethrins. Absorbine® UltraShield® Brand Fly Repellent *(W. F. Young)*, Bronco® Water-Base Equine Fly Spray *(Farnam)*, Durasect® II Long-Acting Livestock Pour-On *(Pfizer Animal Health)*, Flysect® Water-Based Repellent Spray *(Equicare)*, Repel-X® Insecticide & Repellent *(Farnam)*.

permethrin, piperonyl butoxide, pyrethrins, butoxypolypropylene glycol, di-n-propyl isocinchomeronate, n-octyl bicycloheptene dicarboximide. Adams™ Fly Spray and Repellent *(V.P.L.)*, Flysect® Super-7 *(Equicare)*.

permethrin, piperonyl butoxide, pyrethrins, di-n-propyl isocinchomeronate, n-octyl bicycloheptene dicarboximide. Adams™ Fly Repellent Concentrate *(V.P.L.)*, Flysect® Super-C *(Equicare)*.

permethrin, piperonyl butoxide, pyriproxyfen. Sergeant's® PreTect® Flea & Tick Shampoo for Dogs and Puppies *(Sergeant's)*, Virbac KnockOut® IGR Household Pump Spray *(Virbac)*.

permethrin, piperonyl butoxide, pyriproxyfen, d-2-allayl-4-hydroxy-3-methyl-2-cyclopenten-1-one, di-n-propyl isocinchomeronate, n-octyl bicycloheptene dicarboximide. Sergeant's® PreTect® Flea & Tick Spray for Cats & Kittens *(Sergeant's)*, Sergeant's® PreTect® Flea & Tick Spray for Dogs & Puppies *(Sergeant's)*.

permethrin, piperonyl butoxide, pyriproxyfen, linalool. Sergeant's® PreTect® Indoor Flea & Tick Fogger *(Sergeant's)*.

permethrin, pyrethrins. Absorbine® UltraShield® Brand Towelettes *(W. F. Young)*, Happy Jack® DD-33™ Flea & Tick Mist *(Happy Jack)*, Happy Jack® No-Hop Flea-Tick Spray *(Happy Jack)*, Scratchex® Flea & Tick Spray *(Combe)*, SynerKyl® AQ Water-Based Pet Spray *(DVM)*.

permethrin, pyrethrins, n-octyl bicycloheptene dicarboximide. Duocide® L.A. Spray *(Virbac)*.

permethrin, pyrethrins, pyriproxyfen, n-octyl bicycloheptene dicarboximide. Adams™ Room Fogger with Sykillstop™ *(Farnam)*, *(V.P.L.)*, EctoKyl™ IGR Total Release Fogger *(DVM)*, Happy Jack® Flea Flogger Plus *(Happy Jack)*, IGR House & Area Fogger *(Durvet)*, Mycodex® Environmental Control™ Aerosol Room Fogger *(V.P.L.)*, OmniTrol IGR Fogger *(Vedco)*, Virbac KnockOut® ES Area Treatment *(Virbac)*, Virbac KnockOut® Room and Area Fogger *(Virbac)*.

permethrin, pyriproxyfen. Bio Spot® Flea & Tick Control For Dogs (15 lbs. and Under) *(Farnam)*, Bio Spot® Flea & Tick Control For Dogs (Between 15 & 33 lbs.) *(Farnam)*, Bio Spot® Flea & Tick Control For Dogs (33 to 66 lbs.) *(Farnam)*, Bio Spot® Flea & Tick Control For Dogs (Over 66 lbs.) *(Farnam)*, Sergeant's® PreTect® Squeeze-On Flea & Tick Control for Dogs (under 15 lbs) *(Sergeant's)*, Sergeant's® PreTect® Squeeze-On Flea & Tick Control for Dogs (15 to 33 lbs) *(Sergeant's)*, Sergeant's® PreTect® Squeeze-On Flea & Tick Control for Dogs (under 33 lbs) *(Sergeant's)*, Sergeant's® PreTect® Squeeze-On Flea & Tick Control for Dogs (over 33 lbs) *(Sergeant's)*, Virbac® Long Acting KnockOut™ *(Virbac)*.

permethrin, pyriproxyfen, linalool, n-octyl bicycloheptene dicarboximide. Adams™ Inverted Carpet Spray *(Farnam)*, Sergeant's® PreTect® Household Flea & Tick Spray *(Sergeant's)*.

permethrin, pyriproxyfen, n-octyl bicycloheptene dicarboximide. Sergeant's® Flea-Free Breeze™ *(Sergeant's)*.

Permethrin 0.25% Dust *(AgriLabs)*, **permethrin.**
Permethrin 10% *(Durvet)*, **permethrin.**
Petables™ Clean and Heal Povidone Iodine Bath *(A.A.H.)*, **iodine complex (povidone-iodine).**
Petables™ Foaming Silk Bath *(A.A.H.)*, **shampoo formula.**
Pet-Cal™ *(Pfizer Animal Health)*, **calcium, phosphorus, vitamin D.**
Pet Care Ear Mite Lotion & Repellent *(Durvet)*, **di-n-propyl isocinchomeronate, n-octyl bicycloheptene dicarboximide, piperonyl butoxide, pyrethrins.**
Pet Care Ear Mite Solution *(Durvet)*, **rotenone.**
Pet Care Fast Kill Flea & Tick Spray for Dogs & Cats *(Durvet)*, **di-n-propyl isocinchomeronate, n-octyl bicycloheptene dicarboximide, piperonyl butoxide, pyrethrins.**
Pet Care House & Carpet Powder *(Durvet)*, **piperonyl butoxide, pyrethrins.**
Pet Care IGR-House & Carpet Spray *(Durvet)*, **pyriproxyfen, sumethrin, tetramethrin.**
Pet Care Indoor Premise Spray *(Durvet)*, **chlorpyrifos.**
Pet Care Liquid Wormer *(Durvet)*, **pyrantel pamoate.**
Pet Care Liquid Wormer 2X *(Durvet)*, **pyrantel pamoate.**
Pet Care Litter, Kennel and Stall Odor Control Powder *(Durvet)*, **deodorants.**
Pet-F.A. Liquid® *(Pfizer Animal Health)*, **fatty acids (essential), vitamin A, vitamin D, vitamin E, zinc.**
Pet-Form® *(Vet-A-Mix)*, **minerals, vitamins.**
Pet Guard™ Gel *(Virbac)*, **butoxypolypropylene glycol, n-octyl bicycloheptene dicarboximide, piperonyl butoxide, pyrethrins.**
PetLac™ Powder *(Pet-Ag)*, **milk replacing formula.**
petrolatum. Felaxin® *(Schering-Plough)*, Laxatone® & Tuna Flavor Laxatone® *(Evsco)*, Lickables™ Hairball Relief *(A.A.H.)*, Lickables™ Hairball Relief Caviar Flavored *(A.A.H.)*, Petromalt® *(Virbac)*, Puralube® Vet Ophthalmic Ointment *(Pharmaderm)*, Purrge™ Drops *(PPI)*, Sergeant's® Vetscription® Hairball Remedy *(Sergeant's)*, VedaLax™ and VedaLax™ Tuna *(Vedco)*.
petrolatum, 8-hydroxyquinolone, lanolin. Dr. Naylor® Udder Balm *(H.W. Naylor)*.
petrolatum, aloe vera, beeswax, emulsifying wax, glycerine, lanolin. Dealer Select Horse Care Hoof Moisturizer *(Durvet)*.
petrolatum, cod liver oil. Cat Lax® *(Pharmaderm)*, Kat-A-Lax* Feline Laxative *(Veterinary Specialties)*.
petrolatum, glycerine. Hartz® Health measures™ Hairball Remedy *(Hartz Mountain)*.
petrolatum, iron. Lax'aire® *(Pfizer Animal Health)*.
petrolatum, mineral oil. Hairball Preparation *(Vet Solutions)*, Laxa-Stat™ *(Tomlyn)*, Laxatone® for Cats *(Tomlyn)*, Laxatone® for Ferrets & Other Small Animals *(Tomlyn)*.
petrolatum, pine tar. Forshner's® Medicated Hoof Packing *(Equicare)*.
petrolatum, pine tar, turpentine, lanolin, neatsfoot oil. Absorbine® Hooflex® Liquid Conditioner *(W. F. Young)*.
petrolatum, soybean oil, urea, wheat germ oil, cod liver oil, iodine complex (povidone-iodine), lanolin. Vita-Hoof® *(Equicare)*.
petrolatum, vitamin A, vitamin D, benzethonium chloride, cetyl alcohol, lanolin. Udder Ointment™ *(LeGear)*.
petrolatum, zinc oxide, acacia, calamine, castor oil, glycerine. Triple Cast™ *(Neogen)*.
Petromalt® *(Virbac)*, **petrolatum.**
PetroTech 25™ *(Alpha Tech Pet)*, **oil removers.**
Pet-Tabs® *(Pfizer Animal Health)*, **minerals, vitamins.**
Pet-Tabs®/F.A. Granules *(Pfizer Animal Health)*, **fatty acids (essential), minerals, vitamins.**
Pet-Tabs® Jr. *(Pfizer Animal Health)*, **minerals, vitamins.**
Pet-Tabs® Plus *(Pfizer Animal Health)*, **minerals, vitamins.**
Pet-Tinic® *(Pfizer Animal Health)*, **minerals, vitamins.**
Pet Vites *(Vetus)*, **linolenic acid, minerals, vitamins.**
Pet Vites O.F.A. Chewable Tablets *(Vetus)*, **amino acids, fatty acids (omega), vitamins, zinc.**
P.G. 600® Estrus Control *(Intervet)*, **chorionic gonadotropin, serum gonadotropin.**
PHD 22.5 *(Bio-Tek)*, **ortho-benzyl-para-chlorophenol, orthophenylphenol, para-tertiary-amylphenol.**
phenol, pine oil, scarlet red, thymol, camphor, eucalyptus oil, menthol. Scarlet Oil Pump Spray *(Dominion)*.
phenol, piperonyl butoxide, pyrethrins, quaternary ammonia, n-octyl bicycloheptene dicarboximide. Microban® X-580 Institutional Spray Plus *(Microban)*.
phenol, scarlet red, isopropyl alcohol (isopropanol). Dr. Naylor® Red-Kote® *(H.W. Naylor)*.
phenolic disinfectants. 3M™ Phenolic Disinfectant Cleaner Concentrate *(3M)*, Amphyl® Disinfectant Cleaner *(Reckitt Benckiser)*, Pheno-Tek II *(Bio-Tek)*, SynPhenol-3™ *(V.P.L.)*, Tek-Trol® *(Bio-Tek)*.
Pheno-Tek II *(Bio-Tek)*, **phenolic disinfectants.**
phenothrin. Hartz® Advanced Care™ Brand Once-a-Month™ Flea & Tick Drops for Cats and Kittens (10 lbs. & under) *(Hartz Mountain)*, Hartz® Advanced Care™ Brand Once-a-Month™ Flea & Tick Drops for Cats and Kittens (over 10 lbs.) *(Hartz Mountain)*, Hartz® Advanced Care™ Brand Once-a-Month™ Flea & Tick Drops for Dogs and Puppies (16 to 30 lbs.) *(Hartz Mountain)*, Hartz® Advanced Care™ Brand Once-a-Month™ Flea & Tick Drops for Dogs and Puppies (15 lbs. & under) *(Hartz Mountain)*, Hartz® Advanced Care™ Brand Once-a-Month™ Flea & Tick Drops for Dogs and Puppies (31 to 60 lbs.) *(Hartz Mountain)*, Hartz® Advanced Care™ Brand Once-a-Month™ Flea & Tick Drops for Dogs and Puppies (61 to 90 lbs.) *(Hartz Mountain)*, Hartz® Advanced Care™ Brand Once-a-Month™ Flea & Tick Drops for Dogs and Puppies (over 90 lbs.) *(Hartz Mountain)*, Hartz® Advanced Care® Brand Tick Dabber™ Applicator *(Hartz Mountain)*.
phenothrin, d-trans allethrin. Duocide® Shampoo *(Virbac)*.
phenothrin, methoprene. Hartz® Advanced Care™ Brand Flea & Tick Drops Plus+ for Cats and Kittens (10 lbs. & under) *(Hartz Mountain)*, Hartz® Advanced Care™ Brand Flea & Tick Drops Plus+ for Cats and Kittens (over 10 lbs.) *(Hartz Mountain)*, Hartz® Advanced Care™ Brand Flea & Tick Drops Plus+ for Dogs and Puppies (4 to 15 lbs.) *(Hartz Mountain)*, Hartz® Advanced Care™ Brand Flea & Tick Drops Plus+ for Dogs and Puppies (16 to 30 lbs.) *(Hartz Mountain)*, Hartz® Advanced Care™ Brand Flea & Tick Drops Plus+ for Dogs and Puppies (31 to 45 lbs.) *(Hartz Mountain)*, Hartz® Advanced Care™ Brand Flea & Tick Drops Plus+ for Dogs and Puppies (46 to 60 lbs.) *(Hartz Mountain)*, Hartz® Advanced Care™ Brand Flea & Tick Drops Plus+ for Dogs and Puppies (61 to 90 lbs.) *(Hartz Mountain)*, Hartz® Advanced Care™ Brand Flea & Tick Drops Plus+ for Dogs and Puppies (Over 90 lbs.) *(Hartz Mountain)*.
phenothrin, methylcarbamate, n-octyl bicycloheptene dicarboximide. Adams™ Dual Action Flea & Tick Collar for Cats *(Farnam)*, Adams™ Dual Action Flea & Tick Collar for Large Dogs *(Farnam)*, Adams™ Dual Action Flea & Tick Collar for Medium Dogs *(Farnam)*.
phenothrin, piperonyl butoxide, methoprene, n-octyl bicycloheptene dicarboximide, permethrin. Vet-Kem® Siphotrol® Plus II Premise Spray *(Wellmark)*.
phenylbutazone. AmTech Phenylbutazone 20% Injection *(Phoenix Scientific)*, AmTech Phenylbutazone Tablets, USP 100 mg *(Phoenix Scientific)*, AmTech Phenylbutazone Tablets, USP 200 mg *(Phoenix Scientific)*, AmTech Phenylbutazone Tablets, USP 1 gram *(Phoenix Scientific)*, Bizolin®-1 g *(Boehringer Ingelheim)*, Butaject *(Vetus)*, Butapaste *(Vetus)*, Butatabs-D *(Vetus)*, Butatabs-E *(Vetus)*, Butatron™ Tablets *(Bimeda)*, Equi-Phar™ Phenylbutazone 1 gram Tablets *(Vedco)*, Equi-Phar™ Phenylbutazone Injection 20% *(Vedco)*, Equiphen® Paste *(Luitpold)*, Phenylbutazone 20% Injection *(Vet Tek)*, Phenylbutazone Injection 20% *(Aspen)*, *(RXV)*, Phenylbutazone Injection 200 mg/mL *(Butler)*, Phenylbutazone Tablets (Dogs) *(RXV)*, *(Vedco)*, Phenylbutazone Tablets, USP *(Vet Tek)*, Phenylbutazone Tablets, USP 100 mg *(Butler)*, Phenylbutazone Tablets, USP 1 gram *(Butler)*, Phenylbute® Injection 20% *(Phoenix Pharmaceutical)*, Phenylbute® Paste *(Phoenix Pharmaceutical)*, Phenylbute® Tablets 100 mg *(Phoenix Pharmaceutical)*, Phenylbute® Tablets 200 mg *(Phoenix Pharmaceutical)*, Phenylbute® Tablets 1 gram *(Phoenix Pharmaceutical)*, Phenylzone® Paste *(Schering-Plough)*, Pributazone™ Tablets *(First Priority)*, Pro-Bute™ Injection *(AgriLabs)*, Pro-Bute™ Tablets 1 gram *(AgriLabs)*.
Phenylbutazone 20% Injection *(Vet Tek)*, **phenylbutazone.**
Phenylbutazone Injection 20% *(Aspen)*, *(RXV)*, **phenylbutazone.**
Phenylbutazone Injection 200 mg/mL *(Butler)*, **phenylbutazone.**
Phenylbutazone Tablets (Dogs) *(RXV)*, *(Vedco)*, **phenylbutazone.**
Phenylbutazone Tablets, USP *(Vet Tek)*, **phenylbutazone.**
Phenylbutazone Tablets, USP 100 mg *(Butler)*, **phenylbutazone.**
Phenylbutazone Tablets, USP 1 gram *(Butler)*, **phenylbutazone.**
Phenylbute® Injection 20% *(Phoenix Pharmaceutical)*, **phenylbutazone.**
Phenylbute® Paste *(Phoenix Pharmaceutical)*, **phenylbutazone.**
Phenylbute® Tablets 100 mg *(Phoenix Pharmaceutical)*, **phenylbutazone.**
Phenylbute® Tablets 200 mg *(Phoenix Pharmaceutical)*, **phenylbutazone.**
Phenylbute® Tablets 1 gram *(Phoenix Pharmaceutical)*, **phenylbutazone.**
phenylephrine hydrochloride, pyrilamine maleate, sodium chloride, ammonium chloride, guaifenesin (glyceryl guaiacolate, guaiacol). Cough Syrup *(Life Science)*.
phenylephrine hydrochloride, pyrilamine maleate, sodium citrate, ammonium chloride, guaifenesin (glyceryl guaiacolate, guaiacol). Anti-Tussive Syrup with Antihistamine *(Vedco)*, ExpectaHist *(Vetus)*.
phenylephrine hydrochloride, pyrilamine maleate, sodium citrate, guaifenesin (glyceryl guaiacolate, guaiacol). Expectade™ Cough Syrup *(PRN Pharmacal)*.
phenylpropanolamine. Proin™ 50 Chewable Tablets *(PRN Pharmacal)*, Proin™ Drops *(PRN Pharmacal)*.
Phenylzone® Paste *(Schering-Plough)*, **phenylbutazone.**
phenytoin, pentobarbital sodium. Beuthanasia®-D Special *(Schering-Plough)*, Euthasol® *(Delmarva)*.
Phos-Aid *(Butler)*, **phosphoric acid.**
Phos-Aid Solution *(Neogen)*, **phosphinic acid.**
Phos-K™ Gel *(PRN Pharmacal)*, **phosphorus, potassium, propylene glycol.**
phosmet. Del-Phos® Emulsifiable Liquid Insecticide *(Schering-Plough)*, Prolate®/Lintox®-HD *(Wellmark)*, Vet-Kem® Paramite® Sponge-On for Dogs *(Wellmark)*.
Phos P 200 *(Phoenix Pharmaceutical)*, **phosphorus.**
Phosphaid Injection *(Vedco)*, **phosphinic acid.**

phosphatidylcholine, choline. Cholodin® *(MVP)*.

phosphinic acid. Phos-Aid Solution *(Neogen)*, Phosphaid Injection *(Vedco)*.

phospholipids, glycolipids. Dyna-Lode® Supplement for Dogs & Cats *(Harlmen)*.

phospholipids, vitamins, glycolipids, lecithin. Dyna-Lode® Equine Supplement *(Harlmen)*.

phosphoric acid. Phos-Aid *(Butler)*.

phosphoric acid, acetic acid, iodine complex (povidone-iodine). Bou-Matic IO-Wash *(Bou-Matic)*.

phosphoric acid, detergent mixture. Lifegard® 7000 *(Rochester Midland)*, Lifegard® 7500F *(Rochester Midland)*, Lifegard® 7700 *(Rochester Midland)*, Lifegard® 7700ND *(Rochester Midland)*.

phosphoric acid, iodine complex (povidone-iodine). Dineotex *(Stearns)*, Iosan® *(WestAgro)*, K.O. Dyne® *(Westfalia•Surge)*, Metz Iodine Detergent *(Metz)*, Monarch® Mon-O-Dine *(Ecolab Food & Bev. Div.)*, West-Vet® Premise® Disinfectant *(WestAgro)*.

phosphoric acid, potassium, calcium, magnesium. CMPK Oral Solution 33% *(Vedco)*.

phosphoric acid, potassium chloride, calcium, magnesium hydroxide. Cal MPK Gel *(Butler)*.

phosphoric acid, potassium chloride, trisodium phosphate, calcium, magnesium chloride. CMPK Gel *(AgriPharm)*.

phosphoric acid, sulfonic acid. Bac-Drop Udder Wash *(Ecolab Food & Bev. Div.)*.

phosphorus. Phos P 200 *(Phoenix Pharmaceutical)*.

phosphorus, calcium. Di-Calcium Phosphate *(Neogen)*.

phosphorus, calcium, dextrose, magnesium. Cal-Phos #2 Injection *(AgriLabs)*, Cal-Phos Forte *(Bimeda)*.

phosphorus, calcium, dextrose, magnesium borogluconate. Cal Dex #2 *(AgriLabs)*, Cal-Dextro® No. 2 *(Fort Dodge)*, Cal-Dextro® Special *(Fort Dodge)*.

phosphorus, potassium, calcium, magnesium. AmTech CMPK Injection *(Phoenix Scientific)*, CMPK Bolus *(Durvet)*, *(Vets Plus)*, C.M.P.K. Oral Gel *(Phoenix Pharmaceutical)*, Oral CPMK Gel *(First Priority)*.

phosphorus, potassium, propylene glycol. Phos-K™ Gel *(PRN Pharmacal)*.

phosphorus, potassium, sodium chloride, zinc, magnesium. Swine Acid-O-Lite™ *(TechMix)*.

phosphorus, potassium, vitamin D_3, calcium, magnesium. CMPK with D_3 Drench *(Vets Plus)*.

phosphorus, potassium, vitamins, calcium, magnesium. Mega CMPK Bolus *(AgriPharm)*, Slow Release CMPK Bolus *(PRN Pharmacal)*.

phosphorus, potassium chloride, calcium, dextrose, magnesium chloride. Oral Cal MPK *(Durvet)*.

phosphorus, potassium chloride, calcium, magnesium chloride. C.M.P.K. Gel *(AgriLabs)*, CMPK Gel *(Vedco)*.

phosphorus, potassium chloride, calcium, magnesium hydroxide. CMPK Gel *(Durvet)*.

phosphorus, sodium chloride, vitamin A, calcium, iodine, iron. Mo' Milk® Feed Mix and Top Dress *(TechMix)*.

phosphorus, vitamin A, vitamin D_3, calcium. Osteo-Form Powder *(Vet-A-Mix)*, Osteo-Form SA *(Vet-A-Mix)*.

phosphorus, vitamin D, calcium. Calcium Phosphorus Powder *(Pet-Ag)*, Pet-Cal™ *(Pfizer Animal Health)*.

phosphorus, vitamin D_3, calcium. Calcium Phosphorus Tablets *(Pet-Ag)*.

phosphorus, vitamins, calcium. Osteo-Form Tablets *(Vet-A-Mix)*.

phosphorus, vitamins, calcium, milk protein, nutrients. Foal-Lac® Pellets *(Pet-Ag)*.

Physiological Saline Solution *(Butler)*, **sodium chloride.**

Pic-M-Up™ *(AgriPharm)*, **amino acids, electrolytes, energy source(s), vitamins.**

Pig-95 *(Skylabs)*, **electrolytes, iron, vitamins.**

pine oil. 25-Pines™ *(Stearns)*, Bio-Pine 20 *(Bio-Tek)*.

pine oil, quaternary ammonia. Big Pine™ *(Intercon)*, Marcicide II *(M.A.R.C.)*.

pine oil, scarlet red, benzyl alcohol, eucalyptus oil, isopropyl alcohol (isopropanol), methyl salicylate, parachlorometaxylenol. Scarlet Oil *(First Priority)*.

pine oil, scarlet red, benzyl alcohol, eucalyptus oil, methyl salicylate. Scarlet Oil Wound Dressing *(Durvet)*.

pine oil, scarlet red, benzyl alcohol, eucalyptus oil, methyl salicylate, parachlorometaxylenol. Scarlet Oil *(Vedco)*, Scarlet Oil Wound Dressing *(AgriPharm)*.

pine oil, scarlet red, eucalyptus oil, methyl salicylate. Scarlet Oil Smear *(First Priority)*.

pine oil, scarlet red, eucalyptus oil, methyl salicylate, P-chloro-M-xylenol. Scarlex® Scarlet Oil *(Farnam)*.

pine oil, scarlet red, thymol, camphor, eucalyptus oil, menthol, phenol. Scarlet Oil Pump Spray *(Dominion)*.

pine tar, ichthammol, iodide (potassium), iodine. Sole Pack™ Hoof Dressing *(Hawthorne)*, Sole Pack™ Hoof Packing *(Hawthorne)*.

pine tar, iodide (potassium), iodine. Reducine® Absorbent for Horses *(Equicare)*.

pine tar, petrolatum. Forshner's® Medicated Hoof Packing *(Equicare)*.

pine tar, propylene glycol, vitamin A, vitamin C (ascorbic acid), allantoin, benzocaine. A-Plus™ Wound Dressing *(Creative Science)*.

pine tar, turpentine, lanolin, neatsfoot oil. Absorbine® Hooflex® Original Conditioner *(W. F. Young)*.

pine tar, turpentine, lanolin, neatsfoot oil, petrolatum. Absorbine® Hooflex® Liquid Conditioner *(W. F. Young)*.

pine tar, turpentine, wheat germ oil, fish oil, iodine, linseed oil. Dealer Select Horse Care Hoof Dressing With Brush *(Durvet)*.

pine tar, turpentine, wheat germ oil, fish oil, iodine, linseed oil, neatsfoot oil. Shur Hoof™ *(Horse Health)*.

Pipa-Tabs *(Vet-A-Mix)*, **piperazine dihydrochloride.**

piperazine. Alfalfa Pellet Horse Wormer *(Farnam)*, D-Worm™ Liquid Wormer for Cats and Dogs *(Farnam)*, Piperazine-17 Medicated *(Durvet)*, Sergeant's® Vetscription® Sure Shot® Liquid Wormer for Cats & Kittens *(Sergeant's)*, Tasty Paste® Dog & Puppy Wormer *(Farnam)*, Wonder Wormer™ for Horses *(Farnam)*.

Piperazine-17 Medicated *(Durvet)*, **piperazine.**

piperazine adipate. Hartz® Health measures™ Once-a-month® Wormer for Cats and Kittens *(Hartz Mountain)*, Hartz® Health measures™ Once-a-month® Wormer for Dogs *(Hartz Mountain)*, Hartz® Health measures™ Once-a-month® Wormer for Large Dogs *(Hartz Mountain)*, Hartz® Health measures™ Once-a-month® Wormer for Puppies *(Hartz Mountain)*.

piperazine citrate. Hartz® Health measures™ Liquid Wormer *(Hartz Mountain)*, Sergeant's® Vetscription® Worm-Away® for Cats *(Sergeant's)*, Sergeant's® Vetscription® Worm-Away® for Dogs *(Sergeant's)*.

piperazine dihydrochloride. Pipa-Tabs *(Vet-A-Mix)*, Wazine® 17 *(Fleming)*, Wazine® 34 *(Fleming)*, Wazine® Soluble *(Fleming)*.

piperonyl butoxide, cyfluthrin. CyLence® Ultra Insecticide Cattle Ear Tag *(Bayer)*.

piperonyl butoxide, d-2-allayl-4-hydroxy-3-methyl-2-cyclopenten-1-one, di-n-propyl isocinchomeronate, fenoxycarb, n-octyl bicycloheptene dicarboximide, permethrin. Scratchex® Super Spray™ *(Combe)*.

piperonyl butoxide, diazinon. New Z® Diazinon Insecticide Cattle Ear Tags *(Farnam)*.

piperonyl butoxide, d-trans allethrin. Mycodex® SensiCare™ Flea & Tick Shampoo *(V.P.L.)*.

piperonyl butoxide, lambdacyhalothrin. Saber™ Extra Insecticide Ear Tags *(Schering-Plough)*.

piperonyl butoxide, methoprene, n-octyl bicycloheptene dicarboximide, permethrin, phenothrin. Vet-Kem® Siphotrol® Plus II Premise Spray *(Wellmark)*.

piperonyl butoxide, n-octyl bicycloheptene dicarboximide, permethrin. War Paint™ Insecticidal Paste *(Loveland)*.

piperonyl butoxide, permethrin. Atroban® Extra Insecticide Ear Tags *(Schering-Plough)*, Back Side™ Plus *(AgriLabs)*, Buzz Off™ Pour-On *(Boehringer Ingelheim)*, EctoZap™ Plus Pour-On Insecticide *(Aspen)*, Exit™ II Synergized Formula Insecticide *(AgriPharm)*, Happy Jack® Kennel Dip II *(Happy Jack)*, Permectrin™ CDS Pour-On *(Boehringer Ingelheim)*, Poridon™ *(Neogen)*, Synergized DeLice® Pour-On Insecticide *(Schering-Plough)*, Ultra Boss® Pour-On Insecticide *(Schering-Plough)*.

piperonyl butoxide, pyrethrins. 3X Pyrethrin Shampoo *(Vet Solutions)*, Absorbine® Flys-X® Insecticide *(W. F. Young)*, Adams™ Flea & Tick Shampoo *(V.P.L.)*, Brilliance™ Flea & Tick Shampoo *(First Priority)*, Dairy Bomb-50 *(Durvet)*, Dairy Bomb-50Z *(Durvet)*, Dairy Bomb-55Z *(Durvet)*, Davis Pyrethrins *(Davis)*, Ectiban® Synergized DeLice® Pour-On Insecticide *(Durvet)*, Ecto-Soothe™ Shampoo *(Virbac)*, Eradimite™ *(Fort Dodge)*, Grand Champion® Fly Repellent Formula *(Farnam)*, Happy Jack® Mitex™ *(Happy Jack)*, Hartz® Health measures™ Ear Mite Treatment for Cats *(Hartz Mountain)*, Hartz® Health measures™ Ear Mite Treatment for Dogs *(Hartz Mountain)*, Make Your Own Flea & Tick Shampoo *(Davis)*, Mitaplex-P™ *(Tomlyn)*, MoorMan's® Fly Spray *(ADM)*, Mycodex® Pet Shampoo with 3X Pyrethrins *(V.P.L.)*, Mycodex® SensiCare™ Flea & Tick Spray *(V.P.L.)*, Pene-Mite™ *(Farnam)*, Pet Care House & Carpet Powder *(Durvet)*, Prozap® Aqueous Fly Spray *(Loveland)*, Prozap® LD-44Z *(Loveland)*, Pyrethrin Plus *(Durvet)*, Pyrethrins Dip and Spray *(Davis)*, Rabbit Ear Miticide *(Farnam)*, Repel-X®p Emulsifiable Fly Spray *(Farnam)*, Sergeant's® Vetscription® Aloe Ear Mite Treatment *(Sergeant's)*, Sheen II Shampoo *(Butler)*, Sunbugger Carpet Dust *(Sungro)*, Sun-Dust Roach Away *(Sungro)*, Sungro Flea-ZY Pet Shampoo *(Sungro)*, SynerKyl® Pet Dip *(DVM)*.

piperonyl butoxide, pyrethrins, benzocaine, docusate sodium (dioctyl sodium sulfosuccinate). Aurimite® Insecticide *(Schering-Plough)*.

piperonyl butoxide, pyrethrins, butoxypolypropylene glycol. Absorbine® SuperShield® Red Fly Repellent *(W. F. Young)*, Flysect® Citronella Spray *(Equicare)*, Flys-Off® Insect Repellent for Dogs *(Farnam)*, Flys-Off® Lotion Insect Repellent for Dogs *(Farnam)*, VIP® Fly Repellent Ointment *(V.P.L.)*, Wipe® II Brand Fly Spray with Citronella *(Farnam)*.

piperonyl butoxide, pyrethrins, butoxypolypropylene glycol, cypermethrin. Bite Free™ Biting Fly Repellent *(Farnam)*, Endure™ Sweat-Resistant Fly Spray *(Farnam)*, Tri-Tec 14™ Fly Repellent *(Farnam)*.

piperonyl butoxide, pyrethrins, butoxypolypropylene glycol, cypermethrin, di-n-propyl isocinchomeronate. Repel-X® Lotion *(Farnam)*.

piperonyl butoxide, pyrethrins, butoxypolypropylene glycol, di-n-propyl isocinchomeronate. Wipe® Fly Protectant *(Farnam)*.

piperonyl butoxide, pyrethrins, butoxypolypropylene glycol, di-n-propyl isocinchomeronate, n-octyl bicycloheptene dicarboximide, permethrin. Adams™ Fly Spray and Repellent *(V.P.L.)*, Flysect® Super-7 *(Equicare)*.

piperonyl butoxide, pyrethrins, butoxypolypropylene glycol, n-octyl bicycloheptene dicarboximide. Pet Guard™ Gel *(Virbac)*.

piperonyl butoxide, pyrethrins, carbaryl. Adams™ Flea & Tick Dust II *(Farnam)*, *(V.P.L.)*.

piperonyl butoxide, pyrethrins, carbaryl, n-octyl bicycloheptene dicarboximide. Scratchex® Flea & Tick Powder *(Combe)*.

piperonyl butoxide, pyrethrins, diazinon. Sunbugger Residual Ant & Roach Spray Aqueous *(Sungro)*.

piperonyl butoxide, pyrethrins, dicarboximide, n-octyl bicycloheptene dicarboximide. Hartz® 2 in 1® Flea & Tick Killer for Dogs *(Hartz Mountain)*.

piperonyl butoxide, pyrethrins, dichlorvos. Prozap® VIP Insect Spray *(Loveland)*, SK-Surekill® Brand Pyrethrin Plus Fly Spray *(IntAgra)*.

piperonyl butoxide, pyrethrins, dichlorvos, n-octyl bicycloheptene dicarboximide. Super II Dairy & Farm Spray *(Durvet)*.

piperonyl butoxide, pyrethrins, di-n-propyl isocinchomeronate. Happy Jack® Onex *(Happy Jack)*, Relief! Fly Ointment *(Davis)*, Swat® Fly Repellent Ointment *(Farnam)*, VPL Fly Repellent Ointment *(V.P.L.)*.

piperonyl butoxide, pyrethrins, di-n-propyl isocinchomeronate, n-octyl bicycloheptene dicarboximide. Adams™ Flea & Tick Mist *(V.P.L.)*, Adams™ Pyrethrin Dip *(Farnam)*, *(V.P.L.)*, EctoKyl™ 3X Flea & Tick Shampoo *(DVM)*, Flea & Tick Mist *(Davis)*, Flysect® Repellent Spray *(Equicare)*, Flysect® Roll-On Fly Repellent Face Lotion *(Equicare)*, Flys-Off® Fly Repellent Ointment *(Farnam)*, Mita-Clear™ *(Pfizer Animal Health)*, Otomite® Plus *(Virbac)*, Performer® Ear Mite Killer *(AgriLabs)*, Pet Care Ear Mite Lotion & Repellent *(Durvet)*, Pet Care Fast Kill Flea & Tick Spray for Dogs & Cats *(Durvet)*, Roll-On™ Fly Repellent *(Farnam)*, Triple Pyrethrins Flea & Tick Shampoo *(Davis)*, Vet-Kem® Triple Action Flea & Tick Shampoo for Dogs, Cats, & Horses *(Wellmark)*, Virbac Pyrethrin Dip™ *(Virbac)*.

piperonyl butoxide, pyrethrins, di-n-propyl isocinchomeronate, n-octyl bicycloheptene dicarboximide, permethrin. Adams™ Fly Repellent Concentrate *(V.P.L.)*, Flysect® Super-C *(Equicare)*.

piperonyl butoxide, pyrethrins, methoprene. Hartz® Control Pet Care System® Mousse for Cats and Kittens *(Hartz Mountain)*, Vet-Kem® Ovitrol® Plus Flea & Tick Shampoo for Dogs & Cats *(Wellmark)*.

piperonyl butoxide, pyrethrins, methoprene, n-octyl bicycloheptene dicarboximide. Vet-Kem® Ovitrol® Plus Flea, Tick & Bot Spray *(Wellmark)*.

piperonyl butoxide, pyrethrins, n-octyl bicycloheptene dicarboximide. Adams™ Water Based Flea and Tick Mist *(Farnam)*, *(V.P.L.)*, Cerumite 3x *(Evsco)*, Dairy Bomb-55 *(Durvet)*, Ecto-Foam™ *(Virbac)*, Ecto-Soothe™ 3X Shampoo *(Virbac)*, Flea Halt!™ Flea & Tick Repellent Towelettes *(Farnam)*, Flea Halt!™ Flea & Tick Repellent Towelettes for Ferrets *(Farnam)*, Flea, Tick and Lice Shampoo *(Tomlyn)*, Hartz® 2 in 1® Flea & Tick Dip for Dogs and Cats *(Hartz Mountain)*, Hartz® 2 in 1® Luster Bath for Cats *(Hartz Mountain)*, Hartz® 2 in 1® Rid Flea™ Dog Shampoo with Pyrethrin *(Hartz Mountain)*, Hartz® Easy Wash™ Flea & Tick Shampoo for Dogs *(Hartz Mountain)*, Pyrethrin Plus Shampoo *(Vedco)*, Scratchex® Flea & Tick Shampoo *(Combe)*.

piperonyl butoxide, pyrethrins, permethrin. Absorbine® UltraShield® Brand Fly Repellent *(W. F. Young)*, Bronco® Water-Base Equine Fly Spray *(Farnam)*, Durasect® II Long-Acting Livestock Pour-On *(Pfizer Animal Health)*, Flysect® Water-Based Repellent Spray *(Equicare)*, Repel-X® Insecticide & Repellent *(Farnam)*.

piperonyl butoxide, pyrethrins, pyriproxyfen, linalool. Adams™ Carpet Powder *(Farnam)*, Sergeant's® PreTect® Flea & Tick Carpet Powder *(Sergeant's)*.

piperonyl butoxide, pyrethrins, pyriproxyfen, n-octyl bicycloheptene dicarboximide. Adams™ Flea & Tick Mist with Sykillstop™ *(Farnam)*, *(V.P.L.)*, Mycodex® All-In-One™ Spray *(V.P.L.)*, Sergeant's® PreTect® Flea & Tick Shampoo for Cats and Kittens *(Sergeant's)*.

piperonyl butoxide, pyrethrins, quaternary ammonia, n-octyl bicycloheptene dicarboximide, phenol. Microban® X-580 Institutional Spray Plus *(Microban)*.

piperonyl butoxide, pyriproxyfen, d-2-allyl-4-hydroxy-3-methyl-2-cyclopenten-1-one, di-n-propyl isocinchomeronate, n-octyl bicycloheptene dicarboximide, permethrin. Sergeant's® PreTect® Flea & Tick Spray for Cats & Kittens *(Sergeant's)*, Sergeant's® PreTect® Flea & Tick Spray for Dogs & Puppies *(Sergeant's)*.

piperonyl butoxide, pyriproxyfen, linalool, permethrin. Sergeant's® PreTect® Indoor Flea & Tick Fogger *(Sergeant's)*.

piperonyl butoxide, pyriproxyfen, permethrin. Sergeant's® PreTect® Flea & Tick Shampoo for Dogs and Puppies *(Sergeant's)*, Virbac KnockOut® IGR Household Pump Spray *(Virbac)*.

pirimiphos. Dominator® Insecticide Ear Tags *(Schering-Plough)*.

pirimiphos, lambdacyhalothrin. Double Barrel™ VP Insecticide Ear Tags *(Schering-Plough)*.

pirlimycin. Pirsue® Sterile Solution *(Pharmacia & Upjohn)*.

Pirsue® Sterile Solution *(Pharmacia & Upjohn)*, **pirlimycin.**

Plasmune J *(Lake Immunogenics)*, **equine plasma.**

Pleascent® Puppy *(Thornell)*, **deodorants, neutralizer(s).**

Plexadol™ Shampoo *(Butler)*, **iodine complex (povidone-iodine).**

Plexamino® Bolus *(Bimeda)*, **carbohydrates, minerals, protein(s).**

Plex-Sol C *(Vet-A-Mix)*, **vitamins.**

poloxalene. Bloat Guard® Liquid Type A Medicated Article *(Phibro)*, Bloat Guard® Top Dressing Medicated *(Phibro)*, Bloat Guard® Type A Medicated Article *(Phibro)*, Sweetlix® Bloat Guard® Block Medicated *(Sweetlix)*, Therabloat® Drench Concentrate *(Pfizer Animal Health)*.

poloxamer. Combi-Clens® *(G.C. Hanford)*.

Polydine™ Spray *(First Priority)*, **iodine complex (povidone-iodine).**

polyethelene glycol, propionic acid, silicon dioxide, vitamins, cobalt sulfate, magnesium sulfate. Ketopro Oral Gel *(Vedco)*.

polyetheline polymer. Equi-Phar™ Vedlube Dry *(Vedco)*.

Polyflex® *(Fort Dodge)*, **ampicillin.**

Polylites IV *(Butler)*, **dextrose, electrolytes.**

Polymag™ Bolus *(Butler)*, **magnesium hydroxide.**

polymeric dispersant, potassium hydroxide, sodium metasilicate. Lifegard® 800 *(Rochester Midland)*.

Polymune™ *(V.D.I.)*, **equine plasma.**

Polymune-J™ *(V.D.I.)*, **bovine plasma.**

Polymune™ Plus *(V.D.I.)*, **equine plasma.**

polymyxin B, bacitracin, hydrocortisone acetate, neomycin. Neobacimyx®-H *(Schering-Plough)*, TriOptic-S® *(Pfizer Animal Health)*, Vetropolycin® HC Ophthalmic Ointment *(Pharmaderm)*.

polymyxin B, bacitracin, neomycin. Mycitracin® Sterile Ointment *(Pharmacia & Upjohn)*, Neobacimyx® *(Schering-Plough)*, TriOptic-P™ *(Pfizer Animal Health)*, Vetro-Biotic® Ointment *(Pharmaderm)*, Vetropolycin® Ophthalmic Ointment *(Pharmaderm)*.

polymyxin B, oxytetracycline. Terramycin® Ophthalmic Ointment *(Pfizer Animal Health)*.

Polyotic® Soluble Powder *(Fort Dodge)*, **tetracycline.**

Polyox® Powder *(Bimeda)*, **magnesium hydroxide.**

Polyox® II Bolus *(AgriPharm)*, *(Bimeda)*, **magnesium hydroxide.**

polysulfated glycosaminoglycan. Adequan® Canine *(Luitpold)*, Adequan® I.A. *(Luitpold)*, Adequan® I.M. *(Luitpold)*, Chondroprotec® *(Neogen)*.

polyunsaturated fatty acids, vitamin A, vitamin D, vitamin E. Derma-Form Liquid *(Vet-A-Mix)*.

polyvinyl alcohol. Puralube® Vet Tears *(Pharmaderm)*.

polyvinylpyrrolidone. Biozide® Gel *(PPI)*, Biozide® Puffer *(PPI)*, I.O. Dine Complex™ Bolus *(PRN Pharmacal)*, Vedadine Bolus *(Vedco)*.

ponazuril. Marquis™ (15% w/w ponazuril) Antiprotozoal Oral Paste *(Bayer)*.

porcine GI submucosa. Vet BioSISt™ *(Cook)*.

Porcine Maximizer™ *(Novartis Animal Vaccines)*, **fatty acids.**

Poridon™ *(Neogen)*, **permethrin, piperonyl butoxide.**

Posilac 1 Step® *(Monsanto)*, **bovine somatotropin.**

Potassiject *(Vetus)*, **potassium chloride.**

potassium. NutriVed™ Hypo-K Granules *(Vedco)*.

potassium, calcium, magnesium, phosphoric acid. CMPK Oral Solution 33% *(Vedco)*.

potassium, calcium, magnesium, phosphorus. AmTech CMPK Injection *(Phoenix Scientific)*, CMPK Bolus *(Durvet)*, *(Vets Plus)*, C.M.P.K. Oral Gel *(Phoenix Pharmaceutical)*, Oral CPMK Gel *(First Priority)*.

potassium, propylene glycol, phosphorus. Phos-K™ Gel *(PRN Pharmacal)*.

potassium, propylene glycol, vitamin B-complex, calcium, magnesium. Super Calcium Drench *(Vedco)*.

potassium, propylene glycol, vitamins, calcium, magnesium. Calcium Drench Plus Vitamins *(AgriLabs)*, *(Durvet)*.

potassium, protein(s), sodium, vitamin A, vitamin D_3, vitamin E. WGS *(Durvet)*.

potassium, sodium, vitamin A, vitamin D_3, vitamin E. Propack-EXP *(Durvet)*.

potassium, sodium, vitamin E, zinc, microorganisms. Yellow Lite *(AgriPharm)*.

potassium, sodium chloride, zinc, magnesium, phosphorus. Swine Acid-O-Lite™ *(TechMix)*.

potassium, taurine, vitamins, fatty acids (essential), minerals. Felo-Form *(Vet-A-Mix)*.

potassium, vitamin D_3, calcium, magnesium, phosphorus. CMPK with D_3 Drench *(Vets Plus)*.

potassium, vitamins, calcium, magnesium. Calcium Drench *(AgriPharm)*.

potassium, vitamins, calcium, magnesium, phosphorus. Mega CMPK Bolus *(AgriPharm)*, Slow Release CMPK Bolus *(PRN Pharmacal)*.

potassium chloride. Potassiject *(Vetus)*, Potassium Chloride *(Butler)*, *(Phoenix Pharmaceutical)*, *(Vedco)*.

Potassium Chloride *(Butler)*, *(Phoenix Pharmaceutical)*, *(Vedco)*, **potassium chloride.**

potassium chloride, calcium, calcium hypophosphite, dextrose, magnesium borogluconate. Cal-MPK 1234™ *(Butler)*.

potassium chloride, calcium, calcium phosphate, magnesium chloride. CMPK Gel Plus™ *(Vets Plus)*.

potassium chloride, calcium, dextrose. Cal-Dextro® K *(Fort Dodge)*.

potassium chloride, calcium, dextrose, magnesium chloride, phosphorus. Oral Cal MPK *(Durvet)*.

potassium chloride, calcium, magnesium chloride, phosphorus. C.M.P.K. Gel *(AgriLabs)*, CMPK Gel *(Vedco)*.

potassium chloride, calcium, magnesium hydroxide, phosphoric acid. Cal MPK Gel *(Butler)*.

potassium chloride, calcium, magnesium hydroxide, phosphorus. CMPK Gel *(Durvet)*.

potassium chloride, propylene glycol, sodium hypophosphite, calcium, magnesium chloride. 40% CMPK with D_3 Oral Drench *(DVM Formula)*, Oral Calcium Drench *(DVM Formula)*.

potassium chloride, propylene glycol, sodium hypophosphite, vitamin D_3, calcium, magnesium chloride. CMPK D_3 Drench *(Durvet)*.

potassium chloride, sodium acetate, sodium chloride, sodium gluconate, magnesium chloride. AmTech Amisol-R Injection *(Phoenix Scientific)*, Bimesol-R™ Injection *(Bimeda)*, ElectroSol-R *(Phoenix Pharmaceutical)*, Injectrolyte *(Vetus)*.

potassium chloride, sodium chloride, calcium, magnesium sulfate. Electrolyte Supplement *(First Priority)*.

potassium chloride, sodium chloride, sodium lactate, calcium. AmTech Lactated Ringers Injection *(Phoenix Scientific)*, Lactated Ringers *(Vet Tek)*, Lactated Ringers Injection *(Phoenix Pharmaceutical)*, Lactated Ringer's Injection *(Vedco)*, Lactated Ringers Injection *(Vetus)*, Lactated Ringers Injection SC *(Butler)*, Lactated Ringer's Injection, USP *(AgriLabs)*, *(Bimeda)*, Lactated Ringer's Solution *(RXV)*.

potassium chloride, sodium chloride, thiamine hydrochloride (B_1), calcium. Happy Jack® Milkade *(Happy Jack)*.

potassium chloride, sodium hypophosphite, calcium, dextrose, magnesium borogluconate. Cal Dex CMPK Injection *(Aspen)*, C-M-P-K Injection *(Vet Tek)*, Cal-MPK™ 1080 Injection *(Butler)*, Cal-Dex C-M-P-K *(AgriLabs)*, CMPK-Dex *(Vetus)*, CMPK *(RXV)*.

potassium chloride, sodium hypophosphite, calcium, dextrose, magnesium chloride. Cal-Phos #2 with Potassium Injection *(Phoenix Pharmaceutical)*, CMPK Solution *(Vedco)*, *(Aspen)*, M.F.O. Solution *(AgriLabs)*.

potassium chloride, sodium hypophosphite, calcium borogluconate, dextrose, magnesium borogluconate. CMPK Solution *(Bimeda)*.

potassium chloride, sodium phosphate, calcium, dextrose, magnesium chloride. CMPK Oral *(AgriPharm)*.

potassium chloride, tri-calcium phosphate, calcium, magnesium chloride. Oral CMPK Gel *(DVM Formula)*.

potassium chloride, trisodium phosphate, calcium, magnesium chloride, phosphoric acid. CMPK Gel *(AgriPharm)*.

potassium citrate, fatty acids. NutriVed™ Potassium Citrate Granules for Cats and Dogs *(Vedco)*.

potassium dichromate, cobalt sulfate, copper sulfate, hydrochloric acid, manganese sulfate. Ema-Sol™ Concentrate *(Alpharma)*.

Potassium Gel *(Butler)*, **potassium gluconate.**

potassium gluconate. Potassium Gel *(Butler)*, Potassium Powder *(Butler)*, Potassium Tablets *(Butler)*, RenaKare™ *(Neogen)*, Tumil-K® *(King Animal Health)*, Tumil-K® Gel *(King Animal Health)*.

potassium hydroxide, sodium hypochlorite, sodium metasilicate, sodium silicate, detergent mixture. Lifegard® 855 Plus *(Rochester Midland)*.

potassium hydroxide, sodium metasilicate, polymeric dispersant. Lifegard® 800 *(Rochester Midland)*.

potassium iodide, ammonium chloride, guaifenesin (glyceryl guaiacolate, guaiacol). AniTuss *(AHC)*, Spec-Tuss™ *(Neogen)*, Tri-Tussin™ Powder *(Creative Science)*.

potassium iodide, iodine, isopropyl alcohol (isopropanol). Iodine Tincture 7% *(First Priority)*.

potassium nitrate, silver nitrate. Silver Nitrate Stick Applicators *(Vedco)*, Stypt-Stix *(Vetus)*.

potassium peroxymenosulfate. Trifectant™ *(Evsco)*, Virkon®-S *(Farnam, Livestock Div.)*.

Potassium Powder *(Butler)*, **potassium gluconate.**

potassium salts of fatty acids. Ecosect™ Insecticide *(Schering-Plough)*.

Potassium Tablets *(Butler)*, **potassium gluconate.**

Poult Pak *(Alpharma)*, **minerals, vitamins.**

Poviderm Medical Scrub *(Vetus)*, **iodine complex (povidone-iodine).**

Poviderm Medicated Shampoo *(Vetus)*, **iodine complex (povidone-iodine).**

Poviderm Solution *(Vetus)*, **iodine complex (povidone-iodine).**

Povidine *(AgriPharm)*, **iodine complex (povidone-iodine).**

Povidine 0.75% Scrub *(AgriPharm)*, **iodine complex (povidone-iodine).**

Povidine™ Bolus *(Butler)*, **iodine complex (povidone-iodine).**

Povidone Iodine Ointment *(First Priority)*, **iodine complex (povidone-iodine).**

Povidone Iodine Scrub *(First Priority)*, **iodine complex (povidone-iodine).**

Povidone Iodine Shampoo *(First Priority)*, *(Vedco)*, **iodine complex (povidone-iodine).**

Povidone Iodine Solution *(First Priority)*, **iodine complex (povidone-iodine).**

Povidone-Iodine Solution 10% *(Equicare)*, **iodine complex (povidone-iodine).**

Povidone-Iodine Surgical Scrub 7 1/2% *(Equicare)*, **iodine complex (povidone-iodine).**

Povidone Scrub *(Butler)*, **iodine complex (povidone-iodine).**

Povidone Shampoo 5% *(Butler)*, **iodine complex (povidone-iodine).**

Povidone Solution *(Butler)*, **iodine complex (povidone-iodine).**

Power Punch™ *(Vets Plus)*, **microorganisms, minerals, vitamins.**

PP-1 Special Blend *(AgriPharm)*, **lactase enzymes, microorganisms.**

pramoxine hydrochloride. Relief® Creme Rinse *(DVM)*, Relief® Shampoo *(DVM)*, Relief® Spray *(DVM)*, ResiProx™ Leave-on Conditioner *(Virbac)*.

pramoxine hydrochloride, glycerine. Corium-Tx™ *(Virbac)*.

pramoxine hydrochloride, hydrocortisone. Hydrocortisone Solution USP, 1% *(Vet Solutions)*.

praziquantel. Droncit® (praziquantel) Canine Tablets *(Bayer)*, Droncit® (praziquantel) Feline Tablets *(Bayer)*, Droncit® (praziquantel) Injectable for Dogs and Cats *(Bayer)*, Tape Worm Tabs™ for Cats and Kittens *(TradeWinds)*, Tape Worm Tabs™ for Dogs and Puppies *(TradeWinds)*.

praziquantel, pyrantel pamoate. Drontal® (praziquantel/pyrantel pamoate) Tablets *(Bayer)*.

praziquantel, pyrantel pamoate, febantel. Drontal® Plus (praziquantel/pyrantel pamoate/febantel) Tablets *(Bayer)*.

Pre-Conditioning/Receiving Formula Gel *(Durvet)*, **amino acids, bicarbonate, microorganisms, minerals, vitamins.**

Predef® 2X *(Pharmacia & Upjohn)*, **isoflupredone acetate.**

prednisolone. PrednisTab® *(Phoenix Pharmaceutical)*, *(Vedco)*, *(Vet-A-Mix)*, *(Vetus)*.

prednisolone, tetracycline, novobiocin. Delta Albaplex® / Delta Albaplex® 3X *(Pharmacia & Upjohn)*.

prednisolone, trimeprazine tartrate. Temaril-P® Tablets *(Pfizer Animal Health)*.

prednisolone sodium succinate. Solu-Delta-Cortef® *(Pharmacia & Upjohn)*.

PrednisTab® *(Phoenix Pharmaceutical)*, *(Vedco)*, *(Vet-A-Mix)*, *(Vetus)*, **prednisolone.**

Preempt™ *(Milk Specialties)*, *(MS BioScience)*, **microorganisms.**

Preference™ Stain & Odor Remover *(Virbac)*, **deodorants, stain removers.**

Pre-Gold® Germicidal Pre-Milking Teat Dip (Activator) *(Alcide)*, **orthophosphoric acid.**

Pre-Gold® Germicidal Pre-Milking Teat Dip (Base) *(Alcide)*, **sodium chlorite.**

Preventef® Flea and Tick Collar for Cats *(Virbac)*, **diazinon.**

Preventef® Flea and Tick Collar for Dogs *(Virbac)*, **diazinon.**

Preventic® Collar for Dogs *(Virbac)*, **amitraz.**

Preventic® Plus Tick and Flea IGR Collar for Dogs *(Virbac)*, **amitraz, pyriproxyfen.**

Pributazone™ Tablets *(First Priority)*, **phenylbutazone.**

primidone. Neurosyn™ Tablets *(Boehringer Ingelheim)*, Primidone *(Butler)*, *(Fort Dodge)*, Primidone 250 mg Tablets *(Vedco)*, Primitabs *(Vetus)*.

Primidone *(Butler)*, *(Fort Dodge)*, **primidone.**

Primidone 250 mg Tablets *(Vedco)*, **primidone.**

Primitabs *(Vetus)*, **primidone.**

Primor® *(Pfizer Animal Health)*, **ormetoprim, sulfadimethoxine.**

Privasan™ Antiseptic Ointment *(First Priority)*, **chlorhexidine.**

Privermectin™ Drench for Sheep *(First Priority)*, **ivermectin.**

Privermectin™ Equine Oral Liquid *(First Priority)*, **ivermectin.**

PRN Hi-Energy Supplement™ *(PRN Pharmacal)*, **amino acids, minerals, propylene glycol, vitamins.**

PRN High Potency Calcium Gel® *(PRN Pharmacal)*, **calcium.**

Pro 35™ Tearless Shampoo *(Tomlyn)*, **shampoo formula.**

Pro-Bac-C *(AgriLabs)*, **lasalocid sodium.**

Probiocin® Oral Gel for Pets *(Chr. Hansen)*, **microorganisms.**

Probios® Bovine One Oral Gel for Ruminants *(Chr. Hansen)*, **microorganisms.**

Probios® Dispersible Powder *(Chr. Hansen)*, **microorganisms.**

Probios® Equine One Oral Gel *(Chr. Hansen)*, **microorganisms.**

Probios® Feed Granules *(Chr. Hansen)*, **microorganisms.**

Probios® Microbial Calf Pac *(Chr. Hansen)*, **microorganisms.**

Probios® Oral Boluses for Ruminants *(Chr. Hansen)*, **microorganisms.**

Probios® Oral Suspension for Swine *(Chr. Hansen)*, **microorganisms.**

Probios® Plus Natural E Bovine One Oral Gel for Ruminants *(Chr. Hansen)*, **microorganisms, vitamin E.**

Probios® TC *(Chr. Hansen)*, **enzymes.**

Probiotic Plus E for Calves *(Vets Plus)*, **microorganisms, vitamin E.**

Probiotic Plus E for Cattle *(Vets Plus)*, **microorganisms, vitamin E.**

Probiotic Power™ *(Vets Plus)*, **microorganisms, vitamins.**

Pro-Bute™ Injection *(AgriLabs)*, **phenylbutazone.**

Pro-Bute™ Tablets 1 gram *(AgriLabs)*, **phenylbutazone.**

Procal™ Powder *(Butler)*, **amino acids, electrolytes, minerals, torula yeast.**

Prodine Ointment *(Phoenix Pharmaceutical)*, **iodine complex (povidone-iodine).**

Prodine Scrub *(Phoenix Pharmaceutical)*, **iodine complex (povidone-iodine).**

Prodine Solution *(Phoenix Pharmaceutical)*, **iodine complex (povidone-iodine).**

Produmec™ Injection for Cattle and Swine *(TradeWinds)*, **ivermectin.**

Produmec™ Pour-On for Cattle *(TradeWinds)*, **ivermectin.**

Pro-Gen® 20% *(Fleming)*, **arsanilic acid.**

Pro-Gen® 100% *(Fleming)*, **arsanilic acid.**

progesterone. EAZI-Breed™ CIDR® Cattle Insert *(Pharmacia & Upjohn)*.

progesterone, estradiol benzoate. Component® E-C *(VetLife)*, Component® E-S *(VetLife)*, Synovex® C *(Fort Dodge)*, Synovex® S *(Fort Dodge)*.

Proteoseptic Bolus *(Vedco)*, **urea.**

ProTICall® Insecticide for Dogs *(Schering-Plough)*, **permethrin.**

Protobolic™ Bolus Improved *(Butler)*, **minerals, protein(s), vitamins.**

Proud Flesh Powder *(First Priority)*, **copper sulfate, parachlorometaxylenol.**

Proudsoff™ *(Creative Science)*, **copper sulfate.**

Prozap® Aqueous Fly Spray *(Loveland)*, **piperonyl butoxide, pyrethrins.**

Prozap® Beef & Dairy Spray RTU *(Loveland)*, **dichlorvos.**

Prozap® Dairy & Feedlot Insecticide Concentrate *(Loveland)*, **dichlorvos.**

Prozap® Drycide® *(Loveland)*, **permethrin.**

Prozap® Dust'R™ *(Loveland)*, **tetrachlorvinphos.**

Prozap® Garden & Poultry Dust *(Loveland)*, **carbaryl.**

Prozap® Insectrin® Dust *(Loveland)*, **permethrin.**

Prozap® Insectrin® X *(Loveland)*, **permethrin.**

Prozap® Ivermectin Pour-On *(Loveland)*, **ivermectin.**

Prozap® LD-44Z *(Loveland)*, **piperonyl butoxide, pyrethrins.**

Prozap® Residual Insect Spray 2EC *(Loveland)*, **dimethoate.**

Prozap® VIP Insect Spray *(Loveland)*, **dichlorvos, piperonyl butoxide, pyrethrins.**

Prozap® Zipcide® *(Loveland)*, **coumaphos.**

PSD Complex II *(PRN Pharmacal)*, **calcium phosphate.**

pseudoephedrine HCl, pyrilamine maleate. Antihistamine Granules *(Butler)*, Equi-Phar Equi-Hist 1200 Granules *(Vedco)*, EquiPhed *(AHC)*, Tri-Hist® Granules *(Neogen)*.

psyllium. AniPsyll Powder *(AHC)*, Equine Psyllium *(First Priority)*, Equi-Phar™ Sweet Psyllium *(Vedco)*, SandClear™ *(Farnam)*, Sand-Pasture Formula™ *(Horses Prefer)*, Vetasyl™ Fiber Tablets for Cats *(Virbac)*.

psyllium, fermentation extract(s), microorganisms. Equine Enteric Colloid *(TechMix)*.

psyllium, kelp, liver meal, papaya fruit. Fiber Forte® Feline *(Life Science)*.

Pulmotil® 90 *(Elanco)*, **tilmicosin.**

Puppy Drops™ *(Tomlyn)*, **iron, liver extract, vitamins.**

Puppy Formula *(Vet Solutions)*, **milk replacing formula.**

Puralube® Vet Ophthalmic Ointment *(Pharmaderm)*, **petrolatum.**

Puralube® Vet Tears *(Pharmaderm)*, **polyvinyl alcohol.**

Purple Lotion *(Vedco)*, **acriflavine, gentian violet, glycerine, isopropyl alcohol (isopropanol), propylene glycol, urea.**

Purple Lotion Wound Dressing *(Durvet)*, **acriflavine, glycerine, isopropyl alcohol (isopropanol), methyl violet, propylene glycol, urea.**

Purple Lotion Wound Dressing *(First Priority)*, **acriflavine, gentian violet, glycerine, isopropyl alcohol (isopropanol), propylene glycol, urea.**

Purple Spray *(AgriPharm)*, **methyl violet.**

Purrge™ Drops *(PPI)*, **petrolatum.**

PVP Iodine *(Western Chemical)*, **iodine complex (povidone-iodine).**

PVP Iodine Ointment *(Vedco)*, **iodine complex (povidone-iodine).**

Pyoben® Gel *(Virbac)*, **benzoyl peroxide.**

Pyoben® Shampoo *(Virbac)*, **benzoyl peroxide.**

pyrantel pamoate. AmTech Anthelban V *(Phoenix Scientific)*, Anthelban V *(Phoenix Pharmaceutical)*, Champion Protector™ Worm Protector™ 2X *(AgriLabs)*, D-Worm™ 60 Liquid Wormer *(Farnam)*, D-Worm™ 120 Liquid Wormer *(Farnam)*, D-Worm™ Dog Wormer Chewable Tablets for Large Dogs *(Farnam)*, D-Worm™ Dog Wormer Chewable Tablets for Puppies & Small Dogs *(Farnam)*, D-Worm™ Dog Wormer Tablets for Large Dogs *(Farnam)*, D-Worm™ Dog Wormer Tablets for Puppies & Small Dogs *(Farnam)*, Equi-Phar ProTal™ *(Vedco)*, Exodus™ Paste *(Bimeda)*, Happy Jack® Liqui-Vict 2X™ *(Happy Jack)*, Nemex™ Tabs *(Pfizer Animal Health)*, Nemex™-2 Suspension *(Pfizer Animal Health)*, Pet Care Liquid Wormer *(Durvet)*, Pet Care Liquid Wormer 2X *(Durvet)*, RFD® Liquid Wormer *(Pfizer Animal Health)*, Rotectin™ 2 Paste *(Farnam)*, Sergeant's® Vetscription® Sure Shot® Liquid Wormer for Puppies and Dogs *(Sergeant's)*, Strongid® Paste *(Pfizer Animal Health)*, Strongid® T *(Pfizer Animal Health)*.

pyrantel pamoate, febantel, praziquantel. Drontal® Plus (praziquantel/pyrantel pamoate/febantel) Tablets *(Bayer)*.

pyrantel pamoate, ivermectin. Heartgard® Plus Chewables for Dogs *(Merial)*, Iverhart™ Plus Flavored Chewables *(Virbac)*.

pyrantel pamoate, praziquantel. Drontal® (praziquantel/pyrantel pamoate) Tablets *(Bayer)*.

pyrantel tartrate. Banminth® 48 *(Phibro)*, Continuex™ *(Farnam)*, Dealer Select Horse Care Horse & Colt Wormer *(Durvet)*, Equi Aid CW® *(Equi Aid)*, Equi-Phar™ Horse & Colt Wormer *(Vedco)*, Strongid® C *(Pfizer Animal Health)*, Strongid® C 2X™ *(Pfizer Animal Health)*, Strongid® C Thirty *(Pfizer Animal Health)*.

pyrantel tartrate, carbadox. MoorMan's® WDC *(ADM)*.

Pyrethrin Plus *(Durvet)*, **piperonyl butoxide, pyrethrins.**

Pyrethrin Plus Shampoo *(Vedco)*, **n-octyl bicycloheptene dicarboximide, piperonyl butoxide, pyrethrins.**

pyrethrins. Ectrin® Insecticide Cattle Ear Tag *(Boehringer Ingelheim)*.

pyrethrins, benzocaine, docusate sodium (dioctyl sodium sulfosuccinate), piperonyl butoxide. Aurimite® Insecticide *(Schering-Plough)*.

pyrethrins, butoxypolypropylene glycol, cypermethrin, di-n-propyl isocinchomeronate, piperonyl butoxide. Repel-X® Lotion *(Farnam)*.

pyrethrins, butoxypolypropylene glycol, cypermethrin, piperonyl butoxide. Bite Free™ Biting Fly Repellent *(Farnam)*, Endure™ Sweat-Resistant Fly Spray *(Farnam)*, Tri-Tec 14™ Fly Repellent *(Farnam)*.

pyrethrins, butoxypolypropylene glycol, di-n-propyl isocinchomeronate, n-octyl bicycloheptene dicarboximide, permethrin, piperonyl butoxide. Adams™ Fly Spray and Repellent *(V.P.L.)*, Flysect® Super-7 *(Equicare)*.

pyrethrins, butoxypolypropylene glycol, di-n-propyl isocinchomeronate, piperonyl butoxide. Wipe® Fly Protectant *(Farnam)*.

pyrethrins, butoxypolypropylene glycol, n-octyl bicycloheptene dicarboximide, piperonyl butoxide. Pet Guard™ Gel *(Virbac)*.

pyrethrins, butoxypolypropylene glycol, piperonyl butoxide. Absorbine® SuperShield® Red Fly Repellent *(W. F. Young)*, Flysect® Citronella Spray *(Equicare)*, Flys-Off® Insect Repellent for Dogs *(Farnam)*, Flys-Off® Lotion Insect Repellent for Dogs *(Farnam)*, VIP® Fly Repellent Ointment *(V.P.L.)*, Wipe® II Brand Fly Spray with Citronella *(Farnam)*.

pyrethrins, carbaryl, n-octyl bicycloheptene dicarboximide, piperonyl butoxide. Scratchex® Flea & Tick Powder *(Combe)*.

pyrethrins, carbaryl, piperonyl butoxide. Adams™ Flea & Tick Dust II *(Farnam)*, *(V.P.L.)*.

pyrethrins, diazinon, piperonyl butoxide. Sunbugger Residual Ant & Roach Spray Aqueous *(Sungro)*.

pyrethrins, dicarboximide, n-octyl bicycloheptene dicarboximide, piperonyl butoxide. Hartz® 2 in 1® Flea & Tick Killer for Dogs *(Hartz Mountain)*.

pyrethrins, dichlorvos, n-octyl bicycloheptene dicarboximide, piperonyl butoxide. Super II Dairy & Farm Spray *(Durvet)*.

pyrethrins, dichlorvos, piperonyl butoxide. Prozap® VIP Insect Spray *(Loveland)*, SK-Surekill® Brand Pyrethrin Plus Fly Spray *(IntAgra)*.

pyrethrins, di-n-propyl isocinchomeronate, n-octyl bicycloheptene dicarboximide, permethrin, piperonyl butoxide. Adams™ Fly Repellent Concentrate *(V.P.L.)*, Flysect® Super-C *(Equicare)*.

pyrethrins, di-n-propyl isocinchomeronate, n-octyl bicycloheptene dicarboximide, piperonyl butoxide. Adams™ Flea & Tick Mist *(V.P.L.)*, Adams™ Pyrethrin Dip *(Farnam)*, *(V.P.L.)*, EctoKyl™ 3X Flea & Tick Shampoo *(DVM)*, Flea & Tick Mist *(Davis)*, Flysect® Repellent Spray *(Equicare)*, Flysect® Roll-On Fly Repellent Face Lotion *(Equicare)*, Flys-Off® Fly Repellent Ointment *(Farnam)*, Mita-Clear™ *(Pfizer Animal Health)*, Otomite® Plus *(Virbac)*, Performer® Ear Mite Killer *(AgriLabs)*, Pet Care Ear Mite Lotion & Repellent *(Durvet)*, Pet Care Fast Kill Flea & Tick Spray for Dogs & Cats *(Durvet)*, Roll-On™ Fly Repellent *(Farnam)*, Triple Pyrethrins Flea & Tick Shampoo *(Davis)*, Vet-Kem® Triple Action Flea & Tick Shampoo for Dogs, Cats, & Horses *(Wellmark)*, Virbac Pyrethrin Dip™ *(Virbac)*.

pyrethrins, di-n-propyl isocinchomeronate, piperonyl butoxide. Happy Jack® Onex *(Happy Jack)*, Relief! Fly Ointment *(Davis)*, Swat® Fly Repellent Ointment *(Farnam)*, VPL Fly Repellent Ointment *(V.P.L.)*.

pyrethrins, methoprene, n-octyl bicycloheptene dicarboximide, piperonyl butoxide. Vet-Kem® Ovitrol® Plus Flea, Tick & Bot Spray *(Wellmark)*.

pyrethrins, methoprene, piperonyl butoxide. Hartz® Control Pet Care System® Mousse for Cats and Kittens *(Hartz Mountain)*, Vet-Kem® Ovitrol® Plus Flea & Tick Shampoo for Dogs & Cats *(Wellmark)*.

pyrethrins, n-octyl bicycloheptene dicarboximide, permethrin. Duocide® L.A. Spray *(Virbac)*.

pyrethrins, n-octyl bicycloheptene dicarboximide, piperonyl butoxide. Adams™ Water Based Flea and Tick Mist *(Farnam)*, *(V.P.L.)*, Cerumite 3x *(Evsco)*, Dairy Bomb-55 *(Durvet)*, Ecto-Foam™ *(Virbac)*, Ecto-Soothe™ 3X Shampoo *(Virbac)*, Flea Halt!™ Flea & Tick Repellent Towelettes *(Farnam)*, Flea Halt!™ Flea & Tick Repellent Towelettes for Ferrets *(Farnam)*, Flea, Tick and Lice Shampoo *(Tomlyn)*, Hartz® 2 in 1® Flea & Tick Dip for Dogs and Cats *(Hartz Mountain)*, Hartz® 2 in 1® Luster Bath for Cats *(Hartz Mountain)*, Hartz® 2 in 1® Rid Flea™ Dog Shampoo with Pyrethrin *(Hartz Mountain)*, Hartz® Easy Wash™ Flea & Tick Shampoo for Dogs *(Hartz Mountain)*, Pyrethrin Plus Shampoo *(Vedco)*, Scratchex® Flea & Tick Shampoo *(Combe)*.

pyrethrins, permethrin. Absorbine® UltraShield® Brand Towelettes *(W. F. Young)*, Happy Jack® DD-33™ Flea & Tick Mist *(Happy Jack)*, Happy Jack® No-Hop Flea-Tick Spray *(Happy Jack)*, Scratchex® Flea & Tick Spray *(Combe)*, SynerKyl® AQ Water-Based Pet Spray *(DVM)*.

pyrethrins, permethrin, piperonyl butoxide. Absorbine® UltraShield® Brand Fly Repellent *(W. F. Young)*, Bronco® Water-Base Equine Fly Spray *(Farnam)*, Durasect® II Long-Acting Livestock Pour-On *(Pfizer Animal Health)*, Flysect® Water-Based Repellent Spray *(Equicare)*, Repel-X® Insecticide & Repellent *(Farnam)*.

pyrethrins, piperonyl butoxide. 3X Pyrethrin Shampoo *(Vet Solutions)*, Absorbine® Flys-X® Insecticide *(W. F. Young)*, Adams™ Flea & Tick Shampoo *(V.P.L.)*, Brilliance™ Flea & Tick Shampoo *(First Priority)*, Dairy Bomb-50 *(Durvet)*, Dairy Bomb-50Z *(Durvet)*, Dairy Bomb-55Z *(Durvet)*, Davis Pyrethrins *(Davis)*, Ectiban® Synergized DeLice® Pour-On Insecticide *(Durvet)*, Ecto-Soothe™ Shampoo *(Virbac)*, Eradimite™ *(Fort Dodge)*, Grand Champion® Fly Repellent Formula *(Farnam)*, Happy Jack® Mitex™ *(Happy Jack)*, Hartz® Health measures™ Ear Mite Treatment for Cats *(Hartz Mountain)*, Hartz® Health measures™ Ear Mite Treatment for Dogs *(Hartz Mountain)*, Make Your Own Flea & Tick Shampoo *(Davis)*, Mitaplex-P™ *(Tomlyn)*, MoorMan's® Fly Spray *(ADM)*, Mycodex® Pet Shampoo with 3X Pyrethrins *(V.P.L.)*,

Mycodex® SensiCare™ Flea & Tick Spray *(V.P.L.)*, Pene-Mite™ *(Farnam)*, Pet Care House & Carpet Powder *(Durvet)*, Prozap® Aqueous Fly Spray *(Loveland)*, Prozap® LD-44Z *(Loveland)*, Pyrethrin Plus *(Durvet)*, Pyrethrins Dip and Spray *(Davis)*, Rabbit Ear Miticide *(Farnam)*, Repel-X®p Emulsifiable Fly Spray *(Farnam)*, Sergeant's® Vetscription® Aloe Ear Mite Treatment *(Sergeant's)*, Sheen II Shampoo *(Butler)*, Sunbugger Carpet Dust *(Sungro)*, Sun-Dust Roach Away *(Sungro)*, Sungro Flea-ZY Pet Shampoo *(Sungro)*, SynerKyl® Pet Dip *(DVM)*.

pyrethrins, pyriproxyfen, linalool, piperonyl butoxide. Adams™ Carpet Powder *(Farnam)*, Sergeant's® PreTect® Flea & Tick Carpet Powder *(Sergeant's)*.

pyrethrins, pyriproxyfen, n-octyl bicycloheptene dicarboximide, permethrin. Adams™ Room Fogger with Sykillstop™ *(Farnam)*, *(V.P.L.)*, EctoKyl™ IGR Total Release Fogger *(DVM)*, Happy Jack® Flea Flogger Plus *(Happy Jack)*, IGR House & Area Fogger *(Durvet)*, Mycodex® Environmental Control™ Aerosol Room Fogger *(V.P.L.)*, OmniTrol IGR Fogger *(Vedco)*, Virbac KnockOut® ES Area Treatment *(Virbac)*, Virbac KnockOut® Room and Area Fogger *(Virbac)*.

pyrethrins, pyriproxyfen, n-octyl bicycloheptene dicarboximide, piperonyl butoxide. Adams™ Flea & Tick Mist with Sykillstop™ *(Farnam)*, *(V.P.L.)*, Mycodex® All-In-One™ Spray *(V.P.L.)*, Sergeant's® PreTect® Flea & Tick Shampoo for Cats and Kittens *(Sergeant's)*.

pyrethrins, quaternary ammonia, n-octyl bicycloheptene dicarboximide, phenol, piperonyl butoxide. Microban® X-580 Institutional Spray Plus *(Microban)*.

Pyrethrins Dip and Spray *(Davis)*, **piperonyl butoxide, pyrethrins.**

pyrilamine maleate, guaifenesin (glyceryl guaiacolate, guaiacol). AniHist *(AHC)*, Hist-EQ Powder *(Butler)*.

pyrilamine maleate, pseudoephedrine HCl. Antihistamine Granules *(Butler)*, Equi-Phar Equi-Hist 1200 Granules *(Vedco)*, EquiPhed *(AHC)*, Tri-Hist® Granules *(Neogen)*.

pyrilamine maleate, sodium chloride, ammonium chloride, guaifenesin (glyceryl guaiacolate, guaiacol), phenylephrine hydrochloride. Cough Syrup *(Life Science)*.

pyrilamine maleate, sodium citrate, ammonium chloride, guaifenesin (glyceryl guaiacolate, guaiacol), phenylephrine hydrochloride. Anti-Tussive Syrup with Antihistamine *(Vedco)*, ExpectaHist *(Vetus)*.

pyrilamine maleate, sodium citrate, guaifenesin (glyceryl guaiacolate, guaiacol), phenylephrine hydrochloride. Expectade™ Cough Syrup *(PRN Pharmacal)*.

pyriproxyfen. Bio Spot® Stripe-On™ Flea Control For Cats *(Farnam)*, EctoKyl® IGR Emulsifiable Concentrate *(DVM)*, OmniTrol IGR 1.3% Emulsifiable Concentrate *(Vedco)*, Sergeant's® PreTect® Squeeze-On Flea Control for Cats *(Sergeant's)*, Virbac KnockOut® IGR Flea Collar for Cats & Kittens *(Virbac)*, Virbac KnockOut® IGR Flea Collar for Dogs & Puppies *(Virbac)*.

pyriproxyfen, amitraz. Preventic® Plus Tick and Flea IGR Collar for Dogs *(Virbac)*.

pyriproxyfen, d-2-allayl-4-hydroxy-3-methyl-2-cyclopenten-1-one, di-n-propyl isocinchomeronate, n-octyl bicycloheptene dicarboximide, permethrin, piperonyl butoxide. Sergeant's® PreTect® Flea & Tick Spray for Cats & Kittens *(Sergeant's)*, Sergeant's® PreTect® Flea & Tick Spray for Dogs & Puppies *(Sergeant's)*.

pyriproxyfen, linalool, n-octyl bicycloheptene dicarboximide, permethrin. Adams™ Inverted Carpet Spray *(Farnam)*, Sergeant's® PreTect® Household Flea & Tick Spray *(Sergeant's)*.

pyriproxyfen, linalool, permethrin, piperonyl butoxide. Sergeant's® PreTect® Indoor Flea & Tick Fogger *(Sergeant's)*.

pyriproxyfen, linalool, piperonyl butoxide, pyrethrins. Adams™ Carpet Powder *(Farnam)*, Sergeant's® PreTect® Flea & Tick Carpet Powder *(Sergeant's)*.

pyriproxyfen, n-octyl bicycloheptene dicarboximide, permethrin. Sergeant's® Flea-Free Breeze™ *(Sergeant's)*.

pyriproxyfen, n-octyl bicycloheptene dicarboximide, permethrin, pyrethrins. Adams™ Room Fogger with Sykillstop™ *(Farnam)*, *(V.P.L.)*, EctoKyl™ IGR Total Release Fogger *(DVM)*, Happy Jack® Flea Flogger Plus *(Happy Jack)*, IGR House & Area Fogger *(Durvet)*, Mycodex® Environmental Control™ Aerosol Room Fogger *(V.P.L.)*, OmniTrol IGR Fogger *(Vedco)*, Virbac KnockOut® ES Area Treatment *(Virbac)*, Virbac KnockOut® Room and Area Fogger *(Virbac)*.

pyriproxyfen, n-octyl bicycloheptene dicarboximide, piperonyl butoxide, pyrethrins. Adams™ Flea & Tick Mist with Sykillstop™ *(Farnam)*, *(V.P.L.)*, Mycodex® All-In-One™ Spray *(V.P.L.)*, Sergeant's® PreTect® Flea & Tick Shampoo for Cats and Kittens *(Sergeant's)*.

pyriproxyfen, permethrin. Bio Spot® Flea & Tick Control For Dogs (15 lbs. and Under) *(Farnam)*, Bio Spot® Flea & Tick Control For Dogs (Between 15 & 33 lbs.) *(Farnam)*, Bio Spot® Flea & Tick Control For Dogs (33 to 66 lbs.) *(Farnam)*, Bio Spot® Flea & Tick Control For Dogs (Over 66 lbs.) *(Farnam)*, Sergeant's® PreTect® Squeeze-On Flea & Tick Control for Dogs (under 15 lbs) *(Sergeant's)*, Sergeant's® PreTect® Squeeze-On Flea & Tick Control for Dogs (15 to 33 lbs) *(Sergeant's)*, Sergeant's® PreTect® Squeeze-On Flea & Tick Control for Dogs (under 33 lbs) *(Sergeant's)*, Sergeant's® PreTect® Squeeze-On Flea & Tick Control for Dogs (over 33 lbs) *(Sergeant's)*, Virbac® Long Acting KnockOut™ *(Virbac)*.

pyriproxyfen, permethrin, piperonyl butoxide. Sergeant's® PreTect® Flea & Tick Shampoo for Dogs and Puppies *(Sergeant's)*, Virbac KnockOut® IGR Household Pump Spray *(Virbac)*.

pyriproxyfen, sumethrin, tetramethrin. EctoKyl™ IGR Pressurized Spray *(DVM)*, Happy Jack® Flea Zinger Plus *(Happy Jack)*, Mycodex® Environmental Control™ Aerosol Household Spray *(V.P.L.)*, Pet Care IGR-House & Carpet Spray *(Durvet)*, Virbac KnockOut® Area Treatment *(Virbac)*.

PZI Vet® *(Idexx Pharm.)*, **insulin.**

Q

Quadritop™ Cream *(Vetus)*, **neomycin, nystatin, thiostrepton, triamcinolone acetonide.**

Quadritop™ Ointment *(Vetus)*, **neomycin, nystatin, thiostrepton, triamcinolone acetonide.**

Quartermaster® *(Pharmacia & Upjohn)*, **dihydrostreptomycin, penicillin G procaine.**

Quatcide *(Bio-Tek)*, **quaternary ammonia.**

quaternary ammonia. 16% Dual-Quat *(Vet Solutions)*, A-33® Dry *(Ecolab Prof. Prod. Div.)*, Air$_x$® 75 *(Airex)*, Asepticare® TB+II *(Ecolab Prof. Prod. Div.)*, Asepti-HB™ *(Ecolab Prof. Prod. Div.)*, Bacto-Sep *(Interchem)*, D-128 *(Vedco)*, D-256 *(Vedco)*, Dakil *(Davis)*, Di-Quat 10-S *(Butler)*, Disintegrator® *(Phoenix Pharmaceutical)*, D-Trol *(DuBois)*, F-48 *(Rochester Midland)*, Foaming Disinfectant Cleaner *(Davis)*, Foam Quat *(Vet Solutions)*, Germicidal Detergent and Deodorant *(Aire-Mate)*, Germicide Solution *(Phoenix Pharmaceutical)*, Grade A™ *(Intercon)*, KennelSol™ *(Alpha Tech Pet)*, KenneLSol HC™ *(Alpha Tech Pet)*, KenneLSol-NPV™ *(Alpha Tech Pet)*, LDC-19™ *(Intercon)*, Lifegard® 256 Plus *(Rochester Midland)*, Liquatone™ *(Westfalia•Surge)*, Lysol® Brand I.C.™ Quaternary Disinfectant Cleaner *(Reckitt Benckiser)*, Mint Disinfectant *(Air-Tite)*, Multi-Purpose Disinfectant *(LeGear)*, Multi-Quat 128 *(Intercon)*, Multi Quat TB™ *(Intercon)*, P-128 *(First Priority)*, Parr Quat *(Butler)*, Parr Quat 4X *(Butler)*, Parvosol® II RTU *(KenVet)*, Quatcide *(Bio-Tek)*, Quatrol *(Bio-Tek)*, Quatsan *(Bio-Tek)*, Spectrasol™ *(KenVet)*, Steramine *(Stearns)*, Sunkleen 16 *(Sungro)*, Sunkleen 45 *(Sungro)*, Sunkleen 90 *(Sungro)*, Tryad® *(Loveland)*, Udder Cleanitizer® *(Westfalia•Surge)*, Vigilquat *(Alex C. Fergusson)*, V.T.D. *(Interchem)*.

quaternary ammonia, 2-(hydroxymethyl)-2-nitro-1,3 propanediol, formaldehyde. DC&R® Disinfectant *(Loveland)*, Parvosan™ *(KenVet)*.

quaternary ammonia, alcohol. Asepti-Wipe™ *(Ecolab Prof. Prod. Div.)*, MetriWipes® *(Metrex)*.

quaternary ammonia, bis-n-tributyltin oxide. Roccal®-D Plus *(Pharmacia & Upjohn)*.

quaternary ammonia, bronopol, dichloroisocyanurate (sodium). ActaCept™ *(Activon)*.

quaternary ammonia, chlorhexidine digluconate. Spectrum™ *(Westfalia•Surge)*.

quaternary ammonia, chlorhexidine gluconate. Bou-Matic Sprayable Supreme *(Bou-Matic)*, Bou-Matic Supreme *(Bou-Matic)*.

quaternary ammonia, ethanol. Lysol® Brand II I.C.™ Disinfectant Spray *(Reckitt Benckiser)*, Monarch® Super Kabon® *(Ecolab Food & Bev. Div.)*.

quaternary ammonia, glutaraldehyde. Virocid® *(Merial Select)*.

quaternary ammonia, isopropyl alcohol (isopropanol). Cavicide® *(Metrex)*, Kleen-Aseptic® *(Metrex)*.

quaternary ammonia, n-octyl bicycloheptene dicarboximide, phenol, piperonyl butoxide, pyrethrins. Microban® X-580 Institutional Spray Plus *(Microban)*.

quaternary ammonia, pine oil. Big Pine™ *(Intercon)*, Marcicide II *(M.A.R.C.)*.

Quatrol *(Bio-Tek)*, **quaternary ammonia.**

Quatsan *(Bio-Tek)*, **quaternary ammonia.**

Quest® 2% Equine Oral Gel *(Fort Dodge)*, **moxidectin.**

QuickBayt™ Fly Bait *(Bayer)*, **imidacloprid, tricosene.**

QuickHit™ for Dairy Cattle *(SSI Corp.)*, **copper, sulfur, zinc.**

Quick-Start™ *(Vedco)*, **energy source(s), vitamins.**

QuikClean™ Waterless Shampoo *(Fort Dodge)*, **conditioners, lanolin.**

R

Rabbit Ear Miticide *(Farnam)*, **piperonyl butoxide, pyrethrins.**

Rabon® 3% Dust *(AgriLabs)*, **tetrachlorvinphos.**

Rabon® 7.76 Oral Larvicide Premix *(Boehringer Ingelheim)*, **tetrachlorvinphos.**

Rabon® 50% WP *(Boehringer Ingelheim)*, **tetrachlorvinphos.**

Rabon® 97.3 Oral Larvicide Premix *(Boehringer Ingelheim)*, **tetrachlorvinphos.**

racemethionine, vitamin B-complex, choline bitartrate, inositol, liver. Lipocaps *(Vetus)*.

ractopamine hydrochloride. Paylean® 9 *(Elanco)*.

Ralgro® Implants (Cattle) *(Schering-Plough)*, **zeranol.**

Ralgro® Implants (Lamb) *(Schering-Plough)*, **zeranol.**

Ralgro® Magnum™ Implants *(Schering-Plough)*, **zeranol.**

Rally™-20 *(Vedco)*, **tripelennamine hydrochloride.**

RapidVet™ Plasm-ex™ *(DMS Laboratories)*, **electrolytes, oxypolygelatin.**

Rapinovet™ Anesthetic Injection *(Schering-Plough)*, **propofol.**

Ravap® E.C. *(Boehringer Ingelheim)*, **dichlorvos, tetrachlorvinphos.**

RBC's. Canine Packed Red Blood Cells *(P.V.R.)*.

Reashure™ Choline *(Balchem)*, **choline chloride.**

Re-Covr® Injection *(Fort Dodge)*, **tripelennamine hydrochloride.**

Red Alert *(Neogen)*, **vitamins.**

Red Cell® *(Horse Health)*, **iron, minerals, vitamins.**
Redglo® *(Equicare)*, **iron, vitamins.**
Reducine® Absorbent for Horses *(Equicare)*, **iodide (potassium), iodine, pine tar.**
Reducine® Poultice *(Equicare)*, **aloe vera, bentonite, boric acid, ferrous sulfate, glycerine, kaolin.**
ReFresh® Iodine Teat Dip (1.00%) *(Metz)*, **iodine.**
Regressin®-V *(Bioniche Animal Health)*, **Mycobacterium cell wall fraction.**
Regu-Mate® Solution *(Intervet)*, **altrenogest.**
Relief® Creme Rinse *(DVM)*, **pramoxine hydrochloride.**
Relief! Fly Ointment *(Davis)*, **di-n-propyl isocinchomeronate, piperonyl butoxide, pyrethrins.**
Relief® Shampoo *(DVM)*, **pramoxine hydrochloride.**
Relief® Spray *(DVM)*, **pramoxine hydrochloride.**
RenaKare™ *(Neogen)*, **potassium gluconate.**
Ren-O-Sal® Tablets *(Fort Dodge)*, **3-nitro-4-hydroxyphenylarsonic acid (roxarsone).**
Repel-X® Insecticide & Repellent *(Farnam)*, **permethrin, piperonyl butoxide, pyrethrins.**
Repel-X® Lotion *(Farnam)*, **butoxypolypropylene glycol, cypermethrin, di-n-propyl isocinchomeronate, piperonyl butoxide, pyrethrins.**
Repel-X®p Emulsifiable Fly Spray *(Farnam)*, **piperonyl butoxide, pyrethrins.**
ResiChlor™ Leave-on Conditioner *(Virbac)*, **chlorhexidine gluconate.**
ResiCort® Leave-on Conditioner *(Virbac)*, **hydrocortisone.**
ResiHist® Leave-on Conditioner *(Virbac)*, **diphenhydramine.**
resin. Demotec® 95 *(Kane)*, Demotec® Easy Bloc® *(Kane)*.
resin, acetone. Absorbine® SuperShine® Hoof Polish *(W. F. Young)*.
ResiProx™ Leave-on Conditioner *(Virbac)*, **pramoxine hydrochloride.**
ResiSoothe® Leave-on Conditioner *(Virbac)*, **oatmeal.**
ResiZole™ Leave-on Conditioner *(Virbac)*, **miconazole.**
resmethrin. Formula F-500 *(Aire-Mate)*.
resmethrin, botoxylpolypropylene glycol. Absorbine® Concentrated Fly Repellent *(W. F. Young)*.
Re-Sorb® *(Pfizer Animal Health)*, **electrolytes, glucose.**
resorcinol, zinc oxide, bismuth subgallate, bismuth subnitrate, calamine, juniper tar. Pellitol® Ointment *(Veterinary Specialties)*.
Respond *(Jorgensen)*, **calcium, cobalt sulfate, magnesium chloride.**
Response® *(Westfalia•Surge)*, **iodine complex (povidone-iodine).**
Response II™ *(Westfalia•Surge)*, **iodine complex (povidone-iodine).**
Revalor®-200 *(Intervet)*, **estradiol, trenbolone acetate.**
Revalor®-G *(Intervet)*, **estradiol, trenbolone acetate.**
Revalor®-H *(Intervet)*, **estradiol, trenbolone acetate.**
Revalor®-IH *(Intervet)*, **estradiol, trenbolone acetate.**
Revalor®-IS *(Intervet)*, **estradiol, trenbolone acetate.**
Revalor®-S *(Intervet)*, **estradiol, trenbolone acetate.**
Revitilyte™ *(Vets Plus)*, **dextrose, minerals.**
Revitilyte-EQ™ *(Horses Prefer)*, **electrolytes.**
Revitilyte-Gelling™ *(Vets Plus)*, **dextrose, minerals.**
Revitilyte-Plus™ *(Vets Plus)*, **electrolytes, microorganisms, vitamins.**
Revolution® *(Pfizer Animal Health)*, **selamectin.**
RFD® Liquid Wormer *(Pfizer Animal Health)*, **pyrantel pamoate.**
Rhodococcus Equi Antibody *(Lake Immunogenics)*, **immunoglobulin(s) G.**
Rimadyl® Caplets *(Pfizer Animal Health)*, **carprofen.**
Rimadyl® Chewable Tablets *(Pfizer Animal Health)*, **carprofen.**
rinse formula, moisturizer(s). Micro Pearls Advantage™ Hydra-Pearls™ Cream Rinse *(Evsco)*.
Ritter's Tick and Flea Powder *(Ritter)*, **carbaryl, methoxychlor.**
Robamox®-V Oral Suspension *(Fort Dodge)*, **amoxicillin.**
Robamox®-V Tablets *(Fort Dodge)*, **amoxicillin.**
Robaxin®-V Injectable *(Fort Dodge)*, **methocarbamol.**
Robaxin®-V Tablets *(Fort Dodge)*, **methocarbamol.**
robenidine hydrochloride. Robenz® *(Alpharma)*.
Robenz® *(Alpharma)*, **robenidine hydrochloride.**
Robinul®-V *(Fort Dodge)*, **glycopyrrolate.**
Rocadyne *(Rochester Midland)*, **iodine complex (povidone-iodine).**
Roccal®-D Plus *(Pharmacia & Upjohn)*, **bis-n-tributyltin oxide, quaternary ammonia.**
RofenAid® 40 *(Alpharma)*, **ormetoprim, sulfadimethoxine.**
Roll-On™ Fly Repellent *(Farnam)*, **di-n-propyl isocinchomeronate, n-octyl bicycloheptene dicarboximide, piperonyl butoxide, pyrethrins.**
Romet® 30 *(Alpharma)*, **ormetoprim, sulfadimethoxine.**
rosin. OtiCare®-P Ear Powder *(ARC)*.
rosin, Barbadoes aloes, camphor, Churchill's iodine, gum benzoin. Shin-Band *(Dominion)*.
Rotational Zinc™ *(SSI Corp.)*, **sulfur, zinc.**
Rotectin™ 1 Paste 1.87% *(Farnam)*, **ivermectin.**
Rotectin™ 2 Paste *(Farnam)*, **pyrantel pamoate.**
rotenone. Ear Miticide *(Phoenix Pharmaceutical)*, Pet Care Ear Mite Solution *(Durvet)*, Rotenone Shampoo *(Goodwinol)*, Ultra™ Ear Miticide *(Bimeda)*.
rotenone, benzocaine, lanolin. Goodwinol Ointment *(Goodwinol)*.
Rotenone Shampoo *(Goodwinol)*, **rotenone.**
R-Pen *(Alpharma)*, **penicillin G potassium.**
rubeola virus, histamine phosphate. Rubeola Virus Immunomodulator *(Eudaemonic)*.
Rubeola Virus Immunomodulator *(Eudaemonic)*, **histamine phosphate, rubeola virus.**
Rumalax™ Bolus *(AgriLabs)*, **magnesium hydroxide.**
Rumatel® *(Phibro)*, **morantel tartrate.**
Rumen Boluses *(Durvet)*, **magnesium oxide.**
Rumen-Eze *(Vet-A-Mix)*, **emulsifiers, vegetable oil(s).**
Rumensin® 80 *(Elanco)*, **monensin sodium.**
Rumen Yeast Caps Plus *(TechMix)*, **microorganisms.**
Ruminant LactoBac Gel *(Vedco)*, **amino acids, microorganisms, minerals, vitamins.**
Ruminant Lactobacillus Gel *(First Priority)*, **amino acids, bicarbonate, microorganisms, minerals, vitamins.**
RXV-PP-1 (Porcine Probiotic Paste) *(AgriPharm)*, **lactase enzymes, microorganisms.**

S

Saber™ Extra Insecticide Ear Tags *(Schering-Plough)*, **lambdacyhalothrin, piperonyl butoxide.**
Saber™ Pour-On Insecticide *(Schering-Plough)*, **lambdacyhalothrin.**
Sacox® 60 *(Intervet)*, **salinomycin sodium.**
Safe4Hours™ Medical Formula *(Safe4Hours)*, **triclosan.**
SafeCide® IC *(Schering-Plough)*, **orthoboric acid.**
Safe-Guard® 20% Dewormer Type A Medicated Article *(Intervet)*, **fenbendazole.**
Safe-Guard® Beef & Dairy Cattle Dewormer *(Intervet)*, **fenbendazole.**
Safe-Guard® Beef and Dairy Cattle Dewormer (290 g) *(Intervet)*, **fenbendazole.**
Safe-Guard® Cattle Dewormer (92 g) *(Intervet)*, **fenbendazole.**
Safe-Guard® Equine Dewormer (25 g) *(Intervet)*, **fenbendazole.**
Safe-Guard® Horse Dewormer (92 g) *(Intervet)*, **fenbendazole.**
Safe-Guard® Medicated Dewormer for Beef & Dairy Cattle, & Swine *(Intervet)*, **fenbendazole.**
Safe-Guard® Medicated Dewormer for Beef & Dairy Cattle (Flaked Meal) *(Intervet)*, **fenbendazole.**
Safe-Guard® Medicated Dewormer for Beef & Dairy Cattle (Soft Mini-Pellets) *(Intervet)*, **fenbendazole.**
Safe-Guard® Medicated Dewormer for Beef Cattle (20% Protein Block) *(Intervet)*, **fenbendazole.**
Safe-Guard® Medicated Dewormer for Beef Cattle (En-Pro-Al® Molasses Block) *(Intervet)*, **fenbendazole.**
Safe-Guard® Medicated Dewormer for Swine (EZ Scoop®) *(Intervet)*, **fenbendazole.**
safflower oil (linoleic acid), vitamin E, fatty acids. Omega EFA™ Capsules *(Butler)*, Omega EFA™ Capsules XS *(Butler)*, Omega EFA™ Liquid *(Butler)*, Omega EFA™ Liquid XS *(Butler)*.
salicylate (sodium). Liquid Asp-Rin™ *(AgriLabs)*, Liqui-Prin™ *(AgriPharm)*, *(First Priority)*.
salicylic acid. Shurjets *(Jorgensen)*.
salicylic acid, acetic acid, boric acid, glycerine, isopropyl alcohol (isopropanol), lanolin, lidocaine, propylene glycol. Fresh-Ear *(Q.A. Laboratories)*.
salicylic acid, acetic acid, boric acid, glycerine, isopropyl alcohol (isopropanol), lidocaine, propylene glycol. Otic Clear *(Butler)*.
salicylic acid, acetic acid, glycerine, isopropyl alcohol (isopropanol), lanolin, propylene glycol. OtiClean®-A Ear Cleaning and Deodorant Pads *(ARC)*.
salicylic acid, acetic acid, glycerine, isopropyl alcohol (isopropanol), propylene glycol. OtiClean®-A Ear Cleaning Lotion *(ARC)*.
salicylic acid, alcohol base, aromatic vegetable oil(s), methyl salicylate. Bigeloil® *(W. F. Young)*.
salicylic acid, benzoic acid, chlorhexidine, glycerine, malic acid, propylene glycol. Chlor-A-Clens Cleansing Solution *(Vedco)*.
salicylic acid, benzoic acid, chlorhexidine, lidocaine, malic acid. Dermachlor™ Plus *(Butler)*.
salicylic acid, benzoic acid, chlorhexidine, malic acid, propylene glycol. Dermachlor™ Rinse *(Butler)*.
salicylic acid, benzoic acid, eucalyptus oil, malic acid, propylene glycol. Euclens Otic Cleanser *(Vetus)*, OtiCalm™ Cleansing Solution *(DVM)*.
salicylic acid, benzoic acid, malic acid. Derma-Clens® *(Pfizer Animal Health)*.
salicylic acid, benzoic acid, malic acid, propylene glycol. Oti-Clens® *(Pfizer Animal Health)*.
salicylic acid, castor oil. Wartsoff™ *(Creative Science)*.
salicylic acid, chitosanide, docusate sodium (dioctyl sodium sulfosuccinate), lactic acid, propylene glycol. Epi-Otic® *(Virbac)*.
salicylic acid, coal tar, menthol. NuSal-T® Shampoo *(DVM)*.
salicylic acid, eucalyptus oil, glycerine, kaolin, methyl salicylate, peppermint oil. Absorbine® Antiphlogistine® *(W. F. Young)*.

salicylic acid, lactic acid, propylene glycol. Gent-L-Clens™ *(Schering-Plough)*.
salicylic acid, silicon dioxide, zinc oxide, acetic acid, boric acid, isopropyl alcohol (isopropanol), lanolin, propylene glycol. OtiCare®-B Drying Ear Creme *(ARC)*.
salicylic acid, sodium lactate, urea. KeraSolv® Gel *(DVM)*.
salicylic acid, sodium thiosulfate, chloroxylenol. Equine Medicated Shampoo *(Vet Solutions)*, Universal Medicated Shampoo *(Vet Solutions)*.
salicylic acid, sulfur. DermaPet® Seborrheic Shampoo *(DermaPet)*, Micro Pearls Advantage™ Seba-Moist™ Shampoo *(Evsco)*, Nova Pearls™ Antiseborrheic Shampoo *(Tomlyn)*, Nova Pearls™ Dry Skin Bath for Dogs *(Tomlyn)*, Sebolux® Shampoo *(Virbac)*.
salicylic acid, sulfur, coal tar. Allerseb-T® Shampoo *(Virbac)*, LyTar® Shampoo *(DVM)*, Sulfur & Tar Medicated Shampoo *(Davis)*, T-Lux® Shampoo *(Virbac)*.
salicylic acid, sulfur, triclosan. SebaLyt® Shampoo *(DVM)*, SeboRex™ Shampoo *(DVM)*.
salicylic acid, tannic acid, boric acid. Stanisol *(Q.A. Laboratories)*.
salicylic acid, tannic acid, boric acid, camphor, isopropyl alcohol (isopropanol), menthol. Dry-It *(Q.A. Laboratories)*.
salicylic acid, thymol, arnica, bentonite, boric acid, eucalyptus oil, glycerine, isopropyl alcohol (isopropanol), kaolin, methyl salicylate, peppermint oil. Bigeloil® 24-Hour Medicated Poultice *(W. F. Young)*.
Saline 0.9% Solution *(Vetus)*, **sodium chloride.**
Saline Solution *(Vedco)*, **sodium chloride.**
Saline Solution 0.9% *(AgriLabs)*, *(Phoenix Pharmaceutical)*, **sodium chloride.**
salinomycin sodium. Bio-Cox® 60 Granular *(Alpharma)*, Sacox® 60 *(Intervet)*.
Salix™ Injection 5% *(Intervet)*, **furosemide.**
Salix™ Tablets *(Intervet)*, **furosemide.**
SandClear™ *(Farnam)*, **psyllium.**
Sand-Pasture Formula™ *(Horses Prefer)*, **psyllium.**
S aureus, bacteriophage(s), culture medium. Staphage Lysate (SPL)® *(Delmont)*.
Sav-A-Caf® Finisher Iron *(IntAgra)*, **copper, iron.**
Sav-A-Caf® Starter Iron *(IntAgra)*, **copper, iron.**
Sav-A-Pig® Oral Iron *(IntAgra)*, **copper, iron.**
Scarlet Oil *(First Priority)*, **benzyl alcohol, eucalyptus oil, isopropyl alcohol (isopropanol), methyl salicylate, parachlorometaxylenol, pine oil, scarlet red.**
Scarlet Oil *(Vedco)*, **benzyl alcohol, eucalyptus oil, methyl salicylate, parachlorometaxylenol, pine oil, scarlet red.**
scarlet oil, aloe vera. Scarlet Oil with Aloe Vera *(Life Science)*.
Scarlet Oil Pump Spray *(Dominion)*, **camphor, eucalyptus oil, menthol, phenol, pine oil, scarlet red, thymol.**
Scarlet Oil Smear *(First Priority)*, **eucalyptus oil, methyl salicylate, pine oil, scarlet red.**
Scarlet Oil with Aloe Vera *(Life Science)*, **aloe vera, scarlet oil.**
Scarlet Oil Wound Dressing *(AgriPharm)*, **benzyl alcohol, eucalyptus oil, methyl salicylate, parachlorometaxylenol, pine oil, scarlet red.**
Scarlet Oil Wound Dressing *(Durvet)*, **benzyl alcohol, eucalyptus oil, methyl salicylate, pine oil, scarlet red.**
scarlet red, benzyl alcohol, eucalyptus oil, isopropyl alcohol (isopropanol), methyl salicylate, parachlorometaxylenol, pine oil. Scarlet Oil *(First Priority)*.
scarlet red, benzyl alcohol, eucalyptus oil, methyl salicylate, parachlorometaxylenol, pine oil. Scarlet Oil *(Vedco)*, Scarlet Oil Wound Dressing *(AgriPharm)*.
scarlet red, benzyl alcohol, eucalyptus oil, methyl salicylate, pine oil. Scarlet Oil Wound Dressing *(Durvet)*.
scarlet red, eucalyptus oil, methyl salicylate, P-chloro-M-xylenol, pine oil. Scarlex® Scarlet Oil *(Farnam)*.
scarlet red, eucalyptus oil, methyl salicylate, pine oil. Scarlet Oil Smear *(First Priority)*.
scarlet red, isopropyl alcohol (isopropanol), phenol. Dr. Naylor® Red-Kote® *(H.W. Naylor)*.
scarlet red, thuja oil, zinc oxide. Thuja-Zinc Oxide *(Phoenix Pharmaceutical)*, *(Vedco)*.
scarlet red, thymol, camphor, eucalyptus oil, menthol, phenol, pine oil. Scarlet Oil Pump Spray *(Dominion)*.
Scarlex® Scarlet Oil *(Farnam)*, **eucalyptus oil, methyl salicylate, P-chloro-M-xylenol, pine oil, scarlet red.**
Scratchex® 30 Day Flea & Tick Treatment (30 lbs. & under) *(Combe)*, **permethrin.**
Scratchex® 30 Day Flea & Tick Treatment (over 30 lbs.) *(Combe)*, **permethrin.**
Scratchex® Flea & Tick Collar for Cats *(Combe)*, **chlorpyrifos.**
Scratchex® Flea & Tick Collar for Dogs *(Combe)*, **chlorpyrifos.**
Scratchex® Flea & Tick Powder *(Combe)*, **carbaryl, n-octyl bicycloheptene dicarboximide, piperonyl butoxide, pyrethrins.**
Scratchex® Flea & Tick Shampoo *(Combe)*, **n-octyl bicycloheptene dicarboximide, piperonyl butoxide, pyrethrins.**
Scratchex® Flea & Tick Spray *(Combe)*, **permethrin, pyrethrins.**
Scratchex® Super Spray™ *(Combe)*, **d-2-allayl-4-hydroxy-3-methyl-2-cyclopenten-1-one, di-n-propyl isocinchomeronate, fenoxycarb, n-octyl bicycloheptene dicarboximide, permethrin, piperonyl butoxide.**
Screwworm Ear Tick Aerosol *(Durvet)*, **permethrin.**
SDM Injection *(Phoenix Pharmaceutical)*, **sulfadimethoxine.**
SDM Powder *(Bimeda)*, **sulfadimethoxine.**
SDM Solution *(Phoenix Pharmaceutical)*, **sulfadimethoxine.**
SebaLyt® Shampoo *(DVM)*, **salicylic acid, sulfur, triclosan.**
Sebolux® Shampoo *(Virbac)*, **salicylic acid, sulfur.**
SeboRex™ Shampoo *(DVM)*, **salicylic acid, sulfur, triclosan.**
Sedazine® *(Fort Dodge)*, **xylazine hydrochloride.**
See Spot Go!™ *(Tomlyn)*, **2-butoxyethanol, isopropyl alcohol.**
selamectin. Revolution® *(Pfizer Animal Health)*.
selegiline. Anipryl® Tablets *(Pfizer Animal Health)*.
selenium, calcium, cobalt, magnesium. Cal M 64 Plus Se *(Butler)*, Cal-Mag-SE Gel *(Durvet)*.
selenium, tetrachlorvinphos, vitamins, amino acids, minerals. Vita-Plus® with Equitrol® *(Farnam)*.
selenium, vitamin B-complex, calcium, cobalt, magnesium. Calcium SE *(First Priority)*.
selenium, vitamin E. Equ-SeE *(Vet-A-Mix)*, Equ-Se5E *(Vet-A-Mix)*, Prosel-300 *(Durvet)*, Sure E&SE™ *(SureNutrition)*, Vita•E & Selenium Powder *(Horse Health)*, Vita•E & Selenium Crumbles™ *(Horse Health)*, Vita-Min E & Selenium *(Farnam)*, Vitamin E & Selenium Powder *(AHC)*.
selenium, vitamin E, fatty acids. Bovine Maximizer™ *(Novartis Animal Vaccines)*.
selenium, vitamins, calcium, cobalt, magnesium. Cal Ox 64 Plus SE *(AgriPharm)*, Calcium Gel+Selenium *(AgriLabs)*, CalOx 64 SE Oral Gel *(Vedco)*.
selenium, vitamins, calcium, magnesium. Cal-Mag-SV Gel *(Butler)*.
selenium, vitamins, iron, minerals. Go Max™ Liquid *(Farnam)*.
selenium (sodium selenite), vitamin E. BO-SE® *(Schering-Plough)*, E-SE® *(Schering-Plough)*, MU-SE® *(Schering-Plough)*, Velenium™ *(Fort Dodge)*.
semduramicin sodium. Aviax® *(Phibro)*.
Sentinel® Flavor Tabs® *(Novartis)*, **lufenuron, milbemycin oxime.**
Septi-Lube™ *(Boehringer Ingelheim)*, **aqueous base lubricant(s).**
Sergeant's® Flea-Free Breeze™ *(Sergeant's)*, **n-octyl bicycloheptene dicarboximide, permethrin, pyriproxyfen.**
Sergeant's® PreTect® Flea & Tick Carpet Powder *(Sergeant's)*, **linalool, piperonyl butoxide, pyrethrins, pyriproxyfen.**
Sergeant's® PreTect® Flea & Tick Shampoo for Cats and Kittens *(Sergeant's)*, **n-octyl bicycloheptene dicarboximide, piperonyl butoxide, pyrethrins, pyriproxyfen.**
Sergeant's® PreTect® Flea & Tick Shampoo for Dogs and Puppies *(Sergeant's)*, **permethrin, piperonyl butoxide, pyriproxyfen.**
Sergeant's® PreTect® Flea & Tick Spray for Cats & Kittens *(Sergeant's)*, **d-2-allayl-4-hydroxy-3-methyl-2-cyclopenten-1-one, di-n-propyl isocinchomeronate, n-octyl bicycloheptene dicarboximide, permethrin, piperonyl butoxide, pyriproxyfen.**
Sergeant's® PreTect® Flea & Tick Spray for Dogs & Puppies *(Sergeant's)*, **d-2-allayl-4-hydroxy-3-methyl-2-cyclopenten-1-one, di-n-propyl isocinchomeronate, n-octyl bicycloheptene dicarboximide, permethrin, piperonyl butoxide, pyriproxyfen.**
Sergeant's® PreTect® Household Flea & Tick Spray *(Sergeant's)*, **linalool, n-octyl bicycloheptene dicarboximide, permethrin, pyriproxyfen.**
Sergeant's® PreTect® Indoor Flea & Tick Fogger *(Sergeant's)*, **linalool, permethrin, piperonyl butoxide, pyriproxyfen.**
Sergeant's® PreTect® Squeeze-On Flea & Tick Control for Dogs (under 15 lbs) *(Sergeant's)*, **permethrin, pyriproxyfen.**
Sergeant's® PreTect® Squeeze-On Flea & Tick Control for Dogs (15 to 33 lbs) *(Sergeant's)*, **permethrin, pyriproxyfen.**
Sergeant's® PreTect® Squeeze-On Flea & Tick Control for Dogs (under 33 lbs) *(Sergeant's)*, **permethrin, pyriproxyfen.**
Sergeant's® PreTect® Squeeze-On Flea & Tick Control for Dogs (over 33 lbs) *(Sergeant's)*, **permethrin, pyriproxyfen.**
Sergeant's® PreTect® Squeeze-On Flea Control for Cats *(Sergeant's)*, **pyriproxyfen.**
Sergeant's® Vetscription® Aloe Ear Mite Treatment *(Sergeant's)*, **piperonyl butoxide, pyrethrins.**
Sergeant's® Vetscription® Hairball Remedy *(Sergeant's)*, **petrolatum.**
Sergeant's® Vetscription® Sure Shot® Liquid Wormer for Cats & Kittens *(Sergeant's)*, **piperazine.**
Sergeant's® Vetscription® Sure Shot® Liquid Wormer for Puppies and Dogs *(Sergeant's)*, **pyrantel pamoate.**
Sergeant's® Vetscription® Vitamins for Cats & Kittens *(Sergeant's)*, **fatty acids (essential), taurine, vitamins.**
Sergeant's® Vetscription® Vitamins for Dogs & Puppies *(Sergeant's)*, **fatty acids (essential), minerals, vitamins.**
Sergeant's® Vetscription® Worm-Away® for Cats *(Sergeant's)*, **piperazine citrate.**
Sergeant's® Vetscription® Worm-Away® for Dogs *(Sergeant's)*, **piperazine citrate.**
serum gonadotropin, chorionic gonadotropin. P.G. 600® Estrus Control *(Intervet)*.
SevoFlo™ *(Abbott)*, **sevoflurane.**
sevoflurane. SevoFlo™ *(Abbott)*.

shampoo formula. Absorbine® SuperPoo® Conditioning Shampoo *(W. F. Young)*, Bio Guard® Shampoo *(Farnam)*, Cherry Grooming Shampoo *(First Priority)*, DVM Tearless™ Shampoo *(DVM)*, DVM Tearless™ Spray-On Shampoo *(DVM)*, Fast Acting Shampoo *(Davis)*, Grand Champion® Dri-Kleen™ *(Farnam)*, Groom-Aid® 35x *(Evsco)*, Hartz® Groomer's Best™ Conditioning Shampoo *(Hartz Mountain)*, HyLyt*efa® Hypoallergenic Shampoo *(DVM)*, Man O'War™ Shampoo *(Equicare)*, Mycodex® Pearlescent Grooming Shampoo *(V.P.L.)*, PearLyt™ Shampoo *(DVM)*, Petables™ Foaming Silk Bath *(A.A.H.)*, Pro 35™ Tearless Shampoo *(Tomlyn)*, Sho Sno™ Shampoo *(Tomlyn)*, Tearless Ferret Shampoo *(Tomlyn)*, Tearless Puppy Shampoo *(Tomlyn)*, Tearless Shampoo *(Davis)*, UltraGroom™ Shampoo *(Virbac)*.

shampoo formula, aloe vera. AlphaLyte® Premium Pet Shampoo *(Alpha Tech Pet)*.

shampoo formula, coconut oil. Cherryderm™ Grooming Shampoo *(Vetus)*, Cherry Grooming Shampoo *(Butler)*, Cleen Sheen *(Vedco)*, Cocoderm Conditioning Shampoo *(Vetus)*, Grooming Shampoo *(First Priority)*.

shampoo formula, coconut oil, conditioners. Davis Best Luxury Shampoo *(Davis)*.

shampoo formula, deodorants, neutralizer(s). Skunk-Off® Shampoo *(Thornell)*.

shampoo formula, fatty acids. D-Basic™ Shampoo *(DVM)*.

shampoo formula, lanolin. Blue Snow™ *(Schering-Plough)*.

shampoo formula, moisturizer(s). DermaPet® Hypoallergenic Conditioning Shampoo *(DermaPet)*, Micro Pearls Advantage™ Hydra-Pearls™ Shampoo *(Evsco)*, Nova Pearls™ 5 to 1 Concentrate Shampoo *(Tomlyn)*, Nova Pearls™ Sensitive Skin Shampoo *(Tomlyn)*.

shampoo formula, sunscreen formula, conditioners. Vetrolin® Bath *(Equicare)*.

shampoo formula, vitamin E, fatty acids (omega). Omega-Glo E Shampoo *(Vedco)*.

Sheen II Shampoo *(Butler)*, **piperonyl butoxide, pyrethrins.**

SheepPro™ Copper Suspension *(SSI Corp.)*, **copper, sulfur.**

SheepPro™ Zinc Suspension *(SSI Corp.)*, **sulfur, zinc.**

Shin-Band *(Dominion)*, **Barbadoes aloes, camphor, Churchill's iodine, gum benzoin, rosin.**

Shin-O-Gel® *(Hawthorne)*, **camphor, ether, isopropyl alcohol (isopropanol), menthol.**

Sho Sno™ Shampoo *(Tomlyn)*, **shampoo formula.**

Show Winner!™ Cat Vitamins *(Farnam)*, **linolenic acid, minerals, taurine, vitamins.**

Show Winner!™ Dog Vitamins *(Farnam)*, **linolenic acid, minerals, vitamins.**

Show Winner!™ Kitten Vitamins *(Farnam)*, **linolenic acid, minerals, vitamins.**

Show Winner!™ Older Dog Vitamins *(Farnam)*, **linolenic acid, minerals, vitamins.**

Show Winner!™ Puppy Vitamins *(Farnam)*, **linolenic acid, minerals, vitamins.**

Shur Hoof™ *(Horse Health)*, **fish oil, iodine, linseed oil, neatsfoot oil, pine tar, turpentine, wheat germ oil.**

Shurjets *(Jorgensen)*, **salicylic acid.**

silica. EarMed Powder *(Davis)*.

silicon dioxide, vitamins, cobalt sulfate, magnesium sulfate, polyethelene glycol, propionic acid. Ketopro Oral Gel *(Vedco)*.

silicon dioxide, zinc oxide, acetic acid, boric acid, isopropyl alcohol (isopropanol), lanolin, propylene glycol, salicylic acid. OtiCare®-B Drying Ear Creme *(ARC)*.

silver nitrate, potassium nitrate. Silver Nitrate Stick Applicators *(Vedco)*, Stypt-Stix *(Vetus)*.

Silver Nitrate Stick Applicators *(Vedco)*, **potassium nitrate, silver nitrate.**

silver sulfadiazine, enrofloxacin. Baytril® Otic (enrofloxacin/silver sulfadiazine) Antibacterial-Antimycotic Emulsion *(Bayer)*.

simethicone. NutriVed™ FlatuEx Chewable Tablets *(Vedco)*.

skim milk, whey, caseinate. Vaccine Stabilizer *(Alpharma)*.

SK-Surekill® Brand Pyrethrin Plus Fly Spray *(IntAgra)*, **dichlorvos, piperonyl butoxide, pyrethrins.**

Skunk-Off® *(Thornell)*, **deodorants, neutralizer(s).**

Skunk-Off® Shampoo *(Thornell)*, **deodorants, neutralizer(s), shampoo formula.**

Sky-Lytes *(Skylabs)*, **dextrose, electrolytes.**

Sleepaway® *(Fort Dodge)*, **pentobarbital sodium.**

Slow Release CMPK Bolus *(PRN Pharmacal)*, **calcium, magnesium, phosphorus, potassium, vitamins.**

soap formula. Anti-Bacterial Hand Soap *(First Priority)*, Hospital Hand Soap *(Vedco)*.

SOA (Sex Odor Aerosol) *(Intervet)*, **synthetic boar pheromone.**

Socumb™-6 gr *(Butler)*, **pentobarbital sodium.**

sodium, calcium. Cal-Pho-Sol *(Neogen)*.

sodium, vitamin A, vitamin D_3, vitamin E, potassium. Propack-EXP *(Durvet)*.

sodium, vitamin A, vitamin D_3, vitamin E, potassium, protein(s). WGS *(Durvet)*.

sodium, vitamin E, zinc, microorganisms, potassium. Yellow Lite *(AgriPharm)*.

sodium acetate, sodium chloride, sodium gluconate, magnesium chloride, potassium chloride. AmTech Amisol-R Injection *(Phoenix Scientific)*, Bimesol-R™ Injection *(Bimeda)*, ElectroSol-R *(Phoenix Pharmaceutical)*, Injectrolyte *(Vetus)*.

sodium alkyl ether sulfate, sodium lauryl sulfate, propylene glycol. Allermyl™ Shampoo *(Virbac)*.

Sodium Ascorbate *(Neogen)*, *(RXV)*, **vitamin C (ascorbic acid).**

Sodium Ascorbate Injection *(Vedco)*, **vitamin C (ascorbic acid).**

sodium bicarbonate. Bicarboject *(Vetus)*, Sodium Bicarbonate *(Butler)*, Sodium Bicarbonate 8.4% *(Neogen)*, *(Phoenix Pharmaceutical)*, *(Vedco)*.

Sodium Bicarbonate *(Butler)*, **sodium bicarbonate.**

sodium bicarbonate, sodium chloride, ammonium chloride, benzoic acid, calcium phosphate. Expectorant Powder *(First Priority)*.

sodium bicarbonate, vitamin B-complex, magnesium oxide. Buffer Gel™ *(Vets Plus)*.

Sodium Bicarbonate 8.4% *(Neogen)*, *(Phoenix Pharmaceutical)*, *(Vedco)*, **sodium bicarbonate.**

sodium chloride. AmTech Hypertonic Saline Solution 7.2% *(Phoenix Scientific)*, AmTech Saline Solution 0.9% *(Phoenix Scientific)*, Equi-Phar™ Equine 7 HSS *(Vedco)*, Hypersaline E *(Vetus)*, Hyper Saline Solution 8X *(Butler)*, Hypertonic Saline Solution 7.2% *(AgriLabs)*, *(Aspen)*, *(Bimeda)*, *(Phoenix Pharmaceutical)*, *(RXV)*, *(Vet Tek)*, Physiological Saline Solution *(Butler)*, Saline 0.9% Solution *(Vetus)*, Saline Solution *(Vedco)*, Saline Solution 0.9% *(AgriLabs)*, *(Phoenix Pharmaceutical)*, Sterile Saline Solution *(Bimeda)*, *(RXV)*.

sodium chloride, ammonium chloride, benzoic acid, calcium phosphate, sodium bicarbonate. Expectorant Powder *(First Priority)*.

sodium chloride, ammonium chloride, guaifenesin (glyceryl guaiacolate, guaiacol), phenylephrine hydrochloride, pyrilamine maleate. Cough Syrup *(Life Science)*.

sodium chloride, calcium, magnesium sulfate, potassium chloride. Electrolyte Supplement *(First Priority)*.

sodium chloride, sodium citrate. Clear Eyes *(Farnam)*.

sodium chloride, sodium gluconate, magnesium chloride, potassium chloride, sodium acetate. AmTech Amisol-R Injection *(Phoenix Scientific)*, Bimesol-R™ Injection *(Bimeda)*, ElectroSol-R *(Phoenix Pharmaceutical)*, Injectrolyte *(Vetus)*.

sodium chloride, sodium lactate, calcium, potassium chloride. AmTech Lactated Ringers Injection *(Phoenix Scientific)*, Lactated Ringers *(Vet Tek)*, Lactated Ringers Injection *(Phoenix Pharmaceutical)*, Lactated Ringer's Injection *(Vedco)*, Lactated Ringers Injection *(Vetus)*, Lactated Ringers Injection SC *(Butler)*, Lactated Ringer's Injection, USP *(AgriLabs)*, *(Bimeda)*, Lactated Ringer's Solution *(RXV)*.

sodium chloride, sodium phosphate. Opticlear™ Eye Wash Solution *(Tomlyn)*.

sodium chloride, sodium phosphate, hyaluronic acid (sodium hyaluronate). MAP®-5 *(Bioniche Animal Health)*.

sodium chloride, thiamine hydrochloride (B_1), calcium, potassium chloride. Happy Jack® Milkade *(Happy Jack)*.

sodium chloride, vitamin A, calcium, iodine, iron, phosphorus. Mo' Milk® Feed Mix and Top Dress *(TechMix)*.

sodium chloride, zinc, magnesium, phosphorus, potassium. Swine Acid-O-Lite™ *(TechMix)*.

sodium chlorite. 4XLA® Germicidal Pre- & Post-Milking Teat Dip (Base) *(Alcide)*, Bi-Sept™ Base *(Westfalia•*Surge), InterSept™ Base *(Westfalia•*Surge), LD® 1 Udder Wash Base Concentrate *(Alcide)*, Pre-Gold® Germicidal Pre-Milking Teat Dip (Base) *(Alcide)*, Uddergold® Plus Germicidal Barrier Teat Dip (Base) *(Alcide)*.

sodium chlorite (gel). Uddergold® Germicidal Barrier Teat Dip (Base) *(Alcide)*.

sodium citrate, ammonium chloride, guaifenesin (glyceryl guaiacolate, guaiacol), phenylephrine hydrochloride, pyrilamine maleate. Anti-Tussive Syrup with Antihistamine *(Vedco)*, ExpectaHist *(Vetus)*.

sodium citrate, guaifenesin (glyceryl guaiacolate, guaiacol), phenylephrine hydrochloride, pyrilamine maleate. Expectade™ Cough Syrup *(PRN Pharmacal)*.

sodium citrate, sodium chloride. Clear Eyes *(Farnam)*.

sodium citrate, whole blood, adenine, anhydrous lanolin, citric acid, hyaluronic acid (sodium hyaluronate). Canine Plasma *(A.B.B.)*, Canine Red Blood Cells *(A.B.B.)*, Canine Whole Blood *(A.B.B.)*, Feline Plasma *(A.B.B.)*, Feline Red Blood Cells *(A.B.B.)*, Feline Whole Blood *(A.B.B.)*.

sodium gluconate, magnesium chloride, potassium chloride, sodium acetate, sodium chloride. AmTech Amisol-R Injection *(Phoenix Scientific)*, Bimesol-R™ Injection *(Bimeda)*, ElectroSol-R *(Phoenix Pharmaceutical)*, Injectrolyte *(Vetus)*.

sodium hexametaphosphate, acetic acid. DermaPet® DentAcetic™ Wipes/Gel *(DermaPet)*.

sodium hydroxide, calcium hydroxide. Dehorning Paste *(AgriPharm)*, D-Horn Paste *(Dominion)*, Dr. Naylor® Dehorning Paste *(H.W. Naylor)*.

sodium hypochlorite. Hypo-Chlor Formula 6.40 *(Stearns)*.

sodium hypochlorite, sodium metasilicate, sodium silicate, detergent mixture, potassium hydroxide. Lifegard® 855 Plus *(Rochester Midland)*.

sodium hypophosphite, calcium, dextrose, magnesium borogluconate, potassium chloride. Cal-Dex C-M-P-K *(AgriLabs)*, Cal Dex CMPK Injection *(Aspen)*, Cal-MPK™ 1080 Injection *(Butler)*, CMPK *(RXV)*, CMPK-Dex *(Vetus)*, C-M-P-K Injection *(Vet Tek)*.

sodium hypophosphite, calcium, dextrose, magnesium chloride. AmTech Cal-Phos #2 Injection *(Phoenix Scientific)*, Cal MP-1000 *(Butler)*, Cal-Phos #2 *(Vedco)*, Cal-Phos #2 Injection *(Phoenix Pharmaceutical)*.

sodium hypophosphite, calcium, dextrose, magnesium chloride, potassium chloride. Cal-Phos #2 with Potassium Injection *(Phoenix Pharmaceutical)*, CMPK Solution *(Aspen)*, *(Vedco)*, M.F.O. Solution *(AgriLabs)*.

sodium hypophosphite, calcium, magnesium chloride, potassium chloride, propylene glycol. 40% CMPK with D_3 Oral Drench *(DVM Formula)*, Oral Calcium Drench *(DVM Formula)*.

sodium hypophosphite, calcium borogluconate, dextrose, magnesium borogluconate, potassium chloride. CMPK Solution *(Bimeda)*.

sodium hypophosphite, vitamin D_3, calcium, magnesium chloride, potassium chloride, propylene glycol. CMPK D_3 Drench *(Durvet)*.

sodium iodide. AmTech Sodium Iodide 20% Injection *(Phoenix Scientific)*, Iodoject *(Vetus)*, Sodium Iodide *(AgriLabs)*, *(Vet Tek)*, Sodium Iodide 20% *(RXV)*, Sodium Iodide 20% Injection *(Aspen)*, *(Phoenix Pharmaceutical)*, *(Vedco)*, Sodium Iodide Solution 20% *(Butler)*.

Sodium Iodide *(AgriLabs)*, *(Vet Tek)*, **sodium iodide.**

Sodium Iodide 20% *(RXV)*, **sodium iodide.**

Sodium Iodide 20% Injection *(Aspen)*, *(Phoenix Pharmaceutical)*, *(Vedco)*, **sodium iodide.**

Sodium Iodide Solution 20% *(Butler)*, **sodium iodide.**

sodium lactate, calcium, potassium chloride, sodium chloride. AmTech Lactated Ringers Injection *(Phoenix Scientific)*, Lactated Ringers *(Vet Tek)*, Lactated Ringers Injection *(Phoenix Pharmaceutical)*, Lactated Ringer's Injection *(Vedco)*, Lactated Ringers Injection *(Vetus)*, Lactated Ringers Injection SC *(Butler)*, Lactated Ringer's Injection, USP *(AgriLabs)*, *(Bimeda)*, Lactated Ringer's Solution *(RXV)*.

sodium lactate, emollient(s), fatty acids, glycerine, hydrolized animal protein. HyLyt*efa® Hypoallergenic Creme Rinse *(DVM)*.

sodium lactate, urea, salicylic acid. KeraSolv® Gel *(DVM)*.

sodium lauryl sulfate. Degrease Shampoo *(Davis)*.

sodium lauryl sulfate, propylene glycol, sodium alkyl ether sulfate. Allermyl™ Shampoo *(Virbac)*.

sodium lauryl sulfate, zinc sulfate. Dr. Naylor® Hoof 'n Heel® *(H.W. Naylor)*.

sodium linear alkylate sulfonate, hydrogen peroxide, lactic acid. Oxy-Gard™ Activated Peroxide Sanitizing Teat Dip *(Ecolab Food & Bev. Div.)*.

sodium metasilicate, polymeric dispersant, potassium hydroxide. Lifegard® 800 *(Rochester Midland)*.

sodium metasilicate, sodium silicate, detergent mixture, potassium hydroxide, sodium hypochlorite. Lifegard® 855 Plus *(Rochester Midland)*.

Sodium Pentobarbital Injection *(Butler)*, **pentobarbital sodium.**

sodium phosphate, calcium, dextrose, magnesium chloride, potassium chloride. CMPK Oral *(AgriPharm)*.

sodium phosphate, hyaluronic acid (sodium hyaluronate), sodium chloride. MAP®-5 *(Bioniche Animal Health)*.

sodium phosphate, sodium chloride. Opticlear™ Eye Wash Solution *(Tomlyn)*.

sodium propionate, acriflavine, gentian violet. Dr. Naylor® Blu-Kote® *(H.W. Naylor)*.

sodium propionate, urea, acriflavine, furfural, gentian violet, glycerine, isopropyl alcohol (isopropanol), propylene glycol. Blue Lotion *(AgriLabs)*.

sodium propionate, urea, acriflavine, glycerine, methyl violet, propylene glycol. Blue Lotion *(Farnam)*.

sodium silicate, detergent mixture, potassium hydroxide, sodium hypochlorite, sodium metasilicate. Lifegard® 855 Plus *(Rochester Midland)*.

sodium thiosulfate, chloroxylenol, salicylic acid. Equine Medicated Shampoo *(Vet Solutions)*, Universal Medicated Shampoo *(Vet Solutions)*.

SoftGuard™ *(Activon)*, **aloe vera, glycerine, triethanolamine, vitamin E.**

Sole Pack™ Hoof Dressing *(Hawthorne)*, **ichthammol, iodide (potassium), iodine, pine tar.**

Sole Pack™ Hoof Packing *(Hawthorne)*, **ichthammol, iodide (potassium), iodine, pine tar.**

Soloxine® *(King Animal Health)*, **levothyroxine.**

Soluble Colostrum Powder *(Durvet)*, **dried colostrum, microorganisms, vitamins.**

Solu-Delta-Cortef® *(Pharmacia & Upjohn)*, **prednisolone sodium succinate.**

Solumine *(Durvet)*, **vitamin D_3.**

Solu/Tet *(Vedco)*, **tetracycline.**

Solu-Tet® 324 *(Alpharma)*, **tetracycline.**

solvent(s). Natural Solvent™ *(Butler)*.

Somlethol *(Webster)*, **pentobarbital sodium.**

Soothables™ Cool Aid *(A.A.H.)*, **denatonium benzoate, eucalyptus oil, tea tree oil.**

Soothables™ Crystal-Ear *(A.A.H.)*, **ear cleanser formula.**

Soothables™ Tender Foot *(A.A.H.)*, **emollient(s), vitamins.**

sorbitol, activated charcoal. Liqui-Char®-Vet with Sorbitol *(King Animal Health)*.

sorbitol, activated charcoal, kaolin. ToxiBan™ Suspension with Sorbitol *(Vet-A-Mix)*.

sorbitol, vitamins, iron, minerals. Vi-Sorbin® *(Pfizer Animal Health)*.

Sow & Gilt Restart™ One-4 *(TechMix)*, **electrolytes, energy source(s), microorganisms, nutrients, vitamins.**

soybean oil, urea, wheat germ oil, cod liver oil, iodine complex (povidone-iodine), lanolin, petrolatum. Vita-Hoof® *(Equicare)*.

soy protein, vitamins, antioxidants, fatty acids (omega), minerals. Lickables™ Charge Up!™ *(A.A.H.)*.

spearmint oil, witch hazel, alcohol, iodide (potassium), iodine, menthol. Absorbine® RefreshMint® *(W. F. Young)*.

Spectam® Scour-Halt™ *(AgriLabs)*, *(Durvet)*, **spectinomycin.**

Spectam® Water Soluble *(Bimeda)*, **spectinomycin.**

spectinomycin. Adspec® Sterile Solution *(Pharmacia & Upjohn)*, AmTech Spectam® Scour-Halt™ *(Phoenix Scientific)*, BoviSpec™ Sterile Solution *(Vet Tek)*, Spectam® Scour-Halt™ *(AgriLabs)*, *(Durvet)*, Spectam® Water Soluble *(Bimeda)*, Spectinomycin Hydrochloride Injectable *(Durvet)*.

spectinomycin, lincomycin hydrochloride. Linco-Spectin® Sterile Solution *(Pharmacia & Upjohn)*, L-S 50 Water Soluble® Powder *(Pharmacia & Upjohn)*.

Spectinomycin Hydrochloride Injectable *(Durvet)*, **spectinomycin.**

Spectrasol™ *(KenVet)*, **quaternary ammonia.**

Spectrum™ *(Westfalia•Surge)*, **chlorhexidine digluconate, quaternary ammonia.**

Spec-Tuss™ *(Neogen)*, **ammonium chloride, guaifenesin (glyceryl guaiacolate, guaiacol), potassium iodide.**

SPF-Lac® *(Pet-Ag)*, **milk replacing formula.**

squalane. Cerumene™ *(Evsco)*.

Stabilized-C *(Alpharma)*, **vitamin C (ascorbic acid).**

Stafac® 10 *(Phibro)*, **virginiamycin.**

Stafac® 20 *(Phibro)*, **virginiamycin.**

Stafac® 500 *(Phibro)*, **virginiamycin.**

stain removers. Absorbine® ShowClean® Mane & Tail Whitener *(W. F. Young)*.

stain removers, deodorants. Preference™ Stain & Odor Remover *(Virbac)*.

stain removers, neutralizer(s). Elimin • Odor® Pet Stain Eliminator *(Pfizer Animal Health)*.

stain removers, vitamin E, aloe vera, moisturizer(s). CarraVet™ Multi Purpose Cleansing Foam *(V.P.L.)*.

Stam-N-Aid™ *(Neogen)*, **amino acids, minerals, vitamins.**

Stanisol *(Q.A. Laboratories)*, **boric acid, salicylic acid, tannic acid.**

stanozolol. Winstrol®-V Sterile Suspension *(Pharmacia & Upjohn)*, Winstrol®-V Tablets *(Pharmacia & Upjohn)*.

Staphage Lysate (SPL)® *(Delmont)*, **bacteriophage(s), culture medium, S aureus.**

Start To Finish® Energy Pak™ 100 *(Milk Specialties)*, **fat product(s).**

Start To Finish® Mare & Foal Pellets™ *(Milk Specialties)*, **fat product(s), lactose, milk protein, minerals, vitamins, yeast.**

Start To Finish® Mare Replacer™ *(Milk Specialties)*, **fat product(s), lactose, lecithin, minerals, vitamins, whey.**

Start To Finish® Performance Pellets™ *(Milk Specialties)*, **fatty acids, minerals, vitamins, yeast.**

Start To Finish® Sweat Replacer™ *(Milk Specialties)*, **electrolytes.**

Stat *(PRN Pharmacal)*, **energy source(s), minerals, vitamins.**

Steramine *(Stearns)*, **quaternary ammonia.**

Sterile Penicillin G Benzathine and Penicillin G Procaine *(Aspen)*, *(G.C. Hanford)*, **penicillin G benzathine, penicillin G procaine.**

Sterile Penicillin G Procaine *(Aspen)*, **penicillin G procaine.**

Sterile Penicillin G Procaine Aqueous Suspension *(Butler)*, **penicillin G procaine.**

Sterile Saline Solution *(Bimeda)*, *(RXV)*, **sodium chloride.**

sterile water. AmTech Sterile Water for Injection, USP *(Phoenix Scientific)*, Aquaject *(Vetus)*, Sterile Water *(AgriLabs)*, *(G.C. Hanford)*, *(Phoenix Pharmaceutical)*, *(Vedco)*, Sterile Water for Injection *(Butler)*, *(RXV)*, Sterile Water For Injection *(Vet Tek)*, Sterile Water for Injection, USP *(Aspen)*, *(Bimeda)*.

Sterile Water *(AgriLabs)*, *(G.C. Hanford)*, *(Phoenix Pharmaceutical)*, *(Vedco)*, **sterile water.**

Sterile Water for Injection *(Butler)*, *(RXV)*, **sterile water.**

Sterile Water For Injection *(Vet Tek)*, **sterile water.**

Sterile Water for Injection, USP *(Aspen)*, *(Bimeda)*, **sterile water.**

Stock Power *(LeGear)*, **minerals, vitamins.**

Stomadhex™ *(Virbac)*, **chlorhexidine, nicotinamide.**

streptomycin. Streptomycin Oral Solution *(Contemporary Products)*.

Streptomycin Oral Solution *(Contemporary Products)*, **streptomycin.**

Stress-Dex® *(Neogen)*, **dextrose, electrolytes, minerals.**

Stronger Iodine Tincture 7% *(Centaur)*, **iodide (potassium), iodine, isopropyl alcohol (isopropanol).**

Stronghold™ Teat Sealant *(WestAgro)*, **tetrahydrofuran.**

Strongid® C *(Pfizer Animal Health)*, **pyrantel tartrate.**

Strongid® C 2X™ *(Pfizer Animal Health)*, **pyrantel tartrate.**

Strongid® C Thirty *(Pfizer Animal Health)*, **pyrantel tartrate.**

Strongid® Paste *(Pfizer Animal Health)*, **pyrantel pamoate.**

Strongid® T *(Pfizer Animal Health)*, **pyrantel pamoate.**

Strong Iodine Tincture *(Butler)*, **iodide (potassium), iodine, isopropyl alcohol (isopropanol).**

Strong Iodine Tincture 7% *(Durvet)*, **iodide (potassium), iodine, isopropyl alcohol (isopropanol).**

Stypt-Stix *(Vetus)*, **potassium nitrate, silver nitrate.**

sucrose, vitamins, electrolytes, minerals. Dexsolyte Powder *(Neogen)*.

sucrose octyl acetate, isopropyl alcohol, oleoresin capsicum, orange peel bitter, propylene glycol. 3-No-Bite Spray *(Vedco)*, Bitter-3™ *(Butler)*.

sucrose octyl acetate, isopropyl alcohol, oleoresin capsicum, propylene glycol. Bitter Orange™ *(ARC)*.

sulfachlorpyridazine. Vetisulid® Boluses *(Fort Dodge)*, Vetisulid® Injection *(Fort Dodge)*, Vetisulid® Powder *(Fort Dodge)*.

Synovex® C *(Fort Dodge)*, **estradiol benzoate, progesterone.**
Synovex® H *(Fort Dodge)*, **estradiol benzoate, testosterone propionate.**
Synovex® Plus™ *(Fort Dodge)*, **estradiol benzoate, trenbolone acetate.**
Synovex® S *(Fort Dodge)*, **estradiol benzoate, progesterone.**
SynPhenol-3™ *(V.P.L.)*, **phenolic disinfectants.**
synthetic boar pheromone. SOA (Sex Odor Aerosol) *(Intervet)*.

T

T-4 Powder *(Neogen)*, **levothyroxine.**
T8 Solution™ Ear Rinse *(DVM)*, **EDTA (tetrasodium), lanolin, tromethamine.**
tabasco pepper, isopropyl alcohol, orange peel bitter. Triple-No-Chew *(Q.A. Laboratories)*, Triple-No-Chew Spray *(Q.A. Laboratories)*.
Taktic® E.C. *(Intervet)*, **amitraz.**
tannic acid, activated charcoal, alum, copper sulfate, iodoform. Wonder Dust™ Wound Powder *(Farnam)*.
tannic acid, alum, chloroxylenol, ferrous sulfate. Blood Stop Powder *(Aspen)*, *(Durvet)*, *(Vedco)*, Hemostat Powder *(Phoenix Pharmaceutical)*.
tannic acid, benzyl alcohol, crystal violet, isopropyl alcohol (isopropanol). Blue Lotion Aerosol *(Boehringer Ingelheim)*.
tannic acid, boric acid, camphor, isopropyl alcohol (isopropanol), menthol, salicylic acid. Dry-It *(Q.A. Laboratories)*.
tannic acid, boric acid, salicylic acid. Stanisol *(Q.A. Laboratories)*.
tannic acid, chloroxylenol, diphenylamine, ferrous sulfate. Blood Stop Powder *(First Priority)*.
tannic acid, ethylacetate, ethylcellulose, iodine, isopropyl alcohol (isopropanol). Dr. Naylor® Stop-A-Leak *(H.W. Naylor)*.
tannic acid, iodide (potassium), iodine, isopropyl alcohol (isopropanol). Freezex® Hoof Freeze *(Hawthorne)*.
tannic acid, thymol, alum, ferric subsulfate. Blood Stop Powder *(Dominion)*.
tannic acid, thymol, alum, ferric sulfate. Blood Stop Powder *(AgriLabs)*.
tannic acid, turpentine, gentian violet, isopropyl alcohol (isopropanol). Happy Jack® Pad Kote *(Happy Jack)*.
Tape Worm Tabs™ for Cats and Kittens *(TradeWinds)*, **praziquantel.**
Tape Worm Tabs™ for Dogs and Puppies *(TradeWinds)*, **praziquantel.**
Tasty Paste® Dog & Puppy Wormer *(Farnam)*, **piperazine.**
taurine. Dyna-Taurine™ *(Harlmen)*, Formula V™ Taurine Tablets *(Pet-Ag)*.
taurine, methylcellulose. Maxi/Guard® Oral Cleansing Gel *(Addison)*.
taurine, vitamins, amino acids, fatty acids (essential), minerals. NutriVed™ Chewable Vitamins for Cats *(Vedco)*, NutriVed™ Chewable Vitamins for Kittens *(Vedco)*.
taurine, vitamins, amino acids, minerals. Cholodin®-FEL *(MVP)*.
taurine, vitamins, antioxidants, minerals. Lickables™ Hearty Cat™ *(A.A.H.)*.
taurine, vitamins, fatty acids (essential). Sergeant's® Vetscription® Vitamins for Cats & Kittens *(Sergeant's)*.
taurine, vitamins, fatty acids (essential), minerals. NutriVed™ O.F.A. Granules for Cats *(Vedco)*.
taurine, vitamins, fatty acids (essential), minerals, potassium. Felo-Form *(Vet-A-Mix)*.
taurine, vitamins, linolenic acid, minerals. Mrs. Allen's Vita Care® Vitamins for Cats *(Farnam)*, Show Winner!™ Cat Vitamins *(Farnam)*.
taurine, vitamins, minerals. FaVor® *(Pfizer Animal Health)*, Felovite®-II with Taurine *(Evsco)*, Felovite® II with Taurine *(Tomlyn)*, Hartz® Health measures™ Everyday Chewable Vitamins for Cats and Kittens *(Hartz Mountain)*, TunaVite™ *(Vedco)*.
TDC/Teat Dip with Chlorhexidine *(Western Chemical)*, **chlorhexidine gluconate.**
T.D.N. Mini Rockets *(DVM Formula)*, **lactic acid producing bacteria, minerals, vitamins, yeast.**
T.D.N. Mini Rockets™ *(Vets Plus)*, **lactic acid producing bacteria, minerals, vitamins, yeast.**
T.D.N. Rockets *(DVM Formula)*, **lactic acid producing bacteria, minerals, vitamins, yeast.**
T.D.N. Rockets™ *(Vets Plus)*, **lactic acid producing bacteria, minerals, vitamins, yeast.**
Tearless Ferret Shampoo *(Tomlyn)*, **shampoo formula.**
Tearless Puppy Shampoo *(Tomlyn)*, **shampoo formula.**
Tearless Shampoo *(Davis)*, **shampoo formula.**
Teat Dip-Lite *(Western Chemical)*, **glycerine, iodine complex (povidone-iodine).**
Teat Dip with Glycerin *(Western Chemical)*, **glycerine, iodine complex (povidone-iodine).**
Teat Elite *(AgriPharm)*, **moisturizer(s), vitamins.**
Teat Glo® Sanitizing Teat Dip *(Ecolab Food & Bev. Div.)*, **iodine.**
Teat Guard™ *(Ecolab Food & Bev. Div.)*, **iodine complex (povidone-iodine).**
Teat-Kote® *(Westfalia•Surge)*, **glycerine, iodine complex (povidone-iodine).**
Teat Kote 10/III™ *(Westfalia•Surge)*, **iodine complex (povidone-iodine).**
tea tree oil. Excalibur® Sheath Cleaner for Horses *(Equicare)*.
tea tree oil, denatonium benzoate, eucalyptus oil. Soothables™ Cool Aid *(A.A.H.)*.
Tek-Trol® *(Bio-Tek)*, **phenolic disinfectants.**
Telazol® *(Fort Dodge)*, **tiletamine HCl, zolazepam.**
Temaril-P® Tablets *(Pfizer Animal Health)*, **prednisolone, trimeprazine tartrate.**
Tempo® 1% Dust Insecticide *(Bayer)*, **cyfluthrin.**
Tempo® 20 WP Insecticide *(Bayer)*, **cyfluthrin.**
Tempo® SC Ultra Premise Spray *(Bayer)*, **cyfluthrin.**
Terramycin® 10 TM-10® *(Phibro)*, **oxytetracycline.**
Terramycin® 50 *(Phibro)*, **oxytetracycline.**
Terramycin® 100 *(Phibro)*, **oxytetracycline.**
Terramycin® 100 for Fish *(Phibro)*, **oxytetracycline.**
Terramycin® 200 *(Phibro)*, **oxytetracycline.**
Terramycin-343® Soluble Powder *(Pfizer Animal Health)*, **oxytetracycline.**
Terramycin® Ophthalmic Ointment *(Pfizer Animal Health)*, **oxytetracycline, polymyxin B.**
Terramycin® Scours Tablets *(Pfizer Animal Health)*, **oxytetracycline.**
Terramycin® Soluble Powder *(Pfizer Animal Health)*, **oxytetracycline.**
Terra-Vet 100 *(Aspen)*, **oxytetracycline.**
Terra Vet Soluble Powder *(Aspen)*, **oxytetracycline.**
Terra-Vet Soluble Powder 343 *(Aspen)*, **oxytetracycline.**
testosterone propionate, estradiol benzoate. Component® E-H *(VetLife)*, Synovex® H *(Fort Dodge)*.
testosterone propionate, tylosin tartrate, estradiol benzoate. Component® E-H with Tylan® *(VetLife)*.
Tet 324™ *(Bimeda)*, **tetracycline.**
Tet-324 *(Phoenix Pharmaceutical)*, **tetracycline.**
Tetra Bac 324 *(AgriLabs)*, **tetracycline.**
tetracaine, isoflupredone acetate, myristyl-gamma-picolinium chloride, neomycin. Neo-Predef® with Tetracaine Powder *(Pharmacia & Upjohn)*.
tetracaine, isoflupredone acetate, neomycin. Tritop® *(Pharmacia & Upjohn)*.
tetrachlorvinphos. 3% Rabon® Livestock Dust *(Durvet)*, Equitrol® Feed-Thru Fly Control *(Farnam)*, Hartz® 2 in 1® Flea & Tick Collar for Cats and Kittens *(Hartz Mountain)*, Hartz® 2 in 1® Flea & Tick Collar for Dogs and Puppies *(Hartz Mountain)*, Hartz® 2 in 1® Flea & Tick Powder for Cats *(Hartz Mountain)*, Hartz® 2 in 1® Flea & Tick Powder for Dogs *(Hartz Mountain)*, Hartz® 2 in 1® Flea & Tick Spray for Cats *(Hartz Mountain)*, Hartz® 2 in 1® Flea & Tick Spray for Dogs *(Hartz Mountain)*, Hartz® Control Pet Care System® Flea & Tick Dip for Dogs *(Hartz Mountain)*, Hartz® Control Pet Care System® Flea & Tick Repellent for Cats *(Hartz Mountain)*, Hartz® Control Pet Care System® Flea & Tick Repellent for Dogs *(Hartz Mountain)*, Longlife® 90 Day™ Brand Collar for Cats *(Hartz Mountain)*, Longlife® 90 Day™ Brand Collar for Dogs *(Hartz Mountain)*, Louse Powder with Rabon® *(LeGear)*, Prozap® Dust'R™ *(Loveland)*, Rabon® 3% Dust *(AgriLabs)*, Rabon® 7.76 Oral Larvicide Premix *(Boehringer Ingelheim)*, Rabon® 50% WP *(Boehringer Ingelheim)*, Rabon® 97.3 Oral Larvicide Premix *(Boehringer Ingelheim)*.
tetrachlorvinphos, dichlorvos. Ravap® E.C. *(Boehringer Ingelheim)*.
tetrachlorvinphos, methoprene. Hartz® Control Pet Care System® Flea & Flea Egg Killer for Dogs *(Hartz Mountain)*, Hartz® Control Pet Care System® Ultimate Flea Collar® for Cats *(Hartz Mountain)*, Hartz® Control Pet Care System® Ultimate Flea Collar® for Dogs & Puppies *(Hartz Mountain)*.
tetrachlorvinphos, vitamins, amino acids, minerals, selenium. Vita-Plus® with Equitrol® *(Farnam)*.
tetrachlorvinphos, vitamins, minerals. Sweetlix® Rabon® Mineral/Vitamin Molasses Block *(Sweetlix)*.
tetracycline. 5-Way Calf Scour Bolus™ *(AgriLabs)*, AmTech Tetracycline Hydrochloride Soluble Powder-324 *(Phoenix Scientific)*, Calf Scour Bolus Antibiotic *(Durvet)*, Duramycin 10 *(Durvet)*, Duramycin-324 *(Durvet)*, Panmycin Aquadrops® *(Pharmacia & Upjohn)*, Polyotic® Soluble Powder *(Fort Dodge)*, Solu/Tet *(Vedco)*, Solu-Tet® 324 *(Alpharma)*, Tet 324™ *(Bimeda)*, Tet-324 *(Phoenix Pharmaceutical)*, Tetra Bac 324 *(AgriLabs)*, Tetracycline Hydrochloride Soluble Powder-324 *(Butler)*, *(Vedco)*, Tetracycline Soluble Powder 324 *(AgriPharm)*, Tetrasol Soluble Powder *(Med-Pharmex)*, Tet-Sol 10 *(Alpharma)*, Tet-Sol™ 324 *(Alpharma)*.
tetracycline, novobiocin. Albaplex® *(Pharmacia & Upjohn)*.
tetracycline, novobiocin, prednisolone. Delta Albaplex® / Delta Albaplex® 3X *(Pharmacia & Upjohn)*.
Tetracycline Hydrochloride Soluble Powder-324 *(Butler)*, *(Vedco)*, **tetracycline.**
Tetracycline Soluble Powder 324 *(AgriPharm)*, **tetracycline.**
tetrahydrofuran. Stronghold™ Teat Sealant *(WestAgro)*.
tetramethrin, pyriproxyfen, sumethrin. EctoKyl™ IGR Pressurized Spray *(DVM)*, Happy Jack® Flea Zinger Plus *(Happy Jack)*, Mycodex® Environmental Control™ Aerosol Household Spray *(V.P.L.)*, Pet Care IGR-House & Carpet Spray *(Durvet)*, Virbac KnockOut® Area Treatment *(Virbac)*.
Tetrasol Soluble Powder *(Med-Pharmex)*, **tetracycline.**
Tetravet-CA™ *(Alpharma)*, **oxytetracycline.**
Tetroxy®-100 *(Bimeda)*, **oxytetracycline.**
Tetroxy® HCA Soluble Powder *(Bimeda)*, **oxytetracycline.**
Tetroxy® LA *(Bimeda)*, **oxytetracycline.**
Tet-Sol 10 *(Alpharma)*, **tetracycline.**

Tet-Sol™ 324 *(Alpharma)*, **tetracycline.**

Therabloat® Drench Concentrate *(Pfizer Animal Health)*, **poloxalene.**

Theraderm® 2500 *(Westfalia•*Surge), **glycerine, iodine complex (povidone-iodine).**

Theratec™ *(Westfalia•*Surge), **glycerine, iodine complex (povidone-iodine).**

Theratec® Plus *(Westfalia•*Surge), **glycerine, iodine complex (povidone-iodine).**

Theratrate™ *(Westfalia•*Surge), **iodine.**

Therevac®-SB *(King Animal Health)*, **docusate sodium (dioctyl sodium sulfosuccinate), glycerine, medicinal soap base.**

thiabendazole, dexamethasone, neomycin. Tresaderm® *(Merial).*

Thia-Dex *(Neogen)*, **thiamine hydrochloride (B_1).**

Thiamine Hydrochloride *(Vet Tek)*, **thiamine hydrochloride (B_1).**

Thiamine Hydrochloride 200 mg *(Neogen)*, **thiamine hydrochloride (B_1).**

Thiamine Hydrochloride 500 mg *(Neogen)*, **thiamine hydrochloride (B_1).**

thiamine hydrochloride (B_1). AmTech Thiamine Hydrochloride Injection *(Phoenix Scientific)*, B-1 Powder *(SureNutrition)*, Thia-Dex *(Neogen)*, Thiamine Hydrochloride *(Vet Tek)*, Thiamine Hydrochloride 200 mg *(Neogen)*, Thiamine Hydrochloride 500 mg *(Neogen)*, Thiamine Hydrochloride Injection *(Butler)*, *(Phoenix Pharmaceutical)*, *(Vedco)*, Thiamine Hydrochloride Solution *(Phoenix Pharmaceutical)*, Vita•B-1 Crumbles *(Horse Health)*, Vita•B-1 Powder *(Horse Health)*, Vita-Jec® Thiamine HCl *(RXV)*, Vitamin B-1 Powder *(AHC).*

thiamine hydrochloride (B_1), calcium, potassium chloride, sodium chloride. Happy Jack® Milkade *(Happy Jack).*

thiamine hydrochloride (B_1), zinc, biotin, methionine (d-l). Hoof Supplement *(First Priority)*, Integrator™ *(Butler).*

Thiamine Hydrochloride Injection *(Butler)*, *(Phoenix Pharmaceutical)*, *(Vedco)*, **thiamine hydrochloride (B_1).**

Thiamine Hydrochloride Solution *(Phoenix Pharmaceutical)*, **thiamine hydrochloride (B_1).**

thiopental (sodium). Pentothal® Sterile Powder (Veterinary) *(Abbott).*

thiostrepton, triamcinolone acetonide, neomycin, nystatin. Animax® Ointment *(Pharmaderm)*, Dermagen™ Cream *(Butler)*, Dermagen™ Ointment *(Butler)*, Dermalog® Ointment *(RXV)*, Dermalone™ Ointment *(Vedco)*, Derma-Vet™ Cream *(Med-Pharmex)*, Derma-Vet™ Ointment *(Med-Pharmex)*, Panolog® Cream *(Fort Dodge)*, Panolog® Ointment *(Fort Dodge)*, Quadritop™ Cream *(Vetus)*, Quadritop™ Ointment *(Vetus).*

Thrush Treatment *(First Priority)*, **aloe vera, parachlorometaxylenol, propylene glycol.**

Thrush-XX™ *(Farnam)*, **copper naphthenate.**

thuja oil, zinc oxide. Thuja-Zinc Oxide *(Butler).*

thuja oil, zinc oxide, scarlet red. Thuja-Zinc Oxide *(Phoenix Pharmaceutical)*, *(Vedco).*

Thuja-Zinc Oxide *(Butler)*, **thuja oil, zinc oxide.**

Thuja-Zinc Oxide *(Phoenix Pharmaceutical)*, *(Vedco)*, **scarlet red, thuja oil, zinc oxide.**

thymol, alum, ferric subsulfate, tannic acid. Blood Stop Powder *(Dominion).*

thymol, alum, ferric sulfate, tannic acid. Blood Stop Powder *(AgriLabs).*

thymol, arnica, bentonite, boric acid, eucalyptus oil, glycerine, isopropyl alcohol (isopropanol), kaolin, methyl salicylate, peppermint oil, salicylic acid. Bigeloil® 24-Hour Medicated Poultice *(W. F. Young).*

thymol, benzocaine, camphor, iodide (potassium), iodine, menthol. Equi-Phar™ BenzaGel *(Vedco).*

thymol, benzocaine, camphor, isopropyl alcohol (isopropanol), menthol. Liniment Gel with Benzocaine *(First Priority).*

thymol, camphor, eucalyptus oil, menthol, phenol, pine oil, scarlet red. Scarlet Oil Pump Spray *(Dominion).*

thymol, camphor, iodide (potassium), iodine, isopropyl alcohol (isopropanol), menthol. Equi-Phar™ CoolGel *(Vedco).*

thymol, camphor, isopropyl alcohol (isopropanol), menthol. Liniment Gel *(First Priority).*

thymol, witch hazel, benzocaine, camphor, isopropyl alcohol (isopropanol), menthol. Benzo-Gel™ *(Butler).*

thymol, witch hazel, wormwood oil, aloe vera, iodide (potassium), isopropyl alcohol, menthol, parachlorometaxylenol. Veterinary Liniment *(First Priority).*

thyroid. Thyroid Powder™ *(Eudaemonic).*

Thyroid Powder™ *(Eudaemonic)*, **thyroid.**

Thyro-L® *(Vet-A-Mix)*, **levothyroxine.**

Thyrosyn Tablets *(Vedco)*, **levothyroxine.**

Thyro-Tabs® *(Vet-A-Mix)*, **levothyroxine.**

Thyroxine-L Powder *(Butler)*, **levothyroxine.**

Thyroxine-L Tablets *(Butler)*, **levothyroxine.**

Thyrozine *(RXV)*, **levothyroxine.**

Thyrozine Powder *(Phoenix Pharmaceutical)*, **levothyroxine.**

Thyrozine Tablets *(Phoenix Pharmaceutical)*, **levothyroxine.**

tiamulin. Denagard™ 10 *(Boehringer Ingelheim)*, Denagard™ Liquid Concentrate *(Boehringer Ingelheim).*

tiletamine HCl, zolazepam. Telazol® *(Fort Dodge).*

tilmicosin. Micotil® 300 Injection *(Elanco)*, Pulmotil® 90 *(Elanco).*

Tincture Iodine 7% *(Aspen)*, **iodine, isopropyl alcohol (isopropanol).**

Tincture Iodine 7% *(Bimeda)*, **iodide (potassium), iodine, isopropyl alcohol (isopropanol).**

Tissue-Bond™ *(Vedco)*, **cyanoacrylate (formulated).**

Tissumend™ *(V.P.L.)*, **cyanoacrylate (formulated).**

T-Lux® Shampoo *(Virbac)*, **coal tar, salicylic acid, sulfur.**

TM-50® *(Phibro)*, **oxytetracycline.**

TM-50®D *(Phibro)*, **oxytetracycline.**

TM-100® *(Phibro)*, **oxytetracycline.**

TM-100®D *(Phibro)*, **oxytetracycline.**

ToDAY® *(Fort Dodge)*, **cephapirin sodium.**

Tolazine™ Injection *(Lloyd)*, **tolazoline.**

tolazoline. Tolazine™ Injection *(Lloyd).*

ToMORROW® *(Fort Dodge)*, **cephapirin benzathine.**

Topical Fungicide *(Durvet)*, *(First Priority)*, *(Vedco)*, **benzalkonium chloride.**

Top Line™ *(AgriLabs)*, **ivermectin.**

Torbugesic® *(Fort Dodge)*, **butorphanol tartrate.**

Torbugesic®-SA *(Fort Dodge)*, **butorphanol tartrate.**

Torbutrol® Injection *(Fort Dodge)*, **butorphanol tartrate.**

Torbutrol® Tablets *(Fort Dodge)*, **butorphanol tartrate.**

Torpex™ *(Boehringer Ingelheim)*, **albuterol sulfate.**

torula yeast, amino acids, electrolytes, minerals. Procal™ Powder *(Butler).*

Totalon® Pour-On Dewormer *(Schering-Plough)*, **levamisole.**

ToxiBan™ Granules *(Vet-A-Mix)*, **activated charcoal, kaolin.**

ToxiBan™ Suspension *(Vet-A-Mix)*, **activated charcoal, kaolin.**

ToxiBan™ Suspension with Sorbitol *(Vet-A-Mix)*, **activated charcoal, kaolin, sorbitol.**

TranquiVed Injectable (Dogs and Cats) *(Vedco)*, **xylazine hydrochloride.**

TranquiVed Injectable (Horses) *(Vedco)*, **xylazine hydrochloride.**

trenbolone acetate. Component® T-H *(VetLife)*, Component® T-S *(VetLife)*, Finaplix®-H *(Intervet).*

trenbolone acetate, estradiol. Component® TE-G *(VetLife)*, Component® TE-S *(VetLife)*, Revalor®-200 *(Intervet)*, Revalor®-G *(Intervet)*, Revalor®-H *(Intervet)*, Revalor®-IH *(Intervet)*, Revalor®-IS *(Intervet)*, Revalor®-S *(Intervet).*

trenbolone acetate, estradiol benzoate. Synovex® Plus™ *(Fort Dodge).*

trenbolone acetate, tylosin tartrate. Component® T-H with Tylan® *(VetLife)*, Component® T-S with Tylan® *(VetLife).*

trenbolone acetate, tylosin tartrate, estradiol. Component® TE-G with Tylan® *(VetLife)*, Component® TE-S with Tylan® *(VetLife).*

Tresaderm® *(Merial)*, **dexamethasone, neomycin, thiabendazole.**

Trexonil™ *(Wildlife)*, **naltrexone hydrochloride.**

triamcinolone acetonide. Cortalone® Cream *(Vedco)*, Cortalone Tablets *(Vedco)*, Medalone Cream *(Med-Pharmex)*, Triamcinolone Acetonide Tablets *(Boehringer Ingelheim)*, Triamtabs *(Vetus)*, Vetalog® Parenteral *(Fort Dodge).*

triamcinolone acetonide, neomycin, nystatin, thiostrepton. Animax® Ointment *(Pharmaderm)*, Dermagen™ Cream *(Butler)*, Dermagen™ Ointment *(Butler)*, Dermalog® Ointment *(RXV)*, Dermalone™ Ointment *(Vedco)*, Derma-Vet™ Cream *(Med-Pharmex)*, Derma-Vet™ Ointment *(Med-Pharmex)*, Panolog® Cream *(Fort Dodge)*, Panolog® Ointment *(Fort Dodge)*, Quadritop™ Cream *(Vetus)*, Quadritop™ Ointment *(Vetus).*

Triamcinolone Acetonide Tablets *(Boehringer Ingelheim)*, **triamcinolone acetonide.**

Triamtabs *(Vetus)*, **triamcinolone acetonide.**

Tribrissen® 48% Injection *(Schering-Plough)*, **sulfadiazine, trimethoprim.**

Tribrissen® 400 Oral Paste *(Schering-Plough)*, **sulfadiazine, trimethoprim.**

Tribrissen® Tablets *(Schering-Plough)*, **sulfadiazine, trimethoprim.**

tricaine methanesulfonate. Finquel® *(Argent)*, Tricaine-S *(Western Chemical).*

Tricaine-S *(Western Chemical)*, **tricaine methanesulfonate.**

tri-calcium phosphate, calcium, magnesium chloride, potassium chloride. Oral CMPK Gel *(DVM Formula).*

tri-calcium phosphate, vitamins, calcium. Oral Calcium Gel *(DVM Formula).*

tri-calcium phosphate, vitamins, calcium, propylene glycol. Cal-C-Fresh™ *(Vets Plus).*

trichlormethiazide, dexamethasone. Naquasone® Bolus *(Schering-Plough).*

triclosan. DVM Handsoap™ *(DVM)*, Safe4Hours™ Medical Formula *(Safe4Hours)*, Triclosan Deodorizing Shampoo *(Davis)*, Triclosan Hand Soap *(Davis)*, Trisol™ *(KenVet).*

triclosan, chlorhexidine digluconate. Hexadene® Flush *(Virbac).*

triclosan, coal tar, sulfur. Sulfodene® Medicated Shampoo & Conditioner for Dogs *(Combe).*

triclosan, salicylic acid, sulfur. SebaLyt® Shampoo *(DVM)*, SeboRex™ Shampoo *(DVM).*

Triclosan Deodorizing Shampoo *(Davis)*, **triclosan.**

Triclosan Hand Soap *(Davis)*, **triclosan.**

tricosene, imidacloprid. QuickBayt™ Fly Bait *(Bayer).*

tricosene, methomyl. Fly-Zap™ Fly Bait *(Aspen).*

Trienamine™ *(Phoenix Pharmaceutical)*, **tripelennamine hydrochloride.**

triethanolamine, vitamin E, aloe vera, glycerine. SoftGuard™ *(Activon).*

Trifectant™ *(Evsco)*, **potassium peroxymenosulfate.**
Tri-Hist® Granules *(Neogen)*, **pseudoephedrine HCl, pyrilamine maleate.**
trimeprazine tartrate, prednisolone. Temaril-P® Tablets *(Pfizer Animal Health)*.
trimethoprim, sulfadiazine. Tribrissen® 48% Injection *(Schering-Plough)*, Tribrissen® 400 Oral Paste *(Schering-Plough)*, Tribrissen® Tablets *(Schering-Plough)*, Tucoprim® Powder *(Pharmacia & Upjohn)*, Uniprim® Powder *(Macleod)*.
TriOptic-P™ *(Pfizer Animal Health)*, **bacitracin, neomycin, polymyxin B.**
TriOptic-S® *(Pfizer Animal Health)*, **bacitracin, hydrocortisone acetate, neomycin, polymyxin B.**
Tri-Otic® *(Med-Pharmex)*, **betamethasone, clotrimazole, gentamicin.**
tripelennamine hydrochloride. AmTech Tripelennamine Hydrochloride Injection *(Phoenix Scientific)*, Rally™-20 *(Vedco)*, Re-Covr® Injection *(Fort Dodge)*, Trienamine™ *(Phoenix Pharmaceutical)*, Tripelennamine Hydrochloride *(AgriLabs)*, *(Aspen)*, *(Butler)*, *(Vet Tek)*, Triple Histamine *(RXV)*.
Tripelennamine Hydrochloride *(AgriLabs)*, *(Aspen)*, *(Butler)*, *(Vet Tek)*, **tripelennamine hydrochloride.**
Triple Cast™ *(Neogen)*, **acacia, calamine, castor oil, glycerine, petrolatum, zinc oxide.**
Triple Histamine *(RXV)*, **tripelennamine hydrochloride.**
Triple-No-Chew *(Q.A. Laboratories)*, **isopropyl alcohol, orange peel bitter, tabasco pepper.**
Triple-No-Chew Spray *(Q.A. Laboratories)*, **isopropyl alcohol, orange peel bitter, tabasco pepper.**
Triple Pyrethrins Flea & Tick Shampoo *(Davis)*, **di-n-propyl isocinchomeronate, n-octyl bicycloheptene dicarboximide, piperonyl butoxide, pyrethrins.**
trisodium phosphate, calcium, magnesium chloride, phosphoric acid, potassium chloride. CMPK Gel *(AgriPharm)*.
Trisol™ *(KenVet)*, **triclosan.**
Tri-Tec 14™ Fly Repellent *(Farnam)*, **butoxypolypropylene glycol, cypermethrin, piperonyl butoxide, pyrethrins.**
Tritop® *(Pharmacia & Upjohn)*, **isoflupredone acetate, neomycin, tetracaine.**
Tri-Tussin™ Powder *(Creative Science)*, **ammonium chloride, guaifenesin (glyceryl guaiacolate, guaiacol), potassium iodide.**
trizinetrione. DuraCept™ *(Activon)*, EfferSan™ *(Activon)*.
tromethamine, EDTA (edetate disodium dihydrate). DermaPet® TrizEDTA™ Aqueous Flush *(DermaPet)*, DermaPet® TrizEDTA™ Crystals *(DermaPet)*.
tromethamine, EDTA (tetrasodium), lanolin. T8 Solution™ Ear Rinse *(DVM)*.
Tryad® *(Loveland)*, **quaternary ammonia.**
trypsin, balsam peru oil, castor oil. Granulex® V Aerosol Spray *(Pfizer Animal Health)*, Granulex® V Liquid *(Pfizer Animal Health)*, Trypzyme®-V Aerosol Spray *(V.P.L.)*, Trypzyme®-V Liquid *(V.P.L.)*.
Tryptophan Plus Gel™ *(Horses Prefer)*, **amino acids, dextrose, minerals, vitamins.**
Trypzyme®-V Aerosol Spray *(V.P.L.)*, **balsam peru oil, castor oil, trypsin.**
Trypzyme®-V Liquid *(V.P.L.)*, **balsam peru oil, castor oil, trypsin.**
Tucoprim® Powder *(Pharmacia & Upjohn)*, **sulfadiazine, trimethoprim.**
Tumil-K® *(King Animal Health)*, **potassium gluconate.**
Tumil-K® Gel *(King Animal Health)*, **potassium gluconate.**
TunaVite™ *(Vedco)*, **minerals, taurine, vitamins.**
turpentine, ammonium chloride, camphor. White Liniment *(Butler)*, *(Durvet)*.
turpentine, camphor, ether, iodine, isopropyl alcohol (isopropanol). Harold White's® Leg Paint *(Hawthorne)*.
turpentine, gentian violet, isopropyl alcohol (isopropanol), tannic acid. Happy Jack® Pad Kote *(Happy Jack)*.
turpentine, lanolin, neatsfoot oil, petrolatum, pine tar. Absorbine® Hooflex® Liquid Conditioner *(W. F. Young)*.
turpentine, lanolin, neatsfoot oil, pine tar. Absorbine® Hooflex® Original Conditioner *(W. F. Young)*.
turpentine, mineral oil. Vita Oil *(Hawthorne)*.
turpentine, wheat germ oil, fish oil, iodine, linseed oil, neatsfoot oil, pine tar. Shur Hoof™ *(Horse Health)*.
turpentine, wheat germ oil, fish oil, iodine, linseed oil, pine tar. Dealer Select Horse Care Hoof Dressing With Brush *(Durvet)*.
Twin-Pen™ *(AgriLabs)*, **penicillin G benzathine, penicillin G procaine.**
Tylan® 40 *(Elanco)*, **tylosin phosphate.**
Tylan® 40 Sulfa-G™ *(Elanco)*, **sulfamethazine, tylosin phosphate.**
Tylan® 50 Injection *(Elanco)*, **tylosin.**
Tylan® 100 *(Elanco)*, **tylosin phosphate.**
Tylan® 100 Cal *(Elanco)*, **tylosin phosphate.**
Tylan® 200 Injection *(Elanco)*, **tylosin.**
Tylan® Soluble *(Elanco)*, **tylosin tartrate.**
tylosin. Tylan® 50 Injection *(Elanco)*, Tylan® 200 Injection *(Elanco)*, Tylosin Injection *(AgriLabs)*, *(Aspen)*, *(Boehringer Ingelheim)*, TyloVed Injection *(Vedco)*.
Tylosin Injection *(AgriLabs)*, *(Aspen)*, *(Boehringer Ingelheim)*, **tylosin.**
tylosin phosphate. Tylan® 40 *(Elanco)*, Tylan® 100 *(Elanco)*, Tylan® 100 Cal *(Elanco)*.
tylosin phosphate, sulfamethazine. MoorMan's® TYS 5/5 *(ADM)*, Tylan® 40 Sulfa-G™ *(Elanco)*.
tylosin tartrate. Tylan® Soluble *(Elanco)*.
tylosin tartrate, estradiol, trenbolone acetate. Component® TE-G with Tylan® *(VetLife)*, Component® TE-S with Tylan® *(VetLife)*.
tylosin tartrate, estradiol benzoate, progesterone. Component® E-C with Tylan® *(VetLife)*, Component® E-S with Tylan® *(VetLife)*.
tylosin tartrate, estradiol benzoate, testosterone propionate. Component® E-H with Tylan® *(VetLife)*.
tylosin tartrate, trenbolone acetate. Component® T-H with Tylan® *(VetLife)*, Component® T-S with Tylan® *(VetLife)*.
TyloVed Injection *(Vedco)*, **tylosin.**

U

UAA (Universal Animal Antidote) Gel *(Vedco)*, **activated charcoal, attapulgite.**
Udder Balm *(Aspen)*, *(First Priority)*, **aloe vera, emollient(s), vitamins.**
Udder Balm *(Vedco)*, **emollient(s), vitamins.**
Udder Cleanitizer® *(Westfalia•Surge)*, **quaternary ammonia.**
Udder Comfort Cream *(Phoenix Pharmaceutical)*, **emollient(s), vitamins.**
Uddergold® Germicidal Barrier Teat Dip (Activator) *(Alcide)*, **lactic acid.**
Uddergold® Germicidal Barrier Teat Dip (Base) *(Alcide)*, **sodium chlorite (gel).**
Uddergold® Plus Germicidal Barrier Teat Dip (Activator) *(Alcide)*, **mandelic acid.**
Uddergold® Plus Germicidal Barrier Teat Dip (Base) *(Alcide)*, **sodium chlorite.**
Udder Moist *(A.A.H.)*, **emollient(s), moisturizer(s), vitamins.**
Udder Ointment™ *(LeGear)*, **benzethonium chloride, cetyl alcohol, lanolin, petrolatum, vitamin A, vitamin D.**
Ultra Boss® Pour-On Insecticide *(Schering-Plough)*, **permethrin, piperonyl butoxide.**
Ultra-Dyne™ *(Westfalia•Surge)*, **iodine.**
Ultra™ Ear Miticide *(Bimeda)*, **rotenone.**
UltraGroom™ Shampoo *(Virbac)*, **shampoo formula.**
UltraMectrin™ Injection *(RXV)*, **ivermectin.**
UltraMectrin™ Pour-On *(RXV)*, **ivermectin.**
UltraSpot™ by Absorbine® *(W. F. Young)*, **permethrin.**
Unipet Nutritabs® *(Pharmacia & Upjohn)*, **minerals, vitamins.**
Uniprim® Powder *(Macleod)*, **sulfadiazine, trimethoprim.**
Universal Medicated Shampoo *(Vet Solutions)*, **chloroxylenol, salicylic acid, sodium thiosulfate.**
urea. After-Birth Bolus *(AgriPharm)*, AmTech Uterine Bolus *(Phoenix Scientific)*, Intrauterine Bolus *(AgriLabs)*, Proteoseptic Bolus *(Vedco)*, Urea Wound Powder *(First Priority)*, Uterine Bolus *(Butler)*, *(Durvet)*, *(First Priority)*, *(Phoenix Pharmaceutical)*.
urea, acriflavine, furfural, gentian violet, glycerine, isopropyl alcohol (isopropanol), propylene glycol, sodium propionate. Blue Lotion *(AgriLabs)*.
urea, acriflavine, gentian violet, glycerine, isopropyl alcohol (isopropanol), propylene glycol. Purple Lotion *(Vedco)*, Purple Lotion Wound Dressing *(First Priority)*.
urea, acriflavine, glycerine, isopropyl alcohol (isopropanol), methyl violet, propylene glycol. Purple Lotion Wound Dressing *(Durvet)*.
urea, acriflavine, glycerine, methyl violet, propylene glycol. Wound-Kote Gentian Violet *(Farnam)*.
urea, acriflavine, glycerine, methyl violet, propylene glycol, sodium propionate. Blue Lotion *(Farnam)*.
urea, benzalkonium chloride, glycerine, lactic acid, propylene glycol. Humilac® Spray *(Virbac)*.
urea, chitosanide, glycerine, lactic acid. Allergroom® Shampoo *(Virbac)*.
urea, salicylic acid, sodium lactate. KeraSolv® Gel *(DVM)*.
urea, wheat germ oil, cod liver oil, iodine complex (povidone-iodine), lanolin, petrolatum, soybean oil. Vita-Hoof® *(Equicare)*.
urea peroxide, docusate sodium (dioctyl sodium sulfosuccinate). ClearR_x® Ear Cleansing Solution *(DVM)*.
Urea Wound Powder *(First Priority)*, **urea.**
Uroeze® *(King Animal Health)*, **ammonium chloride.**
Uroeze® 200 *(King Animal Health)*, **ammonium chloride.**
Uterine Bolus *(Butler)*, *(Durvet)*, *(First Priority)*, *(Phoenix Pharmaceutical)*, **urea.**

V

Vaccine Stabilizer *(Alpharma)*, **caseinate, skim milk, whey.**
Valbazen® Cattle Dewormer Paste *(Pfizer Animal Health)*, **albendazole.**
Valbazen® Suspension *(Pfizer Animal Health)*, **albendazole.**
V.A.L.® Syrup *(Fort Dodge)*, **vitamin B-complex.**
Vapona® Concentrate Insecticide *(Boehringer Ingelheim)*, **dichlorvos.**
Vedadine Bolus *(Vedco)*, **polyvinylpyrrolidone.**
Veda-K_1 Capsules *(Vedco)*, **vitamin K_1 (phytonadione).**
Veda-K_1 Injection *(Vedco)*, **vitamin K_1 (phytonadione).**
VedaLax™ and VedaLax™ Tuna *(Vedco)*, **petrolatum.**
Vedalyte 8X Powder *(Vedco)*, **dextrose, electrolytes.**
Veda-Sorb Bolus *(Vedco)*, **attapulgite, carob, magnesium trisilicate, pectin.**

Veda-Sorb Jr Bolus *(Vedco)*, **aluminum silicate, attapulgite, carob, magnesium trisilicate, pectin.**

vegetable oil(s), emulsifiers. Bloat Drench™ *(Great States)*, Rumen-Eze *(Vet-A-Mix)*.

vegetable oil(s), glycerine, mineral oil. Hairball Solution *(Pet-Ag)*.

vegetable oil(s), vitamins, amodimethicone, methionine (d-l), minerals. Equ-Aid Plus *(Vet-A-Mix)*.

Velenium™ *(Fort Dodge)*, **selenium (sodium selenite), vitamin E.**

Ventipulmin® Syrup *(Boehringer Ingelheim)*, **clenbuterol hydrochloride.**

Vetadine *(Centaur)*, **iodine complex (povidone-iodine).**

Vetadine Scrub *(Vedco)*, **iodine complex (povidone-iodine).**

Vetadine Solution *(Vedco)*, **iodine complex (povidone-iodine).**

Veta-K_1® Capsules *(Bimeda)*, **vitamin K_1 (phytonadione).**

Veta-K_1® Injection *(Bimeda)*, **vitamin K_1 (phytonadione).**

VetaKet® Injection *(Lloyd)*, **ketamine hydrochloride.**

Veta-Lac® Canine *(Vet-A-Mix)*, **milk replacing formula.**

Veta-Lac® Feline *(Vet-A-Mix)*, **milk replacing formula.**

Vetalar® *(Fort Dodge)*, **ketamine hydrochloride.**

Vetalog® Parenteral *(Fort Dodge)*, **triamcinolone acetonide.**

Vetalyte Plus I.V. Solution *(RXV)*, **dextrose, electrolytes.**

Vetasyl™ Fiber Tablets for Cats *(Virbac)*, **psyllium.**

Vet BioSISt™ *(Cook)*, **porcine GI submucosa.**

Veterinary Liniment *(First Priority)*, **aloe vera, iodide (potassium), isopropyl alcohol, menthol, parachlorometaxylenol, thymol, witch hazel, wormwood oil.**

Veterinary Surfactant *(Vedco)*, **docusate sodium (dioctyl sodium sulfosuccinate), propylene glycol.**

Veterinary Surfactant (D.S.S.) *(First Priority)*, **docusate sodium (dioctyl sodium sulfosuccinate), propylene glycol.**

Vetisulid® Boluses *(Fort Dodge)*, **sulfachlorpyridazine.**

Vetisulid® Injection *(Fort Dodge)*, **sulfachlorpyridazine.**

Vetisulid® Powder *(Fort Dodge)*, **sulfachlorpyridazine.**

Vet-Kem® Breakaway® Flea & Tick Collar for Cats *(Wellmark)*, **propoxur.**

Vet-Kem® Breakaway® Plus Flea & Tick Collar for Cats *(Wellmark)*, **methoprene, propoxur.**

Vet-Kem® Ovitrol® Plus Flea & Tick Shampoo for Dogs & Cats *(Wellmark)*, **methoprene, piperonyl butoxide, pyrethrins.**

Vet-Kem® Ovitrol® Plus Flea, Tick & Bot Spray *(Wellmark)*, **methoprene, n-octyl bicycloheptene dicarboximide, piperonyl butoxide, pyrethrins.**

Vet-Kem® Ovitrol Plus® Spot On® Flea & Tick Control for Dogs & Puppies (under 30 lbs.) *(Wellmark)*, **methoprene, permethrin.**

Vet-Kem® Ovitrol Plus® Spot On® Flea & Tick Control for Dogs & Puppies (over 30 lbs.) *(Wellmark)*, **methoprene, permethrin.**

Vet-Kem® Ovitrol® Spot On® Flea Control for Cats *(Wellmark)*, **methoprene.**

Vet-Kem® Paramite® Sponge-On for Dogs *(Wellmark)*, **phosmet.**

Vet-Kem® Siphotrol® Plus II Premise Spray *(Wellmark)*, **methoprene, n-octyl bicycloheptene dicarboximide, permethrin, phenothrin, piperonyl butoxide.**

Vet-Kem® Siphotrol® Plus Area Treatment for Homes *(Wellmark)*, **methoprene, permethrin.**

Vet-Kem® Siphotrol® Plus Area Treatment Pump Spray for Homes *(Wellmark)*, **methoprene, permethrin.**

Vet-Kem® Siphotrol Plus® Fogger *(Wellmark)*, **methoprene, permethrin.**

Vet-Kem® Tickaway™ Tick Collar for Dogs *(Wellmark)*, **propoxur.**

Vet-Kem® Triple Action Flea & Tick Shampoo for Dogs, Cats, & Horses *(Wellmark)*, **di-n-propyl isocinchomeronate, n-octyl bicycloheptene dicarboximide, piperonyl butoxide, pyrethrins.**

Vet Lube *(Phoenix Pharmaceutical)*, **carboxy methylcellulose, propylene glycol.**

Vetrachloracin® Ophthalmic Ointment *(Pharmaderm)*, **chloramphenicol.**

Vetrin™ Canine Pain Relief Tablets *(Farnam)*, **acetylsalicylic acid.**

Vetro-Biotic® Ointment *(Pharmaderm)*, **bacitracin, neomycin, polymyxin B.**

Vetro-Cort® Lotion *(Pharmaderm)*, **hydrocortisone.**

Vetrolin® Bath *(Equicare)*, **conditioners, shampoo formula, sunscreen formula.**

Vetrolin® Liniment *(Equicare)*, **camphor, methyl salicylate.**

Vetrolin® Shine *(Equicare)*, **conditioners, sunscreen formula, vitamins.**

Vetropolycin® HC Ophthalmic Ointment *(Pharmaderm)*, **bacitracin, hydrocortisone acetate, neomycin, polymyxin B.**

Vetropolycin® Ophthalmic Ointment *(Pharmaderm)*, **bacitracin, neomycin, polymyxin B.**

VetRx™ Caged Bird Remedy *(Goodwinol)*, **alcohol, camphor, Canada balsam, corn oil base, oil origanum, oil rosemary.**

VetRx™ Equine Formula *(Goodwinol)*, **camphor, Canada balsam, corn oil base, milk supplement, oil origanum, oil rosemary.**

VetRx™ for Cats and Kittens *(Goodwinol)*, **alcohol, camphor, Canada balsam, corn oil base, oil origanum, oil rosemary.**

VetRx™ for Dogs and Puppies *(Goodwinol)*, **alcohol, camphor, Canada balsam, corn oil base, oil origanum, oil rosemary.**

VetRx™ Goat & Sheep Remedy *(Goodwinol)*, **alcohol, camphor, Canada balsam, corn oil base, oil origanum, oil rosemary.**

VetRx™ Pigeon Remedy *(Goodwinol)*, **alcohol, camphor, Canada balsam, corn oil base, oil origanum, oil rosemary.**

VetRx™ Poultry Remedy *(Goodwinol)*, **alcohol, camphor, Canada balsam, corn oil base, oil origanum, oil rosemary.**

VetRx™ Rabbit Remedy *(Goodwinol)*, **alcohol, camphor, Canada balsam, corn oil base, oil origanum, oil rosemary.**

VetRx™ Small Fur Animal Remedy *(Goodwinol)*, **alcohol, camphor, Canada balsam.**

Viceton® *(Bimeda)*, **chloramphenicol.**

Victor Gall Remedy *(Fiebing)*, **isopropyl alcohol (isopropanol), methylene blue.**

Vigilquat *(Alex C. Fergusson)*, **quaternary ammonia.**

Viodine™ Medicated Shampoo *(Equicare)*, **iodine complex (povidone-iodine).**

Viokase®-V Powder *(Fort Dodge)*, **amylase, lipase, protease.**

Viokase®-V Tablets *(Fort Dodge)*, **amylase, lipase, protease.**

Vionate® Vitamin Mineral Powder *(ARC)*, **minerals.**

V.I.P.-20™ Iodine Shampoo *(Equicare)*, **iodine complex (povidone-iodine).**

VIP® Flea Control Shampoo *(V.P.L.)*, **limonene.**

VIP® Flea Dip *(V.P.L.)*, **limonene.**

VIP® Fly Repellent Ointment *(V.P.L.)*, **butoxypolypropylene glycol, piperonyl butoxide, pyrethrins.**

Virbac KnockOut® Area Treatment *(Virbac)*, **pyriproxyfen, sumethrin, tetramethrin.**

Virbac KnockOut® ES Area Treatment *(Virbac)*, **n-octyl bicycloheptene dicarboximide, permethrin, pyrethrins, pyriproxyfen.**

Virbac KnockOut® IGR Flea Collar for Cats & Kittens *(Virbac)*, **pyriproxyfen.**

Virbac KnockOut® IGR Flea Collar for Dogs & Puppies *(Virbac)*, **pyriproxyfen.**

Virbac KnockOut® IGR Household Pump Spray *(Virbac)*, **permethrin, piperonyl butoxide, pyriproxyfen.**

Virbac KnockOut® Room and Area Fogger *(Virbac)*, **n-octyl bicycloheptene dicarboximide, permethrin, pyrethrins, pyriproxyfen.**

Virbac® Long Acting KnockOut™ *(Virbac)*, **permethrin, pyriproxyfen.**

Virbac Pyrethrin Dip™ *(Virbac)*, **di-n-propyl isocinchomeronate, n-octyl bicycloheptene dicarboximide, piperonyl butoxide, pyrethrins.**

Virbac® Yard Spray Concentrate *(Virbac)*, **cyano benzeneacetate.**

virginiamycin. Stafac® 10 *(Phibro)*, Stafac® 20 *(Phibro)*, Stafac® 500 *(Phibro)*, V-Max™ M *(Phibro)*.

Virkon®-S *(Farnam, Livestock Div.)*, **potassium peroxymenosulfate.**

Virocid® *(Merial Select)*, **glutaraldehyde, quaternary ammonia.**

Vi-Sorbin® *(Pfizer Animal Health)*, **iron, minerals, sorbitol, vitamins.**

Vi-Sorbits® *(Pfizer Animal Health)*, **iron, vitamins.**

Vita-15™ Injection *(Neogen)*, **minerals, vitamins.**

Vita•B-1 Crumbles *(Horse Health)*, **thiamine hydrochloride (B_1).**

Vita•B-1 Powder *(Horse Health)*, **thiamine hydrochloride (B_1).**

Vita•Biotin™ Crumbles *(Horse Health)*, **biotin.**

Vita Boost Paste™ *(AgriLabs)*, **amino acids, enzymes, microorganisms, vitamins, yeast.**

Vita Charge® 28 Dispersible Powder *(BioZyme)*, **Aspergillus oryzae fermentation extract, minerals, vitamins.**

Vita Charge® Calf Bolus *(BioZyme)*, **Aspergillus oryzae fermentation extract, minerals, vitamins.**

Vita Charge® Equine *(BioZyme)*, **Aspergillus oryzae fermentation extract, minerals, vitamins.**

Vita Charge® Gel Cap *(BioZyme)*, **Aspergillus oryzae fermentation extract, minerals, vitamins.**

Vita Charge® Paste *(BioZyme)*, **Aspergillus oryzae fermentation extract, minerals, vitamins.**

Vita Charge® Power Drench *(BioZyme)*, **Aspergillus oryzae fermentation extract, electrolytes, energy source(s), nutrients, yeast.**

Vita•E & Selenium Powder *(Horse Health)*, **selenium, vitamin E.**

Vita E 300 *(AgriPharm)*, **vitamin E.**

Vita E-AD *(AgriPharm)*, **vitamin A, vitamin D_3, vitamin E.**

Vita•E & Selenium Crumbles™ *(Horse Health)*, **selenium, vitamin E.**

Vita Ferm® Breeder Booster+Mag *(BioZyme)*, **Aspergillus oryzae fermentation extract, minerals, vitamins.**

Vita Ferm® Cattleman's Beefmaker *(BioZyme)*, **Aspergillus oryzae fermentation extract, minerals, vitamins.**

Vita Ferm® Cattleman's Beefmaker+Mag *(BioZyme)*, **Aspergillus oryzae fermentation extract, minerals, vitamins.**

Vita Ferm® Concept-Aid *(BioZyme)*, **Aspergillus oryzae fermentation extract, minerals, vitamins.**

Vita Ferm® Concept-Aid+Mag *(BioZyme)*, **Aspergillus oryzae fermentation extract, minerals, vitamins.**

Vita Ferm® Concept-Aid A•P *(BioZyme)*, **Aspergillus oryzae fermentation extract, minerals, vitamins.**

Vita Ferm® Cow Calf 5 *(BioZyme)*, **Aspergillus oryzae fermentation extract, minerals, vitamins.**

Vita Ferm® Dairy Basemix 12:16 *(BioZyme)*, **Aspergillus oryzae fermentation extract, minerals, vitamins.**

Vita Ferm® Dairy Basemix 18:6 *(BioZyme)*, **Aspergillus oryzae fermentation extract, minerals, vitamins.**
Vita Ferm® Dairy Basemix 18:12 *(BioZyme)*, **Aspergillus oryzae fermentation extract, minerals, vitamins.**
Vita Ferm® Equine *(BioZyme)*, **Aspergillus oryzae fermentation extract, minerals, vitamins.**
Vita Ferm® Ewe and Lamb *(BioZyme)*, **Aspergillus oryzae fermentation extract, minerals, vitamins.**
Vita Ferm® Far Out Dry Cow *(BioZyme)*, **Aspergillus oryzae fermentation extract, minerals, vitamins.**
Vita Ferm® Feedlot Formula *(BioZyme)*, **Aspergillus oryzae fermentation extract, minerals, vitamins.**
Vita Ferm® Fescue Fiber Buster *(BioZyme)*, **Aspergillus oryzae fermentation extract, minerals, vitamins.**
Vita Ferm® Fescue Power Keg *(BioZyme)*, **Aspergillus oryzae fermentation extract, minerals, vitamins.**
Vita Ferm® Formula *(BioZyme)*, **Aspergillus oryzae fermentation extract, minerals, vitamins.**
Vita Ferm® Grass Enhancer *(BioZyme)*, **Aspergillus oryzae fermentation extract, minerals, vitamins.**
Vita Ferm® High Mag *(BioZyme)*, **Aspergillus oryzae fermentation extract, minerals, vitamins.**
Vita Ferm® Milk-N-More Medicated Milk Replacer with Decoquinate *(BioZyme)*, **decoquinate.**
Vita Ferm® Milk-N-More Medicated Milk Replacer with Neo/OTC *(BioZyme)*, **neomycin, oxytetracycline.**
Vita Ferm® Milk-N-More Non-Medicated Milk Replacer *(BioZyme)*, **milk replacing formula.**
Vita Ferm® Natural Protein Pasture Formula (NPPF) *(BioZyme)*, **Aspergillus oryzae fermentation extract, minerals, vitamins.**
Vita Ferm® Pasture Formula *(BioZyme)*, **Aspergillus oryzae fermentation extract, minerals, vitamins.**
Vita Ferm® Power Keg *(BioZyme)*, **Aspergillus oryzae fermentation extract, minerals, vitamins.**
Vita Ferm® Pro-Gest *(BioZyme)*, **Aspergillus oryzae fermentation extract.**
Vita Ferm® Pro-Gest 30 *(BioZyme)*, **Aspergillus oryzae fermentation extract.**
Vita Ferm® Roughage Fortifier *(BioZyme)*, **Aspergillus oryzae fermentation extract, minerals, vitamins.**
Vita Ferm® Sheep & Goat Keg *(BioZyme)*, **Aspergillus oryzae fermentation extract, minerals, vitamins.**
Vita Ferm® Sure Champ and Vita Start Pellets *(BioZyme)*, **Aspergillus oryzae fermentation extract, minerals, vitamins.**
Vita Ferm® Sure Start 2 *(BioZyme)*, **Aspergillus oryzae fermentation extract, minerals, vitamins.**
Vita Ferm® Sure Start Pac *(BioZyme)*, **Aspergillus oryzae fermentation extract, minerals, vitamins.**
Vita Ferm® Up Close Dry Cow *(BioZyme)*, **Aspergillus oryzae fermentation extract, minerals, vitamins.**
Vita Ferm® Vita Grow 32 Natural *(BioZyme)*, **Aspergillus oryzae fermentation extract, minerals, vitamins.**
Vita-Hoof® *(Equicare)*, **cod liver oil, iodine complex (povidone-iodine), lanolin, petrolatum, soybean oil, urea, wheat germ oil.**
Vita-Jec® A & D "500" *(AgriPharm)*, **vitamin A, vitamin D.**
Vita-Jec® B-Complex *(AgriPharm)*, **vitamin B-complex.**
Vita-Jec® B Complex Fortified *(AgriPharm)*, **vitamin B-complex.**
Vita-Jec® B-Complex with Cyano Plus *(AgriPharm)*, **vitamin B-complex, vitamin B_{12} (cyanocobalamin).**
Vita-Jec® Thiamine HCl *(RXV)*, **thiamine hydrochloride (B_1).**
Vita-Jec® Vitamin B_{12} (Cyano 1,000 mcg/mL) *(RXV)*, **vitamin B_{12} (cyanocobalamin).**
Vita-Jec® Vitamin B_{12} (Cyano 3,000 mcg/mL) *(RXV)*, **vitamin B_{12} (cyanocobalamin).**
Vita-Jec® Vitamin K1 Injectable *(RXV)*, **vitamin K_1 (phytonadione).**
Vita-Key® Antioxidant Concentrate *(Vita-Key)*, **amino acids, minerals, vitamins, yeast.**
Vita-Key® Biotin ZM-80 *(Vita-Key)*, **biotin, methionine (d-l), microorganisms, zinc-methionine.**
Vita-Key® Brood Mare Supplement *(Vita-Key)*, **minerals, vitamins.**
Vita-Key® Equine Supplement *(Vita-Key)*, **amino acids, minerals, vitamins, yeast.**
Vita-Key® Mare & Foal Supplement *(Vita-Key)*, **amino acids, minerals, vitamins, yeast.**
Vita-Key® Show Cattle Concentrate, Phase II *(Vita-Key)*, **amino acids, enzymes, microorganisms, minerals, vitamins, yeast.**
Vita-Key® Show Cattle Supplement, Phase I *(Vita-Key)*, **microorganisms, minerals, vitamins.**
Vita-Key® Swine Supplement *(Vita-Key)*, **amino acids, microorganisms, minerals, vitamins, yeast.**
Vi-tal *(Loveland)*, **electrolytes, minerals, vitamins.**
Vital E®-300 *(Schering-Plough)*, **vitamin E.**
Vital E®+A *(Schering-Plough)*, **vitamin A, vitamin E.**
Vital E®-A+D *(Schering-Plough)*, **vitamin A, vitamin D, vitamin E.**
Vita-Lyte *(Phoenix Pharmaceutical)*, **electrolytes, energy source(s), nutrients.**
vitamin A, calcium, iodine, iron, phosphorus, sodium chloride. Mo' Milk® Feed Mix and Top Dress *(TechMix)*.
vitamin A, vitamin B_{12} (cyanocobalamin), vitamin D. Clovite® Conditioner *(Fort Dodge)*, Vitamin A D B_{12} Injection *(Vedco)*.
vitamin A, vitamin B_6, vitamin E, arachidonic acid, linoleic acid, linolenic acid. Mirra-Coat® for Cats *(Pet-Ag)*.
vitamin A, vitamin B_6, vitamin E, biotin, linoleic acid, linolenic acid. Mirra-Coat® Powder and Liquid *(Pet-Ag)*.
vitamin A, vitamin B_6, vitamin E, zinc, linoleic acid. Mirra-Coat® (Equine System) *(Pet-Ag)*.
vitamin A, vitamin C (ascorbic acid), allantoin, benzocaine, pine tar, propylene glycol. A-Plus™ Wound Dressing *(Creative Science)*.
vitamin A, vitamin C (ascorbic acid), vitamin D_3, calcium. NutriVed™ Calcium Plus Chewable Tablets *(Vedco)*.
vitamin A, vitamin D. A-D Injection *(Durvet)*, Happy Jack® Cod Liver Oil *(Happy Jack)*, Vita-Jec® A & D "500" *(AgriPharm)*, Vitamin AD_3 *(AgriLabs)*, Vitamin AD *(Butler)*, Vitamin A & D *(Vedco)*, Vitamin A & D "500" *(AgriPharm)*, Vitamin AD Injection *(Aspen)*, *(Phoenix Pharmaceutical)*, Vitamin AD_3 Injection *(Bimeda)*.
vitamin A, vitamin D, benzethonium chloride, cetyl alcohol, lanolin, petrolatum. Udder Ointment™ *(LeGear)*.
vitamin A, vitamin D, calcium. Calcium Gel + Vitamins *(AgriLabs)*.
vitamin A, vitamin D, vitamin E. EmulsiVit E/A&D *(Vedco)*, Vital E®-A+D *(Schering-Plough)*, Vitamin E+AD *(Durvet)*.
vitamin A, vitamin D, vitamin E, aloe vera. Aloe Heal™ *(Farnam)*.
vitamin A, vitamin D, vitamin E, aloe vera, moisturizer(s). DuraCream *(Durvet)*.
vitamin A, vitamin D, vitamin E, amylase, lipase, protease. PanaKare™ Plus Powder *(Neogen)*, PanaKare™ Plus Tablets *(Neogen)*.
vitamin A, vitamin D, vitamin E, dried colostrum, microorganisms. Colostrum Powder *(Vedco)*.
vitamin A, vitamin D, vitamin E, fat product(s), linoleic acid. Fastbreak™ Plus™ *(Boehringer Ingelheim)*.
vitamin A, vitamin D, vitamin E, fatty acids (omega). 3V Caps™ for Large & Giant Breeds *(DVM)*, 3V Caps™ for Medium & Large Breeds *(DVM)*, 3V Caps™ for Small & Medium Breeds *(DVM)*, 3V Caps™ Liquid *(DVM)*, Omega-3 Fatty Acid Capsules for Large & Giant Breeds *(Vet Solutions)*, Omega-3 Fatty Acid Capsules for Medium Breeds *(Vet Solutions)*, Omega-3 Fatty Acid Capsules for Small Breeds *(Vet Solutions)*, Omega-3 Fatty Acid Liquid *(Vet Solutions)*.
vitamin A, vitamin D, vitamin E, polyunsaturated fatty acids. Derma-Form Liquid *(Vet-A-Mix)*.
vitamin A, vitamin D, vitamin E, zinc, fatty acids (essential). Pet-F.A. Liquid® *(Pfizer Animal Health)*.
vitamin A, vitamin D_3, calcium, phosphorus. Osteo-Form Powder *(Vet-A-Mix)*, Osteo-Form SA *(Vet-A-Mix)*.
vitamin A, vitamin D_3, vitamin E. Vita E-AD *(AgriPharm)*, Vitamin E-AD 300 *(AgriLabs)*, Vitamins AD_3E Dispersible Liquid *(Alpharma)*.
vitamin A, vitamin D_3, vitamin E, fatty acids (essential). NutriVed™ O.F.A. Liquid *(Vedco)*.
vitamin A, vitamin D_3, vitamin E, potassium, protein(s), sodium. WGS *(Durvet)*.
vitamin A, vitamin D_3, vitamin E, potassium, sodium. Propack-EXP *(Durvet)*.
vitamin A, vitamin D_3, vitamin E, vitamin K_3. Vitamins E-K-A Plus D_3 *(Alpharma)*.
vitamin A, vitamin D_3, vitamin E, zinc, fatty acids (essential). NutriVed™ O.F.A. Chewable Tablets for Large Dogs *(Vedco)*.
vitamin A, vitamin D_3, vitamin E, zinc, fatty acids (omega). NutriVed™ O.F.A. Chewable Tablets for Cats *(Vedco)*, NutriVed™ O.F.A. Chewable Tablets for Small and Medium Dogs *(Vedco)*.
vitamin A, vitamin E. Vital E®+A *(Schering-Plough)*.
vitamin A, vitamin E, lactase enzymes, microorganisms. Good Start Calf Bolus *(AgriPharm)*, Good Start Calf Paste *(AgriPharm)*.
vitamin A, vitamin E, yeast, microorganisms. Fastrack® Canine Gel *(Conklin)*, Fastrack® Equine Gel *(Conklin)*.
Vitamin AD_3 *(AgriLabs)*, **vitamin A, vitamin D.**
Vitamin AD *(Butler)*, **vitamin A, vitamin D.**
Vitamin A & D *(Vedco)*, **vitamin A, vitamin D.**
Vitamin A & D "500" *(AgriPharm)*, **vitamin A, vitamin D.**
Vitamin A D B_{12} Injection *(Vedco)*, **vitamin A, vitamin B_{12} (cyanocobalamin), vitamin D.**
Vitamin AD Injection *(Aspen)*, *(Phoenix Pharmaceutical)*, **vitamin A, vitamin D.**
Vitamin AD_3 Injection *(Bimeda)*, **vitamin A, vitamin D.**
Vitamin B-1 Powder *(AHC)*, **thiamine hydrochloride (B_1).**
vitamin B_6, biotin, l-lysine, methionine (d-l). H.B. 15™ *(Farnam)*.
vitamin B_6, vitamin B_{12} (cyanocobalamin), niacin, propylene glycol. Super Keto Drench *(Vedco)*.
vitamin B_6, vitamin E, arachidonic acid, linoleic acid, linolenic acid, vitamin A. Mirra-Coat® for Cats *(Pet-Ag)*.

vitamin E. Dealer Select Horse Care DurVit E Powder *(Durvet)*, Dl-Alpha Tocopherol Acetate Injection *(Vedco)*, EmulsiVit E-300 *(Vedco)*, Vita E 300 *(AgriPharm)*, Vital E®-300 *(Schering-Plough)*, Vitamin E-300 *(AgriLabs)*, Vitamin E 300 *(Durvet)*, Vitamin E Dispersible Liquid *(Alpharma)*.

vitamin E, aloe vera, glycerine, triethanolamine. SoftGuard™ *(Activon)*.

vitamin E, aloe vera, moisturizer(s), stain removers. CarraVet™ Multi Purpose Cleansing Foam *(V.P.L.)*.

vitamin E, aloe vera, moisturizer(s), vitamin A, vitamin D. DuraCream *(Durvet)*.

vitamin E, aloe vera, vitamin A, vitamin D. Aloe Heal™ *(Farnam)*.

vitamin E, amylase, lipase, protease, vitamin A, vitamin D. PanaKare™ Plus Powder *(Neogen)*, PanaKare™ Plus Tablets *(Neogen)*.

vitamin E, arachidonic acid, linoleic acid, linolenic acid, vitamin A, vitamin B_6. Mirra-Coat® for Cats *(Pet-Ag)*.

vitamin E, biotin, linoleic acid, linolenic acid, vitamin A, vitamin B_6. Mirra-Coat® Powder and Liquid *(Pet-Ag)*.

vitamin E, dried colostrum, microorganisms, vitamin A, vitamin D. Colostrum Powder *(Vedco)*.

vitamin E, fat product(s), linoleic acid, vitamin A, vitamin D. Fastbreak™ Plus™ *(Boehringer Ingelheim)*.

vitamin E, fatty acids, safflower oil (linoleic acid). Omega EFA™ Capsules *(Butler)*, Omega EFA™ Capsules XS *(Butler)*, Omega EFA™ Liquid *(Butler)*, Omega EFA™ Liquid XS *(Butler)*.

vitamin E, fatty acids, selenium. Bovine Maximizer™ *(Novartis Animal Vaccines)*.

vitamin E, fatty acids (essential), vitamin A, vitamin D_3. NutriVed™ O.F.A. Liquid *(Vedco)*.

vitamin E, fatty acids (omega), shampoo formula. Omega-Glo E Shampoo *(Vedco)*.

vitamin E, fatty acids (omega), vitamin A, vitamin D. 3V Caps™ for Large & Giant Breeds *(DVM)*, 3V Caps™ for Medium & Large Breeds *(DVM)*, 3V Caps™ for Small & Medium Breeds *(DVM)*, 3V Caps™ Liquid *(DVM)*, Omega-3 Fatty Acid Capsules for Large & Giant Breeds *(Vet Solutions)*, Omega-3 Fatty Acid Capsules for Medium Breeds *(Vet Solutions)*, Omega-3 Fatty Acid Capsules for Small Breeds *(Vet Solutions)*, Omega-3 Fatty Acid Liquid *(Vet Solutions)*.

vitamin E, folic acid. Folic Acid & Vitamin E Powder *(AHC)*.

vitamin E, lactase enzymes, microorganisms, vitamin A. Good Start Calf Bolus *(AgriPharm)*, Good Start Calf Paste *(AgriPharm)*.

vitamin E, microorganisms. Probios® Plus Natural E Bovine One Oral Gel for Ruminants *(Chr. Hansen)*, Probiotic Plus E for Calves *(Vets Plus)*, Probiotic Plus E for Cattle *(Vets Plus)*.

vitamin E, polyunsaturated fatty acids, vitamin A, vitamin D. Derma-Form Liquid *(Vet-A-Mix)*.

vitamin E, potassium, protein(s), sodium, vitamin A, vitamin D_3. WGS *(Durvet)*.

vitamin E, potassium, sodium, vitamin A, vitamin D_3. Propack-EXP *(Durvet)*.

vitamin E, selenium. Equ-SeE *(Vet-A-Mix)*, Equ-Se5E *(Vet-A-Mix)*, Prosel-300 *(Durvet)*, Sure E&SE™ *(SureNutrition)*, Vita•E & Selenium Powder *(Horse Health)*, Vita•E & Selenium Crumbles™ *(Horse Health)*, Vita-Min E & Selenium *(Farnam)*, Vitamin E & Selenium Powder *(AHC)*.

vitamin E, selenium (sodium selenite). BO-SE® *(Schering-Plough)*, E-SE® *(Schering-Plough)*, MU-SE® *(Schering-Plough)*, Velenium™ *(Fort Dodge)*.

vitamin E, vitamin A. Vital E®+A *(Schering-Plough)*.

vitamin E, vitamin A, vitamin D. EmulsiVit E/A&D *(Vedco)*, Vital E®-A+D *(Schering-Plough)*, Vitamin E+AD *(Durvet)*.

vitamin E, vitamin A, vitamin D_3. Vita E-AD *(AgriPharm)*, Vitamin E-AD 300 *(AgriLabs)*, Vitamins AD_3E Dispersible Liquid *(Alpharma)*.

vitamin E, vitamin K_3, vitamin A, vitamin D_3. Vitamins E-K-A Plus D_3 *(Alpharma)*.

vitamin E, yeast, microorganisms, vitamin A. Fastrack® Canine Gel *(Conklin)*, Fastrack® Equine Gel *(Conklin)*.

vitamin E, zinc, fatty acids (essential), vitamin A, vitamin D. Pet-F.A. Liquid® *(Pfizer Animal Health)*.

vitamin E, zinc, fatty acids (essential), vitamin A, vitamin D_3. NutriVed™ O.F.A. Chewable Tablets for Large Dogs *(Vedco)*.

vitamin E, zinc, fatty acids (omega), vitamin A, vitamin D_3. NutriVed™ O.F.A. Chewable Tablets for Cats *(Vedco)*, NutriVed™ O.F.A. Chewable Tablets for Small and Medium Dogs *(Vedco)*.

vitamin E, zinc, fatty acids (omega), vitamin C (ascorbic acid). DermaPet® O.F.A. Plus EZ-C Caps (up to 30 lb.) *(DermaPet)*, DermaPet® O.F.A. Plus EZ-C Caps (50-70 lb.) *(DermaPet)*.

vitamin E, zinc, linoleic acid, vitamin A, vitamin B_6. Mirra-Coat® (Equine System) *(Pet-Ag)*.

vitamin E, zinc, microorganisms, potassium, sodium. Yellow Lite *(AgriPharm)*.

Vitamin E-300 *(AgriLabs)*, **vitamin E.**

Vitamin E 300 *(Durvet)*, **vitamin E.**

Vitamin E+AD *(Durvet)*, **vitamin A, vitamin D, vitamin E.**

Vitamin E-AD 300 *(AgriLabs)*, **vitamin A, vitamin D_3, vitamin E.**

Vita-Min E & Selenium *(Farnam)*, **selenium, vitamin E.**

Vitamin E & Selenium Powder *(AHC)*, **selenium, vitamin E.**

Vitamin E Dispersible Liquid *(Alpharma)*, **vitamin E.**

Vitamin K_1 *(Vet Tek)*, **vitamin K_1 (phytonadione).**

Vitamin K_1 Injection *(Butler)*, *(Neogen)*, *(Phoenix Pharmaceutical)*, **vitamin K_1 (phytonadione).**

Vitamin K_1 Oral Capsules *(Butler)*, *(Phoenix Pharmaceutical)*, **vitamin K_1 (phytonadione).**

Vitamin K-1 Oral Capsules *(RXV)*, **vitamin K_1 (phytonadione).**

vitamin K_1 (phytonadione). AmTech Vitamin K_1 Injection *(Phoenix Scientific)*, K-Caps *(Vetus)*, K-Ject *(Vetus)*, Veda-K_1 Capsules *(Vedco)*, Veda-K_1 Injection *(Vedco)*, Veta-K_1® Capsules *(Bimeda)*, Veta-K_1® Injection *(Bimeda)*, Vita-Jec® Vitamin K1 Injectable *(RXV)*, Vitamin K_1 *(Vet Tek)*, Vitamin K_1 Injection *(Butler)*, *(Neogen)*, *(Phoenix Pharmaceutical)*, Vitamin K_1 Oral Capsules *(Butler)*, *(Phoenix Pharmaceutical)*, Vitamin K-1 Oral Capsules *(RXV)*.

vitamin K_3, vitamin A, vitamin D_3, vitamin E. Vitamins E-K-A Plus D_3 *(Alpharma)*.

vitamin K_3 (menadione). K-Sol *(Alpharma)*.

vitamins. Avi-Con *(Vet-A-Mix)*, B-Plus *(Alpharma)*, Breeder-Pak *(Alpharma)*, Liquid Vitamin Premix *(Alpharma)*, Multi-Pak/256 *(Alpharma)*, Plex-Sol C *(Vet-A-Mix)*, Red Alert *(Neogen)*, Super Vitamins *(Alpharma)*.

vitamins, aloe vera, chloroxylenol, humectant(s). H-Balm Udder Cream *(Centaur)*.

vitamins, aloe vera, emollient(s). Udder Balm *(Aspen)*, *(First Priority)*.

vitamins, aloe vera, lanolin. -50 Below *(AgriPharm)*.

vitamins, aloe vera, lanolin, moisturizer(s), PABA sun screen. Medicated Udder Balm *(First Priority)*.

vitamins, aloe vera, lanolin, neatsfoot oil. Absorbine® Hooflex® Moisturizing Creme *(W. F. Young)*.

vitamins, amino acids. Dealer Select Horse Care Farrier's Select *(Durvet)*.

vitamins, amino acids, bicarbonate, microorganisms, minerals. Pre-Conditioning/Receiving Formula Gel *(Durvet)*, Ruminant Lactobacillus Gel *(First Priority)*.

vitamins, amino acids, biotin. Dealer Select Horse Care NutriHoof *(Durvet)*.

vitamins, amino acids, dextrose, minerals. Tryptophan Plus Gel™ *(Horses Prefer)*.

vitamins, amino acids, electrolytes. Amino Acid Concentrate *(AgriLabs)*, Amino Acid Solution *(AgriLabs)*, OTC™ Jug *(SureNutrition)*.

vitamins, amino acids, electrolytes, energy source(s). Energy+ *(Butler)*, NRG-Plus™ *(Bimeda)*, Pic-M-Up™ *(AgriPharm)*.

vitamins, amino acids, electrolytes, energy source(s), minerals. Energy Drench *(Vedco)*.

vitamins, amino acids, fatty acids (essential), minerals. NutriVed™ Chewable Vitamins for Dogs *(Vedco)*, NutriVed™ Chewable Vitamins for Puppies *(Vedco)*, NutriVed™ Hypo Allergenic Chewable Tablets *(Vedco)*.

vitamins, amino acids, fatty acids (essential), minerals, taurine. NutriVed™ Chewable Vitamins for Cats *(Vedco)*, NutriVed™ Chewable Vitamins for Kittens *(Vedco)*.

vitamins, amino acids, lactic acid producing bacteria, minerals. MultiMax™ *(SureNutrition)*.

vitamins, amino acids, microorganisms, minerals. Ruminant LactoBac Gel *(Vedco)*.

vitamins, amino acids, minerals. Amino Acid Bolus *(Vets Plus)*, Equinime® *(Chariton)*, Maxum® Crumbles *(Horse Health)*, Stam-N-Aid™ *(Neogen)*, Vita Plus® *(Farnam)*.

vitamins, amino acids, minerals, propylene glycol. PRN Hi-Energy Supplement™ *(PRN Pharmacal)*.

vitamins, amino acids, minerals, selenium, tetrachlorvinphos. Vita-Plus® with Equitrol® *(Farnam)*.

vitamins, amino acids, minerals, taurine. Cholodin®-FEL *(MVP)*.

vitamins, amodimethicone, methionine (d-l), minerals, vegetable oil(s). Equ-Aid Plus *(Vet-A-Mix)*.

vitamins, amylase, lipase, protease. Pancreatic Plus Powder *(Butler)*, Pancreatic Plus Tablets *(Butler)*, PancreVed Powder *(Vedco)*, PancreVed Tablets *(Vedco)*.

vitamins, antioxidants, fatty acids (omega), minerals. Lickables™ Super Charger™ *(A.A.H.)*.

vitamins, antioxidants, fatty acids (omega), minerals, soy protein. Lickables™ Charge Up!™ *(A.A.H.)*.

vitamins, antioxidants, minerals. Lickables™ Hearty Dog™ *(A.A.H.)*.

vitamins, antioxidants, minerals, taurine. Lickables™ Hearty Cat™ *(A.A.H.)*.

vitamins, Aspergillus oryzae fermentation extract, minerals. K-Zyme® Cat Granules *(BioZyme)*, K-Zyme® Chewable Dog Tablets *(BioZyme)*, K-Zyme® Dog Granules *(BioZyme)*, Vita Charge® 28 Dispersible Powder *(BioZyme)*, Vita Charge® Calf Bolus *(BioZyme)*, Vita Charge® Equine *(BioZyme)*, Vita Charge® Gel Cap *(BioZyme)*, Vita Charge® Paste *(BioZyme)*, Vita Ferm® Breeder Booster+Mag *(BioZyme)*, Vita Ferm® Cattleman's Beefmaker *(BioZyme)*, Vita Ferm® Cattleman's Beefmaker+Mag *(BioZyme)*, Vita Ferm® Concept-Aid *(BioZyme)*, Vita Ferm® Concept-Aid+Mag *(BioZyme)*, Vita Ferm® Concept-Aid A•P *(BioZyme)*, Vita Ferm® Cow Calf 5 *(BioZyme)*, Vita Ferm® Dairy Basemix 12:16 *(BioZyme)*, Vita Ferm® Dairy Basemix 18:6 *(BioZyme)*, Vita Ferm® Dairy Basemix 18:12 *(BioZyme)*, Vita Ferm® Equine *(BioZyme)*, Vita Ferm® Ewe and Lamb *(BioZyme)*, Vita Ferm® Far Out Dry Cow *(BioZyme)*, Vita Ferm® Feedlot Formula *(BioZyme)*, Vita Ferm® Fescue Fiber Buster *(BioZyme)*, Vita Ferm® Fescue Power Keg *(BioZyme)*, Vita Ferm® Formula *(BioZyme)*, Vita Ferm® Grass Enhancer *(BioZyme)*, Vita Ferm® High Mag *(BioZyme)*,

Vita Ferm® Natural Protein Pasture Formula (NPPF) *(BioZyme)*, Vita Ferm® Pasture Formula *(BioZyme)*, Vita Ferm® Power Keg *(BioZyme)*, Vita Ferm® Roughage Fortifier *(BioZyme)*, Vita Ferm® Sheep & Goat Keg *(BioZyme)*, Vita Ferm® Sure Champ and Vita Start Pellets *(BioZyme)*, Vita Ferm® Sure Start 2 *(BioZyme)*, Vita Ferm® Sure Start Pac *(BioZyme)*, Vita Ferm® Up Close Dry Cow *(BioZyme)*, Vita Ferm® Vita Grow 32 Natural *(BioZyme)*.

vitamins, biotin, methionine, minerals. Bio-Hoof™ *(Horses Prefer)*.

vitamins, bovine origin glycoproteins, microorganisms, minerals. Colostrum-Plus *(Jorgensen)*.

vitamins, calcium, cobalt, magnesium, selenium. Calcium Gel+Selenium *(AgriLabs)*, Cal Ox 64 Plus SE *(AgriPharm)*, CalOx 64 SE Oral Gel *(Vedco)*.

vitamins, calcium, cobalt sulfate, magnesium chloride. Calox 64 Oral Gel *(Vedco)*.

vitamins, calcium, magnesium, phosphorus, potassium. Mega CMPK Bolus *(AgriPharm)*, Slow Release CMPK Bolus *(PRN Pharmacal)*.

vitamins, calcium, magnesium, potassium. Calcium Drench *(AgriPharm)*.

vitamins, calcium, magnesium, potassium, propylene glycol. Calcium Drench Plus Vitamins *(AgriLabs)*, *(Durvet)*.

vitamins, calcium, magnesium, selenium. Cal-Mag-SV Gel *(Butler)*.

vitamins, calcium, milk protein, nutrients, phosphorus. Foal-Lac® Pellets *(Pet-Ag)*.

vitamins, calcium, phosphorus. Osteo-Form Tablets *(Vet-A-Mix)*.

vitamins, calcium, propylene glycol, tri-calcium phosphate. Cal-C-Fresh™ *(Vets Plus)*.

vitamins, calcium, tri-calcium phosphate. Oral Calcium Gel *(DVM Formula)*.

vitamins, choline, fatty acids (essential), methionine (d-l). Lipo-Form *(Vet-A-Mix)*.

vitamins, choline, lipids, minerals. Geri-Form *(Vet-A-Mix)*.

vitamins, cobalt, magnesium, propionic acid, propylene glycol. Keto Oral Gel *(Phoenix Pharmaceutical)*.

vitamins, cobalt, magnesium, propylene glycol. Oral Keto Energel *(First Priority)*.

vitamins, cobalt sulfate, magnesium sulfate, polyethelene glycol, propionic acid, silicon dioxide. Ketopro Oral Gel *(Vedco)*.

vitamins, colostrum whey, microorganisms, minerals. Oral Probiotic Calf Pak *(AgriPharm)*, Sure-Start Plus *(AgriPharm)*.

vitamins, conditioners, sunscreen formula. Vetrolin® Shine *(Equicare)*.

vitamins, dextrose, electrolytes. Ora-Lyte™ Powder *(Butler)*.

vitamins, dextrose, electrolytes, glycine. Electrolyte HE with Vitamins *(DVM Formula)*.

vitamins, dextrose, electrolytes, minerals. Multi-Electrolytes *(Neogen)*.

vitamins, dried colostrum, microorganisms. Soluble Colostrum Powder *(Durvet)*.

vitamins, dried colostrum, microorganisms, minerals. Colostrum Bolus Forte *(Durvet)*.

vitamins, electrolytes. Avian Bluelite® *(TechMix)*, Broiler-Pak *(Alpharma)*, Electro R *(Alpharma)*, High Performance Poultry Pak *(Durvet)*, Hog & Cattle Vitamins and Electrolytes *(Fort Dodge)*, Super B-Plex *(Neogen)*, Vitamins and Electrolytes *(Durvet)*, Vitamins and Electrolytes Concentrate *(Alpharma)*, *(Durvet)*, Vitamins & Electrolytes Concentrate *(Fort Dodge)*, Vitamins & Electrolytes "Plus" *(AgriLabs)*, Vitamins & Electrolytes (Soluble) *(Fort Dodge)*, Vita Pak *(Alpharma)*.

vitamins, electrolytes, energy source(s). Bovine Bluelite® *(TechMix)*, Equine Bluelite® *(TechMix)*, K-9 Bluelite® *(TechMix)*.

vitamins, electrolytes, energy source(s), microorganisms, nutrients. Sow & Gilt Restart™ One-4 *(TechMix)*.

vitamins, electrolytes, energy source(s), nutrients. Advance™ Arrest® *(Milk Specialties)*, Advance™ Pro-Lyte Plus® *(Milk Specialties)*.

vitamins, electrolytes, iron. Pig-95 *(Skylabs)*.

vitamins, electrolytes, microorganisms. Revitilyte-Plus™ *(Vets Plus)*.

vitamins, electrolytes, microorganisms, organic acidifiers. Vit-E-Lyte "Plus" *(Bimeda)*.

vitamins, electrolytes, minerals. Electrolytes-Plus *(Alpharma)*, Vi-tal *(Loveland)*.

vitamins, electrolytes, minerals, sucrose. Dexsolyte Powder *(Neogen)*.

vitamins, emollient(s). Chap-Guard™ Plus *(AgriLabs)*, Soothables™ Tender Foot *(A.A.H.)*, Udder Balm *(Vedco)*, Udder Comfort Cream *(Phoenix Pharmaceutical)*.

vitamins, emollient(s), moisturizer(s). Bova Derm® *(Butler)*, Udder Moist *(A.A.H.)*.

vitamins, energy source(s). Energy Plus *(Q.A. Laboratories)*, Hi-Cal Suspension *(Vedco)*, Liquical™ *(Butler)*, Quick-Start™ *(Vedco)*.

vitamins, energy source(s), fatty acids (omega), minerals. Nutri-Stat™ *(Tomlyn)*.

vitamins, energy source(s), minerals. High-Cal *(Vet Solutions)*, Nutri-Cal® for Ferrets & Other Small Animals *(Tomlyn)*, Stat *(PRN Pharmacal)*.

vitamins, energy source(s), minerals, nutrients. CliniCare® Canine Liquid Diet *(Abbott)*, CliniCare® Feline Liquid Diet *(Abbott)*, CliniCare® RF Specialized Feline Liquid Diet *(Abbott)*.

vitamins, fatty acids, minerals. Super 14™ *(Farnam)*.

vitamins, fatty acids (essential), minerals. Derma-Form Tablets *(Vet-A-Mix)*, NutriVed™ O.F.A. Granules for Dogs *(Vedco)*, Pet-Tabs®/F.A. Granules *(Pfizer Animal Health)*, Sergeant's® Vetscription® Vitamins for Dogs & Puppies *(Sergeant's)*.

vitamins, fatty acids (essential), minerals, potassium, taurine. Felo-Form *(Vet-A-Mix)*.

vitamins, fatty acids (essential), minerals, taurine. NutriVed™ O.F.A. Granules for Cats *(Vedco)*.

vitamins, fatty acids (essential), taurine. Sergeant's® Vetscription® Vitamins for Cats & Kittens *(Sergeant's)*.

vitamins, fatty acids (omega), minerals. Canine F.A./Plus Granules *(Pala-Tech)*, Derma-Form Granules F.A. *(Vet-A-Mix)*, Equine F.A./Plus Granules *(Pala-Tech)*, Feline F.A./Plus Chewable Tablets *(Pala-Tech)*, Mrs. Allen's Shed-Stop® Granules for Cats *(Farnam)*, Mrs. Allen's Shed-Stop® Granules for Dogs *(Farnam)*.

vitamins, fenbendazole, minerals, protein(s). Sweetlix® Safe-Guard® 20% Natural Protein Deworming Block for Beef Cattle *(Sweetlix)*.

vitamins, fermentation extract(s), microorganisms. All-In-One Calf Bolus *(AgriPharm)*, All-In-One Cattle Bolus *(AgriPharm)*.

vitamins, free radical scavengers, vitamin C (ascorbic acid). Electro-Flex™ *(First Priority)*.

vitamins, glycolipids, lecithin, phospholipids. Dyna-Lode® Equine Supplement *(Harlmen)*.

vitamins, goat milk, minerals. GME™ Powder and Liquid (Goat's Milk Esbilac®) *(Pet-Ag)*.

vitamins, iodine. Avian Vitamins Iodized *(ARC)*.

vitamins, iron. Redglo® *(Equicare)*, Vi-Sorbits® *(Pfizer Animal Health)*.

vitamins, iron, liver. Hi-Vite™ Drops *(Evsco)*.

vitamins, iron, liver extract. Ferret Drops™ *(Tomlyn)*, Puppy Drops™ *(Tomlyn)*.

vitamins, iron, minerals. Red Cell® *(Horse Health)*.

vitamins, iron, minerals, selenium. Go Max™ Liquid *(Farnam)*.

vitamins, iron, minerals, sorbitol. Vi-Sorbin® *(Pfizer Animal Health)*.

vitamins, lactose, milk protein, minerals. Multi-Milk™ *(Pet-Ag)*.

vitamins, linolenic acid, minerals. Mrs. Allen's Vita Care® Vitamins for Dogs *(Farnam)*, Nutra-Sure™ Cat Vitamins *(Farnam)*, Pet Vites *(Vetus)*, Show Winner!™ Dog Vitamins *(Farnam)*, Show Winner!™ Kitten Vitamins *(Farnam)*, Show Winner!™ Older Dog Vitamins *(Farnam)*, Show Winner!™ Puppy Vitamins *(Farnam)*.

vitamins, linolenic acid, minerals, taurine. Mrs. Allen's Vita Care® Vitamins for Cats *(Farnam)*, Show Winner!™ Cat Vitamins *(Farnam)*.

vitamins, methionine, propylene glycol. Keto-Gel™ *(Jorgensen)*.

vitamins, microorganisms. Equi-Phar™ LactoBac Gel *(Vedco)*, Innocugel™ Equine *(Butler)*, Probiotic Power™ *(Vets Plus)*.

vitamins, microorganisms, minerals. Equi-Phar™ Equi-Vita-Phos *(Vedco)*, Power Punch™ *(Vets Plus)*, Vita-Key® Show Cattle Supplement, Phase I *(Vita-Key)*.

vitamins, minerals. Energel™ for Cats *(Pet-Ag)*, Energel™ for Dogs *(Pet-Ag)*, Energel™ Powder for Cats *(Pet-Ag)*, Energel™ Powder for Dogs *(Pet-Ag)*, Equi-Phar™ Vita Plex Oral Honey *(Vedco)*, Equivim™ *(Butler)*, Grow Colt® *(Farnam)*, Happy Jack® Vita Tabs *(Happy Jack)*, Hartz® Health measures™ Everyday Chewable Vitamins for Dogs and Puppies *(Hartz Mountain)*, Lixotinic® *(Pfizer Animal Health)*, Mare-Plus® *(Farnam)*, Micro-Vet™ Equine Traditional Blend *(Boehringer Ingelheim)*, Milkin Mix *(Skylabs)*, Pet-Form® *(Vet-A-Mix)*, Pet-Tabs® *(Pfizer Animal Health)*, Pet-Tabs® Jr. *(Pfizer Animal Health)*, Pet-Tabs® Plus *(Pfizer Animal Health)*, Pet-Tinic® *(Pfizer Animal Health)*, Poult Pak *(Alpharma)*, Stock Power *(LeGear)*, Superior-Vita-Min Blend™ *(Horses Prefer)*, Unipet Nutritabs® *(Pharmacia & Upjohn)*, Vita-15™ Injection *(Neogen)*, Vita-Key® Brood Mare Supplement *(Vita-Key)*.

vitamins, minerals, protein(s). Protobolic™ Bolus Improved *(Butler)*.

vitamins, minerals, taurine. FaVor® *(Pfizer Animal Health)*, Felovite®-II with Taurine *(Evsco)*, Felovite® II with Taurine *(Tomlyn)*, Hartz® Health measures™ Everyday Chewable Vitamins for Cats and Kittens *(Hartz Mountain)*, TunaVite™ *(Vedco)*.

vitamins, minerals, tetrachlorvinphos. Sweetlix® Rabon® Mineral/Vitamin Molasses Block *(Sweetlix)*.

vitamins, moisturizer(s). Teat Elite *(AgriPharm)*.

vitamins, neomycin, oxytetracycline. Land O Lakes® Instant Amplifier® Max *(Land O'Lakes)*, Land O Lakes® Instant Amplifier® Select *(Land O'Lakes)*, Land O Lakes® Instant Maxi Care® *(Land O'Lakes)*, Land O Lakes® LitterMilk® *(Land O'Lakes)*.

vitamins, niacin, propylene glycol. Agri Plus Keto-Nia Drench™ *(Vets Plus)*, Niacin-Energy Drench Plus Vitamins *(AgriLabs)*, *(Durvet)*, Oral Keto-Energy Drench *(DVM Formula)*, Oral Keto-Energy Gel *(DVM Formula)*.

vitamins, nutrients. PerforMax™ Ration Maximizer *(Equicare)*.

vitamins, propylene glycol. Keto Plus Gel™ *(AgriLabs)*, Keto-Plus Gel *(AgriPharm)*, Keto "Plus" Gel *(Durvet)*, Keto Plus Oral Gel *(Butler)*.

vitamins, whey, fat product(s), lactose, lecithin, minerals. Start To Finish® Mare Replacer™ *(Milk Specialties)*.

vitamins, yeast, amino acids, enzymes, microorganisms. Vita Boost Paste™ *(AgriLabs)*.

vitamins, yeast, amino acids, enzymes, microorganisms, minerals. Vita-Key® Show Cattle Concentrate, Phase II *(Vita-Key)*.

vitamins, yeast, amino acids, microorganisms, minerals. Vita-Key® Swine Supplement *(Vita-Key)*.

vitamins, yeast, amino acids, minerals. Vita-Key® Antioxidant Concentrate *(Vita-Key)*, Vita-Key® Equine Supplement *(Vita-Key)*, Vita-Key® Mare & Foal Supplement *(Vita-Key)*.

vitamins, yeast, Aspergillus oryzae fermentation extract, minerals. MicroZyme Bolus for Cattle *(Vedco)*.

vitamins, yeast, fat product(s), lactose, milk protein, minerals. Start To Finish® Mare & Foal Pellets™ *(Milk Specialties)*.

W

X

Y

Z

Product Category Index

The Product Category Index (pink pages) serves as a comparison guide for veterinarians and animal health specialists in their product selection.

A trade name will be listed only once, under the product category that best describes it. The index has been divided into several main sections: Pharmaceuticals; Biologicals; Parasiticides; Premise Disinfectants; Foods; Diagnostics; Hospital Supplies; and General Items.

Similar products are likely to appear listed together. However, it should not be assumed that they are interchangeable.

Further information regarding the products listed in the pink pages may be found in the product monograph section (white pages) of the book. The Biologicals section of this index is to be used in conjunction with the Biological Charts (blue pages), where antigens are described in detail.

Every effort has been made to ensure the accuracy of the information published. However, it remains the responsibility of the readers to familiarize themselves with the product information contained on the product label or package insert. The Publisher, Editorial Team and all those involved in the production of this book cannot be held responsible for publication errors or any consequence that could result from the use of published information.

Guide to the Product Category Index

(continued on next page)

PHARMACEUTICALS

ACETONEMIA (KETOSIS) PREPARATIONS

Agri Plus Keto-Nia Drench™ *(Vets Plus)*
Keto-Gel™ *(Jorgensen)*
Keto-Nia-Fresh™ *(Vets Plus)*
Keto Oral Gel *(Phoenix Pharmaceutical)*
Keto Plus Gel™ *(AgriLabs)*
Keto-Plus Gel *(AgriPharm)*
Keto "Plus" Gel *(Durvet)*
Keto Plus Oral Gel *(Butler)*
Ketopro Oral Gel *(Vedco)*
Niacin-Energy Drench Plus Vitamins *(AgriLabs)*
Niacin-Energy Drench Plus Vitamins *(Durvet)*
Oral Keto Energel *(First Priority)*
Oral Keto-Energy Drench *(DVM Formula)*
Oral Keto-Energy Gel *(DVM Formula)*
Propylene Glycol *(AgriLabs)*
Propylene Glycol *(AgriPharm)*
Propylene Glycol *(Aspen)*
Propylene Glycol *(Centaur)*
Propylene Glycol *(Durvet)*
Propylene Glycol *(Vedco)*
Propylene Glycol U.S.P. *(Dominion)*
Propylene Glycol (U.S.P.) *(First Priority)*
Propylene Glycol (U.S.P.) *(Phoenix Pharmaceutical)*
Propylene Glycol, USP *(Vet Tek)*
Super Keto Drench *(Vedco)*

ANABOLIC AGENTS

Injectable
Equipoise® *(Fort Dodge)*
Winstrol®-V Sterile Suspension *(Pharmacia & Upjohn)*

Oral
Winstrol®-V Tablets *(Pharmacia & Upjohn)*

ANALGESICS

Non-opiates

anti-neuralgics, topical
Arthro Ease™ *(Horses Prefer)*
Equine Capsaicin Gel *(Butler)*
Equine Pain Block Gel *(First Priority)*
Sure-Block™ Topical Pain Reliever *(SureNutrition)*

Opiate agonists (narcotics)

injectable
Dolorex® *(Intervet)*
Torbugesic® *(Fort Dodge)*
Torbugesic®-SA *(Fort Dodge)*

ANESTHETICS

Anesthetics, general

aquaculture
Finquel® *(Argent)*
Tricaine-S *(Western Chemical)*

dissociative
AmTech Ketamine Hydrochloride Injection, USP *(Phoenix Scientific)*
KetaFlo™ *(Abbott)*
Ketaject® *(Phoenix Pharmaceutical)*
Ketaset® *(Fort Dodge)*
Keta-Sthetic™ *(RXV)*
Keta-Thesia™ *(Vetus)*
KetaVed™ *(Vedco)*
Telazol® *(Fort Dodge)*
VetaKet® Injection *(Lloyd)*
Vetalar® *(Fort Dodge)*

inhalant
Halothane, USP *(Halocarbon)*
IsoFlo® *(Abbott)*
Isoflurane, USP *(Halocarbon)*
Isoflurane, USP *(Phoenix Pharmaceutical)*
Iso-Thesia *(Vetus)*
SevoFlo™ *(Abbott)*

injectable
Pentothal® Sterile Powder (Veterinary) *(Abbott)*
PropoFlo™ *(Abbott)*
Rapinovet™ Anesthetic Injection *(Schering-Plough)*
Sodium Pentobarbital Injection *(Butler)*

Anesthetics, local
AmTech Lidocaine HCl Injectable-2% *(Phoenix Scientific)*
Carbocaine®-V *(Pharmacia & Upjohn)*
Lidocaine 2% Injectable *(Bimeda)*
Lidocaine 2% Injectable *(Butler)*
Lidocaine HCl 2% *(RXV)*
Lidocaine HCl Injectable 2% *(Aspen)*
Lidocaine Hydrochloride 2% *(Vet Tek)*
Lidocaine Hydrochloride Injectable-2% *(Phoenix Pharmaceutical)*
Lidocaine Hydrochloride Injection 2% *(AgriLabs)*
Lidocaine Injectable 2% *(Vedco)*
Lidoject *(Vetus)*

ANTACID and ADSORBENT PREPARATIONS

Anti-Diarrheal Cattle Bolus *(AgriLabs)*
Anti-Diarrhea Tablets *(ARC)*
BismuKote Paste for Medium & Large Dogs *(Vedco)*
BismuKote Paste for Small Dogs *(Vedco)*
Bismu-Kote Suspension *(Vedco)*
Bismupaste D5 *(Vetus)*
Bismupaste D10 *(Vetus)*
Bismupaste E20 *(Vetus)*
Bismusal *(Bimeda)*
Bismusal *(Durvet)*
Bismusal Suspension *(AgriPharm)*
Bismusol *(First Priority)*
Bismuth Subsalicylate Suspension *(A.A.H.)*
Boltan III™ *(Butler)*
Carmilax® Bolets® *(Pfizer Animal Health)*
Carmilax® Powder *(Pfizer Animal Health)*
Corrective Suspension *(Phoenix Pharmaceutical)*
Diarrhea Tabs *(Butler)*
Endosorb™ Bolus *(PRN Pharmacal)*
Endosorb™ Suspension *(PRN Pharmacal)*
Endosorb™ Tablets *(PRN Pharmacal)*
Equi-Phar™ BismuKote Paste *(Vedco)*
Gastro-Cote *(Butler)*
GastroGard® *(Merial)*
Gastro-Sorb™ Bolus *(Butler)*
Gastro-Sorb™ Calf Bolus *(Butler)*
InstaMag Bolus *(Vedco)*
Intesti-Sorb Bolus *(AgriPharm)*
Intesti-Sorb Calf Bolus *(AgriPharm)*
Kaolin Pectin *(Bimeda)*
Kaolin-Pectin *(Durvet)*
Kaolin-Pectin Plus *(AgriPharm)*
Kaolin Pectin Suspension *(A.A.H.)*
Kaolin Pectin Suspension *(First Priority)*
Kaolin Pectin Suspension *(Vedco)*
Kao-Pec *(AgriLabs)*
Kaopectolin *(Aspen)*
Kaopectolin™ *(Butler)*
Kao-Pect+ *(Phoenix Pharmaceutical)*
Laxade Bolus *(AgriPharm)*
Laxade Powder *(AgriPharm)*
Magnalax Bolus *(Phoenix Pharmaceutical)*
Magnalax Boluses *(Aspen)*
Magnalax Boluses *(Bimeda)*
Magnalax Boluses *(First Priority)*
Magnalax Powder *(Bimeda)*
Magnalax Powder *(Phoenix Pharmaceutical)*
Magnalax Powder *(Vedco)*
Maxi-Sorb Bolus *(Durvet)*
Maxi Sorb Calf Bolus *(Durvet)*
Milk of Magnesia *(Neogen)*
MVT™ Bolus Wet Granulation Formula *(Butler)*
MVT Powder™ *(Butler)*
Neigh-Lox® *(K.P.P.)*
PalaBIS™ *(PharmX)*
Palapectate™ *(PharmX)*
Polymag™ Bolus *(Butler)*
Polyox® Powder *(Bimeda)*
Polyox® II Bolus *(AgriPharm)*
Polyox® II Bolus *(Bimeda)*
Rumalax™ Bolus *(AgriLabs)*
Rumen Boluses *(Durvet)*
Veda-Sorb Bolus *(Vedco)*
Veda-Sorb Jr Bolus *(Vedco)*

ANTICOCCIDIALS

Feed medications
Amprol® 25% Type A Medicated Article *(Merial)*
Amprol Plus® Type A Medicated Article *(Merial)*
Amprovine® 25% Type A Medicated Article *(Merial)*
Avatec® *(Alpharma)*
Aviax® *(Phibro)*
Bio-Cox® 60 Granular *(Alpharma)*
Bovatec® 68 *(Alpharma)*
Bovatec® 150 FP *(Alpharma)*
Bovatec® Liquid 20 *(Alpharma)*
Clinacox™ *(Schering-Plough)*
Coban® 60 *(Elanco)*
Deccox® *(Alpharma)*
Deccox®-L *(Alpharma)*
Deccox®-M *(Alpharma)*
Maxiban® 72 *(Elanco)*
Monteban® 45 *(Elanco)*
Nicarb® 25% *(Phibro)*
Pro-Bac-C *(AgriLabs)*
Robenz® *(Alpharma)*
Sacox® 60 *(Intervet)*
Zoamix® *(Alpharma)*

Milk replacers
Advance™ Calvita® Supreme Medicated A.M. Milk Replacer with Bovatec® *(Milk Specialties)*

Water soluble medications
31.92% Sul-Q-Nox™ /Opti-Med™ *(Alpharma)*
Amprol® 9.6% Oral Solution *(Merial)*
Amprol® 128 20% Soluble Powder *(Merial)*
Corid® 9.6% Oral Solution *(Merial)*
Corid® 20% Soluble Powder *(Merial)*
Ren-O-Sal® Tablets *(Fort Dodge)*

ANTICONVULSANTS

Oral
Neurosyn™ Tablets *(Boehringer Ingelheim)*
Primidone *(Butler)*
Primidone *(Fort Dodge)*
Primidone 250 mg Tablets *(Vedco)*
Primitabs *(Vetus)*

ANTIDOTES

Alcohol dehydrogenase antagonists
Antizol-Vet® *(Orphan Medical)*

Charcoal adsorbents
Liqui-Char®-Vet *(King Animal Health)*
Liqui-Char®-Vet with Sorbitol *(King Animal Health)*
ToxiBan™ Granules *(Vet-A-Mix)*
ToxiBan™ Suspension *(Vet-A-Mix)*
ToxiBan™ Suspension with Sorbitol *(Vet-A-Mix)*
UAA (Universal Animal Antidote) Gel *(Vedco)*

Narcotic antagonists
Antagonil™ *(Wildlife)*
Trexonil™ *(Wildlife)*

Sedative (non-narcotic) antagonists
Antisedan® *(Pfizer Animal Health)*
Tolazine™ Injection *(Lloyd)*
Yobine® Injection *(Lloyd)*

ANTIFLATULENTS

NutriVed™ FlatuEx Chewable Tablets *(Vedco)*

ANTIFUNGALS

Oral
Fulvicin-U/F® Powder *(Schering-Plough)*
Fulvicin-U/F® Tablets *(Schering-Plough)*

Topical
Clotrimazole Solution USP, 1% *(Butler)*
Clotrimazole Solution USP, 1% *(Vet Solutions)*
Clotrimazole Solution USP, 1% *(Vetus)*
Conofite® Cream *(Schering-Plough)*
Conofite® Lotion *(Schering-Plough)*
Conofite® Spray *(Schering-Plough)*
MicaVed® Lotion 1% *(Vedco)*
MicaVed® Spray 1% *(Vedco)*
Micazole Lotion 1% *(Vetus)*
Micazole Spray 1% *(Vetus)*
Miconazole Nitrate Lotion 1% *(Butler)*
Miconazole Nitrate Spray 1% *(Butler)*
Miconosol Lotion 1% *(Med-Pharmex)*
Miconosol Spray 1% *(Med-Pharmex)*
Myosan™ Cream *(Life Science)*
Myosan™ Solution *(Life Science)*
Topical Fungicide *(Durvet)*
Topical Fungicide *(First Priority)*
Topical Fungicide *(Vedco)*

ANTIHISTAMINE

Injectable
AmTech Tripelennamine Hydrochloride Injection *(Phoenix Scientific)*
Rally™ -20 *(Vedco)*
Re-Covr® Injection *(Fort Dodge)*
Trienamine™ *(Phoenix Pharmaceutical)*
Tripelennamine Hydrochloride *(AgriLabs)*
Tripelennamine Hydrochloride *(Aspen)*
Tripelennamine Hydrochloride *(Butler)*
Tripelennamine Hydrochloride *(Vet Tek)*
Triple Histamine *(RXV)*

Please refer to product listings for more complete information.

Please refer to product listings for more complete information.

Please refer to product listings for more complete information.

Calcium Gluconate 23% Solution *(Phoenix Pharmaceutical)*
Calcium Gluconate 23% Solution *(Vet Tek)*
Calcium Gluconate 23% Solution *(Vetus)*
Cal Dex #2 *(AgriLabs)*
Cal-Dex C-M-P-K *(AgriLabs)*
Cal Dex CMPK Injection *(Aspen)*
Cal-Dextro® C *(Fort Dodge)*
Cal-Dextro® K *(Fort Dodge)*
Cal-Dextro® No. 2 *(Fort Dodge)*
Cal-Dextro® Special *(Fort Dodge)*
Cal MP-1000 *(Butler)*
Cal-MP 1700™ *(Butler)*
Cal-MPK™ 1080 Injection *(Butler)*
Cal-MPK 1234™ *(Butler)*
Cal-Nate 1069™ *(Butler)*
Cal-Phos #2 *(Vedco)*
Cal-Phos #2 Injection *(AgriLabs)*
Cal-Phos #2 Injection *(Phoenix Pharmaceutical)*
Cal-Phos #2 with Potassium Injection *(Phoenix Pharmaceutical)*
Calphosan® Solution *(Glenwood)*
Cal-Phos Forte *(Bimeda)*
Cal-Pho-Sol *(Neogen)*
Cal-Pho-Sol Solution SA *(Vedco)*
Ca-P I.V. Therapy *(RXV)*
CMPK *(RXV)*
CMPK-Dex *(Vetus)*
C-M-P-K Injection *(Vet Tek)*
CMPK Solution *(Bimeda)*
CMPK Solution *(Vedco)*
Norcalciphos™ *(Pfizer Animal Health)*

dextrose (main ingredient)

50% Dextrose Injection, USP *(Bimeda)*
AmTech Dextrose Solution 50% *(Phoenix Scientific)*
Dextrose 50% *(AgriLabs)*
Dextrose 50% *(AgriPharm)*
Dextrose 50% *(Durvet)*
Dextrose 50% Solution *(Vedco)*
Dextrose 50% Solution *(Vetus)*
Dextrose Solution *(Aspen)*
Dextrose Solution 50% *(Butler)*
Dextrose Solution 50% *(Phoenix Pharmaceutical)*
Dextrose Solution 50% *(Vet Tek)*
Glucose *(Fort Dodge)*

electrolytes

AmTech Amisol-R Injection *(Phoenix Scientific)*
AmTech Dexolyte Solution Injection *(Phoenix Scientific)*
Bimesol-R™ Injection *(Bimeda)*
Dexalyte *(Butler)*
Dexolyte Solution *(Phoenix Pharmaceutical)*
Electrolyte Solution *(AgriLabs)*
Electrolyte Solution *(Vet Tek)*
Electrolyte Solution with Dextrose *(Vedco)*
Electrolyte w/Dextrose Injection *(Aspen)*
ElectroSol-R *(Phoenix Pharmaceutical)*
E-Lyte *(Vedco)*
Equi-Phar™ Electrolyte with Dextrose *(Vedco)*
Injectrolyte *(Vetus)*
Normosol®-R *(Abbott)*
Vetalyte Plus I.V. Solution *(RXV)*

Lactated Ringer's

AmTech Lactated Ringers Injection *(Phoenix Scientific)*
Lactated Ringers *(Vet Tek)*
Lactated Ringers Injection *(Phoenix Pharmaceutical)*
Lactated Ringer's Injection *(Vedco)*
Lactated Ringers Injection *(Vetus)*
Lactated Ringers Injection SC *(Butler)*
Lactated Ringer's Injection, USP *(AgriLabs)*
Lactated Ringer's Injection, USP *(Bimeda)*
Lactated Ringer's Solution *(RXV)*

potassium chloride

Potassiject *(Vetus)*
Potassium Chloride *(Butler)*
Potassium Chloride *(Phoenix Pharmaceutical)*
Potassium Chloride *(Vedco)*

saline solutions (sodium chloride)

AmTech Hypertonic Saline Solution 7.2% *(Phoenix Scientific)*
AmTech Saline Solution 0.9% *(Phoenix Scientific)*
Equi-Phar™ Equine 7 HSS *(Vedco)*
Hypersaline E *(Vetus)*
Hyper Saline Solution 8X *(Butler)*
Hypertonic Saline Solution 7.2% *(AgriLabs)*
Hypertonic Saline Solution 7.2% *(Aspen)*
Hypertonic Saline Solution 7.2% *(Bimeda)*
Hypertonic Saline Solution 7.2% *(Phoenix Pharmaceutical)*
Hypertonic Saline Solution 7.2% *(RXV)*
Hypertonic Saline Solution 7.2% *(Vet Tek)*
Physiological Saline Solution *(Butler)*
Saline 0.9% Solution *(Vetus)*
Saline Solution *(Vedco)*
Saline Solution 0.9% *(AgriLabs)*
Saline Solution 0.9% *(Phoenix Pharmaceutical)*
Sterile Saline Solution *(Bimeda)*
Sterile Saline Solution *(RXV)*

Oral

electrolytes

Advance™ Pro-Lyte Plus® *(Milk Specialties)*
A-Lyte Concentrate *(Durvet)*
A-Lyte Solution *(Durvet)*
Amcalcilyte Forte *(AgriPharm)*
Amcalcilyte Forte *(Phoenix Pharmaceutical)*
Amcalcilyte Forte *(Vedco)*
AmTech Amcal High Potency Oral Solution *(Phoenix Scientific)*
Apple-Dex® *(Horse Health)*
Avian Bluelite® *(TechMix)*
Baby Pig Restart™ One-4 *(TechMix)*
Biolyte® *(Pharmacia & Upjohn)*
Bluelite® C *(TechMix)*
Bluelite® Swine Formula *(TechMix)*
Bovine Bluelite® *(TechMix)*
Calf Quencher *(Vedco)*
Calf Restart™ One-4 *(TechMix)*
Comeback™ *(AgriPharm)*
Dealer Select Horse Care DurLyte-A *(Durvet)*
Dealer Select Horse Care DurLyte-C *(Durvet)*
Dexalyte 8X Powder *(Butler)*
Dexsolyte Powder *(Neogen)*
Electramine® *(Life Science)*
Electro Dex® *(Horse Health)*
Electro-Flex™ *(First Priority)*
Electrolyte HE with Vitamins *(DVM Formula)*
Electrolyte Pak *(Alpharma)*
Electrolyte Pak Plus Stabilized Vitamin C *(Alpharma)*
Electrolyte Powder 8X *(Phoenix Pharmaceutical)*
Electrolytes-Plus *(Alpharma)*
Electrolyte Supplement *(First Priority)*
Electrolyte with Thickener *(DVM Formula)*
Electro R *(Alpharma)*
Elite™ Electrolyte *(Farnam)*
Elpak™ -G *(Vedco)*
Endura-Lite™ *(Creative Science)*
Endura-Lyte® *(Life Science)*
Entrolyte® *(Pfizer Animal Health)*
Entrolyte® H.E. *(Pfizer Animal Health)*
Equi-Phar™ Electramino Paste *(Vedco)*
Equi-Phar™ Equi-Lyte Powder *(Vedco)*
Glucaminolyte Forte *(AgriPharm)*
Glucaminolyte Forte *(Vedco)*
Gluco-Amino-Forte Oral Solution *(Phoenix Pharmaceutical)*
Gluco Amino Forte Oral Solution *(Vetus)*
Hydra-Lyte *(Vet-A-Mix)*
Hy-Sorb™ *(Bimeda)*
Isotone-SA *(Vet-A-Mix)*
K-9 Bluelite® *(TechMix)*
Keto Amino Forte™ *(Butler)*
Magna-Lyte *(First Priority)*
Multi-Electrolytes *(Neogen)*
Ora-Lyte™ Powder *(Butler)*
OTC™ Jug *(SureNutrition)*
Polylites IV *(Butler)*
Re-Sorb® *(Pfizer Animal Health)*
Revitilyte™ *(Vets Plus)*
Revitilyte-EQ™ *(Horses Prefer)*
Revitilyte-Gelling™ *(Vets Plus)*
Sky-Lytes *(Skylabs)*
Sow & Gilt Restart™ One-4 *(TechMix)*
Start To Finish® Sweat Replacer™ *(Milk Specialties)*
SureLytes™ Plus Carbo Load *(SureNutrition)*
Swine Acid-O-Lite™ *(TechMix)*
Vedalyte 8X Powder *(Vedco)*
Vita Charge® Power Drench *(BioZyme)*

FOOT and HOOF PRODUCTS (non-antimicrobial)

Absorbine® Hooflex® Liquid Conditioner *(W. F. Young)*
Absorbine® Hooflex® Moisturizing Creme *(W. F. Young)*
Absorbine® Hooflex® Original Conditioner *(W. F. Young)*
Absorbine® SuperShine® Hoof Polish *(W. F. Young)*
Dealer Select Horse Care Hoof Dressing With Brush *(Durvet)*
Dealer Select Horse Care Hoof Moisturizer *(Durvet)*
Dr. Naylor® Hoof 'n Heel® *(H.W. Naylor)*
DuraCept™ *(Activon)*
Equi-Phar™ Miracle Heel *(Vedco)*
Forshner's® Medicated Hoof Packing *(Equicare)*
Healthy Foot™ *(SSI Corp.)*
Hoof Conditioner *(First Priority)*
HoofPro+® *(SSI Corp.)*
Improved Hoof Dressing *(Fiebing)*
MagSalt™ *(SSI Corp.)*
New-Hoof™ Concentrate *(Vets Plus)*
New-Hoof Topical™ *(Vets Plus)*
Power Shower Spray™ *(SSI Corp.)*
Rotational Zinc™ *(SSI Corp.)*
SheepPro™ Copper Suspension *(SSI Corp.)*
SheepPro™ Zinc Suspension *(SSI Corp.)*
Shur Hoof™ *(Horse Health)*
Vita-Hoof® *(Equicare)*

HEMATINICS

Injectable, general

Duriron *(Durvet)*

Iron dextran injections

AmTech Iron Dextran Injection *(Phoenix Scientific)*
AmTech Iron Dextran Injection-200 *(Phoenix Scientific)*
Anem-X™ 100 *(AgriPharm)*
Anem-X™ 200 *(AgriPharm)*
Ferrodex™ 100 *(AgriLabs)*
Ferrodex™ 200 *(AgriLabs)*
HemaJect 200 *(Vedco)*
Iron Dextran-200 *(Durvet)*
Iron Dextran Complex *(Premier Farmtech)*
Iron Dextran Injection *(Durvet)*
Iron Dextran Injection *(Phoenix Pharmaceutical)*
Iron Dextran Injection *(Vedco)*
Iron Dextran Injection-200 *(Aspen)*
Iron Dextran Injection-200 *(Butler)*
Iron Dextran Injection-200 *(Phoenix Pharmaceutical)*
Iron Hydrogenated Dextran Injection *(Aspen)*
Iron Hydrogenated Dextran Injection *(V.L.)*

HEMOSTATICS

Topical

Blood Stop Powder *(AgriLabs)*
Blood Stop Powder *(AgriPharm)*
Blood Stop Powder *(Aspen)*
Blood Stop Powder *(Butler)*
Blood Stop Powder *(Centaur)*
Blood Stop Powder *(Davis)*
Blood Stop Powder *(Dominion)*
Blood Stop Powder *(Durvet)*
Blood Stop Powder *(First Priority)*
Blood Stop Powder *(Vedco)*
Caustic Dressing Powder *(Phoenix Pharmaceutical)*
Caustic Powder *(Butler)*
Clotisol® Liquid *(BenePet)*
Clot-It Plus™ *(Evsco)*
Clot Powder *(Q.A. Laboratories)*
Equi-Phar™ Caustic Powder *(Vedco)*
HemaBlock™ *(Abbott)*
Hemostatic Powder *(Butler)*
Hemostat Powder *(Phoenix Pharmaceutical)*
Kwik-Stop® Styptic Powder *(ARC)*
McKillip's Dusting Powder *(Butler)*
McKillip's Dusting Powder *(First Priority)*
Nik Stop® Styptic Powder *(Tomlyn)*
Silver Nitrate Stick Applicators *(Vedco)*
Stypt-Stix *(Vetus)*

HORMONES and ANALOGS

Estrogens / estrogenics

ECP® Sterile Solution *(Pharmacia & Upjohn)*

Gonadotropins (FSH, GnRH, HCG, LH, PMSG)

Chorionic Gonadotropin *(Butler)*
Chorulon® *(Intervet)*
Cystorelin® *(Merial)*
Factrel® *(Fort Dodge)*
Fertagyl® *(Intervet)*
Ovuplant™ *(Fort Dodge)*
P.G. 600® Estrus Control *(Intervet)*

Insulin

PZI Vet® *(Idexx Pharm.)*

Mineralocorticosteroids

Percorten®-V *(Novartis)*

Please refer to product listings for more complete information.

Please refer to product listings for more complete information.

RESPIRATORY STIMULANTS

Dopram®-V Injectable *(Fort Dodge)*

SEDATIVES and TRANQUILIZERS

With analgesic effect

injectable

AmTech Xylazine HCl Injection 20 mg/mL *(Phoenix Scientific)*
AmTech Xylazine HCl Injection 100 mg/mL *(Phoenix Scientific)*
AnaSed® 20 Injection *(Lloyd)*
AnaSed® 100 Injectable *(Lloyd)*
Cervizine® Injectable *(Wildlife)*
Domitor® *(Pfizer Animal Health)*
Dormosedan® *(Pfizer Animal Health)*
Sedazine® *(Fort Dodge)*
TranquiVed Injectable (Dogs and Cats) *(Vedco)*
TranquiVed Injectable (Horses) *(Vedco)*
Wildnil™ *(Wildlife)*
X-Ject E *(Vetus)*
X-Ject SA *(Vetus)*
Xyla-Ject® 20 mg/mL Injectable *(Phoenix Pharmaceutical)*
Xyla-Ject® 100 mg/mL Injectable *(Phoenix Pharmaceutical)*
Xylazine-20 Injection *(Butler)*
Xylazine-100 Injection *(Butler)*
Xylazine HCl Injection *(Boehringer Ingelheim)*
Xylazine HCl Injection *(RXV)*
Xylazine HCl Injection *(Vet Tek)*
Xylazine HCl Injection 100 mg *(AgriLabs)*

Without analgesic effect

injectable

Aceproject *(Vetus)*
Acepromazine Maleate Injection *(AgriLabs)*
Acepromazine Maleate Injection *(Boehringer Ingelheim)*
Acepromazine Maleate Injection *(Butler)*
Acepromazine Maleate Injection *(Phoenix Pharmaceutical)*
Acepromazine Maleate Injection *(RXV)*
Acepromazine Maleate Injection *(Vedco)*
PromAce® Injectable *(Fort Dodge)*

oral

Acepromazine Maleate Tablets *(AgriLabs)*
Acepromazine Maleate Tablets *(Boehringer Ingelheim)*
Acepromazine Maleate Tablets *(Butler)*
Acepromazine Maleate Tablets *(Phoenix Pharmaceutical)*
Acepromazine Maleate Tablets *(Vedco)*
Aceprotabs *(Vetus)*
PromAce® Tablets *(Fort Dodge)*

STERILE WATER, DILUENTS and STABILIZERS

AmTech Sterile Water for Injection, USP *(Phoenix Scientific)*
Aquaject *(Vetus)*
Sterile Water *(AgriLabs)*
Sterile Water *(G.C. Hanford)*
Sterile Water *(Phoenix Pharmaceutical)*
Sterile Water *(Vedco)*
Sterile Water for Injection *(Butler)*
Sterile Water for Injection *(RXV)*
Sterile Water For Injection *(Vet Tek)*
Sterile Water for Injection, USP *(Aspen)*
Sterile Water for Injection, USP *(Bimeda)*
Vaccine Stabilizer *(Alpharma)*

TOPICAL PRODUCTS (non anti-microbial)

Enzymes

Granulex® V Aerosol Spray *(Pfizer Animal Health)*
Granulex® V Liquid *(Pfizer Animal Health)*
Trypzyme®-V Aerosol Spray *(V.P.L.)*
Trypzyme®-V Liquid *(V.P.L.)*

Particles and membranes

Collasate™ *(PRN Pharmacal)*
FasCure™ *(KenVet)*

Various

Allerpet® C *(V.P.L.)*
Allerpet® D *(V.P.L.)*
Aloe Heal™ *(Farnam)*
AluSpray® *(Neogen)*
A-Plus™ Wound Dressing *(Creative Science)*
Biocaine® *(Tomlyn)*
BioDres® Wound Dressing *(DVM)*
CarraSorb™ Freeze-Dried Gel (FDG) *(V.P.L.)*
CarraVet™ Spray-Gel Wound Dressing *(V.P.L.)*
CarraVet™ Wound Dressing *(V.P.L.)*
Chondroprotec® *(Neogen)*
Equi-Phar™ McKillips Powder *(Vedco)*
Excalibur® Sheath Cleaner for Horses *(Equicare)*
Happy Jack® Pad Kote *(Happy Jack)*
HyCoat® *(Neogen)*
KeraSolv® Gel *(DVM)*
Maxi/Guard® Zn7™ Derm *(Addison)*
Natural Solvent™ *(Butler)*
Pad-Tough™ *(Life Science)*
PetroTech 25™ *(Alpha Tech Pet)*
Protecta-Pad® *(Evsco)*
Protecta-Pad® *(Tomlyn)*
Proud Flesh Powder *(First Priority)*
Proudsoff™ *(Creative Science)*
QuickHit™ for Dairy Cattle *(SSI Corp.)*
Soothables™ Tender Foot *(A.A.H.)*
Triple Cast™ *(Neogen)*
Wartsoff™ *(Creative Science)*
Wonder Dust™ Wound Powder *(Farnam)*

URINARY ACIDIFIERS and ANTISEPTICS

Ammonil® Tablets *(King Animal Health)*
d-l-Methionine Powder™ *(Butler)*
DL-Methionine Powder *(First Priority)*
d-l-m Tablets *(Butler)*
Fus-Sol™ Drops *(PPI)*
Methigel® *(Evsco)*
Methio-Form® Chewable Tablets *(Vet-A-Mix)*
Methio-Tabs® *(Vet-A-Mix)*
Uroeze® *(King Animal Health)*
Uroeze® 200 *(King Animal Health)*

UTERINE PREPARATIONS (non-antimicrobial)

After-Birth Bolus *(AgriPharm)*
AmTech Uterine Bolus *(Phoenix Scientific)*
Intrauterine Bolus *(AgriLabs)*
Nolvasan® Cap-Tabs® *(Fort Dodge)*
Nolvasan® Suspension *(Fort Dodge)*
Proteoseptic Bolus *(Vedco)*
Uterine Bolus *(Butler)*
Uterine Bolus *(Durvet)*
Uterine Bolus *(First Priority)*
Uterine Bolus *(Phoenix Pharmaceutical)*

VITAMINS, MINERALS and SUPPLEMENTS

Calcium supplements

oral

40% CMPK with D_3 Oral Drench *(DVM Formula)*
Absorbine® ProCMC® *(W. F. Young)*
Cal "62" Plus Gel *(Aspen)*
Cal-C-Fresh™ *(Vets Plus)*
Calcium Drench *(AgriPharm)*
Calcium Drench™ *(Vets Plus)*
Calcium Drench Plus Vitamins *(AgriLabs)*
Calcium Drench Plus Vitamins *(Durvet)*
Calcium Gel+Selenium *(AgriLabs)*
Calcium Gel + Vitamins *(AgriLabs)*
Calcium Oral Gel *(Phoenix Pharmaceutical)*
Calcium Phosphorus Powder *(Pet-Ag)*
Calcium Phosphorus Tablets *(Pet-Ag)*
Calcium Plus *(First Priority)*
Calcium SE *(First Priority)*
Cal-Gel™ *(Jorgensen)*
Cal-Gel 63 *(Durvet)*
Cal M 64 Plus Se *(Butler)*
Cal-Mag-Co Gel *(Durvet)*
Cal-Mag-SE Gel *(Durvet)*
Cal-Mag-SV Gel *(Butler)*
Cal MPK Gel *(Butler)*
Cal Oral Plus™ *(Butler)*
Calox 64 Oral Gel *(Vedco)*
Cal Ox 64 Plus SE *(AgriPharm)*
CalOx 64 SE Oral Gel *(Vedco)*
Calsorb™ *(PRN Pharmacal)*
Cal Supreme Gel™ *(Bimeda)*
ClearCal 50 *(Vedco)*
CMPK Bolus *(Durvet)*
CMPK Bolus *(Vets Plus)*
CMPK D_3 Drench *(Durvet)*
C.M.P.K. Gel *(AgriLabs)*
CMPK Gel *(AgriPharm)*
CMPK Gel *(Durvet)*
CMPK Gel *(Vedco)*
CMPK Gel Plus™ *(Vets Plus)*
CMPK Oral *(AgriPharm)*
C.M.P.K. Oral Gel *(Phoenix Pharmaceutical)*
CMPK Oral Solution 33% *(Vedco)*
CMPK Solution *(Aspen)*
CMPK with D_3 Drench *(Vets Plus)*
Di-Calcium Phosphate *(Neogen)*
Fresh Cow YMCP Plus *(TechMix)*
Mega CMPK Bolus *(AgriPharm)*
M.F.O. Solution *(AgriLabs)*
Oral Calcium Drench *(DVM Formula)*
Oral Calcium Gel *(DVM Formula)*
Oral Cal MPK *(Durvet)*
Oral CMPK Gel *(DVM Formula)*
Oral CPMK Gel *(First Priority)*
Osteo-Form SA *(Vet-A-Mix)*
Osteo-Form Tablets *(Vet-A-Mix)*
Pet-Cal™ *(Pfizer Animal Health)*
PRN High Potency Calcium Gel® *(PRN Pharmacal)*
PSD Complex II *(PRN Pharmacal)*
Respond *(Jorgensen)*
Slow Release CMPK Bolus *(PRN Pharmacal)*
Super Calcium Drench *(Vedco)*
Super Calcium Gel "62" *(AgriPharm)*

Choline

oral

Reashure™ Choline *(Balchem)*

Cobalt

feed additives

Copro 25 *(Zinpro)*

Copper

oral / feed additives / water additives

Acidified Copper Sulfate *(AgriLabs)*
Acidified Copper Sulfate *(AgriPharm)*
Acidified Copper Sulfate *(Alpharma)*
Availa® Cu 100 *(Zinpro)*
Copasure®-12.5 *(Butler)*
Copasure®-25 *(Butler)*
Copper Blue™ *(AgriLabs)*
Cop-R-Sol™ *(Alpharma)*
Cuplex 50 *(Zinpro)*
Cuplex 100 *(Zinpro)*

D-panthenol

injectable

AmTech d-Panthenol Injection *(Phoenix Scientific)*
D-Panthenol Injectable *(Vedco)*
d-Panthenol Injection *(Butler)*
d-Panthenol Injection *(Phoenix Pharmaceutical)*

Folic acid

oral

Equi-Phar™ Folic 20 *(Vedco)*

Iodine

feed additives

Diamine Iodide-20 (With Salt) *(First Priority)*
Diamine Iodide-40 (With Salt) *(First Priority)*
Diamine Iodide (With Sugar) *(First Priority)*
E.D.D.I. 20 Gr. (Dextrose Base) *(Vedco)*
E.D.D.I. 20 Gr. (Organic Iodine Dextrose) *(Phoenix Pharmaceutical)*
E.D.D.I. 20 Gr. (Organic Iodine Salt) *(Phoenix Pharmaceutical)*
E.D.D.I. 20 Gr. (Salt) *(Vedco)*
E.D.D.I. 40 Gr. (Salt) *(Vedco)*
Hi-Boot® Ethylenediamine Dihydriodide *(WestAgro)*
Iodide Powder *(Neogen)*
Organic Iodide *(Butler)*
Organic Iodide 20 *(Durvet)*
Organic Iodide 40 *(Durvet)*
Organic Iodide Powder *(Neogen)*
Organic Iodine *(AgriLabs)*
Organic Iodine *(AgriPharm)*

oral

EDDI Equine *(Butler)*

Iron

oral

Availa® Fe 60 *(Zinpro)*
Iron-Plus *(Neogen)*
LIB *(Neogen)*
Meth-Iron 65 *(Zinpro)*
Pig-95 *(Skylabs)*
Sav-A-Caf® Finisher Iron *(IntAgra)*
Sav-A-Caf® Starter Iron *(IntAgra)*
Sav-A-Pig® Oral Iron *(IntAgra)*
Vitamin B_{12}-Iron Gel™ *(Horses Prefer)*

Manganese

feed additives

Availa® Mn 80 *(Zinpro)*
Manpro 80 *(Zinpro)*
Manpro 160 *(Zinpro)*

Please refer to product listings for more complete information.

Microorganism supplements

All-Pro Biotic™ *(Vets Plus)*
Bene-Bac™ Pet Gel *(Pet-Ag)*
Bene-Bac™ Powder *(Pet-Ag)*
Bird Bene-Bac™ Powder *(Pet-Ag)*
BP-1 *(AgriPharm)*
Calf RD Formula *(TechMix)*
Digest Aid™ *(Farnam)*
Equine Bene-Bac™ *(Pet-Ag)*
Fastrack® Canine Microbial Supplement *(Conklin)*
Fastrack® Probiotic Pack *(Conklin)*
Lamb & Kid Paste *(Durvet)*
MicroMaster® Equine Gel *(Loveland)*
MicroMaster® Pet Gel *(Loveland)*
Preempt™ *(Milk Specialties)*
Preempt™ *(MS BioScience)*
Probiocin® Oral Gel for Pets *(Chr. Hansen)*
Probios® Dispersible Powder *(Chr. Hansen)*
Probios® Equine One Oral Gel *(Chr. Hansen)*
Probios® Feed Granules *(Chr. Hansen)*
Probios® TC *(Chr. Hansen)*
Zoologic® Bene-Bac™ Large Mammal *(Pet-Ag)*
Zoologic® Bene-Bac™ Powder *(Pet-Ag)*

Multi-supplements

feed additives

4-Plex *(Zinpro)*
4-Plex-C *(Zinpro)*
Availa®-4 *(Zinpro)*
AvailaMin® - Grow/Finish *(Zinpro)*
AvailaMin® - Sow *(Zinpro)*
AvailaMin® - Starter I, II, III *(Zinpro)*
Availa® Z/M *(Zinpro)*
MicroMaster® Avian PAC™ HT *(Loveland)*
MicroMaster® Avian PAC™ Routine *(Loveland)*
MicroMaster® Avian Pulse PAC™ *(Loveland)*
Zinpro+3 *(Zinpro)*

injectable

Multimin™ *(Multimin)*
Vita-15™ Injection *(Neogen)*
Vitamin A D B_{12} Injection *(Vedco)*

oral

3V Caps™ for Large & Giant Breeds *(DVM)*
3V Caps™ for Medium & Large Breeds *(DVM)*
3V Caps™ for Small & Medium Breeds *(DVM)*
3V Caps™ Liquid *(DVM)*
Ab-Sorb™ Bolus *(Bimeda)*
Advance™ Arrest® *(Milk Specialties)*
Advance™ Energy Booster 100® *(Milk Specialties)*
Advance™ RuMin 8™ *(Milk Specialties)*
Amino Acid Bolus *(Vets Plus)*
Amino Acid Concentrate *(AgriLabs)*
Amino Acid Concentrate Oral Solution *(Aspen)*
Amino Acid Concentrate Oral Solution *(Bimeda)*
Amino Acid Oral Concentrate *(Phoenix Pharmaceutical)*
Amino Acid Oral Solution *(Aspen)*
Amino Acid Oral Solution *(Bimeda)*
Amino Acid Oral Solution *(Phoenix Pharmaceutical)*
Amino Acid Solution *(AgriLabs)*
Aminocal Plus™ *(Butler)*
Aminoplex *(Butler)*
Aminoplex Concentrate *(Butler)*
Amino Plus Concentrate *(AgriPharm)*
Amino Plus Solution *(AgriPharm)*
AmTech Amino Acid Oral Concentrate *(Phoenix Scientific)*
AmTech Amino Acid Oral Solution *(Phoenix Scientific)*
Arm & Hammer® Bio-Chlor® *(Church & Dwight)*
Arm & Hammer® Fermenten® *(Church & Dwight)*
Astringent Bolus *(Butler)*
Avian Vitamins Iodized *(ARC)*
Avi-Con *(Vet-A-Mix)*
Bovine Maximizer™ *(Novartis Animal Vaccines)*
Buffer Gel™ *(Vets Plus)*
Canine F.A./Plus Chewable Tablets For Large Dogs *(Pala-Tech)*
Canine F.A./Plus Chewable Tablets For Small and Medium Dogs *(Pala-Tech)*
Canine F.A./Plus Granules *(Pala-Tech)*
Cholodin® *(MVP)*
Cholodin®-FEL *(MVP)*
Clovite® Conditioner *(Fort Dodge)*
Dealer Select Horse Care Farrier's Select *(Durvet)*
Dealer Select Horse Care NutriHoof *(Durvet)*
Deliver® with Dialine™ *(AgriLabs)*
Derma-Form Granules F.A. *(Vet-A-Mix)*
Derma-Form Liquid *(Vet-A-Mix)*
Derma-Form Tablets *(Vet-A-Mix)*
DermaPet® EicosaDerm™ *(DermaPet)*
DermaPet® O.F.A. Plus EZ-C Caps (up to 30 lb.) *(DermaPet)*
DermaPet® O.F.A. Plus EZ-C Caps (50-70 lb.) *(DermaPet)*
DermCaps® *(DVM)*
DermCaps® 10 lb. *(DVM)*
DermCaps® 100 lb. *(DVM)*
DermCaps® Economy Size Liquid *(DVM)*
DermCaps® ES *(DVM)*
DermCaps® ES Liquid *(DVM)*
DermCaps® Liquid *(DVM)*
Double "A" Concentrate *(Vedco)*
Double "A" Solution *(Vedco)*
Dyna-Lode® Equine Supplement *(Harlmen)*
Dyna-Lode® Supplement for Dogs & Cats *(Harlmen)*
Dyna-Taurine™ *(Harlmen)*
EnerCal™ *(Vedco)*
Energel™ for Cats *(Pet-Ag)*
Energel™ for Dogs *(Pet-Ag)*
Energel™ Powder for Cats *(Pet-Ag)*
Energel™ Powder for Dogs *(Pet-Ag)*
Energy Drench *(Vedco)*
Energy+ *(Butler)*
Energy Plus *(Q.A. Laboratories)*
EPIC Daily Feed Supplement for Horses *(Bioniche Animal Health)*
EPIC Neonatal Feed Supplement for Foals *(Bioniche Animal Health)*
Equ-Aid Plus *(Vet-A-Mix)*
Equine Bluelite® *(TechMix)*
Equine F.A./Plus Granules *(Pala-Tech)*
Equinime® *(Chariton)*
Equi-Phar™ Vita Plex Oral Honey *(Vedco)*
Equivim™ *(Butler)*
FaVor® *(Pfizer Animal Health)*
Feline F.A./Plus Chewable Tablets *(Pala-Tech)*
Felo-Form *(Vet-A-Mix)*
Felovite®-II with Taurine *(Evsco)*
Felovite® II with Taurine *(Tomlyn)*
Ferret Drops™ *(Tomlyn)*
Fiber Forte® Feline *(Life Science)*
Foal-Lac® Pellets *(Pet-Ag)*
Formula V™ Taurine Tablets *(Pet-Ag)*
Geri-Form *(Vet-A-Mix)*
Go Max™ Liquid *(Farnam)*
Grow Colt® *(Farnam)*
Happy Jack® Cod Liver Oil *(Happy Jack)*
Happy Jack® Dermaplex™ *(Happy Jack)*
Happy Jack® Milkade *(Happy Jack)*
Happy Jack® ToneKote® *(Happy Jack)*
Happy Jack® Vita Tabs *(Happy Jack)*
Hartz® Health measures™ Everyday Chewable Vitamins for Cats and Kittens *(Hartz Mountain)*
Hartz® Health measures™ Everyday Chewable Vitamins for Dogs and Puppies *(Hartz Mountain)*
H.B. 15™ *(Farnam)*
Heska® F.A. Granules *(Heska)*
Hi-Cal Suspension *(Vedco)*
High-Cal *(Vet Solutions)*
Hi-Vite™ Drops *(Evsco)*
Hog & Cattle Vitamins and Electrolytes *(Fort Dodge)*
Hoof Supplement *(First Priority)*
Integrator™ *(Butler)*
Land O Lakes® Mare's Match® Foal Pellets *(Land O'Lakes)*
Lickables™ Charge Up!™ *(A.A.H.)*
Lickables™ Hearty Cat™ *(A.A.H.)*
Lickables™ Hearty Dog™ *(A.A.H.)*
Lickables™ Super Charger™ *(A.A.H.)*
Lipocaps *(Vetus)*
Lipo-Form *(Vet-A-Mix)*
Liquical™ *(Butler)*
Lixotinic® *(Pfizer Animal Health)*
Mare-Plus® *(Farnam)*
Maxum® Crumbles *(Horse Health)*
Methocol™ Capsules *(Life Science)*
Micro-Vet™ Equine Traditional Blend *(Boehringer Ingelheim)*
Milkin Mix *(Skylabs)*
Mineral Vet 5 *(Neogen)*
Mirra-Coat® (Equine System) *(Pet-Ag)*
Mirra-Coat® for Cats *(Pet-Ag)*
Mirra-Coat® Powder and Liquid *(Pet-Ag)*
Mrs. Allen's Shed-Stop® Granules for Cats *(Farnam)*
Mrs. Allen's Shed-Stop® Granules for Dogs *(Farnam)*
Mrs. Allen's Vita Care® Vitamins for Cats *(Farnam)*
Mrs. Allen's Vita Care® Vitamins for Dogs *(Farnam)*
MultiMax™ *(SureNutrition)*
NRG-Plus™ *(Bimeda)*
Nutra-Sure™ Cat Vitamins *(Farnam)*
Nutri-Cal® *(Evsco)*
Nutri-Cal® for Dogs and Cats *(Tomlyn)*
Nutri-Cal® for Ferrets *(Tomlyn)*
Nutri-Cal® for Ferrets & Other Small Animals *(Tomlyn)*
Nutri-Stat™ *(Tomlyn)*
NutriVed™ B-Complex Plus Iron Liquid *(Vedco)*
NutriVed™ Calcium Plus Chewable Tablets *(Vedco)*
NutriVed™ Chewable Vitamins for Active Dogs *(Vedco)*
NutriVed™ Chewable Vitamins for Cats *(Vedco)*
NutriVed™ Chewable Vitamins for Dogs *(Vedco)*
NutriVed™ Chewable Vitamins for Kittens *(Vedco)*
NutriVed™ Chewable Vitamins for Puppies *(Vedco)*
NutriVed™ Hypo Allergenic Chewable Tablets *(Vedco)*
NutriVed™ O.F.A. Chewable Tablets for Cats *(Vedco)*
NutriVed™ O.F.A. Chewable Tablets for Large Dogs *(Vedco)*
NutriVed™ O.F.A. Chewable Tablets for Small and Medium Dogs *(Vedco)*
NutriVed™ O.F.A. Gel Caps for Large Dogs *(Vedco)*
NutriVed™ O.F.A. Gel Caps for Small and Medium Size Dogs *(Vedco)*
NutriVed™ O.F.A. Granules for Cats *(Vedco)*
NutriVed™ O.F.A. Granules for Dogs *(Vedco)*
NutriVed™ O.F.A. Liquid *(Vedco)*
NutriVed™ Potassium Citrate Granules for Cats and Dogs *(Vedco)*
Omega-3 Fatty Acid Capsules for Large & Giant Breeds *(Vet Solutions)*
Omega-3 Fatty Acid Capsules for Medium Breeds *(Vet Solutions)*
Omega-3 Fatty Acid Capsules for Small Breeds *(Vet Solutions)*
Omega-3 Fatty Acid Liquid *(Vet Solutions)*
Omega EFA™ Capsules *(Butler)*
Omega EFA™ Capsules XS *(Butler)*
Omega EFA™ Liquid *(Butler)*
Omega EFA™ Liquid XS *(Butler)*
One Day Response™ *(Farnam, Livestock Div.)*
Osteo-Form Powder *(Vet-A-Mix)*
Palamega™ Complex Chewable Tablets (Liver Flavor) *(Schering-Plough)*
PerforMax™ Ration Maximizer *(Equicare)*
Pet-F.A. Liquid® *(Pfizer Animal Health)*
Pet-Form® *(Vet-A-Mix)*
Pet-Tabs® *(Pfizer Animal Health)*
Pet-Tabs®/F.A. Granules *(Pfizer Animal Health)*
Pet-Tabs® Jr. *(Pfizer Animal Health)*
Pet-Tabs® Plus *(Pfizer Animal Health)*
Pet-Tinic® *(Pfizer Animal Health)*
Pet Vites *(Vetus)*
Pet Vites O.F.A. Chewable Tablets *(Vetus)*
Phos-K™ Gel *(PRN Pharmacal)*
Pic-M-Up™ *(AgriPharm)*
Plexamino® Bolus *(Bimeda)*
Plex-Sol C *(Vet-A-Mix)*
Porcine Maximizer™ *(Novartis Animal Vaccines)*
PRN Hi-Energy Supplement™ *(PRN Pharmacal)*
Procal™ Powder *(Butler)*
Protobolic™ Bolus Improved *(Butler)*
Puppy Drops™ *(Tomlyn)*
Quick-Start™ *(Vedco)*
Red Alert *(Neogen)*
Red Cell® *(Horse Health)*
Redglo® *(Equicare)*
Rumen Yeast Caps Plus *(TechMix)*
Sergeant's® Vetscription® Vitamins for Cats & Kittens *(Sergeant's)*
Sergeant's® Vetscription® Vitamins for Dogs & Puppies *(Sergeant's)*
Show Winner!™ Cat Vitamins *(Farnam)*
Show Winner!™ Dog Vitamins *(Farnam)*
Show Winner!™ Kitten Vitamins *(Farnam)*
Show Winner!™ Older Dog Vitamins *(Farnam)*
Show Winner!™ Puppy Vitamins *(Farnam)*
Stam-N-Aid™ *(Neogen)*
Start To Finish® Energy Pak™ 100 *(Milk Specialties)*
Start To Finish® Mare & Foal Pellets™ *(Milk Specialties)*
Start To Finish® Performance Pellets™ *(Milk Specialties)*
Stat *(PRN Pharmacal)*

Stock Power *(LeGear)*
Stress-Dex® *(Neogen)*
Super 14™ *(Farnam)*
Super B-Plex *(Neogen)*
Superior-Vita-Min Blend™ *(Horses Prefer)*
Super Vitamins *(Alpharma)*
T.D.N. Mini Rockets *(DVM Formula)*
T.D.N. Mini Rockets™ *(Vets Plus)*
T.D.N. Rockets *(DVM Formula)*
T.D.N. Rockets™ *(Vets Plus)*
Tryptophan Plus Gel™ *(Horses Prefer)*
TunaVite™ *(Vedco)*
Unipet Nutritabs® *(Pharmacia & Upjohn)*
V.A.L.® Syrup *(Fort Dodge)*
Vionate® Vitamin Mineral Powder *(ARC)*
Vi-Sorbin® *(Pfizer Animal Health)*
Vi-Sorbits® *(Pfizer Animal Health)*
Vita-Key® Antioxidant Concentrate *(Vita-Key)*
Vita-Key® Biotin ZM-80 *(Vita-Key)*
Vita-Key® Brood Mare Supplement *(Vita-Key)*
Vita-Key® Equine Supplement *(Vita-Key)*
Vita-Key® Mare & Foal Supplement *(Vita-Key)*
Vitamin E & Selenium Powder *(AHC)*
Vitamins and Electrolytes *(Durvet)*
Vitamins and Electrolytes Concentrate *(Alpharma)*
Vitamins and Electrolytes Concentrate *(Durvet)*
Vitamins & Electrolytes "Plus" *(AgriLabs)*
Vita Plus® *(Farnam)*
Weight Builder™ *(Farnam)*
WGS *(Durvet)*
Zinc Plus™ Tablets *(Butler)*

water additives

B-Plus *(Alpharma)*
Breeder-Pak *(Alpharma)*
Broiler-Pak *(Alpharma)*
Ema-Sol™ Concentrate *(Alpharma)*
High Performance Poultry Pak *(Durvet)*
Liquid Vitamin Premix *(Alpharma)*
Multi-Pak/256 *(Alpharma)*
Poult Pak *(Alpharma)*
Propack-EXP *(Durvet)*
Vi-tal *(Loveland)*
Vitamins AD_3E Dispersible Liquid *(Alpharma)*
Vitamins & Electrolytes Concentrate *(Fort Dodge)*
Vitamins & Electrolytes (Soluble) *(Fort Dodge)*
Vitamins E-K-A Plus D_3 *(Alpharma)*
Vita Pak *(Alpharma)*
Zinpro Sulfate & dl-Methionine Liquid *(Alpharma)*

Multi-supplements with microorganisms

All-In-One Calf Bolus *(AgriPharm)*
All-In-One Cattle Bolus *(AgriPharm)*
Bird Bene-Bac™ Gel *(Pet-Ag)*
BP-1 Special Blend *(AgriPharm)*
Colostrum Bolus Forte *(Durvet)*
Colostrum-Plus *(Jorgensen)*
Colostrum Powder *(Vedco)*
Durazyme Calf Bolus *(Durvet)*
Durazyme Calf Colostrum Supplement *(Durvet)*
Durazyme Energy Pack *(Durvet)*
Durazyme Paste for Calves *(Durvet)*
Ener-Lyte™ *(Aspen)*
EP-1 3X *(RXV)*
Equi-Phar™ Equi-Vita-Phos *(Vedco)*
Equi-Phar™ LactoBac Gel *(Vedco)*
Fastbreak™ Plus™ *(Boehringer Ingelheim)*
Fastrack® Calf Bolus *(Conklin)*
Fastrack® Canine Gel *(Conklin)*
Fastrack® Equine Gel *(Conklin)*
Fastrack® Kick-Off *(Conklin)*
Fastrack® Liquid Dispersible *(Conklin)*
Fastrack® Liquid Dispersible-P *(Conklin)*
Fastrack® Nonruminant Microbial Gel *(Conklin)*
Fastrack® Ruminant Bolus *(Conklin)*
Fastrack® Ruminant Microbial Gel *(Conklin)*
Good Start Calf Bolus *(AgriPharm)*
Good Start Calf Paste *(AgriPharm)*
Greenlyte® *(Bimeda)*
Innocugel™ Equine *(Butler)*
K-Zyme® Cat Granules *(BioZyme)*
K-Zyme® Chewable Dog Tablets *(BioZyme)*
K-Zyme® Dog Granules *(BioZyme)*
MicroMaster® Alert™ Calf Bolus *(Loveland)*
MicroMaster® Avian PAC™ Soluble *(Loveland)*
MicroMaster® Avian PAC™ Soluble Plus *(Loveland)*
MicroMaster® Bovine Paste *(Loveland)*
MicroMaster® Calf PAC™ Soluble *(Loveland)*
MicroMaster® Dairy PAC™ *(Loveland)*
MicroMaster® Porcine PAC™ HT *(Loveland)*
MicroMaster® Porcine Paste *(Loveland)*
MicroMaster® Porcine Starter PAC™ *(Loveland)*
MicroMaster® Porcine Starter PAC™ Soluble *(Loveland)*
MicroZyme Bolus for Cattle *(Vedco)*
NutriVed™ EnerGel Forte *(Vedco)*
Oral Probiotic Calf Pak *(AgriPharm)*
Power Punch™ *(Vets Plus)*
PP-1 Special Blend *(AgriPharm)*
Pre-Conditioning/Receiving Formula Gel *(Durvet)*
Probios® Bovine One Oral Gel for Ruminants *(Chr. Hansen)*
Probios® Microbial Calf Pac *(Chr. Hansen)*
Probios® Oral Boluses for Ruminants *(Chr. Hansen)*
Probios® Oral Suspension for Swine *(Chr. Hansen)*
Probios® Plus Natural E Bovine One Oral Gel for Ruminants *(Chr. Hansen)*
Probiotic Plus E for Calves *(Vets Plus)*
Probiotic Plus E for Cattle *(Vets Plus)*
Probiotic Power™ *(Vets Plus)*
Revitilyte-Plus™ *(Vets Plus)*
Ruminant LactoBac Gel *(Vedco)*
Ruminant Lactobacillus Gel *(First Priority)*
RXV-PP-1 (Porcine Probiotic Paste) *(AgriPharm)*
Soluble Colostrum Powder *(Durvet)*
Sure-Start Plus *(AgriPharm)*
Vita Boost Paste™ *(AgriLabs)*
Vita Charge® 28 Dispersible Powder *(BioZyme)*
Vita Charge® Calf Bolus *(BioZyme)*
Vita Charge® Equine *(BioZyme)*
Vita Charge® Gel Cap *(BioZyme)*
Vita Charge® Paste *(BioZyme)*
Vita Ferm® Breeder Booster+Mag *(BioZyme)*
Vita Ferm® Cattleman's Beefmaker *(BioZyme)*
Vita Ferm® Cattleman's Beefmaker+Mag *(BioZyme)*
Vita Ferm® Concept-Aid *(BioZyme)*
Vita Ferm® Concept-Aid+Mag *(BioZyme)*
Vita Ferm® Concept-Aid A•P *(BioZyme)*
Vita Ferm® Cow Calf 5 *(BioZyme)*
Vita Ferm® Dairy Basemix 12:16 *(BioZyme)*
Vita Ferm® Dairy Basemix 18:6 *(BioZyme)*
Vita Ferm® Dairy Basemix 18:12 *(BioZyme)*
Vita Ferm® Equine *(BioZyme)*
Vita Ferm® Ewe and Lamb *(BioZyme)*
Vita Ferm® Far Out Dry Cow *(BioZyme)*
Vita Ferm® Feedlot Formula *(BioZyme)*
Vita Ferm® Fescue Fiber Buster *(BioZyme)*
Vita Ferm® Fescue Power Keg *(BioZyme)*
Vita Ferm® Formula *(BioZyme)*
Vita Ferm® Grass Enhancer *(BioZyme)*
Vita Ferm® High Mag *(BioZyme)*
Vita Ferm® Natural Protein Pasture Formula (NPPF) *(BioZyme)*
Vita Ferm® Pasture Formula *(BioZyme)*
Vita Ferm® Power Keg *(BioZyme)*
Vita Ferm® Pro-Gest *(BioZyme)*
Vita Ferm® Pro-Gest 30 *(BioZyme)*
Vita Ferm® Roughage Fortifier *(BioZyme)*
Vita Ferm® Sheep & Goat Keg *(BioZyme)*
Vita Ferm® Sure Champ and Vita Start Pellets *(BioZyme)*
Vita Ferm® Sure Start 2 *(BioZyme)*
Vita Ferm® Sure Start Pac *(BioZyme)*
Vita Ferm® Up Close Dry Cow *(BioZyme)*
Vita Ferm® Vita Grow 32 Natural *(BioZyme)*
Vita-Key® Show Cattle Concentrate, Phase II *(Vita-Key)*
Vita-Key® Show Cattle Supplement, Phase I *(Vita-Key)*
Vita-Key® Swine Supplement *(Vita-Key)*
Vita-Lyte *(Phoenix Pharmaceutical)*
Vit-E-Lyte "Plus" *(Bimeda)*
Yellow Lite *(AgriPharm)*

Niacin

oral

Nia-Bol™ *(Great States)*
Niacin Bolus *(Vets Plus)*
Nu-Keto™ Bolus *(Butler)*

Phosphorus

injectable

Phos-Aid *(Butler)*
Phos-Aid Solution *(Neogen)*
Phos P 200 *(Phoenix Pharmaceutical)*
Phosphaid Injection *(Vedco)*

Potassium

oral

NutriVed™ Hypo-K Granules *(Vedco)*
Potassium Gel *(Butler)*
Potassium Powder *(Butler)*
Potassium Tablets *(Butler)*
RenaKare™ *(Neogen)*
Tumil-K® *(King Animal Health)*
Tumil-K® Gel *(King Animal Health)*

Vitamin B - biotin

oral / feed additives / water additives

Bio-Hoof™ *(Horses Prefer)*
Bio-Meth *(Vet-A-Mix)*
Biotin-100 *(Vet-A-Mix)*
Biotin™ Gold *(SureNutrition)*
Dealer Select Horse Care Biotin 800 *(Durvet)*
Equi-Phar™ dl-Methionine with Biotin Powder *(Vedco)*
Horse Care Biotin Crumbles *(Durvet)*
Vita•Biotin™ Crumbles *(Horse Health)*
Vita-Min Biotin *(Farnam)*

Vitamin B complex

injectable

AmTech Vitamin B Complex *(Phoenix Scientific)*
AmTech Vitamin B Complex Fortified *(Phoenix Scientific)*
B-Comject 150 *(Vetus)*
B-Comject Forte *(Vetus)*
B Complex One-Fifty Injection *(Vedco)*
B-Complex-Plus *(AgriLabs)*
Fortified Vitamin B Complex *(AgriLabs)*
Fortified Vitamin B-Complex *(AgriPharm)*
High Level Vitamin B Complex *(Durvet)*
Hi-Po B Complex™ *(Butler)*
Liver 7 Injection *(Neogen)*
Maxi-B 1000 *(Durvet)*
Methaplex Injection *(PRN Pharmacal)*
Super B Complex *(Vedco)*
Vita-Jec® B-Complex *(AgriPharm)*
Vita-Jec® B Complex Fortified *(AgriPharm)*
Vita-Jec® B-Complex with Cyano Plus *(AgriPharm)*
Vitamin B-Complex *(AgriLabs)*
Vitamin B Complex *(AgriPharm)*
Vitamin B Complex *(Aspen)*
Vitamin B Complex *(Butler)*
Vitamin B Complex *(Durvet)*
Vitamin B Complex *(Phoenix Pharmaceutical)*
Vitamin B Complex *(Vedco)*
Vitamin B Complex Forte Injection *(Bimeda)*
Vitamin B Complex Fortified *(Aspen)*
Vitamin B Complex Fortified *(Phoenix Pharmaceutical)*
Vitamin B Complex with Cyano Plus *(AgriPharm)*

oral / feed additives / water additives

Lipotinic *(Vet-A-Mix)*
Liquid B Complex *(Alpharma)*

Vitamin B1 (thiamine)

injectable

AmTech Thiamine Hydrochloride Injection *(Phoenix Scientific)*
Thiamine Hydrochloride *(Vet Tek)*
Thiamine Hydrochloride 200 mg *(Neogen)*
Thiamine Hydrochloride 500 mg *(Neogen)*
Thiamine Hydrochloride Injection *(Butler)*
Thiamine Hydrochloride Injection *(Phoenix Pharmaceutical)*
Thiamine Hydrochloride Injection *(Vedco)*
Thiamine Hydrochloride Solution *(Phoenix Pharmaceutical)*
Vita-Jec® Thiamine HCl *(RXV)*

oral / feed additives / water additives

B-1 Powder *(SureNutrition)*
Thia-Dex *(Neogen)*
Vita•B-1 Crumbles *(Horse Health)*
Vita•B-1 Powder *(Horse Health)*
Vitamin B-1 Powder *(AHC)*

Vitamin B12 (cyanocobalamine)

injectable

AmTech Vitamin B_{12} 1000 mcg *(Phoenix Scientific)*
AmTech Vitamin B_{12} 3000 mcg *(Phoenix Scientific)*
AmTech Vitamin B_{12} 5000 mcg *(Phoenix Scientific)*
B12-Ject 1000 *(Vetus)*
B12-Ject 3000 *(Vetus)*
Vita-Jec® Vitamin B_{12} (Cyano 1,000 mcg/mL) *(RXV)*
Vita-Jec® Vitamin B_{12} (Cyano 3,000 mcg/mL) *(RXV)*
Vitamin B12 *(Butler)*

Please refer to product listings for more complete information.

Vitamin B_{12} *(Vedco)*
Vitamin B_{12} 1000 mcg *(Phoenix Pharmaceutical)*
Vitamin B_{12} 1000 mcg *(Vet Tek)*
Vitamin B_{12} 1000 mcg Injection *(Aspen)*
Vitamin B_{12} 3000 mcg *(Neogen)*
Vitamin B_{12} 3000 mcg *(Phoenix Pharmaceutical)*
Vitamin B_{12} 3000 mcg *(Vet Tek)*
Vitamin B_{12} 5000 mcg *(Neogen)*
Vitamin B_{12} 5000 mcg *(Phoenix Pharmaceutical)*
Vitamin B_{12} Injection 1000 mcg *(Bimeda)*
Vitamin B_{12} Injection (1,000 mcg/mL) *(AgriLabs)*
Vitamin B_{12} Injection 3000 mcg *(Bimeda)*
Vitamin B_{12} Injection (3,000 mcg/mL) *(AgriLabs)*
Vitamin B_{12} Injection 5000 mcg *(Bimeda)*

Vitamin C

injectable
AmTech Vitamin C Injectable Solution *(Phoenix Scientific)*
Sodium Ascorbate *(Neogen)*
Sodium Ascorbate *(RXV)*
Sodium Ascorbate Injection *(Vedco)*
Vitamin C *(AgriLabs)*
Vitamin C *(Butler)*
Vitamin C *(Phoenix Pharmaceutical)*
Vitamin C *(Vet Tek)*

oral / feed additives
Dealer Select Horse Care DurVit C Powder *(Durvet)*
Stabilized-C *(Alpharma)*

Vitamin D

oral / feed additives / water additives
Color-Guard® 500 *(Alpharma)*
Color-Guard® 1000 *(Alpharma)*
High-D 2X Dispersible *(Alpharma)*
Micro-D® 500 *(Alpharma)*
Micro-D® 1000 *(Alpharma)*
Solumine *(Durvet)*

Vitamin E

injection
Dl-Alpha Tocopherol Acetate Injection *(Vedco)*
EmulsiVit E-300 *(Vedco)*
Vita E 300 *(AgriPharm)*
Vital E®-300 *(Schering-Plough)*
Vitamin E-300 *(AgriLabs)*
Vitamin E 300 *(Durvet)*

oral / feed additives / water additives
Dealer Select Horse Care DurVit E Powder *(Durvet)*
Folic Acid & Vitamin E Powder *(AHC)*
Vitamin E Dispersible Liquid *(Alpharma)*

Vitamin E + selenium

injectable
BO-SE® *(Schering-Plough)*
E-SE® *(Schering-Plough)*
MU-SE® *(Schering-Plough)*
Velenium™ *(Fort Dodge)*

oral / feed additives / water additives
Equ-SeE *(Vet-A-Mix)*
Equ-Se5E *(Vet-A-Mix)*
Prosel-300 *(Durvet)*
Sure E&SE™ *(SureNutrition)*
Vita•E & Selenium Powder *(Horse Health)*
Vita•E & Selenium Crumbles™ *(Horse Health)*
Vita-Min E & Selenium *(Farnam)*

Vitamin K

injectable
AmTech Vitamin K_1 Injection *(Phoenix Scientific)*
K-Ject *(Vetus)*
Veda-K_1 Injection *(Vedco)*
Veta-K_1® Injection *(Bimeda)*
Vita-Jec® Vitamin K1 Injectable *(RXV)*
Vitamin K_1 *(Vet Tek)*
Vitamin K_1 Injection *(Butler)*
Vitamin K_1 Injection *(Neogen)*
Vitamin K_1 Injection *(Phoenix Pharmaceutical)*

oral / water additives
K-Caps *(Vetus)*
K-Sol *(Alpharma)*
Veda-K_1 Capsules *(Vedco)*
Veta-K_1® Capsules *(Bimeda)*
Vitamin K_1 Oral Capsules *(Butler)*
Vitamin K_1 Oral Capsules *(Phoenix Pharmaceutical)*
Vitamin K-1 Oral Capsules *(RXV)*

Vitamins A, D, and/or E, injectable combinations
A-D Injection *(Durvet)*
EmulsiVit E/A&D *(Vedco)*
Vita E-AD *(AgriPharm)*
Vita-Jec® A & D "500" *(AgriPharm)*
Vital E®+A *(Schering-Plough)*
Vital E®-A+D *(Schering-Plough)*
Vitamin AD_3 *(AgriLabs)*
Vitamin AD *(Butler)*
Vitamin A & D *(Vedco)*
Vitamin A & D "500" *(AgriPharm)*
Vitamin AD Injection *(Aspen)*
Vitamin AD_3 Injection *(Bimeda)*
Vitamin AD Injection *(Phoenix Pharmaceutical)*
Vitamin E+AD *(Durvet)*
Vitamin E-AD 300 *(AgriLabs)*

Zinc

feed additives
Availa® Zn 40 *(Zinpro)*
Availa® Zn 100 *(Zinpro)*
Zinpro 40 *(Zinpro)*
Zinpro 100 *(Zinpro)*
Zinpro 180 *(Zinpro)*

oral
NutriVed™ Chewable Zinpro® Tablets *(Vedco)*

BIOLOGICALS

ALLERGY ANTIGENS

ANTIBODIES (immunoglobins)

Injectable

Oral

TETANUS TOXOIDS and ANTITOXINS

VACCINES and OTHER BIOLOGICALS

Please refer to product listings for more complete information.

Please refer to product listings for more complete information.

Please refer to product listings for more complete information.

PARASITICIDES

ANTHELMINTICS

Anthelmintics (roundworms / hookworms / whipworms)

Champion Protector™ Worm Protector™ 2X *(AgriLabs)*
D-Worm™ 60 Liquid Wormer *(Farnam)*
D-Worm™ 120 Liquid Wormer *(Farnam)*
D-Worm™ Dog Wormer Chewable Tablets for Large Dogs *(Farnam)*
D-Worm™ Dog Wormer Chewable Tablets for Puppies & Small Dogs *(Farnam)*
D-Worm™ Dog Wormer Tablets for Large Dogs *(Farnam)*
D-Worm™ Dog Wormer Tablets for Puppies & Small Dogs *(Farnam)*
Happy Jack® Liqui-Vict 2X™ *(Happy Jack)*
Nemex™ Tabs *(Pfizer Animal Health)*
Nemex™ -2 Suspension *(Pfizer Animal Health)*
Pet Care Liquid Wormer *(Durvet)*
Pet Care Liquid Wormer 2X *(Durvet)*
RFD® Liquid Wormer *(Pfizer Animal Health)*
Sergeant's® Vetscription® Sure Shot® Liquid Wormer for Puppies and Dogs *(Sergeant's)*

Anthelmintics (roundworms only)

D-Worm™ Liquid Wormer for Cats and Dogs *(Farnam)*
Hartz® Health measures™ Liquid Wormer *(Hartz Mountain)*
Hartz® Health measures™ Once-a-month® Wormer for Cats and Kittens *(Hartz Mountain)*
Hartz® Health measures™ Once-a-month® Wormer for Dogs *(Hartz Mountain)*
Hartz® Health measures™ Once-a-month® Wormer for Large Dogs *(Hartz Mountain)*
Hartz® Health measures™ Once-a-month® Wormer for Puppies *(Hartz Mountain)*
Pipa-Tabs *(Vet-A-Mix)*
Sergeant's® Vetscription® Sure Shot® Liquid Wormer for Cats & Kittens *(Sergeant's)*
Sergeant's® Vetscription® Worm-Away® for Cats *(Sergeant's)*
Sergeant's® Vetscription® Worm-Away® for Dogs *(Sergeant's)*
Tasty Paste® Dog & Puppy Wormer *(Farnam)*

Cestocides

Cestex® *(Pfizer Animal Health)*
Droncit® (praziquantel) Canine Tablets *(Bayer)*
Droncit® (praziquantel) Feline Tablets *(Bayer)*
Droncit® (praziquantel) Injectable for Dogs and Cats *(Bayer)*
Happy Jack® Tapeworm Tablets *(Happy Jack)*
Tape Worm Tabs™ for Cats and Kittens *(TradeWinds)*
Tape Worm Tabs™ for Dogs and Puppies *(TradeWinds)*

Cestocides / anthelmintics

Drontal® (praziquantel/pyrantel pamoate) Tablets *(Bayer)*
Drontal® Plus (praziquantel/pyrantel pamoate/febantel) Tablets *(Bayer)*
Panacur® Granules 22.2% *(Intervet)*
Panacur® Granules 22.2% (Dogs only) *(Intervet)*

Feed medications (Type A)

Atgard® C *(Boehringer Ingelheim)*
Atgard® Swine Wormer *(Boehringer Ingelheim)*
Banminth® 48 *(Phibro)*
Hygromix® 8 (Chickens) *(Elanco)*
Hygromix® 8 (Swine) *(Elanco)*
Ivomec® Premix for Swine Type A Medicated Article *(Merial)*
MoorMan's® Moorguard® Swine Dewormer *(ADM)*
Rumatel® *(Phibro)*
Safe-Guard® 20% Dewormer Type A Medicated Article *(Intervet)*

Feed medications (Type B)

Strongid® C *(Pfizer Animal Health)*
Strongid® C 2X™ *(Pfizer Animal Health)*
Strongid® C Thirty *(Pfizer Animal Health)*

Injectable

AmTech Levamisole Phosphate Injectable Solution *(Phoenix Scientific)*
Levamisole Injectable *(AgriLabs)*
Levamisole Phosphate *(Durvet)*
Levamisole Phosphate Injectable Solution, 13.65% *(AgriPharm)*
Levamisole Phosphate Injectable Solution, 13.65% *(Aspen)*
Levasole® Injectable Solution, 13.65% *(Schering-Plough)*

Oral

Alfalfa Pellet Horse Wormer *(Farnam)*
AmTech Anthelban V *(Phoenix Scientific)*
Anthelban V *(Phoenix Pharmaceutical)*
Anthelcide® EQ Equine Wormer Paste *(Pfizer Animal Health)*
Anthelcide® EQ Equine Wormer Suspension *(Pfizer Animal Health)*
Benzelmin® Paste *(Fort Dodge)*
Continuex™ *(Farnam)*
Curatrem® *(Merial)*
Dealer Select Horse Care Horse & Colt Wormer *(Durvet)*
Equi Aid CW® *(Equi Aid)*
Equi-Phar™ Horse & Colt Wormer *(Vedco)*
Equi-Phar ProTal™ *(Vedco)*
Exodus™ Paste *(Bimeda)*
Ivomec® Sheep Drench *(Merial)*
Ivomec® SR Bolus *(Merial)*
Levasole® Cattle Wormer Boluses *(Schering-Plough)*
Levasole® Sheep Wormer Boluses *(Schering-Plough)*
Levasole® Soluble Drench Powder *(Schering-Plough)*
Levasole® Soluble Drench Powder (Sheep) *(Schering-Plough)*
Panacur® Beef and Dairy Cattle Dewormer *(Intervet)*
Panacur® Cattle Dewormer *(Intervet)*
Panacur® Cattle Dewormer (92 g) *(Intervet)*
Panacur® Granules 22.2% (Horse) *(Intervet)*
Panacur® Horse Dewormer *(Intervet)*
Panacur® Horse Dewormer (25 g) *(Intervet)*
Panacur® Horse Dewormer (57 g) *(Intervet)*
Panacur® Horse Dewormer (92 g) *(Intervet)*
Piperazine-17 Medicated *(Durvet)*
Privermectin™ Drench for Sheep *(First Priority)*
Prohibit® Soluble Drench Powder *(AgriLabs)*
Rotectin™ 2 Paste *(Farnam)*
Safe-Guard® Beef & Dairy Cattle Dewormer *(Intervet)*
Safe-Guard® Beef and Dairy Cattle Dewormer (290 g) *(Intervet)*
Safe-Guard® Cattle Dewormer (92 g) *(Intervet)*
Safe-Guard® Equine Dewormer (25 g) *(Intervet)*
Safe-Guard® Horse Dewormer (92 g) *(Intervet)*
Safe-Guard® Medicated Dewormer for Beef & Dairy Cattle, & Swine *(Intervet)*
Safe-Guard® Medicated Dewormer for Beef & Dairy Cattle (Flaked Meal) *(Intervet)*
Safe-Guard® Medicated Dewormer for Beef & Dairy Cattle (Soft Mini-Pellets) *(Intervet)*
Safe-Guard® Medicated Dewormer for Beef Cattle (20% Protein Block) *(Intervet)*
Safe-Guard® Medicated Dewormer for Beef Cattle (En-Pro-Al® Molasses Block) *(Intervet)*
Safe-Guard® Medicated Dewormer for Swine (EZ Scoop®) *(Intervet)*
Strongid® Paste *(Pfizer Animal Health)*
Strongid® T *(Pfizer Animal Health)*
Sweetlix® Safe-Guard® 20% Natural Protein Deworming Block for Beef Cattle *(Sweetlix)*
Sweetlix® Safe-Guard* Free-Choice Mineral Cattle Dewormer *(Sweetlix)*
Synanthic® Bovine Dewormer Suspension, 9.06% *(Fort Dodge)*
Synanthic® Bovine Dewormer Suspension, 22.5% *(Fort Dodge)*
Valbazen® Cattle Dewormer Paste *(Pfizer Animal Health)*
Valbazen® Suspension *(Pfizer Animal Health)*
Wonder Wormer™ for Horses *(Farnam)*

Topical

Totalon® Pour-On Dewormer *(Schering-Plough)*

Water medications

Levamisole Soluble Pig Wormer *(AgriLabs)*
Levasole® Soluble Pig Wormer *(Schering-Plough)*
Wazine® 17 *(Fleming)*
Wazine® 34 *(Fleming)*
Wazine® Soluble *(Fleming)*

ECTOPARASITE CONTROL, LARGE ANIMALS

Feed medications

MoorMan's® Hi-Mag IGR Minerals® *(ADM)*
MoorMan's® IGR Minerals® *(ADM)*

ENDECTOCIDES (systemic parasiticides)

Injectable

AmTech Phoenectin® Injection for Cattle and Swine *(Phoenix Scientific)*
Dectomax® Injectable Solution *(Pfizer Animal Health)*
Double Impact™ *(AgriLabs)*
Ivercide™ Injection for Cattle and Swine *(Phoenix Pharmaceutical)*
Ivermectin Injection for Cattle and Swine *(Aspen)*
Ivermectin Injection for Cattle and Swine *(Durvet)*
Ivomec® 0.27% Injection for Grower and Feeder Pigs *(Merial)*
Ivomec® 1% Injection for Cattle and Swine *(Merial)*
Ivomec® 1% Injection for Swine *(Merial)*
Ivomec® Plus Injection for Cattle *(Merial)*
Produmec™ Injection for Cattle and Swine *(TradeWinds)*
ProMectin™ Injection for Cattle and Swine *(Vedco)*
UltraMectrin™ Injection *(RXV)*

Oral

Agri-Mectin™ Equine Paste Dewormer 1.87% *(AgriLabs)*
AmTech Phoenectin® Liquid for Horses *(Phoenix Scientific)*
AmTech Phoenectin® Paste 1.87% *(Phoenix Scientific)*
Cooper's® Best Ivermectin Paste 1.87% *(Aspen)*
DVMectin™ Liquid for Horses *(DVM)*
Equimectrin™ Paste 1.87% *(Farnam)*
Equimectrin® Paste 1.87% *(Merial)*
Eqvalan® Liquid *(Merial)*
Eqvalan® Paste 1.87% *(Merial)*
Horse Care Ivermectin Paste 1.87% *(Durvet)*
Ivercide™ Equine Paste 1.87% *(Phoenix Pharmaceutical)*
Ivercide™ Liquid for Horses *(Phoenix Pharmaceutical)*
Iversol *(Med-Pharmex)*
Privermectin™ Equine Oral Liquid *(First Priority)*
ProMectin E™ Liquid for Horses *(Vedco)*
ProMectin E™ Paste *(Vedco)*
Quest® 2% Equine Oral Gel *(Fort Dodge)*
Rotectin™ 1 Paste 1.87% *(Farnam)*
Zimecterin® Paste 1.87% *(Farnam)*
Zimecterin® Paste 1.87% *(Merial)*

Spot treatments

Revolution® *(Pfizer Animal Health)*

Topical insecticides

AmTech Phoenectin® Pour-On for Cattle *(Phoenix Scientific)*
Bimectin™ Pour-On *(Bimeda)*
Cydectin® Pour-On *(Fort Dodge)*
Dectomax® Pour-On *(Pfizer Animal Health)*
Ivercide™ Pour-On for Cattle *(Phoenix Pharmaceutical)*
Ivermectin Pour-On *(Aspen)*
Ivermectin Pour-On *(Durvet)*
Iver-On™ *(Med-Pharmex)*
Ivomec® Eprinex® Pour-On for Beef and Dairy Cattle *(Merial)*
Ivomec® Pour-On for Cattle *(Merial)*
Produmec™ Pour-On for Cattle *(TradeWinds)*
ProMectin B™ Pour-On For Cattle *(Vedco)*
Prozap® Ivermectin Pour-On *(Loveland)*
Top Line™ *(AgriLabs)*
UltraMectrin™ Pour-On *(RXV)*

EXTERNAL PARASITICIDES and INSECTICIDES

External parasiticides, livestock and/or others

insecticide ear tags

Atroban® Extra Insecticide Ear Tags *(Schering-Plough)*
Commando™ Insecticide Cattle Ear Tag *(Boehringer Ingelheim)*
Co-Ral® Plus Insecticide Cattle Ear Tag *(Bayer)*
CyLence® Ultra Insecticide Cattle Ear Tag *(Bayer)*
Dominator® Insecticide Ear Tags *(Schering-Plough)*
Double Barrel™ VP Insecticide Ear Tags *(Schering-Plough)*

Ectrin® Insecticide Cattle Ear Tag *(Boehringer Ingelheim)*
New Z® Diazinon Insecticide Cattle Ear Tags *(Farnam)*
New Z® Permethrin Insecticide Cattle Ear Tags *(Farnam)*
Patriot™ Insecticide Cattle Ear Tags *(Boehringer Ingelheim)*
Saber™ Extra Insecticide Ear Tags *(Schering-Plough)*

topical and premise insecticides

Absorbine® Flys-X® Insecticide *(W. F. Young)*
Absorbine® UltraShield® Brand Fly Repellent *(W. F. Young)*
Animal Insecticide *(Durvet)*
Atroban® 11% EC Insecticide *(Schering-Plough)*
Atroban® 42.5% EC *(Schering-Plough)*
Clean Crop® Malathion 57EC *(Loveland)*
Dairy Bomb-50 *(Durvet)*
Dairy Bomb-50Z *(Durvet)*
Dairy Bomb-55 *(Durvet)*
Dairy Bomb-55Z *(Durvet)*
Ecosect™ Insecticide *(Schering-Plough)*
Ectiban® EC *(Durvet)*
Ectiban® Synergized DeLice® Pour-On Insecticide *(Durvet)*
EctoZap™ Plus Pour-On Insecticide *(Aspen)*
Exit™ II Synergized Formula Insecticide *(AgriPharm)*
Fly-Rid Plus *(Durvet)*
Louse Powder with Rabon® *(LeGear)*
MoorMan's® Fly Spray *(ADM)*
Permectrin™ II *(Aspen)*
Permectrin™ II *(Boehringer Ingelheim)*
Permectrin™ CDS Pour-On *(Boehringer Ingelheim)*
Permethrin 10% *(Durvet)*
Prozap® Aqueous Fly Spray *(Loveland)*
Prozap® Beef & Dairy Spray RTU *(Loveland)*
Prozap® Dairy & Feedlot Insecticide Concentrate *(Loveland)*
Prozap® Drycide® *(Loveland)*
Prozap® Dust'R™ *(Loveland)*
Prozap® Garden & Poultry Dust *(Loveland)*
Prozap® Insectrin® Dust *(Loveland)*
Prozap® Insectrin® X *(Loveland)*
Prozap® VIP Insect Spray *(Loveland)*
Pyrethrin Plus *(Durvet)*
Rabon® 50% WP *(Boehringer Ingelheim)*
Ravap® E.C. *(Boehringer Ingelheim)*
SK-Surekill® Brand Pyrethrin Plus Fly Spray *(IntAgra)*
Super II Dairy & Farm Spray *(Durvet)*
Synergized DeLice® Pour-On Insecticide *(Schering-Plough)*

topical insecticides

1% Permethrin Pour-On *(Durvet)*
3% Rabon® Livestock Dust *(Durvet)*
Absorbine® Concentrated Fly Repellent *(W. F. Young)*
Adams™ Fly Repellent Concentrate *(V.P.L.)*
Adams™ Fly Spray and Repellent *(V.P.L.)*
Atroban® DeLice® Pour-On Insecticide *(Schering-Plough)*
Back Side® *(AgriLabs)*
Back Side™ Plus *(AgriLabs)*
Boss® Pour-On Insecticide *(Schering-Plough)*
Bronco® Water-Base Equine Fly Spray *(Farnam)*
Buzz Off™ Pour-On *(Boehringer Ingelheim)*
Catron™ IV *(Boehringer Ingelheim)*
Co-Ral® 1% *(Durvet)*
Co-Ral® (coumaphos) Emulsifiable Livestock Insecticide Restricted Use Pesticide *(Bayer)*
Co-Ral® Equine and Livestock Dust *(AgriLabs)*
Co-Ral® (coumaphos) Flowable Insecticide Restricted Use Pesticide *(Bayer)*
Co-Ral® (coumaphos) Fly and Tick Spray *(Bayer)*
CyLence® Pour-On Insecticide *(Bayer)*
Dealer Select Horse Care Permeth 5 Fly Spray *(Durvet)*
Del-Phos® Emulsifiable Liquid Insecticide *(Schering-Plough)*
Durasect™ Long-Acting Livestock Pour-On *(Pfizer Animal Health)*
Durasect® II Long-Acting Livestock Pour-On *(Pfizer Animal Health)*
Ectiban® D *(Durvet)*
Ectiban® DeLice® *(Durvet)*
EctoKyl™ 3X Flea & Tick Shampoo *(DVM)*
EctoZap™ Pour-On Insecticide *(Aspen)*
Exit™ Insecticide *(AgriPharm)*
Flea & Tick Mist *(Davis)*
FlyPel® Insecticide Spray for Horses *(Virbac)*
Flysect® Citronella Spray *(Equicare)*
Flysect® Super-7 *(Equicare)*
Flysect® Super-C *(Equicare)*
Flysect® Water-Based Repellent Spray *(Equicare)*
Horse Lice Duster™ III *(Farnam)*
MoorMan's® Dust with Co-Ral® Insecticide *(ADM)*
Permectrin™ Fly & Louse Dust *(Boehringer Ingelheim)*
Permectrin™ Pour-On *(Boehringer Ingelheim)*
Permethrin 0.25% Dust *(AgriLabs)*
Poridon™ *(Neogen)*
Prolate®/Lintox®-HD *(Wellmark)*
Prozap® Zipcide® *(Loveland)*
Rabon® 3% Dust *(AgriLabs)*
Repel-X® Insecticide & Repellent *(Farnam)*
Repel-X®p Emulsifiable Fly Spray *(Farnam)*
Saber™ Pour-On Insecticide *(Schering-Plough)*
Screwworm Ear Tick Aerosol *(Durvet)*
Taktic® E.C. *(Intervet)*
Ultra Boss® Pour-On Insecticide *(Schering-Plough)*
Warbex® Famphur Pour-On for Cattle *(Schering-Plough)*
Wipe® Fly Protectant *(Farnam)*
Wipe® II Brand Fly Spray with Citronella *(Farnam)*

Flea + tick killers

collars

Adams™ Delta Force™ Tick Collar for Dogs *(Farnam)*
Adams™ Dual Action Flea & Tick Collar for Cats *(Farnam)*
Adams™ Dual Action Flea & Tick Collar for Large Dogs *(Farnam)*
Adams™ Dual Action Flea & Tick Collar for Medium Dogs *(Farnam)*
Bansect® Flea & Tick Collar for Cats *(Sergeant's)*
Bansect® Flea & Tick Collar for Dogs *(Sergeant's)*
Happy Jack® Novation™ Flea & Tick Collar for Dogs *(Happy Jack)*
Hartz® 2 in 1® Flea & Tick Collar for Cats and Kittens *(Hartz Mountain)*
Hartz® 2 in 1® Flea & Tick Collar for Dogs and Puppies *(Hartz Mountain)*
Longlife® 90 Day™ Brand Collar for Cats *(Hartz Mountain)*
Longlife® 90 Day™ Brand Collar for Dogs *(Hartz Mountain)*
Preventef® Flea and Tick Collar for Cats *(Virbac)*
Preventef® Flea and Tick Collar for Dogs *(Virbac)*
Scratchex® Flea & Tick Collar for Cats *(Combe)*
Scratchex® Flea & Tick Collar for Dogs *(Combe)*
Vet-Kem® Breakaway® Flea & Tick Collar for Cats *(Wellmark)*
Vet-Kem® Breakaway® Plus Flea & Tick Collar for Cats *(Wellmark)*
Vet-Kem® Tickaway™ Tick Collar for Dogs *(Wellmark)*

dips, lotions and creams

Adams™ Flea & Tick Shampoo *(V.P.L.)*
Brilliance™ Flea & Tick Shampoo *(First Priority)*
Davis Pyrethrins *(Davis)*
Duocide® Shampoo *(Virbac)*
Hartz® 2 in 1® Flea & Tick Dip for Dogs and Cats *(Hartz Mountain)*

powders

Hartz® 2 in 1® Flea & Tick Powder for Cats *(Hartz Mountain)*
Hartz® 2 in 1® Flea & Tick Powder for Dogs *(Hartz Mountain)*
Ritter's Tick and Flea Powder *(Ritter)*

shampoos and foams

Adams™ D-Limonene Flea & Tick Shampoo *(Farnam)*
Ecto-Foam™ *(Virbac)*
Hartz® 2 in 1® Rid Flea™ Dog Shampoo with Allethrin *(Hartz Mountain)*
Hartz® 2 in 1® Rid Flea™ Dog Shampoo with Pyrethrin *(Hartz Mountain)*
Make Your Own Flea & Tick Shampoo *(Davis)*
Mycodex® Pet Shampoo with 3X Pyrethrins *(V.P.L.)*
Mycodex® SensiCare™ Flea & Tick Shampoo *(V.P.L.)*
Scratchex® Flea & Tick Shampoo *(Combe)*
Sheen II Shampoo *(Butler)*
Sungro Flea-ZY Pet Shampoo *(Sungro)*

spot treatments

Bansect® Squeeze-On Flea & Tick Control for Dogs (under 33 lbs) *(Sergeant's)*
Bansect® Squeeze-On Flea & Tick Control for Dogs (over 33 lbs) *(Sergeant's)*
Defend® EXspot® Treatment for Dogs *(Schering-Plough)*
Frontline® Top Spot® for Cats & Kittens *(Merial)*
Frontline® Top Spot® for Dogs & Puppies *(Merial)*
Scratchex® 30 Day Flea & Tick Treatment (30 lbs. & under) *(Combe)*
Scratchex® 30 Day Flea & Tick Treatment (over 30 lbs.) *(Combe)*

sprays

Duocide® L.A. Spray *(Virbac)*
Frontline® Spray Treatment for Cats & Dogs *(Merial)*
Happy Jack® DD-33™ Flea & Tick Mist *(Happy Jack)*
Hartz® 2 in 1® Flea & Tick Spray for Cats *(Hartz Mountain)*
Hartz® 2 in 1® Flea & Tick Spray for Dogs *(Hartz Mountain)*
Hartz® Control Pet Care System® Flea & Tick Repellent for Cats *(Hartz Mountain)*
Hartz® Control Pet Care System® Flea & Tick Repellent for Dogs *(Hartz Mountain)*
Mycodex® SensiCare™ Flea & Tick Spray *(V.P.L.)*
Scratchex® Flea & Tick Spray *(Combe)*
SynerKyl® AQ Water-Based Pet Spray *(DVM)*

Flea control (early stage inhibitors)

collars

Virbac KnockOut® IGR Flea Collar for Cats & Kittens *(Virbac)*
Virbac KnockOut® IGR Flea Collar for Dogs & Puppies *(Virbac)*

injectable

Program® 6 Month Injectable for Cats *(Novartis)*

oral

Hartz® Advanced Care® Brand™ Flea Control Capsules™ for Dogs *(Hartz Mountain)*
Program® Flavor Tabs® *(Novartis)*
Program® Suspension *(Novartis)*

premises

Adams™ Room Fogger with Sykillstop™ *(Farnam)*
Adams™ Room Fogger with Sykillstop™ *(V.P.L.)*
EctoKyl® IGR Emulsifiable Concentrate *(DVM)*

spot treatments

Hartz® Control Pet Care System® OneSpot® for Cats and Kittens *(Hartz Mountain)*
Sergeant's® PreTect® Squeeze-On Flea Control for Cats *(Sergeant's)*
Vet-Kem® Ovitrol® Spot On® Flea Control for Cats *(Wellmark)*

sprays

Adams™ Flea & Tick Mist with Sykillstop™ *(Farnam)*
Adams™ Flea & Tick Mist with Sykillstop™ *(V.P.L.)*
OmniTrol IGR 1.3% Emulsifiable Concentrate *(Vedco)*

Flea control with flea killers

collars

Preventic® Collar for Dogs *(Virbac)*

premises

EctoKyl™ IGR Pressurized Spray *(DVM)*
EctoKyl™ IGR Total Release Fogger *(DVM)*
IGR House & Area Fogger *(Durvet)*
Mycodex® Environmental Control™ Aerosol Room Fogger *(V.P.L.)*

Flea control with heartwormicide and/or anthelmintic

Sentinel® Flavor Tabs® *(Novartis)*

Flea control with tick and/or flea and/or pest killers

collars

Hartz® Advanced Care™ Brand Flea & Tick Drops Plus+ for Cats and Kittens (10 lbs. & under) *(Hartz Mountain)*
Hartz® Advanced Care™ Brand Flea & Tick Drops Plus+ for Dogs and Puppies (4 to 15 lbs.) *(Hartz Mountain)*
Hartz® Advanced Care™ Brand Flea & Tick Drops Plus+ for Dogs and Puppies (16 to 30 lbs.) *(Hartz Mountain)*
Hartz® Advanced Care™ Brand Flea & Tick Drops Plus+ for Dogs and Puppies (31 to 45 lbs.) *(Hartz Mountain)*

Please refer to product listings for more complete information.

Hartz® Advanced Care™ Brand Flea & Tick Drops Plus+ for Dogs and Puppies (46 to 60 lbs.) *(Hartz Mountain)*
Hartz® Advanced Care™ Brand Flea & Tick Drops Plus+ for Dogs and Puppies (61 to 90 lbs.) *(Hartz Mountain)*
Hartz® Advanced Care™ Brand Flea & Tick Drops Plus+ for Dogs and Puppies (Over 90 lbs.) *(Hartz Mountain)*
Hartz® Control Pet Care System® Ultimate Flea Collar® for Cats *(Hartz Mountain)*
Hartz® Control Pet Care System® Ultimate Flea Collar® for Dogs & Puppies *(Hartz Mountain)*
Preventic® Plus Tick and Flea IGR Collar for Dogs *(Virbac)*

dips, lotions and creams
Vet-Kem® Paramite® Sponge-On for Dogs *(Wellmark)*

premises
Adams™ Carpet Powder *(Farnam)*
Adams™ Inverted Carpet Spray *(Farnam)*
Mycodex® Environmental Control™ Aerosol Household Spray *(V.P.L.)*
OmniTrol IGR Fogger *(Vedco)*
Pet Care IGR-House & Carpet Spray *(Durvet)*
Sergeant's® Flea-Free Breeze™ *(Sergeant's)*
Sergeant's® PreTect® Flea & Tick Carpet Powder *(Sergeant's)*
Sergeant's® PreTect® Household Flea & Tick Spray *(Sergeant's)*
Sergeant's® PreTect® Indoor Flea & Tick Fogger *(Sergeant's)*
Sunbugger Carpet Dust *(Sungro)*
Vet-Kem® Siphotrol® Plus II Premise Spray *(Wellmark)*
Vet-Kem® Siphotrol® Plus Area Treatment for Homes *(Wellmark)*
Vet-Kem® Siphotrol® Plus Area Treatment Pump Spray for Homes *(Wellmark)*
Vet-Kem® Siphotrol Plus® Fogger *(Wellmark)*
Virbac KnockOut® IGR Household Pump Spray *(Virbac)*

shampoos / foams
Hartz® Control Pet Care System® Mousse for Cats and Kittens *(Hartz Mountain)*
Sergeant's® PreTect® Flea & Tick Shampoo for Cats and Kittens *(Sergeant's)*
Sergeant's® PreTect® Flea & Tick Shampoo for Dogs and Puppies *(Sergeant's)*
Vet-Kem® Ovitrol® Plus Flea & Tick Shampoo for Dogs & Cats *(Wellmark)*

spot treatments
Bio Spot® Stripe-On™ Flea Control For Cats *(Farnam)*
Frontline® Plus for Cats & Kittens *(Merial)*
Frontline® Plus for Dogs & Puppies *(Merial)*
Hartz® Advanced Care™ Brand Flea & Tick Drops Plus+ for Cats and Kittens (over 10 lbs.) *(Hartz Mountain)*
Sergeant's® PreTect® Squeeze-On Flea & Tick Control for Dogs (under 15 lbs) *(Sergeant's)*
Sergeant's® PreTect® Squeeze-On Flea & Tick Control for Dogs (15 to 33 lbs) *(Sergeant's)*
Sergeant's® PreTect® Squeeze-On Flea & Tick Control for Dogs (under 33 lbs) *(Sergeant's)*
Sergeant's® PreTect® Squeeze-On Flea & Tick Control for Dogs (over 33 lbs) *(Sergeant's)*
Vet-Kem® Ovitrol Plus® Spot On® Flea & Tick Control for Dogs & Puppies (under 30 lbs.) *(Wellmark)*
Vet-Kem® Ovitrol Plus® Spot On® Flea & Tick Control for Dogs & Puppies (over 30 lbs.) *(Wellmark)*

sprays
Hartz® Control Pet Care System® Flea & Flea Egg Killer for Dogs *(Hartz Mountain)*
Mycodex® All-In-One™ Spray *(V.P.L.)*
Scratchex® Super Spray™ *(Combe)*
Sergeant's® PreTect® Flea & Tick Spray for Cats & Kittens *(Sergeant's)*
Sergeant's® PreTect® Flea & Tick Spray for Dogs & Puppies *(Sergeant's)*
Vet-Kem® Ovitrol® Plus Flea, Tick & Bot Spray *(Wellmark)*
Virbac® Long Acting KnockOut™ *(Virbac)*

Flea killers

dips, lotions and creams
Happy Jack® Enduracide® Dip II *(Happy Jack)*
VIP® Flea Dip *(V.P.L.)*

oral
Capstar® *(Novartis)*

shampoos / foams
VIP® Flea Control Shampoo *(V.P.L.)*

spot treatments
Advantage® 9 (imidacloprid) Topical Solution for Cats and Kittens (8 Weeks and Older, 9 lbs. and Under) *(Bayer)*
Advantage® 10 (imidacloprid) Topical Solution for Dogs and Puppies (7 Weeks and Older, Under 10 lbs.) *(Bayer)*
Advantage® 18 (imidacloprid) Topical Solution for Cats and Kittens (8 Weeks and Older, Over 9 lbs.) *(Bayer)*
Advantage® 20 (imidacloprid) Topical Solution for Dogs and Puppies (7 Weeks and Older, 11-20 lbs.) *(Bayer)*
Advantage® 55 (imidacloprid) Topical Solution for Dogs and Puppies (7 Weeks and Older, 21-55 lbs.) *(Bayer)*
Advantage® 100 (imidacloprid) Topical Solution for Dogs and Puppies (7 Weeks and Older, Over 55 lbs.) *(Bayer)*

Flea, tick and/or pest killers

dips, lotions and creams
Adams™ Pyrethrin Dip *(Farnam)*
Adams™ Pyrethrin Dip *(V.P.L.)*
Happy Jack® Kennel Dip II *(Happy Jack)*
Hartz® 2 in 1® Luster Bath for Cats *(Hartz Mountain)*
Hartz® Control Pet Care System® Flea & Tick Dip for Dogs *(Hartz Mountain)*
SynerKyl® Pet Dip *(DVM)*
Virbac Pyrethrin Dip™ *(Virbac)*

powders
Adams™ Flea & Tick Dust II *(Farnam)*
Adams™ Flea & Tick Dust II *(V.P.L.)*
Happy Jack® Flea-Tick Powder II *(Happy Jack)*
Scratchex® Flea & Tick Powder *(Combe)*

shampoos
3X Pyrethrin Shampoo *(Vet Solutions)*
Adams™ Carbaryl Flea & Tick Shampoo *(Farnam)*
Adams™ Carbaryl Flea & Tick Shampoo *(V.P.L.)*
Ecto-Soothe™ Shampoo *(Virbac)*
Ecto-Soothe™ 3X Shampoo *(Virbac)*
Flea, Tick and Lice Shampoo *(Tomlyn)*
Happy Jack® Paracide II Shampoo *(Happy Jack)*
Hartz® Control Pet Care System® Flea & Tick Conditioning Shampoo for Cats *(Hartz Mountain)*
Hartz® Control Pet Care System® Flea & Tick Conditioning Shampoo for Dogs *(Hartz Mountain)*
Hartz® Easy Wash™ Flea & Tick Shampoo for Dogs *(Hartz Mountain)*
Mycodex® Pet Shampoo with Carbaryl *(V.P.L.)*
Pyrethrin Plus Shampoo *(Vedco)*
Triple Pyrethrins Flea & Tick Shampoo *(Davis)*
Vet-Kem® Triple Action Flea & Tick Shampoo for Dogs, Cats, & Horses *(Wellmark)*

spot treatments
Adams™ Spot-On Flea & Tick Control Large Dogs *(Farnam)*
Adams™ Spot-On Flea & Tick Control Small Dogs *(Farnam)*
Advantix™ (see K9 Advantix™) *(Bayer)*
Bio Spot® Flea & Tick Control For Dogs (15 lbs. and Under) *(Farnam)*
Bio Spot® Flea & Tick Control For Dogs (Between 15 & 33 lbs.) *(Farnam)*
Bio Spot® Flea & Tick Control For Dogs (33 to 66 lbs.) *(Farnam)*
Bio Spot® Flea & Tick Control For Dogs (Over 66 lbs.) *(Farnam)*
Equi-Spot™ Spot-On Fly Control for Horses *(Farnam)*
Happy Jack® Kennelspot™ for Dogs (under 33 lbs) *(Happy Jack)*
Happy Jack® Kennelspot™ for Dogs (over 33 lbs) *(Happy Jack)*
Hartz® Advanced Care™ Brand Once-a-Month™ Flea & Tick Drops for Cats and Kittens (10 lbs. & under) *(Hartz Mountain)*
Hartz® Advanced Care™ Brand Once-a-Month™ Flea & Tick Drops for Cats and Kittens (over 10 lbs.) *(Hartz Mountain)*
Hartz® Advanced Care™ Brand Once-a-Month™ Flea & Tick Drops for Dogs and Puppies (16 to 30 lbs.) *(Hartz Mountain)*
Hartz® Advanced Care™ Brand Once-a-Month™ Flea & Tick Drops for Dogs and Puppies (15 lbs. & under) *(Hartz Mountain)*
Hartz® Advanced Care™ Brand Once-a-Month™ Flea & Tick Drops for Dogs and Puppies (31 to 60 lbs.) *(Hartz Mountain)*
Hartz® Advanced Care™ Brand Once-a-Month™ Flea & Tick Drops for Dogs and Puppies (61 to 90 lbs.) *(Hartz Mountain)*
Hartz® Advanced Care™ Brand Once-a-Month™ Flea & Tick Drops for Dogs and Puppies (over 90 lbs.) *(Hartz Mountain)*
K9 Advantix™ 10 (imidacloprid/permethrin) For Dogs and Puppies (7 Weeks and Older, 10 lbs. and Under) *(Bayer)*
K9 Advantix™ 20 (imidacloprid/permethrin) For Dogs and Puppies (7 Weeks and Older, 11-20 lbs.) *(Bayer)*
K9 Advantix™ 55 (imidacloprid/permethrin) For Dogs and Puppies (7 Weeks and Older, 21-55 lbs.) *(Bayer)*
K9 Advantix™ 100 (imidacloprid/permethrin) For Dogs and Puppies (7 Weeks and Older, Over 55 lbs.) *(Bayer)*
Kiltix® Topical Tick Control *(Bayer)*
ProTICall® Insecticide for Dogs *(Schering-Plough)*
UltraSpot™ by Absorbine® *(W. F. Young)*

spray
Adams™ Flea & Tick Mist *(V.P.L.)*
Adams™ Water Based Flea and Tick Mist *(Farnam)*
Adams™ Water Based Flea and Tick Mist *(V.P.L.)*
Happy Jack® No-Hop Flea-Tick Spray *(Happy Jack)*
Hartz® 2 in 1® Flea & Tick Killer for Dogs *(Hartz Mountain)*
Pet Care Fast Kill Flea & Tick Spray for Dogs & Cats *(Durvet)*
Pyrethrins Dip and Spray *(Davis)*

Household and/or premise insecticides
Annihilator™ Insecticide Premise Spray *(Boehringer Ingelheim)*
Annihilator™ WP Wettable Powder Premise Insecticide *(Boehringer Ingelheim)*
Ectiban® WP *(Durvet)*
Fly-Zap™ Fly Bait *(Aspen)*
Formula F-500 *(Aire-Mate)*
Grenade® ER Premise Insecticide *(Schering-Plough)*
Happy Jack® Flea Flogger Plus *(Happy Jack)*
Happy Jack® Flea Zinger Plus *(Happy Jack)*
Larvadex® 2SL *(Novartis)*
Pet Care House & Carpet Powder *(Durvet)*
Pet Care Indoor Premise Spray *(Durvet)*
Prozap® LD-44Z *(Loveland)*
Prozap® Residual Insect Spray 2EC *(Loveland)*
QuickBayt™ Fly Bait *(Bayer)*
SafeCide® IC *(Schering-Plough)*
Sunbugger Residual Ant & Roach Spray Aqueous *(Sungro)*
Sun-Dust Roach Away *(Sungro)*
Sungro Permith *(Sungro)*
Tempo® 1% Dust Insecticide *(Bayer)*
Tempo® 20 WP Insecticide *(Bayer)*
Tempo® SC Ultra Premise Spray *(Bayer)*
Vapona® Concentrate Insecticide *(Boehringer Ingelheim)*
Virbac KnockOut® Area Treatment *(Virbac)*
Virbac KnockOut® ES Area Treatment *(Virbac)*
Virbac KnockOut® Room and Area Fogger *(Virbac)*
Virbac® Yard Spray Concentrate *(Virbac)*

Miticides
CheckMite+™ *(Mann Lake)*
CheckMite+™ Bee Hive Pest Control Strip *(Bayer)*
Happy Jack® Mange Medicine *(Happy Jack)*
Happy Jack® Sardex II® *(Happy Jack)*
Mange Treatment™ *(LeGear)*
Mitaban® *(Pharmacia & Upjohn)*
Rotenone Shampoo *(Goodwinol)*

Repellents
Absorbine® SuperShield® Red Fly Repellent *(W. F. Young)*
Absorbine® UltraShield® Brand Towelettes *(W. F. Young)*
Bite Free™ Biting Fly Repellent *(Farnam)*
Endure™ Sweat-Resistant Fly Spray *(Farnam)*
Flea Halt!™ Flea & Tick Repellent Towelettes *(Farnam)*
Flea Halt!™ Flea & Tick Repellent Towelettes for Ferrets *(Farnam)*
Fly Guard™ Collar/Brow Band *(Farnam)*
Flysect® Repellent Spray *(Equicare)*
Flysect® Roll-On Fly Repellent Face Lotion *(Equicare)*
Flys-Off® Fly Repellent Ointment *(Farnam)*
Flys-Off® Insect Repellent for Dogs *(Farnam)*

Please refer to product listings for more complete information.

PREMISE DISINFECTANTS

ANTIFUNGALS (specific)

Clinafarm® EC *(ASL)*
Clinafarm® SG *(ASL)*

DISINFECTANTS, CLEANERS and SANITIZERS (general)

Benzalkonium chloride
V-Tergent® *(Veterinary Specialties)*

Chlorhexidine
Nolvasan® S *(Fort Dodge)*
Nolvasan® Solution *(Fort Dodge)*

Chlorine / sulfates
EfferSan™ *(Activon)*
Hypo-Chlor Formula 6.40 *(Stearns)*
Lifegard® 855 Plus *(Rochester Midland)*
Trifectant™ *(Evsco)*
Virkon®-S *(Farnam, Livestock Div.)*

Cleaners (general)
25-Pines™ *(Stearns)*
Big Pine™ *(Intercon)*
Bio-Pine 20 *(Bio-Tek)*
Lifegard® 800 *(Rochester Midland)*
Lifegard® 900 *(Rochester Midland)*
Lifegard® 7000 *(Rochester Midland)*
Lifegard® 7500F *(Rochester Midland)*
Lifegard® 7700 *(Rochester Midland)*
Lifegard® 7700ND *(Rochester Midland)*
Pantek® Cleanser *(Loveland)*

Copper
E-Z Copper™ *(SSI Corp.)*

Enzymes
AlphaZyme Plus™ *(Alpha Tech Pet)*
DetergeZyme® *(Metrex)*
EmPower™ *(Metrex)*
Enzymatic Detergent *(Vedco)*
MetriSponge® *(Metrex)*
MetriZyme® *(Metrex)*

Formaldehyde / glutaraldehyde
DC&R® Disinfectant *(Loveland)*
Formaldehyde *(Centaur)*
Formaldehyde Solution *(Vedco)*
Formaldehyde Solution 37% *(Butler)*
Formaldehyde Solution 37% *(First Priority)*
Formaldehyde Solution 37% *(Phoenix Pharmaceutical)*
MetriCide® *(Metrex)*
MetriCide® 28 *(Metrex)*
MetriCide Plus 30® *(Metrex)*

Iodine complex
Dineotex *(Stearns)*
Iodine Disinfectant *(Durvet)*
Iofec®-20 Disinfectant *(Loveland)*
Iosan® *(WestAgro)*
K.O. Dyne® *(Westfalia• Surge)*
Liquatone™ *(Westfalia• Surge)*
Metz Iodine Detergent *(Metz)*
Monarch® Mon-O-Dine *(Ecolab Food & Bev. Div.)*
One Step *(Vedco)*
Parvo Guard™ *(First Priority)*
PVP Iodine *(Western Chemical)*
Rocadyne *(Rochester Midland)*
West-Vet® Premise® Disinfectant *(WestAgro)*

Phenol
3M™ Phenolic Disinfectant Cleaner Concentrate *(3M)*
Amphyl® Disinfectant Cleaner *(Reckitt Benckiser)*
PHD 22.5 *(Bio-Tek)*
Pheno-Tek II *(Bio-Tek)*
SynPhenol-3™ *(V.P.L.)*
Tek-Trol® *(Bio-Tek)*

Quaternary ammonium
16% Dual-Quat *(Vet Solutions)*
A-33® Dry *(Ecolab Prof. Prod. Div.)*
Air$_x$® 75 *(Airex)*
Asepticare® TB+II *(Ecolab Prof. Prod. Div.)*
Asepti-HB™ *(Ecolab Prof. Prod. Div.)*
Asepti-Wipe™ *(Ecolab Prof. Prod. Div.)*
Bacto-Sep *(Interchem)*
Cavicide® *(Metrex)*
D-128 *(Vedco)*
D-256 *(Vedco)*
Dakil *(Davis)*
Di-Quat 10-S *(Butler)*
Disintegrator® *(Phoenix Pharmaceutical)*
D-Trol *(DuBois)*
F-48 *(Rochester Midland)*
Foaming Disinfectant Cleaner *(Davis)*
Foam Quat *(Vet Solutions)*
Germicidal Detergent and Deodorant *(Aire-Mate)*
Germicide Solution *(Phoenix Pharmaceutical)*
Grade A™ *(Intercon)*
KennelSol™ *(Alpha Tech Pet)*
KenneLSol HC™ *(Alpha Tech Pet)*
KenneLSol-NPV™ *(Alpha Tech Pet)*
LDC-19™ *(Intercon)*
Lifegard® 256 Plus *(Rochester Midland)*
Lysol® Brand I.C.™ Quaternary Disinfectant Cleaner *(Reckitt Benckiser)*
Lysol® Brand II I.C.™ Disinfectant Spray *(Reckitt Benckiser)*
Marcicide II *(M.A.R.C.)*
MetriGuard® *(Metrex)*
MetriWipes® *(Metrex)*
Microban® X-580 Institutional Spray Plus *(Microban)*
Mint Disinfectant *(Air-Tite)*
Monarch® Super Kabon® *(Ecolab Food & Bev. Div.)*
Multi-Purpose Disinfectant *(LeGear)*
Multi-Quat 128 *(Intercon)*
Multi Quat TB™ *(Intercon)*
P-128 *(First Priority)*
Parr Quat *(Butler)*
Parr Quat 4X *(Butler)*
Parvosol® II RTU *(KenVet)*
Quatcide *(Bio-Tek)*
Quatrol *(Bio-Tek)*
Quatsan *(Bio-Tek)*
Roccal®-D Plus *(Pharmacia & Upjohn)*
Spectrasol™ *(KenVet)*
Steramine *(Stearns)*
Sunkleen 16 *(Sungro)*
Sunkleen 45 *(Sungro)*
Sunkleen 90 *(Sungro)*
Tryad® *(Loveland)*
Vigilquat *(Alex C. Fergusson)*
Virocid® *(Merial Select)*
V.T.D. *(Interchem)*

Various ingredients
Compliance™ *(Metrex)*
Compliance™ Neutralizing Powder *(Metrex)*
Kleen-Aseptic® *(Metrex)*
MetriClean2® *(Metrex)*
MetriLube® *(Metrex)*
MetriWash™ *(Metrex)*
Parvosan™ *(KenVet)*

Water additives

acidifiers
Citric Acid *(AgriLabs)*
Citric Acid *(Alpharma)*
Citric Acid Soluble Powder *(AgriPharm)*

FOODS

LIQUID DIETS

CliniCare® Canine Liquid Diet *(Abbott)*
CliniCare® Feline Liquid Diet *(Abbott)*
CliniCare® RF Specialized Feline Liquid Diet *(Abbott)*

MILK REPLACERS

Esbilac® Liquid *(Pet-Ag)*
Esbilac® Powder *(Pet-Ag)*
Foal-Lac® Powder *(Pet-Ag)*
GME™ Powder and Liquid (Goat's Milk Esbilac®) *(Pet-Ag)*
Just Born® Milk Replacer for Kittens Powdered Formula *(Farnam)*
Just Born® Milk Replacer for Kittens Ready-To-Use Liquid *(Farnam)*
Just Born® Milk Replacer for Puppies Powdered Formula *(Farnam)*
Just Born® Milk Replacer for Puppies Ready-To-Use Liquid *(Farnam)*
Kitten Formula *(Vet Solutions)*
KMR® Liquid *(Pet-Ag)*
KMR® Powder *(Pet-Ag)*
Land O Lakes® Instant Amplifier® Select Plus *(Land O'Lakes)*
Land O Lakes® Instant Kid Milk Replacer *(Land O'Lakes)*
Land O Lakes® Mare's Match® *(Land O'Lakes)*
Land O Lakes® Ultra Fresh® Lamb Milk Replacer *(Land O'Lakes)*
Multi-Milk™ *(Pet-Ag)*
Nurturall®-C for Kittens *(V.P.L.)*
Nurturall®-C for Puppies *(V.P.L.)*
PetLac™ Powder *(Pet-Ag)*
Puppy Formula *(Vet Solutions)*
SPF-Lac® *(Pet-Ag)*
Start To Finish® Mare Replacer™ *(Milk Specialties)*
Veta-Lac® Canine *(Vet-A-Mix)*
Veta-Lac® Feline *(Vet-A-Mix)*
Vita Ferm® Milk-N-More Non-Medicated Milk Replacer *(BioZyme)*
Zoologic® Milk Matrix 20/14 *(Pet-Ag)*
Zoologic® Milk Matrix 20/20 *(Pet-Ag)*
Zoologic® Milk Matrix 23/30 *(Pet-Ag)*
Zoologic® Milk Matrix 25/13 *(Pet-Ag)*
Zoologic® Milk Matrix 30/55 *(Pet-Ag)*
Zoologic® Milk Matrix 33/40 *(Pet-Ag)*
Zoologic® Milk Matrix 42/25 *(Pet-Ag)*

STARTER FOODS

Intensive Care Gruel™ (ICG) *(TechMix)*

WEANING FORMULAS

Esbilac® 2nd Step™ Puppy Weaning Food *(Pet-Ag)*
KMR® 2nd Step™ Kitten Weaning Food *(Pet-Ag)*

Please refer to product listings for more complete information.

DIAGNOSTICS

DIAGNOSTIC AIDS - CLINICAL

LABORATORY - CHEMICALS and SUPPLIES

HOSPITAL SUPPLIES

ANIMAL IDENTIFICATION SUPPLIES

Marking sticks, pens, sprays
Purple Spray *(AgriPharm)*

BANDAGE MATERIALS

Liquid bandages
Facilitator™ *(Idexx Pharm.)*

BREEDING SUPPLIES

Reproduction supplies

Artificial insemination equipment and supplies
Beltsville Turkey Semen Extender - II *(Intervet)*
Fresh Express® Semen Extender *(Synbiotics)*

Embryo transfer
MAP®-5 *(Bioniche Animal Health)*

HOOF MAINTENANCE

Hoof repair

claw prosthesis
Demotec® 95 *(Kane)*
Demotec® Easy Bloc® *(Kane)*

SURGICAL SUPPLIES

Scrubs and antiseptic hand soaps
Anti-Bacterial Hand Soap *(First Priority)*
Betadine® Surgical Scrub *(Purdue Frederick)*
Chloradine Scrub 4%® *(RXV)*
ChlorhexiDerm™ Plus Scrub *(DVM)*
Chlorhexidine Scrub *(A.A.H.)*
Chlorhexidine Scrub 2% *(First Priority)*
Chlorhexidine Scrub 4% *(First Priority)*
ChlorHex Surgical Scrub *(Vedco)*
Chlor-Scrub 40™ *(Butler)*
DVM Handsoap™ *(DVM)*
Hexascrub Medical Scrub 2% *(Vetus)*
Hexascrub Medical Scrub 4% *(Vetus)*
Hospital Hand Soap *(Vedco)*
Iodine Scrub *(A.A.H.)*
Nolvasan® Surgical Scrub *(Fort Dodge)*
Poviderm Medical Scrub *(Vetus)*
Povidine 0.75% Scrub *(AgriPharm)*
Povidone Iodine Scrub *(First Priority)*
Povidone-Iodine Surgical Scrub 7 1/2% *(Equicare)*
Povidone Scrub *(Butler)*
Prodine Scrub *(Phoenix Pharmaceutical)*
Safe4Hours™ Medical Formula *(Safe4Hours)*
Surgical Scrub and Handwash *(First Priority)*
Surgical Scrub & Handwash *(Vet Solutions)*
Triclosan Hand Soap *(Davis)*
Trisol™ *(KenVet)*
Vetadine Scrub *(Vedco)*
Waterless Antibacterial Hand Cleaner *(Davis)*
West-Vet® Prepodyne® Scrub *(WestAgro)*

Surgical glue
3M™ Vetbond™ Tissue Adhesive *(3M)*
Nexaband® Liquid *(Abbott)*
Nexaband® S/C *(Abbott)*
Tissue-Bond™ *(Vedco)*
Tissumend™ *(V.P.L.)*
Vet BioSISt™ *(Cook)*

UDDER and TEAT CARE MATERIALS

Dilators
Dr. Naylor® Teat Dilators *(H.W. Naylor)*

Please refer to product listings for more complete information.

GENERAL ITEMS

GROOMING EQUIPMENT and SUPPLIES

Allergy relief
Nova Pearls™ Spray On Moisturizer for Cat Dander Relief *(Tomlyn)*

Body washes and braces
Absorbine® RefreshMint® *(W. F. Young)*
Absorbine® ShowSheen® Hair Polish & Detangler *(W. F. Young)*
Tek-Trol® Hog Wash *(Bio-Tek)*

Shampoos and conditioners
Absorbine® ShowClean® Mane & Tail Whitener *(W. F. Young)*
Absorbine® SuperPoo® Conditioning Shampoo *(W. F. Young)*
Allergroom® Shampoo *(Virbac)*
Aloe & Oatmeal Shampoo *(Vet Solutions)*
Aloe & Oatmeal Skin & Coat Conditioner *(Vet Solutions)*
AlphaLyte® Premium Pet Shampoo *(Alpha Tech Pet)*
Bio Guard® Shampoo *(Farnam)*
Blue Snow™ *(Schering-Plough)*
CarraVet™ Multi Purpose Cleansing Foam *(V.P.L.)*
Cherryderm™ Grooming Shampoo *(Vetus)*
Cherry Grooming Shampoo *(Butler)*
Cherry Grooming Shampoo *(First Priority)*
Cleen Sheen *(Vedco)*
Cocoderm Conditioning Shampoo *(Vetus)*
Davis Best Luxury Shampoo *(Davis)*
D-Basic™ Shampoo *(DVM)*
DermaPet® Allay™ Oatmeal Shampoo *(DermaPet)*
DermaPet® Hypoallergenic Conditioning Shampoo *(DermaPet)*
DermaPet® Oatmeal Conditioner *(DermaPet)*
DermaSoothe Oatmeal Leave-On Conditioner *(Davis)*
D'Limonene Dip *(Davis)*
D'Limonene Shampoo *(Davis)*
DVM Tearless™ Shampoo *(DVM)*
DVM Tearless™ Spray-On Shampoo *(DVM)*
Epi-Soothe® Cream Rinse and Conditioner *(Virbac)*
Epi-Soothe® Shampoo *(Virbac)*
Grand Champion® Dri-Kleen™ *(Farnam)*
Groom-Aid® 35x *(Evsco)*
Grooming Shampoo *(First Priority)*
Hartz® Groomer's Best™ Oatmeal Shampoo *(Hartz Mountain)*
HyLyt*efa® Bath Oil/Coat Conditioner *(DVM)*
HyLyt*efa® Hypoallergenic Creme Rinse *(DVM)*
HyLyt*efa® Hypoallergenic Shampoo *(DVM)*
HyLyt*efa® Spray-On Shampoo *(DVM)*
Man O'War™ Shampoo *(Equicare)*
Melaleuca Shampoo *(Davis)*
Micro Pearls Advantage™ Hydra-Pearls™ Cream Rinse *(Evsco)*
Micro Pearls Advantage™ Hydra-Pearls™ Rehydrating Spray *(Evsco)*
Micro Pearls Advantage™ Hydra-Pearls™ Shampoo *(Evsco)*
Mycodex® Pearlescent Grooming Shampoo *(V.P.L.)*
Nova Pearls™ 5 to 1 Concentrate Shampoo *(Tomlyn)*
Nova Pearls™ Sensitive Skin Shampoo *(Tomlyn)*
Oatmeal & Aloe Shampoo *(Davis)*
Omega-Glo E Shampoo *(Vedco)*
PearLyt™ Shampoo *(DVM)*
Pro 35™ Tearless Shampoo *(Tomlyn)*
QuikClean™ Waterless Shampoo *(Fort Dodge)*
ResiSoothe® Leave-on Conditioner *(Virbac)*
Sho Sno™ Shampoo *(Tomlyn)*
Tearless Ferret Shampoo *(Tomlyn)*
Tearless Puppy Shampoo *(Tomlyn)*
Tearless Shampoo *(Davis)*
Triclosan Deodorizing Shampoo *(Davis)*
UltraGroom™ Shampoo *(Virbac)*
Vetrolin® Bath *(Equicare)*
Waterless Spray-On Shampoo *(Davis)*

Sprays
Dealer Select Horse Care Groom 'N Show *(Durvet)*
Groom-Aid® Spray *(Evsco)*
Humilac® Spray *(Virbac)*
Lustre Groom Mist™ *(Butler)*
Melaleuca Mist *(Davis)*
Nova Pearls™ Fresh Scent Deodorant Spray for Dogs and Cats *(Tomlyn)*
Nova Pearls™ Power Moisturizing Spray Mist *(Tomlyn)*
Vetrolin® Shine *(Equicare)*

HOUSEKEEPING

Pest control
Clout™ All Weather Bait *(Bayer)*
Clout™ Place Packs *(Bayer)*

ODOR NEUTRALIZERS

Odor and stain removers
Break-Thru Stain & Odor Remover *(Davis)*
Elimin • Odor® Pet Stain Eliminator *(Pfizer Animal Health)*
Pleascent® Puppy *(Thornell)*
Preference™ Stain & Odor Remover *(Virbac)*
See Spot Go!™ *(Tomlyn)*

Odor neutralizers - oral
Ono™ *(PRN Pharmacal)*

Odor neutralizers - topical
A • O • E™, Animal Odor Eliminator *(Thornell)*
Elimin • Odor® Canine *(Pfizer Animal Health)*
Elimin • Odor® Feline *(Pfizer Animal Health)*
Ferret-Off™ *(Thornell)*
Nova Pearls™ Fresh Scent Deodorant Spray for Ferrets *(Tomlyn)*
Skunk-Off® *(Thornell)*
Skunk-Off® Shampoo *(Thornell)*

Odor neutralizers for use on premises
Cat-Off™ *(Thornell)*
Cat-Off™ Concentrate *(Thornell)*
Dog-Off™ *(Thornell)*
Elimin • Odor® General Purpose *(Pfizer Animal Health)*
Elimin • Odor® Pet Accident *(Pfizer Animal Health)*
Equalizer™ *(Evsco)*
Horse Care Stall Powder *(Durvet)*
K • O • E™, Kennel Odor Eliminator *(Thornell)*
MetriMist® *(Metrex)*
Mycodex® Odor Neutralizer *(V.P.L.)*
Odor Destroyer *(Davis)*
Pet Care Litter, Kennel and Stall Odor Control Powder *(Durvet)*

Please refer to product listings for more complete information.

Biological Charts

The Biological Charts (blue pages) serve as a reference guide for veterinarians in their biological product selection. The vaccines and bacterins are grouped by the appropriate species and delineated by their antigens.

Further information regarding the products listed in the blue pages may be found in the product monograph section (white pages).

Every effort has been made to ensure the accuracy of the information published. However, it remains the responsibility of the readers to familiarize themselves with the product information contained on the product label or package insert. The Publisher, Editorial Team and all those involved in the production of this book, cannot be held responsible for publication errors or any consequence that could result from the use of published information.

Guide to the Biological Charts

BOVINE

K - antibodies
- antitoxin
- extract
- killed
- subunit
- toxoid

M - modified live

Product Name	Actinomyces (C. pyogenes)	Anaplasmosis	Anthrax	BRSV	Brucella spp	BVD Type I	BVD Type II	Campylobacter fetus	Clostridia, 2-way	Clostridia, 4-way	Clostridia, 7-way	Clostridia, 8-way	Clostridium haemolyticum	Clostridium perfringens	Coronavirus	E coli	Fusobacterium	Haemophilus somnus	IBR	L. pomona	Leptospira spp*	Moraxella bovis	Mycoplasma	Neospora caninum	Papillomavirus	Pasteurella haemolytica	Pasteurella multocida	PI3	Rabies	Rotavirus	Salmonella	Serpens spp	Serpulina (Treponema)	Staphylococcus spp	Tetanus Antitoxin	Tetanus Toxoid	Tritrichomonas
Respiragen™ Serum Antibodies *(Colorado Serum)*	K																									K	K										
Bo-Bac-2X™ *(Boehringer Ingelheim)*	K															K											K				K						
Quatracon-2X™ *(Boehringer Ingelheim)*	K															K											K				K						
BovaMune™ *(AgriLabs)*	K															K										K	K				K						
Bovi-Sera™ Serum Antibodies *(Colorado Serum)*	K															K										K	K				K						
Multi Serum *(Durvet)*	K															K										K	K				K						
Poly Serum® *(Novartis Animal Vaccines)*	K															K										K	K				K						
Plazvax® *(Schering-Plough)*		K																																			
Anthrax Spore Vaccine *(Colorado Serum)*			M																																		
Syn Shield™ *(Novartis Animal Vaccines)*				K																																	
Bovi-Shield™ BRSV *(Pfizer Animal Health)*				M																																	
Titanium™ BRSV *(AgriLabs)*				M																																	
Titanium® BRSV *(Intervet)*				M																																	
Vira Shield® 2+BRSV *(Novartis Animal Vaccines)*				K		K	K																														
Resvac® BRSV/Somubac® *(Pfizer Animal Health)*				M														K																			
Titanium® 3+BRSV *(Intervet)*				M		M	M												M																		
Bovi-Shield™ IBR-BRSV-LP *(Pfizer Animal Health)*				M															M	K																	
Bovi-Shield™ IBR-PI$_3$-BRSV *(Pfizer Animal Health)*				M															M									M									
Titanium™ BRSV 3 *(AgriLabs)*				M															M									M									
Titanium® BRSV 3 *(Intervet)*				M															M									M									
Bovi-Shield™ IBR-BVD-BRSV-LP *(Pfizer Animal Health)*				M		M	M												M	K																	
Titanium™ 3+BRSV LP *(AgriLabs)*				M		M	M												M	K																	
Titanium® 3+BRSV LP *(Intervet)*				M		M	M												M	K																	
Conquest™-4K *(Aspen)*				K		K													K									K									
Conquest™-4KW *(Aspen)*				K		K													K									K									
Elite 4™ *(Boehringer Ingelheim)*				K		K													K									K									
Respishield™ 4 *(Merial)*				K		K													K									K									
ResProMune® 4 *(AgriLabs)*				K		K													K									K									
Surround™ 4 *(Biocor)*				K		K													K									K									
Fusion® 4 *(Merial)*				K		K													K/M									M									
Reliant® Plus BVD-K (Dual IBR™) *(Merial)*				K		K													K/M									M									
Reliant® Plus (Dual IBR™) *(Merial)*				K		M													K/M									M									
Bovi-K® 4 *(Pfizer Animal Health)*				M		K													M									M									
CattleMaster® 4 *(Pfizer Animal Health)*				M		K													M									M									
Express 4® *(Boehringer Ingelheim)*				K		M													M									M									
Reliant® 4 *(Merial)*				K		M													M									M									
Bovi-Shield™ 4 *(Pfizer Animal Health)*				M		M													M									M									
Pyramid® MLV 4 *(Fort Dodge)*				M		M													M									M									
Conquest™ 5K (oil base) *(Aspen)*				K		K	K												K									K									
DurGuard™ 5 *(Durvet)*				K		K	K												K									K									
Exalt™ 5 *(AgriPharm)*				K		K	K												K									K									
ResProMune® 4 I-B-P+BRSV *(AgriLabs)*				K		K	K												K									K									
Triangle® 4 + Type II BVD *(Fort Dodge)*				K		K	K												K									K									
Vira Shield® 5 *(Novartis Animal Vaccines)*				K		K	K												K									K									
Master Guard™ Preg 5 *(AgriLabs)*				M		K	K												K									M									
Master Guard® Preg 5 *(Intervet)*				M		K	K												K									M									
Prism™ 4 *(Fort Dodge)*				M		K	K												M									M									
Covert™ 5 *(AgriPharm)*				M		M	M												M									M									
Express™ 5 *(Boehringer Ingelheim)*				M		M	M												M									M									
Jencine® 4 *(Schering-Plough)*				M		M	M												M									M									

2-Way - *Clostridium chauvoei*
- *Cl. septicum*

4-Way - *Clostridium chauvoei*
- *Cl. novyi*
- *Cl. septicum*
- *Cl. sordellii*

7-Way - *Clostridium chauvoei*
- *Cl. perfringens* Types C & D
- *Cl. novyi*
- *Cl. septicum*
- *Cl. sordellii* or *Cl. tetani*

8-Way - *Clostridium chauvoei*
- *Cl. haemolyticum*
- *Cl. novyi*
- *Cl. perfringens* Types C & D
- *Cl. septicum*
- *Cl. sordellii* or *Cl. tetani*

Leptospira spp*
- *L. canicola*
- *L. grippotyphosa*
- *L. hardjo*
- *L. icterohaemorrhagiae*
- *L. pomona*

(continued on next page)

Please refer to product listings for more complete information.

BOVINE *(continued)*

K - antibodies
- antitoxin
- extract
- killed
- subunit
- toxoid

M - modified live

Product Name	Actinomyces (C. pyogenes)	Anaplasmosis	Anthrax	BRSV	Brucella spp	BVD Type I	BVD Type II	Campylobacter fetus	Clostridia, 2-way	Clostridia, 4-way	Clostridia, 7-way	Clostridia, 8-way	Clostridium haemolyticum	Clostridium perfringens	Coronavirus	E coli	Fusobacterium	Haemophilus somnus	IBR	L. pomona	Leptospira spp*	Moraxella bovis	Mycoplasma	Neospora caninum	Papillomavirus	Pasteurella haemolytica	Pasteurella multocida	PI3	Rabies	Rotavirus	Salmonella	Serpens spp	Serpulina (Treponema)	Staphylococcus spp	Tetanus Antitoxin	Tetanus Toxoid	Tritrichomonas
Titanium™ 5 *(AgriLabs)*				M		M	M												M									M									
Titanium® 5 *(Intervet)*				M		M	M												M									M									
TiterVac™ 5 *(Aspen)*				M		M	M												M									M									
Conquest™-4K+H.S. *(Aspen)*				K		K												K	K									K									
Conquest™-4KW+H.S. *(Aspen)*				K		K												K	K									K									
Elite 4-HS™ *(Boehringer Ingelheim)*				K		K												K	K									K									
ResProMune® 4+SomnuMune® (I.M.) *(AgriLabs)*				K		K												K	K									K									
ResProMune® 4+SomnuMune® (I.M., S.C.) *(AgriLabs)*				K		K												K	K									K									
Surround™ 4+HS *(Biocor)*				K		K												K	K									K									
Triangle® 4+HS *(Fort Dodge)*				K		K												K	K									K									
Resvac® 4/Somubac® *(Pfizer Animal Health)*				M		M												K	M									M									
Conquest™-9K *(Aspen)*				K		K													K		K							K									
Elite 9™ *(Boehringer Ingelheim)*				K		K													K		K							K									
Respishield™ 4 L5 *(Merial)*				K		K													K		K							K									
ResProMune™ 9 *(AgriLabs)*				K		K													K		K							K									
Surround™ 9 *(Biocor)*				K		K													K		K							K									
CattleMaster® 4+L5 *(Pfizer Animal Health)*				M		K													M		K							M									
Pyramid® 9 *(Fort Dodge)*				M		M													M		K							M									
Conquest™ 5K+HS (oil base) *(Aspen)*				K		K	K											K	K									K									
DurGuard™ 5HS *(Durvet)*				K		K	K											K	K									K									
Exalt™ 5 + Somnus *(AgriPharm)*				K		K	K											K	K									K									
Vira Shield® 5+Somnus *(Novartis Animal Vaccines)*				K		K	K											K	K									K									
Covert™ 5-HS *(AgriPharm)*				M		M	M											K	M									M									
Express™ 5-HS *(Boehringer Ingelheim)*				M		M	M											K	M									M									
TiterVac™ 5-HS *(Aspen)*				M		M	M											K	M									M									
Triangle® 4+PH-K *(Fort Dodge)*				K		K													K							K		K									
Pyramid® 4+Presponse® SQ *(Fort Dodge)*				M		M													M							K		M									
Conquest™ 10K *(Aspen)*				K		K	K												K		K							K									
DurGuard™ 10 *(Durvet)*				K		K	K												K		K							K									
Exalt™ 5 + L5 *(AgriPharm)*				K		K	K												K		K							K									
Triangle® 9 + Type II BVD *(Fort Dodge)*				K		K	K												K		K							K									
Vira Shield® 5+L5 *(Novartis Animal Vaccines)*				K		K	K												K		K							K									
Master Guard™ 10 *(AgriLabs)*				M		K	K												K		K							M									
Master Guard® 10 *(Intervet)*				M		K	K												K		K							M									
Prism™ 9 *(Fort Dodge)*				M		K	K												M		K							M									
Bovi-Shield® FP 4+L5 *(Pfizer Animal Health)*				M		M	M												M		K							M									
Covert™ 10 *(AgriPharm)*				M		M	M												M		K							M									
Express 10™ *(Boehringer Ingelheim)*				M		M	M												M		K							M									
Titanium™ 5 L5 *(AgriLabs)*				M		M	M												M		K							M									
Titanium® 5 L5 *(Intervet)*				M		M	M												M		K							M									
TiterVac™ 10 *(Aspen)*				M		M	M												M		K							M									
CattleMaster® 4+VL5 *(Pfizer Animal Health)*				M		K		K											M		K							M									
Conquest™ 5K+VL5 (oil base) *(Aspen)*				K		K	K	K											K		K							K									
DurGuard™ 5+VL5 *(Durvet)*				K		K	K	K											K		K							K									
Exalt™ 5 + VL5 *(AgriPharm)*				K		K	K	K											K		K							K									
ResProMune® 5+VL5 *(AgriLabs)*				K		K	K	K											K		K							K									
Vira Shield® 5+VL5 *(Novartis Animal Vaccines)*				K		K	K	K											K		K							K									
Master Guard® 10 + Vibrio *(AgriLabs)*				M		K	K	K											K		K							M									
Cattle-Vac™ 9-Somnus *(Durvet)*				K		K												K	K		K							K									
Conquest™-9K+H.S. *(Aspen)*				K		K												K	K		K							K									
Elite 9-HS™ *(Boehringer Ingelheim)*				K		K												K	K		K							K									

2-Way
- *Clostridium chauvoei*
- *Cl. septicum*

4-Way
- *Clostridium chauvoei*
- *Cl. novyi*
- *Cl. septicum*
- *Cl. sordellii*

7-Way
- *Clostridium chauvoei*
- *Cl. perfringens* Types C & D
- *Cl. novyi*
- *Cl. septicum*
- *Cl. sordellii* or *Cl. tetani*

8-Way
- *Clostridium chauvoei*
- *Cl. haemolyticum*
- *Cl. novyi*
- *Cl. perfringens* Types C & D
- *Cl. septicum*
- *Cl. sordellii* or *Cl. tetani*

*Leptospira spp**
- *L. canicola*
- *L. grippotyphosa*
- *L. hardjo*
- *L. icterohaemorrhagiae*
- *L. pomona*

(continued on next page)

BOVINE *(continued)*

K - antibodies
 - antitoxin
 - extract
 - killed
 - subunit
 - toxoid
M - modified live

Product Name	Actinomyces (C. pyogenes)	Anaplasmosis	Anthrax	BRSV	Brucella spp	BVD Type I	BVD Type II	Campylobacter fetus	Clostridia, 2-way	Clostridia, 4-way	Clostridia, 7-way	Clostridia, 8-way	Clostridium haemolyticum	Clostridium perfringens	Coronavirus	E coli	Fusobacterium	Haemophilus somnus	IBR	L. pomona	Leptospira spp*	Moraxella bovis	Mycoplasma	Neospora caninum	Papillomavirus	Pasteurella haemolytica	Pasteurella multocida	PI3	Rabies	Rotavirus	Salmonella	Serpens spp	Serpulina (Treponema)	Staphylococcus spp	Tetanus Antitoxin	Tetanus Toxoid	Tritrichomonas
ResProMune™ 10 *(AgriLabs)*				K		K												K	K		K							K									
Surround™ 9+HS *(Biocor)*				K		K												K	K		K							K									
Triangle® 9+HS *(Fort Dodge)*				K		K												K	K		K							K									
Triangle® 4+PH/HS *(Fort Dodge)*				K		K												K	K							K		K									
DurGuard™ 10HS *(Durvet)*				K		K	K											K	K		K							K									
Vira Shield® 5+L5 Somnus *(Novartis Animal Vaccines)*				K		K	K											K	K		K							K									
Covert™ 10-HS *(AgriPharm)*				M		M	M											K	M		K							M									
Express™ 10-HS *(Boehringer Ingelheim)*				M		M	M											K	M		K							M									
TiterVac™ 10-HS *(Aspen)*				M		M	M											K	M		K							M									
Triangle® 9+PH-K *(Fort Dodge)*				K		K													K		K					K		K									
DurGuard™ 5HS+VL5 *(Durvet)*				K		K	K	K										K	K		K							K									
Vira Shield® 5+VL5 Somnus *(Novartis Animal Vaccines)*				K		K	K	K										K	K		K							K									
Express™ 5-PHM *(Boehringer Ingelheim)*				M		M	M												M							K	K	M									
Titanium® 5+P.H.M. Bac®-1 *(AgriLabs)*				M		M	M												M							M	M	M									
Titanium® 5+P.H.M. Bac®-1 *(Intervet)*				M		M	M												M							M	M	M									
Brucella Abortus Vaccine (Strain RB-51) *(Professional Biological)*					M																																
CattleMaster® BVD-K *(Pfizer Animal Health)*						K																															
Bovine Virus Diarrhea Vaccine *(Colorado Serum)*						M																															
Triangle® 1 + Type II BVD *(Fort Dodge)*						K	K																														
Vira Shield® 2 *(Novartis Animal Vaccines)*						K	K																														
Bovi-Shield™ IBR-BVD *(Pfizer Animal Health)*						M													M																		
Reliant® IBR/BVD *(Merial)*						M													M																		
Vira Shield® 3 *(Novartis Animal Vaccines)*						K	K												K																		
Express™ 3 *(Boehringer Ingelheim)*						M	M												M																		
Titanium™ 3 *(AgriLabs)*						M	M												M																		
Titanium® 3 *(Intervet)*						M	M												M																		
IBL Vaccine *(Aspen)*						M													M	K																	
Express™ 3/Lp *(Boehringer Ingelheim)*						M	M												M	K																	
Bovi-Shield™ 3 *(Pfizer Animal Health)*						M													M									M									
Bovine 3 *(Durvet)*						M													M									M									
Bovine Rhinotracheitis-Virus Diarrhea-Parainfluenza-3 Vaccine *(Colorado Serum)*						M													M									M									
Express™ IBP *(Boehringer Ingelheim)*						M													M									M									
Herd-Vac™ 3 *(Biocor)*						M													M									M									
IBP Vaccine *(Aspen)*						M													M									M									
Pyramid® MLV 3 *(Fort Dodge)*						M													M									M									
Reliant® 3 *(Merial)*						M													M									M									
DurGuard™ 4 *(Durvet)*						K	K												K									K									
Exalt™ 4 *(AgriPharm)*						K	K												K									K									
Triangle® 3 + Type II BVD *(Fort Dodge)*						K	K												K									K									
Vira Shield® 4 *(Novartis Animal Vaccines)*						K	K												K									K									
Vira Shield® 3+VL5 *(Novartis Animal Vaccines)*						K	K	K											K		K							K									
Titanium™ 4 *(AgriLabs)*						M	M												M									M									
Herd-Vac™ 3 S *(Biocor)*						M												K	M									M									
IBP-SomnuMune® Vaccine *(Aspen)*						M												K	M									M									
Conquest™-8K *(Aspen)*						K													K		K							K									
ResProMune® 8 *(AgriLabs)*						K													K		K							K									
Surround™ 8 *(Biocor)*						K													K		K							K									
Bovine 8 *(Durvet)*						M													M		K							M									
Herd-Vac™ 8 *(Biocor)*						M													M		K							M									

2-Way - *Clostridium chauvoei*
- *Cl. septicum*

4-Way - *Clostridium chauvoei*
- *Cl. novyi*
- *Cl. septicum*
- *Cl. sordellii*

7-Way - *Clostridium chauvoei*
- *Cl. perfringens* Types C & D
- *Cl. novyi*
- *Cl. septicum*
- *Cl. sordellii* or *Cl. tetani*

8-Way - *Clostridium chauvoei*
- *Cl. haemolyticum*
- *Cl. novyi*
- *Cl. perfringens* Types C & D
- *Cl. septicum*
- *Cl. sordellii* or *Cl. tetani*

Leptospira spp*
- *L. canicola*
- *L. grippotyphosa*
- *L. hardjo*
- *L. icterohaemorrhagiae*
- *L. pomona*

(continued on next page)

Please refer to product listings for more complete information.

BOVINE *(continued)*

K - antibodies
- antitoxin
- extract
- killed
- subunit
- toxoid

M - modified live

Product Name	Actinomyces (C. pyogenes)	Anaplasmosis	Anthrax	BRSV	Brucella spp	BVD Type I	BVD Type II	Campylobacter fetus	Clostridia, 2-way	Clostridia, 4-way	Clostridia, 7-way	Clostridia, 8-way	Clostridium haemolyticum	Clostridium perfringens	Coronavirus	E coli	Fusobacterium	Haemophilus somnus	IBR	L. pomona	Leptospira spp*	Moraxella bovis	Mycoplasma	Neospora caninum	Papillomavirus	Pasteurella haemolytica	Pasteurella multocida	PI3	Rabies	Rotavirus	Salmonella	Serpens spp	Serpulina (Treponema)	Staphylococcus spp	Tetanus Antitoxin	Tetanus Toxoid	Tritrichomonas
IBP-L5 Vaccine *(Aspen)*						M													M		K							M									
Pyramid® 8 *(Fort Dodge)*						M													M		K							M									
Reliant® 8 *(Merial)*						M													M		K							M									
Exalt™ 4 + L5 *(AgriPharm)*						K	K												K		K							K									
Triangle® 8 + Type II BVD *(Fort Dodge)*						K	K												K		K							K									
Vira Shield® 4+L5 *(Novartis Animal Vaccines)*						K	K												K		K							K									
Titanium™ 4 L5 *(AgriLabs)*						M	M												M		K							M									
Triangle® 3 V5L *(Fort Dodge)*						K		K											K		K							K									
Bovine 9 *(Durvet)*						M		K											M		K							M									
Cow-Vac® 9 *(Aspen)*						M		K											M		K							M									
Herd-Vac™ 9 *(Biocor)*						M		K											M		K							M									
PregGuard™ FP 9 *(Pfizer Animal Health)*						M	M	K											M		K							M									
Breed-Back-10™ *(Boehringer Ingelheim)*						M		K										K	M		K							M									
Express™ IBP/HS-2P *(Boehringer Ingelheim)*						M												K	M							K	K	M									
Poly-Bac B® 7 *(Texas Vet Lab)*						K												K	K							K	K				K						
Campylobacter Fetus Bacterin-Bovine *(Colorado Serum)*								K																													
Cattle-Vac™ Vibrio-Plus *(Durvet)*								K																													
Vibrin® *(Pfizer Animal Health)*								K																													
Vib Shield® *(Novartis Animal Vaccines)*								K																													
Vib Shield® Plus *(Novartis Animal Vaccines)*								K																													
Pre-Vent 6™ *(AgriLabs)*								K													K																
StayBred™ VL5 *(Pfizer Animal Health)*								K													K																
Surround™ V-L5 *(Biocor)*								K													K																
TriVib 5L® *(Fort Dodge)*								K													K																
TrustGard™ Vibrio/5L *(Vedco)*								K													K																
Vibralone™-L5 *(Intervet)*								K													K																
Vibrio-Lepto-5™ *(Boehringer Ingelheim)*								K													K																
Vibrio-Lepto 5 *(Premier Farmtech)*								K													K																
Vibrio-Lepto 5 *(AgriLabs)*								K													K																
Vibrio-Lepto 5 *(Durvet)*								K													K																
Vibrio-Lepto 5 Vaccine *(Aspen)*								K													K																
Vibrio/Leptoferm-5™ *(Pfizer Animal Health)*								K													K																
Vibrio Lepto 5 (oil base) *(Aspen)*								K													K																
Vib Shield® L5 *(Novartis Animal Vaccines)*								K													K																
Vib Shield® L5 Hardjo Bovis *(Novartis Animal Vaccines)*								K													K																
Vib Shield® Plus L5 *(Novartis Animal Vaccines)*								K													K																
VL5-1X *(Durvet)*								K													K																
VL5-1X Plus™ *(Durvet)*								K													K																
TrichGuard® V5L *(Fort Dodge)*								K													K																K
Clostridium Chauvoei-Septicum Bacterin *(Colorado Serum)*									K																												
Clostridium Chauvoei-Septicum-Pasteurella Haemolytica-Multocida Bacterin *(Colorado Serum)*									K																	K	K										
Clostridium Chauvoei-Septicum-Novyi-Sordellii Bacterin-Toxoid *(Colorado Serum)*										K																											
7 Gauge™ *(AgriPharm)*											K																										
7-Way *(Aspen)*											K																										
Alpha-7™ *(Boehringer Ingelheim)*											K																										
Bar-Vac® 7 *(Boehringer Ingelheim)*											K																										
Caliber® 7 *(Boehringer Ingelheim)*											K																										

2-Way - *Clostridium chauvoei*
- *Cl. septicum*

4-Way - *Clostridium chauvoei*
- *Cl. novyi*
- *Cl. septicum*
- *Cl. sordellii*

7-Way - *Clostridium chauvoei*
- *Cl. perfringens* Types C & D
- *Cl. novyi*
- *Cl. septicum*
- *Cl. sordellii* or *Cl. tetani*

8-Way - *Clostridium chauvoei*
- *Cl. haemolyticum*
- *Cl. novyi*
- *Cl. perfringens* Types C & D
- *Cl. septicum*
- *Cl. sordellii* or *Cl. tetani*

Leptospira spp*
- *L. canicola*
- *L. grippotyphosa*
- *L. hardjo*
- *L. icterohaemorrhagiae*
- *L. pomona*

(continued on next page)

BOVINE *(continued)*

K - antibodies
- antitoxin
- extract
- killed
- subunit
- toxoid

M - modified live

Product Name	Actinomyces (C. pyogenes)	Anaplasmosis	Anthrax	BRSV	Brucella spp	BVD Type I	BVD Type II	Campylobacter fetus	Clostridia, 2-way	Clostridia, 4-way	Clostridia, 7-way	Clostridia, 8-way	Clostridium haemolyticum	Clostridium perfringens	Coronavirus	E coli	Fusobacterium	Haemophilus somnus	IBR	L. pomona	Leptospira spp*	Moraxella bovis	Mycoplasma	Neospora caninum	Papillomavirus	Pasteurella haemolytica	Pasteurella multocida	PI3	Rabies	Rotavirus	Salmonella	Serpens spp	Serpulina (Treponema)	Staphylococcus spp	Tetanus Antitoxin	Tetanus Toxoid	Tritrichomonas
Clostridial 7-Way *(AgriLabs)*											K																										
Electroid® 7 Vaccine *(Schering-Plough)*											K																										
Fortress® 7 *(Pfizer Animal Health)*											K																										
Resist™ 7 *(AgriPharm)*											K																										
TrustGard™ 7 *(Vedco)*											K																										
Ultrabac® 7 *(Pfizer Animal Health)*											K																										
UltraChoice™ 7 *(Pfizer Animal Health)*											K																										
Vision® 7 with Spur® *(Intervet)*											K																										
7-Way/Somnus *(Aspen)*											K							K																			
Bar Vac® 7/Somnus *(Boehringer Ingelheim)*											K							K																			
Clostridial 7-Way plus Somnumune® *(AgriLabs)*											K							K																			
Resist™ 7HS *(AgriPharm)*											K							K																			
TrustGard™ 7/HS *(Vedco)*											K							K																			
Ultrabac® 7/Somubac® *(Pfizer Animal Health)*											K							K																			
Vision® 7 Somnus with Spur® *(Intervet)*											K							K																			
20/20 Vision® 7 with Spur® *(Intervet)*											K											K															
Alpha-7/MB™ *(Boehringer Ingelheim)*											K											K															
Piliguard® Pinkeye + 7 *(Schering-Plough)*											K											K															
One Shot Ultra™ 7 *(Pfizer Animal Health)*											K															K											
8-Way *(Aspen)*												K																									
Bar-Vac® 8 *(Boehringer Ingelheim)*												K																									
Clostridial 8-Way *(AgriLabs)*												K																									
Fortress® 8 *(Pfizer Animal Health)*												K																									
Resist™ 8 *(AgriPharm)*												K																									
Siteguard® MLG Vaccine *(Schering-Plough)*												K																									
Tetni-Vax® *(AgriPharm)*												K																									
TrustGard™ 8 *(Vedco)*												K																									
Ultrabac® 8 *(Pfizer Animal Health)*												K																									
UltraChoice™ 8 *(Pfizer Animal Health)*												K																									
Vision® 8 with Spur® *(Intervet)*												K																									
Vision® 8 Somnus with Spur® *(Intervet)*												K						K																			
One Shot Ultra™ 8 *(Pfizer Animal Health)*												K														K											
Clostridium Haemolyticum Bacterin (Red Water) *(Colorado Serum)*													K																								
Alpha-CD™ *(Boehringer Ingelheim)*														K																							
Bar-Vac® CD *(Boehringer Ingelheim)*														K																							
C & D Antitoxin™ *(Boehringer Ingelheim)*														K																							
C & D Toxoid *(Aspen)*														K																							
Caliber® 3 *(Boehringer Ingelheim)*														K																							
Clostratox® BCD *(Novartis Animal Vaccines)*														K																							
Clostratox® C *(Novartis Animal Vaccines)*														K																							
Clostratox® Ultra C 1300 *(Novartis Animal Vaccines)*														K																							
Clostri Bos™ BCD *(Novartis Animal Vaccines)*														K																							
Clostridial Antitoxin BCD *(Durvet)*														K																							
Clostridial BCD *(Durvet)*														K																							
Clostridium Perfringens Types C & D Antitoxin, Equine Origin *(Colorado Serum)*														K																							
Clostridium Perfringens Types C&D Antitoxin, Equine Origin *(Professional Biological)*														K																							
Clostridium Perfringens Types C & D Toxoid *(Colorado Serum)*														K																							

2-Way - *Clostridium chauvoei*
- *Cl. septicum*

4-Way - *Clostridium chauvoei*
- *Cl. novyi*
- *Cl. septicum*
- *Cl. sordellii*

7-Way - *Clostridium chauvoei*
- *Cl. perfringens* Types C & D
- *Cl. novyi*
- *Cl. septicum*
- *Cl. sordellii* or *Cl. tetani*

8-Way - *Clostridium chauvoei*
- *Cl. haemolyticum*
- *Cl. novyi*
- *Cl. perfringens* Types C & D
- *Cl. septicum*
- *Cl. sordellii* or *Cl. tetani*

*Leptospira spp**
- *L. canicola*
- *L. grippotyphosa*
- *L. hardjo*
- *L. icterohaemorrhagiae*
- *L. pomona*

(continued on next page)

Please refer to product listings for more complete information.

BOVINE *(continued)*

K - antibodies
- antitoxin
- extract
- killed
- subunit
- toxoid

M - modified live

Product Name	Actinomyces (C. pyogenes)	Anaplasmosis	Anthrax	BRSV	Brucella spp	BVD Type I	BVD Type II	Campylobacter fetus	Clostridia, 2-way	Clostridia, 4-way	Clostridia, 7-way	Clostridia, 8-way	Clostridium haemolyticum	Clostridium perfringens	Coronavirus	E coli	Fusobacterium	Haemophilus somnus	IBR	L. pomona	Leptospira spp*	Moraxella bovis	Mycoplasma	Neospora caninum	Papillomavirus	Pasteurella haemolytica	Pasteurella multocida	PI3	Rabies	Rotavirus	Salmonella	Serpens spp	Serpulina (Treponema)	Staphylococcus spp	Tetanus Antitoxin	Tetanus Toxoid	Tritrichomonas
Clostridium Perfringens Types C&D Toxoid *(Professional Biological)*														K																							
Clostri Shield® BCD *(Novartis Animal Vaccines)*														K																							
Electroid® D *(Schering-Plough)*														K																							
Fortress® CD *(Pfizer Animal Health)*														K																							
Gauge™ C&D *(AgriPharm)*														K																							
Siteguard® G *(Schering-Plough)*														K																							
TrustGard™ CD *(Vedco)*														K																							
Ultrabac® CD *(Pfizer Animal Health)*														K																							
UltraChoice™ CD *(Pfizer Animal Health)*														K																							
Vision® CD with Spur® *(Intervet)*														K																							
Bovine Ecolizer®+C *(Novartis Animal Vaccines)*														K		K																					
Bovine Pili Shield™+C *(Novartis Animal Vaccines)*														K		K																					
Cattle-Vac™ E. Coli+C *(Durvet)*														K		K																					
Cattle Vac™ EC+C *(Durvet)*														K		K																					
E-Coli + C Antibody *(AgriPharm)*														K		K																					
Scour Vac™ E Coli + C *(AgriLabs)*														K		K																					
Scour Bos™ 6 *(Novartis Animal Vaccines)*														K	K	K																					
Bar Vac® CD/T *(Boehringer Ingelheim)*														K																						K	
Clostridium Perfringens Types C & D-Tetanus Toxoid *(Colorado Serum)*														K																						K	
Clostridium Perfringens Types C&D-Tetanus Toxoid *(Professional Biological)*														K																						K	
TrustGard™ CD/T *(Vedco)*														K																						K	
Vision® CD•T with Spur® *(Intervet)*														K																						K	
Scour Bos™ 9 *(Novartis Animal Vaccines)*														K	K	K														K							
ScourGuard 3® (K)/C *(Pfizer Animal Health)*														K	K	K														K							
Scour Vac™ 3K+C *(Durvet)*														K	K	K														K							
Scour Vac™ 9 *(AgriLabs)*														K	K	K														K							
First Defense® *(ImmuCell)*															K	K																					
Scour Bos™ 4 *(Novartis Animal Vaccines)*															K															K							
Scour Vac™ 2K *(Durvet)*															K															K							
Scour Vac™ 4 *(AgriLabs)*															K															K							
Calf-Guard® *(Pfizer Animal Health)*															M															M							
ScourGuard 3® (K) *(Pfizer Animal Health)*															K	K														K							
Bar-Guard-99™ *(Boehringer Ingelheim)*																K																					
Bovine Ecolizer® *(Novartis Animal Vaccines)*																K																					
Bovine Pili Shield™ *(Novartis Animal Vaccines)*																K																					
Cattle-Vac™ E. Coli *(Durvet)*																K																					
Cattle-Vac™ EC *(Durvet)*																K																					
Colimune®-Oral *(Bioniche Animal Health)*																K																					
E. Colicin-B™ *(AgriLabs)*																K																					
J-5 Escherichia Coli Bacterin *(Hygieia)*																K																					
J-Vac® *(Merial)*																K																					
Master Guard® J5 *(AgriLabs)*																K																					
Piliguard® E. Coli-1 *(Schering-Plough)*																K																					
ProSystem® Pilimune *(Intervet)*																K																					
Upjohn J-5 Bacterin™ *(Pharmacia & Upjohn)*																K																					
Fusogard™ *(Novartis Animal Vaccines)*																	K																				
Volar® *(Intervet)*																	K																				
Bar Somnus™ *(Boehringer Ingelheim)*																		K																			
Cattle-Vac™ HS *(Durvet)*																		K																			

2-Way - *Clostridium chauvoei*
- *Cl. septicum*

4-Way - *Clostridium chauvoei*
- *Cl. novyi*
- *Cl. septicum*
- *Cl. sordellii*

7-Way - *Clostridium chauvoei*
- *Cl. perfringens* Types C & D
- *Cl. novyi*
- *Cl. septicum*
- *Cl. sordellii* or *Cl. tetani*

8-Way - *Clostridium chauvoei*
- *Cl. haemolyticum*
- *Cl. novyi*
- *Cl. perfringens* Types C & D
- *Cl. septicum*
- *Cl. sordellii* or *Cl. tetani*

*Leptospira spp**
- *L. canicola*
- *L. grippotyphosa*
- *L. hardjo*
- *L. icterohaemorrhagiae*
- *L. pomona*

(continued on next page)

Please refer to product listings for more complete information.

BOVINE *(continued)*

K - antibodies
- antitoxin
- extract
- killed
- subunit
- toxoid

M - modified live

Product Name	Actinomyces (C. pyogenes)	Anaplasmosis	Anthrax	BRSV	Brucella spp	BVD Type I	BVD Type II	Campylobacter fetus	Clostridia, 2-way	Clostridia, 4-way	Clostridia, 7-way	Clostridia, 8-way	Clostridium haemolyticum	Clostridium perfringens	Coronavirus	E coli	Fusobacterium	Haemophilus somnus	IBR	L. pomona	Leptospira spp*	Moraxella bovis	Mycoplasma	Neospora caninum	Papillomavirus	Pasteurella haemolytica	Pasteurella multocida	PI3	Rabies	Rotavirus	Salmonella	Serpens spp	Serpulina (Treponema)	Staphylococcus spp	Tetanus Antitoxin	Tetanus Toxoid	Tritrichomonas
H. Somnus Bacterin *(Aspen)*																		K																			
SomnuMune® *(AgriLabs)*																		K																			
Somnu Shield™ *(Novartis Animal Vaccines)*																		K																			
Somnu Shield™ XT *(Novartis Animal Vaccines)*																		K																			
Somubac® *(Pfizer Animal Health)*																		K																			
Surround™ HS *(Biocor)*																		K																			
TrustGard™ HS *(Vedco)*																		K																			
Bar Somnus 2P™ *(Boehringer Ingelheim)*																		K								K	K										
Poly-Bac B® 3 *(Texas Vet Lab)*																		K								K	K										
Poly-Bac B® Somnus *(Texas Vet Lab)*																		K								K	K				K						
Super Poly-Bac B® Somnus *(Texas Vet Lab)*																		K								K	K				K						
Express™ IP/HS-2P *(Boehringer Ingelheim)*																		K	M							K	K	M									
Bovi-Shield™ IBR *(Pfizer Animal Health)*																			M																		
Bovine Rhinotracheitis Vaccine *(Colorado Serum)*																			M																		
Express™ I *(Boehringer Ingelheim)*																			M																		
Pyramid® IBR *(Fort Dodge)*																			M																		
Reliant® IBR *(Merial)*																			M																		
Titanium™ IBR *(AgriLabs)*																			M																		
Titanium® IBR *(Intervet)*																			M																		
Express™ I/Lp *(Boehringer Ingelheim)*																			M	K																	
IL Vaccine *(Aspen)*																			M	K																	
Reliant® IBR/Lepto *(Merial)*																			M	K																	
Titanium™ IBR-LP *(AgriLabs)*																			M	K																	
Pyramid® IBR+Lepto *(Fort Dodge)*																			M		K																
Bovine Rhinotracheitis-Parainfluenza$_3$ Vaccine *(Colorado Serum)*																			M									M									
Nasal-Vax™ *(AgriPharm)*																			M									M									
Nasalgen® IP Vaccine *(Schering-Plough)*																			M									M									
Quick Shield™ Intranasal IBR-PI3 *(Novartis Animal Vaccines)*																			M									M									
TSV-2® *(Pfizer Animal Health)*																			M									M									
Lepto-5 *(Boehringer Ingelheim)*																					K																
Lepto-5 *(Colorado Serum)*																					K																
Lepto 5 *(Premier Farmtech)*																					K																
Lepto 5 *(AgriLabs)*																					K																
Lepto 5 *(Durvet)*																					K																
Lepto 5 Vaccine *(Aspen)*																					K																
Leptoferm-5® *(Pfizer Animal Health)*																					K																
Lepto Shield™ 5 *(Novartis Animal Vaccines)*																					K																
Lepto Shield™ 5 Hardjo Bovis *(Novartis Animal Vaccines)*																					K																
Surround™ L5 *(Biocor)*																					K																
TrustGard™ 5L *(Vedco)*																					K																
20/20® with Spur® *(Intervet)*																						K															
Cattle-Vac™ Pinkeye 4 *(Durvet)*																						K															
I-Site™ *(AgriLabs)*																						K															
Maxi/Guard® Pinkeye Bacterin *(Addison)*																						K															
Ocu-guard® MB *(Boehringer Ingelheim)*																						K															
Piliguard® Pinkeye-1 *(Schering-Plough)*																						K															
Piliguard® Pinkeye-1 *(Durvet)*																						K															
Pinkeye-3 *(Aspen)*																						K															
Pinkeye Shield™ XT4 *(Novartis Animal Vaccines)*																						K															

2-Way
- *Clostridium chauvoei*
- *Cl. septicum*

4-Way
- *Clostridium chauvoei*
- *Cl. novyi*
- *Cl. septicum*
- *Cl. sordellii*

7-Way
- *Clostridium chauvoei*
- *Cl. perfringens* Types C & D
- *Cl. novyi*
- *Cl. septicum*
- *Cl. sordellii* or *Cl. tetani*

8-Way
- *Clostridium chauvoei*
- *Cl. haemolyticum*
- *Cl. novyi*
- *Cl. perfringens* Types C & D
- *Cl. septicum*
- *Cl. sordellii* or *Cl. tetani*

Leptospira spp*
- *L. canicola*
- *L. grippotyphosa*
- *L. hardjo*
- *L. icterohaemorrhagiae*
- *L. pomona*

(continued on next page)

Please refer to product listings for more complete information.

BOVINE *(continued)*

K - antibodies
- antitoxin
- extract
- killed
- subunit
- toxoid

M - modified live

Product Name	Actinomyces (C. pyogenes)	Anaplasmosis	Anthrax	BRSV	Brucella spp	BVD Type I	BVD Type II	Campylobacter fetus	Clostridia, 2-way	Clostridia, 4-way	Clostridia, 7-way	Clostridia, 8-way	Clostridium haemolyticum	Clostridium perfringens	Coronavirus	E coli	Fusobacterium	Haemophilus somnus	IBR	L. pomona	Leptospira spp*	Moraxella bovis	Mycoplasma	Neospora caninum	Papillomavirus	Pasteurella haemolytica	Pasteurella multocida	PI3	Rabies	Rotavirus	Salmonella	Serpens spp	Serpulina (Treponema)	Staphylococcus spp	Tetanus Antitoxin	Tetanus Toxoid	Tritrichomonas
TrustGard™ MB *(Vedco)*																						K															
Mycoplasma Bovis Bacterin *(Biomune)*																							K														
NeoGuard™ *(Intervet)*																								K													
Papillomune™ *(Biomune)*																									K												
Wart-Vac *(Durvet)*																									K												
Wart Shield™ *(Novartis Animal Vaccines)*																									K												
Wart Vaccine *(AgriLabs)*																									K												
Wart Vaccine *(Colorado Serum)*																									K												
One Shot® *(Pfizer Animal Health)*																										K											
Presponse® SQ *(Fort Dodge)*																										K											
Antidote® PHM *(AgriPharm)*																										K	K										
Pasteurella Haemolytica Multocida Bacterin *(Colorado Serum)*																										K	K										
Presponse® HM *(Fort Dodge)*																										K	K										
Pulmo-guard™ PH-M *(Boehringer Ingelheim)*																										K	K										
Pulmo-guard™ PHM-1 *(Boehringer Ingelheim)*																										K	K										
Once PMH® *(Intervet)*																										M	M										
P.H.M. Bac® 1 *(AgriLabs)*																										M	M										
Defensor® 3 *(Pfizer Animal Health)*																													K								
Imrab® 3 *(Merial)*																													K								
Imrab® Large Animal *(Merial)*																													K								
Rabdomun® Vaccine *(Schering-Plough)*																													K								
Cattle-Vac™ Salmo *(Durvet)*																															K						
ENDOVAC-Bovi® with ImmunePlus® *(Immvac)*																															K						
Salmonella Dublin-Typhimurium Bacterin *(Colorado Serum)*																															K						
Salmo Shield® T *(Novartis Animal Vaccines)*																															K						
Salmo Shield® TD *(Novartis Animal Vaccines)*																															K						
Salmo Vac *(AgriPharm)*																															K						
SDT-Guard™ *(Boehringer Ingelheim)*																															K						
EnterVene™-d *(Fort Dodge)*																															M						
Serpens Species Bacterin *(Hygieia)*																																K					
Treponema Bacterin *(Novartis Animal Vaccines)*																																	K				
Lysigin® *(Boehringer Ingelheim)*																																		K			
Staphylococcus Aureus Bacterin-Toxoid *(Hygieia)*																																		K			
Antitox Tet™ *(Novartis Animal Vaccines)*																																			K		
Tetanus Antitoxin *(Fort Dodge)*																																			K		
Tetanus Antitoxin *(Durvet)*																																			K		
Tetanus Antitoxin, Equine Origin *(Colorado Serum)*																																			K		
Tetanus Antitoxin, Equine Origin *(Professional Biological)*																																			K		
Tetnogen®-AT *(Fort Dodge)*																																			K		
Super-Tet® with Havlogen® *(Intervet)*																																				K	
Tetanus Toxoid-Concentrated *(Colorado Serum)*																																				K	
Tetanus Toxoid-Concentrated *(Professional Biological)*																																				K	
Tetanus Toxoid-Unconcentrated *(Colorado Serum)*																																				K	
Tetguard™ *(Boehringer Ingelheim)*																																				K	
Tetnogen® *(Fort Dodge)*																																				K	
TrichGuard® *(Fort Dodge)*																																					K

2-Way
- *Clostridium chauvoei*
- *Cl. septicum*

4-Way
- *Clostridium chauvoei*
- *Cl. novyi*
- *Cl. septicum*
- *Cl. sordellii*

7-Way
- *Clostridium chauvoei*
- *Cl. perfringens* Types C & D
- *Cl. novyi*
- *Cl. septicum*
- *Cl. sordellii* or *Cl. tetani*

8-Way
- *Clostridium chauvoei*
- *Cl. haemolyticum*
- *Cl. novyi*
- *Cl. perfringens* Types C & D
- *Cl. septicum*
- *Cl. sordellii* or *Cl. tetani*

Leptospira spp*
- *L. canicola*
- *L. grippotyphosa*
- *L. hardjo*
- *L. icterohaemorrhagiae*
- *L. pomona*

(continued on next page)

CANINE

K - antibodies - antitoxin - extract - killed - subunit - toxoid M - modified live Product Name	Bordetella	Borrelia burgdorferi	CAV-1	CAV-2	Coronavirus	Distemper	Giardia	L. canicola	L. grippotyphosa	L. icterohaemorrhagiae	L. pomona	Measles	Parainfluenza	Parvovirus	Rabies	Salmonella
Borde-Vac 1 *(TradeWinds)*	K															
Bronchicine™ CAe *(Biocor)*	K															
CompanionVac™ B *(Aspen)*	K															
CoughGuard® B *(Pfizer Animal Health)*	K															
Performer® Borde-Vac *(AgriLabs)*	K															
Pet Care Canine Kennel Cough Vaccine *(Durvet)*	K															
CoughGuard® CPI/B *(Pfizer Animal Health)*	K												M			
Intra-Trac®-II *(Schering-Plough)*	M												M			
Intra-Trac®-II ADT* *(Schering-Plough)*	M												M			
Kennel-Jec-2™ *(Durvet)*	M												M			
Naramune-2™ *(Boehringer Ingelheim)*	M												M			
Progard®-KC *(Intervet)*	M												M			
Bronchi-Shield® III *(Fort Dodge)*	M			M									M			
Progard®-KC Plus *(Intervet)*	M			M									M			
Vanguard® 5/B *(Pfizer Animal Health)*	K			M		M							M	M		
Galaxy® Lyme *(Schering-Plough)*		K														
LymeVax® *(Fort Dodge)*		K														
ProLyme® *(Intervet)*		K														
Recombitek® Lyme *(Merial)*		K														
Duramune® The Puppyshot® Booster+LymeVax® *(Fort Dodge)*		K		M	K	M		K		K			M	M		
Champion Protector™ Puppy Protector™ *(AgriLabs)*			M			M							M	M		
Paramune™-5 *(Biocor)*			M			M		K		K			M			
Champion Protector™ Canine 7-Way Vaccine *(AgriLabs)*			M			M		K		K			M	M		
First Companion™ Canine 7-Way *(AgriPharm)*			M			M		K		K			M	M		
Solo-Jec-7™ *(Boehringer Ingelheim)*			M			M		K		K			M	M		
Solo-Jec-7™ *(Durvet)*			M			M		K		K			M	M		
Solo-Jec-7™ *(Aspen)*			M			M		K		K			M	M		
Tissuvax® 6 Vaccine *(Schering-Plough)*			M			M		K		K			M	M		
Adenomune™-7 *(Biocor)*			M	K		M		K		K			M	K		
Performer®-Seven *(AgriLabs)*			M	K		M		K		K			M	K		
Adenomune™-7-L *(Biocor)*			M	K		M		K		K			M	M		
Vanguard® DA$_2$P *(Pfizer Animal Health)*				M		M							M			
Vanguard® Plus 4 *(Pfizer Animal Health)*				M		M								M		
Vanguard® DA$_2$MP *(Pfizer Animal Health)*				M		M						M	M			
Commander™ 5 *(Biocor)*				K		M							M	M		
CompanionVac™ 5 *(Aspen)*				K		M							M	M		
Pet Care Puppy 5-Ultra *(Durvet)*				K		M							M	M		
Univac 5 *(TradeWinds)*				K		M							M	M		
Duramune® Max 5 *(Fort Dodge)*				M		M							M	M		
Galaxy® DA2PPv *(Schering-Plough)*				M		M							M	M		
Progard®-5 *(Intervet)*				M		M							M	M		
Recombitek® C4 *(Merial)*				M		M							M	M		
Vanguard® 5 *(Pfizer Animal Health)*				M		M							M	M		
Vanguard® Plus 5 *(Pfizer Animal Health)*				M		M							M	M		
Vanguard® DA$_2$PL *(Pfizer Animal Health)*				M		M		K		K			M			
Vanguard® Plus 4/Lci *(Pfizer Animal Health)*				M		M		K		K				M		
Duramune® Max 5-CvK The Puppyshot® *(Fort Dodge)*				M	K	M							M	M		
Galaxy® DA2PPv+Cv *(Schering-Plough)*				M	K	M							M	M		
Progard®-6 *(Intervet)*				M	K	M							M	M		
Vanguard® 5/CV *(Pfizer Animal Health)*				M	K	M							M	M		
Vanguard® Plus 5/CV *(Pfizer Animal Health)*				M	K	M							M	M		
Recombitek® C4/CV *(Merial)*				M	M	M							M	M		
Commander™ 7 L *(Biocor)*				K		M		K		K			M	M		
CompanionVac™ 7 L *(Aspen)*				K		M		K		K			M	M		
Pet Care Canine 7-Ultra *(Durvet)*				K		M		K		K			M	M		
Univac 7 *(TradeWinds)*				K		M		K		K			M	M		

(continued on next page)

Please refer to product listings for more complete information.

CANINE *(continued)*

K - antibodies
- antitoxin
- extract
- killed
- subunit
- toxoid

M - modified live

Product Name	Bordetella	Borrelia burgdorferi	CAV-1	CAV-2	Coronavirus	Distemper	Giardia	L. canicola	L. grippotyphosa	L. icterohaemorrhagiae	L. pomona	Measles	Parainfluenza	Parvovirus	Rabies	Salmonella
Galaxy® DA2PPvL *(Schering-Plough)*				M		M		K		K			M	M		
Progard®-7 *(Intervet)*				M		M		K		K			M	M		
Recombitek® C6 *(Merial)*				M		M		K		K			M	M		
Vanguard® 5/L *(Pfizer Animal Health)*				M		M		K		K			M	M		
Vanguard® Plus 5/L *(Pfizer Animal Health)*				M		M		K		K			M	M		
Galaxy® DA2PPvL+Cv *(Schering-Plough)*				M	K	M		K		K			M	M		
Progard®-8 *(Intervet)*				M	K	M		K		K			M	M		
Vanguard® 5/CV-L *(Pfizer Animal Health)*				M	K	M		K		K			M	M		
Vanguard® Plus 5/CV-L *(Pfizer Animal Health)*				M	K	M		K		K			M	M		
Recombitek® C6/CV *(Merial)*				M	M	M		K		K			M	M		
Duramune® Max 5/4L *(Fort Dodge)*				M		M		K	K	K	K		M	M		
Duramune® Max 5-CvK/4L The Puppyshot® Booster *(Fort Dodge)*				M	K	M		K	K	K	K		M	M		
Cor-1™ *(VacciCel)*					K											
Duramune® Cv-K *(Fort Dodge)*					K											
FirstDose® CV *(Pfizer Animal Health)*					K											
Galaxy® Cv *(Schering-Plough)*					K											
Progard®-CvK *(Intervet)*					K											
Recombitek® Canine Corona-MLV *(Merial)*					M											
Duramune® Max PC *(Fort Dodge)*					K									M		
FirstDose® CPV/CV *(Pfizer Animal Health)*					K									M		
Progard®-CPv+CvK *(Intervet)*					K									M		
Vanguard® Plus CPV/CV *(Pfizer Animal Health)*					K									M		
Recombitek® Canine Parvo + Corona-MLV *(Merial)*					M									M		
Progard® Puppy-DPv+CvK *(Intervet)*					K	M								M		
Galaxy® D *(Schering-Plough)*						M										
Vanguard® DM *(Pfizer Animal Health)*						M						M				
Progard® Puppy-DPv *(Intervet)*						M								M		
GiardiaVax® *(Fort Dodge)*							K									
Vanguard® Lci *(Pfizer Animal Health)*								K		K						
Duramune® LGP *(Fort Dodge)*									K		K					
Parvocine® *(Biocor)*														K		
Vanguard® CPV (killed) *(Pfizer Animal Health)*														K		
Commander™ Parvo MLV *(Biocor)*														M		
CompanionVac™ Parvo MLV *(Aspen)*														M		
CPV/LP™ *(VacciCel)*														M		
Duramune® Max Pv *(Fort Dodge)*														M		
FirstDose® CPV *(Pfizer Animal Health)*														M		
Galaxy® Pv *(Schering-Plough)*														M		
NeoPar® *(NeoTech)*														M		
Pet Care Canine Parvo-Ultra *(Durvet)*														M		
Progard®-CPv *(Intervet)*														M		
Recombitek® Canine Parvo *(Merial)*														M		
Univac Parvo *(TradeWinds)*														M		
Vanguard® Plus CPV *(Pfizer Animal Health)*														M		
Defensor® 1 *(Pfizer Animal Health)*															K	
Defensor® 3 *(Pfizer Animal Health)*															K	
Imrab® 1 *(Merial)*															K	
Imrab® 3 *(Merial)*															K	
Prorab®-1 *(Intervet)*															K	
Rabdomun® 1 Vaccine *(Schering-Plough)*															K	
Rabdomun® Vaccine *(Schering-Plough)*															K	
Rabvac™ 1 *(Fort Dodge)*															K	
Rabvac™ 3 *(Fort Dodge)*															K	
SEPTI-serum® *(Immvac)*																K

EQUINE

K - antibodies - antitoxin - extract - killed - subunit - toxoid M - modified live Product Name	Anthrax	Cl. botulinum	E. coli	Ehrlichia risticii	Encephalomyelitis	Influenza	Rabies	Rhinopneumonitis	Rhodococcus equi	Rotavirus	Salmonella	Sarcocystis neurona	Streptococcus spp	Tetanus Antitoxin	Tetanus Toxoid	Viral arteritis	West Nile Virus
Anthrax Spore Vaccine *(Colorado Serum)*	J																
BotVax® B *(Neogen)*		K															
Clostridium Botulinum Type B Antitoxin *(V.D.I.)*		K															
E. Colicin-E® *(AgriLabs)*			K														
Equine Coli Endotox® *(Novartis Animal Vaccines)*			K														
Equine Potomavac® *(Merial)*				K													
Mystique® *(Intervet)*				K													
PHF-Vax® *(Schering-Plough)*				K													
PotomacGuard® *(Fort Dodge)*				K													
Potomac Shield™ *(Novartis Animal Vaccines)*				K													
Equine Potomavac® + Imrab® *(Merial)*				K			K										
Mystique® II *(Intervet)*				K			K										
PotomacGuard® EWT *(Fort Dodge)*				K	K										K		
Encephaloid® IM *(Fort Dodge)*					K												
Encephalomyelitis Vaccine Eastern & Western *(Colorado Serum)*					K												
Encevac® with Havlogen® *(Intervet)*					K												
Triple-E® *(Fort Dodge)*					K												
Cephalovac® EWT *(Boehringer Ingelheim)*					K										K		
Cephalovac® VEWT *(Boehringer Ingelheim)*					K										K		
Encephalomyelitis Vaccine Eastern & Western with Tetanus Toxoid *(Colorado Serum)*					K										K		
Encevac®-T with Havlogen® *(Intervet)*					K										K		
Encevac® T + VEE with Havlogen® *(Intervet)*					K										K		
Equiloid® Innovator *(Fort Dodge)*					K										K		
EWT™ *(Schering-Plough)*					K										K		
Triple-E® T Innovator *(Fort Dodge)*					K										K		
Encevac® TC-4 + VEE with Havlogen® *(Intervet)*					K	K									K		
Encevac® TC-4 with Havlogen® *(Intervet)*					K	K									K		
Equi-Flu® EWT *(Boehringer Ingelheim)*					K	K									K		
Equi-Flu® VEWT *(Boehringer Ingelheim)*					K	K									K		
Equine EWTF *(Merial)*					K	K									K		
EWTF™ *(Schering-Plough)*					K	K									K		
Fluvac® Innovator Double-E FT® *(Fort Dodge)*					K	K									K		
Fluvac® Innovator Triple-E® FT *(Fort Dodge)*					K	K									K		
Fluvac® Innovator Double-E FT®+EHV *(Fort Dodge)*					K	K		K							K		
Fluvac® Innovator Triple-E® FT+EHV *(Fort Dodge)*					K	K		K							K		
Prestige® V + VEE with Havlogen® *(Intervet)*					K	K		K							K		
Prestige® V with Havlogen® *(Intervet)*					K	K		K							K		
Calvenza™ EIV *(Boehringer Ingelheim)*						K											
Equicine® II with Havlogen® *(Intervet)*						K											
Flumune® *(Pfizer Animal Health)*						K											
Fluvac® Innovator *(Fort Dodge)*						K											
Flu Avert™ I.N. Vaccine *(Intervet)*						M											
Calvenza™ EIV/EHV *(Boehringer Ingelheim)*						K		K									
Fluvac® Innovator EHV-4/1 *(Fort Dodge)*						K		K									
Prestige® II with Havlogen® *(Intervet)*						K		K									
Imrab® 3 *(Merial)*							K										
Imrab® Large Animal *(Merial)*							K										
Rabvac™ 3 *(Fort Dodge)*							K										

(continued on next page)

Please refer to product listings for more complete information.

EQUINE *(continued)*

K - antibodies
- antitoxin
- extract
- killed
- subunit
- toxoid

M - modified live

Product Name	Anthrax	Cl. botulinum	E. coli	Ehrlichia risticii	Encephalomyelitis	Influenza	Rabies	Rhinopneumonitis	Rhodococcus equi	Rotavirus	Salmonella	Sarcocystis neurona	Streptococcus spp	Tetanus Antitoxin	Tetanus Toxoid	Viral arteritis	West Nile Virus
Calvenza™ EHV *(Boehringer Ingelheim)*								K									
EquiVac™ EHV-1/4 *(Fort Dodge)*								K									
Pneumabort-K®+1b *(Fort Dodge)*								K									
Prestige® with Havlogen® *(Intervet)*								K									
Prodigy® with Havlogen® *(Intervet)*								K									
Rhinomune® *(Pfizer Animal Health)*								M									
Rhodococcus Equi Antibody *(V.D.I.)*									K								
Equine Rotavirus Vaccine *(Fort Dodge)*										K							
ENDOSERUM® *(Immvac)*											K						
ENDOVAC-Equi® with ImmunePlus® *(Immvac)*											K						
Sarcocystis Neurona Vaccine *(Fort Dodge)*												K					
Strepguard® with Havlogen® *(Intervet)*													K				
Strepvax® II *(Boehringer Ingelheim)*													K				
Pinnacle™ I.N. *(Fort Dodge)*													M				
Antitox Tet™ *(Novartis Animal Vaccines)*														K			
Tetanus Antitoxin *(Fort Dodge)*														K			
Tetanus Antitoxin *(Durvet)*														K			
Tetanus Antitoxin, Equine Origin *(Colorado Serum)*														K			
Tetanus Antitoxin, Equine Origin *(Professional Biological)*														K			
Tetnogen®-AT *(Fort Dodge)*														K			
Super-Tet® with Havlogen® *(Intervet)*															K		
Tetanus Toxoid *(Fort Dodge)*															K		
Tetanus Toxoid-Concentrated *(Colorado Serum)*															K		
Tetanus Toxoid-Concentrated *(Professional Biological)*															K		
Tetanus Toxoid-Unconcentrated *(Colorado Serum)*															K		
Tetguard™ *(Boehringer Ingelheim)*															K		
Tetnogen® *(Fort Dodge)*															K		
Arvac® *(Fort Dodge)*																M	
West Nile Virus Vaccine *(Fort Dodge)*																	K

FELINE

K - antibodies
- antitoxin
- extract
- killed
- subunit
- toxoid

M - modified live

Product Name	Bordetella	Calicivirus	Chlamydia	Feline Immunodeficiency Virus	Giardia	Infectious Peritonitis	Leukemia	Microsporum canis	Panleukopenia	Rabies	Rhinotracheitis
Protex®-Bb *(Intervet)*	M										
Fel-O-Guard® Plus 2 *(Fort Dodge)*		M									M
Felocell® RESP-2 *(Pfizer Animal Health)*		M									M
Felomune CVR® *(Pfizer Animal Health)*		M									M
FVR® C Vaccine *(Schering-Plough)*		M									M
Heska® Bivalent Intranasal/Intraocular Vaccine *(Heska)*		M									M
Respomune™ 2 *(Biocor)*		M									M
Felocell® RESP-3 *(Pfizer Animal Health)*		M	M								M
Fel-O-Vax® PCT *(Fort Dodge)*		K							K		K
CompanionVac™ RCP *(Aspen)*		M							K		M
FVR® C-P Vaccine *(Schering-Plough)*		M							K		M
Pet Care Feline 3 Vaccine *(Durvet)*		M							K		M
Respomune®-CP *(Biocor)*		M							K		M
Champion Protector™ Feline *(AgriLabs)*		M							K		M
Eclipse® 3 *(Schering-Plough)*		M							M		M
Fel-O-Guard® Plus 3 *(Fort Dodge)*		M							M		M
Feline 3 Way Vaccine *(TradeWinds)*		M							M		M
Felocell® 3 *(Pfizer Animal Health)*		M							M		M
Heska® Trivalent Intranasal/Intraocular Vaccine *(Heska)*		M							M		M
Protex®-3 *(Intervet)*		M							M		M
PureVax™ Feline 3 *(Merial)*		M							M		M
Rhinopan®-MLV *(Biocor)*		M							M		M
Fel-O-Vax® IV *(Fort Dodge)*		K	K						K		K
Fel-O-Guard® Plus 4 *(Fort Dodge)*		M	K						M		M
Eclipse® 4 *(Schering-Plough)*		M	M						M		M
Feline 4 Way Vaccine *(TradeWinds)*		M	M						M		M
Felocell® 4 *(Pfizer Animal Health)*		M	M						M		M
Performer®-Feline 4 *(AgriLabs)*		M	M						M		M
Pet Care Feline 3-C Vaccine *(Durvet)*		M	M						M		M
Protex®-4 *(Intervet)*		M	M						M		M
PureVax™ Feline 4 *(Merial)*		M	M						M		M
Rhinopan®-4 *(Biocor)*		M	M						M		M
Fel-O-Vax Lv-K® III *(Fort Dodge)*		K					K		K		K
Eclipse® 3 + FeLV *(Schering-Plough)*		M					K		M		M
Fel-O-Guard® Plus 3 + Lv-K *(Fort Dodge)*		M					K		M		M
PureVax™ Feline 3 + Leucat® *(Merial)*		M					K		M		M
Fel-O-Vax Lv-K® IV *(Fort Dodge)*		K	K				K		K		K
Fel-O-Guard® Plus 4 + Lv-K *(Fort Dodge)*		M	K				K		M		M
Eclipse® 4 + FeLV *(Schering-Plough)*		M	M				K		M		M
PureVax™ Feline 4 + Leucat® *(Merial)*		M	M				K		M		M
PureVax™ Feline 3/Rabies *(Merial)*		M							M	M	M
PureVax™ Feline 4/Rabies *(Merial)*		M	M						M	M	M
Eclipse® 3 + FeLV/R *(Schering-Plough)*		M					K		M	K	M
PureVax™ Feline 3/Rabies + Leucat® *(Merial)*		M					K		M	M	M

(continued on next page)

Please refer to product listings for more complete information.

FELINE *(continued)*

K - antibodies
- antitoxin
- extract
- killed
- subunit
- toxoid

M - modified live

Product Name	Bordetella	Calicivirus	Chlamydia	Feline Immunodeficiency Virus	Giardia	Infectious Peritonitis	Leukemia	Microsporum canis	Panleukopenia	Rabies	Rhinotracheitis
Eclipse® 4 + FeLV/R *(Schering-Plough)*		M	M				K		M	K	M
PureVax™ Feline 4/Rabies + Leucat® *(Merial)*		M	M				K		M	M	M
Fel-O-Vax® FIV *(Fort Dodge)*				K							
Fel-O-Vax® Giardia *(Fort Dodge)*					K						
Primucell FIP® *(Pfizer Animal Health)*						M					
Fel-O-Vax Lv-K® *(Fort Dodge)*							K				
Fevaxyn® FeLV *(Schering-Plough)*							K				
Leukocell® 2 *(Pfizer Animal Health)*							K				
Protex®-FeLV *(Intervet)*							K				
PureVax™ Leucat® *(Merial)*							K				
Fel-O-Vax® MC-K *(Fort Dodge)*								K			
FPV-1 *(Biocor)*									K		
Felocell® FPV *(Pfizer Animal Health)*									M		
Defensor® 1 *(Pfizer Animal Health)*										K	
Defensor® 3 *(Pfizer Animal Health)*										K	
Imrab® 1 *(Merial)*										K	
Imrab® 3 *(Merial)*										K	
Prorab®-1 *(Intervet)*										K	
Rabdomun® 1 Vaccine *(Schering-Plough)*										K	
Rabdomun® Vaccine *(Schering-Plough)*										K	
Rabvac™ 1 *(Fort Dodge)*										K	
Rabvac™ 3 *(Fort Dodge)*										K	
PureVax™ Feline Rabies *(Merial)*										M	

Please refer to product listings for more complete information.

OVINE

K - antibodies
- antitoxin
- extract
- killed
- subunit
- toxoid

M - modified live

Product Name	Actinomyces (C. pyogenes)	Anthrax	B. nodosus	Bluetongue	Brucella ovis	Campylobacter fetus	Chlamydia	Clostridia, 2-way	Clostridia, 4-way	Clostridia, 7-way	Clostridia, 8-way	Clostridium haemolyticum	Clostridium perfringens	Corynebacterium	E. coli	Fusobacterium	Parapoxvirus (Orf)	Pasteurella haemolytica	Pasteurella multocida	Rabies	Salmonella	Tetanus Antitoxin	Tetanus Toxoid
Respiragen™ Serum Antibodies *(Colorado Serum)*	K																	K	K				
BovaMune™ *(AgriLabs)*	K														K			K	K		K		
Bovi-Sera™ Serum Antibodies *(Colorado Serum)*	K														K			K	K		K		
Multi Serum *(Durvet)*	K														K			K	K		K		
Poly Serum® *(Novartis Animal Vaccines)*	K														K			K	K		K		
Anthrax Spore Vaccine *(Colorado Serum)*		M																					
Bluetongue Vaccine *(Colorado Serum)*				M																			
Footvax® 10 Strain *(Schering-Plough)*			K																				
Ram Epididymitis Bacterin *(Colorado Serum)*					K																		
Campylobacter Fetus-Jejuni Bacterin *(Hygieia)*						K																	
Campylobacter Fetus Bacterin-Ovine *(Colorado Serum)*						K																	
Chlamydia Psittaci Bacterin *(Colorado Serum)*							K																
Clostridium Chauvoei-Septicum Bacterin *(Colorado Serum)*								K															
Clostridium Chauvoei-Septicum-Pasteurella Haemolytica-Multocida Bacterin *(Colorado Serum)*								K										K	K				
Clostridium Chauvoei-Septicum-Novyi-Sordellii Bacterin-Toxoid *(Colorado Serum)*									K														
7 Gauge™ *(AgriPharm)*										K													
7-Way *(Aspen)*										K													
Bar-Vac® 7 *(Boehringer Ingelheim)*										K													
Caliber® 7 *(Boehringer Ingelheim)*										K													
Electroid® 7 Vaccine *(Schering-Plough)*										K													
Resist™ 7 *(AgriPharm)*										K													
TrustGard™ 7 *(Vedco)*										K													
Ultrabac® 7 *(Pfizer Animal Health)*										K													
UltraChoice™ 7 *(Pfizer Animal Health)*										K													
Vision® 7 with Spur® *(Intervet)*										K													
8-Way *(Aspen)*											K												
Bar-Vac® 8 *(Boehringer Ingelheim)*											K												
Covexin® 8 Vaccine *(Schering-Plough)*											K												
Resist™ 8 *(AgriPharm)*											K												
Siteguard® MLG Vaccine *(Schering-Plough)*											K												
Tetni-Vax® *(AgriPharm)*											K												
TrustGard™ 8 *(Vedco)*											K												
Ultrabac® 8 *(Pfizer Animal Health)*											K												
UltraChoice™ 8 *(Pfizer Animal Health)*											K												
Vision® 8 with Spur® *(Intervet)*											K												
Clostridium Haemolyticum Bacterin (Red Water) *(Colorado Serum)*												K											
Bar-Vac® CD *(Boehringer Ingelheim)*													K										
C & D Antitoxin™ *(Boehringer Ingelheim)*													K										
C & D Toxoid *(Aspen)*													K										
Caliber® 3 *(Boehringer Ingelheim)*													K										
Clostratox® BCD *(Novartis Animal Vaccines)*													K										
Clostratox® C *(Novartis Animal Vaccines)*													K										
Clostratox® Ultra C 1300 *(Novartis Animal Vaccines)*													K										

2-Way
- *Clostridium chauvoei*
- *Cl. septicum*

4-Way
- *Clostridium chauvoei*
- *Cl. novyi*
- *Cl. septicum*
- *Cl. sordellii*

7-Way
- *Clostridium chauvoei*
- *Cl. perfringens* Types C & D
- *Cl. novyi*
- *Cl. septicum*
- *Cl. sordellii* or *Cl. tetani*

8-Way
- *Clostridium chauvoei*
- *Cl. haemolyticum*
- *Cl. novyi*
- *Cl. perfringens* Types C & D
- *Cl. septicum*
- *Cl. sordellii* or *Cl. tetani*

(continued on next page)

Please refer to product listings for more complete information.

OVINE *(continued)*

K - antibodies
- antitoxin
- extract
- killed
- subunit
- toxoid

M - modified live

Product Name	Actinomyces (C. pyogenes)	Anthrax	B. nodosus	Bluetongue	Brucella ovis	Campylobacter fetus	Chlamydia	Clostridia, 2-way	Clostridia, 4-way	Clostridia, 7-way	Clostridia, 8-way	Clostridium haemolyticum	Clostridium perfringens	Corynebacterium	E. coli	Fusobacterium	Parapoxvirus (Orf)	Pasteurella haemolytica	Pasteurella multocida	Rabies	Salmonella	Tetanus Antitoxin	Tetanus Toxoid
Clostridial Antitoxin BCD *(Durvet)*													K										
Clostridial BCD *(Durvet)*													K										
Clostridium Perfringens Types C & D Antitoxin, Equine Origin *(Colorado Serum)*													K										
Clostridium Perfringens Types C&D Antitoxin, Equine Origin *(Professional Biological)*													K										
Clostridium Perfringens Types C & D Toxoid *(Colorado Serum)*													K										
Clostridium Perfringens Types C&D Toxoid *(Professional Biological)*													K										
Clostri Shield® BCD *(Novartis Animal Vaccines)*													K										
Electroid® D *(Schering-Plough)*													K										
Gauge™ C&D *(AgriPharm)*													K										
Siteguard® G *(Schering-Plough)*													K										
TrustGard™ CD *(Vedco)*													K										
Ultrabac® CD *(Pfizer Animal Health)*													K										
UltraChoice™ CD *(Pfizer Animal Health)*													K										
Vision® CD with Spur® *(Intervet)*													K										
Bar Vac® CD/T *(Boehringer Ingelheim)*													K										K
Clostridium Perfringens Types C & D-Tetanus Toxoid *(Colorado Serum)*													K										K
Clostridium Perfringens Types C&D-Tetanus Toxoid *(Professional Biological)*													K										K
TrustGard™ CD/T *(Vedco)*													K										K
Vision® CD•T with Spur® *(Intervet)*													K										K
Caseous D-T™ *(Colorado Serum)*													K	K									K
Case-Bac™ *(Colorado Serum)*														K									
Bar-Guard-99™ *(Boehringer Ingelheim)*															K								
Ovine Ecolizer® *(Novartis Animal Vaccines)*															K								
Volar® *(Intervet)*																K							
Ovine Ecthyma Vaccine *(Colorado Serum)*																	M						
Pasteurella Haemolytica Multocida Bacterin *(Colorado Serum)*																		K	K				
Defensor® 3 *(Pfizer Animal Health)*																				K			
Imrab® 3 *(Merial)*																				K			
Imrab® Large Animal *(Merial)*																				K			
Prorab®-1 *(Intervet)*																				K			
Rabdomun® Vaccine *(Schering-Plough)*																				K			
Antitox Tet™ *(Novartis Animal Vaccines)*																						K	
Tetanus Antitoxin *(Fort Dodge)*																						K	
Tetanus Antitoxin *(Durvet)*																						K	
Tetanus Antitoxin, Equine Origin *(Colorado Serum)*																						K	
Tetanus Antitoxin, Equine Origin *(Professional Biological)*																						K	
Tetnogen®-AT *(Fort Dodge)*																						K	
Ovine Tetanus Shield™ *(Novartis Animal Vaccines)*																							K
Super-Tet® with Havlogen® *(Intervet)*																							K
Tetanus Toxoid *(Fort Dodge)*																							K
Tetanus Toxoid-Concentrated *(Colorado Serum)*																							K
Tetanus Toxoid-Concentrated *(Professional Biological)*																							K
Tetanus Toxoid-Unconcentrated *(Colorado Serum)*																							K
Tetguard™ *(Boehringer Ingelheim)*																							K
Tetnogen® *(Fort Dodge)*																							K

2-Way
- *Clostridium chauvoei*
- *Cl. septicum*

4-Way
- *Clostridium chauvoei*
- *Cl. novyi*
- *Cl. septicum*
- *Cl. sordellii*

7-Way
- *Clostridium chauvoei*
- *Cl. perfringens* Types C & D
- *Cl. novyi*
- *Cl. septicum*
- *Cl. sordellii* or *Cl. tetani*

8-Way
- *Clostridium chauvoei*
- *Cl. haemolyticum*
- *Cl. novyi*
- *Cl. perfringens* Types C & D
- *Cl. septicum*
- *Cl. sordellii* or *Cl. tetani*

Please refer to product listings for more complete information.

PORCINE

K - antibodies
- antitoxin
- extract
- killed
- subunit
- toxoid

M - modified live

Product Name	A. pleuropneumoniae	Actinomyces (C. pyogenes)	Anthrax	Bordetella	Clostridium perfringens	E. coli	Erysipelothrix	Haemophilus parasuis	Influenza	L. bratislava	Lawsonia sp	Leptospira spp*	Mycoplasma	Parvovirus	Pasteurella haemolytica	Pasteurella multocida	PRRS	Pseudorabies	Rotavirus	Salmonella	Streptococcus spp	T.G.E.	Tetanus Antitoxin	Tetanus Toxoid
Emulsibac® APP *(MVP)*	K																							
Pneumosuis® III *(Pfizer Animal Health)*	K																							
Pneu Pac® *(Schering-Plough)*	K																							
Suvaxyn® RespiFend® APP *(Fort Dodge)*	K																							
Ingelvac® APP-ALC *(Boehringer Ingelheim)*	M																							
Pneu Pac®-ER *(Schering-Plough)*	K						K																	
Pneu Parapac®+ER *(Schering-Plough)*	K						K	K																
Haemo Shield® P *(Novartis Animal Vaccines)*	K																							
Parapleuro Shield® P *(Novartis Animal Vaccines)*	K							K								K								
PleuroGuard® 4 *(Pfizer Animal Health)*	K			K			K									K								
DurVac™ Appear-HP *(Durvet)*	K			K			K	K								K								
Parapleuro Shield® P+BE *(Novartis Animal Vaccines)*	K			K			K	K								K								
Prevail™ Para Pleuro Bac+3DT *(Aspen)*	K			K			K	K								K								
Respiragen™ Serum Antibodies *(Colorado Serum)*		K													K	K								
Anthrax Spore Vaccine *(Colorado Serum)*			M																					
Borde-Cell™ *(AgriLabs)*				M																				
Bordetella Bronchiseptica Intranasal Vaccine *(MVP)*				M																				
DurVac™ AR *(Durvet)*				M																				
Maxi/Guard® Nasal Vac *(Addison)*				M																				
Rhinicell® *(Novartis Animal Vaccines)*				M																				
DurVac™ E-AR *(Durvet)*				M			M																	
Rhinicell®+E *(Novartis Animal Vaccines)*				M			M																	
Ingelvac® AR4 *(Boehringer Ingelheim)*				K												K								
Suvaxyn® AR/T *(Fort Dodge)*				K												K								
AR-Pac®-P+ER *(Schering-Plough)*				K			K									K								
AR-Pac®-PD+ER *(Schering-Plough)*				K			K									K								
Atrobac® 3 *(Pfizer Animal Health)*				K			K									K								
Borde Shield® 4 *(Novartis Animal Vaccines)*				K			K									K								
DurVac™ AR-4 *(Durvet)*				K			K									K								
Rhini Shield™ TX4 *(Novartis Animal Vaccines)*				K			K									K								
Rhinogen® BPE *(Intervet)*				K			K									K								
Rhinogen® CTE 5000 *(Intervet)*				K			K									K								
Score® *(Intervet)*				K			K									K								
Suvaxyn® AR/T/E *(Fort Dodge)*				K			K									K								
Toxivac® AD+E *(Boehringer Ingelheim)*				K			K									K								
Sow Bac® E II *(Intervet)*				K		K	K									K								
Suvaxyn® AR/E/EC-4 *(Fort Dodge)*				K		K	K									K								
Myco Silencer® BPM *(Intervet)*				K									K			K								
AR-Parapac®+ER *(Schering-Plough)*				K			K	K								K								
Toxivac® Plus Parasuis *(Boehringer Ingelheim)*				K			K	K								K								
Prefarrow Shield™ 9 *(Novartis Animal Vaccines)*				K	K	K	K									K								
Sow Bac® CE II *(Intervet)*				K	K	K	K									K								
Myco Silencer® BPME *(Intervet)*				K			K						K			K								
Rhinogen® CTSE *(Intervet)*				K			K									K					K			
Sow Bac® TREC *(Intervet)*				K	K	K	K									K			M			M		

Leptospira spp*
- *L. canicola*
- *L. grippotyphosa*
- *L. hardjo*
- *L. icterohaemorrhagiae*
- *L. pomona*

(continued on next page)

Please refer to product listings for more complete information.

PORCINE *(continued)*

K - antibodies
- antitoxin
- extract
- killed
- subunit
- toxoid

M - modified live

Product Name	A. pleuropneumoniae	Actinomyces (C. pyogenes)	Anthrax	Bordetella	Clostridium perfringens	E. coli	Erysipelothrix	Haemophilus parasuis	Influenza	L. bratislava	Lawsonia sp	Leptospira spp*	Mycoplasma	Parvovirus	Pasteurella haemolytica	Pasteurella multocida	PRRS	Pseudorabies	Rotavirus	Salmonella	Streptococcus spp	T.G.E.	Tetanus Antitoxin	Tetanus Toxoid
C & D Antitoxin™ *(Boehringer Ingelheim)*					K																			
C & D Toxoid *(Aspen)*					K																			
Clostratox® BCD *(Novartis Animal Vaccines)*					K																			
Clostratox® C *(Novartis Animal Vaccines)*					K																			
Clostratox® Ultra C 1300 *(Novartis Animal Vaccines)*					K																			
Clostridium Perfringens Types C & D Antitoxin, Equine Origin *(Colorado Serum)*					K																			
Clostridium Perfringens Types C&D Antitoxin, Equine Origin *(Professional Biological)*					K																			
Clostridium Perfringens Types C & D Toxoid *(Colorado Serum)*					K																			
Clostridium Perfringens Types C&D Toxoid *(Professional Biological)*					K																			
DurVac™ E. Coli 3C *(Durvet)*					K	K																		
DurVac™ EC-C *(Durvet)*					K	K																		
E. Colicin-S3+C™ *(AgriLabs)*					K	K																		
LitterGuard® LT-C *(Pfizer Animal Health)*					K	K																		
Porcine Ecolizer® 3+C *(Novartis Animal Vaccines)*					K	K																		
Porcine Pili Shield™+C *(Novartis Animal Vaccines)*					K	K																		
ProSystem® CE *(Intervet)*					K	K																		
Scourmune®-C *(Schering-Plough)*					K	K																		
Clostridium Perfringens Types C & D-Tetanus Toxoid *(Colorado Serum)*					K																			K
Clostridium Perfringens Types C&D-Tetanus Toxoid *(Professional Biological)*					K																			K
Scourmune®-CR *(Schering-Plough)*					K	K													K					
ProSystem® RCE *(Intervet)*					K	K													M					
ProSystem® TREC *(Intervet)*					K	K													M			M		
DurVac™ E. Coli 3 *(Durvet)*						K																		
DurVac™ EC *(Durvet)*						K																		
E. Colicin-S3™ *(AgriLabs)*						K																		
J-5 Escherichia Coli Bacterin *(Hygieia)*						K																		
LitterGuard® *(Pfizer Animal Health)*						K																		
LitterGuard® LT *(Pfizer Animal Health)*						K																		
Porcine Ecolizer® 3 *(Novartis Animal Vaccines)*						K																		
Porcine Pili Shield™ *(Novartis Animal Vaccines)*						K																		
ProSystem® Pilimune *(Intervet)*						K																		
Scourmune® *(Schering-Plough)*						K																		
Suvaxyn® EC-4 *(Fort Dodge)*						K																		
DurVac™ Ery *(Durvet)*							K																	
E-Bac™ *(Intervet)*							K																	
ER Bac® *(Pfizer Animal Health)*							K																	
ER Bac® Plus *(Pfizer Animal Health)*							K																	
Ery Serum™ *(Novartis Animal Vaccines)*							K																	
Ery Shield™ *(Novartis Animal Vaccines)*							K																	
Erysipelas Bacterin *(AgriLabs)*							K																	
Erysipelothrix Rhusiopathiae Serum Antibodies *(Colorado Serum)*							K																	
Erysipelothrix Rhusiopathiae Serum Antibodies *(Professional Biological)*							K																	
Suvaxyn®-E (Swine and Turkey) *(Fort Dodge)*							K																	
Suvaxyn® E *(Fort Dodge)*							K																	

*Leptospira spp**
- *L. canicola*
- *L. grippotyphosa*
- *L. hardjo*
- *L. icterohaemorrhagiae*
- *L. pomona*

(continued on next page)

PORCINE *(continued)*

K - antibodies
- antitoxin
- extract
- killed
- subunit
- toxoid

M - modified live

Product Name	A. pleuropneumoniae	Actinomyces (C. pyogenes)	Anthrax	Bordetella	Clostridium perfringens	E. coli	Erysipelothrix	Haemophilus parasuis	Influenza	L. bratislava	Lawsonia sp	Leptospira spp*	Mycoplasma	Parvovirus	Pasteurella haemolytica	Pasteurella multocida	PRRS	Pseudorabies	Rotavirus	Salmonella	Streptococcus spp	T.G.E.	Tetanus Antitoxin	Tetanus Toxoid
Erycell™ *(Novartis Animal Vaccines)*							M																	
Ery Vac 100 *(Arko)*							M																	
Ery Vac 500 *(Arko)*							M																	
Ingelvac® ERY-ALC *(Boehringer Ingelheim)*							M																	
Suvaxyn® E-oral *(Fort Dodge)*							M																	
FluSure™/ER Bac Plus® *(Pfizer Animal Health)*							K		K															
ER Bac®/Leptoferm-5® *(Pfizer Animal Health)*							K					K												
ER Bac® Plus/Leptoferm-5® *(Pfizer Animal Health)*							K					K												
Ery Shield™+L5 *(Novartis Animal Vaccines)*							K					K												
RespiSure 1 ONE®/ER Bac Plus® *(Pfizer Animal Health)*							K						K											
Myco Silencer® MEH *(Intervet)*							K	K					K											
FluSure™/RespiSure 1 ONE®/ER Bac Plus® *(Pfizer Animal Health)*							K		K				K											
Suvaxyn® LE+B *(Fort Dodge)*							K			K		K												
Ingelvac® PRRS-HPE *(Boehringer Ingelheim)*							K	K									M							
Breed Sow® 7 *(AgriLabs)*							K					K		K										
DurVac™ P-E-L *(Durvet)*							K					K		K										
FarrowSure® *(Pfizer Animal Health)*							K					K		K										
FarrowSure® Plus *(Pfizer Animal Health)*							K					K		K										
MaGESTic™ 7 with Spur® *(Intervet)*							K					K		K										
Parvo Shield® L5E *(Novartis Animal Vaccines)*							K					K		K										
Prevail™ Parvoplex 6-Way+E *(Aspen)*							K					K		K										
Suvaxyn® PLE *(Fort Dodge)*							K					K		K										
FarrowSure® B *(Pfizer Animal Health)*							K			K		K		K										
FarrowSure® Plus B *(Pfizer Animal Health)*							K			K		K		K										
Suvaxyn® PLE+B *(Fort Dodge)*							K			K		K		K										
ReproCyc® PRRS-PLE *(Boehringer Ingelheim)*							K					K		K			M							
FarrowSure® PRV *(Pfizer Animal Health)*							K					K		K				M						
Suvaxyn® PLE/PrV gpI- *(Fort Dodge)*							K					K		K				M						
FarrowSure® B-PRV *(Pfizer Animal Health)*							K			K		K		K				M						
Suvaxyn® PLE+B/PrV gpI- *(Fort Dodge)*							K			K		K		K				M						
Ingelvac® HP-1 *(Boehringer Ingelheim)*								K																
Parapac™ *(Schering-Plough)*								K																
Para Shield® *(Novartis Animal Vaccines)*								K																
Suvaxyn® RespiFend® HPS *(Fort Dodge)*								K																
M+Parapac™ *(Schering-Plough)*								K																
Suvaxyn® RespiFend® MH/HPS *(Fort Dodge)*								K					K											
Ingelvac® PRRS-HP *(Boehringer Ingelheim)*								K					K											
End-FLUence® 2 *(Intervet)*								K									M							
End-FLUence® with Imugen® II *(Intervet)*									K															
FluSure™ *(Pfizer Animal Health)*									K															
FluSure™ RTU *(Pfizer Animal Health)*									K															
MaxiVac®-FLU *(SyntroVet)*									K															
MaxiVac® Excell™ *(SyntroVet)*									K															
Swine Influenza Vaccine (H3N2 Subtype) *(SyntroVet)*									K															
FluSure™/RespiSure 1 ONE® *(Pfizer Animal Health)*									K															
FluSure™/RespiSure® *(Pfizer Animal Health)*									K				K											
FluSure™/RespiSure® RTU *(Pfizer Animal Health)*									K				K											
MaxiVac®-M+ *(SyntroVet)*									K				K											

Leptospira spp*
- *L. canicola*
- *L. grippotyphosa*
- *L. hardjo*
- *L. icterohaemorrhagiae*
- *L. pomona*

(continued on next page)

Please refer to product listings for more complete information.

PORCINE *(continued)*

K - antibodies
- antitoxin
- extract
- killed
- subunit
- toxoid

M - modified live

Product Name	A. pleuropneumoniae	Actinomyces (C. pyogenes)	Anthrax	Bordetella	Clostridium perfringens	E. coli	Erysipelothrix	Haemophilus parasuis	Influenza	L. bratislava	Lawsonia sp	Leptospira spp*	Mycoplasma	Parvovirus	Pasteurella haemolytica	Pasteurella multocida	PRRS	Pseudorabies	Rotavirus	Salmonella	Streptococcus spp	T.G.E.	Tetanus Antitoxin	Tetanus Toxoid
PRV/Marker Gold®-MaxiVac® FLU *(SyntroVet)*									K									M						
BratiVac® *(Pfizer Animal Health)*										K														
BratiVac®-6 *(Pfizer Animal Health)*										K		K												
Enterisol® Ileitis *(Boehringer Ingelheim)*											M													
Lepto-5 *(Boehringer Ingelheim)*												K												
Lepto-5 *(Colorado Serum)*												K												
Lepto 5 *(AgriLabs)*												K												
Lepto 5 *(Durvet)*												K												
Lepto 5 Vaccine *(Aspen)*												K												
Leptoferm-5® *(Pfizer Animal Health)*												K												
Lepto Shield™ 5 *(Novartis Animal Vaccines)*												K												
Surround™ L5 *(Biocor)*												K												
TrustGard™ 5L *(Vedco)*												K												
Breed Sow™ 6 *(AgriLabs)*												K		K										
Parvo-Vac®/Leptoferm-5® *(Pfizer Animal Health)*												K		K										
Parvo Shield® L5 *(Novartis Animal Vaccines)*												K		K										
DurVac™ Myco *(Durvet)*													K											
Ingelvac® M. hyo *(Boehringer Ingelheim)*													K											
M+Pac® *(Schering-Plough)*													K											
Myco Shield™ *(Novartis Animal Vaccines)*													K											
Myco Silencer® M *(Intervet)*													K											
Myco Silencer® Once *(Intervet)*													K											
Prevail MycoPlex™ *(Aspen)*													K											
RespiSure 1 ONE® *(Pfizer Animal Health)*													K											
RespiSure® *(Pfizer Animal Health)*													K											
Suvaxyn® RespiFend® MH *(Fort Dodge)*													K											
Swine Master M Plus™ *(AgriLabs)*													K											
Parvo Shield® *(Novartis Animal Vaccines)*														K										
PRRomiSE® *(Intervet)*																	K							
Ingelvac® PRRS ATP *(Boehringer Ingelheim)*																	M							
Ingelvac® PRRS MLV *(Boehringer Ingelheim)*																	M							
PR-Vac®-Killed *(Pfizer Animal Health)*																		K						
Ingelvac® PRV-G1 *(Boehringer Ingelheim)*																		M						
PR-Vac® *(Pfizer Animal Health)*																		M						
PR-Vac Plus™ *(Pfizer Animal Health)*																		M						
PRV-Begonia with Diluvac Forte® *(Intervet)*																		M						
PRV/Marker Gold® *(SyntroVet)*																		M						
Suvaxyn® PrV gpl- *(Fort Dodge)*																		M						
Rotamune® with Imugen® II *(Intervet)*																			K					
ProSystem® Rota *(Intervet)*																			M					
ProSystem® TG-Emune® Rota with Imugen® II *(Intervet)*																			K			K		
ProSystem® TGE/Rota *(Intervet)*																			M			M		

Leptospira spp*
- *L. canicola*
- *L. grippotyphosa*
- *L. hardjo*
- *L. icterohaemorrhagiae*
- *L. pomona*

(continued on next page)

Please refer to product listings for more complete information.

PORCINE *(continued)*

K - antibodies
- antitoxin
- extract
- killed
- subunit
- toxoid

M - modified live

Product Name	A. pleuropneumoniae	Actinomyces (C. pyogenes)	Anthrax	Bordetella	Clostridium perfringens	E. coli	Erysipelothrix	Haemophilus parasuis	Influenza	L. bratislava	Lawsonia sp	Leptospira spp*	Mycoplasma	Parvovirus	Pasteurella haemolytica	Pasteurella multocida	PRRS	Pseudorabies	Rotavirus	Salmonella	Streptococcus spp	T.G.E.	Tetanus Antitoxin	Tetanus Toxoid
ENDOVAC-Porci® with ImmunePlus® *(Immvac)*																				K				
Salmo Shield® 2 *(Novartis Animal Vaccines)*																				K				
Argus® SC/ST *(Intervet)*																				M				
Enterisol® SC-54 *(Boehringer Ingelheim)*																				M				
Enterisol® SC-54 FF *(Boehringer Ingelheim)*																				M				
Nitro-Sal *(Arko)*																				M				
Nitro-Sal F.D. *(Arko)*																				M				
Salmo Shield® Live *(Novartis Animal Vaccines)*																				M				
DurVac™ Strep *(Durvet)*																					K			
Emulsibac® SS *(MVP)*																					K			
Equisimilis Shield™ *(Novartis Animal Vaccines)*																					K			
Prefarrow Strep Shield® *(Novartis Animal Vaccines)*																					K			
SS Pac® *(Schering-Plough)*																					K			
Strep Bac® with Imugen® II *(Intervet)*																					K			
ProSystem® TG-Emune® with Imugen® II *(Intervet)*																						K		
TGE Shield™ *(Novartis Animal Vaccines)*																						K		
ProSystem® TGE *(Intervet)*																						M		
TGE Cell™ *(Novartis Animal Vaccines)*																						M		
Antitox Tet™ *(Novartis Animal Vaccines)*																							K	
Tetanus Antitoxin *(Fort Dodge)*																							K	
Tetanus Antitoxin *(Durvet)*																							K	
Tetanus Antitoxin, Equine Origin *(Colorado Serum)*																							K	
Tetanus Antitoxin, Equine Origin *(Professional Biological)*																							K	
Tetnogen®-AT *(Fort Dodge)*																							K	
Super-Tet® with Havlogen® *(Intervet)*																								K
Tetanus Toxoid *(Fort Dodge)*																								K
Tetanus Toxoid-Concentrated *(Colorado Serum)*																								K
Tetanus Toxoid-Concentrated *(Professional Biological)*																								K
Tetanus Toxoid-Unconcentrated *(Colorado Serum)*																								K
Tetguard™ *(Boehringer Ingelheim)*																								K
Tetnogen® *(Fort Dodge)*																								K

Leptospira spp*
- *L. canicola*
- *L. grippotyphosa*
- *L. hardjo*
- *L. icterohaemorrhagiae*
- *L. pomona*

Please refer to product listings for more complete information.

POULTRY

K - antibodies
- antitoxin
- extract
- killed
- subunit
- toxoid

M - modified live

Product Name	Adenovirus II-Turkeys	Anemia Virus (CAV)	Bordetella	Bronchitis-Arkansas	Bronchitis-Connecticut	Bronchitis-Delaware	Bronchitis-Florida	Bronchitis-Holland	Bronchitis-Massachusetts	Bursal Disease	Coccidia	E coli	Encephalomyelitis	Erysipelothrix	Fowlpox	H paragallinarum	Herpesvirus-Chicken	Herpesvirus-Turkey	Influenza	Laryngotracheitis	Mycoplasma gallisepticum	Mycoplasma synoviae	Newcastle	Newcastle-B1 strain(s)	Newcastle-C2 strain	Newcastle-LaSota	Paramyxovirus 3	Pasteurella multocida	Pigeonpox	Pneumovirus	Reovirus	Salmonella	Salmonella enteritidis
Bio-Hev™ *(Intervet)*	M																																
H.E. Vac *(Arko)*	M																																
Oralvax-HE™ *(Schering-Plough)*	M																																
Pro'tect™ HE *(Brinton)*	M																																
CAV-Vac® *(Intervet)*		M																															
Circomune™ *(Biomune)*		M																															
Circomune™ W *(Biomune)*		M																															
Tremvac-FP-CAV™ *(Intervet)*		M											M		M																		
Bio-Tella™ *(Intervet)*			K																														
Art Vax® *(Schering-Plough)*			M																														
Acti/Vac® AR *(L.A.H.I. (Maine Biological))*				M																													
Ark Blen® *(Merial Select)*				M																													
Broilerbron®-99 *(ASL)*				M																													
Bronchitis Vaccine (Ark. Type) *(Merial Select)*				M																													
Mildvac-Ark® *(Intervet)*				M																													
Inacti/Vac® IB2 *(L.A.H.I. (Maine Biological))*				K					K																								
Acti/Vac® M48-AR *(L.A.H.I. (Maine Biological))*				M					M																								
Chick Ark Bronc™ *(L.A.H.I. (New Jersey))*				M					M																								
Inacti/Vac® ND-IB2 *(L.A.H.I. (Maine Biological))*				K					K														K										
Acti/Vac® B1-M48-AR *(L.A.H.I. (Maine Biological))*				M					M															M									
Broilerbron®-99 B$_1$ *(ASL)*				M					M															M									
Chick Poly Ark™ *(L.A.H.I. (New Jersey))*				M					M															M									
Newcastle-Bronchitis Vaccine (Mass. & Ark. Types) *(Merial Select)*				M					M															M									
Newcastle B$_1$+Bronchitis Mass+Ark *(Fort Dodge)*				M					M															M									
Trivac-Ark® *(Intervet)*				M					M															M									
Twinvax®-99 *(Schering-Plough)*				M					M															M									
Gallimune™ NC-BR *(Merial Select)*				K					K																	K							
Inacti/Vac® BD3-ND-IB2 *(L.A.H.I. (Maine Biological))*				K					K	K													K										
Bursa Guard N-B *(Merial Select)*				K					K	K																K							
Inacti/Vac® BD3-IB2-REO *(L.A.H.I. (Maine Biological))*				K					K	K																					K		
Inacti/Vac® SE4-ND-IB2 *(L.A.H.I. (Maine Biological))*				K					K														K										K
Inacti/Vac® BD3-ND-IB2-REO *(L.A.H.I. (Maine Biological))*				K					K	K													K								K		
Inacti/Vac® BTO2-ND-IB2-REO *(L.A.H.I. (Maine Biological))*				K					K	K													K								K		
Bursa Guard N-B-R *(Merial Select)*				K					K	K																K					K		
Acti/Vac® CT *(L.A.H.I. (Maine Biological))*					M																												
Newcastle-Bronchitis Vaccine (Conn. Type) *(Merial Select)*					M																			M									
Newcastle B$_1$+Bronchitis Conn *(Fort Dodge)*					M																			M									
Newcastle B$_1$+Bronchitis Conn Mass (5,000 and 10,000 dose) *(Fort Dodge)*					M				M														M										
Acti/Vac® B1-M48-CT *(L.A.H.I. (Maine Biological))*					M				M															M									
Chick Poly Banco™ *(L.A.H.I. (New Jersey))*					M				M															M									
Hatchgard-3™ *(Intervet)*					M				M															M									
Newcastle-Bronchitis Vaccine (Mass. & Conn. Types) *(Merial Select)*					M				M															M									
Newcastle B$_1$+Bronchitis Conn Mass (1,000 dose) *(Fort Dodge)*					M				M															M									
Polybron® B$_1$ *(ASL)*					M				M															M									
Triplevac® *(Intervet)*					M				M															M									
Twinvax®-MR *(Schering-Plough)*					M				M															M									
Newhatch-C2-MC™ *(Intervet)*					M				M																M								
Dublvax® *(Schering-Plough)*					M				M																	M							
LaSota M41 Conn.™ *(L.A.H.I. (New Jersey))*					M				M																	M							
NB Blen® Plus *(Merial Select)*					M				M																	M							
Polybron® N-63 *(ASL)*					M				M																	M							
Bursal Disease-Newcastle Disease-Bronchitis Vaccine (Mass. & Conn. Types) *(Merial Select)*					M				M	M														M									

(continued on next page)

POULTRY *(continued)*

K - antibodies
- antitoxin
- extract
- killed
- subunit
- toxoid

M - modified live

Product Name	Adenovirus II-Turkeys	Anemia Virus (CAV)	Bordetella	Bronchitis-Arkansas	Bronchitis-Connecticut	Bronchitis-Delaware	Bronchitis-Florida	Bronchitis-Holland	Bronchitis-Massachusetts	Bursal Disease	Coccidia	E coli	Encephalomyelitis	Erysipelothrix	Fowlpox	H paragallinarum	Herpesvirus-Chicken	Herpesvirus-Turkey	Influenza	Laryngotracheitis	Mycoplasma gallisepticum	Mycoplasma synoviae	Newcastle	Newcastle-B1 strain(s)	Newcastle-C2 strain	Newcastle-LaSota	Paramyxovirus 3	Pasteurella multocida	Pigeonpox	Pneumovirus	Reovirus	Salmonella	Salmonella enteritidis
Combovac-30® *(Intervet)*					M				M															M		M							
Shor-Bron D *(ASL)*						M																											
Chick Poly Florida™ *(L.A.H.I. (New Jersey))*							M		M															M									
Layermune® IB *(Biomune)*								K																									
Chick Uni Hol™ *(L.A.H.I. (New Jersey))*								M																									
IB-Vac-H® *(Intervet)*								M																									
Ava-Bron-H®-B_1 *(ASL)*								M																M									
Broilerbron®-H-B_1 *(ASL)*								M																M									
Chick Vi Hanco™ *(L.A.H.I. (New Jersey))*								M																M									
Ava-Bron-H®-N-63 *(ASL)*								M																		M							
Newcastle-Bronchitis Vaccine (B1 Type, LaSota Strain and Mass. Type, Holland Strain) *(Merial Select)*								M																		M							
Vi So Hol™ *(L.A.H.I. (New Jersey))*								M																		M							
Repromune™ IBD/ND/IB *(Biomune)*								K	K	K													K										
Repromune™ 4 *(Biomune)*								K	K	K													K								K		
Bronchitis Vaccine *(L.A.H.I. (New Jersey))*									K																								
Acti/Vac® M48 *(L.A.H.I. (Maine Biological))*									M																								
Ava-Bron® *(ASL)*									M																								
Broilerbron® *(ASL)*									M																								
Bronchitis Vaccine (Mass. Type) *(Merial Select)*									M																								
Chick Uni Bronc™ *(L.A.H.I. (New Jersey))*									M																								
Mildvac-Ma5® *(Intervet)*									M																								
Bron-Newcavac-M® *(Intervet)*									K														K										
Inacti/Vac® ND-IB1 *(L.A.H.I. (Maine Biological))*									K														K										
Inacti/Vac® ND-IB1C *(L.A.H.I. (Maine Biological))*									K														K										
Layermune® 2 *(Biomune)*									K														K										
New Bronz® *(Fort Dodge)*									K														K										
Newcastle-Bronchitis Vaccine *(L.A.H.I. (New Jersey))*									K														K										
Acti/Vac® B1 and M48 *(L.A.H.I. (Maine Biological))*									M															M									
Acti/Vac® B1-M48 *(L.A.H.I. (Maine Biological))*									M															M									
Broilerbron® B_1 *(ASL)*									M															M									
Chick Vi Banco™ *(L.A.H.I. (New Jersey))*									M															M									
Chick Vi Banco™ (Drinking Water Use) *(L.A.H.I. (New Jersey))*									M															M									
Newcastle-Bronchitis Vaccine (B_1 Strain, Mass. Type) *(Merial Select)*									M															M									
Newcastle B_1+Bronchitis Mass *(Fort Dodge)*									M															M									
Newhatch-C2-M™ *(Intervet)*									M																M								
Acti/Vac® LAS-MA *(L.A.H.I. (Maine Biological))*									M																	M							
Bio-Sota + Bron MM™ *(Intervet)*									M																	M							
Broilerbron®-H N-79 *(ASL)*									M																	M							
Newcastle-Bronchitis Vaccine (LaSota Strain, Mass. Type) *(Merial Select)*									M																	M							
Newcastle-Bronchitis Vaccine LS Mass II™ *(Fort Dodge)*									M																	M							
Newcastle LaSota+Bronchitis Mass *(Fort Dodge)*									M																	M							
Vi So Bronc® *(L.A.H.I. (New Jersey))*									M																	M							
Vi So Bronc® (Drinking Water Use) *(L.A.H.I. (New Jersey))*									M																	M							
Vi So Hol™ (Drinking Water Use) *(L.A.H.I. (New Jersey))*									M																	M							
Bursal Disease-Newcastle-Bronchitis Vaccine *(L.A.H.I. (New Jersey))*									K	K													K										
Bursal Disease-Newcastle-Bronchitis Vaccine (Standard and Variant) *(L.A.H.I. (New Jersey))*									K	K													K										
Inacti/Vac® BTO1-ND-IB *(L.A.H.I. (Maine Biological))*									K	K													K										
Layermune® 5 *(Biomune)*									K	K													K										
Pro Vac® 3 ACL™ *(Fort Dodge)*									K	K													K										
Breedervac-III-Plus® *(Intervet)*									K	K														K									
New Bronz® MG *(Fort Dodge)*									K												K		K										
Inacti/Vac® BD3-ND-IB1-REO *(L.A.H.I. (Maine Biological))*									K														K								K		

(continued on next page)

Please refer to product listings for more complete information.

POULTRY *(continued)*

K - antibodies
- antitoxin
- extract
- killed
- subunit
- toxoid

M - modified live

Product Name	Adenovirus II-Turkeys	Anemia Virus (CAV)	Bordetella	Bronchitis-Arkansas	Bronchitis-Connecticut	Bronchitis-Delaware	Bronchitis-Florida	Bronchitis-Holland	Bronchitis-Massachusetts	Bursal Disease	Coccidia	E coli	Encephalomyelitis	Erysipelothrix	Fowlpox	H paragallinarum	Herpesvirus-Chicken	Herpesvirus-Turkey	Influenza	Laryngotracheitis	Mycoplasma gallisepticum	Mycoplasma synoviae	Newcastle	Newcastle-B1 strain(s)	Newcastle-C2 strain	Newcastle-LaSota	Paramyxovirus 3	Pasteurella multocida	Pigeonpox	Pneumovirus	Reovirus	Salmonella	Salmonella enteritidis
Layermune® 3 *(Biomune)*									K														K										K
Poulvac® SE-ND-IB *(Fort Dodge)*									K														K										K
Inacti/Vac® BTO1-ND-IB-REO *(L.A.H.I. (Maine Biological))*									K	K													K								K		
Maximune® 8 *(Biomune)*									K	K													K								K		
Optimune® 8 *(Biomune)*									K	K													K								K		
Pro Vac® 4 ACL™ *(Fort Dodge)*									K	K													K								K		
Breedervac-IV-Plus® *(Intervet)*									K	K														K							K		
Bursal Disease-Newcastle Disease-Bronchitis-Reovirus Vaccine *(L.A.H.I. (New Jersey))*									K	K														K							K		
Bursa Guard *(Merial Select)*										K																							
Bursine®-K ACL™ *(Fort Dodge)*										K																							
Inacti/Vac® BD *(L.A.H.I. (Maine Biological))*										K																							
Inacti/Vac® BD3 *(L.A.H.I. (Maine Biological))*										K																							
Inacti/Vac® BTO1 *(L.A.H.I. (Maine Biological))*										K																							
Inacti/Vac® BTO2 *(L.A.H.I. (Maine Biological))*										K																							
Maximune® IBD *(Biomune)*										K																							
Optimune® IBD *(Biomune)*										K																							
Repromune™ IBD *(Biomune)*										K																							
Vi Bursa-K+V *(L.A.H.I. (New Jersey))*										K																							
Vi Bursa-K™ *(L.A.H.I. (New Jersey))*										K																							
89/03® *(Intervet)*										M																							
Bursa-Vac® *(ASL)*										M																							
Bursa-Vac® 3 *(ASL)*										M																							
Bursa-Vac® 4 *(ASL)*										M																							
Bursa Blen® M *(Merial Select)*										M																							
Bursal Disease Vaccine (S-706 Strain) *(Merial Select)*										M																							
Bursal Disease Vaccine (ST-14 Strain) *(Merial Select)*										M																							
Bursal Disease Vaccine (SVS 510) *(Merial Select)*										M																							
Bursaplex® *(Embrex)*										M																							
Bursimune® *(Biomune)*										M																							
Bursine®-2 *(Fort Dodge)*										M																							
Bursine® Plus *(Fort Dodge)*										M																							
Clonevac D-78® *(Intervet)*										M																							
IBD Blen® *(Merial Select)*										M																							
Primevac IBD-3® *(Intervet)*										M																							
Univax-BD® *(Schering-Plough)*										M																							
Univax™ Plus *(Schering-Plough)*										M																							
Variant Vax-BD™ *(Schering-Plough)*										M																							
Vi Bursa-G™ *(L.A.H.I. (New Jersey))*										M																							
Vi Bursa-L™ *(L.A.H.I. (New Jersey))*										M																							
Vi Bursa C.E.™ *(L.A.H.I. (New Jersey))*										M																							
Vivomune® *(Biomune)*										M																							
Bursal Disease-Marek's Disease Vaccine (Standard, Turkey) *(Merial Select)*										M								M															
Bursal Disease-Marek's Disease Vaccine (Standard and Variant, Turkey) *(Merial Select)*										M								M															
Marexine-89/03® *(Intervet)*										M								M															
Vi Mark® Bursal Disease-Marek's Disease Vaccine (Modified Live Virus, Turkey Herpesvirus) *(L.A.H.I. (New Jersey))*										M								M															
Bursine® N-K ACL™ *(Fort Dodge)*										K													K										
Inacti/Vac® BD-ND *(L.A.H.I. (Maine Biological))*										K													K										
Inacti/Vac® BD3-ND *(L.A.H.I. (Maine Biological))*										K													K										
Maximune® 4 *(Biomune)*										K													K										
Optimune® 4 *(Biomune)*										K													K										
Repromune™ IBD/ND *(Biomune)*										K													K										

(continued on next page)

POULTRY *(continued)*

K - antibodies
- antitoxin
- extract
- killed
- subunit
- toxoid

M - modified live

Product Name	Adenovirus II-Turkeys	Anemia Virus (CAV)	Bordetella	Bronchitis-Arkansas	Bronchitis-Connecticut	Bronchitis-Delaware	Bronchitis-Florida	Bronchitis-Holland	Bronchitis-Massachusetts	Bursal Disease	Coccidia	E coli	Encephalomyelitis	Erysipelothrix	Fowlpox	H paragallinarum	Herpesvirus-Chicken	Herpesvirus-Turkey	Influenza	Laryngotracheitis	Mycoplasma gallisepticum	Mycoplasma synoviae	Newcastle	Newcastle-B1 strain(s)	Newcastle-C2 strain	Newcastle-LaSota	Paramyxovirus 3	Pasteurella multocida	Pigeonpox	Pneumovirus	Reovirus	Salmonella	Salmonella enteritidis
Breedervac-Reo-Plus® *(Intervet)*										K																					K		
Bursa Guard Reo *(Merial Select)*										K																					K		
Bursal Disease-Avian Reovirus Vaccine *(L.A.H.I. (New Jersey))*										K																					K		
Bursamate™ *(Intervet)*										K																					K		
Inacti-Vac® BTO2-REOC *(L.A.H.I. (Maine Biological))*										K																					K		
Inacti/Vac® BD3-REO *(L.A.H.I. (Maine Biological))*										K																					K		
Inacti/Vac® BTO1-REO *(L.A.H.I. (Maine Biological))*										K																					K		
Inacti/Vac® BTO2-REO *(L.A.H.I. (Maine Biological))*										K																					K		
Maximune® 6 *(Biomune)*										K																					K		
Optimune® 6 *(Biomune)*										K																					K		
Pro Vac® 2 ACL™ *(Fort Dodge)*										K																					K		
Repromune™ IBD/Reo *(Biomune)*										K																					K		
Bursal Disease-Marek's Disease Vaccine (Standard, Chicken and Turkey) *(Merial Select)*										M							M	M															
Bursal Disease-Marek's Disease Vaccine (Standard and Variant, Chicken and Turkey) *(Merial Select)*										M							M	M															
Marexine-SB-89/03® *(Intervet)*										M							M	M															
Vi Mark® Bursal Disease-Marek's Disease Vaccine (Live Virus, Chicken and Turkey Herpesvirus) *(L.A.H.I. (New Jersey))*										M							M	M															
Bursal Disease-Newcastle Disease Vaccine *(L.A.H.I. (New Jersey))*										M													K	M									
Inacti/Vac® BD-ND-FC3 *(L.A.H.I. (Maine Biological))*										K													K					K					
Inacti/Vac® BD3-ND-REO *(L.A.H.I. (Maine Biological))*										K													K								K		
Inacti/Vac® BTO1-ND-REO *(L.A.H.I. (Maine Biological))*										K													K								K		
Inacti/Vac® BTO2-ND-REO *(L.A.H.I. (Maine Biological))*										K													K								K		
Optimune® 7 *(Biomune)*										K													K								K		
ProVac ND/IBD/Reo ACL™ *(Fort Dodge)*										K													K								K		
Repromune IBD/ND/REO™ *(Biomune)*										K													K								K		
Bursal Disease-Newcastle Disease-Reovirus Vaccine *(L.A.H.I. (New Jersey))*										K														K							K		
Maximune® 7 *(Biomune)*										K														K							K		
Bursa Guard N-R *(Merial Select)*										K																K					K		
Coccivac®-B *(Schering-Plough)*											M																						
Coccivac®-D *(Schering-Plough)*											M																						
Coccivac®-T *(Schering-Plough)*											M																						
Garavax®-T *(Schering-Plough)*												M																					
Inacti/Vac® AE *(L.A.H.I. (Maine Biological))*													K																				
AE-Vac™ *(Fort Dodge)*													M																				
Ava-Trem® *(ASL)*													M																				
Avimune® *(Schering-Plough)*													M																				
Tremblex™ *(L.A.H.I. (New Jersey))*													M																				
Tremor Blen® D *(Merial Select)*													M																				
Tremormune™ AE *(Biomune)*													M																				
Tremvac® *(Intervet)*													M																				
AE + Pox *(ASL)*													M		M																		
AE-Poxine® *(Fort Dodge)*													M		M																		
Avimune®+Pox *(Schering-Plough)*													M		M																		
Poximune® AE *(Biomune)*													M		M																		
PT Blen® *(Merial Select)*													M		M																		
Tremvac-FP® *(Intervet)*													M		M																		
Vi-Trempox™ *(L.A.H.I. (New Jersey))*													M		M																		
Inacti/Vac® ND-AE *(L.A.H.I. (Maine Biological))*													K										K										
Vectormune® FP-LT+AE *(Biomune)*													M		M					M													
Suvaxyn®-E (Swine and Turkey) *(Fort Dodge)*														K																			
Arko Ery Vac FD *(Arko)*														M																			

(continued on next page)

Please refer to product listings for more complete information.

POULTRY *(continued)*

K - antibodies
- antitoxin
- extract
- killed
- subunit
- toxoid

M - modified live

Product Name	Adenovirus II-Turkeys	Anemia Virus (CAV)	Bordetella	Bronchitis-Arkansas	Bronchitis-Connecticut	Bronchitis-Delaware	Bronchitis-Florida	Bronchitis-Holland	Bronchitis-Massachusetts	Bursal Disease	Coccidia	E coli	Encephalomyelitis	Erysipelothrix	Fowlpox	H paragallinarum	Herpesvirus-Chicken	Herpesvirus-Turkey	Influenza	Laryngotracheitis	Mycoplasma gallisepticum	Mycoplasma synoviae	Newcastle	Newcastle-B1 strain(s)	Newcastle-C2 strain	Newcastle-LaSota	Paramyxovirus 3	Pasteurella multocida	Pigeonpox	Pneumovirus	Reovirus	Salmonella	Salmonella enteritidis
Acti/Vac® FP *(L.A.H.I. (Maine Biological))*															M																		
Ava-Pox® CE *(ASL)*															M																		
Bio-Pox M™ *(Intervet)*															M																		
Chick Vi Pox™ *(L.A.H.I. (New Jersey))*															M																		
Fowl Pox Vaccine *(L.A.H.I. (New Jersey))*															M																		
Fowl Pox Vaccine *(Schering-Plough)*															M																		
Fowl Pox Vaccine *(Merial Select)*															M																		
FP-Vac® *(Intervet)*															M																		
FP Blen® *(Merial Select)*															M																		
Pigeon Pox Vaccine *(ASL)*															M																		
Pigeon Pox Vaccine (Chickens and Turkeys) *(L.A.H.I. (New Jersey))*															M																		
Pipovax® *(Schering-Plough)*															M																		
Poulvac® Chick-N-Pox™ *(Fort Dodge)*															M																		
Poximune® *(Biomune)*															M																		
Poxine® *(Fort Dodge)*															M																		
PP-Vac® *(Intervet)*															M																		
Trovac®-AIV H5 *(Merial Select)*															M				M														
Vectormune® FP-LT *(Biomune)*															M					M													
Newcastle Disease-Fowl Pox Vaccine (Recombinant) *(Merial Select)*															M								M										
Vectormune® FP-N *(Biomune)*															M								M										
Corvac-3® *(Intervet)*																K																	
Haemophilus Paragallinarum Bacterin *(L.A.H.I. (New Jersey))*																K																	
Poulvac® Coryza ABC IC_3 *(Fort Dodge)*																K																	
Marek's Disease Vaccine (Rispens CVI 988 Strain) *(Merial Select)*																	M																
Marek's Disease Vaccine (SB-1 Strain) *(Merial Select)*																	M																
MD-Vac® CAF Frozen *(Fort Dodge)*																	M																
MD-Vac® CFL *(Fort Dodge)*																	M																
Poulvac® Marek Rispens CVI+HVT *(Fort Dodge)*																	M																
Rismavac® *(Intervet)*																	M																
SB-1 Frozen *(Intervet)*																	M																
SB-Vac® *(Intervet)*																	M																
Vi Mark® Marek's Disease Vaccine (Live Chicken Herpesvirus) *(L.A.H.I. (New Jersey))*																	M																
HVT + SB-1 *(Intervet)*																	M	M															
Marek's Disease Vaccine (Chicken and Turkey) *(Merial Select)*																	M	M															
Marek's Disease Vaccine (Rispens CVI 988 Strain + FC-126 Strain) *(Merial Select)*																	M	M															
Marexine® SB-Vac® *(Intervet)*																	M	M															
RIS-MA-SB™ *(Intervet)*																	M	M															
RIS-MA™ *(Intervet)*																	M	M															
Vi Mark® Marek's Disease Vaccine (Live Chicken and Turkey Herpesvirus) *(L.A.H.I. (New Jersey))*																	M	M															
VVMD-Vac® *(Fort Dodge)*																	M	M															
HVT *(Intervet)*																		M															
Marek's Disease Vaccine (FC-126 Strain) *(Merial Select)*																		M															
Marexine® *(Intervet)*																		M															
Vi Mark® Marek's Disease Vaccine (Live Turkey Herpesvirus) *(L.A.H.I. (New Jersey))*																		M															

(continued on next page)

POULTRY *(continued)*

K - antibodies
- antitoxin
- extract
- killed
- subunit
- toxoid

M - modified live

Product Name	Adenovirus II-Turkeys	Anemia Virus (CAV)	Bordetella	Bronchitis-Arkansas	Bronchitis-Connecticut	Bronchitis-Delaware	Bronchitis-Florida	Bronchitis-Holland	Bronchitis-Massachusetts	Bursal Disease	Coccidia	E coli	Encephalomyelitis	Erysipelothrix	Fowlpox	H paragallinarum	Herpesvirus-Chicken	Herpesvirus-Turkey	Influenza	Laryngotracheitis	Mycoplasma gallisepticum	Mycoplasma synoviae	Newcastle	Newcastle-B1 strain(s)	Newcastle-C2 strain	Newcastle-LaSota	Paramyxovirus 3	Pasteurella multocida	Pigeonpox	Pneumovirus	Reovirus	Salmonella	Salmonella enteritidis
Bio-Trach™ *(Intervet)*																				M													
Broilertrake® *(ASL)*																				M													
Broilertrake®-M *(ASL)*																				M													
Fowl Laryngotracheitis Vaccine *(L.A.H.I. (New Jersey))*																				M													
Laryngo-Vac™ *(Fort Dodge)*																				M													
LT-Ivax® *(Schering-Plough)*																				M													
LT Blen® *(Merial Select)*																				M													
Ocuvax® *(Schering-Plough)*																				M													
Trachivax® *(Schering-Plough)*																				M													
M.G. Bacterin *(L.A.H.I. (New Jersey))*																					K												
MG-Bac® *(Fort Dodge)*																					K												
F Vax-MG® *(Schering-Plough)*																					M												
Mycoplasma Gallisepticum Vaccine *(Merial Select)*																					M												
Mycovac-L® *(Intervet)*																					M												
MS-Bac™ *(Fort Dodge)*																						K											
Inacti/Vac® Chick-ND *(L.A.H.I. (Maine Biological))*																							K										
Inacti/Vac® ND *(L.A.H.I. (Maine Biological))*																							K										
Inacti/Vac® Pullet-ND *(L.A.H.I. (Maine Biological))*																							K										
Inacti/Vac® Turkey-ND *(L.A.H.I. (Maine Biological))*																							K										
Layermune® ND *(Biomune)*																							K										
Newcastle-K *(Fort Dodge)*																							K										
Newcastle Disease Vaccine *(L.A.H.I. (New Jersey))*																							K										
Newcastle Disease Vaccine (Killed Virus) *(L.A.H.I. (New Jersey))*																							K										
Vi Nu Chick Vac-K™ *(L.A.H.I. (New Jersey))*																							K										
Acti/Vac® RO *(L.A.H.I. (Maine Biological))*																							M										
Clonevac-30® *(Intervet)*																							M										
Respimune™ *(Biomune)*																							M										
Inacti/Vac® ND-PMV3 *(L.A.H.I. (Maine Biological))*																							K				K						
Acti/Vac® B1 *(L.A.H.I. (Maine Biological))*																								M									
B_1 Vac™ *(Intervet)*																								M									
Newcastle Disease Vaccine (B1 Strain) *(Merial Select)*																								M									
Newcastle Disease Vaccine (B1 Type, B1 Strain, Live Virus) *(Fort Dodge)*																								M									
Newcastle Disease Vaccine (B_1 Type, B_1 Strain, Live Virus) *(L.A.H.I. (New Jersey))*																								M									
Newcastle Disease Vaccine (B_1 Type, B_1 Strain, Live Virus) (Drinking Water Use) *(L.A.H.I. (New Jersey))*																								M									
Newvax® *(Schering-Plough)*																								M									
Acti/Vac® LAS *(L.A.H.I. (Maine Biological))*																										M							
Clonevac-30®-T *(Intervet)*																										M							
Newcastle Disease Vaccine (B1 Type, LaSota Strain, Live Virus) *(Fort Dodge)*																										M							
Newcastle Disease Vaccine (B_1 Type, LaSota Strain, Live Virus) *(L.A.H.I. (New Jersey))*																										M							
Newcastle Disease Vaccine (LaSota Strain) *(Merial Select)*																										M							
Singlvax® *(Schering-Plough)*																										M							
Inacti/Vac® PMV3 *(L.A.H.I. (Maine Biological))*																											K						

(continued on next page)

Please refer to product listings for more complete information.

POULTRY *(continued)*

K - antibodies
- antitoxin
- extract
- killed
- subunit
- toxoid

M - modified live

Product Name	Adenovirus II-Turkeys	Anemia Virus (CAV)	Bordetella	Bronchitis-Arkansas	Bronchitis-Connecticut	Bronchitis-Delaware	Bronchitis-Florida	Bronchitis-Holland	Bronchitis-Massachusetts	Bursal Disease	Coccidia	E coli	Encephalomyelitis	Erysipelothrix	Fowlpox	H paragallinarum	Herpesvirus-Chicken	Herpesvirus-Turkey	Influenza	Laryngotracheitis	Mycoplasma gallisepticum	Mycoplasma synoviae	Newcastle	Newcastle-B1 strain(s)	Newcastle-C2 strain	Newcastle-LaSota	Paramyxovirus 3	Pasteurella multocida	Pigeonpox	Pneumovirus	Reovirus	Salmonella	Salmonella enteritidis
Cholervac-IV™ *(Intervet)*																												K					
FC4 Gold *(L.A.H.I. (Maine Biological))*																												K					
Inacti/Vac® FC2 *(L.A.H.I. (Maine Biological))*																												K					
Inacti/Vac® FC2C *(L.A.H.I. (Maine Biological))*																												K					
Inacti/Vac® FC3 *(L.A.H.I. (Maine Biological))*																												K					
Inacti/Vac® FC3-C *(L.A.H.I. (Maine Biological))*																												K					
Inacti/Vac® FC4 *(L.A.H.I. (Maine Biological))*																												K					
Inacti/Vac® FC4C *(L.A.H.I. (Maine Biological))*																												K					
Multimune® K *(Biomune)*																												K					
Multimune® K5 *(Biomune)*																												K					
Pabac® *(Fort Dodge)*																												K					
Pasteurella Multocida Bacterin (Types 1, 3 & 4) *(L.A.H.I. (New Jersey))*																												K					
Pasteurella Multocida Bacterin (Types 1, 3, 4 & 3 x 4) *(L.A.H.I. (New Jersey))*																												K					
Arko Chol Vac FD *(Arko)*																												M					
Avichol® *(Schering-Plough)*																												M					
Choleramune® CU *(Biomune)*																												M					
Choleramune® M *(Biomune)*																												M					
Cholervac-PM-1® *(Intervet)*																												M					
M-Ninevax™ *(Schering-Plough)*																												M					
M-Ninevax®-C *(Schering-Plough)*																												M					
Multimune® CU *(Biomune)*																												M					
Multimune® M *(Biomune)*																												M					
Nitro-Chol® *(Arko)*																												M					
Orachol® *(Schering-Plough)*																												M					
PM-Onevax™ *(Schering-Plough)*																												M					
PM-Onevax®-C *(Schering-Plough)*																												M					
Vi Clemcol-C™ *(L.A.H.I. (New Jersey))*																												M					
Pox Blen® *(Merial Select)*																													M				
Avian Pneumovirus Vaccine *(Biomune)*																														M			
Gallimune™ Reoguard™ *(Merial Select)*																															K		
Inacti/Vac® REO *(L.A.H.I. (Maine Biological))*																															K		
Reomune® 2 *(Biomune)*																															K		
Reomune® 3 *(Biomune)*																															K		
Reomune® SS412 *(Biomune)*																															K		
Tri-Reo® *(Fort Dodge)*																															K		
2177® *(Intervet)*																															M		
Chick Syno Vac™ *(L.A.H.I. (New Jersey))*																															M		
Enterovax™ *(Schering-Plough)*																															M		
Reoguard L *(Merial Select)*																															M		
Teno-Vaxin® *(ASL)*																															M		
Tenosynovitis Vaccine *(Merial Select)*																															M		
Tensynvac® *(Intervet)*																															M		
V.A. ChickVac™ *(Fort Dodge)*																															M		
Megan® Vac 1 *(Megan)*																																M	
Salmune™ *(Biomune)*																																M	
Inacti/Vac® SE4 *(L.A.H.I. (Maine Biological))*																																	K
Inacti/Vac® SE4-C *(L.A.H.I. (Maine Biological))*																																	K
Layermune SE® *(Biomune)*																																	K
Poulvac® SE *(Fort Dodge)*																																	K

WILD, EXOTIC and OTHER SPECIES

K - antibodies
- antitoxin
- extract
- killed
- subunit
- toxoid

M - modified live

Product Name	Species	Aeromonas salmonicida	Arthrobacter sp	CAV-1	Cl botulinum	Distemper	Edwardsiella ictaluri	Flavobacterium columnare	Fowlpox	Mink Enteritis Virus	Pacheco Disease	Polyomavirus	Pseudomonas aeruginosa	Rabies	Salmon Anaemia Virus	Salmonella	Vibrio spp	Yersinia ruckeri
Forte V1 *(Novartis (Aqua Health))*	Salmonids	K													K		K	
Furogen™ *(Novartis (Aqua Health))*	Fish	K																
Furogen b *(Novartis (Aqua Health))*	Carp	K																
Furogen Dip *(Novartis (Aqua Health))*	Salmonids	K																
Lipogen Forte™ *(Novartis (Aqua Health))*	Fish	K															K	
Lipogen Triple *(Novartis (Aqua Health))*	Fish	K															K	
Furogen 2 *(Novartis (Aqua Health))*	Salmonids	M																
Renogen *(Novartis (Aqua Health))*	Salmonids		M															
Cephlopex® *(United)*	Foxes			K														
Biocom® *(United)*	Mink				K					K								
Biocom®-P *(United)*	Mink				K					K			K					
Botumink® *(United)*	Mink				K													
Biocom®-D *(United)*	Mink				K	M				K								
Biocom®-DP *(United)*	Mink				K	M				K			K					
Distox® *(Schering-Plough)*	Mink				K	M				K								
Distox®-Plus *(Schering-Plough)*	Mink				K	M				K			K					
Biovac®-D *(United)*	Mink					M				K								
Distem-R TC® *(Schering-Plough)*	Mink					M												
Distemink® *(United)*	Mink					M												
Fervac®-D *(United)*	Ferrets					M												
Purevax™ Ferret Distemper *(Merial)*	Ferrets					M												
Spravac® *(United)*	Mink					M												
Escogen *(Novartis (Aqua Health))*	Catfish						K											
Aquavac-ESC® *(Intervet)*	Catfish						M											
Fryvacc 1 *(Novartis (Aqua Health))*	Salmonids							K										
Poximune® C *(Biomune)*	Canary								M									
Biovac® *(United)*	Mink									K								
Psittimune® PDV *(Biomune)*	Psittacine birds										K							
Psittimune® APV *(Biomune)*	Psittacine birds											K						
P-Vac™ *(United)*	Mink												K					
Imrab® 3 *(Merial)*	Ferrets													K				
Sal Bac® *(Biomune)*	Pigeons															K		
Typhimune® *(Biomune)*	Doves, Pigeons															K		
Vibrogen *(Novartis (Aqua Health))*	Fish																K	
Vibrogen-2™ *(Novartis (Aqua Health))*	Fish																K	
Ermogen *(Novartis (Aqua Health))*	Fish																	K

Please refer to product listings for more complete information.

Anthelmintic and Parasiticide Charts

The Anthelmintic and Parasiticide Charts (buff pages) serve as a reference guide for veterinarians in their internal parasiticide or endectocide product selection. These products are grouped by the appropriate species and are delineated by the corresponding parasite.

Further information regarding the products listed in the buff pages may be found in the product monograph section (white pages).

Every effort has been made to ensure the accuracy of the information published. However, it remains the responsibility of the readers to familiarize themselves with the product information contained on the product label or package insert. The Publisher, Editorial Team and all those involved in the production of this book, cannot be held responsible for publication errors or any consequence that could result from the use of published information.

Guide to the Anthelmintic and Parasiticide Charts

BOVINE

Product Name	Amblyomma americanum*	Bunostomum spp	Chabertia spp	Chorioptes*	Cooperia spp	Damalinia bovis*	Dictyocaulus spp	Eimeria spp	Fasciola spp	Haematobia irritans*	Haematopinus*	Haemonchus spp	Hypoderma spp*	Linognathus vituli*	Moniezia spp	Nematodirus spp	Oesophagostomum spp	Ostertagia spp	Psoroptes*	Sarcoptes scabei*	Solenopotes*	Strongyloides spp	Thelazia spp	Trichostrongylus spp	Trichuris spp
Ivomec® SR Bolus *(Merial)*	●	●			●		●					●	●	●		●	●	●	●	●	●			●	
Synanthic® Bovine Dewormer Suspension, 9.06% *(Fort Dodge)*		●			●		●					●			●		●	●						●	
Synanthic® Bovine Dewormer Suspension, 22.5% *(Fort Dodge)*		●			●		●					●			●		●	●						●	
Levasole® Cattle Wormer Boluses *(Schering-Plough)*		●			●		●					●				●	●	●						●	
Levasole® Soluble Drench Powder *(Schering-Plough)*		●			●		●					●				●	●	●						●	
Panacur® Cattle Dewormer (92 g) *(Intervet)*		●			●		●					●				●	●	●						●	
Prohibit® Soluble Drench Powder *(AgriLabs)*		●			●		●					●				●	●	●						●	
Safe-Guard® Beef & Dairy Cattle Dewormer *(Intervet)*		●			●		●					●				●	●	●						●	
Safe-Guard® Beef and Dairy Cattle Dewormer (290 g) *(Intervet)*		●			●		●					●				●	●	●						●	
Safe-Guard® Cattle Dewormer (92 g) *(Intervet)*		●			●		●					●				●	●	●						●	
Safe-Guard® Medicated Dewormer for Beef & Dairy Cattle, & Swine *(Intervet)*		●			●		●					●				●	●	●						●	
Safe-Guard® Medicated Dewormer for Beef Cattle (20% Protein Block) *(Intervet)*		●			●		●					●				●	●	●						●	
Safe-Guard® Medicated Dewormer for Beef Cattle (En-Pro-Al® Molasses Block) *(Intervet)*		●			●		●					●				●	●	●						●	
Panacur® Beef and Dairy Cattle Dewormer *(Intervet)*		●			●		●					●			●	●	●	●						●	
Panacur® Cattle Dewormer *(Intervet)*		●			●		●					●			●	●	●	●						●	
Dectomax® Injectable Solution *(Pfizer Animal Health)*		●			●		●				●	●	●	●			●	●	●	●	●	●	●	●	●
AmTech Phoenectin® Injection for Cattle and Swine *(Phoenix Scientific)*		●			●		●				●	●	●	●		●	●	●	●	●	●			●	
Double Impact™ *(AgriLabs)*		●			●		●				●	●	●	●		●	●	●	●	●	●			●	
Ivercide™ Injection for Cattle and Swine *(Phoenix Pharmaceutical)*		●			●		●				●	●	●	●		●	●	●	●	●	●			●	
Ivermectin Injection for Cattle and Swine *(Durvet)*		●			●		●				●	●	●	●		●	●	●	●	●	●			●	
Ivermectin Injection for Cattle and Swine *(Aspen)*		●			●		●				●	●	●	●		●	●	●	●	●	●			●	
Ivomec® 1% Injection for Cattle and Swine *(Merial)*		●			●		●				●	●	●	●		●	●	●	●	●	●			●	
ProMectin™ Injection for Cattle and Swine *(Vedco)*		●			●		●				●	●	●	●		●	●	●	●	●	●			●	
Produmec™ Injection for Cattle and Swine *(TradeWinds)*		●			●		●				●	●	●	●		●	●	●	●	●	●			●	
UltraMectrin™ Injection *(RXV)*		●			●		●				●	●	●	●		●	●	●	●	●	●			●	
Valbazen® Cattle Dewormer Paste *(Pfizer Animal Health)*		●			●		●		●			●			●	●	●	●						●	
Valbazen® Suspension *(Pfizer Animal Health)*		●			●		●		●			●			●	●	●	●						●	
Ivomec® Plus Injection for Cattle *(Merial)*		●			●		●		●		●	●	●	●		●	●	●	●	●	●			●	
Dectomax® Pour-On *(Pfizer Animal Health)*		●		●	●	●	●			●	●	●	●	●			●	●		●	●		●	●	●
Ivomec® Eprinex® Pour-On for Beef and Dairy Cattle *(Merial)*		●		●	●	●	●			●	●	●	●	●		●	●	●		●	●	●		●	●
Cydectin® Pour-On *(Fort Dodge)*		●		●	●	●	●			●	●	●	●	●		●	●	●	●		●			●	

* Arthropod

(continued on next page)

Please refer to product listings for more complete information.

BOVINE *(continued)*

Product Name	Amblyomma americanum*	Bunostomum spp	Chabertia spp	Chorioptes*	Cooperia spp	Damalinia bovis*	Dictyocaulus spp	Eimeria spp	Fasciola spp	Haematobia irritans*	Haematopinus*	Haemonchus spp	Hypoderma spp*	Linognathus vituli*	Moniezia spp	Nematodirus spp	Oesophagostomum spp	Ostertagia spp	Psoroptes*	Sarcoptes scabei*	Solenopotes*	Strongyloides spp	Thelazia spp	Trichostrongylus spp	Trichuris spp
AmTech Levamisole Phosphate Injectable Solution *(Phoenix Scientific)*		●	●		●		●					●				●	●	●						●	
Levamisole Injectable *(AgriLabs)*		●	●		●		●					●				●	●	●						●	
Levamisole Phosphate *(Durvet)*		●	●		●		●					●				●	●	●						●	
Levamisole Phosphate Injectable Solution, 13.65% *(AgriPharm)*		●	●		●		●					●				●	●	●						●	
Levamisole Phosphate Injectable Solution, 13.65% *(Aspen)*		●	●		●		●					●				●	●	●						●	
Levasole® Injectable Solution, 13.65% *(Schering-Plough)*		●	●		●		●					●				●	●	●						●	
Totalon® Pour-On Dewormer *(Schering-Plough)*		●	●		●		●					●				●	●	●						●	
Rumatel® *(Phibro)*					●							●				●	●	●						●	
AmTech Phoenectin® Pour-On for Cattle *(Phoenix Scientific)*					●	●	●			●	●	●	●	●			●	●		●	●	●		●	●
Bimectin™ Pour-On *(Bimeda)*					●	●	●			●	●	●	●	●			●	●		●	●	●		●	●
Iver-On™ *(Med-Pharmex)*					●	●	●			●	●	●	●	●			●	●		●	●	●		●	●
Ivercide™ Pour-On for Cattle *(Phoenix Pharmaceutical)*					●	●	●			●	●	●	●	●			●	●		●	●	●		●	●
Ivermectin Pour-On *(Durvet)*					●	●	●			●	●	●	●	●			●	●		●	●	●		●	●
Ivermectin Pour-On *(Aspen)*					●	●	●			●	●	●	●	●			●	●		●	●	●		●	●
Ivomec® Pour-On for Cattle *(Merial)*					●	●	●			●	●	●	●	●			●	●		●	●	●		●	●
ProMectin B™ Pour-On For Cattle *(Vedco)*					●	●	●			●	●	●	●	●			●	●		●	●	●		●	●
Produmec™ Pour-On for Cattle *(TradeWinds)*					●	●	●			●	●	●	●	●			●	●		●	●	●		●	●
Prozap® Ivermectin Pour-On *(Loveland)*					●	●	●			●	●	●	●	●			●	●		●	●	●		●	●
Top Line™ *(AgriLabs)*					●	●	●			●	●	●	●	●			●	●		●	●	●		●	●
UltraMectrin™ Pour-On *(RXV)*					●	●	●			●	●	●	●	●			●	●		●	●	●		●	●
20% Sulfaquinoxaline Sodium Solution *(Loveland)*								●																	
Amprovine® 25% Type A Medicated Article *(Merial)*								●																	
Bovatec® 150 FP *(Alpharma)*								●																	
Bovatec® 68 *(Alpharma)*								●																	
Bovatec® Liquid 20 *(Alpharma)*								●																	
Corid® 20% Soluble Powder *(Merial)*								●																	
Corid® 9.6% Oral Solution *(Merial)*								●																	
Deccox® *(Alpharma)*								●																	
Deccox®-L *(Alpharma)*								●																	
Rumensin® 80 *(Elanco)*								●																	
Sulfa-Q 20% Concentrate *(AgriPharm)*								●																	
SulfaSURE™ SR Calf Bolus *(Durvet)*								●																	
SulfaSURE™ SR Cattle Bolus *(Durvet)*								●																	
SulfaSure™ SR *(Butler)*								●																	
SulfaSure™ SR Calf Bolus *(Butler)*								●																	
Curatrem® *(Merial)*									●																

* Arthropod

CANINE

Product Name	Ancylostoma spp	Ctenocephalides spp*	Dermacentor variabilis*	Dipylidium spp	Dirofilaria immitis	Echinococcus spp	Otodectes spp*	Sarcoptes scabei*	Taenia spp	Toxascaris leonina	Toxocara canis	Trichuris spp	Trichuris vulpis	Uncinaria stenocephala
ProHeart® 6 *(Fort Dodge)*	●				●									
Champion Protector™ Worm Protector™ 2X *(AgriLabs)*	●									●	●			●
D-Worm™ 120 Liquid Wormer *(Farnam)*	●									●	●			●
D-Worm™ 60 Liquid Wormer *(Farnam)*	●									●	●			●
D-Worm™ Dog Wormer Chewable Tablets for Large Dogs *(Farnam)*	●									●	●			●
D-Worm™ Dog Wormer Chewable Tablets for Puppies & Small Dogs *(Farnam)*	●									●	●			●
D-Worm™ Dog Wormer Tablets for Large Dogs *(Farnam)*	●									●	●			●
D-Worm™ Dog Wormer Tablets for Puppies & Small Dogs *(Farnam)*	●									●	●			●
Happy Jack® Liqui-Vict 2X™ *(Happy Jack)*	●									●	●			●
Nemex™ Tabs *(Pfizer Animal Health)*	●									●	●			●
Nemex™ -2 Suspension *(Pfizer Animal Health)*	●									●	●			●
Pet Care Liquid Wormer *(Durvet)*	●									●	●			●
Pet Care Liquid Wormer 2X *(Durvet)*	●									●	●			●
RFD® Liquid Wormer *(Pfizer Animal Health)*	●									●	●			●
Sergeant's® Vetscription® Sure Shot® Liquid Wormer for Puppies and Dogs *(Sergeant's)*	●									●	●			●
Panacur® Granules 22.2% *(Intervet)*	●								●	●	●	●		●
Panacur® Granules 22.2% (Dogs only) *(Intervet)*	●								●	●	●		●	●
Filaribits Plus® *(Pfizer Animal Health)*	●				●						●		●	
Heartgard® Plus Chewables for Dogs *(Merial)*	●				●					●	●			●
Iverhart™ Plus Flavored Chewables *(Virbac)*	●				●					●	●			●
Interceptor® Flavor Tabs® *(Novartis)*	●				●					●	●		●	
Sentinel® Flavor Tabs® *(Novartis)*	●				●					●	●	●		
Drontal® Plus (praziquantel/pyrantel pamoate/febantel) Tablets *(Bayer)*	●			●		●			●	●	●		●	●
Program® Flavor Tabs® *(Novartis)*		●												
Revolution® *(Pfizer Animal Health)*		●	●		●		●	●						
Cestex® *(Pfizer Animal Health)*				●					●					
Happy Jack® Tapeworm Tablets *(Happy Jack)*				●					●					
Tape Worm Tabs™ for Dogs and Puppies *(TradeWinds)*				●					●					
Droncit® (praziquantel) Canine Tablets *(Bayer)*				●		●			●					
Droncit® (praziquantel) Injectable for Dogs and Cats *(Bayer)*				●		●			●					
Heartgard® Chewables for Dogs *(Merial)*					●									
Heartgard® Tablets for Dogs *(Merial)*					●									
ProHeart® Tablets *(Fort Dodge)*					●									
Filaribits® *(Pfizer Animal Health)*					●					●	●			
Piperazine-17 Medicated *(Durvet)*										●	●			
Sergeant's® Vetscription® Worm-Away® for Dogs *(Sergeant's)*										●	●			
Tasty Paste® Dog & Puppy Wormer *(Farnam)*										●	●			
D-Worm™ Liquid Wormer for Cats and Dogs *(Farnam)*											●			
Hartz® Health measures™ Liquid Wormer *(Hartz Mountain)*											●			
Hartz® Health measures™ Once-a-month® Wormer for Dogs *(Hartz Mountain)*											●			
Hartz® Health measures™ Once-a-month® Wormer for Large Dogs *(Hartz Mountain)*											●			
Hartz® Health measures™ Once-a-month® Wormer for Puppies *(Hartz Mountain)*											●			
Pipa-Tabs *(Vet-A-Mix)*											●			

* Arthropod

Please refer to product listings for more complete information.

EQUINE

Product Name	Dictyocaulus arnfieldi	Draschia megastoma	Gasterophilus spp*	Habronema spp	Onchocerca cervicalis	Oxyuris equi	Parascaris equorum	Sarcocystis neurona	Small Strongyles	Strongyloides spp	Strongylus spp	Trichostrongylus spp
Agri-Mectin™ Equine Paste Dewormer 1.87% *(AgriLabs)*	●	●	●	●	●	●	●		●	●	●	●
AmTech Phoenectin® Liquid for Horses *(Phoenix Scientific)*	●	●	●	●	●	●	●		●	●	●	●
AmTech Phoenectin® Paste 1.87% *(Phoenix Scientific)*	●	●	●	●	●	●	●		●	●	●	●
Cooper's® Best Ivermectin Paste 1.87% *(Aspen)*	●	●	●	●	●	●	●		●	●	●	●
DVMectin™ Liquid for Horses *(DVM)*	●	●	●	●	●	●	●		●	●	●	●
Equimectrin™ Paste 1.87% *(Farnam)*	●	●	●	●	●	●	●		●	●	●	●
Equimectrin® Paste 1.87% *(Merial)*	●	●	●	●	●	●	●		●	●	●	●
Eqvalan® Liquid *(Merial)*	●	●	●	●	●	●	●		●	●	●	●
Eqvalan® Paste 1.87% *(Merial)*	●	●	●	●	●	●	●		●	●	●	●
Horse Care Ivermectin Paste 1.87% *(Durvet)*	●	●	●	●	●	●	●		●	●	●	●
Ivercide™ Equine Paste 1.87% *(Phoenix Pharmaceutical)*	●	●	●	●	●	●	●		●	●	●	●
Ivercide™ Liquid for Horses *(Phoenix Pharmaceutical)*	●	●	●	●	●	●	●		●	●	●	●
Iversol *(Med-Pharmex)*	●	●	●	●	●	●	●		●	●	●	●
Privermectin™ Equine Oral Liquid *(First Priority)*	●	●	●	●	●	●	●		●	●	●	●
ProMectin E™ Liquid for Horses *(Vedco)*	●	●	●	●	●	●	●		●	●	●	●
ProMectin E™ Paste *(Vedco)*	●	●	●	●	●	●	●		●	●	●	●
Rotectin™ 1 Paste 1.87% *(Farnam)*	●	●	●	●	●	●	●		●	●	●	●
Zimecterin® Paste 1.87% *(Farnam)*	●	●	●	●	●	●	●		●	●	●	●
Zimecterin® Paste 1.87% *(Merial)*	●	●	●	●	●	●	●		●	●	●	●
Quest® 2% Equine Oral Gel *(Fort Dodge)*			●	●	●	●	●		●		●	●
Alfalfa Pellet Horse Wormer *(Farnam)*						●	●		●		●	
AmTech Anthelban V *(Phoenix Scientific)*						●	●		●		●	
Anthelban V *(Phoenix Pharmaceutical)*						●	●		●		●	
Benzelmin® Paste *(Fort Dodge)*						●	●		●		●	
Continuex™ *(Farnam)*						●	●		●		●	
Dealer Select Horse Care Horse & Colt Wormer *(Durvet)*						●	●		●		●	
Equi-Phar ProTal™ *(Vedco)*						●	●		●		●	
Equi-Phar™ Horse & Colt Wormer *(Vedco)*						●	●		●		●	
Exodus™ Paste *(Bimeda)*						●	●		●		●	
Panacur® Granules 22.2% (Horse) *(Intervet)*						●	●		●		●	
Panacur® Horse Dewormer *(Intervet)*						●	●		●		●	
Panacur® Horse Dewormer (25 g) *(Intervet)*						●	●		●		●	
Panacur® Horse Dewormer (57 g) *(Intervet)*						●	●		●		●	
Panacur® Horse Dewormer (92 g) *(Intervet)*						●	●		●		●	
Piperazine-17 Medicated *(Durvet)*						●	●		●		●	
Rotectin™ 2 Paste *(Farnam)*						●	●		●		●	
Safe-Guard® Equine Dewormer (25 g) *(Intervet)*						●	●		●		●	
Safe-Guard® Horse Dewormer (92 g) *(Intervet)*						●	●		●		●	
Strongid® C *(Pfizer Animal Health)*						●	●		●		●	
Strongid® C 2X™ *(Pfizer Animal Health)*						●	●		●		●	
Strongid® C Thirty *(Pfizer Animal Health)*						●	●		●		●	
Strongid® Paste *(Pfizer Animal Health)*						●	●		●		●	
Strongid® T *(Pfizer Animal Health)*						●	●		●		●	
Wonder Wormer™ for Horses *(Farnam)*						●	●		●		●	
Anthelcide® EQ Equine Wormer Paste *(Pfizer Animal Health)*						●	●		●	●	●	
Anthelcide® EQ Equine Wormer Suspension *(Pfizer Animal Health)*						●	●		●	●	●	
Marquis™ (15% w/w ponazuril) Antiprotozoal Oral Paste *(Bayer)*								●				

FELINE

Product Name	Ancylostoma spp	Ctenocephalides spp*	Dipylidium spp	Dirofilaria immitis	Otodectes spp*	Taenia spp	Toxascaris leonina	Toxocara cati
Heartgard® Chewables for Cats *(Merial)*	•			•				
Interceptor® Flavor Tabs® *(Novartis)*	•			•				•
Drontal® (praziquantel/pyrantel pamoate) Tablets *(Bayer)*	•		•			•		•
Revolution® *(Pfizer Animal Health)*	•	•		•	•			•
Program® 6 Month Injectable for Cats *(Novartis)*		•						
Program® Flavor Tabs® *(Novartis)*		•						
Program® Suspension *(Novartis)*		•						
Cestex® *(Pfizer Animal Health)*			•			•		
Droncit® (praziquantel) Feline Tablets *(Bayer)*			•			•		
Droncit® (praziquantel) Injectable for Dogs and Cats *(Bayer)*			•			•		
Tape Worm Tabs™ for Cats and Kittens *(TradeWinds)*			•			•		
Hartz® Health measures™ Liquid Wormer *(Hartz Mountain)*							•	
Hartz® Health measures™ Once-a-month® Wormer for Cats and Kittens *(Hartz Mountain)*							•	
Pipa-Tabs *(Vet-A-Mix)*							•	
Piperazine-17 Medicated *(Durvet)*							•	
Sergeant's® Vetscription® Worm-Away® for Cats *(Sergeant's)*							•	
D-Worm™ Liquid Wormer for Cats and Dogs *(Farnam)*							•	•
Sergeant's® Vetscription® Sure Shot® Liquid Wormer for Cats & Kittens *(Sergeant's)*							•	•

* Arthropod

Please refer to product listings for more complete information.

OVINE

Product Name	Bunostomum spp	Chabertia spp	Cooperia spp	Dictyocaulus spp	Eimeria spp	Fasciola spp	Fascioloides magna	Haemonchus spp	Marshallagia spp	Moniezia spp	Nematodirus spp	Oesophagostomum spp	Oestrus ovis*	Ostertagia spp	Strongyloides spp	Thysanosoma spp	Trichostrongylus spp	Trichuris spp
Levasole® Sheep Wormer Boluses *(Schering-Plough)*	•	•	•	•				•			•	•		•			•	
Levasole® Soluble Drench Powder *(Schering-Plough)*	•	•	•	•				•			•	•		•			•	
Levasole® Soluble Drench Powder (Sheep) *(Schering-Plough)*	•	•	•	•				•			•	•		•			•	
Prohibit® Soluble Drench Powder *(AgriLabs)*	•	•	•	•				•			•	•		•			•	
Valbazen® Suspension *(Pfizer Animal Health)*		•	•			•	•	•	•	•	•	•		•		•	•	
Ivomec® Sheep Drench *(Merial)*		•	•	•				•			•	•	•	•	•		•	•
Privermectin™ Drench for Sheep *(First Priority)*		•	•	•				•			•	•	•	•	•		•	•
Bovatec® 150 FP *(Alpharma)*					•													
Bovatec® 68 *(Alpharma)*					•													
Bovatec® Liquid 20 *(Alpharma)*					•													
Deccox® *(Alpharma)*					•													

* Arthropod

PORCINE

Product Name	Ascaris spp	Ascarops spp	Haematopinus*	Hyostrongylus spp	Metastrongylus spp	Oesophagostomum spp	Sarcoptes scabei*	Stephanurus dentatus	Strongyloides spp	Trichuris spp
Banminth® 48 *(Phibro)*	•					•				
MoorMan's® WDC *(ADM)*	•					•				
Wazine® 17 *(Fleming)*	•					•				
Wazine® 34 *(Fleming)*	•					•				
Wazine® Soluble *(Fleming)*	•					•				
Hygromix® 8 (Swine) *(Elanco)*	•					•				•
Levamisole Soluble Pig Wormer *(AgriLabs)*	•				•	•			•	
Levasole® Soluble Pig Wormer *(Schering-Plough)*	•				•	•			•	
MoorMan's® Moorguard® Swine Dewormer *(ADM)*	•			•	•	•		•		•
Safe-Guard® Medicated Dewormer for Beef & Dairy Cattle, & Swine *(Intervet)*	•			•	•	•		•		•
Safe-Guard® Medicated Dewormer for Swine (EZ Scoop®) *(Intervet)*	•			•	•	•		•		•
AmTech Phoenectin® Injection for Cattle and Swine *(Phoenix Scientific)*	•		•	•	•	•	•		•	
Double Impact™ *(AgriLabs)*	•		•	•	•	•	•		•	
Ivercide™ Injection for Cattle and Swine *(Phoenix Pharmaceutical)*	•		•	•	•	•	•		•	
Ivermectin Injection for Cattle and Swine *(Durvet)*	•		•	•	•	•	•		•	
Ivermectin Injection for Cattle and Swine *(Aspen)*	•		•	•	•	•	•		•	
Ivomec® 0.27% Injection for Grower and Feeder Pigs *(Merial)*	•		•	•	•	•	•		•	
Ivomec® 1% Injection for Cattle and Swine *(Merial)*	•		•	•	•	•	•		•	
Ivomec® 1% Injection for Swine *(Merial)*	•		•	•	•	•	•		•	
ProMectin™ Injection for Cattle and Swine *(Vedco)*	•		•	•	•	•	•		•	
Produmec™ Injection for Cattle and Swine *(TradeWinds)*	•		•	•	•	•	•		•	
UltraMectrin™ Injection *(RXV)*	•		•	•	•	•	•		•	
Dectomax® Injectable Solution *(Pfizer Animal Health)*	•		•	•	•	•	•	•	•	
Atgard® C *(Boehringer Ingelheim)*	•	•				•				•
Atgard® Swine Wormer *(Boehringer Ingelheim)*	•	•				•				•
Ivomec® Premix for Swine Type A Medicated Article *(Merial)*	•	•	•	•	•	•	•	•	•	

* Arthropod

POULTRY

Product Name	Ascaridia spp	Capillaria spp	Eimeria spp	Heterakis spp
Wazine® 17 *(Fleming)*	●			
Wazine® 34 *(Fleming)*	●			
Wazine® Soluble *(Fleming)*	●			
Hygromix® 8 (Chickens) *(Elanco)*	●	●		●
20% Sulfaquinoxaline Sodium Solution *(Loveland)*			●	
Albon® Concentrated Solution 12.5% *(Pfizer Animal Health)*			●	
Avatec® *(Alpharma)*			●	
Aviax® *(Phibro)*			●	
Bio-Cox® 60 Granular *(Alpharma)*			●	
Coban® 60 *(Elanco)*			●	
Deccox® *(Alpharma)*			●	
Di-Methox® 12.5% Oral Solution *(AgriLabs)*			●	
Di-Methox® Soluble Powder *(AgriLabs)*			●	
Maxiban® 72 *(Elanco)*			●	
Monteban® 45 *(Elanco)*			●	
Nicarb® 25% *(Phibro)*			●	
OTC 50 *(Durvet)*			●	
Ren-O-Sal® Tablets *(Fort Dodge)*			●	
Robenz® *(Alpharma)*			●	
RofenAid® 40 *(Alpharma)*			●	
Sulfa-Q 20% Concentrate *(AgriPharm)*			●	
Sulfadimethoxine Oral Solution *(Durvet)*			●	
Sulfadimethoxine Oral Solution *(Vedco)*			●	
Sulfadimethoxine Oral Solution *(AgriPharm)*			●	
Sulfadimethoxine Oral Solution *(Aspen)*			●	
Sulfadimethoxine Soluble Powder *(Durvet)*			●	
Sulfadimethoxine Soluble Powder *(Vedco)*			●	
Sulfadimethoxine Soluble Powder *(AgriPharm)*			●	
Sulmet® Drinking Water Solution 12.5% *(Fort Dodge)*			●	
Sulmet® Soluble Powder *(Fort Dodge)*			●	
Zoamix® *(Alpharma)*			●	

WILD, EXOTIC and OTHER SPECIES

Product Name	Species	Dictyocaulus spp	Eimeria spp	Hypoderma (Oedemagena tarandi)*	Hypoderma bovis*	Mazamastrongylus spp	Oesophagostomum spp	Ostertagia-like spp	Otodectes spp*	Trichostrongylus spp
Ivomec® Eprinex® Pour-On for Beef and Dairy Cattle *(Merial)*	Deer	●				●	●	●		●
Avatec® *(Alpharma)*	Partridges, Rabbits		●							
Bovatec® 68 *(Alpharma)*	Rabbits		●							
RofenAid® 40 *(Alpharma)*	Partridges		●							
UltraMectrin™ Injection *(RXV)*	Reindeer			●						
AmTech Phoenectin® Injection for Cattle and Swine *(Phoenix Scientific)*	Bison, Reindeer			●	●					
Ivercide™ Injection for Cattle and Swine *(Phoenix Pharmaceutical)*	Bison, Reindeer			●	●					
Ivermectin Injection for Cattle and Swine *(Durvet)*	Bison, Reindeer			●	●					
Ivermectin Injection for Cattle and Swine *(Aspen)*	Bison, Reindeer			●	●					
Ivomec® 1% Injection for Cattle and Swine *(Merial)*	Bison, Reindeer			●	●					
ProMectin™ Injection for Cattle and Swine *(Vedco)*	Bison, Reindeer			●	●					
Produmec™ Injection for Cattle and Swine *(TradeWinds)*	Bison, Reindeer			●	●					
Ivomec® 0.27% Injection for Grower and Feeder Pigs *(Merial)*	Foxes								●	

* Arthropod

Please refer to product listings for more complete information.

Withdrawal Time Charts

The following pages contain a reference table listing product names alphabetically. This document summarizes information on withdrawal times for food products (meat, milk, fish, eggs, etc.) according to the species and the route of administration.

The withdrawal times listed correspond to label dosages and directions. Deviations from label recommendations may lead to drug residues in food products.

A **zero (0)** indicates that, according to the product label, a withdrawal time is not required when using the products in the dosage and manner recommended by the manufacturer (on-label use).

Note that sometimes the label clearly states that the product requires a 'zero withdrawal time', or that 'no withdrawal time is necessary'. However, it is more often that a product label does not mention anything, unless a withdrawal time is required.

A **blank** field in the withdrawal time column corresponding to meat or milk indicates that a product is not intended for use in animals producing that type of food. For example, the 'Milk' column is left blank when the product is not for use in lactating dairy animals.

Explanatory "Notes" are only included if they contain actual withdrawal statements. Egg and Honey withdrawal information is included in these "Notes".

Further information regarding the products listed here may be found in the product monographs (white section). If there are still doubts after reading the product monograph, contact the manufacturer. Addresses and telephone numbers are listed in the Manufacturer/Distributor Index.

For the sake of clarity, many products known not to require a withdrawal period have been excluded from the listing. Some examples are:

Colostrum and other oral immunoglobulin preparations

EDDI (iodine) presentations for equines

Dehorning and wart-removing pastes

IV solutions used in fluid therapy or to induce diuresis

Lubricants

Microbial culture supplements and probiotics

Most antiseptics, including teat dips and udder washes

Non-cathartic laxatives

Non-medicated topical preparations

Oral preparations of vitamins, minerals, electrolytes, energy, and diverse dietary supplements

Every effort has been made to ensure the accuracy of the information published. However, it remains the responsibility of the readers to familiarize themselves with the information contained on the product label or package insert. The Publisher, Editorial Team, and all those involved in the production of this book, cannot be held responsible for publication errors or any consequence that could result from the use of published information.

Withdrawal Time Chart Abbreviations

aer/sp .... aerosol spray
bd .... beak dip
dw .... drinking water
Epdl. ..... epidural
Imsn. ..... by immersion
Inhl. ...... by Inhalation
Ifltn. ...... by infiltration
I.A. .... intra-articular
I.Derm. ... intradermal
I.M. ...... intramuscular
I.M.M. .... intramammary
I.N. .... intranasal
I.O. .... intra-ocular
I.P. .... intraperitoneal
I.R. .... intraruminal
I.Syn. ..... intrasynovial
I.Ten. ..... intratendinous
I.Tum. .... intratumoral
I.U. .... intra-uterine
I.Vag. ..... intravaginal
I.V. .... intravenous
S.C. ...... subcutaneous
ts .... thigh-stab
ww .... wing web
d. .... days
h. .... hours
w .... weeks

Product Name	Company Name	Species	Route of Administration	Meat	Milk
2% Chlorhexidine Ointment	Davis	Horses	Topical		
Note: Not for use on horses intended for food.					
3-Nitro® 20	Alpharma	Chickens	In the feed	5d	
		Swine	In the feed	5d	
		Turkeys	In the feed	5d	
3-Nitro® Soluble	Alpharma	Chickens	dw	5d	
		Swine	dw	5d	
		Turkeys	dw	5d	
3% Rabon® Livestock Dust	Durvet	Cattle	Topical	0	0
		Swine	Topical	0	
5-Way Calf Scour Bolus™	AgriLabs	Calves	Oral	14d	
7 Gauge™	AgriPharm	Cattle	S.C.	21d	
		Sheep	S.C.	21d	
7-Way	Aspen	Cattle	S.C.	21d	
		Sheep	I.M., S.C.	21d	
7-Way/Somnus	Aspen	Cattle	I.M., S.C.	21d	
8-Way	Aspen	Cattle	S.C.	21d	
		Sheep	S.C.	21d	
20% Sulfaquinoxaline Sodium Solution	Loveland	Cattle	dw	10d	
		Chickens	dw	10d	
		Turkeys	dw	10d	
Note: Do not medicate chickens or turkeys producing eggs for human consumption. Not for use in lactating dairy cows.					
20/20 Vision® 7 with Spur®	Intervet	Cattle	S.C.	21d	
20/20® with Spur®	Intervet	Cattle	S.C.	21d	
31.92% Sul-Q-Nox™ /Opti-Med™	Alpharma	Cattle	dw	10d	
		Chickens	dw	10d	
		Turkeys	dw	10d	
Note: A withdrawal period has not been established for this product in pre-ruminating calves. Do not use in calves to be processed for veal. Do not use in birds producing eggs for food purposes. Not for use in lactating dairy cows.					
89/03®	Intervet	Chickens	S.C.	21d	
2177®	Intervet	Chickens	S.C.	21d	
A180™	Pfizer Animal Health	Beef cattle	S.C.	4d	
Note: A withdrawal period has not been established for this product in pre-ruminating calves. Do not use in calves to be processed for veal. Do not use in cattle intended for dairy production.					
Absorbine® SuperShield® Red Fly Repellent	W. F. Young	Horses	Topical		
Note: Not for use on horses intended for food.					
Acti/Vac® AR	L.A.H.I. (Maine Biological)	Chickens	aer/sp, dw, I.O.	21d	
Acti/Vac® B1	L.A.H.I. (Maine Biological)	Chickens	aer/sp, dw, I.O.	21d	
Acti/Vac® B1 and M48	L.A.H.I. (Maine Biological)	Chickens	aer/sp	21d	
Acti/Vac® B1-M48	L.A.H.I. (Maine Biological)	Chickens	aer/sp, dw, I.O.	21d	
Acti/Vac® B1-M48-AR	L.A.H.I. (Maine Biological)	Chickens	aer/sp, dw, I.O.	21d	
Acti/Vac® B1-M48-CT	L.A.H.I. (Maine Biological)	Chickens	aer/sp, dw, I.O.	21d	
Acti/Vac® CT	L.A.H.I. (Maine Biological)	Chickens	aer/sp, dw, I.O.	21d	
Acti/Vac® FP	L.A.H.I. (Maine Biological)	Chickens	ww	21d	
Acti/Vac® LAS	L.A.H.I. (Maine Biological)	Chickens	aer/sp, dw, I.N., I.O	21d	
Acti/Vac® LAS-MA	L.A.H.I. (Maine Biological)	Chickens	dw, I.O.	21d	
Acti/Vac® M48	L.A.H.I. (Maine Biological)	Chickens	aer/sp, dw, I.O.	21d	
Acti/Vac® M48-AR	L.A.H.I. (Maine Biological)	Chickens	aer/sp, dw, I.O.	21d	
Acti/Vac® RO	L.A.H.I. (Maine Biological)	Chickens	ww	21d	
Adams™ Fly Repellent Concentrate	V.P.L.	Horses	Topical		
Note: Not for use on horses intended for food.					
Adams™ Fly Spray and Repellent	V.P.L.	Horses	Topical		
Note: Not for use on horses intended for food.					
Adequan® I.A.	Luitpold	Horses	I.A.		
Note: Not for use in horses intended for food.					
Adequan® I.M.	Luitpold	Horses	I.M.		
Note: Not for use in horses intended for food.					
A-D Injection	Durvet	Cattle	I.M.	60d	
Adspec® Sterile Solution	Pharmacia & Upjohn	Cattle	S.C.	11d	
Note: A milk discard period has not been established for this product in lactating dairy cattle. Do not use in female dairy cattle 20 months of age or older. A withdrawal period has not been established for this product in pre-ruminating calves. Do not use in calves to be processed for veal.					
Advance™ Calf Medic® Concentrate	Milk Specialties	Cattle	In the feed	30d	
Advance™ Calvita® Deluxe Medicated Milk Replacer	Milk Specialties	Cattle	Oral	30d	
Note: A withdrawal period has not been established for this product in pre-ruminating calves. Do not use in calves to be processed for veal.					

Please refer to product listings for more complete information.

Product Name	Company Name	Species	Route of Administration	Meat	Milk
Advance™ Calvita® Supreme Medicated A.M. Milk Replacer with Bovatec®	Milk Specialties	Cattle	Oral		
Note: A withdrawal period has not been established for this product in pre-ruminating calves. Do not use in calves to be processed for veal. Do not feed to lactating dairy cattle.					
Advance™ Calvita® Supreme Medicated A.M. Milk Replacer with OTC/Neo	Milk Specialties	Cattle	Oral	30d	
Note: A withdrawal period has not been established for this product in pre-ruminating calves. Do not use in calves to be processed for veal.					
AE + Pox	ASL	Chickens	ww	21d	
Note: Do not vaccinate within 4 weeks of initial egg production.					
AE-Poxine®	Fort Dodge	Chickens	ww	21d	
AE-Vac™	Fort Dodge	Chickens	dw	21d	
Note: Do not vaccinate birds in egg production.					
Agri-Cillin™	AgriLabs	Cattle	I.M.	10d	48h
		Horses	I.M.		
		Sheep	I.M.	9d	
		Swine	I.M.	7d	
Note: Not for use in horses intended for food.					
Agri-Mectin™ Equine Paste Dewormer 1.87%	AgriLabs	Horses	Oral		
Note: Not for use in horses intended for food.					
Agrimycin® 100	AgriLabs	Cattle	I.V.	22d	
Note: A withdrawal period has not been established for this product in pre-ruminating calves. Do not use in calves to be processed for veal. Not for use in lactating dairy animals.					
Agrimycin® 200	AgriLabs	Cattle	I.M., I.V., S.C.	28d	
		Swine	I.M.	28d	
Note: Not for use in lactating dairy animals.					
Agrimycin®-343	AgriLabs	Chickens	dw	0	
		Swine	dw	0	
		Turkeys	dw	0	
Note: Do not use in birds producing eggs for food purposes.					
Agrimycin® Powder	AgriLabs	Cattle	dw	5d	
		Chickens	dw		
		Sheep	dw	5d	
		Swine	dw	5d	
		Turkeys	dw	5d	
Note: A milk discard period has not been established for this product in lactating dairy cattle. Do not use in female dairy cattle 20 months of age or older. A withdrawal period has not been established for this product in pre-ruminating calves. Do not use in calves to be processed for veal. Do not administer to chickens or turkeys producing eggs for human consumption.					
Albadry Plus®	Pharmacia & Upjohn	Dairy cattle	I.M.M.	30d	
Note: Do not use less than 30 days prior to calving. Milk from treated cows must not be used for food during the first 72 hours after calving.					
Albamix® Feed Medication	Pharmacia & Upjohn	Chickens	In the feed	4d	
		Ducks	In the feed	3d	
		Turkeys	In the feed	4d	
Note: Not for use in laying chickens or turkeys. Not for use in laying ducks.					
Albon® Boluses	Pfizer Animal Health	Cattle	Oral	7d	60h
Note: A withdrawal period has not been established for this product in pre-ruminating calves. Do not use in calves to be processed for veal.					
Albon® Concentrated Solution 12.5%	Pfizer Animal Health	Cattle	dw	7d	
		Chickens	dw	5d	
		Turkeys	dw	5d	
Note: A withdrawal period has not been established for this product in pre-ruminating calves. Do not use in calves to be processed for veal. Do not administer to chickens over 16 weeks (112 days) of age. Do not administer to turkeys over 24 weeks (168 days) of age.					
Albon® Injection 40%	Pfizer Animal Health	Cattle	I.V.	5d	60h
		Horses	I.V.		
Note: A withdrawal period has not been established for this product in pre-ruminating calves. Do not use in calves to be processed for veal. Not for use in horses intended for food.					
Albon® SR	Pfizer Animal Health	Cattle	Oral	21d	
Note: A withdrawal period has not been established for this product in pre-ruminating calves. Do not use in calves to be processed for veal. Not for use in lactating dairy cows.					
Alfalfa Pellet Horse Wormer	Farnam	Horses	In the feed		
Note: Not for use in horses intended for food.					
Alpha-7™	Boehringer Ingelheim	Cattle	S.C.	60d	
Alpha-7/MB™	Boehringer Ingelheim	Cattle	S.C.	60d	
Alpha-CD™	Boehringer Ingelheim	Cattle	S.C.	60d	
Ambi-Pen™	Butler	Beef cattle	S.C.	30d	
		Horses	I.M.		
Note: Not for use in horses intended for food.					
Amifuse E	Vetus	Horses	I.U.		
Note: Not for use in horses intended for food.					
Amiglyde-V® Intrauterine Solution	Fort Dodge	Horses	I.U.		
Note: Not for use in horses intended for food.					

Product Name	Company Name	Species	Route of Administration	Meat	Milk
Amikacin E Solution	Phoenix Pharmaceutical	Horses	I.U.		
Note: Not for use in horses intended for food.					
Amikacin Sulfate Solution	Vet Tek	Horses	I.U.		
Note: Not for use in horses intended for food.					
Amoxi-Inject® (Cattle)	Pfizer Animal Health	Cattle	I.M., S.C.	25d	96h
Amoxi-Mast®	Pfizer Animal Health	Dairy cattle	I.M.M.	12d	60h
Amprol Plus® Type A Medicated Article	Merial	Chickens	In the feed		
Note: Do not give to laying hens.					
Amprovine® 25% Type A Medicated Article	Merial	Calves	In the feed	24h	
Note: A withdrawal period has not been established for this product in pre-ruminating calves. Do not use in calves to be processed for veal.					
AmTech AmiMax™ E Solution	Phoenix Scientific	Horses	I.U.		
Note: Not for use in horses intended for food.					
AmTech Anthelban V	Phoenix Scientific	Horses	In the feed		
Note: Do not use in horses or ponies intended for food.					
AmTech Chlortetracycline HCl Soluble Powder	Phoenix Scientific	Chickens	dw	1d	
		Swine	dw	5d	
		Turkeys	dw	1d	
Note: Do not feed to chickens producing eggs for human consumption.					
AmTech Dexamethasone Sodium Phosphate Injection	Phoenix Scientific	Horses	I.V.		
Note: Not for use in horses intended for food.					
AmTech Dexamethasone Solution	Phoenix Scientific	Cattle	I.M., I.V.		
Note: A withdrawal period has not been established for this product in pre-ruminating calves. Do not use in calves to be processed for veal.					
AmTech Flunixin Meglumine Injection	Phoenix Scientific	Cattle	I.V.	4d	
		Horses	I.M., I.V.		
Note: A withdrawal period has not been established for this product in pre-ruminating calves. Do not use in calves to be processed for veal. Not for use in horses intended for food. Not for use in lactating or dry dairy cows.					
AmTech Furosemide Injection 5%	Phoenix Scientific	Cattle	I.M., I.V.	48h	48h
		Horses	I.M., I.V.		
Note: Not for use in horses intended for food.					
AmTech GentaMax™ 100	Phoenix Scientific	Horses	I.U.		
Note: Not for use in horses intended for food.					
AmTech Gentamicin Sulfate Pig Pump Oral Solution	Phoenix Scientific	Swine	Oral	14d	
AmTech GentaPoult™	Phoenix Scientific	Chickens	S.C.	35d	
		Turkeys	S.C.	63d	
AmTech Guaifenesin Injection	Phoenix Scientific	Horses	I.V.		
Note: Not for use on horses intended for food.					
AmTech Levamisole Phosphate Injectable Solution	Phoenix Scientific	Cattle	S.C.	7d	
Note: Do not administer to dairy cattle of breeding age.					
AmTech Maxim-100	Phoenix Scientific	Cattle	I.V.	22d	
Note: A withdrawal period has not been established for this product in pre-ruminating calves. Do not use in calves to be processed for veal. Not for use in lactating dairy animals.					
AmTech Maxim-200®	Phoenix Scientific	Cattle	I.M., I.V., S.C.	28d	
		Swine	I.M.	28d	
Note: Not for use in lactating dairy animals.					
AmTech Neomycin Oral Solution	Phoenix Scientific	Cattle	dw	1d	
		Goats	dw	3d	
		Sheep	dw	2d	
		Swine	dw	3d	
Note: A milk discard period has not been established for this product in lactating dairy cattle. Do not use in female dairy cattle 20 months of age or older. A withdrawal period has not been established for this product in pre-ruminating calves. Do not use in calves to be processed for veal.					
AmTech Oxytetracycline HCl Soluble Powder	Phoenix Scientific	Cattle	dw	5d	
		Chickens	dw	0	
		Sheep	dw	5d	
		Swine	dw	5d	
		Turkeys	dw	5d	
Note: A milk discard period has not been established for this product in lactating dairy cattle. Do not use in female dairy cattle 20 months of age or older. A withdrawal period has not been established for this product in pre-ruminating calves. Do not use in calves to be processed for veal. Do not administer to chickens or turkeys producing eggs for human consumption.					
AmTech Oxytetracycline HCl Soluble Powder-343	Phoenix Scientific	Cattle	dw	5d	
		Chickens	dw	0	
		Sheep	dw	5d	
		Swine	dw	5d	
		Turkeys	dw	5d	
Note: A milk discard period has not been established for this product in lactating dairy cattle. Do not use in female dairy cattle 20 months of age or older. A withdrawal period has not been established for this product in pre-ruminating calves. Do not use in calves to be processed for veal. Do not administer to chickens or turkeys producing eggs for human consumption.					
AmTech Phenylbutazone 20% Injection	Phoenix Scientific	Horses	I.V.		
Note: Not for use in horses intended for food.					
AmTech Phenylbutazone Tablets, USP 1 gram	Phoenix Scientific	Horses	Oral		
Note: Not for use in horses intended for food.					

Product Name	Company Name	Species	Route of Administration	Meat	Milk
AmTech Phoenectin® Injection for Cattle and Swine	Phoenix Scientific	Bison	S.C.	56d	
		Cattle	S.C.	35d	
		Reindeer	S.C.	56d	
		Swine	S.C.	18d	
Note: A milk discard period has not been established for this product in lactating dairy cattle. Do not use in female dairy cattle 20 months of age or older.					
AmTech Phoenectin® Liquid for Horses	Phoenix Scientific	Horses	Oral		
Note: Not for use in horses intended for food.					
AmTech Phoenectin® Paste 1.87%	Phoenix Scientific	Horses	Oral		
Note: Not for use in horses intended for food.					
AmTech Phoenectin® Pour-On for Cattle	Phoenix Scientific	Cattle	Topical	48d	
Note: A milk discard period has not been established for this product in lactating dairy cattle. Do not use in female dairy cattle 20 months of age or older.					
AmTech ProstaMate®	Phoenix Scientific	Cattle	I.M.	0	0
		Horses	I.M.		
		Swine	I.M.	0	
Note: Not for use in horses intended for food.					
AmTech Sodium Iodide 20% Injection	Phoenix Scientific	Cattle	I.V.		
Note: Not for use in lactating dairy cows.					
AmTech Spectam® Scour-Halt™	Phoenix Scientific	Swine	Oral	21d	
AmTech Sulfadimethoxine 12.5% Oral Solution	Phoenix Scientific	Cattle	dw	7d	
		Chickens	dw	5d	
		Turkeys	dw	5d	
Note: A withdrawal period has not been established for this product in pre-ruminating calves. Do not use in calves to be processed for veal. Do not administer to chickens over 16 weeks (112 days) of age. Do not administer to turkeys over 24 weeks (168 days) of age.					
AmTech Sulfadimethoxine Injection - 40%	Phoenix Scientific	Cattle	I.V.	5d	60h
Note: A withdrawal period has not been established for this product in pre-ruminating calves. Do not use in calves to be processed for veal.					
AmTech Sulfadimethoxine Soluble Powder	Phoenix Scientific	Cattle	dw	7d	
		Chickens	dw	5d	
		Turkeys	dw	5d	
Note: A withdrawal period has not been established for this product in pre-ruminating calves. Do not use in calves to be processed for veal. Do not administer to chickens over 16 weeks (112 days) of age. Do not administer to turkeys over 24 weeks (168 days) of age.					
AmTech Tetracycline Hydrochloride Soluble Powder-324	Phoenix Scientific	Cattle	dw	5d	
		Chickens	dw	4d	
		Swine	dw	4d	
		Turkeys	dw	4d	
Note: A withdrawal period has not been established for this product in pre-ruminating calves. Do not use in calves to be processed for veal. Do not administer to poultry producing eggs for human consumption.					
AmTech Tripelennamine Hydrochloride Injection	Phoenix Scientific	Cattle	I.M., I.V.	4d	24h
		Horses	I.M.		
Note: A withdrawal period has not been established for this product in pre-ruminating calves. Do not use in calves to be processed for veal. Not for use in horses intended for food.					
AmTech Xylazine HCl Injection 100 mg/mL	Phoenix Scientific	Cervidae	I.M.		
		Horses	I.M., I.V.		
Note: Do not use in *Cervidae* less than 15 days before or during the hunting season. Do not use in domestic food-producing animals. Not for use in horses intended for food.					
AnaSed® 100 Injectable	Lloyd	Cervidae	I.M.		
		Horses	I.M., I.V.		
Note: Not for use in food-producing animals.					
Animal Insecticide	Durvet	Cattle	Topical	0	0
		Swine	Topical	0	
Antagonil™	Wildlife	Cervidae	I.V.		
Note: Do not administer 30 days before or during hunting season. Do not use in domestic food-producing animals.					
Anthelban V	Phoenix Pharmaceutical	Horses	In the feed, Oral		
Note: Do not use in horses or ponies intended for food.					
Anthelcide® EQ Equine Wormer Paste	Pfizer Animal Health	Horses	Oral		
Note: Not for use in horses intended for food.					
Anthelcide® EQ Equine Wormer Suspension	Pfizer Animal Health	Horses	Oral		
Note: Not for use in horses intended for food.					
Anthrax Spore Vaccine	Colorado Serum	Cattle	S.C.	60d	
		Goats	S.C.	60d	
		Horses	S.C.	60d	
		Sheep	S.C.	60d	
		Swine	S.C.	60d	
Note: If emergency conditions require vaccination of animals reaching market age and condition, these should not be offered for slaughter in less than 60 days after administration of the vaccine.					
Antidote® PHM	AgriPharm	Cattle	I.M., S.C.	60d	
Antitox Tet™	Novartis Animal Vaccines	Cattle	I.M., S.C.	21d	
		Horses	I.M., S.C.	21d	
		Sheep	I.M., S.C.	21d	
		Swine	I.M., S.C.	21d	

Product Name	Company Name	Species	Route of Administration	Meat	Milk
A-Plus™ Wound Dressing	Creative Science	Horses	Topical		
Note: Not for use on animals intended for food purposes.					
Apralan® Soluble	Elanco	Swine	dw	28d	
Aquacillin™	Vedco	Cattle	I.M.	10d	48h
		Horses	I.M.		
		Sheep	I.M.	9d	
		Swine	I.M.	7d	
Note: Not for use in horses intended for food.					
Argus® SC/ST	Intervet	Swine	dw	21d	
Ark Blen®	Merial Select	Chickens	dw	21d	
Arko Chol Vac FD	Arko	Turkeys	dw	21d	
Arko Ery Vac FD	Arko	Turkeys	dw	21d	
AR-Pac®-P+ER	Schering-Plough	Swine	S.C.	21d	
AR-Pac®-PD+ER	Schering-Plough	Swine	S.C.	21d	
AR-Parapac®+ER	Schering-Plough	Swine	S.C.	21d	
Arquel® Granules	Fort Dodge	Horses	In the feed		
Note: Not for use in horses intended for food.					
Art Vax®	Schering-Plough	Turkeys	aer/sp, dw	21d	
Arvac®	Fort Dodge	Horses	I.M.	21d	
Aspirin 60 Grain	Butler	Cattle	Oral		
Note: Not for use in lactating dairy animals.					
Aspirin Boluses	Butler	Cattle	Oral		
Note: Not for use in lactating dairy animals.					
Aspirin Boluses	Bimeda	Cattle	Oral		
Note: Not for use in lactating dairy animals.					
Aspirin Boluses-240	AgriLabs	Cattle	Oral		
Note: Not for use in lactating dairy animals.					
Atgard® C	Boehringer Ingelheim	Swine	In the feed	0	
Atgard® Swine Wormer	Boehringer Ingelheim	Swine	In the feed	0	
Atrobac® 3	Pfizer Animal Health	Swine	S.C.	21d	
Atroban® 11% EC Insecticide	Schering-Plough	Horses	Topical		
		Swine	Topical	5d	
Note: Not for use on horses intended for food.					
Atroban® 42.5% EC	Schering-Plough	Swine	Topical	5d	
Atroban® Extra Insecticide Ear Tags	Schering-Plough	Cattle	Ear tags		
Note: Remove tags before slaughter.					
Aureomix® 500 Granular	Alpharma	Swine	In the feed	15d	
Aureomycin® 50 Granular	Alpharma	Cattle	In the feed		
		Ducks	In the feed		
		Turkeys	In the feed		
Note: A withdrawal period has not been established for this product in pre-ruminating calves. Do not use in calves to be processed for veal. Do not feed to ducks producing eggs for food. Do not feed to turkeys producing eggs for food.					
Aureomycin® 90 Granular	Alpharma	Cattle	In the feed		
		Ducks	In the feed		
		Turkeys	In the feed		
Note: A withdrawal period has not been established for this product in pre-ruminating calves. Do not use in calves to be processed for veal. Do not feed to ducks producing eggs for food. Do not feed to turkeys producing eggs for food.					
Aureomycin® 100 Granular	Alpharma	Cattle	In the feed		
		Ducks	In the feed		
		Turkeys	In the feed		
Note: A withdrawal period has not been established for this product in pre-ruminating calves. Do not use in calves to be processed for veal. Do not feed to ducks producing eggs for food. Do not feed to turkeys producing eggs for food.					
Aureomycin® Soluble Powder	Fort Dodge	Calves	dw	24h	
		Chickens	dw	24h	
		Swine	dw	24h	
		Turkeys	dw	24h	
Note: A withdrawal period has not been established for this product in pre-ruminating calves. Do not use in calves to be processed for veal. Do not use in laying chickens.					
Aureomycin® Soluble Powder Concentrate	Fort Dodge	Calves	dw	24h	
		Chickens	dw	24h	
		Swine	dw	24h	
		Turkeys	dw	24h	
Note: A withdrawal period has not been established for this product in pre-ruminating calves. Do not use in calves to be processed for veal. Do not use in laying chickens.					
Aureomycin® Sulmet® Soluble Powder	Fort Dodge	Swine	dw	15d	
Aureo S 700® Granular 10G	Alpharma	Beef cattle	In the feed	7d	
Note: A withdrawal period has not been established for this product in pre-ruminating calves. Do not use in calves to be processed for veal.					

Product Name	Company Name	Species	Route of Administration	Meat	Milk
Aureo S 700® Granular 35G	Alpharma	Beef cattle	In the feed	7d	
Note: A withdrawal period has not been established for this product in pre-ruminating calves. Do not use in calves to be processed for veal.					
AureoZol® 500 Granular	Alpharma	Swine	In the feed	7d	
Ava-Bron®	ASL	Chickens	aer/sp, dw, I.N., I.O	21d	
Ava-Bron-H®-B_1	ASL	Chickens	dw, I.N., I.O	21d	
Ava-Bron-H®-N-63	ASL	Chickens	dw, I.N., I.O	21d	
Ava-Pox® CE	ASL	Chickens Turkeys	ww ts, ww	21d 21d	
Ava-Trem®	ASL	Chickens	dw, ww	21d	
Note: Do not vaccinate within 4 weeks of initial egg production.					
Avian Pneumovirus Vaccine	Biomune	Turkeys	dw, I.O.	21d	
Aviax®	Phibro	Chickens	In the feed	0	
Note: Do not feed to laying chickens.					
Avichol®	Schering-Plough	Chickens	ww	21d	
Avimune®	Schering-Plough	Chickens	dw	21d	
Avimune®+Pox	Schering-Plough	Chickens	ww	21d	
Azium® Powder	Schering-Plough	Horses	Oral		
Note: Not for use in horses intended for food.					
B_1 Vac™	Intervet	Chickens	aer/sp, bd, dw	21d	
Banamine® Granules	Schering-Plough	Horses	In the feed		
Note: Not for use in horses intended for food.					
Banamine® Injectable Solution	Schering-Plough	Cattle Horses	I.V. I.M., I.V.	4d	
Note: A withdrawal period has not been established for this product in pre-ruminating calves. Do not use in calves to be processed for veal. Not for use in horses intended for food. Not for use in lactating or dry dairy cows.					
Banamine® Paste	Schering-Plough	Horses	Oral		
Note: Not for use in horses intended for food.					
Banminth® 48	Phibro	Swine	In the feed	24h	
Bapten® for Injection	PR Pharmaceuticals	Horses	I.Ten.		
Note: Not for use in horses intended for food.					
Bar-Guard-99™	Boehringer Ingelheim	Cattle Sheep	Oral Oral	21d 21d	
Bar Somnus™	Boehringer Ingelheim	Cattle	S.C.	21d	
Bar Somnus 2P™	Boehringer Ingelheim	Cattle	I.M.	21d	
Bar-Vac® 7	Boehringer Ingelheim	Cattle Sheep	S.C. S.C.	21d 21d	
Bar Vac® 7/Somnus	Boehringer Ingelheim	Cattle	S.C.	21d	
Bar-Vac® 8	Boehringer Ingelheim	Cattle Sheep	S.C. S.C.	21d 21d	
Bar-Vac® CD	Boehringer Ingelheim	Cattle Sheep	S.C. S.C.	21d 21d	
Bar Vac® CD/T	Boehringer Ingelheim	Cattle Goats Sheep	S.C. S.C. S.C.	21d 21d 21d	
Baytril® (enrofloxacin) 3.23% Concentrate Antimicrobial Solution	Bayer	Chickens Turkeys	Oral Oral	2d 2d	
Note: Do not use in laying hens producing eggs for human consumption.					
Baytril® 100 (enrofloxacin) 100 mg/mL Antimicrobial Injectable Solution	Bayer	Beef cattle	S.C.	28d	
Note: A withdrawal period has not been established for this product in pre-ruminating calves. Do not use in calves to be processed for veal. Do not use in cattle intended for dairy production.					
Benzelmin® Paste	Fort Dodge	Horses	Oral		
Note: Not for use in horses intended for food.					
Benzo-Gel™	Butler	Horses	Topical		
Note: Not for use on horses intended for food.					
Betadine® Solution	Purdue Frederick	Horses	Topical		
Note: Not for use on animals intended for food purposes.					
Betadine® Surgical Scrub	Purdue Frederick	Horses	Topical		
Note: Not for use on animals intended for food purposes.					
Bimectin™ Pour-On	Bimeda	Cattle	Topical	48d	
Note: Do not administer to dairy cattle of breeding age.					
Bio-Cox® 60 Granular	Alpharma	Chickens	In the feed		
Note: Do not feed to laying hens producing eggs for human consumption.					
Biodry®	Pharmacia & Upjohn	Dairy cattle	I.M.M.	30d	
Note: Do not use less than 30 days prior to calving.					
Bio-Hev™	Intervet	Turkeys	Oral	21d	

Product Name	Company Name	Species	Route of Administration	Meat	Milk
Bio-Mycin® 200	Boehringer Ingelheim	Cattle Swine	I.M., I.V., S.C. I.M.	28d 28d	
Note: Not for use in lactating dairy animals.					
Bio-Pox M™	Intervet	Chickens	ww	21d	
Biosol® Liquid	Pharmacia & Upjohn	Cattle Goats Sheep Swine	dw, In the feed, Oral dw, In the feed, Oral dw, In the feed, Oral dw, In the feed, Oral	1d 3d 2d 3d	
Note: A milk discard period has not been established for this product in lactating dairy cattle. Do not use in female dairy cattle 20 months of age or older. A withdrawal period has not been established for this product in pre-ruminating calves. Do not use in calves to be processed for veal.					
Bio-Sota + Bron MM™	Intervet	Chickens	dw, I.N., I.O	21d	
Bio-Tella™	Intervet	Turkeys	dw	21d	
Bio-Trach™	Intervet	Chickens	aer/sp, dw, I.O.	21d	
Bite Free™ Biting Fly Repellent	Farnam	Horses	Topical		
Note: Not for use on horses intended for food.					
Bizolin®-1 g	Boehringer Ingelheim	Horses	Oral		
Note: Not for use in horses intended for food.					
Bloat-Pac®	Vet-A-Mix	Cattle Goats Sheep	I.R., Oral I.R., Oral I.R., Oral	0 0 0	96h
Bloat Release	AgriLabs	Cattle Goats Sheep	Oral Oral Oral	3d 3d 3d	96h
Bloat Treatment	AgriPharm	Cattle Goats Sheep	Oral Oral Oral	3d 3d 3d	96h
Blood Stop Powder	AgriLabs	Cattle Horses Sheep Swine	Topical Topical Topical Topical		
Note: Not for use on animals intended for food purposes.					
Blood Stop Powder	Centaur	Horses	Topical		
Note: Not for use on animals intended for food purposes.					
Blue Lotion	Farnam	Cattle Horses	Topical Topical		
Note: Not for use on animals intended for food purposes.					
Blue Lotion	AgriLabs	Horses	Topical		
Note: Not for use on horses intended for food.					
Bluetongue Vaccine	Colorado Serum	Goats Sheep	I.M., S.C. I.M., S.C.	21d 21d	
Bo-Bac-2X™	Boehringer Ingelheim	Cattle	S.C.	21d	
Borde-Cell™	AgriLabs	Swine	I.M., I.N.	21d	
Borde Shield® 4	Novartis Animal Vaccines	Swine	I.M., S.C.	21d	
Bordetella Bronchiseptica Intranasal Vaccine	MVP	Swine	I.N.	21d	
BO-SE®	Schering-Plough	Calves Sheep Swine	I.M., S.C. I.M., S.C. I.M., S.C.	30d 14d 14d	
BotVax® B	Neogen	Horses	I.M.	21d	
BovaMune™	AgriLabs	Cattle Sheep	I.M., S.C. I.M., S.C.	21d 21d	
Bovatec® 68	Alpharma	Cattle	In the feed		
Note: A withdrawal period has not been established for this product in pre-ruminating calves. Do not use in calves to be processed for veal.					
Bovatec® 150 FP	Alpharma	Cattle	In the feed		
Note: A withdrawal period has not been established for this product in pre-ruminating calves. Do not use in calves to be processed for veal.					
Bovatec® Liquid 20	Alpharma	Cattle	In the feed		
Note: A withdrawal period has not been established for this product in pre-ruminating calves. Do not use in calves to be processed for veal.					
Bovi-K® 4	Pfizer Animal Health	Cattle	I.M.	21d	
Bovine 3	Durvet	Cattle	I.M., S.C.	21d	
Bovine 8	Durvet	Cattle	I.M., S.C.	21d	
Bovine 9	Durvet	Cattle	I.M., S.C.	21d	
Bovine Ecolizer®	Novartis Animal Vaccines	Calves	Oral	21d	
Bovine Ecolizer®+C	Novartis Animal Vaccines	Calves	Oral	21d	
Bovine Pili Shield™	Novartis Animal Vaccines	Cattle	I.M.	60d	
Bovine Pili Shield™ +C	Novartis Animal Vaccines	Cattle	I.M.	60d	
Bovine Rhinotracheitis-Parainfluenza$_3$ Vaccine	Colorado Serum	Cattle	I.M.	21d	
Bovine Rhinotracheitis Vaccine	Colorado Serum	Cattle	I.M.	21d	
Bovine Rhinotracheitis-Virus Diarrhea-Parainfluenza-3 Vaccine	Colorado Serum	Cattle	I.M.	21d	
Bovine Virus Diarrhea Vaccine	Colorado Serum	Cattle	I.M.	21d	

Product Name	Company Name	Species	Route of Administration	Meat	Milk
Bovi-Sera™ Serum Antibodies	Colorado Serum	Cattle Sheep	I.M., S.C. I.M., S.C.	21d 21d	
Bovi-Shield™ 3	Pfizer Animal Health	Cattle	I.M.	21d	
Bovi-Shield™ 4	Pfizer Animal Health	Cattle	I.M.	21d	
Bovi-Shield™ BRSV	Pfizer Animal Health	Cattle	I.M.	21d	
Bovi-Shield® FP 4+L5	Pfizer Animal Health	Cattle	I.M.	21d	
Bovi-Shield™ IBR	Pfizer Animal Health	Cattle	I.M.	21d	
Bovi-Shield™ IBR-BRSV-LP	Pfizer Animal Health	Cattle	I.M.	21d	
Bovi-Shield™ IBR-BVD	Pfizer Animal Health	Cattle	I.M.	21d	
Bovi-Shield™ IBR-BVD-BRSV-LP	Pfizer Animal Health	Cattle	I.M.	21d	
Bovi-Shield™ IBR-PI_3-BRSV	Pfizer Animal Health	Cattle	I.M.	21d	
BoviSpec™ Sterile Solution	Vet Tek	Cattle	S.C.	11d	
Note: A milk discard period has not been established for this product in lactating dairy cattle. Do not use in female dairy cattle 20 months of age or older. A withdrawal period has not been established for this product in pre-ruminating calves. Do not use in calves to be processed for veal.					
BratiVac®	Pfizer Animal Health	Swine	I.M.	21d	
BratiVac®-6	Pfizer Animal Health	Swine	I.M.	21d	
Breed-Back-10™	Boehringer Ingelheim	Cattle	I.M.	21d	
Breedervac-III-Plus®	Intervet	Chickens	I.M., S.C.	42d	
Breedervac-IV-Plus®	Intervet	Chickens	I.M., S.C.	42d	
Breedervac-Reo-Plus®	Intervet	Chickens	I.M., S.C.	42d	
Breed Sow™ 6	AgriLabs	Swine	I.M.	21d	
Breed Sow® 7	AgriLabs	Swine	I.M., S.C.	21d	
Broilerbron®	ASL	Chickens	aer/sp, I.N., I.O	21d	
Broilerbron®-99	ASL	Chickens	dw, I.N., I.O	21d	
Broilerbron®-99 B_1	ASL	Chickens	aer/sp, I.N., I.O	21d	
Broilerbron® B_1	ASL	Chickens	aer/sp, I.N., I.O	21d	
Broilerbron®-H-B_1	ASL	Chickens	dw, I.N., I.O	21d	
Broilerbron®-H N-79	ASL	Chickens	dw, I.O.	21d	
Broilertrake®	ASL	Chickens	I.O.	21d	
Broilertrake®-M	ASL	Chickens	I.O.	21d	
Bronchitis Vaccine	L.A.H.I. (New Jersey)	Chickens	S.C.	42d	
Bronchitis Vaccine (Ark. Type)	Merial Select	Chickens	aer/sp	21d	
Bronchitis Vaccine (Mass. Type)	Merial Select	Chickens	aer/sp, dw	21d	
Bron-Newcavac-M®	Intervet	Chickens	I.M., S.C.	42d	
Brucella Abortus Vaccine (Strain RB-51)	Professional Biological	Cattle	S.C.	21d	
Bursa Blen® M	Merial Select	Chickens	dw	21d	
Bursa Guard	Merial Select	Chickens	I.M., S.C.	42d	
Bursa Guard N-B	Merial Select	Chickens	S.C.	42d	
Bursa Guard N-B-R	Merial Select	Chickens	S.C.	42d	
Bursa Guard N-R	Merial Select	Chickens	S.C.	42d	
Bursa Guard Reo	Merial Select	Chickens	S.C.	42d	
Bursal Disease-Avian Reovirus Vaccine	L.A.H.I. (New Jersey)	Chickens	S.C.	42d	
Bursal Disease-Marek's Disease Vaccine (Standard and Variant, Chicken and Turkey)	Merial Select	Chickens	S.C.	21d	
Bursal Disease-Marek's Disease Vaccine (Standard and Variant, Turkey)	Merial Select	Chickens	S.C.	21d	
Bursal Disease-Marek's Disease Vaccine (Standard, Chicken and Turkey)	Merial Select	Chickens	S.C.	21d	
Bursal Disease-Marek's Disease Vaccine (Standard, Turkey)	Merial Select	Chickens	S.C.	21d	
Bursal Disease-Newcastle-Bronchitis Vaccine	L.A.H.I. (New Jersey)	Chickens	I.M., S.C.	42d	
Bursal Disease-Newcastle-Bronchitis Vaccine (Standard and Variant)	L.A.H.I. (New Jersey)	Chickens	S.C.	42d	
Bursal Disease-Newcastle Disease-Bronchitis-Reovirus Vaccine	L.A.H.I. (New Jersey)	Chickens	I.M., S.C.	42d	
Bursal Disease-Newcastle Disease-Bronchitis Vaccine (Mass. & Conn. Types)	Merial Select	Chickens	aer/sp	21d	
Bursal Disease-Newcastle Disease-Reovirus Vaccine	L.A.H.I. (New Jersey)	Chickens	S.C.	42d	
Bursal Disease-Newcastle Disease Vaccine	L.A.H.I. (New Jersey)	Chickens	S.C.	42d	
Bursal Disease Vaccine (S-706 Strain)	Merial Select	Chickens	aer/sp, dw	21d	
Bursal Disease Vaccine (ST-14 Strain)	Merial Select	Chickens	S.C.	21d	
Bursal Disease Vaccine (SVS 510)	Merial Select	Chickens	aer/sp, dw	21d	
Bursamate™	Intervet	Chickens	I.M.	42d	

Please refer to product listings for more complete information.

Product Name	Company Name	Species	Route of Administration	Meat	Milk
Bursaplex®	Embrex	Chickens	In ovo, S.C.	21d	
Bursa-Vac®	ASL	Chickens	dw	21d	
Bursa-Vac® 3	ASL	Chickens	aer/sp, dw, I.O.	21d	
Bursa-Vac® 4	ASL	Chickens	dw	21d	
Bursimune®	Biomune	Chickens	dw	21d	
Bursine®-2	Fort Dodge	Chickens	dw	21d	
Bursine®-K ACL™	Fort Dodge	Chickens	I.M., S.C.	42d	
Bursine® N-K ACL™	Fort Dodge	Chickens	I.M., S.C.	42d	
Bursine® Plus	Fort Dodge	Chickens	dw	21d	
Butaject	Vetus	Horses	I.V.		
Note: Not for use in horses intended for food.					
Butapaste	Vetus	Horses	Oral		
Note: Not for use in horses intended for food.					
Butatabs-E	Vetus	Horses	Oral		
Note: Not for use in horses intended for food.					
Butatron™ Tablets	Bimeda	Horses	Oral		
Note: Not for use in horses intended for food.					
Calcium Oral Gel	Phoenix Pharmaceutical	Dairy cattle	Oral	0	
Calf-Guard®	Pfizer Animal Health	Cattle	I.M., Oral	21d	
Calf Scour Bolus Antibiotic	Durvet	Calves	Oral	12d	
Caliber® 3	Boehringer Ingelheim	Cattle	S.C.	21d	
		Sheep	S.C.	21d	
Caliber® 7	Boehringer Ingelheim	Cattle	S.C.	21d	
		Sheep	S.C.	21d	
Cal-Mag-Co Gel	Durvet	Dairy cattle	Oral	0	0
Cal-Mag-SE Gel	Durvet	Dairy cattle	Oral	0	0
Calvenza™ EHV	Boehringer Ingelheim	Horses	I.M., I.N.	21d	
Calvenza™ EIV	Boehringer Ingelheim	Horses	I.M., I.N.	21d	
Calvenza™ EIV/EHV	Boehringer Ingelheim	Horses	I.M., I.N.	21d	
Campylobacter Fetus Bacterin-Bovine	Colorado Serum	Cattle	S.C.	60d	
Campylobacter Fetus Bacterin-Ovine	Colorado Serum	Sheep	S.C.	21d	
Campylobacter Fetus-Jejuni Bacterin	Hygieia	Sheep	S.C.	21d	
Caprine Serum Fraction, Immunomodulator	Professional Biological	Horses	I.M.	21d	
Carbocaine®-V	Pharmacia & Upjohn	Horses	Epdl., I.A., Ifltn., Topical		
Note: Not for use in horses intended for food.					
Carmilax® Bolets®	Pfizer Animal Health	Cattle	Oral	0	12h
Carmilax® Powder	Pfizer Animal Health	Cattle	dw	0	12h
		Sheep	dw	0	
CarraSorb™ Freeze-Dried Gel (FDG)	V.P.L.	Horses	Topical		
Note: Not for use on animals intended for food purposes.					
CarraVet™ Wound Dressing	V.P.L.	Horses	Topical		
Note: Not for use on horses intended for food.					
Case-Bac™	Colorado Serum	Sheep	S.C.	21d	
Caseous D-T™	Colorado Serum	Sheep	S.C.	21d	
Catron™ IV	Boehringer Ingelheim	Swine	Topical	5d	
CattleMaster® 4	Pfizer Animal Health	Cattle	I.M.	21d	
CattleMaster® 4+L5	Pfizer Animal Health	Cattle	I.M.	21d	
CattleMaster® 4+VL5	Pfizer Animal Health	Cattle	I.M.	21d	
CattleMaster® BVD-K	Pfizer Animal Health	Cattle	I.M.	21d	
Cattle-Vac™ 9-Somnus	Durvet	Cattle	I.M., S.C.	21d	
Cattle-Vac™ EC	Durvet	Cattle	I.M.	60d	
Cattle Vac™ EC+C	Durvet	Cattle	I.M.	60d	
Cattle-Vac™ E. Coli	Durvet	Calves	Oral	21d	
Cattle-Vac™ E. Coli+C	Durvet	Calves	Oral	21d	
Cattle-Vac™ HS	Durvet	Cattle	I.M., S.C.	21d	
Cattle-Vac™ Pinkeye 4	Durvet	Cattle	I.M.	60d	
Cattle-Vac™ Salmo	Durvet	Cattle	I.M., S.C.	21d	
Cattle-Vac™ Vibrio-Plus	Durvet	Cattle	I.M.	60d	
Caustic Dressing Powder	Phoenix Pharmaceutical	Horses	Topical		
Note: Not for use on horses intended for food.					
Caustic Powder	Butler	Horses	Topical		
Note: Not for use on horses intended for food.					
CAV-Vac®	Intervet	Chickens	ww	21d	
Note: Do not vaccinate birds in egg production.					

Product Name	Company Name	Species	Route of Administration	Meat	Milk
C & D Antitoxin™	Boehringer Ingelheim	Cattle Sheep Swine	I.V., S.C. I.V., S.C. Oral, S.C.	21d 21d 21d	
C & D Toxoid	Aspen	Cattle Sheep Swine	I.M., S.C. I.M., S.C. I.M., S.C.	21d 21d 21d	
Cefa-Dri®	Fort Dodge	Dairy cattle	I.M.M.	42d	
Note: Milk from treated cows must not be used for food during the first 72 hours after calving. Not to be used within 30 days of calving.					
Cefa-Lak®	Fort Dodge	Dairy cattle	I.M.M.	4d	96h
Cephalovac® EWT	Boehringer Ingelheim	Horses	I.M.	21d	
Cephalovac® VEWT	Boehringer Ingelheim	Horses	I.M.	21d	
Cervizine® Injectable	Wildlife	Cervidae Horses	I.M. I.M., I.V.		
Note: Not for use in food-producing animals.					
Chick Ark Bronc™	L.A.H.I. (New Jersey)	Chickens	dw	21d	
Chick Poly Ark™	L.A.H.I. (New Jersey)	Chickens	dw	21d	
Chick Poly Banco™	L.A.H.I. (New Jersey)	Chickens	dw, I.N., I.O	21d	
Chick Poly Florida™	L.A.H.I. (New Jersey)	Chickens	dw, I.N., I.O	21d	
Chick Syno Vac™	L.A.H.I. (New Jersey)	Chickens	S.C.	21d	
Chick Uni Bronc™	L.A.H.I. (New Jersey)	Chickens	aer/sp, dw, I.N., I.O	21d	
Chick Uni Hol™	L.A.H.I. (New Jersey)	Chickens	aer/sp, dw, I.N., I.O	21d	
Chick Vi Banco™	L.A.H.I. (New Jersey)	Chickens	aer/sp, bd, dw, I.N., I.O.	21d	
Chick Vi Banco™ (Drinking Water Use)	L.A.H.I. (New Jersey)	Chickens	dw	21d	
Chick Vi Hanco™	L.A.H.I. (New Jersey)	Chickens	aer/sp, dw, I.N., I.O	21d	
Chick Vi Pox™	L.A.H.I. (New Jersey)	Chickens	ww	21d	
Chlamydia Psittaci Bacterin	Colorado Serum	Sheep	S.C.	60d	
Chlorasan Antiseptic Ointment	Butler	Horses	Topical		
Note: Not for use on horses intended for food.					
ChlorhexiDerm™ Disinfectant	DVM	Horses	Topical		
Note: Not for use on food-producing animals.					
ChlorhexiDerm™ S Disinfectant	DVM	Horses	Topical		
Note: Not for use on food-producing animals.					
Chlorhexidine Ointment 1%	Phoenix Pharmaceutical	Horses	Topical		
Note: Not for use on horses intended for food.					
ChlorMax™ 50	Alpharma	Beef cattle Cattle Chickens Turkeys	In the feed In the feed In the feed In the feed	48h 24h 24h	
Note: A withdrawal period has not been established for this product in pre-ruminating calves. Do not use on calves to be processed for veal. Do not feed to birds producing eggs for human consumption. For beef cattle being fed at 0.5 mg/lb body weight/day or 350 mg/head/day, withdraw 48 hours prior to slaughter. For calves, beef and non-lactating dairy cattle being fed at 10 mg/lb body weight/day, withdraw 24 hours prior to slaughter.					
Choate's® Liniment	Hawthorne	Horses	Topical		
Note: Not for use on horses intended for food.					
Choleramune® CU	Biomune	Chickens	ww	21d	
Choleramune® M	Biomune	Chickens	ww	21d	
Cholervac-IV™	Intervet	Chickens Turkeys	S.C. S.C.	42d 42d	
Cholervac-PM-1®	Intervet	Chickens	ww	21d	
Note: Do not vaccinate 35 days prior to onset of lay or during egg production.					
Chondroprotec®	Neogen	Horses	Topical		
Note: Not for use on food-producing animals.					
Circomune™	Biomune	Chickens	ww	21d	
Circomune™ W	Biomune	Chickens	dw	21d	
Clean Crop® Malathion 57EC	Loveland	Cattle Goats	Topical Topical		
Note: Do not apply to milk goats.					
Clinacox™	Schering-Plough	Chickens	In the feed		
Note: Do not use in laying hens producing eggs for human consumption.					
Clonevac-30®	Intervet	Chickens	aer/sp, dw	21d	
Clonevac-30®-T	Intervet	Turkeys	dw	21d	
Clonevac D-78®	Intervet	Chickens	aer/sp, dw	21d	
Clostratox® BCD	Novartis Animal Vaccines	Cattle Sheep Swine	S.C. S.C. S.C.	21d 21d 21d	
Clostratox® C	Novartis Animal Vaccines	Cattle Sheep Swine	S.C. S.C. Oral, S.C.	21d 21d 21d	

Product Name	Company Name	Species	Route of Administration	Meat	Milk
Clostratox® Ultra C 1300	Novartis Animal Vaccines	Cattle Sheep Swine	S.C. S.C. Oral, S.C.	21d 21d 21d	
Clostri Bos™ BCD	Novartis Animal Vaccines	Cattle	I.M., S.C.	60d	
Clostridial 7-Way	AgriLabs	Cattle	I.M., S.C.	21d	
Clostridial 7-Way plus Somnumune®	AgriLabs	Cattle	S.C.	21d	
Clostridial 8-Way	AgriLabs	Cattle	I.M., S.C.	21d	
Clostridial Antitoxin BCD	Durvet	Cattle Sheep	S.C. S.C.	21d 21d	
Clostridial BCD	Durvet	Cattle Sheep	I.M. I.M.	21d 21d	
Clostridium Chauvoei-Septicum Bacterin	Colorado Serum	Cattle Goats Sheep	S.C. S.C. S.C.	21d 21d 21d	
Clostridium Chauvoei-Septicum-Novyi-Sordellii Bacterin-Toxoid	Colorado Serum	Cattle Goats Sheep	I.M., S.C. I.M., S.C. I.M., S.C.	21d 21d 21d	
Clostridium Chauvoei-Septicum-Pasteurella Haemolytica-Multocida Bacterin	Colorado Serum	Cattle Goats Sheep	S.C. S.C. S.C.	21d 21d 21d	
Clostridium Haemolyticum Bacterin (Red Water)	Colorado Serum	Cattle Goats Sheep	I.M., S.C. I.M., S.C. I.M., S.C.	21d 21d 21d	
Clostridium Perfringens Types C & D Antitoxin, Equine Origin	Colorado Serum	Cattle Goats Sheep Swine	S.C. S.C. S.C. S.C.	21d 21d 21d 21d	
Note: If emergency conditions require vaccination of animals reaching market age and condition, these should not be offered for slaughter in less than 21 days after administration of the vaccine.					
Clostridium Perfringens Types C&D Antitoxin, Equine Origin	Professional Biological	Cattle Goats Sheep Swine	I.V., S.C. I.V., S.C. I.V., S.C. I.V., S.C.	21d 21d 21d 21d	
Clostridium Perfringens Types C & D-Tetanus Toxoid	Colorado Serum	Cattle Goats Sheep Swine	I.M., S.C. I.M., S.C. I.M., S.C. I.M., S.C.	21d 21d 21d 21d	
Clostridium Perfringens Types C&D-Tetanus Toxoid	Professional Biological	Cattle Goats Sheep Swine	I.M., S.C. I.M., S.C. I.M., S.C. I.M., S.C.	21d 21d 21d 21d	
Clostridium Perfringens Types C & D Toxoid	Colorado Serum	Cattle Goats Sheep Swine	I.M., S.C. I.M., S.C. I.M., S.C. I.M., S.C.	21d 21d 21d 21d	
Clostridium Perfringens Types C&D Toxoid	Professional Biological	Cattle Goats Sheep Swine	I.M., S.C. I.M., S.C. I.M., S.C. I.M., S.C.	21d 21d 21d 21d	
Clostri Shield® BCD	Novartis Animal Vaccines	Cattle Sheep	I.M. I.M.	21d 21d	
CMPK Gel	Durvet	Dairy cattle	Oral	0	0
C.M.P.K. Oral Gel	Phoenix Pharmaceutical	Dairy cattle	Oral	0	
Coban® 60	Elanco	Chickens	In the feed		
Note: Do not administer to chickens over 16 weeks (112 days) of age. Do not feed to laying chickens.					
Coccivac®-B	Schering-Plough	Chickens	aer/sp, In the feed	21d	
Coccivac®-D	Schering-Plough	Chickens	aer/sp, In the feed	21d	
Coccivac®-T	Schering-Plough	Turkeys	aer/sp	21d	
Combicillin	Anthony	Beef cattle Horses	S.C. I.M.	30d	
Note: Not for use in horses intended for food.					
Combicillin-AG	Anthony	Beef cattle	S.C.	30d	
Combovac-30®	Intervet	Chickens	aer/sp, dw	21d	
Commando™ Insecticide Cattle Ear Tag	Boehringer Ingelheim	Cattle	Ear tags		
Note: Remove tags before slaughter.					
Component® E-C	VetLife	Beef cattle	Implant		
Note: Implant in the ear only. Do not attempt to salvage the implanted ear for human or animal food.					
Component® E-C with Tylan®	VetLife	Beef cattle	Implant		
Note: Implant in the ear only. Do not attempt to salvage the implanted ear for human or animal food.					
Component® E-H	VetLife	Beef cattle	Implant		
Note: Implant in the ear only. Do not attempt to salvage the implanted ear for human or animal food.					

Please refer to product listings for more complete information.

Product Name	Company Name	Species	Route of Administration	Meat	Milk
Component® E-H with Tylan®	VetLife	Beef cattle	Implant		
Note: Implant in the ear only. Do not attempt to salvage the implanted ear for human or animal food.					
Component® E-S	VetLife	Beef cattle	Implant		
Note: Implant in the ear only. Do not attempt to salvage the implanted ear for human or animal food.					
Component® E-S with Tylan®	VetLife	Beef cattle	Implant		
Note: Implant in the ear only. Do not attempt to salvage the implanted ear for human or animal food.					
Component® TE-G	VetLife	Beef cattle	Implant		
Note: Implant in the ear only. Do not attempt to salvage the implanted ear for human or animal food.					
Component® TE-G with Tylan®	VetLife	Beef cattle	Implant		
Note: Implant in the ear only. Do not attempt to salvage the implanted ear for human or animal food.					
Component® TE-S	VetLife	Beef cattle	Implant		
Note: Implant in the ear only. Do not attempt to salvage the implanted ear for human or animal food.					
Component® TE-S with Tylan®	VetLife	Beef cattle	Implant		
Note: Implant in the ear only. Do not attempt to salvage the implanted ear for human or animal food.					
Component® T-H	VetLife	Beef cattle	Implant		
Note: Implant in the ear only. Do not attempt to salvage the implanted ear for human or animal food.					
Component® T-H with Tylan®	VetLife	Beef cattle	Implant		
Note: Implant in the ear only. Do not attempt to salvage the implanted ear for human or animal food.					
Component® T-S	VetLife	Beef cattle	Implant		
Note: Implant in the ear only. Do not attempt to salvage the implanted ear for human or animal food.					
Component® T-S with Tylan®	VetLife	Beef cattle	Implant		
Note: Implant in the ear only. Do not attempt to salvage the implanted ear for human or animal food.					
Conquest™ -4K	Aspen	Cattle	I.M., S.C.	21d	
Conquest™ -4K+H.S.	Aspen	Cattle	I.M., S.C.	21d	
Conquest™ -4KW	Aspen	Cattle	I.M.	21d	
Conquest™ -4KW+H.S.	Aspen	Cattle	I.M.	21d	
Conquest™ 5K (oil base)	Aspen	Cattle	I.M.	60d	
Conquest™ 5K+HS (oil base)	Aspen	Cattle	I.M.	60d	
Conquest™ 5K+VL5 (oil base)	Aspen	Cattle	I.M.	60d	
Conquest™ -8K	Aspen	Cattle	I.M., S.C.	21d	
Conquest™ -9K	Aspen	Cattle	I.M., S.C.	21d	
Conquest™ -9K+H.S.	Aspen	Cattle	I.M., S.C.	21d	
Conquest™ 10K	Aspen	Cattle	I.M.	60d	
Continuex™	Farnam	Horses	In the feed		
Note: Not for use in horses intended for food.					
Cooper's® Best Ivermectin Paste 1.87%	Aspen	Horses	Oral		
Note: Not for use in horses intended for food.					
Co-Ral® 1%	Durvet	Cattle	Topical	0	0
Co-Ral® (coumaphos) Emulsifiable Livestock Insecticide Restricted Use Pesticide	Bayer	Cattle Horses	Topical Topical	0	0
Note: Do not spray more than 1 1/4 ounces of product per 4 gallons of water when using on non-lactating cattle within 14 days of freshening. At higher rates, and if freshening should occur within this interval after spraying, the milk should not be used for human food. Not for use on horses intended for food.					
Co-Ral® (coumaphos) Flowable Insecticide Restricted Use Pesticide	Bayer	Cattle Horses	Topical Topical	0 0	
Co-Ral® (coumaphos) Fly and Tick Spray	Bayer	Cattle Horses	Topical Topical		
Note: Do not apply as a spray at rates above 1 quart per 50 gallons of water to lactating dairy cattle or non-lactating dairy cattle within 14 days of freshening. If freshening should occur within the interval after spraying, do not use milk for human food for balance of 14 day interval. Not for use on horses intended for food.					
Co-Ral® Plus Insecticide Cattle Ear Tag	Bayer	Cattle	Ear tags	0	0
Note: Remove tags before slaughter.					
Corid® 9.6% Oral Solution	Merial	Calves	Oral	24h	
Note: A withdrawal period has not been established for this product in pre-ruminating calves. Do not use in calves to be processed for veal.					
Corid® 20% Soluble Powder	Merial	Calves	Oral	24h	
Note: A withdrawal period has not been established for this product in pre-ruminating calves. Do not use in calves to be processed for veal.					
CortiCalm™ Lotion	DVM	Horses	Topical		
Note: Not for use on animals intended for food purposes.					
CortiSpray®	DVM	Horses	Topical		
Note: Not for use on animals intended for food purposes.					
Corvac-3®	Intervet	Chickens	S.C.	42d	
CothiVet®	Neogen	Horses	Topical		
Note: Not for use on horses intended for food.					
Cough Syrup	Life Science	Horses	Oral		
Note: Not for use in food-producing animals.					
Covert™ 5	AgriPharm	Cattle	I.M., S.C.	21d	
Covert™ 5-HS	AgriPharm	Cattle	I.M., S.C.	21d	
Covert™ 10	AgriPharm	Cattle	I.M.	21d	

Product Name	Company Name	Species	Route of Administration	Meat	Milk
Covert™ 10-HS	AgriPharm	Cattle	I.M.	21d	
Covexin® 8 Vaccine	Schering-Plough	Sheep	S.C.	21d	
Cow-Vac® 9	Aspen	Cattle	I.M., S.C.	21d	
CTC 50	Durvet	Cattle	In the feed	0-10d	
		Chickens	In the feed	0-1d	
		Sheep	In the feed	0	
		Swine	In the feed	0	
		Turkeys	In the feed	0	
Note: A withdrawal period has not been established for this product in pre-ruminating calves. Do not use in calves to be processed for veal. A withdrawal period is not required when used in chickens at levels up to 400 g/ton. A withdrawal period is not required when used in growing cattle at a level of 70 mg/head/day or less. Do not feed to chickens producing eggs for human consumption. Do not feed to turkeys producing eggs for human consumption. Withdraw from calves, beef cattle and non-lactating dairy cattle 10 days prior to slaughter when used at levels of 10 mg/lb body weight/day. Withdraw from cattle 2 days prior to slaughter when used at levels of 0.5 mg/lb body weight/day. Withdraw from chickens 24 hours prior to slaughter when used at levels of 500 g/ton.					
CTC Soluble Powder	AgriLabs	Chickens	dw	24h	
		Swine	dw	5d	
		Turkeys	dw	24h	
Note: Do not feed to chickens producing eggs for human consumption.					
CTC Soluble Powder Concentrate	Durvet	Calves	dw	24h	
		Chickens	dw	0-1d	
		Swine	dw	24h	
		Turkeys	dw	0-1d	
Note: Do not administer to poultry at 1,000 mg/gallon of water (1 packet per 25.6 gallons) within 24 hours before slaughter. Do not use in laying chickens.					
Curatrem®	Merial	Cattle	Oral	8d	
Note: A milk discard period has not been established for this product in lactating dairy cattle. Do not use in female dairy cattle 20 months of age or older.					
Cydectin® Pour-On	Fort Dodge	Cattle	Topical		
Note: A withdrawal period has not been established for this product in pre-ruminating calves. Do not use in calves to be processed for veal.					
CyLence® Ultra Insecticide Cattle Ear Tag	Bayer	Cattle	Ear tags		
Note: Remove tags before slaughter.					
Dariclox®	Pfizer Animal Health	Dairy cattle	I.M.M.	10d	48h
Dealer Select Horse Care Horse & Colt Wormer	Durvet	Horses	In the feed		
Note: Not for use in horses intended for food.					
Deccox®	Alpharma	Broilers	In the feed		
		Cattle	In the feed		
		Goats	In the feed		
		Sheep	In the feed		
Note: Do not administer to laying chickens. Do not feed to cows producing milk for food. Do not feed to goats producing milk for food. Do not feed to sheep producing milk for food.					
Deccox®-L	Alpharma	Cattle	In the feed		
Note: Do not feed to cows producing milk for food.					
Dectomax® Injectable Solution	Pfizer Animal Health	Cattle	I.M., S.C.	35d	
		Swine	I.M.	24d	
Note: A withdrawal period has not been established for this product in pre-ruminating calves. Do not use in calves to be processed for veal. Not for use in female dairy cattle 20 months of age or older.					
Dectomax® Pour-On	Pfizer Animal Health	Cattle	Topical	45d	
Note: A withdrawal period has not been established for this product in pre-ruminating calves. Do not use in calves to be processed for veal. Not for use in female dairy cattle 20 months of age or older.					
Defensor® 3	Pfizer Animal Health	Cattle	I.M.	21d	
		Sheep	I.M.	21d	
Del-Phos® Emulsifiable Liquid Insecticide	Schering-Plough	Cattle	Topical	3d	
		Swine	Topical	1d	
Note: Do not treat non-lactating dairy cattle within 28 days of freshening. If freshening should occur within 28 days after treatment, do not use milk as human food for the remainder of the 28-day interval.					
Denagard™ 10	Boehringer Ingelheim	Swine	In the feed	0-7d	
Note: The withdrawal period at the 200 g/ton use level is 7 days. The withdrawal period at the 35 g/ton use level is 2 days.					
Denagard™ Liquid Concentrate	Boehringer Ingelheim	Swine	dw	3-7d	
Note: Withdraw medicated water 3 days before slaughter after treatment at 3.5 mg per lb body weight. Withdraw medicated water 7 days before slaughter after treatment at 10.5 mg per lb body weight.					
Dermacide™	Butler	Horses	Topical		
Note: Not for use on horses intended for food.					
Dexaject	Vetus	Cattle	I.M., I.V.		
		Horses	I.M., I.V.		
Note: A withdrawal period has not been established for this product in pre-ruminating calves. Do not use in calves to be processed for veal. Not for use in horses intended for food.					
Dexamethasone 2.0 mg Injection	Vedco	Horses	I.V.		
Note: Not for use in horses intended for food.					
Dexamethasone 2 mg/mL Injection	RXV	Horses	I.V.		
Note: Not for use in horses intended for food.					

Product Name	Company Name	Species	Route of Administration	Meat	Milk
Dexamethasone Injection	AgriLabs	Horses	I.V.		
Note: Not for use in horses intended for food.					
Dexamethasone Injection	Vet Tek	Horses	I.M., I.V.		
Note: Not for use in horses intended for food.					
Dexamethasone Sodium Phosphate	Phoenix Pharmaceutical	Horses	I.V.		
Note: Not for use in horses intended for food.					
Dexamethasone Sodium Phosphate Injection	Butler	Horses	I.V.		
Note: Not for use in horses intended for food.					
Dexamethasone Sodium Phosphate Injection	Vedco	Horses	I.V.		
Note: Not for use in horses intended for food.					
Dexamethasone Solution	Butler	Cattle	I.M., I.V.		
Note: A withdrawal period has not been established for this product in pre-ruminating calves. Do not use in calves to be processed for veal.					
Dexamethasone Solution	Phoenix Pharmaceutical	Cattle	I.M., I.V.		
Note: A withdrawal period has not been established for this product in pre-ruminating calves. Do not use in calves to be processed for veal.					
Dexamethasone Solution	Aspen	Cattle	I.M., I.V.		
Note: A withdrawal period has not been established for this product in pre-ruminating calves. Do not use in calves to be processed for veal.					
Dexasone	RXV	Horses	I.V.		
Note: Not for use in horses intended for food.					
Dexazone™ 2 mg	Bimeda	Horses	I.V.		
Note: Not for use in horses intended for food.					
Diamine Iodide-20 (With Salt)	First Priority	Cattle	In the feed		
Note: Not to be fed to dairy cattle in production.					
Diamine Iodide-40 (With Salt)	First Priority	Cattle	In the feed		
Note: Not to be fed to dairy cattle in production.					
Di-Methox® 12.5% Oral Solution	AgriLabs	Cattle Chickens Turkeys	dw dw dw	7d 5d 5d	
Note: A withdrawal period has not been established for this product in pre-ruminating calves. Do not use in calves to be processed for veal. Do not administer to chickens over 16 weeks (112 days) of age. Do not administer to turkeys over 24 weeks (168 days) of age.					
Di-Methox® Injection-40%	AgriLabs	Cattle	I.V.	5d	60h
Note: A withdrawal period has not been established for this product in pre-ruminating calves. Do not use in calves to be processed for veal.					
Di-Methox® Soluble Powder	AgriLabs	Cattle Chickens Turkeys	dw dw dw	7d 5d 5d	
Note: A withdrawal period has not been established for this product in pre-ruminating calves. Do not use in calves to be processed for veal. Do not administer to chickens over 16 weeks (112 days) of age. Do not administer to turkeys over 24 weeks (168 days) of age.					
Disal® Injection	Boehringer Ingelheim	Horses	I.M., I.V.		
Note: Not for use in horses intended for food.					
Docusate Solution	Life Science	Horses	Oral		
Note: Not for use in horses intended for food.					
Dolorex®	Intervet	Horses	I.V.		
Note: Not for use in horses intended for food.					
Dominator® Insecticide Ear Tags	Schering-Plough	Cattle	Ear tags		
Note: Remove tags before slaughter.					
Domoso® Gel	Fort Dodge	Horses	Topical		
Note: Not for use on horses intended for food.					
Dormosedan®	Pfizer Animal Health	Horses	I.M., I.V.		
Note: Not for use in horses intended for food.					
Double Barrel™ VP Insecticide Ear Tags	Schering-Plough	Cattle	Ear tags		
Note: Remove tags before slaughter.					
Double Impact™	AgriLabs	Cattle Reindeer Swine	S.C. S.C. S.C.	35d 56d 18d	
Note: A milk discard period has not been established for this product in lactating dairy cattle. Do not use in female dairy cattle 20 months of age or older.					
Dr. Naylor® Blu-Kote®	H.W. Naylor	Horses	Topical		
Note: Not for use on horses intended for food.					
Dr. Naylor® Red-Kote®	H.W. Naylor	Horses	Topical		
Note: Not for use on horses intended for food.					
Dry-Clox®	Fort Dodge	Dairy cattle	I.M.M.	30d	
Note: Not to be used within 30 days of calving.					
Dublvax®	Schering-Plough	Chickens	aer/sp, dw	21d	
Duo-Pen®	AgriPharm	Beef cattle	S.C.	30d	
Duramycin 72-200	Durvet	Cattle Swine	I.M., I.V., S.C. I.M.	28d 28d	
Note: Not for use in lactating dairy animals.					
Duramycin-100	Durvet	Cattle	I.V.	22d	
Note: A withdrawal period has not been established for this product in pre-ruminating calves. Do not use in calves to be processed for veal. Not for use in lactating dairy animals.					

Product Name	Company Name	Species	Route of Administration	Meat	Milk
Duramycin-324	Durvet	Cattle Chickens Swine Turkeys	dw dw dw dw	5d 4d 4d 4d	
Note: A withdrawal period has not been established for this product in pre-ruminating calves. Do not use in calves to be processed for veal. Do not administer to poultry producing eggs for human consumption.					
Duramycin 10	Durvet	Calves Chickens Swine Turkeys	dw dw dw dw	5d 4d 4d 4d	
Note: A withdrawal period has not been established for this product in pre-ruminating calves. Do not use in calves to be processed for veal. Do not administer to chickens or turkeys producing eggs for human consumption.					
Dura-Pen	Durvet	Beef cattle	S.C.	30d	
Durapen™	Vedco	Beef cattle	S.C.	30d	
Durasect® II Long-Acting Livestock Pour-On	Pfizer Animal Health	Cattle	Topical	0	0
DurGuard™ 4	Durvet	Cattle	I.M., S.C.	60d	
DurGuard™ 5	Durvet	Cattle	I.M., S.C.	60d	
DurGuard™ 5HS	Durvet	Cattle	I.M.	60d	
DurGuard™ 5HS+VL5	Durvet	Cattle	I.M.	60d	
DurGuard™ 5+VL5	Durvet	Cattle	I.M.	60d	
DurGuard™ 10	Durvet	Cattle	I.M.	60d	
DurGuard™ 10HS	Durvet	Cattle	I.M.	60d	
DurVac™ Appear-HP	Durvet	Swine	I.M.	21d	
DurVac™ AR	Durvet	Swine	I.M.	21d	
DurVac™ AR-4	Durvet	Swine	I.M., S.C.	21d	
DurVac™ E-AR	Durvet	Piglets Swine	I.N. I.M.	21d 21d	
DurVac™ EC	Durvet	Swine	I.M.	21d	
DurVac™ EC-C	Durvet	Swine	I.M.	21d	
DurVac™ E. Coli 3	Durvet	Swine	Oral	21d	
DurVac™ E. Coli 3C	Durvet	Swine	Oral	21d	
DurVac™ Ery	Durvet	Swine	I.M.	21d	
DurVac™ Myco	Durvet	Swine	I.M.	21d	
DurVac™ P-E-L	Durvet	Swine	I.M.	21d	
DurVac™ Strep	Durvet	Swine	I.M.	21d	
DVMectin™ Liquid for Horses	DVM	Horses	Oral		
Note: Not for use in horses intended for food.					
EAZI-Breed™ CIDR® Cattle Insert	Pharmacia & Upjohn	Cattle	I.Vag.		
Note: Not for use in lactating dairy cows.					
E-Bac™	Intervet	Swine	I.M., S.C.	21d	
E-Coli + C Antibody	AgriPharm	Calves	Oral	21d	
E. Colicin-B™	AgriLabs	Calves	I.N., Oral	21d	
E. Colicin-S$_3$™	AgriLabs	Swine	Oral	21d	
E. Colicin-S$_3$+C™	AgriLabs	Swine	Oral	21d	
Ectiban® D	Durvet	Swine	Topical	5d	
Ectiban® EC	Durvet	Horses Swine	Topical Topical	 5d	
Note: Not for use on horses intended for food.					
Ectrin® Insecticide Cattle Ear Tag	Boehringer Ingelheim	Cattle	Ear tags		
Note: Remove tags before slaughter.					
Electroid® 7 Vaccine	Schering-Plough	Cattle Sheep	I.M., S.C. I.M., S.C.	21d 21d	
Electroid® D	Schering-Plough	Cattle Sheep	I.M., S.C. I.M., S.C.	21d 21d	
Elite 4™	Boehringer Ingelheim	Cattle	I.M.	21d	
Elite 4-HS™	Boehringer Ingelheim	Cattle	I.M.	21d	
Elite 9™	Boehringer Ingelheim	Cattle	I.M.	21d	
Elite 9-HS™	Boehringer Ingelheim	Cattle	I.M.	21d	
Emulsibac® APP	MVP	Swine	I.M., S.C.	60d	
Emulsibac® SS	MVP	Swine	I.M.	60d	
Encephaloid® IM	Fort Dodge	Horses	I.M.	60d	
Encephalomyelitis Vaccine Eastern & Western	Colorado Serum	Horses	I.M.	21d	
Encephalomyelitis Vaccine Eastern & Western with Tetanus Toxoid	Colorado Serum	Horses	I.M.	21d	
Encevac® with Havlogen®	Intervet	Horses	I.M.	21d	
Encevac®-T with Havlogen®	Intervet	Horses	I.M.	21d	

Please refer to product listings for more complete information.

Product Name	Company Name	Species	Route of Administration	Meat	Milk
Encevac® T + VEE with Havlogen®	Intervet	Horses	I.M.	21d	
Encevac® TC-4 with Havlogen®	Intervet	Horses	I.M.	21d	
Encevac® TC-4 + VEE with Havlogen®	Intervet	Horses	I.M.	21d	
End-FLUence® with Imugen® II	Intervet	Swine	I.M.	21d	
End-FLUence® 2	Intervet	Swine	I.M.	21d	
ENDOSERUM®	Immvac	Horses	I.V.	21d	
ENDOVAC-Bovi® with ImmunePlus®	Immvac	Cattle	I.M.	60d	
ENDOVAC-Equi® with ImmunePlus®	Immvac	Horses	I.M.	21d	
ENDOVAC-Porci® with ImmunePlus®	Immvac	Swine	I.M.	60d	
Endura-Lite™ **Note:** Not for use in horses intended for food.	Creative Science	Horses	dw, In the feed, Oral		
Endure™ Sweat-Resistant Fly Spray **Note:** Not for use on horses intended for food.	Farnam	Horses	Topical		
Enterisol® Ileitis	Boehringer Ingelheim	Swine	dw	21d	
Enterisol® SC-54	Boehringer Ingelheim	Swine	dw, I.N.	21d	
Enterisol® SC-54 FF	Boehringer Ingelheim	Swine	dw	21d	
Enterovax™ **Note:** Do not administer to breeders in production.	Schering-Plough	Chickens	dw	21d	
EnterVene™ -d	Fort Dodge	Calves	S.C.	21d	
Equi Aid CW® **Note:** Not for use in horses intended for food.	Equi Aid	Horses	In the feed		
Equicine® II with Havlogen®	Intervet	Horses	I.M.	21d	
Equi-Flu® EWT	Boehringer Ingelheim	Horses	I.M.	21d	
Equi-Flu® VEWT	Boehringer Ingelheim	Horses	I.M.	21d	
Equileve **Note:** Not for use in horses intended for food.	Vetus	Horses	I.M., I.V.		
Equiloid® Innovator	Fort Dodge	Horses	I.M.	21d	
Equimectrin™ Paste 1.87% **Note:** Not for use in horses intended for food.	Farnam	Horses	Oral		
Equimectrin® Paste 1.87% **Note:** Not for use in horses intended for food.	Merial	Horses	Oral		
Equine Coli Endotox® **Note:** Not for use in horses intended for food.	Novartis Animal Vaccines	Horses	Oral		
Equine EWTF	Merial	Horses	I.M.	21d	
Equine Potomavac®	Merial	Horses	I.M.	21d	
Equine Potomavac® + Imrab®	Merial	Horses	I.M.	21d	
Equine Rotavirus Vaccine	Fort Dodge	Horses	I.M.	21d	
Equi-Phar™ BenzaGel **Note:** Not for use on horses intended for food.	Vedco	Horses	Topical		
Equi-Phar™ Caustic Powder **Note:** Not for use on horses intended for food.	Vedco	Horses	Topical		
Equi-Phar™ CoolGel **Note:** Not for use on horses intended for food.	Vedco	Horses	Topical		
Equi-Phar™ Equigesic™ **Note:** Not for use in horses intended for food.	Vedco	Horses	I.M., I.V.		
Equi-Phar EquiGlide™ **Note:** Not for use in horses intended for food.	Vedco	Horses	I.U.		
Equi-Phar Equi-Hist 1200 Granules **Note:** Not for use in horses intended for food.	Vedco	Horses	In the feed		
Equi-Phar™ Furosemide Injection 5% **Note:** Not for use in horses intended for food.	Vedco	Horses	I.M., I.V.		
Equi-Phar™ Horse & Colt Wormer **Note:** Not for use in horses intended for food.	Vedco	Horses	In the feed		
Equi-Phar™ Nitrofurazone Soluble Dressing **Note:** Not for use on horses intended for food.	Vedco	Horses	Topical		
Equi-Phar™ Phenylbutazone 1 gram Tablets **Note:** Not for use in horses intended for food.	Vedco	Horses	Oral		
Equi-Phar™ Phenylbutazone Injection 20% **Note:** Not for use in horses intended for food.	Vedco	Horses	I.V.		
Equi-Phar ProTal™ **Note:** Do not use in horses or ponies intended for food.	Vedco	Horses	In the feed, Oral		
Equi-Phar™ Sweet Psyllium **Note:** Not for use in horses intended for food.	Vedco	Horses	In the feed		
Equiphen® Paste **Note:** Not for use in horses intended for food.	Luitpold	Horses	Oral		
Equipoise® **Note:** Not for use in horses intended for food.	Fort Dodge	Horses	I.M.		

Product Name	Company Name	Species	Route of Administration	Meat	Milk
Equi-Prin™	First Priority	Horses	Oral		
Note: Not for use in animals intended for food purposes.					
Equisimilis Shield™	Novartis Animal Vaccines	Swine	I.M.	21d	
Equi-Spot™ Spot-On Fly Control for Horses	Farnam	Horses	Topical		
Note: Not for use on horses intended for food.					
Equitrol® Feed-Thru Fly Control	Farnam	Horses	In the feed		
Note: Not for use in horses intended for food.					
EquiVac™ EHV-1/4	Fort Dodge	Horses	I.M.	21d	
Eqvalan® Liquid	Merial	Horses	Oral		
Note: Not for use in horses intended for food.					
Eqvalan® Paste 1.87%	Merial	Horses	Oral		
Note: Not for use in horses intended for food.					
ER Bac®	Pfizer Animal Health	Swine	I.M.	21d	
ER Bac®/Leptoferm-5®	Pfizer Animal Health	Swine	I.M.	21d	
ER Bac® Plus	Pfizer Animal Health	Swine	I.M.	21d	
ER Bac® Plus/Leptoferm-5®	Pfizer Animal Health	Swine	I.M.	21d	
Ermogen	Novartis (Aqua Health)	Salmonids	aer/sp, Imsn.	21d	
Erycell™	Novartis Animal Vaccines	Swine	I.M., I.N.	21d	
Ery Serum™	Novartis Animal Vaccines	Swine	S.C.	21d	
Ery Shield™	Novartis Animal Vaccines	Swine	I.M., S.C.	21d	
Ery Shield™ +L5	Novartis Animal Vaccines	Swine	I.M.	21d	
Erysipelas Bacterin	AgriLabs	Swine	S.C.	21d	
Erysipelothrix Rhusiopathiae Serum Antibodies	Colorado Serum	Swine	S.C.	21d	
Erysipelothrix Rhusiopathiae Serum Antibodies	Professional Biological	Swine	S.C.	21d	
Ery Vac 100	Arko	Swine	Oral	21d	
Ery Vac 500	Arko	Swine	Oral	21d	
Escogen	Novartis (Aqua Health)	Catfish	In the feed	21d	
E-SE®	Schering-Plough	Horses	I.M., I.V.		
Note: Not for use in horses intended for food.					
EWT™	Schering-Plough	Horses	I.M.	21d	
EWTF™	Schering-Plough	Horses	I.M.	21d	
Exalt™ 4	AgriPharm	Cattle	I.M., S.C.	60d	
Exalt™ 4 + L5	AgriPharm	Cattle	I.M.	60d	
Exalt™ 5	AgriPharm	Cattle	I.M., S.C.	60d	
Exalt™ 5 + L5	AgriPharm	Cattle	I.M.	60d	
Exalt™ 5 + Somnus	AgriPharm	Cattle	I.M.	60d	
Exalt™ 5 + VL5	AgriPharm	Cattle	I.M.	60d	
Excenel® RTU	Pharmacia & Upjohn	Cattle Swine	I.M., S.C. I.M.	2d 0	0
Note: A withdrawal period has not been established for this product in pre-ruminating calves. Do not use in calves to be processed for veal.					
Exodus™ Paste	Bimeda	Horses	Oral		
Note: Not for use in horses intended for food.					
Expectade™ Cough Syrup	PRN Pharmacal	Horses	Oral		
Note: Not for use in horses intended for food.					
Expectorant Powder	First Priority	Cattle Horses	Oral Oral		
Note: Not for use in animals intended for food purposes.					
Express™ 3	Boehringer Ingelheim	Cattle	S.C.	21d	
Express™ 3/Lp	Boehringer Ingelheim	Cattle	I.M.	21d	
Express 4®	Boehringer Ingelheim	Cattle	I.M.	21d	
Express™ 5	Boehringer Ingelheim	Cattle	S.C.	21d	
Express™ 5-HS	Boehringer Ingelheim	Cattle	S.C.	21d	
Express™ 5-PHM	Boehringer Ingelheim	Cattle	S.C.	60d	
Express 10™	Boehringer Ingelheim	Cattle	I.M.	21d	
Express™ 10-HS	Boehringer Ingelheim	Cattle	I.M.	21d	
Express™ I	Boehringer Ingelheim	Cattle	S.C.	21d	
Express™ IBP	Boehringer Ingelheim	Cattle	S.C.	21d	
Express™ IBP/HS-2P	Boehringer Ingelheim	Cattle	I.M.	21d	
Express™ I/Lp	Boehringer Ingelheim	Cattle	I.M.	21d	
Express™ IP/HS-2P	Boehringer Ingelheim	Cattle	I.M.	21d	
Factrel®	Fort Dodge	Cattle	I.M.	0	0
FarrowSure®	Pfizer Animal Health	Swine	I.M.	21d	
FarrowSure® B	Pfizer Animal Health	Swine	I.M.	21d	
FarrowSure® B-PRV	Pfizer Animal Health	Swine	I.M.	21d	

Please refer to product listings for more complete information.

Product Name	Company Name	Species	Route of Administration	Meat	Milk
FarrowSure® Plus	Pfizer Animal Health	Swine	I.M.	21d	
FarrowSure® Plus B	Pfizer Animal Health	Swine	I.M.	21d	
FarrowSure® PRV	Pfizer Animal Health	Swine	I.M.	21d	
FC4 Gold	L.A.H.I. (Maine Biological)	Chickens Turkeys	I.M., S.C. I.M., S.C.	42d 42d	
Finaplix®-H	Intervet	Beef cattle	Implant		
Note: Implant in the ear only. Do not attempt to salvage the implanted ear for human or animal food.					
Finquel®	Argent	Fish	Imsn.	21d	
FluMeglumine®	Phoenix Pharmaceutical	Cattle Horses	I.V. I.M., I.V.		
Note: A withdrawal period has not been established for this product in pre-ruminating calves. Do not use in calves to be processed for veal. Not for use in horses intended for food. Not for use in lactating or dry dairy cows.					
Flumune®	Pfizer Animal Health	Horses	I.M.	21d	
Flu-Nix™	AgriLabs	Cattle Horses	I.V. I.M., I.V.	4d	
Note: A withdrawal period has not been established for this product in pre-ruminating calves. Do not use in calves to be processed for veal. Not for use in horses intended for food. Not for use in lactating or dry dairy cows.					
Flunixamine™	Fort Dodge	Cattle Horses	I.V. I.M., I.V.	4d	
Note: A withdrawal period has not been established for this product in pre-ruminating calves. Do not use in calves to be processed for veal. Not for use in horses intended for food. Not for use in lactating or dry dairy cows.					
Flunixin Meglumine	Vet Tek	Cattle Horses	I.V. I.M., I.V.	4d	
Note: A withdrawal period has not been established for this product in pre-ruminating calves. Do not use in calves to be processed for veal. Not for use in horses intended for food. Not for use in lactating or dry dairy cows.					
Flunixin Meglumine Injection	Butler	Horses	I.M., I.V.		
Note: Not for use in horses intended for food.					
FluSure™	Pfizer Animal Health	Swine	I.M.	21d	
FluSure™ /ER Bac Plus®	Pfizer Animal Health	Swine	I.M.	21d	
FluSure™ /RespiSure®	Pfizer Animal Health	Swine	I.M.	21d	
FluSure™ /RespiSure 1 ONE®	Pfizer Animal Health	Swine	I.M.	21d	
FluSure™ /RespiSure 1 ONE®/ER Bac Plus®	Pfizer Animal Health	Swine	I.M.	21d	
FluSure™ /RespiSure® RTU	Pfizer Animal Health	Swine	I.M.	21d	
FluSure™ RTU	Pfizer Animal Health	Swine	I.M.	21d	
Fluvac® Innovator	Fort Dodge	Horses	I.M.	21d	
Fluvac® Innovator Double-E FT®	Fort Dodge	Horses	I.M.	21d	
Fluvac® Innovator Double-E FT®+EHV	Fort Dodge	Horses	I.M.	21d	
Fluvac® Innovator EHV-4/1	Fort Dodge	Horses	I.M.	21d	
Fluvac® Innovator Triple-E® FT	Fort Dodge	Horses	I.M.	21d	
Fluvac® Innovator Triple-E® FT+EHV	Fort Dodge	Horses	I.M.	21d	
FlyPel® Insecticide Spray for Horses	Virbac	Horses	Topical		
Note: Not for use on horses intended for food.					
Flysect® Roll-On Fly Repellent Face Lotion	Equicare	Horses	Topical		
Note: Not for use on horses intended for food.					
Flysect® Super-C	Equicare	Horses	Topical		
Note: Not for use on horses intended for food.					
Flysect® Water-Based Repellent Spray	Equicare	Horses	Topical		
Note: Not for use on horses intended for food.					
Flys-Off® Fly Repellent Ointment	Farnam	Horses	Topical		
Note: Not for use on horses intended for food.					
Footvax® 10 Strain	Schering-Plough	Sheep	S.C.	60d	
Forte V1	Novartis (Aqua Health)	Salmonids	I.P.	60d	
Fortress® 7	Pfizer Animal Health	Cattle	S.C.	21d	
Fortress® 8	Pfizer Animal Health	Cattle	S.C.	21d	
Fortress® CD	Pfizer Animal Health	Cattle	S.C.	21d	
Fowl Laryngotracheitis Vaccine	L.A.H.I. (New Jersey)	Chickens	aer/sp, I.N., I.O	21d	
Fowl Pox Vaccine	L.A.H.I. (New Jersey)	Chickens	ww	21d	
Fowl Pox Vaccine	Schering-Plough	Chickens Turkeys	ww ts	21d 21d	
Fowl Pox Vaccine	Merial Select	Chickens	S.C.	21d	
FP Blen®	Merial Select	Chickens	ww	21d	

Please refer to product listings for more complete information.

Withdrawal Time Charts

Withdrawal times listed correspond to label dosages only.

Product Name	Company Name	Species	Route of Administration	Meat	Milk
FP-Vac®	Intervet	Chickens Turkeys	ww ww	21d 21d	
Note: Do not vaccinate birds in egg production. Do not vaccinate within 4 weeks of initial egg production.					
Freezex® Freeze	Hawthorne	Horses	Topical		
Note: Not for use on horses intended for food.					
Freezex® Hoof Freeze	Hawthorne	Horses	Topical		
Note: Not for use on horses intended for food.					
Fryvacc 1	Novartis (Aqua Health)	Salmonids	Imsn.	21d	
Fulvicin-U/F® Powder	Schering-Plough	Horses	In the feed, Oral		
Note: Not for use in horses intended for food.					
Fungisan™	Tomlyn	Horses	Topical		
Note: Not for use on animals intended for food purposes.					
Furall™ (Furazolidone)	Farnam	Horses	Topical		
Note: Not for use on horses intended for food.					
Fura-Ointment®	Farnam	Horses	Topical		
Note: Not for use on horses intended for food.					
Fura-Septin	Anthony	Horses	Topical		
Note: Not for use on horses intended for food.					
Furazolidone Aerosol Powder	V.P.L.	Horses	Topical		
Note: Not for use on horses intended for food.					
Fura-Zone	Neogen	Horses	Topical		
Note: Not for use on horses intended for food.					
Furogen™	Novartis (Aqua Health)	Salmonids	I.P.	21d	
Furogen 2	Novartis (Aqua Health)	Salmonids	I.P.	60d	
Furogen Dip	Novartis (Aqua Health)	Salmonids	Imsn.	21d	
Furoject	Vetus	Horses	I.M., I.V.		
Note: Not for use in horses intended for food.					
Furosemide Injectable 5%	AgriLabs	Cattle Horses	I.M., I.V. I.M., I.V.	48h	48h
Note: Not for use in horses intended for food.					
Furosemide Injection	AgriLabs	Horses	I.M., I.V.		
Note: Not for use in horses intended for food.					
Furosemide Injection 5%	Butler	Horses	I.M., I.V.		
Note: Not for use in horses intended for food.					
Furosemide Injection 5%	Phoenix Pharmaceutical	Cattle Horses	I.M., I.V. I.M., I.V.	48h	48h
Note: Not for use in horses intended for food.					
Fusion® 4	Merial	Cattle	I.M.	21d	
Fusogard™	Novartis Animal Vaccines	Cattle	S.C.	60d	
F Vax-MG®	Schering-Plough	Chickens	aer/sp	21d	
Note: Do not vaccinate birds within 21 days of onset of egg production.					
Gallimune™ NC-BR	Merial Select	Chickens	S.C.	42d	
Gallimune™ Reoguard™	Merial Select	Chickens	S.C.	42d	
Gallimycin®-36	AgriLabs	Dairy cattle	I.M.M.	14d	36h
Gallimycin®-36	Bimeda	Dairy cattle	I.M.M.	14d	36h
Gallimycin®-100 Injection	Bimeda	Cattle Sheep Swine	I.M. I.M. I.M.	14d 3d 7d	72h
Gallimycin®-100P	Bimeda	Chickens Turkeys	In the feed In the feed	1-2d	
Note: Do not use in birds producing eggs for food purposes at the 185 g level. Withdraw from chickens 24 hours prior to slaughter when used at levels of 92.5 g/ton. Withdraw from chickens 48 hours prior to slaughter when used at levels of 185 g/ton.					
Gallimycin®-200 Injection	Bimeda	Cattle	I.M.	6d	
Note: Cattle: If excessive trimming of the injection site is undesirable, do not slaughter animals within 21 days. Not for use in female dairy cattle 20 months of age or older.					
Gallimycin®-Dry Cow	AgriLabs	Dairy cattle	I.M.M.	14d	36h
Note: Calves born to treated cows must not be slaughtered for food at less than 10 days of age. Not for use in lactating dairy cows.					
Gallimycin®-Dry Cow	Bimeda	Dairy cattle	I.M.M.	14d	36h
Note: Animals infused with this product must not be slaughtered for use in food within 96 hours after calving. Calves born to treated cows must not be slaughtered for food at less than 10 days of age.					
Gallimycin® PFC	Bimeda	Chickens Turkeys	dw dw	1d 1d	
Note: Do not administer to chickens or turkeys producing eggs for human consumption.					
Garacin® Piglet Injection	Schering-Plough	Swine	I.M.	40d	
Garacin® Pig Pump	Schering-Plough	Swine	Oral	14d	
Garacin® Soluble Powder	Schering-Plough	Swine	dw	10d	

Please refer to product listings for more complete information.

Product Name	Company Name	Species	Route of Administration	Meat	Milk
Garasol® Injection (100 mg/mL)	Schering-Plough	Chickens Turkeys	S.C. S.C.	35d 63d	
Garavax®-T	Schering-Plough	Turkeys	aer/sp, dw	21d	
GastroGard® ***Note:*** Not for use in horses intended for food.	Merial	Horses	Oral		
Gauge™ C&D	AgriPharm	Cattle Sheep	S.C. S.C.	21d 21d	
Gen-Gard™ Soluble Powder	AgriLabs	Swine	dw	10d	
Gentadip ***Note:*** Not for use in eggs intended for human consumption.	Med-Pharmex	Turkeys	Egg Dip		
Genta-fuse ***Note:*** Not for use in horses intended for food.	Vetus	Horses	I.U.		
GentaMax™ 100 ***Note:*** Not for use in horses intended for food.	Phoenix Pharmaceutical	Horses	I.U.		
Gentamicin Sulfate Solution ***Note:*** Not for use in horses intended for food.	Butler	Horses	I.U.		
Gentamicin Sulfate Solution ***Note:*** Not for use in horses intended for food.	RXV	Horses	I.U.		
Gentamicin Sulfate Solution ***Note:*** Not for use in horses intended for food.	Vet Tek	Horses	I.U.		
Gentamicin Sulfate Solution ***Note:*** Not for use in horses intended for food.	Aspen	Horses	I.U.		
GentaVed™ 100 ***Note:*** Not for use in horses intended for food.	Vedco	Horses	I.U.		
Gentocin® Solution (Equine) ***Note:*** Not for use in horses intended for food.	Schering-Plough	Horses	I.U.		
Go-Dry™ ***Note:*** Discard all milk for 72 hours following calving.	G.C. Hanford	Dairy cattle	I.M.M.	14d	
Grand Champion® Fly Repellent Formula ***Note:*** Not for use on horses intended for food.	Farnam	Horses	Topical		
Guaifenesin Injection ***Note:*** Not for use in horses intended for food.	Butler	Horses	I.V.		
Guaifenesin Injection ***Note:*** Not for use on horses intended for food.	Phoenix Pharmaceutical	Horses	I.V.		
Guailaxin® ***Note:*** Not for use in horses intended for food.	Fort Dodge	Horses	I.V.		
Haemophilus Paragallinarum Bacterin	L.A.H.I. (New Jersey)	Poultry	I.M.	42d	
Haemo Shield® P	Novartis Animal Vaccines	Swine	I.M., S.C.	21d	
Halothane, USP ***Note:*** Not for use on animals intended for food purposes.	Halocarbon	Horses	Inhl.		
Happy Jack® Onex ***Note:*** Not for use on horses intended for food.	Happy Jack	Horses	Topical		
Harold White's® Leg Paint ***Note:*** Not for use on horses intended for food.	Hawthorne	Horses	Topical		
Hatchgard-3™	Intervet	Chickens	aer/sp	21d	
HemaBlock™ ***Note:*** Not for use on animals intended for food purposes.	Abbott	Horses	Topical		
Herd-Vac™ 3	Biocor	Cattle	I.M., S.C.	21d	
Herd-Vac™ 3 S	Biocor	Cattle	I.M., S.C.	21d	
Herd-Vac™ 8	Biocor	Cattle	I.M., S.C.	21d	
Herd-Vac™ 9	Biocor	Cattle	I.M., S.C.	21d	
Hetacin-K® Intramammary Infusion	Fort Dodge	Dairy cattle	I.M.M.	10d	72h
H.E. Vac	Arko	Turkeys	dw	21d	
Histostat® 50	Alpharma	Chickens Turkeys	In the feed In the feed	5d 5d	
Horse Care Ivermectin Paste 1.87% ***Note:*** Not for use in horses intended for food.	Durvet	Horses	Oral		
Horse Lice Duster™ III	Farnam	Swine	Topical	5d	
H. Somnus Bacterin	Aspen	Cattle	I.M., S.C.	21d	
HVT	Intervet	Chickens	S.C.	21d	
HVT + SB-1	Intervet	Chickens	In ovo, S.C.	21d	
Hyalovet® ***Note:*** Not for use in horses intended for food.	Fort Dodge	Horses	I.A.		
HyCoat® ***Note:*** Not for use on horses intended for food.	Neogen	Horses	Topical		
Hygromix® 8 (Chickens)	Elanco	Chickens	In the feed	3d	
Hygromix® 8 (Swine)	Elanco	Swine	In the feed	15d	

Product Name	Company Name	Species	Route of Administration	Meat	Milk
Hylartin® V ***Note:*** Not for use in horses intended for food.	Pharmacia & Upjohn	Horses	I.A.		
Hyvisc® ***Note:*** Not for use in horses intended for food.	Boehringer Ingelheim	Horses	I.A.		
IBD Blen®	Merial Select	Chickens	dw	21d	
IBL Vaccine	Aspen	Cattle	I.M.	21d	
IBP-L5 Vaccine	Aspen	Cattle	I.M., S.C.	21d	
IBP-SomnuMune® Vaccine	Aspen	Cattle	I.M., S.C.	21d	
IBP Vaccine	Aspen	Cattle	I.M., S.C.	21d	
IB-Vac-H®	Intervet	Chickens	aer/sp, dw	21d	
Ice-O-Gel® ***Note:*** Not for use on horses intended for food.	Hawthorne	Horses	Topical		
IL Vaccine	Aspen	Cattle	I.M.	21d	
Immunoboost®	Bioniche Animal Health	Calves	I.V.	21d	
Imrab® 3	Merial	Cattle Horses Sheep	I.M., S.C. I.M., S.C. I.M., S.C.	21d 21d 21d	
Imrab® Large Animal	Merial	Cattle Horses Sheep	I.M., S.C. I.M., S.C. I.M., S.C.	21d 21d 21d	
Inacti/Vac® AE	L.A.H.I. (Maine Biological)	Chickens Turkeys	S.C. S.C.	42d 42d	
Inacti/Vac® BD	L.A.H.I. (Maine Biological)	Chickens	S.C.	42d	
Inacti/Vac® BD-ND	L.A.H.I. (Maine Biological)	Chickens	S.C.	42d	
Inacti/Vac® BD-ND-FC3	L.A.H.I. (Maine Biological)	Chickens	S.C.	42d	
Inacti/Vac® BD3	L.A.H.I. (Maine Biological)	Chickens	S.C.	42d	
Inacti/Vac® BD3-IB2-REO	L.A.H.I. (Maine Biological)	Chickens	S.C.	42d	
Inacti/Vac® BD3-ND	L.A.H.I. (Maine Biological)	Chickens	S.C.	42d	
Inacti/Vac® BD3-ND-IB1-REO	L.A.H.I. (Maine Biological)	Chickens	S.C.	42d	
Inacti/Vac® BD3-ND-IB2	L.A.H.I. (Maine Biological)	Chickens	S.C.	42d	
Inacti/Vac® BD3-ND-IB2-REO	L.A.H.I. (Maine Biological)	Chickens	S.C.	42d	
Inacti/Vac® BD3-ND-REO	L.A.H.I. (Maine Biological)	Chickens	S.C.	42d	
Inacti/Vac® BD3-REO	L.A.H.I. (Maine Biological)	Chickens	S.C.	42d	
Inacti/Vac® BTO1	L.A.H.I. (Maine Biological)	Chickens	S.C.	42d	
Inacti/Vac® BTO1-ND-IB	L.A.H.I. (Maine Biological)	Chickens	S.C.	42d	
Inacti/Vac® BTO1-ND-IB-REO	L.A.H.I. (Maine Biological)	Chickens	S.C.	42d	
Inacti/Vac® BTO1-ND-REO	L.A.H.I. (Maine Biological)	Chickens	S.C.	42d	
Inacti/Vac® BTO1-REO	L.A.H.I. (Maine Biological)	Chickens	S.C.	42d	
Inacti/Vac® BTO2	L.A.H.I. (Maine Biological)	Chickens	S.C.	42d	
Inacti/Vac® BTO2-ND-IB2-REO	L.A.H.I. (Maine Biological)	Chickens	S.C.	42d	
Inacti/Vac® BTO2-ND-REO	L.A.H.I. (Maine Biological)	Chickens	S.C.	42d	
Inacti/Vac® BTO2-REO	L.A.H.I. (Maine Biological)	Chickens	S.C.	42d	
Inacti-Vac® BTO2-REOC	L.A.H.I. (Maine Biological)	Chickens	S.C.	42d	
Inacti/Vac® Chick-ND	L.A.H.I. (Maine Biological)	Chickens	S.C.	42d	
Inacti/Vac® FC2	L.A.H.I. (Maine Biological)	Chickens Turkeys	S.C. S.C.	42d 42d	
Inacti/Vac® FC2C	L.A.H.I. (Maine Biological)	Chickens Turkeys	S.C. S.C.	42d 42d	
Inacti/Vac® FC3	L.A.H.I. (Maine Biological)	Chickens Turkeys	S.C. S.C.	42d 42d	
Inacti/Vac® FC3-C	L.A.H.I. (Maine Biological)	Chickens Turkeys	S.C. S.C.	42d 42d	
Inacti/Vac® FC4	L.A.H.I. (Maine Biological)	Chickens Turkeys	S.C. S.C.	42d 42d	
Inacti/Vac® FC4C	L.A.H.I. (Maine Biological)	Chickens Turkeys	S.C. S.C.	42d 42d	
Inacti/Vac® IB2	L.A.H.I. (Maine Biological)	Chickens	S.C.	42d	
Inacti/Vac® ND	L.A.H.I. (Maine Biological)	Chickens Turkeys	S.C. S.C.	42d 42d	
Inacti/Vac® ND-AE	L.A.H.I. (Maine Biological)	Chickens	S.C.	42d	
Inacti/Vac® ND-IB1	L.A.H.I. (Maine Biological)	Chickens	S.C.	42d	
Inacti/Vac® ND-IB1C	L.A.H.I. (Maine Biological)	Chickens	S.C.	42d	
Inacti/Vac® ND-IB2	L.A.H.I. (Maine Biological)	Chickens	S.C.	42d	
Inacti/Vac® ND-PMV3	L.A.H.I. (Maine Biological)	Turkeys	S.C.	42d	
Inacti/Vac® PMV3	L.A.H.I. (Maine Biological)	Turkeys	S.C.	42d	

Product Name	Company Name	Species	Route of Administration	Meat	Milk
Inacti/Vac® Pullet-ND	L.A.H.I. (Maine Biological)	Chickens	S.C.	42d	
Inacti/Vac® REO	L.A.H.I. (Maine Biological)	Chickens	S.C.	42d	
Inacti/Vac® SE4	L.A.H.I. (Maine Biological)	Chickens	S.C.	42d	
Inacti/Vac® SE4-C	L.A.H.I. (Maine Biological)	Chickens	S.C.	42d	
Inacti/Vac® SE4-ND-IB2	L.A.H.I. (Maine Biological)	Chickens	S.C.	42d	
Inacti/Vac® Turkey-ND	L.A.H.I. (Maine Biological)	Turkeys	S.C.	42d	
Ingelvac® APP-ALC	Boehringer Ingelheim	Swine	I.M.	21d	
Ingelvac® AR4	Boehringer Ingelheim	Swine	I.M., S.C.	21d	
Ingelvac® ERY-ALC	Boehringer Ingelheim	Swine	dw, I.M., S.C.	21d	
Ingelvac® HP-1	Boehringer Ingelheim	Swine	I.M.	60d	
Ingelvac® M. hyo	Boehringer Ingelheim	Swine	I.M.	60d	
Ingelvac® PRRS ATP	Boehringer Ingelheim	Swine	I.M.	21d	
Ingelvac® PRRS-HP	Boehringer Ingelheim	Swine	I.M.	21d	
Ingelvac® PRRS-HPE	Boehringer Ingelheim	Swine	I.M.	21d	
Ingelvac® PRRS MLV	Boehringer Ingelheim	Swine	I.M.	21d	
Ingelvac® PRV-G1	Boehringer Ingelheim	Swine	I.M., I.N.	21d	
In-Synch™	AgriLabs	Cattle Horses Swine	I.M. I.M. I.M.	0 0	0
Note: Not for use in horses intended for food.					
I.O. Dine Complex™ Bolus	PRN Pharmacal	Horses	Topical		
Note: Not for use on horses intended for food.					
Iodoject	Vetus	Cattle	I.V.		
Note: Not for use in lactating dairy cows.					
I-Site™	AgriLabs	Cattle	S.C.	21d	
IsoFlo®	Abbott	Horses	Inhl.		
Note: Not for use in horses intended for food.					
Isoflurane, USP	Halocarbon	Horses	Inhl.		
Note: Not for use in horses intended for food.					
Isoflurane, USP	Phoenix Pharmaceutical	Horses	Inhl.		
Note: Not for use in horses intended for food.					
Iso-Thesia	Vetus	Horses	Inhl.		
Note: Not for use in horses intended for food.					
Ivercide™ Equine Paste 1.87%	Phoenix Pharmaceutical	Horses	Oral		
Note: Not for use in horses intended for food.					
Ivercide™ Injection for Cattle and Swine	Phoenix Pharmaceutical	Bison Cattle Reindeer Swine	S.C. S.C. S.C. S.C.	56d 35d 56d 18d	
Note: A milk discard period has not been established for this product in lactating dairy cattle. Do not use in female dairy cattle 20 months of age or older.					
Ivercide™ Liquid for Horses	Phoenix Pharmaceutical	Horses	Oral		
Note: Not for use in horses intended for food.					
Ivercide™ Pour-On for Cattle	Phoenix Pharmaceutical	Cattle	Topical	48d	
Note: Do not use on female dairy cattle of breeding age.					
Ivermectin Injection for Cattle and Swine	Durvet	Bison Cattle Reindeer Swine	S.C. S.C. S.C. S.C.	56d 35d 56d 18d	
Note: Do not use in female dairy cattle of breeding age.					
Ivermectin Injection for Cattle and Swine	Aspen	Bison Cattle Reindeer Swine	S.C. S.C. S.C. S.C.	56d 35d 56d 18d	
Note: Do not use in female dairy cattle of breeding age.					
Ivermectin Pour-On	Durvet	Cattle	Topical	48d	
Note: Do not use in female dairy cattle of breeding age.					
Ivermectin Pour-On	Aspen	Cattle	Topical	48d	
Note: Do not use in female dairy cattle of breeding age.					
Iver-On™	Med-Pharmex	Cattle	Topical	48d	
Note: Do not use in female dairy cattle of breeding age.					
Iversol	Med-Pharmex	Horses	Oral		
Note: Not for use in horses intended for food.					
Ivomec® 0.27% Injection for Grower and Feeder Pigs	Merial	Swine	S.C.	18d	
Ivomec® 1% Injection for Cattle and Swine	Merial	Bison Cattle Reindeer Swine	S.C. S.C. S.C. S.C.	56d 35d 56d 18d	
Note: Do not use in female dairy cattle of breeding age.					

Product Name	Company Name	Species	Route of Administration	Meat	Milk
Ivomec® 1% Injection for Swine	Merial	Swine	S.C.	18d	
Ivomec® Eprinex® Pour-On for Beef and Dairy Cattle	Merial	Cattle	Topical	0	0
Ivomec® Plus Injection for Cattle	Merial	Cattle	S.C.	49d	
Note: Do not use in female dairy cattle of breeding age.					
Ivomec® Pour-On for Cattle	Merial	Cattle	Topical	48d	
Note: Do not use on female dairy cattle of breeding age.					
Ivomec® Premix for Swine Type A Medicated Article	Merial	Swine	In the feed	5d	
Ivomec® Sheep Drench	Merial	Sheep	Oral	11d	
Ivomec® SR Bolus	Merial	Cattle	Oral	180d	
Note: Do not use in female dairy cattle of breeding age.					
J-5 Escherichia Coli Bacterin	Hygieia	Dairy cattle Goats Swine	S.C. S.C. I.M.	42d 42d 42d	
Jencine® 4	Schering-Plough	Cattle	I.M., S.C.	21d	
J-Vac®	Merial	Dairy cattle	I.M., S.C.	21d	
Ketofen®	Fort Dodge	Horses	I.V.		
Note: Not for use in horses intended for food.					
Keto "Plus" Gel	Durvet	Dairy cattle	Oral	0	
Kopertox®	Fort Dodge	Horses	Topical		
Note: Not for use on horses intended for food.					
KV Wound Powder	KenVet	Horses	Topical		
Note: Not for use on horses intended for food.					
Land O Lakes® Instant Amplifier® Max	Land O'Lakes	Calves	Oral	30d	
Note: A withdrawal period has not been established for this product in pre-ruminating calves. Do not use in calves to be processed for veal.					
Land O Lakes® Instant Amplifier® Select	Land O'Lakes	Calves	Oral	30d	
Note: A withdrawal period has not been established for this product in pre-ruminating calves. Do not use in calves to be processed for veal.					
Land O Lakes® Instant Cow's Match™	Land O'Lakes	Calves	Oral	30d	
Note: A withdrawal period has not been established for this product in pre-ruminating calves. Do not use in calves to be processed for veal.					
Land O Lakes® Instant Maxi Care®	Land O'Lakes	Calves	Oral	30d	
Note: A withdrawal period has not been established for this product in pre-ruminating calves. Do not use in calves to be processed for veal.					
Land O Lakes® Instant Nursing Formula	Land O'Lakes	Calves	Oral	30d	
Note: A withdrawal period has not been established for this product in pre-ruminating calves. Do not use in calves to be processed for veal.					
Land O Lakes® LitterMilk®	Land O'Lakes	Swine	Oral	10d	
Larvadex® 1% Premix	Novartis	Poultry	In the feed	3d	
Note: Not for use in broiler chickens.					
Larvadex® 2SL	Novartis	Poultry	On the premise	24h	
Laryngo-Vac™	Fort Dodge	Chickens	aer/sp, dw, I.O.	21d	
LaSota M41 Conn.™	L.A.H.I. (New Jersey)	Chickens	dw	21d	
Laxade Bolus	AgriPharm	Cattle	Oral	0	24h
Laxade Powder	AgriPharm	Cattle	Oral	0	12h
Layermune® 2	Biomune	Chickens	S.C.	42d	
Layermune® 3	Biomune	Chickens	S.C.	42d	
Layermune® 5	Biomune	Chickens	S.C.	42d	
Layermune® IB	Biomune	Chickens	S.C.	42d	
Layermune® ND	Biomune	Chickens	S.C.	42d	
Layermune SE®	Biomune	Chickens	S.C.	42d	
Legacy®	AgriLabs	Horses	I.U.		
Note: Not for use in horses intended for food.					
Legend® (hyaluronate sodium) Injectable Solution (20 mg)	Bayer	Horses	I.A.		
Note: Not for use in horses intended for food.					
Legend® (hyaluronate sodium) Injectable Solution (40 mg)	Bayer	Horses	I.V.		
Note: Not for use in horses intended for food.					
Lepto-5	Boehringer Ingelheim	Cattle Swine	I.M. I.M.	21d 21d	
Lepto 5	Premier Farmtech	Cattle	S.C.	21d	
Lepto 5	AgriLabs	Cattle Swine	I.M., S.C. I.M., S.C.	21d 21d	
Lepto 5	Durvet	Cattle Swine	I.M. I.M.	21d 21d	
Lepto-5	Colorado Serum	Cattle Swine	I.M., S.C. I.M., S.C.	21d 21d	
Lepto 5 Vaccine	Aspen	Cattle Swine	I.M., S.C. I.M., S.C.	21d 21d	
Leptoferm-5®	Pfizer Animal Health	Cattle Swine	I.M. I.M.	21d 21d	

Please refer to product listings for more complete information.

Product Name	Company Name	Species	Route of Administration	Meat	Milk
Lepto Shield™ 5	Novartis Animal Vaccines	Cattle Swine	I.M. I.M.	21d 21d	
Lepto Shield™ 5 Hardjo Bovis	Novartis Animal Vaccines	Cattle	I.M.	21d	
Levamisole Injectable ***Note:*** Do not administer to dairy cattle of breeding age.	AgriLabs	Cattle	S.C.	7d	
Levamisole Phosphate ***Note:*** Do not administer to dairy cattle of breeding age.	Durvet	Cattle	S.C.	7d	
Levamisole Phosphate Injectable Solution, 13.65% ***Note:*** Do not administer to dairy cattle of breeding age.	AgriPharm	Cattle	S.C.	7d	
Levamisole Phosphate Injectable Solution, 13.65% ***Note:*** Do not administer to dairy cattle of breeding age.	Aspen	Cattle	S.C.	7d	
Levamisole Soluble Pig Wormer	AgriLabs	Swine	dw	72h	
Levasole® Cattle Wormer Boluses ***Note:*** Do not administer to dairy cattle of breeding age.	Schering-Plough	Cattle	Oral	48h	
Levasole® Injectable Solution, 13.65% ***Note:*** Do not administer to dairy cattle of breeding age.	Schering-Plough	Cattle	S.C.	7d	
Levasole® Sheep Wormer Boluses	Schering-Plough	Sheep	Oral	72h	
Levasole® Soluble Drench Powder ***Note:*** Do not administer to dairy cattle of breeding age.	Schering-Plough	Cattle Sheep	Oral Oral	48h 72h	
Levasole® Soluble Drench Powder (Sheep)	Schering-Plough	Sheep	Oral	72h	
Levasole® Soluble Pig Wormer	Schering-Plough	Swine	dw	72h	
Levo-Powder ***Note:*** Not for use in horses intended for food.	Vetus	Horses	Oral		
Lincocin® Injectable	AgriLabs	Swine	I.M.	48h	
Lincocin® Sterile Solution	Durvet	Swine	I.M.	48h	
Lincocin® Sterile Solution (Swine)	Pharmacia & Upjohn	Swine	I.M.	48h	
Lincomix® 20 Feed Medication	Pharmacia & Upjohn	Chickens Swine	In the feed In the feed	0 0	
Lincomix® 50 Feed Medication	Pharmacia & Upjohn	Chickens Swine	In the feed In the feed	0 0	
Lincomix® Injectable	Pharmacia & Upjohn	Swine	I.M.	48h	
Lincomix® Soluble Powder	Pharmacia & Upjohn	Chickens Swine	dw dw	0 0	
Lincomycin Hydrochloride Soluble Powder	Durvet	Chickens Swine	dw dw	0 0	
Lincomycin Soluble	Alpharma	Chickens Swine	dw dw	0 6d	
Lincomycin Soluble Powder	AgriLabs	Chickens Swine	dw dw	0 0	
Lincosol Soluble Powder	Med-Pharmex	Chickens Swine	dw dw	0 6d	
Lipogen Forte™	Novartis (Aqua Health)	Salmonids	I.P.	60d	
Lipogen Triple	Novartis (Aqua Health)	Salmonids	I.P.	60d	
Liquamycin® LA-200®	Pfizer Animal Health	Cattle Swine	I.V., S.C. I.M.	28d 28d	96h
LitterGuard®	Pfizer Animal Health	Swine	I.M., S.C.	21d	
LitterGuard® LT	Pfizer Animal Health	Swine	I.M., S.C.	21d	
LitterGuard® LT-C	Pfizer Animal Health	Swine	I.M., S.C.	21d	
Louse Powder with Rabon®	LeGear	Cattle Horses Poultry Swine	Topical Topical Topical Topical	0 0 0 0	
LT Blen®	Merial Select	Chickens	dw, I.O.	21d	
LT-Ivax®	Schering-Plough	Chickens	I.O.	21d	
Lutalyse® Sterile Solution ***Note:*** Not for use in horses intended for food.	Pharmacia & Upjohn	Cattle Horses Swine	I.M. I.M. I.M.	0 0	0
Lysigin®	Boehringer Ingelheim	Dairy cattle	I.M.	21d	
MaGESTic™ 7 with Spur®	Intervet	Swine	I.M.	21d	
Magnalax Bolus	Phoenix Pharmaceutical	Cattle	Oral		24h
Magnalax Boluses	Bimeda	Cattle	Oral	0	24h
Magnalax Powder	Vedco	Cattle Goats Sheep	Oral Oral Oral	0 0 0	24h 24h

Product Name	Company Name	Species	Route of Administration	Meat	Milk
Magnalax Powder	Phoenix Pharmaceutical	Cattle Goats Sheep	Oral Oral Oral	0 0 0	12h 12h
Magnalax Powder	Bimeda	Cattle Goats Sheep	Oral Oral Oral	0 0 0	24h 24h
Marek's Disease Vaccine (Chicken and Turkey)	Merial Select	Chickens	S.C.	21d	
Marek's Disease Vaccine (FC-126 Strain)	Merial Select	Chickens	S.C.	21d	
Marek's Disease Vaccine (Rispens CVI 988 Strain)	Merial Select	Chickens	S.C.	21d	
Marek's Disease Vaccine (Rispens CVI 988 Strain + FC-126 Strain)	Merial Select	Chickens	S.C.	21d	
Marek's Disease Vaccine (SB-1 Strain)	Merial Select	Chickens	S.C.	21d	
Marexine®	Intervet	Chickens	S.C.	21d	
Marexine-89/03®	Intervet	Chickens	S.C.	21d	
Marexine-SB-89/03®	Intervet	Chickens	S.C.	21d	
Marexine® SB-Vac®	Intervet	Chickens	S.C.	21d	
Marquis™ (15% w/w ponazuril) Antiprotozoal Oral Paste ***Note:*** Not for use in horses intended for food.	Bayer	Horses	Oral		
Master Guard™ 10	AgriLabs	Cattle	I.M., S.C.	21d	
Master Guard® 10	Intervet	Cattle	I.M., S.C.	21d	
Master Guard® 10 + Vibrio	AgriLabs	Cattle	I.M., S.C.	21d	
Master Guard® J5	AgriLabs	Cattle	I.M., S.C.	60d	
Master Guard™ Preg 5	AgriLabs	Cattle	I.M., S.C.	21d	
Master Guard® Preg 5	Intervet	Cattle	I.M., S.C.	21d	
Masti-Clear™	G.C. Hanford	Dairy cattle	I.M.M.	3d	60h
Maxiban® 72	Elanco	Chickens	In the feed	5d	
Maxi/Guard® Nasal Vac	Addison	Swine	I.N.	21d	
Maxi/Guard® Pinkeye Bacterin	Addison	Cattle	S.C.	21d	
Maxim-200® ***Note:*** Not for use in lactating dairy animals.	Phoenix Pharmaceutical	Cattle Swine	I.M., I.V., S.C. I.M.	28d 28d	
Maximune® 4	Biomune	Chickens	S.C.	42d	
Maximune® 6	Biomune	Chickens	S.C.	42d	
Maximune® 7	Biomune	Chickens	S.C.	42d	
Maximune® 8	Biomune	Chickens	S.C.	42d	
Maximune® IBD	Biomune	Chickens	S.C.	42d	
MaxiVac® Excell™	SyntroVet	Swine	I.M.	21d	
MaxiVac®-FLU	SyntroVet	Swine	I.M.	21d	
MaxiVac®-M+	SyntroVet	Swine	I.M.	60d	
MD-Vac® CAF Frozen	Fort Dodge	Chickens	In ovo, S.C.	21d	
MD-Vac® CFL	Fort Dodge	Chickens	S.C.	21d	
Mecadox® 10	Phibro	Swine	In the feed	42d	
Medicated Wound Cream ***Note:*** Not for use on animals intended for food purposes.	First Priority	Horses	Topical		
Medicated Wound Powder ***Note:*** Not for use on animals intended for food purposes.	First Priority	Horses	Topical		
Megan® Vac 1	Megan	Chickens	aer/sp, dw	21d	
MG-Bac®	Fort Dodge	Chickens Turkeys	I.M., S.C. I.M., S.C.	42d 42d	
M.G. Bacterin	L.A.H.I. (New Jersey)	Chickens	S.C.	42d	
Micotil® 300 Injection ***Note:*** Not for use in female dairy cattle 20 months of age or older.	Elanco	Cattle	S.C.	28d	
Microcillin ***Note:*** Not for use in horses intended for food.	Anthony	Cattle Horses Sheep Swine Veal	I.M. I.M. I.M. I.M. I.M.	4d 8d 6d 7d	48h
Micro Pearls Advantage™ Miconazole™ Shampoo ***Note:*** Not for use on animals intended for food purposes.	Evsco	Horses	Topical		
Micro Pearls Advantage™ Miconazole™ Spray ***Note:*** Not for use on animals intended for food purposes.	Evsco	Horses	Topical		
Micro Pearls Advantage™ Seba-Hex™ Shampoo ***Note:*** Not for use on animals intended for food purposes.	Evsco	Horses	Topical		
Mildvac-Ark®	Intervet	Chickens	aer/sp, bd	21d	

Product Name	Company Name	Species	Route of Administration	Meat	Milk
Mildvac-Ma5®	Intervet	Chickens	aer/sp, bd, dw	21d	
M-Ninevax™	Schering-Plough	Turkeys	dw	21d	
M-Ninevax®-C	Schering-Plough	Chickens	ww	21d	
MoorMan's® Beef Cattle Boost® BT	ADM	Beef cattle	Oral		
Note: A withdrawal period has not been established for this product in pre-ruminating calves. Do not use in calves to be processed for veal. Do not feed to lactating dairy cows.					
MoorMan's® CBX	ADM	Swine	In the feed	10w	
MoorMan's® LN 10	ADM	Swine	In the feed	6d	
MoorMan's® NT 10/10	ADM	Calves	In the feed	7d	
		Chickens	In the feed	5-14d	
		Swine	In the feed	5d	
Note: Withdraw from feed 5 days before slaughter of broilers and 14 days before slaughter of laying hens.					
MoorMan's® Special Mix Cattle Boost® BT	ADM	Beef cattle	Oral		
Note: A withdrawal period has not been established for this product in pre-ruminating calves. Do not use in calves to be processed for veal. Do not feed to lactating dairy cows.					
MoorMan's® TYS 5/5	ADM	Swine	In the feed	15d	
MoorMan's® WDC	ADM	Swine	In the feed	10w	
M+Pac®	Schering-Plough	Swine	I.M., S.C.	21d	
M+Parapac™	Schering-Plough	Swine	I.M.	60d	
MS-Bac™	Fort Dodge	Chickens	I.M., S.C.	42d	
		Turkeys	I.M., S.C.	42d	
Multimune® CU	Biomune	Turkeys	dw	21d	
Multimune® K	Biomune	Chickens	S.C.	42d	
		Turkeys	S.C.	42d	
Multimune® K5	Biomune	Chickens	S.C.	42d	
		Turkeys	S.C.	42d	
Multimune® M	Biomune	Turkeys	ww	21d	
Multi Serum	Durvet	Cattle	I.M., S.C.	21d	
		Sheep	I.M., S.C.	21d	
MU-SE®	Schering-Plough	Beef cattle	I.M., S.C.	30d	
		Calves	I.M., S.C.	30d	
MVT Powder™	Butler	Cattle	Oral	0	24h
		Sheep	Oral	0	
Mycoplasma Bovis Bacterin	Biomune	Dairy cattle	S.C.	21d	
Mycoplasma Gallisepticum Vaccine	Merial Select	Chickens	I.O.	21d	
Myco Shield™	Novartis Animal Vaccines	Swine	I.M.	21d	
Myco Silencer® BPM	Intervet	Swine	I.M., S.C.	21d	
Myco Silencer® BPME	Intervet	Swine	I.M., S.C.	21d	
Myco Silencer® M	Intervet	Swine	I.M., S.C.	21d	
Myco Silencer® MEH	Intervet	Swine	I.M.	21d	
Myco Silencer® Once	Intervet	Swine	I.M.	21d	
Mycovac-L®	Intervet	Chickens	aer/sp	21d	
Note: Do not vaccinate chickens within 4 weeks of onset of egg production or during egg production.					
Myosan™ Cream	Life Science	Horses	Topical		
Note: Not for use on animals intended for food purposes.					
Myosan™ Solution	Life Science	Horses	Topical		
Note: Not for use on animals intended for food purposes.					
Mystique®	Intervet	Horses	I.M.	21d	
Mystique® II	Intervet	Horses	I.M.	21d	
Naquasone® Bolus	Schering-Plough	Dairy cattle	Oral	0	72h
Nasalgen® IP Vaccine	Schering-Plough	Cattle	I.N.	21d	
Nasal-Vax™	AgriPharm	Cattle	I.N.	21d	
Naxcel®	Pharmacia & Upjohn	Cattle	I.M., S.C.	0	0
		Chickens	S.C.	0	
		Goats	I.M.	0	0
		Horses	I.M.		
		Sheep	I.M.	0	
		Swine	I.M.	0	
		Turkeys	S.C.	0	
Note: Not for use in horses intended for food.					
NB Blen® Plus	Merial Select	Chickens	dw, I.O.	21d	
Neo-325 Soluble Powder	Bimeda	Cattle	dw	1d	
		Goats	dw	3d	
		Sheep	dw	2d	
		Swine	dw	3d	
		Turkeys	dw	0	
Note: A milk discard period has not been established for this product in lactating dairy cattle. Do not use in female dairy cattle 20 months of age or older. A withdrawal period has not been established for this product in pre-ruminating calves. Do not use in calves to be processed for veal.					

Product Name	Company Name	Species	Route of Administration	Meat	Milk
NeoGuard™	Intervet	Cattle	S.C.	21d	
Neomix® 325 Soluble Powder	Pharmacia & Upjohn	Cattle	dw	1d	
		Goats	dw	3d	
		Sheep	dw	2d	
		Swine	dw	3d	
		Turkeys	dw	0	
Note: A milk discard period has not been established for this product in lactating dairy cattle. Do not use in female dairy cattle 20 months of age or older. A withdrawal period has not been established for this product in pre-ruminating calves. Do not use in calves to be processed for veal.					
Neomix® AG 325 Medicated Premix	Pharmacia & Upjohn	Cattle	In the feed	1d	
		Goats	In the feed	3d	
		Sheep	In the feed	2d	
		Swine	In the feed	3d	
Note: A milk discard period has not been established for this product in lactating dairy cattle. Do not use in female dairy cattle 20 months of age or older. A milk discard period has not been established for this product in lactating dairy goats. Do not use in female dairy goats 12 months of age or older. A withdrawal period has not been established for this product in pre-ruminating calves. Do not use in calves to be processed for veal.					
Neomix® AG 325 Soluble Powder	Pharmacia & Upjohn	Cattle	dw	1d	
		Goats	dw	3d	
		Sheep	dw	2d	
		Swine	dw	3d	
		Turkeys	dw	0	
Note: A milk discard period has not been established for this product in lactating dairy cattle. Do not use in female dairy cattle 20 months of age or older. A withdrawal period has not been established for this product in pre-ruminating calves. Do not use in calves to be processed for veal.					
Neomycin 200	Aspen	Cattle	dw	1d	
		Goats	dw	3d	
		Sheep	dw	2d	
		Swine	dw	3d	
Note: A milk discard period has not been established for this product in lactating dairy cattle. Do not use in female dairy cattle 20 months of age or older. A withdrawal period has not been established for this product in pre-ruminating calves. Do not use in calves to be processed for veal.					
Neomycin 325	AgriLabs	Cattle	dw	30d	
		Goats	dw	30d	
		Sheep	dw	20d	
		Swine	dw	20d	
Note: Not to be used in veal calves.					
Neomycin 325	Durvet	Cattle	dw	1d	
		Goats	dw	3d	
		Sheep	dw	2d	
		Swine	dw	3d	
Note: A milk discard period has not been established for this product in lactating dairy cattle. Do not use in female dairy cattle 20 months of age or older. A withdrawal period has not been established for this product in pre-ruminating calves. Do not use in calves to be processed for veal.					
Neomycin Oral Solution	AgriLabs	Cattle	dw	1d	
		Goats	dw	3d	
		Sheep	dw	2d	
		Swine	dw	3d	
Note: A milk discard period has not been established for this product in lactating dairy cattle. Do not use in female dairy cattle 20 months of age or older. A withdrawal period has not been established for this product in pre-ruminating calves. Do not use in calves to be processed for veal.					
Neomycin Oral Solution	Durvet	Cattle	dw	1d	
		Goats	dw	3d	
		Sheep	dw	2d	
		Swine	dw	3d	
Note: A milk discard period has not been established for this product in lactating dairy cattle. Do not use in female dairy cattle 20 months of age or older. A withdrawal period has not been established for this product in pre-ruminating calves. Do not use in calves to be processed for veal.					
Neomycin Oral Solution	Phoenix Pharmaceutical	Cattle	dw	1d	
		Goats	dw	3d	
		Sheep	dw	2d	
		Swine	dw	3d	
Note: A milk discard period has not been established for this product in lactating dairy cattle. Do not use in female dairy cattle 20 months of age or older. A withdrawal period has not been established for this product in pre-ruminating calves. Do not use in calves to be processed for veal. Not to be used in veal calves.					
Neo-Oxy 10/5 Meal	PennField	Broilers	In the feed	5d	
		Calves	In milk replacer	30d	
		Cattle	In the feed	0-7d	
		Layers	In the feed	14d	
		Swine	In the feed	5d	
		Turkeys	In the feed	14d	
Note: A withdrawal period has not been established for this product in pre-ruminating calves. Do not use in calves to be processed for veal. All use levels in milk replacers require a 30 day withdrawal before slaughter. Withdraw from cattle 7 days before slaughter when used at a level of 1.4 g neomycin base plus 2 g oxytetracycline per head daily.					
Neo-Oxy 10/10 Meal	PennField	Broilers	In the feed	5d	
		Calves	In milk replacer	30d	
		Cattle	In the feed	0-7d	
		Layers	In the feed	14d	
		Swine	In the feed	5d	
		Turkeys	In the feed	14d	
Note: A withdrawal period has not been established for this product in pre-ruminating calves. Do not use in calves to be processed for veal. All use levels in milk replacers require a 30 day withdrawal before slaughter. Withdraw from calves 7 days before slaughter when used at a level of 1.4 g neomycin base plus 2 g oxytetracycline per head daily.					

Product Name	Company Name	Species	Route of Administration	Meat	Milk
Neo-Oxy 50/50 Meal	PennField	Broilers	In the feed	5d	
		Calves	In milk replacer	30d	
		Cattle	In the feed	0-7d	
		Layers	In the feed	14d	
		Swine	In the feed	5d	
		Turkeys	In the feed	14d	
Note: A withdrawal period has not been established for this product in pre-ruminating calves. Do not use in calves to be processed for veal. All use levels in milk replacers require a 30 day withdrawal before slaughter. Withdraw from calves 7 days before slaughter when used at a level of 1.4 g neomycin base plus 2 g oxytetracycline per head daily.					
Neo-Oxy 100/50 Meal	PennField	Broilers	In the feed	5d	
		Calves	In milk replacer	5d	
		Cattle	In the feed	0-7d	
		Layers	In the feed	14d	
		Swine	In the feed	5d	
		Turkeys	In the feed	14d	
Note: A withdrawal period has not been established for this product in pre-ruminating calves. Do not use in calves to be processed for veal. At all use levels in milk replacers for calves, withdraw 5 days before slaughter. Withdraw from calves 7 days before slaughter when used at a level of 1.4 g neomycin base plus 2 g oxytetracycline per head daily.					
Neo-Oxy 100/50 MR	PennField	Cattle	In milk replacer	30d	
		Swine	In milk replacer	5-10d	
Note: A withdrawal period has not been established for this product in pre-ruminating calves. Do not use in calves to be processed for veal. In pigs, when neomycin base level is 140 g/ton, withdraw from feed 10 days before slaughter. In pigs, when neomycin base level is below 140 g/ton, withdraw from feed 5 days before slaughter.					
Neo-Oxy 100/100 Meal	PennField	Broilers	In the feed	5d	
		Calves	In milk replacer	30d	
		Cattle	In the feed	0-7d	
		Layers	In the feed	14d	
		Swine	In the feed	5d	
		Turkeys	In the feed	14d	
Note: A withdrawal period has not been established for this product in pre-ruminating calves. Do not use in calves to be processed for veal. All use levels in milk replacers require a 30 day withdrawal before slaughter. Withdraw from calves 7 days before slaughter when used at a level of 1.4 g neomycin base plus 2 g oxytetracycline per head daily.					
Neo-Sol® 50	Alpharma	Cattle	dw	1d	
		Goats	dw	3d	
		Sheep	dw	2d	
		Swine	dw	3d	
Note: A milk discard period has not been established for this product in lactating dairy cattle. Do not use in female dairy cattle 20 months of age or older. A withdrawal period has not been established for this product in pre-ruminating calves. Do not use in calves to be processed for veal.					
Neosol-Oral	Med-Pharmex	Cattle	dw	1d	
		Goats	dw	3d	
		Sheep	dw	2d	
		Swine	dw	3d	
Note: Not to be used in veal calves.					
Neosol Soluble Powder	Med-Pharmex	Cattle	dw	30d	
		Goats	dw	30d	
		Sheep	dw	20d	
		Swine	dw	20d	
Note: Not to be used in veal calves.					
Neo-Terramycin® 50/50	Phibro	Broilers	In the feed	5d	
		Calves	In the feed	0-7d	
		Layers	In the feed	14d	
		Swine	In the feed	5d	
		Turkeys	In the feed	14d	
Note: When fed at the level of 1.4 g neomycin base plus 2 g oxytetracycline/calf/day requires withdrawal from feed 7 days before slaughter. A withdrawal is not required for calves fed at lower levels.					
Neo-Terramycin® 50/50D	Phibro	Calves	In the feed	30d	
		Swine	In the feed	5-10d	
Note: In pigs, when neomycin base level is 140 g/ton, withdraw from feed 10 days before slaughter. In pigs, when neomycin base level is below 140 g/ton, withdraw from feed 5 days before slaughter.					
Neo-Terramycin® 100/50	Phibro	Broilers	In the feed	5d	
		Calves	In the feed	0-7d	
		Layers	In the feed	14d	
		Swine	In the feed	5d	
		Turkeys	In the feed	14d	
Note: When fed at the level of 1.4 g neomycin base plus 2 g oxytetracycline/calf/day requires withdrawal from feed 7 days before slaughter. A withdrawal is not required for calves fed at lower levels.					
Neo-Terramycin® 100/50D	Phibro	Calves	In the feed	30d	
		Swine	In the feed	5-10d	
Note: In pigs, when neomycin base level is 140 g/ton, withdraw from feed 10 days before slaughter. In pigs, when neomycin base level is below 140 g/ton, withdraw from feed 5 days before slaughter.					
Neoved 200	Vedco	Cattle	dw	30d	
		Goats	dw	30d	
		Sheep	dw	20d	
		Swine	dw	20d	
Note: Not to be used in veal calves.					

Product Name	Company Name	Species	Route of Administration	Meat	Milk
Neovet 325/100	AgriPharm	Cattle Goats Sheep Swine	dw dw dw dw	1d 3d 2d 3d	
Note: A milk discard period has not been established for this product in lactating dairy cattle. Do not use in female dairy cattle 20 months of age or older. A withdrawal period has not been established for this product in pre-ruminating calves. Do not use in calves to be processed for veal.					
Neovet® Neomycin Oral Solution	AgriPharm	Cattle Goats Sheep Swine	dw dw dw dw	30d 30d 20d 20d	
Note: Not to be used in veal calves.					
New Bronz®	Fort Dodge	Chickens	I.M., S.C.	42d	
New Bronz® MG	Fort Dodge	Chickens	I.M., S.C.	42d	
Newcastle B_1+Bronchitis Conn	Fort Dodge	Chickens	aer/sp, dw, I.N., I.O	21d	
Newcastle B_1+Bronchitis Conn Mass (1,000 dose)	Fort Dodge	Chickens	aer/sp, dw, I.N., I.O	21d	
Newcastle B_1+Bronchitis Conn Mass (5,000 and 10,000 dose)	Fort Dodge	Chickens	aer/sp, dw	21d	
Newcastle B_1+Bronchitis Mass	Fort Dodge	Chickens	aer/sp, dw, I.N., I.O	21d	
Newcastle B_1+Bronchitis Mass+Ark	Fort Dodge	Chickens	dw	21d	
Newcastle-Bronchitis Vaccine	L.A.H.I. (New Jersey)	Chickens	S.C.	42d	
Newcastle-Bronchitis Vaccine (B_1 Strain, Mass. Type)	Merial Select	Chickens	aer/sp, dw	21d	
Newcastle-Bronchitis Vaccine (B1 Type, LaSota Strain and Mass. Type, Holland Strain)	Merial Select	Chickens	aer/sp, dw	21d	
Newcastle-Bronchitis Vaccine (Conn. Type)	Merial Select	Chickens	aer/sp, dw	21d	
Newcastle-Bronchitis Vaccine (LaSota Strain, Mass. Type)	Merial Select	Chickens	aer/sp, dw, I.O.	21d	
Newcastle-Bronchitis Vaccine LS Mass II™	Fort Dodge	Chickens	dw, I.N., I.O	21d	
Newcastle-Bronchitis Vaccine (Mass. & Ark. Types)	Merial Select	Chickens	aer/sp, dw	21d	
Newcastle-Bronchitis Vaccine (Mass. & Conn. Types)	Merial Select	Chickens	aer/sp, dw	21d	
Newcastle Disease-Fowl Pox Vaccine (Recombinant)	Merial Select	Chickens	S.C.	21d	
Newcastle Disease Vaccine	L.A.H.I. (New Jersey)	Chickens Turkeys	I.M., S.C. I.M., S.C.	42d 42d	
Newcastle Disease Vaccine (B1 Strain)	Merial Select	Chickens	aer/sp, dw	21d	
Newcastle Disease Vaccine (B1 Type, B1 Strain, Live Virus)	Fort Dodge	Chickens	aer/sp, dw, I.N., I.O	21d	
Newcastle Disease Vaccine (B_1 Type, B_1 Strain, Live Virus)	L.A.H.I. (New Jersey)	Chickens	aer/sp, dw, I.N., I.O	21d	
Newcastle Disease Vaccine (B_1 Type, B_1 Strain, Live Virus) (Drinking Water Use)	L.A.H.I. (New Jersey)	Chickens	dw	21d	
Newcastle Disease Vaccine (B1 Type, LaSota Strain, Live Virus)	Fort Dodge	Chickens	aer/sp, dw, I.N., I.O	21d	
Newcastle Disease Vaccine (B_1 Type, LaSota Strain, Live Virus)	L.A.H.I. (New Jersey)	Chickens	aer/sp, dw, I.N., I.O	21d	
Newcastle Disease Vaccine (Killed Virus)	L.A.H.I. (New Jersey)	Chickens	I.M., S.C.	42d	
Newcastle Disease Vaccine (LaSota Strain)	Merial Select	Chickens	aer/sp, dw	21d	
Newcastle-K	Fort Dodge	Chickens	I.M., S.C.	42d	
Newcastle LaSota+Bronchitis Mass	Fort Dodge	Chickens	aer/sp, dw, I.N., I.O	21d	
Newhatch-C2-M™	Intervet	Chickens	aer/sp	21d	
Newhatch-C2-MC™	Intervet	Chickens	aer/sp	21d	
Newvax®	Schering-Plough	Chickens	aer/sp, dw	21d	
New Z® Diazinon Insecticide Cattle Ear Tags	Farnam	Cattle	Ear tags		
Note: Remove tags before slaughter.					
New Z® Permethrin Insecticide Cattle Ear Tags	Farnam	Cattle	Ear tags		
Note: Remove tags before slaughter.					
NFZ® Puffer	AgriLabs	Cattle	Topical		
Note: A withdrawal period has not been established for this product in pre-ruminating calves. Do not use on calves to be processed for veal.					
NFZ® Puffer	Loveland	Cattle	Topical		
Note: A withdrawal period has not been established for this product in pre-ruminating calves. Do not use on calves to be processed for veal.					
nfz® puffer	AgriPharm	Cattle	Topical		
Note: A withdrawal period has not been established for this product in pre-ruminating calves. Do not use in calves to be processed for veal.					
NFZ® Wound Dressing	Loveland	Horses	Topical		
Note: Not for use on horses intended for food.					
Nicarb® 25%	Phibro	Chickens	In the feed	4d	
Note: Do not feed to laying birds in production.					
Nitro-Chol®	Arko	Turkeys	dw	21d	

Product Name	Company Name	Species	Route of Administration	Meat	Milk
Nitrofurazone	Aspen	Horses	Topical		
Note: Not for use on horses intended for food.					
Nitrofurazone Dressing	Durvet	Horses	Topical		
Note: Not for use on horses intended for food.					
Nitrofurazone Dressing 0.2%	AgriLabs	Horses	Topical		
Note: Not for use on horses intended for food.					
Nitrofurazone Dressing 0.2%	AgriPharm	Horses	Topical		
Note: Not for use on horses intended for food.					
Nitrofurazone Ointment	Phoenix Pharmaceutical	Horses	Topical		
Note: Not for use on horses intended for food.					
Nitrofurazone Soluble Dressing	Med-Pharmex	Horses	Topical		
Note: Not for use on horses intended for food.					
Nitrofurazone Soluble Dressing	Butler	Horses	Topical		
Note: Not for use on horses intended for food.					
Nitro-Sal F.D.	Arko	Swine	dw, S.C.	21d	
Nitrozone™ Ointment	Bimeda	Horses	Topical		
Note: Not for use on horses intended for food.					
Nolvasan® Antiseptic Ointment	Fort Dodge	Horses	Topical		
Note: Not for use on horses intended for food.					
Nolvasan® Cap-Tabs®	Fort Dodge	Horses	I.U.		
Note: Not for use in horses intended for food.					
Nolvasan® Suspension	Fort Dodge	Horses	I.U.		
Note: Not for use in horses intended for food.					
Normal Equine Serum	Colorado Serum	Horses	I.M., I.V., S.C.	21d	
Normal Serum-Equine	Professional Biological	Horses	I.M., I.V., S.C.	21d	
Nuflor® Injectable Solution 300 mg/mL	Schering-Plough	Cattle	I.M. S.C.	28d 38d	
Note: A withdrawal period has not been established for this product in pre-ruminating calves. Do not use in calves to be processed for veal. Not for use in female dairy cattle 20 months of age or older.					
Ocu-guard® MB	Boehringer Ingelheim	Cattle	S.C.	21d	
Ocuvax®	Schering-Plough	Chickens	I.O.	21d	
Once PMH®	Intervet	Cattle	I.M.	21d	
One Shot®	Pfizer Animal Health	Cattle	I.M., S.C.	21d	
One Shot Ultra™ 7	Pfizer Animal Health	Cattle	S.C.	21d	
One Shot Ultra™ 8	Pfizer Animal Health	Cattle	S.C.	21d	
Optimune® 4	Biomune	Chickens	S.C.	42d	
Optimune® 6	Biomune	Chickens	S.C.	42d	
Optimune® 7	Biomune	Chickens	S.C.	42d	
Optimune® 8	Biomune	Chickens	S.C.	42d	
Optimune® IBD	Biomune	Chickens	S.C.	42d	
Orachol®	Schering-Plough	Turkeys	dw	21d	
Oralvax-HE™	Schering-Plough	Turkeys	dw	21d	
Orbenin®-DC	Pfizer Animal Health	Dairy cattle	I.M.M.	28d	
Note: Not to be used within 28 days of calving.					
Organic Iodide	Butler	Cattle	In the feed		
Note: Not to be fed to dairy cattle in production.					
Organic Iodide Powder	Neogen	Cattle	In the feed		
Note: Do not feed to lactating dairy cattle.					
Organic Iodine	AgriLabs	Cattle	In the feed		
Note: Not for use in lactating cows.					
OT 200	Vetus	Cattle Swine	I.M., I.V. I.M.	28d 28d	
Note: Not for use in lactating dairy animals.					
OTC 50	Durvet	Bees Cattle Chickens Sheep Swine Turkeys	In the feed In the feed In the feed In the feed In the feed In the feed	 0-5d 0-3d 0-5d 0-5d 0-5d	
Note: Do not feed to chickens producing eggs for human consumption when used at levels of 400 g/ton and above. Do not feed to turkeys producing eggs for food. In low calcium feeds withdraw from chickens three days before slaughter (at levels of 400 g/ton and above). Remove at least 6 weeks prior to main honey flow. Withdraw from chickens 24 hours prior to slaughter when used at levels of 500 g/ton. Withdraw from sheep, swine and cattle 5 days before slaughter when used at a dose of 10 mg/lb body weight/day. Withdraw from turkeys 5 days before slaughter when used at levels of 200 g/ton or higher.					
Ovine Ecolizer®	Novartis Animal Vaccines	Sheep	Oral	21d	
Ovine Ecthyma Vaccine	Colorado Serum	Goats Sheep	I.Derm. I.Derm.	21d 21d	

Product Name	Company Name	Species	Route of Administration	Meat	Milk
Ovine Tetanus Shield™	Novartis Animal Vaccines	Sheep	I.M., S.C.	21d	
Ovuplant™	Fort Dodge	Horses	Implant		
Note: Not for use in horses intended for food.					
Oxy 500 Calf Bolus	Boehringer Ingelheim	Cattle	Oral	0	
Note: A withdrawal period has not been established for this product in pre-ruminating calves. Do not use in calves to be processed for veal. Not for use in lactating dairy cows.					
Oxy 1000 Calf Bolus	Boehringer Ingelheim	Cattle	Oral	0	
Note: A withdrawal period has not been established for this product in pre-ruminating calves. Do not use in calves to be processed for veal. Not for use in lactating dairy cows.					
Oxybiotic™ -100	Butler	Cattle	I.V.	19d	
Note: Do not use in lactating dairy cattle.					
Oxybiotic™ -200	Butler	Cattle Swine	I.M., I.V. I.M.	28d 28d	
Note: Do not use in lactating dairy cattle.					
OxyCure™ -100	Vedco	Cattle	I.V.	22d	
Note: A withdrawal period has not been established for this product in pre-ruminating calves. Do not use in calves to be processed for veal. Not for use in lactating dairy animals.					
OxyCure™ 200	Vedco	Cattle Swine	I.M., I.V. I.M.	28d 28d	
Note: Not for use in lactating dairy animals.					
Oxy-Mycin® 100	AgriPharm	Cattle	I.V.	19d	
Note: A withdrawal period has not been established for this product in pre-ruminating calves. Do not use in calves to be processed for veal. Not for use in lactating cows.					
Oxy-Mycin® 200	AgriPharm	Cattle Swine	I.M. I.M.	28d 28d	
Note: Not for use in lactating dairy animals.					
Oxytetracycline-343	Durvet	Chickens Swine Turkeys	dw dw dw	 13d 5d	
Note: Do not medicate chickens or turkeys producing eggs for human consumption.					
Oxytet Soluble	Alpharma	Chickens Swine Turkeys	dw dw dw	 13d 5d	
Note: Do not feed to birds producing eggs for human consumption.					
Pabac®	Fort Dodge	Chickens Turkeys	S.C. S.C.	42d 42d	
Panacur® Beef and Dairy Cattle Dewormer	Intervet	Cattle	Oral	8d	0
Note: Do not use at 10 mg/kg in dairy cattle. No milk withdrawal period for milk at 5 mg/kg.					
Panacur® Cattle Dewormer	Intervet	Cattle	Oral	8d	0
Note: Do not use at 10 mg/kg in dairy cattle. No milk withdrawal period for milk at 5 mg/kg.					
Panacur® Cattle Dewormer (92 g)	Intervet	Cattle	Oral	8d	0
Panacur® Granules 22.2%	Intervet	Felidae Ursidae	In the feed In the feed		
Note: Do not use 14 days before or during the hunting season.					
Panacur® Granules 22.2% (Horse)	Intervet	Horses	In the feed		
Note: Not for use in horses intended for food.					
Panacur® Horse Dewormer	Intervet	Horses	Oral		
Note: Not for use in horses intended for food.					
Panacur® Horse Dewormer (25 g)	Intervet	Horses	Oral		
Note: Not for use in horses intended for food.					
Panacur® Horse Dewormer (57 g)	Intervet	Horses	Oral		
Note: Not for use in horses intended for food.					
Panacur® Horse Dewormer (92 g)	Intervet	Horses	Oral		
Note: Not for use in horses intended for food.					
Papillomune™	Biomune	Cattle	S.C.	21d	
Paraguard™ Shampoo	First Priority	Horses	Topical		
Note: Not for use on animals intended for food purposes.					
Parapac™	Schering-Plough	Swine	S.C.	21d	
Parapleuro Shield® P	Novartis Animal Vaccines	Swine	I.M.	21d	
Parapleuro Shield® P+BE	Novartis Animal Vaccines	Swine	I.M.	21d	
Para Shield®	Novartis Animal Vaccines	Swine	I.M.	21d	
Parvo Shield®	Novartis Animal Vaccines	Swine	I.M., S.C.	21d	
Parvo Shield® L5	Novartis Animal Vaccines	Swine	I.M., S.C.	21d	
Parvo Shield® L5E	Novartis Animal Vaccines	Swine	I.M., S.C.	21d	
Parvo-Vac®/Leptoferm-5®	Pfizer Animal Health	Swine	I.M.	21d	
Pasteurella Haemolytica Multocida Bacterin	Colorado Serum	Cattle Goats Sheep	S.C. S.C. S.C.	21d 21d 21d	

Please refer to product listings for more complete information.

Product Name	Company Name	Species	Route of Administration	Meat	Milk
Pasteurella Multocida Bacterin (Types 1, 3 & 4)	L.A.H.I. (New Jersey)	Chickens Turkeys	S.C. S.C.	42d 42d	
Pasteurella Multocida Bacterin (Types 1, 3, 4 & 3 x 4)	L.A.H.I. (New Jersey)	Chickens Turkeys	S.C. S.C.	42d 42d	
Patriot™ Insecticide Cattle Ear Tags	Boehringer Ingelheim	Cattle	Ear tags		
Note: Remove tags before slaughter.					
Pen-Aqueous	Durvet	Cattle Horses Sheep Swine	I.M. I.M. I.M. I.M.	10d 9d 7d	48h
Note: A withdrawal period has not been established for this product in pre-ruminating calves. Do not use in calves to be processed for veal. Not for use in horses intended for food.					
Pen-Aqueous	AgriPharm	Cattle Horses Sheep Swine Veal	I.M. I.M. I.M. I.M. I.M.	4d 8d 6d 7d	48h
Note: Not for use in horses intended for food.					
Penicillin G Potassium	AgriLabs	Turkeys	dw	1d	
Note: Do not feed to turkeys producing eggs for food.					
Penicillin G Potassium USP	Fort Dodge	Turkeys	dw	1d	
Note: Eggs from treated turkeys must not be used in food.					
Penicillin G Potassium, USP	Durvet	Turkeys	dw	1d	
Note: Do not use in birds producing eggs for food purposes.					
Penicillin G Potassium, USP	Bimeda	Turkeys	dw	1d	
Note: Do not use in birds producing eggs for food purposes.					
Penicillin G Potassium, USP	AgriPharm	Turkeys	dw	1d	
Note: Eggs from treated turkeys must not be used in food.					
Penicillin G Procaine	G.C. Hanford	Cattle Horses Sheep Swine	I.M. I.M. I.M. I.M.	10d 9d 7d	48h
Note: Not for use in horses intended for food.					
Pennchlor 50•G®	PennField	Cattle Chickens Sheep Swine Turkeys	In the feed In the feed In the feed In the feed In the feed	0-1d 0-1d 0 0 0	
Note: A withdrawal period has not been established for this product in pre-ruminating calves. Do not use in calves to be processed for veal. A withdrawal period is not required when used in chickens at levels up to 400 g/ton. A withdrawal period is not required when used in growing cattle at a level of 70 mg/head/day or less. Do not feed to chickens producing eggs for human consumption when used at levels above 200 g/ton. Do not feed to turkeys producing eggs for human consumption when used at levels of 25 mg/lb body weight/day. Withdraw from calves, beef cattle and non-lactating dairy cattle 1 day prior to slaughter when used at levels of 10 mg/lb body weight/day. Withdraw from cattle 1 day prior to slaughter when used at levels of 0.5 mg/lb body weight/day. Withdraw from chickens 24 hours prior to slaughter when used at levels of 500 g/ton.					
Pennchlor™ 50 Meal	PennField	Cattle Chickens Sheep Swine Turkeys	In the feed In the feed In the feed In the feed In the feed	0-1d 0-1d 0 0 0	
Note: A withdrawal period has not been established for this product in pre-ruminating calves. Do not use in calves to be processed for veal. A withdrawal period is not required when used in chickens at levels up to 400 g/ton. A withdrawal period is not required when used in growing cattle at a level of 70 mg/head/day or less. Do not feed to chickens producing eggs for human consumption. Do not feed to turkeys producing eggs for human consumption. Withdraw from calves, beef cattle and non-lactating dairy cattle 1 day prior to slaughter when used at levels of 10 mg/lb body weight/day. Withdraw from cattle 1 day prior to slaughter when used at levels of 0.5 mg/lb body weight/day. Withdraw from chickens 24 hours prior to slaughter when used at levels of 500 g/ton.					
Pennchlor™ 64 Soluble Powder	PennField	Calves Chickens Swine	dw dw dw	1d 0-1d 0	
Note: Do not administer to chickens at 1,000 mg/gallon of water within 24 hours before slaughter. Do not administer to laying birds.					
Pennchlor™ 70 Meal	PennField	Cattle Chickens Sheep Swine Turkeys	In the feed In the feed In the feed In the feed In the feed	0-1d 0-1d 0 0 0	
Note: A withdrawal period has not been established for this product in pre-ruminating calves. Do not use in calves to be processed for veal. A withdrawal period is not required when used in chickens at levels up to 400 g/ton. A withdrawal period is not required when used in growing cattle at a level of 70 mg/head/day or less. Do not feed to chickens producing eggs for human consumption when used at levels above 200 g/ton. Do not feed to turkeys producing eggs for human consumption when used at levels of 25 mg/lb body weight/day. Withdraw from calves, beef cattle and non-lactating dairy cattle 1 day prior to slaughter when used at levels of 10 mg/lb body weight/day. Withdraw from cattle 1 day prior to slaughter when used at levels of 0.5 mg/lb body weight/day. Withdraw from chickens 24 hours prior to slaughter when used at levels of 500 g/ton.					

Product Name	Company Name	Species	Route of Administration	Meat	Milk
Pennchlor 90•G®	PennField	Cattle	In the feed	0-1d	
		Chickens	In the feed	0-1d	
		Sheep	In the feed	0	
		Swine	In the feed	0	
		Turkeys	In the feed	0	

Note: A withdrawal period has not been established for this product in pre-ruminating calves. Do not use in calves to be processed for veal.
A withdrawal period is not required when used in chickens at levels up to 400 g/ton.
A withdrawal period is not required when used in growing cattle at a level of 70 mg/head/day or less.
Do not feed to chickens producing eggs for human consumption when used at levels above 200 g/ton.
Do not feed to turkeys producing eggs for human consumption when used at levels of 25 mg/lb body weight/day.
Withdraw from calves, beef cattle and non-lactating dairy cattle 1 day prior to slaughter when used at levels of 10 mg/lb body weight/day.
Withdraw from cattle 1 day prior to slaughter when used at levels of 0.5 mg/lb body weight/day.
Withdraw from chickens 24 hours prior to slaughter when used at levels of 500 g/ton.

Product Name	Company Name	Species	Route of Administration	Meat	Milk
Pennchlor 100 Hi-Flo™ Meal	PennField	Cattle	In the feed	0-1d	
		Chickens	In the feed	0-1d	
		Sheep	In the feed	0	
		Swine	In the feed	0	
		Turkeys	In the feed	0	

Note: A withdrawal period has not been established for this product in pre-ruminating calves. Do not use in calves to be processed for veal.
A withdrawal period is not required when used in growing cattle at a level of 70 mg/head/day or less.
Do not feed to chickens producing eggs for human consumption when used at levels of 10-400 g/ton.
Do not feed to turkeys producing eggs for human consumption.
Withdraw from calves, beef cattle and non-lactating dairy cattle 24 hours prior to slaughter when used at levels of 10 mg/lb body weight/day.
Withdraw from chickens 24 hours prior to slaughter when used at levels of 500 g/ton.

Product Name	Company Name	Species	Route of Administration	Meat	Milk
Pennchlor™ 100-MR	PennField	Cattle	In the feed	0-10d	

Note: A withdrawal period has not been established for this product in pre-ruminating calves. Do not use in calves to be processed for veal.
A withdrawal period is not required when fed at 0.1 mg/lb/day.
Withdraw 10 days before slaughter when fed at 10 mg/lb/day.

Product Name	Company Name	Species	Route of Administration	Meat	Milk
Pennchlor SP 250®	PennField	Swine	In the feed	15d	
Pennchlor SP 500®	PennField	Swine	In the feed	15d	
Pennox™ 50 Meal	PennField	Bees	In the feed		
		Cattle	In the feed	0-5d	
		Chickens	In the feed	0-3d	
		Sheep	In the feed	0-5d	
		Swine	In the feed	0-5d	
		Turkeys	In the feed	0-5d	

Note: Do not feed to chickens producing eggs for human consumption when used at levels of 400 g/ton and above.
Do not feed to turkeys producing eggs for food.
In low calcium feeds withdraw from chickens three days before slaughter (at levels of 400 g/ton and above).
Remove at least 6 weeks prior to main honey flow.
Withdraw from chickens 24 hours prior to slaughter when used at levels of 500 g/ton.
Withdraw from sheep, swine and cattle 5 days before slaughter when used at a dose of 10 mg/lb body weight/day.
Withdraw from turkeys 5 days before slaughter when used at levels of 200 g/ton or higher.

Product Name	Company Name	Species	Route of Administration	Meat	Milk
Pennox 100 Hi-Flo™ Meal	PennField	Bees	In the feed		
		Cattle	In the feed	0-5d	
		Chickens	In the feed	0-3d	
		Sheep	In the feed	0-5d	
		Swine	In the feed	0-5d	
		Turkeys	In the feed	0-5d	

Note: Do not feed to chickens producing eggs for human consumption when used at levels of 400 g/ton and above.
Do not feed to turkeys producing eggs for food.
In low calcium feeds withdraw from chickens three days before slaughter (at levels of 400 g/ton and above).
Remove at least 6 weeks prior to main honey flow.
Withdraw from chickens 24 hours prior to slaughter when used at levels of 500 g/ton.
Withdraw from sheep, swine and cattle 5 days before slaughter when used at a dose of 10 mg/lb body weight/day.
Withdraw from turkeys 5 days before slaughter when used at levels of 200 g/ton or higher.

Product Name	Company Name	Species	Route of Administration	Meat	Milk
Pennox™ 100-MR	PennField	Calves	In the feed	0-5d	

Note: Withdraw from calves 5 days before slaughter when used at a dose of 10 mg/lb body weight/day.

Product Name	Company Name	Species	Route of Administration	Meat	Milk
Pennox 200 Hi-Flo™ Meal	PennField	Bees	In the feed		
		Cattle	In the feed	0-5d	
		Chickens	In the feed	0-3d	
		Sheep	In the feed	0-5d	
		Swine	In the feed	0-5d	
		Turkeys	In the feed	0-5d	

Note: A withdrawal period is not required when used in chickens at levels up to 400 g/ton.
A withdrawal period is not required when used in turkeys at levels lower than 200 g/ton.
Do not feed to chickens producing eggs for human consumption when used at levels of 400 g/ton and above.
Do not feed to turkeys producing eggs for human consumption.
In low calcium feeds withdraw from chickens three days before slaughter (at levels of 400 g/ton and above).
Remove at least 6 weeks prior to main honey flow.
Withdraw from chickens 24 hours prior to slaughter when used at levels of 500 g/ton.
Withdraw from sheep, swine and cattle 5 days before slaughter when used at a dose of 10 mg/lb body weight/day.
Withdraw from turkeys 5 days before slaughter when used at levels of 200 g/ton or higher.

Product Name	Company Name	Species	Route of Administration	Meat	Milk
Pennox™ 200 Injectable	PennField	Calves	I.M., S.C.	28d	
		Cattle	I.M., I.V., S.C.	28d	
		Swine	I.M.	28d	

Note: Not for use in lactating dairy animals.

Product Name	Company Name	Species	Route of Administration	Meat	Milk
Pennox™ 343 Soluble Powder	PennField	Cattle	dw	5d	
		Chickens	dw	0	
		Sheep	dw	5d	
		Swine	dw	0	
		Turkeys	dw	0	
Note: Do not administer to chickens or turkeys producing eggs for human consumption.					
Performer® Ear Mite Killer	AgriLabs	Horses	Topical		
Note: Not for use on horses intended for food.					
Permectrin™ II	Boehringer Ingelheim	Swine	Topical	5d	
Permectrin™ II	Aspen	Swine	Topical	5d	
Permectrin™ Fly & Louse Dust	Boehringer Ingelheim	Swine	Topical	5d	
Permethrin 0.25% Dust	AgriLabs	Swine	Topical	5d	
Permethrin 10%	Durvet	Swine	Topical	5d	
Pet Care Ear Mite Lotion & Repellent	Durvet	Horses	Topical		
Note: Do not use on meat or milk producing animals.					
Phenylbutazone 20% Injection	Vet Tek	Horses	I.V.		
Note: Not for use in horses intended for food.					
Phenylbutazone Injection 20%	RXV	Horses	I.V.		
Note: Not for use in horses intended for food.					
Phenylbutazone Injection 20%	Aspen	Horses	I.V.		
Note: Not for use in horses intended for food.					
Phenylbutazone Injection 200 mg/mL	Butler	Horses	I.V.		
Note: Not for use in horses intended for food.					
Phenylbutazone Tablets, USP	Vet Tek	Horses	Oral		
Note: Not for use in horses intended for food.					
Phenylbutazone Tablets, USP 1 gram	Butler	Horses	Oral		
Note: Not for use in horses intended for food.					
Phenylbute® Injection 20%	Phoenix Pharmaceutical	Horses	I.V.		
Note: Not for use in horses intended for food.					
Phenylbute® Paste	Phoenix Pharmaceutical	Horses	Oral		
Note: Not for use in horses intended for food.					
Phenylbute® Tablets 1 gram	Phoenix Pharmaceutical	Horses	Oral		
Note: Not for use in horses intended for food.					
Phenylzone® Paste	Schering-Plough	Horses	Oral		
Note: Not for use in horses intended for food.					
PHF-Vax®	Schering-Plough	Horses	I.M.	21d	
P.H.M. Bac® 1	AgriLabs	Cattle	I.M.	21d	
Pigeon Pox Vaccine	ASL	Chickens	ww	21d	
Pigeon Pox Vaccine (Chickens and Turkeys)	L.A.H.I. (New Jersey)	Chickens	ww	21d	
		Turkeys	ww	21d	
Piliguard® E. Coli-1	Schering-Plough	Cattle	I.M.	60d	
Piliguard® Pinkeye-1	Schering-Plough	Cattle	I.M.	60d	
Piliguard® Pinkeye-1	Durvet	Cattle	I.M., S.C.	60d	
Piliguard® Pinkeye + 7	Schering-Plough	Cattle	S.C.	21d	
Pinkeye-3	Aspen	Cattle	I.M., S.C.	21d	
Pinkeye Shield™ XT4	Novartis Animal Vaccines	Cattle	I.M.	60d	
Pinnacle™ I.N.	Fort Dodge	Horses	I.N.	30d	
Pipovax®	Schering-Plough	Chickens	ww	21d	
Pirsue® Sterile Solution	Pharmacia & Upjohn	Dairy cattle	I.M.M.	9d	36h
Plazvax®	Schering-Plough	Cattle	S.C.	60d	
PleuroGuard® 4	Pfizer Animal Health	Swine	I.M., S.C.	21d	
PM-Onevax™	Schering-Plough	Turkeys	dw	21d	
PM-Onevax®-C	Schering-Plough	Chickens	ww	21d	
		Turkeys	ww	21d	
Pneumabort-K®+1b	Fort Dodge	Horses	I.M.	60d	
Pneumosuis® III	Pfizer Animal Health	Swine	I.M., S.C.	21d	
Pneu Pac®	Schering-Plough	Swine	I.M., S.C.	60d	
Pneu Pac®-ER	Schering-Plough	Swine	I.M.	60d	
Pneu Parapac®+ER	Schering-Plough	Swine	S.C.	60d	
Poly-Bac B® 3	Texas Vet Lab	Cattle	S.C.	60d	
Poly-Bac B® 7	Texas Vet Lab	Cattle	S.C.	60d	
Poly-Bac B® Somnus	Texas Vet Lab	Cattle	S.C.	60d	
Polybron® B_1	ASL	Chickens	dw, I.O.	21d	
Polybron® N-63	ASL	Chickens	dw, I.O.	21d	
Polyflex®	Fort Dodge	Cattle	I.M.	6d	48h

Please refer to product listings for more complete information.

Product Name	Company Name	Species	Route of Administration	Meat	Milk
Polyotic® Soluble Powder	Fort Dodge	Calves Swine	dw dw	4d 7d	
Note: A withdrawal period has not been established for this product in pre-ruminating calves. Do not use in calves to be processed for veal.					
Poly Serum®	Novartis Animal Vaccines	Cattle Sheep	I.M., S.C. I.M., S.C.	21d 21d	
Porcine Ecolizer® 3	Novartis Animal Vaccines	Swine	Oral	21d	
Porcine Ecolizer® 3+C	Novartis Animal Vaccines	Swine	Oral	21d	
Porcine Pili Shield™	Novartis Animal Vaccines	Swine	I.M.	21d	
Porcine Pili Shield™ +C	Novartis Animal Vaccines	Swine	I.M.	21d	
Poridon™	Neogen	Horses	Topical		
Note: Not for use on horses intended for food.					
Posilac 1 Step®	Monsanto	Dairy cattle	S.C.	0	0
PotomacGuard®	Fort Dodge	Horses	I.M.	60d	
PotomacGuard® EWT	Fort Dodge	Horses	I.M.	60d	
Potomac Shield™	Novartis Animal Vaccines	Horses	I.M.	21d	
Poulvac® Chick-N-Pox™	Fort Dodge	Chickens	ww	21d	
Poulvac® Coryza ABC IC$_3$	Fort Dodge	Chickens	I.M., S.C.	42d	
Poulvac® Marek Rispens CVI+HVT	Fort Dodge	Chicks	S.C.	21d	
Poulvac® SE	Fort Dodge	Chickens	S.C.	21d	
Poulvac® SE-ND-IB	Fort Dodge	Chickens	S.C.	21d	
Pox Blen®	Merial Select	Chickens	ww	21d	
Poximune®	Biomune	Chickens	ww	21d	
Poximune® AE	Biomune	Chickens	ww	21d	
Poxine®	Fort Dodge	Chickens Turkeys	ww ww	21d 21d	
PP-Vac®	Intervet	Chickens	ww	21d	
Note: Do not vaccinate within 4 weeks of initial egg production.					
Pre-Conditioning/Receiving Formula Gel	Durvet	Cattle Goats Sheep	Oral Oral Oral	0 0 0	
Predef® 2X	Pharmacia & Upjohn	Cattle Horses Swine	I.M. I.A., I.M. I.M.	7d 7d 7d	
Note: A withdrawal period has not been established for this product in pre-ruminating calves. Do not use in calves to be processed for veal.					
Prefarrow Shield™ 9	Novartis Animal Vaccines	Swine	I.M.	21d	
Prefarrow Strep Shield®	Novartis Animal Vaccines	Swine	I.M.	21d	
PregGuard™ FP 9	Pfizer Animal Health	Cattle	I.M.	21d	
Presponse® HM	Fort Dodge	Cattle	I.M.	21d	
Presponse® SQ	Fort Dodge	Cattle	S.C.	21d	
Prestige® with Havlogen®	Intervet	Horses	I.M.	21d	
Prestige® II with Havlogen®	Intervet	Horses	I.M.	21d	
Prestige® V with Havlogen®	Intervet	Horses	I.M.	21d	
Prestige® V + VEE with Havlogen®	Intervet	Horses	I.M.	21d	
Prevail MycoPlex™	Aspen	Swine	S.C.	60d	
Prevail™ Para Pleuro Bac+3DT	Aspen	Swine	I.M.	21d	
Prevail™ Parvoplex 6-Way+E	Aspen	Swine	I.M.	21d	
Pre-Vent 6™	AgriLabs	Cattle	I.M., S.C.	21d	
Pributazone™ Tablets	First Priority	Horses	Oral		
Note: Not for use in horses intended for food.					
Primevac IBD-3®	Intervet	Chickens	dw	21d	
Prism™ 4	Fort Dodge	Cattle	I.M., S.C.	21d	
Prism™ 9	Fort Dodge	Cattle	I.M., S.C.	21d	
Privasan™ Antiseptic Ointment	First Priority	Horses	Topical		
Note: Not for use on horses intended for food.					
Privermectin™ Drench for Sheep	First Priority	Sheep	Oral	11d	
Privermectin™ Equine Oral Liquid	First Priority	Horses	Oral		
Note: Not for use in horses intended for food.					
Pro-Bac-C	AgriLabs	Cattle	In milk replacer		
Note: A withdrawal period has not been established for this product in pre-ruminating calves. Do not use in calves to be processed for veal.					
Pro-Bute™ Injection	AgriLabs	Horses	I.V.		
Note: Not for use in horses intended for food.					
Pro-Bute™ Tablets 1 gram	AgriLabs	Horses	Oral		
Note: Not for use in horses intended for food.					
Prodigy® with Havlogen®	Intervet	Horses	I.M.	21d	

Please refer to product listings for more complete information.

Product Name	Company Name	Species	Route of Administration	Meat	Milk
Produmec™ Injection for Cattle and Swine	TradeWinds	Bison Cattle Reindeer Swine	S.C. S.C. S.C. S.C.	56d 35d 56d 18d	
Note: Do not use in female dairy cattle of breeding age.					
Produmec™ Pour-On for Cattle	TradeWinds	Cattle	Topical	48d	
Note: Do not use on female dairy cattle of breeding age.					
Pro-Gen® 20%	Fleming	Chickens Swine Turkeys	In the feed In the feed In the feed	5d 5d 5d	
Pro-Gen® 100%	Fleming	Chickens Swine Turkeys	In the feed In the feed In the feed	5d 5d 5d	
Prohibit® Soluble Drench Powder	AgriLabs	Cattle Sheep	Oral Oral	48h 72h	
Note: Do not administer to dairy cattle of breeding age.					
Prolate®/Lintox®-HD	Wellmark	Cattle Swine	Topical Topical	3d 1d	
Note: Do not treat non-lactating dairy cattle within 28 days of freshening. If freshening should occur within 28 days after treatment, do not use milk as human food for the remainder of the 28-day interval.					
PromAce® Injectable	Fort Dodge	Horses	I.M., I.V., S.C.		
Note: Not for use in horses intended for food.					
ProMectin B™ Pour-On For Cattle	Vedco	Cattle	Topical	48d	
Note: Do not use in female dairy cattle of breeding age.					
ProMectin E™ Liquid for Horses	Vedco	Horses	Oral		
Note: Not for use in horses intended for food.					
ProMectin E™ Paste	Vedco	Horses	Oral		
Note: Not for use in horses intended for food.					
ProMectin™ Injection for Cattle and Swine	Vedco	Bison Cattle Reindeer Swine	S.C. S.C. S.C. S.C.	56d 35d 56d 18d	
Note: A milk discard period has not been established for this product in lactating dairy cattle. Do not use in female dairy cattle 20 months of age or older.					
Promycin™ 100	Phoenix Pharmaceutical	Cattle	I.V.	22d	
Note: A withdrawal period has not been established for this product in pre-ruminating calves. Do not use in calves to be processed for veal. Not for use in lactating dairy animals.					
Prorab®-1	Intervet	Sheep	I.M.	21d	
ProstaMate™	Butler	Cattle Horses Swine	I.M. I.M. I.M.	0 0	0
Note: Not for use in horses intended for food.					
ProstaMate™	RXV	Cattle Horses Swine	I.M. I.M. I.M.	0 0	0
Note: Not for use in horses intended for food.					
ProstaMate™	Vedco	Cattle Horses Swine	I.M. I.M. I.M.	0 0	0
Note: Not for use in horses intended for food.					
ProstaMate®	Phoenix Pharmaceutical	Cattle Horses Swine	I.M. I.M. I.M.	0 0	0
Note: Not for use in horses intended for food.					
ProstaMate™	Vet Tek	Cattle Horses Swine	I.M. I.M. I.M.	0 0	0
Note: Not for use in horses intended for food.					
ProstaMate®	Vetus	Cattle Horses Swine	I.M. I.M. I.M.	0 0	0
Note: Not for use in horses intended for food.					
ProstaMate™	Aspen	Cattle Horses Swine	I.M. I.M. I.M.	0 0	0
Note: Not for use in horses intended for food.					
ProSystem® CE	Intervet	Swine	I.M., S.C.	21d	
ProSystem® Pilimune	Intervet	Cattle Swine	I.M., S.C. I.M., S.C.	21d 21d	
ProSystem® RCE	Intervet	Swine	I.M.	21d	
ProSystem® Rota	Intervet	Swine	I.M., Oral	21d	
ProSystem® TGE	Intervet	Swine	I.M., Oral	21d	
ProSystem® TG-Emune® Rota with Imugen® II	Intervet	Swine	I.M., I.P.	60d	

Please refer to product listings for more complete information.

Product Name	Company Name	Species	Route of Administration	Meat	Milk
ProSystem® TG-Emune® with Imugen® II	Intervet	Swine	I.M., I.P.	60d	
ProSystem® TGE/Rota	Intervet	Swine	I.M., Oral	21d	
ProSystem® TREC	Intervet	Swine	I.M., Oral	21d	
Pro'tect™ HE	Brinton	Turkeys	dw	21d	
Proud Flesh Powder	First Priority	Horses	Topical		
Note: Not for use on horses intended for food.					
Proudsoff™	Creative Science	Cattle Goats Horses Sheep	Topical Topical Topical Topical		
Note: Not for use on animals intended for food purposes.					
Pro Vac® 2 ACL™	Fort Dodge	Chickens	I.M., S.C.	42d	
Pro Vac® 3 ACL™	Fort Dodge	Chickens	I.M., S.C.	42d	
Pro Vac® 4 ACL™	Fort Dodge	Chickens	I.M., S.C.	42d	
ProVac ND/IBD/Reo ACL™	Fort Dodge	Chickens	I.M., S.C.	42d	
Prozap® Drycide®	Loveland	Swine	Topical	5d	
Prozap® Dust'R™	Loveland	Cattle Poultry Swine	Topical Topical Topical	0 0 0	0
Prozap® Garden & Poultry Dust	Loveland	Poultry	Topical	7d	
Prozap® Insectrin® Dust	Loveland	Swine	Topical	5d	
Prozap® Insectrin® X	Loveland	Swine	Topical	5d	
Prozap® Ivermectin Pour-On	Loveland	Cattle	Topical	48d	
Note: Do not use in female dairy cattle of breeding age.					
PRRomiSE®	Intervet	Swine	I.M.	21d	
PR-Vac®	Pfizer Animal Health	Swine	I.M.	21d	
PR-Vac®-Killed	Pfizer Animal Health	Swine	I.M.	21d	
PR-Vac Plus™	Pfizer Animal Health	Swine	I.M.	21d	
PRV-Begonia with Diluvac Forte®	Intervet	Swine	I.M.	21d	
PRV/Marker Gold®	SyntroVet	Swine	I.M., I.N.	21d	
PRV/Marker Gold®-MaxiVac® FLU	SyntroVet	Swine	I.M.	21d	
PT Blen®	Merial Select	Chickens Turkeys	ww ww	21d 21d	
Note: Do not vaccinate chickens within 4 weeks of onset of egg production or during egg production.					
Pulmo-guard™ PH-M	Boehringer Ingelheim	Cattle	S.C.	60d	
Pulmo-guard™ PHM-1	Boehringer Ingelheim	Cattle	S.C.	60d	
Pulmotil® 90	Elanco	Swine	In the feed	7d	
Purple Lotion	Vedco	Horses	Topical		
Note: Not for use on horses intended for food.					
Purple Lotion Wound Dressing	Durvet	Horses	Topical		
Note: Not for use on horses intended for food.					
Purple Lotion Wound Dressing	First Priority	Horses	Topical		
Note: Not for use on horses intended for food.					
Pyramid® 4+Presponse® SQ	Fort Dodge	Cattle	S.C.	21d	
Pyramid® 8	Fort Dodge	Cattle	I.M., S.C.	21d	
Pyramid® 9	Fort Dodge	Cattle	I.M., S.C.	21d	
Pyramid® IBR	Fort Dodge	Cattle	I.M., S.C.	21d	
Pyramid® IBR+Lepto	Fort Dodge	Cattle	I.M., S.C.	21d	
Pyramid® MLV 3	Fort Dodge	Cattle	I.M., S.C.	21d	
Pyramid® MLV 4	Fort Dodge	Cattle	I.M., S.C.	21d	
Quartermaster®	Pharmacia & Upjohn	Dairy cattle	I.M.M.	60d	96h
Note: Animals infused with this product must not be slaughtered for use in food within 96 hours after calving. Not for use in lactating cows. This product must not be used within 6 weeks of the expected date of calving.					
Quatracon-2X™	Boehringer Ingelheim	Cattle	S.C.	21d	
Quest® 2% Equine Oral Gel	Fort Dodge	Horses	Oral		
Note: Do not use in horses or ponies intended for food.					
Quick Shield™ Intranasal IBR-PI3	Novartis Animal Vaccines	Cattle	I.N.	21d	
Rabdomun® Vaccine	Schering-Plough	Cattle Sheep	I.M. I.M.	21d 21d	
Rabon® 3% Dust	AgriLabs	Cattle Swine	Topical Topical	0 0	0
Rabon® 7.76 Oral Larvicide Premix	Boehringer Ingelheim	Horses	In the feed		
Note: This product is not to be used on horses destined for slaughter.					
Rabvac™ 3	Fort Dodge	Horses	I.M.	21d	
Ralgro® Implants (Cattle)	Schering-Plough	Cattle	Implant		
Note: Not for use in lactating dairy animals.					

Please refer to product listings for more complete information.

Product Name	Company Name	Species	Route of Administration	Meat	Milk
Ralgro® Implants (Lamb)	Schering-Plough	Sheep	Implant	40d	
Ralgro® Magnum™ Implants	Schering-Plough	Beef cattle	Implant		
Note: Implant in the ear only. Do not attempt to salvage the implanted ear for human or animal food.					
Rally™ -20	Vedco	Cattle Horses	I.M., I.V. I.M.	4d	24h
Note: A withdrawal period has not been established for this product in pre-ruminating calves. Do not use in calves to be processed for veal. Not for use in horses intended for food.					
Ram Epididymitis Bacterin	Colorado Serum	Sheep	S.C.	21d	
Ravap® E.C.	Boehringer Ingelheim	Cattle	Topical	0	0
Re-Covr® Injection	Fort Dodge	Cattle Horses	I.M., I.V. I.M.	4d	24h
Note: A withdrawal period has not been established for this product in pre-ruminating calves. Do not use in calves to be processed for veal. Not for use in horses intended for food.					
Reducine® Absorbent for Horses	Equicare	Horses	Topical		
Note: Not for use on horses intended for food.					
Regressin®-V	Bioniche Animal Health	Horses	I.Tum.		
Note: Not for use in horses intended for food.					
Regu-Mate® Solution	Intervet	Horses	Oral		
Note: Not for use in horses intended for food.					
Reliant® 3	Merial	Cattle	I.M., S.C.	21d	
Reliant® 4	Merial	Cattle	I.M., S.C.	21d	
Reliant® 8	Merial	Cattle	I.M.	21d	
Reliant® IBR	Merial	Cattle	I.M., S.C.	21d	
Reliant® IBR/BVD	Merial	Cattle	I.M., S.C.	21d	
Reliant® IBR/Lepto	Merial	Cattle	I.M.	21d	
Reliant® Plus BVD-K (Dual IBR™)	Merial	Cattle	I.M.	21d	
Reliant® Plus (Dual IBR™)	Merial	Cattle	I.M., S.C.	21d	
Relief! Fly Ointment	Davis	Horses	Topical		
Note: Not for use on horses intended for food.					
Renogen	Novartis (Aqua Health)	Salmonids	I.P.	60d	
Ren-O-Sal® Tablets	Fort Dodge	Chickens Turkeys	dw dw	5d 5d	
Reoguard L	Merial Select	Chickens	dw	21d	
Reomune® 2	Biomune	Chickens	S.C.	42d	
Reomune® 3	Biomune	Chickens	S.C.	42d	
Reomune® SS412	Biomune	Chickens	S.C.	42d	
Repel-X® Lotion	Farnam	Horses	Topical		
Note: Not for use on horses intended for food.					
Repel-X®p Emulsifiable Fly Spray	Farnam	Horses	Topical		
Note: Not for use on horses intended for food.					
ReproCyc® PRRS-PLE	Boehringer Ingelheim	Swine	I.M.	21d	
Repromune™ 4	Biomune	Chickens	S.C.	42d	
Repromune™ IBD	Biomune	Chickens	S.C.	42d	
Repromune™ IBD/ND	Biomune	Chickens	S.C.	42d	
Repromune™ IBD/ND/IB	Biomune	Chickens	S.C.	42d	
Repromune IBD/ND/REO™	Biomune	Chickens	S.C.	42d	
Repromune™ IBD/Reo	Biomune	Chickens	S.C.	42d	
Resist™ 7	AgriPharm	Cattle Sheep	S.C. S.C.	21d 21d	
Resist™ 7HS	AgriPharm	Cattle	S.C.	21d	
Resist™ 8	AgriPharm	Cattle Sheep	S.C. S.C.	21d 21d	
Respimune™	Biomune	Chickens	aer/sp, dw, I.O.	21d	
Respiragen™ Serum Antibodies	Colorado Serum	Cattle Sheep Swine	I.M., S.C. I.M., S.C. I.M., S.C.	21d 21d 21d	
Respishield™ 4	Merial	Cattle	I.M., S.C.	21d	
Respishield™ 4 L5	Merial	Cattle	I.M., S.C.	21d	
RespiSure®	Pfizer Animal Health	Swine	I.M.	21d	
RespiSure 1 ONE®	Pfizer Animal Health	Swine	I.M.	21d	
RespiSure 1 ONE®/ER Bac Plus®	Pfizer Animal Health	Swine	I.M.	21d	
ResProMune® 4	AgriLabs	Cattle	I.M., S.C.	21d	
ResProMune® 4 I-B-P+BRSV	AgriLabs	Cattle	I.M., S.C.	60d	
ResProMune® 4+SomnuMune® (I.M.)	AgriLabs	Cattle	I.M.	60d	
ResProMune® 4+SomnuMune® (I.M., S.C.)	AgriLabs	Cattle	I.M., S.C.	21d	
ResProMune® 5+VL5	AgriLabs	Cattle	I.M.	60d	

Product Name	Company Name	Species	Route of Administration	Meat	Milk
ResProMune® 8	AgriLabs	Cattle	I.M., S.C.	21d	
ResProMune™ 9	AgriLabs	Cattle	I.M., S.C.	21d	
ResProMune™ 10	AgriLabs	Cattle	I.M., S.C.	21d	
Resvac® 4/Somubac®	Pfizer Animal Health	Cattle	I.M.	21d	
Resvac® BRSV/Somubac®	Pfizer Animal Health	Cattle	I.M.	21d	
Revalor®-200	Intervet	Beef cattle	Implant		
Note: Implant in the ear only. Do not attempt to salvage the implanted ear for human or animal food. Not for use in dairy animals.					
Revalor®-G	Intervet	Beef cattle	Implant		
Note: Implant in the ear only. Do not attempt to salvage the implanted ear for human or animal food. Not for use in dairy animals.					
Revalor®-H	Intervet	Beef cattle	Implant		
Note: Implant in the ear only. Do not attempt to salvage the implanted ear for human or animal food. Not for use in dairy animals.					
Revalor®-IH	Intervet	Beef cattle	Implant		
Note: Implant in the ear only. Do not attempt to salvage the implanted ear for human or animal food. Not for use in dairy animals.					
Revalor®-IS	Intervet	Beef cattle	Implant		
Note: Implant in the ear only. Do not attempt to salvage the implanted ear for human or animal food. Not for use in dairy animals.					
Revalor®-S	Intervet	Beef cattle	Implant		
Note: Implant in the ear only. Do not attempt to salvage the implanted ear for human or animal food. Not for use in dairy animals.					
Rhinicell®	Novartis Animal Vaccines	Swine	I.M., I.N.	21d	
Rhinicell®+E	Novartis Animal Vaccines	Swine	I.M., I.N.	21d	
Rhini Shield™ TX4	Novartis Animal Vaccines	Swine	I.M., S.C.	21d	
Rhinogen® BPE	Intervet	Swine	I.M., S.C.	21d	
Rhinogen® CTE 5000	Intervet	Swine	I.M., S.C.	21d	
Rhinogen® CTSE	Intervet	Swine	I.M., S.C.	21d	
Rhinomune®	Pfizer Animal Health	Horses	I.M.	21d	
RIS-MA™	Intervet	Chickens	S.C.	21d	
RIS-MA-SB™	Intervet	Chickens	S.C.	21d	
Rismavac®	Intervet	Chickens	S.C.	21d	
Note: Do not vaccinate birds within 21 days of onset of egg production.					
Robaxin®-V Injectable	Fort Dodge	Horses	I.V.		
Note: Not for use in horses intended for food.					
Robenz®	Alpharma	Chickens	Oral	5d	
Note: Do not feed to chickens producing eggs for human consumption.					
RofenAid® 40	Alpharma	Chickens Ducks Turkeys	In the feed In the feed In the feed	5d 5d 5d	
Note: Do not feed to ducks producing eggs for food. Do not feed to turkeys producing eggs for food.					
Roll-On™ Fly Repellent	Farnam	Horses	Topical		
Note: Not for use on horses intended for food.					
Romet® 30	Alpharma	Catfish Salmon Trout	In the feed In the feed In the feed	3d 42d 42d	
Rotamune® with Imugen® II	Intervet	Swine	I.M., I.P.	60d	
Rotectin™ 1 Paste 1.87%	Farnam	Horses	Oral		
Note: Not for use in horses intended for food.					
Rotectin™ 2 Paste	Farnam	Horses	Oral		
Note: Not for use in horses intended for food.					
R-Pen	Alpharma	Turkeys	dw	1d	
Note: Do not feed to turkeys producing eggs for food.					
Rubeola Virus Immunomodulator	Eudaemonic	Horses	S.C.		
Note: Not for use in horses intended for food.					
Rumatel®	Phibro	Cattle	In the feed	14d	0
Rumensin® 80	Elanco	Cattle Goats	In the feed In the feed		
Note: A withdrawal period has not been established for this product in pre-ruminating calves. Do not use in calves to be processed for veal. Do not feed to lactating dairy cows. Do not feed to lactating goats.					
Saber™ Extra Insecticide Ear Tags	Schering-Plough	Cattle	Ear tags		
Note: Remove tags before slaughter.					
Saber™ Pour-On Insecticide	Schering-Plough	Beef cattle	Topical		
Note: Do not apply to lactating or dry dairy cows. Not recommended for use on veal calves.					
Sacox® 60	Intervet	Chickens	In the feed	0	
Note: Do not feed to laying birds.					

Product Name	Company Name	Species	Route of Administration	Meat	Milk
Safe-Guard® 20% Dewormer Type A Medicated Article	Intervet	Cattle Swine Wild animals Zoo animals	In the feed In the feed In the feed In the feed	13d 0	0
Note: Do not use 14 days before or during the hunting season.					
Safe-Guard® Beef & Dairy Cattle Dewormer	Intervet	Cattle	Oral	8d	0
Safe-Guard® Beef and Dairy Cattle Dewormer (290 g)	Intervet	Cattle	Oral	8d	0
Safe-Guard® Cattle Dewormer (92 g)	Intervet	Cattle	Oral	8d	0
Safe-Guard® Equine Dewormer (25 g)	Intervet	Horses	Oral		
Note: Not for use in horses intended for food.					
Safe-Guard® Horse Dewormer (92 g)	Intervet	Horses	Oral		
Note: Not for use in horses intended for food.					
Safe-Guard® Medicated Dewormer for Beef & Dairy Cattle, & Swine	Intervet	Cattle Swine	In the feed In the feed	13d 0	0
Safe-Guard® Medicated Dewormer for Beef & Dairy Cattle (Flaked Meal)	Intervet	Cattle	In the feed	13d	0
Safe-Guard® Medicated Dewormer for Beef & Dairy Cattle (Soft Mini-Pellets)	Intervet	Cattle	In the feed	13d	0
Safe-Guard® Medicated Dewormer for Beef Cattle (20% Protein Block)	Intervet	Beef cattle	Oral	16d	
Safe-Guard® Medicated Dewormer for Beef Cattle (En-Pro-Al® Molasses Block)	Intervet	Beef cattle	Oral	11d	
Safe-Guard® Medicated Dewormer for Swine (EZ Scoop®)	Intervet	Swine	In the feed	0	
Sal Bac®	Biomune	Pigeons	S.C.	21d	
Salix™ Injection 5%	Intervet	Cattle Horses	I.M., I.V. I.M., I.V.	48h	48h
Note: Not for use in horses intended for food.					
Salix™ Tablets	Intervet	Cattle Horses	Oral Oral	48h	48h
Note: Not for use in horses intended for food.					
Salmonella Dublin-Typhimurium Bacterin	Colorado Serum	Cattle	S.C.	21d	
Salmo Shield® 2	Novartis Animal Vaccines	Swine	I.M., S.C.	21d	
Salmo Shield® Live	Novartis Animal Vaccines	Swine	I.M.	21d	
Salmo Shield® T	Novartis Animal Vaccines	Cattle	I.M., S.C.	21d	
Salmo Shield® TD	Novartis Animal Vaccines	Cattle	I.M., S.C.	21d	
Salmo Vac	AgriPharm	Cattle	I.M., S.C.	21d	
Salmune™	Biomune	Chickens	aer/sp, dw	28d	
Sarcocystis Neurona Vaccine	Fort Dodge	Horses	I.M.	21d	
SB-1 Frozen	Intervet	Chickens	S.C.	21d	
SB-Vac®	Intervet	Chickens	S.C.	21d	
Scarlet Oil	Vedco	Horses	Topical		
Note: Not for use on horses intended for food.					
Scarlet Oil	First Priority	Horses	Topical		
Note: Not for use on animals intended for food purposes.					
Scarlet Oil Smear	First Priority	Horses	Topical		
Note: Not for use on food-producing animals.					
Scarlet Oil with Aloe Vera	Life Science	Horses	Topical		
Note: Not for use on horses intended for food.					
Scarlet Oil Wound Dressing	Durvet	Horses	Topical		
Note: Not for use on horses intended for food.					
Scarlet Oil Wound Dressing	AgriPharm	Horses	Topical		
Note: Not for use on horses intended for food.					
Scarlex® Scarlet Oil	Farnam	Horses	Topical		
Note: Not for use in animals intended for food purposes.					
Score®	Intervet	Swine	I.M., S.C.	21d	
Scour Bos™ 4	Novartis Animal Vaccines	Cattle	I.M.	60d	
Scour Bos™ 6	Novartis Animal Vaccines	Cattle	I.M.	60d	
Scour Bos™ 9	Novartis Animal Vaccines	Cattle	I.M.	60d	
ScourGuard 3® (K)	Pfizer Animal Health	Cattle	I.M.	21d	
ScourGuard 3® (K)/C	Pfizer Animal Health	Cattle	I.M.	21d	
Scourmune®	Schering-Plough	Swine	S.C.	21d	
Scourmune®-C	Schering-Plough	Swine	S.C.	21d	
Scourmune®-CR	Schering-Plough	Swine	I.M.	60d	
Scour Vac™ 2K	Durvet	Cattle	I.M.	60d	
Scour Vac™ 3K+C	Durvet	Cattle	I.M.	60d	

Product Name	Company Name	Species	Route of Administration	Meat	Milk
Scour Vac™ 4	AgriLabs	Cattle	I.M.	60d	
Scour Vac™ 9	AgriLabs	Cattle	I.M.	60d	
Scour Vac™ E Coli + C	AgriLabs	Cattle	I.M.	60d	
Screwworm Ear Tick Aerosol	Durvet	Swine	Topical	5d	
SDM Injection	Phoenix Pharmaceutical	Cattle	I.V.	5d	60h
Note: A withdrawal period has not been established for this product in pre-ruminating calves. Do not use in calves to be processed for veal.					
SDM Powder	Bimeda	Cattle Chickens Turkeys	dw dw dw	7d 5d 5d	
Note: A withdrawal period has not been established for this product in pre-ruminating calves. Do not use in calves to be processed for veal. Do not administer to chickens over 16 weeks (112 days) of age. Do not administer to turkeys over 24 weeks (168 days) of age.					
SDM Solution	Phoenix Pharmaceutical	Cattle Chickens Turkeys	dw dw dw	7d 5d 5d	
Note: A withdrawal period has not been established for this product in pre-ruminating calves. Do not use in calves to be processed for veal. Do not administer to chickens over 16 weeks (112 days) of age. Do not administer to turkeys over 24 weeks (168 days) of age.					
SDT-Guard™	Boehringer Ingelheim	Cattle	I.M., S.C.	60d	
Sedazine®	Fort Dodge	Cervidae Horses	I.M. I.M., I.V.		
Note: Do not use in *Cervidae* less than 15 days before or during the hunting season. Not for use in food-producing animals. Not for use in horses intended for food.					
Serpens Species Bacterin	Hygieia	Cattle	S.C.	21d	
Shin-O-Gel®	Hawthorne	Horses	Topical		
Note: Not for use on horses intended for food.					
Shor-Bron D	ASL	Chickens	dw	21d	
Shurjets	Jorgensen	Dairy cattle	I.M.M.	0	48h
Singlvax®	Schering-Plough	Chickens	aer/sp, dw	21d	
Siteguard® G	Schering-Plough	Cattle Sheep	I.M., S.C. I.M., S.C.	21d 21d	
Siteguard® MLG Vaccine	Schering-Plough	Cattle Sheep	I.M., S.C. I.M., S.C.	21d 21d	
Sodium Iodide	AgriLabs	Cattle	I.V.		
Note: Not for use in lactating cows.					
Sodium Iodide	Vet Tek	Cattle	I.V.		
Note: Not for use in lactating dairy cows.					
Sodium Iodide 20%	RXV	Cattle	I.V.		
Note: Not for use in lactating dairy cows.					
Sodium Iodide 20% Injection	Vedco	Cattle	I.V.		
Note: Not for use in lactating dairy cows.					
Sodium Iodide 20% Injection	Phoenix Pharmaceutical	Cattle	I.V.		
Note: Not for use in lactating dairy cows.					
Sodium Iodide 20% Injection	Aspen	Cattle	I.V.		
Note: Not for use in lactating dairy cows.					
Sodium Iodide Solution 20%	Butler	Cattle	I.V.		
Note: Not for use in lactating dairy cows.					
Solu/Tet	Vedco	Calves Chickens Swine Turkeys	dw dw dw dw	5d 4d 4d 4d	
Note: Do not administer to laying hens when eggs are destined for human consumption.					
Solu-Tet® 324	Alpharma	Chickens	dw	4d	
Note: Do not use in laying hens producing eggs for human consumption.					
SomnuMune®	AgriLabs	Cattle	I.M., S.C.	21d	
Somnu Shield™	Novartis Animal Vaccines	Cattle	I.M., S.C.	21d	
Somnu Shield™ XT	Novartis Animal Vaccines	Cattle	I.M.	60d	
Somubac®	Pfizer Animal Health	Cattle	S.C.	21d	
Sow Bac® CE II	Intervet	Swine	I.M., S.C.	21d	
Sow Bac® E II	Intervet	Swine	I.M., S.C.	21d	
Sow Bac® TREC	Intervet	Swine	I.M., Oral	21d	
Spectam® Scour-Halt™	AgriLabs	Swine	Oral	21d	
Spectam® Scour-Halt™	Durvet	Swine	Oral	21d	
Spectam® Water Soluble	Bimeda	Chickens	dw	5d	
Note: Do not administer to laying birds.					
SS Pac®	Schering-Plough	Swine	I.M.	60d	

Product Name	Company Name	Species	Route of Administration	Meat	Milk
Stafac® 10	Phibro	Chickens Swine Turkeys	In the feed In the feed In the feed	0 0 0	
Note: Do not use in laying chickens.					
Stafac® 20	Phibro	Chickens Swine Turkeys	In the feed In the feed In the feed	0 0 0	
Note: Do not use in laying chickens.					
Stafac® 500	Phibro	Chickens	In the feed		
Note: Do not use in laying chickens.					
Staphylococcus Aureus Bacterin-Toxoid	Hygieia	Dairy cattle	S.C.	42d	
StayBred™ VL5	Pfizer Animal Health	Cattle	I.M.	21d	
Sterile Penicillin G Benzathine and Penicillin G Procaine	G.C. Hanford	Beef cattle	S.C.	30d	
Note: A withdrawal period has not been established for this product in pre-ruminating calves. Do not use in calves to be processed for veal.					
Sterile Penicillin G Benzathine and Penicillin G Procaine	Aspen	Beef cattle	S.C.	30d	
Note: A withdrawal period has not been established for this product in pre-ruminating calves. Do not use in calves to be processed for veal.					
Sterile Penicillin G Procaine	Aspen	Cattle Horses Sheep Swine Veal	I.M. I.M. I.M. I.M. I.M.	4d 8d 6d 7d	48h
Note: Not for use in horses intended for food.					
Sterile Penicillin G Procaine Aqueous Suspension	Butler	Cattle Horses Sheep Swine Veal	I.M. I.M. I.M. I.M. I.M.	4d 8d 6d 7d	48h
Note: Not for use in horses intended for food.					
Strep Bac® with Imugen® II	Intervet	Swine	I.M.	60d	
Strepguard® with Havlogen®	Intervet	Horses	I.M.	21d	
Streptomycin Oral Solution	Contemporary Products	Cattle Chickens	dw dw	2d 4d	
Note: Do not use in laying hens producing eggs for human consumption.					
Strepvax® II	Boehringer Ingelheim	Horses	I.M.	21d	
Strongid® C	Pfizer Animal Health	Horses	In the feed		
Note: Not for use in horses intended for food.					
Strongid® C 2X™	Pfizer Animal Health	Horses	In the feed		
Note: Not for use in horses intended for food.					
Strongid® C Thirty	Pfizer Animal Health	Horses	In the feed		
Note: Not for use in horses intended for food.					
Strongid® Paste	Pfizer Animal Health	Horses	Oral		
Note: Not for use in horses intended for food.					
Strongid® T	Pfizer Animal Health	Horses	In the feed		
Note: Not for use in horses intended for food.					
Sulfadimethoxine Injection - 40%	Butler	Cattle	I.V.	5d	60h
Sulfadimethoxine Injection-40%	Durvet	Cattle	I.V.	5d	60h
Note: A withdrawal period has not been established for this product in pre-ruminating calves. Do not use in calves to be processed for veal.					
Sulfadimethoxine Injection-40%	Vedco	Cattle	I.V.	5d	60h
Note: A withdrawal period has not been established for this product in pre-ruminating calves. Do not use in calves to be processed for veal.					
Sulfadimethoxine Injection-40%	AgriPharm	Cattle	I.V.	5d	60h
Note: A withdrawal period has not been established for this product in pre-ruminating calves. Do not use in calves to be processed for veal.					
Sulfadimethoxine Injection - 40%	Aspen	Cattle	I.V.	5d	60h
Note: A withdrawal period has not been established for this product in pre-ruminating calves. Do not use in calves to be processed for veal.					
Sulfadimethoxine Oral Solution	Butler	Cattle Chickens Turkeys	dw dw dw	7d 5d 5d	
Note: Do not administer to chickens over 16 weeks (112 days) of age. Do not administer to turkeys over 24 weeks (168 days) of age.					
Sulfadimethoxine Oral Solution	Durvet	Cattle Chickens Turkeys	dw dw dw	7d 5d 5d	
Note: A withdrawal period has not been established for this product in pre-ruminating calves. Do not use in calves to be processed for veal. Do not administer to chickens over 16 weeks (112 days) of age. Do not administer to turkeys over 24 weeks (168 days) of age.					
Sulfadimethoxine Oral Solution	Vedco	Cattle Chickens Turkeys	dw dw dw	7d 5d 5d	
Note: A withdrawal period has not been established for this product in pre-ruminating calves. Do not use in calves to be processed for veal. Do not administer to chickens over 16 weeks (112 days) of age. Do not administer to turkeys over 24 weeks (168 days) of age.					

Product Name	Company Name	Species	Route of Administration	Meat	Milk
Sulfadimethoxine Oral Solution	AgriPharm	Cattle Chickens Turkeys	dw dw dw	7d 5d 5d	
Note: A withdrawal period has not been established for this product in pre-ruminating calves. Do not use in calves to be processed for veal. Do not administer to chickens over 16 weeks (112 days) of age. Do not administer to turkeys over 24 weeks (168 days) of age.					
Sulfadimethoxine Oral Solution	Aspen	Cattle Chickens Turkeys	dw dw dw	7d 5d 5d	
Note: A withdrawal period has not been established for this product in pre-ruminating calves. Do not use in calves to be processed for veal. Do not administer to chickens over 16 weeks (112 days) of age. Do not administer to turkeys over 24 weeks (168 days) of age.					
Sulfadimethoxine Soluble Powder	Durvet	Cattle Chickens Turkeys	dw dw dw	7d 5d 5d	
Note: A withdrawal period has not been established for this product in pre-ruminating calves. Do not use in calves to be processed for veal. Do not administer to chickens over 16 weeks (112 days) of age. Do not administer to turkeys over 24 weeks (168 days) of age.					
Sulfadimethoxine Soluble Powder	Vedco	Cattle Chickens Turkeys	dw dw dw	7d 5d 5d	
Note: A withdrawal period has not been established for this product in pre-ruminating calves. Do not use in calves to be processed for veal. Do not administer to chickens over 16 weeks (112 days) of age. Do not administer to turkeys over 24 weeks (168 days) of age.					
Sulfadimethoxine Soluble Powder	AgriPharm	Cattle Chickens Turkeys	dw dw dw	7d 5d 5d	
Note: A withdrawal period has not been established for this product in pre-ruminating calves. Do not use in calves to be processed for veal. Do not administer to chickens over 16 weeks (112 days) of age. Do not administer to turkeys over 24 weeks (168 days) of age.					
Sulfadimethoxine Soluble Powder	Aspen	Cattle Chickens Turkeys	dw dw dw	7d 5d 5d	
Note: A withdrawal period has not been established for this product in pre-ruminating calves. Do not use in calves to be processed for veal. Do not administer to chickens over 16 weeks (112 days) of age. Do not administer to turkeys over 24 weeks (168 days) of age.					
Sulfa-Max® III Calf Bolus	AgriLabs	Calves	Oral	12d	
Note: Not for use in female dairy cattle 20 months of age or older.					
Sulfa-Max® III Cattle Bolus	AgriLabs	Cattle	Oral	12d	
Note: Not for use in female dairy cattle 20 months of age or older.					
Sulfa-Q 20% Concentrate	AgriPharm	Cattle Chickens Turkeys	dw dw dw	10d 10d 10d	
Note: Do not feed to laying chickens or laying turkeys in production for food. Not for use in lactating dairy cows.					
Sulfasol	Med-Pharmex	Cattle Chickens Turkeys	dw dw dw	7d 5d 5d	
Note: A withdrawal period has not been established for this product in pre-ruminating calves. Do not use in calves to be processed for veal. Do not administer to chickens over 16 weeks (112 days) of age. Do not administer to turkeys over 24 weeks (168 days) of age.					
SulfaSure™ SR	Butler	Cattle	Oral	8d	
Note: Not for use in female dairy cattle 20 months of age or older.					
SulfaSure™ SR Calf Bolus	Butler	Calves	Oral	8d	
Note: Not for use in female dairy cattle 20 months of age or older.					
SulfaSURE™ SR Calf Bolus	Durvet	Calves	Oral	8d	
Note: Not for use in female dairy cattle 20 months of age or older.					
SulfaSURE™ SR Cattle Bolus	Durvet	Cattle	Oral	8d	
Note: Not for use in female dairy cattle 20 months of age or older.					
Sulforal	Med-Pharmex	Cattle Chickens Turkeys	dw dw dw	7d 5d 5d	
Note: Do not administer to chickens over 16 weeks (112 days) of age. Do not administer to turkeys over 24 weeks (168 days) of age.					
Sulmet® Drinking Water Solution 12.5%	Fort Dodge	Cattle Chickens Swine Turkeys	dw dw dw dw	10d 10d 15d 10d	
Note: Do not administer to chickens or turkeys producing eggs for human consumption. Not for use in female dairy cattle 20 months of age or older.					
Sulmet® Oblets®	Fort Dodge	Calves Horses	Oral Oral	10d	
Note: Not for use in female dairy cattle 20 months of age or older. Not for use in horses intended for food.					

Please refer to product listings for more complete information.

Product Name	Company Name	Species	Route of Administration	Meat	Milk
Sulmet® Soluble Powder	Fort Dodge	Cattle Chickens Swine Turkeys	dw dw dw dw	10d 10d 15d 10d	
Note: Do not administer to chickens or turkeys producing eggs for human consumption. Not for use in female dairy cattle 20 months of age or older.					
Super Poly-Bac B® Somnus	Texas Vet Lab	Cattle	S.C.	60d	
Super-Tet® with Havlogen®	Intervet	Cattle Horses Sheep Swine	I.M. I.M. I.M. I.M.	21d 21d 21d 21d	
Suppressor®	RXV	Horses	I.M., I.V.		
Note: Not for use in horses intended for food.					
SupraSulfa III® Calf Bolus	AgriPharm	Calves	Oral	8d	
Note: Not for use in female dairy cattle 20 months of age or older.					
SupraSulfa III® Cattle Bolus	AgriPharm	Cattle	Oral	8d	
Note: Not for use in female dairy cattle 20 months of age or older.					
Sure E&SE™	SureNutrition	Horses	In the feed	0	
Surround™ 4	Biocor	Cattle	I.M., S.C.	21d	
Surround™ 4+HS	Biocor	Cattle	I.M., S.C.	21d	
Surround™ 8	Biocor	Cattle	I.M., S.C.	21d	
Surround™ 9	Biocor	Cattle	I.M., S.C.	21d	
Surround™ 9+HS	Biocor	Cattle	I.M., S.C.	21d	
Surround™ HS	Biocor	Cattle	I.M., S.C.	21d	
Surround™ L5	Biocor	Cattle Swine	I.M., S.C. I.M., S.C.	21d 21d	
Surround™ V-L5	Biocor	Cattle	I.M., S.C.	21d	
Sustain III®	Durvet	Cattle	Oral	12d	
Note: Do not use in lactating dairy cattle. Not for use in female dairy cattle 20 months of age or older.					
Sustain III® Calf Bolus	Durvet	Calves	Oral	12d	
Note: Not for use in female dairy cattle 20 months of age or older.					
Sustain® III Calf Bolus	Bimeda	Calves	Oral	12d	
Note: Not for use in female dairy cattle 20 months of age or older.					
Sustain® III Cattle Bolus	Bimeda	Cattle	Oral	12d	
Note: Do not use in lactating dairy cattle. Not for use in female dairy cattle 20 months of age or older.					
Suvaxyn® AR/E/EC-4	Fort Dodge	Swine	I.M.	21d	
Suvaxyn® AR/T	Fort Dodge	Swine	I.M., S.C.	21d	
Suvaxyn® AR/T/E	Fort Dodge	Swine	I.M.	21d	
Suvaxyn® E	Fort Dodge	Swine	I.M., S.C.	21d	
Suvaxyn® EC-4	Fort Dodge	Swine	I.M.	21d	
Suvaxyn® E-oral	Fort Dodge	Swine	dw	21d	
Suvaxyn®-E (Swine and Turkey)	Fort Dodge	Swine Turkeys	I.M., S.C. S.C.	21d 21d	
Suvaxyn® LE+B	Fort Dodge	Swine	I.M.	21d	
Suvaxyn® PLE	Fort Dodge	Swine	I.M.	21d	
Suvaxyn® PLE+B	Fort Dodge	Swine	I.M.	21d	
Suvaxyn® PLE+B/PrV gpI-	Fort Dodge	Swine	I.M.	21d	
Suvaxyn® PLE/PrV gpI-	Fort Dodge	Swine	I.M.	21d	
Suvaxyn® PrV gpI-	Fort Dodge	Swine	I.M.	21d	
Suvaxyn® RespiFend® APP	Fort Dodge	Swine	I.M.	60d	
Suvaxyn® RespiFend® HPS	Fort Dodge	Swine	I.M.	21d	
Suvaxyn® RespiFend® MH	Fort Dodge	Swine	I.M.	21d	
Suvaxyn® RespiFend® MH/HPS	Fort Dodge	Swine	I.M.	21d	
Swat® Fly Repellent Ointment	Farnam	Horses	Topical		
Note: Not for use on animals intended for food purposes.					
Sweetlix® Rabon® Mineral/Vitamin Molasses Block	Sweetlix	Cattle	Oral	0	0
Sweetlix® Safe-Guard® 20% Natural Protein Deworming Block for Beef Cattle	Sweetlix	Beef cattle	Oral	16d	
Sweetlix® Safe-Guard* Free-Choice Mineral Cattle Dewormer	Sweetlix	Cattle	Oral	13d	
Note: Do not use in female dairy cattle of breeding age.					
Swine Influenza Vaccine (H3N2 Subtype)	SyntroVet	Swine	I.M.	21d	
Swine Master M Plus™	AgriLabs	Swine	I.M., S.C.	21d	
Synanthic® Bovine Dewormer Suspension, 9.06%	Fort Dodge	Cattle	Oral	7d	
Note: Do not use in female dairy cattle of breeding age.					

Product Name	Company Name	Species	Route of Administration	Meat	Milk
Synanthic® Bovine Dewormer Suspension, 22.5%	Fort Dodge	Cattle	I.R., Oral	7d	
Note: Do not use in female dairy cattle of breeding age.					
Synovex® C	Fort Dodge	Beef cattle	Implant		
Note: Implant in the ear only. Do not attempt to salvage the implanted ear for human or animal food.					
Synovex® H	Fort Dodge	Beef cattle	Implant		
Note: Implant in the ear only. Do not attempt to salvage the implanted ear for human or animal food.					
Synovex® Plus™	Fort Dodge	Beef cattle	Implant		
Note: Implant in the ear only. Do not attempt to salvage the implanted ear for human or animal food.					
Synovex® S	Fort Dodge	Beef cattle	Implant		
Note: Implant in the ear only. Do not attempt to salvage the implanted ear for human or animal food.					
Syn Shield™	Novartis Animal Vaccines	Cattle	I.M.	60d	
Taktic® E.C.	Intervet	Cattle	Topical	0	0
		Swine	Topical	3d	
Tenosynovitis Vaccine	Merial Select	Chickens	S.C.	21d	
Teno-Vaxin®	ASL	Chickens	dw	21d	
Note: Do not vaccinate birds in egg production.					
Tensynvac®	Intervet	Chickens	S.C.	21d	
Note: Do not vaccinate after 12 weeks of age.					
Terramycin® 10 TM-10®	Phibro	Cattle	In the feed	5d	
		Chickens	In the feed	0-3d	
		Lobster	In the feed	30d	
		Sheep	In the feed	5d	
		Swine	In the feed	5d	
		Turkeys	In the feed	0-5d	
Note: In chickens at 500 g/ton use level withdraw 24 hours before slaughter. In low calcium feeds withdraw 3 days before slaughter. Do not feed to chickens producing eggs for human consumption. Do not feed to turkeys producing eggs for human consumption. Withdraw from turkeys 5 days before slaughter when used at levels of 200 g/ton or higher.					
Terramycin® 50	Phibro	Cattle	In the feed	5d	
		Chickens	In the feed	0-3d	
		Sheep	In the feed	5d	
		Turkeys	In the feed	0-5d	
Note: In chickens at 500 g/ton use level withdraw 24 hours before slaughter. In low calcium feeds withdraw 3 days before slaughter. Do not feed to chickens producing eggs for human consumption. Do not feed to turkeys producing eggs for human consumption. Withdraw from turkeys 5 days before slaughter when used at levels of 200 g/ton or higher.					
Terramycin® 100	Phibro	Cattle	In the feed	5d	
		Chickens	In the feed	0-3d	
		Sheep	In the feed	5d	
		Turkeys	In the feed	0-5d	
Note: In chickens at 500 g/ton use level withdraw 24 hours before slaughter. In low calcium feeds withdraw 3 days before slaughter. Do not feed to chickens producing eggs for human consumption. Do not feed to turkeys producing eggs for human consumption. Withdraw from turkeys 5 days before slaughter when used at levels of 200 g/ton or higher.					
Terramycin® 100 for Fish	Phibro	Catfish	In the feed	21d	
		Salmonids	In the feed	21d	
Terramycin® 200	Phibro	Cattle	In the feed	5d	
		Chickens	In the feed	0-3d	
		Sheep	In the feed	5d	
		Turkeys	In the feed	0-5d	
Note: In chickens at 500 g/ton use level withdraw 24 hours before slaughter. In low calcium feeds withdraw 3 days before slaughter. Do not feed to chickens producing eggs for human consumption. Do not feed to turkeys producing eggs for human consumption. Withdraw from turkeys 5 days before slaughter when used at levels of 200 g/ton or higher.					
Terramycin-343® Soluble Powder	Pfizer Animal Health	Bees	Oral		
		Cattle	dw	5d	
		Chickens	dw		
		Sheep	dw	5d	
		Swine	dw	0	
		Turkeys	dw	5d	
Note: Do not administer to chickens or turkeys producing eggs for human consumption. Remove at least 6 weeks prior to main honey flow.					
Terramycin® Scours Tablets	Pfizer Animal Health	Calves	Oral	7d	
Note: A withdrawal period has not been established for this product in pre-ruminating calves. Do not use in calves to be processed for veal. Not for use in lactating dairy animals.					
Terramycin® Soluble Powder	Pfizer Animal Health	Bees	Oral		
		Cattle	dw	5d	
		Chickens	dw		
		Sheep	dw	5d	
		Swine	dw	0	
		Turkeys	dw	5d	
Note: Do not administer to chickens or turkeys producing eggs for human consumption. Remove at least 6 weeks prior to main honey flow.					
Terra-Vet 100	Aspen	Cattle	I.V.	22d	
Note: A withdrawal period has not been established for this product in pre-ruminating calves. Do not use in calves to be processed for veal. Do not use in lactating dairy cattle.					

Product Name	Company Name	Species	Route of Administration	Meat	Milk
Terra Vet Soluble Powder	Aspen	Cattle	dw	5d	
		Chickens	dw		
		Sheep	dw	5d	
		Swine	dw	5d	
		Turkeys	dw	5d	
Note: A milk discard period has not been established for this product in lactating dairy cattle. Do not use in female dairy cattle 20 months of age or older. A withdrawal period has not been established for this product in pre-ruminating calves. Do not use in calves to be processed for veal. Do not administer to chickens or turkeys producing eggs for human consumption.					
Terra-Vet Soluble Powder 343	Aspen	Cattle	dw	5d	
		Chickens	dw		
		Sheep	dw	5d	
		Swine	dw	5d	
		Turkeys	dw	5d	
Note: A milk discard period has not been established for this product in lactating dairy cattle. Do not use in female dairy cattle 20 months of age or older. A withdrawal period has not been established for this product in pre-ruminating calves. Do not use in calves to be processed for veal. Do not administer to chickens or turkeys producing eggs for human consumption.					
Tet-324	Phoenix Pharmaceutical	Calves	dw	5d	
		Chickens	dw	4d	
		Swine	dw	4d	
		Turkeys	dw	4d	
Note: A withdrawal period has not been established for this product in pre-ruminating calves. Do not use in calves to be processed for veal. Do not administer to poultry producing eggs for human consumption.					
Tet 324™	Bimeda	Calves	dw	5d	
		Chickens	dw	4d	
		Swine	dw	4d	
		Turkeys	dw	4d	
Note: Do not medicate chickens or turkeys producing eggs for human consumption.					
Tetanus Antitoxin	Fort Dodge	Cattle	I.P., I.V., S.C.	21d	
		Horses	I.P., I.V., S.C.	21d	
		Sheep	I.P., I.V., S.C.	21d	
		Swine	I.P., I.V., S.C.	21d	
Tetanus Antitoxin	Durvet	Cattle	I.M., S.C.	21d	
		Horses	I.M., S.C.	21d	
		Sheep	I.M., S.C.	21d	
		Swine	I.M., S.C.	21d	
Tetanus Antitoxin, Equine Origin	Colorado Serum	Cattle	I.M., S.C.	21d	
		Horses	I.M., S.C.	21d	
		Sheep	I.M., S.C.	21d	
		Swine	I.M., S.C.	21d	
Tetanus Antitoxin, Equine Origin	Professional Biological	Cattle	I.M., S.C.	21d	
		Horses	I.M., S.C.	21d	
		Sheep	I.M., S.C.	21d	
		Swine	I.M., S.C.	21d	
Tetanus Toxoid	Fort Dodge	Horses	I.M.	60d	
		Sheep	I.M.	60d	
		Swine	I.M.	60d	
Tetanus Toxoid-Concentrated	Colorado Serum	Cattle	I.M.	21d	
		Goats	I.M.	21d	
		Horses	I.M.	21d	
		Sheep	I.M.	21d	
		Swine	I.M.	21d	
Tetanus Toxoid-Concentrated	Professional Biological	Cattle	I.M., S.C.	21d	
		Goats	I.M., S.C.	21d	
		Horses	I.M.	21d	
		Sheep	I.M., S.C.	21d	
		Swine	I.M., S.C.	21d	
Tetanus Toxoid-Unconcentrated	Colorado Serum	Cattle	I.M., S.C.	21d	
		Goats	I.M., S.C.	21d	
		Horses	I.M., S.C.	21d	
		Sheep	I.M., S.C.	21d	
		Swine	I.M., S.C.	21d	
Tetguard™	Boehringer Ingelheim	Cattle	I.M., S.C.	21d	
		Horses	I.M., S.C.	21d	
		Sheep	I.M., S.C.	21d	
		Swine	I.M., S.C.	21d	
Tetni-Vax®	AgriPharm	Cattle	S.C.	21d	
		Sheep	S.C.	21d	
Tetnogen®	Fort Dodge	Cattle	I.M., S.C.	21d	
		Horses	I.M., S.C.	21d	
		Sheep	I.M., S.C.	21d	
		Swine	I.M., S.C.	21d	
Tetnogen®-AT	Fort Dodge	Cattle	I.M., S.C.	21d	
		Horses	I.M., S.C.	21d	
		Sheep	I.M., S.C.	21d	
		Swine	I.M., S.C.	21d	

Product Name	Company Name	Species	Route of Administration	Meat	Milk
Tetra Bac 324	AgriLabs	Calves Chickens Swine Turkeys	dw dw dw dw	5d 4d 4d 4d	
Note: Do not administer to poultry producing eggs for human consumption.					
Tetracycline Hydrochloride Soluble Powder-324	Butler	Calves Chickens Swine Turkeys	dw dw dw dw	5d 4d 4d 4d	
Note: Do not administer to poultry producing eggs for human consumption.					
Tetracycline Hydrochloride Soluble Powder-324	Vedco	Calves Chickens Swine Turkeys	dw dw dw dw	5d 4d 4d 4d	
Note: Do not administer to poultry producing eggs for human consumption.					
Tetracycline Soluble Powder 324	AgriPharm	Calves Chickens Swine Turkeys	dw dw dw dw	5d 4d 4d 4d	
Note: A withdrawal period has not been established for this product in pre-ruminating calves. Do not use in calves to be processed for veal. Do not administer to poultry producing eggs for human consumption.					
Tetrasol Soluble Powder	Med-Pharmex	Calves Chickens Swine Turkeys	dw dw dw dw	5d 4d 4d	
Note: A withdrawal period has not been established for this product in pre-ruminating calves. Do not use in calves to be processed for veal. Do not use in birds producing eggs for food purposes.					
Tetroxy®-100	Bimeda	Cattle	I.V.	19d	
Note: Not for use in lactating dairy cows.					
Tetroxy® HCA Soluble Powder	Bimeda	Chickens Swine Turkeys	dw dw dw	0 0 0	
Note: Do not feed to birds producing eggs for human consumption.					
Tetroxy® LA	Bimeda	Cattle Swine	I.M., I.V. I.M.	28d 28d	
Note: Not for use in lactating dairy animals.					
Tet-Sol 10	Alpharma	Calves Chickens Swine Turkeys	dw dw dw dw	5d 4d 4d 4d	
Note: A withdrawal period has not been established for this product in pre-ruminating calves. Do not use in calves to be processed for veal. Do not use in birds producing eggs for food purposes.					
Tet-Sol™ 324	Alpharma	Calves Chickens Swine Turkeys	dw dw dw dw	5d 4d 4d 4d	
Note: A withdrawal period has not been established for this product in pre-ruminating calves. Do not use in calves to be processed for veal. Do not use in birds producing eggs for food purposes.					
TGE Cell™	Novartis Animal Vaccines	Swine	I.M., Oral	21d	
TGE Shield™	Novartis Animal Vaccines	Swine	I.M.	60d	
Thrush Treatment	First Priority	Horses	Topical		
Note: Not for use on animals intended for food purposes.					
Thrush-XX™	Farnam	Horses	Topical		
Note: Not for use on horses intended for food.					
Thuja-Zinc Oxide	Butler	Horses	Topical		
Note: Not for use on horses intended for food.					
Thuja-Zinc Oxide	Vedco	Horses	Topical		
Note: Not for use on horses intended for food.					
Thuja-Zinc Oxide	Phoenix Pharmaceutical	Horses	Topical		
Note: Not for use on horses intended for food.					
Titanium™ 3	AgriLabs	Cattle	I.M., S.C.	21d	
Titanium® 3	Intervet	Cattle	I.M., S.C.	21d	
Titanium® 3+BRSV	Intervet	Cattle	I.M., S.C.	21d	
Titanium™ 3+BRSV LP	AgriLabs	Cattle	I.M., S.C.	21d	
Titanium® 3+BRSV LP	Intervet	Cattle	I.M., S.C.	21d	
Titanium™ 4	AgriLabs	Cattle	I.M., S.C.	21d	
Titanium™ 4 L5	AgriLabs	Cattle	I.M., S.C.	21d	
Titanium™ 5	AgriLabs	Cattle	I.M., S.C.	21d	
Titanium® 5	Intervet	Cattle	I.M., S.C.	21d	
Titanium™ 5 L5	AgriLabs	Cattle	I.M., S.C.	21d	
Titanium® 5 L5	Intervet	Cattle	I.M., S.C.	21d	

Product Name	Company Name	Species	Route of Administration	Meat	Milk
Titanium® 5+P.H.M. Bac®-1	AgriLabs	Cattle	I.M.	21d	
Titanium® 5+P.H.M. Bac®-1	Intervet	Cattle	I.M.	21d	
Titanium™ BRSV	AgriLabs	Cattle	I.M., S.C.	21d	
Titanium® BRSV	Intervet	Cattle	I.M., S.C.	21d	
Titanium™ BRSV 3	AgriLabs	Cattle	I.M., S.C.	21d	
Titanium® BRSV 3	Intervet	Cattle	I.M., S.C.	21d	
Titanium™ IBR	AgriLabs	Cattle	I.M., S.C.	21d	
Titanium® IBR	Intervet	Cattle	I.M., S.C.	21d	
Titanium™ IBR-LP	AgriLabs	Cattle	I.M., S.C.	21d	
TiterVac™ 5	Aspen	Cattle	I.M.	21d	
TiterVac™ 5-HS	Aspen	Cattle	I.M.	21d	
TiterVac™ 10	Aspen	Cattle	I.M.	21d	
TiterVac™ 10-HS	Aspen	Cattle	I.M.	21d	
TM-50®	Phibro	Cattle Chickens Lobster Sheep Turkeys	In the feed In the feed In the feed In the feed In the feed	5d 0-3d 30d 5d 0-5d	
Note: In chickens at 500 g/ton use level withdraw 24 hours before slaughter. In low calcium feeds withdraw 3 days before slaughter. Do not feed to chickens producing eggs for human consumption. Do not feed to turkeys producing eggs for human consumption. Withdraw from turkeys 5 days before slaughter when used at levels of 200 g/ton or higher.					
TM-50®D	Phibro	Bees Cattle Chickens Lobster Sheep Turkeys	In the feed In the feed In the feed In the feed In the feed In the feed	 5d 0-3d 30d 5d 0-5d	
Note: In chickens at 500 g/ton use level withdraw 24 hours before slaughter. In low calcium feeds withdraw 3 days before slaughter. Do not feed to chickens producing eggs for human consumption. Do not feed to turkeys producing eggs for human consumption. Remove at least 6 weeks prior to main honey flow. Withdraw from turkeys 5 days before slaughter when used at levels of 200 g/ton or higher.					
TM-100®	Phibro	Cattle Chickens Lobster Sheep Turkeys	In the feed In the feed In the feed In the feed In the feed	5d 0-3d 30d 5d 0-5d	
Note: In chickens at 500 g/ton use level withdraw 24 hours before slaughter. In low calcium feeds withdraw 3 days before slaughter. Do not feed to chickens producing eggs for human consumption. Do not feed to turkeys producing eggs for human consumption. Withdraw from turkeys 5 days before slaughter when used at levels of 200 g/ton or higher.					
TM-100®D	Phibro	Bees Cattle Chickens Lobster Sheep Turkeys	In the feed In the feed In the feed In the feed In the feed In the feed	 5d 0-3d 30d 5d 0-5d	
Note: In chickens at 500 g/ton use level withdraw 24 hours before slaughter. In low calcium feeds withdraw 3 days before slaughter. Do not feed to chickens producing eggs for human consumption. Do not feed to turkeys producing eggs for human consumption. Remove at least 6 weeks prior to main honey flow. Withdraw from turkeys 5 days before slaughter when used at levels of 200 g/ton or higher.					
ToDAY®	Fort Dodge	Dairy cattle	I.M.M.	4d	96h
Tolazine™ Injection	Lloyd	Horses	I.V.		
Note: Not for use in food-producing animals.					
ToMORROW®	Fort Dodge	Dairy cattle	I.M.M.	42d	
Note: Milk from treated cows must not be used for food during the first 72 hours after calving. Not to be used within 30 days of calving.					
Topical Fungicide	Vedco	Horses	Topical		
Note: Not for use on horses intended for food.					
Topical Fungicide	First Priority	Horses	Topical		
Note: Not for use on horses intended for food.					
Top Line™	AgriLabs	Cattle	Topical	48d	
Note: Do not use in female dairy cattle of breeding age.					
Torbugesic®	Fort Dodge	Horses	I.V.		
Note: Not for use in horses intended for food.					
Torpex™	Boehringer Ingelheim	Horses	I.N.		
Note: Not for use in horses intended for food.					
Totalon® Pour-On Dewormer	Schering-Plough	Cattle	Topical	9d	
Note: Do not use on female dairy cattle of breeding age.					

Product Name	Company Name	Species	Route of Administration	Meat	Milk
Toxivac® AD+E	Boehringer Ingelheim	Swine	I.M.	21d	
Toxivac® Plus Parasuis	Boehringer Ingelheim	Swine	I.M.	21d	
Trachivax®	Schering-Plough	Chickens	I.O.	21d	
TranquiVed Injectable (Horses)	Vedco	Horses	I.M., I.V.		
Note: Not for use in horses intended for food.					
Tremblex™	L.A.H.I. (New Jersey)	Chickens	aer/sp, dw	21d	
Tremor Blen® D	Merial Select	Chickens	dw, ww	21d	
Note: Do not vaccinate chickens within 4 weeks of onset of egg production or during egg production.					
Tremormune™ AE	Biomune	Chickens	ww	21d	
Tremvac®	Intervet	Chickens	dw	21d	
Note: Do not vaccinate 35 days prior to onset of lay or during egg production.					
Tremvac-FP®	Intervet	Chickens Turkeys	ww ww	21d 21d	
Note: Do not vaccinate 35 days prior to onset of lay or during egg production.					
Tremvac-FP-CAV™	Intervet	Chickens	ww	21d	
Note: Do not vaccinate 6 weeks prior to onset of or during lay.					
Treponema Bacterin	Novartis Animal Vaccines	Cattle	S.C.	60d	
Trexonil™	Wildlife	Cervidae	I.V., S.C.		
Note: Do not use 45 days before or during hunting season. Do not use in domestic food-producing animals.					
Triangle® 1 + Type II BVD	Fort Dodge	Cattle	I.M., S.C.	21d	
Triangle® 3 + Type II BVD	Fort Dodge	Cattle	I.M., S.C.	21d	
Triangle® 3 V5L	Fort Dodge	Cattle	S.C.	60d	
Triangle® 4+HS	Fort Dodge	Cattle	I.M., S.C.	21d	
Triangle® 4+PH/HS	Fort Dodge	Cattle	I.M., S.C.	21d	
Triangle® 4+PH-K	Fort Dodge	Cattle	I.M., S.C.	21d	
Triangle® 4 + Type II BVD	Fort Dodge	Cattle	I.M., S.C.	21d	
Triangle® 8 + Type II BVD	Fort Dodge	Cattle	I.M., S.C.	21d	
Triangle® 9+HS	Fort Dodge	Cattle	I.M.	21d	
Triangle® 9+PH-K	Fort Dodge	Cattle	I.M.	21d	
Triangle® 9 + Type II BVD	Fort Dodge	Cattle	I.M., S.C.	21d	
Tribrissen® 48% Injection	Schering-Plough	Horses	I.V.		
Note: Not for use in horses intended for food.					
Tribrissen® 400 Oral Paste	Schering-Plough	Horses	Oral		
Note: Not for use in horses intended for food.					
Tricaine-S	Western Chemical	Fish	Imsn.	21d	
TrichGuard®	Fort Dodge	Cattle	S.C.	60d	
TrichGuard® V5L	Fort Dodge	Cattle	S.C.	60d	
Trienamine™	Phoenix Pharmaceutical	Cattle Horses	I.M., I.V. I.M.	4d	24h
Note: A withdrawal period has not been established for this product in pre-ruminating calves. Do not use in calves to be processed for veal. Not for use in horses intended for food.					
Tripelennamine Hydrochloride	AgriLabs	Cattle Horses	I.M., I.V. I.M.	4d	24h
Note: A withdrawal period has not been established for this product in pre-ruminating calves. Do not use in calves to be processed for veal. Not for use in horses intended for food.					
Tripelennamine Hydrochloride	Butler	Cattle Horses	I.M., I.V. I.M.	4d	24h
Note: A withdrawal period has not been established for this product in pre-ruminating calves. Do not use in calves to be processed for veal. Not for use in horses intended for food.					
Tripelennamine Hydrochloride	Vet Tek	Cattle Horses	I.M., I.V. I.M.	4d	24h
Note: A withdrawal period has not been established for this product in pre-ruminating calves. Do not use in calves to be processed for veal. Not for use in horses intended for food.					
Tripelennamine Hydrochloride	Aspen	Cattle Horses	I.M., I.V. I.M.	4d	24h
Note: A withdrawal period has not been established for this product in pre-ruminating calves. Do not use in calves to be processed for veal. Not for use in horses intended for food.					
Triple-E®	Fort Dodge	Horses	I.M.	21d	
Triple-E® T Innovator	Fort Dodge	Horses	I.M.	21d	
Triple Histamine	RXV	Cattle Horses	I.M., I.V. I.M.	4d	24h
Note: A withdrawal period has not been established for this product in pre-ruminating calves. Do not use in calves to be processed for veal. Not for use in horses intended for food.					
Triplevac®	Intervet	Chickens	aer/sp, bd, dw	21d	
Tri-Reo®	Fort Dodge	Chickens	I.M., S.C.	42d	

Product Name	Company Name	Species	Route of Administration	Meat	Milk
Tri-Tec 14™ Fly Repellent	Farnam	Horses	Topical		
Note: Not for use on horses intended for food.					
Trivac-Ark®	Intervet	Chickens	aer/sp	21d	
TriVib 5L®	Fort Dodge	Cattle	S.C.	60d	
Trovac®-AIV H5	Merial Select	Chickens	S.C.	21d	
TrustGard™ 5L	Vedco	Cattle	I.M.	21d	
		Swine	I.M.	21d	
TrustGard™ 7	Vedco	Cattle	S.C.	21d	
		Sheep	S.C.	21d	
TrustGard™ 7/HS	Vedco	Cattle	S.C.	21d	
TrustGard™ 8	Vedco	Cattle	S.C.	21d	
		Sheep	S.C.	21d	
TrustGard™ CD	Vedco	Cattle	S.C.	21d	
		Sheep	S.C.	21d	
TrustGard™ CD/T	Vedco	Cattle	S.C.	21d	
		Goats	S.C.	21d	
		Sheep	S.C.	21d	
TrustGard™ HS	Vedco	Cattle	I.M.	21d	
TrustGard™ MB	Vedco	Cattle	S.C.	21d	
TrustGard™ Vibrio/5L	Vedco	Cattle	I.M.	21d	
TSV-2®	Pfizer Animal Health	Cattle	I.N.	21d	
Tucoprim® Powder	Pharmacia & Upjohn	Horses	In the feed		
Note: Not for use in horses intended for food.					
Twin-Pen™	AgriLabs	Beef cattle	S.C.	30d	
Twinvax®-99	Schering-Plough	Chickens	aer/sp, dw	21d	
Twinvax®-MR	Schering-Plough	Chickens	aer/sp, bd, dw	21d	
Tylan® 40	Elanco	Chickens	In the feed	0-5d	
Note: Withdraw 5 days before slaughter when fed to chickens at 800 to 1,000 g per ton.					
Tylan® 40 Sulfa-G™	Elanco	Swine	In the feed	15d	
Tylan® 50 Injection	Elanco	Cattle	I.M.	21d	
		Swine	I.M.	14d	
Note: A withdrawal period has not been established for this product in pre-ruminating calves. Do not use in calves to be processed for veal. Do not use in lactating dairy cattle.					
Tylan® 100	Elanco	Chickens	In the feed	0-5d	
Note: Withdraw 5 days before slaughter when fed to chickens at 800 to 1,000 g per ton.					
Tylan® 100 Cal	Elanco	Chickens	In the feed	0-5d	
Note: Withdraw 5 days before slaughter when fed to chickens at 800 to 1,000 g per ton.					
Tylan® 200 Injection	Elanco	Cattle	I.M.	21d	
		Swine	I.M.	14d	
Note: A withdrawal period has not been established for this product in pre-ruminating calves. Do not use in calves to be processed for veal. Do not use in lactating dairy cattle.					
Tylan® Soluble	Elanco	Chickens	dw	24h	
		Swine	dw	2d	
		Turkeys	dw	5d	
Note: Do not use in layers producing eggs for human consumption.					
Tylosin Injection	Boehringer Ingelheim	Cattle	I.M.	21d	
		Swine	I.M.	14d	
Note: Do not use in lactating dairy cattle.					
Tylosin Injection	AgriLabs	Cattle	I.M.	21d	
		Swine	I.M.	14d	
Note: A withdrawal period has not been established for this product in pre-ruminating calves. Do not use in calves to be processed for veal. Do not use in lactating dairy cattle.					
Tylosin Injection	Aspen	Cattle	I.M.	21d	
		Swine	I.M.	14d	
Note: A withdrawal period has not been established for this product in pre-ruminating calves. Do not use in calves to be processed for veal. Do not use in lactating dairy cattle.					
TyloVed Injection	Vedco	Cattle	I.M.	21d	
		Swine	I.M.	14d	
Note: A withdrawal period has not been established for this product in pre-ruminating calves. Do not use in calves to be processed for veal. Do not use in lactating dairy cattle.					
Typhimune®	Biomune	Pigeons	I.M., S.C.	21d	
Ultrabac® 7	Pfizer Animal Health	Cattle	S.C.	21d	
		Sheep	S.C.	21d	
Ultrabac® 7/Somubac®	Pfizer Animal Health	Cattle	S.C.	21d	
Ultrabac® 8	Pfizer Animal Health	Cattle	S.C.	21d	
		Sheep	S.C.	21d	
Ultrabac® CD	Pfizer Animal Health	Cattle	S.C.	21d	
		Sheep	S.C.	21d	

Product Name	Company Name	Species	Route of Administration	Meat	Milk
UltraChoice™ 7	Pfizer Animal Health	Cattle Sheep	S.C. S.C.	21d 21d	
UltraChoice™ 8	Pfizer Animal Health	Cattle Sheep	S.C. S.C.	21d 21d	
UltraChoice™ CD	Pfizer Animal Health	Cattle Sheep	S.C. S.C.	21d 21d	
UltraMectrin™ Injection	RXV	Cattle Reindeer Swine	S.C. S.C. S.C.	35d 56d 18d	
Note: Do not use in female dairy cattle of breeding age.					
UltraMectrin™ Pour-On	RXV	Cattle	Topical	48d	
Note: Do not use in female dairy cattle of breeding age.					
UltraSpot™ by Absorbine®	W. F. Young	Horses	Topical		
Note: Not for use on horses intended for food.					
Uniprim® Powder	Macleod	Horses	In the feed		
Note: Not for use in horses intended for food.					
Univax-BD®	Schering-Plough	Chickens	dw	21d	
Univax™ Plus	Schering-Plough	Chickens	dw, S.C.	21d	
Upjohn J-5 Bacterin™	Pharmacia & Upjohn	Dairy cattle	S.C.	60d	
Urea Wound Powder	First Priority	Horses	Topical		
Note: Not for use on animals intended for food purposes.					
V.A. ChickVac™	Fort Dodge	Chickens	S.C.	21d	
Note: Do not vaccinate birds in egg production.					
Valbazen® Cattle Dewormer Paste	Pfizer Animal Health	Cattle	Oral	27d	
Valbazen® Suspension	Pfizer Animal Health	Cattle Sheep	Oral Oral	27d 7d	
Vapona® Concentrate Insecticide	Boehringer Ingelheim	Cattle	Topical	1d	
Variant Vax-BD™	Schering-Plough	Chickens	dw, S.C.	21d	
Vectormune® FP-LT	Biomune	Chickens	ww	21d	
Vectormune® FP-LT+AE	Biomune	Chickens	ww	21d	
Vectormune® FP-N	Biomune	Chickens	S.C.	21d	
Vedadine Bolus	Vedco	Horses	Topical		
Note: Not for use on horses intended for food.					
Velenium™	Fort Dodge	Beef cattle	I.M., S.C.	30d	
Ventipulmin® Syrup	Boehringer Ingelheim	Horses	Oral		
Note: Not for use in horses intended for food.					
Vetalog® Parenteral	Fort Dodge	Horses	I.A., I.M., I.Syn., S.C.		
Note: Not for use in horses intended for food.					
Vetisulid® Boluses	Fort Dodge	Calves	Oral	7d	
Note: A withdrawal period has not been established for this product in pre-ruminating calves. Do not use in calves to be processed for veal.					
Vetisulid® Injection	Fort Dodge	Calves	I.V.	5d	
Note: A withdrawal period has not been established for this product in pre-ruminating calves. Do not use in calves to be processed for veal.					
Vetisulid® Powder	Fort Dodge	Calves Swine	dw dw	7d 4d	
Note: A withdrawal period has not been established for this product in pre-ruminating calves. Do not use in calves to be processed for veal.					
Vet-Kem® Ovitrol® Plus Flea, Tick & Bot Spray	Wellmark	Horses	Topical		
Note: Not for use on horses intended for food.					
Vet-Kem® Triple Action Flea & Tick Shampoo for Dogs, Cats, & Horses	Wellmark	Horses	Topical		
Note: Not for use on horses intended for food.					
Vetrolin® Liniment	Equicare	Horses	Topical		
Note: Not for use on horses intended for food.					
Vibralone™-L5	Intervet	Cattle	I.M.	21d	
Vibrin®	Pfizer Animal Health	Cattle	S.C.	60d	
Vibrio-Lepto-5™	Boehringer Ingelheim	Cattle	I.M.	21d	
Vibrio-Lepto 5	Premier Farmtech	Cattle	I.M., S.C.	21d	
Vibrio-Lepto 5	AgriLabs	Cattle	I.M., S.C.	21d	
Vibrio-Lepto 5	Durvet	Cattle	I.M., S.C.	21d	
Vibrio Lepto 5 (oil base)	Aspen	Cattle	I.M.	60d	
Vibrio-Lepto 5 Vaccine	Aspen	Cattle	I.M., S.C.	21d	
Vibrio/Leptoferm-5™	Pfizer Animal Health	Cattle	I.M.	21d	
Vibrogen	Novartis (Aqua Health)	Salmonids	aer/sp, Imsn.	21d	
Vibrogen-2™	Novartis (Aqua Health)	Salmonids	aer/sp, Imsn.	21d	
Vib Shield®	Novartis Animal Vaccines	Cattle	I.M., S.C.	21d	
Vib Shield® L5	Novartis Animal Vaccines	Cattle	I.M., S.C.	21d	

Please refer to product listings for more complete information.

Product Name	Company Name	Species	Route of Administration	Meat	Milk
Vib Shield® L5 Hardjo Bovis	Novartis Animal Vaccines	Cattle	I.M.	21d	
Vib Shield® Plus	Novartis Animal Vaccines	Cattle	I.M.	60d	
Vib Shield® Plus L5	Novartis Animal Vaccines	Cattle	I.M.	60d	
Vi Bursa C.E.™	L.A.H.I. (New Jersey)	Chickens	dw	21d	
Vi Bursa-G™	L.A.H.I. (New Jersey)	Chickens	dw	21d	
Vi Bursa-K™	L.A.H.I. (New Jersey)	Chickens	I.M., S.C.	42d	
Vi Bursa-K+V	L.A.H.I. (New Jersey)	Chickens	I.M., S.C.	42d	
Vi Bursa-L™	L.A.H.I. (New Jersey)	Chickens	dw	21d	
Vi Clemcol-C™	L.A.H.I. (New Jersey)	Chickens	ww	21d	
Vi Mark® Bursal Disease-Marek's Disease Vaccine (Live Virus, Chicken and Turkey Herpesvirus)	L.A.H.I. (New Jersey)	Chickens	S.C.	21d	
Vi Mark® Bursal Disease-Marek's Disease Vaccine (Modified Live Virus, Turkey Herpesvirus)	L.A.H.I. (New Jersey)	Chickens	S.C.	21d	
Vi Mark® Marek's Disease Vaccine (Live Chicken and Turkey Herpesvirus)	L.A.H.I. (New Jersey)	Chickens	S.C.	21d	
Vi Mark® Marek's Disease Vaccine (Live Chicken Herpesvirus)	L.A.H.I. (New Jersey)	Chickens	S.C.	21d	
Vi Mark® Marek's Disease Vaccine (Live Turkey Herpesvirus)	L.A.H.I. (New Jersey)	Chickens	S.C.	21d	
Vi Nu Chick Vac-K™	L.A.H.I. (New Jersey)	Chickens	I.M., S.C.	42d	
Vira Shield® 2	Novartis Animal Vaccines	Cattle	I.M.	60d	
Vira Shield® 2+BRSV	Novartis Animal Vaccines	Cattle	I.M.	60d	
Vira Shield® 3	Novartis Animal Vaccines	Cattle	I.M.	60d	
Vira Shield® 3+VL5	Novartis Animal Vaccines	Cattle	I.M.	60d	
Vira Shield® 4	Novartis Animal Vaccines	Cattle	I.M., S.C.	60d	
Vira Shield® 4+L5	Novartis Animal Vaccines	Cattle	I.M.	60d	
Vira Shield® 5	Novartis Animal Vaccines	Cattle	I.M., S.C.	60d	
Vira Shield® 5+L5	Novartis Animal Vaccines	Cattle	I.M.	60d	
Vira Shield® 5+L5 Somnus	Novartis Animal Vaccines	Cattle	I.M.	60d	
Vira Shield® 5+Somnus	Novartis Animal Vaccines	Cattle	I.M.	60d	
Vira Shield® 5+VL5	Novartis Animal Vaccines	Cattle	I.M.	60d	
Vira Shield® 5+VL5 Somnus	Novartis Animal Vaccines	Cattle	I.M.	60d	
Vision® 7 Somnus with Spur®	Intervet	Cattle	S.C.	21d	
Vision® 7 with Spur®	Intervet	Cattle Sheep	S.C. S.C.	21d 21d	
Vision® 8 Somnus with Spur®	Intervet	Cattle	S.C.	21d	
Vision® 8 with Spur®	Intervet	Cattle Sheep	S.C. S.C.	21d 21d	
Vision® CD•T with Spur®	Intervet	Cattle Goats Sheep	S.C. S.C. S.C.	21d 21d 21d	
Vision® CD with Spur®	Intervet	Cattle Goats Sheep	S.C. S.C. S.C.	21d 21d 21d	
Vi So Bronc®	L.A.H.I. (New Jersey)	Chickens	aer/sp, dw, I.N., I.O	21d	
Vi So Bronc® (Drinking Water Use)	L.A.H.I. (New Jersey)	Chickens	dw	21d	
Vi So Hol™	L.A.H.I. (New Jersey)	Chickens	aer/sp, dw, I.N., I.O	21d	
Vi So Hol™ (Drinking Water Use)	L.A.H.I. (New Jersey)	Chickens	dw	21d	
Vita Ferm® Milk-N-More Medicated Milk Replacer with Decoquinate ***Note:*** Do not feed to cows producing milk for food.	BioZyme	Cattle	In milk replacer		
Vita Ferm® Milk-N-More Medicated Milk Replacer with Neo/OTC ***Note:*** A withdrawal period has not been established for this product in pre-ruminating calves. Do not use in calves to be processed for veal.	BioZyme	Cattle	Oral	30d	
Vita-Jec® A & D "500"	AgriPharm	Cattle	I.M.	60d	
Vitamin AD_3	AgriLabs	Cattle	I.M.	60d	
Vitamin AD	Butler	Cattle Sheep Swine	I.M. I.M. I.M.	60d 60d 60d	
Vitamin A & D "500"	AgriPharm	Cattle	I.M.	60d	
Vitamin A D B_{12} Injection	Vedco	Cattle Sheep Swine	I.M. I.M. I.M.	60d 60d 60d	

Product Name	Company Name	Species	Route of Administration	Meat	Milk
Vitamin AD Injection	Phoenix Pharmaceutical	Cattle Sheep Swine	I.M., S.C. I.M., S.C. I.M., S.C.	60d 60d 60d	
Vitamin AD3 Injection	Bimeda	Cattle	I.M.	60d	
Vita-Plus® with Equitrol®	Farnam	Horses	In the feed		
Note: Not for use in horses intended for food.					
Vi-Trempox™	L.A.H.I. (New Jersey)	Chickens	ww	21d	
Vivomune®	Biomune	Chickens	dw	21d	
VL5-1X	Durvet	Cattle	I.M.	21d	
VL5-1X Plus™	Durvet	Cattle	I.M.	60d	
Volar®	Intervet	Cattle Sheep	I.M., S.C. I.M., S.C.	21d 21d	
VPL Fly Repellent Ointment	V.P.L.	Horses	Topical		
Note: Not for use on horses intended for food.					
VVMD-Vac®	Fort Dodge	Chickens	In ovo, S.C.	21d	
Warbex® Famphur Pour-On for Cattle	Schering-Plough	Cattle	Topical	35d	
Note: Do not apply within 21 days of freshening. Do not treat lactating dairy cattle.					
War Paint™ Insecticidal Paste	Loveland	Horses	Topical		
Note: Not for use on horses intended for food.					
Wart Shield™	Novartis Animal Vaccines	Cattle	S.C.	21d	
Wart-Vac	Durvet	Cattle	S.C.	21d	
Wart Vaccine	AgriLabs	Cattle	S.C.	21d	
Wart Vaccine	Colorado Serum	Cattle	S.C.	21d	
Wazine® 17	Fleming	Chickens Swine Turkeys	dw dw dw	14d 21d 14d	
Note: Do not use in laying hens producing eggs for human consumption.					
Wazine® 34	Fleming	Chickens Swine Turkeys	dw dw dw	14d 21d 14d	
Note: Do not use in laying hens producing eggs for human consumption.					
Wazine® Soluble	Fleming	Chickens Swine Turkeys	dw dw dw	14d 21d 14d	
Note: Do not use in laying hens producing eggs for human consumption.					
West Nile Virus Vaccine	Fort Dodge	Horses	I.M.	21d	
White Liniment	Butler	Horses	Topical		
Note: Not for use on horses intended for food.					
White Liniment	Durvet	Horses	Topical		
Note: Not for use on horses intended for food.					
Wildnil™	Wildlife	Cervidae	I.M.		
Note: Do not use 45 days before or during hunting season. Do not use in domestic food-producing animals.					
Winstrol®-V Sterile Suspension	Pharmacia & Upjohn	Horses	I.M.		
Note: Not for use in horses intended for food.					
Wipe® Fly Protectant	Farnam	Horses	Topical		
Note: Not for use on horses intended for food.					
Wonder Wormer™ for Horses	Farnam	Horses	In the feed		
Note: Not for use in horses intended for food.					
X-Ject E	Vetus	Cervidae Horses	I.M. I.M., I.V.		
Note: Do not use in *Cervidae* less than 15 days before or during the hunting season. Do not use in domestic food-producing animals. Not for use in horses intended for food.					
Xyla-Ject® 100 mg/mL Injectable	Phoenix Pharmaceutical	Cervidae Horses	I.M. I.M., I.V.		
Note: Do not use in *Cervidae* less than 15 days before or during the hunting season. Do not use in domestic food-producing animals. Not for use in horses intended for food.					
Xylazine-100 Injection	Butler	Horses	I.M., I.V.		
Note: Not for use in horses intended for food.					
Xylazine HCl Injection	Boehringer Ingelheim	Horses	I.M., I.V.		
Note: Not for use in horses intended for food.					
Xylazine HCl Injection	RXV	Cervidae Horses	I.M. I.M., I.V.		
Note: Do not use in *Cervidae* less than 15 days before or during the hunting season. Do not use in domestic food-producing animals. Not for use in horses intended for food.					

Product Name	Company Name	Species	Route of Administration	Meat	Milk
Xylazine HCl Injection	Vet Tek	Cervidae Horses	I.M. I.M., I.V.		
Note: Do not use in *Cervidae* less than 15 days before or during the hunting season. Not for use in food-producing animals. Not for use in horses intended for food.					
Xylazine HCl Injection 100 mg	AgriLabs	Cervidae Horses	I.M. I.M., I.V.		
Note: Do not use in *Cervidae* less than 15 days before or during the hunting season. Do not use in domestic food-producing animals. Not for use in horses intended for food.					
Zimecterin® Paste 1.87%	Farnam	Horses	Oral		
Note: Not for use in horses intended for food.					
Zimecterin® Paste 1.87%	Merial	Horses	Oral		
Note: Not for use in horses intended for food.					
Zoamix®	Alpharma	Chickens Turkeys	In the feed In the feed		
Note: Not for use in laying chickens or turkeys.					

Product Monographs

The following pages contain the monographs of Biological, Diagnostic, Pharmaceutical, Feed Additive and Pesticide Products.

Every effort has been made to ensure the accuracy of the information published. However it remains the responsibility of the readers to familiarize themselves with the product information contained on the product label or package insert. The publisher, editorial team and all those involved in the production of this book cannot be held responsible for publication errors or any consequences that could result from the use of published information.

1% PERMETHRIN POUR-ON

Durvet **Topical Insecticide**

Cattle and Sheep Insecticide

EPA Reg. No.: 67517-44-12281

Active Ingredient(s):

Permethrin (3-Phenoxyphenyl) methyl (±) cis, trans-3-(2,2-dichloroethenyl)-2,2-dimethylcyclopropanecarboxylate* ... 1.0%
Inert Ingredients: ... 99.0%
Total ... 100.0%

Contains Petroleum distillates

*Cis/trans isomer ratio: Min 35% (±) cis and max. 65% (±) trans

Indications: Controls lice and flies on dairy and beef cattle. Controls keds and lice on sheep.

Directions for Use: It is a violation of Federal law to use this product in a manner inconsistent with its labeling.

Ready to Use: - No dilution necessary.

Application:

Apply To	Target Insects	Application Instructions
Lactating and Non-Lactating Dairy Cattle and Beef Cattle and Calves	Lice Horn flies, Face flies and Aids in Control of: Horse flies, Stable flies, Mosquitoes, Blackflies and Ticks.	Beginning at the head, pour along the center of the back. Apply ½ fluid ounces per 100 pounds body weight of animal up to a maximum of 5 fluid ounces for any one animal.
Sheep	Sheep Keds Lice	Pour along back. Apply ¼ fl oz (7.5 cc) per 50 lbs body wt. of animal up to a maximum of 3 fl oz for any one animal.

For cattle and sheep, repeat treatment as needed, but not more than once every 2 weeks. For optimum lice control two treatments at 14-day intervals are recommended.

Special Note: Durvet 1% PERMETHRIN POUR-ON Insecticide is not effective in controlling cattle grubs.

Precautionary Statements: Hazards to Humans and Domestic Animals:

Caution: Avoid contact with eyes. Harmful if swallowed. Wash thoroughly with soap and water after handling.

Statement of Practical Treatment:

If in eyes: Flush eyes with plenty of water. Call a physician if irritation persists.

If swallowed: Call a doctor or get medical attention. Do not induce vomiting. Do not give anything by mouth to an unconscious person. Avoid alcohol.

Note to Physician: Solvent presents aspiration hazard. Gastric lavage is indicated if material was taken internally.

Environmental Hazards: This pesticide is extremely toxic to fish. Use with care when applying to areas adjacent to any body of water. Do not add directly to water. Do not contaminate water by disposal of equipment washwaters. Apply this product only as specified on the label.

Physical or Chemical Hazards: Do not use or store near heat or open flame.

In case of emergency call: Chemtrec (Poison Control Center) at 1-800-424-9300.

Storage and Disposal: Do not contaminate water, food, or feed by storage or disposal.

Pesticide Storage: Keep container sealed when not in use. Do not store near food or feed.

Pesticide Disposal: Wastes resulting from the use of this product may be disposed of on site or at an approved waste disposal facility.

Container Disposal: Triple rinse (or equivalent). Then offer for recycling or reconditioning or puncture and dispose of in a sanitary landfill or incineration, or if allowed by state and local authorities, by burning. If burned, stay out of smoke.

Warning(s): Keep out of reach of children.

Disclaimer: Notice of Warranty: Durvet, Inc. makes no warranty of merchantability, fitness for any particular purpose, or otherwise, expressed or implied concerning this product or its uses which extend beyond the use of the product under normal conditions in accord with the statements made on the label.

Presentation: One U.S. gallon (3.785 L).

Compendium Code No.: 10840000

2% CHLORHEXIDINE OINTMENT

Davis **Antiseptic**

Active Ingredient(s): Contains 2% chlorhexidine gluconate.

Indications: Davis CHLORHEXIDINE OINTMENT may be used as a soothing topical ointment around surface wounds and sores on dogs, cats and horses.

Dosage and Administration: Carefully cleanse around the wound area and apply as needed. The ointment can be used daily.

Contraindication(s): Do not use for deep or puncture wounds or serious burns.

Precaution(s): Store in original closed container and avoid exposure to heat and/or direct sunlight.

Warning(s): Do not use on horses intended for use as food.

For animal use only.

Keep out of reach of children.

Presentation: 4 oz (56.5 g) and 16 oz (454 g).

Compendium Code No.: 11410002

2% CHLORHEXIDINE SHAMPOO

Davis **Antidermatosis Shampoo**

Active Ingredient(s): Contains 2% chlorhexidine gluconate.

Indications: Davis CHLORHEXIDINE SHAMPOO is a unique formula with special ingredients to increase the effectiveness of chlorhexidine. It is an excellent hygienic shampoo with coat conditioners that cleanses and deodorizes both dogs and cats in a non-irritating formula.

Davis CHLORHEXIDINE SHAMPOO helps soothe skin conditions caused by microorganisms and skin bacteria. It is pleasantly scented with a proven safe 2% chlorhexidine gluconate, and can also be used for routine shampooing.

For conditions associated with: bacteria, fungi, ringworm, and yeast in dogs, cats, puppies and kittens.

Directions for Use: Wet pet's coat thoroughly with warm water. Do not get shampoo into eyes. Apply shampoo on head and ears, then lather. Repeat procedure with neck, chest, middle and hind quarter, finishing legs last. Allow pet to stand for 5 to 10 minutes. Rinse pet thoroughly. For best results, repeat procedure.

Warning(s): For external use only.

Keep out of reach of children.

Presentation: 12 fl. oz. (355 mL) and 1 gallon (3.785 L).

Compendium Code No.: 11410011 Rev. 11/97

3M™ LAURICARE™ MOISTURIZING TEAT DIP CONCENTRATE

3 M **Teat Dip**

Active Ingredient(s): % wt/wt

Lauricidin™ (Glyceryl Monolaurate) Lauric Acid ... 1.0
Caprylic Acid*/Capric Acid* ... 5.0
Lactic Acid ... 6.0

*Including corresponding Propylene Glycol Monofatty Acid Esters

Indications: An aid in reducing the bacteria which cause mastitis.

Directions: Dilution and Mixing Instructions: One gallon of concentrate makes 4 ready-to-use gallons. To mix one gallon of ready-to-use dip, use a clean mixing container such as a distilled/deionized water bottle. Do not use a chemical container that previously contained dips/sanitizers, cleansers, caustic or irritating materials. Carefully pour one quart (one part) of concentrate into the mixing container. Add 3 quarts (3 parts) of clean, potable water slowly to avoid foaming. To obtain good mixing, invert the container several times. Single rinse with clean water between fillings.

Directions for Use:

Pre-Dip — Before each milking, wear disposable gloves, spray or dip teats with diluted LAURICARE™ dip (1 part concentrate plus 3 parts potable water). Clean teats with 3-4 vertical hand motions and then use thumb and forefinger in 1-2 horizontal motions across the teat end to remove dirt and manure. Forestrip to detect mastitis. Spray or dip each teat again. Allow a minimum contact time of 30 seconds, and dry with a single towel prior to milking. Forestripping can be done first in tie stall barns.

Post-Dip — After Each Milking, spray or dip each teat full length (cover entire teat surface) with diluted LAURICARE™ dip (1 part concentrate plus 3 parts potable water). Allow to air dry. Do not wipe dry. To prevent freezing of teats, do not turn cows out in freezing weather until teat dip is dry. If dip cup becomes visibly dirty, discard teat dip and rinse the dip cup. Wash the dip cup well after each milking. Do not return any dip solution to the stock (mixing) container.

Note: LAURICARE™ teat dip is not intended to cure irritated or chapped teats. Consult your veterinarian if these conditions exist.

Precaution(s): Storage: Store concentrate between 40°F and 130°F. If concentrate is accidentally frozen it can be thawed out and used. Allow the dip to return to room temperature before using. Label expiration date is for concentrate.

Diluted Dip: Store between 40°F and 120°F. Do not freeze diluted dip. If diluted LAURICARE™ dip has been frozen, discard. Diluted dip is effective for 90 days. Diluted dip may be cloudy or clear depending upon temperature and age of concentrate. This does not affect performance of the dip.

Caution(s): For external use only on dairy cows. Keep out of the reach of children.

LAURICARE™ concentrate causes eye irritation with direct eye contact; avoid contact with eyes. In case of contact, flush eyes with plenty of water; call a physician if irritation persist. Prolonged skin contact with liquid concentrate or diluted dip may cause skin irritation. Use in an area such as the milking parlor or barn which can be passively ventilated to allow free exchange of inside and outside air.

First Aid: In case of eye contact, flush eyes with plenty of water; call a physician if irritation persists. If skin irritation develops, wash area with water. Call a physician if irritation persists.

Important! Do not use the undiluted concentrate as a teat dip!

Disclaimer: Warranty Information: 3M will replace such quantity of the product proved to be defective. The foregoing warranty is in lieu of all other warranties expressed or implied including the warranty of merchantability or fitness for a particular purpose. 3M shall not be liable for any damages, including special, incidental and/or consequential damages, regardless of the legal theory asserted, including negligence and/or strict liability. Some states do not allow the exclusion or limitation of special, incidental or consequential damages, so the above limitation may not apply to you. This warranty gives you specific legal rights. You may have other rights which vary from state to state.

Presentation: 1 gallon, 4½ gallon pail and 15 gallon drum.

Lauricidin is a trademark of Lauricidin, Inc.

Compendium Code No.: 11380000 34-7042-5691-5

3M™ PHENOLIC DISINFECTANT CLEANER CONCENTRATE

3 M **Disinfectant**

EPA Reg. No.: 6836-252-10350

Active Ingredient(s):

o-benzyl-p-chlorophenol	9.5%
o-phenylphenol	9.5%
Inert Ingredients	81.0%
Total	100.0%

Indications: 3M™ Phenolic Disinfectant Cleaner Concentrate is a multi-purpose germicidal detergent proven effective by the AOAC Use-Dilution Method in 400 ppm hard water (calculated as $CaCO_3$) in the presence of 5% organic bioload (Fetal Bovine Serum). This product disinfects, cleans, and deodorizes in one labor-saving step.

It is a broad spectrum disinfectant with bactericidal, fungicidal, tuberculocidal and virucidal claims.

Antiviral activity includes Canine Parvo Virus, Feline Leukemia Virus, Feline Picornavirus, Infectious Bovine Rhinotracheitis Virus, Newcastle Disease Virus, Avian Influenza Virus.

Directions for Use: It is a violation of Federal law to use this product in a manner inconsistent with its labeling.

For use on hard, non-porous surfaces such as floors, walls, metal surfaces, painted surfaces, exterior bowl surfaces, empty basins, showers, conductive flooring and lavatory fixtures. For use in hospitals, nursing homes, schools, colleges, medical and dental offices, tack shops, kennels, pet shops, veterinary clinics, and animal life science laboratories.

Applications: Use ½ ounce of 3M™ Phenolic Disinfectant Cleaner Concentrate per gallon of water for a minimum contact time of 10 minutes in a single application. For disinfecting, remove gross filth and heavy soil deposits, then thoroughly wet surfaces. This product is extremely versatile and can be applied with a mop, sponge, or cloth as well as soaking. Thoroughly wet surfaces with the recommended use solution for at least 10 minutes. The recommended use solution is used once and discarded on a daily basis. Rinsing is not necessary on floor surfaces unless floors are to be waxed or polished. Tuberculocidal effectiveness is in 10 minutes at 20°C.

Precautionary Statements: Hazards to Humans and Domestic Animals:

Corrosive: Causes eye and skin damage. Do not get in eyes, on skin or clothing. Wear goggles or face shield and rubber gloves when handling. Wash thoroughly with soap and water after handling. Remove and wash contaminated clothing before reuse. Harmful if swallowed. Avoid contamination of food, water, or feed.

Statement of Practical Treatment: In case of skin contact, wash thoroughly with soap and water. In case of eye contact: Immediately flush eyes with water for 15 minutes and get prompt medical attention. If swallowed: Drink promptly a large quantity of water. Avoid alcohol. Call a physician immediately. Note to Physician: Probable mucosal damage may contraindicate the use of gastric lavage. Measures against circulatory shock, respiratory depression, and convulsion may be needed.

Storage and Disposal: Store in original container in areas inaccessible to small children. Do not reuse empty container. Rinse and discard in trash. Refer to Material Safety Data Sheet (MSDS: 07-3145-5) for more information. In case of emergency, call: 1-800-364-3577.

Warning(s): Keep out of reach of children.

Presentation: 0.528 gallons 2 litres. 18 L makes 123 ready-to-use gallons (yield at 70°F).

Compendium Code No.: 11380020 34-8505-5066-5, 34-8505-5064-0, 34-8505-5067-3

3M™ TEAT SHIELD™ WITH GERMICIDE

3 M **Teat Dip**

Mastitis Barrier

Active Ingredient(s): Glyceryl monolaurate 1.0% contained in an acrylic latex composition stabilized to pH 6.7-8.5.

Indications: Forms a protective barrier on the teat, keeping common bacterial organisms known to cause mastitis from entering the teat canal. Kills major mastitis-causing organisms, including staph, strep, and coliform bacteria.

Directions: May be used in place of conventional teat dips.

Directions to apply—Dip teats one half of their length with undiluted TEAT SHIELD™ With Germicide. May take up to 15 minutes to dry, but is an effective germicide and barrier as soon as it is applied.

Before next milking—Wet all the teats thoroughly with warm water during premilking wash. TEAT SHIELD™ with Germicide will turn white.

Pull off the TEAT SHIELD™ With Germicide film with a wetted single service towel. A minimum of 20 second massage of the teats is necessary to promote maximum milk "letdown" and can aid film removal. Any leftover particles that get into the milking system will be caught in the filter.

Important: Occasionally some separation of product may occur. If this occurs, tip container back and forth gently several times until product is remixed.

Note: Do not return TEAT SHIELD™ with Germicide to original stock container once liquid has been poured out. The dip cup solution should be discarded if it becomes visibly dirty.

Precaution(s): TEAT SHIELD™ with Germicide should be transported and stored between 40°F and 120°F. Product that is exposed to temperatures outside the stated range may appear watery with clumps of material, may not provide an adequate barrier to mastitis-causing organisms and should not be used.

Caution(s): Not for internal use. Protect eyes and mucous membranes from contact with this product.

First-Aid: Eyes — immediately flush eyes with plenty of cool, running water for at least 15 minutes. If irritation or discomfort persists, call a physician.

As with any germicide, irritation or sensitization may occur. If irritation occurs, discontinue use immediately; consult your veterinarian if irritation persists.

To prevent freezing of teats, do not turn cows out in freezing weather until TEAT SHIELD™ with Germicide is completely dry.

Keep out of reach of children.

Disclaimer: Warranty Information: 3M will replace such quantity of the product proved to be defective. The foregoing warranty is in lieu of all other warranties expressed or implied including the warranty of merchantability or fitness for a particular purpose. 3M shall not be liable for any damages, including special, incidental and/or consequential damages, regardless of the legal theory asserted, including negligence and/or strict liability. Some states do not allow the exclusion or limitation of special, incidental or consequential damages, so the above limitation may not apply to you. This warranty gives you specific legal rights. You may have other rights which vary from state to state.

Presentation: 1 gallon (3,785 liter).

Compendium Code No.: 11380030 34-7042-5263-3

3M™ VETBOND™ TISSUE ADHESIVE

3 M **Surgical Glue**

Active Ingredient(s): Each vial of VETBOND™ Tissue Adhesive contains 0.1 fl. oz. (3 mL) of product and dispenses approximately 150 drops.

Indications: VETBOND™ Tissue Adhesive is indicated for use by veterinarians in applications including, but not limited to: cat declaws, lacerations and abrasions, sealing surgical incisions, tooth extraction and other oral surgery, and dew claw removal.

VETBOND™ Tissue Adhesive is an n-butyl cyanoacrylate adhesive which can be used to bond tissue together in a variety of veterinary procedures. It contains a blue dye which allows the user to easily see where the product has been applied and gauge the amount used.

Pharmacology: Action: Upon contact with tissue and body fluids, VETBOND™ Tissue Adhesive changes from a liquid to a solid state by polymerizing within seconds to seal a wound. The adhesive stops minor bleeding and binds wound edges, eliminating the need for sutures and/or bandaging in many instances. The thin adhesive coating further acts as a barrier to keep foreign matter from entering the wound. As healing occurs, the tissue adhesive is sloughed off.

Directions: General Instructions for Use:

1. Allow dropper bottle to come to room temperature before using. Cooler adhesive will take longer to polymerize. Do not heat VETBOND™ Tissue Adhesive to bring it to room temperature.
2. Remove bottle cap. To open, cut off tip of bottle with scissors or blade. If any adhesive leaks during the opening of the bottle, clean the bottle tip with clean, dry gauze before placing applicator tip on the bottle. Place flexible applicator tip on the bottle for use. The applicator tip can be removed. Clean the bottle tip with clean, dry gauze before replacing the bottle cap.
3. Application site should be free of excess fluids for best performance of the adhesive. Excessive fluids exert a weakening effect on the bond strength. A saline wash or preparatory solution, e.g. Betadine™*, may be used prior to surgery as long as the surgical site is blotted dry before applying the adhesive.
4. Apply the adhesive sparingly (e.g. one drop per digit in a cat declaw procedure) to the site to form a thin film. This enhances the bonding action. Thick applications tend to crack and lift prematurely.
5. Avoid touching moist surfaces with applicator tip since this could clog the tip.
6. When procedures are complete, remove excess adhesive in vial tip by holding bottle upright and gently squeezing the single drop of adhesive out of the tip onto a paper towel. This will prevent the tip from clogging. To assure that no residual adhesive remains in the applicator tip, attach it to a 3 mL syringe to expel any adhesive out of the tip.
7. Replace bottle cap. Store vial away from heat (in a cool, dry location, if possible). Store bottle upright on a shelf. Do not return bottle to refrigerator.

Recommended Sutureless Cat Declaw Procedure:

1. Anesthetic Recommendations: For optimum product performance, use an anesthetic that allows a smooth recovery and a long-acting tranquilizer that keeps the animal relatively sedated during the post-operative period.
2. Preparation of Surgical Sites:

a. Prepare the foreleg for surgery in your routine manner.

b. Soap and water or antiseptics, such as Betadine™, may be used, provided that the surgical sites are blotted dry before VETBOND™ Tissue Adhesive is applied. These agents must not be applied after the claws are amputated because they could interfere with the polymerization of the adhesive.

3. Surgical Procedure:

a. Squeeze limb to remove venous blood and apply tourniquet tightly above elbow and hock joints. Use appropriate precautions when utilizing the tourniquet for hemostasis.

b. Amputate claws using routine surgical procedure.

c. Treat each wound cavity as follows:

(1) If incision site is quite bloody, remove as much blood as possible by swabbing with a saline-soaked, cotton-tipped applicator.

(2) Hold wound open and apply VETBOND™ Tissue Adhesive to the cut surface and bone within the cavity - use one drop on each digit. See General Instructions for Use. Do not glue hair into site. Preparing the area prior to surgery as described in 2.b. helps hold hair down out of the way. If it is in the way, hair will "wick" the adhesive.

(3) Immediately after the adhesive application, press the skin edges over the bone with forceps and hold together for 5 to 10 seconds.

(4) Remove tourniquet 3 minutes after treating the last cavity. Check for bleeding and reapply a drop of adhesive if necessary, or apply slight pressure to limb to stop oozing. Bleeding will usually stop within 5 to 10 minutes.

(5) Sutures or dressings are generally not needed.

Contraindication(s): Do not use VETBOND™ Tissue Adhesive on infected and/or deep puncture wounds.

Although VETBOND™ Tissue Adhesive is a hemostat, it may not stop the bleeding from large arteries. Further, it is not intended to replace sutures in every case but may be used to approximate wound edges between sutures and also for bandage-free sutureless cat declaw procedures (see directions).

VETBOND™ Tissue Adhesive may be used between stainless steel staples, but application of adhesive on staples may interfere with staple removal.

Precaution(s): Storage: To maximize product performance, store in a cool, dry place. Maintain product at room temperature during use.

Do not use if adhesive, at room temperature, appears thicker than water. Thickened product has partially polymerized and would not be expected to form an acceptable tissue bond.

Caution(s):

1. To prevent adhesion, avoid contact of adhesive with skin and eyes. Should accidental contact occur, the area should be wiped immediately with a paper towel. The adhesive may be removed from skin with dimethylsulfoxide. If the adhesive accidently gets in the eyes, the eyelids should be held open and the eyes flushed thoroughly with water. An ophthalmologist should be consulted. To help avoid such an accident, place a damp towel over the eyes when the material is used on or near the patient's face.
2. Avoid breathing vapors over long periods of time. The adhesive should be used in a well-ventilated area.
3. To prevent adhesion, avoid contact of the adhesive with instruments, gloves, and surgical equipment. Polymerized adhesive on instruments can be removed by soaking in acetone.
4. Avoid unwanted contact of adhesive and animal tissue to prevent undesired adhesion.

Presentation: 3 mL vials.

*Betadine is a trademark of Purdue-Frederick.

Compendium Code No.: 11380040 34-7047-6053-6

3-NITRO® 20

Alpharma **Feed Additive**

Roxarsone-Type A Medicated Article

NADA No.: 007-891

Active Ingredient(s):

3-Nitro-4-hydroxyphenylarsonic acid (roxarsone) 20%
(equivalent to 90.7 grams roxarsone per pound of product)

Inactive ingredient:

Roughage product, calcium carbonate, mineral oil 80%

Indications: For increased rate of weight gain and improved feed efficiency for growing chickens, growing turkeys, and growing-finishing swine.

For improved pigmentation of growing chickens and growing turkeys.

An aid in the treatment of swine dysentery (hemorragic enteritis or bloody scours.)

Dosage and Administration: For increased rate of weight gain, improved feed efficiency, and improved pigmentation for growing chickens and growing turkeys: Mix 4 ounces (113.4 grams) to 8 ounces (226.8 grams) of 3-NITRO® 20 in 2,000 pounds (909 kg) of a complete feed. These mixtures will provide 0.0025% to 0.005% (22.7 grams to 45.4 grams) of 3-Nitro-4-hydroxyphenylarsonic acid (roxarsone) in the feed. Give continuously through the growing period.

For increased rate of weight gain and improved feed efficiency for growing-finishing swine: Mix 4 ounces (113.4 grams) to 6 ounces (170.1 grams) of 3-NITRO® 20 in 2,000 pounds (909 kg) of a complete feed. These mixtures will provide 0.0025% to 0.00375% (22.7 grams to 34.1 grams) of 3-Nitro-4-hydroxyphenylarsonic acid (roxarsone) in the feed. Give continuously through the growing-finishing period.

As an aid in the treatment of swine dysentery (hemorrhagic enteritis or bloody scours): Mix 2 pounds (909 grams) of 3-NITRO® 20 in 2,000 pounds (909 kg) of a complete feed. This mixture will provide 0.02% (181.5 grams) of 3-Nitro-4-hydroxyphenylarsonic acid (roxarsone) in the feed. Give for no more than 6 consecutive days. If improvement is not observed, consult a veterinarian.

Mixing Directions: To obtain a uniform distribution of the active drug ingredient in the finished feed, prepare an intermediate type A medicated article. Then add the appropriate amount of this to 2,000 pounds (909 kg) of finished feed to provide the desired concentration of active drug. Mix thoroughly.

Caution(s): Must be mixed thoroughly in feed before use. Use as the sole source of organic arsenic. Use only as directed. In case of swine dysentery, treated animals must actually consume enough medicated feed to provide a therapeutic dose. Poultry and swine should have access to drinking water at all times. Drug overdosage or lack of water intake may result in leg weakness or paralysis.

Warning(s): Withdraw 5 days before slaughter.

Keep out of reach of children.

In mixing avoid inhaling dust. Avoid contact of product with skin, eyes and clothing. Wash thoroughly after handling.

Poison-Arsenic. Antidote: If swallowed, call a physician, poison control center, or hospital immediately. Induce vomiting by giving Ipecac syrup as directed.

Presentation: 50 lb (22.68 kg) bag.

3-NITRO is a registered trademark of Alpharma Inc.

Compendium Code No.: 10220012 500320 0201

3-NITRO® SOLUBLE

Alpharma **Water Medication**

NADA No.: 093-025

Active Ingredient(s):

Monosodium 3-nitro-4-hydroxyphenlyarsonate........................... 21.7 grams

Inactive ingredient: Dextrose.

Indications: For increased rate of weight gain, improved feed efficiency, and improved pigmentation for growing chickens and growing turkeys; as an aid in the treatment of swine dysentery (hemorrhagic enteritis or bloody scours).

Directions:

For increased rate of weight gain, improved feed efficiency, and improved pigmentation for growing chickens and growing turkeys: Mix contents of the pouch in 250 U.S. gallons (946 liters) of drinking water. Stir vigorously. Give continuously through growing period.

Automatic water proportioner use: To make a concentrated solution, mix pouch contents in 2 U.S. gallons (7.6 liters) water. Set proportioner to deliver 1 fluid ounce (30 mL) of this solution per gallon (3.8 liters) of drinking water. (Either mode of administration provides 0.002% active drug concentration in drinking water.)

As an aid in the treatment of swine dysentery (hemorrhagic enteritis or bloody scours): Mix contents of the pouch in 50 U.S. gallons (189 liters) of drinking water. Stir vigorously. Give for no more than 6 successive days. If no improvement is observed, consult a veterinarian. Treatment may be repeated after 5 days off medication.

Automatic proportioner use: To make a concentrated solution, mix pouch contents in 3 pints (1.4 liters) of water and set proportioner to deliver 1 fluid ounce (30 mL) of this solution per gallon (3.8 liters) of drinking water. (Either mode of administration provides 0.01% drug in water.) Pigs may be treated individually with a drench of 1 fluid ounce (30 mL) of the concentrated solution per 50 pounds (22.7 kg) of body weight, once daily for 1 to 2 days.

Caution(s): In case of swine dysentery, treated animals must consume enough medicated water to provide a therapeutic dose. Drug overdosage may result in leg weakness or paralysis. Use only as directed. Do not administer to birds or animals that have been without water or that have become severely dehydrated.

Use as the sole source of organic arsenic. In mixing, avoid inhaling this powder. Avoid contact of product with eyes, skin, and clothing. Wash thoroughly after handling.

Poison - Arsenic.

Keep out of reach of children.

Antidote(s): If swallowed, call a physician, poison control center or hospital immediately.

Induce vomiting by giving Ipecac Syrup as directed.

Warning(s): Withdraw 5 days before slaughter.

Presentation: 1 oz (28.35 g) pouches.

Compendium Code No.: 10220000

3-NO-BITE SPRAY

Vedco **Topical Product**

Active Ingredient(s): Isopropyl alcohol, deionized water, oleoresin capsicum, sucrose octyl acetate, orange peel bitter, propylene glycol, polysorbate 60, FD&C red #40.

Indications: 3-NO-BITE SPRAY contains three active bittering agents from tabasco pepper, orange peel and denatured alcohol to discourage licking, biting and chewing.

Dosage and Administration: Apply to bandages, casts, hair, or household furniture twice a day or as directed by a veterinarian.

Caution(s): Avoid contact with broken skin, eyes or mucous membranes. If in contact, wash with copious amounts of cool water immediately. If redness or irritation occurs or if accidently swallowed, call a physician or poison control center.

Before applying to extensive areas of furniture, test the effect of the product on a small, inconspicuous area.

Flammable. Keep away from heat or an open flame.

Keep out of the reach of children.

Presentation: 4 oz. container with sprayer.

Compendium Code No.: 10940000

3% RABON® LIVESTOCK DUST

Durvet **Topical Insecticide**

Ready-To-Use Insecticide Dust

EPA Reg. No.: 67517-40-12281

Active Ingredient(s): Contains 3% Rabon®* Insecticide.

By Weight

Tetrachlorvinphos: (CAS #961-11-5) 3.00%
Inert Ingredients 97.00%
100.00%

Indications: For use on livestock. No milk or tissue withdrawal. Controls horn flies, cattle grubs and lice, and aids in the control of face flies on beef and dairy cattle. Controls lice on swine.

Directions for Use: It is a violation of Federal law to use this product in a manner inconsistent with its labeling.

Read entire label before each use.

Application Restriction: Do not apply this product in a way that will contact workers or other persons, either directly or through drift. Only protected handlers may be in the area during application.

For Use on Livestock: Durvet 3% RABON® Dust is a ready-to-use insecticide dust which can be applied by hand or thorough the use of self-treating dust bags. There is no withholding period from last application to slaughter.

Animal	Insect	Remarks
Beef Cattle and Dairy Cattle	Horn Flies, Face Flies and Lice	Hand Dusting — Apply approximately 2 oz of dust by shaking can, rotary duster or by spoon to the upper portions of the back as an aid for the control of face flies. Rub in lightly to carry the dust beneath the hair. Do not treat more often than once every two weeks. Self-Treating Dust Bag Forced Use — Put RABON® Dust in cotton cloth or double burlap bags or use weather-proof cattle dust bags and hang in door exits or alleyways leading from animal buildings, salt or mineral blocks, or watering holes. Protect cloth or burlap bags from weather. Free-Choice Use — Use the same dust bags as above but place in loafing sheds, holding pens, feedlots, near watering holes or other areas where cattle gather. The free choice aids in the control of lice.
	Cattle Grubs	After the grubs have encysted (formed warbles) apply 3-4 oz down the backline and rub in thoroughly, taking care to get the dust into the warble if possible.
Swine	Lice	Hand Dusting — Apply 3-4 oz of dust by conventional hand or power duster to each animal with special attention given to the neck and around the ears. Do not repeat more often than once every 14 days. In severe infestations, both individual animals and bedding may be treated. One lb of RABON® Dust should be applied per 50 sq. ft. of bedding.

Precautionary Statements: Hazard to Humans and Domestic Animals: Caution: Hazard to Humans: Harmful if swallowed or absorbed through the skin. Causes moderate eye irritation. Avoid contact with eyes, skin or clothing. Wash thoroughly with soap and water after handling and before eating, drinking, chewing gum, using tobacco or using the toilet. Avoid contamination of feed and feedstuffs. This product may cause skin sensitization reactions in certain individuals. Wear long sleeved shirt and pants, chemical resistant gloves, shoes and socks. Follow manufacturer's instructions for cleaning/maintaining PPE. If no such instructions for washables, use detergent and hot water. Keep and wash PPE separately from other laundry.

User Safety Recommendations:

Remove clothing immediately if pesticide gets inside. Then wash thoroughly and put on clean clothing.

Remove PPE immediately after handling this product. Wash the outside of gloves.

First Aid:

If Swallowed: Call a physician or Poison Control Center. Drink 1 or 2 glasses of water and induce vomiting by touching the back of the throat with finger, or if available by administering syrup of ipecac. If person is unconscious, do not give anything by mouth and do not induce vomiting.

If In Eyes: Flush eyes with plenty of water. Call a physician if irritation persists.

If On Skin: Wash with plenty of soap and water. Get medical attention if irritation persists.

Note to Physician/Veterinarian: RABON® is an organophosphate insecticide. If symptoms of cholinesterase inhibition are present, atropine sulfate by injection is antidotal. 2-PAM is also antidotal and may be administered, but only in conjunction with atropine.

Symptoms of Exposure: May produce acute cholinesterase depression. Acute cholinesterase depression may be evidenced by headache, nausea, vomiting, diarrhea, abdominal cramps, excessive sweating, salivation and tearing, constricted pupils, blurred vision, tightness in chest, weakness, muscle twitching, and confusion. In extreme cases, unconsciousness, convulsions, and severe respiratory depression may occur.

Environmental Hazards: This product is toxic to fish. Drift and runoff may be hazardous to aquatic organisms in adjacent areas. Do not apply directly to water. Do not contaminate water when disposing of equipment washwater. Apply this product only as specified on this label.

This product is highly toxic to bees exposed to direct treatment on blooming crops or weeds. Do not apply this product or allow it to drift to blooming crops or weeds if bees are visiting the treatment area.

Storage and Disposal: Do not contaminate water, food or feed by storage or disposal.

Pesticide Storage: Store in a dry place in original container.

Container Disposal: Completely empty bag into application equipment. Then dispose of empty bag in a sanitary landfill or by incineration, or, if allowed by State and local authorities, by burning. If burned, stay out of smoke.

Pesticide Disposal: Wastes resulting from the use of this product may be disposed of on-site or at an approved waste disposal facility.

Warning(s): Keep out of reach of children.

Disclaimer: Notice of Warranty: Durvet, Inc. makes no warranty of merchantability, fitness for any particular purpose, or otherwise, expressed or implied concerning this product or its uses which extend beyond the use of the product under normal conditions in accord with the statements made on this label.

Presentation: 12.5 lbs (5.67 kg).

RABON is a registered trademark of Boehringer Ingelheim

Compendium Code No.: 10840011 9712B

3V CAPS™ FOR LARGE & GIANT BREEDS

DVM **Small Animal Dietary Supplement**

Guaranteed Analysis: Nutritional Information (per capsule):

Crude Protein, not less than 7%
Crude Fat, not less than 90%
Crude Fiber, not more than 1%
Moisture, not more than 2%
Eicosapentaenoic Acid (EPA)* ..... 250 mg
Docosahexaenoic Acid (DHA)* ..... 167 mg
Vitamin A ..... 1250 IU
Vitamin D ..... 125 IU
Vitamin E ..... 75 IU

Ingredients: Fish oil, dl-alpha tocopheryl acetate (source of vitamin E), cod liver oil (source of vitamins A and D), gelatin, water, glycerin.

*Not recognized as an essential nutrient by the AAFCO dog nutrient profiles.

Indications: 3V CAPS™ provide a supplemental source of *omega-3 fatty acids plus vitamins A, D and E which are beneficial for the maintenance of healthy skin and coats in large and giant breeds of dogs.

Dosage and Administration: For dogs 60-90 lbs.

Recommended Amounts: 1 to 2 capsules daily.

Note: Capsule may be punctured and liquid contents squeezed onto food, if desired.

Precaution(s): Store the container at room temperature.

Caution(s): For animal use only.

Presentation: 60 and 250 capsules (1488 mg/capsule).

Compendium Code No.: 11420002 Rev 0399

3V CAPS™ FOR MEDIUM & LARGE BREEDS

DVM **Small Animal Dietary Supplement**

Guaranteed Analysis: Nutritional Information (per capsule):

Crude Protein, not less than 7%
Crude Fat, not less than 90%
Crude Fiber, not more than 1%
Moisture, not more than 2%
Eicosapentaenoic Acid (EPA)* ..... 180 mg
Docosahexaenoic Acid (DHA)* ..... 120 mg
Vitamin A ..... 1250 IU
Vitamin D ..... 125 IU
Vitamin E ..... 75 IU

Ingredients: Fish oil, dl-alpha tocopheryl acetate (source of vitamin E), cod liver oil (source of vitamins A and D), gelatin, water, glycerin.

*Not recognized as an essential nutrient by the AAFCO dog nutrient profiles.

Indications: 3V CAPS™ provide a supplemental source of *omega-3 fatty acids plus vitamins A, D and E which are beneficial for the maintenance of healthy skin and coats in medium and large breeds of dogs.

Dosage and Administration: For dogs 30-60 lbs.

Recommended Amounts: 1 to 2 capsules daily.

Note: Capsule may be punctured and liquid contents squeezed onto food, if desired.

Precaution(s): Store the container at room temperature.

Presentation: 60 capsules (1100 mg per capsule).

Compendium Code No.: 11420011 Rev 0499

3V CAPS™ FOR SMALL & MEDIUM BREEDS

DVM **Small Animal Dietary Supplement**

Guaranteed Analysis: Nutritional Information (per capsule):

Crude Protein, not less than 7%
Crude Fat, not less than 90%
Crude Fiber, not more than 1%
Moisture, not more than 2%
Eicosapentaenoic Acid (EPA)* ..... 103 mg
Docosahexaenoic Acid (DHA)* ..... 68 mg
Vitamin A ..... 1250 IU
Vitamin D ..... 125 IU
Vitamin E ..... 75 IU

Ingredients: Fish oil, dl-alpha tocopheryl acetate (source of vitamin E), cod liver oil (source of vitamins A and D), gelatin, water, glycerin.

*Not recognized as an essential nutrient by the AAFCO dog or cat nutrient profiles.

Indications: 3V CAPS™ provide a supplemental source of *omega-3 fatty acids plus vitamins A, D and E which are beneficial for the maintenance of healthy skin and coats in small and medium breeds of dogs, and in cats.

Dosage and Administration: For dogs and cats up to 30 lbs.

Recommended Amounts: 1 to 2 capsules daily.

Note: Capsule may be punctured and liquid contents squeezed onto food, if desired.

Precaution(s): Store the container at room temperature.

Caution(s): For use in dogs and cats.

Presentation: 60 capsules (670 mg/capsule).

Compendium Code No.: 11420021 Rev 0499

3V CAPS™ LIQUID

DVM **Small Animal Dietary Supplement**

Concentrated Dietary Supplement

Guaranteed Analysis: Nutritional Information (per pump; 0.75 mL, 694 mg):

Crude Protein, not less than 7%
Crude Fat, not less than 90%
Crude Fiber, not more than 1%
Moisture, not more than 2%
Eicosapentaenoic Acid (EPA)* ..... 113 mg
Docosahexaenoic Acid (DHA)* ..... 74 mg
Vitamin A ..... 937 IU
Vitamin D ..... 94 IU
Vitamin E ..... 46 IU

Ingredients: Fish oil, dl-alpha tocopheryl acetate (source of vitamin E), cod liver oil (source of vitamins A and D).

*Not recognized as an essential nutrient by the AAFCO dog or cat food nutrient profiles.

Indications: 3V CAPS™ provides a supplemental source of *omega-3 fatty acids plus vitamins A, D and E, which are beneficial for the maintenance of healthy skin and coats in dogs and cats.

Dosage and Administration: Recommended Amounts:

Animal Weight	Recommended Daily Amount
1-19 lbs	One Half (½) Pump**
20-39 lbs	One (1) Pump
40-59 lbs	Two (2) Pumps
60-79 lbs	Three (3) Pumps
80-100 lbs	Four (4) Pumps

**Complete depression of the pump delivers 0.75 mL 3V CAPS™ Liquid.

Precaution(s): Store the container at room temperature.

Caution(s): For use in dogs and cats.

Presentation: 6 fl oz (177 mL).

Compendium Code No.: 11420031 Rev 0399

3X PYRETHRIN SHAMPOO

Vet Solutions **Parasiticide Shampoo**

EPA Reg. No.: 2097-17-72896

Active Ingredient(s):

Pyrethrins 0.15%
*Piperonyl Butoxide technical 1.50%
Inert Ingredients: 98.35%
Total 100.00%

*Equivalent to 1.20% of butylcarbityl (6-propylpiperonyl) ether and .30% of related compounds.

Indications: Kills fleas, ticks and lice on dogs and fleas on cats.

Directions for Use: Read entire label before each use.

It is a violation of Federal Law to use this product in a manner inconsistent with its labeling.

As a precaution, a bland ophthalmic ointment should be placed in the eyes prior to bathing to prevent possible irritation.

Thoroughly wet the entire hair-coat with warm water and then apply enough shampoo to make a lather and work thoroughly into the coat and skin. For best results allow lather to remain in contact with skin for five minutes before rinsing. Rinse thoroughly. Product contains emollient and may be repeated weekly if required. For a complete flee and tick control program consult veterinarian.

Precautionary Statements: Hazards to Humans and Domestic Animals:

Caution: May be harmful if swallowed or absorbed through skin. Avoid skin contact. May cause eye irritation. Avoid contact with eyes. Wash thoroughly after handling. Do not use on animals under 12 weeks of age. Consult a veterinarian before using this product on debilitated, aged, pregnant or nursing animals, or animals on medication. Sensitivities may occur after using any pesticide products for pets. If signs of sensitivity occur bathe your pet with mild soap and rinse with large amounts of water. If signs continue, consult a veterinarian immediately.

First Aid: If in eyes flush with plenty of water. Get medical attention if irritation persists.

If on skin wash thoroughly with soap and water, remove contaminated clothing. If irritation persists consult a physician.

Storage and Disposal:

Storage: Store at room temperature in original container.

Disposal: Do not reuse empty container. Securely wrap original container in several layers of newspaper and discard in trash.

This product is restricted for sale exclusively through veterinary clinics, practices and hospitals.

In case of emergency or for product use information, please call 1-800-285-0508 Monday-Friday, 8:00 a.m.-4:30 p.m. CST.

Warning(s): Keep out of reach of children.

For external use only.

Use only on dogs and cats.

Presentation: 1 gallon (3.79 L).

Compendium Code No.: 10610010 000201

4% MAXIMUM CHLORHEXIDINE SHAMPOO

Davis **Antidermatosis Shampoo**

Active Ingredient(s): 4% Chlorhexidine Gluconate.

Indications: Davis MAXIMUM CHLORHEXIDINE SHAMPOO with 4% Chlorhexidine Gluconate is formulated for moderate to severe skin conditions where a full strength shampoo is required. Proven safe Chlorhexidine Gluconate, combined with deep cleansing agents and moisturizers, works to provide a therapeutic bath and helps to promote healthy skin and coat.

Davis MAXIMUM CHLORHEXIDINE SHAMPOO is effective, yet mild and may even be used for routine shampooing.

For dogs, cats, puppies and kittens.

For moderate to severe conditions associated with bacteria, fungi, ringworm and yeast.

Directions for Use: Wet pet's coat thoroughly with warm water. Apply shampoo to head and ears, then lather. Do not get shampoo into eyes. Repeat procedure with neck, chest, middle and hind quarter, finishing with legs last. Allow pet to stand for 5 to 10 minutes. Rinse thoroughly. For best results, repeat procedure.

Caution(s): If irritation develops, discontinue use and consult a veterinarian. Not for otic use.

Warning(s): For external use only.

Keep out of reach of children.

Presentation: 12 fl. oz. (355 mL) and 1 gallon (3.785 liter) containers.

Compendium Code No.: 11410430 Rev. 1100

4% NON-STING CHLORHEXIDINE SPRAY

Davis **Antidermatosis Spray**

Active Ingredient(s): Contains 4% chlorhexidine. It also contains aloe.

Indications: Davis 4% NON-STING CHLORHEXIDINE SPRAY helps provide quick relief for mild to severe irritations caused by bacteria, ringworm, yeast and fungi in dogs, cats and horses.

This product is also recommended as an aid in the relief of hot spots, itching, inflammation and fleabite dermatitis.

Directions for Use: Shake well before each use. Spray directly on affected areas 2-3 times a day. For added residual activity use in-between medicated shampoos. For best results, use in conjunction with Davis Chlorhexidine Shampoo.

Precaution(s): Store in original closed container away from heat and light.

Caution(s): Avoid contact with eyes. If condition persists or irritation develops, discontinue use and consult your veterinarian.

Warning(s): For external veterinary use only.

Keep out of reach of children.

For topical use only on dogs, cats and horses.

Presentation: 8 fl oz (236.56 mL).

Compendium Code No.: 11410030

4-PLEX

Zinpro **Feed Additive**

Typical Analysis:

Zinc	2.53%
Manganese	1.40%
Copper	0.88%
Cobalt	0.18%
Methionine	8.21%
Lysine	3.80%
Protein	11.5%
Fat	1.5%
Fiber	22.0%
Ash	26.5%

Each ½ ounce of 4-PLEX contains 360 mg zinc from zinc methionine; 200 mg manganese from manganese methionine; 125 mg copper from copper lysine, and 25 mg cobalt from cobalt glucoheptonate.

Indications: Recommended as a nutritional feed additive for livestock.

Physical Description: A light-to-medium brown granular powder. 4-PLEX weighs approximately 27 lbs/cu ft.

Feeding Instructions:

Beef and Dairy Cattle: Feed at the rate of ½ ounce (14 grams) per head daily, or 1 lb per 32 head daily.

Contraindication(s): Do not feed to sheep or related species.

Toxicology: When correctly used, there is no toxicity hazard in the use of 4-PLEX.

Presentation: 4-PLEX is packaged in 50 lb multiwall bags.

Compendium Code No.: 11300000

4-PLEX-C

Zinpro **Feed Additive**

Typical Analysis:

Zinc	5.06%
Manganese	2.80%
Copper	1.76%
Cobalt	0.36%
Methionine	16.42%
Lysine	7.61%
Protein	20.0%
Fat	0.1%
Fiber	2.0%
Ash	51.0%

Each ¼ ounce of 4-PLEX-C contains 360 mg zinc from zinc methionine; 200 mg manganese from manganese methionine; 125 mg copper from copper lysine, and 25 mg cobalt from cobalt glucoheptonate.

Indications: Recommended as a nutritional feed additive for livestock.

Physical Description: A light-to-medium gray powder. 4-PLEX-C weighs approximately 38 lbs/cu ft.

Feeding Instructions:

Beef and Dairy Cattle: Feed at the rate of ¼ ounce (7 grams) per head daily, or 1 lb per 64 head daily.

Contraindication(s): Do not feed to sheep or related species.

Toxicology: When correctly used, there is no toxicity hazard in the use of 4-PLEX-C.

Presentation: 4-PLEX-C is packaged in 50 lb multiwall bags.

Compendium Code No.: 11300010

4XLA® GERMICIDAL PRE- & POST-MILKING TEAT DIP (ACTIVATOR)

Alcide **Teat Dip**

Active Ingredient(s): 2.64% Lactic acid.

Contains: 10% glycerin.

Indications: An aid in reducing the spread of organisms which may cause mastitis.

For use only with 4XLA® Base.

Directions for Use: Measure equal volumes of 4XLA® base and 4XLA® activator into a clean dip cup/container and mix until the color is uniform throughout. Do not dilute. Mix only enough product for one milking of the herd. Dip cups should be washed after each milking.

Application:

Pre-Milking: If teats are visibly dirty, wash and dry teats with a single service towel prior to dipping. Before each cow is milked, dip the teats as far up as possible. Leave 4XLA® Teat Dip on teats for at least 15-30 seconds. Wipe teats dry using a single service towel before milking.

Post-Milking: Immediately after milking, dip teats at least ⅔ to all their length in 4XLA® Teat Dip. Allow to air dry. Do not wipe. 4XLA® Teat Dip can be used as a post-dip alone, or as a pre- and post-milking teat dip.

Always use freshly mixed, full strength 4XLA® Teat Dip. If product in dip cup becomes visibly dirty, discard contents and fill with fresh 4XLA® Teat Dip. 4XLA® Teat Dip may be diluted with water and safely flushed down the drain.

Note 1: If teat irritation occurs, discontinue use until irritation subsides. Consult your veterinarian and milking equipment service personnel if irritation persists.

Note 2: The gold color in the mixed product fades with time. At higher temperatures the fading is more rapid. However, this will not affect the efficacy of the product.

Note 3: 4XLA® should be used only with a compatible pre-dip or udder wash.

Caution(s): For external use only. Not for use in sanitizing dairy equipment. Do not mix with any other teat dip or other product. Avoid contact with food. Avoid contact with eyes. If contact occurs, flush eyes with large quantities of water. See a physician if irritation develops.

Storage and Disposal: Store at room temperature. Protect from heat and freezing. Always store away from continuous artificial light or direct sunlight.

Disposal: Unused teat dip may be diluted with water and flushed down drain. Do not reuse containers. Empty containers should be thoroughly rinsed with water and taken to a recycling center.

Avoid freezing: If product is exposed to freezing temperatures, components must be mixed thoroughly prior to use.

Warning(s): Keep out of the reach of children.

Disclaimer: UMS's and Alcide's liability on any claim, whether in negligence or any other tort or in contract or otherwise, with respect to products delivered hereunder, shall not exceed the purchase price of the products sold or, if UMS and Alcide shall so elect, buyer shall be entitled only to replacement of product. In no event shall UMS and Alcide be liable for buyer's incidental or consequential damages.

Presentation: Available in 1, 5, 15 and 55 gallon sizes.

U.S. Patent 5,384,134

Foreign Patents Issued and Pending

4XLA® is a registered trademark of Alcide Corporation.

Distributed by: Universal Marketing Services, 5545 Avenida de los Robles, Visalia, CA 93291.

Compendium Code No.: 14760000 L8109A Rev. 01 1-99

4XLA® GERMICIDAL PRE- & POST-MILKING TEAT DIP (BASE)

Alcide **Teat Dip**

Active Ingredient(s): 0.64% Sodium chlorite.

Indications: An aid in reducing the spread of organisms which may cause mastitis.

For use only with 4XLA® Activator.

Directions for Use: Measure equal volumes of 4XLA® base and 4XLA® activator into a clean dip cup/container and mix until the color is uniform throughout. Do not dilute. Mix only enough product for one milking of the herd. Dip cups should be washed after each milking.

Application:

Pre-Milking: If teats are visibly dirty, wash and dry teats with a single service towel prior to dipping. Before each cow is milked, dip the teats as far up as possible. Leave 4XLA® Teat Dip on teats for at least 15-30 seconds. Wipe teats dry using a single service towel before milking.

Post-Milking: Immediately after milking, dip teats at least ⅔ to all their length in 4XLA® Teat Dip. Allow to air dry. Do not wipe. 4XLA® Teat Dip can be used as a post-dip alone, or as a pre- and post-milking teat dip.

Always use freshly mixed, full strength 4XLA® Teat Dip. If product in dip cup becomes visibly dirty, discard contents and fill with fresh 4XLA® Teat Dip. 4XLA® Teat Dip may be diluted with water and safely flushed down the drain.

Note 1: If teat irritation occurs, discontinue use until irritation subsides. Consult your veterinarian and milking equipment service personnel if irritation persists.

Note 2: The gold color in the mixed product fades with time. At higher temperatures the fading is more rapid. However, this will not affect the efficacy of the product.

Note 3: 4XLA® should be used only with a compatible pre-dip or udder wash.

Caution(s): For external use only. Not for use in sanitizing dairy equipment. Do not mix with any other teat dip or other product. Avoid contact with food. Avoid contact with eyes. If contact occurs, flush eyes with large quantities of water. See a physician if irritation develops.

Storage and Disposal: Store at room temperature. Protect from heat and freezing. Always store away from continuous artificial light or direct sunlight.

Disposal: Unused teat dip may be diluted with water and flushed down drain. Do not reuse containers. Empty containers should be thoroughly rinsed with water and taken to a recycling center.

Avoid freezing: If product is exposed to freezing temperatures, components must be mixed thoroughly prior to use.

Warning(s): Keep out of the reach of children.

Disclaimer: UMS's and Alcide's liability on any claim, whether in negligence or any other tort or in contract or otherwise, with respect to products delivered hereunder, shall not exceed the purchase price of the products sold or, if UMS and Alcide shall so elect, buyer shall be entitled only to replacement of product. In no event shall UMS and Alcide be liable for buyer's incidental or consequential damages.

Presentation: Available in 1, 5, 15 and 55 gallon sizes.

U.S. Patent 5,384,134

Foreign Patents Issued and Pending

4XLA® is a registered trademark of Alcide Corporation.

Distributed by: Universal Marketing Services, 5545 Avenida de los Robles, Visalia, CA 93291.

Compendium Code No.: 14760010 L8109B Rev. 01 1-99

5-WAY CALF SCOUR BOLUS™

AgriLabs **Tetracycline-Oral**

Tetracycline Hydrochloride Tablets

NADA No.: 011-060

Active Ingredient(s): Each bolus contains:

Tetracycline hydrochloride . . . . 500 mg

Indications: For the control and treatment of bacterial enteritis (scours) caused by *Escherichia coli* and bacterial pneumonia (*Pasteurella* spp., *Hemophilus* spp., and *Klebsiella* spp.) in calves.

Dosage and Administration: Administer orally in divided doses to provide 10 mg of tetracycline per pound of body weight each day for 3-5 days. When feeding milk or milk replacer, administer one (1) hour before or two (2) hours after feeding.

Note: If improvement is not noted in 3-4 days, consult a veterinarian.

Precaution(s): Store at room temperature.

Caution(s): For veterinary use only.

Keep out of the reach of children.

Not for human use.

Use as the sole source of tetracycline.

Warning(s): Do not slaughter for food within 14 days of treatment.

Presentation: 24 and 100 boluses per container.

Compendium Code No.: 10580000

7 GAUGE™

AgriPharm **Bacterin-Toxoid**

Clostridium Chauvoei-Septicum-Novyi-Sordellii-Perfringens Types C & D Bacterin-Toxoid

U.S. Vet. Lic. No.: 124

Contents: This product contains the antigens listed above.

Indications: Recommended for the vaccination of healthy, susceptible sheep and cattle, including bred and/or lactating beef and dairy cattle, as an aid in the reduction of diseases caused by *Clostridium chauvoei, Cl. septicum, Cl. novyi, Cl. sordellii* and *Cl. perfringens* Type C and D. Although *Cl. perfringens* Type B is not a significant problem in the USA, immunity may be provided against the beta and epsilon toxins elaborated by *Cl. perfringens* Type B. This immunity is derived from the combination of Type C (beta) and Type D (epsilon) fractions.

Dosage and Administration: Using aseptic technique, inject 2 mL subcutaneously. Repeat in 21 to 28 days and once annually.

Precaution(s): Store at 35-45 F (2-7 C). Avoid freezing. Shake well before using. Use entire contents when first opened.

Caution(s): Anaphylactoid reactions may occur.

Antidote(s): Epinephrine.

Warning(s): Do not vaccinate within 21 days before slaughter.

For animal use only.

Keep out of reach of children.

Presentation: 10 doses (20 mL), 50 doses (100 mL) and 250 doses (500 mL).

Manufactured by: Boehringer Ingelheim Vetmedica, Inc. St. Joseph, Missouri 64506, U.S.A.

Compendium Code No.: 14571131 33315-00

7-WAY

Aspen **Bacterin-Toxoid**

Clostridium chauvoei-septicum-novyi-sordellii-perfringens Types C and D Bacterin-Toxoid

U.S. Vet. Lic. No.: 124

Composition: Prepared from cultures of the organisms listed. Alum precipitated.

Indications: Recommended for the vaccination of healthy, susceptible cattle and sheep against disease caused by *Clostridium chauvoei, Cl septicum, Cl novyi, Cl sordellii* and *Clostridium perfringens* Types C and D. Although *Clostridium perfringens* Type B is not a significant problem in the U.S.A., immunity may be provided against the beta and epsilon toxins elaborated by *Clostridium perfringens* Type B. This immunity is derived from the combination of Type C (beta) and Type D (epsilon) fractions.

Dosage and Administration:

Cattle: Using aseptic technique, inject 5 mL subcutaneously. Repeat in 21 to 28 days and once annually.

Sheep: Using aseptic technique, inject 2.5 mL subcutaneously or intramuscularly. Repeat in 21 to 28 days and once annually.

Precaution(s): Store out of direct sunlight at a temperature between 35-45°F. Avoid freezing. Shake well before using. Use entire contents when first opened.

Caution(s): Anaphylactoid reactions may occur.

Antidote(s): Administer epinephrine.

Warning(s): Do not vaccinate within 21 days before slaughter.

Presentation: 50 mL, 250 mL and 1,000 mL vials.

(Equivalent to 10, 50 and 200 cattle doses, and to 20, 100 and 400 sheep doses, respectively).

Manufactured by: Boehringer Ingelheim Animal Health, Inc.

Compendium Code No.: 14750000

7-WAY/SOMNUS

Aspen **Bacterin-Toxoid**

Clostridium chauvoei-septicum-novyi-sordellii-perfringens Types C & D-Haemophilus somnus Bacterin-Toxoid

U.S. Vet. Lic. No.: 124

Composition: Prepared from cultures of the organisms listed below. Alum precipitated.

Indications: Recommended for the immunization of healthy susceptible cattle against the diseases caused by *Clostridium chauvoei, Cl septicum, Cl novyi, Cl sordellii, Cl perfringens* types C and D and *Haemophilus somnus.* Although *Clostridium perfringens* type B is not a significant problem in the U.S.A., immunity may be provided against the beta and epsilon toxins elaborated by *Clostridium perfringens* type B. This immunity is derived from the combination of type C (beta) and type D (epsilon) fractions.

Dosage and Administration: Using aseptic technique, inject 5 mL intramuscularly or subcutaneously. Repeat in 21 to 28 days and once annually.

Precaution(s): Store out of direct sunlight at a temperature not over 45°F. Avoid freezing. Shake well before using. Use entire contents when first opened.

Transient swelling at the injection site may occur. Anaphylactoid reactions may occur.

Antidote(s): Administer epinephrine.

Warning(s): Do not vaccinate within 21 days before slaughter.

Presentation: 10, 50 and 200 doses.

Compendium Code No.: 14750010

8-WAY

Aspen **Bacterin-Toxoid**

Clostridium Chauvoei-Septicum-Haemolyticum-Novyi-Sordellii-Perfringens Types C & D Bacterin-Toxoid

U.S. Vet. Lic. No.: 124

Composition: Prepared from cultures of the organisms listed. Alum precipitated.

Indications: Recommended for the vaccination of healthy, susceptible cattle and sheep as an aid in the reduction of diseases caused by *Clostridium chauvoei, Cl. septicum, Cl. haemolyticum, Cl. novyi, Cl. sordellii* and *Clostridium perfringens* Types C and D. Although *Clostridium perfringens* Type B is not a significant problem in the U.S.A., immunity may be provided against the beta and epsilon toxins elaborated by *Clostridium perfringens* Type B. This immunity is derived from the combination of Type C (beta) and Type D (epsilon) fractions.

Dosage and Administration:

Cattle: Using aseptic technique, inject 5 mL subcutaneously. Repeat in 21 to 28 days and once annually.

Sheep: Using aseptic technique, inject 2.5 mL subcutaneously. Repeat in 21 to 28 days and once annually.

Precaution(s): Store out of direct sunlight at a temperature between 35-45°F. Avoid freezing. Shake well before using. Use entire contents when first opened.

Caution(s): Anaphylactoid reactions may occur.

Antidote(s): Epinephrine.

Warning(s): Do not vaccinate within 21 days before slaughter.

Presentation: 50 mL and 250 mL vials.

(Equivalent to 10 and 50 cattle doses, and to 10 and 100 sheep doses, respectively).

Manufactured by: Boehringer Ingelheim Animal Health, Inc., St. Joseph, Missouri 64506 U.S.A.

Compendium Code No.: 14750020 24210-00

16% DUAL-QUAT

Vet Solutions **Disinfectant/Detergent**

One-Step Germicidal Detergent And Deodorant

EPA Reg. No.: 47371-129-72896

Active Ingredient(s):

Didecyl dimethyl ammonium chloride 9.70%

n-Alkyl (C_{14} 50%, C_{12} 40%, C_{16} 10%) dimethyl benzyl ammonium chloride 6.47%

Inert Ingredients: 83.83%

Total 100.00%

Indications: A multi-purpose neutral pH, germicidal detergent and deodorant effective in hard water up to 400 ppm (calculated as $CaCO_3$) in the presence of a moderate amount of soil (5% organic serum) according to the AOAC Use-dilution Test. Disinfects, cleans and deodorizes in one labor-saving step. Effective against the following pathogens: *Pseudomonas aeruginosa*[1], *Staphylococcus aureus*[1], *Salmonella choleraesuis, Acinetobacter calcoaceticus, Bordetella bronchiseptica, Chlamydia psittaci, Enterobacter aerogenes, Enterobacter cloacae, Escherichia coli*[1], *Fusobacterium necrophorum, Klebsiella pneumoniae*[1], *Legionella pneumophila*[1], *Listeria monocytogenes, Pasteurella multocida, Proteus mirabilis, Proteus vulgaris, Salmonella enteritidis, Salmonella typhi, Salmonella typhimurium, Serratia marcescens, Shigella flexneri, Shigella sonnei, Staphylococcus aureus,* (methicillin resistant), *Streptococcus epidermidis*[2], *Streptococcus faecalis*[1], *Streptococcus pyogenes, Enterococcus faecalis* (Vancomycin resistant), *Adenovirus type 4, *Avian polyomavirus, *Canine distemper, *Feline leukemia, *Feline picornavirus, *Herpes simplex type 1, *Herpes simplex type 2, *HIV-1 (AIDS virus), *Infectious bovine rhinotracheitis, *Infectious bronchitis (Avian IBV), *Influenza A/Hong Kong, *Pseudorabies, *Rabies, *Rubella (German Measles), *Transmissible gastroenteritis virus (TGE), *Vaccinia, *Respiratory Syncytial virus (RSV), Aspergillus niger, Candida albicans, Trichophyton mentagrophytes

[1]ATCC and antibiotic-resistant strain

[2]Antibiotic-resistant strain only

Disinfectant, Pseudomonacidal, Staphylocidal, Salmonellacidal, Bactericidal, Fungicidal, Mildewstatic, *Virucidal.

Directions for Use: It is a violation of Federal law to use this product in a manner inconsistent with its labeling.

This product is not to be used as a terminal sterilant/high level disinfectant on any surface or instrument that (1) is introduced directly into the human body, either into or in contact with the bloodstream or normally sterile areas of the body, or (2) contacts intact mucous membranes but which does not ordinarily penetrate the blood barrier or otherwise enter normally sterile areas of the body. This product may be used to preclean or decontaminate critical or semi-critical devices prior to sterilization or high-level disinfection.

General Use Directions: Recommended for use in hospitals, nursing homes, schools, colleges, commercial and industrial institutions, office buildings, veterinary clinics, animal life science laboratories, federally inspected meat and poultry establishments, equine farms, tack shops, pet shops, airports, kennels, hotels, motels, poultry farms, turkey farms, dairy farms, hog farms, breeding establishments, grooming establishments, and households. Disinfects, cleans, and deodorizes floors, walls, metal surfaces, stainless steel surfaces, glazed porcelain, plastic surfaces (such as polypropylene, polystyrene, etc.), and other hard, nonporous surfaces.

Application: Remove heavy soil deposits from surface. Then thoroughly wet surface with a solution of ½ ounce of the concentrate per gallon of water. The solution can be applied with a cloth, mop, sponge, or coarse spray or soaking. Let solution remain on surface for a minimum of 10 minutes. Rinse or allow to air dry. Rinsing of floors is not necessary unless they are to be waxed or polished. Food contact surfaces must be thoroughly rinsed with potable water. Prepare a fresh solution daily on more often if the solution becomes visibly dirty or diluted.

USDA: For use in federally inspected meat and poultry plants on all hard, nonporous surfaces in inedible product processing areas, nonprocessing areas, and/or exterior areas. All surfaces must be thoroughly rinsed with potable water. USDA: For use in federally inspected meat and poultry plants as a floor and wall cleaner for use in all departments. Food products and packaging material must be removed from the room or carefully protected. All surfaces must be thoroughly rinsed with potable water. USDA: For use in federally inspected meat and poultry plants as a disinfectant agent for use in all departments. Food products and packaging materials must be removed from the room or carefully protected. Use product in accordance with its label. All surfaces must be thoroughly rinsed with potable water.

Toilet Bowls: Swab bowl with brush to remove heavy soil prior to cleaning or disinfecting. Clean by applying diluted solution around the bowl and up under the rim. Stubborn stains may require brushing. To disinfect, first remove or expel over the inner trap the residual bowl water. Pour in three ounces of the diluted solution. Swab the bowl completely using a scrub brush or mop, making sure to get under rim. Let stand for 10 minutes or overnight, then flush.

Mildewstatic Instructions: Will effectively control the growth of mold and mildew plus the odors caused by them when applied to hard, nonporous surfaces such as walls, floors, and table tops. Apply solution (½ ounce per gallon of water) with a cloth, mop, sponge, or coarse spray. Make sure to wet all surfaces completely. Let air dry. Repeat application weekly or when growth reappears.

*Kills HIV-1 (AIDS virus) on precleaned, environmental surfaces/objects previously soiled with blood/body fluids in health care settings or other settings in which there is an expected likelihood of soiling of inanimate surfaces/objects with blood/body fluids, and in which the surfaces/objects likely to be soiled with blood/body fluids can be associated with the potential for transmission of Human Immunodeficiency Virus Type I (HIV-1) associated with AIDS.

Special Instructions for Cleaning and Decontamination Against HIV-1 (AIDS Virus) of Surfaces/Objects Soiled with Blood/Body Fluids:

Personal Protection: Disposable latex or vinyl gloves, gowns, face masks, or eye coverings as appropriate must be worn during all cleaning of blood/body fluids and during decontamination procedures.

Cleaning Procedures: Blood/body fluids must be thoroughly cleaned from surfaces/objects before application of disinfectant.

Contact Time: HIV-1 (AIDS virus) is inactivated after a contact time of 4 minutes at 25°C (room temperature). Use a 10-minute contact time for other viruses, fungi, and bacteria listed.

Disposal Of Infectious Materials: Blood/body fluids should be autoclaved and disposed of according to federal, state, and local regulations for infectious waste disposal.

Farm Premise, Livestock, Poultry and Turkey House Disinfectant:

Dilution: 1:256 (630 ppm quat) ½ ounce per gallon of water.

1. Remove all animals and feeds from premises, trucks, coops, crates, and enclosures.
2. Remove all litter and manure from floors, walls, and surfaces of barns, pens, stalls, chutes, vehicles, and other facilities and fixtures occupied or traversed by animals.
3. Empty all troughs, racks, and other feeding and watering appliances.
4. Thoroughly clean all surfaces with soap and detergent, and rinse with water.
5. Saturate all surfaces with the recommended disinfecting solution for a period of 10 minutes.
6. Immerse all halters, ropes, and other types of equipment used in handling and restraining animals, as well as forks, shovels, and scrapers used for removing litter and manure.
7. Ventilate buildings, coops, cars, boats, and other closed spaces. Do not house animals or employ equipment until treatment has been absorbed, set, or dried.
8. After treatment with disinfectant, thoroughly scrub feed racks, troughs, automatic feeders, fountains, and waterers with soap or detergent, and rinse with potable water before reuse.

Precautionary Statements: Hazards to Humans and Domestic Animals:

Danger. Corrosive. Causes irreversible eye damage and skin burns. Harmful if swallowed. Do not get in eyes, on skin, or on clothing. When handling product, protect eyes by wearing goggles or face shield and protect skin by wearing rubber gloves. Wash thoroughly with soap and water after handling. Remove contaminated clothing and wash before reuse.

Statement of Practical Treatment: In case of contact, immediately flush eyes or skin with plenty of water for at least 15 minutes. For eyes, call a physician. If swallowed, call a doctor or get medical attention. Do not induce vomiting or give anything by mouth to an unconscious person. Drink promptly a large quantity of milk, egg whites, gelatin solution, or if these are not available, drink large quantities of water. Avoid alcohol.

Note to Physician: Probable mucosal damage may contraindicate the use of gastric lavage. Measures against circulatory shock, respiratory depression and convulsion may be needed.

Storage and Disposal: Keep product under locked storage, inaccessible to small children. Do not reuse empty container. Rinse thoroughly, securely wrap empty container in several layers of newspaper, and discard in trash.

Warning(s): Keep out of reach of children.

Presentation: 1 gallon (3.79 L).

Compendium Code No.: 10610000 991201

20% CHLORHEXIDINE GLUCONATE ADDITIVE

Davis **Antiseptic Concentrate**

Indications: This product may be used for mixing with non-medicated shampoos.

It is also recommended to make solutions and rinses.

Directions for Use: To make a 1% chlorhexidine shampoo, dilute 6 oz of Davis 20% CHLORHEXIDINE GLUCONATE in one gallon of non-medicated shampoo and mix thoroughly. Wet animal's coat completely with warm water. Do not get shampoo into eyes. Apply shampoo on head and ears, then lather. Repeat procedure with neck, chest, middle and hind quarter, finishing legs last. Allow pet to stand for 5 to 10 minutes. Rinse pet thoroughly. For best results, repeat procedure.

After bathing, a chlorhexidine rinse may result in greater residual activity. To make a .50% solution, dilute 3 oz of Davis 20% CHLORHEXIDINE GLUCONATE in one gallon of water. Mix thoroughly.

To make a 2% chlorhexidine solution, dilute 12 oz of Davis 20% CHLORHEXIDINE GLUCONATE to one gallon of water.

Use under the direction of a licensed veterinarian.

Precautionary Statements: Product may be harmful if swallowed and irritating to eyes, respiratory system and skin.

First Aid:

If Swallowed: Contact a physician immediately. Drink two glasses of water and induce vomiting. Never give anything by mouth to an unconscious person.

If In Eyes or On Skin: Flush affected areas immediately with plenty of water. If irritation persists, consult a physician. Remove contaminated clothing and shoes.

If Inhaled: Remove to fresh air. Give artificial respiration and/or oxygen ff breathing is difficult.

Storage: Avoid exposure to heat and/or direct sunlight.

Warning(s): For external use only. Keep out of reach of children.

Presentation: 32 fl oz (946.25 mL) bottles.

Compendium Code No.: 11410020

20% SULFAQUINOXALINE SODIUM SOLUTION

Loveland **Water Medication**

Antimicrobial

NADA No.: 006-667

Active Ingredient(s):

Sulfaquinoxaline 20%

Indications:

Chickens: For use in the control of coccidiosis caused by *Eimeria tenella, E. necatrix, E. acervulina, E. maxima,* and *E. brunetti.*

Turkeys: For use in the control of coccidiosis caused by *Eimeria meleagrimitis* and *E. adenoeides.*

Chickens and Turkeys: For use in the control of fowl typhoid caused by *Salmonella gallinarum* susceptible to sulfaquinoxaline and acute fowl cholera caused by *Pasteurella multocida* susceptible to sulfaquinoxaline.

Cattle and Calves: For use in the control and treatment of coccidiosis caused by *Eimeria bovis* and *E. zurnii.*

Dosage and Administration: The contents will treat 800 gallons at 8 fl. oz. per 50 gallon level. Suitable for use in medication barrels, tanks and automatic water proportioners.

For automatic drinking water proportioners: Dilute 33 fl. oz. of 20% SULFAQUINOXALINE SODIUM SOLUTION with water to make one (1) gallon of the stock solution. When the stock solution is used in an automatic proportioner that meters 1 fl. oz. of the stock solution per gallon of drinking water, this will provide 128 gallons of medicated water at the 0.04% dose.

For a 0.025% dose, use 21 fl. oz. of 20% SULFAQUINOXALINE SODIUM SOLUTION. The stock solutions for proportioners may be stored in a clean, closed, labeled container for up to three (3) days.

Chickens:

For the control of coccidiosis caused by *Eimeria tenella, E. necatrix, E. acervulina, E. maxima,* and *E. brunetti,* give a 12 fl. oz. (0.04%) dose per 50 gallons of water for two (2) to three (3) days. Stop the treatment for three (3) days. Then give an 8. fl. oz. (0.025%) dose for two (2) more days. If bloody droppings appear, repeat the treatment at this level for two (2) more days.

Do not change the litter unless it is absolutely necessary. Do not give flushing mashes.

Turkeys:

For the control of coccidiosis caused by *Eimeria meleagrimitis* and *E. adenoeides,* give an 8 fl. oz. (0.025%) dose for two (2) days, stop for three (3) days, give for two (2) days, stop for three (3) days and give for two (2) more days. Repeat if necessary.

Do not change the litter unless it is absolutely necessary. Do not give flushing mashes.

Chickens and Turkeys:

For the control of fowl typhoid caused by *Salmonella gallinarum* susceptible to sulfaquinoxaline and acute fowl cholera caused by *Pasteurella multocida* susceptible to sulfaquinoxaline, give a 12 fl. oz. (0.04%) dose for two (2) to three (3) days. Move the birds to clean ground. If the disease recurs, repeat the treatment. If cholera has become established as the respiratory or chronic form, use feed medicated with sulfaquinoxaline.

Cattle and Calves:

For the control and treatment of coccidiosis caused by *Eimeria bovis* and *E. zurnii,* give a 5 fl. oz. (0.015%) dose for three (3) to five (5) days. (Equivalent to 6 mg/lb. body weight.) Cattle and calves will drink approximately one (1) gallon per 100 lbs. of body weight per day. Cattle and calves not eating or drinking should be treated individually.

Make fresh medicated drinking water each day.

1 fl. oz. = 2 measuring tablespoonsful, 16 fl. oz. = 1 pint.

Medicated chickens, turkeys, cattle and calves must consume enough medicated water which provides a recommended dose of approximately 10 to 45.0 mg/lb./day in chickens, 3.5 to 55.0 mg/lb./day in turkeys, and approximately 6 mg/lb./day in cattle and calves, depending upon the age, the class of the animal, the ambient temperature and other factors.

Precaution(s): Keep at a temperature above 41°F (5°C).

Caution(s): Consult a veterinarian or poultry pathologist for a diagnosis.

May cause toxic reactions unless the drug is evenly mixed in water at doses indicated and used according to directions.

Poultry which have survived typhoid outbreaks should not be kept for laying house replacements or breeders unless tests show that they are not carriers.

For the control of outbreaks of disease, the medication should be initiated as soon as the diagnosis is determined.

Prolonged administration of sulfaquinoxaline at higher doses may result in depressed feed intake, deposition of sulfaquinoxaline crystals in the kidney and interference with normal blood clotting.

Hazardous. Causes skin and eye burns. Avoid contact with the eyes, the skin, or clothing. In case of contact, flush immediately with water for at least 15 minutes. For the eyes, get medical attention.

Restricted drug. Use only as directed.

Keep out of the reach of children.

For animal use only.

Warning(s): Not for use in lactating dairy cattle.

Do not give to chickens, turkeys, or cattle and calves within 10 days before slaughter for food.

Do not give to laying chickens or laying turkeys in production for food.

Presentation: 1 gallon (3.785 L) containers.

Compendium Code No.: 10860000

20/20 VISION® 7 WITH SPUR®*

Intervet **Bacterin-Toxoid**

Clostridium Chauvoei-Septicum-Novyi-Sordellii-Perfringens Types C & D-Moraxella Bovis Bacterin-Toxoid

U.S. Vet. Lic. No.: 286

Contents: This product contains the antigens listed above.

Contains formaldehyde as preservative.

Indications: For use in healthy cattle as an aid in preventing disease caused by *Clostridium chauvoei* (Blackleg), *septicum* (Malignant edema), *novyi* (Black disease), *sordellii,* and *perfringens* Types C and D (Enterotoxemia), and *Moraxella bovis* (Pinkeye or Infectious bovine keratoconjunctivitis).

Dosage and Administration: Cattle: 2 mL. Inject subcutaneously. Repeat in 3 to 4 weeks.

Precaution(s): Shake well before using. Store at 35° to 45°F (2° to 7°C). Use entire contents when first opened.

Caution(s): Anaphylactoid reactions may occur.

For use in animals only.

Antidote(s): Epinephrine.

Warning(s): Do not vaccinate within 21 days before slaughter.

Presentation: 10 doses (20 mL) and 50 doses (100 mL).

*Adjuvant—Intervet's Proprietary Technology

Compendium Code No.: 11060010

20/20® WITH SPUR®*

Intervet **Bacterin**

Moraxella Bovis Bacterin

U.S. Vet. Lic. No.: 286

Contents: This product contains the antigen listed above.

Contains formaldehyde as a preservative.

Indications: For use in healthy cattle as an aid in preventing disease caused by *Moraxella bovis* (pinkeye or infectious bovine keratoconjunctivitis).

Dosage and Administration: Cattle: 2 mL. Inject subcutaneously. Repeat in 3 to 4 weeks.

Precaution(s): Shake well before using. Store at 35° to 45°F (2° to 7°C). Use entire contents when first opened.

Caution(s): Anaphylactoid reactions may occur.

For use in animals only.

Antidote(s): Epinephrine.

Warning(s): Do not vaccinate within 21 days before slaughter.

Presentation: 50 doses (100 mL).

*Adjuvant—Intervet's Proprietary Technology

Compendium Code No.: 11060020

25-PINES™

Stearns **Disinfectant**

EPA Reg. No.: 13648-11-3640

Active Ingredient(s):

Pine oil 25%

Inert ingredients 75%

(Includes detergents, isopropanol and other cleaning agents.)

Indications: Cleans, disinfects and deodorizes. Limited disinfectant against intestinal bacteria. Effective against specific gram-negative household germs, such as those causing salmonellosis.

Dosage and Administration: It is a violation of federal law to use the product in a manner inconsistent with its labeling.

To disinfect, clean and deodorize hard nonporous surfaces in one operation: Use a mop or brush to apply a solution of one-quarter (¼) cup (2 fluid ounces) disinfectant to one (1) gallon of water for moderately soiled surfaces such as floors, pet quarters, and garbage cans, maintain a thoroughly wet surface for 10 minutes. Mix a fresh solution before each use; rinsing is not necessary, except on rubber or asphalt tile and on food contact surfaces. Heavily soiled surfaces must be precleaned first, followed by a second application using the above directions to disinfect. Use full strength for cutting grease, crayon, old wax or other heavy-duty cleaning jobs; rinse immediately.

Dog bath: Use 3 tbsp. (1½ fluid ounces) per gallon of water.

Precaution(s): Do not re-use the empty container. Wrap it and put it in the trash collection.

Caution(s): Keep out of the reach of children.

Precautionary Statements:

Hazards to Humans and Domestic Animals: Causes eye irritation. Do not get into the eyes. Avoid contact with the skin or clothing. Harmful if swallowed. Avoid contamination of food and food crops.

Practical Treatment: If eye or skin contact occurs, flush immediately with plenty of water. If irritation persists, get medical attention. If swallowed, do not induce vomiting. Promptly drink large amounts of milk or water and call a physician immediately. Avoid alcohol.

Physical and Chemical Hazards: Keep away from heat, sparks and open flames.

Presentation: 1 gallon containers.

Compendium Code No.: 10170000

31.92% SUL-Q-NOX™/OPTI-MED™

Alpharma **Water Medication**

Antimicrobial-Sulfonamide

NADA No.: 006-891

Active Ingredient(s):

Sulfaquinoxaline (as sodium and potassium salts) 31.92%

Indications: For control or treatment of the following diseases when caused by one or more pathogenic organisms susceptible to sulfaquinoxaline:

Chickens: Control of coccidiosis caused by *Eimeria tenella, E. necatrix, E. maxima, E. brunetti, E. acervulina,* susceptible to sulfaquinoxaline.

Turkeys: Control of coccidiosis caused by *Eimeria meleagrimitis, E. adenoeides,* susceptible to sulfaquinoxaline.

Chickens and Turkeys:

Control of acute fowl cholera caused by *Pasteurella multocida,* susceptible to sulfaquinoxaline.

Control of fowl typhoid caused by *Salmonella gallinarum,* susceptible to sulfaquinoxaline.

Cattle and Calves: For the control and treatment of coccidiosis caused by *Eimeria bovis, E. zurnii,* susceptible to sulfaquinoxaline.

Directions for Use:

Indications	Dosage: Add entire bottle contents to drinking water as follows: 26 fl. oz.	Dosage: Add entire bottle contents to drinking water as follows: 50 fl. oz.	Dosage: Per 128 Gallons of Water 1 Gallon	Treatment
Coccidiosis - Chickens:	163 gal. (0.04%)	312 gal. (0.04%)	20½ fl. oz. (0.04%)	Give for 2-3 days, skip 3 days then
	256 gal. (0.025%)	499 gal. (0.025%)	13 fl. oz. (0.025%)	Give for 2 days more. If bloody droppings appear, repeat treatment at this level for 2 more days. Caution: Do not change litter unless absolutely necessary. Do not give flushing mashes.
Coccidiosis - Turkeys	256 gal. (0.025%)	499 gal. (0.025%)	13 fl. oz. (0.025%)	Give for 2 days - skip 3 days - give for 2 days - skip 3 days and give 2 more days. Repeat if necessary. Caution: Do not change litter unless absolutely necessary. Do not give flushing mashes.
Acute Fowl Cholera - Chickens and Turkeys: Fowl Typhoid - Chickens and Turkeys:	163 gal. (0.04%)	312 gal. (0.04%)	20½ fl. oz. (0.04%)	Use for 2-3 days. Move birds to clean ground. If disease recurs, repeat treatment. Poultry that have survived fowl typhoid outbreaks should not be kept for laying house replacements or breeders unless tests show they are not carriers.
Coccidiosis - Cattle and Calves:	435 gal. (0.015%) 6 mg/lb of body wt.	831 gal. (0.015%) 6 mg/lb of body wt.	7¾ fl. oz. (0.015%) 6 mg/lb of body wt.	Give for 3-5 days. As a generalization, cattle and calves will consume approx. 1 gal/100 lb body weight/day. Cattle or calves not eating or drinking must be treated individually.

Prepare medicated drinking water fresh daily.

Precaution(s): Keep tightly sealed when not in use.

Dispose of any waste or unused portion properly. Store above 41°F (5°C).

Caution(s): Consult a veterinarian or poultry pathologist for diagnosis.

May cause toxic reactions unless drug is evenly mixed in water at dosages indicated and used according to directions.

Levels of sulfaquinoxaline higher than 0.025% in feed or 0.012% in water for more than 24 to 36 hours may result in reduced growth rate in chickens as a result of reduced feed or water intake.

For control of disease outbreaks, medication should be initiated as soon as diagnosis is determined.

Treated animals must actually consume enough medicated water to provide a necessary dosage of approximately 10 to 45 mg/lb/day in chickens and 3.5 to 55 mg/lb/day in turkeys and 6 mg/lb/day in cattle and calves,

depending on class of animal, ambient temperature, age and other factors.

Prolonged administration of sulfaquinoxaline at higher doses may result in depressed feed or water intake, deposition of sulfaquinoxaline crystals in kidney and interference with normal blood clotting.

Do not mix or administer in galvanized containers.

The following word is required on this product to comply with the Agricultural Code of California: Hazardous.

For animal use only. For use in drinking water only.

Restricted Drug - Use only as directed.

Warning(s): Withdraw use of product 10 days before slaughter.

A withdrawal period has not been established for this product in pre-ruminating calves. Do not use in calves to be processed for veal.

Do not medicate chickens or turkeys producing eggs for human consumption.

Not for use in lactating dairy cattle.

Causes skin and eye burns. Avoid contact with eyes, skin or clothing. In case of contact, flush immediately with water for at least 15 minutes; for eye get medical attention.

Keep all medications out of the reach of children. Not for human use.

Presentation: 26 fl oz (OPTI-MED™), 6 x 50 fl oz (SUL-Q-NOX™) and 4 x 1 gallon (128 fl oz) (SUL-Q-NOX™) (for automatic drinking water proportioners).

OPTI-MED is a trademark of Alpharma Inc.

SUL-Q-NOX is a trademark of Alpharma Inc.

Compendium Code No.: 10220022 AHL-302 0106 / AHL-452 0106 / AHL-289 0106

40% CMPK WITH D_3 ORAL DRENCH

DVM Formula **Calcium-Oral**

Guaranteed Analysis: Per Bottle:

Calcium Chloride, Min. 40%

Ingredients: Water, calcium chloride, magnesium chloride, propylene glycol, potassium chloride, sodium hypophosphite, and d-activated animal sterol (vitamin D_3).

Indications: A liquid oral supplement designed to provide calcium, magnesium, phosphorus, potassium, propylene glycol, and vitamin D_3. Vitamin D_3 assists in the absorption of calcium. 40% CMPK WITH D_3 ORAL DRENCH helps reduce the incidence of milk fever, displaced abomassum and retained placenta. Use at calving to stimulate appetite.

Dosage and Administration: Administer one bottle at the first sign of freshening and another bottle 6 to 12 hours after calving, repeat as needed. If the first dose is missed a post calving dose is still beneficial. Shake well before using.

Feeding Directions: Hold the head of the animal in a slightly elevated position and place the neck of the bottle between the teeth and cheek. Administer the entire contents of the bottle slowly, allowing the animal time to swallow. Do not give to animals without a swallowing reflex.

Presentation: 12 oz bottle.

Compendium Code No.: 15030000

-50 BELOW

AgriPharm **Udder Product**

Ingredient(s): Water, mineral oil, cetearyl alcohol, glycol stearate, stearic acid, propylene glycol, glycerin, sorbitol, lanolin, aloe vera, vitamin E, vitamins A and D, ethyl dihydroxypropyl PABA, methylparaben, sodium hydroxide, propylparaben, fragrance, FD&C Blue #1.

Indications: -50 BELOW aids in the protection against the effects of extremes in weather - low humidity, warm and cold temperatures. Daily application of -50 BELOW aids in soothing and softening chapped and irritated skin.

-50 BELOW is recommended for use on teats, udders, hands, and other skin areas that are exposed to frequent washing and temperature changes.

Directions: Thoroughly dry udder and each teat before application of -50 BELOW. Apply -50 BELOW liberally to entire teat and udder area after each milking. Be sure to coat teat orifice.

Caution(s): Before milking, thoroughly wash the entire udder and teat area to avoid contamination of milk.

Warning(s): Keep out of reach of children.

For animal use only.

Presentation: 1 lb and 4 lb containers.

Compendium Code No.: 14570000

50% DEXTROSE INJECTION, USP

Bimeda **Dextrose Therapy**

Active Ingredient(s): Each 100 mL contains:

Dextrose monohydrate . . . . 50 g
Water for injection . . . . q.s.

May contain hydrochloric acid or sodium hydroxide for pH adjustment.

mOsM/L (calc.) 2,525
Caloric value per liter 1,700
Hypertonic . . . . pH 3.5-6.5

The product does not contain any preservatives.

Indications: For use as an aid in the treatment of uncomplicated ketosis in cattle.

Dosage and Administration: For intravenous use only.

Cattle: 100 to 500 mL, depending upon the size and condition of the animal.

The solution should be warmed to body temperature and administered slowly.

Precaution(s): Store at 59°-86°F (15°-30°C).

Caution(s): The product is sterile in the unopened container. If the entire contents are not used, discard the unused portion. It should be handled under aseptic conditions.

For animal use only. Not for human use.

Keep out of the reach of children.

Presentation: 500 mL container.

Compendium Code No.: 13990000

70% ALCOHOL BUFFERED

Butler **Antiseptic**

Active Ingredient(s): 70% Alcohol buffered (isopropanol).

Indications: For external use as an antiseptic and disinfectant.

Directions: Apply to skin directly or with clean gauze, cotton or swab. For rubbing, apply liberally and rub with hands.

Precaution(s): Flammable, keep away from fire or flames.

Danger: Do not transfer this product to unlabeled containers. Dispose of this container properly. Do not reuse this container.

Caution(s): Do not apply to irritated skin. Do not use in eyes or on mucous membranes. If redness, irritation or swelling persists or increases, discontinue use and consult a veterinarian. In case of deep puncture wounds, consult veterinarian.

For external use only. Will produce serious gastric disturbances if taken internally. Not for use in animals food. Use only in well-ventilated area, fumes may be harmful.

Keep out of the reach of children.

In case of accidental ingestion, seek professional assistance or contact a Poison Control Center immediately.

First Aid:

In case of contact: For eyes, immediately flush with water for 15 minutes, call a physician. For skin, if irritation occurs, flush with water, consult physician if necessary. If inhaled, remove to fresh air. If not breathing, give artificial respiration. If breathing is difficult, give oxygen. Call a physician. If ingested, do not give liquids if victim is unconscious or very drowsy. Otherwise give no more than 2 glasses of water and induce vomiting by giving 2 tablespoons syrup of Ipecac. Call a physician.

For animal use only.

Presentation: 128 fluid ounces.

Compendium Code No.: 10820001

70% ISOPROPYL ALCOHOL

Davis **Counterirritant**

Active Ingredient(s): 70% Isopropyl alcohol.

Indications: Use as an invigorating body wash, for diluting liniments, or as an antiseptic.

Dosage and Administration: For rubbing application only.

Precaution(s): Flammable. Keep away from heat or flame.

Caution(s): This preparation is made from isopropyl alcohol and does not contain, nor is it sold as a substitute for ethyl or grain alcohol.

Warning(s): Harmful if swallowed.

Keep out of reach of children.

For external use only. If taken internally, severe gastric disturbances will result. In case of accidental ingestion, call a physician or poison control center immediately. Causes eye irritation. In case of contact, immediately flush eyes with water and call a physician. May cause skin irritation. Avoid contact with eyes, skin, mucous membranes and clothing. Wash hands thoroughly after handling.

Presentation: One Gallon (3.785 L).

Compendium Code No.: 11410041

89/03®

Intervet **Vaccine**

Bursal Disease Vaccine, Live Virus, Variant Strain

U.S. Vet. Lic. No.: 286

Description: 89/03® is a frozen vaccine that contains the Delaware type infectious bursal disease virus, which aids in protection against IBD standard and variant strains.

This vaccine contain Gentamicin as a preservative.

Quality tested for purity, potency, and safety.

Indications: 89/03® is recommended for the vaccination of healthy one-day-old chickens against Infectious Bursal Disease (Standard, Delaware and GLS variants) by subcutaneous injection.

Dosage and Administration: Preparation of Vaccine: Read warning advice on handling vaccine ampule. Sterilize vaccinating equipment by boiling in water for 30 minutes or by autoclaving (20 minutes at 121°C). Do not use chemical disinfectants.

1. Use 1,000 doses with 200 mL sterile diluent per 1,000 chickens.
2. Before withdrawing vaccine from liquid nitrogen canister, protect hands with gloves, wear long sleeves and use a face mask or goggles. It is possible an accident could occur with either the liquid nitrogen or the ampules of vaccine. When removing an ampule from the cane, hold palm of gloved hand away from body and face.
3. When withdrawing a cane of ampules from canister in liquid nitrogen refrigerator, expose only the ampule to be used immediately. The manufacturer recommends handling only one ampule at a time. After removing the ampule from the cane, the remaining ampule(s) should be replaced immediately in the canister of the liquid nitrogen refrigerator.
4. The contents of the ampule are thawed rapidly by immersing them in water at room temperature. Shake ampule to disperse contents. Then break ampule at its neck and immediately proceed as below. 1,000 doses of 89/03® are added for each 200 mL of diluent. Caution: Ampules have been known to explode on sudden temperature changes. Do not thaw in hot or ice cold water.
5. Draw contents of ampule into a sterile 10 mL syringe, mounted with an 18-gauge needle.
6. Dilute immediately by filling the syringe slowly with a portion of the diluent. Important: The diluent should be at room temperature (60°-80°F) at time of mixing.
7. The contents of the filled syringe are then added to remaining diluent. It is important that this be done slowly. Slowly empty the syringe, allowing the vaccine to run down the side of the diluent container. Gently shake the container as the vaccine is being mixed. Withdraw a portion of the diluent with the syringe to flush ampule. Inject the washing back into the diluent bottle. Remove the syringe.
8. Fill the previously sterilized automatic syringe according to the manufacturer's recommendations and set the dose for 0.20 mL.
9. The vaccine is now ready for use.

Method of Vaccination:

Subcutaneous Administration:

1. Hold the chicken by the back of the neck just below the head. The loose skin in the area is raised by gently pinching with the thumb and forefinger. Insert the needle beneath the skin in a downward direction away from the head. Inject 0.20 mL per chicken.
2. Avoid hitting the muscles and bones in the neck.
3. Entire contents of bottle must be used within 1 hour after mixing or discarded.
4. After reconstitution the vaccine should be kept cool and swirled frequently - every 5 minutes.

Records: Keep a record of vaccine, quantity, serial number, expiration date, and place of purchase; the date and time of vaccination; the number, age, breed and locations of chickens; names of operators performing the vaccination and any observed reactions.

Precaution(s): Important - Storage Conditions:

Ampules - Store in liquid nitrogen container.

Diluent - Store at room temperature.

Container - Store liquid nitrogen container securely in upright position in a dry, well-ventilated area and away from incubator intakes and chicken boxes.

Safety Precautions: Liquid nitrogen container and vaccine should be handled only by properly trained personnel who are thoroughly conversant with the Union Carbide publication and instruction booklet regarding the use of, precautions and safe practices for liquified atmospheric gases (particularly liquid nitrogen).

When removing ampule cane, handling frozen ampules, or adding liquid nitrogen, wear long sleeves, a plastic face shield and gloves to protect the skin from contact with the liquid nitrogen. All storage and handling of the liquid nitrogen container must be in a dry, ventilated area. Do not inhale liquid nitrogen vapors. If drowsiness occurs, get fresh air quickly; then ventilate the entire area. If breathing difficulty occurs, apply artificial respiration. If any of these difficulties persist or there is a loss of consciousness, summon a physician immediately. Care should be exercised to prevent contaminating your hands, eyes and clothing with the vaccine.

Do not mix any substance not approved by Intervet, Inc. with this vaccine.

Store vaccine in liquid nitrogen at a temperature below -150°C.

Gloves and visor should be worn when handling liquid nitrogen.

Once thawed, the product should not be refrozen.

Once mixed with diluent, the vaccine should be swirled frequently, every five minutes.

Once mixed with diluent, the vaccine should be used within 1 hour.

Burn the container and all unused contents.

This product is non-returnable.

Caution(s): Use only in localities where permitted and on premises with a history of Infectious Bursal Disease.

Good management practices are recommended to reduce exposure to Infectious Bursal Disease viruses for at least three weeks following vaccination. Therefore, the directions should be followed carefully.

Do not dilute or otherwise stretch the dosage of this vaccine.

Only healthy chickens should be vaccinated.

For veterinary use only.

Read the above directions carefully.

Notice: This vaccine has undergone rigid potency, safety, and purity tests, and meets Intervet Inc. and USDA requirements. It is designed to stimulate effective immunity when used as directed, but the user must be advised that the response to the product depends upon many factors, including, but not limited to, conditions of storage and handling by the user, administration of the vaccine, health and responsiveness of the individual chickens, and the degree of field exposure.

This product is not hazardous when used according to directions supplied. A material safety data sheet (MSDS) is available upon request. This and any other consumer information can be obtained by calling Intervet Customer Service at 1-800-441-8272 or 1-302-934-8051.

The use of this vaccine is subject to applicable local and federal laws and regulations.

Use only as directed.

#

Warning(s): Do not vaccinate within 21 days before slaughter.

Presentation: 1 x 1,000 dose ampule and 1 x 2,000 dose ampule with 200 mL of sterile diluent per 1,000 doses.

89/03® is packaged in two separate units. One is an ampule containing either 1,000 or 2,000 doses of frozen infectious bursal disease virus and the other is a bottle or bag of sterile diluent. The ampules are inserted in metal canes and shipped in a liquid nitrogen (LN) container. The diluent is packaged in separate containers at the rate of 200 mL of diluent per 1,000 doses of vaccine.

U.S. Patent No. 5,919,461

Compendium Code No.: 11060051 27703 AL 157

2177®

Intervet **Vaccine**

Tenosynovitis Vaccine, Live Virus

U.S. Vet. Lic. No.: 286

Description: 2177® is a frozen, live virus vaccine that contains the 2177 strain of avian reovirus. 2177® is a naturally apathogenic avian reovirus originally isolated from commercial chickens.

This vaccine contains Gentamicin as a preservative.

Quality tested for purity, potency, and safety.

Indications: 2177® is recommended for vaccination of healthy one-day-old chickens by subcutaneous injection for the prevention of tenosynovitis/viral arthritis.

Dosage and Administration: Preparation of Vaccine:

Caution: Read warning advice on handling vaccine ampule. Sterilize vaccinating equipment by boiling in water for 30 minutes or by autoclaving (20 minutes at 250°F or 121°C). Do not use chemical disinfectants.

1. Use 1,000 doses of vaccine with 200 mL sterile diluent per 1,000 chickens when administering vaccine by subcutaneous route.
2. Before withdrawing vaccine from liquid nitrogen canister, protect hands with gloves, wear long sleeves and use a face mask or goggles. It is possible an accident could occur with either the liquid nitrogen or the ampules of vaccine. When removing an ampule from the cane, hold palm of gloved hand away from body and face.
3. When withdrawing a cane of ampules from canister in liquid nitrogen container, expose only the ampule to be used immediately. We recommend handling only one ampule at a time. After removing the ampule from the cane, the remaining ampules should be replaced immediately in the canister of the liquid nitrogen container.
4. The contents of the ampule are thawed rapidly by immersing in water at room temperature. Shake ampule to disperse contents. Then break ampule at its neck and immediately proceed as below. Dilute the vaccine with diluent for administration. 1,000 doses of vaccine is added for each 100 or 200 mL of diluent. Caution: Ampules have been known to explode on sudden temperature changes. Do not thaw in hot or ice cold water.
5. Draw contents of ampule into a sterile 10 mL syringe, mounted with an 18-gauge needle.
6. Dilute immediately by filling the syringe slowly with a portion of the diluent. Important: The diluent should be at room temperature (60°-80°F or 16°-27°C) at time of mixing.
7. The contents of the filled syringe are then added to remaining diluent. It is important that this be done slowly. Slowly empty the syringe, allowing the vaccine to run down the side of the diluent container. Gently agitate the container as the vaccine is being mixed. Withdraw a portion of the diluent with the syringe to flush ampule. Remove the remaining diluent from the ampule and inject gently into the diluent container. Remove the syringe.
8. Fill the previously sterilized automatic syringe according to the manufacturer's recommendations.
9. The vaccine is now ready for use.

Method of Vaccination:

Subcutaneous Administration:

1. Hold the chicken by the back of the neck just below the head. The loose skin in the area is raised by gently pinching with the thumb and forefinger. Insert the needle beneath the skin in a downward direction away from the head. Inject 0.2 mL per chicken.
2. Avoid hitting the muscles and bones in the neck.
3. Entire contents of bottle must be used within 1 hour after mixing or discarded according to precaution(s).
4. After reconstitution, the vaccine should be kept cool and gently agitated frequently.

Records: Keep a record of vaccine, quantity, serial number, expiration date, and place of purchase; the date and time of vaccination; the number, age, breed, and locations of chickens; names of operators performing the vaccination and any observed reactions.

Precaution(s): Important: Storage Conditions:

Ampules - Store in liquid nitrogen container.

Diluent - Store at room temperature.

Container - Store liquid nitrogen container securely in upright position in a dry, well-ventilated area and away from incubator intakes and chicken boxes.

Safety Precautions: Liquid nitrogen container and vaccine should be handled only by properly trained personnel who are thoroughly conversant with the Union Carbide publication and instruction booklet regarding the use of, precautions for and safe practices for liquefied atmospheric gases (particularly liquid nitrogen).

When removing ampule cane, handling frozen ampules, or adding liquid nitrogen, wear long sleeves, a plastic face shield and gloves to protect the skin from contact with the liquid nitrogen. All storage and handling of the liquid nitrogen container must be in a dry, ventilated area. Do not inhale liquid nitrogen vapors. If drowsiness occurs, get fresh air quickly; then ventilate entire area. If breathing difficulty occurs, apply artificial respiration. If any of these difficulties persist or there is a loss of consciousness, summon a physician immediately.

Care should be exercised to prevent contaminating your hands, eyes and clothing with the vaccine.

Do not mix any substance, not approved by Intervet Inc., with this vaccine.

Store vaccine in liquid nitrogen at a temperature below -238°F or -150°C.

Gloves and visor should be worn when handling liquid nitrogen.

Once thawed, the product should not be refrozen.

Once mixed with diluent, the vaccine should be gently agitated frequently.

Once mixed with diluent, the vaccine should be used within 1 hour.

Burn the container and all unused contents.

This product is non-returnable.

Caution(s): It is recommended that good management practices be followed to reduce exposure to Reovirus for at least three weeks following vaccination.

Do not dilute or otherwise stretch the dosage of this vaccine.

Only healthy chickens should be vaccinated.

For veterinary use only.

Read the above directions carefully.

Notice: This vaccine has undergone rigid potency, safety and purity tests, and meets Intervet Inc. and USDA requirements. It is designed to stimulate effective immunity when used as directed, but the user must be advised that the response to the product depends upon many factors, including, but not limited to, conditions of storage and handling by the user, administration of the vaccine, health and responsiveness of the individual chickens, and the degree of field exposure.

This product is not hazardous when used according to directions supplied. A material safety data sheet (MSDS) is available upon request. This and any other consumer information can be obtained by calling Intervet Inc. Customer Service at 1-800-441-8272 or 1-302-934-8051.

The use of this vaccine is subject to applicable local and federal laws and regulations.

Use only as directed.

Warning(s): Do not vaccinate within 21 days before slaughter.

Presentation: One 1,000-dose ampule and 200 mL sterile diluent per 1,000 doses for subcutaneous injection.

2177® is packaged in 1,000 dose glass ampules and supplied with diluent packaged in a separate container. The vaccine ampules are inserted in metal canes, stored and shipped in a liquid nitrogen container.

U.S. Patent No. 5,525,342

Compendium Code No.: 11060031 27904 AL156A

A

A-33® DRY

Ecolab Prof. Prod. Div. **Disinfectant/Detergent**

Detergent/Disinfectant/Odor Counteractant

EPA Reg. No.: 42964-25

Active Ingredient(s):

Octyl decyl dimethyl ammonium chloride	1.536%
Dioctyl dimethyl ammonium chloride	0.768%
Didecyl dimethyl ammonium chloride	0.768%
Alkyl (67% C_{12}, 25% C_{14}, 7% C_{16}, 1% C_8, C_{10}, C_{18}) dimethyl benzyl ammonium chloride	12.288%
Inert Ingredients	84.640%
Total	100.000%

(Includes essential oil odor control agents)

Indications: A-33® Dry has been found effective against Human Immunodeficiency Virus, HIV-1, commonly known as the AIDS virus, on inanimate surfaces when tested according to EPA virucidal test requirements.

A-33® Dry is a complete one-step disinfectant cleaner-fungicide-mildewstat-virucide-odor counteractant which is effective in water up to 500 ppm hardness in the presence of 5% blood serum and soap film residue when used as directed.

Airkem's A-33® Dry is a concentrated, premeasured disinfectant odor counteractant. It is low foaming and phosphate free and scientifically formulated with nonionic synthetic detergents and alkaline builders giving it exceptional cleaning and wetting properties.

A-33® Dry with its cleaning and odor counteraction abilities is recommended for disinfecting and cleaning of floors, walls and other hard nonporous environmental surfaces such as tables, chairs, counter tops, bathroom fixtures, sinks, shelves, racks, carts, refrigerators, coolers, tile, linoleum, vinyl, asphalt, porcelain, plastic, metal, glass, or painted, varnished or lacquered surfaces.

Areas of Use: Hospitals, nursing homes, other health-care facilities, schools, colleges, veterinary clinics, animal life science laboratories, industrial facilities, USDA inspected food processing facilities and other food processing plants, restaurants, hotels, motels, office buildings, recreational facilities, retail and wholesale establishments.

When used as directed, this product will deodorize surfaces in toilet areas, behind and under sinks and counters, garbage cans and garbage storage areas, and other places where bacterial growth can cause mal odors.

Directions for Use: It is a violation of federal law to use this product in a manner inconsistent with its labeling.

Prepare a fresh solution daily or when it becomes soiled or diluted.

Effective in hard water up to 500 ppm (calculated as $CaCO_3$) in the presence of 5% blood serum.

Disinfection: For hospital disinfecting and cleaning of nonporous hard surfaces, dilute one packet per gallon of warm water. Stir gently for a uniform solution. Apply solution with cloth, mop, sponge, brush, scrubber, coarse spray device or by soaking, so as to wet all surfaces thoroughly. Allow to remain wet for at least ten minutes. Remove solution and entrapped soil with a clean, wet mop, cloth or wet vacuum pickup. For heavily soiled areas, a precleaning step is required. A-33® Dry may be used at recommended dilution on conductive flooring without any deleterious effect. When used as a hospital disinfectant (½ oz. to 1 gallon), A-33® Dry provides 600 ppm of one of the more potent combinations of germicides commercially available to provide effectiveness in up to 500 ppm hard water, and in the presence of protein (5% blood serum) and dried soap film residues.

Effective as a Virucide: On environmental surfaces A-33® Dry kills viruses such as Human Immunodeficiency Virus, HIV-1 (commonly known as the AIDS virus), Influenza A Japan 305/57 (Asian), Parainfluenza 1, Herpes simplex type 1, Herpes simplex type 2*, Canine distemper*, Canine parvovirus*, Feline pneumonitis*, Feline rhinotraceitis*, Reovirus type 3, and Vaccinia in the presence of 500 ppm hard water and protein provided as 5% blood serum.

*Tested in the presence of residual soap scum.

Kills HIV on pre-cleaned environmental surfaces/objects previously soiled with blood/body fluids in health care settings or other settings in which there is an expected likelihood of soiling of inanimate surfaces/objects with blood or body fluids, and in which the surfaces/objects likely to be soiled with blood or body fluids can be associated with the potential for transmission of human immunodeficiency virus Type 1 (HIV-1) (associated with AIDS).

Special instructions for cleaning and decontamination against HIV on surfaces/objects soiled with blood/body fluids.

A-33® Dry is effective as a virucide against HIV-1 (AIDS virus) on hard, non-porous surfaces in the presence of moderate amounts of organic soil (10% blood serum) when used in health care settings where the potential for the presence of HIV-1 (AIDS virus) on inanimate surfaces is likely.

Personal Protection: When handling items soiled with blood or body fluids, wear personal protection such as disposable latex gloves, gowns, masks, or eye coverings.

Cleaning Procedure: Blood and other body fluids must be thoroughly cleaned from surfaces and objects before application of disinfectant.

Contact Time: 10 minutes.

Mold and Mildewcide: Apply to surface, wetting it thoroughly. If not washed or rubbed off, it will control the growth of mold and mildew and the odors caused by them on environmental surfaces for a period of 14 days. To maintain fungistatic control, repeat application in 14 days or when new growth appears.

Fungicide: Kills *Trichophyton mentagrophytes* (Athletes Foot Fungi), *Candida albicans* (pathogentic yeast), *Geotrichum candidum* (isolated from human), and *Microsporum canis* (human, animal pathogen) in the presence of protein (5% blood serum) and soap scum in 500 ppm hard water when tested according to A.O.A.C. Fungicidal Test. Is an effective fungicide when used on surfaces in areas such as locker rooms, dressing rooms, shower and bath areas, exercise facilities.

Other Organisms: A-33® Dry has been found to be an effective disinfectant against a broad spectrum of bacteria, both gram positive and gram negative organisms under the same severe test conditions listed: *Staphylococcus aureus* ATCC #6538, *Salmonella choleraesuis* ATCC #10708, *Pseudomonas aeruginosa* ATCC #15442, *Proteus vulgaris* ATCC #13315, *Escherichia coli* ATCC #11229, *Enterobacter aerogenes* ATCC #13048, *Micrococcus sendentarius* ATCC #27573, *Pseudomonas cepacia* ATCC #25416, *Salmonella gallinarum* ATCC #9184, *Salmonella typhi* ATCC #6539, *Shigella dysenteriae* ATCC #29026, *Staphylococcus aureus* ATCC #14154, *Streptococcus faecalis* ATCC #828, *Streptococcus pyogenes* ATCC #19615, *Staphylococcus* species ATCC #12715, *Vibrio cholerae* ATCC #25873, *Corynebacterium diptheriae* ATCC #11913, *Neisseria gonorrhea* ATCC #19424, *Serratia marcescens* ATCC #9103, *Shigella flexneri* ATCC #25875, *Klebsiella pneumoniae* ATCC #4352, *Brevibacterium ammoniagenes* ATCC #6872, *Listeria monocytogenes* (clinical isolate), *Staphylococcus aureus HL121* (methicillin resistant), *Proteus mirabilis* ATCC #9240, *Salmonella enteriditis* ATCC #13076, *Salmonella schottmuelleri* ATCC #10719, *Salmonella typhimurium* ATCC #13311, *Shigella sonnei* ATCC #25931, *Staphylococcus epidermidis* ATCC #12228, *Streptococcus mutans* ATCC #25175, *Micrococcus luteus* ATCC #14452, *Escherichia coli* ATCC #29181, *Campylobacter fetus* ATCC #27374, *Haemophilus* influenzae ATCC #19418, *Enterococcus faecalis* (vancomycin resistant) ATCC #51299.

Disinfection and Deodorizing of Animal Housing Facilities (Barns, Kennels, Cages, Hutches, etc): Remove animals and feed from facilities. Remove litter, waste matter and gross soils. Empty all troughs, rack and other feeding and watering equipment.

Thoroughly clean all surfaces with soap or detergent and rinse with water. Immerse all halters, ropes, and other types of equipment used in handling and restraining animals, as well as forks, shovels, and scrapers used for removing litter and manure. Thoroughly scrub all treated feed racks, mangers, troughs, automatic feeders, fountains, and waterers with soap or detergent, and rinse with potable water before reuse. Disinfect surfaces as described under Disinfection. Ventilate buildings and other closed spaces. Allow to air dry before reintroducing animals.

A-33® Dry has been tested and determined acceptable to use on conductive flooring without any deleterious effects.

Contraindication(s): Not to be used on food preparation surfaces, food handling areas, medical devices or on medical equipment surfaces.

Precautionary Statements: Hazards to Humans and Domestic Animals.

Danger: Corrosive. Powder causes irreversible eye damage and skin burns. Do not get into eyes, on skin, or on clothing. Wear protective eyewear (chemical goggles, safety glasses, or face shield), rubber gloves, and protective clothing. Harmful if swallowed. Wash thoroughly with soap and water after handling. Remove contaminated clothing and wash before reuse.

Statement of Practical Treatment:

If In Eyes: Flush immediately with cool water. Remove contact lenses. Continue flushing for 15 minutes, holding eyelids apart. Get prompt medical attention.

If on Skin: Wash with plenty of soap and water. Get medical attention.

If Swallowed: Call a doctor or get medical attention. Do not induce vomiting or give anything by mouth to an unconscious person. Drink promptly a large quantity of milk, eggwhites, gelatin solution, or if these are not available, drink large quantities of water. Avoid alcohol.

For Emergency Medical Information, Call Toll-Free 1-800-328-0026.

Storage and Disposal: Do not contaminate water, food or feed by storage or disposal.

Storage: Store in a cool, dry place. Do not handle packets with wet hands. Do not remove packets before use. Keep container tightly closed when not in use. Do not freeze.

Container Disposal: Triple rinse (or equivalent). Then offer for recycling or reconditioning, or puncture and dispose of in a sanitary landfill, or incineration, or, if allowed by state and local authorities, by burning. If burned, stay out of smoke.

Pesticide Disposal: Pesticide wastes are acutely hazardous. Improper disposal of excess pesticide, spray mixture, or rinsate is a violation of Federal Law. If these wastes cannot be disposed of by use according to label instructions, contact your State Pesticide or Environmental Control Agency, or the Hazardous Waste representative at the nearest EPA Regional Office for guidance.

Disposal of Infectious Materials: Blood and other body fluids should be autoclaved and disposed of according to local regulations for infectious waste disposal.

Warning(s): Keep out of reach of children.

Presentation: 90 x 0.5 oz/14 g (2.81 lb/1.27 kg) water-soluble packets - premeasured ½ oz. packet for hospital and institutional use.

Canister/packet weight is weighed at production site. Packets may gain/lose weight depending on moisture absorption or evaporation. Empty space at the top of the canister could occur due to compaction/settling during shipping.

Manufactured by: Airkem Professional Products, Division of Ecolab Inc., 370 Wabasha Street, St. Paul, MN 55102.

Compendium Code No.: 10160031 745013/8901/0202

A180™ ℞

Pfizer Animal Health **Danofloxacin**

(danofloxacin mesylate) Sterile Antimicrobial Injectable Solution

NADA No.: 141-207

Active Ingredient(s): Each mL contains 180.0 mg of danofloxacin as the mesylate salt, 200.0 mg 2-pyrrolidone, 50.0 mg polyvinyl pyrrolidone, 20.3 mg heavy magnesium oxide, 2.5 mg phenol, 5.0 mg monothioglycerol, hydrochloric acid or sodium hydroxide as needed to adjust pH, nitrogen headspace and water for injection, q.s.

Indications: A180™ (danofloxacin) injectable solution is indicated for the treatment of bovine respiratory disease (BRD) associated with *Mannheimia (Pasteurella) haemolytica* and *Pasteurella multocida*.

Pharmacology: Description: A180™ is a sterile solution containing danofloxacin mesylate, a synthetic fluoroquinolone antimicrobial agent. Danofloxacin mesylate is the non-proprietary designation for (1S)-1cyclopropyl-6-fluoro-1,4-dihydro-7-(5-methyl-2,5-diazabicyclo [2.2.1]hept-2-yl)-4-oxo-3-quinolone carboxylic acid monomethanesulfonate. The empirical formula is $C_{19}H_{20}FN_3O_3 \bullet CH_3SO_3H$ and the molecular weight is 453.49.

Figure 1. The chemical structure of danofloxacin mesylate.

O
COOH
F
N
N
(CH_3SO_3H)
H_3C
N

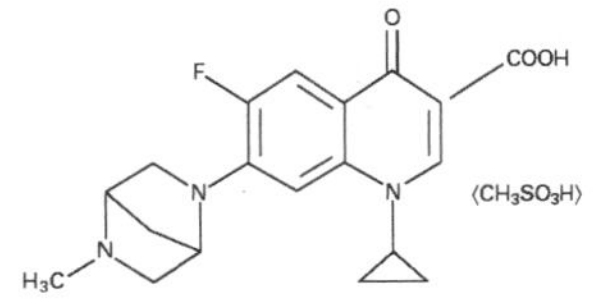

Clinical Pharmacology:

(a) Pharmacokinetics: Danofloxacin distributes extensively throughout the body, as evidenced by a steady state volume of distribution (VDss) exceeding 1 L/kg. Danofloxacin concentrations in the lung homogenates markedly exceed those observed in plasma, further suggesting extensive distribution to the indicated site of infection. Danofloxacin is rapidly eliminated from the body (apparent terminal elimination T1/2 ranging from 3-6 hours), and therefore negligible accumulation is expected to occur when animals are dosed with a q48h-dosing regimen.

Danofloxacin is rapidly absorbed and is highly bioavailable when administered as a subcutaneous injection in the neck. No statistically significant gender difference was observed in peak or total systemic exposure following subcutaneous administration. Linear pharmacokinetics has been demonstrated when danofloxacin is administered by subcutaneous injection at doses up to 10 mg/kg. Pharmacokinetic parameter values associated with a 6-mg/kg dose are provided in Table 1.

Table 1. Danofloxacin pharmacokinetic values (6 mg/kg)

		Steers		Heifers	
		Mean	%CV[e]	Mean	%CV
[a]$AUC_{0\text{-}24}$	μg x hr/mL	9.4	10	8.8	9
[b]F%		92	5	87	3
[a]Cmax	μg/mL	1.25	16	1.27	13
[a,c]Tmax	hr	3.2	42	1.7	31
[d]CL	L/hr	0.54	12	0.62	9
[d]VDss	L/kg	2.7	7	2.6	4
[a]T1/2	hr	4.8	18	4.2	7

[a] Pharmacokinetic estimates based upon a 6-mg/kg subcutaneous injection administered into the lateral neck region. $AUC_{0\text{-}24}$ = area under the plasma concentration versus time curve from hr zero to hr 24 postdose. Cmax = maximum observed concentration. Tmax = time to Cmax.

[b] F% = extent of drug absorption following subcutaneous administration. Within subject F values were determined as the ratio of $AUC_{0\text{-}inf}$ values estimated following a 6-mg/kg dose administered as either a subcutaneous or intravenous injection.

[c] Tmax: statistically significant differences were detected between genders. Given the similarity in Cmax values, these differences are not expected to have any clinical significance.

[d] CL and VDss were determined from data obtained after intravenous administration of a 6-mg/kg dose.

[e] Coefficient of variation %

(b) Microbiology: Danofloxacin exerts its activity by inhibiting the bacterial DNA gyrase enzyme, thereby blocking DNA replication. Inhibition of DNA gyrase is lethal to bacteria and danofloxacin has been shown to be rapidly bactericidal. Danofloxacin is active against gram-negative and gram-positive bacteria.

The Minimum Inhibitory Concentrations (MIC) of danofloxacin for pathogens isolated in natural infections from various clinical studies in North America, 1994-1997, were determined using the standardized microdilution technique (Sensititre/Alamar, Accumed International), and are shown in Table 2.

Table 2. MIC values (μg/mL) of danofloxacin against bacterial isolates from natural infections of cattle

Species	No. Isolates	Range μg/mL	MIC90** μg/mL
Mannheimia			
(Pasteurella) haemolytica	363	≤0.015-0.12	0.06
Pasteurella multocida	301	≤0.015-0.12	0.015
*Haemophilus somnus**	32	≤0.015-0.06	0.06

* The clinical significance of these *in-vitro* data has not been demonstrated.

** The minimum inhibitory concentration for 90% of the isolates.

Dosage and Administration: A180™ is administered as a subcutaneous dose of 6 mg/kg of body weight (1.5 mL/100 lb). Treatment should be repeated once approximately 48 hours following the first injection. Care should be taken to dose accurately. Administered dose volume should not exceed 15 mL per injection site.

A180™ Dosage and Treatment Schedule	
Cattle Weight (lb)	6 mg/kg, given twice, 48 hours apart Dose Volume (mL)
50	0.75
100	1.5
150	2.25
200	3.0
250	3.75
300	4.5
400	6.0
500	7.5
600	9.0
700	10.5
800	12.0
900	13.5
1000	15.0

Precaution(s): Storage Information: Store at or below 30°C (86°F). Protect from light. Protect from freezing. The color is yellow to amber and does not affect potency.

Caution(s): Federal law restricts this drug to use by or on the order of a licensed veterinarian.

Federal law prohibits the extra-label use of this drug in food-producing animals.

The effects of danofloxacin on bovine reproductive performance, pregnancy, and lactation have not been determined.

Subcutaneous injection can cause a transient local tissue reaction that may result in trim loss of edible tissue at slaughter.

Quinolone-class drugs should be used with caution in animals with known or suspected central nervous system (CNS) disorders. In such animals, quinolones have, in rare instances, been associated with CNS stimulation, which may lead to convulsive seizures.

Quinolone-class drugs have been shown to produce erosions of cartilage of weight-bearing joints and other signs of arthropathy in immature, rapidly growing animals of various species. Refer to Animal Safety for information specific to danofloxacin.

For subcutaneous use in cattle only. Use only as directed.

Warning(s): Animals intended for human consumption must not be slaughtered within 4 days from the last treatment. Do not use in cattle intended for dairy production. A withdrawal period has not been established for this product in preruminating calves. Do not use in calves to be processed for veal.

Human Warnings: For use in animals only. Keep out of reach of children. Avoid contact with eyes. In case of contact, immediately flush eyes with copious amounts of water for 15 minutes. In case of dermal contact, wash skin with soap and water. Consult a physician if irritation persists following ocular or dermal exposures. Individuals with a history of hypersensitivity to quinolones should avoid this product. In humans, there is a risk of user photosensitization within a few hours after excessive exposure to quinolones. If excessive accidental exposure occurs, avoid direct sunlight. To report adverse reactions or to obtain a copy of the Material Safety Data Sheet, call 1-800-366-5288.

Toxicology: The approximate oral LD50 for laboratory mice and rats was greater than 2000 mg/kg of body weight. Ninety-day oral gavage studies in dogs and rats established a no observable effect level (NOEL) of 2.4 mg/kg bw/day and 6.25 mg/kg bw/day, respectively. Higher doses in juvenile dogs produced arthropathy, a typical quinolone-associated side effect. In chronic rodent bioassays, no evidence of carcinogenicity was associated with long-term danofloxacin administration in rats and mice. No teratogenic effects were observed in rodents at doses up to 50 mg/kg bw/day (mice) or 100 mg/kg bw/day (rats) or in rabbits at the highest dose tested of 15 mg/kg bw/day. A three-generation rat reproductive toxicity study established a NOEL of 6.25 mg/kg bw/day. Microbial safety analyses indicate that danofloxacin residues present in edible tissues of treated animals will not cause adverse effects on the human intestinal microflora of the consumer.

Adverse Reactions: A hypersensitivity reaction was noted in 2 healthy calves treated with A180™ in a laboratory study. In one location of a multi-site field trial, one out of the 41 calves treated with 6 mg/kg q 48 hours showed lameness on Day 6 only. In this same field trial location one of 38 calves treated with 8 mg/kg once became lame 4 days after treatment and remained lame on the last day of the study (Day 10). Another calf in the same treatment group developed lameness on the last day of the study.

To report suspected adverse effects, and/or obtain a copy of the MSDS, call 1-800-366-5288.

Trial Data: Effectiveness: The effectiveness of the 6 mg/kg BW alternate day regimen was confirmed in 4 well-controlled studies of naturally acquired bacterial respiratory infections in feedlot age cattle. These studies were conducted under commercial conditions at 4 locations in North America. Bacterial pathogens isolated in the clinical field trial are provided in the Microbiology section.

Animal Safety: Safety studies were conducted in feeder calves using single doses of 10, 20, or 30 mg/kg for 6 consecutive days and 18, 24, or 60 mg/kg for 3 consecutive days. No clinical signs of toxicity were observed at doses of 10 and 20 mg/kg when administered for 6 days, nor at doses of 18 and 24 mg/kg when administered for 3 days. Articular cartilage lesions, consistent with fluoroquinolone chondropathy, were observed after examination of joints from animals as follows: one of 5 animals administered 18 mg/kg for 3 days; one of 6 animals administered 20 mg/kg for 6 days; 5 of 6 animals administered 30 mg/kg for 6 days; and in all 4 animals administered 60 mg/kg for 3 days. Clinical signs of inappetance, transient lameness (2/6), ataxia (2/6), tremors (2/6), nystagmus (1/6), exophthalmos (1/6), and recumbency (2/6) were observed when a dose of 30 mg/kg was administered for 6 consecutive days. Recumbency and depression were seen in one out of 4 animals administered 60 mg/kg for 3 days. Swelling at the injection site was noted at each dose level.

Safety was also evaluated in 21-day-old calves. In one group, these immature animals were given injections of 6 mg/kg on study days 0, 2, 3, 5, 6, and 8. A second group of animals received injections of 18 mg/kg for a total of 2 injections 48 hours apart. The only treatment-related sign was erythema of the nasal pad in 3 of 6 calves that received 18 mg/kg. One calf in the 6 mg/kg group had pre-treatment scleral erythema, and developed nasal erythema after treatment that may or may not have been treatment-related. No changes in clinical pathology parameters were observed. No articular cartilage lesions were observed in the joints at any dosage.

An injection site study conducted in feeder calves demonstrated that the product can induce a transient local reaction in the subcutaneous tissue and underlying tissue.

Presentation: A180™ (180 mg danofloxacin/mL) is supplied in 100- and 250-mL, amber-glass, sterile, multi-dose vials.

Compendium Code No.: 36902050 79-9848-00-0

A & L SOFTKOTE

Bou-Matic **Teat Dip**

Post-Milking 1% Iodine Teat Dip

Active Ingredient(s): Active: Nonylphenoxy polyethoxy (12 moles E.O.) ethanol iodine complex providing 1% (w/w) titratable iodine (10,000 ppm w/w).

Contains 12% skin conditioners.

Indications: For use as a post-milking dip and udder wash.

Directions for Use:

Post-Milking Dip: Use full strength.

Immediately after milking, dip teats in undiluted A & L SOFTKOTE. While a cow is being dried up, dip teats in A & L SOFTKOTE once a day for several days following last milking.

Udder Washing: Cows flanks, udder and teats should be washed just prior to milking, using 1 ounce of A & L SOFTKOTE to 2 gallons of water.

Important: Teat Irritation and/or Chapping: Teat dips have the potential to cause irritation of a cow's teats or a milker's hands. Individual tolerance to a particular formulation as well as other factors (dry or cold weather, improper teat dip application, bedding quality, milking equipment, etc.) may also affect skin condition. If you observe abnormal irritation or chapping while using A & L SOFTKOTE, discontinue use and call our technical service department at 1-800-225-3832, or contact your veterinarian.

Contraindication(s): Do not use A & L SOFTKOTE for cleaning or sanitizing equipment.

Caution(s): Keep out of the reach of children. Harmful if swallowed - Eye irritant.

Warning(s): Protect eyes, skin and clothing from contact with product when handling. Wear recommended protective equipment. Keep container tightly closed when not in use. Wash thoroughly after handling product.

First Aid:

Oral Ingestion: Do not induce vomiting. Drink large quantities of water or milk. Never give anything by mouth to an unconscious person. Call a physician.

Skin Contact: Flush with water. Remove contaminated clothing and footwear. If irritation occurs and persists, get medical attention.

Eye Contact: Flush eyes with large quantities of clean, running water. If irritation occurs and persists, get medical attention.

In case of emergency call 1-800-228-5635, ext. 1.

To avoid contamination of milk, wash udders and teats with A & L Hex Udder Wash, A & L Iodine Udder Wash, or A & L SOFTKOTE solution. Then dry each cow's udder and teats with individual clean towels before each milking.

Presentation: 4 X 1 gallon case, 5 gallon pail, 15 and 55 gallon drums and 220 gallon (4 X 55 gallon).

Manufactured by: A & L Laboratories, Inc., 1001 Glenwood Avenue, Minneapolis, MN 55405

Compendium Code No.: 14480001

AB-SORB™ BOLUS

Bimeda **Mineral Supplement**

Source of Trace Minerals (Dietary Supplement)

Guaranteed Analysis:

Calcium, min. . . . . 1.40 g
Calcium, max. . . . . 1.68 g
Copper, min. . . . . 0.98 g
Iron, min. . . . . 1.16 g

Ingredients: Calcium Carbonate, Ferrous sulfate, Iron oxide, Copper sulfate, Lactose, Microcrystalline Cellulose, Dried whey, Corn Starch, Magnesium Stearate, Carob powder.

Indications: AB-SORB™ bolus is a nutritional dietary supplement providing trace minerals for horses, colts, cattle and calves.

Directions for Use: Administer orally following dosage directions. Bolus should be lubricated with mineral oil or petroleum jelly and administered with a balling gun. Boluses can also be crushed and top dressed on feed or given as a drench.

Dosage Directions:

Horses: ½ to 1 Bolus.

Cattle: 1 to 1¼ Bolus.

Colts and Calves: ¼ to ½ Bolus.

Precaution(s): Storage Directions: Keep container tightly closed when not in use. Store in a cool, dry place.

Caution(s): For animal use only.

Warning(s): Keep out of reach of children.

Presentation: 50 x 20 g boluses.

AB-SORB is a Trademark of Bimeda, Inc.

Compendium Code No.: 13990590 Iss. 07-01

ABSORBEN

Allied Monitor **Mycobacterium Test Reagent**

Active Ingredient(s): ABSORBEN is a whole-cell, heat-killed suspension of *Mycobacterium phlei*.

Indications: To be used for ELISA to absorb interfering antibodies.

Presentation: 10 mg.

Compendium Code No.: 10800001

ABSORBINE® ANTIPHLOGISTINE®

W. F. Young **Counterirritant**

Active Ingredient(s): Glycerin, salicylic acid, kaolin, methyl salicylate, oil of peppermint, oil of eucalyptus, glucose and sodium benzoate.

Indications: Medicated clay poultice for horses. For external use only.

For temporary relief of swelling, muscle strain, muscle stiffness, tendon soreness.

Dosage and Administration: Use heated (*) or unheated. Apply to moistened affected area - ½ inch thick - wrap with bandage, cover with Kraft Paper. Stays moist and is long active. It may be kept on the affected area for up to 48 hours.

(*) Loosen lid before heating, but do not remove. Place tub in very hot water, ¾ of the way up. Keep in water until reasonably warm - about 20 minutes.

Caution(s): Avoid getting in eyes or mucous membranes. Do not apply to irritated skin or if irritation develops. If heated, test on back of hand before applying.

Warning(s): Keep out of reach of children.

Presentation: 5 lbs (2.27 kg).

® Trademark owned and licensed by Carter Wallace Inc.

Compendium Code No.: 10990002

ABSORBINE® CONCENTRATED FLY REPELLENT

W. F. Young **Topical Insecticide**

EPA Reg. No.: 1543-9

Active Ingredient(s):

Butoxypolypropylene Glycol 11.0000%
Resmethrin *[5-(phenylmethyl)-3 furanyl)] methyl 2 2-dimethyl-3-(2-methyl-1-propenyl) cyclopropanecarboxylate. 5540%
Related Compounds. 0754%
Inert Ingredients. 88.3706%

*cis/trans isomers ratio: max. 30% (±) cis and min. 70% (±) trans.

Indications: For use on horses.

Kills and repels stable flies, horn flies, house flies, face flies, horse flies, deer flies, bot flies, mosquitoes, ticks and gnats.

Dosage and Administration: For maximum protection, apply 4 to 6 oz of diluted solution to animal.

Directions for Use: It is a violation of Federal Law to use this product in a manner inconsistent with its labeling.

Shake well before diluting and during application.

Dilute before applying to horse. Mix 7 parts water to 1 part concentrate. 4 oz of concentrate makes 1 quart of ready to use repellent.

To Apply: First, remove excess dirt and dust by brushing.

Wipe on Use: Dampen a soft cloth with diluted solution and rub over hair.

Spray Mist: Apply spray mist to horse's coat. Pay particular attention to legs, shoulders and neck, avoiding eyes with spray or wipe. For facial area, wipe on only. For maximum protection apply 4-6 oz of diluted solution to animal. Repeat every 2-3 days, if necessary.

Precaution(s): Storage and Disposal:

Storage: Store in original container only, in a locked storage area. Leaking packages of this product may be disposed of on site or at an approved waste disposal facility.

Disposal: Do not contaminate water, food, or feed by storage or disposal. Wastes resulting from the use of this product may be disposed of on site or at an approved waste disposal facility. Triple rinse (or equivalent). Then offer for recycling or reconditioning, or puncture and dispose of in a sanitary landfill, or incineration, or, if allowed by state and local authorities, by burning. If burned, stay out of smoke.

Environmental Hazard: This product is toxic to fish. Keep out of lakes, streams or ponds. Do not apply where runoff is likely to occur. Do not contaminate water when disposing of equipment washwaters. Apply this product only as specified on the label.

Caution(s): Precautionary Statements:

Hazards to Humans and Domestic Animals: Harmful if swallowed. Avoid contamination of feed and foodstuffs. Avoid contact with eyes. In case of contact immediately flush eyes with plenty of water. Get medical attention if irritation persists. Use on show, race, work, or pleasure horses only. Do not use on horses intended for slaughter.

Warning(s): Buyer assumes all risks of use, storage or handling of this material not in strict accordance with directions given herewith.

Keep out of reach of children.

Presentation: 32 fl oz (1 quart) 946 mL.

Compendium Code No.: 10990010

ABSORBINE® FLYS-X® INSECTICIDE

W. F. Young **Premise and Topical Insecticide**

EPA Reg. No.: 1543-10

Active Ingredient(s):

Pyrethrins 0.1%
*Piperonyl Butoxide, Technical 1.0%
Inert Ingredients 98.9%
100%

*Equivalent to min. 0.8% (butylcarbityl) (6-propylpiperonyl) ether and 0.2% related compounds.

Indications: Can be used on dogs, cats, livestock, and horses applied directly to animals or used as a surface spray.

As a surface spray FLYS-X® controls cockroaches, ants, beetles, spiders, crickets, cadelles, meal worms, and mites.

When applied directly to animals FLYS-X® protects against houseflies, ticks, gnats, mosquitoes, and a host of other insects.

Horse and Livestock:

To protect cattle and horses from horn flies, house flies, mosquitoes and gnats.

To control stable flies, horse flies, deer flies, face flies, and blood sucking lice.

For control of fleas and brown dog ticks on premises and on pets.

Dosage and Administration: Directions for Use: It is a violation of Federal Law to use this product in a manner inconsistent with its labeling.

Horse and Livestock Spray: Effective, fast acting, ready to use insecticide. Apply with conventional sprayers or a cloth.

To protect cattle and horses from horn flies, house files, mosquitoes and gnats, apply a light mist sufficient to wet the surface of the hair.

To control stable flies, horse flies, and deer flies, apply at a rate of 2-4 ounces per adult animal sufficient to wet the hair thoroughly. Repeat treatment daily or at intervals necessary to give continued protection.

To control face flies, apply with a cloth dampened with the spray.

To control blood sucking lice, apply to the infested areas of the animal. Use a stiff brush to get the spray to the base of the hair. Repeat every 2-3 weeks if required.

Pet Insecticide: For control of fleas and brown dog ticks on premises and on pets.

Effective, fast-acting insecticide.

Surface Spraying: Thoroughly spray infested areas, pet beds, resting quarters, nearby cracks and crevices, along and behind baseboards, mouldings, window and door frames and entire areas of floor covering. Fresh bedding should be placed in animal quarters following treatment. Repeat treatment as necessary.

On Pets: Start spraying at the tail, moving the dispenser rapidly and making sure the animal's entire body is covered including the legs and under body. While spraying, fluff the hair so spray will penetrate to the skin.

Do not spray into eyes or face. Avoid contact with genitalia. Repeat as needed.

Household Spray: Effective fast acting ready to use spray for use in homes. Leaves no oily or objectionable residues.

Indoor Application: Use of this product in food processing areas should be limited to periods when the kitchen is not in operation.

Food should be removed or covered during treatment. All food processing surfaces should be covered during treatment or thoroughly cleaned before use. Vacate areas and ventilate before reoccupying. For maximum results, a combination of spot treatment and surface spray is recommended.

Surface Spraying: To control cockroaches, palmetto bugs, ants, silverfish, spiders, crickets, clover mites, cheese mites, granary weevils, confused flour beetles, spider beetles, cigarette beetles, drugstore beetles, meal worms, grain mites and cadelles. Adjust sprayer to a coarse wet spray. Direct the spray into hiding places, cracks and crevices, around containers of stored foods, behind shelves and drawers. For silverfish, spray bookcases. For ants, spray trails, nests, and points of entry. If surface application only is to be used, spray floors and other surfaces at the rate of 1 gallon to 750 square feet of area.

Precaution(s): Storage and Disposal:

Storage: Do not transport or store under 32°F. Store in original container only in a locked storage area. Leaking packages of this product may be disposed of on site or at an approved waste disposal facility.

Disposal: Do not contaminate water, food, or feed by storage or disposal. Wastes resulting from the use of this product may be disposed of on site or at an approved waste disposal facility. Triple rinse (or equivalent). Then offer for recycling or reconditioning, or puncture and dispose of in a sanitary landfill, or incineration, or, if allowed by state and local authorities, by burning. If burned, stay out of smoke.

Environmental Hazard: This product is toxic to fish. Keep out of lakes, streams or ponds. Do not apply where runoff is likely to occur. Do not contaminate water by cleaning of equipment or disposal of wastes. Apply this product only as specified on the label.

Caution(s): Precautionary Statements:

Hazards to Humans and Domestic Animals: Harmful if swallowed. Avoid contamination of feed and foodstuffs. Avoid contact with eyes. In case of contact immediately flush eyes with plenty of water. Get medical attention if irritation persists.

Warning(s): Buyer assumes all risks of use, storage or handling of this material not in strict accordance with directions given herewith.

Keep out of reach of children.

Presentation: 32 fl oz (1 quart) (946 mL) and 1 gallon.

Compendium Code No.: 10990021

ABSORBINE® HOOFLEX® LIQUID CONDITIONER

W. F. Young **Hoof Product**

Active Ingredient(s): Neatsfoot oil 22.0%, lanolin 13.0%, turpentine 7.5%, pine tar 3.5% in a petrolatum, rosin base. Chloroxylenol 1.5% added as a preservative.

Indications: ABSORBINE® HOOFLEX® used on a regular basis aids in maintaining the pliability of the hoof wall, heel, sole, frog, and coronet.

Dosage and Administration: HOOFLEX® is easily applied with convenient applicator. Some horsemen prefer to massage it in, especially around the coronet.

Caution(s): For external veterinary use only.

Warning(s): Keep this and all medications safely out of the reach of children.

Discussion: HOOFLEX® Liquid Conditioner is an easy-to-apply form of the original HOOFLEX® Ointment in a liquid petrolatum base. It contains the same "breathable barrier" to maintain proper moisture balance in the hoof. HOOFLEX® Liquid Conditioner's active ingredients condition the coronary band, hoof wall, frog, and sole so that the hoof can absorb shock without cracking. Because it provides a satin shine while conditioning, HOOFLEX® Liquid Conditioner also makes an excellent showring dressing.

Presentation: 15 oz container with a brush-in-cap applicator and 32 oz refill.

Compendium Code No.: 10990043

ABSORBINE® HOOFLEX® MOISTURIZING CREME

W. F. Young **Hoof Product**

Ingredient(s): Water, lanolin, cetyl alcohol, neatsfoot oil, polysorbate 80, sorbitan oleate, glyceryl stearate, stearic acid, tribehenin, polyoxyethylene (20) sorbitol beeswax, isopropyl myristate, aloe veragel, tea-cocoyl hydrolyzed collagen (and) sorbitol, propylene glycol (and) diazolidinyl urea (and) methylparaben (and) propylparaben, chloroxylenol, (retinyl) palmitate (vitamin A), cholecalciferol (vitamin D), tocopherol (vitamin E), and fragrance.

Indications: Recommended as an aid to help relieve dryness and maintain and build strong, supple hooves.

Directions for Use: Pick and clean the hoof thoroughly. Massage a generous amount of HOOFLEX® Moisturizing Creme directly into the coronary band, hoof wall, sole and frog. Use daily, as often as necessary.

Precaution(s): Store and use at room temperature.

Caution(s): For severe or persistent conditions, consult your farrier or veterinarian.

Presentation: 12 oz (340 g).

Compendium Code No.: 10990050

ABSORBINE® HOOFLEX® ORIGINAL CONDITIONER

W. F. Young **Hoof Product**

Active Ingredient(s): Neatsfoot Oil, Lanolin, Turpentine, Pine Tar, Blended in a Petrolatum, Tallow, Wax, Rosin and Aloe Base, with Chloroxylenol 1.5%.

Indications: ABSORBINE® HOOFLEX® Original Conditioner aids in maintaining the proper moisture balance in all parts of the hoof. HOOFLEX® contains antibacterial and antifungal agents to help prevent infection.

Directions for Use: ABSORBINE® HOOFLEX® is easily applied with a small paint brush. Some horsemen prefer to massage it in, especially around the coronet. Be sure hoof is clean before applying.

Hard, Cracked Hoof Wall and Heel - When cracks occur on the wall and heel it is generally due to excessive dryness. Apply HOOFLEX® to add moisture. Used regularly, HOOFLEX® will provide the moisture balance your horse's hoof needs to stay healthy.

Hard Sole and Frog - The frog is the shock absorber, which when pliable, helps relieve the stress of heavy impact on the leg bones, tendon, and foot. Apply HOOFLEX® directly to the frog and sole daily to heap maintain pliability.

Coronet - Nature intended the coronary band, seat of hoof growth, to be relatively soft and flexible. Help maintain this condition by rubbing HOOFLEX® around the coronet frequently.

Caution(s): For external use only. Do not apply to irritated skin. If excessive irritation develops discontinue treatment. Avoid getting into eyes or mucous membranes.

Warning(s): Keep out of reach of children.

Presentation: 1 pint, 1 quart, and 1 gallon.

Compendium Code No.: 10990220 RM314905/RM314865

ABSORBINE® HOOFLEX® THRUSH REMEDY

W. F. Young **Hoof Product**

Active Ingredient(s): Parachlorometaxylenol; Aluminum Chlorhydroxy Allantoinate.

Indications: HOOFLEX® Thrush Remedy kills imbedded bacteria and fungi, helps eliminate associated odors and promotes normal healing.

Directions for Use:

1. Clean the hoof thoroughly. Remove as much diseased tissue as possible. If necessary, seek the help of a farrier or veterinarian.
2. Saturate the infected area with HOOFLEX® Thrush Remedy twice daily for 3 days, then once daily until the hoof grows out.

For proper hoof maintenance, continue to apply once weekly to help prevent infections.

Caution(s): For external use on livestock only. If condition persists longer than 2 weeks, call your veterinarian. Avoid contact with eyes. In case of contact, immediately flush eyes with plenty of water.

Warning(s): Keep out of reach of children.

Discussion: Thrush and White Line disease are bacterial hoof infections often complicated by fungi. Untreated, they can lead to lameness.

White Line disease is an infection that begins at the white line and extends upward. Cavities form in the hoof and emit a foul odor.

Presentation: 12 fl oz (355 mL).

Compendium Code No.: 10990161 RM342321-5

ABSORBINE® PROCMC®

W. F. Young **Calcium-Oral**

Gastric Relief Formula

Guaranteed Analysis:

Calcium (Min)	1.5%
Calcium (Max)	2.0%
Magnesium (Min)	1.5%
Total Solids (Min)	8.0%

Each ounce provides 0.45 mg of Calcium and Magnesium.

Ingredients Statement: Water, Calcium Carbonate, Magnesium Oxide, Xanthan Gum, Natural Apple Flavor, Methylparaben, Propylparaben, Propylene Glycol, FD&C Red No. 40, FD&C Blue No. 1.

Indications: Horses being fed a high grain, low fiber diet, combined with the physical and emotional stress of training, shipping, weaning or drug therapies are susceptible to equine gastric distress. PROCMC® proactively guards against equine gastric distress and helps to maintain a healthy stomach.

It protects by coating the lining of your horse's stomach and neutralizing stomach acids. Its buffered formula soothes and coats while providing an essential source of calcium and magnesium, which is known to promote strong bones and a healthy cardiovascular system. PROCMC® is highly palatable with a delicious apple flavor.

Important: This product is not a nutritional source of Phosphorous, Copper, Selenium, Zinc, or Vitamin A.

Directions: For Maintenance of All Horses

Feeding Directions: Shake well before use. Thoroughly mix into feed.

For mature horses, feed 1 oz. (30 mL) - 2 oz. (60 mL) once or twice daily.

For foals, feed 1 oz. (30 mL) once or twice daily or as recommended by your veterinarian.

For some horses it may be easiest to dose orally with a syringe.

Safe and effective when used as directed.

Precaution(s): Store in a cool, dry location out of direct sunlight. Do not freeze.

Caution(s): If accidental ingestion should occur, drink plenty of water.

Warning(s): Keep out of reach of children.

Presentation: 64 fl oz (1.89 L) with Tip 'n Measure container.

Compendium Code No.: 10990231 RM 346258

ABSORBINE® REFRESHMINT®

W. F. Young **Grooming Product**

Active Ingredient(s): SD alcohol 40 B (50.0%), witch hazel, water, menthol, spearmint oil, potassium iodide, iodine, FD&C yellow #6, and FD&C blue #1.

Indications: Natural body wash and brace for horses.

Dosage and Administration: Body Wash: Mix two ounces of REFRESHMINT® with one gallon of water. A daily wash helps horses cool out and stay supple.

Brace: Apply full strength to affected areas. REFRESHMINT's® mild formula will not blister, even used under a porous wrap.

Precaution(s): Flammable liquid. Keep away from fire, sparks and heated surfaces.

Caution(s): Replace cap firmly. For external use only. Avoid contact with eyes or mucous membranes. Do not apply to irritated skin. If excessive irritation develops, discontinue use and consult a veterinarian. Use under a porous wrap only.

Warning(s): Keep out of reach of children.

Presentation: 32 fl oz (1 qt) 946 mL and 1 gallon.

Compendium Code No.: 10990071

ABSORBINE® SHOWCLEAN® MANE & TAIL WHITENER

W. F. Young **Grooming Product**

Active Ingredient(s): Water, anionic/nonionic blend (alcohol content 4.0%), coco dimonium phosphate, diazolidinyl urea, methylparaben, propylparaben, propylene glycol, citric acid, sodium chloride, external D&C violet #2 and fragrance.

Indications: A pH balanced, non-irritating solution that lightens, brightens, and highlights your horse's mane, tail, forelocks, and stockings. SHOWCLEAN® is especially effective at removing troublesome stains and discolorations.

SHOWCLEAN® is recommended for all breeds of horses.

Dosage and Administration: For best results, shampoo your horse before using SHOWCLEAN®. To apply combine 8 fluid ounces with one quart of water and mix thoroughly. Using a sponge, saturate areas to be lightened with the mixed solution and let stand for 5 minutes. Rinse thoroughly with water. For heavily stained areas, use at full strength and let stand for 5 minutes. Rinse thoroughly with water.

Warning(s): For external use only. Not for use on humans. Keep out of reach of children.

Presentation: 32 fl oz (1 qt) 946 mL.

Compendium Code No.: 10990082

ABSORBINE® SHOWSHEEN® HAIR POLISH & DETANGLER

W. F. Young **Grooming Product**

Indications: To be used on horses. Produces the finest showring sheen on coat, mane and tail that lasts a full week. Keeps manes and tails tangle free. Not an oil or cream rinse. Spray oils obsolete. Not affected by water and liniment baths.

Dosage and Administration: Shampoo and rinse animal thoroughly. Remove excess water with sweat scraper. Apply small amount of SHOWSHEEN® to one section of coat at a time. Work in well with palm of hand, stroke hair flat. Apply to mane and tail, then comb through. Allow the coat to dry completely before additional grooming. No spray oils necessary.

For Cold Weather Use: Or for touch-ups, curry and brush animal thoroughly. Apply SHOWSHEEN® to the coat, mane and tail while dry. Spray fine mist until hair strands are damp. Then hand stroke in direction of hair. Allow to dry before additional grooming.

Contraindication(s): Do not use on saddle area of the horse.

Presentation: 16 fl oz (1 pt), 32 fl oz sprayer (1 qt) 946 mL, 1 quart refill, and 1 gallon.

Compendium Code No.: 10990111

ABSORBINE® SUPERPOO® CONDITIONING SHAMPOO

W. F. Young **Grooming Shampoo**

Active Ingredient(s): Water, anionic/nonionic blend (alcohol content 4.0%), centrimonium chloride, diazolidinyl urea, methylparaben, propylparaben, propylene glycol, citric acid, sodium chloride, FD&C yellow #6, and fragrance.

Indications: To be used on horses.

Dosage and Administration: Wet horse thoroughly. Pour 1 oz of shampoo into a large pail. Spray one gallon of water into the pail to work up rich suds. Apply lather to mane and tail first, then over the entire body. Work in thoroughly.

Rinse horse completely with clean water. Remove excess water with scraper or by hand toweling. For those "hard to get out" stains, use ABSORBINE® SUPERPOO® concentrate directly, or use Show Clean® whitener and stain remover.

Caution(s): For external use only.

Warning(s): Keep out of the reach of children.

Presentation: 16 fl oz (1 pint) and 32 fl oz (1 quart) 946 mL.

Compendium Code No.: 10990132

ABSORBINE® SUPERSHIELD® RED FLY REPELLENT

W. F. Young **Insect Repellent**

Fly Repellent

EPA Reg. No.: 1543-11

Active Ingredient(s):

Butoxypolypropylene Glycol	10.00%
*Piperonyl Butoxide Technical	1.00%
Pyrethrins	.25%
Inert Ingredients	88.75%

*Equivalent to 0.8% (butylcarbityl)(6 propylpiperonyl)-ether and to 0.2% related compounds.

Indications: For Use on Horses: SUPERSHIELD® Red, the coat conditioning fly repellent, has been developed for use full strength on horses. Its patented formula remains active following wet conditions and perspiration. It is also an excellent grooming aid that conditions and detangles, adding body, vigor and shine to the coat, mane and tail. May be applied with a trigger spray applicator or as a wipe. SUPERSHIELD® Red kills and repels Stable Flies, Horn Flies, House Flies, Face Flies, Horse Flies, Deer Flies, Bot Flies, Mosquitoes and Gnats.

Directions for Use: It is a violation of Federal law to use this product in a manner inconsistent with its labeling.

For maximum protection apply 4 to 6 oz. to animal.

Shake well before and during application.

Wipe On Use: First, brush horse's coat to remove excess dirt and dust. Shake container well and dampen a soft cloth with SUPERSHIELD® Red. Rub over hair with special attention to the legs, shoulders, shanks, neck and facial areas. For maximum protection apply 4 to 6 oz. to animal. Repeat every 2-3 days, if necessary.

Spray Mist: First, remove excess dirt and dust by brushing. Shake container well and apply spray mist to horse's coat, paying particular attention to legs, shoulders, shanks, and neck. Do not spray mist around the head and eyes. Dampen a soft cloth and wipe head, avoiding eyes. For maximum protection apply 4 to 6 oz. to animal. Repeat every 2-3 days, if necessary.

Precautionary Statements: Caution: Hazards to Humans and Domestic Animals: Harmful if swallowed. Avoid contamination of feed and foodstuffs. Avoid contact with eyes. In case of contact immediately flush eyes with plenty of water. Get medical attention if irritation persists. Use on Show, Race, Work, or Pleasure horses only. Environmental Hazard: This product is toxic to fish. Keep out of lakes, streams or ponds. Do not apply where runoff is likely to occur. Do not contaminate water when disposing of equipment washwaters. Apply this product only as specified on this label.

Storage and Disposal:

Storage: Store in original container only, in a locked storage area. Protect from freezing. Leaking packages of this product may be disposed of on site or at an approved waste disposal facility.

Disposal: Do not contaminate water, food, or feed by storage or disposal. Wastes resulting from the use of this product may be disposed of on site or at an approved waste disposal facility. Triple rinse (or equivalent). Then offer for recycling or reconditioning, or puncture and dispose of in a sanitary landfill, or incineration, or, if allowed by state and local authorities, by burning. If burned, stay out of smoke.

Warning(s): Do not use on horses intended for slaughter.

Keep out of reach of children.

Disclaimer: Buyer assumes all risks of use, storage or handling of this material not in strict accordance with directions given herewith.

Presentation: 32 fl oz (946 mL) 1 quart refill, 32 fl oz (946 mL) 1 quart sprayer, and 1 gallon. Licensed under U.S. Pat. 3882824

Compendium Code No.: 10990242 RM346125-1

ABSORBINE® SUPERSHINE® HOOF POLISH

W. F. Young **Hoof Product**

Ingredient(s):

Clear Paste: Acetone, resins.

Black Paste: Acetone, resins, and pigment.

Indications: Fast drying hoof polish and sealer.

To be used on horses.

Dosage and Administration: For best results: Apply 1 or 2 coats to clean, dry hoof. Allow to dry. Close container after use.

Precaution(s): Vapors may ignite explosively. Do not use near heat, sparks or flame. Store and use at room temperature with adequate ventilation. Avoid direct sunlight.

Before reclosing, apply a thin layer of petroleum jelly to neck of container for ease in reopening.

Warning(s): Avoid breathing vapors and contact with skin and eyes. Flush affected area with water for at least 15 minutes. If swallowed induce vomiting and call physician.

Keep out of reach of children.

Presentation: 8 fl oz (236.3 mL) container.

Compendium Code No.: 10990150

ABSORBINE® ULTRASHIELD® BRAND FLY REPELLENT

W. F. Young **External Parasiticide**

EPA Reg. No.: 1543-12

Active Ingredient(s):

*Permethrin	0.50%
Pyrethrins	0.10%
**Piperonyl Butoxide Technical	1.00%
Inert Ingredients	98.40%

*(3-phenoxyphenyl) methyl (±) cis-trans 3-(2,2-dichloroethenyl) 2,2-dimethylcyclopropanecarboxylate cis-trans ratio: Min. 35% (±) cis. Max. 65% (±) trans.

**Equivalent to .80% (butylcarbityl)(6-propylpiperonyl) ether and .20% related compounds.

Indications: Horses and Ponies: Repels flies, mosquitoes and gnats for 3-5 days. Repels and controls house flies, stable flies, horn flies, face flies, horse flies, deer flies, mosquitoes and gnats on horses.

Dogs: Kills fleas and lice on dogs. Also kills fleas and ticks around premises.

Directions for Use: It is a violation of Federal Law to use this product in a manner inconsistent with its labeling. Hold container upright. Shake well before using.

Ready to use. No mixing necessary. This water-based formulation may be applied directly with trigger spray applicator or as a weapon.

Use as a Wipe On: First, brush animal to remove excess dirt and dust. Moisten (but do not wet to the point of dripping) a soft cloth and rub over the hair. It is best to apply by rubbing against the hair growth. Give special attention to the legs, shoulders, shanks, neck and facial areas where flies most often are seen. Only a light application is required. Avoid using an excessive amount on your horses. Do not wet skin. After application, brush thoroughly to bring out bright sheen on the coat. Repeat as required.

Use as a Spray: Apply to face, legs, flanks, top line and other body areas commonly attacked by flies. Do not wet horse's skin or exceed two ounces per application. After application, brush thoroughly to bring out bright sheen on the coat. Repeat treatment as needed.

Dogs: Cover animal's eyes with hands. With a firm stroke to get a proper spray mist, spray head, ears and chest until damp. With fingertips, rub into face around mouth, nose and eyes. Then spray neck, middle and hind quarters, finishing legs last. For best penetration of spray to the skin, direct spray against the natural lay of the hair. On long haired dogs rub your hand against the lay of the hair, spraying the ruffled hair directly behind the hand. Make sure spray thoroughly wets ticks. Repeat treatment as needed. Kills fleas, ticks and lice on dogs and provides up to 28 days protection from reinfestation.

Dogs Sleeping Quarters: Spray around baseboards, window, door frames, wall cracks and local area of floors. Repeat as needed. The pet's bedding areas should be sprayed. Spray old bedding or replace with fresh bedding.

Precautionary Statements: Hazards to Humans and Domestic Animals: Harmful if absorbed through the skin. Avoid contact with skin, eyes or clothing. Wash thoroughly with soap and water after handling.

Statement of Practical Treatment:

If Swallowed: Drink one or two glasses of water and induce vomiting by touching the back of the throat with finger. Repeat until vomit fluid is clear. Call a physician immediately. Do not induce vomiting or give anything to an unconscious person.

If Inhaled: Remove victim to fresh air. Apply artificial respiration if indicated.

If on Skin: Remove contaminated clothing and wash affected areas with soap and water.

If in Eyes: Flush eyes with plenty of water. Call a physician if irritation persists.

Storage and Disposal:

Storage: Store in a cool area above 32°F and protect from freezing.

Disposal: Do not re-use container. Wrap and put in trash.

Environmental Hazard: This product is toxic to fish. Keep out of lakes, streams or ponds. Do not apply where runoff is likely to occur. Do not contaminate water when disposing of equipment washwaters. Apply this product only as specified on the label.

Warning(s): Keep out of reach of children.

Presentation: 32 oz refill, 32 oz sprayer, and 1 gallon.

Compendium Code No.: 10990172

ABSORBINE® ULTRASHIELD® BRAND TOWELETTES

W. F. Young **Insect Repellent**

Residual Insecticide & Repellent Towelettes

EPA Reg. No.: 1543-13

Active Ingredient(s):

*Permethrin	0.40%
Pyrethrins	0.08%
**Piperonyl Butoxide Technical	0.79%
Inert Ingredients:	98.73%
	100.00%

*(3-phenoxyphenyl) methyl (±) cis-trans 3-(2,2-dichloroethenyl) 2,2-dimethylcyclopropane-carboxylate cis-trans ratio: Min. 35% (±) cis, Max. 65% (±) trans

**Equivalent to .63% (butylcarbityl) (6-propylpiperonyl) ether and .16% related compounds

Indications:

Horses and Ponies: Repels and controls house flies, stable flies, horn flies, face flies, horse flies, deer flies, mosquitoes and gnats. Kills fleas and ticks. Repels flies, mosquitoes and gnats for 3-5 days.

Dogs: Kills fleas, ticks and lice on dogs and provides up to 28 days protection from reinfestation.

Directions for Use: It is a violation of Federal Law to use this product in a manner inconsistent with its labeling.

Read entire label before each use.

Use only on horses, ponies and dogs.

This water-based formulation may be applied directly as a wipe-on.

Instructions:

Horses and Ponies: First, brush animal to remove excess dirt and dust. Rub towelette against hair growth. Apply around eyes, ears, nose and under belly. Only a light application is required. Do not wet skin. After application, brush thoroughly to bring out a bright sheen on the coat. Reapply as needed.

Dogs: First, brush animal to remove excess dirt and dust. Rub towelette against the natural lay of the hair. Carefully apply to face around mouth, nose and eyes. Then apply to neck, middle and hind quarters, finishing legs last. Only a light application is required. Do not wet skin. After application, brush thoroughly to bring out a bright sheen on the coat. During the flea season retreat every 3-4 weeks if necessary. Do not use on foals or puppies under 12 weeks.

Precautionary Statements: Caution: Hazards to Humans and Domestic Animals: Harmful if absorbed through the skin. Avoid contact with skin, eyes or clothing. Wash thoroughly with soap and water after handling. Sensitivities may occur after using any pesticide product on pets. If signs of sensitivity occur bathe your pet with mild soap and rinse with large amounts of water. If signs continue, consult a veterinarian immediately.

Consult a veterinarian before using this product on debilitated, aged, pregnant or nursing animals or animals on medication.

Statement of Practical Treatment:

If Swallowed: Drink one or two glasses of water and induce vomiting by touching the back of the throat with finger. Repeat until vomit fluid is clear. Call a physician immediately. Do not induce vomiting or give anything to an unconscious person.

If Inhaled: Remove victim to fresh air. Apply artificial respiration if indicated.

If On Skin: Wash with plenty of soap and water. If irritation persists seek medical attention.

If In Eyes: Flush eyes with plenty of water. Call a physician if irritation persists.

Environmental Hazards: This product is toxic to fish. Keep out of lakes, streams or ponds. Do not apply where runoff is likely to occur. Do not contaminate water when disposing of equipment washwaters. Apply this product only as specified on the label.

Storage and Disposal:

Storage: Store in a cool area above 32°F and protect from freezing.

Disposal: Do not re-use container. Wrap and put in trash.

Warning(s): Keep out of reach of children.

Presentation: 10 x 0.28 oz. (8 g) towelettes.

Compendium Code No.: 10990181

A

ABSORBINE® VETERINARY LINIMENT

W. F. Young **Liniment**

Active Ingredient(s): Menthol 1.27%. Also contains plant extracts of Calendula, Echinacea and Wormwood; Acetone, Chloroxylenol, FD&C Blue No. 1, FD&C Yellow No. 6, Iodine, Potassium Iodide, Thymol, Wormwood Oil and Water.

Indications: Aids in the relief of temporary muscular soreness, stiffness or swelling caused by exposure, overwork or exertion.

Stimulates circulation in the area where applied.

Acts as a bracer and tightener. Treats superficial cuts and abrasions.

Dosage and Administration:

Legs: For relief of temporary muscular soreness and stiffness of the legs, rub ABSORBINE® Liniment in thoroughly. Apply three or more times during the day. To speed up effectiveness wring out a sponge in hot water and hold to the affected area. Repeat for 10 minutes to steam the pores open. Rub dry. Next apply enough ABSORBINE® Liniment to wet the skin. Rub in well. Apply three or more times daily.

Setting Up: Professional trainers recommend "Setting Up" for horses that have temporary leg swelling and muscular stiffness after a workout. After the day's workout "Set Up" by applying ABSORBINE® Liniment to all four legs and wrap lightly. Be careful of bandaging too tightly.

Back, Loin and Shoulder: For relief of soreness and stiffness rub ABSORBINE® Liniment in thoroughly. Apply 3 or more times daily. To speed up effectiveness, steam pores open first with a heavy towel wrung out in hot water. Rub dry and apply ABSORBINE® Liniment. Cover with heavy blanket. Repeat three or four times daily. Take care to protect the horse from drafts

Body Wash: To make a good body wash mix 4 ounces of ABSORBINE® Liniment with 24 ounces of water and 8 ounces of vinegar. A daily wash helps horses cool out and stay supple.

Precaution(s): Danger-Extremely flammable. Keep away from fire, sparks and heated surfaces. Replace cap firmly.

Caution(s): For external use on livestock. Avoid contact with eyes or mucous membranes. Do not apply to irritated skin. If excessive develops, discontinue use and consult a veterinarian. In long standing cases or those not responding to treatment, or in case of puncture or deep wounds, consult a veterinarian.

If you rub - don't wrap.

Warning(s): Keep out of reach of children.

Discussion: Many times a horse incurs temporary muscular soreness and stiffness from a workout. ABSORBINE® Liniment helps relieve these discomforts. Prompt use of ABSORBINE® Liniment can help relieve these discomforts. Prompt use of ABSORBINE® Liniment can help minimize the degree of stiffness and soreness that can settle in. Fatigued muscles need more food, more energy and fast removal of wastes. The blood supplies these needs. A liniment stimulates the blood flow where applied, thus helping meet the muscles' demands. To heighten the stimulating effect, simply massage in ABSORBINE® Liniment. Applied full strength, ABSORBINE® Liniment is antiseptic for superficial cuts and abrasions. Its antiseptic ingredients reduce bacteria of the skin. Either full strength or in a wash ABSORBINE® Liniment is consistently effective and safe. Does not blister, stain or remove hair. Horses can be worked during treatment.

Presentation: 16 fl oz, 32 fl oz, and 1 gallon (3.785 L).

Compendium Code No.: 10990191

ABSORBINE® VETERINARY LINIMENT GEL

W. F. Young **Liniment**

Active Ingredient(s): Menthol 4%. Also Contains: SD alcohol 53%.

Indications: Veterinary Liniment Gel relieves the pain and swelling of joints and muscles due to minor injuries, over exertion and arthritis.

Dosage and Administration:

Legs: To relieve pain and reduce swelling of the legs, rub ABSORBINE® Gel in thoroughly three or more times a day. To speed effectiveness, apply Gel with the lay of the hair and lightly wrap. ABSORBINE® Gel is also effective for pre-workout rubs and post-workout "set up" wraps.

Back, Shoulder, and Flank: For relief of soreness and stiffness, rub ABSORBINE® Gel in thoroughly. Apply three or more times a day. Do not apply Gel under the saddle area if you're going to ride the horse after treatment.

Shipping: During transportation, many horses injure their lower legs in the trailer or they "stock up" from prolonged standing. Shipping wraps are recommended to prevent injuries and ABSORBINE® Gel is safe and effective under porous wraps in reducing swelling.

Arthritis: A common condition in older horses, ABSORBINE® Gel helps to loosen stiff, arthritic joints and reduce the pain and swelling.

Precaution(s): Flammable - Keep away from fire, sparks and heated surfaces.

Store at room temperature.

Caution(s): Use only as directed. For external use only. Avoid contact with eyes and mucous membranes. If skin irritation develops or symptoms persist for more than 10 days, discontinue use. For severe injuries, consult a veterinarian.

Warning(s): Keep out of reach of children.

Discussion: Liniments are mild stimulants to the circulatory system that hasten and assist nature in returning a fatigued muscle, joint or tendon to normal. ABSORBINE® Liniment Gel combines the same time honored blend of Calendula, Echinacea and Wormwood herbs as our trusted Absorbine® Liniment.

Presentation: 12 oz (340 g).

Compendium Code No.: 10990200

ACAREXX™ ℞

Idexx Pharm. **Otic Parasiticide**

(0.01% Ivermectin) Otic Suspension

NADA No.: 141-174

Active Ingredient(s): Each ampule is filled to deliver 0.5 mL of 0.01% ivermectin otic suspension per ear.

Indications: ACAREXX™ (ivermectin) is indicated for the treatment of adult ear mite *(Otodectes cynotis)* infestations in cats and kittens four weeks of age or older. Effectiveness against eggs and immature stages has not been proven.

Pharmacology: Description: Chemical Name: Ivermectin is a mixture of 5-0-demethyl-22, 23-dihydroavermectin A_{1a} (component B_{1a}) and 5-0-demethyl-25-de (1-methylpropyl)-22, 23-dihydro-25-(1-methylethyl)avermectin A_{1b} (component B_{1b}). Empirical formula: $B_{1a} = C_{48}H_{74}O_{14}$, $B_{1b} = C_{47}H_{72}O_{14}$. Molecular weight: $B_{1a} = 875.10$, $B_{1b} = 861.07$.

Dosage and Administration: Dosage: ACAREXX™ is administered topically in the ear canal at an ivermectin concentration of 0.01%. One dose of 0.5 mL is applied in each ear. Repeat treatment one time if necessary, based upon the ear mite life cycle and the response to treatment.

Administration: Tear foil pouch at the notch to remove the two plastic ampules. Use one ampule per ear. Shake well before use. Snap off the cap of the ampule and place the tip into the external ear canal. Squeeze the entire contents of one ampule into the ear and massage the base of the ear to distribute the medication. Repeat the procedure in the other ear using the second ampule. In clinical field trials, ears were not cleaned and many animals still had debris in their ears at the end of the study. Cleaning the ears prior to administration of ACAREXX™ is not necessary to provide effectiveness.

Precaution(s): Storage Conditions: ACAREXX™ should be stored at temperatures below 86°F (30°C). Protect from freezing.

Caution(s): U.S. Federal Law restricts this drug to use by or on the order of a licensed veterinarian.

The safe use of ACAREXX™ in cats used for breeding purposes, during pregnancy, or in lactating queens, has not been evaluated.

Warning(s): Human Warnings: Not for human use. Keep out of reach of children.

Adverse Reactions: In approximately 1% of 80 cats and kittens, pain associated with the pinna and vomiting were observed following treatment with ACAREXX™.

For technical assistance or to report adverse drug reactions, please call 1-800-374-8006.

Trial Data: Effectiveness: One treatment with ACAREXX™ was 92% effective in treating adult ear mite *(Otodectes cynotis)* infestations after 7 days in a dose titration/confirmation study. In a well-controlled clinical field trial, one treatment of ACAREXX™ was 94% effective in clearing cats and kittens of adult ear mite infestations within 7 to 10 days.

Safety: In two Target Animal Safety studies, ACAREXX™ was proven to be safe in kittens four weeks of age or older. Four week old kittens were administered ACAREXX™ at dose rates of 1X, 3X, and 5X the recommended dose for three or six consecutive days and no adverse reactions were observed except one kitten treated at 1X the dose had histologic evidence of minimal, chronic dermal inflammation of the ear. In a well-controlled clinical field trial, ACAREXX™ was used safely in cats and kittens receiving other frequently used veterinary products such as flea control products, vaccines, anthelmintics, antibiotics, and steroids.

Presentation: ACAREXX™ is packaged in two polypropylene ampules per foil pouch, which are packaged 12 foil pouches per display carton.

ACAREXX is a trademark of Idexx Pharmaceuticals, Inc.

Compendium Code No.: 15070021 BRP/ILS/.01/IN/1 06/00

ACCUFIRM™

ImmuCell **Progesterone Test**

Bovine Milk Progesterone Test

Kit Contents: Reagents A, B, C, D; Test tube rack; Tube marker; Test tubes; ACCUFIRM™ rapid test reader (introduction kit only).

Indications: The ACCUFIRM™ bovine milk progesterone test is designed specifically for dairy producers. The test confirms questionable signs of estrus for more accurate heat detection - smarter breeding decisions, identifies open cows 19-24 days after insemination with indirect indication of pregnancy, and indicates cycling/noncycling activity in the postpartum cow.

Test Procedure:

1. After calving, begin regular observation of cows for first signs of estrus. Record any early estrus as an aid to detecting a subsequent estrus when you intend to inseminate.
2. Dairy scientists recommend waiting 45-50 days after calving before inseminating cow. Individual conditions and practices may vary. However, when you see signs of estrus or suspect estrus, test the milk with ACCUFIRM™ to be sure that the cow is in estrus and ready to breed.

   If result is "nonestrus (high progesterone)", do not inseminate. Record the date and the result. Continue to observe the cow for signs of estrus and retest to confirm the observation. If a cow continues to display signs of estrus, but the test results indicate "nonestrus (high progesterone)", arrange for a veterinary examination.

   An "estrus (low progesterone)" result does not indicate the exact time to inseminate, but does serve as a confirmation the cow is in or near estrus. If the decision is made to inseminate, record the date and any appropriate breeding information. Schedule the cow for an ACCUFIRM™ test 19-24 days later.
3. Test milk sample with ACCUFIRM™ 19-24 days after breeding - "open cow" test:

   If the result is "nonestrus (high progesterone)", pregnancy is indirectly indicated.* Because nonpregnant cows have high levels of progesterone during much of their cycle, cows mistakenly inseminated in mid-cycle would test "nonestrus (high progesterone)" 19-24 days later.

   If the result is "estrus (low progesterone)", the cow likely did not conceive. Observe closely for signs of estrus and inseminate again. After insemination, schedule an ACCUFIRM™ test 19-24 days later. It is important to note that a small percentage of pregnant cows may still be pregnant, but have a low progesterone reading. Rebreeding or short-cycling with a prostaglandin product at this time may create the risk of aborting the calf.

   When the breeding heat is accurately identified, an ACCUFIRM™ test 19-24 days later can help identify both pregnant and open cows. Catching open cows (low progesterone) provides the opportunity to observe for heat and reinseminate.

*A "non-estrus (high progesterone)" result on day 19-24 indirectly indicates pregnancy. Ideally, pregnancy should be confirmed by veterinary examination. Because of variable embryonic mortality, which occurs in about 15% of cows properly inseminated, and other reproductive disorders, a "nonestrus (high progesterone)" result does not always predict pregnancy.[7-9]

Collecting Milk Samples:

Prior to milking, take an unused ACCUFIRM™ tube for each cow to be tested. Carry the tubes in a clean pocket. Take care to prevent scratching the tubes.

Write the cow's name or I.D. number on top half of the tube.

After milking, and before dipping teats, manually strip milk from any teat(s) directly into sample tube. Fill tube to within one-half inch of the top and replace cap. Do not use whole milk from a weigh jar or pre-milking strippings. The ACCUFIRM™ kit is designed to give optimal results with post-milking strippings. Using post-milking stripping minimizes the risk of contamination from dirt and manure and also provides a very reliable reading.

You can perform the test immediately or at any time up to four hours after collecting the sample.

How to Use the ACCUFIRM™ Kit:

Test Tubes: Tubes are supplied with caps. Do not remove caps until the tubes are to be used.

Mark the tubes with the marking pen on the top half of the tube. Do not mark on the bottom half, as this will interfere with the ACCUFIRM™ reader.

Tube Rack: The tube rack has a fill mark. You can pour out fluids from the tubes by squeezing the ends of the rack with your fingers and turning the rack upside down. The pressure of your fingers will hold tubes in place when you turn the rack upside down.

Reagents: All reagents are supplied in color-coded bottles. Do not mix caps between bottles. Reagents should be stored in a refrigerator, but they must be warmed to a temperature of at least 65°F/18°C before use. (Do not exceed 90°F/32°C.) For example, at a room temperature of 70°F/21°C, the reagents will require 90 minutes after removal from the refrigerator to warm up.

Reagents may be brought to the correct temperature more quickly by briefly swirling the tightly capped bottles in warm (body temperature) water in a sink or basin until the bottles are no longer cold to the touch.

Always return the reagents to the refrigerator after testing is completed. Never freeze kit components.

Marking Pen: This pen will write smoothly if tubes are dry. Any "permanent-all surface" -type felt tip marker can be used as a replacement.

Reader: Store reader carefully in a clean, dry location (not in refrigerator).

Interpreting Results of the ACCUFIRM™ Test:

Test result:	Day 0	19-24 days after insemination
Low (estrus)	Cow is in or near estrus	Open cow
High (nonestrus)	Nonestrus, do not inseminate	Pregnancy indirectly indicated**

**An "estrus (low progesterone)" result 19-24 days after breeding would normally indicate an open cow. However, there is are small percentage of cows that may still be pregnant but have a low level of progesterone. Re-breeding or short cycling with a prostaglandin product at this time may create the risk of aborting the calf.

Problems and solutions:

1. Rack lost or broken: Mark fill lines can be made on the tubes with the marking pen.
2. Pen lost: Use a "permanent all surface" marking pen, or use tape/labels and a pen/pencil to mark the upper half of the tubes.
3. Too much B or C added to a tube: If overfilled tube is not more than ¼ above the fill mark on the rack, add the reagent to other tubes so that all fluid levels match.
4. More than 2 drops of D added to a tube: If no more than 4 drops are added, add the same number of drops to the other tubes.

Precaution(s): To maximize shelf life, the test kit should be stored in refrigerator at 38°-45°F (4°-8°C). Do not freeze.

Caution(s): If reagents are:

Spilled on skin: Immediately flush skin with cool, running water.

Splashed in eyes: Immediately flush with cool, running water. Remove contact lenses and then continue flushing for at least 15 minutes.

Swallowed: Seek medical attention. Reagents A, B and C contain 0.02% thimerosal. Reagent D contains 3% hydrochloric acid.

Discussion: Progesterone, a hormone found in milk, is a useful indicator of the stages of a cow's reproductive cycle. During estrus, the progesterone level is near zero. If a cow is inseminated and conceives, the progesterone level increases and remains elevated during pregnancy. If conception does not occur, the progesterone level increases, reaches a peak level, and then declines to near zero as the cow approaches return to estrus.

If the milk progesterone level of a cow can be measured on an intended breeding day, confirmation can be made if the cow is in estrus. 19-24 days after breeding, confirmation if a cow is open or if pregnancy is indirectly indicated can be confirmed.[1-5] ACCUFIRM™ provides this valuable information for improved reproductive performance of a herd.

References: Available upon request.

Presentation: 24 or 48 tube test kits.

Compendium Code No.: 11200002

ACEMANNAN IMMUNOSTIMULANT

V.P.L. **Immunostimulant**

Acemannan Immunostimulant

U.S. Vet. Lic. No.: 384

Description: ACEMANNAN IMMUNOSTIMULANT consists of long-chain polydispersed β-(1,4)-linked mannan polymers interspersed with O-acetyl groups. This product is prepared in a lyophilized form. Reconstitution in normal saline produces a solution for intraperitoneal and intralesional injection.

Indications: ACEMANNAN IMMUNOSTIMULANT is indicated for use in the dog and cat as an aid in treatment (i.e. surgery) and clinical management of fibrosarcoma.

Dosage and Administration: Prior to use, reconstitute ACEMANNAN IMMUNOSTIMULANT with 10 mL sterile diluent. Five to 10 minutes may be necessary for complete dissolution. Shake well before using. Use within 4 hours after rehydration.

ACEMANNAN IMMUNOSTIMULANT is administered by concurrent intraperitoneal (IP) and intralesional injections weekly for a minimum of 6 treatments. Recommended IP dose is 1 mg/kg. Recommended intralesional dose is 2 mg injected deep into each tumor mass.

When ACEMANNAN IMMUNOSTIMULANT is used as a prelude to surgery, give concurrent IP and intralesional injections weekly. Continue until delineation, necrosis or maximum tumor enlargement due to edema and immune cellular infiltration occur. Rapid necrosis, which accompanies this response, may happen within 2 to 4 weeks. Surgical excision is recommended immediately upon delineation, necrosis or maximum tumor enlargement.

Benefits of long-term post-surgery treatment have not been clinically established, however, no tumor regrowth has been observed in 5 animals treated with monthly IP injections of 1 mg/kg for 6 months following surgery.

Contraindication(s): There are no known contraindications for use of acemannan.

Precaution(s): Do not store over 35°C. Protect from extremes of heat or light.

Caution(s): The effects of this compound have not been studied in pregnant animals. However, the chemical nature of acemannan and the absence of significant toxicity in several animal species suggest the compound is not a teratogen.

Trial Data: Acemannan is a potent stimulator of macrophage activity. It has been shown to increase TNF-α and IL-1 production in animals. A study was done in 9 dogs and 9 cats with histopathologically confirmed fibrosarcoma. Animals were treated with intraperitoneal and intralesional injections. Eleven of the 18 had surgery in addition to immunotherapy. Twelve of the 18 showed gross tumor necrosis.

Twelve had tumors that increased in size - usually very rapidly (2-4 weeks). This rapid increase suggests an effect attributable to TNF-α. Lymphocytic infiltration and tumor encapsulation were also seen. Benefits of long-term treatment have not been clinically established, however, no tumor regrowth has been observed in 5 animals treated with monthly IP injections of 1 mg/kg for 6 months following surgery.

Presentation: ACEMANNAN IMMUNOSTIMULANT is supplied in kit form. Each kit contains one 10 mg vial of lyophilized acemannan and one 10 mL vial of sterile normal saline diluent for reconstitution or four 10 mg vials of acemannan and four 10 mL vials of diluent.

Manufactured by: Carrington Laboratories, Inc.

Compendium Code No.: 11430000

ACEPROJECT AND ACEPROTABS ℞

Vetus **Tranquilizer**

Acepromazine Maleate 10 mg/mL Injection, and Tabs

NADA No.: 117-531/117-532

Active Ingredient(s): ACEPROJECT: Each mL contains:

Acepromazine maleate	10 mg
Sodium citrate	0.36%
Citric acid	0.075%
Benzyl alcohol	1.0%
Water for injection	q.s.

ACEPROTABS: Each tablet contains either:

Acepromazine maleate	10 or 25 mg

Indications: For use as an aid in tranquilization and as a preanesthetic agent in dogs.

Acepromazine maleate can be used as an aid in controlling intractable animals during examination, treatment, grooming, x-ray and minor surgical procedures.

ACEPROJECT is particularly useful as a preanesthetic agent:

1. To enhance and prolong the effects of barbiturates, thus reducing the requirements for general anesthesia.
2. As an adjunct to surgery under local anesthesia.

Pharmacology: Acepromazine maleate, a potent neuroleptic agent with a low order of toxicity, is of particular value in the tranquilization of dogs. Its rapid action and lack of hypnotic effect are added advantages.

Chemistry: 2-acetyl-10-(3-dimethylaminopropyl) phenothiazine hydrogen maleate.

Mode of Action: Acepromazine maleate has a depressant effect on the central nervous system and therefore causes sedation, muscular relaxation and a reduction in spontaneous activity. It acts rapidly, exerting a prompt and pronounced calming effect. It is an effective preanesthetic agent and lowers the dosage requirement of general anesthetics.

Dosage and Administration: Acepromazine maleate may be given intravenously, intramuscularly or subcutaneously. The dosage should be individualized, depending upon the degree of tranquilization required. As a general rule, the dosage requirement in mg/lb of body weight decreases as the weight of the animal increases. The following schedule may be used as a guide to intravenous, intramuscular or subcutaneous injections:

ACEPROJECT: Dogs 0.25 to 0.5 mg per lb of body weight. Intravenous doses should be administered slowly and a period of at least 15 minutes should be allowed for the drug to take full effect.

ACEPROTABS: 0.25 - 1.0 mg/lb of body weight. Dosage may be repeated as required.

Contraindication(s): Phenothiazines may potentiate the toxicity of organophosphates. Therefore, do not use acepromazine maleate to control tremors associated with organic phosphate poisoning.

Do not use in conjunction with organophosphorus vermifuges or ectoparasiticides, including flea collars.

Do not use with procaine hydrochloride.

Caution(s): Federal law restricts this drug to use by or on the order of a licensed veterinarian.

Tranquilizers are potent central nervous system depressants, and they can cause marked sedation with suppression of the sympathetic nervous system.

Tranquilizers can produce prolonged depression or motor restlessness when given in excessive amounts or when given to sensitive animals.

Tranquilizers are additive in action to the actions of other depressants and will potentiate general anesthesia. Tranquilizers should be administered in smaller doses and with greater care during general anesthesia and also to animals exhibiting symptoms of stress, debilitation, cardiac disease, sympathetic blockade, hypovolemia or shock. Acepromazine, like other phenothiazine derivatives is detoxified in the liver. Therefore, it should be used with caution in animals with a previous history of liver dysfunction or leukopenia.

Hypotension can occur after rapid intravenous injection causing cardiovascular collapse.

Epinephrine is contraindicated for the treatment of acute hypotension produced by phenothiazine derivative tranquilizers since further depression of blood pressure can occur.

Phenothiazines should be used with caution when followed by epidural anesthetic procedures because they may potentiate the arterial hypotensive effects of local anesthetics.

Warning(s): Federal law prohibits the use of this product in animals intended for human consumption.

Toxicology: Acute and chronic toxicity studies have shown a very low order of toxicity for acepromazine maleate.

A safety study using elevated dosages of acepromazine maleate demonstrated no adverse reactions even when administered at three (3) times the upper limit of the recommended daily dosage (ACEPROJECT: 1.5 mg/lb body weight, ACEPROTABS: 3.0 mg/lb body weight). The clinical observation for the high dosage was mild depression which disappeared in most dogs 24 hours after the termination of dosing.

The only occurrence of adverse reaction during numerous clinical trials was a very mild respiratory distress (reverse sneeze) which was transient in nature and did not have an effect on the desired action of the drug.

When administered intramuscularly, acepromazine maleate causes a brief sensation of stinging comparable with that observed with other phenothiazine tranquilizers.

Presentation: ACEPROJECT: 50 mL vials.
ACEPROTABS: Bottles of 100 and 500 tablets.

Compendium Code No.: 14440010

ACEPROMAZINE MALEATE ℞

Boehringer Ingelheim **Tranquilizer**

Preanesthetic and Tranquilizer

NADA No.: 117-531/117-532

Active Ingredient(s): Each mL of injectable sterile solution contains:

Acepromazine maleate	10 mg
Sodium citrate	0.36%
Citric acid	0.075%
Benzyl alcohol	1.0%
Water for injection	q.s.

pH adjusted with 40% sodium hydroxide and/or hydrochloric acid.

Each tablet contains:

Acepromazine maleate	10 mg or 25 mg

Indications: As an aid in tranquilization and as a pre-anesthetic agent in dogs.

ACEPROMAZINE MALEATE INJECTION and TABLETS can be used as an aid in controlling intractable animals during examination, treatment, grooming, x-ray and minor surgical procedures.

ACEPROMAZINE MALEATE INJECTION is particularly useful as a pre-anesthetic agent:

1. To enhance and prolong the effects of barbiturates, thus reducing the requirements for general anesthesia.
2. As an adjunct to surgery under local anesthesia.

Pharmacology: Acepromazine maleate, a potent neuroleptic agent with a low order of toxicity, is of particular value in the tranquilization of dogs.

Chemistry: 2-acetyl-10-(3-dimethylaminopropyl) phenothiazine hydrogen maleate.

Acepromazine Maleate:

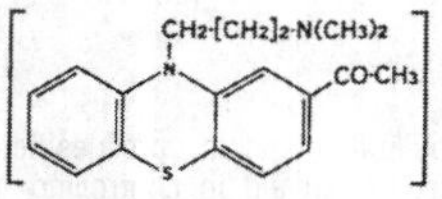

$C_{23}H_{26}N_2O_5S$ = 442.5

Mode of Action: Acepromazine maleate has a depressant effect on the central nervous system and therefore causes sedation, muscular relaxation and a reduction in spontaneous activity. It acts rapidly, exerting a prompt and pronounced calming effect. It is an effective pre-anesthetic agent and lowers the dosage requirement of general anesthetics.

Dosage and Administration:

ACEPROMAZINE MALEATE INJECTION: This sterile solution may be given intravenously, intramuscularly or subcutaneously. The dosage should be individualized, depending upon the degree of tranquilization required. As a general rule, the dosage requirement in mg/lb of body weight decreases as the weight of the animal increases. The following schedule may be used as a guide to intravenous, intramuscular or subcutaneous injections:

Dogs: 0.25-0.5 mg per lb of body weight.

Intravenous doses should be administered slowly, and a period of at least 15 minutes should be allowed for the drug to take full effect.

ACEPROMAZINE MALEATE TABLETS: Dogs: 0.25-1.0 mg lb of body weight. Dosage may be repeated as required.

Contraindication(s): Phenothiazines may potentiate the toxicity of organophosphates. Therefore, do not use acepromazine maleate to control tremors associated with organic phosphate poisoning.

Do not use in conjunction with organophosphorus vermifuges or ectoparasiticides, including flea collars.

Do not use with procaine hydrochloride.

Precaution(s): Store at controlled room temperature 59°-86°F (15°-30°C).

Caution(s): Federal (U.S.A.) law restricts this drug to use by or on the order of a licensed veterinarian.

Tranquilizers are potent central nervous system depressants, and they can cause marked sedation with suppression of the sympathetic nervous system.

Tranquilizers can produce prolonged depression or motor restlessness when given in excessive amounts or when given to sensitive animals.

Tranquilizers are additive in action to the actions of other depressants and will potentiate general anesthesia. Tranquilizers should be administered in smaller doses and with greater care during general anesthesia and also to animals exhibiting symptoms of stress, debilitation, cardiac disease, sympathetic blockade, hypovolemia or shock. Acepromazine, like other phenothiazine derivatives, is detoxified in the liver; therefore, it should be used with caution on animals with a previous history of liver dysfunction or leukopenia.

Hypotension can occur after rapid intravenous injection causing cardiovascular collapse.

Epinephrine is contraindicated for the treatment of acute hypotension produced by phenothiazine-derivative tranquilizers since further depression of blood pressure can occur.

Phenothiazines should be used with caution when followed by epidural anesthetic procedures because they may potentiate the arterial hypotensive effects of local anesthetics.

A few rare but serious occurrences of idiosyncratic reactions to acepromazine may occur in dogs following oral or parenteral administration. These potentially serious adverse reactions include behavioral disorders in dogs such as aggression, biting/chewing, and nervousness.

For use in dogs only.

Warning(s): Federal law prohibits the use of this product in animals intended for human consumption.

Keep out of reach of children.

Toxicology: Acute and chronic toxicity studies have shown a very low order of toxicity for acepromazine maleate.

A safety study using elevated dosages of ACEPROMAZINE MALEATE INJECTION demonstrated no adverse reactions even when administered at three times the upper limit of the recommended daily dosage (1.5 mg/lb of body weight). The clinical observation for this high dosage was mild depression which disappeared in most dogs 24 hours after termination of dosing.

A safety study using elevated dosages of ACEPROMAZINE MALEATE TABLETS demonstrated no adverse reactions even when administered at three times the upper limit of the recommended daily dosage (3.0 mg/lb of body weight). The clinical observation for this high dosage was mild depression which disappeared in most dogs 24 hours after termination of dosing.

The only occurrence of adverse reaction during numerous clinical trials was a very mild respiratory distress (reverse sneeze) which was transient in nature and had no effect on the desired action of the drug.

When administered intramuscularly, acepromazine maleate causes a brief sensation of stinging comparable with that observed with other phenothiazine tranquilizers.

Presentation: Injection: 50 mL vials.

Tablets: Both concentrations are available in bottles of 100 and 500 tablets. Each tablet is quarter scored for convenience of administration.

Compendium Code No.: 10280001

BI 6700-1 4/00

ACEPROMAZINE MALEATE ℞

Butler **Tranquilizer**

NADA No.: 117-531/117-532

Active Ingredient(s): Each mL of sterile solution contains:

Acepromazine maleate	10 mg
Sodium citrate	0.36%
Citric acid	0.075%
Benzyl alcohol	1.0%
Water for injection	q.s.

Each quarter scored tablet contains 10 mg or 25 mg acepromazine maleate.

Indications: ACEPROMAZINE MALEATE, a potent neuroleptic agent with a low order of toxicity, is of particular value in the tranquilization of dogs. Its rapid action and lack of hypnotic effect are added advantages.

As an aid in tranquilization and as a pre-anesthetic agent in dogs. ACEPROMAZINE MALEATE INJECTION and TABLETS can be used as an aid in controlling intractable animals during examination, treatment, grooming, x-ray and minor surgical procedures.

ACEPROMAZINE MALEATE INJECTION is particularly useful as a pre-anesthetic agent:

1. To enhance and prolong the effects of barbiturates, thus reducing the requirements for general anesthesia.
2. As an adjunct to surgery under local anesthesia.

Dosage and Administration:

ACEPROMAZINE MALEATE INJECTION: May be given intravenously, intramuscularly or subcutaneously. The dosage should be individualized, depending upon the degree of tranquilization required. As a general rule, the dosage requirement in mg/lb. of body weight decreases as the weight of the animal increases. The following schedule may be used as a guide to intravenous, intramuscular or subcutaneous injections.

Administer 0.25 mg to 0.5 mg per lb. of body weight. Intravenous doses should be administered slowly, and a period of at least 15 minutes should be allowed for the drug to take full effect.

ACEPROMAZINE MALEATE TABLETS: Give 0.25-1.0 mg per lb. of body weight. The dosage may be repeated as required.

Contraindication(s): Phenothiazines may potentiate the toxicity of organophosphates. Therefore, do not use ACEPROMAZINE MALEATE to control tremors associated with organophosphate poisoning.

Do not use in conjunction with organophosphorus vermifuges or ectoparasiticides, including flea collars.

Do not use with procaine hydrochloride.

Caution(s): Federal law restricts this drug to use by or on the order of a licensed veterinarian.

Keep out of the reach of children.

For use in dogs only.

Tranquilizers are potent central nervous system depressants, and they can cause marked sedation with suppression of the sympathetic nervous system.

Tranquilizers can produce prolonged depression or motor restlessness when given in excessive amounts or when given to sensitive animals.

Tranquilizers are additive to the actions of other depressants and will potentiate general anesthesia. Tranquilizers should be administered in smaller doses and with greater care during general anesthesia and also to animals exhibiting symptoms of stress, debilitation, cardiac disease, sympathetic blockade, hypovolemia or shock. Acepromazine, like other phenothiazine derivatives, is detoxified in the liver; therefore, it should be used with caution in animals with a previous history of liver dysfunction or leukopenia.

Hypotension can occur after rapid intravenous injection causing cardiovascular collapse.

Epinephrine is contraindicated for treatment of acute hypotension produced by phenothiazine derivative tranquilizers since further depression of blood pressure can occur.

Phenothiazines should be used with caution when followed by epidural anesthetic procedures because they may potentiate the arterial hypotensive effects of local anesthetics.

Presentation: Injection: 50 mL vials.
10 mg and 25 mg tablets: Bottles of 100.

Compendium Code No.: 10820010

ACEPROMAZINE MALEATE ℞

Vedco **Tranquilizer**

NADA No.: 117-531 (Injection)/117-532 (Tablets)

Active Ingredient(s): Each mL contains:

Acepromazine maleate	10 mg
Sodium citrate	0.36%
Citric acid	0.075%
Benzyl alcohol	1.0%
Water for injection	q.s.

Each tablet contains:

Acepromazine	10 mg or 25 mg

Indications: As an aid in tranquilization and as a preanesthetic agent in dogs.

ACEPROMAZINE MALEATE INJECTION and TABLETS can be used as an aid in controlling intractable animals during examination, treatment, grooming, x-ray and minor surgical procedures; as a pre-anesthetic agent. Acepromazine maleate has a depressant effect on the central nervous system and therefore causes sedation, muscular relaxation and a reduction in spontaneous activity.

ACEPROMAZINE MALEATE INJECTION is particularly useful as a preanesthetic agent:

1. to enhance and prolong the effects of barbiturates, thus reducing the requirements of general anesthesia;
2. as an adjunct to surgery under local anesthesia.

Pharmacology: Acepromazine maleate, a potent neuroleptic agent with a low order of toxicity, is of particular value in the tranquilization of dogs. Its rapid action and lack of hypnotic effect are added advantages.

Chemistry: 2-acetyl-10-(3-dimethylaminopropyl) phenothiazine hydrogen maleate.

Mode of Action: Acepromazine maleate has a depressant effect on the central nervous system and therefore causes sedation, muscular relaxation and a reduction in spontaneous activity. It acts rapidly, exerting a prompt and pronounced calming effect. It is an effective preanesthetic agent and lowers the dosage requirement of general anesthetics.

Dosage and Administration:

Injection: ACEPROMAZINE MALEATE INJECTION is a sterile solution which may be given intravenously, intramuscularly or subcutaneously. The dosage should be individualized, depending upon the degree of tranquilization required. As a general rule, the dosage requirement in mg/lb of body weight decreases as the weight of the animal increases. The following schedule may be used as a guide to intravenous, intramuscular or subcutaneous injections:

Dogs: 0.25-0.5 mg per lb. of body weight.

Intravenous doses should be administered slowly, and a period of at least 15 minutes should be allowed for the drug to take full effect.

Tablets: The dosage should be individualized, depending upon the degree of tranquilization required. As a general rule, the dosage requirement in mg/lb of body weight decreases as the weight of the animal increases.

Dogs: 0.25-1.0 mg/lb. of body weight.

Contraindication(s): Phenothiazines may potentiate the toxicity of organophosphates. Therefore, do not use acepromazine maleate to control tremors associated with organic phosphate poisoning.

Do not use in conjunction with organophosphorus vermifuges or ectoparasiticides, including flea collars.

Do not use with procaine hydrochloride.

Caution(s): Federal law restricts this drug to use by or on the order of a licensed veterinarian.

Tranquilizers are potent central nervous system depressants, and they can cause marked sedation with suppression of the sympathetic nervous system.

Tranquilizers can produce prolonged depression or motor restlessness when given in excessive amounts or when given to sensitive animals.

Tranquilizers are additive in action to the actions of other depressants and will potentiate general anesthesia. Tranquilizers should be administered in smaller doses and with greater care during general anesthesia and also to animals exhibiting symptoms of stress, debilitation, cardiac disease, sympathetic blockage, hypovolemia or shock. Acepromazine, like other phenothiazine derivatives, is detoxified in the liver; therefore, it should be used with caution on animals with a previous history of liver dysfunction or leukopenia.

Hypotension can occur after rapid intravenous injection causing cardiovascular collapse.

Epinephrine is contraindicated for the treatment of acute hypotension produced by phenothiazine-derivative tranquilizers since further depression of blood pressure can occur.

Phenothiazines should be used with caution when followed by epidural anesthetic procedures because they may potentiate the arterial hypotensive effects of local anesthetics.

Warning(s): Federal law prohibits the use of this product in animals intended for human consumption.

Toxicology: Acute and chronic toxicity studies have shown a very low order of toxicity for acepromazine maleate.

Side Effects: A safety study using elevated dosages of ACEPROMAZINE MALEATE INJECTION demonstrated no adverse reactions even when administered at three times the upper limit of the recommended daily dosage (1.5 mg/lb body weight). The clinical observation for this high dosage was mild depression which disappeared in most dogs 24 hours after termination of dosing.

The only occurrence of adverse reaction during numerous clinical trials was a very mild respiratory distress (reverse sneeze) which was transient in nature and had no effect on the desired action of the drug.

When administered intramuscularly, acepromazine maleate causes a brief sensation of stinging comparable with that observed with other phenothiazine tranquilizers.

Presentation: Injection: 50 mL vials.
Tablets: 10 mg tablets and 25 mg tablets - Bottles of 100 and 500.

Compendium Code No.: 10940021

ACEPROMAZINE MALEATE INJECTION ℞

AgriLabs **Tranquilizer**

NADA No.: 117-531

Active Ingredient(s): Each mL contains 10 mg acepromazine maleate, sodium citrate 0.36%, citric acid 0.075%, benzyl alcohol 1.0% and water for injection q.s., pH adjusted with 40% sodium hydroxide and/or hydrochloric acid.

Indications: As an aid in tranquilization and as a preanesthetic agent in dogs.

ACEPROMAZINE MALEATE INJECTION can be used as an aid in controlling intractable animals during examination, treatment, grooming, x-ray and minor surgical procedures.

ACEPROMAZINE MALEATE INJECTION is particularly useful as a preanesthetic agent: (1) to enhance and prolong the effects of barbiturates, thus reducing the requirements for general anesthesia; (2) as an adjunct to surgery under local anesthesia.

Pharmacology: Description: Acepromazine maleate, a potent neuroleptic agent with a low order of toxicity, is of particular value in the tranquilization of dogs. Its rapid action and lack of hypnotic effect are added advantages.

Chemistry: 2-acetyl-10-(3-dimethylaminopropyl) phenothiazine hydrogen maleate.

Acepromazine Maleate:

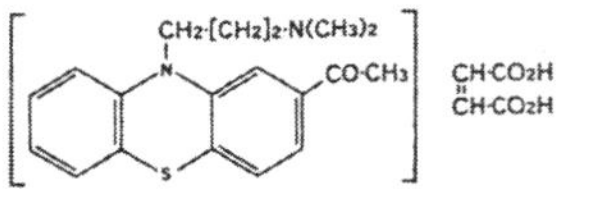

CH_2-$[CH_2]_2$-$N(CH_3)_2$; CO-CH_3 ; CH-CO_2H / CH-CO_2H

$C_{23}H_{26}N_2O_5S$ = 442.5

Mode of Action: Acepromazine maleate has a depressant effect on the central nervous system and therefore causes sedation, muscular relaxation and a reduction in spontaneous activity. It acts rapidly, exerting a prompt and pronounced calming effect. It is an effective preanesthetic agent and lowers the dosage requirement of general anesthetics.

Dosage and Administration: ACEPROMAZINE MALEATE INJECTION is a sterile solution which may be given intravenously, intramuscularly or subcutaneously. The dosage should be individualized, depending upon the degree of tranquilization required. As a general rule, the dosage requirement in mg/lb of body weight decreases as the weight of the animal increases. The following schedule may be used as a guide to intravenous, intramuscular or subcutaneous injections:

Dogs: 0.25-0.5 mg per lb of body weight.

Intravenous doses should be administered slowly, and a period of at least 15 minutes should be allowed for the drug to take full effect.

Contraindication(s): Phenothiazines may potentiate the toxicity of organophosphates. Therefore, do not use acepromazine maleate to control tremors associated with organic phosphate poisoning.

Do not use in conjunction with organophosphorus vermifuges or ectoparasiticides, including flea collars.

Do not use with procaine hydrochloride.

Precaution(s): Store at controlled room temperature, 59°-86°F (15°-30°C).

Caution(s): Federal (U.S.A.) law restricts this drug to use by or on the order of a licensed veterinarian.

Tranquilizers are potent central nervous system depressants, and they can cause marked sedation with suppression of the sympathetic nervous system.

Tranquilizers can produce prolonged depression or motor restlessness when given in excessive amounts or when given to sensitive animals.

Tranquilizers are additive in action to the actions of other depressants and will potentiate general anesthesia. Tranquilizers should be administered in smaller doses and with greater care during general anesthesia and also to animals exhibiting symptoms of stress, debilitation, cardiac disease, sympathetic blockade, hypovolemia or shock. Acepromazine, like other phenothiazine derivatives, is detoxified in the liver; therefore, it should be used with caution on animals with a previous history of liver dysfunction or leukopenia.

Hypotension can occur after rapid intravenous injection causing cardiovascular collapse.

Epinephrine is contraindicated for treatment of acute hypotension produced by phenothiazine-derivative tranquilizers since further depression of blood pressure can occur.

Phenothiazines should be used with caution when followed by epidural anesthetic procedures because they may potentiate the arterial hypotensive effects of local anesthetics.

A few rare but serious occurrences of idiosyncratic reactions to acepromazine may occur in dogs following oral or parenteral administration. These potentially serious adverse reactions include behavioral disorders in dogs such as aggression, biting/chewing, and nervousness.

For use in dogs only.

Keep out of reach of children.

Warning(s): Federal law prohibits the use of this product in animals intended for human consumption.

Toxicology: Acute and chronic toxicity studies have shown a very low order of toxicity for acepromazine maleate.

A safety study using elevated dosages of ACEPROMAZINE MALEATE INJECTION demonstrated no adverse reactions even when administered at three times the upper limit of the recommended daily dosage (1.5 mg/lb body weight). The clinical observation for this high dosage was mild depression which disappeared in most dogs 24 hours after termination of dosing.

The only occurrence of adverse reaction during numerous clinical trials was a very mild respiratory distress (reverse sneeze) which was transient in nature and had no effect on the desired action of the drug.

When administered intramuscularly, acepromazine maleate causes a brief sensation of stinging comparable with that observed with other phenothiazine tranquilizers.

Presentation: 50 mL vials.

Compendium Code No.: 10581500 670010L-00-9909

ACEPROMAZINE MALEATE INJECTION ℞

Phoenix Pharmaceutical **Tranquilizer**

10 mg/mL

NADA No.: 117-531

Active Ingredient(s): Each mL contains: 10 mg acepromazine maleate; sodium citrate 0.36%; citric acid 0.075%, benzyl alcohol 1.0% and water for injection q.s., pH adjusted with 40% sodium hydroxide and/or hydrochloric acid.

Indications: As an aid in tranquilization and as a preanesthetic agent in dogs.

ACEPROMAZINE MALEATE INJECTION can be used as an aid in controlling intractable animals during examination, treatment, grooming, x-ray and minor surgical procedures.

ACEPROMAZINE MALEATE INJECTION is particularly useful as a preanesthetic agent: (1) to enhance and prolong the effects of barbiturates, thus reducing the requirements for general anesthesia; (2) as an adjunct to surgery under local anesthesia.

Pharmacology: Acepromazine maleate, a potent neuroleptic agent with a low order of toxicity, is of particular value in the tranquilization of dogs. Its rapid action and lack of hypnotic effect are added advantages.

Chemistry: 2-acetyl-10-(3-dimethylaminopropyl) phenothiazine hydrogen maleate.

Acepromazine Maleate:

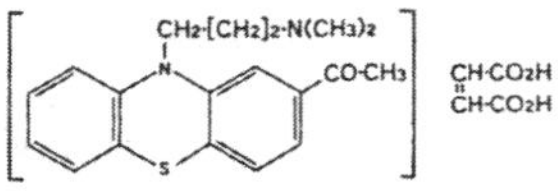

CH_2-$[CH_2]_2$-$N(CH_3)_2$; CO-CH_3 ; CH-CO_2H / CH-CO_2H

$C_{23}H_{26}N_2O_5S$ = 442.5

Mode of Action: Acepromazine maleate has a depressant effect on the central nervous system and therefore causes sedation, muscular relaxation and a reduction in spontaneous activity. It acts rapidly, exerting a prompt and pronounced calming effect. It is an effective preanesthetic agent and lowers the dosage requirement of general anesthetics.

Dosage and Administration: ACEPROMAZINE MALEATE INJECTION is a sterile solution which may be given intravenously, intramuscularly or subcutaneously. The dosage should be individualized, depending upon the degree of tranquilization required. As a general rule, the dosage requirement in mg/lb of body weight decreases as the weight of the animal increases. The following schedule may be used as a guide to intravenous, intramuscular or subcutaneous injections:

Dogs: 0.25-0.5 mg per lb of body weight.

Intravenous doses should be administered slowly, and a period of at least 15 minutes should be allowed for the drug to take full effect.

Contraindication(s): Phenothiazines may potentiate the toxicity of organophosphates. Therefore, do not use acepromazine maleate to control tremors associated with organic phosphate poisoning.

Do not use in conjunction with organophosphorus vermifuges or ectoparasiticides, including flea collars.

Do not use with procaine hydrochloride.

Precaution(s): Store at controlled room temperature, 59°-86°F (15°-30°C).

Caution(s): Federal (U.S.A.) law restricts this drug to use by or on the order of a licensed veterinarian.

Tranquilizers are potent central nervous system depressants, and they can cause marked sedation with suppression of the sympathetic nervous system.

Tranquilizers can produce prolonged depression or motor restlessness when given in excessive amounts or when given to sensitive animals.

Tranquilizers are additive in action to the actions of other depressants and will potentiate general anesthesia. Tranquilizers should be administered in smaller doses and with greater care during general anesthesia and also to animals exhibiting symptoms of stress, debilitation, cardiac disease, sympathetic blockade, hypovolemia or shock. Acepromazine, like other phenothiazine derivatives, is detoxified in the liver; therefore, it should be used with caution on animals with a previous history of liver dysfunction or leukopenia.

Hypotension can occur after rapid intravenous injection causing cardiovascular collapse.

Epinephrine is contraindicated for treatment of acute hypotension produced by phenothiazine-derivative tranquilizers since further depression of blood pressure can occur.

Phenothiazines should be used with caution when followed by epidural anesthetic procedures because they may potentiate the arterial hypotensive effects of local anesthetics.

A few rare but serious occurrences of idiosyncratic reactions to acepromazine may occur in dogs following oral or parenteral administration. These potentially serious adverse reactions include behavioral disorders in dogs such as aggression, biting/chewing, and nervousness.

For use in dogs only.

Warning(s): Federal law prohibits the use of this product in animals intended for human consumption.

Keep out of reach of children.

Toxicology: Acute and chronic toxicity studies have shown a very low order of toxicity for acepromazine maleate.

A safety study using elevated dosages of ACEPROMAZINE MALEATE INJECTION demonstrated no adverse reactions even when administered at three times the upper limit of the recommended daily dosage (1.5 mg/lb body weight). The clinical observation for this high dosage was mild depression which disappeared in most dogs 24 hours after termination of dosing.

The only occurrence of adverse reaction during numerous clinical trials was a very mild respiratory distress (reverse sneeze) which was transient in nature and had no effect on the desired action of the drug.

When administered intramuscularly, acepromazine maleate causes a brief sensation of stinging comparable with that observed with other phenothiazine tranquilizers.

Presentation: 50 mL vials.

Manufactured by: Boehringer Ingelheim Vetmedica, Inc., St. Joseph, MO 64506.

Compendium Code No.: 12560001 67008L-02-0203

ACEPROMAZINE MALEATE INJECTION ℞

RXV **Tranquilizer**

NADA No.: 117-531

Active Ingredient(s): Each mL contains: Acepromazine maleate 10 mg; sodium citrate 0.36%; citric acid 0.075%; benzyl alcohol 1.0%; water for injection q.s., pH adjusted with 40% sodium hydroxide and/or hydrochloric acid.

Indications: As an aid in tranquilization and as a preanesthetic agent in dogs.

ACEPROMAZINE MALEATE INJECTION can be used as an aid in controlling intractable animals during examination, treatment, grooming, x-ray and minor surgical procedures.

ACEPROMAZINE MALEATE INJECTION is particularly useful as a preanesthetic agent: (1) to enhance and prolong the effects of barbiturates, thus reducing the requirements for general anesthesia; (2) as an adjunct to surgery under local anesthesia.

Pharmacology: Acepromazine maleate, a potent neuroleptic agent with a low order of toxicity, is of particular value in the tranquilization of dogs. Its rapid action and lack of hypnotic effect are added advantages.

Chemistry: 2-acetyl-10-(3-dimethylaminopropyl) phenothiazine hydrogen maleate ($C_{23}H_{26}N_2O_2S$ = 442.5).

Acepromazine maleate has a depressant effect on the central nervous system and therefore causes sedation, muscular relaxation and a reduction in spontaneous activity. It acts rapidly, exerting a prompt and pronounced calming effect. It is an effective preanesthetic agent and lowers the dosage requirement of general anesthetics.

Dosage and Administration: ACEPROMAZINE MALEATE INJECTION is a sterile solution which may be given intravenously, intramuscularly or subcutaneously. The dosage should be individualized, depending upon the degree of tranquilization required. As a general rule, the dosage requirement in mg/lb of body weight decreases as the weight of the animal increases. The following schedule may be used as a guide to intravenous, intramuscular or subcutaneous injections:

Dogs: 0.25 - 0.5 mg per lb of body weight.

Intravenous doses should be administered slowly, and a period of at least 15 minutes should be allowed for the drug to take full effect.

Contraindication(s): Phenothiazines may potentiate the toxicity of organophosphates. Therefore, do not use acepromazine maleate to control tremors associated with organic phosphate poisoning.

Do not use in conjunction with organophosphorus vermifuges or ectoparasiticides, including flea collars.

Do not use with procaine hydrochloride.

Caution(s): Federal law restricts this drug to use by or on the order of a licensed veterinarian.

For use in dogs only.

Tranquilizers are potent central nervous system depressants, and they can cause marked sedation with suppression of the sympathetic nervous system.

Tranquilizers can produce prolonged depression or motor restlessness when given in excessive amounts or when given to sensitive animals.

Tranquilizers are additive in action to the actions of other depressants and will potentiate general anesthesia. Tranquilizers should be administered in smaller doses and with greater care during general anesthesia and also to animals exhibiting symptoms of stress, debilitation, cardiac disease, sympathetic blockade, hypovolemia or shock. Acepromazine, like other phenothiazine derivatives, is detoxified in the liver; therefore, it should be used with caution on animals with a previous history of liver dysfunction or leukopenia.

Hypotension can occur after rapid intravenous injection causing cardiovascular collapse.

Epinephrine is contraindicated for treatment of acute hypotension produced by phenothiazine-derivative tranquilizers since further depression of blood pressure can occur.

Phenothiazines should be used with caution when followed by epidural anesthetic procedures because they may potentiate the arterial hypotensive effects of local anesthetics.

Warning(s): Federal law prohibits the use of this product in animals intended for human consumption.

Toxicology: Acute and chronic toxicity studies have shown a very low order of toxicity for acepromazine maleate.

A safety study using elevated dosages of ACEPROMAZINE MALEATE INJECTION demonstrated no adverse reactions even when administered at three times the upper limit of the recommended daily dosage (1.5 mg/lb body weight). The clinical observation for this high dosage was mild depression which disappeared in most dogs 24 hours after termination of dosing.

The only occurrence of adverse reaction during numerous clinical trials was a very mild respiratory distress (reverse sneeze) which was transient in nature and had no effect on the desired action of the drug.

When administered intramuscularly, acepromazine maleate causes a brief sensation of stinging comparable with that observed with other phenothiazine tranquilizers.

Presentation: 50 mL vials.

Compendium Code No.: 10910000

ACEPROMAZINE MALEATE TABLETS ℞

AgriLabs **Tranquilizer**

NADA No.: 117-532

Active Ingredient(s): Each quarter scored tablet contains 10 mg or 25 mg acepromazine maleate.

Indications: As an aid in tranquilization and as a preanesthetic agent in dogs.

ACEPROMAZINE MALEATE TABLETS can be used as an aid in controlling intractable animals during examination, treatment, grooming, x-ray and minor surgical procedures.

Pharmacology: Description: Acepromazine maleate, a potent neuroleptic agent with a low order of toxicity, is of particular value in the tranquilization of dogs. Its rapid action and lack of hypnotic effect are added advantages.

Chemistry: 2-acetyl-10-(3-dimethylaminopropyl) phenothiazine hydrogen maleate.

Acepromazine Maleate:

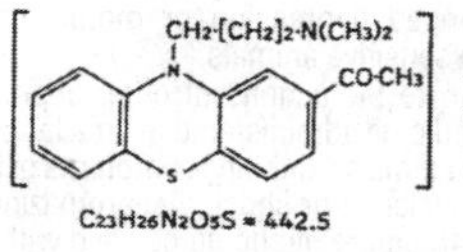

$C_{23}H_{26}N_2O_5S$ = 442.5

Mode of Action: Acepromazine maleate has a depressant effect on the central nervous system and therefore causes sedation, muscular relaxation and a reduction in spontaneous activity. It acts rapidly, exerting a prompt and pronounced calming effect. It is an effective preanesthetic agent and lowers the dosage requirement of general anesthetics.

Dosage and Administration: Dogs: 0.25-1.0 mg/lb of body weight. Dosage may be repeated as required.

Contraindication(s): Phenothiazines may potentiate the toxicity of organophosphates. Therefore, do not use acepromazine maleate to control tremors associated with organic phosphate poisoning.

Do not use in conjunction with organophosphorus vermifuges or ectoparasiticides, including flea collars.

Do not use with procaine hydrochloride.

Caution(s): Federal (U.S.A.) law restricts this drug to use by or on the order of a licensed veterinarian.

Tranquilizers are potent central nervous system depressants, and they can cause marked sedation with suppression of the sympathetic nervous system.

Tranquilizers can produce prolonged depression or motor restlessness when given in excessive amounts or when given to sensitive animals.

Tranquilizers are additive in action to the actions of other depressants and will potentiate general anesthesia. Tranquilizers should be administered in smaller doses and with greater care during general anesthesia and also to animals exhibiting symptoms of stress, debilitation, cardiac disease, sympathetic blockade, hypovolemia or shock. Acepromazine, like other phenothiazine derivatives, is detoxified in the liver; therefore, it should be used with caution on animals with a previous history of liver dysfunction or leukopenia.

Epinephrine is contraindicated for treatment of acute hypotension produced by phenothiazine-derivative tranquilizers since further depression of blood pressure can occur.

Phenothiazines should be used with caution when followed by epidural anesthetic procedures because they may potentiate the arterial hypotensive effects of local anesthetics.

A few rare but serious occurrences of idiosyncratic reactions to Acepromazine may occur in dogs following oral or parenteral administration. These potentially serious adverse reactions include behavioral disorders in dogs such as aggression, biting/chewing, and nervousness.

For use in dogs only.

Keep out of reach of children.

Warning(s): Federal law prohibits the use of this product in animals intended for human consumption.

Toxicology: Acute and chronic toxicity studies have shown a very low order of toxicity for acepromazine maleate.

A safety study using elevated dosages of ACEPROMAZINE MALEATE TABLETS demonstrated no adverse reactions even when administered at three times the upper limit of the recommended daily dosage (3.0 mg/lb body weight). The clinical observation for this high dosage was mild depression which disappeared in most dogs 24 hours after termination of dosing.

The only occurrence of adverse reaction during numerous clinical trials was a very mild respiratory distress (reverse sneeze) which was transient in nature and had no effect on the desired action of the drug.

Presentation: ACEPROMAZINE MALEATE TABLETS are available in 10 and 25 mg concentrations, and are quarter scored for convenience of administration. Both concentrations are available in bottles of 100 and 500 tablets.

Compendium Code No.: 10581510 670122L-00-9909, 670214L-00-9909

ACEPROMAZINE MALEATE TABLETS ℞

Phoenix Pharmaceutical **Tranquilizer**

NADA No.: 117-532

Active Ingredient(s): Composition: Each quarter scored tablet contains 10 mg or 25 mg acepromazine maleate.

Indications: As an aid in tranquilization and as a preanesthetic agent in dogs.

ACEPROMAZINE MALEATE TABLETS can be used as an aid in controlling intractable animals during examination, treatment, grooming, x-ray and minor surgical procedures.

Pharmacology: Description: Acepromazine maleate, a potent neuroleptic agent with a low order of toxicity, is of particular value in the tranquilization of dogs. Its rapid action and lack of hypnotic effect are added advantages.

Chemistry: 2-acetyl-10-(3-dimethylaminopropyl) phenothiazine hydrogen maleate.

Acepromazine Maleate:

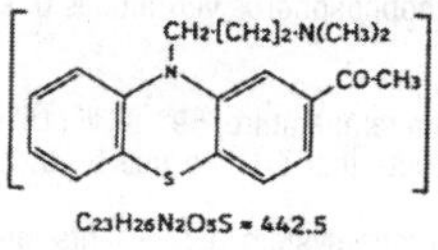

$C_{23}H_{26}N_2O_5S$ = 442.5

Mode of Action: Acepromazine maleate has a depressant effect on the central nervous system and therefore causes sedation, muscular relaxation and a reduction in spontaneous activity. It acts rapidly, exerting a prompt and pronounced calming effect. It is an effective preanesthetic agent and lowers the dosage requirement of general anesthetics.

Dosage and Administration: Dogs: 0.25-1.0 mg/lb of body weight. Dosage may be repeated as required.

Contraindication(s): Phenothiazines may potentiate the toxicity of organophosphates. Therefore, do not use acepromazine maleate to control tremors associated with organic phosphate poisoning.

Do not use in conjunction with organophosphorus vermifuges or ectoparasiticides, including flea collars.

Do not use with procaine hydrochloride.

Caution(s): Federal (U.S.A.) law restricts this drug to use by or on the order of a licensed veterinarian.

Tranquilizers are potent central nervous system depressants, and they can cause marked sedation with suppression of the sympathetic nervous system.

Tranquilizers can produce prolonged depression or motor restlessness when given in excessive amounts or when given to sensitive animals.

Tranquilizers are additive in action to the actions of other depressants and will potentiate general anesthesia. Tranquilizers should be administered in smaller doses and with greater care during general anesthesia and also to animals exhibiting symptoms of stress, debilitation, cardiac disease, sympathetic blockade, hypovolemia or shock. Acepromazine, like other phenothiazine derivatives, is detoxified in the liver; therefore, it should be used with caution on animals with a previous history of liver dysfunction or leukopenia.

Epinephrine is contraindicated for treatment of acute hypotension produced by phenothiazine-derivative tranquilizers since further depression of blood pressure can occur.

Phenothiazines should be used with caution when followed by epidural anesthetic procedures because they may potentiate the arterial hypotensive effects of local anesthetics.

A few rare but serious occurrences of idiosyncratic reactions to Acepromazine may occur in dogs following oral or parenteral administration. These potentially serious adverse reactions include behavioral disorders in dogs such as aggression, biting/chewing, and nervousness.

For use in dogs only.

Warning(s): Federal law prohibits the use of this product in animals intended for human consumption.

Keep out of reach of children.

Toxicology: Acute and chronic toxicity studies have shown a very low order of toxicity for acepromazine maleate.

A safety study using elevated dosages of ACEPROMAZINE MALEATE TABLETS demonstrated no adverse reactions even when administered at three times the upper limit of the recommended daily dosage (3.0 mg/lb body weight). The clinical observation for this high dosage was mild depression which disappeared in most dogs 24 hours after termination of dosing.

The only occurrence of adverse reaction during numerous clinical trials was a very mild respiratory distress (reverse sneeze) which was transient in nature and had no effect on the desired action of the drug.

Presentation: ACEPROMAZINE MALEATE TABLETS are available in 10 and 25 mg concentrations, and are quarter scored for convenience of administration. Both concentrations are available in bottles of 100 and 500 tablets.

Manufactured by: Boehringer Ingelheim Vetmedica, Inc., St. Joseph, MO 64506.

Compendium Code No.: 12560011 670119L-02-0203/670113L-02-0203 / 670115L-02-0203/670117L-02-0203

ACIDIFIED COPPER SULFATE

AgriLabs **Poultry Dietary Supplement**

Soluble Powder

Active Ingredient(s):

Copper sulfate 86.36%

It also contains sodium bicarbonate and citric acid.

Indications: For the nutritional supplementation in the feed or drinking water of poultry and turkeys.

Dosage and Administration: For drinking water add 1 pound per 256 gallons of drinking water or 1 pound per 2 gallons of stock solution when used in proportioners set to deliver 1 oz per gallon of drinking water. In feed add 2 pounds per ton of complete feed.

Caution(s): Use only with glass or plastic containers in preparing concentrated solutions.

Warning(s): Keep out of reach of children.

Presentation: 1 pound.

Compendium Code No.: 10580020

ACIDIFIED COPPER SULFATE

AgriPharm **Mineral Supplement**

Active Ingredient(s): Specifications:

Copper sulfate .... 86.5% per pack

Ingredients: Copper sulfate, sodium bicarbonate, citric acid.

With effervescent action.

Buffered - Soluble.

Dosage and Administration: For drinking water add one (1) pound per 256 gallons of drinking water or one (1) pound per two (2) gallons of stock solution when used in proportioners set to deliver one (1) ounce per gallon of drinking water. In feed add two (2) pounds per ton of complete feed.

Precaution(s): Store in cool dry place.

Caution(s): Use only glass containers in preparing concentrated solutions.

Not for human consumption.

For animal use only.

Keep out of reach of children.

Presentation: 0.454 kg (16 oz.) and 30 x 0.454 kg (16 oz.).

Compendium Code No.: 14570010

ACIDIFIED COPPER SULFATE

Alpharma **Poultry Dietary Supplement**

Ingredient(s): Copper sulfate pentahydrate, citric acid, anhydrous

Indications: A water-soluble source of copper sulfate for nutritional supplementation of chickens, and turkeys.

Directions: Administer for 7 to 10 days.

For Use in Water Proportioners: Add 1 pack of ACIDIFIED COPPER SULFATE to 2 gallons (7570 mL) of stock solution for use in a proportioner set to meter at the rate of 1 oz per gallon.

For Use in Tanks: Add 1 pack of ACIDIFIED COPPER SULFATE to 256 gallons of water. For treating smaller amounts of water: Prepare a stock solution by adding contents of this pack to 1 gallon (3785 mL) of water, then add 1 tablespoon of stock solution to each gallon of drinking water, or add 25 oz (739 mL) of stock solution to 50 gallons of water.

Precaution(s): Store in cool, dry place.

Caution(s): Corrosive to eyes. Exposure to the granular may cause severe eye damage. Hypersensitivity or sensitization can result from copper contact with the skin. May be corrosive to mucous membrane. Avoid inhaling dust. Irritating to the gastric mucosa. Ingestion can cause diarrhea, loss of hair pigment and anemia.

Do not mix stock solutions in metal containers.

For oral animal use only.

Not for human use.

Keep out of reach of children.

Presentation: 16 oz. (453.6 g) pack.

Compendium Code No.: 10220031 AHF-040 0004

ACTACEPT™

Activon **Teat Dip & Spray**

Active Ingredient(s):

Bronopol 29.0%
Quaternary Ammonia 8.0%
Sodium dichloroisocyanurate 7.0%

Indications: Super-concentrated teat dip and spray.

Directions for Use: Directions for Best Results:

1. Using potable water, fill ACTACEPT™ Five Quart Mixing Container up to one gallon line (using warm water will aid in mixing).
2. Empty packet contents into container - use one packet per gallon of water.
3. Secure container cap and shake well until fully blended (solution should be consistent and free from clumps).
4. Gently agitate solution again before each use.

For a thinner teat spray solution, up to one quart of water per gallon of teat spray solution may be added.

Precaution(s): Storage and Handling: ACTACEPT™ must be mixed by shaking or using an automated blending device. Please use ActaCept™ mixing containers (available in multiple sizes).

Solution may be stored for up to seven days after mixing.

Once open, use entire contents of packet (do not attempt to re-seal for later use).

To prevent contamination and evaporation, always secure mixing container caps.

Store in a dry environment.

Caution(s): Keep out of reach of children. Do not drink. For external use on dairy cows only. Do not inhale powder.

If in Eyes: Immediately flush eyes with plenty of cool, running water. Remove contact lens. Continue flushing eyes for at least 15 minutes while holding eyelids apart.

If Swallowed: Rinse mouth and then immediately drink 1-2 large glasses of water. Do not induce vomiting.

If on Skin: Rinse with water.

If irritation or discomfort persists, contact a physician. For emergency medical information, call 1-800-654-6911.

Presentation: 45 g packets (makes 1 gallon), 4 gallon, and 12 gallon.

Compendium Code No.: 10600040

ACTI/VAC® AR

L.A.H.I. (Maine Biological) **Vaccine**

Bronchitis Vaccine, Ark. Type, Live Virus

U.S. Vet. Lic. No.: 196

Active Ingredient(s): A lyophilized bronchitis vaccine, Arkansas type, live virus. Chick embryo origin.

Indications: ACTI/VAC® AR is recommended for vaccination of chickens against infectious bronchitis, Arkansas type. This mild strain is suitable for booster vaccination.

Dosage and Administration: The vaccine is recommended for use at one (1) day of age or older. A second dose should be given at two (2) weeks of age or older. For replacement pullets, a booster vaccination should be given between 16 and 18 weeks of age.

To be administered in the drinking water, intraocularly, or by coarse spray.

Precaution(s): Store below 45°F (7°C).

Caution(s): Federal regulations prohibit the repackaging or sale of the contents of the package in fractional units. Do not accept if the seal is broken.

Use the entire contents of bottle when first opened.

Burn the containers and all unused contents.

Warning(s): Do not vaccinate within 21 days before slaughter.

Presentation: 5 and 10 mL vials, packed 10 vials per box. It is available in 1,000, 3,000, 5,000, 10,000 and 20,000 doses per vial. It is supplied with or without diluent.

Compendium Code No.: 11030002

ACTI/VAC® B1

L.A.H.I. (Maine Biological) **Vaccine**

Newcastle Disease Vaccine, B1 Type, B1 Strain, Live Virus

U.S. Vet. Lic. No.: 196

Active Ingredient(s): ACTI/VAC® B1 is a live virus Newcastle disease vaccine (B1 type, B1 strain) of chick embryo origin. It has been lyophilized (freeze-dried) in vials and sealed under vacuum to preserve stability.

Indications: ACTI/VAC® B1 is recommended for vaccination of chickens against Newcastle disease. B1 strain is a mild one, suitable for primary vaccination.

Dosage and Administration: The vaccine is recommended for use at one (1) day of age or older. A second dose should be given at two (2) weeks of age or older. For replacement pullets, a booster vaccination should be given between 16 and 18 weeks of age.

To be administered in the drinking water, intraocularly, or by coarse spray.

Precaution(s): Store below 45°F (7°C).

Caution(s): Federal regulations prohibit the repackaging or sale of the contents of the package in fractional units. Do not accept if the seal is broken.

Use the entire contents when first opened.

Burn the containers and all unused contents.

Warning(s): Do not vaccinate within 21 days before slaughter.

Presentation: 5 and 10 mL vials, packed 10 vials per box. It is available in 1,000, 2,000, 3,000, 5,000, 10,000 and 20,000 doses per vial. It is supplied with or without diluent.

Compendium Code No.: 11030012

A

ACTI/VAC® B1 AND M48

L.A.H.I. (Maine Biological) **Vaccine**

Newcastle-Bronchitis Vaccine, B1 Type, B1 Strain, Mass. Type, Live Virus

U.S. Vet. Lic. No.: 196

Active Ingredient(s): Newcastle (B1 type, B1 strain) and bronchitis vaccine (Mass. type) live virus. A lyophilized vaccine of chick embryo origin.

Indications: ACTI/VAC® B1 and M48 (combination package) is recommended for vaccination of chickens against Newcastle disease and infectious bronchitis, Massachusetts type. B1 strain and Massachusetts strain are mild strains suitable for primary vaccination.

Dosage and Administration: ACTI/VAC® B1 and M48 (combination package) is designed for use as combination Newcastle disease and bronchitis vaccine in the large drop spray cabinet. Whereas virus titer is very critical when chicks are vaccinated by this method, the two (2) vaccines are produced separately so that the individual titers can be closely controlled.

Coarse spray method: One (1) vial of Newcastle disease vaccine and one (1) vial of bronchitis vaccine should be rehydrated in the same diluent for use as a combination vaccine. Rehydrate with cooled, distilled water in an amount sufficient to vaccinate the required number of chicks according to the directions of the spray cabinet manufacturer.

Precaution(s): Store below 45°F (7°C).

Caution(s): Federal regulations prohibit the repackaging or sale of the contents of the package in fractional units. Do not accept if the seal is broken. Use the entire contents when first opened.

Burn the containers and all unused contents.

Warning(s): Do not vaccinate within 21 days before slaughter.

Presentation: 10 mL vials, 5 vials of Newcastle and 5 vials of bronchitis per box.

Compendium Code No.: 11030022

ACTI/VAC® B1-M48

L.A.H.I. (Maine Biological) **Vaccine**

Newcastle-Bronchitis Vaccine, B1 Type, B1 Strain - Mass. Type, Live Virus

U.S. Vet. Lic. No.: 196

Active Ingredient(s): ACTI/VAC® B1-M48 is a live virus Newcastle (B1 type, B1 strain) and bronchitis (Mass. type) vaccine of chick embryo origin. It has been lyophilized (freeze-dried) in vials and sealed under vacuum to preserve stability.

Indications: ACTI/VAC® B1-M48 is recommended for vaccination of chickens against Newcastle disease and infectious bronchitis, Massachusetts type. B1 strain and Massachusetts strains are mild strains, suitable for primary vaccination.

Dosage and Administration: The vaccine is recommended for use at one (1) day of age or older. A second dose should be given at two (2) weeks of age or older. For replacement pullets, a booster vaccination should be given between 16 and 18 weeks of age.

To be administered in the drinking water, intraocularly, or by coarse spray.

Precaution(s): Store below 45°F (7°C).

Caution(s): Federal regulations prohibit the repackaging or sale of the contents of the package in fractional units. Do not accept if the seal is broken. Use the entire contents when first opened.

Burn the containers and all unused contents.

Warning(s): Do not vaccinate within 21 days before slaughter.

Presentation: 10 mL vials, packed in 10 vials per box. It is available in 100, 500, 1,000, 2,000, 3,000, 5,000 and 10,000 doses per vial. It is supplied with or without diluent.

Compendium Code No.: 11030032

ACTI/VAC® B1-M48-AR

L.A.H.I. (Maine Biological) **Vaccine**

Newcastle-Bronchitis Vaccine, B1 Type, B1 Strain, Mass.-Ark. Type, Live Virus

U.S. Vet. Lic. No.: 196

Active Ingredient(s): ACTI/VAC® B1-M48-AR is a live virus Newcastle (B1 type, B1 strain) and bronchitis (Mass.-Ark. type) vaccine of chicken embryo origin. It has been lyophilized (freeze-dried) in vials and sealed under vacuum to preserve stability.

Indications: ACTI/VAC® B1-M48-AR is recommended for vaccination of chickens against Newcastle disease and infectious bronchitis, Massachusetts and Arkansas types. B1 strain, and Massachusetts and Arkansas strains are mild, suitable for booster vaccination.

Dosage and Administration: The vaccine is recommended for use at one (1) day of age or older. A second dose should be given at two (2) weeks of age or older. For replacement pullets, a booster vaccination should be given between 16 and 18 weeks of age.

To be administered in the drinking water, intraocularly, or by coarse spray.

Precaution(s): Store below 45°F (7°C).

Caution(s): Federal regulations prohibit the repackaging or sale of the contents of the package in fractional units. Do not accept if the seal is broken. Use the entire contents when first opened.

Burn the containers and all unused contents.

Warning(s): Do not vaccinate within 21 days before slaughter.

Presentation: 10 mL vials, packed in 10 vials per box. It is available in 500, 1,000, 3,000, 5,000 and 10,000 doses per vial. It is supplied with or without diluent.

Compendium Code No.: 11030042

ACTI/VAC® B1-M48-CT

L.A.H.I. (Maine Biological) **Vaccine**

Newcastle-Bronchitis Vaccine, B1 Type, B1 Strain, Mass.-Conn. Type, Live Virus

U.S. Vet. Lic. No.: 196

Active Ingredient(s): ACTI/VAC® B1-M48-CT is a live virus Newcastle (B1 type, B1 strain) and bronchitis (Mass.-Conn. type) vaccine of chicken embryo origin. It has been lyophilized (freeze-dried) in vials and sealed under vacuum to preserve stability.

Indications: ACTI/VAC® B1-M48-CT is recommended for vaccination of chickens against Newcastle disease and infectious bronchitis, Massachusetts and Connecticut types. These mild viral strains are suitable for primary vaccination.

Dosage and Administration: The vaccine is recommended for use at one (1) day of age or older. A second dose should be given at two (2) weeks of age or older. For replacement pullets, a booster vaccination should be given between 16 and 18 weeks of age.

To be administered in the drinking water, intraocularly, or by coarse spray.

Precaution(s): Store below 45°F (7°C).

Caution(s): Federal regulations prohibit the repackaging or sale of the contents of the package in fractional units. Do not accept if the seal is broken. Use the entire contents when first opened.

Burn the containers and all unused contents.

Warning(s): Do not vaccinate within 21 days before slaughter.

Presentation: 10 mL vials, packed 10 vials per box. It is available in 1,000, 3,000, 5,000 and 10,000. It is supplied with or without diluent.

Compendium Code No.: 11030052

ACTI/VAC® CT

L.A.H.I (Maine Biological) **Vaccine**

Bronchitis Vaccine, Connecticut Type, Live Virus

U.S. Vet. Lic. No.: 196

Active Ingredient(s): ACTI/VAC® CT is a live virus bronchitis (Conn. type) vaccine of chicken embryo origin. It has been lyophilized (freeze-dried) in vials and sealed under vacuum to preserve stability.

Indications: ACTI/VAC® CT is recommended for vaccination of chickens against infectious bronchitis, Connecticut type. This mild strain is suitable for primary vaccination.

Dosage and Administration: The vaccine is recommended for use at one (1) day of age or older. A second dose should be given at two (2) weeks of age or older. For replacement pullets, a booster vaccination should be given between 16 and 18 weeks of age.

Vaccinate healthy birds only.

Vaccination Methods:

Drinking Water Method: Remove any disinfectant or sanitizers from the drinking water for 24 hours prior to and after vaccination. Rinse all waterers with clean water. Do not use disinfectants. Withhold all water for at least one (1) hour to allow birds to get thirsty before giving the vaccine. Provide ample watering space so that all birds can drink easily.

Intra-ocular Method (for 1,000 dose size): Rehydrate the vaccine with the diluent provided. Insert the control dropper tip into the diluent bottle. Hold the chick with one eye turned up. Put one drop of vaccine into the open eye and hold until the bird swallows.

Spray Method (for 20,000, 10,000 and 5,000 dose size): Rehydrate with cool, distilled water in an amount sufficient to vaccinate the required number of chickens according to the directions of the field sprayer manufacturer. Field spray application should be used only in houses that can be tightly closed. Close all windows, doors, ventilators, etc. and turn off fan. Spray each 1,000 doses of vaccine directly into the faces of 1,000 birds. Leave the house closed for at least 15 minutes after spraying.

Vaccination Reaction: Respiratory symptoms will be more pronounced from the first vaccination and will vary with the age and the level of parental immunity in the chicks. While birds are going through the reaction period, keep them comfortable by providing adequate heat and good ventilation.

Precaution(s): Store below 45°F (7°C).

Caution(s): Always use eye goggles when spraying a live virus vaccine.

Do not rehydrate the vaccine until ready for use.

The use of this vaccine is subject to state laws wherever applicable.

Federal regulations prohibit the repackaging or sale of the contents of the package in fractional units. Do not accept if the seal is broken. Use the entire contents of the bottle when first opened.

Burn the containers and all unused contents.

Warning(s): Do not vaccinate within 21 days before slaughter.

Presentation: 5 mL and 10 mL vials, packed 10 vials per box. It is available in 1,000, 3,000, 5,000, 10,000 and 20,000 doses per vial. It is supplied with or without diluent.

Compendium Code No.: 11030062

ACTI/VAC® FP

L.A.H.I. (Maine Biological) **Vaccine**

Fowl Pox Vaccine, Live Virus

U.S. Vet. Lic. No.: 196

Active Ingredient(s): ACTI/VAC® FP is a live virus fowl pox vaccine of tissue chicken embryo. It has been lyophilized (freeze-dried) in vials and sealed under vacuum to preserve stability.

Indications: ACTI/VAC® FP is recommended for vaccination against fowl pox in chickens.

Dosage and Administration: ACTI/VAC® FP can be administered to day old chicks in areas where fowl pox is prevalent. It can also be used for growing pullets.

Birds may be vaccinated by the wing web method at one (1) day of age or older. For meat birds and laying replacements, this product may be administered from one (1) day to 12 weeks of age. Vaccinate healthy birds only.

Precaution(s): Store in a refrigerator at 45°F (7°C).

Caution(s): Federal regulations prohibit the repackaging or sale of the contents of the package in fractional units. Do not accept if the seal is broken. Use the entire contents when first opened.

Burn the containers and all unused contents.

Warning(s): Do not vaccinate within 21 days before slaughter.

Presentation: Lyophilized in 5 and 10 mL vials, packed 10 vials of vaccine and 10 vials of diluent per box.

Compendium Code No.: 11030072

ACTI/VAC® LAS

L.A.H.I. (Maine Biological) **Vaccine**

Newcastle Disease Vaccine, B1 Type, LaSota Strain, Live Virus

U.S. Vet. Lic. No.: 196

Contents: This product contains the antigen listed above.

Streptomycin and penicillin added as bacteriostatic agents.

This vaccine has been carefully manufactured and has passed all tests for purity and potency according to the requirements of the Company and of the U.S. Department of Agriculture.

Indications: Recommended Vaccination Schedules: Recommended for vaccination against Newcastle disease.

The most satisfactory vaccination schedule may vary from one area to another, depending on such factors as the incidence of disease and concentration of poultry flocks. The following vaccination schedules would be applicable to most areas but may be tailored to local conditions.

Directions for Use:

Drinking Water Method: Remove any disinfectant or sanitizers from the drinking water for 24 hours prior to and after vaccination. Rinse all waterers with clean water. Do not use disinfectants. Withhold all water for at least one hour to allow birds to get thirsty before giving vaccine.

Mix vaccine in the drinking water according to the following schedule:

Age of Birds	Liters of Water to be Used for					
	100 Doses	1000 Doses	2000 Doses	3000 Doses	5000 Doses	10,000 Doses
Under 3 weeks	1	10	20	30	50	100
3 to 8 weeks	2	20	40	60	100	200
Over 8 weeks	4	40	80	120	200	400

Provide ample water space so that all birds can drink easily. Administration through the water lines with a proportioner or medication tank is not recommended.

Intraocular and Intranasal Methods: Rehydrate the vaccine with the diluent provided. Hold the chick with one eye turned up. Put one drop in eye and hold until bird swallows.

Coarse Spray Method: Close all windows, doors, ventilators, etc., and turn off fans. Rehydrate according to the directions of the field sprayer manufacturer. Spray each 1000 doses of vaccine directly into the faces of each 1000 birds. Leave the house closed for at least 15 minutes after spraying.

This vaccine is recommended for use at 2 weeks of age or older. Revaccinate 4 to 6 weeks later. Replacement pullets should be revaccinated between 16 and 18 weeks of age.

Vaccination Reaction: Respiratory symptoms will be more pronounced from the first vaccination and will vary with the age and the level of parental immunity in the chicks. While birds are going through the reaction period, keep them comfortable by providing adequate heat and good ventilation.

Precaution(s): Store not over 45°F (7°C).

Use entire contents when a vial is first opened. Burn all vials and unused contents.

To maintain the quality of this product, it is essential that the directions and precautions for storage, handling and use be carefully followed.

Caution(s): Vaccinate only healthy birds.

Keep permanent vaccination records including vaccine serial number.

Chicks being shipped by parcel post should be vaccinated at their destination so as to not violate postal regulations.

The use of this vaccine is subject to State laws wherever applicable.

Newcastle disease virus can cause an inflammation of the eyes and eyelids of humans; caution should be used not to allow the vaccine to come in contact with the eyes.

Warning(s): Do not vaccinate within 21 days before slaughter.

Presentation: 5 and 10 mL vials, packed 10 vials per box. It is available in 1,000, 2,000, 3,000, 5,000, 10,000 and 20,000 doses per vial. It is supplied with or without diluent.

Compendium Code No.: 11030083 6805

ACTI/VAC® LAS-MA

L.A.H.I. (Maine Biological) **Vaccine**

Newcastle-Bronchitis Vaccine, B1 Type, LaSota Strain, Mass. Type, Live Virus

U.S. Vet. Lic. No.: 196

Contents: This product contains the antigens listed above.

Contains streptomycin and penicillin as preservatives.

This vaccine has been carefully manufactured and has passed all tests for purity and potency according to the requirements of the Company and of the U.S. Department of Agriculture.

Indications: Recommended Vaccination Schedules: This vaccine is recommended for vaccination of chickens against Newcastle disease and infectious bronchitis, Mass. type, for both initial vaccination and revaccination.

The most satisfactory vaccination schedule may vary from one area to another, depending on such factors as the incidence of disease and concentration of poultry flocks. The following vaccination schedules would be applicable to most areas but may be tailored to local conditions.

Directions for Use:

Drinking Water Method: Remove any disinfectant or sanitizers from the drinking water for 24 hours prior to and after vaccination. Rinse all waterers with clean water. Do not use disinfectants. Withhold all water for at least one hour to allow birds to get thirsty before giving vaccine.

Mix vaccine in the drinking water according to the following schedule:

Age of Birds	Liters of Water to be Used for					
	100 Doses	1000 Doses	2000 Doses	3000 Doses	5000 Doses	10,000 Doses
Under 3 weeks	1	10	20	30	50	100
3 to 8 weeks	2	20	40	60	100	200
Over 8 weeks	4	40	80	120	200	400

Provide ample water space so that all birds can drink easily. Administration through the water lines with a proportioner or medication tank is not recommended.

Intraocular (Eye Drop) Method for 1000 and 100 Dose Sizes: Rehydrate the vaccine with the diluent provided. Hold the chick with one eye turned up. Put one drop in eye and hold until bird swallows.

This vaccine is recommended for use at 2 weeks of age or older. Revaccinate 4 to 6 weeks later. Replacement pullets should be revaccinated between 16 and 18 weeks of age.

Vaccination Reaction: Respiratory symptoms will be more pronounced from the first vaccination and will vary with the age and the level of parental immunity in the chicks. While birds are going through the reaction period, keep them comfortable by providing adequate heat and good ventilation.

Precaution(s): Store not over 45°F (7°C).

Use entire contents when a vial is first opened. Burn all vials and unused contents.

To maintain the quality of this product, it is essential that the directions and precautions for storage, handling and use be carefully followed.

Caution(s): Vaccinate only healthy birds.

Keep permanent vaccination records including vaccine serial number.

Chicks being shipped by parcel post should be vaccinated at their destination so as to not violate postal regulations.

The use of this vaccine is subject to State laws wherever applicable.

Newcastle disease virus can cause an inflammation of the eyes and eyelids of humans; caution should be used not to allow the vaccine to come in contact with the eyes.

Warning(s): Do not vaccinate within 21 days before slaughter.

Presentation: 10 mL vials, packed 10 vials per box. It is available in 1,000, 2,000, 3,000, 5,000 and 10,000 doses per vial. It is supplied with or without diluent.

Compendium Code No.: 11030093 6806

ACTI/VAC® M48

L.A.H.I (Maine Biological) **Vaccine**

Bronchitis Vaccine, Mass. Type, Live Virus

U.S. Vet. Lic. No.: 196

Active Ingredient(s): A lyophilized bronchitis vaccine, Mass. type, live virus. Chick embryo origin.

Indications: ACTI/VAC® M48 is recommended for vaccination of chickens against infectious bronchitis, Massachusetts type. Massachusetts strain is a mild strain of vaccine suitable for primary vaccination.

Dosage and Administration: The vaccine is recommended for use at one (1) day of age or older. A second dose should be given at two (2) weeks of age or older. For replacement pullets, a booster vaccination should be given between 16 and 18 weeks of age.

To be administered in the drinking water, intraocularly, or by coarse spray.

Precaution(s): Store below 45°F (7°C).

Caution(s): Federal regulations prohibit the repackaging or sale of the contents of the package in fractional units. Do not accept if the seal is broken. Use the entire contents of bottle when first opened.

Burn the containers and all unused contents.

Warning(s): Do not vaccinate within 21 days before slaughter.

Presentation: 5 and 10 mL vials, packed 10 vials per box. It is available in 1,000, 2,000, 3,000, 5,000, 10,000 and 20,000 doses per vial. It is supplied with or without diluent.

Compendium Code No.: 11030102

ACTI/VAC® M48-AR

L.A.H.I. (Maine Biological) **Vaccine**

Bronchitis Vaccine, Mass.-Ark Type, Live Virus

U.S. Vet. Lic. No.: 196

Active Ingredient(s): A lyophilized bronchitis vaccine, Mass.-Ark type, live virus. Chick embryo origin.

Indications: ACTI/VAC® M48-AR is recommended for vaccination of chickens against infectious bronchitis, Massachusetts and Arkansas types. This is a mild-strained vaccine suitable for booster vaccination.

Dosage and Administration: The vaccine is recommended for use at one (1) day of age or older. A second dose should be given at two (2) weeks of age or older. For replacement pullets, a booster vaccination should be given between 16 and 18 weeks of age.

To be administered in the drinking water, intraocularly, or by coarse spray.

Precaution(s): Store below 45°F (7°C).

Caution(s): Federal regulations prohibit the repackaging or sale of the contents of the package in fractional units. Do not accept if the seal is broken. Use the entire contents of bottle when first opened.

Burn the containers and all unused contents.

Warning(s): Do not vaccinate within 21 days before slaughter.

Presentation: 5 and 10 mL vials, packed 10 vials per box. It is available in 1,000, 3,000, 5,000, 10,000 and 20,000 doses per vial. It is supplied with or without diluent.

Compendium Code No.: 11030112

ACTI/VAC® RO

L.A.H.I. (Maine Biological) **Vaccine**

Newcastle Disease Vaccine, Roakin Type, Live Virus

U.S. Vet. Lic. No.: 196

Active Ingredient(s): ACTI/VAC® RO is a lyophilized live virus Newcastle disease vaccine (Roakin type) of chicken embryo origin.

Indications: ACTI/VAC® RO is recommended for vaccination of chickens against Newcastle disease where highly pathogenic Newcastle disease is prevalent.

Dosage and Administration: Birds may be vaccinated by the wing web method at any time after four (4) weeks of age but not later than one (1) month before they come into production.

It is recommended for use as the last vaccination after the use of B1 Strain or LaSota Strain.

Vaccinate healthy birds only.

Precaution(s): Store below 45°F (7°C).

Caution(s): Federal regulations prohibit the repackaging or sale of the contents of the package in fractional units. Do not accept if the seal is broken. Use the entire contents when first opened.

Burn the containers and all unused contents.

Warning(s): Do not vaccinate within 21 days before slaughter.

Presentation: 5 mL vials, packed 5 vials of vaccine and 5 vials of diluent per box with 5 double needles for wing web application. It is available in 500 and 1,000 doses per vial.

Compendium Code No.: 11030122

ADAMS™ CARBARYL FLEA & TICK SHAMPOO

Farnam **Parasiticide Shampoo**

EPA Reg. No.: 2097-8

Active Ingredient(s):

Carbaryl (1-Naphthyl N-Methylcarbamate) 0.50%
Inert Ingredients 99.50%
Total 100.00%

Indications: A routine cleansing shampoo to restore natural luster to the hair coat of dogs and cats. Kills fleas, lice and ticks.

Directions for Use: It is a violation of Federal law to use this product in a manner inconsistent with its labeling.

Read entire label before each use.

Use only on dogs, puppies, cats and kittens.

For external use only.

User Safety Requirements: Wear long-sleeved shirts, long pants, shoes plus socks and household latex or rubber gloves when applying this product. Change clothing as soon as possible after use. Wash the outside of gloves before removing. As with any pesticide product, wash hands thoroughly immediately after handling and before eating, smoking or using the toilet.

Use product only outside or in a well-ventilated area. Wear household latex or rubber gloves.

This product should not be applied by children.

As a precaution, a bland ophthalmic ointment should be placed in the eyes prior to bathing to prevent possible irritation.

Thoroughly soak animal with warm water taking 2-3 minutes to wet hair. Apply Shampoo on head and ears and lather, then repeat procedure with neck, chest, middle, and hindquarters, finishing legs last. For best effects, allow lather to remain in contact with skin for 5 minutes before rinsing. Rinse thoroughly. Repeat every 2 weeks. Do not allow to get into eyes or on scrotum. For a complete flea and tick control program consult your veterinarian.

Precautionary Statements: Hazards to Humans and Domestic Animals:

Caution:

Human: Avoid contact with eyes, skin, or clothing. In case of contact immediately flush eyes or skin with water. Obtain medical attention if irritation persists. Harmful if swallowed.

Animal: Do not use on animals under 12 weeks of age. Consult a veterinarian before using this product on debilitated, aged, medicated, pregnant or nursing animals. Sensitivities may occur after using any pesticide product for pets. If signs of sensitivity occur, bathe your pet with mild soap and rinse with large amounts of water. If signs continue, consult a veterinarian immediately.

First Aid:

If in Eyes: Flush eyes with plenty of water. Call a physician if irritation persists.

If on Skin: Wash with plenty of soap and water. See physician if irritation persists.

If Swallowed: Call physician or Poison Control Center.

Environmental Hazards: This product is extremely toxic to aquatic invertebrates. Do not contaminate water by cleaning of equipment or disposal of waste.

In case of emergency, or for product use information, call (602) 285-1660 Monday-Friday, 7:00 am to 4:45 pm, MST.

Storage and Disposal:

Storage: Store in a cool, dry area.

Disposal: Do not reuse container. Rinse thoroughly and wrap container in several layers of newspaper and discard in trash.

Warning(s): Keep out of reach of children.

Presentation: 12 fl oz (355 mL) bottle.

Compendium Code No.: 10000510 9701 85-6646-02

ADAMS™ CARBARYL FLEA & TICK SHAMPOO

V.P.L. **Parasiticide Shampoo**

EPA Reg. No.: 2097-8

Active Ingredient(s):

Carbaryl (1-Naphthyl N-Methylcarbamate) 0.50%
Inert Ingredients 99.50%
Total 100.00%

Indications: A routine cleansing shampoo to restore natural luster to the hair coat of dogs and cats. Kills fleas, lice and ticks.

Directions for Use: It is a violation of Federal law to use this product in a manner inconsistent with its labeling.

Read entire label before each use.

Use only on dogs, puppies, cats and kittens.

For external use only.

User Safety Requirements: Wear long-sleeved shirts, long pants, shoes plus socks and household latex or rubber gloves when applying this product. Change clothing as soon as possible after use. Wash the outside of gloves before removing. As with any pesticide product, wash hands thoroughly immediately after handling and before eating, smoking or using the toilet.

Use product only outside or in a well-ventilated area. Wear household latex or rubber gloves. This product should not be applied by children.

As a precaution, a bland ophthalmic ointment should be placed in the eyes prior to bathing to prevent possible irritation.

Thoroughly soak animal with warm water taking 2-3 minutes to wet hair. Apply Shampoo on head and ears and lather, then repeat procedure with neck, chest, middle, and hindquarters, finishing legs last. For best effects, allow lather to remain in contact with skin for 5 minutes before rinsing. Rinse thoroughly. Repeat every 2 weeks. Do not allow to get into eyes or on scrotum. For a complete flea and tick control program consult your veterinarian.

Precautionary Statements: Hazards to Humans and Domestic Animals:

Caution:

Human: Avoid contact with eyes, skin, or clothing. In case of contact immediately flush eyes or skin with water. Obtain medical attention if irritation persists. Harmful if swallowed.

Animal: Do not use on animals under 12 weeks of age. Consult a veterinarian before using this product on debilitated, aged, medicated, pregnant or nursing animals. Sensitivities may occur after using any pesticide product for pets. If signs of sensitivity occur, bathe your pet with mild soap and rinse with large amounts of water. If signs continue, consult a veterinarian immediately.

First Aid:

If in Eyes: Flush eyes with plenty of water. Call a physician if irritation persists.

If on Skin: Wash with plenty of soap and water. See physician if irritation persists.

If Swallowed: Call physician or Poison Control Center.

Environmental Hazards: This product is extremely toxic to aquatic invertebrates. Do not contaminate water by cleaning of equipment or disposal of waste.

In case of emergency, or for product use information, call (602) 285-1660 Monday-Friday, 7:00 am to 4:45 pm, MST.

Storage and Disposal:

Storage: Store in a cool, dry area.

Disposal: Do not reuse container. Rinse thoroughly and wrap container in several layers of newspaper and discard in trash.

Warning(s): Keep out of reach of children.

Presentation: 12 fl oz (355 mL) bottle.

Compendium Code No.: 11430510 9701 85-6646-02

ADAMS™ CARPET POWDER

Farnam **Flea Control & Premise Insecticide**

Carpet Powder with Linalool and Nylar®

EPA Reg. No.: 4758-175

Active Ingredient(s):

Linalool 2.500%
Piperonyl Butoxide, Technical* 0.500%
Pyrethrins 0.075%
Nylar®: 2-(1-methyl-2-(4-phenoxyphenoxy)ethoxy) pyridine** 0.020%
Other Ingredients: 96.905%

*Equivalent to 0.4% (Butylcarbityl)(6-propylpiperonyl) ether and 0.1% related compounds.

**Nylar® is a registered trademark of McLaughlin Gormley King Co.

Indications: Kills fleas and ticks on carpet. Contains Nylar® Insect Growth Regulator. Contains the botanically derived insecticide Linalool. Treats up to 400 square feet. Kills all four stages of the flea - adults, eggs, larvae, and pupae. Breaks the flea life cycle and controls reinfestation for up to 365 days.

Directions for Use: It is a violation of Federal law to use this product in a manner inconsistent with its labeling.

Shake well before using.

One 16-ounce canister contains enough powder to treat 1 to 2 rooms (200-400 square feet). When using this product at the lower rate, allow the powder to remain in place for 24 hours before vacuuming. Apply powder more heavily to areas of flooring on which pets spend most of their time. Apply to dry surfaces only. Do not wet powder.

Carpets: Shake powder evenly across surface. Brush lightly with broom to force powder deep into carpet where fleas and their larvae exist. Wait at least 60 minutes before (lightly) vacuuming to remove visible surface powder. For maximum efficacy, delay vacuuming for up to 24 hours. When emptying vacuum bag after use, wrap contents or disposable bag in several layers of newspaper and discard in trash.

Treat pets with a registered flea and tick control product prior to re-entry.

Precautionary Statements: Hazards to Humans and Domestic Animals:

Caution: Causes moderate eye irritation. Avoid contact with eyes or clothing. Wash thoroughly with soap and water after handling and before eating or smoking. Do not contaminate feed, water or foodstuffs. Do not apply to food processing surfaces or use in food processing areas where food is exposed. Cover fish aquariums before use. Keep children and pets off treated carpet during treatment and while powder is still visible on its surface.

First Aid:

If in eyes: Flush eyes with plenty of water. Get medical attention if irritation persists.

In case of emergency or for product use information please call 602-285-1660 Monday - Friday, 7:00 - 3:45 pm MST.

Storage and Disposal:

Storage: Store in a cool, dry area inaccessible to children and pets.

Disposal: Do not reuse empty container. Wrap container and put in trash collection.

Warning(s): Keep out of reach of children.

Presentation: 16 oz. (454 g).

Compendium Code No.: 10000790

ADAMS™ DELTA FORCE™ TICK COLLAR FOR DOGS

Farnam **Parasiticide Collar**

EPA Reg. No.: 68451-1-4758

Active Ingredient(s): Percentage by Weight

Deltamethrin 4.0%
Inert Ingredients: 96.0%
Total 100.00%

Indications: ADAMS™ DELTA FORCE™ Tick Collar for Dogs provides full season, up to 6 months protection against fleas and ticks.

Kills Ticks (including Deer ticks which may carry Lyme disease), also kills fleas.

Directions for Use: It is a violation of Federal law to use this product in a manner inconsistent with its labeling.

Read entire label before each use.

Use only on dogs.

ADAMS™ DELTA FORCE™ Tick Collar for Dogs, containing deltamethrin insecticide, has been specially formulated using patented insecticide-release technology. Maximum effectiveness may not occur for 2-3 weeks after collar placement. Fleas *(Clenocephalides* sp.) on the dog will be killed and ones which are present in the dog's environment that may appear on your pet will be killed. Collar will kill ticks including Brown dog tick *(Rhipicephalus sanguineus)*, American dog tick *(Dermacentor variabilis)* and deer ticks *(Ixodes scapularis* and *I. pacificus)* which may carry the Lyme disease. This collar should be worn continuously. Reapply a new collar every 6 months.

Place the collar around the dog's neck, buckle and adjust for proper fit. Cut off approximately 2 inches from the buckle and dispose of excess length by wrapping in newspaper and placing in trash. The collar must be worn loosely so that two fingers may be placed between collar and dog's neck. Living and rest areas of pet must also be treated with appropriate pest control measures to ensure control of pests. Wetting will not impair the collar's effectiveness or the pet's protection. If the dog goes swimming or is out in the rain, it is not necessary to remove the collar. ADAMS™ DELTA FORCE™ Tick Collar for Dogs may be used in addition to a lead or constraint collar. Use only one ADAMS™ DELTA FORCE™ Tick Collar for Dogs at a time.

Precautionary Statements: Hazards to Humans and Domestic Animals:

Caution: Do not open protective pouch until ready to use. Do not let children play with this collar. Harmful if swallowed or absorbed through skin. Causes moderate eye irritation. Avoid contact with skin, eyes, or clothing. Wash thoroughly with soap and water after handling. Do not use on puppies under 12 weeks. Consult a veterinarian before using this product on debilitated, aged, pregnant, medicated, or nursing animals. Sensitivities may occur after using any pesticide product for pets. If signs of sensitivity occur, remove collar and bathe your pet with mild soap and rinse with large amounts of water. If signs continue, consult a veterinarian immediately.

First Aid:

If Swallowed: Call a physician or poison control center. Do not induce vomiting or give anything by mouth to an unconscious person.

If on Skin: Wash with plenty of soap and water. Get medical attention.

If in Eyes: Flush eyes with plenty of water. Call a physician if irritation persists.

Collar is intended for use only as an insecticide generator and is not to be taken internally by man or animals. Applying other pesticides on the dog may not be necessary while the collar is being worn.

In case of emergency call: 1-800-228-5635, extension 233.

Storage and Disposal: Store in original, unopened container, away from children. Do not reuse container or used collar. Wrap in newspaper and put in trash.

Warning(s): Do not let children play with this collar.

Presentation: 1 x 0.9 oz. collar (adjustable - one size fits all).

DELTA FORCE™ is a trademark of Farnam Companies, Inc.

Distributed by: Pet Chemicals, P.O. Box 18993, Memphis, TN 38181-0993.

Compendium Code No.: 10000800 01-1322/0CC1

ADAMS™ D-LIMONENE FLEA & TICK SHAMPOO

Farnam **Parasiticide Shampoo**

EPA Reg. No.: 4758-141

Active Ingredient(s):

D-Limonene 5.00%
Inert Ingredients: 95.00%
Total 100.00%

Indications: For dogs, cats, puppies, and kittens.

Kills fleas and ticks. Conditions coat and deodorizes.

Contains a botanically derived insecticide.

ADAMS™ D-Limonene Flea & Tick Shampoo is highly regarded not only as an effective flea and tick killer, but also as a superior grooming product. Its non-alkaline formula contains the key active ingredient d-Limonene, a pleasant citrus-scented insecticide, plus cleansing agents, lanolin, and special conditioners. As a result, tangles brush out easily, leaving the pet with a clean, soft, shiny, healthier looking coat and a fresh, clean smell.

Directions for Use: It is a violation of Federal law to use this product in a manner inconsistent with its labeling.

Read entire label before each use.

Use only on dogs, cats, puppies, and kittens.

Wet dog or cat with warm water and apply a small amount of shampoo along the back of the animal. Work well into coat, starting at head and working back. Include legs and feet. When lather is desired consistency, continue to work into coat for 10 minutes to kill fleas. Rinse thoroughly with warm water and dry. When washing cats, kittens or puppies, dry with cloth immediately after rinsing to prevent chilling. Do not use on puppies or kittens under 12 weeks of age. Do not reapply product for one week.

For added protection against fleas and ticks, use Adams™ Flea & Tick Dip and Spray as part of pet grooming. As with any quality product, be sure to read all label instructions carefully.

Precautionary Statements: Hazards to Humans and Domestic Animals:

Warning: Causes eye irritation. Do not get in eyes. Harmful if swallowed. While washing dogs, cats, kittens, or puppies, avoid getting shampoo in animal's eyes. Do not use on kittens or puppies under 12 weeks of age. Consult a veterinarian before using this product on debilitated, aged, pregnant, or nursing animals, or animals on medication.

Applicators of flea shampoo products are to use protective gloves to reduce the risk of dermal irritation or dermal sensitization.

Sensitivities may occur after using any pesticide product for pets. If signs of sensitivity occur, bathe your pet with mild soap and rinse with large amounts of water. If signs continue, consult a veterinarian immediately. Individual animals may exhibit one or more of the following symptoms: hypothermia, tremors, ataxia, excess salivation, agitation, and vocalization followed by lethargic behavior, and skin and eye irritation in varying degrees. Discontinue use if one or more of the above symptoms develops. May be used in conjunction with organophosphates and carbamate based insecticides. Does not inhibit acetylcholinesterase activity.

First Aid:

If Swallowed: Call a physician or Poison Control Center. Give a glass or two of water and induce vomiting by touching the back of throat with finger, or, if available, by administration of syrup of ipecac. Never give anything by mouth or induce vomiting in an unconscious person.

If in Eyes: Flush eyes with plenty of water. Get medical attention.

Environmental Hazards: Do not apply directly to water, or to areas where surface water is present or to intertidal areas below the mean high water mark. Do not contaminate water when disposing of equipment washwater or rinsate.

In case of emergency or for product use information please call 602-285-1660 Monday - Friday, 7:00 - 3:45 pm MST.

Storage and Disposal: Disposal: Do not reuse container. Wrap container and discard in trash.

Warning(s): Keep out of reach of children.

Presentation: 12 fl oz (354 mL).

Compendium Code No.: 10000810 0CC1

ADAMS™ DUAL ACTION FLEA & TICK COLLAR FOR CATS

Farnam **Parasiticide Collar**

EPA Reg. No.: 2517-61-37425

Active Ingredient(s):

O-Isopropoxyphenyl methylcarbamate 9.00%
*3-Phenooxybenzyl d-cis and trans **2,2 dimethyl-3-(2-methylpropenyl) cyclopropanecarboxylate 3.00%
N-Octyl bicycloheptene diacarboximide 3.00%
Other Ingredients 85.00%

*dis-(cis/trans)phenothrin

**cis/trans isomer ratio: Max. 25% (±) cis and Min. 75% (±) trans

Indications: This collar kills fleas and ticks for 6 months. The collar has the effect of simultaneous usage of a spray and a powder in the control of fleas and ticks, including ticks that may carry Rocky Mountain Spotted Fever, Lyme Disease and Ehrlichiosis.

Directions for Use: It is a violation of Federal Law to use this product in a manner inconsistent with its labeling.

Read entire label before each use.

Use only on cats.

Place collar around pet's neck, adjust for fit and buckle in place. The collar must be worn loosely to allow for growth of the pet and to permit the collar to move about the neck. Generally, a properly fitted collar is one that when fastened, will snugly slide over pet's head. Leave 2 or 3 inches for extra adjustment. Cut off and dispose of excess length. Wash hands after installing collar on pet. Under normal conditions, replace collar every 6 months. Under conditions of severe infestation and where continued rapid kill is desired, collar may be replaced more often.

Precautionary Statements: Hazards to Humans and Domestic Animals:

Caution: Do not open until ready to use. Dust will form on collar during storage. Do not get dust in mouth or eyes. Harmful if swallowed. If in eyes will cause eye irritation. In case of contact, flush eyes with water. If irritation persists, get medical attention. Collar is intended for external use only, not to be taken internally. Some animals may become irritated by any collar. If this occurs, remove collar. If condition persists, consult a veterinarian. Consult a veterinarian before using this product on debilitated, aged, pregnant, medicated, or nursing animals. Do not use on pets under 12 weeks of age. Sensitivities may occur after using any pesticide product for pets. If signs of sensitivity occur remove collar and bathe your pet with mild soap and rinse with large amounts of water.

First Aid:

Note to Physician/Veterinarian: Dust released by this collar is a cholinesterase inhibitor. Atropine is antidotal. Do not use this product on animals simultaneously or within 30 days before or after treatment with, or exposure to, cholinesterase inhibiting drugs, pesticides or chemicals. However, flea and tick collars may be immediately replaced.

Storage and Disposal: Store unopened collar in a cool, dry place. Dispose of empty pouch and expired collar in trash.

Warning(s): Do not allow children to play with collar.

Discussion: Important Consumer Information: This collar kills fleas and ticks for 6 months. The collar is a double layer sustained-release system containing three active agents combining the insecticidal actions of vapors and powders, working in two ways to provide fast-acting quick kill and long-lasting head-to-tail protection. Thus, collar has the effect of simultaneous usage of a spray and a powder in the control of fleas and ticks, including ticks that may carry Rocky Mountain Spotted Fever, Lyme Disease and Ehrlichiosis. Wetting collar will not impair collar's effectiveness. It is not necessary to remove collar if pets go swimming or are out in the rain. Use ADAMS™ Dual Action Flea & Tick Collar year round for most effective control. Reapply every 6 months.

Presentation: 0.5 oz (14 g) collar (green).

Compendium Code No.: 10000520

A

ADAMS™ DUAL ACTION FLEA & TICK COLLAR FOR LARGE DOGS

Farnam **Parasiticide Collar**

EPA Reg. No.: 2517-61-37425

Active Ingredient(s):

O-Isopropoxyphenyl methylcarbamate 9.00%
*3-Phenooxybenzyl d-cis and trans **2,2 dimethyl-3-(2-methylpropenyl) cyclopropanecarboxylate 3.00%
N-Octyl bicycloheptene diacarboximide 3.00%
Other Ingredients 85.00%

*dis-(cis/trans)phenothrin

**cis/trans isomer ratio: Max. 25% (±) cis and Min. 75% (±) trans

Indications: This collar kills fleas and ticks for 6 months. The collar has the effect of simultaneous usage of a spray and a powder in the control of fleas and ticks, including ticks that may carry Rocky Mountain Spotted Fever, Lyme Disease and Ehrlichiosis.

Directions for Use: It is a violation of Federal Law to use this product in a manner inconsistent with its labeling.

Read entire label before each use.

Use only on large dogs.

Place collar around pet's neck, adjust for fit and buckle in place. The collar must be worn loosely to allow for growth of the pet and to permit the collar to move about the neck. Generally, a properly fitted collar is one that when fastened, will snugly slide over pet's head. Leave 2 or 3 inches for extra adjustment. Cut off and dispose of excess length. Wash hands after installing collar on pet. Under normal conditions, replace collar every 6 months. Under conditions of severe infestation and where continued rapid kill is desired, collar may be replaced more often.

Precautionary Statements: Hazards to Humans and Domestic Animals:

Caution: Do not open until ready to use. Dust will form on collar during storage. Do not get dust in mouth or eyes. Harmful if swallowed. If in eyes will cause eye irritation. In case of contact, flush eyes with water. If irritation persists, get medical attention. Collar is intended for external use only, not to be taken internally. Some animals may become irritated by any collar. If this occurs, remove collar. If condition persists, consult a veterinarian. Consult a veterinarian before using this product on debilitated, aged, pregnant, medicated, or nursing animals. Do not use on pets under 12 weeks of age. Sensitivities may occur after using any pesticide product for pets. If signs of sensitivity occur remove collar and bathe your pet with mild soap and rinse with large amounts of water.

First Aid:

Note to Physician/Veterinarian: Dust released by this collar is a cholinesterase inhibitor. Atropine is antidotal. Do not use this product on animals simultaneously or within 30 days before or after treatment with, or exposure to, cholinesterase inhibiting drugs, pesticides or chemicals. However, flea and tick collars may be immediately replaced.

Storage and Disposal: Store unopened collar in a cool, dry place. Dispose of empty pouch and expired collar in trash.

Warning(s): Do not allow children to play with collar.

Discussion: Important Consumer Information: This collar kills fleas and ticks for 6 months. The collar is a double layer sustained-release system containing three active agents combining the insecticidal actions of vapors and powders, working in two ways to provide fast-acting quick kill and long-lasting head-to-tail protection. Thus, collar has the effect of simultaneous usage of a spray and a powder in the control of fleas and ticks, including ticks that may carry Rocky Mountain Spotted Fever, Lyme Disease and Ehrlichiosis. Wetting collar will not impair collar's effectiveness. It is not necessary to remove collar if pets go swimming or are out in the rain. Use ADAMS™ Dual Action Flea & Tick Collar year round for most effective control. Reapply every 6 months.

Presentation: 1.2 oz (34 g) collar (blue) and 1.2 oz (34 g) collar (red). Fits necks up to 26".

Compendium Code No.: 10000530

ADAMS™ DUAL ACTION FLEA & TICK COLLAR FOR MEDIUM DOGS

Farnam **Parasiticide Collar**

EPA Reg. No.: 2517-61-37425

Active Ingredient(s):

O-Isopropoxyphenyl methylcarbamate 9.00%
*3-Phenooxybenzyl d-cis and trans **2,2 dimethyl-3-(2-methylpropenyl) cyclopropanecarboxylate 3.00%
N-Octyl bicycloheptene diacarboximide 3.00%
Other Ingredients 85.00%

*dis-(cis/trans)phenothrin

**cis/trans isomer ratio: Max. 25% (±) cis and Min. 75% (±) trans

Indications: This collar kills fleas and ticks for 6 months. The collar has the effect of simultaneous usage of a spray and a powder in the control of fleas and ticks, including ticks that may carry Rocky Mountain Spotted Fever, Lyme Disease and Ehrlichiosis.

Directions for Use: It is a violation of Federal Law to use this product in a manner inconsistent with its labeling.

Read entire label before each use.

Use only on medium dogs.

Place collar around pet's neck, adjust for fit and buckle in place. The collar must be worn loosely to allow for growth of the pet and to permit the collar to move about the neck. Generally, a properly fitted collar is one that when fastened, will snugly slide over pet's head. Leave 2 or 3 inches for extra adjustment. Cut off and dispose of excess length. Wash hands after installing collar on pet. Under normal conditions, replace collar every 6 months. Under conditions of severe infestation and where continued rapid kill is desired, collar may be replaced more often.

Precautionary Statements: Hazards to Humans and Domestic Animals:

Caution: Do not open until ready to use. Dust will form on collar during storage. Do not get dust in mouth or eyes. Harmful if swallowed. If in eyes will cause eye irritation. In case of contact, flush eyes with water. If irritation persists, get medical attention. Collar is intended for external use only, not to be taken internally. Some animals may become irritated by any collar. If this occurs, remove collar. If condition persists, consult a veterinarian. Consult a veterinarian before using this product on debilitated, aged, pregnant, medicated, or nursing animals. Do not use on pets under 12 weeks of age. Sensitivities may occur after using any pesticide product for pets.

If signs of sensitivity occur remove collar and bathe your pet with mild soap and rinse with large amounts of water.

First Aid:

Note to Physician/Veterinarian: Dust released by this collar is a cholinesterase inhibitor. Atropine is antidotal. Do not use this product on animals simultaneously or within 30 days before or after treatment with, or exposure to, cholinesterase inhibiting drugs, pesticides or chemicals. However, flea and tick collars may be immediately replaced.

A

Storage and Disposal: Store unopened collar in a cool, dry place. Dispose of empty pouch and expired collar in trash.

Warning(s): Do not allow children to play with collar.

Discussion: Important Consumer Information: This collar kills fleas and ticks for 6 months. The collar is a double layer sustained-release system containing three active agents combining the insecticidal actions of vapors and powders, working in two ways to provide fast-acting quick kill and long-lasting head-to-tail protection. Thus, collar has the effect of simultaneous usage of a spray and a powder in the control of fleas and ticks, including ticks that may carry Rocky Mountain Spotted Fever, Lyme Disease and Ehrlichiosis. Wetting collar will not impair collar's effectiveness. It is not necessary to remove collar if pets go swimming or are out in the rain. Use ADAMS™ Dual Action Flea & Tick Collar year round for most effective control. Reapply every 6 months.

Presentation: 0.90 oz (25 g) collar (blue) and 0.90 oz (25 g) collar (red). Fits necks up to 20".

Compendium Code No.: 10000540

ADAMS™ FLEA & TICK DUST II

Farnam **Parasiticide Powder**

Odorless Residual Insecticide Powder

EPA Reg. No.: 37425-13

Active Ingredient(s):

Pyrethrins	0.10%
*Piperonyl Butoxide, technical	1.00%
**Carbaryl (1-Naphthyl N-Methylcarbamate)	12.50%
Silica Gel	10.00%
Inert Ingredients:	76.40%
Total	100.00%

*Equivalent to 0.8% of butylcarbityl (6-propyl piperonyl) ether and 0.2% related compounds.

**Sevin-Trademark of Union Carbide Corporation for Carbaryl.

Indications: Kills fleas, ticks and lice on dogs, puppies, cats and kittens over 12 weeks of age.

Directions for Use: It is a violation of Federal Law to use this product in a manner inconsistent with its labeling.

Read entire label before each use.

Use only on dogs, cats, puppies and kittens.

Dogs and Cats: Use product only outside or in a well-ventilated area. Wearing household latex or rubber gloves, dust entire animal, avoiding pet's eyes, nose, mouth and genital areas. Rub or brush pet's hair to work dust down to the skin. Consult a veterinarian before using this product on debilitated, aged, nursing animals or animals on medication. Do not use on pregnant animals. Do not use on animals under 12 weeks of age. Do not repeat treatment for one week. Dust pet bedding and doghouse using a shake can or other dust applicator. This product should not be applied by children.

Precautionary Statements: Hazards to Humans and Domestic Animals:

Caution:

Humans: Harmful if swallowed or absorbed through skin. Avoid contact with eyes, skin or clothing. Wash thoroughly with soap and water after handling.

Animals: Avoid contaminating animal's food or water. Avoid treatment of nursing animals. Do not treat puppies or kittens under 12 weeks of age. Sensitivities may occur after using any pesticide product for pets. If signs of sensitivity occur, bathe your pet with mild soap and rinse with large amounts of water. If signs continue, consult a veterinarian immediately.

This product contains cholinesterase. Do not use this product on animals simultaneously or within 30 days before or after treatment with or exposure to cholinesterase inhibiting drugs, pesticides or chemicals. However, flea and tick collars may be immediately replaced.

First Aid:

If Swallowed: Call a physician or Poison Control Center. Drink 1 or 2 glasses of water and induce vomiting by touching the back of throat with finger. If person is unconscious, do not give anything by mouth and do not induce vomiting.

If on Skin: Wash with plenty of soap and water. Get medical attention.

User Safety Requirements: Wear long-sleeved shirt, long pants, shoes plus socks and household latex or rubber gloves when applying this product. Change clothing as soon as possible after use. Wash the outside of gloves before removing. As with any pesticide product, wash hands thoroughly immediately after handling and before eating, smoking or using the toilet.

Note to Physician/Veterinarian: Carbaryl is a cholinesterase inhibitor. Atropine by injection is antidotal.

In case of emergency, or for product use information, call (602) 285-1660 Monday-Friday, 7:00 am to 3:45 pm, MST.

Storage and Disposal:

Storage: Store in a cool, dry area. Do not contaminate water, food or feed by storage or disposal. Keep cap tightly closed when not in use to avoid moisture absorption. Do not transfer contents to other containers.

Disposal: Do not reuse empty container. Wrap container in newspaper and put in trash.

Warning(s): Keep out of reach of children.

Presentation: 3 oz (85 g).

*U.S. Patent No. 4,668,666

Compendium Code No.: 10000550

9F9

ADAMS™ FLEA & TICK DUST II

V.P.L. **Parasiticide Powder**

Odorless Residual Insecticide Powder

EPA Reg. No.: 37425-13

Active Ingredient(s):

Pyrethrins	0.10%
*Piperonyl Butoxide, technical	1.00%
**Carbaryl (1-Naphthyl N-Methylcarbamate)	12.50%
Silica Gel	10.00%
Inert Ingredients:	76.40%
Total	100.00%

*Equivalent to 0.8% of butylcarbityl (6-propyl piperonyl) ether and 0.2% related compounds.

**Sevin-Trademark of Union Carbide Corporation for Carbaryl.

Indications: Kills fleas, ticks and lice on dogs, puppies, cats and kittens over 12 weeks of age.

Directions for Use: It is a violation of Federal Law to use this product in a manner inconsistent with its labeling.

Read entire label before each use.

Use only on dogs, cats, puppies and kittens.

Dogs and Cats: Use product only outside or in a well-ventilated area. Wearing household latex or rubber gloves, dust entire animal, avoiding pet's eyes, nose, mouth and genital areas. Rub or brush pet's hair to work dust down to the skin. Consult a veterinarian before using this product on debilitated, aged, nursing animals or animals on medication. Do not use on pregnant animals. Do not use on animals under 12 weeks of age. Do not repeat treatment for one week. Dust pet bedding and doghouse using a shake can or other dust applicator. This product should not be applied by children.

Precautionary Statements: Hazards to Humans and Domestic Animals:

Caution:

Humans: Harmful if swallowed or absorbed through skin. Avoid contact with eyes, skin or clothing. Wash thoroughly with soap and water after handling.

Animals: Avoid contaminating animal's food or water. Avoid treatment of nursing animals. Do not treat puppies or kittens under 12 weeks of age. Sensitivities may occur after using any pesticide product for pets. If signs of sensitivity occur, bathe your pet with mild soap and rinse with large amounts of water. If signs continue, consult a veterinarian immediately.

This product contains cholinesterase. Do not use this product on animals simultaneously or within 30 days before or after treatment with or exposure to cholinesterase inhibiting drugs, pesticides or chemicals. However, flea and tick collars may be immediately replaced.

First Aid:

If Swallowed: Call a physician or Poison Control Center. Drink 1 or 2 glasses of water and induce vomiting by touching the back of throat with finger. If person is unconscious, do not give anything by mouth and do not induce vomiting.

If on Skin: Wash with plenty of soap and water. Get medical attention.

User Safety Requirements: Wear long-sleeved shirt, long pants, shoes plus socks and household latex or rubber gloves when applying this product. Change clothing as soon as possible after use. Wash the outside of gloves before removing. As with any pesticide product, wash hands thoroughly immediately after handling and before eating, smoking or using the toilet.

Note to Physician/Veterinarian: Carbaryl is a cholinesterase inhibitor. Atropine by injection is antidotal.

In case of emergency, or for product use information, call (602) 285-1660 Monday-Friday, 7:00 am to 3:45 pm, MST.

Storage and Disposal:

Storage: Store in a cool, dry area. Do not contaminate water, food or feed by storage or disposal. Keep cap tightly closed when not in use to avoid moisture absorption. Do not transfer contents to other containers.

Disposal: Do not reuse empty container. Wrap container in newspaper and put in trash.

Warning(s): Keep out of reach of children.

Presentation: 3 oz (85 g).

*U.S. Patent No. 4,668,666

Compendium Code No.: 11430520

9F9

ADAMS™ FLEA & TICK MIST

V.P.L. **Parasiticide Spray**

EPA Reg. No.: 37425-12

Active Ingredient(s):

Pyrethrins	0.15%
Piperonyl butoxide, technical*	1.50%
N-octyl bicycloheptene dicarboximide	0.50%
Di-n-propyl isocinchomeronate	0.50%
Inert Ingredients**	97.35%
Total	100.00%

*Equivalent to 1.20% of butylcarbityl (6-propylpiperonyl) ether and .30% of related compounds.

**Inert ingredients include grooming additives to ease combing and brushing of the coat to remove dead fleas, ticks and lice.

Indications: The "quick kill" insecticide, repellent, and deodorant spray for dogs, puppies, cats, and kittens.

Directions for Use: It is a violation of Federal law to use this product in a manner inconsistent with its labeling.

Use only in a well ventilated area.

Dogs and Cats: Cover animal's eyes with hand and with a firm, fast stroke to get a proper spray mist, spray head, ears and chest until damp. With fingertips, rub into face around mouth, nose and eyes. Then spray neck, middle and hindquarters, finishing legs last. For best penetration of spray to the skin, direct spray against the natural lay of hair. On long haired dogs, rub your hand against the lay of the hair, spraying the ruffled hair directly behind the hand. Make sure spray thoroughly wets ticks. Repeat treatment as needed.

Nursing Puppies and Kittens: Spray only along back or on your fingertips and rub into coat.

Precautionary Statements: Hazards to Humans and Domestic Animals:

Caution: Keep out of reach of children.

Human: Harmful if swallowed or inhaled. Avoid breathing mist. Avoid contamination of food. Wash hands with soap and water after using.

Animal: Avoid treatment of nursing puppies and kittens. If treatment is necessary, follow special instructions. Do not oversaturate, especially on cats. Avoid spraying of genital areas.

Environmental Hazards: This product is toxic to fish. Do not add directly to water. Do not apply where runoff is likely to occur.

Physical or Chemical Hazards:

Flammable: Keep away from heat and open flame. Contains alcohol. Do not apply to painted or finished wood surfaces.

Storage and Disposal:

Storage: Store in a cool, dry area away from heat and open flame. Do not contaminate water, food or feed by disposal. Do not transfer to other containers.

Disposal: Do not reuse container. Rinse thoroughly and wrap container in several layers of newspaper and discard in trash.

Presentation: Available in 16 oz and 32 oz plastic bottles with trigger sprayer.

Compendium Code No.: 11430010

ADAMS™ FLEA & TICK MIST WITH SYKILLSTOP™

Farnam **Parasiticide Spray**

Insecticide, Insect Growth Regulator, Repellant & Deodorant

EPA Reg. No.: 37425-12

Active Ingredient(s):

Pyrethrins	0.15%
Nylar† 2-[1-methyl-2-(4-phenoxy-phenoxy) ethoxy] pyridine	0.15%
Piperonyl butoxide, technical*	1.50%
N-octyl bicycloheptene dicarboximide	0.50%
Inert Ingredients**	97.70%
Total	100.00%

*Equivalent to 1.20% of butylcarbityl (6-propylpiperonyl) ether and .30% related compounds.

**Inert ingredients include grooming additives to ease combing and brushing of the coat to remove dead fleas and ticks.

†Nylar is a registered trademark of McLaughlin, Gormley, King Co.

Indications: Kills adult fleas and ticks. Controls immature fleas for 18 weeks. Repels gnats, flies, and mosquitoes.

Egg-control formula: A fast-acting flea and tick spray for dogs, cats, puppies and kittens. Kills adult fleas and ticks. Controls immature fleas for 126 days.

Directions for Use: It is a violation of Federal law to use this product in a manner inconsistent with its labeling.

Read entire label before each use.

Use only on dogs, puppies, cats and kittens.

Use only in a well ventilated area.

Dogs and Cats: Remove safety cap and insert sprayer. Cover animal's eyes with hand and with a firm, fast stroke to get a proper spray mist, spray head, ears and chest until damp. With fingertips, rub into face around mouth, nose and eyes. Then spray neck, middle and hindquarters, finishing legs last. For best penetration of spray to the skin, direct spray against the natural lay of the hair. On long-haired dogs, rub your hand against the lay of the hair, spraying the ruffled hair directly behind the hand. Make sure spray thoroughly wets ticks. Reapply every 3 weeks.

Precautionary Statements: Hazards to Humans and Domestic Animals:

Warning:

Human: Causes substantial but temporary eye injury. Harmful if swallowed or absorbed through skin. Do not get in eyes or on clothing. Avoid contact with skin. Wash thoroughly with soap and water after handling. Remove contaminated clothing and wash before reuse.

Animal: Consult a veterinarian before using this product on debilitated, aged, medicated, pregnant, or nursing animals or animals under 12 weeks of age. Do not oversaturate, especially on cats. Avoid spraying of genital areas. Sensitivities may occur after using any pesticide product for pets. If signs of sensitivity occur, bathe your pet with mild soap and rinse with large amounts of water. If signs continue, consult a veterinarian immediately.

First Aid:

If in Eyes: Call physician. Flush eyes with gentle stream of water for 15 minutes.

If Swallowed: Call physician or Poison Control Center. Drink promptly a large quantity of milk, egg white, or gelatin mixture, or if these are unavailable, a large quantity of water.

If on Skin: Wash with plenty of soap and water. Get medical attention if irritation persists.

In case of emergency, or for product use information, call (602) 285-1660 Monday-Friday, 7:00 am to 4:45 pm, MST.

Environmental Hazards: This product is toxic to fish. Do not add directly to water. Do not apply where runoff is likely to occur.

Physical or Chemical Hazards: Flammable. Keep away from heat and open flame. Contains alcohol. Do not apply to painted or finished wood surfaces.

Storage and Disposal:

Storage: Store in a cool, dry area away from heat and open flame.

Disposal: Do not reuse container. Rinse thoroughly and wrap container in several layers of newspaper and discard in trash.

Warning(s): Keep out of reach of children.

Sold only to licensed veterinarians.

This product is restricted for sale exclusively through veterinary clinics, practices and hospitals.

Presentation: 16 fl oz (473 mL) and 32 fl oz (946 mL).

Compendium Code No.: 10000560 9609 85-6852-01

ADAMS™ FLEA & TICK MIST WITH SYKILLSTOP™

V.P.L. **Parasiticide Spray**

Insecticide, Insect Growth Regulator, Repellant & Deodorant

EPA Reg. No.: 37425-12

Active Ingredient(s):

Pyrethrins	0.15%
Nylar† 2-[1-methyl-2-(4-phenoxy-phenoxy) ethoxy] pyridine	0.15%
Piperonyl butoxide, technical*	1.50%
N-octyl bicycloheptene dicarboximide	0.50%
Inert Ingredients**	97.70%
Total	100.00%

*Equivalent to 1.20% of butylcarbityl (6-propylpiperonyl) ether and .30% related compounds.

**Inert ingredients include grooming additives to ease combing and brushing of the coat to remove dead fleas and ticks.

†Nylar is a registered trademark of McLaughlin, Gormley, King Co.

Indications: Kills adult fleas and ticks. Controls immature fleas for 18 weeks. Repels gnats, flies, and mosquitoes.

Egg-control formula: A fast-acting flea and tick spray for dogs, cats, puppies and kittens. Kills adult fleas and ticks. Controls immature fleas for 126 days.

Directions for Use: It is a violation of Federal law to use this product in a manner inconsistent with its labeling.

Read entire label before each use.

Use only on dogs, puppies, cats and kittens.

Use only in a well ventilated area.

Dogs and Cats: Remove safety cap and insert sprayer. Cover animal's eyes with hand and with a firm, fast stroke to get a proper spray mist, spray head, ears and chest until damp. With fingertips, rub into face around mouth, nose and eyes. Then spray neck, middle and hindquarters, finishing legs last. For best penetration of spray to the skin, direct spray against the natural lay of the hair. On long-haired dogs, rub your hand against the lay of the hair, spraying the ruffled hair directly behind the hand. Make sure spray thoroughly wets ticks. Reapply every 3 weeks.

Precautionary Statements: Hazards to Humans and Domestic Animals:

Warning:

Human: Causes substantial but temporary eye injury. Harmful if swallowed or absorbed through skin. Do not get in eyes or on clothing. Avoid contact with skin. Wash thoroughly with soap and water after handling. Remove contaminated clothing and wash before reuse.

Animal: Consult a veterinarian before using this product on debilitated, aged, medicated, pregnant, or nursing animals or animals under 12 weeks of age. Do not oversaturate, especially on cats. Avoid spraying of genital areas. Sensitivities may occur after using any pesticide product for pets. If signs of sensitivity occur, bathe your pet with mild soap and rinse with large amounts of water. If signs continue, consult a veterinarian immediately.

First Aid:

If in Eyes: Call physician. Flush eyes with gentle stream of water for 15 minutes.

If Swallowed: Call physician or Poison Control Center. Drink promptly a large quantity of milk, egg white, or gelatin mixture, or if these are unavailable, a large quantity of water.

If on Skin: Wash with plenty of soap and water. Get medical attention if irritation persists.

In case of emergency, or for product use information, call (602) 285-1660 Monday-Friday, 7:00 am to 4:45 pm, MST.

Environmental Hazards: This product is toxic to fish. Do not add directly to water. Do not apply where runoff is likely to occur.

Physical or Chemical Hazards: Flammable. Keep away from heat and open flame. Contains alcohol. Do not apply to painted or finished wood surfaces.

Storage and Disposal:

Storage: Store in a cool, dry area away from heat and open flame.

Disposal: Do not reuse container. Rinse thoroughly and wrap container in several layers of newspaper and discard in trash.

Warning(s): Keep out of reach of children.

Sold only to licensed veterinarians.

This product is restricted for sale exclusively through veterinary clinics, practices and hospitals.

Presentation: 16 fl oz (473 mL) and 32 fl oz (946 mL).

Compendium Code No.: 11430530 9609 85-6852-01

ADAMS™ FLEA & TICK SHAMPOO

V.P.L. **Parasiticide Shampoo**

EPA Reg. No.: 37425-4

Active Ingredient(s):

Pyrethrins	0.15%
Piperonyl butoxide, technical*	1.50%
N-octyl bicyclopheptene dicarboximide	0.50%
Inert Ingredients**	97.85%
Total	100.00%

*Equivalent to 1.20% of butylcarbityl (6-propylpiperonyl) ether and 0.30% of related compounds.

**Inert ingredients include a concentrated, rich lathering shampoo enriched with coconut extract and lanolin.

Indications: Quickly kills fleas and ticks. Cleans, conditions, and deodorizes skin and coat. Removes loose dandruff, dirt, and scales. Leaves the coat soft and shining.

Directions for Use: It is a violation of Federal law to use this product in a manner inconsistent with its labeling.

Thoroughly soak animal with warm water taking 2-3 minutes to wet hair. Apply ADAMS™ Flea & Tick Shampoo on head and ears and lather, then repeat procedure with neck, chest, middle, and hindquarters, finishing legs last. Let animal stand 3-5 minutes (this is an important part of grooming procedure), then rinse animal thoroughly.

For extremely dirty or scaly animals the above procedure may be repeated. ADAMS™ Flea & Tick Shampoo may be used every 7-10 days.

Precautionary Statements: Hazards to Humans and Domestic Animals: Caution:

Human: Harmful if swallowed. Avoid contact with eyes. In case of contact, flush with water. Avoid contact with food and food serving areas. Wash thoroughly after using with soap and warm water.

Animals: Do not use on puppies and kittens less than twelve weeks of age.

Environmental Hazards: This product is toxic to fish. Do not add directly to water. Do not wash animal where runoff is likely to occur.

Storage and Disposal:

Storage: Store in a cool, dry area away from heat and open flame. Do not contaminate water, food or feed by disposal. Do not transfer to other containers.

Disposal: Do not reuse container. Rinse thoroughly and wrap container in several layers of newspaper and discard in trash.

Presentation: Available in 6 oz, 12 oz and 1 gallon plastic bottles.

Compendium Code No.: 11430020

ADAMS™ FLY REPELLENT CONCENTRATE

V.P.L. **Parasiticide Spray**

Insecticide and Repellent

EPA Reg. No.: 37425-21

Active Ingredient(s):

Permethrin I (3-phenoxyphenol) methyl (±) cis, trans-3 (2,2-dichloroethyenyl) 2,2-dimethyl cyclopropane carboxylate	1.00%
Pyrethrins	0.50%
*Piperonyl butoxide, technical	1.85%
N-Octyl bicycloheptene dicarboximide	3.10%
Di-n-propyl isocinchomeronate	1.25%
Inert Ingredients	92.30%
Total	100.00%

*Equivalent to 1.48% of butylcarbityl (6-propylpiperonyl) ether and 0.37% of related compounds.

Indications: ADAMS™ Fly Repellent Concentrate contains two insecticide systems and a repellent for use on horses for immediate and temporary control of face flies, stable flies, horse flies, deer flies, ticks, mosquitoes, gnats and house flies.

Directions for Use: It is a violation of Federal law to use this product in a manner inconsistent with its labeling.

Thoroughly brush the horse's coat, prior to application, to remove loose dirt and debris. For dirty horses, and as a preparation for show grooming, clean the coat with a good cleansing shampoo. Use at a 1 to 4 ratio with water. Put required amount of concentrate into sprayer or mixing container and add appropriate amount of water (one pint of concentrate makes five pints of spray).

Cover entire surface of animal with spray, but avoid getting product into horse's eyes or other sensitive areas such as mouth or nose. Spray horse's coat especially around shoulders, flanks, neck and legs. Brush coat against grain while spraying to ensure adequate penetration of product. Make sure application has completely dried on hair coat before covering with tack. As a wipe, apply liberally with a clean cloth or sponge. For initial treatment, apply ADAMS™ Fly Repellent Concentrate daily. As infestation subsides and protection builds, reapply every 2-3 days as needed. Also, reapply every time animal is washed or exposed to a heavy rain.

Precautionary Statements: Hazards to Humans and Domestic Animals: Caution:

Human: May cause eye injury. Harmful if swallowed or inhaled. Avoid breathing mist. Avoid contact with skin, eyes or clothing. Remove contaminated clothing and wash before reuse. Wash hands with soap and water after using. Do not contaminate foodstuffs. Do not smoke while using. If accidental contact occurs, see Statement of Practical Treatment.

Animal: Avoid contact with eyes or mucous membranes. Avoid treatment of foals under six weeks of age.

Physical or Chemical Hazards: Keep away from heat and open flame. Do not apply to painted or finished wood surfaces.

Environmental Hazards: Do not apply directly to any body of water. Do not contaminate water when disposing of equipment wash waters.

Statement of Practical Treatment:

If in Eyes: Flush with plenty of water. Get medical attention if irritation persists.

If on Skin: Wash with plenty of soap and water. Get medical attention if irritation persists.

Storage and Disposal:

Storage: Store in a cool, dry area away from heat and open flame. Do not contaminate water, food or feed by storage or disposal. Do not transfer contents to other containers.

Disposal: Do not reuse empty container. Rinse thoroughly and wrap container in several layers of newspaper and discard in trash.

Warning(s): Do not use on horses intended for food. Keep out of reach of children.

Presentation: Available in 32 oz (946 mL) concentrate.

Compendium Code No.: 11430030

ADAMS™ FLY SPRAY AND REPELLENT

V.P.L. — **Parasiticide Spray**

EPA Reg. No.: 37425-17-622

Active Ingredient(s):

Permethrin (3-phenoxyphenol) methyl (±) cis, trans-3 (2,2-dichloroethyenyl) 2,2-dimethyl cyclopropane carboxylate	0.20%
Pyrethrins	0.20%
*Piperonyl butoxide, technical	0.50%
N-Octyl bicycloheptene dicarboximide	2.00%
Di-n-propyl isocinchomeronate	1.00%
Butoxypolypropylene glycol	5.00%
Inert Ingredients	91.10%
Total	100.00%

*Equivalent to 0.40% butylcarbityl (6-propyl piperonyl) ether and 0.10% of related compounds.

Indications: ADAMS™ Fly Spray and Repellent combines oil of aloe with other emollients to moisturize the skin and produce a show condition coat.

Contains two insecticide systems and two repellents for use on horses for immediate and residual control of face flies, stable flies, house flies, mosquitoes, gnats, mites, chiggers, lice, and ticks.

Directions for Use: It is a violation of Federal law to use this product in a manner inconsistent with its labeling.

Thoroughly brush the horse's coat, prior to application, to remove loose dirt and debris. For dirty horses, and as a preparation for show grooming, clean the coat with a good cleansing shampoo. Wait until coat is completely dry before applying ADAMS™ Fly Spray and Repellent.

Cover entire surface of animal with spray, but avoid getting product into horse's eyes or other sensitive areas such as mouth or nose. Brush coat against grain while spraying to ensure adequate penetration of product. As a wipe, apply liberally with a clean cloth or sponge. Make sure spray has completely dried before covering with any tack.

For initial treatment, apply ADAMS™ Fly Spray and Repellent daily for 2-3 days. As infestation subsides, repeat treatment every 5-10 days or as prescribed by a veterinarian. Also, reapply every time animal is washed or exposed to a heavy rain.

Precautionary Statements: Hazards to Humans and Domestic Animals:

Human: Do not get in eyes, on skin or clothing. May cause eye injury. Wear safety glasses or other appropriate eye protection. Harmful if swallowed. Avoid breathing vapors. Wash hands with soap and water after using. Do not contaminate foodstuffs. Remove contaminated clothing and wash before reuse. Do not smoke while using. If accidental contact occurs, see Statement of Practical Treatment.

Animal: Avoid contact with eyes or mucous membranes. Avoid treatment of foals under six weeks of age unless prescribed by a veterinarian.

Physical or Chemical Hazards: Flammable. Keep away from heat and open flame. Contains alcohol. Do not apply to painted or finished wood surfaces.

Environmental Hazards: Do not apply directly to any body of water. Do not contaminate water when disposing of equipment wash waters.

Storage and Disposal:

Storage: Store in a cool, dry area away from heat and open flame. Do not contaminate water, food or feed by storage or disposal. Do not transfer contents to other containers.

Disposal: Do not reuse empty container. Rinse thoroughly and wrap container in several layers of newspaper and discard in trash.

Statement of Practical Treatment:

If in Eyes: Flush with plenty of water. Get medical attention if irritation persists.

If Swallowed: Call a physician or Poison Control Center. Drink 1 or 2 glasses of water and induce vomiting by touching back of throat with finger. Do not induce vomiting or give anything by mouth to an unconscious person.

If on Skin: Wash with plenty of soap and water. Get medical attention if irritation persists.

Warning(s): Do not use on horses intended for food. Keep out of reach of children.

Presentation: Available in 32 oz (946 mL) RTU spray bottle.

Compendium Code No.: 11430040

ADAMS™ INVERTED CARPET SPRAY

Farnam — **Flea Control & Premise Insecticide**

EPA Reg. No.: 4758-169

Active Ingredient(s):

Linalool	1.000%
N-Octyl bicycloheptene dicarboximide*	1.000%
Nylar®: 2-[1-Methyl-2-(4-phenoxyphenoxy) ethoxy] pyridine	0.015%
Permethrin**	0.200%
Other Ingredients	97.785%

*MGK 264 (Insecticide Synergist)

**(3-phenoxyphenyl) methyl (±) cis-trans-3-(2,2-dichloroethenyl)-2,2-dimethylcyclopropanecarboxylate. Cis-trans ratio: 35% (±) cis and max 65% (±) trans.

Indications: Kills all four stages of the flea: Adults, eggs, pupae and larvae. Breaks the flea life cycle and controls reinfestation for up to 210 days. Also kills ticks, roaches, ants, spiders, lice, crickets, centipedes, waterbugs, silverfish and sowbugs.

Directions for Use: It is a violation of Federal law to use this product in a manner inconsistent with its labeling. Do not allow children or pets to contact treated surfaces until spray has dried.

Indoors: Thoroughly vacuum all carpeting, upholstered furniture, drapes, along baseboards, under furniture and in closets. Seal vacuum bag and dispose of in outdoor trash. Spray ADAMS™ Inverted Carpet Spray from a distance of two to three feet from surface being treated. Apply with a smooth back-and-forth motion to carpets, drapes, rugs and upholstered furniture. Avoid wetting or saturating carpets or furniture. An evenly applied fine mist spray is sufficient. Do not spray wood furniture, floors or trim as water spotting may occur. Repeat treatment as necessary to eliminate fleas and ticks. Apply directly to exposed insects: roaches, ants, spiders, crickets, centipedes, waterbugs, silverfish and sowbugs.

Pet Bedding: Treat bed bedding and resting places. Apply a uniform spray to nearby cracks and crevices, along baseboards, window and door sills and localized areas where fleas, ticks or lice may be present as these are primary hiding places for these pests. Removal and replacement of pet bedding after treatment is not necessary.

Precautionary Statements: Hazards to Humans and Domestic Animals:

Caution: May be harmful if absorbed through skin. Causes moderate eye irritation. Avoid contact with eyes, skin, or clothing. Wash thoroughly with soap and water after handling. Remove pets, birds and cover fish aquariums before spraying. In the home, food processing surfaces should be covered before treatment or thoroughly washed before use. Do not apply while food processing, preparation or serving is underway.

Statement of Practical Treatment:

If in Eyes: Flush eyes with plenty of water. Get medical attention if irritation persists.

If on Skin: Wash with plenty of soap and water. Get medical attention.

Physical or Chemical Hazards: Contents under pressure. Do not use or store near heat or open flame. Do not puncture or incinerate container. Exposure to temperatures above 130°F may cause bursting. Provide adequate ventilation during use. Do not use in or around electrical equipment due to possibility of shock hazard. Protect from freezing.

In case of emergency or for product use information please call 602-285-1660 Monday - Friday, 7:00 - 3:45 pm MST.

Storage and Disposal:

Storage: Store in a cool, dry area out of reach of children. Protect from freezing.

Disposal: Do not puncture or incinerate container. Wrap container in several layers of newspaper and dispose of in trash collection.

Warning(s): Keep out of reach of children.

Presentation: 16 oz (454 g).

®Nylar is a registered trademark of McLaughlin Gormley King Co.

Compendium Code No.: 10000821

ADAMS™ PYRETHRIN DIP

Farnam — **Topical Insecticide**

EPA Reg. No.: 37425-19

Active Ingredient(s):

Pyrethrins	0.97%
Piperonyl Butoxide, Technical*	3.74%
N-Octyl Bicycloheptene Dicarboximide	5.70%
Di-N-Propyl Isocinchomeronate	1.94%
Inert Ingredients*	87.65%
Total	100.00%

With aloe vera extract, lanolin and sunscreens.

*Equivalent to 2.992% of butylcarbityl (6-propylpiperonyl) ether and 0.748% of related compounds.

Indications: Kills and repels fleas, ticks, lice, gnats, mosquitoes and flies on dogs and cats.

Directions for Use: It is a violation of Federal law to use this product in a manner inconsistent with its labeling.

Read entire label before each use.

Use only on dogs and cats.

Shake well before every use.

Dogs and Cats: To kill fleas and ticks, thoroughly mix ½ oz (1 tablespoon) of ADAMS™ Pyrethrin Dip with 1 gal. of warm water. For outdoor animals in areas of severe infestations 2 oz (4 tablespoons) per gal. may be used. Do not dilute more than will be used in a 24 hour period. If animal's coat is very dirty, bathe first with Adams™ Shampoo.

Dip should be applied to dry or damp (not wet) coat. Sponge or dip animal with diluted ADAMS™ Pyrethrin Dip making sure all areas are soaked to the skin. Let drip dry on animal. Do not rinse off. Repeat treatment every 7 days if necessary. Dependant on reinfestation levels in the animal's environment, extended insecticide and repellent activity, has been demonstrated with ADAMS™ Pyrethrin Dip*.

Precautionary Statements: Hazards to Humans and Domestic Animals:

Warning:

Human: Causes substantial but temporary eye injury. Do not get in eyes or on clothing. Wash thoroughly with soap and water after handling. Remove contaminated clothing and wash before reuse. Harmful if swallowed or inhaled. Avoid contamination of food. Wash hands with soap and water after using.

Animal: Do not use on puppies, kittens or foals less than 12 weeks old. Consult a veterinarian before using this product on debilitated, aged, medicated, pregnant, or nursing animals. Sensitivities may occur after using any pesticide product for pets. If signs of sensitivity occur, bathe your pet with mild soap and rinse with large amounts of water. If signs continue, consult a veterinarian immediately.

First Aid:

If Swallowed: Call a physician or poison control center. Do not induce vomiting. Drink promptly a large quantity of milk, egg whites, gelatin solution, or if these are not available, drink large quantities of water. Avoid alcohol. Probable mucosal damage may contraindicate the use of gastric lavage.

If in Eyes: Hold eyelids open and flush with a steady, gentle stream of water for 15 minutes. Get medical attention.

In case of emergency, or for product use information, call (602) 285-1660 Monday-Friday, 7:00 am to 4:45 pm, MST.

Environmental Hazards: This product is toxic to fish. Do not add directly to water. Do not apply where runoff is likely to occur.

Storage and Disposal:

Storage: Store in a cool, dry area away from heat or open flame. Do not contaminate water, food or feed by storage or disposal.

Disposal: Do not reuse container. Rinse thoroughly and wrap container in several layers of newspaper and discard in trash.

Warning(s): Keep out of reach of children.

Presentation: 4 fl oz (118 mL).

*U.S. Patent No. 4,668,666

Compendium Code No.: 10000570 9704 85-6630-02

ADAMS™ PYRETHRIN DIP

V.P.L. **Topical Insecticide**

EPA Reg. No.: 37425-19

Active Ingredient(s):

Pyrethrins	0.97%
Piperonyl Butoxide, Technical*	3.74%
N-Octyl Bicycloheptene Dicarboximide	5.70%
Di-N-Propyl Isocinchomeronate	1.94%
Inert Ingredients*	87.65%
Total	100.00%

With aloe vera extract, lanolin and sunscreens.

*Equivalent to 2.992% of butylcarbityl (6-propylpiperonyl) ether and 0.748% of related compounds.

Indications: Kills and repels fleas, ticks, lice, gnats, mosquitoes and flies on dogs and cats.

Directions for Use: It is a violation of Federal law to use this product in a manner inconsistent with its labeling.

Read entire label before each use.

Use only on dogs and cats.

Shake well before every use.

Dogs and Cats: To kill fleas and ticks, thoroughly mix ½ oz (1 tablespoon) of ADAMS™ Pyrethrin Dip with 1 gal. of warm water. For outdoor animals in areas of severe infestations 2 oz (4 tablespoons) per gal. may be used. Do not dilute more than will be used in a 24 hour period. If animal's coat is very dirty, bathe first with Adams™ Shampoo.

Dip should be applied to dry or damp (not wet) coat. Sponge or dip animal with diluted ADAMS™ Pyrethrin Dip making sure all areas are soaked to the skin. Let drip dry on animal. Do not rinse off. Repeat treatment every 7 days if necessary. Dependant on reinfestation levels in the animal's environment, extended insecticide and repellent activity, has been demonstrated with ADAMS™ Pyrethrin Dip*.

Precautionary Statements: Hazards to Humans and Domestic Animals:

Warning:

Human: Causes substantial but temporary eye injury. Do not get in eyes or on clothing. Wash thoroughly with soap and water after handling. Remove contaminated clothing and wash before reuse. Harmful if swallowed or inhaled. Avoid contamination of food. Wash hands with soap and water after using.

Animal: Do not use on puppies, kittens or foals less than 12 weeks old. Consult a veterinarian before using this product on debilitated, aged, medicated, pregnant, or nursing animals. Sensitivities may occur after using any pesticide product for pets. If signs of sensitivity occur, bathe your pet with mild soap and rinse with large amounts of water. If signs continue, consult a veterinarian immediately.

First Aid:

If Swallowed: Call a physician or poison control center. Do not induce vomiting. Drink promptly a large quantity of milk, egg whites, gelatin solution, or if these are not available, drink large quantities of water. Avoid alcohol. Probable mucosal damage may contraindicate the use of gastric lavage.

If in Eyes: Hold eyelids open and flush with a steady, gentle stream of water for 15 minutes. Get medical attention.

In case of emergency, or for product use information, call (602) 285-1660 Monday-Friday, 7:00 am to 4:45 pm, MST.

Environmental Hazards: This product is toxic to fish. Do not add directly to water. Do not apply where runoff is likely to occur.

Storage and Disposal:

Storage: Store in a cool, dry area away from heat or open flame. Do not contaminate water, food or feed by storage or disposal.

Disposal: Do not reuse container. Rinse thoroughly and wrap container in several layers of newspaper and discard in trash.

Warning(s): Keep out of reach of children.

Presentation: 4 fl oz (118 mL).

*U.S. Patent No. 4,668,666

Compendium Code No.: 11430540 9704 85-6630-02

ADAMS™ ROOM FOGGER WITH SYKILLSTOP™

Farnam **Premise Insecticide**

EPA Reg. No.: 37425-37

Active Ingredient(s):

2-[1-Methyl-2-(4-phenoxyphenoxy) ethoxy] pyridine	0.100%
Pyrethrins	0.050%
N-Octyl bicycloheptenedicarboximide*	0.400%
Permethrin [**(3-Phenoxyphenyl) methyl ± cis, trans-3-(2,2-dichloroethenyl) 2,2-dimethylcyclopropanecarboxylate]	0.400%
Related Compounds	0.035%
Other Ingredients	99.015%
Total	100.000%

*MGK 264, Insecticide Synergist **cis-trans isomer ratio: Min. 25% ± cis Max 65% ± trans

Indications: A ready to use, water-based, automatic room fogger that contains adulticides to kill adult and pre-adult fleas, and an insect growth regulator to kill larval fleas for 210 days. For use in rooms, apartments, homes, attics, basements, campers, boats, household storage areas, garages, pet sleeping areas, cabins.

Directions for Use: It is a violation of Federal law to use this product in a manner inconsistent with its labelling. Shake well before use. Keep container upright.

This product will kill ants, cockroaches, crickets, fleas, houseflies, mosquitos, rice weevils, saw-toothed grain beetles, small flying moths, and ticks. It will also prevent pre-adult fleas from developing into the adult biting stage up to 210 days. Cover exposed food, dishes and food-handling equipment. Open cabinets and doors of area to be treated. Shut off fans and air conditioners. Close doors and windows. Point valve opening away from face and eyes when releasing. Use one unit for each 6,000 cubic feet of area. Do not use more than one fogger per room. Do not use in small, enclosed spaces such as closets, cabinets or under counters or tables. Do not use in a room 5 ft x 5 ft or smaller; instead, allow fog to enter from other rooms. Turn off all ignition sources such as pilot lights (shut off gas valves), other open flames, or running electrical appliances that cycle off and one (i.e., refrigerators, thermostats, etc.). Call your gas utility or management company if you need assistance with your pilot lights. Do not remain in the area during treatment and ventilate thoroughly before re-entry.

To Operate Valve: To lock valve in open position for automatic discharge, press the valve button all the way down, hooking the catch. Then place fogger on stand or table in the center of the room with valve locked open, placing several layers of newspaper or pad under fogger. Leave building at once and keep building closed for two hours before airing out. Open all doors and windows and allow to air for 30 minutes. Repeat spraying in two weeks or when necessary.

To Control Ticks and Fleas: Old bedding should be removed and replaced with fresh, clean bedding after treatment. Pets should be treated with a registered Adams™ product for flea and tick control in conjunction with this treatment.

Precautionary Statements: Hazards to Humans and Domestic Animals:

Caution: Harmful if swallowed or absorbed through skin. Do not breathe vapors or spray mist. Avoid contact with skin or eyes. In case of contact, flush with water. Wash with soap and water after use. Obtain medical attention if irritation persists. Avoid contamination of food.

Statement of Practical Treatment:

If Swallowed: Call a physician or Poison Control Center immediately.

If in Eyes: Flush with water. Get medical attention if irritation persists.

If on Skin or Clothing: Remove contaminated clothing and wash before reuse. Wash skin with soap and warm water. Get medical attention if irritation persists.

If Inhaled: Remove victim to fresh air if effects occur and call a physician.

Environmental Hazards: Do not contaminate water when disposing of equipment washwaters.

Physical or Chemical Hazards: This product contains a highly flammable ingredient. It may cause a fire or explosion if not used properly. Follow the "Directions for Use" on the label very carefully.

Extremely flammable. Contents under pressure. Keep away from heat, sparks and open flame. Do not puncture or incinerate container. Exposure to temperatures above 130°F may cause bursting.

Storage and Disposal:

Storage: Store in cool, dry area away from heat or open flame.

Disposal: Replace cap and discard container in trash. Do not incinerate or puncture.

Warning(s): Keep out of reach of children.

Presentation: 6 oz (170 g) aerosol can.

Compendium Code No.: 10000580

ADAMS™ ROOM FOGGER WITH SYKILLSTOP™

V.P.L. **Premise Insecticide**

EPA Reg. No.: 37425-37

Active Ingredient(s):

2-[1-Methyl-2-(4-phenoxyphenoxy) ethoxy] pyridine	0.100%
Pyrethrins	0.050%
N-Octyl bicycloheptenedicarboximide*	0.400%
Permethrin [**(3-Phenoxyphenyl) methyl ± cis, trans-3-(2,2-dichloroethenyl) 2,2-dimethylcyclopropanecarboxylate]	0.400%
Related Compounds	0.035%
Other Ingredients	99.015%
Total	100.000%

*MGK 264, Insecticide Synergist

**cis-trans isomer ratio: Min. 25% ± cis Max 65% ± trans

Indications: A ready to use, water-based, automatic room fogger that contains adulticides to kill adult and pre-adult fleas, and an insect growth regulator to kill larval fleas for 210 days. For use in rooms, apartments, homes, attics, basements, campers, boats, household storage areas, garages, pet sleeping areas, cabins.

Directions for Use: It is a violation of Federal law to use this product in a manner inconsistent with its labelling.

Shake well before use.

Keep container upright.

This product will kill ants, cockroaches, crickets, fleas, houseflies, mosquitos, rice weevils, saw-toothed grain beetles, small flying moths, and ticks. It will also prevent pre-adult fleas from developing into the adult biting stage up to 210 days. Cover exposed food, dishes and food-handling equipment. Open cabinets and doors of area to be treated. Shut off fans and air conditioners. Close doors and windows. Point valve opening away from face and eyes when releasing. Use one unit for each 6,000 cubic feet of area. Do not use more than one fogger per room. Do not use in small, enclosed spaces such as closets, cabinets or under counters or tables. Do not use in a room 5 ft x 5 ft or smaller; instead, allow fog to enter from other rooms. Turn off all ignition sources such as pilot lights (shut off gas valves), other open flames, or running electrical appliances that cycle off and one (i.e., refrigerators, thermostats, etc.). Call your gas utility or management company if you need assistance with your pilot lights. Do not remain in the area during treatment and ventilate thoroughly before re-entry.

To Operate Valve: To lock valve in open position for automatic discharge, press the valve button all the way down, hooking the catch. Then place fogger on stand or table in the center of the room with valve locked open, placing several layers of newspaper or pad under fogger. Leave building at once and keep building closed for two hours before airing out. Open all doors and windows and allow to air for 30 minutes. Repeat spraying in two weeks or when necessary.

To Control Ticks and Fleas: Old bedding should be removed and replaced with fresh, clean bedding after treatment. Pets should be treated with a registered Adams™ product for flea and tick control in conjunction with this treatment.

Precautionary Statements: Hazards to Humans and Domestic Animals:

Caution: Harmful if swallowed or absorbed through skin. Do not breathe vapors or spray mist. Avoid contact with skin or eyes. In case of contact, flush with water. Wash with soap and water after use. Obtain medical attention if irritation persists. Avoid contamination of food.

Statement of Practical Treatment:

If Swallowed: Call a physician or Poison Control Center immediately.

If in Eyes: Flush with water. Get medical attention if irritation persists.

If on Skin or Clothing: Remove contaminated clothing and wash before reuse. Wash skin with soap and warm water. Get medical attention if irritation persists.

If Inhaled: Remove victim to fresh air if effects occur and call a physician.

Environmental Hazards: Do not contaminate water when disposing of equipment washwaters.

Physical or Chemical Hazards: This product contains a highly flammable ingredient. It may cause a fire or explosion if not used properly. Follow the "Directions for Use" on the label very carefully.

Extremely flammable. Contents under pressure. Keep away from heat, sparks and open flame. Do not puncture or incinerate container. Exposure to temperatures above 130°F may cause bursting.

Storage and Disposal:

Storage: Store in cool, dry area away from heat or open flame.

Disposal: Replace cap and discard container in trash. Do not incinerate or puncture.

Warning(s): Keep out of reach of children.

Presentation: 6 oz (170 g) aerosol can.

Compendium Code No.: 11430550

ADAMS™ SPOT-ON FLEA & TICK CONTROL FOR LARGE DOGS

Farnam **Topical Insecticide**

EPA Reg. No.: 270-279-37425

Active Ingredient(s):

Permethrin*: 45.0%
Inert Ingredients: 55.0%
Total 100.0%

*(3-phenoxyphenyl) methyl (±)-cis, trans-3-(2,2-dichloroethenyl)-2,2-dimethylcyclopropane-carboxylate

cis/trans ratio: Max 55% (±) cis and min 45% (±) trans

Indications: Kills and repels adult fleas for up to 3 to 4 weeks. Kills and repels ticks, including Deer Ticks (vector of Lyme Disease), Brown Dog Ticks and American Dog Ticks, for up to 4 weeks. Protects against blood feeding by mosquitoes (vector of heartworm) for up to 4 weeks. For use on large dogs (over 33 pounds).

Directions for Use: It is a violation of Federal law to use this product in a manner inconsistent with its labeling.

Read entire label before each use.

Use only on dogs over 6 months of age.

Do not use on cats or animals other than dogs. Do not get this product in your dog's eyes or mouth. Repeat applications may be made, if necessary, but do not apply more often than once every 3 weeks, except to reapply after shampooing the dog.

For Dogs Weighing More Than 33 Pounds: Apply approximately half of the tube (1.5 mL) of ADAMS™ Spot-On Flea & Tick Control for Dogs solution as a spot or stripe to the dogs back between the shoulder blades and apply the rest of the tube's contents (1.5 mL) as a spot or stripe to the dog's back directly in front of the base of the tail. Or, apply the entire tube (3.0 mL) as a continuous stripe on the dog's back starting between the shoulder blades and ending directly in front of the base of the tail.

How To Apply: Remove product tube from package. Holding tube with notched end pointing up and away from face and body, cut narrow end at notches. Invert tube over dog and use open end to part dog's hair. Squeeze tube firmly to apply all of the solution to the dog's skin. Wrap tube and put in trash.

Contraindication(s): Do not use on cats or animals other than dogs. Do not use on dogs less than 6 months of age.

Precautionary Statements: Hazards to Humans and Domestic Animals:

Caution:

Hazards to Humans: Harmful if swallowed. Avoid contact with eyes or clothing. Causes moderate eye irritation. Wash thoroughly with soap and water after handling.

Hazards to Domestic Animals: For external use on dogs only. Do not use on dogs less than 6 months of age. Consult a veterinarian before using this product on debilitated, aged, medicated, pregnant, or nursing dogs. Consult a veterinarian before using on dogs with known organ dysfunction. Do not use on cats or animals other than dogs. Cats which actively groom or engage in close physical contact with recently treated dogs may be at risk of toxic exposure. Certain medications can interact with pesticides. It is advisable to consult a veterinarian before using this product with any other pesticide or drug.

First Aid:

If Swallowed: Call a physician or Poison Control Center. Drink 1 or 2 glasses of water and induce vomiting by touching back of throat with finger or, if available, by administration of syrup of ipecac. Do not induce vomiting or give anything by mouth to an unconscious person.

If in Eyes: Flush eyes with plenty of water. Call a physician if irritation persists.

Adverse Reactions: Some animals may be sensitive to ingredients in this product. Reactions in dogs may include skin sensitivity. Dogs may show lethargy, increased pruritis (itchiness), erythema (redness), rash and hair discoloration or hair loss at the application site. Observe the dog following treatment. Sensitivity may occur after using any pesticide product on pets. If signs of sensitivity occur, bathe your dog with a mild, non-insecticidal shampoo and rinse with large amounts of water. If signs continue, consult a veterinarian immediately.

In case of emergency, or for product information, call (602) 285-1660 Monday - Friday, 7:00 am - 3:45 pm, MST.

Environmental Hazards: This product is extremely toxic to fish. Do not add directly to water. Do not contaminate water when disposing of product or packaging.

Physical or Chemical Hazards: Do not use or store near heat or open flames.

Storage and Disposal: Do not contaminate water, food or feed by storage or disposal.

Storage: Store in a cool, dry place. Protect from freezing. Pesticide Disposal: Securely wrap original container in several layers of newspaper and discard in trash.

Container Disposal: Do not reuse empty container, Wrap container and put in trash.

Warning(s): Keep out of reach of children.

Disclaimer: Notice of Warranty: The manufacturer makes no warranty of merchantability, fitness for any particular purpose, or otherwise, expressed or implied concerning this product or its uses which extend beyond the use of the product under normal conditions in accordance with the statements made on the label.

Discussion: ADAMS™ Spot-On Flea & Tick Control for Dogs is an effective and easy to use product. ADAMS™ Spot-On Flea & Tick Control for Dogs has demonstrated greater then 92% control of fleas within one day of application. As with all flea and tick control products, ADAMS™ Spot-On Flea & Tick Control for Dogs should be used as part of a program aimed at reducing flea populations in the dog's environment (bedding, carpets, kennel, yard). Consult your veterinarian, entomologist, or retailer for program recommendations.

Presentation: 1 x 3.0 mL applicator and 3 x 3.0 mL applicators.

Compendium Code No.: 10000590

9C9

ADAMS™ SPOT-ON FLEA & TICK CONTROL FOR SMALL DOGS

Farnam **Topical Insecticide**

EPA Reg. No.: 270-279-37425

Active Ingredient(s):

Permethrin*: 45.0%
Inert Ingredients: 55.0%
Total 100.0%

*(3-phenoxyphenyl) methyl (±)-cis, trans-3-(2,2-dichloroethenyl)-2,2-dimethylcyclopropane-carboxylate

cis/trans ratio: Max 55% (±) cis and min 45% (±) trans

Indications: Kills and repels adult fleas for up to 3 to 4 weeks. Kills and repels ticks, including Deer Ticks (vector of Lyme Disease), Brown Dog Ticks and American Dog Ticks, for up to 4 weeks. Protects against blood feeding by mosquitoes (vector of heartworm) for up to 4 weeks. For use on small dogs (under 33 pounds).

Directions for Use: It is a violation of Federal law to use this product in a manner inconsistent with its labeling.

Read entire label before each use.

Use only on dogs over 6 months of age.

Do not use on cats or animals other than dogs. Do not get this product in your dog's eyes or mouth. Repeat applications may be made, if necessary, but do not apply more often than once every 3 weeks, except to reapply after shampooing the dog.

For Dogs Weighing Less Than 33 Pounds: Apply one tube (1.5 mL) of ADAMS™ Spot-On Flea & Tick Control for Dogs solution as a spot between the shoulder blades or as a stripe to the dog's back.

How To Apply: Remove product tube from package. Holding tube with notched end pointing up and away from face and body, cut narrow end at notches. Invert tube over dog and use open end to part dog's hair. Squeeze tube firmly to apply all of the solution to the dog's skin. Wrap tube and put in trash.

Contraindication(s): Do not use on cats or animals other than dogs. Do not use on dogs less than 6 months of age.

Precautionary Statements: Hazards to Humans and Domestic Animals:

Caution:

Hazards to Humans: Harmful if swallowed. Avoid contact with eyes or clothing. Causes moderate eye irritation. Wash thoroughly with soap and water after handling.

Hazards to Domestic Animals: For external use on dogs only. Do not use on dogs less than 6 months of age. Consult a veterinarian before using this product on debilitated, aged, medicated, pregnant, or nursing dogs. Consult a veterinarian before using on dogs with known organ dysfunction. Do not use on cats or animals other than dogs. Cats which actively groom or engage in close physical contact with recently treated dogs may be at risk of toxic exposure. Certain medications can interact with pesticides. It is advisable to consult a veterinarian before using this product with any other pesticide or drug.

First Aid:

If Swallowed: Call a physician or Poison Control Center. Drink 1 or 2 glasses of water and induce vomiting by touching back of throat with finger or, if available, by administration of syrup of ipecac. Do not induce vomiting or give anything by mouth to an unconscious person.

If in Eyes: Flush eyes with plenty of water. Call a physician if irritation persists.

Adverse Reactions: Some animals may be sensitive to ingredients in this product. Reactions in dogs may include skin sensitivity. Dogs may show lethargy, increased pruritis (itchiness), erythema (redness), rash and hair discoloration or hair loss at the application site. Observe the dog following treatment. Sensitivity may occur after using any pesticide product on pets. If signs of sensitivity occur, bathe your dog with a mild, non-insecticidal shampoo and rinse with large amounts of water. If signs continue, consult a veterinarian immediately.

In case of emergency, or for product information, call (602) 285-1660 Monday - Friday, 7:00 am - 3:45 pm, MST.

Environmental Hazards: This product is extremely toxic to fish. Do not add directly to water. Do not contaminate water when disposing of product or packaging.

Physical or Chemical Hazards: Do not use or store near heat or open flames.

Storage and Disposal: Do not contaminate water, food or feed by storage or disposal.

Storage: Store in a cool, dry place. Protect from freezing. Pesticide Disposal: Securely wrap original container in several layers of newspaper and discard in trash.

Container Disposal: Do not reuse empty container, Wrap container and put in trash.

Warning(s): Keep out of reach of children.

Disclaimer: Notice of Warranty: The manufacturer makes no warranty of merchantability, fitness for any particular purpose, or otherwise, expressed or implied concerning this product or its uses which extend beyond the use of the product under normal conditions in accordance with the statements made on the label.

Discussion: ADAMS™ Spot-On Flea & Tick Control for Dogs is an effective and easy to use product. ADAMS™ Spot-On Flea & Tick Control for Dogs has demonstrated greater then 92% control of fleas within one day of application. As with all flea and tick control products, ADAMS™ Spot-On Flea & Tick Control for Dogs should be used as part of a program aimed at reducing flea populations in the dog's environment (bedding, carpets, kennel, yard). Consult your veterinarian, entomologist, or retailer for program recommendations.

Presentation: 1 x 1.5 mL applicator and 3 x 1.5 mL applicators.

Compendium Code No.: 10000600

9C9

ADAMS™ WATER BASED FLEA AND TICK MIST

Farnam **Parasiticide Spray**

EPA Reg. No.: 37425-18

Active Ingredient(s):

Pyrethrins 0.20%
Piperonyl Butoxide, Technical* 0.75%
N-Octyl Bicycloheptene Dicarboximide 2.00%
Inert Ingredients** 97.05%
Total 100.00%

*Equivalent to 0.60% of butylcarbityl (6-propylpiperonyl) ether and 0.15% of related compounds.

**Inert ingredients include: Concentrated aloe vera gel, aloe vera extract, natural woolfat (lanolin) and other grooming and cleansing agents.

Indications: Kills and temporarily repels fleas, ticks, lice, flies, gnats, mosquitoes and chiggers on dogs, puppies, cats and kittens.

Directions for Use: It is a violation of Federal law to use this product in a manner inconsistent with its labeling.

Read entire label before each use.

Use only on dogs, cats, puppies and kittens.

Shake well before use. Use only in a well ventilated area.

Dogs, Puppies, Cats, Kittens: Cover animal's eyes with hand and with a firm, fast stroke to get a proper spray mist, spray head, ears and chest until damp. With fingertips, rub into face and around mouth, nose and eyes. Next spray neck, middle and hindquarters, finishing legs last. For best penetration of spray to the skin, direct spray against the natural lay of the hair. On long haired animals, rub your hand against the lay of the hair, spraying the ruffled hair directly behind the hand. Make sure spray thoroughly wets ticks. Allow ADAMS™ Water Based Flea and Tick Mist to remain on animal for 5 minutes then towel dry, brush and comb to remove dead fleas and ticks. Do not reapply product for one week.

Precautionary Statements: Hazards to Humans and Domestic Animals:

Caution:

Human: Harmful if swallowed or inhaled. Avoid breathing mist. Avoid contamination of food. Wash hands with soap and water after using.

Animal: Do not use on animals under 12 weeks of age. Consult a veterinarian before using this product on debilitated, aged, pregnant, or nursing animals, or animals on medication. Sensitivities may occur after using any pesticide product for pets. If signs of sensitivity occur, bathe your pet with mild soap and rinse with large amounts of water. If signs continue, consult a veterinarian immediately.

First Aid:

If in Eyes: Call a physician. Flush eyes with gentle stream of water for 15 minutes.

If Swallowed: Call physician or Poison Control Center. Drink promptly a large quantity of milk, egg white, gelatin mixture, or if these are unavailable, a large quantity of water.

If on Skin: Wash with plenty of soap and water. See physician if irritation persists.

In case of emergency, or for product use information, call (602) 285-1660 Monday-Friday, 7:00 am to 3:45 pm, MST.

Environmental Hazards: This product is toxic to fish. Do not add directly to water. Do not apply where runoff is likely to occur.

Physical or Chemical Hazards: Do not use or store near heat or open flame.

Storage and Disposal:

Storage: Store in a cool, dry area away from heat or open flame. Do not contaminate water, food or feed by storage or disposal. Do not transfer contents to other containers.

Disposal: Do not reuse container. Rinse thoroughly and wrap container in several layers of newspaper and discard in trash.

Warning(s): Keep out of reach of children.

Presentation: 16 fl oz (473 mL) and 32 fl oz (946 mL).

Compendium Code No.: 10000610

ADAMS™ WATER BASED FLEA AND TICK MIST

V.P.L. **Parasiticide Spray**

EPA Reg. No.: 37425-18

Active Ingredient(s):

Pyrethrins	0.20%
Piperonyl Butoxide, Technical*	0.75%
N-Octyl Bicycloheptene Dicarboximide	2.00%
Inert Ingredients**	97.05%
Total	100.00%

*Equivalent to 0.60% of butylcarbityl (6-propylpiperonyl) ether and 0.15% of related compounds.

**Inert ingredients include: Concentrated aloe vera gel, aloe vera extract, natural woolfat (lanolin) and other grooming and cleansing agents.

Indications: Kills and temporarily repels fleas, ticks, lice, flies, gnats, mosquitoes and chiggers on dogs, puppies, cats and kittens.

Directions for Use: It is a violation of Federal law to use this product in a manner inconsistent with its labeling.

Read entire label before each use.

Use only on dogs, cats, puppies and kittens.

Shake well before use. Use only in a well ventilated area.

Dogs, Puppies, Cats, Kittens: Cover animal's eyes with hand and with a firm, fast stroke to get a proper spray mist, spray head, ears and chest until damp. With fingertips, rub into face and around mouth, nose and eyes. Next spray neck, middle and hindquarters, finishing legs last. For best penetration of spray to the skin, direct spray against the natural lay of the hair. On long haired animals, rub your hand against the lay of the hair, spraying the ruffled hair directly behind the hand. Make sure spray thoroughly wets ticks. Allow ADAMS™ Water Based Flea and Tick Mist to remain on animal for 5 minutes then towel dry, brush and comb to remove dead fleas and ticks. Do not reapply product for one week.

Precautionary Statements: Hazards to Humans and Domestic Animals:

Caution:

Human: Harmful if swallowed or inhaled. Avoid breathing mist. Avoid contamination of food. Wash hands with soap and water after using.

Animal: Do not use on animals under 12 weeks of age. Consult a veterinarian before using this product on debilitated, aged, pregnant, or nursing animals, or animals on medication. Sensitivities may occur after using any pesticide product for pets. If signs of sensitivity occur, bathe your pet with mild soap and rinse with large amounts of water. If signs continue, consult a veterinarian immediately.

First Aid:

If in Eyes: Call a physician. Flush eyes with gentle stream of water for 15 minutes.

If Swallowed: Call physician or Poison Control Center. Drink promptly a large quantity of milk, egg white, gelatin mixture, or if these are unavailable, a large quantity of water.

If on Skin: Wash with plenty of soap and water. See physician if irritation persists.

In case of emergency, or for product use information, call (602) 285-1660 Monday-Friday, 7:00 am to 3:45 pm, MST.

Environmental Hazards: This product is toxic to fish. Do not add directly to water. Do not apply where runoff is likely to occur.

Physical or Chemical Hazards: Do not use or store near heat or open flame.

Storage and Disposal:

Storage: Store in a cool, dry area away from heat or open flame. Do not contaminate water, food or feed by storage or disposal. Do not transfer contents to other containers.

Disposal: Do not reuse container. Rinse thoroughly and wrap container in several layers of newspaper and discard in trash.

Warning(s): Keep out of reach of children.

Presentation: 16 fl oz (473 mL) and 32 fl oz (946 mL).

Compendium Code No.: 11430560

AD™ ANTIGEN

United **Aleutian Disease Test**

U.S. Vet. Lic. No.: 245

Indications: Aleutian disease (AD) is a virus disease of mink characterized by glomerulonephritis, arteritis, generalized plasmacytosis, hypergammaglobulinemia and infectious immune complexes. This cell culture propagated antigen, when used in the counterelectrophoresis (CEP) test, provides a rapid serological test for detecting the presence of antibody to AD.[1] It contains 8 or 16 "units" per 0.01 mL.

Test Principles: Detection procedure: AD may be manifested at certain stages by exhibiting elevated globulin levels. This observation led to the first detection procedure, the iodine agglutination test.[2] A more specific test was developed which detects antibody to AD by CEP,[1] and this method provides a reliable and rapid diagnostic tool throughout the life span of the mink.[3]

Principal: Mink blood, obtained by clipping a toenail and collecting the blood in a capillary tube, is centrifuged to obtain serum. Antigen prepared by extraction from AD infected mink,[1] or cell culture,[5] will combine with specific antibody to form a visible precipitin line in an agarose gel.[4,6] The CEP test utilizes the relatively rapid electrophoretic mobility of the antigen and the electroendosmotic properties of the antibody in agarose gel. The antigen migrates toward the anode, whereas, the antibody migrates toward the cathode, resulting in the development of the precipitin lines within 60 minutes.

Test Procedure: Equipment: The CEP test for AD may be performed on a variety of commercially available CEP equipment. A power supply compatible with the electrophoresis cell and test plate, chosen on the basis of convenience, reliability, and in keeping with the number of samples to be run per day, constitute the basic tools. A number of manufacturers also provide viewers. These provide oblique illumination against dark background for easier observation of precipitin lines. A bacteria colony counter may also serve this purpose.

Expendable supplies: CEP test plates are prepared from a high quality grade of agarose (not agar) with tris barbital buffer of ionic strength compatible with the balance of the test system. They may require wicks or be of the self-wicking type. Suitable test slides in a variety of sizes may be prepared by the user. Wells, usually 3.0 mm in diameter and a 10 microliter capacity, may be punched with commercially available or custom made punches. Specific information on sources for supplies may be obtained by writing United Vaccines.

Directions for use:

A. Titer (strength): The AD reagent has been prepared to contain eight (8) or 16 "units" of antigen per 10 mcL (0.01 mL) using a control serum which is positive at a 1:160 dilution. One hundred CEP assays may be performed per 1 mL of eight (8) "units" reagent. 200 tests may be performed per 1 mL of concentrated 16 "units" reagent (recommended dilution); for example (16 "units" only), in 10 microliter wells use one part antigen plus one (1) part saline or CEP buffer; maximum recovery of antigen may be made by rinsing the vial with physiological saline or CEP buffer; for convenience, the appropriate diluent may be added directly to the reagent vial. The titer of the antigen can be influenced by buffer, pH, and the quality of the agarose used for test plates.

B. Procedure:

1. CEP plates (slides) should be prepared as follows:
   a. Place clean slides on a leveling table.
   b. Prepare agarose by dissolving in distilled water to make a 1.4% to 1.8% solution (the grade and concentration of agarose influences the migration rate of the antigen and antibody). Add warm (approximately 60°C) buffer (gelman buffer at 18 g/1,200 mL H_2O) in a volume equal to the agarose. This results in 0.7% to 0.9% agarose in buffer, pH 8.6. Sodium Azide (NaN_3) at 0.03% may be added as a preservative. Hold in water bath (60°-70°C) with occasional stirring.
   c. Dispense the maximum amount of agarose per slide which will not spill over the slides, producing a layer approximately 3 mm deep (17.0 mL per slide, 82 x 101 mm). Allow to gel and store in a humidified container.
   d. Punch wells in pairs, 3 mm in diameter and 3 mm to 7 mm apart (inside edge to inside edge). Remove plugs by vacuum aspiration or other mechanical means.
2. Centrifuge the blood, which has been collected in a capillary tube, for three (3) to five (5) minutes.
3. To load the sample into the CEP plate, break the capillary tube at the serum/clot interface and touch the serum containing portion to the bottom of the well on the anode (+) side of the plate. If the serum does not leave the tube by capillary attraction, a small rubber bulb may be used to expel it.
4. Add the AD™ Antigen to the test wells on the cathode (-) side of the plate. This may be accomplished manually with a capillary tube or with a semi-automatic dispensing syringe.
5. Positive control serum should be placed in one well on each plate. Users wishing to gain experience in performing the CEP test should use strongly and weakly positive, as well as negative, control sera. These are available upon request from United Vaccines.
6. Fill the reservoirs with an appropriate volume of buffer, place the test plate on the CEP apparatus in accordance with the manufacturer's directions, and position wicks if the system requires this manner of contact. Adjust power to four (4) to six (6) volts per cm to obtain clear precipitin lines in 40 to 60 minutes.

Reading and interpretation of results:

A. When the migration of reactants is complete, a precipitin line will be visible at the positive control position and at other wells which contain AD positive serum.

B. Precipitin lines will be clearly visible if the plate is illuminated bilaterally from below and viewed against a dark background. Staining or rinsing are optional.

C. Precipitin lines will generally appear as sharp, gray lines halfway between the serum and antigen well, or closer to the serum well. The position of the lines (as well as titer of the reagents) is influenced by buffer, pH, and the qualities of the agarose. Lines may be straight or slightly curved.

D. If the results are obscured by hemolysis, the precipitin lines will become more clearly visible by soaking the plates 15 minutes to 18 hours in 2% saline solution.

Precaution(s): Stability of antigen: The antigen may be stored in an upright position at 2°-7°C. For extended storage after first use, it may be frozen in an upright position. Freezing and thawing should be limited to not more than two cycles.

Caution(s):

A. Incinerate or autoclave final container and all unused contents. Disinfect test plates after each use.
B. AD® Antigen is potentially infectious to mink of all genotypes and should be used only as an *in vitro* diagnostic reagent.
C. Use only high quality agarose (Bio-Rad Standard Low-mr, Sea Kem ME, Litex HSA). Pretest in the 0.7 to 0.9% range to determine the concentration for optimum sensitivity.
D. Buffer should be in the range of pH 8.6 to 8.8.
E. Use clean glassware and avoid contamination of the antigen with mink serum or the mink serum with antigen.
F. Excessive voltage across the CEP plate will distort the precipitin lines or melt the agarose. Four (4) to six (6) volts per cm will generally produce precipitin lines from strongly positive sera in 30 minutes and from weakly positive sera in 60 minutes.

References: Available upon request.
Presentation: 2x1,000 test vials.
Compendium Code No.: 11040121

ADENOMUNE™-7

Biocor **Bacterin-Vaccine**

Canine Distemper-Adenovirus Type 2-Hepatitis-Parainfluenza-Parvovirus Vaccine-Leptospira Bacterin, Modified Live and Killed Virus

U.S. Vet. Lic. No.: 462

Contents: This product contains the antigens listed above.

This product contains gentamicin and amphotericin B as preservatives.

All live virus fractions contained are attenuated to assure safety. The Adenovirus Type 2 and Parvovirus are inactivated to assure safety.

Indications: ADENOMUNE™-7 is a multivalent vaccine recommended for use in the vaccination of healthy dogs against disease caused by the viral and bacterial fractions of canine distemper, canine hepatitis, canine parainfluenza, canine parvovirus, canine adenovirus type 2 and leptospirosis caused by either *Leptospira canicola* or *Leptospira icterohaemorrhagiae.*

Directions: Aseptically rehydrate the vial of desiccated virus with the accompanying vial of killed virus and bacterin. Shake well. Administer entire contents (1 mL) IM or SC.

Persistence of maternal origin antibody in puppies should receive consideration in determining vaccination programs. Ideally puppies should be vaccinated at 9 weeks of age with revaccination every 2-4 weeks until at least 18 weeks of age. Dogs vaccinated over 18 weeks of age should receive a 1 mL dose followed by a second dose 2-4 weeks later. Annual revaccination with a single 1 mL dose is recommended.

Precaution(s): Store at 35°-45°F (2°-7°C). Do not freeze.

Use entire contents when first rehydrated.

Burn these containers and all unused contents.

Caution(s): Do not vaccinate pregnant bitches.

In case of anaphylactoid reactions, epinephrine should be administered immediately.

For use in dogs only.

For veterinary use only.

Presentation: Code 60211B - 25 x 1 dose (1 mL) vials with diluent.
Compendium Code No.: 13940011 BAH9125-1098

ADENOMUNE™-7-L

Biocor **Bacterin-Vaccine**

Canine Distemper-Adenovirus Type 2-Hepatitis-Parainfluenza-Parvovirus Vaccine-Leptospira Bacterin, Modified Live and Killed Virus

U.S. Vet. Lic. No.: 462

Contents: This product contains the antigens listed above.

This product contains gentamicin and amphotericin B as preservatives.

All live virus fractions contained are attenuated to assure safety. The Adenovirus Type 2 is inactivated to assure safety.

Indications: ADENOMUNE™-7-L is a multivalent vaccine recommended for use in the vaccination of healthy dogs against disease caused by the viral and bacterial fractions of canine distemper, canine hepatitis, canine adenovirus type 2, canine parainfluenza, canine parvovirus and leptospirosis caused by *Leptospira canicola* and *Leptospira icterohaemorrhagiae.*

Directions: Aseptically rehydrate the vial of desiccated virus with the accompanying vial of liquid product. Shake well. Administer entire contents (1 mL) IM or SC.

Persistence of maternal origin antibody in puppies should receive consideration in determining vaccination programs. Ideally puppies should be vaccinated at 9 weeks of age with revaccination every 2-4 weeks until at least 18 weeks of age. Dogs vaccinated over 18 weeks of age should receive a 1 mL dose followed by a second dose 2-4 weeks later. Annual revaccination with a single 1 mL dose is recommended.

Precaution(s): Store at 35°-45°F (2°-7°C). Do not freeze.

Use entire contents when first rehydrated.

Burn these containers and all unused contents.

Caution(s): Do not vaccinate pregnant bitches.

In case of anaphylactoid reactions, epinephrine should be administered immediately.

For use in dogs only.

For veterinary use only.

Presentation: Code 60411B - 25 x 1 dose (1 mL) vials with diluent.
Compendium Code No.: 13940021 BAH9325-1098

ADEQUAN® CANINE ℞

Luitpold **Polysulfated Glycosaminoglycan**

(Polysulfated Glycosaminoglycan) (PSGAG) Solution 100 mg/mL

NADA No.: 141-038

Active Ingredient(s): Each mL of ADEQUAN® Canine contains 100 mg of PSGAG, 0.9% v/v benzyl alcohol as a preservative, and water for injection q.s. to 1 mL. Sodium hydroxide and/or hydrochloric acid added when necessary to adjust pH.

Indications: ADEQUAN® Canine is recommended for intramuscular injection for the control of signs associated with non-infectious degenerative and/or traumatic arthritis of canine synovial joints.

Pharmacology: The active ingredient in ADEQUAN® Canine is polysulfated glycosaminoglycan (PSGAG). Polysulfated glycosaminoglycan is a semi-synthetic glycosaminoglycan prepared by extracting glycosaminoglycans (GAGs) from bovine tracheal cartilage. GAGs are polysaccharides composed of repeating disaccharide units. The GAG present in PSGAG is principally chondroitin sulfate containing 3 to 4 sulfate esters per disaccharide unit. The molecular weight for PSGAG used in the manufacture of ADEQUAN® is 3,000 to 15,000 daltons.

The specific mechanism of action of ADEQUAN® in canine joints is not known. PSGAG is characterized as a "disease modifying osteoarthritis drug". Experiments conducted *in vitro* have shown PSGAG to inhibit certain catabolic enzymes which have increased activity in inflamed joints, and to enhance the activity of some anabolic enzymes. For example, PSGAG has been shown to significantly inhibit serine proteinases. Serine proteinases have been demonstrated to play a role in the Interleukin-1 mediated degradation of cartilage proteoglycans and collagen. PSGAG is reported to be an inhibitor of Prostaglandin E2 (PGE2) synthesis. PGE2 has been shown to increase the loss of proteoglycan from cartilage. PSGAG has been reported to inhibit some catabolic enzymes such as elastase, stromelysin, metalloproteases, cathepsin B1, and hyaluronidases, which degrade collagen, proteoglycans, and hyaluronic acid in degenerative joint disease. Anabolic effects studied include ability to stimulate the synthesis of protein, collagen, proteoglycans, and hyaluronic acid in various cells and tissues *in vitro.* Cultured human and rabbit chondrocytes have shown increased synthesis of proteoglycan and hyaluronic acid in the presence of PSGAG. PSGAGs have shown a specific potentiating effect on hyaluronic acid synthesis by synovial membrane cells *in vitro.*

Absorption, distribution, metabolism, and excretion of PSGAG following intramuscular injection have been studied in several species, including rats, rabbits, humans, horses and dogs.

Studies in rabbits showed maximum blood concentrations of PSGAG following IM injection were reached between 20 to 40 minutes following injection, and that the drug was distributed to all tissues studied, including articular cartilage, synovial fluid, adrenals, thyroid, peritoneal fluid, lungs, eyes, spinal cord, kidneys, brain, liver, spleen, bone marrow, skin, and heart.

Following intramuscular injection of PSGAG in humans, the drug was found to be bound to serum proteins. PSGAG binds to both albumin and chi- and beta-globulins and the extent of the binding is suggested to be 30 to 40%. Therefore, the drug may be present in both bound and free form in the bloodstream. Because of its relatively low molecular weight, the synovial membrane is not a significant barrier to distribution of PSGAG from the bloodstream to the synovial fluid. Distribution from the synovial fluid to the cartilage takes place by diffusion. In the articular cartilage the drug is deposited into the cartilage matrix.

Serum and synovial fluid distribution curves of PSGAG have been studied in dogs and appear similar to those found in humans and rabbits.

In rabbits, metabolism of PSGAG is reported to take place in the liver, spleen, and bone marrow. Metabolism may also occur in the kidneys. PSGAG administered intramuscularly and not protein bound or bound to other tissues is excreted primarily via the kidneys, with a small proportion excreted in the feces.

Dosage and Administration: The recommended dose of ADEQUAN® Canine is 2 mg/lb body weight (.02 mL/lb, or 1 mL per 50 lb), by intramuscular injection only, twice weekly for up to 4 weeks (maximum of 8 injections). Do not exceed the recommended dose or therapeutic regimen. Do not mix ADEQUAN® Canine with other drugs or solvents.

Contraindication(s): Do not use in dogs showing hypersensitivity to PSGAG. PSGAG is a synthetic heparinoid; do not use in dogs with known or suspected bleeding disorders.

Precaution(s): Storage Conditions: Store at room temperature 18°-25°C (64°-77°F).

Caution(s): Federal law restricts this drug to use by or on the order of a licensed veterinarian.

Use with caution in dogs with renal or hepatic impairment.

Warning(s): Human Warning: Keep this and all medications out of reach of children.

Adverse Reactions: In the clinical efficacy trial, 24 dogs were treated with ADEQUAN® Canine twice weekly for 4 weeks. Possible adverse reactions were reported after 2.1% of the injections. These included transient pain at the injection site (1 incident), transient diarrhea (1 incident each in 2 dogs), and abnormal bleeding (1 incident). These effects were mild and self-limiting and did not require interruption of therapy. To report suspected adverse reactions or for a copy of the Material Safety Data Sheet for this product, contact Luitpold Pharmaceuticals, Inc. at 1-800-458-0163.

Toxicology: Toxicity: In a subacute toxicity study, 32 adult beagle dogs (4 males and 4 females per treatment group) received either 0.9% saline solution or PSGAG at a dose of 5 mg, 15 mg, or 50 mg per kg of body weight (approximately 2.3, 6.8, or 22.7 mg/lb), via intramuscular injection twice weekly for 13 weeks. PSGAG doses represent approximately 1X, 3X, and 10X the recommended dosage of 2 mg/lb, and more than 3 times the recommended 4-week duration of treatment. Necropsies were performed 24 hours after the final treatment. During week 12, one dog in the 50 mg/kg dosage group developed a large hematoma at the injection site which necessitated euthanasia. No other mortalities occurred during the treatment period. Statistically significant changes in the 50 mg/kg group included increased prothrombin time, reduced platelet count, an increase in ALT and cholesterol, and increased liver and kidney weights. Increased cholesterol and kidney weights were also noted in the 15 mg/kg group. Microscopic lesions were noted in the liver (Kupffer cells containing eosinophilic foamy cytoplasm), kidneys (swollen, foamy cells in the proximal convoluted tubules), and lymph nodes (macrophages with eosinophilic foamy cytoplasm) in the 15 mg/kg and 50 mg/kg groups. Intramuscular inflammation, hemorrhage, and degeneration were seen in all 3 PSGAG treated groups; the incidence and severity appeared dose related.

Trial Data: Efficacy: Efficacy of ADEQUAN® Canine was demonstrated in two studies. A laboratory study using radiolabeled PSGAG established distribution of PSGAG into canine serum and synovial fluid following a single intramuscular injection of 2 mg/lb. A clinical field trial was conducted in dogs diagnosed with radiographically-confirmed traumatic and/or degenerative joint disease of 1 or 2 joints. Joints evaluated included hips, stifles, shoulders, hocks and elbows. Fifty-one dogs were randomly assigned to receive either ADEQUAN® Canine at 2 mg/lb of body weight or 0.9% saline. Both treatments were administered by intramuscular injection twice weekly for 4 weeks (8 injections total). Investigators administering treatment and evaluating the dogs were unaware of the treatment assignment. A total of 71 limbs in 51 dogs were evaluated. Of these, 35 limbs in 24 dogs were in the ADEQUAN® Canine treated group. Each lame limb was scored for lameness at a walk, lameness at a trot, pain, range of motion, and functional disability. The scores for the individual parameters were combined to determine a total orthopedic score. At the end of the treatment period, dogs treated with ADEQUAN® Canine showed a statistically significant improvement in range of motion and total orthopedic score over placebo treated control dogs.

Reproductive Safety: Studies to establish the safety of ADEQUAN® Canine in breeding, pregnant, or lactating dogs have not been conducted.

Presentation: ADEQUAN® Canine Solution 100 mg/mL in a 5 mL preserved multiple dose vial, packaged in boxes of 2 (NDC 10797-975-02).

Compendium Code No.: 10390001 Rev. 4/00

ADEQUAN® I.A. ℞

Luitpold **Polysulfated Glycosaminoglycan**

(Polysulfated Glycosaminoglycan) (PSGAG) Solution 250 mg/mL

NADA No.: 136-383

Active Ingredient(s): Description: Each milliliter of ADEQUAN® I.A. contains 250 mg of polysulfated glycosaminoglycan and water for injection q.s. Sodium hydroxide and/or hydrochloric acid added when necessary to adjust pH.

Indications: ADEQUAN® I.A. is recommended for the treatment of non-infectious degenerative and/or traumatic joint dysfunction and associated lameness of the carpal joints in horses.

Pharmacology: Polysulfated glycosaminoglycan is chemically similar to the mucopolysaccharides of cartilagenous tissue. It is a potent proteolytic enzyme inhibitor and diminishes or reverses the processes which result in the loss of cartilagenous mucopolysaccharides. PSGAG improves joint function by stimulating synovial membrane activity, reducing synovial protein levels and increasing synovial fluid viscosity in traumatized equine carpal joints.

Dosage and Administration: The recommended dose of ADEQUAN® I.A. in horses is 250 mg (1 ampule or vial) once a week for five weeks, intra-articularly. The joint area must be shaved, cleansed and sterilized as in a surgical procedure prior to injection. Do not mix ADEQUAN® I.A. with any other drugs or solvents.

Contraindication(s): Do not use in horses showing hypersensitivity to polysulfated glycosaminoglycan. Do not administer ADEQUAN® I.A. in the face of joint sepsis.

Precaution(s): Store at controlled room temperature 18°-25°C (64°-77°F).

Caution(s): Federal law restricts this drug to use by or on the order of a licensed veterinarian.

ADEQUAN® I.A. is indicated for use only in the carpal joint of horses. Do not mix ADEQUAN® I.A. with other drugs or solvents.

Reactions in the joint may occasionally occur within 48 hours after intra-articular treatment. If the reaction involves excessive inflammation, cease therapy with ADEQUAN® I.A.

Post-injection inflammation may result from possible sensitivity to ADEQUAN® I.A.; traumatic injection technique; exceeding the recommended dose, frequency of administration or number of ADEQUAN® I.A. injections; and from combining ADEQUAN® I.A. with other drugs. Excessive joint inflammation may be manifested by rapid onset, tenderness, swelling and warmth over the injected carpus. Inflammatory joint reactions may successfully be treated by systemic anti-inflammatory drugs, cold hydrotherapy, and rest. Serious reactions of this type may indicate the presence of joint sepsis.

Joint sepsis is a rare, but potentially life-threatening complication of intra-articular injection. It usually results from the deposition of skin organisms into the joint space by the needle tip. Gustafson et al., (1989) have demonstrated that ADEQUAN® I.A. may potentiate a subinfective dose of contaminant bacteria.[2,3] Hence, strict aseptic injection technique is of the utmost importance.

Successful resolution of joint sepsis depends upon prompt recognition and rigorous antimicrobial treatment.[1,4,5,6] Early diagnosis of septic arthritis may be complicated by the similar appearance of joint inflammation. Excessive inflammation accompanied by lameness, swelling, and edema extending beyond the joint limits should alert the practitioner to the possibility of sepsis. Synovial fluid analysis with cytology and bacterial culture of the fluid or a section of synovial membrane are valuable diagnostic aids. Upon suspicion of joint sepsis, broad spectrum antibiotic therapy should be instituted without delay and joint lavage considered. It is recommended that samples used for bacterial culture be taken prior to initiating antibiotic therapy.

The concomitant use of ADEQUAN® I.A. with steroidal or non-steroidal anti-inflammatory agents may mask the symptoms of joint sepsis, thereby delaying the diagnosis and reducing the likelihood of a satisfactory resolution.

Intra-articular injections should not be performed when the overlying skin is scurfed or blistered, as this precludes adherence to aseptic injection technique.

Impairment of Fertility: Fertility impairment studies in mares and stallions have not been conducted. Do not use in horses intended for breeding.

Warning(s): Not for use in horses intended for food.

Toxicology: Toxicity: Toxicity studies were conducted in horses. Doses as high as 1,250 mg were administered intracarpally to six horses once a week for 18 weeks. This dosage is five times the recommended dosage and 3.6 times the recommended therapeutic regimen. Clinical observations revealed soreness and swelling in 1.8% (2 of 109 animals) at the injection site which was mild, self limiting and lasted less than one day. There was a dose related elevation on partial thromboplastin time, creatinine and glucose. No animal had any clinical illness during the trial and none showed clinical evidence of toxicity except for transient swelling at the injection site, possibly due to mechanical invasion of the joint.

Adverse Reactions: Two major categories of adverse reactions have been reported following the intra-articular administration of ADEQUAN® I.A.:

1. Inflammatory joint reactions consisting of joint pain, effusion, and swelling with associated lameness.
2. Septic arthritis.

Less frequently, nonseptic arthritis, hemarthrosis, and cellulitis at the injection site and surrounding tissues have been reported.

References: Available upon request.

Presentation: ADEQUAN® I.A. solution, 250 mg/mL is available as: 1 mL single dose vials (packaged in boxes of 6) (NDC 10797-991-72).

Compendium Code No.: 10390012 Rev. 04/00

ADEQUAN® I.M. ℞

Luitpold **Polysulfated Glycosaminoglycan**

Brand of Polysulfated Glycosaminoglycan (PSGAG) Solution 500 mg/5 mL

NADA No.: 140-901

Active Ingredient(s): Description: Each 5 mL of ADEQUAN® I.M. contains 500 mg of Polysulfated Glycosaminoglycan and water for injection q.s. Sodium Hydroxide and/or Hydrochloric Acid added when necessary to adjust pH. Sodium Chloride may be added to adjust tonicity.

Indications: ADEQUAN® I.M. is recommended for the intramuscular treatment of noninfectious degenerative and/or traumatic joint dysfunction and associated lameness of the carpal and hock joints in horses.

Pharmacology: Polysulfated Glycosaminoglycan is chemically similar to the glycosaminoglycans in articular cartilage matrix. PSGAG is a potent proteolytic enzyme inhibitor and diminishes or reverses the pathologic processes of traumatic or degenerative joint disease which result in a net loss of cartilage matrix components. PSGAG improves joint function by reducing synovial fluid protein levels and increasing synovial fluid hyaluronic acid concentration in traumatized equine carpal and hock joints.

Dosage and Administration: The recommended dose of ADEQUAN® I.M. in horses is 500 mg every four (4) days for 28 days intramuscularly. The injection site must be thoroughly cleansed prior to injection. Do not mix ADEQUAN® I.M. with other drugs or solvents.

Contraindication(s): There are no known contraindications to the use of intramuscular Polysulfated Glycosaminoglycan.

Precaution(s): Storage Conditions: Store at controlled room temperature 18°-25°C (64°-77°F). Discard unused portion.

Dispose of spent needles in accordance with all federal, state and local environmental laws.

Caution(s): Federal law restricts this drug to use by or on the order of a licensed veterinarian.

Warning(s): Not for use in horses intended for food.

Keep this and all medications out of the reach of children.

Toxicology: Toxicity: Toxicity studies were conducted in horses. Doses as high as 2,500 mg were administered intramuscularly to six horses twice a week for 12 weeks. This dosage is five times the recommended dosage and three times the recommended therapeutic regimen. Clinical observations revealed no soreness or swelling at the injection site or in the affected joint. No animal had any clinical or laboratory evidence of toxicity.

Reproductive Safety: Studies have not been conducted to establish safety in breeding horses.

Presentation: ADEQUAN® I.M. solution, 500 mg/5 mL is available in 5 mL single dose vials, packaged in boxes of 4.

Compendium Code No.: 10390022 Rev. 4/00

A-D INJECTION

Durvet **Vitamins A-D**

Vitamins A and D-Sterile

Active Ingredient(s): Compositions: Each mL sterile solution contains:

Vitamin A .... 500,000 IU
Vitamin D_3 .... 75,000 IU

In an emulsifiable base with vitamin E (antioxidant) 5 IU per mL, ethyl alcohol 8% v/v, benzyl alcohol 2% v/v, BHA 0.75% and BHT 0.75% (preservatives).

Indications: For use as a supplemental nutritive source of vitamins A and D in cattle.

Dosage and Administration: Inject intramuscularly using a sterile 14 to 18 gauge needle 1 to 2 inches long. Injection should be made into a heavily muscled area, preferably high on the rump, using aseptic technique.

Calves- ½ to 1 mL
Yearling Cattle- 1 to 2 mL
Adult Cattle- 2 to 4 mL

These suggested dosages may be repeated after 60 days, if necessary.

Precaution(s): Store between 15°C-30°C (59°F-86°F). Protect from light and excessive heat. Keep partially used vial under refrigeration. Keep from freezing.

Caution(s): For animal use only.

Keep out of reach of children.

Warning(s): Do not inject into meat animals within 60 days of marketing.

Presentation: 100 mL (NDC 30798-036-10), 250 mL (NDC 30798-036-13), and 500 mL (NDC 30798-036-17).

Compendium Code No.: 10840021 Rev. 5-95

ADSPEC® STERILE SOLUTION ℞

Pharmacia & Upjohn **Spectinomycin Injection**

brand of spectinomycin sulfate sterile solution

NADA No.: 141-077

Active Ingredient(s): Each mL of ADSPEC® Sterile Solution contains spectinomycin sulfate tetrahydrate equivalent to 100 mg spectinomycin; and 9.45 mg benzyl alcohol, added as preservative. The pH was adjusted with hydrochloric acid or sodium hydroxide.

Indications: ADSPEC® Sterile Solution is indicated for the treatment of bovine respiratory disease (pneumonia) associated with *Pasteurella haemolytica, Pasteurella multocida,* and *Haemophilus somnus.*

Pharmacology: Description: ADSPEC® Sterile Solution contains the sulfate salt of spectinomycin, an aminocyclitol antibiotic produced by *Streptomyces spectabilis.*

Figure 1. Chemical structure of spectinomycin sulfate tetrahydrate

The chemical name of spectinomycin sulfate tetrahydrate is: Decahydro-4a,7,9-trihydroxy-2-methyl-6,8-bis(methylamino)-4*H*-pyrano[2,3-*b*] [1,4]benzodioxin-4-one sulfate, tetrahydrate.

Microbiology: Spectinomycin is bacteriostatic and exerts its antibacterial effect by binding to the 30S ribosome and inhibiting bacterial protein synthesis. Spectinomycin has activity against a variety of gram-negative bacteria, some mycoplasma, and a limited number of gram-positive bacteria. Generally, it is not active against anaerobic bacteria.

Spectinomycin has demonstrated *in vitro* and *in vivo* activity against the three major pathogenic bacteria *(Pasteurella haemolytica, Pasteurella multocida,* and *Haemophilus somnus)* associated with bovine respiratory disease (pneumonia).

Spectinomycin has also demonstrated *in vitro* activity against *Actinomyces pyogenes, Mycoplasma bovis,* and *Mycoplasma dispar.* The clinical significance of this *in vitro* activity in cattle has not been demonstrated.

Dosage and Administration: ADSPEC® Sterile Solution is to be administered to cattle at a daily dose of 10 to 15 mg spectinomycin per kg of body weight (4.5 to 6.8 mL per 100 lb body weight). Treatment should be administered at 24-hour intervals for 3 to 5 consecutive days. Selection of dose (10 to 15 mg/kg/day) and duration of treatment (3 to 5 days) should be based on an assessment of the severity of disease, pathogen susceptibility, and clinical response. Do not inject more than 50 mL per site.

ADSPEC® Sterile Solution is to be administered to cattle by subcutaneous injection in the neck.

Contraindication(s): As with all drugs, the use of ADSPEC® Sterile Solution is contraindicated in animals previously found to be hypersensitive to the drug.

Precaution(s): Storage Conditions: Store at controlled room temperature 20° to 25°C (68° to 77°F) [for additional information see USP]. Protect from freezing.

Caution(s): Federal (USA) law restricts this drug to use by or on the order of a licensed veterinarian.

The safety of ADSPEC® Sterile Solution has not been determined for cattle intended for breeding.

Discoloration at the injection site may persist beyond 11 days after injection. This may necessitate trimming of the injection site and surrounding tissues at slaughter.

Warning(s): Residue Warnings: Treated cattle must not be slaughtered for 11 days following last treatment. Dosages administered either in excess of the approved maximum dose or by unapproved routes may result in illegal residues in edible tissues.

A withdrawal period has not been established for this product in pre-ruminating calves. Do not use in calves to be processed for veal.

A milk discard period has not been established for this product in lactating dairy cattle. Do not use in female dairy cattle 20 months of age or older. Use of spectinomycin in this class of cattle may cause drug residues in milk.

Human Warnings: Not for human use. Keep out of reach of children.

As with other antibiotics, allergic reactions may occur in previously sensitized individuals. Repeated or prolonged exposure may lead to sensitization. Avoid direct contact with skin, eyes, mouth, and clothing. Persons with a known hypersensitivity to spectinomycin should avoid exposure to this product.

In case of accidental eye exposure, flush with water for 15 minutes. In case of accidental skin exposure, wash with soap and water. Seek medical attention if allergic reactions occur.

The material safety data sheet contains more detailed occupational safety information. To report adverse effects in users, to obtain more information or obtain a material safety data sheet, call 1-800-253-8600.

Trial Data: Animal Safety: Cattle: When spectinomycin sulfate sterile solution was administered at 10 times (150 mg/kg/day) the maximum daily recommended therapeutic dose for 5 days, treatment-related effects included increased relative kidney weights in heifers and steers, squamous and transitional epithelial cells in the urine of steers, and decreased urinary pH in steers. Urinalysis was not performed on the heifers in this study. Minimal injection site reactions were also present at 1 day and 4 days post injection.

When spectinomycin sulfate sterile solution was administered at doses of 15, 45, or 75 mg/kg/day (1X, 3X, or 5X the maximum daily recommended therapeutic dose) for 15 days, treatment-related effects included decreased urinary pH and mild swelling at injection sites. At necropsy, labeled injection sites examined at 1 day and 8 days after injection of 30 mL of spectinomycin sulfate sterile solution had dark red, tan, brown, and/or dark brown areas, often with some expansion (thickening) of the subcutis. Only mild discoloration was observed on gross examination of injection sites at 15 days after injection.

When spectinomycin sulfate sterile solution was administered subcutaneously at a dose of 15 mg/kg/day to 152 crossbred beef calves with naturally occurring BRD in clinical field trials, one calf died following the second daily injection. The cause of death following a gross necropsy was reported as an anaphylactic reaction.

Adverse Reactions: The use of ADSPEC® Sterile Solution may result in mild swelling at the injection site. Anaphylactic reactions may occur in animals previously sensitized.

Presentation: ADSPEC® Sterile Solution is available in 500 mL vials (NDC 0009-7383-05).

Manufactured by: Pharmacia & Upjohn, S.A. de C.V., Calzada de Tlalpan #2962, 04870 Mexico, D.F.

Compendium Code No.: 10490002 801 760 002

ADVANCE™ ARREST®

Milk Specialties **Electrolytes-Oral**

Nutritional Energy Supplement and Electrolytes for Calves, Pigs, Foals, Lambs, and Kids

Guaranteed Analysis:

Sodium, not less than 2.00%
Potassium, not less than 0.50%
Magnesium, not less than 0.05%
Dextrose, not less than 33.00%

It contains electrolytes, minerals, energy sources, dextrose, fiber, gums, acids, vitamin C and calcium pantothenate.

Indications: ADVANCE™ ARREST® is designed for use with young animals that require supplemental energy, nutrients and electrolytes.

To be effective, it must be used as soon as possible when animals require the nutrients mentioned above.

Dosage and Administration: Feeding Directions:

Calves (replacement heifers, bull calves, or veal calves):

Normal Feeding: At first sign of requiring supplemental energy, nutrients and electrolytes, feed ADVANCE™ ARREST® to replace a portion of the regular milk replacer feeding program according to the Feeding and Use Table. Continue feeding ADVANCE™ ARREST® twice per day (10-12 hour intervals) for 4 days or 8 feedings. Return calf to full milk feeding over a 2 day period according to the Feeding and Use Table.

Accelerated Feeding: For calves requiring an increased frequency of feeding of supplemental energy, nutrients, and electrolytes, 4 quarts of ADVANCE™ ARREST® should be fed each 24 hour period with a portion of the milk replacer in an accelerated feeding program. Return calf to full milk feeding over a 2 day period according to the Feeding and Use Table.

Newly arrived, shipped-in calves: Animals newly arrived at a rearing unit and requiring supplemental energy, nutrients, and electrolytes should be fed 1 quart milk replacer and 2 quarts of ADVANCE™ ARREST® twice a day. Follow directions provided in the Feeding and Use Table.

Feeding/Management Recommendations for All Calves: At each feeding, feed the milk replacer first followed by ADVANCE™ ARREST® 15 minutes later. Any ADVANCE™ ARREST® not voluntarily consumed within 15 minutes should be given by esophageal feeder.

Provide water free choice.

Feed from an open pail or nipple.

Pigs: For individual baby pigs, use a syringe with a small plastic tube for force feeding or a dose bottle/pump. Baby pigs still with the sow should be group fed mixed ADVANCE™ ARREST® ad-libitum for 24-48 hours using a suitable feeder. Weaned pigs should be fed mixed ADVANCE™ ARREST® ad-libitum for 12 hours and access to normal water source limited during this period. If mixed product gets too thick for water systems, mix at ½ strength (½ measure per 2 quarts or one measure per 4 quarts).

Lamb/Kid: If lamb/kid is being fed milk from a nipple bottle, feed mixed product in the bottle or feed through normal feeders or tube.

Foal: Feed from an open pail or with a tube.

Discussion: ADVANCE™ ARREST® is a free flowing buff colored powder that easily mixes in warm water. A gelling agent helps hold insoluble fiber in suspension.

ADVANCE™ ARREST® was developed through a research program in conjunction with the University of Illinois and extensive data on its use available.*

*For further information on why electrolyte balance is so important for young animals, contact Milk Specialties Company.

Presentation: 100 g foil packets and 10 lb pails with measuring cup included.

Compendium Code No.: 10850010

ADVANCE™ CALF MEDIC® CONCENTRATE

Milk Specialties **Feed Medication**

Medicated Scour Control Supplement

Active Ingredient(s):

Oxytetracycline .... 6,400 grams/ton (3.2 g/lb)
Neomycin Base .... 12,800 grams/ton (6.4 g/lb)

Guaranteed Analysis:

Crude Protein, not less than 8.0%
Crude Fat, not less than 0.5%
Crude Fiber, not more than 0.2%
Ash, not more than 20.0%
Added minerals, not more than 10.0%
Vitamin A, not more than .... 800,000 IU/lb
Vitamin D_3, not less than .... 160,000 IU/lb
Vitamin E, not less than .... 525 IU/lb
Energy, ME (Calculated) .... 2600 Kcal/kg

Indications: As an aid in the prevention or treatment of bacterial diarrhea (scours).

Dosage and Administration: Feeding Directions:

Prevention: Mix one half jar (1.67 pounds or 26.7 net oz) of ADVANCE™ CALF MEDIC® Concentrate with 50 pounds of dry, non-medicated milk replacer or feed ingredients to make a type C medicated milk replacer containing dry levels as indicated below under directions for use.

Direction's for Use (Type C Feed): As an aid in the prevention of bacterial enteritis (scours).

Oxytetracycline .... 200 g/t
Neomycin Base .... 400 g/t

Feed as complete ration. Reconstitute this medicated milk replacer at 1 lb powder per 1 gallon of water to provide 100 milligrams of oxytetracycline plus 200 milligrams of neomycin base per gallon of milk replacer.

Treatment: Mix one jar (3.34 pounds or 53.4 net oz) of ADVANCE™ CALF MEDIC® Concentrate with 50 pounds of dry, non-medicated milk replacer or feed ingredients to make a type C medicated milk replacer containing drug levels as indicated below under directions for use.

Directions for Use (Type C Feed): As an aid in the treatment of bacterial enteritis (scours).

Oxytetracycline .... 400 g/t
Neomycin Sulfate .... 800 g/t

Feed as complete ration. Reconstitute this medicated milk replacer at 1 lb powder per 1 gallon of water to provide 200 milligrams of oxytetracycline plus 400 milligrams of neomycin base per gallon of milk replacer.

Warning(s): Withdraw this feed 30 days before slaughter.

Presentation: Available in 3.34 lb pail.

Compendium Code No.: 10850030

ADVANCE™ CALVITA® DELUXE MEDICATED MILK REPLACER

Milk Specialties **Milk Replacer**

Active Ingredient(s):

Oxytetracycline .... 100 grams/ton
Neomycin Base (from Neomycin Sulfate) .... 200 grams/ton

Guaranteed Analysis:

Crude Protein, not less than 22.00%
Crude Fat, not less than 10.00%
Crude Fiber, not more than 1.0%
Calcium, not less than 0.75%
Calcium, not more than 1.25%
Phosphorus, not less than 0.70%
Vitamin A, not less than .... 30,000 IU/lb
Vitamin D_3, not less than .... 10,000 IU/lb
Vitamin E, not less than .... 100 IU/lb

Ingredients: Dried whey, dried whey product, soy flour, animal and vegetable fat (preserved with BHA and BHT), lecithin, dried skimmed milk, dried milk protein, dicalcium phosphate, calcium carbonate, vitamin A supplement, vitamin D_3 supplement, vitamin E supplement, ascorbic acid, magnesium oxide, zinc sulfate, ferrous sulfate, niacin supplement, manganese sulfate, calcium pantothenate, vitamin B_5 supplement, thiamine mononitrate, riboflavin supplement, copper sulfate, pyridoxine hydrochloride, ethylenediamine dihydriodide, folic acid, choline chloride, cobalt sulfate, sodium selenite, sodium silico aluminate, polyoxyethylene glycol (400) mono and dioleates, artificial flavor.

Indications: A dairy herd and dairy beef calf milk replacer for aid in the prevention of bacterial diarrhea (scours).

Feeding Instructions: In any calf raising program, it is important that calves receive colostrum for the first 3 days. Feed first milk colostrum during the first 24 hours of life (first feeding within 1 hour following birth). For Days 2-3 feed transitional colostrum, then on Day 4 feed CALVITA® Milk Replacer. If transitional colostrum is not available, feed CALVITA® Milk Replacer starting on Day 2.

Mixing: Sprinkle ½ lb* of milk replacer into a bucket of warm water (110°F) and bring to a total volume of 2 quarts.

Cold Weather Mixing: Feed three times a day at equal intervals. Sprinkle ½ lb of milk replacer into a bucket of warm water (110°F) and bring to a total volume of 2 quarts.

Always make reconstituted milk replacer as needed for immediate feeding.

Feeding: Beginning on day 4, introduce milk replacer.

Light Breed Calves: 1½ to 2 quarts liquid milk replacer twice per day.

Heavy Breed Calves: 2 to 2½ quarts of liquid milk replacer twice per day.

Management Tips: For best mixing, sprinkle milk replacer powder onto water.

Use a wire whisk to agitate powder and water.

Fresh, clean water should be available at all times.

Feeding and mixing equipment should be cleaned after each feeding.

Introduce a good quality calf starter at 7 days of age.

Offer free choice hay after weaning.

Wean calves when eating at least 1½ to 2 lbs calf starter per head per day.

One measuring cup (enclosed in bag) holds approximately ½ lb of dry milk replacer. Check cup quantity periodically.

Caution(s): This product contains quality soy flour which contributes protein and fiber, therefore, this product is not recommended as sole source of milk replacement for animals less than three (3) weeks of age.

Warning(s): Withdraw this feed 30 days before slaughter.

A withdrawal period has not been established for this medication in pre-ruminating calves. Do not use in calves to be processed for veal.

Presentation: 25 lb (11.36 kg) and 50 lb (22.72 kg) bags.

Compendium Code No.: 10850040

ADVANCE™ CALVITA® SUPREME MEDICATED A.M. MILK REPLACER WITH BOVATEC®

Milk Specialties **Milk Replacer**

Active Ingredient(s):

Lasalocid (as lasalocid sodium) .... 90 g/ton

Guaranteed Analysis:

Crude Protein, not less than 18.00%
Crude Fat, not less than 21.00%
Crude Fiber, not more than 0.15%
Calcium, not less than 0.75%
Calcium, not more than 1.25%
Phosphorus, not less than 0.70%
Vitamin A, not less than .... 30,000 IU/lb
Vitamin D_3, not less than .... 10,000 IU/lb
Vitamin E, not less than .... 200 IU/lb

Ingredients: Dried whey, dried whey protein concentrate, dried whey product, animal and vegetable fat (preserved with BHA and BHT), dried skimmed milk, lecithin, dried milk protein, dicalcium phosphate, calcium carbonate, L-lysine, DL-methionine, vitamin A supplement, vitamin D_3 supplement, vitamin E supplement, ascorbic acid, magnesium oxide, zinc sulfate, ferrous sulfate, niacin supplement, manganese sulfate, calcium pantothenate, vitamin B_{12} supplement, thiamine mononitrate, riboflavin supplement, copper sulfate, pyridoxine hydrochloride, ethylenediamine dihydriodide, folic acid, choline chloride, cobalt sulfate, sodium selenite, sodium silico aluminate, polyoxyethylene glycol (400) mono and dioleates, artificial flavor.

Indications: A dairy herd and dairy beef calf milk replacer for the control of coccidiosis caused by *Eimeria bovis* and *Eimeria zurnii* in replacement calves.

Feeding Instructions: In any calf raising program, it is important that calves receive colostrum for the first 3 days. Feed first milk colostrum during the first 24 hours of life (first feeding within 1 hour following birth). For Days 2-3 feed transitional colostrum, then on Day 4 feed CALVITA® Milk Replacer. If transitional colostrum is not available, feed CALVITA® Milk Replacer starting on Day 2.

Mixing: Sprinkle ½ lb* of milk replacer into a bucket of warm water (110°F) and bring to a total volume of 2 quarts.

Feeding: Beginning on day 4, introduce milk replacer.

Light Breed Calves: 1½ to 2 quarts liquid milk replacer twice per day.

Heavy Breed Calves: 2 to 2½ quarts of liquid milk replacer twice per day.

Management Tips: For best mixing, sprinkle milk replacer powder onto water.

Use a wire whisk to agitate powder and water.

Fresh, clean water should be available at all times.

Feeding and mixing equipment should be cleaned after each feeding.

Introduce a good quality calf starter at 7 days of age.

Offer free choice hay after weaning.

Wean calves when eating at least 1½ to 2 lbs calf starter per head per day.

One measuring cup (enclosed in bag) holds approximately ½ lb of dry milk replacer. Check cup quantity periodically.

This product contains 45 milligrams of lasalocid per pound. Feed to provide 45 milligrams of lasalocid per 100 pounds (1 mg/2.2 lbs) of body weight daily. Feed during periods of coccidiosis exposure or when experience indicates coccidiosis is likely to be a problem.

Caution(s): The safety of lasalocid in unapproved species has not been established.

Warning(s): Withdrawal period has not been established for lasalocid in pre-ruminating calves.

Do not feed to lactating cows.

Do not use in calves to be processed for veal.

Do not feed to foals, dogs, and cats.

Presentation: 50 lb (22.72 kg) bag.

Compendium Code No.: 10850050

ADVANCE™ CALVITA® SUPREME MEDICATED A.M. MILK REPLACER WITH OTC/NEO

Milk Specialties **Milk Replacer**

Active Ingredient(s):

Oxytetracycline .... 200 grams/ton
Neomycin Base (from Neomycin Sulfate) .... 400 grams/ton

Guaranteed Analysis:

Crude Protein, not less than 18.00%
Crude Fat, not less than 21.00%
Crude Fiber, not more than 0.15%
Calcium, not less than 0.75%
Calcium, not more than 1.25%
Phosphorus, not less than 0.70%
Vitamin A, not less than .... 30,000 IU/lb
Vitamin D_3, not less than .... 10,000 IU/lb
Vitamin E, not less than .... 200 IU/lb

Ingredients: Dried whey, dried whey protein concentrate, dried whey product, animal and vegetable fat (preserved with BHA and BHT), dried skimmed milk, lecithin, dried milk protein, dicalcium phosphate, calcium carbonate, L-lysine, DL-methionine, vitamin A supplement, vitamin D_3 supplement, vitamin E supplement, ascorbic acid, magnesium oxide, zinc sulfate, ferrous sulfate, niacin supplement, manganese sulfate, calcium pantothenate, vitamin B_{12} supplement, thiamine mononitrate, riboflavin supplement, copper sulfate, pyridoxine hydrochloride, ethylenediamine dihydriodide, folic acid, choline chloride, cobalt sulfate, sodium selenite, sodium silico aluminate, polyoxyethylene glycol (400) mono and dioleates, artificial flavor.

Indications: A dairy herd and dairy beef calf milk replacer for aid in the treatment of bacterial diarrhea (scours).

Feeding Instructions: In any calf raising program, it is important that calves receive colostrum for the first 3 days. Feed first milk colostrum during the first 24 hours of life (first feeding within 1 hour following birth). For Days 2-3 feed transitional colostrum, then on Day 4 feed CALVITA® Milk Replacer. If transitional colostrum is not available, feed CALVITA® Milk Replacer starting on Day 2.

Mixing: Sprinkle ½ lb* of milk replacer into a bucket of warm water (110°F) and bring to a total volume of 2 quarts.

Cold Weather Mixing: Feed three times a day at equal intervals. Sprinkle ½ lb of milk replacer into a bucket of warm water (110°F) and bring to a total volume of 2 quarts.

Always make reconstituted milk replacer as needed for immediate feeding.

Feeding: Beginning on day 4, introduce milk replacer.

Light Breed Calves: 1½ to 2 quarts liquid milk replacer twice per day.

Heavy Breed Calves: 2 to 2½ quarts of liquid milk replacer twice per day.

Management Tips: For best mixing, sprinkle milk replacer powder onto water.

Use a wire whisk to agitate powder and water.

Fresh, clean water should be available at all times.

Feeding and mixing equipment should be cleaned after each feeding.

Introduce a good quality calf starter at 7 days of age.

Offer free choice hay after weaning.

Wean calves when eating at least 1½ to 2 lbs calf starter per head per day.

One measuring cup (enclosed in bag) holds approximately ½ lb of dry milk replacer. Check cup quantity periodically.

Warning(s): Withdraw this feed 30 days before slaughter.

A withdrawal period has not been established for this medication in pre-ruminating calves. Do not use in calves to be processed for veal.

Presentation: 50 lb (22.72 kg) bag.

Compendium Code No.: 10850060

ADVANCE™ ENERGY BOOSTER 100®

Milk Specialties **Large Animal Dietary Supplement**

98% pure bypass fatty acids

Guaranteed Analysis:

Total Fatty Acids, not less than 98.00%
Unsaponifiable Matter, not more than 2.00%
Insoluble Impurities, not more than 1.00%
Moisture, not more than 1.00%

Ingredient Listing: Hydrolyzed animal fat (preserved with BHT), sodium silico aluminate.

Indications: A high energy density dietary supplement for dairy cows.

Feeding Directions: ENERGY BOOSTER 100® has been proven as the most palatable rumen inert or bypass fat and can be fed as a top dress, in a total mixed ration or in a grain mix.

The recommended feeding rate is ¼ lb to 1 lb per cow per day depending on stage of lactation. The following table will assist choosing the right amount of ENERGY BOOSTER 100® to feed.

Production Level		Early Lactation	Mid-Lactation	Late Lactation
>24,000 lbs	% Total fat in the diet	5.0-6.0	4.5-6.0	max 4.5
	lb of ENERGY BOOSTER 100® in the diet*	0.5-1.0	0.5-1.0	0.3-0.5
<18-24,000 lbs	% Total fat in the diet	approx. 5.0	4.0-5.0	max 4.5
	lb of ENERGY BOOSTER 100® in the diet	0.5-1.0	0.5-0.75	0.25
<18,000 lbs	% Total fat in the diet	4.5-5.0	4.5	4.0
	lb of ENERGY BOOSTER 100® in the diet	0.5-1.0	0.25-0.50	0.25
Dry and Pre-Fresh Cows	lb of ENERGY BOOSTER 100® in the diet		0.1-0.2	

*Beneficial in grazing herds and high forage diets.

For best results with dairy cows: Restrict the use of free fats (such as tallow, grease) to 1.0% or less of the dry matter.

Restrict the amount of fat from oilseeds (cottonseed, soybeans) to less than 1% of the dry matter.

Use ENERGY BOOSTER 100® to add up to 2% fat units in the diet.

Keep total fat level in the diet below 5.0 or 5.5%.

Start feeding ENERGY BOOSTER 100® at 2 oz per cow per day three weeks prior to calving and then increase as necessary during first weeks of lactation as appetite and intake increase.

Precaution(s): Do not store in direct sunlight or in temperatures exceeding 115°F.

Discussion: ENERGY BOOSTER 100® is a blend of specific free fatty acids which provide the dairy cow with a pure energy that does not interfere with rumen fermentation and fiber digestion. It was developed by Milk Specialties Company.

When added to the ration of the dairy cow, ENERGY BOOSTER 100® increases the energy density of the diet. The extra energy provided supports higher milk production, improves body condition leading to better reproduction and less heat stress.

Presentation: 50 lb bags.

Compendium Code No.: 10850070

ADVANCE™ PRO-LYTE PLUS®

Milk Specialties **Electrolytes-Oral**

Nutritional Energy Supplement and Electrolytes

Guaranteed Analysis:

Sodium, not less than 4.8%
Potassium, not less than 1.8%
Magnesium, not less than 0.16%

This product contains electrolytes, acetate, vitamin C and calcium pantothenate, glycine, alkalizing agents and salts of organic acids in a powder form.

Indications: PRO-LYTE PLUS® is a nutritional energy supplement supplying electrolytes for calves, piglets, foals, lambs and kids. It provides rapidly available energy and essential electrolytes

A

and fluids when mixed with water and should be fed as soon as possible when the animal requires supplemental energy, nutrients and electrolytes.

Dosage and Administration: Feeding Directions:

Calves (replacement heifers, bull calves, or veal calves):

Normal Feeding: At first sign of requiring supplemental energy, nutrients and electrolytes, feed PRO-LYTE PLUS® to replace a portion of the regular milk replacer feeding program according to the Feeding and Use Table. Continue feeding PRO-LYTE PLUS® twice per day (10-12 hour intervals) for 4 days or 8 feedings. Return calf to full milk feeding over a 2 day period according to the Feeding and Use Table.

Accelerated Feeding: For calves requiring an increased frequency of feeding of supplemental energy, nutrients, and electrolytes, 4 quarts of PRO-LYTE PLUS® should be fed each 24 hour period with a portion of the milk replacer in an accelerated feeding program. Return calf to full milk feeding over a 2 day period according to the Feeding and Use Table.

Newly arrived, shipped-in calves: Animals newly arrived at a rearing unit and requiring supplemental energy, nutrients, and electrolytes should be fed 1 quart milk replacer and 2 quarts of PRO-LYTE PLUS® twice a day. Follow directions provided in the Feeding and Use Table.

Feeding/Management Recommendations for All Calves: At each feeding, feed the milk replacer first followed by PRO-LYTE PLUS® 15 minutes later. Any PRO-LYTE PLUS® not voluntarily consumed within 15 minutes should be given by esophageal feeder.

Provide water free choice.

Feed from an open pail or nipple.

Pigs: For individual baby pigs, use a syringe with a small plastic tube for force feeding or a dose bottle/pump. Baby pigs still with the sow should be group fed mixed PRO-LYTE PLUS® ad-libitum for 24-48 hours using a suitable feeder. Weaned pigs should be fed mixed PRO-LYTE PLUS® ad-libitum for 12 hours and access to normal water source limited during this period.

Lamb/Kid: If lamb/kid is being fed milk from a nipple bottle, feed mixed product in the bottle or feed through normal feeders or tube.

Foal: Feed from an open pail or with a tube.

Discussion: Neonatal diarrhea is generally accompanied by losses of water, sodium, potassium and bicarbonate. Losses of these nutrients result in dehydration, acidosis and depletion of potassium. The key attributes of an oral electrolyte are to correct the dehydration and acidosis of the young animal. In addition, the oral electrolyte should replenish the lost electrolytes and provide energy.

Rehydrating the neonate is the most critical and is usually achieved by providing water and salt. The absorption of water and salt can be enhanced with the inclusion of glycines, acetate and citrate into the solution. PRO-LYTE PLUS® contains all three ingredients.

The next critical area to correct is acidosis. Research shows that young animals treated with an oral electrolyte that provides an alkalizing agent have a more complete recovery. Sodium bicarbonate, an alkalizing agent, raises the abomassal pH when fed. Acetate and citrate act as alkalizing agents within the cell tissues. The inclusion of these metabolizing bases can reduce the burden on the kidneys to correct acidosis.

PRO-LYTE PLUS® is formulated with sodium bicarbonate, acetate and citrate to increase system pH. In addition, oral electrolytes with a strong ion difference (Na^+ K^- Cl^-), greater than plasma will have a tendency to alkalinize. PRO-LYTE PLUS® has a specific ion difference (SID) of 70 mEq/L.

Presentation: Available in 4 oz (113.5 g) foil packets and 8 lb pails with measuring cup included.

Compendium Code No.: 10850080

ADVANCE™ RUMIN 8™

Milk Specialties **Large Animal Dietary Supplement**

Guaranteed Analysis:

Crude Protein, not less than	2.50%
Crude Fat, not less than	0.50%
Crude Fiber, not more than	0.20%
Carbohydrate, not less than	70.00%
ADF, not more than	0.20%
Ash, not more than	14.00%
Calcium, not less than	1.00%
Calcium, not more than	1.50%
Phosphorus, not less than	0.65%
Potassium, not less than	2.25%

Ingredient Listing: Dried corn syrup, dried whey product, malic acid, fumaric acid, maltodextrins, dextrose, artificial flavor 797.

Indications: A nutritional supplement (soluble sugars) for use in lactating dairy cows.

Recommended to promote rumen microbial activity and to increase energy and protein availability.

Feeding Directions: RUMIN 8™ is a highly palatable nutritional supplement that can be fed as a top dress, in a total mixed ration (TMR), in a grain mix (concentrate) and/or in pelleted feed.

The recommended feeding rate is ⅓ to ½ lb per cow per day. However, it is suggested that producers start their cows at the ½ lb rate to insure a positive response.

The types of diets that have shown the greatest responses to RUMIN 8™ supplementation are:

Dry, mature corn silage and corn grain (kernels passing thru undigested).

Diets containing supplemented urea.

The feeding rate of RUMIN 8™ will depend on 2 factors: (1) the level of soluble protein in the diet and (2) the sugar and starch concentration in the feedstuffs and their relative availability. Diets low in sugar and high in soluble protein, especially if supplemented with urea, will probably require the ½ lb per cow per day use.

Discussion: The advantages of supplementing soluble sugars and organic acids to lactating dairy cows are greater uptake of rumen ammonia, lower blood urea and greater microbial protein. Adequate soluble sugar levels will allow for maximum milk production and economical use of microbial protein.

Presentation: 50 lbs (22.67 kg).

Compendium Code No.: 10850090

ADVANTAGE®

(imidacloprid) Topical Solution

Bayer

Once-a-month topical flea treatment for cats and kittens 8 weeks and older, and dogs and puppies 7 weeks and older.

READ THE ENTIRE LABEL BEFORE EACH USE

For the Prevention and Treatment of Flea Infestations

- Available only through licensed practicing veterinarians
- Kills 98-100% of the fleas on cats and dogs within 12 hours
- One treatment prevents further flea infestation for up to four weeks on cats and at least four weeks on dogs
- Kills fleas before they lay eggs
- Convenient, easy to apply

Active Ingredient	% By Weight
Imidacloprid; 1-[(6-Chloro-3-pyridinyl) methyl]-N-nitro-2-imidazolidinimine	9.1%
Inert Ingredients	90.9%
Total	100.0%

KEEP OUT OF REACH OF CHILDREN

WARNING

See Below for First Aid and Precautionary Statements

Precautionary Statements

Hazards to Humans

Causes eye irritation. Harmful if swallowed. Do not get in eyes or on clothing. Avoid contact with skin. Wash hands thoroughly with soap and warm water after handling. Keep out of reach of children. Do not contaminate feed or food.

Hazards to Domestic Animals

For external use only. Do not use on kittens under eight weeks of age or puppies under seven weeks of age. As with any product, consult your veterinarian before using this product on debilitated, aged, pregnant or nursing animals. Individual sensitivities, while rare, may occur after using ANY pesticide product for pets. If signs persist, or become more severe, consult a veterinarian immediately. If your animal is on medication, consult your veterinarian before using this or any other product. For consumer questions call 1-800-255-6826. For medical emergencies call 1-877-258-2280.

First Aid

If in eyes: Hold eyelids open and flush with plenty of water. Get medical attention if irritation persists.

If swallowed: Call a physician or Poison Control Center.

If on skin: Wash with plenty of soap and water.

To Physician: Treat the patient symptomatically.

Directions for Use

It is a violation of Federal Law to use this product in a manner inconsistent with its labeling.

How to Apply

1. Use Advantage® 9 and Advantage® 18 only on cats. Use Advantage® 10, Advantage® 20, Advantage® 55 and Advantage® 100 only on dogs. Do not use on other animals.
2. Remove one applicator tube from the package.

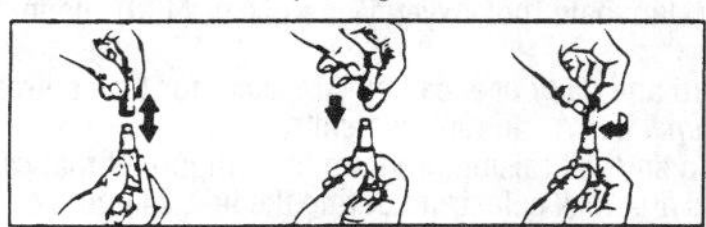

3. Hold applicator tube in an upright position. Pull cap off tube.
4. Turn the cap around and place other end of cap back on tube.
5. Twist cap to break seal, then remove cap from tube.
6. Cats:

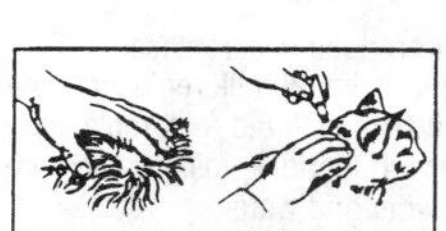

Part the hair in the neck at the base of the skull until the skin is visible. Place the tip of the tube on the skin and squeeze the tube twice to *expel the entire contents of the tube directly on the skin. Do not get this product in your pet's eyes or mouth.* The product is bitter tasting and salivation may occur for a short time if the cat licks the product immediately after treatment. Treatment at the base of the skull will minimize the opportunity for the cat to lick the product.

Dogs:

10 lbs. and under:

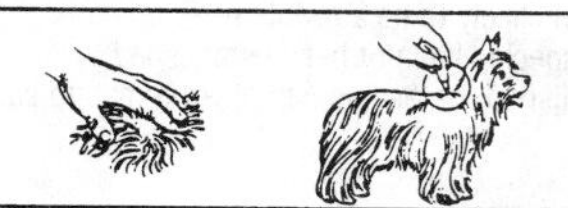

11-20 lbs.:

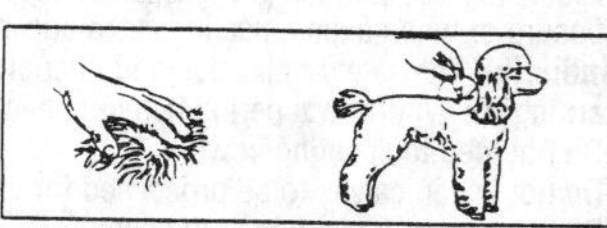

The dog should be standing for easy application. Part the hair on the dog's back, between the shoulder blades, until the skin is visible. Place the tip of the tube on the skin and squeeze the tube twice to *expel the entire contents directly on the skin. Do not get this product in your pet's eyes or mouth.*

21-55 lbs.:

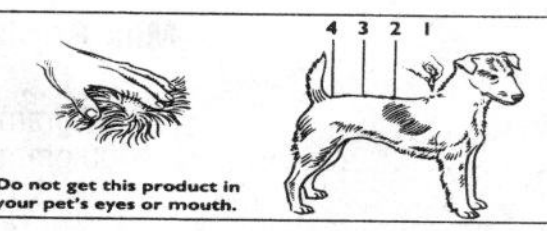

Over 55 lbs.:

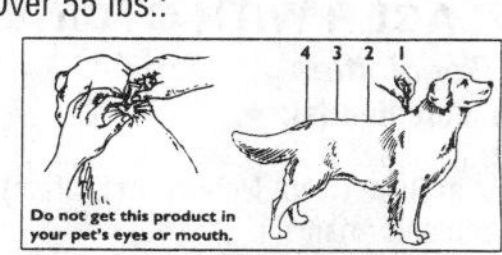

The dog should be standing for easy application. The entire contents of the Advantage® tube should be applied evenly to three or four spots on the top of the back from the shoulder to the base of the tail. At each spot, part the hair until the skin is visible. Place the tip of the tube on the skin and gently squeeze to expel a portion of the solution on the skin. Do not apply an excessive amount of solution at any one spot that could cause some of the solution to run off the side of the dog.

7. Discard empty tube as described in Storage and Disposal.

Use the calendar stickers to remind you when your pet is due for its next monthly application of Advantage®.

The successive feeding activity of fleas on pets may elicit a hypersensitivity skin disorder known as flea allergy dermatitis (FAD). Treatment of pets with Advantage® rapidly kills fleas and may reduce the incidence of this condition.

Advantage® kills 98-100% of the existing fleas on pets within 12 hours. Reinfesting fleas are killed within 2 hours with protection against further flea infestation lasting for up to four (4) weeks on cats and at least four (4) weeks on dogs. Pre-existing pupae in the environment may continue to emerge for six (6) weeks or longer depending upon the climatic conditions.

Larval flea stages in the pet's surroundings are killed following contact with an Advantage® treated pet. Advantage® remains efficacious following a shampoo treatment, swimming or after exposure to rain or sunlight.

Monthly treatments are required for optimal control and prevention of fleas.

If re-treatment becomes necessary earlier than four weeks, do not re-treat more than once weekly.

Storage and Disposal

Do not contaminate water, food or feed by storage or disposal.

Storage: Store in a cool, dry place.

Pesticide Disposal: Securely wrap original container in several layers of newspaper and discard in trash.

Container Disposal: Do not reuse empty container. Wrap container and put in trash.

Limited Warranty and Limitation of Damages

Bayer Corporation, Agriculture Division, Animal Health warrants that this material conforms to the chemical description on the label. BAYER CORPORATION MAKES NO OTHER EXPRESS OR IMPLIED WARRANTY, INCLUDING ANY OTHER EXPRESS OR IMPLIED WARRANTY OF FITNESS OR MERCHANTABILITY, and no agent of Bayer Corporation is authorized to do so except in writing with a specific reference to this warranty. Any damages arising from a breach of this warranty shall be limited to direct damages and shall not include consequential commercial damages such as loss of profits or values, etc.

Orange/9 For Cats and Kittens 8 Weeks and Older and 9 lbs. and Under.
Code 0326—Four 0.4 mL Tubes
Code 0536—Six 0.4 mL Tubes
EPA Est. 11556-DEU-1 EPA Reg. No. 11556-116 0536, R.1

Purple/18 For Cats and Kittens 8 Weeks and Older and Over 9 lbs.
Code 0327—Four 0.8 mL Tubes
Code 0537—Six 0.8 mL Tubes
EPA Est. 11556-DEU-1 EPA Reg. No. 11556-118 0537, R.1

Green/10 For Small Dogs and Puppies 7 Weeks and Older and 10 lbs. and Under
Code 0328—Four 0.4 mL Tubes
Code 0538—Six 0.4 mL Tubes
EPA Est. 11556-DEU-1 EPA Reg. No. 11556-117 0328/0538, R.7

Teal/20 For Dogs and Puppies 7 Weeks and Older and 11-20 lbs.
Code 0329—Four 1.0 mL Tubes
Code 0539—Six 1.0 mL Tubes
EPA Est. 11556-DEU-1 EPA Reg. No. 11556-119 0329/0539, R.7

Red/55 For Dogs and Puppies 7 Weeks and Older and 21-55 lbs.
Code 0330—Four 2.5 mL Tubes
Code 0540—Six 2.5 mL Tubes
EPA Est. 11556-DEU-1 EPA Reg. No. 11556-120 0330/0540, R.7

Blue/100 For Dogs and Puppies 7 Weeks and Older and Over 55 lbs.
Code 0331—Four 4.0 mL Tubes
Code 0541—Six 4.0 mL Tubes
EPA Est. 11556-DEU-1 EPA Reg. No. 11556-122 0331/0541, R.6

Made in Germany

Manufactured For Bayer Corporation, Agriculture Division, Animal Health, Shawnee Mission, Kansas 66201 U.S.A.

Compendium Code No.: 10400051

ADVANTIX™

(see **K9 ADVANTIX™** *– page 1673)*

AE + POX

ASL **Vaccine**

U.S. Vet. Lic. No.: 226

Active Ingredient(s): AE + POX is a live virus vaccine of chicken embryo origin containing both AE and pox viruses. The AE virus was selected for its affinity for the chicken's intestinal tract and immunizing capability.

The strain of fowl pox virus contained in the AE + POX has the ability to give good takes and immunity in chickens 10 to 18 weeks of age. One vaccination usually lasts through the laying period.

Indications: For the vaccination of healthy, susceptible chickens between 10 and 18 weeks of age, intended for use as breeder or commercial layer replacements against avian encephalomyelitis (AE) and fowl pox.

Dosage and Administration: AE + POX is administered by wing-web stab. Vaccinated birds should be examined in 7-10 days for fowl pox "takes." Small inflamed wart-like swellings will be seen at the site of inoculation on susceptible birds if the vaccine was properly applied. If for any reason the birds do not have the reaction, they should be revaccinated immediately in order to ensure flock immunity.

Wing-Web Administration:

1. Rehydrate the vaccine according to the package insert. Do not break off any of the needles on the applicator.
2. Hold the chicken and spread the underside of one wing outward.
3. Dip the applicator into the vaccine bottle, wetting both needles.
4. Pierce the web of the exposed wing with the charged applicator.
5. Redip the applicator in the vaccine vial and proceed to the next bird.
6. Avoid hitting blood vessels, bones and the wing muscle.
7. Be careful not to touch any part of the bird with the vaccine except the area to be inoculated.
8. Examine and record takes on 10% of the flock 7-10 days following vaccination. A normal take shows a slight swelling and scab formation at the site of vaccination. Takes generally disappear two (2) weeks following vaccination.

Precaution(s): Refrigerator under 45°F (7°C) until ready for use. Vaccines are perishable unless properly stored.

Caution(s): Careless handling of the vaccine may result in contamination of unfeathered parts of the chickens. The vaccine should only be used on healthy, susceptible birds between the ages of 10 and 18 weeks. Do not use less than one dose per bird.

If the breeder birds are vaccinated, hatching eggs should not be saved until at least six weeks after vaccination. In susceptible layers, the vaccine could cause a 5 to 15% drop in egg production for two or three weeks. The virus will pass to the progeny hatched from eggs produced during this period.

Vaccinated pullets should not be added to nonvaccinated flocks in production.

Consult a poultry pathologist for further recommendations, based on conditions existing in a designated area at any given time.

Do not open and mix the vaccine until ready to begin vaccination. Use the entire contents immediately after mixing. Burn the containers and all unused contents.

The capacity of the vaccine to produce satisfactory results depends upon many factors, including, but not limited to, conditions of storage and handling by the user, administration of the vaccine, health and responsiveness of individual animals and the degree of field exposure. Therefore, directions for use should be followed carefully.

Consult an American Scientific Laboratories representative or local poultry pathologist for a monitoring program to determine the effectiveness of the vaccine application. The use of the vaccine is subject to applicable state and federal laws and regulations.

Warning(s): Do not vaccinate within four (4) weeks of initial egg production, nor within 21 days before slaughter.

Do not vaccinate on premises with susceptible laying birds or young chickens. The virus may spread from the vaccinated birds and affect egg production of the layers or the health of young susceptible chickens.

Presentation: Wing-web use: 1,000 dose vials.

Compendium Code No.: 11020000

AE-POXINE®

Fort Dodge **Vaccine**

Avian Encephalomyelitis-Fowl Pox Vaccine, Live Virus

U.S. Vet. Lic. No.: 112

Contents: This product contains the antigens listed above.

Contains gentamicin as a preservative.

Indications: AE-POXINE® is recommended for the prevention of avian encephalomyelitis and fowl pox when it is administered as directed to healthy pullets between the ages of eight weeks and four weeks before the start of egg production.

Directions: Read in full, follow directions carefully.

1. Rehydrate 1 vial of this vaccine with 1 vial of diluent.
2. Remove aluminum seal and rubber stopper from vaccine vial and from diluent vial. Avoid contamination of the stoppers and the vials' contents.

1,000 Doses:

3. Pour approximately one-half the diluent into the vaccine vial. Replace stopper and shake gently until contents are dissolved.
4. Pour all the reconstituted vaccine back into the remaining diluent in the diluent bottle. Replace diluent stopper and gently mix. The vaccine is then ready for use.
5. Hold individual bird and spread wing with the underside facing upwards.
6. Dip the vaccinator tool into the vaccine. Take care that the channels of the needles are immersed.
7. Stick the vaccine-laden needles through the membrane, or web, of the wing, avoiding blood vessels, bones, and wing muscles.
8. Attempt to use all of the vaccine from 1 vial within 1 hour after rehydrating.

Takes: The usual take consists of some swelling at the site of the puncture as early as the fourth day following vaccination. The swelling may increase during the next 5 days, and a scab may form at the site.

Records: Keep a record of vaccine serial number and expiration date; date of receipt and date of vaccination; where vaccination took place; and any reactions observed.

Precaution(s): Store this vaccine at not over 45°F (7°C). Use entire contents when vial is first opened. Burn vaccine container and all unused contents.

Do not expose the vaccine to either direct sunlight or extreme heat during the vaccinating period.

This product should be stored, transported, and administered in accordance with the directions.

This vaccine is nonreturnable.

Caution(s): The vaccine should not be allowed to touch the feathers, the head of the chicken, or the bird's skin (except at the site of vaccination).

The use of this vaccine is subject to state laws, wherever applicable.

Warning(s): Do not vaccinate within 21 days before slaughter.

If given to laying flocks, this live virus vaccine could cause a significant or even serious drop in egg production - often lasting 10 days to 2 weeks. Eggs for hatching should not be taken from the flock until 4 weeks have passed following vaccination. Do not vaccinate or expose chicks under 3 weeks of age, sick or debilitated birds, or birds under stress.

For wing-web stab administration only.

For veterinary use only.

Presentation: 10 x 1,000 dose vials.

Compendium Code No.: 10030022 10450A

AE-VAC™

Fort Dodge **Vaccine**

Avian Encephalomyelitis Vaccine, Live Virus

U.S. Vet. Lic. No.: 112

Contents: This product contains the antigens listed above.

Contains gentamicin as a preservative.

Indications: AE-VAC™ is recommended for chicken replacement pullets as an aid in the prevention of avian encephalomyelitis.

Directions: Read in full, follow directions carefully.

Vaccination Recommendations: Vaccinate healthy chickens when they are at least 10 weeks of age but no later than 4 weeks before they start to lay.

For drinking-water administration:

1. Discontinue use of medications or sanitizing agents in the drinking water 24 hours before vaccinating. Do not resume use for 24 hours following vaccination.
2. Water used for the drinking-water administration of a live virus vaccine must be non-chlorinated.
3. Provide enough waterers so two-thirds of the birds may drink at one time. Scrub waterers with fresh, clean, non-chlorinated water, and use no disinfectant. Let the waterers drain dry.
4. Turn off automatic waterers, so the only available water is the vaccine water. Do not give vaccine water through medication tanks.

5. Withhold water for 2 to 4 hours before vaccinating. Do not deprive the birds of water if the temperature is extremely high.
6. Remove seal from vaccine vial.
7. Remove stopper and half-fill vial with clean, cool, non-chlorinated water.
8. Replace stopper and shake until dissolved.
9. Use a clean container two-thirds filled with cool, clean, non-chlorinated water. Add dried milk. Use 2 ounces (56.8 grams) dried milk if final volume of water is to be 4 gallons (15.2 liters) or 12.5 ounces (355 grams) dried milk if final volume of water is to be 25 gallons (95 liters). Stir the mixture until the dried milk is dissolved.
10. Add the rehydrated vaccine from the vial and again stir the contents thoroughly.
11. Next, add the mixture to the final volume of water, as follows:

Add this amount of vaccine	To this final volume of water
1,000 doses	4 gallons (15.2 liters)

12. Give 1 dose of vaccine per bird.
13. Distribute the final volume of vaccine water evenly among the clean waterers. Do not place the waterers in direct sunlight. Resume regular water administration only after all the vaccine water has been consumed.

Records: Keep a record of vaccine serial number and expiration date; date of receipt and date of vaccination; where vaccination took place; and any reactions observed.

Precaution(s): Store this vaccine at not over 45°F (7°C). Use entire contents when vial is first opened. Burn vaccine container and all unused contents.

This product should be stored, transported, and administered in accordance with the directions.

This product is nonreturnable.

Caution(s): The use of this vaccine is subject to state laws , wherever applicable.

Warning(s): Do not vaccinate within 21 days before slaughter.

Do not vaccinate birds in egg production. If given to laying flocks, this live virus vaccine could cause a 10% to 15% drop in production for 10 days to 2 weeks. Eggs for hatching should not be taken from the flock until 4 weeks have passed following vaccination.

For veterinary use only.

Presentation: 10 x 1,000 dose vials.

Compendium Code No.: 10030031 10440A

AFTER-BIRTH BOLUS

AgriPharm **Uterine Bolus**

Active Ingredient(s): Each bolus contains:

Urea .... 13.4 g

Indications: For use as an antiseptic and proteolytic aid in beef, dairy cattle and sheep.

Dosage and Administration: For intrauterine or topical use only. Insert boluses into the uterus or dissolve in one (1) pint warm water to make a flush.

Cattle: Two (2) to four (4) boluses.

Sheep: One-half (½) to one (1) boluses.

For topical application, dissolve four (4) boluses in one pint of warm water and thoroughly flush the wound.

Repeat treatment in 24 to 48 hours if necessary.

Precaution(s): Store in a cool dry place.

Keep the container tightly closed when not in use.

Caution(s): Do not administer orally.

Strict cleanliness must be observed to prevent the introduction of further infections. Thoroughly cleanse hands and arms of operator and external genital parts of the animal with soap and water before inserting boluses or flush.

Do not use in deep or puncture wounds or for serious burns. For animal use only.

Presentation: Bottles of 50 boluses.

Compendium Code No.: 14570021

AGRI-CILLIN™

AgriLabs **Penicillin Injection**

NADA No.: 065-493

Active Ingredient(s): Each mL contains:

Penicillin G procaine	300,000 units
Sodium citrate	10 mg
Povidone	5.0 mg
Lecithin	6.0 mg
Procaine hydrochloride	20 mg (2.0%)
Potassium phosphate monobasic	3.0 mg
Potassium phosphate dibasic	6.0 mg
Sodium formaldehyde sulfoxylate	0.2 mg (0.4%)
Polysorbate-80	0.4 mg
Sorbitan monolaurate (span 20)	0.2%
Polyoxyethylene sorbitan (tween 20)	0.1 mg
Methyl paraben	1.3 mg (0.1%)
Propyl paraben	0.2 mg (0.1%)
Sodium carboxymethylcellulose	1 mg (0.15%)
Procaine hydrochloride	20 mg
Water for injection	q.s.

Indications: For use in the treatment of disease organisms susceptible to penicillin in cattle, sheep and swine.

Dosage and Administration: For intramuscular injection only. Shake well before using.

AGRI-CILLIN™ should be administered by the intramuscular route. The product is ready for injection after warming the vial to room temperature and shaking to ensure a uniform suspension. The recommended daily dosage of penicillin is 3,000 units per pound of body weight (1 mL per 100 lbs. of body weight). Continue treatment until recovery is apparent and for at least one (1) day after symptoms disappear, usually in two (2) to three (3) days. Treatment should not exceed four (4) consecutive days. Not more than 10 mL should be injected at any one (1) site in adult livestock. Rotate injection sites for each treatment.

Precaution(s): Store between 2-8°C (36-46°F).

Caution(s): Keep out of the reach of children. Livestock remedy. Not for human use.

Warning(s): Exceeding the recommended dosage of 3,000 units per pound of body weight per day, administration at the recommended level for more than four (4) consecutive days, and/or exceeding 10 mL intramuscularly per injection site, may result in antibiotic residues beyond the withdrawal time.

Not for use in horses intended for food.

Milk taken from animals during treatment and for 48 hours (4 milkings) after the last treatment must not be used for food. Discontinue use of this drug for the following time periods before treated animals are slaughtered for food:

Cattle	10 days
Sheep	9 days
Swine	7 days

Treatment should not exceed four (4) consecutive days.

Presentation: 100 mL, 250 mL, and 500 mL multiple dose sterile vials.

Compendium Code No.: 10580030

AGRI-MECTIN™ EQUINE PASTE DEWORMER 1.87%

AgriLabs **Parasiticide-Oral**

(ivermectin) Paste 1.87%-Anthelmintic & Boticide

ANADA No.: 200-286

Active Ingredient(s): Each Syringe Contains:

Ivermectin 1.87%

Indications: Consult a veterinarian for assistance in the diagnosis, treatment, and control of parasitism. AGRI-MECTIN™ Equine Paste Dewormer (ivermectin) Paste 1.87% provides effective control of the following parasites in horses: Large Strongyles (adults): *Strongylus vulgaris* (also early forms in blood vessels), *S. edentatus* (also tissue stages), *S. equinus, Triodontophorus* spp.; Small Strongyles including those resistant to some benzimidazole class compounds (adults and fourth-stage larvae): *Cyathostomum* spp., *Cylicocyclus* spp., *Cylicostephanus* spp., *Cylicodontophorus* spp.; Pinworms (adults and fourth-stage larvae): *Oxyuris equi*; Ascarids (adults and third- and fourth-stage larvae): *Parascaris equorum*; Hairworms (adults): *Trichostrongylus axei*; Large-mouth Stomach Worms (adults): *Habronema muscae*; Bots (oral and gastric stages): *Gasterophilus* spp.; Lungworms (adults and fourth-stage larvae): *Dictyocaulus arnfieldi*; Intestinal Threadworms (adults): *Strongyloides westeri*; Summer Sores caused by *Habronema* and *Draschia* spp. cutaneous third-stage larvae; Dermatitis caused by neck threadworm microfilariae, *Onchocerca* sp.

Dosage and Administration: The syringe contains sufficient paste to treat one 1250 lb horse at the recommended dose rate of 91 mcg ivermectin per lb (200 mcg/kg) of body weight. Each weight marking on the syringe plunger delivers enough paste to treat 250 lb of body weight. (1) While holding plunger, turn the knurled ring on the plunger to the right so the side nearest the barrel is at the prescribed weight marking. (2) Make sure that horse's mouth contains no feed. (3) Remove the cover from the tip of the syringe. (4) Insert the syringe tip into the horse's mouth at the space between the teeth. (5) Depress the plunger as far as it will go, depositing paste on the back of the tongue. (6) Immediately raise the horse's head for a few seconds after dosing.

Parasite Control Program: All horses should be included in a regular parasite control program with particular attention being paid to mares, foals and yearlings. Foals should be treated initially at 6 to 8 weeks of age, and routine treatment repeated as appropriate. Consult a veterinarian for a control program to meet your specific needs. AGRI-MECTIN™ Paste effectively controls gastrointestinal nematodes and bots of horses. Regular treatment will reduce the chances of verminous arteritis caused by *S. vulgaris.*

Precaution(s): Store at controlled room temperature, 20° to 25°C (68° to 77°F).

Caution(s): AGRI-MECTIN™ Equine Paste Dewormer (ivermectin) Paste 1.87% has been formulated specifically for use in horses only. This product should not be used in other animal species as severe adverse reactions, including fatalities in dogs, may result. Refrain from smoking and eating when handling. Wash hands after use. Avoid contact with eyes. Keep this and all drugs out of the reach of children. Ivermectin and excreted ivermectin residues may adversely affect aquatic organisms. Do not contaminate ground or surface water. Dispose of the syringe in approved landfill or by incineration.

Note to User: Swelling and itching reactions after treatment with AGRI-MECTIN™ Paste have occurred in horses carrying heavy infections of neck threadworm *(Onchocera* sp.) microfilariae. These reactions were most likely the result of microfilariae dying in large numbers. Symptomatic treatment may be advisable. Consult a veterinarian should any such reactions occur. Healing of summer sores involving extensive tissue changes may require other appropriate therapy in conjunction with treatment with AGRI-MECTIN™ Paste. Reinfection, and measures for its prevention should also be considered. Consult a veterinarian if the condition does not improve.

For oral use in horses only.

Warning(s): Residue Warning: Do not use in horses intended for food purposes.

Toxicology: Safety: AGRI-MECTIN™ Paste may be used in horses of all ages, including mares at any stage of pregnancy. Stallions may be treated without adversely affecting their fertility.

Discussion: Product Advantages: Broad-Spectrum Control - AGRI-MECTIN™ Paste kills important internal parasites, including bots and the arterial stages of *Strongylus vulgaris*, with a single dose. AGRI-MECTIN™ Paste is a potent antiparasitic agent that is neither a benzimidazole nor an organophosphate.

Presentation: 12 x 6.08 g (0.21 oz) syringes.

Compendium Code No.: 10581260 Iss. 01-00

AGRIMYCIN® 100

AgriLabs **Oxytetracycline Injection**

(Oxytetracycline Hydrochloride Injection) Antibiotic

ANADA No.: 200-068

Active Ingredient(s): Each mL Contains:

Oxytetracycline base (as HCl)	100 mg
Magnesium Chloride • $6H_2O$	5.76% w/v
Water For Injection	17% v/v
Propylene Glycol	q.s.

with Sodium Formaldehyde Sulfoxylate, 1.3% w/v as a preservative and Monoethanolamine for pH adjustment.

Indications: Diseases for Which AGRIMYCIN® 100 (Oxytetracycline Hydrochloride Injection) is Indicated: The use of AGRIMYCIN® 100 (Oxytetracycline Hydrochloride Injection) is indicated in beef cattle, beef calves, non-lactating dairy cattle and dairy calves for treatment of the following disease conditions caused by one or more of the Oxytetracycline sensitive pathogens listed as follows:

Disease	Causative Organism(s) Which Show Sensitivity to AGRIMYCIN® 100 (Oxytetracycline Hydrochloride Injection)
Bacterial Pneumonia and Shipping Fever Complex Associated with *Pasteurella* spp.	*Pasteurella* spp.
Bacterial Enteritis (scours)	*Escherichia coli*
Necrotic Pododermatitis (Foot Rot)	*Fusobacterium necrophorum*
Calf Diphtheria	*Fusobacterium necrophorum*
Wooden Tongue	*Actinobacillus lignieresii*
Wound Infections; Acute Metritis; Traumatic Injury	Caused by oxytetracycline-susceptible strains of streptococcal and staphylococcal organisms.

Pharmacology: Description: AGRIMYCIN® 100 (Oxytetracycline Hydrochloride Injection) is a sterile ready-to-use preparation containing 100 mg/mL Oxytetracycline HCl, for administration of the broad spectrum antibiotic, Oxytetracycline, by injection.

Antibiotic Action of Oxytetracycline: Oxytetracycline is effective against a wide range of gram-negative and gram-positive organisms that are pathogenic for cattle. The antibiotic is primarily bacteriostatic in effect, and is believed to exert its antimicrobial action by the inhibition of microbial protein synthesis. The antibiotic activity of Oxytetracycline is not appreciably diminished in the presence of body fluids, serum or exudates. Since the drugs in the tetracycline class have similar antimicrobial spectra, organisms can develop cross resistance among them. Oxytetracycline is concentrated by the liver in the bile and excreted in the urine and feces at high concentrations and in a biologically active form.

Dosage and Administration: Recommended Daily Dosages:

Treat at the first clinical signs of disease.

The intravenous injection of 3 to 5 mg of Oxytetracycline Hydrochloride per pound of body weight per day (3 to 5 mL per 100 lbs body weight) is the recommended dosage.

Severe foot-rot and the severe forms of the indicated diseases should be treated with 5 mg per pound of body weight. Surgical procedures may be indicated in some forms of foot-rot or other conditions.

In disease treatment, the daily dose of AGRIMYCIN® 100 (Oxytetracycline Hydrochloride Injection) should be continued 24 to 48 hours following remission of disease symptoms; however, not to exceed a total of 4 consecutive days.

Directions for Making an Intravenous Injection in Cattle:

Equipment Recommended:

1. Choke rope — a rope or cord about 5 feet long, with a loop in one end, to be used as a tourniquet.
2. Syringe and needles; gravity flow intravenous set.
3. Use new, very sharp hypodermic needles, 16-gauge, 1½ to 2 inches long. Dull needles will not work. Extra needles should be available in case the one being used becomes clogged.
4. Scissors or clippers.
5. 70% rubbing alcohol compound or other equally effective antiseptic for disinfecting the skin.
6. The medication to be given.

Preparation of Equipment: Thoroughly clean the needles, syringe and intravenous set and disinfect them by boiling in water for twenty minutes or by immersing in a suitable chemical disinfectant such as 70% alcohol for a period of not less than 30 minutes. Warm the bottle of medication to approximately body temperature and keep warm until used.

It is recommended that the correct dose be diluted in water for injection, sodium chloride injection or other suitable vehicle immediately prior to administration. Doses up to 50 mL may be diluted in 250 mL. Larger doses may be diluted in 500 mL of one of the diluents. Adverse reactions may be minimized and the drug dose can be better regulated by this method of administration.

Avoid touching the needle with the hands at all times.

In case of the syringe method of administration, disinfect the vial cap by wiping with 70% alcohol or other suitable antiseptic. Touching a sterile needle only by the hub, attach it to the syringe and push the plunger down the barrel to empty it of air. Puncture the rubber cap of the vial and withdraw the plunger upward in the syringe to draw up a volume of AGRIMYCIN® 100 (Oxytetracycline Hydrochloride Injection), 100 mg/mL of about 5 mL more than is needed for injection. Withdraw from the vial and, pointing the needle upward, remove all air bubbles from the syringe by pushing the plunger upward to the volume required.

If the injection cannot be made immediately, the tip of the needle may be covered with cotton soaked in 70% alcohol to prevent contamination.

Preparation of the Animal for Injection:

1. Approximate location of vein. The jugular vein runs in the jugular groove on each side of the neck from the angle of the jaw to just above the brisket and slightly above and to the side of the windpipe.
2. Method of restraint — A stanchion or chute is ideal for restraining the animal. With a halter, rope or cattle leader (nose tongs), pull the animal's head around the side of the stanchion, cattle chute or post in such a manner to form a bow in the neck, then snub the head securely to prevent movement. By forming the bow in the neck, the outside curvature of the bow tends to expose the jugular vein and make it easily accessible. Caution: Avoid a tight rope or halter around the throat or upper neck which might impede blood flow. Animals that are down present no problem so far as restraint is concerned.
3. Clip hair in area where injection is to be made (over the vein in the upper third of the neck). Clean and disinfect the skin with alcohol or other suitable antiseptic.

Dosage for Injection: Refer to the table below for proper dosage according to body weight of the animal.

Weight of Animals, Lbs (Beef Cattle, Beef Calves, Non-Lactating Dairy Cattle, Dairy Calves)	Milligrams of Oxytetracycline Hydrochloride per 100 lbs of Body Weight Per Day	Daily Dosage of AGRIMYCIN® 100 (Oxytetracycline Hydrochloride Injection) (mL)
50 lbs	300-500 mg	1.5-2.5 mL
100 lbs	300-500 mg	3-5 mL
200 lbs	300-500 mg	6-10 mL
300 lbs	300-500 mg	9-15 mL
400 lbs	300-500 mg	12-20 mL
500 lbs	300-500 mg	15-25 mL
600 lbs	300-500 mg	18-30 mL
800 lbs	300-500 mg	24-40 mL
1000 lbs	300-500 mg	30-50 mL
1200 lbs	300-500 mg	36-60 mL
1400 lbs	300-500 mg	42-70 mL

Caution: If no improvement is noted within 24 to 48 hours consult a veterinarian. For intravenous use only.

Entering the Vein and Making the Injection:

1. Raise the vein: This is accomplished by tying the choke rope tightly around the neck, close to the shoulder. The rope should be tied in such a way that it will not come loose and so that it can be untied quickly by pulling the loose end. In thick-necked animals, a block of wood placed in the jugular groove between the rope and hide will help considerably in applying the desired pressure at the right point. The vein is a soft flexible tube through which blood flows back to the heart. Under ordinary conditions it cannot be seen or felt with the fingers. When the flow of blood is blocked at the base of the neck by the choke rope, the vein becomes enlarged and rigid because of the back pressure. If the choke rope is sufficiently tight, the vein stands out and can be easily seen and felt in thick-necked animals. As a further check in identifying the vein, tap it with the fingers in front of the choke rope. Pulsations that can be seen or felt with the fingers in front of the point being tapped will confirm the fact that the vein is properly distended. It is impossible to put the needle into the vein unless it is distended. Experienced operators are able to raise the vein simply by hand pressure, but the use of a choke rope is more certain.
2. Inserting the needle. This involves three distinct steps. First, insert the needle through the hide. Second, insert the needle into the vein. This may require two or three attempts before the vein is entered. The vein has a tendency to roll away from the point of the needle, especially if the needle is not sharp. The vein can be steadied with the thumb and finger of one hand. With the other hand, the needle point is placed directly over the vein, slanting it so that its direction is along the length of the vein, either toward the head or toward the heart. Properly positioned this way, a quick thrust of the needle will be followed by a spurt of blood through the needle, which indicates that the vein has been entered. Third, once in the vein, the needle should be inserted along the length of the vein all the way to the hub, exercising caution to see that the needle does not penetrate the opposite side of the vein. Continuous steady flow of blood through the needle indicates that the needle is still in the vein. If blood does not flow continuously, the needle is out of the vein (or clogged) and another attempt must be made. If difficulty is encountered, it may be advisable to use the vein on the other side of the neck.
3. While the needle is being placed in proper position in the vein, an assistant should get the medication ready so that the injection can be started without delay after the vein has been entered. Remove the rubber stopper from the bottle of intravenous solution, connect the intravenous tube to the neck of the bottle, invert the bottle and allow some of the solution to run through the tube to eliminate all air bubbles.
4. Making the injection. With needle in proper position as indicated by continuous flow of blood, release the choke rope by a quick pull on the free end. This is essential — the medication cannot flow into the vein while the vein is blocked. Immediately connect the intravenous tube to the needle, and raise the bottle. The solution will flow by gravity. Rapid injection may occasionally produce shock. Administer slowly. The animal should be observed at all times during the injection in order not to give the solution too fast. This may be determined by watching the respiration of the animal and feeling or listening to the heart beat. If the heart beat and respiration increase markedly, the rate of injection should be immediately stopped by pinching the tube until the animal recovers approximately to its previous respiration or heart beat rate, when the injection can be resumed at a slower rate. The rate of flow can be controlled by pinching the tube between the thumb and forefinger or by raising and lowering the bottle.

   Bubbles entering the bottle through the air tube or valve indicate the rate at which the medication is flowing. If the flow should stop, this means the needle has slipped out of the vein (or is clogged) and the operation will have to be repeated. If using the syringe technique, pull back gently on the plunger: if blood flows into the syringe, the needle is in proper position. Depress the plunger slowly. If there is any resistance to the depression of the plunger, stop and repeat insertion procedure. The resistance indicates that either the needle is clogged or it has slipped out of the vein. With either method of administration, syringe or gravity flow, watch for any swelling under the skin near the needle, which would indicate that the medication is not going into the vein. Should this occur, it is best to try the vein on the opposite side of the neck. Sudden movement of the animal, especially twisting of the neck or raising or lowering the head, may sometimes cause the needle to slip out of the vein. To prevent this, tape the needle hub to the skin of the neck to hold the needle in position. Whenever there is any doubt as to the position of the needle, this should be checked in the following manner: Pinch off the intravenous tube to stop flow, disconnect the tube from the needle and re-apply pressure to the vein. Free flow of blood through the needle indicates that it is in proper position and the injection can then be continued. If using the syringe, gently pull back on the plunger. Blood should flow into the syringe.
5. Removing the needle. When the injection is complete, remove needle with a straight pull. Then apply pressure over area of injection momentarily to control any bleeding through needle puncture, using cotton soaked in alcohol or other suitable antiseptic.

Precaution(s): Store between 15°C and 30°C (59°-86°F).

Note: Solution may darken on storage but potency remains unaffected.

Caution(s): Rapid intravenous administration may result in animal collapse. Oxytetracycline should be administered intravenously slowly over a period of at least 5 minutes.

If no improvement occurs within 24 to 48 hours, consult a veterinarian. Do not use the drug for more than 4 consecutive days. Use beyond 4 days or doses higher than maximum recommended dose may result in antibiotic tissue residues beyond the withdrawal period.

The improper or accidental injection of the drug outside of the vein will cause local tissue irritation manifested by temporary swelling and discoloration at the injection site.

Shortly after injection, treated animals may have a transient hemoglobinuria (darkened urine).

Consult with a veterinarian prior to administering this product in order to determine the proper treatment required in the event of an adverse reaction. At the first sign of any adverse reaction, discontinue use of product and seek the advice of a veterinarian. Some of the reactions may be attributed either to anaphylaxis (an allergic reaction) or to cardiovascular collapse of unknown cause.

Because bacteriostatic drugs interfere with the bactericidal action of Penicillin, do not give Oxytetracycline Hydrochloride in conjunction with Penicillin.

As with other antibiotics, use of this drug may result in over-growth of nonsusceptible organisms. If any unusual symptoms occur or in the absence of a favorable response following treatment, discontinue use immediately and call a veterinarian.

For use in animals only.

Warning(s): Discontinue treatment with AGRIMYCIN® 100 (Oxytetracycline Hydrochloride Injection) at least 22 days prior to slaughter of the animal. Not for use in lactating dairy animals.

A withdrawal period has not been established for this product in pre-ruminating calves. Do not use in calves to be processed for veal.

Restricted Drug (California) — Use only as directed.

Keep out of reach of children.

Adverse Reactions: Reports of adverse reactions associated with oxytetracycline administration include injection site swelling, restlessness, ataxia, trembling, swelling of eyelids, ears, muzzle, anus and vulva (or scrotum and sheath in males), respiratory abnormalities (labored breathing), frothing at the mouth, collapse and possibly death. Some of these reactions may be attributed either to anaphylaxis (an allergic reaction) or to cardiovascular collapse of unknown cause.

Discussion: General Indications for Use: A great many of the pathogens involved in cattle diseases are known to be susceptible to Oxytetracycline Hydrochloride therapy. Many strains of organisms, however, have shown resistance to Oxytetracycline. In the case of certain coliforms, streptococci and staphylococci, it may be advisable to conduct culture and sensitivity testing to determine susceptibility of the infecting organism to Oxytetracycline. In this manner, the likelihood of successful treatment with AGRIMYCIN® 100 (Oxytetracycline Hydrochloride Injection) solution can be determined in advance.

Instructions for Care of Sick Animals: The use of antibiotics, as with most medications used in the management of diseases, is based on accurate diagnosis and adequate treatment. When properly used in the treatment of diseases caused by oxytetracycline-susceptible organisms, animals usually show a noticeable improvement within 24 to 48 hours. If improvement does not occur within this period of time, the diagnosis and treatment of animal diseases should be carried out by a veterinarian. The use of professional veterinary and laboratory services can reduce treatment costs, time and needless losses. Good management, housing, sanitation and nutrition are essential in the care of animals and in the successful treatment of disease.

Presentation: AGRIMYCIN® 100 (Oxytetracycline Hydrochloride Injection) is available in 500 mL multidose vials containing 100 mg Oxytetracycline Hydrochloride per mL.

Compendium Code No.: 10580051 Rev. 11-00

AGRIMYCIN® 200

AgriLabs **Oxytetracycline Injection**

(Oxytetracycline Injection) Antibiotic

ANADA No.: 200-123

Active Ingredient(s): AGRIMYCIN® 200 (oxytetracycline injection) is a sterile preconstituted solution of the broad-spectrum antibiotic oxytetracycline. Each mL contains 200 mg of oxytetracycline base as amphoteric oxytetracycline and, on a w/v basis, 40.0% 2-pyrrolidone, 5.0% povidone, 1.8% magnesium oxide, 0.2% sodium formaldehyde sulfoxylate (as a preservative), monoethanolamine and/or hydrochloric acid as required to adjust pH.

Indications: AGRIMYCIN® 200 is intended for use in the treatment of the following diseases in beef cattle, nonlactating dairy cattle; calves, including preruminating (veal) calves; and swine when due to oxytetracycline-susceptible organisms:

Cattle: In cattle, AGRIMYCIN® 200 is indicated in the treatment of pneumonia and shipping fever complex associated with *Pasteurella* spp. and *Hemophilus* spp; infectious bovine keratoconjunctivitis (pinkeye) caused by *Moraxella bovis;* foot-rot and diphtheria caused by *Fusobacterium necrophorum;* bacterial enteritis (scours) caused by *Escherichia coli;* wooden tongue caused by *Actinobacillus lignieresii;* leptospirosis caused by *Leptospira pomona* and wound infections and acute metritis caused by strains of staphylococci and streptococci organisms sensitive to oxytetracycline.

Swine: In swine, AGRIMYCIN® 200 (oxytetracycline injection) is indicated in the treatment of bacterial enteritis (scours, colibacillosis) caused by *Escherichia coli;* pneumonia caused by *Pasteurella multocida;* and leptospirosis caused by *Leptospira pomona.*

In sows, AGRIMYCIN® 200 is indicated as an aid in the control of infectious enteritis (baby pig scours, colibacillosis) in suckling pigs caused by *Escherichia coli.*

Pharmacology: AGRIMYCIN® 200 (oxytetracycline injection) is a sterile, ready-to-use solution for the administration of the broad-spectrum antibiotic oxytetracycline by injection. Oxytetracycline is an antimicrobial agent that is effective in the treatment of a wide range of diseases caused by susceptible gram-positive and gram-negative bacteria.

Dosage and Administration: Dosage:

Cattle: AGRIMYCIN® 200 is to be administered by intramuscular, subcutaneous or intravenous injection to beef cattle, nonlactating dairy cattle, and calves, including preruminating (veal) calves.

A single dosage of 9 milligrams of AGRIMYCIN® 200 per pound of body weight administered intramuscularly or subcutaneously is recommended in the treatment of the following conditions: 1) bacterial pneumonia caused by *Pasteurella* spp. (shipping fever) in calves and yearlings, where re-treatment is impractical due to husbandry conditions, such as cattle on range, or where their repeated restraint is inadvisable; 2) infectious bovine keratoconjunctivitis (pinkeye) caused by *Moraxella bovis.*

AGRIMYCIN® 200 can also be administered by intravenous, subcutaneous or intramuscular injection at a level of 3 to 5 milligrams of oxytetracycline per pound of body weight per day. In the treatment of severe foot-rot and advanced cases of other indicated diseases, dosage level of 5 milligrams per pound of body weight per day is recommended. Treatment should be continued 24 to 48 hours following remission of disease signs; however, not to exceed a total of four consecutive days. Consult your veterinarian if improvement is not noted within 24 to 48 hours of the beginning of treatment.

Swine: In swine a single dosage of 9 milligrams of AGRIMYCIN® 200 per pound of body weight administered intramuscularly is recommended in the treatment of bacterial pneumonia caused by *Pasteurella multocida* in swine, where re-treatment is impractical due to husbandry conditions or where repeated restraint is inadvisable.

AGRIMYCIN® 200 can also be administered by intramuscular injection at a level of 3 to 5 milligrams of oxytetracycline per pound of body weight per day. Treatment should be continued 24 to 48 hours following remission of disease signs; however, not to exceed a total of four consecutive days. Consult your veterinarian if improvement is not noted within 24 to 48 hours of the beginning of treatment.

For sows, administer once intramuscularly 3 milligrams of oxytetracycline per pound of body weight approximately 8 hours before farrowing or immediately after completion of farrowing.

For swine weighing 25 lb of body weight and under, AGRIMYCIN® 200 should be administered undiluted for treatment at 9 mg/lb but should be administered diluted for treatment at 3 to 5 mg/lb body weight.

	9 mg/lb Dosage Volume of Undiluted AGRIMYCIN® 200	3 or 5 mg/lb Dosage Volume of Diluted AGRIMYCIN® 200		
Body Weight	9 mg/lb	3 mg/lb	Dilution*	5 mg/lb
5 lb	0.2 mL	0.6 mL	1:7	1.0 mL
10 lb	0.5 mL	0.9 mL	1:5	1.5 mL
25 lb	1.1 mL	1.5 mL	1:3	2.5 mL

* To prepare dilutions, add one part AGRIMYCIN® 200 to three, five or seven parts of sterile water, or 5 percent dextrose solution as indicated; the diluted product should be used immediately.

Directions for Use: AGRIMYCIN® 200 is intended for use in the treatment of disease due to oxytetracycline-susceptible organisms in beef cattle, nonlactating dairy cattle; calves, including preruminating (veal) calves; and swine. A thoroughly cleaned, sterile needle and syringe should be used for each injection (needles and syringes may be sterilized by boiling in water for 15 minutes). In cold weather, AGRIMYCIN® 200 should be warmed to room temperature before administration to animals. Before withdrawing the solution from the bottle, disinfect the rubber cap on the bottle with suitable disinfectant, such as 70 percent alcohol. The injection site should be similarly cleaned with the disinfectant. Needles of 16 to 18 gauge and 1 to 1½ inches long are adequate for intramuscular injections. Needles 2 to 3 inches are recommended for intravenous use.

Intramuscular Administration: Intramuscular injections should be made by directing the needle of suitable gauge and length into the fleshy part of a thick muscle such as in the rump, hip, or thigh regions; avoid blood vessels and major nerves. Before injecting the solution, pull back gently on the plunger. If blood appears in the syringe, a blood vessel has been entered; withdraw the needle and select a different site. No more than 10 mL should be injected intramuscularly at any one site in adult beef cattle and nonlactating dairy cattle, and not more than 5 mL per site in adult swine; rotate injection sites for each succeeding treatment. The volume administered per injection site should be reduced according to age and body size so that 1 to 2 mL per site is injected in small calves.

Subcutaneous Administration: Subcutaneous injections in beef cattle, nonlactating dairy cattle, and calves, including preruminating (veal) calves, should be made by directing the needle of suitable gauge and length through the loose folds of the neck skin in front of the shoulder. Care should be taken to ensure that the tip of the needle has penetrated the skin but is not lodged in muscle. Before injecting the solution, pull back gently on the plunger. If blood appears in the syringe, a blood vessel has been entered; withdraw the needle and select a different site. The solution should be injected slowly into the area between the skin and muscles. No more than 10 mL should be injected subcutaneously at any one site in adult beef cattle and nonlactating dairy cattle; rotate injection sites for each succeeding treatment. The volume administered per injection site should be reduced according to age and body size so that 1-2 mL per site is injected in small calves.

Intravenous Administration: AGRIMYCIN® 200 (oxytetracycline injection) may be administered intravenously to beef cattle and nonlactating dairy cattle. As with all highly concentrated materials, AGRIMYCIN® 200 should be administered slowly by the intravenous route.

Preparation of the Animal for Injection:

1. Approximate location of vein. The jugular vein runs in the jugular groove on each side of the neck from the angle of the jaw to just above the brisket and slightly above and to the side of the windpipe. (See Fig. I)
2. Restraint. A stanchion or chute is ideal for restraining the animal. With a halter, rope, or cattle leader (nose tongs), pull the animal's head around the side of the stanchion, cattle chute, or post in such a manner to form a bow in the neck (See Fig. II), then snub the head securely to prevent movement. By forming the bow in the neck, the outside curvature of the bow tends to expose the jugular vein and make it easily accessible. Caution: Avoid restraining the animal with a tight rope or halter around the throat or upper neck which might impede blood flow. Animals that are down present no problem so far as restraint is concerned.
3. Clip hair in area where injection is to be made (over the vein in the upper third of the neck). Clean and disinfect the skin with alcohol or other suitable antiseptic.

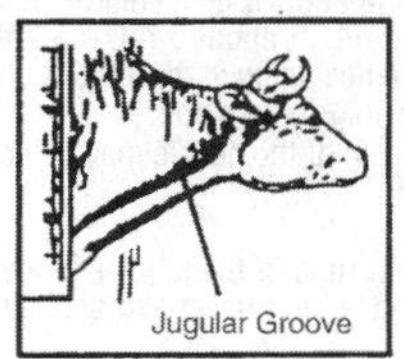

Figure I

Figure II

Entering the Vein and Making the Injection:

1. Raise the vein. This is accomplished by tying the choke rope tightly around the neck close to the shoulder. The rope should be tied in such a way that it will not come loose and so that it can be untied quickly by pulling the loose end (See Fig. II). In thick-necked animals, a block of wood placed in the jugular groove between the rope and the hide will help considerably in applying the desired pressure at the right point. The vein is a soft flexible tube through which blood flows back to the heart. Under ordinary conditions it cannot be seen or felt with the fingers. When the flow of blood is blocked at the base of the neck by the choke rope, the vein becomes enlarged and rigid because of the back pressure. If the choke rope is sufficiently tight, the vein stands out and can be easily seen and felt in thin-necked animals. As a further check in identifying the vein, tap it with the fingers in front of the choke rope. Pulsations that can be seen or felt with the fingers in front of the point being tapped will confirm the fact that the vein is properly distended. It is impossible to put the needle into the vein unless it is distended. Experienced operators are able to raise the vein simply by hand pressure, but the use of a choke rope is more certain.
2. Inserting the needle. This involves three distinct steps. First, insert the needle through the hide. Second, insert the needle into the vein. This may require two or three attempts before the vein is entered. The vein has a tendency to roll away from the point of the needle, especially if the needle is not sharp. The vein can be steadied with the thumb and finger of one hand. With the other hand, the needle point is placed directly over the vein, slanting it so that its direction is along the length of the vein, either toward the head or toward the heart. Properly positioned this way, a quick thrust of the needle will be followed by a spurt of blood through the needle, which indicates that the vein has been entered. Third, once in the vein, the needle should be inserted along the length of the vein all the way to the hub

exercising caution to see that the needle does not penetrate the opposite side of the vein. Continuous steady flow of blood through the needle indicates that the needle is still in the vein. If blood does not flow continuously, the needle is out of the vein (or clogged) and another attempt must be made. If difficulty is encountered, it may be advisable to use the vein on the other side of the neck.

3. While the needle is being placed in proper position in the vein, an assistant should get the medication ready so that the injection can be started without delay after the vein has been entered.
4. Making the injection. With the needle in position as indicated by continuous flow of blood, release the choke rope by a quick pull on the free end. This is essential - the medication cannot flow into the vein while it is blocked. Immediately connect the syringe containing AGRIMYCIN® 200 (oxytetracycline injection) to the needle and slowly depress the plunger. If there is resistance to depression of the plunger, this indicates that the needle has slipped out of the vein (or is clogged) and the procedure will have to be repeated. Watch for any swelling under the skin near the needle which would indicate that the medication is not going into the vein. Should this occur, it is best to try the vein on the opposite side of the neck.
5. Removing the needle. When injection is complete, remove needle with straight pull. Then apply pressure over the area of injection momentarily to control any bleeding through needle puncture, using cotton soaked in alcohol or other suitable antiseptic.

Precaution(s): AGRIMYCIN® 200 does not require refrigeration; however, it is recommended that it be stored at room temperature, 15°-30°C (59°-86°F). The antibiotic activity of oxytetracycline is not appreciably diminished in the presence of body fluids, serum, or exudates. Keep from freezing.

Caution(s): Exceeding the highest recommended dosage level of drug per pound of body weight per day, administering more than the recommended number of treatments, and/or exceeding 10 mL intramuscularly or subcutaneously per injection site in adult beef cattle and nonlactating dairy cattle, and 5 mL intramuscularly per injection site in adult swine, may result in antibiotic residues beyond the withdrawal period.

Consult with your veterinarian prior to administering this product in order to determine the proper treatment required in the event of an adverse reaction. At the first sign of any adverse reaction, discontinue use of product and seek the advice of your veterinarian. Some of the reactions may be attributed either to anaphylaxis (an allergic reaction) or to cardiovascular collapse of unknown cause.

Shock may be observed following intravenous administration, especially where highly concentrated materials are involved. To minimize this occurrence, it is recommended that AGRIMYCIN® 200 be administered slowly by this route.

Shortly after injection, treated animals may have transient hemoglobinuria resulting in darkened urine.

As with all antibiotic preparations, use of the drug may result in overgrowth of nonsusceptible organisms, including fungi. A lack of response by the treated animal, or the development of new signs, may suggest that an overgrowth of nonsusceptible organisms has occurred. If any of these conditions occur, consult your veterinarian.

Since bacteriostatic drugs may interfere with the bactericidal action of penicillin, it is advisable to avoid giving AGRIMYCIN® 200 in conjunction with penicillin.

For animal use only.

Livestock drug, not for human use.

Restricted drug (California), use only as directed.

Warning(s): Discontinue treatment at least 28 days prior to slaughter of cattle and swine. Not for use in lactating dairy animals. Rapid intravenous administration may result in animal collapse. Oxytetracycline should be administered intravenously slowly over a period of at least 5 minutes.

Keep out of reach of children.

Adverse Reactions: Reports of adverse reactions associated with Oxytetracycline administration include injection site swelling, restlessness, ataxia, trembling, swelling of eyelids, ears, muzzle, anus and vulva (or scrotum and sheath in males), respiratory abnormalities (labored breathing), frothing at the mouth, collapse and possibly death. Some of these reactions may be attributed either to anaphylaxis (an allergic reaction) or to cardiovascular collapse of unknown cause.

Discussion: Care of Sick Animals: The use of antibiotics in the management of diseases is based on an accurate diagnosis and an adequate course of treatment. When properly used in the treatment of diseases caused by oxytetracycline-susceptible organisms, most animals that have been treated with oxytetracycline injection show a noticeable improvement within 24 to 48 hours. It is recommended that the diagnosis and treatment of animal diseases be carried out by a veterinarian. Since many diseases look alike but require different types of treatment, the use of professional veterinary and laboratory services can reduce treatment time, costs and needless losses. Good housing, sanitation and nutrition are important in the maintenance of healthy animals, and are essential in the treatment of diseased animals.

Presentation: 100 mL, 250 mL and 500 mL.

Compendium Code No.: 10580042 Rev. 7-01

AGRIMYCIN®-343

AgriLabs **Water Medication**

Oxytetracycline Hydrochloride Soluble Powder

ANADA No.: 200-066

Active Ingredient(s): The packet contains 102.4 grams of oxytetracycline HCl and will make:

512 gallons (1,938 L) containing 200 mg oxytetracycline HCl per gallon.

256 gallons (969 L) containing 400 mg oxytetracycline HCl per gallon.

128 gallons (484 L) containing 800 mg oxytetracycline HCl per gallon.

The packet will treat 10,240 pounds of swine.

Each pail contains 1.715 kilograms of oxytetracycline HCl and will make:

8,576 gallons (32,460 L) containing 200 mg oxytetracycline HCl per gallon.

4,288 gallons (16,230 L) containing 400 mg oxytetracycline HCl per gallon.

2,144 gallons (8,115 L) containing 800 mg oxytetracycline HCl per gallon.

Each pail will treat 171,500 pounds of swine.

Indications: Antibiotic for control of specific diseases in poultry and swine.

Dosage and Administration: Mixing Instructions for Water Medication (Chicken—Turkeys—Swine):

For Use in Water Proportioners—

For Packets: Add the following amount to one gallon of stock solution when proportioner is set to meter at the rate of one ounce per gallon.

For Pail: Use the enclosed scoop to add the following amount to one gallon of stock solution when proportioner is set to meter at the rate of one ounce per gallon. One level scoop is equal to approximately 34 grams.

Chickens:

Disease	Treatment Level	Packs/Gal. Stock Sol.	Scoops/Gal. Stock Sol.
Control of infectious synovitis caused by *Mycoplasma synoviae*, susceptible to oxytetracycline.	200-400 mg	¼-½ (34-68 g)	1-2 (34-68 g)
Control of chronic respiratory disease (CRD) and air sac infections caused by *Mycoplasma gallisepticum* and *Escherichia coli*, susceptible to oxytetracycline.	400-800 mg	½-1 (68-135.5 g)	2-4 (68-135.5 g)
Control of fowl cholera caused by *Pasteurella multocida*, susceptible to oxytetracycline.	400-800 mg	½-1 (68-135.5 g)	2-4 (68-135.5 g)

Turkeys:

Disease	Treatment Level	Packs/Gal. Stock Sol.	Scoops/Gal. Stock Sol.
Control of hexamitiasis caused by *Hexamita meleagridis* susceptible to oxytetracycline.	200-400 mg	¼-½ (34-68 g)	1-2 (34-68 g)
Control of infectious synovitis caused by *Mycoplasma synoviae* susceptible to oxytetracycline.	400 mg	½ (68 g)	2 (68 g)
Growing Turkeys — Control of complicating bacterial organisms associated with bluecomb (transmissible enteritis, coronaviral enteritis) susceptible to oxytetracycline.	25 mg/lb. body weight	Varies with age & water consumption	Varies with age & water consumption

Swine:

Disease	Treatment Level	Packs/Gal. Stock Sol.	Scoops/Gal. Stock Sol.
For the Control and Treatment of the Following Diseases in Swine: Bacterial enteritis caused by *Escherichia coli* and *Salmonella choleraesuis*, susceptible to oxytetracycline. Bacterial pneumonia caused by *Pasteurella multocida*, susceptible to oxytetracycline. For Breeding Swine: Leptospirosis (reducing the incidence of abortions and shedding of leptospira) caused by *Leptospira pomona*, susceptible to oxytetracycline.	10 mg/lb. body weight	Varies with age & water consumption	Varies with age & water consumption

Directions for Use: Mix fresh solutions daily - Use as sole source of drinking water - Do not mix this product directly with milk or milk replacers. Administer one hour before or two hours after feeding milk or milk replacers.

If improvement is not noted within 24 to 48 hours, consult a poultry veterinarian or poultry diagnostic laboratory. As a generalization, 200 chickens will drink one gallon of water per day for each week of age. Turkeys will consume twice that amount. Administer up to 5 days to swine and 7 to 14 days for chickens and turkeys.

Note: The concentration of drug required in medicated water must be adequate to compensate for variation in the age of the animals, feed consumption rate, and the environmental temperature and humidity, each of which affects water consumption.

Precaution(s): Recommended Storage: Store below 77°F (25°C).

Caution(s): Use as sole source of oxytetracycline—Not to be used for more than 5 consecutive days in swine and 14 consecutive days in chickens and turkeys.

For use in drinking water only—Not for use in liquid feed supplements.

For use in animals only.

Warning(s): Do not feed to birds producing eggs for human consumption. Discontinue treatment of chickens, turkeys and swine 0 days prior to slaughter.

Keep out of reach of children.

Presentation: 4.78 oz (135.5 g) packet and 5 lb (2.27 kg) pail.

Compendium Code No.: 10580062 Rev. 1001

AGRIMYCIN® POWDER

AgriLabs **Water Medication**

Oxytetracycline HCl Soluble Powder-Antibiotic

ANADA No.: 200-146

Active Ingredient(s): Each packet contains 10 grams of oxytetracycline HCl.

Indications: A broad spectrum antibiotic for control and treatment of specific diseases in poultry, cattle, sheep and swine.

Directions for Use:

For the control of the following poultry diseases caused by organisms susceptible to oxytetracycline: Add the following amount to two gallons of stock solution when proportioner is set to meter at the rate of one ounce per gallon.

	Dosage	Packets/2 Gallons Stock Solution
Chickens		
Infectious synovitis caused by *Mycoplasma synoviae*	200-400 mg/gal	5-10
Chronic respiratory disease (CRD) and air sac infection caused by *Mycoplasma gallisepticum* and *Escherichia coli*	400-800 mg/gal	10-20
Fowl cholera caused by *Pasteurella multocida*	400-800 mg/gal	10-20
Turkeys		
Hexamitiasis caused by *Hexamita meleagridis*	200-400 mg/gal	5-10
Infectious synovitis caused by *Mycoplasma synoviae*	400 mg/gal	10
Growing Turkeys—Complicating bacterial organisms associated with bluecomb (transmissible enteritis, coronaviral enteritis)	25 mg/lb body weight daily	varies with age & water consumption (1 packet will treat 400 pounds of turkeys.)

Medicate continuously at the first clinical signs of disease and continue for 7 to 14 consecutive days. If improvement is not noted within 24-48 hours, consult a poultry diagnostic laboratory or poultry pathologist to determine diagnosis and advice on dosage.

For the control and treatment of the following diseases caused by organisms susceptible to oxytetracycline:

	Dosage
Swine	
Bacterial enteritis caused by *Escherichia coli* and *Salmonella choleraesuis*	Administer in the drinking water at a level of 10 mg oxytetracycline HCl per pound of body weight daily. Administer up to 14 days.
Bacterial pneumonia caused by *Pasteurella multocida* For Breeding Swine: Leptospirosis (reducing the incidence of abortions and shedding of leptospira) caused by *Leptospira pomona*.	
Calves, Beef Cattle and Non-Lactating Dairy Cattle	
Bacterial enteritis caused by *Escherichia coli*	Administer in the drinking water at a level of 10 mg oxytetracycline HCl per pound of body weight daily. Administer up to 14 days.
Bacterial pneumonia (shipping fever complex) caused by *Pasteurella multocida*.	
Sheep	
Bacterial enteritis caused by *Escherichia coli*	Administer in the drinking water at a level of 10 mg oxytetracycline HCl per pound of body weight daily. Administer up to 14 days.
Bacterial pneumonia (shipping fever complex) caused by *Pasteurella multocida*.	

Each packet will treat 1000 pounds of swine, cattle or sheep at 10 mg/pound.

Special Note: The concentration of drug required in medicated water must be adequate to compensate for variation in the age of the animal, feed consumption rate and the environmental temperature and humidity, each of which affects water consumption.

Precaution(s): Recommended Storage: Store below 77°F (25°C).

Caution(s): Use as sole source of oxytetracycline. Prepare fresh solutions every 24 hours.

For use in drinking water only. Not for use in liquid feed supplements. For animal use only.

Restricted Drug(s) (California). Not for human use, use only as directed. For oral use only.

Warning(s): Do not administer to turkeys, swine, cattle or sheep within 5 days of slaughter. Do not administer to chickens or turkeys producing eggs for human consumption. Do not administer this product with milk or milk replacers. Administer 1 hour before or 2 hours after feeding milk or milk replacers.

A withdrawal period has not been established for this product in pre-ruminating calves. Do not use in calves to be processed for veal.

A milk discard period has not been established for this product in lactating dairy cattle. Do not use in female dairy cattle 20 months of age or older. Keep out of reach of children.

Presentation: 181.5 g (6.4 oz) packet.

Compendium Code No.: 10581270 Iss. 10/99

AGRI PLUS KETO-NIA DRENCH™

Vets Plus **Acetonemia Preparation**

Oral High Energy Nutrient Supplement

Guaranteed Analysis: (min. per 200 mL):

Niacin........ 11,500 mg
Vitamin B_6........ 60 mg
Vitamin B_{12}........ 600 mcg

Ingredients: Propylene Glycol, Niacinamide, Dextrose, Cyanocobalamin (Vitamin B_{12}), Pyridoxine Hydrochloride (Vitamin B_6), Choline Bitartrate, Vitamin A Acetate, D-Activated Animal Sterol (Vitamin D_3), d-Calcium Pantothenate, DL-alpha-Tocopheryl Acetate (Vitamin E), Ascorbic Acid (Vitamin C), Riboflavin, Folic Acid and Silica.

Indications: Use on every fresh cow or heifer before and after calving. AGRI PLUS KETO-NIA DRENCH™ provides propylene glycol, niacin, and other B complex vitamins to lower the incidence of ketosis, boost energy, and stimulate appetite.

Dosage and Administration: Provide 200 mL at the first sign of freshening and another 200 mL 6 to 12 hours post calving, repeat as needed. If first dose is missed, a post calving dose is still beneficial. Shake well before using. 1 gallon provides nineteen 200 mL feedings.

Feeding Directions: Administer orally using a drench gun. Hold the head of the cow in a slightly elevated position and carefully place the nozzle into the back of the mouth between the cheek and teeth. Administer the recommended dosage. Do not give to cows that are unable to swallow.

Precaution(s): Keep in a cool dry place. Avoid freezing.

Caution(s): Keep out of the reach of children. Contact with eyes or wounds or prolonged contact with skin, can cause irritation.

Animal use only.

Presentation: 4x1 gallon (3.8 liter) containers per case, 5 gallon pail, and 15 gallon drum.

Compendium Code No.: 10730020

AG-TEK® POLY-LUBE™

Kane **Lubricant**

Ingredient(s): Lubricating powder

Indications: A powder formulated to make a liquid lubricant for use during obstetrical and artificial insemination procedures. It can also be used as a powdered hand soap.

Presentation: 12 x 8 oz (226 g) containers.

Compendium Code No.: 10660001

AIR$_X$® 75

Airex **Disinfectant**

Antibacterial Heavy Duty Cleaner & Odor Counteractant

EPA Reg. No.: 1839-83-44089

Active Ingredient(s):

N-Alkyl (60% C14, 30% C16, 5% C12, 5% C18) dimethyl benzyl ammonium chlorides........ 0.105%
N-Alkyl (68% C12, 32% C14) dimethyl ethylbenzyl ammonium chlorides........ 0.105%
Inert Ingredients........ 99.790%
Total........ 100.000%

Indications: Designed specifically as a general non-acid cleaner and disinfectant for use in hospitals, nursing homes, schools and hotels. It is formulated to disinfect hard, non-porous inanimate environmental surfaces such as floors, walls, metal surfaces, stainless steel surfaces, porcelain, glazed ceramic tile, plastic surfaces, bathrooms, shower stalls, bathtubs and cabinets.

Tuberculocidal Activity - This product exhibits disinfectant efficacy against *Mycobacterium tuberculosis* (BCG) in 10 minutes at 20 degrees Centigrade when used as directed on previously cleaned hard nonporous inanimate surfaces.

Bactericidal Activity - When used as directed, this product exhibits effective disinfectant activity against the organisms: *Staphyloccocus aureus, Salmonella choleraesuis, Pseudomonas aeruginosa, Escherichia coli* 0157:H7, Methicillin resistant *Staphyloccocus aureus* (MRSA), Vancomycin resistant *Staphyloccus aureus* (VRSA), Vancomycin resistant *Enterococcus aureus* (VRE) and meets the requirements for hospital use.

*Virucidal Activity - This product, when used on environmental, inanimate, non-porous surfaces, exhibits effective virucidal activity against HIV-1 (associated with AIDS), Canine Parvovirus and Poliovirus Type 1.

Efficacy tests have demonstrated that this product is an effective bactericide, fungicide, and virucide in the presence of organic soil (5% blood serum).

Directions for Use: It is a violation of Federal law to use this product in a manner inconsistent with its labeling.

For plastic and painted surface, spot test on an inconspicuous area before use. May be used in the kitchen on counters, sinks, appliances, and stove tops. A rinse with potable water is required for surfaces in direct contact with food. In addition this product deodorizes those areas which generally are hard to keep fresh smelling, such as garbage storage areas, empty garbage bins and cans, restrooms and other areas which are prone to odors caused by microorganisms.

This product is not to be used as a terminal sterilant/high-level disinfectant on any surface or instrument that (1) is introduced directly into the human body, either into or in contact with the bloodstream or in contact with bloodstream or normally sterile areas of the body, or (2) contacts intact mucous membranes but which does not ordinary penetrate the blood barrier or otherwise enter normally sterile areas of the body.

Disinfection, Deodorizing and Cleaning - Remove gross filth or heavy soil prior to application of the product. Hold container six to eight inches from surface to be treated. Spray area until it is covered with the solution. Allow product to penetrate and remain wet for 10 minutes. No scrubbing is necessary. Wipe off with a clean cloth, mop or sponge. The product will not leave grit or soap scum.

Precautionary Statements:

Hazards to Humans and Domestic Animals: Causes eye and skin irritation. Do not get in eyes, on skin or on clothing. Harmful if swallowed. Avoid contamination of food. Remove contaminated clothing and wash before reuse. Wash thoroughly with soap and water after handling.

Statement of Practical Treatment - In case of contact, immediately flush eyes or skin with plenty of water for at least 15 minutes. For eyes, call a physician. If swallowed, drink egg whites or gelatin solution, or if these are not available, drink large quantities of water. Call a physician immediately.

Note to Physician - Probable mucosal damage may contraindicate the use of gastric lavage.

Storage and Disposal: Do not contaminate water, food or feed by storage or disposal.

Pesticide Storage - Store in a dry place no lower in temperature than 50°F or higher than 120°F.

Container Disposal - Do not reuse empty bottle. Wrap container and put in trash.

Warning(s): Keep out of reach of children.

Presentation: 1 quart, 6x1 gallon, 5 gallon and 55 gallon drums.

U.S. Patent No. 5,444,094

Compendium Code No.: 10040001

ALBAC® 50

Alpharma **Feed Medication**

Bacitracin Zinc-Type A Medicated Article-Antibacterial

ANADA No.: 200-233

Active Ingredient(s): Each pound contains feed grade zinc bacitracin equivalent to 50 grams bacitracin (Master Standard).

Composition: The zinc salt of a dried fermentation product obtained by culturing *B. licheniformis* Tracy on a media adapted for microbiological production of bacitracin, and calcium carbonate.

Indications: For supplementing rations of chickens, turkeys, pheasants, quail, swine and cattle.

Increase rate of weight gain and improved feed efficiency in growing chickens, turkeys, pheasants, growing quail (not over 5 weeks of age), laying chickens, growing-finishing swine, and feedlot cattle.

Increased egg production and improved feed efficiency in laying chickens.

Dosage and Administration: Mixing Directions: Prepare an intermediate premix containing 5 grams per pound by mixing 1.0 lb of ALBAC® 50 in 9.0 lbs of soybean meal or ground corn. Then add 0.8 to 10 lbs of intermediate premix per ton of Type C medicated feed.

Usage levels for bacitracin from ALBAC® 50:

Species	Grams bacitracin per ton	
	Min.	Max.
Growing chickens, turkeys and pheasants	4	50
Growing quail (not over 5 weeks of age)	5	20
Laying chickens	10	25
Growing-finishing swine	10	50
Feedlot cattle	35-70 mg/head/day	

Levels shown are minimum and maximum quantities.

The bacitracin zinc concentration may be varied between these levels.

Caution(s): For manufacturing registered livestock and poultry feeds only.

Restricted drug: Use only as directed.

For use in dry feeds only. Not for use in liquid Type B medicated feed.

Warning(s): Not for use in feeds for breeder chickens.

Presentation: 50 lb (22.67 kg) bags.

Compendium Code No.: 10220041

ALBADRY PLUS®

Pharmacia & Upjohn **Mastitis Therapy**

brand of penicillin G procaine and novobiocin sodium suspension

NADA No.: 055-098

Active Ingredient(s): Description: Each 10 mL Plastet® Disposable Syringe contains:

Novobiocin sodium equiv. to novobiocin........ 400 mg
Penicillin G procaine........ 200,000 IU
Chlorobutanol anhydrous (chloral derivative - used as a preservative)........ 50 mg

in a special bland vehicle.
Manufactured by a non-sterilizing process.

Indications: ALBADRY PLUS® Suspension is indicated for the treatment, in dry cows only, of subclinical mastitis caused by susceptible strains of *Staphylococcus aureus* and *Streptococcus agalactiae*.

Dosage and Administration:

Dosage: Infuse one tube per quarter at start of dry period (but not less than 30 days prior to calving).

Shake well before using.

Directions for Using the Flexi-Tube™ System: The Flexi-Tube™ is designed to provide the choice of either insertion of the full cannula, as has traditionally been practiced, or insertion of no more than ⅛ inch of the cannula, as recommended by the National Mastitis Council.

a. Full Insertion: Remove the blue end cap by pulling straight up. Gently insert the full cannula into the teat canal; carefully infuse the product.
b. Partial Insertion: Remove both the blue end cap and the red cannula by pushing sideways. Gently insert the exposed blue tip into the teat canal; carefully infuse the product.

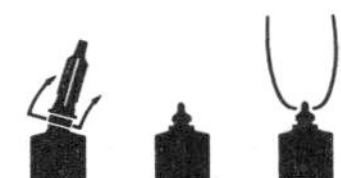

Administration: At the time of drying off, but not less than 30 days prior to calving, milk the udder dry. Wash the teats and udder thoroughly with warm water containing a suitable dairy antiseptic. Dry the teats and udder thoroughly. Infuse each quarter using the following procedure. Using the alcohol pads provided, scrub each teat end clean using a separate pad for each teat. Warm ALBADRY PLUS® Suspension to body temperature and shake thoroughly. Choose the desired insertion length (full or partial) and insert tip into teat canal. Instill entire contents into the quarter. Massage the udder after treatment to distribute the ALBADRY PLUS® Suspension throughout the quarters. Using a suitable teat dip, dip all teats following treatment.

Precaution(s): Storage Conditions: Store at controlled room temperature 20° to 25°C (68° to 77°F) [see USP].

Caution(s): Administration of this product in any manner other than shown under Dosage may result in drug residues.

Discard empty container; do not reuse.

Keep out of reach of children.

For use in animals only — Not for human use.

Restricted drug — Use only as directed (California).

Warning(s):

1. Do not use less than 30 days prior to calving.
2. Milk from treated cows must not be used for food during the first 72 hours after calving.
3. Treated animals must not be slaughtered for food for 30 days following udder infusion.

Presentation: ALBADRY PLUS® Suspension is available in unbroken packages of 12-10 mL Plastet® Disposable Syringes with 12 individually wrapped 70% isopropyl alcohol pads and unbroken packages of 144-10 mL Plastet® Disposable Syringes with 144 individually wrapped 70% isopropyl alcohol pads.

Manufactured by: Norbrook Laboratories Limited, Newry, BT35 6JP, Northern Ireland.

Compendium Code No.: 10490010 812 404 007

ALBAMIX® FEED MEDICATION

Pharmacia & Upjohn **Feed Medication**

(Novobiocin mixture) (Type A Medicated Article)

NADA No.: 012-375

Active Ingredient(s): Each pound contains:

Novobiocin . . . . 25 grams

Amorphous fractions from novobiocin manufacture.

Ingredients—Soybean hulls, #20 grind; mineral oil, USP.

Indications:

Chickens and Turkeys—For use in feed for the treatment of staphylococcal synovitis, generalized staphylococcal infections, and as an aid in the treatment of breast blisters associated with staphylococcal infections susceptible to novobiocin.

Turkeys Only—For use in feed for the treatment of acute outbreaks of fowl cholera and as an aid in the control of recurring outbreaks of fowl cholera caused by strains of *Pasteurella multocida* susceptible to novobiocin.

Mink—For use in moist feed for the treatment of generalized staphylococcal infections, staphylococcal abscesses, and urinary infections of staphylococcal origin. Also for urinary or generalized infections caused by organisms shown to be novobiocin-sensitive based upon laboratory diagnosis. When fed as directed (200 grams per ton of wet feed) novobiocin is safe in pregnant and lactating females, males and growing kits of all color phases.

Ducks—For the control of infectious serositis and fowl cholera in ducks caused by stains of *Pasteurella anapestifer* and *P. multocida* respectively, susceptible to novobiocin.

Dosage and Administration:

Important: Must be thoroughly mixed with feed before use.

Sick animals need the full dosage recommended. All dosage recommendations are based on an animal's usual daily intake; if the animal is not eating normally, put the recommended amount of drug in a smaller amount of feed or treat individually. It is important that each animal get the full dosage as follows:

Directions for Use:

Type C Medicated Feeds:

Turkeys—350 grams novobiocin (14 lb ALBAMIX®) per ton of feed to provide approximately 8 mg/lb body weight daily for the average 16-week-old heavy-breed turkey. Since younger birds consume more feed proportionally than older birds, the daily drug intake will decrease as the birds get older. The minimum effective dose in turkeys has been found to be approximately 7 mg/lb body weight per day for staphylococcal synovitis and generalized staph infections; and 5 mg/lb for fowl cholera.

Use 200 grams novobiocin (8 lb ALBAMIX®) per ton of feed to provide approximately 5 mg/lb body weight daily for the average 16-week-old bird. The minimum effective dose of novobiocin for turkeys in the treatment of staphylococcal-associated breast blisters is approximately 4 mg/lb body weight daily.

Chickens—Use 350 grams novobiocin (14 lb ALBAMIX®) per ton of feed to provide approximately 14 mg/lb body weight daily for the 4- to 8-week-old bird. As with turkeys, feed consumption per pound of body weight declines with increasing age. The minimum effective dose for chickens for treatment of staph synovitis and generalized staph infections is approximately 10 mg/lb body weight daily.

Use 200 grams novobiocin (8 lb ALBAMIX®) to provide 4- to 8-week-old chickens with about 7 mg/lb body weight daily. The minimum effective dose for chickens in the treatment of staphylococcal-associated breast blisters is approximately 6 mg/lb body weight daily.

Note: Type C Medicated Feed containing ALBAMIX® Feed Medication (Type A Medicated Article) should be fed to the flock for 5 to 7 days. Start feeding at the first signs of infection or recurrence of the disease.

Treatment may be repeated at a later date if necessary.

Ducks—Use 350 grams novobiocin (14 lb ALBAMIX®) per ton of feed. Mix thoroughly. The medicated feed should be the sole ration for the infected ducks. Medication should be started at the first signs of infection and continued for 5 to 7 days. Medication may be continued for 14 days if necessary, or repeated if the infection recurs.

Mink—Use 200 grams novobiocin (8 lb ALBAMIX®) per ton of wet feed for the treatment of staphylococcal or other novobiocin-sensitive organisms causing generalized infection, abscesses or urinary infection.

Mixing Instructions and Administration: After mixing the ground meat, cereal fraction and water to prepare the standard wet ration, add 8 pounds of ALBAMIX® per ton of the wet feed mixture. Mix thoroughly.

Type C Medicated Feed containing ALBAMIX® Feed Medication (Type A Medicated Article) should be fed to the herd for 7 days. Treatment may be repeated at a later date, if necessary.

Precaution(s): Store at room temperature and in a dry place to prevent caking.

Caution(s): As with most bacterial diseases, it is important that a diagnosis and bacteriological examination be made prior to or early in the treatment of the disease and the antibiotic sensitivity of the causative organism determined. If antibiotic sensitivity tests demonstrate that the causative organism is not sensitive to novobiocin, other appropriate antibacterial therapy should be used.

Not for human use.

Restricted Drug—Use only as directed (California).

Warning(s): Discontinue therapy with ALBAMIX® 4 days before slaughter of turkeys and chickens.

Not for use in laying chickens and laying turkeys.

Discontinue therapy with ALBAMIX® 3 days before slaughter of ducks.

Not for use in laying ducks.

Presentation: 50 pounds (22.6 kg).

Compendium Code No.: 10490020

ALBAPLEX® ℞

Pharmacia & Upjohn **Tetracycline-Novobiocin**

Tetracycline hydrochloride and novobiocin sodium tablets

NADA No.: 055-076

Active Ingredient(s): ALBAPLEX® Tablets, designed for use in dogs, contain a combination of two antibiotics—tetracycline hydrochloride and novobiocin sodium—which supply additive antibacterial effects against certain bacterial pathogens. Each tablet contains:

	ALBAPLEX®
Tetracycline hydrochloride	60 mg
Novobiocin sodium	60 mg

Indications: ALBAPLEX® Tablets are indicated for use in the treatment of acute or chronic canine respiratory infections such as tonsillitis, bronchitis, and tracheobronchitis when caused by pathogens susceptible to tetracycline hydrochloride and/or novobiocin sodium such as *Staphylococcus* spp. and *E. coli*. As with all antibiotics, appropriate *in vitro* culturing and susceptibility tests of samples taken before treatment should be conducted.

Pharmacology:

Tetracycline Hydrochloride: Tetracycline hydrochloride is an odorless, yellow, fine crystalline powder which is freely soluble in water and gastric juice. Tetracycline hydrochloride is absorbed readily from the gastrointestinal tract. Following oral administration to dogs, peak blood concentrations are obtained within two to four hours, effective concentrations are found at 12 hours and detectable amounts remain in the serum for at least 24 hours. The antibiotic is excreted principally through the kidney.

The range of antimicrobial activity of tetracycline hydrochloride includes a broad range of gram-positive and gram-negative bacteria such as alpha and beta streptococci; some strains of staphylococci, *Klebsiella pneumoniae*, certain clostridia, Shigella, *Aerobacter aerogenes* and some strains of Salmonella. The clinical significance of this has not been determined.

In an *in vivo* study, it was shown that tetracycline was significantly less effective than novobiocin in eliminating pathogenic staphylococci organisms from the throats of dogs suffering from upper respiratory infections. However, it was also shown that tetracycline was significantly more effective than novobiocin in eliminating pathogenic streptococci.

Studies show that tetracycline hydrochloride has a low order of toxicity comparable to that of other tetracyclines.

Novobiocin Sodium: Novobiocin sodium is an antibiotic produced by *Streptomyces niveus* and developed in the Research Laboratories of The Upjohn Company. The crystalline antibiotic has a light yellow to white color depending upon the state of subdivision. In contrast to most antibiotics produced by actinomycetes, novobiocin sodium, like penicillin, is acidic in nature and is stable to the degree of acidity or alkalinity present in the gastrointestinal tract.

Following oral administration to dogs, peak blood concentrations are obtained within one to two hours and significant levels are found at twelve hours. When appreciable amounts of novobiocin sodium are present in the serum, the drug diffuses into the pleural and ascitic fluids. Novobiocin sodium does not diffuse into the cerebrospinal fluid. The antibiotic is concentrated in the liver and bile and is excreted in the feces and urine. As determined by tests in animals, novobiocin sodium has a relatively low order of toxicity.

In vitro studies show that novobiocin sodium is active against both gram-positive and gram-negative bacteria, including some strains of *Staphylococcus aureus, Streptococcus hemolyticus, Diplococcus pneumoniae*, and some strains of *Proteus vulgaris*. The clinical significance of this has not been determined. Novobiocin sodium shows no cross-resistance with penicillin against resistant strains of *Staphylococcus aureus*. However, *in vitro* studies indicate that *Staphylococcus aureus* may develop resistance to novobiocin sodium as with other antibiotics.

Combined Antibiotic Therapy: Therapy with ALBAPLEX® Tablets offers a wider range of antimicrobial activity than does therapy with either single antibiotic.

An *in vivo* clinical study in dogs with upper respiratory infections showed ALBAPLEX® Tablets were significantly more effective in eliminating *Staphylococcus* spp. and *E. coli* organisms from throat tissues than was tetracycline hydrochloride or novobiocin sodium administered singly. Treatment failure was significantly reduced by use of ALBAPLEX® Tablets when compared to treatment with either single antibiotic. This *in vivo* clinical study demonstrated that the two antibiotics had complementary spectra of activities with significantly fewer organisms resistant to the combination of tetracycline hydrochloride and novobiocin sodium than to either single antibiotic.

Dosage and Administration: The recommended dose of ALBAPLEX® Tablets for dogs is:

10 mg of each antibiotic per lb of body weight repeated at 12 hour intervals. This dose can be given as follows:

ALBAPLEX® Tablets (one tablet for each 6 lbs of body weight):

Body Weight	ALBAPLEX® Tablets every 12 Hours
2.5 to 4 lb	½
5 to 8 lb	1
9 to 15 lb	2
16 to 24 lb	3
25 to 40 lb	5
41 to 65 lb	8

Treatment should be continued for at least 48 hours after the temperature has returned to normal and all evidence of infection has disappeared. Treatment with ALBAPLEX® Tablets may be continued for a period as long as 10 days if clinical judgement indicates.

Precaution(s): Store at controlled room temperature 20° to 25°C (68° to 77°F) [see USP].

Caution(s): Federal (USA) law restricts this drug to use by or on the order of a licensed veterinarian.

For use in animals only.

Warning(s): Not for human use.

Side Effects: Since the use of any broad spectrum antibiotic may result in overgrowth of nonsusceptible organisms, constant observation of the animal patient is essential. If new infections appear during therapy, appropriate measures should be taken.

Because of the wide antibacterial effect of this antibiotic combination on intestinal flora, a change in the character of the stools may be anticipated in certain animals; however, administration of novobiocin sodium and tetracycline hydrochloride, combined, to dogs at exaggerated dosages daily for six months caused no significant toxic effects. If allergic reactions develop during treatment with ALBAPLEX® Tablets, use should be discontinued.

Presentation: ALBAPLEX® Tablets are supplied in bottles of 500.

Compendium Code No.: 10490030

ALBON® BOLUSES

Pfizer Animal Health **Sulfadimethoxine**

(sulfadimethoxine)

NADA No.: 031-715

Active Ingredient(s): Each bolus contains 5 g or 15 g of sulfadimethoxine.

Indications: ALBON® is effective in the treatment of shipping fever complex and bacterial pneumonia associated with *Pasteurella* spp. sensitive to sulfadimethoxine; and calf diphtheria and foot rot associated with *Fusobacterium necrophorum (Sphaerophorus necrophorus)* sensitive to sulfadimethoxine in cattle.

Pharmacology: Description: ALBON® is a low-dose, rapidly absorbed, long-acting sulfonamide.

Actions: Sulfadimethoxine has been demonstrated in laboratory studies to be effective against a wide variety of organisms, such as streptococci, staphylococci and members of the *E. coli*-salmonella group of bacteria.

Comparatively low doses of ALBON® give rapid, sustained blood levels required for effective disease therapy.

Dosage and Administration: ALBON® should be administered to cattle so that the initial dose is equivalent to 25 mg/lb of body weight and each subsequent daily dose is equivalent to 12.5 mg/lb of body weight. Length of treatment will depend on clinical response. In most cases, treatment for 3-4 days is adequate. Treatment should not be continued beyond 5 days.

The following tables show the dosage and dosage forms to be used for cattle of different weights.

ALBON® Boluses, 5 g

Dosage Schedule for Cattle: 200-600 lb of body weight

Animal Weight, lb	First Day	Daily for the Following 3-4 Days
200	1 bolus	½ bolus
300	1½ boluses	1 bolus
400	2 boluses	1 bolus
500	2½ boluses	1½ boluses
600	3 boluses	1½ boluses

ALBON® Boluses, 15 g

Dosage Schedule for Cattle: 600-1,200 lb of body weight

Animal Weight, lb	First Day	Daily for the Following 3-4 Days
600	1 bolus	½ bolus
800	1½ boluses	1 bolus
1,000-1,200	2 boluses	1½ boluses

Precaution(s): Store at controlled room temperature 15°-30°C (59°-86°F).

Caution(s): During treatment period, make certain that animals maintain adequate water intake.

If animals show no improvement within 2-3 days, reevaluate your diagnosis. Treatment should not be continued beyond 5 days.

Restricted drug (California)—Use only as directed.

Not for human use.

Warning(s): Milk taken from animals during treatment and for 60 hours (5 milkings) after the latest treatment must not be used for food.

Do not slaughter animals for food purposes within 7 days following the last treatment.

A withdrawal period has not been established for this product in preruminating calves.

Do not use in calves to be processed for veal

Toxicology: Toxicity and Safety: ALBON® has been shown to be a well-tolerated sulfonamide with relatively high solubility at the pH normally occurring in the kidney and with a low degree of toxicity. Following the administration of ALBON® at the recommended dosage, no undesirable side effects have been observed.

Presentation: ALBON® Boluses, 5 g - 50 boluses per bottle.
ALBON® Boluses, 15 g - 12 and 50 boluses per bottle.

Compendium Code No.: 36900040 75-8448-04

ALBON® CONCENTRATED SOLUTION 12.5%

Pfizer Animal Health **Water Medication**

(sulfadimethoxine) Antibacterial for use in drinking water

NADA No.: 031-205

Active Ingredient(s): Each fl oz contains 3.75 g sulfadimethoxine.

Indications: For oral use in chickens, turkeys, and cattle.

Broiler and Replacement Chickens—Use for the treatment of disease outbreaks of coccidiosis, fowl cholera, and infectious coryza.

Meat-producing Turkeys—Use for the treatment of disease outbreaks of coccidiosis and fowl cholera.

Dairy Calves, Dairy Heifers, and Beef Cattle—Use for the treatment of shipping fever complex and bacterial pneumonia associated with *Pasteurella* spp. sensitive to sulfadimethoxine; and calf diphtheria and foot rot associated with *Fusobacterium necrophorum (Sphaerophorus necrophorus)* sensitive to sulfadimethoxine.

Dosage and Administration:

Chickens and Turkeys

Treatment Period: 6 consecutive days.

Recommended Concentration: Chickens—0.05%; Turkeys—0.025%

Chickens: Add 1 fl oz (30 mL) to 2 gal of drinking water or 25 fl oz to 50 gal of drinking water.

Turkeys: Add 1 fl oz (30 mL) to 4 gal of drinking water or 25 fl oz to 100 gal of drinking water.

Automatic Proportioners* Stock Solution—To make 2 gal of stock solution:

Chickens: Add 1 gal of ALBON® Concentrated Solution 12.5% to 1 gal of water.

Turkeys: Add 2 qt of ALBON® Concentrated Solution 12.5% to 6 qt of water.

*Set proportioner to a feed rate of 1 fl oz of stock solution per gal of water.

Dairy Calves, Dairy Heifers, and Beef Cattle

Treatment Period: 5 consecutive days.

Dosage: Initial dose of 25 mg/lb followed by four maintenance doses of 12.5 mg/lb/day.

Summer Administration: Dosage recommendations for summer are based on an estimated water intake of 1 gal of water for every 100 lb of body weight per day.

Daily Drinking Water Supply	ALBON® Concentrated Solution 12.5%	
	Initial Dose	Maintenance Dose
25 gal	1 pt (16 fl oz)	1 cup (8 fl oz)
50 gal	1 qt (32 fl oz)	1 pt (16 fl oz)
200 gal	1 gal (128 fl oz)	2 qt (64 fl oz)

Water Administration: Dosage recommendations for winter are based on an estimated water intake of 1 gal of water for every 150 lb of body weight per day.

Daily Drinking Water Supply	ALBON® Concentrated Solution 12.5%	
	Initial Dose	Maintenance
16 gal	1 pt (16 fl oz)	1 cup (8 fl oz)
33 gal	1 qt (32 fl oz)	1 pt (16 fl oz)
127 gal	1 gal (128 fl oz)	2 qt (64 fl oz)

For individual treatment of cattle, ALBON® Concentrated Solution 12.5% may be given as a drench. Administer using an initial dose of 25 mg/lb followed by 4 maintenance doses of 12.5 mg/lb/day. One fl oz will medicate one 150-lb animal initially and ½ fl oz will medicate one 150-lb animal on maintenance dose.

Precaution(s): Store at controlled room temperature 15°-30°C (59°-86°F). If freezing occurs, thaw before using. Protect from light; direct sunlight may cause discoloration. Freezing or discoloration does not affect potency.

Caution(s): Restricted drug (California)—Use only as directed.

Chickens and Turkeys—If animals show no improvement within 5 days, discontinue treatment and reevaluate diagnosis. Handle the recommended dilutions (chickens 0.05% and turkeys 0.025%) as regular drinking water. Administer as sole source of drinking water and sulfonamide medication.

Chickens and turkeys that have survived fowl cholera outbreaks should not be kept for replacements or breeders.

Cattle—During treatment period, make certain that animals maintain adequate water intake. If animals show no improvement within 2 or 3 days, reevaluate diagnosis. Treatment should not be continued beyond 5 days.

Prepare a fresh stock solution daily.

Warning(s):

Chickens and Turkeys—Withdraw 5 days before slaughter. Do not administer to chickens over 16 weeks (112 days) of age or to turkeys over 24 weeks (168 days) of age.

Cattle—Withdraw 7 days before slaughter. For dairy calves, dairy heifers, and beef cattle only.

A withdrawal period has not been established for this product in preruminating calves.

Do not use in calves to be processed for veal.

Not for human use.

Presentation: 1 gal (3.8 L).

Compendium Code No.: 36900050 85-8445-03

ALBON® INJECTION 40% ℞

Pfizer Animal Health **Sulfadimethoxine**

(sulfadimethoxine)

NADA No.: 041-245

Active Ingredient(s): Each mL contains 400 mg of sulfadimethoxine compounded with 20% propylene glycol, 1% benzyl alcohol, 0.1 mg disodium edetate, 1.0 mg sodium formaldehyde sulfoxylate, and pH adjusted with sodium hydroxide.

Indications: Dogs and Cats: ALBON® Injection 40% is indicated for the treatment of a wide range of respiratory, genitourinary tract, enteric, and soft tissue infections. For example: tonsillitis, pustular dermatitis, pharyngitis, anal gland infections, bronchitis, abscesses, pneumonia, wound infections, cystitis, bacterial enteritis, nephritis, canine salmonellosis, metritis, bacterial enteritis associated with coccidiosis in dogs, and pyometra when caused by streptococci, staphylococci, escherichia, salmonella, klebsiella, proteus or shigella organisms sensitive to sulfadimethoxine.

Limitations: Dogs and Cats: Sulfadimethoxine is not effective in viral or rickettsial infections, and as with any antibacterial agent, occasional failures in therapy may occur due to resistant microorganisms. The usual precautions in sulfonamide therapy should be observed.

Horses: ALBON® Injection 40% is indicated for the treatment of respiratory disease caused by *Streptococcus equi* (strangles).

Cattle: ALBON® Injection 40% is indicated for the treatment of bovine respiratory disease complex (shipping fever complex) and bacterial pneumonia associated with *Pasteurella* spp. sensitive to sulfadimethoxine; necrotic pododermatitis (foot rot) and calf diphtheria caused by *Fusobacterium necrophorum (Sphaerophorus necrophorus)* sensitive to sulfadimethoxine.

Limitations: See Dogs and Cats, under Limitations.

Pharmacology: Description: ALBON® Injection 40% is a low-dosage, rapidly absorbed, long-acting sulfonamide, effective for the treatment of a wide range of bacterial infections commonly encountered in dogs and cats; the treatment of respiratory disease of horses, and the treatment of shipping fever complex, bacterial pneumonia, calf diphtheria, and foot rot in cattle.

Sulfadimethoxine is a white, almost tasteless and odorless compound. Chemically, it is N1-(2,6-dimethoxy-4-pyrimidinyl) sulfanilamide. The structural formula is:

$$H_2N-C_6H_4-SO_2-NH-C_4HN_2(OCH_3)_2$$

Actions: Dogs and Cats: Sulfadimethoxine has been demonstrated clinically or in the laboratory to be effective against a variety of organisms, such as streptococci, klebsiella, proteus, shigella, staphylococci, escherichia, and salmonella.[1,2] These organisms have been demonstrated in respiratory, genitourinary, enteric, and soft tissue infections of dogs and cats.

The systemic sulfonamides which include sulfadimethoxine are bacteriostatic agents. Sulfonamides competitively inhibit bacterial synthesis of folic acid (pteroylglutamic acid) from para-aminobenzoic acid. Mammalian cells are capable of utilizing folic acid in the presence of sulfonamides.

The tissue distribution of sulfadimethoxine, as with all sulfonamides, is a function of plasma levels, degree of plasma protein binding, and subsequent passive distribution in the tissues of the lipid-soluble un-ionized form. The relative amounts are determined by both its pKa and by the pH of each tissue. Therefore, levels tend to be higher in less acid tissue and body fluids or those diseased tissues having high concentrations of leucocytes.[2]

In the dog, sulfadimethoxine is not acetylated as in most other animals, and it is excreted predominantly as the unchanged drug.[3] Sulfadimethoxine has a relatively high solubility at the pH normally occurring in the kidney, precluding the possibility of precipitation and crystalluria. Slow renal excretion results from a high degree of tubular reabsorption,[4] and plasma protein binding is very high, providing a blood reservoir of the drug. Thus, sulfadimethoxine maintains higher blood levels than most other long-acting sulfonamides. Single, comparatively low doses of Albon give rapid and sustained therapeutic blood levels.[1]

To assure successful sulfonamide therapy (1) the drug must be given early in the course of the disease, and it must produce a high sulfonamide level in the body rapidly after administration, (2) therapeutically effective sulfonamide levels must be maintained in the body throughout the treatment period, (3) treatment should continue for a short period of time after the clinical signs have disappeared, and (4) the causative organisms must be sensitive to this class of drugs.

Horses and Cattle:

Actions: General principles of sulfonamide treatment, antibacterial spectrum of activity, and the tissue distribution of sulfadimethoxine are discussed under Actions, Dogs and Cats.

In the horse, the concentration of sulfadimeth-oxine has been determined to be higher in the wall of the duodenum than in any other part of the intestine. This, together with the high drug concentration in the bile, suggests enterohepatic cycling of the drug. Significant drug concentrations were also present in the cerebro-spinal fluid.[5] Single, comparatively low doses of Albon give rapid and sustained therapeutic blood levels.[1]

Dosage and Administration: Dogs and Cats: ALBON® Injection 40% is recommended only for administration by the intravenous route. Usually the injectable formulation may be used to obtain effective blood levels almost immediately or to facilitate treatment of the fractious animal, and the oral formulations utilized for maintenance therapy. However, the injectable formulation may be used for the entire course of Albon therapy when indicated.

Dogs and cats should receive 1 mL of ALBON® Injection 40% per 16 lb of body weight (55 mg/kg) as an initial dose, followed by ½ mL per 16 lb of body weight (27.5 mg/kg) every 24 hours thereafter. Representative weights and doses are indicated in the following table:

Each mL contains 400 mg of sulfadimethoxine.

Animal Weight	Initial Dose 25 mg/lb (55 mg/kg)	Subsequent Daily Doses 12.5 mg/lb (27.5 mg/kg)
8 lb (3.6 kg)	½ mL	¼ mL
16 lb (7.3 kg)	1 mL	½ mL
32 lb (14.5 kg)	2 mL	1 mL
64 lb (29.1 kg)	4 mL	2 mL

Horses and Cattle: ALBON® Injection 40% must be administered only by the intravenous route in horses and cattle. Horses and cattle should receive 1 mL of Albon Injection 40% per 16 lb of body weight (55 mg/kg) as an initial dose, followed by ½ mL per 16 lb of body weight (27.5 mg/kg) every 24 hours thereafter. Albon® Boluses may be utilized for maintenance therapy in cattle. Representative weights and doses are indicated in the following table:

Each mL contains 400 mg of sulfadimethoxine.

Animal Weight	Initial Dose 25 mg/lb (55 mg/kg)	Subsequent Daily Doses 12.5 mg/lb (27.5 mg/kg)
250 lb (113.6 kg)	15.6 mL	7.8 mL
500 lb (227.2 kg)	31.2 mL	15.6 mL
750 lb (340.9 kg)	46.9 mL	23.5 mL
1000 lb (454.5 kg)	62.5 mL	31.3 mL

Length of treatment depends on the clinical response. In most cases treatment for 3-5 days is adequate. Treatment should be continued until the animal is asymptomatic for 48 hours.

For storage information, see Note under Precautions.

Precaution(s): Note: Store at room temperature. Should crystallization occur at cold temperatures, crystals will dissolve either by storing at room temperature for several days or by heating the vial in warm water. Crystallization and redissolution do not impair the efficacy of the product.

Caution(s): Federal law restricts this drug to use by or on the order of a licensed veterinarian.

Dogs and Cats: During treatment period, make certain that animals maintain adequate water intake.

If animals show no improvement within 2 or 3 days, consult your veterinarian.

Intramuscular administration is not recommended. Some animals treated by the intramuscular route exhibit signs of pain during and for a few minutes following such injections, and in dogs blood levels are lower than those obtained by intravenous treatment.

Horses and Cattle: During treatment period, make certain that animals maintain adequate water intake.

If animals show no improvement within 2 or 3 days, reevaluate your diagnosis.

Warning(s): Milk taken from animals during treatment and for 60 hours (5 milkings) after the latest treatment must not be used for food.

Do not administer within 5 days of slaughter. Not for use in horses intended for food.

A withdrawal period has not been established for this product in preruminating calves.

Do not use in calves to be processed for veal.

Not for human use.

Toxicology: Toxicity and Safety:

Dogs and Cats: Data regarding acute and chronic toxicities of sulfadimethoxine indicate the drug is very safe. The LD50 in mice is greater than 2 g/kg of body weight when administered intraperitoneally and greater than 16 g/kg when administered orally. In dogs receiving massive single oral doses of 3.2 g/kg of body weight, diarrhea was the only adverse effect observed. Dogs given 160 mg/kg of body weight orally daily for 13 weeks showed no signs of toxicity.

Cattle and Horses: No toxic effects were noted in horses receiving up to 3 times the recommended dosage as a single injection or twice the recommended dosage for an entire course of therapy. In cattle sulfadimethoxine has been shown to be safe through extensive clinical use with other dosage forms. In addition, studies with intravenous administration of ALBON® Injection 40% have demonstrated that hemolysis of erythrocytes does not occur by this route of administration. Sulfadimethoxine has a high solubility at the pH normally occurring in the kidney, precluding the possibility of precipitation and crystalluria. Toxicity data in laboratory animals is discussed under Toxicity and Safety, Dogs and Cats.

References: Available upon request.

Presentation: ALBON® Injection 40% is available in 100-mL, multiple-dose vials.

Manufactured by: Boehringer Ingelheim Vetmedica, Inc., St. Joseph, Missouri 64506, USA

Compendium Code No.: 36900030 85-8434-03

ALBON® TABLETS AND ORAL SUSPENSION 5% ℞

Pfizer Animal Health **Sulfadimethoxine**

(sulfadimethoxine)

NADA No.: 015-102 (Tablets) / 043-785 (Suspension)

Active Ingredient(s):

ALBON® Tablets: 125 mg, 250 mg, or 500 mg sulfadimethoxine per tablet.

ALBON® Oral Suspension 5%: Each teaspoon (5 mL) contains 250 mg sulfadimethoxine.

Indications: For the treatment of sulfadimethoxine-sensitive bacterial infections in dogs and cats and bacterial enteritis associated with coccidiosis in dogs.

ALBON® is indicated for the treatment of respiratory, genitourinary tract, enteric, and soft tissue infections in dogs and cats: tonsillitis, pharyngitis, bronchitis, pneumonia, cystitis, nephritis, metritis, pyometra, pustular dermatitis, anal gland infections, abscesses, wound infections, bacterial enteritis, canine salmonellosis, bacterial enteritis associated with coccidiosis in dogs, when caused by streptococci, staphylococci, escherichia, salmonella, klebsiella, proteus or shigella organisms sensitive to sulfadimethoxine.

Limitations: Sulfadimethoxine is not effective in viral or rickettsial infections, and as with any antibacterial agent, occasional failures in therapy may occur due to resistant microorganisms. The usual precautions in sulfonamide therapy should be observed.

Pharmacology: Description: ALBON® is a low-dosage, rapidly absorbed, long-acting sulfonamide, effective for the treatment of a wide range of bacterial infections commonly encountered in dogs and cats.

Sulfadimethoxine is a white, almost tasteless and odorless compound. Chemically, it is N^1-(2,6-dimethoxy-4-pyrimidinyl) sulfanilamide. The structural formula is:

$$H_2N-C_6H_4-SO_2-NH-C_4HN_2(OCH_3)_2$$

Actions: Sulfadimethoxine has been demonstrated clinically or in the laboratory to be effective against a variety of organisms, such as streptococci, klebsiella, proteus, shigella, staphylococci, escherichia, and salmonella.[1,2] These organisms have been demonstrated in respiratory, genitourinary, enteric, and soft tissue infections of dogs and cats.

The systemic sulfonamides which include sulfadimethoxine are bacteriostatic agents. Sulfonamides competitively inhibit bacterial synthesis of folic acid (pteroylglutamic acid) from para-aminobenzoic acid. Mammalian cells are capable of utilizing folic acid in the presence of sulfonamides.

The tissue distribution of sulfadimethoxine, as with all sulfonamides, is a function of plasma levels, degree of plasma protein binding, and subsequent passive distribution in the tissues of the lipid-soluble un-ionized form. The relative amounts are determined by both its pKa and by the pH of each tissue. Therefore, levels tend to be higher in less acid tissue and body fluids or those diseased tissues having high concentrations of leucocytes.[2]

In the dog, sulfadimethoxine is not acetylated as in most other animals, and it is excreted predominantly as the unchanged drug.[3] Sulfadimethoxine has a relatively high solubility at the pH normally occurring in the kidney, precluding the possibility of precipitation and crystalluria. Slow renal excretion results from a high degree of tubular reabsorption,[4] and plasma protein binding is very high, providing a blood reservoir of the drug. Thus, sulfadimethoxine maintains higher blood levels than most other long-acting sulfonamides. Single, comparatively low doses of ALBON® give rapid and sustained therapeutic blood levels.[1]

To assure successful sulfonamide therapy (1) the drug must be given early in the course of the disease, and it must produce a high sulfonamide level in the body rapidly after administration, (2) therapeutically effective sulfonamide levels must be maintained in the body throughout the treatment period, (3) treatment should continue for a short period of time after the clinical signs have disappeared, and (4) the causative organisms must be sensitive to this class of drugs.

Dosage and Administration:
Initial dose: 25 mg/lb (55 mg/kg) of animal body weight.
Subsequent Daily Doses: 12.5 mg/lb (27.5 mg/kg) of animal body weight.
ALBON® Tablets: For ease of administration in animals of varying weights, 3 tablet sizes are provided. The following table indicates how dosage may be adjusted depending on tablet size and body weight. Subsequent doses should be given at 24-hour intervals.

Tablet Size	Approximate Animal Weight	Initial Dose 25 mg/lb (55 mg/kg)	Subsequent Daily Doses 12.5 mg/lb (27.5 mg/kg)
125 mg	5 lb (2.2 kg)	1 tablet	½ tablet
250 mg	10 lb (4.5 kg)	1 tablet	½ tablet
500 mg	20 lb (9.1 kg)	1 tablet	½ tablet

ALBON® Oral Suspension 5%: Dogs and cats should receive 1 teaspoonful of ALBON® Oral Suspension 5% per 10 lb of body weight (25 mg/lb or 55 mg/kg) as an initial dose, followed by ½ teaspoonful per 10 lb of body weight (12.5 mg/lb or 27.5 mg/kg) every 24 hours thereafter. Representative weights and doses are indicated in the following table:

Animal Weight	Initial Dose 25 mg/lb (55 mg/kg)	Subsequent Daily Doses 12.5 mg/lb (27.5 mg/kg)
5 lb (2.2 kg)	½ tsp (2½ mL)	¼ tsp (1¼ mL)
10 lb (4.5 kg)	1 tsp (5 mL)	½ tsp (2½ mL)
20 lb (9.1 kg)	2 tsp (10 mL)	1 tsp (5 mL)
40 lb (18.2 kg)	4 tsp (20 mL)	2 tsp (10 mL)
80 lb (36.4 kg)	8 tsp (40 mL)	4 tsp (20 mL)

Treatment may be initiated with Albon® Injection 40% to obtain effective blood levels almost immediately or to facilitate treatment of the fractious animal.

Length of treatment depends on the clinical response. In most cases treatment for 3-5 days is adequate. Treatment should be continued until the animal is asymptomatic for 48 hours.

Precaution(s): Storage: Store at controlled room temperature 15°-30°C (59°-86°F).

Caution(s): Federal law restricts this drug to use by or on the order of a licensed veterinarian.
During treatment period, make certain that animals maintain adequate water intake.
If animals show no improvement within 2 or 3 days, reevaluate your diagnosis.
Not for human use.

Toxicology: Toxicity and Safety: Data regarding acute and chronic toxicities of sulfadimethoxine indicate the drug is very safe. The LD_{50} in mice is greater than 2 g/kg of body weight when administered intraperitoneally and greater than 16 g/kg when administered orally. In dogs receiving massive single oral doses of 3.2 g/kg of body weight, diarrhea was the only adverse effect observed. Dogs given 160 mg/kg of body weight orally daily for 13 weeks showed no signs of toxicity.

References: Available upon request.

Presentation: ALBON® is available in the following dosage forms for dogs and cats:
ALBON® Tablets: 125 mg, 250 mg, or 500 mg sulfadimethoxine per tablet.
ALBON® Oral Suspension 5%: 2- and 16-oz bottles; each tsp (5 mL) contains 250 mg sulfadimethoxine in a custard-flavored carrier.

Compendium Code No.: 36901771 75-8430-07

ALBON® SR ℞

Pfizer Animal Health **Sulfadimethoxine**

(sulfadimethoxine) Sustained Release Bolus

NADA No.: 093-107

Active Ingredient(s): Each bolus contains 12.5 g sulfadimethoxine.

Indications: ALBON® SR is effective in the treatment of shipping fever complex and bacterial pneumonia associated with organisms such as *Pasteurella* spp. sensitive to sulfadimethoxine; and calf diphtheria and foot rot associated with *Fusobacterium necrophorum (Sphaerophorus necrophorus)* sensitive to sulfadimethoxine in beef cattle and nonlactating dairy cattle.

Pharmacology: Description: The ALBON® SR Bolus is a slow-release formulation of the low-dose, rapidly absorbed, long-acting sulfonamide, sulfadimethoxine.

Sulfadimethoxine is a white, almost tasteless and odorless compound. Chemically, it is N^1-(2,6-dimethoxy-4-pyrimidinyl) sulfanilamide. The structural formula is:

OCH_3
H_2N–(benzene ring)–SO_2–NH–(pyrimidine ring, N, N)
OCH_3

Actions: Sulfadimethoxine has been demonstrated in laboratory studies to be effective against a wide variety of organisms, such as streptococci, staphylococci, klebsiella, proteus, shigella, and members of the *E. coli*-salmonella group of bacteria.[1,2]

The systemic sulfonamides which include sulfadimethoxine are bacteriostatic agents. Sulfonamides competitively inhibit bacterial synthesis of folic acid (pteroylglutamic acid) from para-aminobenzoic acid. Mammalian cells are capable of utilizing folic acid in the presence of sulfonamides.

The tissue distribution of sulfadimethoxine, as with all sulfonamides, is a function of plasma levels, degree of plasma protein binding, and subsequent passive distribution in the tissues of the lipid-soluble un-ionized form. The relative amounts are determined by both its pKa and by the pH of each tissue. Therefore, levels tend to be higher in less acid tissue and body fluids or those diseased tissues having high concentrations of leucocytes.[2]

Dosage and Administration: ALBON® SR Boluses are to be orally administered to beef cattle and nonlactating dairy cattle. Care should be taken to make certain the boluses are swallowed before releasing the animal. As with any orally administered bolus, occasional regurgitation will occur in ruminants. To fully maintain the sustained release effect, the boluses must not be divided. Animals should receive 1 bolus for the nearest 200 lb of body weight, i.e., 62.5 mg/lb of body weight. Representative weights and doses are indicated in the following table:

Animal Weight, lb	200	400	600	800	1,000
Number of Boluses	1	2	3	4	5

To assure successful sulfonamide therapy (1) the drug must be given early in the course of the disease, and it must produce a high sulfonamide level in the body rapidly after administration, (2) therapeutically effective sulfonamide levels must be maintained in the body throughout the treatment period, (3) treatment should continue for a short period of time after the clinical signs have disappeared, and (4) the causative organisms must be sensitive to this class of drugs.

Precaution(s): Store at controlled room temperature 15°-30°C (59°-86°F).

Caution(s): Federal law restricts this drug to use by or on the order of a licensed veterinarian.
During treatment period, make certain that animals maintain adequate water intake.
Do not repeat treatment for 7 days.
Not for human use.

Warning(s): Do not use in lactating dairy cattle.
Do not administer within 21 days of slaughter.
A withdrawal period has not been established for this product in preruminating calves.
Do not use in calves to be processed for veal.

Toxicology: Toxicity and Safety: Data regarding acute and chronic toxicities of sulfadimethoxine indicate the drug is very safe. The LD_{50} in mice is greater than 2 g/kg of body weight when administered intraperitoneally and greater than 16 g/kg when administered orally. In dogs receiving massive single oral doses of 3.2 g/kg of body weight, diarrhea was the only adverse effect observed. Dogs given 160 mg/kg of body weight orally daily for 13 weeks showed no signs of toxicity.

Sulfadimethoxine has a relatively high solubility at the pH normally occurring in the kidney, precluding the possibility of precipitation and crystalluria. Following the administration of ALBON® (sulfadimethoxine) at the recommended dosage, no undesirable side effects have been observed.

Sustained Action: Use of ALBON® SR Boluses facilitates treatment and assures effective sulfonamide levels. Since only 1 treatment is required, both stress due to handling in acutely sick animals and labor costs are reduced. Sulfadimethoxine in itself maintains higher blood levels than most other long-acting sulfonamides.[3] Slow renal excretion results from a high degree of tubular reabsorption and plasma protein binding is very high, providing a blood reservoir of the drug.[3,4] In addition, the greatly prolonged rumen dissolution rate of ALBON® SR Boluses assures that the drug will be available for continued absorption over an extended period of time.

Blood Levels: ALBON® SR given once to cattle at the recommended dose level of sulfadimethoxine of 62.5 mg/lb (137.5 mg/kg) of body weight provides rapid, therapeutically effective plasma sulfonamide levels for a period of 4 days. As shown in the following chart, a single administration of ALBON® SR maintains higher plasma levels for 76 hours than repeated treatment with the regular ALBON® Bolus at the recommended levels.

Sulfadimethoxine Plasma Levels in Bovines

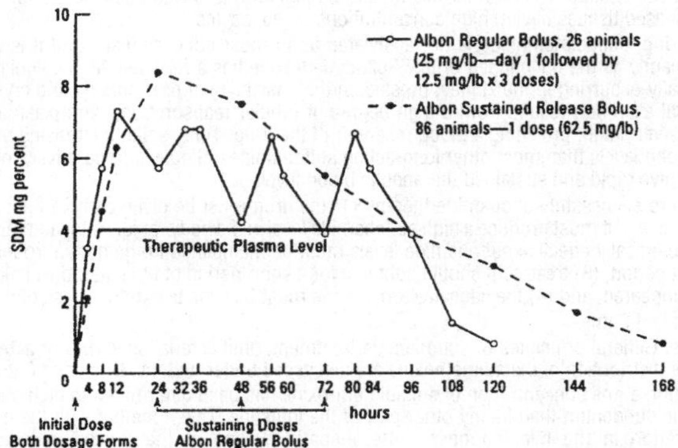

References: Available upon request.

Presentation: 50 boluses per bottle.

Compendium Code No.: 36900061 75-8447-06

ALFALFA PELLET HORSE WORMER

Farnam **Parasiticide-Oral**

Active Ingredient(s): Piperazine, dehydrated alfalfa and artificial flavors.
Piperazine phosphate monohydrate 50%
Equivalent to 21% (44.69 g) piperazine base.

Indications: For the control of the four major species of internal parasites: Large strongyles or bloodworms *(Strongylus vulgaris)*, large roundworms or ascarids *(Parascaris equorum)*, small strongyles and pinworms *(Oxyuris equi)*. Recommended for the treatment of all horses and ponies. Can be used on foals over three months of age. Can be used on mares until foaling time. Excellent for horses in heavy training and valuable race and show horses.

Dosage and Administration: The prescribed dosage for horses is 50 mg of piperazine base (119 mg of piperazine phosphate) per pound of body weight. Each pack contains 7.5 oz. by weight, enough to treat an adult horse weighing 900 lbs.

Table of Recommended Dosages		
Foals	Approx. 300 lbs.	2.50 oz.
Yearlings	Approx. 600 lbs.	5.00 oz.
Adult Horses	Approx. 900 lbs.	7.50 oz.

For horses over 900 lbs. in weight, increase the dosage proportionately according to the above table.

Treatment: Dose each horse individually. Carefully determine the weight of the animal to be treated and determine the correct dosage. Mix ALFALFA PELLET WORMER thoroughly with the amount of grain the horse will consume in a single feeding. Do not give the horse additional feed that day until the treated feed is fully consumed. Most horses will take the medicated feed readily and should be given plenty of good hay when all grain is consumed. If the horse won't eat the medication, add liquid molasses.

Note: Horses are constantly subject to reinfestation, particularly through grazing in confined pastures. Therefore, periodic worming and good stable sanitation are essential. For the most effective control of internal parasites, use ALFALFA PELLET WORMER every 8-10 weeks.

Precaution(s): Store out of direct sunlight.

Caution(s): Recommended dosages should be followed carefully. Animals with known kidney pathology should be treated only by a veterinarian.

Warning(s): This drug is not to be administered to horses that are to be slaughtered for use in food. Keep out of reach of children. Not for human use.

Presentation: 7.5 oz. packet.

Compendium Code No.: 10000000

ALLERCAINE™

Tomlyn **Topical Anesthetic**

Antiseptic Anti-Itch Spray

Active Ingredient(s):

Lidocaine Hydrochloride 2.4%
Benzalkonium Chloride 0.1%

Compounded in a vanishing liquid base containing PEG-75 lanolin, aloe vera gel, allantoin and denatonium benzoate (Bittran™ II) among other ingredients. Stabilized at a pH of normal animal skin.

Indications: Recommended for the temporary relief of pain and itching of insect bites and other minor allergic problems in dogs.

Directions: ALLERCAINE™ can be sprayed on localized irritated areas as required. Animals that are highly allergic should be bathed regularly for optimum skin and tissue health.

Precaution(s): Store at room temperature.

Caution(s): Consult your veterinarian immediately if swelling occurs, or redness and irritation persists for five days or more. Care must be taken to avoid getting into eyes. Avoid excessive application. Do not apply to entire body or to large areas of broken skin. Wash hands after use. Do not use on cats.

For external animal use only.

Keep out of reach of children and pets.

Presentation: 4 fl oz (118 mL) and 12 fl oz (355 mL).

Compendium Code No.: 11220001 615-1 4/617-1 7

ALLERGENIC EXTRACT - FLEA ANTIGEN

Greer **Allergy Diagnostic**

U.S. Vet. Lic. No.: 294

Active Ingredient(s): FLEA ANTIGEN is an aqueous extract of the whole bodies of *Ctenocephalides* spp. with phenol added as a preservative.

Indications:

1. Diagnostic: FLEA ANTIGEN is a valuable aid in the diagnosis of flea bite allergy. Compatible clinical signs and documented exposure to fleas are also necessary to establish the diagnosis.
2. Therapeutic: FLEA ANTIGEN EXTRACT is indicated as an aid in alleviating the symptoms associated with flea bite allergy. A program of controlling the flea population by breaking the life cycle and minimizing flea infestation on the animal should be initiated before or concurrent with hyposensitization treatment. Concomitant antibiotic therapy and an appropriate bathing program should be given where significant secondary bacterial infection is evident. Short-term corticosteroid therapy may be used as an adjunct in the early stages of therapy.

The exact mechanism by which flea antigen elicits an allergic response is still under investigation. It has been demonstrated however, that successful hyposensitization treatment decreases specific IgE antibody levels, theoretically by increasing the level of blocking IgG antibodies. These blocking IgG antibodies are believed to complex with the circulating antigen before it can reach the IgE present on the skin and trigger the allergic response.

Test Procedure: Skin Testing:

1. Materials Needed:
   a. Sterile 1 mL tuberculin type syringes with 25- to 26-gauge needles, ⅜ to ½ inch in length.
   b. FLEA ANTIGEN at 1:1,000 w/v (final concentration).
   c. Diluent control (negative control).
   d. 1:100,000 w/v histamine phosphate (positive control).
2. Suggested Procedure:
   a. Prepare the test area by clipping and cleansing the testing site (lateral thorax or inguinal area).
   b. Five (5) minutes prior to the test, the site may be flooded with alcohol which is allowed to dry by evaporation.
   c. Using a separate syringe for each solution, load the 1 mL tuberculin syringe with 0.1 mL of control solution or flea extract.
   d. Ensure that all air bubbles have been expelled from the loaded syringe, because the injection of air bubbles may force dermal cells apart and create false reactions.
   e. The injection sites should be at least 2.5 cm from each other and the injections should be atraumatic.
   f. After gently stretching the skin around the test site, the needle is inserted into the skin at an angle of approximately 10° with the bevel upwards.
   g. Stop inserting the needle when the entire bevel is buried in the skin (ideally the bevel should be visible through the superficial layers of the skin).
   h. Inject 0.05 mL of the control solution of flea extract and gently remove the needle to prevent traumatic hemorrhage.
   i. Retain the remaining 0.05 mL of control solution or flea extract in case the wheal is unsatisfactory due to the movement of the patient or poor injection technique.
   j. The skin test should be completed as soon as possible to allow simultaneous comparison of the flea antigen wheal against the controls.
3. Interpretation:
   a. Immediate (IgE mediated) reactivity will cause a wheal within 15 minutes.
   b. A wheal that is five (5) or more millimeters greater than the negative control denotes a positive reaction. However, a strong positive is likely to be close to the histamine injection in size, and will be a minimum of 1 cm in diameter.
   c. If the patient is negative at 15 minutes, re-examine after 24 hours to check for delayed reactions.
   d. See Overdose procedure if adverse reactions occur.

Hyposensitization:

Discussion: The optimum dosage and route of administration of FLEA ANTIGEN has not been clearly established and currently many dosage schedules are in use.

Subcutaneous or intradermal injections have been administered with success,[6,7] but it has been noted that if at least part of each injection is intradermal the response seems improved.[1]

A suggested treatment schedule is offered below, however; in the final analysis, the dosage and length of treatment will depend upon the sensitivity and responsiveness of the patient.

Treatment: The suggested hyposensitization dose is 0.1-0.5 mL of FLEA ANTIGEN at a 1:100 w/v per 25 lbs. of body weight. Treatments should be initiated with a 0.1 mL/25 lbs. dose and gradually increased to a maintenance dose of 0.5 mL/25 lbs. The treatment should continue for a 6- to 24-week period.

The injection is administered intradermally at a number of sites with a 1.0 mL sterile tuberculin syringe, using a 25- or 26-gauge needle ⅜ to ½ inch in length. Intradermal injections should not exceed 0.2 mL per site or adverse reactions may occur.

Suggested Dosage Schedule:

Week	Volume of 1:100 w/v FLEA ANTIGEN per 25 lbs. of body weight
1	0.1 mL
2	0.2 mL
3	0.3 mL
4	0.4 mL
5	0.5 mL
6	0.5 mL
Biweekly to 24 weeks if necessary	etc.

Boosters can be given if symptoms re-occur or as a prophylactic measure before flea season. The booster dose should not exceed the last dose given.

Contraindication(s):

1. Diagnostic: Corticosteroids will inhibit the histamine mediated immediate skin test. Any patient that has undergone continual corticosteroid treatment should discontinue the treatment for a period of one week for every month of the treatment before the patient is skin tested. However, animals with severe skin problems should be treated with antibiotics, soothing baths and possibly a short-term oral cortisone until their skin conditions will not interfere with skin testing.
2. Therapeutic: FLEA ANTIGEN is indicated for hyposensitization only when flea bite hypersensitivity has been unequivocally demonstrated both clinically and by intradermal skin testing.

Caution(s): Have in stock the following:

1. A hydrocortisone (such as Solu-Cortef® or a prednisolone (such as Solu-Delta-Cortef®).
2. An antihistamine such as diphenhydramine hydrochloride (Benadryl®).
3. Epinephrine diluted 1:1,000.

Keep the patient under observation for a period of at least 30 minutes after administration.

Note: Animals prone to severe reactions should be given diphenhydramine hydrochloride (Benadryl®) 30 minutes prior to treatment dose administration.

Overdose: If symptoms of overdosage occur (see Side Effects section below), treatment employing (a), (b) or (c) below, or a combination thereof can be effective in combating an adverse reaction.

a) Intravenous injection of hydrocortisone (i.e. Solu-Cortef®) in a dosage of 10-15 mg/lb., or alternatively, a prednisolone (i.e. Solu-Delta-Cortef®) in a dosage of 5 mg/lb.
b) Intramuscular or subcutaneous injection of epinephrine in a dosage of 0.5-1.0 mL at 1:1,000.
c) Intravenous injection of an antihistamine such as diphenhydramine hydrochloride (Benadryl®) in a dosage of 0.5-1.0 mg/lb.

Note: In a crisis situation epinephrine may be administered intravenously. Use 0.5 to 1.0 mL of a 1:1,000 dilution.

Side Effects: Adverse reactions are very rarely seen and usually consist of an exacerbation of clinical signs if too large a dose is given. However, in the event of an overdose or alternatively, exquisite sensitivity of the animal, the patient may exhibit restlessness, panting, generalized hives, vomiting, circulatory collapse and diarrhea (see Overdose section above for treatment).

There are also several normal reactions that may occur and the owner should be advised of these prior to administration of the allergen. Temporary pain and discomfort may be experienced at the time of injection, with some stiffness and soreness occurring later. A small area of ulceration may occur where intradermal administration is employed.

References: Available upon request.

Presentation: FLEA ANTIGEN is supplied in sterile 10 mL vials at a concentration of 1:100 w/v (aqueous only).

Compendium Code No.: 11100000

ALLERGENIC EXTRACTS - MIXED

Greer **Allergy Diagnostic**

U.S. Vet. Lic. No.: 294

Active Ingredient(s):

Pollens: Pure dry pollens are defatted in ether and extracted in an aqueous buffered solution. Grass pollen, which is a common cause of canine inhalant dermatitis, is more prevalent in late spring and early summer. The weeds, notably the ragweeds, are prolific producers of pollen and can cause animal allergies especially in the late summer and early fall periods. Tree pollens can also cause canine allergies although the pollination season for each species is relatively short.

Fungi: Fungal antigens are extracts of the cells and spores of pure culture fungi (molds) including yeasts, or of rusts and smuts, collected from their natural environments. Aqueous extracts of fungi are prepared from defatted material extracted in an aqueous buffered solution. Airborne fungi are an important cause of animal allergy, especially since they are present in the house throughout the year. Outdoors, fungi can also be found in large numbers from May to December with peak periods varying according to genus and climate conditions.

Dust: Screened dust from private homes is extracted in an aqueous buffered solution and dialyzed to remove irritants. House dust extract is concentrated to an extract ration of 1:1 w/v to achieve adequate Protein Nitrogen Units (PNU). House dust is a common cause of canine inhalant dermatitis because of its ubiquity in the home and its heterogeneous composition.

Epidermals, Miscellaneous Inhalants, and Foods: Epidermal extracts are made individually from the hide, hair, or feathers and contain the natural dander. Epidermals, other inhalants, and foods* are prepared using defatted materials obtained from sources as near the natural inhalant or edible food as possible.

*A small group of foods, primarily cereal grains, are extracted with fluid containing 0.1% sodium formaldehyde sulfoxylate (SFS), an anti-oxidant. This results in a light-colored extract which avoids the tattoo effect which may occur after skin testing with oxidized extracts. Extracts containing SFS are labeled for diagnostic use only.

Insects: Insects are made from the whole bodies of the insects collected from their natural habitats or are grown in laboratory colonies, such as the dust mites, *Dermatophagoides farinae* and *D. pteronyssinus*.

Indications:

1. Diagnostic: Greer allergen extracts are aids in the skin test diagnosis of animal allergies. Compatible clinical signs and history are necessary to establish the diagnosis.
2. Therapeutic: Greer ALLERGENIC EXTRACTS are indicated for immunotherapy (hyposensitization) to aid in alleviating the symptoms associated with allergic dermatitis. A program of reducing or avoiding exposure to the offending allergen, if possible, should be initiated before or concurrent with hyposensitization treatment. Concomitant antibiotic therapy and an appropriate bathing program should be given where significant secondary

bacterial infection of the skin is evident. Food extracts are not recommended in immunotherapy, but may be useful diagnostically.

Allergens interact with immunoglobulin E (IgE) to stimulate the release of mediators such as histamine from the surface of mast cells and cause skin induration and erythema reactions upon skin testing, along with other allergic symptoms which are indicative of the subject's hypersensitivity to the antigen. The allergy skin test is useful to confirm the diagnosis of allergic dermatitis. Upon a course of immunotherapy, there is generally an increase in immunoglobin G (IgG) antibodies which have been surmised to complex with the circulating antigen before it can reach the IgE present in the tissues and trigger the allergic response. Clinical improvement, however, does not correlate well with increased levels of IgG antibodies, and IgG levels vary during long-term therapy. Thus, other mechanisms following immunotherapy are probably involved in the relief of symptoms upon further exposure to the antigen.

Test Procedure: Intradermal Skin Testing:

Discussion: The signs of atopic disease may be seasonal or perennial depending upon the animal's sensitivities. Selection of the appropriate seasonal allergens for testing should be tailored to the region of the country where the animal resides. In addition, allergens which are encountered year-round in the home (e.g., house dust, mites, and molds) and in the external environment should be included in the testing scheme, where suspect. Although food extracts may be helpful in affirming or ruling out suspected food allergies, they are not recommended for definitive differential diagnosis; elimination diets remain the best method of diagnosis for food allergies. Positive intradermal skin test information or other specific allergen test results should be weighed along with clinical signs and patient history before a decision on treatment is made.

1. Materials Needed:

a. Sterile 1 mL tuberculin type syringes with ⅜ to ½ inch, 26- or 27-gauge needles.

b. Allergen at 1,000 PNU/mL or 1:1,000 w/v (final concentration).*

c. Negative control (saline diluent).

d. Positive control: The available histamine phosphate 0.275 mg/mL should be diluted 1:10 to yield 0.0275 mg/mL.

*The following allergens may give more consistent results when tested at concentrations lower than 1,000 PNU/mL:

149	Corn (Zea Mays)	250 PNU/mL
B04	4 Insect Mix	250 PNU/mL
M23	Rhizopus nigricans	100 PNU/mL
M012	Rhizopus mix	100 PNU/mL
M02	Mold Mix #2	250 PNU/mL
D9	House Dust	100 PNU/mL
D01	HMRU Dust Mix	100 PNU/mL
E27	Sheep Wool	500 PNU/mL
H7	Silk	500 PNU/mL
B51	Mite, *D. farinae*	1:1,000 to 1:5,000 w/v
B58	Mite, *D. pteronyssinus*	1:1,000 to 1:5,000 w/v
B060	House Dust Mite Mix	1:1,000 to 1:5,000 w/v

2. Suggested Procedure: Before testing, the veterinarian may wish to sedate or tranquilize the patient. Care must be taken to avoid sedatives with antihistaminic activity such as acetylpromazine. Xylazine may be used.

a. Prepare the test area (usually the lateral thorax) by clipping and gently cleansing the testing site with a moist towel if necessary. Sites may be marked for easy reading.

b. Using a separate syringe for each solution, load separate 1 mL tuberculin syringes with 0.1 mL of control solutions and the test allergen extracts.*

c. Ensure that all air bubbles have been expelled from the loaded syringe, because the injection of air bubbles may force dermal cells apart and create false reactions.

d. The injection sites should be at least 2.5 cm from each other and the injections should be atraumatic.

e. After gently stretching the skin around the test site, the needle is inserted into the skin at an angle of approximately 10° with the bevel upwards.

f. Stop inserting the needle when the entire bevel is buried in the skin (ideally the bevel should be visible through the superficial layers of the skin).

g. Inject 0.05 mL of the control solution or allergen extract forming a bleb in the skin. Gently remove the needle to prevent traumatic hemorrhage.

h. Retain the remaining 0.05 mL of control solution or allergen extract in case the wheal is unsatisfactory due to the movement of the patient or poor injection technique.

i. The skin test should be completed as soon as possible to allow simultaneous comparison of the allergen wheal against the controls.

*Mixes for skin testing should not contain more than eight (8) related antigens (up to 8 grass pollens, weed pollens, tree pollens, or molds, etc. As examples of preferred mixes, see the standard Greer Stock Mixes in the catalog.). If unrelated antigens or more than eight (8) antigens are included, specific antigens may be masked or diluted by others in the mix, causing a false negative test.

3. Interpretation:

a. The skin test site is read 15 minutes after injection. The wheal is best observed by oblique or side lighting in a darkened room. Immediate (IgE mediated) reactivity will cause a wheal within 15 minutes. 24 to 48 hour reactions are occasionally seen for reasons not known at this time.

b. A wheal diameter significantly greater than the negative control denotes a positive reaction. A strong positive reaction may be approximately the size of the histamine response. Graded responses may be determined subjectively, or an objective scale of 1+ to 4+ may be used with 3+ being the size of the positive control.

c. See Overdose section below if adverse reactions occur.

Immunotherapy:

Discussion: The optimum dosage and route of administration of allergens has not been clearly established and currently many dosage schedules are in use. Subcutaneous or intradermal injections can be administered, but the subcutaneous route is more routinely employed.

It is recommended that if clinical signs of atopy are present and the animal skin tests are positive to a particular allergen or allergens, which cannot be avoided, then hyposensitization immunotherapy is indicated. However, in animals whose seasonal involvement is short, or for an old animal, an alternate-day short-acting oral corticosteroid or an antihistamine may be the treatment of choice.

Hyposensitization is accomplished by injecting therapeutic allergens in a low enough dosage to be tolerated, with a slightly increased dosage at each subsequent treatment interval, attempting to reach, but not to exceed, a maximum tolerated dose as determined by increasing the dosage until signs of overdose are seen and then reducing to the maximum tolerated dose. At this point, the patient is kept at the maintenance dosage level with injections repeated at 20- to 40-day intervals.

During the course of therapy, a few patients may develop allergy to other antigens, even though allergy to the original antigens are controlled. Thus, additional testing and treatment may become necessary.

Boosters may be administered if symptoms recur after treatment.

A suggested treatment schedule is offered below, however, the final choice of the dosage and length of treatment will depend upon the sensitivity and responsiveness of the patient.

Treatment: Antigen selection is based on (a) the degree of reaction to a specific allergen test (size of wheal) (b) the clinical signs relative to patient history. However, if the patient exhibits numerous sensitivities (at the time of the first testing or at a later date), the veterinarian may administer two (2) vaccines alternately. Allergens may be administered singly, or combined into a vaccine mixture.* The allergens selected for the vaccine (treatment vial) should be limited to not more than 12. If a new antigen is added to an existing vaccine, the administration of the vaccine should proceed as if it were a new vaccine (start at day 0).

*If the patient has flea sensitivity also, the veterinarian may treat with Flea Antigen Extract. Food extracts are not recommended for treatment since their efficacy in immunotherapy has not been established.

The injection usually is administered subcutaneously with a 1.0 mL sterile tuberculin syringe, using a ⅜ to ½ inch, 25- to 27-gauge needle. If intradermal injections are administered, the dose should not exceed 0.2 mL per site or adverse reactions may occur.

Dosages for immunotherapy usually start at 0.1 mL of a dilution that is 1/100 to 1/10 of the concentrate. If it is suspected that the patient is extremely sensitive, lower doses or more dilute solutions may be used initially with gradually increasing doses similar to the suggested dosage schedule. If the patient can tolerate higher dosages, the schedule may be accelerated (such as starting at a higher dose or concentration, or by administering doses every 2 days rather than every 3 days) to reach a maintenance dose of 1.0 mL of the concentrate in fewer days. Dosages more dilute (less concentrated) than the purchased strengths may be made by appropriate one-to-ten dilutions in the office with a commercial saline, buffered saline, or glycero-saline diluent containing phenol preservative, 0.5 mL of extract to 4.5 mL of diluent.

Suggested Dosage Schedule:

Day	2,000 PNU/mL	20,000 PNU/mL
0	0.1 mL	
3	0.2 mL	
6	0.4 mL	
9	0.8 mL	
12	1.0 mL	
15		0.1 mL
18		0.2 mL
21		0.4 mL
24		0.8 mL
27		1.0 mL*
30		1.0 mL
33		1.0 mL
36		1.0 mL
46		1.0 mL
56		1.0 mL
76		1.0 mL
96		1.0 mL

*Maintenance dose if tolerated; otherwise maintain at the tolerated level of a lower volume or a lower concentration.

(For smaller or more sensitive animals, the starting dosage concentrations may be 1/10 those in the above table, beginning with 200 PNU/mL).

Thereafter: Keep the maintenance dose schedule at approximately 20-day intervals until relief is evident, at which time the interval may be increased to greater than 20 days, or the schedule may be modified to administer the doses preseasonally if the allergy is seasonal. If the relief wanes, the intervals may be shortened. A maximum period of immunotherapy has not been determined. Occasionally patients may have to undergo treatment indefinitely. If relief upon immunotherapy does not occur within nine (9) months to one (1) year, the treatment should be stopped and the animal re-evaluated.

Contraindication(s):

1. Diagnostic: Diagnostic skin testing is contraindicated in patients on corticosteroids or drugs with antihistamine activity which will cause inhibition of the histamine-mediated skin test reaction. These drugs should be withdrawn for a period sufficient that the patient exhibits a positive skin test response to a control skin test with histamine. The withdrawal time for antihistamines is based on their biological half-life. The withdrawal time for corticosteroids is about one week for each month of continual corticosteroid administration.
   Animals with severe skin problems should not be skin tested.
2. Therapeutic: Because of the potential for *de novo* sensitization, allergens are not indicated for hyposensitization treatment unless specific allergen hypersensitivity has been identified by means of intradermal skin testing, or *in vitro* specific allergen sensitivity testing, accompanied by compatible clinical signs, history, and a differential diagnosis to rule out other etiologic conditions.

Precaution(s): Extracts should be stored at 2-8°C. Do not freeze.

Caution(s): Do not inject intravenously.

Have the following available:

1. Epinephrine diluted 1:1,000.
2. A fast-acting, water-soluble corticosteroid injection such as hydrocortisone, prednisolone, or dexamethasone.
3. An injectable antihistamine such as diphenhydramine.

Keep the animal under observation for at least 30 minutes after the administration of a testing or treatment dose. Animals prone to severe reactions should be given diphenhydramine or another appropriate antihistamine 30 minutes prior to the treatment dose administration.

Extracts in 50% glycerin should be diluted with an aqueous diluent before use to avoid pain or stinging due to the high concentration of glycerin.

Overdose: If symptoms of overdosage occur (see Side Effects section below), treatment employing (a), (b) or (c) below, or a combination thereof can be effective in combating an adverse reaction.

a) The immediate intramuscular injection of epinephrine at a dosage of 0.01 mL/kg at a 1:1,000 dilution, or in the case of a severe reaction, administer a 1:10,000 dilution intravenously in increments of 0.5 mL to 1.0 mL to a total dosage of 0.5 mL to 5.0 mL. Epinephrine administration can be repeated every 15 to 30 minutes as needed.

b) Intravenous injection of an appropriate corticosteroid such as prednisolone sodium succinate 35 mg/kg, or dexamethasone sodium phosphate 5 mg/kg.

c) Intravenous injection of an antihistamine such as diphenhydramine hydrochloride in a dosage of 1.0 to 2.0 mg/kg, slowly.

Side Effects: Adverse reactions are very rarely seen and usually consist of an exacerbation of clinical signs if too large a dose is given. However, in the event of an overdose or alternatively, exquisite sensitivity of the animal, the patient may exhibit restlessness, panting, generalized hives, vomiting, circulatory collapse, and/or diarrhea (see Overdose section above for treatment).

There are also several normal reactions that may occur and the owner should be advised of these prior to administration of the allergen. Temporary pain and discomfort may be experienced at the time of injection, with some stiffness and soreness occurring later. A small area of ulceration may occur where intradermal administration is employed.

References: Available upon request.

Presentation: Greer ALLERGENIC EXTRACTS for veterinary use are available as sterile aqueous solutions labeled on a PNU/mL basis (10,000, 20,000 and 40,000 PNU/mL for pollens* and fungi; 10,000 and 20,000 PNU/mL for epidermals, foods, miscellaneous inhalants and insects; and at 10,000 PNU/mL for house dust). On a weight/volume concentration, extracts are formulated at 1:10, 1:20, 1:40, or 1:50 w/v for most pollens,* fungi, epidermals, foods and inhalants; and 1:20 and 1:100 for insects. Special dust (HMRU mix) is 1:1, 1:2, and 1:5 w/v. House dust is 1:1 and 1:2 w/v and 10,000 PNU/mL. House dust mites, *Dermatophagoides farinae* and *D. pteronyssinus* are 1:100 w/v singly or mixed. Extracts usually are supplied in volumes of 5, 10, 30, and 50 mL. Intradermal tests are 1,000 PNU/mL or 1:1,000 w/v in 5 mL vials only. Individual prescription mixes are also available upon request.

* Short ragweed (Ambrosia artemisiifolia) pollen extracts have potency states in terms of antigen E units/mL as well as a PNU/mL or w/v concentration.

Glycerinated extract concentrations are available for certain extracts. The dosages are the same as aqueous extracts. Glycerin 50% concentrates should be diluted before use and are not appropriate as concentrates for diagnostic skin testing. While glycerin 50% enhances, stability, when given in a concentrated solution it will sting upon injection.

Compendium Code No.: 11100011

ALLERGROOM® SHAMPOO

Virbac **Grooming Shampoo**

Routine and Dry Seborrhea Shampoo

Ingredient(s): Contains: Chitosanide, urea 5%, glycerin 1%, and lactic acid in a shampoo base also containing water, TEA lauryl sulfate, lauramide DEA, imidazolidinyl urea, and fragrance. May also contain sodium hydroxide and sodium chloride.

Chitosanide, urea and glycerin are present in encapsulated (Spherulites®) and free forms.

Indications: A shampoo for normal or dry skin in dogs and cats of any age.

Directions: Shake well before use. Wet the coat with warm water and apply sufficient shampoo to create a rich lather. Massage ALLERGROOM® into wet coat, lather freely. Rinse and repeat. Allow to remain on hair for 5 to 10 minutes, then rinse thoroughly with clean water.

Frequency of use: Once weekly or as directed by your veterinarian.

Caution(s): For topical use only. Avoid contact with eyes. In case of contact, flush eyes with water and seek medical attention if irritation persists.

Available through licensed veterinarians only.

Warning(s): Keep out of reach of children.

Discussion: ALLERGROOM® contains Spherulites®, an exclusive and patented encapsulation system developed by Virbac to provide slow release of ingredients long after the shampoo is rinsed off.

ALLERGROOM® also contains Chitosanide, a natural biopolymer creating a protective film on the skin and hair.

Presentation: 8 oz (237 mL), 16 oz (473 mL), and 1 gallon (3.79 L) containers.

Compendium Code No.: 10230000

ALLERMYL™ SHAMPOO

Virbac **Antidermatosis Shampoo**

Soothing-Cleansing-Anti-Pruritic-Micro-Emulsion

Active Ingredient(s): Contains: Water, cocoamphodiacetate, sodium lauryl sulfate, sodium alkyl ether sulfate, propylene glycol, PEG-8 caprylic/capric glycerides, propylene glycol laurate, vitamin F (source of essential fatty acids), tocopheryl acetate, piroctone olamine, sodium chloride, L-rhamnose, chlorhexidine gluconate.

Dye and fragrance free.

Indications: Uses: ALLERMYL™ Shampoo is used for the topical management of allergic skin conditions. It relieves irritation and itching, has a beneficial effect on damaged skin, and cleanses the epidermis. It is specially formulated to meet the needs of dogs and cats with allergic skin disease, by combining ingredients that help maintain skin integrity and natural balance.

ALLERMYL™ Shampoo is a unique foaming micro-emulsion formulated for the management of allergic skin conditions in dogs and cats. It contains a soothing combination of natural anti-inflammatory ingredients, mild cleansing agents, and essential fatty acids. The foaming micro-emulsion helps the ingredients penetrate the skin for deep, soothing relief.

Directions for Use: Shake well before use. Due to the fluid nature of the product, pouring ALLERMYL™ Shampoo onto your hand prior to application is not recommended. Wet the hair coat with warm water, invert bottle and apply a thin line of shampoo from the base of the neck to the base of the tail. Massage ALLERMYL™ Shampoo into wet hair coat, lather well. Allow ALLERMYL™ Shampoo to remain on the hair coat for 5 to 10 minutes. Rinse thoroughly with water.

Frequency of use: Initially 2 to 3 applications per week for 2 weeks, then as directed by your veterinarian.

Precaution(s): Storage: Store at room temperature. Avoid prolonged exposure to excessive heat.

Caution(s): For animal use only. For topical use only. Avoid contact with eyes. In case of contact, flush eyes with water and seek medical attention if irritation persists.

Warning(s): Keep out of the reach of children. Wash hands after using.

Presentation: 8 fl oz (237 mL) and 16 fl oz (473 mL).

Available through licensed veterinarians only.

Compendium Code No.: 10230730 231130-01 / 251133-01

ALLERPET® C

V.P.L. **Allergy Relief Aid**

Active Ingredient(s): DI UV water, quaternium-26, hydrolyzed wheat protein, glycerin, quaternium-22, cocamidopropylbetaine, allantoin, d-panthenol, aloe vera gel, imidazolidinyl urea and collagen.

Indications: ALLERPET® C is formulated to aid in the reduction of the major causes of allergies due to cats.

ALLERPET® C cleanses the hair of dander and saliva, is non-irritating, and can also be used on rabbits, hamsters, gerbils, guinea pigs, mice, rats and ferrets.

Dosage and Administration: Remove the cap and peel off the inner protective seal from the bottle.

Before using ALLERPET® C, comb the cat thoroughly (brush all other small animals) to remove as much dead hair as possible.

Moisten a washcloth with ALLERPET® C and drywash the pet by rubbing the fur both with and against the lay of the hair, making certain that the pet is dampened to the skin. Do not saturate the hair. Pay attention to areas of the body that the cat licks most often and to the genital areas of all animals. Dry with a towel. Repeat the procedure once a week. For the best results, the first application should be performed by a non-allergic person.

Caution(s): Antigens are considered to be the prime causes of allergic reactions to cats.

Presentation: 12 U.S. fl. oz. (355 mL) containers.

* ALLERPET is a registered trademark of Allerpet, Inc.

Compendium Code No.: 11430060

ALLERPET® D

V.P.L. **Allergy Relief Aid**

Active Ingredient(s): DI UV water, quaternium-26, hydrolyzed wheat protein, glycerin, quaternium-22, cocamidopropylbetaine, allantoin, d-panthenol, aloe vera gel, imidazolidinyl urea and collagen.

Indications: ALLERPET® D is formulated to aid in the reduction of the major causes of allergies due to dogs.

ALLERPET® D cleanses the hair of dander and saliva, and is non-irritating.

Dosage and Administration: Remove the cap and peel off the inner protective seal from the bottle.

Before using ALLERPET® D, brush or comb the dog thoroughly to remove as much dead hair as possible.

Moisten a washcloth with ALLERPET® D and 'drywash' the dog by rubbing the fur both with and against the lay of the hair, making certain that the pet is dampened to the skin. Do not saturate the hair. Pay attention to areas of the body that the dog licks most often and to the genital area. Dry with a towel. Repeat the procedure once a week. For the best results, the first application should be performed by a non-allergic person.

Caution(s): Antigens are considered to be the prime causes of allergic reactions to dogs.

Presentation: 12 U.S. fl. oz. (355 mL) containers.

* ALLERPET is a registered trademark of Allerpet, Inc.

Compendium Code No.: 11430070

ALLERSEB-T® SHAMPOO

Virbac **Antidermatosis Shampoo**

with Spherulites®

Ingredient(s): Contains: Solubilized tar equivalent to 4% coal tar U.S.P., sulfur 2% and salicylic acid 2% in a shampoo base also containing water, sodium lauryl sulfate, Spherulites, triethanolamine, magnesium aluminum silicate, hydroxypropyl methylcellulose and fragrance. Sulfur and salicylic acid are present in encapsulated (Spherulites) and free forms. Chitosanide, glycerin and urea are present in encapsulated form.

Indications: ALLERSEB-T® is an antiseborrheic, keratolytic and antiseptic shampoo for removing scales, crusts and excessive oil associated with seborrhea and moist eczema in dogs. It leaves the coat clean, soft and lustrous.

ALLERSEB-T® is an antiseborrheic, keratolytic and antiseptic shampoo for use on dogs of any age.

Directions: Shake well before use. Wet the coat with warm water and apply sufficient shampoo to create a rich lather. Massage ALLERSEB-T® into wet coat, lather freely. Rinse and repeat. Allow to remain on hair for 5 to 10 minutes, then rinse thoroughly with clean water.

Frequency of use: initially two to three times a week for four weeks, then reducing to once a week, or as directed by your veterinarian.

Caution(s): For topical use only. Not for use on cats. Avoid contact with eyes. If irritation occurs, decrease frequency of use or discontinue use entirely. Wash hands and exposed skin after use.

Available through licensed veterinarians only.

Warning(s): Keep out of reach of children.

Discussion: ALLERSEB-T® contains Spherulites, an exclusive and patented encapsulation system developed by Virbac to provide slow release of ingredients long after the shampoo is rinsed off.

ALLERSEB-T® also contains Chitosanide, a natural biopolymer creating a protective film on the skin and hair.

Presentation: 8 fl oz (237 mL) containers.

Compendium Code No.: 10230010

ALLERSPRAY™

Evsco **Topical Antipruritic**

Active Ingredient(s):

Lidocaine Hydrochloride 2.4%
Benzalkonium Chloride 0.1%

Compounded in a vanishing liquid base containing PEG-75 lanolin, aloe vera gel, allantoin and denatonium benzoate (Bittran II™) among other ingredients. Stabilized at a pH of normal animal skin.

Indications: ALLERSPRAY™ with Bittran II™ is an antiseptic spray that calms, soothes and helps give temporary relief of pain and itching of insect bites and other minor allergic problems. ALLERSPRAY™ can be used daily as an aid for compulsive scratching and biting problems. Provides an anti-septic/analgesic spray for symptomatic relief of itching and pain due to the following: Hot spots, flea bites, contact allergies (grass, carpets, synthetics, etc.), insect bites (bees, mosquitoes, ants, etc.)

ALLERSPRAY™ provides a fine mist to the sensitive area, adheres easily to the skin (no messy run-off), and vanishes, leaving the skin and coat dry, non-sticky.

Directions: ALLERSPRAY™ can be sprayed on localized irritated areas as required. Dogs that are highly allergic should be bathed regularly for optimum skin and tissue health.

Precaution(s): Store at room temperature.
Caution(s): Consult your veterinarian immediately if swelling occurs, or redness and irritation persists for five days or more. Care must be taken to avoid spraying into animal's eyes. Avoid excessive application, do not apply to entire body or to large areas of broken skin. Wash hands after use. Not for use on cats.
For external animal use only.
Keep out of reach of children and pets.
Presentation: 4 fl oz (118 mL) and 12 X 4 oz (118 mL).
Compendium Code No.: 10050000

ALL-IN-ONE CALF BOLUS

AgriPharm **Large Animal Dietary Supplement**

Guaranteed Analysis: Per Bolus:

Vitamin A	200,000 U.S.P. Units
Vitamin D_3	20,000 U.S.P. Units
Vitamin E	250 I.U.
Niacin	1,000 mg
Calcium Pantothenate	40 mg
Riboflavin	50 mg
Choline Chloride	50 mg
Lactobacillus acidophilus, (LA88)	1.5 X 10^9 CFU/Bolus

Ingredients: Calcium meal, dried egg, dried *Aspergillus niger* fermentation product, dried *Bacillus Subtilus* fermentation product: Contains a source of viable naturally occurring microorganism *Lactobacillus acidophilus* (LA88), Whey, Vitamin A (stability improved), Vitamin D_3, Riboflavin, Choline Chloride, Vitamin C, Vitamin B_{12}, Sulfur, Magnesium Oxide Carbonate, Copper Sulfate, Ethylene Diamine Dihydroiodide, Potassium Iodide, Iron Sulfate, Selenium, DL Methionine, and Ethoxyquin as preservative.
Indications: A nutritional bolus.
Dosage and Administration: Newborn Calves: Two (2) boluses 1st day as soon after birth as possible.
Caution(s): For animal use only.
This product contains no medication.
No withdrawal necessary.
Keep out of reach of children.
Presentation: 50 X 7 g (¼ oz) boluses, 12 per case.
Compendium Code No.: 14570030

ALL-IN-ONE CATTLE BOLUS

AgriPharm **Large Animal Dietary Supplement**

Guaranteed Analysis: Per Bolus:

Vitamin A	600,000 U.S.P. Units
Vitamin D_3	60,000 U.S.P. Units
Vitamin E	750 I.U.
Niacin	3,000 mg
Calcium Pantothenate	120 mg
Riboflavin	150 mg
Choline Chloride	150 mg
Lactobacillus acidophilus, (LA88)	3 X 10^9 CFU/Bolus

Ingredients: Calcium meal, dried egg, dried *Aspergillus niger* fermentation product, dried *Bacillus Subtilus* fermentation product: Contains a source of viable naturally occurring microorganism *Lactobacillus acidophilus* (LA88), Whey, Vitamin A (stability improved), Vitamin D_3, Riboflavin, Choline Chloride, Vitamin C, Vitamin B_{12}, Sulfur, Magnesium Oxide Carbonate, Copper Sulfate, Ethylene Diamine Dihydroiodide, Potassium Iodide, Iron Sulfate, Selenium, DL Methionine, and Ethoxyquin as preservative.
Indications: A nutritional bolus.
Dosage and Administration: Two (2) boluses as needed.
Caution(s): For animal use only.
This product contains no medication.
No withdrawal necessary.
Keep out of reach of children.
Presentation: 50 X 21 g (¾ oz) boluses, 8 per case.
Compendium Code No.: 14570040

ALL-PRO BIOTIC™

Vets Plus **Dietary Supplement**

Guaranteed Analysis: (min. per lb.):

Lactic Acid Bacteria	200 billion CFU

Ingredients: *Lactobacillus acidophilus* DDS-1, *Lactobacillus casei, Lactobacillus fermentum, Lactobacillus plantarum, Streptococcus faecium*, Distiller Grain, Yeast and Artificial Flavor.
Indications: Contains a source of live (viable) naturally occurring microorganisms for all species.
Directions for Use:
Swine:
Market Hogs: Starter - 2.5 lbs/ton; Grower - 2.5 lbs/ton
Gestating Sows: 30 days prior to farrowing - 2.5 lbs/ton or 14 days prior to farrowing - 5 lbs/ton
Lactating Sows: During lactation - 2.5 lbs/ton
Cattle:
Calf Conditioner: Starter - Mix 5 lbs into the amount of feed normally consumed by 100 head on a daily basis or top dress at the rate of 1 oz/head/day; Grower/Growing Heifer - Mix 2.5 lbs into the amount of feed normally consumed by 100 head on a daily basis or top dress at the rate of ½ oz/head/day.
Dairy Cattle:
Lactating Cows: Mix 2.5 lbs into the amount of feed normally consumed by 100 head on a daily basis or top dress at the rate of ½ oz/head/day. Feedlot Receiving Program Starter (0-28 days) - Mix 2.5 lbs. into the amount of feed normally consumed by 250 head on a daily basis or top dress at the rate of ½ oz/head/day.
Sheep/Lambs:
Starter-Creep Feed (12-120 days): Mix 2.5 lbs into the amount of feed normally consumed by 250 head on a daily basis or top dress at the rate of ½ oz/head/day.
Fattening (60-100 lbs): Mix 2.5 lbs into the amount of feed normally consumed by 250 head on a daily basis or top dress at the rate of ¼ oz/head/day
Poultry:
Chickens: Layers - 2.5 lbs/ton; Broilers - 1.25 lbs/ton
Turkeys: Starter - 5 lbs/ton; Grower - 2.5 lbs/ton; Finisher - 1.25 lbs/ton
Horses:
Foals: 4 gm per head at birth; 1 gm/head/day thereafter
Adults: Maintenance - 2 gm/head/day; Breeding & Performance - Top dress 4 gm/head/day
Precaution(s): Keep in cool, dry place.
Caution(s): Keep out of reach of children. For animal use only.
Presentation: 6x5 lb pails per case and 25 lb pails.
Compendium Code No.: 10730030

ALL PURPOSE LUBRICANT

Durvet **Lubricant**

Non Spermicidal
Active Ingredient(s): Contains: A bland aqueous lotion with methylparaben and propylparaben as preservatives.
Indications: Lubrication of the arm or glove for rectal and obstetrical procedures in large or small animals; for lubrication of devices such as stomach tubes, enema nozzles, catheters and obstetrical instruments before insertion into body cavities; as an aid in delivery at dry birth.
Directions: Apply 7 to 10 mL to prewetted or dry glove, arm, or instruments. Distribute evenly.
To prepare a bulk lubricant to aid in dry birth, add lubricant to two quarts of water until the desired viscosity is reached. Formulated to function even if water is not available.
Caution(s): For animal use only.
Warning(s): Keep out of reach of children.
Presentation: 8 oz (NDC 30798-461-28) and 1 gallon (3.785 L) (NDC 30798-461-35).
Compendium Code No.: 10840052 Rev. 08/01

ALOCETIC™ EAR RINSE

DVM **Otic Cleanser**

Acetic Acid and Aloe
Ingredients: Water, acetic acid, nonoxynol-12, fragrance, methylparaben, DMDM hydantoin, aloe vera gel, FD&C yellow #5, FD&C blue #1.
ALOCETIC™ Ear Rinse is an antimicrobial, antiseptic, alcohol free cleansing formulation in a soothing aloe base.
Indications: For treatment of moisture in ear. Also, for routine cleansing where an antimicrobial agent is required in dogs and cats.
Directions for Use: Apply ALOCETIC™ liberally into ear canal. Gently massage base of ear to help break up internal wax and crust. Use cotton or absorbent material to clean excess solution and debris from open area of ear. Apply once or twice weekly or as directed by veterinarian.
Precaution(s): Store at room temperature.
Caution(s): For external use on animals only.
Warning(s): Keep out of reach of children.
Presentation: 4 fl oz (118 mL) and 12 fl oz (355 mL).
Compendium Code No.: 11420041 Rev 0597

ALOE & OATMEAL SHAMPOO

Vet Solutions **Grooming Shampoo**

Soap Free Grooming Shampoo Formulated with Moisturizers for Normal, Sensitive or Dry Skin
Ingredient(s): Deionized Water, Sodium C14-16 Olefin Sulfonate, Glycerin, Lauramido Propyl Betaine, Lauramide DEA, Aloe Vera Gel, Oat Flour, Lactic Acid, Fragrance, Polyquaternium-10, Sodium Hydroxymethylglycinate.
Indications: Vet Solutions ALOE & OATMEAL SHAMPOO is specially formulated to soothe dry skin. Its formulation adds essential moisture while providing a deep rich lather that gently cleans the skin without removing natural skin oils. For dogs and cats.
Directions: Shake well. With tepid water thoroughly wet animal's coat. Massage small amounts of shampoo into the coat while continuously adding water to get better dispersion. Continue until a generous lather is generated. Rinse well. Shampoo may be used weekly.
Precaution(s): Storage: Store at controlled room temperature.
Caution(s): For topical use only. Avoid contact with eyes and ears.
Sold exclusively through veterinarians.
Presentation: 473 mL (16 fl. oz.) and 1 gallon.
Compendium Code No.: 10610020 000102

ALOE & OATMEAL SKIN & COAT CONDITIONER

Vet Solutions **Coat Conditioner**

Ingredient(s): Deionized Water, Aloe Vera Gel, Cetearyl Alcohol, PEG-40 Hydrogenated Castor Oil, Stearalkonium Chloride, Glycerin, Oat flour, Chamomile Extract, Fragrance, Lactic Acid, Retinyl Palmitate, Tocopheryl Acetate, Cholecalciferol, Tetrasodium EDTA, Methylchloroisothiazolinone, Methylisothiazolinone.
Indications: Soothing conditioner formulated with moisturizers vitamins A, D and E and chamomile. For dogs and cats.
Vet Solutions ALOE & OATMEAL SKIN & COAT CONDITIONER contains a unique combination of natural soothing agents, moisturizers and vitamins.
Directions: Shake well. After shampooing the animal, massage conditioner into the coat working it down to the skin. For optimal soothing and conditioning, do not rinse. As a routine conditioner, lightly rinse. Conditioner may be used after every bath.
Precaution(s): Storage: Store at controlled room temperature.
Caution(s): For topical use only. Avoid contact with eyes and ears.
Sold exclusively through veterinarians.
Presentation: 473 mL (16 fl. oz.) and 1 gallon.
Compendium Code No.: 10610030 000102

ALOECLENS OTIC CLEANSER

Vetus **Otic Cleanser**

Ear Cleansing Solution
Ingredient(s): Deionized Water, Propylene Glycol, Aloe Vera Gel, SD Alcohol 40-2, Lactic Acid, Glycerin, Dioctyl Sodium Sulfosuccinate, Salicylic Acid, Fragrance, Benzoic Acid, Benzyl Alcohol.
Indications: Vetus ALOECLENS OTIC CLEANSER is specially formulated to deodorize and gently clean, dry and acidify the ear canal. This provides an ideal environment for healthy ears. For dogs and cats.
Directions: Apply liberally into the ear canal. Massage the base of the ear. Allow pet to shake head. Clean excess with a cotton ball. If excessively dirty ears; apply 2-3 times daily over several days. For maintenance of healthy ears; 1-2 times weekly or as often as recommended by your veterinarian. Always apply after swimming.

Precaution(s): Storage: Store at controlled room temperature.
Caution(s): For topical use only. Avoid contact with eyes.
Presentation: 8 oz (236.5 mL) (NDC: 47611-365-59).
Sold exclusively to veterinarians.
Distributed by: Burns Veterinary Supply, Inc., Westbury, NY 11590.
Compendium Code No.: 14441030

ALOEDINE® MEDICATED SHAMPOO

Farnam **Antidermatosis Shampoo**

Active Ingredient(s):

Poloxamer iodine complex 1% yielding 0.2% titratable iodine in an aloe vera base shampoo

Indications: For horses, ponies and dogs.
Dosage and Administration: Wet animal with warm water. Apply one to two ounces of ALOEDINE® to the entire body. Work into a rich lather and rinse. Repeat application for maximum effectiveness and then rinse again.
Precaution(s): Store out of direct sunlight.
Caution(s): Animals: For external use only. Not for use on puppies, cats or kittens. Care should be taken to keep shampoo out of the animal's eyes.
Warning(s): Keep out of reach of children. For animal use only. May be harmful if swallowed.
Discussion: Horses have a variety of skin problems, most of which are extremely difficult to diagnose even for veterinarians. We recommend use of a deep cleaning medicated shampoo on a regular basis to help prevent skin conditions that can develop in horses, particularly in the summer. Skin problems in horses are extremely difficult to treat once started, but the regular use of ALOEDINE® will aid in preventing many of these problems. ALOEDINE® develops a rich lather which penetrates deep and cleanses contaminated areas.

ALOEDINE® contains aloe vera gel to moisturize and enrich skin and hair. Aloe Vera is found in the leaves of the succulent aloe vera plant. Aloe vera has been used for hundreds of years as a natural aid to healthy hair.

This product is also excellent for use on adult dogs, but not for use on puppies, cats or kittens.

Presentation: 473 mL (16 fl. oz.) bottle.
Compendium Code No.: 10000020

ALOE HEAL™

Farnam **Topical Wound Dressing**

Active Ingredient(s): Aloe vera gel, glyceryl stearate (and) PEG-100, stearic acid, cetyl alcohol, glycerine, triethanolamine, safflower oil, vitamin A palmitate, cholecalciferol, allantoin, herbal fragrance, dl-alpha tocopheryl acetate, sunflower oil, dl-panthenol, grapefruit juice concentrate, propylene glycol (and) diazolidinyl urea (and) methylparaben (and) propyl paraben FD&C blue #1 and FD&C yellow #5.
Indications: Farnam's ALOE HEAL™ is a first aid cream especially formulated for use on minor cuts and abrasions, skin irritations, proud flesh, and cracked heals. The high percentage of aloe vera gel, vitamins A, D, and E, safflower and sunflower seed oils in a rich, creamy base combine to make ALOE HEAL™'s soothing and healing action unsurpassed for minor cuts, abrasions and skin irritations.

For use on horses and dogs.

Dosage and Administration: Cleanse all wounds or intended areas of application thoroughly with a mild soap and water. If necessary, clip or shave hair from around the wound area. Cover the affected and surrounding areas with ALOE HEAL™ and bandage lightly if possible with several layers of gauze. Apply several times daily for best results. Continue treatment until wound is completely healed.
Caution(s): Not for use on deep or puncture wounds. If irritation develops or persists, discontinue use and consult your veterinarian.
Warning(s): Keep out of reach of children.
Presentation: 4 oz (113 g) and 16 oz.
Compendium Code No.: 10000011

ALPHA-7™

Boehringer Ingelheim **Bacterin-Toxoid**

Clostridium Chauvoei-Septicum-Novyi-Sordellii-Perfringens Types C & D Bacterin-Toxoid

U.S. Vet. Lic. No.: 124
Contents: This product contains the antigens listed above.

Preservative: Gentamicin.

Indications: Recommended for the vaccination of healthy susceptible cattle, including bred and/or lactating beef and dairy cattle, against disease caused by the organisms listed above.
Dosage and Administration: Using aseptic technique, inject a single 2 mL dose subcutaneously. A 2 mL booster dose is recommended annually. Calves vaccinated under 3 months of age should be vaccinated at weaning or 4-6 months of age.
Precaution(s): Store at 35-45°F (2-7°C). Avoid freezing. Shake well before using. Use entire contents when first opened.
Caution(s): Swelling at the injection site may occur. Anaphylactoid reactions may occur.
Antidote(s): Epinephrine.
Warning(s): Do not vaccinate within 60 days of slaughter.

Animal inoculation only. Accidental injection to humans can cause serious local reactions. Contact a physician immediately if accidental injection occurs.

Presentation: 10 dose (20 mL), 50 dose (100 mL), 250 dose (500 mL) vials.
Compendium Code No.: 10280031 13501-07

ALPHA-7/MB™

Boehringer Ingelheim **Bacterin-Toxoid**

Clostridium Chauvoei-Septicum-Novyi-Sordellii-Perfringens Types C & D-Moraxella Bovis Bacterin-Toxoid

U.S. Vet. Lic. No.: 124
Composition: Prepared from chemically inactivated cultures of the above organisms with a special DD-2 adjuvant system to maximize immune response. Contains gentamicin as a preservative.
Indications: Recommended as an aid in the reduction of diseases caused by *Clostridium chauvoei, Cl septicum, Cl novyi, Cl sordellii, Cl perfringens* Types C and D, and *Moraxella bovis*. Immunity may be provided against the beta and epsilon toxins elaborated by *Clostridium perfringens* Type B. This immunity is derived from the combination of Type C (beta) and Type D (epsilon) fractions.
Dosage and Administration: Using aseptic technique, inject a single 2 mL dose subcutaneously. Vaccinate calves at 3 months of age or older prior to the infectious bovine kerotoconjunctivitis (IBK) season. Revaccinate after 21 days with *Moraxella Bovis* Bacterin. A 2 mL booster dose of ALPHA-7/MB™ is recommended annually.
Precaution(s): Store at a temperature of 35-45°F (2-7°C). Avoid freezing. Shake well before using. Use entire contents when first opened.
Caution(s): Injection site swellings will often occur that may persist. Anaphylactoid reactions may occur.

The use of a biological product in lactating dairy cattle can cause reduced milk production.

Antidote(s): Epinephrine.
Warning(s): Do not vaccinate within 60 days of slaughter.

Animal inoculation only. Accidental injection to humans can cause serious local reactions. Contact a physician immediately if accidental injection occurs.

Presentation: 10 dose (20 mL) and 50 dose (100 mL) vials.
Compendium Code No.: 10280021 15301-03 / 15302-02

ALPHA-CD™

Boehringer Ingelheim **Toxoid**

Clostridium Perfringens Types C & D Toxoid

U.S. Vet. Lic. No.: 124
Composition: ALPHA-CD™ toxoid is prepared from chemically detoxified cultures of the above organisms with the special DD-2 adjuvant system to maximize immune response. Contains gentamicin as a preservative.
Indications: ALPHA-CD™ toxoid is recommended for the vaccination of healthy, susceptible cattle as an aid in the reduction of enterotoxemia caused by *Clostridium perfringens* Types C and D toxins. Immunity may be provided against the beta and epsilon toxins elaborated by *Clostridium perfringens* Type B. This immunity is derived from the combination of Type C (beta) and Type D (epsilon) fractions.
Dosage and Administration: Using aseptic technique, inject a single 2 mL dose subcutaneously. Calves vaccinated under 3 months of age should be revaccinated at weaning or 4-6 months of age. A 2 mL booster dose is recommended annually.
Precaution(s): Store at a temperature between 35-45°F (2-7°C). Avoid freezing. Shake well before using. Use entire contents when first opened.
Caution(s): Swelling at the injection site may occur. The use of a biological product in lactating dairy cattle may cause reduced milk production. Anaphylactoid reactions may occur.
Antidote(s): Epinephrine.
Warning(s): Do not vaccinate within 60 days of slaughter.

Animal inoculation only. Accidental injection to humans can cause serious local reactions. Contact a physician immediately if accidental injection occurs.

Presentation: 10 doses (20 mL), 50 doses (100 mL) and 250 doses (500 mL).
Compendium Code No.: 10280041 15101-04 / 15102-03 / 15103-03

ALPHALYTE® PREMIUM PET SHAMPOO

Alpha Tech Pet **Grooming Shampoo**

Ingredient(s): Cocamide DEA (derived from coconut oil), cocoamido betaine, glycerine, aloe vera, vitamin E, triazinyl stilbene, sodium chloride, citric acid, additional ingredients are proprietary and confidential (fragrance, dyes, and other additives).
Indications: Hypoallergenic shampoo for dogs, cats, puppies, and kittens.
Directions for Use: Wet hair coat thoroughly. Massage ALPHALYTE® Premium Pet Shampoo liberally throughout the hair coat. Lather and massage hair coat for about 5 minutes. Rinse thoroughly until your pet's hair coat is completely clean. Avoid contact with eyes. Towel dry and comb out your pet's hair coat. Repeat as necessary, bathe as often as needed to control skin problems.
Presentation: Available in pints (12 to a case) and gallons (2 to a case).
Compendium Code No.: 10140000

ALPHAZYME PLUS™

Alpha Tech Pet **Presoak**

Bio-Active Odor Counteractant & Enzyme Based Cleaner

Ingredient(s): ALPHAZYME PLUS™ is a concentrated, biodegradable, enzyme-based odor counteractant and cleaner combined in a stabilized bacterial spore system. It is totally organic with no deleterious ingredients, has a near neutral pH, and is biodegradable.
Indications: For Animal Care Facilities:

Effective Bio-Active Enzymatic Action - Formulated for veterinary clinics and animal care facilities. ALPHAZYME PLUS™ is a concentrated, biodegradable, enzyme-based odor counteractant and cleaner combined in a stabilized bacterial spore system for breaking down organic waste and eliminating odors in veterinary clinics and animal care facilities. It breaks down and removes dried-on fecal debris, urine, blood, tissue, mucous, and proteinaceous materials completely and effectively. This intelligently bio-active and environmentally safe process allows stabilized bacterial spores to produce fat and starch-splitting enzymes that work on organic debris, reducing it to an odor free solution of CO_2 and water.

Long Acting - ALPHAZYME PLUS™ acts within minutes to eliminate odors through its patent pending powerful odor counteractant and continues working as its intelligent stabilized bacterial spores produce just the right amount of odor eating enzyme to remove the cause of the odors.

Animals are not subjected to harmful cleaning agents or fumes because this is an environmentally safe process. ALPHAZYME PLUS™ is specifically designed for the animal care industry.

ALPHAZYME PLUS™ is a concentrated, bio-active enzyme-based odor counteractant and cleaner for cages, runs, floors, drains, and room deodorizing. The timed-release bio-active protease enzymes in ALPHAZYME PLUS™ are especially effective in the removal of protein, blood, mucus, feces, and urine; from cages, runs, floors, drains, and other odor producing areas in your facility. The environmentally safe process allows fat and starch-splitting enzymes to work on organic debris, reducing it to CO_2 and water. ALPHAZYME PLUS™ is ideal for use on concrete surfaces, grout, tile, plastic, metal, rubber, stainless steel and galvanized steel, and as a room deodorizer.

ALPHAZYME PLUS™ is also safe for use around any household furnishings.

Many Uses - A superior product to break down organic waste and associated odors. May be used on cages and other animal accommodations where odor producing debris builds up, making cleaning and appropriate disinfection difficult to manage. ALPHAZYME PLUS™ may be used on cat litter to control odors, is especially effective against the odor of tomcat spray, and may also be used for blood, urine, and fecal stain removal from clothing, uniforms, rugs, and pet bedding. ALPHAZYME PLUS™ is also an outstanding choice for use as a room spray air freshener containing a fresh black cherry fragrance, eliminating odors at their source.

Safe - ALPHAZYME PLUS™ is easily measured and dispensed, absolutely harmless to humans and animals, and will not produce hazardous dust or harm soft metals, including aluminum.

Directions for Use: Shake well before using. ALPHAZYME PLUS™ works best when allowed to work uninterrupted in a moist environment. For cages and other animal accommodations use 1 part ALPHAZYME PLUS™ to 4 parts lukewarm water around (170 degrees). For optimal use on heavily soiled areas apply solution and allow to air dry over a 4 hour period prior to disinfecting. May also be used following disinfection to provide long term odor control - simply apply and allow to air dry. For vomitus, urine, tomcat spray, cat litter, room deodorizing, and stain removal, a more concentrated solution as needed may be used to dissipate odors immediately, breaking down offending odor producing substrates to CO_2 and water. Repeat as needed. The use of ammonia or vinegar prior to using ALPHAZYME PLUS™ will greatly diminish its effectiveness.

Important Note - ALPHAZYME PLUS™ is not a sterilant or disinfectant and is intended to be used as a supplement to the normal cleaning and disinfection routine of animal care facilities. ALPHAZYME PLUS™ may be used as often as needed to control stains and odors associated with organic debris. For normal cleaning and disinfection of animal care facilities the manufacturer highly recommends the use of KennelSol™ Disinfectant on a daily basis, Alpha Sani-Wipes™ to sanitize hands between handling of animals, and Alpha Drain-X™ for drain maintenance.

Warning(s): Keep out of reach of children. If ingested, induce vomiting. If splashed into eyes, rinse with cold water.

Presentation: ALPHAZYME PLUS™ is available in ½ gallon containers packaged 3 to a case and 2½ gallon pails.

Compendium Code No.: 10140011

ALTOSID® CATTLE CUSTOM BLENDING PREMIX

Wellmark **Feed Additive**

EPA Reg. No.: 2724-473

Active Ingredient(s):

Methoprene [Isopropyl (*E,E*)-11-methoxy-3,7,11-trimethyl-2,4-dodecadienoate] 10.5%
Inert Ingredients: 89.5%
Total 100.0%

Indications: To prevent the breeding of horn flies in the manure of treated cattle.

Directions for Use: It is a violation of Federal Law to use this product in a manner inconsistent with its labeling.

Blending and Feeding ALTOSID® Cattle Premix: ALTOSID® Cattle Premix interrupts the development of the horn fly in the manure of treated cattle. Begin use in the spring before horn flies appear on cattle and continue feeding until cold weather restricts horn fly activity.

ALTOSID® Cattle Premix rations may be fed to beef and dairy cattle, including breeding cattle, lactating cattle, and calves. When used as directed, rations containing ALTOSID® Cattle Premix may be fed up to slaughter, and to lactating dairy cows without withholding milk.

This product can be used in complete feeds, concentrates, hand feeds, or mineral supplements.

ALTOSID® Cattle Premix is fed to cattle at the level of 340 mg/100 lb body weight/month to achieve horn fly control. This rate is equal to 11.3 mg ALTOSID® Cattle Premix/100 lb body weight/day. The calculations in the following chart assume a 1000 pound animal as the head weight; see chart for mixing directions:

Feed Product	Daily Feeding Rate	Ratio of Supplement to Feedstuffs	ALTOSID® Cattle Premix in Supplement mg/lb (%)	ALTOSID® Cattle Premix in Feed mg/lb (%)	Grams ALTOSID® Cattle Premix/Ton of Feed Product g/ton
Complete Feed	2.6 lb/cwt	-	-	4.3 (0.001)	8.7
Supplement or Premix for Preparing Complete Feeds	-	1:9	44 (0.01)	4.3 (0.001)	87
	-	1:19	87 (0.02)	4.3 (0.001)	174
	-	1:39	174 (0.04)	4.3 (0.001)	348
	-	1:79	348 (0.08)	4.3 (0.001)	696
Complete Feed	3.5 lb/cwt*	-	-	3.2 (0.0007)	6.5
Supplement or Premix for Preparing Complete Feeds	-	1:9	32 (0.007)	3.2 (0.0007)	65
	-	1:19	65 (0.014)	3.2 (0.0007)	130
	-	1:39	129 (0.028)	3.2 (0.0007)	260
	-	1:79	258 (0.056)	3.2 (0.0007)	520
Concentrate Fed with Roughage	1.0 lb/cwt	-	-	11.3 (0.0025)	22.6
Supplement or Premix for Preparing Complete Feeds	-	1:9	113 (0.025)	11.3 (0.0025)	226
	-	1:19	226 (0.05)	11.3 (0.0025)	452
	-	1:39	452 (0.10)	11.3 (0.0025)	904
	-	1:79	904 (0.20)	11.3 (0.0025)	1808
Supplement for Hand Feeding	2.0 lb/head	-	57 (0.013)	-	113
	1.5 lb/head	-	75 (0.017)	-	151
	1.0 lb/head	-	113 (0.025)	-	226
	0.5 lb/head	-	226 (0.050)	-	452
Mineral Mix	4.0 oz/head	-	452 (0.10)	-	904
	3.0 oz/head	-	603 (0.13)	-	1206
	2.0 oz/head	-	904 (0.20)	-	1808
	1.0 oz/250 lb	-	452 (0.10)	-	904
	1.0 oz/500 lb	-	904 (0.20)	-	1808
	1.0 oz/750 lb	-	1356 (0.30)	-	2712

* Consumption level of total ration formulated for lactating dairy cattle at 3.5% body weight intake.

Important Note to Feed Mill Operators:

ALTOSID® Cattle Premix is a light, fluffy product and therefore, whenever possible, the material should be added directly to the mixer. Elevators, long free-fall gravity chutes, etc. should be avoided.

It is critical, in order to avoid loss of the low density premix, that additions be made under conditions of low air turbulence or flow (shut off exhaust systems during ALTOSID® Cattle Premix addition).

Whenever possible, add the ALTOSID® Cattle Premix after the addition of the liquid components and blend to homogeneity.

When and How to Use ALTOSID® Cattle Premix: Use ALTOSID® Cattle Premix to break the life cycle of the horn fly. When fed to cattle, ALTOSID® Cattle Premix passes through the digestive system and is deposited throughout the manure. Here it stops the development of immature horn flies, before they can emerge as new adult flies. ALTOSID® Cattle Premix does not affect existing adult flies.

Start feeding ALTOSID® Cattle Premix early in the spring before horn flies appear. Continue feeding throughout the summer and into the fall until cold weather restricts fly activity.

If significant numbers of adult horn flies are already present when ALTOSID® Cattle Premix is introduced, it may take 3 to 5 weeks for an effect on the adult horn fly population to be clearly observed. For fast relief from existing fly burdens, consider the use of adulticide sprays, dusts, back-rubbers, or pour-ons.

Adult horn flies remain feeding on cattle day and night and leave the animal only to lay eggs in freshly passed manure. Without ALTOSID® Cattle Premix, eggs hatch and develop in the manure, resulting in a new generation of adult flies. These newly emerged flies may be carried downwind to a neighboring herd. Area wide fly control to include neighboring herds reduces the numbers of migrating flies.

ALTOSID® Cattle Premix may be fed up to slaughter and to lactating dairy cows without withholding milk.

Precautionary Statements: Hazards to Humans and Domestic Animals:

Caution: Causes eye and skin irritation. Avoid contact with eyes, skin, or clothing. Avoid breathing dust. Wash thoroughly with soap and water after handling.

Statement of Practical Treatment:

If in Eyes: Flush eyes with plenty of water. Get medical attention if irritations persists.

If on Skin: Wash with plenty of soap and water. Get medical attention if irritations persists.

Storage and Disposal:

Storage: Store ALTOSID® Cattle Premix in a cool, dry place. Do not contaminate water, food, or feed by storage or disposal.

Disposal: Wastes resulting from the use of this product may be disposed of on site or at an approved waste disposal facility.

Container Disposal: Completely empty bag into mixer. Dispose of empty bag in a sanitary landfill or by incineration, or by burning if allowed by state and local authorities. If burned, stay out of smoke.

Warning(s): ALTOSID® Cattle Premix is intended for use only in cattle.

Keep out of reach of children.

Disclaimer: Seller makes no warranty, express or implied, concerning the use of this product other than indicated on the label. Buyer assumes all risk of use and handling of this material.

Presentation: 6 lb bag in a box.

ALTOSID® is a registered trademark of Wellmark International.

Compendium Code No.: 10930000

ALTOSID® PREMIX

Wellmark **Feed Additive**

Methoprene (insect growth regulator)

EPA Reg. No.: 2724-474

Active Ingredient(s):

Methoprene [Isopropyl (E,E)-11-methoxy-3,7,11-trimethyl-2,4-dodecadienoate] 0.4%
Other Ingredients: 99.6%
Total 100.0%

Guaranteed Analysis:

Crude Protein, not less than ..... .35%
Crude Fat, not less than 5%
Crude Fiber, not more than 6%

Feed Ingredients: Soybean meal, dehulled soybean meal, corn distillers, dried grains with solubles, corn gluten feed, mineral oil, cane molasses.

Indications: To prevent the breeding of horn flies in the manure of treated cattle. A pesticidally active feed concentrate for continuous feeding during the fly season.

Directions for Use: It is a violation of Federal Law to use this product in a manner inconsistent with its labeling.

This product prevents emergence of adult horn flies from the manure of the treated cattle. Begin use in the spring before horn flies appear on cattle and continue feeding until cold weather restricts horn fly activity. Introduction of the product when significant numbers of adult flies are present requires the use of adulticide sprays or dusts.

The dosage of ALTOSID® Premix is proportional to body weight. The recommended consumption of this product is 0.0125 lb to 0.025 lb per 100 lb of body weight per month (30 days). Feed by either of the following methods.

Mixed with Free-Choice-Fed Minerals: Mix ALTOSID® Premix with free-choice-fed minerals to produce an ALTOSID® Premix and mineral mixture containing 0.02% active ingredient (methoprene) as shown in the following table.

ALTOSID® Premix. ..... 5 lb (5%)
Free-Choice Minerals ..... 95 lb (95%)
Total ..... 100 lb (100%)

Place the mixture of ALTOSID® Premix and minerals near watering or loafing areas and provide one feeder for each 15 to 20 head. Put out only a 5 to 7 day supply of the mixture at one time and protect it from the rain.

When the recommended mixture of ALTOSID® Premix and minerals is consumed at the rate of 0.25 lb to 0.5 lb per 100 lb of body weight per month, this mixture provides 0.0125 lb to 0.025 lb of ALTOSID® Premix per 100 lb of body weight per month.

Mixed-Ration Feeding: Thoroughly mix ALTOSID® Premix with grain or supplement to provide 0.0125 lb to 0.025 lb of ALTOSID® Premix per 100 lb of body weight per month.

Use the following table as a guide for determining the proper mixing rate.
Daily Grain or Supplement Consumption:

Body Weight (pounds)	Pounds of ALTOSID Premix Needed per Ton of Grain or Supplemental Feed	
	2 to 4 lb	5 to 10 lb
500	2.1	-
600	2.5	1.0
700	2.9	1.2
800	3.3	1.3
900	3.8	1.5
1000	4.1	1.7
1100	4.6	1.8
1200	5.0	2.0
1300	5.4	2.2
1400	5.8	2.3
1500	6.3	2.5
1600	6.7	2.7

Storage and Disposal: Do not contaminate water or feed by storage or disposal.

Storage: Store in dry area. Do not contaminate with pesticides or fertilizer.

Pesticide Disposal: Wastes resulting from the use of this product may be disposed of on site or at an approved waste disposal facility.

Container Disposal: Completely empty bag by shaking and tapping sides and bottom to loosen clinging particles. Empty residue into application equipment. Then dispose of empty bag in a sanitary landfill or by incineration, or if allowed by state and local authorities, by burning. If burned, stay out of smoke.

Warning(s): Use this product only as specified. Keep out of reach of children.

Presentation: 25 bag.

ALTOSID® Premix is a registered trademark of Wellmark International.

Compendium Code No.: 10930010

ALUSPRAY®

Neogen **Topical Wound Dressing**

Aerosol Bandage

Active Ingredient(s): Each gram contains:

Aluminum powder .... 40 mg

Indications: ALUSPRAY® is recommended as a protective barrier against external irritant agents in wounds in small and large animals.

Directions for Use: Shake well before use. Clean the area to be sprayed. Apply ALUSPRAY® to cover the area to be protected with a thin layer of powder.

Precaution(s): Contents under pressure. Do not use in the presence of an open flame or spark. Do not place in hot water or near radiators, stoves or other sources of heat. Do not puncture or incinerate the container or store at a temperature over 50°C (122°F).

Container may explode if heated. Propellant is flammable.

Caution(s): Avoid spraying in animal's eyes.

This product stains. Avoid contact with hands and clothes.

For veterinary use only. External use only.

Warning(s): Keep out of reach of children.

Presentation: 75 g containers (NDC#59051-9100-0).

Manufactured by: Vetoquinol SA.

Compendium Code No.: 14910011 696-1101

A-LYTE CONCENTRATE

Durvet **Electrolytes-Oral**

Active Ingredient(s): Contents: Each 500 mL of aqueous solution contains:

Dextrose .... 25 g
Calcium .... 204 mg
Sodium .... 211 mg
Magnesium .... 98.6 mg
Potassium .... 524 mg
Cyanocobalamin (B_{12}) .... 25 mcg
Niacinamide .... 750 mg
Pyridoxine (B_6) .... 41 mg
Thiamine (B_1) .... 44 mg
Riboflavin (B_2) .... 20 mg
d-Pantothenic Acid .... 25 mg
L-Leucine .... 935 mg
L-Lysine Hydrochloride .... 850 mg
L-Glutamic Acid .... 680 mg
L-Valine .... 680 mg
L-Phenylalanine .... 595 mg
L-Arginine Hydrochloride .... 425 mg
L-Isoleucine .... 425 mg
L-Threonine .... 391 mg
L-Histidine HCl • H_2O .... 297.5 mg
L-Methionine .... 255 mg
L-Cysteine HCl • H_2O .... 250 mg

Ingredients: Calcium Chloride, Dextrose Monohydrate, Magnesium Sulfate, Potassium Chloride, Sodium Acetate, Cyanocobalamin, Niacinamide, Riboflavin 5 Sodium Phosphate, d-Pantothenic Acid, Thiamine Hydrochloride, Pyridoxine Hydrochloride, L-Arginine HCl, L-Cysteine HCl, L-Glutamic Acid, L-Histidine HCl, L-Isoleucine, L-Leucine, L-Lysine HCl, L-Methionine, L-Phenylalanine, L-Threonine, L-Valine, Propylene Glycol, Lactic Acid, Sorbitol, Citric Acid, Methylparaben, Ethylparaben, and Propylparaben.

Indications: An oral source of vitamins, amino acids and electrolytes for cattle, swine, sheep and horses when dietary intake is reduced.

Dosage and Administration: For use in drinking water.

A-LYTE CONCENTRATE may be used undiluted or diluted with water. Supply fresh drinking water daily.

Dosage: Undiluted.

Cattle: Administer 1 oz. A-LYTE CONCENTRATE per 100 pounds body weight in the drinking water to be consumed in one day.

Horses: Administer 10 oz. A-LYTE CONCENTRATE per 1000 pounds body weight in the drinking water to be consumed in one day.

Sheep and Swine: Administer ½ oz. A-LYTE CONCENTRATE per 50 pounds body weight in the drinking water to be consumed in one day.

Precaution(s): Protect from freezing.

Caution(s): For animal use only. Keep out of reach of children.

Presentation: 500 mL (16.9 fl oz) (NDC 30798-002-17).

Compendium Code No.: 10840031 Iss. 03-00

A-LYTE SOLUTION

Durvet **Electrolytes-Oral**

Active Ingredient(s): Composition: Each 100 mL of aqueous solution contains:

Dextrose • H_2O .... 5 g
Sodium Acetate • $3H_2O$ .... 250 mg
Magnesium Sulfate • $7H_2O$ .... 20 mg
Potassium Chloride .... 20 mg
Calcium Chloride $2H_2O$ .... 15 mg
Niacinamide .... 150 mg
Pyridoxine Hydrochloride (B_6) .... 10 mg
Thiamine Hydrochloride (B_1) .... 10 mg
Riboflavin (B_2) .... 4 mg
Total Protein .... 28.5 mg

Containing amino acids: L-Valine, L-Glutamic Acid, L-Leucine, L-Lysine Hydrochloride, L-Phenylalanine, L-Arginine Hydrochloride, L-Isoleucine, L-Threonine, L-Cysteine Hydrochloride • H_2O, L-Histidine Hydrochloride • H_2O, L-Methionine.

With methylparaben 0.18%, propylparaben 0.02%, and ethylparaben 0.01% (preservatives).

Indications: For use as a supplemental nutritive source of amino acids, electrolytes, B complex vitamins, and dextrose in cattle and horses.

Dosage and Administration: Administer orally as a drench. The usual recommended dose in adult cattle and horses is 500 to 3000 mL, depending on size and condition.

Precaution(s): Store between 15° and 30°C (59°-86°F).

Caution(s): For animal use only. Keep out of the reach of children.

Presentation: 500 mL (NDC 30798-024-17).

Compendium Code No.: 10840041 Rev. 5-95

AMBI-PEN™ ℞

Butler **Penicillin Injection**

Sterile Penicillin G Benzathine and Penicillin G Procaine in Aqueous Suspension

NADA No.: 065-500

Active Ingredient(s): Each mL of suspension contains:

Penicillin G benzathine .... 150,000 units
Penicillin G procaine .... 150,000 units
Lecithin .... 11.7 mg
Sodium formaldehyde sulfoxylate .... 1.75 mg
Methylparaben (as preservative) .... 1.20 mg
Propylparaben (as preservative) .... 0.14 mg
Tween 40 .... 8.19 mg
Span 40 .... 11.3 mg
Sodium citrate anhydrous .... 3.98 mg
Procaine hydrochloride .... 20.0 mg
Sodium carboxymethylcellulose .... 1.04 mg
Water for injection .... q.s.

Indications: AMBI-PEN™ is indicated for treatment of the following bacterial infections in dogs, horses, and beef cattle due to penicillin susceptible micro-organisms that are susceptible to the serum levels common to this particular dosage form, such as:

1. Bacterial pneumonia *(Streptococcus* spp., *Corynebacterium pyogenes, Staphylococcus aureus).*
2. Upper respiratory infections such as rhinitis or pharyngitis *(Corynebacterium pyogenes).*
3. Equine strangles *(Streptococcus equi).*
4. Blackleg *(Clostridium chauvoei).*

Pharmacology: Penicillin G is an antibiotic which shows a marked bactericidal effect against certain organisms during their growth phase. It is relatively specific in its action against gram-positive bacteria but is usually ineffective against gram-negative organisms.

When treating an animal for a bacterial infection, it is advisable to isolate and identify the causative organisms and conduct appropriate *in vitro* susceptibility tests. In cases where organisms other than those susceptible to penicillin are present, a re-evaluation of treatment should be made. Organisms normally considered susceptible to penicillin include *Clostridium septicum, Corynebacterium pyogenes, Staphylococcus aureus, Streptococcus canis, Streptococcus equi* and *Streptococcus pyogenes.*

Dosage and Administration: Shake well before each use.

Horses: 2 mL per 150 lbs. of body weight given intramuscularly (2,000 units penicillin G procaine and 2,000 units penicillin G benzathine per lb. of body weight). The treatment should be repeated in 48 hours.

Beef Cattle: 2 mL per 150 lbs. of body weight given subcutaneously only (2,000 units penicillin G procaine and 2,000 units penicillin G benzathine per lb. of body weight). The treatment should be repeated in 48 hours.

Important: Treatment in beef cattle should be limited to two (2) doses given by subcutaneous injection only.

Dogs: 1 mL per 10-20 lbs. of body weight given intramuscularly or subcutaneously (6,000 to 15,000 units penicillin G procaine and 6,000 to 15,000 units penicillin G benzathine per lb. of body weight). The treatment should be repeated in 48 hours.

Sterile penicillin G benzathine and penicillin G procaine in aqueous suspension should be given by intramuscular injection to horses. In beef cattle, the recommended dosage should be administered by subcutaneous injection only. Dogs may be injected by either the intramuscular or subcutaneous route.

It is normally recommended that any bacterial infection be treated as early as possible and with a dosage that will give effective blood levels. Although the recommended dosage will give longer detectable penicillin blood levels than penicillin G procaine alone, it is recommended that a second dose be administered at 48 hours when treating a penicillin susceptible-bacterial infection.

If definite improvement is not noted following the second dose, the diagnosis should be re-evaluated and use of another chemotherapeutic agent considered.

Contraindication(s): Sterile penicillin G benzathine and penicillin G procaine in aqueous suspension is contraindicated in patients which have shown hypersensitivity to penicillin.

Precaution(s): Store under refrigeration below 59°F (15°C). Protect from freezing.
Caution(s): Federal law restricts this drug to use by or on the order of a licensed veterinarian.
Warning(s): Beef cattle should be withheld from slaughter for food use for 30 days following the last treatment with this drug. Treatment in beef cattle must be limited to two (2) doses.
Not to be used for horses intended for slaughter for food purposes.
Side Effects: Anaphylactic reactions have been reported in cattle given penicillin. Treated animals should be closely observed and if allergic or anaphylactic reactions occur, administer epinephrine or antihistamines immediately.
Presentation: 100 mL and 250 mL vials.
Compendium Code No.: 10820031

AMCALCILYTE FORTE

AgriPharm — **Electrolytes-Oral**

Oral Solution

Active Ingredient(s): Each 1000 mL of aqueous solution contains:

Dextrose - H2O	275.0 g
Calcium Hypophosphite	36.5 g
Potassium Chloride	15.0 g
Sodium Chloride	2.0 g
Potassium Phosphate, monobasic	0.5 g
L-Glutamic Acid	560.0 mg
L-Arginine Hydrochloride	450.0 mg
L-Proline	400.0 mg
L-Lysine Hydrochloride	240.0 mg
L-Leucine	160.0 mg
L-Phenylalanine	110.0 mg
L-Valine	110.0 mg
L-Threonine	100.0 mg
L-Isoleucine	70.0 mg
L-Histidine Hydrochloride	40.0 mg
L-Methionine	40.0 mg
L-Tyrosine	24.0 mg
Methylparaben (preservative)	0.0896%
Propylparaben (preservative)	0.0196%

Indications: For use as a supplemental nutritive source of electrolytes, dextrose, and amino acids in cattle.
Dosage and Administration: Administer orally as a drench or by use of a stomach tube. The usual recommended dose in adult cattle is 500 to 1000 mL, depending on size and condition.
Precaution(s): Store at controlled room temperature between 15°C and 30°C (59°F-86°F).
Caution(s): For animal use only.
Warning(s): Keep out of reach of children.
Presentation: 1000 mL.
Compendium Code No.: 14571140

AMCALCILYTE FORTE

Phoenix Pharmaceutical — **Electrolytes-Oral**

Oral Solution-Electrolytes-Dextrose-Amino Acids

Active Ingredient(s): Composition: Each 1000 mL of aqueous solution contains:

Dextrose • H_2O	275.0 g
Calcium Hypophosphite	36.5 g
Potassium Chloride	15.0 g
Sodium Chloride	2.0 g
Potassium Phosphate, monobasic	0.5 g
Total protein	2.3 g

Containing amino acids: L-glutamic acid, L-arginine hydrochloride, L-proline, L-lysine hydrochloride, L-leucine, L-phenylalanine, L-valine, L-threonine, L-isoleucine, L-histidine hydrochloride, L-methionine, and L-tyrosine.

Methylparaben (preservative)	0.09%
Propylparben (preservative)	0.01%

Indications: For use as a supplemental nutritive source of electrolytes, dextrose, and amino acids in cattle.
Dosage and Administration: Administer orally as a drench. The usual recommended dose in adult cattle is 500 to 1000 mL, depending on size and condition.
Precaution(s): Store between 15° and 30°C (59° and 86°F).
Caution(s): For animal use only.
Warning(s): Keep out of reach of children.
Presentation: 1,000 mL bottles (NDC 57319-067-08).
Manufactured by: Phoenix Scientific, Inc., St. Joseph, MO 64503.
Compendium Code No.: 12560022 Rev. 3-02

AMCALCILYTE FORTE

Vedco — **Electrolytes-Oral**

Active Ingredient(s): Each 1,000 mL contains:

Dextrose H_2O	275.0 g
Calcium hyposphosphite	36.5 g
Potassium chloride	15.0 g
Sodium chloride	2.0 g
Potassium phosphate monobasic	0.5 g
L-glutamic acid	560.0 mg
L-arginine hydrochloride	450.0 mg
L-proline	400.0 mg
L-lysine hydrochloride	240.0 mg
L-leucine	160.0 mg
L-phenylalanine	110.0 mg
L-valine	110.0 mg
L-threonine	100.0 mg
L-isoleucine	70.0 mg
L-histidine hydrochloride	40.0 mg
L-methionine	40.0 mg
L-tyrosine	24.0 mg
Preservatives:	
Methylparaben	0.09%
Propylparaben	0.01%

Indications: For use as a supplemental source of electrolyes, dextrose, and amino acids in cattle.
Dosage and Administration: Administer orally as a drench or by use of a stomach tube. The usual recommended dose in adult cattle is 500 to 1,000 mL depending upon the size and the condition of the animal.
Precaution(s): Store at a controlled room temperature between 59-86°F (15-30°C).
Caution(s): Keep out of the reach of children. Not for human use.
Presentation: 1,000 mL containers.
Compendium Code No.: 10940030

AMFOROL® ℞

Fort Dodge — **Antidiarrheal Antibiotic-Adsorbent**

Oral Suspension and Tablets

NADA No.: 042-548 (Suspension)/042-841 (Tablets)

Active Ingredient(s): Each 5 mL of suspension and each tablet contains:

Kanamycin activity (as the sulfate)	100 mg
Bismuth subcarbonate	250 mg
Activated attapulgite (aluminum magnesium silicate)	500 mg

Indications: AMFOROL® is indicated for the treatment of bacterial enteritis in dogs (caused by organisms susceptible to kanamycin) and the symptomatic relief of the associated diarrhea.
Pharmacology:
Therapeutic action of ingredients: Kanamycin Sulfate (Kantrim®): Kanamycin is active against Salmonella, Shigella, *Alcaligenes faecalis, E. coli,* Proteus and *Staphylococcus aureus*, all species associated with bacterial enteric infections. Most of the dose is not absorbed from the gastrointestinal tract, providing bactericidal action at the site of infection.
Bismuth subcarbonate and activated attapulgite (aluminum magnesium silicate) are antidiarrheals.
Dosage and Administration: Dogs - The following dosage schedule is recommended, based upon a simple estimation of animal size:
Oral Suspension: Five mL (5 mL) per 20 lbs body weight every 8 hours. Maximum dose, 15 mL every 8 hours. For animals under 10 lbs, 2.5 mL every 8 hours.
Oral Tablets: One tablet per 20 lbs body weight every 8 hours. Maximum dose, three tablets every 8 hours. For animals under 10 lbs, one-half tablet every 8 hours.
It is recommended that an initial loading dose preceded the above schedule, consisting of twice the amount of a single dose.
Contraindication(s): AMFOROL® is contraindicated in treatment of Salmonella septicemias.
Precaution(s):
AMFOROL® Veterinary Oral Suspension - Store below 25°C (77°F).
AMFOROL® Veterinary Oral Tablets - Store at controlled room temperature 15° to 30°C (59° to 86°F).
Because of the bactericidal activity of kanamycin, prolonged treatment may permit overgrowth of nonsusceptible organisms (e.g., fungi). If remission of symptoms is not evident after 2 to 3 days treatment, the diagnosis should be re-established. Do not treat for longer than 5 days.
Dogs, especially those weighing less than 5 lbs, when treated with oral kanamycin should be under close clinical observation for potential nephrotoxic and ototoxic side effects, as the recommended dosage may produce systemic levels of this aminoglycoside. Kanamycin should be used cautiously if the dog is also receiving other nephrotoxic or ototoxic drugs.
Caution(s): Federal law restricts this drug to use by or on the order of a licensed veterinarian.
Warning(s): Treatment of Salmonella infections confined to the gastrointestinal tract with kanamycin may result in prolonged shedding of this microorganism. Follow-up cultures after treatment are strongly advised.
Side Effects: The bismuth subcarbonate in AMFOROL® may produce darkening of the tongue and stools which can be confused with melena. Prolonged exposure to orally administered bismuth salts has been associated with encephalopathies in other species. Signs may include lack of energy, muscle twitching, confusion, convulsions and comas.
Presentation:
AMFOROL® Veterinary Oral Suspension is available in bottles of 474 mL (16 fl oz) (NDC 0856-2005-60).
AMFOROL® Veterinary Oral Tablets are available in bottles of 100 (NDC 0856-2006-60).
Compendium Code No.: 10030040 6020H

AMIFUSE E ℞

Vetus — **Intrauterine Antibiotic**

(Amikacin Sulfate Solution)

ANADA No.: 200-181

Active Ingredient(s): Each mL contains:

Amikacin sulfate	250 mg

The solution contains, in addition to amikacin sulfate, 2.5% sodium citrate with pH adjusted to 4.5 with sulfuric acid and 0.66% sodium bisulfite added. The multi-dose 12 gram vial contains 0.01% benzethonium chloride as a preservative.
Indications: AMIFUSE E (Amikacin Sulfate Solution) is indicated for the treatment of uterine infections (endometritis, metritis and pyometra) in mares, when caused by susceptible organisms including *Escherichia coli, Pseudomonas* sp, and *Klebsiella* sp. The use of amikacin sulfate in eliminating infections caused by the above organisms has been shown clinically to improve fertility in infected mares.
While nearly all strains of *Escherichia coli, Pseudomonas* sp and *Klebsiella* sp, including those that are resistant to gentamicin, kanamycin or other aminoglycosides, are susceptible to amikacin at levels achieved following treatment, it is recommended that the invading organism be cultured and its susceptibility demonstrated as a guide to therapy. Amikacin susceptibility discs, 30 mcg, should be used for determining *in vitro* susceptibility.
Pharmacology: Description: Amikacin sulfate is a semisynthetic aminoglycoside antibiotic derived from kanamycin. It is $C_{22}H_{43}N_5O_{13}{\bullet}2H_2SO_4$,D-streptamine, 0-3-amino-3-deoxy-α-D-glucopyranosyl-(1-6)-0-[6-amino-6-deoxy-α-D-glucopyranosyl-(1-4)-N1-(4-amino-2-hydroxy-1-oxobutyl)-2-deoxy-, (S)-, sulfate (1:2)(salt).
Action:
Antibacterial Activity: The effectiveness of AMIFUSE E (Amikacin Sulfate Solution) in infections caused by *Escherichia coli, Pseudomonas* sp, and *Klebsiella* sp has been demonstrated clinically in the horse. In addition, the following microorganisms have been shown to be susceptible to amikacin *in vitro*,[1] although the clinical significance of this action has not been demonstrated in animals: *Enterobacter* sp, *Proteus mirabilis, Proteus* sp (indole positive), *Serratia marcescens, Salmonella* sp, *Shigella* sp, *Providencia* sp, *Citrobacter freundii, Listeria monocytogenes, Staphylococcus aureus* (both penicillin resistant and penicillin sensitive).
The aminoglycoside antibiotics in general have limited activity against gram-positive pathogens, although *Staphylococcus aureus* and *Listeria monocytogenes* are susceptible to amikacin as noted above.
Amikacin has been shown to be effective against many aminoglycoside-resistant strains due

to its ability to resist degradation by aminoglycoside inactivating enzymes known to affect gentamicin, tobramycin and kanamycin.[2]

Clinical Pharmacology:

Endometrial Tissue Concentrations: Comparisons of amikacin activity in endometrial biopsy tissue following intrauterine infusion with that following intramuscular injection of amikacin sulfate in mares demonstrate superior endometrial tissue concentrations when the drug is administered by the intrauterine route. Intrauterine infusion of 2 grams AMIFUSE E (Amikacin Sulfate Solution) daily for three consecutive days in mares results in peak concentrations typically exceeding 40 mcg/g of endometrial biopsy tissue within one hour after infusion. Twenty-four hours after each treatment amikacin activity is still detectable at concentrations averaging 2 to 4 mcg/g. However, the drug is not appreciably absorbed systemically following intrauterine infusion. Endometrial tissue concentrations following intramuscular injection roughly parallel, but are typically somewhat lower than corresponding serum concentrations of amikacin.

Dosage and Administration: For treatment of uterine infections in mares, 2 grams (8 mL) of AMIFUSE E (Amikacin Sulfate Solution), mixed with 200 mL 0.9% Sodium Chloride Injection, USP and aseptically infused into the uterus daily for three consecutive days, has been found to be the most efficacious dosage.

Contraindication(s): There are no known contraindications for the use of amikacin sulfate in horses other than a history of hypersensitivity to amikacin.

Precaution(s): AMIFUSE E (Amikacin Sulfate Solution) is supplied as a colorless solution which is stable at room temperature. At times the solution may become pale yellow in color. This does not indicate a decrease in potency.

Store at controlled room temperature 15°-30°C (59°-86°F).

Caution(s): Federal law restricts this drug to use by or on the order of a licensed veterinarian.

Although amikacin sulfate is not absorbed to an appreciable extent following intrauterine infusion, concurrent use of other aminoglycosides should be avoided because of the potential additive effects.

Warning(s): Not to be used in horses intended for food. *In vitro* studies have demonstrated that when sperm are exposed to the preservative which is present in the 48 mL vials (250 mg/mL) sperm viability is impaired.

Adverse Reactions: No adverse reactions or other side effects have been reported.

Trial Data: Safety: AMIFUSE E (Amikacin Sulfate Solution) is non-irritating to equine endometrial tissue when infused into the uterus as directed (see "Dosage and Administration"). In laboratory animals as well as equine studies, the drug was generally found not to be irritating when injected intravenously, subcutaneously or intramuscularly.

Although amikacin, like other aminoglycosides, is potentially nephrotoxic, ototoxic and neurotoxic, parenteral (intravenous) administration of amikacin sulfate twice daily at dosages of up to 10 mg/lb for 15 consecutive days in horses resulted in no clinical, laboratory or histopathologic evidence of toxicity.

Intrauterine infusion of 2 grams of AMIFUSE E (Amikacin Sulfate Solution) 8 hours prior to breeding by natural service did not impair fertility in mares. Therefore, mares should not be bred for at least 8 hours following uterine infusion.

References: Available upon request.

Presentation: 48 mL vial.

Compendium Code No.: 14440030

AMIGLYDE-V® INJECTION ℞

Fort Dodge **Amikacin Injection**

Amikacin Sulfate, Sterile

NADA No.: 127-892

Active Ingredient(s): The dosage form is supplied as a sterile, colorless to straw colored solution containing, in addition to amikacin sulfate, 2.5% sodium citrate, USP; pH adjusted with sulfuric acid, 0.66% sodium bisulfite added, and 0.1 mg benzethonium chloride, USP per mL as a preservative.

Indications: AMIGLYDE-V® (amikacin sulfate) is indicated for the treatment of the following conditions in dogs:

Genitourinary tract infections (cystitis) caused by susceptible strains of *Escherichia coli* and *Proteus* sp.

Skin and soft tissue infections caused by susceptible strains of *Pseudomonas* sp. and *Escherichia coli.*

While nearly all strains of *Escherichia coli, Pseudomonas* sp., and *Proteus* sp., including those that are resistant to gentamicin, kanamycin or other aminoglycosides, are susceptible to amikacin at levels achieved following treatment, it is recommended that the invading organism be cultured and its susceptibility demonstrated as a guide to therapy. Amikacin susceptibility discs, 30 mcg, should be used for determining *in vitro* susceptibility.

Pharmacology:

Description: Amikacin sulfate is a semi-synthetic aminoglycoside antibiotic derived from kanamycin. It is $C_{22}H_{43}N_5O_{13} \bullet 2H_2SO_4$, D-streptamine, 0-3-amino-3-deoxy-α-D-glucopyranosyl - (1→6) - 0 - [6-amino-6-deoxy-α-D-glucopyranosyl-(1→4)] - N[1]-(4-amino-2-hydroxy-1-oxobutyl)-2-deoxy-,(S)-,sulfate(1:2)(salt).

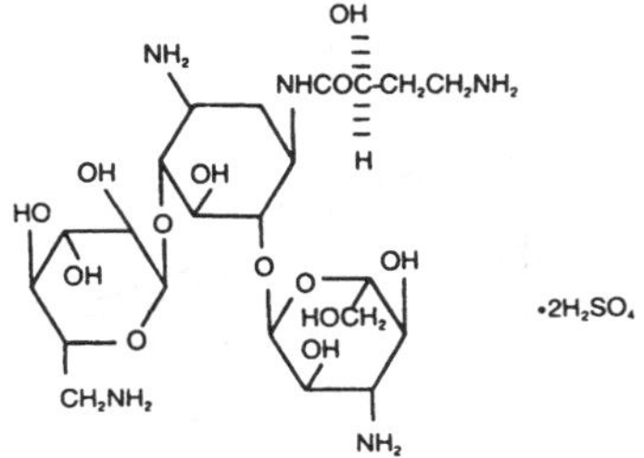

Action: Amikacin, like other aminoglycoside antibiotics, is a bactericidal agent that exerts its action at the level of the bacterial ribosome. Amikacin has been shown to be effective against many aminoglycoside-resistant strains due to its ability to resist degradation by aminoglycoside inactivating enzymes known to affect gentamicin, tobramycin and kanamycin.[1]

Microbiology: Amikacin has been shown to be effective in the treatment of skin and soft tissue infections caused by *Pseudomonas* sp. and *Escherichia coli* and in urinary tract infections caused by *Escherichia coli* and *Proteus* sp. The susceptibility of veterinary isolates to amikacin is summarized in the following table:

Organism (No. of Isolates)	Minimum Inhibitory Concentration (mcg/mL)	
	Range	MIC_{90}*
Escherichia coli (50)	1-32	4
Proteus mirabilis (50)	1-128	6
Enterobacter sp. (50)	0.5-128	4
Staphylococcus aureus (50)	1-128	2
Klebsiella pneumoniae (50)	0.5-16	2
Pseudomonas aeruginosa (50)	1-64	8

*Concentration at which 90% of the isolates are susceptible.

In addition, the following microorganisms have been shown to be susceptible to amikacin *in vitro*,[2] although the clinical significance of this action has not been demonstrated in animals: *Serratia marcescens, Salmonella* sp., *Shigella* sp., *Providencia* sp., *Citrobacter freundii, Listeria monocytogenes.*

The aminoglycoside antibiotics in general have limited activity against gram-positive pathogens, although *Staphylococcus aureus* and *Listeria monocytogenes* are susceptible to amikacin as noted above.

Pharmacokinetics: Amikacin is well absorbed following intravenous, subcutaneous, or intramuscular injection but is not appreciably absorbed orally. The serum half-life ($T\frac{1}{2}$) averages from 1 to 2 hours in dogs depending on the route of administration.[3] Amikacin is excreted unchanged in urine, concentrations in excess of 1,000 mcg/mL typically being achieved within three hours in dogs. Serum concentration-time profiles in dogs following subcutaneous administration are illustrated graphically in Figure 1.

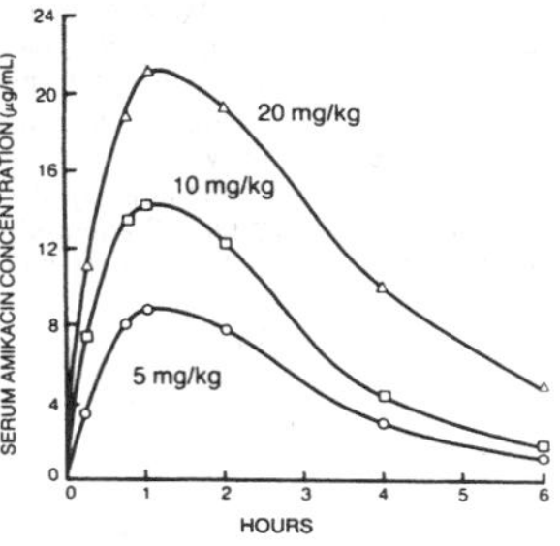

Figure 1: Amikacin Concentration-Time Curves in Dogs (n=6) Following Subcutaneous Injection

Dosage and Administration: AMIGLYDE-V® (amikacin sulfate) Injection should be administered subcutaneously or intramuscularly at a dosage of 10 mg/kg (5 mg/lb) twice daily. Dogs with skin and soft tissue infections should be treated for a minimum of 7 days and those with genitourinary infections should be treated for 7 to 21 days or until culture negative and asymptomatic. If no response is observed after three days of treatment, therapy should be discontinued and the case re-evaluated. Maximum duration of therapy should not exceed 30 days.

Contraindication(s): Systemic aminoglycoside therapy is contraindicated in dogs with seriously impaired renal function.

Precaution(s): Store vials at controlled room temperature 15° to 30°C (59° to 86°F). At times the solution may become pale yellow in color. This does not indicate a decrease in potency.

Caution(s): Federal law restricts this drug to use by or on the order of a licensed veterinarian.

The following conditions have been found to contribute to the toxicity of aminoglycosides in dogs: Prior renal damage (most commonly found in dogs of advanced age) and dogs infected with heartworm microfilaria;[5] and hypovolemic dehydration (dehydrated patients should be rehydrated prior to initiating therapy).

In dogs where decreased renal function is suspected prior to treatment, BUN or serum creatinine levels may not indicate the degree of kidney impairment. A creatinine clearance determination may be more useful.

Monitoring of renal function during treatment is recommended. Although there is not a completely reliable monitoring program for aminoglycoside toxicity, urinalysis may indicate early nephrotoxicity. Unfavorable changes in the urinalysis which may indicate toxicity include: Decreased specific gravity in the absence of fluid therapy; and appearance in the urine of casts, albumin, glucose or blood.

Continued use of aminoglycosides where any functional renal impairment has occurred may lead to enhanced renal damage as well as increased likelihood of ototoxicity and/or neuromuscular blockade.[6]

Concurrent or sequential use of topically or systemically administered nephrotoxic, ototoxic, or neuromuscular blocking drugs, particularly other aminoglycosides such as streptomycin, gentamicin, kanamycin and neomycin should be avoided because of the potential for additive effects.

Concurrent administration of furosemide with aminoglycosides may enhance nephrotoxicity.[7]

Not for use in breeding dogs as reproductive studies have not been conducted.

Neurotoxic and nephrotoxic antibiotics may be absorbed in significant quantities from body surfaces after local irrigation or application. The potential toxic effect of antibiotics administered in this fashion should be considered.[8]

If hypersensitivity develops, treatment with AMIGLYDE-V® Injection should be discontinued and appropriate therapy instituted.

Warning(s): Amikacin should be used with extreme caution in dogs, in which hearing acuity is required for functioning, such as seeing eye, hearing ear or military patrol, as the auditory and vestibular impairment tends not to be reversible.[6]

Aminoglycosides, including amikacin, are not indicated in uncomplicated episodes of cystitis unless causative agents are susceptible to them and are not susceptible to antibiotics having less potential for toxicity.

Early signs of ototoxicity can include ataxia, nausea and vomiting. Auditory and vestibular impairment may be reversible in the very early stages, but if treatment is continued, the conditions will become irreversible.[6]

For veterinary use only.

Toxicology: The intravenous and intramuscular LD_{50} in dogs is greater than 250 mg/kg. Like other aminoglycosides, amikacin has nephrotoxic, neurotoxic and ototoxic potential. In dogs, minimal to mild renal changes were detectable histopathologically after amikacin dosage of 45 mg/kg/day for two weeks, and dogs receiving a dosage of 30 mg/kg/day for 90 days had minimal renal alterations which were believed to be entirely reversible. Urinary casts were not observed in dogs receiving a 30 mg/kg dose for 90 days. In efficacy studies involving 80 infected dogs treated with amikacin at the recommended dosage rate of 10 mg/kg b.i.d. for 8-21 consecutive days, no evidence of nephrotoxicity or any other toxicity was encountered. Regarding ototoxicity, studies in cats reveal that amikacin has less potential for ototoxicity than gentamicin.[4]

Adverse Reactions: In clinical studies in dogs, transient pain on injection has been reported as well as rare cases of vomiting or diarrhea following amikacin therapy. In 90 day intramuscular toxicology studies, evidence of muscle damage was detected histologically as well as by elevated creatinine phosphokinase.

References: Available upon request.

Presentation: AMIGLYDE-V® Injection (50 mg/mL) is supplied in 50 mL vials (NDC 0856-2326-20).

Compendium Code No.: 10030060 4100D

AMIGLYDE-V® INTRAUTERINE SOLUTION ℞

Fort Dodge **Intrauterine Antibiotic**

Amikacin Sulfate Injection, USP-Veterinary Solution

NADA No.: 127-892

Active Ingredient(s): The dosage form supplied is a sterile, colorless to light straw-colored solution. The solution contains, in addition to amikacin sulfate USP, 2.5% sodium citrate, USP with pH adjusted to 4.5 with sulfuric acid and 0.66% sodium bisulfite added. The multi-dose 12 gram—48 mL vial contains 0.01% benzethonium chloride, USP as a preservative.

Indications: AMIGLYDE-V® is indicated for the treatment of uterine infections (endometritis, metritis and pyometra) in mares, when caused by susceptible organisms including *Escherichia coli, Pseudomonas* sp and *Klebsiella* sp. The use of AMIGLYDE-V® in eliminating infections caused by the above organisms has been shown clinically to improve fertility in infected mares.

While nearly all strains of *Escherichia coli, Pseudomonas* sp and *Klebsiella* sp, including those that are resistant to gentamicin, kanamycin or other aminoglycosides, are susceptible to amikacin at levels achieved following treatment, it is recommended that the invading organism be cultured and its susceptibility demonstrated as a guide to therapy. Amikacin susceptibility discs, 30 mcg, should be used for determining *in vitro* susceptibility.

Pharmacology: Amikacin sulfate is a semi-synthetic aminoglycoside antibiotic derived from kanamycin. It is $C_{22}H_{43}N_5O_{13}{\bullet}2H_2SO_4$, D-streptamine, 0-3-amino-3-deoxy-α-D-glucopyranosyl-(1→6)-0-[6-amino-6-deoxy-α-D-glucopyranosyl-(1→4)-N[1]-(4-amino-2-hydroxy-1-oxobutyl) -2-deoxy-, (S)-, sulfate (1:2) (salt).

Action:

Antibacterial Activity: The effectiveness of AMIGLYDE-V® (amikacin sulfate injection, USP) in infections caused by *Escherichia coli, Pseudomonas* sp and *Klebsiella* sp has been demonstrated clinically in the horse. In addition, the following microorganisms have been shown to be susceptible to amikacin *in vitro*,[1] although the clinical significance of this action has not been demonstrated in animals: *Enterobacter* sp, *Proteus mirabilis, Proteus* sp (indole positive), *Serratia marcescens, Salmonella* sp, *Shigella* sp, *Providencia* sp, *Citrobacter freundii, Listeria monocytogenes, Staphylococcus aureus* (both penicillin-resistant and penicillin-sensitive).

The aminoglycoside antibiotics in general have limited activity against gram-positive pathogens, although *Staphylococcus aureus* and *Listeria monocytogenes* are susceptible to amikacin as noted above.

Amikacin has been shown to be effective against many aminoglycoside-resistant strains due to its ability to resist degradation by aminoglycoside inactivating enzymes known to affect gentamicin, tobramycin and kanamycin.[2]

Clinical Pharmacology:

Endometrial Tissue Concentrations: Comparisons of amikacin activity in endometrial biopsy tissue following intrauterine infusion with that following intramuscular injection of AMIGLYDE-V® in mares demonstrate superior endometrial tissue concentrations when the drug is administered by the intrauterine route.

Intrauterine infusion of 2 grams AMIGLYDE-V® daily for three consecutive days in mares results in peak concentrations typically exceeding 40 mcg/g of endometrial biopsy tissue within one hour after infusion. Twenty-four hours after each treatment amikacin activity is still detectable at concentrations averaging 2 to 4 mcg/g. However, the drug is not appreciably absorbed systemically following intrauterine infusion. Endometrial tissue concentrations following intramuscular injection are roughly parallel, but are typically somewhat lower than corresponding serum concentrations of amikacin.

Dosage and Administration: For treatment of uterine infections in mares, 2 grams (8 mL) of AMIGLYDE-V®, mixed with 200 mL 0.9% Sodium chloride injection, USP and aseptically infused into the uterus daily for three consecutive days, has been found to be the most efficacious dosage.

Contraindication(s): There are no known contraindications for the use of AMIGLYDE-V® in horses other than a history of hypersensitivity to amikacin.

Precaution(s): AMIGLYDE-V® (amikacin sulfate injection, USP) Veterinary Solution is supplied as a colorless solution which is stable at room temperature. At times the solution may become pale yellow in color. This does not indicate a decrease in potency.

Store at controlled room temperature 15° to 30°C (59° to 86°F).

Caution(s): Federal law restricts this drug to use by or on the order of a licensed veterinarian.

Although AMIGLYDE-V® is not absorbed to an appreciable extent following intrauterine infusion, concurrent use of other aminoglycosides should be avoided because of the potential additive effects.

In vitro studies have demonstrated that when sperm are exposed to the preservative which is present in the 48 mL vials (250 mg/mL) sperm viability is impaired.

Warning(s): Not to be used in horses intended for food.

Toxicology: Safety: AMIGLYDE-V® is non-irritating to equine endometrial tissue when infused into the uterus as directed (see Dosage and Administration). In laboratory animals as well as the equine studies, the drug was generally found not to be irritating when injected intravenously, subcutaneously or intramuscularly.

Although amikacin, like other aminoglycosides, is potentially nephrotoxic, ototoxic and neurotoxic, parenteral (intravenous) administration of AMIGLYDE-V® (amikacin sulfate injection, USP) twice daily at dosages of up to 10 mg/lb for 15 consecutive days in horses resulted in no clinical, laboratory nor histopathologic evidence of toxicity.

Intrauterine infusion of 2 grams of AMIGLYDE-V® 8 hours prior to breeding by natural service did not impair fertility in mares. Therefore, mares should not be bred for at least 8 hours following uterine infusion.

Adverse Reactions: No adverse reactions or other side effects have been reported.

References: Available upon request.

Presentation: 48 mL vial, 250 mg/mL (NDC 0856-2332-20).

Compendium Code No.: 10030071 4120G

AMIJECT D ℞

Vetus **Amikacin Injection**

(Amikacin Sulfate Injection)

ANADA No.: 200-178

Active Ingredient(s): Each mL contains:

Amikacin sulfate . . . . 50 mg

The dosage form supplied is a sterile, colorless to straw colored solution containing, in addition to amikacin sulfate, 2.5% sodium citrate, pH adjusted with sulfuric acid, 0.66% sodium bisulfite added, and 0.1 mg benzethonium chloride per mL as a preservative.

Indications: AMIJECT D (Amikacin Sulfate Injection) is indicated for the treatment of the following conditions in dogs:

Genitourinary tract infections (cystitis) caused by susceptible strains of *Escherichia coli* and *Proteus* sp.

Skin and soft tissue infections caused by susceptible strains of *Pseudomonas* sp and *Escherichia coli.*

While nearly all strains of *Escherichia coli, Pseudomonas* sp and *Proteus* sp, including those that are resistant to gentamicin, kanamycin or other aminoglycosides, are susceptible to amikacin at levels achieved following treatment, it is recommended that the invading organism be cultured and its susceptibility demonstrated as a guide to therapy. Amikacin susceptibility discs, 30 mcg, should be used for determining *in vitro* susceptibility.

Pharmacology: Description: Amikacin sulfate is a semi-synthetic aminoglycoside antibiotic derived from kanamycin. It is $C_{22}H_{43}N_5O_{13}{\bullet}2H_2SO_4$, D-streptamine, 0-3-amino-3-deoxy-α-D-glucopyranosyl - (1-6)-0-[6-amino-6-deoxy-α-D-glucopyranosyl-(1-4)]-N1-(4-amino-2-hydroxy-1-oxobutyl)-2-deoxy-, (S)-, sulfate (1:2)(salt).

Action: Amikacin, like other aminoglycoside antibiotics, is a bactericidal agent that exerts its action at the level of the bacterial ribosome. Amikacin has been shown to be effective against many aminoglycoside-resistant strains due to its ability to resist degradation by aminoglycoside inactivating enzymes known to affect gentamicin, tobramycin and kanamycin.[1]

Microbiology: Amikacin has been shown to be effective in the treatment of skin and soft tissue infections caused by *Pseudomonas* sp and *Escherichia coli* and in urinary tract infections caused by *Escherichia coli* and *Proteus* sp. The susceptibility of veterinary isolates to amikacin is summarized in the following table:

Organism (No. of Isolates)	Minimum Inhibitory Concentration (mcg/mL)	
	Range	MIC_{90}*
Escherichia coli (50)	1-32	4
Proteus mirabilis (50)	1-128	6
Enterobacter sp (50)	0.5-128	4
Staphylococcus aureus (50)	1-128	2
Klebsiella pneumoniae (50)	0.5-16	2
Pseudomonas aeruginosa (50)	1-64	8

*Concentration at which 90% of the isolates are susceptible

In addition, the following microorganisms have been shown to be susceptible to amikacin *in vitro*,[2] although the clinical significance of this action has not been demonstrated in animals: *Serratia marcescens, Salmonella* sp, *Shigella* sp, *Providencia* sp, *Citrobacter freundii, Listeria monocytogenes.*

The aminoglycoside antibiotics in general have limited activity against gram-positive pathogens, although *Staphylococcus aureus* and *Listeria monocytogenes* are susceptible to amikacin as noted above.

Pharmacokinetics: Amikacin is well absorbed following intravenous, subcutaneous, or intramuscular injection but is not appreciably absorbed orally. The serum half-life (T1/2) averages from 1 to 2 hours in dogs depending on the route of administration.[3] Amikacin is excreted unchanged in urine, concentrations in excess of 1,000 mcg/mL typically being achieved within three hours in dogs. Serum concentration-time profiles in dogs following subcutaneous administration are illustrated graphically in Figure 1.

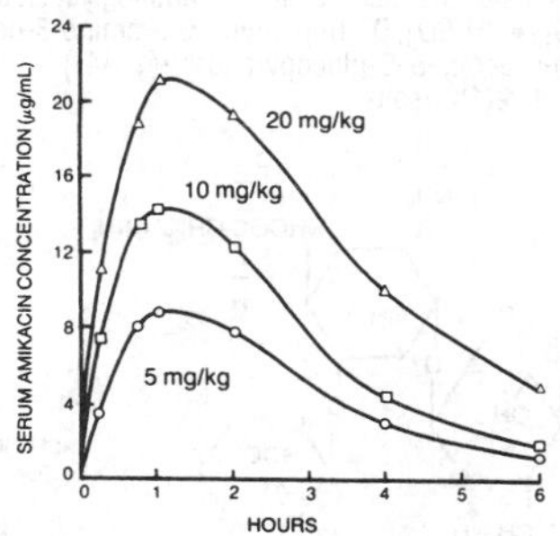

Figure 1: Amikacin Concentration-Time Curves in Dogs (n=6) Following Subcutaneous Injection

Dosage and Administration: AMIJECT D (Amikacin Sulfate Injection) should be administered subcutaneously or intramuscularly at a dosage of 10 mg/kg (5 mg/lb) twice daily. Dogs with skin and soft tissue infections should be treated for a minimum of 7 days and those with genitourinary infections should be treated for 7 to 21 days or until culture negative and asymptomatic. If no response is observed after three days of treatment, therapy should be discontinued and the case re-evaluated. Maximum duration of therapy should not exceed 30 days.

Contraindication(s): Systemic aminoglycoside therapy is contraindicated in dogs with seriously impaired renal function.

Precaution(s): Store vials at controlled room temperature (15°-30°C, 59°-86°F). At times the solution may become pale yellow in color. This does not indicate a decrease in potency.

Caution(s): Federal law restricts this drug to use by or on the order of a licensed veterinarian.

For use in dogs only.

The following conditions have been found to contribute to the toxicity of aminoglycosides in dogs:

-Prior renal damage (most commonly found in dogs of advanced age) and dogs infected with heartworm microfilaria.[5]

-Hypovolemic dehydration (dehydrated patients should be rehydrated prior to initiating therapy).

In dogs where decreased renal function is suspected prior to treatment, BUN or serum creatinine levels may not indicate the degree of kidney impairment. A creatinine clearance determination may be more useful.

Monitoring of renal function during treatment is recommended. Although there is not a completely reliable monitoring program for aminoglycoside toxicity, urinalysis may indicate early nephrotoxicity. Unfavorable changes in the urinalysis which may indicate toxicity include:

-Decreased specific gravity in the absence of fluid therapy.

-Appearance in the urine of casts, albumin, glucose or blood.

Continued use of aminoglycosides where any functional renal impairment has occurred may lead to enhanced renal damage as well as increased likelihood of ototoxicity and/or neuromuscular blockade.[6]

Concurrent or sequential use of topically or systemically administered nephrotoxic, ototoxic, or neuromuscular blocking drugs, particularly other aminoglycosides such as streptomycin, gentamicin, kanamycin and neomycin should be avoided because of the potential for additive effects.

Concurrent administration of furosemide with aminoglycosides may enhance nephrotoxicity.[7]

Not for use in breeding dogs as reproductive studies have not been conducted.

Neurotoxic and nephrotoxic antibiotics may be absorbed in significant quantities from body surfaces after local irrigation or application. The potential toxic effect of antibiotics administered in this fashion should be considered.[8]

If hypersensitivity develops, treatment with AMIJECT D (Amikacin Sulfate Injection) should be discontinued and appropriate therapy instituted.

Amikacin should be used with extreme caution in dogs, in which hearing acuity is required for functioning, such as seeing eye, hearing ear or military patrol, as the auditory and vestibular impairment tends not to be reversible.[6]

Aminoglycosides, including amikacin, are not indicated in uncomplicated episodes of cystitis unless causative agents are susceptible to them and are not susceptible to antibiotics having less potential for toxicity.

Early signs of ototoxicity can include ataxia, nausea and vomiting. Auditory and vestibular impairment may be reversible in the very early stages, but if treatment is continued, the conditions will become irreversible.[6]

Toxicology: The intravenous and intramuscular LD_{50} in dogs is greater than 250 mg/kg. Like other aminoglycosides, amikacin has nephrotoxic, neurotoxic, and ototoxic potential. In dogs, minimal to mild renal changes were detectable histopathologically after amikacin dosage of 45 mg/kg/day for two weeks, and dogs receiving a dosage of 30 mg/kg/day for 90 days had minimal renal alterations which were believed to be entirely reversible. Urinary casts were not observed in dogs receiving a 30 mg/kg dose for 90 days. In efficacy studies involving 80 infected dogs treated with amikacin at the recommended dosage rate of 10 mg/kg b.i.d. for 8-21 consecutive days, no evidence of nephrotoxicity or any other toxicity was encountered. Regarding ototoxicity, studies in cats reveal that amikacin has less potential for ototoxicity than gentamicin.[4]

Adverse Reactions: In clinical studies in dogs, transient pain on injection has been reported as well as rare cases of vomiting or diarrhea following amikacin therapy. In 90 day intramuscular toxicology studies, evidence of muscle damage was detected histologically as well as by elevated creatinine phosphokinase.

References: Available upon request.

Presentation: 50 mL vial.

Compendium Code No.: 14440040

AMIKACIN C INJECTION ℞

Phoenix Pharmaceutical **Amikacin Injection**

(Amikacin Sulfate Injection) Sterile-50 mg/mL

ANADA No.: 200-178

Active Ingredient(s): Each mL of solution contains:

Amikacin (as the sulfate) .... 50 mg
Sodium citrate, USP (as buffer) .... 25.1 mg
Sodium bisulfite .... 6.6 mg
Benzethonium chloride, USP (as preservative) .... 0.1 mg
Water for injection, USP .... q.s.

pH adjusted with sulfuric acid.

The dosage form supplied is a sterile, colorless to straw colored solution containing, in addition to amikacin sulfate, 2.5% sodium citrate, pH adjusted with sulfuric acid, 0.66% sodium bisulfite added, and 0.1 mg benzethonium chloride per mL as a preservative.

Indications: AMIKACIN C INJECTION (Amikacin Sulfate Injection) is indicated for the treatment of the following conditions in dogs:

Genitourinary tract infections (cystitis) caused by susceptible strains of *Escherichia coli* and *Proteus* sp.

Skin and soft tissue infections caused by susceptible strains of *Pseudomonas* sp and *Escherichia coli.*

While nearly all strains of *Escherichia coli, Pseudomonas* sp, and *Proteus* sp, including those that are resistant to gentamicin, kanamycin or other aminoglycosides, are susceptible to amikacin at levels achieved following treatment, it is recommended that the invading organism be cultured and its susceptibility demonstrated as a guide to therapy. Amikacin susceptibility discs, 30 mcg, should be used for determining *in vitro* susceptibility.

Pharmacology: Description: Amikacin sulfate is a semi-synthetic aminoglycoside antibiotic derived from kanamycin. It is $C_{22}H_{43}N_5O_{13}\bullet 2H_2SO_4$,D-streptamine, 0-3-amino-3-deoxy-α-D-glucopyranosyl - (1→6) - 0 - [6-amino-6-deoxy-α-D-glucopyranosyl - (1→4)]-N[1]-(4-amino-2-hydroxy-1-oxobutyl)-2-deoxy-,(S)-,sulfate(1:2)(salt).

$\bullet 2H_2SO_4$

Action: Amikacin, like other aminoglycoside antibiotics, is a bactericidal agent that exerts its action at the level of the bacterial ribosome. Amikacin has been shown to be effective against many aminoglycoside-resistant strains due to its ability to resist degradation by aminoglycoside inactivating enzymes known to affect gentamicin, tobramycin and kanamycin.[1]

Microbiology: Amikacin has been shown to be effective in the treatment of skin and soft tissue infections caused by *Pseudomonas* sp and *Escherichia coli* and in urinary tract infections caused by *Escherichia coli* and *Proteus* sp. The susceptibility of veterinary isolates to amikacin is summarized in the following table:

Organism (No. of Isolates)	Minimum Inhibitory Concentration (mcg/mL)	
	Range	MIC_{90}*
Escherichia coli (50)	1-32	4
Proteus mirabilis (50)	1-128	6
Enterobacter sp (50)	0.5-128	4
Staphylococcus aureus (50)	1-128	2
Klebsiella pneumoniae (50)	0.5-16	2
Pseudomonas aeruginosa (50)	1-64	8

*Concentration at which 90% of the isolates are susceptible

In addition, the following microorganisms have been shown to be susceptible to amikacin *in vitro*,[2] although the clinical significance of this action has not been demonstrated in animals: *Serratia marcescens, Salmonella* sp, *Shigella* sp, *Providencia* sp, *Citrobacter freundii, Listeria monocytogenes.*

The aminoglycoside antibiotics in general have limited activity against gram-positive pathogens, although *Staphylococcus aureus* and *Listeria monocytogenes* are susceptible to amikacin as noted above.

Pharmacokinetics: Amikacin is well absorbed following intravenous, subcutaneous, or intramuscular injection but is not appreciably absorbed orally. The serum half-life ($T\frac{1}{2}$) averages from 1 to 2 hours in dogs depending on the route of administration.[3] Amikacin is excreted unchanged in urine, concentrations in excess of 1,000 mcg/mL typically being achieved within three hours in dogs. Serum concentration-time profiles in dogs following subcutaneous administration are illustrated graphically in Figure 1.

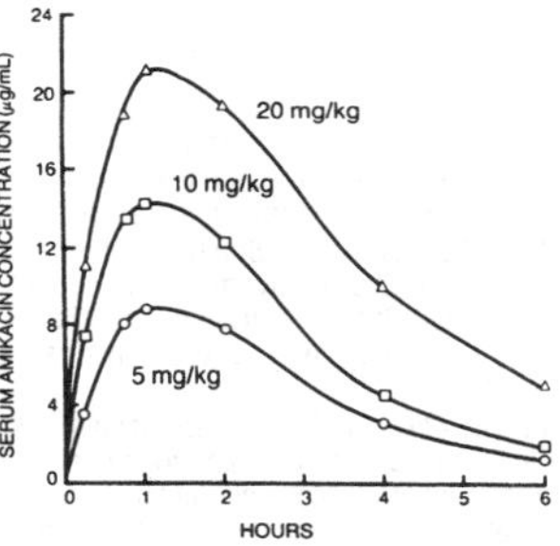

Figure 1: Amikacin Concentration-Time Curves in Dogs (n=6) Following Subcutaneous Injection

Dosage and Administration: AMIKACIN C INJECTION (Amikacin Sulfate Injection) should be administered subcutaneously or intramuscularly at a dosage of 10 mg/kg (5 mg/lb) twice daily. Dogs with skin and soft tissue infections should be treated for a minimum of 7 days and those with genitourinary infections should be treated for 7 to 21 days or until culture negative and asymptomatic. If no response is observed after three days of treatment, therapy should be discontinued and the case re-evaluated. Maximum duration of therapy should not exceed 30 days.

Contraindication(s): Systemic aminoglycoside therapy is contraindicated in dogs with seriously impaired renal function.

Precaution(s): Store vials at controlled room temperature (15°-30°C, 59°-86°F). At times the solution may become pale yellow in color. This does not indicate a decrease in potency.

Caution(s): Federal law restricts this drug to use by or on the order of a licensed veterinarian.

Amikacin should be used with extreme caution in dogs, in which hearing acuity is required for functioning, such as seeing eye, hearing ear or military patrol, as the auditory and vestibular impairment tends not to be reversible.[6]

Aminoglycosides, including amikacin, are not indicated in uncomplicated episodes of cystitis unless the causative agents are susceptible to them and are not susceptible to antibiotics having less potential for toxicity.

Early signs of ototoxicity can include ataxia, nausea and vomiting. Auditory and vestibular impairment may be reversible in the very early stages, but if treatment is continued, the conditions will become irreversible.[6]

The following conditions have been found to contribute to the toxicity of aminoglycosides in dogs:

-Prior renal damage (most commonly found in dogs of advanced age) and dogs infected with heartworm microfilaria.[5]

-Hypovolemic dehydration (dehydrated patients should be rehydrated prior to initiating therapy).

In dogs where decreased renal function is suspected prior to treatment, BUN or serum creatinine levels may not indicate the degree of kidney impairment. A creatinine clearance determination may be more useful.

Monitoring of renal function during treatment is recommended. Although there is not a completely reliable monitoring program for aminoglycoside toxicity, urinalysis may indicate early nephrotoxicity. Unfavorable changes in the urinalysis which may indicate toxicity include:

-Decreased specific gravity in the absence of fluid therapy.

-Appearance in the urine of casts, albumin, glucose or blood.

Continued use of aminoglycosides where any functional renal impairment has occurred may lead to enhanced renal damage as well as increased likelihood of ototoxicity and/or neuromuscular blockade.[6]

Concurrent or sequential use of topically or systemically administered nephrotoxic, ototoxic, or neuromuscular blocking drugs, particularly other aminoglycosides such as streptomycin, gentamicin, kanamycin and neomycin should be avoided because of the potential for additive effects.

Concurrent administration of furosemide with aminoglycosides may enhance nephrotoxicity.[7]

Not for use in breeding dogs as reproductive studies have not been conducted.

Neurotoxic and nephrotoxic antibiotics may be absorbed in significant quantities from body surfaces after local irrigation or application. The potential toxic effect of antibiotics administered in this fashion should be considered.[8]

If hypersensitivity develops, treatment with AMIKACIN C INJECTION (Amikacin Sulfate Injection) should be discontinued and appropriate therapy instituted.

For subcutaneous or intramuscular use in the dog only.

Warning(s): Not for human use. Keep out of reach of children.

Toxicology: The intravenous and intramuscular LD_{50} in dogs is greater than 250 mg/kg. Like other aminoglycosides, amikacin has nephrotoxic, neurotoxic, and ototoxic potential. In dogs, minimal to mild renal changes were detectable histopathologically after amikacin dosage of 45 mg/kg/day for two weeks, and dogs receiving a dosage of 30 mg/kg/day for 90 days had minimal renal alterations which were believed to be entirely reversible. Urinary casts were not observed in dogs receiving a 30 mg/kg dose for 90 days. In efficacy studies involving 80 infected dogs treated with amikacin at the recommended dosage rate of 10 mg/kg b.i.d. for 8-21 consecutive days, no evidence of nephrotoxicity or any other toxicity was encountered. Regarding ototoxicity, studies in cats reveal that amikacin has less potential for ototoxicity than gentamicin.[4]

Adverse Reactions: In clinical studies in dogs, transient pain on injection has been reported as well as rare cases of vomiting or diarrhea following amikacin therapy. In 90 day intramuscular toxicology studies, evidence of muscle damage was detected histologically as well as by elevated creatinine phosphokinase.

References: Available upon request.

Presentation: 50 mL vials (NDC 57319-372-04).

Manufactured by: Phoenix Scientific, Inc., St. Joseph, MO 64503.

Compendium Code No.: 12560032 Rev. 8-01/Rev. 2/01

AMIKACIN E SOLUTION ℞

Phoenix Pharmaceutical **Intrauterine Antibiotic**

(Amikacin Sulfate Solution) Sterile-250 mg/mL

ANADA No.: 200-181

Active Ingredient(s): Each mL contains:

Amikacin (as the sulfate)	250 mg
Sodium citrate (as buffer)	25.1 mg
Sodium bisulfite	6.6 mg
Benzethonium chloride (as preservative)	0.1 mg
Water for injection	q.s.

pH adjusted with sulfuric acid

The dosage form supplied is a sterile, colorless to straw colored solution containing, in addition to amikacin sulfate, 2.5% sodium citrate, pH adjusted with sulfuric acid, 0.66% sodium bisulfite added, and 0.1 mg benzethonium chloride per mL as a preservative.

Indications: AMIKACIN E SOLUTION (Amikacin Sulfate Solution) is indicated for the treatment of uterine infections (endometritis, metritis and pyometra) in mares, when caused by susceptible organisms including *Escherichia coli, Pseudomonas* sp, and *Klebsiella* sp. The use of amikacin sulfate in eliminating infections caused by the above organisms has been shown clinically to improve fertility in infected mares.

While nearly all strains of *Escherichia coli, Pseudomonas* sp and *Klebsiella* sp, including those that are resistant to gentamicin, kanamycin or other aminoglycosides, are susceptible to amikacin at levels achieved following treatment, it is recommended that the invading organism be cultured and its susceptibility demonstrated as a guide to therapy. Amikacin susceptibility discs, 30 mcg, should be used for determining *in vitro* susceptibility.

Pharmacology: Description: Amikacin sulfate is a semisynthetic aminoglycoside antibiotic derived from kanamycin. It is $C_{22}H_{43}N_5O_{13}\bullet 2H_2SO_4$,D-streptamine, 0-3-amino-3-deoxy-α-D-glucopyranosyl - (1→6) - 0 - [6-amino-6-deoxy-α-D-glucopyranosyl - (1→4)-N[1]-(4-amino-2-hydroxy-1-oxobutyl)-2-deoxy-,(S)-,sulfate (1:2) (salt).

NH₂ OH NHCOC-CH₂CH₂NH₂ H OH OH HO O OH O O OH HOCH₂ OH ·2H₂SO₄ CH₂NH₂ NH₂

Action:

Antibacterial Activity: The effectiveness of AMIKACIN E SOLUTION (Amikacin Sulfate Solution) in infections caused by *Escherichia coli, Pseudomonas* sp, and *Klebsiella* sp has been demonstrated clinically in the horse. In addition, the following microorganisms have been shown to be susceptible to amikacin *in vitro*,[1] although the clinical significance of this action has not been demonstrated in animals: *Enterobacter* sp, *Proteus mirabilis, Proteus* sp (indole positive), *Serratia marcescens, Salmonella* sp, *Shigella* sp, *Providencia* sp, *Citrobacter freundii, Listeria monocytogenes, Staphylococcus aureus* (both penicillin resistant and penicillin sensitive).

The aminoglycoside antibiotics in general have limited activity against gram-positive pathogens, although *Staphylococcus aureus* and *Listeria monocytogenes* are susceptible to amikacin as noted above.

Amikacin has been shown to be effective against many aminoglycoside-resistant strains due to its ability to resist degradation by aminoglycoside inactivating enzymes known to affect gentamicin, tobramycin and kanamycin.[2]

Clinical Pharmacology:

Endometrial Tissue Concentrations: Comparisons of amikacin activity in endometrial biopsy tissue following intrauterine infusion with that following intramuscular injection of amikacin sulfate in mares demonstrate superior endometrial tissue concentrations when the drug is administered by the intrauterine route.

Intrauterine infusion of 2 grams AMIKACIN E SOLUTION (Amikacin Sulfate Solution) daily for three consecutive days in mares results in peak concentrations typically exceeding 40 mcg/g of endometrial biopsy tissue within one hour after infusion. Twenty-four hours after each treatment amikacin activity is still detectable at concentrations averaging 2 to 4 mcg/g. However, the drug is not appreciably absorbed systemically following intrauterine infusion. Endometrial tissue concentrations following intramuscular injection roughly parallel, but are typically somewhat lower than corresponding serum concentrations of amikacin.

Dosage and Administration: For treatment of uterine infections in mares, 2 grams (8 mL) of AMIKACIN E SOLUTION (Amikacin Sulfate Solution), mixed with 200 mL 0.9% Sodium Chloride Injection, USP and aseptically infused into the uterus daily for three consecutive days, has been found to be the most efficacious dosage.

Contraindication(s): There are no known contraindications for the use of amikacin sulfate in horses other than a history of hypersensitivity to amikacin.

Precaution(s): AMIKACIN E SOLUTION (Amikacin Sulfate Solution) is supplied as a colorless solution which is stable at room temperature. At times the solution may become pale yellow in color. This does not indicate a decrease in potency.

Store between 15°-30°C (59°-86°F).

Caution(s): Federal law restricts this drug to use by or on the order of a licensed veterinarian.

Although amikacin sulfate is not absorbed to an appreciable extent following intrauterine infusion, concurrent use of other aminoglycosides should be avoided because of the potential additive effects.

For intrauterine use in the horse only.

Warning(s): Not to be used in horses intended for food. *In vitro* studies have demonstrated that when sperm are exposed to the preservative which is present in the 48 mL vials (250 mg/mL) sperm viability is impaired.

Not for human use. Keep out of reach of children.

Adverse Reactions: No adverse reactions or other side effects have been reported.

Trial Data: Safety: AMIKACIN E SOLUTION (Amikacin Sulfate Solution) is non-irritating to equine endometrial tissue when infused into the uterus as directed (see "Dosage and Administration"). In laboratory animals as well as equine studies, the drug was generally found not to be irritating when injected intravenously, subcutaneously or intramuscularly.

Although amikacin, like other aminoglycosides, is potentially nephrotoxic, ototoxic and neurotoxic, parenteral (intravenous) administration of amikacin sulfate twice daily at dosages of up to 10 mg/lb for 15 consecutive days in horses resulted in no clinical, laboratory or histopathologic evidence of toxicity.

Intrauterine infusion of 2 grams of AMIKACIN E SOLUTION (Amikacin Sulfate Solution) 8 hours prior to breeding by natural service did not impair fertility in mares. Therefore, mares should not be bred for at least 8 hours following uterine infusion.

References: Available upon request.

Presentation: 48 mL/12 g vial (NDC 57319-373-04).

Manufactured by: Phoenix Scientific, Inc., St. Joseph, MO 64503.

Compendium Code No.: 12560042 Rev. 8/01

AMIKACIN SULFATE INJECTION ℞

Butler **Amikacin Injection**

ANADA No.: 200-178

Active Ingredient(s): Each mL of solution contains:

Amikacin (as the sulfate)	50 mg
Sodium citrate, USP (as buffer)	25.1 mg
Sodium bisulfite	6.6 mg
Benzethonium chloride, USP (as preservative)	0.1 mg
Water for injection, USP	q.s.

pH adjusted with sulfuric acid.

The dosage form supplied is a sterile, colorless to straw colored solution containing, in addition to amikacin sulfate, 2.5% sodium citrate, pH adjusted with sulfuric acid, 0.66% sodium bisulfite added, and 0.1 mg benzethonium chloride per mL as a preservative.

Indications: AMIKACIN SULFATE INJECTION is indicated for the treatment of the following conditions in dogs:

Genitourinary tract infections (cystitis) caused by susceptible strains of *Escherichia coli* and *Proteus* sp.

Skin and soft tissue infections caused by susceptible strains of *Pseudomonas* sp. and *Escherichia coli*.

While nearly all strains of *Escherichia coli, Pseudomonas* sp., and *Proteus* sp., including those that are resistant to gentamicin, kanamycin or other aminoglycosides, are susceptible to amikacin at levels achieved following treatment, it is recommended that the invading organism be cultured and its susceptibility demonstrated as a guide to therapy. Amikacin susceptibility discs, 30 mcg, should be used for determining *in vitro* susceptibility.

Pharmacology: Description: Amikacin sulfate is a semi-synthetic aminoglycoside antibiotic derived from kanamycin. It is $C_{22}H_{43}N_5O_{13}\bullet 2H_2SO_4$,D-streptamine, 0-3-amino-3-deoxy-α-D-glucopyranosyl - (1→6) - 0 - [6-amino-6-deoxy-α-D-glucopyranosyl - (1→4)]-N[1]-(4-amino-2-hydroxy-1-oxobutyl)-2-deoxy-,(S)-,sulfate(1:2)(salt).

NH₂ OH NHCOC-CH₂CH₂NH₂ H OH OH HO O OH O O OH HOCH₂ OH ·2H₂SO₄ CH₂NH₂ NH₂

Action: Amikacin, like other aminoglycoside antibiotics, is a bactericidal agent that exerts its action at the level of the bacterial ribosome. Amikacin has been shown to be effective against many aminoglycoside-resistant strains due to its ability to resist degradation by aminoglycoside inactivating enzymes known to affect gentamicin, tobramycin and kanamycin.[1]

Microbiology: Amikacin has been shown to be effective in the treatment of skin and soft tissue infections caused by *Pseudomonas* sp. and *Escherichia coli* and in urinary tract infections caused by *Escherichia coli* and *Proteus* sp. The susceptibility of veterinary isolates to amikacin is summarized in the following table:

Organism (No. of Isolates)	Minimum Inhibitory Concentration (mcg/mL)	
	Range	MIC_{90}*
Escherichia coli (50)	1-32	4
Proteus mirabilis (50)	1-128	6
Enterobacter sp. (50)	0.5-128	4
Staphylococcus aureus (50)	1-128	2
Klebsiella pneumoniae (50)	0.5-16	2
Pseudomonas aeruginosa (50)	1-64	8
*Concentration at which 90% of the isolates are susceptible		

In addition, the following microorganisms have been shown to be susceptible to amikacin *in vitro*,[2] although the clinical significance of this action has not been demonstrated in animals: *Serratia marcescens, Salmonella* sp., *Shigella* sp., *Providencia* sp., *Citrobacter freundii, Listeria monocytogenes.*

The aminoglycoside antibiotics in general have limited activity against gram-positive pathogens, although *Staphylococcus aureus* and *Listeria monocytogenes* are susceptible to amikacin as noted above.

Pharmacokinetics: Amikacin is well absorbed following intravenous, subcutaneous, or intramuscular injection but is not appreciably absorbed orally. The serum half-life (T½) averages from 1 to 2 hours in dogs depending on the route of administration.[3] Amikacin is excreted unchanged in urine, concentrations in excess of 1,000 mcg/mL typically being achieved within three hours in dogs. Serum concentration-time profiles in dogs following subcutaneous administration are illustrated graphically in Figure 1.

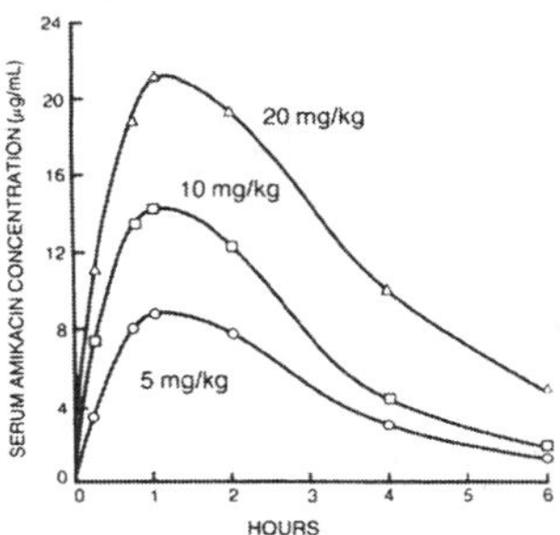

Figure 1: Amikacin Concentration-Time Curves in Dogs (n=6) Following Subcutaneous Injection

Dosage and Administration: AMIKACIN SULFATE INJECTION should be administered subcutaneously or intramuscularly at a dosage of 10 mg/kg (5 mg/lb) twice daily. Dogs with skin and soft tissue infections should be treated for a minimum of 7 days and those with genitourinary infections should be treated for 7 to 21 days or until culture negative and asymptomatic. If no response is observed after three days of treatment, therapy should be discontinued and the case re-evaluated. Maximum duration of therapy should not exceed 30 days.

Contraindication(s): Systemic aminoglycoside therapy is contraindicated in dogs with seriously impaired renal function.

Precaution(s): Store vials at controlled room temperature (15°-30°C, 59°-86°F). At times the solution may become pale yellow in color. This does not indicate a decrease in potency.

Caution(s): Federal law restricts this drug to use by or on the order of a licensed veterinarian.

Amikacin should be used with extreme caution in dogs, in which hearing acuity is required for functioning, such as seeing eye, hearing ear or military patrol, as the auditory and vestibular impairment tends not to be reversible.[6]

Aminoglycosides, including amikacin, are not indicated in uncomplicated episodes of cystitis unless the causative agents are susceptible to them and are not susceptible to antibiotics having less potential for toxicity.

Early signs of ototoxicity can include ataxia, nausea and vomiting. Auditory and vestibular impairment may be reversible in the very early stages, but if treatment is continued, the conditions will become irreversible.[6]

The following conditions have been found to contribute to the toxicity of aminoglycosides in dogs:

-Prior renal damage (most commonly found in dogs of advanced age) and dogs infected with heartworm microfilaria.[5]

-Hypovolemic dehydration (dehydrated patients should be rehydrated prior to initiating therapy).

In dogs where decreased renal function is suspected prior to treatment, BUN or serum creatinine levels may not indicate the degree of kidney impairment. A creatinine clearance determination may be more useful.

Monitoring of renal function during treatment is recommended. Although there is not a completely reliable monitoring program for aminoglycoside toxicity, urinalysis may indicate early nephrotoxicity. Unfavorable changes in the urinalysis which may indicate toxicity include:

-Decreased specific gravity in the absence of fluid therapy.

-Appearance in the urine of casts, albumin, glucose or blood.

Continued use of aminoglycosides where any functional renal impairment has occurred may lead to enhanced renal damage as well as increased likelihood of ototoxicity and/or neuromuscular blockade.[6]

Concurrent or sequential use of topically or systemically administered nephrotoxic, ototoxic, or neuromuscular blocking drugs, particularly other aminoglycosides such as streptomycin, gentamicin, kanamycin and neomycin should be avoided because of the potential for additive effects.

Concurrent administration of furosemide with aminoglycosides may enhance nephrotoxicity.[7]

Not for use in breeding dogs as reproductive studies have not been conducted.

Neurotoxic and nephrotoxic antibiotics may be absorbed in significant quantities from body surfaces after local irrigation or application. The potential toxic effect of antibiotics administered in this fashion should be considered.[8]

If hypersensitivity develops, treatment with AMIKACIN SULFATE INJECTION should be discontinued and appropriate therapy instituted.

For subcutaneous or intramuscular use in the dog only.

For animal use only.

Not for human use.

Keep out of reach of children.

Toxicology: The intravenous and intramuscular LD_{50} in dogs is greater than 250 mg/kg. Like other aminoglycosides, amikacin has nephrotoxic, neurotoxic, and ototoxic potential. In dogs, minimal to mild renal changes were detectable histopathologically after amikacin dosage of 45 mg/kg/day for two weeks, and dogs receiving a dosage of 30 mg/kg/day for 90 days had minimal renal alterations which were believed to be entirely reversible. Urinary casts were not observed in dogs receiving a 30 mg/kg dose for 90 days. In efficacy studies involving 80 infected dogs treated with amikacin at the recommended dosage rate of 10 mg/kg b.i.d. for 8-21 consecutive days, no evidence of nephrotoxicity or any other toxicity was encountered. Regarding ototoxicity, studies in cats reveal that amikacin has less potential for ototoxicity than gentamicin.[4]

Adverse Reactions: In clinical studies in dogs, transient pain on injection has been reported as well as rare cases of vomiting or diarrhea following amikacin therapy. In 90 day intramuscular toxicology studies, evidence of muscle damage was detected histologically as well as by elevated creatinine phosphokinase.

References: Available upon request.

Presentation: 50 mL vials (NDC 11695-3543-10).

Manufactured by: Phoenix Scientific, Inc., St. Joseph, MO 64506

Compendium Code No.: 10820040 Iss. 6-97

AMIKACIN SULFATE INJECTION ℞

Vet Tek **Amikacin Injection**

50 mg/mL

ANADA No.: 200-178

Active Ingredient(s): Each mL of solution contains:

Amikacin (as the sulfate) .... 50 mg
Sodium citrate, USP (as buffer) .... 25.1 mg
Sodium bisulfite .... 6.6 mg
Benzethonium chloride, USP (as preservative) .... 0.1 mg
Water for injection, USP .... q.s.

pH adjusted with sulfuric acid.

Indications: AMIKACIN SULFATE INJECTION is indicated for the treatment of the following conditions in dogs:

Genitourinary tract infections (cystitis) caused by susceptible strains of *Escherichia coli* and *Proteus* sp.

Skin and soft tissue infections caused by susceptible strains of *Pseudomonas* sp and *Escherichia coli.*

While nearly all strains of *Escherichia coli, Pseudomonas* sp, and *Proteus* sp, including those that are resistant to gentamicin, kanamycin or other aminoglycosides, are susceptible to amikacin at levels achieved following treatment, it is recommended that the invading organism be cultured and its susceptibility demonstrated as a guide to therapy. Amikacin susceptibility discs, 30 mcg, should be used for determining *in vitro* susceptibility.

Pharmacology: Description: Amikacin sulfate is a semi-synthetic aminoglycoside antibiotic derived from kanamycin. It is $C_{22}H_{43}N_5O_{13} \bullet 2H_2SO_4$,D-streptamine, 0-3-amino-3-deoxy-α-D-glucopyranosyl - (1→6)-0-[6-amino-6-deoxy-α-D-glucopyranosyl-(1→4)]-N^1-(4-amino-2-hydroxy-1-oxobutyl)-2-deoxy-,(S)-,sulfate(1:2)(salt).

The dosage form supplied is a sterile, colorless to straw colored solution containing, in addition to amikacin sulfate, 2.5% sodium citrate, pH adjusted with sulfuric acid, 0.66% sodium bisulfite added, and 0.1 mg benzethonium chloride per mL as a preservative.

Action: Amikacin, like other aminoglycoside antibiotics, is a bactericidal agent that exerts its action at the level of the bacterial ribosome. Amikacin has been shown to be effective against many aminoglycoside-resistant strains due to its ability to resist degradation by aminoglycoside inactivating enzymes known to affect gentamicin, tobramycin and kanamycin.[1]

Microbiology: Amikacin has been shown to be effective in the treatment of skin and soft tissue infections caused by *Pseudomonas* sp and *Escherichia coli* and in urinary tract infections caused by *Escherichia coli* and *Proteus* sp. The susceptibility of veterinary isolates to amikacin is summarized in the following table:

Organism (No. of Isolates)	Minimum Inhibitory Concentration (mcg/mL)	
	Range	MIC_{90}*
Escherichia coli (50)	1-32	4
Proteus mirabilis (50)	1-128	6
Enterobacter sp (50)	0.5-128	4
Staphylococcus aureus (50)	1-128	2
Klebsiella pneumoniae (50)	0.5-16	2
Pseudomonas aeruginosa (50)	1-64	8
*Concentration at which 90% of the isolates are susceptible		

In addition, the following microorganisms have been shown to be susceptible to amikacin *in vitro*,[2] although the clinical significance of this action has not been demonstrated in animals: *Serratia marcescens, Salmonella* sp, *Shigella* sp, *Providencia* sp, *Citrobacter freundii, Listeria monocytogenes.*

The aminoglycoside antibiotics in general have limited activity against gram-positive pathogens, although *Staphylococcus aureus* and *Listeria monocytogenes* are susceptible to amikacin as noted above.

Pharmacokinetics: Amikacin is well absorbed following intravenous, subcutaneous, or intramuscular injection but is not appreciably absorbed orally. The serum half-life (T 1/2) averages from 1 to 2 hours in dogs depending on the route of administration.[3] Amikacin is excreted unchanged in urine, concentrations in excess of 1,000 mcg/mL typically being achieved within three hours in dogs. Serum concentration-time profiles in dogs following subcutaneous administration are illustrated graphically in Figure 1.

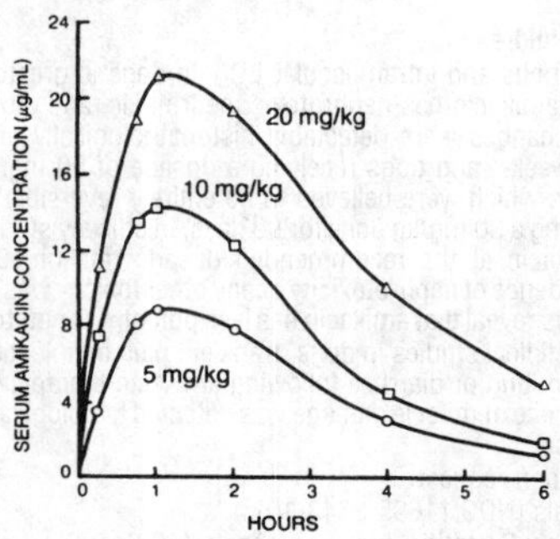

Figure 1: Amikacin Concentration-Time Curves in Dogs (n=6) Following Subcutaneous Injection

Dosage and Administration: AMIKACIN SULFATE INJECTION should be administered subcutaneously or intramuscularly at a dosage of 10 mg/kg (5 mg/lb) twice daily. Dogs with skin and soft tissue infections should be treated for a minimum of 7 days and those with genitourinary infections should be treated for 7 to 21 days or until culture negative and asymptomatic. If no response is observed after three days of treatment, therapy should be discontinued and the case re-evaluated. Maximum duration of therapy should not exceed 30 days.

Contraindication(s): Systemic aminoglycoside therapy is contraindicated in dogs with seriously impaired renal function.

Amikacin should be used with extreme caution in dogs, in which hearing acuity is required for functioning, such as seeing eye, hearing ear or military patrol, as the auditory and vestibular impairment tends not to be reversible.[6]

Aminoglycosides, including amikacin, are not indicated in uncomplicated episodes of cystitis unless the causative agents are susceptible to them and are not susceptible to antibiotics having less potential for toxicity.

Early signs of ototoxicity can include ataxia, nausea and vomiting. Auditory and vestibular impairment may be reversible in the very early stages, but if treatment is continued, the conditions will become irreversible.[6]

Precaution(s): Store vials at controlled room temperature (15°-30°C, 59°-86°F). At times the solution may become pale yellow in color. This does not indicate a decrease in potency.

Caution(s): Federal law restricts this drug to use by or on the order of a licensed veterinarian.

The following conditions have been found to contribute to the toxicity of aminoglycosides in dogs:

-Prior renal damage (most commonly found in dogs of advanced age) and dogs infected with heartworm microfilaria.[5]

-Hypovolemic dehydration (dehydrated patients should be rehydrated prior to initiating therapy).

In dogs where decreased renal function is suspected prior to treatment, BUN or serum creatinine levels may not indicate the degree of kidney impairment. A creatinine clearance determination may be more useful.

Monitoring of renal function during treatment is recommended. Although there is not a completely reliable monitoring program for aminoglycoside toxicity, urinalysis may indicate early nephrotoxicity. Unfavorable changes in the urinalysis which may indicate toxicity include:

-Decreased specific gravity in the absence of fluid therapy.

-Appearance in the urine of casts, albumin, glucose or blood.

Continued use of aminoglycosides where any functional renal impairment has occurred may lead to enhanced renal damage as well as increased likelihood of ototoxicity and/or neuromuscular blockade.[6]

Concurrent or sequential use of topically or systemically administered nephrotoxic, ototoxic, or neuromuscular blocking drugs, particularly other aminoglycosides such as streptomycin, gentamicin, kanamycin and neomycin should be avoided because of the potential for additive effects.

Concurrent administration of furosemide with aminoglycosides may enhance nephrotoxicity.[7]

Not for use in breeding dogs as reproductive studies have not been conducted.

Neurotoxic and nephrotoxic antibiotics may be absorbed in significant quantities from body surfaces after local irrigation or application. The potential toxic effect of antibiotics administered in this fashion should be considered.[8]

If hypersensitivity develops, treatment with AMIKACIN SULFATE INJECTION should be discontinued and appropriate therapy instituted.

Warning(s): For subcutaneous or intramuscular use in the dog only.

Not for human use. Keep out of reach of children.

Toxicology: The intravenous and intramuscular LD_{50} in dogs is greater than 250 mg/kg. Like other aminoglycosides, amikacin has nephrotoxic, neurotoxic, and ototoxic potential. In dogs, minimal to mild renal changes were detectable histopathologically after amikacin dosage of 45 mg/kg/day for two weeks, and dogs receiving a dosage of 30 mg/kg/day for 90 days had minimal renal alterations which were believed to be entirely reversible. Urinary casts were not observed in dogs receiving a 30 mg/kg dose for 90 days. In efficacy studies involving 80 infected dogs treated with amikacin at the recommended dosage rate of 10 mg/kg b.i.d. for 8-21 consecutive days, no evidence of nephrotoxicity or any other toxicity was encountered. Regarding ototoxicity, studies in cats reveal that amikacin has less potential for ototoxicity than gentamicin.[4]

Adverse Reactions: In clinical studies in dogs, transient pain on injection has been reported as well as rare cases of vomiting or diarrhea following amikacin therapy. In 90 day intramuscular toxicology studies, evidence of muscle damage was detected histologically as well as by elevated creatinine phosphokinase.

References: Available upon request.

Presentation: 50 mL vials.

Manufactured by: Phoenix Scientific, Inc.

Compendium Code No.: 14200000

AMIKACIN SULFATE SOLUTION ℞

Vet Tek **Intrauterine Antibiotic**

250 mg/mL

ANADA No.: 200-181

Active Ingredient(s): Each mL contains:

Amikacin (as the sulfate) .... 250 mg
Sodium citrate, USP (as buffer) .... 25.1 mg
Sodium bisulfite .... 6.6 mg
Benzethonium chloride (as preservative) .... 0.1 mg
pH adjusted with sulfuric acid.
Water for injection .... q.s.

Indications: AMIKACIN SULFATE SOLUTION is indicated for the treatment of uterine infections (endometritis, metritis and pyometra) in mares, when caused by susceptible organisms including *Escherichia coli, Pseudomonas* sp, and *Klebsiella* sp. The use of amikacin sulfate in eliminating infections caused by the above organisms has been shown clinically to improve fertility in infected mares.

While nearly all strains of *Escherichia coli, Pseudomonas* sp and *Klebsiella* sp, including those that are resistant to gentamicin, kanamycin or other aminoglycosides, are susceptible to amikacin at levels achieved following treatment, it is recommended that the invading organism be cultured and its susceptibility demonstrated as a guide to therapy. Amikacin susceptibility discs, 30 mcg, should be used for determining *in vitro* susceptibility.

Pharmacology: Description: Amikacin sulfate is a semisynthetic aminoglycoside antibiotic derived from kanamycin. It is $C_{22}H_{43}N_5O_{13} \bullet 2H_2SO_4$,D-streptamine, 0-3-amino-3-deoxy-α-D-glucopyranosyl-(1→6)-0-[6-amino-6-deoxy-α-D-glucopyranosyl-(1→4)-N[1]-(4-amino-2-hydroxy-1-oxobutyl)-2-deoxy-,(S)-,sulfate (1:2) (salt).

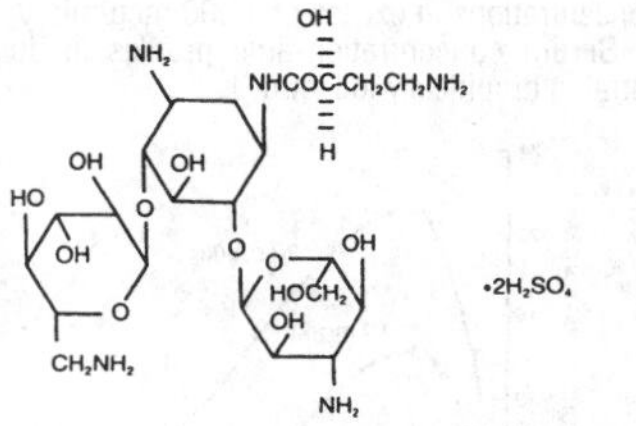

The dosage form supplied is a sterile, colorless to light straw colored solution.

Action:

Antibacterial Activity: The effectiveness of AMIKACIN SULFATE SOLUTION in infections caused by *Escherichia coli, Pseudomonas* sp, and *Klebsiella* sp has been demonstrated clinically in the horse. In addition, the following microorganisms have been shown to be susceptible to amikacin *in vitro*,[1] although the clinical significance of this action has not been demonstrated in animals: *Enterobacter* sp, *Proteus mirabilis, Proteus* sp (indole positive), *Serratia marcescens, Salmonella* sp, *Shigella* sp, *Providencia* sp, *Citrobacter freundii, Listeria monocytogenes, Staphylococcus aureus* (both penicillin resistant and penicillin sensitive).

The aminoglycoside antibiotics in general have limited activity against gram-positive pathogens, although *Staphylococcus aureus* and *Listeria monocytogenes* are susceptible to amikacin as noted above.

Amikacin has been shown to be effective against many aminoglycoside-resistant strains due to its ability to resist degradation by aminoglycoside inactivating enzymes known to affect gentamicin, tobramycin and kanamycin.[2]

Clinical Pharmacology:

Endometrial Tissue Concentrations: Comparisons of amikacin activity in endometrial biopsy tissue following intrauterine infusion with that following intramuscular injection of amikacin sulfate in mares demonstrate superior endometrial tissue concentrations when the drug is administered by the intrauterine route.

Intrauterine infusion of 2 grams AMIKACIN SULFATE SOLUTION daily for three consecutive days in mares results in peak concentrations typically exceeding 40 mcg/g of endometrial biopsy tissue within one hour after infusion. Twenty-four hours after each treatment amikacin activity is still detectable at concentrations averaging 2 to 4 mcg/g. However, the drug is not appreciably absorbed systemically following intrauterine infusion. Endometrial tissue concentrations following intramuscular injection roughly parallel, but are typically somewhat lower than corresponding serum concentrations of amikacin.

Dosage and Administration: For treatment of uterine infections in mares, 2 grams (8 mL) of AMIKACIN SULFATE SOLUTION, mixed with 200 mL 0.9% Sodium Chloride Injection, USP and aseptically infused into the uterus daily for three consecutive days, has been found to be the most efficacious dosage.

Contraindication(s): There are no known contraindications for the use of amikacin sulfate in horses other than a history of hypersensitivity to amikacin.

Precaution(s): AMIKACIN SULFATE SOLUTION is supplied as a colorless solution which is stable at room temperature. At times the solution may become pale yellow in color. This does not indicate a decrease in potency.

Store at controlled room temperature 15°-30°C (59°-86°F).

Caution(s): Federal law restricts this drug to use by or on the order of a licensed veterinarian.

Although amikacin sulfate is not absorbed to an appreciable extent following intrauterine infusion, concurrent use of other aminoglycosides should be avoided because of the potential for additive effects.

In vitro studies have demonstrated that when sperm are exposed to the preservative which is present in the 48 mL vials (250 mg/mL) sperm viability is impaired.

Warning(s): Not to be used in horses intended for food.

For intrauterine use in the horse only.

Not for human use. Keep out of reach of children.

Safety: AMIKACIN SULFATE SOLUTION is non-irritating to equine endometrial tissue when infused into the uterus as directed (see "Dosage and Administration"). In laboratory animals as well as equine studies, the drug was generally found not to be irritating when injected intravenously, subcutaneously or intramuscularly.

Although amikacin, like other aminoglycosides, is potentially nephrotoxic, ototoxic and neurotoxic, parenteral (intravenous) administration of amikacin sulfate twice daily at dosages of up to 10 mg/lb for 15 consecutive days in horses resulted in no clinical, laboratory or histopathologic evidence of toxicity.

Intrauterine infusion of 2 grams of AMIKACIN SULFATE SOLUTION 8 hours prior to breeding by natural service did not impair fertility in mares. Therefore, mares should not be bred for at least 8 hours following uterine infusion.

Adverse Reactions: No adverse reactions or other side effects have been reported.

References: Available upon request.

Presentation: 48 mL vial.

Manufactured by: Phoenix Scientific, Inc.

Compendium Code No.: 14200010

AMINO ACID BOLUS

Vets Plus **Large Animal Dietary Supplement**

Guaranteed Analysis: Per bolus:

Protein	12 g
Brewer's Yeast	2 g
Dextrose	2.5 g
Vitamin A	10,000 IU
Vitamin D_3	1,000 IU
Vitamin E	100 IU
Niacin	100 mg
Thiamin HCl	100 mg
Riboflavin	25 mg
Pyridoxine HCl	25 mg
Vitamin B_{12}	100 mcg
Calcium Pantothenate	100 mg
Biotin	100 mcg
Choline Chloride	50 mg
Sodium	300 mg
Potassium	200 mg
Calcium	1,250 mg
Phosphorus	930 mg
Iodide	50 mcg
Selenium	10 mcg
Magnesium	50 mg
Manganese	5 mg
Iron	10 mg
Cobalt	200 mcg
Copper	3 mg
Zinc	50 mg

Ingredients: Soy protein concentrate, animal plasma, dicalcium phosphate, dextrose, dried brewer's yeast, corn starch, sodium chloride, silicon dioxide, calcium proteinate, magnesium proteinate, potassium chloride, zinc proteinate, dl-alpha-tocopherol, magnesium stearate, nicotinic acid, thiamine HCl, calcium pantothenate, choline chloride, iron proteinate, manganese proteinate, copper proteinate, riboflavin, pyridoxine HCl, vitamin A acetate, vitamin B_{12} supplement, biotin, cobalt proteinate, d-activated animal sterol (vitamin D_3), potassium iodide, selenium yeast.

Indications: AMINO ACID BOLUS is a nutritional supplement providing protein, vitamins, chelated minerals and dextrose for cattle, horses, sheep and swine.

Dosage and Administration: Administer orally 1 to 4 boluses for each 250 pounds of body weight per day, depending on the condition of the animal. Lubricate bolus with mineral oil or petroleum jelly and administer with a balling gun. Boluses may be crushed and top dressed on feed, or given as a drench.

Precaution(s): Keep lid tightly closed. Store in a cool, dry place.

Caution(s): Keep out of reach of children.

For animal use only.

Presentation: 50 boluses, 34 g each.

Compendium Code No.: 10730040

AMINO ACID CONCENTRATE

AgriLabs **Large Animal Dietary Supplement**

Active Ingredient(s):

Amino acids: L-arginine HCl, L-histidine HCl H_2O, L-leucine, L-isoleucine, L-lysine HCl, methionine, L-phenylalanine, L-threonine, L-tryptophane, L-valine and L-cysteine HCl H_2O.

Vitamins: Riboflavin 5' $NaPO_4$, dexpanthenol, thiamine HCl, pyridoxine HCl, vitamin B_{12} and niacinamide.

Electrolytes: Potassium chloride, magnesium sulfate $7H_2O$, sodium glutamate, sodium acetate $3H_2O$, and calcium chloride $2H_2O$.

Indications: An oral source of vitamins, amino acids, and electrolytes for cattle, swine, sheep and horses when dietary intake of these nutrients is reduced.

Dosage and Administration: For use in drinking water. AMINO ACID CONCENTRATE may be used undiluted or diluted with water. Supply fresh drinking water each day.

Cattle: Administer 1 oz. AMINO ACID CONCENTRATE per 100 lbs. of body weight in drinking water to be consumed in one (1) day.

Horses: Administer 10 oz. AMINO ACID CONCENTRATE per 1,000 lbs. of body weight in drinking water to be consumed in one (1) day.

Sheep and Swine: Administer ½ oz. AMINO ACID CONCENTRATE per 50 lbs. of body weight in drinking water to be consumed in one (1) day.

Precaution(s): Protect from freezing.

Caution(s): Keep out of the reach of children.

Presentation: 16 oz. (473 mL) bottles.

Compendium Code No.: 10580080

AMINO ACID CONCENTRATE ORAL SOLUTION

Aspen **Large Animal Dietary Supplement**

Active Ingredient(s): Each 100 mL of aqueous solution contains:

Dextrose • H_2O	5 g
Sodium acetate • $3H_2O$	250 mg
Magnesium sulfate • $7H_2O$	200 mg
Potassium chloride	200 mg
Calcium chloride • $2H_2O$	150 mg
Niacinamide	150 mg
Pyridoxine hydrochloride (B_6)	10 mg
Thiamine hydrochloride (B_1)	10 mg
d-panthenol	5 mg
Riboflavin (B_2)	4 mg
Cyanocobalamin (B_{12})	5 mcg
L-leucine	187 mg
L-lysine hydrochloride	170 mg
L-glutamic acid	136 mg
L-valine	136 mg
L-phenylalanine	119 mg
L-arginine hydrochloride	85 mg
L-isoleucine	85 mg
L-threonine	78.2 mg
L-histidine hydrochloride • H_2O	59.5 mg
L-methionine	51 mg
L-cysteine hydrochloride • H_2O	50 mg
L-tryptophan	34 mg

Preservatives:

Propylene glycol	2.5%
Sorbitol	2.5%
Lactic acid	0.16%
Citric acid	0.1%
BHA	0.005%
Methylparaben	0.18%
Propylparaben	0.02%
Ethylparaben	0.01%

Indications: For use as a supplemental source of concentrated amino acids, electrolytes, B-complex vitamins, and dextrose in cattle.

Dosage and Administration: Cattle: Administer 1 oz AMINO ACID CONCENTRATE per 100 pounds body weight in drinking water to be consumed in one day.

Horses: Administer 10 oz AMINO ACID CONCENTRATE per 1000 pounds body weight in drinking water to be consumed in one day.

Sheep and Swine: Administer ½ oz AMINO ACID CONCENTRATE per 50 pounds body weight in drinking water to be consumed in one day.

Precaution(s): Store at a controlled room temperature, between 59° and 86°F (15°-30°C).

Caution(s): Keep out of the reach of children.

Presentation: 500 mL containers.

Compendium Code No.: 14750030

AMINO ACID CONCENTRATE ORAL SOLUTION

Bimeda **Large Animal Dietary Supplement**

Active Ingredient(s): Each 100 mL contains:

Dextrose • H_2O	5 g
Sodium acetate • $3H_2O$	250 mg
Magnesium sulfate • $7H_2O$	200 mg
Potassium chloride	200 mg
Calcium chloride • $2H_2O$	150 mg
Niacinamide	150 mg
Pyridoxine HCl	10 mg
Thiamine HCl	10 mg
d-Panthenol	5 mg
Riboflavin	4 mg
Cyanocobalamine (B_{12})	5 mcg
L-argenine HCl	85 mg
L-cysteine HCl • H_2O	50 mg
L-glutamic acid	136 mg
L-histidine HCl • H_2O	59.5 mg
L-isoleucine	85 mg
L-leucine	187 mg
L-lysine HCl	170 mg
L-methionine	51 mg
L-phenylalanine	119 mg
L-threonine	78.2 mg
L-valine	136 mg
Methylparaben	0.18%
Ethylparaben	0.01%
Propylparaben	0.02%

Indications: An oral source of B-complex vitamins, amino acids, electrolytes, and dextrose for cattle, swine, sheep and horses when daily intake is reduced.

Dosage and Administration: For cattle, horses, sheep and swine: Administer 1 oz. per 100 lbs. of body weight in the drinking water to be consumed in one (1) day.

Precaution(s): Store at a controlled room temperature between 59°-86°F (15°-30°C).

Protect from light and freezing.

Caution(s): Not for human use. Keep out of the reach of children.

Presentation: 500 mL bottles.

Compendium Code No.: 13990010

AMINO ACID ORAL CONCENTRATE

Phoenix Pharmaceutical **Large Animal Dietary Supplement**

Active Ingredient(s): Composition: Each 100 mL of aqueous solution contains:

Dextrose • H_2O	5 g
Sodium Acetate • $3H_2O$	250 mg
Magnesium Sulfate • $7H_2O$	200 mg
Potassium Chloride	200 mg
Calcium Chloride • $2H_2O$	150 mg
Niacinamide	150 mg
Pyridoxine Hydrochloride (B_6)	10 mg
Thiamine Hydrochloride (B_1)	10 mg
Riboflavin (B_2)	4 mg
Total Protein	1156.7 mg

Comprised of: L-valine, L-glutamic acid, L-leucine, L-lysine hydrochloride, L-phenylalanine, L-arginine hydrochloride, L-isoleucine, L-threonine, L-cysteine hydrochloride • H_2O, L-histidine hydrochloride • H_2O, and L-methionine.

Preservatives:

Methylparaben	0.18%
Propylparaben	0.02%
Ethylparaben	0.01%

Indications: For use as a supplemental nutritive source of concentrated amino acids, electrolytes, B complex vitamins, and dextrose in cattle and horses.
Dosage and Administration: Administer orally as a drench. The usual recommended dose in adult cattle and horses is 50 to 500 mL, depending on size and condition.
Precaution(s): Store between 15° and 30°C (59°-86°F).
Caution(s): For animal use only.
Warning(s): Keep out of reach of children.
Presentation: 500 mL bottles (NDC 57319-082-07).
Compendium Code No.: 12560051 Rev. 2-01

AMINO ACID ORAL SOLUTION

Aspen **Large Animal Dietary Supplement**

Composition: Each 100 mL of aqueous solution contains:

Dextrose • H_2O ... 5 g
Sodium acetate • $3H_2O$ ... 250 mg
Magnesium sulfate • $7H_2O$ ... 20 mg
Potassium chloride ... 20 mg
Calcium chloride • $2H_2O$ ... 15 mg
Niacinamide ... 150 mg
Pyridoxine hydrochloride (B_6) ... 10 mg
Thiamine hydrochloride (B_1) ... 10 mg
d-panthenol ... 5 mg
Riboflavin (B_2) ... 4 mg
Cyanocobalamin (B_{12}) ... 5 mcg
L-valine ... 5 mg
L-glutamic acid ... 4 mg
L-leucine ... 4 mg
L-lysine hydrochloride ... 3 mg
L-phenylalanine ... 3 mg
L-arginine hydrochloride ... 2.5 mg
L-isoleucine ... 2 mg
L-threonine ... 2 mg
L-cysteine hydrochloride • H_2O ... 1 mg
L-histidine hydrochloride • H_2O ... 1 mg
L-methionine ... 1 mg
L-tryptophan ... 1 mg

Preservatives:

Propylene glycol ... 2.5%
Sorbitol ... 2.5%
Lactic acid ... 0.16%
Citric acid ... 0.1%
BHA ... 0.005%
Methylparaben ... 0.18%
Propylparaben ... 0.02%
Ethylparaben ... 0.01%

Indications: For use as a supplemental source of amino acids, electrolytes, B-complex vitamins, and dextrose in cattle and horses.
Dosage and Administration: Administer orally as a drench. The usual recommended dose in adult cattle and horses is 500 to 3,000 mL, depending upon the size and the condition.
Precaution(s): Store between 15° and 30°C (59°-86°F).
Warning(s): For animal use only. Keep out of the reach of children.
Presentation: 500 mL and 1000 mL.
Compendium Code No.: 14750040

AMINO ACID ORAL SOLUTION

Bimeda **Large Animal Dietary Supplement**

Active Ingredient(s): Each 100 mL contains:

Dextrose • H_2O ... 5 g
Sodium acetate • $3H_2O$ ... 250 mg
Magnesium sulfate • $7H_2O$ ... 20 mg
Potassium chloride ... 20 mg
Calcium chloride • $2H_2O$ ... 15 mg
Niacinamide ... 150 mg
Pyridoxine HCl ... 10 mg
Thiamine HCl ... 10 mg
d-Panthenol ... 5 mg
Riboflavin ... 4 mg
Cyanocobalamine (B_{12}) ... 5 mcg
L-argenine HCl ... 2.5 mg
L-cysteine HCl • H_2O ... 1 mg
L-glutamic acid ... 4 mg
L-histidine HCl • H_2O ... 1 mg
L-isoleucine ... 2 mg
L-leucine ... 4 mg
L-lysine HCl ... 3 mg
L-methionine ... 1 mg
L-phenylalanine ... 3 mg
L-threonine ... 2 mg
L-valine ... 5 mg
Methylparaben ... 0.18%
Ethylparaben ... 0.01%
Propylparaben ... 0.02%

Indications: An oral source of B-complex vitamins, amino acids, electrolytes, and dextrose for cattle, swine, sheep and horses when daily intake is reduced.
Dosage and Administration: For cattle, horses, sheep and swine: Administer 1 oz. per 10 lbs. of body weight in the drinking water to be consumed in one (1) day.
Precaution(s): Store at a controlled room temperature between 59°-86°F (15°-30°C).
Protect from light and freezing.
Caution(s): Not for human use. Keep out of the reach of children.
Presentation: 500 mL and 1,000 mL bottles.
Compendium Code No.: 13990020

AMINO ACID ORAL SOLUTION

Phoenix Pharmaceutical **Large Animal Dietary Supplement**

Active Ingredient(s): Composition: Each 100 mL of aqueous solution contains:

Dextrose • H_2O ... 5 g
Sodium Acetate • $3H_2O$ ... 250 mg
Magnesium Sulfate • $7H_2O$ ... 20 mg
Potassium Chloride ... 20 mg
Calcium Chloride • $2H_2O$ ... 15 mg
Niacinamide ... 150 mg
Pyridoxine Hydrochloride (B_6) ... 10 mg
Thiamine Hydrochloride (B_1) ... 10 mg
Riboflavin (B_2) ... 4 mg
Total Protein ... 28.5 mg

Containing Amino Acids: L-valine, L-glutamic acid, L-leucine, L-lysine hydrochloride, L-phenylalanine, L-arginine hydrochloride, L-isoleucine, L-threonine, L-cysteine hydrochloride • H_2O, L-histidine hydrochloride • H_2O, and L-methionine

Preservatives:

Methylparaben ... 0.18%
Propylparaben ... 0.02%
Ethylparaben ... 0.01%

Indications: For use as a supplemental nutritive source of amino acids, electrolytes, B complex vitamins, and dextrose in cattle and horses.
Dosage and Administration: Administer orally as a drench. The usual recommended dose in adult cattle and horses is 500 to 3000 mL, depending on size and condition.
Precaution(s): Store between 15° and 30°C (59°-86°F).
Caution(s): For animal use only.
Warning(s): Keep out of reach of children.
Presentation: 500 mL bottles (NDC 57319-081-07).
Compendium Code No.: 12560061 Rev. 3-99

AMINO ACID SOLUTION

AgriLabs **Large Animal Dietary Supplement**

Active Ingredient(s):

Amino acids: L-arginine HCl, L-histidine HCl H_2O, L-leucine, L-isoleucine, L-lysine HCl, methionine, L-phenylalanine, L-threonine, L-tryptophane, L-valine and L-cysteine HCl H_2O.

Vitamins: Riboflavin 5' NaPO4, dexpanthenol, thiamine HCl, pyridoxine HCl, vitamin B_{12} and niacinamide.

Electrolytes: Potassium chloride, magnesium sulfate 7H20, sodium glutamate, sodium acetate $3H_2O$, and calcium chloride $2H_2O$.

Indications: An oral source of vitamins, amino acids, and electrolytes for cattle, swine, sheep and horses when dietary intake of these nutrients is reduced.
Dosage and Administration: For use in drinking water. Supply fresh drinking water daily.

Dosage: Undiluted.

Cattle: Administer 1 oz. AMINO ACID SOLUTION per 100 lbs. of body weight in drinking water to be consumed in one (1) day.

Horses: Administer 10 oz. AMINO ACID SOLUTION per 100 lbs. of body weight in drinking water to be consumed in one (1) day.

Sheep and Swine: Administer ½ oz. AMINO ACID SOLUTION per 5 lbs. of body weight in drinking water to be consumed in one (1) day.

Precaution(s): Protect from freezing.
Caution(s): Keep out of the reach of children.
Presentation: 16 oz. (473 mL) bottles.
Compendium Code No.: 10580090

AMINOCAL PLUS™

Butler **Fluid Therapy**

Active Ingredient(s): Each 1,000 mL of aseptically filled aqueous solution contains:

Dextrose • H_2O ... 275.0 g
Calcium hypophosphite ... 36.5 g
Potassium chloride ... 15.0 g
Sodium chloride ... 2.0 g
Potassium phosphate, monobasic ... 0.5 g
L-glutamic acid ... 560.0 mg
L-arginine hydrochloride ... 450.0 mg
L-proline ... 400.0 mg
L-lysine hydrochloride ... 240.0 mg
L-leucine ... 160.0 mg
L-phenylalanine ... 110.0 mg
L-valine ... 110.0 mg
L-threonine ... 100.0 mg
L-isoleucine ... 70.0 mg
L-histidine hydrochloride ... 40.0 mg
L-methionine ... 40.0 mg
L-tyrosine ... 24.0 mg
Methylparaben (preservative) ... 0.09%
Propylparaben (preservative) ... 0.01%

Indications: For use as a supplemental source of electrolytes, dextrose, and amino acids in cattle.
Dosage and Administration: Administer orally as a drench or by the use of a stomach tube. The usual recommended dose in adult cattle is 500 to 1,000 mL, depending upon the size and condition of the animal.
Precaution(s): Store at a controlled room temperature between 15° and 30°C (59°-86°F).
Caution(s): Not for human use. Keep out of the reach of children.
Presentation: 1,000 mL.
Compendium Code No.: 10820051

AMINOPLEX ℞

Butler **Fluid Therapy**

Active Ingredient(s): Each 100 mL of aseptically filled aqueous solution contains:

Dextrose • H_2O ... 5 g
Sodium acetate • $3H_2O$ ... 250 mg
Magnesium sulfate • $7H_2O$ ... 20 mg
Potassium chloride ... 20 mg
Calcium chloride • $2H_2O$ ... 15 mg

Niacinamide . . . 150 mg
Pyridoxine hydrochloride (B_6) . . . 10 mg
Thiamine hydrochloride (B_1) . . . 10 mg
d-Panthenol . . . 5 mg
Riboflavin (B_2) . . . 4 mg
Cyanocobalamin (B_{12}) . . . 5 mcg
L-valine . . . 5 mg
L-glutamic acid . . . 4 mg
L-leucine . . . 4 mg
L-lysine hydrochloride . . . 3 mg
L-phenylalanine . . . 3 mg
L-arginine hydrochloride . . . 2.5 mg
L-isoleucine . . . 2 mg
L-threonine . . . 2 mg
L-cysteine hydrochloride • H_2O . . . 1 mg
L-histidine hydrochloride • H_2O . . . 1 mg
L-methionine . . . 1 mg
L-tryptophan . . . 1 mg

With propylene glycol 2.5%, sorbitol 2.5%, lactic acid 0.16%, citric acid 0.1%, BHA 0.005%; methylparaben 0.18%, propylparaben 0.02%, and ethylparaben 0.01% (preservatives).

Indications: For use as a supplemental source of amino acids, electrolytes, B-complex vitamins, and dextrose in cattle and horses.

Dosage and Administration: Administer orally as a drench or by the use of a stomach tube. The usual recommended dose in adult cattle and horses is 500 to 3,000 mL, depending upon the size and condition of the animal.

Precaution(s): Store at a controlled room temperature between 15° and 30°C (59°-86°F).

Caution(s): Federal law restricts this drug to use by or on the order of a licensed veterinarian.

Not for human use. Keep out of the reach of children.

Presentation: 500 mL and 1,000 mL vials.

Compendium Code No.: 10820061

AMINOPLEX CONCENTRATE ℞

Butler — **Fluid Therapy**

Active Ingredient(s): Each 100 mL of aseptically filled aqueous solution contains:

Dextrose • H_2O . . . 5 g
Sodium acetate • $3H_2O$ . . . 250 mg
Magnesium sulfate • $7H_2O$ . . . 200 mg
Potassium chloride . . . 200 mg
Calcium chloride • $2H_2O$ . . . 150 mg
Niacinamide . . . 150 mg
Pyridoxine hydrochloride (B_6) . . . 10 mg
Thiamine hydrochloride (B_1) . . . 10 mg
d-Panthenol . . . 5 mg
Riboflavin (B_2) . . . 4 mg
Cyanocobalamin (B_{12}) . . . 5 mcg
L-leucine . . . 187 mg
L-lysine hydrochloride . . . 170 mg
L-glutamic acid . . . 136 mg
L-valine . . . 136 mg
L-phenylalanine . . . 119 mg
L-arginine hydrochloride . . . 85 mg
L-isoleucine . . . 85 mg
L-threonine . . . 78.2 mg
L-histidine hydrochloride • H_2O . . . 59.5 mg
L-methionine . . . 51 mg
L-cysteine hydrochloride • H_2O . . . 50 mg
L-tryptophan . . . 34 mg

With propylene glycol 2.5%, sorbitol 2.5%, lactic acid 0.16%, citric acid 0.1%, BHA 0.005%; methylparaben 0.18%, propylparaben 0.02%, and ethylparaben 0.01% (preservatives).

Indications: For use as a supplemental source of concentrated amino acids, electrolytes, B-complex vitamins, and dextrose in cattle and horses.

Dosage and Administration: Administer orally as a drench or by the use of a stomach tube. The usual recommended dose in adult cattle and horses is 50 to 500 mL, depending upon the size and condition of the animal.

Precaution(s): Store at a controlled room temperature between 15° and 30°C (59°-86°F).

Caution(s): Federal law restricts this drug to use by or on the order of a licensed veterinarian.

Not for human use. Keep out of the reach of children.

Presentation: 500 mL vials.

Compendium Code No.: 10820071

AMINO PLUS CONCENTRATE

AgriPharm — **Large Animal Dietary Supplement**

Active Ingredient(s): Each 100 mL of aqueous solution contains:

Dextrose • H_2O . . . 5 g
Sodium acetate • $3H_2O$ . . . 250 mg
Magnesium sulfate • $7H_2O$ . . . 200 mg
Potassium chloride . . . 200 mg
Calcium chloride • $2H_2O$ . . . 150 mg
Niacinamide . . . 150 mg
Pyridoxine hydrochloride (B_6) . . . 10 mg
Thiamine hydrochloride (B_1) . . . 10 mg
d-panthenol . . . 5 mg
Riboflavin (B_2) . . . 4 mg
Cyanocobalamin (B_{12}) . . . 5 mcg
L-leucine . . . 187 mg
L-lysine hydrochloride . . . 170 mg
L-glutamic acid . . . 136 mg
L-valine . . . 136mg
L-phenylalanine . . . 119 mg
L-arginine hydrochloride . . . 85 mg
L-isoleucine . . . 85 mg
L-threonine . . . 78.2 mg
L-histidine hydrochloride • H_2O . . . 59.5 mg
L-methionine . . . 51 mg
L-cysteine hydrochloride • H_2O . . . 50 mg

With methylparaben 0.18%, propylparaben 0.02%, and ethylparaben 0.01% (preservatives).

Indications: For use as a supplemental source of concentrated amino acids, electrolytes, B complex vitamins, and dextrose in cattle.

Dosage and Administration: Administer orally as a drench.

The usual recommended dose in adult cattle is 50 to 500 mL, depending upon the size and condition of the animal.

Precaution(s): Store at a controlled room temperature between 59°-86°F (15°-30°C).

Caution(s): For animal use only. Keep out of the reach of children.

Presentation: 500 mL containers.

Compendium Code No.: 14570050

AMINO PLUS SOLUTION

AgriPharm — **Large Animal Dietary Supplement**

Active Ingredient(s): Each 100 mL of aqueous solution contains:

Dextrose • H_2O . . . 5 g
Sodium acetate • $3H_2O$ . . . 250 mg
Magnesium sulfate • $7H_2O$ . . . 20 mg
Potassium chloride . . . 20 mg
Calcium chloride • $2H_2O$ . . . 15 mg
Niacinamide . . . 150 mg
Pyridoxine hydrochloride (B_6) . . . 10 mg
Thiamine hydrochloride (B_1) . . . 10 mg
d-panthenol . . . 5 mg
Riboflavin (B_9) . . . 5 mg
Cyanocobalamin (B_{12}) . . . 5 mcg
L-valine . . . 5 mg
L-glutamic acid . . . 4 mg
L-leucine . . . 4 mg
L-lysine hydrochloride . . . 3 mg
L-phenylalanine . . . 3 mg
L-arginine hydrochloride . . . 2.5 mg
L-isoleucine . . . 2 mg
L-threonine . . . 2 mg
L-cysteine hydrochloride • H_2O . . . 1 mg
L-histidine hydrochloride • H_2O . . . 1 mg
L-methionine . . . 1 mg

With methylparaben 0.18%, propylparaben 0.02%, and ethylparaben 0.01% (preservatives).

Indications: For use as a supplemental source of amino acids, electrolytes, B complex vitamins, and dextrose in cattle and horses.

Dosage and Administration: Administer orally as a drench.

The usual recommended dose in adult cattle and horses is 500 to 3,000 mL, depending upon the size and condition of the animal.

Precaution(s): Store at a controlled room temperature between 59°-86°F (15°-30°C).

Caution(s): For animal use only. Keep out of the reach of children.

Presentation: 500 mL containers.

Compendium Code No.: 14570060

AMMONIL® TABLETS ℞

King Animal Health — **Urinary Acidifier**

Active Ingredient(s): dl-Methionine in 200 mg and 500 mg tablets.

Indications: For use as a urinary acidifier in cats and dogs.

Dosage and Administration: The suggested dose of AMMONIL® 200 mg tablet for adult cats is one (1) tablet per 10 lbs. (4.5 kg) of body weight three (3) or four (4) times a day with food.

For dogs one (1) tablet per 10 lbs. (4.5 kg) of body weight once or twice a day with food. The dosage may then be adjusted to attain the desired urine pH (approximately 6).

Not intended for use in kittens.

The suggested dose of AMMONIL® 500 mg tablet for adult cats is one (1) tablet per 10 lbs. (4.5 kg) of body weight once or twice a day with food.

For dogs one-half (½) tablet per 10 lbs. (4.5 kg) of body weight once or twice a day with food. The dosage may then be adjusted to attain the desired urine pH (approximately 6).

Not intended for use in kittens.

Contraindication(s): Do not administer to animals with severe liver or kidney damage or to animals exhibiting acidosis.

Precaution(s): Store at a controlled room temperature of 15°-30°C (59°-86°F).

Caution(s): Federal law restricts this drug to use by or on the order of a licensed veterinarian.

Warning(s): Keep this and all medications out of the reach of children.

Presentation: Bottles of 1,000 tablets.

Compendium Code No.: 11320001

AMOXI-DROP® ℞

Pfizer Animal Health — **Amoxicillin Oral**

(amoxicillin) Veterinary Oral Suspension

NADA No.: 055-085

Active Ingredient(s): Each 15-mL bottle contains 0.75 g and each 30-mL bottle contains 1.5 g of amoxicillin activity. When reconstituted with required amount of water, each mL contains 50 mg of amoxicillin as the trihydrate.

Indications:

Dogs: AMOXI-DROP® is indicated in the treatment of susceptible strains of the organisms causing the following infections:

Respiratory tract infections (tonsillitis, tracheobronchitis) due to *Staphylococcus aureus, Streptococcus* spp., *E. coli*, and *Proteus mirabilis.*

Genitourinary tract infections (cystitis) due to *Staphylococcus aureus, Streptococcus* spp., *E. coli*, and *Proteus mirabilis.*

Gastrointestinal tract infections (bacterial gastroenteritis) due to *Staphylococcus aureus, Streptococcus* spp., *E. coli*, and *Proteus mirabilis.*

Bacterial dermatitis due to *Staphylococcus aureus, Streptococcus* spp., and *Proteus mirabilis.*

Soft tissue infections (abscesses, lacerations, and wounds) due to *Staphylococcus aureus, Streptococcus* spp., *E. coli*, and *Proteus mirabilis.*

Cats: AMOXI-DROP® is indicated in the treatment of susceptible strains of the organisms causing the following infections:

Upper respiratory tract infections due to *Staphylococcus aureus, Staphylococcus* spp., *Streptococcus* spp., *Haemophilus* spp., *E. coli, Pasteurella* spp., and *Proteus mirabilis.*

Genitourinary tract infections (cystitis) due to *Staphylococcus aureus, Streptococcus* spp., *E. coli, Proteus mirabilis,* and *Corynebacterium* spp.

Gastrointestinal tract infections due to *E. coli, Proteus* spp., *Staphylococcus* spp., and *Streptococcus* spp.

Skin and soft tissue infections (abscesses, lacerations, and wounds) due to *Staphylococcus aureus, Staphylococcus* spp., *Streptococcus* spp., *E. coli,* and *Pasteurella multocida.*

Pharmacology: Description: AMOXI-DROP® (amoxicillin) is a semisynthetic antibiotic with a broad spectrum of activity. It provides bactericidal activity against a wide range of common gram-positive and gram-negative pathogens. Chemically, it is d(-)-α-amino-p-hydroxybenzyl penicillin trihydrate.

Action: AMOXI-DROP® is stable in the presence of gastric acid and may be given without regard to meals. It is rapidly absorbed after oral administration. It diffuses readily into most body tissues and fluids with the exception of brain and spinal fluid, except when meninges are inflamed. Most of the amoxicillin is excreted unchanged in the urine.

Amoxicillin is similar to ampicillin in its bactericidal action against susceptible organisms. It acts through the inhibition of biosynthesis of cell wall mucopeptide. *In vitro* and/or *in vivo* studies have demonstrated the susceptibility of most strains of the following gram-positive and gram-negative bacteria: α- and β-haemolytic streptococci, nonpenicillinase-producing staphylococci, *Streptococcus faecalis, Escherichia coli,* and *Proteus mirabilis.* Because it does not resist destruction by penicillinase, it is not effective against penicillinase-producing bacteria, particularly resistant staphylococci. All strains of Pseudomonas and most strains of Klebsiella and Enterobacter are resistant.

Dosage and Administration:

Dogs: The recommended dosage is 5 mg/lb of body weight. Administer twice daily for 5-7 days. Continue for 48 hours after all symptoms have subsided.

Cats: The recommended dosage is 50 mg (5-10 mg/lb). Administer once daily for 5-7 days. Continue for 48 hours after all symptoms have subsided.

Directions for mixing oral suspension: Add required amount of water (see table below) to the bottle and shake vigorously. Each mL of suspension will contain 50 mg of amoxicillin as the trihydrate.

Bottle Size	Amount of Water Required for Reconstitution
15 mL	12 mL
30 mL	23 mL

Note: Any unused portion of the reconstituted suspension must be discarded after 14 days. After mixing, refrigeration preferable, but not required.

Contraindication(s): The use of this drug is contraindicated in animals with a history of an allergic reaction to penicillin.

Precaution(s): Do not store dry powder at temperatures above 25°C (77°F).

Caution(s): Federal law restricts this drug to use by or on the order of a licensed veterinarian.

Warning(s): For use in dogs and cats only. Not for use in animals which are raised for food production.

Adverse Reactions: Amoxicillin is a semisynthetic penicillin and has the potential for producing allergic reactions. If an allergic reaction occurs, administer epinephrine and/or steroids.

Presentation: AMOXI-DROP® is supplied in 15-mL and 30-mL bottles.

Manufactured by: SmithKline Beecham Pharmaceuticals, Philadelphia, PA 19101

Compendium Code No.: 36901660 75-8000-04

AMOXI-INJECT® (Cattle) ℞

Pfizer Animal Health **Amoxicillin Injection**

NADA No.: 055-089

Active Ingredient(s): AMOXI-INJECT® (amoxicillin) is supplied in vials containing 25 grams of amoxicillin activity as the trihydrate.

Indications: AMOXI-INJECT® (amoxicillin) is indicated in the treatment of susceptible strains of the organisms causing the following infections in cattle:

Respiratory tract infections (shipping fever, pneumonia) due to *Pasteurella multocida, Pasteurella hemolytica, Hemophilus* spp., *Streptococci* spp., and *Staphylococci* spp.

Acute necrotic pododermatitis (foot rot) due to *Fusobacterium necrophorum* susceptible to amoxicillin.

As with all antibiotics, appropriate *in vitro* culturing and susceptibility testing of samples taken before treatment should be conducted.

Pharmacology: Description: AMOXI-INJECT® (amoxicillin) is a semisynthetic antibiotic with a broad spectrum of activity. Amoxicillin provides bactericidal activity against a wide range of common Gram-positive and Gram-negative pathogens. Chemically, it is D-(-)-α amino-p-hydroxybenzyl penicillin trihydrate.

Actions: Amoxicillin is rapidly absorbed following intramuscular or subcutaneous administration. It diffuses readily into most body tissues and fluids with the exception of brain and spinal fluid except when meninges are inflamed. Most of amoxicillin is excreted unchanged in the urine.

Amoxicillin is a bactericidal antibiotic. It acts through the inhibition of biosynthesis of cell wall mucopeptides. The following *in vitro* data are available but their clinical significance has not been demonstrated. These *in vitro* data have shown the susceptibility of most strains of the following Gram-positive and Gram-negative bacteria: alpha- and beta-hemolytic streptococci, non-penicillinase-producing staphylococci, *Streptococcus faecalis, Escherichia coli* and *Proteus mirabilis.* Because amoxicillin does not resist destruction by penicillinase, it is not effective against penicillinase-producing bacteria, particularly resistant staphylococci. All strains of *Pseudomonas* and most strains of *Klebsiella* and *Enterobacter* are resistant.

Dosage and Administration: Dosage: The dosage of AMOXI-INJECT® (amoxicillin) for veterinary aqueous injection will vary according to the animal being treated, the severity of infection, and the animal's response.

The recommended dosage for cattle is 3 to 5 mg per pound of body weight once daily by intramuscular or subcutaneous injection. Treatment should be continued 48 to 72 hours after the animal has become afebrile or asymptomatic. Do not continue treatment beyond 5 days. Maximum volume per injection site should not exceed 30 mL.

Directions for Use: AMOXI-INJECT® (amoxicillin) is packaged as a multi-dose dry-filled vial and requires reconstitution prior to use. It should be reconstituted to the desired concentration by adding the recommended amount of Sterile Water for Injection, U.S.P. according to labeled directions.

25 Gram Vial (250 mg/mL Concentration): Add 77 mL of Sterile Water for Injection.

Contraindications: The use of this drug is contraindicated in animals with a history of an allergic reaction to penicillin.

Precaution(s): After reconstitution, the product is stable for 12 months under refrigeration or for 3 months at room temperature (72°F). Date and concentration should be noted on the label at the time of reconstitution.

Caution(s): Federal law restricts this drug to use by or on the order of a licensed veterinarian.

Warning(s): For use in cattle only. Treated animals must not be slaughtered for food during treatment and for 25 days after the last treatment. Milk from treated cows must not be used for food during treatment and for 96 hours (8 milkings) after the last treatment. Treatment should not exceed 5 days.

Adverse Reactions: Amoxicillin is a semisynthetic penicillin and has the potential to produce an allergic reaction. If an allergic reaction occurs, administer epinephrine and/or steroids.

Presentation: 25 g vial.

Compendium Code No.: 36900800 75-8024 / 34-002-LO-1/91

AMOXI-INJECT® (Dogs and Cats) ℞

Pfizer Animal Health **Amoxicillin Injection**

Sterile Amoxicillin for Suspension

NADA No.: 055-091

Active Ingredient(s): Each vial contains 3 grams of amoxicillin activity as the trihydrate.

Indications: AMOXI-INJECT® is indicated in the treatment of susceptible strains of the organisms causing the following infections:

Dogs:

Respiratory tract infections (tonsillitis, tracheobronchitis) due to *Staphylococcus aureus, Streptococcus* spp., *E. coli,* and *Proteus mirabilis.*

Genitourinary tract infections (cystitis) due to *Staphylococcus aureus, Streptococcus* spp., *E. coli,* and *Proteus mirabilis.*

Gastrointestinal tract infections (bacterial gastroenteritis) due to *Staphylococcus aureus, Streptococcus* spp., *E. coli,* and *Proteus mirabilis.*

Bacterial dermatitis due to *Staphylococcus aureus, Streptococcus* spp., and *Proteus mirabilis.*

Soft tissue infections (abscesses, lacerations, wounds) due to *Staphylococcus aureus, Streptococcus* spp., *E. coli,* and *Proteus mirabilis.*

Cats:

Upper respiratory tract infections due to *Staphylococcus aureus, Staphylococcus* spp., *Streptococcus* spp., *Hemophilus* spp., *E. coli, Pasteurella* spp., and *Proteus mirabilis.*

Genitourinary tract infections (cystitis) due to *Staphylococcus aureus, Streptococcus* spp., *E. coli, Proteus mirabilis,* and *Corynebacterium* spp.

Gastrointestinal tract infections due to *E. coli, Proteus* spp., *Staphylococcus* spp., and *Streptococcus* spp.

Skin and soft tissue infections (abscesses, lacerations, wounds) due to *Staphylococcus aureus, Staphylococcus* spp., *Streptococcus* spp., *E. coli,* and *Pasteurella multocida.*

As with all antibiotics, appropriate *in vitro* culturing and susceptibility testing of samples taken before treatment should be conducted.

Pharmacology: Description: AMOXI-INJECT® (amoxicillin) is a semisynthetic antibiotic with a broad spectrum of activity. It provides bactericidal activity against a wide range of common gram-positive and gram-negative pathogens. Chemically it is d-(-)-α-amino-p-hydroxybenzyl penicillin trihydrate.

Action: Amoxicillin is rapidly absorbed following intramuscular or subcutaneous administration. It diffuses readily into most body tissues and fluids with the exception of brain and spinal fluid, except when meninges are inflamed. Most of the amoxicillin is excreted unchanged in the urine.

Amoxicillin is a bactericidal antibiotic. It acts through the inhibition of biosynthesis of cell wall mucopeptide. *In vivo* and/or *in vitro* studies have demonstrated the susceptibility of most strains of the following gram-positive and gram-negative bacteria: α- and β-hemolytic streptococci, nonpenicillinase-producing staphylococci, *Streptococcus* spp., *Escherichia coli,* and *Proteus mirabilis.* Because amoxicillin does not resist destruction by penicillinase, it is not effective against penicillinase-producing bacteria, particularly resistant staphylococci. All strains of Pseudomonas and most strains of Klebsiella and Enterobacter are resistant.

Dosage and Administration: Dosage: The recommended dosage for dogs and cats is 5 mg/lb of body weight. Administer once daily by intramuscular or subcutaneous injection. Treatment should be continued for 48 hours after the animal has become afebrile or asymptomatic. If no improvement is seen within 5 days, review the diagnosis and change therapy.

Directions for Use: AMOXI-INJECT® is packaged as a multi-dose, dry-filled vial and requires reconstitution prior to use. It should be reconstituted to the desired concentration by adding the recommended amount of sterile water for injection, USP according to label directions.

100 mg/mL concentration: Add 27 mL of sterile water for injection

250 mg/mL concentration: Add 9 mL of sterile water for injection

After reconstitution, the product is stable for 12 months under refrigeration or 3 months at controlled room temperature (20°-25°C/68°-77°F). Date and concentration should be noted on the label at the time of reconstitution.

Contraindication(s): The use of this drug is contraindicated in animals with a history of an allergic reaction to penicillin.

Precaution(s): Storage: Store at controlled room temperature 15°-30°C (59°-86°F).

Caution(s): Federal law restricts this drug to use by or on the order of a licensed veterinarian.

Warning(s): For use in dogs and cats only.

Adverse Reactions: Amoxicillin is a semisynthetic penicillin and has the potential for producing allergic reactions. If an allergic reaction occurs, administer epinephrine and/or steroids. Possible minor irritation at the injection site may occur.

Presentation: 3 grams vials.

Manufactured by: G.C. Hanford Mfg. Co., Syracuse, NY 13201

Compendium Code No.: 36901670 75-8025-03

AMOXI-MAST® ℞

Pfizer Animal Health **Mastitis Therapy**

(amoxicillin) Lactating Cow Formula-Intramammary Infusion

NADA No.: 055-100

Active Ingredient(s): AMOXI-MAST® is a stable, nonirritating suspension of amoxicillin trihydrate containing the equivalent of 62.5 mg of amoxicillin per disposable syringe. AMOXI-MAST® is manufactured by a nonsterilizing process.

Indications: AMOXI-MAST® is indicated in the treatment of subclinical infectious bovine mastitis in lactating cows due to *Streptococcus agalactiae* and penicillin-sensitive *Staphylococcus aureus.* Early detection and treatment of mastitis is advised.

Pharmacology: Amoxicillin trihydrate is a semisynthetic penicillin derived from the penicillin nucleus, 6-amino-penicillanic acid. Chemically, it is d(-)-α-amino-p-hydroxybenzyl penicillin trihydrate.

Action: Amoxicillin is bactericidal in action against susceptible organisms. It is a broad-spectrum antibiotic which is effective against common infectious mastitis pathogens, namely *Streptococcus agalactiae* and penicillin-sensitive *Staphylococcus aureus.*

In vitro studies have demonstrated the susceptibility of the following strains of bacteria: α- and β-haemolytic streptococci, nonpenicillinase-producing staphylococci, and *Escherichia coli.*

Susceptibility has not been demonstrated against penicillinase-producing bacteria, particularly resistant staphylococci. Most strains of Pseudomonas, Klebsiella, and Enterobacter are resistant. The clinical or subclinical significance of these *in vitro* studies is not known.

Dosage and Administration: Milk out udder completely. Wash udder and teats thoroughly with warm water containing a suitable dairy antiseptic. Dry thoroughly. Clean and disinfect the teat with alcohol swabs provided in the carton. Remove the syringe tip cover and insert the tip of the syringe into the teat orifice. Express the suspension into the quarter with gentle and continuous pressure. Withdraw the syringe and grasp the end of the teat firmly. Massage the medication up into the milk cistern.

For optimum response, the drug should be administered by intramammary infusion in each infected quarter as described above. Treatment should be repeated at 12-hour intervals for a total of 3 doses. At the next routine milking after the last dose, the treated quarter should be milked out and the milk discarded.

Each carton contains 12 alcohol swabs to facilitate proper cleaning and disinfecting of the teat orifice.

Precaution(s): Do not store above 24°C (75°F).

Caution(s): Federal law restricts this drug to use by or on the order of a licensed veterinarian.

Because it is a derivative of 6-amino-penicillanic acid, AMOXI-MAST® has the potential for producing allergic reactions. Such reactions are rare; however, should they occur, the subject should be treated with the usual agents (antihistamines, pressor amines).

Warning(s): Milk taken from animals during treatment and for 60 hours (5 milkings) after the last treatment must not be used for food. Treated animals must not be slaughtered for food purposes within 12 days after the last treatment.

Presentation: AMOXI-MAST® is supplied in cartons of 12 single-dose syringes with 12 alcohol swabs. Each 10-mL, disposable syringe contains amoxicillin trihydrate equivalent to 62.5 mg of amoxicillin activity.

Manufactured by: G.C. Hanford Mfg. Co., Syracuse, NY 13201

Compendium Code No.: 36900071 75-8161-00

AMOXI-TABS® ℞

Pfizer Animal Health **Amoxicillin Oral**

(amoxicillin)

NADA No.: 055-078 (Dogs)/055-081 (Dogs/Cats)

Active Ingredient(s): Each tablet contains either:

Amoxicillin .... 50 mg
Amoxicillin .... 100 mg
Amoxicillin .... 150 mg
Amoxicillin .... 200 mg
Amoxicillin .... 400 mg

Indications:

Dogs: AMOXI-TABS® are indicated in the treatment of susceptible strains of the organisms causing the following infections:

Respiratory tract infections (tonsillitis, tracheobronchitis) due to *Staphylococcus aureus, Streptococcus* spp., *E. coli,* and *Proteus mirabilis.*

Genitourinary tract infections (cystitis) due to *Staphylococcus aureus, Streptococcus* spp., *E. coli,* and *Proteus mirabilis.*

Gastrointestinal tract infections (bacterial gastroenteritis) due to *Staphylococcus aureus, Streptococcus* spp., *E. coli,* and *Proteus mirabilis.*

Bacterial dermatitis due to *Staphylococcus aureus, Streptococcus* spp., and *Proteus mirabilis.*

Soft tissue infections (abscesses, lacerations, and wounds) due to *Staphylococcus aureus, Streptococcus* spp., *E. coli,* and *Proteus mirabilis.*

Cats: AMOXI-TABS® are indicated in the treatment of susceptible strains of the organisms causing the following infections:

Upper respiratory tract infections due to *Staphylococcus aureus, Streptococcus* spp., and *E. coli.*

Genitourinary tract infections (cystitis) due to *Staphylococcus aureus, Streptococcus* spp., *E. coli,* and *Proteus mirabilis.*

Gastrointestinal tract infections due to *E. coli.*

Skin and soft tissue infections (abscesses, lacerations, and wounds) due to *Staphylococcus aureus, Streptococcus* spp., *E. coli,* and *Pasteurella multocida.*

As with all antibiotics, appropriate *in vitro* culturing and susceptibility testing of samples taken before treatment should be conducted.

Pharmacology: Description: AMOXI-TABS® (amoxicillin) is a semisynthetic antibiotic with a broad spectrum of activity. It provides bactericidal activity against a wide range of common gram-positive and gram-negative pathogens. Chemically, it is d(-)-α-amino-p-hydroxybenzyl penicillin trihydrate.

Action: AMOXI-TABS® is stable in the presence of gastric acid and may be given without regard to meals. It is rapidly absorbed after oral administration. It diffuses readily into most body tissues and fluids with the exception of brain and spinal fluid, except when meninges are inflamed. Most of the amoxicillin is excreted unchanged in the urine.

Amoxicillin is similar to ampicillin in its bactericidal action against susceptible organisms. It acts through the inhibition of biosynthesis of cell wall mucopeptide. *In vitro* and/or *in vivo* studies have demonstrated the susceptibility of most strains of the following gram-positive and gram-negative bacteria: α- and β-haemolytic streptococci, nonpenicillinase-producing staphylococci, *Streptococcus faecalis, Escherichia coli,* and *Proteus mirabilis.* Because it does not resist destruction by penicillinase, it is not effective against penicillinase-producing bacteria, particularly resistant staphylococci. All strains of Pseudomonas and most strains of Klebsiella and Enterobacter are resistant.

Dosage and Administration:

Dogs: The recommended dosage is 5 mg/lb of body weight twice a day.

Cats: The recommended dosage is 50 mg (5-10 mg/lb) once a day.

Dosage should be continued for 5-7 days or 48 hours after all symptoms have subsided. If no improvement is seen in 5 days, review diagnosis and change therapy.

Contraindication(s): The use of this drug is contraindicated in animals with a history of an allergic reaction to penicillin.

Precaution(s): Do not store at temperatures above 25°C (77°F).

Caution(s): Federal law restricts this drug to use by or on the order of a licensed veterinarian.

Warning(s): For use in dogs and cats only.

Adverse Reactions: Amoxicillin is a semisynthetic penicillin and has the potential for producing allergic reactions. If an allergic reaction occurs, administer epinephrine and/or steroids.

Presentation: AMOXI-TABS® are supplied in 5 strengths: 50 mg, 100 mg, 150 mg, and 200 mg in bottles of 500 tablets; 400 mg in bottles of 250 tablets.

Manufactured by: SmithKline Beecham Pharmaceuticals, Philadelphia, PA 19101

Compendium Code No.: 36901680 75-8004-04

AMPHICOL® FILM-COATED TABLETS ℞

Butler **Chloramphenicol**

Chloramphenicol Tablets

NADA No.: 055-059

Active Ingredient(s): Each tablet contains either:

Chloramphenicol .... 250 mg
Chloramphenicol .... 500 mg
Chloramphenicol .... 1 g

Indications: Chloramphenicol tablets are recommended for oral treatment of the following conditions in dogs:

1. Bacterial pulmonary infections caused by susceptible micro-organisms such as: *Staphylococcus aureus, Streptococcus pyogenes,* and *Brucella bronchiseptica.*
2. Infections of the urinary tract caused by susceptible micro-organisms such as: *Escherichia coli, Proteus vulgaris, Corynebacterium renale, Streptococcus* spp., and hemolytic Staphylococcus.
3. Enteritis caused by susceptible micro-organisms such as: *E. coli, Proteus* spp., *Salmonella* spp., and *Pseudomonas* spp.
4. Infections associated with canine distemper caused by susceptible micro-organisms such as: *B. bronchiseptica, E. coli, P. aeruginosa, Proteus* spp., *Shigella* spp. and *Neisseria catarrhalis.*

Pharmacology: Chloramphenicol is a broad-spectrum antibiotic shown to have specific therapeutic activity against a wide variety of organisms. Its activity was first demonstrated in culture filtrates from a species of soil organism collected in Venezuela, later designated as *Streptomyces venezualae.* The antibiotic was subsequently isolated from culture filtrates[1], identified chemically[2], and later synthesized.[3]

Aqueous solutions of chloramphenicol are neutral in pH. Chloramphenicol is stable for several years at room temperature and forms colorless to yellowish-white crystals in the shape of elongated plates or fine needles. It is only slightly soluble in water, but soluble in alcohol and propylene glycol.

Chloramphenicol is exceptionally stable in the presence of extremely high pH, although it is destroyed at pH's in excess of 10. Dissolved in distilled water, it can withstand boiling for five hours.[1]

At low concentrations, chloramphenicol exerts a bacteriostatic effect on a wide range of pathogenic organisms, including many gram-positive and gram-negative bacteria, spirochetes, several rickettsiae and certain large viruses and mycoplasma (PPLO).[4-13,13a] At high concentrations, it inhibits growth of animal and plant cells.

Chloramphenicol exerts its bacteriostatic action by inhibiting protein synthesis in susceptible organisms. Complete suppression of the assimilation of ammonia and of the incorporation of amino acids, particularly glutamic acid, together with an increased formation of ribonucleic acid (RNA), lead to an inhibition of bacterial growth.[4,14-17]

Chloramphenicol antagonizes the action of such antibiotics as penicillin and streptomycin, which act only on growing cells, but is synergistic to tetracycline which also acts by inhibiting protein synthesis.[18] It is possible that chloramphenicol would produce similar synergism with other antibiotics which act by inhibiting protein synthesis.

In this respect, the experimentally demonstrated synergistic action between chloramphenicol and gamma-globulins should be mentioned. Clinical observations in man and corresponding investigations in laboratory animals experimentally infected with various pathogenic bacteria have shown that a combination of chloramphenicol with gamma-globulin or specific antisera has a greater therapeutic effect than would be expected from a mere addition of the individual effects.[19-22]

Many experiments have revealed that the development of resistance to chloramphenicol is rare compared with that occurring with other important antibiotics.[23-34] Bacterial resistance may develop in some strains against chloramphenicol, but it has been encountered infrequently in clinical usage.

Chloramphenicol achieves maximum serum levels very rapidly following oral, intravenous and intraperitoneal administration. Intramuscular injection with chloramphenicol, except certain soluble forms, results in a somewhat delayed absorption and lower serum levels than when given by the oral, intravenous or intraperitoneal route.

Chloramphenicol diffuses readily into all body tissues, but at different concentrations. Highest concentrations are found in the liver and kidney of dogs indicating that these organs are the main route of inactivation and excretion for the metabolites. The lungs, spleen, heart and skeletal muscles contain concentrations similar to that of the blood.[27,35-39]

Chloramphenicol reaches a significant concentration in the aqueous and vitreous humors of the eye from the blood.[4]

A significant difference from other antibiotics is its marked ability to diffuse into the cerebrospinal fluid. Within three to four hours after administration, the concentration in the cerebrospinal fluid has reached, on the average, 50% of the concentration in the serum. If the meninges are inflamed, the percentage may be even higher.[4,27,29,40-43]

Chloramphenicol diffuses readily into milk, pleural and ascitic fluids and crosses the placenta attaining concentrations of about 75% of that of the maternal blood.[36,44]

Chloramphenicol is rather rapidly metabolized, mainly in the liver, by conjugation with glucuronic acid.

Dosage and Administration: Dogs: 25 mg/lb. of body weight every six (6) hours for oral administration.

Additional adjunctive therapy should be used when indicated. Most susceptible infectious disease organisms will respond to chloramphenicol therapy in three (3) to five (5) days when the recommended dosage regimen is followed. If a response to chloramphenicol therapy is not obtained in three (3) to five (5) days, discontinue its use and review the diagnosis. Also, a change of therapy should be considered.

Laboratory tests should be conducted including *in vitro* culturing and susceptibility tests on samples collected prior to treatment.

Contraindication(s): Because of potential antagonism, chloramphenicol should not be administered simultaneously with penicillin or streptomycin.

Precaution(s): Store at or below 77°F (25°C).

Caution(s): Federal law restricts this drug to use by or on the order of a licensed veterinarian.

For animal use only.

The product is for use in dogs only.

1. The antibiotic contains a chemical structure (nitrobenzene group) that is characteristic of a group of drugs long known to depress hematopoietic activity of the bone marrow.[54]
2. *In vitro* tissue culture studies using canine bone marrow cells have demonstrated that extremely high concentrations of chloramphenicol inhibit both uptake of iron by the nucleated red cells and incorporation of iron into heme.[55]
3. Chloramphenicol products should not be administered in conjunction with or two hours

prior to the induction of general anesthesia with pentobarbital because of prolonged recovery time.

4. Chloramphenicol products should not be administered to dogs maintained for breeding purposes. Some experiments indicate that chloramphenicol causes, in experimental animals, particularly females, significant disorders in morphology as well as in function of the gonads.

Warning(s): Not for use in animals which are raised for food production.

Not for human use. Keep out of reach of children.

Toxicology: Approximately 55% of a single daily dose can be recovered from the urine of a treated dog. A small fraction of this is in the form of unchanged chloramphenicol.[36]

A single intravenous dose of 150 mg/kg (approximately 68 mg/lb.) in propylene glycol is the maximum dose tolerated by the dog.[45] Toxic effects were not observed when dogs were administered orally, 200 mg/kg (approximately 91 mg/lb.) a day for over four months.[40] In the mouse, the LD_{50} is 150-250 mg/kg (68 to 114 mg/lb.) of body weight by intravenous injection and 1,500 mg/kg (approximately 681 mg/lb.) by the oral administration.[1,46]

Side Effects: Certain individual dogs may exhibit transient vomiting or diarrhea after an oral dose of 25 mg/lb. of body weight.[49]

References: Available upon request.

Presentation: 250 mg: Bottles of 500 tablets.
500 mg: Bottles of 500 tablets.
1 g: Bottles of 100 tablets.

AMPHICOL is a Registered Trademark of The Butler Company.

Compendium Code No.: 10820081

AMPHYL® DISINFECTANT CLEANER

Reckitt Benckiser **Disinfectant**

Tuberculocidal*-Pseudomonacidal*-Germicidal*-Fungicidal*-Virucidal*

EPA Reg. No.: 675-43

Active Ingredient(s):

o-Phenylphenol 10.5%
o-Benzyl-p-chlorophenol 5.0%
Inert Ingredients: 84.5%

*Includes detergent, other cleaning agents, and no phosphorus compounds.

Indications: Professional AMPHYL® Disinfectant Cleaner is recommended for use in hospitals, nursing homes, dental and doctor offices, and other institutional facilities.

Professional AMPHYL® Disinfectant Cleaner disinfects and deodorizes in one operation.

Germicidal*: Staphylocidal (including methicillin and gentamicin resistant staphylococcus), Pseudomonacidal, Turerculocidal.

Fungicidal*: Against pathogenic fungi.

Veridical*: Against the following viruses - Human Immunodeficiency Virus Type 1 [AIDS Virus], Herpes Simplex Type 1, Influenza A_2 [Hong Kong], and Vaccinia).

*On environmental surfaces.

Directions for Use: It is a violation of Federal law to use this product in a manner inconsistent with its labeling.

Professional AMPHYL® Disinfectant Cleaner is a concentrate. Always dilute in accordance with label instructions. Thoroughly preclean all soiled surfaces with Professional AMPHYL® Disinfectant Cleaner prior to disinfecting, as described below.

Note: Prepare fresh Professional AMPHYL® Disinfectant Cleaner solution for each use. If a freshly prepared 0.5% Professional AMPHYL® Disinfectant Cleaner solution is not to be utilized immediately, add 2 oz. of isopropyl alcohol to each quart of product solution to maintain clarity.

For General Cleaning: Use 0.5% solution for lightly soiled areas and 1% solution for more difficult soil conditions.

For General Disinfection: (including tuberculocidal effectiveness). When required, remove heavy soil and gross filth prior to disinfection, as per above cleaning instructions. Floors, walls, and environmental surfaces should be mopped, wiped, or scrubbed with the recommended solution (1:200), maintaining a thoroughly wet surface for 10 minutes and allowed to air dry. Discard used solution daily or more often if soiling is evident. Professional AMPHYL® Disinfectant Cleaner is effective in 10 minutes at 20°C (68°F).

To prepare proper dilutions in required quantities, add full strength Professional AMPHYL® Disinfectant Cleaner to water as below:

Correct Dilution Strength	Professional AMPHYL® Disinfectant Cleaner	Water
0.5% (1:200)	5 cc (1 tsp.)	1 quart
	20 cc (4 tsp.)	1 gallon
	40 cc (1⅓ oz.)	2 gallons

One tablespoonful equals about ½ fluid ounce or 15 cc.

Precautionary Statements: Hazards to Humans and Domestic Animals: Danger: Corrosive. Causes eye damage and skin irritation. Do not get in eyes, on skin, or on clothing. Wear goggles or face shield and rubber gloves when handling. Harmful if swallowed. Avoid contamination of food.

First Aid:

In case of eye contact, immediately flush eyes thoroughly with plenty of water. Remove any contact lenses and continue to flush eyes with plenty of water for at least 15 minutes. Get medical attention.

If on skin, wash with plenty of soap and water. If irritation persists, get medical attention.

If swallowed, do not induce vomiting. Drink a large amount of water. Call a physician.

Storage and Disposal:

Storage: Store in original container in areas inaccessible to small children. Keep securely closed.

Disposal: Do not reuse empty container. Wrap and discard in trash.

Warning(s): Keep out of reach of children.

Notice: This product contains a chemical known to the State of California to cause cancer.

Presentation: 1 gallon (3.79 liters).

Compendium Code No.: 10011011 372412

AMPROL® 9.6% ORAL SOLUTION

Merial **Water Medication**

(amprolium) Coccidiostat

NADA No.: 013-149

Active Ingredient(s): AMPROL® 9.6% Solution contains 9.6% amprolium.

Benzoic acid 0.1% added as preservative.

Indications: AMPROL® (amprolium) 9.6% Oral Solution is intended for the treatment of coccidiosis in growing chickens, turkeys and laying hens.

Water-soluble treatment for coccidiosis.

Directions: Give amprolium at the 0.012% level (8 fl oz per 50 gallons) as soon as coccidiosis is diagnosed and continue for 3 to 5 days. (In severe outbreaks, give amprolium at the 0.024% level.) Continue with 0.006% amprolium medicated water for an additional 1 to 2 weeks. No other source of drinking water should be available to the birds during this time. Use as the sole source of amprolium.

To Prepare 50 Gallons of Medicated Water:

Dosage Level	Mixing Directions
0.024%	Add 1 pint (16 fluid ounces) of AMPROL® (amprolium) 9.6% Oral Solution to about 5 gallons of water in a 50 gallon medication barrel. Stir, then add water to the 50 gallon mark. Stir thoroughly.
0.012%	Follow same directions as above but use ½ pint (8 fluid ounces) of AMPROL® 9.6% Oral Solution.
0.006%	Follow same directions as above but use 4 fluid ounces of AMPROL® 9.6% Oral Solution.

For Automatic Water Proportioners: For automatic water proportioners that meter 1 fluid ounce of stock solution per gallon of drinking water.

Dosage Level	AMPROL® 9.6% Oral Solution per Gallon of Stock Solution
0.024%	41 fl oz
0.012%	20.5 fl oz
0.006%	10.25 fl oz

Note: Make drinking water fresh daily. Stock solutions for proportioners may be stored in a clean, closed, labeled container for up to 3 days.

Precaution(s): Store at temperatures above 41°F (5°C).

Caution(s): If no improvement is noted within 3 days, have the diagnosis confirmed and follow the directions of your veterinarian or poultry pathologist. Losses may result from intercurrent disease or other conditions affecting drug intake which can contribute to the virulence of coccidiosis under field conditions.

For oral use in animals only.

For animal use only.

Warning(s): May cause eye irritation. For irritation, flush with plenty of water; get medical attention.

Keep this and all drugs out of the reach of children.

Presentation: 128 fl oz (1 gal) (3.785 L) plastic bottle and 4 x 128 fl oz (1 gal) (3.785 L) plastic bottles per case.

AMPROL is a registered trademark of Merial.

Distributed by: Phibro Animal Health, Fairfield, NJ 07004.

Compendium Code No.: 11110870 69035700 / 69035600

AMPROL® 25% TYPE A MEDICATED ARTICLE

Merial **Feed Medication**

(amprolium)

NADA No.: 012-350

Active Ingredient(s):

Amprolium 25%

Ingredients: Corn Gluten Feed and Soybean Oil.

Indications: AMPROL® (amprolium) 25% when fed continuously is intended for use as an aid in (1) preventing outbreaks of coccidiosis in growing chickens, turkeys and pheasants and (2) development of active immunity to coccidiosis in replacement chickens. AMPROL® 25% is also intended for use as an aid in the prevention and treatment of coccidiosis in laying chickens.

Directions: Mixing Directions: AMPROL® (amprolium) 25% should be thoroughly and evenly mixed in the feed in accordance with current good manufacturing practice for medicated feed.

The table below shows the amount of AMPROL® 25% to be used in each ton (2,000 lb) of feed to obtain desired levels of amprolium in the Type C medicated feed.

Feeding Level of Amprolium in Type C Medicated Feed	Use This Amount of AMPROL® 25% Per Ton
0.004%	5 oz
0.006%	8 oz
0.008%	10 oz
0.0125%	1 lb
0.0175%	1 lb 6½ oz
0.025%	2 lb

Suggested Directions for Feed Tags:

Use Directions:

Chickens:

Broilers:

Aid in Prevention: Use 0.0125% amprolium Type C medicated feeds continuously for most field conditions as they exist under modern management practices. Where severe coccidiosis conditions exist, use 0.025% amprolium Type C medicated feed. For field conditions where only *E. tenella* is the major problem, use 0.008%-0.0125% amprolium Type C medicated feed.

Replacements:

Aid in Immunity Development or Prevention:

Prevention Program: Where immunity development is not desirable, use 0.0125%-0.025% amprolium Type C medicated feed continuously from day old until onset of production.

Immunity Development Program: Use 0.004%-0.0125% amprolium Type C medicated feed continuously until onset of production.

Selection of the level to be used should be based upon comparative hazard of infection with cecal and intestinal species. the higher levels will interfere with the development of immunity to *E. tenella* (cecal).

The following are suggested feeding schedules for various conditions of coccidial exposure. The planning and evaluation of any program should be in the hands of a veterinarian or poultry pathologist who is familiar with the specific operation and with the general nature of disease problems in the area.

1. Severe exposure:
   0-5 weeks of age: 0.0125%
   5-8 weeks of age: 0.008%-0.0125%
   over 8 weeks of age: 0.004%-0.0125%
2. Moderate exposure:
   0-5 weeks of age: 0.008%-0.0125%
   5-8 weeks of age: 0.006%-0.0125%
   over 8 weeks of age: 0.004%-0.0125%
3. Slight exposure:
   0-5 weeks of age: 0.004%-0.0125%
   5-8 weeks of age: 0.004%-0.0125%
   over 8 weeks of age: 0.004%-0.0125%

Laying Hens:

Treatment: Use 0.025% amprolium Type C medicated feed for two weeks in severe outbreaks or 0.0125% amprolium Type C medicated feed for two weeks in moderate outbreaks.

Aid in Prevention: Use 0.0125% amprolium Type C medicated feed continuously.

Turkeys:

Aid in Prevention: Use 0.0125%-0.025% amprolium Type C medicated feed continuously.

Pheasants: For the prevention of coccidiosis in growing pheasants caused by *Eimeria colchici, E. duodenalis,* and *E. phasiani.*

Type C medicated feed with 0.0175% amprolium should be fed continuously as the sole ration. Mix 1.4 pounds (1 lb 6½ oz) AMPROL® 25% per ton of feed.

Caution(s): To be used only in the manufacture of registered feeds.

Use as the sole source of amprolium.

Do not change the litter while giving this feed unless absolutely necessary.

If losses exceed 0.5% in a 2-day period, obtain an accurate diagnosis, and follow the instructions of your veterinarian or poultry pathologist. Losses may result from intercurrent disease or other conditions affecting drug intake which can contribute to the virulence of coccidiosis under field conditions.

In replacement flocks the grower must expect that excessive exposure to one or more species may overwhelm the drug in some flocks and prompt treatment will be required.

Fertility, hatchability and other reproductive data are not available on amprolium in breeding pheasants.

Do not use in feeds containing bentonite.

Warning(s): Keep this and all drugs out of the reach of children.

Presentation: 50 lb (22.68 kg) bag.

® AMPROL is a registered trademark of Merial.

Merial Limited: Registered in England and Wales (No. 3332751) with registered offices at 27 Knightsbridge, London SW1X 7QT, England and domesticated in Delaware, USA as Merial LLC.

Distributed by: Koffolk, Inc., Fort Lee, NJ 07024.

Compendium Code No.: 11110880 607200

AMPROL® 128 20% SOLUBLE POWDER

Merial **Water Medication**

(amprolium) Coccidiostat

NADA No.: 033-165

Active Ingredient(s): AMPROL® 128 20% Soluble Powder contains 20% amprolium.

Indications: AMPROL® 128 (amprolium) 20% Soluble Powder is intended for the treatment of coccidiosis in growing chickens, turkeys and laying hens.

Water-soluble treatment for coccidiosis.

Directions: Give amprolium at the 0.012% level (10 oz AMPROL® 128 20% Soluble Powder per 128 gallons) as soon as coccidiosis is diagnosed and continue for three to five days. (In severe outbreaks, give amprolium at the 0.024% level.) Continue with 0.006% amprolium medicated water for an additional 1 to 2 weeks. No other source of drinking water should be available to the birds during this time.

Use as the sole source of amprolium.

Premeasured for 50-Gallon Medication Barrel: For use in automatic water proportioners that meter 1 fluid ounce of stock solution per gallon of drinking water.

To prepare dosage levels of:	Dissolve AMPROL® 128 (amprolium) 20% Soluble Powder in one gallon of water. (Makes 1 gallon of stock solution.)
0.024%	2 bags (20 oz) in 1 gallon
0.012%	1 bag (10 oz) in 1 gallon
0.006%	½ bag (5 oz) in 1 gallon

To Prepare 50 Gallons of Medicated Water:

Dosage Level	Mixing Directions
0.024%	Dissolve 8 ounces of AMPROL® 128 20% Soluble Powder in about 5 gallons of water in a 50 gallon medication barrel. Stir, then add water to the 50 gallon mark. Stir thoroughly.
0.012%	Follow same directions as above but use 4 ounces of AMPROL® 128 20% Soluble Powder.
0.006%	Follow same directions as above but use 2 ounces of AMPROL® 128 20% Soluble Powder.

Note: Make drinking water fresh daily. Stock solutions for proportioners may be stored in a clean, closed, labeled container for up to 3 days.

Caution(s): If no improvement is noted within 3 days, have the diagnosis confirmed and follow the directions of your veterinarian or poultry pathologist. Losses may result from intercurrent disease or other conditions affecting drug intake which can contribute to the virulence of coccidiosis under field conditions.

For animal use only.

Warning(s): Keep this and all drugs out of the reach of children.

Presentation: 10 oz bag and 24 x 10 oz bags per pail.

AMPROL is a registered trademark of Merial.

Distributed by: Phibro Animal Health, 710 Route 46 East - Suite 401, Fairfield, NJ 07004.

(Merial Limited: Registered in England and Wales [Reg. No. 3332751] with registered offices at 27 Knightsbridge, London, SW1X 7QT, England and domesticated in Delaware, USA as Merial LLC).

Compendium Code No.: 11110890 668009 / 6845409

AMPROL PLUS® TYPE A MEDICATED ARTICLE

Merial **Feed Medication**

(amprolium with ethopabate)

NADA No.: 013-461

Active Ingredient(s):

Amprolium 25%

Ethopabate 0.8%

Ingredients: Corn Gluten Feed and Soybean Oil.

Indications: AMPROL PLUS® (amprolium, ethopabate) is intended for use as an aid in prevention of coccidiosis (1) in broiler chickens and (2) in replacement chickens where immunity to coccidiosis is not desired.

Directions: Mixing Directions: AMPROL PLUS® (amprolium, ethopabate) should be thoroughly and evenly mixed in the feed in accordance with current good manufacturing practice for medicated feed. One pound of AMPROL PLUS® per ton of Type C medicated feed will produce a feed mixture containing 0.0125% amprolium and 0.0004% ethopabate. One pound of AMPROL PLUS® and one pound of Amprol® (amprolium) 25% per ton of Type C medicated feed will produce a feed mixture containing 0.025% amprolium and 0.0004% ethopabate.

Suggested Directions for Feed Tags:

Use Directions:

Chickens: For most field conditions as they exist under modern management practices use 0.0125% amprolium-0.0004% ethopabate Type C medicated feed. Where severe coccidiosis conditions exist, use 0.025% amprolium-0.0004% ethopabate Type C medicated feed.

Use amprolium-ethopabate Type C medicated feed as the only ration from the time birds are placed on litter until past the time when coccidiosis is ordinarily a hazard.

Caution(s): Use as the sole source of amprolium.

Do not use amprolium-ethopabate Type C medicated feed as a treatment for outbreaks of coccidiosis.

Do not change the litter while giving this feed unless absolutely necessary.

If losses exceed 0.5% in a 2-day period, obtain an accurate diagnosis, and follow the instructions of your veterinarian or poultry pathologist. Losses may result from intercurrent disease or other conditions affecting drug intake which can contribute to the virulence of coccidiosis under field conditions.

Do not use in feeds containing bentonite. To be used only in the manufacture of registered feeds.

Warning(s): Not for laying hens. Keep this and all drugs out of the reach of children.

Presentation: 50 lb (22.68 kg) bag.

® AMPROL PLUS and AMPROL are registered trademarks of Merial.

Merial Limited - Registered in England and Wales (No. 3332751) with registered offices at 27 Knightsbridge, London SW1X 7QT, England and domesticated in Delaware, USA as Merial LLC.

Compendium Code No.: 11110900 611230

AMPROVINE® 25%

Merial **Feed Medication**

(amprolium) Type A Medicated Article-Coccidiostat

NADA No.: 012-350

Active Ingredient(s):

Amprolium 25%

Ingredients: Corn Gluten Feed and Soybean Oil.

Indications: An aid in the prevention and treatment of coccidiosis caused by *Eimeria bovis* and *E. zurnii* in calves.

To be used in the preparation of medicated feed.

Directions: Mixing Directions: AMPROVINE® 25% should be thoroughly and evenly mixed in the feed in accordance with current good manufacturing practice for medicated feed. AMPROVINE® 25% may be used to manufacture a Type B medicated feed in the concentration range of 0.05% to 1.25% amprolium.

For example, 100 lb of AMPROVINE® 25% may be mixed to make one ton of 1.25% Type B medicated feed.

Dosage and Use Directions:

Prevention: 227 mg amprolium/100 lb (5 mg/kg) body weight per day for 21 days during period of exposure or when experience indicates that coccidiosis is likely to be a hazard.

Treatment: 454 mg amprolium/100 lb (10 mg/kg) body weight per day for 5 days. Use on a herd basis only; when one or more calves show signs of coccidiosis, it is likely that the rest of the group have been exposed and all calves in the group should be treated.

The proper amount of amprolium supplement is mixed with the amount of ration usually consumed in one day. The tables give suggested directions for using the 1.25% Type B medicated feed.

Animal Weight lb	Animal Weight kg	Type B Feed Fed at Rate of (lb/Head/Day)	Daily Type B Feed Contains (mg amprolium)	Total Pounds of 1.25% Type B Feed for 100 Head
For 21 Day Preventive Program				
200	90.7	0.08	453.6	168
300	136.1	0.12	680.4	252
400	181.4	0.16	907.2	336
500	226.8	0.20	1134.0	420
600	272.2	0.24	1360.8	504
For 5 Day Treatment Program				
200	90.7	0.16	907.2	80
300	136.1	0.24	1360.8	120
400	181.4	0.32	1814.4	160
500	226.8	0.40	2268.0	200
600	272.2	0.48	2721.6	240

Caution(s): To be used only in the manufacture of registered feeds.

For a satisfactory diagnosis a microscopic examination of the feces should be done by a veterinarian or diagnostic laboratory before treatment. When treating outbreaks, drug should be administered promptly after diagnosis is determined.

Do not use in feeds containing bentonite. Use as the sole source of amprolium.

Warning(s): Residue Information: Withdraw 24 hours before slaughter. A withdrawal period has not been established for this product in pre-ruminating calves. Do not use in calves to be processed for veal.

Keep this and all drugs out of the reach of children.

The Material Safety Data Sheet (MSDS) contains more detailed occupational safety information. To report adverse effects, obtain an MSDS, or for assistance, contact Merial at 1-888-637-4251.

Presentation: 50 lb (22.68 kg) bag.

® AMPROVINE is a registered trademark of Merial.

Merial Limited - Registered in England and Wales (No. 3332751) with registered offices at 27 Knightsbridge, London SW1X 7QT, England and domesticated in Delaware, USA as Merial LLC.

Compendium Code No.: 11110001 61122

AMTECH AMCAL HIGH POTENCY ORAL SOLUTION

Phoenix Scientific **Electrolytes-Oral**

Electrolytes-Dextrose-Amino Acids

Active Ingredient(s): Composition: Each 1000 mL of aqueous solution contains:

Dextrose • H_2O	275.0 g
Calcium hypophosphite	36.5 g
Potassium chloride	15.0 g
Sodium chloride	2.0 g
Potassium phosphate, monobasic	0.5 g
Total protein	2.3 g
Methylparaben (preservative)	0.09%
Propylparben (preservative)	0.01%

Containing Amino Acids: L-glutamic acid, L-arginine hydrochloride, L-proline, L-lysine hydrochloride, L-leucine, L-phenylalanine, L-valine, L-threonine, L-isoleucine, L-histidine hydrochloride, L-methionine, L-tyrosine.

Indications: For use as a supplemental nutritive source of electrolytes, dextrose, and amino acids in cattle.

Dosage and Administration: Administer orally as a drench. The usual recommended dose in adult cattle is 500 to 1000 mL, depending on size and condition.

Precaution(s): Store between 15° and 30°C (59°-86°F).

Caution(s): For animal use only. Keep out of reach of children.

Presentation: 1000 mL (NDC 59130-600-04).

Compendium Code No.: 10740000 Rev. 4-95

AMTECH AMIMAX™ C INJECTION ℞

Phoenix Scientific **Antimicrobial Injection**

(Amikacin Sulfate Injection)

ANADA No.: 200-178

Active Ingredient(s): Each mL of solution contains:

Amikacin (as the sulfate)	50 mg
Sodium citrate, USP (as buffer)	25.1 mg
Sodium bisulfite	6.6 mg
Benzethonium chloride, USP (as preservative)	0.1 mg
Water for injection, USP	q.s.

pH adjusted with sulfuric acid.

The dosage form supplied is a sterile, colorless to straw colored solution containing, in addition to amikacin sulfate, 2.5% sodium citrate, pH adjusted with sulfuric acid, 0.66% sodium bisulfite added, and 0.1 mg benzethonium chloride per mL as a preservative.

Indications: AMIMAX™ C Injection (Amikacin Sulfate Injection) is indicated for the treatment of the following conditions in dogs:

Genitourinary tract infections (cystitis) caused by susceptible strains of *Escherichia coli* and *Proteus* sp.

Skin and soft tissue infections caused by susceptible strains of *Pseudomonas* sp and *Escherichia coli*.

While nearly all strains of *Escherichia coli*, *Pseudomonas* sp, and *Proteus* sp, including those that are resistant to gentamicin, kanamycin or other aminoglycosides, are susceptible to amikacin at levels achieved following treatment, it is recommended that the invading organism be cultured and its susceptibility demonstrated as a guide to therapy. Amikacin susceptibility discs, 30 mcg, should be used for determining *in vitro* susceptibility.

Pharmacology: Description: Amikacin sulfate is a semi-synthetic aminoglycoside antibiotic derived from kanamycin. It is $C_{22}H_{43}N_5O_{13}{\bullet}2H_2SO_4$,D-streptamine, 0-3-amino-3-deoxy-α-D-glucopyranosyl - (1→6) - 0 - [6-amino-6-deoxy-α-D-glucopyranosyl - (1→4)]-N¹-(4-amino-2-hydroxy-1-oxobutyl)-2-deoxy-,(S)-,sulfate (1:2) (salt).

Action: Amikacin, like other aminoglycoside antibiotics, is a bactericidal agent that exerts its action at the level of the bacterial ribosome. Amikacin has been shown to be effective against many aminoglycoside-resistant strains due to its ability to resist degradation by aminoglycoside inactivating enzymes known to affect gentamicin, tobramycin and kanamycin.(1)

Microbiology: Amikacin has been shown to be effective in the treatment of skin and soft tissue infections caused by *Pseudomonas* sp and *Escherichia coli* and in urinary tract infections caused by *Escherichia coli* and *Proteus* sp. The susceptibility of veterinary isolates to amikacin is summarized in the following table:

Organism (No. of Isolates)	Minimum Inhibitory Concentration (mcg/mL)	
	Range	MIC_{90}*
Escherichia coli (50)	1-32	4
Proteus mirabilis (50)	1-128	6
Enterobacter sp. (50)	0.5-128	4
Staphylococcus aureus (50)	1-128	2
Klebsiella pneumoniae (50)	0.5-16	2
Pseudomonas aeruginosa (50)	1-64	8

*Concentration at which 90% of the isolates are susceptible

In addition, the following microorganisms have been shown to be susceptible to amikacin *in vitro*,(2) although the clinical significance of this action has not been demonstrated in animals: *Serratia marcescens*, *Salmonella* sp, *Shigella* sp, *Providencia* sp, *Citrobacter freundii*, *Listeria monocytogenes*.

The aminoglycoside antibiotics in general have limited activity against gram-positive pathogens, although *Staphylococcus aureus* and *Listeria monocytogenes* are susceptible to amikacin as noted above.

Pharmacokinetics: Amikacin is well absorbed following intravenous, subcutaneous, or intramuscular injection but is not appreciably absorbed orally. The serum half-life (T½) averages from 1 to 2 hours in dogs depending on the route of administration.(3) Amikacin is excreted unchanged in urine, concentrations in excess of 1,000 mcg/mL typically being achieved within three hours in dogs. Serum concentration-time profiles in dogs following subcutaneous administration are illustrated graphically in Figure 1.

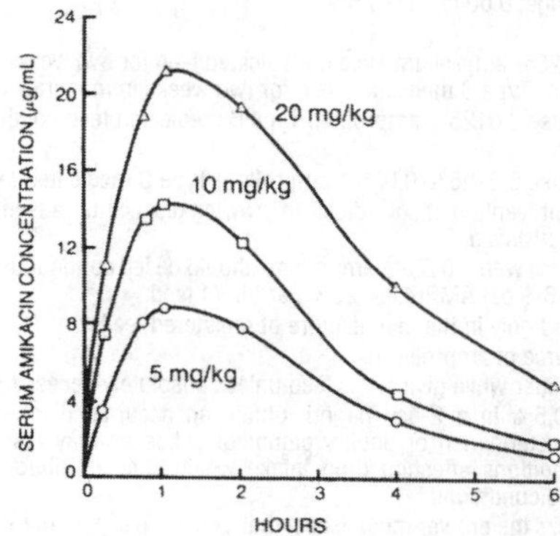

Figure 1: Amikacin Concentration-Time Curves in Dogs (n=6) Following Subcutaneous Injection

Dosage and Administration: AMIMAX® C Injection (Amikacin Sulfate Injection) should be administered subcutaneously or intramuscularly at a dosage of 10 mg/kg (5 mg/lb) twice daily. Dogs with skin and soft tissue infections should be treated for a minimum of 7 days and those with genitourinary infections should be treated for 7 to 21 days or until culture negative and asymptomatic. If no response is observed after three days of treatment, therapy should be discontinued and the case re-evaluated. Maximum duration of therapy should not exceed 30 days.

Contraindication(s): Systemic aminoglycoside therapy is contraindicated in dogs with seriously impaired renal function.

Precaution(s): Store vials at controlled room temperature (15°-30°C, 59°-86°F). At times the solution may become pale yellow in color. This does not indicate a decrease in potency.

Caution(s): Federal law restricts this drug to use by or on the order of a licensed veterinarian.

Amikacin should be used with extreme caution in dogs, in which hearing acuity is required for functioning, such as seeing eye, hearing ear or military patrol, as the auditory and vestibular impairment tends not to be reversible.(6)

Aminoglycosides, including amikacin, are not indicated in uncomplicated episodes of cystitis unless causative agents are susceptible to them and are not susceptible to antibiotics having less potential for toxicity.

Early signs of ototoxicity can include ataxia, nausea and vomiting. Auditory and vestibular impairment may be reversible in the very early stages, but if treatment is continued, the conditions will become irreversible.(6)

The following conditions have been found to contribute to the toxicity of aminoglycosides in dogs:

-Prior renal damage (most commonly found in dogs of advanced age) and dogs infected with heartworm microfilaria.(5)

-Hypovolemic dehydration (dehydrated patients should be rehydrated prior to initiating therapy).

In dogs where decreased renal function is suspected prior to treatment, BUN or serum creatinine levels may not indicate the degree of kidney impairment. A creatinine clearance determination may be more useful.

Monitoring of renal function during treatment is recommended. Although there is not a completely reliable monitoring program for aminoglycoside toxicity, urinalysis may indicate early nephrotoxicity. Unfavorable changes in the urinalysis which may indicate toxicity include:

-Decreased specific gravity in the absence of fluid therapy.

-Appearance in the urine of casts, albumin, glucose or blood.

Continued use of aminoglycosides where any functional renal impairment has occurred may lead to enhanced renal damage as well as increased likelihood of ototoxicity and/or neuromuscular blockade.(6)

Concurrent or sequential use of topically or systemically administered nephrotoxic, ototoxic, or neuromuscular blocking drugs, particularly other aminoglycosides such as streptomycin, gentamicin, kanamycin and neomycin should be avoided because of the potential for additive effects.

Concurrent administration of furosemide with aminoglycosides may enhance nephrotoxicity.(7)

Not for use in breeding dogs as reproductive studies have not been conducted.

Neurotoxic and nephrotoxic antibiotics may be absorbed in significant quantities from body surfaces after local irrigation or application. The potential toxic effect of antibiotics administered in this fashion should be considered.(8)

If hypersensitivity develops, treatment with AMIMAX™ C Injection (Amikacin Sulfate Injection) should be discontinued and appropriate therapy instituted.

Warning(s): Not for human use. Keep out of reach of children.

For subcutaneous or intramuscular use in the dog only.

Toxicology: The intravenous and intramuscular LD_{50} in dogs is greater than 250 mg/kg. Like other aminoglycosides, amikacin has nephrotoxic, neurotoxic, and ototoxic potential. In dogs, minimal to mild renal changes were detectable histopathologically after amikacin dosage of 45 mg/kg/day for two weeks, and dogs receiving a dosage of 30 mg/kg/day for 90 days had minimal renal alterations which were believed to be entirely reversible. Urinary casts were not observed in dogs receiving a 30 mg/kg dose for 90 days. In efficacy studies involving 80 infected dogs treated with amikacin at the recommended dosage rate of 10 mg/kg b.i.d. for 8-21 consecutive days, no evidence of nephrotoxicity or any other toxicity was encountered. Regarding ototoxicity, studies in cats reveal that amikacin has less potential for ototoxicity than gentamicin.(4)

Adverse Reactions: In clinical studies in dogs, transient pain on injection has been reported as well as rare cases of vomiting or diarrhea following amikacin therapy. In 90 day intramuscular toxicology studies, evidence of muscle damage was detected histologically as well as by elevated creatinine phosphokinase.

References: Available upon request.

Presentation: 50 mL vials (NDC 59130-658-11).

Compendium Code No.: 10740011 Rev. 3-97

AMTECH AMIMAX™ E SOLUTION ℞

Phoenix Scientific **Intrauterine Antibiotic**

(Amikacin Sulfate Solution)

ANADA No.: 200-181

Active Ingredient(s): Each mL contains:

Amikacin (as the sulfate)	250 mg
Sodium citrate (as buffer)	25.1 mg
Sodium bisulfite	6.6 mg
Benzethonium chloride (as preservative)	0.1 mg
Water for injection	q.s.

pH adjusted with sulfuric acid.

The dosage form supplied is a sterile, colorless to light straw colored solution. The solution contains, in addition to amikacin sulfate, 2.5% sodium citrate with pH adjusted to 4.5 with sulfuric acid and 0.66% sodium bisulfite added. The multi-dose 12 gram vial contains 0.01% benzethonium chloride as a preservative.

Indications: AMIMAX™ E Solution (Amikacin Sulfate Solution) is indicated for the treatment of uterine infections (endometritis, metritis and pyometra) in mares, when caused by susceptible organisms including *Escherichia coli, Pseudomonas* sp, and *Klebsiella* sp. The use of amikacin sulfate in eliminating infections caused by the above organisms has been shown clinically to improve fertility in infected mares.

While nearly all strains of *Escherichia coli, Pseudomonas* sp and *Klebsiella* sp, including those that are resistant to gentamicin, kanamycin or other aminoglycosides, are susceptible to amikacin at levels achieved following treatment, it is recommended that the invading organism be cultured and its susceptibility demonstrated as a guide to therapy. Amikacin susceptibility discs, 30 mcg, should be used for determining *in vitro* susceptibility.

Pharmacology: Description: Amikacin sulfate is a semisynthetic aminoglycoside antibiotic derived from kanamycin. It is $C_{22}H_{43}N_5O_{13} \bullet 2H_2SO_4$,D-streptamine, 0-3-amino-3-deoxy-α-D-glucopyranosyl - (1$\rightarrow$6) - 0 - [6-amino-6-deoxy-α-D-glucopyranosyl - (1$\rightarrow$4)-N[1]-(4-amino-2-hydroxy-1-oxobutyl)-2-deoxy-,(S)-,sulfate (1:2) (salt).

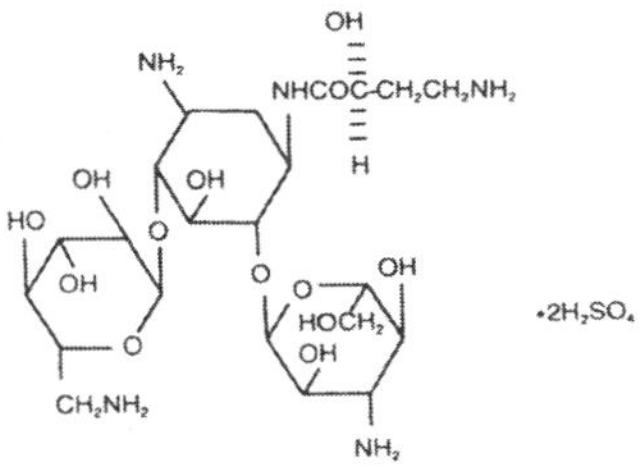

Action:

Antibacterial Activity: The effectiveness of AMIMAX™ E Solution (Amikacin Sulfate Solution) in infections caused by *Escherichia coli, Pseudomonas* sp, and *Klebsiella* sp has been demonstrated clinically in the horse. In addition, the following microorganisms have been shown to be susceptible to amikacin *in vitro*,(1) although the clinical significance of this action has not been demonstrated in animals: *Enterobacter* sp, *Proteus mirabilis, Proteus* sp (indole positive), *Serratia marcescens, Salmonella* sp, *Shigella* sp, *Providencia* sp, *Citrobacter freundii, Listeria monocytogenes, Staphylococcus aureus* (both penicillin resistant and penicillin sensitive).

The aminoglycoside antibiotics in general have limited activity against gram-positive pathogens, although *Staphylococcus aureus* and *Listeria monocytogenes* are susceptible to amikacin as noted above.

Amikacin has been shown to be effective against many aminoglycoside-resistant strains due to its ability to resist degradation by aminoglycoside inactivating enzymes known to affect gentamicin, tobramycin and kanamycin.(2)

Clinical Pharmacology:

Endometrial Tissue Concentrations: Comparisons of amikacin activity in endometrial biopsy tissue following intrauterine infusion with that following intramuscular injection of amikacin sulfate in mares demonstrate superior endometrial tissue concentrations when the drug is administered by the intrauterine route.

Intrauterine infusion of 2 grams AMIMAX™ E Solution (Amikacin Sulfate Solution) daily for three consecutive days in mares results in peak concentrations typically exceeding 40 mcg/g of endometrial biopsy tissue within one hour after infusion. Twenty-four hours after each treatment amikacin activity is still detectable at concentrations averaging 2 to 4 mcg/g. However, the drug is not appreciably absorbed systemically following intrauterine infusion. Endometrial tissue concentrations following intramuscular injection roughly parallel, but are typically somewhat lower than corresponding serum concentrations of amikacin.

Safety: AMIMAX™ E Solution (Amikacin Sulfate Solution) is non-irritating to equine endometrial tissue when infused into the uterus as directed (see "Dosage and Administration"). In laboratory animals as well as equine studies, the drug was generally found not to be irritating when injected intravenously, subcutaneously or intramuscularly.

Although amikacin, like other aminoglycosides, is potentially nephrotoxic, ototoxic and neurotoxic, parenteral (intravenous) administration of amikacin sulfate twice daily at dosages of up to 10 mg/lb for 15 consecutive days in horses resulted in no clinical, laboratory or histopathologic evidence of toxicity.

Intrauterine infusion of 2 grams of AMIMAX™ E Solution (Amikacin Sulfate Solution) 8 hours prior to breeding by natural service did not impair fertility in mares. Therefore, mares should not be bred for at least 8 hours following uterine infusion.

Dosage and Administration: For treatment of uterine infections in mares, 2 grams (8 mL) of AMIMAX™ E Solution (Amikacin Sulfate Solution), mixed with 200 mL 0.9% Sodium Chloride Injection, USP and aseptically infused into the uterus daily for three consecutive days, has been found to be the most efficacious dosage.

Contraindication(s): There are no known contraindications for the use of amikacin sulfate in horses other than a history of hypersensitivity to amikacin.

Precaution(s): AMIMAX™ E Solution (Amikacin Sulfate Solution) is supplied as a colorless solution which is stable at room temperature. At times the solution may become pale yellow in color. This does not indicate a decrease in potency.

Store at controlled room temperature 15°-30°C (59°-86°F).

Caution(s): Federal law restricts this drug to use by or on the order of a licensed veterinarian.

Although amikacin sulfate is not absorbed to an appreciable extent following intrauterine infusion, concurrent use of other aminoglycosides should be avoided because of the potential additive effects.

Warning(s): Not to be used in horses intended for food. *In vitro* studies have demonstrated that when sperm are exposed to the preservative which is present in the 48 mL vials (250 mg/mL) sperm viability is impaired.

For intrauterine use in the horse only.

Not for human use. Keep out of reach of children.

Side Effects: No adverse reactions or other side effects have been reported.

References: Available upon request.

Presentation: 48 mL vial (NDC 59130-657-11).

Compendium Code No.: 10740022 Rev. 3-97

AMTECH AMINO ACID ORAL CONCENTRATE

Phoenix Scientific **Large Animal Dietary Supplement**

Active Ingredient(s): Composition: Each 100 mL of aqueous solution contains:

Dextrose • H_2O	5 g
Sodium acetate • $3H_2O$	250 mg
Magnesium sulfate • $7H_2O$	200 mg
Potassium chloride	200 mg
Calcium chloride • $2H_2O$	150 mg
Niacinamide	150 mg
Pyridoxine hydrochloride (B_6)	10 mg
Thiamine hydrochloride (B_1)	10 mg
Riboflavin (B_2)	4 mg
Total protein	1156.7 mg

Comprised of: L-valine, L-glutamic acid, L-leucine, L-lysine hydrochloride, L-phenylalanine, L-arginine hydrochloride, L-isoleucine, L-threonine, L-cysteine hydrochloride • H_2O, L-histidine hydrochloride • H_2O, L-methionine.

With methylparaben 0.18%, propylparaben 0.02%, and ethylparaben 0.01% (preservatives).

Indications: For use as a supplemental nutritive source of concentrated amino acids, electrolytes, B complex vitamins, and dextrose in cattle and horses.

Dosage and Administration: Administer orally as a drench. The usual recommended dose in adult cattle and horses is 50 to 500 mL, depending on size and condition .

Precaution(s): Store between 15°C-30°C (59°F-86°F).

Caution(s): For animal use only.

Keep out of the reach of children.

Presentation: 500 mL (NDC 59130-602-03).

Compendium Code No.: 10740030 Rev. 4-95

AMTECH AMINO ACID ORAL SOLUTION

Phoenix Scientific **Large Animal Dietary Supplement**

Active Ingredient(s): Each 100 mL of aqueous solution contains:

Dextrose • H_2O	5 g
Sodium Acetate • $3H_2O$	250 mg
Magnesium Sulfate • $7H_2O$	20 mg
Potassium Chloride	20 mg
Calcium Chloride • $2H_2O$	15 mg
Niacinamide	150 mg
Pyridoxine Hydrochloride (B_6)	10 mg
Thiamine Hydrochloride (B_1)	10 mg
Riboflavin (B_2)	4 mg
Total Protein	28.5 mg

Containing amino acids: L-valine, L-glutamic acid, L-leucine, L-lysine hydrochloride, L-phenylalanine, L-arginine hydrochloride, L-isoleucine, L-threonine, L-cysteine hydrochloride • H_2O, L-histidine hydrochloride • H_2O, L-methionine.

With methylparaben 0.18%, propylparaben 0.02%, and ethylparaben 0.01% (preservatives).

Indications: For use as a supplemental nutritive source of amino acids, electrolytes, B complex vitamins, and dextrose in cattle and horses.

Dosage and Administration: Administer orally as a drench. The usual recommended dose in adult cattle and horses is 500 to 3000 mL, depending on size and condition.

Precaution(s): Store between 15° and 30°C (59°-86°F).

Caution(s): For animal use only.

Keep out of reach of children.

Presentation: 500 mL and 1000 mL (NDC 59130-601-04) bottles.

Compendium Code No.: 10740040 Rev. 4-95

AMTECH AMISOL-R INJECTION ℞

Phoenix Scientific **Fluid Therapy**

Replacement Electrolytes (Sterile Solution-Nonpyrogenic)

Active Ingredient(s): Each 100 mL Contains:

Sodium Chloride	526 mg
Sodium Acetate	222 mg
Sodium Gluconate	502 mg
Potassium Chloride	37 mg
Magnesium Chloride Hexahydrate	30 mg
Water for Injection	q.s.

May contain hydrochloric acid or sodium hydroxide for pH adjustment.

Electrolytes per 1000 mL (not including ions for pH adjustment): Sodium 140 mEq; Potassium 5 mEq; Magnesium 3 mEq; Chloride 98 mEq; Acetate 27 mEq; Gluconate 23 mEq.

295 mOsm/liter (Calc.)

pH 5.5-7.5 Isotonic

Contains no preservative.

Indications: AMISOL-R is a sterile, nonpyrogenic solution of balanced electrolytes indicated for

A

replacing acute losses of extracellular fluid and electrolytes, and for correcting moderate to severe acidosis.

Dosage and Administration: Contents or lesser amount as determined by veterinarian as a single dose; usually 3-10% of body weight. In shock, up to 10% of body weight in 1-2 hours. For intravenous or subcutaneous use. Solution should be warmed to body temperature and administered slowly.

Precaution(s): Do not use this product if seal is broken or solution is not clear. If entire contents are not used, discard unused portion. Additives may be incompatible. When introducing additives, use aseptic technique, mix thoroughly and do not store.

Protect from freezing.

Caution(s): Federal law restricts this drug to use by or on the order of a licensed veterinarian.

For animal use only.

Not for human use.

Warning(s): Keep out of reach of children.

Presentation: 1000 mL (NDC 59130-654-04).

Compendium Code No.: 10740650 Rev. 12-96

AMTECH ANTHELBAN V ℞

Phoenix Scientific **Parasiticide-Oral**

(pyrantel pamoate) Equine Anthelmintic Suspension

ANADA No.: 200-246

Active Ingredient(s): ANTHELBAN V is a suspension of pyrantel pamoate in a palatable vanilla-flavored vehicle. Each mL contains 50 mg of pyrantel base as pyrantel pamoate.

Indications: For the removal and control of mature infections of large strongyles *(Strongylus vulgaris, S. edentatus, S. equinus);* pinworms *(Oxyuris equi);* large roundworms *(Parascaris equorum);* and small strongyles in horses and ponies.

Pharmacology: Pyrantel pamoate is a compound belonging to a family classified chemically as tetrahydro-pyrimidines. It is a yellow, water-insoluble crystalline salt of the tetrahydropyrimidine base and pamoic acid containing 34.7% base activity. The chemical structure and name are given below:

(E)-1,4,5,6-Tetrahydro-1-methyl-2-[2-(2-thienyl) vinyl] pyrimidine 4, 4' methylenebis [3-hydroxy-2-naphthoate] (1:1)

Dosage and Administration: Administer 3 mg pyrantel base per pound of body weight (6 mL ANTHELBAN V) per 100 lb body weight).

For maximum control of parasitism, it is recommended that foals (2-8 months of age) be dosed every 4 weeks. To minimize potential hazard that the mare may pose to the foal, she should be treated 1 month prior to anticipated foaling date followed by retreatment 10 days to 2 weeks after birth of foal. Horses over 8 months of age should be routinely dosed every 6 weeks.

Directions for Use: ANTHELBAN V may be administered by means of a stomach tube, dose syringe or by mixing into the feed.

Stomach Tube - Measure the appropriate dosage of ANTHELBAN V and mix in the desired quantity of water. Protect drench from direct sunlight and administer to the animal immediately following mixing. Do not attempt to store diluted suspension.

ANTHELBAN V is inactive against the common horse bot (*Gasterophilus* sp.). However, ANTHELBAN V may be administered concurrently with carbon disulfide observing the usual precautions with carbon disulfide.

Dose Syringe - Draw the appropriate dosage of ANTHELBAN V into a dose syringe and administer to the animal. Do not expose ANTHELBAN V to direct sunlight.

Feed - Mix the appropriate dosage of ANTHELBAN V in the normal grain ration. Fasting of animals prior to or following treatment is not required.

Precaution(s): Store below 86°F (30°C).

This product is a suspension and as such will separate. To insure uniform re-suspension and to achieve proper dosage, it is extremely important that the product be shaken and stirred thoroughly before every use.

Caution(s): Federal law restricts this drug to use by or on the order of a licensed veterinarian.

It is recommended that severely debilitated animals not be treated with this preparation.

Warning(s): Not for horses or ponies intended for food. Keep out of reach of children.

Trial Data: Efficacy: Critical (worm-count) studies in horses demonstrated that pyrantel pamoate administered at the recommended dosage was efficacious against mature infections of *Strongylus vulgaris* (>90%), *S. edentatus* (69%), *S. equinus* (>90%), *Oxyuris equi* (81%), *Parascaris equorum* (>90%), and small strongyles (>90%).

Safety: ANTHELBAN V (pyrantel pamoate) is well tolerated by horses and ponies of all ages. No adverse drug response was observed when dose rates up to 60 mg pyrantel base per pound of body weight were administered by stomach tube nor when 3 mg base per pound was given by intratracheal injection. The reproductive performance of pregnant mares and stud horses dosed with ANTHELBAN V has not been affected.

Presentation: 473 mL (1 pint) 16 oz (NDC 59130-692-06) and 946 mL (1 qt) 32 oz (NDC 59130-692-18).

Compendium Code No.: 10740053 Iss. 5-98

AMTECH ASPIRIN BOLUS

Phoenix Scientific **Non-Steroidal Anti-Inflammatory**

Active Ingredient(s): Each bolus contains:

Acetylsalicylic Acid .... 240 grains (15.6 g)

Indications: To be used orally as an aid in reducing fever and in relief of minor muscular aches and joint pains in cattle and horses.

Dosage and Administration: Administer orally.

To mature horses and cattle give 2 to 4 boluses; to foals and calves, 1 to 2 boluses. Allow animals to drink water after administration.

Precaution(s): Do not store above 30°C (86°F). Keep lid tightly closed and store in a dry place.

Warning(s): For animal use only. Keep out of reach of children.

Presentation: 50 boluses (NDC 59130-674-15).

Compendium Code No.: 10740061 Iss. 1-96

AMTECH ATROPINE SULFATE INJECTION 1/120 GRAIN ℞

Phoenix Scientific **Anticholinergic**

Active Ingredient(s): Each mL contains:

Atropine Sulfate .... 0.54 mg
Sodium Chloride .... 9 mg
Benzyl Alcohol (preservative) 1.5%
Water for Injection .... q.s.

pH adjusted with sulfuric acid when necessary.

Indications: As a pre-anesthetic adjuvant or to reduce salivation, bronchial secretion or internal peristalsis associated with colic or diarrhea in dogs and cats. As an antidote for parasympathomimetic drugs.

Dosage and Administration: For intravenous, intramuscular or subcutaneous use.

Dogs and Cats: Inject 1 mL for each 20 lbs of body weight as a pre-anesthetic adjuvant or to reduce salivation, bronchial secretion or internal peristalsis associated with colic or diarrhea.

As an antidote for parasympathomimetic drugs, 1 mL for each 7.5 lbs of body weight. It is suggested that ¼ of the dosage be injected intravenous and the remainder intramuscular or subcutaneous.

Precaution(s): Store between 15°C-30°C (59°F-86°F).

Caution(s): Federal law restricts this drug to use by or on the order of a licensed veterinarian.

Warning(s): Poisonous alkaloid. Keep out of reach of children. Antidotes: Warmth, emetics, cholinergics.

For animal use only.

Presentation: 100 mL sterile multiple dose vials (NDC 59130-671-01).

Compendium Code No.: 10740071 Iss. 12-95

AMTECH CALCIUM GLUCONATE 23% SOLUTION

Phoenix Scientific **Calcium Therapy**

Active Ingredient(s): Each 100 mL contains:

Calcium gluconate (provides 2.14 grams calcium) .... 23 grams
Water for injection .... q.s.

Contains boric acid as a solubilizing agent.

Electrolytes per 1000 mL:

Calcium .... 1069 mEq; Hypertonic
Osmolarity (cal.) .... 6,782 mOsmol/L

This product is sterile in unopened container. It contains no preservative.

Indications: To be used as an aid in the treatment of parturient paresis (milk fever) in cattle.

Dosage and Administration:

Cattle: 250 to 500 mL.

Administer intravenously or intraperitoneally.

Solution should be warmed to body temperature and administered slowly.

Precaution(s): Store between 15°C-30°C (59°F-86°F).

Use entire contents when first opened. It should be handled under aseptic conditions.

Caution(s): If there is no apparent improvement in the animal's condition within 24 hours, consult a veterinarian.

For animal use only.

Keep out of reach of children.

Presentation: 500 mL (NDC 59130-605-03).

Compendium Code No.: 10740090 Rev. 5-95

AMTECH CAL-PHOS #2 INJECTION ℞

Phoenix Scientific **Calcium-Combination Therapy**

Active Ingredient(s): Composition: Each 500 mL contains:

Calcium (complexed as boryl esters of gluconic acid) .... 10.00 grams
Magnesium (obtained from 23.07 grams of magnesium chloride hexahydrate) ... 2.76 grams
Phosphorus (obtained from 20.65 grams of sodium hypophosphite • H_2O) ..... 6.03 grams
Dextrose • H_2O .... 75.00 grams
Water for injection .... q.s.
Osmolarity (cal.) .... 11,760 mOsmol/L

This product contains no preservatives.

Indications: For use as an aid in the treatment of hypocalcemia (parturient paresis, milk fever), hypomagnesemia (grass tetany), and other conditions associated with calcium, phosphorous and magnesium deficiencies in cattle.

Dosage and Administration: Warm solution to body temperature. The usual intravenous dose in cattle is 500 mL per 800 to 1,000 pounds of body weight.

Contraindication(s): Do not administer this product to animals showing signs of cardiac distress.

Precaution(s): Store between 15°C and 30°C (59°F-86°F).

Use entire contents when first opened. Discard any unused solution.

Caution(s): Federal law restricts this drug to use by or on the order of a licensed veterinarian.

Administration should be made slowly and with care to avoid adverse effects such as heart block or shock. Perivascular or subcutaneous deposition of hypertonic solutions may result in severe inflammation at the injection site.

For animal use only.

Keep out of reach of children.

Presentation: 500 mL (NDC 59130-603-03).

Compendium Code No.: 10740080 Rev. 5-95

AMTECH CHLORHEXIDINE SOLUTION

Phoenix Scientific **Antiseptic**

Active Ingredient(s): Contains 2% Chlorhexidine Gluconate.

Indications: A topical aqueous cleaning solution for use on horses and dogs for application to superficial cuts, abrasions or insect stings.

Directions for Use: Rinse skin area to be treated with CHLORHEXIDINE SOLUTION. Wipe away excess and pat dry with a sterile gauze or sponge.

Dilute: 1 ounce (2 tablespoons) of CHLORHEXIDINE SOLUTION per gallon of clean water.

Caution(s): Avoid contact with eyes and mucous membranes. This product is not to be used in ears. If contact is made, flush immediately and thoroughly with clean water. Keep out of reach of children. For use on horses and dogs.

For animal use only.

For external use only.

Presentation: 3.785 L (1 gallon) (NDC 59130-717-05).

Compendium Code No.: 10740100 Iss. 10-98

AMTECH CHLORTETRACYCLINE HCL SOLUBLE POWDER

Phoenix Scientific **Antimicrobial Water Medication**

Antibiotic

ANADA No.: 200-236

Active Ingredient(s): The packet contains 102.4 grams of chlortetracycline hydrochloride (64 g/lb).

Indications: Chickens: Control of infectious synovitis caused by *M. synoviae*, chronic respiratory disease (CRD) and air sac infections caused by *M. gallisepticum* and *E. coli*.

Turkeys: Control of infectious synovitis caused by *M. synoviae* and complicating bacterial organisms associated with bluecomb (transmissible enteritis, coronaviral enteritis).

Swine: Control and treatment of bacterial enteritis (scours) caused by *E. coli* and *Salmonella* spp. and bacterial pneumonia associated with *Pasteurella* spp., *Hemophilus* spp., *Klebsiella* spp.

Directions for Use: For use in drinking water of chickens, turkeys and swine.

Dissolve the contents of one packet of CHLORTETRACYCLINE HCL SOLUBLE POWDER in four (4) gallons of water to prepare a stock solution, when metered at the rate of 1 oz of stock solution per gallon of drinking water, will deliver 200 mg chlortetracycline HCl per gallon of drinking water. One level measuring teaspoon contains approximately 575 mg chlortetracycline hydrochloride which will treat 57.5 lbs (26 kg) of animal at 10 mg/lb for one day. Not to be used for more than 14 consecutive days in chickens and turkeys and five days in swine. The concentration of drug required in drinking water must be adjusted to provide a correct dosage in order to compensate for variations in the age of the animal, class of poultry, environmental temperature and humidity; each of which affects water consumption.

Chickens and Turkeys: Administer for 7 to 14 days. Medicate continuously at the first clinical signs of disease. The dosage range permitted provides for different levels based on the severity of the infection. Consult a poultry diagnostic laboratory or a poultry pathologist to determine the diagnosis and advice regarding the optimum level of the drug where ranges are permitted. As a generalization, 100 turkeys will drink one gallon of water per day for each week of age. Chickens will consume one half this amount.

Dosage:

Chickens: Control of infectious synovitis caused by *M. synoviae* - 200 to 400 mg chlortetracycline hydrochloride per gallon drinking water (5.0-13.4 mg/lb body weight per day). Control of chronic respiratory disease (CRD) and air sac infections caused by *M. gallisepticum* and *E. coli* - 400 to 800 mg chlortetracycline hydrochloride per gallon drinking water (10.0-26.8 mg/lb body weight per day).

Turkeys: Control of infectious synovitis caused by *M. synoviae* - 400 mg chlortetracycline hydrochloride per gallon drinking water (3.2-16.8 mg/lb body weight per day). Control of complicating bacterial organisms associated with bluecomb (transmissible enteritis, coronaviral enteritis)-25 mg chlortetracycline hydrochloride per body weight daily.

Swine: Control and treatment of bacterial enteritis (scours) caused by *E. coli* and *Salmonella* spp. and bacterial pneumonia associated with *Pasteurella* spp., *Hemophilus* spp., *Klebsiella* spp. - 10 mg chlortetracycline hydrochloride per pound body weight daily in divided doses for 3 to 5 days

Precaution(s): Store in cool, dry place.

Caution(s): Prepare a fresh solution daily. When using galvanized waterer, prepare fresh solution every 12 hours. Use only against organisms sensitive to chlortetracycline. Use as the sole source of chlortetracycline. Do not mix in liquid feed supplements, milk or milk replacers. Administer 1 hour before or 2 hours after feeding with milk or milk replacers.

For animal use only.

Restricted Drug(s) (California). Not for human use.

For use in drinking water only.

Use as the sole source of drinking water.

Warning(s): Withdraw 24 hours before slaughter of chickens, turkeys and five days for swine. Do not feed to chickens producing eggs for human consumption. For growing turkeys only.

Keep out of reach of children.

Presentation: 725.8 g (25.6 oz) (NDC 59130-682-29) packets.

Compendium Code No.: 10740113 Iss. 9-01

AMTECH CLINDAMYCIN HYDROCHLORIDE ORAL LIQUID ℞

Phoenix Scientific **Clindamycin**

Antibiotic

ANADA No.: 200-193

Active Ingredient(s): Each mL of CLINDAMYCIN HYDROCHLORIDE ORAL LIQUID contains clindamycin hydrochloride equivalent to 25 mg clindamycin; and ethyl alcohol, 8.64%.

Indications:

Dogs: Aerobic bacteria: CLINDAMYCIN HYDROCHLORIDE ORAL LIQUID is indicated for the treatment of soft tissue infections (wounds and abscesses), dental infections and osteomyelitis caused by susceptible strains of *Staphylococcus aureus*.

Anaerobic bacteria: CLINDAMYCIN HYDROCHLORIDE ORAL LIQUID is indicated for the treatment of soft tissue infections (deep wounds and abscesses), dental infections and osteomyelitis caused by or associated with susceptible strains of *Bacteroides fragilis, Bacteroides melaninogenicus, Fusobacterium necrophorum* and *Clostridium perfringens*. (See Microbiology section for additional information.)

Cats: Aerobic bacteria: CLINDAMYCIN HYDROCHLORIDE ORAL LIQUID is indicated for the treatment of soft tissue infections (wounds and abscesses), and dental infections caused by or associated with susceptible strains of *Staphylococcus aureus, Staphylococcus intermedius* and *Streptococcus* spp.

Anaerobic bacteria: CLINDAMYCIN HYDROCHLORIDE ORAL LIQUID is indicated for the treatment of soft tissue infections (deep wounds and abscesses) and dental infections caused by or associated with susceptible strains of *Clostridium* perfringens and *Bacteroides fragilis*. (See Microbiology section for additional information).

Pharmacology: Description: CLINDAMYCIN HYDROCHLORIDE ORAL LIQUID contains clindamycin hydrochloride which is the hydrated salt of clindamycin. Clindamycin is a semi-synthetic antibiotic produced by a 7(S)-chlorosubstitution of the 7(R)-hydroxyl group of a naturally produced antibiotic produced by *Streptomyces lincolnensis var. lincolnensis*.

CLINDAMYCIN HYDROCHLORIDE ORAL LIQUID is a palatable formulation intended for oral administration to dogs and cats.

Actions:

Site and Mode of Action: Clindamycin is an inhibitor of protein synthesis in the bacterial cell. The site of binding appears to be in the 50S sub-unit of the ribosome. Binding occurs to the soluble RNA fraction of certain ribosomes, thereby inhibiting the binding of amino acids to those ribosomes. Clindamycin differs from cell wall inhibitors in that it causes irreversible modification of the protein-synthesizing subcellular elements at the ribosomal level.

Microbiology: The following clindamycin *in vitro* data are available but their clinical significance is unknown. Clindamycin has been shown to have *in vitro* activity against the following organisms isolated from animals:

Aerobic gram positive cocci, including: *Staphylococcus aureus* (penicillinase and non-penicillinase producing strains), *Staphylococcus intermedius, Staphylococcus simulans, Staphylococcus epidermidis*, Streptococci (except *Enterococcus faecalis)*.

Anaerobic gram negative bacilli, including: *Bacteroides* species, *Fusobacterium* species.

Anaerobic gram positive nonsporeforming bacilli, including: *Propionibacterium, Eubacterium, Actinomyces* species.

Anaerobic and microaerophilic gram positive cocci, including: *Peptococcus* species, *Peptostreptococcus* species, Microaerophilic streptococci.

Clostridia: Most *Cl. perfringens* are susceptible, but other species may be resistant to clindamycin.

Overall Susceptibility to Clindamycin of Anaerobes Isolated from Canine Lesions. Data Obtained from Three Veterinary Diagnostic Laboratories.

	Susceptible ≤3.2 µg/mL	Resistant ≥4.0 µg/mL
All Isolates	122/137 (89%)	15/137 (11%)
Clostridium spp.	41/49 (84%)	8/49 (16%)
Bacteroides spp.	42/46 (91%)	4/46 (9%)
Fusobacterium spp.	16/16 (100%)	0/16 (0%)
Peptostreptococcus spp.	15/16 (94%)	1/16 (6%)
Actinomyces spp.	5/6 (83%)	1/6 (17%)
Proprionibacterium spp.	3/4 (75%)	1/4 (25%)

The MIC values for the anaerobes isolated from feline lesions are not different from the MIC values for the anaerobes isolated from canine lesions.

Mycoplasma species: Most mycoplasma species are susceptible to clindamycin.

Clindamycin and erythromycin show parallel resistance. Partial cross resistance has been demonstrated between clindamycin, erythromycin and macrolide antibiotics.

Absorption: Clindamycin hydrochloride is rapidly absorbed from the canine and feline gastrointestinal tract. Dogs and cats orally dosed with therapeutic amounts of clindamycin hydrochloride demonstrated antibacterial serum levels of the drug within 15 minutes post-dosing.

Canine Serum Levels: Therapeutically effective serum levels of clindamycin hydrochloride can be maintained by oral dosing at the rate of 2.5 mg/lb every 12 hours. Dogs orally dosed with clindamycin hydrochloride at 2.5 mg/lb every 12 hours during a 72 hours dosing regimen continuously maintained antibacterial serum levels of the drug. This same study revealed that average peak serum concentrations occurred 1 hour and 15 minutes after dosing. The biological half-life for clindamycin hydrochloride in dog serum was about 5 hours. There was no bioactivity accumulation after a regimen of multiple oral doses.

Feline Serum Levels: Therapeutically effective serum levels of clindamycin can be maintained by oral dosing at the rate of 5 to 10 mg/lb body weight once every 24 hours. The average peak serum concentration of clindamycin occurs about 1 hour after oral administration. The terminal half-life of clindamycin in feline serum is approximately 7.5 hours. Minimal accumulation occurs after multiple oral doses of clindamycin hydrochloride, and steady-state should be achieved by the third dose.

Clindamycin Serum Concentrations 5 mg/lb (11 mg/kg) After Single Oral Dose of Antirobe Aquadrops:

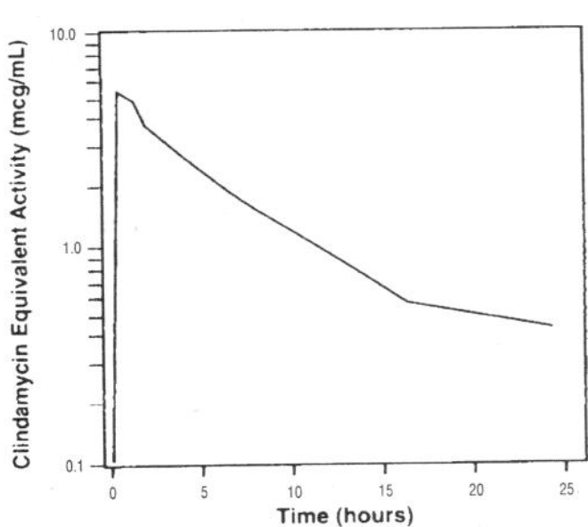

Feline Tissue levels: Tissue concentrations measured at 10 days (µg/g; means) of clindamycin hydrochloride liquid in cats 2 hours after oral administration at 10 mg/lb body weight once every 24 hours for 10 days.

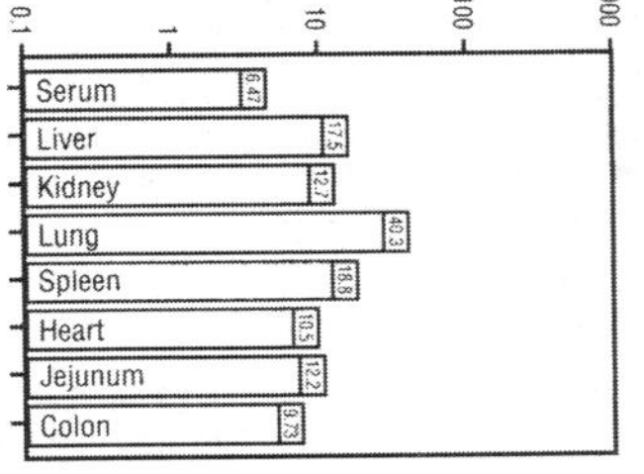

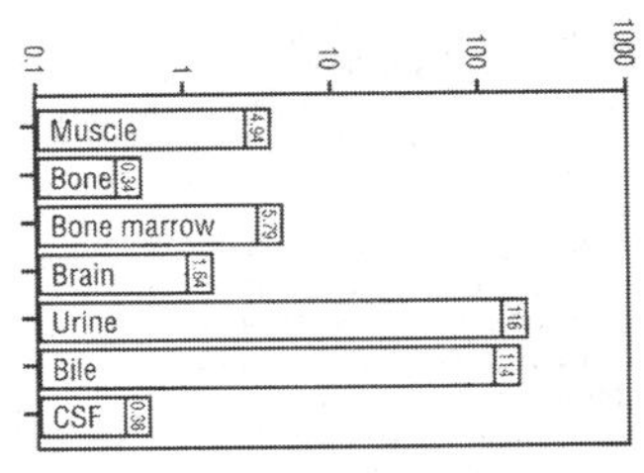

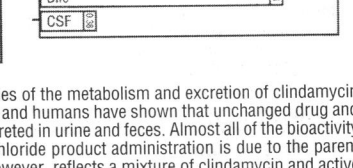

Metabolism and Excretion: Extensive studies of the metabolism and excretion of clindamycin hydrochloride administered orally in animals and humans have shown that unchanged drug and bioactive and bioinactive metabolites are excreted in urine and feces. Almost all of the bioactivity detected in serum after clindamycin hydrochloride product administration is due to the parent molecule (clindamycin). Urine bioactivity, however, reflects a mixture of clindamycin and active metabolites, especially N-demethyl clindamycin and clindamycin sulfoxide.

Dosage and Administration:

Canine Infected Wounds, Abscesses and Dental Infections:

Oral: 2.5 mg/lb body weight every 12 hours.

Duration: Treatment with clindamycin hydrochloride products may be continued up to a maximum of 28 days if clinical judgment indicates. Treatment of acute infections should not be continued for more than three or four days if no response to therapy is seen.

Dosage Schedule:

CLINDAMYCIN HYDROCHLORIDE ORAL LIQUID: Administer 1 mL/10 lbs body weight every 12 hours.

Canine Osteomyelitis:

Oral: 5.0 mg/lb body weight every 12 hours.

Duration: Treatment with CLINDAMYCIN HYDROCHLORIDE ORAL LIQUID is recommended for a minimum of 28 days. Treatment should not be continued for longer than 28 days if no response to therapy is seen.

Dosage Schedule:

CLINDAMYCIN HYDROCHLORIDE ORAL LIQUID: Administer 2 mL/10 lbs body weight every 12 hours.

Feline Infected Wounds and Abscesses and Dental Infections:

Oral: 5.0 to 10.0 mg/lb body weight once every 24 hours depending on the severity of the condition.

Duration: Treatment with CLINDAMYCIN HYDROCHLORIDE ORAL LIQUID may be continued up to a maximum of 14 days if clinical judgment indicates. Treatment of acute infections should not be continued for more than three to four days if no clinical response to therapy is seen.

Dosage Schedule: CLINDAMYCIN HYDROCHLORIDE ORAL LIQUID, to provide 5.0 mg/lb, administer 1 mL/5 lb body weight once every 24 hours; to provide 10.0 mg/lb, administer 2 mL/5 lb body weight once every 24 hours.

Contraindication(s): CLINDAMYCIN HYDROCHLORIDE ORAL LIQUID is contraindicated in animals with a history of hypersensitivity to preparations containing clindamycin or lincomycin.

Because of potential adverse gastrointestinal effects, do not administer to rabbits, hamsters, guinea pigs, horses, chinchillas or ruminating animals.

Precaution(s): Store at controlled room temperature 20°-25°C (68°-77°F).

Caution(s): Federal (USA) law restricts this drug to use by or on the order of a licensed veterinarian.

CLINDAMYCIN HYDROCHLORIDE ORAL LIQUID should be prescribed with caution in atopic animals.

During prolonged therapy of one month or greater, periodic liver and kidney function tests and blood counts should be performed.

The use of clindamycin hydrochloride occasionally results in overgrowth of non-susceptible organisms such as clostridia and yeasts. Therefore, the administration of clindamycin hydrochloride should be avoided in those species sensitive to the gastrointestinal effects of clindamycin (see Contraindications). Should superinfections occur, appropriate measures should be taken as indicated by the clinical situation.

Patients with very severe renal disease and/or very severe hepatic disease accompanied by severe metabolic aberrations should be dosed with caution, and serum clindamycin levels monitored during high-dose therapy.

Clindamycin hydrochloride has been shown to have neuromuscular blocking properties that may enhance the action of other neuromuscular blocking agents. Therefore, clindamycin hydrochloride should be used with caution in animals receiving such agents.

Safety in gestating bitches and queens or breeding male dogs and cats has not been established.

Warning(s): Not for human use.

Toxicology: Toxicology and Safety:

Rat and Dog Data: One year oral toxicity studies in rats and dogs at doses of 30, 100 and 300 mg/kg/day (13.6, 45.5 and 136.4 mg/lb/day) have shown clindamycin hydrochloride to be well tolerated. Differences did not occur in the parameters evaluated to assess toxicity when comparing groups of treated animals with contemporary controls. Rats administered clindamycin hydrochloride at 600 mg/kg/day (272.7 mg/lb/day) for six months tolerated the drug well; however, dogs orally dosed at 600 mg/kg/day (272.7 mg/lb/day) vomited, had anorexia, and subsequently lost weight.

Safety in gestating bitches or breeding males has not been established.

Cat Data: The recommended daily therapeutic dose range for CLINDAMYCIN HYDROCHLORIDE ORAL LIQUID is 11 to 22 mg/kg/day (5 to 10 mg/lb/day) depending on the severity of the condition. CLINDAMYCIN HYDROCHLORIDE ORAL LIQUID was tolerated with little evidence of toxicity in domestic shorthair cats when administered orally at 10x the minimum recommended therapeutic daily dose (11 mg/kg; 5 mg/lb) for 15 days, and at doses up to 5x the minimum recommended therapeutic dose for 42 days. Gastrointestinal tract upset (soft feces to diarrhea) occurred in control and treated cats with emesis occurring at doses 3x or greater than the minimum recommended therapeutic dose (11 mg/kg/day; 5 mg/lb/day). Lymphocytic inflammation of the gallbladder was noted in a greater number of treated cats at the 110 mg/kg/day (50 mg/lb/day) dose level than for control cats. No other effects were noted. Safety in gestating queens or breeding male cats has not been established.

Side Effects: Side effects occasionally observed in either clinical trials or during clinical use were vomiting and diarrhea.

Discussion: *In Vitro* Susceptibility Testing: Susceptibility tests should be done on samples collected prior to initiation of therapy with CLINDAMYCIN HYDROCHLORIDE ORAL LIQUID. Clindamycin susceptibility testing is performed by using Cleocin® Susceptibility Disks (clindamycin 2 mcg) and Cleocin® Susceptibility Powder 20 mg. A standardized disk testing procedure* is recommended for determining susceptibility of aerobic bacteria to clindamycin. A description is contained in the Cleocin® Susceptibility Disk insert. Using this method, the laboratory can designate isolates as resistant, intermediate, or susceptible. Tube or agar dilution methods may be used for aerobic and anaerobic bacteria. When the directions in the Cleocin® Susceptibility Powder insert are followed, a MIC (minimal inhibitory concentration) of 1.6 mcg/mL may be considered susceptible; MICs of 1.6 to 4.8 mcg/mL may be considered intermediate and MICs greater than 4.8 mcg/mL may be considered resistant.

References: *Available upon request.

Presentation: CLINDAMYCIN HYDROCHLORIDE ORAL LIQUID is available as 20 mL filled in 30 mL bottles (25 mg/mL) supplied in packers containing 12 cartoned bottles with direction labels and calibrated dosing droppers.

Compendium Code No.: 10740124

Rev. 6-00

AMTECH CMPK INJECTION ℞

Phoenix Scientific — **Calcium Therapy**

Active Ingredient(s): Composition: Each 500 mL of sterile aqueous solution contains:

Calcium (as calcium borogluconate, equivalent to calcium gluconate 23.2%)	10.8 g
Potassium (as potassium chloride)	8.0 g
Phosphorus (as sodium hypophosphite • H_2O)	2.5 g
Magnesium (as magnesium borogluconate)	1.6 g
Dextrose • H_2O	75.0 g

Milliequivalents per liter:

Cations	
Calcium	1,080 mEq/L
Potassium	410 mEq/L
Magnesium	261 mEq/L
Sodium	161 mEq/L
Anions	
Borogluconate	1,341 mEq/L
Chloride	410 mEq/L
Hypophosphite	161 mEq/L
Osmolarity (calc.)	11,597 mOsmol/L

This product contains no preservatives.

Indications: For use as an aid in the treatment of hypocalcemia (parturient paresis, milk fever), hypomagnesemia (grass tetany), and other conditions associated with calcium, magnesium, phosphorus and potassium deficiencies in cattle.

Dosage and Administration: Warm solution to body temperature. The usual intravenous dose in cattle is 500 mL per 800 to 1,000 pounds of body weight.

Contraindication(s): Do not administer this product to animals showing signs of cardiac distress.

Precaution(s): Store between 15°C and 30°C (59°F - 86°F).

Use entire contents when first opened. Discard any unused solution.

Caution(s): Federal law restricts this drug to use by or on the order of a licensed veterinarian.

Administration should be made slowly and with care to avoid adverse effects such as heart block or shock. Perivascular or subcutaneous deposition of hypertonic solutions may result in severe inflammation at the injection site.

Warning(s): For animal use only.

Keep out of reach of children.

Presentation: 500 mL (NDC 59130-604-03).

Compendium Code No.: 10740131

Rev. 5-95

AMTECH DEXAMETHASONE SODIUM PHOSPHATE INJECTION ℞

Phoenix Scientific — **Corticosteroid Injection**

4 mg/mL

NADA No.: 123-815

Active Ingredient(s): Each mL of sterile aqueous solution contains: Dexamethasone sodium phosphate, 4 mg; sodium citrate, 10 mg; sodium bisulfite, 2 mg; benzyl alcohol, 1.5%; sodium hydroxide and/or hydrochloric acid to adjust pH; water for injection, q.s.

Indications: DEXAMETHASONE SODIUM PHOSPHATE is indicated for use as an anti-inflammatory or glucocorticoid agent in conditions as acute arthritis.

DSP may be used as supportive therapy in non-specific dermatoses such as summer eczema and atopy, provided proper therapy is also instituted to correct the cause of the underlying dermatosis. It may also be used prior to or after surgery to enhance recovery of poor surgical risks, provided that it is used in conjunction with full antibiotic coverage.

Pharmacology: DEXAMETHASONE SODIUM PHOSPHATE (DSP) is a salt of dexamethasone, a synthetic corticosteroid which possesses glucocorticoid activity. DSP is a white or slightly yellow crystalline powder which is particularly suitable for intravenous administration because it is highly water soluble.

Actions: Dexamethasone as a steroid is equivalent in potency to some established steroids and considerably more potent than others. In the case of the dog, dexamethasone is approximately equivalent in dosage to prednisone, but about 30 to 40 times more potent that prednisolone. DSP is especially well suited for intravenous use in situations requiring a rapid and intense glucocorticoid and/or anti-inflammatory effect.

Dosage and Administration: For intravenous use only.

Dogs: 0.25 to 1 mg intravenously as the initial dosage. (Based on 3 mg per mL of dexamethasone). The dose may be repeated for three to five days or until a response is noted.

Horses: 2.5 to 5 mg intravenously. (Based on 3 mg per mL of dexamethasone). If permanent corticosteroid effect is required, oral therapy with dexamethasone may be substituted. When therapy is to be withdrawn after prolonged corticosteroid administration, the daily dose should be reduced gradually over a number of days, in a stepwise fashion.

Contraindication(s): Do not use in viral infections. Except when used for emergency therapy, DSP is contraindicated in animals with tuberculosis, chronic nephritis, Cushing's disease and peptic ulcers. Existence of congestive heart failure, osteoporosis and diabetes are relative contraindications.

When administered in the presence of infections, appropriate antibacterial agents should also be administered and continued for at least 3 days after discontinuance of the steroid.

Precaution(s): Store between 15°C and 30°C (59°F and 86°F).

Caution(s): Federal law restricts this drug to use by or on the order of a licensed veterinarian.

Clinical and experimental data have demonstrated that corticosteroids administered orally or parenterally to animals may induce the first stage of parturition when administered during the last trimester of pregnancy and may precipitate premature parturition followed by dystocia, fetal death, retained placenta and metritis. Additionally, corticosteroids administered in dogs, rabbits, and rodents during pregnancy have resulted in cleft palate in offspring. Corticosteroids administered to dogs during pregnancy have also resulted in other congenital anomalies, including deformed forelegs.

Because of the anti-inflammatory action of corticosteroids, signs of infection may be hidden. It may therefore be necessary to stop treatment until diagnosis is made. Overdosage of some glucocorticoids may result in sodium and fluid retention, potassium loss and weight gains.

In infections characterized by overwhelming toxicity, DSP therapy in conjunction with indicated antibacterial therapy is effective in reducing mortality and morbidity. It is essential that the causative organism be known and an effective anti-bacterial agent be administered concurrently. The injudicious use of adrenal hormones in animals with infections can be hazardous.

Use of corticosteroids, depending on dose, duration and specific steroid, may result in inhibition of endogenous steroid production following drug withdrawal. In patients presently receiving or recently withdrawn from systemic steroid treatments, therapy with a rapid acting corticosteroid should be considered in unusually stressful situations.

Warning(s): Do not use in horses intended for food.

Keep out of reach of children.

Adverse Reactions: The therapeutic use of DSP is unlikely to cause undesired accentuation of metabolic effects. However, if continued corticosteroid therapy is anticipated, a high protein intake should be provided to keep the animal in positive nitrogen balance. A retardant effect on wound healing should be considered when it is used in conjunction with surgery. Euphoria, or an improvement of attitude, and increased appetite are the usual manifestations. The intra-articular injection in leg injuries in the horse may lead to osseous metaplasia.

Side reactions such as glycosuria, hyperglycemia, diarrhea, polydipsia and polyuria have been observed in some species.

- Elevated levels of SGPT and SAP
- Vomiting and diarrhea (occasionally bloody)
- Cushing's syndrome in dogs has been reported in association with prolonged or repeated steroid therapy.
- Corticosteroids reportedly cause laminitis in horses.

Presentation: DEXAMETHASONE SODIUM PHOSPHATE INJECTION is supplied in 30 mL (NDC 59130-755-14) and 100 mL (NDC 59130-755-01) vials containing 4 mg of dexamethasone sodium phosphate per mL. (Equivalent to 3 mg per mL of dexamethasone).
Compendium Code No.: 10740710 Iss. 12-01

AMTECH DEXAMETHASONE SOLUTION ℞

Phoenix Scientific **Corticosteroid Injection**

2 mg per mL

ANADA No.: 200-108
Active Ingredient(s): Each mL contains 2 mg dexamethasone, 500 mg polyethylene glycol 400, 9 mg benzyl alcohol, 1.8 mg methylparaben and 0.2 mg propylparaben as preservatives, 4.75% alcohol, HCl to adjust pH to approximately 4.9, water for injection q.s.
Indications: DEXAMETHASONE SOLUTION is indicated for the treatment of primary bovine ketosis and as an anti-inflammatory agent in the bovine and equine.

As supportive therapy, dexamethasone may be used in the management of various rheumatic, allergic, dermatologic, and other diseases known to be responsive to anti-inflammatory corticosteroids.

DEXAMETHASONE SOLUTION may be used intravenously as supportive therapy when an immediate hormonal response is required.

Bovine Ketosis: DEXAMETHASONE SOLUTION is offered for the treatment of primary ketosis. The gluconeogenic effects of dexamethasone, when administered intramuscularly, are generally noted within the first 6 to 12 hours. When DEXAMETHASONE SOLUTION is used intravenously, the effects may be noted sooner. Blood sugar levels rise to normal levels rapidly and generally rise to above normal levels within 12 to 24 hours. Acetone bodies are reduced to normal concentrations usually within 24 hours. The physical attitude of animals treated with dexamethasone brightens and appetite improves, usually within 12 hours. Milk production, which is suppressed as a compensatory reaction in this condition, begins to increase. In some instances, it may even surpass previous peaks. The recovery process usually takes from three to seven days.

Supportive Therapy: Dexamethasone may be used as supportive therapy in mastitis, metritis, traumatic gastritis, and pyelonephritis, while appropriate primary therapy is administered. In these cases, the corticosteroid combats accompanying stress and enhances the feeling of general well-being.

Dexamethasone may also be used as supportive therapy in inflammatory conditions, such as arthritic conditions, snake bite, acute mastitis, shipping fever, pneumonia, laminitis, and retained placenta.

Equine: Dexamethasone is indicated for the treatment of acute musculoskeletal inflammations, such as bursitis, carpitis, osselets, tendonitis, myositis, and sprains. If boney changes exist in any of these conditions, joints, or accessory structures, responses to dexamethasone cannot be expected. In addition, dexamethasone may be used as supportive therapy in fatigue, heat exhaustion, influenza, laminitis, and retained placenta provided that the primary cause is determined and corrected.
Dosage and Administration: DEXAMETHASONE SOLUTION is intended for intravenous or intramuscular administration.

Therapy with dexamethasone as with any other potent corticosteroid, should be individualized according to the severity of the condition being treated, anticipated duration of steroid therapy, and the animal's threshold or tolerance for steroid excess.

Treatment may be changed over to dexamethasone from any other glucocorticoid with proper reduction or adjustment of dosage.

Bovine:
DEXAMETHASONE SOLUTION - 5 to 20 mg intravenously or intramuscularly.
Equine:
DEXAMETHASONE SOLUTION - 2.5 to 5 mg intravenously or intramuscularly.

Contraindication(s): Except for emergency therapy, do not use in animals with chronic nephritis and hypercorticalism (Cushing's syndrome). Existence of congestive heart failure, diabetes, and osteoporosis are relative contraindications. Do not use in viral infections during the viremic stage.
Precaution(s): Store between 2° and 30<198C (36° and 86°F).
Caution(s): Federal law restricts this drug to use by or on the order of a licensed veterinarian.

Animals receiving Dexamethasone should be under close observation. Because of the anti-inflammatory action of corticosteroids, signs of infection may be masked and it may be necessary to stop treatment until further diagnosis is made. Overdosage of some glucocorticoids may result in sodium retention, fluid retention, potassium loss, and weight gain.

Dexamethasone may be administered to animals with acute or chronic bacterial infections providing the infections are controlled with appropriate antibiotic or chemotherapeutic agents.

Doses greater than those recommended in horses may produce a transient drowsiness or lethargy in some horses. The lethargy usually abates in 24 hours.

Use of corticosteroids, depending on dose, duration, and specific steroid, may result in inhibition of endogenous steroid production following drug withdrawal. In patients presently receiving or recently withdrawn from systemic corticosteroid treatments, therapy with a rapidly acting corticosteroid should be considered in unusually stressful situations.
Warning(s): A withdrawal period has not been established for this product in preruminal calves. Do not use in calves to be processed for veal.
Toxicology: Clinical and experimental data have demonstrated that corticosteroids administered orally or parenterally to animals may induce the first stage of parturition when administered during the last trimester of pregnancy and may precipitate parturition followed by dystocia, fetal death, retained placenta, and metritis.

Additionally, corticosteroids administered to dogs, rabbits, and rodents during pregnancy have produced cleft palate. Other congenital anomalies including deformed forelegs, phocomelia, and anascara have been reported in offspring of dogs which received corticosteroids during pregnancy.
Side Effects: Corticosteroids reportedly cause laminitis in horses.
Discussion: Description: Dexamethasone is a synthetic analogue of prednisolone, having similar but more potent anti-inflammatory therapeutic action and diversified hormonal and metabolic effects. Modification of the basic corticoid structure as achieved in dexamethasone offers enhanced anti-inflammatory effect compared to older corticosteroids. The dosage of dexamethasone required is markedly lower than that of prednisone and prednisolone.

Dexamethasone is not species-specific; however, the veterinarian should read the sections on Indications, Dosage, Side Effects, Contraindications, Cautions and Toxicology before this drug is used.
Trial Data: Experimental Studies: Experimental animal studies on dexamethasone have revealed it possesses greater anti-inflammatory activity than many steroids. Veterinary clinical evidence indicates dexamethasone has approximately twenty times the anti-inflammatory activity of prednisolone and seventy to eighty times that of hydrocortisone. Thymus involution studies show dexamethasone possesses twenty-five times the activity of prednisolone. In reference to mineralcorticoid activity, dexamethasone does not cause significant sodium or water retention. Metabolic balance studies show that animals on controlled and limited protein intake will exhibit nitrogen losses on exceedingly high dosages.
Presentation: DEXAMETHASONE SOLUTION, 2 mg per mL, 100 mL multiple dose vial (NDC 59130-666-01).
Compendium Code No.: 10740152 Rev. 3-01

A

AMTECH DEXOLYTE SOLUTION INJECTION ℞

Phoenix Scientific **Electrolyte Injection**

Electrolytes-Dextrose

Active Ingredient(s): Composition: Each 500 mL of sterile aqueous solution contains:

Dextrose • H_2O	12.50 g
Sorbitol	12.50 g
Sodium lactate	3.95 g
Sodium chloride	2.40 g
Potassium chloride	0.37 g
Magnesium chloride • $6H_2O$	0.21 g
Calcium chloride • $2H_2O$	0.19 g

Milliequivalents per liter:
Cations:

Sodium	153 mEq/L
Potassium	9 mEq/L
Calcium	6 mEq/L
Magnesium	4 mEq/L

Anions:

Chloride	101 mEq/L
Lactate	71 mEq/L
Osmolarity (calc.)	617 mOsmol/L

This product contains no preservatives.
Indications: For use in conditions associated with fluid and electrolyte loss, such as dehydration, shock, vomiting and diarrhea, particularly when an immediate source of energy is also indicated.
Dosage and Administration: Warm solution to body temperature and administer slowly (10 to 30 mL per minute) by intravenous or intraperitoneal injection, using strict aseptic procedures.

Adult Cattle and Horses - 1000 to 2000 mL
Calves, Ponies and Foals - 500 to 1000 mL
Adult Sheep and Swine - 500 to 1000 mL

These are suggested dosages. The actual amount and rate of fluid administration must be judged by the veterinarian in relation to the condition being treated and the clinical response of the animal, being careful to avoid overhydration.
Contraindication(s): Do not administer intraperitoneally to horses.
Precaution(s): Store between 15°C and 30°C (59°F-86°F).

Use entire contents when first opened. Discard any unused solution.
Caution(s): Federal law restricts this drug to use by or on the order of a licensed veterinarian.

For animal use only.
Keep out of reach of children.
Presentation: 500 mL (NDC 59130-606-03) and 1000 mL (NDC 59130-606-04).
Compendium Code No.: 10740161 Rev. 5-95

AMTECH DEXTROSE SOLUTION 50%

Phoenix Scientific **Fluid Therapy**

Active Ingredient(s): Each 100 mL contains:

Dextrose • H_2O	50 g

This product contains no preservatives.
Indications: For use as an aid in the treatment of acetonemia (Ketosis) in cattle.
Dosage and Administration: For intravenous administration only.

Intravenous administration must be done slowly and made under strict aseptic conditions. Solution should be warmed to body temperature prior to administration.

Cattle: 100 to 500 mL depending on size and condition. Treatment may be repeated in several hours or on successive days as needed.
Precaution(s): Store at 15°C-30°C (59°F-86°F).

After a quantity has been withdrawn for injection, the remainder should be discarded.
Caution(s): Do not administer intraperitoneally.

Keep out of reach of children.
For animal use only.
Presentation: 500 mL single dose container (NDC 59130-607-03).
Compendium Code No.: 10740170

AMTECH D-PANTHENOL INJECTION ℞

Phoenix Scientific **Vitamin Injection**

Active Ingredient(s): Each mL contains:

Dexpanthenol	250 mg
Benzyl alcohol	1% w/v
Water for injection	q.s.
Acetic acid, glacial, U.S.P.	to adjust pH

Indications: For use as a nutritional source of d-panthenol.
Dosage and Administration:

Dogs and Cats: 25 mg per 5 lbs. body weight intramuscularly.
Horses: Initial dose 10 mL intravenously or intramuscularly.
Contraindication(s): In therapy of colic resulting from administration of cholinergic type anthelmintics.
Caution(s): Federal law restricts this drug to use by or on the order of a licensed veterinarian.

Following the administration of succinylcholine chloride, a one-hour waiting period is advisable before initiation of dexpanthenol therapy.

For animal use only.
Keep out of reach of children.
Presentation: 100 mL (NDC 59130-650-01).
Compendium Code No.: 10740141 Iss. 2-94

A

AMTECH EPINEPHRINE INJECTION USP ℞

Phoenix Scientific **Epinephrine**

Active Ingredient(s): Each mL contains:

Epinephrine	1 mg
Sodium chloride	9 mg
Sodium metabisulfite	1 mg
Chlorobutanol (preservative)	5 mg
Water for injection	q.s.

With hydrochloric acid to adjust pH.

Indications: Epinephrine is a powerful, quick-acting vasoconstrictor for emergency use only in the treatment of anaphylactic shock.

Dosage and Administration:

Cattle, Horses, Sheep and Swine - Inject subcutaneously or intramuscularly 1 mL per 100 pounds of body weight.

Intravenous injection is not recommended, but if it is found to be clinically necessary, ¼ to ½ of the intramuscular dose should be used.

Precaution(s): Protect from light. Store in refrigerator at 2°-8°C (36°-46°F). Do not freeze.

Do not use injection if it is pinkish or darker than slightly yellow or if it contains precipitate.

Caution(s): Federal law restricts this drug to use by or on the order of a licensed veterinarian.

The symptoms of anaphylactoid shock include glassy eyes, increased salivation, grinding of the teeth, rapid breathing, muscular tremors, staggering gait, and collapse with death following. These symptoms may appear shortly after injection of a bacterin, vaccine, or antibiotic.

Hazardous: Not for human use. Use only as directed.

Keep out of reach of children.

For animal use only.

Presentation: 30 mL sterile multiple dose vial (NDC 59130-672-14).

Compendium Code No.: 10740180

Iss. 12-95

AMTECH FLUNIXIN MEGLUMINE INJECTION ℞

Phoenix Scientific **Analgesic-Anti-inflammatory**

ANADA No.: 200-124

Active Ingredient(s): Description: Each milliliter of FLUNIXIN MEGLUMINE INJECTION contains flunixin meglumine equivalent to 50 mg flunixin, 0.1 mg edetate disodium, 2.5 mg sodium formaldehyde sulfoxylate, 4.0 mg diethanolamine, 207.2 mg propylene glycol; 5.0 mg phenol as preservative, hydrochloric acid, water for injection q.s.

Indications: Horse: FLUNIXIN MEGLUMINE INJECTION is recommended for the alleviation of inflammation and pain associated with musculoskeletal disorders in the horse. It is also recommended for the alleviation of visceral pain associated with colic in the horse.

Cattle: FLUNIXIN MEGLUMINE INJECTION is indicated for the control of pyrexia associated with bovine respiratory disease and endotoxemia. FLUNIXIN MEGLUMINE INJECTION is also indicated for the control of inflammation in endotoxemia.

Pharmacology: Flunixin meglumine is a potent non-narcotic, nonsteroidal analgesic agent with anti-inflammatory and antipyretic activity. It is significantly more potent than pentazocine, meperidine and codeine as an analgesic in the rat yeast paw test.

Horse: Flunixin is four times as potent on a mg per mg basis as phenylbutazone as measured by the reduction in lameness and swelling in the horse. Plasma half-life in horse serum is 1.6 hours following a single dose of 1.1 mg/kg. Measurable amounts are detectable in horse plasma at 8 hours post injection.

Cattle: Flunixin meglumine is a weak acid (pKa=5.82)[1] which exhibits a high degree of plasma protein binding (approximately 99%).[2] However, free (unbound) drug appears to readily partition into body tissues (V_{ss}predictions range from 297 to 782 mL/kg.[2-5] Total body water is approximately equal to 570 mL/kg.[6] In cattle, elimination occurs primarily through biliary excretion.[7] This may, at least in part, explain the presence of multiple peaks in the blood concentration/time profile following IV administration.[2]

In healthy cattle, total body clearance has been reported to range from 90 to 151 mL/kg/hr.[2-5] These studies also report a large discrepancy between the volume of distribution at a steady state (V_{ss}) and the volume of distribution associated with the terminal elimination phase (V_β). This discrepancy appears to be attributable to extended drug elimination from a deep compartment.[8] The terminal half-life has been shown to vary from 3.14 to 8.12 hours.[2-5]

Flunixin persists in inflammatory tissues[9] and is associated with anti-flammatory properties which extend well beyond the period associated with detectable plasma drug concentrations.[4,9] These observations account for the counterclockwise hysteresis associated with flunixin's pharmacokinetic/pharmacodynamic relationships.[10] Therefore, prediction of drug concentrations based upon the estimated plasma terminal elimination half-life will likely underestimate both the duration of drug action and the concentration of drug remaining at the site of activity.

Dosage and Administration: Horse: The recommended dose for musculoskeletal disorders is 0.5 mg per pound (1 mL/100 lbs) of body weight once daily. Treatment may be given by intravenous or intramuscular injection and repeated for up to 5 days. Studies show onset of activity is within 2 hours. Peak response occurs between 12 and 16 hours and duration of activity is 24-36 hours.

The recommended dose for the alleviation of pain associated with equine colic is 0.5 mg per pound of body weight. Intravenous administration is recommended for prompt relief. Clinical studies show pain is alleviated in less than 15 minutes in many cases. Treatment may be repeated when signs of colic recur. During clinical studies approximately 10% of the horses required one or two additional treatments. The cause of colic should be determined and treated with concomitant therapy.

Cattle: The recommended dose for cattle is 1.1 to 2.2 mg/kg (0.5 to 1 mg/lb; 1 to 2 mL per 100 lbs) given by slow intravenous administration either once a day as a single dose or divided into two doses administered at 12-hour intervals for up to 3 days. The total daily dose should not exceed 2.2 mg/kg (1.0 mg/lb) of body weight. Avoid rapid intravenous administration of the drug.

Contraindication(s): Horse: There are no known contraindications to this drug when used as directed. Intra-arterial injection should be avoided. Horses inadvertently injected intra-arterially can show adverse reactions. Signs can be ataxia, incoordination, hyperventilation, hysteria, and muscle weakness. Signs are transient and disappear without antidotal medication within a few minutes. Do not use in horses showing hypersensitivity to flunixin meglumine.

Cattle: There are no known contraindications to this drug in cattle when used as directed. Do not use in animals showing hypersensitivity to flunixin meglumine. Use judiciously when renal impairment or gastric ulceration are suspected.

Precaution(s): Store between 2° and 30°C (36° and 86°F).

Caution(s): Federal law restricts this drug to use by or on the order of a licensed veterinarian.

As a class, cyclo-oxygenase inhibitory NSAIDs may be associated with gastrointestinal and renal toxicity. Sensitivity to drug-associated adverse effects varies with the individual patient. Patients at greatest risk for renal toxicity are those that are dehydrated, on concomitant diuretic therapy, or those with renal, cardiovascular, and/or hepatic dysfunction.

Since many NSAIDs possess the potential to induce gastrointestinal ulceration, concomitant use of FLUNIXIN MEGLUMINE INJECTION with other anti-inflammatory drugs, such as other NSAIDs and corticosteroids, should be avoided or closely monitored.

Horse: The effect of FLUNIXIN MEGLUMINE INJECTION on pregnancy has not been determined. Studies to determine activity of FLUNIXIN MEGLUMINE INJECTION when administered concomitantly with other drugs have not been conducted. Drug compatibility should be monitored closely in patients requiring adjunctive therapy.

Cattle: Do not use in bulls intended for breeding, as reproductive effects of FLUNIXIN MEGLUMINE INJECTION in these classes of cattle have not been investigated. NSAIDS are known to have potential effects on both parturition and the estrous cycle. There may be a delay in the onset of estrus if flunixin is administered during the prostaglandin phase of the estrous cycle. The effects of flunixin on imminent parturition have not been evaluated in a controlled study. NSAIDs are known to have the potential to delay parturition through a tocolytic effect. Do not exceed the recommended dose.

For intravenous or intramuscular use in horses and for intravenous use in beef and nonlactating dairy cattle only. Not for use in lactating and dry dairy cows. Not for use in veal calves.

Warning(s): Residue Warnings: Cattle must not be slaughtered for human consumption within 4 days of the last treatment. Not for use in lactating or dry dairy cows. A withdrawal period has not been established for this product in preruminating calves. Do not use in calves to be processed for veal. Not for use in horses intended for food.

Toxicology: Safety:

Horse: A 3-fold intramuscular dose of 1.5 mg/lb of body weight daily for 10 consecutive days was safe. No changes were observed in hematology, serum chemistry, or urinalysis values. Intravenous dosages of 0.5 mg/lb daily for 15 days; 1.5 mg/lb daily for 10 days; and 2.5 mg/lb daily for 5 days produced no changes in blood or urine parameters. No injection site irritation was observed following intramuscular injection of the 0.5 mg/lb recommended dose. Some irritation was observed following a 3-fold dose administered intramuscularly.

Cattle: No flunixin-related changes (adverse reactions) were noted in cattle administered a 1X (22 mg/kg; 1.0 mg/lb) dose for 9 days (three times the maximum clinical duration). Minimal toxicity manifested itself at moderately elevated doses (3X and 5X) when flunixin was administered daily for 9 days, with occasional findings of blood in the feces and/or urine. Discontinue use if hematuria or fecal blood are observed.

Adverse Reactions: In horses, isolated reports of local reactions following intramuscular injection, particularly in the neck, have been received. These include localized swelling, sweating, induration, and stiffness. In rare instances in horses, fatal or nonfatal clostridial infections or other infections have been reported in association with intramuscular use of Flunixin Meglumine Injectable Solution. In horses and cattle, rare instances of anaphylactic-like reactions, some of which have been fatal, have been reported primarily following intravenous use.

References: Available upon request.

Presentation: FLUNIXIN MEGLUMINE INJECTION, 50 mg/mL, is available in 100 mL and 250 mL multidose vials.

Compendium Code No.: 10740193

Rev. 11-00

AMTECH FUROSEMIDE INJECTION 5% ℞

Phoenix Scientific **Diuretic**

Diuretic-Saluretic

ANADA No.: 200-293

Active Ingredient(s): Each mL contains 50 mg furosemide as a diethanolamine salt preserved and stabilized with myristyl-gamma-picolinium chloride 0.02%, EDTA sodium 0.1%, sodium metasulfite 0.1% with sodium chloride 0.2% in Water For Injection, USP, pH adjusted with sodium hydroxide.

Indications:

Dogs, Cats & Horses: FUROSEMIDE INJECTION 5% is an effective diuretic possessing a wide therapeutic range. Pharmacologically it promotes the rapid removal of abnormally retained extracellular fluids. The rationale for the efficacious use of diuretic therapy is determined by the clinical pathology producing the edema. FUROSEMIDE INJECTION 5% is indicated for the treatment of edema, (pulmonary congestion, ascites) associated with cardiac insufficiency and acute noninflammatory tissue edema.

The continued use of heart stimulants, such as digitalis or its glycosides is indicated in cases of edema involving cardiac insufficiency.

Cattle: FUROSEMIDE INJECTION 5% is indicated for the treatment of physiological parturient edema of the mammary gland and associated structures.

Pharmacology: Description: FUROSEMIDE INJECTION 5% is a chemically distinct diuretic and saluretic pharmacodynamically characterized by the following:

1) A high degree of efficacy, low-inherent toxicity and a high therapeutic index.
2) A rapid onset of action of comparatively short duration.
3) A pharmacological action in the functional area of the nephron, i.e., proximal and distal tubules and the ascending limb of the loop of Henle.
4) A dose-response relationship and a ratio of minimum to maximum effective dose range greater than tenfold.

The intravenous route produces the most rapid diuretic response.

The CAS Registry Number is 54-31-9.

FUROSEMIDE INJECTION 5%, a diuretic, is an anthranilic acid derivative with the following structural formula:

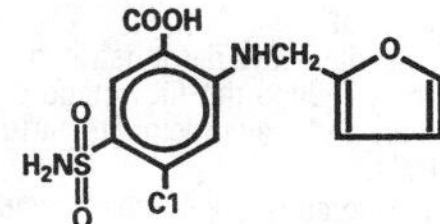

Generic name: Furosemide (except in United Kingdom-furosemide). Chemical name: 4-chloro-N-furfuryl-5-sulfamoylanthranilic acid.

Actions: The therapeutic efficacy of FUROSEMIDE INJECTION 5% is from the activity of the intact and unaltered molecule throughout the nephron, inhibiting the reabsorption of sodium not only in the proximal and distal tubule but also in the ascending limb of the loop of Henle. The prompt onset of action is a result of the drug's rapid absorption and a poor lipid solubility. The low lipid solubility and a rapid renal excretion minimize the possibility of its accumulation in tissues and organs or crystalluria. FUROSEMIDE INJECTION 5% has no inhibitory effect on carbonic anhydrase or aldosterone activity in the distal tubule. The drug possesses diuretic activity either in the presence of acidosis or alkalosis.

Dosage and Administration: The usual dosage of FUROSEMIDE INJECTION 5% is 1 to 2 mg/lb.

body weight (approximately 2.5 to 5 mg/kg). The lower dose is suggested for cats. Administer once or twice daily at 6- to 8-hour intervals either intravenously or intramuscularly. A prompt diuresis usually ensues from the initial treatment. Diuresis may be initiated by the parenteral administration of FUROSEMIDE INJECTION 5%.

The dosage should be adjusted to the individual's response. In severe edematous or refractory cases, the dose may be doubled or increased by increments of 1 mg per pound body weight. The established effective dose should be administered once or twice daily. The daily schedule of administration can be timed to control the period of micturition for the convenience of the client or veterinarian. Mobilization of the edema may be most efficiently and safely accomplished by utilizing an intermittent daily dosage schedule, i.e., every other day or 2 to 4 consecutive days weekly.

Diuretic therapy should be discontinued after reduction of the edema, or maintained after determining a carefully programmed dosage schedule to prevent recurrence of edema. For long-term treatment, the dose can generally be lowered after the edema has once been reduced. Re-examination and consultations with client will enhance the establishment of a satisfactorily programmed dosage schedule. Clinical examination and serum BUN, CO_2 and electrolyte determinations should be performed during the early period of therapy and periodically thereafter, especially in refractory cases. Abnormalities should be corrected or the drug temporarily withdrawn.

Dosage: Parenteral:

Dogs & Cats: Administer intramuscularly or intravenously ¼ to ½ mL per 10 pounds body weight. Administer one or twice daily, permitting a 6- to 8-hour interval between treatments. In refractory or severe edematous cases the dosage may be doubled or increased by increments of 1 mg per pound body weight as recommended in preceding paragraphs. "Dosage and Administration".

Horse: The individual dose is 250 to 500 mg (5 to 10 mL) administered intramuscularly or intravenously once or twice daily at 6- to 8-hour intervals until desired results are achieved. The veterinarian should evaluate the degree of edema present and adjust dosage schedule accordingly.

Cattle: The individual dose administered intramuscularly or intravenously is 500 mg (10 mL) once daily or 250 g (5 mL) twice daily at 12-hour intervals. Treatment not to exceed 48 hours postparturition.

Contraindication(s): FUROSEMIDE INJECTION 5% is a highly effective diuretic-saluretic which if given in excessive amounts may result in dehydration and electrolyte imbalance. Therefore, the dosage and schedule may have to be adjusted to the patient's needs. The animal should be observed for early signs of electrolyte imbalance, and corrective measures administered. Early signs of electrolyte imbalance are: increased thirst, lethargy, drowsiness or restlessness, fatigue, oliguria, gastro-intestinal disturbances and tachycardia. Special attention should be given to potassium levels. FUROSEMIDE INJECTION 5% may lower serum calcium levels and cause tetany in rare cases of animals having an existing hypocalcemic tendency.

Although diabetes mellitus is a rarely reported disease in animals, active or latent diabetes mellitus may on rare occasions be exacerbated by FUROSEMIDE INJECTION 5%. While it has not been reported in animals the use of high doses of salicylates, as in rheumatic diseases, in conjunction with FUROSEMIDE INJECTION 5% may result in salicylate toxicity because of competition for renal excretory sites.

Transient loss of auditory capacity has been experimentally produced in cats following intravenous injection of excessive doses of FUROSEMIDE INJECTION 5% at a very rapid rate.

Electrolyte balance should be monitored prior to surgery in patients receiving FUROSEMIDE INJECTION 5%. Imbalances must be corrected by administration of suitable fluid therapy.

FUROSEMIDE INJECTION 5% is contraindicated in anuria. Therapy should be discontinued in cases of progressive renal disease if increasing azotemia and oliguria occur during the treatment. Sudden alterations of fluid and electrolyte imbalance in an animal with cirrhosis may precipitate hepatic coma, therefore observation during period of therapy is necessary. In hepatic coma and in states of electrolyte depletion, therapy should not be instituted until the basic condition is improved or corrected. Potassium supplementation may be necessary in cases routinely treated with potassium-depleting steroids.

Precaution(s): Store between 15°C and 30°C (59°-86°F).

Caution(s): Federal law restricts this drug to use by or on the order of a licensed veterinarian.

FUROSEMIDE INJECTION 5% is a highly effective diuretic and if given in excessive amounts as with any diuretic may lead to excessive diuresis which could result in electrolyte imbalance, dehydration and reduction of plasma volume enhancing the risk of circulatory collapse, thrombosis, and embolism. Therefore, the animal should be observed for early signs of fluid depletion with electrolyte imbalance, and corrective measures administered. Excessive loss of potassium in patients receiving digitalis or its glycosides may precipitate digitalis toxicity. Caution should be exercised in animals administered potassium-depleting steroids.

It is important to correct potassium deficiency with dietary supplementation. Caution should be exercised in prescribing enteric-coated potassium tablets.

There have been several reports in human literature, published and unpublished, concerning nonspecific small-bowel lesions consisting of stenosis, with or without ulceration, associated with the administration of enteric-coated thiazides with potassium salts. These lesions may occur with enteric-coated potassium tablets alone or when they are used with nonenteric-coated thiazides, or certain other oral diuretics. These small-bowel lesions may have caused obstruction, hemorrhage, and perforation. Surgery was frequently required, and deaths have occurred. Available information tends to implicate enteric-coated potassium salts, although lesions of this type also occur spontaneously. Therefore, coated potassium-containing formulations should be administered only when indicated and should be discontinued immediately if abdominal pain, distension, nausea, vomiting, or gastro-intestinal bleeding occurs.

Human patients with known sulfonamide sensitivity may show allergic reactions to FUROSEMIDE INJECTION 5%, however, these reactions have not been reported in animals.

Sulfonamide diuretics have been reported to decrease arterial responsiveness to pressor amines and to enhance the effect of tubocurarine. Caution should be exercised in administering curare or its derivatives to patients undergoing therapy with FUROSEMIDE INJECTION 5% and it is advisable to discontinue FUROSEMIDE INJECTION 5% for one day prior to any elective surgery.

For animal use only.

Warning(s):

Cattle: Milk taken from animals during treatment and for 48 hours (four milkings) after the last treatment must not be used for food. Cattle must not be slaughtered for food within 48 hours following last treatment.

Horses: Do not use in horses intended for food.

Keep out of reach of children.

Toxicology: Acute Toxicity: The following table illustrates low acute toxicity of FUROSEMIDE INJECTION 5% in three different species. (Two values indicate two different studies.)

LD50 of FUROSEMIDE INJECTION 5% in mg/kg body weight:

Species	Oral	Intravenous
Mouse	1050-1500	308
Rat	2650-4600*	680
Dog	>1000 and >4640	>300 and >464

*Note: The lower value for the rat oral LD50 was obtained in a group of fasted animals; the higher figure is from a study performed in fed rats.

Toxic doses lead to convulsions, ataxia, paralysis and collapse. Animals surviving toxic dosages may become dehydrated and depleted of electrolytes due to the massive diuresis and saluresis.

Chronic Toxicity: Chronic toxicity studies with FUROSEMIDE INJECTION 5% were done in a one-year study in rats and dogs. In a one-year study in rats, renal tubular degeneration occurred with all doses higher than 50 mg/kg. A six-month study in dogs revealed calcification and scarring of the renal parenchyma at all doses above 10 mg/kg.

Reproductive Studies: Reproductive studies were conducted in mice, rats and rabbits. Only in rabbits administered high doses (equivalent to 10 to 25 times the recommended average dose of 2 mg/kg for dogs, cats, horses, and cattle) of furosemide during the second trimester period did unexplained maternal deaths and abortions occur. The administration of FUROSEMIDE INJECTION 5% is not recommended during the second trimester of pregnancy.

Presentation: Available in 50 mL multidose vials for dogs, cats, horses and cattle (NDC 59130-709-11) and 100 mL multidose vials for horses and cattle (NDC 59130-709-01).

Compendium Code No.: 10740660 Rev. 01-00

AMTECH GENTAMAX™ 100 ℞

Phoenix Scientific **Gentamicin**

(Gentamicin Sulfate Solution) 100 mg/mL

ANADA No.: 200-137

Active Ingredient(s): Each mL of GENTAMAX™ 100 (Gentamicin Sulfate Solution) contains: Gentamicin sulfate equivalent to 100 mg gentamicin base; 3.2 mg sodium metabisulfite; 0.1 mg edetate disodium; 1.8 mg methylparaben and 0.2 mg propylparaben as preservatives; water for injection q.s.

Indications: GENTAMAX™ 100 (Gentamicin Sulfate Solution) is recommended for the control of bacterial infections of the uterus (metritis) in horses and as an aid in improving conception in mares with uterine infections caused by bacteria sensitive to gentamicin.

Bacteriologic studies should be conducted to identify the causative organism and to determine its sensitivity to gentamicin sulfate. Sensitivity discs of the drug are available for this purpose.

Pharmacology: Chemistry: Gentamicin is a mixture of aminoglycoside antibiotics derived from the fermentation of *Micromonospora purpurea*. Gentamicin sulfate is a mixture of sulfate salts of the antibiotics produced in this fermentation. The salts are weakly acidic, freely soluble in water, and stable in solution.

Antibacterial Activity: *In vitro* antibacterial activity has shown that gentamicin is active against most gram-negative and gram-positive bacteria isolated from domestic animals.[1] Gentamicin is active against *Pseudomonas aeruginosa*, indole-positive and -negative *Proteus* species, *Escherichia coli*, *Klebsiella* species, *Enterobacter* species, *Alcaligenes* species, *Staphylococcus* species, and *Streptococcus* species.

Studies in man indicate that recommended doses of gentamicin produce serum concentrations bactericidal for most bacteria sensitive to gentamicin within an hour after intramuscular injection; these concentrations last for 6 to 12 hours.[2] Some 30% of the administered dose of gentamicin is bound by serum proteins and released as the drug is excreted.

Gentamicin is excreted almost entirely by glomerular filtration. High concentrations of the active form are found in the urine. Fifty to 100% of the gentamicin injected can be recovered unchanged within 24 hours from the urine of patients with normal renal function. A small amount is excreted into the bile.

Dosage and Administration: The recommended dose is 20 to 25 mL (2.0-2.5 grams) gentamicin sulfate solution per day for 3 to 5 days during estrus. Each dose should be diluted with 200-500 mL of sterile physiological saline before aseptic uterine infusion.

Contraindication(s): There are no known contraindications to this drug when used as directed.

Precaution(s): Store between 2° and 30°C (36° and 86°F). Protect from freezing.

Caution(s): Federal law restricts this drug to use by or on the order of a licensed veterinarian.

If hypersensitivity to any of the components develops, or if an overgrowth of nonsusceptible bacteria, fungi, or yeasts occurs, treatment with GENTAMAX™ 100 (Gentamicin Sulfate Solution) should be discontinued and appropriate therapy instituted. Although GENTAMAX™ 100 (Gentamicin Sulfate Solution) is not spermicidal, treatment should not be given the day of breeding.

For intra-uterine use in horses only.

Not for human use.

Warning(s): Not for use in horses intended for food.

Toxicology: Toxicity Studies: No toxic effects were observed in rats given gentamicin sulfate 20 mg/kg/day for 24 days; in cats given 10 mg/kg/day for 40 days. Gentamicin sulfate given to dogs at 6 mg/lb/day, 6 days weekly for 3 weeks, caused no detectable kidney damage. At higher doses, impairment of equilibrium and renal function were observed in these species.

Side Effects: There have been no reports of drug hypersensitivity or adverse side effects following the recommended intrauterine infusion of gentamicin sulfate solution combined with sterile physiological saline in mares.

References: Available upon request.

Presentation: GENTAMAX™ 100 (Gentamicin Sulfate Solution), 100 mg per mL for intrauterine use, is available in 100 mL (NDC 59130-667-01) and 250 mL (NDC 59130-667-02) multiple dose vials.

Compendium Code No.: 10740201 Rev. 4-97

AMTECH GENTAMICIN SULFATE PIG PUMP ORAL SOLUTION ℞

Phoenix Scientific **Gentamicin Oral**

Antibacterial

ANADA No.: 200-174

Active Ingredient(s): Description: Each milliliter of GENTAMICIN SULFATE PIG PUMP ORAL SOLUTION contains gentamicin sulfate, equivalent to 5 mg gentamicin.

Indications: GENTAMICIN SULFATE PIG PUMP ORAL SOLUTION is recommended for the control and treatment of colibacillosis in neonatal pigs 1-3 days of age, caused by strains of *E. Coli* sensitive to gentamicin.

Pharmacology: Chemistry: Gentamicin is a mixture of aminoglycoside antibiotics derived from the fermentation of *Micromonospora purpurea*. Gentamicin sulfate is a mixture of sulfate salts of the antibiotics produced in this fermentation. The salts are weakly acidic and freely soluble in water. Gentamicin sulfate is stable in the subject solution under usual storage conditions for periods indicated by the expiration date.

Dosage and Administration: Administer orally to baby pigs. Recommended dose is one full pump per pig one time at the first sign of disease. One pump delivers 1 mL of GENTAMICIN SULFATE PIG PUMP SOLUTION (5 mg gentamicin).

Directions for Use: Unlock pump with counterclockwise turn, and press plunger down two times to fill delivery unit. A separate extension tube is enclosed for administration convenience. Administer 1 full pump (plunger depression) directly into the mouth of each affected pig.

Contraindication(s): There are no known contraindications to this drug when used as directed.

Precaution(s): Store between 2° and 30°C (36° and 86°F).

Destroy partially used contents 90 days after opening.

Warning(s): For use in neonatal swine only.

Pigs treated with the recommended dose of GENTAMICIN SULFATE PIG PUMP ORAL SOLUTION must not be slaughtered for food at least 14 days following treatment.

Presentation: GENTAMICIN SULFATE PIG PUMP ORAL SOLUTION, 5 mg per mL is available in 118 mL (4 fl oz) bottles (approximately 118 doses) with pump applicator (NDC 59130-663-07).

Compendium Code No.: 10740210 Iss. 4-97

AMTECH GENTAPOULT™

Phoenix Scientific **Gentamicin**

(Gentamicin Sulfate Injection) Sterile Injection Veterinary

ANADA No.: 200-147

Active Ingredient(s): Description: Each milliliter of GENTAPOULT™ (Gentamicin Sulfate Injection) contains gentamicin sulfate veterinary, equivalent to 100 mg gentamicin base; 3.2 mg sodium metabisulfite; 0.1 mg edetate disodium; 4.5 mg sodium acetate anhydrous; 3.0 mg glacial acetic acid; 0.8 mg methylparaben and 0.1 mg propylparaben as preservatives; water for injection q.s.

Indications: GENTAPOULT™ (Gentamicin Sulfate Injection) is recommended for the prevention of early mortality in day-old chickens associated with *Escherichia coli, Salmonella typhimurium,* and *Pseudomonas aeruginosa* susceptible to gentamicin sulfate. Turkeys — as an aid in the prevention of early mortality of 1 to 3 day-old turkeys associated with *Arizona paracolon* infections susceptible to gentamicin sulfate.

Pharmacology: Chemistry: Gentamicin sulfate veterinary is a bactericidal aminoglycoside antibiotic derived from *Micromonospora purpurea* of the Actinomycetes group. It is a powder, readily soluble in water and basic in nature. Gentamicin aqueous solutions do not require refrigeration and are stable over a wide range of temperatures and pH.

Dosage and Administration:

Chickens: Each day-old chicken should be aseptically injected subcutaneously in the neck with GENTAPOULT™ (Gentamicin Sulfate Injection) diluted with sterile, physiological saline solution to provide 0.2 mg gentamicin in a 0.2 mL dose. This concentration can be provided by diluting GENTAPOULT™ (Gentamicin Sulfate Injection) as follows:

GENTAPOULT™ (Gentamicin Sulfate Injection) mL	Sterile Saline mL	No. of Doses	Dose/Chicken mL
1	99	500	0.2
2	198	1000	0.2
4	396	2000	0.2
10	990	5000	0.2
100 (1 vial)	9900	50000	0.2

Turkeys: Each 1 to 3 day-old turkey should be aseptically injected subcutaneously in the neck with GENTAPOULT™ (Gentamicin Sulfate Injection) diluted with sterile, physiologic saline solution to provide 1 mg gentamicin in a 0.2 mL dose. The dose should be injected under the loose skin on top of the neck, halfway between the head and the base of the neck. This concentration can be provided by diluting GENTAPOULT™ (Gentamicin Sulfate Injection) as follows:

GENTAPOULT™ (Gentamicin Sulfate Injection) mL	Sterile Saline mL	No. of Doses	Dose/Turkey mL
1	19	100	0.2
2	38	200	0.2
4	76	400	0.2
10	190	1000	0.2
100 (1 vial)	1900	10000	0.2

Clean and sterilize needles and syringes by boiling in water for 15 minutes prior to use. Disinfect the injection site and top of the bottle with a suitable disinfectant, such as 70% isopropyl alcohol. Use all precautions to prevent contamination of vial contents.

Precaution(s): Protect from freezing.

Store between 15°C and 30°C (59°F and 86°F).

Caution(s): For use in day-old chickens and 1 to 3-day old turkeys only.

For subcutaneous use only.

Warning(s): Chickens injected with GENTAPOULT™ (Gentamicin Sulfate Injection) must not be slaughtered for food for a least five (5) weeks following treatment. Turkeys injected with GENTAPOULT™ (Gentamicin Sulfate Injection) must not be slaughtered for food for at least nine (9) weeks following treatment.

Presentation: GENTAPOULT™ (Gentamicin Sulfate Injection) 100 mg/mL is available in 100 mL vials (NDC 59130-742-01).

Compendium Code No.: 10740670 Iss. 4-01

AMTECH GUAIFENESIN INJECTION ℞

Phoenix Scientific **Muscle Relaxant**

ANADA No.: 200-230

Active Ingredient(s): Each mL of the injection contains: 50 mg guaifenesin, 50 mg dextrose (anhydrous), 20 mg propylene glycol, 50 mg dimethylacetamide (parenteral grade), 0.75 mg edetate disodium, water for injection q.s.

This is a single dose vial, containing no preservative.

Indications: For intravenous use as a skeletal muscle relaxant for horses.

Pharmacology: Description: Guaifenesin, 3 - (o-Methoxyphenoxy) 1,2-propanediol, is a white to slightly gray, crystalline powder having a bitter taste. It may have a slight characteristic odor.

Actions: Guaifenesin is a guaiacol derivative closely related to mephenesin. The propanediol derivatives are central-acting skeletal muscle relaxants which selectively depress transmission of nerve impulses at the internuncial neurons of the spinal cord, brainstem, and subcortical regions of the brain.

Propanediol derivatives have a wide margin of safety, the toxic dose is three times greater than the recommended dose. Respiration is not severely depressed, and the function of the diaphragm is uninterrupted.[1,2] Tidal volume is slightly decreased and minute volume remains normal. In addition to skeletal muscle, the pharyngeal and laryngeal muscles are sufficiently relaxed for easier surgical intubation procedures. At the beginning of relaxation, there is a slight fall in blood pressure, however, throughout the relaxation period the heart function is unchanged. There is a slight increase in gastrointestinal activity. There is no apparent impairment of lung and kidney functions.

With the recommended administration and dosage of GUAIFENESIN INJECTION, induction is usually smooth and rapid (two to four minutes) providing a duration of action between 15 to 25 minutes. A slightly transient hemolysis occurs at a 5% concentration.[3,4] Higher concentrations cause intravascular hemolysis.[3,5]

The 5% dextrose minimizes the hemolytic action of guaifenesin alone and reduces the tendency to form thrombi at the intravenous injection site.[6] Guaifenesin appears safe when administered to pregnant mares[7] and in human studies did not pass the placental barrier.[2]

Metabolism and excretion of guaifenesin is not well understood. Oxidation products are excreted in the urine as a glycuronimide.

Dosage and Administration: For intravenous use only. Administer rapidly with a positive pressure system or gravity flow using a 12 to 14 gauge needle at the dose rate of 1 mL/pound of body weight. From a standing position the patient will begin to relax and gradually fall when approximately ½ the total dose has been given. Continue the remaining calculated dose for complete relaxation. Average duration of muscle relaxation is 10-25 minutes. For continued relaxation time, additional GUAIFENESIN INJECTION may be administered as determined by the veterinarian at a rate necessary to achieve the desired plane of relaxation. Recovery is usually smooth and uneventful with the horse regaining an upright position usually within 45 minutes after the medication is discontinued.

Contraindication(s): Do not administer physostigmire to horses receiving GUAIFENESIN INJECTION.

Precaution(s): Store between 2° and 30°C (36° and 86°F). Do not freeze.

Destroy partially used vials.

Caution(s): Federal law restricts this drug to use by or on the order of a licensed veterinarian.

Avoid perivascular leakage to prevent local tissue irritation.

If used for prolonged periods, such as in tetanus, serum hemoglobin levels should be monitored.

Oxygen or sustained artificial respiration facilities should be available when the drug is employed.

Additional care should be employed when administering the drug to anemic or hypovolemic animals with cardiac or respiratory problems.

Extreme care should be exercised at all times in handling this product to prevent the introduction of microbial contamination.

For intravenous use in horses only.

For animal use only.

Not for human use.

Keep out of the reach of children.

Warning(s): Not to be used in horses intended for food.

References: Available upon request.

Presentation: 1,000 mL sterile, single dose plastic vial (NDC 59130-690-04).

Compendium Code No.: 10740221 Rev. 5-98

AMTECH HYPERTONIC SALINE SOLUTION 7.2% ℞

Phoenix Scientific **Saline Solution**

Active Ingredient(s): Composition: Each 100 mL of sterile aqueous solution contains:

Sodium chloride . . . . 7.2 g

Milliequivalents per liter:

Cations:

Sodium . . . . 1232 mEq/L

Anions:

Chloride . . . . 1232 mEq/L

Total osmolarity is 2464 milliosmoles per liter.

This product contains no preservatives.

Indications: For use in replacement therapy of sodium, chloride and water which may become depleted in many diseases.

Dosage and Administration: Warm to body temperature and administer slowly by intravenous or subcutaneous injection. The amount and rate of administration must be judged in relation to the condition being treated and the clinical response of the animal, being careful to avoid overhydration.

Precaution(s): Store between 15°C-30°C (59°F-86°F).

Use entire contents when first opened. Discard any unused solution.

Caution(s): Federal law restricts this drug to use by or on the order of a licensed veterinarian.

For animal use only.

Keep out of reach of children.

Presentation: 1000 mL (NDC 59130-628-04).

Compendium Code No.: 10740230

AMTECH IRON DEXTRAN INJECTION

Phoenix Scientific **Iron Injection**

(Iron Hydrogenated Dextran)

ANADA No.: 200-254

Active Ingredient(s): IRON DEXTRAN INJECTION is a sterile solution containing ferric hydroxide in complex with a low molecular weight dextran fraction equivalent to 100 mg elemental iron per mL with 0.5% phenol as a preservative.

Indications: IRON DEXTRAN INJECTION is intended for the prevention or treatment of iron deficiency anemia in baby pigs.

Dosage and Administration: Intramuscular injection.

Prevention: 1 mL (100 mg) at 2-4 days of age.

Treatment: 1 mL (100 mg).

May be repeated in approximately 10 days.

Directions for Use: Disinfect rubber stopper of vial as well as site of injection. Use small needle

(20 gauge, ⅝ inch) that has been sterilized (boiled in water for 20 minutes). Injection should be intramuscular into the back of the ham.

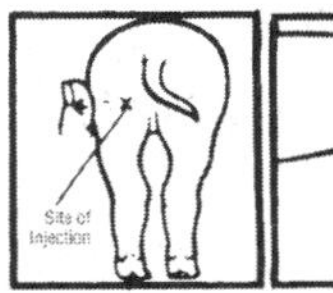

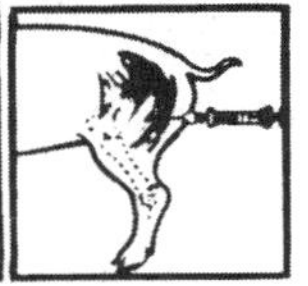

Notice: Organic iron preparation injected intramuscularly into pigs beyond 4 weeks of age may cause staining of muscle tissue.

Precaution(s): Store at controlled room temperature 59°-86°F (15°-30°C).

Caution(s): IRON DEXTRAN INJECTION cannot be considered a substitute for sound animal husbandry. If disease is present in the litter consult a veterinarian.

For intramuscular use only. For use in animals only. Keep out of reach of children.

Side Effects: Occasionally pigs may show a reaction to injectable iron, clinically characterized by prostration with muscular weakness. In extreme cases, death may result.

Discussion: IRON DEXTRAN INJECTION is easy and economical to use. Injection into the ham is rapid, safe, effective, quickly absorbed by the blood and goes to work immediately. With IRON DEXTRAN INJECTION the right dosage can be given to every animal with assurance that it will be utilized.

Iron deficiency anemia occurs commonly in the suckling pig, often within the first few days following birth. As body size and blood volume increase rapidly from the first few days following birth, hemoglobin levels in the blood fall due to diminishing iron reserves which cannot be replaced adequately from iron in the sow's milk. This natural deficiency lowers the resistance of the pig and scours, pneumonia or other infections may develop and lead to death of the animal. Pigs not hampered by iron deficiency anemia are more likely to experience normal growth and to maintain their normal level of resistance to disease.

Presentation: IRON DEXTRAN INJECTION is available in 100 mL multidose vials (NDC 59130-705-01).

Compendium Code No.: 10740240 Rev. 7-99

AMTECH IRON DEXTRAN INJECTION-200

Phoenix Scientific **Iron Injection**

Hematinic 200 mg/mL

ANADA No.: 200-256

Active Ingredient(s): Description: IRON DEXTRAN INJECTION-200 is a sterile solution containing ferric hydroxide in complex with a low molecular weight dextran fraction equivalent to 200 mg elemental iron per mL with 0.5% phenol as a preservative.

Indications: IRON DEXTRAN INJECTION-200 is intended for the prevention or treatment of anemia in baby pigs due to iron deficiency.

Dosage and Administration: For intramuscular injection only.

For the prevention of anemia due to iron deficiency, administer an intramuscular injection of 200 milligrams of elemental iron (1 mL) at 1 to 3 days of age. For the treatment of anemia due to iron deficiency, administer an intramuscular injection of 200 milligrams of elemental iron (1 mL) at the first signs of anemia.

Directions for Use: Disinfect rubber stopper of vial as well as site of injection. Use small needle (20 gauge, ⅝ inch) that has been sterilized (boiled in water for 20 minutes). Injection should be intramuscular into the back of the ham. Place tension on the skin over the rear of the ham and inject to a depth of ½" or slightly more.

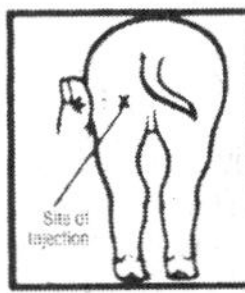

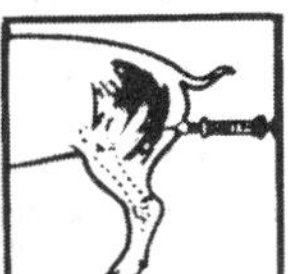

IRON DEXTRAN INJECTION-200 cannot be considered a substitute for sound animal husbandry. If disease is present in the litter, consult a veterinarian.

Precaution(s): Store at controlled room temperature 59°-86°F (15°-30°C).

Caution(s): For animal use only. Keep out of reach of children.

Side Effects: Occasionally pigs may show a reaction to injectable iron, clinically characterized by prostration with muscular weakness. In extreme cases, death may result.

Notice: Organic iron preparation injected intramuscularly into pigs beyond 4 weeks of age may cause staining of the ham muscle.

Discussion: Actions: IRON DEXTRAN INJECTION-200 is easy and economical to use. Injection into the ham is rapid, safe, effective, quickly absorbed by the blood and goes to work immediately. With IRON DEXTRAN INJECTION-200, the right dosage can be given to every animal with assurance that it will be utilized. Iron deficiency anemia occurs commonly in the suckling pig, often within the first few days following birth. As body size and blood volume increase rapidly from the first few days following birth, hemoglobin levels in the blood fall due to diminishing iron reserves which cannot be replaced adequately from iron in the sow's milk. This natural deficiency lowers the resistance of the pig and scours, pneumonia or other infections may develop and lead to death of the animal. Pigs not hampered by iron deficiency anemia are more likely to experience normal growth and to maintain their normal level of resistance to disease. Adequate iron is necessary for normal, healthy, vigorous growth.

Presentation: IRON DEXTRAN INJECTION-200, 200 mg/mL is available in 100 mL multidose vials.

Compendium Code No.: 10740250 Rev. 9-99

AMTECH KETAMINE HYDROCHLORIDE INJECTION, USP Ⓒⅲ

Phoenix Scientific **General Anesthetic**

ANADA No.: 200-042

Active Ingredient(s): KETAMINE HYDROCHLORIDE INJECTION, USP is supplied as a slightly acid (pH 3.5 to 5.5) solution for intramuscular injection in a concentration containing the equivalent of 100 mg ketamine base per milliliter and contains 0.1 mg/mL benzethonium chloride as a preservative.

Indications: KETAMINE HYDROCHLORIDE INJECTION, USP may be used in cats for restraint or as the sole anesthetic agent for diagnostic or minor, brief, surgical procedures that do not require skeletal muscle relaxation. It may be used in subhuman primates for restraint.

Pharmacology: KETAMINE HYDROCHLORIDE INJECTION, USP is chemically designated dl 2-(o-chlorophenyl)-2-(methylamino) cyclohexanone hydrochloride.

Action: KETAMINE HYDROCHLORIDE INJECTION, USP is a rapid-acting agent whose pharmacological action is characterized by profound analgesia, normal pharyngeal-laryngeal reflexes, mild cardiac stimulation and respiratory depression. Skeletal muscle tone is variable and may be normal, enhanced or diminished. The anesthetic state produced does not fit into the conventional classification of stages of anesthesia, but instead KETAMINE HYDROCHLORIDE INJECTION, USP produces a state of unconsciousness which has been termed "dissociative" anesthesia in that it appears to selectively interrupt association pathways to the brain before producing somesthetic sensory blockade.

In contrast to other anesthetics, protective reflexes, such as coughing and swallowing are maintained under KETAMINE HYDROCHLORIDE INJECTION, USP anesthesia. The degree of muscle tone is dependent upon level of dose; therefore, variations in body temperature may occur. At low dosage levels there may be an increase in muscle tone and a concomitant slight increase in body temperature. However, at high dosage levels there is some diminution in muscle tone and a resultant decrease in body temperature, to the point where supplemental heat may be advisable.

In cats, there is usually some transient cardiovascular stimulation, increased cardiac output with slight increase in mean systolic pressure with little or no change in total peripheral resistance. At higher doses respiratory rate is usually decreased.

The assurance of a patent airway is greatly enhanced by virtue of maintained pharyngeal-laryngeal reflexes. Although some salivation is occasionally noted, the persistence of the swallowing reflex aids in minimizing the hazards associated with ptyalism. Salivation may be effectively controlled with atropine sulfate in dosages of 0.04 mg/kg (0.02 mg/lb) in cats and 0.01 to 0.05 mg/kg (0.005 to 0.025 mg/lb) in subhuman primates.

Other reflexes, e.g., corneal, pedal, etc., are maintained during KETAMINE HYDROCHLORIDE INJECTION, USP anesthesia, and should not be used as criteria for judging depth of anesthesia. The eyes normally remain open with the pupils dilated. It is suggested that a bland ophthalmic ointment be applied to the cornea if anesthesia is to be prolonged.

Following the administration of recommended doses, cats become ataxic in about 5 minutes with anesthesia usually lasting from 30 to 45 minutes at higher doses. At the lower doses, complete recovery usually occurs in 4 to 5 hours but with higher doses recovery time is more prolonged and may be as long as 24 hours.

In studies involving 14 species of subhuman primates represented by at least ten anesthetic episodes for each species, the median time to restraint ranged from 1.5 [*Aotus trivirgatus* (night monkey) and *Cebus capucinus* (white throated capuchin)] to 5.3 minutes [*Macaca nemestrina* (pig tailed macaque)]. The median duration of restraint ranged between 20 and 55 minutes in all but five of the species studied. Total time from injection to end of restraint ranged from 43 [*Saimiri sciureus* (squirrel monkey)] to 183 minutes [*Macaca nemestrina* (pig tailed macaque)] after injection. Recovery is generally smooth and uneventful. The duration is dose related.

By single intramuscular injection, KETAMINE HYDROCHLORIDE INJECTION, USP usually has a wide margin of safety in cats and subhuman primates. In cats, cases of prolonged recovery and death have been reported.

Dosage and Administration: KETAMINE HYDROCHLORIDE INJECTION, USP is well tolerated by cats and subhuman primates when administered by intramuscular injection.

Fasting prior to induction of anesthesia or restraint with KETAMINE HYDROCHLORIDE INJECTION, USP is not essential; however, when preparing for elective surgery, it is advisable to withhold food for at least six hours prior to administration of KETAMINE HYDROCHLORIDE INJECTION, USP.

Anesthesia may be of shorter duration in immature cats. Restraint in subhuman primate neonates (less than 24 hours of age) is difficult to achieve.

As with other anesthetic agents, the individual response to KETAMINE HYDROCHLORIDE INJECTION, USP is somewhat varied depending upon the dose, general condition and age of the subject so that dosage recommendations cannot be absolutely fixed.

Dosage:

Cats: A dose of 11 mg/kg (5 mg/lb) is recommended to produce restraint. Dosages from 22 to 33 mg/kg (10 to 15 mg/lb) produce anesthesia that is suitable for diagnostic or minor surgical procedures that do not require skeletal muscle relaxation.

Subhuman Primates: The recommended restraint dosages of KETAMINE HYDROCHLORIDE INJECTION, USP for the following species are: *Cercocebus torquatus* (white-collared mangabey), *Papio cynocephalus* (yellow baboon), *Pan troglodytes verus* (chimpanzee), *Papio anubis* (olive baboon), *Pongo pygmaeus* (orangutan), *Macaca nemestrina* (pig-tailed macaque) 5 to 7.5 mg/kg; *Presbytis entellus* (entellus langur) 3 to 5 mg/kg: *Gorilla gorilla gorilla* (gorilla) 7 to 10 mg/kg; *Aotus trivirgatus* (night monkey) 10 to 12 mg/kg; *Macaca mulatta* (rhesus monkey) 5 to 10 mg/kg; *Cebus capucinus* (white-throated capuchin) 13 to 15 mg/kg; and *Macaca fascicularis* (crab-eating macaque), *Macaca radiata* (bonnet macaque) and *Saimiri sciureus* (squirrel monkey) 12 to 15 mg/kg.

A single intramuscular injection produces restraint suitable for TB testing, radiography, physical examination or blood collection.

Contraindication(s): KETAMINE HYDROCHLORIDE INJECTION, USP is contraindicated in cats and subhuman primates suffering from renal or hepatic insufficiency.

KETAMINE HYDROCHLORIDE INJECTION, USP is detoxified by the liver and excreted by the kidneys; therefore, any pre-existent hepatic or renal pathology or impairment of function can be expected to result in prolonged anesthesia; related fatalities have been reported.

Precaution(s): Store at controlled room temperature 15°-30°C (59°-86°F). Protect from light.

Color of solution may vary from colorless to very slightly yellowish and may darken upon prolonged exposure to light. This darkening does not affect potency. Do not use if precipitate appears.

Caution(s): Federal law restricts the drug to use by or on the order of a licensed veterinarian.

In cats, doses in excess of 50 mg/kg during any single procedure should not be used. The maximum recommended dose in subhuman primates is 40 mg/kg.

To reduce the incidence of emergence reactions, animals should not be stimulated by sound or handling during the recovery period. However, this does not preclude the monitoring of vital signs.

Apnea, respiratory arrest, cardiac arrest and death have occasionally been reported with ketamine used alone, and more frequently when used in conjunction with sedatives or other anesthetics. Close monitoring of patients is strongly advised during induction, maintenance and recovery from anesthesia.

For intramuscular use in cats and subhuman primates only.

Adverse Reactions: Respiratory depression may occur following administration of high doses of KETAMINE HYDROCHLORIDE INJECTION, USP. If at any time respiration becomes excessively depressed and the animal becomes cyanotic, resuscitative measures should be instituted promptly. Adequate pulmonary ventilation using either oxygen or room air is recommended as a resuscitative measure.

Adverse reactions reported have included emesis, salivation, vocalization, erratic recovery, spastic jerking movements, convulsions, muscular tremors, hypertonicity, opisthotonos, dyspnea and cardiac arrest. In the cat, myoclonic jerking and/or mild tonic convulsions can be controlled by ultrashort-acting barbiturates which should be given to effect. The barbiturates should be administered intravenously at a dose level of one-sixth to one-fourth the usual dose for the product being used. Acepromazine may also be used. However, recent information indicates that some phenothiazine derivatives may potentiate the toxic effects of organic phosphate compounds such as found in flea collars and certain anthelmintics. A study has indicated that ketamine hydrochloride alone does not potentiate the toxic effects of organic phosphate compounds.

Trial Data: Clinical Studies: KETAMINE HYDROCHLORIDE INJECTION, USP has been clinically studied in subhuman primates in addition to those species listed under Dosage and Administration. Dosages for restraint in these additional species, based on limited clinical data, are: *Cercopithecus aethiops* (grivet), *Papio papio* (guinea baboon) 10 to 12 mg/kg; *Erythrocebus patas patas* (patas monkey) 3 to 5 mg/kg; *Hylobates lar* (white-handed gibbon) 5 to 10 mg/kg; *Lemur catta* (ringtailed lemur) 7.5 to 10 mg/kg; Macaca fuscata (Japanese macaque) 5 mg/kg; *Maccaca speciosa* (stumptailed macaque) and *Miopithecus talapoin* (mangrove monkey) 5 to 7.5 mg/kg; and *Symphalangus syndactylus* (siamangs) 5 to 7 mg/kg.

Presentation: KETAMINE HYDROCHLORIDE INJECTION, USP is supplied in 10 mL vials (NDC 59130-659-10).

Compendium Code No.: 10740260 Rev. 4-99

AMTECH LACTATED RINGERS INJECTION ℞

Phoenix Scientific **Fluid Therapy**

Sterile Nonpyrogenic Solution

Active Ingredient(s): Each 100 mL contains:

Sodium Chloride	600 mg
Sodium Lactate	310 mg
Potassium Chloride	30 mg
Calcium Chloride Dihydrate	20 mg
Water for Injection	q.s.

The Calcium, Potassium and Sodium contents are approximately 2.7, 4.0, and 130 mEq/liter, respectively. Total Osmolar Concentration: 269 mOsm per liter (calculated).

It contains no preservatives.

Indications: For the correction of electrolyte depletion, metabolic acidosis and dehydration of cattle, calves, horses, sheep and swine.

Dosage and Administration: May be injected intravenously, subcutaneously or intraperitoneally (except in horses) using strict aseptic technique.

Cattle and Horses: 2 to 5 mL per pound of body weight depending on size and condition of animal, repeated 1 to 3 times daily or as needed.

Swine and Sheep: 2 to 5 mL per pound of body weight depending on size and condition of animal, repeated 1 to 3 times daily or as needed.

If administered subcutaneously divide the dosage into several sites of injection and massage points of injection to aid in absorption and help prevent inflammation and/or sloughing.

Contraindication(s): Do not administer to horses by intraperitoneal injection. Do not administer to animals with inadequate renal function. Not for use in lactic acidosis.

Precaution(s): Store at between 15°C and 30°C (59°F-86°F).

Use entire contents when first opened.

Caution(s): Federal law restricts this drug to use by or on the order of a licensed veterinarian.

Solution should be warmed to body temperature prior to administration and administered at a slow rate. This is a single dose unit. For animal use only.

Warning(s): Keep out of reach of children.

Presentation: 1000 mL single dose units (NDC 59130-610-04).

Compendium Code No.: 10740680 Rev. 5-94

AMTECH LEVAMISOLE PHOSPHATE INJECTABLE SOLUTION

Phoenix Scientific **Parasiticide Injection**

Sterile Anthelmintic

ANADA No.: 200-271

Active Ingredient(s): Each mL of solution contains levamisole phosphate equivalent to 136.5 mg of levamisole hydrochloride.

Indications: LEVAMISOLE PHOSPHATE is a sterile solution recommended for the treatment of cattle infected with the following parasites:

Stomach Worms: *Haemonchus, Ostertagia, Trichostrongylus.*

Intestinal Worms: *Trichostrongylus, Cooperia, Nematodirus, Bunostomum, Oesophagostomum, Chabertia.*

Lungworms: *Dictyocaulus.*

Dosage and Administration: Dosage: Inject subcutaneously in the mid-neck region at the rate of 2 mL per 100 lb body weight. It is recommended that no more than 10 mL be injected at one site.

Consult your veterinarian for assistance in the diagnosis, treatment, and control of parasitism.

The maturation of some helminth species may be arrested at pre-adult stage when adult worm populations are heavy.

Cattle that are severely parasitized or maintained under conditions of constant helminth exposure may require retreatment with two to four weeks after the first treatment.

Administration: Thoroughly clean and disinfect syringes and needles by boiling in water for twenty minutes. Use 14 or 16 gauge ½ to 1 inch needles.

Do not remove rubber stopper from the bottle, but clean and disinfect it with 70% alcohol. With syringe attached to needle, insert needle through the rubber stopper and withdraw the required dose.

The proper method of injection site preparation by swabbing with 70% alcohol or other suitable disinfectant, and the proper method of administration under a fold of skin in the mid-neck region are demonstrated below. A clean, sterile needle should be used for each animal to avoid spreading infection.

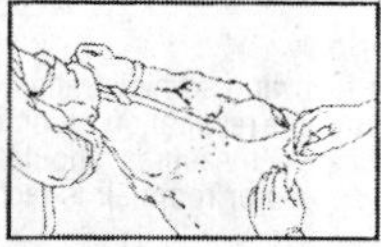

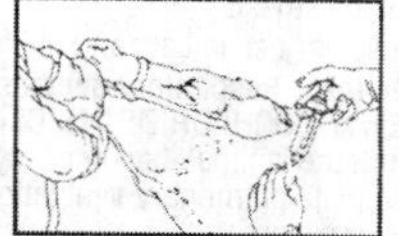

Precaution(s): Storage Conditions: To assure maximum potency and efficacy, store at or below 70°F. Refrigeration advisable. Avoid freezing.

Caution(s): Careful cattle weight estimates are essential for proper performance of this product. It is recommended that LEVAMISOLE PHOSPHATE be injected only in cattle in stocker or feeder condition. Cattle nearing slaughter weight and condition may show objectionable reactions at the site of injection. An occasional animal in stocker or feeder flesh may show swelling at the injection site. The swelling will subside in 7 to 14 days and is no more severe than that observed from commonly used vaccines and bacterins.

The mid-neck region is the preferred injection site. Always use sterile needles and syringes. Non-sterile equipment may cause abscesses at the site of injection. Contents should be used as soon as possible after the seal has been broken. It is recommended that the cap be wiped with alcohol prior to withdrawing solution. Also, skin at injection site should be swabbed with alcohol to avoid infection.

Muzzle foam may be observed; however, this reaction will disappear within a few hours. If this condition persists, a veterinarian should be consulted. Follow recommended dosage carefully.

Experience under field conditions indicates that stressful procedures such as vaccination, castration, dehorning, concurrent exposure to cholinesterase-inhibiting drugs, pesticides, or chemicals, may increase the risk associated with the use of this product. Such concurrent stress should be avoided when using this product.

Consult veterinarian before using in severely debilitated animals.

Warning(s): Do not administer to cattle within 7 days of slaughter for food to avoid tissue residues. To prevent residues in milk, do not administer to dairy animals of breeding age.

Keep this and all drugs out of the reach of children.

Presentation: Available in 500 mL vials (NDC 59130-736-03).

Compendium Code No.: 10740690 Iss. 8-00

AMTECH LEVOTHYROXINE SODIUM TABLETS ℞

Phoenix Scientific **Thyroid Therapy**

Active Ingredient(s): Each tablet contains either:

Levothyroxine sodium, USP	0.2 mg - pink
Levothyroxine sodium, USP	0.5 mg - white
Levothyroxine sodium, USP	0.8 mg - light blue

Indications: Provides thyroid replacement therapy in all conditions of inadequate production of thyroid hormones in the dog.

Pharmacology: Description: Each LEVOTHYROXINE SODIUM TABLET provides synthetic crystalline levothyroxine sodium (L-Thyroxine).

Action: Levothyroxine sodium acts as does endogenous thyroxine, to stimulate metabolism, growth, development and differentiation on tissues. It increases the rate of energy exchange and increases the maturation rate of the epiphyses. Levothyroxine sodium is absorbed rapidly from the gastrointestinal tract after oral administration. Following absorption, the compound becomes bound to the serum alpha globulin fraction. For purposes of comparison, 0.1 mg of levothyroxine sodium elicits a clinical response approximately equal to that produced by one grain (65 mg) of desiccated thyroid.

Dosage and Administration: The initial recommended daily dose is 0.1 mg/10 lb body weight. Dosage is then adjusted according to patient's response by monitoring T4 blood levels at time intervals of four weeks.

Thyroxine tablets may be administered orally or placed in the food.

Contraindication(s): Levothyroxine sodium therapy is contraindicated in thyrotoxicosis, acute myocardial infraction and uncorrected adrenal insufficiency. Use in pregnant bitches has not been evaluated.

Precaution(s): Storage: Store between 15°C and 30°C (59°F-86°F).

Tightly close the container after each use.

Caution(s): Federal law restricts this drug to use by or on the order of a licensed veterinarian.

The effects of levothyroxine sodium therapy are slow in being manifested. Overdosage of any thyroid drug may produce the signs and symptoms of thyrotoxicosis including but not limited to polydipsia, polyuria, polyphagia, reduced heat tolerance and hyperactivity or personality change. Administer with caution to animals with clinically significant heart disease, hypertension or other complications for which a sharply increased metabolic rate might prove hazardous.

Complies with USP Dissolution Test 2.

For animal use only.

Warning(s): Keep out of reach of children.

Adverse Reactions: There are no particular adverse reactions connected with L-Thyroxine therapy at the recommended dosage levels. Overdose will result in the signs of thyrotoxicosis listed above under Cautions.

Discussion: Hypothyroidism is the generalized metabolic disease resulting from deficiency of the thyroid hormones levothyroxine (T4) and liothyronine (T3). Levothyroxine sodium will provide levothyroxine (T4) as a substrate for the physiologic deiodination to liothyronine (T3). Administration of levothyroxine sodium alone will result in complete physiologic thyroid replacement.

Canine hypothyroidism is usually primary, ie., due to atrophy of the thyroid gland. In the majority of cases the atrophy is associated with lymphocytic thyroiditis and in the remainder it is non-inflammatory and as of yet unknown etiology. Less than 10 percent of cases of hypothyroidism are secondary, i.e., due to deficiency of thyroid stimulating hormone (TSH). TSH deficiency may occur as a component of congenital hypopituitarism or as an acquired disorder in adult dogs, in which case it is invariably due to the growth of a pituitary tumor.

Hypothyroidism in the Dog: Hypothyroidism usually occurs in middle-aged and older dogs although the condition will sometimes be seen in younger dogs of the larger breeds. Neutered animals of either sex are also frequently affected, regardless of age. The following are clinical signs of hypothyroidism in dogs: Lethargy, lack of endurance, increased sleeping; Reduced interest, alertness and excitability; Slow heart rate, weak apex beat and pulse, low voltage on ECG; Preference for warmth, low body temperature, cool skin; Increased body weight; Stiff and slow movements, dragging of front feet; Head tilt, disturbed balance, unilateral facial paralysis; Atrophy of epidermis, thickening of dermis; Surface and follicular hyperkeratosis, pigmentation; Puffy face, blepharoptosis, tragic expression; Dry, coarse, sparse coat, slow regrowth after clipping; Retarded turnover of hair (carpet coat of boxers); Shortening or absence of estrus, lack of libido; Dry feces, occasional diarrhea; Hypercholesterolemia; Normochromic, normocytic anemia; Elevated serum creatinine phosphokinase.

Presentation: Bottles of 180 and 1000 tablets.

Compendium Code No.: 10740271 Rev. 5-01

AMTECH LIDOCAINE HCL INJECTABLE-2% ℞

Phoenix Scientific **Local Anesthetic**

Active Ingredient(s): Composition: Each mL of sterile aqueous solution contains:

Lidocaine hydrochloride 2.0%
Sodium chloride 0.2%
Potassium phosphate monobasic 0.2%
Potassium phosphate dibasic 0.2%
Methylparaben (preservative) 0.1%
Water for injection .... q.s.

Indications: Lidocaine is a potent local anesthetic for producing epidural and nerve conduction anesthesia.

Dosage and Administration:

Epidural:

Cattle and Horses - 5 to 15 mL.

Dogs and Cats - 1 mL per 10 pounds of body weight.

Nerve Block:

Cattle and Horses - 5 to 20 mL.

Contraindication(s): Lidocaine is contraindicated in animals with a known hypersensitivity to the drug.

Precaution(s): Store between 15°C and 30°C (59°F-86°F).

Caution(s): Federal law restricts this drug to use by or on the order of a licensed veterinarian.

Lidocaine is usually well tolerated. Nevertheless, as with all local anesthetics, untoward effects may occur due to hypersensitivity, faulty technique, overdosage and inadvertent intravascular or subarachnoid injection. In case of respiratory arrest, immediate resuscitation with oxygen is indicated. For animal use only. Keep out of reach of children.

Presentation: 100 mL (NDC 59130-611-01) and 250 mL (NDC 59130-611-02).

Compendium Code No.: 10740281 Rev. 10-95 / Iss. 1-02

AMTECH MANNITOL INJECTION 20% ℞

Phoenix Scientific **Diuretic**

Sterile Solution

Active Ingredient(s): Each 100 mL contains:

Mannitol USP .... 20 g
Water for Injection .... q.s.

This solution contains 1098 mOsmols/Liter.

This is a single dose vial that contains no preservatives.

Indications: MANNITOL INJECTION 20% is indicated for use as an osmotic diuretic in canine species. Mannitol is essentially inert metabolically. When given parenterally, it is freely filtered at the glomerulus which produces osmotic diuresis as more than 90% of the mannitol injected escapes reabsorption.

Dosage and Administration: The usual canine dosage administered intravenously is 1.5-2.0 g per kg body weight given over a 30 minute period. This is approximately 3.4-4.5 mL/lb of body weight.

Precaution(s): Store at between 15° and 30°C (59° and 86°F).

Use entire contents when first opened.

Caution(s): Federal law restricts this drug to use by or on the order of a licensed veterinarian.

For animal use only.

Note: Crystals of mannitol may form in a 20% saturated solution of mannitol. Dissolve the crystals by warming in hot water or autoclaving for 15 minutes. Cool to body temperature before administering.

Warning(s): Keep out of reach of children.

Presentation: 100 mL single dose vials (NDC 59130-757-01).

Compendium Code No.: 10740700 Iss. 1-02

AMTECH MAXIM-100

Phoenix Scientific **Oxytetracycline Injection**

(Oxytetracycline Hydrochloride Injection) Antibiotic

ANADA No.: 200-068

Active Ingredient(s): Each mL contains:

Oxytetracycline base (as HCl) .... 100 mg
Magnesium Chloride • $6H_2O$ .... 5.76% w/v
Water For Injection .... 17% v/v
Propylene Glycol .... q.s.

with Sodium Formaldehyde Sulfoxylate, 1.3% w/v as a preservative and Monoethanolamine for pH adjustment.

Indications: Diseases for Which MAXIM-100 (Oxytetracycline Hydrochloride Injection) is Indicated: The use of MAXIM-100 (Oxytetracycline Hydrochloride Injection) is indicated in beef cattle, beef calves, non-lactating dairy cattle and dairy calves for treatment of the following disease conditions caused by one or more of the Oxytetracycline sensitive pathogens listed as follows:

Disease	Causative Organism(s) Which Show Sensitivity to MAXIM-100 (Oxytetracycline Hydrochloride Injection)
Bacterial Pneumonia and Shipping Fever Complex Associated with *Pasteurella* spp.	*Pasteurella* spp.
Bacterial Enteritis (scours)	*Escherichia coli*
Necrotic Pododermatitis (Foot Rot)	*Fusobacterium necrophorum*
Calf Diphtheria	*Fusobacterium necrophorum*
Wooden Tongue	*Actinobacillus lignieresii*
Wound Infections; Acute Metritis; Traumatic Injury	Caused by oxytetracycline-susceptible strains of streptococcal and staphylococcal organisms.

Pharmacology: General Indications for Use: A great many of the pathogens involved in cattle diseases are known to be susceptible to Oxytetracycline Hydrochloride therapy. Many strains of organisms, however, have shown resistance to Oxytetracycline. In the case of certain coliforms, streptococci and staphylococci, it may be advisable to conduct culture and sensitivity testing to determine susceptibility of the infecting organism to Oxytetracycline. In this manner, the likelihood of successful treatment with MAXIM-100 (Oxytetracycline Hydrochloride Injection) solution can be determined in advance.

Description: MAXIM-100 (Oxytetracycline Hydrochloride Injection) is a sterile ready-to-use preparation containing 100 mg/mL Oxytetracycline HCl, for administration of the broad spectrum antibiotic, Oxytetracycline, by injection.

Antibiotic Action of Oxytetracycline: Oxytetracycline is effective against a wide range of gram-negative and gram-positive organisms that are pathogenic for cattle. The antibiotic is primarily bacteriostatic in effect, and is believed to exert its antimicrobial action by the inhibition of microbial protein synthesis. The antibiotic activity of Oxytetracycline is not appreciably diminished in the presence of body fluids, serum or exudates. Since the drugs in the tetracycline class have similar antimicrobial spectra, organisms can develop cross resistance among them. Oxytetracycline is concentrated by the liver in the bile and excreted in the urine and feces at high concentrations and in a biologically active form.

Dosage and Administration: Recommended Daily Dosages:

Treat at the first clinical signs of disease.

The intravenous injection of 3 to 5 mg of Oxytetracycline Hydrochloride per pound of body weight per day (3 to 5 mL per 100 lbs body weight) is the recommended dosage.

Severe foot-rot and the severe forms of the indicated diseases should be treated with 5 mg per pound of body weight. Surgical procedures may be indicated in some forms of Foot-Rot or other conditions.

In disease treatment, the daily dose of MAXIM-100 (Oxytetracycline Hydrochloride Injection) should be continued 24 to 48 hours following remission of disease symptoms; however, not to exceed a total of 4 consecutive days.

Directions for Making an Intravenous Injection in Cattle:

Equipment Recommended:

1. Choke rope — a rope or cord about 5 feet long, with a loop in one end, to be used as a tourniquet.
2. Syringe and needles; gravity flow intravenous set.
3. Use new, very sharp hypodermic needles, 16-gauge, 1½ to 2 inches long. Dull needles will not work. Extra needles should be available in case the one being used becomes clogged.
4. Scissors or clippers.
5. 70% rubbing alcohol compound or other equally effective antiseptic for disinfecting the skin.
6. The medication to be given.

Preparation of Equipment: Thoroughly clean the needles, syringe and intravenous set and disinfect them by boiling in water for twenty minutes or by immersing in a suitable chemical disinfectant such as 70% alcohol for a period of not less than 30 minutes. Warm the bottle of medication to approximately body temperature and keep warm until used.

It is recommended that the correct dose be diluted in water for injection, sodium chloride injection or other suitable vehicle immediately prior to administration. Doses up to 50 mL may be diluted in 250 mL. Larger doses may be diluted in 500 mL of one of the diluents. Adverse reactions may be minimized and the drug dose can be better regulated by this method of administration.

Avoid touching the needle with the hands at all times.

In case of the syringe method of administration, disinfect the vial cap by wiping with 70% alcohol or other suitable antiseptic. Touching a sterile needle only by the hub, attach it to the syringe and push the plunger down the barrel to empty it of air. Puncture the rubber cap of the vial and withdraw the plunger upward in the syringe to draw up a volume of MAXIM-100 (Oxytetracycline Hydrochloride Injection), 100 mg/mL of about 5 mL more than is needed for injection. Withdraw from the vial and, pointing the needle upward, remove all air bubbles from the syringe by pushing the plunger upward to the volume required.

If the injection cannot be made immediately, the tip of the needle may be covered with cotton soaked in 70% alcohol to prevent contamination.

Preparation of the Animal for Injection:

1. Approximate location of vein. The jugular vein runs in the jugular groove on each side of the neck from the angle of the jaw to just above the brisket and slightly above and to the side of the windpipe.
2. Method of restraint — A stanchion or chute is ideal for restraining the animal. With a halter, rope or cattle leader (nose tongs), pull the animal's head around the side of the stanchion, cattle chute or post in such a manner to form a bow in the neck, then snub the head securely to prevent movement. By forming the bow in the neck, the outside curvature of the bow tends to expose the jugular vein and make it easily accessible. Caution: Avoid a tight rope or halter around the throat or upper neck which might impede blood flow. Animals that are down present no problem so far as restraint is concerned.
3. Clip hair in area where injection is to be made (over the vein in the upper third of the neck). Clean and disinfect the skin with alcohol or other suitable antiseptic.

Dosage for Injection:

Refer to the table below for proper dosage according to body weight of the animal.

Weight of Animals, Lbs (Beef Cattle, Beef Calves, Non-Lactating Dairy Cattle, Dairy Calves)	Milligrams of Oxytetracycline Hydrochloride per 100 lbs of Body Weight Per Day	Daily Dosage of MAXIM-100 (Oxytetracycline Hydrochloride Injection) (mL)
50 lbs	300-500 mg	1.5-2.5 mL
100 lbs	300-500 mg	3-5 mL
200 lbs	300-500 mg	6-10 mL
300 lbs	300-500 mg	9-15 mL
400 lbs	300-500 mg	12-20 mL
500 lbs	300-500 mg	15-25 mL
600 lbs	300-500 mg	18-30 mL
800 lbs	300-500 mg	24-40 mL
1000 lbs	300-500 mg	30-50 mL
1200 lbs	300-500 mg	36-60 mL
1400 lbs	300-500 mg	42-70 mL

Caution: If no improvement is noted within 24 to 48 hours consult a veterinarian. For intravenous use only.

Entering the Vein and Making the Injection:

1. Raise the vein: this is accomplished by tying the choke rope tightly around the neck, close to the shoulder. The rope should be tied in such a way that it will not come loose and so that it can be untied quickly by pulling the loose end. In thick-necked animals, a block of wood placed in the jugular groove between the rope and hide will help considerably in applying the desired pressure at the right point. The vein is a soft flexible tube through which blood flows back to the heart. Under ordinary conditions it cannot be seen or felt with the fingers. When the flow of blood is blocked at the base of the neck by the choke rope, the vein becomes enlarged and rigid because of the back pressure. If the choke rope is sufficiently tight, the vein stands out and can be easily seen and felt in thick-necked animals. As a further check in identifying the vein, tap it with the fingers in front of the choke rope.

A

Pulsations that can be seen or felt with the fingers in front of the point being tapped will confirm the fact that the vein is properly distended. It is impossible to put the needle into the vein unless it is distended. Experienced operators are able to raise the vein simply by hand pressure, but the use of a choke rope is more certain.

2. Inserting the needle. This involves three distinct steps. First, insert the needle through the hide. Second, insert the needle into the vein. This may require two or three attempts before the vein is entered. The vein has a tendency to roll away from the point of the needle, especially if the needle is not sharp. The vein can be steadied with the thumb and finger of one hand. With the other hand, the needle point is placed directly over the vein, slanting it so that its direction is along the length of the vein, either toward the head or toward the heart. Properly positioned this way, a quick thrust of the needle will be followed by a spurt of blood through the needle, which indicates that the vein has been entered. Third, once in the vein, the needle should be inserted along the length of the vein all the way to the hub, exercising caution to see that the needle does not penetrate the opposite side of the vein. Continuous steady flow of blood through the needle indicates that the needle is still in the vein. If blood does not flow continuously, the needle is out of the vein (or clogged) and another attempt must be made. If difficulty is encountered, it may be advisable to use the vein on the other side of the neck.
3. While the needle is being placed in proper position in the vein, an assistant should get the medication ready so that the injection can be started without delay after the vein has been entered. Remove the rubber stopper from the bottle of intravenous solution, connect the intravenous tube to the neck of the bottle, invert the bottle and allow some of the solution to run through the tube to eliminate all air bubbles.
4. Making the injection. With needle in proper position as indicated by continuous flow of blood, release the choke rope by a quick pull on the free end. This is essential — the medication cannot flow into the vein while the vein is blocked. Immediately connect the intravenous tube to the needle, and raise the bottle. The solution will flow by gravity. Rapid injection may occasionally produce shock. Administer slowly. The animal should be observed at all times during the injection in order not to give the solution too fast. This may be determined by watching the respiration of the animal and feeling or listening to the heart beat. If the heart beat and respiration increase markedly, the rate of injection should be immediately stopped by pinching the tube until the animal recovers approximately to its previous respiration or heart beat rate, when the injection can be resumed at a slower rate. The rate of flow can be controlled by pinching the tube between the thumb and forefinger or by raising and lowering the bottle.

   Bubbles entering the bottle through the air tube or valve indicate the rate at which the medication is flowing. If the flow should stop, this means the needle has slipped out of the vein (or is clogged) and the operation will have to be repeated. If using the syringe technique, pull back gently on the plunger: if blood flows into the syringe, the needle is in proper position. Depress the plunger slowly. If there is any resistance to the depression of the plunger, stop and repeat insertion procedure. The resistance indicates that either the needle is clogged or it has slipped out of the vein. With either method of administration, syringe or gravity flow, watch for any swelling under the skin near the needle, which would indicate that the medication is not going into the vein. Should this occur, it is best to try the vein on the opposite side of the neck. Sudden movement of the animal, especially twisting of the neck or raising or lowering the head, may sometimes cause the needle to slip out of the vein. To prevent this, tape the needle hub to the skin of the neck to hold the needle in position. Whenever there is any doubt as to the position of the needle, this should be checked in the following manner: Pinch off the intravenous tube to stop flow, disconnect the tube from the needle and re-apply pressure to the vein. Free flow of blood through the needle indicates that it is in proper position and the injection can then be continued. If using the syringe, gently pull back on the plunger. Blood should flow into the syringe.
5. Removing the needle. When the injection is complete, remove needle with a straight pull. Then apply pressure over area of injection momentarily to control any bleeding through needle puncture, using cotton soaked in alcohol or other suitable antiseptic.

Instructions for Care of Sick Animals: The use of antibiotics, as with most medications used in the management of diseases, is based on accurate diagnosis and adequate treatment. When properly used in the treatment of diseases caused by oxytetracycline-susceptible organisms, animals usually show a noticeable improvement within 24 to 48 hours. If improvement does not occur within this period of time, the diagnosis and treatment of animal diseases should be carried out by a veterinarian. The use of professional veterinary and laboratory services can reduce treatment costs, time and needless losses. Good management, housing, sanitation and nutrition are essential in the care of animals and in the successful treatment of disease.

Precaution(s): Store at 59°-86°F.

Note: The solution may darken on storage but potency remains unaffected.

Caution(s): If no improvement occurs within 24 to 48 hours, consult a veterinarian. Do not use the drug for more than 4 consecutive days. Use beyond 4 days or doses higher than maximum recommended dose may result in antibiotic tissue residues beyond the withdrawal period.

For use in animals only.

Restricted Drug (California) — Use only as directed.

Keep out of reach of children.

Warning(s): Discontinue treatment with MAXIM-100 (Oxytetracycline Hydrochloride Injection) at least 22 days prior to slaughter of the animal. Not for use in lactating dairy animals.

A withdrawal period has not been established for this product in pre-ruminating calves. Do not use in calves to be processed for veal.

Side Effects: The improper or accidental injection of the drug outside of the vein will cause local tissue irritation manifested by temporary swelling and discoloration at the injection site.

Shortly after injection, treated animals may have a transient hemoglobinuria (darkened urine).

Reactions of an allergic or anaphylactic nature, sometimes fatal, have been known to occur in hypersensitive animals following the injection of Oxytetracycline solutions, but such reactions are rare.

At the first sign of any adverse reaction or anaphylactic shock (noted by glassy eyes, increased salivation, grinding of the teeth, rapid breathing, muscular tremors, staggering, swelling of the eyelids or collapse), the product should be discontinued. Epinephrine solution at the recommended dosage levels should be administered and a veterinarian should be called immediately.

Because bacteriostatic drugs interfere with the bactericidal action of Penicillin, do not give Oxytetracycline Hydrochloride in conjunction with Penicillin.

As with other antibiotics, use of this drug may result in over-growth of nonsusceptible organisms. If any unusual symptoms occur or in the absence of a favorable response following treatment, discontinue use immediately and call a veterinarian.

Presentation: MAXIM-100 (Oxytetracycline Hydrochloride Injection) is available in 500 mL multidose vials containing 100 mg Oxytetracycline Hydrochloride per mL (NDC 59130-673-03).

Compendium Code No.: 10740290 Rev. 9-96

AMTECH MAXIM-200®

Phoenix Scientific **Oxytetracycline Injection**

(Oxytetracycline Injection) Antibiotic

ANADA No.: 200-123

Active Ingredient(s): MAXIM-200® (oxytetracycline injection) is a sterile preconstituted solution of the broad spectrum antibiotic oxytetracycline. Each mL contains 200 mg of oxytetracycline base as amphoteric oxytetracycline and, on a w/v basis, 40.0% 2-pyrrolidone, 5.0% povidone, 1.8% magnesium oxide, 0.2% sodium formaldehyde sulfoxylate (as a preservative), monoethanolamine and/or hydrochloric acid as required to adjust pH.

Indications: MAXIM-200® is intended for use in the treatment of the following diseases in beef cattle, nonlactating dairy cattle; calves, including preruminating (veal) calves; and swine when due to oxytetracycline-susceptible organisms:

Cattle: In cattle, MAXIM-200® is indicated in the treatment of pneumonia and shipping fever complex associated with *Pasteurella* spp. and *Hemophilus* spp; infectious bovine keratoconjunctivitis (pinkeye) caused by *Moraxella bovis;* foot-rot and diphtheria caused by *Fusobacterium necrophorum;* bacterial enteritis (scours) caused by *Escherichia coli;* wooden tongue caused by *Actinobacillus ligniersii;* leptospirosis caused by *Leptospira pomona;* and wound infections and acute metritis caused by strains of staphylococci and streptococci organisms sensitive to oxytetracycline.

Swine: In swine, MAXIM-200® (oxytetracycline injection) is indicated in the treatment of bacterial enteritis (scours, colibacillosis) caused by *Escherichia coli;* pneumonia caused by *Pasteurella multocida;* and leptospirosis caused by *Leptospira pomona.*

In sows, MAXIM-200® is indicated as an aid in the control of infectious enteritis (baby pig scours, colibacillosis) in suckling pigs caused by *Escherichia coli.*

Pharmacology: MAXIM-200® (oxytetracycline injection) is a sterile, ready-to-use solution for the administration of the broad-spectrum antibiotic oxytetracycline by injection. Oxytetracycline is an antimicrobial agent that is effective in the treatment of a wide range of diseases caused by susceptible gram-positive and gram-negative bacteria.

Dosage and Administration: Dosage:

Cattle: MAXIM-200® is to be administered by intramuscular, subcutaneous or intravenous injection to beef cattle, nonlactating dairy cattle and calves, including preruminating (veal) calves.

A single dosage of 9 milligrams of MAXIM-200® per pound of body weight administered intramuscularly or subcutaneously is recommended in the treatment of the following conditions: 1) bacterial pneumonia caused by *Pasteurella* spp. (shipping fever) in calves and yearlings, where re-treatment is impractical due to husbandry conditions, such as cattle on range, or where their repeated restraint is inadvisable; 2) infectious bovine keratoconjunctivitis (pinkeye) caused by *Moraxella bovis.*

MAXIM-200® can also be administered by intravenous, subcutaneous or intramuscular injection at a level of 3 to 5 milligrams of oxytetracycline per pound of body weight per day. In the treatment of severe foot-rot and advanced cases of other indicated diseases, dosage level of 5 milligrams per pound of body weight per day is recommended. Treatment should be continued 24 to 48 hours following remission of disease signs; however, not to exceed a total of four consecutive days. Consult your veterinarian if improvement is not noted within 24 to 48 hours of the beginning of treatment.

Swine: In swine a single dosage of 9 milligrams of MAXIM-200® per pound of body weight administered intramuscularly is recommended in the treatment of bacterial pneumonia caused by *Pasteurella multocida* in swine, where re-treatment is impractical due to husbandry conditions or where repeated restraint is inadvisable.

MAXIM-200® can also be administered by intramuscular injection at a level of 3 to 5 milligrams of oxytetracycline per pound of body weight per day. Treatment should be continued 24 to 48 hours following remission of the disease signs; however, not to exceed a total of four consecutive days. Consult your veterinarian if improvement is not noted within 24 to 48 hours of the beginning of treatment.

For sows, administer once intramuscularly 3 milligrams of oxytetracycline per pound of body weight approximately 8 hours before farrowing or immediately after completion of farrowing.

For swine weighing 25 lb of body weight and under, MAXIM-200® should be administered undiluted for treatment at 9 mg/lb but should be administered diluted for treatment at 3 to 5 mg/lb body weight.

	9 mg/lb Dosage Volume of Undiluted MAXIM-200®	3 or 5 mg/lb Dosage Volume of Diluted MAXIM-200®		
Body Weight	9 mg/lb	3 mg/lb	Dilution*	5 mg/lb
5 lb	0.2 mL	0.6 mL	1:7	1.0 mL
10 lb	0.5 mL	0.9 mL	1:5	1.5 mL
25 lb	1.1 mL	1.5 mL	1:3	2.5 mL

*To prepare dilutions, add one part MAXIM-200® to three, five or seven parts of sterile water, or 5 percent dextrose solution as indicated; the diluted product should be used immediately.

Directions for Use: MAXIM-200® is intended for use in the treatment of disease due to oxytetracycline-susceptible organisms in beef cattle, nonlactating dairy cattle; calves, including preruminating (veal) calves; and swine. A thoroughly cleaned, sterile needle and syringe should be used for each injection (needles and syringes may be sterilized by boiling in water for 15 minutes). In cold weather, MAXIM-200® should be warmed to room temperature before administration to animals. Before withdrawing the solution from the bottle, disinfect the rubber cap on the bottle with suitable disinfectant, such as 70 percent alcohol. The injection site should be similarly cleaned with the disinfectant. Needles of 16 to 18 gauge and 1 to 1½ inches long are adequate for intramuscular injections. Needles 2 to 3 inches are recommended for intravenous use.

Intramuscular Administration: Intramuscular injections should be made by directing the needle of suitable gauge length into the fleshy part of a thick muscle such as in the rump, hip, or thigh regions; avoid blood vessels and major nerves. Before injecting the solution, pull back gently on the plunger. If blood appears in the syringe, a blood vessel has been entered; withdraw the needle and select a different site. No more than 10 mL should be injected intramuscularly at any one site in adult beef cattle and nonlactating dairy cattle, and not more than 5 mL per site in adult swine; rotate injection sites for each succeeding treatment. The volume administered per injection site should be reduced according to age and body size so that 1 to 2 mL per site is injected in small calves.

Subcutaneous Administration: Subcutaneous injections in beef cattle, nonlactating dairy cattle, and calves, including preruminating (veal) calves, should be made by directing the needle of suitable gauge and length through the loose folds of the neck skin in front of the shoulder. Care should be taken to ensure that the tip of the needle has penetrated the skin but is not lodged in muscle. Before injecting the solution, pull back gently on the plunger. If blood appears in the syringe, a blood vessel has been entered; withdraw the needle and select a different site. The solution should be injected slowly into the area between the skin and muscles. No more than

10 mL should be injected subcutaneously at any one site in adult beef cattle and nonlactating dairy cattle; rotate injection sites for each succeeding treatment. The volume administered per injection site should be reduced according to age and body size so that 1-2 mL per site is injected in small calves.

Intravenous Administration: MAXIM-200® (oxytetracycline injection) may be administered intravenously to beef cattle and nonlactating dairy cattle. As with all highly concentrated materials, MAXIM-200® should be administered slowly by the intravenous route.

Preparation of the Animal for Injection:

1. Approximate location of vein. The jugular vein runs in the jugular groove on each side of the neck from the angle of the jaw to just above the brisket and slightly above and to the side of the windpipe. (See Fig. I)
2. Restraint. A stanchion or chute is ideal for restraining the animal. With a halter, rope, or cattle leader (nose tongs), pull the animal's head around the side of the stanchion, cattle chute, or post in such a manner to form a bow in the neck (See Fig. II), then snub the head securely to prevent movement. By forming the bow in the neck, the outside curvature of the bow tends to expose the jugular vein and make it easily accessible. Caution: Avoid restraining the animal with a tight rope or halter around the throat or upper neck which might impede blood flow. Animals that are down present no problem so far as restraint is concerned.
3. Clip hair in area where injection is to be made (over the vein in the upper third of the neck). Clean and disinfect the skin with alcohol or other suitable antiseptic.

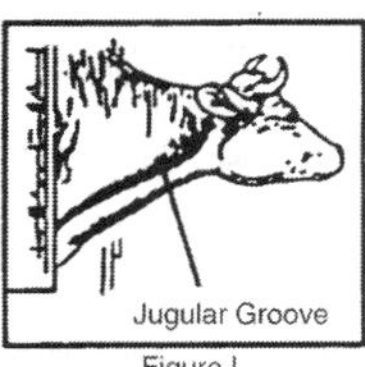

Figure I

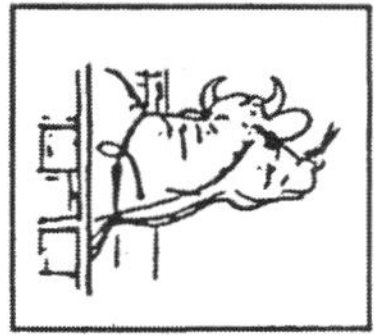
Figure II

Entering the Vein and Making the Injection:

1. Raise the vein. This is accomplished by tying the choke rope tightly around the neck close to the shoulder. The rope should be tied in such a way that it will not come loose and so that it can be untied quickly by pulling the loose end (See Fig. II). In thick-necked animals, a block of wood placed in the jugular groove between the rope and hide will help considerably in applying the desired pressure at the right point. The vein is a soft flexible tube through which blood flows back to the heart. Under ordinary conditions it cannot be seen or felt with the fingers. When the flow of blood is blocked at the base of the neck by the choke rope, the vein becomes enlarged and rigid because of the back pressure. If the choke rope is sufficiently tight, the vein stands out and can be easily seen and felt in thin-necked animals. As a further check in identifying the vein, tap it with the fingers in front of the choke rope. Pulsations that can be seen or felt with the fingers in front of the point being tapped will confirm the fact that the vein is properly distended. It is impossible to put the needle into the vein unless it is distended. Experienced operators are able to raise the vein simply by hand pressure, but the use of a choke rope is more certain.
2. Inserting the needle. This involves three distinct steps. First, insert the needle through the hide. Second, insert the needle into the vein. This may require two or three attempts before the vein is entered. The vein has a tendency to roll away from the point of the needle, especially if the needle is not sharp. The vein can be steadied with the thumb and finger of one hand. With the other hand, the needle point is placed directly over the vein, slanting it so that its direction is along the length of the vein, either toward the head or toward the heart. Properly positioned this way, a quick thrust of the needle will be followed by a spurt of blood through the needle, which indicates that the vein has been entered. Third, once in the vein, the needle should be inserted along the length of the vein all the way to the hub exercising caution to see that the needle does not penetrate the opposite side of the vein. Continuous steady flow of blood through the needle indicates that the needle is still in the vein. If blood does not flow continuously, the needle is out of the vein (or clogged) and another attempt must be made. If difficulty is encountered, it may be advisable to use the vein on the other side of the neck.
3. While the needle is being placed in proper position in the vein, an assistant should get the medication ready so that the injection can be started without delay after the vein has been entered.
4. Making the injection. With the needle in position as indicated by continuous flow of blood, release the choke rope by a quick pull on the free end. This is essential - the medication cannot flow into the vein while it is blocked. Immediately connect the syringe containing MAXIM-200® (oxytetracycline injection) to the needle and slowly depress the plunger. If there is resistance to depression of the plunger, this indicates that the needle has slipped out of the vein (or is clogged) and the procedure will have to be repeated. Watch for any swelling under the skin near the needle which would indicate that the medication is not going into the vein. Should this occur, it is best to try the vein on the opposite side of the neck.
5. Removing the needle. When injection is complete, remove needle with straight pull. Then apply pressure over the area of injection momentarily to control any bleeding through needle puncture, using cotton soaked in alcohol or other suitable antiseptic.

Precaution(s): MAXIM-200® does not require refrigeration; however, it is recommended that it be stored at room temperature, 15°-30°C (59°-86°F). The antibiotic activity of oxytetracycline is not appreciably diminished in the presence of body fluids, serum, or exudates. Keep from freezing.

Caution(s): Exceeding the highest recommended dosage level of drug per pound of body weight per day, administering more than the recommended number of treatments, and/or exceeding 10 mL intramuscularly or subcutaneously per injection site in adult beef cattle and nonlactating dairy cattle, and 5 mL intramuscularly per injection site in adult swine, may result in antibiotic residues beyond the withdrawal period.

Consult with your veterinarian prior to administering this product in order to determine the proper treatment required in the event of an adverse reaction. At the first sign of any adverse reaction, discontinue use of product and seek the advice of your veterinarian. Some of the reactions may be attributed either to anaphylaxis (an allergic reaction) or to cardiovascular collapse of unknown cause.

Shock may be observed following intravenous administration, especially where highly concentrated materials are involved. To minimize this occurrence, it is recommended that MAXIM-200® be administered slowly by this route. Shortly after injection, treated animals may have transient hemoglobinuria resulting in darkened urine.

As with all antibiotic preparations, use of the drug may result in overgrowth of nonsusceptible organisms, including fungi. A lack of response by the treated animal, or the development of new signs, may suggest that an overgrowth of nonsusceptible organisms has occurred. If any of these conditions occur, consult your veterinarian.

Since bacteriostatic drugs may interfere with the bactericidal action of penicillin, it is advisable to avoid giving MAXIM-200® in conjunction with penicillin.

Livestock drug, not for human use.

Restricted drug (California), use only as directed.

For animal use only.

Keep out of reach of children.

Warning(s): Discontinue treatment at least 28 days prior to slaughter of cattle and swine. Not for use in lactating dairy animals. Rapid intravenous administration may result in animal collapse. Oxytetracycline should be administered intravenously slowly over a period of at least 5 minutes.

Adverse Reactions: Reports of adverse reactions associated with oxytetracycline administration include injection site swelling, restlessness, ataxia, trembling, swelling of eyelids, ears, muzzle, anus and vulva (or scrotum and sheath in males), respiratory abnormalities (labored breathing), frothing at the mouth, collapse and possibly death. Some of these reactions may be attributed either to anaphylaxis (an allergic reaction) or to cardiovascular collapse of unknown cause.

Discussion: Care of Sick Animals: The use of antibiotics in the management of diseases is based on an accurate diagnosis and an adequate course of treatment. When properly used in the treatment of diseases caused by oxytetracycline susceptible organisms, most animals that have been treated with oxytetracycline injection show a noticeable improvement within 24 to 48 hours. It is recommended that the diagnosis and treatment of animal diseases be carried out by a veterinarian. Since many diseases look alike but require different types of treatment, the use of professional veterinary and laboratory services can reduce treatment time, costs and needless losses. Good housing, sanitation and nutrition are important in the maintenance of healthy animals, and are essential in the treatment of diseased animals.

Presentation: 100 mL, 250 mL and 500 mL.

Compendium Code No.: 10740303 Rev. 2-01

AMTECH NEOMYCIN ORAL SOLUTION

Phoenix Scientific **Water Medication**

Antibacterial

ANADA No.: 200-118

Active Ingredient(s): Each mL contains:

Neomycin Sulfate .... 200 mg

(equivalent to 140 mg neomycin base)

Indications: For the treatment and control of colibacillosis (bacterial enteritis) caused by *Escherichia coli* susceptible to neomycin sulfate in cattle (excluding veal calves), swine, sheep and goats.

Dosage and Administration: Administer to cattle (excluding veal calves), swine, sheep and goats at a dose of 10 mg neomycin sulfate per pound of body weight in divided doses for a maximum of 14 days.

Dosage Schedule for Treatment of Colibacillosis:

Pounds of Body Weight	Amount of NEOMYCIN ORAL SOLUTION per Day in Divided Doses
25 Lb	1.2 mL (¼ tsp*)
50 Lb	2.5 mL (½ tsp*)
100 Lb	5 mL (1 tsp*)
300 Lb	15 mL (1 tbsp*)
591.5 Lb	29.5 mL (1 fl oz)

* Teaspoon (tsp)/Tablespoon (tbsp) is equal to U.S. Standard Measure.

NEOMYCIN ORAL SOLUTION may be given undiluted or diluted with water.

Herd Treatment: Each 3.785 L (1 Gal) will treat 75700 pounds of body weight. Therefore, estimate the total number of pounds of body weight of the animals to be treated and administer 28.5 mL (1 fl oz) for 591.5 pounds. The product should be added to the amount of drinking water estimated to be consumed in 12-24 hours. Provide medicated water as the sole source of drinking water each day until consumed, followed by non-medicated water as required. Fresh medicated water should be prepared each day.

Individual Animal Treatment: To provide 10 mg neomycin sulfate per pound of body weight, mix 5 mL (1 tsp*) in water or milk for each 100 pounds of body weight. Administer daily either as a drench in divided dosages or in the drinking water to be consumed in 12-24 hours.

Precaution(s): Store at controlled room temperature between 15° and 30°C (59°-86°F).

Caution(s): To administer the stated dosage, the concentration of neomycin required in medicated water must be adjusted to compensate for variation in age and weight of animal, the nature and severity of disease signs, and environmental temperature and humidity, each of which affects water consumption.

If symptoms persist after using this preparation for 2 or 3 days, consult a veterinarian. If symptoms such as fever, depression, or going off feed develop, oral neomycin is not indicated as the sole treatment since systemic levels of neomycin are not obtained due to poor absorption from the gastrointestinal tract.

Important: Treatment should continue 24 to 48 hours beyond remission of disease symptoms, but not to exceed a total of 14 consecutive days. Animals not drinking or eating should be treated individually by drench.

Restricted Drug - Use only as directed (California).

For oral use only.

For animal use only.

Keep out of reach of children.

Warning(s): Discontinue treatment prior to slaughter by at least the number of days listed below for appropriate species:

Cattle.. 1 day
(not to be used in veal calves)

Sheep .... 2 days

Swine and Goats.. 3 days

A withdrawal period has not been established for this product in pre-ruminating calves. Do not use in calves to be processed for veal.

A milk discard period has not been established for this product in lactating dairy cattle. Do not use in female dairy cattle 20 months of age or older.

Presentation: 473.1 mL (1 pint) and 3.785 L (1 Gal) (NDC 59130-640-05).

Compendium Code No.: 10740311 Rev. 3-98

A

AMTECH OXYTETRACYCLINE HCL SOLUBLE POWDER

Phoenix Scientific **Water Medication**

(Oxytetracycline HCl)

ANADA No.: 200-146

Active Ingredient(s): Each packet contains 10 grams of oxytetracycline HCl.

Indications: A broad spectrum antibiotic for control and treatment of specific diseases in poultry, cattle, sheep and swine.

Directions for Use:

For the control of the following poultry diseases caused by organisms susceptible to oxytetracycline: Add the following amount to two gallons of stock solution when proportioner is set to meter at the rate of one ounce per gallon.

	Dosage	Packets/2 Gallons Stock Solution
Chickens		
Infectious synovitis caused by *Mycoplasma synoviae*	200-400 mg/gal	5-10
Chronic respiratory disease (CRD) and air sac infection caused by *Mycoplasma gallisepticum* and *Escherichia coli*	400-800 mg/gal	10-20
Fowl cholera caused by *Pasteurella multocida*	400-800 mg/gal	10-20
Turkeys		
Hexamitiasis caused by *Hexamita meleagridis*	200-400 mg/gal	5-10
Infectious synovitis caused by *Mycoplasma synoviae*	400 mg/gal	10
Growing Turkeys—Complicating bacterial organisms associated with bluecomb (transmissible enteritis, coronaviral enteritis)	25 mg/lb body weight daily	varies with age & water consumption (1 packet will treat 400 pounds of turkeys.)

Medicate continuously at the first clinical signs of disease and continue for 7 to 14 consecutive days. If improvement is not noted within 24-48 hours, consult a poultry diagnostic laboratory or poultry pathologist to determine diagnosis and advice on dosage.

For the control and treatment of the following diseases caused by organisms susceptible to oxytetracycline:

	Dosage
Swine	
Bacterial enteritis caused by *Escherichia coli* and *Salmonella choleraesuis*	Administer in the drinking water at a level of 10 mg oxytetracycline HCl per pound of body weight daily. Administer up to 14 days.
Bacterial pneumonia caused by *Pasteurella multocida* For Breeding Swine: Leptospirosis (reducing the incidence of abortions and shedding of leptospira) caused by *Leptospira pomona.*	
Calves, Beef Cattle and Non-lactating Dairy Cattle	
Bacterial enteritis caused by *Escherichia coli*	Administer in the drinking water at a level of 10 mg oxytetracycline HCl per pound of body weight daily. Administer up to 14 days.
Bacterial pneumonia (shipping fever complex) caused by *Pasteurella multocida.*	
Sheep	
Bacterial enteritis caused by *Escherichia coli*	Administer in the drinking water at a level of 10 mg oxytetracycline HCl per pound of body weight daily. Administer up to 14 days.
Bacterial pneumonia (shipping fever complex) caused by *Pasteurella multocida.*	

Each packet will treat 1000 pounds of swine, cattle or sheep at 10 mg/pound.

Special Note: The concentration of drug required in medicated water must be adequate to compensate for variation in the age of the animal, feed consumption rate and the environmental temperature and humidity, each of which affects water consumption.

Precaution(s): Recommended Storage: Store below 77°F (25°C).

Caution(s): Use as sole source of oxytetracycline. Prepare fresh solutions every 24 hours.

For use in drinking water only.

Not for use in liquid feed supplements.

For animal use only.

Keep out of reach of children.

Restricted Drug(s) (California). Not for human use. Use only as directed.

Warning(s): Do not administer to turkeys, swine, cattle or sheep within 5 days of slaughter. Do not administer to chickens or turkeys producing eggs for human consumption. Do not administer this product with milk or milk replacers. Administer 1 hour before or 2 hours after feeding milk or milk replacers.

A withdrawal period has not been established for this product in pre-ruminating calves. Do not use in calves to be processed for veal.

A milk discard period has not been established for this product in lactating dairy cattle. Do not use in female dairy cattle 20 months of age or older.

Presentation: 25 x 181.5 g (6.4 oz) packet.

Compendium Code No.: 10740320 Iss. 9-99

AMTECH OXYTETRACYCLINE HCL SOLUBLE POWDER-343

Phoenix Scientific **Water Medication**

A broad spectrum Antibiotic

ANADA No.: 200-247

Active Ingredient(s): Each packet contains 204.8 grams of oxytetracycline HCl. Each packet will make: 1,024 gallons (3,876 L) containing 200 mg oxytetracycline HCl per gallon; 512 gallons (1,938 L) containing 400 mg oxytetracycline HCl per gallon; 256 gallons (969 L) containing 800 mg oxytetracycline HCl per gallon.

Indications: A broad spectrum antibiotic for control and treatment of specific diseases in poultry, cattle, sheep and swine.

Directions for Use: For the control of the following poultry diseases caused by organisms susceptible to oxytetracycline: Add the following amount to two gallons of stock solution when proportioner is set to meter at the rate of one ounce per gallon.

	Dosage	Packets/2 Gallons Stock Solution
Chickens		
Infectious synovitis caused by *Mycoplasma synoviae*	200-400 mg/gal	¼-½
Chronic respiratory disease (CRD) and air sac infection caused by *Mycoplasma gallisepticum* and *Escherichia coli*	400-800 mg/gal	½-1
Fowl cholera caused by *Pasteurella multocida*	400-800 mg/gal	½-1
Turkeys		
Hexamitiasis caused by *Hexamita meleagridis*	200-400 mg/gal	¼-½
Infectious synovitis caused by *Mycoplasma synoviae*	400 mg/gal	½
Growing Turkeys—Complicating bacterial organisms associated with bluecomb (transmissible enteritis, coronaviral enteritis)	25 mg/lb body weight daily	varies with age & water consumption (1 packet will treat 8192 pounds of turkeys.)

Medicate continuously at the first clinical signs of disease and continue for 7 to 14 consecutive days. If improvement is not noted within 24-48 hours, consult a poultry diagnostic laboratory or poultry pathologist to determine diagnosis and advice on dosage.

For the control and treatment of the following diseases caused by organisms susceptible to oxytetracycline.

	Dosage
Swine	
Bacterial enteritis caused by *Escherichia coli* and *Salmonella choleraesuis*	Administer in the drinking water at a level of 10 mg oxytetracycline HCl per pound of body weight daily. Administer up to 5 days.
Bacterial pneumonia caused by *Pasteurella multocida* For Breeding Swine: Leptospirosis (reducing the incidence of abortions and shedding of leptospira) caused by *Leptospira pomona.*	
Calves, Beef Cattle and Non-Lactating Dairy Cattle	
Bacterial enteritis caused by *Escherichia coli*	Administer in the drinking water at a level of 10 mg oxytetracycline HCl per pound of body weight daily. Administer up to 5 days.
Bacterial pneumonia (shipping fever complex) caused by *Pasteurella multocida.*	
Sheep	
Bacterial enteritis caused by *Escherichia coli*	Administer in the drinking water at a level of 10 mg oxytetracycline HCl per pound of body weight daily. Administer up to 5 days.
Bacterial pneumonia (shipping fever complex) caused by *Pasteurella multocida.*	

Each packet will treat 20,480 pounds of swine, cattle or sheep at 10 mg/pound.

Special Note: The concentration of drug required in medicated water must be adequate to compensate for variation in the age of the animal, feed consumption rate and the environmental temperature and humidity, each of which affects water consumption.

Precaution(s): Recommended Storage: Store below 77°F (25°C).

Caution(s): Use as sole source of oxytetracycline. Not to be used for more than 14 consecutive days in chickens and turkeys or 5 consecutive days in cattle, swine or sheep. Prepare fresh solutions every 24 hours.

For use in drinking water only.

Not for use in liquid feed supplements.

Restricted Drug(s) (California). Not for human use. Use only as directed.

For oral use only. For animal use only.

Warning(s): Do not administer to turkeys, swine, cattle or sheep within 5 days of slaughter.

Do not administer to chickens or turkeys producing eggs for human consumption.

Do not administer this product with milk or milk replacers. Administer 1 hour before or 2 hours after feeding milk or milk replacers.

A withdrawal period has not been established for this product in preruminating calves. Do not use in calves to be processed for veal.

A milk discard period has not been established for this product in lactating dairy cattle. Do not use in female dairy cattle 20 months of age or older.

Keep out of reach of children.

Presentation: 25 x 272.2 g (9.6 oz) packets (NDC 59130-704-27).

Compendium Code No.: 10740331 Rev. 03-00

AMTECH OXYTOCIN INJECTION ℞

Phoenix Scientific **Oxytocin**

Active Ingredient(s): Each mL contains:

Oxytocic Activity Equivalent to 20 USP Posterior Pituitary units with Sodium Hydroxide/Acetic Acid for pH adjustment.

Chlorobutanol (as preservative) . . . . 2.4 mg

Water For Injection . . . . q.s.

Indications: Oxytocin may be used as a uterine contractor to precipitate and accelerate normal parturition and postpartum evacuation of uterine debris. In surgery it may be used postoperatively following cesarian section to facilitate involution and resistance to the large inflow of blood. It will contract smooth muscle cells of the mammary gland for milk letdown if the udder is in proper physiological state.

Dosage and Administration: (Intravenous, intramuscular or subcutaneous)

For obstetrical use:

Horses and Cows . . . . 100 U.S.P. units (5 mL)

Sows and Ewes. . . . . 30-50 U.S.P. units (1½ to 2½ mL)

For milk letdown:

Cows. . . . . 10-20 U.S.P. units (½-1 mL)

Sows. . . . . 5-20 U.S.P. units (¼ to 1 mL)

Contraindication(s): Do not use in dystocia due to abnormal presentation of fetus, until correction is accomplished.

Precaution(s): Store at controlled room temperature between 15°C and 30°C (59°F-86°F). Do not freeze.

Note: As this is a multi-dose container, this preparation should be handled under aseptic conditions.

Caution(s): Federal law restricts this drug to use by or on the order of a licensed veterinarian.

For prepartum usage, full relaxation of the cervix should be accomplished either naturally or by the administration of estrogen prior to oxytocin therapy.

Hazardous - Not for human use (California).

For animal use only. Keep out of reach of children.

Presentation: 100 mL (NDC 59130-639-01).

Compendium Code No.: 10740340 Rev. 10-95

AMTECH PHENYLBUTAZONE 20% INJECTION ℞

Phoenix Scientific **NSAID Injection**

(Phenylbutazone)

ANADA No.: 200-126

Active Ingredient(s): Each mL contains 200 mg of phenylbutazone, 10.45 mg of benzyl alcohol as preservative, sodium hydroxide to adjust pH to 9.5 to 10.0, and water for injection, q.s.

Indications: For relief of inflammatory conditions associated with the musculoskeletal system in horses.

Pharmacology: Description: PHENYLBUTAZONE 20% INJECTION (phenylbutazone) is a synthetic, nonhormonal anti-inflammatory, antipyretic compound useful in the management of inflammatory conditions. The apparent analgesic effect is probably related mainly to the compound's anti-inflammatory properties.

Chemically, phenylbutazone is 4-butyl-1,2-diphenyl- 3,5-pyrazolidinedione. It is a pyrazolon derivative entirely unrelated to the steroid hormones, and has the following structural formula:

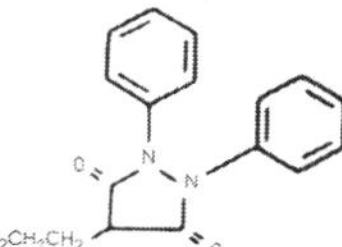

Background Pharmacology: Kuzell,[1,2,3] Payne,[4] Fleming,[5] and Denko[6] demonstrated clinical effectiveness of phenylbutazone in acute rheumatism, gout, gouty arthritis, and various other rheumatoid disorders in man. Anti-rheumatic and anti-inflammatory activity has been well established by Fabre, Domenjoz,[8] Wilhelmi,[9] and Yourish.[10]

Camberos[14] reported favorable results with phenylbutazone following intermittent treatment of Thoroughbred horses for arthritis and chronic arthrosis (e.g., osteoarthritis of medial and distal bones of the hock, arthritis of the stifle and hip, arthrosis of the spine, chronic hip pains, chronic pain in trapezius muscles, and generalized arthritis). Results were less favorable in cases of traumatism, muscle rupture, strains and inflammations of the third phalanx. Sutter[15] reported favorable response in chronic equine arthritis, fair results in a severely bruised mare, and poor results in two cases where the condition was limited to the third phalanx.

Dosage and Administration: Horses:

Intravenously: 1 to 2 g per 1,000 lbs of body weight (5 to 10 mL/1,000 lbs) daily. Injection should be given slowly and with care. Limit intravenous administration to a maximum of 5 successive days, which may be followed by oral phenylbutazone dosage forms.

Guidelines to Successful Therapy:

1. Use a relatively high dose for the first 48 hours, then reduce gradually to a maintenance dose. Maintain lowest dose capable of producing desired clinical response.
2. Response to phenylbutazone therapy is prompt, usually occurring within 24 hours. If no significant clinical response is evident after 5 days, reevaluate diagnosis and therapeutic approach.
3. In animals, phenylbutazone is largely metabolized in 8 hours. It is recommended that a third of the daily dose be administered at 8 hour intervals. Reduce dosage as symptoms regress. In some cases, treatment may be given only when symptoms appear with no need for continuous medication. If long-term therapy is planned, oral administration is suggested.
4. Many chronic conditions will respond to phenylbutazone therapy, but discontinuance of treatment may result in recurrence of symptoms.

Contraindication(s): Parenteral injections should be made intravenously only; do not inject subcutaneously or intramuscularly. Use with caution in patients who have a history of drug allergy.

Precaution(s): Store in a refrigerator between 2°C and 8°C (36°F and 46°F).

Caution(s): Federal law restricts this drug to use by or on the order of a licensed veterinarian.

Stop medication at the first sign of gastrointestinal upset, jaundice, or blood dyscrasia. Authenticated cases of agranulocytosis associated with the drug have occurred in man; fatal reactions, although rare, have been reported in dogs after long-term therapy. To guard against this possibility, conduct routine blood counts at weekly intervals during the early phase of therapy and at intervals of two weeks thereafter. Any significant fall in the total white count, relative decrease in granulocytes, or black or tarry stools, should be regarded as a signal for immediate cessation of therapy and institution of appropriate countermeasures.

In the treatment of inflammatory conditions associated with infections, specific anti-infective therapy is required.

Warning(s): Treated animals should not be slaughtered for food purposes. For horses only.

References: Available upon request.

Presentation: For Horses only: 100 mL vials, 200 mg/mL (1 g/5 mL).

Compendium Code No.: 10740352 Rev. 10-99

AMTECH PHENYLBUTAZONE TABLETS, USP 100 MG ℞

Phoenix Scientific **NSAID-Oral**

Anti-inflammatory

NADA No.: 094-170

Active Ingredient(s): Each tablet contains:

Phenylbutazone, USP . . . . 100 mg

Indications: For relief of inflammatory conditions associated with the musculoskeletal system in dogs.

Pharmacology: Description: Phenylbutazone is a synthetic, non-hormonal anti-inflammatory compound useful in the management of inflammatory conditions. The apparent analgesic effect is probably related to the compound's anti-inflammatory properties.

Chemically, Phenylbutazone is 4-butyl-1,2-diphenyl-3,5-pyrazolidinedione. It is a pyrazolon derivative, entirely unrelated to the Steroid hormones, and has the following structural formula:

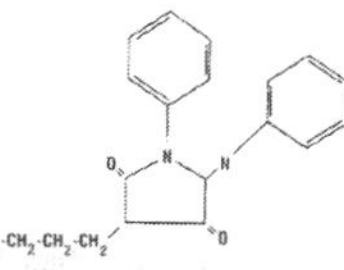

Background Pharmacology: Kuzell, (1,2,3) Payne, (4) Fleming, (5) and Denko, (6) demonstrated clinical effectiveness of Phenylbutazone in acute rheumatism, gout, gouty, arthritis, and various other rheumatoid disorders in man. Anti-inflammatory activity has been well established by Fabre, (7), Domenjoz, (8) Wilhelmi, (9) and Yourish, (10).

Lieberman (11) reported on the effective use of phenylbutazone in the treatment of painful conditions of the musculoskeletal system in dogs. Joshua (12) observed objective improvement without toxicity following long term therapy of two aged arthritic dogs. Ogilvie and Sutter (13) reported rapid response to phenylbutazone therapy in a review of 19 clinical cases including arthritis, rheumatism, and other conditions associated with lameness and musculoskeletal weakness. Camberos (14) reported favorable results with phenylbutazone following intermittent treatment of Thoroughbred horses for arthritis and chronic arthrosis (e.g., osteoarthritis of medial, and distal bones of the hock, arthritis of stifle and hip, arthrosis of the spine, chronic hip pains, chronic pain in trapezius muscles, and generalized arthritis). Results were less favorable in cases of traumatism, muscle rupture, strains, and inflammations of the third phalanx. Sutter (15) reported favorable response in chronic equine arthritis, fair results in a severely bruised mare, and poor results in two cases where the condition was limited to the third phalanx.

Dosage and Administration: Orally—20 mg per lb of body weight (100 mg/5 lb) in three divided doses daily. Maximum dose is 800 mg per day regardless of weight. Use a relatively high dose for the first 48 hours, then reduce gradually to a maintenance dose. Maintain lowest dose capable of producing desired clinical response.

Guidelines to Successful Therapy:

1. Response to Phenylbutazone therapy is prompt, usually occurring within 24 hours. If no significant clinical response is evident after 5 days, re-evalutate diagnosis and therapeutic approach.
2. In animals, Phenylbutazone is largely metabolized in 8 hours. It is recommended that a third of the daily dose be administered at 8 hour intervals. Reduce dosage as symptoms regress. In some cases, treatment may be given only when symptoms appear with no need for continuous medication. If long term therapy is planned, oral administration is suggested.
3. In many cases, tablets may be crushed and given with feed.
4. Many chronic conditions will respond to Phenylbutazone therapy, but discontinuance of treatment may result in recurrence of symptoms.
5. The duration of treatment will depend upon the degree of severity of the condition and generally ranges from 6 to 14 days with retreatment given only to control recurring symptoms. If there is no improvement in 5 days, discontinue treatment.

Contraindication(s): Animals showing evidence of cardiac, hepatic, or renal damage or a history of blood dyscrasia, or those with signs or history of anemia.

Precaution(s): Store at controlled room temperature, 20° to 25°C (68° to 77°F).

Dispense in a tight container with child-resistant closure.

Caution(s): Federal (U.S.A.) law restricts this drug to use by or on the order of a licensed veterinarian.

Stop medication at first sign of gastrointestinal upset, jaundice, or blood dyscrasia. Authenticated cases of agranulocytosis associated with the drug have occurred in man; fatal reactions, although rare, have been reported in dogs after long-term therapy. To guard against this possibility, conduct routine blood counts at weekly intervals during the early phase of therapy and at intervals of two weeks thereafter. Any significant fall in the total white count, relative decrease in granulocytes, or black or tarry stools, should be regarded as a signal for immediate cessation of therapy and institution of appropriate counter measures.

In the treatment of inflammatory conditions associated with infections, specific anti-infective therapy is required.

For oral use in dogs only.

Keep out of reach of children.

References: Available upon request.

Presentation: PHENYLBUTAZONE TABLETS, USP 100 mg are supplied in bottles of 500 and 1000 tablets.

Compendium Code No.: 10740371 Iss. 7-98

AMTECH PHENYLBUTAZONE TABLETS, USP 200 MG ℞

Phoenix Scientific **Phenylbutazone-Oral**

Anti-inflammatory

NADA No.: 094-170

Active Ingredient(s): Each tablet contains:

Phenylbutazone, USP . . . . 200 mg

Indications: For relief of inflammatory conditions associated with the musculoskeletal system in dogs.

Pharmacology: Description: Phenylbutazone is a synthetic, non-hormonal anti-inflammatory compound useful in the management of inflammatory conditions. The apparent analgesic effect is probably related to the compound's anti-inflammatory properties.

Chemically, Phenylbutazone is 4-butyl-1,2-diphenyl-3,5-pyrazolidinedione. It is a pyrazolon derivative, entirely unrelated to the Steroid hormones, and has the following structural formula:

Background Pharmacology: Kuzell, (1,2,3) Payne, (4) Fleming, (5) and Denko, (6) demonstrated clinical effectiveness of Phenylbutazone in acute rheumatism, gout, gouty, arthritis, and various other rheumatoid disorders in man. Anti-inflammatory activity has been well established by Fabre, (7), Domenjoz, (8) Wilhelmi, (9) and Yourish, (10).

Lieberman (11) reported on the effective use of phenylbutazone in the treatment of painful conditions of the musculoskeletal system in dogs. Joshua (12) observed objective improvement without toxicity following long term therapy of two aged arthritic dogs. Ogilvie and Sutter (13) reported rapid response to phenylbutazone therapy in a review of 19 clinical cases including arthritis, rheumatism, and other conditions associated with lameness and musculoskeletal weakness. Camberos (14) reported favorable results with phenylbutazone following intermittent treatment of Thoroughbred horses for arthritis and chronic arthrosis (e.g., osteoarthritis of medial, and distal bones of the hock, arthritis of stifle and hip, arthrosis of the spine, chronic hip pains, chronic pain in trapezius muscles, and generalized arthritis). Results were less favorable in cases of traumatism, muscle rupture, strains, and inflammations of the third phalanx. Sutter (15) reported favorable response in chronic equine arthritis, fair results in a severely bruised mare, and poor results in two cases where the condition was limited to the third phalanx.

Dosage and Administration: Orally—20 mg per lb of body weight (200 mg/10 lb) in three divided doses daily. Maximum dose is 800 mg per day regardless of weight. Use a relatively high dose for the first 48 hours, then reduce gradually to a maintenance dose. Maintain lowest dose capable of producing desired clinical response.

Guidelines to Successful Therapy:

1. Response to Phenylbutazone therapy is prompt, usually occurring within 24 hours. If no significant clinical response is evident after 5 days, re-evalutate diagnosis and therapeutic approach.
2. In animals, Phenylbutazone is largely metabolized in 8 hours. It is recommended that a third of the daily dose be administered at 8 hour intervals. Reduce dosage as symptoms regress. In some cases, treatment may be given only when symptoms appear with no need for continuous medication. If long term therapy is planned, oral administration is suggested.
3. In many cases, tablets may be crushed and given with feed.
4. Many chronic conditions will respond to Phenylbutazone therapy, but discontinuance of treatment may result in recurrence of symptoms.
5. The duration of treatment will depend upon the degree of severity of the condition and generally ranges from 6 to 14 days with retreatment given only to control recurring symptoms. If there is no improvement in 5 days, discontinue treatment.

Contraindication(s): Animals showing evidence of cardiac, hepatic, or renal damage or a history of blood dyscrasia, or those with signs or history of anemia.

Precaution(s): Store at controlled room temperature, 20° to 25°C (68° to 77°F).

Dispense in a tight container with child-resistant closure.

Caution(s): Federal (U.S.A.) law restricts this drug to use by or on the order of a licensed veterinarian.

Stop medication at first sign of gastrointestinal upset, jaundice, or blood dyscrasia. Authenticated cases of agranulocytosis associated with the drug have occurred in man; fatal reactions, although rare, have been reported in dogs after long-term therapy. To guard against this possibility, conduct routine blood counts at weekly intervals during the early phase of therapy and at intervals of two weeks thereafter. Any significant fall in the total white count, relative decrease in granulocytes, or black or tarry stools, should be regarded as a signal for immediate cessation of therapy and institution of appropriate counter measures.

In the treatment of inflammatory conditions associated with infections, specific anti-infective therapy is required. For oral use in dogs only. Keep out of reach of children.

References: Available upon request.

Presentation: PHENYLBUTAZONE TABLETS, USP 200 mg are supplied in bottles of 100 and 500 tablets.

Compendium Code No.: 10740640 801025 Iss. 1-99

AMTECH PHENYLBUTAZONE TABLETS, USP 1 GRAM ℞

Phoenix Scientific **NSAID-Oral**

Anti-inflammatory

NADA No.: 091-818

Active Ingredient(s): Each tablet contains 1 g of phenylbutazone.

Indications: Phenylbutazone is for the relief of inflammatory conditions associated with the musculoskeletal system in horses.

Pharmacology: Phenylbutazone chemically is 4-butyl-1, 2 diphenyl-3, 5-pyrazolidinedione.

$C_{19}H_{20}N_2O_2$

Mol. Wt. 308.38

Background Pharmacology: Phenylbutazone was first synthesized in 1948 and introduced into human medicine in 1949. Kuzell (1), (2), (3), Payne, (4), Fleming, (5) and Denko, (6) demonstrated the clinical effectiveness of phenylbutazone in gout, gouty arthritis, acute arthritis, acute rheumatism and various other rheumatoid disorders in humans. Fabre (7), Domenjoz, (8), Wilhelmi, (9) and Yourish, (10), have established the anti-rheumatic and anti-inflammatory activity of phenylbutazone. It is entirely unrelated to the steroid hormones.

Toxicity of phenylbutazone has been investigated in rats and mice (11), and dogs (12).

Phenylbutazone has been used by Camberos (13), in thoroughbred horses. Favorable results were reported in cases of traumatism, muscle rupture, strains and inflammations of the third phalanx. Results were not as favorable in the periodic treatment of osteoarthritis of the stifle and hip, arthrosis of the trapezious muscles and general arthritis. Sutter, (14) reported a favorable response in chronic equine arthritis of long duration, fair results in severely bruised mare and poor results in two cases where the condition was limited to the third phalanx.

Dosage and Administration: For Horses Only: Orally 1 to 2 tablets per 500 pounds of body weight, but not to exceed 4 g per animal daily. Use high dose for the first 48 hours, then gradually reduce to a maintenance dose.

Precaution(s): Store at controlled room temperature, 20° to 25°C (68° to 77°F).

Dispense in tight, child resistant containers.

Caution(s): Federal law restricts this drug to use by or on the order of a licensed veterinarian.

Use with caution in patients who have history of drug allergy.

In the treatment of inflammatory conditions associated with infections, specific anti-infective therapy should be used concurrently. Keep out of reach of children.

Warning(s): Not for use in horses intended for food. For oral use in horses only.

References: Available upon request.

Presentation: Tablets containing 1 gram of phenylbutazone are supplied in bottles of 100 tablets (NDC 59130-715-34).

Compendium Code No.: 10740361 Rev. 04-00

AMTECH PHOENECTIN® INJECTION FOR CATTLE AND SWINE

Phoenix Scientific **Parasiticide Injection**

(ivermectin) Injection 1% Sterile Solution

ANADA No.: 200-228

Active Ingredient(s): PHOENECTIN® Injection is a clear, ready-to-use, sterile solution containing 1% ivermectin, 40% glycerol formal, 1.5% benzyl alcohol (preservative), and propylene glycol, q.s. ad 100%. It is formulated to deliver the recommended dose level of 200 mcg ivermectin/kilogram of body weight in cattle when given subcutaneously at the rate of 1 mL/110 lb (50 kg).

In swine, PHOENECTIN® Injection is formulated to deliver the recommended dose level of 300 mcg ivermectin/kilogram body weight when given subcutaneously in the neck at the rate of 1 mL/75 lb (33 kg).

Indications: A parasiticide for the treatment and control of internal and external parasites of cattle and swine.

Cattle: PHOENECTIN® Injection is indicated for the effective treatment and control of the following harmful species of gastrointestinal roundworms, lungworms, grubs, sucking lice, and mange mites in cattle:

Gastrointestinal Roundworms (adults and fourth-stage larvae): *Ostertagia ostertagi* (including inhibited *O. ostertagi), O. lyrata, Haemonchus placei, Trichostrongylus axei, T. colubriformis, Cooperia oncophora, C. punctata, C. pectinata, Oesophagostomum radiatum, Bunostomum phlebotomum, Nematodirus helvetianus* (adults only), *N. spathiger* (adults only).

Lungworms (adults and fourth-stage larvae): *Dictyocaulus viviparus.*

Cattle Grubs (parasitic stages): *Hypoderma bovis, H. lineatum.*

Sucking Lice: *Linognathus vituli, Haematopinus eurysternus, Solenopotes capillatus.*

Mites (Scabies): *Psoroptes ovis* (syn. *P. communis* var. *bovis), Sarcoptes scabiei* var. *bovis.*

Persistent Activity: PHOENECTIN® Injection has been proved to effectively control infections and to protect cattle from reinfection with *Dictyocaulus viviparus* for 21 days after treatment; *Ostertagia ostertagi* for 21 days after treatment; *Oesophagostomum radiatum, Haemonchus placei, Trichostrongylus axei, Cooperia punctata,* and *Cooperia oncophora* for 14 days after treatment.

Swine: PHOENECTIN® Injection is indicated for the effective treatment and control of the following harmful species of gastrointestinal roundworms, lungworms, lice, and mange mites in swine:

Gastrointestinal Roundworms (adults and fourth-stage larvae): Large roundworm: *Ascaris suum.*

Red stomach worm: *Hyostrongylus rubidus.* Nodular worm: *Oesophagostomum* spp.

Threadworm: *Strongyloides ransomi* (adults only). Somatic Roundworm Larvae:

Threadworm: *Strongyloides ransomi* (somatic larvae).

Sows must be treated at least seven days before farrowing to prevent infection in piglets.

Lungworms: *Metastrongylus* spp (adults).

Lice: *Haematopinus suis.*

Mange Mites: *Sarcoptes scabiei* var. *suis.*

Reindeer: For the treatment and control of warbles *(Oedemagena tarandi)* in reindeer (see Special Minor Use section under "Dosage and Administration").

American Bison: For the treatment and control of grubs *(Hypoderma bovis)* in American bison (see Special Minor Use section under "Dosage and Administration").

Pharmacology: Ivermectin is derived from the avermectins, a family of potent, broad-spectrum antiparasitic agents isolated from fermentation of *Streptomyces avermitilis.*

Mode of Action: Ivermectin is a member of the macrocyclic lactone class of endectocides which have a unique mode of action. Compounds of the class bind selectively and with high affinity to glutamate-gated chloride ion channels which occur in invertebrate nerve and muscle cells. This leads to an increase in the permeability of the cell membrane to chloride ions with hyperpolarization of the nerve or muscle cell, resulting in paralysis and death of the parasite. Compounds of this class may also interact with other ligand-gated chloride channels, such as those gated by the neurotransmitter gamma-aminobutyric acid (GABA).

The wide margin of safety is attributable to the fact that mammals do not have glutamate-gated chloride channels, the macrocyclic lactones have a low affinity for other mammalian ligand-gated chloride channels and they do not readily cross the blood-brain barrier.

Dosage and Administration: Dosage:

Cattle: PHOENECTIN® should be given only by subcutaneous injection under the loose skin in front or behind the shoulder at the recommended dose level of 200 mcg ivermectin per kilogram of body weight. Each mL of PHOENECTIN® contains 10 mg of ivermectin, sufficient to treat 110 lb (50 kg) of body weight (maximum 10 mL per injection site).

Body Weight (lb)	Dose (mL)
220	2
330	3
440	4
550	5
660	6
770	7
880	8
990	9
1100	10

Swine: PHOENECTIN® should be given only by subcutaneous injection in the neck of swine at the recommended dose level of 300 mcg of ivermectin per kilogram (2.2 lb) of body weight. Each mL of PHOENECTIN® contains 10 mg of ivermectin, sufficient to treat 75 lb of body weight.

	Body Weight (lb)	Dose (mL)
Growing Pigs	19	¼
	38	½
	75	1
	150	2
Breeding Animals (Sows, Gilts, and Boars)	225	3
	300	4
	375	5
	450	6

Administration:

Cattle: PHOENECTIN® Injection is to be given subcutaneously only, to reduce risk of potentially fatal clostridial infection of the injection site. Animals should be appropriately restrained to achieve the proper route of administration. Use of a 16-gauge ½ to ¾" needle is suggested. Inject under the loose skin in front of or behind the shoulder (see illustration).

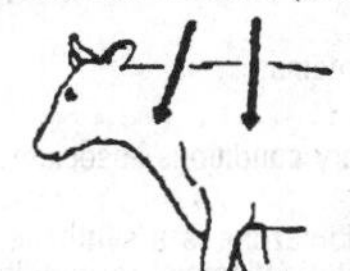

Any single-dose syringe or standard automatic syringe equipment may be used with the 50 mL package size. When using the 200 mL or 500 mL package size, use only automatic syringe equipment.

Use sterile equipment and sanitize the injection site by applying a suitable disinfectant. Clean, properly disinfected needles should be used to reduce the potential for injection site infections. No special handling or protective clothing is necessary.

Swine: PHOENECTIN® (ivermectin) Injection is to be given subcutaneously in the neck. Animals should be appropriately restrained to achieve the proper route of administration. Use of a 16- or 18-gauge needle is suggested for sows and boars, while an 18- or 20-gauge needle may be appropriate for young animals. Inject under the skin, immediately behind the ear (see illustration).

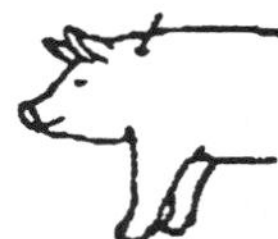

Any single-dose syringe or standard automatic syringe equipment may be used with the 50 mL package size. When using the 200 mL or 500 mL package size, use only automatic syringe equipment. As with any injection, sterile equipment should be used. The injection site should be cleaned and disinfected with alcohol before injection. The rubber stopper should also be disinfected with alcohol to prevent contamination of the contents. Mild and transient pain reactions may be seen in some swine following subcutaneous administration.

Recommended Treatment Program:

Swine: At the time of initiating any parasite control program, it is important to treat all breeding animals in the herd. After the initial treatment, use PHOENECTIN® (ivermectin) Injection regularly as follows:

Breeding Animals:

Sows: Treat prior to farrowing, preferably 7-14 days before, to minimize infection of piglets.

Gilts: Treat 7-14 days prior to breeding. Treat 7-14 days prior to farrowing.

Boars: Frequency and need for treatments are dependent upon exposure. Treat at least two times a year.

Feeder Pigs (Weaners/Growers/Finishers): All weaner/feeder pigs should be treated before placement in clean quarters.

Pigs exposed to contaminated soil or pasture may need retreatment if reinfection occurs.

Note:

1. PHOENECTIN® Injection has a persistent drug level sufficient to control mite infestations throughout the egg to adult life cycle. However, since the ivermectin effect is not immediate, care must be taken to prevent reinfestation from exposure to untreated animals or contaminated facilities. Generally, pigs should not be moved to clean quarters or exposed to uninfested pigs for approximately one week after treatment. Sows should be treated at least one week before farrowing to minimize transfer of mites to newborn baby pigs.
2. Louse eggs are unaffected by PHOENECTIN® Injection and may require up to three weeks to hatch. Louse infestations developing from hatching eggs may require retreatment.
3. Consult a veterinarian for aid in the diagnosis and control of internal and external parasites of swine.

Special Minor Use:

Reindeer: For the treatment and control of warbles *(Oedemagena tarandi)* in reindeer, inject 200 micrograms ivermectin per kilogram of body weight, subcutaneously. Follow use directions for cattle as described under Administration.

American Bison: For the treatment and control of grubs *(Hypoderma bovis)* in American Bison, inject 200 micrograms ivermectin per kilogram of body weight, subcutaneously. Follow use directions for cattle as described under Administration.

Consult your veterinarian for assistance in the diagnosis, treatment and control of parasitism.

Contraindication(s): PHOENECTIN® Injection for Cattle and Swine has been developed specifically for use in cattle, swine, reindeer and American bison only. This product should not be used in other animal species as severe adverse reactions, including fatalities in dogs, may result.

Precaution(s): Store between 15°C and 30°C (59°F and 86°F).

Protect product from light.

Environmental Safety: Studies indicate that when ivermectin comes in contact with the soil, it readily and tightly binds to the soil and becomes inactive over time. Free ivermectin may adversely affect fish and certain water-borne organisms on which they feed. Do not permit water runoff from feedlots or production sites to enter lakes, streams, or ponds. Do not contaminate water by direct application or by the improper disposal of drug containers. Dispose of containers in an approved landfill or by incineration.

Caution(s): This product is not for intravenous or intramuscular use.

Use sterile equipment and sanitize the injection site by applying a suitable disinfectant. Clean, properly disinfected needles should be used to reduce the potential for injection site infections.

Transitory discomfort has been observed in some cattle following subcutaneous administration. A low incidence of soft tissue swelling at the injection site has been observed. These reactions have disappeared without treatment. For cattle, divide doses greater than 10 mL between two injection sites to reduce occasional discomfort or site reaction.

Observe cattle for injection site reactions. Reactions may be due to clostridial infection and should be aggressively treated with appropriate antibiotics. If injection site infections are suspected, consult your veterinarian.

Warning(s): Residue Warning: Do not treat cattle within 35 days of slaughter. Because a withdrawal time in milk has not been established, do not use in female dairy cattle of breeding age.

Do not treat swine within 18 days of slaughter.

Do not treat reindeer or American bison within 8 weeks (56 days) of slaughter.

Keep this and all drugs out of the reach of children.

Not for use in humans.

Discussion: PHOENECTIN® (ivermectin) is an injectable parasiticide for cattle and swine. One low-volume dose effectively treats and controls the following internal and external parasites that may impair the health of cattle and swine: gastrointestinal roundworms (including inhibited *Ostertagia ostertagi* in cattle), lungworms, grubs, sucking lice, and mange mites of cattle; and gastrointestinal roundworms, lungworms, lice, and mange mites of swine.

When to Treat Cattle with Grubs: PHOENECTIN® effectively controls all stages of cattle grubs. However, proper timing of treatment is important. For most effective results, cattle should be treated as soon as possible after the end of the heel fly (warble fly) season. Destruction of *Hypoderma* larvae (cattle grubs) at the period when these grubs are in vital areas may cause undesirable host-parasite reactions including the possibility of fatalities. Killing *Hypoderma lineatum* when it is in the tissue surrounding the esophagus (gullet) may cause salivation and bloat, killing *H. bovis* when it is in the vertebral canal may cause staggering or paralysis. These reactions are not specific to treatment with PHOENECTIN®, but can occur with any successful treatment of grubs. Cattle should be treated either before or after these stages of grub development. Consult your veterinarian concerning the proper time for treatment.

Cattle treated with PHOENECTIN® after the end of the heel fly season may be retreated with PHOENECTIN® during the winter for internal parasites, mange mites, or sucking lice without danger of grub-related reactions. A planned parasite control program is recommended.

Presentation: PHOENECTIN® Injection for Cattle and Swine is available in three ready-to-use sizes:

The 50 mL (NDC 59130-685-11) bottle contains sufficient solution to treat 10 head of 550 lb (250 kg) cattle or 100 head of 38 lb (17.3 kg) swine.

The 200 mL bottle contains sufficient solution to treat 40 head of 550 lb (250 kg) cattle or 400 head of 38 lb (17.3 kg) swine. Use automatic syringe equipment only.

The 500 mL bottle contains sufficient solution to treat 100 head of 550 lb (250 kg) cattle or 1000 head of 38 lb (17.3 kg) swine. Use automatic syringe equipment only.

Compendium Code No.: 10740621

Rev. 3-02

AMTECH PHOENECTIN® LIQUID FOR HORSES ℞

Phoenix Scientific **Parasiticide-Oral**

(ivermectin) 10 mg per mL

ANADA No.: 200-202

Active Ingredient(s): PHOENECTIN® (ivermectin) Liquid is a clear, ready-to-use solution with each mL containing 1% ivermectin (10 mg), 0.2 mL propylene glycol, 80 mg polysorbate 80, 9 mg sodium phosphate monobasic monohydrate, 1.3 mg sodium phosphate dibasic anhydrous, 1 mg butylated hydroxytoluene, 0.1 mg disodium edetate, 3% benzyl alcohol and water for injection q.s. ad 100%.

Indications: PHOENECTIN® (ivermectin) Liquid is indicated for the effective treatment and control of the following parasites or parasitic conditions in horses:

Large Strongyles: *Strongylus vulgaris* (adults and arterial larval stages), *S. edentatus* (adults and tissue stages), *S. equinus* (adults), *Triodontophorus* spp (adults).

Small Strongyles - including those resistant to some benzimidazole class compounds (adults and fourth-stage larvae): *Cyathostomum* spp, *Cylicocyclus* spp, *Cylicostephanus* spp, *Cylicodontophorus* spp.

Pinworms (adults and fourth-stage larvae): *Oxyuris equi.*

Ascarids (adults and third- and fourth-stage larvae): *Parascaris equorum.*

Hairworms (adults): *Trichostrongylus axei.*

Large-mouth Stomach Worms (adults): *Habronema muscae.*

Bots (oral and gastric stages): *Gasterophilus* spp.

Lungworms (adults and fourth-stage larvae): *Dictyocaulus arnfieldi.*

Intestinal Threadworms (adults): *Strongyloides westeri.*

Summer Sores caused by *Habronema* and *Draschia* spp cutaneous third-stage larvae.

Dermatitis caused by neck threadworm microfilariae, *Onchocerca* sp.

Pharmacology: Ivermectin is derived from the avermectins, a family of potent, broad-spectrum antiparasitic agents, which are isolated from fermentation of *Streptomyces avermitilis.*

Mode of Action: Ivermectin, one of the avermectins, kills certain parasitic roundworms and ectoparasites such as mites and lice. The avermectins are different in their action from other antiparasitic agents. This action involves a chemical that serves as a signal from one nerve cell to another, or from a nerve cell to a muscle cell. This chemical, a neurotransmitter, is called gamma-aminobutyric acid or GABA.

In roundworms, ivermectin stimulates the release of GABA from nerve endings and enhances binding of GABA to special receptors at nerve junctions, thus interrupting nerve impulses - thereby paralyzing and killing the parasite.

The enhancement of the GABA effect in arthropods such as mites and lice resembles that in roundworms except that nerve impulses are interrupted between the nerve ending and the muscle cell. Again, this leads to paralysis and death.

The principal peripheral neurotransmitter in mammals, acetylcholine, is unaffected by ivermectin. Ivermectin does not readily penetrate the central nervous system of mammals where GABA functions as a neurotransmitter.

Dosage and Administration: Dosage: PHOENECTIN® (ivermectin) Liquid for Horses is formulated for administration by stomach tube (nasogastric intubation) or as an oral drench. The recommended dose is 200 mcg of ivermectin per kilogram (91 mcg/lb) of body weight. Each mL contains sufficient ivermectin to treat 110 lb (50 kg) of body weight: 10 mL will treat an 1100 lb (500 kg) horse.

Administration: Use a calibrated dosing syringe inserted into the bottle to measure the appropriate dose, or pour the PHOENECTIN® (ivermectin) Liquid into a graduated cylinder for dose measurement. Use a clean syringe if accessing the bottle to avoid contaminating the remaining product.

Administration by stomach tube (gravity or positive flow): The recommended dose can be used undiluted or diluted up to 40 times with clean tepid water (see Notes to Veterinarian). Use tepid water to flush any drug remaining in the tube into the horse's stomach.

Administration by drench: For administration by this method, an undiluted dose is usually preferred. Clear the horse's mouth of any food material, elevate the horse's head, and using a syringe, deposit the appropriate dose in the back of the mouth. In order to avoid unnecessary coughing or the potential for material to enter the trachea and lungs, do not use excessive pressure (squirting), do not use a large (diluted) dose volume, and do not deposit the dose in the laryngeal area. Increased dose rejection may occur if the dose is deposited in the buccal space. Keep the horse's head elevated and observe the horse to insure the dose is retained.

Suggested Parasite Control Program: All horses should be included in a regular parasite control program with particular attention being paid to mares, foals and yearlings. Foals should be treated initially at 6 to 8 weeks of age, and routine treatment repeated as appropriate. PHOENECTIN® (ivermectin) effectively controls gastrointestinal nematodes and bots in horses. Regular treatment will reduce the chances of verminous arteritis and colic caused by *S. vulgaris.* With its broad spectrum, PHOENECTIN® (ivermectin) is well suited to be the major product in a parasite control program.

Contraindication(s): PHOENECTIN® (ivermectin) Liquid has been formulated specifically for use in horses only. This product should not be used in other animal species as severe adverse reactions, including fatalities in dogs, may result.

Precaution(s): Store in a tightly closed container at room temperature.

Protect PHOENECTIN® (ivermectin) Liquid (undiluted or diluted) from light.

Environmental Safety: Studies indicate that when ivermectin comes in contact with the soil, it readily and tightly binds to the soil and becomes inactive over time. Free ivermectin may adversely affect fish and certain water-borne organisms on which they feed. Do not contaminate lakes, streams, or ground water by direct application or by improper disposal of drug containers. Dispose of drug container in an approved landfill or by incineration.

Caution(s): Federal (U.S.A.) law restricts this drug to use by or on the order of a licensed veterinarian.

For veterinary use only.

Warning(s): Do not use in horses intended for food purposes.

Refrain from smoking and eating when handling. Wash hands after use. Avoid contact with eyes. Keep this and all drugs out of the reach of children.

Safety: PHOENECTIN® (ivermectin) Liquid may be used in horses of all ages including mares at any stage of pregnancy. Stallions may be treated without adversely affecting their fertility. These horses have been treated with no adverse effects other than those noted under Notes to Veterinarian.

Discussion: PHOENECTIN® (ivermectin) Liquid for Horses has been formulated for professional administration by stomach tube or oral drench. One low-volume dose is effective against important internal parasites, including the arterial stages of *Strongylus vulgaris*, and bots.

Ivermectin is a potent antiparasitic agent whose chemical structure is different from those of other antiparasitic agents. Its convenience, broad-spectrum efficiency and safety margin make PHOENECTIN® (ivermectin) Liquid an ideal parasite control product for horses.

Notes to Veterinarian: Swelling and itching reactions after treatment with PHOENECTIN® (ivermectin) have occurred in horses carrying heavy infections of neck threadworm microfilariae, *Onchocerca* sp. These reactions were most likely the result of microfilariae dying in large numbers. Symptomatic treatment may be advisable.

Healing of summer sores involving extensive tissue changes may require other therapy in conjunction with PHOENECTIN® (ivermectin). Reinfection, and measures for its prevention, should also be considered.

Special consideration should be given to the effects or potential for injury from handling, restraint, and placement of the tube during administration by stomach tube. PHOENECTIN® (ivermectin) Liquid should be administered by drench if the risks associated with tubing are of concern. Due to the consequences of improper administration (also see Dosage and Administration), PHOENECTIN® (ivermectin) Liquid is intended for use by a veterinarian only and is not recommended for dispensing.

PHOENECTIN® (ivermectin) Liquid in 1 to 20 and 1 to 40 dilutions with tap water has been shown to be stable for 72 hours under the conditions recommended for the product (i.e., at room temperature, in a tightly closed container, protected from light). The diluted product does not promote the growth of common organisms. However, prolonged storage of the diluted product cannot be recommended, as the effects of possible contaminants and interactions with untested materials are unknown.

Presentation: PHOENECTIN® (ivermectin) Liquid for Horses is available in 100 mL (NDC 59130-680-01) and 200 mL (NDC 59130-680-22) plastic bottles. The 100 mL bottle contains sufficient ivermectin to treat 10-500 kg (1,100 lb) horses. The 200 mL bottle contains sufficient ivermectin to treat 20-500 kg (1,100 lb) horses. Contents may be poured into a graduated cylinder for dose measurement. Alternatively, a clean syringe may be inserted directly into the bottle to draw off the appropriate dose.

Compendium Code No.: 10740384 Rev. 2-00 / Iss. 2-00

AMTECH PHOENECTIN® PASTE 1.87%

Phoenix Scientific **Parasiticide-Oral**

(ivermectin) Anthelmintic and Boticide

ANADA No.: 200-286

Active Ingredient(s): Each syringe contains:

Ivermectin 1.87%

Indications: PHOENECTIN® (ivermectin) Paste 1.87% provides effective control of the following parasites in horses:

Large Strongyles (adults): *Strongylus vulgaris* (also early forms in blood vessels), *S. edentatus* (also tissue stages), *S. equinus, Triodontophorus* spp.

Small Strongyles including those resistant to some benzimidazole class compounds (adults and fourth-stage larvae): *Cyathostomum* spp., *Cylicocyclus* spp., *Cylicostephanus* spp., *Cylicodontophorus* spp.

Pinworms (adults and fourth-stage larvae): *Oxyuris equi.*

Ascarids (adults and third- and fourth-stage larvae): *Parascaris equorum.*

Hairworms (adults): *Trichostrongylus axei.*

Large-mouth Stomach Worms (adults): *Habronema muscae.*

Bots (oral and gastric stages): *Gasterophilus* spp.

Lungworms (adults and fourth-stage larvae): *Dictyocaulus arnfieldi.*

Intestinal Threadworms (adults): *Strongyloides westeri.*

Summer Sores caused by *Habronema* and *Draschia* spp. cutaneous third-stage larvae.

Dermatitis caused by neck threadworm microfilariae, *Onchocerca* sp.

Dosage and Administration: The syringe contains sufficient paste to treat one 1250 lb horse at the recommended dose rate of 91 mcg ivermectin per lb (200 mcg/kg) of body weight. Each weight marking on the syringe plunger delivers enough paste to treat 250 lb of body weight. (1) While holding plunger, turn the knurled ring on the plunger to the right so the side nearest the barrel is at the prescribed weight marking. (2) Make sure that horse's mouth contains no feed. (3) Remove the cover from the tip of the syringe. (4) Insert the syringe tip into the horse's mouth at the space between the teeth. (5) Depress the plunger as far as it will go, depositing paste on the back of the tongue. (6) Immediately raise the horse's head for a few seconds after dosing.

Parasite Control Program: All horses should be included in a regular parasite control program with particular attention being paid to mares, foals and yearlings. Foals should be treated initially at 6 to 8 weeks of age, and routine treatment repeated as appropriate. Consult your veterinarian for a control program to meet your specific needs. PHOENECTIN® (ivermectin) Paste 1.87% effectively controls gastrointestinal nematodes and bots of horses. Regular treatment will reduce the chances of verminous arteritis caused by *S. vulgaris.*

Consult your veterinarian for assistance in the diagnosis, treatment, and control of parasitism.

Precaution(s): Store at controlled room temperature, 20° to 25°C (68° to 77°F).

Dispose of the syringe in approved landfill or by incineration.

Caution(s): PHOENECTIN® (ivermectin) Paste 1.87% has been formulated specifically for use in horses only. This product should not be used in other animal species as severe adverse reactions, including fatalities in dogs, may result. Ivermectin and excreted ivermectin residues may adversely affect aquatic organisms. Do not contaminate ground or surface water.

Note to User: Swelling and itching reactions after treatment with PHOENECTIN® (ivermectin) Paste 1.87% have occurred in horses carrying heavy infections of neck threadworm *(Onchocera* sp.) microfilariae. These reactions were most likely the result of microfilariae dying in large numbers. Symptomatic treatment may be advisable. Consult your veterinarian should any such reactions occur. Healing of summer sores involving extensive tissue changes may require other appropriate therapy in conjunction with treatment with PHOENECTIN® (ivermectin) Paste 1.87%. Reinfection, and measures for its prevention should also be considered. Consult your veterinarian if the condition does not improve.

For oral use in horses only.

Warning(s): Residue Warning: Do not use in horses intended for food purposes.

Refrain from smoking and eating when handling. Wash hands after use. Avoid contact with eyes. Keep this and all drugs out of the reach of children.

Side Effects: Safety: PHOENECTIN® (ivermectin) Paste 1.87% may be used in horses of all ages including mares at any stage of pregnancy. Stallions may be treated without adversely affecting their fertility.

Presentation: 6.08 g (0.21 oz) syringe (NDC 59130-712-31).

Compendium Code No.: 10740632 Rev. 1-01

AMTECH PHOENECTIN® POUR-ON FOR CATTLE

Phoenix Scientific **Parasiticide-Topical**

(ivermectin) 5 mg per mL-Parasiticide

ANADA No.: 200-219

Active Ingredient(s): Contains 5 mg ivermectin/mL.

Indications: PHOENECTIN® Pour-On applied at the recommended dose level of 500 mcg/kg is indicated for the effective control of these parasites.

Gastrointestinal Roundworms: *Ostertagia ostertagi* (including inhibited stage) (adults and L_4), *Haemonchus placei* (adults and L_4), *Trichostrongylus axei* (adults and L_4), *T. colubriformis* (adults and L_4), *Cooperia* spp (adults and L_4), *Strongyloides papillosus* (adults), *Oesophagostomum radiatum* (adults and L_4), *Trichuris* spp (adults).

Lungworms: *Dictyocaulus viviparus* (adults and L_4).

Cattle Grubs (parasitic stages): *Hypoderma bovis, H. lineatum.*

Mites: *Sarcoptes scabiei* var. *bovis.*

Lice: *Linognathus vituli, Haematopinus eurysternus, Damalinia bovis, Solenopotes capillatus.*

Horn Flies: *Haematobia irritans.*

Pharmacology: Persistent Activity: PHOENECTIN® Pour-On has been proved to effectively control infections and to protect cattle from re-infection with *Ostertagia ostertagi, Oesophagostomum radiatum, Haemonchus placei, Trichostrongylus axei, Cooperia punctata* and *Cooperia oncophora* for 14 days after treatment.

Mode of Action: Ivermectin as a member of the avermectin family kills certain parasitic roundworms and ectoparasites, such as mites, lice, horn flies and other insects. Its action is unique to the avermectin class of antiparasitic agents. This action involves a chemical that serves as a signal from one nerve cell to another, or from a nerve cell to a muscle cell. This chemical, a neurotransmitter, is called gamma-aminobutyric acid or GABA.

In roundworms, ivermectin stimulates the release of GABA from nerve endings and enhances binding of GABA to special receptors at nerve junctions, thus interrupting nerve impulses - thereby paralyzing and killing the parasite.

The enhancement of the GABA effect in arthropods such as mites, lice, and horn flies resembles that in roundworms except that nerve impulses are interrupted between the nerve ending and the muscle cell. Again, this leads to paralysis and death.

Ivermectin has no measurable effect against flukes or tapeworms, presumably because they do not have GABA as a nerve impulse transmitter.

The principal peripheral neurotransmitter in mammals, acetylcholine, is unaffected by ivermectin. Ivermectin does not readily penetrate the central nervous system of mammals where GABA functions as a neurotransmitter.

Dosage and Administration: Treatment for Cattle for Horn Flies: PHOENECTIN® Pour-On controls horn flies *(Haematobia irritans)* for up to 28 days after dosing. For best results PHOENECTIN® Pour-On should be part of a parasite control program for both internal and external parasites based on the epidemiology of these parasites. Consult your veterinarian or an entomologist for the most effective timing of applications.

Dosage: The dose rate is 1 mL for each 22 lb of body weight. The formulation should be applied along the topline in a narrow strip extending from the withers to the tailhead.

Administration:

Dispensing Cap (250 mL, 500 mL and 1 L bottles): The enclosed dispensing cap is graduated in 5 mL increments. Each 5 mL will treat 110 lbs body weight. When body weight is between markings, use the next higher increment.

Attach the dispensing cap to the bottle.

Select the correct dose rate by rotating the adjuster top in either direction to position the dose indicator to the appropriate level.

Hold the bottle upright and gently squeeze it to deliver a slight excess of the required dose as indicated by the calibration lines.

By releasing the pressure, the dose automatically adjusts to the correct level. Tilt the bottle to deliver the dose. The off (stop) position will close the system between dosing.

Applicator Gun* (3.785 L bottle, 5 L backpack and 25 L carboy): Because of the solvents used in PHOENECTIN® Pour-On, only the PHOENECTIN® applicator gun from Simcro Tech Limited, or equivalent, is recommended. Other applicators may exhibit compatibility problems, resulting in locking, incorrect dosage or leakage.

Insert the brass end of the draw tube into the larger hole on the back side of the cap with the stem.

Slide one of the coil springs over one end of the draw-off tubing. Attach that end of the draw-off tubing to the stem on the applicator gun and slide the spring up to the connection. Slide the other coil spring over the other end of the draw-off tubing and connect that end to the cap that has the stem. Slide the spring to the connection. Replace the shipping cap with the cap having the draw-off tubing attached. Tighten this draw-off cap to the bottle.

Follow the applicator gun manufacturer's directions for priming the gun, adjusting the dose, and care of the applicator gun following use.

Directions for Use - PHOENECTIN® (ivermectin) Pour-On Applicator:

This applicator has been designed for use with PHOENECTIN® Pour-On only, and is not recommended to be used with other products.

To Prime Applicator: Connect the delivery tube to the applicator and PHOENECTIN® Pour-On gallon bottle, squeeze the handle of the applicator several times until the pour-on is drawn through the tube filling the barrel. Point the applicator nozzle upwards and gently squeeze the handle several times until all air has been expelled from the applicator barrel.

To Set Dose: Turn the dose adjuster band clockwise to move the piston forward to the required dose setting marked on the barrel. Turning the dosage adjuster band clockwise decreases the dose while counter-clockwise increases the dose. The system is now ready for use.

*Important - when adjusting the piston forward or back to a new dose setting, make sure the front face of the piston lines up with the printed mark on the barrel.

Cleaning Instructions:

1. Carefully remove the tubing from the PHOENECTIN® Pour-On container and rinse applicator and tubing thoroughly with clean water.

2. Occasionally disassemble applicator by unscrewing barrel from handle mounting.
3. Lubricate the piston "O" ring and the felt washer with vegetable oil.
4. Reassemble applicator.
5. Squeeze the applicator a few times to spread the oil throughout the barrel.
6. Store the applicator in a plastic bag to keep it dust free for reuse.

Replacement parts for the PHOENECTIN® Pour-On applicator can be purchased directly from: Felton Medical Inc., 11535 West 83rd Terrace, Lenexa, KS 66214, Ph: 800-448-8522 - Fax: (913) 599-0909 U.S. Agents for Manufacturer, Simcro Tech Ltd. NZ.

If breakage occurs, under normal use, call (913) 599-5959 for free replacement.

Weight	Dose
220 lb (100 kg)	10 mL
330 lb (150 kg)	15 mL
440 lb (200 kg)	20 mL
550 lb (250 kg)	25 mL
660 lb (300 kg)	30 mL
770 lb (350 kg)	35 mL
880 lb (400 kg)	40 mL
990 lb (450 kg)	45 mL
1100 lb (500 kg)	50 mL

*Additional Applicator Guns and Draw Tubes may be purchased from your local retail dealer or through Phoenix Scientific, Inc., St. Joseph, MO (816) 364-3777.

When to Treat Cattle with Grubs: PHOENECTIN® Pour-On effectively controls all stages of cattle grubs. However, proper timing of treatment is important. For the most effective results, cattle should be treated as soon as possible after the end of the heel fly (warble fly) season. While this is not peculiar to ivermectin, destruction of *Hypoderma* larvae (cattle grubs) at the period when these grubs are in vital areas may cause undesirable host-parasite reactions. Killing *Hypoderma lineatum* when it is in the esophageal tissues may cause bloat; killing *H. bovis* when it is in the vertebral canal may cause staggering or paralysis. Cattle should be treated either before or after these stages of grub development.

Cattle treated with PHOENECTIN® Pour-On at the end of the fly season may be re-treated with PHOENECTIN® during the winter without danger of grub-related reactions. For further information and advice on a planned parasite control program, consult your veterinarian.

Consult your veterinarian for assistance in the diagnosis, treatment and control of parasitism.

Precaution(s): Flammable! Keep away from heat, sparks, open flame, and other sources of ignition.

Store at controlled room temperature 15°-30°C (59°-86°F).

Store away from excessive heat (104°F/40°C) and protect from light.

Use only in well-ventilated areas or outdoors.

Close container tightly when not in use.

Cloudiness in the formulation may occur when PHOENECTIN® (ivermectin) Pour-On is stored at temperatures below 32°F. Allowing to warm at room temperature will restore the normal appearance without affecting efficacy.

Environmental Safety: Studies indicate that when ivermectin comes in contact with the soil, it readily and tightly binds to the soil and becomes inactive over time. Free ivermectin may adversely affect fish or certain water-borne organisms on which they feed. Do not permit cattle to enter lakes, streams or ponds for at least six hours after treatment. Do not contaminate water by direct application or by the improper disposal of drug containers. Dispose of containers in an approved landfill or by incineration.

Caution(s): Cattle should not be treated when hair or hide is wet since reduced efficacy may be experienced.

Do not use when rain is expected to wet cattle within six hours after treatment.

This product is for application to skin surface only. Do not give orally or parenterally.

Antiparasitic activity of ivermectin will be impaired if the formulation is applied to areas of the skin with mange scabs or lesions, or with dermatoses or adherent materials, e.g., caked mud or manure.

Ivermectin has been associated with adverse reaction in sensitive dogs; therefore, PHOENECTIN® Pour-On is not recommended for use in species other than cattle.

Warning(s): Residue Warning: Cattle must not be treated within 48 days of slaughter for human consumption. Because a withdrawal time in milk has not been established, do not use in female dairy cattle of breeding age.

Not for use in humans.

This product should not be applied to self or others because it may be irritating to human skin and eyes and absorbed through the skin. To minimize accidental skin contact, the user should wear a long-sleeved shirt and rubber gloves. If accidental skin contact occurs, wash immediately with soap and water. If accidental eye exposure occurs, flush eyes immediately with water and seek medical attention.

Keep this and all drugs out of the reach of children.

Safety: Studies conducted in the U.S.A. have demonstrated the safety margin for ivermectin. Based on plasma levels, the topically applied formulation is expected to be at least as well tolerated by breeding animals as is the subcutaneous formulation which had no effect on breeding performance.

Discussion: PHOENECTIN® (ivermectin) Pour-On delivers internal and external parasite control in one convenient low-volume application. Ivermectin is a potent antiparasitic agent whose chemical structure is different from those of other antiparasitic agents.

Presentation: PHOENECTIN® Pour-On is available in a 250 mL (8.5 fl oz) (NDC 59130-681-02) bottle, a 500 mL (16.9 fl oz) (NDC 59130-681-03) bottle, a 1 L (33.8 fl oz) (NDC 59130-681-04) bottle for use with the dispensing cap provided, or in a 3.785 L (1 gal) (NDC 59130-681-05) bottle, a 5.0 L (169 fl oz) backpack and a 25 L (6.6 gal) (NDC 59130-681-48) carboy for use with the appropriate automatic dosing applicator.

Compendium Code No.: 10740392 Rev. 11-00

AMTECH PROSTAMATE® ℞

Phoenix Scientific **Prostaglandin**

(dinoprost tromethamine injection) Sterile Solution

ANADA No.: 200-253

Active Ingredient(s): This product contains the naturally occurring prostaglandin F2 alpha (dinoprost) as the tromethamine salt. Each mL contains dinoprost tromethamine equivalent to 5 mg dinoprost: also, benzyl alcohol, 9.45 mg added as preservative. When necessary, pH was adjusted with sodium hydroxide and/or hydrochloric acid. Dinoprost tromethamine is a white or slightly off-white crystalline powder that is readily soluble in water at room temperature in concentrations to at least 200 mg/mL.

Indications: For intramuscular use for estrus synchronization, treatment of unobserved (silent) estrus and pyometra (chronic endometritis) in cattle; for abortion of feedlot and other non-lactating cattle; for parturition induction in swine; and for controlling the timing of estrus in estrous cycling mares and clinically anestrous mares that have a corpus luteum.

Cattle: PROSTAMATE® Sterile Solution is indicated as a luteolytic agent.

PROSTAMATE® is effective only in those cattle having a corpus luteum, i.e., those which ovulated at least five days prior to treatment. Future reproductive performance of animals that are not cycling will be unaffected by injection of PROSTAMATE®.

Swine: For intramuscular use for parturition induction in swine. PROSTAMATE® Sterile Solution is indicated for parturition induction in swine when injected within 3 days of normal predicted farrowing.

Mares: PROSTAMATE® Sterile Solution is indicated for its luteolytic effect in mares. This luteolytic effect can be utilized to control the timing of estrus in estrous cycling and clinically anestrous mares that have a corpus luteum.

Pharmacology: General Biologic Activity: Prostaglandins occur in nearly all mammalian tissues. Prostaglandins, especially PGE's and PGF's, have been shown, in certain species, to 1) increase at time of parturition in amniotic fluid, maternal placenta, myometrium, and blood, 2) stimulate myometrial activity, and 3) to induce either abortion or parturition. Prostaglandins, especially PGF2α, have been shown to 1) increase in the uterus and blood to levels similar to levels achieved by exogenous administration which elicited luteolysis, 2) be capable of crossing from the uterine vein to the ovarian artery (sheep), 3) be related to IUD induced luteal regression (sheep), and 4) be capable of regressing the corpus luteum of most mammalian species studied to date. Prostaglandins have been reported to result in release of pituitary tropic hormones. Data suggest prostaglandins, especially PGE's and PGF's, may be involved in the process of ovulation and gamete transport. Also PGF2α have been reported to cause increase in blood pressure, bronchoconstriction, and smooth muscle stimulation in certain species.

Metabolism: A number of metabolism studies have been done in laboratory animals. The metabolism of tritium labeled dinoprost (^{3}H PGF2 alpha) in the rat and in the monkey was similar. Although quantitative differences were observed, qualitatively similar metabolites were produced. A study demonstrated that equimolar doses of ^{3}H PGF2 alpha Tham and ^{3}H PGF2 alpha free acid administered intravenously to rats demonstrated no significant differences in blood concentration of dinoprost. An interesting observation in the above study was that the radioactive dose of ^{3}H PGF2 alpha rapidly distributed in tissues and dissipated in tissues with almost the same curve as it did in the serum. The half-life of dinoprost in bovine blood has been reported to be on the order of minutes. A complete study on the distribution of decline of ^{3}H PGF2 alpha Tham in the tissue of rats was well correlated with the work done in the cow. Cattle serum collected during 24 hours after doses of 0 to 250 mg dinoprost have been assayed by RIA for dinoprost and the 15-keto metabolites. These data support previous reports that dinoprost has a half-life of minutes. Dinoprost is a natural prostaglandin. All systems associated with dinoprost metabolism exist in the body; therefore, no new metabolic, transport, excretory, binding or other systems need be established by the body to metabolize injected dinoprost.

Dosage and Administration: Cattle: PROSTAMATE® Sterile Solution is supplied at a concentration of 5 mg dinoprost per mL. PROSTAMATE® is luteolytic in cattle at 25 mg (5 mL) administered intramuscularly. As with any multidose vial, practice aseptic techniques in withdrawing each dose. Adequately clean and disinfect the vial closure prior to entry with a sterile needle.

Instructions for Use:

1. For Intramuscular Use for Estrus Synchronization in Beef Cattle and Non-Lactating Dairy Heifers. PROSTAMATE® is used to control the timing of estrus and ovulation in estrous cycling cattle that have a corpus luteum.

   Inject a dose of 5 mL PROSTAMATE® (25 mg PGF2α) intramuscularly either once or twice at a 10 to 12 day interval.

   With the single injection, cattle should be bred at the usual time relative to estrus. With the two injections cattle can be bred after the second injection either at the usual time relative to detected estrus or at about 80 hours after the second injection of PROSTAMATE®.

   Estrus is expected to occur 1 to 5 days after injection if a corpus luteum was present. Cattle that do not become pregnant to breeding at estrus on days 1 to 5 after injection will be expected to return to estrus in about 18 to 24 days.
2. For Intramuscular Use for Unobserved (Silent) Estrus in Lactating Dairy Cows with a Corpus Luteum. Inject a dose of 5 mL PROSTAMATE® (25 mg PGF2α) intramuscularly. Breed cows as they are detected in estrus. If estrus has not been observed by 80 hours after injection, breed at 80 hours. If the cow returns to estrus breed at the usual time relative to estrus.

Management Considerations: Many factors contribute to success and failure of reproduction management, and these factors are important also when time of breeding is to be regulated with PROSTAMATE® Sterile Solution. Some of these factors are:

a. Cattle must be ready to breed-they must have a corpus luteum and be healthy;
b. Nutritional status must be adequate as this has a direct effect on conception and the initiation of estrus in heifers or return of estrous cycles in cows following calving;
c. Physical facilities must be adequate to allow cattle handling without being detrimental to the animal;
d. Estrus must be detected accurately if timed A1 is not employed;
e. Semen of high fertility must be used;
f. Semen must be inseminated properly.

A successful breeding program can employ PROSTAMATE® effectively, but a poorly managed breeding program will continue to be poor when PROSTAMATE® is employed unless other management deficiencies are remedied first.

Cattle expressing estrus following PROSTAMATE® are receptive to breeding by a bull. Using bulls to breed large numbers of cattle in heat following PROSTAMATE® will require proper management of bulls and cattle.

3. For Intramuscular Use for Treatment of Pyometra (chronic endometritis) in Cattle. Inject a dose of 5 mL PROSTAMATE® (25 mg PGF2α) intramuscularly. In studies conducted with dinoprost tromethamine sterile solution, pyometra was defined as presence of a corpus luteum in the ovary and uterine horns containing fluid but not a conceptus based on palpation *per rectum*. Return to normal was defined as evacuation of fluid and return of the uterine horn size to 40 mm or less based on palpation *per rectum* at 14 and 28 days. Most cattle that recovered in response to PROSTAMATE® recovered within 14 days after injection. After 14 days, recovery rate of treated cattle was no different than that of non-treated cattle.
4. For Intramuscular Use for Abortion of Feedlot and Other Non-Lactating Cattle. PROSTAMATE® is indicated for its abortifacient effect in feedlot and other non-lactating cattle during the first 100 days of gestation. Inject a dose of 25 mg intramuscularly. Cattle that abort will abort within 35 days of injection.

   Commercial cattle were palpated *per rectum* for pregnancy in six feedlots. The percent of pregnant cattle in each feedlot less than 100 days of gestation ranged between 26 and 84; 80% or more of the pregnant cattle were less than 150 days of gestation. The abortion rates following injection of dinoprost tromethamine sterile solution increased with increasing doses up to about 25 mg. As examples, the abortion rates, over 7 feedlots on the dose titration study, were 22%, 50%, 71%, 90% and 78% for cattle up to 100 days of gestation when injected IM with dinoprost tromethamine sterile solution doses of 0, 1 (5 mg), 2 (10 mg), 4 (20 mg) and 8 (40 mg) mL, respectively. The statistical predicted relative abortion rate based on the dose titration data, was about 93% for the 5 mL (25 mg) dinoprost tromethamine sterile solution dose for cattle injected up to 100 days of gestation.

Swine: PROSTAMATE® Sterile Solution will induce parturition in swine at 10 mg (2 mL) when injected intramuscularly.

As with any multidose vial, practice aseptic techniques in withdrawing each dose. Adequately clean and disinfect the vial closure prior to entry with a sterile needle.

Instructions for Use: The response to treatment varies by individual animals with a mean interval from administration of 2 mL PROSTAMATE® (10 mg dinoprost) to parturition of approximately 30 hours. This can be employed to control the time of farrowing in sows and gilts in late gestation.

Management Considerations: Several factors must be considered for the successful use of PROSTAMATE® Sterile Solution for parturition induction in swine. The product must be administered at a relatively specific time (treatment earlier than 3 days prior to normal predicted farrowing may result in increased piglet mortality). It is important that adequate records be maintained on (1) the average length of gestation period for the animals on a specific location, and (2) the breeding and projected farrowing dates for each animal. This information is essential to determine the appropriate time for administration of PROSTAMATE®.

Mares:

1. Evaluate the reproductive status of the mare.
2. Administer a single intramuscular injection of 1 mg per 100 lbs (45.5 kg) body weight which is usually 1 mL to 2 mL PROSTAMATE® Sterile Solution.
3. Observe for signs of estrus by means of daily teasing with a stallion, and evaluate follicular changes on the ovary by palpation of the ovary *per rectum*.
4. Some clinically anestrous mares will not express estrus but will develop a follicle which will ovulate. These mares may become pregnant if inseminated at the appropriate time relative to rupture of the follicle.
5. Breed mares in estrus in a manner consistent with normal management.

Dinoprost tromethamine is administered once as a single intramuscular injection of 1 mg per 100 lbs (45.5 kg) body weight which is usually 1 mL to 2 mL of PROSTAMATE® containing 5 mg dinoprost as the tromethamine salt per milliliter.

Instructions for Use: PROSTAMATE® Sterile Solution is indicated for its luteolytic effect in mares. This luteolytic effect can be utilized to control the timing of estrus in estrous cycling and clinically anestrous mares that have a corpus luteum in the following circumstances:

1. Controlling Time of Estrus of Estrous Cycling Mares: Mares treated with PROSTAMATE® during diestrus (4 or more days after ovulation) will return to estrus within 2 to 4 days in most cases and ovulate 8 to 12 days after treatment. This procedure may be utilized as an aid to scheduling the use of stallions.
2. Difficult-to-Breed Mares: In extended diestrus there is failure to exhibit regular estrous cycles which is different from true anestrus. Many mares described as anestrus during the breeding season have serum progesterone levels consistent with the presence of a functional corpus luteum.

   A proportion of "barren", maiden, and lactating mares do not exhibit regular estrous cycles and may be in extended diestrus. Following abortion, early fetal death and resorption, or as a result of "pseudopregnancy", there may be serum progesterone levels consistent with a functional corpus luteum.

   Treatment of such mares with PROSTAMATE® usually results in regression of the corpus luteum followed by estrus and/or ovulation. In one study with 122 Standardbred and Thoroughbred mares in clinical anestrus for an average of 58 days and treated during the breeding season, behavioral estrus was detected in 81 percent at an average time of 3.7 days after injection with 5 mg dinoprost tromethamine sterile solution; ovulation occurred an average of 7.0 days after treatment. Of those mares bred, 59% were pregnant following an average of 1.4 services during that estrus.

   Treatment of "anestrous" mares which abort subsequent to 36 days of pregnancy may not result in return to estrus due to presence of functional endometrial cups.

Precaution(s): Storage Conditions: Store at controlled room temperature 20° to 25°C (68° to 77°F).

Caution(s): Federal (USA) law restricts this drug to use by or on the order of a licensed veterinarian.

Cattle: Do not administer to pregnant cattle unless abortion is desired.

Do not administer intravenously (I.V.), as this route might potentiate adverse reactions.

Cattle administered a progestogen would be expected to have a reduced response to PROSTAMATE® Sterile Solution.

Aggressive antibiotic therapy should be employed at the first sign of infection at the injection site whether localized or diffuse. As with all parenteral products careful aseptic techniques should be employed to decrease the possibility of post injection bacterial infections.

Swine: Do not administer to sows and/or gilts prior to 3 days of normal predicted farrowing, as increased number of stillborn and postnatal mortality may result.

Mares: PROSTAMATE® Sterile Solution is ineffective when administered prior to day-5 after ovulation.

Pregnancy status should be determined prior to treatment, since PROSTAMATE® has been reported to induce abortion and parturition when sufficient doses were administered.

Mares should not be treated if they suffer from either acute or subacute disorders of the vascular system, gastrointestinal tract, respiratory system, or reproductive tract.

Do not administer by intravenous route.

Nonsteroidal anti-inflammatory drugs (i.e., indomethacin) may inhibit prostaglandin synthesis, therefore these drugs should not be administered concurrently.

Restricted Drug - Use only as directed (California).

For use in animals only.

Warning(s): Important:

Cattle: No milk discard or preslaughter drug withdrawal period is required for labeled uses.

Swine: No preslaughter drug withdrawal period is required for labeled uses.

Mares: Not for use in horses intended for food.

Not for human use.

Women of child-bearing age, asthmatics, and persons with bronchial and other respiratory problems should exercise extreme caution when handling this product. In the early stages, women may be unaware of their pregnancies. Dinoprost tromethamine is readily absorbed through the skin and can cause abortion and/or bronchiospasms. Direct contact with the skin should, therefore, be avoided. Accidental spillage on the skin should be washed off immediately with soap and water.

Use of this product in excess of the approved dose may result in drug residues.

Keep out of reach of children.

Toxicology: Safety and Toxicity:

Laboratory Animals: Dinoprost was non-teratogenic in rats when administered orally at 1.25, 3.2, 10.0 and 20.0 mg/kg/day from day 6th-15th of gestation or when administered subcutaneously at 0.5 and 1.0 mg/kg/day on gestation days 6, 7 and 8 or 9, 10 and 11 or 12, 13 and 14. Dinoprost was non-teratogenic in the rabbit when administered either subcutaneously at doses of 0.5 and 1.0 mg/kg/day on gestation days 6, 7 and 8 or 9, 10 and 11 or 12, 13 and 14 or 15, 16 and 17 or orally at doses of 0.01, 0.1 and 1.0 mg/kg/day on days 6-18 or 5.0 mg/kg/day on days 8-18 of gestation. A slight and marked embryo lethal effect was observed in dams given 1.0 and 5.0 mg/kg/day respectively. This was due to the expected luteolytic properties of the drug.

A 14-day continuous intravenous infusion study in rats at 20 mg PGF2α per kg body weight indicated prostaglandins of the F series could induce bone deposition. However, such bone changes were not observed in monkeys similarly administered dinoprost tromethamine sterile solution at 15 mg PGF2α per kg body weight for 14 days.

Cattle: In cattle, evaluation was made of clinical observations, clinical chemistry, hematology, urinalysis, organ weights, and gross plus microscopic measurements following treatment with various doses up to 250 mg dinoprost administered twice intramuscularly at a 10 day interval or doses of 25 mg administered daily for 10 days. There was no unequivocal effect of dinoprost on the hematology or clinical chemistry parameters measured. Clinically, a slight transitory increase in heart rate was detected. Rectal temperature was elevated about 1.5°F through the 6th hour after injection with 250 mg dinoprost, but had returned to baseline at 24 hours after injection. No dinoprost associated gross lesions were detected. There was no evidence of toxicological effects. Thus, dinoprost had a safety factor of at least 10X on injection (25 mg luteolytic dose vs. 250 mg safe dose), based on studies conducted with cattle. At luteolytic doses, dinoprost had no effect on progeny. If given to a pregnant cow, it may cause abortion; the dose required for abortion varies considerably with the stage of gestation.

Induction of abortion in feedlot cattle at stages of gestation up to 100 days of gestation did not result in dystocia, retained placenta or death of heifers in the field studies. The smallness of the fetus at this early stage of gestation should not lead to complications at abortion. However, induction of parturition or abortion with any exogenous compound may precipitate dystocia, fetal death, retained placenta and/or metritis, especially at latter stages of gestation.

Swine: In pigs, evaluation was made of clinical observations, food consumption, clinical pathologic determinations, body weight changes, urinalysis, organ weights, and gross and microscopic observations following treatment with single doses of 10, 30, 50 and 100 mg dinoprost administered intramuscularly. The results indicated no treatment related effects from dinoprost treatment that were deleterious to the health of the animals or to their offspring.

Mares: Dinoprost tromethamine was administered to adult mares (weighing 320 to 485 kg; 2 to 20 years old), at the rates of 0, 100, 200, 400, and 800 mg per mare per day for 8 days. Route of administration for each dose group was both intramuscularly (2 mares) and subcutaneously (2 mares). Changes were detected in all treated groups for clinical (reduced sensitivity to pain; locomotor incoordination; hypergastromotility; sweating; hyperthermia; labored respiration), blood chemistry (elevated cholesterol, total bilirubin, LDH, and glucose), and hematology (decreased eosinophils; increased hemoglobin, hematocrit, and erythrocytes) measurements. The effects in the 100 mg dose, and to a lesser extent, the 200 mg dose groups were transient in nature, lasting for a few minutes to several hours. Mares did not appear to sustain adverse effects following termination of the side effects.

Mares treated with either 400 mg or 800 mg exhibited more profound symptoms. The excessive hyperstimulation of the gastrointestinal tract caused a protracted diarrhea, slight electrolyte imbalance (decreased sodium and potassium), dehydration, gastrointestinal irritation, and slight liver malfunction (elevated SGOT, SGPT at 800 mg only). Heart rate was increased but pH of the urine was decreased. Other measurements evaluated in the study remained within normal limits. No mortality occurred in any of the groups. No apparent differences were observed between the intramuscular and subcutaneous routes of administration. Luteolytic doses of dinoprost tromethamine are on the order of 5 to 10 mg administered on one day, therefore, dinoprost tromethamine sterile solution was demonstrated to have a wide margin of safety. Thus, the 100 mg dose gave a safety margin of 10 to 20X for a single injection or 80 to 160X for the 8 daily injections.

Additional studies investigated the effects in the mare of single intramuscular doses of 0, 0.25, 1.0, 2.5, 3.0, 5.0, and 10.0 mg dinoprost tromethamine. Heart rate, respiration rate, rectal temperature, and sweating were measured at 0, 0.25, 0.50, 0.75, 1.0, 1.5, 2.0, 3.0, 4.0, 5.0, and 6.0 hr. after injection. Neither heart rate nor respiration rates were significantly altered ($P > 0.05$) when compared to contemporary control values. Sweating was observed for 0 of 9, 2 of 9, 7 of 9, 9 of 9, and 8 of 9 mares injected with 0.25, 1.0, 2.5, 3.0, 5.0, or 10.0 mg dinoprost tromethamine, respectively. Sweating was temporary in all cases and was mild for doses of 3.0 mg or less but was extensive (beads of sweat over the entire body and dripping) for the 10 mg dose. Sweating after the 5.0 mg dose was intermediate between that seen for mares treated with 3.0 and 10.0 mg. Sweating began within 15 minutes after injection and ceased by 45 to 60 minutes after injection. Rectal temperature was decreased during the interval 0.5 until 1.0, 3 to 4, or 5 hours after injection for 0.25 and 1.0 mg, 2.5 and 3.0, or 5.0 and 10.0 mg dose groups, respectively. Average rectal temperature during the periods of decreased temperature was on the order of 97.5 to 99.6, with the greatest decreases observed in the 10 mg dose group.

Adverse Reactions: Cattle:

1. The most frequently observed side effect is increased rectal temperature at a 5X or 10X overdose. However, rectal temperature change has been transient in all cases observed and has not been detrimental to the animal.
2. Limited salivation has been reported in some instances.
3. Intravenous administration might increase heart rate.
4. Localized post injection bacterial infections that may become generalized have been reported. In rare instances such infections have terminated fatally. See Cautions.

Swine: The most frequently observed side effects were erythema and pruritus, slight incoordination, nesting behavior, itching, urination, defecation, abdominal muscle spasms, tail movements, hyperpnea or dyspnea, increased vocalization, salivation, and at the 100 mg (10X) dose only, vomition. These side effects are transitory, lasting from 10 minutes to 3 hours, and were not detrimental to the health of the animal.

Mares: The most frequently observed side effects are sweating and decreased rectal temperature. However, these have been transient in all cases observed and have not been detrimental to the animal. Other reactions seen have been increase in heart rate, increase in respiration rate, some abdominal discomfort, locomotor incoordination, and lying down. These effects are usually seen within 15 minutes of injection and disappear within one hour. Mares usually continue to eat during the period of expression of side effects. One anaphylactic reaction of several hundred mares treated with dinoprost tromethamine sterile solution was reported but was not confirmed.

Presentation: PROSTAMATE® Sterile Solution is available in 30 mL glass vials (NDC 59130-702-14).

Compendium Code No.: 10740402 Rev. 11-99

AMTECH SALINE SOLUTION 0.9% ℞

Phoenix Scientific **Saline Solution**

Active Ingredient(s): Composition: Each 100 mL of sterile aqueous solution contains:
Sodium chloride . . . . . 0.9 g
Milliequivalents per liter:
Cations:
Sodium chloride . . . . . 154 mEq/L
Anions:
Chloride . . . . . 154 mEq/L
Total osmolarity is 308 milliosmoles per liter.
This product contains no preservatives.

Indications: For use in replacement therapy of sodium, chloride and water which may become depleted in many diseases. Because this solution is isotonic with body fluids, it may also be used as a solvent or diluent, for antibiotics and other pharmaceuticals and biologicals where compatible, and for washing mucous membranes and other tissue surfaces.

Dosage and Administration: Warm to body temperature and administer slowly by intravenous or subcutaneous injection. The amount and rate of administration must be judged by the veterinarian in relation to the condition being treated and the clinical response of the animal, being careful to avoid overhydration. When used as a solvent or diluent for pharmaceuticals and biologicals, follow the manufacturer's directions.

Precaution(s): Store between 15°C and 30°C (59°F-86°F).
Use entire contents when first opened. Discard any unused solution.

Caution(s): Federal law restricts this drug to use by or on the order of a licensed veterinarian.
For animal use only.
Keep out of reach of children.

Presentation: 250 mL, 500 mL (NDC 59130-613-03) and 1000 mL.

Compendium Code No.: 10740411 Rev. 4-95

AMTECH SODIUM IODIDE 20% INJECTION ℞

Phoenix Scientific **Sodium Iodide**

Active Ingredient(s): Composition: Each 100 mL of sterile aqueous solution contains:
Sodium iodide . . . . . 20 grams
Water for injection . . . . . q.s.

Indications: For use as an aid in the treatment of actinomycosis (lumpy jaw), actinobacillosis (wooden tongue) and necrotic stomatitis in cattle.

Dosage and Administration: Using aseptic procedures, administer slowly by intravenous injection. Inject carefully to avoid deposition outside of the vein. The usual dose is 30 mg per pound of body weight (15 mL/100 lb). May be repeated at weekly intervals, if necessary.

Contraindication(s): The use of sodium iodide is contraindicated in pregnancy and hyperthyroidism.

Precaution(s): Store between 15°C and 30°C (59°F-86°F).

Caution(s): Federal law restricts this drug to use by or on the order of a licensed veterinarian.
Animals vary in their susceptibility of iodides. Administer with caution until the animal's tolerance is determined. Discontinue treatment if adverse reactions occur.
For animal use only.
Keep out of reach of children.

Warning(s): Not for use in lactating dairy cows.

Presentation: 250 mL (NDC 59130-614-02).

Compendium Code No.: 10740420 Rev. 12-95

AMTECH SPECTAM® SCOUR-HALT™

Phoenix Scientific **Spectinomycin**

(spectinomycin) Oral Solution-Anti-Infective

NADA No.: 033-157

Active Ingredient(s): Each mL contains:
Spectinomycin (from spectinomycin dihydrochloride pentahydrate) . . . . . 50 mg

Indications: For use in pigs under four (4) weeks of age for treatment and control of porcine enteric colibacillosis (scours) caused by *E. coli* susceptible to spectinomycin.

Dosage and Administration: Dose: Pigs under 10 lbs - 1 pump (1 mL) twice daily. Pigs over 10 lbs - 2 pumps (2 mL) twice daily.

Each pump of the plunger delivers 1 mL of solution containing 50 mg of spectinomycin. Treatment may be continued twice daily for 3 to 5 days. If pigs do not improve within 48 hours, rediagnosis is suggested.

Administration: The plastic doser supplied in each package with SPECTAM® SCOUR-HALT™ makes treatment easy. After inserting the doser in the bottle, screw the top on tightly to avoid spilling. Push the piece of clear plastic tubing over the end of the pump. Then press the plunger a few times to fill the pump and the clear plastic tube with medication. To administer SPECTAM® SCOUR-HALT™, insert the plastic tube in the pig's mouth and press the plunger to obtain the desired dose.

Directions for Use: The 1000 mL bottle of SPECTAM® SCOUR-HALT™ should be used only to refill the 240 mL container in the following manner.

1. Remove the cap and doser from the 240 mL bottle.
2. Unscrew the cap from the 1000 mL bottle.
3. Pour (from the 1000 mL bottle) the volume desired.
4. Reinsert the doser in the 240 mL bottle and screw the top on tightly.
5. Screw the top tightly on the 1000 mL bottle.

Precaution(s): Store at controlled room temperature, 20°-25°C (68°-77°F).
When not in use remove the plunger from the bottle. Put the clear plastic tube in the neck of the bottle and press the plunger a few times to remove the medication from the pump. Replace the original cap on the bottle and always rinse out the dose with water to prevent sticking.

Caution(s): This product is only intended for use in pigs under four weeks of age or weighing less than 15 lbs.
Restricted Drug - Use only as directed (California).
For animal use only.

Warning(s): Do not administer within 21 days of slaughter.
Not for human use.
Keep out of reach of children.

Presentation: SPECTAM® SCOUR-HALT™ is supplied in 240 mL (8 fl oz) multiple-dose plastic bottles. Each bottle is individually packed in a carton with a convenient plastic doser. Also available in 500 mL and 1,000 mL refill bottles with plastic doser and 1 gal (128 fl oz) refill.
® Registered Trademark Merial Limited
™ Trademark of Merial Limited

Compendium Code No.: 10740612 Iss. 3-00 / Rev. 2-02 / Iss. 2-01

AMTECH STERILE WATER FOR INJECTION, USP

Phoenix Scientific **Sterile Water**

Sterile-Nonpyrogenic

Active Ingredient(s): Contains:
Water for injection, USP 100%
pH . . . . . 5.0-7.0 Hypotonic
This product contains no preservative.

Indications: This sterile water for injection is made by distillation and is suitable for use as a diluent for preparation of pharmaceutical solutions when made isotonic by addition of suitable solutes.

Dosage and Administration: Use as required.

Precaution(s): Store between 15°C-30°C (59°F-86°F).
Do not use this product if seal is broken or solution is not clear. If entire contents are not used, discard unused portion. Additives may be incompatible. When introducing additives, use aseptic technique, mix thoroughly, and do not store.
Solutions made from this water should be used promptly or sterilized with adequate precautions for maintaining sterility.

Caution(s): Federal law restricts this drug to use by or on the order of a licensed veterinarian.
For animal use only.
Keep out of reach of children.

Presentation: 100 mL, 250 mL (NDC 59130-615-02) 500 mL and 1000 mL vials.

Compendium Code No.: 10740431 Rev. 11-97

AMTECH SULFADIMETHOXINE 12.5% ORAL SOLUTION

Phoenix Scientific **Water Medication**

Antibacterial

ANADA No.: 200-192

Active Ingredient(s): Each fluid ounce contains 3.75 g sulfadimethoxine solubilized with sodium hydroxide.

Indications:
Broiler and Replacement Chickens: Use for the treatment of disease outbreaks of coccidiosis, fowl cholera, and infectious coryza.
Meat Producing Turkeys: Use for the treatment of disease outbreaks of coccidiosis and fowl cholera.
Dairy Calves, Dairy Heifers and Beef Cattle: Use in the treatment of shipping fever complex, bacterial pneumonia, calf diphtheria, and foot rot.

Dosage and Administration: Prepare a fresh stock solution daily.

Species	Concentration	Use Directions
Chickens	0.05%	Add 1 fl oz* to 2 gallons of drinking water -or- 25 fl oz to 50 gallons of drinking water
Turkeys	0.025%	Add 1 fl oz* to 4 gallons of drinking water -or- 25 fl oz to 100 gallons of drinking water

Automatic Proportioners** Stock Solution — To make 2 gallons of stock solution use:

Chickens	1 gal Sulfadimethoxine 12.5% Drinking Water Solution Concentrate - plus - 1 gal of water
Turkeys	2 qts Sulfadimethoxine 12.5% Drinking Water Solution Concentrate - plus - 6 qts of water

Treatment Period: 6 consecutive days.
Dairy Calves, Dairy Heifers and Beef Cattle:
Dosage: 25 mg/lb first day followed by 12.5 mg/lb/day for 4 days.

	Sulfadimethoxine in Water		
		Water Consumption	
		(Summer) 1 gallon/† 100 lb b.w.	(Winter) 1 gallon/† 150 lb b.w.
First Day Add:	1 pint (16 fl oz) to:	25 gallons	16 gallons
	1 quart (32 fl oz) to:	50 gallons	33 gallons
	1 gallon (128 fl oz) to:	200 gallons	127 gallons
Next 4 Days Add:	1 pint (16 fl oz) to:	50 gallons	33 gallons
	1 quart (32 fl oz) to:	100 gallons	66 gallons
	1 gallon (128 fl oz) to:	400 gallons	266 gallons

†This dosage recommendation is based on a water consumption of 1 gallon per 100 lb of body weight per day, the expected water consumption rate for summer. Water consumption during cold months (winter) may drop markedly (30-40%). Accordingly, adjustments in drug concentration in drinking water must be made to insure proper drug intake.

For individual treatment of cattle, Sulfadimethoxine 12.5% Drinking Water Solution may be given as a drench. Administer using same mg/lb dose as outlined above. Four fluid ounces will medicate one-600 lb animal initially or two-600 lb animals on maintenance dose.

Treatment Period: 5 consecutive days.

*1 fl oz Sulfadimethoxine 12.5% Drinking Water Solution = 30 mL or 2 tablespoonfuls.

**Set proportioner to a feed rate of 1 fl oz of Sulfadimethoxine Stock Solution per gallon of water.

Precaution(s): Store at room temperature; if freezing occurs, thaw before using. Protect from light; direct sunlight may cause discoloration. Freezing or discoloration does not affect potency.

Caution(s):
Chickens and Turkeys: If animals show no improvement within 5 days, discontinue treatment and re-evaluate diagnosis. Handle the recommended dilutions (chickens 0.05% and turkeys 0.025%) as regular drinking water. Administer as sole source of drinking water and sulfonamide medication.
Chickens and turkeys that have survived fowl cholera outbreaks should not be kept for replacements or breeders.
Cattle: During treatment period, make certain that animals maintain adequate water intake. If

animals show no improvement within 2 or 3 days, re-evaluate diagnosis. Treatment should not be continued beyond 5 days.

Warning(s):

Chickens and Turkeys: Withdraw 5 days before slaughter.

Do not administer to chickens over 16 weeks (112 days) of age or to turkeys over 24 weeks (168 days) of age.

Cattle: Withdraw 7 days before slaughter. For dairy calves, dairy heifers and beef cattle only. A withdrawal period has not been established for this product in pre-ruminating calves. Do not use in calves to be processed for veal.

For use in animals only. Restricted drug (California). Use only as directed. Not for human use. Keep out of reach of children.

Presentation: 3.785 L (1 gal) (128 fl oz) containers (NDC 59130-662-05).

Compendium Code No.: 10740440 Iss. 3-97

AMTECH SULFADIMETHOXINE INJECTION - 40%

Phoenix Scientific **Sulfadimethoxine**

Antibacterial

ANADA No.: 200-177

Active Ingredient(s): Composition: Each mL contains 400 mg sulfadimethoxine compounded with 20% propylene glycol, 1% benzyl alcohol (preservative), 0.1 mg disodium edetate, 1 mg sodium formaldehyde sulfoxylate, and pH adjusted with sodium hydroxide.

Indications: Cattle: For the treatment of bovine respiratory disease complex (shipping fever complex) and bacterial pneumonia associated with *Pasteurella* spp sensitive to sulfadimethoxine; necrotic pododermatitis (foot rot) and calf diphtheria caused by *Fusobacterium necrophorum (Sphaerophorus necrophorus)*, sensitive to sulfadimethoxine.

Pharmacology: Description: SULFADIMETHOXINE INJECTION 40% is a low-dosage, rapidly absorbed, long-acting sulfonamide, effective for the treatment of shipping fever complex, bacterial pneumonia, calf diphtheria and foot rot in cattle.

Sulfadimethoxine is a white, almost tasteless and odorless compound. Chemically, it is N^1-(2,6-dimethoxy-4-pyrimidinyl) sulfanilamide. The structural formula is:

H_2N–C_6H_4–SO_2•NH–(pyrimidine ring, N, N)–OCH_3, OCH_3

Actions: Sulfadimethoxine has been demonstrated clinically or in the laboratory to be effective against a variety of organisms, such as streptococci, klebsiella, proteus, shigella, staphylococci, escherichia, and salmonella.[1,2]

The systemic sulfonamides which include sulfadimethoxine are bacteriostatic agents. Sulfonamides competitively inhibit bacterial synthesis of folic acid (pteroylglutamic acid) from para-aminobenzoic acid. Mammalian cells are capable of utilizing folic acid in the presence of sulfonamides.

The tissue distribution of sulfadimethoxine, as with all sulfonamides, is a function of plasma levels, degree of plasma protein binding, and subsequent passive distribution in the tissues of the lipid-soluble un-ionized form. The relative amounts are determined by both its pKa and by the pH of each tissue. Therefore, levels tend to be higher in less acid tissue and body fluids or those diseased tissues having high concentrations of leucocytes.[2]

Slow renal excretion results from a high degree of tubular reabsorption,[3] and plasma protein binding is very high, providing a blood reservoir of the drug. Thus, sulfadimethoxine maintains higher blood levels than most other long-acting sulfonamides. Single, comparatively low doses of SULFADIMETHOXINE INJECTION 40% give rapid and sustained therapeutic blood levels.[1]

To assure successful sulfonamide therapy (1) the drug must be given early in the course of the disease, and it must produce a high sulfonamide level in the body rapidly after administration, (2) therapeutically effective sulfonamide levels must be maintained in the body throughout the treatment period, (3) treatment should continue for a short period of time after the clinical signs have disappeared, and (4) the causative organisms must be sensitive to this class of drugs.

Dosage and Administration: SULFADIMETHOXINE INJECTION 40% must be administered only by the intravenous route in cattle. Cattle should receive 1 mL of SULFADIMETHOXINE INJECTION 40% per 16 pounds of body weight (55 mg/kg) as an initial dose, followed by 0.5 mL per 16 pounds of body weight (27.5 mg/kg) every 24 hours thereafter. Sulfadimethoxine Boluses may be utilized for maintenance therapy in cattle. Representative weights and doses are indicated in the following table:

Animal Weight	Initial Dose 25 mg/lb. (55 mg/kg)	Subsequent Daily Doses 12.5 mg/lb. (27.5 mg/kg)
250 lb (113.6 kg)	15.6 mL	7.8 mL
500 lb (227.2 kg)	31.2 mL	15.6 mL
750 lb (340.9 kg)	46.9 mL	23.5 mL
1000 lb (454.5 kg)	62.5 mL	31.3 mL

Length of treatment depends on the clinical response. In most cases treatment for 3 to 5 days is adequate. Treatment should be continued until the animal is asymptomatic for 48 hours.

Directions for Intravenous Injection:

Equipment needed:

1. A nose lead and/or halter sufficiently strong enough to effectively restrain or hold the animal's head steady so that the intravenous injection can be made with ease.
2. Hypodermic needles, 16 or 18 gauge and 2 inches long. Only new, sharp and sterile hypodermic needles should be used. Dull needles should be discarded. Extra needles should always be available in case the needle being used should become clogged.
3. Hypodermic syringes, 40 or 50 mL sterile disposable or reusable glass syringes should be available.
4. Alcohol (70%) or equally effective antiseptic for disinfecting the skin.

Preparation of equipment: Glass syringes and regular hypodermic needles should be thoroughly cleaned and washed. Following this, the needles and syringes should be immersed in boiling water for 30 minutes prior to each injection. Regular hypodermic needles should not be used more than 3-4 times as repeated skin puncturing and boiling of the needles causes them to become quite dull. Disposable hypodermic needles and syringes should not be used more than once.

Restraint of animal: The cow should preferably be in a stanchion for maximum restraint. If this is not possible, the animal should be restrained in a manner to prevent excessive movement. A nose lead should be applied and the animal's head turned sidewise to stretch the skin and tense the muscles of the neck region.

Locating the jugular vein: When the animal has been restrained (as above), you will notice a long depression of the skin from below the angle of the jaw to just above the shoulder. This is known as the jugular furrow or jugular groove. The jugular vein is located just under the jugular groove.

Preparation of SULFADIMETHOXINE INJECTION 40% for injection: The rubber cap of the bottle should be thoroughly cleaned with 70% alcohol or other satisfactory antiseptic. The correct amount of SULFADIMETHOXINE INJECTION 40% for treatment should be calculated (see dosage directions) and that amount withdrawn into a syringe. One or two syringefuls of air should be injected into the bottle first to make withdrawing the drug easier. SULFADIMETHOXINE INJECTION 40% should preferably be at room temperature when filling syringes and when injecting intravenously.

Entering the vein: The skin of the injection area should be clean and free of dirt. Cotton saturated with 70% alcohol (or suitable antiseptic) should be used to wipe the injection site.

Apply pressure over the jugular vein close to the shoulder. This will reduce the flow of blood to the heart and cause the jugular vein to bulge or enlarge. (See Figure 1). When the jugular vein has been "raised", insert the hypodermic needle at a 45 degree angle through the skin just underneath the jugular vein. The beveled edge of the hypodermic needles should be up.

After the skin has been punctured, the point of the needle should be directed toward the side of the vein and pushed into the center of the vein (See Figure 2). When the needle is in the center of the vein, there will be a free flow of blood back through the needle. Release external pressure when you are sure the needle is within the vein.

Injecting the SULFADIMETHOXINE INJECTION 40%: After the needle has been accurately inserted into the jugular vein, firmly attach the syringe containing SULFADIMETHOXINE INJECTION 40% to the inserted hypodermic needle. Caution, be sure syringe is free of air. Exert firm pressure on the plunger of the syringe to inject the SULFADIMETHOXINE INJECTION 40% while the barrel is held firmly. The injection should be made moderately slow - never rapidly.

If the animal moves, causing resistance in pushing the plunger of the syringe, or if a bubble of the drug is noted under the skin, the needle is no longer within the vein. The needle should be repositioned.

When the injection is completed, quickly withdraw the syringe and needle with a quick pull and apply light pressure over the injection site with alcohol and cotton to minimize bleeding from the puncture site.

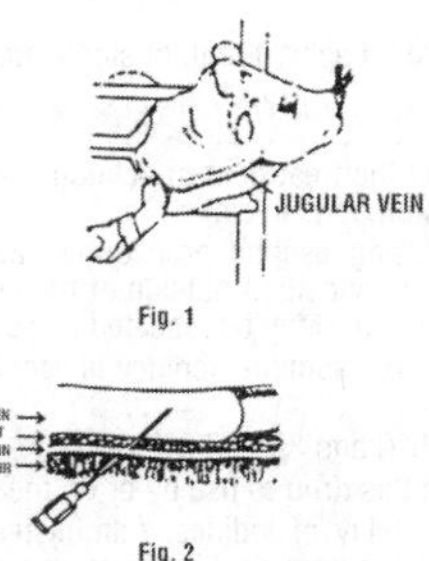

Fig. 1

Fig. 2

Precaution(s): Store at room temperature between 15° and 30°C (59° and 86°F). Should crystallization occur at cold temperatures, crystals will dissolve either by storing at room temperature for several days or by heating the vial in warm water. Crystallization and redissolution do not impair the efficacy of the product.

Caution(s): During treatment period, make certain that animals maintain adequate water intake.

If animals show no improvement within 2 or 3 days, consult your veterinarian.

Tissue damage may result from perivascular infiltration.

Limitations: Sulfadimethoxine is not effective in viral or rickettsial infections, and as with any anti-bacterial agent, occasional failures in therapy may occur due to resistant microorganisms. The usual precautions in sulfonamide therapy should be observed.

Warning(s): Milk taken from animals during treatment and for 60 hours (5 milkings) after the latest treatment must not be used for food.

Do not administer within 5 days of slaughter.

A withdrawal period has not been established for this product in preruminating calves. Do not use in calves to be processed for veal.

For intravenous use only in cattle.

Restricted drug (California) - Use only as directed.

Not for human use .

For animal use only. Keep out of reach of children.

Toxicology: Toxicity and Safety: Data regarding acute (LD_{50}) and chronic toxicities of sulfadimethoxine indicate the drug is safe. The LD_{50} in mice is greater than 2 g/kg body weight when administered intraperitoneally and greater than 16 g/kg when administered orally. In dogs receiving massive single oral doses of 3.2 g/kg body weight, diarrhea was the only adverse effect observed. Dogs given 160 mg/kg body weight orally daily for 13 weeks showed no signs of toxicity.

In cattle sulfadimethoxine has been shown to be safe through extensive clinical use with other dosage forms. In addition, studies with intravenous administration of SULFADIMETHOXINE INJECTION 40% have demonstrated that hemolysis of erythrocytes does not occur by this route of administration. Sulfadimethoxine has a relatively high solubility at the pH normally occurring in the kidney, precluding the possibility of precipitation and crystalluria.

References: Available upon request.

Presentation: 250 mL multiple dose vial (NDC 59130-661-02).

Compendium Code No.: 10740450 Rev. 9-99

AMTECH SULFADIMETHOXINE SOLUBLE POWDER

Phoenix Scientific **Water Medication**

Antibacterial

ANADA No.: 200-258

Active Ingredient(s): Each packet contains 94.6 g (3.34 oz) sulfadimethoxine as sodium sulfadimethoxine.

Indications: For Broiler and Replacement Chickens Only: Use for the treatment of disease outbreaks of coccidiosis, fowl cholera, and infectious coryza.

For Meat-producing Turkeys Only: Use for the treatment of disease outbreaks of coccidiosis and fowl cholera.

For Dairy Calves, Dairy Heifers, and Beef Cattle: Use for the treatment of shipping fever complex and bacterial pneumonia associated with *Pasteurella* spp. sensitive to sulfadimethoxine; and calf diphtheria and foot rot associated with *Sphaerophorus necrophorus* sensitive to sulfadimethoxine.

Dosage and Administration:

Species	Concentration	Use Direction
Chickens	0.05%	Contents of packet to 50 gal of water
Turkeys	0.025%	Contents of packet to 100 gal of water

Automatic Proportioners: To make stock solution, add contents of 5 packets to 2 gal of water for chickens and to 4 gal of water for turkeys. Set proportioner to feed at rate of 1 fl oz stock solution per gal of water.

Treatment Period: 6 consecutive days.

Dairy Calves, Dairy Heifers, and Beef Cattle:

Dosage: 25 mg/lb the first day followed by 12.5 mg/lb/day for 4 days.

Sulfadimethoxine in Water:

	Amount of Stock Solution for Cattle*	Water Consumption	
		(Summer) 1 gal/100 lb body wt**	(Winter) 1 gal/150 lb body wt**
First Day Add	1 qt	10 gal	7 gal
	2 qt	20 gal	14 gal
	1 gal	40 gal	28 gal
Next 4 Days Add	1 qt	20 gal	14 gal
	2 qt	40 gal	28 gal
	1 gal	80 gal	56 gal

*Note: Make a cattle stock solution by adding 1 packet of SULFADIMETHOXINE SOLUBLE POWDER to 1 gal of water.

*Twenty fl oz of cattle stock solution will medicate 1 600-lb animal initially or 2 600-lb animals on maintenance dose. Contents of packet will medicate 6 600-lb animals initially or 12 600-lb animals on maintenance dose.

**This dosage recommendation is based on a water consumption of 1 gal per 100 lb of body weight per day, the expected water consumption rate for summer. Water consumption during cold months (winter) may drop markedly (30-40%). Accordingly, adjustments must be made in the dilution rates to compensate for this and insure proper drug intake.

For treatment of individual cattle, SULFADIMETHOXINE SOLUBLE POWDER stock solution for cattle may be given as a drench. Administer using same mg/lb dosage as outlined above.

Treatment Period: 5 consecutive days.

Caution(s): Chickens and Turkeys: If animals show no improvement within 5 days, discontinue treatment and reevaluate diagnosis. Prepare a fresh stock solution daily. Handle the recommended dilutions (chickens 0.05% and turkeys 0.025%) as regular drinking water. Administer as sole source of drinking water and sulfonamide medication.

Chickens and turkeys that have survived fowl cholera outbreaks should not be kept for replacements or breeders.

Cattle: During treatment period, make certain that animals maintain adequate water intake. If animals show no improvement within 2 or 3 days, reevaluate diagnosis. Treatment should not be continued beyond 5 days.

Warning(s): Chickens and Turkeys: Withdraw 5 days before slaughter. Do not administer to chickens over 16 weeks (112 days) of age or to turkeys over 24 weeks (168 days) of age.

Cattle: Withdraw 7 days before slaughter. For dairy calves, dairy heifers, and beef cattle only. A withdrawal period has not been established for this product in pre-ruminating calves. Do not use in calves to be processed for veal.

Restricted drug (California) - Use only as directed.

Not for human use.

Presentation: 25 x 107 g (3.77 oz) packets (NDC 59130-706-28).

Compendium Code No.: 10740461 Rev. 3-99

AMTECH TETRACYCLINE HYDROCHLORIDE SOLUBLE POWDER-324

Phoenix Scientific **Antimicrobial Water Medication**

Antibiotic

ANADA No.: 200-136

Active Ingredient(s): Each pound contains 324 g of tetracycline hydrochloride.

Indications: For use in the control and treatment of the following conditions in swine, calves and poultry.

Swine: Bacterial enteritis (scours) caused by *Escherichia coli* and bacterial pneumonia associated with *Pasteurella* spp., *Hemophilus* spp. and *Klebsiella* spp. susceptible to tetracycline.

Calves: Bacterial enteritis (scours) caused by *Escherichia coli* and bacterial pneumonia (shipping fever complex) associated with *Pasteurella* spp., *Hemophilus* spp., and *Klebsiella* spp. susceptible to tetracycline.

Chickens: Control of chronic respiratory disease (CRD) and air sac infection caused by *Mycoplasma gallisepticum* and *Escherichia coli;* infectious synovitis caused by *Mycoplasma synoviae* susceptible to tetracycline.

Turkeys: Control of infectious synovitis caused by *Mycoplasma synoviae* and bluecomb (transmissible enteritis, coronaviral enteritis) caused by complicating bacterial organisms susceptible to tetracycline.

Dosage and Administration: Administer TETRACYCLINE HYDROCHLORIDE SOLUBLE POWDER-324 in the drinking water of swine and calves at a drug level of tetracycline hydrochloride per gallon to provide approximately 10 mg/lb of body weight, daily, for 3 to 5 days.

Administer TETRACYCLINE HYDROCHLORIDE SOLUBLE POWDER-324 in the drinking water of chickens and turkeys at a level of 25 mg/lb of body weight, daily, for 7 to 14 days.

Do not mix this product with milk or milk replacers. Administer one hour before or two hours after feeding milk or milk replacers. Drug use level must be adjusted to provide 10 mg/lb body weight daily in divided doses for swine and calves or, in the case of chickens and turkeys, 25 mg/lb.

Mixing Instructions: The enclosed 43 cc cup, when level full twice provides approximately 71.4 g (2.52 oz) of finished product which contains 51.0 g of tetracycline hydrochloride.

Swine: A stock solution of 71.4 g of product dissolved in 1500 mL (approximately 50 fl oz or 3 pints) of warm water provides about 34 mg of tetracycline hydrochloride activity per mL.

This stock solution metered at 1 oz/gallon will provide drinking water which contains approximately 1000 mg of tetracycline hydrochloride activity per gallon.

Calves: For individual dosing, prepare a solution of 71.4 g of product dissolved in 500 mL (approximately 16 fl oz or 1 pint) of warm water which provides about 100 mg of tetracycline hydrochloride activity per mL.

Administer 5 mL (1 measuring teaspoonful) of the stock solution (100 mg/mL) twice daily for each 100 lb of body weight as a drench or by dose syringe. This will provide the recommended dosage level of 10 mg/lb body weight daily in divided doses.

Chickens and Turkeys: A stock solution of 71.4 g of product dissolved in 1500 mL (approximately 50 fl oz or 3 pints) of warm water provides about 34 mg of tetracycline hydrochloride activity per mL.

This stock solution metered at 1 oz./gallon will provide drinking water which contains approximately 1000 mg of tetracycline hydrochloride activity per gallon.

The contents of the 2 lb container will provide sufficient drug to treat 64,800 total pounds of swine or calves for a single day at the recommended dosage level of 10 mg/lb of body weight in divided doses. The same container will treat 25,920 lb of poultry when supplied at 25 mg/lb.

The contents of the 5 lb container will provide sufficient drug to treat 162,000 total pounds of swine or calves for a single day at the recommended dosage level of 10 mg/lb of body weight in divided doses. The same container will treat 64,800 lb of poultry when supplied at 25 mg/lb.

The contents of the 25 lb container will provide sufficient drug to treat 810,000 total pounds of swine or calves for a single day at the recommended dosage level of 10 mg/lb of body weight in divided doses. The same container will treat 324,000 lb of poultry when supplied at 25 mg/lb.

Note: The concentration of the drug required in medicated water must be adequate to compensate for variation in the age of the animal, feed consumption and the environmental temperature and humidity, each of which affects water consumption.

Caution(s): Use as sole source of tetracycline. Not to be used in swine or calves for more than 5 days. Not to be used in chickens or turkeys for more than 14 consecutive days. When used in plastic or stainless steel waterers or automatic medicators, prepare fresh solution every 24 hours. When used in galvanized waterers, prepare fresh solution every 12 hours. If condition does not improve within 2 to 3 days, consult your veterinarian.

Restricted drug, use only as directed - Not for human use (California). For animal use only.

Warning(s): Do not slaughter swine for food purposes within 4 days of treatment.

Do not slaughter cattle for food purposes within 5 days of treatment.

Do not slaughter poultry for food within 4 days of treatment.

Not for use in poultry producing eggs for human consumption.

A withdrawal period has not been established for this product in pre-ruminating calves. Do not use in calves to be processed for veal.

Keep out of reach of children.

Presentation: 907.2 kg (2 lb) (NDC 59130-647-08), 2.26 kg (5 lb) (NDC 59130-647-09) plastic bucket, and 11.34 kg (25 lb) (NDC 59130-647-39).

Compendium Code No.: 10740473 Rev. 12-98 / Rev. 12-98 / Iss. 12-98

AMTECH THIAMINE HYDROCHLORIDE INJECTION ℞

Phoenix Scientific **Thiamine**

Active Ingredient(s): Composition: Each mL of sterile aqueous solution contains:

Thiamine HCl .... 200 mg
Disodium edetate 0.01%
Benzyl alcohol........ 1.5%
Water for injection .... q.s.

Indications: For the treatment of vitamin B_1 deficiencies.

Dosage and Administration: To be determined by the veterinarian. For intramuscular use.

Precaution(s): Store between 15°C and 30°C (59°F-86°F). Do not expose to excessive heat.

Caution(s): Federal law restricts this drug to use by or on the order of a licensed veterinarian.

Anaphylactogenesis to parenteral Thiamine HCl has been reported.

Administer slowly with caution in doses over 500 mg.

For animal use only.

Keep out of reach of children.

Presentation: 100 mL (NDC 59130-631-01) and 250 mL (NDC 59130-631-02).

Compendium Code No.: 10740482 Rev. 11-94 / Rev. 9-95

AMTECH TRIPELENNAMINE HYDROCHLORIDE INJECTION ℞

Phoenix Scientific **Antihistamine**

ANADA No.: 200-162

Active Ingredient(s): TRIPELENNAMINE HYDROCHLORIDE INJECTION is supplied in multiple dose vials containing 20 mg of Tripelennamine Hydrochloride USP per mL.

Indications: For use in cattle and horses in conditions in which antihistaminic therapy may be expected to lead to alleviation of some signs of disease.

Pharmacology: Tripelennamine hydrochloride is a white, crystalline material which is stable, nonhygroscopic, and readily soluble in water.

Action: Tripelennamine hydrochloride is characterized by its capacity to antagonize many of the pharmacologic effects of histamine.

Dosage and Administration: Warm the solution to near body temperature.

Using aseptic precautions, administer intravenously or intramuscularly as specified below. Intramuscular injections should be made into the heavy musculature of the hind leg or cervical area.

The doses specified below may be repeated in 6 to 12 hours if necessary.

Cattle: Administer intravenously or intramuscularly at a dose of 0.5 mg per lb of body weight (2.5 mL for each 100 lbs. of body weight). For a more rapid onset of action, the intravenous route of administration is recommended.

Horses: Administer intramuscularly only at a dose of 0.5 mg per lb of body weight (2.5 mL for each 100 lbs of body weight).

Precaution(s): Storage: Protect from light. Store between 15°C and 30°C (59°F-86°F). Avoid excessive heat (104°F).

Caution(s): Federal law restricts this drug to use by or on the order of a licensed veterinarian.

Central nervous system stimulation in the form of hyperexcitability, nervousness, and muscle tremors lasting up to 20 minutes have been noted in horses, particularly following intravenous administration; therefore, only the intramuscular route of administration should be used in horses.

Overdosage of tripelennamine hydrochloride may give rise to excitement, ataxia, and convulsions.

Depression of the central nervous system and incoordination may occur when the drug is used at therapeutic dose levels.

Disturbances in gastrointestinal function may occur in some instances.

While poisonous snake bites have been treated with antihistaminic drugs, other conjunctive therapy is required because of toxic reactions associated with the protein complex of venom.

Warning(s): Do not use in horses intended for food purposes.

Milk that has been taken during treatment and for 24 hours (two milkings) after the last treatment must not be used for food.

Treated cattle must not be slaughtered for food during treatment and for four days following the last treatment.

A withdrawal period has not been established for this product in pre-ruminating calves. Do not use in calves to be processed for veal. For animal use only. Keep out of reach of children.

Presentation: TRIPELENNAMINE HYDROCHLORIDE INJECTION is supplied in 100 mL (NDC 59130-660-01), 250 mL (NDC 59130-660-02), and 500 mL (NDC 59130-660-03) multiple dose vials.

Compendium Code No.: 10740491 Rev. 8-97

AMTECH UTERINE BOLUS

Phoenix Scientific **Intrauterine Antiseptic**

Active Ingredient(s): Composition: Each bolus contains:

Urea . . . 13.4 g

Indications: For use as an antiseptic and proteolytic aid in beef, dairy cattle and sheep.

Dosage and Administration: For intrauterine or topical use only. Insert boluses into uterus or dissolve in one pint warm water to make a flush.

Cattle: 2-4 boluses.

Sheep: ½-1 bolus.

For topical application, dissolve 4 boluses in one pint of warm water and thoroughly flush wound.

Repeat treatment in 24 to 48 hours if necessary.

Precaution(s): Store in a cool, dry place.

Keep container tightly closed when not in use.

Caution(s): Do not administer orally.

Strict cleanliness must be observed to prevent introduction of further infections. Thoroughly cleanse hands and arms of operator and external genital parts of the animal with soap and water before inserting boluses or flush.

Do not use in deep or puncture wounds or for serious burns.

For animal use only. Keep out of reach of children.

Presentation: 50 boluses (NDC 59130-693-15).

Compendium Code No.: 10740501 Iss. 10-97

AMTECH VITAMIN B COMPLEX

Phoenix Scientific **Vitamin B-Complex**

Active Ingredient(s): Each mL contains:

Thiamine HCl . . . 12.5 mg
Riboflavin 5' phosphate sodium . . . 2 mg
Niacinamide . . . 12.5 mg
d-Panthenol . . . 5 mg
Pyridoxine HCl . . . 5 mg
Cobalt (as cyanocobalamin) . . . 0.2 ppm
Benzyl alcohol (preservative) . . . 1.5%
Water for injection . . . q.s.

Indications: An aqueous solution of B-vitamins to provide a supplemental nutritional supply of these vitamins and complexed cobalt to cattle, sheep and swine.

Dosage and Administration: Administer intramuscularly.

Sheep and Swine: 5 to 10 mL. Cattle: 10 to 20 mL. Repeat daily as indicated.

Precaution(s): Store between 15°C and 30°C (59°F-86°F). Keep from freezing.

Caution(s): Anaphylactogenesis to parenteral thiamine HCl has been reported. Administer slowly and with caution in doses over 50 mg. For animal use only. Keep out of reach of children.

Presentation: 100 mL (NDC 59130-618-01), 250 mL (NDC 59130-618-02) and 500 mL (NDC 59130-618-03).

Compendium Code No.: 10740512 Rev. 9-94 / Rev. 12-94 / Rev. 10-95

AMTECH VITAMIN B COMPLEX FORTIFIED

Phoenix Scientific **Vitamin B-Complex**

Active Ingredient(s): Each mL contains:

Thiamine HCl . . . 100 mg
Riboflavin 5' phosphate sodium . . . 5 mg
Niacinamide . . . 100 mg
d-Panthenol . . . 10 mg
Pyridoxine HCl . . . 10 mg
Cobalt (as cyanocobalamin) . . . 4.0 ppm
Benzyl alcohol (preservative) . . . 1.5%
Citric acid . . . 5 mg
Water for injection . . . q.s.

Indications: An aqueous solution of B complex vitamins to provide a supplemental nutritional supply of these vitamins and complexed cobalt to cattle, sheep and swine.

Dosage and Administration: Administer intramuscularly or subcutaneously.

Sheep and Swine: 5 to 10 mL.

Cattle: 10 to 20 mL.

Repeat daily as indicated.

Precaution(s): Store between 15°C and 30°C (59°F-86°F). Keep from freezing.

Caution(s): Anaphylactogenesis to parenteral thiamine HCl has been reported. Administer slowly and with caution in doses over 50 mg. For animal use only. Keep out of reach of children.

Presentation: 100 mL (NDC 59130-619-01), 250 mL (NDC 59130-619-02) and 500 mL (NDC 59130-619-03).

Compendium Code No.: 10740522 Rev. 7-94 / Rev. 4-94 / Rev. 10-95

AMTECH VITAMIN B_{12} 1000 mcg ℞

Phoenix Scientific **Vitamin B_{12}**

(Cyanocobalamin Injection)

Active Ingredient(s): Composition: Each mL of sterile aqueous solution contains:

Cyanocobalamin (B_{12}) . . . 1000 mcg
Sodium chloride . . . 0.8% w/v
Benzyl alcohol (preservative) . . . 1.5% v/v

Indications: For use as an aid in the management of vitamin B_{12} deficiencies in cattle, horses, dogs, and cats.

Dosage and Administration: Inject subcutaneously or intramuscularly.

Cattle and Horses - 1 to 2 mL

Dogs and Cats - 0.25 to 0.5 mL

May be repeated once or twice weekly, as indicated by condition and response.

Precaution(s): Store between 15°C and 30°C (59°F-86°F). Avoid exposure to light.

Caution(s): Federal law restricts this drug to use by or on the order of a licensed veterinarian.

For animal use only.

Keep out of reach of children.

Presentation: 100 mL (NDC 59130-620-01), 250 mL (NDC 59130-620-02), and 500 mL (NDC 59130-620-03).

Compendium Code No.: 10740532 Rev. 8-94 / Rev. 9-95 / Rev. 10-95

AMTECH VITAMIN B_{12} 3000 mcg ℞

Phoenix Scientific **Vitamin B_{12}**

(Cyanocobalamin Injection)

Active Ingredient(s): Composition: Each mL of sterile aqueous solution contains:

Cyanocobalamin (B_{12}) . . . 3000 mcg
Sodium chloride . . . 0.8% w/v
Benzyl alcohol (preservative) . . . 1.5% v/v

Indications: For use as a supplemental nutritive source of vitamin B_{12} in cattle, horses, sheep, swine, dogs and cats.

Dosage and Administration: Inject subcutaneously or intramuscularly.

Cattle, Horses, Sheep and Swine - 1 to 2 mL

Dogs and Cats - 0.25 to 0.5 mL

Suggested dosage may be repeated at 1 to 2 week intervals, as indicated by condition and response.

Precaution(s): Store between 15°C and 30°C (59°F-86°F). Avoid exposure to light.

Caution(s): Federal law restricts this drug to use by or on the order of a licensed veterinarian.

For animal use only.

Keep out of reach of children.

Presentation: 100 mL (NDC 59130-621-01) and 250 mL (NDC 59130-621-02).

Compendium Code No.: 10740542 Rev. 11-95 / Rev. 8-94

AMTECH VITAMIN B_{12} 5000 mcg ℞

Phoenix Scientific **Vitamin B_{12}**

(Cyanocobalamin Injection)

Active Ingredient(s): Each mL of sterile aqueous solution contains:

Cyanocobalamin . . . 5000 mcg
Benzyl alcohol (as preservative) . . . 1.5% w/v
Sodium chloride . . . 0.8% w/v
Water for injection . . . q.s.

Indications: For use in vitamin B_{12} deficiency associated with cobalt deficiency in cattle and sheep and for vitamin B_{12} deficiency associated with inadequate vitamin B_{12} intake or intestinal malabsorption in swine.

Dosage and Administration: Inject intramuscularly or subcutaneously. Dosage may be repeated in weekly intervals if necessary.

Cattle and Sheep: 0.2 to 0.4 mL

Swine: 0.1 to 0.4 mL

Precaution(s): Store between 15°C and 30°C (59°F-86°F). Avoid exposure to light.

Caution(s): Federal law restricts this drug to use by or on the order of a licensed veterinarian.

For animal use only.

Keep out of reach of children.

Presentation: 100 mL (NDC 59130-622-01).

Compendium Code No.: 10740551 Iss. 3-95

AMTECH VITAMIN C INJECTABLE SOLUTION ℞

Phoenix Scientific **Vitamin C**

Active Ingredient(s): Composition: Each mL of sterile aqueous solution contains:

Sodium ascorbate . . . 250 mg
Benzyl alcohol (preservative) . . . 1.5% v/v
Sodium metabisulfite . . . 0.2% w/v

Indications: For use as a nutritive supplement of vitamin C in guinea pigs and primates.

Dosage and Administration: Administer intramuscularly 1 to 10 mL, depending on condition, species, and body weight. Repeat daily or as indicated by desired response.

Precaution(s): Store between 15°C and 30°C (59°F-86°F). Protect from light.

Since pressure may develop on long storage, precautions should be taken to release pressure before use. Storage under refrigeration will reduce possibility of pressure buildup.

Caution(s): Federal law restricts this drug to use by or on the order of a licensed veterinarian.

For animal use only. Keep out of reach of children.

Presentation: 100 mL (NDC 59130-623-01) and 250 mL (NDC 59130-623-02).

Compendium Code No.: 10740562 Rev. 6-95 / Rev. 8-94

AMTECH VITAMIN K_1 INJECTION ℞

Phoenix Scientific **Vitamin K_1-Injection**

(phytonadione injection) 10 mg/mL Aqueous Colloidal Solution

Active Ingredient(s): Each milliliter contains:

Phytonadione . . . 10 mg

Inactive ingredients:

Polyoxyethylated fatty acid derivative . . . 70 mg
Dextrose . . . 37.5 mg
Water for Injection, q.s. . . . 1 mL

Added as preservative:

Benzyl alcohol . . . 0.9%

Indications: VITAMIN K_1 INJECTION is indicated in coagulation disorders which are due to faulty formation of factors II, VII, IX and X when caused by vitamin K deficiency or interference with vitamin K activity.

VITAMIN K_1 INJECTION is indicated in cattle, calves, horses, swine, sheep, goats, dogs, and cats to counter hypoprothrombinemia induced by ingestion of anticoagulant rodenticides.

VITAMIN K_1 INJECTION is also indicated to counter hypoprothrombinemia caused by consumption of bishydroxycoumarin found in spoiled and moldy sweet clover.

Pharmacology: Phytonadione is a vitamin, which is a clear, yellow to amber, viscous, odorless or nearly odorless liquid. It is insoluble in water, soluble in chloroform and slightly in ethanol. It has a molecular weight of 450.70.

Phytonadione is 2-methyl-3-phytyl-1, 4-naphthoquinone. Its empirical formula is $C_{31}H_{46}O_2$.

VITAMIN K_1 INJECTION is a yellow, sterile, aqueous colloidal solution of vitamin K_1, with a pH of 5.0 to 7.0, available for injection by the intravenous, intramuscular, and subcutaneous routes.

Clinical Pharmacology: VITAMIN K_1 INJECTION aqueous colloidal solution of vitamin K_1 for parenteral injection, possesses the same type and degree of activity as does naturally-occurring vitamin K, which is necessary for the production via the liver of active prothrombin (factor II), proconvertin (factor VII), plasma thromboplastin component (factor IX), and Stuart factor (factor X). The prothrombin test is sensitive to the levels of three of these four factors -- II, VII, and X. Vitamin K is an essential cofactor for a microsomal enzyme that catalyzes the post-translational carboxylation of multiple, specific, peptide-bound glutamic acid residues in inactive hepatic precursors of factors II, VII, IX, and X. The resulting gamma-carboxyglutamic acid residues convert the precursors into active coagulation factors that are subsequently secreted by liver cells into the blood.

Phytonadione is readily absorbed following intramuscular administration. After absorption, phytonadione is initially concentrated in the liver, but the concentration declines rapidly. Very little vitamin K accumulates in tissues. Little is known about the metabolic fate of vitamin K. Almost no free unmetabolized vitamin K appears in bile or urine.

In normal animals, phytonadione is virtually devoid of pharmacodynamic activity. However, in animals deficient in vitamin K, the pharmacological action of vitamin K is related to its normal physiological function, that is, to promote the hepatic biosynthesis of vitamin K dependent clotting factors.

The action of the aqueous colloidal solution, when administered intravenously, is generally detectable within an hour or two and hemorrhage is usually controlled within 3 to 6 hours. A normal prothrombin level may often be obtained in 12 to 14 hours.

Dosage and Administration:

Cattle, Calves, Horses, Swine, Sheep, and Goats: Acute hypoprothrombinemia (with hemorrhage) and Non-acute hypoprothrombinemia — 0.5-2.5 mg/kg subcutaneously or intramuscularly.

Dogs and Cats: Acute hypoprothrombinemia (with hemorrhage) and Non-acute hypoprothrombinemia — 0.25-2.5 mg/kg subcutaneously or intramuscularly. Use higher end of dose for second generation rodenticides.

Whenever possible, VITAMIN K_1 INJECTION should be given by the subcutaneous or intramuscular route. When intravenous administration is considered unavoidable, the drug should be diluted and injected very slowly, not exceeding 1 mg per minute.

Directions For Dilution: VITAMIN K_1 INJECTION may be diluted with 0.9% Sodium Chloride Injection, 5% Dextrose Injection, or 5% Dextrose and Sodium Chloride Injection. Other diluents should not be used. When dilutions are indicated, administration should be started immediately after mixture with the diluent, and unused portions of the dilution should be discarded.

Whole blood or component therapy may be indicated if bleeding is excessive. This therapy, however, does not correct the underlying disorder and VITAMIN K_1 INJECTION should be given concurrently. In the event of shock or excessive blood loss, the use of whole blood or component therapy is indicated.

Contraindication(s): Hypersensitivity to any component of this medication.

Precaution(s): Protect from light at all times. Store in a dark place. Store at controlled room temperature 15°C-30°C (59°-86°F).

Caution(s): Federal law restricts this drug to use by or on the order of a licensed veterinarian.

Drug Interactions: Temporary resistance to prothrombin-depressing anticoagulants may result, especially when larger doses of phytonadione are used. If relatively large doses have been employed, it may be necessary when reinstituting anticoagulant therapy to use somewhat larger doses of the prothrombin-depressing anticoagulant, or to use one which acts on a different principle, such as heparin sodium.

Laboratory Tests: Prothrombin time should be checked regularly as clinical conditions indicate.

Parenteral drug products should be inspected visually for particulate matter and discoloration prior to administration, whenever solution and container permit.

An immediate coagulant effect should not be expected after administration of phytonadione. It takes a minimum of 1 to 2 hours for measurable improvement in the prothrombin time. Whole blood or component therapy may also be necessary if the bleeding is severe.

Phytonadione will not counteract the anticoagulant action of heparin.

When vitamin K_1 is used to correct excessive anticoagulant-induced hypoprothrombinemia, anticoagulant therapy still being indicated, the patient is again faced with the clotting hazards existing prior to starting the anticoagulant therapy. Phytonadione is not a clotting agent, but overzealous therapy with vitamin K_1 may restore conditions which originally permitted thromboembolic phenomena. Dosage should be kept as low as possible, and prothrombin time should be checked regularly as clinical conditions indicate.

Repeated large doses of vitamin K are not warranted in hepatic disease if the response to the initial therapy is unsatisfactory. Failure to respond to vitamin K may indicate that the condition being treated is inherently unresponsive to vitamin K.

For animal use only.

Warning(s): Keep out of reach of children.

Adverse Reactions: Deaths have occurred after intravenous administration. (See Intravenous Use.)

Pain, swelling, and tenderness at the injection site may occur. Intramuscular injection may result in hematomas.

The possibility of allergic sensitivity, including an anaphylactoid reaction, should be kept in mind.

Intravenous Use: Severe reactions, including fatalities, have occurred during and immediately after intravenous injection of phytonadione, even when precautions have been taken to dilute the phytonadione and to avoid rapid infusion. Typically these severe reactions have resembled hypersensitivity or anaphylaxis, including shock and cardiac and/or respiratory arrest. Some patients have exhibited these severe reactions on receiving phytonadione for the first time. Therefore the intravenous route should be restricted to those situations where other routes are not feasible and the serious risk involved is considered justified.

Presentation: VITAMIN K_1 INJECTION is supplied in 100 mL bottles (NDC 59130-633-01).

Compendium Code No.: 10740571 Rev. 2-01

AMTECH XYLAZINE HCL INJECTION 20 mg/mL ℞

Phoenix Scientific **Analgesic-Sedative**

(xylazine)

ANADA No.: 200-184

Active Ingredient(s): Each mL contains 20 mg xylazine (base equivalent), 0.9 mg methylparaben, 0.1 mg propylparaben, water for injection; citric acid and sodium citrate for pH adjustment to 5.5 ± 0.3.

Xylazine hydrochloride (equivalent to 2% base)	2.3%
Inert ingredients	97.7%
	100.0%

Indications: XYLAZINE HCL INJECTION (xylazine) should be used in dogs and cats when it is desirable to produce a state of sedation accompanied by a shorter period of analgesia. XYLAZINE HCL INJECTION (xylazine) has been used successfully as follows:

1. Diagnostic procedures - Examination of mouth and ears, abdominal palpation, rectal palpation, vaginal examination, catheterization of the bladder and radiographic examinations.
2. Orthopedic procedures, such as application of casting materials and splints.
3. Dental procedures.
4. Minor surgical procedures of short duration such as debridement, removal of cutaneous neoplasms and suturing of lacerations.
5. To calm and facilitate restraint of fractious animals.
6. Therapeutic medication for sedation and relief of pain following injury or surgery.
7. Major surgical procedures:
   a. When used as a preanesthetic to general anesthesia.
   b. When used in conjunction with local anesthetics.

Pharmacology: XYLAZINE HCL INJECTION (xylazine), a non-narcotic compound, is a sedative and analgesic as well as muscle relaxant. Its sedative and analgesic activity is related to central nervous system depression. Its muscle-relaxant effect is based on inhibition of the intraneural transmission of impulses in the central nervous system. The principal pharmacological activities develop within 10 to 15 minutes after intramuscular or subcutaneous injection, and within 3 to 5 minutes following intravenous administration.

A sleeplike state, the depth of which is dose-dependent, is usually maintained for 1 to 2 hours, while analgesia lasts from 15 to 30 minutes. The centrally-acting muscle relaxant effect causes relaxation of the skeletal musculature complementing sedation and analgesia.

In animals under the influence of XYLAZINE HCL INJECTION (xylazine), the respiratory rate is reduced as in natural sleep. Following treatment with XYLAZINE HCL INJECTION (xylazine), the heart rate is decreased and a transient change in the conductivity of the cardiac muscle may occur as evidenced by a partial atrioventricular block. This resembles the atrioventricular block often observed in apparently normal animals.[1] Intravenous administration of XYLAZINE HCL INJECTION (xylazine) causes a transient rise in blood pressure, followed by a slight decrease.

XYLAZINE HCL INJECTION (xylazine) has no effect on blood clotting time or other hematologic parameters.

Dosage and Administration:

1. Dosage:

   Intravenously - 0.5 mL/20 lbs. body weight (0.5 mg/lb.).

   Intramuscularly or Subcutaneously - 1 mL/20 lbs. body weight (1 mg/lb.).

   In large dogs (over 50 lbs.), a dosage of 0.5 mg/lb. administered intramuscularly may provide sufficient sedation and/or analgesia for most procedures.

   Since vomiting may occur (see Side Effects), fasting for 6-24 hours prior to the use of XYLAZINE HCL INJECTION (xylazine) may reduce the incidence; the I.V. route results in the least vomiting.

   Following injection of XYLAZINE HCL INJECTION (xylazine), the animal should be allowed to rest quietly until the full effect has been reached.

   These dosages produce sedation which is usually maintained for 1 to 2 hours and analgesia which lasts for 15 to 30 minutes.
2. Preanesthetic to Local Anesthesia: XYLAZINE HCL INJECTION (xylazine) at the recommended dosages can be used in conjunction with local anesthetics, such as procaine or lidocaine.
3. Preanesthetic to General Anesthesia: XYLAZINE HCL INJECTION (xylazine) at the recommended dosage rates, produces an additive effect to central nervous system depressants such as pentobarbital sodium, thiopental sodium and thiamylal sodium. Therefore, the dosage of such compounds should be reduced and administered to the desired effect. In general, ⅓ to ½ of the calculated dosage of the barbiturates will be needed to produce a surgical plane of anesthesia. Post-anesthetic or emergence excitement has not been observed in animals preanesthetized with XYLAZINE HCL INJECTION (xylazine).

   XYLAZINE HCL INJECTION (xylazine) has been used successfully as a preanesthetic agent for pentobarbital sodium, thiopental sodium, thiamylal sodium, nitrous oxide, ether, halothane and methoxyflurane anesthesia.

Precaution(s): Store at controlled room temperature (15° to 30°C or 59° to 86°F).

Caution(s): Federal law restricts this drug to use by or on the order of a licensed veterinarian.

Clinical results with xylazine have not revealed any detrimental effects when the compound is administered to pregnant dogs or cats. However, until more definitive studies are completed, XYLAZINE HCL INJECTION (xylazine) is not recommended for use in these animals.

Careful consideration should be given before administering to dogs or cats with significantly depressed respiration, severe pathologic heart disease, advanced liver or kidney disease, severe endotoxic or traumatic shock and stress conditions such as extreme heat, cold, or fatigue.

Analgesic effect is variable, and depth should be carefully assayed prior to surgical/clinical procedures. In spite of sedation, the practitioner and handlers should proceed with caution since defense reactions may not be diminished.

Do not use XYLAZINE HCL INJECTION (xylazine) in conjunction with tranquilizers.

Since an additive effect results from the use of XYLAZINE HCL INJECTION (xylazine) and the barbiturate compounds, it should be used with caution with these central nervous system depressants. Products known to produce respiratory depression or apnea, such as thiamylal sodium, should be given at a reduced dosage and, when injected intravenously, should be administered slowly.

When intravenous administration is desired, avoid perivascular injection in order to achieve the desired effect. Studies have shown negligible evidence of tissue irritationm, however, following perivascular injection of xylazine.

Bradycardia and an arrhythmia in the form of incomplete atrioventricular block have been reported following xylazine administration. Although clinically the importance of this effect is questioned,[1] a standard dose of atropine given prior to or following XYLAZINE HCL INJECTION (xylazine) (xylazine) will greatly decrease the incidence.

While sedation usually lasts from 1 to 2 hours, recovery periods in excess of 4 to 5 hours have been reported in both dogs and cats.

Warning(s): This drug is for use in dogs and cats only.

Not for human use.

Keep out of reach of children.

Side Effects: Emesis occurs occasionally in dogs, and frequently in cats, soon after the administration of XYLAZINE HCL INJECTION (xylazine), but before clinical sedation is evident. When observed, emesis usually occurs only a single time, after which there is no further emetic effect. The use of antiemetics may delay this phenomenon. The occurrence of emesis may be considered a desirable effect when XYLAZINE HCL INJECTION (xylazine) is administered as a preanesthetic to general anesthesia.

XYLAZINE HCL INJECTION (xylazine) used at recommended dosage levels may occasionally cause slight muscle tremors, bradycardia with partial A-V heart block and a reduced respiratory rate. Should excessive respiratory depression occur following the use of XYLAZINE HCL INJECTION (xylazine), administer respiratory stimulants and provide artificial respiration.

Movement in response to sharp auditory stimuli may be observed.

Increased urination may occur in cats following the use of XYLAZINE HCL INJECTION (xylazine).

Trial Data: Safety: XYLAZINE HCL INJECTION (xylazine) is tolerated in dogs and cats at 10 times the recommended dose. However, doses of this magnitude produced muscle tremors, emesis and long periods of sedation.

References: Available upon request.

Presentation: XYLAZINE HCL INJECTION (xylazine) is supplied in 20 mL multiple-dose vials as a sterile solution (NDC 59130-678-13).

Compendium Code No.: 10740590 Rev. 3-00

AMTECH XYLAZINE HCL INJECTION 100 mg/mL ℞

Phoenix Scientific **Analgesic-Sedative**

(Xylazine)

ANADA No.: 200-139

Active Ingredient(s): Each mL contains 100 mg xylazine, (base equivalent), 0.9 mg methylparaben, 0.1 mg propylparaben, water for injection; citric acid and sodium citrate for pH adjustment to 5.5 ± 0.3.

Xylazine hydrochloride (equivalent to 10% base)	11.4%
Inert ingredients	88.6%
	100.0%

Indications: XYLAZINE HCL INJECTION (xylazine) should be used in horses and *Cervidae* (Fallow Deer, Mule Deer, Sika Deer, White-Tailed Deer and Elk) when it is desirable to produce a state of sedation accompanied by a shorter period of analgesia.

Horses: XYLAZINE HCL INJECTION (xylazine) has been used successfully as follows:

1. Diagnostic procedures - oral and ophthalmic examinations, abdominal palpation, rectal palpation, vaginal examination, catheterization of the bladder and radiographic examinations.
2. Orthopedic procedures, such as application of casting materials and splints.
3. Dental procedures.
4. Minor surgical procedures of short duration such as debridement, removal of cutaneous neoplasms and suturing of lacerations.
5. To calm and facilitate handling of fractious animals.
6. Therapeutic medication for sedation and relief of pain following injury or surgery.
7. Major surgical procedures:
   a. When used as a preanesthetic to general anesthesia.
   b. When used in conjunction with local anesthetics.

Cervidae: XYLAZINE HCL INJECTION (xylazine) may be used for the following:

1. To calm and facilitate handling of fractious animals.
2. Diagnostic procedures.
3. Minor surgical procedures.
4. Therapeutic medication for sedation and relief of pain following injury or surgery.
5. As a preanesthetic to local anesthesia. XYLAZINE HCL INJECTION (xylazine) at the recommended dosages can be used in conjunction with local anesthetics, such as procaine or lidocaine.

Pharmacology: XYLAZINE HCL INJECTION (xylazine), a non-narcotic compound, is a sedative and analgesic as well as muscle relaxant. Its sedative and analgesic activity is related to central nervous system depression. Its muscle relaxant effect is based on inhibition of the intraneural transmission of impulses in the central nervous system. The principal pharmacological activities develop within 10 to 15 minutes after intramuscular injection in horses and *Cervidae*, and within 3 to 5 minutes following intravenous administration in horses.

A sleeplike state, the depth of which is dose-dependent, is usually maintained for 1 to 2 hours, while analgesia lasts from 15 to 30 minutes. The centrally-acting muscle relaxant effect causes relaxation of the skeletal musculature, complementing sedation and analgesia.

In horses and *Cervidae* under the influence of XYLAZINE HCL INJECTION (xylazine), the respiratory rate is reduced as in natural sleep. Following treatment with XYLAZINE HCL INJECTION (xylazine), the heart rate is decreased and a transient change in the conductivity of the cardiac muscle may occur, as evidenced by a partial atrioventricular block. This resembles the atrioventricular block often observed in normal horses.[1,2,3,4] Partial A-V block may occasionally occur following intramuscular injection of XYLAZINE HCL INJECTION (xylazine). When given intravenously in horses, the incidence of partial A-V block is higher. Intravenous administration causes a transient rise in blood pressure in horses, followed by a slight decrease.

XYLAZINE HCL INJECTION (xylazine) has no effect on blood clotting time or other hematologic parameters.

Dosage and Administration:

Horses:

1. Dosage:
   Intravenously - 0.5 mL/100 lbs body weight (0.5 mg/lb).
   Intramuscularly - 1.0 mL/100 lbs body weight (1.0 mg/lb).
   Following injection of XYLAZINE HCL INJECTION (xylazine) the animal should be allowed to rest quietly until the full effect has been reached.
   These dosages produce sedation which is usually maintained for 1 to 2 hours, and analgesia which lasts for 15 to 30 minutes.
2. Preanesthetic to Local Anesthesia: XYLAZINE HCL INJECTION (xylazine) at the recommended dosages can be used in conjunction with local anesthetics, such as procaine or lidocaine.
3. Preanesthetic to General Anesthesia: XYLAZINE HCL INJECTION (xylazine) at the recommended dosage rates produces an additive effect to central nervous system depressants such as pentobarbital sodium, thiopental sodium and thiamyl sodium. Therefore, the dosage of such compounds should be reduced and administered to the desired effect. In general, only ⅓ to ½ of the calculated dosage of the barbiturates will be needed to produce a surgical plane of anesthesia. Post-anesthetic or emergence excitement has not been observed in animals preanesthetized with XYLAZINE HCL INJECTION (xylazine).
   XYLAZINE HCL INJECTION (xylazine) has been used successfully as a preanesthetic agent for pentobarbital sodium, thiopental sodium, thiamylal sodium, nitrous oxide, ether, halothane, glyceryl guaiacolate and methoxyflurane anesthesia.

Cervidae: Administer intramuscularly, either by hand syringe or syringe dart, in the heavy muscles of the croup or shoulder.

Dosage Range:

Fallow Deer *(Dama dama)* - 2.0 to 4.0 mL/100 lbs body weight (2.0 to 4.0 mg/lb).

Mule Deer *(Odocoileus hemionus)* - 1.0 to 2.0 mL/100 lbs body weight (1.0 to 2.0 mg/lb).

Sika Deer *(Cervus nippon)* - 1.0 to 2.0 mL/100 lbs body weight (1.0 to 2.0 mg/lb).

White-Tailed Deer *(Odocoileus virginianus)* - 1.0 to 2.0 mL/100 lbs body weight (1.0 to 2.0 mg/lb).

Elk *(Cervus canadensis)* - 0.25 to 0.5 mL/100 lbs body weight (0.25 to 0.5 mg/lb).

Following injection of XYLAZINE HCL INJECTION (xylazine) the animal should be allowed to rest quietly until the full effect has been reached. These dosages produce sedation which is usually maintained for 1 to 2 hours and analgesia which lasts for 15 to 30 minutes.

Precaution(s): Store at controlled room temperature (15° to 30°C or 59° to 86°F).

Caution(s): Federal law restricts this drug to use by or on the order of a licensed veterinarian.

Careful consideration should be given before administering to horses and *Cervidae* with significantly depressed respiration, severe pathologic heart disease, advanced liver or kidney disease, severe endotoxic or traumatic shock and stress conditions such as extreme heat, cold, high altitude or fatigue.

Do not use XYLAZINE HCL INJECTION (xylazine) in conjunction with tranquilizers.

Analgesic effect is variable, and depth should be carefully assayed prior to surgical/clinical procedures. Variability of analgesia occurs most frequently at the distal extremities of horses and *Cervidae*. In spite of sedation, the practitioner and handlers should proceed with caution since defense reactions may not be diminished.

Horses: Since an additive effect results from the use of XYLAZINE HCL INJECTION (xylazine) and the barbiturate compounds, it should be used with caution with these central nervous system depressants. Products known to produce respiratory depression or apnea, such as thiamylal sodium should be given at a reduced dosage and, when injected intravenously, should be administered slowly. When intravenous administration of XYLAZINE HCL INJECTION (xylazine) is desired, avoid perivascular injection in order to achieve the desired effect. Studies have shown negligible evidence of tissue irritation, however, following perivascular injection of xylazine.

Intracarotid Arterial Injection Should be Avoided. As with many compounds, including tranquilizers, immediate violent seizures followed by collapse may result from inadvertent administration into the carotid artery. Although the reaction with XYLAZINE HCL INJECTION (xylazine) is usually transient and recovery may be rapid and complete, special care should be taken to assure that the needle is in the jugular vein rather than the carotid artery.

Bradycardia and arrhythmia in the form of incomplete atrioventricular block have been reported following xylazine administration. Although clinically the importance of this effect is questioned,[1,2,3,4] a standard dose of atropine given prior to or following xylazine will greatly decrease the incidence.

Sedation for transport is most successful if actual transportation is begun after the full effect of the drug has been reached and the animal's stability is maintained while standing. In addition, it should be noted that animals under the influence of xylazine can be aroused by noise or other stimuli and this may increase the risk of injury.

Cervidae: As in all ruminants, it is preferable to administer XYLAZINE HCL INJECTION (xylazine) to fasted *Cervidae* as a safeguard against aspiration of food material into the lungs and/or bloat during deep sedation.

Care should be taken to administer XYLAZINE HCL INJECTION (xylazine) in the heavy muscles of the croup or shoulder. Injections given subcutaneously, intraperitoneally or into fat deposits will give unpredictable results.

Intra-arterial injection should be avoided, as with many compounds, including tranquilizers, immediate violent seizures followed by collapse may result from inadvertent administration into an artery.

The animal should not be disturbed during induction or until the full effect of the drug has been reached which is usually 10 to 15 minutes following injection.

The usual time to initial effect of the drug is 2 to 5 minutes. The administrator of the drug should be fully cognizant of this interval prior to administration of drug to free-ranging deer or elk, especially at night or in heavily wooded areas.

If the animal has been underdosed (faulty injection or miscalculation on weight) it is advisable to wait one hour before administering a second dose.

Adequate ventilation- especially in cages or crates- is mandatory; keep head and neck in position to insure patient air passage and to prevent aspiration of stomach contents.

During sedation, animals should be prevented from assuming lateral recumbency. A sternal recumbent position is desirable.

While under the effects of XYLAZINE HCL INJECTION (xylazine) the animal should be protected from extreme hot or cold environments.

Efforts should be made to prevent patient from rising until almost complete recovery is attained.

The transportation of *Cervidae* given XYLAZINE HCL INJECTION (xylazine) should be carefully monitored to prevent excessive struggling, injury or death.

Hyperthermic reactions may occur, especially if the subject is in a highly excited state when the drug is administered. Hosing the head and entire body with cold water has usually proven to be an effective deterrent.

The safety of XYLAZINE HCL INJECTION (xylazine) has not been demonstrated in pregnant *Cervidae*. Avoid use during the breeding season.

Cervidae should be observed closely until all of the sedative effects of XYLAZINE HCL INJECTION (xylazine) are gone.

Care should be taken at all times when administering XYLAZINE HCL INJECTION (xylazine) to *Cervidae*. This is due to the method of administration (usually darting), the difficulty in estimating body weights and the accepted theory that wild animals are more unpredictable in their response to sedatives and analgesics than the domesticated species.

Keep out of reach of children.

Warning(s): Do not use in *Cervidae* less than 15 days before or during the hunting season.

This drug should not be administered to domestic food-producing animals. Not for use in horses intended for food.

Avoid accidental administration to humans. Should such exposure occur, notify a physician immediately. Artificial respiration may be indicated.

In *Cervidae*, occasional capture-associated deaths occur. Clinical trials reveal a mortality rate of approximately 3.5% attendant with the administration of xylazine.

Side Effects: XYLAZINE HCL INJECTION (xylazine) in horses and *Cervidae*, used at recommended dosage levels may occasionally cause slight muscle tremors, bradycardia with partial A-V heart block and a reduced respiratory rate. Movement in response to sharp auditory stimuli may be observed.

In horses, sweating, rarely profuse, has been reported following administration. In *Cervidae*, salivation, various vocalizations (bellowing, bleating, groaning, grunting, snoring) on expiration, audible grinding of molar teeth, protruding tongue and elevated temperatures have also been noted in some cases.

Trial Data: Safety: XYLAZINE HCL INJECTION (xylazine) is tolerated at 10 times the recommended dose in horses and at doses above the recommended range in *Cervidae.* However, some elevated doses produced muscle tremors and long periods of sedation.

References: Available upon request.

Presentation: XYLAZINE HCL INJECTION (xylazine) is available in 50 mL multiple dose vials (NDC 59130-668-11).

Compendium Code No.: 10740580 Rev. 4-00

ANASED® 20 INJECTION ℞

Lloyd **Analgesic-Sedative**

(Xylazine Sterile Solution) 20 mg/mL

NADA No.: 139-236

Active Ingredient(s): ANASED® is supplied as a sterile solution.

Each mL contains xylazine hydrochloride equivalent to 20 mg base activity, methylparaben 0.9 mg, propylparaben 0.1 mg, and water for injection. pH adjusted with citric acid and sodium citrate.

Indications: Xylazine should be used in dogs and cats when it is desirable to produce a state of sedation accompanied by a shorter period of analgesia. Xylazine has been used successfully as follows:

1. Diagnostic procedures - examination of mouth and ears, abdominal palpation, rectal palpation, vaginal examination, catheterization of the bladder and radiographic examinations of the head and extremities.
2. Orthopedic procedures, such as application of casting materials and splints.
3. Dental procedures.
4. Minor surgical procedures of short duration such as debridement, removal of cutaneous neoplasms and suturing of lacerations.
5. To calm and facilitate the handling of fractious animals.
6. Major surgical procedures:
   a. Used as a pre-anesthetic to general anesthesia.
   b. Used in conjunction with local anesthetics.

Pharmacology: Xylazine, a nonnarcotic compound, is a sedative and analgesic as well as a muscle relaxant. Its sedative and analgesic activity is related to central nervous system depression. Its muscle relaxant effect is based upon inhibition of the intraneural transmission of impulses in the central nervous system. The principal pharmacological activities develop within 10 to 15 minutes after intramuscular or subcutaneous injection, and within three to five minutes following intravenous administration.

A sleeplike state, the depth of which is dose-dependent, is usually maintained for one to two hours, while analgesia lasts from 15 to 30 minutes. The centrally acting muscle relaxant effect causes relaxation of the skeletal musculature complementing sedation and analgesia.

In animals under the influence of xylazine, the respiratory rate is reduced as in natural sleep. Following treatment with xylazine, the heart rate is decreased and a transient change in the conductivity of the cardiac muscle may occur as evidenced by a partial atrioventricular block. This resembles the atrioventricular block often observed in apparently normal animals. Intravenous administration of xylazine causes a transient rise in blood pressure, followed by a slight decrease.

Xylazine does not have an effect on blood clotting time or other hematologic parameters.

Dosage and Administration:

1. Dosage:
   Intravenous - 0.5 mL/20 lbs body weight (0.5 mg/lb, or 1.1 mg/kg).
   Intramuscular or subcutaneous - 1.0 mL/20 lbs body weight (1.0 mg/lb or 2.2 mg/kg).
   In large dogs (over 50 lbs) a dosage of 0.5 mg/lb administered intramuscularly may provide sufficient sedation and/or analgesia for most procedures.
   Since vomiting may occur (see side effects), fasting for 6-24 hours prior to the use of xylazine may reduce the incidence; the I.V. route results in the least vomiting.
   Following the injection of xylazine, the animal should be allowed to rest quietly until the full effect has been reached.
   These dosages produce sedation which is usually maintained for 1 to 2 hours and analgesia which lasts for 15 to 30 minutes.
2. Pre-anesthetic to local anesthesia:
   Xylazine at the recommended dosages can be used in conjunction with local anesthetics, such as procaine or lidocaine.
3. Pre-anesthetic to general anesthesia:
   Xylazine, at the recommended dosage rates, produces an additive effect to central nervous system depressants such as pentobarbital sodium, thiopental sodium and thiamylal sodium. Therefore, the dosage of such compounds should be reduced and administered to the desired effect. In general, ⅓ to ½ of the calculated dosage of the barbiturates will be needed to produce a surgical plane of anesthesia. Postanesthetic or emergence excitement has not been observed in animals pre-anesthetized with xylazine.
   Xylazine has been used successfully as a pre-anesthetic agent for pentobarbital sodium, thiopental sodium, thiamylal sodium, nitrous oxide, ether, halothane and methoxyflurane anesthesia.

Precaution(s): Protect from heat. Do not store over 30°C (86°F).

Caution(s): Federal law restricts this drug to use by or on the order of a licensed veterinarian.

Clinical results with xylazine have not revealed any detrimental effects when the compound is administered to pregnant dogs or cats. However, until more definitive studies are completed, xylazine is not recommended for use in these animals.

Careful consideration should be given before administering to dogs or cats with significantly depressed respiration, severe pathologic heart disease, advanced liver or kidney disease, severe endotoxic or traumatic shock and stress conditions such as extreme heat, cold, or fatigue.

Analgesic effect is variable, and depth should be carefully assayed prior to surgical/clinical procedures. In spite of sedation, the practitioner and handlers should proceed with caution since defense reactions may not be diminished.

Do not use xylazine in conjunction with tranquilizers.

Since an additive effect results from the use of xylazine and the barbiturate compounds, it should be used with caution with these central nervous system depressants. Products known to produce respiratory depression or apnea, such as thiamylal sodium, should be given at a reduced dosage and, when injected intravenously, should be administered slowly.

When intravenous administration is desired, avoid perivascular injection in order to achieve the desired effect. Studies have shown negligible evidence of tissue irritation, however, following the perivascular injection of xylazine.

Bradycardia and an arrhythmia in the form of incomplete atrioventricular block have been reported following xylazine administration. Although clinically the importance of this effect is questioned, a standard dose of atropine given prior to or following xylazine will greatly decrease the incidence.

While sedation usually lasts from 1 to 2 hours, recovery periods in excess of 4 to 5 hours have been reported in dogs and cats.

Warning(s): The drug is for use in dogs and cats only.

Toxicology: Xylazine has been tested in dogs at 4 times the recommended dose. Doses of this magnitude produced muscle tremors, emesis and long periods of sedation.

Side Effects: Emesis occurs occasionally in dogs, and frequently in cats, soon after the administration of xylazine, but before clinical sedation is evident. When observed, emesis usually occurs only a single time, after which there is no further emetic effect. The use of anti-emetics may delay this phenomenon. The occurrence of emesis may be considered a desirable effect when xylazine is administered as a pre-anesthetic to general anesthesia.

Xylazine used at the recommended dosage levels may occasionally cause slight muscle tremors, bradycardia with partial A-V heart block and a reduced respiratory rate. Should excessive respiratory depression or bradycardia occur following the use of ANASED® (xylazine), administer yohimbine to rapidly reverse the xylazine-induced effects.

Gaseous extension of the stomach may occur in dogs treated with xylazine making radiographic interpretation more difficult.

Movement in response to sharp auditory stimuli may be observed.

Increased urination may occur in cats following the use of xylazine.

References: Available upon request.

Presentation: 20 mL multiple-dose vials.

Compendium Code No.: 11350010

ANASED® 100 INJECTABLE ℞

Lloyd **Analgesic-Sedative**

(Xylazine) 100 mg/mL

NADA No.: 139-236

Active Ingredient(s): Each mL contains: Xylazine hydrochloride equivalent to 100 mg of base activity, methylparaben 0.9 mg, propylparaben 0.1 mg, sodium citrate dihydrate 5.0 mg and water for injection. pH adjusted with citric acid and sodium citrate.

Indications: Xylazine should be used in horses and *Cervidae* (Fallow Deer, Mule Deer, Sika Deer, White-Tailed Deer and Elk) when it is desirable to produce a state of sedation accompanied by a shorter period of analgesia. Horses: Xylazine has been used successfully as follows:

1. Diagnostic procedures - oral and ophthalmic examinations, abdominal palpation, rectal palpation, vaginal examination, catheterization of the bladder and radiographic examinations.
2. Orthopedic procedures, such as the application of casting materials and splints.
3. Dental procedures.
4. Minor surgical procedures of short duration such as debridement, removal of cutaneous neoplasms and suturing of lacerations.
5. To calm and facilitate the handling of fractious animals.
6. Major surgical procedures:
   a. When used as a pre-anesthetic to general anesthesia.
   b. When used in conjunction with local anesthetics.

Cervidae: Xylazine may be used for the following:

1. To calm and facilitate the handling of fractious animals.
2. Diagnostic procedures.
3. Minor surgical procedures.
4. Therapeutic medication for sedation and relief of pain following injury or surgery.
5. As a preanesthetic to local anesthesia. ANASED® at the recommended dosages can be used in conjunction with local anesthetics, such as procaine or lidocaine.

Pharmacology: Xylazine, a nonnarcotic compound, is a sedative and analgesic as well as a muscle relaxant. Its sedative and analgesic activity is related to central nervous system depression. Its muscle-relaxant effect is based upon inhibition of the intraneural transmission of impulses in the central nervous system. The principal pharmacological activities develop within 10 to 15 minutes after intramuscular injection in horses and *Cervidae,* and within 3 to 5 minutes following intravenous administration in horses.

A sleeplike state, the depth of which is dose-dependent, is usually maintained for one to two hours, while analgesia lasts from 15 to 30 minutes. The centrally acting muscle-relaxant effect causes relaxation of the skeletal musculature complementing sedation and analgesia.

In horses and *Cervidae* under the influence of xylazine, the respiratory rate is reduced as in natural sleep. Following treatment with xylazine, the heart rate is decreased and a transient change in the conductivity of the cardiac muscle may occur, as evidenced by a partial atrioventricular block. This resembles the atrioventricular block often observed in normal horses. Although a partial A-V block may occasionally occur following intramuscular injection of xylazine, the incidence is less than when it is administered intravenously. Intravenous administration of xylazine causes a transient rise in blood pressure, followed by a slight decrease.

Xylazine does not have an effect on blood clotting time or other hematologic parameters.

Dosage and Administration:

1. Dosage: Horses:
   Intravenous - 0.5 mL/100 lb body weight (0.5 mg/lb, or 1.1 mg/kg).
   Intramuscular - 1.0 mL/100 lb body weight (1 mg/lb, or 2.2 mg/kg).
   Cervidae:
   Administer intramuscularly, by either hand syringe or syringe dart, in the heavy muscles of the croup or shoulder.
   Fallow Deer *(Dama dama)* — 2.0 to 4.0 mL/100 lbs body weight (2.0 to 4.0 mg/lb or 4.4 to 8.8 mg/kg).
   Mule Deer *(Odocoileus hemionus)* — 1.0 to 2.0 mL/100 lbs body weight (1.0 to 2.0 mg/lb or 2.2 to 4.4 mg/kg).
   Sika Deer *(Cervus nippon)* — 1.0 to 2.0 mL/100 lbs body weight (1.0 to 2.0 mg/lb or 2.2 to 4.4 mg/kg).
   White-Tailed Deer *(Odocoileus virginianus)* — 1.0 to 2.0 mL/100 lbs body weight (1.0 to 2.0 mg/lb or 2.2 to 4.4 mg/kg).
   Elk *(Cervus canadensis)* — 0.25 to 0.5 mL/100 lbs body weight (0.25 to 0.5 mg/lb or 0.55 to 1.1 mg/kg).
   Following injection of xylazine, the animal should be allowed to rest quietly until the full effect has been reached.
   These dosages produce sedation which is usually maintained for 1 to 2 hours, and analgesia which lasts for 15 to 30 minutes.
2. Pre-anesthetic to local anesthesia:
   Xylazine at the recommended dosages can be used in conjunction with local anesthetics, such as procaine or lidocaine.

3. Pre-anesthetic to general anesthesia:

   Xylazine, at the recommended dosage rates, produces an additive effect to central nervous system depressants such as pentobarbital sodium, thiopental sodium and thiamylal sodium. Therefore, the dosage of such compounds should be reduced and administered to the desired effect. In general, only ⅓ to ½ of the calculated dosage of the barbiturates will be needed to produce a surgical plane of anesthesia. Post-anesthetic or emergence excitement has not been observed in animals pre-anesthetized with xylazine.

   Xylazine has been used successfully as a pre-anesthetic agent for pentobarbital sodium, thiopental sodium, thiamylal sodium, nitrous oxide, ether, halothane, glyceryl guaiacolate and methoxyflurane anesthesia.

Precaution(s): Protect from heat. Do not store over 30°C (86°F).

Caution(s): Federal law restricts this drug to use by or on the order of a licensed veterinarian.

Careful consideration should be given before administering to horses and *Cervidae* with significantly depressed respiration, severe pathologic heart disease, advanced liver or kidney disease, severe endotoxic or traumatic shock and stress conditions such as extreme heat, cold, high altitude or fatigue.

Do not use xylazine in conjunction with tranquilizers.

Analgesic effect is variable, and depth should be carefully assayed prior to surgical/clinical procedures. Variability of analgesia occurs most frequently at the distal extremities of horses and *Cervidae*. In spite of sedation, the practitioner and handlers should proceed with caution since defense reactions may not be diminished.

Intracarotid arterial injection should be avoided. As with many compounds, including tranquilizers, immediate violent seizures followed by collapse may result from inadvertent administration into the carotid artery. Although the reaction with xylazine is usually transient and recovery may be rapid and complete, special care should be taken to ensure that the needle is in the jugular vein rather than the carotid artery.

Horses: Since an additive effect results from the use of xylazine and the barbiturate compounds, it should be used with caution with these central nervous system depressants. Products known to produce respiratory depression or apnea, such as thiamylal sodium, should be given at a reduced dosage and, when injected intravenously, should be administered slowly. When intravenous administration is desired, avoid perivascular injection in order to achieve the desired effect. Studies have shown negligible evidence of tissue irritation, however, following perivascular injection of xylazine.

Bradycardia and an arrhythmia in the form of incomplete atrioventricular block have been reported following xylazine administration. Although clinically the importance of this effect is questioned, a standard dose of atropine given prior to or following xylazine will greatly decrease the incidence.

Sedation for transport is most successful if actual transportation is begun after the full effect of the drug has been reached and the animal's stability is maintained while standing. In addition, it should be noted that animals under the influence of xylazine can be aroused by noise or other stimuli and this may increase the risk of injury.

Cervidae: It is preferable to administer ANASED® to fasted *Cervidae.* As in all ruminants a safeguard against aspiration of food material into the lungs and/or bloat during deep sedation is necessary.

Care should be taken to administer ANASED® in the heavy muscles of the croup or shoulder. Injections given subcutaneously, intraperitoneally or into fat deposits will give unpredictable results.

Cervidae should not be disturbed during induction or until the full effect of the drug has been reached which is usually 10 to 15 minutes following injection.

The usual time to initial effect of the drug is 2 to 5 minutes. The administrator of the drug should be fully cognizant of this interval prior to administration of drug to free-ranging deer elk, especially at night or in heavily wooded areas.

If the animal has been underdosed (faulty injection or miscalculation on weight) it is advisable to wait one hour before administering a second dose.

Adequate ventilation - especially in cages or crates - is mandatory; keep head and neck in position to insure patent air passage and to prevent aspiration of stomach contents.

During sedation *Cervidae* should be prevented from assuming lateral recumbency. A sternal recumbent position is desirable.

While under the effects of xylazine, the animal should be protected from an extremely hot or cold environment.

Efforts should be made to prevent patient from rising until almost complete recovery is attained.

The transportation of *Cervidae* given ANASED® should be carefully monitored to prevent excessive struggling, injury or death.

Hyperthemic reactions may occur, especially if the subject is in a highly excited state when the drug is administered. Hosing the head and the entire body with cold water has usually proven to be an effective deterrent.

Data are presently inadequate to recommend ANASED® use in pregnant *Cervidae.* Avoid use during breeding season.

Cervidae should be observed closely until all of the sedative effects of ANASED® are gone.

Care should be taken at all times when administering ANASED® to *Cervidae.* This is due to the difficulty in estimating body weights and the accepted theory that wild animals are more unpredictable in their response to sedatives and analgesics than the domesticated species.

Warning(s): This drug is for use in horses and *Cervidae* only and should not be administered to food-producing animals.

Avoid accidental administration to humans. Should such exposure occur, notify a physician immediately. Artificial respiration may be indicated.

In *Cervidae,* occasional capture-associated deaths occur. Clinical trials reveal a mortality rate of approximately 3.5% attendant with the administration of xylazine.

Toxicology: Xylazine has been tested in horses at 5 times the recommended dose, and at doses above the recommended range in *Cervidae.* However, doses of this magnitude may produce convulsions and long periods of sedation in horses and muscle tremors and long periods of sedation in *Cervidae.*

Side Effects: Xylazine in horses and *Cervidae* used at recommended dosage levels may occasionally cause slight muscle tremors, bradycardia with partial A-V heart block and a reduced respiratory rate. Movement in response to sharp auditory stimuli may be observed. In horses, sweating, rarely profuse, has been reported following administration. In *Cervidae,* salivation, various vocalizations (bellowing, bleating, groaning, grunting, snoring) on expiration, audible grinding of molar teeth, protruding tongue and elevated temperatures have also been noted in some cases.

References: Available upon request.

Presentation: 50 mL multiple-dose vials.

Compendium Code No.: 11350000

ANEM-X™ 100

AgriPharm — **Iron Injection**

Injection Iron Hydrogenated Dextran

NADA No.: 106-772

Active Ingredient(s): ANEM-X™ 100 is a sterile solution containing ferric hydroxide in complex with a low molecular weight dextran fraction equivalent to 100 mg elemental iron per mL with 0.5% phenol as a preservative.

Indications: For the prevention or treatment of baby-pig anemia due to iron deficiency.

Dosage and Administration: Intramuscular injection.

Prevention: 1 mL (100 mg) at one (1) to three (3) days of age.

Treatment: 1 mL (100 mg). May be repeated in approximately 10 days.

For intramuscular use only.

Caution(s): Use of the product after four weeks of age may cause staining of the ham muscle.

Warning(s): Keep out of reach of children. For animal use only.

Presentation: 100 mL containers.

Compendium Code No.: 14570070

ANEM-X™ 200

AgriPharm — **Iron Injection**

Injection Iron Hydrogenated Dextran

NADA No.: 106-772

Active Ingredient(s): ANEM-X™ 200 is a sterile solution containing ferric hydroxide in complex with a low molecular weight dextran fraction equivalent to 200 mg elemental iron per mL with 0.5% phenol as a preservative.

Indications: For the prevention or treatment of baby-pig anemia due to iron deficiency.

Dosage and Administration: Intramuscular injection.

Prevention: 1 mL (200 mg) at one (1) to three (3) days of age.

Treatment: 1 mL (200 mg). May be repeated in approximately 10 days.

For intramuscular use only.

Caution(s): Use of the product after four weeks of age may cause staining of the ham muscle.

Warning(s): Keep out of reach of children. For animal use only.

Presentation: 100 mL containers.

Compendium Code No.: 14570080

ANIHIST

AHC — **Antihistamine**

Antihistamine Granules

Active Ingredient(s): Each ounce contains:

Guaifenesin, USP . . . . 2400 mg
Pyrilamine Maleate, USP . . . . 600 mg
in a palatable base.

Indications: For use as an antihistamine and expectorant.

Dosage and Administration: Usual Dosage: ½ ounce (1 level tablespoon) per 1,000 pound body weight or as recommended by a veterinarian. Can be mixed with feed and repeated at 12 hour intervals as needed.

Shake well before use.

Precaution(s): Keep lid tightly closed and store in a dry place.

Do not store above 30°C (86°F).

Caution(s): For use in horses only.

For animal use only.

Keep out of reach of children.

For veterinary use only.

Warning(s): Do not use at least 72 hours prior to sporting event.

Presentation: 20 ounces (NDC 65090-001-15), 5 pounds (NDC 65090-001-30), and 25 pounds (NDC 65090-001-50).

Compendium Code No.: 10770000

ANIMAL INSECTICIDE

Durvet — **Premise and Topical Insecticide**

Shaker Duster Contains Co-Ral®

EPA Reg. No.: 67517-21-12281

Active Ingredient(s):

O,O-Diethyl O-(3-chloro-4-methyl-2-oxo-2H-1-benzopyran-7-yl) phosphorothioate 1.0%
Inert Ingredients 99.0%
100.0%

Indications: For dairy or beef cattle and swine for control of hornflies and lice.

A ready-to-use insecticide dusting powder. Effective in controlling hornflies and lice; aids in controlling face flies. No withdrawal period required: may be used with dairy cattle in production or beef cattle being fed for slaughter.

Directions for Use: It is a violation of Federal law to use this product in a manner inconsistent with its labeling.

To Control Lice on Swine: Apply not more than 1 oz (3 level tablespoonfuls) per head as a uniform coat to the head, shoulders, and back by use of shaker can or suitable mechanical dust applicator. Repeat as necessary but not more often than once every ten days. Treat no more than 6 times per season.

Bedding Treatment: Apply 2 oz (6 level tablespoonfuls) uniformly over each 30 square feet of fresh, dry bedding by use of a shaker can or suitable mechanical dust applicator. Repeat as necessary but not more often than once every ten days. Treat no more than 6 times per season.

Note: In severe infestations both individual animals and the bedding may be treated as directed above.

To Control Hornflies and Lice on Beef and Dairy Cattle: Apply not more than 2 oz (6 level tablespoonfuls) evenly into the hair over the head, neck, shoulders, back and tailhead. Repeat as necessary, but not more often than every 14 days. (Maximum Seasonal Application Rate: 26 applications/year).

Precautionary Statements: Hazards to Humans and Domestic Animals:

Caution: Harmful if swallowed, inhaled or absorbed through skin. Avoid breathing dusts. Avoid contact with eyes, skin and clothing. Wash thoroughly with soap and water after handling. Remove contaminated clothing and wash clothing before reuse.

Statement of Practical Treatment:

If Swallowed: Call a physician or Poison Control Center. Drink 1 or 2 glasses of water and induce vomiting by touching the back of throat with finger. Do not induce vomiting or give anything by mouth to an unconscious person.

If Inhaled: Remove victim to fresh air. If not breathing give artificial respiration preferably mouth-to-mouth. Get medical attention.

If on Skin: Wash with plenty of soap and water. Get medical attention if irritation persists.

If in Eyes: Flush eyes with plenty of water. Call a physician if irritation persists.

Note to Physician: Atropine sulfate by injection is antidotal. 2-PAM is also antidotal and may be administered in conjunction with atropine.

Environmental Hazards: This product is toxic to birds, fish, and aquatic invertebrates. Do not apply directly to water. Do not contaminate water when disposing of equipment washwater or rinsate.

Restrictions: For external, insecticidal use on above specified animals only. Avoid contamination of feed, troughs, water and water utensils. Provide thorough ventilation while dusting. Do not apply to sick, stressed or convalescent animals.

Storage and Disposal: Do not contaminate water, food or feed by storage or disposal.

Pesticide Disposal: Wastes resulting from the use of this product may be disposed of on site or at an approved waste disposal facility.

Container Disposal: Completely empty container into application equipment. Then dispose of empty container in a sanitary landfill or by incineration, or, if allowed by State and local authorities, by burning. If burned, stay out of smoke.

Warning(s): No interval is required between treatment and slaughter or between treatment and use of milk as feed.

Keep out of reach of children.

Disclaimer: Notice of Warranty: Durvet, Inc. makes no warranty of merchantability, fitness for any particular purpose, or otherwise, expressed or implied concerning this product or its uses which extend beyond the use of the product or its uses which extend beyond the use of the product under normal conditions in accord with the statements made on this label.

Presentation: 2 lb (907 g) and 25 lb (11.34 kg).

® A Reg. TM of the parent company of Miles, Inc.

*U.S. Patent No. 2,748,146

Compendium Code No.: 10840061 1/99

ANIMAX® OINTMENT ℞

Pharmaderm **Topical Antimicrobial-Corticosteroid**

Nystatin-Neomycin Sulfate-Thiostrepton-Triamcinolone Acetonide Ointment

NADA No.: 140-847

Active Ingredient(s): ANIMAX® Ointment combines nystatin, neomycin sulfate, thiostrepton and triamcinolone acetonide in a non-irritating polyethylene and mineral oil base.

Each mL contains:

Nystatin .... 100,000 units
Neomycin sulfate equivalent to neomycin base .... 2.5 mg
Thiostrepton .... 2,500 units
Triamcinolone acetonide .... 1.0 mg

The preparation is intended for local therapy in a variety of cutaneous disorders of cats and dogs; it is especially useful in disorders caused, complicated or threatened by bacterial and/or candidal (monilial) infection.

Indications: ANIMAX® Ointment is particularly useful in the treatment of acute and chronic otitis of varied etiologies, in interdigital cysts in cats and dogs and in anal gland infections in dogs.

The preparation is also indicated in the management of dermatologic disorders characterized by inflammation and dry or exudative dermatitis, particularly those caused, complicated, or threatened by bacterial or candidal *(Candida albicans)* infections. It is also of value in eczematous dermatitis, contact dermatitis, and seborrheic dermatitis; and as an adjunct in the treatment of dermatitis due to parasitic infestation.

Pharmacology: Actions: By virtue of its four active ingredients, ANIMAX® Ointment provides four basic therapeutic effects: anti-inflammatory, antipruritic, antifungal and antibacterial. Triamcinolone acetonide is a potent synthetic corticosteroid providing rapid and prolonged symptomatic relief on topical administration. Inflammation, edema, and pruritus promptly subside, and lesions are permitted to heal. Nystatin is the first well-tolerated antifungal antibiotic of dependable efficacy for the treatment of cutaneous infections caused by *Candida albicans* (Monilia). Nystatin is fungistatic *in vitro* against a variety of yeast and yeast-like fungi including many fungi pathogenic to animals. No appreciable activity is exhibited against bacteria. Thiostrepton has a high order of activity against gram-positive organisms, including many which are resistant to other antibiotics; neomycin exerts antimicrobial action against a wide range of gram-positive and gram-negative bacteria. Together they provide comprehensive therapy against those organisms responsible for most superficial bacterial infections.

Dosage and Administration: Frequency of administration is dependent on the severity of the condition. For mild inflammations, application may range from once daily to once a week; for severe conditions ANIMAX® Ointment may be applied as often as two to three times daily, if necessary. Frequency of treatment may be decreased as improvement occurs.

Wear gloves during the administration of the ointment or wash hands immediately after application.

Otitis: Clean canal of impacted cerumen. Inspect canal and remove any foreign bodies such as grass awns, ticks, etc. Instill three to five drops of ANIMAX® Ointment.

Preliminary use of a local anesthetic may be advisable.

Infected Anal Glands, Cystic Areas, etc.: Drain gland or cyst and then fill with ANIMAX® Ointment.

Other Dermatologic Disorders: Clean affected areas, removing any encrusted discharge or exudate. Apply ANIMAX® Ointment (Nystatin-Neomycin Sulfate-Thiostrepton-Triamcinolone Acetonide Ointment) sparingly in a thin film.

Precaution(s):

240 mL bottle: Do not store above 86°F.

7.5 mL, 15 mL, and 30 mL tubes: Store at room temperature; avoid excessive heat (104°F).

Caution(s): Federal law restricts this drug to use by or on the order of a licensed veterinarian.

ANIMAX® Ointment is not intended for the treatment of deep abscesses or deep-seated infections such as inflammation of the lymphatic vessels. Parenteral antibiotic therapy is indicated in these infections.

ANIMAX® Ointment (Nystatin-Neomycin Sulfate-Thiostrepton-Triamcinolone Acetonide Ointment) has been extremely well tolerated. Cutaneous reactions attributable to its use have been extremely rare. The occurrence of systemic reactions is rarely a problem with topical administration. There is some evidence that corticosteroids can be absorbed after topical application and cause systemic effects. Therefore, an animal receiving ANIMAX® Ointment therapy should be observed closely for signs such as polydipsia, polyuria, and increased weight gain.

ANIMAX® Ointment is not generally recommended for the treatment of deep or puncture wounds or serious burns.

Sensitivity to neomycin may occur. If redness, irritation, or swelling persists or increases, discontinue use. Do not use if pus is present since the drug may allow the infection to spread. Keep this and all medications out of the reach of children. Avoid ingestion. Oral or parenteral use of corticosteroids (depending on dose, duration of use, and specific steroid) may result in inhibition of endogenous steroid production following drug withdrawal.

Before instilling any medication into the ear, examine the external ear canal thoroughly to be certain the tympanic membrane is not ruptured in order to avoid the possibility of transmitting infection to the middle ear as well as damaging the cochlea or vestibular apparatus from prolonged contact. If hearing or vestibular dysfunction is noted during the course of treatment, discontinue the use of ANIMAX® Ointment.

Warning(s): Clinical and experimental data have demonstrated that corticosteroids administered orally or by injection to animals may induce the first stage of parturition if used during the last trimester of pregnancy and may precipitate premature parturition followed by dystocia, fetal death, retained placenta, and metritis.

Additionally, corticosteroids administered to dogs, rabbits and rodents during pregnancy have resulted in cleft palate in the offspring. In dogs, other congenital anomalies have resulted: deformed forelegs, phocomelia, and anasarca.

For use in dogs and cats only.

Side Effects: SAP and SGPT (ALT) enzyme elevations, polydypsia and polyuria, vomiting and diarrhea (occasionally bloody) have been observed following parenteral or systemic use of synthetic corticosteroids in dogs.

Cushing's syndrome has been reported in association with prolonged or repeated steroid therapy in dogs.

Temporary hearing loss has been reported in conjunction with treatment of otitis with products containing corticosteroids. However, regression usually occurred following withdrawal of the drug. If hearing dysfunction is noted during the course of treatment with ANIMAX® Ointment, discontinue its use.

Presentation: ANIMAX® Ointment is supplied in 7.5 mL, 15 mL and 30 mL tubes, and 240 mL or 8 oz. bottles.

Compendium Code No.: 10880000

ANIPRIN F

AHC **Non-Steroidal Anti-Inflammatory**

Molasses-Flavored Aspirin Powder

Active Ingredient(s):

	Each ounce contains:	Each pound contains:
Acetylsalicylic Acid	50%	225,000 mg

in a palatable base.

Indications: To be used orally as an aid in reducing fever and in relief of minor muscular aches and joint pains in horses and cattle.

Dosage and Administration: Administer orally. Can be mixed with feed.

To mature horses and cattle give 4 to 8 tablespoons two to three times daily. Or, as recommended by a veterinarian. Allow animals ample supply of fresh, clean water after administration.

Precaution(s): Shake well before use.

Keep lid tightly closed and store in a dry place.

Do not store above 30°C (85°F).

Caution(s): Keep this and all medication out of the reach of children.

For animal use only.

For veterinary use only.

Presentation: 16 oz jar, 2.5 lb jar and 5 lb pail.

Compendium Code No.: 10770010

ANIPRYL® TABLETS ℞

Pfizer Animal Health **MAO Inhibitor**

(selegiline hydrochloride, L-deprenyl hydrochloride)

NADA No.: 141-080

Active Ingredient(s): ANIPRYL® (selegiline hydrochloride) tablets are white, convex tablets containing 2, 5, 10, 15, and 30 mg of selegiline HCl. It is commonly referred to in the clinical and pharmacological literature as L-deprenyl (the levorotatory form of deprenyl HCl).

Indications: ANIPRYL® tablets are indicated for the control of clinical signs associated with canine cognitive dysfunction syndrome (CDS) and control of clinical signs associated with uncomplicated canine pituitary dependent hyperadrenocorticism (PDH).

Pharmacology: Selegiline hydrochloride is (—)-*(R)*-*N*,α-Dimethyl-*N*-2-propynylphenethylamine hydrochloride.

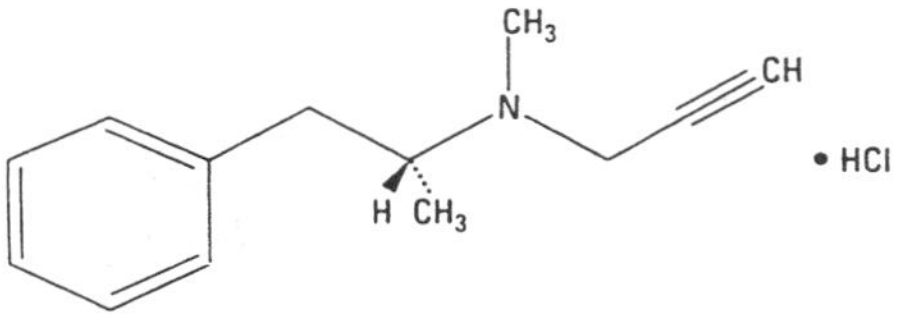

Molecular Formula: $C_{13}H_{17}N$ HCl

Molecular Weight: 223.75

Selegiline is an irreversible inhibitor of monoamine oxidase (MAO).[1,2] MAOs are widely distributed throughout the body and are subclassified into 2 types, A and B, which differ in their substrate specificity and tissue distribution. Selegiline is believed to be a selective inhibitor of MAO-B at recommended dosages in the dog due to its greater affinity for type B enzyme active sites compared to type A sites.[1] In CNS neurons, MAO plays an important role in the catabolism of catecholamines, (dopamine, and, to a lesser extent, norepinephrine and epinephrine) and serotonin.[1,2] Selegiline may have pharmacologic effects unrelated to MAO-B inhibition. There is some evidence that it may increase dopaminergic activity by other mechanisms, including increasing synthesis and release of dopamine into the synapse as well as interfering with dopamine re-uptake from the synapse.[2-4] Effects resulting from selegiline administration may also be mediated through its metabolites. Two of its 3 principal metabolites, L-amphetamine and L-methamphetamine, have pharmacological actions of their own. However, the extent to which these metabolites contribute to the effects of selegiline is unknown.

Therapeutic effects of selegiline are thought to result in part from enhanced catecholaminergic nerve function and increased dopamine levels in the CNS.[5,6] The pathogenesis of the development of clinical signs associated with cognitive decline is considered to be partly a result of a decrease in the level of catecholamines in the CNS and deficiencies in neurotransmission.[7] There is

A

evidence which points to hypothalamic dopamine deficiency playing a role in the pathogenesis of pituitary dependent hyperadrenocorticism in the dog.[8,9]

Based upon IV administration of selegiline to 4 mixed breed female dogs, the plasma elimination half-life was estimated to be 60 ± 10 minutes (mean ± SD) and the volume of distribution at steady-state (Vss) was estimated to be 9.4 ± 1.6 L/kg (mean ± SD). The relatively large Vss suggests that the selegiline is extensively distributed to body tissues. The absolute bioavailability, F, of an oral solution was less than 10%.[10]

Dosage and Administration:

CDS: The recommended dosage for oral administration for the control of clinical signs associated with CDS is 0.5-1.0 mg/kg once daily, preferably administered in the morning. Initially, dogs should be dosed to the nearest whole tablet. Adjustments should then be made based on response and tolerance to the drug.

PDH: The recommended dosage for the control of clinical signs associated with canine PDH is 1.0 mg/kg once daily, preferably administered in the morning. If no improvement is observed after 2 months of therapy, dosage may be increased to a maximum of 2.0 mg/kg once daily. If no improvement is seen after 1 month at the higher dose or if at any time clinical signs progress, the dog should be re-evaluated. In dogs whose clinical signs of PDH progress despite ANIPRYL® therapy in the absence of concurrent disease, alternative therapy should be considered.

Dogs should be monitored closely for possible adverse events associated with any increase in dose.

Clinical Use of ANIPRYL® in CDS: CDS is an age-related deterioration of cognitive abilities characterized by behavioral changes not wholly attributable to a general medical condition such as neoplasia, infection, or organ failure. CDS is typified by multiple cognitive impairments which affect the dog's function. In clinical trials, the observed behavioral changes associated with CDS in older dogs included: disorientation, decreased activity level, abnormal sleep/wake cycles, loss of housetraining, decreased or altered responsiveness to family members, and decreased or altered greeting behavior. In clinical trials, ANIPRYL® was shown to be effective in controlling clinical signs associated with CDS. After 4 weeks of treatment, dogs treated with ANIPRYL® showed significant improvement when compared to placebo-treated controls in sleeping patterns, housetraining, and activity level. Some dogs showed increased improvement up to 3 months, however, onset, duration and magnitude of response varied with individual dogs.

The diagnosis of CDS in dogs is a diagnosis of exclusion, based on thorough behavioral and medical histories, in conjunction with appropriate diagnostic work-up and testing.[11] Periodic patient monitoring to evaluate the response and tolerance to the drug and for the presence of concurrent or new disease is recommended.

Clinical Use of ANIPRYL® in PDH: Clinical signs of PDH seen in clinical trials included panting, reduced activity, polydipsia, polyuria, changes in sleep patterns, altered appetite, obesity, alopecia, abdominal distention, reduced skin elasticity, thin skin, poor hair growth, pyoderma, decreased responsiveness to attention, and decreased enthusiasm of greeting. In clinical studies involving 125 evaluable cases of naturally occurring PDH, ANIPRYL® was shown to be effective in controlling clinical signs associated with the disease. On physical examination, abdominal distention was the parameter which most consistently improved following treatment with ANIPRYL®. Based on owner assessments, activity level was the parameter most consistently evaluated as "improved". Approximately 60% of the dogs were evaluated by the veterinarians and owners to be "slightly improved" to "improved" after 1 month of ANIPRYL® therapy. By month 2, veterinarians reported that approximately 77% were "slightly improved" to "improved". Approximately 20% of dogs did not respond to ANIPRYL® and were deemed treatment failures.

Those dogs that responded to ANIPRYL® tended to do so within 1-2 months after treatment was initiated. Response to therapy varied between patients with some dogs showing improvement in all presenting clinical signs and others showing improvement in only 1-2 parameters. Duration of response was also variable, with some dogs continuing on ANIPRYL® for over 1 year with good control of clinical signs and others showing an initial response to therapy only to be followed within several months by recurrence of clinical signs of PDH. There was no correlation demonstrated between an individual dog's clinical response to ANIPRYL® and that dog's low dose dexamethasone suppression test results, therefore, monitoring should be based on history and physical examination findings.

Contraindication(s): ANIPRYL® is contraindicated in patients with known hypersensitivity to this drug.

In humans, selegiline is contraindicated for use with meperidine and this contraindication is often extended to other opioids.

ANIPRYL® should not be administered at doses exceeding those recommended (0.5-2.0 mg/kg once daily).

In humans, concurrent use of MAO inhibitors with alpha-2 agonists has resulted in extreme fluctuations of blood pressure; therefore, blood pressure monitoring is recommended with concurrent use in dogs. Also, in humans, severe CNS toxicity including death has been reported with the combination of selegiline and tricyclic antidepressants, and selegiline and selective serotonin reuptake inhibitors. Although no such adverse drug interactions were reported in the clinical trials in dogs, it seems prudent to avoid the combination of ANIPRYL® and selective serotonin reuptake inhibitors (e.g., fluoxetine) as well as ANIPRYL® and tricyclic (e.g., clomipramine, amitriptyline, imipramine) or other antidepressants.

At least 14 days should elapse between discontinuation of ANIPRYL® and initiation of treatment with a tricyclic antidepressant or selective serotonin reuptake inhibitor. Because of the long half-life of fluoxetine and its active metabolites, at least 5 weeks should elapse between discontinuation of fluoxetine and initiation of treatment with ANIPRYL®.

Concurrent use of ANIPRYL® with ephedrine or potential MAO inhibitors, such as amitraz, is not recommended.

Precaution(s): Store at controlled room temperature 20°-25°C (68°-77°F).

Caution(s): Federal law restricts this drug to use by or on the order of a licensed veterinarian.

General: ANIPRYL® is not recommended for other behavior problems such as aggression. In the clinical trials, 3 dogs showed an increase in aggression while on this drug. The safety and efficacy of ANIPRYL® has not been evaluated in dogs with debilitating systemic diseases other than PDH.

The decision to prescribe ANIPRYL® should take into consideration that the MAO system of enzymes is complex and incompletely understood and there is only a limited amount of carefully documented clinical experience with selegiline. Consequently, the full spectrum of possible responses to selegiline may not have been observed in pre-marketing evaluation of the drug. It is advisable, therefore, to observe patients carefully for atypical responses.

Endocrine function testing to confirm pituitary dependent hyperadrenocorticism should be performed prior to ANIPRYL® administration for that condition. ANIPRYL® is not recommended for treatment of patients with hyperadrenocorticism not of pituitary origin such as those due to an adrenal tumor or administration of glucocorticoids. If complications of PDH are evident at the time of diagnosis or emerge during ANIPRYL® therapy, the patient should be evaluated and, if warranted, alternative therapy considered. Concurrent use of ANIPRYL® in conjunction with other therapies of canine PDH has not been reported.

Laboratory Tests: No specific laboratory tests are deemed essential for the management of patients on ANIPRYL®, as response to therapy should be based on the history and physical examinations for both PDH and CDS. In clinical trials for PDH, no correlation was found between an individual patient's clinical response and results of the low dose dexamethasone suppression (LDDS) test. There was no evidence of adrenal insufficiency in these trials.

In the 12 week clinical trial for CDS, a small number of dogs had a drop in hematocrit; some dropping within the normal range and some dropping below 37%. The clinical significance of this is unknown at this time. It is advisable to conduct a thorough physical examination and to consider appropriate laboratory tests to establish hematological and serum biochemical baseline data prior to administration of ANIPRYL®.

Reproductive Safety: The safety of ANIPRYL® in breeding, pregnant and lactating bitches, and breeding dogs has not been determined.

For a copy of the Material Safety Data Sheet (MSDS) or to report adverse reactions call Pfizer Animal Health at 1-800-366-5288.

Warning(s): Keep out of reach of children. Not for human use.

For use in dogs only.

Toxicology: Safety: In a laboratory safety study, ANIPRYL® was administered orally to healthy adult beagles once daily for 6 months at doses of 0, 1, 2, 3, or 6 mg/kg (0.5x, 1x, 1.5x and 3x the maximum recommended daily dose of 2.0 mg/kg). The drug was demonstrated to be safe at the recommended dose range of 0.5-2.0 mg/kg. The following statistically significant clinical observations were noted in dogs in the 1.5x and 3x group: salivation, decreased pupillary response, and decreased body weight despite normal to increased feed consumption. Additional reactions seen at the 3x dose included panting, decreased skin elasticity (dehydration) and stereotypic behaviors, i.e., weaving (repetitive left to right movement) in the cage. This repetitive movement started several hours after dosing but was no longer present at the time of the next morning dose. There were no changes noted in blood pressure, heart rate and ECG parameters, nor were there any ophthalmic changes.

Adverse Reactions: In clinical trials, 404 dogs treated with ANIPRYL® for as long as 18 months were monitored for the occurrence of adverse events. Many of the observations listed in the following table may be associated with the underlying disease (PDH or CDS), the advanced age of the patients or the development of unrelated concurrent disease. One index of relative importance, however is whether or not a reaction caused treatment discontinuation. Eighteen dogs (4%) experienced one or more of the following adverse events that led either to discontinuation of therapy with ANIPRYL®, dismissal from the study, or a reduction in dose: restlessness/agitation, vomiting, disorientation, diarrhea, diminished hearing, possible drug interaction (weakness, confusion, incoordination and "seizure-like" activity while being treated concurrently with metronidazole, prednisone, and trimethoprim sulfa), increase in destructive behavior in a dog with separation anxiety, anorexia, anemia, stiffness and polydipsia.

Percentage of Dogs with Adverse Events Reported in Clinical Field Trials

Adverse Event	ANIPRYL® (n=404)	Placebo (n=67)
vomiting	26%	21%
diarrhea	18%	10%
hyperactive/restless*	12%	6%
anorexia	8%	1%
neurologic**	6%	1%
lethargy	6%	1%
salivation	5%	4%
urinary tract infection	4%	1%
pruritus/dermatologic	4%	1%
weakness	4%	0
pale gums	3%	1%
polyuria/polydipsia	3%	1%
weight loss	3%	0
diminished hearing	2%	0
panting	2%	1%
cardiovascular/respiratory***	2%	0
licking	2%	1%

*This includes hyperactivity, irritability, abnormal repetitive movements, anxiousness, and restlessness.

**This includes ataxia, incoordination, staggering, disorientation, decreased proprioception, and seizure.

***This includes heart murmurs, tachycardia, collapse, dyspnea, pleural effusion, and sneezing.

References: Available upon request.

Presentation: Five tablet strengths are available in blister-packs of 30 tablets each: 2 mg, 5 mg, 10 mg, 15 mg, and 30 mg. Each box contains 1 blister pack (30 tablets).

Compendium Code No.: 36900000 75-0000-00

ANIPSYLL POWDER

AHC **Laxative**

Psyllium Feed Supplement

Ingredient(s): Psyllium, roughage.

Indications: ANIPSYLL is a source of psyllium and dietary fiber. ANIPSYLL aids in the treatment and prevention of constipation, sluggish intestines and sand colic.

Dosage and Administration: Recommended Dosage:

Therapeutic Dose: Feed 9 ounces twice daily for up to 20 days.

Maintenance Dose: Feed 3 ounces daily for 14 days, followed by 1 ounce daily as a preventative.

Precaution(s): Store in a cool, dry place. Reseal after each use.

Caution(s): For animal use only. Keep out of reach of children.

Presentation: 3 lb pail, 10 lb bucket and 20 lb bucket.

Compendium Code No.: 10770020

ANITUSS

AHC **Antitussive**

Palatable Expectorant Granules

Guaranteed Analysis:

Guaifenesin USP 7%
Ammonium Chloride 75%
Potassium Iodide USP 2%
in a sweet, palatable base.

Indications: A sweet, palatable granule mixed in water as an expectorant in large animals.

Dosage and Administration: Usual Dosage: Dissolve one pound of ANITUSS in 1 gallon of water to make stock solution.

Horses, Cattle and Sheep: Mix 1 pint of stock solution with 15 to 25 gallons of drinking water, or ½ to 1 ounce stock solution three times daily. For horses and cattle, ½ to 1 ounce of ANITUSS may be given in feed or drinking water daily. Swine and Poultry: Mix 1 pint of stock solution with 25 to 50 gallons of drinking water.

Animals should be kept on medication feed or water for 3-4 days, or as recommended by a veterinarian. Allow no other sources of drinking water during treatment.

Precaution(s): Keep lid tightly closed and store in a cool, dry place.

Do not store above 30°C (86°F).

Caution(s): For animal use only. Keep out of reach of children. For veterinary use only.

Presentation: 16 ounces and 25 pounds.

Compendium Code No.: 10770030

ANNIHILATOR™ INSECTICIDE PREMISE SPRAY

Boehringer Ingelheim **Premise Insecticide**

EPA Reg. No.: 4691-164

Active Ingredient(s):

Deltamethrin: (s)-cyano-3-phenoxybenzyl-(1R,3R)-3-(2,2-dibromovinyl)-2,2-dimethyl-cyclopropanecarboxylate 0.02%
Other Ingredients 99.98%
Total 100.00%

Indications: ANNIHILATOR™ Insecticide Premise Spray is intended to be used in and around residences and their immediate surroundings such as (but not limited to): apartments, atriums, attics, automobiles, basements, bathrooms, boats, cabins, campers, carports, clothes storage, condominiums, decks, dens, driveways, garages, gazebos, homes, kitchens, lanai, living rooms, parlors, patios, pet sleeping areas, play rooms, porches, recreational vehicles, solariums, storage areas, sun rooms, utility rooms and verandahs. Do not use in commercial food handling establishments, restaurants or other places where food is commercially prepared or processed.

ANNIHILATOR™ Insecticide Premise Spray's long-lasting action keeps on killing for up to 30 days after you spray. Contact kill gives you immediate results when spraying insects directly, while residual activity kills insects when they return to treated areas. ANNIHILATOR™ Insecticide Premise Spray will not stain surfaces or fabrics.

Directions for Use: It is a violation of Federal law to use this product in a manner inconsistent with its labeling.

Hold container upright. Do not spray up into air. Apply to surfaces only as a spot and crack and crevice treatment. Turn sprayer nozzle to "open" or "on" position. Hold approximately 12 inches from surface to be sprayed. Squeeze trigger to spray until surface is slightly moist.

Indoors:

Cockroaches (including adult and immature stages of both non-resistant and organophosphate and carbamate resistant strains), ants, booklice, boxelder bugs, centipedes, crickets, dermestids, firebrats, fleas, palmetto bugs, silverfish, sowbugs, ticks and waterbugs: Apply as a spot and crack crevice treatment to areas where these pests crawl and hide, especially in hidden areas around sinks and storage areas, behind baseboards, around doors and windows, behind and under refrigerators, cabinets, sinks and stoves, the underside of shelves, drawers, bookcases, and similar areas. Cover all food handling surfaces and cover or remove all food and cooking utensils or wash thoroughly after treatment. Exposed food should be covered or removed. Repeat as necessary but not more than once per week.

Ants: Spray ant trails and around doors and windows and other places where ants enter the house. Repeat as necessary but not more than once per week.

Carpenter Ants: For effective control, locate and treat nests and surrounding areas. Apply around doors and windows and other places where ants enter premises and where they crawl and hide. Spray into infested wood through existing openings.

Ticks and Fleas on Surfaces: Remove pet bedding and destroy or clean thoroughly. Spray pet resting quarters. Adult fleas and larvae contacted by spray will be killed. Put fresh bedding down once spray has dried. Do not spray animals directly. For best results, pets should be treated with an appropriate flea and/or tick control product registered for use on pets before allowing them to return to the treated area. Spray rugs and carpets where infestations are bad. Delicate fabrics should be tested for staining in an inconspicuous area prior to use.

Silverfish, Crickets, Spiders: Apply along and behind baseboards, to window and door frames, corners, pipes, storage localities, attics, crawl spaces and other areas over which these pests may crawl.

Centipedes, Ground Beetles, Pillbugs, Sowbugs, Scorpions and Ticks: Apply around doors and windows and other places where these pests may enter premises. Treat baseboards, storage areas and other locations where these pests are found.

Bedbugs and Lice: Remove linens and wash before reuse. Lightly spray mattresses, especially tufts, folds and edges. Apply to the interior of the frame. Allow to dry before remaking bed.

Flying Insects: House flies, gnats, mosquitoes and small flying moths: Spray localized resting areas, such as under eaves, porches, inside surfaces of windows and door frames, surfaces around light fixtures and cords, railings, etc. and anywhere these insects may rest. Insects coming to rest on treated surfaces will be killed.

Horse Stables and/or Livestock Facilities: To control stable flies, horn flies, house flies, face flies, horse flies, deer flies, mosquitoes and gnats. Apply thoroughly to surfaces until wet. Insects coming to rest on treated surfaces will be killed or repelled. Repeat as necessary but not more than once per week. Do not spray animals or humans, or apply to animal feed or watering equipment.

Outdoors:

Paint sprayer away from face. Hold sprayer on a slight downward angle, approximately 12 inches from surface to be sprayed. Spray with wind if breeze is blowing. Do not contaminate fish ponds or apply directly to water.

Pests on Outside Surfaces of Buildings: For control of building infestation with ants, clover mites crickets and sowbugs (pillbugs). Spray foundation of building where insects are active and may find entrance up to a height of 2 to 3 feet. Apply to outside surfaces of buildings where insects tend to congregate. Spray areas include (but are not limited to) screens, window frames, eaves, porches, patios, garages and refuse dumps. Repeat treatment as necessary but not more than once per week.

Crawling Insects: ants, cockroaches (including Asian cockroaches), centipedes, crickets, mole crickets, water bugs and silverfish. Spray infested surface of patio or picnic area. Also spray legs of tables and chairs.

Ants: Spray freely around ant trails and hills. Spray around nests hidden under steps, brickwork, concrete, etc. Break apart accessible nests and spray freely on and around debris. Repeat as necessary but not more than once per week.

Lone Star Ticks, Dog Ticks, Crickets and Fleas: Apply thoroughly to infestation in bushes, grass or weeds.

Wasps, Mud-daubers, Hornets, Yellow Jackets and Bees: Spray nests and other surfaces where bees may rest. Aim spray at nest openings. Applications should be made late in the evening when insects are at rest.

Flying Insects: House flies, gnats, mosquitoes and small flying moths: Spray outside surfaces of window and door frames and other areas where these pests may enter the home. Also spray localized resting areas, such as under eaves porches, surfaces around light fixtures and cords, railings, etc. where these insects may rest. Insects coming to rest on treated surfaces will be killed.

Termites, Carpenter Ants and Carpenter Bees: (for localized control only). Apply ANNIHILATOR™ Insecticide Premise Spray to voids or channels in damaged wood of a structure, or to cracks, crevices and spaces in and between wooden portions of structure or between wood and the foundation, in locations vulnerable to attack such as crawl spaces. Retreat if needed but not more than once per week.

For termites, the purpose of such applications is to kill workers or winged forms which may be present in the treated areas at the time of application. Not recommended as sole protection against termites. For active infestations, get a professional inspection. Such applications are not a substitute for mechanical alteration, soil treatment or foundation treatment but are merely a supplement. For severe termite infestation contact a professional pest control operator in your area.

Precautionary Statements: Hazards to Humans and Domestic Animals:

Caution: Contact with product may result in transient tingling and reddening of the skin. Avoid contact with skin or clothing.

Environmental Hazards: This product is extremely toxic to fish and aquatic invertebrates. Do not apply directly to water. Do not contaminate water when disposing of washwater or rinsate. This product is highly toxic to bees exposed to direct treatment or residues on blooming crops or weeds. Do not apply this product or allow it to drift to blooming crops or weeds if bees are visiting the treatment area.

Physical/Chemical Hazards: Do not apply this product in or on electrical equipment due to the possibility of shock hazard.

Storage and Disposal:

Storage: Store in a cool, dry area away from children. Keep from freezing.

Container Disposal: Use product until container is empty. Offer for recycling if possible. If recycling is not available or if the container is not empty, wrap the container in several layers of paper and discard in the trash or by other procedures approved by State and local authorities.

Warning(s): Keep out of reach of children.

Disclaimer: Warranty and Limitation of Damages: Seller warrants that this material conforms to its chemical description and is reasonably fit for the purposes stated on the label when used in accordance with directions under normal conditions of use and Buyer assumes the risk of any use contrary to such directions. Seller makes no other express or implied warranty, including any other express or implied warranty of Fitness or of Merchantability, and no agent of Seller is authorized to do so except in writing and with specific reference to this warranty. In no event shall Seller's liability for any breach of warranty exceed the purchase price of the material as to which a claim is made.

Presentation: 1 qt (0.946 L) and 1 U.S. gal (3.785 L).

Pat. 4488922

Compendium Code No.: 10281241 626705L-00-0111

ANNIHILATOR™ WP WETTABLE POWDER PREMISE INSECTICIDE

Boehringer Ingelheim **Premise Insecticide**

EPA Reg. No.: 4691-163

Active Ingredient(s):

Deltamethrin: (s)-cyano-3-phenoxybenzyl-(IR,3R)-3-(2,2-dibromovinyl)-2,2-dimethyl-cyclopranecarboxylate 5.00%
Other Ingredients 95.00%
Total 100.00%

Indications: For use by individuals/firms licensed or registered by the state to apply pesticide products.

For industrial control of major nuisance pests.

Controls numerous pests in and around unoccupied poultry houses, horse stalls, cattle barns, and swine and other livestock buildings.

For use in non-food/non-feed areas of food/feed processing plants.

Directions for Use: It is a violation of Federal law to use this product in a manner inconsistent with its labeling.

Indoors: ANNIHILATOR™ WP is intended to be mixed with water and applied indoors as crack and crevice, spot and broadcast treatments with pressurized sprayers or other equipment suitable for applying insecticides to localized areas. To minimize airborne particles, spray pressure should not exceed 30 psi at the nozzle tip.

Handling Procedures: Wear protective clothing when using or handling this product to help avoid exposure to eyes and skin. As a minimum, eye protection and chemically resistant gloves, a long-sleeved shirt and long-legged pants or coveralls are recommended. To avoid breathing spray mist during application in confined areas, wear a mask or respirator of a type recommended by NIOSH for filtering spray mists.

Adults, children and pets should not contact treated surfaces until spray has dried. Do not treat pets with this product. Before spraying, remove pets, cover aquaria and turn off air pump. Do not apply where electrical short circuits could occur. Do not use indoors as a space spray or in fogging equipment. It is recommended that eye protection be worn when making applications overhead.

Treatment Sites: When used in accordance with label directions, ANNIHILATOR™ WP may be applied in and around non-residential buildings and structures. This product can be applied to walls, floors, ceilings, in and around cabinets, between, behind and beneath equipment and appliances, around floor drains, window and door frames, and around plumbing, sinks and other possible pest harborage sites. Permitted areas of use include, but are not limited to, the non-food/non-feed areas of: buses, food manufacturing, processing and servicing establishments, warehouses, laboratories, railcars, trucks, unoccupied poultry houses, horse stalls, cattle barns, industrial buildings and installations.

Treatments may be applied at 21-day intervals or as necessary to maintain adequate control.

Mixing Instructions: ANNIHILATOR™ WP is intended to be mixed with water and applied with hand pressurized or power operated sprayers as a coarse spray. When diluting, add water to the spray tank and the appropriate amount of ANNIHILATOR™ WP. Thoroughly agitate the sprayer before using to insure proper suspension of the wettable powder. Re-invert sprayer before use if spraying is interrupted. If spray screens are used, they should be 50 mesh or larger. Dilute ANNIHILATOR™ WP insecticide only with water.

Dosage Chart: This product is intended for dilution prior to applications as directed in the following table. Use the scoop provided for measuring from tile jar. Each level scoopful contains 0.8 oz ANNIHILATOR™ WP.

Pests	Concentration of Active Ingredient	Dilution Rate Per Gallon of Final Spray
ants, bees, centipedes, cockroaches (maintenance rate), flies (including such flies as stable, house, cluster and horse flies), firebrats, gnats, hornets, killer bees, midges, mosquitoes, silverfish, yellow jackets, wasps	0.03% w/w	1 scoop
bedbugs, carpet beetles, cockroaches (clean out rate), crickets, fleas, lice, pillbugs, scorpions, sowbugs, spiders, ticks	0.06% w/w	2 scoops
carpenter ants	0.03% w/w	1 scoop

Tank Mixing: Unless prohibited by a product's label, users at their own discretion can tank-mix pesticides such as insect growth regulators currently labeled for similar use patterns. It is always recommended that a small jar compatibility test using proper proportions of chemicals and water be run to check for physical compatibility prior to tank-mixing.

Application Methods: This product may be applied as crack and crevice, spot, general surface and broadcast treatments. Treat where pests are found or normally occur.

Crack and Crevice Applications: Use a low pressure system with a pinpoint or variable pattern nozzle to apply the spray mixture to areas such as floors, cracks and crevices in and around baseboards, walls, expansion joints, areas around water and sewer pipes, and voids formed by equipment or appliances.

Spot and Broadcast Applications: Use a low pressure system with fan-type nozzle to uniformly apply spot treatments between, beneath and behind equipment or appliances.

Premise Pest Control: Apply as a coarse, low pressure spot or crack and crevice spray to areas that pests normally inhabit. Pay particular attention to dark corners of rooms and closets; floor drains; crack and crevices in walls; along and behind baseboards; around plumbing and other utility installations, doors, windows and in attics and crawl spaces. Applications may be made to floor surfaces along baseboards and around air ducts.

Pet Kennels: For residual control of crawling and flying insects in and around these structures, apply as a general surface and/or crack and crevice spray. Optimal control results if facilities to be treated are clean and if the exterior perimeter is concurrently treated with ANNIHILATOR™ WP. Apply only to areas of facility where animals are not present. Allow spray to dry before allowing re-entry of animals into treated areas. Do not apply to animal feed or watering equipment.

Non-Food/Non-Feed Areas: ANNIHILATOR™ WP may be applied as a general, spot or crack and crevice treatment in non-food/non-feed areas. Non-food/non-feed establishment areas are areas such as garbage rooms, lavatories, floor drains (to sewers), entries and vestibules, offices, locker rooms, machine rooms, boiler rooms, mop closets and storage (after packaging, canning or bottling). All areas that insects inhabit or through which insects may enter should be treated.

Indoor Pests Controlled by ANNIHILATOR™ WP: Ants[1], Beetles, Brown dogs ticks[2], Centipedes, Cockroaches[3] (American), (Asian), (brown-banded), (German), (oriental), (smoky brown), Crickets, Firebrats, Fleas[4], Mosquitoes, Silverfish, Scorpions, Sowbugs, Spiders, Ticks and other insect pests.

Numbers refer to "Specific Indoor use Directions".

Specific Indoor Use Directions:

1. Ants may be controlled by treating ant trails and wherever else these pests may find entrance; for example, around doors and windows.
2. For control of brown dog ticks, thoroughly apply the spray to infested areas, such as cracks and crevices, along baseboards, windows and door frames, and areas of floor and floor coverings where these pests may be present. Non-carpeted flooring should only be treated wit spot applications as necessary. Spots are defined as areas not exceeding two square feet. use a 0.06% spray at the rate of 1 gallon of diluted spray per 1600 square feet. Do not treat pets with this product. Adults, children and pets should not contact treated surfaces until spray has dried.
3. Cockroaches can be controlled by making crack and crevice, spot or general surface treatments. Treat where insects are found or normally occur including, but not limited to, floors, cracks and crevices in walls, along and behind baseboards; around plumbing, floor drains and other utility installations; and beneath and behind sinks, cabinets or other fixtures.
4. To control fleas, thoroughly apply a fine-particle spray to infested areas. An insect growth regulator may be added to achieve extended control of developing flea larvae and pupae. Non-carpeted flooring should only be treated with spot applications as necessary. Spots are defined as areas not to exceed two square feet.

Treated areas should be vacated during application, except for the applicator. Cover aquaria and fish bowls and remove other pets. Adults, children and pets should not contact treated surfaces until spray has dried. Old bedding should be replaced or thoroughly washed. Do not treat pets with this product. To control the source of flea infestations, pets inhabiting the treated premises should be treated with a flea control product registered for application to animals.

Outdoors: ANNIHILATOR™ WP is intended to be mixed with water and applied outdoors with pressurized sprayers as a general surface spray. The active ingredient in this product will provide effective residual control of pests listed on this label.

Handling Procedures for General Use Outdoors: Do not allow adults, children or pets on treated surfaces until spray has dried. Keep out of fish pools or other bodies of water. Do not treat vegetable gardens. Do not allow livestock to graze in treated areas.

Treatment Sites: When used in accordance with label directions. ANNIHILATOR™ WP may be applied to and around outside surfaces of residential and non-residential buildings and structures. Permitted areas of use include, but are not limited to: Crawl Spaces, Decks, Driveways, Eaves, Fences, Foundations, Garages, Lawns, Refuse dumps, Walkways, Walls, Window and door frames.

Mixing Instructions: ANNIHILATOR™ WP is intended to be mixed with water and applied with hand pressurized or power operated sprayers as a coarse spray. When diluting, add water to the spray tank and the appropriate amount of ANNIHILATOR™ WP. Thoroughly agitate the sprayer before using. Re-invert sprayer before use if spraying is interrupted. If spray screens are used, they should be 50 mesh or larger. Dilute ANNIHILATOR™ WP insecticide only with water.

Dosage Chart: This product is intended for dilution prior to application as directed in the following table. Use the scoop provided for measuring from the jar. Each level scoopful contains 0.8 oz ANNIHILATOR™ WP.

Concentration of Spray Mixture		Amount of ANNIHILATOR™ WP (ounce)	Amount of water (gal)	
High Conc.	0.03%	0.08	1	low volume
	0.06%	1.60	1	
Low Conc.	0.003%	0.80	10	high volume
		4.00	50	
		8.00	100	
	0.006%	1.60	10	
		8.00	50	
		16.00	100	

Tank Mixing: Unless prohibited by a product's label, users at their own discretion, can tank-mix pesticides, such as insect growth regulators, currently labeled for similar use patterns. It is always recommended that a small jar compatibility test using proper proportions of chemicals and water be run to check for physical compatibility prior to tank-mixing.

Application Methods: This product may be applied outdoors as a general surface spray. Treat where pests are found or normally occur.

Low Volume Directed Sprays: Application of low volume, high concentration (0.03 - 0.06%), sprays can quickly reduce localized heavy pest infestations on outside surfaces. Use a low pressure system with a pinpoint or variable pattern nozzle, such as a hand pump sprayer or backpack sprayer, and apply the spray mixture to specific areas such as cracks and crevices along walkways, patios, windows and door frames or other areas where insects may congregate or gain entrance to the structure.

High Volume Broadcast Sprays: Application of high volume, low concentration (0.003 - 0.006%) sprays, such as with power spraying equipment, can help prevent infestations of buildings by reducing pests in outdoor areas. Longer residual is achieved at the higher rates (about 0.006%). This type of treatment provides more thorough coverage over large areas than low volume directed sprays. Treat by applying spray mixture directly to areas such as flower beds, junctions of soil and structural walls, under shrubs along base of fences and under eaves. Apply as a coarse spray at the rate of about 10 gallons spray mixture per 1000 square feet. Thoroughly and uniformly wet the treated area. use sufficient amount of spray dilution to cover the area to the point of wetness but avoid applying to the point of runoff.

Outdoor Pests Controlled by ANNIHILATOR™ WP: Ants, Bees[1], Beetles, Carpenter ants, Centipedes, Cockroaches (American), (Asian), (brown-banded), (German), (oriental), (smoky brown), Crickets, Fire ants[2], Fleas[3], Hornets[1], Midges[3], Mosquitoes[3], Moths, Pillbugs, Scorpions[4], Sowbugs, Spiders, Ticks, Wasps[1], Yellow Jackets[1] and other outdoor insects.

Numbers refer to "Specific Outdoor Use Directions".

Specific Outdoor Use Directions:

1. Wasps, Hornets, Yellow Jackets and Bees - Application should be made late in the evening when insects are at rest. Aim spray at nest openings in ground, bushes, in cracks and crevices and under attic rafters which may harbor nests. Saturate nest and contact as many insects as possible.
2. Fire ant mounds may be controlled by applying ANNIHILATOR™ WP as a drench. Dilute 1.6 oz per 2 gallons of water. Gently sprinkle 1 to 2 gallons of the diluted insecticide over the surface of each mount and surrounding area to a 2 foot diameter. For best results, apply in cool weather 65 to 80°F, or in early morning or late evening hours. Treat new mounds as they appear. Pressurized sprays may disturb the ants and cause migration, reducing product effectiveness.
3. Flies, midges and mosquitoes may be controlled by spraying outside surfaces of doors, screens, window frames, or wherever these insects may enter the room. Also, spray surfaces around light fixtures on porches, in garages and other places where these insects alight or congregate.
4. Scorpions may be controlled by removing accumulations of lumber, firewood and other materials serving as harborage sites. Before stacking firewood or lumber, apply ANNIHILATOR™ WP as a localized spray to surfaces immediately below such materials. Do not treat firewood directly. Broadcast sprays outdoors may assist in reducing pests migrating from surrounding areas.

For Control of Wood-Infesting Insects: ANNIHILATOR™ WP is intended to be mixed with water and applied as a general surface or localized injection treatment with pressurized sprayers or other equipment suitable for applying insecticides to localized areas.

Handling Procedures: Contact with treated surfaces should be avoided until spray has dried. Cover or remove exposed foods before treatment. Before spraying, remove pets, cover aquaria and turn off air pump. Do not apply where electrical short circuits could occur.

Treatment Sites: When used in accordance with label directions, ANNIHILATOR™ WP can be applied to residential and non-residential buildings and structures for control of wood-infesting insects. Permitted areas of use include but are not limited to: crawl spaces, gaps between wooden members, junctions between wood and foundation, voids and channels in damaged wood, wall voids and wood surfaces.

Mixing Directions: To make a 0.03% water-based spray, mix 0.8 ounces (1 scoop) of ANNIHILATOR™ WP per gallon of spray mixture. To make a 0.06% water-based spray, mix 1.6 ounces (2 scoops) of ANNIHILATOR™ WP per gallon of spray mixture. When diluting, add water to the spray tank and the appropriate amount of ANNIHILATOR™ WP. Thoroughly agitate the sprayer before using to insure proper suspension of the wettable powder. Re-invert sprayer before use if spraying is interrupted. If spray screens are used, they should be 50 mesh or larger. Dilute ANNIHILATOR™ WP insecticide only with water.

Dosage Rates: Applications of 0.03% to 0.06% ANNIHILATOR™ WP can be made depending on pest species and method of application. Expect increased residual control of higher rates. See "Specific Use Directions for Control of Wood-Infesting Insects" for additional information.

Tank Mixing: Unless prohibited by a product's label, users at their own discretion can tank-mix pesticides such as insect growth regulators currently labeled for similar use patterns. It is always recommended that a small jar compatibility test using proper proportions of chemicals and water be run to check for physical compatibility prior to tank-mixing.

Application Methods: This product may be applied either as a coarse spray or by brushing onto targeted surfaces. Equipment capable of delivering a coarse, low pressure (about 20 psi) spray is recommended for treatment of large or overhead areas. Inaccessible areas such as wall voids can be treated by injecting the spray mixture under low pressure (about 20 psi) through drilled openings. Use sufficient amount of spray dilution to cover the area to the point of wetness but avoid applying to the point of runoff.

Drilling may be necessary prior to applying ANNIHILATOR™ WP to avoid cracks or joint spaces in vulnerable locations and to channeled section of wood but it must be recognized that such drilling and treating may not result in complete coverage of infested and vulnerable voids. All treatment holes drilled in construction elements in commonly occupied areas of structures must be securely plugged. Inspect at 6 months and 1 year to insure that the colony has been killed. Retreat if needed.

Overhead Areas: It is recommended that, when spraying overhead ares, care should be taken to avoid dripping or runoff from contacting applicator.

Wood-Infesting Insects Controlled by ANNIHILATOR™ WP: Beetles[1] (Anobiidae), (Bostrichidae), (Cerambycidae), (Lyctidae), Carpenter ants and other wood-infesting ants[2], Carpenter bees.

1. Beetles may be controlled by applying spray mixture to infested areas, or areas where infestations are likely to occur. This includes, but is not limited to, wood surfaces, voids and channels in damaged wood, spaces between wooden members of a structure and junctions between wood and foundations. Apply to wetness but avoid runoff.
2. Wood-infesting ants may be controlled by applying spray mixture around doors and windows, cracks or crevices, or other areas where ants may enter, crawl or hide.

Primary colonies are typically found outside through an exterior inspection. Correction of sanitation and structural deficiencies or landscape modifications may be necessary for effective control.

Precautionary Statements: Hazards to Humans and Domestic Animals:

Caution: Causes moderate eye irritation. Contact with product may cause transient tingling and reddening of the skin. Avoid contact with eyes, skin or clothing. Wash thoroughly with soap and water after handling.

First Aid:

If in Eyes: Flush eyes with plenty of water. Call a physician if irritation persists.

Handling Procedures: Wear protective clothing when using or handling this product to help avoid exposure to eyes and skin. As a minimum, eye protection and chemically resistant gloves, a long-sleeved shirt and long-legged pants or coveralls are recommended. To avoid breathing spray mist during application in confined areas, wear a mask or respirator of a type recommended by NIOSH for filtering spray mists.

Adults, children and pets should not contact treated surfaces until spray has dried. Do not treat pets with this product. Before spraying, remove pets, cover aquaria and turn off air pump. Do not apply where electrical short circuits could occur. Do not use indoors as a space spray or in fogging equipment. It is recommended that eye protection be worn when making applications overhead.

Environmental Hazards: This product is extremely toxic to fish and other aquatic organisms. Do not apply directly to water, to areas where surface water is present or to intertidal areas below the mean high water mark. Use with care when applying in areas adjacent to any body of water. Do not contaminate water when disposing of equipment wash waters. Remove pets and cover aquariums and terrariums before spraying.

Physical and Chemical Hazards: Do not use water based sprays of ANNIHILATOR™ WP in conduits, motor housings, junction boxes, or other electrical equipment because of the possible shock hazard.

Storage and Disposal: Do not contaminate water, food or feed by storage or disposal.

Storage: Mix as needed. Do not store diluted material. Store in original container in secured dry storage area. Prevent cross-contamination with other pesticides and fertilizers. If the container is leaking and/or material is spilled on floor or paved surfaces, sweep up and remove to chemical waste area.

Pesticide Disposal: Wastes resulting from use of this product may be disposed of on site or at an approved waste disposal facility.

Container Disposal: Empty container completely into application equipment. Do not reuse empty container. Triple rinse (or equivalent). Then offer for recycling or reconditioning, or puncture and dispose of in a sanitary landfill, or by incineration, or if allowed by state and local authorities, by burning. If burned, stay out of smoke.

Warning(s): Keep out of reach of children.

Disclaimer: Warranty and Limitation of Damages: Sellers warrants that this material conforms to its chemical description and is reasonably fit for the purpose stated on the label when used in accordance with directions under normal conditions of use and Buyer assumes the risk of any use contrary to such directions. Seller makes no other express or implied warranty, including any other express or implied warranty of Fitness or of Merchantability, and no agent of Seller is authorized to do so except in writing and with specific reference to this warranty. In no event shall Seller's liability for any breach of warranty exceed the purchase price of the material as to which a claim is made.

Discussion: General Information: ANNIHILATOR™ WP is a wettable powder insecticide containing 5.0% by weight active ingredient which will provide effective knockdown and long residual control up to 60 days of flies in and around non-residential buildings and structures and on various modes of transport.

ANNIHILATOR™ WP does not damage paints, plastics, fabrics or other surfaces where water alone causes no damage. To ensure against possible damage to delicate material, test a small inconspicuous area before treatment.

Presentation: 1 pound (453.59 grams).

Compendium Code No.: 10281251 BI 6265-1 4/01

ANTAGONIL™ ℞

Wildlife **Narcotic Antagonist**

(Yohimbine Hydrochloride) Sterile Injection

NADA No.: 140-874

Active Ingredient(s): ANTAGONIL™ is a sterile injection which contains yohimbine hydrochloride as the active ingredient. Each mL contains:

Yohimbine hydrochloride	5 mg
Methylparaben as a preservative	1 mg
Ethyl alcohol	0.30%
Water for injection	

The pH is adjusted with hydrochloride acid or sodium hydroxide.

Indications: For use as an antagonist to xylazine sedation in free-ranging or confined members of the family Cervidae (deer and elk).

Pharmacology: ANTAGONIL™ (yohimbine hydrochloride) is a synthetic indole alkaloid which is an alpha-2-antagonist producing rapid reversal of the effects of xylazine sedation.

Dosage and Administration: 0.2 to 0.3 mg/kg body weight administered intravenously. When using ANTAGONIL™ in wild or exotic species, one must be prepared and knowledgeable about proper procedures to handle problems resulting from having animals in lateral and sternal recumbency for extended periods of time. Users must also have necessary equipment, supplies and experienced personnel to handle such situations that may occur during or following immobilization and reversal procedures to minimize possible injury to the animal and personnel.

Reversal of the effects of xylazine sedation in members of the deer family is usually accomplished within 2 to 10 minutes after intravenous administration of ANTAGONIL™ at a dose rate of 0.2 to 0.3 mg/kg body weight. The antagonism of xylazine sedation was most consistent at this dose range. In field trials, occasional animals did require longer periods for reversal to be accomplished without regard to the dose of xylazine administered or the species.

Precaution(s): Protect from light. Store in a refrigerator (2° to 8°C [34° to 46°F]).

Caution(s): Federal law restricts this drug to use by or on the order of a licensed veterinarian.

Intrathoracic, intra-abdominal, subcutaneous or intramuscular injection is to be avoided.

Warning(s): Do not use in domestic food-producing animals. Do not use 30 days before or during hunting season.

Side Effects: Side effects observed in clinical studies with yohimbine hydrochloride are hypotension and transient excitement.

Presentation: ANTAGONIL™ is supplied in 20 mL multiple use vials.

Compendium Code No.: 10520000

A

ANTHELBAN V ℞

Phoenix Pharmaceutical **Parasiticide-Oral**

(pyrantel pamoate) Equine Anthelmintic Suspension

ANADA No.: 200-246

Active Ingredient(s): ANTHELBAN V is a suspension of pyrantel pamoate in a palatable vanilla-flavored vehicle. Each mL contains 50 mg of pyrantel base as pyrantel pamoate.

Indications: For the removal and control of mature infections of large strongyles *(Strongylus vulgaris, S. edentatus, S. equinus)*; pinworms *(Oxyuris equi)*; large roundworms *(Parascaris equorum)*; and small strongyles in horses and ponies.

Pharmacology: Pyrantel pamoate is a compound belonging to a family classified chemically as tetrahydro-pyrimidines. It is a yellow, water-insoluble crystalline salt of the tetrahydropyrimidine base and pamoic acid containing 34.7% base activity. The chemical structure and name are given below:

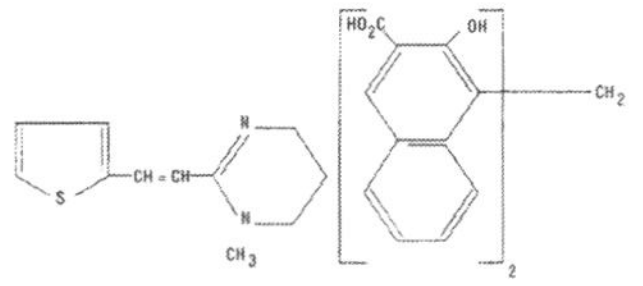

(E)-1,4,5,6-Tetrahydro-1-methyl-2-[2-(2-thienyl) vinyl] pyrimidine 4, 4' methylenebis [3-hydroxy-2-naphthoate] (1:1)

Dosage and Administration: Shake well before use. Administer 3 mg pyrantel base per pound of body weight [6 mL ANTHELBAN V (pyrantel pamoate)] per 100 lb body weight).

For maximum control of parasitism, it is recommended that foals (2-8 months of age) be dosed every 4 weeks. To minimize potential hazard that the mare may pose to the foal, she should be treated 1 month prior to anticipated foaling date followed by retreatment 10 days to 2 weeks after birth of foal. Horses over 8 months of age should be routinely dosed every 6 weeks.

Directions for Use: ANTHELBAN V (pyrantel pamoate) may be administered by means of a stomach tube, dose syringe or by mixing into the feed.

Stomach Tube - Measure the appropriate dosage of ANTHELBAN V and mix in the desired quantity of water. Protect drench from direct sunlight and administer to the animal immediately following mixing. Do not attempt to store diluted suspension. ANTHELBAN V is inactive against the common horse bot *(Gasterophilus* sp.). However, ANTHELBAN V may be administered concurrently with carbon disulfide observing the usual precautions with carbon disulfide.

Dose Syringe - Draw the appropriate dosage of ANTHELBAN V into a dose syringe and administer to the animal. Do not expose ANTHELBAN V to direct sunlight.

Feed - Mix the appropriate dosage of ANTHELBAN V in the normal grain ration. Fasting of animals prior to or following treatment is not required.

Precaution(s): Recommended Storage: Store below 86°F (30°C).

This product is a suspension and as such will separate. To insure uniform re-suspension and to achieve proper dosage, it is extremely important that the product be shaken and stirred thoroughly before every use.

Caution(s): Federal law restricts this drug to use by or on the order of a licensed veterinarian.

It is recommended that severely debilitated animals not be treated with this preparation.

Warning(s): Not for horses or ponies intended for food. Keep out of reach of children.

Trial Data: Efficacy: Critical (worm-count) studies in horses demonstrated that pyrantel pamoate administered at the recommended dosage was efficacious against mature infections of *Strongylus vulgaris* (>90%), *S. edentatus* (69%), *S. equinus* (>90%), *Oxyuris equi* (81%), *Parascaris equorum* (>90%), and small strongyles (>90%).

Safety: ANTHELBAN V (pyrantel pamoate) is well tolerated by horses and ponies of all ages. No adverse drug response was observed when dose rates up to 60 mg pyrantel base per pound of body weight were administered by stomach tube nor when 3 mg base per pound was given by intratracheal injection. The reproductive performance of pregnant mares and stud horses dosed with ANTHELBAN V has not been affected.

Presentation: 473 mL (1 pint) (NDC 57319-420-21) and 946 mL (1 quart) (NDC 57319-420-22).

Manufactured by: Phoenix Scientific, Inc., St. Joseph, MO 64503.

Compendium Code No.: 12560073 Rev. 2-01 / Rev. 7-01

ANTHELCIDE® EQ EQUINE WORMER PASTE

Pfizer Animal Health **Parasiticide-Oral**

(oxibendazole)

NADA No.: 121-042

Description: ANTHELCIDE® EQ Paste is a paste formulation of oxibendazole, a broad-spectrum benzimidazole anthelmintic. This formulation has been developed for ease of administration. Each syringe contains 0.85 oz (24 g) of paste.

ANTHELCIDE® EQ Paste contains:

Oxibendazole	22.7%

Indications: ANTHELCIDE® EQ Paste is indicated for removal and control of: large strongylids *(Strongylus edenatus, S. equinus, S. vulgaris)*; small strongylids (species of the genera *Cylicostephanus, Cylicocyclus, Cyathostomum, Triodontophorus, Cylicodontophorus,* and *Gyalocephalus)*; large roundworms *(Parascaris equorum)*; pinworms *(Oxyuris equi)* including various larval stages; and threadworms *(Strongyloides westeri)*.

Dosage and Administration: The dosage of oxibendazole is 10 mg/kg (2.2 lb) of body weight (15 mg/kg for strongyloides). Each mark on the syringe delivers ANTHELCIDE® EQ to treat 100 lb (67 lb for strongyloides). Horses maintained on premises where reinfection is likely to occur should be retreated in 6-8 weeks.

Dosage Table

10 mg/kg		15 mg/kg	
Syringe Mark	Horse Weight (lb)	Syringe Mark	Horse Weight (lb)
100	100	300	200
200	200	600	400
400	400	900	600
600	600	1200	800
800	800		
1000	1000		
1200	1200		

ANTHELCIDE® EQ is compatible with carbon disulfide, which can be used concurrently for bot control *(Gasterophilus* spp.) when administered by a veterinarian. Routine carbon disulfide cautions must be observed.

Use of syringe: Determine the weight of the horse and dial the correct setting on the plunger, having the side of the wheel nearest the barrel on the desired mark. Remove the cap from the syringe. Insert the tip of the syringe into the side of the animal's mouth between the incisor and molar teeth and press the plunger down as far as it will go, depositing the paste on the back of the tongue.

Contraindication(s): ANTHELCIDE® EQ is contraindicated in severely debilitated horses or horses suffering from infectious disease, toxemia, or colic.

Precaution(s): Store at controlled room temperature 15°-30°C (59°-86°F).

Caution(s): Consult your veterinarian for assistance in the diagnosis, treatment, and control of parasitism.

Warning(s): Not for use in horses intended for food. For use in horses only.

Keep out of reach of children.

Presentation: ANTHELCIDE® EQ Paste is supplied in 12 0.85-oz (24-g) syringes.

U.S. Patent Nos. 3,480,642 and 3,574,845

Compendium Code No.: 36901710

75-6045-09

ANTHELCIDE® EQ EQUINE WORMER SUSPENSION ℞

Pfizer Animal Health **Parasiticide-Oral**

(oxibendazole)

NADA No.: 109-722

Active Ingredient:

Oxibendazole 10%

Oxibendazole is a broad-spectrum benzimidazole anthelmintic.

Indications: ANTHELCIDE® EQ Suspension is indicated for removal and control of: large strongyles *(Strongylus edentatus, S. equinus, S. vulgaris);* small stronglyes (species of the genera *Cylicostephanus, Cylicocyclus, Cyathostomum, Triodontophorus, Cylicodontophorus,* and *Gyalocephalus);* large roundworms *(Parascaris equorum);* pinworms *(Oxyuris equi)* including various larval stages; and threadworms *(Strongyloides westeri).*

ANTHELCIDE® EQ is compatible with carbon disulfide, which can be used concurrently for bot control *(Gasterophilus* spp.). Routine carbon disulfide cautions must be observed.

Dosage and Administration: Shake well before using. The dosage of oxibendazole for the horse is 10 mg/kg of body weight (15 mg/kg for strongyloides). Each mL of suspension contains 100 mg of oxibendazole. Administer by stomach tube in 3-4 pints of warm water, or if preferred, by top dressing or mixing into a portion of the normal grain ration. Prepare individual doses to assure that each animal receives the correct amount. Horses maintained on premises where reinfection is likely to occur should be retreated in 6-8 weeks.

Dosage Table

Body Weight (lb)	Dosage of 10% Suspension*	
	10 mg/kg (mL)	15 mg/kg (mL)
220	10	15
440	20	30
660	30	45
880	40	60
1100	50	75
1320	60	90

*Contains 100 mg oxibendazole per mL of suspension.

Precaution(s): Store at controlled room temperature 15°-30°C (59°-86°F). Protect from freezing.

Caution: U.S. Federal law restricts this drug to use by or on the order of a licensed veterinarian.

For use in horses only.

Warning: Not for use in horses intended for food. Keep out of reach of children.

Presentation: 1 gal (3.785 L).

U.S. Patent Nos. 3,480,642 and 3,574,845

Compendium Code No.: 36901721

85-6056-09

ANTHRAX SPORE VACCINE

Colorado Serum **Vaccine**

Anthrax Spore Vaccine, Nonencapsulated Live Culture

U.S. Vet. Lic. No.: 188

Active Ingredient(s): Contains anthrax spore vaccine nonencapsulated live culture.

ANTHRAX SPORE VACCINE is prepared with a relatively nonpathogenic, uncapsulated variant strain of *B. anthracis,* originally developed at the Onderstepoort Laboratory, Pretoria, South Africa and used with excellent results throughout South Africa, England, India and in many other countries. The vaccine consists of viable spores suspended in diluent containing saponin. It is fully tested for purity, dissociation, spore count, safety and potency prior to release for sale.

Indications: For the vaccination of all healthy domestic farm animals, against anthrax.

Dosage and Administration: Inject 1 mL subcutaneously into each animal.

When to Vaccinate: In those areas where anthrax is an annual problem, it is advisable to vaccinate at about four (4) weeks prior to the time the disease usually appears. If an outbreak occurs, all animals not showing clinical symptoms should be vaccinated. Not all such animals may be fully protected but further spread of the disease may be stopped by promptly following this procedure.

The recommended dose for all domestic farm animals is 1 mL. In heavily contaminated regions a booster in injection two (2) to three (3) weeks after the first dose is administered is recommended.

The region of the neck just in front of the shoulder is a convenient site for administering the vaccine to cattle and sheep. Horses and mules may be vaccinated subcutaneously in the middle portion of the neck or in the brisket at a time when the animals are not being heavily worked. A light to moderate swelling may appear at the site of injection. This will disappear after several days.

Precaution(s): Store in the dark at 2-7°C. Shake well before using.

Sterilize needles and syringes by boiling in clean water.

Use the entire contents when first opened. Burn the container and all unused contents.

Caution(s): Anaphylactic reactions sometimes follow administration of products of this nature. If noted, administer adrenaline or an equivalent drug. For veterinary use only.

Accidental Human Exposure: ANTHRAX SPORE VACCINE is a live nonencapsulated variant of *Bacillus anthracis* that has been shown to be pure, safe and immunogenic. However, because humans are susceptible to anthrax the product should be carefully handled to avoid exposure. If the vaccine should be accidentally injected, ingested, or if exposure should occur otherwise through the conjunctiva or broken skin, consult a physician immediately.

Warning(s): Do not vaccinate within 60 days before slaughter. If emergency conditions require the vaccination of animals reaching market age and condition these should not be offered for slaughter in less than 60 days after administration of the vaccine.

Discussion: Anthrax occurs in all parts of the world. It is an acute, febrile infection that has a rapidly fatal course. It is one of the oldest and most destructive disease of livestock and has caused the loss of many human lives as well.

The specific case of anthrax is a micro-organism known as *Bacillus anthracis.* The organsims are highly virulent and once access to the animal body is gained, they multiply quickly, invade the blood stream and produce a rapidly fatal blood infection. In the presence of oxygen the bacilli form spores which are remarkably tenacious, highly resistant to heat, low temperatures and chemical disinfectants, retaining viability for many years in both soil and water and upon hides or contaminated objects held in storage. Animals of all species are susceptible to anthrax to some degree. Cattle, horses, sheep and goats are those most frequently affected. Swine apparently possess some natural resistance but anthrax does occasionally appear in hogs. Dogs, cats and wild animals may become infected under some conditions. Mice and guinea pigs are highly susceptible.

The symptoms of anthrax vary according to the species of animals and the acuteness of the attack. The average period of incubation under natural causes is indefinite ranging from 24 hours to as much as five days or more. The acute form, most common in cattle, sheep and goats is characterized by its sudden onset and rapidly fatal course. Affected animals present a picture of cerebral apoplexy - sudden staggering, difficult respiration, trembling, collapse with convulsive movements and death which may occur without evidence of illness. Swelling sometimes appear in different parts of the body, such as the throat and tongue, particularly in affected swine.

Presentation: 10 dose (10 mL) and 50 dose (50 mL) vials.

Compendium Code No.: 11010001

ANTI-BACTERIAL HAND SOAP

First Priority **Hand Soap**

Active Ingredient(s): Water, sodium lauryl sulfate, cocamide DEA, ethylene glycol monostearate, methylparaben, aloe vera, citric acid, sodium chloride, fragrance, FD&C color, PCMX and lanolin.

Indications: A soap for frequent hand washing. Helps eliminate animal odors from the skin. Moisturizer enriched formulation helps prevent skin from drying and cracking while cleaning. PCMX acts as an antibacterial agent.

Directions: Use as frequently as necessary.

Presentation: 16 fl oz (473 mL) and 1 gallon (3.785 L).

Compendium Code No.: 11390002

Rev. 5-99 / Rev. 5-98

ANTI-DIARRHEAL CATTLE BOLUS

AgriLabs **Antidiarrheal-Adsorbent**

Antidiarrheal-Demulcent

Active Ingredient(s): Each bolus contains: Activated attapulgite, carob flour, pectin, and magnesium trisilicate, in a palatable base.

Indications: For use as an aid in relief of simple non-infectious diarrhea in horses and cattle.

Dosage and Administration: Administer orally. Give two (2) boluses to adult cattle and horses. Give one (1) bolus to calves and foals.

Repeat treatment at 4 to 6 hour intervals as needed. Discontinue use of product after 3 days. If symptoms persist after using this preparation for 3 days, consult a veterinarian.

Precaution(s): Store at controlled room temperature between 15° and 30°C (59°-86°F).

Warning(s): For animal use only. Keep out of reach of children.

Presentation: 50 boluses.

Compendium Code No.: 10580100

ANTI-DIARRHEA TABLETS

ARC **Adsorbent**

Active Ingredient(s): Each tablet contains:

Kaolin .... 8 grains

Aluminum Hydroxide .... 2 grains

Pectin .... 1.5 grains

Desiccated Liver

Indications: A soothing and protective aid for simple diarrhea when antibiotics or anticholinergic drugs are not needed. Safe for long term use for dogs and cats with a sensitive digestive system.

Directions: Give 2 tablets for each 10 lbs. body weight, 3 times daily. Withhold food for at least 12-24 hours and then feed bland low-fat foods such as boiled rice and low-fat cottage cheese.

Caution(s): Available only from veterinarians.

Presentation: Contains 100 and 500 tablets.

Compendium Code No.: 10960000

ANTIDOTE® PHM

AgriPharm **Bacterin-Toxoid**

Pasteurella haemolytica-multocida Bacterin-Toxoid

U.S. Vet. Lic. No.: 315

Contents: This product contains a toxoid as well as cell associated antigens from multiple isolates of *Pasteurella haemolytica* Type A-1 and cell associated antigens from *Pasteurella multocida.*

Indications: For use in cattle 30 days of age or older, as an aid in the prevention of respiratory disease due to *P haemolytica* and *P multocida.*

Dosage and Administration: Shake well. Inject 2 mL I.M. or S.C. in the neck. Repeat in 14 to 28 days. Annual revaccination is recommended.

Precaution(s): Store at 45°F (7°C). Do not freeze. Use entire contents when first opened.

Caution(s): In case of anaphylactoid or hypersensitivity reactions, administer epinephrine and symptomatic treatments immediately. Hypersensitivity reactions, including delayed

hypersensitivity, or death may occur with a biological product and can cause reduced milk production in lactating dairy cattle. Following subcutaneous use, persistent swelling may occur at the injection site.
Warning(s): Do not vaccinate within 60 days of slaughter.
Presentation: 10 dose (20 mL) and 50 dose (100 mL) vials.
Compendium Code No.: 14571280

ANTIHISTAMINE GRANULES ℞

Butler **Antihistamine**

Active Ingredient(s): Each ounce contains:
Pyrilamine Maleate . . . . 600 mg
Pseudoephedrine Hydrochloride . . . . 600 mg
in a palatable base (sucrose).
Indications: For use when a histamine antagonizing preparation is required.
Dosage and Administration: 1/2 ounce (1 level tablespoonful) per 1,000 pounds body weight. Can be mixed with feed and repeated at 12 hour intervals if needed.
Precaution(s): Store at controlled room temperature 15°-30°C (59°-86°F).
Caution(s): Federal law restricts this drug to use by or on the order of a licensed veterinarian.
Keep out of reach of children. For animal use only.
Warning(s): Do not use at least 72 hours prior to sporting events.
Presentation: 20 ounce containers / 12 per case (NDC-11695-1234-6).
Manufactured by: Sparhawk Labs, Lenexa, KS 66215
Compendium Code No.: 10820090 Revised 07-98

ANTI-ITCH SPRAY

Vetus **Topical Corticosteroid**

1% Hydrocortisone-Anti-Inflammatory-Anti-Pruritic
Ingredient(s): Hydrocortisone USP (1% w/v), Alcohol, Glycerin, Allantoin, Hamamelis Distillate, Aloe Vera, Fragrance, FD&C Blue #1.
Indications: For the temporary relief of itching associated with minor skin irritations and rashes of dogs and cats.
Directions: Shake well before use, for adult dogs and cats apply ANTI-ITCH SPRAY 3-4 times daily, directly onto the affected area for temporary relief or as directed by a veterinarian. For puppies and kittens, follow directions of a veterinarian.
Precaution(s): Store at room temperature and out of sunlight.
Caution(s): If condition worsens, or if symptoms persist for more than 7 days or clear up and occur again within a few days, discontinue use of this product and consult a veterinarian.
For external use only.
Warning(s): Keep out of the reach of children.
Presentation: 2 fl oz (60 mL) and 4 fl oz (120 mL) containers.
Distributed by: Burns Veterinary Supply, Inc., Westbury, NY 11590.
Compendium Code No.: 14440940

ANTIROBE® ℞

Pharmacia & Upjohn **Clindamycin**

brand of clindamycin hydrochloride capsules, USP and liquid
NADA No.: 120-161 (capsules) / 135-940 (liquid)
Active Ingredient(s):
ANTIROBE® Capsules (For Use in Dogs Only):
25 mg Capsule, each yellow and white capsule contains clindamycin hydrochloride equivalent to 25 mg of clindamycin.
75 mg Capsule, each green capsule contains clindamycin hydrochloride equivalent to 75 mg of clindamycin.
150 mg Capsule, each light blue and green capsule contains clindamycin hydrochloride equivalent to 150 mg of clindamycin.
300 mg Capsule, each light blue capsule contains clindamycin hydrochloride equivalent to 300 mg of clindamycin.
ANTIROBE AQUADROPS® Liquid (For Use in Dogs and Cats) is a palatable formulation intended for oral administration. Each mL of ANTIROBE AQUADROPS® contains clindamycin hydrochloride equivalent to 25 mg clindamycin; and ethyl alcohol, 8.64%.
Indications: ANTIROBE® (brand of clindamycin hydrochloride) Capsules (for use in dogs only) and AQUADROPS® Liquid (for use in dogs and cats) are indicated for the treatment of infections caused by susceptible strains of the designated microorganisms in the specific conditions listed below:
Dogs: Skin infections (wounds and abscesses) due to coagulase positive staphylococci (*Staphylococcus aureus* or *Staphylococcus intermedius*). Deep wounds and abscesses due to *Bacteroides fragilis, Prevotella melaninogenicus, Fusobacterium necrophorum* and *Clostridium perfringens.* Dental infections due to *Staphylococcus aureus, Bacteroides fragilis, Prevotella melaninogenicus, Fusobacterium necrophorum* and *Clostridium perfringens.* Osteomyelitis due to *Staphylococcus aureus, Bacteroides fragilis, Prevotella melaninogenicus, Fusobacterium necrophorum* and *Clostridium perfringens.*
Cats: Skin infections (wounds and abscesses) due to *Staphylococcus aureus, Staphylococcus intermedius* and *Streptococcus* spp. Deep wounds and infections due to *Clostridium perfringens* and *Bacteroides fragilis.* Dental infections due to *Staphylococcus aureus, Staphylococcus intermedius, Streptococcus* spp., *Clostridium perfringens* and *Bacteroides fragilis.*
Pharmacology: ANTIROBE® Capsules and ANTIROBE AQUADROPS® Liquid contain clindamycin hydrochloride which is the hydrated salt of clindamycin. Clindamycin is a semisynthetic antibiotic produced by a 7(S)-chlorosubstitution of the 7(R)-hydroxyl group of a naturally produced antibiotic produced by *Streptomyces lincolnensis var. lincolnensis.*
Actions:
Site and Mode of Action: Clindamycin is an inhibitor of protein synthesis in the bacterial cell. The site of binding appears to be in the 50S sub-unit of the ribosome. Binding occurs to the soluble RNA fraction of certain ribosomes, thereby inhibiting the binding of amino acids to those ribosomes. Clindamycin differs from cell wall inhibitors in that it causes irreversible modification of the protein-synthesizing subcellular elements at the ribosomal level.
Microbiology: Clindamycin is a lincosaminide antimicrobial agent with activity against a wide variety of aerobic and anaerobic bacterial pathogens. Clindamycin is a bacteriostatic compound that inhibits bacterial protein synthesis by binding to the 50S ribosomal subunit. The minimum inhibitory concentrations (MICs) of Gram-positive and obligate anaerobic pathogens isolated from dogs and cats in the United States are presented in Table 1 and Table 2. Bacteria were isolated in 1998-1999. All MICs were performed in accordance with the National Committee for Clinical Laboratory Standards (NCCLS).

Table 1. Clindamycin MIC Values (μg/mL) from Diagnostic Laboratory Survey Data Evaluating Canine Pathogens in the U.S. During 1998-99[1]

Organism	Number of Isolates	MIC_{50}	MIC_{85}	MIC_{90}	Range
Soft Tissue/Wound[2]					
Staphylococcus aureus	17	0.5	0.5	≥4.0	0.25-≥4.0
Staphylococcus intermedius	28	0.25	0.5	≥4.0	0.125-≥4.0
Staphylococcus spp.	18	0.5	0.5	≥4.0	0.25-≥4.0
Beta-hemolytic streptococci	46	0.5	0.5	≥4.0	0.25-≥4.0
Streptococcus spp.	11	0.5	≥4.0	≥4.0	0.25-≥4.0
Osteomyelitis/Bone[3]					
Staphylococcus aureus	20	0.5	0.5	0.5	0.5[4]
Staphylococcus intermedius	15	0.5	≥4.0	≥4.0	0.25-≥4.0
Staphylococcus spp.	18	0.5	≥4.0	≥4.0	0.25-≥4.0
Beta-hemolytic streptococci	21	0.5	2.0	2.0	0.25-≥4.0
Streptococcus spp.	21	≥4.0	≥4.0	≥4.0	0.25-≥4.0
Dermal/Skin[5]					
Staphylococcus aureus	25	0.5	≥4.0	≥4.0	0.25-≥4.0
Staphylococcus intermedius	48	0.5	≥4.0	≥4.0	0.125-≥4.0
Staphylococcus spp.	32	0.5	≥4.0	≥4.0	0.25-≥4.0
Beta-hemolytic streptococci	17	0.5	0.5	0.5	0.25-0.5

[1] The correlation between the *in vitro* susceptibility data and clinical response has not been determined.
[2] Soft Tissue/Wound: includes samples labeled wound, abscess, aspirate, exudates, draining tract, lesion, and mass
[3] Osteomyelitis/Bone: includes samples labeled bone, fracture, joint, tendon
[4] No range, all isolates yielded the same value
[5] Dermal/Skin: includes samples labeled skin, skin swab, biopsy, incision, lip

Table 2. Clindamycin MIC Values (μg/mL) from Diagnostic Laboratory Survey Data Evaluating Feline Pathogens from Wound and Abscess Samples in the U.S. During 1998[1]

Organism	Number of Isolates	MIC_{50}	MIC_{90}	Range
Bacteroides/Prevotella	30	0.06	4.0	≤0.015-4.0
Fusobacterium spp.	17	0.25	0.25	≤0.015-0.5
Peptostreptococcus spp.	18	0.13	0.5	≤0.015-8.0
Porphyromonas spp.	13	0.06	0.25	≤0.015-8.0

[1] The correlation between the *in vitro* susceptibility data and clinical response has not been determined.

Absorption: Clindamycin hydrochloride is rapidly absorbed from the canine and feline gastrointestinal tract.
Dog Serum Levels: Serum levels at or above 0.5 μg/mL can be maintained by oral dosing at a rate of 2.5 mg/lb of clindamycin hydrochloride every 12 hours. This same study revealed that average peak serum concentrations of clindamycin occur 1 hour and 15 minutes after oral dosing. The elimination half-life for clindamycin in dog serum was approximately 5 hours. There was no bioactivity accumulation after a regimen of multiple oral doses in healthy dogs.
Clindamycin Serum Concentrations 2.5 mg/lb (5.5 mg/kg) After B.I.D. Oral Dose of ANTIROBE® Capsules to Dogs

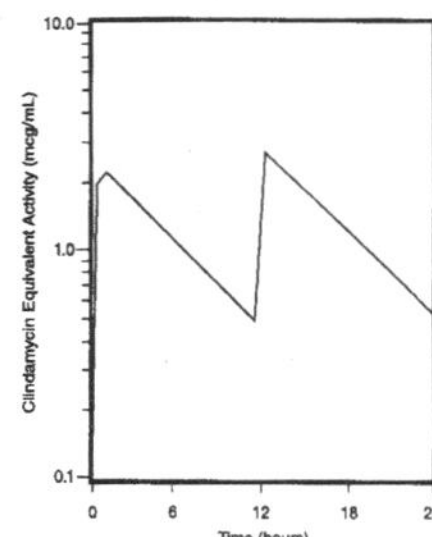

Cat Serum Levels: Serum levels at or above 0.5 μg/mL can be maintained by oral dosing at a rate of 2.5 mg/lb of clindamycin hydrochloride every 24 hours. The average peak serum concentration of clindamycin occurs approximately 1 hour after oral dosing. The elimination half-life of clindamycin in feline serum is approximately 7.5 hours. In healthy cats, minimal accumulation occurs after multiple oral doses of clindamycin hydrochloride, and steady-state should be achieved by the third dose.
Clindamycin Serum Concentrations 5 mg/lb (11 mg/kg) After Single Oral Dose of ANTIROBE AQUADROPS® to Cats

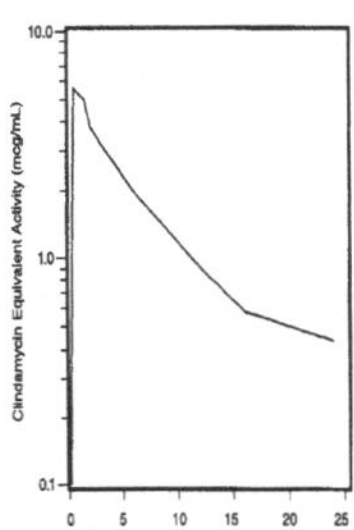

Metabolism and Excretion: Extensive studies of the metabolism and excretion of clindamycin hydrochloride administered orally in animals and humans have shown that unchanged drug and bioactive and bioinactive metabolites are excreted in urine and feces. Almost all of the bioactivity detected in serum after ANTIROBE® product administration is due to the parent molecule (clindamycin). Urine bioactivity, however, reflects a mixture of clindamycin and active metabolites, especially N-dimethyl clindamycin and clindamycin sulfoxide.

Dosage and Administration:

Dogs: Infected Wounds, Abscesses and Dental Infections:

Oral: 2.5-15.0 mg/lb body weight every 12 hours.

Duration: Treatment with ANTIROBE® products may be continued up to a maximum of 28 days if clinical judgment indicates. Treatment of acute infections should not be continued for more than three or four days if no response to therapy is seen.

Dosage Schedule:

Capsules:

ANTIROBE® 25 mg, administer 1-6 capsules every 12 hours for each 10 pounds of body weight.

ANTIROBE® 75 mg, administer 1-6 capsules every 12 hours for each 30 pounds of body weight.

ANTIROBE® 150 mg, administer 1-6 capsules every 12 hours for each 60 pounds of body weight.

ANTIROBE® 300 mg, administer 1-6 capsules every 12 hours for each 120 pounds of body weight.

Liquid:

ANTIROBE AQUADROPS®, administer 1-6 mL/10 lbs body weight every 12 hours.

Dogs: Osteomyelitis:

Oral: 5.0-15.0 mg/lb body weight every 12 hours.

Duration: Treatment with ANTIROBE® is recommended for a minimum of 28 days. Treatment should not be continued for longer than 28 days if no response to therapy is seen.

Dosage Schedule:

Capsules:

ANTIROBE® 25 mg, administer 2-6 capsules every 12 hours for each 10 pounds of body weight.

ANTIROBE® 75 mg, administer 2-6 capsules every 12 hours for each 30 pounds of body weight.

ANTIROBE® 150 mg, administer 2-6 capsules every 12 hours for each 60 pounds of body weight.

ANTIROBE® 300 mg, administer 2-6 capsules every 12 hours for each 120 pounds of body weight.

Liquid:

ANTIROBE AQUADROPS®, administer 2-6 mL/10 lbs body weight every 12 hours.

Cats: Infected Wounds and Abscesses, and Dental Infections:

5.0-15.0 mg/lb body weight once every 24 hours depending on the severity of the condition.

Duration: Treatment with ANTIROBE AQUADROPS® Liquid may be continued up to a maximum of 14 days if clinical judgment indicates. Treatment of acute infections should not be continued for more than three to four days if no clinical response to therapy is seen.

Dosage Schedule:

ANTIROBE AQUADROPS®, to provide 5.0 mg/lb, administer 1 mL/5 lbs body weight once every 24 hours; to provide 15.0 mg/lb, administer 3 mL/5 lbs body weight once every 24 hours.

Contraindication(s): ANTIROBE® Capsules and ANTIROBE AQUADROPS® Liquid are contraindicated in animals with a history of hypersensitivity to preparations containing clindamycin or lincomycin.

Because of potential adverse gastrointestinal effects, do not administer to rabbits, hamsters, guinea pigs, horses, chinchillas or ruminating animals.

Precaution(s): Store at controlled room temperature 20° to 25°C (68° to 77°F) [see USP].

Caution(s): Federal (USA) law restricts this drug to use by or on the order of a licensed veterinarian.

During prolonged therapy of one month or greater, periodic liver and kidney function tests and blood counts should be performed.

The use of ANTIROBE® occasionally results in overgrowth of non-susceptible organisms such as clostridia and yeasts. Therefore, the administration of ANTIROBE® should be avoided in those species sensitive to the gastrointestinal effects of clindamycin (see Contraindications). Should superinfections occur, appropriate measures should be taken as indicated by the clinical situation.

Patients with very severe renal disease and/or very severe hepatic disease accompanied by severe metabolic aberrations should be dosed with caution, and serum clindamycin levels monitored during high-dose therapy.

Clindamycin hydrochloride has been shown to have neuromuscular blocking properties that may enhance the action of other neuromuscular blocking agents. Therefore, ANTIROBE® should be used with caution in animals receiving such agents.

Safety in gestating bitches and queens or breeding male dogs and cats has not been established.

Warning(s): Keep out of reach of children. Not for human use.

Toxicology: Toxicology and Safety:

Rat and Dog Data: One year oral toxicity studies in rats and dogs at doses of 30, 100 and 300 mg/kg/day (13.6, 45.5 and 136.4 mg/lb/day) have shown clindamycin hydrochloride to be well tolerated. Differences did not occur in the parameters evaluated to assess toxicity when comparing groups of treated animals with contemporary controls. Rats administered clindamycin hydrochloride at 600 mg/kg/day (272.7 mg/lb/day) for six months tolerated the drug well; however, dogs orally dosed at 600 mg/kg/day (272.7 mg/lb/day) vomited, had anorexia, and subsequently lost weight. At necropsy these dogs had erosive gastritis and focal areas of necrosis of the mucosa of the gall bladder.

Safety in gestating bitches or breeding males has not been established.

Cat Data: The recommended daily therapeutic dose range for clindamycin hydrochloride (ANTIROBE AQUADROPS® Liquid) is 11 to 33 mg/kg/day (5 to 15 mg/lb/day) depending on the severity of the condition. Clindamycin hydrochloride (ANTIROBE AQUADROPS® Liquid) was tolerated with little evidence of toxicity in domestic shorthair cats when administered orally at 10x the minimum recommended therapeutic daily dose (11 mg/kg; 5 mg/lb) for 15 days, and at doses up to 5x the minimum recommended therapeutic dose for 42 days. Gastrointestinal tract upset (soft feces to diarrhea) occurred in control and treated cats with emesis occurring at doses 3x or greater than the minimum recommended therapeutic dose (11 mg/kg/day; 5 mg/lb/day). Lymphocytic inflammation of the gallbladder was noted in a greater number of treated cats at the 110 mg/kg/day (50 mg/lb/day) dose level than for control cats. No other effects were noted. Safety in gestating queens or breeding male cats has not been established.

Adverse Reactions: Side effects occasionally observed in either clinical trials or during clinical use were vomiting and diarrhea.

To report adverse reactions or a suspected adverse reaction, or to request a material safety data sheet (MSDS), call 1-800-793-0596.

Presentation: ANTIROBE® Capsules are available as:

25 mg - bottles of 600 (NDC 0009-3043-01)
75 mg - bottles of 200 (NDC 0009-3044-01)
150 mg - bottles of 100 (NDC 0009-3045-01)
150 mg - blister packages of 100 (NDC 0009-3045-08)
300 mg - blister packages of 100 (NDC 0009-5015-01)

ANTIROBE AQUADROPS® Liquid is available as 20 mL filled in 30 mL bottles (25 mg/mL) supplied in packers containing 12 cartoned bottles with direction labels and calibrated dosing droppers (NDC 0009-3179-01).

ANTIROBE® Capsules - Made by Patheon YM Inc., Toronto, Ontario, M3B 1Y5, Canada

Compendium Code No.: 10490052 813 805 711E

ANTISEDAN® ℞

Pfizer Animal Health **Medetomidine Reversing Agent**

(atipamezole hydrochloride) Sterile Injectable Solution–5.0 mg/mL

NADA No.: 141-033

Active Ingredient(s): Each mL of ANTISEDAN® contains 5.0 mg atipamezole hydrochloride, 1.0 mg methylparaben (NF), 8.5 mg sodium chloride (USP), and water for injection (USP).

Indications: ANTISEDAN® is indicated for the reversal of the clinical effects of the sedative and analgesic agent, Domitor® (medetomidine hydrochloride), in dogs.

Pharmacology: ANTISEDAN® (atipamezole hydrochloride) is a synthetic alpha$_2$-adrenergic antagonist which reverses the effects of Domitor® (medetomidine hydrochloride) in dogs. The chemical name is 4-(2-ethyl-2,3-dihydro-1H-inden-2-yl)-1H-imidazole hydrochloride. The molecular formula is $C_{14}H_{16}N_2$•HCl and the structural formula is:

Clinical Pharmacology: Activation of peripheral and central alpha$_2$-adrenergic receptors is known to induce a pattern of pharmacological responses including sedation, reduction of anxiety, analgesia, bradycardia, and transient hypertension with a subsequently reduced blood pressure. Atipamezole is a potent alpha$_2$-antagonist which selectively and competitively inhibits alpha$_2$-adrenergic receptors. The result of atipamezole administration in the dog is the rapid recovery from the sedation and other clinical effects produced by the alpha$_2$-adrenergic agonist, medetomidine. Atipamezole is not expected to reverse the effects of other classes of sedatives, anesthetics, or analgesics.

Rapid absorption occurs following intramuscular injection, with a maximum serum concentration reached in approximately 10 minutes. Onset of arousal is usually apparent within 5 to 10 minutes of injection, depending on the depth and duration of medetomidine-induced sedation. Elimination half-life from serum is less than 3 hours. Atipamezole undergoes extensive hepatic biotransformation, with excretion of metabolites primarily in urine.

A transient, approximately 10% decrease in systolic blood pressure occurs immediately after administration of atipamezole to medetomidine-sedated dogs, followed by an increase in pressure within 10 minutes to the pre-atipamezole level. This is the opposite of the response to alpha$_2$-agonist therapy, and is probably due to peripheral vasodilation.

Atipamezole will produce a rapid improvement in medetomidine-induced bradycardia. An increase in heart rate is usually apparent within approximately 3 minutes of injection, but approximately 40% of dogs are not expected to immediately return to presedative rate. Some dogs may experience brief heart rate elevations above baseline. Respiratory rate also increases following atipamezole injection.

Dosage and Administration: ANTISEDAN® is administered intramuscularly regardless of the route used for Domitor®. The concentration of ANTISEDAN® has been formulated such that the volume of injection is the same (mL for mL) as the recommended dose volume of Domitor®, and may be given at any time following Domitor® administration. Although injection volumes are the same, the concentration of ANTISEDAN® (5.0 mg/mL) is 5 times that of Domitor® (1.0 mg/mL). Dogs that are sedated but ambulatory may be treated with ANTISEDAN®, if warranted.

The dosage of ANTISEDAN® is calculated based upon body surface area. Use the table below to determine the proper injection volume based on bodyweight:

ANTISEDAN® Injection Volume (mL) IM	Body Wt (lb) If Domitor® Given IM*	Body Wt (lb) If Domitor® Given IV*
0.1		3-4
0.15	4-5	5-7
0.2	6-7	8-11
0.25	8-9	12-15
0.3	10-14	16-21
0.4	15-20	22-31
0.5	21-27	32-43
0.6	28-35	44-55
0.7	36-44	56-68
0.8	45-53	69-82
0.9	54-63	83-97
1.0	64-78	98-121
1.2	79-101	122-156
1.4	102-126	157-194
1.6	127-165	195+
2.0	166+	

*The IM dose of Domitor® is 1.0 mg/m^2 of body surface area and the IV dose is 0.75 mg/m^2.

Precaution(s): Storage: Store protected from light at controlled room temperature 15°-30°C (59°-86°F).

Caution(s): Federal law restricts this drug to use by or on the order of a licensed veterinarian.

ANTISEDAN® can produce an abrupt reversal of sedation and, presumably, analgesia. The potential for apprehensive or aggressive behavior should be considered in the handling of dogs emerging from sedation, especially those individuals predisposed to nervousness or fright.

Persons handling dogs that have recently received ANTISEDAN® should use caution and also avoid situations where a dog could fall.

Information on use of atipamezole with concurrent drugs is inadequate; therefore, caution should be exercised when administering multiple drugs. Animals should be monitored closely, particularly for persistent hypothermia, bradycardia, and depressed respiration, until the animal has recovered completely. Caution should be used in administration of anesthetic agents to elderly or debilitated animals.

While atipamezole does reverse the clinical signs associated with medetomidine sedation, complete physiologic return to pretreatment status may not be immediate and should be monitored.

ANTISEDAN® has not been evaluated in breeding animals; therefore, the drug is not recommended for use in pregnant or lactating animals, or in animals intended for breeding.

Warning(s): For intramuscular use in dogs only.

Keep out of reach of children. Not for human use.

Atipamezole hydrochloride can be absorbed and may cause irritation following direct exposure to skin, eyes, or mouth. In case of accidental eye exposure, flush with water for 15 minutes. In case of accidental skin exposure, wash with soap and water. Remove contaminated clothing. If irritation or other adverse reaction occurs (e.g., increased heart rate, tremor, muscle cramps), seek medical attention. In case of accidental oral exposure or injection, seek medical attention. Precaution should be used while handling and using filled syringes.

Users with cardiovascular disease (e.g., hypertension or ischemic heart disease) should take special precautions to avoid any exposure to this product.

The material safety data sheet (MSDS) contains more detailed occupational safety information.

To report adverse reactions in users or to obtain a copy of the MSDS for this product call 1-800-366-5288.

Note to Physician: This product contains an alpha-2-adrenergic antagonist.

Side Effects: Occasional vomiting may occur. Rarely, a brief state of excitement or apprehensiveness may be seen in treated dogs. Other potential side effects of $alpha_2$-antagonists include hypersalivation, diarrhea, and tremors.

Trial Data: Animal Safety: Atipamezole was tolerated in healthy dogs receiving doses 10-fold the recommended dose and in dogs receiving repeated doses at 1-, 3-, and 5-fold doses, in the absence of medetomidine. Signs of overdose were dose-related and consistent with those expected in nonsedated dogs having received a stimulant. Signs seen at elevated doses included excitement, panting, trembling, vomiting, soft or liquid feces or vasodilation (injection) of the sclera. Some localized skeletal muscle injury was seen at the injection site; but no associated clinical signs or complications were observed. Dogs receiving the proper dose in the absence of medetomidine, or 3-fold overdose after medetomidine sedation, exhibited no significant clinical signs.

Presentation: ANTISEDAN® is supplied in 10-mL, multidose vials containing 5.0 mg of atipamezole hydrochloride per mL.

U.S. Patent No. 4,689,399

ANTISEDAN® and Domitor® are trademarks of Orion Corporation.

Developed and manufactured by: Orion Corporation, Orion-Farmos, Espoo, Finland

Compendium Code No.: 36901730 75-6298-00

ANTISEPTIC IODINE SPRAY

Dominion **Topical Wound Dressing**

Active Ingredient(s): Contents:

Povidone Iodine (equivalent to Titratable Iodine 1%) 10%
Isopropanol 99% 65.0%
Inert ingredients . . . . . qs

Description: ANTISEPTIC IODINE SPRAY contains an iodine complex which provides the active iodine in a non-staining, non-stinging form upon topical application. The alcohol base aids in producing a quick drying product, which does not delay wound healing.

Indications: As an aid in the treatment and control of bacterial infections of superficial wounds, cuts and abrasions, navel stumps, dockings, and castration wounds. Also for disinfection of skin areas prior to injections or surgical procedures.

Directions: Remove cap from the pump top. Holding the bottle upright and 15 cm from the skin, spray a thin film over the affected area by depressing the pump.

Precaution(s): Contents are flammable. Do not store near heat or flame. Keep tightly closed.

Caution(s): If redness, irritation, or swelling persists or increases, discontinue use and consult a veterinarian.

Do not use on deep or puncture wounds or on serious burns. Avoid contact with eyes or mucous membranes. Keep out of reach of children.

Presentation: 500 mL bottle; 12 bottles/carton.

Compendium Code No.: 15080000

ANTITOX TET™

Novartis Animal Vaccines **Antitoxin**

Tetanus Antitoxin, Equine Origin

U.S. Vet. Lic. No.: 303

Composition: This product is prepared from the blood of horses hyperimmunized with *Clostridium tetani* toxoid. Contains gentamicin and thimerosal as preservatives.

Indications: For use in cattle, horses, sheep, and swine as an aid in the prevention and treatment of tetanus caused by *Clostridium tetani*.

Dosage and Administration: Shake well before using. Administer the following doses intramuscularly or subcutaneously:

	Prevention	Treatment
Cattle and horses	1500 units	10,000-25,000 units
Sheep and swine	500 units	5,000-12,500 units

The maximum volume recommended per injection site is 25 mL for cattle or horses and 10 mL for sheep or swine.

Precaution(s): Store in the dark at 35°-45°F (2°-7°C). Do not freeze. Use entire contents when first opened.

Caution(s): Horses - the preventative dose may cause injection site reactions. All species - The treatment dose may cause severe injection site reactions and/or systemic reactions. Symptomatic treatment: epinephrine.

Warning(s): Do not administer within 21 days prior to slaughter.

Discussion: Technical Disease Information: Tetanus is a sporadic disease that affects a wide variety of domestic animals as well as man. The causative agent, *Clostridium tetani* is an obligate anaerobe. It only grows where there is no oxygen present. The bacteria are present in manure and soil as spores, which are highly resistant to destruction. When these spores are carried into a wound such as a puncture (e.g. castration or docking wound), tissue damage can produce an area devoid of oxygen, which allows the spores to begin growing. These growing bacteria produce a potent neurotoxin which travels along nerve tissue to the central nervous system (CNS), which results in the visible symptoms of tetanus. If large amounts of toxin are produced at the wound site, this toxin can also diffuse in the blood lymph system and be carried to the CNS in this manner. There is also some evidence that preformed toxin can be absorbed through wounds in the mouth when eating toxin-contaminated feeds.

Tetanus usually affects animals less than six months of age because this is the time when procedures such as tail docking and castration are normally performed. Symptoms usually appear after a 4-10 day incubation period. The first symptoms noticed are erect ears, a stiff tail, and prolapsed third eyelids. These progress to generalized muscle spasms and a tightly clenched jaw (hence the name "lockjaw"). All four limbs will be rigid and extended, causing the animal to assume a "sawhorse" stance. The animal is overly sensitive to touch and sound, either of which can precipitate severe spasms. Death is caused by respiratory failure and usually occurs within 3-10 days after symptoms appear. The mortality rate approaches 100% of affected animals.

In the early stages of the disease, tetanus may be confused with strychnine poisoning, hypomagnesemia, or acute laminitis. Prevention includes removal of any sharp objects that may cause puncture wounds. Use clean techniques when performing surgeries such as castration and tail docking. In addition, ANTITOX TET™ should be routinely administered at the prevention dosage anytime animals receive any surgery (such as tail docking and castration) that may allow the growth of tetanus organisms. Attempted treatment of tetanus in an affected animal is usually futile, which is why prevention is so important. In some cases, a large dose of ANTITOX TET™ in conjunction with aggressive therapeutic treatment has been beneficial.

References: Available upon request.

Presentation: 1,500 and 10,000 units.

Compendium Code No.: 11140002

ANTI-TUSSIVE SYRUP WITH ANTIHISTAMINE

Vedco **Antitussive**

Active Ingredient(s): Each fluid ounce contains:

Guaifenesin . . . . . 8 grs.
Ammonium chloride . . . . . 8 grs.
Sodium citrate . . . . . 8 grs.
Pyrilamine maleate . . . . . 50 mg
Phenylephrine hydrochloride . . . . . 50 mg

In a flavored syrup base.

Indications: A decongestant, expectorant and antihistamine for the relief of cough symptoms related to upper respiratory conditions.

Dosage and Administration: Administer orally: Horses: Two (2) to four (4) ounces.

Sheep, Swine and Young Animals: One (1) to two (2) ounces.

Dogs and Cats: One (1) to two (2) teaspoonfuls, depending upon size. Repeat every two (2) hours if necessary.

Caution(s): For veterinary use only. Not for human use. Keep out of the reach of children.

Presentation: 1 gallon containers.

Compendium Code No.: 10940040

ANTIVENIN

Fort Dodge **Antivenin**

(Crotalidae) Polyvalent (North and South American Snakebite Antiserum)

U.S. Vet. Lic. No.: 112

Composition: ANTIVENIN is a refined and concentrated preparation of equine serum globulins obtained by fractionating blood from healthy horses that have been immunized with the following venoms: Eastern diamondback *(C. adamanteus)*, Western diamondback *(C. atrox)*, Central and South American rattlesnake *(C. terrificus)*, and fer-de-lance *(B. atrox)*. 0.25% phenol and 0.005% thimerosal (mercury derivative) are added as preservatives.

Indications: For use in dogs which have received bites from viperine snakes, such as rattlesnakes, copperheads and cottonmouth water moccasins.

Dosage and Administration: The dose varies from 10 to 50 mL (1 to 5 vials), intravenously, of rehydrated ANTIVENIN, depending on the severity of symptoms, lapse of time after the bite, size of snake and size of patient (the smaller the body of the victim, the larger the dose required). Additional doses should be given every 2 hours as required, if symptoms such as swelling and pain persist or recur.

In emergency, when exposure is such that intravenous administration of ANTIVENIN is not practical, the product may be administered intramuscularly as close to the site of exposure as practical.

General supportive therapy should be instituted whenever required. Corticosteroids should be given to suppress systemic reactions or delayed serum sickness. They also exert a beneficial effect on shock that invariably accompanies a snake bite. There is no evidence to indicate that corticosteroids will neutralize venom or inhibit the accompanying necrosis. However, they may minimize tissue destruction. Antibiotics, fluid therapy, blood transfusions and tetanus prophylaxis may be indicated.

Contraindication(s): The use of excessive heat or cold is contraindicated. Antihistamines and tranquilizers are also contraindicated, and may potentiate the effect of snake venom.

Precaution(s): Storage temperature not to exceed 98°F (37°C). Avoid freezing and excessive heat. Use immediately after rehydration.

This package is not returnable for credit or exchange.

Caution(s): Attempts should be made to immobilize the patient until treatment is initiated. Sedatives and analgesics should also be employed with discretion, because large doses may mask important clinical signs.

In case of anaphylactoid reaction, administer epinephrine. Restricted to use by or on the order of a licensed veterinarian.

Discussion: ANTIVENIN neutralizes the venom of the viperine snakes, including all North American species of rattlesnakes, copperheads and cottonmouth moccasins. It contains a protective substance against the venoms of the related species in Central and South America, including the bushmaster and the fer-de-lance, and the habu and Mamushi of the Pacific Islands and Asiatic mainland.

ANTIVENIN is standardized by its ability to neutralize in mice the toxic action of a standard venom injected intravenously.

General Information: ANTIVENIN is specific against the viperine class of snakes, whose venom is hemotoxic. The elapine are the second class of poisonous snakes and include the coral snake, the cobra and the mamba. Their venom is mainly neurotoxic. Both classes of poisonous snakes contain some neurotoxic and hemotoxic factors. However, horses from which ANTIVENIN is derived have not been immunized against elapine venom.

The death incidence, worldwide, from snake bite is greater in dogs than in any other domestic animal. They most frequently are bitten in the head region; occasionally on the shoulders, thighs or legs. Fatalities in horses and cattle are less common. However, they do occur, particularly when bitten about the head or neck.

Symptoms from viperine envenomation are swelling, pain, muscular weakness, impaired vision, cyanosis, hemolytic anemia, bleeding tendencies, dyspnea, shock and subsequently tissue necrosis.

Some clinical evaluators of ANTIVENIN reported the diamondback as the most lethal snake to dogs, and the ground or pygmy rattler the least dangerous. Sloughing or tissue necrosis was most frequently associated with, but not limited to, the water moccasin.

Trial Data: Sixteen practicing veterinarians had uniformly successful results with ANTIVENIN in patients having mild symptoms at time of treatment. Of 103 dogs treated with acute symptoms, 72% survived following a single 10 mL dose; there was a higher percentage (83%) of recovery when 20 to 70 mL was given. Overall, 82% of ANTIVENIN-treated animals survived; the majority not receiving ANTIVENIN succumbed. The success of ANTIVENIN appears to be directly related to the time interval before treatment. Only 45% of dogs survived if there was at least a four-hour lag period between time of bite and ANTIVENIN treatment. The survival rate doubled if less than four hours elapsed before ANTIVENIN was administered.

Presentation: 1 dose (10 mL) vials.

Compendium Code No.: 10030081 2100F

ANTIZOL-VET® ℞

Orphan Medical **Antidote for Ethylene Glycol Poisoning**

(Fomepizole) for injection

NADA No.: 141-075

Active Ingredient(s): One single use vial (1.5 mL) of ANTIZOL-VET® sterile solution contains 1.5 grams of fomepizole without excipients. 1 vial, when reconstituted with 30 mL of sodium chloride for injection (provided) contains 50 mg/mL of active ingredient.

Indications: ANTIZOL-VET® is indicated as an antidote for ethylene glycol (antifreeze) poisoning in dogs who have ingested or are suspected of having ingested ethylene glycol.

Pharmacology: ANTIZOL-VET® for injection is a synthetic alcohol dehydrogenase inhibitor. It is a 4-methyl substituted five membered ring structure with the molecular formula $C_4H_6N_2$ and a molecular weight of 82.1 grams per mole. The chemical name is 4-methylpyrazole. ANTIZOL-VET® acts as a competitive inhibitor of the liver enzyme alcohol dehydrogenase. The oxidation of ethylene glycol to glycoaldehyde by alcohol dehydrogenase is a critical step in the metabolism of this compound. Alcohol dehydrogenase is also involved in the metabolism of ethanol, methanol, and other hydrocarbon alcohols. Glycolic, glyoxalic, and oxalic acids, the metabolites of ethylene glycol, are the substances responsible for the severe metabolic acidosis and renal tubular epithelial damage present in poisoned dogs. Once inhibition of alcohol dehydrogenase has been achieved by treatment with ANTIZOL-VET®, the remaining unchanged ethylene glycol and its metabolites are excreted in the urine.

Dosage and Administration:

Directions for Reconstitution: A 30 mL vial of 0.9% sodium chloride injection is included with the 1.5 mL vial of ANTIZOL-VET® in the antidote kit. If the ANTIZOL-VET® solution has become solid in the vial, the solution should be liquefied by running the vial under warm water or holding in the hand. Solidification does not affect the efficacy, safety, or stability of ANTIZOL-VET®. While using good sterile technique, remove the entire contents of the ANTIZOL-VET® vial with a syringe and inject it into the 30 mL vial of 0.9% sodium chloride. Shake the solution very well to mix. In the space provided on the label of the constitution vial, write in the date and time that the dilution was prepared. Store the reconstituted vial at room temperature. Discard the reconstituted solution 72 hours following reconstitution.

Directions for Dosing: An initial loading dose of 20 mg/kg should be administered intravenously (IV) as soon as practical upon suspicion of ethylene glycol poisoning (use Table 1 below to determine the number of mL to inject). At 12, 24, and 36 hours following the initial loading dose of ANTIZOL-VET®, doses of 15, 15, and 5 mg/kg should be administered respectively. If the animal has not recovered following this regimen and there is a suspicion or documentation of remaining ethylene glycol in the bloodstream of the affected animal, the practitioner should continue to dose the animal with 5 mg/kg every 12 hours until ethylene glycol does not remain in the bloodstream or the animal has visibly recovered.

Table 1: Volume of Reconstituted (50 mg/mL) ANTIZOL-VET® Needed to Dose a Dog of the Following Body Weights at the Indicated Dose:

	Inject IV At:		
	Initial Loading Dose	12 and 24 Hours After Initial Dose	36 Hours After Initial Dose
Animal Body Weight (kg)	Milliliters of Reconstituted ANTIZOL-VET® Needed for a Dose of 20 mg/kg	Milliliters of Reconstituted ANTIZOL-VET® Needed for a Dose of 15 mg/kg	Milliliters of Reconstituted ANTIZOL-VET® Needed for a Dose of 5 mg/kg
5	2.0 mL	1.5 mL	0.5 mL
10	4.0 mL	3.0 mL	1.0 mL
15	6.0 mL	4.5 mL	1.5 mL
20	8.0 mL	6.0 mL	2.0 mL
25	10.0 mL	7.5 mL	2.5 mL
30	12.0 mL	9.0 mL	3.0 mL
35	14.0 mL	10.5 mL	3.5 mL
40	16.0 mL	12.0 mL	4.0 mL
45	18.0 mL	13.5 mL	4.5 mL
50	20.0 mL	15.0 mL	5.0 mL
55	22.0 mL	16.5 mL	5.5 mL
60	24.0 mL	18.0 mL	6.0 mL
65	26.0 mL	19.5 mL	6.5 mL
70	28.0 mL	21.0 mL	7.0 mL

Example calculation: Use the 50 mg/mL solution of reconstituted ANTIZOL-VET® for the 20 mg/kg dose. The number of milliliters of the reconstituted ANTIZOL-VET® needed for an animal weighing 7.6 kg =

$$\frac{\text{20 mg/kg (dose required) x 7.6 kg (body weight in kg)}}{\text{50 mg/mL (ANTIZOL–VET® concentration)}} = \text{3.04 mL.}$$

Additional Therapy: Supportive care to correct fluid, acid-base, and electrolyte imbalances may also be necessary. If ingestion of antifreeze is witnessed, vomiting should be induced. Gastric lavage with activated charcoal is indicated within 1 to 2 hours of ingestion; beyond this time, the procedure is of little benefit.

Contraindication(s): There are no known contraindications to ANTIZOL-VET®. However, ANTIZOL-VET® can cause central nervous system depression at doses much higher than recommended. For this reason, additional monitoring of the dog may be necessary when concomitantly administering drugs which cause central nervous system depression.

Precaution(s): Store the antidote kit at room temperature 15° to 30°C (59° to 86°F).

Caution(s): Federal Law restricts this drug to use by or on the order of a licensed veterinarian.

Dilute 1:20 in 0.9% sodium chloride injection prior to intravenous injection.

ANTIZOL-VET® should not be administered without dilution into sodium chloride. Any competitive substrate (such as ethanol) given concurrently with ANTIZOL-VET® may contribute to central nervous system depression and respiration should be monitored. Other pyrazoles may be marrow and hepatotoxic and should not be substituted for fomepizole. Overdosage of ANTIZOL-VET® may cause additional central nervous system depression. Follow the dosing regimen carefully.

Warning(s): For use in dogs only. Safety for use in breeding animals and lactating or pregnant bitches has not been demonstrated.

Human Warnings: Not for use in humans. Keep out of reach of children. Irritant. Avoid ocular, dermal or inhalation exposures. In case of eye or skin exposure, flush immediately with copious amounts of water. Seek medical attention if irritation persists. Use product only in a well ventilated area. If accidental inhalation occurs, move to fresh air. The material safety data sheet (MSDS) contains additional information regarding the safe use of this product.

Toxicology: Safety: A subacute toxicity study was conducted in dogs for 14 days with dose levels of 10, 20, and 30 mg/kg of ANTIZOL-VET® administered intravenously twice per day in 0.9% sodium chloride injection, USP. A two phase overdosing toxicity study was conducted in dogs for 14 days. Dose levels of 150 and 75 (phase I) and 25 and 50 (phase II) mg/kg of ANTIZOL-VET® were administered intravenously twice per day in 0.9% sodium chloride injection. ANTIZOL-VET® administered at 25 mg/kg resulted in decreased food consumption, body weight loss, and breaths with sweet odors. At 30 mg/kg, ANTIZOL-VET® administration resulted in hypoactivity and increased liver weights at necropsy. At 50 mg/kg or greater, ANTIZOL-VET® resulted in ataxia, hypoactivity, hypothermia, tremors and/or prostration, injected sclera, ptosis, decreased defecation, and protruding tongues.

Side Effects: Adverse Reactions: In the clinical field study, one of 105 dogs experienced an anaphylactic type reaction following the second dose of ANTIZOL-VET®. Clinical signs included tachypnea, gagging, excessive salivation and trembling. Dosing with ANTIZOL-VET® was discontinued and the animal survived.

Trial Data: Pharmacokinetics: Results from a twice daily 14 day intravenous study evaluating doses of 10, 20, and 30 mg/kg in dogs showed a dose proportional increase in plasma levels of fomepizole after a single (first) dose. In this same study it was noted that there was a non-linear increase in plasma levels of fomepizole after the fourteenth day of dosing that was particularly evident in the 30 mg/kg dose group. The non-linear accumulation in plasma is assumed to be a result of a saturable elimination process. At 10 mg/kg there was no plasma accumulation and no fomepizole detectable in plasma prior to the last (28th) dose. Fifty percent of the dogs dosed at 20 mg/kg showed some plasma accumulation after 14 days of dosing. In general, dogs dosed below 20 mg/kg should have no detectable fomepizole in their plasma by 12 hours following intravenous dose administration.

Discussion: Prognosis: ANTIZOL-VET® is only effective if injected into the bloodstream prior to complete metabolism of ethylene glycol. To evaluate whether ethylene glycol has been completely metabolized, it is advisable to measure serum BUN and creatinine, and to monitor urine output. Correction of dehydration is essential to obtain accurate serum BUN and creatinine values. Serum concentrations of blood urea nitrogen >40 mg/dl and creatinine >1.8 mg/dl that do not resolve after dehydration is corrected indicate that ethylene glycol has been fully metabolized and significant renal damage may exist. However, if urine flow is maintained, benefit to risk considerations suggest that treatment with ANTIZOL-VET® is warranted.

Presentation: ANTIZOL-VET® is provided as an antidote kit containing two sterile vials. The smaller vial is a sterile single-use vial with 1.5 mL (1.5 g) of ANTIZOL-VET® without excipients. In addition, a 30 mL vial of 0.9% sodium chloride injection is provided for ANTIZOL-VET® reconstitution.

Distributed by: The Butler Company.

Compendium Code No.: 14840000

A • O • E™, ANIMAL ODOR ELIMINATOR

Thornell **Deodorant Product**

Description: Does not contain enzymes, bacteria, nor oxidizers. Nontoxic, nonirritating, biodegradable, nonflammable. Water soluble for easy cleanup.

Indications: To eliminate animal odors from anal and other glandular secretions, urine, feces, tomcat spray, emesis, necrotic tissue etc.

For use on animals and their accidents, bedding, cages, litter - any companion animal odor.

A • O • E™ works chemically through bonding, absorption and counteraction. It contains inhibitors to control odors caused by further biological (organic) decomposition (putrefaction), and residuals that re-activate after the initial application to combat and prevent odors.

A • O • E™ is used principally on accidents in examining and waiting rooms; however, it is frequently dispensed for home use on cat litter boxes and animal accidents.

Dosage and Administration: Spray directly on the source of the odor. If the odor persists after the A • O • E™ has dried, the source of the odor has not been reached. Re-apply.

Use as an air freshener for quick but temporary relief by spraying two (2) or three (3) times into the air.

One (1) ounce bottle of concentrate when diluted with water makes 16 ounces.

Precaution(s): A • O • E™ has an indefinite shelf life.

Caution(s): Although safe, as with all chemicals, it should be kept out of the reach of children. For external use only. When used on fabrics always spot test for color fastness.

Presentation: 1 oz. bottle and 8 oz. spray bottle.

Compendium Code No.: 11210000

A-PLUS™ WOUND DRESSING

Creative Science **Topical Wound Dressing**

Active Ingredient(s): Contains: Allantoin 1.25%, Benzocaine 2.00%, Vitamin A 200,000 I.U., Ascorbic acid 2,000 mg, Pine tar 1.00%, Vitamin E (as antioxidant) in a propylene glycol hydrogenated oil base.

Indications: For use on cuts, abrasions, saddle sores and other skin and flesh wounds as an aid in treatment and fly repellent. A-PLUS™ Wound Dressing allows regrowth of hair to natural color in wound area.

Aid in healing; prevents white hair; minimizes scar tissue; relieves pain; sticks to wound.

Directions: Cover the entire wound including ½ inch around the edges once daily. As healing begins, applications every other day may be desirable. A-PLUS™ Wound Dressing ointment may be used under a bandage.

Note: For very large and deep, penetrating wounds, consult your veterinarian.

Precaution(s): Store in a cool, dry place.

Warning(s): Not for use on animals intended for food use.

Not for human use.

Keep out of reach of children.

Presentation: 8 oz (226 g) container.

Compendium Code No.: 13760002

APPLE-DEX™

Horse Health **Electrolytes-Oral**

Guaranteed Analysis:

Calcium, Min. 0.25%
Calcium, Max. 0.75%
Salt (NaCl), Min. 68.00%
Salt (NaCl), Max. 73.00%
Potassium, Min. 11.00%
Magnesium, Min. 0.40%

Ingredients: Salt (Sodium Chloride), Potassium Chloride, Magnesium Sulfate, Calcium Lactate Pentahydrate, Potassium Sulfate, Artificial Apple Flavor, Artificial Coloring.

Apple flavored.

Indications: APPLE-DEX™ supplements horses to provide additional electrolyte salts that may be lost by dehydration.

Electrolytes for all classes of horses.

Directions: Dosage: APPLE-DEX™ may be administered in the horse's feed or drinking water at the rate of 2 ounces per 10 gallons of fresh water, or 2 ounces in the horse's daily feed ration in place of regular salt.

Important: When administered in water allow no other source of drinking water.

Precaution(s): Keep container tightly closed. Store in a cool, dry place.

Caution(s): For animal use only.

For veterinary use only.

Warning(s): Not for use in animals intended for human consumption.

Keep out of reach of children.

Presentation: 2.27 kg (5 lb), 9.07 kg (20 lb) and 13.6 kg (30 lb).

Compendium Code No.: 15000060 9CC5 / 9FF6 / 9B7

APRALAN® SOLUBLE

Elanco **Water Medication**

NADA No.: 106-964

Active Ingredient(s): Contains apramycin sulfate equivalent to 48 g apramycin activity (medicates 128 gallons or 486 liters of drinking water, 8448 lbs body weight).

Indications: For the control of porcine colibacillosis (weanling pig scours) caused by strains of *E. coli* sensitive to apramycin.

Dosage and Administration: Treated pigs should consume enough medicated water to receive 12.5 mg of apramycin per kg of body weight per day (5.67 mg/lb/day). Continue treatment for 7 days.

Mixing Directions: Use the plastic spoon for measuring the amount of powder to be used. Add to the drinking water at the rate of 375 mg of apramycin per gallon according to the following table. Stir on addition, let stand for 15 minutes to allow particles to dissolve. Stir again to dispense medication.

Total Body Weight to be Treated*		APRALAN® Soluble Per Day (Plastic spoon leveled full)	Approximate Daily Water Consumption (Gallon)	Apramycin (mg)
lb	kg			
264	120	1	4	1,500
1320	600	5	20	7,500
8448	3840	Entire Contents	128	48,000

*Number of pigs X average weight

Water consumption should be monitored closely to determine that the recommended dosage is being consumed. The drug concentration should be adjusted according to water consumption. Water consumption varies considerably with ambient temperature, humidity and other factors. Prepare fresh medicated water daily. Rusty waterers may cause rapid loss of potency.

Notice: Organisms vary in their degree of sensitivity to chemotherapeutics. If no improvement is observed after recommended treatment, diagnosis and sensitivity should be reconfirmed.

Precaution(s): Storage: Protect from moisture. Keep tightly closed. Store in a cool, dry place.

Warning(s): Do not slaughter treated swine for 28 days following treatment.

Keep out of the reach of children.

Presentation: 48 g.

Compendium Code No.: 10310001 WS 1651 AMX

AQUACILLIN™

Vedco **Penicillin Injection**

(Penicillin G Procaine-Injectable Antibiotic in Aqueous Suspension)

NADA No.: 065-493

Active Ingredient(s): Each mL contains:

Penicillin G procaine .... 300,000 units
Sodium citrate .... 10 mg
Povidone .... 5 mg
Lecithin .... 6 mg
Sodium carboxymethylcellulose .... 1 mg
Methyl paraben .... 1.3 mg
Propyl paraben .... 0.2 mg
Sodium formaldehyde sulfoxylate .... 0.2 mg
Procaine hydrochloride .... 20 mg
Water for injection .... q.s.

Indications: For the treatment of bacteria pneumonia (shipping fever) caused by *Pasteurella multocida* in cattle and sheep; erysipelas caused by *Erysipelothrix rhusiopathiae (insidiosa)* in swine; and strangles caused by *Streptococcus equi* in horses.

Dosage and Administration: Shake well before using.

Cattle, Sheep, Swine and Horses: 3,000 units per pound of body weight or 1 mL for each 100 pounds of body weight once a day. Continue the treatment for at least one (1) day after the symptoms disappear (usually 2 or 3 days). Treatment should not exceed four (4) consecutive days. If improvement is not observed, consult a veterinarian.

Penicillin G procaine suspension should be injected deep within the fleshy muscles of the hip, rump, round or thigh. Do not inject subcutaneously, into a blood vessel or near a major nerve. The site of each injection should be changed. Use a 16 or 18 gauge needle, 1½ inches long. The needle and syringe should be washed thoroughly before use and sterilized in boiling water for 15 or 20 minutes before use. The injection site should be washed with soap and water and painted with a disinfectant such as 70% alcohol. Warm the product to room temperature and shake well. Wipe the rubber stopper in the vial with 70% alcohol. Withdraw the suspension from the vial and inject deep into the muscle. Do not inject more than 10 mL into one site.

Precaution(s): Store in a refrigerator (36-46°F, 2-8°C).

Caution(s): Keep out of the reach of children.

Use only as directed. For veterinary use only. Not for human use.

Sensitivity reactions to penicillin or procaine such as hives or respiratory distress, sometimes fatal, have been known to occur in some animals. If signs of sensitivity do occur, stop the use of the medication and call a veterinarian. If respiratory distress is severe, the immediate injection of epinephrine may be helpful.

As with any antibiotic preparation, prolonged use may result in the overgrowth of nonsusceptible organisms, including fungi. If this condition is suspected, stop the use of the medication and consult a veterinarian. The milk withholding time for the product is based on human safety standards. The milk plant may advise additional testing to ensure compliance with industry requirements.

Warning(s): Not for use in horses intended for food.

Milk that has been taken from animals during treatment and for 48 hours (4 milkings) after the last treatment with this drug must not be used for food.

Discontinue the use of this drug for the following time periods before treated animals are slaughtered for food:

Cattle .... 10 days
Sheep .... 9 days
Swine .... 7 days

Presentation: 100 mL, 250 mL and 500 mL sterile multiple dose vials.

Compendium Code No.: 10490050

AQUAJECT

Vetus **Sterile Water**

Contents:

Water for Injection USP 100%

Sterile, nonpyrogenic, hypotonic.

pH 5.0-7.0

Indications: This is a single dose vial. After a quantity has been withdrawn for use the remainder should be discarded.

This sterile water for injection is made by distillation and is suitable for use as a diluent for preparation of pharmaceutical solutions when made isotonic by addition of suitable solutes. This product contains no preservative; solutions made from this water should be used promptly or sterilized with adequate precautions for maintaining sterility.

Precaution(s): Store between 15°C and 30°C (59°-86°F).

Caution(s): Do not use this product if seal is broken or solution is not clear. Contains no preservative. If entire contents are not used, discard unused portion. Additives may be incompatible. When introducing additives, use aseptic technique, mix thoroughly, and do not store. For animal use only.

Presentation: 100 mL, 250 mL, and 500 mL vials.

Compendium Code No.: 14440050

AQUAVAC-ESC®

Intervet **Vaccine**

Edwardsiella Ictaluri Vaccine, Avirulent Live Culture

U.S. Vet. Lic. No.: 286

Description: AQUAVAC-ESC® contains the known avirulent strain of *Edwardsiella ictaluri*, designated RE-33, as a freeze-dried preparation sealed under vacuum.

Indications: AQUAVAC-ESC® is indicated for the prevention of ESC disease (enteric septicemia of catfish) in catfish due to *E. ictaluri* infection. Catfish should be healthy and free of disease at the time of vaccination. Sick or weak catfish may not develop adequate immunity. Catfish should be at least 7 days of age post hatch or older at the time of vaccination. For maximum benefit, catfish should be vaccinated for a minimum of two minutes at least 14 days prior to anticipated exposure to ESC disease. Vaccination is not recommended when water temperatures are below 21°C (70°F) or above 29°C (85°F). AQUAVAC-ESC® is administered to catfish as a timed bath treatment.

Dosage and Administration: Dosage: The dosage of AQUAVAC-ESC® is based on total catfish weight and the volume of water in which they are vaccinated. Each vial of AQUAVAC-ESC® is sufficient to vaccinate 1.5 pounds of catfish in 1 gallon of water. When applied to fry at 7 days of age post hatch (an average size of 13,000 catfish per pound or 29 catfish/gram or 812 catfish per fluid ounce), each vial of vaccine is sufficient to vaccinate 20,000 fry in 1 gallon of water.

When vaccinating 7 days post hatch fry, the following tables should be used to determine the proper dosage and use of AQUAVAC-ESC®.

Table A:

	Number of 7 Day Post Hatch Fry to be Vaccinated as a Single Group				
	200,000	400,000	600,000	800,000	1,000,000
Vials of Vaccine	10	20	30	40	50
Gallons of Water	10	20	30	40	50

When vaccinating catfish older than 7 day post hatch fry, each ten-pack of AQUAVAC-ESC® vaccine is sufficient to vaccinate 15 pounds of catfish in 10 gallons of water as described in "Administration", (7), below. The following table can be used to help determine the proper dosage and use of AQUAVAC-ESC®.

Table B:

	Pounds of Catfish to be Vaccinated as a Single Group				
	15	30	45	60	75
Vials of Vaccine	10	20	30	40	50
Gallons of Water	10	20	30	40	50

Administration: Prior to vaccination, ensure that all nets, buckets, tanks and other equipment are thoroughly cleaned and properly disinfected prior to use. Ensure that all troughs or hauling tanks have been cleaned and flushed free of any excess feces or feed. To reduce stress, it is recommended that the catfish not be fed for 3 to 4 hours prior to vaccination. Use standard methods to determine the total weight of each group of catfish to be vaccinated.

Caution - because the dosage of AQUAVAC-ESC® is based on total catfish weight, it is important that the catfish be inventoried as accurately as possible immediately prior to vaccination to ensure full efficacy of the vaccine. Refer to Table A or Table B as guidelines to determine the amount of vaccine and volume of water needed for vaccinating each group of catfish.

AQUAVAC-ESC® should be kept refrigerated between 2° and 7°C (35° and 45°F) at all times prior to use. Caution - do not rehydrate AQUAVAC-ESC® until immediately prior to use.

Tank Vaccination During Transport:

1. Calculate the water volume of transport tank and determine the volume of water for vaccination based on guidelines in Table A or Table B. Fill the transport tank with clean water to this level.
2. Turn on oxygen to transport tank. Ensure the air stones are all working and adequate oxygenation is being provided to all areas of the tank.
3. Add catfish to be vaccinated to the transport tank.
4. Rehydrate the number of vials of vaccine needed by removing the tear-off seal and stopper from each vial and filling each to approximately two-thirds full with clean well water. Reinsert the rubber stopper and, while covering the stopper, invert each vial several times until the contents are completely dissolved.
5. Immediately add vaccine to transport tank, pouring evenly across the surface of the tank. Mix gently but thoroughly.
6. Wait at least two minutes.
7. After two minutes, fill the transport tank with at least an equal amount of water and do not dilute further for at least 15 minutes. Haul to the nursery or fingerling pond for stocking. The usual precautions must be taken to ensure fish in the transport tank are properly tempered to the pond water temperature before discharge.
8. Discharge catfish and vaccine solution into pond and observe for any signs of stress.
9. Begin feeding as usual.

Records: The user is advised to keep a written record of vaccination including vaccine, quantity, serial number, expiration date, and place of purchase; the date and time of vaccination; the breed, lot number, pond number, population, age, average size and total weight of catfish vaccinated; names of operators administering the vaccine; water temperature and environmental conditions as well as observations on the general health of the animals at the time of vaccination; and any unusual reactions or conditions observed.

Precaution(s): Storage Conditions: AQUAVAC-ESC® should be stored in a refrigerator between 2° and 7°C (35° and 45°F) prior to use. Once AQUAVAC-ESC® has been rehydrated, it must be used immediately. At no time should AQUAVAC-ESC® be frozen or exposed to direct sunlight or excessive heat above ambient air or water temperatures.

Use AQUAVAC-ESC® vaccine immediately following rehydration.

Do not attempt to store or reuse the vaccine once it has been rehydrated. Each vial of AQUAVAC-ESC® vaccine is designed and intended for use in a single application.

Dilute AQUAVAC-ESC® vaccine only as directed. Any changes in the recommended dilution rate may cause the product to become ineffective.

Use the entire contents of each vial when first opened and rehydrated.

When vaccination has been completed, burn all containers and any unused contents.

Caution(s): Vaccinate only healthy catfish. Although disease may not be evident, concurrent disease and adverse environmental conditions may cause complications or reduce effectiveness of AQUAVAC-ESC® vaccine.

Withhold all chemical or antibiotic treatments in the water or feed for 3 days before and 5 days after vaccination.

Ensure accuracy of inventories prior to vaccination. Because the dosage of AQUAVAC-ESC® is based on total catfish weight, it is important that the catfish be inventoried as accurately as possible immediately prior to vaccination to ensure full efficacy and safety of the vaccine.

Do not attempt to vaccinate more catfish than directed or otherwise change the dosage of AQUAVAC-ESC®. To do otherwise can cause the product to become ineffective.

AQUAVAC-ESC® is intended for veterinary use only.

The use of this vaccine is subject to applicable federal, state and local laws and regulations.

Use only as directed.

Notice: AQUAVAC-ESC® has undergone rigid potency, safety and purity tests, and meets Intervet Inc. and USDA requirements. It is designed to stimulate effective immunity when used as directed, but the user must be advised that the response to the product depends upon many factors, including, but not limited to, conditions of storage and handling by the user, administration of the vaccine, health and responsiveness of the individual catfish, environmental conditions following vaccination and the severity and timing of field exposure to *E. ictaluri* and ESC disease following vaccination. Therefore, directions should be followed carefully to ensure safe use and optimum performance.

AQUAVAC-ESC® is not hazardous when used according to directions and poses no known human health risk for healthy individuals. A material safety data sheet (MSDS) is available upon request. This and any other consumer information can be obtained by calling Intervet Customer Service at 1-800-441-8272 or 1-302-934-8051.

Warning(s): Avoid contact of open wounds with the vaccine. Wash hands thoroughly after using the vaccine.

Any adverse or unusual effects associated with the use of AQUAVAC-ESC® should be immediately reported to Intervet Inc. at the following telephone number: 1-800-441-8272.

Trial Data: AQUAVAC-ESC® has been shown to provide significant protection from disease and mortality when vaccinated catfish are challenged with common virulent or wild-type isolates of *E. ictaluri*.

Discussion: Vaccination Programs: AQUAVAC-ESC® is intended for use in a comprehensive program of catfish health management and producers are encouraged to consult with their veterinarian or other fish health professionals before use. AQUAVAC-ESC® can be applied as a bath at any time during the production cycle. AQUAVAC-ESC® is easily administered at any time catfish are being handled and can be integrated into routine catfish handling practices such as grading, inventorying, sorting, splitting, hauling, moving or ponding. The most common application is a bath treatment of 7 days post hatch fry in a transport tank before stocking catfish into nursery or fingerling ponds.

Presentation: 10 vials per pack.

U.S. Patent No. 6,019,981

Compendium Code No.: 11062610 AL193

ARGUS®* SC/ST

Intervet **Vaccine**

Salmonella Choleraesuis Vaccine, Avirulent Live Culture

U.S. Vet. Lic. No.: 286

Contents: This product contains the antigen listed above.

Indications: *Salmonella choleraesuis* vaccine is used as an aid in the prevention of pneumonia, diarrhea, septicemia and mortality caused by *S. choleraesuis* and as an aid in control of disease caused by *S. typhimurium* and an aid in control of *S. typhimurium* shedding.

Dosage and Administration: Administer to healthy swine 3 weeks of age or older.

Water Administration: This product was developed to be used exclusively by the oral route. Aseptically rehydrate the contents of the desiccated vial with enclosed diluent. Shake well. Add to the water delivery system using the appropriate ratio to achieve the delivery of 1 mL of vaccine per pig (see detailed instructions below). Water may be withheld for 1-2 hours before vaccination. Occasional remixing of the vaccine solution 2 to 3 times during the vaccination procedure aids in assuring a uniform dose for all swine.

Water Delivery of Vaccine:

Do not open or mix ARGUS® SC/ST until ready to vaccinate.

Remove all medications, sanitizers and disinfectants from drinking water before initiating oral vaccination.

Flush watering system with non-chlorinated/non-treated clean water to eliminate any antibacterial agents.

Withhold water for one to two (1-2) hours before vaccination.

Rehydrate ARGUS® SC/ST with accompanying 50 mL or 100 mL diluent, depending on the dose size.

Set proportioner to deliver 1 oz. (30 mL) of hydrated ARGUS® SC/ST per 1 gallon (3.75 L) of water.

If necessary, make a dilution, according to the table below, using a clean container with clean non-treated water.

Insert proportioner hose into the stock solution with the ARGUS® SC/ST (diluted or undiluted) and start water flow until all vaccine solution has been consumed. Flush the vaccine container with clean non-treated water. The pigs should consume vaccine within the first 3-4 hours after hydration of the vaccine.

Once the ARGUS® SC/ST has been dispensed and the proportioner has delivered all fluids, return to non-treated water flow. Do not medicate or use disinfectants within 24 hours after vaccination.

Body Weight lb.	Average Water Consumption in Gallons Per 100 animals a 4 Hour Period[1]	Dilution for stock solution (after in hydration of vaccine with 1 diluent)
10	3.0	Undiluted[2]
15	4.5	Undiluted[2]
20	6.0	6.0 oz.
25	7.5	7.5 oz.
50	15.0	15.0 oz.
75	22.5	22.5 oz.
100	30.0	30.0 oz.
150	45.0	45.0 oz.
200	60.0	60.0 oz.
250 and up	75.0	75.0 oz.

[1]Calculations are based on an average daily water consumption of 15% of body weight. Young animals and lactating sows may consume up to 20% of body weight.

[2]Mixing one vial of ARGUS® SC/ST with one vial of diluent makes a stock solution. (Hint: A 100-dose vial will treat 100 pigs).

Example:

For vaccination of 100 pigs, average weight 25 lbs.: Identify the row for 25 lb. pigs and then select the average water consumption values for 25 lb. pigs (7.5 gallons per 100 pigs per 4 hours). Rehydrate ARGUS® SC/ST with the provided diluent. Add the rehydrated ARGUS® SC/ST to enough clean water (approximately 4 oz.) to make 7.5 ounces of final stock solution. Deliver the stock solution at the rate of one ounce per gallon.

If you require additional assistance please call 1-800-835-0541.

Precaution(s): Store at 2°C-7°C (35°F-45°F). Do not freeze. Use entire contents when first opened. Burn containers and all unused contents.

Caution(s): Do not use antibiotics, sulfonamides or furans in feed or water for 3 days before and 3 days after vaccination. In case of anaphylactoid reaction, epinephrine should be administered immediately.

For veterinary use only.

Warning(s): Do not vaccinate within 21 days before slaughter.

Presentation: 50 doses (50 mL) and 100 doses (100 mL).

*U.S. Patent Registration Nos. 5,468,485 and 5,378,744.

Compendium Code No.: 11062760 78610002/91878601

ARK BLEN®

Merial Select **Vaccine**

Bronchitis Vaccine, Arkansas Type, Live Virus

U.S. Vet. Lic. No.: 279

Contents: This product contains the antigen listed above.

This vaccine is composed of live viruses in a lyophilized preparation sealed under vacuum.

Contains gentamicin as a bacteriostatic agent.

Notice: Merial Select's vaccines have met the requirements of the USDA in regard to safety, purity, potency, and the capability to protect susceptible chickens. This vaccine has been tested by the Master Seed immunogenicity test for efficacy.

Indications: This vaccine is recommended for the vaccination of healthy chickens at least 21 days of age by drinking water as an aid in the prevention of Arkansas type bronchitis.

This vaccine is recommended for the protection of healthy chickens. It is essential that the chickens be maintained under good environmental conditions and that exposure to disease viruses be reduced as much as possible.

Dosage and Administration:

Drinking Water Vaccination Using Pouring Application: Drinking water revaccination is recommended for healthy chickens at least 21 days of age.

1. Remove all medications, sanitizers and disinfectants from the drinking water 72 hours (three days) prior to vaccination.
2. Provide sufficient waterers so that all the chickens can drink at one time. Shut off water supply and allow chickens to consume all the water in the lines.

3. Raise water lines above the chickens' heads. Clean and rinse the waterers thoroughly.
4. Withhold all water from the chickens for a minimum of two hours in warm weather to four hours in cool weather prior to vaccination to stimulate thirst. Withdrawal time should be reduced if half-house brooding is in process.
5. Do not open or mix vaccine until ready to vaccinate.
6. Drinking water for vaccine delivery should contain one ounce (29 gram) of non-fat dry milk per gallon (3.8 liters) of non-chlorinated water, or should contain milk product based stabilizer prepared according to the manufacturer's instructions.
7. Reconstitute the vaccine in 3 gallons (11 liters) of milk-water during cool weather or 4 gallons (15 liters) of milk-water during warm weather for each 1,000 doses.
8. Distribute vaccine solution among waterers. Avoid direct sunlight.
9. Lower waterers and allow the chickens to drink freely. Add the remaining vaccine solution to the water lines as the chickens drink.
10. Do not provide additional drinking water until all the vaccine is consumed.

Drinking Water Vaccination Using Proportioner Application: Drinking water revaccination is recommended for healthy chickens at least 21 days of age. Several types of medicator/proportioners are commercially available. Set proportioner to deliver one ounce (30 mL) of vaccine concentrate per one gallon (3.8 liters) of water.

1. Remove all medications, sanitizers and disinfectants from the drinking water 72 hours (three days) prior to vaccination.
2. Clean all containers, hoses and waterers prior to vaccination.
3. Withhold all water from the chickens for a minimum of two hours in warm weather to four hours in cool weather prior to vaccination to stimulate thirst. Withdrawal time should be reduced if half-house brooding is in process.
4. Do not open or mix vaccine until ready to vaccinate.
5. Calculate to supply vaccine solution at a rate of 3 gallons (11 liters) per 1,000 chickens in cool weather and 4 gallons (15 liters) per 1,000 chickens in warm weather. The age of the chickens should be considered when calculating water supply. Always use non-chlorinated water when vaccinating chickens.
   Example:
   1,000 chickens in cool weather x 3 gallons (11 liters) = 3 gallons (11 liters).
   1,000 chickens in warm weather x 4 gallons (15 liters) = 4 gallons (15 liters).
6. Prepare vaccine stock solution as follows:
   a. Determine the quantity of vaccine concentrate required by multiplying one ounce (30 mL) x gallons of water needed for vaccine/drinking water.
   Example:
   For 1,000 chickens: 3 gallons x 1 ounce (30 mL) = 3 ounces (90 mL).
   b. Add 3 ounces (85 gm) of non-fat dry milk per 16 ounces (480 mL) of cool water, or use a commercial milk product based stabilizer according to the manufacturer's instructions. For 1,000 chickens add 0.5 ounces (16 gm) non-fat dry milk to the 3 ounces (90 mL) of water.
   c. Reconstitute the dried vaccine with the milk solution. Rinse the vaccine vial to remove all the vaccine.
7. Insert proportioner hose into the vaccine stock solution and start water flow. Continue until all solution has been consumed before changing water supply to direct flow.
8. Do not medicate or use disinfectants for 24 hours after vaccination.

Precaution(s): Store vaccine at 35-45°F (2-7°C). Do not freeze. Improper storage or handling of the vaccine may result in loss of potency.

Mix only the amount of vaccine to be used immediately and use promptly. Use all at one time and do not stretch the dosage. Use entire vial contents when first opened. Burn the container and all unused contents.

Caution(s): Birds should be vaccinated before they reach maturity since bronchitis virus may cause permanent damage to the reproductive tract of mature birds, resulting in eggs with poor interior quality and shell texture.

Infectious bronchitis is highly contagious when non-vaccinated birds are kept in close contact with vaccinated birds during the period of respiratory signs. The vaccine should be used with caution around non-vaccinated laying birds.

Do not vaccinate diseased chickens.

Administer a minimum of one dose per chicken.

Avoid stress conditions during and following vaccination.

Do not place chickens in contaminated facilities.

Exposure to disease must be minimized as much as possible.

The capability of this vaccine to produce satisfactory results depends upon many factors, including, but not limited to, conditions of storage and handling by the user, administration of the vaccine, health and responsiveness of individual chickens, and degree of field exposure. Therefore, directions for use should be followed carefully. The use of this vaccine is subject to applicable state and federal laws and regulations.

Use only in localities where permitted.

For veterinary use only.

Warning(s): Do not vaccinate within 21 days of slaughter.

Presentation: ARK BLEN® is supplied without a diluent for drinking water administration in 25 x 5,000 dose vials.

Compendium Code No.: 11050002 0699

ARKO CHOL VAC FD

Arko **Vaccine**

Pasteurella multocida Avirulent Live Culture, Avian Isolate

U.S. Vet. Lic. No.: 337

Active Ingredient(s): ARKO CHOL VAC FD is a live bacterial vaccine offering protection to turkeys against naturally occurring field strains of *P. multocida*.

Potency: ARKO CHOL VAC FD is freeze dried to protect potency.

Indications: ARKO CHOL VAC FD is recommended for oral immunization in healthy turkeys to reduce losses due to fowl cholera.

Dosage and Administration: This is a two (2) dose vaccine. The first dose should be given at six (6) weeks of age. The second dose should be given at 9-11 weeks of age. Subsequent revaccination may be given every 3-5 weeks thereafter as needed. Turkeys must be healthy and free from any outside stresses at the time of vaccination. ARKO CHOL VAC FD will provide a successful vaccination, but the immune response in the birds also depends on administration techniques, previous exposure to immunosuppressing agents and the environment. Prevaccination exposure to field coryza, Newcastle, hemorrhagic enteritis and other diseases can influence the birds ability to respond to vaccination. Do not use ARKO CHOL VAC FD within 14 days of vaccinating for Newcastle.

The first dose of vaccine should be administered in the drinking water at six (6) weeks of age. A repeat vaccination should be given every 3-5 weeks.

1. Medications and disinfecting products in the drinking water are not compatible with ARKO CHOL VAC FD. Discontinue their use for at least three (3) days before vaccinating and do not resume their use for three (3) days after vaccination.
2. Do not use chlorinated water for vaccination. Scrub and clean all waterers before vaccination with nonchlorinated water.
3. Flush the water lines with one (1) pound of powdered milk per 100 gallons of water prior to vaccinating to protect the vaccine and prevent possible inactivation from chlorine.
4. Rehydrate the vaccine just prior to use. Remove the aluminum seal and the stopper. Rehydrate the vaccine with milk or distilled water to a level of 20 mL. Milk diluent can be made by adding powdered milk to cool, clean, nonchlorinated water at a rate of one (1) teaspoon per gallon. After reconstitution, reseat the stopper and shake to thoroughly dissolve the vaccine. Do not mix the vaccine into the drinking water until just before vaccination.
5. The vaccine is to be used at a rate of one (1) vial of vaccine for every 1,000 birds. Generally water may be withheld for up to two (2) hours prior to vaccinating to assure that all the turkeys will drink. The vaccine should be administered in an amount of drinking water (milk added) that would be consumed by thirsty turkeys in approximately two (2) hours. Provide ample watering space so that all turkeys can drink easily.
6. The daily water consumption for each flock needs to be determined just prior to vaccination. Water consumption is affected by weather, management conditions and the age of the birds. When specific water consumption information is not available, please refer to the reference table below which will serve as a general guideline to determine the amount of water to be used with the vaccine if more specific information is not available.

Water consumption per 1,000 doses:

Age in weeks	Gallons of water consumed by 1,000 turkeys per day (average temperatures)
4	40
5	50
6	60
7	75
8	95
9	115
10	125
12	150
15	165

Vaccinate only healthy birds. Do not vaccinate in the face of a challenge due to cholera or any other disease. Vaccination during a challenge can cause complications and reduce immunity. Do not use this vaccine within two (2) weeks on either side of a vaccination with live Newcastle virus vaccine. Discontinue all medications and antibiotics three (3) days prior to vaccination. Resume medications three (3) days post-vaccination if needed.

Precaution(s): Store this vaccine at not over 45°F (7°C). Protect from sunlight.

It is advisable to record the vaccine serial number, the expiration date, the date of vaccination and any reactions observed. This product should be stored, transported, and administered in accordance with the instructions and directions.

Caution(s): Use only proper hygiene when handling the vaccine. Use the entire contents when first opened. Burn all the containers and unused portions of the vaccine. Clean any spills with disinfectants. Keep the vaccine away from open wounds. Wear gloves if necessary. Consult a physician if contamination occurs. Wash hands thoroughly after using the vaccine.

Warning(s): Do not vaccinate within 21 days before slaughter.

Discussion: Fowl cholera is a contagious, widely distributed disease in turkeys occurring as a septicemia with a sudden onset. Pneumonia is particularly common in turkeys resulting in high morbidity and mortality.

Product Safety: This vaccine will produce effective immunity. It has passed potency, safety and purity tests meeting all the requirements set forth by Arko Laboratories Ltd. and the USDA. The response to the product, the stimulation of antibodies within the turkey and the resultant level of immunity may be affected by other factors: Management conditions, concurrent infections and stress levels at vaccination.

Trial Data: Challenge: ARKO CHOL VAC FD protected isolated turkeys in controlled laboratory experimentation against challenge with the P1059 (type 3) strain of *Pasteurella multocida*.

Presentation: 1,000 dose vials.

Compendium Code No.: 11230000

ARKO ERY VAC FD

Arko **Vaccine**

Erysipelothrix rhusiopathiae Vaccine, Avirulent Live Culture

U.S. Vet. Lic. No.: 337

Active Ingredient(s): ARKO ERY VAC FD is a live bacterial vaccine offering protection to turkeys against naturally occurring field strains of erysipelas.

Potency: ARKO ERY VAC FD is freeze dried to protect potency.

Indications: ARKO ERY VAC FD is recommended for oral immunization in healthy turkeys to reduce losses due to erysipelas.

Dosage and Administration: This is a two (2) dose vaccine. The first dose should be given at eight (8) weeks of age. The second dose should be given at 10-11 weeks of age. Subsequent revaccination may be given every three (3) weeks thereafter as needed. Turkeys must be healthy and free from any outside stresses at the time of vaccination. ARKO ERY VAC FD will provide a successful vaccination, but the immune response in the birds also depends on administration techniques, previous exposure to immunosuppressing agents and the environment. Prevaccination exposure to field coryza, Newcastle, hemorrhagic enteritis and other diseases can influence the birds ability to respond to vaccination.

The first dose of vaccine should be administered in the drinking water at eight (8) weeks of age. A repeat vaccination should be given 2-3 weeks following the initial vaccination.

1. Medications and disinfecting products in the drinking water are not compatible with ARKO ERY VAC FD. Discontinue their use for at least three (3) days before vaccinating and do not resume their use for three (3) days after vaccination.
2. Do not use chlorinated water for vaccination. Scrub and clean all waterers before vaccination with nonchlorinated water.

3. Flush the water lines with one (1) pound of powdered milk per 100 gallons of water prior to vaccinating to protect the vaccine and prevent possible inactivation from chlorine.
4. Rehydrate the vaccine just prior to use. Remove the aluminum seal and the stopper. Rehydrate the vaccine with milk or distilled water to a level of 20 mL. Milk diluent can be made by adding powdered milk to cool, clean, nonchlorinated water at a rate of one (1) teaspoon per gallon. After reconstitution, reseat the stopper and shake to thoroughly dissolve the vaccine. Do not mix the vaccine into the drinking water until just before vaccination.
5. The vaccine is to be used at a rate of one (1) vial of vaccine for every 1,000 birds. Generally water may be withheld for up to two (2) hours prior to vaccinating to assure that all the turkeys will drink. The vaccine should be administered in an amount of drinking water (milk added) that would be consumed by thirsty turkeys in approximately two (2) hours. Provide ample watering space so that all turkeys can drink easily.
6. The daily water consumption for each flock needs to be determined just prior to vaccination. Water consumption is affected by weather, management conditions and the age of the birds. When specific water consumption information is not available, please refer to the reference table below which will serve as a general guideline to determine the amount of water to be used with the vaccine if more specific information is not available.

Water consumption per 1,000 doses:

Age in weeks	Gallons of water consumed by 1,000 turkeys per day (average temperatures)
8	95
9	115
10	125
12	150
15	165

Vaccinate only healthy birds. Do not vaccinate in the face of a challenge due to erysipelas or any other disease. Vaccination during a challenge can cause complications and reduce immunity. Do not use this vaccine within two (2) weeks on either side of a vaccination with live Newcastle virus vaccine. Discontinue all medications and antibiotics three (3) days prior to vaccination. Resume medications three (3) days post-vaccination if needed.

Precaution(s): Store this vaccine at not over 45°F (7°C). Protect from sunlight.

It is advisable to record the vaccine serial number, the expiration date, the date of vaccination and any reactions observed. This product should be stored, transported, and administered in accordance with the instructions and directions.

Caution(s): Use only proper hygiene when handling the vaccine. Use the entire contents when first opened. Burn all the containers and unused portions of the vaccine. Clean any spills with disinfectants. Keep the vaccine away from open wounds. Wear gloves if necessary. Consult a physician if contamination occurs. Wash hands thoroughly after using the vaccine.

Warning(s): Do not vaccinate within 21 days before slaughter.

Discussion: Erysipelas is a contagious, widely distributed disease occurring as a septicemia with a sudden onset. Acute erysipelas is particularly common in turkeys resulting in high morbidity and mortality.

Product Safety: This vaccine will produce effective immunity. It has passed potency, safety and purity tests meeting all the requirements set forth by Arko Laboratories Ltd. and the USDA. The response to the product, the stimulation of antibodies within the turkey and the resultant level of immunity may be affected by other factors: Management conditions, concurrent infections and stress levels at vaccination.

Trial Data: Challenge: ARKO ERY VAC FD protected isolated turkeys in controlled laboratory experimentation against challenge with virulent erysipelas.

Presentation: 1,000 dose vials.

Compendium Code No.: 11230010

ARM & HAMMER® BIO-CHLOR®

Church & Dwight **Large Animal Dietary Supplement**

Rumen Fermentation Enhancer

Guaranteed Analysis: As Fed

Crude Protein (min.) 43.00%*
Crude Fiber 6.80%
Crude Fat 1.95%
NEL (Mcal/lb) 0.69%
Sulphur (S) (min.) 2.04%
Chloride (Cl-) (min.) 7.31%

*Includes not more than 28.0% equivalent crude protein from non-protein nitrogen.

Ingredients: Dried condensed corn fermentation solubles, processed grain by-products, natural and artificial flavors.

DCAD (Dietary Cation-Anion Difference): BIO-CHLOR® provides a source of dietary anions with a DCAD of -296 meq/100 grams. Research indicates that the optimum DCAD for transition rations is -10 to -15.

Bulk Density:

Farm Ready: 29-32 lbs/cu. ft.

Mill Mix: 32-35 lbs/cu. ft.

Indications: BIO-CHLOR® Rumen Fermentation Enhancer is a patented feed supplement for prepartum transition cows.

Dosage and Administration: Feeding Recommendations: BIO-CHLOR® should be fed as the primary protein source in prepartum cow diets. Though feeding rates will vary based on the dietary cation content of the diet, amounts of 2.0 to 2.5 pounds per cow per day should provide sufficient anionic activity for DCAD balancing in most prepartum cow rations.

For specific feeding recommendations, always consult with a nutrition advisor.

Precaution(s): Storage: BIO-CHLOR® should be stored in a cool, dry area.

Discussion: BIO-CHLOR® offers a unique solution for your transition cows' dietary needs: palatable sources of anions to balance DCAD and amino acids, peptides and non-protein nitrogen (NPN). By formulating these dietary essentials within an organic complex, they are released into the rumen at a desirable rate. This slow-release formulation allows for a more stable rumen environment and increases microbial protein production. Research shows that a stable rumen environment leads to improved dry matter intake and increased milk production.

Presentation: BIO-CHLOR® is available in 50 lb bags and two granulations: Farm Ready or Mill Mix.

ARM & HAMMER is a registered trademark of Church & Dwight Company.

Compendium Code No.: 10720001

ARM & HAMMER® FERMENTEN®

Church & Dwight **Large Animal Dietary Supplement**

Rumen Fermentation Enhancer

Guaranteed Analysis: As Fed

Crude Protein (min.) 43.00%*
Crude Fiber 8.00%
Crude Fat 2.10%
NEL (Mcal/lb) 0.74%

*Includes not more than 28.0% equivalent crude protein from non-protein nitrogen.

Ingredients: Dried condensed corn fermentation solubles, processed grain by-products, glutamic acid, natural and artificial flavors.

Bulk Density: 32-35 lbs/cu. ft.

Indications: FERMENTEN® Rumen Fermentation Enhancer is a unique feed supplement for lactating cows and growing heifers.

Dosage and Administration: Feeding Recommendations: FERMENTEN® should be fed as a protein source in both lactating cow and heifer diets.

For specific feeding recommendations, always consult with a nutrition advisor.

Lactating Cows: Feed at a rate of 1.75 to 2.00 pounds per head per day.

Heifers: Feed at a rate of 0.50 pounds per head per day for heifers up to 400 pounds and 0.75 pounds per head per day for heifers over 400 pounds.

Discussion: FERMENTEN® provides a palatable source of amino acids, peptides and non-protein nitrogen (NPN) bound within an organic complex and formulated for maximum utilization by the rumen bacteria. The patented process allows for a desirable rate of nutrient release, and FERMENTEN® provides rumen bacteria with a steady supply of this unique nutrient combination. By minimizing the nutrient level peaks and valleys, FERMENTEN® allows for a steady state environment in the rumen promoting bacterial growth and efficiency. Research shows that a stable rumen environment leads to improved dry matter intake and increased milk production in lactating cows, as well as overall heifer growth improvement.

Presentation: FERMENTEN® is available in 50 lb bags and bulk trucks.

ARM & HAMMER is a registered trademark of Church & Dwight Company.

Compendium Code No.: 10720011

ARMOR®

Westfalia•Surge **Teat Dip**

Active Ingredient(s): 0.4% (wt/wt) titratable iodine.

Non-medicinal ingredients: 5% emollient package.

Indications: A sanitizing iodine barrier teat dip.

This product aids in reducing the spread of organisms which may cause mastitis.

Directions for Use: Use at full strength. Do not dilute.

Pre Dipping: Before milking, dip or spray each teat with an approved pre-dip product. After 15 to 30 seconds, dry each teat thoroughly with a single service paper towel. If the udder and teats are heavily soiled, wash with a sanitizing solution and dry before pre-dip application.

Post-Dipping: Immediately after milking, dip each teat with ARMOR®. Allow teats to air dry.

If a common teat cup is used for application, a fresh solution should always be used at each milking. The teat dip cup should be emptied, cleaned and rinsed with potable water after each milking session or when cup becomes contaminated during milking. Do not pour remaining solution from dip cup back into original container.

Precautionary Statements: May be harmful or fatal if swallowed. Protect eyes and skin when handling. Do not take internally. Avoid breathing vapors.

Refer to Material Safety Data Sheet (MSDS).

First Aid:

If in Eyes: Flush immediately with large volumes of water for at least 15 minutes. Call a physician.

If Swallowed: Do not induce vomiting. Rinse mouth promptly then give a small amount/glass of milk or water. Avoid alcohol. Call a physician. Do not give anything by mouth to an unconscious or convulsing person.

If on Skin: Flush immediately with large volumes of water for at least 15 minutes while removing contaminated clothing and shoes. If irritation develops, get medical attention.

Inhalation of Vapors: If breathing difficulty or irritation occurs, remove to fresh air. If symptoms persist, get medical attention.

For Assistance with Medical Emergency, Call: 1-800-228-5635 ext. 149 or 1-612-851-8180 ext. 149.

Storage and Disposal: Keep from freezing. If frozen, separation may occur. Thaw completely and mix thoroughly before use.

Store this product in a cool dry area away from direct sunlight and heat to avoid deterioration.

Keep containers closed to prevent contamination of this product.

Warning(s): Danger: Keep out of reach of children. Can cause eye damage.

Presentation: Contact the company for container sizes available.

Compendium Code No.: 10020001

AR-PAC®-P+ER

Schering-Plough **Bacterin**

Bordetella bronchiseptica-Erysipelothrix rhusiopathiae-Pasteurella multocida Bacterin

U.S. Vet. Lic. No.: 165A

Active Ingredient(s): The product contains chemically-inactivated cultures of *Bordetella bronchiseptica* (piliated), *Erysipelothrix rhusiopathiae* and *Pasteurella multocida.*

Preservatives: Formaldehyde and gentamicin.

Indications: For use as an aid in the control and prevention of *Bordetella bronchiseptica* and *Erysipelothrix rhusiopathiae* and *Pasteurella multocida* infections in swine.

Dosage and Administration: Shake well before using. Inject subcutaneously using aseptic technique according to the following dosage schedule:

Sows and Gilts:

2 mL, at time of breeding.

2 mL, 7-14 days prior to first farrowing.

2 mL, 7-14 days prior to each subsequent farrowing.

Newborn:

2 mL, at seven (7) days of age.

2 mL, between 17 and 28 days of age.

Precaution(s): Store at 2-7°C (35-45°F). Do not freeze.
Caution(s): Use the entire contents when first opened. Transient local reactions may be observed at the injection site. If an allergic response occurs, administer epinephrine or its equivalent.
Warning(s): Do not vaccinate within 21 days before slaughter.
Presentation: 50 dose (100 mL) and 125 dose (250 mL) plastic vials.
Compendium Code No.: 10470020

AR-PAC®-PD+ER

Schering-Plough **Bacterin-Toxoid**

Bordetella bronchiseptica-Erysipelothrix rhusiopathiae-Pasteurella multocida Bacterin-Toxoid

U.S. Vet. Lic. No.: 165A
Active Ingredient(s): This product contains chemically-inactivated cultures of *B. bronchiseptica* (piliated), *E. rhusiopathiae* and *P. multocida* types A and D and chemically inactivated toxin of *P. multocida* type D.

Preservatives: Gentamicin.

Indications: For use in healthy swine as an aid in the control and prevention of atrophic rhinitis caused by *B. bronchiseptica* and *P. multocida* type D toxin, erysipelas caused by *E. rhusiopathiae,* and pneumonia caused by *P. multocida* type A.
Dosage and Administration: Shake well. Using aseptic technique, inject sows and gilts with 2 mL subcutaneously six (6) to seven (7) weeks and two (2) to three (3) weeks prior to the first farrowing. Inject piglets with 2 mL subcutaneously at seven (7) days of age and between 17 and 28 days of age.
Precaution(s): Store at 2-7°C (35-45°F). Do not freeze.
Caution(s): Use the entire contents when first opened. Transient local reactions may be observed at the injection site. If an allergic response occurs, administer epinephrine or its equivalent.
Warning(s): Do not vaccinate within 21 days before slaughter.
Presentation: 50 dose (100 mL) and 125 dose (250 mL) plastic vials.
Compendium Code No.: 10470030

AR-PARAPAC®+ER

Schering-Plough **Bacterin-Toxoid**

Bordetella bronchiseptica-Erysipelothrix rhusiopathiae-Haemophilus parasuis-Pasteurella multocida Bacterin-Toxoid

U.S. Vet. Lic. No.: 165A
Contents: Contains chemically-inactivated cultures of *H parasuis, B bronchiseptica, P multocida* Types A and D, and *E rhusiopathiae,* and chemically-inactivated toxin common to *P multocida* Types A and D.

Preservatives: Gentamicin and amphotericin B.

Indications: For use in healthy swine for the prevention of Glasser's disease caused by *H parasuis,* atrophic rhinitis associated with *B bronchiseptica* and *P multocida* Types A and D toxin, pneumonia caused by *P multocida* Type A, and erysipelas caused by *E rhusiopathiae.*
Dosage and Administration: Shake well. Using aseptic technique, inject sows/gilts with 2 mL subcutaneously 6 to 7 weeks and 2 to 3 weeks prior to the first farrowing, and 2 to 3 weeks prior to each subsequent farrowing. Inject piglets from vaccinated dams with 2 mL subcutaneously at 7 days of age and between 17 and 28 days of age.
Precaution(s): Store at 2° to 7°C (35° to 45°F). Do not freeze. Use entire contents when first opened.
Caution(s): Transient local reaction may occur at the injection site. If allergic response occurs, administer epinephrine.
Antidote(s): Epinephrine.
Warning(s): Do not vaccinate within 21 days prior to slaughter.

For veterinary use only.

Presentation: 25 dose (50 mL) and 50 dose (100 mL) vials.
Compendium Code No.: 10470040

ARQUEL® GRANULES ℞

Fort Dodge **Anti-inflammatory**

Meclofenamic Acid

NADA No.: 095-641
Active Ingredient(s): Each packet contains 500 mg of meclofenamic acid.
Indications: ARQUEL® is indicated for the oral treatment of acute or chronic inflammatory diseases involving the musculoskeletal system of the horse.
Pharmacology:

Description: ARQUEL® (meclofenamic acid) is a member of the fenamate group of compounds synthesized by the research laboratories of Warner Lambert. Chemically, ARQUEL® is unrelated to the corticosteroids, salicylates, indomethacin, or pyrazolones (e.g., phenylbutazone, dipyrone). Meclofenamic acid is a white, crystalline solid, almost insoluble in water, with a molecular weight of 296.2 and a melting point of 257° to 259°C. Chemically, meclofenamic acid is described as N-(2,6-dichloro-m-tolyl) anthranilic acid and is represented by the following structural formula:

COOH, Cl, NH, CH_3, Cl

Action: ARQUEL® is a nonsteroidal drug with anti-inflammatory, analgesic and antipyretic properties. Clinical studies have demonstrated the drug's ability to reduce inflammation. The analgesic effect is a result of its anti-inflammatory properties.

The mode of pharmacodynamic action has not been determined. It is believed that fenamates and certain other nonsteroidal anti-inflammatory drugs act peripherally, to inhibit the migration of monocytes from inflamed vessels inhibiting phagocytic activity, thereby preventing prostaglandin release, and centrally, via thalamocortical projection, to raise pain threshold.

Dosage and Administration: The recommended dosage for ARQUEL® (meclofenamic acid) is 1 mg/lb (2.2 mg/kg) or, in other words, 1 g (two packets) per 1,000 pounds, once daily for five to seven days for both acute and chronic conditions.

When clinical judgment indicates treatment beyond the initial five- to seven-day period, a maintenance dosage level should be individualized for each animal and may be repeated at appropriate intervals. The goal is to determine the lowest reasonable dosage for the shortest duration at a time interval which provides anti-inflammatory effect as indicated by normal locomotion and activity.

The contents of the packets can be added to the daily grain ration (a moist feed, molasses added, is suggested to prevent separation of medication from the feed).

Initial clinical signs of relief are usually noted in 72 to 96 hours.

Experimentally, horses have been maintained on the drug up to 42 days, or intermittently for as long as six months or more, without signs of intolerance or toxicity.

Contraindication(s): Meclofenamic acid should not be administered to animals with active gastrointestinal, hepatic or renal diseases.
Precaution(s): Store at controlled room temperature 15° to 30°C (59° to 86°F). Protect from moisture.
Caution(s): Federal law restricts this drug to use by or on the order of a licensed veterinarian.

This drug should be discontinued at the first signs of intolerance (e.g., gastrointestinal distress [colic], diarrhea, appetite suppression, change in stool consistency). In the treatment of inflammatory conditions associated with infections, specific anti-infective therapy is required.

Warning(s): Not for use in horses intended for food.
Adverse Reactions: At recommended dosages, side effects have been rarely reported. However, at higher dosages, a lower hematocrit was observed, as was positive occult blood in the feces. Mild colic and change in stool consistency have been observed in horses that have heavy concurrent *Gasterophilus* (bot) infestations.
Trial Data: Clinical studies, performed without benefit of placebo control, with 304 horses were undertaken by 18 investigators who conducted 14 field trials with ARQUEL® (meclofenamic acid). The drug was used in the treatment of a variety of acute or chronic inflammatory diseases of the musculoskeletal system. The horses represented a variety of breeds, with quarter horses, thoroughbreds and standardbreds the most common. ARQUEL® was consumed readily by 88.2% of the horses; those that did not accept the drug were mainly those unaccustomed to eating grain or a commercial equine feed.

The majority of the cases were diagnosed (and confirmed radiographically) as osteoarthritis, navicular disease and laminitis. Of the 279 cases in which the actual disease condition was specified, 77.8% of the animals with navicular disease improved, and 76.4% of those with laminitis improved. Of 123 animals with a poor prognosis, 72.3% showed an improvement in normal locomotion and activity.

Clinical observations by the investigators indicate that the first signs of improvement usually occur 72 to 96 hours after treatment is started.

References: Available upon request.
Presentation: ARQUEL® (meclofenamic acid) is supplied as a 5% granulation packed in 10-g packets. Boxes of 10 packets (NDC 0856-2051-01).
Manufactured by: Trillium Health Care Manufacturing Inc., Brockville, Ontario K6V 5W5
Compendium Code No.: 10030090 2050F

ARQUEL® TABLETS ℞

Fort Dodge **Analgesic-Antipyretic**

Meclofenamic Acid

NADA No.: 110-201
Active Ingredient(s): ARQUEL® Tablets contain 20 mg meclofenamic acid.
Indications: ARQUEL® is indicated for relief of signs of chronic inflammatory diseases involving the musculoskeletal system of the dog. ARQUEL® is not recommended as the initial mode of therapy because the canine gastrointestinal system is extremely sensitive to the effects of ARQUEL® and other nonsteroidal antiinflammatory drugs. Selection of ARQUEL® requires a careful assessment of the benefit/risk ratio (see Cautions, Warnings and Adverse Reactions sections).
Pharmacology: Description: ARQUEL® (meclofenamic acid) is described as N-(2,6-dichloro-m-tolyl) anthranilic acid. It is an antiinflammatory drug for oral administration. The structural formula of ARQUEL® is:

COOH, Cl, NH, CH_3, Cl

It is a white, crystalline solid, almost insoluble in water, with a molecular weight of 296.2 and a melting point of 257° to 259°C.

ARQUEL® is a nonsteroidal drug with antiinflammatory, analgesic and antipyretic properties. The mode of pharmacodynamic action has not been determined, but it is believed that fenamates and other nonsteroidal antiinflammatory drugs act to inhibit prostaglandin synthesis and to compete for binding at the prostaglandin receptor site. The exact mechanism is not understood, but it has been clearly demonstrated that it occurs before the production of the endoperoxide intermediates in the chain of reactions that leads from arachidonic acid to the production of prostaglandins. Therapeutic action does not result from pituitary adrenal stimulation. There is no evidence that ARQUEL® alters the course of the underlying disease.

Dosage and Administration: Recommended dosage of ARQUEL® for dogs is 1.1 mg/kg (0.5 mg/lb) daily for five to seven days for the relief of signs and symptoms of chronic inflammatory diseases involving the musculoskeletal system.

When clinical judgment indicates treatment beyond the initial five to seven-day period, a maintenance dosage level should be individualized for each animal and may be repeated at appropriate intervals. The ideal maintenance goal is to determine the lowest dosage for the shortest duration of time, at an interval which provides antiinflammatory effect as evidenced by normal locomotion and activity. If the duration of therapy is extended, periodic evaluations should be made to insure that the drug is still necessary and well tolerated.

Initial clinical signs of relief are usually noted in 72 to 96 hours.

Contraindication(s): ARQUEL® should not be administered to animals with congestive heart failure or active gastrointestinal, hepatic or renal disease.
Precaution(s): Store at controlled room temperature 15° to 30°C (59° to 86°F). Protect from moisture.
Caution(s): Federal law restricts this drug to use by or on the order of a licensed veterinarian.

The dosage should not exceed 0.5 mg/lb.

The dog should be carefully observed for signs of bloody (red) or tarry (black) stools or diarrhea. The veterinarian should be contacted immediately if any of these conditions are observed.

Animals receiving nonsteroidal antiinflammatory agents, such as ARQUEL®, should be evaluated periodically to ensure that the drug is still necessary and well tolerated. These periodic evaluations should include fecal examinations for the presence of occult blood and, if positive, a determination of hemoglobin and hematocrit values to assess possible chronic blood loss.

Caution should be exercised in prescribing NSAIDs to animals at risk of renal complications. This high risk group comprises animals with chronic renal insufficiency, congestive heart failure, hepatic cirrhosis and volume contraction secondary to nephrotic syndrome or diuretic use. NSAID therapy should also be withheld from animals that are about to undergo surgery because of the risk of acute renal failure due to decreased renal blood flow, as well as of impaired homeostasis due to the effects of these agents on platelet function.[1]

Fertility impairment studies have not been conducted in the dog with ARQUEL® (meclofenamic acid). It is not known if ARQUEL® can cause impairment of fertility in the dog. ARQUEL® should be given to the dog only if clearly needed, and the possibility of a risk of impaired fertility is accepted.

Reproduction studies during pregnancy have not been conducted with ARQUEL®. It is not known if ARQUEL® can cause harm to the embryo or fetus. ARQUEL® should be used in pregnant dogs only if the potential benefit justifies a potential risk to the unborn.

The safety and effectiveness of the drug have not been established for dogs below the age of 8 months.

Warning(s): The canine species has a gastrointestinal tract that is extremely sensitive to nonsteroidal antiinflammatory drugs (NSAIDs). It is approximately four times more sensitive than the human and twice as sensitive as the horse based on maximum tolerated dose.

Dosage should not exceed 1.1 mg/kg (0.5 mg/lb) or signs of gastrointestinal intolerance (diarrhea, bloody or tarry stools) will become evident in most animals.

If signs of intolerance (e.g., gastrointestinal distress, diarrhea, appetite suppression, change in stool consistency) are severe, the drug should be discontinued until the signs subside. Therapy can then be restarted at a lower dose and gradually increased. If the above signs of intolerance are not severe, therapy may be continued at a lower dose to determine the dog's response to this regimen of therapy. In the treatment of inflammatory conditions associated with infections, specific antiinfective therapy must be administered (see Adverse Reactions and Dosage and Administration sections).

For oral use in dogs only.

Adverse Reactions: In the controlled clinical studies there were 102 dogs treated with ARQUEL®.

The following adverse reactions were reported.

Gastrointestinal: The most frequently reported adverse reactions associated with ARQUEL® involved the gastrointestinal system. These disturbances occurred in the following decreasing order of frequency with the approximate incidences in parentheses: vomiting (6%), bloody diarrhea (5%), diarrhea (4%), anorexia (3%). Other gastrointestinal reactions reported at incidences less than 1% included tarry stool and constipation.

Central Nervous System: Malaise, lassitude, drowsiness (4%).

Integumentary: Dermatitis (<1%).

Urinary System: Incontinence (<1%), inability to urinate (<1%), polyuria (<1%), increased thirst (<1%).

Fatalities: One fatality occurred during the clinical studies; the cause of death was not determined.

In the uncontrolled clinical studies 517 dogs were treated with ARQUEL®.

The following adverse reactions were reported.

Gastrointestinal: The most frequently reported adverse reactions involved the gastrointestinal system. These disturbances occurred in the following decreasing order of frequency with the approximate incidences in parentheses: vomiting (5%), diarrhea (4%), anorexia (1.7%), bloody diarrhea (0.8%), tarry stools (0.4%), constipation (0.2%).

Central Nervous System: Fatigue, depression (<1%), personality change (<1%), hyperthermia, hyperventilation (<1%).

Cardiovascular: Edema (<1%).

Urinary System: Incontinence (<1%).

Fatalities: One fatality occurred; the cause of death was not determined.

References: Available upon request.

Presentation: ARQUEL® (meclofenamic acid) 20 mg - Each white round scored tablet contains 20 mg of meclofenamic acid. Available in bottles of 500.

NDC 0856-5474-01 - 20 mg - bottles of 500

Compendium Code No.: 10030101 5470F

ARREST® DIP/SPRAY

Westfalia•Surge **Teat Dip**

Active Ingredient(s): Contains:

Chlorhexidine digluconate 0.50%

Contains skin conditioning agents in a stable pH aqueous base.

Indications: This product has been tested according to recognized protocols under farm conditions of exposure to known mastitis causing organisms and has been proven effective in reducing new infections of mastitis.

Dosage and Administration: Thoroughly cover at least the lower one-third (⅓) of each teat immediately after milking with ARREST®. At the end of lactation, apply ARREST® daily for one (1) week after milking. In addition, begin application of ARREST® about one (1) week prior to parturition.

A fresh solution of teat dip should always be used at each milking. The teat dip cup should be emptied, cleaned and rinsed with potable water after each milking session or when cup becomes contaminated during milking. Do not pour remaining solution from dip cup back into the original container.

Precaution(s): Store ARREST® in cool, dry place. Keep from freezing. If frozen, thaw completely and mix well prior to use. Keep containers closed to prevent contamination of teat dip.

Caution(s): Danger - Keep out of the reach of children. Can cause eye damage. Protect eyes when handling. Do not get in eyes or on clothing. Harmful if swallowed. Avoid contamination of food.

First Aid:

Eyes: In case of contact with eyes, flush immediately with plenty of water for at least 15 minutes. Call a physician.

Internal: Do not take internally. If swallowed, promptly drink a large quantity of milk, egg whites, gelatin solution. If these are not available, drink large quantities of water. Avoid alcohol. Call a physician.

General Chemical Warnings: Always read label directions completely before using product. Always exercise caution when handling any chemicals. Avoid contact with eyes, skin and clothing. Never dispense any chemical product from its original container into another container for storage or resale. Never mix two or more products together. Mixing of products could result in release of toxic gases and/or render product ineffective for recommended use application.

Always use product in ventilated area. Avoid inhaling vapors or fumes. Always use product according to recommendations for particular application. Never exceed recommended usage without consulting trained personnel.

Presentation: Contact the company for container sizes available.

* ARREST is a registered trademark of Westfalia•Surge, Inc.

Compendium Code No.: 10020021

ARTEC™

Ecolab Food & Bev. Div. **Teat Dip**

Active Ingredient(s):

Heptanoic Acid 1.5%

Inert Ingredients 98.5%

Formula ingredients contain no phosphorus.

Contains 78% emollient system including glycerin and lanolin.

Indications: ARTEC™ is a unique, patent pending, fatty acid based teat dip that provides protection against mastitis-causing pathogens.

Equally effective against both contagious and environmental mastitis organisms, such as *Escherichia coli, Streptococcus agalactiae, Streptococcus uberis* and *Staphylococcus aureus.*

Pharmacology: Properties:

Form .... liquid

Color .... blue

Odor .... mint

Spec. Grav. @ 68°F (20°C) 1.071

Pounds per gallon........ 8.92 (4.05 kg)

100% pH........ 4.5

Directions for Use:

Pre-Milking: Ecolab recommends the use of an approved pre-dip.

Post-Milking: Immediately after milking, use ARTEC™ at full strength. Submerge teat ⅔ their length in ARTEC™ teat dip. Allow to air dry. Do not wipe. Always use fresh, full strength ARTEC™ teat dip. If the product in the dip cup becomes visibly dirty, discard contents and replenish with fresh product. Do not reuse or return unused product to the original container Do not turn cows into freezing weather until ARTEC™ teat dip is completely dry or wiped.

Expanding Usage: End of lactation - use daily for one week. Prior to parturition - use daily for one week. Follow post-milking instructions for complete use directions.

Caution(s): Important: Do not add ARTEC™ to any other teat dip or other product. If transferred from this container to any other, make sure the other container is thoroughly pre-cleaned and bears the proper container labeling for ARTEC™. Use of a complete cow care program including both pre- and post- dipping may aid reducing the spread of organisms which may cause mastitis.

Presentation: 4x1 gallon, 5 gallons, 15 gallons, and 55 gallons.

Patent Pending

Compendium Code No.: 14490160 30862/0300/0900

ARTHRICARE™ CHEWABLE TABLETS FOR LARGE DOGS ℞

V.P.L. **Non-Steroidal Anti-Inflammatory**

Active Ingredient(s): Each tablet contains 273 mg of buffered, microencapsulated aspirin.

Other Ingredients: Calcium phosphate, microcrystalline cellulose, sucrose, aspirin, liver powder, hydrolyzed vegetable oil, stearic acid, silicon dioxide, zinc oxide, iron oxide, fish oil, vitamin E, beta carotene, ascorbic acid (vitamin C), copper sulfate, manganese sulfate, calcium pantothenate, vitamin A, riboflavin (vitamin B_2), pyridoxine HCl (vitamin B_6), thiamine mononitrate (vitamin B_1), niacin (vitamin B_3), TBHQ (a preservative), menadione (vitamin K), folic acid, biotin, selenium, cyanocobalamin (vitamin B_{12}).

Blended in a roast beef and liver flavor enhancing base.

Indications: Aids in the temporary relief of pain and inflammation associated with arthritis and joint problems in dogs.

Dosage and Administration: Recommended aspirin dosage is 15 mg/kg body weight (6.82 mg/lb) every 12 hours.

1 tablet per 40 pounds body weight every 12 hours. Recommended dosage levels may be increased or decreased at the discretion of a veterinarian.

For dogs only. ARTHRICARE™ Chewable Tablets may be offered free choice or crumbled and mixed with food. Give at or immediately before mealtime.

Contraindication(s): Not for use in cats.

Precaution(s): Store at or below 86°F.

Caution(s): Federal law restricts this drug to use by or on the order of a licensed veterinarian.

If vomiting or diarrhea occur, stop administration or decrease dosage and consult your veterinarian. Not for use in cats.

Warning(s): Keep out of reach of children.

Presentation: 60 tablets (for large dogs).

Compendium Code No.: 11430081

ARTHRO EASE™

Horses Prefer **Analgesic-Topical**

Fast Acting Topical Pain Reliever

Ingredient(s): D.I. Water, Mineral Oil, Glycerin, Capsaicin, Wintergreen Oil, Laureth, Polyacrelamide, Polysorbate, DMDM Hydantoin, Methyl Paraben, Propyl Paraben, Propylene glycol, FD and C Blue #1, FD and C Yellow #5.

No artificial fragrance added.

Indications: For temporary relief of joint aches and pains.

Directions: Apply ARTHRO EASE™ liberally to the affected areas 2-3 times a day, but do not rub vigorously. Clip hair of the area to be treated, if hair is excessively long. Apply to all sides of a joint where applicable. Wash hands thoroughly after application.

Do not apply to open cuts.

Caution(s): Avoid contact with eyes, nose, and mucus membrane. In the event of contact, rinse with water. Wash hands thoroughly after each application. Discontinue use, if excessive irritation occurs and if conditions persists contact your veterinarian.

For animal use.

For external use only.

Warning(s): Keep out of reach of children.

Presentation: 8 oz.

Compendium Code No.: 36950002

ART VAX®

Schering-Plough **Vaccine**

Bordetella Avium Vaccine, Avirulent Live Culture

U.S. Vet. Lic. No.: 165A

Contents: ART VAX® vaccine is a live bacterial vaccine containing a chemically-induced mutant of *Bordetella avium* which is immunogenic for turkeys when given by spray at one day of age, then in the drinking water at 2 weeks of age.

Indications: For use in turkeys as an aid in preventing *B. avium* rhinotracheitis (turkey coryza) through vaccination by spray application and in the drinking water.

Dosage and Administration: When to Vaccinate: Vaccinate by spray at one day of age, then in the drinking water at 2 weeks of age. Revaccinate every 4 to 6 weeks thereafter as necessary according to exposure conditions. Good management practices must be followed to reduce exposure of birds to virulent *B. avium* during the first several weeks of life. Vaccination after infection with a field strain of *B. avium* is ineffective.

Your Vaccination Program: The development of a durable, strong protection to this disease depends upon the use of an effective vaccination program as well as many circumstances such as administration techniques, environment and flock health at the time of vaccination. Also, the immune response to one vaccination under field conditions is seldom complete for all animals within a given flock. Even when vaccination is successful, the protection stimulated in individual animals against different diseases may not be life long. Therefore, a program of periodic revaccination may be necessary.

Preparation of the Vaccine:

For Drinking Water:

1. Assemble the vaccine and equipment needed to vaccinate the entire flock at one time.
2. Do not open and rehydrate the vaccine until ready for use.
3. Remove the tear-off aluminum seal from the vaccine vial without disturbing the rubber stopper.
4. Use cool, clean, non-chlorinated tap water to which powdered milk has been added as directed under How to Vaccinate.
5. Remove the rubber stopper from the vaccine vial and rehydrate the vaccine by filling the vial about half-full with tap water (milk added).
6. Reseat the stopper and shake the vial to thoroughly dissolve the vaccine.

For Spray: Rehydrate each 1000 doses of vaccine to 140 mL using sterile water as diluent.

How to Vaccinate:

By Spray: Use this method for one day of age vaccination. Proper coarse spray application of this vaccine is best accomplished through use of a clean spray cabinet, such as the ASL Spramark II, which delivers 7 mL per shot. Spray each poult box twice for a total of 14 mL of vaccine per 100 poults.

By Drinking Water: Do not mix the vaccine into the drinking water until ready for use. Drinking water for vaccination should be mixed with powdered milk to prevent possible inactivation from chlorine or other water additives and also to stabilize the vaccine bacteria. The powdered milk should be added to the water at the rate of 3 grams per 11 liters (one heaped teaspoon per 3 U.S. gallons or 2.5 Imp. gallons); or 87 grams per 190 liters (one heaped cupful per 50 U.S. gallons or 41 Imp. gallons).

Use only clean waterers and equipment free of disinfectants or sanitizers. All water must be withheld for at least 2 hours prior to vaccination to assure that all turkeys drink. Mix the rehydrated vaccine in the quantity of drinking water (milk added) which will be consumed by thirsty turkeys in approximately 2 hours.

The following schedule is a general guideline for the amount of water to use with the vaccine. These amounts will vary depending upon the individual management conditions, climate, age and sex of the birds.

Each 1,000 Birds:

Age	Liters	U.S. Gal	Imperial Gal
2 wks.	30	8	7
3 wks.	45	12	10
4 wks.	61	16	14
5 wks.	76	20	17
6 wks.	99	26	22
7 wks.	121	32	27
8 wks.	152	40	34
9 wks.	182	48	41

Another helpful guideline for daily water consumption is 3.8 liters (one U.S. gallon or 0.8 Imp. gallon) of water per week of age per 100 poults; figure 40% of this amount. This 40% is about a 3 hour supply for the flock.

Distribute 1,000 doses of vaccine in water as used by 1,000 turkeys. Provide ample water space so that all turkeys can drink easily. Do not administer through the water lines with a proportioner or medication tank.

Records: Keep a record of vaccine type, quantity, serial number, expiration date and place of purchase; the date and time of vaccination; the number, age, breed, and location of the birds; names of operators performing the vaccination and any observed reactions.

Contraindication(s): Turkeys must be healthy and free of environmental or physical stress at the time of vaccination. Do not use this vaccine within 10 days before or 10 days after vaccinating turkeys with live virus or live bacterial vaccines.

Precaution(s): Store at 2° to 7°C (35° to 45°F).

Do not spill or spatter the vaccine. Burn empty bottles, caps and all unused vaccine and accessories. Use entire contents of vial when first opened.

Caution(s):

1. For veterinary use only.
2. To avoid interference with the development of protection, turkeys to be water vaccinated should not be given any antibiotic and/or sulfonamide medication used in the prevention or treatment of *B. avium* rhinotracheitis for 3 days before and 5 days after vaccination.
3. Vaccinate only healthy birds. Coccidiosis, respiratory disease, mycoplasma infection, or other disease conditions may cause serious complications or reduce protection. Avoid exposing birds other than turkeys to the vaccine.
4. All birds within a flock should be vaccinated on the same day. Isolate other susceptible birds on the premises from the birds being vaccinated.
5. In outbreak situations, vaccinate houses of healthy birds first, progressing toward houses of affected birds. Vaccination of affected house of birds is not recommended. Under these conditions, use an effective treatment.
6. Wash hands thoroughly after using the vaccine.
7. Do not dilute the vaccine or otherwise stretch the dosage.

Warning(s): Do not vaccinate within 21 days of slaughter.

Presentation: Supplied in 10 x 1,000 dose units.

Compendium Code No.: 10470061

ARVAC®

Fort Dodge **Vaccine**

Equine Arteritis Vaccine, Modified Live Virus

U.S. Vet. Lic. No.: 112

Composition: ARVAC® is a dessicated preparation containing viable modified Equine Arteritis virus propagated on an equine cell line culture system.

This vaccine has been tested and shown to be satisfactory for marketing in accordance with procedures required by the U.S. Department of Agriculture.

Neomycin, polymyxin B and amphotericin B added as preservatives.

Indications: For the vaccination of healthy non-stressed horses to stimulate the development of protection against viral abortion and respiratory infection due to equine arteritis virus.

Dosage and Administration: Aseptically rehydrate to liquid form using the diluent supplied. Administer one 1 mL dose intramuscularly. Vaccinate males and young animals at any time, but stallions should be vaccinated not less than 3 weeks prior to breeding. Vaccinate mares preferably as maidens or when open. Mares in foal should not be vaccinated until after foaling and then not less than 3 weeks prior to breeding. Maiden and barren mares may be vaccinated anytime but should be vaccinated not less than 3 weeks prior to breeding. See section on Cautions. Repeat with annual booster dose.

Precaution(s): Store in dark at 2° to 7°C (35° to 45°F). Use entire contents within 60 minutes after rehydration. Burn container and unused contents.

Caution(s): In case of anaphylactic reaction, administer epinephrine.

The vaccinal virus has been modified to the extent that it may be irregularly infective when given by natural portraits of entry. A high degree of safety has been demonstrated for horses of any age and pregnant mares.[1] However, the vaccination of foals under six weeks of age is not recommended except in emergency situations when threatened by natural exposure.

Pregnant mares should not be vaccinated during the last two months of gestation since a few instances of fetal invasion by vaccinal virus have been demonstrated during this period. It is preferable to immunize mares during the maiden or open periods; however, when pregnant mares are threatened by known natural exposure, vaccination may be undertaken with considerably less risk than is inherent in natural infection. Owners are to be advised of the possibility of fetal infection before vaccinating pregnant mares.

Mild post-vaccinal febrile reactions and normal total white counts with mild transient lymphopenia have occurred in some vaccinates. Vaccinated horses will serologically convert, a condition that should be kept in mind in the case of animals intended for export to countries with regulations regarding EAV.

Distribution shall be limited to those States where authorized by proper State officials and under such additional conditions as these authorities may require. For veterinary use only.

Warning(s): Do not vaccinate within 21 days before slaughter.

Discussion: Disease Information: Equine Arteritis Virus (EAV) is known to infect only equines. The severity of the disease is variable ranging from highly acute to subclinical in nature. The acute disease is characterized clinically by fever, leukopenia, depression, nasal discharge, lacrimation, conjunctivitis, photophobia, edema of the face, limbs, transient maculopapular skin rash and produces abortion in pregnant mares. The most consistent clinical signs have been hyperthermia, leukopenia and edema of the eye. There may be colic, diarrhea and severe loss of weight with dehydration.

References: Available upon request.

Presentation: Package of 10 dose (10 x 1 mL) vials.

Compendium Code No.: 10030112 1700F

ASEPTICARE® TB+II

Ecolab Prof. Prod. Div. **Disinfectant**

Germicidal Solution-One-step cleaner, disinfectant & deodorizer

EPA Reg. No.: 1130-15-1677

Active Ingredient(s):

N-Alkyl (68% C_{12}, 32% C_{14}) dimethyl ethylbenzyl ammonium chloride 0.154%
N-Alkyl (60% C_{14}, 30% C_{16}, 5% C_{12}, 5% C_{18}) dimethyl benzyl ammonium chloride ... 0.154%
Isopropanol 21.000%
Inert Ingredients: 78.692%

Indications: A novel way to effectively clean, deodorize and sanitize against odor-causing organisms and disinfect hard surfaces. Kills dangerous germs such as *Salmonella choleraesuis, Staphylococcus aureus, Pseudomonas aeruginosa* and *Klebsiella pneumoniae* in 10 minutes. Kills dangerous viruses such as Influenza A2/HK and Herpes Simplex Type II in 30 seconds. Kills Mycobacterium bovis BCG (Tuberculosis) in 6 minutes at 20°C. Kills Polio I Virus and Rhinovirus (associated with common colds) in 3 minutes. Kills HIV-1 (AIDS Virus) on pre-cleaned environmental surfaces or objects previously soiled with blood or body fluids in 30 seconds at room temperature (20-25°C) in health care settings or other settings in which there is an expected likelihood of soiling of inanimate surfaces/objects with blood or body fluids and in which the surfaces/objects likely to be soiled with blood or body fluids can be associated with the potential for transmission of the human immunodeficiency virus Type 1 (HIV-1) associated with AIDS.

Kills *Trichophyton mentagrophytes, Aspergillus niger* and *Candida albicans* in 5 minutes at 20°C. Kills pathogenic fungi in 5 minutes at 20°C.

Bactericidal, Tuberculocidal, Fungicidal and Virucidal.

For use in hospitals — veterinary clinics; on toilet seats and bathroom fixtures; bedpans: sickrooms; offices; on telephones. For use on stainless steel, chrome, porcelain, glass, Formica, vinyl, plastic and other hard, non-porous surfaces of respirators and respirator facepieces and CPR training mannequins.

Directions for Use: To Disinfect Non-Food Contact Surfaces: It is a violation of Federal law to use this in a manner inconsistent with its labeling. This product is not to be used as a terminal sterilant/high level disinfectant on any surface or instrument that (1) is introduced directly into the human body, either into or in contact with the bloodstream or normally sterile areas of the body, or (2) contacts intact mucous membranes but which does not ordinarily penetrate the blood barrier or otherwise enter normally sterile areas of the body. This product may be used to preclean or decontaminate critical or semi-critical medical devices prior to sterilization or high level disinfection. Remove gross filth. Use solution as is. Do not dilute. Soak items to be disinfected or apply solution with cloth or sponge so as to thoroughly wet surface. Allow to remain wet for 10 minutes, let air dry.

Special Instructions for Cleaning and Decontamination Against HIV-1 (AIDS Virus) for Surfaces or Objects Soiled with Blood or Body Fluids.

Personal Protection: When using this product, wear disposable latex gloves, protective gown, face masks or eye coverings as appropriate when handling HIV-1 infected blood or body fluids.

Cleaning Procedure: All blood and other body fluids must be thoroughly cleaned from surfaces and objects before application of this product.

Contact Time: Thoroughly wet surface. Allow to remain wet 30 seconds, let air dry. Although efficacy at a 30 second contact time has been shown to be adequate against HIV-1 (AIDS virus) this contact time would not be sufficient for other organisms. Use a 10 minute contact time for disinfection against all of the organisms claimed.

Precautionary Statements: Hazards to Humans and Domestic Animals:

Caution: Harmful if absorbed through skin. Causes moderate eye irritation. Avoid contact with eyes, skin, or clothing. Wash thoroughly with soap and water after handling.

Statement of Practical Treatment:

If on Skin: Wash with plenty of soap and water.

If in Eyes: Flush eyes with plenty of water. Call a physician if irritation persists.

Physical or Chemical Hazards: Do not store near heat or open flame.

Storage and Disposal: Store in cool, well-ventilated area.

Disposal: Wastes resulting from the use of this product may be discarded by pouring down drain and flushing with large quantity of water.

Container Disposal: Do not reuse empty container. Wrap container and put in trash.

Disposal of Infectious Material: Dispose of used solution in accordance with local regulations for infectious waste disposal.

Warning(s): Keep out of reach of children.

Presentation: 32 fl oz (946 mL) and 2.5 gallons.

Compendium Code No.: 10160021 722374/8902/0801

ASEPTI-HB™

Ecolab Prof. Prod. Div. **Disinfectant**

Disinfectant Spray

EPA Reg. No.: 61178-2-1677

Active Ingredient(s):

Alkyl (C_{14} 60%, C_{16} 30%, C_{12} 5%, C_{18} 5%) Dimethyl Benzyl Ammonium Chloride..... 0.07%
Alkyl (C_{12} 68%, C_{14} 32%) Dimethyl Ethylbenzyl Ammonium Chloride 0.07%
Inert Ingredients: 99.86%
Total: 100 00%

Indications: A disinfectant spray for use on hard, non-porous inanimate environmental surfaces in hospitals, clinics, day care centers, vet centers, homes, restaurants, hotels, motels, health clubs, and spas.

Directions for Use: It is a violation of Federal Law to use this product in a manner inconsistent with its labeling. To clean, deodorize, and disinfect, hold dispenser 10 inches from the surface, press atomizer with quick short strokes, spraying evenly until wet. Wait for the appropriate contact time. Controls cross contamination from treated inanimate environmental surfaces as a disinfectant spray. For use on toilet seats, telephones, door knobs and similar hard, nonporous inanimate environmental surfaces.

*Kills HIV-1 (AIDS, human immunodeficiency virus Type 1), Herpes simplex Type 1 and Type 2, Parainfluenza Type 1, Influenza B (Allen) virus, Measles virus and Pseudorabies in 30 seconds. Kills Influenza A2 (Asian) in 50 seconds. Kills HBV (Hepatitis B Virus) in 10 minutes. (For California use only; HBV contact time is 15 minutes). Kills *Pseudomonas aeruginosa, Neisseria gonorrhoeae, Salmonella choleraesuis, Staphylococcus aureus, Legionella pneumophila, Treponema pallidum* (ATCC #27087) and *Aspergillus niger* in 10 minutes.

Kills HIV-1 and HBV on precleaned environmental surfaces/objects previously soiled with blood/body fluids in health care settings or other settings in which there is an expected likelihood of soiling of inanimate surfaces/objects with blood or body fluids, and in which the surfaces/objects likely to be soiled with blood or body fluids can be associated with the potential for transmission of Human Immunodeficiency virus Type 1 (H1V-1 associated with AIDS virus) or Hepatitis B Virus (HBV).

Special Instructions for Cleaning and Decontamination Against HIV-1 and HBV for Surfaces/Objects Soiled with Blood or Body Fluids.

Personal Protection: Specific barrier protection items to be used when handling items soiled with blood or body fluids are disposable latex gloves, gown, masks, or eye coverings.

Cleaning Procedure: Blood and other body fluids must be thoroughly cleaned from surfaces and objects before application of this disinfectant.

Disposal of Infectious Materials: Blood and other body fluids should be autoclaved and disposed of according to federal, state and local regulations for infectious waste disposal.

Contact Time: Leave surfaces wet for 30 seconds and 10 minutes for HIV-1 and HBV, respectively. The 30 second contact time will not control other common types of viruses and bacteria. (For California use only: HBV contact time is 15 minutes).

Kills Herpes simplex Types 1 and 2 and Influenza B in 30 seconds (Influenza A2 in 50 seconds) on inanimate environmental surfaces, cleans as it disinfects.

Spray: Furniture, toilet seats, telephones, door knobs, light switches and shower stalls. For Use In: Hospitals and sickrooms, public restrooms, fast food chains, airplanes, hotels, motels, day care centers, veterinary clinics and health clubs/spas. For: Doctors, nurses, paramedics, CPR instructors, firefighters, police, vacationers and business travelers.

This product is not to be used as a terminal sterilant/high level disinfectant on any surface or instrument that (1) is introduced directly into the human body, either into or in contact with the bloodstream or normally sterile areas of the body, or (2) contacts intact mucous membranes but which does not ordinarily penetrate the blood barrier or otherwise enter normally sterile areas of the body. This product may he used to preclean or decontaminate critical or semi-critical medical devices prior to sterilization or high level disinfection.

Kills	Contact Time
HBV (Hepatitis B virus) (For California Use Only: HBV contact time is 15 minutes)	10 minutes
HIV-1 (AIDS virus, human immunodeficiency virus Type 1)	30 seconds
Herpes simplex virus type	30 seconds
Herpes simplex virus type 2	30 seconds
Parainfluenza type 1 virus	30 seconds
Pseudorabies virus	30 seconds
Influenza A2 (Asian) virus	50 seconds
Influenza A/Brazil virus	10 minutes
Influenza B (Allen) virus	30 seconds
Measles virus	30 seconds
Pseudomonas aeruginosa	10 minutes
Salmonella choleraesuis	10 minutes
Staphylococcus aureus	10 minutes
Aspergillus niger	10 minutes
Legionella pneumophila	10 minutes
Neisseria gonorrhoeae	10 minutes
Streptococcus pyogenes	10 minutes
Treponema pallidum (ATCC #27087)	10 minutes

Precautionary Statements: Hazard to Humans and Domestic Animals: Avoid contact with eyes. In case of contact flush eyes with water. Get medical attention if irritation persists.

Storage and Disposal: Wrap empty container and dispose in trash container.

Warning(s): Keep out of reach of children.

Presentation: 32 fl. oz./946 mL.

Compendium Code No.: 10160000 726987/8901/1298

ASEPTI-WIPE™

Ecolab Prof. Prod. Div. **Disinfectant**

Germicidal Disposable Cloth

EPA Reg. No.: 9480-5-303

Active Ingredient(s):

n-Alkyl (68% C_{12}, 32% C_{14}) dimethyl ethylbenzyl ammonium chlorides............ 0.14%
n-Alkyl (60% C_{14}, 30% C_{16}, 5% C_{12}, 5% C_{18}) dimethyl benzyl ammonium chlorides ... 0.14%
Isopropyl Alcohol 8.00%
Inert Ingredients 91.72%
Total:........ 100.00%

Indications: Disinfects Environmental Surfaces:

- Effective against *Staphylococcus aureus, Salmonella choleraesuis, Pseudomonas aeruginosa, Klebsiella pneumoniae* in 5 minutes.
- Kills dangerous viruses such as Influenza A2/HK and Herpes Simplex Type II in 30 seconds.
- Kills *Mycobacterium bovis* BCG (Tuberculosis) in 10 minutes at 20°C.
- Kills HIV on pre-cleaned environmental surfaces/objects previously soiled with blood/body fluids in 30 seconds at room temperature (20-25°C) in healthcare or other settings in which there is an expected likelihood of soiling of inanimate surfaces/objects with blood or body fluids, and in which the surfaces/objects likely to be soiled with blood or body fluids can be associated with the potential for transmission of human immunodeficiency virus Type I (HIV-1).

A dual chain quaternary/alcohol solution impregnated in a wiping cloth.

A non woven disposable cloth for use in hospitals and other critical care areas where control of the hazards of cross-contamination is required. Use on surfaces and equipment such as stainless steel, Formica, glass tables, carts, baskets, counters, cabinets, telephones and other hard non-porous surfaces.

Some Areas of Use: Hard surfaces in Surgery, Recovery, Anesthesia, X-Ray Cat. Lab, E.R., Orthopedics, New Born Nursery, Respiratory Therapy, Radiology, Central Supply.

Directions for Use: To Disinfect Non-Food Contact Surfaces: It is a violation of Federal Law to use this product in a manner inconsistent with its labeling.

Dispenser: To start feed: Remove large cover and discard seal from container. From center of towelette roll, pull up towelette corner, twist it into a point and thread it through the hole in the container cover. Pull through about one inch. Replace cover. Pull out first towelette and snap off at a 90° angle. Remaining towelettes feed automatically ready for next use. When through using, keep small center cap closed to prevent moisture loss.

Open, unfold, wipe to remove gross filth. Use second towel to thoroughly wet surface. Allow to remain wet for 5 minutes where required let air dry.

"This product is not to be used as a terminal sterilant/high level disinfectant on any surface or instrument that (1) is introduced directly into the human body, either into or in contact with the bloodstream or normally sterile areas of the body, or (2) contacts intact mucous membranes but which does not originally penetrate the blood barrier or otherwise enter normally sterile areas of the body. This product may be used to preclean or decontaminate critical or semi-critical medical devices prior to sterilization or high level disinfection".

Special Instructions for Cleaning and Decontamination Against HIV-1 for Surfaces or Objects Soiled with Blood or Body Fluids:

Personal Protection: When using the germicidal cloth, wear disposable protective gloves, protective gowns, face masks, or eye coverings as appropriate when handling HIV-1 infected blood or body fluids.

Cleaning Procedure: All blood and other body fluids must be thoroughly cleaned from surface and objects before disinfection by the germicidal cloth. Open, unfold first germicidal cloth to remove gross filth.

Contact Time: Use second germicidal cloth to thoroughly wet surface. Allow to remain wet 30 seconds, let air dry. Although efficacy at a 30 second contact time has been shown to be adequate against HIV-1 (AIDS Virus) this time would not be sufficient for other organisms. Use listed disinfection times against all of the organisms claimed.

Precautionary Statements: Hazards to Humans and Domestic Animals:

Caution: Avoid contact with eyes. In case of eye contact, flush with plenty of water for at least 15 minutes. If irritation persists, call a physician.

Storage and Disposal:

Towelette: Do not reuse towel. Dispose of used towel in trash.

Dispenser: Do not reuse empty container. Wrap container and put in trash collection.

Do not use or store near heat or open flame.

Disposal of Infectious Materials: Dispose of used towelette in accordance with local regulations for infectious waste disposal.

Warning(s): Keep out of reach of children.

Presentation: 180 wipes/unit - 6 x 6.75".

Compendium Code No.: 10160011 739447/8901/0301; 718912/8900/0697

ASPIRIN 60 GRAIN

Butler **Non-Steroidal Anti-Inflammatory**

Active Ingredient(s): Each tablet contains:
Acetylsalicylic acid (aspirin) . . . . . 60 grains

Indications: To be used orally as an aid in reducing fever and as an aid in the relief of minor muscular aches and joint pain.

Dosage and Administration: Administer orally.
To mature horses and cattle, give 6-12 tablets; to foals and calves, 2-4 tablets; to sheep and swine, ¼-1 tablet, as indicated. Allow the animals to drink water after administration.

Precaution(s): Do not store above 30°C (86°F).
Caution(s): For veterinary use only.
Warning(s): Not for use in lactating dairy animals.
Presentation: Bottles of 100 tablets.
Compendium Code No.: 10820101

ASPIRIN 240 GRAIN BOLUSES

Vedco **Non-Steroidal Anti-Inflammatory**

Active Ingredient(s): Each bolus contains:
Acetylsalicylic acid . . . . . 240 gr.

Indications: To be used orally as an aid in reducing fever and for the relief of minor muscular aches and joint pain.

Dosage and Administration: Horses and Cattle: One (1) to three (3) boluses, two (2) or three (3) times a day. Discontinue if any unusual symptoms should appear.

Precaution(s): Do not store above 86°F (30°C).
Caution(s): Keep out of the reach of children.
Warning(s): Not for use in lactating dairy animals.
Presentation: 50 boluses per container.
Compendium Code No.: 10940061

ASPIRIN 480 GRAIN BOLUSES

Vedco **Non-Steroidal Anti-Inflammatory**

Active Ingredient(s): Each bolus contains: Acetylsalicylic acid 480 grains (31.2 g).

Indications: To be used orally as an aid in reducing fever and in relief of minor aches and joint pains in cattle and horses.

Dosage and Administration: Mature horses and cattle, administer orally ½ to 1½ boluses 2 to 3 times daily. Lubricate bolus and administer with balling gun. Allow animals ample supply of fresh water after administration.

Precaution(s): Keep lid tightly closed and store in a dry place.
Do not store above 30°C (86°F).

Warning(s): For veterinary use only. Keep out of reach of children.
Presentation: 50 boluses.
Compendium Code No.: 10940071

ASPIRIN BOLUS

Aspen **Non-Steroidal Anti-Inflammatory**

Analgesic-Antipyretic

Active Ingredient(s): Each bolus contains:
Acetylsalicylic Acid . . . . . 240 grains (15.6 g)

Indications: To be used orally as an aid in reducing fever and in relief of minor muscular aches and joint pains in cattle and horses.

Dosage and Administration: Mature Horses and Cattle, administer orally 1 to 3 boluses two to three times daily. Lubricate bolus and administer with balling gun.
Allow animals ample supply of fresh clean water after administration.

Precaution(s): Keep lid tightly closed and store in a dry place.
Do not store above 30°C (86°F).

Warning(s): For animal use only. Keep out of reach of children.
Presentation: 50 boluses.
Compendium Code No.: 14750051

ASPIRIN BOLUS

Durvet **Non-Steroidal Anti-Inflammatory**

NDC No.: 30798-003-69

Active Ingredient(s): Each bolus contains:
Acetylsalicylic acid . . . . . 240 grains (15.6 g)

Indications: For use as an aid in the reduction of fever, and for the relief of minor muscular aches and joint pains in cattle and horses.

Dosage and Administration: Administer orally.
Mature horses and cattle: Give two (2) to four (4) boluses.
Foals and calves: Give one (1) to two (2) boluses.
Allow the animal to drink water after administration.

Precaution(s): Keep the lid tightly closed and store in a dry place. Do not store above 86°F (30°C).
Caution(s): Keep out of the reach of children. For animal use only.
Presentation: 50 boluses.
Compendium Code No.: 10840071

ASPIRIN BOLUS 240 GRAINS

Phoenix Pharmaceutical **Non-Steroidal Anti-Inflammatory**

240 Grains-Analgesic Antipyretic

Active Ingredient(s): Contents: Each Bolus contains:
Acetylsalicylic Acid . . . . . 240 gr (15.6 g)

Indications: To be used orally as an aid in reducing fever and in relief of minor muscular aches and joint pains in cattle and horses.

Dosage and Administration: Administer orally.
To mature horses and cattle give 2 to 4 boluses; to foals and calves, 1 to 2 boluses. Allow animals to drink water after administration.

Precaution(s): Do not store above 30°C (86°F). Keep lid tightly closed and store in a dry place.
Caution(s): For animal use only.
Warning(s): Keep out of reach of children.
Presentation: 50 boluses (NDC 57319-354-12).
Manufactured by: Phoenix Scientific, St. Joseph, MO 64503.
Compendium Code No.: 12560082 Rev. 02-02

ASPIRIN BOLUS-480

AgriLabs **Non-Steroidal Anti-Inflammatory**

Analgesic-Antipyretic

Active Ingredient(s): Each bolus contains:
Acetylsalicylic Acid . . . . . 480 grains (31.2 g)

Indications: To be used orally as an aid in reducing fever and in relief of minor muscular aches and joint pains in cattle and horses.

Dosage and Administration: Mature Horses and Cattle, administer orally ½ to 1½ boluses two to three times daily. Lubricate bolus and administer with balling gun. Allow animals ample supply of fresh clean water after administration.

Precaution(s): Keep lid tightly closed and store in a dry place.
Do not store above 30°C (86°F).

Warning(s): For animal use only. Keep out of reach of children.
Presentation: 50 boluses.
Compendium Code No.: 10580111

ASPIRIN BOLUSES

Bimeda **Non-Steroidal Anti-Inflammatory**

Active Ingredient(s): Each bolus contains:
Acetylsalicylic acid (aspirin) . . . . . 240 grains

Indications: For use as an aid in reducing fever and for mild analgesia.

Dosage and Administration: Administer orally.
Mature Horses and Cattle . . . . . 2 to 4 boluses
Foals and Calves . . . . . 1 to 2 boluses
Allow the animals to drink water after administration.

Caution(s): For animal use only. Not for human use. Keep out of the reach of children.
Warning(s): Not for use in lactating dairy animals.
Presentation: Jars of 50 boluses.
Compendium Code No.: 13990041

ASPIRIN BOLUSES

Butler **Non-Steroidal Anti-Inflammatory**

Active Ingredient(s): Each bolus contains:
Acetylsalicylic acid . . . . . 240 grains

Indications: To be used orally as an aid in reducing fever and as an aid in the relief of minor muscular aches and joint pain.

Dosage and Administration: Horses and Cattle: One (1) to three (3) boluses two (2) or three (3) times a day. Discontinue use if any unusual symptoms should appear.

Precaution(s): Do not store above 30°C (86°F).
Caution(s): Keep out of the reach of children. For veterinary use only.
Warning(s): Not for use in lactating dairy animals.
Presentation: Boxes of 50 boluses.
Compendium Code No.: 10820111

ASPIRIN BOLUSES-240

AgriLabs **Non-Steroidal Anti-Inflammatory**

Active Ingredient(s): Each bolus contains:
Acetylsalicylic acid (aspirin) . . . . . 240 grains

Indications: For use as an aid in reducing fever and for mild analgesia in horses and cattle.

Dosage and Administration: Administer orally. To mature horses and cattle give two (2) to four (4) boluses. To foals and calves, give one (1) to two (2) boluses.

Caution(s): Keep out of the reach of children. Not for human use.
Warning(s): Not for use in lactating dairy animals.
Presentation: Boxes of 50 boluses.
Compendium Code No.: 10580121

ASPIRIN BOLUSES 240 GRAINS

AgriPharm **Non-Steroidal Anti-Inflammatory**

Active Ingredient(s): Each bolus contains:
Acetylsalicylic acid (aspirin) . . . . . 240 gr (15.6 g)

Indications: For use as an aid in relieving minor muscular aches and joint pain, and in reducing fever in cattle and horses.

Dosage and Administration: For oral use only.
Horses and Cattle: . . . . . 1 to 3 boluses
Lubricate boluses and administer two to three times daily using a balling gun. Allow animals to drink water after administration. Discontinue use if any unusual symptoms should appear.

Precaution(s): Do not store above 30°C (86°F). Store in a cool, dry place. Keep tightly closed when not in use.
Caution(s): For animal use only. Keep out of reach of children.
Warning(s): Not for use in lactating dairy animals.
Presentation: Jars of 50 boluses.
Compendium Code No.: 14570091

ASPIRIN BOLUSES 240 GRAINS

First Priority **Non-Steroidal Anti-Inflammatory**

240 grains

Active Ingredient(s): Each bolus contains:
Acetylsalicylic Acid (Aspirin) . . . . . 240 gr (15.552 g)

Indications: For use as an aid in reducing fever and for mild analgesia in beef cattle, non-lactating dairy cattle, horses, calves and foals.

Dosage and Administration: Administer 1 to 2 ASPIRIN BOLUSES to mature beef cattle, non-lactating dairy cattle and horses two times daily and 1 ASPIRIN BOLUS to calves and foals two times daily. Lubricate each bolus with mineral oil prior to oral administration.
Discontinue treatment if any unusual symptoms should appear. Provide treated animals with fresh drinking water following administration of ASPIRIN BOLUS.

Precaution(s): Do not store above 30°C (86°F). Keep lid tightly closed and store in a dry location.
Keep tightly closed when not in use. Use only as directed.

Warning(s): For use in animals only. Keep out of reach of children.
Presentation: 50 boluses.
Compendium Code No.: 11390011

A

ASPIRIN BOLUSES 480 GRAINS

AgriPharm **Non-Steroidal Anti-Inflammatory**

Active Ingredient(s): Each bolus contains:
Acetylsalicylic acid (aspirin) .... 480 gr (31.2 g)

Indications: For use as an aid in relieving minor muscular aches and joint pain, and in reducing fever in cattle and horses.

Dosage and Administration: For oral use only.
Horses and Cattle: .... ½ to 1½ boluses
Lubricate boluses and administer two to three times daily using a balling gun. Allow animals to drink water after administration. Discontinue use if any unusual symptoms should appear.

Precaution(s): Do not store above 30°C (86°F). Store in a cool, dry place. Keep tightly closed when not in use.

Caution(s): For animal use only. Keep out of reach of children.

Presentation: Jars of 50 boluses, 12 jars/case.

Compendium Code No.: 14570101

ASPIRIN LIQUID CONCENTRATE

AgriPharm **Water Medication**

Active Ingredient(s): Contains 12% Acetylsalicylic Acid (Aspirin).

Indications: Product Description: A concentrated solution for use in livestock drinking water.
For use in swine, poultry, beef and dairy cattle.

Directions for Use: Open container and add 1 oz. of product to 1 gallon of water. Stir stock solution and meter with proportioner at a rate of 1:128 ratio. For seven-day continuous rate, use 4 oz. of product to 1 gallon of water on day one and 1 oz. of product to 1 gallon of water for the remaining six days.

Precaution(s): Keep container closed when not in use. Store in a cool, dry place.

Caution(s): Flammable - use with caution.
For animal use only.

Warning(s): Keep out of reach of children.

Presentation: 32 oz (960 mL) and 6x32 oz (960 mL).

Compendium Code No.: 14571150 Iss. 4-01

ASPIRIN LIQUID CONCENTRATE

First Priority **Water Medication**

Active Ingredient(s): Contains 12% Acetylsalicylic Acid (Aspirin).

Indications: Product Description: A concentrated solution for use in livestock drinking water.
For use in swine, poultry, beef and dairy cattle.

Directions for Use: Open container and add 1 oz. of product to 1 gallon of water. Stir stock solution and meter with proportioner at a rate of 1:128 ratio. For seven-day continuous rate, use 4 oz. of product to 1 gallon of water on day one and 1 oz. of product to 1 gallon of water for the remaining six days.

Precaution(s): Keep container closed when not in use. Store in a cool, dry place.

Caution(s): Flammable - use with caution.
For animal use only.

Warning(s): Keep out of reach of children.

Presentation: 32 fl oz (960 mL) (NDC# 58829-311-32).

Compendium Code No.: 11390780 Iss. 04-01

ASPIRIN POWDER

AgriLabs **Non-Steroidal Anti-Inflammatory**

Relief of body pain and fever.

Active Ingredient(s): Each pound contains:
Acetylsalicylic Acid (Aspirin) .... 1 lb

Indications: For use as an aid in reducing fever and for mild analgesia.

Dosage and Administration: Administer orally.
Cattle, Horses: 5-60 gm (¼-2 oz).
Calves, Foals: 3-6 gm (⅛-⅕ oz).
Sheep, Swine: 1-3 gm (approx. ⅛ oz).
Poultry: 0.15% level in ration.
Dogs: 0.15-1.0 gm.

Precaution(s): Store in a cool dry place not above 30°C (86°F).

Warning(s): For animal use only. Keep out of reach of children.

Presentation: 1 lb.

Compendium Code No.: 10580131

ASPIRIN POWDER

AgriPharm **Non-Steroidal Anti-Inflammatory**

Active Ingredient(s): Each pound contains:
Acetylsalicylic acid (aspirin) .... 1 lb.

Indications: For use as an aid in reducing fever and for mild analgesia.

Dosage and Administration: Administer orally.
Cattle, Horses: 5-60 g (0.2 oz)
Calves, Foals: 0.5-6.0 g
Sheep, Swine: 1-3 g
Poultry: 0.15% level in ration
Cats: 30-65 mg (0.03-0.065 g)
Dogs: 0.15 - 1.0 g

Precaution(s): Store in a cool, dry place not above 30°C (86°F).

Caution(s): For animal use only. Keep out of reach of children.

Presentation: 11.34 kg (25 lb.).

Compendium Code No.: 14570111

ASPIRIN POWDER

Bimeda **Non-Steroidal Anti-Inflammatory**

Analgesic-Antipyretic

Active Ingredient(s): Contents: Each pound contains:
Acetylsalicylic Acid .... 1 lb

Indications: To be used orally as an aid in reducing fever and in relief of minor muscular aches and joint pain.

Dosage and Administration: Administer orally.
Cattle, Horses: 5-60 g (¼-2 oz).
Calves, Foals: 3-6 g (⅛-⅕ oz).
Sheep, Swine: 1-3 g (approx. ⅛ oz).
Poultry: 0.15% level ration.
Dogs: 0.15%-1.0 g.

Precaution(s): Keep lid tightly closed and store in a dry place. Do not store above 30°C (86°F).

Caution(s): For animal use only.

Warning(s): Keep out of reach of children.

Presentation: 1 lb (453.6 g) and 25 lb.

Compendium Code No.: 13990500 8ASP007-801

ASPIRIN POWDER

Butler **Non-Steroidal Anti-Inflammatory**

NDC No.: 11695-4100-4

Active Ingredient(s): Each pound contains:
Acetylsalicylic acid (aspirin) .... 1 lb.

Indications: For use as an aid in reducing fever and for mild analgesia.

Dosage and Administration: Administer orally.
Cattle and Horses .... 5-60 g
Calves and Foals .... 0.5-6.0 g
Sheep and Swine .... 1-3 g
Poultry .... 0.15% level in ration
Cats .... 30-65 mg (0.03-0.065 g)
Dogs .... 0.15-1.0 g

Precaution(s): Store in a cool, dry place at not above 30°C (86°F).

Caution(s): For animal use only. Keep out of the reach of children.

Presentation: 1 lb. (16 oz.) container.

Compendium Code No.: 10820121

ASPIRIN POWDER

First Priority **Non-Steroidal Anti-Inflammatory**

Active Ingredient(s): Each pound contains:
Acetylsalicylic Acid (Aspirin) .... 1 lb

Indications: For use as an aid in reducing fever and for mild analgesia. For relief of body pain and fever.

Directions for Use: Administer orally.
Cattle, Horses: 5-60 g (¼-2 oz)
Calves, Foals: 3-6 g (⅛-⅕ oz)
Sheep, Swine: 1-3 g (approx. ⅛ oz)
Poultry: 0.15% level in ration
Dogs: 0.15% - 1.0 g

Precaution(s): Storage: Store at controlled room temperature between 15°-30°C (59°-86°F). Keep container tightly closed when not in use.

Caution(s): For animal use only.

Warning(s): Keep out of reach of children.

Presentation: 1 lb (453.6 g) jar (NDC# 58829-187-16), 1 lb (453.6 g) bag and 25 lb (11.34 kg) pail (NDC# 58829-187-26).

Compendium Code No.: 11390023 Rev. 09-01 / Rev. 09-01 / Rev. 6-01

ASPIRIN POWDER

Vedco **Non-Steroidal Anti-Inflammatory**

Active Ingredient(s): Each pound contains:
Acetylsalicylic acid (aspirin) .... 1 lb.

Indications: For use as an aid in reducing fever and for mild analgesia.

Dosage and Administration: Administer orally.
Cattle and Horses: 5-60 g (approx. ⅓ to 4 tablespoons).
Calves and Foals: 0.5-6.0 g (approx. 1⁄10 to 1 teaspoon).
Sheep and Swine: 1-3 g (approx. 1⁄10 to ½ teaspoon).
Poultry: 0.15% level in ration.
Cats: 30-65 mg (0.03-0.065 g).
Dogs: 0.15-1.0 g.

Precaution(s): Store in a cool, dry place at not above 30°C (86°F).

Caution(s): For animal use only.

Warning(s): Keep out of reach of children.

Presentation: 1 lb (16 oz) (NDC 50919-263-26) and 25 lb pail.

Compendium Code No.: 10940092

ASPIRIN POWDER MOLASSES-FLAVORED

Butler **Non-Steroidal Anti-Inflammatory**

Active Ingredient(s): Each ounce contains:
Acetylsalicylic Acid 50%
In a palatable base.

Indications: To be used orally as an aid in reducing fever and in relief of minor muscular aches and joint pains in horses and cattle.

Dosage and Administration: Administer orally. Can be mixed with feed.
To mature horses and cattle give 4 to 8 tablespoons two to three times daily, or as recommended by a veterinarian.
Allow animals ample supply of fresh, clean water after administration.

Precaution(s): Keep lid tightly closed and store in a dry place. Do not store above 30°C (86°F).
Shake well before use.

Caution(s): For use in animals only. For veterinary use only.

Warning(s): Keep this and all medication out of the reach of children.

Presentation: 5 lb (NDC 11695-1301-4).

Compendium Code No.: 10820132

ASPIRIN U.S.P.

Neogen **Non-Steroidal Anti-Inflammatory**

Active Ingredient(s):
Acetylsalicylic Acid (Aspirin) .... 226 g
Sucrose (Apple Flavored) .... q.s.
1 level tablespoon is approximately ½ oz.
½ oz contains approximately 7080 mg of Aspirin.

Indications: For use as an aid in reducing fever and for mild analgesia.
Directions: As per veterinarian's instructions.
Caution(s): For animal use only.
Warning(s): Keep out of reach of children.
Presentation: 1 lb.
Compendium Code No.: 14910500 L200-0598 Rev 11/01

ASPIRIN U.S.P POWDER

Neogen **Non-Steroidal Anti-Inflammatory**
Powder Form
Active Ingredient(s):
Acetylsalicylic Acid U.S.P. (Aspirin) 99.9%
28,321 mg/oz (453 g/lb)
Indications: For use as an aid in reducing fever and for mild analgesia.
Directions: Administer orally, as per veterinarian's instructions.
Caution(s): Sold to licensed veterinarians only.
For animal use only.
Warning(s): Keep out of reach of children.
Presentation: 1 lb.
Compendium Code No.: 14910193 L108-0997 Rev. 11/01

ASP-RIN CONCENTRATE

AgriLabs **Water Medication**
Active Ingredient(s): Contains 12% Acetylsalicylic Acid.
Indications: Product Description: A concentrated solution for use in livestock drinking water.
For use in swine, poultry, beef and dairy cattle.
Directions for Use: Open container and add 1 oz. of product to 1 gallon of water. Stir stock solution and meter with proportioner at a rate of 1:128 ratio. For seven-day continuous rate, use 4 oz. of product to 1 gallon of water on day one and 1 oz. of product to 1 gallon of water for the remaining six days.
Precaution(s): Keep container closed when not in use. Store in a cool, dry place.
Caution(s): Flammable - use with caution. For animal use only.
Warning(s): Keep out of reach of children.
Presentation: 32 oz (960 mL).
Compendium Code No.: 10581280

ASSURE®/FeLV

Synbiotics **FeLV Test**
U.S. Vet. Lic. No.: 312
Contents:
Anti-FeLV antibody coated sticks .... 25 sticks
Predispensed HRP-monoclonal antibody conjugate (A - blue stripe) .... 25 tubes
Predispensed substrate buffer (B - white stripe) .... 25 tubes
Chromogen (C - white cap) .... 3.0 mL
S.E.R. (D - blue cap) .... 3.0 mL
Transfer pipettes 25
Indications: A feline leukemia virus antigen test kit.
Test Principle: The bulbous ends of the plastic sticks are coated with an antibody directed against a specific FeLV antigen, p27. A second antibody directed against the p27 antigen is conjugated to the enzyme horseradish peroxidase. The specimen is incubated in a single step with both the antibody coated stick and enzyme labeled antibodies. If antigen is present, it is captured by the stick. The enzyme labeled antibodies are captured in turn by the antigen on the stick. The unbound enzyme labeled antibody is washed away and the stick is placed into a chromogenic substrate. The development of a distinct blue color in the solution indicates the presence of FeLV antigen. In the absence of FeLV antigen, no color will develop.
Test Procedure: Materials required, but not provided:
1. Marking pen.
2. Timer.
3. Normal saline (whole blood specimens).
4. Distilled or deionized water.

Procedure: Saliva, whole blood, plasma or serum specimens may be used as samples in the ASSURE®/FeLV test kit. Whole blood or plasma should contain an anticoagulant. Whole blood, serum and plasma specimens may be stored at 2-8°C for up to seven (7) days. If longer storage is required, plasma and serum may be frozen. Whole blood should not be used beyond seven (7) days. Hemolysis in the plasma or serum does not interfere with the test as long as adequate washing is performed.

Saliva should be collected from the buccal cavity (between the cheek and gum). Do not induce salivation with drugs as this can invalidate the test results.

Test procedure:

A. Whole blood/plasma/serum procedure:

Preparation: For each cat to be tested, remove one (1) test tube of predispensed conjugate from box A (blue stripe) and one (1) test tube of predispensed substrate buffer from box B (white stripe). Mark each test tube with the cat's name or identification number. Place the test tubes in the appropriate positions in the workstation. Remove the stopper(s) from the tube(s) of conjugate in row A.

Obtain one (1) stick for each cat to be tested. Open the plastic bag at the non-bulbous end of the stick. Pull the stick partway out of the bag to write the cat's name or I.D. number on the stick.

Step 1. Using a clean transfer pipette for each specimen, add three (3) drops (100 mcg) of whole blood, plasma or serum to the appropriate tube in row A. Mix gently by tapping the bottom of the tubes several times. Place the stick into the corresponding tube of conjugate in row A. Wait for five (5) minutes (may be left for up to 20 minutes).

During the waiting period, prepare the test tube(s) in row B by removing the stopper(s) and adding three (3) drops of chromogen (bottle C) to each tube of predispensed substrate buffer. Mix gently by tapping the bottom of each tube several times.

Step 2. After five (5) minutes, remove the stick(s) from the tube(s) in row A, being careful not to drip any liquid into the tube(s) in row B. Immediately wash under a forceful stream of distilled or deionized water. Wash all surfaces of the ball and the lower third of the stick, giving attention to the areas between the ball and the stick, and the ball and the tip. Alternatively, place at least 50 mL of distilled or deionized water into a disposable cup and vigorously swirl the stick to remove unbound conjugate. Complete washing is necessary to produce accurate test results. It is impossible to wash the stick too much.

Note: For whole blood samples, the sticks should be rinsed with normal saline until no red is visible before proceeding with water wash. (Saline helps remove hemoglobin residues which may cause nonspecific color development.)

Step 3. Shake off any excess liquid. Place each stick into the corresponding tube of prepared substrate in row B of the workstation. Wait for five (5) minutes. (Weak positives may be verified by waiting for up to 10 minutes.) Remove the stick from the tube and observe the color of the solution in each tube against a white background. A distinct blue color indicates a positive test result. Negative test results will be free of any color development.

B. Saliva procedure:

Preparation: For each cat to be tested remove one (1) test tube of the predispensed conjugate from box A (blue stripe) and one (1) test tube of the predispensed substrate from box B (white stripe). Place the test tubes in an appropriate place in the work station.

Step 1. Remove the stopper(s) from the conjugate tube(s) A. Dispense three (3) drops of reagent D/SER to each conjugate tube A. Gently tap the tube on the bottom for several seconds to mix SER with the conjugate solution.

Obtain one (1) stick for each cat to be tested. Open the plastic bag at the non-bulbous end of the stick. Pull the stick partway out of the bag to write the cat's name or I.D. number on the stick. Wet the bulbous end of the stick(s) under a stream of distilled or deionized water, or swirl the stick in a cup or beaker filled with distilled or deionized water for five (5) seconds.

Step 2. Place the bulbous end of the stick under the upper lip of the cat and slide the stick to the back of the mouth between the cheek and the gum. Gently rotate the stick for 5-10 seconds in the cat's mouth. (Abrasions to the stick's surface or cellular debris obtained during sampling do not affect test performance.) Immediately place the saliva coated dipstick into the corresponding tube of conjugate, tube A. Twirl the stick gently for three (3) to five (5) seconds to mix. Wait for 10 minutes.

During the waiting period, prepare the test tube(s) in row B by removing the stopper(s) and adding three (3) drops of chromogen (bottle C) to each tube of predispensed substrate buffer. Mix gently by tapping the bottom of each tube several times.

Step 3. After 10 minutes, remove the stick(s) from the conjugate tube(s) in row A, being careful not to drip the liquid from the sticks into the substrate tubes in row B. Immediately wash the stick(s) under a forceful stream of distilled or deionized water. Wash all surfaces of the ball and the lower third of the stick, giving attention to the areas between the ball and the stick, and the ball and the tip. Complete washing is necessary to produce accurate test results. It is impossible to wash the stick too much.

Step 4. Shake off any excess liquid. Place each stick into the corresponding tube of prepared substrate in row B of the work station. Wait for five (5) minutes. (Weak positives may be verified by waiting for up to 10 minutes.) Remove the stick from the tube and observe the color of the solution in each tube against a white background. A distinct blue color indicates a positive test result. Negative test results will be free of any color development.

Interpretation of results:

Whole blood, plasma or serum positive: Following exposure, a cat may test positive (i.e., be viremic) within 1-14 days.[4] Because infection may be transient in cats that develop immunity, all animals with positive results should be confirmed. Immediate confirmation may be obtained with saliva or IFA. Positive results with these modalities indicate persistent infection, in the majority of cases. Alternatively, positive reactors may be isolated and retested in three (3) to four (4) weeks. A positive test at that time would indicate persistent infection, while a negative test would indicate immune clearance of the virus.

Saliva positive: A positive test result with saliva, in the majority of cases, indicates a persistent infection. A saliva test will not be strongly positive until the virus is amplified in the bone marrow, released into the circulation, and finally has infected the epithelial tissues. Therefore, a period from one (1) to two (2) months following exposure may be required for the detection of antigen in saliva.[4] Consequently, saliva test results correlate closely with IFA, regarded as the "gold standard" in FeLV testing.

Note: It should be emphasized that there are rare times when cats that are transiently infected will have positive results for FeLV by IFA and blood, plasma, serum or saliva ELISA assays. Repeat testing should be performed in three (3) to four (4) weeks.

Precaution(s):
1. Store the test kit at 35-45°F (2-8°C). Do not freeze.
2. Properly stored reagents are stable until the expiration date.
3. Allow the components to come to room temperature (70-77°F/21-25°C) before use.
4. Use only distilled or deionized water. Do not use tap water.
5. All specimens should be considered potentially infectious and disposed of accordingly.

Caution(s):
1. Do not mix materials from different test kit lots.
2. Follow the instructions carefully.
3. For veterinary use only.

Discussion: Feline leukemia virus (FeLV) is a contagious oncogenic RNA virus that causes both neoplastic and non-neoplastic diseases in cats.[1] Because FeLV is immunosuppressive, it also predisposes cats to a number of secondary infections.[2]

ASSURE®/FeLV uses highly specific antibodies to quickly identify FeLV infected cats. ASSURE®/FeLV has been optimized to use saliva, whole blood, plasma or serum specimens. When saliva is used as a sample, cats actively shedding virus may be identified within 15-20 minutes without invasive sampling techniques. Rapid identification of these animals allows them to be separated from noninfected cats to prevent the spread of FeLV. Whole blood, plasma or serum specimens may be used in a 7-10 minute format for detection of circulating antigen at any stage in the disease cycle, even before clinical signs of infection are apparent.[3]
References: Available upon request.
Presentation: 25 tests/kit.
Compendium Code No.: 11150011

ASSURE®/FH

Synbiotics **Heartworm Test**
Feline Heartworm Antibody Test Kit
U.S. Vet. Lic. No.: 312
Contents:

	10 Tests/Kit	25 Tests/Kit
Protein A Coated Wands	10 ea.	25 ea.
Predispensed FH Antigen - HRP Conjugate (A tubes)	10 ea.	25 ea.
Predispensed Substrate buffer (B tubes)	10 ea.	25 ea.
Predispensed Wash solution (W tubes)	10 ea.	25 ea.
Chromogen (C)	1 vial	1 vial

Transfer Pipets

Work Station

Additional material required, but not provided: Stopwatch, marking pen, distilled or deionized water, squirt bottle or cup.

Indications: For the detection of antibodies to feline heartworm.

Test Principles: The plastic wands are coated with Protein A. A highly specific antigen of *Dirofilaria immitis* is labeled with horseradish peroxidase (HRP). The specimen (either plasma or serum) is incubated simultaneously with the coated wands and the enzyme-labeled FH antigen. Antibodies to FH, if present in the cat sample, are bound to the wand and enzyme-linked FH antigen at the same time. The free enzyme-linked antigen is washed away and a chromogenic substrate is added. The development of a distinct blue color indicates the presence of antibody to FH. In the absence of FH antibody, no color change will be observed.

ASSURE®/FH is highly specific, sensitive and simple to perform. Test results can be obtained in 10 minutes.

Test Procedure: Plasma or serum specimens may be used as samples in the ASSURE®/FH test kit. Plasma should contain an anticoagulant. Serum and plasma specimens may be stored at 2°-7°C for up to seven days. If longer storage is required, plasma and serum may be frozen. Moderate hemolysis or lipemia in plasma or serum should not affect performance as long as adequate washing is performed. When in doubt, collect a new sample.

Prior to use, allow kit components to come to room temperature (72° to 78°F; 21° to 25°C).

For each sample you will need:

Transfer pipette (one use only).

FH antibody capturing coated wand. Label with pet's name.

Predispensed FH antigen Conjugate A tube.

Predispensed substrate Buffer B tube.

Predispensed Wash Solution W tube.

Work station with Reagent C.

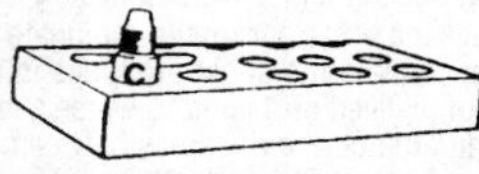

Squirt bottle with distilled or deionized water.

A. Sample and Conjugate:

1. Add 1 drop (40 µL) of sample to Tube A.
   Tap to mix.
   Proceed to Step 2.

B. Conjugate Incubation:

2. Place bulbous end of the labeled Wand in Tube A.
   Twirl 1-3 seconds to mix.
   Wait 5 minutes (may be left up to 10 minutes).

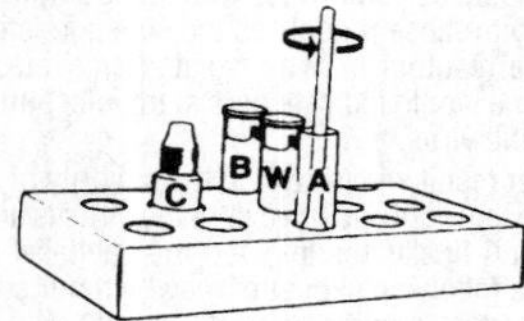

C. Prepare Tube B:

3. During waiting period:
   Remove stopper from Tube B.
   Add 3 drops Bottle C (white cap) to Tube B.
   Tap to mix.
   Set aside for use in Step 5.

D. Wash Step:

4. Transfer Wand to Tube W.
   Pre-Wash by dipping vigorously 20-25 times.

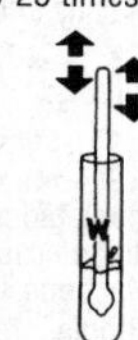

Then wash Wand by using Method A or B:

A. Squirt Bottle Method

Direct a forceful stream of distilled or deionized water against bulbous end and tip of Wand and work up handle.

Shake off excess water.

Repeat 5-7 times totaling approximately 8 oz of water per Wand.

B. Cup Method

Swirl/Swish vigorously in 100 ml distilled or deionized water for a minimum of 30 seconds.

Shake off excess water.

Replace water between Wands.

Note: It is impossible to overwash the Wand!

E. Color Development:

Place washed Wand in Tube B.

Twirl 1-3 seconds to mix.

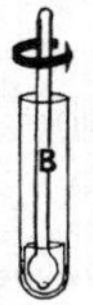

Wait 5 minutes.

Remove Wand.

Good Techniques = Accurate Results:

Plasma samples must contain an anticoagulant.

Severely hemolyzed and lipemic samples may produce non-specific color. When in doubt, obtain a better quality sample.

Washing is the most important step. Wands cannot be overwashed. Underwashing will result in non-specific blue color development in Tube B.

Prolonged incubation for more than 5 minutes in Step 5 may result in non-specific blue color development. If no color is seen at 5 minutes, the sample is negative.

Do not use the test kit past the expiration date and do not intermix components from different serial numbers.

Test Interpretation: Observe solution against workstation window or a white background for color.

A blue color indicates the presence of antibody to heartworm.

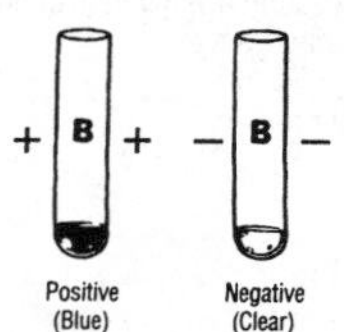

Positive Procedural Control (Optional): After completion of test, if a negative/clear result is obtained.

Place Wand back into Tube A.

Twirl to mix for 1-3 seconds.

Remove from Tube A.

Do not wash.

Place back into Tube B.

Blue color should develop within 1 minute indicating reagents were added correctly and kit is performing properly. If color does not develop, repeat the test.

Storage: Store the test kit at 2°-7°C (36°-45°F). Do not freeze. Properly stored reagents are stable until the expiration date.

Caution(s):

1. Allow kit to come to room temperature (21°-25°C; 70°-78°F) prior to use.
2. Do not expose kit to direct sunlight.
3. Do not use expired reagents or mix from different kit lots.
4. Hold reagent vials vertically for proper drop volume.
5. Dispose of potentially infected specimens appropriately.
6. For veterinary use only.

Discussion: Feline heartworm disease (FHD) is becoming a more common diagnosis in cats presenting with coughing, intermittent vomiting and abnormal heart and lung sounds. Heartworm infection is often more difficult to diagnose in the cat as there are fewer worms present and circulating microfilaria are rare. The life span of the parasite is typically shorter in cats and infections tend to be self limiting after 2 to 3 years although heartworms are capable of causing severe disease. Cats with low worm burdens can be considered heavily infected due to their smaller body size. Male cats are more frequently and generally more heavily infected. A large percentage of naturally infected cats test antigen negative. Other clinical signs and serology must be considered in the event of a negative antigen assay. An ELISA test for host antibody is a valuable screening tool. When used in conjunction with other tests and the evaluation of clinical symptoms, the antibody test aids in the correct diagnosis of infection.

ASSURE®/FH uses a highly specific recombinant antigen to quickly identity antibodies to heartworm in infected cats.

ASSURE®/FH has been optimized to use plasma or serum specimens.

Presentation: 10 and 25 test kits.

ASSURE®/FH is a registered trademark of Synbiotics Corporation.

Compendium Code No.: 11150020

ASSURE®/PARVO

Synbiotics **Parvovirus Test**

U.S. Vet. Lic. No.: 312

Description: Canine parvovirus antigen test kit.

Components:

	10 Test Kit	25 Test Kit
Anti-CPV Antibody Coated Wands	10 ea	25 ea
Predispensed HRP-Monoclonal Antibody Conjugate (A Tubes)	10 ea	25 ea
Predispensed Substrate Buffer (B Tubes)	10 ea	25 ea
Bottle C-Chromogen (White Cap)	2.5 mL	3.0 mL

Materials required, but not provided: Marking pen, timer, distilled or deionized water, wash bottle.

Indications: For the detection of canine parvovirus antigen.

Test Principles: The bulbous ends of the plastic wands have been coated with antibody to CPV. A second antibody directed against a specific CPV antigen is conjugated to the enzyme horseradish peroxidase (HRP). The fecal sample is incubated simultaneously with both the antibody-coated wand and enzyme-labeled antibodies. If antigen is present, it is captured by the wand. The enzyme-labeled antibodies are in turn captured by the antigen bound to the wand. The unbound enzyme-labeled antibody and feces are removed during the wash step and the wand is placed into a chromogenic substrate.

The development of a distinct blue color in the solution indicates the presence of CPV antigen. In the absence of CPV, no color will develop.

Test Procedure: Sample Information: Canine fecal material is required. Stool samples may be stored at 2°-7°C (36°-45°F) for 48 hours. If longer storage is required the samples may be stored frozen.

Prior to use, allow kit components to come to room temperature (70° to 78°F; 21° to 25°C).

For each sample you will need:

1. Anti-CPV Antibody Coated Wand. Label with dog's ID.

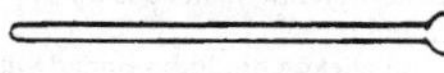

2. Predispensed HRP-Monoclonal Antibody Conjugate Tube A.
3. Predispensed Substrate Buffer Tube B. Label with dog's ID.
4. Workstation with Reagent C.
5. Squirt Bottle with Distilled or Deionized Water.

A. Sample Collection

1_A. Pre-wet bulbous end of wand with deionized or distilled water for 3-5 seconds.

1_B. Swirl wand in fecal material 3-5 seconds to cover bulbous end with a thin coat of feces.

Note: A specimen may be obtained rectally by inserting bulbous end of wand into rectum and gently swirling 3-5 seconds. Do not use a lubricant.

B. Conjugate Incubation

2. Place bulbous end of wand in tube A.

Twirl wand vigorously until fecal material is suspended in the liquid.

Wait 5 minutes.

C. Prepare B Tube

3. During waiting period:

Remove stopper from tube B.

Add 3 drops bottle C (White Cap) to tube B.

Tap to mix.

Set tube aside for use in step 5.

D. Wash Step

4. Remove wand from tube A.

Wash bulbous end and tip of wand by swirling/swishing vigorously in a cup containing at least 250 mL of deionized or distilled water for a minimum of 15 seconds.

After swirling in cup, continue to wash wand by directing a forceful stream of deionized or distilled water against bulbous end and tip of wand and work up handle.

Shake off excess water.

Repeat washing with a forceful stream 5-7 times until all fecal material is removed from the wand.

Replace liquid in cup between wands.

Note: Bloody samples may require saline rinse.

E. Color Development

5. Place washed wand in tube B.

Twirl 1-3 seconds to mix.

Wait 5 minutes.

Remove wand.

Read results.

Notes:

A thin coat of fecal material on the bulbous end is required. Swirl bulbous end of wand in material for 3-5 seconds.

In step 2, feces should be removed from the wand and suspended in the liquid.

Washing is the most important step. Wands cannot be overwashed. Underwashing will result in non-specific color development in the tube B.

Read results at 5 minutes. If no color is seen at 5 minutes, the sample is negative.

Do not use the test kit past the expiration date and do not intermix components from different serial numbers.

Store kit at 2° to 7°C (36° to 45°F). Allow kit to come to room temperature before use. Do not expose kit to direct sunlight.

Failure to change wash solution in step 4 can lead to false color development.

Test Interpretation: Observe solution against work-station window or a white background for blue color.

Positive = Blue

Negative = Clear

Note: Color intensity will vary with level of CPV present.

Optional Procedural Control

To verify technique and kit performance when a negative result is obtained:

Place wand back into tube A.

Twirl to mix for 1-3 seconds.

Remove wand.

Do not wash.

Place back into tube B.

Blue color will develop within 1 minute indicating reagents were added correctly and kit is performing properly. If color does not develop, repeat the test. (This is a procedure and reagent check only. CPV antigen is not present.)

Storage: Store the test kit at 2°-7°C (36°-45°F). Do not freeze. Properly stored reagents are stable until the expiration date.

Caution(s):

1. Allow kit to come to room temperature (21°-25°C, 70°-78°F) prior to use; approximately one hour.
2. Do not expose kit to direct sunlight.
3. Do not use expired reagents or mix from different kit serials.
4. Hold reagent vial vertically for proper drop volume.
5. Vaccination with modified live CPV vaccines may cause shedding of viral particles in the feces 4-10 days post-vaccination. This can cause a weak positive result.
6. Dispose of potentially infected specimens appropriately.

For use in testing canine specimens only.

Discussion: Canine Parvovirus (CPV) is a member of the feline parvovirus subgroup. It is closely related to feline panleukopenia virus and mink enteritis virus. CPV was first recognized as a virus in dogs in 1978 in North America. It has since spread globally and is considered endemic to nearly all populations of domesticated and wild canines.

CPV causes two forms of disease: Myocarditis and enteritis. Due to maternal antibody protection the myocardial form is rare. The enteric form, however, is prevalent and can be fatal to puppies and geriatric dogs. CPV enteritis causes severe, often bloody diarrhea, vomiting, leukopenia and dehydration.

Transmission is fecal-oral and most infections occur from exposure to contaminated feces. CPV is highly contagious and stable under a variety of environmental conditions.

Rapid diagnosis of CPV allows for quarantine and prompt treatment of infected dogs. Diagnosis may be difficult in milder cases. ASSURE®/Parvo is an enzyme linked immunosorbent assay (ELISA) which detects all strains of Canine Parvovirus shed in the feces. Positive results with the fecal ELISA indicate the presence of canine parvovirus.

References:

Parrish, C.R. *et al:* Antigenic relationships between canine parvovirus type 2, feline panleukopenia virus and mink enteritis virus using conventional antisera and monoclonal antibodies. *Arch. Viral.* 72:267-278; 1982.

Studdart, M. J. *et al:* Aspects of the diagnosis, pathogenesis and epidemiology of canine parvovirus. *Aust. Vet. J.* 60:197-200; 1983.

Siegl, G. *et al:* Characteristics and Taxonomy of Parvoviridae. *Intervirology.* 23:61-73; 1985.

Parrish, C.R.: Emergence and natural history of canine, mink and feline parvoviruses. *Adv. Virus Res.* 38:403-450; 1990.

Presentation: 10 and 25 test kits.

Compendium Code No.: 11150030

ASTRINGENT BOLUS

Butler **Large Animal Dietary Supplement**

Guaranteed Analysis:

	Per Bolus	Per Pound
Calcium (Ca) min.	1.4 g	7.0%
Calcium (Ca) max.	1.68 g	8.4%
Copper (Cu) min.	0.98 g	4.9%
Iron (Fe) min.	1.16 g	5.8%

Ingredients: Calcium Carbonate, Ferrous Sulfate, Copper Sulfate, Hemicellulose Extract, Dried Whey, Corn Starch and Magnesium Stearate.

Indications: A supplemental nutritive bolus that provides trace minerals and minerals for horses, colts, cattle and calves.

Directions for Use:

Horses: ½ to 1 bolus.

Cattle: 1 to 1¼ bolus.

Colts and Calves: ¼ to ½ bolus.

Precaution(s): Keep container tightly closed when not in use. Store in a cool, dry place.

Caution(s): For animal use only. Not for human use.

Presentation: 50 boluses (20.0 g per bolus).

Compendium Code No.: 10820141

ATGARD® C

Boehringer Ingelheim **Feed Medication**

(dichlorvos) Swine Wormer-Type A Medicated Article

NADA No.: 040-848

Active Ingredient(s): By Weight

Dichlorvos. 9.6%

Inactive Ingredients: Stabilized polyvinyl chloride/plasticizer resin pellet with a coating of talc, natural carbohydrates and resin 90.4%

Total 100.0%

ATGARD® C is a broad spectrum swine anthelmintic in the form of resin pellets containing the active ingredient dichlorvos. The pellets are covered by a soluble protective coating.

Indications: ATGARD® C is effective against whipworms *(Trichuris suis)*, nodular worms *(Oesophagostomum* spp.), large roundworms *(Ascaris suum)*, and thick stomach worms *(Ascarops strongylina)*. When fed for the last 30 days of gestation, this product improves litter production efficiency by increasing the number of pigs born alive, birth weights, survival to market, and the rate of weight gain.

To Deworm Swine: For the removal and control of mature, immature, and/or 4th stage larvae of the whipworm *(Trichuris suis)*, nodular worm *(Oesophagostomum* spp.), large roundworm *(Ascaris suum)*, and thick stomach worm *(Ascarops strongylina)* occurring in the gastrointestinal tracts of pigs, boars, open or bred gilts and sows.

Dosage and Administration: Use Directions: There are a variety of dosage regimens for the administration of ATGARD® C in worming programs or for the improvement of litter production efficiency. Choose the program that best fits your operation and objectives.

ATGARD® C "Scoop" Program (One day-top dress)

Recommended dewormer dosage for swine over 70 lbs: To deworm one open or bred gilt or sow, boar, or pig from 70 lbs to market weight, thoroughly mix one level scoop of ATGARD® C (use scoop provided in the 8 lb package) into the daily ration of each animal. After the allotted medicated feed has been consumed, resume feeding regular rations.

Medicated Feeds Containing 0.0384% Dichlorvos (Two day - complete feed): For swine up to 70 pounds bodyweight, feed as sole ration for two consecutive days. For swine from 70 pounds to market weight, feed as sole ration at the rate of 8.4 pounds of feed per head until the medicated feed has been consumed. For boars, open or bred gilts and sows, feed as sole ration at the rate of 4.2 pounds of feed per head per day for 2 consecutive days.

Prepare a complete feed containing 0.0384% dichlorvos (174 mg/lb) according to the following mixing chart.

Pounds of Complete Feed	Pounds of ATGARD® C to be Added to Feed
550	2
1000	4
2000	8

For Swine up to 70 lbs Body Weight: Feed as the sole ration for 2 consecutive days. Use the following table as a guide for estimating consumption of the medicated feed:

Weight of Pigs (lbs)	Amount of Medicated Feed to be Fed in 2 Days (lbs per Pig)
30	4.0
40	5.5
50	6.5
60	7.5
70	8.4

Medicated Feeds Containing 0.0528% Dichlorvos (One day - complete feed): For boars, open or bred gilts and sows, feed as sole ration at the rate of 6 pounds per head for one feeding.

In all cases, after the allotted medicated feed has been consumed, resume feeding regular rations.

A

ATGARD® C can be mixed in meal or crumble feeds after crumbles have been manufactured. Use the following table as a guide for preparing medicated swine feeds for deworming.

Deworming: Mixing Directions - Complete Feeds

Pounds Complete Feed	Dichlorvos		Pounds ATGARD® C to be Added Per Ton of Feed
	mg/lb.	%	
2000	174	0.0384	8.0
2000	239	0.0528	11.0

To Improve Litter Production Efficiency: For administration to pregnant swine as an aid in improving litter production efficiency by increasing pigs born alive, birth weights, survival to market, and rate of weight gain. Treatment also removes and controls mature, immature and/or 4th stage larvae of the whipworm *(Trichuris suis)*, nodular worm *(Oesophagostomum* spp.), large roundworm *(Ascaris suum)*, and thick stomach worm *(Ascarops strongylina)* occurring in the gastrointestinal tract of the sow or gilt.

1. Incorporate ATGARD® C into gestation feed for pregnant swine containing no other drugs at the rate to provide 1000 mg dichlorvos per head per day during the last 30 days of gestation.
2. ATGARD® C can be mixed in meal or crumbled feeds after crumbles have been manufactured. Do not mix in feeds to be pelleted nor with pelleted feed. Use the following table as a guide for preparing medicated swine gestation feeds.

To Improve Litter Production Efficiency: Mixing Directions - Complete Feeds

Pounds Complete Feed per Head Daily	Dichlorvos in Feed		Pounds ATGARD® C to be Added Per Ton of Feed
	mg/lb	%	
4	250	0.0552	11.5
5	200	0.0442	9.2
6	167	0.0368	7.7

Individual Rations: Each package of ATGARD® C (dichlorvos) Swine Wormer contains a plastic scoop. A level scoop holds 15.2 grams ATGARD® C (1460 mg dichlorvos), the recommended dewormer dosage for swine over 70 lbs.

To deworm one open or bred gilt or sow, boar, or pig from 70 lbs to market weight, thoroughly mix one level scoop of ATGARD® C into the usual daily ration of each animal. After the allotted medicated feed has been consumed, resume feeding regular rations.

This package (8 lbs/3.6 kg) contains sufficient ATGARD® C (dichlorvos) Swine Wormer to individually deworm 239 sows.

Precaution(s): Store between 0°C and 27°C (32°-81°F).

Caution(s): For the manufacture of medicated swine feeds only.

Warning(s): There is no pre-slaughter withdrawal period when used at the recommended dosage level.

Medicated feeds containing ATGARD® C must bear the following statements:

Note: Consult your veterinarian for assistance in the diagnosis, treatment, and control of parasitism.

1. Do not use in any animals other than swine.
2. Do not mix in feeds to be pelleted nor with pelleted feed. (Required only on medicated feed supplements.)
3. Do not allow fowl access to this feed or to feces from treated animals.
4. Do not soak feed or feed as wet mash. Feed must be fed dry.
5. Dichlorvos is a cholinesterase inhibitor. Do not use this product in animals simultaneously or within a few days before or after treatment with or exposure to cholinesterase-inhibiting drugs, pesticides, or chemicals. If human or animal poisoning should occur, immediately consult a physician or a veterinarian. Atropine is antidotal.
6. Do not reuse any of the containers or container materials used in packaging (product). All packaging materials must be destroyed after (product) has been used. (Required only on medicated feed supplements.)

Keep out of the reach of children. Avoid contact with skin. ATGARD® C is a cholinesterase inhibitor. If human or animal poisoning should occur, immediately consult a physician or a veterinarian. Atropine is antidotal.

Presentation: 4 x 8 lb (3.6 kg) drum.

ATGARD® is a Registered Trademark of Boehringer Ingelheim Vetmedica, Inc.

Compendium Code No.: 10280050 610101L-01-9801, 610103L-01-9801

ATGARD® SWINE WORMER

Boehringer Ingelheim **Feed Medication**

(dichlorvos)

NADA No.: 043-606

Active Ingredient(s): ATGARD® is a broad-spectrum swine anthelmintic in the form of non-digestible, rice shaped resin pellets impregnated with the active ingredient dichlorvos.

The packet contains 0.40 oz of dichlorvos (2,2-dichlorovinyl dimethyl phosphate) in a stabilized polyvinyl chloride/plasticizer resin pellet.

Indications: For the removal and control of the sexually mature (adult), sexually immature, and/or 4th stage larvae of the whipworm *(Trichuris suis)*, nodular worms *(Oesophagostomum* sp.), large roundworm *(Ascaris suum)* and the mature thick stomach worm *(Ascarops stongylina)* occurring in the lumen of the gastro-intestinal tract of pigs, boars, and open or bred gilts and sows.

Pharmacology: The preparation is an uncoated, rice-shaped resin pellet, approximating one-eighth inch in length and one-sixteenth inch in diameter, the active ingredient of which is dichlorvos (2, 2-dichlorovinyl dimethyl phosphate). It is designed to be administered to swine in limited amounts of a meal-type (non-pelleted) ration. When used according to directions, the active ingredient (dichlorvos) release rate is sufficient to provide for high anthelmintic efficiency but not of such magnitude as to exceed the degrading (detoxification) capacity of the pig. This characteristic provides a wide margin of safety comparable to or exceeding many drugs used in the field of animal health.

Anthelmintic Spectrum and Activity:

Common Name	Scientific Name	Developmental stages shown susceptible to dichlorvos
Roundworm	*Ascaris suum*	Sexually mature (a), sexually immature (b), and/or 4th stage larvae (c).
Nodular worms	*Oesophagostomum* sp.	Sexually mature (a), sexually immature (b), and/or 4th stage larvae (c).
Whipworm	*Trichuris suis*	Sexually mature (a), sexually immature (b), and/or 4th stage larvae (c).
Stomach worm	*Ascarops strongylina*	Sexually mature (a).

(a) Full sized parasite; produces eggs.
(b) Sometimes called 5th stage larvae, incapable of egg production.
(c) Minute in size, much too young for egg production.

Dosage and Administration: The preparation is designed to be mixed into a dry meal or crumble-type rations. The product cannot be adequately mixed into pelleted feeds nor should it be used in liquid or semi-liquid rations. The contents of the two (2) packet sizes provide for a single anthelmintic treatment for the number of pigs in various weight classes and for breeding swine as follows:

Pig Dosage Table:

Pig Weight (lbs)	Number of Pigs/Packet	Pounds Feed/Packet	Pounds Feed/Pig
20-30	60	20	0.33
31-40	45	25	0.56
41-60	30	30	1.00
61-80	25	25	1.00
81-100	20	20	1.00
Adult Gilts, Sows, Boars	20	80	4.00

To incorporate in the ration, open packet(s), pour the contents on the feed and mix thoroughly on a clean, impervious surface.

Administer medicated feed shortly after mixing. Do not allow swine access to feed other than that containing the preparation until the treatment is complete, after which normal feeding should be resumed. Preconditioning swine by overnight fasting is not necessary nor recommended. Do not treat swine with signs of increased peristalsis (diarrhea, scours) until these signs subside or are brought under control by proper medication. Consult a veterinarian for assistance in the diagnosis, treatment and control of parasitism.

In feeder pigs, the best results will be obtained by treating at five (5) to six (6) weeks of age on an individual litter basis, prior to the time when dichlorvos-sensitive gastro-intestinal nematodes have had the opportunity to reach full egg-laying potential. Repeating the treatment four (4) to five (5) weeks later will afford the maximum anthelmintic value from the product and will help to minimize premise contamination. The utilization of specially constructed pens which are used only for deworming purposes and that can be thoroughly cleaned after each use will further reduce such contamination.

In those instances where lots of pigs of mixed sizes are to be treated, maximum anthelmintic efficiency will be obtained by segregating comparable sized pigs into individual lots.

In gilts and sows, optimum results will be obtained by treatment approximately one (1) week in advance of breeding and farrowing. Preferably these treatments should be given away from the farrowing and nursing areas.

Example: Separate similar sized pigs into individual lots or pens for treatment.

Do not allow swine access to feed other than that containing ATGARD® Swine Wormer. Waterers do not have to be shut off. Normal feeding should be resumed after the treatment is completed. Do not store unused feed containing ATGARD® Swine Wormer.

Precaution(s): Store at less than 80°F. Do not store unused packet(s) contents or medicated feed.

Unused contents and feed containing ATGARD® Swine Wormer should be buried 18 inches deep in the ground and covered in a manner rendering it unavailable to man, animals, or fowl. Avoid contact with the skin.

Caution(s): Do not use in any animals other than swine. Do not allow fowl access to feed containing the preparation or to manure from treated animals. ATGARD® Swine Wormer (dichlorvos) is a cholinesterase inhibitor. Do not use this product on animals simultaneously or within a few days before or after treatment with or exposure to cholinesterase inhibiting drugs, pesticides or chemicals.

If human or animal poisoning should occur, immediately consult a physician or veterinarian respectively. Atropine is antidotal.

For use in animals only.

Warning(s): There is no pre-slaughter withdrawal period when used at the recommended dosage level.

Keep out of the reach of children.

Toxicology: Extensive field and laboratory trials with various formulations of dichlorvos have shown that the preparation, as recommended, is safe to use. The wide margin of safety is comparable to or exceeds most drugs used in the field of animal health.

ATGARD® Swine Wormer given at the recommended dosages to breeding swine has been shown not to have any adverse effects on production. It does not cause abortion or premature births, impaired fertility, fewer pigs per litter, or decreased litter survival or performance.

Discussion: Parasites and Herd Health: Whipworms, nodular worms, large roundworms and stomach worms do not cause death in pigs unless present in very large numbers. Seldom do pigs harbor a single species, thus the infections are usually mixed. Under modern methods of swine production (concentration and confinement), unless control measures are taken, each group of pigs tend to harbor more worms than its ancestors. These infections adversely affect herd health and performance as follows:

1. Chronic blood loss.
2. Tissue destruction (especially during migratory stages of roundworms).
3. Chronic and sometimes severe inflammation of the intestinal lining.
4. Blockage of secretory ducts (liver, pancreas).
5. Reduced absorptive capacity of the gastro-intestinal tract.
6. Toxin production and release.
7. Enhancement of other diseases.

Improved growth rates, feed efficiency and general herd health have been observed following the use of formulated dichlorvos. The best opportunity for receiving such benefits will be afforded by treating pigs as early in life as is practical, i.e., five to six weeks of age and again four to five weeks later. Additional treatments to feeder pigs may be dictated by extreme re-exposure rates on the premises and other management practices which favor rapid parasite development.

Gilts, sows and boars should not be ignored in a general parasite control program. These animals can serve as constant sources of infective eggs and larvae. To minimize contamination from the breeding stock, it is recommended to treat these animals routinely one week prior to breeding and again one week prior to farrowing.

Clear economic responses will not always be obtained by the use of the product. Variablility in such responses will be directly related to the degree of dichlorovs-sensitive parasite populations present in the treated animals.

Parasite Control: Push-button swine parasite control is the dream of some, but it is yet to be accomplished. One is working with an animal that has been thousands of years in the making and a host-parasite relationship that has come about over eons (geological ages) of adjustment. The parasite's life is one of a large income without work, security without effort and protection without fear. In order to perpetuate this type of life, nature has amply provided mechanisms to ensure continuation of the species. The primary mechanism is concerned with massive egg production and the ability of these eggs to remain infective under a variety of conditions.

In order to obtain the maximum benefits from the ATGARD® preparation, the following general points will be helpful.

1. Establish or maintain proper nutrition, care, housing and sanitation.
2. Worm control is similar to weed control - never let a parasite go to seed.
3. Consider every pig as an individual and meet its needs.
   a. Provide adequate feeder space.
   b. Separate small pigs from larger pigs and treat both lots separately.
   c. Follow dosage directions.
   d. Estimate the weights of pigs correctly.
   e. Remove normal rations before initiating treatment.
   f. Do not treat pigs with an appetite impaired due to disease. Correct the deficiency by proper treatment first.
   g. Do not treat pigs showing signs of increased peristalsis (scours, diarrhea). Correct with proper therapy and then treat for worm removal.
4. Treat pigs as early in life as is practical, i.e., five to six weeks of age and repeat the treatment four to five weeks later.
5. Treat sows 7-10 days before breeding and farrowing. In the Midwest where nodular worms are a problem the infective eggs do not survive freezing. Carrier sows maintain infection from season to season. The treatment of sows during the winter months will minimize warm season contamination rates.
6. Frequently consult a practicing veterinarian, extension specialist, or university parasitologist on how to best meet special parasite control needs.

Trial Data: Table 1 illustrates the preparation's efficacy against sexually immature and/or 4th stage larvae of the roundworm, nodular worms, and whipworm respectively in naturally infected pigs individually treated with the recommended dose in feed. In all trials, the anthelmintic efficacy was well over 90%.

Table 1:

Ref.	No. Pigs	Avg. Body Weight (lbs)	Worms eliminated/Worms at necropsy (Percent efficacy)		
			Roundworms	Nodular worms	Whipworms
1	64	31.8	410/0 (100%)	66/4 (94.3%)	1,693/9 (99.5%)
2	6	46.5	69/0 (100%)	63/0 (100%)	119/7 (94.4%)
9	98	36.9	652/13 (98%)	826/55 (93.8%)	1,545/9 (99.4%)

Table 2 illustrates the preparation's efficacy against sexually mature adults of the roundworm, nodular worms, whipworm and stomach worm respectively in naturally infected pigs individually treated with the recommended dose in feed. The anthelmintic efficacy in all trials was consistently greater than 97%.

Table 2:

Ref.	No. Pigs	Avg. Body Weight (lbs)	Worms eliminated/Worms at necropsy (percent efficacy)			
			Roundworms	Nodular worms	Whipworms	Stomach worms
1	64	31.8	723/7 (99%)	1,955/45 (97.8%)	13,006/51 (99.6%)	5/0 (100%)
9	98	36.9	423/10 (97.7%)	525/9 (98.3%)	1,259/18 (98.6%)	738/0 (100%)

Table 3 illustrates the ability of ATGARD® Swine Wormer (dichlorvos) to reduce the fecal parasite egg counts in breeding swine, thus helping to minimize premise contamination. When ATGARD® Swine Wormer is used as part of a regular parasite treatment program in young growing pigs and in breeding stock on a given farm, it becomes an important management factor by gradually lowering the overall parasite exposure rate and subsequent infection levels.

Table 3: Effects of ATGARD® Swine Wormer on fecal passage of parasite eggs when given to breeding stock.

Breeding Class	Trial Location No.	Total No. Animals	Avg. Body Weight (lbs)	Results of individual fecal examinations for parasite eggs.					
				Roundworms		Nodular Worms		Whipworms	
				No. Infected	No. Cleared	No. Infected	No. Cleared	No. Infected	No. Cleared
Gilts	1	25	350	25	25	0	—	2	2
Gilts	3	2	400	0	—	2	2	0	—
Gilts	2	24	275	12	12	6	6	17	17
Gilts	5	43	300	37	36	28	23	0	—
Sows	2	53	400	1	1	53	53	0	—
Sows	3	4	400	1	1	4	3	0	—
Sows	5	26	400	8	8	21	21	0	—
Sows	10	24	275	24	24	24	24	24	24
Boars	5	5	400	4	4	4	4	0	—
Boar	1	1	375	1	1	0	—	0	—
Totals (all locations)				113	112	142	136	43	43

References: Available upon request.

Presentation: 1.92 oz (54.6 g) packets, 5 packets to a box, 12 boxes to a carton.

ATGARD® is a Registered Trademark of Boehringer Ingelheim Vetmedica, Inc.

Compendium Code No.: 10280061 610701F-01-9909

ATROBAC® 3

Pfizer Animal Health **Bacterin-Toxoid**

Bordetella Bronchiseptica-Erysipelothrix Rhusiopathiae-Pasteurella Multocida Bacterin-Toxoid

U.S. Vet. Lic. No.: 189

Contents: ATROBAC® 3 consists of killed, standardized cultures of *B. bronchiseptica, Erysipelothrix rhusiopathiae,* and toxigenic *P. multocida,* with adjuvants added.

Indications: For use in healthy swine as an aid in the prevention and control of erysipelas, and atrophic rhinitis due to *Bordetella bronchiseptica* and toxigenic *Pasteurella multocida* (type A or D).

Directions: For protection against atrophic rhinitis it is advisable to vaccinate sows and gilts and their litters. Shake well.

Sows and Gilts: Aseptically administer a single 5-mL dose subcutaneously to healthy sows and gilts 7 weeks before farrowing, followed by a second dose 4 weeks later. Revaccination with a single dose 3 weeks before subsequent farrowings is recommended.

Pigs: Aseptically administer a single 2-mL dose subcutaneously to healthy pigs 1 week of age, followed by a second dose 3 weeks later.

Precaution(s): Store at 2°-7°C. Do not freeze. Use entire contents when first opened.

Caution(s): As with many vaccines, anaphylaxis may occur after use. Initial antidote of epinephrine is recommended and should be followed with appropriate supportive therapy.

Warning(s): Do not vaccinate within 21 days before slaughter. For veterinary use only.

Presentation: 20 mL and 100 mL vials.

Compendium Code No.: 36900170 85-4004-04

ATROBAN® 11% EC INSECTICIDE

Schering-Plough **Premise and Topical Insecticide**

Emulsifiable Concentrate Long-Lasting Insecticidal Spray

EPA Reg. No.: 773-59

Active Ingredient(s):

Permethrin: 3-(phenoxyphenyl)methyl (±)-cis, trans-3-(2,2-dichloroethenyl)-2, 2-dimethylcyclopropanecarboxylate* 11.0%
Other Ingredients 89.0%
100.0%

*cis/trans ratio: Max. 55% (±) cis and min. 45% (±) trans.

Contains petroleum distillates.

The product contains 0.107 lbs (48.5 g) of permethrin per pint (473 mL).

Indications: ATROBAN® 11% EC Insecticide is an emulsifiable concentrate long-lasting insecticidal spray for livestock and their premises.

For the control of horn flies, face flies, stable flies, house flies, horse flies, black flies, mosquitoes, eye gnats, mange mites, scabies mites, ticks, lice, and sheep keds on lactating and non-lactating dairy cattle and goats, beef cattle, horses and sheep.

For the control of Northern fowl mites on poultry.

For the control of lice and mange on swine.

For use in and around horse, beef, dairy, swine, sheep and poultry premises, animal hospital pens and kennels and outside meat processing premises to control house flies, stable flies, little house flies *(Fannia* spp.). It also aids in the control of cockroaches, ants, spiders, mosquitoes, crickets, face flies.

Directions for Use: It is a violation of Federal law to use this product in a manner inconsistent with its labeling.

Mix ATROBAN® 11% EC Insecticidal Spray thoroughly as follows:

Repeat applications as needed, but not more often than once every 2 weeks. Spray lactating dairy animals only after milking is completed. Use as needed on horses not intended for human consumption.

Lactating and Non-Lactating Dairy Cattle and Goats, Beef Cattle, Horses and Sheep:

1. Horn flies, Face flies, Stable flies, House flies, Horse flies, Black flies, Mosquitoes, Eye gnats, Mange mites, Scabies mites, Ticks, Lice, Sheep keds (Sprayer): Dilute 1 pt to 25 gals water (3 tbsp/2.5 gals). Apply 1-2 qts of coarse spray per animal over whole body surface. For mange, scabies, ticks and lice, thoroughly wet animal. Repeat application in 10-14 days for mites.
2. Horn flies only (Sprayer): Dilute 1 pt to 50 gals water (3 tbsp/2.5 gals). Apply 1 qt of coarse spray per animal.
3. Horn flies, Face flies, Stable flies, Ear ticks (Low Pressure Sprayer): Dilute 1 pt to 2.5 gals water (3 tbsp/qt). Apply 1-2 oz spray per animal. Spot treat back, face, legs and ears.
4. Horn flies, Face flies, Stable flies (Back Rubber/Self oiler): Dilute 1 pt to 10 gals diesel oil (3 tbsp/gal). Keep rubbing device charged. Results are improved by daily forced use.

Poultry:

Northern fowl mites (Sprayer): Dilute 1 pt to 25 gals water (3 tbsp/2.5 gals). Apply 1 gal of coarse spray per 100 birds, paying particular attention to vent area.

Swine:

Lice, Mange (Sprayer): Dilute 1 pt to 25 gals water (3 tbsp/2.5 gals). Thoroughly wet animals, including ears. For mange, repeat at 14 days.

Premises — In and around Horse, Beef, Dairy, Swine, Sheep and Poultry Premises, Animal Hospital Pens and Kennels and outside Meat Processing Premises. Note: This product is not recommended for use on vinyl or plastic surfaces.

House Flies, Stable Flies, Little House Flies *(Fannia* spp.). Aids in control of cockroaches, ants, spiders, mosquitoes, crickets, Face flies:

a. Sprayer: Dilute 1 pt to 10 gals water (3 tbsp/gal). Spray to point of runoff or 1 gal per 750-1000 sq. ft.
b. Overhead space spray system: Dilute 1 pt to 10 gals diesel or mineral oil (3 tbsp/gal). Apply 4 oz spray per 1000 cu. ft. of air space.

Do not apply dilutions for premise treatment directly on livestock or poultry. Ensure that feed and water are not contaminated by spray drift. For space spraying, do not remain in treated areas and ventilate the areas before reoccupying. Animals should be removed from areas prior to treatment. Do not use in milk rooms. The use of any residual fly spray should be supplemented with proper manure management and general sanitation to reduce or eliminate fly breeding sites.

Precautionary Statements: Hazards to Humans and Domestic Animals:

Caution: Harmful if swallowed or absorbed through the skin. Avoid contact with skin, eyes or clothing. Avoid breathing spray mist. Remove contaminated clothing and wash clothing before reuse.

Statement of Practical Treatment:

If Swallowed: Call a doctor or get medical attention. Do not induce vomiting. Do not give anything by mouth to an unconscious person. Avoid alcohol.

If on Skin: Remove contaminated clothing and wash skin thoroughly with soap and water after handling.

If in Eyes: Immediately flush eyes with plenty of water. Get medical attention if irritation persists.

If Inhaled: Remove victim to fresh air. Apply artificial respiration if needed. Get medical attention.

Note to Physician: Vomiting may cause aspiration pneumonia.

Environmental Hazards: Do not apply directly to water, or to areas where surface water is present, or to intertidal areas below the mean high water mark. Do not contaminate water when cleaning equipment or disposing of equipment washwaters.

Physical or Chemical Hazard: Do not use or store near heat or open flame.

Storage and Disposal: Do not contaminate water, food or feed by storage or disposal.

Storage: Store in a cool, dry place.

Pesticide Disposal: Pesticide wastes are toxic. Improper disposal of excess pesticide, spray mixture, or rinsate is a violation of Federal law. If these wastes cannot be disposed of by use according to label instructions, contact your State Pesticide or Environmental Control Agency, or the Hazardous Waste Representative at the nearest EPA Regional Office for guidance.

Container Disposal: Triple rinse (or equivalent). Then offer for recycling or reconditioning, or puncture and dispose of in a sanitary landfill, or by incineration, or if allowed by State and local authorities by burning. If burned, stay out of smoke.

Warning(s): For swine allow 5 days between last treatment and slaughter.

Use as needed on horses not intended for human consumption. Keep out of reach of children.

Disclaimer: Notice of Warranty: Schering-Plough Animal Health Corp. makes no warranty of merchantability, fitness for any particular purpose or otherwise, expressed or implied, concerning this product or its uses which extend beyond the use of the product under normal conditions in accord with the statements made on the label.

Presentation 1 pint (473 mL) and 1 U.S. quart (946 mL).

Compendium Code No.: 10470072 Rev. 3/00

ATROBAN® 42.5% EC

Schering-Plough **Topical Insecticide**

Insecticidal Spray

EPA Reg. No.: 773-60

Active Ingredient(s):

Permethrin (3-phenoxyphenyl) methyl (±) cis, trans-3-(2,2-dichloroethenyl)-2,2-dimethylcyclopropanecarboxylate* 42.5%

Inert Ingredients: 57.5%

Total 100.0%

This product contains xylene.

*cis/trans ratio: Max 55% (±) cis and min 45% (±) trans

This product contains 0.45 lbs (204 g) of permethrin per pint (473 mL).

Indications: Insecticidal spray for livestock, horses, cattle, swine, sheep, poultry and their premises.

Directions for Use: It is a violation of Federal law to use this product in a manner inconsistent with its labeling.

Dip Treatment General Instructions: Charge dip vats with recommended application concentration by using quantities of ATROBAN® 42.5% EC insecticidal spray and clean water as directed below. Mix thoroughly before each use. Dip to thoroughly wet animals to ensure complete coverage.

Spray Treatment General Instructions: For all sprays intended for direct application to animals and building surfaces, add ATROBAN® 42.5% EC insecticidal spray to clean water as directed below, mix thoroughly and apply as a coarse spray. Spray lactating dairy cows only after milking is completed.

Recommended Applications: The use of ATROBAN® 42.5% EC insecticidal spray requires no withdrawal period between last application and slaughter.

For Control of Horn flies on Beef, Dairy Cattle (Lactating and Non-Lactating), and Horses: Dilute ATROBAN® 42.5% EC insecticidal spray with clean water at a ratio of 1:1600 (½ pint/100 gal). A 1:1600 dilution gives a 0.027% permethrin concentration. Apply sufficient spray (approximately 1 qt/animal) or dip to thoroughly wet animals to ensure complete coverage. Repeat applications as needed but not more often than once every 2 weeks.

For Control of Horn flies, Face flies, Stable flies, House flies, Horse flies, Mosquitoes, and Lice on Beef, Dairy Cattle (Lactating and Non-Lactating), Sheep, Goats, and Horses: Dilute ATROBAN® 42.5% EC insecticidal spray with clean water at a ratio of 1:800 (1 pint/100 gal). A 1:800 dilution gives a 0.054% permethrin concentration. Apply sufficient spray (approximately 2 qts/animal) or dip to thoroughly wet animals to ensure complete coverage. Repeat applications as needed but not more often than once every 2 weeks.

For Control of Ticks (including the genera *Boophilus* spp., *Amblyomma, Dermacentor, and Rhipicephalus),* Chorioptic mites, and Psoroptic (Scabies) mites on Beef, Dairy Cattle (Lactating and Non-Lactating), Sheep, Goats, and Horses: Dilute ATROBAN® 42.5% EC insecticidal spray with clean water at a ratio of 1:800 (1 pint/100 gal). A 1:800 dilution gives a 0.054% concentration. Apply sufficient spray (approximately 2 qts/animal) or dip to thoroughly wet animals to ensure complete coverage. Repeat applications as needed but not more often than once every 10 to 14 days.

For Control of Northern fowl mites and Lice on Poultry in Cages or Houses: Dilute ATROBAN® 42.5% EC insecticidal spray with clean water at a ratio of 1:800 (¼ pint/25 gal). A 1:800 dilution gives a 0.054% permethrin concentration. Apply sufficient spray (approximately 1 gal/100 birds). One application should control an infestation. Do not treat more often than once every 2 weeks and do not apply more than four treatments.

For Control of Hog lice on Swine: Dilute ATROBAN® 42.5% EC insecticidal spray with clean water at a ratio of 1:800 (¼ pint/25 gal). A 1:800 dilution gives a 0.054% permethrin concentration. Apply sufficient spray to thoroughly wet animals to ensure complete coverage (approximately 1 pint/animal). One application should control an infestation. Do not treat swine 5 days prior to slaughter.

For Control of Mange mites on Swine: Dilute ATROBAN® 42.5% EC insecticidal spray with clean water at a ratio of 1:400 (¼ pint/12½ gal). A 1:400 dilution gives a 0.108% permethrin concentration. Apply sufficient spray to thoroughly wet animals to ensure complete coverage (approximately 1 pint/animal). Repeat application in 14 days. Do not treat swine 5 days prior to slaughter.

For use in and around Horse, Beef, Dairy, Swine, Sheep, and Poultry Premises and Outside Meat Processing Premises for Control of House flies, Stable flies, and Little house flies *(Fannia* spp.):

Note: This product is not recommended for use on vinyl or plastic surfaces.

Dilute ATROBAN® 42.5% EC insecticidal spray with clean water at a ratio of 1:320 (¼ pint/10 gal). A 1:320 dilution gives a 0.128% permethrin concentration. For small amounts of finished spray, mix 1½ teaspoonfuls in a gallon of water. Apply finished spray to surfaces where flies rest at the rate of one gallon per 750-1000 sq ft, but do not allow runoff to occur. Timing and frequency of application should be based upon flies reaching nuisance levels, but not more often than once every 2 weeks. If, under conditions of heavy fly pressure, longer residual control is desired, it is permissible to double the above concentration for premise application. Do not apply dilution for premise treatment directly on livestock or poultry. Ensure that animals' feed and water are not contaminated by spray drift. Do not use in milk rooms.

Precautionary Statements: Hazards to Humans and Domestic Animals:

Danger. Corrosive. Causes skin burns and severe eye irritation. Do not get in eyes, on skin, or on clothing. Harmful if swallowed. Avoid breathing spray mist. Wear goggles or face shield, rubber gloves, and protective clothing (i.e., coveralls worn over long sleeved shirt and long pants, socks, and chemical resistant footwear) when handling this concentrate. Wash thoroughly with soap and water after handling. Remove contaminated clothing and wash before reuse.

First Aid:

If Swallowed: Call a poison control center or doctor immediately for treatment advice. Have person sip a glass of water if able to swallow. Do not induce vomiting unless told to do so by a poison control center or doctor.

If on Skin or Clothing: Take off contaminated clothing. Rinse skin immediately with plenty of water for 15-20 minutes. Call a poison control center or doctor for treatment advice.

If in Eyes: Hold eye open and rinse gently with water 15-20 minutes. Remove contact lenses, if present, after the first 5 minutes, then continue rinsing eyes. Call a poison control center for treatment advice.

If Inhaled: Move person to fresh air. If person is not breathing, call 911 or an ambulance, then give artificial respiration, preferably mouth-to-mouth, if possible. Call a poison control center or doctor for further advice.

Note to Physician: Probable mucosal damage may contraindicate the use of gastric lavage. Vomiting may cause aspiration pneumonia.

Have the product container or label with you when calling a poison control center or doctor or going for treatment.

Environmental Hazards: This pesticide is toxic to fish and other aquatic organisms. Do not apply directly to water, or to areas where surface water is present, or to intertidal areas below the mean high water mark. Do not contaminate water when cleaning equipment or disposing of equipment washwaters.

Physical or Chemical Hazard: Do not use or store near heat or open flame.

Storage and Disposal: Do not contaminate water, food, or feed by storage or disposal.

Storage: Store in cool, dry place away from heat or open flame.

Pesticide Disposal: Pesticide wastes are acutely hazardous. Improper disposal of excess pesticide, spray mixture, or rinsate is a violation of Federal law. If these wastes cannot be disposed of by use according to label instructions, contact your State Pesticide or Environmental Control Agency or the Hazardous Waste Representative at the nearest EPA Regional Office for guidance.

Container Disposal: Triple rinse (or equivalent). Then offer for recycling or reconditioning, or puncture and dispose of in a sanitary landfill, or incineration, or if allowed by State and local authorities, by burning. If burned, stay out of smoke.

Warning(s): The use of ATROBAN® 42.5% EC insecticidal spray requires no withdrawal period between last application and slaughter.

Do not treat swine 5 days prior to slaughter.

Presentation: 1 U.S. Pint (473 mL).

Compendium Code No.: 10470081 Rev. 7/00

ATROBAN® DELICE® POUR-ON INSECTICIDE

Schering-Plough **Topical Insecticide**

EPA Reg. No.: 773-66

Active Ingredient(s):

Permethrin: 3-(phenoxyphenyl)methyl (±) cis, trans-3-(2,2-dichloroethenyl-2,2-dimethylcyclopropanecarboxylate* 1.0%

Other Ingredients** 99.0%

100.0%

*cis/trans ratio: Min. 35% (±) cis and max. 65% (±) trans.

**Contains petroleum distillates.

Indications: Non-systemic pour-on insecticide for beef, lactating and non-lactating dairy cattle; controls lice and flies on cattle and keds and lice on sheep.

Directions for Use: It is a violation of Federal law to use the product in a manner inconsistent with its labeling.

Ready to use—No dilution necessary.

Lactating and Non-Lactating Dairy Cattle and Beef Cattle and Calves:

Target Insects: Lice, horn flies, face flies and aids in the control of: horse flies, stable flies, mosquitoes, blackflies, and ticks.

Application Instructions: Pour along back and down face. Apply ½ fl oz (15 cc) per 100 lbs body wt of animal, up to a maximum of 5 fl oz for any one animal.

Sheep:

Target Insects: Sheep keds and lice.

Application Instructions: Pour along back. Apply ¼ fl oz (7.5 cc) per 50 lb body wt of animal, up to a maximum of 3 fl oz for any one animal.

For cattle and sheep, repeat treatment as needed, but not more often than once every 2 weeks. For optimum lice control, two treatments at 14-day intervals are recommended.

Special Note: ATROBAN® DELICE® Pour-On Insecticide is not effective in controlling cattle grubs.

Precautionary Statements: Hazards to Humans and Domestic Animals:

Caution—Avoid contact with the eyes.

Statement of Practical Treatment:

If In Eyes: Immediately flush eyes with plenty of water. Get medical attention if discomfort persists.

If Swallowed: Call a physician immediately. Do not induce vomiting unless under medical attention.

Note to Physician: The solvent presents an aspiration hazard. Gastric lavage is indicated if material was taken internally.

Environmental Hazards: The pesticide is extremely toxic to fish. Use with care when applying to areas adjacent to any body of water. Do not add directly to water. Do not contaminate water by cleaning of equipment or disposal of wastes. Apply this product only as specified on the label.

Physical or Chemical Hazards: Do not use or store near heat or open flame.

Storage and Disposal: Do not contaminate water, food or feed by storage or disposal.

Storage: Keep the container sealed when not in use. Do not store near food or feed.

Pesticide Disposal: Wastes resulting from the use of the product may be disposed of on site or at an approved waste disposal facility.

Container Disposal: Triple rinse (or equivalent). Then offer for recycling or reconditioning, or puncture and dispose of in a sanitary landfill or by incineration, or, if allowed by state and local authorities, by burning. If burned, stay out of smoke.

Warning(s): Keep out of reach of children.

Disclaimer: Notice of Warranty: Schering-Plough Animal Health Corp. makes no warranty of merchantability, fitness for any particular purpose or otherwise expressed or implied concerning this product or its uses which extend beyond the use of the product under normal conditions in accord with the statements made on this label.

Presentation: 1 U.S. gallon (3.785 L), 2.5 gallons and 55 gallons.

Compendium Code No.: 10470091 20722916 Rev. 8/00

ATROBAN® EXTRA INSECTICIDE EAR TAGS

Schering-Plough **Insecticide Ear Tags**

EPA Reg. No.: 773-78

Active Ingredient(s): % by wt

Permethrin: (3-phenoxyphenyl) methyl (±)-cis,trans-3-(2,2-dichloroethenyl)-2,2-dimethylcyclopropanecarboxylate* 10.0
Piperonyl Butoxide Technical** 13.0
Other Ingredients: 77.0
Total 100.0

*cis/trans ratio: Max 55% (±)cis and min 45% (±) trans

**Equivalent to min 10.4% (butycarbityl)(6-propylpiperonyl) ether and 2.6% related compounds.

Indications: For use on dairy (lactating and non-lactating) and beef cattle and calves to control horn flies, face flies, gulf coast ticks, spinose ear ticks, and as an aid to control lice, stable flies and house flies.

Directions for Use: It is a violation of Federal law to use this product in a manner inconsistent with its labeling.

1. Place male button onto pin until it projects through the tip.
2. Dip tag button into disinfectant solution.
3. Press female tag under the clip by depressing lever.
4. Apply through ear between second and third rib, halfway between ear tip and head.

For control of horn flies, attach one tag to each ear of each animal. Tags remain effective up to 5 months. For season-long control of gulf coast ticks and face flies and as an aid in the control of lice, stable flies, and house flies, attach two tags per animal (one in each ear). Apply when flies first appear in spring. Replace as necessary. Apply with Allflex® Tagging System.

Precautionary Statements: Hazards to Humans and Domestic Animals:

Caution: Wash thoroughly with soap and water after handling and before eating or smoking. Avoid contamination of feed and foodstuffs.

First Aid:

If on Skin or Clothing: Take off contaminated clothing. Rinse skin immediately with plenty of water for 15-20 minutes. Call a poison control center or doctor for treatment advice.

If Inhaled: Move person to fresh air. If person is not breathing, call 911 or an ambulance, then give artificial respiration, preferably mouth-to-mouth if possible. Call a poison control center or doctor for further treatment advice.

If Swallowed: Call a poison control center or doctor immediately for treatment advice. Have person sip a glass of water if able to swallow. Do not induce vomiting unless told to do so by the poison control center or doctor. Do not induce vomiting or give anything by mouth to any unconscious person.

Hotline Number: Have the product container or label with you when calling the poison control center or doctor or going for treatment. You may also contact the Rocky Mountain Poison Center at 1-303-595-4869 for emergency medical treatment information.

Environmental Hazards: This pesticide is toxic to fish. Do not add directly to water. Do not contaminate water by disposal of used tags. Use this product only as specified on the label.

Storage and Disposal: Do not contaminate water, food or feed by storage or disposal.

Storage: Store in cool place away from direct sunlight.

Pesticide Disposal: Remove tags before slaughter. Wastes resulting from the use of this product may be disposed of on site or at an approved waste disposal facility.

Container Disposal: Dispose of empty bag in a sanitary landfill or by incineration, or, if allowed by State and local authorities, by burning. If burned, stay out of smoke.

Warning(s): Remove tags before slaughter.

Keep out of reach of children.

Disclaimer: Notice of Warranty: Schering-Plough Animal Health Corp. makes no warranty of merchantability, fitness for any particular purpose or otherwise expressed or implied concerning this product or its uses beyond the use of this product under normal conditions in accord with the statements made on the label.

Presentation: 20 x 9.5 g tags and buttons.

Allflex is a registered trademark of AllFlex USA, Inc.

Compendium Code No.: 10470101 Rev. 3/01

ATROJECT ℞

Vetus **Anticholinergic**

Active Ingredient(s): Each mL contains:

Atropine sulfate .... 0.54 mg
Sodium chloride .... 9 mg
Benzyl alcohol (preservative) 1.5%
Water for injection .... q.s.

The pH is adjusted with sulfuric acid when necessary.

Indications: For use as a preanesthetic adjuvant.

Dosage and Administration: For intravenous, intramuscular or subcutaneous use.

Dogs and Cats: Inject 1 mL for each 20 lbs. of body weight as a preanesthetic adjuvant or to reduce salivation, bronchial secretion, or internal peristalsis associated with colic or diarrhea.

As an antidote for parasympathomimetic drugs, inject 1 mL for each 7.5 lbs. of body weight.

It is suggested that one-quarter (¼) of the dose should be injected intravenously, and the remainder either by intramuscular or subcutaneous injection.

Caution(s): Federal law restricts this drug to use by or on the order of a licensed veterinarian.

For veterinary use only.

Antidote(s): Warmth, emetics, cholinergics.

Warning(s): Poisonous alkaloid. Keep out of reach of children.

Presentation: 100 mL multiple dose vials.

Compendium Code No.: 14440060

ATROPINE L.A. ℞

Butler **Anticholinergic**

Active Ingredient(s): Each mL contains:

Atropine sulfate .... 15 mg
Sodium chloride .... 9 mg
Benzyl alcohol (preservative) 1%
Water for injection .... q.s.

The pH is adjusted with sulfuric acid and/or sodium hydroxide if necessary.

Indications: For use as an antidote in the treatment of organophosphate insecticide poisoning in cattle, horses, and sheep.

Dosage and Administration: Initial dose:

Cattle: 30 mg per 100 lbs. of body weight.
Horses: 6.5 mg per 100 lbs. of body weight.
Sheep: 50 mg per 100 lbs. of body weight.

The recommended average initial dose should be split, injecting one-quarter (¼) to one-third (⅓) slowly I.V. and the remainder I.M. or S.C. After the symptoms appear to be under control, repeated maintenance doses should be administered based on the individual response of the animal.

Caution(s): Federal (USA) law restricts this drug to use by or on the order of a licensed veterinarian For veterinary use only. Poisonous alkaloid. Keep out of the reach of children.

Antidote(s): Warmth, emetics, cholinergics.

Presentation: 100 mL sterile multiple dose vials.

Compendium Code No.: 10820150

ATROPINE SA ℞

Butler **Anticholinergic**

Active Ingredient(s): Each mL contains:

Atropine sulfate .... 0.54 mg
Sodium chloride .... 9 mg
Benzyl alcohol (preservative) 1.5%
Water for injection .... q.s.

The pH is adjusted with sulfuric acid when necessary.

Indications: For use as a pre-anesthetic adjuvant or to reduce salivation, bronchial secretion or internal peristalsis associated with colic or diarrhea. Also for use as an antidote for parasympathomimetic drugs.

Dosage and Administration:

Dogs and Cats: Inject 1 mL for each 20 lbs. of body weight as a pre-anesthetic adjuvant or to reduce salivation, bronchial secretion or internal peristalsis associated with colic or diarrhea.

As an antidote for parasympathomimetic drugs: 1 mL for each 7.5 lbs. of body weight. It is suggested that one-quarter (¼) of the dosage be injected I.V. and the remainder I.M. or S.C.

Caution(s): Federal (USA) law restricts this drug to use by or on the order of a licensed veterinarian. For veterinary use only.

Antidote(s): Warmth, emetics, cholinergics.

Warning(s): Poisonous alkaloid. Keep out of the reach of children.

Presentation: 100 mL sterile multiple dose vial.

Compendium Code No.: 10820161

ATROPINE SULFATE 1/120 ℞

Neogen **Anticholinergic**

Sterile Solution

Active Ingredient(s): Each mL contains:

Atropine sulfate .... 0.54 mg
Sodium chloride .... 9 mg
Benzyl Alcohol 1.5%
Water for Injection .... q.s.

Indications: For use in dogs and cats as an antidote in the treatment of organophosphate insecticide poisoning; to reduce salivation, bronchial secretions or intestinal peristalsis associated with colic or diarrhea, and as a preanesthetic adjuvant.

Dosage and Administration: Dogs and Cats: Inject intravenously, intramuscularly, or subcutaneously, 1 mL for each 20 lb of body weight as a preanesthetic adjuvant, or to reduce salivation, bronchial secretions, or intestinal peristalsis associated with colic or diarrhea.

As an antidote for parasympathomimetic drugs, inject 1 mL for each 5 lbs of body weight administered to effect and repeat as necessary. It is suggested that ¼ of the dosage be injected intravenously and the remainder intramuscularly or subcutaneously.

Precaution(s): Store at controlled room temperature between 15°-30°C (59°-86°F).

Caution(s): Federal law restricts this drug to use by or on the order of a licensed veterinarian.

For animal use only.

Warning(s): Poisonous alkaloid. Keep out of reach of children.

Antidote(s): Warmth, emetics, cholinergics.

Presentation: 12 x 100 mL multi-dose vials per carton (NDC: 59051-9051-5).

Manufactured by: Sparhawk Laboratories, Lenexa, KS 66215.

Compendium Code No.: 14910022 0501

ATROPINE SULFATE 1/120 ℞

Vet Tek **Anticholinergic**

Injection 1/120 Grain

Active Ingredient(s): Each mL Contains:

Atropine Sulfate .... 0.54 mg
Sodium Chloride .... 9 mg
Benzyl Alcohol (preservative) 1.5%
Water For Injection .... q.s.

pH adjusted with sulfuric acid when necessary.

Indications: For use as a pre-anesthetic adjuvant or to reduce salivation, bronchial secretion or internal peristalsis associated with colic or diarrhea in dogs and cats. It is also used as an antidote for parasympathomimetic drugs.

Dosage and Administration: For intravenous, intramuscular or subcutaneous use.

Dogs and cats: Inject 1 mL for each 20 lbs of body weight as a pre-anesthetic adjuvant or to reduce salivation, bronchial secretion or internal peristalsis associated with colic or diarrhea.

As an antidote for parasympathomimetic drugs, 1 mL for each 7.5 lbs of body weight It is suggested that ¼ of the dosage be injected intravenous and the remainder intramuscular or subcutaneous.

Precaution(s): Store between 15°C-30°C (59°F-86°F).

Caution(s): Federal law restricts this drug to use by or on the order of a licensed veterinarian. For animal use only.
Antidote(s): Warmth, emetic, cholinergics.
Warning(s): Poisonous alkaloid. Keep out of reach of children.
Presentation: 100 mL vials (NDC 60270-022-10).
Compendium Code No.: 14200021 Iss. 8-95

ATROPINE SULFATE INJECTION ℞

Vedco **Anticholinergic**

Active Ingredient(s): Each mL contains:
Atropine sulfate .... 0.54 mg
Sodium chloride .... 9 mg
Benzyl alcohol (preservative) 1.5%
Water for injection .... q.s.

Indications: ATROPINE SULFATE INJECTION is used as a pre-anesthetic adjuvant or to reduce salivation, bronchial secretion or internal peristalis associated with colic or diarrhea.

Dosage and Administration:
Dogs and Cats: Inject 1 mL for each 20 lbs. of body weight.
As an antidote for parasymphathomimetic drugs, 1 mL for each 7.5 lbs. of body weight. It is suggested that one-quarter (¼) of the dosage be inject intravenously and the remainder intramuscularly or subcutaneously.

Caution(s): Federal law restricts this drug to use by or on the order of a licensed veterinarian. Poisonous alkaloid. Keep out of the reach of children.
Antidote(s): Warmth, emetics, cholinergics.
Presentation: 100 mL sterile multiple dose vial.
Compendium Code No.: 10940101

ATROPINE SULFATE INJECTION 1/120 GRAIN ℞

Phoenix Pharmaceutical **Anticholinergic**

1/120 Grain
Active Ingredient(s): Each mL contains:
Atropine Sulfate .... 0.54 mg
Sodium Chloride .... 9 mg
Benzyl Alcohol (preservative) 1.5%
Water for Injection .... q.s.
pH adjusted with sulfuric acid when necessary.

Indications: For use in dogs and cats as a pre-anesthetic adjuvant or to reduce salivation, bronchial secretion or internal peristalis associated with colic or diarrhea.
This product is also used as an antidote for parasympathomimetic drugs.

Dosage and Administration: For intravenous, intramuscular or subcutaneous use.
Dogs and Cats: Inject 1 mL for each 20 lbs of body weight as a pre-anesthetic adjuvant or to reduce salivation, bronchial secretion or internal peristalis associated with colic or diarrhea.
As an antidote for parasympathomimetic drugs, 1 mL for each 7.5 lbs of body weight. It is suggested that ¼ of the dosage be injected intravenous and the remainder intramuscular or subcutaneous.

Precaution(s): Store between 15°C and 30°C (59°F and 86°F).
Caution(s): Federal law restricts this drug to use by or on the order of a licensed veterinarian. For animal use only.
Warning(s): Poisonous alkaloid. Keep out of reach of children. Antidotes: Warmth, emetics, cholinergics.
Presentation: 100 mL sterile multiple dose vials (NDC 57319-340-05).
Manufactured by: Phoenix Scientific, St. Joseph, MO 64503.
Compendium Code No.: 12560092 Rev. 8/01

ATROPINE SULFATE INJECTION 15 MG/ML L.A. ℞

RXV **Anticholinergic**

Active Ingredient(s): Each mL contains:
Atropine sulfate .... 15 mg
Sodium chloride .... 9 mg
Benzyl alcohol (preservative) 1%
Water for injection .... q.s.
pH adjusted with sulfuric acid and/or sodium hydroxide if necessary.

Indications: For use as an antidote in the treatment of organophosphate insecticide poisoning of cattle, horses, and sheep.

Dosage and Administration: Initial Dose:
Cattle - 30 mg per 100 lbs of body weight.
Horses - 6.5 mg per 100 lbs of body weight.
Sheep - 50 mg per 100 lbs of body weight.
The recommended average initial dose should be split, injecting ¼ to ⅓ slowly I.V. and the remainder I.M. or S.C. After symptoms appear to be under control, repeated maintenance doses should be administered based on the individual response of the animal.

Precaution(s): Store at controlled room temperature between 15°-30°C (59°-86°F).
Caution(s): Federal law restricts this drug to use by or on the order of a licensed veterinarian.
Antidote(s): Warmth, emetics, cholinergics.
Warning(s): Poisonous alkaloid. Keep out of the reach of children. For animal use only.
Presentation: 100 mL sterile multiple dose vials.
Compendium Code No.: 10910011

ATROPINE SULFATE L.A. 15 MG/ML ℞

Neogen **Anticholinergic**

Sterile Solution
Active Ingredient(s): Each mL contains:
Atropine Sulfate .... 15 mg
Sodium Chloride .... 9 mg
Methylparaben .... 1.8 mg
Propylparaben .... 0.2 mg
Water for Injection .... q.s.
pH adjusted with Hydrochloric Acid and/or Sodium Hydroxide if necessary.

Indications: For use as an antidote in the treatment of organophosphate insecticide poisoning of cattle, horses and sheep.

Dosage and Administration: Initial Dose:
Cattle: 30 mg per 100 lbs. of body weight.
Horses: 6.5 mg per 100 lbs. of body weight.
Sheep: 50 mg per 100 lbs. of body weight.
The recommended average initial dose should be split, injecting one quarter (¼) to one-third (⅓) slowly I.V. and the remainder I.M. or S.C. After symptoms appear to be under control, repeated maintenance doses should be administered based on the individual response of the animal.

Precaution(s): Store at controlled room temperature between 15°-30°C (59°-86°F).
Caution(s): Federal law restricts this drug to use by or on the order of a licensed veterinarian. For animal use only.
Warning(s): Poisonous alkaloid. Keep out of reach of children.
Antidote(s): Warmth, emetics, cholinergics.
Presentation: 12 x 100 mL multi-dose vials per carton (NDC: 59051-9050-5).
Manufactured by: Omega Laboratories, Montreal, Quebec, H3M 3E4.
Compendium Code No.: 14910032 0201

AUREOMIX® 500 GRANULAR

Alpharma **Feed Medication**

Chlortetracycline, sulfamethazine, penicillin-Type A Medicated Article
NADA No.: 035-688
Active Ingredient(s):
Chlortetracycline calcium complex equivalent to chlortetracycline HCl .... 40 g/lb
Sulfamethazine .... 8.8% (40 g/lb)
Penicillin (from procaine penicillin) .... 20 g/lb
Ingredients: Calcium sulfate and dried *Streptomyces aureofaciens* fermentation product.

Indications: For reduction of the incidence of cervical abscesses; treatment of bacterial swine enteritis (salmonellosis or necrotic enteritis caused by *Salmonella choleraesuis* and vibrionic dysentery); prevention of these diseases during times of stress; maintenance of weight gains in the presence of atrophic rhinitis; growth promotion and increased feed efficiency in swine weighing up to 75 pounds.
For use in the manufacture of swine feeds.

Directions: Mixing directions: Use 2.5 lb AUREOMIX® 500 per 1 ton (907.2 kg) of final feed. Make a preblend of 2.5 lb of AUREOMIX® 500 with part (15-20 lb) of the feed ingredients. Mix thoroughly with the remainder of the ingredients to give a final concentration of 100 g chlortetracycline, 100 g sulfamethazine and 50 g penicillin per ton of feed.

Warning(s): Withdraw 15 days prior to slaughter.
Presentation: 50 lb (22.68 kg) bag.
Compendium Code No.: 10220081 AHG-024 0104

AUREOMYCIN® 50 GRANULAR

Alpharma **Feed Medication**

Chlortetracycline-Type A Medicated Article
NADA No.: 048-761
Active Ingredient(s): Chlortetracycline calcium complex equivalent to 50 g chlortetracycline hydrochloride per lb.
Ingredients: Dried *Streptomyces aureofaciens* Fermentation Product and Calcium Sulfate.

Indications: For use in the manufacture of medicated animal feeds for cattle, swine, sheep, turkeys, chickens, ducks and psittacine birds.

Directions: Use directions: Mix sufficient AUREOMYCIN® 50 Granular Medicated Article to supply desired concentration of chlortetracycline per ton with part of the feed ingredients to make a preblend.
Add the remainder of the ingredients and mix thoroughly. For specific use levels, see below.
Mixing directions:

Level desired, grams per ton	Amount of medicated article per ton †
10	⅕ lb
50	1 lb
100	2 lb
200	4 lb
400	8 lb
500	10 lb

† It is recommended that 1 pound of AUREOMYCIN® 50 Granular Type A Medicated Article be diluted with 4 pounds of one of the feed ingredients to form a 5 pound working premix. Use 1 pound of the working premix to make a preblend (see Use directions) for a Type C feed containing 10 g AUREOMYCIN® chlortetracycline/ton of feed.

Cattle:
Calves (up to 250 lb): Increased rate of weight gain and improved feed efficiency. - 0.1 mg/lb Chlortetracycline body wt/day.
Beef Cattle (over 700 lb): Control of active infection of anaplasmosis caused by *Anaplasma marginale* susceptible to chlortetracycline. - 0.5 mg/lb Chlortetracycline body wt/day.
Beef and Non-Lactating Dairy Cattle (over 700 lb): Control of active infection of anaplasmosis caused by *Anaplasma marginale* susceptible to chlortetracycline when delivered in a free-choice feed. Free-choice feed must be manufactured under a feed mill license utilizing an FDA approved formulation. - 0.5 to 2.0 mg/lb Chlortetracycline body wt/day.
Calves, Beef and Non-Lactating Dairy Cattle: Treatment of bacterial enteritis caused by *Escherichia coli* and bacterial pneumonia caused by *Pasteurella multocida* organisms susceptible to chlortetracycline. Feed for not more than 5 days. The appropriate amount of AUREOMYCIN®-containing feed supplement may be mixed in the cattle's daily ration or administered as a top-dress. It must be spread uniformly on top of the ration and sufficient space must be provided so that all cattle can eat at the same time. - 10 mg/lb Chlortetracycline body wt/day.
Calves (250 to 400 lb): Increased rate of weight gain and improved feed efficiency. - 25 to 70 mg/head/day.
Growing Cattle (over 400 lb): Increased rate of weight gain, improved feed efficiency, and reduction of liver condemnation due to liver abscesses. - 70 mg/head/day.
Beef Cattle: Control of bacterial pneumonia associated with shipping fever complex caused by *Pasteurella* spp. susceptible to chlortetracycline. - 350 mg/head/day.
Beef Cattle (under 700 lb): Control of active infection of anaplasmosis caused by *Anaplasma marginale* susceptible to chlortetracycline. - 350 mg/head/day.
Swine:
Control of porcine proliferative enteropathies (ileitis) caused by *Lawsonia intracellularis* susceptible to chlortetracycline. - 10 mg/lb Chlortetracycline body wt/day.
Treatment of bacterial enteritis caused by *Escherichia coli* and *Salmonella choleraesuis* and bacterial pneumonia caused by *Pasteurella multocida* susceptible to chlortetracycline. (Note: This

dose is equivalent to 400 grams per ton, depending on feed consumption and body weight.) Feed for not more than 14 days. - 10 mg/lb Chlortetracycline body wt/day.

Increased rate of weight gain and improved feed efficiency. - 10 to 50 g/ton Chlortetracycline in complete feed.

Reduction in the incidence of cervical lymphadenitis (jowl abscesses) caused by Group E *Streptococci* susceptible to chlortetracycline. - 50 to 100 g/ton Chlortetracycline in complete feed.

Breeding Swine: Control of leptospirosis (reducing the incidence of abortion and shedding of leptospirae) caused by *Leptospira pomona* susceptible to chlortetracycline. Feed continuously for not more than 14 days. - 400 g/ton Chlortetracycline in complete feed.

Sheep:

Breeding Sheep: Reduction in the incidence of (vibrionic) abortions caused by *Campylobacter fetus* infection susceptible to chlortetracycline. - 80 mg/head/day.

Increased rate of weight gain and improved feed efficiency. - 20 to 50 g/ton Chlortetracycline in complete feed.

Turkeys:

Control of complicating bacterial organisms associated with bluecomb (transmissible enteritis; coronaviral enteritis) susceptible to chlortetracycline. Feed continuously for 7 to 14 days. - 25 mg/lb Chlortetracycline body wt/day.

Increased rate of weight gain and improved feed efficiency. - 10 to 50 g/ton Chlortetracycline in complete feed.

Control of infectious synovitis caused by *Mycoplasma synoviae* susceptible to chlortetracycline. Feed continuously for 7 to 14 days. - 200 g/ton Chlortetracycline in complete feed.

Control of hexamitiasis caused by *Hexamita meleagrides* susceptible to chlortetracycline. Feed continuously for 7 to 14 days. - 400 g/ton Chlortetracycline in complete feed.

Turkey Poults not over 4 weeks of age: Reduction of mortality due to paratyphoid caused by *Salmonella typhimurium* susceptible to chlortetracycline. - 400 g/ton Chlortetracycline in complete feed.

Chickens:

Increased rate of weight gain and improved feed efficiency. - 10 to 50 g/ton Chlortetracycline in complete feed.

Control of infectious synovitis caused by *Mycoplasma synoviae* susceptible to chlortetracycline. Feed continuously for 7 to 14 days. - 100 to 200 g/ton Chlortetracycline in complete feed.

Control of chronic respiratory disease (CRD) and air sac infection caused by *Mycoplasma gallisepticum* and *Escherichia coli* susceptible to chlortetracycline. Feed continuously for 7 to 14 days. - 200 to 400 g/ton Chlortetracycline in complete feed.

Reduction of mortality due to *Escherichia coli* infections susceptible to chlortetracycline. Feed for 5 days. - 500 g/ton Chlortetracycline in complete feed.

Ducks:

Control and treatment of fowl cholera caused by *Pasteurella multocida* susceptible to chlortetracycline. Feed in complete ration to provide from 8 to 28 mg per pound of body weight per day depending upon age and severity of disease. Feed for not more than 21 days. - 200 to 400 g/ton Chlortetracycline in complete feed.

Psittacine birds:

Treatment of psittacine birds (parrots, macaws, cockatoos) suspected or known to be infected with psittacosis caused by *Chlamydia psittaci* sensitive to chlortetracycline. Feed continuously for 45 days. Each bird should consume an amount of medicated feed equal to one-fifth of its body weight daily. During treatment, parrots, macaws, and cockatoos should be kept individually or in pairs in clean cages. - 10 mg/g feed.

Caution(s): For use in dry feed only. Not for use in liquid type B medicated feeds.

Aspergilliosis may occur following prolonged treatment.

Warning(s): A withdrawal period has not been established for this product in pre-ruminating calves. Do not use in calves to be processed for veal. Not to be fed to ducks or turkeys producing eggs for human consumption.

Psittacosis, avian chlamydiosis, or ornithosis is a reportable communicable disease, transmissible between wild and domestic birds, other animals and man. Contact appropriate public health and regulatory officials.

Presentation: 50 lb (22.68 kg) bag.

AUREOMYCIN is a registered trademark of Alpharma Inc.

Compendium Code No.: 10220103 700334 0203

AUREOMYCIN® 90 GRANULAR

Alpharma **Feed Medication**

Chlortetracycline-Type A Medicated Article

NADA No.: 048-761

Active Ingredient(s): Chlortetracycline calcium complex equivalent to 90 g chlortetracycline hydrochloride per lb.

Ingredients: Dried *Streptomyces aureofaciens* Fermentation Product and Calcium Sulfate.

Indications: For use in the manufacture of medicated animal feeds for cattle, swine, sheep, turkeys, chickens, ducks and psittacine birds.

Directions: Use directions: Mix sufficient AUREOMYCIN® 90 Granular Medicated Article to supply desired concentration of chlortetracycline per ton with part of the feed ingredients to make a preblend.

Add the remainder of the ingredients and mix thoroughly. For specific use levels, see below.

Mixing directions:

Level desired, grams per ton	Amount of medicated article per ton †
50	9 oz
100	1 lb 2 oz
200	2 lb 4 oz
400	4 lb 8 oz
500	5 lb 9 oz

† It is recommended that 1 pound 2 ounces of AUREOMYCIN® 90 Granular Type A Medicated Article be diluted with 2 pounds 14 ounces of one of the feed ingredients to form a 4 pound working premix. Use 2 pounds of the working premix to make a preblend (see Use directions) for a Type C feed containing 50 g AUREOMYCIN® chlortetracycline/ton of feed.

Cattle:

Calves (up to 250 lb): Increased rate of weight gain and improved feed efficiency. - 0.1 mg/lb Chlortetracycline body wt/day.

Beef Cattle (over 700 lb): Control of active infection of anaplasmosis caused by *Anaplasma marginale* susceptible to chlortetracycline. - 0.5 mg/lb Chlortetracycline body wt/day.

Beef and Non-Lactating Dairy Cattle (over 700 lb): Control of active infection of anaplasmosis caused by *Anaplasma marginale* susceptible to chlortetracycline when delivered in a free-choice feed. Free-choice feed must be manufactured under a feed mill license utilizing an FDA approved formulation. - 0.5 to 2.0 mg/lb Chlortetracycline body wt/day.

Calves, Beef and Non-Lactating Dairy Cattle: Treatment of bacterial enteritis caused by *Escherichia coli* and bacterial pneumonia caused by *Pasteurella multocida* organisms susceptible to chlortetracycline. Feed for not more than 5 days. The appropriate amount of AUREOMYCIN®-containing feed supplement may be mixed in the cattle's daily ration or administered as a top-dress. If the AUREOMYCIN®-containing feed supplement is administered as a top-dress, it must be spread uniformly on top of the ration and sufficient space must be provided so that all cattle can eat at the same time. - 10 mg/lb Chlortetracycline body wt/day.

Calves (250 to 400 lb): Increased rate of weight gain and improved feed efficiency. - 25 to 70 mg/head/day.

Growing Cattle (over 400 lb): Increased rate of weight gain, improved feed efficiency, and reduction of liver condemnation due to liver abscesses. - 70 mg/head/day.

Beef Cattle: Control of bacterial pneumonia associated with shipping fever complex caused by *Pasteurella* spp. susceptible to chlortetracycline. - 350 mg/head/day.

Beef Cattle (under 700 lb): Control of active infection of anaplasmosis caused by *Anaplasma marginale* susceptible to chlortetracycline. - 350 mg/head/day.

Swine:

Control of porcine proliferative enteropathies (ileitis) caused by *Lawsonia intracellularis* susceptible to clortetracycline. - 10 mg/lb Chlortetracycline body wt/day.

Treatment of bacterial enteritis caused by *Escherichia coli* and *Salmonella choleraesuis* and bacterial pneumonia caused by *Pasteurella multocida* susceptible to chlortetracycline. (Note: This dose is equivalent to 400 grams per ton, depending on feed consumption and body weight.) Feed for not more than 14 days. - 10 mg/lb Chlortetracycline body wt/day.

Increased rate of weight gain and improved feed efficiency. - 10 to 50 g/ton Chlortetracycline in complete feed.

Reduction in the incidence of cervical lymphadenitis (jowl abscesses) caused by Group E *Streptococci* susceptible to chlortetracycline. - 50 to 100 g/ton Chlortetracycline in complete feed.

Breeding Swine: Control of leptospirosis (reducing the incidence of abortion and shedding of leptospirae) caused by *Leptospira pomona* susceptible to chlortetracycline. Feed continuously for not more than 14 days. - 400 g/ton Chlortetracycline in complete feed.

Sheep:

Breeding Sheep: Reduction in the incidence of (vibrionic) abortions caused by *Campylobacter fetus* infection susceptible to chlortetracycline. - 80 mg/head/day.

Increased rate of weight gain and improved feed efficiency. - 20 to 50 g/ton Chlortetracycline in complete feed.

Turkeys:

Control of complicating bacterial organisms associated with bluecomb (transmissible enteritis; coronaviral enteritis) susceptible to chlortetracycline. Feed continuously for 7 to 14 days. - 25 mg/lb Chlortetracycline body wt/day.

Increased rate of weight gain and improved feed efficiency. - 10 to 50 g/ton Chlortetracycline in complete feed.

Control of infectious synovitis caused by *Mycoplasma synoviae* susceptible to chlortetracycline. Feed continuously for 7 to 14 days. - 200 g/ton Chlortetracycline in complete feed.

Control of hexamitiasis caused by *Hexamita meleagrides* susceptible to chlortetracycline. Feed continuously for 7 to 14 days. - 400 g/ton Chlortetracycline in complete feed.

Turkey Poults not over 4 weeks of age: Reduction of mortality due to paratyphoid caused by *Salmonella typhimurium* susceptible to chlortetracycline. - 400 g/ton Chlortetracycline in complete feed.

Chickens:

Increased rate of weight gain and improved feed efficiency. - 10 to 50 g/ton Chlortetracycline in complete feed.

Control of infectious synovitis caused by *Mycoplasma synoviae* susceptible to chlortetracycline. Feed continuously for 7 to 14 days. - 100 to 200 g/ton Chlortetracycline in complete feed.

Control of chronic respiratory disease (CRD) and air sac infection caused by *Mycoplasma gallisepticum* and *Escherichia coli* susceptible to chlortetracycline. Feed continuously for 7 to 14 days. - 200 to 400 g/ton Chlortetracycline in complete feed.

Reduction of mortality due to *Escherichia coli* infections susceptible to chlortetracycline. Feed for 5 days. - 500 g/ton Chlortetracycline in complete feed.

Ducks:

Control and treatment of fowl cholera caused by *Pasteurella multocida* susceptible to chlortetracycline. Feed in complete ration to provide from 8 to 28 mg per pound of body weight per day depending upon age and severity of disease. Feed for not more than 21 days. - 200 to 400 g/ton Chlortetracycline in complete feed.

Psittacine birds:

Treatment of psittacine birds (parrots, macaws, cockatoos) suspected or known to be infected with psittacosis caused by *Chlamydia psittaci* sensitive to chlortetracycline. Feed continuously for 45 days. Each bird should consume an amount of medicated feed equal to one-fifth of its body weight daily. During treatment, parrots, macaws, and cockatoos should be kept individually or in pairs in clean cages. - 10 mg/g feed.

Caution(s): For use in dry feed only. Not for use in liquid type B medicated feeds.

Aspergilliosis may occur following prolonged treatment.

Warning(s): A withdrawal period has not been established for this product in pre-ruminating calves. Do not use in calves to be processed for veal. Not to be fed to ducks or turkeys producing eggs for human consumption.

Psittacosis, avian chlamydiosis, or ornithosis is a reportable communicable disease, transmissible between wild and domestic birds, other animals and man. Contact appropriate public health and regulatory officials.

Presentation: 50 lb (22.68 kg) bag.

AUREOMYCIN is a registered trademark of Alpharma Inc.

Compendium Code No.: 10220113 700335 0203

AUREOMYCIN® 100 GRANULAR

Alpharma **Feed Medication**

Chlortetracycline-Type A Medicated Article

NADA No.: 048-761

Active Ingredient(s): Chlortetracycline calcium complex equivalent to 100 g chlortetracycline hydrochloride per lb.

Ingredients: Dried *Streptomyces aureofaciens* Fermentation Product and Calcium Sulfate.

Indications: For use in the manufacture of medicated animal feeds for cattle, swine, sheep, turkeys, chickens, ducks and psittacine birds.

Directions: Use directions: Mix sufficient AUREOMYCIN® 100 Granular Medicated Article to supply desired concentration of chlortetracycline per ton with part of the feed ingredients to make a preblend.

Add the remainder of the ingredients and mix thoroughly. For specific use levels, see below.

Mixing directions:

Level desired, grams per ton	Amount of medicated article per ton †
50	½ lb
100	1 lb
200	2 lb
400	4 lb
500	5 lb

† It is recommended that 1 pound of AUREOMYCIN® 100 Granular Type A Medicated Article be diluted with 3 pounds of one of the feed ingredients to form a 4 pound working premix. Use 2 pounds of the working premix to make a preblend (see Use directions) for a Type C feed containing 50 g AUREOMYCIN® chlortetracycline/ton of feed.

Cattle:

Calves (up to 250 lb): Increased rate of weight gain and improved feed efficiency. - 0.1 mg/lb Chlortetracycline body wt/day.

Beef Cattle (over 700 lb): Control of active infection of anaplasmosis caused by *Anaplasma marginale* susceptible to chlortetracycline. - 0.5 mg/lb Chlortetracycline body wt/day.

Beef and Non-Lactating Dairy Cattle (over 700 lb): Control of active infection of anaplasmosis caused by *Anaplasma marginale* susceptible to chlortetracycline when delivered in a free-choice feed. Free-choice feed must be manufactured under a feed mill license utilizing an FDA approved formulation. - 0.5 to 2.0 mg/lb Chlortetracycline body wt/day.

Calves, Beef and Non-Lactating Dairy Cattle: Treatment of bacterial enteritis caused by *Escherichia coli* and bacterial pneumonia caused by *Pasteurella multocida* organisms susceptible to chlortetracycline. Feed for not more than 5 days. The appropriate amount of AUREOMYCIN®-containing feed supplement may be mixed in the cattle's daily ration or administered as a top-dress. If the AUREOMYCIN®-containing feed supplement is administered as a top-dress, it must be spread uniformly on top of the ration and sufficient space must be provided so that all cattle can eat at the same time. - 10 mg/lb Chlortetracycline body wt/day.

Calves (250 to 400 lb): Increased rate of weight gain and improved feed efficiency. - 25 to 70 mg/head/day.

Growing Cattle (over 400 lb): Increased rate of weight gain, improved feed efficiency, and reduction of liver condemnation due to liver abscesses. - 70 mg/head/day.

Beef Cattle: Control of bacterial pneumonia associated with shipping fever complex caused by *Pasteurella* spp. susceptible to chlortetracycline. - 350 mg/head/day.

Beef Cattle (under 700 lb): Control of active infection of anaplasmosis caused by *Anaplasma marginale* susceptible to chlortetracycline. - 350 mg/head/day.

Swine:

Control of porcine proliferative enteropathies (ileitis caused by *Lawsonia intracellularis* susceptible to chlortetracycline. - 10 mg/lb Chlortetracycline body wt/day.

Treatment of bacterial enteritis caused by *Escherichia coli* and *Salmonella choleraesuis* and bacterial pneumonia caused by *Pasteurella multocida* susceptible to chlortetracycline. (Note: This dose is equivalent to 400 grams per ton, depending on feed consumption and body weight.) Feed for not more than 14 days. - 10 mg/lb Chlortetracycline body wt/day.

Increased rate of weight gain and improved feed efficiency. - 10 to 50 g/ton Chlortetracycline in complete feed.

Reduction in the incidence of cervical lymphadenitis (jowl abscesses) caused by Group E *Streptococci* susceptible to chlortetracycline. - 50 to 100 g/ton Chlortetracycline in complete feed.

Breeding Swine: Control of leptospirosis (reducing the incidence of abortion and shedding of leptospirae) caused by *Leptospira pomona* susceptible to chlortetracycline. Feed continuously for not more than 14 days. - 400 g/ton Chlortetracycline in complete feed.

Sheep:

Breeding Sheep: Reduction in the incidence of (vibrionic) abortions caused by *Campylobacter fetus* infection susceptible to chlortetracycline. - 80 mg/head/day.

Increased rate of weight gain and improved feed efficiency. - 20 to 50 g/ton Chlortetracycline in complete feed.

Turkeys:

Control of complicating bacterial organisms associated with bluecomb (transmissible enteritis; coronaviral enteritis) susceptible to chlortetracycline. Feed continuously for 7 to 14 days. - 25 mg/lb Chlortetracycline body wt/day.

Increased rate of weight gain and improved feed efficiency. - 10 to 50 g/ton Chlortetracycline in complete feed.

Control of infectious synovitis caused by *Mycoplasma synoviae* susceptible to chlortetracycline. Feed continuously for 7 to 14 days. - 200 g/ton Chlortetracycline in complete feed.

Control of hexamitiasis caused by *Hexamita meleagrides* susceptible to chlortetracycline. Feed continuously for 7 to 14 days. - 400 g/ton Chlortetracycline in complete feed.

Turkey Poults not over 4 weeks of age: Reduction of mortality due to paratyphoid caused by *Salmonella typhimurium* susceptible to chlortetracycline. - 400 g/ton Chlortetracycline in complete feed.

Chickens:

Increased rate of weight gain and improved feed efficiency. - 10 to 50 g/ton Chlortetracycline in complete feed.

Control of infectious synovitis caused by *Mycoplasma synoviae* susceptible to chlortetracycline. Feed continuously for 7 to 14 days. - 100 to 200 g/ton Chlortetracycline in complete feed.

Control of chronic respiratory disease (CRD) and air sac infection caused by *Mycoplasma gallisepticum* and *Escherichia coli* susceptible to chlortetracycline. Feed continuously for 7 to 14 days. - 200 to 400 g/ton Chlortetracycline in complete feed.

Reduction of mortality due to *Escherichia coli* infections susceptible to chlortetracycline. Feed for 5 days. - 500 g/ton Chlortetracycline in complete feed.

Ducks:

Control and treatment of fowl cholera caused by *Pasteurella multocida* susceptible to chlortetracycline. Feed in complete ration to provide from 8 to 28 mg per pound of body weight per day depending upon age and severity of disease. Feed for not more than 21 days. - 200 to 400 g/ton Chlortetracycline in complete feed.

Psittacine birds:

Treatment of psittacine birds (parrots, macaws, cockatoos) suspected or known to be infected with psittacosis caused by *Chlamydia psittaci* sensitive to chlortetracycline. Feed continuously for 45 days. Each bird should consume an amount of medicated feed equal to one-fifth of its body weight daily. During treatment, parrots, macaws, and cockatoos should be kept individually or in pairs in clean cages. - 10 mg/g feed.

Caution(s): For use in dry feed only. Not for use in liquid type B medicated feeds.

Aspergilliosis may occur following prolonged treatment.

Warning(s): A withdrawal period has not been established for this product in pre-ruminating calves. Do not use in calves to be processed for veal. Not to be fed to ducks or turkeys producing eggs for human consumption.

Psittacosis, avian chlamydiosis, or ornithosis is a reportable communicable disease, transmissible between wild and domestic birds, other animals and man. Contact appropriate public health and regulatory officials.

Presentation: 50 lb (22.68 kg) bag.

AUREOMYCIN is a registered trademark of Alpharma Inc.

Compendium Code No.: 10220093 700336 0203

AUREOMYCIN® SOLUBLE POWDER

Fort Dodge **Tetracycline-Oral**

Chlortetracycline-Antibiotic

NADA No.: 065-071

Active Ingredient(s):

Chlortetracycline hydrochloride. . . . . 25 g per pound

Note: One standard measuring teaspoonful of AUREOMYCIN® Soluble Powder contains approximately 200 mg of chlortetracycline hydrochloride.

Indications:

For the control or treatment of the following poultry diseases caused by organisms sensitive to chlortetracycline:

Chickens: Chronic respiratory disease (air-sac infection), *(Mycoplasma gallisepticum, Escherichia coli);* infectious synovitis *(Mycoplasma synoviae);* for the control of mortality due to fowl cholera *(Pasteurella multocida)* in growing chickens.

Turkeys: Complicated blue comb (transmissible enteritis); infectious synovitis *(Mycoplasma synoviae).*

For the control or treatment of the following diseases caused by organisms sensitive to chlortetracycline:

Swine: Bacterial enteritis (scours), *(Escherichia coli, Salmonella* spp.); bacterial pneumonia (*Pasteurella* spp., *Hemophilus* spp., *Klebsiella* spp.).

Calves: Bacterial pneumonia (*Pasteurella* spp., *Hemophilus* spp., *Klebsiella* spp.); bacterial enteritis (*Escherichia coli, Salmonella* spp.).

Dosage and Administration:

For the control or treatment of the following poultry diseases caused by organisms sensitive to chlortetracycline:

Chickens	Dose
Chronic respiratory disease (air-sac infection) *(Mycoplasma gallisepticum, Escherichia coli)*	4-8 packets per 100 gallons
Infectious synovitis *(Mycoplasma synoviae)*	2-4 packets per 100 gallons
For the control of mortality due to fowl cholera *(Pasteurella multocida)* in growing chickens	10 packets per 100 gallons
Administer at the indicated rates in the total water consumed over a full, 24-hour period.	
Turkeys	**Dose**
Complicated blue comb (transmissible enteritis)	25 mg/lb body weight/day. Administer 1 packet for every 400 lbs of turkeys in the total water consumed over a full, 24-hour period.
Infectious synovitis *(Mycoplasma synoviae)*	4 packets per 100 gallons. Administer at this rate in the total water consumed over a full, 24-hour period.

Medicate continuously at the first clinical signs of disease and continue for 7 to 14 consecutive days. The dosage ranges permitted provide for different levels based on the severity of the infection. Consult a poultry diagnostic laboratory or a poultry pathologist to determine the diagnosis and for advice regarding the optimal level of the drug where ranges are permitted.

For the control or treatment of the following diseases caused by organisms sensitive to chlortetracycline:

Swine	Dose - 10 mg/lb body weight/day
Bacterial enteritis (scours), *(Escherichia coli, Salmonella* spp.), bacterial pneumonia (*Pasteurella* spp., *Hemophilus* spp., *Klebsiella* spp.)	10 packets per 100 gallons. (This will treat 10,000 lbs of pigs for one day; that is one hundred 100-lb pigs; providing 10 mg/lb body weight.) Administer at this rate in the total water consumed over a full, 24-hour period; do not administer for more than 5 days.
Calves	**Dose - 10 mg/lb body weight/day**
Bacterial pneumonia (*Pasteurella* spp., *Hemophilus* spp., *Klebsiella* spp.), bacterial enteritis (*Escherichia coli, Salmonella* spp.)	One standard measuring teaspoonful of powder contains 200 mg. Administer 5 such teaspoonfuls in solution to a 100-lb calf daily in divided doses; do not administer for more than 5 days.

This packet contains 10 g chlortetracycline HCl and will make:

100 gallons containing 100 mg Aureomycin® chlortetracycline HCl per gallon;
50 gallons containing 200 mg Aureomycin® chlortetracycline HCl per gallon;
25 gallons containing 400 mg Aureomycin® chlortetracycline HCl per gallon;
10 gallons containing 1000 mg Aureomycin® chlortetracycline HCl per gallon.

General information on dosage: Dosages in terms of packets per 100 gallons are based on stated dosages per unit of body weight and average water consumption of the species. Weather conditions, ambient temperature, humidity, age, class of livestock, and other factors may affect consumption and, except where calves are drenched, the unit dosage should be used as a guide to effective use in drinking water. Animal must actually consume enough medicated water to provide the desired therapeutic dose under the conditions that prevail.

Precaution(s): Store at controlled room temperature 15° to 30°C (59° to 86°F).

Caution(s): When used in plastic or stainless steel waterers or automatic water medicators, prepare fresh solutions every 24 hours. When used in galvanized waterers, prepare fresh solutions every 12 hours.

Warning(s): Use as the sole source of chlortetracycline. Not to be used for more than 14 consecutive days in chickens and turkeys, 5 days in calves, or 5 days in swine. Do not use in laying chickens. For growing turkeys only. Do not administer this product with milk or milk replacers. Administer one hour before or two hours after feeding milk or milk replacers. Do not administer to swine within 24 hours of slaughter. Do not administer to calves within 24 hours of slaughter. A withdrawal period has not been established for this product in pre-ruminating calves. Do not use in calves to be processed for veal. Do not administer to poultry at 1000 mg/gallon of water (10 packets per 100 gallons) within 24 hours of slaughter.

Presentation: 24.8 lb. pail containing 62 x 6.4 oz (181.4 g) packets (NDC 0856-8742-28).

Compendium Code No.: 10030120

AUREOMYCIN® SOLUBLE POWDER CONCENTRATE

Fort Dodge **Water Medication**

Chlortetracycline-Antibiotic

NADA No.: 065-440

Active Ingredient(s):

Chlortetracycline hydrochloride - 25.6 g per 6.4 oz packet (64 g/lb)

Chlortetracycline hydrochloride - 102.4 g per 25.6 oz packet (64 g/lb)

Indications: For the control or treatment of the following diseases caused by organisms susceptible to chlortetracycline:

Swine: Bacterial enteritis (scours) *(Escherichia coli, Salmonella* spp.); bacterial pneumonia *(Pasteurella* spp., *Hemophilus* spp., *Klebsiella* spp.).

Calves: Bacterial pneumonia *(Pasteurella* spp., *Hemophilus* spp., *Klebsiella* spp.); bacterial enteritis *(Escherichia coli, Salmonella* spp.).

Chickens: Chronic respiratory disease (CRD) and air-sac infection *(Mycoplasma gallisepticum, Escherichia coli);* infectious synovitis *(Mycoplasma synoviae);* for the control of mortality due to fowl cholera *(Pasteurella multocida)* in growing chickens.

Turkeys: Control of complicating bacterial organisms associated with bluecomb (transmissible enteritis or coronavirus enteritis) susceptible to chlortetracycline; infectious synovitis *(Mycoplasma synoviae).*

Directions for Use:

	6.4 oz packet	25.6 oz packet
Swine	Dose — 10 mg/lb body weight/day	
Bacterial enteritis (scours) *(Escherichia coli, Salmonella* spp.)	10 packets per 256 gallons. (This will treat 25,600 lbs of pigs for one day; that is two hundred fifty-six 100 lb pigs; providing 10 mg/lb body weight).	5 packets per 512 gallons. (This will treat 51,200 lbs of pigs for one day; that is five hundred twelve 100 lb pigs; providing 10 mg/lb body weight.)
Bacterial pneumonia *(Pasteurella* spp., *Hemophilus* spp., *Klebsiella* spp.	Administer at this rate in the total water consumed over a full, 24-hour period; do not administer for more than 5 days.	
Calves	Dose — 10 mg/lb body weight/day	
Bacterial pneumonia *(Pasteurella* spp., *Hemophilus* spp., *Klebsiella* spp.)	One standard measuring teaspoonful of powder contains 500 mg. Administer 4 such teaspoonfuls in solution to a 200-lb calf daily in divided doses.	
Bacterial enteritis *(Escherichia coli, Salmonella* spp.)	Administer at this rate in the total water consumed over a full 24-hour period, or as a drench in divided doses. Do not administer for more than 5 days.	
Chickens	Dose	
Chronic respiratory disease (CRD) and air-sac infection *(Mycoplasma gallisepticum, Escherichia coli)*	4-8 packets per 256 gallons (400-800 mg/gallon)	2-4 packets per 512 gallons (400-800 mg/gallon)
Infectious synovitis *(Mycoplasma synoviae)*	2-4 packets per 256 gallons (200-400 mg/gallon)	1-2 packets per 512 gallons (200-400 mg/gallon)
For the control of mortality due to fowl cholera *(Pasteurella multocida)* in growing chickens	10 packets per 256 gallons (1000 mg/gallon)	5 packets per 512 gallons (1000 mg/gallon)
Administer at the indicated rates in the total water consumed over a full, 24-hour period.		
Turkeys	Dose	
Control of complicating bacterial organisms associated with bluecomb (transmissible enteritis or coronavirus enteritis) susceptible to chlortetracycline	25 mg/lb body weight/day. Administer 1 packet for every 1,024 lbs of turkeys in the total water consumed over a full, 24-hour period.	Administer 1 packet for every 4,096 lbs of turkeys in the total water consumed over a full, 24-hour period.
Infectious synovitis *(Mycoplasma synoviae)*	4 packets per 256 gallons (400 mg/gallon). Administer at this rate in the total water consumed over a full, 24-hour period.	2 packets per 512 gallons (400 mg/gallon).

Medicate chickens and turkeys continuously at the first clinical signs of disease and continue for 7 to 14 consecutive days. The dosage ranges permitted provide for different levels based on the severity of the infection. If improvement is not noted in 24-48 hours, consult a veterinarian or a diagnostic laboratory to determine diagnosis and for advice regarding the optimal level of the drug where ranges are permitted.

The 6.4 oz packet contains 25.6 g chlortetracycline HCl and will make:

256 gallons containing 100 mg Aureomycin chlortetracycline HCl per gallon
128 gallons containing 200 mg Aureomycin chlortetracycline HCl per gallon
64 gallons containing 400 mg Aureomycin chlortetracycline HCl per gallon
25.6 gallons containing 1000 mg Aureomycin chlortetracycline HCl per gallon

The 25.6 oz packet contains 102.4 g chlortetracycline HCl and will make:

1024 gallons containing 100 mg Aureomycin chlortetracycline HCl per gallon
512 gallons containing 200 mg Aureomycin chlortetracycline HCl per gallon
256 gallons containing 400 mg Aureomycin chlortetracycline HCl per gallon
102.4 gallons containing 1000 mg Aureomycin chlortetracycline HCl per gallon

General Information on Dosage: Dosages in terms of 6.4 oz packets per 256 gallons and 25.6 oz packets per 512 gallons are based on stated dosages per unit of body weight and average water consumption of the species. Weather conditions, ambient temperature, humidity, age, class of livestock and other factors may affect consumption and, except where calves are drenched, the unit dosage should be used as a guide to effective use in drinking water. Animal must actually consume enough medicated water to provide the desired therapeutic dose under the conditions that prevail.

Precaution(s): Store at controlled room temperature 15° to 30°C (59° to 86°F).

Caution(s): When used in plastic or stainless steel waterers or automatic waterers, prepare fresh solutions every 24 hours. When used in galvanized waterers, prepare fresh solutions every 12 hours.

When feeding milk or milk replacers, administration one hour before or two hours after feeding is recommended.

Warning(s): Use as the sole source of chlortetracycline. Not to be used for more than 14 consecutive days in chickens and turkeys, 5 days in calves, or 5 days in swine. Do not use in laying chickens. For growing turkeys only. Do not administer this product with milk or milk replacers. Administer one hour before or two hours after feeding milk or milk replacers. Do not administer to swine within 24 hours of slaughter. Do not administer to calves within 1 day of slaughter. A withdrawal period has not been established for this product in pre-ruminating calves. Do not use in calves to be processed for veal. Do not administer to chickens at 1000 mg/gallon of water (one 6.4 oz packet per 25.6 gallons; one 25.6 oz packet per 102.4 gallons) within 24 hours of slaughter.

Presentation: 24.8 lb pail containing 62 x 6.4 oz (181.4 g) packets (NDC 0856-8751-28) and a 40 lb pail containing 25 x 25.6 oz (725.7 g) packets (NDC 0856-8751-43).

Manufactured by: PM Resources, Inc., Bridgeton, MO 63044

Compendium Code No.: 10030130 6621B (6.4 oz), 6631B (25.6 oz)

AUREOMYCIN® SULMET® SOLUBLE POWDER

Fort Dodge **Water Medication**

Chlortetracycline Bisulfate and Sulfamethazine Bisulfate

NADA No.: 055-012

Active Ingredient(s): Each pound contains chlortetracycline bisulfate equivalent to 102.4 g chlortetracycline hydrochloride activity and sulfamethazine bisulfate equivalent to 102.4 g sulfamethazine.

Indications: For prevention and treatment of bacterial swine enteritis and for maintenance of weight gains in the presence of bacterial swine enteritis; aid in the maintenance of weight gains in the presence of atrophic rhinitis; aid in the reduction of incidence of cervical abscesses.

Dosage and Administration:

Dosage:

One level standard measuring teaspoon per 2 gallons of water or ¼ lb per 102 gallons. This will provide 250 mg chlortetracycline activity and 250 mg sulfamethazine per gallon. To insure adequate and uniform intake of drug, medicated water should be available at all times during the treatment period and should be the only water source available. When used in plastic or stainless steel waterers or automatic water medicators, prepare fresh solutions every 24 hours. When used in galvanized waterers, prepare fresh solutions every 12 hours.

One level standard measuring teaspoon contains approximately 500 mg chlortetracycline activity and 500 mg sulfamethazine.

Administration:

Bacterial swine enteritis: For prevention and treatment of bacterial swine enteritis and for maintenance of weight gains in the presence of bacterial swine enteritis, use above dosage continuously, but no longer than 28 days. If symptoms persist after using this preparation for 2 or 3 days, consult a veterinarian.

Aid in the maintenance of weight gains in the presence of atrophic rhinitis: Use above dosage continuously, but not longer than 28 days.

Aid in the reduction of incidence of cervical abscesses: Use of above dosage must be continuous during period of possible exposure, but not longer than 28 days.

For best advice on the control of diseases, consult your veterinarian.

Precaution(s): Store at controlled room temperature 15° to 30°C (59° to 86°F).

Caution(s): AUREOMYCIN® SULMET® Soluble Powder may cause eye irritation. In case of contact, flush eyes with plenty of water.

No other tetracycline or sulfonamide should be used during medication with this product.

For oral veterinary use in swine only.

Warning(s): Discontinue medication 15 days before slaughter for human consumption.

Presentation: 40 x 4 oz (113.4 g) packets per pail (NDC 0856-8729-30).

Compendium Code No.: 10030140 6641B

AUREO S 700® GRANULAR 10G

Alpharma **Feed Medication**

Aureomycin® chlortetracycline plus sulfamethazine

Active Ingredient(s):

Chlortetracycline calcium complex equivalent to chlortetracycline HCl . . . . 10 g/Lb.
Sulfamethazine . . . . 2.2% (10 g/Lb.)

Ingredients: Roughage Products, Calcium Carbonate, Calcium Sulfate, Dried *Streptomyces aureofaciens* Fermentation Product and Mineral Oil.

Indications: As an aid in the maintenance of weight gains in the presence of respiratory disease such as shipping fever in beef cattle.

For use in the manufacture of beef cattle feeds.

Directions: Thoroughly mix with grain and/or protein to make Type C feed that will supply 350 mg of chlortetracycline and 350 mg of sulfamethazine per head per day. The following chart allows the amounts of AUREO S 700® 10G needed for various quantities fed.

AUREO S 700® 10G (Lb./Ton Feed)	Feed Will Contain (g/Ton)		Feed at Lb./Head/Day
	Chlortetracycline	Sulfamethazine	
140	1400	1400	0.5
70	700	700	1
35	350	350	2
17.5	175	175	4
14	140	140	5
7	70	70	10
3.5	35	35	20

Feed for 28 days.

Warning(s): Withdraw 7 days prior to slaughter.

A withdrawal period has not been established for this product in pre-ruminating calves. Do not use in calves to be processed for veal.

Presentation: 50 Lb. (22.7 kg).

Compendium Code No.: 10220061 XPM0009077

A

AUREO S 700® GRANULAR 35G

Alpharma **Feed Medication**

Chlortetracycline, sulfamethazine 35G Type A Medicated Article

NADA No.: 035-805

Active Ingredient(s):

Chlortetracycline calcium complex (equivalent to chlortetracycline HCl) .... 35 g/lb
Sulfamethazine... 7.7% (35 g/lb)

Ingredients: Calcium sulfate and dried *Streptomyces aureofaciens* fermentation product.

Indications: As an aid in the maintenance of weight gains in the presence of respiratory disease such as shipping fever.

For use in the manufacture of beef cattle feeds.

Directions: Mixing directions: Mix sufficient AUREO S 700® in the feed to supply 350 mg of Aureomycin chlortetracycline and 350 mg of sulfamethazine per head per day. The following table shows the amounts of AUREO S 700® needed for various quantities of supplement.

AUREO S 700® (lb/ton Supplement)	Supplement Will Contain (g/ton)		Feed Supplement at (lb/head/day)
	Chlortetracycline	Sulfamethazine	
40	1400	1400	0.5
20	700	700	1
10	350	350	2
5	175	175	4
4	140	140	5
2	70	70	10
1	35	35	20

Feed for 28 days.

Warning(s): Withdraw 7 days prior to slaughter. A withdrawal period has not been established for this product in pre-ruminating calves. Do not use in calves to be processed for veal.

Presentation: 50 lb (22.7 kg) bag.

Compendium Code No.: 10220072 AHG-031a 0104

AUREOZOL® 500 GRANULAR

Alpharma **Feed Medication**

Aureomycin® chlortetracycline, sulfathiazole and penicillin-Type A Medicated Article

ANADA No.: 200-167

Active Ingredient(s):

Chlortetracycline calcium complex equivalent to chlortetracycline HCl............. 40 g/lb
Sulfathiazole.. 8.8% (40 g/lb)
Penicillin (from procaine penicillin) .... 20 g/lb

Ingredients: Dried *Streptomyces aureofaciens* Fermentation Product and calcium sulfate.

Indications: For use in the manufacture of medicated swine feeds.

Directions: Use directions: Provide 100 g/ton chlortetracycline, 100 g/ton sulfathiazole, and 50 g/ton of penicillin by thoroughly mixing 2.5 lb (1.14 kg) of AUREOZOL® 500 Granular into each ton (907.2 kg) of complete swine feed for the following indications.

Type of swine feed-permitted claims and limitations: For Use in Swine Feeds as Specified Below:

Pre-starter and Starter Feeds: Administer to swine in a complete medicated feed for reduction of the incidence of cervical abscesses; treatment of bacterial enteritis (salmonellosis or necrotic enteritis caused by *Salmonella choleraesuis* and vibrionic dysentery); maintenance of weight gains in the presence of atrophic rhinitis; increased rate of weight gain and improved feed efficiency from 10 pounds of body weight to 6 weeks post-weaning. For swine raised in confinement (dry-lot) or on limited pasture.

Grower and Finisher Feeds: Administer to swine in a complete medicated feed for reduction of the incidence of cervical abscesses; treatment of bacterial enteritis (salmonellosis or necrotic enteritis caused by *Salmonella choleraesuis* and vibrionic dysentery); maintenance of weight gains in the presence of atrophic rhinitis; increased rate of weight gain from 6 to 16 weeks post-weaning. For swine raised in confinement (dry-lot) or on limited pasture.

Caution(s): In order to achieve the desired performance results, feed as the sole ration.

Note: Manufacture of Type B or C feeds from this product requires a Medicated Feed License Application approved by FDA.

For animal use only.

Warning(s): Withdraw 7 days prior to slaughter.

Presentation: 50 lb (22.68 kg) bag.

Compendium Code No.: 10220123 AHG-028 0103

AURIMITE® INSECTICIDE

Schering-Plough **Otic Parasiticide**

EPA Reg. No.: 773-87

Active Ingredient(s): 0.04% pyrethrins, 0.49% piperonyl butoxide technical.*

Other Ingredients: 99.47%

*Equivalent to 0.392% of (butylcarbityl) (6-propylpiperonyl) ether and 0.098% of related compounds.

Indications: For use as an aid in controlling ear mites in the ears of dogs and cats.

Directions for Use: It is a violation of Federal law to use this product in a manner inconsistent with its labeling.

Read entire label before each use.

Use only on dogs and cats.

Shake well before using. Cleanse ear thoroughly. Apply the recommended drops into ears twice daily for 7 to 10 days. Repeat treatment in 2 weeks if necessary.

Body Weight	Dosage
5 to 15 lbs	4 to 5 drops
15 to 30 lbs	5 to 10 drops
30 lbs or over	10 to 15 drops

Do not reapply product for 2 weeks.

Do not use on dogs or cats under 12 weeks of age.

Consult a veterinarian before using this product on debilitated, aged, pregnant, nursing animals, or animals on medication.

Discontinue use and consult a veterinarian if infestation persists.

Precautionary Statements: Hazards to Humans and Domestic Animals:

Caution: Harmful if swallowed. Avoid inhalation of vapors. Avoid contact with skin. Avoid contact with eyes. Flush eyes with plenty of water. Get medical attention if irritation persists. Wash contaminated skin promptly with soap and water. Avoid contamination of food and water.

Sensitivities may occur after using any pesticide product for pets. If signs of sensitivity occur, bathe your pet with mild soap and rinse with large amounts of water. If signs continue, consult a veterinarian immediately.

First Aid:

If on skin or clothing: Take off contaminated clothing. Rinse skin immediately with plenty of water for 15-20 minutes. Call a poison control center or doctor for treatment advice.

If in eyes: Hold eye open and rinse slowly and gently with water for 15-20 minutes. Remove contact lenses, if present, after the first 5 minutes, then continue rinsing eye. Call a poison control center or doctor for further treatment advice.

Hotline Number: Have the product container or label with you when calling the poison control center or doctor, or going for treatment. You may also contact the Rocky Mountain Poison Center at 1-303-595-4869 for emergency medical treatment information.

Storage and Disposal: Store in original bottle in locked storage areas. Do not reuse bottle. Rinse thoroughly before discarding in trash.

Warning(s): Keep out of reach of children.

Presentation: 1 fl oz (NDC 0061-0733-01) and 16 fl oz (1 pt) (NDC 0061-0733-03) bottles.

Compendium Code No.: 10470111 Rev. 9/01 / Rev. 11/00

AVA-BRON®

ASL **Vaccine**

U.S. Vet. Lic. No.: 226

Active Ingredient(s): A live virus vaccine containing a modified strain of infectious bronchitis virus of the Massachusetts type. The virus is grown under exacting standards of quality control in eggs produced by healthy chickens in closely supervised flocks.

Indications: For the vaccination of healthy chickens against Massachusetts type infectious bronchitis. The vaccine has a broad-spectrum of usage, as it is recommended for both initial vaccination and revaccination of broilers and replacement chickens.

In susceptible chickens, AVA-BRON® stimulates high levels of protection with a moderate respiratory reaction.

Dosage and Administration: AVA-BRON® may be given by intranasal, eyedrop, or drinking water methods. AVA-BRON® may be used on healthy broilers at one (1) day of age by coarse spray.

Intranasal Administration:

1. The sterile diluent supplied should be used to reconstitute the vaccine. (See the package insert for complete mixing instructions.)
2. The mixed solution should be stored on ice until used.
3. All of the vaccine should be used within 30 minutes after mixing.
4. To administer, hold the chicks beak shut and place a finger over the lower nostril. Place a full drop of the vaccine on the other nostril. Release the bird after the drop of vaccine has been inhaled.

Intraocular (eye drop) Administration:

1. The sterile diluent supplied should be used to reconstitute the vaccine. (See the package insert for complete mixing instructions.)
2. The mixed solution should be stored on ice until used.
3. All of the vaccine should be used within 30 minutes after mixing.
4. Hold the chicken to be vaccinated with the head tilted to one side giving clear access to one eye.
5. Hold the plastic bottle containing the vaccine in a vertical position. Gently press the sides of the bottle releasing one drop of vaccine onto the eye of the chicken.
6. Be sure that the vaccine spreads over the eye before releasing the chicken. There is usually an automatic reflex action that serves to spread the vaccine over the eye surface as soon as the vaccine is dropped into the eye.

Drinking Water Administration:

1. Remove all medications, sanitizers, and disinfectants from the drinking water, preferably 72 hours before vaccinating, and 24 hours after vaccinating.
2. Provide enough watering space so that at least two-thirds (⅔) of the chickens can drink at one time.
3. Scrub waterers thoroughly and rinse with fresh, clean water.
4. Withhold water for two (2) hours before vaccinating to stimulate thirst. (The time can be varied depending upon climatic conditions.)
5. Waterers should be raised to a height such that the chickens cannot drink and that lends itself to filling the waterers with the vaccine.
6. Rehydrate the vaccine according to the package insert.
7. Add the rehydrated vaccine to clean, cool, nonchlorinated tap water and mix in accordance with the following chart:

Age of Chickens	1,000 doses added to this amount of water	10,000 doses added to this amount of water
2-4 wks.	2.5 gal. (9.5 L)	25 gal. (95 L)
4-8 wks.	5 gal. (19 L)	50 gal. (190 L)
Over 8 wks.	10 gal. (38 L)	100 gal. (380 L)

8. Nonfat powdered milk may be beneficial to help maintain the virus. A 3.2 oz. measure is added to each 10 gallons of water used to prepare the vaccine.
9. Distribute the solution among the waterers. Avoid placing the waterers in direct sunlight.
10. Do not provide any other drinking water until all of the vaccine treated water has been consumed.
11. Lower waterers to the correct height so that chickens may drink.
12. It is recommended to walk the chickens after lowering the waterers so that all of the chickens will drink and receive a uniform dose of the vaccine.

Coarse Spray for Biojector Plus Administration:

1. Caution. When the machine is turned on and the metal switch on the microvalve plate is touched, the machine is activated, resulting in a needle projecting out. This can cause damage to the needle and/or what is activating the switch, if other than a baby chick.
2. The Biojector Plus is metered to deliver a 0.03 mL dose of vaccine.
3. The vaccine is rehydrated with a sterile water diluent at the rate of 30 mL per 1,000 doses.

4. Turn the machine on to check the adjustment of the spray nozzle. The air flow from the nozzle will blow the down away from the eye area if adjusted correctly. Minor adjustments can be made by moving the arm which holds the spray nozzle attachment. (See American Scientific Laboratories' Hatchery Equipment Manual.)
5. The machine must be properly primed with vaccine before vaccinating chicks. See an American Scientific Laboratories' Hatchery Equipment Manual for proper procedure for priming Biojector Plus.
6. The chick is positioned such that the beak is pointed away from the microvalve plate, with one eye facing up, and the head resting against the head rest protrusion of the microvalve plate. When the head is placed in this position, it will contact the switch which activates the Biojector Plus nozzle and the Biojector syringe with needle.
7. The maximum recommended speed of vaccination is 3,000 birds per hour.

Precaution(s): Refrigerate under 45°F (7°C) until ready for use. Vaccines are perishable unless properly stored.

Caution(s): The capacity of the vaccine to produce satisfactory results depends upon many factors, including, but not limited to, conditions of storage and handling by the user, administration of the vaccine, health and responsiveness of individual animals and degree of field exposure.

Consult a poultry pathologist for further recommendations based on conditions existing in a designated area at any given time.

The vaccine program for replacement pullets should not be started after chickens are 15 weeks of age.

Chickens should not be placed on contaminated premises. Exposure should be avoided immediately after vaccination because it takes up to 10 days to develop resistance.

All susceptible chickens on the same premises should be vaccinated at the same time. If this is not possible, then strict isolation and separate caretakers should be employed for nonvaccinated units. Efforts should be taken to reduce stress conditions at the time the vaccine is administered.

Warning(s): Do not vaccinate within 21 days before slaughter.

Presentation: Intranasal, intraocular, or coarse spray use: 1,000 dose vials.
Drinking water or coarse spray use: 1,000 dose vials.

Compendium Code No.: 11020030

AVA-BRON-H®-B1

ASL **Vaccine**

U.S. Vet. Lic. No.: 226

Active Ingredient(s): The vaccine contains a Holland strain of infectious bronchitis virus (Mass. serotype) that has low disease producing properties, yet stimulates high serological titers. The B_1 Newcastle virus fraction of the vaccine is very mild. The viruses are grown in specific pathogen free eggs under rigid quality control and vacuum dried in the final container.

Indications: Recommended as a booster vaccination for healthy chickens that have previously received a mild Newcastle and a mild Holland strain of bronchitis virus.

Dosage and Administration: For intranasal or eye drop methods (H-107), rehydrate the vaccine with the diluent provided; use the applicator tip. May also be administered by the drinking water method.

Intranasal Administration:
1. The sterile diluent supplied should be used to reconstitute the vaccine. (See the package insert for complete mixing instructions.)
2. The mixed solution should be stored on ice until used.
3. All of the vaccine should be used within 30 minutes after mixing.
4. To administer, hold the chicks beak shut and place a finger over the lower nostril. Place a full drop of the vaccine on the other nostril. Release the bird after the drop of vaccine has been inhaled.

Intraocular (eye drop) Administration:
1. The sterile diluent supplied should be used to reconstitute the vaccine. (See the package insert for complete mixing instructions.)
2. The mixed solution should be stored on ice until used.
3. All of the vaccine should be used within 30 minutes after mixing.
4. Hold the chicken to be vaccinated with the head tilted to one side giving clear access to one eye.
5. Hold the plastic bottle containing the vaccine in a vertical position. Gently press the sides of the bottle releasing one drop of vaccine onto the eye of the chicken.
6. Be sure that the vaccine spreads over the eye before releasing the chicken. There is usually an automatic reflex action that serves to spread the vaccine over the eye surface as soon as the vaccine is dropped into the eye.

Drinking Water Administration:
1. Remove all medications, sanitizers, and disinfectants from the drinking water, preferably 72 hours before vaccinating, and 24 hours after vaccination.
2. Provide enough watering space so that at least two-thirds (⅔) of the chickens can drink at one time.
3. Scrub waterers thoroughly and rinse with fresh, clean water.
4. Withhold water for two (2) hours before vaccinating to stimulate thirst. (The time can be varied depending upon climatic conditions.)
5. Waterers should be raised to a height such that the chickens cannot drink and that lends itself to filling the waterers with the vaccine.
6. Rehydrate the vaccine according to the package insert.
7. Add the rehydrated vaccine to clean, cool, nonchlorinated tap water and mix in accordance with the following chart:

Age of Chickens	1,000 doses added to this amount of water	10,000 doses added to this amount of water
2-4 wks.	2.5 gal. (9.5 L)	25 gal. (95 L)
4-8 wks.	5 gal. (19 L)	50 gal. (190 L)
Over 8 wks.	10 gal. (38 L)	100 gal. (380 L)

8. Nonfat powdered milk may be beneficial to help maintain the virus. A 3.2 oz. measure is added to each 10 gallons of water used to prepare the vaccine.
9. Distribute the solution among the waterers provided. Avoid placing the waterers in direct sunlight.
10. Do not provide any other drinking water until all of the vaccine treated water has been consumed.
11. Lower waterers to the correct height so that chickens may drink.
12. It is recommended to walk the chickens after lowering the waterers so that all of the chickens will drink and receive a uniform dose of the vaccine.

Precaution(s): Refrigerate under 45°F (7°C) until ready for use. Vaccines are perishable unless properly stored.

Caution(s): Revaccination of laying hens with a Holland strain of bronchitis may cause a slight drop in egg production, unless adequate levels of immunity have been maintained prior to revaccination.

Newcastle disease vaccine can cause inflammation of the eyelids of humans, lasting two or three days. The user should avoid contaminating the hands, eyes or clothing with the vaccine.

Warning(s): Do not vaccinate within 21 days of slaughter.

Presentation: Intranasal, drinking water, or eyedrop: 1,000 dose vials.
Drinking water only: 1,000 dose vials.

Compendium Code No.: 10220010

AVA-BRON-H®-N-63

ASL **Vaccine**

U.S. Vet. Lic. No.: 226

Active Ingredient(s): The vaccine contains a Holland strain of infectious bronchitis virus (Mass. serotype) and a LaSota strain of Newcastle virus that stimulate high levels of immunity that persist for long periods of time.

Indications: Recommended as a booster vaccination where maximum protection for Newcastle disease and a broader spectrum of protection for infectious bronchitis are desired, as in breeder hens or commercial layers.

Dosage and Administration: For intranasal or eye drop methods (H-207), rehydrate the vaccine with the diluent provided; use the applicator tip. May also be administered by the drinking water method.

Intranasal Administration:
1. The sterile diluent supplied should be used to reconstitute the vaccine. (See the package insert for complete mixing instructions.)
2. The mixed solution should be stored on ice until used.
3. All of the vaccine should be used within 30 minutes after mixing.
4. To administer, hold the chicks beak shut and place a finger over the lower nostril. Place a full drop of the vaccine on the other nostril. Release the bird after the drop of vaccine has been inhaled.

Intraocular (eye drop) Administration:
1. The sterile diluent supplied should be used to reconstitute the vaccine. (See the package insert for complete mixing instructions.)
2. The mixed solution should be stored on ice until used.
3. All of the vaccine should be used within 30 minutes after mixing.
4. Hold the chicken to be vaccinated with the head tilted to one side giving clear access to one eye.
5. Hold the plastic bottle containing the vaccine in a vertical position. Gently press the sides of the bottle releasing one drop of vaccine onto the eye of the chicken.
6. Be sure that the vaccine spreads over the eye before releasing the chicken. There is usually an automatic reflex action that serves to spread the vaccine over the eye surface as soon as the vaccine is dropped into the eye.

Drinking Water Administration:
1. Remove all medications, sanitizers, and disinfectants from the drinking water, preferably 72 hours before vaccinating, and 24 hours after vaccination.
2. Provide enough watering space so that at least two-thirds (⅔) of the chickens can drink at one time.
3. Scrub waterers thoroughly and rinse with fresh, clean water.
4. Withhold water for two (2) hours before vaccinating to stimulate thirst. (The time can be varied depending upon climatic conditions.)
5. Waterers should be raised to a height such that the chickens cannot drink and that lends itself to filling the waterers with the vaccine.
6. Rehydrate the vaccine according to the package insert.
7. Add the rehydrated vaccine to clean, cool, nonchlorinated tap water and mix in accordance with the following chart:

Age of Chickens	1,000 doses added to this amount of water	10,000 doses added to this amount of water
2-4 wks.	2.5 gal. (9.5 L)	25 gal. (95 L)
4-8 wks.	5 gal. (19 L)	50 gal. (190 L)
Over 8 wks.	10 gal. (38 L)	100 gal. (380 L)

8. Nonfat powdered milk may be beneficial to help maintain the virus. A 3.2 oz. measure is added to each 10 gallons of water used to prepare the vaccine.
9. Distribute the solution among the waterers provided. Avoid placing the waterers in direct sunlight.
10. Do not provide any other drinking water until all of the vaccine treated water has been consumed.
11. Lower waterers to correct height so chickens may drink.
12. It is recommended to walk the chickens after lowering the waterers so that all of the chickens will drink and receive a uniform dose of the vaccine.

Precaution(s): Refrigerate under 45°F (7°C) until ready for use. Vaccines are perishable unless properly stored.

Caution(s): Revaccination of laying hens with a Holland strain of bronchitis may cause a slight drop in egg production, unless adequate levels of immunity have been maintained prior to revaccination.

A delay in revaccination may result in some layers becoming susceptible to bronchitis. Exposure to the virus in these birds can cause a drop in egg production.

Newcastle disease vaccine can cause inflammation of the eyelids of humans, lasting two or three days. The user should avoid contaminating hands, eyes or clothing with the vaccine.

Warning(s): Do not vaccinate within 21 days of slaughter.

Presentation: Intranasal, drinking water, or intraocular: 1,000 dose vials.
Drinking water use only: 1,000 dose vials.

Compendium Code No.: 11020020

A

AVAILA®-4

Zinpro **Feed Additive**

Typical Analysis:

Zinc . . . 5.06%
Manganese . . . 2.80%
Copper . . . 1.76%
Cobalt . . . 0.18%
Total Amino Acid . . . 10.24%
Aspartic Acid . . . 0.66%
Threonine . . . 0.48%
Serine . . . 1.17%
Glutamic Acid . . . 1.19%
Proline . . . 0.99%
Glycine . . . 0.89%
Alanine . . . 0.53%
Cystine . . . 0.49%
Valine . . . 0.75%
Methionine . . . 0.07%
Isoleucine . . . 0.48%
Leucine . . . 0.80%
Tyrosine . . . 0.28%
Phenylalanine . . . 0.48%
Histidine . . . 0.11%
Lysine . . . 0.20%
Arginine . . . 0.67%

Indications: A nutritional feed additive for livestock. It combines zinc, manganese and copper amino acid complexes.

Physical Description: A light brown granular powder. AVAILA®-4 weighs approximately 38 lbs/cu ft.

Dosage and Administration:

Beef and Dairy Cattle: Feed at the rate of ¼ ounce (7 grams) per head daily, or 1 lb per 64 head daily.

Each ¼ ounce of AVAILA®-4 will supply 360 mg zinc from zinc amino acid complex; 200 mg manganese from manganese amino acid complex; 125 mg, copper from copper amino acid complex and 12 mg cobalt from cobalt glucoheptonate.

Contraindication(s): Do not feed to sheep or related species.

Toxicology: When correctly used, there is no toxicity hazard in the use of AVAILA®-4.

Presentation: AVAILA®-4 is packaged in 50 lb multiwall bags.

Compendium Code No.: 11300070

AVAILA® Cu 100

Zinpro **Feed Additive**

Copper Amino Acid Complex

Typical Analysis:

Copper . . . 10.00%
Total Amino Acid . . . 20.62%
Aspartic Acid . . . 1.33%
Threonine . . . 0.97%
Serine . . . 2.35%
Glutamic Acid . . . 2.40%
Proline . . . 2.00%
Glycine . . . 1.80%
Alanine . . . 1.06%
Cystine . . . 0.98%
Valine . . . 1.51%
Methionine . . . 0.15%
Isoleucine . . . 0.96%
Leucine . . . 1.61%
Tyrosine . . . 0.56%
Phenylalanine . . . 0.96%
Histidine . . . 0.23%
Lysine . . . 0.41%
Arginine . . . 1.35%

Indications: A nutritional feed additive for livestock and poultry. When used as a commercial feed ingredient it must be declared as copper amino acid complex.

Physical Description: A dark green granular powder. AVAILA® Cu 100 copper amino acid complex weighs approximately 35 lbs/cu ft.

Dosage and Administration:

Swine: Add 0.5 lb (227 grams) per ton of complete ration.
Laying Hens, Broilers and Turkeys: Add 0.5 lb (227 grams) per ton of complete ration.
Dairy Cattle: Feed 1.25 grams per head daily, or 1 ounce per 24 head daily.
Beef Cattle: Feed 1.25 grams per head daily, or 1 ounce per 24 head daily.
Horses: Feed 1.25 grams per head daily.

Contraindication(s): Contains high levels of copper: do not feed to sheep or related species.

Toxicology: When correctly used, there is no toxicity hazard in the use of AVAILA® Cu 100.

Presentation: AVAILA® Cu 100 is packaged in 50 lb multiwall bags.

Compendium Code No.: 11300020

AVAILA® Fe 60

Zinpro **Feed Additive**

Iron Amino Acid Complex

Typical Analysis:

Iron . . . 6.00%
Total Amino Acid . . . 13.93%
Aspartic Acid . . . 0.90%
Threonine . . . 0.65%
Serine . . . 1.59%
Glutamic Acid . . . 1.62%
Proline . . . 1.35%
Glycine . . . 1.22%
Alanine . . . 0.71%
Cystine . . . 0.66%
Valine . . . 1.02%
Methionine . . . 0.10%
Isoleucine . . . 0.65%
Leucine . . . 1.09%
Tyrosine . . . 0.38%
Phenylalanine . . . 0.65%
Histidine . . . 0.16%
Lysine . . . 0.27%
Arginine . . . 1.91%

Indications: A nutritional feed additive for livestock and poultry. When used as a commercial feed ingredient it must be declared as iron amino acid complex.

Physical Description: A light brown granular powder. AVAILA® Fe 60 iron amino acid complex weighs approximately 35 lbs/cu ft and is packaged in 50 lb. multiwall bags.

Dosage and Administration:

Swine:
Sows: Add 5 lbs per ton of gestation-farrowing-lactation ration.
Pig Starters: Add 5 lbs per ton of complete ration.
Growing and Finishing Swine: Add 2½ lbs per ton of complete ration.
Dairy Cattle: Feed 10 grams per head daily, or 1 lb per 45 head daily.
Beef Cattle: Feed 10 grams per head daily, or 1 lb per 45 head daily.
Calves: Feed 1 lb (454 grams) per 225 head daily.
Sheep: Feed 1 lb (454 grams) per 225 head daily.
Chickens and Turkeys: Add 5 lbs per ton of complete ration.
Horses: Feed 10 grams per head daily.

Toxicology: When correctly used, there is no toxicity hazard in the use of AVAILA® Fe 60.

Presentation: AVAILA® Fe 60 is packaged in 50 lb multiwall bags.

Compendium Code No.: 11300030

AVAILAMIN® - GROW/FINISH

Zinpro **Feed Additive**

Typical Analysis:

Zinc . . . 4.00%
Copper . . . 4.00%
Total Amino Acid . . . 16.22%
Aspartic Acid . . . 1.05%
Threonine . . . 0.76%
Serine . . . 1.85%
Glutamic Acid . . . 1.89%
Proline . . . 1.58%
Glycine . . . 1.42%
Alanine . . . 0.83%
Cystine . . . 0.77%
Valine . . . 1.19%
Methionine . . . 0.12%
Isoleucine . . . 0.75%
Leucine . . . 1.27%
Tyrosine . . . 0.44%
Phenylalanine . . . 0.75%
Histidine . . . 0.18%
Lysine . . . 0.32%
Arginine . . . 1.06%

Indications: A nutritional feed additive for swine. It combines zinc and copper amino acid complexes.

Physical Description: A greenish-brown granular powder. AVAILAMIN® - Grow/Finish weighs approximately 35 lb per cu ft and is packaged in 50-lb multiwall bags.

Dosage and Administration:

Swine: Feed at the rate of 1 lb per ton of complete feed.*

This feeding rate provides 20 ppm zinc from zinc amino acid complex and 20 ppm copper from copper amino acid complex.

*Double recommended feeding rates during periods of reduced feed intake.

Caution(s): Do not feed to sheep or related species.

Toxicology: When correctly used, there is no toxicity hazard in the use of AVAILAMIN® - Grow/Finish.

Presentation: AVAILAMIN® - Grow/Finish is packaged in 50-lb multiwall bags.

Compendium Code No.: 11300080

AVAILAMIN® - SOW

Zinpro **Feed Additive**

Typical Analysis:

Zinc . . . 3.20%
Manganese . . . 1.60%
Copper . . . 2.00%
Iron . . . 1.60%
Total Amino Acids . . . 18.18%
Aspartic Acid . . . 1.18%
Threonine . . . 0.85%
Serine . . . 2.08%
Glutamic Acid . . . 2.12%
Proline . . . 1.77%
Glycine . . . 1.59%
Alanine . . . 0.93%
Cystine . . . 0.87%
Valine . . . 1.33%
Methionine . . . 0.13%
Isoleucine . . . 0.85%
Leucine . . . 1.42%
Tyrosine . . . 0.49%
Phenylalanine . . . 0.84%
Histidine . . . 0.20%
Lysine . . . 0.36%
Arginine . . . 1.19%

Indications: A nutritional feed additive for swine. It combines zinc, copper, iron and manganese amino acid complexes.

Physical Description: A gray-brown granular powder. AVAILAMIN® - Sow weighs approximately 35 lb per cu ft.

Dosage and Administration:

Sows: Feed at the rate of 2.5 lbs per ton of complete feed.

This feeding rate provides 40 ppm zinc from zinc amino acid complex, 25 ppm copper from copper amino acid complex, 20 ppm manganese from manganese amino acid complex and 20 ppm iron from iron amino acid complex.

Contraindication(s): Do not feed to sheep or related species.

Toxicology: When correctly used, there is no toxicity hazard in the use of AVAILAMIN® - Sow.

Presentation: AVAILAMIN® - Sow is packaged in 50-lb multiwall bags.

Compendium Code No.: 11300090

AVAILAMIN® - STARTER I, II, III

Zinpro **Feed Additive**

Typical Analysis:

Zinc	2.28%
Manganese	0.57%
Copper	2.85%
Iron	2.28%
Total Amino Acids	17.08%
Aspartic Acid	1.10%
Threonine	0.80%
Serine	1.95%
Glutamic Acid	1.99%
Proline	1.66%
Glycine	1.49%
Alanine	0.88%
Cystine	0.81%
Valine	1.25%
Methionine	0.12%
Isoleucine	0.79%
Leucine	1.33%
Tyrosine	0.46%
Phenylalanine	0.79%
Histidine	0.19%
Lysine	0.34%
Arginine	1.12%

Indications: A nutritional feed additive for young pigs. It combines copper, zinc, iron and manganese amino acid complexes.

Physical Description: A tannish-brown granular powder. AVAILAMIN® - Starter I, II, III weighs approximately 35 lb per cu ft.

Dosage and Administration:

Creep/Starter/Nursery: Feed at the rate of 3.5 lbs per ton of complete feed.

This feeding rate provides 50 ppm copper from copper amino acid complex, 40 ppm from zinc from zinc amino acid complex, 40 ppm iron from iron amino acid complex and 10 ppm manganese from manganese amino acid complex.

Contraindication(s): Do not feed to sheep or related species.

Toxicology: When correctly used, there is no toxicity hazard in the use of AVAILAMIN® - Starter I, II, III.

Presentation: AVAILAMIN® - Starter I, II, III is packaged in 50-lb multiwall bags.

Compendium Code No.: 11300100

AVAILA® Mn 80

Zinpro **Feed Additive**

Manganese Amino Acid Complex

Typical Analysis:

Manganese	8.00%
Total Amino Acid	19.15%
Aspartic Acid	1.24%
Threonine	0.90%
Serine	2.19%
Glutamic Acid	2.23%
Proline	1.86%
Glycine	1.67%
Alanine	0.98%
Cystine	0.91%
Valine	1.40%
Methionine	0.14%
Isoleucine	0.89%
Leucine	1.50%
Tyrosine	0.52%
Phenylalanine	0.89%
Histidine	0.21%
Lysine	0.38%
Arginine	1.25%

Indications: A nutritional feed additive for livestock and poultry. When used as a commercial feed ingredient it must be declared as manganese amino acid complex.

Physical Description: A light brown granular powder. AVAILA® Mn 80 manganese amino acid complex weighs approximately 35 lbs/cu ft.

Dosage and Administration:

Swine: Add 1 lb (454 grams) per ton of complete ration.

Laying Hens, Broilers and Turkeys: Add 1 lb (454 grams) per ton of complete ration.

Dairy Cattle: Feed 2.5 grams per head daily, or 1 ounce per 12 head daily.

Beef Cattle: Feed 2.5 grams per head daily, or 1 ounce per 12 head daily.

Sheep: Feed 0.50 grams per head daily, or 1 ounce per 60 head daily.

Horses: Feed 2.5 grams per head daily.

Toxicology: When correctly used, there is no toxicity hazard in the use of AVAILA® Mn 80.

Presentation: AVAILA® Mn 80 is packaged in 50 lb multiwall bags.

Compendium Code No.: 11300040

AVAILA® Z/M

Zinpro **Feed Additive**

Typical Analysis:

Zinc	4.00%
Manganese	4.00%
Total Amino Acid	17.58%
Aspartic Acid	1.14%
Threonine	0.83%
Serine	2.01%
Glutamic Acid	2.05%
Proline	1.71%
Glycine	1.54%
Alanine	0.89%
Cystine	0.84%
Valine	1.28%
Methionine	0.13%
Isoleucine	0.82%
Leucine	1.37%
Tyrosine	0.48%
Phenylalanine	0.82%
Histidine	0.20%
Lysine	0.35%
Arginine	1.15%

Ingredients: Zinc amino acid complex, manganese amino acid complex.

When used as a commercial feed ingredient it must be declared as zinc and manganese amino acid complex. Association of American Feed Control Officials (AAFCO) No. 57.150. International Feed Number (IFN) 6-32-054.

Indications: A nutritional feed additive for all poultry rations.

Pharmacology: Physical Description: A light brown granular powder. AVAILA® Z/M Amino Acid Complex weighs approximately 35 lb./cu. ft.

Directions for Use: Feeding Instructions:

Laying Hens, Broilers and Turkeys: Add 2 lbs (908 grams) per ton of complete ration to provide 40 parts per million zinc from zinc amino acid complex and 40 parts per million manganese from manganese amino acid complex.

Toxicology: Toxicity and Safe Handling: When used correctly, there is no toxicity hazard in the use of AVAILA® Z/M.

Presentation: AVAILA® Z/M is packaged in 22.68 kg (50 lbs) multiwall bags.

U.S. Patent No. 5,698,724.

Compendium Code No.: 11300221

AVAILA® Zn 40

Zinpro **Feed Additive**

Zinc Amino Acid Complex

Typical Analysis:

Zinc	4.00%
Total Amino Acid	8.03%
Aspartic Acid	0.52%
Threonine	0.38%
Serine	0.92%
Glutamic Acid	0.93%
Proline	0.78%
Glycine	0.70%
Alanine	0.41%
Cystine	0.38%
Valine	0.59%
Methionine	0.06%
Isoleucine	0.37%
Leucine	0.63%
Tyrosine	0.22%
Phenylalanine	0.37%
Histidine	0.09%
Lysine	0.16%
Arginine	0.52%

Indications: A nutritional feed additive for livestock and poultry. When used as a commercial feed ingredient it must be declared as zinc amino acid complex.

Physical Description: A light brown granular powder. AVAILA® Zn 40 zinc amino acid complex weighs approximately 35 lb/cu ft.

Dosage and Administration:

*Swine: Add 2 lbs (908 grams) per ton of complete ration.

Laying Hens, Broilers And Turkeys: Add 2 lbs (908 grams) per ton of complete ration.

Dairy Cattle: Feed 9 grams per head daily, or 2 lbs per 100 head daily.

Beef Cattle: Feed 9 grams per head daily, or 2 lbs per 100 head daily.

*Sheep: Feed 1 gram per head daily, or 1 lb per 454 head daily.

Horses: Feed 4.5 grams per head daily.

*Double recommended levels during periods of reduced feed intake.

Toxicology: When correctly used, there is no toxicity hazard in the use of AVAILA® Zn 40.

Presentation: AVAILA® Zn 40 is packaged in 50 lb multiwall bags.

Compendium Code No.: 11300060

AVAILA® Zn 100

Zinpro **Feed Additive**

Zinc Amino Acid Complex

Typical Analysis:

Zinc	10.00%
Total Amino Acid	20.00%
Aspartic Acid	1.29%
Threonine	0.94%
Serine	2.28%
Glutamic Acid	2.33%
Proline	1.94%
Glycine	1.75%
Alanine	1.03%
Cystine	0.95%
Valine	1.46%

Methionine.......... 0.15%
Isoleucine.......... 0.93%
Leucine.......... 1.56%
Tyrosine.......... 0.54%
Phenylalanine.......... 0.93%
Histidine.......... 0.22%
Lysine.......... 0.39%
Arginine.......... 1.31%

Indications: A nutritional feed additive for livestock and poultry. When used as a commercial feed ingredient it must be declared as zinc amino acid complex.

Physical Description: A light brown granular powder. AVAILA® Zn 100 zinc amino acid complex weighs approximately 35 lb/cu ft.

Dosage and Administration:

*Swine: Add 0.8 lb (360 grams) per ton of complete ration.

Laying Hens, Broilers And Turkeys: Add 0.8 lb (360 grams) per ton of complete ration.

Dairy Cattle: Feed 3.6 grams per head daily, or 1 lb per 125 head daily.

Beef Cattle: Feed 3.6 grams per head daily, or 1 lb per 125 head daily.

*Sheep: Feed 0.4 gram per head daily, or 1 lb per 1,250 head daily.

Horses: Feed 2.0 grams per head daily.

*Double recommended levels during periods of reduced feed intake.

Toxicology: When correctly used, there is no toxicity hazard in the use of AVAILA® Zn 100.

Presentation: AVAILA® Zn 100 is packaged in 50 lb multiwall bags.

Compendium Code No.: 11300050

AVA-POX® CE

ASL **Vaccine**

U.S. Vet. Lic. No.: 226

Active Ingredient(s): A fowl pox virus grown in specific pathogen-free eggs under rigid quality control, and vacuum dried in the final container.

Indications: The vaccine is recommended for the vaccination of healthy chickens and turkeys 8-18 weeks of age against fowl pox.

Dosage and Administration: AVA-POX® CE is administered by the wing-web stab method of administration in chickens. In turkeys, AVA-POX® CE can be administered by wing-web stab or the thigh stab method of administration.

Vaccinated birds should be examined in 7-10 days for fowl pox "takes." Small inflamed wart-like swellings will be seen at the site of inoculation on susceptible birds if the vaccine was properly applied. If for any reason the birds do not have this reaction, they should be revaccinated immediately in order to ensure flock immunity.

Wing Web Application in Chickens:

1. Rehydrate the vaccine according to the package insert. Do not break off any of the needles on the applicator.
2. Hold the chicken and spread the underside of one wing outward.
3. Dip the applicator into the vaccine bottle, wetting both needles.
4. Pierce the web of the exposed wing with the charged applicator.
5. Redip the applicator in the vaccine vial and proceed to the next bird.
6. Avoid hitting blood vessels, bones and the wing muscle.
7. Be careful not to touch any part of the bird with the vaccine except the area to be inoculated.
8. Examine and record takes 7-10 days following vaccination. A normal take shows a slight swelling and scab formation at the site of vaccination. Takes generally disappear two (2) weeks following vaccination.
9. Special note: The wing-web vaccination can be applied in turkeys, but may occasionally lead to unwanted virus spread to head parts. The problem can be avoided by the thigh-stab method.

Thigh-stab Administration in Turkeys:

1. Rehydrate the vaccine according to the package insert. Do not break off any of the needles on the applicator.
2. As an assistant holds the legs of the turkey with one hand and holds the bird's head downward with its back toward him, he then passes his other hand downwards on the outside of one thigh, turning the feathers back and exposing a bare spot.
3. The vaccinator dips the applicator into the vaccine bottle and stabs it into the thigh muscles.
4. Be careful not to pierce the tendons, but go deep enough to break the skin and deliver the vaccine.
5. Redip the applicator in the vaccine vial and proceed to the next bird.
6. Be careful not to touch any part of the bird with the vaccine except the area to be inoculated.
7. Examine and record takes on 10% of the flock 7-10 days following vaccination. A normal take shows slight swelling and scab formation at the site of vaccination. Takes generally disappear two (2) weeks following vaccination.

Precaution(s): Refrigerate under 45°F (7°C) until ready for use. Vaccines are perishable unless properly stored.

Caution(s): Careless handling of the vaccine may result in the contamination of the unfeathered part of the birds.

Consult a poultry pathologist for further recommendations, based on conditions existing in a designated area at any given time.

Do not open and mix the vaccine until ready to commence vaccination. Use the entire contents immediately after mixing. Burn the containers and all unused contents.

The capacity of the vaccine to produce satisfactory results depends on many factors, including, but not limited to, conditions of storage and handling by the user, administration of the vaccine, health and responsiveness of individual animals and degree of field exposure. Therefore, directions for use should be followed carefully.

The vaccine program for replacement pullets should not be started after chickens are 15 weeks of age.

Consult an American Scientific Laboratories' representative or local poultry pathologist for a monitoring program to determine the effectiveness of the vaccine application. The use of the vaccine is subject to applicable state and federal laws and regulations.

Warning(s): Do not vaccinate within 21 days of slaughter.

Presentation: Wing-web use: 1,000 dose vials.

Compendium Code No.: 11020041

AVATEC®

Alpharma **Feed Medication**

Lasalocid Sodium-Type A Medicated Article (medicated premix)-Coccidiocidal

NADA No.: 096-298

Active Ingredient(s): Each pound contains 90.7 g (20%) of lasalocid sodium activity in a carrier suitable for incorporation in feed.

Indications: For the prevention of coccidiosis in:

Target Species:	Caused by:
Broiler or Fryer Chickens:	*Eimeria tenella, E. necatrix, E. acervulina, E. brunetti, E. mivati* and *E. maxima*
Growing Turkeys:	*E. meleagrimitis, E. gallopavonis, E. adenoeides*
Rabbits:	*Eimeria stiedae*
Chukar Partridges:	*Eimeria legionensis*

Directions for Use:

Broiler, Fryer Chickens and Growing Turkeys: Use AVATEC® continuously in the feed to provide from 68 g per ton (0.0075%) to 113 g per ton (0.0125%) lasalocid sodium concentration. The dosage range allows adjustment of drug level to severity of exposure. The higher levels are indicated for severe exposure. Consult a poultry disease diagnostician for advice regarding the optimal level of drug.

Rabbits: Use AVATEC® continuously in the feed for rabbits up to 6½ weeks of age to provide 113 g per ton (0.0125%) lasalocid sodium concentration.

Chukar Partridges: Use AVATEC® continuously in the feed for young birds up to 8 weeks of age to provide 113 g per ton (0.0125%) lasalocid sodium concentration.

Mixing directions: Thoroughly mix the following amounts of AVATEC® to make one ton of feed to provide from 68 g per ton (0.0075%) to 113 g per ton (0.0125%) lasalocid sodium concentration. When adding less than one pound of premix per ton of feed, it is recommended that the premix first be mixed with a small amount of feed (10-25 lbs.) prior to incorporation into the final feed.

Dosage for use in target species	Concentration % in Feed	Lasalocid grams/ton	lbs AVATEC® per ton feed
Broiler, Fryer Chickens and Growing Turkeys	0.0075%	68	¾
	0.0100%	90.7	1
	0.01125%	102	1⅛
Broiler, Fryer Chickens, Growing Turkeys, Rabbits, Chukar Partridges	0.0125%	113	1¼

Caution(s): Note: In addition to label statements of identity, ingredients and directions for use, labeling of feeds containing AVATEC® must contain the following statements:

For Broiler Or Fryer Chickens Only and/or

For Growing Turkeys Only and/or

For Chukar Partridges (Up To Eight Weeks Of Age) Only and/or

For Rabbits (Up To Six And One Half Weeks Of Age) Only.

Additionally, all feed labeling must state: Feed Continuously As The Sole Ration.

Warning(s): When mixing and handling lasalocid premix, use protective clothing, impervious gloves and a dust mask. Avoid contact with eyes. Operators should wash thoroughly with soap and water after handling.

For use in the manufacture of medicated feeds only.

Presentation: 50 lb (22.68 kg) bag.

Compendium Code No.: 10220132 710309 0103

AVA-TREM®

ASL **Vaccine**

U.S. Vet. Lic. No.: 226

Active Ingredient(s): AVA-TREM® contains a live, freeze-dried virus of chicken embryo origin selected for its affinity for the birds' intestinal tract and high immunizing capability.

The virus is propagated and processed under exacting standards of production and quality control in accordance with existing USDA regulations. A stabilizer was developed by American Scientific Laboratories to ensure maximum stability of the virus.

Indications: For the vaccination of healthy pullets for avian encephalomyelitis (epidemic tremor).

The vaccine should be used on susceptible birds between 10 and 18 weeks of age, intended for use as breeder or commercial layer replacements.

Dosage and Administration: AVA-TREM® may be administered by the wing-web or the drinking water method.

Wing-Web Administration:

1. Rehydrate the vaccine according to the package insert. Do not break off any of the needles on the applicator.
2. Hold the chicken and spread the underside of one wing outward.
3. Dip the applicator into the vaccine bottle, wetting both needles.
4. Pierce the web of the exposed wing with the charged applicator.
5. Redip the applicator in the vaccine vial and proceed to the next bird.
6. Avoid hitting blood vessels, bones and the wing muscle.
7. Be careful not to touch any part of the chicken with the vaccine except the area to be inoculated.
8. Examine and record takes on 10% of the flock 7-10 days following vaccination. A normal take shows a slight swelling and scab formation at the site of vaccination. Takes generally disappear two (2) weeks following vaccination.

Drinking Water Administration:

1. Remove all medications, sanitizers, and disinfectants from the drinking water, preferably 72 hours before vaccinating, and 24 hours after vaccinating.
2. Provide enough watering space so that at least two-thirds (⅔) of the chickens can drink at one time.
3. Scrub waterers thoroughly and rinse with fresh, clean water.
4. Withhold water for two (2) hours before vaccinating to stimulate thirst. (The time can be varied depending upon climatic conditions.)
5. Waterers should be raised to a height such that the chickens cannot drink and that lends itself to filling the waterers with vaccine.
6. Rehydrate the vaccine according to package insert.

7. Add rehydrated vaccine to clean, cool, nonchlorinated tap water and mix in accordance with the following chart:

Age of Chickens	1,000 doses added to this amount of water	10,000 doses added to this amount of water
2-4 wks.	2.5 gal. (9.5 L)	25 gal. (95 L)
4-8 wks.	5 gal. (19 L)	50 gal. (190 L)
Over 8 wks.	10 gal. (38 L)	100 gal. (380 L)

8. Nonfat powdered milk may be beneficial to help maintain the virus. A 3.2 oz. measure is added to each 10 gallons of water used to prepare the vaccine.
9. Distribute the solution among the waterers. Avoid placing the waterers in direct sunlight.
10. Do not provide any other drinking water until all of the vaccine treated water has been consumed.
11. Lower waterers to the correct height so that chickens may drink.
12. It is recommended to walk the chickens after lowering the waterers so that all of the chickens will drink and receive a uniform dose of vaccine.

Precaution(s): Refrigerate under (45°F) 7°C until ready for use. Vaccines are perishable unless properly stored.

Caution(s): The vaccine should be used only on healthy, susceptible birds between 10 and 18 weeks of age, intended for use as breeder or commercial layer replacements.

Do not use less than one dose per bird.

If breeder birds are vaccinated, hatching eggs should not be saved until at least six weeks after vaccination. If used on susceptible layers, the vaccine could cause a 5 to 15% drop in egg production for two or three weeks. The virus will pass to the progeny hatched from eggs produced during this period.

Vaccinated pullets should not be added to nonvaccinated flocks in production.

Consult a poultry pathologist for further recommendations based on conditions existing in the designated treatment area at any given time.

Do not open and mix the vaccine until ready to begin vaccination. Use the entire contents immediately after mixing. Burn the containers and all unused contents.

The capacity of the vaccine to produce satisfactory results depends upon many factors, including, but not limited to, the conditions of storage and handling by the user, the administration of the vaccine, the health and responsiveness of individual animals and the degree of field exposure. Therefore, directions for use should be followed carefully.

Consult an American Scientific Laboratories technical representative or local poultry pathologist for a monitoring program to determine the effectiveness of the vaccine application. The use of the vaccine is subject to applicable state and federal laws and regulations.

Warning(s): Do not vaccinate within four (4) weeks of initial egg production nor within 21 days of slaughter.

Do not vaccinate birds under 10 weeks of age.

Do not vaccinate on premises with susceptible laying birds or young chickens. The virus may spread from the vaccinated birds and affect egg production of the layers or the health of the young susceptible chickens.

Presentation: Water use only: 1,000 dose vials.
Wing-web use: 1,000 dose vials.

Compendium Code No.: 11020050

AVIAN BLUELITE®

TechMix **Electrolytes-Oral**

Active Ingredient(s): Guaranteed Analysis (not less than):

	Per lb.	Per oz.
Vitamin A, I.U.	5,000,000.0	312,400.00
Vitamin D_3, I.C.U.	1,000,000.0	62,500.00
Vitamin E, I.U.	6,700.0	419.00
Choline bitartrate, mg	10,000.0	625.00
Niacin, mg	2,000.0	125.00
d-Pantothenic acid, mg	837.0	52.00
Riboflavin, mg	500.0	31.00
Menadione, mg	33.5	2.10
Thiamine, mg	119.3	7.50
Pyridoxine, mg	110.0	6.90
Folic acid, mg	33.5	2.10
d-Biotin, mg	13.4	0.84
Vitamin B_{12}, mg	1,675.0	0.11
Potassium (K)	12.120%	3,436.00 mg
Sodium (Na)	3.000%	850.00 mg
Calcium (Ca)	0.920%	261.00 mg
Phosphorus (P)	0.450%	128.00 mg
Magnesium (Mg)	0.270%	76.60 mg
Zinc (Zn)	0.040%	11.34 mg
Manganese (Mn)	0.032%	9.10 mg

Ingredients: Dipotassium phosphate, potassium sulfate, sodium bicarbonate, calcium lactate, magnesium gluconate, citric acid, glycine, zinc methionine, manganese methionine, vitamin A acetate (stability improved), D-activated animal sterol (source of vitamin D_3), dl-alpha tocopheryl acetate (source of vitamin E activity), choline bitartrate, niacin supplement, ascorbic acid (vitamin C), d-pantothenic acid, riboflavin supplement, pyridoxine HCl, thiamine HCl, folic acid, d-biotin, menadione dimethylpyrimidinol bisulfite (source of vitamin K activity), vitamin B_{12} supplement, and FD&C certified color added.

Indications: A concentrated source of buffered electrolytes and vitamins on a palatable, acidified, readily soluble carrier intended for use in chicks, broilers, layers, turkeys, ducks, geese and game birds as an aid in reducing dehydration (shrink), as a result of hot weather, handling, moving, or when starting recently hatched birds.

Dosage and Administration: Administer AVIAN BLUELITE® in the drinking water or feed for five (5) to seven (7) days in one of the following ways:

I. Water Administration:

A. Stock Solution: In birds with severe dehydration, mix and dissolve one (1) packet (1 lb.) of AVIAN BLUELITE® in one (1) gallon of stock solution and administer 1 oz. of stock solution to each gallon of drinking water. The dosage can be reduced in half for birds with signs of mild dehydration.

B. Waterer or Fountain: For holding tank use, mix 1 oz. (approximately 2 heaping tablespoons) of AVIAN BLUELITE® to each eight (8) gallons of drinking water or one (1) packet (1 lb.) of AVIAN BLUELITE® to each 128 gallons of drinking water for birds with severe signs of dehydration. The dosage can be reduced in half for birds with signs of mild dehydration.

II. Feed Administration: Mix two (2) packets of AVIAN BLUELITE® per ton of complete feed.

Precaution(s): Store in a dry room at temperatures between 40°-86°F (4°C-30°C). Unused bag portions should be resealed with tape or binders.

Caution(s): For exclusive use in water or feed, intended for the avian species.

Keep out of the reach of children.

Birds showing symptoms of severe depression, coma or those that are too weak and dehydrated to drink normally should be treated as directed by a veterinarian and under the observation of a veterinarian and designated poultry service person. Provide fresh feed and water on a free-choice basis at all times.

Trial Data: AVIAN BLUELITE® has been field tested in geese, ducks, and game birds under farm-field conditions and in trials at the University of Minnesota under veterinary supervision to evaluate the potential benefits of AVIAN BLUELITE® as a rehydration drinking water additive for turkeys and chickens. In the university trials, young chicks and turkey poults were stressed with systemic infections or were deprived of feed and water for 48 hours to determine their response to AVIAN BLUELITE® in minimizing dehydration, morbidity and mortality. Chicks and poults were individually weighed throughout the trial period to determine and evaluate the responses of the AVIAN BLUELITE® in regard to total body weight, average body weight and individual size variation in the trials.

Chick Trial - Feed and Water Deprivation: In a trial to determine the potential value of AVIAN BLUELITE® in starting baby chicks that might be deprived of feed and water for a period of time after hatching, 80 broiler chicks were divided into two groups and subjected to total feed and water deprivation for 48 hours. The results of this trial indicated that AVIAN BLUELITE® helped reduce the losses of dehydration or body weight when feed and water were withheld for a period of time.

	Mean Hatching Weight/Chick	Mean 7-Day Weight/Chick	Mean 14-Day Weight/Chick
Group I: Feed and water withheld 48 hours after hatching, then chicks given feed and plain water.	43.60 g	134.5 g	353.8 g
Group II: Feed and water withheld 48 hours as in Group I after hatching, then chicks were placed on feed and water with AVIAN BLUELITE®.	43.14 g	133.0 g	359.5 g

Note: Group I chicks had a mortality of three birds at two weeks of age and Group II had one bird die during the two-week trial. Group II birds were slightly heavier and showed significantly less size variation in their range of body weight at two weeks of age.

Chick Trial with Systemic Infection: Two hundred broiler chicks were divided into four groups of 50 birds. All birds were fed a medicated prestarter containing 500 g of chlortetracycline per ton. Chicks in Groups III and IV were injected subcutaneously in the cervical region with viable *Salmonella arizoniae* (10^6) bacteria shortly after hatching. The body weight rehydration response with AVIAN BLUELITE® in this trial was as follows:

	Mean Hatching Weight/Chick	Mean 7-Day Weight/Chick	Mean 14-Day Weight/Chick
Group I: Noninfected plain water	43.0 g	163.5 g	439.4 g
Group II: Noninfected with AVIAN BLUELITE®	43.0 g	163.7 g	441.9 g
Group III: Infected plain water	42.5 g	139.5 g	387.9 g
Group IV: Infected with AVIAN BLUELITE®	43.4 g	147.4 g	403.2 g

Note: Birds in Groups III and IV showed good evidence of systemic infection as compared to birds in Groups I and II, as illustrated by their lower body weight. Group IV birds showed improved body weights and less size variation in body weight than Group III.

Turkey and Poult Trial - Feed and Water Deprivation: In a trial to determine the potential value of AVIAN BLUELITE® in starting male turkey poults, 100 young poults were divided into two groups and deprived of water and feed for 48 hours immediately after hatching. The results of this trial indicate that AVIAN BLUELITE® will help reduce variability of body weight or dehydration under many brooding conditions.

	Mean Hatching Weight/Poult	Mean 7-Day Weight/Poult	Mean 14-Day Weight/Poult
Group I: Feed and water withheld 48 hours after hatching, poults were then given feed and plain water.	58.9 g	117.3 g	268.0 g
Group II: Feed and water withheld 48 hours after hatching, poults were then placed on feed and water with AVIAN BLUELITE®.	59.6 g	120.8 g	277.5 g

Note: Both groups had a mortality of two birds at two weeks of age. Poults given AVIAN BLUELITE® had less weight or size variation within the group at both 7 and 14 days of age.

Turkey Poults with Systemic Infections: Two hundred turkey poults were divided into four groups of 50 poults and were fed a medicated prestarter containing 400 g of chlortetracycline per ton. Poults in Groups III and IV were injected subcutaneously in the cervical region with viable *Salmonella arizoniae* (10^6) bacteria shortly after hatching. The response to AVIAN BLUELITE® as measured by body weight response was as follows:

	Mean Hatching Weight/Poult	Mean 7-Day Weight/Poult	Mean 14-Day Weight/Poult
Group I: Noninfected plain water	56.6 g	198.3 g	466.3 g
Group II: Noninfected with AVIAN BLUELITE®	57.6 g	191,2 g	473.8 g
Group III: Infected plain water	57.0 g	191.1 g	430.9 g
Group IV: Infected with AVIAN BLUELITE®	56.6 g	189.3 g	442.3 g

Trial Conclusions: AVIAN BLUELITE® has been evaluated and tested under a variety of university and field conditions. When used as directed, it will reduce losses of body weight or dehydration associated with systemic infections as shown in these trials. AVIAN BLUELITE® is for use when brooding or starting birds after hatching. Its rehydration action helps reduce stunting or the incidence of peewees as shown by its efficacy in reducing the variability of body size when starting birds that do not receive feed or water within 24-48 hours after hatching.

AVIAN BLUELITE® is readily consumed and highly soluble in both stock solutions for medicators and in holding tanks and waterers. Its broad formulation of electrolytes, vitamins and buffered acidified action makes it ideal for use under a wide variety of field conditions.

Presentation: 25 lb. pail.

Compendium Code No.: 11440000

AVIAN PNEUMOVIRUS VACCINE

Biomune **Vaccine**

Avian Pneumovirus Vaccine, Modified Live Virus

U.S. Vet. Lic. No.: 368

Description: This vaccine contains live avian pneumovirus in a freeze-dried form. The application of this vaccine to one-week-old susceptible turkeys will aid in the prevention of respiratory disease caused by avian pneumovirus infection.

Contains gentamicin and amphotericin B as preservatives.

Warranty: This vaccine was thoroughly tested before sale and meets the requirements of the U.S. Department of Agriculture.

Indications: This vaccine is recommended for vaccination of healthy turkeys at one week of age or older using either drinking water or intraocular routes of administration. Revaccination is recommended four weeks later. Turkeys should be maintained in good environmental conditions and exposure to infectious diseases should be reduced as much as possible.

Directions for Use: For drinking water or intraocular use.

Drinking Water Application:

1. Do not open or rehydrate the vaccine until ready to vaccinate.
2. Do not use any medications, sanitizers or disinfectants in the drinking water for 48 hours before vaccination and for 24 hours after vaccination.
3. Thoroughly rinse water lines or waterers with fresh clean water.
4. Prior to administration of the vaccine, withhold water from the turkeys for approximately 2 hours to stimulate thirst. Be careful in hot weather.
5. Rehydrate the vaccine as follows:
   Note: As an aid in preserving the vaccine, 30 mL (1 ounce) of rehydrated non-fat powdered milk may be added to each 3.8 liters (1 gallon) of clean, cool, non-chlorinated water used for hydrating and mixing the vaccine.
   a. Remove the aluminum seal and rubber stopper from the vial containing the freeze-dried vaccine.
   b. Carefully pour the milk/water into the vaccine vial until the vial is approximately two-thirds full.
   c. Insert the stopper and shake vigorously until all vaccine is rehydrated.
   d. Pour vaccine into medicator or reservoir.
   e. Rinse vaccine vial to remove all vaccine and add to the vaccine solution to be administered.
6. The vaccine is to be mixed with an appropriate volume of water to be consumed over a one-hour period depending on the age of the turkeys, ambient temperature and the type of watering system used. For 1,000 one-week-old turkeys, it is recommended to mix the rehydrated vaccine with 15.2 liters (4 gallons) of water.
7. Distribute the vaccine to ensure all to turkeys have access to water.
8. Avoid placing vaccine in direct sunlight.
9. Provide no other drinking water until all the vaccine has been consumed.

Intraocular Application:

1. Remove the aluminum seal and rubber stopper from the vial containing the freeze-dried vaccine and pour part of the diluent supplied with the vaccine into the vial.
2. Insert the rubber stopper and shake well until all vaccine is rehydrated. Pour the rehydrated vaccine back into the remaining diluent in the diluent vial and mix. Allow 30 mL of diluent for each 1,000 turkeys.
3. Place the dropper tip in the diluent vial. The vaccine is now ready for intraocular administration.
4. Hold the bird on its side and allow one drop of the mixed vaccine to fall onto the open eye.
5. Hold the bird until the drop of vaccine disappears. Care must be taken to avoid injury to the eye with the dropper tip.

Precaution(s): Store the vaccine at 35-45°F (2-7°C).

Do not open and mix the vaccine until ready to begin vaccination.

Use entire contents of vial immediately after mixing.

Burn the container and all unused contents. This vaccine is not returnable to the manufacturer.

Caution(s): Notice: This vaccine is conditionally licensed. Potency and efficacy studies are in progess.

Do not dilute or otherwise extend the dosage.

Vaccinate all turkeys on the premises at the same time. Vaccinate only healthy turkeys.

Warning(s): Do not vaccinate within 21 days of slaughter.

Presentation: 10 x 500 doses, 10 x 1,000 doses, 10 x 2,000 doses, 10 x 5,000 doses and 10 x 10,000 doses.

Patent pending

Compendium Code No.: 11290510 305

AVIAN VITAMINS IODIZED

ARC **Small Animal Dietary Supplement**

Active Ingredient(s): Guaranteed Analysis (per fl. oz., 29 mL):

Vitamin A	31,000 I.U.
Vitamin B_1	22 mg
Vitamin B_2	34 mg
Vitamin B_6	42 mg
Vitamin B_{12}	0.90 mg
Vitamin C	1,900 mg
Vitamin D_3	5,200 I.U.
Vitamin E	55 I.U.
Vitamin K	10.2 mg
Niacinamide	325 mg
Folic acid	150 mcg
d-Pantothenic acid	88 mg
Choline	82 mg
Iodine	8 mg
Biotin	15 mcg

Contents: Vitamin A palmitate, d-activated animal sterol, alpha tocopheryl acetate, riboflavin phosphate sodium, d-panthenol, pyridoxine HCl, thiamine HCl, niacinamide, cyanocobalamin, phytonadione, ascorbic acid, folic acid, biotin, polysorbate 80, sodium benzoate (preservative), propylene glycol, choline dihydrogen citrate, potassium iodide (source of iodine), sucrose, sorbitol, sodium saccharin, BHA and disodium EDTA (preservatives), and deionized water.

Indications: A liquid water soluble supplement for caged and aviary birds.

Dosage and Administration: Mix in fresh water each day.

Add to drinking water. Replace each day with fresh solution.

Use eight (8) drops per tablespoon of water, 16 drops per fluid ounce of water, or one (1) tablespoon per quart of water.

Caution(s): Keep out of the reach of children.

Presentation: 1 oz. size.

Compendium Code No.: 10960010

AVIAX®

Phibro **Feed Medication**

Semduramicin Sodium-Type A Medicated Article

NADA No.: 140-940

Active Ingredient(s):

Semduramicin sodium 5.13%

Equivalent to 5% semduramicin or 22.7 g/lb.

Indications: For the prevention of coccidiosis in broiler chickens caused by *Eimeria tenella, E. acervulina, E. maxima, E. brunetti, E. necatrix* and *E. mivati/mitis.*

Type A medicated article.

Dosage and Administration: Thoroughly mix 1.0 lb of AVIAX® Type A Medicated Article per 2000 lb of feed ingredients to provide 25 ppm (22.7 g) of semduramicin per ton of Type C finished broiler feeds. Feed continuously as the sole ration to broiler chickens.

Precaution(s): Store in dry cool place.

Warning(s): Do not feed to laying hens.

For use in the manufacture of broiler chicken feed. Do not feed undiluted.

Certain components of animal feeds including medicated premixes possess properties that may be a potential health hazard or a source of personal discomfort to certain individuals who are exposed to them. Human exposure should, therefore, be minimized by observing the general industry standards for occupational health and safety.

Precautions such as the following should be considered: dust masks or respirators and protective clothing should be worn; dust-arresting equipment and adequate ventilation should be utilized; personal hygiene should be observed; wash before eating or leaving a work site; be alert for signs of allergic reactions—seek prompt medical treatment if such reactions are suspected.

Presentation: 40 lb (18.2 kg) bag.

AVIAX is a registered trademark of Phibro Animal Health, for semduramicin sodium.

Compendium Code No.: 36930002

AVICHOL®

Schering-Plough **Vaccine**

Pasteurella multocida Vaccine, Avirulent Live Culture, Avian Isolate

U.S. Vet. Lic. No.: 165A

Active Ingredient(s): AVICHOL® is a live bacterial vaccine containing the known avirulent isolate of *Pasteurella multocida* type 3, Clemson University strain, in a freeze-dried preparation sealed under vacuum.

The seed culture used to make the vaccine has been laboratory tested for protection against challenge with the X-73 (type 1) strain of *P. multocida.*

Indications: For the vaccination of healthy chickens six weeks of age or older as an aid in preventing pasteurellosis (fowl cholera) due to *P. multocida* type 1.

Dosage and Administration:

When to Vaccinate: The best results are obtained when the vaccine is administered initially to chickens at 10 to 12 weeks of age and repeated once at about 18 to 20 weeks of age. There should be at least six (6) weeks and not more than 10 weeks between vaccinations.

Vaccination Program: The development of a durable, strong protection to the disease depends upon the use of an effective vaccination program as well as many other circumstances such as administration techniques, environment and flock health at the time of vaccination. Also, the immune response to one (1) vaccination under field conditions is seldom complete for all animals within a given flock. Even when vaccination is successful, the protection stimulated in individual animals against different diseases may not be life-long. Therefore, a program of revaccination may be necessary.

Preparation of the Vaccine:

1. Do not open and mix the vaccine until ready for use.
2. Mix only one (1) vial at a time and use the entire contents within two (2) hours.
3. Remove the tear-off aluminum seal and stopper from the vial containing the dried vaccine.
4. Remove the tear-off aluminum seal and stopper from the bottle containing the diluent.
5. Hold the diluent bottle firmly in an upright position and insert the neck of the vaccine vial on the adapter of the diluent bottle. The neck of the vaccine vial should snap into position and should be seated securely on the adapter on the diluent bottle.
6. Invert the two (2) containers so that the vaccine vial is on the bottom and allow the diluent to flow into the vaccine vial. If the diluent does not flow freely, squeeze the diluent bottle gently and the diluent will flow into the vaccine vial. The vaccine vial should be completely filled with diluent to prevent excess foaming.
7. Hold the joined containers by the ends and shake vigorously until the vaccine plug is completely dissolved.
8. Return the joined containers to their original position (diluent bottle on the bottom). Allow the vaccine to flow into the diluent bottle. If the vaccine does not flow into the diluent bottle, tap or squeeze the diluent bottle gently and release to draw the vaccine into the diluent bottle. Be sure that all of the product is removed from the vaccine vial.
9. Remove the vaccine vial and adapter from the neck of the diluent bottle.
10. The vaccine is now ready to use.

How to Vaccinate: Vaccination is accomplished by dipping the needle applicator into the mixed vaccine and piercing the webbed portion of the underside of the wing. Avoid piercing through feathers which may wipe off the vaccine, and avoid hitting the wing muscle or bone to minimize reaction. The applicator is designed to pick up the proper amount of vaccine on the needle, which is deposited in the tissues when the wing is pierced. Redip the applicator in the vaccine before each application. Excess vaccine adhering to the applicator should be removed by touching the applicator to the inside of the vial.

Reactions: Examination for Takes: Normally, no overall clinical reaction is observed. At 5-10 days following vaccination, a swelling of the skin (subcutaneous granuloma) will develop on the wing-web at the point of inoculation. The absence of this local reaction may mean that the birds were immune before vaccination or that improper vaccination methods were used. Examination for these takes may be used to ensure that proper vaccination has been conducted. Immunity will normally develop within four (4) days after vaccination.

Records: Keep a record of the vaccine type, quantity, serial number, expiration date, and place of purchase; the date and time of vaccination; the number, age, breed, and location of the birds; the names of operators performing the vaccination and any observed reactions.

Contraindication(s): Initial vaccination in chickens over 12 weeks of age may be undesirable because larger granulomas may develop at the site of inoculation and this may result in the downgrading of carcasses at slaughter.

Precaution(s): Store at 35° to 45°F (2° to 7°C).

Caution(s): For veterinary use only.

1. Vaccinate healthy birds only. Although disease may not be evident, coccidiosis, chronic respiratory disease, mycoplasma infection, lymphoid leukosis, infectious bursal disease, Marek's disease, or other disease conditions may cause serious complications or reduce protection.
2. To avoid interference with the development of immunity, chickens to be vaccinated should not be given any antibiotic and/or sulfonamide medication used in the prevention or treatment of fowl cholera for three days before and five days after vaccination.
3. All birds within a flock should be vaccinated on the same day. Isolate other susceptible birds on the premises from the birds being vaccinated.
4. In outbreak situations, vaccinate healthy birds first, progressing toward outbreak areas in order to vaccinate diseased birds last.
5. Do not spill or spatter the vaccine. Use the entire contents of the vial when first opened. Burn the empty bottles, caps and all unused vaccine and accessories.
6. Avoid contact of open wounds or inoculation of vaccinating personnel with the vaccine since this might cause a bacterial infection. If this occurs, consult a physician immediately to obtain proper treatment. The vaccine organism, as with any *P. multocida* strain, may accidently act as a human pathogen and precaution should be taken to avoid exposure.
7. Wash hands thoroughly after using the vaccine.
8. Do not dilute the vaccine or otherwise stretch the dosage.

Warning(s): Do not vaccinate within 21 days before slaughter.

Presentation: Supplied in 10 x 500 dose units.

Compendium Code No.: 10470120

AVI-CON

Vet-A-Mix **Small Animal Dietary Supplement**

Active Ingredient(s): Guaranteed analysis per 200 mg dose:

Vitamin A	200 I.U.
Vitamin D_3	25 I.U.
Vitamin E	1 I.U.
Thiamine	100 mcg
Riboflavin	300 mcg
Pyridoxine	100 mcg
Vitamin B_{12}	1 mcg
Biotin	4 mcg
Choline	4,000 mcg
Folic acid	60 mcg
Niacin	1,000 mcg
Pantothenic acid	300 mcg
Menadione (K_3)	200 mcg

Indications: A dietary supplement for pet birds designed to provide the vitamins necessary for normal health and feathering.

Dosage and Administration: For dietary supplementation, mix two (2) measures in each fluid ounce of drinking water each day.

For young, ailing or aged birds, mix four (4) measures in each fluid ounce of drinking water each day.

To ensure freshness, prepare a water/vitamin mixture each day.

Each measure contains 100 mg AVI-CON.

Due to the special water soluble base, AVI-CON will remain a fresh, free flowing powder as long as the container is kept tightly closed when not in use. Accelerated tests show optimum vitamin stability when compared to other vitamin preparations for birds.

Note: AVI-CON, like all other bird vitamins, will remain potent for a limited period when mixed with drinking water. Do not mix more than the amount of drinking water that will be consumed in one (1) day.

Caution(s): Keep out of the reach of children.

Presentation: 50 g and 250 g bottles.

Compendium Code No.: 10500000

AVIMUNE®

Schering-Plough **Vaccine**

Avian Encephalomyelitis Vaccine, Live Virus

U.S. Vet. Lic. No.: 165A

Active Ingredient(s): Avian encephalomyelitis vaccine, chicken embryo origin, live virus, freeze dried (lyophilized). The vaccine contains gentamicin as a preservative.

Indications: For vaccinating healthy chickens between 10 weeks of age and four weeks prior to the onset of egg production, as an aid in the prevention and vertical transmission of avian encephalomyelitis infection (AE or epidemic tremors).

Dosage and Administration:

When to Vaccinate: Between 10 weeks of age and four (4) weeks before egg production.

Vaccination Program: The development of a durable, strong protection depends upon the use of an effective vaccination program as well as many circumstances such as administration techniques, environment and flock health at the time of vaccination.

Preparation of the Vaccine:

1. Assemble the vaccine and equipment needed to vaccinate the entire flock at one time.
2. Do not open and mix the vaccine until ready for use.
3. Remove the tear-off aluminum seal from the vaccine vial without disturbing the rubber stopper.
4. Use cool, clean, nonchlorinated tap water to which powdered milk has been added as directed under How to Vaccinate.
5. Holding the vial submerged in a pail of water (milk added) or under a running stream of water, lift the lip of the rubber stopper so that the water is sucked into the vial.
6. Reseat the stopper and shake the vial to thoroughly dissolve the vaccine.

How to Vaccinate: Do not mix the vaccine into the drinking water until ready for use. Drinking water for vaccination should be mixed with powdered milk to prevent inactivation from chlorine or other water additives and also to stabilize the vaccine virus. The powdered milk should be added to the water at the rate of one (1) heaped teaspoon per three (3) U.S. gallons or 2.5 imperial gallons (3 g per 11 L); or one (1) heaped cupful per 80 U.S. gallons or 66 imperial gallons (90 g per 300 L).

Withhold water from the birds for several hours before vaccinating so that the birds are thirsty. Thoroughly clean and rinse all watering containers so that no residual disinfectants remain. Dilute the vaccine immediately before use with cool, clean, nonchlorinated water (milk added). Pour the dissolved vaccine material into the following amounts of water and mix thoroughly.

Each 1,000 Birds	U.S. Gallons	Imperial Gallons	Metric Liters
Between 10 weeks of age and 4 weeks before egg production.	10	8	40

Distribute the diluted vaccine so that all of the birds are able to drink within a one (1) hour period and do not add any more water until the vaccine is consumed. Avoid placing water in direct sunlight.

Records: Keep a record of the vaccine type, quantity, serial number, expiration date, and place of purchase; the date and time of vaccination; the number, age, breed, and location of the birds; the names of operators performing the vaccination; and any observed reactions.

Precaution(s): Store at 35° to 45° F (2° to 7°C).

Caution(s):

1. For veterinary use only.
2. Vaccinate healthy birds only.
3. All birds within a house should be vaccinated on the same day. Isolate other susceptible birds on the premises from the birds being vaccinated.
4. In outbreak situations, vaccinate healthy birds first, progressing toward outbreak areas in order to vaccinate diseased birds last.
5. Do not spill or spatter the vaccine. Use the entire contents of the vial when first opened. Burn the empty bottles, caps, and all unused vaccine and accessories.
6. Wash hands thoroughly after using the vaccine.
7. Do not dilute the vaccine or otherwise stretch the dosage.
8. Do not mix vaccinated pullets with layers from a nonvaccinated flock.

Warning(s): Do not vaccinate within 21 days before slaughter.

Presentation: Supplied in 10 x 5,000 dose units.

Compendium Code No.: 10470130

AVIMUNE®+POX

Schering-Plough **Vaccine**

Avian Encephalomyelitis-Fowl Pox Vaccine, Live Virus

U.S. Vet. Lic. No.: 165A

Active Ingredient(s): AVIMUNE®+POX is a combination live virus vaccine of chicken embryo origin containing a fowl pox virus selected for its ability to stimulate strong protection against a wide variety of fowl pox strains and avian encephalomyelitis virus. The vaccine contains gentamicin as a preservative.

Indications: For the vaccination of healthy chickens 10 weeks of age or older, as an aid in the prevention of avian encephalomyelitis and fowl pox through vaccination by the wing-web method.

Dosage and Administration:

When to Vaccinate: Between 10 weeks of age and four (4) weeks before egg production.

Vaccination Program: The development of a durable, strong protection depends upon the use of an effective vaccination program as well as many circumstances such as administration techniques, environment and flock health at the time of vaccination. Also, the immune response to one (1) vaccination under field conditions is seldom complete for all animals within a given flock. Even when vaccination is successful, the protection stimulated in individual animals against different diseases may not be life-long. Therefore, under certain circumstances revaccination may be necessary.

Preparation of the Vaccine:

1. Do not open and mix the vaccine until ready for use.
2. Mix only one (1) vial at a time and use the entire contents within two (2) hours.
3. Remove the tear-off aluminum seal and stopper from the vial containing the dried vaccine.
4. Remove the tear-off aluminum seal and stopper from the bottle containing the diluent.
5. Hold the diluent bottle firmly in an upright position and insert the vaccine vial on the adapter of the diluent bottle. The neck of the vaccine vial should snap into position and should be seated securely on the adapter on the diluent bottle.
6. Invert the two (2) containers so that the vaccine vial is on the bottom and allow the diluent to flow into the vaccine vial. If the diluent does not flow freely, squeeze the bottle gently and the diluent will flow into the vaccine vial. The vaccine vial should be completely filled with diluent to prevent excess foaming.
7. Hold the joined containers by the ends and shake vigorously until the vaccine plug is completely dissolved.
8. Return the joined containers to their original position (diluent bottle on the bottom). Allow the vaccine to flow into the diluent bottle. If the vaccine does not flow into the diluent bottle, tap or squeeze the diluent bottle gently and release to draw the vaccine into the diluent bottle. Be sure that all of the product is removed from the vaccine vial.
9. Remove the vaccine vial and adapter from the neck of the diluent bottle.
10. The vaccine is now ready for use.

How to Vaccinate: Vaccination is accomplished by dipping the needle applicator into the mixed vaccine and piercing the webbed portion of the underside of the wing. Avoid piercing through feathers which may wipe off the vaccine, and avoid hitting the wing muscle or bone to minimize reaction. The applicator is designed to pick up the proper amount of vaccine on the needle, which is deposited in the tissues when the wing is pierced. Redip the applicator in the vaccine before each application. Excess vaccine adhering to the applicator should be removed by touching the applicator to the side of the vaccine vial.

Examine for Takes: Examine the birds for takes six (6) to eight (8) days following vaccination. A positive take, showing that the vaccination was successful, is indicated by swelling of the skin or scab formation at the point of inoculation. The absence of takes may mean that birds were immune before vaccination or that improper vaccination methods were used. Protection will normally develop within about 10 to 14 days after vaccination. Swelling and scabs will disappear two (2) to three (3) weeks following vaccination.

Records: Keep a record of the vaccine type, quantity, serial number, expiration date, and place of purchase; the date and time of vaccination; the number, age, breed, and location of the birds; the names of operators performing the vaccination; and any observed reactions.

Precaution(s): Store at 35° to 45° F (2° to 7°C).

Caution(s): For veterinary use only.

1. Vaccinate healthy birds only. Although disease may not be evident, coccidiosis, chronic respiratory disease, mycoplasma infection, lymphoid leukosis, infectious bursal disease,

Marek's disease, or other disease conditions may cause serious complications or reduce protection.

2. All birds within a house should be vaccinated on the same day. Isolate other susceptible birds on the premises from the birds being vaccinated.
3. In outbreak situations, vaccinate healthy birds first, progressing toward outbreak areas in order to vaccinate diseased birds last.
4. Do not spill or spatter the vaccine. Use the entire contents of the vial when first opened. Burn the empty bottles, caps, and all unused vaccine and accessories.
5. Do not dilute the vaccine or otherwise stretch the dosage.
6. Wash hands thoroughly after using the vaccine.
7. Do not mix vaccinated pullets with layers from a nonvaccinated flock.

Warning(s): Do not vaccinate within 21 days before slaughter.

Presentation: Supplied in 10 x 1,000 dose units.

Compendium Code No.: 10470140

AZIUM® POWDER ℞

Schering-Plough **Corticosteroid-Oral**

(Dexamethasone) 10 mg

NADA No.: 030-434

Active Ingredient(s): AZIUM® Powder is available in packets containing 10 mg crystalline dexamethasone.

Indications: Cattle and Horses: AZIUM® is indicated for treatment of primary ketosis in cattle and as an anti-inflammatory agent in both cattle and horses. AZIUM® Powder is indicated in cases where cattle and horses require additional steroid therapy following parenteral administration. These oral forms may be used as supportive therapy for the management of inflammatory conditions such as acute arthritic lameness, and for various stress conditions when corticosteroids are required while the animal is being treated for a specific condition.

AZIUM® is not species-specific, therefore, the veterinarian should read the sections on Indications, Dosage, Side Effects, Contraindications and Precautions and Warning before the drug is used.

Pharmacology: AZIUM® is a synthetic analogue of prednisolone, having similar but more potent anti-inflammatory therapeutic action and diversified hormonal and metabolic effects. Modification of the basic corticoid structure as achieved in AZIUM® offers an enhanced anti-inflammatory effect compared to older corticosteroids. The dosage of AZIUM® required is markedly lower than that of prednisone and prednisolone.

Experimental animal studies on dexamethasone have revealed that it possesses greater anti-inflammatory activity than many steroids. Veterinary clinical evidence indicates that dexamethasone has approximately 20 times the anti-inflammatory activity of prednisolone and 70 to 80 times that of hydrocortisone. Thymus involution studies show dexamethasone possesses 25 times the activity of prednisolone. In reference to mineralocorticoid activity, dexamethasone does not cause significant sodium or water retention. Metabolic balance studies show that animals on controlled and limited protein intake will exhibit nitrogen loss on exceedingly high dosages.

Dosage and Administration: Therapy with AZIUM®, as with any other potent corticosteroid, should be individualized according to the severity of the condition being treated, anticipated duration of steroid therapy, and the animal's threshold or tolerance for steroid excess.

Treatment may be changed over to AZIUM® from any other glucocorticoid with the proper reduction or adjustment of the dosage.

AZIUM® Powder is intended for oral administration to cattle and horses. The powder is easily administered by drench or by sprinkling on a small amount of feed.

Cattle and Horses: 5 to 10 mg the first day then 5 mg per day as required. If a response is not achieved in five (5) days, the condition may not be amenable to AZIUM® therapy.

In cases where animals have been treated with parenteral forms of AZIUM®, the powder may be given, if required, at doses of 5 mg per day 24 to 48 hours after injections. Treatment may be repeated if necessary.

Contraindication(s): Except for emergency therapy, do not use in animals with chronic nephritis and hypercorticalism (Cushing's syndrome). The existence of congestive heart failure, diabetes and osteoporosis are relative contraindications. Do not use in viral infections during the viremic stage.

Precaution(s): Animals receiving AZIUM® should be under close observation. Because of the anti-inflammatory action of corticosteroids, signs of infection may be masked and it may be necessary to stop treatment until a further diagnosis is made. Overdosage of some glucocorticoids may result in sodium retention, (fluid retention), potassium loss and weight gain.

AZIUM® may be administered to animals with acute or chronic bacterial infections providing that the infections are controlled with the appropriate antibiotics or chemotherapeutic agents.

The use of corticosteroids, depending upon dose, duration and specific steroid, may result in the inhibition of endogenous steroid production following drug withdrawal. In patients presently receiving or recently withdrawn from systemic corticosteroid treatments, therapy with a rapidly acting corticosteroid should be considered in unusually stressful situations.

Store between 2-30°C (36-86°F).

Caution(s): Federal law restricts this drug to use by or on the order of a licensed veterinarian.

Warning(s): Clinical and experimental data have demonstrated that corticosteroids administered orally or parenterally to animals may induce the first stage of parturition when administered during the last trimester of pregnancy and may precipitate premature parturition followed by dystocia, fetal death, retained placenta and metritis.

Additionally, corticosteroids administered to dogs, rabbits, and rodents during pregnancy have produced cleft palate. Other congenital anomalies including deformed forelegs, phocomelia, and anasarca have been reported in offspring of dogs which received corticosteroids during pregnancy. Not for use in horses intended for food.

Side Effects: Side effects such as SAP and SGPT enzyme elevations, weight loss, anorexia, polydipsia, and polyuria have occurred following the use of synthetic corticosteroids in dogs. Vomiting and diarrhea (occasionally bloody) have been observed in cats and dogs.

Cushing's syndrome in dogs has been reported in association with prolonged or repeated steroid therapy. Corticosteroids reportedly cause laminitis in horses.

Presentation: 10 mg packets, boxes of 30 and 100.

Compendium Code No.: 10470151

AZIUM® SOLUTION ℞

Schering-Plough **Corticosteroid Injection**

(Dexamethasone) 2 mg/mL-Sterile

NADA No.: 012-559

Active Ingredient(s): Each mL contains 2 mg dexamethasone, 500 mg polyethylene glycol 400, 9 mg benzyl alcohol, 1.8 mg methylparaben and 0.2 mg propylparaben as preservatives, 4.75% alcohol, HCl to adjust pH to approximately 4.9 and water for injection q.s.

Indications: AZIUM® Solution is indicated for the treatment of primary bovine ketosis and as an anti-inflammatory agent in the bovine and equine.

As supportive therapy, AZIUM® Solution may be used in the management of various rheumatic, allergic, dermatologic and other diseases known to be responsive to anti-inflammatory corticosteroids. AZIUM® Solution may be used intravenously as supportive therapy when an immediate hormonal response is required.

Bovine Ketosis: AZIUM® Solution is offered for the treatment of primary ketosis. The gluconeogenic effects of AZIUM®, when administered intramuscularly, are generally noted within the first 6 to 12 hours. When AZIUM® Solution is used intravenously, the effects may be noted sooner. Blood sugar levels rise to normal levels within 12 to 24 hours. Acetone bodies are reduced to normal concentrations usually within 24 hours. The physical attitude of animals treated with AZIUM® Solution brightens and appetite improves, usually within 12 hours. Milk production, which is suppressed as a compensatory reaction in this condition, begins to increase. In some instances, it may even surpass previous peaks. The recovery process usually takes from 3 to 7 days.

Supportive Therapy: AZIUM® Solution may be used as supportive therapy in mastitis, metritis, traumatic gastritis and pyelonephritis, while appropriate primary therapy is administered. In these cases, the corticosteroid combats accompanying stress and enhances the feeling of general well-being.

AZIUM® Solution may also be used as supportive therapy in inflammatory conditions, such as arthritic conditions, snake bite, acute mastitis, shipping fever, pneumonia, laminitis and retained placenta.

Equine: AZIUM® Solution is indicated for the treatment of acute musculoskeletal inflammations such as bursitis, carpitis, osselets, tendonitis, myositis and sprains. If boney changes exist in any of these conditions, joints, or accessory structures, a response to AZIUM® Solution cannot be expected. In addition, AZIUM® Solution may be used as a supportive therapy in fatigue, heat exhaustion, influenza, laminitis and retained placenta provided that the primary cause is determined and corrected.

AZIUM® Solution is not species-specific, however, the veterinarian should read the sections on Indications, Dosage, Side Effects, Contraindications and Cautions and Warnings before the drug is used.

Pharmacology: AZIUM® (dexamethasone) Solution is a synthetic analogue of prednisolone, having similar but more potent anti-inflammatory therapeutic action and diversified hormonal and metabolic effects. Modification of the basic corticoid structure as achieved in AZIUM® Solution offers enhanced anti-inflammatory effect compared to older corticosteroids. The dosage of AZIUM® Solution required is markedly lower than that of prednisone and prednisolone.

Dosage and Administration: Therapy with AZIUM® Solution, as with any other potent corticosteroid, should be individualized according to the severity of the condition being treated, anticipated duration of steroid therapy, and the animal's threshold or tolerance for steroid excess.

Treatment may be changed over to AZIUM® Solution from any other glucocorticoid with proper reduction or adjustment of dosage.

Bovine: AZIUM® Solution - 5 to 20 mg intravenously or intramuscularly.

Azium® Powder may be administered or the parenteral dose repeated as needed.

Equine: AZIUM® Solution - 2.5 to 5 mg intravenously or intramuscularly.

Azium® Powder may be administered or the parenteral dose repeated as needed.

Contraindication(s): Except for emergency therapy, do not use in animals with chronic nephritis and hypercorticalism (Cushing's syndrome). The existence of congestive heart failure, diabetes and osteoporosis are relative contraindications. Do not use in viral infections during the viremic stage.

Precaution(s): Store between 2° and 30°C (36° and 86°F).

Caution(s): Federal law restricts this drug to use by or on the order of a licensed veterinarian.

Animals receiving AZIUM® Solution should be under close observation. Because of the anti-inflammatory action of corticosteroids, signs of infection may be masked and it may be necessary to stop treatment until a further diagnosis is made. Overdosage of some glucocorticoids may result in sodium retention, fluid retention, potassium loss and weight gain.

AZIUM® Solution may be administered to animals with acute or chronic bacterial infections providing that the infections are controlled with appropriate antibiotics or chemotherapeutic agents.

Doses greater than those recommended in horses may produce a transient drowsiness or lethargy in some horses. The lethargy usually abates in 24 hours.

The use of corticosteroids, depending on dose, duration and specific steroid, may result in the inhibition of endogenous steroid production following drug withdrawal. In patients presently receiving or recently withdrawn from systemic corticosteroid treatments, therapy with a rapidly acting corticosteroid should be considered in unusually stressful situations.

Clinical and experimental data have demonstrated that corticosteroids administered orally or parenterally to animals may induce the first stage of parturition when administered during the last trimester of pregnancy and may precipitate premature parturition followed by dystocia, fetal death, retained placenta and metritis.

Additionally, corticosteroids administered to dogs, rabbits, and rodents during pregnancy have produced cleft palate. Other congenital anomalies including deformed forelegs, phocomelia, and anasarca have been reported in offspring of dogs which received corticosteroids during pregnancy.

Warning(s): A withdrawal period has not been established for this product in pre-ruminating calves. Do not use in calves to be processed for veal.

Side Effects: Side effects such as SAP and SGPT enzyme elevations, weight loss, anorexia, polydipsia, and polyuria have occurred following the use of synthetic corticosteroids in dogs. Vomiting and diarrhea (occasionally bloody) have been observed in cats and dogs.

Cushing's syndrome in dogs has been reported in association with prolonged or repeated steroid therapy.

Corticosteroids reportedly cause laminitis in horses.

Trial Data: Experimental Studies: Experimental animal studies on dexamethasone have revealed that it possesses greater anti-inflammatory activity than many steroids. Veterinary clinical evidence indicates that dexamethasone has approximately twenty times the anti-inflammatory activity of prednisolone and seventy to eighty times that of hydrocortisone. Thymus involution studies show dexamethasone possesses twenty-five times the activity of prednisolone. In reference to mineralocorticoid activity, dexamethasone does not cause significant sodium or water retention. Metabolic balance studies show that animals on controlled and limited protein intake will exhibit nitrogen losses on exceedingly high dosages.

Presentation: 100 mL multiple dose vials (NDC 0061-0884-01).

Compendium Code No.: 10470161 Rev. 3/00

B

B-1 POWDER

SureNutrition **Thiamine**

Guaranteed Analysis:

Thiamine (B_1) . . . . 8,000 mg/lb (500 mg/oz)

Ingredients: Sucrose, Thiamine Mononitrate, Calcium Silicate (Anti-Caking Agent) and Artificial Color.

Indications: A palatable source of B-1 for horses.

Dosage and Administration: Feeding Directions: Mix ½ to 1 ounce daily in the feed.

The enclosed scoop holds 1 oz.

Precaution(s): Store in a cool, dry place and keep tightly closed when not in use.

Caution(s): For animal use only.

Warning(s): Keep out of reach of children.

Presentation: 5 lb (2.2 kg) and 20 lb (9 kg) pails.

Compendium Code No.: 12060000 0BB1 / 0A1

B_1 VAC™

Intervet **Vaccine**

Newcastle Disease Vaccine, B_1 Type, B_1 Strain, Live Virus

U.S. Vet. Lic. No.: 286

Description: B_1 VAC™, a live virus vaccine, is prepared from a proven B_1 strain of Newcastle disease virus. The virus has been propagated using SPF substrates. The immunizing capability has also been proven by Master Seed Immunogenicity Test.

This vaccine contains gentamicin as a preservative.

Quality tested for purity, potency, and safety.

Indications: Drinking Water - Vaccination of healthy chickens two weeks of age or older for protection against Newcastle disease.

Beak-O-Vac or Coarse Spray - Vaccination of healthy chickens one day of age for protection against Newcastle disease.

If chickens are vaccinated earlier than two weeks of age, revaccination at four weeks is recommended for optimum protection.

Dosage and Administration: Vaccination Programs: Many factors must be considered in determining a sound vaccination program for a particular farm or poultry complex. To be fully effective, the vaccine must be administered properly to healthy, receptive animals maintained in a proper environment under good management. In addition, the response may be influenced by the age of the animals and their immune status. Seldom does one live virus vaccination under field conditions produce lifetime protection for all individuals in a given flock. The level of immunity required will vary with operational practices and the degree of exposure. Therefore, a program of periodic revaccinations may be necessary.

Preparation of Vaccine:

For Beak-O-Vac Use: Do not open and mix the vaccine until ready to begin vaccination. Use vaccine immediately after mixing.

1. Remove the tear-off seal and stopper from the vial containing the dried vaccine.
2. Remove the seal and stopper from the bottle of diluent.
3. Pour a small amount of diluent into the vial of vaccine.
4. Insert the rubber stopper and shake.
5. Pour the rehydrated vaccine into the bottle containing the rest of the diluent. Replace the stopper and shake.

The vaccine is now ready for use by the following methods. For best results, be sure to follow the directions carefully!

Beak-O-Vac Administration - For Chickens One Day of Age:

1. Rehydrate the vaccine as directed.
2. Attach the container holding the vaccine to the machine and adjust for delivery of 33-35 doses per mL.
3. Hold the chicken in such a manner that the chicken's beak is opened in the direction of the nozzle so the vaccine is deposited on the roof of the mouth as the beak is turned.

Preparation of Vaccine:

For Drinking Water or Coarse Spray Use: Do not open and mix the vaccine until ready to begin vaccination. Use vaccine immediately after mixing.

1. Remove the tear-off seal and stopper from the vial containing the dried vaccine.
2. Carefully pour clean, cool, non-chlorinated water into the vaccine vial until the vial is approximately two-thirds full.
3. Insert the rubber stopper and shake vigorously until all material is dissolved.
4. The vaccine is now ready for drinking water or coarse spray use in accordance with the following directions. For best results, be sure to follow directions carefully!

Drinking Water Administration - For Chickens Two Weeks of Age or Older:

1. Do not use any disinfectants in the drinking water for 48 hours before vaccinating and for 24 hours after vaccination.
2. Withhold water from the chickens until they are thirsty. Withholding periods will vary from 2 to 8 hours according to the age of the chickens and the weather. Be careful in hot weather.
3. Scrub waterers and rinse thoroughly with fresh, clean water. Do not use disinfectants for cleaning the waterers.
4. Rehydrate the vaccine as directed above.
5. Mix rehydrated vaccine with clean, cool, non-chlorinated water in accordance with chart below.

Water Per Age of Chickens	Water Per 1,000 Doses Vaccine
2-4 Weeks	6 gal. (23 liters)
4-8 Weeks	10 gal. (38 liters)
8 Weeks or Older	16 gal. (60 liters)

As an aid in preserving the virus, 85 mL (3.2 ounces) of non-fat powdered milk may be added with each 38 liters (10 gallons) of water used for mixing vaccine. Add the dried milk first and agitate thoroughly. Then add the rehydrated vaccine from the vial and again mix thoroughly.

6. Distribute the vaccine solution, as prepared above, among the waterers provided for the chickens. Avoid placing waterers in direct sunlight.
7. Provide no other drinking water until all the vaccine-water solution has been consumed.

Coarse Spray Vaccination - For Chickens One Day of Age:

1. Use rehydrated vaccine as indicated for specific coarse spray vaccination machines. For example, a machine which dispenses 20 mL in 3 seconds to a box of 100 chickens; - total volume for 10,000 doses is 2,000 mL of deionized water. Mix thoroughly.
2. Add the prepared vaccine solution to the reservoir on the machine.
3. Prime and adjust machine as instructed in manual accompanying the specific machine.
4. Place boxes holding 100 chickens each on the conveyor belt or in machine. Activate spray head.

Coarse Spray Vaccination - For Chickens Two Days of Age or Older:

1. Initial spray vaccination should be by coarse spray, i.e., Hardi®.
2. Do not use any disinfectants or skim milk in sprayer.
3. Use sprayer only for administration of vaccine. Clean thoroughly after each use.
4. Shut off all fans while spray vaccinating. Turn on fans immediately after spraying. Be careful in hot weather.
5. Spray chickens by walking slowly through the house.
6. Follow the recommendation of the manufacturer of the sprayer regarding water volume.
7. Use only clean, cool, deionized water.
8. Individual(s) spraying chickens should wear a face mask and goggles.

Records: Keep a record of vaccine, quantity, serial number, expiration date, and place of purchase; the date and time of vaccination; the number, age, breed, and locations of chickens; names of operators performing the vaccination and any observed reactions.

Precaution(s): Store vaccine in refrigerator between 2 and 7°C (35 and 45°F).

Do not spill or splash the vaccine.

Use entire contents when first opened.

Burn containers and all unused contents.

This product is non-returnable.

Caution(s): Vaccinate only healthy chickens. Although disease may not be evident, coccidiosis, mycoplasma infection, infectious bursal disease, reovirus infection, Marek's disease, and other disease conditions may cause complications or reduce immunity.

All susceptible chickens on the same premises should be vaccinated at the same time.

The revaccination of laying hens with live Newcastle vaccine may be detrimental to the flock and cannot be generally recommended. Consult your Intervet representative for more information.

Efforts should be taken to reduce stress conditions at the time of vaccination and during the reaction period.

Do not dilute the vaccine or otherwise stretch the dosage. For veterinary use only.

Notice: This vaccine has undergone rigid potency, safety and purity tests, and meets Intervet Inc. and USDA requirements. It is designed to stimulate effective immunity when used as directed, but the user must be advised that the response to the product depends upon many factors, including, but not limited to, conditions of storage and handling by the user, administration of the vaccine, health and responsiveness of individual chickens, and the degree of field exposure. Therefore, directions should be followed carefully.

This product is not hazardous when used according to directions supplied. A material safety data sheet (MSDS) is available upon request. This and any other consmer informaiton can be obtained by calling Intervet Customer Service at 1-800-441-8272 or 1-302-934-8051.

The use of the vaccine is subject to applicable federal and local laws and regulations.

Use only as directed.

Warning(s): Do not vaccinate within 21 days before slaughter.

Newcastle virus occasionally causes conjunctivitis in humans lasting two or three days. Avoid any contact of vaccine with eyes.

Presentation: 10 x 2,000 doses for drinking water or coarse spray use.
10 x 10,000 doses for drinking water or coarse spray use.
10 x 10,000 doses with diluent for Beak-O-Vac use.

Compendium Code No.: 11060071 IAI 00110 AL 138

B12-JECT 1000 ℞

Vetus **Vitamin B_{12}**

Active Ingredient(s): Each mL of sterile aqueous solution contains:

Cyanocobalamin (B_{12}) . . . . 1,000 mcg
Sodium chloride . . . . 0.8% w/v
Benzyl alcohol (preservative) . . . . 1.5% w/v

Indications: For use as an aid in the management of vitamin B_{12} deficiencies in cattle, horses, dogs and cats.

Dosage and Administration: Inject subcutaneously or intramuscularly.

Cattle and Horses . . . . 1-2 mL
Dogs and Cats. . . . . 0.25-0.50 mL

May be repeated once or twice a week, as indicated by the condition and response of the animal.

Precaution(s): Store at a controlled room temperature between 59°-86°F (15°-30°C). Avoid exposure to light.

Caution(s): Federal law restricts this drug to use by or on the order of a licensed veterinarian.

For animal use only.

Warning(s): Keep out of reach of children.

Presentation: 100 mL vials.

Compendium Code No.: 14440851

B12-JECT 3000 ℞

Vetus **Vitamin B_{12}**

Active Ingredient(s): Each mL of sterile aqueous solution contains:

Cyanocobalamin (B_{12}) . . . . 3,000 mcg
Sodium chloride . . . . 0.8% w/v
Benzyl alcohol (preservative) . . . . 1.5% w/v

Indications: For use as a supplemental source of vitamin B_{12} in cattle, horses, sheep, swine, dogs and cats.

Dosage and Administration: Inject subcutaneously or intramuscularly.

Cattle, Horses, Sheep and Swine. . . . . 1-2 mL
Dogs and Cats. . . . . 0.25-0.50 mL

The suggested dosage may be repeated at one- to two-week intervals, as indicated by the condition and response of the animal.

Precaution(s): Store at a controlled room temperature between 59°-86°F (15°-30°C). Avoid exposure to light.

Caution(s): Federal law restricts this drug to use by or on the order of a licensed veterinarian.

For animal use only.

Warning(s): Keep out of reach of children.

Presentation: 100 mL vials.

Compendium Code No.: 14440861

B

BABY PIG RESTART™ ONE-4

TechMix **Electrolytes-Oral**

Guaranteed Analysis:

Crude Protein ... not less than 16.00%
Crude Fat ... not less than 10.00%
Crude Fiber ... not more than 0.50%
Vitamin A ... not less than 20,000 I.Units/lb
Vitamin D ... not less than 4,000 I.Units/lb
Vitamin E ... not less than 25 I.Units/lb
Sodium (Na) ... not less than 0.77% (218.0 mg/oz)
Potassium (K) ... not less than 0.66% (186.0 mg/oz)
Calcium (Ca) ... not less than 0.59% (167.0 mg/oz)
Calcium (Ca) ... not more than 1.09% (309.0 mg/oz)
Phosphorus (P) ... not less than 0.48% (135.0 mg/oz)
Magnesium (Mg) ... not less than 0.06% (16.0 mg/oz)

Ingredients: Dried skim milk, dried whey, animal and vegetable fat (stabilized with BHA and lecithin), animal plasma, dextrose, fructose, sucrose, lactose, dibasic potassium phosphate, glycine, sodium bicarbonate, calcium lactate, magnesium gluconate, citric acid, potassium chloride, dried *Lactobacillus acidophilus* fermentation product, dried *Lactobacillus lactis* fermentation product, dried *Lactobacillus plantarum* fermentation product, dried *Streptococcus diacetylactim* fermentation product, dried *Streptococcus faecium* fermentation product, dried *Bacillus subtilis* fermentation product, dried *Bacillis subtilis* fermentation extract, dried *Aspergillus oryzae* fermentation extract, dl-alpha tocopheryl acetate (source of Vitamin E activity), choline bitartrate, vitamin A acetate, niacin supplement, d-activated animal sterol (source of vitamin D_3), ascorbic acid (vitamin C), d-calcium pantothenate, d-biotin, riboflavin supplement, vitamin B_{12} supplement, menadione dimethylpyrimidinol bisulfite (source of vitamin K activity), thiamin hydrochloride, pyridoxine hydrochloride, folic acid, natural and artificial flavors added.

Indications: A blend of milk fat, milk sugars, animal fat, blood plasma and electrolytes intended to provide essential nutrients for the energy-deficient young piglet.

Dosage and Administration: Top Dressing: Top dress eight ounces of BABY PIG RESTART™ ONE-4 on the pig starter twice a day for every eight to ten pigs during the first 48 hours after weaning.

Drinking Water: For pigs of any age, showing signs of stunting or starving, mix eight ounces of BABY PIG RESTART™ ONE-4 in two quarts of water and feed continuously in flat pan or drinking bowl.

Oral Drenching for One- to Five-Day-Old Pigs: Mix four ounces of BABY PIG RESTART™ ONE-4 (one part) with eight ounces of water (two parts). Shake or stir well to make a suspension. Slowly administer 15 millimeters (½ ounce) of the suspension on the back of the tongue and repeat as needed for severely stunted or starved one- to five-day-old piglets.

Precaution(s): Store in a dry room at temperatures between 4°C and 30°C (40°F-86°F). Once bag is opened, seal bag with tape or binder and place unused portion in a dry air sealable container.

Caution(s): Pigs showing symptoms of coma, shock or are too weak and dehydrated to eat and drink normally should be treated as directed by a veterinarian. This product is not nutritionally complete if administered by itself for long periods of time. It should not be administered beyond the recommended period without the addition of milk, milk replacers and pig starters.

Warning(s): Livestock product.

Keep out of reach of children.

Discussion: BABY PIG RESTART™ ONE-4 is specifically designed to help prevent starveouts and stunting in young pigs that are not consuming sufficient or adequate energy from their milk or pig starter intake.

Why Baby Pigs Starve and Stunt: When a pig is born, it has a short six to twelve hour energy reserve within its body. Most healthy farrowed pigs have a two to four hour blood, liver and tissue energy supply and a body fat reserve equivalent to about 1½ percent of its body weight.

If a baby pig doesn't receive fat and lactose rich milk within two to three hours after farrowing, it will use up its limited energy reserve very quickly. From birth to four weeks of age, pigs require substantial amounts of energy to maintain their body temperature. Chilling, diarrhea and environmental stress burn up the young pig's energy reserve at an increased rate, predisposing the pig to hypoglycemia and starvation. Primary causes of baby pig mortality are dehydration and the hypoglycemia associated with inadequate milk intake during nursing or the lack of sufficient energy intake after weaning.

Fast growing, healthy pigs reach 12-14 pounds body weight between 21 and 24 days of age and normally develop a body fat content of 12-15 percent of their body weight as they approach weaning age. The normal stress of weaning causes a rapid depletion of energy and body fat. Recent research has shown that normal pigs, without the stress of diarrhea, utilize or burn up 35-50 percent of their body fat within 36 hours after weaning. To reduce weaning stress, even normal, healthy pigs require quick energy within hours after weaning. Their body fat reserves frequently drop to seven to nine percent of their body weight with just normal weaning stresses.

Pigs with added diarrhea stress at weaning are significantly more susceptible to dehydration, stunting and starving as their energy and electrolyte intake and fat reserves are not sufficient to maintain normal body temperature and metabolism.

Presentation: 12x2 lb (.90 kg) bags (24 lb pail) and 25 lb pail.

Compendium Code No.: 11440010

BAC-DROP UDDER WASH

Ecolab Food & Bev. Div. **Udder Wash**

Active Ingredient(s):

Phosphoric acid ... 41.25%
Dodecylbenzene sulfonic acid ... 6.8%

Indications: A germicidal udder wash.

Dosage and Administration:

1. Prepare the udder washing solution in a plastic pail, using 30 mL of BAC-DROP per 18 L of warm water, 110°-115°F or use a Klenzade™ Sprayer*.
2. Approximately one (1) minute before application of the machine, wash and massage the teats and udder with the solution, using a paper towel, which has been soaked in the solution.
3. After gentle washing and massage of the udder, press the excess solution from the towel and use the reverse side to dry the teats and udder.
4. Discard the used towel and use a clean towel for each cow.
5. Check the udder with a strip cup or screening paddle before applying the machine.

*The Klenzade™ sprayer may be used to wash the udder in place of a pail. Ask your Klenzade™ dealer for details.

Table of dilution: 30 mL BAC-DROP per 18 L of water - 10 mL BAC-DROP per 6 L of water - 5 mL BAC-DROP per 3 L of water provides a minimum of 100 ppm dodecylbenzene sulfonic acid.

Caution(s): For industrial use only. Use only at the recommended use dilution.

Antidote(s): External: Immediately flush skin with plenty of cool running water for at least 15 minutes. Remove contaminated clothing and wash before reuse.

Eyes: Immediately flush eyes with plenty of cool running water for at least 15 minutes.

Internal: If swallowed, do not induce vomiting. Immediately drink a large quantity of water, then drink milk or milk of magnesia. Follow with olive, mineral or vegetable oil, or raw eggs.

Get medical attention immediately.

After use, rinse the empty container thoroughly with water and discard it.

Warning(s): Corrosive. Causes eye damage and skin irritation. Do not get in eyes, on skin or on clothing when handling. Harmful if swallowed. Avoid the contamination of food.

Presentation: 4 x 1 gallon case and 15 gallon.

Compendium Code No.: 14490002

BACIFERM® GRANULAR 50

Alpharma **Feed Medication**

Bacitracin Zinc Premix-Type A Medicated Article

NADA No.: 046-920

Active Ingredient(s): Each pound contains bacitracin zinc equivalent to 50.0 grams of bacitracin (master standard).

Composition: A dried fermentation product obtained by culturing *B. licheniformis* Tracy on media adapted for microbiological production of bacitracin and calcium carbonate.

Indications: Increased rate of weight gain and improved feed efficiency in growing broiler chickens, turkeys, pheasants; growing quails; growing-finishing swine; and feedlot cattle.

Dosage and Administration: Growth and feed efficiency:

Animal	Indication	lb/ton*		grams+ per ton Type C Feed (range)
		Min.	Max.	
Growing broiler chickens, turkeys, pheasants	Increased rate of weight gain and improved feed efficiency.	0.08	1.0	4-50
Growing quail	Increased rate of weight gain and improved feed efficiency. Feed as the Type C feed to starting quail through 5 weeks of age.	0.1	0.4	5-20
Growing - finishing swine	Increased rate of weight gain.	0.4	0.4	20
	Improved feed efficiency.	0.4	0.8	20-40
Feedlot cattle	Increased rate of weight gain and improved feed efficiency.	35-70 mg/head/day		

* Amount listed represents lb BACIFERM® 50 Granular per ton of Type C feed

+ Amount listed represents g bacitracin zinc per ton of Type C feed

Mixing directions: Mix BACIFERM® 50 Granular along with the other ingredients; 0.2 lb of BACIFERM® 50 Granular supplies 10 grams of bacitracin zinc; 1 lb of BACIFERM® 50 Granular supplies 50 grams of bacitracin zinc; 2 lb of BACIFERM® 50 Granular supplies 100 grams of bacitracin zinc. Levels shown are minimum and maximum levels. Vary the antibiotic concentration when necessary to fit the feeding program to insure adequate level of antibiotic in total ration.

In order to assure equal distribution of bacitracin zinc use an intermediate premix; mix one 50 lb bag of BACIFERM® 50 Granular premix with 1950 lb of unmedicated feedstuff(s) to make one ton of intermediate premix. One 50 lb bag of BACIFERM® 50 Granular supplies 2500 grams of bacitracin zinc. Use 8 lb of this intermediate premix to supply 10 g of bacitracin zinc in one ton of Type C feed.

Caution(s): For use in dry feeds only. Not for use in liquid feed supplements.

For use in manufacturing poultry and livestock feeds only.

Presentation: 50 lb (22.68 kg) bags.

Compendium Code No.: 10220690 AHG-038 0104

BACK SIDE®

AgriLabs **Topical Insecticide**

Insecticide-Non-Systemic Pour-On

EPA Reg. No.: 773-66-53302

Active Ingredient(s):

Permethrin (3-phenoxyphenyl) methyl (±) cis, trans-3-(2,2-dichloroethenyl)-2,2-dimethylcyclopropanecarboxylate* ... 1.0%
Inert Ingredients** ... 99.0%
Total 100.0%

*cis/trans ratio: Min 35% (±) cis and max 65% (±) trans

**Contains petroleum distillates.

Indications: BACK SIDE® Insecticide is a non-systemic pour-on for beef, lactating and non-lactating dairy cattle. It controls lice and flies on cattle and controls keds and lice on sheep.

Directions for Use: It is a violation of Federal law to use this product in a manner inconsistent with its labeling.

Ready To Use - No dilution necessary.

Apply To	Target Insects	Application Instructions
Lactating and Non-Lactating Dairy Cattle, Beef Cattle and Calves	Lice, Horn Flies, Face Flies. Aids in control of Horse flies, Stable flies, Mosquitoes Black flies, and Ticks.	Pour along back and down face. Apply ½ fl oz (15 cc) per 100 lbs body weight of animal, up to a maximum of 5 fl oz for any one animal.
Sheep	Sheep Keds, Lice	Pour along back. Apply ¼ fl oz (7.5 cc) per 50 lbs body wt of animal, up to a maximum of 3 fl oz for any one animal.

For cattle and sheep, repeat treatment as needed, but not more than once every 2 weeks. For optimum lice control, two treatments at 14-day intervals are recommended.

Special Note: BACK SIDE® Insecticide is not effective in controlling cattle grubs.

Precautionary Statements: Hazards to Humans and Domestic Animals: Caution: Avoid contact with eyes.

Statement of Practical Treatment:

If in Eyes: Immediately flush eyes with plenty of water. Get medical attention if discomfort persists.

If Swallowed: Call a physician immediately. Do not induce vomiting unless under medical attention.

Note to Physician: Solvent presents aspiration hazard. Gastric lavage is indicated if material was taken internally.

Environmental Hazards: This pesticide is extremely toxic to fish. Use with care when applying to areas adjacent to any body of water. Do not add directly to water. Do not contaminate water by cleaning of equipment or disposal of wastes. Apply this product only as specified on the label.

Physical or Chemical Hazards: Do not use or store near heat or open flame.

Storage and Disposal: Do not contaminate water, food or feed by storage or disposal.

Storage: Keep container sealed when not in use. Do not store near food or feed.

Pesticide Disposal: Wastes resulting from the use of this product may be disposed of on site or at an approved waste disposal facility.

Container Disposal: Triple rinse (or equivalent). Then offer for recycling or reconditioning, or puncture and dispose of in a sanitary landfill or incineration, or if allowed by State and local authorities, by burning. If burned, stay out of smoke.

Containers One Gallon and Under: Do not reuse empty container. Rinse thoroughly, wrap in several layers of newspaper and place in trash.

Warning(s): Keep out of reach of children.

Disclaimer: Notice of Warranty: AgriLabs, Ltd. makes no warranty or merchantability for any particular purpose, or otherwise, expressed or implied concerning this product or its uses which extend beyond the use of the product under normal conditions in accordance with the statements made on this label.

Presentation: 1 gallon (3.785 L) and 2.5 gallons (9.5 L).

Compendium Code No.: 10580151 1/00

BACK SIDE™ PLUS

AgriLabs **Topical Insecticide**

Pour-On

EPA Reg. No.: 28293-259-53302

Active Ingredient(s):

Permethrin (3-phenoxyphenyl) methyl (±) cis, trans-3-(2,2-dichloroethenyl) 2,2-dimethylcyclopropanecarboxylate* 1.0%
Piperonyl Butoxide Technical** 1.0%
Inert Ingredients*** 98.0%

*cis/trans ratio: Min 35% (±) cis and max 65% (±) trans

**Equivalent to Min. 0.8% (butylcarbityl) (6-propylpiperonyl) ether and 0.2% related compounds.

***Contains petroleum distillate

Indications: The synergized formula kills lice and flies on cattle. It also kills keds on sheep.

Directions for Use: It is a violation of Federal law to use this product in a manner inconsistent with its labeling.

Ready To Use - No dilution necessary.

Apply To	Target Insects	Application Instructions
Lactating and Non-Lactating Dairy Cattle, Beef Cattle and Calves	Lice, Horn Flies, Face Flies. Aids in control of horse flies, stable flies, house flies, mosquitoes and black flies.	Dosage: Apply ½ fl oz (15 cc) per 100 lbs body wt. of animal up to a maximum of 5 fl oz for any one animal. Pour-On: Pour correct dose along back line and down face. Ready-to-Use Spray: Use undiluted in a mist sprayer to apply correct dose. Apply directly to neck, face, back, legs and ears. Back Rubber Use: Mix one pint per gallon of mineral oil. Keep rubbing device charged. Results improved by daily forced use.
Sheep	Sheep Keds, Lice	Pour along back. Apply ¼ fl oz (7.5 cc) per 50 lbs body wt. of animal, up to a maximum of 3 fl oz for any one animal. For optimum control, all animals in the flock should be treated after shearing.
Premises — in and around horse, beef, dairy, swine, sheep and poultry premises, animal hospital pens and kennels and "outside" meat processing premises.	House Flies, Stable Flies, Face Flies, Gnats, Mosquitoes, Black Flies, Fleas and Little House Flies. Aids in control of cockroaches, ants, spiders, crickets.	For use as a ready-to-use spot spray or premise spray, use undiluted in a mist sprayer. Apply directly to surface to leave a residual insecticidal coating, paying particular attention to areas where insects crawl or alight. One gallon will treat approximately 7,300 square feet.

For cattle and sheep, repeat treatment as needed, but no more than once every two weeks. For optimum lice control, two treatments at a 14-day interval are recommended.

Special Note: This product is not effective in controlling on cattle grubs. This is an oil-base, ready-to-use product that may leave an oily appearance on the hair coat of some animals. This product should be used in an integrated pest management system which may involve repeat treatments and the use of other pest control practices.

Precautionary Statements: Hazards to Humans and Domestic Animals:

Caution: Harmful if absorbed through skin. Avoid contact with skin, eyes and clothing. Prolonged or frequently repeated skin contact may cause allergic reactions in some individuals. Wash thoroughly with soap and water after handling.

Statement of Practical Treatment:

If Swallowed: Call a physician immediately. Do not induce vomiting unless under medical attention.

If in Eyes: Immediately flush eyes with plenty of water. Get medical attention if discomfort persists.

If on Skin: Wash skin with soap and water. Get medical attention.

Environmental Hazards: This product is extremely toxic to fish and other aquatic invertebrates. Do not add directly to water, or to areas where surface waters are present or to intertidal areas below the mean high water mark. Do not contaminate water when disposing of equipment washwaters. Apply this product only as specified on the label.

Physical or Chemical Hazards: Do not use or store near heat or open flame.

Storage and Disposal: Do not contaminate water, food or feed by storage or disposal.

Storage: Keep container sealed when not in use. Do not store near food or feed.

Pesticide Disposal: Wastes resulting from the use of this product may be disposed of on site or at an approved waste disposal facility.

Container Disposal: Triple rinse (or equivalent). Then offer for recycling or reconditioning, or puncture and dispose of in a sanitary landfill or incineration, or, if allowed by State and local authorities, by burning. If burned, stay out of smoke.

Warning(s): Keep out of reach of children.

Disclaimer: Buyer assumes all risks of use, storage or handling of this product not in strict accordance with directions given herewith.

Presentation: Available in gallons and 2.5 gallons.

Compendium Code No.: 10580160

BACTODERM® ℞

Pfizer Animal Health **Topical Antibacterial**

(mupirocin) Ointment 2%

NADA No.: 140-839

Active Ingredient(s): Each gram of BACTODERM® ointment contains 20 mg of mupirocin in a bland, water-washable ointment base consisting of polyethylene glycol 400 and polyethylene glycol 3350 (polyethylene glycol ointment, NF).

Indications: BACTODERM® ointment is indicated for the topical treatment of canine bacterial infections of the skin, including superficial pyoderma, caused by susceptible strains of *Staphylococcus aureus* and *Staphylococcus intermedius.*

Pharmacology: Mupirocin is a naturally-occurring, broad-spectrum antibiotic. The chemical name is 9-4-[5S-(2S,3S-epoxy-5S-hydroxy-4S-methylhexyl)-3R,4R-dihydroxytetrahydropyran-2S-yl]-3-methylbut-2(E)-enoyloxy-nonanoic acid. The chemical structure is:

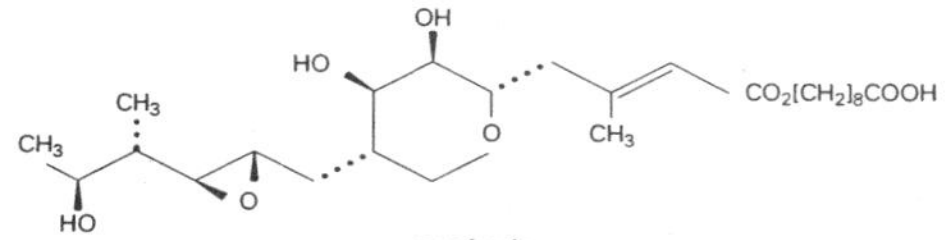

mupirocin

Clinical Pharmacology: Mupirocin is a chemical entity produced by fermentation of the organism *Pseudomonas fluorescens.* Mupirocin inhibits bacterial protein synthesis by reversibly and specifically binding to bacterial isoleucyl transfer-RNA synthetase. Due to this mode of action, mupirocin shows no cross resistance with chloramphenicol, erythromycin, gentamicin, lincomycin, neomycin, novobiocin, penicillin, streptomycin, and tetracycline. Mupirocin is an antimicrobial agent that inhibits the growth of gram-positive and gram-negative bacteria.

Bacteria susceptible to the action of mupirocin *in vitro* include the aerobic isolates of *Staphylococcus aureus* (including methicillin-resistant strains and β-lactamase-producing strains), *Staphylococcus intermedius, Staphylococcus epidermidis,* other coagulase positive or negative Staphylococci, α-hemolytic Streptococci, β group A Streptococci (including *S. pyogenes),* other β Streptococci (including *S. agalactiae),* group D Streptococci (including *S. faecalis* and *S. faecium),* group Viridans Streptococci, *Streptococcus pneumoniae, Corynebacterium hofmanii, Bacillus subtilis, Escherichia coli, Klebsiella pneumoniae, Proteus mirabilis, Proteus vulgaris, Enterobacter cloacae, Enterobacter aerogenes, Citrobacter freundii, Hemophilus influenzae* (including β-lactamase-producing strains), *Neisseria gonorrheae* (including β-lactamase-producing strains), *Neisseria meningitidis, Branhamella catarrhalis* and *Pasteurella multocida,* and the anaerobic isolates of *Peptostreptococcus anaerobius, Clostridium difficile,* and *Clostridium sporogenes.*

Clinical significance of the *in vitro* data is unknown except for susceptible strains of *Staphylococcus aureus* and *Staphylococcus intermedius.*

Dosage and Administration: Prior to treatment, the lesion should be cleansed. BACTODERM® ointment should be applied to the affected area twice a day. Apply a sufficient amount of ointment to completely cover the infected area. Maximum duration of treatment should not exceed 30 days.

Contraindication(s): This drug is contraindicated in animals with a history of sensitivity reactions to any of its components.

Precaution(s): Store between 15° and 30°C (59° and 86°F).

Caution(s): Federal law restricts this drug to use by or on the order of a licensed veterinarian.

Warning(s): Because of the potential hazard of nephrotoxicity due to the polyethylene glycol content of the base, care should be exercised when using this product in treating extensive deep lesions where absorption of large quantities of polyethylene glycol is possible.

Safety of use in pregnant or breeding animals has not been determined.

Bactoderm ointment is not for ophthalmic use.

For dermatologic use on dogs.

Keep out of reach of children.

Adverse Reactions: No adverse reactions have been reported with this product. If a skin reaction such as irritation should occur, treatment should be discontinued and appropriate therapy instituted.

Presentation: BACTODERM® ointment is supplied in 15-gram tubes.

Manufactured by: SmithKline Beecham Pharmaceuticals, Philadelphia, PA 19101

Compendium Code No.: 36901740 75-8030-02

BACTO-SEP

Interchem **Disinfectant**

EPA Reg. No.: 33431-6

Active Ingredient(s):

Didecyl dimethyl ammonium chloride 7.5%
Inert ingredients 92.5%
Total 100.0%

Indications: Disinfectant-sanitizer-fungicide deodorizer for hospitals, institutional, dairy and other farm use.

At 1 oz./four gallons, BACTO-SEP fulfills the criteria of appendix F of the Grade "A" pasteurized milk ordinances 1978 recommendations of the U.S. Public Health Services in waters up to 1,000 ppm of hardness calculated as $CaCO_3$ when evaluated by the AOAC Germicidal and Detergent Sanitizer Method against *Escherichia coli* and *Staphylococcus aureus.*

Dosage and Administration:

General Classification: It is a violation of federal law to use the product in a manner inconsistent with its labeling.

Apply BACTO-SEP with a cloth, mop or mechanical spray device. When applied with a mechanical spray device, the surface must be sprayed until thoroughly wetted. Treated surfaces must remain wet for 10 minutes, fresh solutions should be prepared each day or when the use solution becomes visibly dirty.

Disinfection in hospitals, and other health care institutions: For disinfecting floors, walls, countertops, bathing areas, lavatories, tables, chairs, garbage pails and other hard nonporous surfaces:

Add 3½ oz. BACTO-SEP to four (4) gallons water. Apply to previously cleaned hard surfaces with a mop or cloth.

At this use-level, BACTO-SEP is effective against *Pseudomonas aeruginosa.*

Disinfection in institutions, industries and schools: For disinfecting floors, walls, bedframes, countertops, tables, chairs, garbage pails, bathroom fixtures and other hard nonporous surfaces:

Add 2 oz. of BACTO-SEP to four (4) gallons of water. Apply to previously cleaned hard surfaces with a mop or cloth.

At 2 oz./four (4) gallon use-level BACTO-SEP is effective against *Staphylococcus aureus, Salmonella choleraesuis* and *Trichophyton interdigitale* (the athlete's foot fungus).

Disinfection of poultry equipment, animal quarters and kennels: Poultry brooders, watering founts, feeding equipment and other animal quarters (such as stalls and kennel areas) can be disinfected after thorough cleaning by applying a solution of 2 oz. BACTO-SEP in four (4) gallons of water with a mop, cloth or brush. Small utensils should be immersed in this solution.

Prior to disinfection, all poultry, other animals and their feeds must be removed from the premises. This includes emptying all troughs, racks and other feeding and watering appliances. Remove all litter and droppings from floors, walls and other surfaces occupied or traversed by poultry or other animals.

After disinfection, ventilate buildings, coops and other closed spaces. Do not house poultry, or other animals, or employ equipment until the treatment has been absorbed, set or dried.

All treated equipment that will contact feed or drinking water must be rinsed with potable water before re-use.

Sanitizing of food processing equipment, dairy equipment, food utensils, dishes, glasses, sink tops, countertops, refrigerated storage and display equipment and other hard nonporous surfaces. No potable water rinse is required.

Wash and rinse all articles thoroughly, then apply a solution of 1 oz. BACTO-SEP in four (4) gallons of water (150 ppm active). Surfaces should remain wet for a least one (1) minute followed by adequate draining and air drying. Fresh solutions should be prepared each day or when the use solution becomes visibly dirty. For mechanical application, the use solution may not be re-used for sanitizing applications.

Apply to sink tops, countertops, refrigerated storage and display equipment and other stationary hard surfaces with a cloth or brush. No potable water rinse is required.

Dishes, glasses, cooking utensils and other similar size food processing equipment can be sanitized by immersion in a 1 oz./four (4) gallon dilution of BACTO-SEP.

No potable water rinse is required.

The udders, flanks and teats of dairy cows can be sanitized by washing them with a solution of 1 oz. BACTO-SEP in four (4) gallons of warm water. No potable water rise is required.

Use a fresh towel for each cow. Avoid contamination of sanitizing solution by dirt and soil. Do not dip the used towel back into the sanitizing solution. When the solution becomes visibly dirty, discard it and provide a fresh solution.

Precaution(s): Do not contaminate water, food, or feed by storage and disposal. Open dumping is prohibited. Do not re-use the empty container.

Pesticide Disposal: Pesticide, spray mixture, or rinsate that can not be used or chemically processed should be disposed of in a landfill site approved for pesticides or buried in a safe place away from water supplies.

Container Disposal: Reseal the container and offer for reconditioning or triple rinse (or equivalent) and offer for recycling, reconditioning or disposal in an approved landfill site or bury in a safe place.

General: Consult federal, state or local disposal authorities for approved alternate procedures.

Caution(s): Precautionary Statements:

Hazard to Humans and Domestic Animals:

Danger - Keep out of the reach of children. Corrosive. Causes eye and skin irritation. Do not get in eyes, on skin or on clothing. Protect eyes and skin when handling. Harmful if swallowed. Avoid the contamination of food.

Statement of Practical Treatment: In case of contact, immediately flush eyes or skin with plenty of water for at least 15 minutes. For eyes, call a physician. Remove and wash all contaminated clothing before re-use.

If swallowed, drink milk, egg whites, gelatin solution or if these are not available, drink large quantities of water. Avoid alcohol. Call a physician.

Note to Physician: Probable muscosal damage may contraindicate the use of gastric lavage. Measures against circulatory shock, respiratory depression and convulsion may be needed.

Presentation: 1 gallon, 5 gallon, 30 gallon, and 55 gallon containers.

Compendium Code No.: 10200000

BACTRASAN™ SOLUTION

Aspen **Teat Dip**

Active Ingredient(s): This product is a chlorhexidine solution that contains:

1,6-di (N-p-chlorophenyldiguanido) hexane digluconate	2.0% w/w
Isopropyl alcohol	1.0% w/w
Inert Ingredients	97.0% w/w

Contains artificial color.

Indications: For use in preparation of a 0.5% solution for dipping teats as an aid in the control of mastitis-causing bacteria, such as *Streptococcus agalactiae, Streptococcus dysgalactiae, Streptococcus uberis, Staphylococcus aureus, E coli* and *Pseudomonas aeruginosa* on teats.

Dosage and Administration: Directions for Dilution:

To prepare 1 gallon of a 0.5% solution for dipping teats, mix 32 fluid ounces (1 qt) of BACTRASAN™ Solution with 96 fluid ounces (3 qts) of clean water* or distilled water in a clean 1-gallon container.

Alternatively, mix 32 fluid ounces (1 qt) of BACTRASAN™ Solution with 90 fluid ounces of clean water* or distilled water and 6 fluid ounces of glycerin in a clean 1-gallon container.

*Precipitate may occur with certain types of water used for dilution. It is preferable to use distilled water or deionized water.

Directions for Use of the 0.5% Solution: Dip each teat into the 0.5% solution immediately after each milking. Thoroughly wash teats and udder immediately prior to next milking.

Teat dipping should start at least one week before the cow freshens and continue until four days or more after drying off.

Precaution(s): Store at room temperature.

Do not allow to freeze.

Avoid contamination of feed and foodstuffs. Rinse empty container thoroughly with water and properly destroy by crushing or burial.

Caution(s): Dilute with the proper amount of water before use as a teat dip. Do not use the concentrate as a teat dip.

Warning(s): May be irritating to eyes and mucous membranes. If contact occurs, flush with copious amounts of water. Call a physician for treatment of eyes. May be harmful if swallowed.

For external animal use only.

Keep out of reach of children.

Presentation: 3.7 L (128 fl oz) (1 gal).

Compendium Code No.: 14750060

BAG BALM® OINTMENT

Dairy Association **Udder Product**

Ingredient(s): 8-Hydroxy quinoline sulfate 0.3% in a petrolatum lanolin base.

Indications: For chapped conditions and superficial abrasions. After each milking apply thoroughly and allow coating to remain on surface. This protective ointment helps to keep superficial tissue moist and soft.

Directions: Massage thoroughly and allow ointment to remain for full softening effect.

For pets, apply BAG BALM® liberally to the affected area. For use on cows, thoroughly wash treated teats and udder with separate towels before each milking. To avoid contamination after each milking, bathe the udder with plenty of hot water, strip milk out and dry skin. Apply BAG BALM® freely and massage gently with this proven ointment twice daily. This product contains no alcohol.

Caution(s): In case of deep or puncture wounds seek medical help. Discontinue use if rash or irritation occurs. Keep this, and all medications, away from children.

Presentation: 1 oz, 10 oz and 4.5 lb pail.

Compendium Code No.: 10480001

BAG SALVE

First Priority **Udder Product**

Emollient, Antiseptic

Active Ingredient(s): 8-Hydroxyquinoline sulfate 0.2% and Methyl Salicylate. In a petrolatum and lanolin base.

Indications: For chapped teats, superficial scratches, abrasions, windburn and sunburn. This antiseptic protective ointment helps to keep superficial tissue soft. For minor congestion of the udder due to calving, high feeding, bruising or chilling.

Directions for Use: Using individual towels, thoroughly wash treated teats and udder before each milking to avoid contamination of milk. After each milking, bathe with plenty of hot water, strip milk out clean, dry skin and apply BAG SALVE freely. Massage gently fifteen minutes twice daily or more often as necessary. Allow a coating to remain on surface for full antiseptic and softening effect on the udder.

Precaution(s): Storage: Store at controlled room temperature between 15° and 30°C (59°-86°F). Keep container tightly closed when not in use.

Caution(s): In case of deep or puncture wounds or if rash or irritation develops, discontinue use and consult a veterinarian. For animal use only.

Warning(s): Keep out of reach of children.

Presentation: 1 lb (453.6 g) and 4.5 lb (2043 g) (NDC 58829-290-45).

Compendium Code No.: 11390032 Rev. 06-01

BANAMINE® GRANULES ℞

Schering-Plough **Analgesic-Anti-inflammatory**

(Flunixin meglumine)

NADA No.: 106-616

Active Ingredient(s): Each 10 g packet of BANAMINE® Granules contains flunixin meglumine equivalent to 250 mg flunixin and each 20 g packet of BANAMINE® Granules contains flunixin meglumine equivalent to 500 mg flunixin.

Indications: BANAMINE® is recommended for the alleviation of inflammation and pain associated with musculoskeletal disorders in the horse.

Pharmacology: Flunixin meglumine is a potent non-narcotic, non-steroidal, analgesic agent with anti-inflammatory and anti-pyretic activity. It is significantly more potent than pentazocine, meperidine or codeine as an analgesic in the rat yeast paw test. Oral studies in the horse show the onset of flunixin activity occurs within two hours of administration. Peak response occurs between 12 and 16 hours and the duration of activity is 24-36 hours.

Dosage and Administration: The recommended dose of flunixin is 0.5 mg per pound of body weight once a day, i.e. one (1) 10 g packet treats 500 pounds and one (1) 20 g packet treats 1,000 pounds. The granules are easily administered by sprinkling on a small amount of feed. Treatment may be given initially by intravenous or intramuscular injection of BANAMINE® Solution, followed by BANAMINE® Granules on days two (2) to five (5). BANAMINE® treatment should not exceed five (5) consecutive days.

Contraindication(s): There are not any known contraindications to the drug when used as directed.

Precaution(s): The effect of BANAMINE® on pregnancy has not been determined. Studies to date show that there is not a detrimental effect on stallion spermatogenesis with or following the recommended dose of BANAMINE®. Store between 2-30°C (36-86°F).

Caution(s): Federal law restricts this drug to use by or on the order of a licensed veterinarian.

Warning(s): Not for use in horses intended for food.

Toxicology: Toxic effects were not observed in rats given oral flunixin 2 mg/kg per day for 42 days. Higher doses produced ulceration of the gastro-intestinal tract. The emetic dose in dogs is between 150 and 250 mg/kg. Flunixin was well tolerated in monkeys dosed daily with 4 mg/kg for 56 days. Adverse effects did not occur in horses dosed orally with 1.0 or 1.5 mg/lb. for 15 consecutive days.

Side Effects: During clinical studies, significant side effects were not reported.

Presentation: BANAMINE® Granules, 250 mg are available in 10 g packets, box of 50 and BANAMINE® Granules, 500 mg are available in 20 g packets, box of 25.

Compendium Code No.: 10470170

BANAMINE® INJECTABLE SOLUTION ℞

Schering-Plough **Analgesic-Anti-inflammatory**

(Flunixin meglumine) 50 mg/mL

NADA No.: 101-479

Active Ingredient(s): Each milliliter of BANAMINE® Injectable Solution contains flunixin meglumine equivalent to 50 mg flunixin, 0.1 mg edetate disodium, 2.5 mg sodium formaldehyde sulfoxylate, 4.0 mg diethanolamine, 207.2 mg propylene glycol; 5.0 mg phenol as preservative, hydrochloric acid, water for injection q.s.

Indications:

Horse: BANAMINE® Injectable Solution is recommended for the alleviation of inflammation and pain associated with musculoskeletal disorders in the horse. It is also recommended for the alleviation of visceral pain associated with colic in the horse.

Cattle: BANAMINE® Injectable Solution is indicated for the control of pyrexia associated with bovine respiratory disease and endotoxemia. BANAMINE® Injectable Solution is also indicated for the control of inflammation in endotoxemia.

Pharmacology: Flunixin meglumine is a potent, non-narcotic, non-steroidal, analgesic agent with anti-inflammatory and antipyretic activity. It is significantly more potent than pentazocine, meperidine, and codeine as an analgesic in the rat yeast paw test.

Horse: Flunixin is four times as potent on a mg-per-mg basis as phenylbutazone as measured by the reduction in lameness and swelling in the horse. Plasma half-life in horse serum is 1.6 hours following a single dose of 1.1 mg/kg. Measurable amounts are detectable in horse plasma at 8 hours postinjection.

Cattle: Flunixin meglumine is a weak acid (pKa=5.82) which exhibits a high degree of plasma protein binding (approximately 99%). However, free (unbound) drug appears to readily partition into body issues (V_{SS} predictions range from 297 to 782 mL/kg. Total body water is approximately equal to 570 mL/kg). In cattle, elimination occurs primarily through biliary excretion. This may, at least in part, explain the presence of multiple peaks in the blood concentration/time profile following IV administration.

In healthy cattle, total body clearance has been reported to range from 90 to 151 mL/kg/hr. These studies also report a large discrepancy between the volume of distribution at steady state (V_{SS}) and the volume of distribution associated with the terminal elimination phase (V_{β}). This discrepancy appears to be attributable to extended drug elimination from a deep compartment. The terminal half-life has been shown to vary from 3.14 to 8.12 hours.

Flunixin persists in inflammatory tissues and is associated with anti-inflammatory properties which extend well beyond the period associated with detectable plasma drug concentrations. These observations account for the counterclockwise hysteresis associated with flunixin's pharmacokinetic/pharmacodynamic relationships. Therefore, prediction of drug concentrations based upon the estimated plasma terminal elimination half-life will likely underestimate both the duration of drug action and the concentration of drug remaining at the site of activity.

Dosage and Administration:

Horse: The recommended dose for musculoskeletal disorders is 0.5 mg per pound (1 mL/100 lbs) of body weight once daily. Treatment may be given by intravenous or intramuscular injection and repeated for up to 5 days. Studies show onset of activity is within 2 hours. Peak response occurs between 12 and 16 hours and duration of activity is 24-36 hours.

The recommended dose for the alleviation of pain associated with equine colic is 0.5 mg per pound of body weight. Intravenous administration is recommended for prompt relief. Clinical studies show pain is alleviated in less than 15 minutes in many cases. Treatment may be repeated when signs of colic recur. During clinical studies approximately 10% of the horses required one or two additional treatments. The cause of colic should be determined and treated with concomitant therapy.

Cattle: The recommended dose for cattle is 1.1 to 2.2 mg/kg (0.5 to 1 mg/lb; 1 to 2 mL per 100 lbs) given by slow intravenous administration either once a day as a single dose or divided into two doses administered at 12-hour intervals for up to 3 days. The total daily dose should not exceed 2.2 mg/kg (1.0 mg/lb) of body weight. Avoid rapid intravenous administration of the drug.

Contraindication(s):

Horse: There are not any known contraindications to this drug when used as directed. Intra-arterial injection should be avoided. Horses inadvertently injected intra-arterially can show adverse reactions. Signs can be ataxia, incoordination, hyperventilation, hysteria, and muscle weakness. Signs are transient and disappear without antidotal medication within a few minutes. Do not use in horses showing hypersensitivity to flunixin meglumine.

Cattle: There are no known contraindications to this drug in cattle when used as directed. Do not use in animals showing hypersensitivity to flunixin meglumine. Use judiciously when renal impairment or gastric ulceration are suspected.

Precaution(s): Store between 2° and 30°C (36° and 86°F).

Caution(s): Federal law restricts this drug to use by or on the order of a licensed veterinarian.

As a class, cyclo-oxygenase inhibitory NSAIDs may be associated with gastrointestinal and renal toxicity. Sensitivity to drug-associated adverse effects varies with the individual patient. Patients at greatest risk for renal toxicity are those that are dehydrated, on concomitant diuretic therapy, or those with renal, cardiovascular, and/or hepatic dysfunction.

Since many NSAIDs possess the potential to induce gastrointestinal ulceration, concomitant use of BANAMINE® Injectable Solution with other anti-inflammatory drugs, such as other NSAIDs and corticosteroids, should be avoided or closely monitored.

Horse: The effect of BANAMINE® Injectable Solution on pregnancy has not been determined. Studies to determine the activity of BANAMINE® Injectable Solution when administered concomitantly with other drugs have not been conducted. Drug compatibility should be monitored closely in patients requiring adjunctive therapy.

Cattle: Do not use in bulls intended for breeding, as reproductive effects of BANAMINE® Injectable Solution in these classes of cattle have not been investigated. NSAIDs are known to have potential effects on both parturition and the estrous cycle. There may be a delay in the onset of estrus if flunixin is administered during the prostaglandin phase of the estrous cycle. The effects of flunixin on imminent parturition have not been evaluated in a controlled study. NSAIDs are known to have the potential to delay parturition through a tocolytic effect. Do not exceed the recommended dose.

Warning(s): Cattle must not be slaughtered for human consumption within 4 days of the last treatment. Not for use in lactating or dry dairy cows. A withdrawal period has not been established for this product in preruminating calves. Do not use in calves to be processed for veal. Not for use in horses intended for food.

For intravenous or intramuscular use in horses and for intravenous use in beef and nonlactating dairy cattle only.

Adverse Reactions: In horses, isolated reports of local reactions following intramuscular injection, particularly in the neck, have been received. These include localized swelling, sweating, induration, and stiffness. In rare instances in horses, fatal or nonfatal clostridial infections or other infections have been reported in association with intramuscular use of BANAMINE® Injectable Solution. In horses and cattle, rare instances of anaphylactic-like reactions, some of which have been fatal, have been reported, primarily following intravenous use.

Safety:

Horse: A 3-fold intramuscular dose of 1.5 mg/lb of body weight daily for 10 consecutive days was safe. No changes were observed in hematology, serum chemistry, or urinalysis values. Intravenous dosages of 0.5 mg/lb daily for 15 days; 1.5 mg/lb daily for 10 days; and 2.5 mg/lb daily for 5 days produced no changes in blood or urine parameters. No injection site irritation was observed following intramuscular injection of the 0.5 mg/lb recommended dose. Some irritation was observed following a 3-fold dose administered intramuscularly.

Cattle: No flunixin-related changes (adverse reactions) were noted in cattle administered a 1X (2.2 mg/kg; 1.0 mg/lb) dose for 9 days (three times the maximum clinical duration). Minimal toxicity manifested itself at moderately elevated doses (3X and 5X) when flunixin was administered daily for 9 days, with occasional findings of blood in the feces and/or urine. Discontinue use if hematuria or fecal blood are observed.

References: Available upon request.

Presentation: BANAMINE® Injectable Solution, 50 mg/mL, is available in 50-mL, 100-mL, and 250-mL multi-dose vials.

Compendium Code No.: 10470180

BANAMINE® PASTE ℞

Schering-Plough **Analgesic-Anti-inflammatory**

(Flunixin Meglumine)—1500 mg flunixin/syringe

NADA No.: 137-409

Active Ingredient(s): Each 30 g syringe of BANAMINE® Paste contains flunixin meglumine equivalent to 1500 mg flunixin.

Indications: BANAMINE® Paste is recommended for the alleviation of inflammation and pain associated with musculoskeletal disorders in the horse.

B

Pharmacology: Activity: Flunixin meglumine is a potent non-narcotic, non-steroidal, analgesic agent with anti-inflammatory and anti-pyretic activity. It is significantly more potent than pentazocine, meperidine or codeine as an analgesic in the rat yeast paw test. Oral studies in the horse show the onset of flunixin activity occurs within 2 hours of administration. Peak response occurs between 12 and 16 hours and the duration of activity is 24 to 36 hours.

Dosage and Administration: The recommended dose of flunixin is 0.5 mg per pound of body weight once daily. The BANAMINE® Paste syringe, calibrated in twelve 250-pound weight increments, delivers 125 mg of flunixin for each 250 pounds (see dosage table). One syringe will treat a 1000 pound horse once daily for 3 days, or three 1000 pound horses one time.

Dosage Table:

Syringe Mark*	Horse Weight (lbs)	BANAMINE® Paste Delivered (g)	Mg Flunixin Delivered
0	—	—	—
250	250	2.5	125
500	500	5.0	250
750	750	7.5	375
1000	1000	10.0	500

* Use dial edge nearest syringe barrel to mark dose.

The paste is orally administered by inserting the nozzle of the syringe through the interdental space, and depositing the required amount of paste on the back of the tongue by depressing the plunger.

Treatment may be given initially by intravenous or intramuscular injection of BANAMINE® Solution, followed by BANAMINE® Granules or BANAMINE® Paste on days 2-5. BANAMINE® treatment should not exceed 5 consecutive days.

Contraindication(s): There are no known contraindications to this drug when used as directed.

Precaution(s): Store between 2° and 30°C (36° and 86°F).

Caution(s): Federal law restricts this drug to use by or on the order of a licensed veterinarian.

The effect of BANAMINE® on pregnancy has not been determined. Studies to date show that there is no detrimental effect on stallion spermatogenesis with or following the recommended dose of BANAMINE® Paste. For oral use in horses only.

Warning(s): Not for use in horses intended for food.

Toxicology: No toxic effects were observed in rats given oral flunixin 2 mg/kg per day for 42 days. Higher doses produced ulceration of the gastrointestinal tract. The emetic dose in dogs is between 150 and 250 mg/kg. Flunixin was well tolerated in monkeys dosed daily with 4 mg/kg for 56 days. No adverse effects occurred in horses dosed orally with 1.0 or 1.5 mg/lb. for 5 consecutive days.

Side Effects: During field studies with BANAMINE® Paste, no significant side effects were reported.

Presentation: 30 g syringes, box of six.

Compendium Code No.: 10470191 13407339 Jan. 1999

BANDGUARD® CREAM 2%

Schering-Plough **Bandage Protectant**

Active Ingredient(s): Contains: Diphemanil methylsulfate.

Indications: An unpleasant-tasting preparation for application on bandages, casts, tape, and other wound dressings to deter self-mutilation.

Dosage and Administration: Apply BANDGUARD® Cream directly on bandages, casts, tape, and other wound dressings to deter self-mutilation.

Precaution(s): Store between 2-30°C (36-89°F).

Caution(s): For veterinary use only.

Warning(s): Not for use on skin or wound surfaces.

Presentation: 20 g tubes (boxes of 12) and 50 g tubes.

Compendium Code No.: 10470200

BANDGUARD® SPRAY

Schering-Plough **Bandage Protectant**

Active Ingredient(s): Contains: Dephemanil methylsulfate (an anticholinergic).

Indications: An unpleasant tasting preparation for application on bandages, casts, tape and other wound dressing to deter self-mutilation. Not approved for use on skin or wound surfaces.

Dosage and Administration: Hold bottle 6-8 inches away from dressing and spray until slightly wet. Use as needed.

Precaution(s): Store between 2-30°C (36-86°F).

Presentation: Carton of 12 x 2 fl. oz. plastic spray bottles.

Compendium Code No.: 10470210

BANMINTH® 48

Phibro **Feed Medication**

Pyrantel tartrate (anthelmintic)-Type A Medicated Article

NADA No.: 043-290

Active Ingredient(s):

Pyrantel Tartrate . . . . 10.6% (48 grams per pound)

Indications: For the removal and control of large roundworm *(Ascaris suum)* and nodular worm *(Oesophagostomum)* infections of swine.

Aid in the prevention of migration and establishment of large roundworm *(Ascaris suum)* infections; aid in the prevention of establishment of nodular worm *(Oesophagostomum)* infections of swine.

For the removal and control of large roundworm *(Ascaris suum)* infections of swine.

Directions:

Mixing and Use Directions: Complete swine feeds containing 0.0881% (800 g/t) pyrantel tartrate:

Amount of BANMINTH® 48 Per Ton of Complete Feed	Resultant Use Level of Pyrantel Tartrate in Complete Feed	Indications for Use
16.67 lb	0.0881% (800 g/t)	For the removal and control of large roundworm *(Ascaris suum)* and nodular worm *(Oesophagostomum)* infections of swine.†

Directions for Use: As a single therapeutic treatment in complete feed; feed at the rate of 1 lb of feed per 40 lb of body weight for animals up to 200 lb. For animals 200 lb or over, feed 5 lb of feed per head. Quantity of medicated feed required to treat pigs of various body weight is shown below:

Pig Weight (lb)	Quantity of Feed Per Pig
20	½ lb
40	1 lb
60	1½ lb
80	2 lb
100	2½ lb
200 and over	5 lb

Fast pigs overnight for optimum results. Pigs will generally consume this quantity of medicated feed within a few hours time after which regular feeding should be resumed. Better worming is achieved when pigs are separated by size into different lots or pens for treatment. Water should be made available to animals during fasting and treatment periods.

Complete swine feeds containing 0.0106% (96 g/t) pyrantel tartrate:

Amount of BANMINTH® 48 Per Ton of Complete Feed	Resultant Use Level of Pyrantel Tartrate in Complete Feed	Indications for Use	Directions for Use
2 lb	0.0106% (96 g/t)	Aid in the prevention of migration and establishment of large roundworm *(Ascaris suum)* infections; aid in the prevention of establishment of nodular worm *(Oesophagostomum)* infections of swine.	Feed continuously as the sole ration.
2 lb	0.0106% (96 g/t)	For the removal and control of large roundworm *(Ascaris suum)* infections of swine.†	Feed for 3 days as the sole ration.

Swine protein supplements for further dilution to feed containing 0.0106% (96 g/t) pyrantel tartrate:

Amount of BANMINTH® 48 Per Ton of Protein Supplement*	Indications for Use	Directions for Use
To calculate the amount of BANMINTH® 48 per ton of protein supplement, divide 4,000 by the quantity (lb) of protein supplement that will be mixed with grain(s) to produce a ton of complete feed, that is: 4,000 ÷ X = pounds of BANMINTH® 48 per ton of protein supplement. where X = quantity (lb) of protein supplement that will be mixed with grain(s) to produce a ton of complete feed. Example Calculation: Directions for use of the protein supplement require that 500 pounds are to be mixed with grain(s) to produce a ton of complete feed. 4,000 ÷ 500 = 8 pounds of BANMINTH® 48 per ton of protein supplement.	Aid in the prevention of migration and establishment of large roundworm *(Ascaris suum)* infections; aid in the prevention of establishment of nodular worm *(Oesophagostomum)* infections of swine.	Prepare a complete feed by mixing proper quantities of protein supplement with grain(s). If pelleted, grind pellets before or during mixing. The resultant complete feed contains 0.0106% (96 g/t) pyrantel tartrate and is to be fed continuously as the sole ration.
	For the removal and control of large roundworm *(Ascaris suum)* infections of swine.†	Prepare a complete feed by mixing proper quantities of protein supplement with grain(s). If pelleted, grind pellets before or during mixing. The resultant complete feed contains 0.0106% (96 g/t) pyrantel tartrate and is to be fed for 3 days as the sole ration.

Swine protein supplements for further dilution to feed containing 0.0881% (800 g/t) pyrantel tartrate:

Amount of BANMINTH® 48 Per Ton of Protein Supplement*	Indications for Use	Directions for Use
To calculate the amount of BANMINTH® 48 per ton of protein supplement, divide 33,333 by the quantity (lb) of protein supplement that will be mixed with grain(s) to produce a ton of complete feed, that is: 33,333 ÷ X = pounds of BANMINTH® 48 per ton of protein supplement. where X = quantity (lb) of protein supplement that will be mixed with grain(s) to produce a ton of complete feed. Example Calculation: Directions for use of the protein supplement require that 333 pounds are to be mixed with grain(s) to produce a ton of complete feed. 33,333 ÷ 333 = 100 pounds of BANMINTH® 48 per ton of protein supplement.	For the removal and control of large roundworm *(Ascaris suum)* and nodular worm *(Oesophagostomum)* infections of swine.†	Prepare a complete feed by mixing proper quantities of protein supplement with grain(s). If pelleted, grind pellets before or during mixing. The resultant complete feed contains 0.0881% (800 g/t) pyrantel tartrate and is to be fed as a single therapeutic treatment at the rate of 1 lb of feed per 40 lb of body weight for animals up to 200 lb. For animals 200 lb or over, feed 5 lb of feed per head. Fast pigs overnight for optimum results. Pigs will generally consume this quantity of medicated feed within a few hours time, after which regular feeding should be resumed. Better worming is achieved when pigs are separated by size into different lots or pens for treatment. Water should be made available to animals during fasting and treatment periods.

*To find grams of pyrantel tartrate, multiply pounds of Banminth by forty-eight (48).

†Consult your veterinarian for assistance in the diagnosis, treatment and control of parasitism.

Precaution(s): Store in a dry, cool place.

Caution(s): For use in the manufacture of complete swine feeds and/or swine protein supplement feeds only.

Consult your veterinarian before using in severely debilitated animals. Do not mix in feeds containing bentonite.

Warning(s): Withdraw 24 hours prior to slaughter.

Certain components of animal feeds, including medicated premixes, possess properties that may be a potential health hazard or a source of personal discomfort to certain individuals who are exposed to them. Human exposure should, therefore, be minimized by observing the general industry standards for occupational health and safety.

Precautions such as the following should be considered: dust masks or respirators and protective clothing should be worn; dust-arresting equipment and adequate ventilation should be utilized; personal hygiene should be observed; wash before eating or leaving a work site; be alert for signs of allergic reactions—seek prompt medical treatment if such reactions are suspected.

Presentation: 50 lb (22.6 kg) bags.

BANMINTH is a registered trademark of Phibro Animal Health, for pyrantel tartrate.

U.S. Patent No. 3,549,624

Compendium Code No.: 36930011

BANSECT® FLEA AND TICK COLLAR FOR CATS

Sergeant's **Parasiticide Collar**

EPA Reg. No.: 2517-44

Active Ingredient(s):

Naled (1,2-dibromo-2,2-dichloroethyl dimethyl phosphate) 10%
Other Ingredients: 90%

Indications: This collar kills all types of fleas common to cats, and should be worn continuously to help reduce flea infestations.

It kills fleas for up to 120 days and aids in tick control for up to 30 days.

This product is fast acting and unaffected by water.

It also kills the ticks that carry Lyme Disease.

Directions for Use: It is a violation of Federal Law to use this product in a manner inconsistent with its labeling. Read entire label before each use.

Buckle collar securely but not tightly around cat's neck. Collar should be worn loosely. Cut off and dispose of excess length in trash. Collar will start killing fleas on cat immediately. New fleas temporarily appearing will be killed during four months collar is worn. When bathing cat, remove collar until cat is dry. Replace every four months. This collar kills ticks more slowly, but ticks will usually be dead in one to five days. Although ticks are only an occasional problem on cats, collar will continue to aid in tick control for thirty days. Dead ticks occasionally remaining in cat's coat are easily detached. For best results, remove hard-to-kill ticks inside ears when collar is put on.

Contraindication(s): Do not use on cats under 12 weeks. Do not use this product on animals simultaneously or within 30 days before or after treatment with or exposure to cholinesterase inhibiting drugs, pesticides or chemicals.

Precautionary Statements:

Hazards to Humans and Domestic Animals: Caution: Do not open inner envelope until ready to use. Collar is intended for use only as an insecticide generator and is not to be taken internally by man or animals. Even with the BANSECT® Collar, some cats may be sensitive and may develop neck irritation and loss of hair under the collar. When Collar is first worn, observe neck area for irritation every few days. Sensitivities may occur after using any pesticide product for pets. If signs of sensitivity occur remove collar and bathe your pet with mild soap and rinse with large amounts of water. If signs continue, consult a veterinarian immediately. Consult a veterinarian before using this product on debilitated, aged, pregnant, medicated or nursing animals.

Flea and tick collars may be immediately replaced.

Use only on cats.

In case of emergency, call: 1-800-224-PETS.

Storage and Disposal:

Storage: Store only in original container, in a cool dry place inaccessible to children and pets.

Disposal: Discard in the trash the empty pouch, the expired collar and any trimmed excess collar.

Warning(s): Do not allow children to play with collar.

Presentation: 0.5 oz (14 g) collar.

Patent No. 3,918,407

Compendium Code No.: 10830070 OVD KCO6851

BANSECT® FLEA AND TICK COLLAR FOR DOGS

Sergeant's **Parasiticide Collar**

EPA Reg. No.: 2517-43

Active Ingredient(s):

Naled (1,2-dibromo-2,2-dichloroethyl dimethyl phosphate) 15%
Other Ingredients: 85%

Indications: This collar kills all types of fleas common to dogs, and should be worn continuously to help reduce flea infestations.

It kills fleas for up to 120 days and aids in tick control for up to 30 days.

This product is fast acting and unaffected by water.

It also kills the ticks that carry Lyme Disease.

Directions for Use: It is a violation of Federal Law to use this product in a manner inconsistent with its labeling.

Read entire label before each use.

Buckle collar securely but not tightly around dog's neck. Collar should be worn loosely. Cut off and dispose of excess length in trash. Collar will start killing fleas on dog immediately. New fleas temporarily appearing will be killed during four months collar is worn. When bathing dog, remove collar until dog is dry. Replace every four months. This collar kills ticks more slowly, but ticks will usually be dead in one to five days. Collar will continue to aid in tick control for thirty days, killing American Dog Tick and even Rocky Mountain Wood Tick, carrier of Rocky Mountain Spotted Fever. Dead ticks occasionally remaining in dog's coat are easily detached. For best results, remove hard-to-kill ticks inside ears when collar is put on.

Contraindication(s): Do not use on cats.

Do not use on puppies under 12 weeks. Do not use this product on animals simultaneously or within 30 days before or after treatment with or exposure to cholinesterase inhibiting drugs, pesticides or chemicals.

Precautionary Statements:

Hazards to Humans and Domestic Animals: Caution: Do not open inner envelope until ready to use. Collar is intended for use only as an insecticide generator and is not to be taken internally by man or animals. Even with the BANSECT® Collar, some dogs may be sensitive and may develop neck irritation and loss of hair under the collar. When collar is first worn, observe neck area for irritation every few days. Sensitivities may occur after using any pesticide product for pets. If signs of sensitivity occur remove collar and bathe your pet with mild soap and rinse with large amounts of water. If signs continue, consult a veterinarian immediately. Consult a veterinarian before using this product on debilitated, aged, pregnant, medicated or nursing animals.

Flea and tick collars may be immediately replaced.

Use only on dogs.

In case of emergency, call: 1-800-224-PETS.

Storage and Disposal:

Storage: Store only in original container, in a cool dry place inaccessible to children and pets.

Disposal: Discard in the trash the empty pouch, the expired collar and any trimmed excess collar.

Warning(s): Do not allow children to play with collar.

Presentation: 0.9 oz (25 g) collar.

Patent No. 3,918,407

Compendium Code No.: 10830080 CVD 995555P

BANSECT® SQUEEZE-ON FLEA AND TICK CONTROL FOR DOGS (UNDER 33 LBS)

Sergeant's **Parasiticide-Topical**

EPA Reg. No.: 270-279-2517

Active Ingredient(s):

*Permethrin: 45.0%
Other Ingredients: 55.0%
Total 100.0%

*(3-phenoxyphenyl) methyl (±)-cis, trans-3-(2,2-dichloroethenyl)-2,2-dimethylcyclopropane-carboxylate

cis/trans ratio: Max 55% (±) cis and min 45% (±) trans

Indications: BANSECT® Squeeze-On Flea and Tick Control for Dogs is an effective and easy to use product. BANSECT® Squeeze-On Flea and Tick Control for Dogs has demonstrated greater than 92% control of fleas within one day of application. As with all flea and tick control products, BANSECT® Squeeze-On should be used as part of a program aimed at reducing flea populations in the dog's environment (bedding, carpets, kennel, yard). Consult your veterinarian, entomologist or retailer for program recommendations.

Kills adult fleas for up to 30 days.

Use only on dogs over 6 months of age.

Directions for Use: It is a violation of Federal law to use this product in a manner inconsistent with its labelling.

Read entire label before each use.

Do not get this product in your dog's eyes or mouth. Repeat applications may be made if necessary, but don't apply more often than once every 3 weeks, except to reapply after shampooing the dog.

For Dogs Weighing Less Than 33 Pounds: Apply one tube (1.5 mL) of BANSECT® Squeeze-On Flea and Tick Control solution as a spot between the shoulder blades or as a stripe to the dog's back.

How To Apply: Remove product tube from package. Holding tube with notched end pointing up and away from face and body, cut off narrow end at notches. Invert tube over dog and use open end to part dog's hair. Squeeze tube firmly to apply all of the solution to the dog's skin. Wrap tube and put in trash.

Contraindication(s): Do not use on cats or animals other than dogs.

Do not use on dogs less than 6 months of age.

Certain medications can interact with pesticides. It is advisable to consult a veterinarian before using this product with any other pesticide or drug.

Precautionary Statements: Hazards to Humans and Domestic Animals: Caution:

Hazards to Humans: Harmful if swallowed. Avoid contact with eyes or clothing. Causes moderate eye irritation. Wash thoroughly with soap and water after handling.

Hazards to Domestic Animals: For external use on dogs only. Consult a veterinarian before using this product on debilitated, aged, medicated, pregnant, or nursing dogs. Consult a veterinarian before using on dogs with known organ dysfunction. Cats which actively groom or engage in close physical contact with recently treated dogs may be at risk of toxic exposure.

First Aid:

If Swallowed: Call a physician or Poison Control Center. Drink 1 or 2 glasses of water and induce vomiting by touching back of throat with finger or, if available, by administration of syrup of Ipecac. Do not induce vomiting or give anything by mouth to an unconscious person.

If In Eyes: Flush eyes with plenty of water. Call a physician if irritation persists.

Adverse Reactions: Some animals may be sensitive to ingredients in this product. Reactions in dogs may include skin sensitivity. Dogs may show lethargy, increased pruritus (itchiness), erythema (redness), rash and hair discoloration or hair loss at the applications site. Observe the dog following treatment. Sensitivity may occur after using any pesticide product on pets. If signs of sensitivity occur, bathe your dog with a mild, non-insecticidal shampoo and rinse with large amounts of water. If signs continue, consult a veterinarian immediately.

Environmental Hazards: This product is extremely toxic to fish. Do not add directly to water. Do not contaminate water when disposing of product or packaging.

Physical or Chemical Hazards: Do not use or store near heat or open flames.

In case of emergency, call: 1-800-228-5635 ext. 233.

Storage and Disposal: Do not contaminate water, food or feed by storage or disposal.

Storage: Store in a cool, dry place. Protect from freezing.

Pesticide Disposal: Securely wrap original container in several layers of newspaper and discard in trash.

Container Disposal: Do not reuse empty container. Wrap container and put in trash.

Warning(s): Keep out of reach of children.

Presentation: Three 1.5 mL applicators (0.1 fl oz) (3 month supply).

Compendium Code No.: 10830120 RIVD P002105

BANSECT® SQUEEZE-ON FLEA AND TICK CONTROL FOR DOGS (OVER 33 LBS)

Sergeant's **Parasiticide-Topical**

EPA Reg. No.: 270-279-2517

Active Ingredient(s):

*Permethrin: 45.0%
Other Ingredients: 55.0%
Total 100.0%

*(3-phenoxyphenyl) methyl (±)-cis, trans-3-(2,2-dichloroethenyl)-2,2-dimethylcyclopropane-carboxylate

cis/trans ratio: Max 55% (±) cis and min 45% (±) trans

Indications: BANSECT® Squeeze-On Flea and Tick Control for Dogs is an effective and easy to use product. BANSECT® Squeeze-On Flea and Tick Control for Dogs has demonstrated greater than 92% control of fleas within one day of application. As with all flea and tick control products, BANSECT® Squeeze-On should be used as part of a program aimed at reducing flea populations in the dog's environment (bedding, carpets, kennel, yard). Consult your veterinarian, entomologist or retailer for program recommendations.

Kills adult fleas for up to 30 days.

Use only on dogs over 6 months of age.

Directions for Use: It is a violation of Federal law to use this product in a manner inconsistent with its labelling.

Read entire label before each use.

Do not get this product in your dog's eyes or mouth. Repeat applications may be made if necessary, but don't apply more often than once every 3 weeks, except to reapply after shampooing the dog.

For Dogs Weighing More Than 33 Pounds: Apply approximately half of the tube (1.5 mL) of BANSECT® Squeeze-On Flea and Tick Control solution as a spot or stripe to the dog's back between the shoulder blades and apply the rest of the tube's contents (1.5 mL) as a spot or stripe to the dog's back directly in front of the base of the tail. Or, apply the entire tube (3.0 mL) as a continuous stripe on the dog's back starting between the shoulder blades and ending directly in front of the base of the tail.

How To Apply: Remove product tube from package. Holding tube with notched end pointing up and away from face and body, cut off narrow end at notches. Invert tube over dog and use open end to part dog's hair. Squeeze tube firmly to apply all of the solution to the dog's skin. Wrap tube and put in trash.

Contraindication(s): Do not use on cats or animals other than dogs.

Do not use on dogs less than 6 months of age.

Certain medications can interact with pesticides. It is advisable to consult a veterinarian before using this product with any other pesticide or drug.

Precautionary Statements: Hazards to Humans and Domestic Animals: Caution:

Hazards to Humans: Harmful if swallowed. Avoid contact with eyes or clothing. Causes moderate eye irritation. Wash thoroughly with soap and water after handling.

Hazards to Domestic Animals: For external use on dogs only. Consult a veterinarian before using this product on debilitated, aged, medicated, pregnant, or nursing dogs. Consult a veterinarian before using on dogs with known organ dysfunction. Cats which actively groom or engage in close physical contact with recently treated dogs may be at risk of toxic exposure.

First Aid:

If Swallowed: Call a physician or Poison Control Center. Drink 1 or 2 glasses of water and induce vomiting by touching back of throat with finger or, if available, by administration of syrup of Ipecac. Do not induce vomiting or give anything by mouth to an unconscious person.

If In Eyes: Flush eyes with plenty of water. Call a physician if irritation persists.

Adverse Reactions: Some animals may be sensitive to ingredients in this product. Reactions in dogs may include skin sensitivity. Dogs may show lethargy, increased pruritus (itchiness), erythema (redness), rash and hair discoloration or hair loss at the applications site. Observe the dog following treatment. Sensitivity may occur after using any pesticide product on pets. If signs of sensitivity occur, bathe your dog with a mild, non-insecticidal shampoo and rinse with large amounts of water. If signs continue, consult a veterinarian immediately.

Environmental Hazards: This product is extremely toxic to fish. Do not add directly to water. Do not contaminate water when disposing of product or packaging.

Physical or Chemical Hazards: Do not use or store near heat or open flames.

In case of emergency, call: 1-800-228-5635 ext. 233.

Storage and Disposal: Do not contaminate water, food or feed by storage or disposal.

Storage: Store in a cool, dry place. Protect from freezing.

Pesticide Disposal: Securely wrap original container in several layers of newspaper and discard in trash.

Container Disposal: Do not reuse empty container. Wrap container and put in trash.

Warning(s): Keep out of reach of children.

Presentation: Three 3.0 mL applicators (0.207 fl oz) (3 month supply).

Compendium Code No.: 10830130 RIVD P002106

BAPTEN® FOR INJECTION ℞

PR Pharmaceuticals **Lysyl Oxidase Inhibitor**

beta-aminopropionitrile fumarate

NADA No.: 141-107

Active Ingredient(s): Each package contains BAPTEN® as a sterile lyophilized powder accompanied by a vial of sterile saline diluent. Each vial contains 7.0 mg of sterile beta-aminopropionitrile fumarate (BAPTEN®) powder. Following reconstitution with 10 mL of sterile saline diluent, each vial contains 0.7 mg/mL of BAPTEN®. The lyophilized powder dissolves rapidly for immediate treatment.

Indications: For treatment of tendinitis of the superficial digital flexor tendon (SDFT) in the adult horse where there is sonographic evidence of fiber tearing.

Pharmacology: Mechanism of Action: BAPTEN® is a specific inhibitor of the enzyme, lysyl oxidase, involved in the polymerization/crosslinking of individual collagen fibrils.[1,2]

BAPTEN® inhibits the crosslinking of new collagen fibers that form as a result of injury to the tendon. Temporary inhibition of random collagen crosslinking, followed by conservative exercise, theoretically allows the subsequent formation of physiologically aligned crosslinked collagen fibers. Although collagen synthesis proceeds at the same rate and the healing process is not shortened by the use of BAPTEN®, the remodeled tendon should be stronger. Due to BAPTEN®'s inhibition of collagen crosslinking, tendon lesions could worsen if exercise recommendations are exceeded and lesion status is not monitored by ultrasound.

Dosage and Administration: Each reconstituted vial contains 7 mg of BAPTEN® in a volume of 10 mL. BAPTEN® should be injected intralesionally every other day for 5 treatments. The volume injected will vary with the size of the lesion.

B

Following lesion evaluation using diagnostic ultrasound (DUS), begin treatment approximately 30 days after the initial tendon injury. Sedation and restraint is essential during injections to avoid injury to both horse and handlers. Hair over the affected tendon should be clipped; care should be taken to avoid irritating or damaging the skin. The area should be aseptically prepared for injection.

BAPTEN® is administered at 0.2 mL per site into multiple sites of the sonographically defined lesion at 1.5 cm intervals beginning 1.5 cm distal to the lesion and continuing 1.5 cm proximal to the lesion. Injections are placed medially, laterally and on the palmar surface of the tendon at each level, directly into the tendon to a maximum of 10 mL (up to 50 injections per treatment).

The use of a small gauge (27x½"-1") needle is recommended. Injections should be made with the horse in a weight bearing position. This helps discriminate between uninjured tendon (difficult to penetrate with needle) and the lesion area (easier to penetrate with needle).

The entire procedure, to a maximum of 7 mg = 10 mL is repeated every other day for a series of five treatments.

The contents of each reconstituted vial must be used immediately or discarded.

Diagnostic Ultrasound (DUS) and Conservative Exercise: Sonographic monitoring is essential for the management of BAPTEN® treated tendon injuries. DUS is used to diagnose the extent of the lesion and provide guidance for the intralesional injections during the treatment period.

Stall rest is recommended during the injection treatment period. DUS also determines the progressive level of exercise for each horse. Using the pretreatment sonographic evaluation to establish a baseline, subsequent advances in exercise (tendon loading) should be preceded by decreases in lesion cross-sectional area (CSA), and improved echogenicity and fiber alignment. Clinical evaluation alone (lameness, pain on palpation, heat, swelling) cannot safely determine the progression of exercise.

Avoid advancing exercise beyond walking unless diagnostic ultrasound shows decreased total tendon cross-sectional area, and improved echogenicity and fiber alignment. Immediately return to lower exercise level when these criteria are not met at new loading levels.

It is recommended that horses be handwalked for 30-45 minutes during the first four months following BAPTEN® treatment. During the clinical study conducted in the field, 70% of the 27 tendon lesions that increased in size by the end of the 16 week study had had their exercise levels increased without the necessary concomitant decrease in tendon CSA. Only 15% of the 52 improved tendons broke the exercise recommendations during that time. Clients should be informed that clinical evidence of increased lameness, heat, or swelling warrants immediate cessation of exercise, veterinary examination, and DUS evaluation.

Successful DUS parameters at 16 weeks do not preclude the susceptibility of the tendon to reinjury when subjected to an inappropriate rehabilitation program. Each horse should be individually monitored and conservatively exercised for 10 months or longer.

Contraindication(s): Do not use in horses with dermal irritation or open skin lesions in the injection area. Do not administer intraarticularly, into the tendon sheath, or in the presence of concurrent limb fractures.

Precaution(s): Store at controlled room temperature 15-30°C (59-86°F).

Caution(s): Federal law restricts this drug to use by or on the order of a licensed veterinarian.

Not for use in humans. Keep out of reach of children.

May cause irritation to skin, eyes or mucous membranes. Avoid accidental injection. In case of accidental exposure to skin, wash with plenty of soap and water. In case of contact with eyes, flush immediately with plenty of water. Seek medical attention if irritation becomes severe or persists.

The material safety data sheet (MSDS) contains more detailed occupational safety information.

To report adverse effects in users or to obtain a copy of the MSDS 1-888-484-9249.

Concomitant medication: Do not use any irritants or penetrating substances on the affected area for 10 days prior to, or for 8 weeks after BAPTEN® injection. Steroids are not recommended during this period since they may decrease the production of collagen.

Breeding animals: Do not use in breeding animals since the effects of BAPTEN® on fertility, pregnancy, or fetal health have not been determined.

Return to function: The safety and efficacy of BAPTEN® have been determined in clinical studies conducted over a 4 month period. The ultimate evaluation of tendon healing based on the return to successful performance remains undetermined.

For intratendinous injection in the horse.

Warning(s): Not to be used in horses intended for food.

Adverse Reactions: Increased swelling, heat, pain on palpation, and occasional lameness are commonly observed during and after the BAPTEN® treatment period. Inflammation is due to the injection procedure as well as BAPTEN®. Most reactions are transient and subside within 2 weeks; some may persist for as long as four months. When excessive swelling or lameness occurs after a BAPTEN® injection, it may be necessary to delay subsequent injections and treat the inflammation.

Information regarding reactions during the BAPTEN® injection period are based on data from nearly 200 horses that took part in clinical studies. During the BAPTEN® clinical studies, 2 horses experienced severe adverse reactions subsequent to BAPTEN® injections, resulting in chronic peritendinous and tendinous inflammation.

During the studies, no infections occurred secondary to BAPTEN® injections.

Trial Data: Evaluation of Efficacy: In the BAPTEN® studies, tendon remodeling was evaluated using the following diagnostic ultrasound (DUS) measurements: tendon cross-sectional area (CSA), echogenicity of the lesion, and parallelism of newly formed collagen fiber bundles (fiber alignment). The percent change in CSA for the total tendon, the total injured zone, and the maximum injured zone were evaluated over a four month period. Following initial BAPTEN® injections, a low level exercise regimen was initiated during the four month study period. Increases in exercise were scheduled to occur only after improvement in ultrasound parameters.

References: Available upon request.

Presentation: Each package contains five vials of sterile lyophilized BAPTEN® powder (10 mL) and five vials of sterile saline diluent for reconstitution. The entire package constitutes one course of five treatments.

BAPTEN® is a registered trademark licensed to PR Pharmaceuticals, Inc.

Compendium Code No.: 10570000

BAR-GUARD-99™

Boehringer Ingelheim **Antiserum**

Escherichia Coli Antibody, Equine Origin

U.S. Vet. Lic. No.: 124

Composition: BAR-GUARD-99™ is prepared from the blood of horses hyperimmunized with a whole culture of *Escherichia coli,* 0101:K30:K99, containing the K99 pilus antigen. Contains cresol as a preservative.

Indications: Uses: BAR-GUARD-99™ is recommended for the prevention of colibacillosis caused by K99 strains of *Escherichia coli* in neonatal calves and lambs. It is also effective when administered in the early stages of infection characterized by milk diarrhea but no dehydration or depression.

Directions: Colostrum should be fed to the animal prior to administration of BAR-GUARD-99™ antibody product.

Dosage:

Calves: Using aseptic technique, administer 10 mL orally as soon as possible after birth. For optimal results BAR-GUARD-99™ should be administered within 12 hours after birth and preferably within 6 hours of birth. BAR-GUARD-99™ may also be administered within 8 hours of exposure, not to exceed 20 hours of age.

Lambs: Using aseptic technique, administer 2 mL orally as soon as possible after birth. BAR-GUARD-99™ should be administered within 12 hours after birth and preferably within 6 hours of birth.

Precaution(s): Store out of direct sunlight at a temperature between 35°-45°F (2°-7°C). Avoid freezing. Shake well and use immediately.

Caution(s): For oral use only. The efficacy of BAR-GUARD-99™ may be reduced if administered to calves showing signs of severe diarrhea, mild dehydration and depression. The product is not effective against diarrhea caused by infectious agents other than K99 strains of *E. coli.* As a good management practice, colostrum should be administered to calves and lambs as soon as possible after birth. Anaphylactoid reactions may occur.

Antidote(s): Epinephrine.

Warning(s): Do not administer within 21 day of slaughter.

Presentation: 1 dose (10 mL) syringe and 5 dose (50 mL) vials.

Compendium Code No.: 10280121 BI 1081-1 4/00

BAR SOMNUS™

Boehringer Ingelheim **Bacterin**

Haemophilus Somnus Bacterin

U.S. Vet. Lic. No.: 124

Composition: Contains inactivated cultures of *Haemophilus somnus.*

Preservative: Neomycin.

Indications: Recommended for the vaccination of healthy susceptible cattle, as an aid in the reduction of disease caused by *Haemophilus somnus.*

Dosage and Administration: Using aseptic technique, inject 2 mL subcutaneously. Repeat in 21 days and once annually. Calves vaccinated before 6 months of age should be revaccinated at 6 months of age.

Precaution(s): Store out of direct sunlight at a temperature between 35-45°F (2-7°C). Avoid freezing. Shake well before using. Use entire contents when first opened.

Caution(s): Anaphylactoid reactions may occur.

Antidote(s): Epinephrine.

Warning(s): Do not vaccinate within 21 days before slaughter.

Presentation: 10 dose (20 mL) and 50 dose (100 mL) vials.

Compendium Code No.: 10280081 15001-03 / 15002-03

BAR SOMNUS 2P™

Boehringer Ingelheim **Bacterin**

Haemophilus Somnus-Pasteurella Haemolytica-Multocida Bacterin

U.S. Vet. Lic. No.: 124

Composition: Chemically inactivated aluminum hydroxide adsorbed whole cultures of the organisms listed. Contains neomycin as a preservative.

Indications: Recommended for the vaccination of healthy susceptible cattle against diseases caused by *Haemophilus somnus, Pasteurella haemolytica* and *Pasteurella multocida.*

Dosage and Administration: Using aseptic technique, inject 2 mL intramuscularly in healthy cattle of any age. Repeat in 21 days and once annually. Calves vaccinated before six months of age should be revaccinated after 6 months of age.

Precaution(s): Store out of direct sunlight at a temperature between 35-45°F (2-7°C). Avoid freezing. Shake well before using. Use entire contents when first opened.

Caution(s): Anaphylactic reactions may occur.

Antidote(s): Epinephrine.

Warning(s): Do not vaccinate within 21 days before slaughter.

Presentation: 10 doses (20 mL) and 50 doses (100 mL).

Compendium Code No.: 10280071 15607-00 / 15602-02

BAR-VAC® 7

Boehringer Ingelheim **Bacterin-Toxoid**

Clostridium Chauvoei-Septicum-Novyi-Sordellii-Perfringens Types C & D Bacterin-Toxoid

U.S. Vet. Lic. No.: 124

Composition: Prepared from cultures of the organisms listed. Alum precipitated.

Indications: Recommended for the vaccination of healthy, susceptible cattle and sheep against disease caused by *Clostridium chauvoei, Cl. septicum, Cl. novyi, Cl. sordellii* and *Cl. perfringens* Types C and D. Although *Clostridium perfringens* Type B is not a significant problem in the U.S.A., immunity may be provided against the beta and epsilon toxins elaborated by *Clostridium perfringens* Type B. This immunity is derived from the combination of Type C (beta) and Type D (epsilon) fractions.

Dosage and Administration:

Cattle: Using aseptic technique, inject 5 mL subcutaneously. Repeat in 21 to 28 days and once annually.

Sheep: Using aseptic technique, inject 2.5 mL subcutaneously. Repeat in 21 to 28 days and once annually.

Precaution(s): Store out of direct sunlight at a temperature between 35-45°F (2-7°). Avoid freezing. Shake well before using. Use entire contents when first opened.

Caution(s): Anaphylactoid reactions may occur.

Antidote(s): Administer epinephrine.

Warning(s): Do not vaccinate within 21 days before slaughter.

Animal inoculation only.

Presentation: 10 cattle doses or 20 sheep doses (50 mL), 50 cattle doses or 100 sheep doses (250 mL), and 200 cattle doses or 400 sheep doses (1000 mL).

Compendium Code No.: 10280141 13301-01 / 13302-04 / 13303-04

BAR VAC® 7/SOMNUS

Boehringer Ingelheim **Bacterin-Toxoid**

Clostridium Chauvoei-Septicum-Novyi-Sordellii-Perfringens Types C & D-Haemophilus Somnus Bacterin-Toxoid

U.S. Vet. Lic. No.: 124

Composition: Prepared from cultures of the organisms listed. Alum precipitated.

Indications: Recommended for the vaccination of healthy, susceptible cattle against diseases caused by *Clostridium chauvoei, Cl. septicum, Cl. novyi, Cl. sordellii, Cl. perfringens* Types C and D and *Haemophilus somnus.* Although *Clostridium perfringens* Type B is not a significant problem in the U.S.A., immunity may be provided against the beta and epsilon toxins elaborated by *Clostridium perfringens* Type B. This immunity is derived from the combination of Type C (beta) and Type D (epsilon) fractions.

Dosage and Administration: Using aseptic technique, inject 5 mL subcutaneously. Repeat in 21 to 28 days and once annually.

Precaution(s): Store out of direct sunlight at a temperature between 35-45°F (2-7°). Avoid freezing. Shake well before using. Use entire contents when first opened.

Caution(s): Transient swelling at the injection site may occur. Anaphylactoid reactions may occur.

Antidote(s): Administer epinephrine.

Warning(s): Do not vaccinate within 21 days before slaughter.

Presentation: 10 doses (50 mL), 50 doses (250 mL), and 200 doses (500 mL).

Compendium Code No.: 10280091 18701-03 / 18702-03 / 18703-03

BAR-VAC® 8

Boehringer Ingelheim **Bacterin-Toxoid**

Clostridium Chauvoei-Septicum-Haemolyticum-Novyi-Sordellii-Perfringens Types C & D Bacterin-Toxoid

U.S. Vet. Lic. No.: 124

Composition: Prepared from cultures of the organisms listed. Alum precipitated.

Indications: Recommended for the vaccination of healthy, susceptible cattle and sheep against diseases caused by *Clostridium chauvoei, Cl. septicum, Cl. haemolyticum, Cl. novyi, Cl. sordellii* and *Cl. perfringens* Types C and D. Although *Clostridium perfringens* Type B is not a significant problem in the U.S.A., immunity may be provided against the beta and epsilon toxins elaborated by *Clostridium perfringens* Type B. This immunity is derived from the combination of Type C (beta) and Type D (epsilon) fractions.

Dosage and Administration:

Cattle: Using aseptic technique, inject 5 mL subcutaneously. Repeat in 21 to 28 days and once annually.

Sheep: Using aseptic technique, inject 2.5 mL subcutaneously. Repeat in 21 to 28 days and once annually.

Precaution(s): Store out of direct sunlight at a temperature between 35-45°F (2-7°C). Avoid freezing. Shake well before using. Use entire contents when first opened.

Caution(s): Anaphylactoid reactions may occur.

Antidote(s): Epinephrine.

Warning(s): Do not vaccinate within 21 days before slaughter.

Presentation: 10 cattle doses or 20 sheep doses (50 mL) and 50 cattle doses or 100 sheep doses (250 mL).

Compendium Code No.: 10280152 24201-02 / 24202-02

BAR VAC® CD

Boehringer Ingelheim **Toxoid**

Clostridium Perfringens Types C & D Toxoid

U.S. Vet. Lic. No.: 124

Composition: Prepared from cultures of *Clostridium perfringens* Types C and D. Alum precipitated.

Indications: Recommended for the vaccination of healthy, susceptible sheep and cattle against enterotoxemia caused by the toxins of *Clostridium perfringens* Types C and D. Although *Cl. perfringens* Type B is not a significant problem in the U.S.A., immunity may be provided against the beta and epsilon toxins elaborated by *Cl. perfringens* Type B. This immunity is derived from the combination of Type C (beta) and Type D (epsilon) fractions.

Dosage and Administration:

Sheep: Using aseptic technique, inject 2 mL subcutaneously. Repeat in 21 to 28 days and annually.

Cattle: Using aseptic technique, inject 5 mL subcutaneously. Repeat in 21 to 28 days and annually.

Precaution(s): Store out of direct sunlight at a temperature between 35-45°F (2-7°C). Avoid freezing. Shake well before using. Use entire contents when first opened.

Caution(s): Anaphylactoid reactions may occur.

Antidote(s): Administer epinephrine.

Warning(s): Do not vaccinate within 21 days before slaughter.

Presentation: 10 cattle doses or 25 sheep doses (50 mL) and 50 cattle doses or 125 sheep doses (250 mL).

Compendium Code No.: 10280102 BI 1109-1 3/02

BAR VAC® CD/T

Boehringer Ingelheim **Toxoid**

Clostridium Perfringens Types C & D-Tetanus Toxoid

U.S. Vet. Lic. No.: 124

Composition: Prepared from cultures of the organisms listed. Alum precipitated.

Indications: Recommended for the vaccination of healthy, susceptible sheep, goats and cattle against enterotoxemia and tetanus caused by the toxins of *Clostridium perfringens* Types C and D and *Clostridium tetani.* Although *Cl. perfringens* Type B is not a significant problem in the U.S.A., immunity may be provided against the beta and epsilon toxins elaborated by *Cl. perfringens* Type B. This immunity is derived from the combination of Type C (beta) and Type D (epsilon) fractions.

Dosage and Administration:

Cattle: Using aseptic technique, inject 5 mL subcutaneously. Repeat in 21 to 28 days and once annually.

Sheep and Goats: Using aseptic technique, inject 2 mL subcutaneously. Repeat in 21 to 28 days and once annually.

Precaution(s): Store out of direct sunlight at 35-45°F (2-7°C). Avoid freezing. Shake well before using. Use entire contents when first opened.

Caution(s): Anaphylactoid reactions may occur.

Antidote(s): Administer epinephrine.

Warning(s): Do not vaccinate within 21 days before slaughter.

Presentation: 10 cattle doses or 25 sheep/goat doses (50 mL) and 50 cattle doses or 125 sheep/goat doses (250 mL).

Compendium Code No.: 10280111 BI 1203-1 3/01

BAYTRIL® ℞

(enrofloxacin) 3.23% Concentrate Antimicrobial Solution

Bayer

For Use In Chicken And Turkey Drinking Water Only

Not For Use In Laying Hens Producing Eggs For Human Consumption

Each mL contains: 32.3 mg enrofloxacin.

Indicated for the control of mortality associated with *E. coli* in chickens and mortality associated with *E. coli* and *P. multocida* (fowl cholera) in turkeys.

CAUTION: Federal (U.S.A.) law restricts this drug to use by or on the order of a licensed veterinarian.

Federal law prohibits the extralabel use of this drug in food producing animals.

DESCRIPTION: Enrofloxacin is a synthetic chemotherapeutic agent from the class of quinolone carboxylic acid derivatives. It has antibacterial activity against a broad spectrum of gram-negative and gram-positive bacteria. Each milliliter (mL) of Baytril Antimicrobial Solution contains 32.3 mg enrofloxacin.

CHEMICAL NOMENCLATURE AND STRUCTURAL FORMULA: 1- cyclopropyl-7-(4-ethyl-1-piperazinyl)-6-fluoro-1,4-dihydro-4-oxo-3-quinolinecarboxylic acid

MICROBIOLOGY:

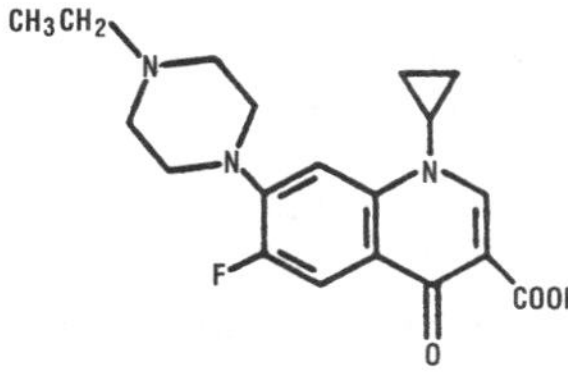

The mode of action of enrofloxacin is bactericidal by inhibition of DNA-gyrase, an essential bacterial enzyme. *In vitro* and *in vivo* activity has been demonstrated against *Escherichia coli* in chickens and against *Escherichia coli* and *Pasteurella multocida* in turkeys, major pathogens associated with mortality.

The minimum inhibitory concentrations (MICs) of enrofloxacin were determined for isolates obtained from natural infections in chickens and turkeys from 1994 through 1996. The ranges of MIC values along with the MIC_{50} (minimum inhibitory concentration for 50% of the isolates) and the MIC_{90} (minimum inhibitory concentration for 90% of the isolates) are shown in Table 1.

Table 1. MIC Values of Enrofloxacin Against Bacterial Isolates from Natural Infections (μg/mL)

Pathogen	Source	No. isolates	MIC range	MIC_{50}	MIC_{90}
Escherichia coli	chicken	82	0.015-1	0.03	0.06
Escherichia coli	turkey	59	0.015-0.06	0.03	0.06
Pasteurella multocida	turkey	45	≤0.008-0.125	0.03	0.03

Isolates for susceptibility testing should be collected prior to initiation of enrofloxacin therapy and subjected to standardized susceptibility tests. Disk diffusion and broth or agar dilution techniques performed according to the National Committee for Clinical Laboratory Standards (NCCLS) may be used. With the disk diffusion method, use only disks containing 5 mcg enrofloxacin.

PHARMACOLOGY: Pharmacokinetic studies were conducted in healthy growing broiler chickens and turkeys using an HPLC assay for parent enrofloxacin. Enrofloxacin was provided in the drinking water at the rate of 25 and 50 ppm continuously for seven days. Following initiation of medication at either the 25 or 50 ppm treatment rate, the first plasma levels measured (at 6 hours) were more than 8x and 15x the MIC_{50} values*, respectively, for *E. coli* isolates from chickens and more than 6x and 11x the MIC_{50} values*, respectively, for *E. coli* and *P. multocida* isolates from turkeys.

* Reflects MIC values from Table 1 above for isolates obtained from 1994 through 1996.

All pharmacokinetic measures were obtained from birds which were maintained at temperatures of 80°F. The concentrations determined are presented in Table 2 for chickens and Table 3 for turkeys.

Table 2. Mean Plasma Concentrations of Enrofloxacin in Chickens

Dose Level (ppm)	Mean Plasma Concentration at 6 Hours** (μg/mL)	Mean Plasma Concentration at 12 Hours** (μg/mL)	Mean Plasma Concentration at 24 to 168 Hours** (μg/mL)
25	0.241	0.317	0.381
50	0.464	0.653	0.712

**Represents numbers of hours after medication was initiated.

Table 3. Mean Plasma Concentrations of Enrofloxacin in Turkeys.

Dose Level (ppm)	Mean Plasma Concentration at 6 Hours ** (μg/mL)	Mean Plasma Concentration at 24 to 168 Hours ** (μg/mL)
25	0.204	0.240
50	0.352	0.458

**Represents numbers of hours after medication was initiated.

Based upon comparisons of intravenous versus oral gavage doses of enrofloxacin solution, data from bioassays conducted in chickens and turkeys indicate that the bioavailability of oral enrofloxacin exceeds 84% in both species. The volume of the central (vascular) compartment was less than 40% of the estimated steady-state volume of distribution (vascular, intracellular and extracellular compartments).

INDICATIONS:

Chickens - Baytril® (enrofloxacin) 3.23% Concentrate Antimicrobial Solution is indicated for the control of mortality associated with *E. coli* susceptible to enrofloxacin.

Turkeys - Baytril® (enrofloxacin) 3.23% Concentrate Antimicrobial Solution is indicated for the control of mortality associated with *E. coli* and *P. multocida* (fowl cholera) susceptible to enrofloxacin.

CONTRAINDICATIONS: As with all drugs, the use of Baytril® (enrofloxacin) 3.23% Concentrate Antimicrobial Solution is contraindicated in animals previously found to be hypersensitive to the drug.

WARNINGS: For use in animals only. Keep out of the reach of children. Avoid contact with eyes. In case of contact, immediately flush eyes with copious amounts of water for 15 minutes. Wash hands with soap and water after handling. Consult a physician if irritation develops or persists following ocular or dermal exposures. Individuals with a history of hypersensitivity to quinolones should avoid exposure to this product. In humans, there is a risk of user photosensitization within a few hours after excessive exposure to quinolones. If accidental exposure occurs, avoid direct sunlight. To report adverse reactions and/or to obtain a copy of the Material Safety Data Sheet, call 1-800-633-3796.

RESIDUE WARNING: Chickens and turkeys intended for human consumption must not be slaughtered within **two days** of the last treatment. Do not use in laying hens producing eggs for human consumption. Use of this product in a manner other than indicated or with dosages in excess of those included on this label may result in illegal drug residues in edible tissues.

PRECAUTIONS: This product is not recommended for use in automatic water proportioners if water hardness is greater than 196 ppm. Water proportioners should be tested for accuracy before use.

Fresh stock solutions should be prepared daily.

Do not use or store Baytril® (enrofloxacin) 3.23% Concentrate Antimicrobial Solution in galvanized metal watering systems or containers.

Do not operate chlorinators while administering medication.

The effects of Baytril Antimicrobial Solution on the reproductive function of treated turkeys have not been determined.

Poultry litter from treated flocks should not be used in cattle feed.

Poultry litter from treated flocks spread on agricultural land should be incorporated into the soil whenever possible.

The following practices are recommended: 10- to 14-day interval between flocks, top dressing with clean litter, and more frequent removal of caked litter from the house.

EFFICACY: A total of 1537 chickens was treated with enrofloxacin at 3 field study locations in flocks naturally infected with *Escherichia coli*. A total of 2292 turkeys was treated at 3 study locations undergoing a natural *E. coli* outbreak. In addition, there were 3 field study locations with fowl cholera *(Pasteurella multocida)* involving 612 turkeys treated with enrofloxacin.

In each study the birds received a water concentration of 25 ppm enrofloxacin for 3 days. In all cases mortality was significantly reduced when compared to unmedicated control birds. No adverse effects were reported in treated birds.

TOXICOLOGY: The oral LD_{50} for laboratory rats was greater than 5000 mg/kg of body weight. Ninety-day feeding studies in dogs and rats revealed no observable effects at treatment rates of 3 and 40 mg/kg respectively. Chronic studies in rats and mice revealed no adverse effects at 5.3 mg/kg and 323 mg/kg respectively. There was no evidence of carcinogenic effects in laboratory animal models. A two-generation rat reproduction study revealed no adverse effects following treatments with 10 mg/kg. Teratogenicity studies in rabbits and rats revealed no teratogenic effects at doses of 25 mg/kg and 50 mg/kg respectively.

ANIMAL SAFETY: There were no significant findings when day old chicks were treated for 21 consecutive days at either 25, 125, or 625 ppm except for minimal histological changes described as atrophy of the testicles which were not dose related.

In two studies in which growing turkeys received 125 ppm in the water for 21 consecutive days beginning at either one or twenty-one days of age, there were no significant effects on clinical signs, body weights, water consumption, feed conversion, clinical pathology or histopathology. Turkey poults which received 625 ppm exhibited decreased activity, listlessness, decreased body weight gain, and some mortality.

No adverse effects upon reproductive parameters occurred when male and female chickens were treated at the rate of 150 ppm for 7 consecutive days at 5 intervals between one and 206 days of age.

DOSAGE AND ADMINISTRATION: Baytril Antimicrobial Solution should be added to clean drinking water to provide a final concentration of 25 to 50 ppm. The medication should be administered as the only source of drinking water. Medication should be initiated promptly when colibacillosis or fowl cholera is diagnosed and should be administered continuously for 3 to 7 days. Selection of dosage and duration should be based on the veterinarian's judgement of disease severity. The presence of Baytril Antimicrobial Solution in drinking water does not affect water consumption. However, the inherent relationship between ambient temperature and water intake should be considered when determining an appropriate dosing regimen. Final concentrations of 25 ppm and 50 ppm can be obtained by using the following mixing schedule:

For Direct Water Application to make 10 gallons of final concentration:		
Final Concentration	**Baytril 3.23%**	**Water**
25 ppm	1 fl oz	10 gallons
50 ppm	2 fl oz	10 gallons

For Water Proportioners that meter 1 fl oz of Stock Solution per gallon of drinking water:		
To Produce Drinking Water with a Final Concentration of:	**Use a Stock Solution Made by Combining:**	
	Baytril 3.23%	**Water**
25 ppm	1 volume	9 volumes
50 ppm	2 volumes	8 volumes

STORAGE: Store in an upright position. Protect stock solutions and medicated drinking water from freezing and direct sunlight.

HOW SUPPLIED:

Code 0247 - 946 mL (one quart) containers

71002471, R.7 Insert July 1999; 71002472, R.6 Label

Code 0248 - 3.8 L (one gallon) containers

71002481, R.7 Insert July 1999; 71002482, R.6 Label

U.S. Patent No. 4,670,444

Bayer Corporation, Agriculture Division, Animal Health, Shawnee Mission, Kansas 66201 U.S.A.

NADA 140-828, Approved by FDA

Compendium Code No.: 10400080

BAYTRIL® 100 ℞

(enrofloxacin) 100 mg/mL Antimicrobial Injectable Solution

Bayer

For Subcutaneous Use In Cattle Only

Not For Use In Cattle Intended For Dairy Production Or In Calves To Be Processed For Veal

CAUTION: Federal (U.S.A.) law restricts this drug to use by or on the order of a licensed veterinarian.

Federal (U.S.A.) law prohibits the extra-label use of this drug in food producing animals.

PRODUCT DESCRIPTION: Baytril® 100 is a sterile, ready-to-use injectable antimicrobial solution that contains enrofloxacin, a broad-spectrum fluoroquinolone antimicrobial agent.

Therapeutic treatment with Baytril® 100 injectable solution may be administered as a single-dose or as a multiple-day therapy.

Each milliliter of Baytril® 100 injectable solution contains 100 mg of enrofloxacin. Excipients are L-arginine base 200 mg, n-butyl alcohol 30 mg, benzyl alcohol (as a preservative) 20 mg, and water for injection, q.s.

CHEMICAL NOMENCLATURE AND STRUCTURE: 1-cyclopropyl-7-(4-ethyl-1-piperazinyl)-6-fluoro-1, 4-dihydro-4-oxo-3-quinolinecarboxylic acid.

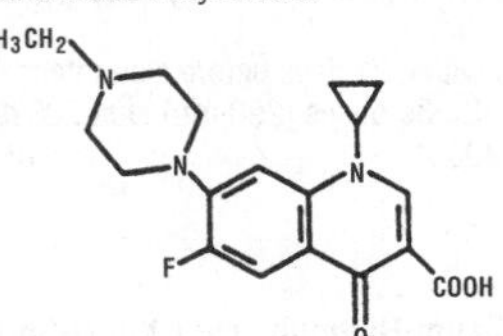

PHARMACOLOGY:

Microbiology: Enrofloxacin is bactericidal and exerts its antibacterial effect by inhibiting bacterial DNA gyrase (a type II topoisomerase) thereby preventing DNA supercoiling and replication, which leads to cell death.[1] Enrofloxacin is active against gram-negative and gram-positive bacteria. Activity against *Mycoplasma* spp. has also been detected.

Enrofloxacin has demonstrated *in vivo* and *in vitro* activity against *Pasteurella haemolytica, Pasteurella multocida*, and *Haemophilus somnus*, the major pathogenic bacteria associated with bovine respiratory disease.

The Minimum Inhibitory Concentrations (MICs) of enrofloxacin were determined[2] for isolates obtained from natural infections in cattle during 1994 and 1995 (see Table I).

Table I - MIC Values (μg/mL) of Enrofloxacin Against Bacteria and Mycoplasma Isolated from Natural Infections

ISOLATE	No. Isolates	MIC_{50}**	MIC_{90}**
Haemophilus somnus	104	0.015	0.03
Mycoplasma spp*	124	0.25	0.5
Pasteurella haemolytica	121	0.06	0.06
Pasteurella multocida	108	0.015	0.03

* The clinical significance of these *in vitro* data has not been demonstrated.

** The MIC for 50% and 90% of the isolates.

EFFICACY: A total of 845 calves with naturally-occurring bovine respiratory disease (BRD) were treated with Baytril® 100 in eight field trials located in five cattle-feeding states. Response to treatment was compared to non-treated controls. Single-dose and multiple-day therapy regimens were evaluated. BRD and mortality were significantly reduced in enrofloxacin-treated calves. No adverse reactions were reported in treated animals.

INDICATIONS: Baytril® 100 (enrofloxacin) injectable solution is indicated for the treatment of bovine respiratory disease (BRD) associated with *Pasteurella haemolytica, Pasteurella multocida* and *Haemophilus somnus*.

WARNING:
Animals intended for human consumption must not be slaughtered within 28 days from the last treatment.
Do not use in cattle intended for dairy production.
A withdrawal period has not been established for this product in pre-ruminating calves.
Do not use in calves to be processed for veal.

HUMAN WARNINGS: For use in animals only. Keep out of the reach of children. Avoid contact with eyes. In case of contact, immediately flush eyes with copious amounts of water for 15 minutes. In case of dermal contact, wash skin with soap and water. Consult a physician if irritation persists following ocular or dermal exposures. Individuals with a history of hypersensitivity to quinolones should avoid this product. In humans, there is a risk of user photosensitization within a few hours after excessive exposure to quinolones. If excessive accidental exposure occurs, avoid direct sunlight. To report adverse reactions or to obtain a copy of the Material Safety Data Sheet, call 1-800-633-3796.

PRECAUTIONS: The effects of enrofloxacin on bovine reproductive performance, pregnancy, and lactation have not been adequately determined.

Subcutaneous injection can cause a transient local tissue reaction that may result in trim loss of edible tissue at slaughter.

Baytril® 100 contains different excipients than other Baytril® products. The safety and efficacy of this formulation in species other than cattle have not been determined.

Quinolone-class drugs should be used with caution in animals with known or suspected Central Nervous System (CNS) disorders. In such animals, quinolones have, in rare instances, been associated with CNS stimulation which may lead to convulsive seizures.

Quinolone-class drugs have been shown to produce erosions of cartilage of weight-bearing joints and other signs of arthropathy in immature animals of various species. No articular cartilage lesions were observed in the stifle joints of 23-day-old calves at 2 days and 9 days following treatment with enrofloxacin at doses up to 25 mg/kg for 15 consecutive days.

ADVERSE REACTIONS: No adverse reactions were observed during clinical trials.

TOXICOLOGY: The oral LD50 for laboratory rats was greater than 5000 mg/kg of body weight. Ninety-day feeding studies in dogs and rats revealed no observable adverse effects at treatment rates of 3 and 40 mg/kg respectively. Chronic studies in rats and mice revealed no observable adverse effects at 5.3 mg/kg and 323 mg/kg respectively. There was no evidence of carcinogenic effect in laboratory animal models. A two-generation rat reproduction study revealed no effect with 10 mg/kg treatments. No teratogenic effects were observed in rabbits at doses of 25 mg/kg or in rats at 50 mg/kg.

ANIMAL SAFETY: Safety studies were conducted in feeder calves using single doses of 5, 15, and 25 mg/kg for 15 consecutive days and 50 mg/kg for 5 consecutive days. No clinical signs of toxicity were observed when a dose of 5 mg/kg was administered for 15 days. Clinical signs of depression, incoordination, and muscle fasciculation were observed in calves when doses of

15 or 25 mg/kg were administered for 10 to 15 days. Clinical signs of depression, inappetence, and incoordination were observed when a dose of 50 mg/kg had been administered for 3 days. No drug-related abnormalities in clinical pathology parameters were identified. No articular cartilage lesions were observed after examination of stifle joints from animals administered 25 mg/kg for 15 days.

A safety study was conducted in 23-day-old calves using doses of 5, 15, and 25 mg/kg for 15 consecutive days. No clinical signs of toxicity or changes in clinical pathology parameters were observed. No articular cartilage lesions were observed in the stifle joints at any dose level at 2 days and 9 days following 15 days of drug administration.

An injection site study conducted in feeder calves demonstrated that the formulation may induce transient reaction in the subcutaneous tissue and underlying muscle. No painful responses to administration were observed.

DOSAGE AND ADMINISTRATION: Baytril® 100 injectable solution provides flexible dosages and durations of therapy. Baytril® 100 may be administered as a single dose for one day or for multiple days of therapy. Selection of the appropriate dose and duration of therapy should be based on an assessment of the severity of disease, pathogen susceptibility and clinical response. Administered dose volume should not exceed 20 mL per injection site.

Single-Dose Therapy: Administer once, a subcutaneous dose of 7.5-12.5 mg/kg of body weight (3.4-5.7 mL/100 lb).

Multiple-Day Therapy: Administer daily, a subcutaneous dose of 2.5-5.0 mg/kg of body weight (1.1-2.3 mL/100 lb). Treatment should be repeated at 24-hour intervals for three days. Additional treatments may be given on days 4 and 5 to animals which have shown clinical improvement but not total recovery.

Table II - Baytril® 100 Dose and Treatment Schedule*

CATTLE WEIGHT (lb)	Single-Dose Therapy 7.5-12.5 mg/kg Dose Size (mL)	Multiple-Day Therapy 2.5-5.0 mg/kg Dose Size (mL)
100	3.5-5.5	1.5-2.0
200	7.0-11.0	2.5-4.5
300	10.5-17.0	3.5-6.5
400	14.0-22.5	4.5-9.0
500	17.0-28.0	5.5-11.5
600	20.5-34.0	7.0-13.5
700	24.0-40.0	8.0-16.0
800	27.5-45.5	9.0-18.0
900	31.0-51.0	10.5-20.5
1000	34.0-56.5	11.5-22.5
1100	37.5-62.5	12.5-25.0

*Dose volumes have been rounded to the nearest 0.5 mL within the dose range.

Note: Subcutaneous injection can cause a transient local tissue reaction that may result in trim loss of edible tissue at slaughter.

STORAGE CONDITIONS: Protect from direct sunlight. Do not refrigerate, freeze or store at or above 40°C (104°F). Precipitation may occur due to cold temperature. To redissolve, warm and then shake the vial.

HOW SUPPLIED: Baytril® 100 (enrofloxacin) Antimicrobial Injectable Solution:

Code: 0236 100 mg/mL 100 mL Bottle

Code: 0321 100 mg/mL 250 mL Bottle

REFERENCES:

1. Hooper, D.C., Wolfson, J.S., *Quinolone Antimicrobial Agents,* 2nd ed, 59-75, 1993.
2. National Committee for Clinical Laboratory Standards, Performance Standards for Antimicrobial Disk and Dilution Susceptibility Tests for Bacteria Isolated from Animals; Proposed Standard, Document M31-P, 1994.

U.S. Patent No. 4,670,444

For customer service, to obtain product information, including the Material Safety Data Sheet, or to report adverse reactions call (800) 633-3796.

80002360, R.8 November, 2000

Bayer Corporation, Agriculture Division, Animal Health, Shawnee Mission, Kansas 66201 U.S.A.

NADA #141-068, Approved by FDA

Compendium Code No.: 10400071

BAYTRIL® ℞

(enrofloxacin) Antibacterial Injectable Solution 2.27%

Bayer

For Dogs Only

CAUTION:

Federal (U.S.A.) law restricts this drug to use by or on the order of a licensed veterinarian.

▶ Federal law prohibits the extralabel use of this drug in food-producing animals. ◀

DESCRIPTION:

Enrofloxacin is a synthetic chemotherapeutic agent from the class of the quinolone carboxylic acid derivatives. It has antibacterial activity against a broad spectrum of Gram negative and Gram positive bacteria (See Tables I and II). Each mL of injectable solution contains: enrofloxacin 22.7 mg, n-butyl alcohol 30 mg, potassium hydroxide for pH adjustment and water for injection, q.s.

CHEMICAL NOMENCLATURE AND STRUCTURAL FORMULA:

1-cyclopropyl-7-(4-ethyl-1-piperazinyl)-6-fluoro-1,4-dihydro-4-oxo-3-quinolinecarboxylic acid.

CH_3CH_2 N N N F COOH O

ACTIONS:

Microbiology: Quinolone carboxylic acid derivatives are classified as DNA gyrase inhibitors. The mechanism of action of these compounds is very complex and not yet fully understood. The site of action is bacterial gyrase, a synthesis promoting enzyme. The effect on *Escherichia coli* is the inhibition of DNA synthesis through prevention of DNA supercoiling. Among other things, such compounds lead to the cessation of cell respiration and division. They may also interrupt bacterial membrane integrity.[1]

Enrofloxacin is bactericidal, with activity against both Gram negative and Gram positive bacteria. The minimum inhibitory concentrations (MICs) were determined for a series of 37 isolates representing 9 genera of bacteria from natural infections in dogs, selected principally because of resistance to one or more of the following antibiotics: ampicillin, cephalothin, colistin, chloramphenicol, erythromycin, gentamicin, kanamycin, penicillin, streptomycin, tetracycline, triple sulfa and sulfa/trimethoprim. The MIC values for enrofloxacin against these isolates are presented in Table I. Most strains of these organisms were found to be susceptible to enrofloxacin *in vitro* but the clinical significance has not been determined for some of the isolates.

The susceptibility of organisms to enrofloxacin should be determined using enrofloxacin 5 mcg disks. Specimens for susceptibility testing should be collected prior to the initiation of enrofloxacin therapy.

Table I — MIC Values for Enrofloxacin Against Canine Pathogens (Diagnostic laboratory isolates, 1984)

Organisms	Isolates	MIC Range (mcg/mL)
Bacteroides spp.	2	2
Bordetella bronchiseptica	3	0.125-0.5
Brucella canis	2	0.125-0.25
Clostridium perfringens	1	0.5
Escherichia coli	4	≤0.016-0.031
Klebsiella spp.	10	0.031-0.5
Proteus mirabilis	6	0.062-0.125
Pseudomonas aeruginosa	4	0.5-8
Staphylococcus spp.	5	0.125

The inhibitory activity on 120 isolates of seven canine urinary pathogens was also investigated and is listed in Table II.

Table II — MIC Values for Enrofloxacin Against Canine Urinary Pathogens (Diagnostic laboratory isolates, 1985)

Organisms	Isolates	MIC Range (mcg/mL)
E. coli	30	0.06-2.0
P. mirabilis	20	0.125-2.0
K. pneumoniae	20	0.06-0.5
P. aeruginosa	10	1.0-8.0
Enterobacter spp.	10	0.06-1.0
Staph. (coag. +)	20	0.125-0.5
Strep. (alpha hemol.)	10	0.5-8.0

Distribution in the Body: Enrofloxacin penetrates into all canine tissues and body fluids. Concentrations of drug equal to or greater than the MIC for many pathogens (See Tables I, II and III) are reached in most tissues by two hours after dosing at 2.5 mg/kg and are maintained for 8-12 hours after dosing. Particularly high levels of enrofloxacin are found in urine. A summary of the body fluid/tissue drug levels at 2 to 12 hours after dosing at 2.5 mg/kg is given in Table III.

Table III — Body Fluid/Tissue distribution of Enrofloxacin in Dogs
Single Oral Dose = 2.5 mg/kg (1.13 mg/lb)

	Post-treatment Enrofloxacin Levels Canine (n=2)	
Body Fluids (mcg/mL)	**2 Hr.**	**8 Hr.**
Urine	43.05	55.35
Eye Fluids	0.53	0.66
Whole Blood	1.01	0.36
Plasma	0.67	0.33
Tissues (mcg/g) Hematopoietic System		
Liver	3.02	1.36
Spleen	1.45	0.85
Bone Marrow	2.10	1.22
Lymph Node	1.32	0.91
Urogenital System		
Kidney	1.87	0.99
Bladder Wall	1.36	0.98
Testes	1.36	1.10
Prostate	1.36	2.20
Uterine Wall	1.59	0.29
Gastrointestinal and Cardiopulmonary Systems		
Lung	1.34	0.82
Heart	1.88	0.78
Stomach	3.24	2.16
Small Intestine	2.10	1.11
Other		
Fat	0.52	0.40
Skin	0.66	0.48
Muscle	1.62	0.77
Brain	0.25	0.24
Mammary Gland	0.45	0.21
Feces	1.65	9.97

Pharmacokinetics: In dogs, the absorption and elimination characteristics of the oral formulation are linear (plasma concentrations increase proportionally with dose) when enrofloxacin is administered at up to 11.5 mg/kg, twice daily.[2] Approximately 80% of the orally administered dose enters the systemic circulation unchanged. The eliminating organs, based on the drug's body clearance time, can readily remove the drug with no indication that the eliminating mechanisms are saturated. The primary route of excretion is via the urine. The absorption and elimination characteristics beyond this point are unknown. Saturable absorption and/or elimination processes may occur at greater doses. When saturation of the absorption process occurs, the plasma concentration of the active moiety will be less than predicted, based on the concept of dose proportionality.

Following an oral dose in dogs of 2.5 mg/kg (1.13 mg/lb), enrofloxacin reached 50% of its maximum serum concentration in 15 minutes and peak serum level was reached in one hour. The elimination half-life in dogs is approximately 2½-3 hours at that dose.

A graph indicating the mean serum levels following a dose of 2.5 mg/kg (1.13 mg/lb) in dogs (oral and intramuscular) is shown in Figure 1.

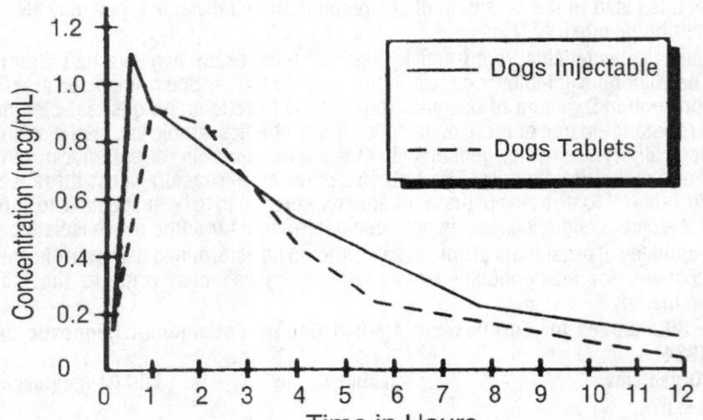

Figure 1 - Serum Concentrations of Enrofloxacin Following a Single Oral or Intramuscular Dose at 2.5 mg/kg in Dogs

Breakpoint: Based on pharmacokinetic studies of enrofloxacin in dogs after a single oral administration of 2.5 mg enrofloxacin/kg BW (i.e. half of the lowest-end single daily dose range) and the data listed in Tables I and II, the following breakpoints are recommended for canine isolates.

Zone Diameter (mm)	MIC (μg/mL)	Interpretation
≥ 21	≤ 0.5	Susceptible (S)
18 - 20	1	Intermediate (I)
≤ 17	≥ 2	Resistant (R)

A report of "Susceptible" indicates that the pathogen is likely to be inhibited by generally achievable plasma levels. A report of "intermediate" is a technical buffer and isolates falling into this category should be retested. Alternatively the organism may be successfully treated if the infection is in a body site where drug is physiologically concentrated. A report of "resistant" indicates that the achievable drug concentrations are unlikely to be inhibitory and other therapy should be selected.

Standardized procedures require the use of laboratory control organisms for both standardized disk diffusion assays and standardized dilution assays. The 5 μg enrofloxacin disk should give the following zone diameters and enrofloxacin powder should provide the following MIC values for reference strains.

QC strain	MIC (μg/mL)	Zone Diameter (mm)
E. coli ATCC 25922	0.008 - 0.03	32 - 40
P. aeruginosa ATCC 27853	1 - 4	15 - 19
S. aureus ATCC 25923		27 - 31
S. aureus ATCC 29213	0.03 - 0.12	

INDICATIONS:

Baytril® (brand of enrofloxacin) Injectable Solution is indicated for the management of diseases in dogs associated with bacteria susceptible to enrofloxacin.

EFFICACY CONFIRMATION:

Clinical efficacy was established in dermal infections (wounds and abscesses) associated with susceptible strains of *Escherichia coli, Klebsiella pneumoniae, Proteus mirabilis,* and *Staphylococcus intermedius;* respiratory infections (pneumonia, tonsillitis, rhinitis) associated with susceptible strains of *Escherichia coli* and *Staphylococcus aureus;* and urinary cystitis associated with susceptible strains of *Escherichia coli, Proteus mirabilis,* and *Staphylococcus aureus.*

CONTRAINDICATIONS:

Enrofloxacin is contraindicated in dogs known to be hypersensitive to quinolones.

Based on the studies discussed under the section on Animal Safety Summary, the use of enrofloxacin is contraindicated in small and medium breeds of dogs during the rapid growth phase (between 2 and 8 months of age). The safe use of enrofloxacin has not been established in large and giant breeds during the rapid growth phase. Large breeds may be in this phase for up to one year of age and the giant breeds for up to 18 months. In clinical field trials utilizing a daily oral dose of 5.0 mg/kg, there were no reports of lameness or joint problems in any breed. However, controlled studies with histological examination of the articular cartilage have not been conducted in the large or giant breeds.

ADVERSE REACTIONS:

No drug related side effects were reported in 122 clinical cases treated with Baytril® (enrofloxacin) Injectable Solution followed by Baytril® Tablets at 5.0 mg/kg per day.

To report adverse reactions or a suspected adverse reaction call 1-800-633-8405.

ANIMAL SAFETY SUMMARY:

Adult dogs receiving enrofloxacin orally at a daily dosage rate 52 mg/kg for 13 weeks had only isolated incidences of vomition and inappetence. Adult dogs receiving the tablet formulation for 30 consecutive days at a daily treatment of 25 mg/kg did not exhibit significant clinical signs nor were there effects upon the clinical chemistry, hematological or histological parameters. Daily doses of 125 mg/kg for up to 11 days induced vomition, inappetence, depression, difficult locomotion and death while adult dogs receiving 50 mg/kg/day for 14 days had clinical signs of vomition and inappetence.

Adult dogs dosed intramuscularly for three treatments at 12.5 mg/kg followed by 57 oral treatments at 12.5 mg/kg, all at 12 hour intervals, did not exhibit either significant clinical signs or effects upon the clinical chemistry, hematological or histological parameters.

Oral treatment of 15 to 28 week old growing puppies with daily dosage rates of 25 mg/kg has induced abnormal carriage of the carpal joint and weakness in the hindquarters. Significant improvement of clinical signs is observed following drug withdrawal. Microscopic studies have identified lesions of the articular cartilage following 30 day treatments at either 5, 15 or 25 mg/kg in this age group. Clinical signs of difficult ambulation or associated cartilage lesions have not been observed in 29 to 34 week old puppies following daily treatments of 25 mg/kg for 30 consecutive days nor in 2 week old puppies with the same treatment schedule.

Tests indicated no effect on circulating microfilariae or adult heartworms *(Dirofilaria immitis)* when dogs were treated at a daily dosage rate of 15 mg/kg for 30 days. No effect on cholinesterase values was observed.

No adverse effects were observed on reproductive parameters when male dogs received 10 consecutive daily treatments of 15 mg/kg/day at 3 intervals (90, 45 and 14 days) prior to breeding or when female dogs received 10 consecutive daily treatments of 15 mg/kg/day at 4 intervals; between 30 and 0 days prior to breeding, early pregnancy (between 10th & 30th days), late pregnancy (between 40th & 60th days), and during lactation (the first 28 days).

DRUG INTERACTIONS:

Concomitant therapy with other drugs that are metabolized in the liver may reduce the clearance rates of the quinolone and the other drug.

Enrofloxacin has been administered to dogs at a daily dosage rate of 10 mg/kg concurrently with a wide variety of other health products including anthelmintics (praziquantel, febantel), insecticides (pyrethrins), heartworm preventatives (diethylcarbamazine) and other antibiotics (ampicillin, gentamicin sulfate, penicillin). No incompatibilities with other drugs are known at this time.

WARNINGS:

For use in animals only. The use of this product in cats may result in retinal toxicity. Keep out of reach of children.

Avoid contact with eyes. In case of contact, immediately flush eyes with copious amounts of water for 15 minutes. In case of dermal contact, wash skin with soap and water. Consult a physician if irritation persists following ocular or dermal exposure. Individuals with a history of hypersensitivity to quinolones should avoid this product. In humans, there is a risk of user photosensitization within a few hours after excessive exposure to quinolones. If excessive accidental exposure occurs, avoid direct sunlight.

For a copy of the Material Safety Data Sheet (MSDS), call 1-800-633-8405.

PRECAUTION:

Quinolone-class drugs should be used with caution in animals with known or suspected Central Nervous System (CNS) disorders. In such animals, quinolones have, in rare instances, been associated with CNS stimulation which may lead to convulsive seizures.

Quinolone-class drugs have been associated with cartilage erosions in weight-bearing joints and other forms of arthropathy in immature animals of various species.

The use of fluoroquinolones in cats has been reported to adversely affect the retina. Such products should be used with caution in cats.

DOSAGE AND ADMINISTRATION:

Baytril Injectable Solution may be used as the initial dose at 2.5 mg/kg. It should be administered intramuscularly (IM) as a single dose, followed by initiation of Baytril Tablet therapy.

Baytril Injectable Solution may be administered as follows:

Weight of Animal	Baytril Injectable Solution* 2.5 mg/kg
9.1 kg (20 lb)	1.00 mL
27.2 kg (60 lb)	3.00 mL

* The initial Baytril Injectable administration should be followed 12 hours later by initiation of Baytril Tablet therapy.

The lower limit of the dose range was based on efficacy studies in dogs where enrofloxacin was administered at 2.5 mg/kg twice daily. Target animal safety and toxicology studies were used to establish the upper limit of the dose range and treatment duration.

STORAGE:

Protect from direct sunlight. Do not freeze.

HOW SUPPLIED:

Code Number	Baytril Injectable Solution 22.7 mg/mL Vial Size
1865	20 mL

REFERENCES:

1 Dougherty, T.J. and Saukkonen, J.J. Membrane Permeability Changes Associated with DNA Gyrase Inhibitors in *Escherichia coli.* Antimicrob. Agents and Chemoth., V. 28, Aug. 1985; 200-206.

2 Walker, R.D., *et al,* Pharmacokinetic Evaluation of Enrofloxacin Administered Orally to Healthy Dogs. Am. J. Res., V. 53, No. 12, Dec. 1992; 2315-2319.

For a copy of the Material Safety Data Sheet or to report adverse reactions, call 1-800-633-8405.

U.S. Patent No. 4,670,444 80003870 R.6/January, 2001

Bayer Corporation, Agriculture Division, Animal Health, Shawnee Mission, Kansas 66201 U.S.A.

NADA 140-913, Approved by FDA

Compendium Code No.: 10400091

BAYTRIL® ℞

(enrofloxacin) Antibacterial Tablets For Dogs and Cats

Bayer

CAUTION:

Federal (U.S.A.) law restricts this drug to use by or on the order of a licensed veterinarian.

▶ Federal law prohibits the extralabel use of this drug in food-producing animals. ◀

DESCRIPTION:

Enrofloxacin is a synthetic chemotherapeutic agent from the class of the quinolone carboxylic acid derivatives. It has antibacterial activity against a broad spectrum of Gram negative and Gram positive bacteria (See Tables I and II). It is rapidly absorbed from the digestive tract, penetrating into all measured body tissues and fluids (See Table III). Tablets are available in three tablet sizes (22.7, 68.0 and 136.0 mg enrofloxacin).

CHEMICAL NOMENCLATURE AND STRUCTURAL FORMULA:

1-cyclopropyl-7-(4-ethyl-1-piperazinyl)-6-fluoro-1,4-dihydro-4-oxo-3-quinolinecarboxylic acid.

CH_3CH_2 N N F COOH O

ACTIONS:

Microbiology: Quinolone carboxylic acid derivatives are classified as DNA gyrase inhibitors.

The mechanism of action of these compounds is very complex and not yet fully understood. The site of action is bacterial gyrase, a synthesis promoting enzyme. The effect on *Escherichia coli* is the inhibition of DNA synthesis through prevention of DNA supercoiling. Among other things, such compounds lead to the cessation of cell respiration and division. They may also interrupt bacterial membrane integrity.[1]

Enrofloxacin is bactericidal, with activity against both Gram negative and Gram positive bacteria. The minimum inhibitory concentrations (MICs) were determined for a series of 39 isolates representing 9 genera of bacteria from natural infections in dogs and cats, selected principally because of resistance to one or more of the following antibiotics: ampicillin, cephalothin, colistin, chloramphenicol, erythromycin, gentamicin, kanamycin, penicillin, streptomycin, tetracycline, triple sulfa and sulfa/trimethoprim. The MIC values for enrofloxacin against these isolates are presented in Table I. Most strains of these organisms were found to be susceptible to enrofloxacin *in vitro* but the clinical significance has not been determined for some of the isolates.

The susceptibility of organisms to enrofloxacin should be determined using enrofloxacin 5 mcg disks. Specimens for susceptibility testing should be collected prior to the initiation of enrofloxacin therapy.

TABLE I — MIC Values for Enrofloxacin Against Canine and Feline Pathogens (Diagnostic laboratory isolates, 1984)

Organisms	Isolates	MIC Range (mcg/mL)
Bacteroides spp.	2	2
Bordetella bronchiseptica	3	0.125-0.5
Brucella canis	2	0.125-0.25
Clostridium perfringens	1	0.5
Escherichia coli	5*	≤0.016-0.031
Klebsiella spp.	11*	0.031-0.5
Proteus mirabilis	6	0.062-0.125
Pseudomonas aeruginosa	4	0.5-8
Staphylococcus spp.	5	0.125

*Includes feline isolates.

The inhibitory activity on 120 isolates of seven canine urinary pathogens was also investigated and is listed in Table II.

TABLE II — MIC Values for Enrofloxacin Against Canine Urinary Pathogens (Diagnostic laboratory isolates, 1985)

Organisms	Isolates	MIC Range (mcg/mL)
E. coli	30	0.06-2.0
P. mirabilis	20	0.125-2.0
K. pneumoniae	20	0.06-0.5
P. aeruginosa	10	1.0-8.0
Enterobacter spp.	10	0.06-1.0
Staph. (coag. +)	20	0.125-0.5
Strep. (alpha hemol.)	10	0.5-8.0

Distribution in the Body: Enrofloxacin penetrates into all canine and feline tissues and body fluids. Concentrations of drug equal to or greater than the MIC for many pathogens (See Tables I, II and III) are reached in most tissues by two hours after dosing at 2.5 mg/kg and are maintained for 8-12 hours after dosing. Particularly high levels of enrofloxacin are found in urine. A summary of the body fluid/tissue drug levels at 2 to 12 hours after dosing at 2.5 mg/kg is given in Table III.

TABLE III — Body Fluid/Tissue Distribution of Enrofloxacin in Dogs and Cats
Single Oral Dose = 2.5 mg/kg (1.13 mg/lb)

	Post-treatment Enrofloxacin Levels			
	Canine (n = 2)		Feline (n = 4)	
Body Fluids (mcg/mL)	**2 Hr.**	**8 Hr.**	**2 Hr.**	**12 Hr.**
Bile	—	—	2.13	1.97
Cerebrospinal Fluid	—	—	0.37	0.10
Urine	43.05	55.35	12.81	26.41
Eye Fluids	0.53	0.66	0.45	0.65
Whole Blood	1.01	0.36	—	—
Plasma	0.67	0.33	—	—
Serum	—	—	0.48	0.18
Tissues (mcg/g) Hematopoietic System				
Liver	3.02	1.36	1.84	0.37
Spleen	1.45	0.85	1.33	0.52
Bone Marrow	2.10	1.22	1.68	0.64
Lymph Node	1.32	0.91	0.49	0.21
Urogenital System				
Kidney	1.87	0.99	1.43	0.37
Bladder Wall	1.36	0.98	1.16	0.55
Testes	1.36	1.10	1.01	0.28
Prostate	1.36	2.20	1.88	0.55
Ovaries	—	—	0.78	0.56
Uterine Wall	1.59	0.29	0.81	1.05
Gastrointestinal and Cardiopulmonary Systems				
Lung	1.34	0.82	0.91	0.33
Heart	1.88	0.78	0.84	0.32
Stomach	3.24	2.16	3.26	0.27
Small Intestine	2.10	1.11	2.72	0.40
Large Intestine	—	—	0.94	1.10
Other				
Fat	0.52	0.40	0.24	0.11
Skin	0.66	0.48	0.46	0.17
Muscle	1.62	0.77	0.53	0.29
Brain	0.25	0.24	0.22	0.12
Mammary Gland	0.45	0.21	0.36	0.30
Feces	1.65	9.97	0.37	4.18

Pharmacokinetics: In dogs, the absorption and elimination characteristics of the oral formulation are linear (plasma concentrations increase proportionally with dose) when enrofloxacin is administered at up to 11.5 mg/kg, twice daily.[2] Approximately 80% of the orally administered dose enters the systemic circulation unchanged. The eliminating organs, based on the drug's body clearance time, can readily remove the drug with no indication that the eliminating mechanisms are saturated. The primary route of excretion is via the urine. The absorption and elimination characteristics beyond this point are unknown. In cats, no oral absorption information is available at other than 2.5 mg/kg, administered orally as a single dose. Saturable absorption and/or elimination processes may occur at greater doses. When saturation of the absorption process occurs, the plasma concentration of the active moiety will be less than predicted, based on the concept of dose proportionality.

Following an oral dose in dogs of 2.5 mg/kg (1.13 mg/lb) enrofloxacin reached 50% of its maximum serum concentration in 15 minutes and peak serum level was reached in one hour. The elimination half-life in dogs is approximately 2½-3 hours at that dose, while in cats it is greater than 4 hours. In a study comparing dogs and cats, the peak concentration and the time to peak concentration were not different. A graph indicating the mean serum levels following a dose of 2.5 mg/kg (1.13 mg/lb) in dogs (oral and intramuscular) and cats (oral) is shown in Figure 1.

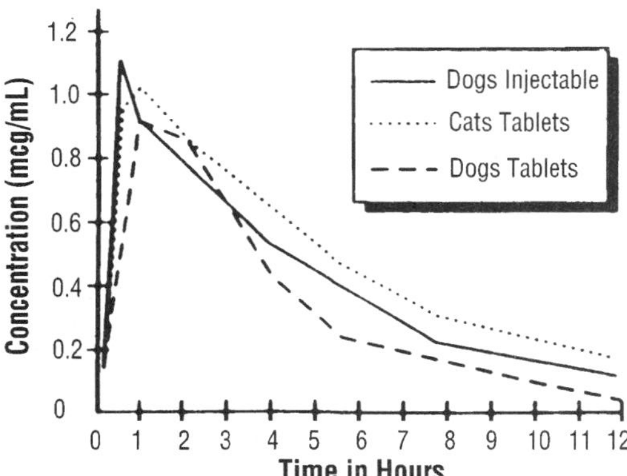

Figure 1 - Serum Concentrations of Enrofloxacin Following a Single Oral or Intramuscular Dose at 2.5 mg/kg in Dogs and a Single Oral Dose at 2.5 mg/kg in Cats.

Breakpoint: Based on pharmacokinetic studies of enrofloxacin in dogs and cats after a single oral administration of 2.5 mg enrofloxacin/kg BW (i.e. half of the lowest-end single daily dose range) and the data listed in Tables I and II, the following breakpoints are recommended for canine and feline isolates.

Zone Diameter (mm)	MIC (µg/mL)	Interpretation
≥ 21	≤ 0.5	Susceptible (S)
18 - 20	1	Intermediate (I)
≤ 17	≥ 2	Resistant (R)

A report of "Susceptible" indicates that the pathogen is likely to be inhibited by generally achievable plasma levels. A report of "Intermediate" is a technical buffer and isolates falling into this category should be retested. Alternatively the organism may be successfully treated if the infection is in a body site where drug is physiologically concentrated. A report of "Resistant" indicates that the achievable drug concentrations are unlikely to be inhibitory and other therapy should be selected.

Standardized procedures require the use of laboratory control organisms for both standardized disk diffusion assays and standardized dilution assays. The 5 µg enrofloxacin disk should give the following zone diameters and enrofloxacin powder should provide the following MIC values for reference strains.

QC strain	MIC (µg/mL)	Zone Diameter (mm)
E. coli ATCC 25922	0.008 - 0.03	32 - 40
P. aeruginosa ATCC 27853	1 - 4	15 - 19
S. aureus ATCC 25923		27 - 31
S. aureus ATCC 29213	0.03 - 0.12	

INDICATIONS:

Baytril (brand of enrofloxacin) Antibacterial Tablets are indicated for the management of diseases associated with bacteria susceptible to enrofloxacin. Baytril Antibacterial Tablets are indicated for use in dogs and cats.

EFFICACY CONFIRMATION:

Dogs: Clinical efficacy was established in dermal infections (wounds and abscesses) associated with susceptible strains of *Escherichia coli, Klebsiella pneumoniae, Proteus mirabilis,* and *Staphylococcus intermedius;* respiratory infections (pneumonia, tonsillitis, rhinitis) associated with susceptible strains of *Escherichia coli* and *Staphylococcus aureus;* and urinary cystitis associated with susceptible strains of *Escherichia coli, Proteus mirabilis,* and *Staphylococcus aureus.*

Palatability: Free choice palatability of Baytril® Taste Tabs® Tablets in dogs was confirmed in a study in which 350 individual dosings resulted in a voluntary ingestion rate of 73%.

Cats: Clinical efficacy was established in dermal infections (wounds and abscesses) associated with susceptible strains of *Pasteurella multocida, Staphylococcus aureus,* and *Staphylococcus epidermidis.*

CONTRAINDICATIONS:

Enrofloxacin is contraindicated in dogs and cats known to be hypersensitive to quinolones.

Dogs: Based on the studies discussed under the section on Animal Safety Summary, the use of enrofloxacin is contraindicated in small and medium breeds of dogs during the rapid growth phase (between 2 and 8 months of age). The safe use of enrofloxacin has not been established in large and giant breeds during the rapid growth phase. Large breeds may be in this phase for up to one year of age and the giant breeds for up to 18 months. In clinical field trials utilizing a daily oral dose of 5.0 mg/kg there were no reports of lameness or joint problems in any breed. However, controlled studies with histological examination of the articular cartilage have not been conducted in the large or giant breeds.

ADVERSE REACTIONS:

Dogs: Two of the 270 (0.7%) dogs treated with Baytril® (brand of enrofloxacin) Tablets at 5.0 mg/kg per day in the clinical field studies exhibited side effects, which were apparently drug related. These two cases of vomition were self-limiting.

Post Approval Experience: The following adverse experiences, although rare, are based on voluntary post-approval adverse drug experience reporting. The categories of reactions are listed in decreasing order of frequency by body system.

Gastrointestinal: Anorexia, diarrhea, vomiting, elevated liver enzymes

Neurologic: ataxia, seizures

Behavioral: Depression, lethargy, nervousness

Cats: No drug-related side effects were reported in 124 cats treated with Baytril® (brand of enrofloxacin) Tablets at 5.0 mg/kg per day for 10 days, in clinical field studies.

Post Approval Experience: The following adverse experiences, although rare, are based on voluntary post-approval adverse drug experience reporting. The categories of reactions are listed in decreasing order of frequency by body system.

Ocular: Mydriasis, retinal degeneration (retinal atrophy, attenuated retinal vessels, and hyperreflective tapeta have been reported), loss of vision. Mydriasis may be an indication of impending or existing retinal changes.

Gastrointestinal: vomiting, anorexia, elevated liver enzymes, diarrhea

Neurologic: ataxia, seizures

Behavioral: Depression, lethargy, vocalization, aggression

To report adverse reactions or a suspected adverse reaction call 1-800-633-8405.

ANIMAL SAFETY SUMMARY:

Dogs: Adult dogs receiving enrofloxacin orally at a daily dosage rate of 52 mg/kg for 13 weeks had only isolated incidences of vomition and inappetence. Adult dogs receiving the tablet formulation for 30 consecutive days at a daily treatment of 25 mg/kg did not exhibit significant clinical signs nor were there effects upon the clinical chemistry, hematological or histological parameters. Daily doses of 125 mg/kg for up to 11 days induced vomition, inappetence, depression, difficult locomotion and death while adult dogs receiving 50 mg/kg/day for 14 days had clinical signs of vomition and inappetence.

Adult dogs dosed intramuscularly for three treatments at 12.5 mg/kg followed by 57 oral treatments at 12.5 mg/kg, all at 12 hour intervals, did not exhibit either significant clinical signs or effects upon the clinical chemistry, hematological or histological parameters.

Oral treatment of 15 to 28 week old growing puppies with daily dosage rates of 25 mg/kg has induced abnormal carriage of the carpal joint and weakness in the hindquarters. Significant improvement of clinical signs is observed following drug withdrawal. Microscopic studies have identified lesions of the articular cartilage following 30 day treatments at either 5, 15 or 25 mg/kg in this age group. Clinical signs of difficult ambulation or associated cartilage lesions have not been observed in 29 to 34 week old puppies following daily treatments of 25 mg/kg for 30 consecutive days nor in 2 week old puppies with the same treatment schedule.

Tests indicated no effect on circulating microfilariae or adult heartworms *(Dirofilaria immitis)* when dogs were treated at a daily dosage rate of 15 mg/kg for 30 days. No effect on cholinesterase values was observed.

No adverse effects were observed on reproductive parameters when male dogs received 10 consecutive daily treatments of 15 mg/kg/day at 3 intervals (90, 45 and 14 days) prior to breeding or when female dogs received 10 consecutive daily treatments of 15 mg/kg/day at 4 intervals; between 30 and 0 days prior to breeding, early pregnancy (between 10th & 30th days), late pregnancy (between 40th & 60th days), and during lactation (the first 28 days).

Cats: Cats in age ranges of 3 to 4 months and 7 to 10 months received daily treatments of 25 mg/kg for 30 consecutive days with no adverse effects upon the clinical chemistry, hematological or histological parameters. In cats 7-10 months of age treated daily for 30 consecutive days, 2 of 4 receiving 5 mg/kg, 3 of 4 receiving 15 mg/kg, 2 of 4 receiving 25 mg/kg and 1 of 4 nontreated controls experienced occasional vomition. Five to 7 month old cats had no side effects with daily treatments of 15 mg/kg for 30 days, but 2 of 4 animals had articular cartilage lesions when administered 25 mg/kg/day for 30 days.

Doses of 125 mg/kg for 5 consecutive days to adult cats induced vomition, depression, incoordination and death while those receiving 50 mg/kg for 6 days had clinical signs of vomition, inappetence, incoordination and convulsions, but they returned to normal.

Enrofloxacin was administered to thirty-two (8 per group), six- to eight- month-old cats at doses of 0, 5, 20, and 50 mg/kg of body weight once a day for 21 consecutive days. There were no adverse effects observed in cats that received 5 mg/kg body weight of enrofloxacin. The administration of enrofloxacin at 20 mg/kg body weight or greater caused salivation, vomition, and depression. Additionally, dosing at 20 mg/kg body weight or greater resulted in mild to severe fundic lesions on ophthalmologic examination (change in color of the fundus, central or generalized retinal degeneration), abnormal electroretinograms (including blindness), and diffuse light microscopic changes in the retina.

DRUG INTERACTIONS:

Compounds that contain metal cations (e.g., aluminum, calcium, iron, magnesium) may reduce the absorption of some quinolone-class drugs from the intestinal tract. Concomitant therapy with other drugs that are metabolized in the liver may reduce the clearance rates of the quinolone and the other drug.

Dogs: Enrofloxacin has been administered to dogs at a daily dosage rate of 10 mg/kg concurrently with a wide variety of other health products including anthelmintics (praziquantel, febantel), insecticides (pyrethrins), heartworm preventatives (diethylcarbamazine) and other antibiotics (ampicillin, gentamicin sulfate, penicillin, dihydrostreptomycin). No incompatibilities with other drugs are known at this time.

Cats: Enrofloxacin was administered at a daily dosage rate of 5 mg/kg concurrently with anthelmintics (praziquantel, febantel), an insecticide (propoxur) and another antibacterial (ampicillin). No incompatibilities with other drugs are known at this time.

WARNINGS:

For Use in Animals Only. In Rare Instances, Use of this Product in Cats has been associated with Retinal Toxicity. Do not exceed 5 mg/kg of body weight per day in cats. Safety in Breeding or Pregnant Cats has not Been Established. Keep Out of Reach of Children.

Avoid contact with eyes. In case of contact, immediately flush eyes with copious amounts of water for 15 minutes. In case of dermal contact, wash skin with soap and water. Consult a physician if irritation persists following ocular or dermal exposure. Individuals with a history of hypersensitivity to quinolones should avoid this product. In humans, there is a risk of user photosensitization within a few hours after excessive exposure to quinolones. If excessive accidental exposure occurs, avoid direct sunlight.

For a copy of the Material Safety Data Sheet, call 1-800-633-8405.

PRECAUTION:

Quinolone-class drugs should be used with caution in animals with known or suspected Central Nervous System (CNS) disorders. In such animals, quinolones have, in rare instances, been associated with CNS stimulation which may lead to convulsive seizures.

Quinolone-class drugs have been associated with cartilage erosions in weight-bearing joints and other forms of arthropathy in immature animals of various species.

The use of fluoroquinolones in cats has been reported to adversely effect the retina. Such products should be used with caution in cats.

DOSAGE AND ADMINISTRATION:

Dogs: Administer orally at a rate to provide 5-20 mg/kg (2.27 to 9.07 mg/lb) of body weight. Selection of a dose within this range should be based on clinical experience, the severity of disease, and susceptibility of the pathogen. Animals which receive doses in the upper-end of the dose range should be carefully monitored for clinical signs that may include inappetence, depression, and vomition.

Weight of Dog	Once Daily Dosing Chart			
	5.0 mg/kg	10.0 mg/kg	15.0 mg/kg	20.0 mg/kg
9.1 kg (20 lb)	2 x 22.7 mg tablets	1 x 22.7 mg plus 1 x 68 mg tablets	1 x 136 mg tablet	1 x 136 mg plus 2 x 22.7 mg tablets
27.2 kg (60 lb)	1 x 136 mg tablet	2 x 136 mg tablets	3 x 136 mg tablets	4 x 136 mg tablets

All tablet sizes are double scored for accurate dosing.

Cats: Administer orally at 5 mg/kg (2.27 mg/lb) of body weight. The dose for dogs and cats may be administered either as a single daily dose or divided into two (2) equal daily doses administered at twelve (12) hour intervals. The dose should be continued for at least 2-3 days beyond cessation of clinical signs, to a maximum of 30 days.

Weight of Cat	Once Daily Dosing Chart (5 mg/kg/day)
5 lb (2.27 kg)	1/2 x 22.7 mg tablet
10 lb (4.5 kg)	1 x 22.7 mg tablet
15 lb (6.8 kg)	1 and 1/2 x 22.7 mg tablets or 1/2 x 68 mg tablet

All tablet sizes are double scored for accurate dosing.

Palatability: Most dogs will consume Baytril® Taste Tabs® Tablets willingly when offered by hand. Alternatively the tablet(s) may be offered in food or hand-administered (pilled) as with other oral tablet medications. In cats, Baytril® Taste Tabs® Tablets should be pilled. After administration, watch the animal closely to be certain the entire dose has been consumed.

Dogs & Cats: The duration of treatment should be selected based on clinical evidence. Generally, administration of Baytril Tablets should continue for at least 2-3 days beyond cessation of clinical signs. For severe and/or complicated infections, more prolonged therapy, up to 30 days, may be required. If no improvement is seen within five days, the diagnosis should be reevaluated and a different course of therapy considered.

The lower limit of the dose range in dogs and the daily dose for cats was based on efficacy studies in dogs and cats where enrofloxacin was administered at 2.5 mg/kg twice daily. Target animal safety and toxicology were used to establish the upper limit of the dose range for dogs and treatment duration for dogs and cats.

STORAGE:

Dispense tablets in tight containers only.

HOW SUPPLIED:

Taste Tabs® Code Number	Film Coated Code Number	Baytril Tablets Tablet Size	Tablets/Bottle
0387	1868	22.7 mg	100 Double Scored
0388	1881	22.7 mg	500 Double Scored
0389	1869	68.0 mg	50 Double Scored
0390	1882	68.0 mg	250 Double Scored
0417	—	136.0 mg	50 Double Scored
0391	—	136.0 mg	200 Double Scored

U.S. Patent No. 4,670,444

REFERENCES:

[1] Dougherty, T.J. and Saukkonen, J.J. Membrane Permeability Changes Associated with DNA Gyrase Inhibitors in *Escherichia coli* Antimicrob. Agents and Chemoth., V. 28, Aug. 1985, 200-206.

[2] Walker, R.D. *et al*, Pharmacokinetic Evaluation of Enrofloxacin Administered Orally to Healthy Dogs. Am. J. Res., V. 53, No. 12, Dec. 1992; 2315-2319.

March, 2001

Bayer Corporation, Agriculture Division, Animal Health, Shawnee Mission, Kansas 66201, U.S.A.

NADA 140-441, Approved by FDA

Compendium Code No.: 10400122

BAYTRIL® OTIC ℞

(enrofloxacin/silver sulfadiazine) Antibacterial-Antimycotic Emulsion

Bayer

For Ototopical Use In Dogs

Caution: Federal (U.S.A.) Law restricts this drug to use by or on the order of a licensed veterinarian.

▶ Federal law prohibits the extralabel use of this drug in food-producing animals. ◀

PRODUCT DESCRIPTION:

Each milliliter of Baytril® Otic contains: enrofloxacin 5 mg (0.5% w/v), silver sulfadiazine (SSD) 10 mg (1.0% w/v), benzyl alcohol (as a preservative) and cetylstearyl alcohol (as a stabilizer) in a neutral oil and purified water emulsion. The active ingredients are delivered via a physiological carrier (a nonirritating emulsion).

CHEMICAL NOMENCLATURE AND STRUCTURE:

Enrofloxacin

1-Cyclopropyl-7-(4-ethyl-1-piperazinyl)-6-fluoro-1, 4-dihydro-4-oxo-3-quinolinecarboxylic acid.

CH_3 H_2C N N N F O O HO

Silver Sulfadiazine

Benzenesulfonamide, 4-amino-N-2-pyrimidinyl-monosilver

ACTIONS:

Enrofloxacin, a 4-fluoroquinolone compound, is bactericidal with activity against a broad spectrum of both Gram negative and Gram positive bacteria. Fluoroquinolones elicit their bactericidal activities through interactions with two intracellular enzymes, DNA gyrase (DNA topoisomerase II) and DNA topoisomerase IV, which are essential for bacterial DNA transcription, synthesis and replication. It is believed that fluoroquinolones actively bind with bacterial DNA:ENZYME complexes and thereby inhibit the essential processes catalyzed by the enzymes (DNA supercoiling and chromosomal decatenation).[1] The ultimate outcome of the fluoroquinolone intervention is DNA fragmentation and bacterial cell death.[2,3]

Silver sulfadiazine (SSD) is synthesized from silver nitrate and sodium sulfadiazine.[4] This compound has a wide spectrum of antimicrobial activity against Gram negative and Gram positive bacteria and is also an effective antimycotic.[5,6] SSD suppresses microbial growth through inhibition of DNA replication and modification of the cell membrane.

MICROBIOLOGY:

In clinical field trials, Baytril® Otic demonstrated elimination or reduction of clinical signs associated with otitis externa and *in vitro* activity against cultured organisms. Baytril® Otic is effective when used as a treatment for canine otitis externa associated with one or more of the following organisms: *Malassezia pachydermatis, coagulase-positive Staphylococcus spp., Pseudomonas aeruginosa, Enterobacter spp., Proteus mirabilis, Streptococci spp., Aeromonas hydrophila, Aspergillus spp., Klebsiella pneumoniae,* and *Candida albicans.*

In vitro assays, such as disk-diffusion and agar/broth-dilution, are used to determine the susceptibilities of microbes to antimicrobial therapies. Results of agar/broth-dilution assays are reported as a Minimal Inhibitory Concentration (MIC) which represents the lowest antimicrobial concentration, expressed in μg/mL, capable of inhibiting the growth of a pathogenic microorganism. MICs are used in conjunction with pharmacokinetics to predict the *in vivo* efficacy of systemically administered antimicrobials. Topical administration of Baytril® Otic to an exudate and debris-free canal, however, will generally result in local antimicrobial concentrations that greatly exceed serum and tissue levels resulting from systemic therapy. Therefore, when using Baytril® Otic as a treatment for canine otitis externa, interpret susceptibility data cautiously.

INDICATIONS:

Baytril® Otic is indicated as a treatment for canine otitis externa complicated by bacterial and fungal organisms susceptible to enrofloxacin and/or silver sulfadiazine (see Microbiology section).

EFFECTIVENESS:

Due to its combination of active ingredients, Baytril® Otic provides antimicrobial therapy against bacteria and fungi (which includes yeast) commonly encountered in cases of canine otitis externa.

The effectiveness of Baytril® Otic was evaluated in a controlled, double-blind, multi-site clinical trial. One hundred and sixty-nine dogs (n=169), with naturally occurring active otitis externa participated in the study. The presence of active disease was verified by aural cytology, microbial culture and otoscopy/clinical scoring. Qualified cases were randomly assigned to either Baytril Otic treatment (n=113) or to a comparable placebo-based regimen (n=56). Treatments were administered twice daily for up to 14 days. Assessment of effectiveness was based on continued resolution of clinical signs 3 to 4 days following administration of the last dose.

At study conclusion, Baytril® Otic was found to be a significantly more effective treatment for canine otitis externa than the placebo regimen. Based on the scoring system used to assess treatment response, therapeutic success occurred in 67% of Baytril® Otic-treated infections compared to 14% with placebo (r-value^2 0.001) after 14 days of treatment.

CONTRAINDICATIONS:

Baytril® Otic is contraindicated in dogs with suspected or known hypersensitivity to quinolones and/or sulfonamides.

HUMAN WARNINGS:

Not for human use. Keep out of the reach of children. Avoid contact with eyes. In case of contact, immediately flush eyes with copious amounts of water for 15 minutes. In case of dermal contact, wash skin with soap and water. Consult a physician if irritation develops or persists following ocular or dermal exposures. Individuals with a history of hypersensitivity to quinolone compounds or antibacterials should avoid handling this product. In humans, there is a risk of user photosensitization within a few hours after excessive exposure to quinolones. If excessive accidental exposure occurs, avoid direct sunlight.

PRECAUTIONS:

The use of Baytril® Otic in dogs with perforated tympanic membranes has not been evaluated. Therefore, the integrity of the tympanic membrane should be evaluated before administering this product. If hearing or vestibular dysfunction is noted during the course of treatment, discontinue use of Baytril® Otic.

Quinolone-class drugs should be used with caution in animals with known or suspected Central Nervous System (CNS) disorders. In such animals, quinolones have, in rare instances, been associated with CNS stimulation which may lead to convulsive seizures.

Quinolone-class drugs have been associated with cartilage erosions in weightbearing joints and other forms of arthropathy in immature animals of various species.

The safe use of Baytril® Otic in dogs used for breeding purposes, during pregnancy, or in lactating bitches, has not been evaluated.

ADVERSE REACTIONS:

During clinical trials, 2 of 113 (1.7%) dogs exhibited reactions that may have resulted from treatment with Baytril® Otic. Both cases displayed local hypersensitivity responses of the aural epithelium to some component within the Baytril® Otic formulation. The reactions were characterized by acute inflammation of the ear canal and pinna.

To report a suspected adverse reaction call 1-800-633-3796.

SAFETY:

General Safety Study:

In a target animal safety study, Baytril® Otic was administered in both ears of 24 clinically normal beagle dogs at either recommended or exaggerated dosages: 10, 30 or 50 drops applied twice daily for 42 consecutive days. A control group of 8 beagle dogs was treated by administering 50 drops of vehicle in one ear twice daily for 42 consecutive days, with the contralateral ear untreated. Erythema was noted in all groups, including both treated and untreated ears in the controls, which resolved following termination of treatment.

Oral Safety Study:

In order to test safety in case of ingestion, Baytril® Otic was administered, twice daily for 14 consecutive days, to the dorsum of the tongue and to the left buccal mucosa of 6 clinically normal dogs. No adverse local or systemic reactions were reported.

DOSAGE AND ADMINISTRATION:

Shake well before each use.

Tilt head so that the affected ear is presented in an upward orientation. Administer a sufficient quantity of Baytril® Otic to coat the aural lesions and the external auditory canal. As a general guide, administer 5-10 drops per treatment in dogs weighing 35 lbs. or less and 10-15 drops per treatment in dogs weighing more than 35 lbs. Following treatment, gently massage the ear so as to ensure complete and uniform distribution of the medication throughout the external ear canal. Apply twice daily for a duration of up to 14 days.

STORAGE:

Store between 4 and 25°C (40 - 77°F). Store in an upright position. Do not store in direct sunlight.

HOW SUPPLIED:

Baytril® Otic (enrofloxacin/silver sulfadiazine)

Code Number	Size	Presentation
0420	15 mL	Oval plastic bottle with dropper tip and extended tip closure
0421	30 mL	Oval plastic bottle with dropper tip and extended tip closure

REFERENCES:

1. Hooper DC and Wolfson JS. Mechanisms of quinolone action and bacterial killing, in Quinolone Antimicrobial Agents. Washington DC, American Society for Microbiology, 2nd ed., 1993, 53-75.
2. Gootz TD and Brightly KE. Fluoroquinolone antibacterial: mechanism of action, resistance and clinical aspects. Medicinal Research Reviews 1996; 16 (5): 433-486.
3. Drlica K and Zhoa X. DNA gyrase, topoisomerase IV and the 4-quinolones. Microbiology and Molecular Biology Reviews 1997; 61(3): 377-392.
4. Fox CL. Silver sulfadiazine: a new topical therapy for *Pseudomonas* in burns. Archives of Surgery 1968; 96:184-188.
5. Wlodkowski TJ and Rosenkranz HS. Antifungal activity of silver sulfadiazine. Lancet 1973; 2:739-740.
6. Schmidt A. *In vitro* activity of climbazole, clotrimazole and silver sulfadiazine against isolates of *Malassezia pachydermatis.* J of Vet Medicine Series B 1997; 44: 193-197.

For a copy of the Material Safety Data Sheet (MSDS) or to report Adverse Reactions call Bayer Customer Service at 1-800-633-3796.

Bayer Corporation, Agriculture Division, Animal Health, Shawnee Mission, Kansas 66201 U.S.A.

U.S. Patent No: 5,753,269 — 80004200 R.0, August, 2000

NADA # 141-176, Approved by FDA

Compendium Code No.: 10400100

B-COMJECT 150 ℞

Vetus — **Vitamin B-Complex**

NDC No.: 47611-056-82

Active Ingredient(s): Each mL of sterile solution contains:

Thiamine HCl (vitamin B_1)	150 mg
Riboflavin 5' phosphate sodium	2 mg
Niacinamide	150 mg
Panthenol	10 mg
Pyridoxine HCl	10 mg
Inositol	20 mg
Choline chloride	20 mg
Benzyl alcohol (as preservative)	2%
Water for injection	q.s.

Indications: For prevention of vitamin B deficiencies in pigs, sheep, cattle and horses.

Dosage and Administration: For intramuscular or intravenous use. Administer 1-5 mg per 100 lbs. of body weight.

Precaution(s): Avoid undue exposure to light.

Caution(s): Federal law restricts this drug to use by or on the order of a licensed veterinarian.

For animal use only.

Presentation: 100 mL multiple dose vials.

Compendium Code No.: 14440070

B-COMJECT FORTE

Vetus — **Vitamin B-Complex**

Active Ingredient(s): Each mL contains:

Thiamine HCl	100 mg
Riboflavin 5' Phosphate Sodium	5 mg
Niacinamide	100 mg
d-Panthenol	10 mg
Pyridoxine HCl	10 mg
Cobalt (as Cyanocobalamin)	4.0 ppm
Benzyl Alcohol (preservative)	1.5%
Citric Acid	5 mg
Water for Injection	q.s.

Indications: An aqueous solution of B Complex vitamins to provide a supplemental nutritional supply of these vitamins and Complexed Cobalt to cattle, sheep and swine.

Dosage and Administration: Administer intramuscularly or subcutaneously.

Sheep and Swine: 5 to 10 mL.

Cattle: 10 to 20 mL.

Repeat daily as indicated.

Precaution(s): Store between 15°C and 30°C (59°F-86°F). Keep from freezing.

Caution(s): Anaphylactogenesis to parenteral Thiamine HCl has been reported. Administer slowly and with caution in doses over 50 mg. For animal use only.

Warning(s): Keep out of reach of children.

Presentation: 100 mL vials (NDC 47611-762-82).

Distributed by: Burns Veterinary Supply, Inc.

Compendium Code No.: 14440081 — Rev. 6-97

B

B COMPLEX ONE-FIFTY INJECTION ℞

Vedco **Vitamin B-Complex**

Active Ingredient(s): Each mL contains:

Thiamine HCl (vitamin B_1)	150 mg
Riboflavin 5' phosphate sodium	2 mg
Niacinamide	150 mg
Panthenol	20 mg
Pyridoxine HCl	10 mg
Inositol	20 mg
Choline chloride	20 mg
Preservative:	
Benzyl alcohol	2%
Water for injection	q.s.

Indications: For prevention of deficiencies of vitamin B compound in pigs, sheep, cattle and horses.

Dosage and Administration: For intravenous or intramuscular use.

Administer 1 to 5 mL per 100 lbs. of body weight.

Precaution(s): Avoid undue exposure to light.

Caution(s): Federal law restricts this drug to use by or on the order of a licensed veterinarian.

Keep out of the reach of children. Not for human use.

Presentation: 100 mL sterile multiple dose vials.

Compendium Code No.: 10940110

B-COMPLEX-PLUS

AgriLabs **Vitamin B-Complex**

Active Ingredient(s): Each mL of sterile aqueous solution contains:

Thiamine Hydrochloride (B_1)	12.5 mg
Niacinamide	12.5 mg
Pyridoxine Hydrochloride (B_6)	5.0 mg
d-Panthenol	5.0 mg
Riboflavin (B_2) (as Riboflavin 5' phosphate sodium)	2.0 mg
Cyanocobalamin (B_{12})	1000 mcg

with benzyl alcohol 1.5% v/v as a preservative, ammonium sulfate, 0.1%.

Indications: For use as a supplemental source of B complex vitamins in cattle, swine and sheep.

Dosage and Administration: Subcutaneous or intramuscular injection is recommended. May be administered intravenously at the discretion of a veterinarian. The following are suggested dosages, depending on the condition of the animal and the desired response.

Adult Cattle: 1 to 2 mL per 500 pounds of body weight.

Calves, Swine and Sheep: 1 to 2 mL.

May be repeated once or twice weekly.

Precaution(s): Store at controlled room temperature between 15° to 30°C (59°-86°F).

Protect from light.

Caution(s): Hypersensitivity reactions to the parenteral administration of products containing thiamine have been reported. Administer with caution and keep treated animals under close observation.

Warning(s): For animal use only. Keep out of reach of children.

Presentation: Available in 100 mL and 250 mL.

Compendium Code No.: 10580140

BELTSVILLE TURKEY SEMEN EXTENDER - II

Intervet **Semen Extender**

Indications: For use as a turkey semen extender.

Dosage and Administration: Dilution Directions:

1. Collect the semen and make the dilutions at room temperature, 68° to 75°F.
2. Dilute the semen and the extender at a ratio of 1:1.
3. Do not use mixers to blend the semen and extender. The semen should be mixed gently using a pipet.

A.I. Schedule:

1. Gently mix the sample to make sure the semen and extender are well mixed.
2. Each insemination dose should contain a minimum of 200 million sperm.
3. Inseminate each hen three (3) times within the first 10 days, then every seven (7) days.
4. For the best results, the first insemination should be made before the lay of the first egg.

Precaution(s):

1. The diluted semen can be stored in either a test tube or an erlenmeyer flask.
2. Allow plenty of air space in the tube or flask.
3. Cover the tube or flask with aluminum foil. Do not stopper with a cotton plug, rubber stopper, etc.
4. Place the tube or flask in a beaker containing a small volume of water at 77°F (25°C).
5. Place the beaker with the tube or flask in it into a 41°F (5°C) cooler or refrigerator.
6. The storage of the diluted semen should not exceed six hours and should be gently agitated during this time to avoid settling of the sperm cells.
7. Refrigeration is not required for storage of the extender.

Notice: The product has been manufactured under strict sanitary standards and conditions. Every lot has been carefully tested and determined to be free of microbial contamination. The product should be handled and stored per label or other instructions to ensure product integrity.

Disclaimer: The information contained herein, is to the best of Intervet Inc.'s knowledge, considered reliable. The use of the product is intended by persons having skill and at their own discretion and risk. No representation or warranty, expressed or implied, including the warranties of merchantability and fitness for a particular purpose is made with respect to the information contained herein.

Presentation: The product is presented in liquid form. It is available for use in 2.5 mL, 10 mL and 50 mL sizes (with or without gentamicin).

Compendium Code No.: 11060081

BEMACOL® ℞

Pfizer Animal Health **Ophthalmic Antibiotic**

(chloramphenicol 1%) Sterile Veterinary Ophthalmic Ointment

NADA No.: 065-460

Active Ingredient(s): Description: Each gram contains chloramphenicol USP 10 mg, in a light mineral oil USP, white petrolatum USP, polyoxyethylene sorbitan monostearate base.

Indications: BEMACOL® (chloramphenicol) Veterinary Ophthalmic Ointment 1% is appropriate for use in dogs and cats for the topical treatment of bacterial conjunctivitis caused by pathogens susceptible to chloramphenicol.

Pharmacology: Action: Chloramphenicol is a broad-spectrum antibiotic providing rapid clinical response and having therapeutic activity against susceptible strains of a number of gram-positive and gram-negative organisms including *Escherichia coli, Staphylococcus aureus* and *Streptococcus hemolyticus.*

Dosage and Administration: Application of the ointment should be preceded by cleansing to remove discharge and crusts. The ointment is applied every 3 hours around the clock for 48 hours, after which night instillations may be omitted. A small amount of ointment should be placed in the lower conjunctival sac. Treatment should be continued for 2 days after the eye appears normal. Therapy for cats should not exceed 7 days.

Contraindication(s): Chloramphenicol products must not be used in meat, egg, or milk-producing animals. The length of time that residues persist in milk or tissue has not been determined.

Precaution(s): Store at room temperature.

Caution(s): Federal law restricts this drug to use by or on the order of a licensed veterinarian.

Most susceptible bacteria will respond to chloramphenicol therapy in a few days. If improvement is not noted in this period of time, a change of therapy should be considered.

When infection is suspected as the cause of a disease process, especially in purulent or catarrhal conjunctivitis, attempts should be made to determine which antibiotics will be effective through susceptibility testing prior to applying ophthalmic preparations.

Warning(s): Not for use in animals which are raised for food production.

Prolonged use in cats may produce blood dyscrasias.

For veterinary use only.

Presentation: 3.5-gram (1/8-oz), sterile, tamper-proof tubes.

Manufactured by: Altana Inc., Melville, NY 11747, USA

Compendium Code No.: 36901750 75-8250-02

BENE-BAC™ PET GEL

Pet-Ag **Small Animal Dietary Supplement**

Ingredient(s): Guaranteed Total (viable) Lactic Acid Producing Bacteria: 10 million colony forming units per gram *(Lactobacillus acidophilus, Lactobacillus plantarum, Streptococcus faecium, Lactobacillus casei).*

Dried *Lactobacillus acidophilus* fermentation product, dried *L. plantarum* fermentation product, dried *Streptococcus faecium* fermentation product, dried *L. casei* fermentation product, vegetable oils, sugar, silicon dioxide, artificial color, Polysorbate 80 preserved with tertiary butyl hydroquinone, and ethoxyquin.

Indications: A source of live naturally occurring microorganisms for dogs, cats, and other small mammals.

Directions for Use: A source of live naturally occurring microorganisms for small mammals subjected to changing environment, training, working, transporting or hand feeding. Place gel on back of tongue or on food.

Newborns: ½ g at birth; ½ g on days 3, 5, and 7 and at weaning. Hand fed orphans, increase to 1 g on days 7, 14, and at introduction to solid food.

Maintenance: 1 g for each 10 lbs of body weight up to 50 lbs. 5 g for 50 lbs body weight and over. Administer 1 day prior and 1 day following conditions above.

Precaution(s): Store at room temperature.

Presentation: 0.53 oz (15 g) syringes (12 per case) and 4 x 1 g tubes (12 per case).

Compendium Code No.: 10970011

BENE-BAC™ POWDER

Pet-Ag **Dietary Supplement**

Beneficial Bacteria

Ingredient(s): Guaranteed total live (viable) Lactic Acid Product Bacteria: 10 million Colony Forming Units (CFU) per gram *(Lactobacillus fermentum, Enterococcus faecium, Lactobacillus plantarum, Lactobacillus acidophilus).*

Sucrose, maltodextrin, silicon dioxide, dried *lactobacillus fermentum,* dried *enterococcus faecium,* dried *L. plantarum,* and dried *L. acidophilus* fermentation products.

Indications: For domestic, exotic and wildlife mammals.

A source of live naturally-occurring microorganisms.

Recommended as part of the management program for all mammals subjected to changing environmental or nutritional conditions or after antibiotic therapy.

Help for animals under adverse conditions such as: simple intestinal stress, antibiotic therapy, post surgery, birth, weaning, worming, traveling.

Directions for Use: Initial Treatment: Provide one dosage from table below on days 1, 3, 5 and 7, and then one dosage per week until weaned.

Body Weight	Amount of BBP
< ½ lb (227 g)	¼ level teaspoon
½ - 1 lb	½ level teaspoon
1 lb - 5 lbs	1 level teaspoon
5 lbs - 20 lbs	2 level teaspoons
20 lbs+	3 level teaspoons

For Maintenance: Use above recommended daily dosage once weekly. Treat animals by top dressing BENE-BAC™ Powder on moistened or oiled dry food or fresh fruits or vegetables. Discard uneaten food after no more than 8 hours and thoroughly wash dishes.

Regular use of BBP for normal maintenance is recommended.

General Information: If several animals are maintained in a common cage, use the approximate total weight of all animals to determine feeding level. Mix with feed so that all animals receive appropriate dose.

One level teaspoon equals approximately 2.7 grams of BENE-BAC™ Powder.

Wash all feeding dishes, water bottles or water dishes, thoroughly with hot, soapy water and rinse well after each use.

Be sure to contact your veterinarian for any illness.

Precaution(s): Store in cool, dry conditions.

Presentation: 16 oz (454 g).

Compendium Code No.: 10970340

BENZELMIN® PASTE

Fort Dodge **Parasiticide-Oral**

Oxfendazole, Equine Anthelmintic Paste

NADA No.: 132-105

Active Ingredient(s): Each 12 g syringe contains:

Oxfendazole . . . . 4.5 g

Indications: Description: BENZELMIN® Equine Anthelmintic Paste is a broad-spectrum anthelmintic which has been specially developed to provide maximum efficacy, ease of administration and safety.

BENZELMIN® Equine Anthelmintic Paste is effective in horses for the removal of most gastrointestinal worms: Ascarids (large roundworms): *Parascaris equorum*

Pinworms (mature and 4th stage larvae): *Oxyuris equi*

Large Strongyles (blood worms, red worms, or palisade worms): *Strongylus edentatus, Strongylus vulgaris, Strongylus equinus*

Small Strongyles

Dosage and Administration: The recommended dose of oxfendazole is 10 mg/kg of body weight. BENZELMIN® Equine Anthelmintic Paste is formulated to deliver 4.5 g of oxfendazole or 12 g of paste per 1000 lb of body weight.

Horses maintained on premises where reinfection is likely to occur should be retreated in 6-8 weeks.

Method of Administration: The paste is readily administered directly into the horse's mouth. Withholding feed or water prior to administration is not necessary. The recommendations for administration are as follows:

1. Remove cap from the end of the syringe.
2. "Zero" the syringe by turning the dial ring (the side of the ring facing the barrel) to zero, and advancing the plunger.
3. Following determination of the weight of the horse, select the proper dosage to administer (one mark on the plunger for each 250 lbs of body weight).
4. Confirm that the horse's mouth is free of grass, hay or grain.
5. Insert the syringe tip into the side of the horse's mouth, direct tip through the interdental space (space between incisor and premolar teeth) and quickly deposit the drug as far back on the base of the tongue as possible.

Precaution(s): Partially Used Syringes — Multi-dose syringes that are partially used, if recapped, may be stored for up to six months provided the expiration date on the labeling is not exceeded.

Caution(s): It is recommended that this drug be administered with caution to sick or severely debilitated horses. Consult your veterinarian for assistance in the diagnosis, treatment and control of parasitism.

Warning(s): Use strictly as directed. Keep out of reach of children. Not for human use. Not for use in horses intended for food.

Toxicology: Safety: When used as directed, BENZELMIN® (oxfendazole) Equine Anthelmintic Paste has an ample safety margin for all practical conditions of use in horses.

Presentation: 0.42 oz (12 g) syringe (NDC 0856-0805-05).

U.S. Patent No. 3,929,821; 4,080,461; and others.

Compendium Code No.: 10030160 0080B

BENZO-GEL™ ℞

Butler **Liniment**

NDC No.: 11695-2160-6

Active Ingredient(s): Benzocaine, camphor, menthol, thymol, witch hazel, isopropyl alcohol in a specially prepared base.

Indications: A topical anesthetic, this liniment gel with benzocaine is to be used for temporary relief of minor muscle stiffness and soreness due to overexertion in horses.

Dosage and Administration: May be used concentrated or diluted depending on the condition. It will not burn or blister.

For horses in training: Use before and after workouts, under bandages, either wet or dry.

In shipping horses: Apply on legs and use a cotton bandage. Liniment Gel with Benzocaine will not burn or blister under bandages.

Method of Use: Be certain skin and hair are clean. It is advised that the area to be treated be washed first. Apply by rubbing deeply into hair in the first application, assuring contact with the skin. Following first application, apply a generous amount for the second application. Use as often as indicated.

For using as a diluted application the indications are: Use after strenuous exercise for any type of performance animal.

Use as a therapeutic bodywash when coolant is indicated.

Mix 2 tablespoons of gel to a quart of warm water. Apply with a sponge, covering the horse's entire body. Use a brisk rubbing motion when applying. Guard against creating heat or irritation by overrubbing.

Racetracks: When saliva and urine tests are to be conducted, do not administer before or after racing as horses may pick up components by licking and the ingredients may show up in testing.

Precaution(s): It is important to keep the cap on tight, thereby avoiding evaporation.

Store in a cool dry area. Do not store near heat.

Caution(s): Federal law restricts this drug to use by or on the order of a licensed veterinarian.

Do not apply any other type of external medicants to the same area where this product has been administered.

Avoid contact with eyes and mucous membranes. If the condition for which this preparation is used or persists, or if a rash develops, discontinue use and consult your veterinarian.

Warning(s): Not for use on food producing animals.

For animal use only.

Keep out of reach of children.

Presentation: 1 lb.

Compendium Code No.: 10820180

BENZOYL PEROXIDE SHAMPOO

Butler **Antidermatosis Shampoo**

Ingredient(s): Sodium lauryl sulfate, Deionized water, Benzoyl peroxide 2.5%, Magnesium aluminim silicate, quaternium 33 and Ethyl hexanediol, Lauramide DEA, Steartrimonium hydrolyzed animal protein, Laureth 4, Citric acid, Fragrance.

Indications: BENZOYL PEROXIDE SHAMPOO is used for the topical treatment of conditions where an antibacterial, keratolytic agent is of benefit or for routine antiseptic shampooing of dogs and cats.

Directions: Shake well before using.

Wet coat thoroughly with water. Using 2-3 cc at a time, work up a lather over as large an area as possible. Continue process until entire coat is lathered. When entire coat is treated, allow BENZOYL PEROXIDE SHAMPOO to remain on the coat for 5-10 minutes. Rinse thoroughly with water. May be used daily to once every one or two weeks depending on severity of condition.

Precaution(s): Store below 80°F.

Caution(s): If irritation develops, discontinue use. Contact sensitivity to Benzoyl peroxide has been observed in humans. The use of BENZOYL PEROXIDE SHAMPOO does not eliminate the possible requirement for appropriate systemic treatment.

For external use only on dogs or cats. Keep away from eye area. May bleach colored fabrics.

Keep out of reach of children.

Presentation: 6 oz.

Compendium Code No.: 10820190

B

BENZOYL PEROXIDE SHAMPOO

Davis **Antidermatosis Shampoo**

Active Ingredient(s): Davis BENZOYL PEROXIDE SHAMPOO contains 2.5% Benzoyl Peroxide in a deep cleansing shampoo base.

Indications: This synergistic shampoo is formulated to help with conditions associated with seborrhea dermatitis, canine and feline acne, and for conditions where a keratolytic vehicle may be beneficial.

An excellent degreaser for problem coats, Davis BENZOYL PEROXIDE SHAMPOO also aids in the opening and flushing of hair follicles. Contains natural moisturizers to promote hydration of the coat and skin.

Directions for Use: Wet pet's coat thoroughly with warm water. Apply shampoo to head and ears, then lather. Be careful not to get shampoo into eyes. Repeat procedure with neck, chest, middle and hind quarters, finishing legs last. Allow pet to stand for 5 to 10 minutes. Rinse thoroughly. May be used daily or as directed by a veterinarian. If irritation develops, discontinue use and bathe pet with Davis Hypoallergenic Tearless Shampoo.

Caution(s): Rubber gloves are recommended when using Benzoyl Peroxide. Avoid contact with eyes or mucous membranes.

For external use only.

For veterinary use only.

Warning(s): Do not get shampoo into eyes.

Keep out of reach of children.

Presentation: 12 fl oz (355 mL) and 1 gallon (3.785 L).

Compendium Code No.: 11400051 Rev. 5/99

BETADINE® SOLUTION

Purdue Frederick **Surgical Preparation**

Antiseptic Microbicide

Active Ingredient(s): Povidone-iodine 5% — equal to 0.5% available iodine.

Inactive ingredients: citric acid, dibasic sodium phosphate, glycerin, nonoxynol-9, purified water.

Indications: Uses

- for preparation of the skin prior to surgery.
- helps to reduce bacteria that potentially can cause skin infection warnings.

Use full strength for:

- Preoperative prepping of skin and mucous membranes.
- Preventing bacterial infection.
- Emergency antisepsis of minor lacerations, abrasions, and burns.
- Postoperative application to surgical incisions.

Directions: Apply full strength, once or twice daily until healed, as a paint, wet soak or spray. May be covered with a gauze bandage.

Precaution(s): Avoid storing at excessive heat. Store in original container. Nonstaining to skin, hair and natural fabrics.

Caution(s): When using this product

- in pre-operative prepping, avoid "pooling" beneath the animal.
- prolonged exposure to wet solution may cause irritation or, rarely, severe skin reactions.
- do not heat prior to application

Stop using this product in rare instances of local irritation or sensitivity.

If swallowed, get medical help or contact a Poison Control Center right away.

External use only.

For professional and hospital veterinary use only.

Warning(s): Do not use this product on food-producing animals.

Keep out of reach of children.

Presentation: 16 oz. (NDC 0034-9100-88) and 32 oz. (NDC 0034-9100-90) plastic bottles with flip-up dispenser cap and 1 gallon plastic containers (NDC 0034-9100-01).

Compendium Code No.: 11370001

BETADINE® SURGICAL SCRUB

Purdue Frederick **Surgical Scrub**

Antiseptic Sudsing Skin Cleanser

Active Ingredient(s): Povidone-iodine, 7.5% — equal to 0.75% available iodine.

Inactive Ingredients: ammonium nonoxynol-4-sulfate, purified water.

Indications: Uses

for preparation of the skin prior to surgery.

- helps to reduce bacteria that potentially can cause skin infection.
- for handwashing to reduce bacteria on the skin.
- significantly reduces the number of microorganisms on the hands and forearms prior to surgery or patient care.

A Microbicidal Cleanser:

For the Veterinarian: Pre- and postoperative scrubbing and washing.

For the Animal: Preoperative prepping.

Directions:

A. Surgical hand scrub:

- wet hands with water.
- pour about 5 cc (1 teaspoonful) of Scrub on the palm of the hand and spread over both hands.
- without adding more water, scrub thoroughly for about five minutes.
- use a brush if desired. Clean thoroughly under fingernails.
- add a little water and develop copious suds. Rinse thoroughly under running water.
- repeat the entire procedure using another 5 cc of Scrub.

B. Patient pre-op skin preparation:

- after the surgical area is clipped, wet it with water.

- apply Scrub (1 cc is sufficient to cover an area of 20-30 square inches), develop lather and scrub thoroughly for about 5 minutes.
- rinse off using sterile gauze saturated with water.
- the area may then be painted with Betadine® Solution Veterinary and allowed to dry.

Precaution(s): Do not store at excessive heat.

Caution(s): For external use only.

Stop using this product and ask a doctor
- if irritation and redness develop.
- in rare instances of local irritation or sensitivity.

When using this product do not heat prior to application.

If swallowed, get medical help or contact a Poison Control Center right away.

For professional and hospital veterinary use only.

Warning(s): Do not use this product on food-producing animals.

Keep out of reach of children.

Presentation: 16 oz. (NDC 0034-9200-88) and 32 oz. (NDC 0034-9200-90) plastic bottles with flip-up dispenser cap and 1 gallon plastic containers (NDC 0034-9200-01).

Compendium Code No.: 11370011

BETAGEN™ OTIC SOLUTION ℞

Med-Pharmex **Otic Antimicrobial-Corticosteroid**

(Gentamicin Sulfate with Betamethasone Valerate)

ANADA No.: 200-183

Active Ingredient(s): Each mL of BETAGEN™ Otic Solution contains gentamicin sulfate equivalent to 3 mg gentamicin base, betamethasone valerate equivalent to 1 mg betamethasone, 1.0 mg hydroxyethylcellulose, 2.5 mg glacial acetic acid, 200 mg purified water, 19% ethanol, 9.4 mg benzyl alcohol as preservative, 300 mg glycerin and propylene glycol q.s.

Indications: BETAGEN™ Otic Solution is indicated for the treatment of acute and chronic canine otitis externa and canine and feline superficial infected lesions caused by bacteria sensitive to gentamicin.

Pharmacology: Gentamicin is a bactericidal antibiotic of the aminoglycoside group derived from *Micromonospora purpurea* of the *Actinomyces* group. It is a powder, white to buff in color, basic in nature, readily soluble in water and highly stable in solution.

Betamethasone valerate is a synthetic corticosteroid derivative of prednisolone.

BETAGEN™ Otic Solution combines the broad-spectrum activity of gentamicin sulfate with the anti-inflammatory and antipruritic activity of betamethasone valerate. *In vitro* antibacterial activity[1] has shown that gentamicin is active against most gram-negative bacteria including *Pseudomonas aeruginosa*, indole-positive and negative *Proteus* sp., *Escherichia coli, Klebsiella pneumoniae, Aerobacter aerogenes*, and *Neisseria*. Gentamicin is also active against strains of gram-positive bacteria including *Staphylococcus* species and some *Streptococcus* species.

Betamethasone valerate has emerged from intensive research as the most promising of some 50 newly synthesized corticosteroids in the experimental model described by McKenzie[2] *et al.* This human bioassay technique has been found reliable for evaluating the vasoconstrictor properties of new topical corticosteroids and is useful in predicting clinical efficacy.

Betamethasone valerate in human medicine has been shown to provide anti-inflammatory and antipruritic activity in the topical management of corticosteroid-responsive dermatoses. In the responsive cases, the local anti-inflammatory activity is sustained by the vasoconstrictor properties of the steroid.

Dosage and Administration: Duration of treatment will depend upon the severity of the condition and the response obtained. The duration of treatment and/or frequency of the dosage may be reduced, but care should be taken not to discontinue therapy prematurely.

Otitis externa: The external ear and ear canal should be properly cleaned and dried before treatment. Remove foreign material, debris, crusted exudates, etc., with suitable nonirritating solutions. Excessive hair should be clipped from the treatment area of the external ear. Instill 3 to 8 drops of BETAGEN™ Otic Solution (approximately room temperature) into the ear canal twice daily for seven to fourteen days.

Superficial infected lesions: The lesion and adjacent area should be properly cleaned before treatment. Excessive hair should be removed. Apply a sufficient amount of BETAGEN™ Otic Solution to cover the treatment area twice daily for seven to fourteen days.

Contraindication(s): If hypersensitivity to any of the components occurs, treatment with this product should be discontinued and appropriate therapy instituted.

Concomitant use of drugs known to induce ototoxicity should be avoided.

This preparation should not be used in conditions where corticosteroids are contraindicated.

Do not administer parenteral corticosteroids during treatment with BETAGEN™ Otic Solution.

Precaution(s): Store between 2°C and 25°C (36°F and 77°F).

Caution(s): Federal law restricts this drug to use by or on the order of a licensed veterinarian.

Clinical and experimental data have demonstrated that corticosteroids administered orally or parenterally to animals may induce the first stage of parturition when administered during the last trimester of pregnancy and may precipitate premature parturition followed by dystocia, fetal death, retained placenta, and metritis. Additionally, corticosteroids can induce cleft palates in offspring when given to pregnant animals during the period of palate closure of the embryos. Other congenital anomalies including deformed forelegs, phocomelia, and anasarca have been reported in offspring of dogs which received corticosteroids during pregnancy.

Avoid ingestion.

Before instilling any medication into the ear, examine the external ear canal thoroughly to be certain the tympanic membrane is not ruptured in order to avoid the possibility of transmitting infection to the middle ear as well as damaging the cochlea or vestibular apparatus from prolonged contact. If hearing or vestibular dysfunction is noted during the course of treatment, discontinue use of BETAGEN™ Otic Solution.

The antibiotic sensitivity of the pathogenic organism should be determined prior to the use of this preparation. Use of topical antibiotics occasionally allows overgrowth of non-susceptible bacteria, fungi, or yeasts. In these cases, treatment should be instituted with other appropriate agents as indicated.

Adverse systemic reactions have been observed following the oral ingestion of some topical corticosteroid preparations. Patients should be closely observed for the usual signs of adrenocorticosteroid overdosage which include sodium retention, potassium loss, fluid retention, weight gains, polydipsia and/or polyuria. Prolonged use or overdosage may produce adverse immunosuppressive effects.

Experimentally it has been demonstrated that corticosteroids, especially at high dosage levels, may result in delayed wound healing. An increase in the incidence of osteoporosis may be noted, mainly in the elderly, with prolonged use of these compounds. Their use in older dogs during the healing stages of bone fracture is not indicated for the reason listed above.

Use of corticosteroids, depending on dose, duration, and specific steroid, may result in inhibition of endogenous steroid production following drug withdrawal. In patients presently receiving or recently withdrawn from systemic corticosteroid treatments, therapy with a rapidly acting corticosteroid should be considered in unusually stressful situations.

For use in dogs and cats only.

Toxicology: Parenterally, no toxic effects were observed in rats given gentamicin sulfate 20 mg/kg/day for twenty-four days; in cats given 10 mg/kg/day for forty days. Gentamicin sulfate given to dogs at 6 mg/lb/day, 6 days weekly for three weeks, caused no detectable kidney damage. At higher doses, impairment of equilibrium and of renal function were observed in these species.

Subacute otic toxicity study in dogs showed gentamicin sulfate with betamethasone valerate solution to be well tolerated locally with no adverse systemic effects when administered 5 drops twice a day for 21 consecutive days.

Gentamicin sulfate solution in a 21-day subacute dermal toxicity study in dogs was shown to be well tolerated when applied topically to abraded skin. There were no meaningful findings except a reduction in eosinophil count attributable to absorption of the corticosteroid component.

Side Effects: Side, effects such as SAP and SGPT enzyme elevations, weight loss, anorexia, polydipsia, and polyuria have occurred following the use of parenteral or systemic synthetic corticosteroids in dogs. Vomiting and diarrhea (occasionally bloody) have been observed in dogs and cats.

Cushing's Syndrome in dogs has been reported in association with prolonged or repeated steroid therapy.

References: Available upon request.

Presentation: BETAGEN™ Otic Solution, squeeze bottles of 7.5 mL, 15 mL, and 240 mL (8 fl oz).

Compendium Code No.: 10270010

BETAGEN™ TOPICAL SPRAY ℞

Med-Pharmex **Topical Antimicrobial-Corticosteroid**

(Gentamicin Sulfate with Betamethasone Valerate)

ANADA No.: 200-188

Active Ingredient(s): Each mL contains: gentamicin sulfate equivalent to 0.57 mg gentamicin base, betamethasone valerate equivalent to 0.284 mg betamethasone, 163 mg isopropyl alcohol, propylene glycol, methylparaben and propylparaben as preservatives, purified water q.s. Hydrochloric acid may be added to adjust pH.

Indications: For the treatment of infected superficial lesions in dogs caused by bacteria sensitive to gentamicin.

Pharmacology: Gentamicin is a mixture of aminoglycoside antibiotics derived from the fermentation of *Micromonospora purpurea*. Gentamicin sulfate is a mixture of sulfate salts of the antibiotics produced in this fermentation. The salts are weakly acidic and freely soluble in water.

Gentamicin sulfate contains not less than 500 micrograms of gentamicin base per milligram.

Betamethasone valerate is a synthetic glucocorticoid.

Gentamicin, a broad-spectrum antibiotic, is a highly effective topical treatment for bacterial infections of the skin. *In vitro*, gentamicin is bactericidal against a wide variety of gram-positive and gram-negative bacteria isolated from domestic animals.[1,2] Specifically, gentamicin is active against the following organisms isolated from canine skin: *Alcaligenes* sp., *Citrobacter* sp., *Klebsiella* sp., *Pseudomonas aeruginosa*, indole-positive and negative *Proteus* sp., *Escherichia coli*, *Enterobacter* sp., *Staphylococcus* sp., and *Streptococcus* sp.

Betamethasone valerate emerged from intensive research as the most promising of some 50 newly synthesized corticosteroids in the experimental model described by McKenzie[3], *et al.* This human bioassay technique has been found reliable for evaluating the vasoconstrictor properties of new topical corticosteroids and is useful in predicting clinical efficacy.

Betamethasone valerate in veterinary medicine has been shown to provide anti-inflammatory and antipruritic activity in the topical management of corticosteroid responsive infected superficial lesions in dogs.

Dosage and Administration: Prior to treatment, remove excessive hair and clean the lesion and adjacent area. Hold bottle upright 3 to 6 inches from the lesion and depress the sprayer head twice. Administer 2 to 4 times daily for 7 days.

Each depression of the sprayer head delivers 0.7 mL of BETAGEN™ Topical Spray.

Contraindication(s): If hypersensitivity to any of the components occurs, treatment with this product should be discontinued and appropriate therapy instituted.

Precaution(s): Store upright between 2°C and 30°C (36°F and 86°F).

Caution(s): Federal law restricts this drug to use by or on the order of a licensed veterinarian.

Clinical and experimental data have demonstrated that corticosteroids administered orally or parenterally to animals may induce the first stage of parturition when administered during the last trimester of pregnancy and may precipitate premature parturition followed by dystocia, fetal death, retained placenta, and metritis.

Additionally, corticosteroids administered to dogs, rabbits and rodents during pregnancy have produced cleft palate. Other congenital anomalies including deformed forelegs, phocomelia, and anasarca have been reported in offspring of dogs which received corticosteroids during pregnancy.

Antibiotic susceptibility of the pathogenic organism(s) should be determined prior to the use of this preparation. Use of topical antibiotics may permit overgrowth of non-susceptible bacteria, fungi, or yeasts. If this occurs, treatment should be instituted with other appropriate agents as indicated.

Administration of recommended dose beyond 7 days may result in delayed wound healing. Animals treated longer than 7 days should be monitored closely.

Avoid ingestion. Oral or parenteral use of corticosteroids, depending on dose, duration, and specific steroid may result in inhibition of endogenous steroid production following drug withdrawal.

In patients presently receiving or recently withdrawn from systemic corticosteroid treatments, therapy with a rapidly acting corticosteroid should be considered in especially stressful situations.

If ingestion should occur, patients should be closely observed for the usual signs of adrenocorticoid overdosage which include sodium retention, potassium loss, fluid retention, weight gains, polydipsia, and/or polyuria. Prolonged use or overdosage may produce adverse immunosuppressive effects.

For topical use in dogs only.

Toxicology: Gentamicin sulfate with betamethasone valerate topical spray was well tolerated in an abraded skin study in dogs. No treatment-related toxicological changes in the skin were observed.

Systemic effects directly related to treatment were confined to histological changes in the adrenals, liver, and kidney and to organ-to-body weight ratios of adrenals. All were dose related, were typical for or not unexpected with corticosteroid therapy, and were considered reversible with cessation of treatment.

Side Effects: Side effects such as SAP and SGPT enzyme elevations, weight loss, anorexia, polydipsia, and polyuria have occurred following parenteral or systemic use of synthetic corticosteroids in dogs. Vomiting and diarrhea (occasionally bloody) have been observed in dogs.

Cushings syndrome in dogs has been reported in association with prolonged or repeated steroid therapy.

References: Available upon request.

Presentation: Plastic spray bottle containing 60 mL, 120 mL or 240 mL of BETAGEN™ Topical Spray.

Compendium Code No.: 10270001

BETASONE® ℞

Schering-Plough **Corticosteroid Injection**

(Betamethasone dipropionate and betamethasone sodium phosphate) Aqueous Suspension

NADA No.: 049-185

Active Ingredient(s): Each mL of BETASONE® Aqueous Suspension contains the equivalent of 5 mg betamethasone as betamethasone dipropionate and 2 mg betamethasone as betamethasone sodium phosphate, dibasic sodium phosphate 2 mg, sodium chloride 5 mg, edetate sodium 0.1 mg, polysorbate-80 0.5 mg, sodium carboxymethylcellulose 5 mg, benzyl alcohol 9 mg, methylparaben 1.8 mg and propylparaben 0.2 mg as preservatives, polyethylene glycol-4000 20 mg, hydrochloric acid to adjust pH to 7.2 in water for injection q.s.

Indications: BETASONE® Aqueous Suspension is recommended as an aid in the control of pruritus associated with dermatoses in the dog.

Pharmacology: BETASONE® Aqueous Suspension is a sterile parenteral combination of two esters of betamethasone. The highly soluble betamethasone sodium phosphate is in solution and is rapidly hydrolyzed within the body to provide prompt anti-inflammatory and antipruritic effects. Sustained anti-inflammatory and antipruritic activity is provided by the less soluble ester, betamethasone dipropionate which is in suspension in the formulation. Administration of the product containing the combined esters results in a rapid and continuous relief of pruritus associated with dermatoses.

Dosage and Administration: BETASONE® Aqueous Suspension should be administered aseptically by intramuscular injection. The usual recommended dose is 0.25-0.5 mL per 20 lbs. of body weight depending on the severity of the condition. The dose may be repeated when necessary.

The frequency of dosage depends upon the recurrence of pruritic symptoms. Clinical studies indicate that the relief of pruritus averaged three (3) weeks with a range of one (1) to six (6) weeks, and in many cases only one (1) injection was required. Therefore, the dosage may be repeated every three (3) weeks, or when symptoms recur, for a total of four (4) injections.

Contraindication(s): BETASONE® has a primarily glucocorticoid action and should not be used as replacement therapy when mineralocorticoid action is desired.

Corticosteroids are contraindicated in animals with acute or chronic bacterial infections unless therapeutic doses of an effective antimicrobial agent are used. BETASONE® like all corticosteroids, may mask the signs of infection such as elevation of temperature.

Although not absolute contraindications, caution should be taken in the administration of betamethasone to dogs with congestive heart failure, diabetes, and chronic nephritis.

Precaution(s): Shake well before using. Store between 2-30°C (36-86°F). Protect from light. Do not freeze.

Caution(s): Federal law restricts this drug to use by or on the order of a licensed veterinarian.

An increase in the incidence of osteoporosis may be noted, mainly in older dogs, with the prolonged use of corticosteroids. Their use in older dogs during the healing stages of bone fracture are not indicated.

The use of corticosteroids, depending upon dose duration, and specific steroid, may result in the inhibition of endogenous steroid production following drug withdrawal. In patients presently receiving or recently withdrawn from systemic corticosteroid treatments, therapy with a rapidly acting corticosteroid should be considered only in unusually stressful situations.

Warning(s): Clinical and experimental data have demonstrated that corticosteroids administered orally or parenterally to animals may induce the first stage of parturition when administered during the last trimester of pregnancy and may precipitate premature parturition followed by dystocia, fetal death, retained placenta and metritis.

Additionally, corticosteroids administered to dogs, rabbits, and rodents during pregnancy have produced cleft palate. Other congenital anomalies including deformed forelegs, phocomelia, and anasarca have been reported in the offspring of dogs which received corticosteroids during pregnancy.

Side Effects: For all the beneficial effects of the corticosteroids, one should be aware of the possible untoward reactions which may occur. BETASONE®, like cortisone and all other corticosteroid derivatives when given systemically, is capable of causing side effects, especially during long continued use and/or high dosage. Some of these are: suppression of inflammation, reduction of fever, increased protein degradation and its conversion to carbohydrate leading to a negative nitrogen balance, sodium retention and potassium diuresis, retardation of wound healing; lowered resistance to many infectious agents such as bacteria or fungi, reduction in numbers of circulating lymphocytes.

Side effects such as SAP and SGPT enzyme elevations, weight loss, anorexia, polydipsia, and polyuria have occurred following use of synthetic corticosteroids in dogs. Vomiting and diarrhea (occasionally blood) have been observed in dogs and cats.

Cushing's syndrome in dogs has been reported in association with prolonged or repeated steroid therapy.

Corticosteroids reportedly cause laminitis in horses.

Presentation: 5 mL multiple dose vials in packages of 6.

Compendium Code No.: 10470220

BEUTHANASIA®-D SPECIAL Ⓒ III

Schering-Plough **Euthanasia Agent**

Euthanasia Solution

NADA No.: 119-807

Active Ingredient(s): Description: A non-sterile solution containing pentobarbital sodium and phenytoin sodium as the active ingredients. Rhodamine B, a bluish-red fluorescent dye, is included in the formulation to help distinguish it from parenteral drugs intended for therapeutic use. Although this solution is not sterile, benzyl alcohol, a bacteriostat is included to retard the growth of microorganisms.

Each mL contains: active ingredients: 390 mg pentobarbital sodium (barbituric acid derivative), 50 mg phenytoin sodium; inactive ingredients: 10% ethyl alcohol, 18% propylene glycol, 0.003688 mg rhodamine B, 2% benzyl alcohol (preservative), purified water q.s. Sodium hydroxide and/or hydrochloric acid may be added to adjust pH.

Manufactured by a nonsterilizing process.

Indications: For use in dogs for humane, painless, and rapid euthanasia.

Pharmacology: Actions: BEUTHANASIA®-D Special contains two active ingredients which are chemically compatible but pharmacologically different. Each ingredient acts in such a manner so as to cause humane, painless, and rapid euthanasia. Euthanasia is due to cerebral death in conjunction with respiratory arrest and circulatory collapse. Cerebral death occurs prior to cessation of cardiac activity.

When administered intravenously, pentobarbital sodium produces rapid anesthetic action. There is a smooth and rapid onset of unconsciousness. At the lethal dose, there is depression of vital medullary respiratory and vasomotor centers.

When administered intravenously phenytoin sodium produces toxicity signs of cardiovascular collapse and/or central nervous system depression. Hypotension occurs when the drug is administered rapidly.

Pharmacodynamic Activity: The sequence of events leading to humane, painless, and rapid euthanasia following intravenous injection of BEUTHANASIA®-D Special is similar to that following intravenous injection of pentobarbital sodium, or other barbituric acid derivatives. Within seconds, unconsciousness is induced with simultaneous collapse of the dog. This stage rapidly progresses to deep anesthesia with concomitant reduction in the blood pressure. A few seconds later, breathing stops, due to depression of the medullary respiratory center; encephalographic activity becomes isoelectric, indicating cerebral death; and then cardiac activity ceases.

Phenytoin sodium exerts its effect during the deep anesthesia stage caused by the pentobarbital sodium. This ingredient, due to its cardiotoxic properties, hastens the stoppage of electrical activity in the heart.

Dosage and Administration: Dosage: Dogs, 1 mL for each 10 pounds of body weight.

Administration: Intravenous injection is preferred. Intracardiac injection may be made when intravenous injection is impractical, as in a very small dog, or in a comatose dog with impaired vascular functions. Good injection skill is necessary for intracardiac injection.

The calculated dose should be given in a single bolus injection.

For intravenous injection, a needle of sufficient gauge to ensure intravenous placement of the entire dose should be used. The use of a Luer-Lock® syringe is recommended to prevent accidental exposure due to needle/syringe separation.

Precaution(s): Store between 15° and 30°C (59° and 86°F).

Caution(s): Federal law restricts this drug to use by or on the order of a licensed veterinarian.

Caution should be exercised to avoid contact of the drug with open wounds or accidental self-inflicted injections. Keep out of reach of children. If eye contact, flush eyes with water and seek medical attention.

Euthanasia may sometimes be delayed in dogs with severe cardiac or circulatory deficiencies. This may be explained by the impaired movement of the drug to its site of action. An occasional dog may elicit reflex responses manifested by motor movement; however, an unconscious animal does not experience pain, because the cerebral cortex is not functioning.

When restraint may cause the dog pain, injury, or anxiety, or danger to the person making the injection, prior use of tranquilizing or immobilizing drugs may be necessary.

Warning(s): For canine euthanasia only. Must not be used for therapeutic purposes. Do not use in animals intended for food.

Presentation: BEUTHANASIA®-D Special is available in 100 mL multiple-dose vials, NDC 0061-0473-05.

Compendium Code No.: 10470231 81-482043

BICARBOJECT ℞

Vetus **Fluid Therapy**

Active Ingredient(s): BICARBOJECT is a sterile nonpyrogenic preparation of sodium bicarbonate ($NaHCO_3$) in water for injection.

Each mL contains:

Sodium bicarbonate (equal to 1 mEq/mL) .... 84 mg

Water for injection .... q.s.

The total osmolar concentration of the product is approximately 2,000 mOsm/L.

Preservatives have not been added.

Indications: Sodium bicarbonate is indicated in the treatment of metabolic acidosis which may be due to severe renal disease, uncontrolled diabetes, circulatory insufficiency due to shock or severe dehydration, cardiac arrest and severe primary lactic acidosis. Sodium bicarbonate is also indicated in severe diarrhea which is often accompanied by a significant loss of bicarbonate. Sodium bicarbonate 8.4% is indicated in the treatment of metabolic acidosis in cattle, horses, sheep, swine and dogs depending upon causative factor.

Sodium bicarbonate is useful in the treatment of metabolic acidosis due to a wide variety of causes. Sodium bicarbonate therapy increases plasma bicarbonate, buffers excess hydrogen ion concentration, raises blood pH and reverses the clinical manifestations of acidosis.

Dosage and Administration: Sodium bicarbonate 8.4% is injected intravenously. Caution should be taken in emergencies where very rapid infusion of large quantities of bicarbonate is indicated, such as in cardiac arrest. Sodium bicarbonate solutions are hypertonic and may produce an undesirable rise in plasma sodium concentration during the process of correction of metabolic acidosis. During cardiac arrest, however, the risks from acidosis exceed those of hypernatremia. In cattle and horses, 200 to 300 mL of 8.4% solution may be given undiluted by rapid infusion using a needle and syringe.

Sodium bicarbonate 8.4% solution is often added to other intravenous fluids for the less urgent forms of metabolic acidosis. The amount of bicarbonate to be given over a four (4) to eight (8) hour period is approximately 2 to 5 mEq per kg of body weight (1-2.5 mL/lb. body weight) depending upon the severity of the acidosis as judged by the lowering of total CO_2 content, blood pH and clinical condition of the animal.

Bicarbonate therapy should always be planned in a stepwise fashion since the degree of response from a given dose is not precisely predictable. Initially, an infusion of 2 to 5 mEq per kg of body weight over a period of four (4) to eight (8) hours will produce a measurable improvement in the abnormal acid-base status of the blood. Completion of therapy is dependent upon the clinical response of the animal. If severe symptoms have abated, then the frequency of administration and size of the dose should be reduced.

Contraindication(s): Sodium bicarbonate is contraindicated in animals losing chloride by vomiting and in animals receiving diuretics known to produce a hypochloremic alkalosis.

Precaution(s): Store at a temperature between 59°F-86°F (15°C-30°C).

The product is in a sterile single dose vial. Discard the unused portion after use. Do not use if the solution is hazy, cloudy or contains a precipitate.

Caution(s): Federal law restricts the drug to use by or on the order of a licensed veterinarian.

Bicarbonate therapy is directed at producing a substantial correction of low total CO_2 content and blood pH, but risks of over-dosage and alkalosis should be avoided. Repeated fractional doses and periodic monitoring by appropriate laboratory tests are therefore recommended to minimize the possibility of overdosage. Sodium bicarbonate addition to parenteral solutions containing calcium should be avoided except where compatibility has been previously established. Precipitation or haze may result from sodium bicarbonate-calcium admixtures, and the resulting solution should not be administered.

In case alkalosis occurs, the bicarbonate should be stopped and the animal managed according to the degree of alkalosis present. Sodium chloride injection (0.9%) may be given intravenously. Potassium chloride may be indicated if there is hypokalemia. Severe alkalosis may be accompanied by hyperirritability or tetany, and these symptoms may be controlled by calcium gluconate. An acidifying agent such as ammonium chloride may also be indicated in severe alkalosis.

For veterinary use only.

Warning(s): Keep out of the reach of children.

Presentation: 100 mL single dose vial (NDC 47611-652-82).

Compendium Code No.: 14440091

BIGELOIL®

W. F. Young **Counterirritant**

Active Ingredient(s): Thymol, menthol, methyl salicylate, capsicum, salicylic acid 0.65%, oils of juniper and pine, alcohol 75%.

Indications: BIGELOIL® is recommended as a rubbing application for sore knees, bucked shins, strained and wrenched tendons and other temporary injuries of this type.

As an antiseptic BIGELOIL® is useful in the field of superficial irritations and minor injuries to the skin.

Diluted with water BIGELOIL® makes a refreshing brace or body wash for tired overheated animals.

Directions for Use: For bruises, minor injuries, superficial wounds, pain and stiffness caused by exposure, sprains or strains use full strength applying liberally over the affected area and rubbing until dry. Repeat as necessary. For broken skin or irritations apply without rubbing. As a brace or body wash 2 or 3 ounces in a quart of tepid water.

Precaution(s): Keep away from open flame.

Caution(s): BIGELOIL® is a counter-irritant and should be kept away from eyes and mucous membrane. Discontinue if excessive irritation develops after use.

Warning(s): Restricted livestock drug. For external use only. Not for human use.

Keep out of reach of children.

Presentation: 16 oz, 32 oz and 128 oz.

Compendium Code No.: 10990210

BIGELOIL® 24-HOUR MEDICATED POULTICE

W. F. Young **Poultice**

Ingredient(s): Water, Bentonite, Kaolin, Isopropyl Alcohol, Glycerine, Boric Acid, Oils of Eucalyptus and Peppermint, Methyl Salicylate, Salicylic Acid, Tincture of Arnica, Thymol.

Indications: BIGELOIL® 24-Hour Medicated Poultice is a natural dual clay poultice that helps reduce pain and swelling which may be caused by overexertion in tendons, muscles and hooves.

Directions for Use: Apply directly to affected area ½-inch thick, extending over area to be covered. Promptly cover with a thick layer of absorbent cloth. For hooves, pack in around frog, and spread a layer over the sole and cover with paper. Removes easily with water.

Precaution(s): Avoid freezing.

Caution(s): For external use only. Use only as directed. Avoid contact with eyes and mucous membranes. If skin irritation develops or symptoms persist for more than 7 days, discontinue use. For severe injuries, consult a veterinarian. For animal use only.

Warning(s): Keep out of reach of children.

Presentation: 5 lb.

Compendium Code No.: 10990250 RM 346210

BIGELOIL® LIQUID GEL

W. F. Young **Liniment**

Topical Pain Relieving Gel

Active Ingredient(s):

Menthol 2.0%

Indications: A topical analgesic for temporary relief of aches and pains of muscles and joints associated with: Arthritis, Sprains, Strains, Bruises, Superficial wounds and Bucked shins.

Directions: Apply to the affected area three or more times per day. Rub until absorbed.

For faster relief, rub with hair and wrap lightly.

For minor cuts, scrapes or irritations, apply without rubbing.

Precaution(s): Keep away from open flame.

Caution(s): When Using This Product: Avoid contact with eyes and mucous membranes.

Stop Using this Product If: Skin irritation develops or symptoms persist for more than 10 days.

Do Not Use: On severe injuries, consult a veterinarian.

For external use only.

Warning(s): Keep out of reach of children.

Presentation: 14 fl oz (397 mL).

Compendium Code No.: 10990260 RM 342360-1

BIG PINE™

Intercon **Disinfectant**

EPA Reg. No.: 48211-11

Active Ingredient(s):

Pine oil	3.95%
Alkyl (C_{14}, 58%; C_{16}, 28%; C_{12}, 14%) dimethyl benzyl ammonium chloride	1.97%
Inert ingredients	94.08%
Total ingredients	100.00%

Indications: This product may be used for cleaning and deodorizing, one-step cleaning and disinfection, or disinfection of precleaned, nonporous, inanimate hard surfaces. This disinfectant is effective against a wide variety of gram-positive and gram-negative bacteria. it is also an excellent deodorant and is especially effective in controlling odors that are bacterial in origin.

This disinfectant is effective at 6 oz. per gallon against *Pseudomonas aeruginosa* PRD-10, *Salmonella choleraesuis* ATCC 10708, and *Staphylococcus aureus* ATCC 6538 when tested by the A.O.A.C. use dilution test method for precleaned, hard nonporous surfaces.

This disinfectant is also an effective virucide at 6 oz. per gallon for influenza virus, type A, Brazil on inanimate environmental surfaces.

This product may be used for cleaning and disinfecting hard, nonporous, inanimate environmental surfaces (glass, metal, glazed porcelain, linoleum, tile, smooth leather, vinyl, enameled and finished wood surfaces) on walls, floors, appliances and furnishings.

This disinfectant mixes with water to form clear, stable use solutions. Use solutions are noncorrosive and nonstaining to plastic, vinyl, synthetics, enamel, tile and most common metals. Has a pleasant pine odor.

Dosage and Administration:

General Classification: It is a violation of federal law to use the product in a manner inconsistent with its labeling.

Application Information: Select the proper dilution of this product for the required use from the directions below. Apply the use solution with a clean mop, sponge, cloth, squeegee, or mechanical scrubber.

Prepare fresh use solutions daily. Do not re-use solutions. Discard solutions when they become visibly soiled. For disinfection, thoroughly wet the surfaces to be treated. Surfaces must remain moist for at least 10 minutes to assure proper germicidal action.

Cleaning: To clean and deodorize or to preclean prior to disinfection. Depending on the soil level of the area to be cleaned, use 3 to 12 oz. of this product per gallon of water.

Disinfecting: Hospitals, veterinary clinics, nursing homes: Use 7½ oz. of this product per gallon of water (1 part to 16 parts water) for one-step cleaning and disinfection of areas with light to medium soil loads. For heavily soiled areas, preclean as described above and then disinfect with this product at 6 oz. per gallon (1 part to 20 parts water).

Industrial areas, restaurants, food and meat processing plants (nonfood processing areas), other nonmedical uses: Preclean surfaces. Then, disinfect with a solution of 4 oz. of this product in a gallon of water (1 part to 31 parts water). Alternatively, clean and disinfect in one operation using 7½ oz. of this product per gallon of water.

For mildew control: Follow directions for hospital disinfection. Repeat treatment every seven (7) days, or when new growth appears.

This product may be used through automatic floor scrubbing equipment.

This product must not be used on food contact surfaces.

Precaution(s): Store only in tightly closed, original container in a secure area inaccessible to children. Do not contaminate water, food, or feed by storage or disposal. Pesticide wastes are acutely hazardous. Improper disposal of excess pesticide, spray mixture, or rinsate is a violation of federal law. If these wastes cannot be disposed of by use according to label instructions, contact the nearest State Pesticide or Environmental Control Agency, or the hazardous waste representative at the nearest EPA Regional Office for guidance. Do not re-use empty container. Triple rinse empty container with water. Return metal drums to reconditioner or puncture and dispose of in a sanitary landfill or by other procedures approved by state and local authorities. Plastic containers may be disposed of in a sanitary landfill, incinerated or, if allowed by local authorities, by burning. If burned, stay out of smoke.

(If container is one gallon or less, use this container disposal statement: Do not re-use empty container. Rinse thoroughly before discarding in trash.)

Caution(s): Keep out of the reach of children.

Avoid contamination of food. Wear goggles or face mask and rubber gloves when handling.

Precautionary Statements: Hazard to Humans and Domestic Animals:

Practical Treatment (First Aid): In case of contact, immediately flush eyes or skin with plenty of water for at least 15 minutes. For eyes, call a physician. Remove and wash contaminated clothing before re-use.

If swallowed, drink promptly a large quantity of milk, raw egg whites, gelatin solution or, if these are not available, drink a large quantity of water. Avoid alcohol. Call a physician immediately.

Environmental Hazards: This product is toxic to fish. Do not discharge into lakes, streams, ponds, or public water unless in accordance with an NPDES permit.

Physical or Chemical Hazards: Do not use or store near heat or open flame.

Presentation: 4x1 gallon (3.785 L), 5 gallon containers, and 55 gallon drums.

Compendium Code No.: 10130000

BIMECTIN™ POUR-ON

Bimeda **Parasiticide-Topical**

(ivermectin)

ANADA No.: 200-219

Active Ingredient(s): Contains 5 mg ivermectin per mL.

Indications: BIMECTIN™ Pour-On at the recommended dose level of 500 mcg/kg is indicated for the effective control of these parasites.

Gastrointestinal Roundworms: *Ostertagia ostertagi* (including inhibited stage) (adults and L_4), *Haemonchus placei* (adults and L_4), *Trichostrongylus axei* (adults and L_4), *T. colubriformis* (adults and L_4), *Cooperia* spp (adults and L_4), *Strongyloides papillosus* (adults), *Oesophagostomum radiatum* (adults and L_4), *Trichuris* spp (adults).

Lungworms: *Dictyocaulus viviparus* (adults and L_4).

Cattle Grubs (parasitic stages): *Hypoderma bovis, H. lineatum.*

Mites: *Sarcoptes scabiei* var. *bovis.*

Lice: *Linognathus vituli, Haematopinus eurysternus, Damalinia bovis, Solenopotes capillatus.*

Horn Flies: *Haematobia irritans.*

Dosage and Administration:

Treatment for Cattle for Horn Flies: BIMECTIN™ Pour-On controls horn flies *(Haematobia irritans)* for up to 28 days after dosing. For best results, BIMECTIN™ Pour-On should be part of a parasite control program for both internal and external parasites based on the epidemiology of these parasites. Consult your veterinarian or an entomologist for the most effective timing of applications.

Dosage: The dose rate is 1 mL for each 22 lb of body weight. The formulation should be applied along the topline in a narrow strip extending from the withers to the tailhead.

Administration:

Measuring Cup (250 mL, 500 mL and 1 L bottles): The enclosed measuring cup is graduated in 5 mL increments. Each 5 mL will treat 110 lbs body weight. When body weight is between markings, use the next higher increment.

Applicator Gun* (3.785 L bottle): Because of the solvents used in BIMECTIN™ Pour-On, only the BIMECTIN™ applicator gun from Simcro Tech Limited, or equivalent, is recommended. Other applicators may exhibit compatibility problems, resulting in locking, incorrect dosage or leakage.

Insert the brass end of the draw tube into the larger hole on the back side of the cap with the stem.

Slide one of the coil springs over one end of the draw-off tubing. Attach that end of the draw-off tubing to the stem on the applicator gun and slide the spring up to the connection. Slide the other coil spring over the other end of the draw-off tubing and connect that end to the cap that has the stem. Slide the spring to the connection. Replace the shipping cap with the cap having the draw-off tubing attached. Tighten this draw-off cap and draw tube to the bottle.

Follow the applicator gun manufacturer's directions for priming the gun, adjusting the dose, and care of the applicator gun following use.

Weight	Dose
220 lb (100 kg)	10 mL
330 lb (150 kg)	15 mL
440 lb (200 kg)	20 mL
550 lb (250 kg)	25 mL
660 lb (300 kg)	30 mL
770 lb (350 kg)	35 mL
880 lb (400 kg)	40 mL
990 lb (450 kg)	45 mL
1100 lb (500 kg)	50 mL

*Additional Applicator Guns and Draw Tubes may be purchased from your Phoenix Pharmaceutical Distributor or through Phoenix Pharmaceutical, Inc.

When to Treat Cattle with Grubs: BIMECTIN™ Pour-On effectively controls all stages of cattle grubs. However, proper timing of treatment is important. For the most effective results, cattle should be treated as soon as possible after the end of the heel fly (warble fly) season. While this is not peculiar to ivermectin, destruction of *Hypoderma* larvae (cattle grubs) at the period when these grubs are in vital areas may cause undesirable host-parasite reactions. Killing *Hypoderma lineatum* when it is in the esophageal tissues may cause bloat; killing *H. bovis* when it is in the vertebral canal may cause staggering or paralysis. Cattle should be treated either before or after these stages of grub development.

Cattle treated with BIMECTIN™ Pour-On at the end of the fly season may be re-treated with BIMECTIN™ during the winter without danger of grub-related reactions. For further information and advice on a planned parasite control program, consult your veterinarian.

Safety: Studies conducted in the U.S.A. have demonstrated the safety margin for ivermectin. Based on plasma levels, the topically applied formulation is expected to be at least as well tolerated by breeding animals as is the subcutaneous formulation which had no effect on breeding performance.

Consult your veterinarian for assistance in the diagnosis, treatment and control of parasitism.

Precaution(s): Flammable! Keep away from heat, sparks, open flame, and other sources of ignition.

Store at controlled room temperature 15°-30°C (59°-86°F).

Store away from excessive heat (104°F/40°C) and protect from light.

Use only in well-ventilated areas or outdoors.

Close container tightly when not in use.

Cloudiness in the formulation may occur when BIMECTIN™ (ivermectin) Pour-On is stored at temperatures below 32°F. Allowing to warm at room temperature will restore the normal appearance without affecting efficacy.

Do not contaminate water by direct application or by the improper disposal of drug containers. Dispose of containers in an approved landfill or by incineration.

Caution(s): This product should not be applied to self or others because it may be irritating to human skin and eyes and absorbed through the skin. To minimize accidental skin contact, the user should wear a long-sleeved shirt and rubber gloves. If accidental skin contact occurs, wash immediately with soap and water. If accidental eye exposure occurs, flush eyes immediately with water and seek medical attention.

Cattle should not be treated when hair or hide is wet since reduced efficacy may be experienced.

Do not use when rain is expected to wet cattle within six hours after treatment.

This product is for application to skin surface only. Do not give orally or parenterally.

Antiparasitic activity of ivermectin will be impaired if the formulation is applied to areas of the skin with mange scabs or lesions, or with dermatoses or adherent materials, e.g., caked mud or manure.

Ivermectin has been associated with adverse reaction in sensitive dogs; therefore, BIMECTIN™ (ivermectin) Pour-On is not recommended for use in species other than cattle.

Consult your veterinarian for assistance in the diagnosis, treatment and control of parasitism.

Warning(s): Cattle must not be treated within 48 days of slaughter for human consumption. Because a withdrawal time in milk has not been established, do not use in female dairy cattle of breeding age.

Not for use in humans.

Keep this and all drugs out of the reach of children.

Presentation: 250 mL (8.5 fl oz) bottle, 500 mL (16.9 fl oz) bottle, 1 L (33.8 fl oz) bottle, 3.785 L (1 gal) bottle, 5 L bottle, or 25 L bottle.

Manufactured by: Phoenix Scientific, Inc., St. Joseph, MO 84503

Compendium Code No.: 13990050 Iss. 3-99

BIMESOL-R™ INJECTION ℞

Bimeda **Fluid Therapy**

Replacement Electrolytes-Sterile Solution-Nonpyrogenic

Active Ingredient(s): Each 100 mL Contains:

Sodium Chloride . . . . . 526 mg
Sodium Acetate . . . . . 222 mg
Sodium Gluconate . . . . . 502 mg
Potassium Chloride . . . . . 37 mg
Magnesium Chloride Hexahydrate . . . . . 30 mg

May contain hydrochloric acid or sodium hydroxide for pH adjustment.

Electrolytes per 1000 mL (not including ions for pH adjustment): Sodium 140 mEq; Potassium 5 mEq; Magnesium 3 mEq; Chloride 98 mEq; Acetate 27 mEq; Gluconate 23 mEq.

295 mOsm/Liter (Calc.)

pH 5.5-7.5 Isotonic

Contains no preservative.

Indications: BIMESOL-R™ is a sterile, nonpyrogenic solution of balanced electrolytes indicated for replacing acute losses of extracellular fluid and electrolytes, and for correcting moderate to severe acidosis.

Dosage and Administration: Contents or lesser amount as determined by a veterinarian as a single dose; usually 3-10% of body weight in 1-2 hours. For intravenous or subcutaneous use. Solution should be warmed to body temperature and administered slowly.

Precaution(s): Do not use this product if seal is broken or solution is not clear. If the entire contents are not used, discard unused portion. Additives may be incompatible. When introducing additives, use aseptic technique, mix thoroughly and do not store.

Protect from freezing.

Caution(s): Federal law restricts this drug to use by or on the order of a licensed veterinarian.

For animal use only.

Warning(s): Keep out of reach of children.

Presentation: 1000 mL (NDC# 61133-0106-0).

™ BIMESOL-R is a Trademark of Bimeda, Inc.

Manufactured by: Bimeda-MTC Animal Health Inc., Cambridge, Ontario, Canada N3C 2W4.

Compendium Code No.: 13990510 Iss. 8.00

B

BIOCAINE®

Tomlyn **Topical Anesthetic**

Active Ingredient(s):

Lidocaine 2.0%

Compounded in a vanishing lotion base containing urea, lanolin, myristalkonium chloride and quaternium-14, chloroxylenol, allantoin and denatonium benzoate (Bittran™ II).

Indications: A lotion formulated to soothe irritated skin and relieve pain associated with minor cuts, burns and abrasions on dogs and cats. The bitter component discourages pet from chewing on lesions.

Directions: Cleanse injured area thoroughly before applying BIOCAINE®. Apply daily until lesion is healed.

Precaution(s): Store at room temperature.

Caution(s): Consult your veterinarian if redness, irritation or swelling occurs or persists.

For external animal use only.

Keep out of reach of children and pets.

Presentation: 12 x 2 fl oz (59 mL) and 12 x 4 fl oz (118 mL).

Compendium Code No.: 11220010 092-1, 093-1

BIOCOM®

United **Bacterin-Toxoid-Vaccine**

Mink Enteritis Vaccine, Killed Virus-Clostridium botulinum Type C Bacterin-Toxoid

U.S. Vet. Lic. No.: 245

Active Ingredient(s): An inactivated vaccine which contains MEV types 1 and 2 and *Cl. botulinum* type C.

Preservatives: Gentamicin and thimerosal.

Indications: BIOCOM® is for use as an aid in the prevention of viral enteritis and botulism in healthy, susceptible mink.

Dosage and Administration: Inject 1 mL under the loose skin of the armpit of mink of at least six (6) weeks of age. For a proper suspension, shake before and occasionally during use. Revaccinate all adults at the time of kit vaccination.

Precaution(s): Store at 35-45°F (2-7°C).

Caution(s): Do not use as a diluent for live virus vaccines.

Use the entire contents when the container is first opened.

Consult a veterinarian or United Vaccines Inc. for an alternate vaccinating schedule and before using this vaccine on a farm where disease exists or has occurred in the last 18 months.

Presentation: 100 dose, 250 dose and 500 dose vials.

Compendium Code No.: 11040001

BIOCOM®-D

United **Bacterin-Toxoid-Vaccine**

Mink Distemper-Enteritis Vaccine, Modified Live and Killed Virus-Clostridium botulinum Type C Bacterin-Toxoid

U.S. Vet. Lic. No.: 245

Active Ingredient(s): The vaccine consists of two components: A freeze-dried distemper vaccine consisting of modified live canine distemper virus (Distemink®) and a liquid inactivated vaccine consisting of MEV types 1 and 2 and *Cl. botulinum* type C (Biocom®). The liquid is used to dissolve the Distemink®.

Preservatives: Gentamicin and thimerosal.

Indications: BIOCOM®-D is for use as an aid in the prevention of distemper, viral enteritis, and botulism in healthy, susceptible mink.

Dosage and Administration: Mixing of the Vaccines:

1. Do not mix the vaccines until ready to use.
2. Mix only one pair of vials at a time, and use the entire contents within two (2) hours.
3. Disinfect rubber stoppers with alcohol.
4. Using a sterile transfer needle, transfer the Biocom® into the bottle of Distemink®.
5. To do this, shake the Biocom® to obtain a uniform suspension. Insert the short end of the double-pointed transfer needle into the Biocom® and turn the bottle upside down; then, insert the other end of the transfer needle into the Distemink®. The Biocom® will be drawn into the Distemink® bottle by vacuum.
6. After all the Biocom® has been transferred, shake gently to suspend evenly.
7. Do not transfer the vaccine to other containers.

Use sharp, sterile needles and sterile syringes. Inject 1 mL under the loose skin of the armpit of mink of at least 10 weeks of age. For a proper suspension, shake before and occasionally during use. Revaccinate all adults at the time of kit vaccination.

Keep a record of brand name, quantity, serial number, expiration date, and place of purchase. Record the date of vaccination, the number, age and location of the mink.

Precaution(s): Store at 35-45°F (2-7°C).

Caution(s): Consult a veterinarian or United Vaccines Inc. for an alternate vaccinating schedule and before using the vaccine on a farm where disease exists or has occurred in the last 18 months or where earlier botulism protection is desired.

1. Burn the empty containers and any unused portion of the vaccine.
2. Syringes and reusable, stainless steel needles may be sterilized by boiling them in distilled water for 15 to 20 minutes. Do not disinfect them with chemicals as these can destroy the vaccine.
3. Incubating diseases (such as Aleutian disease), parasites, nutritional deficiencies (anemia), maternal antibodies and poor management practices (dehydration, adverse temperatures) will reduce the effectiveness of the vaccine.
4. If shock occurs after vaccination, use atropine sulfate or epinephrine.

5. Should disease occur in an unvaccinated herd, the losses may be minimized by promptly vaccinating those animals which are not showing signs of the disease. The best procedure is to first vaccinate the mink located the farthest distance from those showing symptoms. Care should be taken to use a sterile needle for each animal and to disinfect handling gloves as often as is practical. Consult a veterinarian regarding the treatment and handling of sick animals.
6. Animals infected, yet not showing signs of disease at the time of vaccination, will not be protected by the vaccine. Symptoms of the disease may continue to develop for as long as two months after vaccination.

Presentation: 100 dose and 250 dose vials.
Compendium Code No.: 11040011

BIOCOM®-DP

United **Bacterin-Toxoid-Vaccine**

Mink Distemper-Enteritis Vaccine, Modified Live and Killed Virus-Clostridium botulinum Type C-Pseudomonas aeruginosa Bacterin-Toxoid

U.S. Vet. Lic. No.: 245

Active Ingredient(s): The vaccine consists of two components: A freeze-dried distemper vaccine consisting of modified live canine distemper virus (Distemink) and a liquid inactivated vaccine consisting of MEV types 1 and 2, *Cl. botulinum* type C, and *Pseudomonas aeruginosa* serotypes 5, 6, and 7-8 (IATS). The liquid is used to dissolve the Distemink®.

Preservatives: Gentamicin and thimerosal.

Indications: BIOCOM®-DP is for use as an aid in the prevention of distemper, viral enteritis, botulism and Pseudomonas pneumonia in healthy, susceptible mink.

Dosage and Administration: Mixing of the Vaccines:
1. Do not mix the vaccines until ready to use.
2. Mix only one pair of vials at a time, and use the entire contents within two (2) hours.
3. Disinfect rubber stoppers with alcohol.
4. Using a sterile transfer needle, transfer the Biocom®-P into the bottle of Distemink®.
5. To do this, shake the Biocom®-P to obtain a uniform suspension. Insert the short end of the double-pointed transfer needle into the Biocom®-P and turn the bottle upside down; then, insert the other end of the transfer needle into the Distemink. The Biocom®-P will be drawn into the Distemink® bottle by vacuum.
6. After all the Biocom®-P has been transferred, shake gently to suspend evenly.
7. Do not transfer the vaccine to other containers.

Use sharp, sterile needles and sterile syringes. Inject 1 mL under the loose skin of the armpit of min ofk at least 10 weeks of age. For a proper suspension, shake before and occasionally during use. Revaccinate all adults at the time of kit vaccination.

Keep a record of brand name, quantity, serial number, expiration date, and place of purchase. Record the date of vaccination, the number, age and location of the mink.

Precaution(s): Store at 35-45°F (2-7°C).

Caution(s): Consult a veterinarian or United Vaccines Inc. for an alternate vaccinating schedule and before using the vaccine on a farm where disease exists or has occurred in the last 18 months or where earlier botulism protection is desired.
1. Burn the empty containers and any unused portion of the vaccine.
2. Syringes and reusable, stainless steel needles may be sterilized by boiling them in distilled water for 15 to 20 minutes. Do not disinfect them with chemicals as these can destroy the vaccine.
3. Incubating diseases (such as Aleutian disease), parasites, nutritional deficiencies (anemia), maternal antibodies and poor management practices (dehydration, adverse temperatures) will reduce the effectiveness of the vaccine.
4. If shock occurs after vaccination, use atropine sulfate or epinephrine.
5. Should disease occur in an unvaccinated herd, the losses may be minimized by promptly vaccinating those animals which are not showing signs of the disease. The best procedure is to first vaccinate the mink located the farthest distance from those showing symptoms. Care should be taken to use a sterile needle for each animal and to disinfect handling gloves as often as is practical. Consult a veterinarian regarding the treatment and handling of sick animals.
6. Animals infected, yet not showing signs of disease at the time of vaccination, will not be protected by the vaccine. Symptoms of the disease may continue to develop for as long as two months after vaccination.

Presentation: 100 dose and 250 dose vials.
Compendium Code No.: 11040021

BIOCOM®-P

United **Bacterin-Toxoid-Vaccine**

Mink Enteritis Vaccine, Killed Virus-Clostridium botulinum Type C-Pseudomonas aeruginosa Bacterin-Toxoid

U.S. Vet. Lic. No.: 245

Active Ingredient(s): An inactivated vaccine which contains MEV types 1 and 2 and *Cl. botulinum* type C and *Pseudomonas aeruginosa* serotypes 5, 6, and 7-8 (IATS).

Preservatives: Gentamicin and thimerosal.

Indications: BIOCOM®-P is for use as an aid in the prevention of viral enteritis, botulism and Pseudomonas pneumonia in healthy, susceptible mink.

Dosage and Administration: Inject 1 mL under the loose skin of the armpit of mink of at least six (6) weeks of age. For a proper suspension, shake before and occasionally during use. Revaccinate all adults at the time of kit vaccination.

Precaution(s): Store at 35-45°F (2-7°C).

Caution(s): Do not use as a diluent for live virus vaccines.

Use the entire contents when the container is first opened.

Consult a veterinarian or United Vaccines Inc. for an alternate vaccinating schedule and before using the vaccine on a farm where disease exists or has occurred in the last 18 months.

Presentation: 100 dose, 250 dose and 500 dose vials.
Compendium Code No.: 11040031

BIO-COX® 60 GRANULAR

Alpharma **Feed Medication**

Brand of salinomycin sodium-Type A Medicated Article

NADA No.: 128-686

Active Ingredient(s): Salinomycin equivalent to 60 grams salinomycin sodium activity per pound.

Indications: Broiler, roaster and replacement (breeder and layer) chickens: For the prevention of coccidiosis caused by *Eimeria tenella, E. necatrix, E. acervulina, E. maxima, E. brunetti* and *E. mivati.*

Quail: For the prevention of coccidiosis caused by *Eimeria dispersa* and *E. lettyae.*

Directions:

Broiler, roaster and replacement (breeder and layer) chickens: Use BIO-COX® 60 Granular to provide salinomycin sodium concentrations ranging from 40-60 g/ton (0.0044% to 0.0066%) for the prevention of coccidiosis in broiler, roaster and replacement chickens caused by *Eimeria tenella, E. necatrix, E. acervulina, E. maxima, E. brunetti* and *E. mivati.* The dosage should be adjusted to meet the severity of the coccidial challenge, which varies with environmental and management conditions.

Quail: Use BIO-COX® 60 Granular to provide salinomycin sodium concentration of 50 g/ton (0.0055%) for the prevention of coccidiosis in quail caused by *Eimeria dispersa* and *E. lettyae.*

Mixing directions: Thoroughly mix BIO-COX® 60 Granular with non-medicated feed to provide the level of salinomycin sodium per ton as indicated in the table below.

Salinomycin Sodium Activity	Amount of BIO-COX® 60 Granular Type A Medicated Article (60 g/lb) Per Ton of Feed	
(grams per ton)	lb	grams
40	0.67	304
45	0.75	341
50	0.83	377
55	0.92	418
60	1.00	454

Feeding Directions: Feed continuously as the sole ration.

Important: Must be thoroughly mixed in feeds before use. Not approved for use with pellet binders.

Precaution(s): Store in a cool, dry place.

Caution(s): May be fatal if fed to adult turkeys or to horses.

Warning(s): Do not feed to laying hens producing eggs for human consumption.

When mixing and handling BIO-COX® 60 Granular premix, use protective clothing, impervious gloves, eye protection, and an approved dust respirator. Operators should wash thoroughly with soap and water after handling. If accidental eye contact occurs, immediately rinse thoroughly with water.

For use in broiler, roaster, replacement (breeder and layer) chickens, and quail only.

For use in manufacturing medicated feeds only.

Presentation: 50 lb (22.68 kg) bag.
Compendium Code No.: 10220151

AHG-029 0103

BIODRES® WOUND DRESSING

DVM **Topical Wound Dressing**

Indications: A sterile biosynthetic absorbent wound dressing.

Dosage and Administration: Opening instructions for resealable ziplock pouch:
1. Tear off the top side of the ziplock pouch.
2. Pull open the ziplock pouch and remove a sterile dressing pack.
3. Immediately reseal the pouch by pressing along the ziplock.

Instructions for the use of BIODRES® Wound Dressing:
1. Peel open the sterile dressing pack and remove BIODRES using aseptic technique.
2. Hold BIODRES by overlapping the edges and remove the blue film liner only. Discard the blue liner.
3. Apply the uncovered (hydrogel) side to the wound. Allow BIODRES to overlap intact skin.
4. Secure BIODRES by covering with a piece of gauze or a wrap bandage.
5. Change BIODRES every 48 hours, or as often as necessary until the wound is healed.
6. Gently cleanse the wound prior to the application of fresh BIODRES.

Caution(s): For animal use only.

Presentation: 4" X 4" (10.2 cm sq.), box of 12.
Compendium Code No.: 11420050

BIODRY®

Pharmacia & Upjohn **Mastitis Therapy**

brand of novobiocin suspension

NADA No.: 102-511

Active Ingredient(s): Description: Each 10 mL Plastet® Disposable Syringe contains:
Novobiocin sodium.......... 400 mg
Chlorobutanol anhydrous (chloral derivative—used as a preservative)........ 50 mg

In a special bland vehicle.

Manufactured by a non-sterilizing process.

Indications: BIODRY® Suspension is indicated for the treatment, in dry cows only, of mastitis caused by susceptible strains of *Staphylococcus aureus* and *Streptococcus agalactiae.*

Dosage and Administration:

Dosage: Infuse one tube per quarter at start of dry period (but not less than 30 days prior to calving).

Shake well before using.

Directions for Using the Flexi-Tube® System: The Flexi-Tube® is designed to provide the choice of either insertion of the full cannula, as has traditionally been practiced, or insertion of no more than ⅛ inch of the cannula, as recommended by the National Mastitis Council.

a. Full Insertion: Remove the blue end cap by pulling straight up as shown. Gently insert the full cannula into the teat canal; carefully infuse the product.

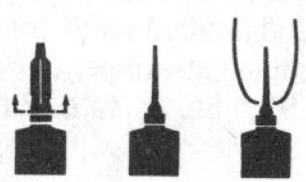

b. Partial Insertion: Remove both the blue end cap and the red cannula by pushing sideways as shown. Gently insert the exposed blue tip into the teat canal; carefully infuse the product.

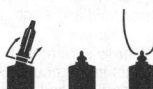

Administration: At the time of drying off, but not less than 30 days prior to calving, milk the udder dry. Wash the teats and udder thoroughly with warm water containing a suitable dairy antiseptic. Dry the teats and udder thoroughly. Infuse each quarter using the following procedure. Using the alcohol pads provided, wipe each teat end clean using a separate pad for each teat. Warm BIODRY® Suspension to body temperature and shake thoroughly. Choose the desired insertion length (full or partial) and insert tip into teat canal. Instill entire contents into the quarter. Massage the udder after treatment to distribute the BIODRY® throughout the quarters. Using a suitable teat dip, dip all teats following treatment.

Precaution(s): Storage Conditions: Store at controlled room temperature 20° to 25°C (68° to 77°F) [see USP].

Discard empty container; Do not reuse.

Caution(s): Administration of this product in any manner other than shown under Dosage may result in drug residues.

For udder instillation in dry cows only.

For use in animals only — Not for human use.

Restricted Drug — Use only as directed (California).

Keep out of reach of children.

Warning(s):

1. Do not use less than 30 days prior to calving.
2. Treated animals must not be slaughtered for human consumption for 30 days following udder infusion.

Presentation: BIODRY® Suspension is available in unbroken packages of 12-10 mL Plastet® Disposable Syringes with 12 individually wrapped 70% isopropyl alcohol pads (NDC 0009-0924-10).

Compendium Code No.: 10490061 810 920 210

BIO GUARD® SHAMPOO

Farnam **Grooming Shampoo**

Indications: BIO GUARD®'s gentle, water-based formula lathers up quickly, rinses out easily, yet won't wash out the protection of your pet's flea and tick control. Non-irritating, pH-balanced formula cleans and conditions the coat and leaves a fresh, clean scent. Safe for dogs, cats, kittens and puppies of all ages.

Safe for people, too.

Also for use as a regular grooming shampoo.

Use with Bio Spot®, Advantage®, Frontline®, FleaTrol™ and Onespot™ flea and tick control treatments.

Won't wash out spot-on flea and tick protection.

Directions:

1. Wet pet thoroughly with warm water.
2. Work shampoo well into coat.
3. Rinse pet thoroughly and towel dry.

Note: When washing puppies and kittens, towel dry them immediately after rinsing to prevent a chill.

Precaution(s): Keep from freezing.

Caution(s): Not for internal use.

Warning(s): Keep out of reach of children.

Presentation: 12 fl oz (355 mL) and 1 gallon (3.785 L).

Bio Spot® is a registered trademark of Farnam Companies, Inc.; FleaTrol™ is a trademark of Wellmark International; Onespot™ is a trademark of the Hartz Mountain Corporation; Advantage® is a registered trademark of Bayer Corporation; and Frontline® is a registered trademark of Merial.

Compendium Code No.: 10001000 0A1 / 0CC0

BIO-HEV™

Intervet **Vaccine**

Hemorrhagic Enteritis Vaccine, Live Virus

U.S. Vet. Lic. No.: 286

Contents: BIO-HEV™ contains lyophilized, live pheasant origin avian adenovirus II.

Indications: The vaccine has been shown effective in preventing clinical hemorrhagic enteritis in growing turkeys.

Dosage and Administration: Method of Preparation of the Vaccine:

1. Match the dose size of container to the number of birds to be vaccinated.
2. The vaccine should be rehydrated with chlorine-free water (e.g. distilled or powdered milk solution) prior to mixing.
   a. Remove the metal cap.
   b. Remove the rubber stopper and add about one-half (½) teaspoon (4 mL) of water.
   c. Replace the rubber stopper and agitate contents.
3. Add the contents of the vial(s) to the mixing container.
4. Rinse the vaccine container(s) once.
5. Agitate the vaccine contained in the mixing tank to obtain a uniform concentration of virus.
6. Proceed immediately to vaccinate the flock.

Method of Vaccination:

1. All birds should be vaccinated by oral administration at 28 to 35 days of age.
2. Remove chlorinated water for 48 hours prior to vaccination.
3. Use powdered milk in the water the day preceding vaccination at the rate of one (1) cup per 25 gallons of water.
4. By 6 a.m. on the day of vaccination, raise waterers above bird height. All water must be removed from drinkers and overhead lines.
5. Withhold water for one (1) to two (2) hours before vaccination depending upon the temperature.
6. Room temperature should be around 80°F. Overhead fans may be turned off during vaccination to increase thirst in the flock.
7. Mix vaccine in large barrels or use a proportioner. Use powdered milk at the rate of one (1) cup per 25 gallons of water along with the vaccine when mixing in barrels. When using a proportioner, the stock solution should be sufficient to provide dosing for over two (2) to three (3) hours.
8. Use approximately 10 gallons of water per 1,000 birds. This should require two (2) to three (3) hours to consume.
9. Stir the vaccine solution before filling each bucket.
10. Keep the birds active to stimulate drinking.
11. Keep the waterers out of direct sunlight.

Precaution(s): Store vaccine at not over 45°F or 7°C.

Use the entire contents when first opened.

Burn the vaccine container and all unused contents.

Caution(s):

1. BIO-HEV™ is to be used in turkeys only.
2. The flock should appear clinically healthy before vaccinating.
3. Other infections, notably respiratory diseases, can increase the likelihood of adverse reactions.
4. Optimum results are obtained when the vaccine is given to turkeys at 28 to 35 days of age through the drinking water.
5. Water should be withheld long enough prior to vaccination to cause a mild to moderate thirst in the turkeys.
6. A bucket or proportioner may be used to deliver the vaccine.
7. The water must be free of chlorine, iodine, disinfectants or medications that could inactivate the virus.
8. Vaccination is dependent upon the birds ingesting enough live virus to produce a mild infection.
9. Do not use more vaccine than recommended because this will increase the risk of an adverse reaction.
10. Do not use any other vaccine for one to two weeks after giving H.E. Vaccine.
11. In six to seven days after vaccination, a mild reaction to the virus may be observed.
12. Follow all directions closely.

Warning(s): Do not vaccinate within 21 days before slaughter.

Presentation: Each box of vaccine contains 10 vials of vaccine (1,000 or 5,000 doses per vial), and a directions for use circular.

Compendium Code No.: 11060141

BIO-HOOF™

Horses Prefer **Equine Dietary Supplement**

Guaranteed Analysis:

	Per oz.	Per lb.
Biotin	20 mg	320 mg
Pyridoxine (Vit. B_6)	30 mg	480 mg
Vitamin A	14,250 IU	228,000 IU
Vitamin D_3	3,875 IU	62,000 IU
Vitamin E	125 IU	2,000 IU
Lysine	190 mg	3.04 gm
Methionine	85 mg	1.36 gm
Zinc	85 mg	1.36 gm

Ingredients: Corn Distiller Solubles, Wheat Middlings, Yeast Culture, Dried Molasses, Vitamin A Acetate (stability improved), D-activated Animal Sterol (Source of Vitamin D_3), DL- alpha tocopheryl Acetate (source of Vitamin E), Pyridoxine Hydro Chloride, Biotin, L-Methionine, L-Lysine, Zinc Sulfate, Zinc Methionine, Oil and Apple Flavor.

Indications: Suggested Use: BIO-HOOF™ is carefully formulated to help support hoof strength and condition, maintain normal hoof growth and promote normal hair growth.

Directions: Feeding Directions: Feed 1 ounce of BIO-HOOF™ daily for every 1,000 lbs. of body weight. Close container after each use.

Caution(s): For animal use only.

Warning(s): Keep out of reach of children.

Presentation: 5 lbs. (2.27 g).

Compendium Code No.: 36950011

BIOLYTE®

Pharmacia & Upjohn **Electrolytes-Oral**

Calf Electrolyte Formula

Active Ingredient(s): Contains: Dextrose anhydrous, sodium bicarbonate, sodium chloride, potassium chloride, magnesium sulfate anhydrous.

Each 110 gram packet of BIOLYTE® Calf Electrolyte Formula contains: dextrose anhydrous, sodium bicarbonate, sodium chloride, potassium chloride, magnesium sulfate anhydrous. Each packet provides: sodium, 184.25 mEq; potassium, 31.35 mEq; magnesium, 9.1 mEq; bicarbonate, 111.38 mEq; chloride, 104.23 mEq; dextrose, 93.5 grams.

Each 800 gram bottle of BIOLYTE® Calf Electrolyte Formula contains: dextrose anhydrous, sodium bicarbonate, sodium chloride, potassium chloride, magnesium sulfate anhydrous. Each 80 grams of BIOLYTE® provides: sodium, 134.0 mEq; potassium, 22.8 mEq; magnesium, 6.6 mEq; bicarbonate, 81.0 mEq; chloride, 75.8 mEq; dextrose, 68 grams.

Each 9600 gram pail of BIOLYTE® Calf Electrolyte Formula contains: dextrose anhydrous, sodium bicarbonate, sodium chloride, potassium chloride, magnesium sulfate anhydrous. Each 80 grams of BIOLYTE® provides: sodium, 134.0 mEq; potassium, 22.8 mEq; magnesium, 6.6 mEq; bicarbonate, 81.0 mEq; chloride, 75.8 mEq; dextrose, 68 grams.

Indications: Indicated for oral use for nutritional support and re-establishment and maintenance of electrolyte balance in neonatal calves.

Dosage and Administration: Preparation of Solution:

3.85 oz (110 grams): Dissolve one packet of BIOLYTE® Calf Electrolyte Formula in water and dilute to a total volume of 1 quart.

28 oz (800 gm) and 21 lbs (9600 grams): Dissolve 80 grams (⅓ cup)* BIOLYTE® Calf Electrolyte Formula in water and dilute to a total volume of 1 quart or dissolve 240 grams (1 cup) of BIOLYTE® in water and dilute to a total volume of 3 quarts.

*Enclosed dose cup measures 80 grams (⅓ cup) at the recess marks.

Administer the solution by feeding or drench at the rate of 1 quart per 60 pounds bodyweight 3-4 times daily for 2 days as the only source of oral fluids. For the following 2 days the solution should be diluted 1:1 with milk replacer and given at feeding time.

Precaution(s): Avoid exposure to excessive heat.

Keep container tightly closed.

Store in a dry place.

Warning(s): For use in animals only.

Not for human use.

Presentation: 3.85 oz (110 grams) packets (NDC 0009-3281-08), 28 oz (800 gm) bottles (NDC 0009-3281-05) and 21 lb (9600 gram) pails (NDC 0009-3281-06).

Compendium Code No.: 10490071 814 359 002 / 813 166 210 / 813 801 208

B

BIO-METH

Vet-A-Mix **Equine Dietary Supplement**

Active Ingredient(s): Guaranteed Analysis:

	Per 400 g
D-biotin	900 mg (0.225%)
DL-methionine	300,000 mg (75.0%)

Ingredients: DL-methionine, D-biotin, roughage products, calcium carbonate, and mineral oil.

Indications: For use as a nutritional supplement in horses when biotin and methionine deficiencies exist.

Dosage and Administration: The usual dose for a 1,000 to 1,200 lb. (500 kg) horse is 15 mg of D-biotin and 5 g of DL-methionine (2 slightly rounded teaspoonfuls) per day. For heavier horses, double the above dosage. The dosage for ponies is one (1) slightly rounded teaspoonful per day. Supplementation may be necessary for six (6) to nine (9) months.

BIO-METH can be administered by mixing the daily dose in the concentrate or by top dressing on grain, preferably rolled or ground. To facilitate the proper adhesion of BIO-METH to the ration, slightly moisten the grain with water or a liquid supplement.

Note: One (1) slightly rounded teaspoonful of BIO-METH weighs approximately 3.3 g and contains 7.5 mg of D-biotin and 2.5 g DL-methionine.

Precaution(s): Store at room temperature and protect from light. Avoid excessive heat (104°F).

Caution(s): Keep out of the reach of children.

Presentation: 400 g and 2,000 g bottles. A teaspoon measure is enclosed in each package of BIO-METH.

Compendium Code No.: 10500011

BIOMOX® ORAL SUSPENSION ℞

Delmarva **Amoxicillin Oral**

Amoxicillin

NADA No.: 065-495

Active Ingredient(s): Contains 0.75 g or 1.5 g of amoxicillin activity. After reconstitution with the required amount of water, each mL will contain 50 mg of amoxicillin as the trihydrate.

Indications: BIOMOX® (amoxicillin) oral suspension is indicated in the treatment of the following infections in dogs when caused by susceptible strains of organisms:

Bacterial dermatitis due to *Staphylococcus aureus, Streptococcus* spp., *Staphylococcus* spp., and *E. coli.*

Soft tissue infections (abscesses, wounds, lacerations) due to *Staphylococcus aureus, Streptococcus* spp., *E. coli, Proteus mirabilis* and *Staphylococcus* spp.

As is true with all antibiotic therapy, appropriate *in vitro* cultures and sensitivities should be conducted prior to treatment.

Pharmacology: BIOMOX® (amoxicillin) is a broad-spectrum, semisynthetic antibiotic which provides bactericidal activity against a wide range of common gram-positive and gram-negative pathogens. Amoxicillin chemically is D-(-)a-amino-p-hydroxybenzyl penicillin trihydrate.

Amoxicillin has bactericidal activity against susceptible organisms similar to that of ampicillin. It acts by inhibiting the biosynthesis of bacterial cell wall mucopeptide. Most strains of the following gram-positive and gram-negative bacteria have demonstrated susceptibility to amoxicillin, both *in vitro* and *in vivo:* Non-penicillinase-producing staphylococci, alpha- and beta-hemolytic streptococci, *Streptococcus faecalis, Escherichia coli* and *Proteus mirabilis.* Amoxicillin does not resist destruction by penicillinase; therefore, it is not effective against penicillinase-producing bacteria, particularly resistant staphylococci. Most strains of Enterobacter and Klebsiella and all strains of Pseudomonas are resistant.

Amoxicillin may be given without regard to meals because it is stable in gastric acid. It is rapidly absorbed following oral administration and diffuses readily into most body fluids and tissues. It diffuses poorly into the brain and spinal fluid except when the meninges are inflamed. Most of amoxicillin is excreted in the urine unchanged.

Dosage and Administration: The recommended dosage is 5 mg per pound of body weight administered twice a day for five (5) to seven (7) days. Continue for 48 hours after all symptoms have subsided. If improvement is not noted within five (5) days, the diagnosis should be reconsidered and therapy changed.

Directions for Mixing Oral Suspension: Add sufficient water to the bottle as indicated in the table below and shake vigorously. Each mL of suspension will contain 50 mg of amoxicillin as the trihydrate.

Bottle Size	Amount of water to add for reconstitution
15 mL	11 mL
30 mL	21 mL

Note: When stored at room temperature or in a refrigerator, discard the unused portion of the reconstituted suspension after 14 days.

Contraindication(s): The use of amoxicillin is contraindicated in animals with a history of an allergic reaction to penicillin.

Precaution(s): Until adequate reproductive studies are accomplished, BIOMOX® (amoxicillin) oral suspension should not be used in pregnant or breeding animals.

Caution(s): Federal law restricts this drug to use by or on the order of a licensed veterinarian.

Warning(s): For use in dogs only.

Side Effects: Amoxicillin is a semisynthetic penicillin and,therefore, has the potential for producing allergic reactions. Epinephrine and/or steroids should be administered if an allergic reaction occurs.

Presentation: 15 mL bottles of 0.75 g amoxicillin activity and 30 mL bottles of 1.5 g amoxicillin activity.

Compendium Code No.: 14260000

BIOMOX® TABLETS ℞

Delmarva **Amoxicillin Oral**

Amoxicillin

NADA No.: 065-492

Active Ingredient(s): Each tablet contains:

Amoxicillin	50 mg
Amoxicillin	100 mg
Amoxicillin	200 mg
Amoxicillin	400 mg

Indications: BIOMOX® (amoxicillin) tablets are indicated in the treatment of the following infections in dogs when caused by susceptible strains of organisms:

Bacterial dermatitis due to *Staphylococcus aureus, Streptococcus* spp., *Staphylococcus* spp., and *E. coli.*

Soft tissue infections (abscesses, wounds, lacerations) due to *Staphylococcus aureus, Streptococcus* spp., *E. coli, Proteus mirabilis* and *Staphylococcus* spp.

As is true with all antibiotic therapy, appropriate *in vitro* cultures and sensitivities should be conducted prior to treatment.

Pharmacology: BIOMOX® (amoxicillin) is a broad-spectrum, semisynthetic antibiotic which provides bactericidal activity against a wide range of common gram-positive and gram-negative pathogens. Amoxicillin chemically is D-(-)a-amino-p-hydroxybenzyl penicillin trihydrate.

Amoxicillin has bactericidal activity against susceptible organisms similar to that of ampicillin. It acts by inhibiting the biosynthesis of bacterial cell wall mucopeptide. Most strains of the following gram-positive and gram-negative bacteria have demonstrated susceptibility to amoxicillin, both *in vitro* and *in vivo:* Non-penicillinase-producing staphylococci, alpha- and beta-hemolytic streptococci, *Streptococcus faecalis, Escherichia coli* and *Proteus mirabilis.* Amoxicillin does not resist destruction by penicillinase; therefore, it is not effective against penicillinase-producing bacteria, particularly resistant staphylococci. Most strains of Enterobacter and Klebsiella and all strains of Pseudomonas are resistant.

Amoxicillin may be given without regard to meals because it is stable in gastric acid. It is rapidly absorbed following oral administration and diffuses readily into most body fluids and tissues. It diffuses poorly into the brain and spinal fluid except when the meninges are inflamed. Most of amoxicillin is excreted in the urine unchanged.

Dosage and Administration: The recommended dosage is 5 mg per pound of body weight administered twice a day for five (5) to seven (7) days or for 48 hours after all symptoms have subsided. If improvement is not noted within five (5) days, the diagnosis should be reconsidered and therapy changed.

Contraindication(s): The use of amoxicillin is contraindicated in animals with a history of an allergic reaction to penicillin.

Precaution(s): Until adequate reproductive studies are accomplished, BIOMOX® (amoxicillin) tablets should not be used in pregnant or breeding animals.

Caution(s): Federal law restricts this drug to use by or on the order of a licensed veterinarian.

Warning(s): For use in dogs only.

Side Effects: Amoxicillin is a semisynthetic penicillin and, therefore, has the potential for producing allergic reactions. Epinephrine and/or steroids should be administered if an allergic reaction occurs.

Presentation: 50 mg, 100 mg, and 200 mg: Bottles of 500 and 1,000 tablets.
400 mg: Bottles of 250 and 500 tablets.

Compendium Code No.: 14260010

BIO-MYCIN® 200

Boehringer Ingelheim **Oxytetracycline Injection**

(Oxytetracycline) Injection Antibiotic

ANADA No.: 200-008

Active Ingredient(s): BIO-MYCIN® 200 (oxytetracycline injection) is a sterile, ready-to-use solution of the broad spectrum antibiotic oxytetracycline by injection. Each mL contains 200 mg of oxytetracycline base as oxytetracycline amphoteric; magnesium oxide 1.7% w/v; sodium formaldehyde sulfoxylate 0.5% w/v; polyethylene glycol 400 30% w/v; monoethanolamine to adjust pH; water for injection USP qs.

Indications: For the treatment of disease in beef cattle, non-lactating dairy cattle and swine.

BIO-MYCIN® 200 is intended for use in the treatment of the following diseases in beef cattle, non-lactating dairy cattle and swine when due to oxytetracycline-susceptible organisms:

Cattle: In cattle, BIO-MYCIN® 200 is indicated in the treatment of pneumonia and shipping fever complex associated with *Pasteurella* spp. and *Hemophilus* spp.; infectious bovine keratoconjunctivitis (pinkeye) caused by *Moraxella bovis;* footrot and diphtheria caused by *Fusobacterium necrophorum;* bacterial enteritis (scours) caused by *Escherichia coli;* wooden tongue caused by *Actinobacillus lignieresii;* leptospirosis caused by *Leptospira pomona;* and wound infections and acute metritis caused by strains of staphylococci and streptococci organisms sensitive to oxytetracycline.

Swine: In swine, BIO-MYCIN® 200 is indicated in the treatment of bacterial enteritis (scours, colibacillosis) caused by *Escherichia coli;* pneumonia caused by *Pasteurella multocida;* and leptospirosis caused by *Leptospira pomona.*

In sows, BIO-MYCIN® 200 is indicated as an aid in the control of infectious enteritis (baby pig scours, colibacillosis) in suckling pigs caused by *Escherichia coli.*

Dosage and Administration: Read entire insert carefully before using this product.

Cattle: BIO-MYCIN® 200 is to be administered by intramuscular, subcutaneous, or intravenous injection to beef cattle and non-lactating dairy cattle.

A single dosage of 9 milligrams of BIO-MYCIN® 200 per pound of body weight administered intramuscularly or subcutaneously is recommended in the treatment of the following conditions: 1) bacterial pneumonia caused by *Pasteurella* spp. (shipping fever) in calves and yearlings, where retreatment is impractical due to husbandry conditions, such as cattle on range, or where their repeated restraint is inadvisable; 2) infectious bovine keratoconjuctivitis (pinkeye) caused by *Moraxella bovis.*

Cattle Dosage Guide: At the first signs of pneumonia or pinkeye* administer a single dose of BIO-MYCIN® 200 by deep intramuscular injection or subcutaneous injection according to the following weight categories**:

Animal weight (lb)	Number of mL or cc
100	4.5
200	9.0
300	13.5
400	18.0
500	22.5
600	27.0
700	31.5
800	36.0
900	40.5
1000	45.0
1100	49.5
1200	54.0

*See package insert for dosing instructions for other indicated diseases and full product information.

**Do not administer more than 10 mL at any one injection site (1 to 2 mL per site in small calves).

BIO-MYCIN® 200 can also be administered by intravenous, subcutaneous, or intramuscular injection at a level of 3 to 5 milligrams of oxytetracycline per pound of body weight per day. In the treatment of severe footrot and advanced cases of other indicated diseases, a dosage level of 5 milligrams per pound of body weight per day is recommended. Treatment should be continued 24 to 48 hours following remission of disease signs; however, not to exceed a total of four consecutive days. Consult your veterinarian if improvement is not noted within 24 to 48 hours of the beginning of treatment.

Swine: In swine a single dosage of 9 milligrams of BIO-MYCIN® 200 per pound of body weight administered intramuscularly is recommended in the treatment of bacterial pneumonia caused by *Pasteurella multocida* in swine, where retreatment is impractical due to husbandry conditions or where repeated restraint is inadvisable.

Swine Dosage Guide: At the first signs of pneumonia* administer a single dose of BIO-MYCIN® 200 by deep intramuscular injection according to the following weight categories**:

Animal weight (lb)	Number of mL or cc
10	0.5
25	1.1
50	2.3
75	3.4
100	4.5
125	5.6
150	6.8
175	7.9
200	9.0
225	10.1
250	11.3
275	12.4
300	13.5
325	14.6

*See package insert for dosing instructions for other indicated diseases and full product information.

**Do not administer more than 5 mL at any one injection site.

BIO-MYCIN® 200 can also be administered by intramuscular injection at a level of 3 to 5 milligrams of oxytetracycline per pound of body weight per day.

Treatment should be continued 24 to 48 hours following remission of disease signs; however, not to exceed a total of four consecutive days. Consult your veterinarian if improvement is not noted within 24 to 48 hours of the beginning of treatment.

For sows, administer once intramuscularly 3 milligrams of oxytetracycline per pound of body weight approximately 8 hours before farrowing or immediately after completion of farrowing.

For swine weighing 25 lb of body weight and under, BIO-MYCIN® 200 should be administered undiluted for treatment at 9 mg/lb but should be administered diluted for treatment at 3 or 5 mg/lb.

Body Weight	9 mg/lb Dosage		3 or 5 mg/lb Dosage	
	Volume of Undiluted BIO-MYCIN® 200		Volume of Diluted BIO-MYCIN® 200	
	9 mg/lb	3 mg/lb	Dilution*	5 mg/lb
5 lb	0.2 mL	0.6 mL	1:7	1.0 mL
10 lb	0.5 mL	0.9 mL	1:5	1.5 mL
25 lb	1.1 mL	1.5 mL	1:3	2.5 mL

*To prepare dilutions, add one part BIO-MYCIN® 200 to three, five or seven parts of sterile water; or 5 percent dextrose solution as indicated; the diluted product should be used immediately.

Directions for Use: BIO-MYCIN® 200 is intended for use in the treatment of disease due to oxytetracycline susceptible organisms in beef cattle, non-lactating dairy cattle and swine. A thoroughly cleaned, sterile needle and syringe should be used for each injection (needles and syringes may be sterilized by boiling in water for 15 minutes). In cold weather, BIO-MYCIN® 200 should be warmed to room temperature before administration to animals. Before withdrawing the solution from the bottle, disinfect the rubber cap on the bottle with a suitable disinfectant, such as 70% alcohol. The injection site should be similarly cleaned with the disinfectant. Needles of 16 to 18 gauge and 1 to 1½ inches long are adequate for intramuscular injections. Needles 2 to 3 inches are recommended for intravenous use.

Intramuscular Administration: Intramuscular injections should be made by directing the needle of suitable gauge and length into the fleshy part of a thick muscle such as in the rump, hip or thigh regions; avoid blood vessels and major nerves. Before injecting the solution, pull back gently on the plunger. If blood appears in the syringe, a blood vessel has been entered; withdraw the needle and select a different site.

No more than 10 mL should be injected intramuscularly at any one site in adult beef cattle and non-lactating dairy cattle, and not more than 5 mL per site in adult swine; rotate injection sites for each succeeding treatment. The volume administered per injection site should be reduced according to age and body size so that 1 to 2 mL per site is injected in small calves.

Subcutaneous Administration: Subcutaneous injections in beef cattle and non-lactating dairy cattle should be made by directing the needle of suitable gauge and length through the loose folds of the neck skin in front of the shoulder. Care should be taken to ensure that the tip of the needle has penetrated the skin but is not lodged in muscle. Before injecting the solution, pull back gently on the plunger. If blood appears in the syringe, a blood vessel has been entered; withdraw the needle and select a different site. The solution should be injected slowly into the area between the skin and muscles.

No more than 10 mL should be injected subcutaneously at any one site in adult beef cattle and non-lactating dairy cattle; rotate injection sites for each succeeding treatment. The volume administered per injection site should be reduced according to age and body size so that 1 to 2 mL per site is injected in small calves.

Intravenous Administration: BIO-MYCIN® 200 (oxytetracycline injection) may be administered intravenously to beef cattle and non-lactating dairy cattle. As with all highly concentrated materials, BIO-MYCIN® 200 should be administered slowly by the intravenous route.

Preparation of the Animal for Injection:

1. Approximate location of vein. The jugular vein runs in the jugular groove on each side of the neck from the angle of the jaw to just above the brisket and slightly above and to the side of the windpipe. (See Fig. I).
2. Restraint. A stanchion or chute is ideal for restraining the animal. With a halter, rope, or cattle leader (nose tongs), pull the animal's head around the side of the stanchion, cattle chute, or post in such a manner to form a bow in the neck (See Fig. II), then snub the head securely to prevent movement. By forming the bow in the neck, the outside curvature of the bow tends to expose the jugular vein and make it easily accessible. Caution: Avoid restraining the animal with a tight rope or halter around the throat or upper neck which might impede blood flow. Animals that are down present no problem so far as restraint is concerned.
3. Clip hair in area where injection is to be made (over the vein in the upper third of the neck). Clean and disinfect the skin with alcohol or other suitable antiseptic.

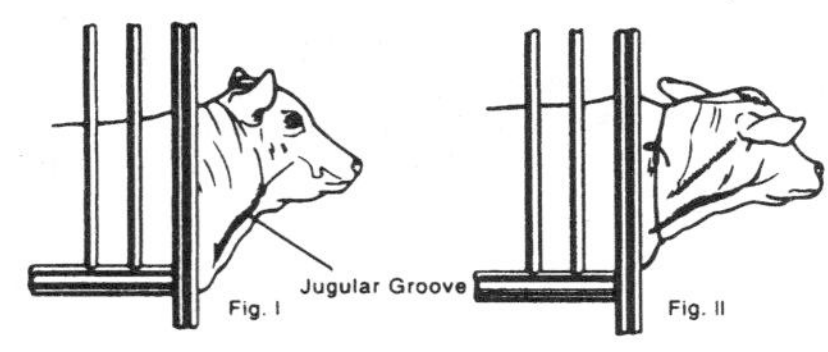

Entering the Vein and Making the Injection:

1. Raise the vein. This is accomplished by tying the choke rope tightly around the neck close to the shoulder. The rope should be tied in such a way that it will not come loose and so that it can be untied quickly by pulling the loose end (See Fig. II). In thick-necked animals, a block of wood placed in the jugular groove between the rope and the hide will help considerably in applying the desired pressure at the right point. The vein is a soft flexible tube through which the blood flows back to the heart. Under ordinary conditions, it cannot be seen or felt with the fingers. When the flow of blood is blocked at the base of the neck by the choke rope, the vein becomes enlarged and rigid because of the back pressure. If the choke rope is sufficiently tight, the vein stands out and can be easily seen and felt in thin-necked animals. As a further check in identifying the vein, tap it with the fingers in front of the choke rope. Pulsations that can be seen or felt with the fingers in front of the point being tapped will confirm the fact that the vein is properly distended. It is impossible to put the needle into the vein unless it is distended. Experienced operators are able to raise the vein simply by hand pressure, but the use of a choke rope is more certain.
2. Inserting the needle. This involves three distinct steps. First, insert the needle through the hide. Second, insert the needle into the vein. This may require two or three attempts before the vein is entered. The vein has a tendency to roll away from the point of the needle, especially if the needle is not sharp. The vein can be steadied with the thumb and finger of one hand. With the other hand, the needle point is placed directly over the vein, slanting it so that its direction is along the length of the vein, either toward the head or toward the heart. Properly positioned this way, a quick thrust of the needle will be followed by a spurt of blood through the needle, which indicates that the vein has been entered. Third, once in the vein, the needle should be inserted along the length of the vein all the way to the hub, exercising caution to see that the needle does not penetrate the opposite side of the vein. Continuous steady flow of blood through the needle indicates that the needle is still in the vein. If blood does not flow continuously, the needle is out of the vein (or clogged) and another attempt must be made. If difficulty is encountered, it may be advisable to use the vein on the other side of the neck.
3. While the needle is being placed in proper position in the vein, an assistant should get the medication ready so that the injection can be started without delay after the vein has been entered.
4. Making the injection. With the needle in position as indicated by continuous flow of blood, release the choke rope by a quick pull on the free end. This is essential—the medication cannot flow into the vein while it is blocked. Immediately connect the syringe containing BIO-MYCIN® 200 (oxytetracycline injection) to the needle and slowly depress the plunger. If there is resistance to depression of the plunger, this indicates that the needle has slipped out of the vein (or is clogged) and the procedure will have to be repeated. Watch for any swelling under the skin near the needle, which would indicate that the medication is not going into the vein. Should this occur, it is best to try the vein on the opposite side of the neck.
5. Removing the needle. When injection is complete, remove needle with straight pull. Then apply pressure over area of injection momentarily to control any bleeding through needle puncture, using cotton soaked in alcohol or other suitable antiseptic.

Precaution(s): BIO-MYCIN® 200 does not require refrigeration; however, it is recommended that it be stored at controlled room temperature, 15°-30°C (59°-86°F). Keep from freezing. Handle aseptically.

Caution(s): When administered to cattle, muscle discoloration may necessitate trimming of the injection site(s) and surrounding tissues during the dressing procedure.

Exceeding the highest recommended dosage level of drug per pound of body weight per day, administering more than the recommended number of treatments and/or exceeding 10 mL intramuscularly or subcutaneously per injection site in adult beef cattle and non-lactating dairy cattle, and 5 mL intramuscularly per injection site in adult swine, may result in antibiotic residues beyond the withdrawal period.

Reactions of an allergic or anaphylactic nature, sometimes fatal, have been known to occur in hypersensitive animals following the injection of oxytetracycline. Such adverse reactions can be characterized by signs such as restlessness, erection of hair, muscle trembling; swelling of eyelids, ears, muzzle, anus and vulva (or scrotum and sheath in males); labored breathing, defecation and urination, glassy-eyed appearance, eruption of skin plaques, frothing from the mouth, and prostration. Pregnant animals that recover may subsequently abort. At the first sign of any adverse reaction, discontinue use of this product and administer epinephrine at the recommended dosage levels. Call a veterinarian immediately.

Shock may be observed following intravenous administration, especially where highly concentrated materials are involved. To minimize this occurrence, it is recommended that BIO-MYCIN® 200 be administered slowly by this route.

Shortly after injection treated animals may have transient hemoglobinuria resulting in darkened urine.

As with all antibiotic preparations, use of this drug may result in overgrowth of nonsusceptible organisms, including fungi. A lack of response by the treated animal, or the development of new signs, may suggest that an overgrowth of nonsusceptible organisms has occurred. If any of these conditions occur, consult your veterinarian.

Since bacteriostatic drugs may interfere with the bactericidal action of penicillin, it is advisable to avoid giving BIO-MYCIN® 200 in conjunction with penicillin.

Warning(s): Discontinue treatment for at least 28 days prior to slaughter of cattle and swine. Not for use in lactating dairy animals.

Restricted Drug (California): Use only as directed. Keep out of reach of children.

For use in animals only.

Discussion: Oxytetracycline is an antimicrobial agent that is effective in the treatment of a wide range of diseases caused by susceptible gram-positive and gram-negative bacteria.

The antibiotic activity of oxytetracycline is not appreciably diminished in the presence of body fluids, serum or exudates.

Care of Sick Animals: The use of antibiotics in the management of diseases is based on an accurate diagnosis and an adequate course of treatment. When properly used in the treatment of diseases caused by oxytetracycline susceptible organisms most animals that have been treated with oxytetracycline injection show a noticeable improvement within 24 to 48 hours. It is recommended that the diagnosis and treatment of animal diseases be carried out by a veterinarian. Since many diseases look alike but require different types of treatment, the use of professional veterinary and laboratory services can reduce treatment time, costs and needless losses. Good housing, sanitation and nutrition are important in the maintenance of healthy animals, and are essential in the treatment of diseased animals.

Presentation: BIO-MYCIN® 200 is available in 100 mL, 250 mL and 500 mL bottles containing 200 mg oxytetracycline per mL.
U.S. Patent No. 5,075,295

Compendium Code No.: 10280161 BI 3495-23R-1 1/01

BIO-PINE 20

Bio-Tek **Disinfectant**

20% Pine Type Disinfectant

EPA Reg. No.: 13648-19-11725

Active Ingredient(s):

Pine Oil. 20%
Inert Ingredients: 80%

Indications: Heavy duty cleaner and disinfectant that cleans, deodorizes and disinfects*.

Limited disinfectant against intestinal bacteria.

Effective against specific gram-negative household germs, such as those causing Salmonellosis (food poisoning). This product is a heavy duty cleaner, disinfectant and deodorizer; leaves a lasting fresh smell.

Directions for Use: It is a violation of Federal law to use this product in a manner inconsistent with its labeling

To Disinfect, Clean and Deodorize Hard, Non-Porous Surfaces In One Operation: Use a mop or brush to apply a solution of ¼ cup disinfectant to one gallon of water for moderately soiled surfaces such as floors, tubs, toilets, sinks, locker rooms, walls, pet quarters and garbage cans, maintaining a thoroughly wet surface for 10 minutes. Mix fresh solution before each use; no rinsing necessary except on rubber or asphalt tile and on food contact surfaces. Heavily soiled surfaces must be pre-cleaned first, followed by a second application using directions above to disinfect. Use full strength for cutting grease, crayon, old wax or other heavy duty cleaning jobs; rinse immediately.

Laundry: Use full strength on heavily soiled areas such as collars, cuffs and grease stains. Rub in well and use ½ cup in washer along with regular detergent as a cleaning booster and deodorizer.

Pre-Soaking: To kill odor-causing bacteria, use ½ cup per gallon of water for diapers, baby clothes and bedding.

Dog Bath: Use 3 tsp. per gallon of water.

Precautionary Statements: Hazards to Humans and Domestic Animals:

Warning: Causes eye and skin irritation. Do not get in eyes, on skin or on clothing. Harmful if swallowed. Avoid contamination of food/food crops.

Statement of Practical Treatment:

If In Eyes: Flush with plenty of water. Get medical attention. If Swallowed: Drink promptly a large quantity of water. Do not induce vomiting. Avoid alcohol. Get medical attention. If On Skin: Wash with plenty of soap and water. Get medical attention if irritation persists. Note to Physician: Probable mucosal damage may contraindicate the use of gastric lavage.

Environmental Hazards: This product is toxic to fish. Do not discharge effluent containing this product into lakes, streams, ponds, estuaries, oceans or other waters unless in accordance with the requirements of a National Pollutant Discharge Elimination System (NPDES) permit and the permitting authority has been notified in writing prior to discharge. Do not discharge effluent containing this product to sewer systems without previously notifying the local sewage treatment plant authority. For guidance contact your State Water Board or regional office of the E.P.A.

Physical or Chemical Hazards: Do not use or store near heat or open flame.

Storage and Disposal: Do not contaminate water, food, or feed by storage or disposal.

Storage: Keep container closed when not in use. Do not store near heat or open flame. Pesticide Disposal: Do not clean equipment or dispose of equipment wastewaters in a manner that will contaminate water resources. Wastes resulting from the use of this product may be disposed of on site or at an approved waste disposal facility. Container Disposal: Triple rinse (or equivalent). Then offer for recycling or reconditioning, or puncture and dispose of in a sanitary landfill, or incineration, or if allowed by state and local authorities, by burning. If burned, stay out of smoke.

Warning(s): Keep out of reach of children.

Presentation: 4x1 gallon cases and 55 gallon drums.

Compendium Code No.: 13700000

BIO-POX M™

Intervet **Vaccine**

Fowl Pox Vaccine, Live Virus

U.S. Vet. Lic. No.: 286

Contents: BIO-POX M™ (fowl pox vaccine - mild) contains a mild strain of fowl pox virus especially adapted to cell culture. To improve the ease of handling in the field, the product is lyophilized as it is packaged.

The vaccine is thoroughly tested before sale and meets the requirements of the U.S. Department of Agriculture.

Contains penicillin and streptomycin as preservatives.

Indications: The vaccine is recommended for the prevention of fowl pox and fowl pox diphtheria in young chickens (one day to 10 weeks of age). It is administered by the wing web method in chickens, using a two-needle applicator.

Dosage and Administration: Do not open and mix the vaccine until ready to commence vaccination. Use the vaccine immediately after mixing.

1. Tear off the aluminum seal from the vial containing the dried vaccine.
2. Lift off the rubber stopper.
3. Remove the seal and stopper from the bottle of diluent.
4. Pour a small amount of the diluent into the vial of dried vaccine.
5. Replace the rubber stopper and shake the bottle.
6. Pour the partially dissolved vaccine into the bottle containing the rest of the diluent.
7. Replace the rubber stopper and shake vigorously until all the material is dissolved.
8. The vaccine is now ready for use by the following vaccination method. For the best results, follow the directions carefully.

Wing web application in chickens:

1. Rehydrate the vaccine, as directed.
2. Hold the bird and spread the underside of one (1) wing outward.
3. Dip the applicator into the vaccine vial, wetting both needles.
4. Pierce the web of the exposed wing with the charged applicator.
5. Redip the applicator in the vaccine vial and proceed to the next bird.
6. Avoid hitting blood vessels, bones and the wing muscle.
7. Be careful not to touch any part of the bird with the vaccine except the area to be inoculated.

Examination of takes: Examine for takes 7-10 days following vaccination. A positive take, showing that the vaccination was successful, is indicated by swelling of the skin or scab formation at the point of inoculation. Swelling and scabs will disappear two (2) weeks following vaccination. The absence of takes may mean that birds were immune before vaccination or that improper vaccination methods were used. Immunity will normally develop about 10 to 14 days after vaccination.

Records: Keep a record of vaccine type, quantity, and serial number; the date and time of vaccination; the number, age, breed, and location of the birds; names of operators performing the vaccination and any observed reactions.

Contraindication(s): Birds to be vaccinated should be free of all kinds of diseases, including latent form of chronic respiratory disease (CRD), clinical coccidiosis, blackhead, parasite infections, etc. and maintained under good environmental conditions.

Precaution(s): Store vaccine at not over 7°C (45°F). Do not spill or spatter the vaccine. Burn or boil the empty bottles, and the unused vaccine and accessories.

Caution(s): Do not overdilute the vaccine or otherwise extend the dosage.

Birds should not be placed on contaminated premises. Exposure should be avoided immediately following vaccination because it takes up to 10 days to develop resistance.

All susceptible birds on the premises should be vaccinated at the same time. If this is not possible, then strict isolation and separate caretakers should be employed for nonvaccinated units. Efforts should be taken to reduce stress conditions at the time the vaccine is administered.

Warning(s): Do not vaccinate within 21 days of slaughter.

Presentation: Available in 500 or 1,000 dose vials with diluent.

Compendium Code No.: 11060151

BIOSOL® LIQUID

Pharmacia & Upjohn **Water Medication**

Neomycin Sulfate (commercial grade)-Antibacterial

ANADA No.: 200-113

Active Ingredient(s): Contains per mL: neomycin sulfate (commercial grade) 200 mg equivalent to 140 mg neomycin.

Indications: Indicated for the treatment and control of colibacillosis (bacterial enteritis) caused by *Escherichia coli* susceptible to neomycin sulfate in cattle (excluding veal calves), swine, sheep and goats.

Dosage and Administration: Administer to cattle, swine, sheep and goats at a dose of 10 mg neomycin sulfate per pound of body weight in divided doses for a maximum of 14 days.

Dosage Schedule for treatment of colibacillosis:

Pounds of Body Weight	Amount of BIOSOL® Liquid Per Day in Divided Doses
25 lbs	¼ teaspoonful
50 lbs	½ teaspoonful
100 lbs	1 teaspoonful
300 lbs	1 tablespoonful
600 lbs	1 fluid ounce

Teaspoon = U.S. Standard Measure

BIOSOL® Liquid may be given undiluted or diluted with water. Herd Treatment: Each bottle will treat 9,600 pounds body weight. Therefore, estimate the total number of pounds body weight of the animals to be treated and administer one (1) fluid ounce for each 600 pounds. The product should be added to the amount of drinking water to be consumed in 12-24 hours. Provide medicated water as the sole source of water each day until consumed, followed by non-medicated water as required. Fresh medicated water should be prepared each day. Individual Animal Treatment: To provide 10 mg neomycin sulfate per pound of body weight, mix one (1) teaspoon in water or milk for each 100 pounds body weight. Administer daily either as a drench in divided doses or in the drinking water to be consumed in 12-24 hours.

Important: Treatment should continue 24 to 48 hours beyond remission of disease symptoms, but not to exceed a total of 14 consecutive days. Animals not drinking or eating should be treated individually by drench.

Precaution(s): Store at controlled room temperature 20° to 25°C (68° to 77°F) [see USP].

Caution(s): To administer the stated dosage, the concentration of neomycin required in medicated water must be adjusted to compensate for variation in age and weight of animal, the nature and severity of disease signs, and environmental temperature and humidity, each of which affects water consumption.

If symptoms persist after using this preparation for 2 or 3 days, consult a veterinarian. If symptoms such as fever, depression, or going off feed develop, oral neomycin is not indicated as the sole treatment since systemic levels of neomycin are not obtained due to low absorption from the gastrointestinal tract.

Restricted Drug—Use only as directed (California).

For oral use in animals only.

Not for human use. Keep out of reach of children.

Warning(s): Discontinue treatment prior to slaughter by at least the number of days listed below for appropriate species:

Cattle. . . . . 1 day
Sheep . . . . 2 days
Swine and goats . . . . 3 days

A withdrawal period has not been established for this product in pre-ruminating calves. Do not use in calves to be processed for veal.

A milk discard period has not been established for this product in lactating dairy cattle. Do not use in female dairy cattle 20 months of age or older.

Presentation: 16 fl oz (473 mL) bottles.

Compendium Code No.: 10490080

BIO-SOTA + BRON MM™

Intervet **Vaccine**

Newcastle-Bronchitis Vaccine, B_1 Type, LaSota Strain, Mass. Type, Live Virus

U.S. Vet. Lic. No.: 286

Contents: The vaccine contains LaSota strain of Newcastle virus, and infectious bronchitis virus of the Massachusetts type. The embryonated chicken eggs used in the production were obtained from specific pathogen free flocks (SPF).

The vaccine is thoroughly tested before sale and meets the requirements of the U.S. Department of Agriculture.

Contains gentamicin as a preservative.

Indications: BIO-SOTA + BRON MM™, offering high levels of protection with mild reaction, is ideal for use on broilers and replacement pullets where disease exposure indicates.

Use for both initial vaccination and revaccination of healthy chickens, broilers and replacement birds. The most satisfactory vaccination schedule may vary from one area to another, depending on incidence of disease, progeny maternal antibodies and other management considerations.

Dosage and Administration: Vaccinate healthy chickens with Newcastle disease vaccine in water at two (2) weeks of age or older when maternal antibody subsides. Vaccinate with Newcastle vaccine by intra-ocular or intranasal route of healthy chickens at one (1) day of age or older in disease enzootic area.

Revaccinate healthy chickens at least 21 days after the first vaccination in drinking water or by spray method. Booster vaccination by spray method every three (3) months.

Preparation and Use of the Vaccine:

Intra-ocular/intranasal administration for birds as early as one (1) day old:

1. Rehydrate the vaccine by adding the diluent to half fill the vial. Replace the rubber stopper and shake well to dissolve the lyophilized vaccine. Pour the vaccine into the remaining diluent and shake well. Mix a 1,000 dose vial into 30 mL.
2. Fit the dropper/dispenser on the diluent bottle.
3. Allow one (1) drop of the vaccine to fall into one (1) eye/nostril.

Drinking water administration for birds 14 days or older:

1. Discontinue medication 48 hours before vaccination. The waterers should be thoroughly cleaned before use. Do not use disinfecting solutions during cleaning as disinfectant residue may destroy the virus.
2. Deprive the birds of water about two (2) hours prior to vaccination.
3. Tear off the aluminum seal from the vial containing the lyophilized vaccine and remove the stopper. Use clean, cold, nonchlorinated water for rehydration of the dried vaccine. Mix a 1,000 dose vial with two (2) gallons of water.
4. Dried milk powder can be used as a stabilizer. It is added at the rate of one (1) teaspoon (15 g) per two (2) gallons of water. Add the dried milk powder before adding the vaccine.
5. Provide enough waterers so that all birds may have an opportunity to drink the vaccine-treated water.
6. Avoid exposure of the waterers to direct sunlight.
7. Do not resume watering until the vaccine-treated water has been consumed. Then continue watering with untreated water for 24 hours before resuming the normal watering practice.
8. Vaccination with less than one (1) dose per bird may fail to immunize satisfactorily.

Precaution(s): Store the vaccine at not over 7°C (45°F). Use the entire contents of the vial immediately after mixing. Do not spill or spatter the vaccine. Burn the empty bottles and the unused vaccine. The vaccine is not returnable to the manufacturer.

Caution(s): Do not overdilute or otherwise extend the dosage.

The vaccine is not recommended for chickens that are sick or debilitated due to disease or stress. Chickens should not be placed on contaminated premises. Exposure should be avoided immediately following vaccination because it takes up to 10 days to develop resistance.

All susceptible chickens on the premises should be vaccinated at the same time. Efforts should be taken to reduce stress conditions at the time the vaccine is administered.

Warning(s): Do not vaccinate within 21 days of slaughter.

Newcastle disease vaccine can cause inflammation of the eyes and eyelids of humans. Caution should be used to avoid contamination of the eyes with this vaccine.

Presentation: Available in 10,000 dose vials with diluent.

Compendium Code No.: 11060161

BIO SPOT® FLEA & TICK CONTROL FOR DOGS (15 LBS. & UNDER)

Farnam **Parasiticide-Topical**

EPA Reg. No.: 270-278

Active Ingredient(s):

Permethrin: (CAS #52645-53-1)	45.0%
Pyriproxyfen: (CAS #95737-68-1) (Nylar®)	5.0%
Other Ingredients:	50.0%
Total	100.0%

Indications: Kills and repels adult fleas for up to 3 to 4 weeks. Kills flea eggs and larvae for up to 4 months. Kills and repels ticks for up to 4 weeks, including Deer Ticks (vector of Lyme Disease), Brown Dog Ticks and American Dog Ticks. It also protects against blood feeding by mosquitoes (vector of heartworm) for up to 4 weeks. Use only on dogs over 12 weeks of age.

Directions for Use: It is a violation of Federal law to use this product in a manner inconsistent with its labeling.

Read entire label before each use.

Use only on dogs over 12 weeks of age.

Do not use on cats or animals other than dogs. May be toxic and potentially fatal if applied to or ingested by cats. Do not get this product in your dog's eyes or mouth. Repeat applications may be made if necessary, but do not apply more often than once every 3 weeks, except to reapply after shampooing the dog.

For Dogs Weighing 15 lbs. and Under: Apply one tube (1.0 mL) of BIO SPOT® solution as a spot or stripe to the dog's back between the shoulder blades.

How To Apply: Remove product tube from package. Holding tube with notched end pointing up and away from face and body, snap or cut off narrow end at notches. Invert tube over dog and use open end to part dog's hair. Squeeze tube firmly to apply all of the solution to the dog's skin. Wrap tube and put in trash.

BIO SPOT® is an effective and easy to use product. BIO SPOT® has demonstrated greater than 92% control of fleas within one day of application. BIO SPOT® prevents eggs from fleas on treated dogs from developing into biting adults for up to 4 months. BIO SPOT® kills and repels Deer Ticks (vector of Lyme Disease), Brown Dog Ticks, and American Dog Ticks for up to 4 weeks. BIO SPOT® also kills and repels mosquitoes and protects against bloodfeeding by mosquitoes (vector of heartworm) for up to 4 weeks.

Contraindication(s): Do not use on cats or animals other than dogs. Do not use on puppies under 12 weeks of age.

Precautionary Statements: Hazards to Humans and Domestic Animals:

Caution:

Hazards to Humans: Harmful if swallowed. Avoid contact with eyes or clothing. Causes moderate eye irritation. Wash thoroughly with soap and water after handling.

Hazards to Domestic Animals: For external use on dogs only. Do not use on puppies under 12 weeks of age. Consult a veterinarian before using this product on debilitated, aged, medicated, pregnant, or nursing dogs. Consult a veterinarian before using on dogs with known organ dysfunction. Do not use on cats or animals other than dogs. Cats which actively groom or engage in close physical contact with treated dogs may be at risk of serious harmful effect. Certain medications can interact with pesticides. It is advisable to consult a veterinarian before using this product with any other pesticide or drug.

First Aid:

If Swallowed: Call a Poison Control Center or doctor immediately for treatment advice. Have person sip a glass of water if able to swallow. Do not induce vomiting unless told to do so by a Poison Control Center or doctor. Do not give anything by mouth to an unconscious person.

If in Eyes: Hold eye open and rinse slowly and gently with water for 15-20 minutes. Remove contact lenses, if present, after the first 5 minutes, then continue rinsing eye. Call a Poison Control Center or doctor for treatment advice.

In case of emergency or for product information, call (602) 285-1660, Monday-Friday, 7:00 AM - 3:45 PM MST.

Have the product container or label with you when calling a Poison Control Center or doctor, or going for treatment.

Adverse Reactions: Some animals may be sensitive to ingredients in this product. Reactions in dogs may include skin sensitivity. Dogs may show lethargy, increased pruritus (itchiness), erythema (redness), rash and hair discoloration or hair loss at the application site. Observe the dog following treatment. Sensitivity may occur after using any pesticide product on pets. If signs of sensitivity occur, bathe your dog with a mild, non-insecticidal shampoo and rinse with large amounts of water. If signs continue, consult a veterinarian immediately.

Environmental Hazards: This product is extremely toxic to fish. Do not add directly to water. Do not contaminate water when disposing of product or packaging.

Storage and Disposal: Do not contaminate water, food or feed by storage or disposal.

Storage: Store in a cool, dry place. Protect from freezing.

Pesticide Disposal: Securely wrap original container in several layers of newspaper and discard in trash.

Container Disposal: Do not reuse empty container. Wrap container and put in trash.

Warning(s): Keep out of reach of children.

Disclaimer: Notice of Warranty: Farnam Companies, Inc. makes no warranty of merchantability, fitness for any particular purpose, or otherwise, expressed or implied concerning this product or its uses which extend beyond the use of the product under normal conditions in accordance with the statements made on the label.

Presentation: 3 x 1.0 mL applicators.

Nylar® is a registered trademark of McLaughlin Gormley King Company.

U.S. Patent No. 5,942,525

Compendium Code No.: 10000770 02-0134

BIO SPOT® FLEA & TICK CONTROL FOR DOGS (BETWEEN 15 & 33 LBS.)

Farnam **Parasiticide-Topical**

EPA Reg. No.: 270-278

Active Ingredient(s):

Permethrin: (CAS #52645-53-1)	45.0%
Pyriproxyfen: (CAS #95737-68-1) (Nylar®)	5.0%
Other Ingredients:	50.0%
Total	100.0%

Indications: Kills and repels adult fleas for up to 3 to 4 weeks. Kills flea eggs and larvae for up to 4 months. Kills and repels ticks for up to 4 weeks, including deer ticks (vector of Lyme Disease), Brown dog ticks and American dog ticks. It also protects against blood feeding by mosquitoes (vector of heartworm) for up to 4 weeks. Use only on dogs over 12 weeks of age.

Directions for Use: It is a violation of Federal law to use this product in a manner inconsistent with its labeling.

Read entire label before each use. Use only on dogs over 12 weeks of age.

Do not use on cats or animals other than dogs. May be toxic and potentially fatal if applied to or ingested by cats. Do not get this product in your dog's eyes or mouth. Repeat applications may be made if necessary, but do not apply more often than once every 3 weeks, except to reapply after shampooing the dog.

For Dogs Weighing Between 15 and 33 lbs.: Apply one tube (1.5 mL) of BIO SPOT® solution as a spot or stripe to the dog's back between the shoulder blades.

How To Apply: Remove product tube from package. Holding tube with notched end pointing up and away from face and body, snap or cut off narrow end at notches. Invert tube over dog and use open end to part dog's hair. Squeeze tube firmly to apply all of the solution to the dog's skin. Wrap tube and put in trash.

BIO SPOT® is an effective and easy to use product. BIO SPOT® has demonstrated greater than 92% control of fleas within one day of application. BIO SPOT® prevents eggs from fleas on treated dogs from developing into biting adults for up to 4 months. BIO SPOT® kills and repels Deer Ticks (vector of Lyme Disease), Brown Dog Ticks, and American Dog Ticks for up to 4 weeks. BIO SPOT® also kills and repels mosquitoes and protects against bloodfeeding by mosquitoes (vector of heartworm) for up to 4 weeks.

Contraindication(s): Do not use on cats or animals other than dogs. Do not use on puppies under 12 weeks of age.

Precautionary Statements: Hazards to Humans and Domestic Animals:

Caution:

Hazards to Humans: Harmful if swallowed. Avoid contact with eyes or clothing. Causes moderate eye irritation. Wash thoroughly with soap and water after handling.

Hazards to Domestic Animals: For external use on dogs only. Do not use on puppies under 12 weeks of age. Consult a veterinarian before using this product on debilitated, aged, medicated, pregnant, or nursing dogs. Consult a veterinarian before using on dogs with known organ dysfunction. Do not use on cats or animals other than dogs. Cats which actively groom or engage in close physical contact with treated dogs may be at risk of serious harmful effect. Certain medications can interact with pesticides. It is advisable to consult a veterinarian before using this product with any other pesticide or drug.

First Aid:

If Swallowed: Call a Poison Control Center or doctor immediately for treatment advice. Have person sip a glass of water if able to swallow. Do not induce vomiting unless told to do so by a Poison Control Center or doctor. Do not give anything by mouth to an unconscious person.

If in Eyes: Hold eye open and rinse slowly and gently with water for 15-20 minutes. Remove contact lenses, if present, after the first 5 minutes, then continue rinsing eye. Call a Poison Control Center or doctor for treatment advice.

In case of emergency or for product information, call (602) 285-1660, Monday-Friday, 7:00 AM-3:45 PM MST.

Have the product container or label with you when calling a Poison Control Center or doctor, or going for treatment.

Adverse Reactions: Some animals may be sensitive to ingredients in this product. Reactions in dogs may include skin sensitivity. Dogs may show lethargy, increased pruritus (itchiness), erythema (redness), rash and hair discoloration or hair loss at the application site. Observe the dog following treatment. Sensitivity may occur after using any pesticide product on pets. If signs of sensitivity occur, bathe your dog with a mild, non-insecticidal shampoo and rinse with large amounts of water. If signs continue, consult a veterinarian immediately.

Environmental Hazards: This product is extremely toxic to fish. Do not add directly to water. Do not contaminate water when disposing of product or packaging.

Storage and Disposal: Do not contaminate water, food or feed by storage or disposal.

Storage: Store in a cool, dry place. Protect from freezing.

Pesticide Disposal: Securely wrap original container in several layers of newspaper and discard in trash.

Container Disposal: Do not reuse empty container. Wrap container and put in trash.

Warning(s): Keep out of reach of children.

Disclaimer: Notice of Warranty: Farnam Companies, Inc. makes no warranty of merchantability, fitness for any particular purpose, or otherwise, expressed or implied concerning this product or its uses which extend beyond the use of the product under normal conditions in accordance with the statements made on the label.

Presentation: Available in packages of 1 x 1.5 mL and 3 x 1.5 mL applicators.

Nylar® is a registered trademark of McLaughlin Gormley King Company.

U.S. Patent No. 5,942,525

Compendium Code No.: 10000051 9DD8 / 02-0136

BIO SPOT® FLEA & TICK CONTROL FOR DOGS (33 TO 66 LBS.)

Farnam **Parasiticide-Topical**

EPA Reg. No.: 270-278

Active Ingredient(s):

Permethrin: (CAS #52645-53-1) 45.0%
Pyriproxyfen: (CAS #95737-68-1) (Nylar®) 5.0%
Other Ingredients: 50.0%
Total 100.0%

Indications: Kills and repels adult fleas for up to 3 to 4 weeks. Kills flea eggs and larvae for up to 4 months. Kills and repels ticks for up to 4 weeks, including deer ticks (vector of Lyme Disease), Brown dog ticks and American dog ticks. It also protects against blood feeding by mosquitoes (vector of heartworm) for up to 4 weeks. Use only on dogs over 12 weeks of age.

Directions for Use: It is a violation of Federal law to use this product in a manner inconsistent with its labeling.

Read entire label before each use.

Use only on dogs over 12 weeks of age.

Do not use on cats or animals other than dogs. May be toxic and potentially fatal if applied to or ingested by cats. Do not get this product in your dog's eyes or mouth. Repeat applications may be made if necessary, but do not apply more often than once every 3 weeks, except to reapply after shampooing the dog.

For Dogs Weighing 33 lbs. to 66 lbs.: Apply approximately half of the tube (1.5 mL) of BIO SPOT® solution as a spot or stripe to the dog's back between the shoulder blades and apply the rest of the tube's contents (1.5 mL) as a spot or stripe to the dog's back directly in front of the base of the tail. Or apply the entire tube (3.0 mL) as a continuous stripe on the dog's back starting between the shoulder blades and ending directly in front of the base of the tail.

How To Apply: Remove product tube from package. Holding tube with notched end pointing up and away from face and body, snap or cut off narrow end at notches. Invert tube over dog and use open end to part dog's hair. Squeeze tube firmly to apply all of the solution to the dog's skin. Wrap tube and put in trash.

BIO SPOT® is an effective and easy to use product. BIO SPOT® has demonstrated greater than 92% control of fleas within one day of application. BIO SPOT® prevents eggs from fleas on treated dogs from developing into biting adults for up to 4 months. BIO SPOT® kills and repels Deer Ticks (vector of Lyme Disease), Brown Dog Ticks, and American Dog Ticks for up to 4 weeks. BIO SPOT® also kills and repels mosquitoes and protects against bloodfeeding by mosquitoes (vector of heartworm) for up to 4 weeks.

Contraindication(s): Do not use on cats or animals other than dogs. Do not use on puppies under 12 weeks of age.

Precautionary Statements: Hazards to Humans and Domestic Animals:

Caution:

Hazards to Humans: Harmful if swallowed. Avoid contact with eyes or clothing. Causes moderate eye irritation. Wash thoroughly with soap and water after handling.

Hazards to Domestic Animals: For external use on dogs only. Do not use on puppies under 12 weeks of age. Consult a veterinarian before using this product on debilitated, aged, medicated, pregnant, or nursing dogs. Consult a veterinarian before using on dogs with known organ dysfunction. Do not use on cats or animals other than dogs. Cats which actively groom or engage in close physical contact with treated dogs may be at risk of serious harmful effect. Certain medications can interact with pesticides. It is advisable to consult a veterinarian before using this product with any other pesticide or drug.

First Aid:

If Swallowed: Call a Poison Control Center or doctor immediately for treatment advice. Have person sip a glass of water if able to swallow. Do not induce vomiting unless told to do so by a Poison Control Center or doctor. Do not give anything by mouth to an unconscious person.

If in Eyes: Hold eye open and rinse slowly and gently with water for 15-20 minutes. Remove contact lenses, if present, after the first 5 minutes, then continue rinsing eye. Call a Poison Control Center or doctor for treatment advice.

In case of emergency or for product information, call (602) 285-1660, Monday-Friday, 7:00 AM-3:45 PM MST.

Have the product container or label with you when calling a Poison Control Center or doctor, or going for treatment.

Adverse Reactions: Some animals may be sensitive to ingredients in this product. Reactions in dogs may include skin sensitivity. Dogs may show lethargy, increased pruritus (itchiness), erythema (redness), rash and hair discoloration or hair loss at the application site. Observe the dog following treatment. Sensitivity may occur after using any pesticide product on pets. If signs of sensitivity occur, bathe your dog with a mild, non-insecticidal shampoo and rinse with large amounts of water. If signs continue, consult a veterinarian immediately.

Environmental Hazards: This product is extremely toxic to fish. Do not add directly to water. Do not contaminate water when disposing of product or packaging.

Storage and Disposal: Do not contaminate water, food or feed by storage or disposal.

Storage: Store in a cool, dry place. Protect from freezing. Pesticide Disposal: Securely wrap original container in several layers of newspaper and discard in trash.

Container Disposal: Do not reuse empty container. Wrap container and put in trash.

Warning(s): Keep out of reach of children.

Disclaimer: Notice of Warranty: Farnam Companies, Inc. makes no warranty of merchantability, fitness for any particular purpose, or otherwise, expressed or implied concerning this product or its uses which extend beyond the use of the product under normal conditions in accordance with the statements made on the label.

Presentation: Available in packages of 1 x 3.0 mL and 3 x 3.0 mL applicators.

Nylar® is a registered trademark of McLaughlin Gormley King Company.

U.S. Patent No. 5,942,525

Compendium Code No.: 10000041 9DD8 / 01-1401

BIO SPOT® FLEA & TICK CONTROL FOR DOGS (OVER 66 LBS.)

Farnam **Parasiticide-Topical**

EPA Reg. No.: 270-278

Active Ingredient(s):

Permethrin: (CAS #52645-53-1) 45.0%
Pyriproxyfen: (CAS #95737-68-1) (Nylar®) 5.0%
Other Ingredients: 50.0%
Total 100.0%

Indications: Kills and repels adult fleas for up to 3 to 4 weeks. Kills flea eggs and larvae for up to 4 months. Kills and repels ticks for up to 4 weeks, including Deer Ticks (vector of Lyme Disease), Brown Dog Ticks and American Dog Ticks. It also protects against blood feeding by mosquitoes (vector of heartworm) for up to 4 weeks. Use only on dogs over 12 weeks of age.

Directions for Use: It is a violation of Federal law to use this product in a manner inconsistent with its labeling.

Read entire label before each use.

Use only on dogs over 12 weeks of age.

Do not use on cats or animals other than dogs. May be toxic and potentially fatal if applied to or ingested by cats. Do not get this product in your dog's eyes or mouth. Repeat applications may be made if necessary, but do not apply more often than once every 3 weeks, except to reapply after shampooing the dog.

For Dogs Weighing Over 66 lbs.: Apply approximately half of the tube (2.25 mL) of BIO SPOT® solution as a spot or stripe to the dog's back between the shoulder blades and apply the rest of the tube's contents (2.25 mL) as a spot or stripe to the dog's back directly in front of the base of the tail. Or apply the entire tube (4.5 mL) as a continuous stripe on the dog's back starting between the shoulder blades and ending directly in front of the base of the tail.

How To Apply: Remove product tube from package. Holding tube with notched end pointing up and away from face and body, snap or cut off narrow end at notches. Invert tube over dog and use open end to part dog's hair. Squeeze tube firmly to apply all of the solution to the dog's skin. Wrap tube and put in trash.

BIO SPOT® is an effective and easy to use product. BIO SPOT® has demonstrated greater than 92% control of fleas within one day of application. BIO SPOT® prevents eggs from fleas on treated dogs from developing into biting adults for up to 4 months. BIO SPOT® kills and repels Deer Ticks (vector of Lyme Disease), Brown Dog Ticks, and American Dog Ticks for up to 4 weeks. BIO SPOT® also kills and repels mosquitoes and protects against bloodfeeding by mosquitoes (vector of heartworm) for up to 4 weeks.

Contraindication(s): Do not use on cats or animals other than dogs. Do not use on puppies under 12 weeks of age.

Precautionary Statements: Hazards to Humans and Domestic Animals:

Caution:

Hazards to Humans: Harmful if swallowed. Avoid contact with eyes or clothing. Causes moderate eye irritation. Wash thoroughly with soap and water after handling.

Hazards to Domestic Animals: For external use on dogs only. Do not use on puppies under 12 weeks of age. Consult a veterinarian before using this product on debilitated, aged, medicated, pregnant, or nursing dogs. Consult a veterinarian before using on dogs with known organ dysfunction. Do not use on cats or animals other than dogs. Cats which actively groom or engage in close physical contact with treated dogs may be at risk of serious harmful effect. Certain medications can interact with pesticides. It is advisable to consult a veterinarian before using this product with any other pesticide or drug.

First Aid:

If Swallowed: Call a Poison Control Center or doctor immediately for treatment advice. Have person sip a glass of water if able to swallow. Do not induce vomiting unless told to do so by a Poison Control Center or doctor. Do not give anything by mouth to an unconscious person.

If in Eyes: Hold eye open and rinse slowly and gently with water for 15-20 minutes. Remove contact lenses, if present, after the first 5 minutes, then continue rinsing eye. Call a Poison Control Center or doctor for treatment advice.

In case of emergency or for product information, call (602) 285-1660, Monday-Friday, 7:00 AM-3:45 PM MST.

Have the product container or label with you when calling a Poison Control Center or doctor, or going for treatment.

Adverse Reactions: Some animals may be sensitive to ingredients in this product. Reactions in dogs may include skin sensitivity. Dogs may show lethargy, increased pruritus (itchiness), erythema (redness), rash and hair discoloration or hair loss at the application site. Observe the dog following treatment. Sensitivity may occur after using any pesticide product on pets. If signs of sensitivity occur, bathe your dog with a mild, non-insecticidal shampoo and rinse with large amounts of water. If signs continue, consult a veterinarian immediately.

Environmental Hazards: This product is extremely toxic to fish. Do not add directly to water. Do not contaminate water when disposing of product or packaging.

Storage and Disposal: Do not contaminate water, food or feed by storage or disposal.

Storage: Store in a cool, dry place. Protect from freezing. Pesticide Disposal: Securely wrap original container in several layers of newspaper and discard in trash.

Container Disposal: Do not reuse empty container. Wrap container and put in trash.

Warning(s): Keep out of reach of children.

Disclaimer: Notice of Warranty: Farnam Companies, Inc. makes no warranty of merchantability, fitness for any particular purpose, or otherwise, expressed or implied concerning this product

or its uses which extend beyond the use of the product under normal conditions in accordance with the statements made on the label.
Presentation: Available in packages of 1 x 4.5 mL and 3 x 4.5 mL applicators.
Nylar® is a registered trademark of McLaughlin Gormley King Company.
U.S. Patent No. 5,942,525
Compendium Code No.: 10000780 01-1400

BIO SPOT® STRIPE-ON™ FLEA CONTROL FOR CATS

Farnam **Flea Control**

EPA Reg. No.: 270-308
Active Ingredient(s):
Pyriproxyfen: 2-[1-methyl-2-(4-phenoxyphenoxy) ethoxy] pyridine . . . 5.3%
Inert Ingredients: . . . 94.7%
Total . . . 100.0%
Indications: A topical solution for use on cats.
Prevents flea eggs from developing into biting adults for 3 months.
Directions for Use: It is a violation of Federal law to use this product in a manner inconsistent with its labeling.
Read entire label completely before using. Do not get this product in your pet's eyes or mouth. Repeat applications may be made if necessary, but do not apply more often than once every 3 weeks. Do not use this product in or on electrical equipment due to the possibility of shock hazard.
How to Apply: Remove product tab by tearing along perforation. Holding tab with tube end pointed up and away from face and body, cut along dotted line. While gently holding cat, use the narrow end of the tab to part cat's hair, and apply product as a narrow stripe down cat's back from back of head to base of tail. Squeeze tube firmly to apply all of the solution directly to cat's skin. Continue to gently restrain cat for a few seconds until product absorbs into cat's coat. Wrap tab and put in trash.
Contraindication(s): Do not use on kittens under 12 weeks of age.
Precautionary Statements: Hazards to Humans and Domestic Animals: Caution:
Hazards to Humans: Causes moderate eye irritation. Avoid contact with eyes or clothing. Wash thoroughly with soap and water after handling.
Hazards to Domestic Animals: For external use only. Do not use on cats under 12 weeks of age. Consult a veterinarian before using this product on debilitated, aged, pregnant, or nursing animals.
Sensitivities may occur after using any pesticide, product for pets. If signs of sensitivity occur, bathe your pet with mild soap and rinse with large amounts of water. If signs continue, consult a veterinarian immediately.
Certain medications can interact with pesticides. Consult a veterinarian before using on medicated animals.
First Aid:
If Swallowed: Call a physician or Poison Control Center. Drink 1 or 2 glasses of water and induce vomiting by touching back of throat with finger, or, if available, by administering syrup of ipecac. If person is unconscious, do not give anything by mouth and do not induce vomiting.
If in Eyes: Flush eyes with plenty of water. Call a physician if irritation persists.
Storage and Disposal: Storage: Store in a cool, dry place. Protect from freezing. Pesticide Disposal: Securely wrap original container in several layers of newspaper and discard in trash. Container Disposal: Do not reuse empty container. Wrap container and put in trash.
Warning(s): Keep out of reach of children.
Disclaimer: Farnam Companies, Inc. makes no warranty of merchantability, fitness for any particular purpose, or otherwise, expressed or implied concerning this product or its uses which extend beyond the use of the product under normal conditions in accordance with the statements made on the label.
Presentation: Two 1.5 mL applicators.
Nylar® is a registered trademark of McLaughlin Gormley King Company.
Compendium Code No.: 10000030

BIO-TELLA™

Intervet **Bacterin**

Bordetella Avium Bacterin
U.S. Vet. Lic. No.: 286
Contents: *Bordetella avium* bacterin (Turkey Coryza) consists of an antigenic preparation of inactivated *Bordetella avium* mixed in a specially formulated immunostimulating solution. Extensive laboratory and field studies proved the vaccine to be safe and efficacious in preventing clinical disease caused by virulent strains of *Bordetella avium* in turkeys.
Indications: This vaccine is recommended for vaccination of healthy turkeys for prevention of upper respiratory disease caused by *Bordetella avium.*
For oral administration through drinking water.
Dosage and Administration: The bacterin is to be administered orally through drinking water and can be given as early as one week, however, the recommended age of vaccination is two to six weeks. Revaccination should be done at an interval of two to three weeks post initial vaccination.
Directions for Use:
1. Shake the vaccine well before use.
2. For initial vaccination of one-week-old turkeys, mix the contents of one bottle (2,000 doses) with approximately six gallons of drinking water.
3. For revaccination at three weeks of age, mix the contents of one bottle of vaccine with approximately 18 gallons of drinking water.
4. Birds should be water starved prior to administering the vaccine.
5. Allow sufficient time to drink the vaccine completely before adding fresh water.
6. Repeat the vaccination 2 to 3 weeks after the initial vaccination. Turkeys may be vaccinated as early as 1 week, however, the recommended age of vaccination is 2 to 6 weeks.

Precaution(s):
1. Use entire contents of the bottle when first opened.
2. Store at below 45°F (7°C); do not freeze.

Discussion: Turkey coryza in an acute, highly contagious upper respiratory disease of turkeys caused by *Bordetella avium.* The disease is of great economic importance to the turkey industry. *Bordetella avium* primarily affects young turkeys between the ages of one to six weeks. Outbreaks of turkey coryza occur in almost all major turkey producing areas all over the world. Farms with continuous confinement production and multi-age flocks have the greatest problems with the disease.
Clinical signs of turkey coryza in young turkeys include an abrupt onset of sneezing accompanied by profuse oculonasal discharge, open-mouth breathing, submandibular swelling and tracheal collapse. The clinical signs are usually mild in older turkeys. During the course of the disease, the oculonasal discharge changes from watery and foamy to a yellowish-brown, sticky exudate that stains the face. Although the morbidity may be as high as 100%, the mortality usually remains low.
Older flocks serve as recovered carriers and are thought to be the most prevalent source of infection for younger, susceptible flocks on multi-age farms. Contaminated litter and water are the potential sources of infection for new flocks. The *Bordetella avium* organism persists for at least six months in moist litter.
Proper sanitation procedures will greatly reduce the *Bordetella avium* organisms from the environment. They are readily susceptible to most common disinfectants and drying. Birds can also be immunized by vaccination.
Extensive testing has shown this product to be safe and efficacious when administered orally through drinking water. More than 80% of the laboratory tested and more than 70% of the field tested turkeys vaccinated orally with a normal (1x) dose of the vaccine were protected against challenge with a virulent strain of the *Bordetella* organism.
Presentation: This product is available for use in 2,000 dose size units.
Compendium Code No.: 11060171

BIOTIN-100

Vet-A-Mix **Biotin**

Active Ingredient(s): Guaranteed Analysis: Per Pound
D-Biotin . . . 100 mg
Ingredients: D-Biotin, rice hulls and mineral oil.
Indications: For use as a nutritional supplement in horses.
Dosage and Administration: The usual dose for a 1,100 lb. (500 kg) horse is 2 heaping measures per day. The dosage for ponies is 1 heaping measure daily. Top dress or mix with the daily ration. One heaping measure of BIOTIN-100 weighs 1.2 ounces and contains 7.5 mg of d-biotin.
To facilitate the proper adhesion of BIOTIN-100 to the ration, slightly moisten the grain with water or a liquid supplement.
Presentation: 5 lb. bags and 20 lb. pails. Measure cup enclosed.
Compendium Code No.: 10500020

BIOTIN™ GOLD

SureNutrition **Biotin**

Guaranteed Analysis: Minimum:

	per lb:	per oz:
Lysine, min.	3.55%	1,000 mg
Methionine, min.	7.10%	2,000 mg
Zinc (Zn), min.	1,850 ppm	52 mg
Biotin, min.	320 mg	20 mg
Gelatin, min.	40,000 mg	2,500 mg

Ingredients: Corn Distiller's Dried Grains with Solubles, Yeast Culture, Alfalfa Meal, Gelatin, DL-Methionine, L-Lysine Monohydrochloride, D-Biotin, Zinc Proteinate, Corn Oil and Artificial Color.
Dosage and Administration: Feeding Directions: Feed two scoops per head per day for 10 days and then one scoop per head per day. Horses with chronic Biotin deficiency problems may stay on two scoops per day.
The enclosed scoop holds 1 oz.
Caution(s): For animal use only.
Warning(s): Keep out of reach of children.
Presentation: 3 lb (1.36 kg), 5 lb (2.2 kg), 10 lb (4.5 kg) and 20 lb (9 kg) pails.
Compendium Code No.: 12060010 0BB1 / 0A1

BIO-TRACH™

Intervet **Vaccine**

Fowl Laryngotracheitis Vaccine, Modified Live Virus
U.S. Vet. Lic. No.: 286
Contents: The vaccine consists of a freeze-dried (lyophilized) preparation of modified live virus strain of fowl laryngotracheitis propagated in chicken embryos.
The vaccine contains gentamicin as a preservative.
Quality Assurance: The vaccine is manufactured using USDA a approved production outline. Only COFAL negative, specific pathogen free (SPF) eggs are used for production of the vaccine. The seed virus is derived from a master seed lot which has been fully tested for purity, safety and immunogenicity. The vaccine is presented in lyophilized form under vacuum and is fully tested for purity, safety and potency according to the standard requirements of the USDA.
Indications: For the prevention of laryngotracheitis in chickens by oral administration through the drinking water. When administered through drinking water, the vaccine induces the development of protective antibodies against infections caused by virulent strains of the virus. The level and duration of immunity, however, depend upon several factors such as the health and nutritional status of the birds, stress factors, concurrent diseases and climatic conditions.
Dosage and Administration: Preparation of the Vaccine:
A. Oral Administration through Drinking Water:
1. Match the dose size of the container to the number of birds to be vaccinated.
2. Tear off the aluminum seal(s) and carefully remove the rubber stopper(s) from the vaccine vial(s).
3. Pour enough clean, nonsanitized water into the vials to fill them approximately three-quarters (¾) full. Replace the stoppers and shake well. The water used should be free of chlorine, iodine or other disinfectants that could kill the virus in the vaccine. Dry skim milk powder may be added to the water at the rate of one (1) cup per 25 gallons of water or approximately 8.0 g per gallon of water prior to mixing with the vaccine. For proper mixing, the reconstituted vaccine from all the vials should be added to a mixing container with the right amount of skim milk solution.
4. Agitate the vaccine in the mixing container to obtain a uniform concentration of the vaccine virus.
5. Proceed immediately to vaccinate the flock as follows:
   a. Withhold chlorinated water for 24 hours before and 24 hours after vaccination and substitute the skim milk/water solution.
   b. Withhold water for four (4) to six (6) hours prior to vaccination to induce thirst.
   c. On the day of vaccination, rinse the waterers with clean, nonsanitized water or milk solution in order to remove residual disinfectants. Mix the vaccine with enough water to last the birds for approximately two (2) to three (3) hours. Provide adequate space

so that at least two-thirds (⅔) of the birds can drink at the same time. Allow sufficient time to consume the vaccine. Soon after the vaccine is consumed the water troughs and tanks should be flushed with a milk solution and rinsed with clean, nonsanitized water.

B. Eye Drop Application - For 1,000 dose size only: The vaccine may be administered by the eye drop method when the chickens are 14 to 16 weeks of age. The preferable age for vaccination is 16 weeks.

1. Tear off the aluminum seal(s) and carefully remove the stopper(s) from the vaccine vial(s).
2. Remove the aluminum seal and rubber stopper from the diluent bottle and transfer enough diluent to the vaccine vial to fill them approximately three-quarters (¾) full. Replace the rubber stopper and shake vigorously for uniform mixing.
3. Transfer the mixed virus suspension from the vaccine vial into the diluent bottle containing the remaining diluent. Replace the rubber stopper and shake well to mix. Replace the rubber stopper with the dropper tip provided in the diluent carton. The vaccine is now ready for use by the following vaccination method:

   Hold the bird on its side and squeeze out one (1) drop (approximately 0.03 mL) of the vaccine to fall into the open eye. Hold the bird until the drop of the vaccine disappears.

C. Spray Application: Birds may be vaccinated by the coarse spray method when they are six (6) weeks of age or older. Revaccination may be done later at 16 to 18 weeks of age.

1. Match the dose size of the container to the number of birds to be vaccinated.
2. Tear off the aluminum seal(s) and carefully remove the rubber stopper(s) from the vaccine vial(s).
3. Pour enough cool, distilled water into the vials to fill them approximately three-quarters (¾) full. Replace the stoppers and shake well. Put the reconstituted vaccine in the sprayer tank and add distilled water proportioned to the number of chickens to be vaccinated. Mix the vaccine thoroughly in the mixing container to obtain uniform concentration of the vaccine virus. The amount of water per 1,000 chickens will vary with house types, density, etc. (normally, 2-3 gal. of water is needed to vaccinate 20,000 chickens). The vaccine should be prepared according to the directions in the spray cabinet or by the directions given by the manufacturer of the field sprayer.

   Spray vaccination method should be done only in houses that can be closed tightly. Close all windows, doors, ventilators, etc. Turn off the fans. Spray the vaccine directly onto the birds. Leave the house closed for at least 15 minutes after spraying.

Precaution(s): The vaccine should be stored in a refrigerator between 35-45°F (2-7°C). If the diluent is included, (for eye drop application), it should be stored at room temperature.

Use all of the vaccine immediately after mixing. Do not store any unused reconstituted vaccine for future use.

Burn the vaccine containers, packaging materials and unused vaccine, if any, when the vaccination is completed.

Caution(s):

1. Mix the vaccine thoroughly with the drinking water (milk/water solution) prior to use.
2. Vaccinate all of the birds on the farm at one time.
3. Vaccinate healthy birds only. The vaccine must be prepared and administered as directed to obtain the best results. Improper handling or administration may result in variable responses.
4. Use goggles when spraying a live virus vaccine.

Warning(s): Do not vaccinate within 21 days before slaughter.

Presentation: Drinking water administered vaccine: Each box of vaccine contains 10 vials of vaccine (1,000, 5,000 or 10,000 doses per vial), and a directions for use circular.

Coarse spray administered vaccine: Each box of vaccine contains 10 vials of vaccine (5,000 or 10,000 doses per vial), and a directions for use circular.

Eye drop administered vaccine: Each box of vaccine contains 10 vials of vaccine (1,000 doses per vial). Each box of diluent contains 10 diluent bottles (30 mL per bottle) and 10 dropper tips. A directions for use circular is enclosed in both the vaccine and diluent boxes.

Compendium Code No.: 11060181

BIOVAC®

United **Vaccine**

Mink Enteritis Vaccine, Killed Virus

U.S. Vet. Lic. No.: 245

Active Ingredient(s): An inactivated vaccine which contains MEV types 1 and 2.

Preservatives: Gentamicin and thimerosal.

Indications: BIOVAC® is for use as an aid in the prevention of viral enteritis in healthy, susceptible mink.

Dosage and Administration: Inject 1 mL under the loose skin of the armpit of mink of at least six (6) weeks of age. For a proper suspension, shake before and occasionally during use. Revaccinate all adults at the time of kit vaccination.

Precaution(s): Store at 35-45°F (2-7°C).

Caution(s): Do not use as a diluent for live virus vaccines.

Use the entire contents when the container is first opened.

Consult a veterinarian or United Vaccines Inc. for an alternate vaccinating schedule and before using the vaccine on a farm where disease exists or has occurred in the last 18 months.

Presentation: 100 dose and 250 dose vials.

Compendium Code No.: 11040041

BIOVAC®-D

United **Vaccine**

Mink Distemper-Enteritis Vaccine, Modified Live and Killed Virus

U.S. Vet. Lic. No.: 245

Active Ingredient(s): The vaccine consists of two components: A freeze-dried distemper vaccine consisting of modified live canine distemper virus (Distemink®) and a liquid inactivated vaccine consisting of MEV types 1 and 2 (Biovac®). The liquid is used to dissolve the Distemink®.

Preservatives: Gentamicin and thimerosal.

Indications: BIOVAC®-D is for use as an aid in the prevention of distemper and viral enteritis in healthy, susceptible mink.

Dosage and Administration: Mixing of the Vaccines:

1. Do not mix the vaccines until ready to use.
2. Mix only one pair of vials at a time, and use the entire contents within two (2) hours.
3. Disinfect rubber stoppers with alcohol.
4. Using a sterile transfer needle, transfer Biovac® into the bottle of Distemink®.
5. To do this, shake Biovac® to obtain a uniform suspension. Insert the short end of the double-pointed transfer needle into Biovac® and turn the bottle upside down; then, insert the other end of the transfer needle into the Distemink®. Biovac® will be drawn into the Distemink® bottle by vacuum.
6. After all the Biovac® has been transferred, shake gently to suspend evenly.
7. Do not transfer the vaccine to other containers.

Use sharp, sterile needles and sterile syringes. Inject 1 mL under the loose skin of the armpit of mink of at least 10 weeks of age. For a proper suspension,shake before and occasionally during use. Revaccinate all adults at the time of kit vaccination.

Keep a record of brand name, quantity, serial number, expiration date, and place of purchase. Record the date of vaccination, the number, age and location of the mink.

Precaution(s): Store at 35-45°F (2-7°C).

Caution(s): Consult a veterinarian or United Vaccines Inc. for an alternate vaccinating schedule and before using the vaccine on a farm where disease exists or has occurred in the last 18 months or where earlier botulism protection is desired.

1. Burn the empty containers and any unused portion of the vaccine.
2. Syringes and reusable, stainless steel needles may be sterilized by boiling them in distilled water for 15 to 20 minutes. Do not disinfect them with chemicals as these can destroy the vaccine.
3. Incubating diseases (such as Aleutian disease), parasites, nutritional deficiencies (anemia), maternal antibodies and poor management practices (dehydration, adverse temperatures) will reduce the vaccine's effectiveness.
4. If shock occurs after vaccination, use atropine sulfate or epinephrine.
5. Should disease occur in an unvaccinated herd, the losses may be minimized by promptly vaccinating those animals which are not showing signs of the disease. The best procedure is to first vaccinate the mink located the farthest distance from those showing symptoms. Care should be taken to use a sterile needle for each animal and to disinfect handling gloves as often as is practical. Consult a veterinarian regarding the treatment and handling of sick animals.
6. Animals infected, yet not showing signs of disease at the time of vaccination, will not be protected by the vaccine. Symptoms of the disease may continue to develop for as long as two months after vaccination.

Presentation: 100 dose and 250 dose vials.

Compendium Code No.: 11040051

BIOZIDE® GEL

PPI **Topical Wound Dressing**

Fungicidal-Bactericidal

Active Ingredient(s): This product is manufactured with a water washable nonirritating gel base. It contains BIOZIDE® polyvinylpyrrolidone-iodine complex supplying 1.0% available iodine.

Indications: For topical antiinfective treatment of wounds, cuts, ulcers, abrasions, and postoperative wound protection.

Directions for Use:

Wounds — cleanse wound with soap and water. Dry with clean towel and gauze. Apply BIOZIDE® Gel directly on the cleansed wound with a spatula or piece of gauze. Bandage over wound if desired. If necessary, change dressing several times daily. For deep or puncture wounds, use as directed by veterinarian. If redness, irritation, or swelling increases, discontinue use and consult veterinarian.

Precaution(s): Keep closed when not in use.

Caution(s): For veterinary use only.

Warning(s): Keep out of reach of children.

Presentation: 2 oz. and 20 oz. jar.

Compendium Code No.: 12270001

BIOZIDE® PUFFER

PPI **Topical Wound Dressing**

Bactericidal Fungicidal

Active Ingredient(s): Contains BIOZIDE® polyvinylpyrrolidone-iodine complex in a water soluble base, 0.75% available iodine.

Indications: For topical antiinfective treatment of wounds, cuts, ulcers, abrasions, and for postoperative wound protection.

Directions for Use:

Wounds - cleanse wound with soap and water. Dry with clean towel or gauze. Apply BIOZIDE® powder. Repeat several times daily as necessary, a bandage may be used if desired.

For deep puncture wounds, use as directed by veterinarian. If redness, irritation or swelling increases; discontinue use and reconsult veterinarian.

Caution(s): For veterinary use only.

Warning(s): Keep out of reach of children.

Presentation: 60 gram puffer.

Compendium Code No.: 12270011

BIRD BENE-BAC™ GEL

Pet-Ag **Small Animal Dietary Supplement**

Active Ingredient(s): Dried *Lactobacillus fermentum*, dried *L. casei* (avian strain), dried *Streptococcus faecium*, *L. plantarum* and *L. acidophilus* fermentation products, vegetable oils, sugar, silicon dioxide, artificial color, polysorbate 80 preserved with TBHQ, and ethoxyquin.

The guaranteed total (viable) lactic acid producing bacteria is 10 million colony forming units (CFU) per gram.

Indications: The product is recommended as part of the management program for birds and reptiles subjected to changing environmental or nutritional conditions or after antibiotic therapy.

Dosage and Administration: Directions for Use with Birds:

Hand Feeding: Administer ½ g on days 1, 3, 5, and 7 and then once per week until after weaning from hand feeding. Mix with formula after heating, or dose directly into the feeding syringe or mouth.

Growing Phase: Administer ½ g once per week for the first three (3) months.

Maintenance: Administer every other week. Use ½ g for small species and 1 g for large species.

Changing Conditions: Administer two (2) treatments, three (3) days apart before and after periods of environmental or nutritional changes. Use the levels recommended above.

For Use with Reptiles:

Growing and Maintenance: ½-1 g, 12-24 hours before feeding and 2-12 hours after feeding.

Administer by placing the gel on food or directly into the mouth.

Precaution(s): Store under cool, dry conditions.

Presentation: 12x15 g syringe (professional pack), 6x15 g syringe (carded merchandise), and 4x1 g syringe.

Compendium Code No.: 10970021

BIRD BENE-BAC™ POWDER

Pet-Ag **Small Animal Dietary Supplement**

Active Ingredient(s): Dextrose, maltodextrin, dried *Lactobacillus fermentum*, dried *L. casei* (avian strain), dried *Streptococcus faecium*, dried *L. plantarum*, and dried *L. acidophilus* fermentation products.

The guaranteed total (viable) lactic acid producing bacteria is 25 million colony forming units (CFU) per gram.

Indications: The product is recommended as part of the management program for birds and reptiles subjected to changing environmental or nutritional conditions or after antibiotic therapy.

Dosage and Administration:

Hand Feeding: Mix with formula after cooling to 100°F or less. Provide one (1) feeding on days 1,3,5 and 7, and then one (1) feeding per week until weaned from hand feeding formula.

Body Weight	Amount of BIRD BENE-BAC™ Powder
10-30 g	1/8 level teaspoon
30-250 g	1/4 level teaspoon
250-450 g	1/2 level teaspoon

Growing and Maintenance: Treat birds once a week by top dressing BIRD BENE-BAC™ Powder on moistened or oiled dry food or fresh fruits or vegetables. Use 1/8 teaspoon for birds 1 lb. or less and 1/8 teaspoon for every pound thereafter up to a maximum of one (1) teaspoon per treatment. Discard uneaten food after no more than eight (8) hours and thoroughly wash dishes.

Changing Conditions: Use the quantities indicated for growing and maintenance, but provide two (2) feedings, three (3) days apart, before and after periods of environmental or nutritional changes. If the bird is anorexic, consult a veterinarian.

General Information: If several birds are maintained in a common cage or flyway, use the approximate total weight of all birds to determine the feeding level. Mix with the feed so that all of the birds receive the appropriate dose.

For large ratites, use one (1) teaspoon for growing birds and two (2) teaspoons for mature stock. Follow the frequency directions indicated above. One (1) level teaspoon equals approximately 2.7 g of BIRD BENE-BAC™ Powder.

Wash all feeding dishes, water bottles, or water dishes thoroughly with hot, soapy water and rinse well after each use.

Reptiles should be provided BIRD BENE-BAC™ Powder on the same weight basis as birds.

Be sure to contact a veterinarian for any illness.

Precaution(s): Store in cool, dry conditions.

Presentation: 4.5 oz. jar (12 per box) and 10 oz. jar (6 per case).

Compendium Code No.: 10970031

BI-SEPT™ ACTIVATOR

Westfalia•Surge **Teat Dip**

Pre-Post Milking Non-Iodine Teat Dip

Active Ingredient(s): Contents:

Lactic Acid 2.9%
Inactive Ingredients: 97.1%*

*Contains 8% Glycerin.

Indications: This topical liquid product, when properly mixed with BI-SEPT™ Base and used undiluted as a pre and post teat dip, effectively aids in reducing the spread of mastitis.

Directions for Use: Use only when properly mixed with BI-SEPT™ Base. Do not dilute.

Always prepare mixture in a ventilated area: add one volume of BI-SEPT™ Activator to one volume of BI-SEPT™ Base to a clean container. Mix thoroughly. Prepare only enough product for one milking of the herd.

Pre Dipping: Before milking, dip each teat with BI-SEPT™. After 15 to 30 seconds, dry each teat thoroughly with a single service towel. If the udder and teats are heavily soiled, wash with a sanitizing solution and dry before application of BI-SEPT™ teat dip.

Post Dipping: Immediately after milking, dip each teat with BI-SEPT™. Allow teats to air dry. Do not wipe. If outside temperature is below freezing, allow to air dry on the teat before the cow leaves the parlor to prevent freezing. At the end of lactation, apply this product daily for one week after the last milking. In addition, begin application of this product about one week prior to calving. If a common teat dip cup is used for application, a fresh solution should always be used at each milking. The teat dip cup should be emptied, cleaned and rinsed with potable water after each milking session or when cup becomes contaminated during milking. Do not pour remaining solution from dip cup back into original container.

Precaution(s): Storage Instructions: Store this product in a cool dry area away from direct sunlight and heat to avoid deterioration. Keep containers closed to prevent contamination of this product. Keep from freezing.

Precautionary Statements: Danger. Contains materials which may irritate or burn eyes. May be harmful or fatal if swallowed. May cause skin irritation. Protect eyes and skin when handling. Do not take internally. Avoid breathing vapors when mixing this product with BI-SEPT™ Base. Do not mix with any other chemical products. Refer to Material Safety Data Sheet (MSDS).

First Aid:

If in Eyes: Flush with large volumes of water for at least 15 minutes. Call a physician immediately.

If Swallowed: Do not induce vomiting. Rinse mouth promptly then give small amount/glass of milk or water (4-6 oz. child/10-12 oz. adult) (120-180 mL child/300-360 mL adult). Avoid alcohol. Call a physician immediately. Do not give anything by mouth to an unconscious or convulsing person.

If on Skin: While removing contaminated clothing and shoes, flush with large volumes of water for at least 15 minutes. If irritation develops and persists, get medical attention.

Inhalation of Vapors: If breathing difficulty or irritation occurs, remove to fresh air. If symptoms persist, get medical attention.

For assistance with medical emergency, call 1-800-451-8346.

For farm, commercial and industrial use only.

Warning(s): Keep out of reach of children.

Presentation: Contact the company for container sizes available.

BI-SEPT is a trademark of Westfalia•Surge, Inc.

Compendium Code No.: 10020210 Rev. 10-00

BI-SEPT™ BASE

Westfalia•Surge **Teat Dip**

Pre-Post Milking Non-Iodine Teat Dip

Active Ingredient(s): Contents:

Sodium Chlorite 0.7%
Inactive Ingredients: 99.3%*

*Contains 2% Glycerin.

Indications: This topical liquid product, when properly mixed with BI-SEPT™ Activator and used undiluted as a pre and post teat dip, effectively aids in reducing the spread of mastitis.

Directions for Use: Use only when properly mixed with BI-SEPT™ Activator. Do not dilute.

Always prepare mixture in a ventilated area: add one volume of BI-SEPT™ Base to one volume of BI-SEPT™ Activator to a clean container. Mix thoroughly. Prepare only enough product for one milking of the herd.

Pre Dipping: Before milking, dip each teat with BI-SEPT™. After 15 to 30 seconds, dry each teat thoroughly with a single service towel. If the udder and teats are heavily soiled, wash with a sanitizing solution and dry before application of BI-SEPT™ teat dip.

Post Dipping: Immediately after milking, dip each teat with BI-SEPT™. Allow teats to air dry. Do not wipe. If outside temperature is below freezing, allow to air dry on the teat before the cow leaves the parlor to prevent freezing. At the end of lactation, apply this product daily for one week after the last milking. In addition, begin application of this product about one week prior to calving. If a common teat dip cup is used for application, a fresh solution should always be used at each milking. The teat dip cup should be emptied, cleaned and rinsed with potable water after each milking session or when cup becomes contaminated during milking. Do not pour remaining solution from dip cup back into original container.

Precaution(s): Storage Instructions: Store this product in a cool dry area away from direct sunlight and heat to avoid deterioration. Keep containers closed to prevent contamination of this product. Keep from freezing.

Precautionary Statements: Danger. Contains materials which may irritate or burn eyes. May be harmful or fatal if swallowed. Protect eyes and skin when handling. Do not take internally. Avoid breathing vapors when mixing this product with BI-SEPT™ Activator. Do not mix with any other chemical products. Refer to Material Safety Data Sheet (MSDS).

First Aid:

If in Eyes: Flush with large volumes of water for at least 15 minutes. Call a physician immediately.

If Swallowed: Do not induce vomiting. Rinse mouth promptly then give small amount/glass of milk or water (4-6 oz. child/10-12 oz. adult) (120-180 mL child/300-360 mL adult). Avoid alcohol. Call a physician immediately. Do not give anything by mouth to an unconscious or convulsing person.

If on Skin: While removing contaminated clothing and shoes, flush with large volumes of water for at least 15 minutes. If irritation develops and persists, get medical attention.

Inhalation of Vapors: If breathing difficulty or irritation occurs, remove to fresh air. If symptoms persist, get medical attention.

For assistance with medical emergency call 1-800-451-8346.

For farm, commercial and industrial use only.

Warning(s): Keep out of reach of children.

Presentation: Contact the company for container sizes available.

BI-SEPT is a trademark of Westfalia•Surge, Inc.

Compendium Code No.: 10020220 Rev. 10-00

BISMUKOTE PASTE FOR MEDIUM & LARGE DOGS

Vedco **Antidiarrheal-Adsorbent**

Active Ingredient(s): Bismuth subsalicylate, magnesium aluminum silicate, benzoic acid, sorbic acid, sucrose, bacon flavor, artificial colors, salicylic acid, sodium salicylate, sodium saccharine.

Indications: For medium and large dogs, as an aid in the treatment and prevention of diarrhea or gastrointestinal inflammation.

Dosage and Administration: 1cc per 10 pounds of body weight 3 to 4 times per day, administered on the tongue. 1cc InnoBiz-10 = 100 mg bismuth subsalicylate.

Caution(s): Hospitalization, oral and intravenous hydration may be necessary in cases of diarrhea or gastrointestinal inflammation. Consult your veterinarian if signs of depression, fever, vomiting, diarrhea, or abdominal discomfort persist. This beneficial medication may cause a temporary and harmless darkening of the tongue or stool.

Warning(s): For animal use only.

Presentation: 30cc/30g tube.

Compendium Code No.: 10940130

BISMUKOTE PASTE FOR SMALL DOGS

Vedco **Antidiarrheal-Adsorbent**

Active Ingredient(s): Bismuth subsalicylate, magnesium aluminum silicate, xanthan, bezoic acid, sorbic acid, sucrose, bacon flavor, artificial colors, salicylic acid, sodium salicylate, sodium saccharine.

Indications: For small dogs, as an aid in the treatment and prevention of diarrhea or gastrointestinal inflammation.

Dosage and Administration: 1cc per 5 pounds of body weight 3 to 4 times per day, administered on the tongue. 1cc BISMUKOTE PASTE = 50 mg bismuth subsalicylate.

Caution(s): Hospitalization, oral and intravenous hydration may be necessary in cases of diarrhea or gastrointestinal inflammation. Consult your veterinarian if signs of depression, fever, vomiting, diarrhea, or abdominal discomfort persist. This medication may cause a temporary and harmless darkening of the tongue or stool.

Warning(s): For animal use only.

Presentation: 15cc/15g tube.

Compendium Code No.: 10940140

BISMU-KOTE SUSPENSION

Vedco **Antidiarrheal-Adsorbent**

Active Ingredient(s): Contains:

Bismuth subsalicylate 1.75%

Indications: A palatable oral suspension for use in controlling nonspecific diarrhea by coating intestinal mucosa, thereby decreasing hyperperistalsis and irritation.

By absorbing toxins in the gastro-intestinal tracts of cattle, horses, dogs and cats, BISMU-KOTE acts as a counterirritant.

Dosage and Administration: Shake well before using.

Horses and Cattle: 6-10 oz. every two (2) to three (3) hours.

Foals and Calves: 3-4 oz. every two (2) to three (3) hours.

Dogs and Cats: 1-3 tbsp. every one (1) to three (3) hours.
Precaution(s): Keep from freezing.
Caution(s): Keep out of the reach of children.
Continue treatment until the condition improves. If symptoms persist for two days or longer, consult a veterinarian.
Presentation: 1 gallon containers.
Compendium Code No.: 10940120

B

BISMUPASTE D5

Vetus **Antidiarrheal-Adsorbent**

Contents: Bismuth subsalicylate 5%, magnesium aluminum silicate, xanthan, benzoic acid, sorbic acid, sucrose, bacon flavor, artificial colors, salicylic acid, sodium salicylate, sodium saccharine.
Indications: For small dogs, as an aid in the treatment and prevention of diarrhea or gastrointestinal inflammation.
Dosage and Administration: Directions: Use 1 cc per 5 pounds of body weight 3 to 4 times per day, administered on the back of the tongue.
1 cc BISMUPASTE D5 = 50 mg bismuth subsalicylate.
Caution(s): Hospitalization, and oral or intravenous hydration may be necessary in cases of diarrhea or gastrointestinal inflammation. Consult your veterinarian if signs of depression, fever, vomiting, diarrhea, or abdominal discomfort persist. This beneficial medication may cause a temporary and harmless darkening of the tongue and stool.
Warning(s): For animal use only.
Presentation: 15 cc/15 g tube.
Compendium Code No.: 14440110

BISMUPASTE D10

Vetus **Antidiarrheal-Adsorbent**

Contents: Bismuth subsalicylate 10%, magnesium aluminum silicate, xanthan, benzoic acid, sorbic acid, sucrose, bacon flavor, artificial colors, salicylic acid, sodium salicylate, sodium saccharine.
Indications: For medium and large dogs, as an aid in the treatment and prevention of diarrhea or gastrointestinal inflammation.
Dosage and Administration: Directions: Use 1 cc per 10 pounds of body weight 3 to 4 times per day, administered on the back of the tongue.
1 cc BISMUPASTE D10 = 100 mg bismuth subsalicylate.
Caution(s): Hospitalization, and oral or intravenous hydration may be necessary in cases of diarrhea or gastrointestinal inflammation. Consult your veterinarian if signs of depression, fever, vomiting, diarrhea, or abdominal discomfort persist. This beneficial medication may cause a temporary and harmless darkening of the tongue and stool.
Warning(s): For animal use only.
Presentation: 30 cc/30 g tube.
Compendium Code No.: 14440100

BISMUPASTE E20

Vetus **Antidiarrheal-Adsorbent**

Contents: Bismuth subsalicylate 20%, magnesium aluminum silicate, xanthan, benzoic acid, sorbic acid, sucrose, apple flavor, artificial colors, salicylic acid, sodium salicylate, sodium saccharine.
Indications: For horses, as an aid in the treatment and prevention of diarrhea or gastrointestinal inflammation.
Dosage and Administration: Directions: Use 5 cc per 100 pounds of body weight 3 to 4 times per day, or as directed by a veterinarian.
5 cc BISMUPASTE E20 = 1 g bismuth subsalicylate.
Caution(s): Hospitalization, and oral or intravenous hydration may be necessary in cases of diarrhea or gastrointestinal inflammation. Consult your veterinarian if signs of depression, fever, vomiting, diarrhea, or abdominal discomfort persist. This beneficial medication may cause a temporary and harmless darkening of the tongue and stool.
Warning(s): For animal use only.
Presentation: 60 cc/60 g tube.
Compendium Code No.: 14440120

BISMUSAL

Bimeda **Antidiarrheal-Adsorbent**

Active Ingredient(s): Contains:
Bismuth subsalicylate 1.75%
Indications: An oral suspension for use in controlling nonspecific diarrhea by coating the intestinal mucosa, thereby decreasing hyperperistalsis and irritation. By absorbing toxins in the gastro-intestinal tract of cattle, horses, dogs and cats, BISMUSAL acts as a counter-irritant.
Dosage and Administration: Shake well before using.
Horses and Cattle: 6-10 oz. every two (2) to three (3) hours.
Foals and Calves: 3-4 oz. every two (2) to three (3) hours.
Dogs and Cats: 1-3 tablespoons every one (1) to three (3) hours.
Precaution(s): Keep from freezing.
Caution(s): Not for human use. Keep out of the reach of children.
Warning(s): Continue treatment until the condition improves. If symptoms persist for two (2) days or longer, consult a veterinarian.
Presentation: 1 gallon containers.
Compendium Code No.: 13990060

BISMUSAL

Durvet **Antidiarrheal-Adsorbent**

Palatable Anti-Diarrheal Suspension
Active Ingredient(s): Composition:
Bismuth Subsalicylate 1.75%
in a palatable aqueous suspension.
Flavoring and coloring added.
Indications: A palatable oral suspension for use as an aid in the control of simple diarrhea in cattle, horses and dogs.
Dosage and Administration: Shake well before using.
Administer orally after the first sign of diarrhea and after each loose bowel movement or as needed.
Dogs: 1 to 3 tablespoons.
Calves and Foals: 3 to 4 ounces.
Cattle and Horses: 6 to 10 ounces.
Contraindication(s): Not recommended for use in cats.
This product contains salicylate, do not administer with other salicylate containing products such as aspirin. Do not administer to pregnant animals unless prescribed by a licensed veterinarian.
Precaution(s): Store at room temperature not above 37°C (98.6°F). Protect from freezing.
Caution(s): This product may cause stools to darken.
If diarrhea persists after using this product for 2 days contact a veterinarian.
For animal use only. For oral use only.
Warning(s): Keep out of reach of children.
Presentation: 1 gallon (3.785 L) (NDC 30798-831-35).
Compendium Code No.: 10841920 Rev. 11-00

BISMUSAL SUSPENSION

AgriPharm **Antidiarrheal-Adsorbent**

Antidiarrheal Liquid
Active Ingredient(s): Contains:
Bismuth subsalicylate 1.75%
In a palatable aqueous suspension. Flavoring and coloring added.
Indications: A palatable oral solution for use as an aid in the control of non-specific diarrhea of cattle, horses, dogs and cats.
Dosage and Administration: For oral administration.
Horses and Cattle .... 6 to 10 oz every 2 to 3 hours
Foals and Calves .... 3 to 4 oz every 2 to 3 hours
Dogs and Cats .... 1 to 3 tablespoons every 1 to 3 hours
May be repeated until condition improves.
Precaution(s): Shake well before using. Keep from freezing.
Store at controlled room temperature between 15°-37°C (59°-98.6°F).
Caution(s): For animal use only. Keep out of reach of children.
This product contains salicylate, do not administer with other salicylate containing products, such as aspirin.
If symptoms persist after using this product for 2 to 3 days consult a veterinarian.
Presentation: 1 gallon containers.
Compendium Code No.: 14570120

BISMUSOL

First Priority **Antidiarrheal-Adsorbent**

Anti-Diarrheal Liquid-Palatable Oral Suspension
Active Ingredient(s):
Bismuth Subsalicylate 1.75%
In a palatable aqueous suspension. Flavoring and coloring are added.
Indications: A palatable oral suspension for use as an aid in controlling simple diarrhea in cattle, horses, dogs and cats.
Dosage and Administration: Shake well before using.
Administer orally.
Dogs and Cats: 1 to 3 tablespoonfuls every 1-3 hours.
Calves and Foals: 3 to 4 ounces every 2-3 hours.
Horses and Cattle: 6-10 ounces every 2-3 hours.
Contraindication(s): This product contains salicylate; do not administer with other salicylate containing products, such as aspirin. Do not administer to pregnant animals unless prescribed by a licensed veterinarian.
Precaution(s): Storage: Store at room temperature not above 37°C (98.6°F). Keep from freezing.
Caution(s): If diarrhea persists after using this product for 2 days, consult veterinarian.
For animal use only. For oral use only.
Warning(s): Keep out of reach of children.
Presentation: 1 gallon (3.785 L) (NDC 58829-221-01).
Compendium Code No.: 11390041 Rev. 06-01

BISMUTH SUBSALICYLATE SUSPENSION

A.A.H. **Antidiarrheal-Adsorbent**

Anti-Diarrheal Palatable Oral Suspension
Active Ingredient(s): Composition:
Bismuth Subsalicylate 1.75%
In a palatable aqueous suspension. Flavoring and coloring added.
Indications: A palatable oral suspension for use as an aid in controlling simple diarrhea in cattle, horses, dogs and cats.
Dosage and Administration: Administer orally.
Dogs and Cats: 1 to 3 tablespoonfuls every 1-3 hours.
Calves and Foals: 3 to 4 ounces every 2-3 hours.
Horses and Cattle: 6 to 10 ounces every 2-3 hours.
Precaution(s): Shake well before using. Keep from freezing.
Store at room temperature not above 37°C (98.6°F).
Caution(s): This product contains salicylate; do not administer with other salicylate containing products, such as aspirin.
If diarrhea persists after using this product for 2 days, consult veterinarian.
For animal use only.
Warning(s): Keep out of reach of children.
Presentation: 4 x 3.78 L (128 fl oz) (1 gal) jugs per case.
Compendium Code No.: 11180190 1201

BITE FREE™ BITING FLY REPELLENT

Farnam **Insect Repellent**

EPA Reg. No.: 270-251
Active Ingredient(s):
Cypermethrin [(±)-alpha-cyano-(3-phenoxyphenyl) methyl-(±)-cis, trans 3-(2,2-dichloroethenyl)-2,2-dimethylcyclopropanecarboxylate] 0.150%
Pyrethrins 0.200%
Piperonyl Butoxide Technical* 1.600%
Butoxy Polypropylene Glycol 5.000%
Inert Ingredients 93.05%

*Equivalent to 1.28% (butylcarbityl) (6-propylpiperonyl) ether and 0.32% of related compounds.
Indications: Biting fly repellent for horses and ponies that protects against biting and nuisance flies, gnats, mosquitoes, deer ticks and lice.
Directions for Use: It is a violation of Federal law to use this product in a manner inconsistent with its labeling.

Wash hands with soap and water after use. Shake well before using. To protect horses from horse flies, house flies, stable flies, face flies, horn flies, deer flies, gnats, mosquitoes, lice and deer ticks that may transmit Lyme Disease: Thoroughly brush the horse's coat prior to application to remove loose dirt and debris. For dirty horses, shampoo and rinse thoroughly.

Wait until coat is completely dry before applying BITE FREE™ Biting Fly Repellent.

BITE FREE™ may be applied either as a spray or as a wipe. For horse's face, always apply as a wipe using a piece of clean, absorbent cloth, toweling (Turkish) or sponge. Wear rubber glove or mitt when applying as a wipe. Spray or wipe horse's entire body while brushing against the lay of the coat to ensure adequate coverage. Avoid getting spray into horse's eyes, nose or mouth. Application should be liberal for best residual results. Reapply every 5 to 7 days under normal conditions for initial applications. As protection builds, reapply every 10 to 14 days as needed. Also, reapply each time animal is washed or exposed to heavy rain.
Precautionary Statements: Hazards to Humans and Domestic Animals: Caution:

Humans: For animal use only. Not for use on humans. Harmful if swallowed. Avoid contact with eyes, skin or clothing. Avoid breathing spray mist. Avoid contamination of food. Wash hands with soap and water after use.

Horses: Avoid contact with eyes or mucous membranes. Harmful if swallowed. Avoid breathing spray mist. Avoid contamination of food.

Statement of Practical Treatment:

If Swallowed: Contact a physician or Poison Control Center immediately. Drink 1 or 2 glasses of water and induce vomiting by touching back of throat with finger or by administering syrup of ipecac. Do not induce vomiting or give anything by mouth to an unconscious person.

If Inhaled: Remove victim to fresh air. Apply artificial respiration and/or seen medical attention if indicated.

If on Skin: Remove contaminated clothing and wash skin thoroughly with soap and water.

If in Eyes: Immediately flush eyes with plenty of water. Get medical attention if irritation persists.

Environmental Hazards: This product is toxic to fish. Keep out of lakes, streams and ponds. Do not contaminate water by cleaning of equipment or disposal of wastes. Do not apply to any body of water. Do not contaminate water when disposing of equipment washwaters.
Storage and Disposal:

Storage: Store in a cool, dry place.

Pesticide Disposal: Securely wrap empty original container in several layers of newspaper and discard in trash.

Container Disposal: Do not reuse empty container. Wrap container and put in trash.
Warning(s): Not for use on horses intended for human consumption. Keep out of reach of children.
Presentation: 32 fl. oz. (0.946 L).
Compendium Code No.: 10000060

BITTER-3™

Butler — **Topical Product**

Active Ingredient(s): Isopropyl alcohol, deionized water, oleoresin capsicum, sucrose octyl acetate, orange peel bitter, propylene glycol, polysorbate 60, FD&C red #40.
Indications: BITTER-3 contains three active bittering agents from tabasco pepper, orange peel and denatured alcohol to discourage licking, biting and chewing.
Dosage and Administration: Shake well before using. Apply to bandages, casts, hair, or household furniture twice daily or as directed by a veterinarian.
Precaution(s): Keep away from heat or open flame.
Caution(s): Avoid contact with broken skin, eyes or mucous membranes. If in contact, wash with copious amounts of cool water immediately. If redness or irritation occurs or if accidentally swallowed, call a physician or poison control center.

Before applying to extensive areas of furniture, test on a small inconspicuous area.

Sold only through veterinarians. Keep out of reach of children.
Presentation: 2 oz. gel (12/box) and 4 oz. mister (12/box).
Compendium Code No.: 10820210

BITTER ORANGE™

ARC — **Topical Product**

Ingredients: Water, isopropyl alcohol (22% by volume), oleoresin capsicum, sucrose octa acetate, propylene glycol, polysorbate 60.
Indications: Double strength creme for dogs. Extremely bitter tasting to discourage licking, biting and chewing.
Dosage and Administration: Apply to bandages, casts, or hair three times daily or as otherwise directed by your veterinarian.
Caution(s): Avoid contact with broken skin, eyes or mucous membranes. If eyes are contacted, wash with warm water immediately. Use carefully as may cause staining.

First Aid (Animals) call a veterinarian.
Warning(s): Harmful if swallowed. First Aid (Human) call a physician or poison control center. Keep out of reach of children.
Presentation: 1 fl oz and 2 fl oz.
Compendium Code No.: 10960020

BITTER SAFE MIST

Butler — **Topical Product**

Active Ingredient(s): Water, propylene glycol, Bitrex® (denatonium benzoate NF), and fragrance.
Indications: BITTER SAFE MIST discourages licking, biting and chewing.
Dosage and Administration: Apply to bandages, casts, hair or household furniture twice daily or as directed by a veterinarian.
Caution(s): Avoid contact with broken skin, eyes or mucous membranes. If in contact, wash with copious amounts of cool water.

Before applying to extensive areas of furniture, test the effect of the product on a small inconspicuous area.

Sold only through veterinarians.

Keep out of reach of children.
Presentation: 4 fl. oz. mister, 12/box (NDC 11695-108-04).
Compendium Code No.: 10820200

BIZOLIN®-1 G ℞

Boehringer Ingelheim — **Non-Steroidal Anti-Inflammatory**

(Phenylbutazone) 1 gram per Tablet
NADA No.: 099-618
Active Ingredient(s): Each tablet contains: Phenylbutazone (4-butyl-1, 2-diphenyl-3, 5-pyrazolidinedione) 1 gram; inert ingredients (as excipients) - q.s.
Indications: BIZOLIN® Tablets have non-hormonal anti-inflammatory properties in the management of musculoskeletal conditions in horses, such as generalized arthritis.
Dosage and Administration: Horses: 2 to 4 mg per lb of body weight (equivalent to 1 to 2 grams per 500 lb of body weight) or 2 to 4 BIZOLIN® Tablets, 1 g for 1000 lb of body weight per day. Do not exceed 4 grams per animal per day. As symptoms regress, reduce dosage 25% to 50% of initial dose as needed to control symptoms. If there is no improvement in 5 days discontinue treatment. Infective conditions should be treated concurrently with the proper anti-infectives. Response to treatment is variable, as is also the tolerance for the drug. Withdrawal of the drug may be followed by reappearance of symptoms, after which it may be given intermittently to control symptoms. The drug is symptomatic in action and not curative.

Recommendations: Use up to the maximum recommended dose for the first 48 hours. As symptoms regress, reduce dosage 25% to 50% of the initial "loading dose" as needed to control symptoms. Because of the more rapid metabolism in animals, administer BIZOLIN® Tablets in 3 divided daily doses (at 8-hour intervals) to maintain therapeutic blood level. Response to BIZOLIN® Tablets treatment usually occurs within 24 hours after the initial dose. If no response is evident after 5 days of dosing, treatment should be discontinued.

While many chronic conditions, such as chronic osteoarthritis, will respond to BIZOLIN® therapy, no permanent cure can be effected owing to the advance tissue changes. In such cases discontinuance of treatment often will result in recurrence of symptoms. However, intermittent therapy may be extremely valuable to alleviate symptoms of chronic inflammatory lesions.
Contraindication(s): Animals showing evidence of cardiac, hepatic, or renal damage or a history of blood dyscrasia, or those with signs or history of anemia. Treated animals should not be slaughtered for food purposes.
Precaution(s): Store at controlled room temperature, 59°-86°F (15°-30°C).
Caution(s): Federal (U.S.A.) law restricts this drug to use by or on the order of a licensed veterinarian.

Stop medication at first sign of gastrointestinal upset, blood dyscrasia, jaundice, or black or tarry stools. Agranulocytosis associated with the drug has occurred in man and was reversible upon discontinuance of treatment. Fatal reactions, although rare, have been reported in dogs after long-term therapy. Routine blood counts should be made at weekly intervals during the early phase of therapy and thereafter at intervals of two weeks. A significant fall in total white count, or a relative decrease in granulocytes, or black or tarry stools indicate that therapy with BIZOLIN® Tablets, 1 gram should be immediately discontinued. In the treatment of inflammatory conditions associated with infection specific anti-infective therapy is required. Caution should be observed when administering to patients with a history of drug allergy.
Warning(s): Treated animals should not be used for food purposes.

Keep out of the reach of children.

For use in animals only.
Trial Data: The clinical effectiveness of phenylbutazone in acute rheumatism, gout, gouty arthritis, and various other rheumatoid disorders in man was demonstrated by Kuzell[1,2,3], Payne[4], Fleming[5], and Denko[6]. Anti-inflammatory activity has been well-established by Fabre[7], Domenjoz[8], Wilhelmi[9], and Yourish[10]. The effective use of phenylbutazone in the treatment of painful conditions of the musculoskeletal system in dogs, including arthritis and painful injuries to the limbs and joints has been reported by Lieberman[11]. Joshua[12] observed objective improvement without toxicity following long-term therapy of two aged arthritic dogs. Ogilvie and Sutter[13] reported rapid response to phenylbutazone therapy in a review of 19 clinical cases including posterior weakness, arthritis, rheumatism, and other conditions associated with lameness and musculoskeletal weakness.

Favorable results have been reported by Camberos[14] following intermittent treatment of horses in generalized arthritis, chronic pain in trapezius muscles, osteoarthritis of the medial and distal bones of the hock, chronic hip pains, arthritis of stifle and hip, arthrosis of the spine. In cases of traumatism, muscle rupture, inflammation of the third phalanx, and strains, results were less favorable. Sutter[15] reported favorable response to chronic equine arthritis.
References: Available upon request.
Presentation: Bottles of 100 tablets.
Compendium Code No.: 10280170

BLOAT DRENCH™

Great States — **Bloat Preparation**

Ingredients: Vegetable oil, polyethylene glycol, poly glycerol oleate, sodium benzoate, methylparabens, propylparabens.
Indications: For use as an aid in the treatment of frothy bloat in cattle and sheep.
Dosage and Administration: Shake well before using.

Administer the contents of this dosing container orally as a drench to aid in the relief of bloated conditions in average size mature cattle. Young cattle and sheep should receive 6 to 12 fluid ounces as the severity of the condition indicates. Should condition persist, consult your veterinarian immediately.
Caution(s): For animal use only.
Warning(s): Keep out of reach of children.
Presentation: 12 x 12 fl oz (355 mL) long-necked, plastic bottles per case.
Compendium Code No.: 14110001

BLOAT GUARD® LIQUID TYPE A MEDICATED ARTICLE

Phibro — **Bloat Preparation**

Brand of Poloxalene
NADA No.: 038-281
Active Ingredient(s):
Poloxalene 99.5%

Inert Ingredients: Ethoxyquin (a preservative), 0.12%; BHT (butylated hydroxytoluene, a preservative), 0.38%
Indications: For use in the manufacture of liquid feed supplements. For control of legume (alfalfa, clover) and wheat pasture bloat in cattle.

B

Directions:

Directions for Use in Liquid Feeds:

BLOAT GUARD® Liquid Type A Medicated Article must be thoroughly blended and evenly distributed into a liquid feed supplement and offered to cattle in a covered liquid feed supplement feeder with lick wheels. The formula for the liquid feed supplement is as follows:

	% w/w
Ammonium Polyphosphate	2.660
Phosphoric Acid (75%)	3.370
Sulfuric Acid	1.000
Water	10.000
Molasses—Sufficient to make	100.000

Vitamins A & D and Trace Minerals may be added.

The concentration of BLOAT GUARD® Liquid per pound of liquid feed supplement is as follows:

Indications for Use	Required Level of BLOAT GUARD® Liquid
For control of legume (alfalfa, clover) and wheat pasture bloat in cattle.	7.5 grams per pound (1.65% w/w)
For control of legume (alfalfa, clover) bloat in cattle grazing pre-bloom legumes.	10.0 grams per pound (2.2% w/w)

Important: To maintain proper distribution of BLOAT GUARD® Liquid in liquid feed supplements, the viscosity of the medicated liquid supplement must be no less than 275 cps. During storage the medicated liquid may separate out of liquid supplements within five days if not agitated. It is essential that all of the stored mixture be thoroughly remixed (for example, by using a recirculating pump) before being transferred to feeders with free-turning lick wheels. Movement of the lick wheels is sufficient to prevent separation in the feeders.

Feeding and Management Directions for Liquid Feed Supplement Medicated with BLOAT GUARD® Liquid

These medicated supplements are effective for the control of legume (alfalfa, clover) and wheat pasture bloat in cattle, when consumed as recommended.

1. Use a covered liquid feeder with one free-turning lick wheel per 25 head at a height so that all cattle can conveniently lick the wheel.
2. The location of the liquid feeder is extremely important for adequate consumption. Place feeder where cattle congregate (for example, near drinking water), thus providing ready access to the medicated liquid feed supplement. In large pastures, additional feeders should be placed so that cattle are never more than 500 feet from a feeder while grazing.
3. For adequate protection, it is essential that each animal consume the total recommended dosage of medication daily.
4. If grazing on pre-bloom legumes, use a liquid feed supplement containing 10 grams of BLOAT GUARD® Liquid per pound (2.2% w/w). Each animal must consume the medicated liquid feed supplement at a rate of 0.15 pounds per 100 pounds body weight per day for adequate protection. Example: 1.5 pounds of 2.2% medicated supplement for a 1000-pound animal daily. If consumption exceeds 0.2 pounds per 100 pounds body weight per day, cattle should be changed to a liquid feed supplement containing 7.5 grams of BLOAT GUARD® Liquid per pound (1.65% w/w).
5. If grazing legumes or wheat pasture, use a liquid feed supplement containing 7.5 grams of BLOAT GUARD® Liquid per pound (1.65% w/w). Each animal must consume the medicated liquid feed supplement at a rate of 0.2 pounds per 100 pounds body weight per day for adequate protection. Example: 2 pounds of the 1.65% medicated supplement for a 1000-pound animal daily.
6. Introduce the feeding of the medicated liquid feed supplement at least 2-5 days before pasturing on legume or wheat to accustom the cattle to the medicated liquid supplement and to lick wheel feeding. If the medicated liquid feed supplement feeding is interrupted, this 2-5 day introductory feeding should be repeated.

Precaution(s): Keep container closed when not in use.

Cold Weather Note: At temperatures below 50°F, this product will thicken and may appear cloudy, but is not damaged.

Presentation: 450 lb (204.12 kg).

BLOAT GUARD is a registered trademark of Phibro Animal Health, for poloxalene.

Compendium Code No.: 36930021

BLOAT GUARD® TOP DRESSING MEDICATED

Phibro **Bloat Preparation**

Brand of Poloxalene

NADA No.: 032-704

Active Ingredient(s):

Poloxalene 53%

Inert ingredient:

Verxite #4 .... 47%

Each ⅔ oz. by weight of top dressing contains 10 g of poloxalene.

Indications: For prevention of legume (alfalfa, clover) and wheat pasture bloat in cattle.

Dosage and Administration: Daily Dosage: Use the measure in the BLOAT GUARD® package, which is equal to one-quarter of a standard measuring cup and holds approximately ⅔ ounce of BLOAT GUARD® by weight. Each ⅔ ounce by weight contains 10 grams of poloxalen (the active ingredient).

It is essential that each animal consume the total recommended dosage of BLOAT GUARD® daily for adequate protection.

Animal Weight Pounds	Number of Measures
Less than 500	½ to 1
500 to 1,000	1 to 2
1,000 to 1,500	1½ to 3
Over 1,500	2 to 4

BLOAT GUARD® is to be consumed daily. BLOAT GUARD® should be fed as a top dressing on individual rations of ground feed, starting two or three days before animals are exposed to bloat-producing conditions. The higher dosage levels are recommended when bloat-producing conditions are severe.

Repeat the feeding of BLOAT GUARD® when animals are exposed to bloat-producing conditions for more than 12 hours from the last feeding of BLOAT GUARD®. But do not exceed the higher dosage levels in any 24-hour period.

If animals do not accept BLOAT GUARD® readily, stir the recommended amount into their feed. After animals become accustomed to the change in diet, use BLOAT GUARD® as a top dressing.

Precaution(s): Reclose the bag after each use. Store in a cool place.

The normal shelf-life of this product is at least 24 months. However, when the product is subjected to extreme temperatures (100°F) for long periods of time (6 months), spontaneous combustion may occur. The product is not combustible unless it develops a strong, irritating odor. If this occurs, flush with water and discard immediately.

Presentation: 20-pound bags.

BLOAT GUARD is a registered trademark of Phibro Animal Health, for poloxalene, U.S. patent 3,465,083.

Verxite is a trademark of W.R. Grace & Company.

Compendium Code No.: 36930031

BLOAT GUARD® TYPE A MEDICATED ARTICLE

Phibro **Bloat Preparation**

Brand of Poloxalene

NADA No.: 032-704

Active Ingredient(s):

Poloxalene 53%

(Equivalent to 240 grams per pound)

Inert Ingredients: Ethoxyquin (a preservative), 0.064%; BHT (butylated hydroxy toluene, a preservative), 0.20%; Vexrite (nonnutritive), approximately 47%.

Indications: For prevention of legume (alfalfa, clover) and wheat pasture bloat in cattle. For use in the manufacture of feed.

Directions:

Mixing Directions: BLOAT GUARD® Type A Medicated Article must be thoroughly and evenly distributed into feedstuffs. A mixture of BLOAT GUARD® and one common feed ingredient should be made prior to final mixing when less than 25 pounds of BLOAT GUARD® is to be blended into a ton of feed.

Possible Mixing Ratios: Each pound of BLOAT GUARD® contains 240 grams of poloxalene, the active drug ingredient. The following table illustrates various amounts of BLOAT GUARD® which may be added to feeds—the resulting concentration of poloxalene, the active drug ingredient, is also shown.

Pounds of BLOAT GUARD® Per Ton of Type C Medicated Feed	Grams of Poloxalene Per Pound of Type C Medicated Feed	% W/W of Poloxalene in Type C Medicated Feed
8.3 lb	1	0.22
16.6 lb	2	0.44
33.2 lb	4	0.88
50.0 lb	6	1.32
83.3 lb	10	2.20
100.0 lb	12	2.64
208.3 lb	25	5.50
416.6 lb	50	11.00
625.0 lb	75	16.50
833.3 lb	100	22.00

For example: 50 pounds of BLOAT GUARD®, when added to 1 ton of feed, results in a final concentration of 6 grams poloxalene per pound of Type C Medicated Feed (1.32% by weight).

Feeding Directions: It is essential that each animal consume the total recommended dosage of BLOAT GUARD® daily for adequate protection.

The dosage of BLOAT GUARD® is proportional to body weight and also depends upon the severity of the bloat-producing conditions. The normal dosage of BLOAT GUARD® (1 gram of poloxalene per 100 pounds of body weight) is recommended for cattle under moderate bloat-producing conditions. For cattle under severe bloat-producing conditions, the normal dose should be doubled (2 grams of poloxalene per 100 pounds of body weight).

Repeat the feeding of the normal dosage of BLOAT GUARD® when animals are exposed to bloat-producing conditions more than 12 hours from the last feeding of the bloat preventive feed. But do not exceed the double dosage of BLOAT GUARD® in any 24-hour period. Animals should be fed the recommended amounts of bloat preventive feed starting two or three days before they are exposed to bloat-producing conditions.

Precaution(s): Store in a cool place.

The normal life of this product is at least 24 months. However, when the product is subjected to extreme temperatures (100°F) for long periods of time (6 months), spontaneous combustion may occur. The product is not combustible unless it develops a strong, irritating odor; if this occurs, flush with water and discard immediately.

Presentation: 50 lb (22.7 kg).

BLOAT GUARD is a registered trademark of Phibro Animal Health, for poloxalene.

Verxite is a registered trademark of W.R. Grace & Co.

Compendium Code No.: 36930041

BLOAT-PAC®

Vet-A-Mix **Bloat Preparation**

Active Ingredient(s): Vegetable oil, polyglycerol oleate, polyethylene glycol monooleate, butylated hydroxyanisole, butylated hydroxytoluene, citric acid, ethoxyquin, propylene glycol and propyl gallate.

Indications: For the treatment of acute forage or frothy bloat of cattle, sheep and goats.

Dosage and Administration: The usual recommended dosages are as follows:

Mature Cattle	150-300 mL
Heifers	125-250 mL
Calves	100-200 mL
Lambs and Kids	50-100 mL

Administer orally or by direct injection into the rumen with a large gauge needle between the hip bone and rib cage in the left flank areas. BLOAT-PAC® may be given orally as a drench.

Warning(s): If administered to milking dairy cows, do not market milk for 96 hours after treatment.

Presentation: 500 mL bottles, and 1 gallon containers.

Compendium Code No.: 10500030

BLOAT RELEASE

AgriLabs **Bloat Preparation**

Active Ingredient(s): Each fl oz contains:
Docusate Sodium 240 mg
in an emulsified soybean oil base.

Indications: For use as an aid in the treatment of frothy bloat in ruminants and as a fecal softener.

Dosage and Administration: Administer as a drench or via stomach tube.
Adult Cattle . . . 12 fl oz
Young Cattle, Sheep and Goats . . . 6 fl oz

Contraindication(s): Do not use concurrently with mineral oil or other drugs.

Precaution(s): Store at controlled room temperature between 15° and 30°C (59°-86°F).
Shake well before using.

Warning(s): Milk taken from animals during treatment and within 96 hours (8 milkings) after latest treatment must not be used for food. Do not treat animals within 3 days of slaughter.
For animal use only.
Keep out of reach of children.

Presentation: 12 fl oz.

Compendium Code No.: 10580170

BLOAT TREATMENT

AgriPharm **Bloat Preparation**

Active Ingredient(s): Each fl. oz. contains:
Docusate sodium . . . 240 mg
In an emulsified soybean oil base.

Indications: For use as an aid in the treatment of frothy bloat in ruminants and as a fecal softener.

Dosage and Administration: Shake well before using.
Administer as a drench or via stomach tube.
Adult cattle . . . 12 fl. oz.
Young cattle, sheep and goats . . . 6 fl. oz.

Contraindication(s): Do not use concurrently with mineral oil or other drugs.

Precaution(s): Store at a controlled room temperature between 59°-86°F (15°-30°C).

Caution(s): For animal use only. Keep out of the reach of children.

Warning(s): Milk taken from animals during treatment and within 96 hours (8 milkings) after the last treatment with this drug must not be used for food. Do not treat animals within three (3) days of slaughter.

Presentation: 12 fl. oz. containers.

Compendium Code No.: 14570130

BLOAT TREATMENT

Butler **Bloat Preparation**

Active Ingredient(s): Each fluid ounce contains:
Dioctyl sodium sulfosuccinate . . . 240 mg
In an emulsified soybean oil base.

Indications: For use as an aid in the treatment of frothy bloat in ruminants and for use as a fecal softener.

Dosage and Administration: Shake well before using.
Administer orally as a drench or via a stomach tube.
Adult Cattle: 12 fl. oz.
Young Cattle, Sheep and Goats: 6 fl. oz.

Precaution(s): Store at a controlled room temperature between 15° and 30°C (59°-86°F).

Caution(s): For veterinary use only. Keep out of the reach of children.
Restricted drug; use only as directed.

Presentation: 12 fl. oz. containers

Compendium Code No.: 10820220

BLOAT TREATMENT

Durvet **Bloat Preparation**

Active Ingredient(s): Each fl. oz. contains:
Docusate Sodium . . . 240 mg
in an emulsified soybean oil base.

Indications: For use as an aid in the treatment of frothy bloat in ruminants and as a fecal softener.

Dosage and Administration: Administer as a drench or via stomach tube.
Adult Cattle . . . 12 fl. oz.
Young Cattle, Sheep and Goats . . . 6 fl. oz.

Contraindication(s): Do not use concurrently with mineral oil or other drugs.

Precaution(s): Store at controlled room temperature between 15° and 30°C (59°-86°F).
Shake well before using.

Caution(s): For animal use only.
Keep out of reach of children.

Presentation: 12 fl. oz.

Compendium Code No.: 10840090

BLOOD STOP POWDER

AgriLabs **Hemostatic**

Active Ingredient(s): Contains:
Tannic acid . . . 1.0%
Alum ammonium . . . 5.0%
Iron sulfate . . . 84.0%
Thymol iodide . . . 0.1%
Talc . . . 9.9%

Indications: To check bleeding of minor cuts and wounds.

Dosage and Administration: Apply BLOOD STOP POWDER freely to wound area. Bandage if necessary. After bleeding has stopped, apply BLOOD STOP POWDER again to prevent outbreak of bleeding. Do not disturb scab formed over the wound or bleeding may start again.
The product is not sterilized. Do not apply or use in deep wounds or in body cavities.

Precaution(s): Keep the container tightly closed when not in use.

Caution(s): Not for human use. For external use on livestock. Keep out of the reach of children.

Warning(s): Not to be used on animals intended for food.

Presentation: 16 oz. (454 g) containers.

Compendium Code No.: 10580180

BLOOD STOP POWDER

AgriPharm **Hemostatic**

Active Ingredient(s): Contains:
Iron sulfate . . . 84%
Carboxy methylcellulose . . . 5%
Diphenylamine . . . 1%
Corn starch . . . 10%

Indications: For use as an aid in checking capillary bleeding after dehorning in cattle or superficial cuts and wounds on cattle, horses, sheep and swine.

Dosage and Administration: Apply topically to the bleeding area as often as necessary.

Caution(s): Not for human use. Keep out of the reach of children.
In case of deep or puncture wounds or severe burns, consult a veterinarian. If redness, irritation, or swelling persists or increase, discontinue use of the product and consult a veterinarian.

Presentation: 16 oz. (l lb.) containers.

Compendium Code No.: 14570140

BLOOD STOP POWDER

Aspen **Hemostatic**

Active Ingredient(s):
Ferrous sulfate • $7H_2O$ . . . 0.84%
Ammonium alum . . . 5%
Chloroxylenol . . . 1%
Tannic acid . . . 1%
In a free-flowing absorbent base, not sterilized.

Indications: For use as an aid in controlling minor bleeding from superficial cuts and wounds and after dehorning.

Dosage and Administration: Apply the powder freely to the bleeding surface. Repeat as needed. Bandage, if necessary.

Precaution(s): Store at a controlled room temperature, between 59° and 86°F (15°-30°C).
Keep the container tightly closed when not in use.

Caution(s): Keep out of the reach of children.
In case of deep or puncture wounds or serious burns, consult a veterinarian. If redness, irritation, or swelling persists or increases, discontinue use and consult a veterinarian.

Presentation: 453.6 g (1 lb).

Compendium Code No.: 14750070

BLOOD STOP POWDER

Butler **Hemostatic**

Active Ingredient(s): BLOOD STOP POWDER contains: Ferric Subsulfate, Aluminum Chloride, Diatomite, Bentonite, Copper Sulfate, Ammonium Chloride, Iodophore complex.

Indications: An aid to stop bleeding caused by clipping nails, docking tails and trimming beaks and minor cuts. Pressure bandaging to be used in conjunction with product following tail docking.
For external veterinary use only to control bleeding for dogs, cats and birds.

Directions: Apply with moistened cotton tipped applicator to the cut nail or other superficial bleeding area using moderate constant pressure for five to ten seconds. Do not use in deep wounds or body cavities or on burns.

Caution(s): Keep out of reach of children.

Presentation: 14 gms.

Compendium Code No.: 10820230

BLOOD STOP POWDER

Centaur **Hemostatic**

Active Ingredient(s):
Iron Sulfate . . . 84%
Carboxy Methylcellulose . . . 5%
Diphenylamine . . . 1%
Corn Starch . . . 10%

Indications: For use as an aid in checking capillary bleeding.
*Contains diphenylamine to protect against screw worms and maggots.

Directions: Apply moderate amounts to affected area. Surface should be thoroughly covered with the powder. May be applied under a bandage.

Caution(s): For animal use only.
For external use only. Not to be taken by mouth.

Warning(s): Not to be used on animals intended for food.
If accidental eye contamination occurs flood with water and contact a physician immediately. If accidental ingestion occurs contact a physician immediately. Keep out of reach of children.

Presentation: 20 oz containers.

Manufactured by: Unavet, North Kansas City, MO 64116.

Compendium Code No.: 14880130 Rev. 10-93

BLOOD STOP POWDER

Davis **Hemostatic**

Active Ingredient(s): Ferric subsulfate.

Indications: Helps stop bleeding caused by nail cutting.
For use on dogs and cats.

Dosage and Administration: Apply Davis BLOOD STOP POWDER freely with a moistened cotton-tipped applicator to the area being treated. The surface should be thoroughly covered with the powder. Apply moderate pressure for 5 to 10 seconds. Repeat as needed.

Contraindication(s): Not for use on burns or open wounds.

Precaution(s): Keep the container tightly closed when not in use.

Caution(s): If redness, irritation or swelling persists or increases, discontinue use and consult a veterinarian. For external use only. Do not get into eyes.

Warning(s): Keep out of reach of children.

Presentation: 1.5 oz (42.6 g) containers.

Compendium Code No.: 11410060

BLOOD STOP POWDER

Dominion **Hemostatic**

Active Ingredient(s): Contents:

Iron Sulfate 84%
Tannic Acid 1%
Ammonium Alum........ 5%
Thymol Iodide 0.1%
in a talc base.

Indications: BLOOD STOP POWDER is indicated to check bleeding of minor cuts and wounds.

Dosage and Administration: Apply freely to the wound area. Bandage in place if necessary. After bleeding has stopped, apply again to prevent further bleeding. Do not disturb the scab formed, as this might start the bleeding process again.

Caution(s): It is advised to give tetanus antitoxin as a precautionary measure.

For external use only. Keep out of reach of children.

Presentation: 60 gram, 200 gram and 400 gram bottles; 12 bottles/carton.

Compendium Code No.: 15080010

BLOOD STOP POWDER

Durvet **Hemostatic**

Active Ingredient(s): Contents: Ferrous Sulfate • $7H_2O$ 0.84%, Ammonium Alum 5%, Chloroxylenol 1%, Tannic Acid 1%. In a free-flowing absorbent base. Not sterilized.

Indications: For use as an aid in controlling minor bleeding from superficial cuts and wounds and after dehorning.

Dosage and Administration: Apply powder freely to bleeding surface. Repeat as needed. Bandage if necessary.

Precaution(s): Store at controlled room temperature between 15° and 30°C (59°-86°F). Keep container tightly closed when not in use.

Caution(s): In case of deep or puncture wounds or serious burns, consult veterinarian. If redness, irritation, or swelling persists or increases, discontinue use and consult veterinarian.

For external use only. For animal use only. Keep out of reach of children.

Presentation: 6 oz (NDC 30798-023-26) and 16 oz (NDC 30798-023-31).

Compendium Code No.: 10840101

Iss. 12-94

BLOOD STOP POWDER

First Priority **Hemostatic**

Ingredient(s): Ferrous Sulfate, Tannic Acid, Chloroxylenol, Diphenylamine Intermediate, Sodium Carboxymethylcellulose, Cornstarch.

Indications: To check bleeding of minor cuts and wounds.

Directions for Use: Apply BLOOD STOP POWDER freely to wound area. Bandage in place if necessary. After bleeding has stopped apply BLOOD STOP again to prevent outbreak of bleeding. Do not disturb scab formed over the wound or bleeding may start again.

Precaution(s): Storage: Store at controlled room temperature between 15°-30°C (59°-86°F). Keep container tightly closed when not in use.

Caution(s): This product is not sterilized. Do not apply or use in deep wounds or body cavities.

For external use on animals. For animal use only.

Warning(s): Not for use on humans or food producing animals. Keep out of reach of children.

Presentation: 6 oz (170 g) (NDC# 58829-185-06) and 16 oz (453.6 g) (NDC# 58829-185-16).

Compendium Code No.: 11390053

Rev. 01-02 / Rev. 05-01

BLOOD STOP POWDER

Vedco **Hemostatic**

Topical Antiseptic-Styptic

Active Ingredient(s):

Ferrous sulfate • $7H_2O$........ 0.84%
Ammonium alum........ 5%
Chloroxylenol........ 1%
Tannic acid........ 1%

In a free-flowing absorbent base. Not sterilized.

Indications: For use as an aid in controlling capillary bleeding after dehorning cattle, or from superficial cuts and wounds in cattle, sheep, horses, and swine.

Directions for Use: Apply powder freely to bleeding surface. Repeat as needed. Bandage if necessary.

Precaution(s): Store at controlled room temperature between 15° and 30°C (59°-86°F).

Keep container tightly closed when not in use.

Caution(s): In case of deep or puncture wounds or serious burns consult veterinarian. If redness, irritation, or swelling persists or increases, discontinue use and consult veterinarian.

Warning(s): For external use only. For animal use only. Keep out of reach of children.

Presentation: 6 oz and 16 oz containers.

Compendium Code No.: 10940150

BLUELITE® C

TechMix **Electrolytes-Oral**

Active Ingredient(s): Guaranteed Analysis (not less than):

		Per oz.
Potassium (K)	2.200%	623.70 mg
Sodium (Na)	1.850%	524.50 mg
Calcium (Ca)	0.650%	184.30 mg
Phosphorus (P)	0.180%	51.00 mg
Magnesium (Mg)	0.055%	15.60 mg

Ingredients: Dextrose, fructose, lactose monohydrate, sucrose, glycine, citric acid, potassium chloride, sodium chloride, calcium lactate, magnesium gluconate, dibasic potassium phosphate, artificial flavors and FD&C certified color added.

Indications: BLUELITE® C is designed for oral use in young calves prior to weaning. Mix BLUELITE® C into all fluids (water, milk or milk replacer) fed to calves showing signs of dehydration or body shrink as a result of disease, moving, handling or sorting.

Dosage and Administration:

1. Administer one (1) full measure (approximately 4 oz.) of BLUELITE® C to each half gallon or two (2) quarts of milk, water, or milk replacer fed to the calf on a daily basis.
2. Daily feed calves a minimum amount of milk, water, and milk replacer fluids to equal 10% of the calves' weight. Increase fluid intake of severely dehydrated calves through additional feedings to help alleviate dehydration. Severely dehydrated calves should be fed 20-50% more fluid on a daily basis through two (2) or three (3) additional daily feedings. Do not overfeed calves at any one feeding.
3. Dehydrated calves with severe diarrhea should not be fed any, or very little, milk or milk replacer during the first 24-48 hours of treatment as excessive milk may lead to additional digestive disturbances or stress. Resume milk feeding gradually after the first 24-48 hours of treatment. Calves with mild diarrhea can be given some diluted milk throughout treatment. Calves withheld from milk too long tend to become stunted and should be gradually returned to milk diets as soon as possible following treatment.
4. BLUELITE® C may be administered via esophageal tube or as a drench at the rate of 1 oz. of BLUELITE® C for each 10 lbs. of body weight on a daily basis. Continue to administer BLUELITE® C into all fluids administered to the calf as long as signs of dehydration persist.
5. Calves that do not appear to be responding within 8-12 hours after receiving BLUELITE® C or that are too weak and dehydrated to drink fluids normally should be treated as directed by a veterinarian.

Precaution(s): Store in a dry room at temperatures between 40°-86°F (4°-30°C). Once the pail is opened, seal the bag with binder and keep the unused portion in a dry, sealed container.

Caution(s): For calf and veterinary use only.

Keep out of the reach of children.

Discussion: Water or tissue fluid represents over 75% of the young calf's body weight. Older calves or mature cattle have a lower percentage of body fluid because of a greater concentration of solid tissue mass. This higher fluid content in the young calf predisposes it to a more severe dehydration or shrink than that encountered by the adult bovine when exposed to the stress of handling, hauling, and disease.

Electrolytes serve as the primary way in which the body balances its fluids. Through the electrolytes and their osmotic pressure, the body fluids are maintained at proper levels or balance between intracellular fluid in relation to the fluid of the interstitial tissue outside the cells and blood vascular fluid. Without adequate water and electrolytes, the body cannot maintain its proper fluid balance and the tissues start to dehydrate.

Young calves require a constant source of readily available energy as they have less energy reserves than the older calf or adult bovine which carries vast energy reserves in the form of body fat. The young calf, with little body fat, has a very limited source of energy to call on from the blood and liver. These blood and liver reserves are frequently depleted in 24-48 hours following stresses that result in dehydration. Calves suffering from diarrhea quickly lose their reserves of energy and develop hypoglycemia (low blood sugar) which is evidenced by listlessness and depression. Calves in this condition require a readily available source of energy and electrolytes in ample volumes of fluid to avoid further depression which, if not corrected, leads to coma and death.

Calves losing 5-8% of their body fluid and electrolytes as a result of dehydration encounter impaired growth and tissue maintenance. Fluid losses equalling 10-15% of the body weight result in severe tissue damage and may result in death if not corrected. Enteric infections caused by viruses and *E. coli* can quickly dehydrate the calf as fluids are lost via the stools through hypermotility of the digestive tract.

Acidification Action: Calves prior to weaning are essentially a monogastric, nonruminating animal in that almost all of the digestion in the stomach occurs in the abomasum. This digestion in the abomasum is conducted in an acid media. Calves drinking milk or milk replacer require extensive acidification action to lower the pH of the recently ingested milk and milk replacer. Under an ideal digestive environment in the abomasum, milk forms a clot and coagulates shortly after ingestion. This clot formation is initiated, in part, by the acid properties of the gastric fluid. When BLUELITE® C is added to whole milk, it aids the digestion process by initiating clotting action with the solid nutrients of the milk in a short period of time. BLUELITE® C is a palatable acidifier and helps lower the pH of the milk and milk replacer so that it can be digested by the young calf. Research reports indicate that calves with poor acidification action in the abomasum are prone to digestive upsets and some enteric infections that may lead to scours.

Trial Data: BLUELITE® C has been field tested on farms raising calves born on the farm and on farms where young calves were purchased and moved onto the farm. In a field trial where 34 calves were bought and moved onto the farm, the 17 calves fed BLUELITE® C rehydrated by 2.3% of their body weight in 48 hours and 5.8% after 96 hours. The control calves were fed exactly the same as the BLUELITE® C calves mentioned above, except the control calves did not receive BLUELITE® C and rehydrated by only 0.2% after 48 hours and 2.4% after 96 hours.

In a series of comparative evaluations regarding the rehydration value of BLUELITE® C, the body weights of calves suffering from dehydration and scours were recorded to determine the value of extra fluid feeding or intake. In these trials, calves were given milk replacer in the morning and evening and an additional feeding of water at noon equal to the amount of fluid fed in the morning or night. Calves receiving BLUELITE® C in all three feedings rehydrated by 10.2% of their body weight after 48 hours, while the control calves not receiving the BLUELITE® C rehydrated by 6.3%. These comparisons indicated that dehydrated calves would benefit by the feeding of BLUELITE® C and the additional fluid.

Presentation: 4x6 lb. (2.72 kg) pails with 4 oz. measures (24 lb. case).

Compendium Code No.: 11440020

BLUELITE® SWINE FORMULA

TechMix **Electrolytes-Oral**

Active Ingredient(s): BLUELITE® Swine Formula is a multiple electrolyte formula, it provides seven electrolytes to help maintain fluid in the cells.

BLUELITE® Swine Formula provides four essential cations - potassium, magnesium, sodium and calcium - which are required by the fluids in the tissue and three anions - bicarbonate, phosphate and chloride.

BLUELITE® Swine Formula also contains dextrose, fructose, sucrose, lactose, and glycine.

Indications: BLUELITE® Swine Formula is an electrolyte water acidifier in combination with multiple energy sources designed for swine and can be given to swine of any age as an aid to reduce losses of dehydration, and hypoglycemia associated with stress, scours, weaning, or management.

BLUELITE® Swine Formula can be fed to nursing pigs or newly weaned pigs to help combat dehydration and may be used in conjunction with most medicants. Stresses such as severe changes in weather, environment, housing, or production management can lead to reduced feed and water intake. BLUELITE® Swine Formula should be administered in the water or feed intended for finishing hogs, lactating sows and gilts whenever water or feed intake is reduced.

Dosage and Administration: Always administer BLUELITE® Swine Formula in the drinking water whenever pigs show the above symptoms for 5-7 days and maintain in the feed for 7-14 days according to the following schedule:

Administer BLUELITE® Swine Formula in the drinking water in one of the following ways:

1. One (1) ounce (3 level tablespoons) of BLUELITE® Swine Formula powder for each four (4) gallons of drinking water, or
2. One (1) cup of BLUELITE® Swine Formula powder for each 24 gallons of drinking water, or

3. One (1) pound (2.5 cups) of BLUELITE® Swine Formula powder for each 64 gallons of drinking water, or
4. Stock solution: Mix 2 lbs. or five (5) cups of BLUELITE® Swine Formula powder in enough water to make one (1) gallon of stock solution. Administer 1 oz. of stock solution in each gallon of drinking water.

Feed Mixing: Add one (1) bag (6 lbs. or 2.72 kg) of BLUELITE® Swine Formula to each ton of complete swine feed. Keep BLUELITE® Swine Formula in the feed or ration for seven (7) days or until pigs no longer show signs of dehydration, or until the feed intake has returned to normal.

Discussion: Water represents over 50% of the body weight of the mature pig, and since fat is almost free of water, the young piglet has a much higher percentage of water in his body than the mature pig. Water represents almost 75% of the young piglet's body weight.

Electrolytes serve as the primary way in which the body balances its fluids. Through the electrolytes and their osmotic pressure, the body fluids are maintained at proper levels or balance between intracellular fluid in relation to the fluid of the interstitial tissue outside the cells and blood vascular fluid. Without adequate water and electrolytes, the body cannot maintain its proper fluid balance between the compartments and the tissues start to dehydrate.

Dehydration of the cells and tissue leads to reduced growth, impaired maintenance and may result in death when the body loses between 7-15% of its normal body fluid. Young pigs which have a high percentage of their body weight in fluid are very subject to severe dehydration which contributes to high mortality wherever they are exposed to stress or disease. Enteric infections caused by *E. coli*, TGE and rotavirus quickly dehydrate the body as the fluids are lost via the stools. This dehydration from diarrhea makes the young piglet subject to shock and death in a matter of minutes or several hours.

Water Acidification Action: The young pig has a limited ability to secrete acid in its digestive tract. *E. coli*, which are a primary cause of neonatal infections and death in the young piglet are known to proliferate and grow in the digestive tract when the pig does not produce enough acid to maintain the proper pH.

Many acidifiers have been tested to inhibit the growth of the E. coli in regard to their acidification action and palatability. BLUELITE® Swine Formula was designed to promote acidification action in a palatable, safe manner. The palatable buffered acidifier in BLUELITE® Swine Formula has been tested and proven effective in its ability to provide an acidification action.

Trial Data: BLUELITE® Swine Formula has been field tested in normal pigs at weaning and as a tool for supportive therapy in enteric *E. coli* infections. The results of these field tests indicate:

1. BLUELITE® Swine Formula can increase weight gain under normal farm conditions when weaning.
2. Pigs will consume more water when BLUELITE® Swine Formula is added to the water to reduce dehydration.
3. BLUELITE® Swine Formula is supportive therapy when treating pigs for scours or pneumonia.

Presentation: 14x2 lb. (0.90 kg) (28 lb. pail) and 8x6 lb. (2.72 kg) bags (48 lb. case).

Compendium Code No.: 11440030

BLUE LOTION

AgriLabs — **Topical Wound Dressing**

Active Ingredient(s): Contains isopropyl alcohol (73.4% v/v), propylene glycol, glycerine, urea, sodium propionate, furfural, gentian violet and acriflavine.

Indications: A germicidal, fungicidal, antiseptic, and protective wound dressing for use in the treatment of minor cuts, scratches and superficial abrasions.

Dosage and Administration: Remove pus and exudate from the infected area. When spraying hold the container approximately six (6) inches from the area to be treated. Spray an amount sufficient to cover the wound. One (1) application is usually sufficient. Severe cases may be treated once or twice a day.

Precaution(s): Store in a cool place. Flammable. Do not expose to heat or store at a temperature above 120°F. Do not use near an open flame.

Caution(s): Keep out of the reach of children. In case of deep or puncture wounds or serious burns, consult a veterinarian. If redness, irritation, or swelling persists or increases, discontinue use and consult a veterinarian. Keep away from eyes and mucous membranes.

Hazardous. Livestock remedy. Not for human use.

Warning(s): Not for use on horses intended for food use.

Presentation: 1 pint sprayer bottles.

Compendium Code No.: 10580190

BLUE LOTION

Farnam — **Topical Wound Dressing**

Active Ingredient(s):

Propylene glycol	32.29%
Glycerine	10.52%
Urea	3.00%
Sodium propionate	2.33%
Methyl violet	0.85%
Acriflavine	0.05%

Indications: A quick-drying, penetrating antiseptic wound dressing and gall lotion. Effective against bacterial infections most common in the skin lesions of horses, cattle and dogs. For use as an aid in treatment of surface wounds, minor cuts, skin abrasions, harness galls and saddle sores.

Dosage and Administration: First clean and dry the affected area to be treated. Then apply BLUE LOTION generously with the dauber cap directly onto lesions. Repeat the applications once a day or more often until healing takes place.

Caution(s): Not for human use.

Keep out of reach of children.

For external use only. Livestock remedy. In case of deep or puncture wounds or serious burns, consult a veterinarian. If redness, irritation or swelling persists or increases, discontinue use and consult a veterinarian. Avoid contact with the eyes and mucous membranes. Do not apply to large areas of the body. Do not apply at all to cats.

Note that this product will stain clothing.

Flammable! Keep away from heat or open flame.

Warning(s): Not for use on animals intended for food.

Presentation: 4 fl. oz. (118 mL).

Compendium Code No.: 10000070

BLUE LOTION AEROSOL

Boehringer Ingelheim — **Topical Wound Dressing**

Active Ingredient(s): Contains: Crystal violet, benzyl alcohol, tannic acid, and isopropyl alcohol 62.39% w/w.

Indications: For use prior to surgical procedures such as castrating or docking; for disinfection of injection sites; and for sores, minor cuts, bruises and abrasions.

Dosage and Administration: Thoroughly clean and dry the affected area removing all secretions and dirt before each application. Then shake well. Depress valve and direct the spray at the wound. Spray the affected area thoroughly. Repeat the treatment two (2) or more times a day if necessary until healing takes place.

Disinfection of injection site: Clip the hair at the site of injection. Briefly spray to disinfect and mark the injection site.

Working and hunting dogs: For sore abraded foot pads, spray once or twice a day to control the infection and to dry and toughen the pads for hard running.

If redness, irritation, or swelling persists or increases, discontinue use and consult a veterinarian. Not for use on burns or in body cavities or deep wounds.

Note: When used on or near the teats or udders of dairy animals the teats and udders should be thoroughly washed before the next milking to prevent contamination of milk.

Precaution(s): Extremely flammable, contents under pressure. Do not use near fire, sparks or flame. Do not puncture or incinerate container. Exposure to temperatures above 120°F may cause bursting. Store at room temperature. Use only as directed.

Caution(s): Livestock drug. Not for human use. For external animal use only. Keep out of the reach of children.

Avoid spraying in eyes. Avoid inhalation. Harmful if swallowed. Do not contaminate milk or milk handling equipment with this spray. Do not apply to large areas of the animal's body. Do not spray on cats.

Discussion: Crystal violet is an organic dye with known antiseptic qualities. It is beneficial in reducing light strain on the wound. Isopropyl alcohol is highly bactericidal while benzyl alcohol is an anesthetic and aids in the control of itching.

The tannic acid acts as an astringent to dry the wound and to promote healing. It also works to precipitate protein and aids in the toughening of the pads of working dogs.

The blue color of crystal violet identifies the treated area and is also useful to mark animals for identification purposes.

Presentation: 10 oz. aerosol sprayers.

Compendium Code No.: 10280200

BLUE LOTION TOPICAL ANTISEPTIC

Aspen — **Topical Wound Dressing**

Active Ingredient(s):

Benzalkonium Chloride	0.5%
Chlorothymol	0.2%
Isopropyl Alcohol	12.48%

And inert ingredients.

Indications: An antiseptic spray for the treatment of cowpox sores, cuts and abrasions. An aid in the prevention of superficial infections. A pre-injection topical antiseptic.

Directions for Use: Thoroughly clean and dry affected area, removing all dirt and secretions before each application. Shake product well. Apply BLUE LOTION to the wound, assuring thorough coverage of affected area. Repeat treatment 2 or more times daily if necessary until healing takes place.

Injection Sites: Clip hair at injection site. Apply BLUE LOTION to disinfect and mark injection site.

Working and Hunting Dogs: Apply BLUE LOTION to sore, abraded foot pads once or twice daily to help control infection.

Contraindication(s): Do not spray on cats.

Caution(s): Avoid spraying in eyes. Avoid inhalation. Harmful if swallowed. Do not contaminate milk or milk handling equipment with this spray. Do not apply to large areas of animal's body.

Warning(s): For animal use only.

Use only as directed. Livestock drug. Not for human use. For external animal use only. Keep out of reach of children.

Presentation: 16 oz.

Compendium Code No.: 14750080

BLUE LOTION TOPICAL ANTISEPTIC

First Priority — **Topical Wound Dressing**

Active Ingredient(s):

Benzalkonium Chloride	0.5%
Chlorothymol	0.2%
Isopropyl Alcohol	12.48%

And inert ingredients.

Indications: An antiseptic spray for the treatment of cowpox sores, cuts and abrasions. An aid in the prevention of superficial infections. A pre-injection topical antiseptic.

Directions for Use: Thoroughly clean and dry affected area, removing all dirt and secretions before each application. Shake product well. Apply BLUE LOTION to the wound, assuring thorough coverage of affected area. Repeat treatment 2 or more times daily if necessary until healing takes place.

Injection Sites: Clip hair at injection site. Apply BLUE LOTION to disinfect and mark injection site.

Working and Hunting Dogs: Apply BLUE LOTION to sore, abraded foot pads once or twice daily to help control infection.

Contraindication(s): Do not spray on cats.

Caution(s): Avoid spraying in eyes. Avoid inhalation. Harmful if swallowed. Do not contaminate milk or milk handling equipment with this spray. Do not apply to large areas of animal's body.

For animal use only. Use only as directed. Livestock drug.

For external animal use only.

Warning(s): Not for human use. Keep out of reach of children.

Presentation: 16 fl oz (473 mL) (NDC# 58829-196-16).

Compendium Code No.: 11390062 Rev. 3-98

B

BLUE SNOW™

Schering-Plough **Grooming Shampoo**

Indications: A rich, biodegradable shampoo for pets and show animals of all hair colors, especially white; prevents and counteracts the yellowing of the hair. Lanolin added for a soft, lustrous coat.

Dosage and Administration: Shake well. Wet the coat thoroughly with warm water and apply the shampoo. Work in thoroughly and rinse. A second application may be necessary, if the coat is excessively dirty.

Presentation: 1 gallon bottles.

Compendium Code No.: 10470240

BLUETONGUE VACCINE

Colorado Serum **Vaccine**

Bluetongue Vaccine, Modified Live Virus, Type 10

U.S. Vet. Lic. No.: 188

Active Ingredient(s): Contains bluetongue vaccine modified live virus, type 10.

Penicillin and streptomycin are added as preservatives.

The advantages of the tissue culture technique for viral vaccine production are well understood and widely accepted in medical circles. The successful propagation of bluetongue virus in a tissue culture system has made it possible to obtain a relatively tissue-free suspension with a high virus titer and permits a more accurate determination of virus yield.

Indications: For the vaccination of healthy sheep and goats against type 10 bluetongue infections.

Dosage and Administration: The incidence of bluetongue is seasonal, with animals usually contracting the disease in August and September due to the virus being transmitted by biting insects. Treatment is almost totally ineffective and preventive vaccination, late in the spring or in the early summer is not only recommended but becomes vitally important.

Lambs from immune ewes carry a degree of resistance to bluetongue which may last as long as three (3) months. As lambs approach weaning time the maternal antibody disappears and the acquired resistance can breakdown in the face of field exposure. It is at this time that lambs should be vaccinated. If vaccinated too young the "maternal antibody" may interfere with the proper active immune response.

The vaccination of pregnant ewes could result in births of abnormal lambs and this practice is not recommended. Instead, all breeding stock should be protected with BLUETONGUE VACCINE approximately three (3) weeks prior to the breeding season or after lambing.

The entire contents of the accompanying vial of diluent should be withdrawn with a syringe and needle and transferred into the vial of dried vaccine. Do not remove the stoppers from either vial. Shake the vaccine bottle until the dried material is completely rehydrated. Live virus products contain a stabilizer that may slow rehydration slightly but complete liquefaction will take place within a few moments. The vaccine is then ready to use. Use only the diluent furnished with the product to rehydrate the vaccine.

Shake to ensure proper rehydration and inject 2 mL of the rehydrated vaccine intramuscularly or subcutaneously into each animal. The axillary space (between foreleg and body) is a convenient site. Sterile technique should be used.

Precaution(s): Store in the dark at 2-7°C. Shake gently after rehydrating.

Sterilize needles and syringes by boiling in clean water. Do not use chemical disinfectants or detergents for this purpose.

Use the entire contents when the bottle is first opened. Burn the container and all unused contents.

Caution(s): Anaphylaxis (shock) may sometimes follow the use of products of this nature. Epinephrine or an equivalent drug should be available for immediate use in these instances. Artificial respiration is also helpful.

Do not administer to pregnant animals.

For veterinary use only.

Warning(s): Do not vaccinate within 21 days before slaughter.

Discussion: Bluetongue, originally known as sore muzzle, is a disease of sheep and goats caused by a filterable virus. In addition to serotype 10 types 11, 13 and 17 have been isolated in sheep in the United States. The disease encompasses a wide range of symptoms, including a high temperature and dullness. Mucous membranes of the nasal cavity and of the mouth take on a bluish or purplish color, leading to the bluetongue terminology applied to the disease.

Ulcers may appear on the gums, lips, face, ears and on the neck. Affected animals are often stiff and some may die. Mortality is occasionally high but usually does not exceed 15% of the affected animals. The greatest economic loss results from poor condition, long convalescence, interruption of breeding schedules and lowered wool value.

Presentation: Each package contains one bottle containing dried BLUETONGUE VACCINE serotype 10, and a second bottle of sterile diluent in 50 dose (100 mL) vials.

Compendium Code No.: 11010011

BLU-GARD™ SPRAY

Ecolab Food & Bev. Div. **Teat Spray**

Active Ingredient(s):

Linear dodecyl benzene sulfonic acid 1.94%

Indications: Reduces new mastitis infection caused by *Staphylococcus aureus* and *Streptococcus agalactiae.*

Dosage and Administration: Use a post-milking teat spray on each teat as an aid in a complete cow care programme to help reduce the spread of organisms which may cause mastitis.

Immediately after milking, spray teat with full strength BLU-GARD™ Spray ensuring the teat orifice is completely covered. Allow to air dry. Do not wipe. Always use fresh full strength product. Do not turn cows out in freezing weather until BLU-GARD™ Spray is completely dry.

Wash entire udder and teats thoroughly just prior to next milking with an appropriate udder wash product solution.

M.S.D.S. available.

Precaution(s): Keep from freezing.

Caution(s): BLU-GARD™ Spray is not intended to cure or help the healing of chapped or irritated teats. In case of teat irritation or chapping, have the condition examined and if necessary, treated by veterinarian.

Keep out of the reach of children.

First Aid:

Eyes: Flush immediately with plenty of clean water for at least 15 minutes.

Internal: If swallowed, do not induce vomiting. Rinse mouth with clean water; then drink one or two glasses of water or milk.

Get medical attention immediately.

Important: Do not mix BLU-GARD™ Spray with any other teat spray, dip or other products. If transferred from this container to any other, make sure the other container is thoroughly pre-cleaned and bears the proper container labelling - BLU-GARD™ Spray.

Presentation: 5 gallon pail and 15 gallon drum.

Compendium Code No.: 14490011

BLU-GARD™ TEAT DIP

Ecolab Food & Bev. Div. **Teat Dip**

Active Ingredient(s): Linear dodecyl benzene sulfonic acid 1.94% in an emollient base.

Indications: Reduces new mastitis infections caused by *Staphylococcus aureus.*

Dosage and Administration: Immediately after each cow is milked, submerge each teat in undiluted Klenzade™ BLU-GARD™. Allow to air dry. Do not wipe teats.

Always use fresh, full strength BLU-GARD™. If product in dip cup becomes visibly dirty, discard contents, rinse cup and replenish with undiluted BLU-GARD™.

Wash the entire udder and teats thoroughly just prior to milking with a suitable udder wash solution. Use the proper procedures for udder washing.

Precaution(s): Keep from freezing. If frozen, thaw completely and shake well before use.

Caution(s): For industrial use only.

Consult a veterinarian if the cow's teats are sore, or chapped, before starting or using BLU-GARD™.

Warning(s): Keep out of the reach of children.

Harmful if swallowed. Protect the eyes and skin from contact with the product. Contact may cause irritation. Wear rubber gloves and splash-proof glasses, goggles or a face shield when handling the product. Do not contaminate food.

First Aid:

Eyes: Flush immediately with plenty of cool running water. Remove contact lenses. Continue flushing for 15 minutes holding eyelids apart to ensure rinsing of the entire eye.

Skin: Flush immediately with plenty of cool running water. Wash thoroughly with soap and water.

If swallowed: Do not induce vomiting. Rinse mouth immediately; then drink one or two large glasses of water or milk.

Never give anything by mouth to an unconscious person.

If irritation or discomfort persists, call a physician.

Presentation: 4 x 1 gallon case, 5 gallon pail, 15 gallon and 55 gallon drums.

M.S.D.S. available.

Compendium Code No.: 14490022

BLU-SHIELD™ SANITIZING BARRIER TEAT DIP

Ecolab Food & Bev. Div. **Teat Dip**

Active Ingredient(s): Linear dodecyl benzene sulfonic acid, 1.0%. Contains glycerin plus other emollients.

Indications: BLU-GUARD is a non-iodine, germicidal teat dip that forms a protective barrier on the teat. Helps prevent common bacterial organisms known to cause mastitis from entering the teat canal and provides extended anti-microbial protection after dipping.

Benefits

Effective:

- Unique, patented teat dip-provides both a barrier and a germicide proven to prevent new mastitis infections.
- The active ingredient, linear dodecyl benzene sulfonic acid, is 99.99% effective in killing colioform, staph and strep organisms by the AOAC germicidal and Detergent Sanitizer Test.
- Unique barrier properties provide milking to milking protection.
- Barrier helps to prevent new invasions of bacteria from entering the teat canal.
- Anti-microbial protection for the important hours after dipping.
- The active ingredient in BLU-SHIELD™ has been proven effective in reducing colioform infections - in addition to *Staph aureus* and *Strep agalactiae* infections

Gentle

- Non-iodine - won't stain teats or hands.
- Helps protect cows from teat irritation while keeping soft and pliable
- The active ingredient - LAS, for short - is carried in an emollient base that contains glycerin - helps improve teat condition.

Convenient to Use

- Easier to remove than latex barrier type teat dips.
- Highly visible on teat unlike some latex barrier dips.
- Ready-to-use - no mixing.

Pharmacology: Properties:

Form	liquid
Color	blue
Odor	mild
Wetting Ability	excellent
Specific gravity	1.03
Pounds per Gallon	8.6

Formula contains no phosphorus.

Dosage and Administration: Immediately after milking, use Klenzade dip cup with BLU-SHIELD™ at full strength. Submerge one-half length of teat in solution. Allow to air dry. Do not wipe. Always use fresh, full strength BLU-SHIELD™. If product in cup becomes visibly dirty, discard contents and replenish with undiluted product. Do not return any used product to original container. Do not dip wet teats. Do not turn cows out in freezing weather until BLU-SHIELD™ is completely dry.

Wash entire udder and teats thoroughly just prior to next milking with appropriate udder wash product solution to avoid contamination of milk. Use proper procedures for udder washing.

Precaution(s): Transport and store between 40°F (4°C) and 100°F (37.8°C). Do not freeze. Product damaged if frozen. Product that has been frozen and thawed may appear watery with clumps of material and will not produce a uniform film on the teat.

Presentation: 4 x 1 gallon cases, 5 gallon pail, and 15 gallon drum.

Compendium Code No.: 14490030

BMD® 30

Alpharma **Feed Medication**

Bacitracin Methylene Disalicylate-Type A Medicated Article-Antibacterial

NADA No.: 046-592

Active Ingredient(s): Each pound contains feed grade bacitracin methylene disalicylate equivalent to 30 grams bacitracin (Master Standard).

Composition: A dried precipitated fermentation product obtained by culturing *B. licheniformis* Tracy on media adapted for microbiological production of bacitracin; calcium carbonate.

Indications: For supplementing rations of swine, chickens, turkeys, pheasants, quail and feedlot beef cattle.

Directions: Mixing directions: Prepare an intermediate premix containing 5 grams per pound by mixing 1.0 lb of BMD® 30 with 5.0 lbs of soybean meal or ground corn. Then add 0.8 to 50 lbs of intermediate premix per ton of finished feed.

Growing/finishing swine:

For increased rate of weight gain and improved feed efficiency: 10-30 grams bacitracin per ton of feed.

For control of swine dysentery (bloody scours) associated with *Brachyspira hyodysenteriae* in pigs up to 250 lbs body weight. Feed 250 grams per ton of complete feed on premises with a history of swine dysentery, but where signs of the disease have not yet occurred or following an approved treatment of the disease condition: 250 grams bacitracin per ton of feed.

The 250 g/ton level will provide 5 to 7 mg/lb in swine weighing 40 to 250 lbs.

Pregnant sows:

For control of clostridial enteritis caused by *C. perfringens* in suckling piglets when fed to sows from 14 days before through 21 days after farrowing on premises with a history of clostridial scours: 250 grams bacitracin per ton of feed.

Broiler and replacement chickens:

For increased rate of weight gain and improved feed efficiency: 4-50 grams bacitracin per ton of feed.

As an aid in prevention of necrotic enteritis caused or complicated by *Clostridium* spp. or other organisms susceptible to bacitracin methylene disalicylate: 50 grams bacitracin per ton of feed.

As an aid in control of necrotic enteritis caused or complicated by *Clostridium* spp. or other organisms susceptible to bacitracin methylene disalicylate: 100-200 grams bacitracin per ton of feed.

Laying hens:

For increased egg production and improved feed efficiency during the first seven months of production: 10-25 grams bacitracin per ton of feed.

Growing turkeys:

For increased rate of weight gain and improved feed efficiency: 4-50 grams bacitracin per ton of feed.

As an aid in control of transmissible enteritis in growing turkeys complicated by organisms susceptible to bacitracin methylene disalicylate: 200 grams bacitracin per ton of feed.

Pheasants:

For increased rate of weight gain and improved feed efficiency: 4-50 grams bacitracin per ton of feed.

Quail:

For increased rate of weight gain and improved feed efficiency in quail not over 5 weeks of age: 5-20 grams bacitracin per ton of feed.

For prevention of ulcerative enteritis in growing quail due to *Clostridium colinum* susceptible to bacitracin methylene disalicylate. Feed continuously as the sole ration: 200 grams bacitracin per ton of feed.

Feedlot beef cattle:

For reduction in the number of liver condemnations due to abscesses in feedlot beef cattle: 70 mg per head per day (continuously), 250 mg per head per day (5 days in 30).

Note: Where minimum levels are shown, increase the antibiotic concentration within approved range when necessary to fit the feeding program, and to insure adequate levels of antibiotic in the complete ration.

Caution(s): For manufacturing registered livestock and poultry feeds only.

Growing/finishing swine and Pregnant sows: Diagnosis should be confirmed by a veterinarian when results are not satisfactory. Feed containing an approved level of bacitracin methylene disalicylate should be the sole ration.

Broiler and replacement chickens: To control a necrotic enteritis outbreak, start medication at the first clinical signs of disease. The dosage range permitted provides for different levels based on severity of the infection. Consult a poultry diagnostic laboratory or pathologist to determine the diagnosis and advice regarding the optimal level of drug. Administer continuously for 5-7 days or as long as clinical signs persist, and then reduce medication to prevention level (50 g/ton).

Restricted Drug: Use only as directed. (CA)

For use in animals only.

For use in dry feeds only.

Not for use in liquid type B medicated feeds.

Presentation: 50 lb (22.68 kg) bag.

Compendium Code No.: 10220162 AHG-001 0104

BMD® 50

Alpharma **Feed Medication**

Bacitracin Methylene Disalicylate-Type A Medicated Article-Antibacterial

NADA No.: 046-592

Active Ingredient(s): Each pound contains feed grade bacitracin methylene disalicylate equivalent to 50 grams bacitracin (Master Standard).

Composition: A dried precipitated fermentation product obtained by culturing *B. licheniformis* Tracy on media adapted for microbiological production of bacitracin; calcium carbonate.

Indications: For supplementing rations of swine, chickens, turkeys, pheasants, quail and feedlot beef cattle.

Directions: Mixing Directions: Prepare an intermediate premix containing 5 grams per pound by mixing 1.0 lb of BMD® 50 with 9.0 lbs of soybean meal or ground corn. Then add 0.8 to 50 lbs of intermediate premix per ton of finished feed.

Broiler and replacement chickens:

For increased rate of weight gain and improved feed efficiency: 4-50 grams bacitracin per ton of feed.

As an aid in the prevention of necrotic enteritis caused or complicated by *Clostridium* spp. or other organisms susceptible to bacitracin methylene disalicylate: 50 grams bacitracin per ton of feed.

As an aid in control of necrotic enteritis caused or complicated by *Clostridium* spp. or other organisms susceptible to bacitracin methylene disalicylate: 100-200 grams bacitracin per ton of feed.

Laying hens:

For increased egg production and improved feed efficiency during the first seven months of production: 10-25 grams bacitracin per ton of feed.

Growing turkeys:

For increased rate of weight gain and improved feed efficiency: 4-50 grams bacitracin per ton of feed.

As an aid in control of transmissible enteritis in growing turkeys complicated by organisms susceptible to bacitracin methylene disalicylate: 200 grams bacitracin per ton of feed.

Pheasants:

For increased rate of weight gain and improved feed efficiency: 4-50 grams bacitracin per ton of feed.

Quail:

For increased rate of weight gain and improved feed efficiency in quail not over 5 weeks of age: 5-20 grams bacitracin per ton of feed.

For prevention of ulcerative enteritis in growing quail due to *Clostridium colinum* susceptible to bacitracin methylene disalicylate. Feed continuously as the sole ration: 200 grams bacitracin per ton of feed.

Growing/finishing swine:

For increased rate of weight gain and improved feed efficiency: 10-30 grams bacitracin per ton of feed.

For control of swine dysentery (bloody scours) associated with *Treponema hyodysenteriae* in pigs up to 250 lbs body weight. Feed 250 grams per ton of complete feed on premises with a history of swine dysentery, but where signs of the disease have not yet occurred or following an approved treatment of the disease condition: 250 grams bacitracin per ton of feed.

The 250 g/ton level will provide 5 to 7 mg/lb in swine weighing 40 to 250 lbs.

Pregnant sows:

For control of clostridial enteritis caused by *C. perfringens* in suckling piglets when fed to sows from 14 days before through 21 days after farrowing on premises with a history of clostridial scours: 250 grams bacitracin per ton of feed.

Feedlot beef cattle:

For reduction in the number of liver condemnations due to abscesses in feedlot beef cattle: 70 mg/head/day (continuously) or 250 mg/head/day (5 days in 30).

Note: Where minimum levels are shown, increase the antibiotic concentration within approved range when necessary to fit the feeding program, and to insure adequate levels of antibiotic in the complete ration.

Caution(s): For manufacturing registered poultry and livestock feeds only.

Broiler and replacement chickens: To control a necrotic enteritis outbreak, start medication at the first clinical signs of disease. The dosage range permitted provides for different levels based on severity of the infection. Consult a poultry diagnostic laboratory or pathologist to determine the diagnosis and advice regarding the optimal level of drug. Administer continuously for 5-7 days or as long as clinical signs persist, and then reduce medication to prevention level (50 g/ton).

Growing/finishing swine and Pregnant sows: Diagnosis should be confirmed by a veterinarian when results are not satisfactory. Feed containing an approved level of bacitracin methylene disalicylate should be the sole ration.

Restricted drug - Use only as directed (CA).

For use in animals only.

For use in dry feeds only.

Not for use in liquid Type B medicated feeds.

Presentation: 50 lb (22.68 kg) bags.

Compendium Code No.: 10220172 0991310 0106

BMD® 60

Alpharma **Feed Medication**

Bacitracin Methylene Disalicylate-Type A Medicated Article-Antibacterial

NADA No.: 046-592

Active Ingredient(s): Each pound contains feed grade bacitracin methylene disalicylate equivalent to 60 grams bacitracin (Master Standard).

Composition: A dried precipitated fermentation product obtained by culturing *B. licheniformis* Tracy on media adapted for microbiological production of bacitracin; calcium carbonate.

Indications: For supplementing rations of swine, chickens, turkeys, pheasants, quail and feedlot beef cattle.

Directions: Mixing Directions: Prepare an intermediate premix containing 5 grams per pound by mixing 1.0 lb of BMD® 60 with 11.0 lbs of soybean meal or ground corn. Then add 0.8 to 50 lbs of intermediate premix per ton of finished feed.

Growing/finishing swine:

For increased rate of weight gain and improved feed efficiency: 10-30 grams bacitracin per ton of feed.

For control of swine dysentery (bloody scours) associated with *Brachyspira hyodysenteriae* in pigs up to 250 lbs body weight. Feed 250 grams per ton of complete feed on premises with a history of swine dysentery, but where signs of the disease have not yet occurred or following an approved treatment of the disease condition: 250 grams bacitracin per ton of feed.

The 250 g/ton level will provide 5 to 7 mg/lb in swine weighing 40 to 250 lbs.

Pregnant sows:

For control of clostridial enteritis caused by *C. perfringens* in suckling piglets when fed to sows from 14 days before through 21 days after farrowing on premises with a history of clostridial scours: 250 grams bacitracin per ton of feed.

Broiler and replacement chickens:

For increased rate of weight gain and improved feed efficiency: 4-50 grams bacitracin per ton of feed.

As an aid in prevention of necrotic enteritis caused or complicated by *Clostridium* spp. or other organisms susceptible to bacitracin methylene disalicylate: 50 grams bacitracin per ton of feed.

As an aid in control of necrotic enteritis caused or complicated by *Clostridium* spp. or other organisms susceptible to bacitracin methylene disalicylate: 100-200 grams bacitracin per ton of feed.

Laying hens:

For increased egg production and improved feed efficiency during the first seven months of production: 10-25 grams bacitracin per ton of feed.

Growing turkeys:

For increased rate of weight gain and improved feed efficiency: 4-50 grams bacitracin per ton of feed.

As an aid in control of transmissible enteritis in growing turkeys complicated by organisms susceptible to bacitracin methylene disalicylate: 200 grams bacitracin per ton of feed.

Pheasants:

For increased rate of weight gain and improved feed efficiency: 4-50 grams bacitracin per ton of feed.

Quail:

For increased rate of weight gain and improved feed efficiency in quail not over 5 weeks of age: 5-20 grams bacitracin per ton of feed.

For prevention of ulcerative enteritis in growing quail due to *Clostridium colinum* susceptible to bacitracin methylene disalicylate. Feed continuously as the sole ration: 200 grams bacitracin per ton of feed.

Feedlot beef cattle:

For reduction in the number of liver condemnations due to abscesses in feedlot beef cattle: 70 mg per head per day (continuously), 250 mg per head per day (5 days in 30).

Note: Where minimum levels are shown, increase the antibiotic concentration within approved range when necessary to fit the feeding program, and to insure adequate levels of antibiotic in the complete ration.

Caution(s): For manufacturing registered livestock and poultry feeds only.

Growing/finishing swine and Pregnant sows: Diagnosis should be confirmed by a veterinarian when results are not satisfactory. Feed containing an approved level of bacitracin methylene disalicylate should be the sole ration.

Broiler and replacement chickens: To control a necrotic enteritis outbreak, start medication at the first clinical signs of disease. The dosage range permitted provides for different levels based on severity of the infection. Consult a poultry diagnostic laboratory or pathologist to determine the diagnosis and advice regarding the optimal level of drug. Administer continuously for 5-7 days or as long as clinical signs persist, and then reduce medication to prevention level (50 g/ton).

Restricted Drug: Use only as directed. (CA) For use in animals only.

For use in dry feeds only. Not for use in liquid type B medicated feeds.

Presentation: 50 lb (22.68 kg) bag.

Compendium Code No.: 10220182 AHG-003 0104

BMD® SOLUBLE

Alpharma **Water Medication**

Bacitracin methylene disalicylate oral veterinary (soluble powder)

NADA No.: 065-470

Active Ingredient(s): Contains 51.2 g bacitracin activity from bacitracin methylene disalicylate equivalent to 200 g bacitracin activity per pound or to 18,520 units bacitracin (master standard) per gram.

Ingredients: Fruit granulated sugar, bicarbonate of soda, petro ag. anti caking agent.

Indications:

Broiler and replacement chickens: An aid in prevention and control of necrotic enteritis caused by *Clostridium perfringens* susceptible to bacitracin methylene disalicylate.

Growing turkeys: An aid in control of transmissible enteritis (blue comb, mud fever) in growing turkeys complicated by organisms susceptible to bacitracin methylene disalicylate.

Growing quail: For the prevention of ulcerative enteritis due to *Clostridium colinum* susceptible to bacitracin methylene disalicylate.

Swine: For use in the treatment of swine dysentery associated with *Treponema (Serpulina) hyodysenteriae.*

Directions for Use:

Animal	Condition	Prevention	Control
Broiler and replacement chickens	Necrotic enteritis caused by *Clostridium perfringens* susceptible to bacitracin methylene disalicylate.	100 mg/gal	200-400 mg/gal
Growing turkeys	Transmissible enteritis (blue comb, mud fever) complicated by organisms susceptible to bacitracin methylene disalicylate.	—	400 mg/gal
Growing quail	Ulcerative enteritis due to *Clostridium colinum* susceptible to bacitracin methylene disalicylate.	400 mg/gal	—
Swine	Swine dysentery (bloody scours) associated with *Treponema (Serpulina) hyodysenteriae.*	—	1000 mg/gal

Prepare a fresh solution daily and use as sole source of drinking water.

Mixing Instructions:

For Proportioners: Select the treatment dosage. Set the proportioner at the desired delivery rate. To prepare the proportioner's stock solution, place the indicated quantity of BMD® Soluble in a 2-gallon container, fill with water and stir until dissolved.

For Tanks: One package of BMD® Soluble will medicate approximately 50 gallons of water at a dosage of 1000 mg/gallon.

	Proportioner setting	
Treatment dosage	1 ounce/gallon	2 ounce/gallon
100 mg/gal	½ pack	¼ pack
200 mg/gal*	1 pack	½ pack
400 mg/gal	2 packs	1 pack
1000 mg/gal	5 packs	2½ packs

* 200 mg/gallon is equivalent to about 100 g of feed grade BMD per ton of feed.

To control an outbreak, start medication at first clinical signs of disease. Consult a diagnostic laboratory or veterinarian to determine the diagnosis and advice regarding the optimal level of drug to use. For necrotic enteritis in broiler and replacement chickens, administer continuously 5-7 days or as long as clinical signs persist, then reduce medication to prevention level (100 mg/gal). For transmissible enteritis in turkeys, administer continuously as long as clinical signs persist. For swine dysentery start medication at first signs of the disease or at time of exposure and administer continuously for 7 days or until signs of dysentery disappear. Treatment not to exceed 14 days.

Precaution(s): Store in a cool, dry place.

Caution(s): Not for use in swine weighing more than 250 lb.

Not for human use. For oral use in animals only. Restricted drug. Use only as directed.

For poultry and livestock drinking water. Concentrated - For water medicators.

Presentation: 4.1 oz (116.2 g) packages.

Compendium Code No.: 10220191 AHF-002H 0002

BO-BAC-2X™

Boehringer Ingelheim **Antiserum**

Actinomyces Pyogenes-Escherichia Coli-Pasteurella Multocida-Salmonella Typhimurium Antibody, Bovine Origin

U.S. Vet. Lic. No.: 124

Composition: The concentrated serum is prepared from the blood of cattle hyperimmunized with *Actinomyces pyogenes, Pasteurella multocida* Carter's Serotype A, *Escherichia coli* serotype 78:K80:NM, and *Salmonella typhimurium.*

Contains 0.2% cresol as a preservative.

Indications: Recommended for the prophylaxis and treatment of diseases caused by *Actinomyces pyogenes, Pasteurella multocida, Escherichia coli* and *Salmonella typhimurium* in cattle.

Dosage and Administration: Prophylactic: 15 mL per 50 lbs. of body weight administered subcutaneously as soon as possible after birth.

Therapeutic: 30 mL per 50 lbs. of body weight, repeat every 12 to 24 hours (depending upon condition of the animal) until improvement is satisfactory.

Precaution(s): Store out of direct sunlight at a temperature between 35-45°F (2-7°C). Avoid freezing. Shake well before using. Use the entire contents when first opened.

Caution(s): Anaphylactoid reactions may occur.

Antidote(s): Epinephrine.

Warning(s): Do not vaccinate within 21 days before slaughter.

Do not vaccinate with bovine virus diarrhea vaccine, bovine rhinotracheitis vaccine or bovine parainfluenza$_3$ vaccine, or *Haemophilus somnus* or *Pasteurella haemolytica* bacterins within 21 days after use of this serum.

Presentation: 250 mL vial.

Compendium Code No.: 10280212 BI 1137-1 2/01, 13701-05

BOLTAN III™

Butler **Antidiarrheal-Adsorbent**

NDC No.: 11695-3022-2

Active Ingredient(s): Each bolus contains: Kaolin colloidal 160 grains, in a base containing aluminum hydroxide, carob flour, pectin, albumen tannate and electrolytes sodium chloride, potassium chloride, and magnesium sulfate.

Indications: An adsorbent, demulcent bolus for use as an aid in the treatment of simple diarrheas in horses and cattle.

Dosage and Administration: Horses and Cattle: Two or three boluses orally 2 or 3 times daily, or as directed by veterinarian.

Precaution(s): Do not store over 30°C (86°F).

Caution(s): If symptoms persist after using the preparation for 2 or 3 days, reconsult veterinarian.

Horses and cattle being treated should have access to clean, fresh drinking water, ad lib.

Warning(s): For veterinary use only. Livestock drug.

Keep out of the reach of children.

Presentation: 50 boluses.

Compendium Code No.: 10820250

BORDE-CELL™

AgriLabs **Vaccine**

Bordetella bronchiseptica Vaccine, Avirulent Live Culture

U.S. Vet. Lic. No.: 303

Active Ingredient(s): The vaccine contains an avirulent live culture of *Bordetella bronchiseptica.*

Indications: For use in healthy swine as an aid in the prevention and control of diseases caused by *Bordetella bronchiseptica.*

Dosage and Administration: Shake well before using. Administer 2 mL intramuscularly to sows and gilts five (5) and two (2) weeks prior to farrowing. Administer 1 mL intranasally (½ mL into each nostril) to piglets one (1) day of age.

Precaution(s): Store in the dark at 35°-45°F (2°-7°C). Do not freeze.

Caution(s): Needles and syringes should not be sterilized with chemicals. Use the entire contents when first opened. Do not use the vaccine in conjunction with antibiotics effective against *Bordetella bronchiseptica.* Burn the container and any unused contents. Anaphylactic reactions may occur following the use of the biological. Symptomatic treatment: Epinephrine.

For veterinary use only.

Warning(s): Do not vaccinate within 21 days before slaughter.

Presentation: 30 mL (30 piglet doses, 15 sow doses) and 100 mL (100 piglet doses, 50 sow doses) bottles.

Compendium Code No.: 10580200

BORDE SHIELD® 4

Novartis Animal Vaccines **Bacterin**

Bordetella bronchiseptica-Erysipelothrix rhusiopathiae-Pasteurella multocida Bacterin

U.S. Vet. Lic. No.: 303

Composition: The bacterin contains chemically inactivated highly antigenic cultures of *Bordetella bronchiseptica, Erysipelothrix rhusiopathiae* and two strains of *Pasteurella multocida* adjuvanted with aluminum hydroxide. Contains penicillin and streptomycin as preservatives.

Indications: For use in healthy swine as an aid in the prevention and control of atrophic rhinitis, erysipelas, pasteurellosis and other diseases caused by *Bordetella bronchiseptica, Erysipelothrix rhusiopathiae,* and *Pasteurella multocida.*

Dosage and Administration: Shake well before using. Inoculate sows and gilts intramuscularly or subcutaneously with two (2) 5 mL doses five (5) and two (2) weeks prior to farrowing. Vaccinate piglets with 1 mL at 7-10 days of age and 2 mL at 21-28 days of age.

Precaution(s): Store between 35°-45°F (2°-7°C). Do not freeze.

Caution(s): Use the entire contents when first opened. Anaphylactic reactions may occur following the use of this biological. Symptomatic treatment: Epinephrine.

Warning(s): Do not vaccinate within 21 days before slaughter.

Discussion: *Erysipelothrix rhusiopathiae* is the cause of swine erysipelas (SE) or diamond skin disease. The disease is worldwide in distribution and many apparently normal animals can carry and shed the organism. SE is generally divided into three general classifications - peracute, subacute, and chronic. The peracute septicemic form may be seen as sudden death, fever, lameness, and depression. Skin changes may occur as purplish-red discoloration of the ears and abdomen. There may in some cases be the characteristic diamond-shaped skin lesions. The subacute form is a milder manifestation of the acute form. The chronic form will usually follow recovery of acute or subacute cases, or appear in animals where immunity is not completely protective. The chronic form will most often appear as lameness and bacterial growths in the heart. The diagnosis of SE should be made by bacterial isolation from tissues of aborted fetuses.

Bordetella bronchiseptica has long been established as a primary cause of atrophic rhinitis (AR) and pneumonia. In the case of AR, *B. bronchiseptica* may act as a primary invader and, depending upon the virulence of the strain, may act alone or may compromise the nasal epithelium so that secondary Pasteurella organisms can invade and cause more extensive damage.

The most common clinical signs of AR are sneezing, snuffling, rubbing the nose, black tear streaks from the eye and excessive nasal discharge.

A more severe clinical situation associated with *B. bronchiseptica* is bronchopneumonia. This can occur in piglets as young as three to five days of age and is considered a primary infection. The clinical signs of *B. bronchiseptica* bronchopneumonia are coughing and labored breathing. Morbidity and mortality can be high.

Pasteurella multocida is another important cause of pneumonia and atrophic rhinitis in swine. It is found worldwide, and it is a common inhabitant of the respiratory tract of healthy animals. It can affect animals of any age.

P. multocida is divided into two types, A and D. Type A is a common cause of pneumonia. Its importance is as a secondary invader. Lungs damaged by other causes such as poor air quality, ascarid (roundworm) migrations, or other infectious agents, can be invaded by Pasteurella, which causes further lung damage and culminates in a severe pneumonia. These animals will show typical pneumonia symptoms - coughing, shortness of breath, labored breathing ("thumping"), and fevers up to 107°F. If not treated in the early stages, many animals become chronic cases. Death losses, while typically low, may be high in some cases.

Toxin-producing strains of *P. multocida* type D are an important cause of atrophic rhinitis. The bacteria colonize the nasal turbinates, then release a toxin which causes damage to the tissues and results in the typical signs of AR - sneezing, sniffling, teary eyes and crooked snouts. An important feature with type D is that it can infect older pigs and cause severe AR, whereas piglets normally have to be infected with *B. bronchiseptica* within a few days after birth in order to develop AR.

Nasal turbinates damaged by AR are not able to do an effective job of filtering the air the pig breathes, allowing more bacteria access to the lungs. This, in turn, makes it more likely that the pig will develop severe pneumonia.

Presentation: Available in 100 mL bottles.

Compendium Code No.: 11140012

BORDETELLA BRONCHISEPTICA INTRANASAL VACCINE

MVP **Vaccine**

Bordetella bronchiseptica Vaccine (Avirulent Live Culture)

U.S. Vet. Lic. No.: 301

Active Ingredient(s): The vaccine contains cultures of avirulent live *Bordetella bronchiseptica*.

Indications: For use as an aid in the prevention of respiratory disease associated with virulent *Bordetella bronchiseptica* in swine.

Dosage and Administration: Shake well before and occasionally during use. Administer ½ mL into each nostril of piglets within 24 hours of birth.

Precaution(s): Store at 35°-45°F (2°-7°C). Do not freeze.

Caution(s): Use the entire contents when first opened. Burn the container and any unused contents after use.

For veterinary use only.

Warning(s): Do not use within 21 days before slaughter.

Presentation: 30 mL (30 dose) and 100 mL (100 dose) vials.

Compendium Code No.: 11120000

BORDE-VAC 1

TradeWinds **Bacterin**

Bordetella Bronchiseptica Bacterin, Cellular Antigen Extract

U.S. Vet. Lic. No.: 462

Contents: BORDE-VAC 1 is a nonadjuvanted antigenic extract prepared from the cells of *Bordetella bronchiseptica*.

This product contains thimerosal (merthiolate) as a preservative.

Indications: Recommended for use as an aid in the control of Canine Infectious Tracheobronchitis (Kennel Cough) caused by the organism represented.

Directions: Shake well. Aseptically remove entire contents into the syringe. Push out any air trapped in the syringe. Administer entire contents (1 mL) subcutaneously under loose skin (back of neck) to healthy dogs at least 8 weeks of age. Do not vaccinate into blood vessels. If blood enters the syringe, choose another injection site. For initial vaccination, a second dose is required 2-4 weeks later. This product should be administered by subcutaneous injection only. Annual revaccination with a single 1 mL dose is recommended.

Precaution(s): Store at 35°F-45°F (2°C-8°C). Do not freeze. Use entire contents when first opened.

Caution(s): Care should be taken to avoid microbial contamination of the product. In case of anaphylactoid reactions, epinephrine should be administered immediately. Transient local irritation at the site of injection, though rare, may occur subsequent to use of this product.

For veterinary use only.

Discussion: The effect of persisting *B. bronchiseptica* maternal antibody on the immune response in puppies to this bacterin has not been determined. Puppies from bitches immune to the organism usually have low antibody titers that are dissipated by 4-6 weeks of age. Although kennel cough is considered a disease of complex etiology, it can be reproduced by challenge with *B. bronchiseptica* alone. A close association and/or confinement of dogs facilitates spread of the disease syndrome. Antibiotic therapy has been shown to be generally unsuccessful in reducing or eliminating *B. bronchiseptica* infection in dogs.

Presentation: 1 dose (1 mL).

Manufactured by: Biocor Animal Health Inc., Omaha, NE 68134 U.S.A.

Compendium Code No.: 12610000 TW7001-1001

BO-SE® ℞

Schering-Plough **Vitamin E-Selenium**

(Selenium, Vitamin E) Injection

NADA No.: 012-635

Active Ingredient(s): Description: BO-SE® (selenium, vitamin E) is an emulsion of selenium-tocopherol. Each mL contains: 2.19 mg sodium selenite (equivalent to 1 mg selenium), 50 mg (68 USP units) vitamin E (as d-alpha tocopheryl acetate), 250 mg polysorbate 80, 2% benzyl alcohol (preservative), water for injection q.s. Sodium hydroxide and/or hydrochloric acid may be added to adjust pH.

Indications: BO-SE® (selenium, vitamin E) is recommended for the prevention and treatment of white muscle disease (Selenium-Tocopherol Deficiency) syndrome in calves, lambs, and ewes. Clinical signs are: Stiffness and lameness, diarrhea and unthriftiness, pulmonary distress and/or cardiac arrest. In sows and weanling pigs, as an aid in the prevention and treatment of diseases associated with Selenium-Tocopherol Deficiency such as hepatic necrosis, mulberry heart disease, and white muscle disease. Where known deficiencies of selenium and/or vitamin E exist, it is advisable, from the prevention and control standpoint, to inject the sow during the last week of pregnancy.

Pharmacology: It has been demonstrated that selenium and tocopherol exert physiological effects and that these effects are intertwined with sulfur metabolism. Additionally, tocopherol appears to have a significant role in the oxidation process, thus suggesting an interrelationship between selenium and tocopherol in overcoming sulfur-induced depletion and restoring normal metabolism. Although oral ingestion of adequate amounts of selenium and tocopherol would seemingly restore normal metabolism, it is apparent that the presence of sulfur and perhaps other factors interfere during the digestive process with the proper utilization of selenium and tocopherol. When selenium and tocopherol are injected, they bypass the digestive process and exert their full metabolic effects promptly on cell metabolism. Anti-inflammatory action has been demonstrated by selenium-tocopherol in the Selye Pouch Technique and experimentally induced polyarthritis study in rats.

B

Dosage and Administration: Inject subcutaneously or intramuscularly.

Calves: 2.5-3.75 mL per 100 pounds of body weight depending on the severity of the condition and the geographical area.

Lambs 2 weeks of age and older: 1 mL per 40 pounds of body weight (minimum, 1 mL).

Ewes: 2.5 mL per 100 pounds of body weight.

Sows: 1 mL per 40 pounds of body weight.

Weanling pigs: 1 mL per 40 pounds of body weight (minimum 1 mL). Not for use in newborn pigs.

Contraindication(s): Do not use in pregnant ewes. Deaths and abortions have been reported in pregnant ewes injected with this product.

Precaution(s): Storage: Store between 2° and 30°C (36° and 86°F). Protect from freezing.

Caution(s): Federal law restricts this drug to use by or on the order of a licensed veterinarian.

Selenium-Tocopherol Deficiency (STD) syndrome produces a variety and complexity of symptoms often interfering with a proper diagnosis. Even in selenium deficient areas there are other disease conditions which produce similar clinical signs. It is imperative that all these conditions be carefully considered prior to the treatment of STD syndrome. Serum selenium levels, elevated SGOT, and creatine serum levels may serve as aids in arriving at a diagnosis of STD, when associated with other indices. Selenium is toxic if administered in excess. A fixed dose schedule is therefore important (read the package insert for each selenium-tocopherol product carefully before using).

Important: Use only the selenium-tocopherol product recommended for each species. Each formulation is designed for the species indicated to produce the maximum efficacy and safety.

Anaphylactoid reactions, some of which have been fatal, have been reported in animals administered BO-SE® Injection. Signs include excitement, sweating, trembling, ataxia, respiratory distress and cardiac dysfunction.

For veterinary use only.

Warning(s): Discontinue use 30 days before the treated calves are slaughtered for human consumption. Discontinue use 14 days before the treated lambs, ewes, sows and pigs are slaughtered for human consumption.

Adverse Reactions: Reactions, including acute respiratory distress, frothing from the nose and mouth, bloating, severe depression, abortions and deaths have occurred in pregnant ewes. No known treatment exists because at this time the cause of the reaction is unknown.

Presentation: 100 mL sterile, multiple dose vials (NDC 0061-0807-05).

Compendium Code No.: 10470251 Rev. 10/98

BOSS® POUR-ON INSECTICIDE

Schering-Plough **Topical Insecticide**

EPA No.: 773-82

Active Ingredient(s):

Permethrin: (3-phenoxyphenyl)-methyl (±) cis, trans-3-(2,2-dichloroethenyl-2,2-dimethylcyclopropanecarboxylate* 5.00%

Inert Ingredients** 95.00%

Total 100.00%

*cis/trans ratio: Min. 35% (±) cis and Max. 65% (±) trans.

**contains petroleum distillates

Indications: Pour-on insecticide for beef and dairy cattle and sheep.

For lactating and non-lactating dairy cattle and beef cattle and calves.

Controls flies and lice on cattle. Controls keds and lice on sheep.

Directions for Use: It is a violation of Federal law to use the product in a manner inconsistent with its labeling.

Ready To Use—No dilution necessary.

Apply to	Target Species	Dosage
Lactating and Non-Lactating Dairy Cattle, Beef Cattle and Calves	Lice, Horn flies, Face flies, Aids in control of Horse flies, Stable flies, Mosquitoes, Black flies and Ticks	Apply 3 mL per 100 lbs body weight of animal up to a maximum of 30 mL for any one animal. Pour along back and down face.
Sheep	Sheep keds, Lice	Pour along back. Apply 1.5 mL per 50 lbs of body weight of animal up to a maximum of 18 mL for any one animal.

For cattle and sheep, repeat treatment as needed but not more than once every 2 weeks. For optimum lice control, two treatments at 14 day intervals are recommended.

Special Note: BOSS® Pour-On Insecticide is not effective against cattle grubs. BOSS® Pour-On Insecticide should be used in an integrated pest management system which may involve repeat treatments and the use of other pest control practices.

Precautionary Statements: Hazards to Humans and Domestic Animals:

Caution — Harmful if swallowed or absorbed through the skin. Avoid contact with skin, eyes, or clothing. Wash thoroughly with soap and water after handling. Prolonged or frequently repeated skin contact may cause allergic reactions in some individuals.

Statement of Practical Treatment:

If Swallowed: Call a physician immediately. Do not induce vomiting unless under medical attention.

Note to Physician: Solvent presents aspiration hazard. Gastric lavage is indicated if material was taken internally.

B

If in Eyes: Immediately flush eyes with plenty of water. Get medical attention if discomfort persists.

If on Skin: Wash skin with soap and water. Get medical attention.

Environmental Hazards: This product is extremely toxic to fish and other aquatic invertebrates. Do not add directly to water. Do not contaminate water by cleaning of equipment or disposal of wastes. Apply this product only as specified on label.

Storage and Disposal: Do not contaminate water, food or feed by storage or disposal.

Storage: Keep container sealed when not in use. Do not store near food or feed.

Pesticide Disposal: Wastes resulting from the use of this product may be disposed of on-site or at an approved waste-disposal facility.

Container Disposal: Triple rinse (or equivalent). Then offer for recycling or reconditioning, or puncture and dispose of in a sanitary landfill or incinerator, or, if allowed by State and local authorities, by burning. If burned, stay out of smoke.

Warning(s): Keep out of reach of children.

Disclaimer: Notice of Warranty: Schering-Plough Animal Health Corporation makes no warranty of merchantability, fitness for any particular purpose, or otherwise expressed or implied concerning this product or its uses which extend beyond the use of this product under normal conditions and in accord with the statement on the label.

Presentation: 1 U.S. quart (0.968 L) (NDC 0061-5030-01) and 1 U.S. gallon (3.78 L) (NDC 0061-5030-02).

Compendium Code No.: 10470262 Rev. 9/99 / Rev. 2/99

BOTUMINK®

United **Bacterin-Toxoid**

Clostridium botulinum Type C Bacterin-Toxoid

U.S. Vet. Lic. No.: 245

Active Ingredient(s): An inactivated vaccine which contains *Cl. botulinum* type C.

Preservative: Thimerosal.

Indications: BOTUMINK® is for use as an aid in the prevention of botulism in healthy, susceptible mink.

Dosage and Administration: Inject 1 mL under the loose skin of the armpit of mink of at least six (6) weeks of age. For a proper suspension, shake before and occasionally during use. Revaccinate all adults at the time of kit vaccination.

Precaution(s): Store at 35-45°F (2-7°C).

Caution(s): Do not use as a diluent for live virus vaccines.

Use the entire contents when the container is first opened.

Consult a veterinarian or United Vaccines Inc. for an alternate vaccinating schedule and before using the vaccine on a farm where disease exists or has occurred in the last 18 months.

Presentation: 100 dose, 250 dose and 500 dose vials.

Compendium Code No.: 11040061

BOTVAX® B

Neogen **Toxoid**

Clostridium Botulinum Type B Toxoid

U.S. Vet. Lic. No.: 302

Contents: Purified botulinum type B toxoid aluminum phosphate adsorbed.

Preservative: 0.01% Thimerosal.

Contains no more than 0.2% formaldehyde as inactivating solution.

Indications: For the prevention of equine botulism due to *Clostridium botulinum* Type B in healthy horses.

Dosage and Administration: Dosage: Inject 2.0 mL intramuscularly at monthly intervals for a total of 3 doses. Booster annually with a single 2.0 mL intramuscular dose.

Research has demonstrated that pregnant mares immunized during the third trimester of gestation, with the third dose (booster) given 2-4 weeks before parturition, respond with antibody. This antibody is concentrated in colostrum and results in significant passively acquired antibody in normal sulking foals.

Administration: Inject intramuscularly using aseptic technique. Shake well before use.

Precaution(s): Store at 2-7°C (35-45°F). Do not freeze. Use the entire contents when opened.

Caution(s): Transitory local reactions at the injection site such as heat and minor swelling may occur. Anaphylactoid reactions may occur. Epinephrine is antidotal.

This is a conditionally licensed vaccine. Efficacy and potency have not been determined. These studies are in progress.

For veterinary use only.

Warning(s): Do not vaccinate food producing animals within 21 days of slaughter.

Presentation: 5 dose (10 mL) vials.

Compendium Code No.: 14910202 L309-0300

BOU-MATIC ALOE-SOFT

Bou-Matic **Teat Dip & Spray**

Active Ingredient(s): Nonylphenoxy polyethoxy (12 moles E.O.) ethanol-iodine complex providing 1.0% w/w titratable iodine (10,000 ppm. w/w).

Contains 10% skin conditioners.

Indications: 1% iodine post-milking teat dip and udder wash with ESP™ skin conditioning technology.

Directions: Usage Directions:

Post-Dipping/Spraying: Dip/spray teats with undiluted ALOE-SOFT immediately after milking. Allow to air dry. Replace the solution if it becomes visibly dirty. With freshening cows, begin dipping teats twice daily for about 10 days before calving. For dry cows, dip/spray teats with undiluted ALOE-SOFT once a day for several days following the last milking. During the cold weather do not turn cows out until teats are dry to prevent chapping and freezing. If necessary, wipe dry with a single paper towel.

Udder Washing: If necessary, wash cow teats prior to milking. Use a dilution ratio of 1 oz (30 mL) of undiluted ALOE-SOFT per two gallons (8 L) of lukewarm water (110°F-115°F, 40°C-45°C). After udder washing, dry each teat with individual clean towels or use Bou-Matic Kleen & Dri, a single step pre-milking udder prep.

Important—Teat Irritation and/or Chapping: Teat dips have the potential to cause irritation of a cow's teats or milker's hands. Individual tolerance to a particular formulation as well as other factors (dry or cold weather, improper teat dip application, bedding quality, milking equipment, etc.) may also affect skin condition. If you observe abnormal irritation or chapping while using ALOE-SOFT, discontinue use and call the technical service department at 1-800-225-3832, or contact your Bou-Matic dealer.

Contraindication(s): Do not use for cleaning and/or sanitizing equipment.

Precaution(s):

Storage and Disposal: Store this product in a cool, dry area away from direct sunlight and heat to avoid deterioration. Dispose of only in compliance with federal, state, and local laws.

Spillage: In case of small spill (less than one gallon), flood area with a large quantity of water. For larger spills, contain and remove with inert absorbent and dispose of according to federal, state, and local laws.

Keep from freezing.

Caution(s): Keep out of the reach of children.

Harmful if swallowed. Harmful if inhaled. Causes eye irritation.

Warning(s): Protect eyes, skin and clothing from contact with product. Keep container tightly closed when not in use. Use with adequate ventilation. Wash thoroughly after handling product.

First Aid:

External: In case of contact, immediately flush contaminated skin with plenty of water. If irritation occurs and persists, call a physician.

Internal: If swallowed, dilute by giving several glasses of water or milk. Do not induce vomiting. If vomiting does occur, repeat giving several glasses of water or milk. Get prompt medical attention. Never give anything by mouth to an unconscious person.

Eyes: Immediately flush with plenty of clean, running water for at least 15 minutes, holding eyelids apart to ensure flushing of the entire eye surface. If irritation persists, call a physician.

For additional precautions consult Material Safety Data Sheet.

Medical personnel familiar with this product are available 24 hours a day, 7 days a week.

Toll-Free Emergency Number: 1/800-424-9300

Presentation: 5, 15, 30 and 55 gallon drums.

Compendium Code No.: 14480020

BOU-MATIC BOVI-KOTE

Bou-Matic **Teat Dip**

Active Ingredient(s): Iodine 1% (10,000 ppm titratable iodine). Humectant, plasticizer, emollient, moisturizer and filming agents: 10.0%. pH 4.5 +/- 0.3.

Indications: A post-milking barrier teat dip with skin conditioning properties and extended protection against mastitis-causing organisms. This product washes off easily with normal teat prep. It forms a flexible, non-tacky film on the teat and closes the teat orifice to help prevent micro-organisms from entering the teat canal between and after milking.

Dosage and Administration: Immediately after milking, dip teats with undiluted solution. While cow is being dried up, dip teats with this product once a day for several days following last milking.

Presentation: 4x1 gallon case, 5 gallon pail, 15, 30 and 55 gallon drums, and 220 gallon (4x55 gallon).

Compendium Code No.: 14480030

BOU-MATIC BOVI-KOTE 5

Bou-Matic **Teat Dip**

0.5% Iodine Post-Milking Barrier Teat Dip

Active Ingredient(s): Nonylphenoxy polyethoxy (12 moles E.O.) ethanol iodine complex providing 0.5% w/w titratable iodine (5,000 ppm w/w). Contains 5% skin conditioners.

Indications: For use as a post-milking teat dip.

Directions for Use:

Post Dipping: Dip teats with undiluted BOVI-KOTE 5 immediately after milking. Allow to air dry. Replace the solution if it becomes visibly dirty. With freshening cows, begin dipping teats twice daily for about 10 days before calving. For dry cows, dip teats with undiluted BOVI-KOTE once a day for several days following last milking. During cold weather, do not turn cows out until teats are dry to prevent chapping and freezing. If necessary, wipe dry with a single paper towel.

Important: Teat Irritation and/or Chapping: Teat dips have the potential to cause irritation of a cow's teats or milker's hands. Individual tolerance to a particular formulation as well as other factors (dry or cold weather, improper teat dip application, bedding quality, milking equipment, etc.) may also affect skin condition. If you observe irritation or chapping while using BOVI-KOTE 5, discontinue use and call the technical service department at 1-800-225-3832, or contact your Bou-Matic dealer.

Precaution(s): Keep from freezing.

Storage and Disposal: Store this product in a cool dry area away from direct sunlight and heat to avoid deterioration. Store in a locked cabinet or room to keep it out of the reach of children. Dispose of only in compliance with federal, state, and local laws.

Spillage: In case of a small spill (less than 1 gallon), flood area with a large quantity of water. For larger spills, contain and remove with inert absorbent and dispose of according to provincial and local laws.

Contraindication(s): Do not use for cleaning and/or sanitizing equipment.

Caution(s): Keep out of reach of children.

Harmful if swallowed - Harmful if inhaled - Causes eye irritation.

Warning(s): Protect eyes, skin and clothing from contact with product. Keep container tightly closed when not in use. Use with adequate ventilation. Wash thoroughly after handling product.

First Aid:

External: In case of contact, flush contaminated skin with plenty of water. If irritation occurs and persists, call a physician.

Internal: If swallowed, dilute by giving several glasses of water or milk. Do not induce vomiting. If vomiting does occur, repeat giving several glasses of water or milk. Get prompt medical attention. Never give anything by mouth to an unconscious person.

Eyes: Immediately flush with plenty of clean, running water for at least 15 minutes, holding eyelids apart to ensure flushing of the entire eye surface. If irritation persists, call a physician.

To avoid contamination of milk, before milking thoroughly wash udders and teats with Bou-Matic 10-Wash or Bou-Matic Micro-Wash, then dry each cow's udder and teats with individual clean towels, or use Bou-Matic Kleen & Dri, ready to use pre-dip wipes.

For additional precautions consult Material Safety Data Sheet.

Medical personnel familiar with this product are available 24 hours a day, 7 days a week.

Toll-Free Emergency Number: 1/800-424-9300

Presentation: 4 X 1 gallon case, 5 gallon pail, 15 and 55 gallon drums, and 220 gallon (4 X 55 gallon).

Compendium Code No.: 14480040 822213-1 11/99

BOU-MATIC BOVISOFT

Bou-Matic **Teat Dip & Spray**

1% Iodine Post-Milking Teat Dip or Spray and Udder Wash

Active Ingredient(s): Nonylphenoxy polyethoxy (12 moles E.O.) ethanol-iodine complex providing 1.0% w/w titratable iodine (10,000 ppm. w/w). Contains 12% skin conditioners.

Indications: 1% iodine pre- and post-milking teat dip or spray and udder wash.

Directions for Use:

Post-Dipping/Spraying: Dip/spray teats with undiluted BOVISOFT immediately after milking. Allow to air dry. Replace the solution if it becomes visibly dirty. With freshening cows, begin dipping teats twice daily for about 10 days before calving. For dry cows, dip/spray teats with undiluted BOVISOFT once a day for several days following the last milking. During the cold weather do not turn cows out until teats are dry to prevent chapping and freezing. If necessary, wipe dry with a single paper towel.

Udder Washing: If necessary, wash cow teats prior to milking. Use a dilution ratio of 1 oz (30 mL) of undiluted BOVISOFT per two gallons (8 L) of lukewarm water (110°F-115°F, 40°C-45°C). After udder washing, dry each teat with individual clean towels or Bou-Matic Kleen & Dry, a single step pre-milking udder prep.

Contraindication(s): Do not use for cleaning and/or sanitizing equipment.

Storage and Disposal: Store this product in a cool, dry area away from direct sunlight and heat to avoid deterioration. Dispose of only in compliance with federal, state, and local laws.

Spillage: In case of small spill (less than one gallon), flood area with a large quantity of water. For larger spills, contain and remove with inert absorbent and dispose of according to federal, state, and local laws. Keep from freezing.

Caution(s): Medical personnel familiar with this product are available 24 hours a day, 7 days a week at the toll-free emergency number.

Protect eyes, skin and clothing from contact with product. Keep container tightly closed when not in use. Use with adequate ventilation. Wash thoroughly after handling product.

First Aid:

External: In case of contact, flush contaminated skin with plenty of water. If irritation occurs and persists, call a physician.

Internal: If swallowed, dilute by giving several glasses of water or milk. Do not induce vomiting. If vomiting does occur, repeat giving several glasses of water or milk. Get prompt medical attention. Never give anything by mouth to an unconscious person.

Eyes: Immediately flush with plenty of clean, running water for at least 15 minutes, holding eyelids apart to ensure flushing of the entire eye surface. If irritation persists, call a physician.

Teat Irritation and/or Chapping: Teat dips have the potential to cause irritation of a cow's teats or milker's hands. Individual tolerance to a particular formulation as well as other factors (dry or cold weather, improper teat dip application, bedding quality, milking equipment, etc.) may also affect skin condition. If you observe abnormal irritation or chapping while using BOVISOFT, discontinue use and call the technical service department, or contact your Bou-Matic dealer.

Warning(s): Keep out of the reach of children.

Harmful if swallowed. Harmful if inhaled. Causes eye irritation.

Presentation: 5 gallon pail, 15 and 55 gallon drums.

Compendium Code No.: 14480050

BOU-MATIC DERMA-GUARD

Bou-Matic **Teat Dip & Spray**

Active Ingredient(s):

Capric/Caprylic acids 1.0%

With 8.5% ESP™ Skin Conditioning Technology.

Indications: Teat dip or spray with ESP™ skin conditioning technology.

Directions: Usage Directions:

Pre-Dipping/Spraying: Teats should be clean and dry before dipping. If needed, wash and dry with a single service towel. Dip/spray with undiluted product and allow 20-60 seconds contact time. Wipe the teats dry before applying the milking unit.

Post-Dipping/Spraying: Dip/spray teats with undiluted product immediately after milking. Allow to air dry. With freshening cows, begin dipping teats twice daily for about 10 days before calving. For dry cows, dip/spray teats once a day for several days following the last milking. During cold weather, do not turn out cows until teats are dry to prevent chapping and freezing. If necessary, wipe dry with a single service towel.

Precaution(s): Keep container tightly closed when not in use.

Storage and Disposal: Store this product in a cool, dry area away from direct sunlight and heat to avoid deterioration. Store in a locked cabinet or room to keep it out of the reach of children. Dispose of according to Federal State and local laws.

Spillage: In case of small spill (less than one gallon), flood area with a large quantity of water. For larger spills, contain and remove with inert absorbent and dispose of according to Federal, State, and local laws.

Keep from freezing.

Caution(s): Do not use this product for cleaning and/or sanitizing equipment.

Important: Teat Irritation or Chapping: Teat dips have the potential to cause irritation of a cow's teats or milker's hands. Individual tolerance to a particular formulation as well as other factors (dry or cold weather, improper teat dip application, bedding quality, milking equipment, etc.) may also affect teat condition. If you observe abnormal irritation or chapping, discontinue use and call the technical service department at 1-800-225-3832, or contact your dealer.

Warning(s): Keep out of the reach of children.

Harmful if swallowed. Harmful if inhaled. Causes eye irritation.

Medical personnel familiar with this product are available 24 hours a day, 7 days a week.

Toll Free Emergency Number: 1-800-424-9300

Protect eyes from contact with this product. Use with adequate ventilation. Wash thoroughly after handling product.

First Aid:

External: In case of contact, immediately flush contaminated skin with plenty of water. If irritation occurs and persists, call a physician.

Internal: If conscious, dilute by giving several glasses of water or milk. Do not induce vomiting. If vomiting does occur, repeat giving several glasses of water or milk. Get prompt medical attention. Never give anything by mouth to an unconscious person.

Eyes: Immediately flush with plenty of clean, running water for at least 15 minutes holding eyelids apart to ensure flushing of the entire eye surface. If irritation persists, call a physician.

Presentation: 2.5 gallon, 5 gallon, 15 gallon, 55 gallon and 275 gallon containers.

Manufactured by: A & L Laboratories, Inc., A Company of DEC International, Inc., P.O. Box 8050, Madison, WI 53708.

Compendium Code No.: 14480170

BOU-MATIC EXTRA-GUARD

Bou-Matic **Teat Dip**

Active Ingredient(s):

Capric/Caprylic acids. 1.0%

With 11% ESP™ Skin Conditioning Technology.

Indications: Non-iodine post-milking barrier teat dip.

Directions: Usage Directions:

Post-Dipping: Dip teats with undiluted product immediately after milking. Allow to air dry. Replace the solution if it becomes visibly dirty. With freshening cows, begin dipping teats twice daily for about 10 days before calving. For dry cows, dip teats once a day for several days following the last milking. During cold weather, do not turn out cows until teats are dry to prevent chapping and freezing. If necessary, wipe dry with a single service towel.

Precaution(s): Keep container tightly closed when not in use.

Storage and Disposal: Store this product in a cool, dry area away from direct sunlight and heat to avoid deterioration. Storage temperature should not be less than 40°F (4°C) or more than 105°F (40°C). Store in a locked cabinet or room to keep it out of the reach of children. Dispose of according to Federal, State and local laws.

Spillage: In case of small spill (less than one gallon), flood area with a large quantity of water. For larger spills, contain and remove with inert absorbent and dispose of according to Federal, State, and local laws.

Keep from freezing.

Caution(s): Do not use this product for cleaning and/or sanitizing equipment.

Important: Teat Irritation or Chapping: Teat dips have the potential to cause irritation of a cow's teats or milker's hands. Individual tolerance to a particular formulation as well as other factors (dry or cold weather, improper teat dip application, bedding quality, milking equipment, etc.) may also affect teat condition. If you observe abnormal irritation or chapping, discontinue use and call the technical service department at 1-800-225-3832, or contact your dealer.

Warning(s): To avoid contamination of milk, wash udder and teats with an effective udder wash, or pre-dip with an effective teat dip, then dry each cow's udder and teats with individual clean towels.

Keep out of the reach of children.

Harmful if swallowed. Harmful if inhaled. Causes eye irritation.

Medical personnel familiar with this product are available 24 hours a day, 7 days a week.

For emergencies call 1-800-424-9300.

Protect eyes from contact with this product. Use with adequate ventilation. Wash thoroughly after handling product.

First Aid:

External: In case of contact, immediately flush contaminated skin with plenty of water. If irritation occurs and persists, call a physician.

Internal: If conscious, dilute by giving several glasses of water or milk. Do not induce vomiting. If vomiting does occur, repeat giving several glasses of water or milk. Get prompt medical attention. Never give anything by mouth to an unconscious person.

Eyes: Immediately flush with plenty of clean running water for at least 15 minutes, holding eyelids apart to ensure flushing of the entire eye surface. If irritation persists, call a physician.

Presentation: 5 gallon, 15 gallon, 55 gallon and 275 gallon containers.

Manufactured by: A & L Laboratories, Inc., A Company of DEC International, Inc., P.O. Box 8050, Madison, WI 53708.

Compendium Code No.: 14480180

BOU-MATIC IO-WASH

Bou-Matic **Udder Wash**

Active Ingredient(s):

Nonylphenoxy polyethoxy (12 moles E.O.) ethanol-iodine complex . . . . . 8.75% (w/w)
(providing 1.75% w/w titratable iodine).

Phosphoric Acid . . . . 3.00% (w/w)

Acetic Acid . . . . 3.00% (w/w)

Inert Ingredients: . . . . 85.25% (w/w)

Indications: A concentrated product to prepare udder wash solution.

Dosage and Administration:

1. Prepare the udder wash solution in a plastic pail using 1 ounce of IO-WASH per 5 gallons of warm water (110°F-115°F), or ½ ounce to each 2½ gallons.
   IO-WASH may also be applied as a spray by using an in-line proportioner to meter the proper amount of udder wash into the spray.
2. Approximately one minute before applying milking unit, wash teats with a clean paper towel wetted with the udder wash solution. Dry with another clean, single-service towel.
3. Discard the used towel. Do not reuse towels or dip used towels back into the udder wash solution.

Precaution(s):

Storage and Disposal: Store this product in a cool, dry area away from direct sunlight and heat to avoid deterioration. Dispose of only in compliance with federal, state, and local laws.

Spillage: In case of a small spill (less than one gallon), flood area with a large quantity of water. For larger spills, contain and remove with inert absorbent and dispose of according to federal, state, and local laws.

Physical and Chemical Hazards: Do not mix this product with chlorinated cleaners or sanitizers, as this will release toxic chlorine gas.

Keep from freezing.

Caution(s): Danger. Contains phosphoric and acetic acids.

May be fatal if swallowed. Harmful if inhaled.

Causes severe eye and skin irritations or burns.

A concentrated product - Must be diluted before using.

Warning(s): For additional precautions consult Material Safety Data Sheet.

Medical personnel familiar with this product are available 24 hours a day, 7 days a week at the toll-free emergency number.

Protect eyes, skin and clothing from contact with product. When handling, wear chemical goggles, rubber boots, rubber apron and rubber gloves. Keep container tightly closed when not in use. Use with adequate ventilation. Wash thoroughly after handling product.

First Aid:

External: In case of contact, flush contaminated skin with plenty of water for at least 15 minutes. Remove contaminated clothing and shoes while flushing with water. If irritation or burn occurs, call a physician.

Internal: If swallowed, dilute by giving several glasses of water or milk. Do not induce vomiting. If vomiting does occur, repeat giving several glasses of water or milk. Get prompt medical attention.

Never give anything by mouth to an unconscious person.

Eyes: Immediately flush with plenty of clean, running water for at least 15 minutes, holding eyelids apart to ensure flushing of the entire eye surface. Call a physician.

Presentation: 4x1 gallon case, 5 gallon pail, and 15 gallon drum.

Compendium Code No.: 14480060

BOU-MATIC KLEEN & DRI

Bou-Matic **Teat Preparation**

Ingredient(s): Ethanol (50%). Water, cetrimide (0.16%) and chlorhexidine gluconate (0.1%).

Indications: Ready-to-use pre-dip wipes.

KLEEN & DRI wipes contain a non-irritating, instant-killing disinfectant, which is effective against broad range of mastitis-causing organisms.

Other Applications: Disinfection of the cow teats before intravenous injections or any other form of treatment involving penetration of the teat.

General disinfection for veterinarians before treating animals.

Dosage and Administration: Direction for use as a pre-milking teat preparation:

Strip each teat.

Pull out a KLEEN & DRI wipe from the pail. When the perforation appears, give a snap sideways to separate from the next towel.

Use one single KLEEN & DRI wipe per cow to clean and sanitize each teat for 3 to 4 seconds, including the teat end.

Note: The ingredients used to moisturize KLEEN & DRI are fast drying and do not require the use of a paper towel to dry teats prior to applying the milking unit.

Important: For best results, the teats should be free of heavy dirt.

Precaution(s): Keep away from fire or flame and heat. Close pail opening between milking.

Warning(s): For external use only. Avoid contact with eyes. Toll Free Emergency Number: 1-800-228-5635, Ext. 1

Keep out of reach of children.

Presentation: Package contains 700 premoistened wipes.

Compendium Code No.: 14480071

BOU-MATIC MAXI-SOFT

Bou-Matic **Teat Dip**

Active Ingredient(s): Iodine 0.5% (5000 ppm w/w). Emollient, humectant and filmogene agents: 6%. pH 4.4 +/- 0.5.

Indications: A high viscosity teat dip for extended protection and high visibility to be used before and/or after milking.

Dosage and Administration:

Pre-Milking Teat Dipping: After teats have been cleaned, examine each quarter with strip cup. Dip each quarter in undiluted solution. Allow product to stay on teat 20 to 40 seconds, then wipe dry with individual clean towel.

Post-Milking Teat Dipping: Immediately after milking, dip teats in undiluted product. While a cow is being dried, dip teats in the solution once a day for several days following last milking.

Udder Washing: Use diluted at 1 oz per gallon of lukewarm water. Wash udder and teats with the solution, then dry each cow's udder and teats with individual clean towels before milking.

Presentation: 5 gallon pail, 15, 30 and 55 gallon drums, and 220 gallon (4x55 gallon).

Compendium Code No.: 14480080

BOU-MATIC NOVA BLEND VI

Bou-Matic **Teat Dip & Spray**

Active Ingredient(s): Nonylphenoxy polyethoxy (12 moles E.O.) ethanol-iodine complex providing 3% w/w titratable iodine (30,000 ppm. w/w).

Indications: An iodine concentrated product to prepare teat dip. A ready-to-use dip/spray presentation is also available.

Dosage and Administration: To make:

1% Iodine teat dip, 8% skin conditioners, mix 1 part of NOVA BLEND VI with 2 parts of potable water.

0.5% Iodine teat dip, 4% skin conditioners, mix 1 part of NOVA BLEND VI with 5 parts of potable water.

0.25% Iodine teat dip, 2% skin conditioners, mix 1 part of NOVA BLEND VI with 1 parts of potable water.

Usage Directions for Ready-to-Use NOVA BLEND VI:

Premilking Teat Dipping/Spraying: After teats have been properly cleaned, examine each quarter with strip cup. Dip or spray each teat with ready-to-use NOVA BLEND VI. Allow product to stay on teats 20-45 seconds, then wipe dry with a clean towel.

Teat Dipping/Spraying: Immediately after milker unit is removed, dip or spray each teat in ready-to-use NOVA BLEND VI. Allow to air dry. Replace the solution if it becomes visibly dirty. With freshening cows, begin dipping teats daily for about 10 days before calving.

Udder Washing: Cow's teats should be washed just prior to milking, using ready-to-use NOVA BLEND VI at the following dilutions:

0.25% Iodine	2 oz/gal (60 mL/4 L)
0.5% Iodine	1 oz/gal (30 mL/4 L)
1.0% Iodine	1 oz/2 gal (30 mL/8 L)

For Dry Cows: Dip/spray teats with ready-to-use NOVA BLEND VI once a day for several days following the last milking.

Iodine Concentrate Teat Dip: 3% Iodine-1 gallon (4 L) makes 3 gallons (11 L) of 1% or 6 gallons (23 L) of 0.5% or 12 gallons (45 L) of 0.25% iodine teat dip/spray, with a high level of skin conditioners.

Do not use as is.

Important: When mixing, always use containers completely free of any residue.

Contraindication(s): Do not use for cleaning and/or sanitizing equipment.

Precaution(s): Keep from freezing.

Storage and Disposal: Store concentrated and diluted product in a cool, dry area away from direct sunlight and heat at temperature between 40°F and 100°F to avoid deterioration. Dispose of only in compliance with federal, state, and local laws.

Spillage: In case of a small spill (less than one gallon), flood area with a large quantity of water. For larger spills, contain and remove with inert absorbent material and dispose of according to federal, state, and local laws.

Caution(s): Keep out of the reach of children.

Harmful if swallowed. Harmful if inhaled. Causes eye irritation.

Warning(s): Protect eyes, skin and clothing from contact with product. When handling, concentrate, wear chemical goggles, rubber boots, rubber apron and rubber gloves. Keep container tightly closed when not in use. Use with adequate ventilation. Wash thoroughly after handling product.

First Aid:

External: In case of contact, immediately flush contaminated skin with plenty of water for at least 15 minutes. Remove contaminated clothing and shoes while flushing with water. If irritation or burn occurs, call a physician.

Internal: If conscious, dilute by giving several glasses of water or milk. Do not induce vomiting. It vomiting does occur, repeat giving several glasses of water or milk. Got prompt medical attention. Never give anything by mouth to an unconscious person.

Eyes: Immediately flush with plenty of clean, running water for at least 15 minutes, holding eyelids apart to ensure flushing of the entire eye surface. Call a physician.

For additional precautions consult Material Safety Data Sheet.

Medical personnel familiar with this product are available 24 hours a day, 7 days a week at the toll-free emergency number.

Presentation: 2.5 and 5 gallon pails, 8.3 and 55 gallon drums, and 220 gallon (4x55 gallon).

Compendium Code No.: 14480091

BOU-MATIC NOVABLEND 10

Bou-Matic **Teat Preparation**

Active Ingredient(s): Nonylphenoxy polyethoxy (12 moles E.O.) ethanol-iodine complex providing either 0.5 or 1.0% w/w titratable iodine.

Indications: A ready-to-use iodine solution to be used as a teat dip, teat spray or udder wash in dairy cattle.

Directions for Use:

Premilking Teat Dipping/Spraying: After teats have been properly cleaned, examine each quarter with strip cup. Dip or spray each teat with ready-to-use NOVABLEND 10. Allow product to stay on teats 20-45 seconds, then wipe dry with a clean towel.

Postmilking Teat Dipping/Spraying: Immediately after milker unit is removed, dip or spray each teat in ready-to-use NOVABLEND 10. Allow to air dry. Replace the solution if it becomes visibly dirty. With freshening cows, begin dipping teats daily for about 10 days before calving.

Udder Washing: Cow's teats should be washed just prior to milking, using ready-to-use NOVABLEND 10 at the following dilutions: 0.5% Iodine - 1 oz/gal; 1.0% Iodine - 1 oz/gal.

For Dry Cows: Dip/spray teats with ready-to-use NOVABLEND 10 once a day for several days following the last milking.

Contraindication(s): Do not use for cleaning and/or sanitizing equipment.

Storage and Disposal: Store this product in a cool, dry area away from direct sunlight and heat at temperature between 40°F and 100°F to avoid deterioration. Dispose of only in compliance with federal, state, and local laws.

Spillage: In case of small spill (less than one gallon), flood area with a large quantity of water. For larger spills, contain and remove with inert absorbent and dispose of according to federal, state, and local laws.

Caution(s): Contains nonylphenoxy (12 moles E.O.) ethanol-iodine complex.

See below for additional precautions and/or consult Material Safety Data Sheet.

Precautions: Protect eyes, skin and clothing from contact with product. When handling concentrate, wear goggles, and rubber gloves. Keep container tightly closed when not in use. Use with adequate ventilation. Wash thoroughly after handling product.

First Aid:

External: In case of contact, rinse off with water. Remove contaminated clothing and shoes while flushing with water. If irritation occurs, call a physician.

Internal: If swallowed, dilute by giving several glasses of water or milk. Do not induce vomiting. It vomiting does occur, repeat giving several glasses of water or milk. Get prompt medical attention. Never give anything by mouth to an unconscious person.

Eyes: Immediately flush with plenty of clean, running water for at least 15 minutes, holding eyelids apart to ensure flushing of the entire eye surface. Call a physician.

Warning(s): Keep out of the reach of children.

Harmful if swallowed. Harmful if inhaled. Causes eye irritation.

Presentation: 5 gallon pail, 15 and 55 gallon drums, and 220 gallon (4x55 gallon).

Compendium Code No.: 14480100

BOU-MATIC PENETRATE

Bou-Matic **Teat Dip & Spray**

Teat Dip-Teat Spray-Udder Wash

Active Ingredient(s): Nonylphenoxypolyethoxy (12 moles EO) ethanol-iodine complex providing 1.0% titratable iodine (10,000 ppm).

Contains 10% skin conditioners.

Indications: 1% iodine post-milking teat dip or spray or udder wash.

Directions: Usage Directions:

Post-Dipping/Spraying: Dip/spray teats with undiluted product immediately after milking. Allow to air dry. Replace the solution if it becomes visibly dirty. With freshening cows, begin dipping teats twice daily for about 10 days before calving. For dry cows, dip/spray teats once a day for several days following the last milking. During cold weather, do not turn out cows until teats are dry to prevent chapping and freezing. If necessary, wipe dry with a single service towel.

Udder Wash: To avoid contamination of milk, wash teats with this product diluted at 1 oz (30 mL) per 2 gal (8 L) of lukewarm water. Then, dry each cow's udder and teats with individual clean towels.

Precaution(s): Keep container tightly closed when not in use.

Storage and Disposal: Store this product in a cool, dry area away from direct sunlight and heat to avoid deterioration. Store in a locked cabinet or room to keep it out of the reach of children. Dispose of according to Federal, State, and local laws.

Spillage: In case of small spill (less than one gallon), flood area with a large quantity of water. For large spills, contain and remove with inert absorbent and dispose of according to Federal, State, and local laws.

Keep from freezing.

Caution(s): Do not use this product for cleaning and/or sanitizing equipment.

Important: Teat Irritation or Chapping: Teat dips have the potential to cause irritation of a cow's teats or milker's hands. Individual tolerance to a particular formulation as well as other factors (dry or cold weather, improper teat dip application, bedding quality, milking equipment, etc.) may also affect teat condition. If you observe abnormal irritation or chapping, discontinue use and call the technical service department at 1-800-225-3832, or contact your dealer.

Warning(s): Keep out of the reach of children.
Harmful if swallowed. Harmful if inhaled. Causes eye irritation.
Medical personnel familiar with this product are available 24 hours a day, 7 days a week.
For emergencies call 1-800-424-9300.
Protect eyes from contact with this product. Use with adequate ventilation. Wash thoroughly after handling product.
First Aid:
External: In case of contact, immediately flush contaminated skin with plenty of water. If irritation occurs and persists, call a physician.
Internal: If conscious, dilute by giving several glasses of water or milk. Do not induce vomiting. If vomiting does occur, repeat giving several glasses of water or milk. Get prompt medical attention. Never give anything by mouth to an unconscious person.
Eyes: Immediately flush with plenty of clean, running water for at least 15 minutes, holding eyelids apart to ensure flushing of the entire eye surface. If irritation persists, call a physician.
Presentation: 275 gallon container.
Manufactured by: A & L Laboratories, Inc., A Company of DEC International, Inc., P.O. Box 8050, Madison, WI 53708.
Compendium Code No.: 14480190

BOU-MATIC SUPREME

Bou-Matic **Teat Dip & Spray**

Active Ingredient(s): This ready to use formulation contains:
Chlorhexidine gluconate 0.5%
Quaternary ammonium .... 400 ppm
Other ingredients: 5% skin emollient. This product has been pasteurized to assure purity.
Indications: For pre- and post-milking applications as a teat dip, udder wash, or spray.
Note: This formulation is manufactured following the federally regulated Good Manufacturing Practices in a Food and Drug Administration registered facility.
Dosage and Administration: Pre-milking teat dipping or spraying: Teats should be clean and dry before dipping. If needed, wash the teats and dry with a single service towel. Dip teats in undiluted product and allow 30-60 seconds contact time. Wipe the teats dry before applying the milker unit.
Post-milking teat dipping: Immediately after milking, dip teats in undiluted product. Allow to air dry. With freshening cows, begin dipping teats twice daily for about 10 days before calving. When a cow is being dried up, dip or spray teats with undiluted product once a day for 10 days before calving.
Udder Wash: Wash teats with this product at 1 oz to 2 gallons of lukewarm water. Then dry each cow's udder with individual clean towels before each milking.
Presentation: 4x1 gallon case, 5 gallon pail, 15, 30 and 55 gallon drums, and 220 gallon (4x55 gallon).
Compendium Code No.: 14480110

BOU-MATIC SUPER DIP

Bou-Matic **Teat Dip**

Full Strength Teat Dip with Skin Conditioners
Active Ingredient(s):
Chlorhexidine gluconate .... 0.35% (w/w)
With 2.5% ESP™ Skin Conditioning Technology, purified water, and colorants.
Indications: This product is formulated to be used full strength as a pre- and post-milking teat dip.
Directions: Usage Directions:
Pre-Dipping: Teats should be clean and dry before dipping. If needed, wash the teats and dry with a single service towel. Dip teats in undiluted product and allow 30-60 seconds contact time. Wipe the teats dry before applying the milker unit.
Post-Dipping: Dip teats with undiluted SUPER DIP immediately after milking. Allow to air dry. Replace the solution if it becomes visibly dirty. With freshening cows, begin dipping teats twice daily for about 10 days before calving. For dry cows, dip teats with undiluted SUPER DIP once a day for several days following the last milking. During cold weather do not turn cows out until teats are dry to prevent chapping and freezing. If necessary, wipe dry with a single paper towel.
Udder Wash: To avoid contamination of milk, wash teats with SUPER DIP at 2 oz (60 mL) per 1-2 gallons (4-8 L) of lukewarm (110°F-115°F, 40°C-45°C) water. The dry each cow's udder and teats with individual clean towels before each milking.
Important—Teat Irritation and/or Chapping: Teat dips have the potential to cause irritation of a cow's teats or milker's hands. Individual tolerance to a particular formulation as well as other factors (dry or cold weather, improper teat dip application, bedding quality, milking equipment, etc.) may also affect skin condition. If you observe abnormal irritation or chapping while using SUPER DIP, discontinue use and call the technical service department at 1-800-225-3832, or contact your Bou-Matic dealer.
Contraindication(s): Do not use for cleaning and/or sanitizing equipment.
Precaution(s):
Storage and Disposal: Store this product in a cool, dry area away from direct sunlight and heat to avoid deterioration. Dispose of only in compliance with federal, state, and local laws.
Spillage: In case of small spill (less than one gallon), flood area with a large quantity of water. For larger spills, contain and remove with inert absorbent and dispose of according to federal, state, and local laws.
Keep from freezing.
Caution(s): Keep out of the reach of children.
Harmful if swallowed. Causes eye irritation.
Warning(s): Protect eyes from contact with product. Keep container tightly closed when not in use. Wash thoroughly after handling product.
First Aid:
External: In case of contact, immediately flush contaminated skin with plenty of water. If irritation occurs and persists, call a physician.
Internal: If swallowed, dilute by giving several glasses of water or milk. Do not induce vomiting. If vomiting does occur, repeat giving several glasses of water or milk. Get prompt medical attention. Never give anything by mouth to an unconscious person.
Eyes: Immediately flush with plenty of clean, running water for at least 15 minutes, holding eyelids apart to ensure flushing of the entire eye surface. If irritation persists, call a physician.
For additional precautions consult Material Safety Data Sheet.
Medical personnel familiar with this product are available 24 hours a day, 7 days a week.
Toll-Free Emergency Number: 1/800-424-9300
Presentation: 4x1 gallon case, 5 gallon pail, 15, 30, 55 and 220 gallon drums.
Compendium Code No.: 14480120

BOU-MATIC UDDERDINE-5

Bou-Matic **Teat Dip & Spray**

Teat Dip-Teat Spray-Udder Wash
Active Ingredient(s): Nonylphenoxypolyethoxy (12 moles EO) ethanol-iodine complex providing 0.5% titratable iodine (5000 ppm).
Contains 4.5% skin conditioners.
Indications: 0.5% iodine pre- and post-milking teat dip or spray or udder wash.
Directions: Usage Directions:
Pre-Dipping/Spraying: Teats should be clean and dry before dipping. If needed, wash and dry with a single service towel. Dip/spray with undiluted product and allow 20-40 seconds contact time. Wipe the teats dry before applying the milking unit.
Post-Dipping/Spraying: Dip/spray teats with undiluted product immediately after milking. Allow to air dry. With freshening cows, begin dipping teats twice daily for about 10 days before calving. For dry cows, dip/spray teats once a day for several days following last milking. During cold weather, do not turn out cows until teats are dry to prevent chapping and freezing. If necessary, wipe dry with a single service towel.
Udder Wash: To avoid contamination of milk, wash teats with this product diluted at 1 oz (30 mL) per 1 gal (4 L) of lukewarm water. Then dry each cow's udder and teats with individual clean towels before each milking.
Precaution(s): Keep container tightly closed when not in use.
Storage and Disposal: Store this product in a cool, dry area away from direct sunlight and heat to avoid deterioration. Store in a locked cabinet or room to keep it out of the reach of children. Dispose of according to Federal, State, and local laws.
Spillage: In case of small spill (less than one gallon), flood area with a large quantity of water. For larger spills, contain and remove with inert absorbent and dispose of according to Federal, State, and local laws.
Keep from freezing.
Caution(s): Do not use this product for cleaning and/or sanitizing equipment.
Important: Teat Irritation or Chapping: Teat dips have the potential to cause irritation of a cow's teats or milker's hands. Individual tolerance to a particular formulation as well as other factors (dry or cold weather, improper teat dip application, bedding quality, milking equipment, etc.) may also affect teat condition. If you observe abnormal irritation or chapping, discontinue use and call the technical service department at 1-800-225-3832, or contact your dealer.
Warning(s): Keep out of the reach of children.
Harmful if swallowed. Harmful if inhaled. Causes eye irritation.
Medical personnel familiar with this product are available 24 hours a day, 7 days a week.
For emergencies call 1-800-424-9300.
Protect eyes from contact with this product. Use with adequate ventilation. Wash thoroughly after handling product.
First Aid:
External: In case of contact, immediately flush contaminated skin with plenty of water. If irritation occurs and persists, call a physician.
Internal: If conscious, dilute by giving several glasses of water or milk. Do not induce vomiting. If vomiting does occur, repeat giving several glasses of water or milk. Get prompt medical attention. Never give anything by mouth to an unconscious person.
Eyes: Immediately flush with plenty of clean, running water for at least 15 minutes, holding eyelids apart to ensure flushing of the entire eye surface. If irritation persists, call a physician.
Presentation: 2.5 gallon, 5 gallon, 15 gallon, 55 gallon, and 275 gallon containers.
Manufactured by: A & L Laboratories, Inc., A Company of DEC International, Inc., P.O. Box 8050 Madison, WI 53708.
Compendium Code No.: 14480151

BOU-MATIC UDDERDINE-10

Bou-Matic **Teat Dip & Spray**

Teat Dip-Teat Spray-Udder Wash
Active Ingredient(s): Nonylphenoxypolyethoxy (12 moles EO) ethanol-iodine complex providing 1.0% titratable iodine (10,000 ppm).
Contains 8% skin conditioners.
Indications: 1% iodine post-milking teat dip or spray or udder wash.
Directions: Usage Directions:
Post-Dipping/Spraying: Dip/spray teats with undiluted product immediately after milking. Allow to air dry. Replace the solution if it becomes visibly dirty. With freshening cows, begin dipping teats twice daily for about 10 days before calving. For dry cows, dip/spray teats once a day for several days following the last milking. During cold weather, do not turn out cows until teats are dry to prevent chapping and freezing. If necessary, wipe dry with a single service towel.
Udder Wash: To avoid contamination of milk, wash teats with this product diluted at 1 oz (30 mL) per 2 gal (8 L) of lukewarm water. Then, dry each cow's udder and teats with individual clean towels.
Precaution(s): Keep container tightly closed when not in use.
Storage and Disposal: Store this product in a cool, dry area away from direct sunlight and heat to avoid deterioration. Store in a locked cabinet or room to keep it out of the reach of children. Dispose of according to Federal, State, and local laws.
Spillage: In case of small spill (less than one gallon), flood area with a large quantity of water. For larger spills, contain and remove with inert absorbent and dispose of according to Federal, State and local laws.
Keep from freezing.
Caution(s): Do not use this product for cleaning and/or sanitizing equipment.
Important: Teat Irritation or Chapping: Teat dips have the potential to cause irritation of a cow's teats or milker's hands. Individual tolerance to a particular formulation as well as other factors (dry or cold weather, improper teat dip application, bedding quality, milking equipment, etc.) may also affect teat condition. If you observe abnormal irritation or chapping, discontinue use and call the technical service department at 1-800-225-3832, or contact your dealer.
Warning(s): Keep out of the reach of children.
Harmful if swallowed. Harmful if inhaled. Causes eye irritation.
Medical personnel familiar with this product are available 24 hours a day, 7 days a week.
For emergencies call 1-800-424-9300.
Protect eyes from contact with this product. Use with adequate ventilation. Wash thoroughly after handling product.
First Aid:
External: In case of contact, immediately flush contaminated skin with plenty of water. If irritation occurs and persists, call a physician.
Internal: If conscious, dilute by giving several glasses of water or milk. Do not induce vomiting.

If vomiting does occur, repeat giving several glasses of water or milk. Get prompt medical attention. Never give anything by mouth to an unconscious person.

Eyes: Immediately flush with plenty of clean, running water for at least 15 minutes, holding eyelids apart to ensure flushing of the entire eye surface. If irritation persists, call a physician.

Presentation: 2.5 gallon, 5 gallon, 15 gallon, 55 gallon and 275 gallon containers.

Manufactured by: A & L Laboratories, Inc., A Company of DEC International, Inc., P.O. Box 8050, Madison, WI 53708.

Compendium Code No.: 14480200

BOU-MATIC UDDERDINE-12

Bou-Matic **Teat Dip & Spray**

Active Ingredient(s): Nonylphenoxy polyethoxy (12 moles E.O.) ethanol-iodine complex providing 1.0% w/w titratable iodine (10,000 ppm. w/w). Contains 2.5% skin conditioners.

Indications: 1% iodine pre- and post-milking teat dip or spray and udder wash.

Dosage and Administration:

Pre-Dipping/Spraying: First clean teats properly and examine each quarter with a strip cup. Then dip or spray each teat in undiluted UDDERDINE-12. Ensure that product stays on teats for 20 to 40 seconds, then dry with individual clean towel to reduce the risk of residual iodine on the teat.

Post-Dipping/Spraying: Dip/spray teats with undiluted UDDERDINE-12 immediately after milking. Allow to air dry. Replace the solution if it becomes visibly dirty. With freshening cows, begin dipping teats twice daily for about 10 days before calving. For dry cows, dip/spray teats with undiluted UDDERDINE-12 once a day for several days following the last milking. During the cold weather do not turn cows out until teats are dry to prevent chapping and freezing. If necessary, wipe dry with a single paper towel.

Udder Washing: If necessary, wash cow teats prior to milking. Use a dilution ratio of 1 oz (30 mL) of undiluted UDDERDINE-12 per two gallons (8 L) of lukewarm water (110°F-115°F, 40°C-45°C). After udder washing, dry each teat with individual clean towels.

Teat Irritation and/or Chapping: Teat dips have the potential to cause irritation of a cow's teats or milker's hands. Individual tolerance to a particular formulation as well as other factors (dry or cold weather, improper teat dip application, bedding quality, milking equipment, etc.) may also affect skin condition. If you observe abnormal irritation or chapping while using UDDERDINE-12, discontinue use and call the technical service department at 1-800-225-3832, or contact your Bou-Matic dealer.

Contraindication(s): Do not use for cleaning and/or sanitizing equipment.

Precaution(s):

Storage and Disposal: Store this product in a cool, dry area away from direct sunlight and heat to avoid deterioration. Dispose of only in compliance with federal, state, and local laws.

Spillage: In case of small spill (less than one gallon), flood area with a large quantity of water. For larger spills, contain and remove with inert absorbent and dispose of according to federal, state, and local laws.

Keep from freezing.

Caution(s): Keep out of the reach of children.

Harmful if swallowed. Harmful if inhaled. Causes eye irritation.

Warning(s): Protect eyes, skin and clothing from contact with product. When handling, wear chemical goggles, rubber boots, rubber apron and rubber gloves. Keep container tightly closed when not in use. Use with adequate ventilation. Wash thoroughly after handling product.

First Aid:

External: In case of contact, flush contaminated skin with plenty of water for at least 15 minutes. Remove contaminated clothing and shoes while flushing with water. If irritation occurs and persists, call a physician.

Internal: If swallowed, dilute by giving several glasses of water or milk. Do not induce vomiting. If vomiting does occur, repeat giving several glasses of water or milk. Get prompt medical attention. Never give anything by mouth to an unconscious person.

Eyes: Immediately flush with plenty of clean, running water for at least 15 minutes, holding eyelids apart to ensure flushing of the entire eye surface. If irritation persists, call a physician.

For additional precautions consult Material Safety Data Sheet.

Medical personnel familiar with this product are available 24 hours a day, 7 days a week at the toll-free emergency number.

Presentation: 15, 30 and 55 gallon drums, and 220 gallon (4x55 gallon).

Compendium Code No.: 14480140

BOU-MATIC UDDERDINE-502

Bou-Matic **Teat Dip & Spray**

Active Ingredient(s): Nonylphenoxy polyethoxy (12 moles E.O.) ethanol-iodine complex providing 0.5% w/w titratable iodine (5,000 ppm. w/w). Contains 2.5% skin conditioners.

Indications: 0.5% iodine pre- and post-milking teat dip or spray and udder wash.

Dosage and Administration:

Pre-Dipping/Spraying: First clean teats properly and examine each quarter with a strip cup. Then dip or spray each teat in undiluted UDDERDINE-502. Ensure that product stays on teats for 20 to 40 seconds, then dry with individual clean towel.

Post-Dipping/Spraying: Dip/spray teats with undiluted UDDERDINE-502 immediately after milking. Allow to air dry. Replace the solution if it becomes visibly dirty. With freshening cows, begin dipping teats twice daily for about 10 days before calving. For dry cows, dip/spray teats with undiluted UDDERDINE-502 once a day for several days following the last milking. During the cold weather do not turn cows out until teats are dry to prevent chapping and freezing. If necessary, wipe dry with a single paper towel.

Udder Washing: If necessary, wash cow teats prior to milking. Use a dilution ratio of 1 oz (30 mL) of undiluted UDDERDINE-502 per 1 gallon (4 L) of lukewarm water (110°F-115°F, 40°C-45°C). After udder washing, dry each teat with individual clean towels.

Teat Irritation and/or Chapping: Teat dips have the potential to cause irritation of a cow's teats or milker's hands. Individual tolerance to a particular formulation as well as other factors (dry or cold weather, improper teat dip application, bedding quality, milking equipment, etc.) may also affect skin condition. If you observe abnormal irritation or chapping while using UDDERDINE-502, discontinue use and call the technical service department at 1-800-225-3832, or contact your Bou-Matic dealer.

Contraindication(s): Do not use for cleaning and/or sanitizing equipment.

Precaution(s):

Storage and Disposal: Store this product in a cool, dry area away from direct sunlight and heat to avoid deterioration. Dispose of only in compliance with federal, state, and local laws.

Spillage: In case of small spill (less than one gallon), flood area with a large quantity of water. For larger spills, contain and remove with inert absorbent and dispose of according to federal, state, and local laws.

Keep from freezing.

Caution(s): Keep out of the reach of children.

Harmful if swallowed. Harmful if inhaled. Causes eye irritation.

Warning(s): For additional precautions consult Material Safety Data Sheet.

Medical personnel familiar with this product are available 24 hours a day, 7 days a week at the toll-free emergency number.

Protect eyes, skin and clothing from contact with product. When handling, wear chemical goggles, rubber boots, rubber apron and rubber gloves. Keep container tightly closed when not in use. Use with adequate ventilation. Wash thoroughly after handling product.

First Aid:

External: In case of contact, flush contaminated skin with plenty of water for at least 15 minutes. Remove contaminated clothing and shoes while flushing with water. If irritation occurs and persists, call a physician.

Internal: If swallowed, dilute by giving several glasses of water or milk. Do not induce vomiting. If vomiting does occur, repeat giving several glasses of water or milk. Get prompt medical attention. Never give anything by mouth to an unconscious person.

Eyes: Immediately flush with plenty of clean, running water for at least 15 minutes, holding eyelids apart to ensure flushing of the entire eye surface. If irritation persists, call a physician.

Presentation: 5 gallon pail, 15 gallon drum, and 220 gallon (4x55 gallon).

Compendium Code No.: 14480160

BOVA DERM®

Butler **Udder Cream**

Active Ingredient(s): Contains: Vitamins A, D_3, E, B_2 (riboflavin), B_5 (panthenol), B_6 (pyridoxine), H (d-biotin) and B_3 (Niacinamide) in a specially compounded base stabilized at the pH of normal animal skin.

Indications: BOVA DERM® with multi-vitamins is for use as an aid in reducing dry, cracked and chapped udders in cattle. It contains humectants which assist in maintaining skin and tissue in a natural moisture balance.

The nonsticky, disappearing cream base discourages dirt and manure from sticking to udders.

Dosage and Administration: Apply once a day or as needed after milking to aid in reducing dryness, cracking and chapping associated with chapped udders in cattle.

Precaution(s): BOVA DERM® is not a substitute for balanced nutrition. Animals with signs of nutritional deficiency in the skin may require injections of therapeutic levels of vitamins. Consult a veterinarian for assistance in the diagnosis and treatment of nutritional deficiency.

Caution(s): If an animal shows signs of uncontrolled generalized infections, consult a veterinarian. Wash the teats and udder thoroughly before milking.

For veterinary use only. Keep out of the reach of children.

Presentation: 16 oz. (454 g) containers.

Compendium Code No.: 10820260

BOVAMUNE™

AgriLabs **Antiserum**

Corynebacterium pyogenes-Escherichia coli-Pasteurella haemolytica-multocida-Salmonella typhimurium Antiserum, Bovine Origin

U.S. Vet. Lic. No.: 303

Active Ingredient(s): The antiserum is prepared from the blood of cattle hyperimmunized with *Corynebacterium pyogenes, Escherichia coli, Pasteurella haemolytica, Pasteurella multocida* and *Salmonella typhimurium.*

Indications: For use as an aid in the prevention and treatment of enteric and respiratory conditions in calves, cattle and sheep when caused by *Corynebacterium pyogenes, Escherichia coli, Pasteurella haemolytica, Pasteurella multocida* and *Salmonella typhimurium.*

Dosage and Administration: Shake well before using. Administer the following doses subcutaneously or intramuscularly.

	Prevention	Treatment
Calves (as soon after birth as possible)	20-40 mL	40-100 mL
Cattle	50-75 mL	75-150 mL
Sheep	10-15 mL	20-40 mL

The recommended dose for treatment is to be administered at 12-24 hour intervals until improvement is noted.

Precaution(s): Store in the dark at 35°-45°F (2°-7°C). Do not freeze.

Caution(s): Use the entire contents when first opened. Anaphylactic reactions may occur following the use of this biological. Symptomatic treatment: Epinephrine.

Warning(s): Do not administer within 21 days prior to slaughter.

Presentation: 250 mL vials.

Compendium Code No.: 10580210

BOVATEC® 68

Alpharma **Feed Additive**

Lasalocid Sodium-Type A Medicated Article (medicated premix)

NADA No.: 096-298

Active Ingredient(s): Each pound contains 68 grams (15%) of lasalocid (as lasalocid sodium activity) in a carrier suitable for incorporation in feed.

Indications:

Cattle: For improved feed efficiency and increased rate of weight gain and for control of coccidiosis caused by *Eimeria bovis* and *E. zuernii* in feedlot cattle being fed in confinement for slaughter.

For increased rate of weight gain and for control of coccidiosis caused by *Eimeria bovis* and *E. zuernii* in pasture cattle (slaughter, stocker, feeder cattle, and dairy and beef replacement heifers).

Sheep: For prevention of coccidiosis caused by *Eimeria ovina, E. crandallis, E. ovinoidalis (E. ninakohlyakimovae), E. parva* and *E. intricata* in sheep maintained in confinement.

Rabbits: For the prevention of coccidiosis caused by *Eimeria stiedae.*

Directions:

Important: Must be thoroughly mixed in feeds before use. BOVATEC® premix should be further diluted before mixing in complete feed.

Mixing directions: The product should be further diluted in an intermediate blending step prior to mixing in final feed. Do not feed undiluted.

A. Feedlot cattle being fed in confinement for slaughter - For improved feed efficiency and increased rate of weight gain and for control of coccidiosis caused by *Eimeria bovis* and *E. zuernii.*

Sheep - For prevention of coccidiosis caused by *Eimeria ovina, E. crandallis, E. ovinoidalis (E. ninakohlyakimovae), E. parva* and *E. intricata* in sheep maintained in confinement.

Feeding directions:

For improved feed efficiency in cattle: Feed continuously at the rate of not less than 10 grams nor more than 30 grams of lasalocid per ton of total ration (90% dry matter) to provide not less than 100 mg nor more than 360 mg per head per day.

For improved feed efficiency and increased rate of weight gain in cattle: Feed continuously at the rate of not less than 25 grams nor more than 30 grams of lasalocid per ton of total ration (90% dry matter) to provide not less than 250 mg nor more than 360 mg per head per day.

For control of coccidiosis in cattle: Feed continuously at the rate of 30 grams of lasalocid per ton of total ration (90% dry matter) to provide an intake of 1 mg of lasalocid per 2.2 pounds of body weight per day in cattle up to 800 pounds (maximum 360 mg per day).

For prevention of coccidiosis in sheep: Feed continuously at the rate of not less than 20 grams nor more than 30 grams of lasalocid per ton of total ration (90% dry matter) to provide not less than 15 mg nor more than 70 mg per head per day depending on body weight.

1. Complete feeds for feedlot cattle and sheep in confinement:

a. Intermediate blending: Mix 1 part of BOVATEC® 68 premix (Type A Medicated Article) with 12.5 parts of finely ground non-medicated feedstuffs to provide an intermediate premix containing 5 grams of lasalocid per pound.

b. Using this intermediate premix, the following table would apply to the manufacture of complete feeds:

Intended lasalocid concentration in the complete feed:		Add the following amounts of 5 grams per pound intermediate premix per ton of complete feed mixed:
grams/ton	mg/lb	pounds/ton
10	5	2
20	10	4
25	12.5	5
30*	15	6

*Maximum approved concentration in complete feeds.

2. Supplements for feedlot cattle and sheep in confinement:

a. Dry supplements:

(1) Intermediate Blending: Mix 1 part of BOVATEC® 68 premix (Type A Medicated Article) with 2.4 parts of finely ground non-medicated feedstuffs to provide an intermediate premix containing 20 grams of lasalocid per pound. For example, mix one 50 lb bag of BOVATEC® 68 premix with 120 lbs of non-medicated feedstuffs.

(2) Using this intermediate premix, the following table would apply to the manufacture of feedlot supplements:

Feedlot supplements		
Intended lasalocid concentration in the supplement:		Add the following amounts of 20 grams per pound intermediate premix per ton of supplement mixed:
grams/ton	mg/lb	pounds/ton
100	50	5
200	100	10
300	150	15
360	180	18
400	200	20
500	250	25
600	300	30
720	360	36
800	400	40
1200	600	60
1440	720	72

(3) Thoroughly mix supplement with grain and roughage to provide 10 to 30 grams per ton for cattle and 20 to 30 grams per ton for sheep in the complete feed.

b. Liquid supplements intended for addition to dry feeds:

(1) Supplements with suspending agent(s) should be in a pH range of 4-8 and maintain positional stability for up to three months with a viscosity of not less than 300 cps.

(2) Conventional liquid supplements should be in a pH range of 4-8. Ten minute recirculation required daily and prior to use.

B. Pasture cattle (slaughter, stocker, feeder cattle, and dairy and beef replacement heifers) - For increased rate of weight gain and for control of coccidiosis caused by *Eimeria bovis* and *E. zuernii.*

Feeding directions:

For increased rate of weight gain: Feed at the rate of not less than 60 mg nor more than 200 mg per head per day.

For control of coccidiosis: Hand feed continuously at the rate of 1 mg of lasalocid per 2.2 pounds of body weight per day in cattle up to 800 pounds (maximum 360 mg per day).

1. Feeds and supplements requiring no further dilution before use:

a. Intermediate blending: Mix 1 part of BOVATEC® 68 premix (Type A Medicated Article) with 12.5 parts of finely ground non-medicated feedstuffs to provide an intermediate premix containing 5 grams of lasalocid per pound.

b. Final blending: See table below:

In feeds or supplements fed at the rate of:	To achieve a lasalocid intake of:	Add the following amounts of 5 grams per pound intermediate premix per ton of feed or supplement mixed:	Lasalocid will be present in the feed or supplement at the following concentrations:
lb/head/day	mg/head/day	pounds per ton	grams/ton
1	60	24	120
	100	40	200
	200	80	400
2	60	12	60
	100	20	100
	200	40	200
3	60	8	40
	100	13.3	66.5
	200	26.7	133.5
4	60	6	30
	100	10	50
	200	20	100

B

2. Supplements requiring further dilution before use: Sufficient non-medicated feedstuffs must be thoroughly mixed with the supplement in accordance with the feeding rates listed in section B.1.b. above.

a. Intermediate blending: Mix 1 part of BOVATEC® 68 premix (Type A medicated article) with 2.4 parts of finely ground non-medicated feedstuffs to provide an intermediate premix containing 20 grams of lasalocid per pound. For example, mix one 50 lb bag of BOVATEC® 68 premix with 120 lbs of non-medicated feedstuffs.

b. Using this intermediate premix, the following table would apply to the manufacture of pasture supplements:

Intended lasalocid concentration in the supplement:	Add the following amounts of 20 grams per pound intermediate premix per ton of supplement mixed:
grams/ton	pounds/ton
400	20
600	30
800	40
1000	50
1200	60
1440	72

3. Free choice (self-fed) supplements: Free choice supplements must be formulated to provide not less than 60 mg nor more than 200 mg of lasalocid per head per day. (Manufacture of Type C free-choice feeds from this product requires a Medicated Feed License Application approved by FDA.)

Note: Coccidiosis may occur when young pasture cattle are co-mingled with adult cattle passing coccidial occysts.

C. Rabbits - For the prevention of coccidiosis caused by *Eimeria stiedae.*

Type A Medicated Article to be mixed with feed to produce a Type C medicated feed. The Type C is formulated to provide 113 g lasalocid/ton to be fed as the sole ration for up to 6 and ½ weeks of age.

Caution(s): Do not allow horses or other equines access to premixes or supplements containing lasalocid, as ingestion may be fatal. The safety of lasalocid in unapproved species has not been established. Feeding undiluted or mixing errors resulting in excessive concentration of lasalocid could be fatal to cattle and sheep.

Warning(s): A withdrawal period has not been established for the product in pre-ruminating calves. Do not use in calves to be processed for veal.

When mixing and handling lasalocid premix, use protective clothing, impervious gloves and a dust mask. Avoid contact with eyes. Operators should wash thoroughly with soap and water after handling.

Presentation: 50 lb (22.68 kg) bag.

Compendium Code No.: 10220222 710310 0104

BOVATEC® 150 FP

Alpharma **Feed Additive**

Brand of Lasalocid-Type A Medicated Article (medicated premix)

NADA No.: 096-298

Active Ingredient(s): Each pound contains 150 grams (33.1%) of lasalocid (as lasalocid sodium activity) in a carrier suitable for incorporation in feed.

Indications:

Feedlot cattle being fed in confinement for slaughter: For improved feed efficiency and increased rate of weight gain and for control of coccidiosis caused by *Eimeria bovis* and *E. zuernii.*

Pasture cattle (slaughter, stocker, feeder cattle, and dairy and beef replacement heifers): For increased rate of weight gain and for control of coccidiosis caused by *Eimeria bovis* and *E. zuernii.*

Sheep: For prevention of coccidiosis caused by *Eimeria ovina, E. crandallis, E. ovinoidalis (E. ninakohlyakimovae), E. parva* and *E. intricata* in sheep maintained in confinement.

Dosage and Administration: Important: Must be thoroughly mixed in feeds before use.

Mixing Directions: This product should be further diluted in an intermediate blending step prior to mixing in final feed. Do not feed undiluted.

A. Feeding Directions for Feedlot Cattle Fed in Confinement for Slaughter, and Sheep:

For improved feed efficiency in cattle: Feed continuously at the rate of not less than 10 grams nor more than 30 grams of lasalocid per ton of total ration (90% dry matter) to provide not less than 100 mg nor more than 360 mg per head per day.

For improved feed efficiency and increased rate of weight gain in cattle: Feed continuously at the rate of not less than 25 grams nor more than 30 grams of lasalocid per ton of total ration (90% dry matter) to provide not less than 250 mg nor more than 360 mg per head per day.

For control of coccidiosis in cattle: Feed continuously at the rate of 30 grams of lasalocid per ton of total ration (90% dry matter) to provide an intake of 1 mg of lasalocid per 2.2 pounds of body weight per day in cattle up to 800 pounds (maximum 360 mg per day).

For prevention of coccidiosis in sheep: Feed continuously at the rate of not less than 20 grams nor more than 30 grams of lasalocid per ton of total ration (90% dry matter) to provide not less than 15 mg nor more than 70 mg per head per day depending on body weight.

1. Complete feeds for feedlot cattle and sheep in confinement:

a. Intermediate Blending: Mix 1 part of BOVATEC® 150 FP Premix (Type A Medicated Article) with 29 parts of finely ground non-medicated feedstuffs to provide an intermediate premix containing 5 grams of lasalocid per pound.

b. Using this intermediate premix, the following table would apply to the manufacture of complete feeds:

Intended lasalocid concentration in the complete feed:		Add the following amounts of 5 g/lb intermediate premix per ton of complete feed mixed:
grams/ton	mg/lb	pounds/ton
10	5.0	2
20	10.0	4
25	12.5	5
30*	15.0	6

*Maximum approved concentration in complete feeds.

2. Supplements for feedlot cattle and sheep in confinement:
   a. Dry Supplements:
   (1) Intermediate Blending: Mix 1 part of BOVATEC® 150 FP Premix (Type A Medicated Article) with 6.5 parts of finely ground non-medicated feedstuffs to provide an intermediate premix containing 20 grams of lasalocid per pound.
   (2) Using this intermediate premix, the following table would apply to the manufacture of feedlot supplements:

Feedlot Supplements		
Intended lasalocid concentration in the supplement:		Add the following amounts of 20 g/lb intermediate premix per ton of supplement mixed:
grams/ton	mg/lb	pounds/ton
100	50	5
200	100	10
300	150	15
360	180	18
400	200	20
500	250	25
600	300	30
720	360	35
800	400	40
1200	600	60
1440	720	72

   (3) Thoroughly mix supplement with grain and roughage to provide 10 to 30 grams per ton for cattle and 20 to 30 grams per ton for sheep in the complete feed.
   b. Liquid Supplements Intended for Addition to Dry Feeds:
   (1) Supplements with suspending agent(s) should be in a pH range of 4-8 and maintain positional stability for up to three months with a viscosity not less than 300 cps.
   (2) Conventional liquid supplements should be in a pH range of 4-8. Ten minute recirculation required daily and prior to use.

B. Feeding Directions for Pasture Cattle (Slaughter, Stocker, Feeder Cattle, and Dairy and Beef Replacement Heifers):

For increased rate of weight gain: Feed at the rate of not less than 60 mg nor more than 200 mg per head per day.

For control of coccidiosis: Hand feed continuously at the rate of 1 mg of lasalocid per 2.2 pounds of body weight per day in cattle up to 800 pounds (maximum 360 mg per day).

1. Feeds and supplements requiring no further dilution before use:
   a. Intermediate Blending: Mix 1 part of BOVATEC® 150 FP Premix (Type A Medicated Article) with 29 parts of finely ground non-medicated feedstuffs to provide an intermediate premix containing 5 grams of lasalocid per pound.
   b. Final Blending: See table below:

In feeds or supplements fed at the rate of:	To achieve a lasalocid intake of:	Add the following amounts of 5 grams per pound intermediate premix per ton of feed or supplement mixed:	Lasalocid will be present in the feed or supplement at the following concentrations:
lb/head/day	mg/head/day	pounds per ton	grams/ton
1	60	24	120
	100	40	200
	200	80	400
2	60	12	60
	100	20	100
	200	40	200
3	60	8	40
	100	13.3	66.5
	200	26.7	133.5
4	60	6	30
	100	10	50
	200	20	100

2. Supplements requiring further dilution before use: Sufficient non-medicated feedstuffs must be thoroughly mixed with the supplement in accordance with the feeding rates listed in Section B.1.b. above.
   a. Intermediate Blending: Mix 1 part of BOVATEC® 150 FP premix (Type A Medicated Article) with 6.5 parts of finely ground non-medicated feedstuffs to provide an intermediate premix containing 20 grams of lasalocid per pound. For example, mix one 50 lb bag of BOVATEC® 150 FP Premix with 325 lbs of non-medicated feedstuffs.
   b. Using this intermediate premix, the following table would apply to the manufacture of pasture supplements:

Intended lasalocid concentration in the supplement:	Add the following amounts of 20 g/lb intermediate premix per ton of supplement mixed:
grams/ton	pounds per ton
400	20
600	30
800	40
1000	50
1200	60
1440	72

3. Free choice (self-fed) supplements: Free choice supplements must be formulated to provide not less than 60 mg nor more than 200 mg of lasalocid per head per day. (Manufacture of Type C free-choice feeds from this product requires a Medicated Feed License Application approved by FDA.)

Note: Coccidiosis may occur when young pasture cattle are co-mingled with adult cattle passing coccidial occysts.

Caution(s): Do not allow horses or other equines access to premixes or supplements containing lasalocid, as ingestion may be fatal.

The safety of lasalocid in unapproved species has not been established.

Feeding undiluted or mixing errors resulting in excessive concentrations of lasalocid could be fatal to cattle and sheep.

Warning(s): A withdrawal period has not been established for this product in pre-ruminating calves.

Do not use in calves to be processed for veal.

When mixing and handling lasalocid premix, use protective clothing, impervious gloves and a dust mask. Avoid contact with eyes. Operators should wash thoroughly with soap and water after handling.

Presentation: 50 lb (22.68 kg) bags.

Compendium Code No.: 10220202 710316 0105

BOVATEC® LIQUID 20

Alpharma **Feed Medication**

Brand of lasalocid-Type A Medicated Article (medicated premix)

NADA No.: 096-298

Active Ingredient(s): Each pound contains 90.7 grams (20%) of lasalocid (as lasalocid sodium activity) in a carrier suitable for incorporation in liquid feed supplements.

Indications:

Cattle: For improved feed efficiency and increased rate of weight gain when used in medicated feeds for cattle fed in confinement for slaughter. For increased rate of weight gain when used in medicated feeds for pasture cattle (slaughter, stocker, feeder cattle, and dairy and beef replacement heifers).

For control of coccidiosis caused by *Eimeria bovis* and *E. zuernii* in cattle up to 800 lbs.

Sheep: For prevention of coccidiosis caused by *Eimeria ovina, E. crandallis, E. ovinoidalis (E. ninakohlyakimovae), E. parva* and *E. intricata* in sheep maintained in confinement.

Directions for Use: Important: Must be thoroughly mixed in feeds before use.

Do not feed undiluted.

Use Directions:

A. Feedlot Cattle Being Fed in Confinement for Slaughter - For improved feed efficiency and increased rate of weight gain and for control of coccidiosis caused by *Eimeria bovis* and *E. zuernii.*

Sheep - For prevention of coccidiosis caused by *Eimeria ovina, E. crandallis, E. ovinoidalis (E. ninakohlyakimovae), E. parva* and *E. intricata* in sheep maintained in confinement.

Feeding Directions:

For Improved Feed Efficiency in Cattle: Feed continuously at the rate of not less than 10 grams nor more than 30 grams of lasalocid per ton of total ration (90% dry matter) to provide not less than 100 mg nor more than 360 mg per head per day.

For Improved Feed Efficiency and Increased Rate of Weight Gain in Cattle: Feed continuously at the rate of not less than 25 grams nor more than 30 grams of lasalocid per ton of total ration (90% dry matter) to provide not less than 250 mg nor more than 360 mg per head per day.

For Control of Coccidiosis in Cattle: Feed continuously at the rate of 30 grams of lasalocid per ton of total ration (90% dry matter) to provide an intake of 1 mg of lasalocid per 2.2 pounds of body weight per day in cattle up to 800 pounds (maximum 360 mg per day).

For Prevention of Coccidiosis in Sheep: Feed continuously at the rate of not less than 20 grams nor more than 30 grams of lasalocid per ton of total ration (90% dry matter) to provide not less than 15 mg nor more than 70 mg per head per day depending on body weight.

B. Pasture Cattle (Slaughter, Stocker, Feeder Cattle, and Dairy and Beef Replacement Heifers) - For increased rate of weight gain and for control of coccidiosis caused by *Eimeria bovis* and *E. zuernii.*

Feeding Directions:

For Increased Rate of Weight Gain: Feed at the rate of not less than 60 mg nor more than 200 mg per head per day. Hand-fed: The drug must be contained in at least one pound of feed. Self-fed: Free-choice feed must be manufactured under a feed mill license utilizing an FDA approved formulation.

For Control of Coccidiosis: Hand feed continuously at the rate of 1 mg of lasalocid per 2.2 pounds of body weight per day in cattle up to 800 pounds (maximum 360 mg per day).

Mixing Directions - for incorporation into liquid feed supplements:

(1) Agitate BOVATEC® Liquid 20 before use.
(2) Supplements with suspending agent(s) should be in a pH range of 4-8 and maintain positional stability for up to three months with a viscosity not less than 300 cps.
(3) Conventional liquid supplements should be in a pH range of 4-8. Ten minute recirculation required daily and prior to use.

The following is provided as a guide in determining the quantity of BOVATEC® Liquid 20 (Type A Medicated Article) to be added in preparing liquid feed supplements (LFS). Preparation of intermediate liquid premix is not recommended.

LFS To Be Fed Undiluted: As a Type C Medicated Feed - Hand-Fed or Top Dressed:

Amount of LFS to be fed	To achieve a lasalocid intake of	BOVATEC® Liquid 20 per Ton LFS	
(Lb./Head/Day)	(Mg/Head/Day)	Pounds	Fluid Ounce*
0.5	15	0.67	9.8
0.5	60	2.65	39.2
0.5	70	3.09	45.7
0.5	100	4.41	65.3
0.5	200	8.83	130.6
0.5	360	15.88	235.0
1.0	15	.34	4.9
1.0	60	1.33	19.6
1.0	70	1.55	22.9
1.0	100	2.21	32.7
1.0	200	4.41	65.3
1.0	360	7.94	117.5

LFS To Be Diluted: As a Type B Medicated Feed - Mixed into a Feed:

Amount of LFS to be added to final feed	Lasalocid in final feed	BOVATEC® Liquid 20 per Ton LFS	
(Lb./Ton)	(Gram/Ton)	Pounds	Fluid Ounce*
100	10	2.21	32.7
100	20	4.42	65.3
100	25	5.52	81.6
100	30	6.62	97.9
150	10	1.48	21.8
150	20	2.96	43.6
150	25	3.68	54.4
150	30	4.42	65.3
200	10	1.11	16.4
200	20	2.21	32.7
200	25	2.76	40.8
200	30	3.31	49.0

* 6.13 gm lasalocid per fluid ounce (BOVATEC® Liquid 20 specific gravity is 1.035)

Note: Coccidiosis may occur when young pasture cattle are co-mingled with adult cattle passing coccidial oocysts.

Caution(s): Do not allow horses or other equines access to premixes or supplements containing lasalocid, as ingestion may be fatal. The safety of lasalocid in unapproved species has not been established. Feeding undiluted or mixing errors resulting in excessive concentrations of lasalocid could be fatal to cattle and sheep.

Warning(s): A withdrawal period has not been established for this product in pre-ruminating calves. Do not use in calves to be processed for veal.

When mixing and handling lasalocid liquid premix, use protective clothing and impervious gloves. Avoid contact with eyes. Operators should wash thoroughly with soap and water after handling.

Presentation: 50 lb. (22.68 kg).

Compendium Code No.: 10220212 AHL-295 0009

BOVIGAM™-TB

Biocor **Tuberculosis Test**

Mycobacterium bovis Gamma Interferon Test Kit for Cattle

U.S. Vet. Lic. No.: 462A

Test Description: BOVIGAM™-TB is a rapid *in vitro* blood-based assay of cell mediated response to *M. bovis* PPD tuberculin for the diagnosis of bovine tuberculosis (TB) infection in cattle.

Tuberculin PPD antigens are presented to lymphocytes in whole blood culture. The production of IFN-γ from the cells is then detected using a monoclonal antibody-based sandwich enzyme immunoassay (EIA). Lymphocytes from cattle not infected with *M. bovis* do not produce IFN-γ. Therefore, detection of IFN-γ correlates to *M. bovis* infection.

BOVIGAM™-TB is intended for use post tuberculin skin testing in cattle. The IFN-γ assay is used as a confirmatory test for positive and negative reactors within 3 to 30 days after application of the skin test.

Kit Components: Table 1

1. Microplates coated with antibody to IFN-γ.	10 x 96 wells with lids	30 x 96 wells with lids	Ready for use.
2. Positive bovine IFN-γ control. Contains 0.01% w/v thimerosal.	2 x 1 mL	3 x 2 mL	Freeze dried. Reconstitute with deionised or distilled water.
3. Negative bovine IFN-γ control. Contains 0.01% w/v thimerosal.	2 x 1 mL	3 x 2 mL	Freeze dried. Reconstitute with deionised or distilled water.
4. Green Diluent: Plasma diluent buffer. Contains 0.01% w/v thimerosal.	1 x 60 mL	1 x 175 mL	Ready for use.
5. Wash Buffer — 20X Concentrate. Contains 0.01% w/v thimerosal.	3 x 125 mL	2 x 500 mL	Dilute with deionised or distilled water.
6. Conjugate — 100X Concentrate. (Horseradish peroxidase labeled antibovine IFN-γ.) Contains 0.01% w/v thimerosal.	1 x 1.5 mL	2 x 2 mL	Freeze dried. Reconstitute with deionised or distilled water.
7a. Blue Diluent: Conjugate diluent buffer — 5X Concentrate. Contains 0.05% w/v thimerosal.	1 x 25 mL	N/A	Dilute with deionised or distilled water.
7b. Blue Diluent: Conjugate diluent buffer. Contains 0.01% w/v thimerosal.	N/A	2 x 175 mL	Ready for use.
8. Enzyme substrate buffer solution. Contains H_2O_2.	1 x 125 mL	2 x 175 mL	Ready for use.
9. Chromogen Solution — 100X Concentrate. Contains TMB in DMSO.	1 x 1.5 mL	2 x 2 mL	Dilute in enzyme substrate buffer solution.
10. Enzyme stopping solution. (0.5M H_2SO_4).	1 x 75 mL	1 x 175 mL	Ready for use.
11. Avian PPD	1 x 20 mL	3 x 20 mL	Ready for use.
12. Bovine PPD	1 x 20 mL	3 x 20 mL	Ready for use.

Materials Required But Not Provided

A Blood Collection

1. Lithium heparin Vacutainers: 1 / animal
2. 18G Vacutainer needles — 1 inch: 1 / animal
3. Needle holders: 2-3 / blood collector

B Blood Culture

1. Sterile graduated 5 or 10 mL pipettes: 1 / animal
2. Sterile 24-well tissue culture trays: 1 / 8 animals
3. Tips for "Combitip" dispenser (5 mL): 3 / herd
4. Sterile phosphate buffered saline (0.01M, pH 7.2): 100 μL / animal

C Plasma Harvesting

1. Tips to fit 100-1000 μL pipette: 3 / animal
2. 1 mL microtubes in 96-well format racks and caps for plasma storage: 1 rack / 30 animals

D Bovine IFN-γ EIA

1. Tips to fit 12-channel pipette.: 3 / animal
2. Various polypropylene tubes, EIA reagent troughs, and tips.

Equipment:

- 37°C humidified incubator.
- Accurate, replaceable-tip variable-volume pipettes (to deliver up to 1 mL).
- Graduated 1, 5 and 10 mL pipettes.
- Measuring cylinders - 100 mL, 1 L and 2 L.
- Deionised or distilled water - 6 L.
- 12-channel pipette (to deliver 50 μL and 100 μL).
- Microplate shaker (optional).
- Microplate/strip washer.
- Microplate reader. This reader MUST be fitted with a 450 nm and 620-650 nm filters.

Test Procedure: Preparation of Reagents

1. Antigens: Mix thoroughly before use. Use as supplied (0.3 mg/mL). May be used directly from refrigerator.
2. Plates: Allow plate(s) to equilibrate to room temperature before unsealing plastic pouch. Allow at least 30 minutes.
3. Positive and Negative Controls: Reconstitute appropriate vials with 1 mL (10 Plate) or 2 mL (30 Plate) of deionised or distilled water. Ensure complete resolubilisation. Reconstituted controls may be stored at 35° to 45°F (2° to 7°C) for up to 3 months, but must be brought to room temperature and mixed thoroughly before used again.
4. Green Diluent: Bring to room temperature and mix thoroughly. Use undiluted as plasma diluent buffer.
5. Conjugate: Reconstitute freeze dried Conjugate 100X Concentrate with 1.5 mL (10 Plate) or 2 mL (30 Plate) of deionised or distilled water. Ensure complete resolubilisation. Mixing should be performed with a minimum of frothing. Conjugate 100X Concentrate Must be kept at 35° to 45°F (2° to 7°C) at all times and used within 3 months of reconstitution.
   Note: Excessive frothing of conjugate may cause denaturation and reduce its performance in the EIA.

For The 10 Plate BOVIGAM™-TB Kit Only

Bring Blue Diluent (Conjugate Diluent Buffer) 5X Concentrate to room temperature and mix thoroughly. Prepare working strength Blue Diluent (conjugate diluent buffer) by mixing one part 5X concentrate with 4 parts deionised or distilled water. Working strength Blue Diluent may be stored at 35° to 45°F (2° to 7°C) for up to 3 months but must be brought to room temperature and mixed thoroughly before being used again.

For The 30 Plate BOVIGAM™-TB Kit Only

The Blue Diluent is supplied pre-diluted and ready for use. Prepare working strength Conjugate Reagent combining appropriate volumes of working strength Blue Diluent and reconstituted Conjugate 100X Concentrate as set out in the Reagent Preparation Table shown below. Mix thoroughly but gently. Avoid frothing. The working strength Conjugate Reagent should be used within 5 minutes of preparation and unused reagent immediately discarded. Return any unused Conjugate 100X Concentrate to 35° to 45°F (2° to 7°C) immediately after use.

Reagent Preparation Table for Diluting Conjugate and Chromogen

Table 2

Number of Plates	Volume of Concentrate Conjugate (100X) or Chromogen (100X)	Volume of Diluent Blue Diluent or Enzyme Substrate Buffer
1	0.12 mL	12 mL
2	0.24 mL	24 mL
3	0.36 mL	36 mL
4	0.48 mL	48 mL
5	0.60 mL	60 mL
6	0.72 mL	72 mL
7	0.84 mL	84 mL
8	0.96 mL	96 mL
9	1.08 mL	108 mL
10	1.20 mL	120 mL
20	2.0 mL	200 mL
30	3.0 mL	300 mL

6. Wash Buffer: Prepare working strength wash buffer by adding one part 20X Concentrate with 19 parts deionised or distilled water. Mix thoroughly. Working strength wash buffer may be stored at room temperature for up to 2 weeks. Unused Wash Buffer 20X Concentrate should be returned to 35° to 45°F (2° to 7°C) after use.
   Note: Wash Buffer 20X Concentrate may contain salt crystals. Redissolve crystals by warming to 37°C. Mix thoroughly before dilution.
7. Enzyme Substrate Solution: Bring the Enzyme Substrate Buffer and Chromogen Solution 100X Concentrate to room temperature and ensure each is thoroughly mixed before dilution. Prepare enzyme substrate solution just prior to use by combining appropriate volumes of Chromogen Solution concentrate and Enzyme Substrate Buffer as shown in the Reagent Preparation Table. Enzyme substrate solution must be completely mixed and should be colourless. Discard if blue coloration occurs.
   Use within 10 minutes of preparation.
   Note: If possible use plastic polypropylene disposable containers sterilised by irradiation to prepare the enzyme substrate solution. Do not use polystyrene containers or pipettes. Any glassware used with the enzyme substrate reagents should be rinsed thoroughly with 1N H_2SO_4 or HCl followed by at least three washes of deionised or distilled water, ensuring no acid residue remains on the glassware.
8. Safe Disposal of Reagents: All waste and unused portions of prepared reagents should be disposed of in accordance with State and local requirements.

Procedural Notes

1. All test plasmas and reagents except the Conjugate 100X Concentrate must be brought to

room temperature (22 ± 5°C) before use. Thawed test samples should be mixed thoroughly by carefully vortexing each tube.

Do not warm above 37°C.

Note: Several hours may be required to ensure a full bottle of reagent has reached room temperature. If a shorter equilibration time is desired, an ambient temperature water bath must be used.

2. All kit components are to be stored at 35° to 45°F (2° to 7°C). Return to 35° to 45°F (2° to 7°C) immediately after use. Working strength wash buffer may be stored at room temperature (22 ± 5°C) for up to 2 weeks.
3. The Conjugate 100X Concentrate must be left at 35° to 45°F (2° to 7°C) at all times, even during reconstitution.
4. Complete reconstitution of freeze dried components is essential for valid performance of the assay. To ensure this, reconstitute reagents and allow vials to sit for at least 15 minutes, then mix by gently inverting each vial 4 or 5 times. A roller-rocker apparatus may be used. Mix again just prior to use.

   Note: It is important that high quality deionised or distilled water is used to reconstitute and dilute reagents as horseradish peroxidase is readily inactivated by pollutants common in laboratory water supplies.
5. Once the assay has been started it should be completed without interruption.
6. Use a separate disposable tip for each sample to prevent cross contamination.
7. Test plasmas from individual animals should be added simultaneously to EIA wells using a 12-channel pipette.
8. EIA plates should be incubated elevated on an inverted test-tube rack (or similar) to minimise inter-well variations.
9. Each test plasma should be assayed in duplicate in adjacent wells (e.g. rows A and B) starting at the top of column 1 of the microplate.
10. Positive and negative bovine IFN-γ controls should be assayed in triplicate in serial wells of Columns 4, 5 and 6 (e.g. row F for positive and row E for negative controls).

Following these recommendations allows 45 test plasmas from 15 animals to be assayed in duplicate per EIA microplate.

Stage One — Whole Blood Culture Method

Step:-

1. Blood Collection:

   Blood is collected within 3-30 days from cattle reacting positively to the single intradermal skin test.

   Collect a minimum volume of 5 mL of blood from each animal into a blood collection tube containing heparin as anti-coagulant and gently mix blood by inversion several times to dissolve the heparin. Blood samples should be transported to the laboratory at ambient temperature (22 ± 5°C, avoid extremes) and put into culture within 30 hours of collection. Under no circumstances should blood be stored in refrigerator.
2. Dispensing Blood:

   Blood samples must be evenly mixed before aliquoting. Use a roller-rocker or gently invert tubes about 10 times immediately prior to dispensing.

   Note: It is important to keep cell damage to an absolute minimum as the test requires viable lymphocytes.

   Dispense three 1.5 mL aliquots of heparinised blood from each animal into wells of a 24-well tissue culture tray (see Table 3 below for recommended layout). This should be performed under aseptic conditions using either sterile disposable pipettes with automatic pipette filler or sterile transfer pipettes.

Recommended Layout for Dispensing Blood and Antigens into 24-Well Culture Trays

Table 3

Animal 1	NIL A1	AvPPD A2	BoPPD A3	NIL A4	AvPPD A5	BoPPD A6	Animal 2
Animal 3	NIL B1	AvPPD B2	BoPPD B3	NIL B4	AvPPD B5	BoPPD B6	Animal 4
Animal 5	NIL C1	AvPPD C2	BoPPD C3	NIL C4	AvPPD C5	BoPPD C6	Animal 6
Animal 7	NIL D1	AvPPD D2	BoPPD D3	NIL D4	AvPPD D5	BoPPD D6	Animal 8

NIL=Nil Control Antigen (PBS); AvPPD=Avian PPD; BoPPD=Bovine PPD

3. Addition of Stimulation Antigens:

   Add 100 µL of either PBS (nil antigen control), avian PPD or bovine PPD using aseptic technique to the appropriate 3 wells containing the blood previously dispensed in Step 1 of the procedure above. Antigens are best dispensed using a repetitive delivery pipette such as the Eppendorf "Combitip" system, fitted with sterile 5 mL tips and set on 1.

   The antigens must be mixed thoroughly into the aliquoted blood. Preferably use a microplate shaker set for 1 minute on high. If a suitable machine is not available, swirl each 24-well culture tray ten times both clockwise and counterclockwise on a flat smooth surface. Hold the lid and plate firmly together. Use sufficient force to raise the meniscus several millimeters while being careful not to cross contaminate wells or to get blood on the lid. Avoid frothing of blood.

   Optimal performance of this test is dependent on the stimulation antigens being completely mixed in with the blood.
4. Incubation:

   Incubate tissue culture trays, containing blood and antigens, for 16-24 hours at 37°C in a humidified atmosphere.
5. Harvesting of Plasma Samples:

   Plasma collection may be facilitated by centrifuging the 24-well trays at 500 g for approximately 10 minutes at room temperature (22° ± 5°C).

   After the incubation, carefully remove approximately 500 µL of plasma from above the sedimented red cells using a variable-volume pipette (100-1,000 µL) and transfer to separate storage tubes as outlined in the Recommended Plasma Storage Layout Table (Table 4). It is convenient to use 1 mL microtubes in 96-well format storage racks. Use a new pipette tip for each plasma sample.

   Note: It is important to minimise harvest of any cellular material along with the plasma. However, contamination of the plasma with a very small amount of erythrocytes during harvesting has no effect on the IFN-γ EIA. Similarly, slight hemolysis of blood samples has little effect on the IFN-γ EIA.

   Recommended Plasma Storage Layout

   Table 4

Row	1	2	3	4	5	6	7	8	9	10	11	12
A	1N	1A	1B	2N	2A	2B	3N	3A	3B	4N	4A	4B
B	5N	5A	5B	6N	6A	6B	7N	7A	7B	8N	8A	8B
C	9N	9A	9B	X	X	X	10N	10A	10B	11N	11A	11B
D	12N	12A	12B	13N	13A	13B	14N	14A	14B	15N	15A	15B
E	16N	16A	16B	17N	17A	17B	18N	18A	18B	19N	19A	19B
F	20N	20A	20B	21N	21A	21B	22N	22A	22B	23N	23A	23B
G	24N	24A	24B	X	X	X	25N	25A	25B	26N	26A	26B
H	27N	27A	27B	28N	28A	28B	29N	29A	29B	30N	30A	30B

   The nil antigen sample for animal No. 1 is stored in well A1, the avian sample in A2 and the bovine sample in A3, and so on for each other animal. Wells C4, C5, C6, G4, G5 and G6 should be left empty. This storage pattern is convenient as it allows transfer of the assay samples from the storage racks directly into the EIA trays using a 12-channel pipette. The empty wells in the EIA plate, after the samples have been transferred, are used for assaying positive and negative controls supplied with the EIA kit.

   Samples should be assayed in duplicate. Plasma in row A of the storage rack should be transferred to rows A and B of the EIA microplate, row B to C and D, row C to E and F and row D to G and H. The samples in one full storage rack will require two EIA microplates to assay.
6. Plasma Storage:

   Plasma may be stored at 35° to 45°F (2° to 7°C) for up to 7 days if not required for assays on the day of collection. Each microtube must be sealed with an appropriate cap before storage. Label sample racks with all relevant information including date, operator initials, tube contents and animal numbers and herd details. For longer periods, samples may be stored frozen at -20°C for several months.

   Note: Samples must be allowed to equilibrate to room temperature prior to testing by EIA. Carefully vortex each tube several times immediately prior to assay for IFN-γ.

   Caution: Plasma may clot during thawing. Clots do not affect the ELISA, as long as there is no blockage to the volume of plasma being aspirated by the pipette.

Stage Two — Bovine IFN-γ EIA

Step:-

1. Reconstitute freeze dried components, if required, while equilibrating other reagents according to the guidelines outlined in "Procedural Notes".
2. Add 50 µL of Green Diluent to the required wells.
3. Add 50 µL of test and control samples to the appropriate wells containing Green Diluent. Control samples should be added last to each plate. Mix thoroughly by vortexing plates for 1 minute on a microplate shaker, or if not available, by pipetting up and down 5 times.
4. Cover each plate with a lid and incubate at room temperature (22° ± 5°C) for 60 ± 5 minutes.
5. Shake out contents and wash wells 6 times at room temperature. Fill wells with wash buffer taking care not to cross contaminate adjacent wells. Shake out wash fluid and repeat operation a further 5 times. After the sixth wash, place plate(s) face down on clean filter paper and allow to drain, and flick several times over absorbent paper to remove as much remaining wash buffer as possible.

   Note: Automatic microplate washers may be used providing the number of wash cycles and the delay period between each wash has been optimised to remove background reactions. Ensure that unbound conjugate has been adequately removed from the wells to prevent invalid results.
6. Add 100 µL of freshly prepared conjugate reagent to wells. The reagent is 1X conjugate diluted in working strength Blue Diluent according to the Reagent Preparation Table (Table 2). Mix thoroughly as in Step 3.
7. Cover each plate and incubate as in Step 4 for 60 ± 5 minutes.
8. Wash wells as in Step 5.

   Note: The enzyme substrate solution is best prepared after this wash step.
9. Add 100 µL of freshly prepared enzyme substrate solution to wells. Mix thoroughly as in Step 3.
10. Cover each plate with a lid and incubate as in Step 4 for 30 minutes. Protect from direct sunlight.

    Note: Commence incubation time as you add substrate to the first well(s).
11. Add 50 µL of enzyme stopping solution to each well, being careful not to transfer chromogen from well to well, then mix by gentle agitation.

    Note: The stopping solution should be added to wells in the same order and at the same speed as the enzyme substrate solution.
12. Read the absorbance of each well within 5 minutes of terminating the reaction using a 450 nm filter with a 620-650 nm reference filter. The absorbance values will then be used to calculate results.

Quality Control (Valid Assay)

The control results must be examined before the sample results can be interpreted. Determine the mean absorbance of negative and positive controls.

Acceptable range of means:

- negative bovine IFN-γ control < 0.130

Note: The negative control replicates must not vary by more than 0.040.

- positive bovine IFN-γ control > 0.700

Note: The positive control replicates must not deviate by more than 30% from their mean absorbance.

If either of the above criteria is not met, the EIA run is invalid and must be repeated.

Abbreviated Test Procedure

Day 1 — Whole Blood Culture

1. Collect blood.
2. Aliquot heparinised blood.
3. Add antigens.
4. Incubate overnight.
5. Harvest plasmas.
6. Store plasmas (if necessary).

Day 2 — Bovine IFN-γ EIA

1. Reconstitute freeze dried components.
2. Add Green Diluent to required wells.
3. Add test plasmas (simultaneously for each animal) and controls to wells.
4. Incubate for 60 minutes.
5. Wash wells.

6. Prepare Conjugate Reagent and add to wells.
7. Incubate for 60 minutes.
8. Wash wells.
9. Prepare Substrate Solution.
10. Add Substrate to wells.
11. Incubate for 30 minutes.
12. Stop reaction.
13. Read results with 450 / 620-650 nm filters.
14. Validate and interpret results.

Interpretation of Results:

1. Calculate mean nil antigen, avian and bovine PPD absorbance values for each sample.
2. Compare the mean absorbance values of the nil antigen, avian and bovine PPD samples for each animal.

Positive = OD Bovine PPD - nil antigen ≥ 0.1; and OD Bovine PPD - avian ≥ 0.1
Negative = OD Bovine PPD - nil antigen < 0.1; or OD Bovine PPD - avian PPD < 0.1
3. Blood plasma collected from cattle, within 3-30 days post application of the skin test, having an OD value greater than 0.100 above that of avian PPD and nil (PBS) antigen, indicates the presence of *Mycobacterium bovis* infection.

Caution: Immunosuppression caused by recent dexamethasone treatment or parturition may depress IFN-γ responses to mycobacterial antigens. Animals that have received an injection of dexamethasone within one week, or that have calved within 4 weeks, should be retested to reduce the possibility of a false-negative result.

As with any biological test, this test may give a false positive or false negative result due to local conditions. A test should be interpreted in the context of all available clinical, historical and epidemiological information relevant to the animal(s) under test. Further confirmatory testing may be required in certain circumstances.

Responsibility for the test interpretation and consequent animal husbandry decisions rests solely on the user, and any consulting veterinarian and appropriate health advisors or authorities. CSL Limited accepts no responsibility for any loss or damage, howsoever caused, arising from the interpretation of test results.

Limitations of Procedure: False results may occur due to:

1. Incorrect technique;
2. Use of any anticoagulant other than heparin;
3. Excessive levels of circulating IFN-γ;
4. Immunosuppression;
5. Use of contaminated reagents;
6. Other deviations from the recommended test procedure.

Storage: Store kit at 35° to 45°F (2° to 7°C). Bring all reagents except Conjugate Concentrate to room temperature (22° ± 5°C) before use. Return to 35° to 45°F (2° to 7°C) immediately after use.

Discussion: Tuberculosis, a disease caused by *Mycobacterium bovis* infection of cattle, occurs in every country of the world and is of major importance to the dairy cattle industry. In some countries, the overall incidence of disease in individual dairy herds may approach a morbidity rate of 60-70%.

Trial Data: Field Studies: Field trials in over 13,000 head of cattle in Australia, USA, Ireland, New Zealand, Italy and Spain have shown that BOVIGAM™-TB is more sensitive than the intradermal tuberculin test for the diagnosis of bovine tuberculosis and may even detect *M. bovis*-infected cattle at an earlier stage.

A controlled laboratory study was conducted at the USDA/ARS/National Animal Disease Center, Bacterial Diseases of Livestock Research Unit, Ames, IA, USA. The study was carried out in 20 head of Hereford steers sensitized with killed *M. bovis* and compared BOVIGAM™-TB responses to USA sourced PPD and CSL PPD. Essentially the study showed that positive diagnosis of sensitized cattle occurred in all cattle stimulated with either USA's PPD or CSL's PPD. In addition, studies in New Zealand indicate that the specificity of the assay was not affected by skin testing and it is more sensitive than the Comparative Cervical Skin Test (CCT) when used between 3 and 30 days after the Caudal Fold Skin Test (CFT).

References: Available upon request.

Presentation: 10 plate test kit.

™ Trademark of CSL Limited

Manufactured by: CSL Limited, 45 Poplar Rd Parkville, Victoria 3052 Australia

Compendium Code No.: 13940290 BI7062-202

BOVI-K® 4

Pfizer Animal Health **Vaccine**

Bovine Rhinotracheitis-Virus Diarrhea-Parainfluenza$_3$-Respiratory Syncytial Virus Vaccine, Modified Live and Killed Virus

U.S. Vet. Lic. No.: 189

Description: BOVI-K® 4 is a freeze-dried preparation of modified live virus (MLV) strains of IBR, PI$_3$, and BRSV viruses, plus a liquid vaccine of inactivated BVD virus (both cytopathic and noncytopathic strains), which is used to rehydrate the freeze-dried vaccine. Modified live viral antigens are propagated on established cell lines. This product is adjuvanted with aluminum hydroxide to enhance immune response.

Contains gentamicin as preservative.

Indications: BOVI-K® 4 is for vaccination of healthy, nonpregnant cattle as an aid in preventing infectious bovine rhinotracheitis caused by infectious bovine rhinotracheitis (IBR) virus, bovine viral diarrhea caused by bovine viral diarrhea (BVD) virus, and disease caused by parainfluenza$_3$ (PI$_3$) virus and bovine respiratory syncytial virus (BRSV).

Directions:

1. General Directions: Vaccination of healthy, nonpregnant cattle 3 months of age or older is recommended. Aseptically rehydrate the freeze-dried vaccine (Bovi-Shield™ IBR-PI$_3$-BRSV) with the accompanying vial of liquid vaccine (BVD vaccine), shake well, and administer 2 mL intramuscularly. In accordance with Beef Quality Assurance guidelines, this product should be administered in the muscular region of the neck.
2. Primary Vaccination: Administer a single 2-mL dose to healthy cattle, followed by a second dose of CattleMaster® BVD-K and Bovi-Shield™ BRSV 3-4 weeks later.
3. Revaccination: Annual revaccination with a single dose is recommended.
4. Good animal husbandry and herd health management practices should be employed.

Precaution(s): Store at 2°C-7°C. Prolonged exposure to higher temperatures and/or direct sunlight may adversely affect potency. Do not freeze.

Use entire contents when first opened.

Sterilized syringes and needles should be used to administer this vaccine. Do not sterilize with chemicals because traces of disinfectant may inactivate the vaccine.

Burn containers and all unused contents.

Caution(s): Do not use in pregnant cows (abortions can result) or in calves nursing pregnant cows.

As with many vaccines, anaphylaxis may occur after use. Initial antidote of epinephrine is recommended and should be followed with appropriate supportive therapy.

This product has been shown to be efficacious in healthy animals. A protective immune response may not be elicited if animals are incubating an infectious disease, are malnourished or parasitized, are stressed due

to shipment or environmental conditions, are otherwise immunocompromised, or the vaccine is not administered in accordance with label directions.

Warning(s): Do not vaccinate within 21 days before slaughter.

For veterinary use only.

Discussion: Disease Description: IBR, BVD, PI$_3$, and BRSV viruses are commonly associated with respiratory disease and/or reproductive failure in cattle. IBR virus infection is characterized by high temperature, excessive nasal discharge, conjunctivitis and ocular discharge, inflamed nose ("red nose"), increased rate of respiration, coughing, loss of appetite, and depression. Infection is spread by direct contact, by contaminated respiratory droplets transmitted through feed, water, and by air, and through breeding by infected bulls. Cattle infected during pregnancy may abort.

BVD virus may be transmitted in nasal secretions, saliva, blood, feces, and/or urine, and by direct contact with contaminated objects; it invades through the nose and mouth and replicates systemically. Infection during pregnancy may result in abortion, fetal resorption, or congenital malformation of the fetus. Moreover, if susceptible cows are infected with noncytopathic BVD virus during the first trimester of pregnancy, their calves may be born persistently infected with the virus. Exposure of those calves to certain virulent cytopathic BVD virus strains may precipitate BVD-mucosal disease. Clinical signs of BVD include loss of appetite, ulcerations in the mouth, profuse salivation, elevated temperature, diarrhea, dehydration, and lameness.

PI$_3$ virus usually localizes in the upper respiratory tract, causing elevated temperature and moderate nasal and ocular discharge. Although clinical signs typically are mild, PI$_3$ infection weakens respiratory tissues. Invasion and replication of other pathogens, particularly *Pasteurella* spp., is thereby facilitated and may result in pneumonia.

BRSV is the etiologic agent of a specific viral respiratory disease of cattle of all ages, including nursing calves. Infection is characterized by rapid breathing, coughing, loss of appetite, discharge from the nose and eyes, fever, and swelling around the throat and neck. In an acute outbreak, deaths may follow within 48 hours after onset of signs. Clinically, BRSV infection may be indistinguishable from other viral infections associated with the bovine respiratory disease complex. BRSV infection, like PI$_3$, facilitates invasion and replication of other respiratory pathogens. Exacerbation of clinical signs has been documented when concurrent BRSV and BVD or IBR infection exists.

Trial Data: Safety and Efficacy: In safety studies of the fractions of BOVI-K® 4, no adverse reactions to vaccination were observed.

Efficacy of each fraction of BOVI-K® 4 was demonstrated in challenge-of-immunity studies. Cattle vaccinated with any fraction of BOVI-K® 4, followed by challenge with a disease-causing strain of that fraction, showed no signs or had significantly fewer clinical signs than nonvaccinated control cattle. Serologic studies demonstrated no immunologic interference among the fractions of BOVI-K® 4.

Presentation: 10 dose and 50 dose vials.

Compendium Code No.: 36901810 75-4095-04

BOVINE 3

Durvet **Vaccine**

Bovine Rhinotracheitis-Virus Diarrhea-Parainfluenza 3 Vaccine, Modified Live Virus

U.S. Vet. Lic. No.: 272

Active Ingredient(s): Bovine rhinotracheitis, virus diarrhea, parainfluenza 3 vaccine, modified live virus.

The product contains gentamicin and amphotericin B as preservatives.

Indications: BOVINE 3 is recommended for the vaccination of healthy cattle against disease caused by the organisms represented.

Dosage and Administration: Aseptically rehydrate vial of dessicated virus with the accompanying vial of diluent. Shake well. Administer 2 mL IM or SC to healthy cattle.

Persistence of maternal antibody in calves may interfere with development of active immunity following vaccination. Calves vaccinated before 3 months of age should be revaccinated at 4-6 months of age or at weaning. Annual revaccination with a single 2 mL dose is recommended.

Precaution(s): Store at 35°F-45°F (2°C-7°C). Do not freeze. Protect the vaccine from the direct rays of the sun. Use entire contents when first opened. Care should be taken to avoid chemical or microbial contamination of the product. Burn these containers and all unused contents.

Caution(s): Do not use in pregnant cows or calves nursing pregnant cows. In case of anaphylactoid reactions, epinephrine should be administered immediately.

Scientific evidence demonstrates the inability of some animals of an occasional herd to develop antibodies to Bovine Virus Diarrhea after vaccination. The affected animal may exhibit symptoms similar to mucosal disease.

Antidote(s): Epinephrine.

Warning(s): Do not vaccinate within 21 days before slaughter.

For veterinary use only.

Presentation: 10 dose (20 mL) and 50 dose (100 mL) vials.

Compendium Code No.: 10840110

BOVINE 8

Durvet **Bacterin-Vaccine**

Bovine Rhinotracheitis-Virus Diarrhea-Parainfluenza 3 Vaccine, Modified Live Virus-Leptospira canicola-grippotyphosa-hardjo-icterohaemorrhagiae-pomona Bacterin

U.S. Vet. Lic. No.: 272

Active Ingredient(s): Bovine rhinotracheitis, virus diarrhea, parainfluenza 3 vaccine, modified live virus, with *Leptospira canicola, L grippotyphosa, L hardjo, L icterohaemorrhagiae* and *L pomona* bacterin.

This product contains gentamicin and amphotericin B as preservatives.

Indications: BOVINE 8 is recommended for use in the vaccination of healthy cattle against disease caused by the viral and bacterial fractions represented.

Dosage and Administration: Aseptically rehydrate vial of desiccated virus with the accompanying vial of bacterin. Shake well. Administer 2 mL IM or SC to healthy cattle. Calves vaccinated under 3 months of age should be revaccinated at 4-6 months of age or at weaning because of the persistence of maternal antibody that may interfere with development of active immunity. Annual revaccination with a single 2 mL dose is recommended.

Precaution(s): Store at 35°F-45°F (2°C-7°C). Do not freeze. Protect the vaccine from the direct

rays of the sun. Use entire contents when first rehydrated. Care should be taken to avoid chemical or microbial contamination of the product. Burn these containers and all unused contents.
Caution(s): Do not use in pregnant cows or calves nursing pregnant cows. In case of anaphylactoid reactions, epinephrine should be administered immediately.

Scientific evidence demonstrates the inability of some animals of an occasional herd to develop antibodies to bovine virus diarrhea after vaccination. The affected animal may exhibit symptoms similar to mucosal disease.
Antidote(s): Epinephrine.
Warning(s): Do not vaccinate within 21 days before slaughter.

For veterinary use only.
Presentation: 10 dose (20 mL) and 50 dose (100 mL) vials.
Compendium Code No.: 10840130

BOVINE 9

Durvet **Bacterin-Vaccine**

Bovine Rhinotracheitis-Virus Diarrhea-Parainfluenza 3 Vaccine, Modified Live Virus-Campylobacter Fetus-Leptospira Canicola-Grippotyphosa-Hardjo-Icterohaemorrhagiae-Pomona Bacterin

U.S. Vet. Lic. No.: 272
Contents: This product contains the antigens listed above.

This product contains gentamicin and amphotericin B as preservatives.
Indications: BOVINE 9 is recommended for use in the vaccination of healthy cattle against diseases caused by the viral and bacterial fractions represented.
Directions: Aseptically rehydrate the vial of desiccated virus with the accompanying vial of bacterin. Shake well. Administer 5 mL intramuscularly or subcutaneously to healthy cattle. In *Campylobacter fetus* infected herds or endemic areas, a second vaccination in 21 days is required.

Persistence of maternal antibody in calves may interfere with the development of active immunity following vaccination. Calves vaccinated before 3 months of age should be revaccinated at 4-6 months of age or at weaning. Annual revaccination with a single 5 mL dose is recommended.
Precaution(s): Store at 35°F-45°F (2°C-7°C). Protect the vaccine from direct rays of the sun. Use entire contents when first rehydrated. Care should be taken to avoid chemical or microbial contamination of the product. Burn the container and all unused contents.
Caution(s): In case of an anaphylactoid reactions, epinephrine should be administered immediately.

For veterinary use only.
Warning(s): Do not vaccinate within 21 days before slaughter.

Do not use in pregnant cows or calves nursing pregnant cows.
Trial Data: Scientific evidence demonstrates the inability of some animals of an occasional herd to develop antibodies to Bovine Virus Diarrhea after vaccination. The affected animal may exhibit symptoms similar to mucosal disease.
Presentation: 10 dose and 20 dose vials.
Manufactured by: Biocor, Inc., Omaha, NE 68134.
Compendium Code No.: 10840141 11/92 / 10/92

BOVINE BLUELITE®

TechMix **Electrolytes-Oral**

Active Ingredient(s): BOVINE BLUELITE® contains buffered electrolytes, fat-water soluble vitamins (A, D, E, K, B-complex, ascorbic acid), and multiple energy sources with a pH regulating action. The buffered electrolytes in BOVINE BLUELITE® are nonirritating.

BOVINE BLUELITE® also contains aromatic and flavoring agents.
Indications:

Dairy cows: Supportive rehydration therapy for winter dysentery, following surgical correction of displaced abomasums, rumenotomics and severe dehydration related to calving or toxic infections. BOVINE BLUELITE® is readily consumed by dairy calves and lactating dairy cows. It encourages water intake to help maintain body fluids when dairy cattle encounter dehydration as a result of winter dysentery, bacterial diarrhea, pneumonia, or moldy feeds.

Feedlot and growing calves: Calves off feed and pulled into sickpens out of feedlot.

Feedlot cattle: BOVINE BLUELITE® should be added to the drinking water whenever cattle are dehydrated as a result of shipping, sorting, moving and for supportive therapy in calves pneumonia, shipping fever, diarrhea, vaccination or processing.

Sheep and feedlot lambs: BOVINE BLUELITE® helps lambs get started on water and feed when shipping into the feedlot. BOVINE BLUELITE® should be used in the water or feed whenever lambs are dehydrated as a result of bacterial diarrhea, coccidiosis, or during stresses related to sorting, handling and shipping. BOVINE BLUELITE® can be used to help stimulate water intake.
Dosage and Administration:

I. Water Administration:

A. Administer BOVINE BLUELITE® in the drinking water for 5-7 days or as long as the animals show evidence of dehydration or until animals are consuming their normal amount of feed ration on a daily basis. Allow cattle or sheep to drink water with the BOVINE BLUELITE® on a free choice basis.

B. Administer BOVINE BLUELITE® in the drinking water for cattle or sheep in one of the following ways:

1. Individual Administration: One (1) heaping tablespoon of BOVINE BLUELITE® to each gallon of drinking water.
   Dairy cows: 12-16 oz. of BOVINE BLUELITE® powder per head on a daily basis as a drench or in 2-3 gallons of water administered via a stomach pump.
   Feedlot and growing calves: 1 to 1½ oz. of BOVINE BLUELITE® powder per 100 lbs. of body weight.
   After initial drench administration, continue BOVINE BLUELITE® in the drinking water at normal dosage rates for 3-5 days.
2. Water Tank Administration:
   a. One (1) level 8 oz. cup of BOVINE BLUELITE® to each 32 gallons of drinking water, or
   b. One (1) pound (or 2¼ cups) of BOVINE BLUELITE® to 64 gallons of drinking water, or
   c. One (1) 6 lb. bag of BOVINE BLUELITE® to each 384 gallons of drinking water.
3. Stock Solution Drenching: Mix 2 lbs. of BOVINE BLUELITE® (4½ cups) in a gallon of stock solution. Administer 1 oz. of stock solution to each gallon of drinking water.
   Dairy cows: Administer 32-40 oz. of BOVINE BLUELITE® stock solution per animal.
   Beef and growing calves: Administer 4-6 oz. of BOVINE BLUELITE® stock solution per each 100 lbs. of body weight.
4. Drinking Water Dosage for Severe Dehydration:
   Dairy cows: Mix 12-16 oz. of BOVINE BLUELITE® powder in 3-5 gallons of drinking water, or 1-2 oz. of BOVINE BLUELITE® powder in the drinking cup 4-6 times a day.
   Feedlot and growing calves: Mix 4-6 oz. of BOVINE BLUELITE® powder in 2-3 gallons of drinking water.
   After initial loading dose in the drinking water, maintain animals on BOVINE BLUELITE® at normal dosages in the drinking water for an additional 3-5 days.

II. Feed Administration:

A. Top Dressing for Cattle:

1. Individual Topdress: Two (2) heaping tablespoons of BOVINE BLUELITE® on the feed consumed by a 400 lb. calf on a daily basis.
2. Flock Topdress: One-half (½) cup of BOVINE BLUELITE® on the amount of feed consumed daily for a 1,000 lb. animal. Example: Four (4), 500 lb. calves should be fed one (1) cupful of BOVINE BLUELITE® on a daily basis.

B. Top Dressing for Sheep:

1. Individual Topdress: One (1) heaping teaspoon of BOVINE BLUELITE® on the feed consumed by a 60 lb. lamb on a daily basis.
2. Flock Topdress: One-half (½) cup of BOVINE BLUELITE® on the feed consumed by 10, 60 lb. lambs on a daily basis.

III. Water Intake: Cattle on dry forages and grains normally consume water equivalent to 9-11% of their body weight on a daily basis depending upon temperature, stress and water availability. Lactating cows should be offered additional water with BOVINE BLUELITE® equivalent to their daily volume of milk production.
Compatibilities: BOVINE BLUELITE® in water is compatible with most antibiotics, coccidiostats and microbial cultures and may be added to the drinking water in tanks or troughs.
Discussion: BOVINE BLUELITE® is an oral rehydration formula specifically designed for ruminating animals such as feedlot steers and heifers, lactating dairy cows, and sheep. Ruminant animals possess an ability to efficiently utilize both roughage and grain through bacterial fermentation in the rumen as compared to simple stomached animals like swine, poultry and young nursing calves that cannot utilize or digest roughage on an efficient basis.
Presentation: 14x2 lb. (0.90 kg) (28 lb. pail) and 8x6 lb. (2.72 kg) bags (48 lb. case).
Compendium Code No.: 11440040

BOVINE ECOLIZER®

Novartis Animal Vaccines **Antibodies**

Escherichia coli Antibody, Equine Origin

U.S. Vet. Lic. No.: 303
Composition: This product is prepared from the blood of horses hyperimmunized with K99 piliated *Escherichia coli*. Contains oxytetracycline, phenol, and thimerosal as preservatives.
Indications: For use in newborn calves as an aid in the prevention of colibacillosis caused by K99 piliated *Escherichia coli*.
Dosage and Administration: Shake well before using. Administer 10 mL orally to calves less than 12 hours old. Slowly syringe toward the back of the calf's mouth. Colostrum should be fed to each calf.
Precaution(s): Store in the dark at 35°-45°F (2°-7°C). Do not freeze.
Caution(s): Use entire contents when first opened. Anaphylactic reactions may occur following the use of this biological. Symptomatic treatment: Epinephrine.

For veterinary use only.
Warning(s): Do not administer within 21 days prior to slaughter.
Discussion: Despite advances in sanitation, vaccination, and antibiotics, baby calf scours caused by *Escherichia coli* (colibacillosis) is still the number one killer of newborn calves. It causes 50% of the deaths of newborn dairy calves and 75% of the deaths in beef calves.

The K99 pilus is the main virulence factor found on enterotoxigenic strains of *E coli* (ETEC) that are isolated from calves. This pilus has been shown to be one of the main attachment mechanisms which allow the ETEC to colonize on the microvilli in the lower small intestine. Colonization and irritation interfere with absorption of fluids from the gut. This produces hypermotility and diarrhea. The production of enterotoxins also contributes to the diarrhea by causing hypersecretion of fluids from the intestinal cells.
Presentation: Available in single dose syringes and 100 mL (10 dose) bottles.
Compendium Code No.: 11140022

BOVINE ECOLIZER®+C

Novartis Animal Vaccines **Antibodies-Antitoxin**

Clostridium Perfringens Type C Antitoxin-Escherichia coli Antibody, Equine Origin

U.S. Vet. Lic. No.: 303
Composition: This product is prepared from the blood of horses hyperimmunized with *Clostridium perfringens* Type C and K99 piliated *Escherichia coli*. Contains oxytetracycline, phenol, and thimerosal as preservatives.
Indications: For use in newborn calves as an aid in the prevention of disease caused by *Clostridium perfringens* Type C and K99 piliated *Escherichia coli*.
Dosage and Administration: Shake well before using. Administer 10 mL orally to calves less than 4 hours old. Slowly syringe toward the back of the calf's mouth. Colostrum should be fed to each calf.
Precaution(s): Store in the dark at 35°-45°F (2°-7°C). Do not freeze. Use entire contents when first opened.
Caution(s): Anaphylactic reactions may occur following the use of this biological. Symptomatic treatment: Epinephrine.

For veterinary use only.
Warning(s): Do not administer within 21 days prior to slaughter.
Discussion: Despite advances in sanitation, vaccination, and antibiotics, baby calf scours caused by *Escherichia coli* (colibacillosis) is still the number one killer of newborn calves. It causes 50% of the deaths of newborn dairy calves and 75% of the deaths in beef calves.

The K99 pilus is the main virulence factor found on enterotoxigenic strains of *E coli* (ETEC) that are isolated from calves. This pilus has been shown to be one of the main attachment mechanisms which allow the ETEC to colonize on the microvilli in the lower small intestine. Colonization and irritation interfere with absorption of fluids from the gut. This produces hypermotility and diarrhea. The production of enterotoxins also contributes to the diarrhea by causing hypersecretion of fluids from the intestinal cells.

Type C enterotoxemia is caused by an intestinal overgrowth of *Clostridium perfringens* Type C which produces primarily beta and some alpha exotoxins. *Clostridium perfringens* Type C is widely distributed in the soil and is a common inhabitant of the intestinal tract.

Calves may be found dead without previously showing symptoms. Symptoms seen in affected animals include abdominal pain, diarrhea (sometimes blood-tinged), and depression.

Engorgement with milk or grain is considered a predisposing factor for enterotoxemia. It is believed that a large intake of milk may slow the digestive processes, allowing the clostridial bacteria time to multiply. In addition, the enzyme trypsin, which can inactivate the beta toxin, may not be present in adequate concentrations under these circumstances. It is usually the healthy, vigorous offspring of high-producing mothers which are affected by the disease.

Postmortem lesions vary according to the predominating type of exotoxin. If alpha toxin predominates, there will be extensive hemorrhage in the jejunum and ileum as well as the mesenteric and intestinal lymph nodes. There will be blood-stained contents in the lower intestine and the colon. If beta toxin predominates, there will be necrosis of the jejunum and ileum and peritonitis. Petechial hemorrhages will be found on the spleen, heart, thymus and serosal surfaces.

Presentation: Available in single dose syringes (10 mL) and 100 mL (10 dose) bottles.

Compendium Code No.: 11140032

BOVINE MAXIMIZER™

Novartis Animal Vaccines **Large Animal Dietary Supplement**

Active Ingredient(s): A combination of fatty acids, vitamin E and selenium.

Indications: Newborn calves have very low energy reserves. The fatty acids in MAXIMIZER™ provide a readily available source of the extra energy needed by so many calves. In addition, MAXIMIZER™ provides guaranteed levels of both vitamin E and selenium, to help prevent diseases caused by deficiencies of these agents.

Dosage and Administration: Administer one (1) 80 mL tube orally to each calf at birth or upon arrival to the farm. Individual calves can be retreated at a later date if they require additional energy.

Discussion: Newborn calves have only limited energy reserves to draw upon; as a result, they are very susceptible to stresses caused by even short-term starvation. Many things can upset this delicate energy balance, including poor-milking dams, low ambient temperatures, and stresses of moving young dairy calves. Upsetting this balance can result in deaths directly from starvation, but can also cause indirect deaths due to rendering calves more prone to secondary infections such as colibacillosis or viral scours. All in all, these losses contribute to a very significant profit loss for the average calf producer.

The fatty acids in MAXIMIZER™ are an important energy source for young calves, supplied in a convenient, easy-to-administer form. The vitamin E and selenium are designed to provide additional sources of these vital substances, which are often deficient in young calves.

Trial Data: Much of the economic loss connected with raising young calves is related, either directly or indirectly, to energy shortages in the calves. Calves that are energy deficient can die as a direct result of starvation, and they are also more prone to develop problems such as bacterial scours.

To demonstrate the effectiveness of MAXIMIZER™ in young calves, 136 purchased dairy calves, ranging in age from 2-5 days, were divided into two groups, MAXIMIZER™-treated and controls, and monitored over a 28-day period. The MAXIMIZER™ calves showed definite advantages both in rate of gain and in feed efficiency.

Calves (2-5 days old) were treated on arrival with MAXIMIZER™. The biggest weight gain advantage, 16.71 lbs., was seen in calves that weighed between 80 and 90 lbs. on arrival. Calves with a beginning weight of 90-100 lbs. gained an average of 10.96 lbs., and calves weighing 100-110 lbs. gained an average of 4.19 lbs. more than equivalent control groups. As a whole, the MAXIMIZER™-treated calves showed a weight gain advantage of 10.37 lbs. over the control group of calves.

Calves treated with MAXIMIZER™ consumed more dry feed, averaging an additional 9.79 lbs. of dry matter over the 28-day trial period. Since all calves were offered free choice dry feed, this indicates that MAXIMIZER™-treated calves acclimate faster to dry feed consumption.

While MAXIMIZER™-treated calves were consuming more dry feed, they were also converting this feed to pounds of gain more efficiently than control calves. On average, treated calves showed an advantage of 0.28 lbs. less feed consumed for every pound of gain when compared to the control calves.

Presentation: 1 dose (80 mL) tube.

Compendium Code No.: 11140043

BOVINE PILI SHIELD™

Novartis Animal Vaccines **Bacterin**

Escherichia Coli Bacterin

U.S. Vet. Lic. No.: 303

Composition: This bacterin contains inactivated cultures of K99 piliated *Escherichia coli* adjuvanted with Xtend III®. Contains penicillin, streptomycin, and thimerosal as preservatives.

Indications: For use in healthy heifers and cows as an aid in the prevention and control of colibacillosis in calves caused by K99 piliated *Escherichia coli.*

Dosage and Administration: Shake well before using. Administer 1 mL intramuscularly 2 weeks to 12 months prior to calving. Vaccinate dairy cows during the dry off period. Revaccinate annually.

Precaution(s): Store in the dark at 35°-45°F (2°-7°C). Do not freeze. Use entire contents when first opened.

Caution(s): It is essential that calves receive colostrum from the vaccinated dam within 8 hours of birth. Anaphylactic reactions may occur following the use of this biological. Symptomatic treatment: Epinephrine.

For veterinary use only.

Warning(s): Do not vaccinate within 60 days prior to slaughter.

This product causes persistent swelling at the site of injection.

Discussion: Technical Disease Information: *Escherichia coli: E. coli* (colibacillosis) is primarily an enteric disease of calves from birth to 7 days of age. It may cause a severe diarrhea. Pathogenic *E. coli* are commonly found in the manure of healthy cows, which results in most calves being exposed shortly after birth. Unless the calf has received some type of protection immediately following birth, it is very susceptible to developing colibacillosis. The bacteria attach to the lining cells of the intestine by means of projections called pili. After attachment, the bacteria produce toxins which cause the intestine to secrete large amounts of fluid which results in diarrhea, dehydration and possible death.

Prevention: Oral antibodies are an economical and effective method of preventing diarrheas caused by *E. coli.* Cows and heifers are vaccinated once a year with a 1 mL dose of BOVINE PILI SHIELD™. This causes antibodies to be formed in the colostrum. When the calf receives colostrum it receives these antibodies, which will act to prevent the bacteria from causing diarrhea. Therefore, the simple and economical prevention of scours can be achieved with a single, yearly dose of BOVINE PILI SHIELD™ to the dam, along with a calf-management program that makes sure calves receive adequate colostrum following birth.

Trial Data: *E. coli* Challenge:

Group	% Mortality	Avg. Clinical Score
Vaccinates	0%	1.5
Controls	70% p = 0.0002	82.9 p = 0.0000
	Extremely Significant	

Presentation: Available in 20 dose (20 mL) and 100 dose (100 mL) bottles.

Compendium Code No.: 11140052 MP-F200-APR00

BOVINE PILI SHIELD™+C

Novartis Animal Vaccines **Bacterin-Toxoid**

Clostridium Perfringens Type C-Escherichia Coli Bacterin-Toxoid

U.S. Vet. Lic. No.: 303

Composition: This bacterin contains inactivated cultures of *Clostridium perfringens* Type C and K99 piliated *Escherichia coli* adjuvanted with Xtend III®. Contains thimerosal as a preservative.

Indications: For use in healthy pregnant cattle as an aid in the prevention and control of enterotoxemia in calves caused by *Clostridium perfringens* Type C and colibacillosis in calves caused by K99 piliated *Escherichia coli.*

Dosage and Administration: Shake well before using. Administer 1 mL intramuscularly 1-3 months prior to calving. Vaccinate dairy cows during the dry off period. Revaccinate prior to each subsequent calving.

Precaution(s): Store in the dark at 35°-45°F (2°-7°C). Do not freeze. Use entire contents when first opened.

Caution(s): It is essential that calves receive colostrum from the vaccinated dam within 8 hours of birth. Anaphylactic reactions may occur following the use of this biological. Symptomatic treatment: Epinephrine.

For veterinary use only.

Warning(s): Do not vaccinate within 60 days prior to slaughter.

This product causes persistent swelling at the site of injection.

Discussion: Technical Disease Information: *Escherichia coli: E. coli* (colibacillosis) is primarily an enteric disease of calves from birth to 7 days of age. It may cause a severe diarrhea. Pathogenic *E. coli* are commonly found in the manure of healthy cows, which results in most calves being exposed shortly after birth. Unless the calf has received some type of protection immediately following birth, it is very susceptible to developing colibacillosis. The bacteria attach to the lining cells of the intestine by means of projections called pili. After attachment, the bacteria produce toxins which cause the intestine to secrete large amounts of fluid which results in diarrhea, dehydration and possible death.

Clostridium perfringens Type C: *Clostridium perfringens* Type C is commonly found in soil. It is also a common inhabitant of the intestinal tract in healthy animals. Engorgement with milk is often a predisposing factor. Type C enterotoxemia is caused by an overgrowth of these bacteria in the calf's intestine. This results in severe toxemia and high mortality rates. Calves may be found dead without showing any symptoms. They may show signs including bloating, abdominal pain, hemorrhagic diarrhea or extreme weakness.

Prevention: Oral antibodies are an economical and effective method of preventing diarrheas caused by *E. coli* and *Clostridium perfringens* Type C. Cows and heifers are vaccinated once a year with a 1 mL dose of BOVINE PILI SHIELD™+C. This causes antibodies to be formed in the colostrum. When the calf receives colostrum it receives these antibodies, which will act to prevent the bacteria from causing diarrhea. Therefore, the simple and economical prevention of scours can be achieved with a single, yearly dose of BOVINE PILI SHIELD™+C to the dam, along with a calf-management program that makes sure calves receive adequate colostrum following birth.

Trial Data: *E. coli* Challenge:

Group	% Mortality	Avg. Clinical Score
Vaccinates	0%	1.5
Controls	70% p = 0.0002	82.9 p = 0.0000
	Extremely Significant	

Cl. perfringens Type C Antitoxin Titers:

Group (pooled samples)	Titer (AU/mL)
Dam's colostrum	$\geq 50 < 100$
Calf serum (3 days of age)	≥ 10
Calf serum (10 days of age)	≥ 10

Presentation: Available in 20 dose (20 mL) and 100 dose (100 mL) bottles.

Compendium Code No.: 11140062 MP-F200-APR00

BOVINE POSITIVE REAGENT

Allied Monitor **Mycobacterium Test Reagent**

Active Ingredient(s): Serum obtained from adult bovine, confirmed paratuberculous by fecal culture and necropsy. It is sterile-filtered and lyophilized.

Indications: For use as a positive control in ELISA and AGID against PPA antigen.

Presentation: 1 mL.

Compendium Code No.: 10800011

BOVINE RHINOTRACHEITIS-PARAINFLUENZA$_3$ VACCINE

Colorado Serum **Vaccine**

Bovine Rhinotracheitis-Parainfluenza$_3$ Vaccine, Modified Live Virus

U.S. Vet. Lic. No.: 188

Active Ingredient(s): Bovine rhinotracheitis, parainfluenza-3 vaccine, modified live virus.

Penicillin and streptomycin have been added as preservatives.

Indications: When the vaccine is rehydrated by adding the diluent as directed, the resulting single product is recommended for the vaccination of healthy cattle against bovine rhinotracheitis and parainfluenza-3 infections.

Dosage and Administration: Cattle should be vaccinated before or at the time of admission to feedlots or dairy areas. Yearly booster injections are recommended for breeding stock. Maternal antibodies in young calves may interfere with the development of an active immunity. If emergency conditions require vaccination these calves should be revaccinated one (1) month after weaning.

B

Be sure that breeding stock is immunized on a regular basis when cows are open.

Needle punctures and tissue damage at the site of injection may result in the condemnation of carcasses.

Rehydrate the vaccine just prior to use. To rehydrate the BOVINE RHINOTRACHEITIS-PARAINFLUENZA$_3$ VACCINE, withdraw the entire contents of the accompanying diluent vial with a sterile syringe and needle, without removing the stopper, and transfer it to the vial of dried vaccine. Shake the vaccine bottle until the dried material is completely rehydrated. Live virus products contain a stabilizer that may slow rehydration slightly but complete liquefaction will take place within a few moments. The vaccine is then ready to use. Use only the diluent furnished with the product for rehydrating the vaccine.

The recommended dose is 2 mL to be administered immediately after rehydrating. Injection should be intramuscular, preferably in the neck region to avoid areas of prime meat cuts.

If it is necessary to vaccinate young calves, revaccinate these animals at six (6) months of age.

Precaution(s): Store in the dark at 2° to 7°C. Sterilize needles and syringes by boiling in clean water. Do not use chemical disinfectants or detergents for this purpose.

Use the entire contents when the bottle is first opened. Burn the container and all unused contents.

Caution(s): Anaphylaxis (shock) may sometimes follow the use of products of this nature. Epinephrine (adrenalin) or an equivalent drug should be available for immediate use in these instances. Artificial respiration is also helpful.

Do not use in pregnant cows or in calves nursing pregnant cows.

Do not administer to calves of less than four weeks of age.

For veterinary use only.

Warning(s): Do not vaccinate within 21 days before slaughter.

Discussion: Bovine rhinotracheitis is normally sudden and mild in nature. Salivation, congestion of the nasal mucosa, serous nasal discharge, rapid respiration, coughing, and depression, are some of the symptoms frequently observed. Temperatures may vary from slightly above normal to as high as 108°F (42°C).

Parainfluenza-3 infection is symptomized by coughing, mucopurulent oculonasal discharge, difficult respiration, and dehydration. Temperatures may range from a little above normal to 104°F (40°C). Diarrhea is not usually present. Dry scabs appear on the muzzle.

Both of the above virus infections are herd diseases. Both produce high morbidity and low mortality. Substantial weight loss is a serious economic factor.

Presentation: Packaged in 10 dose (20 mL) and 50 dose (100 mL) vials.

Compendium Code No.: 11010031

BOVINE RHINOTRACHEITIS VACCINE

Colorado Serum **Vaccine**

Bovine Rhinotracheitis Vaccine, Modified Live Virus

U.S. Vet. Lic. No.: 188

Contents: This product contains the antigen listed above.

Penicillin and streptomycin have been added as preservatives.

Indications: When the vaccine is rehydrated by adding the diluent as directed the resulting single product is recommended for the vaccination of healthy cattle against bovine rhinotracheitis.

Dosage and Administration: Rehydrate vaccine just prior to use. To rehydrate the vaccine, withdraw the entire contents of the accompanying diluent vial with a sterile syringe and needle, without removing the stopper, and transfer it to the vial of dried vaccine. Shake the vaccine bottle until dried material is completely rehydrated. Live virus products contain a stabilizer that may slow rehydration slightly but complete liquefaction will take place within a few moments. The vaccine is then ready to use. Use only the diluent furnished with this product for rehydrating the vaccine.

Recommended dose is 2 mL to be administered immediately after rehydrating. Injection should be intramuscular preferably in the neck region to avoid areas of prime meat cuts.

Precaution(s): Store in the dark at 2° to 7°C.

Sterilize needles and syringes by boiling in clean water. Do not use chemical disinfectants or detergents for this purpose.

Use entire contents when bottle is first opened.

Burn the container and all unused contents.

Caution(s): Cattle should be vaccinated before or at the time of admission to feed lots or dairy areas. Yearly booster injections are recommended for breeding stock. Maternal antibodies in young calves may interfere with development of an active immunity. If emergency conditions require vaccination these calves should be revaccinated one month after weaning.

Do not use in pregnant cows or in calves nursing pregnant cows. Be sure that breeding stock is immunized on a regular basis when cows are open.

Anaphylaxis (shock) may sometimes follow the use of products of this nature. Epinephrine or equivalent should be available for immediate use in these instances. Artificial respiration is also helpful.

For veterinary use only.

Warning(s): Do not vaccinate within 21 days before slaughter. Needle punctures and tissue damage at the site of injection may result in condemnation of carcasses.

Discussion: Similarity of symptoms of IBR infection and other virus diseases commonly found in feed lot cattle must be taken into consideration when planning an effective vaccination program.

Bovine rhinotracheitis sometimes referred to as "Red Nose" or "Rhino", is caused by a specific virus which attacks the upper respiratory passages (trachea, mucous membranes, and larynx). Salivation congestion of the nasal mucosa, serous nasal discharge, rapid respiration, coughing, and depression, are some of the symptoms frequently observed. Temperatures may vary from a little above normal to as high as 108°F (42°C). High morbidity with low mortality is the usual pattern. The most serious economic factor in the feed lot is the substantial weight loss of affected animals. In dairy cows milk production is lowered or stopped.

Usually the disease appears three or more weeks after animals are started on feed in the corrals, when they are reaching full feed and starting to take on considerable flesh. Outbreaks may also appear in beef cattle in prime condition and almost ready for market. Weight loss in these instances is very costly. The number of affected animals, in any feed lot group, is quite variable. This disease does not respond readily or satisfactorily to therapy. Prevention is the only practical way to avoid the losses that accompany outbreaks. Regular use of BOVINE RHINOTRACHEITIS VACCINE is good practice.

Presentation: Packaged is one bottle containing dried BOVINE RHINOTRACHEITIS VACCINE and a second bottle of sterile diluent available in 10 dose (20 mL) and 50 dose (100 mL) sizes.

Compendium Code No.: 11010361

BOVINE RHINOTRACHEITIS-VIRUS DIARRHEA-PARAINFLUENZA-3 VACCINE

Colorado Serum **Vaccine**

Bovine Rhinotracheitis-Virus Diarrhea-Parainfluenza$_3$ Vaccine, Modified Live Virus

U.S. Vet. Lic. No.: 188

Active Ingredient(s): Contains dried bovine rhinotracheitis, virus diarrhea, parainfluenza-3 vaccine and a second bottle of sterile diluent.

Penicillin and streptomycin are added as preservatives.

Indications: The product is recommended for the vaccination of healthy cattle against bovine rhinotracheitis, bovine virus diarrhea, and parainfluenza-3 infection.

Dosage and Administration: Cattle should be vaccinated before or at the time of admission to feedlots or dairy areas. Yearly booster injections are recommended for breeding stock. Maternal antibodies in young calves may interfere with the development of an active immunity. If emergency conditions require vaccination these calves should be revaccinated one (1) month after weaning.

Be sure that breeding stock is immunized on a regular basis when cows are open.

Needle punctures and tissue damage at the site of injection may result in the condemnation of carcasses.

Rehydrate the vaccine just prior to use. To rehydrate the vaccine, withdraw the entire contents of the accompanying diluent vial with a sterile syringe and needle, without removing the stopper, and transfer it to the vial of dried vaccine. Shake the vaccine bottle until the dried material is completely rehydrated. Live virus products contain a stabilizer that may slow rehydration slightly but complete liquefaction will take place within a few moments. The vaccine is then ready to use. Use only the diluent furnished with the product for rehydrating the vaccine.

Recommended dose is 2 mL to be administered immediately after rehydrating. Injection should be intramuscular, preferably in the neck region to avoid areas of prime meat cuts.

If it is necessary to vaccinate young calves, revaccinate these animals at six (6) months of age.

Precaution(s): Store in the dark at 2-7°C. Sterilize needles and syringes by boiling in clean water. Do not use chemical disinfectants or detergents for this purpose.

Use the entire contents when bottle is first opened. Burn the container and all unused contents.

Caution(s): Anaphylaxis (shock) may sometimes follow the use of products of this nature. Epinephrine or an equivalent drug should be available for immediate use in these instances. Artificial respiration is also helpful.

Do not use in pregnant cows or in calves nursing pregnant cows. Do not administer to calves under four weeks of age. For veterinary use only.

Warning(s): Do not vaccinate within 21 days before slaughter.

Discussion: Bovine rhinotracheitis is normally sudden and mild in nature. Salivation, congestion of the nasal mucosa, serous nasal discharge, rapid respiration, coughing and depression, are some of the symptoms frequently observed. Temperatures may vary from slightly above normal to as high as 108°F (42°C).

Bovine virus diarrhea appears suddenly and most of the animals in a herd will become involved. Affected animals develop abnormal temperatures, become depressed, go off feed, and there is a mucous oculonasal discharge with a dry nonproductive cough. Most of the time diarrhea is noted. Lameness will also develop in a considerable number of the animals.

Parainfluenza-3 infection is symptomized by coughing, mucopurulent oculonasal discharge, difficult respiration, and dehydration. Temperatures may range from a little above normal to 104°F (40°C). Diarrhea is not usually present. Dry scabs appear on the muzzle.

All three of the above virus infections (IBR, BVD, and PI$_3$) are herd diseases. All produce high morbidity and low mortality. Substantial weight loss is a serious economic factor.

Presentation: 10 dose (20 mL) and 50 dose (100 mL) vials.

Compendium Code No.: 11010050

BOVINE VIRUS DIARRHEA VACCINE

Colorado Serum **Vaccine**

Bovine Virus Diarrhea Vaccine, Modified Live Virus

U.S. Vet. Lic. No.: 188

Contents: Packaged herewith is one bottle containing dried Bovine Virus Diarrhea Vaccine and a second bottle of sterile diluent.

Penicillin and streptomycin are added as preservatives.

Indications: When the vaccine is rehydrated by adding the diluent as directed the resulting single product is recommended for the vaccination of healthy cattle as an aid in prevention of disease due to Bovine Virus Diarrhea virus.

Dosage and Administration: Rehydrate vaccine just prior to use. To rehydrate the vaccine, withdraw the entire contents of the accompanying diluent vial with a sterile syringe and needle, without removing the stopper, and transfer it to the vial of dried vaccine. Shake the vaccine bottle until dried material is completely rehydrated. Live virus products contain a stabilizer that may slow rehydration slightly but complete liquefaction will take place within a few moments. The vaccine is then ready to use.

Use only the diluent furnished with this product for rehydrating the vaccine.

Recommended dose is 2 mL to be administered immediately after rehydrating. Injection should be intramuscular, preferably in the neck region to avoid areas of prime meat cuts.

Directions:

When to Vaccinate: Cattle should be vaccinated before or at the time of admission to feed lots or dairy areas. Yearly booster injections are recommended for breeding stock. Maternal antibodies in young calves may interfere with development of an active immunity. If emergency conditions require vaccination these calves should be revaccinated one month after weaning.

Be sure that breeding stock is immunized on a regular basis when cows are open.

Contraindication(s): Do not vaccinate pregnant cows or calves nursing susceptible pregnant cows.

Precaution(s): Store in dark at 2° to 7°C. Sterilize needles and syringes by boiling in clean water. Do not use chemical disinfectants or detergents for this purpose. Use entire contents when bottle is first opened. Burn this container and all unused contents.

Caution(s): Anaphylaxis (shock) may sometimes follow the use of products of this nature. Adrenalin or equivalent should be available for immediate use in these instances.

Warning(s): Do not vaccinate within 21 days before slaughter.

Discussion: Bovine virus diarrhea appears suddenly and most of the animals in a herd will become involved. Affected animals develop abnormal temperatures, become depressed, go off feed, and there is a mucous oculonasal discharge with a dry non-productive cough. Most of the time diarrhea is noted. Lameness will also develop in a considerable number of the animals.

Abortions are caused by this disease. BVD infections are usually no accompanied by high mortality but morbidity and heavy loss of weight are serious factors.

Presentation: Conveniently packaged in 10 dose (20 mL) and 50 dose (100 mL) sizes.

Compendium Code No.: 11010061

BOVI-SERA™ SERUM ANTIBODIES

Colorado Serum **Antiserum**

Corynebacterium pyogenes-Escherichia coli-Pasteurella haemolytica-multocida-Salmonella typhimurium Antiserum, Bovine Isolates, Bovine Origin

U.S. Vet. Lic. No.: 188

Active Ingredient(s): Prepared from the blood of cattle hyperimmunized with repeated injections of live cultures of *Corynebacterium pyogenes, Escherichia coli,* (including K-99) *Pasteurella haemolytica, Pasteurella multocida,* and *Salmonella typhimurium,* isolated from cattle.

Contains thimerosal and phenol as preservatives.

Indications: For use as an aid in the prevention and treatment of enteric and respiratory conditions in cattle and sheep when caused by the micro-organsims used to hyperimmunize the animals in which the antiserum has been produced.

Dosage and Administration: Injections may be subcutaneous or intramuscular.

For prevention:

Calves: 20 mL to 40 mL, as soon after birth as possible.

Cattle: 50 mL to 75 mL.

Sheep: 10 mL to 15 mL.

For treatment:

Calves: 40 mL to 100 mL.

Cattle: 75 mL to 150 mL.

Sheep: 20 mL to 40 mL.

The recommended dose is to be administered at 12 to 24 hour intervals until an improvement is noted.

Precaution(s): Store in the dark at 2-7°C.

Caution(s): Anaphylactic reactions sometimes follow administration of products of this nature. If noted, administer adrenaline or an equivalent drug.

Use the entire contents when the bottle is first opened. For veterinary use only.

Warning(s): Do not vaccinate within 21 days before slaughter.

Presentation: 20 mL, 250 mL and 1,000 mL bottles.

Compendium Code No.: 11010020

BOVI-SHIELD™ 3

Pfizer Animal Health **Vaccine**

Bovine Rhinotracheitis-Virus Diarrhea-Parainfluenza$_3$ Vaccine, Modified Live Virus

U.S. Vet. Lic. No.: 189

Description: BOVI-SHIELD™ 3 is a freeze-dried preparation of modified live virus (MLV) strains of IBR, BVD, and PI$_3$ viruses, plus a sterile diluent used to rehydrate the freeze-dried vaccine. Viral antigens are propagated on established cell lines.

Contains gentamicin as preservative.

Indications: BOVI-SHIELD™ 3 is for vaccination of healthy, nonpregnant cattle as an aid in preventing infectious bovine rhinotracheitis caused by infectious bovine rhinotracheitis (IBR) virus, bovine viral diarrhea (Type 1 and Type 2) caused by bovine viral diarrhea (BVD) virus, and disease caused by parainfluenza$_3$ (PI$_3$) virus.

Directions:

1. General Directions: Vaccination of healthy, nonpregnant cattle is recommended. Aseptically rehydrate the freeze-dried vaccine with the sterile diluent provided, shake well, and administer 2 mL intramuscularly. In accordance with Beef Quality Assurance guidelines, this product should be administered in the muscular region of the neck.
2. Primary Vaccination: Administer a single 2 mL dose to healthy cattle.
3. Revaccination: Annual revaccination with a single dose is recommended.
4. Good animal husbandry and herd health management practices should be employed.

Precaution(s): Store at 2°-7°C. Prolonged exposure to higher temperatures and/or direct sunlight may adversely affect potency. Do not freeze.

Use entire contents when first opened.

Sterilized syringes and needles should be used to administer this vaccine. Do not sterilize with chemicals because traces of disinfectant may inactivate the vaccine.

Burn containers and all unused contents.

Caution(s): Do not use in pregnant cows (abortions can result) or in calves nursing pregnant calves.

As with many vaccines, anaphylaxis may occur after use. Initial antidote of epinephrine is recommended and should be followed with appropriate supportive therapy.

This product has been shown to be efficacious in healthy animals. A protective immune response may not be elicited if animals are incubating an infectious disease, are malnourished or parasitized, are stressed due to shipment or environmental conditions, are otherwise immunocompromised, or the vaccine is not administered in accordance with label directions.

Warning(s): Do not vaccinate within 21 days before slaughter.

For veterinary use only.

Discussion: Disease Description: IBR, BVD, and PI$_3$ viruses are commonly associated with respiratory disease and/or reproductive failure in cattle. IBR virus infection is characterized by high temperature, excessive nasal discharge, conjunctivitis and ocular discharge, inflamed nose ("red nose"), increased rate of respiration, coughing, loss of appetite, and depression. Cattle infected during pregnancy may abort.

BVD virus may be transmitted in nasal secretions, saliva, blood, feces, and/or urine, and by direct contact with contaminated objects; it invades through the nose and mouth and replicates systemically. Infection during pregnancy may result in abortion, fetal resorption, or congenital malformation of the fetus. Moreover, if susceptible cows are infected with noncytopathic BVD virus during the first trimester of pregnancy, their calves may be born persistently infected with the virus. Exposure of those calves to certain virulent cytopathic BVD virus strains may precipitate BVD-mucosal disease. Clinical signs of BVD include loss of appetite, ulcerations in the mouth, profuse salivation, elevated temperature, diarrhea, dehydration, and lameness.

PI$_3$ virus usually localizes in the upper respiratory tract, causing elevated temperature and moderate nasal and ocular discharge. Although clinical signs typically are mild, PI$_3$ infection weakens respiratory tissues. Invasion and replication of other pathogens, particularly *Pasteurella* spp., is thereby facilitated and may result in pneumonia.

Trial Data: Safety and Efficacy: In safety studies of the fractions of BOVI-SHIELD™ 3, no adverse reactions to vaccination were observed.

Efficacy of each fraction of BOVI-SHIELD™ 3 was demonstrated in challenge-of-immunity studies. Cattle vaccinated with any fraction of BOVI-SHIELD™ 3, followed by challenge with a disease-causing strain of that fraction, showed no signs or had significantly fewer clinical signs than nonvaccinated control cattle. Serologic studies demonstrated no immunologic interference among the fractions of BOVI-SHIELD™ 3.

Presentation: 10 dose and 50 dose vials.

Compendium Code No.: 36900430 75-4148-01

BOVI-SHIELD™ 4

Pfizer Animal Health **Vaccine**

Bovine Rhinotracheitis-Virus Diarrhea-Parainfluenza$_3$-Respiratory Syncytial Virus Vaccine, Modified Live Virus

U.S. Vet. Lic. No.: 189

Description: BOVI-SHIELD™ 4 is a freeze-dried preparation of modified live virus (MLV) strains of IBR, BVD, PI$_3$, and BRSV viruses, plus a sterile diluent used to rehydrate the freeze-dried vaccine. Viral antigens are propagated on established cell lines.

Contains gentamicin as preservative.

Indications: BOVI-SHIELD™ 4 is for vaccination of healthy, nonpregnant cattle as an aid in preventing infectious bovine rhinotracheitis caused by infectious bovine rhinotracheitis (IBR) virus, bovine viral diarrhea (Type 1 and Type 2) caused by bovine viral diarrhea (BVD) virus, and disease caused by parainfluenza$_3$ (PI$_3$) virus and bovine respiratory syncytial virus (BRSV).

Directions:

1. General Directions: Vaccination of healthy, nonpregnant cattle is recommended. Aseptically rehydrate the freeze-dried vaccine with the sterile diluent provided, shake well, and administer 2 mL intramuscularly. In accordance with Beef Quality Assurance guidelines, this product should be administered in the muscular region of the neck.
2. Primary Vaccination: Administer a single 2 mL dose to healthy cattle, followed by a second dose of Bovi-Shield™ BRSV 3-4 weeks later.
3. Revaccination: Annual revaccination with a single dose is recommended.
4. Good animal husbandry and herd health management practices should be employed.

Precaution(s): Store at 2°-7°C. Prolonged exposure to higher temperatures and/or direct sunlight may adversely affect potency. Do not freeze.

Use entire contents when first opened.

Sterilized syringes and needles should be used to administer this vaccine. Do not sterilize with chemicals because traces of disinfectant may inactivate the vaccine.

Burn containers and all unused contents.

Caution(s): Do not use in pregnant cows (abortions can result) or in calves nursing pregnant cows.

As with many vaccines, anaphylaxis may occur after use. Initial antidote of epinephrine is recommended and should be followed with appropriate supportive therapy.

This product has been shown to be efficacious in healthy animals. A protective immune response may not be elicited if animals are incubating an infectious disease, are malnourished or parasitized, are stressed due to shipment or environmental conditions, are otherwise immunocompromised, or the vaccine is not administered in accordance with label directions.

Warning(s): Do not vaccinate within 21 days before slaughter.

For veterinary use only.

Discussion: Disease Description: IBR, BVD, PI$_3$, and BRSV viruses are commonly associated with respiratory disease and/or reproductive failure in cattle. IBR virus infection is characterized by high temperature, excessive nasal discharge, conjunctivitis and ocular discharge, inflamed nose ("red nose"), increased rate of respiration, coughing, loss of appetite, and depression. Cattle infected during pregnancy may abort.

BVD virus may be transmitted in nasal secretions, saliva, blood, feces, and/or urine, and by direct contact with contaminated objects; it invades through the nose and mouth and replicates systemically. Infection during pregnancy may result in abortion, fetal resorption, or congenital malformation of the fetus. Moreover, if susceptible cows are infected with noncytopathic BVD virus during the first trimester of pregnancy, their calves may be born persistently infected with the virus. Exposure of those calves to certain virulent cytopathic BVD virus strains may precipitate BVD-mucosal disease. Clinical signs of BVD include loss of appetite, ulcerations in the mouth, profuse salivation, elevated temperature, diarrhea, dehydration, and lameness.

PI$_3$ virus usually localizes in the upper respiratory tract, causing elevated temperature and moderate nasal and ocular discharge. Although clinical signs typically are mild, PI$_3$ infection weakens respiratory tissues. Invasion and replication of other pathogens, particularly *Pasteurella* spp., is thereby facilitated and may result in pneumonia.

BRSV is the etiologic agent of a specific viral respiratory disease of cattle of all ages, including nursing calves. Infection is characterized by rapid breathing, coughing, loss of appetite, discharge from the nose and eyes, fever, and swelling around the throat and neck. In an acute outbreak, deaths may follow within 48 hours after onset of signs. Clinically, BRSV infection may be indistinguishable from other viral infections associated with the bovine respiratory disease complex. BRSV infection, like PI$_3$, facilitates invasion and replication of other respiratory pathogens. Exacerbation of clinical signs has been documented when concurrent BRSV and BVD or IBR infection exists.

Trial Data: Safety and Efficacy: In safety studies of the fractions of BOVI-SHIELD™ 4, no adverse reactions to vaccination were observed.

Efficacy of each fraction of BOVI-SHIELD™ 4 was demonstrated in challenge-of-immunity studies. Cattle vaccinated with any fraction of BOVI-SHIELD™ 4, followed by challenge with a disease-causing strain of that fraction, showed no signs or had significantly fewer clinical signs than nonvaccinated control cattle. Serologic studies demonstrated no immunologic interference among the fractions of BOVI-SHIELD™ 4.

Presentation: 5 dose, 10 dose and 50 dose vials.

Compendium Code No.: 36900441 75-4156-02

BOVI-SHIELD™ BRSV

Pfizer Animal Health **Vaccine**

Bovine Respiratory Syncytial Virus Vaccine, Modified Live Virus

U.S. Vet. Lic. No.: 189

Description: BOVI-SHIELD™ BRSV is a freeze-dried preparation of an attenuated strain of BRSV propagated on an established bovine cell line, plus a sterile diluent used to rehydrate the freeze-dried vaccine.

Contains gentamicin as preservative.

Indications: BOVI-SHIELD™ BRSV is for vaccination of healthy cattle, including pregnant cows, as an aid in preventing disease caused by bovine respiratory syncytial virus (BRSV).

Directions:

1. General Directions: Vaccination of healthy cattle, including pregnant cows, is recommended. Aseptically rehydrate the freeze-dried vaccine with the sterile diluent provided, shake well, and administer 2 mL intramuscularly. In accordance with Beef Quality Assurance guidelines, this product should be administered in the muscular region of the neck.
2. Primary Vaccination: Healthy cattle should receive 2 doses administered 3-4 weeks apart. To avoid possible maternal antibody interference with active immunization, calves vaccinated before the age of 6 months should be revaccinated after 6 months of age.
3. Revaccination: Annual revaccination with a single dose is recommended.
4. Good animal husbandry and herd health management practices should be employed.

Precaution(s): Store at 2°-7°C. Prolonged exposure to higher temperatures and/or direct sunlight may adversely affect potency. Do not freeze.

Use entire contents when first opened.

Sterilized syringes and needles should be used to administer this vaccine. Do not sterilize with chemicals because traces of disinfectant may inactivate the vaccine.

Burn containers and all unused contents.

Caution(s): As with many vaccines, anaphylaxis may occur after use. Initial antidote of epinephrine is recommended and should be followed with appropriate supportive therapy.

This product has been shown to be efficacious in healthy animals. A protective immune response may not be elicited if animals are incubating an infectious disease, are malnourished or parasitized, are stressed due to shipment or environmental conditions, are otherwise immunocompromised, or the vaccine is not administered in accordance with label directions.

Warning(s): Do not vaccinate within 21 days before slaughter.

For veterinary use only.

Discussion: Disease Description: BRSV is the etiologic agent of a specific viral respiratory disease of cattle of all ages, including nursing calves.[1-4] Infection is characterized by rapid breathing, coughing, loss of appetite, discharge from the nose and eyes, fever, and swelling around the throat and neck. In an acute outbreak, deaths may follow within 48 hours after onset of signs. Pathology typically consists of subpleural and interstitial emphysema with consolidating lesions characteristic of pneumonia. Clinically, BRSV infection may be indistinguishable from other viral infections associated with the bovine respiratory disease complex. Exacerbation of clinical signs has been documented when concurrent BRSV and BVD or IBR infection exists.

Trial Data: Safety and Efficacy: Safety of BOVI-SHIELD™ BRSV was demonstrated by controlled testing in a comprehensive cross-section of over 28,000 healthy cattle under a variety of typical field conditions.[5,6] Test animals included calves ranging in age from 1-4 months old, bulls ranging in age from 5-9 months old, feeder cattle ranging in weight from 500-900 lb, dairy cows, and over 1,000 pregnant cows in all trimesters of pregnancy. BOVI-SHIELD™ BRSV was administered to test animals in two 2-mL intramuscular doses given 4 weeks apart, and the cattle were then observed over a 14-day period following each dose. The overall abortion rate for vaccinated pregnant cows was no greater than the generally referenced spontaneous abortion rate.[7-9] At conclusion of the studies, participating veterinarians reported no local or systemic adverse reactions related to use of the vaccine.

Efficacy of BOVI-SHIELD™ BRSV was demonstrated in challenge-of-immunity tests conducted under federally approved protocol. All vaccinated cattle remained clinically normal following challenge which produced typical signs of disease in nonvaccinated control cattle.

References: Available upon request.

Presentation: 10 dose and 50 dose vials.

Compendium Code No.: 36900380 75-4252-00

BOVI-SHIELD® FP 4+L5

Pfizer Animal Health **Bacterin-Vaccine**

Bovine Rhinotracheitis-Virus Diarrhea-Parainfluenza$_3$-Respiratory Syncytial Virus Vaccine, Modified Live Virus-Leptospira Canicola-Grippotyphosa-Hardjo-Icterohaemorrhagiae-Pomona Bacterin

U.S. Vet. Lic. No.: 189

Description: BOVI-SHIELD® FP 4+L5 is a freeze-dried preparation of modified live virus (MLV) strains of IBR, BVD, PI_3, and BRSV viruses, plus a liquid bacterin containing the 5 *Leptospira* serovars identified above. The liquid bacterin is used to rehydrate the freeze-dried vaccine. Viral antigens are propagated on established cell lines.

Contains gentamicin as preservative.

Indications: BOVI-SHIELD® FP 4+L5 is for vaccination of healthy cows and heifers prior to breeding as an aid in preventing abortion caused by infectious bovine rhinotracheitis (IBR, bovine herpesvirus Type 1) virus; persistent infection caused by bovine virus diarrhea (BVD) virus Types 1 and 2 fetal infection; respiratory disease caused by IBR, BVD Types 1 and 2, parainfluenza$_3$ (PI_3) and bovine respiratory syncytial virus (BRSV); and leptospirosis caused by *Leptospira canicola, L. grippotyphosa, L. hardjo, L. icterohaemorrhagiae,* and *L. pomona.*

Directions:

1. General Directions: Vaccination of healthy, non-pregnant cattle is recommended. Aseptically rehydrate the freeze-dried vaccine (Bovi-Shield™ 4) with the liquid bacterin provided (Leptoferm-5®+A), shake well, and administer 2 mL intramuscularly. In accordance with Beef Quality Assurance guidelines, this product should be administered in the muscular region of the neck.
2. Primary Vaccination: Administer a single 2 mL dose to healthy cattle, followed by a single dose of Bovi-Shield™ BRSV 3-4 weeks later. As an aid in preventing IBR and BVD fetal infections, administer a 2 mL dose approximately 1 month prior to breeding.
3. Revaccination: Annual revaccination with a single dose of BOVI-SHIELD® FP 4+L5 is recommended.
4. Good animal husbandry and herd health management practices should be employed.

Precaution(s): Store at 2°-7°C. Prolonged exposure to higher temperatures and/or direct sunlight may adversely affect potency. Do not freeze.

Use entire contents when first opened.

Sterilized syringes and needles should be used to administer this vaccine. Do not sterilize with chemicals because traces of disinfectant may inactivate the vaccine.

Burn containers and all unused contents.

Caution(s): Do not use in pregnant cows (abortions can result) or in calves nursing pregnant cows.

As with many vaccines, anaphylaxis may occur after use. Initial antidote of epinephrine is recommended and should be followed with appropriate supportive therapy.

This product has been shown to be efficacious in healthy animals. A protective immune response may not be elicited if animals are incubating an infectious disease, are malnourished or parasitized, are stressed due to shipment or environmental conditions, are otherwise immunocompromised, or the vaccine is not administered in accordance with label directions.

For veterinary use only.

Warning(s): Do not vaccinate within 21 days before slaughter.

Discussion: Disease Description: IBR, BVD, PI_3, and BRSV viruses are commonly associated with respiratory disease and/or reproductive failure in cattle. IBR virus infection is characterized by high temperature, excessive nasal discharge, conjunctivitis and ocular discharge, inflamed nose ("red nose"), increased rate of respiration, coughing, loss of appetite, and depression. Cattle infected during pregnancy may abort.

BVD virus may be transmitted in nasal secretions, saliva, blood, feces, and/or urine, and by direct contact with contaminated objects; it invades through the nose and mouth and replicates systemically. Infection during pregnancy may result in abortion, fetal resorption, or congenital malformation of the fetus. Moreover, if susceptible cows are infected with non-cytopathic BVD virus during the first trimester of pregnancy, their calves may be born persistently infected with the virus. Exposure of those calves to certain virulent cytopathic BVD virus strains may precipitate BVD-mucosal disease. Clinical signs of BVD include loss of appetite, ulcerations in the mouth, profuse salivation, elevated temperature, diarrhea, dehydration, and lameness.

PI_3 virus usually localizes in the upper respiratory tract, causing elevated temperature and moderate nasal and ocular discharge. Although clinical signs typically are mild, PI_3 infection weakens respiratory tissues. Invasion and replication of other pathogens, particularly *Pasteurella* spp., is thereby facilitated and may result in pneumonia.

BRSV is the etiologic agent of a specific viral respiratory disease of cattle of all ages, including nursing calves. Infection is characterized by rapid breathing, coughing, loss of appetite, discharge from the nose and eyes, fever, and swelling around the throat and neck. In an acute outbreak, deaths may follow within 48 hours after onset of signs. Clinically, BRSV infection may be indistinguishable from other viral infections associated with the bovine respiratory disease complex. BRSV infection, like PI_3, facilitates invasion and replication of other respiratory pathogens. Exacerbation of clinical signs has been documented when concurrent BRSV and BVD or IBR infection exists.

Leptospirosis may be caused by several serovars of *Leptospira*, of which *L. canicola, L. grippotyphosa, L. hardjo, L. icterohaemorrhagiae*, and *L. pomona* are the most common affecting cattle. *Leptospira* localize in the kidneys, are shed in the urine, and cause anaemia, bloody urine, fever, loss of appetite, and prostration in calves. Signs are usually subclinical in adult cattle. Infected pregnant cows, however, often abort, and dairy cows may exhibit a marked decrease in milk production. *Leptospira* spp. are known zoonotic pathogens.

Trial Data: Safety and Efficacy: In safety studies of the fractions of BOVI-SHIELD® FP 4+L5, no adverse reactions to vaccination were observed.

Efficacy of each fraction of BOVI-SHIELD® FP 4+L5 was demonstrated in challenge-of-immunity studies. Cattle vaccinated with any fraction of BOVI-SHIELD® FP 4+L5, followed by challenge with a disease-causing strain of that fraction, showed no signs or had significantly fewer clinical signs than non-vaccinated control cattle. Serologic studies demonstrated no immunologic interference among the fractions of BOVI-SHIELD® FP 4+L5. The effectiveness of BOVI-SHIELD® FP 4+L5 in preventing IBR-induced abortion was demonstrated by vaccinating susceptible heifers approximately 4 weeks prior to breeding. The vaccinated heifers, along with a group of non-vaccinated controls, were challenged with virulent IBR virus (Cooper strain) at approximately 190 days post-breeding. Results are summarized in the following table.

Group	No. of Pregnant Heifers	No. of Abortions[3,4]	Percent of Abortions[4]
Vaccinates[1]	20	1/20[3]	5.0%
Vaccinates[2]	20	0/20	0.0%
Controls	11	10/11[4]	91.0%[4]

[1] Vaccination with a single dose 1 month prior to breeding. Seronegative heifers with no history of vaccination with any product containing IBR or BVD vaccine viruses were selected for use in the efficacy studies.

[2] Vaccination with 2 doses at 5 months and 1 month prior to breeding.

[3] One stillbirth (IBR positive). Nineteen of 20 normal.

[4] Nine abortions (IBR positive). One calf appeared healthy at birth, subsequently became ill (IBR positive). One of 11 animals normal.

Similar study designs were used to demonstrate the effectiveness of the BVD fraction contained in BOVI-SHIELD® FP 4+L5 in preventing fetal infections associated with both Types 1 and 2 BVD. In these studies, vaccinated heifers, along with a group of non-vaccinated control heifers, were challenged with virulent strains of either BVD Type 1 or 2 viruses when fetal ages ranged from approximately 73-98 days. Results of these studies are summarized in the following table.

Group	Challenge	No. of Heifers Challenged	Viremia Heifers[3]	No. of Calves Evaluated	Calves BVD Positive[4]
Vaccinates[1]	BVD1	19	0/19 (0.0%)	19	1/19 (5.3%)
Vaccinates[2]	BVD1	19	0/19 (0.0%)	19	0/19 (0.0%)
Controls	BVD1	10	9/10 (90.0%)	10	7/10 (70.0%)
Vaccinates[1]	BVD2	20	1/20 (5.0%)	18	6/18 (33.3%)
Vaccinates[2]	BVD2	20	1/20 (5.0%)	19	7/19 (36.8%)
Controls	BVD2	10	9/10 (90.0%)	10	9/10 (90.0%)

[1] Vaccination with a single dose 1 month prior to breeding. Seronegative heifers with no history of vaccination with any product containing IBR or BVD vaccine viruses were selected for use in the efficacy studies.

[2] Vaccination with 2 doses at 5 months and 1 month prior to breeding.

[3] Virus isolations performed on whole blood samples collected on days 0, 2, 4, 6, 8, 10, and 14 post-challenge of heifers.

[4] Whole blood collected from calves on the day of calving and prior to nursing (pre-colostral) was tested for BVD virus. Full-thickness ear notch and skin sample biopsies were tested by immunocytochemistry evaluation for the presence of BVD virus. If any sample was determined to be positive, the fetus was considered persistently infected with BVD virus.

Presentation: 5 dose, 10 dose and 50 dose vials.

Compendium Code No.: 36900611 75-4168-03

BOVI-SHIELD™ IBR

Pfizer Animal Health **Vaccine**

Bovine Rhinotracheitis Vaccine, Modified Live Virus

U.S. Vet. Lic. No.: 189

Description: BOVI-SHIELD™ IBR is a freeze-dried preparation of a modified live virus (MLV) strain of the IBR virus, plus a sterile diluent used to rehydrate the freeze-dried vaccine. The viral antigen is propagated on an established cell line.

Contains gentamicin as preservative.

Indications: BOVI-SHIELD™ IBR is for vaccination of healthy, nonpregnant cattle as an aid in preventing infectious bovine rhinotracheitis caused by infectious bovine rhinotracheitis (IBR) virus.

Directions:

1. General Directions: Vaccination of healthy, nonpregnant cattle is recommended. Aseptically rehydrate the freeze-dried vaccine with the sterile diluent provided, shake well, and administer 2 mL intramuscularly. In accordance with Beef Quality Assurance guidelines, this product should be administered in the muscular region of the neck.

2. Primary Vaccination: Administer a single 2 mL dose to healthy cattle. To avoid possible maternal antibody interference with active immunization, calves vaccinated before the age of 6 months should be revaccinated after 6 months of age.
3. Revaccination: Annual revaccination with a single dose is recommended.
4. Good animal husbandry and herd health management practices should be employed.

Precaution(s): Store at 2°-7°C. Prolonged exposure to higher temperatures and/or direct sunlight may adversely affect potency. Do not freeze.

Use entire contents when first opened.

Sterilized syringes and needles should be used to administer this vaccine. Do not sterilize with chemicals because traces of disinfectant may inactivate the vaccine.

Burn containers and all unused contents.

Caution(s): Do not use in pregnant cows (abortions can result) or in calves nursing pregnant cows.

As with many vaccines, anaphylaxis may occur after use. Initial antidote of epinephrine is recommended and should be followed with appropriate supportive therapy.

This product has been shown to be efficacious in healthy animals. A protective immune response may not be elicited if animals are incubating an infectious disease, are malnourished or parasitized, are stressed due to shipment or environmental conditions, are otherwise immunocompromised, or the vaccine is not administered in accordance with label directions.

Warning(s): Do not vaccinate within 21 days before slaughter.

For veterinary use only.

Discussion: Disease Description: IBR virus is commonly associated with respiratory disease and/or reproductive failure in cattle. Infection is characterized by high temperature, excessive nasal discharge, conjunctivitis and ocular discharge, inflamed nose ("red nose"), increased rate of respiration, coughing, loss of appetite, and depression. Cattle infected during pregnancy may abort.

Trial Data: Safety and Efficacy: In safety studies with the IBR fraction of BOVI-SHIELD™ IBR, no adverse reactions to vaccination were observed.

Efficacy of the IBR fraction of BOVI-SHIELD™ IBR was demonstrated in a challenge-of-immunity study. Cattle vaccinated with the IBR fraction, followed by challenge with a disease-causing strain of IBR virus, had significantly fewer clinical signs than nonvaccinated control cattle.

Presentation: 50 dose vial.

Compendium Code No.: 36900720 75-4179-00

BOVI-SHIELD™ IBR-BRSV-LP

Pfizer Animal Health **Bacterin-Vaccine**

Bovine Rhinotracheitis-Respiratory Syncytial Virus Vaccine, Modified Live Virus-Leptospira Pomona Bacterin

U.S. Vet. Lic. No.: 189

Description: BOVI-SHIELD™ IBR-BRSV-LP is a freeze-dried preparation of modified live virus (MLV) strains of IBR and BRSV viruses, plus a liquid bacterin containing *L. pomona.* The liquid bacterin is used to rehydrate the freeze-dried vaccine. Viral antigens are propagated on established cell lines.

Contains gentamicin as preservative.

Indications: BOVI-SHIELD™ IBR-BRSV-LP is for vaccination of healthy, nonpregnant cattle as an aid in preventing infectious bovine rhinotracheitis caused by infectious bovine rhinotracheitis (IBR) virus, disease caused by infectious bovine respiratory syncytial virus (BRSV), and leptospirosis caused by *Leptospira pomona.*

Directions:

1. General Directions: Vaccination of healthy, nonpregnant cattle is recommended. Aseptically rehydrate the freeze-dried vaccine with the liquid bacterin provided, shake well, and administer 2 mL intramuscularly. In accordance with Beef Quality Assurance guidelines, this product should be administered in the muscular region of the neck.
2. Primary Vaccination: Administer a single 2 mL dose to healthy cattle, followed by a second dose of Bovi-Shield™ BRSV 3-4 weeks later.
3. Revaccination: Annual revaccination with a single dose is recommended.
4. Good animal husbandry and herd health management practices should be employed.

Precaution(s): Store at 2°-7°C. Prolonged exposure to higher temperatures and/or direct sunlight may adversely affect potency. Do not freeze.

Use entire contents when first opened.

Sterilized syringes and needles should be used to administer this vaccine. Do not sterilize with chemicals because traces of disinfectant may inactivate the vaccine.

Burn containers and all unused contents.

Caution(s): Do not use in pregnant cows (abortions can result) or in calves nursing pregnant cows.

As with many vaccines, anaphylaxis may occur after use. Initial antidote of epinephrine is recommended and should be followed with appropriate supportive therapy.

This product has been shown to be efficacious in healthy animals. A protective immune response may not be elicited if animals are incubating an infectious disease, are malnourished or parasitized, are stressed due to shipment or environmental conditions, are otherwise immunocompromised, or the vaccine is not administered in accordance with label directions.

Warning(s): Do not vaccinate within 21 days before slaughter.

For veterinary use only.

Discussion: Disease Description: IBR and BRSV viruses are commonly associated with respiratory disease and/or reproductive failure in cattle. IBR virus infection is characterized by high temperature, excessive nasal discharge, conjunctivitis and ocular discharge, inflamed nose ("red nose"), increased rate of respiration, coughing, loss of appetite, and depression. Cattle infected during pregnancy may abort.

BRSV is the etiologic agent of a specific viral respiratory disease of cattle of all ages, including nursing calves. Infection is characterized by rapid breathing, coughing, loss of appetite, discharge from the nose and eyes, fever, and swelling around the throat and neck. In an acute outbreak, deaths may follow within 48 hours after onset of signs. Clinically, BRSV infection may be indistinguishable from other viral infections associated with the bovine respiratory disease complex. BRSV infection facilitates invasion and replication of other respiratory pathogens. Exacerbation of clinical signs has been documented when concurrent BRSV and BVD or IBR infection exists.

Leptospirosis may be caused by several serovars of *Leptospira*, of which *L. pomona* is one of the most common affecting cattle. *Leptospira* localize in the kidneys, are shed in the urine, and cause anaemia, bloody urine, fever, loss of appetite, and prostration in calves. Signs are usually subclinical in adult cattle. Infected pregnant cows, however, often abort, and dairy cows may exhibit a marked decrease in milk production. *Leptospira* spp. are known zoonotic pathogens.

Trial Data: Safety and Efficacy: In safety studies of the fractions of BOVI-SHIELD™ IBR-BRSV-LP, no adverse reactions to vaccination were observed.

Efficacy of each fraction of BOVI-SHIELD™ IBR-BRSV-LP was demonstrated in challenge-of-immunity studies. Cattle vaccinated with any fraction of BOVI-SHIELD™ IBR-BRSV-LP, followed by challenge with a disease-causing strain of that fraction, showed no signs or had significantly fewer clinical signs than nonvaccinated control cattle. Serologic studies demonstrated no immunologic interference among the fractions of BOVI-SHIELD™ IBR-BRSV-LP.

Presentation: 10 dose and 50 dose vials.

Compendium Code No.: 36900590 75-4180-00

B

BOVI-SHIELD™ IBR-BVD

Pfizer Animal Health **Vaccine**

Bovine Rhinotracheitis-Virus Diarrhea Vaccine, Modified Live Virus

U.S. Vet. Lic. No.: 189

Description: BOVI-SHIELD™ IBR-BVD is a freeze-dried preparation of modified live virus (MLV) strains of IBR and BVD viruses. The sterile diluent is used to rehydrate the freeze-dried vaccine. Viral antigens are propagated on established cell lines.

Contains gentamicin as preservative.

Indications: BOVI-SHIELD™ IBR-BVD is for vaccination of healthy, nonpregnant cattle as an aid in preventing infectious bovine rhinotracheitis caused by infectious bovine rhinotracheitis (IBR) virus and bovine viral diarrhea (Type 1 and Type 2) caused by bovine viral diarrhea (BVD) virus.

Directions:

1. General Directions: Vaccination of healthy, nonpregnant cattle is recommended. Aseptically rehydrate the freeze-dried vaccine with the sterile diluent provided, shake well, and administer 2 mL intramuscularly. In accordance with Beef Quality Assurance guidelines, this product should be administered in the muscular region of the neck.
2. Primary Vaccination: Administer a single 2 mL dose to healthy cattle. To avoid possible maternal antibody interference with active immunization, calves vaccinated before the age of 6 months should be revaccinated after 6 months of age.
3. Revaccination: Annual revaccination with a single dose is recommended.
4. Good animal husbandry and herd health management practices should be employed.

Precaution(s): Store at 2°-7°C. Prolonged exposure to higher temperatures and/or direct sunlight may adversely affect potency. Do not freeze.

Use entire contents when first opened.

Sterilized syringes and needles should be used to administer this vaccine. Do not sterilize with chemicals because traces of disinfectant may inactivate the vaccine.

Burn containers and all unused contents.

Caution(s): Do not use in pregnant cows (abortions can result) or in calves nursing pregnant cows.

As with many vaccines, anaphylaxis may occur after use. Initial antidote of epinephrine is recommended and should be followed with appropriate supportive therapy.

This product has been shown to be efficacious in healthy animals. A protective immune response may not be elicited if animals are incubating an infectious disease, are malnourished or parasitized, are stressed due to shipment or environmental conditions, are otherwise immunocompromised, or the vaccine is not administered in accordance with label directions.

Warning(s): Do not vaccinate within 21 days before slaughter.

For veterinary use only.

Discussion: Disease Description: IBR and BVD viruses are commonly associated with respiratory disease and/or reproductive failure in cattle. IBR virus infection is characterized by high temperature, excessive nasal discharge, conjunctivitis and ocular discharge, inflamed nose ("red nose"), increased rate of respiration, coughing, loss of appetite, and depression. Cattle infected during pregnancy may abort.

BVD virus may be transmitted in nasal secretions, saliva, blood, feces, and/or urine, and by direct contact with contaminated objects; it invades through the nose and mouth and replicates systemically. Infection during pregnancy may result in abortion, fetal resorption, or congenital malformation of the fetus. Moreover, if susceptible cows are infected with noncytopathic BVD virus during the first trimester of pregnancy, their calves may be born persistently infected with the virus. Exposure of those calves to certain virulent cytopathic BVD virus strains may precipitate BVD-mucosal disease. Clinical signs of BVD include loss of appetite, ulcerations in the mouth, profuse salivation, elevated temperature, diarrhea, dehydration, and lameness.

Trial Data: Safety and Efficacy: In safety studies of the fractions of BOVI-SHIELD™ IBR-BVD, no adverse reactions to vaccination were observed.

Efficacy of each fraction of BOVI-SHIELD™ IBR-BVD was demonstrated in challenge-of-immunity studies. Cattle vaccinated with either fraction of BOVI-SHIELD™ IBR-BVD, followed by challenge with a disease-causing strain of that fraction, showed no signs or had significantly fewer clinical signs than nonvaccinated control cattle. Serologic studies demonstrated no immunologic interference between the fractions of BOVI-SHIELD™ IBR-BVD.

Presentation: 10 dose and 50 dose vials.

Compendium Code No.: 36900420 75-4124-01

BOVI-SHIELD™ IBR-BVD-BRSV-LP

Pfizer Animal Health **Bacterin-Vaccine**

Bovine Rhinotracheitis-Virus Diarrhea-Respiratory Syncytial Virus Vaccine, Modified Live Virus-Leptospira Pomona Bacterin

U.S. Vet. Lic. No.: 189

Description: BOVI-SHIELD™ IBR-BVD-BRSV-LP is a freeze-dried preparation of modified live virus (MLV) strains of IBR, BVD, and BRSV viruses, plus a liquid bacterin containing *L. pomona.* The liquid bacterin is used to rehydrate the freeze-dried vaccine. Viral antigens are propagated on established cell lines.

Contains gentamicin as preservative.

Indications: BOVI-SHIELD™ IBR-BVD-BRSV-LP is for vaccination of healthy, nonpregnant cattle as an aid in preventing infectious bovine rhinotracheitis caused by infectious bovine rhinotracheitis (IBR) virus, bovine viral diarrhea (Type 1 and Type 2) caused by bovine viral diarrhea (BVD) virus, disease caused by bovine respiratory syncytial virus (BRSV), and leptospirosis caused by *Leptospira pomona.*

Directions:

1. General Directions: Vaccination of healthy, nonpregnant cattle is recommended. Aseptically rehydrate the freeze-dried vaccine with the liquid bacterin provided, shake well, and administer 2 mL intramuscularly. In accordance with Beef Quality Assurance guidelines, this product should be administered in the muscular region of the neck.
2. Primary Vaccination: Administer a single 2 mL dose to healthy cattle, followed by a second dose of Bovi-Shield™ BRSV 3-4 weeks later.
3. Revaccination: Annual revaccination with a single dose is recommended.
4. Good animal husbandry and herd health management practices should be employed.

Precaution(s): Store at 2°-7°C. Prolonged exposure to higher temperatures and/or direct sunlight may adversely affect potency. Do not freeze.

Use entire contents when first opened.

Sterilized syringes and needles should be used to administer this vaccine. Do not sterilize with chemicals because traces of disinfectant may inactivate the vaccine.

Burn containers and all unused contents.

Caution(s): Do not use in pregnant cows (abortions can result) or in calves nursing pregnant cows.

As with many vaccines, anaphylaxis may occur after use. Initial antidote of epinephrine is recommended and should be followed with appropriate supportive therapy.

This product has been shown to be efficacious in healthy animals. A protective immune response may not be elicited if animals are incubating an infectious disease, are malnourished or parasitized, are stressed due to shipment or environmental conditions, are otherwise immunocompromised, or the vaccine is not administered in accordance with label directions.

Warning(s): Do not vaccinate within 21 days before slaughter.

For veterinary use only.

Discussion: Disease Description: IBR, BVD, and BRSV viruses are commonly associated with respiratory disease and/or reproductive failure in cattle. IBR virus infection is characterized by high temperature, excessive nasal discharge, conjunctivitis and ocular discharge, inflamed nose ("red nose"), increased rate of respiration, coughing, loss of appetite, and depression. Cattle infected during pregnancy may abort.

BVD virus may be transmitted in nasal secretions, saliva, blood, feces, and/or urine, and by direct contact with contaminated objects; it invades through the nose and mouth and replicates systemically. Infection during pregnancy may result in abortion, fetal resorption, or congenital malformation of the fetus. Moreover, if susceptible cows are infected with noncytopathic BVD virus during the first trimester of pregnancy, their calves may be born persistently infected with the virus. Exposure of those calves to certain virulent cytopathic BVD virus strains may precipitate BVD-mucosal disease. Clinical signs of BVD include loss of appetite, ulcerations in the mouth, profuse salivation, elevated temperature, diarrhea, dehydration, and lameness.

BRSV is the etiologic agent of a specific viral respiratory disease of cattle of all ages, including nursing calves. Disease is characterized by rapid breathing, coughing, loss of appetite, discharge from the nose and eyes, fever, and swelling around the throat and neck. In an acute outbreak, deaths may follow within 48 hours after onset of signs. Clinically, BRSV infection may be indistinguishable from other viral infections associated with the bovine respiratory disease complex. BRSV infection facilitates invasion and replication of other respiratory pathogens. Exacerbation of clinical signs has been documented when concurrent BRSV and BVD or IBR infection exists.

Leptospirosis may be caused by several serovars of *Leptospira*, of which *L. pomona* is one of the most common affecting cattle. *Leptospira* localize in the kidneys, are shed in the urine, and cause anaemia, bloody urine, fever, loss of appetite, and prostration in calves. Signs are usually subclinical in adult cattle. Infected pregnant cows, however, often abort, and dairy cows may exhibit a marked decrease in milk production. *Leptospira* spp. are known zoonotic pathogens.

Trial Data: Safety and Efficacy: In safety studies of the fractions of BOVI-SHIELD™ IBR-BVD-BRSV-LP, no adverse reactions to vaccination were observed.

Efficacy of each fraction of BOVI-SHIELD™ IBR-BVD-BRSV-LP was demonstrated in challenge-of-immunity studies. Cattle vaccinated with any fraction of BOVI-SHIELD™ IBR-BVD-BRSV-LP, followed by challenge with a disease-causing strain of that fraction, showed no signs or had significantly fewer clinical signs than nonvaccinated control cattle. Serologic studies demonstrated no immunologic interference among the fractions of BOVI-SHIELD™ IBR-BVD-BRSV-LP.

Presentation: 10 dose and 50 dose vials.

Compendium Code No.: 36900600 75-4129-01

BOVI-SHIELD™ IBR-PI_3-BRSV

Pfizer Animal Health **Vaccine**

Bovine Rhinotracheitis-Parainfluenza$_3$-Respiratory Syncytial Virus Vaccine, Modified Live Virus

U.S. Vet. Lic. No.: 189

Description: BOVI-SHIELD™ IBR-PI_3-BRSV is a freeze-dried preparation of modified live virus (MLV) strains of IBR, PI_3, and BRSV viruses, plus a sterile diluent used to rehydrate the freeze-dried vaccine. Viral antigens are propagated on established cell lines.

Contains gentamicin as preservative.

Indications: BOVI-SHIELD™ IBR-PI_3-BRSV is for vaccination of healthy, nonpregnant cattle as an aid in preventing infectious bovine rhinotracheitis caused by infectious bovine rhinotracheitis (IBR) virus, and disease caused by parainfluenza$_3$ (PI_3) virus and bovine respiratory syncytial virus (BRSV).

Directions:

1. General Directions: Vaccination of healthy, nonpregnant cattle is recommended. Aseptically rehydrate the freeze-dried vaccine with the sterile diluent provided, shake well, and administer 2 mL intramuscularly. In accordance with Beef Quality Assurance guidelines, this product should be administered in the muscular region of the neck.
2. Primary Vaccination: Administer a single 2 mL dose to healthy cattle, followed by a second dose of Bovi-Shield™ BRSV 3-4 weeks later.
3. Revaccination: Annual revaccination with a single dose is recommended.
4. Good animal husbandry and herd health management practices should be employed.

Precaution(s): Store at 2°-7°C. Prolonged exposure to higher temperatures and/or direct sunlight may adversely affect potency. Do not freeze.

Use entire contents when first opened.

Sterilized syringes and needles should be used to administer this vaccine. Do not sterilize with chemicals because traces of disinfectant may inactivate the vaccine.

Burn containers and all unused contents.

Caution(s): Do not use in pregnant cows (abortions can result) or in calves nursing pregnant cows.

As with many vaccines, anaphylaxis may occur after use. Initial antidote of epinephrine is recommended and should be followed with appropriate supportive therapy.

This product has been shown to be efficacious in healthy animals. A protective immune response may not be elicited if animals are incubating an infectious disease, are malnourished or parasitized, are stressed due to shipment or environmental conditions, are otherwise immunocompromised, or the vaccine is not administered in accordance with label directions.

Warning(s): Do not vaccinate within 21 days before slaughter.

For veterinary use only.

Discussion: Disease Description: IBR, PI_3, and BRSV viruses are commonly associated with respiratory disease and/or reproductive failure in cattle. IBR virus infection is characterized by high temperature, excessive nasal discharge, conjunctivitis and ocular discharge, inflamed nose ("red nose"), increased rate of respiration, coughing, loss of appetite, and depression. Cattle infected during pregnancy may abort.

PI_3 virus usually localizes in the upper respiratory tract, causing elevated temperature and moderate nasal and ocular discharge. Although clinical signs typically are mild, PI_3 infection weakens respiratory tissues. Invasion and replication of other pathogens, particularly *Pasteurella* spp., is thereby facilitated and may result in pneumonia.

BRSV is the etiologic agent of a specific viral respiratory disease of cattle of all ages, including nursing calves. Infection is characterized by rapid breathing, coughing, loss of appetite, discharge from the nose and eyes, fever, and swelling around the throat and neck. In an acute outbreak, deaths may follow within 48 hours after onset of signs. Clinically, BRSV infection may be indistinguishable from other viral infections associated with the bovine respiratory disease complex. BRSV infection, like PI_3, facilitates invasion and replication of other respiratory pathogens. Exacerbation of clinical signs has been documented when concurrent BRSV and BVD or IBR infection exists.

Trial Data: Safety and Efficacy: In safety studies of the fractions of BOVI-SHIELD™ IBR-PI_3-BRSV, no adverse reactions to vaccination were observed.

Efficacy of each fraction of BOVI-SHIELD™ IBR-PI_3-BRSV was demonstrated in challenge-of-immunity studies. Cattle vaccinated with any fraction of BOVI-SHIELD™ IBR-PI_3-BRSV, followed by challenge with a disease-causing strain of that fraction, showed no signs or had significantly fewer clinical signs than nonvaccinated control cattle. Serologic studies demonstrated no immunologic interference among the fractions of BOVI-SHIELD™ IBR-PI_3-BRSV.

Presentation: 10 dose and 50 dose vials.

Compendium Code No.: 36900400 75-4194-00

BOVISPEC™* STERILE SOLUTION ℞

Vet Tek **Spectinomycin Injection**

Brand of spectinomycin sulfate sterile solution

NADA No.: 141-077

Active Ingredient(s): Each mL of BOVISPEC™ Sterile Solution contains spectinomycin sulfate tetrahydrate equivalent to 100 mg spectinomycin; and 9.45 mg benzyl alcohol, added as preservative. The pH was adjusted with hydrochloric acid or sodium hydroxide.

Indications: BOVISPEC™ Sterile Solution is indicated for the treatment of bovine respiratory disease (pneumonia) associated with *Pasteurella haemolytica, Pasteurella multocida,* and *Haemophilus somnus.*

Pharmacology: BOVISPEC™ Sterile Solution contains the sulfate salt of spectinomycin, an aminocyclitol antibiotic produced by *Streptomyces spectabilis.*

Figure 1. Chemical structure of spectinomycin sulfate tetrahydrate

The chemical name of spectinomycin sulfate tetrahydrate is: Decahydro-4a,7,9-trihydroxy-2-methyl-6,8-bis (methylamino)-4*H*-pyrano [2,3-*b*][1,4]benzodioxin-4-one sulfate, tetrahydrate.

Microbiology: Spectinomycin is bacteriostatic and exerts its antibacterial effect by binding to the 30S ribosome and inhibiting bacterial protein synthesis. Spectinomycin has activity against a variety of gram-negative bacteria, some mycoplasma, and a limited number of gram-positive bacteria. Generally, it is not active against anaerobic bacteria.

Spectinomycin has demonstrated *in vitro* and *in vivo* activity against the three major pathogenic bacteria *(Pasteurella haemolytica, Pasteurella multocida,* and *Haemophilus somnus)* associated with bovine respiratory disease (pneumonia).

Spectinomycin has also demonstrated *in vitro* activity against *Actinomyces pyogenes, Mycoplasma bovis,* and *Mycoplasma dispar.* The clinical significance of this *in vitro* activity in cattle has not been demonstrated.

Dosage and Administration: BOVISPEC™ Sterile Solution is to be administered to cattle at a daily dose of 10 to 15 mg spectinomycin per kg of body weight (4.5 to 6.8 mL per 100 lb body weight). Treatment should be administered at 24-hour intervals for 3 to 5 consecutive days. Selection of dose (10 to 15 mg/kg/day) and duration of treatment (3 to 5 days) should be based on an assessment of the severity of disease, pathogen susceptibility, and clinical response. Do not inject more than 50 mL per site.

BOVISPEC™ Sterile Solution is to be administered to cattle by subcutaneous injection in the neck.

Contraindication(s): As with all drugs, the use of BOVISPEC™ Sterile Solution is contraindicated in animals previously found to be hypersensitive to the drug.

Precaution(s): Storage Conditions: Store at controlled room temperature 20° to 25°C (68° to 77°F) [for additional information see USP]. Protect from freezing.

Caution(s): Federal (USA) law restricts this drug to use by or on the order of a licensed veterinarian.

The safety of BOVISPEC™ Sterile Solution has not been determined for cattle intended for breeding.

Discoloration at the injection site may persist beyond 11 days after injection. This may necessitate trimming of the injection site and surrounding tissues at slaughter.

For use in animals only.

Restricted drug—Use only as directed (California).

Warning(s): Residue Warnings: Treated cattle must not be slaughtered for 11 days following last treatment. Dosages administered either in excess of the approved maximum dose or by unapproved routes may result in illegal residues in edible tissues.

A withdrawal period has not been established for this product in pre-ruminating calves. Do not use in calves to be processed for veal.

A milk discard period has not been established for this product in lactating dairy cattle. Do not use in female dairy cattle 20 months of age or older. Use of spectinomycin in this class of cattle may cause drug residues in milk.

Human Warnings: Not for human use. Keep out of reach of children.

As with other antibiotics, allergic reactions may occur in previously sensitized individuals. Repeated or prolonged exposure may lead to sensitization. Avoid direct contact with skin, eyes, mouth, and clothing. Persons with a known hypersensitivity to spectinomycin should avoid exposure to this product.

In case of accidental eye exposure, flush with water for 15 minutes. In case of accidental skin exposure, wash with soap and water. Seek medical attention if allergic reactions occur.

The material safety data sheet contains more detailed occupational safety information. To report adverse effects in users, to obtain more information or obtain a material safety data sheet, call 1-800-253-8600.

Trial Data: Animal Safety: Cattle: When spectinomycin sulfate sterile solution was administered at 10 times (150 mg/kg/day) the maximum daily recommended therapeutic dose for 5 days, treatment-related effects included increased relative kidney weights in heifers and steers, squamous and transitional epithelial cells in the urine of steers, and decreased urinary pH in steers. Urinalysis was not performed on the heifers in this study. Minimal injection site reactions were also present at 1 day and 4 days post injection.

When spectinomycin sulfate sterile solution was administered at doses of 15, 45, or 75 mg/kg/day (1X, 3X, or 5X the maximum daily recommended therapeutic dose) for 15 days, treatment-related effects included decreased urinary pH and mild swelling at injection sites. At necropsy, labeled injection sites examined at 1 day and 8 days after injection of 30 mL of spectinomycin sulfate sterile solution had dark red, tan, brown, and/or dark brown areas, often with some expansion (thickening) of the subcutis. Only mild discoloration was observed on gross examination of injection sites at 15 days after injection.

When spectinomycin sulfate sterile solution was administered subcutaneously at a dose of 15 mg/kg/day to 152 crossbred beef calves with naturally occurring BRD in clinical field trials, one calf died following the second daily injection. The cause of death following a gross necropsy was reported as an anaphylactic reaction.

Adverse Reactions: The use of BOVISPEC™ Sterile Solution may result in mild swelling at the injection site.

Anaphylactic reactions may occur in animals previously sensitized.

Presentation: BOVISPEC™ Sterile Solution is available in the following package size: 500 mL vial (NDC 30798-678-17).

Manufactured by: Pharmacia & Upjohn, S.A. de C.V., Calzada de Tlalpan # 2962, 04870 Mexico, D.F.

*Trademark of Pharmacia & Upjohn Animal Health

Compendium Code No.: 14200270 7373-07-000

BP-1

AgriPharm **Large Animal Dietary Supplement**

Active Ingredient(s): Vegetable oil, dextrose, dried egg, sorbitan monostearate, *Lactobacillus acidophilus, Bifidobacterium thermophilum, Bifidobacterium longum, Streptococcus faecium,* and Lactase enzymes.

Guaranteed analysis: Represented as total colony forming units. 20 billion colony forming units per pound, equivalent to approximately 44 million colony forming units per gram.

Indications: BP-1 contains bovine host specific lactic acid producing bacteria to provide an oral source of these bacteria. The bacteria were selected for their ability to be compatible in a wide range of gut conditions.

Dosage and Administration: Administer orally on the back of the tongue.

Beef cattle; incoming/stockers/weanings:

Preshipment:

Under 400 lbs.	10 g
Over 400 lbs.	15 g
First and last day of clinical therapy	15 g
Newborn calves	5 g at birth

Dairy cattle:

Cows:

Freshening	30 g
First and last day of clinical therapy	15 g
Newborn calves	5 g at birth

The product does not contain medication.

Precaution(s): Store in a cool place.

Refrigeration is recommended for extended storage periods.

Caution(s): For animal use only. Keep out of the reach of children.

Not intended for use as a source of antibodies.

Presentation: 60 g and 300 g containers.

Compendium Code No.: 14570150

BP-1 SPECIAL BLEND

AgriPharm **Large Animal Dietary Supplement**

Guaranteed Analysis: Represented as total colony forming units. 20 x 10^9 colony forming units per pound, equivalent to approximately 4.4 x 10^7 colony forming units per gram.

Ingredients: Vegetable oil, dextrose, dried egg, sorbitan monostearate, *Lactobacillus acidophilus, Bifidobacterium thermophilum, Bifidobacterium longum, Streptococcus faecium,* and lactase enzymes.

Indications: BP-1 SPECIAL BLEND contains bovine host specific lactic acid producing bacteria providing an oral source of these bacteria. These bacteria were selected for their ability to be compatible in a wide range of gut conditions.

This product contains a source of live naturally occurring microorganisms.

Dosage and Administration: Administer orally on back of tongue.

Beef Cattle (Incoming/Stockers/Weanlings):

Preshipment:

Under 400 lbs	10 gm
Over 400 lbs.	15 gm
1st and Last Day of Clinical Therapy	15 gm
Newborn Calves	5 gm at birth

Dairy cattle:

Cows:

Freshening	30 gm
1st and Last Day of Clinical Therapy	15 gm
Newborn Calves	5 gm at birth

Precaution(s): Store in a cool place. Refrigeration recommended for extended storage periods.

Warning(s): For animal use only. Keep out of reach of children.

Presentation: 60 g and 300 g.

Compendium Code No.: 14570160

B-PLUS

Alpharma **Water Additive**

Guaranteed Analysis: Per Pound:

Riboflavin	13,200 mg
d-Pantothenic Acid	56,000 mg
Niacinamide	132,000 mg
Vitamin B_{12}	40 mg
Ascorbic Acid	40,000 mg
Folic Acid	1,680 mg
Biotin	200 mg
Thiamine	8,000 mg
Pyridoxine	4,000 mg

Ingredients: Niacinamide, sodium chloride, potassium chloride, d-calcium pantothenic acid, ascorbic acid, riboflavin, biotin supplement, thiamine HCl, vitamin B_{12} supplement, pyridoxine HCl, folic acid.

Indications: Use water-soluble B-PLUS in poultry drinking water during periods of stress such as extremes in temperature (high or low), before and after transportation, or when conditions interfere with normal routine.

Directions: Mix 1 pack in 256 gallons of water.

Precaution(s): Store in cool, dry place.

Caution(s): For oral animal use only.

Not for human use.

Keep out of reach of children.

Presentation: 4 oz (113.4 g).

Compendium Code No.: 10220140 AHF-033A 0003

BRATIVAC®

Pfizer Animal Health **Bacterin**

Leptospira Bratislava Bacterin

U.S. Vet. Lic. No.: 189

Description: BRATIVAC® contains chemically inactivated whole cultures of the *Leptospira* serovar listed above.

Indications: BRATIVAC® is for vaccination of healthy swine as an aid in the prevention of leptospirosis caused by *Leptospira bratislava.*

Directions:

1. General Directions: Shake well. Aseptically administer 2 mL intramuscularly.
2. Primary Vaccination: Healthy swine should receive 2 doses administered 2-6 weeks apart, beginning 2-6 weeks before breeding.
3. Revaccination: Revaccination with a single dose is recommended prior to or at breeding.
4. Good animal husbandry and herd health management practices should be employed.

Precaution(s): Store at 2°-7°C. Prolonged exposure to higher temperatures may adversely affect potency. Do not freeze.

Use entire contents when first opened.

Sterilized syringes and needles should be used to administer this vaccine.

Caution(s): As with many vaccines, anaphylaxis may occur after use. Initial antidote of epinephrine is recommended and should be followed with appropriate supportive therapy.

This product has been shown to be efficacious in healthy animals. A protective immune response may not be elicited if animals are incubating an infectious disease, are malnourished or parasitized, are stressed due to shipment or environmental conditions, are otherwise immunocompromised, or the vaccine is not administered in accordance with label directions.

Warning(s): Do not vaccinate within 21 days before slaughter.

For use in swine only. For veterinary use only.

Discussion: Disease Description: Leptospirosis is a worldwide disease of animals and humans and causes serious economic loss to the swine industry.[1] The disease is usually transmitted by direct or indirect contact with leptospiral-infected urine, but there is substantial evidence for venereal transmission of *L. bratislava.*[2-4]

Leptospirosis in swine is characterized by poor productivity, fever, anemia, kidney inflammation, and abortions. Late-term abortions are the most important effect. *Leptospira* serovars produce similar clinical signs, yet immunity to leptospirosis is serovar-specific.[1] Recent studies on the epidemiology and pathogenesis of *L. bratislava* provide evidence for an association between infection of swine and poor reproductive performance.[5]

Trial Data: Safety and Efficacy: During developmental tests and in field use of BRATIVAC®, no significant postvaccination reactions were reported.

L. bratislava is fastidious in its growth requirements and has proven difficult to isolate. However, *L. bratislava* has been isolated in aborted pigs and fetuses in European studies; and in 1986, Ellis and Thiermann reported the isolation of *L. bratislava* from the kidney and genital tract of 2 sows in the United States.[2,3] Subsequently, *L. bratislava* was also isolated in the United States from weak pigs, stillborn pigs, and swine placental tissues.[6,7] Recent serological surveys show that infections of swine by *L. bratislava* are prevalent. Antibody to *L. bratislava,* detectable by the microscopic agglutination test (MAT), has been shown to be present in sera from greater than 30% of finishing pigs and 50% of adult pigs.[4,5] Furthermore, controlled vaccination studies conducted in swine herds showing evidence of infection and poor reproductive performance support the conclusion that *L. bratislava* can be controlled through vaccination.[5]

Challenge-of-immunity tests were conducted by scientists at the Veterinary Research Laboratories, Belfast, Northern Ireland to determine the efficacy of BRATIVAC® against virulent isolates of *L. bratislava.* Fifteen pigs were divided into 2 groups. Ten pigs were administered 2 doses of BRATIVAC® in 2-mL doses given 2 weeks apart, and a group of 5 pigs was used as nonvaccinated controls. Subsequently, all pigs were challenged with virulent strains of *L. bratislava.* After challenge, *L. bratislava* was recovered from the kidneys of all 5 control pigs and from the oviduct of one of them. In contrast, leptospires were not recovered from the kidneys or genital tracts of the 10 vaccinated pigs. Leptospiraemia was demonstrated in the blood of all 5 control pigs beginning on the third postchallenge day. Leptospiraemia was demonstrated in only 2 of the 10 vaccinated pigs on the third postchallenge day. Two controls also experienced a rise in rectal temperature after challenge. Vaccinated animals remained healthy after challenge, while nonvaccinated animals developed clinical signs of leptospirosis.

References: Available upon request.

Presentation: 10 dose and 50 dose vials.

Compendium Code No.: 36900580 75-4483-05

B

BRATIVAC®-6

Pfizer Animal Health — Bacterin

Leptospira Bratislava-Canicola-Grippotyphosa-Hardjo-Icterohaemorrhagiae-Pomona Bacterin

U.S. Vet. Lic. No.: 189

Description: BRATIVAC®-6 contains chemically inactivated whole cultures of the 6 *Leptospira* serovars listed above.

Indications: BRATIVAC®-6 is for vaccination of healthy swine as an aid in the prevention of leptospirosis caused by *Leptospira bratislava, L. canicola, L. grippotyphosa, L. hardjo, L. icterohaemorrhagiae,* and *L. pomona.*

Directions:

1. General Directions: Shake well. Aseptically administer 2 mL intramuscularly.
2. Primary Vaccination: Healthy swine should receive 2 doses administered 2-6 weeks apart, beginning 2-6 weeks before breeding.
3. Revaccination: Revaccination with a single dose is recommended prior to or at breeding.
4. Good animal husbandry and herd health management practices should be employed.

Precaution(s): Store at 2°-7°C. Prolonged exposure to higher temperatures may adversely affect potency. Do not freeze.

Use entire contents when first opened.

Sterilized syringes and needles should be used to administer this vaccine.

Caution(s): As with many vaccines, anaphylaxis may occur after use. Initial antidote of epinephrine is recommended and should be followed with appropriate supportive therapy.

This product has been shown to be efficacious in healthy animals. A protective immune response may not be elicited if animals are incubating an infectious disease, are malnourished or parasitized, are stressed due to shipment or environmental conditions, are otherwise immunocompromised, or the vaccine is not administered in accordance with label directions.

Warning(s): Do not vaccinate within 21 days before slaughter.

For use in swine only.

For veterinary use only.

Discussion: Disease Description: Leptospirosis is a worldwide disease of animals and humans and causes serious economic loss to the swine industry.[1] The disease is usually transmitted by direct or indirect contact with leptospiral-infected urine, but there is substantial evidence for venereal transmission of *L. bratislava.*[2-4]

Leptospirosis in swine is characterized by poor productivity, fever, anemia, kidney inflammation, and abortions. Late-term abortions are the most important effect. All of the above *Leptospira* serovars produce similar clinical signs, yet immunity to leptospirosis is serovar-specific.[1] Studies on the epidemiology and pathogenesis of *L. bratislava* provide evidence for an association between infection of swine and poor reproductive performance.[5]

Trial Data: Safety and Efficacy: During developmental tests and in field use of BRATIVAC®-6, no significant postvaccination reactions were reported.

L. bratislava is fastidious in its growth requirements and has proven difficult to isolate. However, *L. bratislava* has been isolated in aborted pigs and fetuses in European studies; and in 1986, Ellis and Thiermann reported the isolation of *L. bratislava* from the kidney and genital tract of 2 sows in the United States.[2,3] Subsequently, *L. bratislava* was also isolated in the United States from weak pigs, stillborn pigs, and swine placental tissues.[6,7] Recent serological surveys show that infections of swine by *L. bratislava* are prevalent. Antibody to *L. bratislava,* detectable by the microscopic agglutination test (MAT), has been shown to be present in sera from greater than 30% of finishing pigs and 50% of adult pigs.[4,5] Furthermore, controlled vaccination studies conducted in swine herds showing evidence of infection and poor reproductive performance support the conclusion that *L. bratislava* can be controlled through vaccination.[5]

Challenge-of-immunity tests were conducted by scientists at the Veterinary Research Laboratories, Belfast, Northern Ireland to determine the efficacy of BratiVac® against virulent isolates of *L. bratislava.* Fifteen pigs were divided into 2 groups. Ten pigs were administered 2 doses of BratiVac® in 2-mL doses given 2 weeks apart, and a group of 5 pigs was used as nonvaccinated controls. Subsequently, all pigs were challenged with virulent strains of *L. bratislava.* After challenge, *L. bratislava* was recovered from the kidneys of all 5 control pigs and from the oviduct of one of them. In contrast, leptospires were not recovered from the kidneys or genital tracts of the 10 vaccinated pigs. Leptospiraemia was demonstrated in the blood of all 5 control pigs beginning on the third postchallenge day. Leptospiraemia was demonstrated in only 2 of the 10 vaccinated pigs on the third postchallenge day. Two controls also experienced a rise in rectal temperature after challenge.

These results are similar to results of previously conducted challenge-of-immunity tests on the other 5 fractions of BRATIVAC®-6. In those studies also, vaccinated animals remained healthy after challenge, while nonvaccinated animals developed clinical signs of leptospirosis. In interference-of-immunity studies conducted in swine, no interference between all serovars in BRATIVAC®-6 was reported.

References: Available upon request.

Presentation: 50 dose vials.

Compendium Code No.: 36901760 — 75-4486-06

BREAK-THRU STAIN & ODOR REMOVER

Davis — Cleaning Product

Ingredients: Enzymes, surfactants, inert ingredients and water.

Indications: This product is recommended to speed up the biodegradation process on new and old stains and odors caused by wine, feces, blood, vomit and other organic fluids.

It may be used on carpets, upholstery, drapery, fabrics, mattresses and other water-safe surfaces.

Directions for Use: Shake container well before each use. Test an inconspicuous area for colorfastness.

To eliminate stains, saturate the problem area with Davis BREAK-THRU STAIN & ODOR REMOVER, allowing the product to penetrate into the surface for 5 or more minutes. Gently blot or rub with a clean cloth or paper towel. If discoloration remains, repeat process allowing the product to work up to one hour before blotting away.

For odors, be sure to apply product directly to the source. Davis BREAK-THRU STAIN & ODOR REMOVER must reach into the carpet pads and backing if the odor is deep within your carpeting. Allow area to dry completely for best results. This may take several days. If odor remains, repeat process.

If stains or odors remain after using Davis BREAK-THRU STAIN & ODOR REMOVER, it is most likely that the product did not reach the source of the stain or odor. Reapply product to the problem area.

Warning(s): For external use only. Keep out of reach of children.

Presentation: 32 fl oz (946.25 mL) and one gallon (3.785 L) containers.

Compendium Code No.: 11410071

BREED-BACK-10™

Boehringer Ingelheim — Bacterin-Vaccine

Bovine Rhinotracheitis-Virus Diarrhea-Parainfluenza$_3$ Vaccine, Modified Live Virus-Haemophilus Somnus-Campylobacter Fetus-Leptospira Canicola-Grippotyphosa-Hardjo-Icterohaemorrhagiae-Pomona Bacterin

U.S. Vet. Lic. No.: 124

Contents: This product contains the antigens listed above.

Preservative: Neomycin.

Indications: Recommended for the vaccination of healthy, susceptible cattle four months of age or older against disease caused by bovine rhinotracheitis, virus diarrhea, parainfluenza$_3$ viruses, *Haemophilus somnus,* the prevention of infertility, delayed conception or abortion caused by *Campylobacter fetus* and against leptospirosis caused by *Leptospira canicola, L. grippotyphosa, L. hardjo, L. icterohaemorrhagiae* and *L. pomona.*

The following predisposing conditions are reported as possible causes of post-vaccinal reactions or inadequate immune response:

1. Vaccine administered during the incubation period of a virulent BVD virus infection.
2. Stimulation of latent virulent BVD virus infection induced by stress of handling, shipping, etc. followed by administration of the vaccine.
3. Complete or partial incompetence of the animal's immune system against BVD virus antigen.
4. Cattle persistently infected with non-cytopathic BVD virus becoming superinfected with a second cytopathic virus either from natural infection or MLV BVD vaccination.

Directions: Rehydrate the vaccine with the accompanying bottle of bacterin. Shake well and use immediately.

Dosage: Using aseptic technique, inject 5 mL intramuscularly. Repeat bacterin dose in 14 to 21 days and once annually. Animals vaccinated before 6 months of age when maternal antibody may interfere should be revaccinated at 6 months or at weaning.

Precaution(s): Store out of direct sunlight at a temperature not over 45°F. Avoid freezing. Use entire contents when first opened. Burn containers and all unused contents.

Caution(s): Stressed cattle should not be vaccinated.

Do not use in pregnant cows or in calves nursing pregnant cows.

Anaphylactoid reactions may occur.

Note: It is possible that healthy appearing cattle can be persistently infected with or incubating virulent BVD virus at time of vaccination. In view of these findings and suggested causes, BVD Vaccine is contraindicated in persistently infected cattle and use should be limited only to healthy, immunocompetent, unstressed, non-pregnant cattle.

Antidote(s): Epinephrine.

Warning(s): Do not vaccinate within 21 days before slaughter.

Presentation: Available in packages of one 5 dose vial of vaccine with one 25 mL vial of bacterin and one 20 dose vial of vaccine with one 100 mL vial of bacterin.

Compendium Code No.: 10280221 — 20901-01 / 20902-01

BREEDER-PAK

Alpharma — Water Additive

Guaranteed Analysis: Per Pound:

Vitamin D_3	14,000,000 IU
Vitamin E	50,000 IU
Biotin	400 mg
d-Pantothenic Acid	56,000 mg
Thiamine	10,000 mg
Pyridoxine	4,000 mg
MSBC	16,000 mg
Vitamin B_{12}	75 mg
Riboflavin	16,000 mg
Niacinamide	132,000 mg
Folic Acid	2,000 mg

Ingredients: Niacinamide, vitamin E supplement, d-calcium pantothenic acid, sodium chloride, vitamin D_3 supplement, biotin supplement, vitamin B_{12} supplement, riboflavin, menadione sodium bisulfite complex, thiamine HCl, potassium chloride, pyridoxine HCl, folic acid.

Indications: BREEDER-PAK is designed for use as a vitamin supplement for broiler and turkey breeders.

Directions: Mix 1 pack in 256 gallons of drinking water.

Precaution(s): Store in cool, dry place.

Caution(s): For oral animal use only.

Not for human use.

Keep out of reach of children.

Presentation: 4 oz (113.4 g).

Compendium Code No.: 10220230 — AHF-027A 0003

BREEDERVAC-III-PLUS®

Intervet — Vaccine

Bursal Disease-Newcastle-Bronchitis Vaccine, Standard and Variant, Mass. Type, Killed Virus

U.S. Vet. Lic. No.: 286

Description: BREEDERVAC-III-PLUS® is prepared using specific pathogen free (SPF) or approved substrates and contains Newcastle disease virus, infectious bronchitis disease virus, and Standard, GLS, and Delaware (A and E) strains of infectious bursal disease virus, inactivated and suspended in the aqueous phase of an oil adjuvant emulsion.

Quality tested for purity, potency and safety.

Indications: BREEDERVAC-III-PLUS® is indicated for the vaccination of breeder replacement chickens against Newcastle disease, infectious bursal disease, (Standard; Delaware and GLS variants), and Mass. type infectious bronchitis. Chickens should be in good health when vaccinated. Sick or weak chickens will not develop adequate immunity.

The use of any inactivated vaccine may cause false positive results on Mycoplasma plate tests. Avoid Mycoplasma testing prior to ten weeks post-vaccination.

Dosage and Administration: Allow the vaccine to reach ambient temperature 16-27°C (60-80°F), before use and shake vigorously before and periodically during use. Inject 0.5 mL intramuscularly or subcutaneously in chickens at least 3 weeks old, using an 18 gauge x ½" or ¼" needle.

Vaccination Program: Although this vaccine can be used for primary vaccination at three weeks of age or older, available evidence suggests that the best protection is obtained when it is used for the revaccination of chickens previously immunized (primed) with the same type of live virus vaccines. Do not administer this vaccine during the critical laying period from onset until after peak production.

Example: Breeder chickens.
Primary vaccination with a live bursal disease vaccine (Clonevac-D78® and/or Primevac IBD-3®) on at least one occasion prior to 12 weeks of age.
Primary vaccination with a live Newcastle and bronchitis vaccines on at least two occasions prior to 12 weeks of age.
These primary vaccinations would then be followed by vaccination with BREEDERVAC-III-PLUS® at 16-22 weeks of age. A minimum of four weeks should elapse between the last live virus priming and injection with BREEDERVAC-III-PLUS®. Local conditions must be taken into consideration and, where necessary, veterinary advice should be sought.
Immunity: It is evident that for optimal protection, preceding vaccination with live vaccines (priming) should have taken place. Generally, in flocks vaccinated with BREEDERVAC-III-PLUS®, a protective level of immunity will be achieved with only small variations between individual chickens. Revaccination during molt is recommended.
Vaccination Reaction: This vaccine does not provoke clinical reactions in chickens. If shock is observed, this must usually be ascribed to the stress of handling.
Records: Keep a record of vaccine, quantity, serial number, expiration date, and place of purchase; the date and time of vaccination; the number, age, breed, and locations of chickens; names of operators performing the vaccination and any observed reactions.
Precaution(s): Storage Conditions: Store in the dark in a refrigerator between 2-7°C (35-45°F). Do not freeze or expose to direct sunlight.
Do not mix this vaccine with any other substances.
Use entire contents when first opened.
This product is non-returnable.
Caution(s): If it is desired to vaccinate birds during lay, a drop in egg production may occur.
Vaccinate market chickens by subcutaneous route only.
Injection of inactivated vaccine into breast muscle may create processing plant problems under certain conditions.
Ensure that vaccination equipment is clean and sterile before use.
Do not use vaccination equipment with rubber parts, as the oil emulsion may attack certain types of rubber.
For veterinary use only.
Notice: This vaccine has undergone rigid potency, safety and purity tests, and meets Intervet Inc. and USDA requirements. It is designed to stimulate effective immunity when used as directed, but the user must be advised that the response to the product depends upon many factors, including, but not limited to, conditions of storage and handling by the user, administration of the vaccine, health and responsiveness of the individual chickens, and the degree of field exposure. Therefore, directions should be followed carefully.
This product is not hazardous when used according to directions supplied. A material safety data sheet (MSDS) is available upon request. This and any other consumer information can be obtained by calling Intervet Customer Service at 1-800-441-8272 or 1-302-934-8051.
The use of this vaccine is subject to applicable local and federal laws and regulations.
Use only as directed.
Warning(s): Do not vaccinate chickens within 42 days before slaughter.
Do not administer this vaccine during the critical egg laying period from onset until after peak production.
To avoid human injection, extreme caution should be used when injecting any oil emulsion vaccine. Accidental human injection may cause serious local reactions. Contact a physician immediately if accidental human injection occurs.
Presentation: 1,000 doses (500 mL).
U.S. Patent Nos. 4,530,831, 5,064,646
Other Patents Pending
Compendium Code No.: 11060201 Intervet 11306 AL 131

BREEDERVAC-IV-PLUS®

Intervet **Vaccine**

Bursal Disease-Newcastle Disease-Bronchitis-Reovirus Vaccine, Standard and Variant, Mass. Type, Killed Virus

U.S. Vet. Lic. No.: 286

Description: BREEDERVAC-IV-PLUS® is prepared using specific pathogen free (SPF) or approved substrates and contains Newcastle disease virus, infectious bronchitis disease virus (Massachusetts type), two strains of avian reovirus (1733 and 2408), and Standard, GLS, and Delaware (A and E) strains of infectious bursal disease virus, inactivated and suspended in the aqueous phase of an oil adjuvant emulsion.
Quality tested for purity, potency and safety.
Indications: BREEDERVAC-IV-PLUS® is indicated for the vaccination of breeder replacement chickens against Newcastle disease, Infectious Bursal Disease (Standard, Delaware and GLS variants), Massachusetts type infectious bronchitis and diseases caused by avian reoviruses. The Newcastle and bronchitis fractions of BREEDERVAC-IV-PLUS® are used primarily for protection of the breeder hen. The IBD fraction is used primarily for early protection of progeny with maternal antibodies, and the Reovirus fraction is used to protect the breeder hen against tenosynovitis and the progeny against malabsorption. Chickens should be in good health when vaccinated. Sick or weak chickens will not develop adequate immunity.
The use of any inactivated vaccine may cause false positive results on Mycoplasma plate tests. Avoid Mycoplasma testing prior to 10 weeks post-vaccination.
Dosage and Administration: Allow the vaccine to reach ambient temperature, 16-27°C (60-80°F) before use and shake vigorously before and periodically during use. Inject 0.5 mL intramuscularly or subcutaneously in chickens at least 3 weeks old, using an 18 gauge x ½" or ¼" needle.
Vaccination Program: Although this vaccine can be used for primary vaccination at three weeks of age or older, available evidence suggests that the best protection is obtained when it is used for the revaccination of chickens previously immunized (primed) with the same type of live virus vaccines. Do not administer this vaccine during the critical egg laying period from onset until after peak production.
Example: Breeder chickens.
Primary vaccination with a modified live avian reovirus (Tensynvac®) vaccine prior to 12 weeks of age.
Primary vaccination with a live bursal disease vaccine (Clonevac-D78®) prior to 12 weeks of age.
Primary vaccination with live Newcastle and bronchitis vaccines on at least two occasions prior to 12 weeks of age. These primary vaccinations would then be followed by vaccination with BREEDERVAC-IV-PLUS® at 16-22 weeks of age. A minimum of four weeks should elapse between the last live virus priming and injection with BREEDERVAC-IV-PLUS®. Local conditions must be taken into consideration and, where necessary, veterinary advice should be sought.
Immunity: It is evident that for optimal protection, preceding vaccination with live vaccines (priming) should have taken place. Generally, in flocks vaccinated with BREEDERVAC-IV-PLUS®, a protective level of immunity will be achieved with only small variations between individual chickens. Revaccination during molt is recommended.
Vaccination Reaction: This vaccine does not provoke clinical reactions in chickens. If shock is observed, this must usually be ascribed to the stress of handling.
Records: Keep a record of vaccine, quantity, serial number, expiration date, place of purchase; the date and time of vaccination; the number, age, breed, and locations of chickens; names of operators performing the vaccination and any observed reactions.
Precaution(s): Storage Conditions: Store in the dark in a refrigerator between 2-7°C (35-45°F). Do not freeze or expose to direct sunlight.
Do not mix this vaccine with any other substances.
Use entire contents when first opened.
This product is non-returnable.
Caution(s): If it is desired to vaccinate birds during lay, a drop in egg production may occur.
Vaccinate market chickens by subcutaneous route only.
Injection of inactivated vaccine into breast muscle may create processing plant problems under certain conditions.
Ensure that vaccination equipment is clean and sterile before use.
Do not use vaccination equipment with rubber parts as the oil emulsion may attack certain types of rubber.
For veterinary use only.
Notice: This vaccine has undergone rigid potency, safety and purity tests, and meets Intervet Inc. and USDA requirements. It is designed to stimulate effective immunity when used as directed, but the user must be advised that the response to the product depends upon many factors, including, but not limited to, conditions of storage and handling by the user, administration of the vaccine, health and responsiveness of the individual chickens, and the degree of field exposure. Therefore, directions should be followed carefully.
This product is not hazardous when used according to directions supplied. A material safety data sheet (MSDS) is available upon request. This and any other consumer information can be obtained by calling Intervet Customer Service at 1-800-441-8272 or 1-302-934-8051.
The use of this vaccine is subject to applicable local and federal laws and regulations.
Use only as directed.
Warning(s): Do not vaccinate chickens within 42 days before slaughter.
Do not administer this vaccine during the critical egg laying period from onset until after peak production.
To avoid human injection, extreme caution should be used when injecting any oil emulsion vaccine. Accidental human injection may cause serious local reactions. Contact a physician immediately if accidental human injection occurs.
Presentation: 1,000 doses (500 mL).
U.S. Patent No. 4,530,831
Other Patents Pending
Compendium Code No.: 11060211 Intervet 11411 AL 124

BREEDERVAC-REO-PLUS®

Intervet **Vaccine**

Bursal Disease-Reovirus Vaccine, Standard and Variant, Killed Virus

U.S. Vet. Lic. No.: 286

Description: BREEDERVAC-REO-PLUS® is prepared using specific pathogen free (SPF) or approved substrates and contains Standard, GLS, and Delaware (A and E) strains of Infectious Bursal Disease virus, and two strains of avian reovirus (1733 and 2408) inactivated and suspended in the aqueous phase of an oil adjuvant emulsion.
Quality tested for purity, potency and safety.
Indications: BREEDERVAC-REO-PLUS® is indicated for the vaccination of breeder replacement chickens against Infectious Bursal Disease, (Standard, Delaware and GLS variants) and disease caused by avian reoviruses. The IBD fraction is used primarily for early protection of progency with maternal antibodies, and the Reovirus fraction is used to protect the breeder hen against tenosynovitis and the progeny against malabsorption. Chickens should be in good health when vaccinated. Sick or weak chickens will not develop adequate immunity.
The use of any inactivated vaccine may cause false positive results on Mycoplasma plate tests. Avoid Mycoplasma testing prior to 10 weeks post-vaccination.
Dosage and Administration: Allow the vaccine to reach ambient temperature, 16-27°C (60-80°F) before use and shake vigorously before and periodically during use. Inject 0.5 mL intramuscularly or subcutaneously in chickens at least 3 weeks old, using an 18 gauge x ½" or ¼" needle.
Vaccination Programs: Although this vaccine can be used for primary vaccination at three weeks of age or older, available evidence suggests that the best protection is obtained when it is used for the revaccination of chickens previously immunized (primed) with the same type of live virus vaccines. Do not administer this vaccine during the critical egg laying period from onset until after peak production.
Examples: Breeder chickens.
Primary vaccination with modified live mild avian reovirus vaccine (Tensynvac®) prior to 12 weeks of age.
Primary vaccination with live bursal disease vaccine (Clonevac-D78®) prior to 12 weeks of age.
These primary vaccinations would then be followed by vaccination with BREEDERVAC-REO-PLUS® at 16-22 weeks of age. A minimum of four weeks should elapse between the last live virus priming and injection with BREEDERVAC-REO-PLUS®. Local conditions must be taken into consideration and, where necessary, veterinary advice should be sought.
Immunity: It is evident that for optimal protection, preceding vaccination with live vaccines (priming) should have taken place. Generally, in flocks vaccinated with BREEDERVAC-REO-PLUS®, a protective level of immunity will be achieved with only small variations between individual chickens.
Vaccination Reaction: This vaccine does not provoke clinical reactions in chickens. If shock is observed, this must usually be ascribed to the stress of handling.
Records: Keep a record of vaccine, quantity, serial number, expiration date, place of purchase; the date and time of vaccination; the number, age, breed, and locations of chickens; names of operators performing the vaccination and any observed reactions.
Precaution(s): Storage Conditions: Store in the dark in a refrigerator between 2-7°C (35-45°F). Do not freeze or expose to direct sunlight.
Do not mix this vaccine with any other substances.
Use entire contents when first opened.
This product is non-returnable.
Caution(s): If it is desired to vaccinate birds during lay, a drop in egg production may occur.
Vaccinate market chickens by subcutaneous route only.
Injection of inactivated vaccine into the breast muscle may create processing plant problems under certain conditions.

Ensure that vaccination equipment is clean and sterile before use.

Do not use vaccination equipment with rubber parts as the oil emulsion may attack certain types of rubber.

For veterinary use only.

Notice: This vaccine has undergone rigid potency, safety and purity tests, and meets Intervet Inc. and USDA requirements. It is designed to stimulate effective immunity when used as directed, but the user must be advised that the response to the product depends upon many factors, including, but not limited to, conditions of storage and handling by the user, administration of the vaccine, health and responsiveness of the individual chickens, and the degree of field exposure. Therefore, directions should be followed carefully.

This product is not hazardous when used according to direction supplied. A material safety data sheet (MSDS) is available upon request. This and any other consumer information can be obtained by calling Intervet Customer Service at 1-800-441-8272 or 1-302-934-8051.

The use of this vaccine is subject to applicable federal and local laws and regulations.

Use only as directed.

Warning(s): Do not vaccinate chickens within 42 days before slaughter.

Do not administer this vaccine during the critical egg laying period from onset until after peak production.

To avoid human injection, extreme caution should be used when injecting any oil emulsion vaccine. Accidental human injection may cause serious local reactions. Contact a physician immediately if accidental human injection occurs.

Presentation: 1,000 doses (500 mL).

U.S. Patent No. 4,530,831 Other Patents Pending

Compendium Code No.: 11060221 Intervet 11509 AL 123

BREED SOW™ 6

AgriLabs **Bacterin-Vaccine**

Parvovirus Vaccine-Leptospira Canicola-Grippotyphosa-hardjo-Icterohaemorrhagiae-Pomona Bacterin, Killed Virus

U.S. Vet. Lic. No.: 272

Contents: Parvovirus vaccine, porcine cell line origin, killed virus, *Leptospira canicola, L. grippotyphosa, L. hardjo, L. icterohaemorrhagiae* and *L. pomona* bacterin.

Contains gentamicin and amphotericin B as a preservatives.

Indications: BREED SOW™ 6 is a killed virus, adjuvanted product recommended for the immunization of swine against infection by swine parvovirus and the leptospira serovars *Leptospira canicola, L. grippotyphosa, L. hardjo, L. icterohaemorrhagiae* and *L. pomona.*

Dosage and Administration: Shake well. Inject 2 mL intramuscularly to sows and gilts four (4) to six (6) weeks prior to breeding, followed by a second vaccination two (2) to four (4) weeks later. A single revaccination two (2) to six (6) weeks prior to subsequent breeding is recommended.

Make intramuscular injections deeply into a large muscle (thigh). Cleanse the area and insert needle. Needle should be at least ¾" in length.

Precaution(s): Store at 35-45°F (2-7°C).

Caution(s): Use the entire contents when the vial is first opened. Anaphylactic reactions, although rare, may occur. In such instances epinephrine should be administered immediately.

Warning(s): Do not vaccinate within 21 days of slaughter.

Presentation: 50 dose (100 mL) vials.

Compendium Code No.: 10580231

BREED SOW® 7

AgriLabs **Bacterin-Vaccine**

Parvovirus Vaccine-Killed Virus-Erysipelothrix rhusiopathiae-Leptospira canicola-grippotyphosa-hardjo-icterohaemorrhagiae-pomona Bacterin

U.S. Vet. Lic. No.: 272

Active Ingredient(s): Parvovirus vaccine killed virus vaccine, *Erysipelothrix rhusiopathiae, Leptospira canicola, L. grippotyphosa, L. hardjo, L. icterohaemorrhagiae* and *L. pomona* bacterin.

Indications: Killed bacterin and vaccine for use as an aid in the prevention of porcine parvovirus, leptospirosis caused by *Leptospira canicola, L. grippotyphosa, L. hardjo, L. icterohaemorrhagiae, L. pomona* and *Erysipelothrix rhusiopathiae* (erysipelas).

Dosage and Administration: Administer 5 mL intramuscularly or subcutaneously to sows and gilts four (4) to six (6) weeks prior to breeding and again in three (3) to four (4) weeks. Revaccinate with a single dose four (4) to six (6) weeks prior to each subsequent breeding. Vaccinate boars semi-annually.

Precaution(s): Store at 35-45°F (2-7°C).

Caution(s): Use the entire contents when the vial is first opened. Anaphylactic reactions, although rare, may occur. In such instances epinephrine should be administered immediately.

Warning(s): Do not vaccinate within 21 days of slaughter.

Presentation: 100 mL (20 dose) and 250 mL (50 dose) vials.

Compendium Code No.: 10580220

BRILLIANCE™ FLEA & TICK SHAMPOO

First Priority **Parasiticide Shampoo**

EPA Reg. No.: 68077-1

Active Ingredient(s):

Pyrethrins	0.10%
*Piperonyl Butoxide, Technical	1.00%
Inert Ingredients:	98.90%
	100.00%

*Equivalent to 0.4% (butylcarbityl) (6-propylpiperonyl) ether and 0.1% of related compounds.

Indications: An insecticide shampoo for use on dogs and cats that kills fleas and ticks.

Directions for Use: Read entire label before each use.

It is a violation of Federal law to use this product in a manner inconsistent with its labeling.

As a shampoo to kill fleas and ticks, wet the pet's coat with warm water. Starting at the head, work shampoo thoroughly into the hair. Allow the lather to penetrate the fur for five minutes before rinsing. Dry with a towel. The pet will have a clear lustrous coat, free of fleas and ticks. Repeat every week if necessary.

Pet bedding and quarters should be treated simultaneously with an approved product.

Consult a veterinarian before using this product on debilitated, aged, pregnant or nursing animals, or animals on medication. Sensitivities may occur after using any pesticide product for pets. If signs of sensitivity occur bathe your pet with mild soap and rinse with large amounts of water. If signs continue, consult a veterinarian immediately.

Contraindication(s): Do not use on puppies or kittens under 12 weeks of age.

Precautionary Statements: Hazards to Humans and Domestic Animals:

Caution: Harmful if swallowed. Causes eye irritation. Avoid contact with skin, eyes or clothing. Wash thoroughly with soap and water after handling.

First Aid:

If swallowed: Call a physician or Poison Control Center. Drink 1 or 2 glasses of water and induce vomiting by touching back of throat with finger. If person is unconscious, do not give anything by mouth and do not induce vomiting.

If on skin: Wash with plenty of soap and water. Get medical attention if irritation persists.

If in eyes: Flush eyes with plenty of water. Get medical attention if irritation persists.

Storage and Disposal: Store in a cool, dry place, inaccessible to children and pets.

Do not reuse container. Wrap container in several layers of newspaper and discard in trash.

Warning(s): Use only on dogs or cats. Keep out of reach of children.

Disclaimer: Buyer assumes all risks of use, storage or handling of this material not in strict accordance with directions given herewith.

Presentation: 16 fl oz (473 mL), 1 gallon (3.785 L) and 2.5 gallon (9.46 L).

Compendium Code No.: 11390071

BROILERBRON®

ASL **Vaccine**

Bronchitis Vaccine, Mass. Type, Live Virus

U.S. Vet. Lic. No.: 226

Active Ingredient(s): The vaccine is formulated from a very mild strain of infectious bronchitis virus of the Mass. type. The virus is grown under exacting standards of quality control in eggs produced by healthy chickens in closely supervised flocks.

Gentamicin is added as a bacteriostatic agent.

Indications: The vaccine is recommended for the vaccination of broilers or the initial vaccination of chickens at two weeks of age or older against infectious bronchitis (Mass. type). When this vaccine is used for the initial vaccination of replacement chickens, then less mild vaccines should be given at least eight weeks after the first vaccination and not later than 16 weeks of age initially.

BROILERBRON®, producing a mild reaction, is designed for broilers or for the initial vaccination of chickens. The degree of protection produced may not be as great as that stimulated by less modified vaccines.

Dosage and Administration:

Vaccination Programs: Many factors must be considered in determining the proper vaccination program for a particular farm or poultry operation. To be fully effective, the vaccine must be administered to healthy receptive chickens held in a proper environment under good management. In addition, the response may be modified by the age of the chickens and their immune status. Seldom does one vaccination under field conditions produce complete protection for all individuals in a given flock. The amount of protection required will vary with the type of operation and the degree of exposure that a flock is likely to encounter. For these reasons, a program of periodic revaccination may be required.

Preparation of the Vaccine (for intranasal or intraocular use): Do not open and mix the vaccine until ready to begin vaccination. Use the vaccine immediately after mixing.

1. Tear off the aluminum seal from the vial containing the dried vaccine.
2. Lift off the rubber stopper.
3. Remove the plastic screw-cap and applicator insert from the polyethylene bottle of diluent.
4. Carefully pour the diluent into the vaccine vial until it is approximately two-thirds (⅔) full.
5. Put back the rubber stopper and shake.
6. Pour the partly dissolved vaccine into the bottle containing the rest of the diluent.
7. Replace the plastic applicator insert and screw-cap and shake vigorously until all of the material is dissolved. Use the applicator insert for intranasal or intraocular administration.

The vaccine is now ready for use by the following methods. For the best results, be sure to follow the directions carefully.

Intranasal or Intraocular Administration: For chickens two (2) weeks of age or older. Rehydrate the vaccine as directed above.

Intranasally: Hold the chicken's beak shut and place a finger over the lower nostril. Place a full drop of the vaccine on the other nostril. Release the chicken after the drop of vaccine has been inhaled.

Intraocularly: Place one (1) full drop of the vaccine into an open eye. Do not release the chicken until after it has swallowed.

Preparation of the Vaccine (for spray use): Do not open and mix the vaccine until ready to begin vaccination. Use the vaccine immediately after mixing.

1. Tear off the aluminum seal from the vial containing the dried vaccine.
2. Lift off the rubber stopper.
3. Carefully pour clean, cool tap water into the vaccine vial until the vial is approximately two-thirds (⅔) full.
4. Put back the rubber stopper and shake vigorously until all of the material is dissolved.
5. The vaccine is now ready for spray use in accordance with the directions below. For the best results, be sure to follow the directions carefully.

Spray Administration: Recommended for the vaccination of healthy chickens at one (1) day of age. Full directions for use of the American Scientific Laboratories' Spray Cabinet are available from the company.

Coarse Spray for Biojector Plus Administration:

1. Caution. When the machine is turned on and the metal switch on the microvalve plate is touched, the machine is activated, resulting in a needle projecting out. This can cause damage to the needle and/or the switch activator, if other than a baby chick.
2. The Biojector Plus is metered to deliver a 0.03 mL dose of vaccine.
3. The vaccine is rehydrated with a sterile water diluent at the rate of 30 mL per 1,000 doses.
4. Turn the machine on to check the adjustment of the spray nozzle. The air flow from the nozzle will blow the down away from the eye area if adjusted correctly. Minor adjustments can be made by moving the arm which holds the spray nozzle attachment. (See American Scientific Laboratories' Hatchery Equipment Manual.)
5. The machine must be properly primed with vaccine before vaccinating chicks. See an American Scientific Laboratories' Hatchery Equipment Manual for proper procedure for priming Biojector Plus.
6. The chick is positioned such that the beak is pointed away from the microvalve plate, with one eye facing up, and the head resting against the head rest protrusion of the microvalve plate. When the head is placed in this position, it will contact the switch which activates the Biojector Plus nozzle and the Biojector syringe with needle.
7. The maximum recommended speed of vaccination is 3,000 birds per hour.

Precaution(s): The product is not returnable. Store the vaccine in the refrigerator under 45°F (7°C).

Federal regulations prohibit the repackaging or sale of the contents of the package in fractional units. Do not accept if the seal is broken.

Caution(s): Use the entire contents of each vial when first opened.

Burn the containers and all unused contents.

Chickens to be vaccinated should be free of all diseases, including the latent form of chronic respiratory disease (CRD), clinical coccidiosis, blackhead, parasite infestations, etc., and maintained under good environmental conditions.

Consult a poultry pathologist for further recommendations based on conditions existing in a designated area at any given time.

The vaccination program for replacement pullets should not be started after chickens are 16 weeks of age.

Chickens should not be placed on contaminated premises. Exposure should be avoided immediately after vaccination because it takes up to 10 days to develop resistance.

All susceptible chickens on the same premises should be vaccinated at the same time. If this is not possible, then strict isolation and separate caretakers should be employed for nonvaccinated groups. Efforts should be taken to reduce stress conditions at the time the vaccine is administered.

Notice: All American Scientific Laboratories' vaccines released for sale meet the requirements of the licensing authority (U.S. Department of Agriculture) in regard to safety, purity, potency and the capacity to immunize normal, susceptible chickens.

The capacity of the vaccine to produce satisfactory results depends upon many factors including, but not limited to, conditions of storage and handling by the user, administration of the vaccine, the health and responsiveness of individual animals and the degree of field exposure. Therefore, the directions for use should be followed carefully.

The use of the vaccine is subject to applicable state and federal laws and regulations.

Warning(s): Do not vaccinate within 21 days before slaughter.

Presentation: Intranasal, intraocular or coarse spray: 10 x 1,000 dose vials.
Coarse spray for mass administration only: 10,000 dose vials.

Compendium Code No.: 11020060

BROILERBRON®-99

ASL **Vaccine**

U.S. Vet. Lic. No.: 226

Active Ingredient(s): The vaccine is formulated from the modified DPI strain of Arkansas type infectious bronchitis virus. The virus is grown under exacting standards of quality control in eggs produced by healthy chickens in closely supervised flocks.

Indications: Recommended for the vaccination of broilers or the initial vaccination of replacement chickens against the Ark. type of infectious bronchitis. The frequency of occurrence of the various types of infectious bronchitis virus should be considered in planning a vaccination program.

The strain of virus was received from the University of Delaware and was selected for its high immunizing capability and mild reaction. @P1 = **Dosage and Administration:** BROILERBRON®-99 is administered by intranasal, intraocular, or drinking water application. @BTKWN = Intranasal Administration:

1. The sterile diluent supplied should be used to reconstitute the vaccine. (See the package insert for complete mixing instructions.)
2. The mixed solution should be stored on ice until used.
3. All of the vaccine should be used within 30 minutes after mixing.
4. To administer, hold the chicks beak shut and place a finger over the lower nostril. Place a full drop of the vaccine on the other nostril. Release the bird after the drop of vaccine has been inhaled.

Intraocular (eye drop) Administration:

1. The sterile diluent supplied should be used to reconstitute the vaccine. (See the package insert for complete mixing instructions.)
2. The mixed solution should be stored on ice until used.
3. All of the vaccine should be used within 30 minutes after mixing.
4. Hold the chicken to be vaccinated with the head tilted to one side giving clear access to one eye.
5. Hold the plastic bottle containing the vaccine in a vertical position. Gently press the sides of the bottle releasing one drop of vaccine onto the eye of the chicken.
6. Be sure that the vaccine spreads over the eye before releasing the chicken. There is usually an automatic reflex action that serves to spread the vaccine over the eye surface as soon as the vaccine is dropped into the eye.

Drinking Water Administration:

1. Remove all medications, sanitizers, and disinfectants from the drinking water, preferably 72 hours before vaccinating, and 24 hours after vaccinating.
2. Provide enough watering space so that at least two-thirds (⅔) of the chickens can drink at one time.
3. Scrub waterers thoroughly and rinse with fresh, clean water.
4. Withhold water for two (2) hours before vaccinating to stimulate thirst. (The time can be varied depending upon climatic conditions.)
5. Waterers should be raised to a height such that the chickens cannot drink and that lends itself to filling the waterers with the vaccine.
6. Rehydrate the vaccine according to the package insert.
7. Add the rehydrated vaccine to clean, cool, nonchlorinated tap water and mix in accordance to the following chart:

Age of Chickens	1,000 doses added to this amount of water	10,000 doses added to this amount of water
2-4 wks.	2.5 gal. (9.5 L)	25 gal. (95 L)
4-8 wks.	5 gal. (19 L)	50 gal. (190 L)
Over 8 wks.	10 gal. (38 L)	100 gal. (380 L)

8. Nonfat powdered milk may be beneficial to help maintain the virus. A 3.2 oz. measure is added to each 10 gallons of water used to prepare the vaccine.
9. Distribute the solution among the waterers. Avoid placing the waterers in direct sunlight.
10. Do not provide any other drinking water until all of the vaccine treated water has been consumed.
11. Lower waterers to the correct height so that chickens may drink.
12. It is recommended to walk the chickens after lowering the waterers so that all of the chickens will drink and receive a uniform dose of the vaccine.

Precaution(s): Refrigerate under 45°F (7°C) until ready for use. Vaccines are perishable unless properly stored.

Caution(s): The capacity of the vaccine to produce satisfactory results depends upon many factors, including, but not limited to, conditions of storage and handling by the user, administration of the vaccine, health and responsiveness of individual animals and the degree of field exposure.

Consult a poultry pathologist for further recommendations based on conditions existing in a designated area at any given time.

The vaccination program for replacement pullets should not be started after chickens are 15 weeks of age.

Chickens should not be placed on contaminated premises. Exposure should be avoided immediately after vaccination because it takes up to 10 days to develop resistance.

All susceptible chickens on the same premises should be vaccinated at the same time. If this is not possible, then strict isolation and separate caretakers should be employed for nonvaccinated units. Efforts should be taken to reduce stress conditions at the time the vaccine is administered.

Chickens to be vaccinated should be free of all diseases, including the latent form of chronic respiratory disease (CRD), clinical coccidiosis, blackhead, parasite infestations, etc. and maintained under good environmental conditions.

Warning(s): Do not vaccinate within 21 days of slaughter.

Presentation: Intranasal or intraocular use: 1,000 dose vials.
Drinking water use: 1,000 and 10,000 dose vials.

Compendium Code No.: 11020080

BROILERBRON®-99 B_1

ASL **Vaccine**

Newcastle-Bronchitis Vaccine, B_1 Type, B_1 Strain, Mass. & Ark. Types, Live Virus

U.S. Vet. Lic. No.: 226

Active Ingredient(s): The freeze-dried vaccine is a live virus vaccine containing the B_1 strain of Newcastle and modified strains of Massachusetts and Arkansas type infectious bronchitis viruses. The viruses are grown under exacting standards of quality control in specific pathogen free eggs produced by healthy chickens in closely supervised flocks.

The vaccine is distributed in freeze-dried and frozen form.

Gentamicin is added as a bacteriostatic agent.

Indications: Freeze-dried Vaccine:

The mild freeze-dried vaccine is recommended for the vaccination of broilers or the initial vaccination of replacement chickens against Newcastle disease and infectious bronchitis (Mass. and Ark. types).

The frequency of occurrence of the various types of infectious bronchitis virus should be considered in planning a vaccination program. For replacements, a second vaccination with a less mild vaccine should be given at least eight weeks after the first vaccination, but not later than at 15 weeks of age.

BROILERBRON®-99 B_1 produces a very mild reaction and is intended for broilers or the initial vaccination of other chickens. The degree of protection produced may not be as great as that stimulated by less mild vaccines.

BROILERBRON®-99 B_1 may be administered by intraocular, intranasal, or coarse spray.

Frozen Vaccine:

The mild frozen vaccine is recommended for the initial vaccination of broilers or replacement chickens against Newcastle disease and infectious bronchitis (Mass. and Ark. types). When the frozen vaccine is used for initial vaccination, other vaccines should be given as a booster to stimulate high levels of immunity that persist for a longer period of time.

Broilers may be vaccinated at one day of age by coarse spray application. Do not administer to one day old chicks to be raised as layers. The frozen product formulation was developed for those individuals desiring a mild reacting day old vaccination.

BROILERBRON®-99 B_1 (Frozen) may be administered by coarse spray.

Dosage and Administration:

Vaccination Programs: Many factors must be considered in determining the proper vaccination program for a particular farm or poultry operation. To be fully effective, the vaccine must be administered to healthy receptive chickens held in a proper environment under good management. In addition, the response may be modified by the age of the chickens and their immune status. Seldom does one vaccination under field conditions produce complete protection for all individuals in a given flock. The amount of protection required will vary with the type of operation and the degree of exposure that a flock is likely to encounter. For these reasons, a program of periodic revaccination may be required.

Freeze-dried Vaccine:

Preparation of the Vaccine (for intranasal or intraocular use): Do not open and mix the vaccine until ready to begin vaccination. Use the vaccine immediately after mixing.

1. Tear off the aluminum seal from the vial containing the dried vaccine.
2. Lift off the rubber stopper.
3. Remove the plastic screw-cap and applicator insert from the polyethylene bottle of diluent.
4. Carefully pour the diluent into the vaccine vial until it is approximately two-thirds (⅔) full.
5. Put back the rubber stopper and shake.
6. Pour the partly dissolved vaccine into the bottle containing the rest of the diluent.
7. Replace the plastic applicator insert and screw-cap and shake vigorously until all of the material is dissolved. Use the applicator insert for intranasal or intraocular administration.

The vaccine is now ready for use by the following methods. For the best results, be sure to follow the directions carefully.

Intranasal or Intraocular Administration: For chickens four (4) weeks of age or older. Rehydrate the vaccine as directed above.

Intranasally: Hold the chicken's beak shut and place a finger over the lower nostril. Place a full drop of the vaccine on the other nostril. Release the chicken after the drop of vaccine has been inhaled.

Intraocularly: Place one (1) full drop of the vaccine into the open eye. Do not release the chicken until after it has swallowed.

Preparation of the Vaccine (for coarse spray use): 10,000 dose vials are for mass administration use only.

Do not open and mix the vaccine until ready to begin vaccination. Use the vaccine immediately after mixing.

1. Tear off the aluminum seal from the vial containing the dried vaccine.
2. Lift off the rubber stopper.
3. Carefully pour clean, cool distilled water into the vaccine vial until the vial is approximately two-thirds (⅔) full.
4. Replace the rubber stopper and shake vigorously until all material is dissolved.

5. Pour the vaccine into a bottle containing sufficient distilled water to vaccinate the required number of chickens.
6. Follow the directions of the spray cabinet manufacturer when mixing and administering the vaccine.

Frozen Vaccine:

Preparation of the Vaccine (for coarse spray use): 10,000 dose vials are for mass administration use only.

Do not open and mix the vaccine until ready to begin vaccination. Use the vaccine immediately after mixing.

B

1. Use one (1) ampule in 300 mL of water for each 10,000 chickens to be vaccinated.
2. The contents of the ampule are thawed rapidly by immersing in water at room temperature. Shake the ampule to disperse the contents. Then break the ampule at its neck and immediately proceed as follows.
   Caution: Ampules have been known to explode on sudden temperature changes. Do not thaw in hot or ice cold water.
3. Draw the contents of the ampule into a sterile 10 mL syringe.
4. Dilute immediately by filling the syringe slowly from a portion of the water.
   Important: The water should be cool (below 60°F) at the time of mixing.
5. The contents of the filled syringe are then added to the remaining water diluent. Shake the bottle as the vaccine is being mixed. Withdraw a portion of the diluent with the syringe to flush the ampule. Inject the washing back into the diluent bottle.
6. The vaccine is now ready for use.

Coarse Spray Administration: Recommended for the vaccination of healthy chickens at one (1) day of age. Full directions for use of the American Scientific Laboratories' Spray Cabinet are available from the company.

Coarse Spray for Biojector Plus Administration:

1. Caution. When the machine is turned on and the metal switch on the microvalve plate is touched, the machine is activated, resulting in a needle projecting out. This can cause damage to the needle and/or what is activating the switch, if other than a baby chick.
2. The Biojector Plus is metered to deliver a 0.03 mL dose of vaccine.
3. The vaccine is rehydrated with sterile water diluent at the rate of 30 mL per 1,000 doses.
4. Turn the machine on to check the adjustment of the spray nozzle. The air flow from the nozzle will blow the down away from the eye area if adjusted correctly. Minor adjustments can be made by moving the arm which holds the spray nozzle attachment. (See American Scientific Laboratories' Hatchery Equipment Manual.)
5. The machine must be properly primed with vaccine before vaccinating chicks. See an American Scientific Laboratories' Hatchery Equipment Manual for proper procedure for priming Biojector Plus.
6. The chick is positioned such that the beak is pointed away from the microvalve plate, with one eye facing up, and the head resting against the head rest protrusion of the microvalve plate. When the head is placed in this position, it will contact the switch which activates the Biojector Plus nozzle and the Biojector syringe with needle.
7. The maximum recommended speed of vaccination is 3,000 birds per hour.

Precaution(s): Freeze-dried Vaccine:

Store the vaccine in the refrigerator at under 45°F (7°C) until ready for use. Vaccines are perishable unless properly stored.

Frozen Vaccine:

Keep in liquid nitrogen until ready for use. Vaccines are perishable unless properly stored. Liquid nitrogen containers and vaccine should be handled by properly trained personnel only. See Form 0888K "Precautions and Safe Practices-Liquefied Atmospheric Gases", published by the Linde Division of Union Carbide Corp., New York, N.Y.

Proper storage is essential to maintain potency of the vaccine.

Ampule: Store in liquid nitrogen.

Container: Store the liquid nitrogen container securely in an upright position in a dry, well-ventilated area away from incubator intakes and chicken boxes.

Important: Follow the directions on the container for checking liquid nitrogen levels.

Caution(s): Freeze-dried Vaccine:

Use the entire contents when first opened. Use only in states where permitted.

The capacity of the vaccine to produce satisfactory results depends upon many factors, including, but not limited to, conditions of storage and handling by the user, administration of the vaccine, health and responsiveness of individual animals and degree of field exposure. Therefore, directions for use should be followed carefully.

Consult a poultry pathologist for further recommendations based on the conditions existing in a designated area at any given time.

A bronchitis vaccination program for replacement pullets should not be started after the chickens are 15 weeks of age.

Chickens should not be placed on contaminated premises. Exposure should be avoided immediately after vaccination because it takes up to 10 days to develop resistance.

All susceptible chickens on the same premises should be vaccinated at the same time. If this is not possible, then strict isolation and separate caretakers should be employed for nonvaccinated units.

Efforts should be taken to reduce stress conditions at the time the vaccine is administered.

Chickens to be vaccinated should be free of all diseases, including the latent form of chronic respiratory disease (CRD), clinical coccidiosis, blackhead, parasite infestations, etc. and maintained under good environmental conditions.

Newcastle disease vaccine can cause inflammation of the eyelids of humans, lasting two or three days. The user should avoid contaminating hands, eyes or clothing with the vaccine.

See the package for full product information and directions for use. It is imperative that the user of the product comply with the indications for use, contraindications, precautions and warnings stated. The vaccine must be prepared and administered as directed to obtain the best results.

Frozen Vaccine:

Use the entire contents when first opened. Use only in states where permitted.

Liquid nitrogen containers and vaccines should be handled by properly trained personnel only. Ampules have been known to explode on sudden temperature changes. Do not thaw in hot or cold water. Precautions should be taken to protect one's self from flying glass. When removing the ampule cane, handling frozen ampules or adding liquid nitrogen, wear long sleeves, a plastic face shield, and gloves to protect the skin from contact with the liquid nitrogen.

All storage and handling of the liquid nitrogen container must be in a well-ventilated area. Do not inhale liquid nitrogen vapors. If drowsiness occurs, get fresh air immediately and ventilate the entire area. If breathing difficulty occurs or if there is a loss of consciousness, apply artificial respiration and summon a physician at once.

The capacity of the vaccine to produce satisfactory results depends upon many factors, including, but not limited to, conditions of storage and handling by the user, administration of the vaccine, health and responsiveness of individual animals and degree of field exposure. Therefore, directions for use should be followed carefully.

Consult a poultry pathologist for further recommendations based on the conditions existing in a designated area at any given time.

Chickens to be vaccinated should be free of all diseases, including the latent form of chronic respiratory disease (CRD), clinical coccidiosis, blackhead, parasite infestations, etc. and maintained under good environmental conditions.

Newcastle disease vaccine can cause inflammation of the eyelids of humans, lasting two or three days. The user should avoid contaminating hands, eyes or clothing with the vaccine.

See the package for full product information and directions for use. It is imperative that the user of the product comply with indications for use, contraindications, precautions and warnings stated. The vaccine must be prepared and administered as directed to obtain the best results.

Notice: All American Scientific Laboratories' vaccines released for sale meet the requirements of the licensing authority (U.S. Department of Agriculture) in regard to safety, purity, potency and the capacity to immunize normal, susceptible chickens.

The use of these vaccines are subject to applicable state and federal laws and regulations.

Warning(s): Do not vaccinate within 21 days before slaughter.

Presentation: Freeze-dried Vaccine:
Intranasal or intraocular: 1,000 dose vials.
Coarse spray: 1,000 dose vials.
Coarse spray for mass administration only: 10,000 dose vials.
Frozen Vaccine (coarse spray): 10,000 dose vials.

Compendium Code No.: 11020090

BROILERBRON® B_1

ASL **Vaccine**

U.S. Vet. Lic. No.: 226

Active Ingredient(s): BROILERBRON® B_1 is formulated from a mild strain of infectious bronchitis virus of the Mass. type and the B_1 strain of Newcastle virus. The viruses are grown under exacting standards of quality control in eggs produced by healthy chickens in closely supervised flocks.

BROILERBRON® B_1 produces a mild reaction and is intended for broilers or initial vaccination of other chickens.

Indications: Recommended for the vaccination of broilers or the initial vaccination of replacement chickens against Newcastle disease and infectious bronchitis (Mass. type).

Dosage and Administration: BROILERBRON® B_1 may be administered by intraocular, intranasal and coarse spray methods.

BROILERBRON® B_1 may be administered to healthy one-day-old chickens by coarse spray application.

Intraocular (eye drop) Administration:

1. The sterile diluent supplied should be used to reconstitute the vaccine. (See the package insert for complete mixing instructions.)
2. The mixed solution should be stored on ice until used.
3. All of the vaccine should be used within 30 minutes after mixing.
4. Hold the chicken to be vaccinated with the head tilted to one side giving clear access to one eye.
5. Hold the plastic bottle containing the vaccine in a vertical position. Gently press the sides of the bottle releasing one drop of vaccine onto the eye of the chicken.
6. Be sure that the vaccine spreads over the eye before releasing the chicken. There is usually an automatic reflex action that serves to spread the vaccine over the eye surface as soon as the vaccine is dropped into the eye.

Intranasal Administration:

1. The sterile diluent supplied should be used to reconstitute the vaccine. (See the package insert for complete mixing instructions.)
2. The mixed solution should be stored on ice until used.
3. All of the vaccine should be used within 30 minutes after mixing.
4. To administer, hold the chicks beak shut and place a finger over the lower nostril. Place a full drop of the vaccine on the other nostril. Release the bird after the drop of vaccine has been inhaled.

Coarse Spray for Biojector Plus Administration:

1. Caution. When the machine is turned on and the metal switch on the microvalve plate is touched, the machine is activated, resulting in a needle projecting out. This can cause damage to the needle and/or what is activating the switch, if other than a baby chick.
2. The Biojector Plus is metered to deliver a 0.03 mL dose of vaccine.
3. The vaccine is rehydrated with sterile water diluent at the rate of 30 mL per 1,000 doses.
4. Turn the machine on to check the adjustment of the spray nozzle. The air flow from the nozzle will blow the down away from the eye area if adjusted correctly. Minor adjustments can be made by moving the arm which holds the spray nozzle attachment. (See American Scientific Laboratories' Hatchery Equipment Manual.)
5. The machine must be properly primed with vaccine before vaccinating chicks. See an American Scientific Laboratories' Hatchery Equipment Manual for proper procedure for priming Biojector Plus.
6. The chick is positioned such that the beak is pointed away from the microvalve plate, with one eye facing up, and the head resting against the head rest protrution of the microvalve plate. When the head is placed in this position, it will contact the switch which activates the Biojector Plus nozzle and the Biojector syringe with needle.
7. Maximum recommended speed of vaccination is 3,000 birds per hour.

Precaution(s): Refrigerate under 45°F (7°C) until ready for use. Vaccines are perishable unless properly stored.

Caution(s): The capacity of the vaccine to produce satisfactory results depends upon many factors including, but not limited to, conditions of storage and handling by the user, administration of the vaccine, health and responsiveness of individual animals and the degree of field exposure.

Consult a poultry pathologist for further recommendations based on conditions existing in a designated area at any given time.

A bronchitis vaccination program for replacement pullets should not be started after the chickens are 15 weeks of age.

Chickens should not be placed on contaminated premises. Exposure should be avoided immediately after vaccination because it takes up to 10 days to develop resistance.

All susceptible chickens on the same premises should be vaccinated at the same time. If this is not possible, then strict isolation and separate caretakers should be employed for nonvaccinated units.

Efforts should be taken to reduce stress conditions at the time the vaccine is administered.

Chickens to be vaccinated should be free of all diseases, including latent form of chronic respiratory disease (CRD), clinical coccidiosis, blackhead, parasite infestations, etc., and maintained under good environmental conditions.

Newcastle disease vaccine can cause inflammation of the eyelids of humans, lasting two or three days. The user should avoid contaminating hands, eyes or clothing with the vaccine.

Warning(s): Do not vaccinate within 21 days before slaughter.

Presentation: Intranasal or intraocular: 1,000 dose vials.
Coarse spray: 1,000 dose vials.
Coarse spray for mass administration only: 10,000 dose vials.

Compendium Code No.: 11020070

BROILERBRON®-H-B_1

ASL **Vaccine**

U.S. Vet. Lic. No.: 226

Active Ingredient(s): The vaccine is formulated from a modified Holland strain of infectious bronchitis virus of the Massachusetts type which offers a broad spectrum of protection for infectious bronchitis, while the B_1 Newcastle fraction of the vaccine is very mild.

The strain of bronchitis virus was received from APHIS and further modified to reduce its potential for producing respiratory side effects and yet retain a high immunizing capability.

The Newcastle strain has been passed through specific pathogen free (SPF) chickens to enhance their level of transmission which is necessary for better protection when used for drinking water vaccination. The viruses are grown under exacting standards of quality control in SPF embryos produced by healthy birds in closely supervised flocks.

Indications: The vaccine is recommended for the initial vaccination of replacement chickens or the vaccination of broilers which are two weeks of age or older against Newcastle disease and infectious bronchitis (Mass. type).

Dosage and Administration: For intranasal, or eye drop methods, rehydrate the vaccine with the diluent provided; use the applicator insert. May also be administered by the drinking water method.

Intranasal Administration:
1. The sterile diluent supplied should be used to reconstitute the vaccine. (See the package insert for complete mixing instructions.)
2. The mixed solution should be stored on ice until used.
3. All of the vaccine should be used within 30 minutes after mixing.
4. To administer, hold the chicks beak shut and place a finger over the lower nostril. Place a full drop of the vaccine on the other nostril. Release the bird after the drop of vaccine has been inhaled.

Intraocular (eye drop) Administration:
1. The sterile diluent supplied should be used to reconstitute the vaccine. (See the package insert for complete mixing instructions.)
2. The mixed solution should be stored on ice until used.
3. All of the vaccine should be used within 30 minutes after mixing.
4. Hold the chicken to be vaccinated with the head tilted to one side giving clear access to one eye.
5. Hold the plastic bottle containing the vaccine in a vertical position. Gently press the sides of the bottle releasing one drop of vaccine onto the eye of the chicken.
6. Be sure that the vaccine spreads over the eye before releasing the chicken. There is usually an automatic reflex action that serves to spread the vaccine over the eye surface as soon as the vaccine is dropped into the eye.

Drinking Water Administration:
1. Remove all medications, sanitizers, and disinfectants from the drinking water, preferably 72 hours before vaccinating, and 24 hours after vaccination.
2. Provide enough watering space so that at least two-thirds (⅔) of the chickens can drink at one time.
3. Scrub waterers thoroughly and rinse with fresh, clean water.
4. Withhold water for two (2) hours before vaccinating to stimulate thirst. (The time can be varied depending upon climatic conditions.)
5. Waterers should be raised to a height such that the chickens cannot drink and that lends itself to filling the waterers with the vaccine.
6. Rehydrate the vaccine according to the package insert.
7. Add the rehydrated vaccine to clean, cool, nonchlorinated tap water and mix in accordance to the following chart:

Age of Chickens	1,000 doses added to this amount of water	10,000 doses added to this amount of water
2-4 wks.	2.5 gal. (9.5 L)	25 gal. (95 L)
4-8 wks.	5 gal. (19 L)	50 gal. (190 L)
Over 8 wks.	10 gal. (38 L)	100 gal. (380 L)

8. Nonfat powdered milk may be beneficial to help maintain the virus. A 3.2 oz. measure is added to each 10 gallons of water used to prepare the vaccine.
9. Distribute the solution among the waterers provided. Avoid placing the waterers in direct sunlight.
10. Do not provide any other drinking water until all of the vaccine treated water has been consumed.
11. Lower waterers to the correct height so that chickens may drink.
12. It is recommended to walk the chickens after lowering the waterers so that all of the chickens will drink and receive a uniform dose of the vaccine.

Precaution(s): Refrigerate under 45°F (7°C) until ready for use. Vaccines are perishable unless properly stored.

Caution(s): Chickens less than two weeks of age should not be vaccinated with the product.

The capacity of the vaccine to produce satisfactory results depends upon many factors including, but not limited to, conditions of storage and handling by the user, administration of the vaccine, health and responsiveness of individual animals and the degree of field exposure.

Consult a poultry pathologist for further recommendations based on conditions existing in a designated area at any given time.

A bronchitis vaccination program for replacement pullets should not be started after the chickens are 15 weeks of age.

Chickens should not be placed on contaminated premises. Exposure should be avoided immediately after vaccination because it takes up to 10 days to develop resistance.

All susceptible chickens on the same premises should be vaccinated at the same time. If this is not possible, then strict isolation and separate caretakers should be employed for nonvaccinated units.

Efforts should be taken to reduce stress conditions at the time the vaccine is administered.

Chickens to be vaccinated should be free of all diseases, including latent form of chronic respiratory disease (CRD), clinical coccidiosis, parasite infestations, etc., and maintained under good environmental conditions.

Revaccination of laying hens with a Holland strain of bronchitis may cause a slight drop in egg production, unless adequate levels of immunity have been maintained prior to revaccinction. Any delay in revaccination may result in a few birds becoming susceptible to bronchitis. Exposure of these birds to the virus can cause a drop in production and affect egg quality.

Newcastle disease vaccine can cause inflammation of the eyelids of humans, lasting two or three days. The user should avoid contaminating hands, eyes or clothing with the vaccine.

Warning(s): Do not vaccinate within 21 days before slaughter.

Presentation: Intranasal, drinking water, or eyedrop: 1,000 dose vials.
Drinking water use only: 1,000 dose vials.

Compendium Code No.: 11020110

BROILERBRON®-H N-79

ASL **Vaccine**

Newcastle-Bronchitis Vaccine, B_1 Type, LaSota Strain, Mass. Type, Live Virus

U.S. Vet. Lic. No.: 226

Contents: Newcastle-bronchitis vaccine (B_1 type, LaSota strain, Mass. type), live virus. Gentamicin is added as a bacteriostatic agent.

Indications: This vaccine is recommended for initial vaccination of healthy chickens 2 weeks of age or older by intraocular or drinking water methods of application against Newcastle disease and infectious bronchitis (Mass. type). For use in broilers or initial vaccination of replacement chickens.

Dosage and Administration: Rehydration of the Vaccine: For Intraocular use

Do not open and mix the vaccine until ready to begin vaccination. Use vaccine immediately after mixing.
1. Tear off the aluminum seal from the vial containing the dried vaccine.
2. Lift off the rubber stopper.
3. Remove the plastic screw-cap and applicator insert from the polyethylene bottle of diluent.
4. Pour a small amount of diluent into the vial of dried vaccine.
5. Replace the rubber stopper and shake.
6. Pour the partly dissolved vaccine into the bottle containing the rest of the diluent.
7. Replace the plastic applicator insert and screw-cap and shake vigorously until all of the material is dissolved.

The vaccine is now ready for use by the following method.

Intraocular Administration: For chickens 2 weeks of age or older.

Place one full drop of vaccine into the open eye. Do not release the chicken until after it has swallowed.

Rehydration of the Vaccine: For Drinking Water Use.

Do not open and mix the vaccine until ready to begin vaccination. Use vaccine immediately after mixing.
1. Tear off the aluminum seal from the vial containing the dried vaccine.
2. Lift off the rubber stopper.
3. Carefully pour clean, cool tap water into the vaccine vial until the vial is approximately two-thirds full.
4. Replace the rubber stopper and shake vigorously until all material is dissolved.
5. The vaccine is now ready for drinking water use in accordance with directions below. For best results be sure to follow directions carefully.

Drinking Water Administration: For chickens 2 weeks of age or older.
1. Remove all medication, sanitizers, and disinfectants from the drinking water, preferably 72 hours before vaccinating, and for 24 hours after vaccination.
2. Provide enough watering space so that at least two-thirds of the chickens can drink at one time.
3. Scrub waterers thoroughly and rinse with fresh, clean water.
4. Withhold water for 2 hours before vaccinating to stimulate thirst.
5. Rehydrate the vaccine as directed above.
6. Add rehydrated vaccine to clean, cool tap water and mix in accordance with the following chart:

Age of chickens	1,000 doses added to this amount of water
2 weeks to 4 weeks	2½ Gallons (9.5 liters)
4 weeks to 8 weeks	5 Gallons (18.9 liters)
8 weeks or older	10 gallons (37.9 liters)

7. Distribute the vaccine solution, as prepared above, among the waterers provided for the chickens. Avoid placing the waterers in direct sunlight.
8. Provide no other drinking water until all the vaccine treated water has been consumed.

Contraindication(s): Chickens to be vaccinated should be free of all diseases including latent form of chronic respiratory disease (CRD), clinical coccidiosis, blackhead, parasite infestations, etc. and maintained under good environmental conditions.

Precaution(s): Store vaccine in refrigerator under 45°F (7°C).

Use entire contents when first opened. Burn containers and all unused contents.

Caution(s): Consult your poultry pathologist for further recommendations based on conditions existing in a designated area at any given time.

The vaccination program for replacement pullets should not be started after chickens are 16 weeks of age.

Different vaccines should not be mixed for single application.

Chickens should not be placed on contaminated premises. Exposure should be avoided immediately after vaccination, because it takes up to 10 days to develop resistance.

All susceptible chickens on the same premises should be vaccinated at the same time. If this is not possible, then strict isolation and separate caretakers should be employed for non-vaccinated units. Efforts should be taken to reduce stressful conditions at the time the vaccine is administered.

The capacity of the vaccine to produce satisfactory results depends upon many factors including, but not limited to, conditions of storage and handling by the user, administration of the vaccine, health and responsiveness of individual animals and the degree of field exposure. Therefore, directions for use should be followed carefully.

B

The use of the vaccine is subject to applicable state and federal laws and regulations.

Warning(s): Do not vaccinate within 21 days before slaughter.

Newcastle disease virus can cause inflammation of the eyelids of humans, lasting two or three days. The user should avoid contaminating his hands, eyes and clothing with this vaccine.

Discussion: The vaccine is formulated from a clone-selected LaSota strain of Newcastle disease virus (N-79) and a special modified Holland strain of infectious bronchitis virus of Mass. type (BROILERBRON®-H). It has been demonstrated that clone-selected LaSota strain (N-79) offers the same protection as the regular LaSota strain and yet at the same time gives a mild reaction comparable to the B_1 strain. The strain of bronchitis virus was received from APHIS and further modified to reduce its potential for producing respiratory side effects and yet retain high immunizing capability. The viruses are grown under exacting standards of quality control in eggs produced by healthy chickens in closely supervised flocks.

Vaccination Programs: Many factors must be considered in determining the proper vaccination program for a particular farm or poultry operation. To be fully effective, the vaccine must be administered to healthy receptive chickens held in a proper environment under good management. In addition, the response may be modified by the age of the chickens and their immune status. Seldom does one vaccination under field conditions produce complete protection for all individuals in a given flock. The amount of protection required will vary with the type of operation and the degree of exposure that a flock is likely to encounter. For these reasons, a program of periodic revaccination may be required.

Notice: All American Scientific Laboratories' vaccines released for sale meet the requirements of the licensing authority (U.S. Department of Agriculture) in regard to safety, purity, potency and the capacity to immunize normal, susceptible chickens.

Presentation: 10 x 1000 dose-vials.

Compendium Code No.: 11020101

BROILER-PAK

Alpharma **Water Additive**

Vitamin and Electrolyte Concentrate

Guaranteed Analysis: Per Pound:

Vitamin A	20,000,000 IU
Vitamin D_3	3,000,000 IU
Vitamin E	10,000 IU
Riboflavin	2,000 mg
Folic Acid	500 mg
Thiamine HCl	1,200 mg
Biotin	25 mg
d-Pantothenic Acid	16,000 mg
MSBC (source of vitamin K)	8,000 mg

Contains citric acid and the electrolytes of sodium and potassium.

Ingredients: Citric acid, potassium chloride, sodium chloride, vitamin A supplement, vitamin E supplement, d-calcium pantothenic acid, menadione sodium bisulfite complex, vitamin D_3 supplement, riboflavin, thiamine HCl, biotin supplement, folic acid

Indications: For use in broilers and other poultry to assure adequate intake of vitamins and electrolytes.

Directions: Mix one 4 oz pack in 256 gallons of drinking water or one 8 oz pack in 512 gallons of drinking water . Administer for 3 to 5 days and repeat as necessary.

Automatic water proportioner use: Mix one 4 oz pack's contents in 2 gallons of stock or one 8 oz pack's contents in 4 gallons of stock. Set proportioner to deliver 1 fluid ounce of this solution per gallon of water.

Precaution(s): Store in cool, dry place.

Caution(s): For oral animal use only. Not for human use. Keep out of reach of children.

Presentation: 4 oz (113.5 g) and 8 oz (226.8 g).

Compendium Code No.: 10220241 AHF-024A 0005, AHF-025A 0005

BROILERTRAKE®

ASL **Vaccine**

U.S. Vet. Lic. No.: 226

Active Ingredient(s): BROILERTRAKE® contains a modified live laryngotracheitis virus.

Indications: BROILERTRAKE® is a laryngotracheitis vaccine recommended for the immunization of healthy broilers. It is effective in the face of a disease outbreak or as a booster vaccination in breeder flocks or commercial layers.

In the event of emergency conditions or an outbreak of laryngotracheitis, chickens as young as two weeks of age may be vaccinated. If used in an attempt to check an outbreak of laryngotracheitis on a farm, those pens not showing symptoms should be vaccinated first.

The vaccine is for eye drop application on healthy chickens for the prevention of infectious laryngotracheitis. When applied to susceptible chickens, this product produces a mild conjunctivitis in some of the chickens. The eye reaction occurs on the fourth or fifth day post-vaccination. The eye reaction is more noticeable in housing areas with excess ammonia or heavy dust in the air. The vaccine stimulates the chicken's immune system, giving protection against the disease.

Dosage and Administration: BROILERTRAKE® is administered by intraocular application to chickens four (4) weeks of age or older. Replacement chickens should be vaccinated at four (4) or five (5) weeks of age and again at 16 to 20 weeks of age.

Intraocular (eye drop) Administration:

1. The sterile diluent supplied should be used to reconstitute the vaccine. (See the package insert for complete mixing instructions.)
2. The mixed solution should be stored on ice until used.
3. All of the vaccine should be used within 30 minutes after mixing.
4. Hold the chicken to be vaccinated with the head tilted to one side giving clear access to one eye.
5. Hold the plastic bottle containing the vaccine in a vertical position. Gently press the sides of the bottle releasing one drop of vaccine onto the eye of the chicken.
6. Be sure that the vaccine spreads over the eye before releasing the chicken. There is usually an automatic reflex action that serves to spread the vaccine over the eye surface as soon as the vaccine is dropped into the eye.

Precaution(s): Refrigerate under 45°F (7°C) until ready to use. Vaccines are perishable unless properly stored.

Caution(s): The capacity of the vaccine to produce satisfactory results depends upon many factors, including, but not limited to, conditions of storage and handling by the user, administration of the vaccine, health and responsiveness of individual animals and degree of field exposure.

All susceptible chickens on the same premises should be vaccinated at the same time. If this is not possible, then strict isolation and separate caretakers should be employed for nonvaccinated units. Efforts should be taken to reduce stress conditions at the time the vaccine is administered.

Chickens to be vaccinated should be free of all diseases, including the latent form of chronic respiratory disease (CRD), clinical coccidiosis, blackhead, parasite infestations, etc. and maintained under good environmental conditions.

Warning(s): Do not vaccinate within 21 days of slaughter.

Presentation: Intraocular: 1,000 dose vials.

Compendium Code No.: 11020120

BROILERTRAKE®-M

ASL **Vaccine**

U.S. Vet. Lic. No.: 226

Active Ingredient(s): BROILERTRAKE®-M contains an attenuated, modified live laryngotracheitis virus.

Indications: BROILERTRAKE®-M is recommended for the immunization of healthy broilers or as an initial vaccination for breeders or commercial layers.

The vaccine is for eye drop application of healthy chickens for the prevention of infectious laryngotracheitis. When applied to susceptible chickens, the product produces a mild conjunctivitis in some of the chickens. The eye reaction occurs on the fourth or fifth day of post-vaccination. The eye reaction is more noticeable in housing areas with excess ammonia or heavy dust in the air. The vaccine stimulates the chicken's immune system, giving protection against the disease.

Dosage and Administration: BROILERTRAKE®-M is administered by intraocular application to chickens four (4) weeks of age or older. Replacement chickens should be vaccinated at four (4) to five (5) weeks of age and again at 16 to 20 weeks of age.

In the event of emergency conditions or an outbreak of laryngotracheitis, chickens as young as two (2) weeks of age may be vaccinated. If used in an attempt to check an outbreak of laryngotracheitis on a farm, those pens not showing symptoms should be vaccinated first.

Intraocular (eye drop) Administration:

1. The sterile diluent supplied should be used to reconstitute the vaccine. (See the package insert for complete mixing instructions.)
2. The mixed solution should be stored on ice until used.
3. All of the vaccine should be used within 30 minutes after mixing.
4. Hold the chicken to be vaccinated with the head tilted to one side giving clear access to one eye.
5. Hold the plastic bottle containing the vaccine in a vertical position. Gently press the sides of the bottle releasing one drop of vaccine onto the eye of the chicken.
6. Be sure that the vaccine spreads over the eye before releasing the chicken. There is usually an automatic reflex action that serves to spread the vaccine over the eye surface as soon as the vaccine is dropped into the eye.

Precaution(s): Refrigerate under 45°F (7°C) until ready to use. Vaccines are perishable unless properly stored.

Caution(s): The capacity of the vaccine to produce satisfactory results depends upon many factors, including, but not limited to, conditions of storage and handling by the user, administration of the vaccine, health and responsiveness of individual animals and degree of field exposure.

Consult a poultry pathologist for further recommendations based on conditions existing in a designated area at any given time.

Chickens should not be placed on contaminated premises. Exposure should be avoided immediately after vaccination because it takes up to 10 days to develop resistance.

All susceptible chickens on the same premises should be vaccinated at the same time. If this is not possible, then strict isolation and separate caretakers should be employed for nonvaccinated units. Efforts should be taken to reduce stress conditions at the time the vaccine is administered.

Chickens to be vaccinated should be free of all diseases, including the latent form of chronic respiratory disease (CRD), clinical coccidiosis, blackhead, parasite infestations, etc. and maintained under good environmental conditions.

Warning(s): Do not vaccinate within 21 days of slaughter.

Presentation: Intraocular: 1,000 dose vials.

Compendium Code No.: 11020130

BRONCHICINE™ CAe

Biocor **Bacterin**

Bordetella Bronchiseptica Bacterin, Cellular Antigen Extract

U.S. Vet. Lic. No.: 462

Contents: BRONCHICINE™ CAe is a nonadjuvanted antigenic extract prepared from the cells of *Bordetella bronchiseptica*.

This product contains thimerosal (merthiolate) as a preservative.

Indications: Recommended for use as an aid in the control of Canine Infectious Tracheobronchitis (Kennel Cough) caused by the organism represented.

Directions: Shake well. Aseptically remove entire contents into the syringe. Push out any air trapped in the syringe. Administer 1 mL subcutaneously under loose skin (back of neck) to healthy dogs at least 8 weeks of age. Do not vaccinate into blood vessels. If blood enters the syringe, choose another injection site. For initial vaccination, a second dose is required 2-4 weeks later. This product should be administered by subcutaneous injection only. Annual revaccination with a single 1 mL dose is recommended.

Precaution(s): Store at 35°F-45°F (2°C-8°C). Do not freeze. Use entire contents when first opened.

Caution(s): Care should be taken to avoid microbial contamination of the product. In case of anaphylactoid reactions, epinephrine should be administered immediately. Transient local irritation at the site of injection, though rare, may occur subsequent to use of this product.

For use in dogs only.

Discussion: The effect of persisting *B. bronchiseptica* maternal antibody on the immune response in puppies to this bacterin has not been determined. Puppies from bitches immune to the organism usually have low antibody titers that are dissipated by 4-6 weeks of age. Although kennel cough is considered a disease of complex etiology, it can be reproduced by challenge with *B. bronchiseptica* alone. A close association and/or confinement of dogs facilitates spread of the disease syndrome. Antibiotic therapy has been shown to be generally unsuccessful in reducing or eliminating *B. bronchiseptica* in dogs.

Presentation: Code 61412B - 10 x 1 dose (1 mL) vials with syringe.
Code 61411B - 25 x 1 dose (1 mL) vials.
Code 61454B - 10 dose (10 mL) vials.

™ Trademark of Biocor Animal Health Inc.

Compendium Code No.: 13940241 BAH7001-1001 / BAH7025-1001 / BAH708-1001

BRONCHI-SHIELD® III

Fort Dodge **Vaccine**

Canine Adenovirus Type 2-Parainfluenza-Bordetella Bronchiseptica Vaccine, Modified Live Virus and Avirulent Live Culture

U.S. Vet. Lic. No.: 112

Contents: This product contains the antigens listed above.

Indications: For vaccination of healthy dogs and puppies eight weeks of age or older as an aid in prevention of diseases caused by *Bordetella bronchiseptica,* canine parainfluenza virus and canine adenovirus type 2.

Dosage and Administration:

Preparation of the Vaccine: Rehydrate with the accompanying sterile diluent. Shake well and draw back into the syringe the required amount. Remove needle from syringe and attach enclosed applicator tip. Use immediately.

Instill 0.5 mL of rehydrated vaccine into each nostril using a syringe with applicator tip. Annual revaccination is recommended.

InfoVax-ID® System: The InfoVax-ID® System provides a simple and effective method of recording pertinent information on the vaccines administered to animals in a veterinary practice.

For vaccines requiring reconstitution, remove label from both vials and affix both labels to the animal's medical chart.

Using the InfoVax-ID® System:

1. Grasp the lower right hand corner of the tab at the arrow marked "Peel Here" between your thumb and forefinger.
2. Pull steadily at a slight upward angle until the top portion of the label is separated from the vial.
3. Place the label on the animal's medical chart. Press down on the label to ensure adhesion.

Precaution(s): Store in dark at 2° to 7°C (35° to 45°F). Avoid freezing. Shake well after rehydration. Burn container and all unused contents.

Caution(s): In the absence of a veterinarian-client-patient relationship, Federal law prohibits the relabeling, repackaging, resale, or redistribution of the individual contents of this package. (9 CFR 112.6)

This product is designed for intranasal use only. Do not vaccinate dogs parenterally. A very small percentage of animals may show sneezing, coughing or nasal discharge following vaccination. These signs are usually transient. In case of anaphylactoid reaction, administer epinephrine.

Warning(s): For intranasal use only.

Do not vaccinate dogs parenterally. For veterinary use only.

Presentation: 25 doses (25-1 mL vials of vaccine plus 25-1 mL vials of diluent), featuring the InfoVax-ID® System.

U.S. Pat. No. 5,704,648 (InfoVax-ID® System)

Compendium Code No.: 10030181 1122C

BRONCHITIS VACCINE

L.A.H.I. (New Jersey) **Vaccine**

Bronchitis Vaccine, Mass. Type, Killed Virus

U.S. Vet. Lic. No.: 196

Active Ingredient(s): This product is an inactivated viral vaccine used as an aid in the prevention of Massachusetts type infectious bronchitis in chickens. The vaccine is presented as an oil emulsion.

The vaccine is manufactured in accordance with a detailed production outline, which has been filed with the Veterinary Services of the USDA. Only specific pathogen free (SPF) eggs are used for production purposes. Seed virus is derived from a master seed virus lot which has been fully tested for purity, safety and immunogenicity. The fill volume for these products is 500 mL in a 625 mL plastic bottle. The bottles are sealed with a rubber stopper and an aluminum overseal.

Quality Control: The flocks producing SPF eggs are under constant observation by experienced personnel and routinely sampled and tested serologically to confirm absence of exposure to a large variety of avian pathogens. Shipments from the supplier are accompanied by regular reports on test results for each flock from which eggs were obtained.

These products are fully tested for purity, safety and potency according to the standard requirements for infectious bronchitis vaccines published as part 113, in particular, sections 113.120 of title 9 of the federal regulations by the Animal and Plant Health Inspection Service of the USDA, and according to the production outline submitted to the U.S. Department of Agriculture.

Each serial is tested for: Bacteria and fungi and salmonella.

Potency is tested according to the outline approved by the USDA.

Indications: This product is packaged for subcutaneous vaccination in chickens three weeks of age or older. The recommended age for vaccination is 18 to 20 weeks of age. At least three weeks prior to the administration of the killed vaccine, a live Mass. type bronchitis vaccine should be used in any of the recommended methods of application for priming. Prevaccination with live vaccine is an absolute necessity for the effective use of the inactivated vaccine. If birds are to be kept for a second year of production, they should be revaccinated during molt.

Dosage and Administration: Immediately prior to use, shake the vaccine vigorously for 30 seconds to one (1) minute. Remove the aluminum overseal and the vaccine is ready to use.

Method of Vaccination: It is recommended that the inoculation be given subcutaneously in the mid-portion of the neck. Each bird should receive 0.5 mL of vaccine in this manner.

Precaution(s): The vaccine shall be stored in the dark in a refrigerator between 2-7°C (35-45°F).

Expiration date: 24 months.

Caution(s): It is imperative that the user of this product comply with the indications for use, contraindications, cautions and method of vaccination stated on the directions sheet packed with the product. The vaccine must be prepared and administered as directed to obtain the best results. For veterinary use only.

Warning(s): Do not market birds for at least six (6) weeks after vaccinating so that there is not swelling at the site of vaccine administration.

Presentation: 1,000 dose bottles.

Compendium Code No.: 10080012

BRONCHITIS VACCINE (Ark. Type)

Merial Select **Vaccine**

Bronchitis Vaccine, Arkansas Type, Live Virus

U.S. Vet. Lic. No.: 279

Contents: This vaccine contains the bronchitis virus of the Arkansas type.

Penicillin and streptomycin sulfate are added as bacteriostatic agents.

Contains fungizone as a fungistatic agent.

Notice: Merial Select's vaccines have met the requirements of the USDA in regard to safety, purity, potency and the capability to protect susceptible chickens. This vaccine has been tested by the Master Seed immunogenicity test for efficacy.

Indications: This vaccine is recommended for coarse spray vaccination of healthy, one day old chickens to aid in the prevention of bronchitis. It is essential that the chickens be maintained under good environmental conditions, and that exposure to disease viruses be reduced as much as possible.

Dosage and Administration: Read directions carefully.

Preparation of Vaccine:

1. Dilute the vaccine only as directed, observing all precautions and warnings for handling.
2. Remove from the liquid nitrogen only the ampules that are going to be used immediately. Move quickly, but carefully.
3. Place the ampule(s) in a large, clean container of water at 68° to 86°F (20° to 30°C) to thaw ampule quickly. Thaw the entire contents. Gently swirl the ampule to disperse contents. Break ampule at its neck and quickly proceed as described below.
4. Mix the contents of the ampule with cool, non-chlorinated water using 10,000 doses of vaccine to 700 mL of water.
5. Use the vaccine mixture immediately as described below.

Use of Vaccine for Coarse Spray Administration: Coarse spray vaccination is recommended for healthy chickens at one day of age or older.

1. Each box of 100 chickens should receive approximately 7 mL of vaccine. The exact amount can be determined by spraying into a calibrated tube or container to arrive at the number of applications needed to deliver 7 mL of vaccine.
2. Take care to administer a full dose to each chicken.
3. Allow chicks to dry; avoid chilling.

Precaution(s): Storage Conditions:

Ampules: Store in liquid nitrogen container.

Diluent: Store at room temperature.

Liquid Nitrogen Container: Carefully observe all liquid nitrogen precautions, including wearing eye protection and gloves. Store in a cool, well-ventilated area. Check liquid nitrogen level daily. Keep container away from incubator intakes and chicken boxes. Do not hold ampule toward face when removing from a liquid nitrogen container. Never refreeze a vaccine ampule after thawing.

Liquid Nitrogen Precautions: The liquid nitrogen containers and vaccines should be handled only by properly trained personnel. These persons should be familiar with the Union Carbide publication "Precautions and Safe Practices - Liquid Atmospheric Gasses", form #9888.

Liquid nitrogen is extremely cold. Protect eyes with goggles or face shield. Wear gloves and long sleeves when removing and handling frozen ampules or when adding liquid nitrogen to the container.

Storage and handling of liquid nitrogen containers should be in a well-ventilated area. Excessive amounts of nitrogen reduces the concentration of oxygen in the air of an unventilated space and can cause asphyxiation. If drowsiness occurs, get fresh air quickly and ventilate the entire area. If a person becomes groggy or loses consciousness while working with liquid nitrogen, get the person to a well-ventilated area immediately. If breathing has stopped, begin artificial respiration. Call a physician immediately.

Use entire contents when first opened.

Burn the container and all unused contents.

Caution(s): Do not vaccinate diseased birds.

Vaccinate all birds on the premises at one time.

Administer a full dose to each bird.

Avoid stress conditions during and following vaccination.

Do not place chickens in contaminated facilities.

Exposure to disease must be minimized as much as possible.

For veterinary use only.

Administer only as recommended.

The capability of this vaccine to produce satisfactory results depends upon many factors, including, but not limited to, conditions of storage and handling by the user, administration of the vaccine, health and responsiveness of individual animals and degree of field exposure. Therefore, directions for use should be followed carefully. The use of this vaccine is subject to applicable local and federal laws and regulations.

Warning(s): Do not vaccinate within 21 days before slaughter.

Presentation: 5 x 10,000 dose vials.

Compendium Code No.: 11050011 0399

BRONCHITIS VACCINE (Mass. Type)

Merial Select **Vaccine**

Bronchitis Vaccine, Massachusetts Type, Live Virus

U.S. Vet. Lic. No.: 279

Contents: These vaccines contain the bronchitis virus of the Massachusetts type.

Penicillin and streptomycin sulfate are added as bacteriostatic agents.

Contains amphotericin B as a fungistatic agent.

Notice: Merial Select's vaccines have met the requirement of the USDA in regard to safety, purity, potency and the capability to protect susceptible chickens. These vaccines have been tested by the Master Seed immunogenicity test for efficacy.

Indications: These vaccines are recommended for the vaccination of healthy chickens as an aid in the prevention of bronchitis.

The frozen vaccine is recommended for use as a coarse spray in healthy one day old chickens.

The 5,000 dose size of the freeze-dried vaccine is recommended for the vaccination of healthy chickens seven days of age or older.

It is essential that the chickens be maintained under good environmental conditions, and that exposure to disease viruses be reduced as much as possible.

Dosage and Administration: Read directions carefully.

A. Frozen Vaccine: For one (1) day old chickens.

Preparation of Vaccine:

1. Dilute the vaccine only as directed, observing all precautions and warnings for handling.
2. Remove from the liquid nitrogen only the ampules that are going to be used immediately. Move quickly, but carefully.
3. Place the ampule(s) in a large, clean container of water at 68° to 86°F (20° to 30°C) to thaw ampule quickly. Thaw the entire contents. Gently swirl the ampule to disperse contents. Break ampule at its neck and quickly proceed as described below.
4. Mix the contents of the ampule with cool, non-chlorinated water using 10,000 doses of vaccine to 700 mL of water.
5. Use the vaccine mixture immediately as described below.

Use of Vaccine for Coarse Spray Administration: Coarse spray vaccination is recommended for healthy chickens at one day of age or older.

1. Each box of 100 chickens should receive approximately 7 mL of vaccine. The exact amount can be determined by spraying into a calibrated tube or container to arrive at the number of applications needed to deliver 7 mL of vaccine.
2. Take care to administer a full dose to each chicken.
3. Allow chicks to dry; avoid chilling.

B. Freeze-dried Vaccine (5,000 doses): For seven (7) day old chickens.

Drinking Water Vaccination - Pouring Application:

1. Do not open or mix the vaccine until ready to vaccinate.
2. Remove all medications, sanitizers and disinfectants from the drinking water 72 hours (three days) prior to vaccination.
3. Provide sufficient waterers so that all of the chickens can drink at one time. Shut off the water supply and allow the chickens to drink the troughs dry.
4. Raise the water troughs above chickens' heads. Clean and rinse the waterers thoroughly.
5. Withhold all water from the chickens for a minimum of two (2) hours in warm weather to four (4) hours in cool weather prior to vaccination to stimulate thirst. The water withdrawal time should be reduced if half-house brooding is in process.
6. Calculate to supply vaccine solution at a rate of three (3) gallons (11 L) per 1,000 chickens in cool weather and four (4) gallons (15 L) per 1,000 chickens in warm weather. The age of the chickens should be considered when calculating the water supply. Always use non-chlorinated water when vaccinating chickens.
   Example:
   10,000 chickens in cool weather x 3 gallons (11 L) = 30 gallons (114 L).
   14,500 chickens in warm weather x 4 gallons (15 L) = 58 gallons (220 L).
7. Add one of the following to pouring water for vaccine distribution:
   a. One (1) ounce (30 mL) of non-fat, dry milk per gallon (4 L) of water, or
   b. Four (4) ounces (118 mL) of fresh skim milk per gallon (4 L) of water.
8. Prepare the vaccine concentrate as follows:
   a. Prepare a container of milk/water figuring one (1) ounce (30 mL) of concentrate for one (1) gallon (4 L) of water to be used.
   b. Add cool milk/water to the vial until the dried vaccine is dissolved. Add the vaccine to the container of milk/water to make the vaccine concentrate. Rinse the vaccine vial to remove all of the vaccine.
9. To make the vaccine solution, add one (1) ounce (30 mL) of concentrate for each gallon (4 L) of water needed.
10. Distribute the vaccine solution among waterers. Avoid direct sunlight.
11. Lower the water troughs and allow the birds to drink freely. Add the remaining vaccine solution to the troughs as the birds drink.
12. Do not provide any additional drinking water until all of the vaccine solution is consumed.

Drinking Water Vaccination - Proportioner Application: Several types of medicator/proportioners are commercially available. Set the proportioner to deliver one (1) ounce (30 mL) of vaccine concentrate per one (1) gallon (4 L) of water.

1. Do not open or mix the vaccine until ready to vaccinate.
2. Remove all medications, sanitizers and disinfectants from the proportioner 72 hours (three days) prior to vaccination.
3. Clean all containers, hoses, and waterers prior to vaccination.
4. Withhold all water from the chickens for a minimum of two (2) hours in warm weather to four (4) hours in cool weather prior to vaccination to stimulate thirst.
5. Calculate to supply the vaccine solution at a rate of three (3) gallons (11 L) per 1,000 chickens in cool weather and four (4) gallons (15 L) per 1,000 chickens in warm weather. The age of the chickens should be considered when calculating the water supply. Always use non-chlorinated water when vaccinating chickens.
   Example:
   10,000 chickens in cool weather x 3 gallons (11 L) = 30 gallons (114 L).
   14,500 chickens in warm weather x 4 gallons (15 L) = 58 gallons (220 L).
6. Prepare the vaccine concentrate as follows:
   a. Add three (3) ounces (90 mL) of non-fat, dry milk per 16 ounces (473 mL) of cool water, or
   b. Use undiluted, cool, fresh skim milk.
7. To make the vaccine solution, add one (1) ounce (30 mL) of concentrate for each gallon (4 L) of water needed.
8. Add the milk solution to the vial until the dried vaccine is dissolved. Rinse the vaccine vial to remove all of the vaccine.
9. Insert the proportioner hose into the vaccine concentrate and start the water flow. Continue until all of the concentrate has been consumed before changing the water supply to direct flow.
10. Do not medicate or use disinfectants for 24 hours after vaccination.

Coarse Spray Application: Coarse spray application is recommended for revaccination only and not as a primary vaccination. Use a sprayer delivering a coarse spray pattern to dispense the rehydrated vaccine quickly and evenly throughout a house of chickens.

1. Prior to spraying, reduce the air flow by raising curtains or stopping fans. Air movement should be limited for 15 minutes following vaccination.
2. Fill the vaccine container with cool, distilled, de-ionized water.
3. Pour the reconstituted vaccine into a clean container and add five (5) ounces (150 mL) of cool water for each 1,000 chickens to be vaccinated.
4. Place the vaccine solution into a spray canister and walk through the house spraying at the rate of 1,000 chickens per minute. Direct the spray directly above the heads of the chickens.
5. Avoid direct contact with the vaccine solution. Wear goggles and a face mask while spraying.
6. Do not use vaccinating equipment for any other purpose.

Precaution(s):

A. Storage Conditions for Frozen Vaccine:

Ampules: Store in a liquid nitrogen container.

Diluent: Store at room temperature.

Liquid Nitrogen Container: Carefully observe all liquid nitrogen precautions, including wearing eye protection and gloves. Store in a cool, well-ventilated area. Check the liquid nitrogen level daily. Keep the container away from incubator intakes and chicken boxes. Do not hold ampule toward face when removing from a liquid nitrogen container. Never refreeze a vaccine ampule after thawing.

Liquid Nitrogen Precautions: The liquid nitrogen containers and vaccines should be handled only by properly trained personnel. These persons should be familiar with the Union Carbide publication "Precautions and Safe Practices - Liquid Atmospheric Gasses", form #9888.

Liquid nitrogen is extremely cold. Accidental contact with the skin or eyes can cause serious frostbite. Protect the eyes with goggles or a face shield. Wear gloves and long sleeves when removing and handling frozen ampules or when adding liquid nitrogen to the container.

Storage and handling of liquid nitrogen containers should be in a well-ventilated area. Excessive amounts of nitrogen reduce the concentration of oxygen in the air of an unventilated space and can cause asphyxiation. If drowsiness occurs, get fresh air quickly and ventilate the entire area. If a person becomes groggy or loses consciousness while working with liquid nitrogen, get the person to a well-ventilated area immediately. If breathing has stopped, begin artificial respiration. Call a physician immediately.

Use the entire contents when first opened.

Burn the container and all unused contents.

B. Storage Conditions for Freeze-dried Vaccine:

Store the freeze-dried vaccine at 35-45°F (2-7°C). Do not freeze.

Caution(s):

A. Frozen Vaccine:

Administer only as recommended.

Do not vaccinate diseased birds.

Vaccinate all of the birds on the premises at one time.

Administer a full dose to each bird.

Avoid stress conditions during and following vaccination.

Do not place chickens in contaminated facilities.

Exposure to disease must be minimized as much as possible.

For veterinary use only.

The capability of the vaccine to produce satisfactory results depends upon many factors, including, but not limited to, conditions of storage and handling by the user, administration of the vaccine, health and the responsiveness of individual animals and the degree of field exposure. Therefore, directions for use should be followed carefully. The use of the vaccine is subject to applicable state and federal laws and regulations.

B. Freeze-dried Vaccine:

Do not vaccinate diseased birds.

Vaccinate all of the birds on the premises at one time.

Administer a minimum of one dose for each bird.

Avoid stress conditions during and following vaccination.

Do not place chickens in contaminated facilities.

Exposure to disease must be minimized as much as possible.

For veterinary use only.

The capability of the vaccine to produce satisfactory results depends upon many factors, including, but not limited to, conditions of storage and handling by the user, administration of the vaccine, health and the responsiveness of individual animals and the degree of field exposure. Therefore, directions for use should be followed carefully.

The use of the vaccine is subject to applicable state and federal laws and regulations.

Use the entire vial contents when first opened.

Burn the container and all unused contents.

Use only in states where permitted.

Warning(s): Do not vaccinate within 21 days before slaughter.

Presentation: Frozen vaccine: 5 x 10,000 dose vials.
Freeze-dried vaccine: 25 x 5,000 dose vials.

Compendium Code No.: 11050021 1298

BRONCO® WATER-BASE EQUINE FLY SPRAY

Farnam **Parasiticide-Topical**

EPA Reg. No.: 270-294

Active Ingredient(s):

Pyrethrins	0.05%
Piperonyl Butoxide Technical*	0.50%
Permethrin**	0.10%
Other Ingredients	99.35%
Total	100.00%

*Equivalent to 0.4% (butylcarbityl) (6-propylpiperonyl) ether and to 0.1% of related compounds.

**(3-phenoxyphenyl) methyl (±) cis/trans 3-(2,2-dichloroethenyl) 2,2-dimethyl cyclopropane carboxylate.

cis/trans ratio: min. 35% (±) cis and max. 65% (±) trans

Indications: Water based insecticide and repellent for use on horses and dogs and their premises. Kills and repels six fly species, ticks, gnats and mosquitoes.

Kills and Repels: Stable files, horse files, face files, deer flies, house flies, horn flies, mosquitoes, gnats, ticks, fleas, chiggers and lice.

Directions for Use: It is a violation of Federal law to use this product in a manner inconsistent with its labeling.

For horses use full strength. This non-oily insecticide repellent may be applied with a trigger spray applicator or as a wipe. Kills and repels stable files, horse files, face files, deer flies, house flies, horn flies, mosquitoes, gnats, ticks, fleas, chiggers and lice.

Directions for Wipe-on Use: Thoroughly brush horse to remove excess dirt and dust. Extremely dirty horses should be shampooed, rinsed and allowed to dry before applying wipe. Use a sponge or clean soft cloth or mitt. Apply liberally over areas to be protected. Pay special attention to legs, belly, shoulders, neck, and facial areas. Avoid eyes and mucous membranes.

Directions for Trigger Spray Use: Remove excess dirt and dust. Apply light spray mist to coat while brushing lightly against lay of the hair. Avoid spray in eyes and mucous membranes. Apply with sponge or cloth to those areas.

To Kill and Repel Flying Insects in Animal Quarters: Spray in areas where insects congregate. Direct spray to contact insects for rapid knockdown and kill. Spray around outside of door facings and screens to render area unattractive to insects. This helps to repel insects and prevent entrance into building.

Fleas and Ticks on Dogs: Start spraying at the animal's head avoiding the eyes, nose and mouth as you spray. Make sure the animal's entire body is covered including the legs, under body and tail. While spraying, fluff the hair so that the spray will penetrate to the skin. Make sure spray wets thoroughly. Avoid contact with genitalia. Reapply everyday.

Pet Areas: To control Fleas and Brown Dog Ticks on premise: Thoroughly spray infested areas, pet beds, resting quarters, nearby cracks and crevices, along and behind baseboards, moldings, window and door frames, and local areas of floor and floor covering. Fresh bedding should be placed in animal's quarters following treatment. Concurrent treatment of animals is recommended. Reapply everyday.

Precautionary Statements: Hazards to Humans and Domestic Animals:

Caution: For animal use only. Do not use on animals under three months of age. Consult a veterinarian before using this product on debilitated, aged, medicated, pregnant or nursing animals. Do not use on cats. Not for use on humans. Harmful if swallowed, inhaled, or absorbed through skin. Avoid breathing spray mist. Avoid contact with eyes, skin or clothing. Wash thoroughly with soap and water after handling. Remove contaminated clothing and wash before reuse. Sensitivities may occur after using Any pesticide product for pets. If signs of sensitivity occur, bathe your pet with mild soap and rinse with large amounts of water. If signs continue, consult a veterinarian immediately.

First Aid:

If Swallowed: Drink 1 or 2 glasses of water and induce vomiting by touching the back of throat with finger. Repeat until vomit fluid is clear. Do not induce vomiting or give anything by mouth to an unconscious person. Call a physician or Poison Control Center immediately.

If Inhaled: Remove affected person to fresh air. Apply artificial respiration if indicated. Get medical attention if irritation persists.

If on Skin: Remove contaminated clothing and wash affected areas with soap and water. Get medical attention if irritation persists.

If in Eyes: Immediately flush eyes with plenty of water. Get medical attention if irritation persists.

Environmental Hazards: This product is toxic to fish. Do not apply directly to water. Do not contaminate water when disposing of equipment washwaters.

Physical and Chemical Hazards: Do not use this product in or on electrical equipment due to the possibility of shock hazard.

Storage and Disposal:

Storage: Store in a cool, dry place. Do not store near heat or open flame.

Disposal: Securely wrap original container in several layers of newspaper and discard in trash.

Container Disposal: Do not reuse empty container. Wrap container and put in trash.

Warning(s): Use only on dogs or horses.

Presentation: 32 fl oz (946.4 mL) with sprayer and 1 gallon.

Compendium Code No.: 10000082

BRON-NEWCAVAC-M®

Intervet — **Vaccine**

Newcastle-Bronchitis Vaccine, Mass. Type, Killed Virus

U.S. Vet. Lic. No.: 286

Description: This vaccine is prepared from a single strain of Newcastle disease virus and a single strain of bronchitis virus, Massachusetts Type, inactivated with formalin and suspended in the aqueous phase of an oil adjuvant emulsion.

Quality tested for purity, potency and safety.

Indications: The vaccine is indicated for the vaccination of chickens against Newcastle disease and infectious Bronchitis caused by Massachusetts Type virus. Chickens should be in good health when vaccinated. Sick or weak chickens will not develop adequate immunity.

The use of any inactivated vaccine may cause false positive results on Mycoplasma plate tests. Avoid Mycoplasma testing prior to 10 weeks post-vaccination.

Dosage and Administration: Allow the vaccine to reach ambient temperature 16-27°C (60-80°F), before use and shake vigorously before and periodically during use. Inject 0.5 mL intramuscularly or subcutaneously in at least 3 week old chickens using a medium-sized needle. Do not vaccinate within 42 days before slaughter.

Vaccination Program: Although BRON-NEWCAVAC-M® can be used for primary vaccination at any age, available evidence suggests that the best protection is obtained when BRON-NEWCAVAC-M® is used for the revaccination of chickens previously immunized with live Newcastle and Bronchitis vaccines. Do not administer this vaccine during the critical egg laying period from onset until after peak production.

Examples: Breeder and layer pullets.

Primary vaccination with live Newcastle and Bronchitis vaccines on at least two occasions before the age of 12 weeks, with at least 4 weeks between the last live vaccine and BRON-NEWCAVAC-M® and followed by BRON-NEWCAVAC-M® (Newcastle-Bronchitis Vaccine, Inactivated) at 16-20 weeks.

Local conditions must be taken into consideration, and where necessary, veterinary advice should be sought.

Immunity: If the chickens are primed with live Newcastle and Mass. Bronchitis vaccine, the antibody response will be detectable after three or four weeks. Generally, in flocks vaccinated with BRON-NEWCAVAC-M® a protective level of immunity will be achieved with only small variations between individual chickens.

It is evident that for optimal protection preceding vaccinations with live vaccines should have taken place.

Vaccination Reaction: This vaccine does not provoke clinical reactions. If shock is observed, this must usually be ascribed to stress by handling.

Records: Keep a record of vaccine, quantity, serial number, expiration date, place of purchase; the date and time of vaccination; the number, age, breed, and locations of chickens; names of operators performing the vaccination and any observed reactions.

Precaution(s): Storage Conditions: Store in the dark in a refrigerator between 2 and 7°C (35 and 45°F). Do not freeze.

Do not mix this vaccine with any other substances.

Use entire contents when first opened.

This product is non-returnable.

Caution(s): If it is desired to vaccinate birds during lay, a drop in egg production may occur.

Vaccinate market chickens by subcutaneous route only.

Injection of inactivated vaccine into breast muscle may create processing plant problems under certain conditions.

Ensure that vaccination equipment is clean and sterile before use.

Do not use vaccination equipment with rubber parts, as the oil emulsion may attack certain types of rubber.

For veterinary use only.

Notice: This vaccine has undergone rigid potency, safety and purity tests, and meets Intervet Inc. and USDA requirements. It is designed to stimulate effective immunity when used as directed, but the user must be advised that the response to the product depends upon many factors, including, but not limited to, conditions of storage and handling by the user, administration of the vaccine, health and responsiveness of the individual chickens, and the degree of field exposure. Therefore, directions should be followed carefully.

This product is not hazardous when used according to directions supplied. A material safety data sheet (MSDS) is available upon request. This and any other consumer information can be obtained by calling Intervet Customer Service at 1-800-441-8272 or 1-302-934-8051.

The use of this vaccine is subject to applicable local and federal laws and regulations.

Use only as directed.

Warning(s): Do not vaccinate chickens within 42 days before slaughter.

Do not administer this vaccine during the critical egg laying period from onset until after peak production.

To avoid human injection, extreme caution should be used when injecting any oil emulsion vaccine. Accidental human injection may cause serious local reactions. Contact a physician immediately if accidental human injection occurs.

Presentation: 1,000 doses (500 mL).

Compendium Code No.: 11060232 — Intervet 10008 AL118

BRUCELLA ABORTUS VACCINE (STRAIN RB-51)

Professional Biological — **Vaccine**

Brucella abortus Vaccine, Strain RB-51, Live Culture

U.S. Vet. Lic. No.: 188

Contents: *Brucella abortus* vaccine, strain RB-51, live culture.

Indication(s): For use in the bovine as an aid in the prevention of infection and abortion caused by *Brucella abortus*. For vaccination of female cattle only.

Dosage and Administration: Rehydrate vaccine with accompanying diluent. Mix well before use.

Calves 4 to 12 months of age: Administer a 2.0 mL subcutaneous injection.

Cows over 12 months of age: Vaccination of cows over 12 months of age may be done only under authorization from State or Federal Animal Health Officials. Thereafter user should obtain a separate buffered diluent solution available from Professional Biological Company to prepare the final vaccine dilution.

Precaution(s): Store in the dark at 2° to 7°C. Use entire contents when first rehydrated.

Burn or sterilize this container and any remaining contents.

Caution(s): Diluent is buffered solution specifically prepared for use with this vaccine. Use only this diluent to assure viability of the vaccine.

If anaphylactoid reaction occurs administer adrenalin or equivalent.

Antidote(s): Adrenalin.

Warning(s): Do not vaccinate within 3 weeks of slaughter.

The use and distribution of this vaccine may be subject to conditions and restrictions in the United States by State and Federal regulatory authorities.

In the case of accidental human exposure contact your physician. Warning: This organism is Rifampin resistant.

For veterinary use only.

Discussion: Brucellosis or "Bangs Disease" is a contagious disease of cattle caused by the gram negative bacterium *Brucella abortus*. This organism causes abortion and infertility in animals and Undulant fever in humans. Control and elimination of this disease in cattle involves testing and culling reactors and vaccinating healthy females.

This *BRUCELLA ABORTUS* VACCINE, RB-51, is the result of research, development and production efforts by both the public and private sectors, selected as a stable strain which produces protective immunity while not inducing antibodies which react in standard serological tests. RB-51 has been tested to verify safety, efficacy and to demonstrate that there is no serological reaction in standard tests.

Presentation: 10 mL (5 dose) and 50 mL (25 dose) vials.

Compendium Code No.: 14250000

BUFFER GEL™

Vets Plus — **Dietary Supplement**

Oral Gel for Acidosis

Guaranteed Analysis: (min):

	Per Tube	Per lb.
Sodium Bicarbonate	140 g	174 g
Magnesium Oxide	46 g	58 g
Riboflavin	5 g	6 g
d-Calcium Pantothenate	10 mg	12 mg
Niacin	125 mg	155 mg
Vitamin B_{12}	100 mcg	124 mcg
Vitamin C	5 g	6 g
Vitamin E	50 IU	62 IU

Ingredients: Sodium Bicarbonate, Magnesium Oxide, DL-alpha-Tocopherol Acetate (Vitamin E), Riboflavin, Niacinamide, d-Calcium Pantothenate, Pyridoxine Hydrochloride (Vitamin B_6), Cyanocobalamin (Vitamin B_{12}), Ascorbic Acid (Vitamin C), Vegetable Oil, Silica, and preservative.

Indications: Administer to any animal when changing their ration, feeding wet grain or silage, off feed, or freshening. BUFFER GEL™ provides sodium bicarbonate, magnesium oxide, and vitamin B complex to lower the incidence of acidosis and stimulate appetite.

Dosage and Administration: Give one tube per head per day, as needed, maximum of two tubes per head per day. If conditions do not improve, consult your veterinarian.

Feeding Directions: Place the tube in a dosing gun and remove the cap. Hold the head of the animal in a slightly elevated position and place the nozzle on the back of the tongue. Administer the entire contents of the tube slowly, allowing the animal time to swallow. Do not give to animals that are unable to swallow.

Precaution(s): Keep in a cool dry place. Avoid freezing.

Caution(s): Keep out of the reach of children. Contact with eyes or wounds or prolonged contact with skin can cause irritation. Single dose unit. Properly dispose of unused portion.

Animal use only.

Presentation: 12x300 cc (365 gm) tubes per case.

Compendium Code No.: 10730050

BURO-O-CORT 2:1

Q.A. Laboratories — **Topical Corticosteroid**

Active Ingredient(s): Each mL contains:

Burow's solution (astringent) . . . . 20 mg

Hydrocortisone (anti-inflammatory, antipruritic) . . . . 10 mg

In a water miscible propylene glycol base.

Indications: A topical treatment for the relief of inflammatory pruritic conditions in dogs.

Dosage and Administration: Apply three (3) to four (4) times a day.
Contraindication(s): As with any hydrocortisone product, BUR-O-CORT 2:1 should not be used in the presence of tuberculosis of the skin.
Precaution(s): Store in a cool area.
Caution(s): Keep out of the reach of children.
For topical use only. Not for ophthalmic use. Not for deep-seated infections.
Presentation: 1 oz. and 16 oz. containers.
Compendium Code No.: 13680000

B

BUR-OTIC® HC EAR TREATMENT ℞

Virbac **Otic Corticosteroid**
NDC No.: 51311-035-01
Active Ingredient(s): Hydrocortisone, 1%.
Other Ingredients: Propylene glycol, water, burow's solution, acetic acid, benzalkonium chloride.
Indications: For inflammatory manifestations of corticosteroid-responsive ear conditions in dogs and cats.
Dosage and Administration: Apply five to ten drops in each affected ear twice a day for five days or as directed by your veterinarian. If condition persists, discontinue use of this product and consult your veterinarian.
Caution(s): Federal law (USA) restricts this drug to use by or on the order of a licensed veterinarian.
Warning(s): Avoid contact with eyes. Keep out of reach of children.
Presentation: 1 fl oz (30 mL).
Compendium Code No.: 10230020

BUROWS H SOLUTION

Vetus **Topical Corticosteroid**
Active Ingredient(s):
Hydrocortisone 1.0%
Burows solution 2.0%
In a base containing propylene glycol.
Indications: BUROWS H SOLUTION exhibits astringent, anti-inflammatory and antipruritic action when used as an aid in the treatment of moist dermatitis in dogs.
Dosage and Administration: Shake well before using. Apply three (3) or four (4) times a day.
Contraindication(s): As with any hydrocortisone product, do not use in the presence of tuberculosis of the skin.
Precaution(s): Store in a cool, dry place.
Caution(s): For external use only. Do not use around the eyes. Not for deep-seated infections.
For veterinary use only. Keep out of the reach of children.
Presentation: 1 oz squeeze bottles, 2 oz sprayer and 16 oz bottles.
Compendium Code No.: 14440130

BURSA BLEN® M

Merial Select **Vaccine**
Bursal Disease Vaccine, Live Virus
U.S. Vet. Lic. No.: 279
Contents: This vaccine contains live bursal disease virus.
Contains gentamicin as a bacteriostatic agent.
Notice: Merial Select's vaccines have met the requirements of the USDA in regard to safety, purity, potency, and the capability to protect susceptible chickens. This vaccine has been tested by the Master Seed immunogenicity test for efficacy.
Indications: For the initial vaccination of healthy meat-type chickens at least nine days of age by drinking water as an aid in the prevention of infectious bursal disease.
This vaccine is recommended for the protection of healthy chickens. It is essential that the chickens be maintained under good environmental conditions and that exposure to disease viruses be reduced as much as possible.
Dosage and Administration:
Drinking Water Vaccination Using Pouring Application: Drinking water vaccination is recommended for healthy chickens at least nine days of age.
1. Remove all medications, sanitizers and disinfectants from the drinking water 72 hours (three days) prior to vaccination.
2. Provide sufficient waterers so that all the chickens can drink at one time. Shut off water supply and allow chickens to consume all the water in the lines.
3. Raise water lines above the chickens' heads. Clean and rinse the waterers thoroughly.
4. Withhold all water from the chickens for a minimum of two hours in warm weather to four hours in cool weather prior to vaccination to stimulate thirst. Withdrawal time should be reduced if half-house brooding is in process.
5. Do not open or mix vaccine until ready to vaccinate.
6. Drinking water for vaccine delivery should contain one ounce (29 gram) of non-fat dry milk per gallon (3.8 liters) of non-chlorinated water, or should contain milk product based stabilizer prepared according to the manufacturer's instructions.
7. Reconstitute the vaccine in 3 gallons (11 liters) of milk-water during cool weather or 4 gallons (15 liters) of milk-water during warm weather for each 1,000 doses.
8. Distribute vaccine solution among waterers. Avoid direct sunlight.
9. Lower waterers and allow the chickens to drink freely. Add the remaining vaccine solution to the water lines as the chickens drink.
10. Do not provide additional drinking water until all the vaccine is consumed.

Drinking Water Vaccination Using Proportioner Application: Drinking water vaccination is recommended for healthy chickens at least nine days of age. Several types of medicator/proportioners are commercially available. Set proportioner to deliver one ounce (30 mL) of vaccine concentrate per one gallon (3.8 liters) of water.
1. Remove all medications, sanitizers and disinfectants from the drinking water 72 hours (three days) prior to vaccination.
2. Clean all containers, hoses and waterers prior to vaccination.
3. Withhold all water from the chickens for a minimum of two hours in warm weather to four hours in cool weather prior to vaccination to stimulate thirst. Withdrawal time should be reduced if half-house brooding is in process.
4. Do not open or mix vaccine until ready to vaccinate.
5. Calculate to supply vaccine solution at a rate of 3 gallons (11 liters) per 1,000 chickens in cool weather and 4 gallons (15 liters) per 1,000 chickens in warm weather. The age of the chickens should be considered when calculating water supply. Always use non-chlorinated water when vaccinating chickens.
Example:
1,000 chickens in cool weather x 3 gallons (11 liters) = 3 gallons (11 liters).
1,000 chickens in warm weather x 4 gallons (15 liters) = 4 gallons (15 liters).
6. Prepare vaccine stock solution as follows:
   a. Determine the quantity of vaccine concentrate required by multiplying one ounce (30 mL) x gallons of water needed for vaccine/drinking water.
   Example:
   For 1,000 chickens: 3 gallons x 1 ounce (30 mL) = 3 ounces (90 mL).
   b. Add 3 ounces (85 gm) of non-fat dry milk per 16 ounces (480 mL) of cool water, or use a commercial milk product based stabilizer according to the manufacturer's instructions. For 1,000 chickens add 0.5 ounces (16 gm) non-fat dry milk to the 3 ounces (90 mL) of water.
   c. Reconstitute the dried vaccine with the milk solution. Rinse the vaccine vial to remove all the vaccine.
7. Insert proportioner hose into the vaccine stock solution and start water flow. Continue until all solution has been consumed before changing water supply to direct flow.
8. Do not medicate or use disinfectants for 24 hours after vaccination.

Precaution(s): Store vaccine at 35-45°F (2-7°C). Do not freeze. Use entire vial contents when first opened. Burn the container and all unused contents.
Caution(s): Do not vaccinate diseased chickens.
Vaccinate all chickens on the premises at one time.
Administer a minimum of one dose per chicken.
Avoid stress conditions during and following vaccination.
Do not place chickens in contaminated facilities.
Exposure to disease must be minimized as much as possible.
The capability of this vaccine to produce satisfactory results depends upon many factors, including, but not limited to, conditions of storage and handling by the user, administration of the vaccine, health and responsiveness of individual chickens, and degree of field exposure. Therefore, directions for use should be followed carefully. The use of this vaccine is subject to applicable state and federal laws and regulations.
For veterinary use only.
Warning(s): Do not vaccinate within 21 days of slaughter.
Presentation: BURSA BLEN® M is supplied without a diluent for water administration only (25 x 2,000 doses and 15 x 10,000 doses).
Compendium Code No.: 11050032 0699

BURSA GUARD

Merial Select **Vaccine**
Bursal Disease Vaccine, Killed Virus, Standard & Variant
U.S. Vet. Lic. No.: 279
Composition: This product is a suspension of bursal disease virus emulsified in oil. It contains the Standard and Variant E strains of bursal virus.
Bursal Disease Virus Origin: Bursal Tissue 100%
Indications: Use in chicken replacement pullets or breeder hens to stimulate an increased level of passive immunity in their progeny against bursal disease virus, standard and variant strains.
Directions: Warm vaccine to room temperature. Shake well. Inject 0.5 mL intramuscularly or subcutaneously using aseptic technique. Vaccinate at 16 weeks of age or older. Birds should be primed with a live bursal disease vaccine at least 4 weeks prior to the first use of this product.
Precaution(s): Store in the dark between 36-45°F (2-7°C). Do not freeze. Use entire contents when first opened.
Caution(s): For veterinary use only.
Warning(s): Do not vaccinate within 42 days before slaughter.
Humans injected with this vaccine should seek immediate medical attention. Advise medical personnel that the vaccine is an oil emulsion type.
Presentation: 10 x 1,000 dose (500 mL) bottles.
Compendium Code No.: 11050042

BURSA GUARD N-B

Merial Select **Vaccine**
Bursal Disease-Newcastle Disease-Bronchitis Vaccine, Standard & Variant, Mass & Ark Types, Killed Virus
U.S. Vet. Lic. No.: 279
Composition: This product is a suspension of bursal disease, Newcastle disease, and bronchitis viruses emulsified in oil. The following strains are utilized:
Bursal - Standard and Variant E
Newcastle - LaSota
Bronchitis - Mass and Ark
Bursal Virus Origin: Bursal Tissue 100%
Newcastle, Bronchitis Virus Origin: Chick Embryo 100%
Indications: Use in chicken pullet/hens to protect them against Newcastle disease and bronchitis and to stimulate passive immunity in their progeny against bursal disease.
Directions: Warm vaccine to room temperature. Shake well. Inject 0.5 mL subcutaneously using aseptic technique. Vaccinate at 12-13 weeks of age and repeat at 20-21 weeks of age. Birds should be primed with live bursal disease and bronchitis vaccines at least 4 weeks prior to the first use of this product.
Precaution(s): Store in the dark between 36-45°F (2-7°C). Do not freeze. Use entire contents when first opened.
Caution(s): For veterinary use only.
Warning(s): Do not vaccinate within 42 days before slaughter.
Humans injected with this vaccine should seek immediate medical attention. Advise medical personnel that the vaccine is an oil emulsion type.
Presentation: 10 x 1,000 dose (500 mL) bottles.
Compendium Code No.: 11050052

BURSA GUARD N-B-R

Merial Select **Vaccine**
Bursal Disease-Newcastle Disease-Bronchitis-Reovirus Vaccine, Standard & Variant, Mass & Ark Types, Killed Virus
U.S. Vet. Lic. No.: 279
Composition: This product is a suspension of bursal disease and Newcastle disease, bronchitis and reovirus viruses emulsified in oil. The following strains are utilized:
Bursal - Standard and Variant E
Newcastle - LaSota

Bronchitis - Mass and Ark
Reo - 1133, 2408, MSB
Bursal Virus Origin: Bursal Tissue 100%
Newcastle, Bronchitis, Reovirus Origin: Chick Embryo 100%

Indications: Use in chicken pullet/hens to protect them against Newcastle disease and bronchitis and to stimulate passive immunity in their progeny against bursal disease and reovirus.
Directions: Warm vaccine to room temperature. Shake well. Inject 0.5 mL subcutaneously using aseptic technique. Vaccinate at 12-13 weeks of age and repeat at 20-21 weeks of age. Birds should be primed with live reovirus, bronchitis and bursal disease vaccines at least 4 weeks prior to the first use of this product.
Precaution(s): Store in the dark between 36-45°F (2-7°C). Do not freeze. Use entire contents when first opened.
Caution(s): For veterinary use only.
Warning(s): Do not vaccinate within 42 days before slaughter.
Humans injected with this vaccine should seek immediate medical attention. Advise medical personnel that the vaccine is an oil emulsion type.
Presentation: 10 x 1,000 dose (500 mL) bottles.
Compendium Code No.: 11050062

BURSA GUARD N-R

Merial Select **Vaccine**

Bursal Disease-Newcastle Disease-Reovirus Vaccine, Standard & Variant, Killed Virus
U.S. Vet. Lic. No.: 279
Composition: This product is a suspension of bursal disease and Newcastle disease viruses, and reovirus emulsified in oil. The following strains are utilized:
Bursal - Standard and Variant E
Newcastle - LaSota
Reo - 1133, 2408, MSB
Bursal Virus Origin: Bursal Tissue 100%
Newcastle, Reovirus Origin: Chick Embryo 100%

Indications: Use in chicken pullet/hens to protect them against Newcastle disease and to stimulate passive immunity in their progeny against bursal disease and reovirus.
Directions: Warm vaccine to room temperature. Shake well. Inject 0.5 mL subcutaneously using aseptic technique. Vaccinate at 12-13 weeks of age and repeat at 20-21 weeks of age. Birds should be primed with live reovirus and bursal disease vaccines at least 4 weeks prior to the first use of this product.
Precaution(s): Store in the dark between 36-45°F (2-7°C). Do not freeze. Use entire contents when first opened.
Caution(s): For veterinary use only.
Warning(s): Do not vaccinate within 42 days before slaughter.
Humans injected with this vaccine should seek immediate medical attention. Advise medical personnel that the vaccine is an oil emulsion type.
Presentation: 10 x 1,000 dose (500 mL) bottles.
Compendium Code No.: 11050072

BURSA GUARD REO

Merial Select **Vaccine**

Bursal Disease-Reovirus Vaccine, Killed Virus, Standard & Variant
U.S. Vet. Lic. No.: 279
Composition: This product is a suspension of bursal disease virus and avian reovirus emulsified in oil. It contains the Standard and Variant E strains of bursal disease virus and the 1133, 2408, and MSB strains of reovirus.
Bursal Disease Virus Origin: Bursal Tissue 100%
Reovirus Origin: Chick Embryo 100%

Indications: Use in chicken pullet/hens to stimulate an increased level of passive immunity in their progeny against bursal disease virus and tenosynovitis or malabsorption caused by avian reoviruses.
Directions: Warm vaccine to room temperature. Shake well. Inject 0.5 mL subcutaneously using aseptic technique. Vaccinate at 12-13 weeks of age and repeat at 20-21 weeks of age. Birds should be primed with live reovirus and bursal disease vaccines at least 4 weeks prior to the first use of this product.
Precaution(s): Store in the dark between 36-45°F (2-7°C). Do not freeze. Use entire contents when first opened.
Caution(s): For veterinary use only.
Warning(s): Do not vaccinate within 42 days before slaughter.
Humans injected with this vaccine should seek immediate medical attention. Advise medical personnel that the vaccine is an oil emulsion type.
Presentation: 10 x 1,000 dose (500 mL) bottles.
Compendium Code No.: 11050082

BURSAL DISEASE-AVIAN REOVIRUS VACCINE

L.A.H.I. (New Jersey) **Vaccine**

Bursal Disease-Avian Reovirus Vaccine, Standard and Variant, Killed Virus
U.S. Vet. Lic. No.: 196
Active Ingredient(s): This product is a suspension of killed infectious bursal disease viruses of chicken tissue culture, chicken embryo and bursal tissue origin and avian reovirus of chicken tissue culture origin.

The vaccine is manufactured in accordance with a detailed production outline, which has been filed with the Veterinary Services of the USDA. Seed virus is derived from a master seed lot, which has been fully tested for purity, safety and immunogenicity. The fill volume is 500 mL in a 625 mL plastic bottle. The bottles are sealed with a rubber stopper and an aluminum overseal.

Quality Control: The flocks producing SPF eggs are under constant observation by experienced personnel and routinely sampled and tested serologically to confirm absence of exposure to a large variety of avian pathogens. Shipments from the supplier are accompanied by regular reports on test results for each flock from which eggs were obtained.

The products are fully tested for purity and safety according to the standard requirements as published in the federal regulations by the Animal and Plant Health Inspection Service of the U.S. Department of Agriculture.

Each serial is tested for: Bacterial and fungi; extraneous viruses; safety and potency tests in chickens according to the production outline filed with the USDA.

Samples and complete test reports on each serial are submitted to the Veterinary Services of the USDA and no merchandise is released for shipment until this government agency has given its release agreement.

Indications: This product is used for vaccination and revaccination of breeder chickens for the passive protection of baby chicks against standard and variant bursal disease and reovirus infection. Breeders can be vaccinated when they are 15-22 weeks of age. At the time of vaccination, they should have an SN titer of 15 against reovirus. To obtain satisfactory results, the birds should be primed with live tenosynovitis vaccine. Good results have been obtained when tenosynovitis vaccine is given at five to seven days and revaccinated four to five weeks later.
Dosage and Administration: Immediately prior to use, shake the vaccine vigorously for 30 seconds to one (1) minute. Remove the aluminum overseal and the vaccine is ready to use.
Method of Vaccination: The vaccine should be administered subcutaneously in the middle portion of the neck.
Each bird should receive 1.0 mL of vaccine.
Precaution(s): The vaccine shall be stored in the dark in a refrigerator between 35-45°F (2-7°C).
Expiration dating: 24 months.
Caution(s): It is imperative that the user of this product comply with the indications for use, contraindications, cautions and methods of vaccination stated in the direction sheet packed with each product. The vaccine must be prepared and administered as directed to obtain the best results. For veterinary use only.
Warning(s): Do not market birds for at least six (6) weeks after vaccinating so that there is not swelling at the site of vaccine administration.
Presentation: 1,000 dose bottles.
Compendium Code No.: 10080022

B

BURSAL DISEASE-MAREK'S DISEASE VACCINE (Standard and Variant, Chicken and Turkey)

Merial Select **Vaccine**

Bursal Disease-Marek's Vaccine, Live Virus, Standard and Variant, Live Chicken and Turkey Herpesvirus
U.S. Vet. Lic. No.: 279
Contents: The vaccine contains the ST-14 strain and the 1084A strains of live bursal disease virus, and the FC-126 strain of turkey herpesvirus, and the SB-1 strain of chicken herpesvirus.
Penicillin and streptomycin sulfate are added as bacteriostatic agents.
Contains fungizone as a fungistatic agent.
Notice: The vaccine has met the requirements of the USDA in regards to safety, purity, potency and the ability to protect normally susceptible chickens. The vaccine has been tested by the master seed immunogenicity test for efficacy.
Indications: The vaccine is recommended for use in healthy one day old chickens as an aid in the prevention of infectious bursal disease (gumboro) and Marek's disease. Chickens to be vaccinated must be healthy and free of all diseases. It is essential that the chickens be maintained under good environmental conditions, and that exposure to disease viruses be reduced as much as possible in the field.
Dosage and Administration: Frozen Vaccine:
Preparation of the Vaccine for Use:
Important: Sterilize the vaccinating equipment by autoclaving for a minimum of 15 minutes at 250°F (121°C) or by boiling in water for at least 20 minutes. Never allow chemical disinfectants to come into contact with the vaccinating equipment.

1. Use 200 mL of sterile diluent for each 1,000 doses of vaccine indicated on the ampule.
2. Remove only one (1) ampule of vaccine at a time from the liquid nitrogen container. Thaw and use immediately. Do not hold the ampule toward the face when removing it from a liquid nitrogen container. Never refreeze a vaccine ampule after thawing.
3. Rapidly thaw the ampule by immersing it in water at room temperature (15-25°C). Gently swirl the ampule to disperse contents. Break the ampule at its neck and quickly proceed as described below.
4. Remove the cover from the diluent container. Draw the contents of the ampule into a sterile 10 mL syringe fitted with an 18 to 20 gauge needle. Slowly add the contents of the vaccine ampule to the appropriate volume of diluent. Withdraw a small amount of the diluent, rinse the ampule once and add this to the vaccine-diluent mixture. Mix the contents of the diluent container thoroughly by swirling and inverting the container. Do not shake vigorously.
5. Use the vaccine-diluent mixture immediately as described below.

Method of Vaccination:

1. Give subcutaneously only.
2. Use a sterile automatic syringe with a 20-22 gauge, ⅜"-½" needle which is set to accurately deliver 0.2 mL per dose. Check the accuracy of delivery several times during the vaccination procedure.
3. Dilute the vaccine only as directed observing all precautions and warnings for handling.
4. Keep the bottle of diluted vaccine in an ice bath and agitate continuously.
5. Inject chickens under the loose skin at the back of the neck (subcutaneously), holding the chicken by the back of the neck just below the head. The loose skin in this area is raised by gently pinching with the thumb and forefinger. Insert the needle beneath the skin in a direction away from the head. Inject 0.2 mL per chicken. Avoid hitting the muscles and bones in the neck.
6. Use the entire contents of the vaccine container within one (1) hour after mixing the vaccine with the diluent.

Precaution(s):
Ampules: Store in a liquid nitrogen container.
Diluent: Store at room temperature.
Liquid nitrogen container: Store in a cool, well-ventilated area. Check the liquid nitrogen level once a day. Keep the container away from incubator intakes and chicken boxes.
Liquid Nitrogen Precautions: The liquid nitrogen containers and vaccines should be handled by properly trained personnel only. These persons should be familiar with the Union Carbide publication "Precautions and Safe Practices - Liquid Atmospheric Gases", form #9888. Liquid nitrogen is extremely cold. Accidental contact with the skin or eyes can cause serious frostbite. Protect the eyes with goggles or a face shield. Wear gloves and long sleeves when removing and handling frozen ampules or when adding liquid nitrogen to the container. Storage and handling of liquid nitrogen containers should be in a well-ventilated area. Excessive amounts of nitrogen reduce the concentration of oxygen in the air of an unventilated space and can cause asphyxiation. If drowsiness occurs, get fresh air quickly and ventilate the entire area. If a person becomes groggy or loses consciousness while working with liquid nitrogen, get the person to a well-ventilated area immediately. If breathing has stopped, begin artificial respiration. Call a physician immediately.
Caution(s): Use only in localities where permitted.
Use only in flocks with a history of infectious bursal disease.

Do not vaccinate diseased birds.
Vaccinate all of the birds on the premises at one time.
Administer a minimum of one dose for each bird.
Avoid stress conditions during and following vaccination.
Do not place chickens in contaminated facilities.
Exposure to disease must be minimized as much as possible.
For veterinary use only.
Administer only as recommended.
Use the entire contents when first opened.
Burn the container and all unused contents.

The capability of the vaccine to produce satisfactory results depends upon many factors, including, but not limited to, conditions of storage and handling by the user, administration of the vaccine, health and the responsiveness of individual animals and the degree of field exposure. Directions for use should be followed carefully.

The use of the vaccine is subject to applicable local and federal laws and regulations.

Warning(s): Do not vaccinate within 21 days before slaughter.

Presentation: 5 x 1,000 doses.

Compendium Code No.: 11050132

BURSAL DISEASE-MAREK'S DISEASE VACCINE (Standard and Variant, Turkey)

Merial Select **Vaccine**

Bursal Disease-Marek's Disease Vaccine, Live Virus, Standard and Variant, Live Turkey Herpesvirus

U.S. Vet. Lic. No.: 279

Active Ingredient(s): The vaccine contains the ST-14 and the 1084A strains of the live bursal disease virus and the FC-126 strain of the turkey herpesvirus.

Penicillin and streptomycin sulfate are added as bacteriostatic agents.

Contains fungizone as a fungistatic agent.

Notice: The vaccine has met the requirements of the USDA in regards to safety, purity, potency and the capability to protect normally susceptible chickens. The vaccine has been tested by the master seed immunogenicity test for efficacy.

Indications: The vaccine is recommended for use in healthy one day old chickens to aid in the prevention of infectious bursal disease (gumboro) and Marek's disease.

Chickens to be vaccinated must be healthy and free of all diseases. It is essential that the chickens be maintained under good environmental conditions, and that exposure to disease viruses be reduced as much as possible in the field.

Dosage and Administration: Frozen Vaccine:
Preparation of the Vaccine for Use:

Important: Sterilize the vaccinating equipment by autoclaving for a minimum of 15 minutes at 250°F (121°C) or by boiling in water for at least 20 minutes. Never allow chemical disinfectants to come into contact with the vaccinating equipment.

1. Use 200 mL of sterile diluent for each 1,000 doses of vaccine indicated on the ampule.
2. Remove only one (1) ampule of vaccine at a time from the liquid nitrogen container. Thaw and use immediately. Do not hold the ampule toward the face when removing it from a liquid nitrogen container. Never refreeze a vaccine ampule after thawing.
3. The contents of the ampule are thawed rapidly by immersing it in water at room temperature (15-25°C). Gently swirl the ampule to disperse the contents. Break the ampule at its neck and quickly proceed as described below.
4. Remove the cover from the diluent container. Draw the contents of the ampule into a sterile 10 mL syringe fitted with an 18 to 20 gauge needle. Slowly add the contents of the vaccine ampule to the appropriate volume of diluent. Withdraw a small amount of the diluent, rinse the ampule once and add this to the vaccine diluent mixture. Mix the contents of the diluent container thoroughly by swirling and inverting the container. Do not shake vigorously.
5. Use the vaccine-diluent mixture immediately as described below.

Method of Vaccination:

1. Give subcutaneously only.
2. Use a sterile automatic syringe with a 20-22 gauge, ⅜"-½" needle which is set to accurately deliver 0.2 mL per dose. Check the accuracy of delivery several times during the vaccination procedure.
3. Dilute the vaccine only as directed observing all precautions and warnings for handling.
4. Keep the bottle of diluted vaccine in an ice bath and agitate continuously.
5. Inject chickens under the loose skin at the back of the neck (subcutaneously), holding the chickens by the back of the neck just below the head. The loose skin in this area is raised by gently pinching with the thumb and forefinger. Insert the needle beneath the skin in a direction away from the head. Inject 0.2 mL per chicken. Avoid hitting the muscles and bones in the neck.
6. Use the entire contents of the vaccine container within one (1) hour after mixing the vaccine with the diluent.

Precaution(s):

Ampules: Store in a liquid nitrogen container.

Diluent: Store at room temperature.

Liquid nitrogen container: Store in a cool, well-ventilated area. Check the liquid nitrogen level once a day. Keep the container away from incubator intakes and chicken boxes.

Liquid Nitrogen Precautions: The liquid nitrogen containers and vaccines should be handled by properly trained personnel only. These persons should be familiar with the Union Carbide publication "Precautions and Safe Practices - Liquid Atmospheric Gases", form #9888. Liquid nitrogen is extremely cold. Accidental contact with the skin or eyes can cause serious frostbite. Protect the eyes with goggles or a face shield. Wear gloves and long sleeves when removing and handling frozen ampules or when adding liquid nitrogen to the container. Storage and handling of liquid nitrogen containers should be in a well-ventilated area. Excessive amounts of nitrogen reduces the concentration of oxygen in the air of an unventilated space and can cause asphyxiation. If drowsiness occurs, get fresh air quickly and ventilate the entire area. If a person becomes groggy or loses consciousness while working with liquid nitrogen, get the person to a well-ventilated area immediately. If breathing has stopped, begin artificial respiration. Call a physician immediately.

Caution(s): Use only in localities where permitted.
Use only in flocks with a history of infectious bursal disease.
Do not vaccinate diseased birds.
Vaccinate all of the birds on the premises at one time.
Administer a minimum of one dose for each bird.
Avoid stress conditions during and following vaccination.
Do not place chickens in contaminated facilities.
Exposure to disease must be minimized as much as possible.
For veterinary use only.
Administer only as recommended.
Use the entire contents when first opened.
Burn the container and all unused contents.

The capability of the vaccine to produce satisfactory results depends upon many factors, including, but not limited to, conditions of storage and handling by the user, administration of the vaccine, health and the responsiveness of individual animals and the degree of field exposure. Directions for use should be followed carefully.

The use of the vaccine is subject to applicable local and federal laws and regulations.

Warning(s): Do not vaccinate within 21 days before slaughter.

Presentation: 5 x 1,000 doses and 5 x 2,000 doses.

Compendium Code No.: 11050141

BURSAL DISEASE-MAREK'S DISEASE VACCINE (Standard, Chicken and Turkey)

Merial Select **Vaccine**

Bursal Disease-Marek's Disease Vaccine, Live Virus, Live Chicken and Turkey Herpesvirus

U.S. Vet. Lic. No.: 279

Active Ingredient(s): The vaccine contains the ST-14 strain of the live bursal disease virus, the FC-126 strain of turkey herpesvirus and the SB-I strain of chicken herpesvirus.

Penicillin and streptomycin sulfate are added as bacteriostatic agents.

Contains fungizone as a fungistatic agent.

Notice: The vaccine has met the requirements of the USDA in regards to safety, purity, potency and the capability to protect normally susceptible chickens. The vaccine has been tested by the master seed immunogenicity test for efficacy.

Indications: The vaccine is recommended for use in healthy one day old chickens as an aid in the prevention of infectious bursal disease (gumboro) and Marek's disease. Chickens to be vaccinated must be healthy and free of all diseases. It is essential that the chickens be maintained under good environmental conditions, and that exposure to disease viruses be reduced as much as possible in the field.

Dosage and Administration: Frozen Vaccine:
Preparation of the Vaccine for Use:

Important: Sterilize the vaccinating equipment by autoclaving for a minimum of 15 minutes at 250°F (121°C) or by boiling in water for at least 20 minutes. Never allow chemical disinfectants to come into contact with the vaccinating equipment.

1. Use 200 mL of sterile diluent for each 1,000 doses of vaccine indicated on the ampule.
2. Remove only one (1) ampule of vaccine at a time from the liquid nitrogen container. Thaw and use immediately. Do not hold the ampule toward the face when removing it from a liquid nitrogen container. Never refreeze a vaccine ampule after thawing.
3. The contents of the ampule are thawed rapidly by immersing it in water at room temperature (15-25°C). Gently swirl the ampule to disperse the contents. Break the ampule at its neck and quickly proceed as described below.
4. Remove the cover from the diluent container. Draw the contents of the ampule into a sterile 10 mL syringe fitted with an 18 to 20 gauge needle. Slowly add the contents of the vaccine ampule to the appropriate volume of diluent. Withdraw a small amount of the diluent, rinse the ampule once and add this to the vaccine diluent mixture. Mix the contents of the diluent container thoroughly by swirling and inverting the container. Do not shake vigorously.
5. Use the vaccine-diluent mixture immediately as described below.

Method of Vaccination:

1. Give subcutaneously only.
2. Use a sterile automatic syringe with a 20-22 gauge, ⅜"-½" needle which is set to accurately deliver 0.2 mL per dose. Check the accuracy of delivery several times during the vaccination procedure.
3. Dilute the vaccine only as directed observing all precautions and warnings for handling.
4. Keep the bottle of diluted vaccine in an ice bath and agitate continuously.
5. Inject chickens under the loose skin at the back of the neck (subcutaneously), holding the chickens by the back of the neck just below the head. The loose skin in this area is raised by gently pinching with the thumb and forefinger. Insert the needle beneath the skin in a direction away from the head. Inject 0.2 mL per chicken. Avoid hitting the muscles and bones in the neck.
6. Use the entire contents of the vaccine container within one (1) hour after mixing the vaccine with the diluent.

Precaution(s):

Ampules: Store in a liquid nitrogen container.

Diluent: Store at room temperature.

Liquid nitrogen container: Store in a cool, well-ventilated area. Check the liquid nitrogen level once a day. Keep the container away from incubator intakes and chicken boxes.

Liquid Nitrogen Precautions: The liquid nitrogen containers and vaccines should be handled by properly trained personnel only. These persons should be familiar with the Union Carbide publication "Precautions and Safe Practices - Liquid Atmospheric Gases", form #9888. Liquid nitrogen is extremely cold. Accidental contact with the skin or eyes can cause serious frostbite. Protect the eyes with goggles or a face shield. Wear gloves and long sleeves when removing and handling frozen ampules or when adding liquid nitrogen to the container. Storage and handling of liquid nitrogen containers should be in a well-ventilated area. Excessive amounts of nitrogen reduces the concentration of oxygen in the air of an unventilated space and can cause asphyxiation. If drowsiness occurs, get fresh air quickly and ventilate the entire area. If a person becomes groggy or loses consciousness while working with liquid nitrogen, get the person to a well-ventilated area immediately. If breathing has stopped, begin artificial respiration. Call a physician immediately.

Caution(s): Use only in localities where permitted.
Use only in flocks with a history of infectious bursal disease.
Do not vaccinate diseased birds.
Vaccinate all of the birds on the premises at one time.
Administer a minimum of one dose for each bird.
Avoid stress conditions during and following vaccination.
Do not place chickens in contaminated facilities.
Exposure to disease must be minimized as much as possible.
For veterinary use only.
Administer only as recommended.
Use the entire contents when first opened.
Burn the container and all unused contents.

The capability of the vaccine to produce satisfactory results depends upon many factors, including, but not limited to, conditions of storage and handling by the user, administration of the vaccine, health and the responsiveness of individual animals and the degree of field exposure. Directions for use should be followed carefully.

The use of the vaccine is subject to applicable local and federal laws and regulations.

Warning(s): Do not vaccinate within 21 days before slaughter.

Presentation: 5 x 1,000 doses and 5 x 2,000 doses.

Compendium Code No.: 11050151

BURSAL DISEASE-MAREK'S DISEASE VACCINE (Standard, Turkey)

Merial Select **Vaccine**

Bursal Disease-Marek's Disease Vaccine, Live Virus, Live Turkey Herpesvirus

U.S. Vet. Lic. No.: 279

Active Ingredient(s): The vaccine contains the ST-14 strain of live bursal disease virus and the FC-126 strain of turkey herpesvirus.

Penicillin and streptomycin sulfate are added as bacteriostatic agents.

Contains fungizone as a fungistatic agent.

Notice: The vaccine has met the requirements of the USDA in regard to safety, purity, potency and the capability to protect normally susceptible chickens. This vaccine has been tested by the master seed immunogenicity test for efficacy.

Indications: The vaccine is recommended for use in healthy one day old chickens to aid in the prevention of infectious bursal disease (gumboro) and Marek's disease.

Chickens to be vaccinated must be healthy and free of all diseases. It is essential that the chickens be maintained under good environmental conditions, and that exposure to disease viruses be reduced as much as possible in the field.

Dosage and Administration: Frozen Vaccine:

Preparation of the Vaccine for Use:

Important: Sterilize the vaccinating equipment by autoclaving for a minimum of 15 minutes at 250°F (121°C) or by boiling in water for at least 20 minutes. Never allow chemical disinfectants to come into contact with the vaccinating equipment.

1. Use 200 mL of sterile diluent for each 1,000 doses of vaccine indicated on the ampule.
2. Remove only one (1) ampule of vaccine at a time from the liquid nitrogen container. Thaw and use immediately. Do not hold the ampule toward the face when removing it from a liquid nitrogen container. Never refreeze a vaccine ampule after thawing.
3. The contents of the ampule are thawed rapidly by immersing it in water at room temperature (15-25°C). Gently swirl the ampule to disperse contents. Break the ampule at its neck and quickly proceed as described below.
4. Remove the cover from the diluent container. Draw the contents of the ampule into a sterile 10 mL syringe fitted with an 18 to 20 gauge needle. Slowly add the contents of the vaccine ampule to the appropriate volume of diluent. Withdraw a small amount of the diluent, rinse the ampule once and add this to the vaccine diluent mixture. Mix the contents of the diluent container thoroughly by swirling and inverting the container. Do not shake vigorously.
5. Use the vaccine-diluent mixture immediately as described below.

Method of Vaccination:

1. Give subcutaneously only.
2. Use a sterile automatic syringe with a 20-22 gauge, ⅜"-½" needle which is set to accurately deliver 0.2 mL per dose. Check the accuracy of delivery several times during the vaccination procedure.
3. Dilute the vaccine only as directed, observing all precautions and warnings for handling.
4. Keep the bottle of diluted vaccine in an ice bath and agitate continuously.
5. Inject chickens under the loose skin at the back of the neck (subcutaneously), holding the chickens by the back of the neck just below the head. The loose skin in this area is raised by gently pinching with the thumb and forefinger. Insert the needle beneath the skin in a direction away from the head. Inject 0.2 mL per chicken. Avoid hitting the muscles and bones in the neck.
6. Use the entire contents of the vaccine container within one (1) hour after mixing the vaccine with the diluent.

Precaution(s):

Ampules: Store in a liquid nitrogen container.

Diluent: Store at room temperature.

Liquid nitrogen container: Store in a cool, well-ventilated area.

Check the liquid nitrogen level once a day. Keep the container away from incubator intakes and chicken boxes.

Liquid Nitrogen Precautions: The liquid nitrogen containers and vaccines should be handled by properly trained personnel only. These persons should be familiar with the Union Carbide publication "Precautions and Safe Practices - Liquid Atmospheric Gases", form #9888. Liquid nitrogen is extremely cold. Accidental contact with the skin or eyes can cause serious frostbite. Protect the eyes with goggles or a face shield. Wear gloves and long sleeves when removing and handling frozen ampules or when adding liquid nitrogen to the container. Storage and handling of liquid nitrogen containers should be in a well-ventilated area. Excessive amounts of nitrogen reduces the concentration of oxygen in the air of an unventilated space and can cause asphyxiation. If drowsiness occurs, get fresh air quickly and ventilate the entire area. If a person becomes groggy or loses consciousness while working with liquid nitrogen, get the person to a well-ventilated area immediately. If breathing has stopped, begin artificial respiration. Call a physician immediately.

Caution(s): Use only in localities where permitted.

Use only in flocks with a history of infectious bursal disease.

Do not vaccinate diseased birds.

Vaccinate all of the birds on the premises at one time.

Administer a minimum of one dose for each bird.

Avoid stress conditions during and following vaccination.

Do not place chickens in contaminated facilities.

Exposure to disease must be minimized as much as possible.

For veterinary use only.

Administer only as recommended.

Use the entire contents when first opened.

Burn the container and all unused contents.

The capability of the vaccine to produce satisfactory results depends upon many factors, including, but not limited to, conditions of storage and handling by the user, administration of the vaccine, health and the responsiveness of individual animals and the degree of field exposure. Directions for use should be followed carefully.

The use of the vaccine is subject to applicable local and federal laws and regulations.

Warning(s): Do not vaccinate within 21 days before slaughter.

Presentation: 5 x 1,000 doses and 5 x 2,000 doses.

Compendium Code No.: 11050161

BURSAL DISEASE-NEWCASTLE-BRONCHITIS VACCINE

L.A.H.I. (New Jersey) **Vaccine**

Bursal Disease-Newcastle-Bronchitis Vaccine, Mass. Type, Killed Virus, Standard and Variant

U.S. Vet. Lic. No.: 196

Active Ingredient(s): This product is a suspension of killed bursal disease, Newcastle disease and infectious bronchitis viruses. The vaccine is presented as an oil emulsion.

The vaccine is manufactured in accordance with a detailed production outline, which has been filed with the Veterinary Services of the USDA. Only specific pathogen free (SPF) eggs are used for production purposes. Seed virus is derived from a master seed virus lot which has been fully tested for purity, safety and immunogenicity. The fill volume for this product is 500 mL in a 625 mL plastic bottle. The bottles are sealed with a rubber stopper and an aluminum overseal.

Quality Control: The flocks producing SPF eggs are under constant observation by experienced personnel and routinely sampled and tested serologically to confirm absence of exposure to a large variety of avian pathogens. Shipments from the supplier are accompanied by regular reports on test results for each flock from which eggs were obtained.

The product is fully tested for purity, safety and potency according to the standard requirements for bursal disease vaccine and Newcastle/infectious bronchitis disease vaccine, killed virus, published as part 113, in particular, 113.120, 113.125 and 113.132 of title 9 of the federal regulations by the Animal and Plant Health Inspection Service of the U.S. Department of Agriculture.

Each serial is tested for: Bacteria and fungi; safety and potency tests in chickens.

Samples and complete test reports on each serial are submitted to the Veterinary Services of the USDA and no merchandise is released for shipment until this government agency has given its release agreement.

Indications: This product is packaged for subcutaneous or intramuscular vaccination in chickens three weeks of age or older. It is recommended as an aid in the prevention of bursal disease, Newcastle disease and Massachusetts type infectious bronchitis in chickens. The recommended age for vaccination is 18 to 20 weeks of age. At least three weeks prior to the administration of the killed vaccine, a live Newcastle disease and Massachusetts type bronchitis vaccine should be used in any of the recommended methods of application for priming. Prevaccination with a live vaccine is an absolute necessity for the effective use of the killed vaccine. If birds are to be kept for a second year of production, they should be revaccinated during molt.

Dosage and Administration: Immediately prior to use, shake the vaccine vigorously for 30 seconds to one (1) minute. Remove the aluminum overseal and the vaccine is ready for use.

Method of Vaccination: The inoculation should be given subcutaneously in the mid-portion of the neck or intramuscularly in the breast or leg muscles. Each bird should receive 1.0 mL of vaccine in this manner.

Precaution(s): The vaccine shall be stored in the dark in a refrigerator between 35-45°F (2-7°C).

Expiration date: 24 months.

Caution(s): It is imperative that the user of this product comply with the indications for use, contraindications, cautions and method of vaccination stated on the direction sheet packed with the product. The vaccine must be prepared and administered as directed to obtain the best results. For veterinary use only.

Warning(s): Do not market birds for at least six (6) weeks after vaccinating so that there is no swelling at the site of vaccine administration.

Presentation: 1,000 doses (500 mL).

Compendium Code No.: 10080062

BURSAL DISEASE-NEWCASTLE-BRONCHITIS VACCINE (Standard and Variant)

L.A.H.I. (New Jersey) **Vaccine**

Bursal Disease-Newcastle-Bronchitis Vaccine, Mass. Type, Killed Virus, Standard and Variant

U.S. Vet. Lic. No.: 196

Active Ingredient(s): This product is a suspension of killed bursal disease, Newcastle disease and infectious bronchitis viruses. The vaccine is presented as an oil emulsion.

The vaccine is manufactured in accordance with a detailed production outline, which has been filed with the Veterinary Services of the USDA. Seed virus is derived from a master seed lot, which has been fully tested for purity, safety and immunogenicity. The fill volume is 500 mL in a 625 mL plastic bottle. The bottles are sealed with a rubber stopper and an aluminum overseal.

Quality Control: The flocks producing SPF eggs are under constant observation by experienced personnel and routinely sampled and tested serologically to confirm absence of exposure to a large variety of avian pathogens. Shipments from the supplier are accompanied by regular reports on test results for each flock from which eggs were obtained.

The products are fully tested for purity and safety according to the standard requirements as published in the federal regulations by the Animal and Plant Health Inspection Service of the U.S. Department of Agriculture.

Each serial is tested for: Bacteria and fungi; extraneous viruses; safety and potency tests in chickens according to the production outline filed with the USDA.

Samples and complete test reports on each serial are submitted to the Veterinary Services of the USDA and no merchandise is released for shipment until this government agency has given its release agreement.

Indications: This product is recommended as an aid in the prevention of bursal disease, Newcastle disease and Massachusetts type infectious bronchitis in chickens.

This product is used for revaccination of chickens for the prevention of Newcastle disease and infectious bursal disease caused by standard or variant virus strains. It also serves as an aid in preventing infectious bronchitis (Mass. type). Birds should be three weeks of age or older. The recommended age is 18 to 20 weeks of age. At least three weeks prior to the administration of the killed vaccine, a live Newcastle disease and Massachusetts type bronchitis vaccine should be used in any of the recommended methods of application for priming. Prevaccination with live vaccine is an absolute necessity for the effective use of the killed vaccine. If birds are to be kept for a second year of production, they should be revaccinated during molt.

Dosage and Administration: Immediately prior to use, shake the vaccine vigorously for 30 seconds to one (1) minute. Remove the aluminum overseal and the vaccine is ready for use.

Method of Vaccination: The inoculation should be given subcutaneously in the mid portion of the neck. Each bird should receive 1.0 mL of the vaccine in this manner.

Precaution(s): The vaccine shall be stored in the dark in a refrigerator between 35-45°F (2-7°C).

Expiration dating: 24 months.

Caution(s): It is imperative that the user of this product comply with the indications for use, contraindications, cautions and methods of vaccination stated in the direction sheet packed with each product. The vaccine must be prepared and administered as directed to obtain the best results. For veterinary use only.

Warning(s): Do not market birds for at least six (6) weeks after vaccinating so that there is no swelling at the site of vaccine administration.

Presentation: 10,000 doses.

Compendium Code No.: 10080072

BURSAL DISEASE-NEWCASTLE DISEASE-BRONCHITIS-REOVIRUS VACCINE

L.A.H.I. (New Jersey) **Vaccine**

Bursal Disease-Newcastle Disease-Bronchitis-Reovirus Vaccine, Mass. Type, Killed Virus

U.S. Vet. Lic. No.: 196

Contents: This product is a suspension of killed standard type infectious bursal disease viruses of chicken tissue culture and bursal tissue origin, infectious bronchitis and Newcastle disease of chicken embryo origin, and avian reoviruses of chicken tissue culture origin emulsified in an oil base.

This vaccine was carefully produced and passes all tests in accordance with the U.S. Government requirements.

Indications: The vaccine is used to protect vaccinated chickens against Newcastle disease and infectious bronchitis (Mass. type) and to passively protect the progeny of vaccinated chickens against bursal disease and against malabsorption syndrome caused by avian reovirus infection. The breeders can be vaccinated when they are 15-22 weeks of age. At the time of vaccination, they should have an SN titer of ≥ 15 against reovirus. To obtain satisfactory results, chickens should be primed with live tenosynovitis vaccine at 5-7 days of age and then 4-5 weeks later. The chickens should also be primed with live mild infectious bronchitis vaccine, Mass. type, 6-8 weeks before the killed vaccine is given.

Dosage and Administration: Shake for two minutes before use.

Preparation of Vaccine: Remove the aluminum overseal and the vaccine is ready to use. Should greater than four hours elapse between the first and last use of the vaccine from any one container, it is recommended that the vaccine be shaken again before continuing with the vaccinations.

Dosage: Intramuscularly or subcutaneously; inject each chicken with a 0.5 mL dose of the vaccine.

Contraindication(s): Vaccinate only healthy birds. Consult your poultry pathologist before vaccinating.

Precaution(s): Do not freeze. Store vaccine between 2-7°C (35-45°F).

Burn vaccine containers and all unused contents.

Use entire contents when first opened.

Use aseptic precautions. Sterilize needles, syringes and stopper.

Warning(s): Do not market chickens for at least six weeks after vaccinating. Make sure that the chickens marketed do not have swellings at the site of vaccine administration since this may result in condemnation of the chickens.

It is imperative that the user of this product comply with the instructions stated. The vaccine must be prepared and administered as directed to obtain the best results. Under certain conditions, injecting this vaccine into the breast muscle may create processing problems.

Use of non-sterile needles to administer the vaccine may result in abscess formation and condemnation of chickens. Avoid self-injection with the vaccine. Consult physician immediately if self-injection with vaccine occurs.

For veterinary use only.

Presentation: 500 mL (1000 dose) bottles.

Compendium Code No.: 10080042

BURSAL DISEASE-NEWCASTLE DISEASE-BRONCHITIS VACCINE (Mass. & Conn. Types)

Merial Select **Vaccine**

Bursal Disease-Newcastle Disease-Bronchitis Vaccine, B1 Type, B1 Strain, Mass. & Conn. Types, Live Virus

U.S. Vet. Lic. No.: 279

Active Ingredient(s): The vaccine contains the S-706 strain of live bursal disease virus, the B_1 strain of the Newcastle disease virus and selected strains of infectious bronchitis virus of the Massachusetts and Connecticut type.

Penicillin and streptomycin sulfate are added as bacteriostatic agents.

Contains fungizone as a fungistatic agent.

Notice: The vaccine has met the requirements of the USDA in regard to safety, purity, potency and the capability to immunize normally susceptible chickens. The vaccine has been tested by the master seed immunogenicity test for efficacy.

Indications: The vaccine is recommended for the vaccination of healthy one day old chickens against bursal disease, Newcastle disease and infectious bronchitis.

Chickens to be vaccinated must be healthy and free of all diseases. It is essential that the chickens be maintained under good environmental conditions, and that exposure to disease viruses be reduced as much as possible in the field.

Dosage and Administration: Frozen Vaccine:

Preparation of the Vaccine for Use:

Important: Sterilize the vaccinating equipment by autoclaving for a minimum of 15 minutes at 250°F (121°C) or by boiling in water for at least 20 minutes. Never allow chemical disinfectants to come into contact with the vaccinating equipment.

1. Remove only one (1) ampule of vaccine at a time from the liquid nitrogen container. Thaw and use immediately. Do not hold the ampule toward the face when removing it from a liquid nitrogen container. Never refreeze a vaccine ampule after thawing.
2. The contents of the ampule are thawed rapidly by immersing it in water at room temperature (15-25°C). Gently swirl the ampule to disperse the contents. Break the ampule at its neck and quickly proceed as described below.
3. Transfer the contents of the ampule into a sterile 2 mL or 5 mL syringe fitted with an 18 to 20 gauge needle to cool, distilled, de-ionized water (10,000 doses to 700 mL of water).
4. Use the vaccine mixture immediately as described below.

Method of Vaccination:

1. Use the coarse spray application method.
2. Attach the spray head to the container and set the nozzle at a coarse spray setting.
3. To each box of 100 chickens, administer the vaccine by spraying 18-24 inches above the box.
4. Each box of 100 chickens should receive approximately 7 mL of vaccine. The exact amount can be determined by spraying into a calibrated tube or container to arrive at the number of applications needed to deliver 7 mL of vaccine.
5. Whatever the volume of vaccine used, take care to administer 1,000 doses to 1,000 chickens.

Precaution(s):

Ampules: Store in a liquid nitrogen container.

Liquid nitrogen container: Carefully observe all liquid nitrogen precautions, including wearing eye protection and gloves. Store in a cool, well-ventilated area. Check the liquid nitrogen level once a day. Keep the container away from incubator intakes and chicken boxes.

Liquid Nitrogen Precautions: The liquid nitrogen containers and vaccines should be handled by properly trained personnel only. These persons should be familiar with the Union Carbide publication "Precautions and Safe Practices - Liquid Atmospheric Gases", form #9888. Liquid nitrogen is extremely cold. Accidental contact with the skin or eyes can cause serious frostbite. Protect the eyes with goggles or a face shield. Wear gloves and long sleeves when removing and handling frozen ampules or when adding liquid nitrogen to the container. Storage and handling of liquid nitrogen containers should be in a well-ventilated area. Excessive amounts of nitrogen reduces the concentration of oxygen in the air of an unventilated space and can cause asphyxiation. If drowsiness occurs, get fresh air quickly and ventilate the entire area. If a person becomes groggy or loses consciousness while working with liquid nitrogen, get the person to a well-ventilated area immediately. If breathing has stopped, begin artificial respiration. Call a physician immediately.

Caution(s): Use only in localities where permitted.

Use only in localities with a history of infectious bursal disease.

Do not vaccinate diseased birds.

Vaccinate all of the birds on the premise at one time.

Administer a minimum of one dose for each bird.

Avoid stress conditions during and following vaccination.

Do not place chickens in contaminated facilities.

Exposure to disease must be minimized as much as possible.

For veterinary use only.

Since Newcastle disease virus can cause inflammation to the eyelids of humans lasting up to three days, care should be taken to avoid contamination of the eyes, hands and clothing with the vaccine.

Administer only as recommended.

Use the entire contents when first opened.

Burn the container and all unused contents.

The capability of the vaccine to produce satisfactory results depends upon many factors, including, but not limited to, conditions of storage and handling by the user, administration of the vaccine, health and the responsiveness of individual animals and the degree of field exposure. Therefore, directions for use should be followed carefully.

The use of the vaccine is subject to applicable local and federal laws and regulations.

Warning(s): Do not vaccinate within 21 days before slaughter.

Presentation: 5 x 10,000 dose vials.

Compendium Code No.: 11050181

BURSAL DISEASE-NEWCASTLE DISEASE-REOVIRUS VACCINE

L.A.H.I. (New Jersey) **Vaccine**

Bursal Disease-Newcastle Disease-Reovirus Vaccine, Killed Virus, Standard and Variant

U.S. Vet. Lic. No.: 196

Active Ingredient(s): The product is a suspension of killed infectious bursal disease viruses of chicken tissue culture, chicken embryo and bursal tissue origin, Newcastle disease virus and avian reoviruses of chicken tissue culture origin emulsified in an oil base.

The vaccine was carefully produced and passed all tests in accordance with the U.S. government requirements.

Indications: The vaccine is used for protection against standard and variant bursal disease, Newcastle disease virus and reovirus infections.

Dosage and Administration: Shake the vaccine for two (2) minutes before use.

Inject each bird with a 1.0 mL dose subcutaneously in the mid portion of the neck.

The breeders can be vaccinated when they are 15-22 weeks of age. At the time of vaccination, they should have an SN titer of ± 15 against reovirus. To obtain satisfactory results, the birds should be primed with live tenosynovitis vaccine at 5-7 days and then 4-5 weeks later.

Preparation of Vaccine: Remove the aluminum overseal and the vaccine is ready to use. Should greater than four (4) hours elapse between the first and last use of the vaccine from any one container, it is recommended that the vaccine be shaken again before continuing with the vaccinations.

Precaution(s): Keep the vaccine in the dark between 35-45°F (2-7°C). Do not freeze.

Caution(s): For veterinary use only.

Use aseptic precautions. Sterilize needles, syringes and stopper.

Vaccinate healthy birds only. Consult a poultry pathologist before vaccinating.

Burn the vaccine containers and all unused contents.

Use the entire contents when first opened.

It is imperative that the user of this product comply with the instructions stated in the direction sheet packed with each product. The vaccine must be prepared and administered as directed to obtain the best results.

The use of nonsterile needles under field vaccination may result in abscess formation and condemnation of the birds.

Warning(s): Do not market birds for at least six (6) weeks after vaccinating. Make sure that the birds marketed do not have swellings at the site of vaccine administration since this may result in condemnations of the birds.

Presentation: 1,000 dose (500 mL) bottles.

Compendium Code No.: 10080052

BURSAL DISEASE-NEWCASTLE DISEASE VACCINE

L.A.H.I. (New Jersey) **Vaccine**

Bursal Disease-Newcastle Disease Vaccine, Killed Virus, Standard and Variant

U.S. Vet. Lic. No.: 196

Active Ingredient(s): This product is a suspension of killed infectious bursal disease viruses of chicken tissue culture, chicken embryo and bursal tissue origin and Newcastle disease virus of chicken embryo origin emulsified in an oil base.

Indications: The product is recommended for the initial vaccination and revaccination of broiler breeders for the passive protection of progeny broilers against standard and variant infectious bursal disease and Newcastle disease.

Dosage and Administration: The initial vaccination is administered to pullets at three weeks of age or older. Revaccination is recommended between 16-20 weeks of age.

Shake for two (2) minutes before use.

Inject each bird with a 0.5 mL dose subcutaneously in the mid portion of the neck.

Preparation of Vaccine: Remove the aluminum overseal and the vaccine is ready to use. Should greater than four (4) hours elapse between the first and last use of the product from any one container, it is recommended that the vaccine be shaken again before continuing with the vaccinations.

Precaution(s): Keep the vaccine in the dark at between 35-45°F (2-7°C). Do not freeze.

Caution(s): For veterinary use only.

Use aseptic precautions. Sterilize needles, syringes and stopper.

Vaccinate only healthy birds. Consult a poultry pathologist before vaccinating.

Burn the vaccine containers and all unused contents.

Use the entire contents when first opened.

It is imperative that the user of this product comply with the indications for use, cautions and method of vaccination stated on the label. The vaccine must be prepared and administered as directed to obtain the best results.

The use of nonsterile needles in field vaccination may result in abscess formation and condemnation of birds.

Warning(s): Do not market birds for at least six (6) weeks after vaccinating. Make sure that the birds marketed do not have swellings at the site of vaccine administration since this may result in condemnations of the birds.

Discussion: The vaccine is manufactured in accordance with a detailed production outline, which has been filed with the Veterinary Services of USDA. Only specific pathogen free (SPF) eggs are used for production purposes. The seed virus is derived from a master seed virus lot which has been fully tested for purity, safety and immunogenicity.

Quality Control: The flocks producing SPF eggs are under constant observation by experienced personnel and are routinely sampled and tested serologically to confirm the absence of exposure to a large variety of avian pathogens. Shipments from the supplier are accompanied by regular reports on test results for each flock from which eggs are obtained.

This product is fully tested for purity, safety and potency according to the standard requirements for bursal disease vaccine, killed virus, chicken tissue culture origin, published as part 113, in particular, section 113.212 of title 9 and also the standard requirements for Newcastle disease vaccine, killed virus, chicken embryo origin, published in section 113.205 of title 9 of the federal regulations by the Animal and Plant Health Inspection Service of the U.S. Department of Agriculture.

Each serial is tested for: Bacteria, fungi and salmonella.

Safety and potency tests in chickens according to 9CFR 113.212 (challenge against standard and variant IBD viruses).

Newcastle potency testing is conducted according to the outline approved by the USDA.

Presentation: 10 x 500 mL bottles.

Compendium Code No.: 10080032

BURSAL DISEASE VACCINE (S-706 Strain)

Merial Select **Vaccine**

Bursal Disease Vaccine, Live Virus

U.S. Vet. Lic. No.: 279

Active Ingredient(s): These vaccines contain the S-706 strain of live bursal disease virus.

Penicillin and streptomycin sulfate are added as bacteriostatic agents.

Contains fungizone as a fungistatic agent.

Notice: These vaccines have met the requirements of the USDA in regard to safety, purity, potency and the capability to immunize normally susceptible chickens. These vaccines have been tested by the master seed immunogenicity test for efficacy.

Indications: These vaccines are recommended for the vaccination of healthy chickens against bursal disease.

The frozen vaccine is recommended for use in healthy one day old chickens.

The freeze-dried vaccine is recommended for the vaccination of seven day old chickens using drinking water or spray vaccination.

Chickens to be vaccinated must be healthy and free of all diseases. It is essential that the chickens be maintained under good environmental conditions, and that exposure to disease viruses be reduced as much as possible in the field.

Dosage and Administration:

A. Frozen Vaccine: For use in one (1) day old chickens.

Preparation of the Vaccine for Use:

Important: Sterilize the vaccinating equipment by autoclaving for a minimum of 15 minutes at 250°F (121°C) or by boiling in water for at least 20 minutes. Never allow chemical disinfectants to come into contact with the vaccinating equipment.

1. Remove only one (1) ampule of vaccine at a time from the liquid nitrogen container. Thaw and use immediately. Do not hold the ampule towards the face when removing it from a liquid nitrogen container. Never refreeze a vaccine ampule after thawing.
2. The contents of the ampule are thawed rapidly by immersing it in water at room temperature (15-25°C). Gently swirl the ampule to disperse the contents. Break the ampule at its neck and quickly proceed as described below.
3. Transfer the contents of the ampule into a sterile 2 mL or 5 mL syringe fitted with an 18 to 20 gauge needle to cool, distilled, de-ionized water (10,000 doses to 700 mL of water).
4. Use the vaccine mixture immediately as described below.

Method of Vaccination:

1. Use the coarse spray application method.
2. Attach the spray head to the container and set the nozzle at a coarse spray setting.
3. To each box of 100 chickens, administer the vaccine by spraying 18-24 inches above the box.
4. Each box of 100 chickens should receive approximately 7 mL of vaccine. The exact amount can be determined by spraying into a calibrated tube or container to arrive at the number of applications needed to deliver 7 mL of vaccine.
5. Whatever the volume of vaccine used, take care to administer 1,000 doses to 1,000 chickens.

B. Freeze-dried Vaccine: For use in seven (7) day old chickens.

Drinking Water Vaccination - Pouring Application: For use in houses containing between 10,000 and 15,000 chickens.

1. Do not open or mix the vaccine until ready to vaccinate.
2. Remove all medications, sanitizers and disinfectants from the drinking water 72 hours (three days) prior to vaccination.
3. Provide sufficient waterers so that all of the chickens can drink at one time. Shut off the water supply and allow the chickens to drink the troughs dry.
4. Raise the water troughs above chickens' heads. Clean and rinse the waterers thoroughly.
5. Withhold all water from the chickens for a minimum of two (2) hours in warm weather to four (4) hours in cool weather prior to vaccination to stimulate thirst. The water withdrawal time should be reduced if half-house brooding is in process.
6. Calculate to supply the vaccine solution at at rate of three (3) gallons (11 L) per 1,000 chickens in cool weather and four (4) gallons (15 L) per 1,000 chickens in warm weather. The age of the chickens should be considered when calculating the water supply. Always use nonchlorinated water when vaccinating chickens.
   Example:
   10,000 chickens in cool weather x 3 gallons (11 L) = 30 gallons (114 L).
   14,500 chickens in warm weather x 4 gallons (15 L) = 58 gallons (220 L).
7. Add one of the following to pouring water for vaccine distribution:
   a. One (1) ounce (30 mL) of nonfat, dry milk per gallon (4 L) of water, or
   b. Four (4) ounces (118 mL) of fresh skim milk per gallon (4 L) of water.
8. Prepare the vaccine concentrate as follows:
   a. Prepare a container of milk/water figuring one (1) ounce (30 mL) of concentrate for one (1) gallon (4 L) of water to be used.
   b. Add cool milk/water to the vial until the dried vaccine is dissolved. Add the vaccine to the container of milk/water to make the vaccine concentrate. Rinse the vaccine vial to remove all of the vaccine.
9. To make the vaccine solution, add one (1) ounce (30 mL) of concentrate for each gallon (4 L) of water needed.
10. Distribute the vaccine solution among the waterers. Avoid direct sunlight.
11. Lower the water troughs and allow the birds to drink freely. Add the remaining vaccine solution to the troughs as the birds drink.
12. Do not provide any additional drinking water until all of the vaccine solution is consumed.

Drinking Water Vaccination - Proportioner Application: Several types of medicator/ proportioners are commercially available. Set the proportioner to deliver one (1) ounce (30 mL) of the vaccine concentrate per one (1) gallon (4 L) of water.

1. Do not open or mix the vaccine until ready to vaccinate.
2. Remove all medications, sanitizers and disinfectants from the proportioner 72 hours (three days) prior to vaccination.
3. Clean all containers, hoses and waterers prior to vaccination.
4. Withhold all water from the chickens for a minimum of two (2) hours in warm weather to four (4) hours in cool weather prior to vaccination to stimulate thirst.
5. Calculate to supply the vaccine solution at a rate of three (3) gallons (11 L) per 1,000 chickens in cool weather and four (4) gallons (15 L) per 1,000 chickens in warm weather. The age of the chickens should be considered when calculating the water supply. Always use nonchlorinated water when vaccinating chickens.
   Example:
   10,000 chickens in cool weather x 3 gallons (11 L) = 30 gallons (114 L).
   14,500 chickens in warm weather x 4 gallons (15 L) = 58 gallons (220 L).
6. Prepare the vaccine concentrate as follows:
   a. Add three (3) ounces (90 mL) of nonfat, dry milk per 16 ounces (473 mL) of cool water, or
   b. Use undiluted cool, fresh skim milk.
7. To make the vaccine solution, add one (1) ounce (30 mL) of the concentrate for each gallon (4 L) of water needed.
8. Add the milk solution to the vial until the dried vaccine is dissolved. Rinse the vaccine vial to remove all of the vaccine.
9. Insert the proportioner hose into the vaccine concentrate and start the water flow. Continue until all of the concentrate has been consumed before changing the water supply to direct flow.
10. Do not medicate or use disinfectants for 24 hours after vaccination.

Spray Application: For use in houses containing between 10,000 and 15,000 chickens. Spray application is recommended for revaccination only and not as a primary vaccination. Use a sprayer delivering a coarse spray pattern to dispense the rehydrated vaccine quickly and evenly throughout a house of chickens.

1. Prior to spraying, reduce the air flow by raising curtains or stopping fans. Air movement should be limited for 15 minutes following vaccination.
2. Fill the vaccine container with cool, distilled, de-ionized water.
3. Pour the reconstituted vaccine into a clean container and add five (5) ounces (150 mL) of cool water for each 1,000 chickens to be vaccinated.
4. Place the vaccine solution into the spray canister and walk through the house spraying at the rate of 1,000 chickens per minute. Direct the spray directly above the heads of the chickens.
5. Avoid direct contact with the vaccine solution. Wear goggles and a face mask while spraying.
6. Do not use vaccinating equipment for any other purposes.

Precaution(s):

A. Storage Conditions for Frozen Vaccine:

Ampules: Store in a liquid nitrogen container.

Liquid nitrogen container: Carefully observe all liquid nitrogen precautions, including wearing eye protection and gloves. Store in a cool, well-ventilated area. Check the liquid nitrogen level once a day. Keep the container away from incubator intakes and chicken boxes.

Liquid Nitrogen Precautions: The liquid nitrogen containers and vaccines should be handled by properly trained personnel only. These persons should be familiar with the Union Carbide publication "Precautions and Safe Practices - Liquid Atmospheric Gases", form #9888. Liquid nitrogen is extremely cold. Accidental contact with the skin or eyes can cause serious frostbite. Protect the eyes with goggles or a face shield. Wear gloves and long sleeves when removing and handling frozen ampules or when adding liquid nitrogen to the container. Storage and handling of liquid nitrogen containers should be in a well-ventilated area. Excessive amounts of nitrogen reduces the concentration of oxygen in the air of an unventilated space and can cause asphyxiation. If drowsiness occurs, get fresh air quickly and ventilate the entire area. If a person becomes groggy or loses consciousness while working with liquid nitrogen, get the person to a well-ventilated area immediately. If breathing has stopped, begin artificial respiration. Call a physician immediately.

B. Storage Conditions for Freeze-dried Vaccine:

Store the freeze-dried vaccine at 35-45°F (2-7°C). Do not freeze.

Caution(s):

A. Frozen Vaccine:

Do not vaccinate diseased birds.

Vaccinate all of the birds on the premises at one time.

Administer a minimum of one dose for each bird.

Avoid stress conditions during and following vaccination.

Do not place chickens in contaminated facilities.

Exposure to disease must be minimized as much as possible.

For veterinary use only.

The capability of the vaccine to produce satisfactory results depends upon many factors, including, but not limited to, conditions of storage and handling by the user, administration of the vaccine, health and the responsiveness of individual animals and the degree of field exposure. Therefore, directions for use should be followed carefully.

The use of the vaccine is subject to applicable state and federal laws and regulations.

Use only in localities where permitted.

Use only in localities with a history of infectious bursal disease.

Administer only as recommended.

Use the entire contents when first opened.

Burn the container and all unused contents.

B. Freeze-dried Vaccine:

Do not vaccinate diseased birds.

Vaccinate all of the birds on the premises at one time.

Administer a minimum of one dose for each bird.

Avoid stress conditions during and following vaccination.

Do not place chickens in contaminated facilities.

Exposure to disease must be minimized as much as possible.

For veterinary use only.

The capability of the vaccine to produce satisfactory results depends upon many factors, including, but not limited to, conditions of storage and handling by the user, administration of the vaccine, health and the responsiveness of individual animals and the degree of field exposure. Therefore, directions for use should be followed carefully.

The use of the vaccine is subject to applicable state and federal laws and regulations.

Use the entire vial contents when first opened.

Burn the container and all unused contents.

Use only in localities where permitted.

Use only in flocks with a history of infectious bursal disease.

Warning(s): Do not vaccinate within 21 days before slaughter.

Presentation: Frozen vaccine: 5x10,000 dose vials, 200 mL sterile diluent included per 1,000 doses.

Freeze-dried vaccine: 25x2,500 dose, 25x5,000 dose, 10x15,000 dose and 15x25,000 dose vials.

Compendium Code No.: 11050091

BURSAL DISEASE VACCINE (ST-14 Strain)

Merial Select **Vaccine**

Bursal Disease Vaccine, Live Virus

U.S. Vet. Lic. No.: 279

Active Ingredient(s): The vaccine contains the ST-14 strain of live bursal disease virus.

Penicillin and streptomycin sulfate are added as bacteriostatic agents.

Contains fungizone as a fungistatic agent.

Notice: The vaccine has met the requirements of the USDA in regard to safety, purity, potency and the capability to protect normally susceptible chickens. The vaccine has been tested by the master seed immunogenicity test for efficacy.

Indications: The vaccine is recommended for use in healthy one day old chickens to aid in the prevention of infectious bursal disease (gumboro).

Chickens to be vaccinated must be healthy and free of all diseases. It is essential that the chickens be maintained under good environmental conditions, and that exposure to disease viruses be reduced as much as possible in the field.

Dosage and Administration: Frozen Vaccine:

Preparation of the Vaccine for Use:

Important: Sterilize the vaccinating equipment by autoclaving for a minimum of 15 minutes at 250°F (121°C) or by boiling in water for at least 20 minutes. Never allow chemical disinfectants to come into contact with the vaccinating equipment.

1. Use 200 mL of sterile diluent for each 1,000 doses of vaccine indicated on the ampule.
2. Remove only one (1) ampule of vaccine at a time from the liquid nitrogen container. Thaw and use immediately. Do not hold the ampule toward the face when removing it from a liquid nitrogen container. Never refreeze a vaccine ampule after thawing.
3. The contents of the ampule are thawed rapidly by immersing it in water at room temperature (15-25°C). Gently swirl the ampule to disperse the contents. Break the ampule at its neck and quickly proceed as described below.
4. Remove the cover from the diluent container. Draw the contents of the ampule into a sterile 10 mL syringe fitted with an 18 to 20 gauge needle. Slowly add the contents of the vaccine ampule to the appropriate volume of diluent. Withdraw a small amount of the diluent, rinse the ampule once and add this to the vaccine-diluent mixture. Mix the contents of the diluent container thoroughly by swirling and inverting the container. Do not shake vigorously.
5. Use the vaccine-diluent mixture immediately as described below.

Method of Vaccination:

1. Give subcutaneously only.
2. Use a sterile automatic syringe with a 20-22 gauge, ⅜"-½" needle which is set to accurately deliver 0.2 mL per dose. Check the accuracy of delivery several times during the vaccination procedure.
3. Dilute the vaccine only as directed observing all precautions and warnings for handling.
4. Keep the bottle of diluted vaccine in an ice bath and agitate continuously.
5. Inject chickens under the loose skin at the back of the neck (subcutaneously), holding the chickens by the back of the neck just below the head. The loose skin in this area is raised by gently pinching with the thumb and forefinger. Insert the needle beneath the skin in a direction away from the head. Inject 0.2 mL per chicken. Avoid hitting the muscles and bones in the neck.
6. Use the entire contents of the vaccine container within one (1) hour after mixing the vaccine with the diluent.

Precaution(s):

Ampules: Store in a liquid nitrogen container.

Diluent: Store at room temperature.

Liquid nitrogen container: Store in a cool, well-ventilated area. Check the liquid nitrogen level once a day. Keep the container away from incubator intakes and chicken boxes.

Liquid Nitrogen Precautions: The liquid nitrogen containers and vaccines should be handled by properly trained personnel only. These persons should be familiar with the Union Carbide publication "Precautions and Safe Practices - Liquid Atmospheric Gases", form #9888. Liquid nitrogen is extremely cold. Accidental contact with the skin or eyes can cause serious frostbite. Protect the eyes with goggles or a face shield. Wear gloves and long sleeves when removing and handling frozen ampules or when adding liquid nitrogen to the container. Storage and handling of liquid nitrogen containers should be in a well-ventilated area. Excessive amounts of nitrogen reduces the concentration of oxygen in the air of an unventilated space and can cause asphyxiation. If drowsiness occurs, get fresh air quickly and ventilate the entire area. If a person becomes groggy or loses consciousness while working with liquid nitrogen, get the person to a well-ventilated area immediately. If breathing has stopped, begin artificial respiration. Call a physician immediately.

Caution(s): Use only in localities where permitted. Use only in flocks with a history of infectious bursal disease. Do not vaccinate diseased birds. Vaccinate all of the birds on the premise at one time. Administer a minimum of one dose for each bird. Avoid stress conditions during and following vaccination. Do not place chickens in contaminated facilities. Exposure to disease must be minimized as much as possible. For veterinary use only. Administer only as recommended. Use the entire contents when first opened. Burn the container and all unused contents.

The capability of the vaccine to produce satisfactory results depends upon many factors, including, but not limited to, conditions of storage and handling by the user, administration of the vaccine, health and the responsiveness of individual animals and the degree of field exposure. Directions for use should be followed carefully.

The use of the vaccine is subject to applicable local and federal laws and regulations.

Warning(s): Do not vaccinate within 21 days before slaughter.

Presentation: 5 x 1,000 doses and 5 x 2,000 doses.

Compendium Code No.: 11050101

BURSAL DISEASE VACCINE (SVS 510)

Merial Select **Vaccine**

Bursal Disease Vaccine, Live Virus, Standard and Variant, SVS 510

U.S. Vet. Lic. No.: 279

Active Ingredient(s): The vaccine contains selected strains of live bursal disease virus for the vaccination of healthy chickens seven days of age or older.

Contains streptomycin sulfate and penicillin as bacteriostatic agents.

Contains fungizone as a fungistatic agent.

Notice: The vaccine has met the requirements of the USDA in regard to safety, purity, potency and the capability to protect normally susceptible chickens. The vaccine has been tested by the master seed immunogenicity test for efficacy.

Indications: The vaccine is recommended as an aid in the prevention of bursal disease in healthy seven day old chickens.

Chickens to be vaccinated must be free of all diseases. It is essential that the chickens be maintained under good environmental conditions and that exposure to disease viruses be reduced as much as possible in the field.

Dosage and Administration: Freeze-dried Vaccine:

Drinking Water Vaccination - Pouring Application:

1. Do not open or mix the vaccine until ready to vaccinate.
2. Remove all medications, sanitizers and disinfectants from the drinking water 72 hours (three days) prior to vaccination.
3. Provide sufficient waterers so that all of the chickens can drink at one time. Shut off the water supply and allow the chickens to drink the troughs dry.
4. Raise the water troughs above the chickens' heads. Clean and rinse all containers, hoses, and waterers thoroughly prior to vaccination.
5. Withhold all water from the chickens for a minimum of two (2) hours in warm weather to four (4) hours in cool weather prior to vaccination to stimulate thirst. The water withdrawal time should be reduced if half-house brooding is in process.
6. Calculate to supply the vaccine solution at a rate of three (3) gallons (11 L) per 1,000 chickens in warm weather. The age of the chickens should be considered when calculating the water supply. Always use nonchlorinated water when vaccinating chickens.
   Example:
   2,500 chickens in cool weather x 3 gallons (11 L) = 7.5 gallons (28 L).
   5,000 chickens in warm weather x 4 gallons (15 L) = 20 gallons (76 L).
7. Add one of the following to pouring water for vaccine distribution:
   a. One (1) ounce (30 mL) of nonfat, dry skim milk per gallon (4 L) of water, or
   b. Four (4) ounces (118 mL) of fresh skim milk per gallon (4 L) of water.
8. Prepare the vaccine concentrate as follows:
   a. Prepare a container of milk/water figuring one (1) ounce (30 mL) of concentrate for one (1) gallon (4 L) of water to be used.
   b. Add cool milk/water to the vial until the dried vaccine is dissolved. Add the vaccine to the container of milk/water to make the vaccine concentrate. Rinse the vaccine vial to remove all of the vaccine.
9. To make the vaccine solution, add one (1) ounce (30 mL) of concentrate for each gallon (4 L) of water needed.
10. Distribute the vaccine solution among the waterers. Avoid direct sunlight.
11. Lower the water troughs and allow the birds to drink freely. Add the remaining vaccine solution to the troughs as the birds drink.
12. Do not provide any additional drinking water until all of the vaccine solution is consumed.

Drinking Water Vaccination - Proportioner Application: Several types of medicator/ proportioners are commercially available. Set the proportioner to deliver one (1) ounce (30 mL) of vaccine concentrate per one (1) gallon (4 L) of water.

1. Do not open or mix the vaccine until ready to vaccinate.
2. Remove all medications, sanitizers and disinfectants from the proportioner 72 hours (three days) prior to vaccination.
3. Provide sufficient waterers so that all of the chickens can drink at one time. Shut off the water supply and allow the chickens to drink the troughs dry.
4. Raise the water troughs above the chickens' heads. Clean and rinse all containers, hoses, and waterers thoroughly prior to vaccination.
5. Withhold all water from the chickens for a minimum of two (2) hours in warm weather to

four (4) hours in cool weather prior to vaccination to stimulate thirst.The water withdrawal times should be reduced if half-house brooding is in process.

6. Calculate to supply the vaccine solution at a rate of three (3) gallons (11 L) per 1,000 chickens in cool weather and four (4) gallons (15 L) per 1,000 chickens in warm weather. The age of the chickens should be considered when calculating the water supply. Always use nonchlorinated water when vaccinating chickens.
   Example:
   2,500 chickens in cool weather x 3 gallons (11 L) = 7.5 gallons (28 L).
   5,000 chickens in warm weather x 4 gallons (15 L) = 20 gallons (78 L).
7. Prepare the vaccine concentrate as follows:
   a. Add three (3) ounces (90 mL) of dried, nonfat skim milk per 16 ounces (473 mL) of cool water, or
   b. Use undiluted, cool, fresh skim milk.
8. To make the vaccine solution, add one (1) ounce (30 mL) of concentrate for each gallon (4 L) of water needed.
9. Add the milk solution to the vial until the dried vaccine is dissolved. Rinse the vaccine vial to remove all of the vaccine.
10. Insert the proportioner hose into the vaccine concentrate and start the water flow. Continue until all of the concentrate has been consumed before changing the water supply to direct flow.
11. Do not medicate or use disinfectants for 24 hours after vaccination.

Coarse Spray Application: Coarse spray application is recommended for revaccination only and not as a primary vaccination. Use a sprayer delivering a coarse spray pattern to dispense the rehydrated vaccine quickly and evenly throughout a house of chickens.

1. Prior to spraying, reduce the air flow by raising curtains or stopping fans. Air movement should be limited for 15 minutes following vaccination.
2. Fill the vaccine container with cool, distilled, de-ionized water.
3. Pour the reconstituted vaccine into a clean container and add five (5) ounces (150 mL) of cool, distilled, de-ionized water for each 1,000 chickens to be vaccinated.
4. Place the vaccine solution into a spray canister and walk through the house spraying at the rate of 1,000 chickens per minute. Direct the spray directly above the heads of the chickens.
5. Avoid direct contact with the vaccine solution. Wear goggles and a mask while spraying.
6. Do not use vaccinating equipment for any other purpose.

Precaution(s): Store at 35-45°F (2-7°C). Do not freeze.

Caution(s): Use only in localities where permitted.

Use only in flocks with a history of infectious bursal disease.

Do not vaccinate diseased birds.

Vaccinate all of the birds on the premises at one time.

Administer a minimum of one dose for each bird.

Avoid stress conditions during and following the vaccination.

Do not place chickens in contaminated facilities.

Exposure to disease must be minimized as much as possible.

For veterinary use only.

Use the entire contents when first opened.

Burn the container and all unused contents.

The capability of the vaccine to produce satisfactory results depends upon many factors, including, but not limited to, conditions of storage and handling by the user, administration of the vaccine, health and the responsiveness of individual animals and the degree of field exposure. Directions for use should be followed carefully.

The use of the vaccine is subject to applicable local and federal laws and regulations.

Warning(s): Do not vaccinate within 21 days before slaughter.

Presentation: 10 x 5,000 dose and 15 x 25,000 dose vials.

Compendium Code No.: 11050111

BURSAMATE™

Intervet **Vaccine**

Bursal Disease-Reovirus Vaccine, Standard and Variant Killed Virus

U.S. Vet. Lic. No.: 286

Description: BURSAMATE™ is prepared using specific pathogen free or approved substrates and contains Standard, GLS, and Delaware E strains of Infectious Bursal Disease virus and two strains of avian reovirus (1733 and 2408) inactivated and suspended in the aqueous phase of an oil adjuvant emulsion.

Quality tested for purity, potency and safety.

Indications: BURSAMATE™ is indicated for the vaccination of healthy chickens at least 21 weeks of age by the intramuscular route (0.5 mL) as an aid in the prevention of Infectious Bursal Disease virus (Standard, Delaware, and GLS variants) and disease caused by avian reoviruses.

Dosage and Administration: Allow the vaccine to reach ambient temperature, 16-27°C (60-80°F), before use and shake vigorously before and periodically during use. Inject 0.5 mL intramuscularly in chickens at least 21 weeks old, using an 18 gauge x ½" or ¼" needle.

Vaccination Programs: The best protection is obtained when this vaccine is used for revaccination of chickens previously immunized (primed) with the same type of live virus vaccines. A minimum of four weeks should elapse between the last live virus priming and injection with BURSAMATE™. Local conditions must be taken into consideration and, where necessary, veterinary advice should be sought.

Immunity: It is evident that for optimal protection, preceding vaccination with live vaccines (priming) should have taken place. Generally, in flocks vaccinated with BURSAMATE™, a protective level of immunity will be achieved with only small variations between individual chickens.

Vaccination Reaction: This vaccine does not provoke clinical reactions in chickens. If shock is observed, this must usually be ascribed to the stress of handling.

Records: Keep a record of vaccine, quantity, serial number, expiration date, place of purchase; the date and time of vaccination; the number, age, breed, and locations of chickens; names of operators performing the vaccination, and any observed reactions.

Precaution(s): Storage Conditions: Store in the dark in a refrigerator between 2-7°C (35-45°F). Do not freeze or expose to direct sunlight.

Do not mix this vaccine with any other substances.

Use entire contents when first opened.

This product is non-returnable.

Caution(s): Chickens should be in good health when vaccinated. Sick or weak chickens may not develop adequate immunity.

Do not administer this vaccine during the critical egg laying period from onset until after peak production. Administration of this product during the lay period may result in a drop in egg production.

Ensure that vaccination equipment is clean and sterile before use.

Do not use vaccination equipment with rubber parts, as the oil emulsion may attack certain types of rubber.

For veterinary use only.

Notice: This vaccine has undergone rigid potency, safety and purity tests, and meets Intervet Inc. and USDA requirements. It is designed to stimulate effective immunity when used as directed, but the user must be advised that the response to the product depends upon many factors, including, but not limited to, conditions of storage and handling by the user, administration of the vaccine, health and responsiveness of the individual chickens, and the degree of field exposure. Therefore, directions should be followed carefully.

This product is not hazardous when used according to directions supplied. A material safety data sheet (MSDS) is available upon request. This and any other consumer information can be obtained by calling Intervet Customer Service at 1-800-441-8272 or 1-302-934-8051.

The, use of this vaccine is subject to applicable local and federal laws and regulations.

Use only as directed.

Warning(s): Do not vaccinate chickens within 42 days before slaughter.

To avoid human injection, extreme caution should be used when injecting any oil emulsion vaccine. Accidental human injection may cause serious local reactions. Contact a physician immediately if accidental human injection occurs.

Presentation: 1,000 doses (500 mL).

Compendium Code No.: 11062820 Rev. 12301 AL198

BURSAPLEX®

Embrex **Vaccine**

Bursal Disease Vaccine, Live Virus

U.S. Vet. Lic. No.: 279

Description: BURSAPLEX® contains a live strain of bursal disease virus of chicken embryo origin in conjunction with bursal disease antiserum.

Contains gentamicin as a bacteriostatic agent.

Indications: This vaccine is recommended for vaccination of healthy chickens as an aid in the prevention of Bursal Disease. It is recommended for subcutaneous injection of chickens at one day of age or *in ovo* vaccination of 18- to 19-day old embryonated chicken eggs using the Embrex Inovoject® Egg Injection System. It is essential that the birds be maintained under good environmental conditions and that exposure to disease viruses be reduced as much as possible.

Dosage and Administration: Rehydration of Vaccine:

1. Dilute the vaccine only as directed, observing all precautions and warnings for handling.
2. Rehydrate only the vials of vaccine that are to be used immediately.
3. For each 1,000 doses of vaccine to be administered by subcutaneous injection, use 200 mL of sterile diluent. For each 4,000 doses of vaccine to be administered *in ovo,* use 200 mL of sterile diluent.
4. Transfer enough diluent to the vial containing the lyophilized virus to fill it about ¾ full. Replace the stopper and shake the contents vigorously until the vaccine is evenly suspended.
5. Pour the virus suspension into the remaining diluent. Replace the stopper and thoroughly mix the vaccine and diluent by swirling and inverting.
6. Rinse the vial to be sure of removing all the vaccine.
7. Use the vaccine-diluent mixture immediately as described for subcutaneous injection or *in ovo* administration.
8. Keep the bottle of diluted vaccine in an ice bath and agitate continuously.

In Ovo Administration: Before initiating *in ovo* vaccination, carefully read and follow the Inovoject® operator's manual. Failure to follow instructions may result in personal injury, embryonic morbidity and mortality. Only healthy embryonated eggs should be used.

1. Sanitize the Inovoject® Egg Injection System before and after use.
2. Inject a 0.05 mL dose into each embryonated egg.
3. Use the entire contents of the vaccine container within one hour after mixing.

Subcutaneous Injection Method:

Important: Sterilize vaccinating equipment by autoclaving 15 minutes at 121°C or by boiling in water for 20 minutes. Never allow any chemical disinfectant to come in contact with vaccinating equipment.

1. Use a sterile automatic syringe with a 20-22 gauge, ⅜-½ inch needle that is set to accurately deliver 0.2 mL. Check the accuracy of delivery several times during the vaccination procedure.
2. Hold the chicken by the back of the neck, just below the head. The loose skin in this area is raised by gently pinching with the thumb and forefinger. Insert the needle beneath the skin in a direction away from the head. Inject 0.2 mL per chicken. Avoid hitting the muscles and bones in the neck.
3. Use entire contents of bottle within one hour after mixing.

Contraindication(s): Do not vaccinate diseased embryonated eggs or diseased birds.

Precaution(s): Store at 35-45°F (2-7°C). Do not freeze. Use entire vial contents when first opened. Burn this container and all unused contents.

Diluent: Store at room temperature.

Caution(s): Use only in localities where permitted.

Use only in flocks with a history of Infectious Bursal Disease.

When using *in ovo* vaccination, this vaccine may be combined only with Merial Select's Marek's Disease Vaccine, Serotypes 2 and 3, Live Virus (List No. MHSF-3115 and MHSF-3175).

Administer a full dose to each embryonated egg or to each bird.

Vaccinate all birds on the premises at one time.

Avoid stress conditions during and following vaccination.

Do not place chickens in contaminated facilities.

Exposure to disease must be minimized as much as possible.

For veterinary use only.

Warning(s): Do not vaccinate within 21 days before slaughter.

Discussion: Notice: BURSAPLEX® has met the requirements of the USDA in regard to safety, purity, potency and the capability to protect normally susceptible chickens. This vaccine has been tested by the Master Seed immunogenicity test for efficacy.

The ability of this vaccine to produce satisfactory results may depend on many factors, including, but not limited to, conditions of storage and handling by the user; administration of the vaccine; health and responsiveness of individual chickens; and the degree of exposure. Therefore, directions for use should be followed carefully. The use of this vaccine is subject to applicable state and federal laws and regulations.

Presentation: 1,000 doses, 2,000 doses and 8,000 doses.

Inovoject® is a registered trademark of Embrex, Inc.

Manufactured by: Merial Select, Inc., Gainseville, GA 30503.

Compendium Code No.: 11470000

BURSA-VAC®

ASL **Vaccine**

Bursal Disease Vaccine, Live Virus

U.S. Vet. Lic. No.: 226

Description: BURSA-VAC® contains an attenuated strain of infectious bursal disease (IBD) virus.

Gentamicin is added as a preservative.

Indications: When administered properly to healthy, susceptible chickens, this vaccine is used as an aid in the prevention of Bursal Disease.

BURSA-VAC® is recommended for vaccination of healthy chickens 7-14 days of age, only on premises with a history of IBD infection. However, if chickens are from immune parents, vaccination should be delayed until they are at least 10 days of age, for best protection.

Dosage and Administration: Read full directions below carefully.

Rehydration of the Vaccine:

1. Tear off the aluminum seal from the vial containing the dried vaccine.
2. Lift off the rubber stopper.
3. Carefully pour clean, non-chlorinated water into the vaccine vial until the vial is approximately ⅔ full.
4. Put back the rubber stopper and shake vigorously until all material is dissolved.
5. The vaccine is now ready for use in accordance with directions below.

Drinking Water Administration:

For vaccination of healthy chickens from 7 to 14 days age by the drinking water method of administration:

1. Remove all medications, sanitizers, and disinfectants from the drinking water, preferably 72 hours before vaccinating, and 24 hours following vaccination.
2. Provide enough watering space so that at least ⅔ of the chickens can drink at one time.
3. Scrub waterers thoroughly and rinse with fresh, clean water.
4. Withhold water for 2 hours before vaccinating to stimulate thirst.
5. Rehydrate the vaccine as directed above.
6. Add rehydrated vaccine at the rate of 1½ gallons (5.7 L) per 1,000 doses to clean, non-chlorinated water.

Age of Chickens	Water per 1,000 Doses
7-14 days	1.5 gal (5.7 L)
2-4 wks	2.5 gal (8.5 L)
4-8 wks	5 gal (19 L)
Over 8 wks	10 gal (38 L)

7. Distribute the vaccine solution as prepared above, among the waterers provided for the chickens. Avoid placing the waterers in direct sunlight.
8. Provide no other drinking water until all the vaccine treated water has been consumed.

Precaution(s): Store vaccine in refrigerator under 45°F (7°C). Use entire contents when first opened. Burn containers and all unused contents.

Caution(s): Use only in states where permitted and in chickens to be placed on premises with a history of infectious bursal disease.

Only vaccinate healthy chickens.

Consult your poultry pathologist for further recommendations based on conditions existing in your area at any given time. All susceptible chickens on the same premises should be vaccinated at the same time. If this is not possible, then strict isolation and separate caretakers should be employed for non-vaccinated units.

Efforts should be taken to reduce stress conditions at the time the vaccine is administered.

Care should be taken to avoid the spread of virus from vaccinated flocks to clean premises.

The capacity of this vaccine to produce satisfactory results depends on many factors, including, but not limited to, conditions of storage and handling by the user, administration of the vaccine, health and responsiveness of individual animals and degree of field exposure. Therefore, directions for use should be followed carefully.

The use of this vaccine is subject to applicable state and federal laws and regulations.

Warning(s): Do not vaccinate within 21 days before slaughter.

Discussion: A few vaccinated chickens will usually develop symptoms, i.e. depression, anorexia and diarrhea, and occasionally chickens may die with typical lesions. In most instances, the total mortality in the vaccinated flocks is under 1%.

Field observations indicate that natural outbreaks of IBD in unvaccinated flocks will approximate at least 3% mortality, with numerous culls produced.

Presentation: Drinking water application: 10 x 1,000 dose (NDC 0138-5163-01), 10 x 2,500 dose and 10 x 5,000 dose vials.

Compendium Code No.: 11020151

BURSA-VAC® 3

ASL **Vaccine**

Bursal Disease Vaccine, Live Virus

U.S. Vet. Lic. No.: 226

Description: BURSA-VAC® 3 contains an attenuated strain of infectious bursal disease (IBD) virus.

Gentamicin is added as a preservative.

Indications: When administered properly to healthy, susceptible chickens, this vaccine is used as an aid in the prevention of bursal disease.

BURSA-VAC® 3 is recommended for vaccination of healthy chickens only on premises with a history of IBD infection. However, if chickens are from immune parents, vaccination should be delayed until they are at least 10 days of age, for best protection.

Dosage and Administration: Read full directions below carefully.

Rehydration of the Vaccine (for intraocular use): Do not open and mix the vaccine until ready to begin vaccination. Use vaccine immediately after mixing.

1. Tear off the aluminum seal from the vial containing the dried vaccine.
2. Lift off the rubber stopper.
3. Remove the plastic screw-cap and applicator insert from the polyethylene bottle of diluent.
4. Pour a small amount of diluent into the vial of dried vaccine.
5. Replace the rubber stopper and shake.
6. Pour the partly dissolved vaccine into the bottle containing the rest of the diluent.
7. Replace the plastic applicator insert and screw-cap and shake vigorously until all material is dissolved.

The vaccine is now ready for use by the following method.

For best results be sure to follow directions carefully.

Intraocular Administration:

For chickens one day of age or older. Rehydrate vaccine as directed above. Place one full drop of vaccine into the open eye. Do not release the chicken until after it has swallowed.

Coarse Spray and Drinking Water Administration:

For vaccination of healthy, susceptible chickens at one day of age by coarse spray; and 14 days of age by drinking water.

Rehydration of the Vaccine:

1. Tear off the aluminum seal from the vial containing the dried vaccine.
2. Lift off the rubber stopper.
3. Carefully pour clean, cool, non-chlorinated water into the vaccine vial until the vial is approximately ⅔ full.
4. Put back the rubber stopper and shake vigorously until all the material is dissolved.
5. The vaccine is now ready for drinking water or coarse spray use in accordance with directions below.

Coarse Spray Administration: The vaccine should be rehydrated at the rate of 80 mL of distilled water per 1,000 doses of vaccine. Each 100 chicks should receive 7 mL of vaccine solution.

Drinking Water Administration:

1. Remove all medications, sanitizers, and disinfectants from the drinking water, preferably 72 hours before vaccinating and 24 hours following vaccination.
2. Provide enough watering space so that at least ⅔ of the chickens can drink at one time.
3. Scrub waterers thoroughly and rinse with fresh, clean water.
4. Withhold water for 2 hours before vaccinating to stimulate thirst.
5. Rehydrate the vaccine as directed above.
6. Add rehydrated vaccine at the rate of 2½ gallons (9.5 L) per 1,000 doses to clean, cool, tap water.
7. Distribute the vaccine solution, as prepared abaove, among the waterers provided for the chickens. Avoid placing the waterers in direct sunlight.
8. Provide no other drinking water until all of the vaccine treated water has been consumed.

Precaution(s): Store vaccine in refrigerator under 45°F (7°C). Use entire contents when first opened. Burn containers and all unused contents.

Caution(s): Use only in states where permitted and in chickens to be placed on premises with a history of infectious bursal disease.

Only vaccinate healthy chickens.

Consult your poultry pathologist for further recommendations based on conditions existing in your area at any given time.

All susceptible chickens on the same premise should be vaccinated at the same time. If this is not possible, then strict isolation and separate caretakers should be employed for non-vaccinated units. Efforts should be taken to reduce stress conditions at the time the vaccine is administered.

Care should be taken to avoid the spread of virus from vaccinated flocks to clean premises.

Notice: All American Scientific Laboratories, Inc. vaccines released for sale meet the requirements of the licensing authority (U.S. Department of Agriculture) in regard to safety, purity, potency, and the capacity to immunize normal, susceptible chickens.

The capacity of this vaccine to produce satisfactory results depends on many factors, including, but not limited to, conditions of storage and handling by the user, administration of the vaccine, health and responsiveness of individual animals and degree of field exposure. Therefore, directions for use should be followed carefully.

The use of this vaccine is subject to applicable state and federal laws and regulations.

Warning(s): Do not vaccinate within 21 days before slaughter.

Discussion: Vaccination Programs: Many factors must be considered in determining the proper vaccination program for a particular term or poultry operation. To be fully effective, the vaccine must administered to healthy, receptive chickens held in a proper environment under good management. In addition, the response may be modified by the age of the chickens and their immune status. Seldom does one vaccination under field conditions produce complete protection for all individuals in a given flock. The amount of protection required will vary with the type of operation and the degree of exposure that a flock is likely to encounter. For these reasons a program of periodic revaccination may be required.

Presentation: Intraocular, drinking water or coarse spray use: 10 x 1,000 dose vials.

Drinking water or coarse spray use: 1,000 dose, 10 x 5,000 dose and 10 x 10,000 dose vials.

Compendium Code No.: 11020161

BURSA-VAC® 4

ASL **Vaccine**

Bursal Disease Vaccine, Live Virus Variant

U.S. Vet. Lic. No.: 226

Description: BURSA-VAC® 4 contains a variant strain of infectious bursal disease (IBD) virus.

The variant strain in BURSA-VAC® 4 is an attenuation of the 1084E Strain isolated at the University of Delaware.

Gentamicin is added as a bacteriostatic agent.

Indications: BURSA-VAC® 4 is recommended for the vaccination of healthy chickens only on premises with a history of IBD infection at 14 days of age or older, by drinking water.

When administered properly to healthy, susceptible chickens, it will usually provide flock protection against a more virulent natural infection of Bursal Disease.

Dosage and Administration: Read full directions below carefully.

Rehydration of the Vaccine:

1. Tear off the aluminum seal from the vial containing the dried vaccine.
2. Lift off the rubber stopper.
3. Carefully pour clean, cool, non-chlorinated water into the vaccine vial until the vial is approximately ⅔ full.
4. Replace the rubber stopper and shake vigorously until all the material is dissolved.
5. The vaccine is now ready for drinking water use in accordance with directions below.

Drinking Water Administration: For vaccination of healthy susceptible chickens 14 days of age or older by the drinking water method of administration.

1. Remove all medications, sanitizers, and disinfectants from the drinking water, preferably 72 hours before vaccinating and 24 hours following vaccination.
2. Provide enough watering space so that at least ⅔ of the chickens can drink at one time.
3. Scrub waterers thoroughly and rinse with fresh, clean water.
4. Withhold water for 2 hours before vaccinating to stimulate thirst.
5. Rehydrate the vaccine as directed above.
6. Add rehydrated vaccine to clean, cool, non-chlorinated water in accordance with the chart below:

Age of Chickens	Water per 1000 doses
2-4 wks	2.5 gal. (9.5 L)
4-8 wks	5 gal. (19 L)
Over 8 wks	10 gal. (38 L)

7. Distribute the solution, as prepared above, among the waterers provided for the chickens. Avoid placing the waterers in direct sunlight.
8. Provide no other drinking water until all of the vaccine treated water has been consumed.

Contraindication(s): Chickens to be vaccinated should be free of all diseases, including latent forms of chronic respiratory disease (CRD). Clinical coccidiosis, blackhead, parasite infestation, etc. and maintained under good environmental conditions.

Precaution(s): Store vaccine in refrigerator under 45°F (7°C). Use entire contents of each vial when first opened. Burn containers and all unused contents.

Caution(s): Use only in states where permitted and in chickens to be placed on premises with a history of infectious bursal disease.

Consult your poultry pathologist for further recommendations based on conditions existing in your area at any given time.

All susceptible chickens on the same premises should be vaccinated at the same time. If this is not possible, then strict isolation and separate caretakers should be employed for non-vaccinated units. Efforts should be taken to reduce stress conditions at the time the vaccine is administered.

Care should be taken to avoid the spread of virus from vaccinated flocks to clean premises.

Notice: All American Scientific Laboratories, Inc. vaccines released for sale meet the requirements of the licensing authority (U.S. Department of Agriculture) in regard to safety, purity, potency, and the capacity to immunize normal, susceptible chickens.

The capacity of this vaccine to produce satisfactory results depends on many factors, including, but not limited to, conditions of storage and handling by the user, administration of the vaccine, health and responsiveness of individual animals and degree of field exposure. Therefore, directions for use should be followed carefully.

The use of this vaccine is subject to applicable state and federal laws and regulations.

Warning(s): Do not vaccinate within 21 days before slaughter.

Discussion: Vaccination Programs: Many factors must be considered in determining the proper vaccination program for a particular term or poultry operation. To be fully effective, the vaccine must administered to healthy, receptive chickens held in a proper environment under good management. In addition, the response may be modified by the age of the chickens and their immune status. Seldom does one vaccination under field conditions produce complete protection for all individuals in a given flock. The amount of protection required will vary with the type of operation and the degree of exposure that a flock is likely to encounter. For these reasons a program of periodic revaccination may be required.

Presentation: Drinking water use: 10 x 1,000 dose and 10 x 5,000 dose vials.

Patent 4,824,668

Compendium Code No.: 11020171 0125R8/0125R9 / R0130R6

BURSIMUNE®

Biomune **Vaccine**

Bursal Disease Vaccine, Live Virus

U.S. Vet. Lic. No.: 368

Contents: This vaccine contains a live strain of bursal disease virus.

Contains gentamicin and amphotericin B as preservatives.

This vaccine is thoroughly tested before sale and meets the requirements of U.S. Department of Agriculture.

Indications: This vaccine is recommended for the vaccination of healthy chickens at two-weeks of age. Careful consideration and determination of the immune status of the flock to be vaccinated is recommended. Vaccinate when passive resistance (parental antibody) to infectious bursal disease subsides.

Directions for Use: Read before rehydrating the vaccine. For drinking water use.

1. Discontinue water medication 48 hours before vaccination. Do not resume any medication in the water for 24 hours after all vaccine water has been consumed. The waterers should be thoroughly cleaned before use. Do not use disinfecting solutions during cleaning as the disinfectant residue may destroy the virus. Drinking containers must be free of all disinfecting solutions and medicants for 48 hours prior to vaccination and for 24 hours after vaccination.
2. Deprive the birds of water two hours prior to vaccination.
3. Tear off the aluminum seal from the vial containing the dried vaccine and remove the stopper.
4. Use clean, cold, nonchlorinated water for rehydration of the dried vaccine. Mix a 1,000 dose vial with 2 gallons (7.6 L), a 2,000 dose vial with 4 gallons (15.2 L) of water, a 5,000 dose vial with 10 gallons (38 L), a 10,000 dose vial with 20 gallons (76 L) of water, or a 25,000 dose vial of vaccine with 50 gallons (190 L) of water.
5. A dried milk powder may be beneficial as a stabilizer. It is used in the water at the rate of 7.5 grams per gallon (3.8 L) as follows: 15 grams per 2 gallons (7.6 L), 30 grams per 4 gallons (15.2 L), 75 grams per 10 gallons (38 L), 150 grams per 20 gallons (76 L), or 375 grams per 50 gallons (190 L). Add the milk powder before the vaccine is added.
6. Provide enough waterers so that all birds may have an opportunity to drink the vaccine-treated water.
7. Avoid exposure of the waterers to direct sunlight.
8. Do not resume watering until water containing vaccine has been consumed. Then continue watering with untreated water for 24 hours before resuming the normal watering practice.
9. Vaccinating with less than one dose per bird may fail to protect satisfactorily.

Precaution(s): Store the vaccine at 35°-45°F (2°-7°C).

Use entire contents of vial immediately after mixing.

Do not dilute or otherwise extend the dosage.

Do not spill or splatter the vaccine. Burn empty bottles and unused vaccine.

Caution(s): Distribution in each State shall be limited to authorized recipients designated by proper State officials and under such additional conditions as these authorities may require.

Recommended use shall be restricted to premises having a history of the disease.

This vaccine is not returnable to the manufacturer.

Warning(s): Do not vaccinate within 21 days of slaughter.

Presentation: 10 x 1,000 doses/box, 10 x 2,000 doses/box, 10 x 5,000 doses/box, 10 x 10,000 doses/box, 1 x 25,000 doses/box, and 10 x 25,000 doses/box.

Compendium Code No.: 11290012 102R

BURSINE®-2

Fort Dodge **Vaccine**

Bursal Disease Vaccine, Live Virus

U.S. Vet. Lic. No.: 112

Contents: This product contains the antigen listed above.

Contains gentamicin as a preservative.

Indications: BURSINE®-2 is a modified live virus vaccine to aid in the prevention of infectious bursal disease (IBD or gumboro disease) of chickens.

BURSINE®-2 is particularly suited for use in flocks where maternal antibodies have interfered in active immunization using the milder live virus vaccines. BURSINE®-2 is well suited for the priming of breeder replacement pullets prior to the vaccination with an inactivated IBD vaccine.

B

Directions: Read in full, follow directions carefully.

Vaccination Recommendations:

Chickens: Vaccinate healthy chickens via the drinking water at 7 days of age or older.

Breeders: When used as a primer for an inactivated IBD vaccine, BURSINE®-2 should be administered via the drinking water 6-8 weeks prior to administration of an inactivated product.

1. Discontinue use of medications or sanitizing agents in the drinking water 24 hours before vaccinating. Do not resume use for 24 hours following vaccination.
2. Water used for the drinking-water administration of a live virus vaccine must be non-chlorinated.
3. Provide enough waterers so two-thirds of the birds may drink at one time. Scrub waterers with fresh, clean, non-chlorinated water, and use no disinfectant. Let waterers drain dry.
4. Turn off automatic waterers, so the only available water is the vaccine water. Do not give vaccine water through medication tanks.
5. Withhold water for 2 to 4 hours before vaccinating. Do not deprive the birds of water if the temperature is extremely high.
6. Remove seal from vaccine vial.
7. Remove stopper and half-fill vial with clean, cool, non-chlorinated water.
8. Replace stopper and shake until dissolved.
9. Use a clean container two-thirds filled with cool, clean, non-chlorinated water. Add dried milk at the rate of one ounce (28.4 gm) per 2 U.S. gallons (7.6 liters). Use 1-2 gallons (3.8-7.6 liters) of this solution for 1,000 doses of vaccine.
10. Add the rehydrated vaccine to the powdered milk solution and stir thoroughly.
11. Distribute the final volume of vaccine water evenly among the clean waterers. Do not place the waterers in direct sunlight. Resume regular water administration only after all the vaccine water has been consumed.

Records: Keep a record of vaccine serial number and expiration date, date of receipt and date of vaccination, where vaccination takes place, and any reactions observed.

Precaution(s): Store vaccine at not over 45°F (7°C). Use entire contents of vial when first opened. Burn vaccine container and all unused contents.

This product should be stored, transported, and administered in accordance with the instructions and directions. This product is nonreturnable.

Caution(s): Use only in states where permitted and on premises with a history of infectious bursal disease.

Warning(s): Do not vaccinate within 21 days before slaughter.

For veterinary use only.

Presentation: 10 x 1,000 doses, 10 x 2,500 doses, 10 x 5,000 doses, 10 x 10,000 doses and 25,000 doses.

Compendium Code No.: 10030221 10520B

BURSINE®-K ACL™

Fort Dodge **Vaccine**

Bursal Disease Vaccine, Killed Virus

U.S. Vet. Lic. No.: 112

Contents: This product contains the antigen listed above.

Gentamicin added as a preservative.

Indications: For the revaccination of healthy chickens as an aid in the prevention of the signs associated with infectious bursal disease caused by standard and variant strains. Progeny of vaccinates are aided in the prevention of signs and lesions associated with infectious bursal disease.

Dosage and Administration: Inject 0.5 mL (0.5 cc) intramuscularly or subcutaneously (in the lower neck region), using aseptic technique. Vaccinate only healthy birds. For primed birds, a single dose between 16 and 22 weeks (approximately 4 weeks prior to lay) is indicated.

Precaution(s): Store in the dark at 36° to 45°F (2° to 7°C). Do not freeze. Warm to 72°F (22°C) and shake well before using. Use entire contents when first opened.

Warning(s): Do not vaccinate within 42 days before slaughter.

In case of accidental human injection seek immediate medical attention.

For veterinary use only.

Presentation: 1,000 doses (500 mL).

Compendium Code No.: 10030231 10051C

BURSINE® N-K ACL™

Fort Dodge **Vaccine**

Bursal Disease-Newcastle Disease Vaccine, Killed Virus

U.S. Vet. Lic. No.: 112

Contents: This product contains the antigens listed above.

Gentamicin added as a preservative.

Indications: For subcutaneous or intramuscular revaccination of healthy chickens 3 weeks of age or older, as an aid in the prevention of the signs and lesions associated with infectious bursal disease caused by standard and variant strains and newcastle disease. Progeny of vaccinates are aided in the prevention of signs and lesions associated with infectious bursal disease and newcastle disease.

Dosage and Administration: Inject 0.5 mL (0.5 cc) intramuscularly or subcutaneously (in the lower neck region), using aseptic technique. Vaccinate only healthy birds. For primed birds, a single dose between 16 and 22 weeks (approximately 4 weeks prior to lay) is indicated.

Precaution(s): Store in the dark at 36° to 45°F (2° to 7°C). Do not freeze. Warm to 72°F (22°C) and shake well before using. Use entire contents when first opened.

Warning(s): Do not vaccinate within 42 days before slaughter.

In case of accidental human injection seek immediate medical attention.

For veterinary use only.

Presentation: 1,000 doses (500 mL).

Compendium Code No.: 10030201 10071C

BURSINE® PLUS

Fort Dodge **Vaccine**

Bursal Disease Vaccine, Live Virus

U.S. Vet. Lic. No.: 112

Contents: This product contains the antigen listed above.

Contains gentamicin as a preservative.

B

Indications: BURSINE® Plus is a live virus vaccine to aid in the prevention of infectious bursal disease (IBD or Gumboro disease) of chickens.

BURSINE® Plus is well suited for the priming of breeder replacement pullets prior to the vaccination with an inactivated IBD vaccine.

For drinking water administration to healthy growing chickens as young as 7 days of age as an aid in the prevention of infectious bursal disease.

Directions: Read in full, follow directions carefully.

Directions for drinking water administration:

Chickens: Vaccinate healthy chickens via the drinking water at 7 days of age or older.

Breeders: When used as a primer for an inactivated IBD vaccine, BURSINE® Plus should be administered via the drinking water 6 to 8 weeks prior to administration of an inactivated product.

1. Discontinue use of medication or sanitizing agents in the drinking water 4 hours before vaccinating. Do not resume use for 24 hours following vaccination.
2. Water used for the drinking water administration of a live virus vaccine must be non-chlorinated.
3. Provide enough waterers so two-thirds of the birds may drink at one time. Scrub waterers with fresh, clean, non-chlorinated water and use no disinfectant. Let waterers drain dry.
4. Turn off automatic waterers, so the only available water is the vaccine water. Do not give vaccine water through medication tanks.
5. Withhold water for 2 to 4 hours before vaccinating. Do not deprive the birds of water if the temperature is extremely high.
6. Remove seal from vaccine vial.
7. Remove stopper and half-fill vial with clean, cool, non-chlorinated water.
8. Replace stopper and shake until dissolved.
9. Use a clean container two thirds filled with cool, clean, non-chlorinated water. Add dried milk at the rate of one ounce (28.4 gm) per 2 U.S. gallons (7.6 liters). Use 1 to 2 gallons (3.8-7.6 liters) of this solution for 1,000 doses of vaccine.
10. Add the rehydrated vaccine to the powdered milk solution and stir thoroughly.
11. Distribute the final volume of vaccine water evenly among the clean waterers. Do not place the waterers in direct sunlight. Resume regular water administration only after all the vaccine water has been consumed.

Records: Keep a record of vaccine serial number and expiration date, date of receipt and date of vaccination, where vaccination takes place, and any reactions observed.

Precaution(s): Store vaccine at not over 45°F (7°C). Use entire contents of vial when first opened. Burn vaccine container and all unused contents.

This product should be stored, transported, and administered in accordance with the instructions and directions.

This product is nonreturnable.

Caution(s): Use only in states where permitted and on premises with a history of infectious bursal disease.

Warning(s): Do not vaccinate within 21 days before slaughter.

For veterinary use only.

Presentation: 10 x 1,000 doses, 10 x 2,500 doses, 10 x 5,000 doses, 10 x 10,000 doses and 25,000 doses.

Compendium Code No.: 10030211 10530E

BUTAJECT ℞

Vetus **Phenylbutazone-Injection**

(Phenylbutazone)

ANADA No.: 200-126

Active Ingredient(s): Each mL contains 200 mg of phenylbutazone, 10.45 mg of benzyl alcohol as preservative, sodium hydroxide to adjust pH to 9.5 to 10.0 and water for injection, q.s.

Indications: For relief of inflammatory conditions associated with the musculoskeletal system in horses.

Pharmacology: Description: BUTAJECT (phenylbutazone) is a synthetic, non-hormonal anti-inflammatory, antipyretic compound useful in the management of inflammatory conditions. The apparent analgesic effect is probably related mainly to the compound's anti-inflammatory properties.

Chemically, phenylbutazone is 4-butyl-1, 2-diphenyl-3, 5-pyrazolidinedione. It is a pyrazolon derivative entirely unrelated to the steroid hormones.

Background Pharmacology: Kuzell, Payne, Fleming and Denko demonstrated clinical effectiveness of phenylbutazone in acute rheumatism, gout, gouty arthritis, and various other rheumatoid disorders in man. Anti-rheumatic and anti-inflammatory activity has been well established by Fabre, Domenjoz, Wilhelmi, and Yourish.

Lieberman reported on the effective use of phenylbutazone in the treatment of painful conditions of the musculoskeletal system in dogs; including posterior paralysis associated with intervertebral disc syndrome, painful fractures, arthritis, and painful injuries to the limbs and joints. Joshua observed objective improvement without toxicity following long-term therapy of two aged arthritic dogs. Ogilivie and Sutter reported rapid response to phenylbutazone therapy in a review of 19 clinical cases including posterior paralysis, posterior weakness, arthritis, rheumatism, and other conditions associated with lameness and musculoskeletal weakness.

Camberos reported favorable results with phenylbutazone following intermittent treatment of thoroughbred horses for arthritis and chronic arthrosis (e.g. osteoarthritis of medial and distal bones of the hock, arthritis of stifle and hip, arthrosis of the spine, chronic hip pains, chronic pain in the trapezius muscles, and generalized arthritis). Results were less favorable in cases of traumatism, muscle rupture, strains and inflammations of the third phalanx. Sutter reported favorable response in chronic equine arthritis, fair results in a severely bruised mare, and poor results in two cases where the condition was limited to the third phalanx.

Dosage and Administration: For horses only.

Intravenously: 1 to 2 g per 1,000 lbs of body weight (5 to 10 mL/1,000 lbs) daily. Injection should be given slowly and with care. Limit intravenous administration to a maximum of 5 successive days, which may be followed by oral phenylbutazone dosage forms.

Guidelines to Successful Therapy:

1. Use a relatively high dose for the first 48 hours, then reduce gradually to a maintenance dose. Maintain lowest dose capable of producing desired clinical response.
2. Response to phenylbutazone therapy is prompt, usually occurring within 24 hours. If no significant clinical response is evident after 5 days, reevaluate diagnosis and therapeutic approach.
3. In animals, phenylbutazone is largely metabolized in 8 hours. It is recommended that a third of the daily dose be administered at 8 hour intervals. Reduce dosage as symptoms regress. In some cases, treatment may be given only when symptoms appear with no need for continuous medication. If long-term therapy is planned, oral administration is suggested.
4. Many chronic conditions will respond to phenybutazone therapy, but discontinuance of treatment may result in recurrence of symptoms.

Contraindication(s): Parenteral injections should be made intravenously only; do not inject subcutaneously or intramuscularly. Use with caution in patients who have a history of drug allergy.

Precaution(s): Store in refrigerator between 2°C and 8°C (36°F and 46°F).

Caution(s): Federal law restricts this drug to use by or on the order of a licensed veterinarian.

Stop medication at the first sign of gastrointestinal upset, jaundice, or blood dyscrasia. Authenticated cases of agaranulocytosis associated with the drug have occurred in man; fatal reactions, although rare, have been reported in dogs after long-term therapy. To guard against this possibility, conduct routing blood counts at weekly intervals during the early phase of therapy and at intervals of two weeks thereafter. Any significant fall in the total white count, relative decrease in granulocytes, or black or tarry stools, should be regarded as a signal for immediate cessation of therapy and institution of appropriate countermeasures. In the treatment of inflammatory conditions associated with infections, specific anti-infective therapy is required.

Warning(s): Not for use in horses intended for food.

References: Available upon request.

Presentation: 100 mL vials.

Compendium Code No.: 14440140

BUTAPASTE ℞

Vetus **Phenylbutazone-Oral**

phenylbutazone

NADA No.: 116-087

Active Ingredient(s): Each syringe contains 12 g phenylbutazone.

Each 1 g marking on the plunger contains:

Phenylbutazone. . . . . 1 g

Indications: For the relief of inflammatory conditions associated with the musculoskeletal system in horses.

Pharmacology: Description: BUTAPASTE is a synthetic, nonhormonal anti-inflammatory, antipyretic compound useful in the management of inflammatory conditions. The apparent analgesic effect is probably related mainly to the compound's anti-inflammatory properties.

Chemically, phenylbutazone is 4-butyl-1,2-diphenyl-3,5-pyrazolidinedione. It is a pyrazolone derivative, entirely unrelated to the steroid hormones, and has the following structural formula:

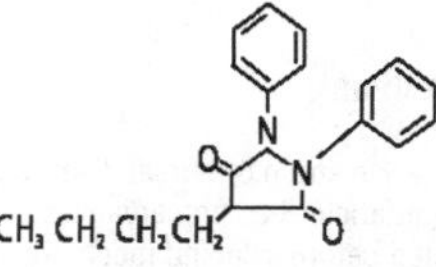

Dosage and Administration: Orally - 1 to 2 g of phenylbutazone per 500 lb of body weight, but not to exceed 4 g daily. Use a relatively high dose for the first 48 hours, then reduce gradually to a maintenance dose. Maintain lowest dose capable of producing desired clinical response.

Guidelines to Successful Therapy:

1. Use a relative high dose for the first 48 hours, then reduce gradually to a maintenance dose. Maintain lowest dose capable of producing desired clinical response.
2. Response to BUTAPASTE therapy is prompt, usually occurring within 24 hours. If no significant clinical response is evident after 5 days, reevaluate diagnosis and therapeutic approach.
3. When administering BUTAPASTE the oral cavity should be empty. Deposit paste on back of tongue by depressing plunger that has been previously set to deliver the correct dose.
4. Many chronic conditions will respond to BUTAPASTE therapy but discontinuance of treatment may result in recurrence of symptoms.

Contraindication(s): Use with caution in patients who have a history of drug allergy.

Precaution(s): Storage: Store at 15°-30°C (59°-86°F).

Caution(s): Federal (U.S.A.) law restricts this drug to use by or on the order of a licensed veterinarian.

Stop medication at the first sign of gastrointestinal upset, jaundice, or blood dyscrasia. Authenticated cases of agranulocytosis associated with the drug have occurred in man; fatal reactions, although rare, have been reported in dogs after long-term therapy. To guard against this possibility, conduct routine blood counts at weekly intervals during the early phase of therapy and at intervals of 2 weeks thereafter. Any significant fall in the total white count, relative decrease in granulocytes, or black or tarry stools, should be regarded as a signal for immediate cessation of therapy and institution of appropriate countermeasures.

In the treatment of inflammatory conditions associated with infections, specific anti-infective therapy is required.

For horses only.

Warning(s): Not for use in horses intended for food.

Keep out of reach of children.

Presentation: Syringe containing 12 g of phenylbutazone, NDC 47611-870-61 (12 g).

Distributed by: Burns Veterinary Supply, Inc., Westbury, NY 11590.

Compendium Code No.: 14441010

BUTATABS-D ℞

Vetus **Phenylbutazone-Oral**

Active Ingredient(s): Each tablet contains:

Phenylbutazone. . . . . 100 mg

Indications: Phenylbutazone is used for the treatment of inflammatory conditions of the musculoskeletal system in dogs.

Pharmacology: Phenylbutazone is the generic name of the drug known chemically as 4-butyl 1,2-diphenyl-3,5-pyrazolidinedione.

Phenylbutazone is a white crystalline solid, slightly soluble in water, and soluble in some organic solvents. It does not have an odor, but has a slightly bitter taste.

Phenylbutazone is a nonhormonal anti-inflammatory agent. It is unrelated to the corticosteroid anti-inflammatory agents. The anti-inflammatory activity of phenylbutazone has been shown in lower animals[1] and in man.[2] The greatest amount of data on efficacy is in man.[3-6] Studies in dogs have reported useful anti-inflammatory activity in the treatment of painful conditions of the musculoskeletal system.[1,7] These conditions include painful fractures, arthritis, and painful injuries to the limbs and joints.

Dosage and Administration: Administer 20 mg per lb. of body weight orally (100 mg/5 lbs.) once a day in three (3) divided doses, not to exceed 800 mg a day, regardless of body weight.

Administration:

1. Use a high dose for the first 48 hours, then reduce it gradually to a maintenance dose. Maintain the lowest dose capable of producing the desired clinical response.
2. In many cases, the tablets may be crushed and given with food. Reduce the dose as symptoms regress. In some cases, treatment may be given only when symptoms appear, without need for continuous medications. If a long term therapy is planned, oral administration is suggested.
3. In animals, phenylbutazone is mostly metabolized within eight (8) hours. It is recommended that one-third (⅓) of the daily dose be administered at 8-hour intervals.
4. Many chronic conditions will respond to phenylbutazone therapy but discontinuance of the treatment may result in the recurrence of symptoms.

Contraindication(s): Phenylbutazone should not be administered to patients with serious hepatic, renal or cardiac pathology, or those with a history of blood dyscrasia.

Caution(s): Federal law restricts this drug to use by or on the order of a licensed veterinarian.

1. Use with caution in patients with a history of drug allergies.
2. Stop the medication at the first sign of gastrointestinal upset, jaundice or blood dyscrasia. Cases of agranulocytosis associated with phenylbutazone have occurred in man. Only one case has been reported in veterinary medicine in a dog on high level, long-term therapy.
3. To guard against this possibility, conduct routine blood counts at not more than seven-day intervals during the early course of therapy. Any significant fall in the total white count, relative decrease in granuloctyes or black or tarry stool should be a sign for immediate cessation of therapy and the institution of appropriate treatment.
4. When treating inflammatory conditions associated with infections, anti-infective therapy is required.
5. The response to phenylbutazone therapy occurs within 24 hours. If a significant clinical response is not evident after five days of therapy, re-evaluate the diagnosis and therapeutic regimen.

References: Available upon request.

Presentation: Bottles of 1,000 tablets.

Compendium Code No.: 14440151

BUTATABS-E ℞

Vetus **Phenylbutazone-Oral**

NDC No.: 47611-002-01

Active Ingredient(s): Each tablet contains:

Phenylbutazone . . . . 1.0 g

Indications: Phenylbutazone is used for the treatment of inflammatory conditions of horses associated with the musculoskeletal system.

Pharmacology: Phenylbutazone is the generic name of the drug known chemically as 4-butyl-1,2-diphenyl-3,5-pyrazolidinedione.

Phenylbutazone is a white crystalline solid, slightly soluble in water, and soluble in some organic solvents. It does not have an odor, but has a slightly bitter taste.

Phenylbutazone is a nonhormonal, anti-inflammatory agent. It is unrelated to the corticosteroid anti-inflammatory agents. The anti-inflammatory activity of phenylbutazone has been shown in lower animals and in man. The greatest amount of data on efficacy is in man. Studies in horses have shown that the drug is well absorbed when administered orally with a balling gun. The apparent half-life is 3.5 hours.

Dosage and Administration: The oral dose for horses is two (2) to four (4) tablets (2 to 4 g) per 1,000 lbs. per day.

The total daily dose should be limited to four (4) tablets per day. Because of the relatively short half-life of the drug, administration every eight (8) hours is the most satisfactory schedule.

The response to phenylbutazone is usually prompt. If there is not a significant clinical effect in five (5) days, a re-evaluation of the diagnosis and the treatment should be made.

Precaution(s): Store the product in a cool place (46° to 59°F) or alternatively store in a refrigerator.

Caution(s): Federal (USA) law restricts this drug to use by or on the order of a licensed veterinarian.

Use with caution in patients with a history of drug allergies.

When treating inflammatory conditions associated with infections, anti-infective therapy is required.

Warning(s): Not for use in horses intended for food purposes.

Side Effects: Doses of phenylbutazone higher than those recommended have produced intestinal ulcerative lesions. Necrotizing phlebitis in the portal vein has been observed in horses receiving high doses for extended periods of time.

Presentation: Bottles of 100 tablets.

Compendium Code No.: 14440160

BUTATRON™ TABLETS ℞

Bimeda **Phenylbutazone-Oral**

(Phenylbutazone Tablets, USP) Anti-Inflammatory

NADA No.: 044-756

Active Ingredient(s): Each tablet contains either:

Phenylbutazone U.S.P. . . . . 100 mg
Phenylbutazone U.S.P. . . . . 1 g

Indications: Phenylbutazone possesses non-hormonal, anti-inflammatory activity of value in the management of musculoskeletal conditions in dogs and horses such as the arthritides, including osteoarthritis, and as an aid in the relief of inflammation associated with intervertebral disc syndrome in dogs.

Pharmacology: Description: Phenylbutazone is a non-hormonal, anti-inflammatory agent. Chemically, it is described as 4-Butyl-1,2 diphenyl-3,5-pyrazolidinedione, a synthetic pyrazolone derivative, entirely unrelated to the steroid compounds.

Actions and Uses: Kuzell,[1,2,3] Payne,[4] Fleming,[5] and Denko,[6] demonstrated clinical effectiveness of phenylbutazone in acute rheumatism, gout, gouty arthritis, and various other rheumatoid disorders in man. Anti-inflammatory activity has been well established by Fabre,[7] Domenjoz,[8] Wilhelmi,[9] and Yourish.[10]

Lieberman[11] reported on the effective use of phenylbutazone in the treatment of conditions of the musculoskeletal system in dogs, including posterior paralysis associated with intervertebral disc syndrome, fracture, arthritis and injuries to the limbs and joints. Joshua[12] observed objective improvement without toxicity following long-term therapy of two aged arthritic dogs. Ogilvie and Sutter[13] reported rapid response to phenylbutazone therapy in a review of 19 clinical cases including posterior paralysis, posterior weakness, arthritis, rheumatism and other conditions associated with lameness and musculoskeletal weakness.

Camberos[14] reported favorable results with phenylbutazone following intermittent treatment of thoroughbred horses for arthritis and chronic arthrosis (e.g. osteoarthritis of medial and distal bones of the hock, arthritis of the stifle and hip, arthrosis of the spine and generalized arthritis). Results were less favorable in cases of traumatism, muscle rupture, strains and inflammatory conditions if the third phalanx. Sutter[15] reported favorable responses in chronic equine arthritis, fair results in a severely bruised mare and poor results in two cases where the condition was limited to the third phalanx.

Dosage and Administration: Dosage:

Dogs: Orally - 20 mg per pound body weight (100 mg/5 lbs) daily in 3 divided doses, not to exceed 800 mg daily regardless of body weight.

Horses: Orally - 1-2 grams per 500 lbs body weight, not to exceed 4 g daily.

Administration:

1. Use a relatively high dose for the first 48 hours, then reduce gradually to a maintenance dose. Maintain lowest dose capable of producing the desired clinical response.
2. In many cases, tablets may be crushed and given with feed. Reduce the dosage as symptoms regress. In some cases treatment may be given only when symptoms appear with no need for continuous medication.
3. In animals, phenylbutazone is largely metabolized in 8 hours. It is recommended that a third of the daily dose be administered at 8 hour intervals.
4. Many chronic conditions will respond to phenylbutazone therapy, but discontinuance of treatment may result in recurrence of symptoms.

Contraindication(s): Phenylbutazone should not be administered to animals with serious heptic, renal or cardiac pathology, or those with a history of blood dyscrasia.

Precaution(s): Storage: Store at controlled room temperature, 20°-25°C (68°-77°F).

Caution(s): Federal (USA) law restricts this drug to use by or on the order of a licensed veterinarian.

1. Use with caution in animals with a history of drug allergy.
2. Stop medication at the first sign of gastrointestinal upset, jaundice, or blood dyscrasia. Authenticated cases of agranulocytosis associated with phenylbutazone have occurred in man. Phenylbutazone induced blood dyscrasias have been reported in dogs. Thrombocytopenia and leukopenia are early manifestations followed by nonregenerative anemia. The occurrence of this reaction is not dose dependent and is unpredictable. To guard against this possibility, conduct routine blood counts at not more than 7 day intervals during the early course of therapy, and at intervals of not more than 14 days throughout the course of therapy. Any significant fall in the total white count, relative decrease in granulocytes, or black or tarry stools, should be regarded as a signal for immediate cessation of therapy and institution of appropriate treatment.
3. When treating inflammatory conditions associated with infection, specific anti-infective therapy is required.
4. Response to phenylbutazone therapy is prompt, usually occurring within 24 hours. If no significant clinical response is evident after 5 days of therapy, re-evaluate diagnosis and therapeutic regimen.

For animal use only.

Warning(s): Phenylbutazone should not be administered to meat, egg or milk producing animals because the status of residues of drug remaining in edible tissues has not been determined.

Not for human use.

Keep out of reach of children.

References: Available upon request.

Presentation: BUTATRON™ (Phenylbutazone Tablets, U.S.P.) are supplied in the following tablet concentrations and package sizes:

100 mg tablets . . . . Bottles of 1000 tablets
1 g tablets . . . . Bottles of 100 tablets

BUTATRON is a Trademark of Bimeda, Inc.

Compendium Code No.: 13990520 8BUT003-1001

BUZZ OFF™ POUR-ON

Boehringer Ingelheim **Premise and Topical Insecticide**

EPA Reg. No.: 4691-121

Active Ingredient(s):

Permethrin (CAS No. 52645-53-1) 7.4%
Piperonyl Butoxide Technical (CAS No. 51-03-6) 7.4%
Other Ingredients* 85.2%
Total 100.0%

*Contains Petroleum Distillate

Indications: Controls flies, ticks and lice on horses.

Horses and Foals: Target pests include stable flies, horn flies, face flies, deer flies, house flies, eye gnats, lice and ticks. Aids in the control of horse flies, mosquitoes, black flies.

Mature Horses: Target pests include stable flies, horn flies, face flies, deer flies, house flies, eye gnats, lice and ticks. Aids in the control of horse flies, mosquitoes, black flies.

Premises: Target pests include house flies, stable flies, face flies, gnats, mosquitoes, black flies, fleas, little house flies (*Fannia* spp.). Aids in control of cockroaches, ants, spiders and crickets.

Directions for Use: It is a violation of Federal law to use this product in a manner inconsistent with its labeling.

Important: This is a highly concentrated formulation. Use only with an accurate measuring container or applicator.

Ready to Use - no dilution necessary.

Apply To:	Target Pests:	Application Instructions:
Horses and Foals	Stable Flies, Horn Flies, Face Flies, Deer Flies, House Flies, Eye Gnats, Lice and Ticks. Aids in the control of Horse Flies, Mosquitoes and Black Flies.	Wipe-On: Apply 8 mL to 16 mL as a wipe-on. Dampen an applicator mitt, cloth or toweling (turkish) with BUZZ OFF™ Pour-On. Rub over hair with special attention to the legs, shoulders, neck and facial areas where flies tend to congregate. Be especially careful not to get in horse's eyes. Repeat treatment as needed. Ready-To-Use Spray: Use BUZZ OFF™ Pour-On after riding or exercise. Use undiluted in a mist sprayer, applying 8 mL to 16 mL per animal. Apply directly onto attached ticks. Repeat as needed.
Horses	Stable Flies, Horn Flies, Face Flies, Deer Flies, House Flies, Eye Gnats, Lice and Ticks. Aids in the control of Horse Flies, Mosquitoes and Black Flies.	Pour-On: After riding or exercise, pour 8 mL to 16 mL of BUZZ OFF™ Pour-On along the back and down the face of mature horses, being careful to avoid the eyes. Do not use this method of application on foals. Repeat treatment as needed.
Premises - in and around Horse Premises	House Flies, Stable Flies, Face Flies, Gnats, Mosquitoes, Black Flies, Fleas, Little House Flies (*Fannia* spp.). Aids in control of Cockroaches, Ants, Spiders and Crickets.	Ready-To-Use Spot or Premise Spray: Use undiluted in a mist sprayer. Apply directly to surface to leave a residual insecticidal coating, paying particular attention to areas where insects crawl or alight. 500 mL will treat approximately 7,200 square feet.

Special Note: BUZZ OFF™ Pour-On is an oil-base, ready-to-use product that may leave an oily appearance on the hair coat of some animals.

BUZZ OFF™ Pour-On should be used in an integrated pest management system which may involve repeat treatments and the use of other pest control practices.

Precautionary Statements: Hazards to Humans and Domestic Animals:

Caution: Harmful if absorbed through the skin. Avoid contact with skin, eyes, or clothing. Avoid breathing vapor or mist. Prolonged or frequently repeated skin contact may cause allergic reactions in some individuals. Remove contaminated clothing and wash contaminated clothing before reuse. Wash thoroughly with soap and water after handling.

First Aid:

If on Skin: Wash with plenty of soap and water. Get medical attention.

Environmental Hazards: This pesticide is extremely toxic to fish and other aquatic invertebrates. Do not add directly to water. Do not contaminate water when disposing of equipment washwaters.

Physical or Chemical Hazards: Do not use or store near heat or open flame.

Storage and Disposal: Do not contaminate water, food or feed by storage or disposal.

Storage: Keep container sealed when not in use. Do not store near food or feed.

Pesticide Disposal: Waste resulting from the use of this product may be disposed of on site or at an approved waste disposal facility.

Container Disposal: Triple rinse (or equivalent). Then offer for recycling or reconditioning, or puncture and dispose of in a sanitary landfill or incineration, or, if allowed by State and local authorities, by burning. If burned, stay out of smoke.

Warning(s): Keep out of reach of children.

Disclaimer: Warranty and Limitation of Damages: Seller warrants that this material conforms to its chemical description and is reasonably fit for the purposes stated on the label when used in accordance with directions under normal conditions of use and Buyer assumes the risk of any use contrary to such directions. Seller makes no other express or implied warranty, including any other expressed or implied warranty of Fitness or of Merchantability, and no agent of Seller is authorized to do so except in writing and with a specific reference to this warranty. In no event shall Seller's liability for any breach of warranty exceed the purchase price of the material as to which a claim is made.

Presentation: 1 pint (473 mL) containers.

Compendium Code No.: 10280241 BI 4083-8R-1 10/99

C

CAL "62" PLUS GEL

Aspen **Calcium-Oral**

Active Ingredient(s): Each tube contains 537 mg/mL (384 mg/gm) of a unique base of calcium chloride and calcium carbonate.

Minimum contents of 300 mL dose

Calcium .... 60.0 gm - 14.3% minimum
62.8 gm - 14.8% maximum

Magnesium .... 6.8 gm - 1.7%

Cobalt 0.6 gm - 0.1%

Ingredients: Water, calcium chloride, calcium carbonate, dextrose, magnesium chloride, sodium citrate, cobalt sulfate, silicon dioxide.

Indications: A nutritional supplement containing calcium, magnesium, and cobalt for dairy cattle during calving.

Dosage and Administration: Give one tube prior to or after calving and second tube 12 to 24 hours after calving.

1. Hold head of the cow in a slightly elevated position.
2. Place nozzle near rear of mouth. Use of hook nozzle is recommended.
3. Discharge entire contents of tube.
4. Hold head up and allow animal time to swallow.

No withdrawal time is necessary.

Precaution(s): Do not freeze.

Presentation: 300 mL (420 g) tube.

Compendium Code No.: 14750100

CAL-C-FRESH™

Vets Plus **Calcium-Oral**

Oral Calcium and B-Vitamin Gel with Buffer

Guaranteed Analysis: (min):

	Per Tube	Per lb.
Calcium	54 g	65 g
Calcium (max)	58 g	70 g
Thiamine Hydrochloride	100 mg	121 mg
Riboflavin	5 mg	6 mg
d-Calcium Pantothenate	10 mg	12 mg
Niacin	100 mg	121 mg
Vitamin B_{12}	100 mcg	121 mcg
Ascorbic Acid	5 mg	6 mg
Vitamin E	50 IU	60 IU

Ingredients: Calcium Chloride, Tri-Calcium Phosphate, DL-alpha-Tocopherol Acetate (Vitamin E), Propylene Glycol, Thiamine Hydrochloride, Riboflavin, Sodium Bicarbonate, Niacinamide, d-Calcium Pantothenate, Cyanocobalamin (Vitamin B_{12}), Ascorbic Acid (Vitamin C), and Xanthan Gum.

Indications: Administer to every fresh cow or heifer before and after calving. CAL-C-FRESH™ provides calcium to lower the incidence of milk fever, propylene glycol for energy, and vitamins to stimulate appetite. CAL-C-FRESH™ can also be used as a follow up to IV treatment.

Dosage and Administration: Give one tube at the first sign of freshening and give another tube 6 to 12 hours post calving, repeat every 12 hours as needed. If the first dose is missed, a post calving dose is still beneficial. If conditions do not improve, consult your veterinarian.

Feeding Directions: Place the tube in a dosing gun and remove the cap. Hold the head of the cow in a slightly elevated position and place the nozzle on the back of the tongue. Administer the entire contents of the tube slowly, allowing the cow time to swallow. Do not give to cows that are unable to swallow.

Precaution(s): Keep in a cool dry place. Avoid freezing.

Caution(s): Keep out of the reach of children. Contact with eyes or wounds or prolonged contact with skin can cause irritation. Single dose unit. Properly dispose of unused portion.

Animal use only.

Presentation: 12x300 cc (375 gm) tubes per case.

Compendium Code No.: 10730060

CALCIUM 23% SOLUTION ℞

Vedco **Calcium Therapy**

Active Ingredient(s): Each 500 mL contains:

Calcium (as calcium borogluconate - equivalent to calcium gluconate) .... 10.7 g

Cations:

Calcium .... 1,069 mEq/L

Anions:

Gluconate .... 1,069 mEq/L

This product contains no preservatives.

Indications: For use as an aid in the treatment of hypocalcemia (parturient paresis, milk fever) in cattle.

Dosage and Administration: Warm the solution to body temperature before administration. The usual intravenous dose in cattle is 500 mL per 800 to 1,000 pounds of body weight. If given intramuscularly or subcutaneously, divide the dosage among several injection sites and massage to aid in absorption. If improvement does not occur after the use of the product, consult a veterinarian.

Precaution(s): Store at a controlled room temperature between 59-86°F (15-30°C).

Caution(s): Federal law restricts this drug to use by or on the order of a licensed veterinarian.

Keep out of the reach of children.

Follow strict sterile procedures when using the product. Intravenous administration should be made slowly to avoid adverse effects such as heart block or shock.

Use the entire contents when first opened. Discard any unused solution.

Presentation: 500 mL containers.

Compendium Code No.: 10940200

CALCIUM DRENCH

AgriPharm **Calcium-Oral**

A Ready to use blend of Ca, Mg, Vitamin D, B complex Vitamins and Propylene Glycol

Active Ingredient(s): Minimum contents of 200 mL dose:

Calcium .... 34 g/dose - 12.8% minimum (wt/wt)
40.8 g/dose - 15.4% maximum (wt/wt)

Potassium .... 0.6 g/dose
Magnesium .... 2.05 g/dose
Riboflavin .... 5 mg/dose
Pyridoxine HCl .... 10 mg/dose
Calcium Pantothenate .... 10 mg/dose
Vitamin B_{12} .... 100 mcg/dose
Vitamin D_3 .... 100,000 IU/dose

Ingredients: Calcium chloride, magnesium chloride, propylene glycol, vitamin D_3, potassium chloride, riboflavin, pyridoxine HCl, calcium pantothenate, vitamin B_{12}, water.

Indications: For use as a high calcium nutritional supplement for dairy cattle during calving.

Dosage and Administration: Shake well before using.

Administer in cheek with drench gun as needed.

Cows:

Pre-Calving .... 200 mL
Post-Calving .... 200 mL

The container will provide 18-200 mL feedings.

Precaution(s): Store drench above 40°F. Do not freeze.

Warning(s): For animal use only. Keep out of reach of children.

Presentation: 3785 mL.

Compendium Code No.: 14570180

CALCIUM DRENCH™

Vets Plus **Calcium-Oral**

Oral Nutrient Supplement

Guaranteed Analysis: (Per 200 mL):

Calcium min. .... 25 g
Calcium max. .... 32 g

Ingredients: Water, Calcium Chloride, Propylene Glycol, Magnesium Chloride, Potassium Chloride, Dextrose, Choline Bitartrate, Niacinamide, Silica, Vitamin A Acetate, DL-alpha-Tocopheryl Acetate (Vitamin E), d-Activated Animal Sterol (Vitamin D_3), d-Calcium Pantothenate, Ascorbic Acid (Vitamin C), Riboflavin, Cyanocobalamin (Vitamin B_{12}), Folic Acid, Pyridoxine Hydrochloride (Vitamin B_6), and FD&C red color #40.

Indications: Use on every fresh cow or heifer before and after calving. CALCIUM DRENCH™ provides calcium to lower the incidence of milk fever, propylene glycol for energy, and vitamin B complex to stimulate appetite. CALCIUM DRENCH™ can also be used as a follow up to IV treatment.

Dosage and Administration: Provide 200 mL at the first sign of freshening and another 200 mL 6 to 12 hours after calving, repeat as needed. If the first dose is missed, a post calving dose is still beneficial. Shake well before using. If conditions do not improve, consult your veterinarian. 1 gallon provides nineteen 200 mL feedings.

Feeding Directions: Administer orally using a drench gun. Hold the head of the cowl in a slightly elevated position and carefully place nozzle into the back of the mouth between the cheek and teeth. Slowly administer recommended dosage. Do not give to cows that are unable to swallow.

Precaution(s): Keep in a cool dry place. Avoid freezing.

Caution(s): For animal use only.

Warning(s): Keep out of the reach of children. Contact with eyes or wounds or prolonged contact with skin, can cause irritation.

Presentation: 4 x 1 gallon (3.8 L) containers per case, 5 gallon pail, and 15 gallon drum.

Compendium Code No.: 10730001

CALCIUM DRENCH PLUS VITAMINS

AgriLabs **Calcium-Oral**

Oral Calcium Supplement for Pre & Post Calving Use

Guaranteed Analysis: (per 200 mL feeding)

Calcium (Ca), Min. 12.7%
Calcium (Ca), Max. 15.2%

Indications: Use CALCIUM DRENCH PLUS VITAMINS before and after freshening as a milk fever preventative. It can also be used after calving as an appetite stimulant.

Dosage and Administration: Provide one 200 mL feeding immediately following calving. Give additional feedings as needed. Administer using a drench gun. The drench should be administered slowly between the cheek and the teeth. Do not administer to a cow without a swallowing reflex.

Presentation: 1 gallon.

Compendium Code No.: 10580250

CALCIUM DRENCH PLUS VITAMINS

Durvet **Calcium-Oral**

NDC No.: 30798-556-35/30798-556-36

Guaranteed Analysis:

Calcium (Ca), Min. 12.7%
Calcium (Ca), Max. 15.2%

Ingredients: Calcium chloride, magnesium chloride, propylene glycol, potassium chloride, riboflavin supplement, vitamin B_{12} supplement, thiamin HCl, pyridoxin HCl and d-calcium pantothenate.

Indications: Use CALCIUM DRENCH with Vitamins before and after freshening as a milk fever preventative. It can also be used after calving as an appetite stimulant.

Dosage and Administration: Shake well before use.

Provide 200 mL precalving and another 200 mL post calving. Administer using a drench gun. The drench should be administered slowly between the teeth. Do not administer to a cow without a swallowing reflex.

Warning(s): Not for human use. For animal use only. Keep out of the reach of children.

Presentation: 3.785 L (1 gal) and 9.463 L (2½ gal).

Compendium Code No.: 10840170

CALCIUM GEL+SELENIUM

AgriLabs **Calcium-Oral**

A Nutritional Supplement for Dairy Cattle

Guaranteed Analysis: Per Tube:

Calcium	64 g - 16.7% minimum
Calcium	67 g - 17.2% maximum
Magnesium	62 g - 1.6%
Cobalt	0.7 g - 0.2%
Thiamine	100 mg
Niacin	100 mg
Pantothenic Acid	10 mg
Pyridoxine	10 mg
Vitamin E	5 mg
Riboflavin	5 mg
Citric Acid	5 mg
Selenium	2.6 mg
Vitamin B_{12}	100 mcg
Vitamin D_3	100,000 IU

Ingredients: Polyethylene glycol, calcium hydroxide, calcium propionate, magnesium oxide, vitamin D_3, cobalt chloride, sodium selenite, thiamine hydrochloride, niacin, calcium pantothenate, pyridoxine hydrochloride, riboflavin, alpha-tocopheryl acetate (source of vitamin E), citric acid, cyanocobalamin (vitamin B_{12}).

Indications: This preparation supplies calcium and selenium to ensure normal nutritional levels before, during and after calving.

Dosage and Administration: Give one tube prior to or after calving and second tube 12 to 24 hours after calving. Never administer more than one tube in 24 hour period.

Place the tube in a dosing gun and remove the cap. Hold the head of the cow in a normal to slightly elevated position and carefully place the nozzle into the back of the mouth. Administer the entire contents of one tube per feeding. Do not give to cows that are unable to swallow.

Precaution(s): This product is supplied in a single dose unit.

Discard unused portion.

Do not freeze.

Caution(s): Contact with eyes or wounds or prolonged contact with skin can cause irritation.

Warning(s): Keep out of reach of children.

Presentation: 14 ounce (400 g) tube.

Compendium Code No.: 10580270

CALCIUM GEL + VITAMINS

AgriLabs **Calcium-Oral**

Active Ingredient(s): Each tube contains:

Calcium (min.)	16%
Calcium (max.)	20% (54 g)
Vitamin A	600,000 I.U.
Vitamin D_3	100,000 I.U.

Contains calcium chloride, water, vitamin A, vitamin D_3, starch and guar gum.

Indications: A nutritional supplement preparation that supplies calcium to ensure normal levels in the blood before, during and after calving.

Dosage and Administration: Give one (1) tube within 6-12 hours prior to calving. Give another tube within 6-12 hours after calving.

Hold the head of the cow in a normal to slightly elevated position. Place the tube in the cow's mouth directly over the tongue. The product is carefully pressed out of the 300 mL tube. Hold the cow's mouth closed and allow time to swallow. Administer the entire 300 mL tube for each dose.

Caution(s): Follow label directions. Keep out of the reach of children.

Contact with the eyes or wounds, or prolonged contact with the skin can cause irritation.

Presentation: 14 oz. (400 g) tubes.

Compendium Code No.: 10580260

CALCIUM GLUCONATE 23%

AgriPharm **Calcium Therapy**

Active Ingredient(s): Each 500 mL contains:

Calcium gluconate	23% w/v
(provides 10.71 g of calcium* per 500 mL)	
Water for injection	q.s.

*Present as salts of boryl esters of gluconic acid.

Indications: For use in cattle as an aid in treating uncomplicated milk fever (parturient paresis).

Dosage and Administration: For intravenous administration only.

Cattle	250-500 mL

The dosage may be repeated at 8- to 12-hour intervals if required.

Presentation: Store at a controlled room temperature between 59°-86°F (15°-30°C).

Caution(s): Keep out of the reach of children.

For animal use only.

The solution should be warmed to room temperature and administered slowly. The entire contents should be used upon entering, as the product does not contain preservatives. Discard any unused portion. Do not use if the solution is cloudy or contains a precipitate.

Note: Monitor the animal's condition closely. Retreatment may be necessary. If there is not noticeable improvement within 24 hours following treatment, consult a veterinarian. Aseptic precautions should be observed such as using sterile needles and syringes.

Disinfect the site of injection.

Presentation: 500 mL containers.

Compendium Code No.: 14570190

CALCIUM GLUCONATE 23% SOLUTION

AgriLabs **Calcium Therapy**

Active Ingredient(s): Each 100 mL contains:

Calcium gluconate	23 g

(Calcium present as the boryl esters of gluconic acid.)

This product contains no preservatives.

Indications: To be used as an aid in the treatment of parturient paresis (milk fever) in cattle.

Dosage and Administration: Cattle: 250 to 500 mL.

Administer intravenously or intraperitoneally.

The solution should be warmed to body temperature and administered slowly. This product should be handled under aseptic conditions.

If there is no apparent improvement in the condition of the animal within 24 hours, consult a veterinarian.

Precaution(s): Store at a controlled room temperature between 2-30°C (36-86°F).

Caution(s): Livestock drug. Use only as directed. Use the entire contents when first opened.

Presentation: 500 mL bottles.

Compendium Code No.: 10580280

CALCIUM GLUCONATE 23% SOLUTION

Aspen **Calcium Therapy**

Active Ingredient(s): Each mL contains:

Calcium Gluconate (provides 2.14 grams Calcium)	23 grams
Water for Injection	q.s.

Contains boric acid as a solubilizing agent.

Electrolytes per 1000 mL: Calcium 1069 mEq;

Hypertonic

Osmolarity (calc.) 6,782 mOsmol/L.

Indications: To be used as an aid in the treatment of parturient paresis (milk fever) in cattle.

Dosage and Administration: Administer intravenously or intraperitoneally.

Solution should be warmed to body temperature and administered slowly. This product is sterile in unopened container. It contains no preservative. Use entire contents when first opened. It should be handled under aseptic conditions. If there is no apparent improvement in the animal's condition within 24 hours, consult a veterinarian.

Precaution(s): Store between 15°C-30°C (59°F-86°F).

Warning(s): For animal use only.

Keep out of reach of children.

Presentation: 500 mL.

Compendium Code No.: 14750120

CALCIUM GLUCONATE 23% SOLUTION

Bimeda **Calcium Therapy**

Active Ingredient(s): Each 100 mL contains:

Calcium gluconate (provides 2.14 g calcium)	23 g
Water for injection	q.s.

Contains boric acid as a solubilizing agent.

Electrolytes per 1,000 mL:

Calcium	1,069 mEq
Hypertonic	pH 3.0-5.0

The product does not contain any preservatives.

Indications: To be used as an aid in the treatment of parturient paresis (milk fever) in cattle.

Dosage and Administration: For intravenous use only.

Cattle: 250 to 500 mL.

The solution should be warmed to body temperature and administered slowly.

If there is no apparent improvement in the animals condition within 24 hours, consult a veterinarian.

Precaution(s): Store at 36°-86°F (2°-30°C).

Caution(s): The product is sterile in the unopened container. Use the entire contents when first opened. It should be handled under aseptic conditions.

For animal use only. Not for human use. Keep out of the reach of children.

Presentation: 500 mL bottles.

Compendium Code No.: 13990100

CALCIUM GLUCONATE 23% SOLUTION

Durvet **Calcium Therapy**

Active Ingredient(s): Each 100 mL contains:

Calcium Gluconate	23 grams
(Calcium present as the boryl esters of gluconic acid)	
Osmolarity (calc.)	6,782 mOsmol/L

It contains no preservative.

Indications: To be used as an aid in the treatment of parturient paresis (milk fever) in cattle.

Dosage and Administration: Cattle: 250 to 500 mL.

Administer intravenously or intraperitoneally. Solution should be warmed to body temperature and administered slowly.

Precaution(s): Store between 15°C-30°C (59°F-86°F). Keep from freezing.

Use entire contents when first opened.

Caution(s): It should be handled under aseptic conditions. If there is no apparent improvement in the animal's condition within 24 hours; consult a veterinarian.

For animal use only. Livestock drug. Keep out of reach of children.

Presentation: 500 mL bottles (NDC 30798-027-17).

Compendium Code No.: 10840181 Rev. 5-95

CALCIUM GLUCONATE 23% SOLUTION

Phoenix Pharmaceutical **Calcium Therapy**

Active Ingredient(s): Each 100 mL contains:

Calcium Gluconate (provides 2.14 g Calcium)	23 g
Water for injection	q.s.

Contains boric acid as a solubilizing agent.

Electrolytes per 1,000 mL:

Calcium	1,069 mEq

Hypertonic.

Osmolarity (calc.)	6,782 mOsmol/L

The product contains no preservatives.

Indications: To be used as an aid in the treatment of parturient paresis (milk fever) in cattle.

Dosage and Administration:

Cattle: 250 to 500 mL.

Administer intravenously or intraperitoneally.

The solution should be warmed to body temperature and administered slowly.

Precaution(s): Store at 15°-30°C (59°-86°F).

The product is sterile in an unopened container. Use the entire contents when first opened. It should be handled under aseptic conditions.

Caution(s): If there is not apparent improvement in the animal's condition within 24 hours, consult a veterinarian.

For animal use only.

Not for human use.

Warning(s): Keep out of reach of children.

Presentation: 500 mL vials (NDC 57319-072-07).

Compendium Code No.: 12560131 Rev. 1-99

CALCIUM GLUCONATE 23% SOLUTION

Vet Tek **Calcium Therapy**

Active Ingredient(s): Each 100 mL contains:

Calcium Gluconate (provides 2.14 g Calcium) .... 23 grams
Water For Injection .... q.s.

Contains boric acid as a solubilizing agent.

Electrolytes per 1,000 mL:

Calcium .... 1,069 mEq

Hypertonic.

Osmolarity (calc.) .... 6,782 mOsmol/L

The product is sterile in an unopened container. It contains no preservatives.

Indications: To be used as an aid in the treatment of parturient paresis (milk fever) in cattle.

Dosage and Administration:

Cattle: 250 to 500 mL.

Administer intravenously or intraperitoneally.

The solution should be warmed to body temperature and administered slowly.

Precaution(s): Store at controlled room temperature 15°C-30°C (59°F-86°F). Use entire contents when first opened. It should be handled under aseptic conditions.

Caution(s): For animal use only.

Warning(s): Keep out of reach of children.

If there is no apparent improvement in the animal's condition within 24 hours, consult a veterinarian.

Presentation: 500 mL vials. (NDC 60270-027-17).

Compendium Code No.: 14200041 Rev. 8-96

CALCIUM GLUCONATE 23% SOLUTION

Vetus **Calcium Therapy**

Active Ingredient(s): Each 100 mL contains: Calcium gluconate 23 g (provides 2.14 g calcium), water for injection q.s.

Contains boric acid as a solubilizing agent.

Electrolytes per 1,000 mL: Calcium 1,069 mEq

Hypertonic.

Osmolarity (calc.) 6,782 mOsmol/L.

Indications: To be used as an aid in the treatment of parturient paresis (milk fever) in cattle.

This product is sterile in the unopened container. It contains no preservatives. Use the entire contents when first opened.

It should be handled under aseptic conditions.

If there is no apparent improvement in the animal's condition within 24 hours, consult a veterinarian.

Dosage and Administration: Cattle: 250 to 500 mL.

Administer intravenously or intraperitoneally.

The solution should be warmed to body temperature and administered slowly.

Precaution(s): Store at 59°-86°F (15°-30°C).

Caution(s): For animal use only.

Warning(s): Keep out of the reach of children.

Presentation: 500 mL vials.

Compendium Code No.: 14440180

CALCIUM ORAL GEL

Phoenix Pharmaceutical **Calcium-Oral**

Nutritional Supplement

Guaranteed Analysis: Per Tube: mg/dose

Calcium (Min)	64 g (16.2%)
(Max)	76 g (19.2%)
Magnesium	6.3 g (1.6%)
Cobalt	0.7 g (0.2%)
Vitamin D_3	100,000 IU
Thiamine HCl	100 mg
Niacinamide	100 mg
d-Panthenol	10 mg
Pyridoxine HCl	10 mg
Vitamin E	5 mg
Riboflavin	5 mg
Citric Acid	5 mg
Cyanocobalamin	100 mg

Ingredients: Polyethylene Glycol, Calcium Propionate, Calcium Hydroxide, Magnesium Oxide, Cobalt Sulfate, Thiamine HCl, Niacinamide, Pyridoxine HCl, Riboflavin, Cyanocobalamin, Citric Acid, Purified Water, d-Panthenol, Mineral Oil, Vitamin D_3, Vitamin E.

Indications: A nutritional supplement for dairy cattle during and after calving.

Directions for Use: Hold the head of the cow in a slightly elevated position. Place nozzle near rear of mouth. Use of a hook nozzle is recommended. Discharge entire contents of the tube. Hold head up and allow animal time to swallow.

Give one tube prior to calving or after calving and the second tube 12 to 24 hours after calving.

Precaution(s): Store at room temperature.

Caution(s): For animal use only.

Warning(s): Not a drug. No withdrawal time.

Keep out of reach of children.

Presentation: 300 mL dose (NDC 57139-457-29).

Manufactured by: First Priority, Inc., Elgin, IL 60123-1146.

Compendium Code No.: 12560142 Rev. 03-02

CALCIUM PHOSPHORUS POWDER

Pet-Ag **Small Animal Dietary Supplement**

Guaranteed Analysis:

Calcium, min.	19%
Calcium, max.	22%
Phosphorus, min.	14.5%
Vitamin D_3, min.	8250 IU/kg

Ingredients: Dicalcium phosphate, dehydrated cheese, calcium carbonate, soy flour, artificial colors, ethoxyquin, vitamin D_3 supplement.

Indications: CALCIUM PHOSPHORUS is a palatable cheese-flavored source of supplemental calcium and phosphorus for dogs and cats. When your pet requires additional calcium and phosphorus, PetAg CALCIUM PHOSPHORUS provides these two minerals in a biologically available formulation.

CALCIUM PHOSPHORUS supplies calcium and phosphorus in a ratio similar to the AAFCO recommendations for cats and dogs. The ratio of calcium and phosphorus in the diet is important for the efficient utilization of the minerals by dogs and cats. CALCIUM PHOSPHORUS is fortified with vitamin D necessary for calcium and phosphorus utilization by the animal.

Calcium, phosphorus and vitamin D are essential nutrients for proper bone and teeth development. Correct supply of these nutrients might help prevent development of osteoporosis in older dogs and cats.

Dosage and Administration: The following is a guideline for feeding CALCIUM PHOSPHORUS. The feeding level may be adjusted to the pet's requirement for additional calcium and phosphorus or to your veterinarian's advice on the feeding of additional calcium and phosphorus.

Dogs:

Adult Maintenance — Feed 1 teaspoon per 10 lbs. (4.5 kg) body weight daily.

Growing Puppies — Feed 1 teaspoon per 5 lbs. (2.2 kg) body weight daily.

Cats:

Cats and Kittens — Feed ½ teaspoon per 8 lbs. (3.6 kg) body weight daily.

Precaution(s): Store in a cool, dry place.

Presentation: 24 oz. (1 lb., 8 oz.) 681 g (12 per case) and 56 oz. (6 per case) cans.

Compendium Code No.: 10970041 0998

CALCIUM PHOSPHORUS TABLETS

Pet-Ag **Small Animal Dietary Supplement**

Active Ingredient(s): Each Tablet Contains: Calcium 580 mg; Phosphorus 450 mg (from Dicalcium Phosphate); Vitamin D_3 400 I.U. in a protein chewable base.

Indications: Uses: CALCIUM PHOSPHORUS TABLETS provide a supplemental source of calcium, phosphorus and vitamin D_3, especially during periods of rapid growth, pregnancy and lactation.

Dosage and Administration: CALCIUM PHOSPHORUS TABLETS are scored for easy dosage.

CALCIUM PHOSPHORUS TABLETS can be hand fed or crumbled and offered with food.

Dogs:

Maintenance: ½ tablet per day per 10 kilograms body weight.

Growth, late gestation, lactation: 1 tablet per day per 10 kilograms body weight. It is recommended that dogs larger than 30 kilograms receive no more than 3 tablets per day.

Cats:

Maintenance: ¼ tablet per day per 2 kilograms body weight.

Growth, late gestation, lactation: ½ tablet per day per 2 kilograms body weight. It is recommended that cats larger than 3 kilograms receive no more than 1 tablet per day.

Caution(s): Use only as directed by your veterinarian.

Presentation: Jars of 50 tablets, 12 per case.

Compendium Code No.: 10970051 0996

CALCIUM PLUS

First Priority **Calcium-Oral**

Guaranteed Analysis: Per tube/dose:

Calcium (Min)	64 g (16.2%)
(Max)	76 g (19.2%)
Magnesium	6.3 g (1.6%)
Cobalt	0.7 g (0.2%)
Vitamin D_3	100,000 IU
Thiamine HCl	100 mg
Niacinamide	100 mg
d-Panthenol	10 mg
Pyridoxine HCl	10 mg
Vitamin E	5 mg
Riboflavin	5 mg
Citric Acid	5 mg
Cyanocobalamin	100 mcg

Ingredients: Polyethylene Glycol, Calcium Propionate, Calcium Hydroxide, Magnesium Oxide, Cobalt Sulfate, Thiamine HCl, Niacinamide, Pyridoxine HCl, Riboflavin, Cyanocobalamin, Citric Acid, Purified Water, d-Panthenol, Mineral Oil, Vitamin D_3, Vitamin E.

Indications: A nutritional supplement for dairy cattle during and after calving.

Directions for Use: Hold the head of the cow in a slightly elevated position. Place nozzle near rear of mouth. Use of hook nozzle recommended. Discharge entire contents of the tube. Hold head up and allow animal time to swallow.

Give one tube prior to or after calving and second tube 12 to 24 hours after calving.

Precaution(s): Storage: Store at controlled room temperature between 15°-30°C (59°-86°F). Keep container tightly closed when not in use.

Caution(s): For animal use only.

Warning(s): Keep out of reach of children.

Presentation: 300 mL tube (NDC# 58829-274-30).

Compendium Code No.: 11390081 Rev. 04-02

CALCIUM SE

First Priority **Calcium-Oral**

Guaranteed Analysis: Per tube:

Calcium (Min)	64 g (16.2%)
(Max)	76 g (19.2%)
Magnesium	6.3 g (1.6%)
Cobalt	0.7 g (0.2%)
Vitamin D_3	100,000 IU
Thiamine HCl	100 mg
Niacinamide	100 mg
d-Panthenol	10 mg
Pyridoxine HCl	10 mg
Riboflavin	5 mg
Vitamin E	5 mg
Citric Acid	5 mg
Selenite (from yeast)	3 mg
Cyanocobalamin (Vitamin B_{12})	100 mcg

Ingredients: Polyethylene Glycol, Calcium Propionate, Calcium Hydroxide, Magnesium Oxide, Cobalt Sulfate, Selenium Yeast 0.2%, Thiamine HCl, Niacinamide, Pyridoxine, HCl, Riboflavin, Cyanocobalamin, Citric Acid, Purified Water, d-Panthenol, Mineral Oil, Vitamin D_3, Vitamin E.

Indications: A nutritional supplement for dairy cattle during and after calving.

Directions for Use: Hold the head of the cow in a slightly elevated position. Place nozzle near rear of mouth. Use of hook nozzle recommended. Discharge entire contents of the tube. Hold head up and allow animal time to swallow.

Give one tube prior to or after calving and second tube 12 to 24 hours after calving.

Precaution(s): Storage: Store at controlled room temperature between 15°-30°C (59°-86°F). Keep tightly closed when not in use.

Caution(s): Follow label directions. Dairy cattle feeding of selenium more than 0.3 ppm is not permitted.

For animal use only.

Warning(s): Keep out of reach of children.

Presentation: 300 mL tube (NDC# 58829-276-30).

Compendium Code No.: 11390091 Rev. 04-02

CAL DEX #2 ℞

AgriLabs **Calcium-Combination Therapy**

Active Ingredient(s): Composition: Each mL contains:

Calcium (as gluconate salt)	16.84 mg (8.42 g/500 mL)
Phosphorus	9.6 mg (4.8 g/500 mL)
Magnesium	3.76 mg (1.88 g/500 mL)
Dextrose	165.0 mg (82.5 g/500 mL)
Water for Injection	q.s.
Osmolarity (calc.)	6,741 mOsmol/L

Indications: A source of sterile injectable calcium, phosphorus, magnesium and dextrose for use in the treatment of milk fever (parturient paresis), grass tetany and other conditions in cattle (including lactating dairy cows), swine and sheep where calcium, phosphorus and magnesium deficiencies may occur.

Dosage and Administration: Administer intravenously, intramuscularly, subcutaneously or intraperitoneally. Warm to body temperature before administration to reduce any likelihood of shock reaction.

Cattle: 500 mL to 750 mL.

Swine and Sheep: 50 mL to 125 mL.

This product should be administered using aseptic technique. Administration should be made slowly and to effect, with monitoring of the animal during administration. In cases where accelerated respiration rate or heart rate is observed during treatment, the administration should be stopped until these vital signs return to an acceptable rate at which time injection can be continued. If part or all dosage is given by subcutaneous or intramuscular administration, it is advised that a maximum of 25 mL per injection site be used. Any unused portion should be discarded. Do not use if material has precipitated.

Precaution(s): Store between 15°C-30°C (59°F-86°F).

Caution(s): Federal law restricts this drug to use by or on the order of a licensed veterinarian.

For animal use only.

Warning(s): Keep out of reach of children.

Presentation: 500 mL bottle.

Compendium Code No.: 10581520 Iss. 5-01

CAL-DEX C-M-P-K ℞

AgriLabs **Calcium-Combination Therapy**

Active Ingredient(s): Composition: Each 500 mL of sterile aqueous solution contains:

Calcium	10.8 g
(as calcium borogluconate, equivalent to calcium gluconate 23.2%)	
Potassium	8.0 g
(as potassium chloride)	
Phosphorus	2.5 g
(as sodium hypophosphite • H_2O)	
Magnesium	1.6 g
(as magnesium borogloconate)	
Dextrose • H_2O	75.0 g

Millequivalents per liter

Cations	
Calcium	1,080 mEq/L
Potassium	410 mEq/L
Magnesium	261 mEq/L
Sodium	161 mEq/L
Anions	
Borogluconate	1,341 mEq/L
Chloride	410 mEq/L
Hypophosphite	161 mEq/L

Indications: For use as an aid in the treatment of hypocalcemia (parturient paresis, milk fever), hypomagnesemia (grass tetany), and other conditions associated with calcium, magnesium, phosphorus and potassium deficiencies in cattle.

Dosage and Administration: Warm solution to body temperature. The usual intravenous dose in cattle is 500 mL per 800 to 1,000 pounds of body weight.

Contraindication(s): Do not administer this product to animals showing signs of cardiac distress.

Precaution(s): Store at room temperature between 15° and 30°C (59°-86°F).

This product contains no preservatives. Use entire contents when first opened. Discard any unused solution.

Caution(s): Federal law restricts this drug to use by or on the order of a licensed veterinarian.

Administration should be made slowly and with care to avoid adverse effects such as heart block or shock. Perivascular or subcutaneous deposition of hypertonic solutions may result in severe inflammation at the injection site.

Warning(s): Not for human use.

Keep out of reach of children.

Presentation: 500 mL.

Compendium Code No.: 10581530 Rev. 06-90

CAL DEX CMPK INJECTION ℞

Aspen **Calcium-Combination Therapy**

Composition: Each 500 mL of sterile aqueous solution contains:

Calcium	10.8 g
(as calcium borogluconate, equivalent to calcium gluconate 23.2%)	
Potassium	8.0 g
(as potassium chloride)	
Phosphorus	2.5 g
(as sodium hypophosphite • H_2O)	
Magnesium	1.6 g
(as magnesium borogluconate)	
Dextrose • H_2O	75.0 g

Millequivalents per liter

Cations	
Calcium	1,080 mEq/L
Potassium	410 mEq/L
Magnesium	261 mEq/L
Sodium	161 mEq/L
Anions	
Borogluconate	1,341 mEq/L
Chloride	410 mEq/L
Hypophosphite	161 mEq/L
Osmolarity (calc.)	11,597 mOsmol/L

Indications: For use as an aid in the treatment of hypocalcemia (parturient paresis, milk fever), hypomagnesemia (grass tetany), and other conditions associated with calcium, magnesium, phosphorus and potassium deficiencies in cattle.

Dosage and Administration: Warm solution to body temperature. The usual intravenous dose in cattle is 500 mL per 800 to 1,000 pounds of body weight.

Contraindication(s): Do not administer this product to animals showing signs of cardiac distress.

Precaution(s): Store between 15°C and 30°C (59°F-86°F).

This product contains no preservatives. Use entire contents when first opened. Discard any unused solution.

Caution(s): Federal law restricts this drug to use by or on the order of a licensed veterinarian.

Administration should be made slowly and with care to avoid adverse effects such as heart block or shock. Perivascular or subcutaneous deposition of hypertonic solutions may result in severe inflammation at the injection site.

Warning(s): For animal use only.

Keep out of the reach of children.

Presentation: 500 mL size.

Compendium Code No.: 14750110

CAL-DEXTRO® C ℞

Fort Dodge **Calcium-Combination Therapy**

Sterile Solution

Active Ingredient(s): Each mL contains:

Calcium (as gluconate salt)	22 mg (11 g/500 mL)

With dextrose not more than 44.9 mg; boric acid not more than 25.2 mg; bromine (as bromide) not more than 7 mg; sodium 2 mg; water for injection, USP, q.s.

Indications: A source of sterile injectable calcium for use in the treatment of milk fever (parturient paresis) in cattle (including lactating dairy cows), or in treatment of hypocalcemia in cattle, sheep, swine and horses.

Dosage and Administration: Administer intravenously, intramuscularly, subcutaneously or intraperitoneally. Warm to body temperature before administration to reduce any likelihood of a shock reaction.

Cattle and Horses — 500 mL to 750 mL.

Swine and Sheep — 50 mL to 125 mL.

This product should be administered using aseptic technique. Administration should be made slowly and to effect, with monitoring of the animal during administration. In cases where accelerated respiration rate or heart rate is observed during treatment, the administration should be stopped until these vital signs return to an acceptable rate at which time injection can be continued. If part or all dosage is given by subcutaneous or intramuscular administration, it is advised that a maximum of 25 mL per injection site be used. Any unused portion should be discarded. Do not use if material has precipitated.

To Open Container: Wipe cap, top and neck of bottle with 70% alcohol. Screw down cap until a snap is heard indicating bottle top seal is broken. Carefully unscrew cap removing top of bottle. Attach sterile IV administration unit.

Precaution(s): Store at controlled room temperature 15° to 30°C (59° to 86°F). Protect from freezing.

Caution(s): Federal law restricts this drug to use by or on the order of a licensed veterinarian.

Keep out of reach of children.

Presentation: 500 mL bottles, package of 12 (NDC 0856-0235-01).

Compendium Code No.: 10030240 2355I

CAL-DEXTRO® K ℞

Fort Dodge **Calcium-Combination Therapy**

Sterile Solution

Active Ingredient(s): Each mL contains:

Calcium (as gluconate salt)	16.84 mg (8.42 g/500 mL)
Potassium	1.04 mg (0.52 g/500 mL)
Dextrose	165.0 mg (82.5 g/500 mL)

With boric acid not more than 21.14 mg; bromine (as bromide) not more than 7 mg; sodium 2 mg; chloride 0.9 mg; water for injection, USP, q.s.

Indications: A source of sterile injectable calcium, potassium and dextrose for use in the treatment of milk fever (parturient paresis) in cattle (including lactating dairy cows).

Dosage and Administration: Administer intravenously, intramuscularly, subcutaneously or intraperitoneally. Warm to body temperature before administration to reduce any likelihood of a shock reaction.

Cattle — 500 mL to 750 mL.

This product should be administered using aseptic technique. Administration should be made slowly and to effect, with monitoring of the animal during administration. In cases where accelerated respiration rate or heart rate is observed during treatment, the administration should be stopped until these vital signs return to an acceptable rate at which time injection can be continued. If part or all dosage is given by subcutaneous or intramuscular administration, it is advised that a maximum of 25 mL per injection site be used. Any unused portion should be discarded. Do not use if material has precipitated.

To Open Container: Wipe cap, top and neck of bottle with 70% alcohol. Screw down cap until a snap is heard indicating bottle top seal is broken. Carefully unscrew cap removing top of bottle. Attach sterile IV administration unit.

Precaution(s): Store at controlled room temperature 15° to 30°C (59° to 86°F). Protect from freezing.

Caution(s): Federal law restricts this drug to use by or on the order of a licensed veterinarian.

Keep out of reach of children.

Presentation: 500 mL bottles, package of 12 (NDC 0856-0231-01).

Compendium Code No.: 10030250 2315Q

CAL-DEXTRO® NO. 2 ℞

Fort Dodge **Calcium-Combination Therapy**

Sterile Solution

Active Ingredient(s): Each mL contains:

Calcium (as gluconate salt)	16.84 mg (8.42 g/500 mL)
Phosphorus	9.8 mg (4.9 g/500 mL)
Magnesium	3.84 mg (1.92 g/500 mL)
Dextrose	165.0 mg (82.5 g/500 mL)

With boric acid not more than 21.14 mg; bromine (as bromide) not more than 7 mg; sodium 2 mg; water for injection, USP q.s.

Indications: A source of sterile injectable calcium, phosphorus, magnesium and dextrose for use in the treatment of milk fever (parturient paresis), grass tetany and other conditions in cattle (including lactating dairy cows), swine and sheep where calcium, phosphorus and magnesium deficiencies may occur.

Dosage and Administration: Administer intravenously, intramuscularly, subcutaneously or intraperitoneally. Warm to body temperature before administration to reduce any likelihood of shock reaction.

Cattle — 500 mL to 750 mL.

Swine and Sheep — 50 mL to 125 mL.

This product should be administered using aseptic technique. Administration should be made slowly and to effect, with monitoring of the animal during administration. In cases where accelerated respiration rate or heart rate is observed during treatment, the administration should be stopped until these vital signs return to an acceptable rate at which time injection can be continued. If part or all dosage is given by subcutaneous or intramuscular administration, it is advised that a maximum of 25 mL per injection site be used. Any unused portion should be discarded. Do not use if material has precipitated.

To Open Container: Wipe cap, top and neck of bottle with 70% alcohol. Screw down cap until a snap is heard indicating bottle top seal is broken. Carefully unscrew cap removing top of bottle. Attach sterile IV administration unit.

Precaution(s): Store at controlled room temperature of 15° to 30°C (59° to 86°F). Protect from freezing.

Caution(s): Federal law restricts this drug to use by or on the order of a licensed veterinarian.

Keep out of reach of children.

Presentation: 500 mL bottles, package of 12 (NDC 0856-0263-01).

Compendium Code No.: 10030260 2635T

CAL-DEXTRO® SPECIAL ℞

Fort Dodge **Calcium-Combination Therapy**

Sterile Solution

Active Ingredient(s): Each mL contains:

Calcium (as gluconate salt)	22 mg (11 g/500 mL)
Phosphorus	1.022 mg (511 mg/500 mL)
Magnesium	0.402 mg (201 mg/500 mL)
Dextrose	150 mg (75 g/500 mL)

With boric acid not more than 25.17 mg; bromine (as bromide) not more than 7 mg; sodium 2 mg; water for injection, USP q.s.

Indications: A source of sterile injectable calcium, phosphorus, magnesium and dextrose for use in the treatment of milk fever (parturient paresis) in cattle (including lactating dairy cows).

Dosage and Administration: Administer intravenously, intramuscularly, subcutaneously or intraperitoneally. Warm to body temperature before administration to reduce any likelihood of shock reaction.

Cattle — 500 mL to 750 mL.

This product should be administered using aseptic technique. Administration should be made slowly and to effect, with monitoring of the animal during administration. In cases where accelerated respiration rate or heart rate is observed during treatment, the administration should be stopped until these vital signs return to an acceptable rate at which time injection can be continued. If part or all dosage is given by subcutaneous or intramuscular administration, it is advised that a maximum of 25 mL per injection site be used. Any unused portion should be discarded. Do not use if material has precipitated.

To Open Container: Wipe cap, top and neck of bottle with 70% alcohol. Screw down cap until a snap is heard indicating bottle top seal is broken. Carefully unscrew cap removing top of bottle. Attach sterile IV administration unit.

Precaution(s): Store at controlled room temperature of 15° to 30°C (59° to 86°F). Protect from freezing.

Caution(s): Federal law restricts this drug to use by or on the order of a licensed veterinarian.

Keep out of reach of children.

Presentation: 500 mL bottles, package of 12 (NDC 0856-0271-01).

Compendium Code No.: 10030270 2715P

CALF-GUARD®

Pfizer Animal Health **Vaccine**

Bovine Rota-Coronavirus Vaccine, Modified Live Virus

U.S. Vet. Lic. No.: 189

Description: CALF-GUARD® contains attenuated strains of bovine rotavirus and bovine coronavirus propagated on established cell lines and freeze-dried to preserve stability.

Contains penicillin and streptomycin as preservatives.

Indications: CALF-GUARD® is for vaccination of healthy newborn calves or pregnant cows as an aid in preventing diarrhea (scours) caused by bovine rotavirus and bovine coronavirus.

Directions:

1. General Directions: Vaccination of healthy newborn calves or pregnant cows is recommended. Aseptically rehydrate the freeze-dried vaccine with the sterile diluent provided, shake well, and administer 3 mL without delay.
2. Calf Vaccination: Remove needle from syringe and administer a single 3 mL dose into the back of the calf's mouth. Vaccination should occur as soon as possible after birth because susceptible calves are at risk as soon as they are born. Vaccination of calves older than 1 day may not be effective.
3. Cow Vaccination: Healthy cows should receive 2 intramuscular doses administered 3-6 weeks apart during late pregnancy. Ideally, the second dose should be administered within 30 days prior to calving. In accordance with Beef Quality Assurance guidelines, this product should be administered in the muscular region of the neck.
4. Cow Revaccination: Cows should be revaccinated with 2 doses during each subsequent pregnancy.
5. Good animal husbandry and herd health management practices should be employed.

Precaution(s): Store at 2°-7°C. Prolonged exposure to higher temperatures and/or direct sunlight may adversely affect potency. Do not freeze.

Use entire contents when first opened.

Sterilized syringes and needles should be used to administer this vaccine. Do not sterilize with chemicals because traces of disinfectant may inactivate the vaccine.

Burn containers and all unused contents.

Caution(s): As with many vaccines, anaphylaxis may occur after use. Initial antidote of epinephrine is recommended and should be followed with appropriate supportive therapy.

This product has been shown to be efficacious in healthy animals. A protective immune response may not be elicited if animals are incubating an infectious disease, are malnourished or parasitized, are stressed due to shipment or environmental conditions, are otherwise immunocompromised, or the vaccine is not administered in accordance with label directions.

For veterinary use only.

Warning(s): Do not vaccinate within 21 days before slaughter.

Discussion: Disease Description: Neonatal calf diarrhea has a complex etiology, but bovine rota- and coronavirus have been found to be 2 of its most common causative agents.[1-3] Experimental studies have demonstrated that either virus can initiate calf diarrhea.[4-5] Viral diarrhea is often complicated by secondary infection with *Escherichia coli* or other enteric pathogens.

Trial Data: Safety and Efficacy: Immunization must precede natural exposure in order to be effective. Thus, immunization during the first 24 hours of life, the earlier the better, is strongly recommended. Data indicates that the effectiveness of CALF-GUARD® declines when some animals in a herd are left unprotected.[6] In such cases, infected calves may seed the premises with virus, and expose other calves prior to immunization. All calves should be vaccinated for best results. Vaccination with CALF-GUARD® may be accomplished by oral vaccination of calves at birth, or by intramuscular vaccination of cows during pregnancy; vaccinated cows provide immunity to their calves via protective antibodies transmitted in colostrum and milk.

CALF-GUARD® was evaluated in field studies where calves in 21 herds and cows in 5 herds were vaccinated and compared with nonvaccinated calves and calves from nonvaccinated cows during corresponding test periods. Incidence of scours was 25.7% among 1,598 vaccinated calves, while incidence among 1,035 nonvaccinated calves was 47.8%. Death loss from scours was 2.9% among vaccinated calves and 19.0% among nonvaccinated calves. Among 2,927 calves from vaccinated cows, incidence of scours was 11.3%, with 0.9% death loss. In contrast, 21.7% of 2,801 calves from nonvaccinated cows developed scours, and death loss was 4.1%. These results indicate that vaccination with CALF-GUARD® significantly reduces incidence and death loss from neonatal calf diarrhea. Because the disease has a variety of causes, however, the vaccine should not be expected to entirely eliminate its occurrence.

Experimental calves remained normal following oral administration of CALF-GUARD®, and adverse reactions in vaccinated calves were not reported during extensive field trials. Similarly, in field trials with vaccinated pregnant cows, abortions or other adverse reactions were not reported.

References: Available upon request.

Presentation: 25 x 1 dose vials.

U.S. Patent Nos. 3,838,004; 3,839,556; and 3,869,547

Compendium Code No.: 36900523 75-4002-06

CALF QUENCHER

Vedco **Electrolytes-Oral**

Ingredient(s): Dextrose anhydrous, sodium bicarbonate, sodium chloride, potassium chloride, magnesium sulfate anhydrous. Each 80 grams of CALF QUENCHER provides: Sodium, 134 mEq; potassium, 22.8 mEq; magnesium, 6.6 mEq; bicarbonate, 81 mEq; chloride 75.8 mEq; dextrose, 68 grams.

Indications: CALF QUENCHER calf electrolyte formula is recommended for oral use for nutritional support and re-establishment and maintenance of electrolyte balance in neonatal calves with moderate to severe electrolyte loss and dehydration as a result of diarrhea.

Dosage and Administration: Preparation of Oral Solution: Dissolve 80 g (⅓ cup) of CALF QUENCHER calf electrolyte formula in water and dilute to a total volume of 1 quart or dissolve 240 g (1 cup) of CALF QUENCHER in water and dilute to a total volume of 3 quarts.

Administer the oral solution by feeding or drench at the rate of 1 quart per 60 pounds bodyweight 3-4 times a day for 2 days as the only source or oral fluids. For the following 2 days the oral solution should be diluted 1:1 with milk replacer and given at feeding time.

Precaution(s): Avoid exposure to excessive heat. Store in a cool, dry place. Keep container tightly closed.

Warning(s): Keep this and all medicines out of the reach of children. Not for human use. For veterinary use only.

Presentation: 800 g and 21 lb containers.

Compendium Code No.: 10940210

CALF RD FORMULA

TechMix **Large Animal Dietary Supplement**

Guaranteed Analysis:

Lactic Acid Bacteria*, Minimum.................................. $2.5x10^8$ CFU*/gram

*CFU (Colony-Forming Units)

* *Lactobacillus acidophilus, Lactobacillus lactis, Lactobacillus casei, Enterococcus faecium*

Ingredients: Dried Whey, Lactose, Dried *Saccharomyces cervisiae* Fermentation Product, Dried *Lactobacillus acidophilus* Fermentation Product, Dried *Lactobacillus lactis* Fermentation Product, Dried *Lactobacillus casei* Fermentation Product, Dried *Enterococcus faecium* Fermentation Product, Animal Digest, Dried *Aspergillus oryzae* Fermentation Extract, Vitamin A Acetate, d-Activated Animal Sterol (source of Vitamin D_3), dl-Alpha Tocopheryl Actetate (source of Vitamin E Activity), Ascorbic Acid, Niacin Supplement, Sodium Silico Aluminate, Soybean Oil and Natural Artificial Flavors added.

C

Indications: CALF RD FORMULA contains a source of live (viable) naturally occurring microorganisms and a fermentation extract for dairy, beef, or veal calves.

Directions for Use:

Dairy, Beef or Veal Calves: Mix one level scoop (4 grams) with the milk, milk replacer or rehydration product per calf per day from day 1 to weaning. For large volume feeding, mix 200 grams (0.44 lb.) of CALF RD FORMULA with 50 gallons of milk or milk replacer in each feeding (when 2 quarts of milk or milk replacer are fed at each of two feedings per day).

Precaution(s): Storage: Store in a cool dry place to maintain maximum shelf life of culture.

Caution(s): Intended for animal use only. This product is intended as a source of microbial cultures only.

Disclaimer: Buyer assumes all responsibility for use, storage, and handling of this product. TechMix makes no other claims or warranties expressed or implied.

Presentation: CALF RD FORMULA is available in a 800 gram jar and a 25 pound pail.

Compendium Code No.: 11440140 991208

CALF RESTART™ ONE-4

TechMix **Electrolytes-Oral**

Guaranteed Analysis:

Crude Protein.......................... not less than 10.00%
Crude Fat.......................... not less than 2.50%
Crude Fiber.......................... not more than 0.50%
Calcium (Ca).......................... not less than 0.65% (184.4 mg/oz)
Calcium (Ca).......................... not more than 1.15% (326.3 mg/oz)
Phosphorus (P).......................... not less than 0.35% (99.3 mg/oz)
Sodium (Na).......................... not less than 1.50% (452.0 mg/oz)
Potassium (K).......................... not less than 1.50% (425.6 mg/oz)
Magnesium (Mg).......................... not less than 0.04% (11.3 mg/oz)
Vitamin A.......................... not less than 50,000 I.Units/lb
Vitamin D_3.......................... not less than 5,000 I.Units/lb
Vitamin E.......................... not less than 50 I.Units/lb

Ingredients: Bovine animal plasma, dried skim milk, dried whey, animal fat (preserved with BHA), dextrose, fructose, lactose monohydrate, sucrose, glycine, citric acid, potassium chloride, sodium chloride, calcium lactate, magnesium gluconate, dibasic potassium phosphate, dried *Lactobacillus acidophilus* fermentation product, dried *Lactobacillus lactis* fermentation product, dried *Streptococcus diacetylactis* fermentation product, dried *Streptococcus faecium* fermentation product, dried *Bacillus subtilis* fermentation product, dried *Bacillus subtilis* fermentation extract, dried *Aspergillus oryzae* fermentation extract, vitamin A acetate, d-activated animal sterol (source of vitamin D_3), dl-alpha tocopheryl acetate (source of vitamin E activity), artificial flavor and FD&C certified color added.

Indications: A supplemental blend of acidified milk sugars, electrolytes, bovine animal plasma and animal fat specifically intended to provide essential nutrients for the energy-deficient young calf.

Dosage and Administration:

1. Fill bottle to the bottom of the neck with warm water, shake well and slowly drench calf.
2. To provide additional water or fluid for the dehydrated calf, refill bottle with warm water and drench calf a second time.
3. CALF RESTART™ ONE-4 is specifically intended for calves that are energy deficient as a result of inadequate milk consumption or calves that have lost normal body condition as a result of diarrhea and dehydration.
4. If calves are not consuming any milk or milk replacer, administer one bottle every six to eight hours for up to four feedings and then gradually start calves on milk or a high quality milk replacer.
5. When fed in conjunction with milk or additional water at one feeding, do not feed more than two quarts of total fluid at a feeding to prevent fluid overload.

Caution(s): Drench carefully and slowly to avoid inhalation or spillover into the windpipe or trachea. Calves showing symptoms of coma, shock or too weak to stand should be treated as directed by a veterinarian.

Warning(s): Livestock product.

Keep out of reach of children.

Discussion: CALF RESTART™ ONE-4 was specifically designed for use as a drench in young calves that are in a nutrient deficient conditions as a result of dehydration or not consuming sufficient milk or milk replacer. CALF RESTART™ ONE-4 provides a broad spectrum of nutrients that are highly digestible and readily metabolized by the young calf. After extensive field testing and evaluation, CALF RESTART™ ONE-4 has been shown to be of benefit in reducing losses due to starvation when calves are not nursing or voluntarily drinking enough milk replacer to meet their metabolic needs.

Presentation: 30x5 oz (140 gram) drench bottles, 10 lb and 25 lb pails.

Compendium Code No.: 11440051

CALF SCOUR BOLUS ANTIBIOTIC

Durvet **Tetracycline-Oral**

tetracycline hydrochloride

NADA No.: 065-004

Active Ingredient(s): Contains: 500 mg of tetracycline hydrochloride per bolus.

Indications: Indicated for oral use in calves for the treatment of bacterial pneumonia caused by organisms susceptible to tetracycline and bacterial enteritis caused by *E. coli* and *Salmonella* organisms susceptible to tetracycline.

Dosage and Administration: Dosage: Administer orally 10 mg per pound of body weight per day divided into two daily doses (one bolus per 100 lb twice daily).

Contraindication(s): Antidiarrheal products containing aluminum hydroxide or salts of calcium or magnesium should not be used concurrently with tetracycline hydrochloride bolus.

Precaution(s): Store at controlled room temperature 15° to 30°C (59° to 86°F).

Caution(s): If no improvement is noted in two to three days, consult a veterinarian.

Not for human use. Keep out of reach of children. Do not use for more than five days. Use as the sole source of tetracycline.

Restricted Drug—Use only as directed (California). For use in animals only.

Warning(s): Do not slaughter animals for food within 12 days of treatment.

Side Effects: The use of broad-spectrum antibiotics may result in gastrointestinal disturbances. They may be minimized by reducing the individual dose and administering the drug at more frequent intervals. Allergic manifestations are rare. If adverse reactions occur, discontinue medication.

Presentation: 25 (NDC 30798-668-66) and 100 (NDC 30798-668-70) boluses.

Compendium Code No.: 10840191 0599-11-000/0599-12-000

CAL-GEL™

Jorgensen **Calcium-Oral**

Mineral Supplement

Guaranteed Analysis:

Calcium: 53 grams or 11.9%
Magnesium: 5.54 grams or 1.24%
Cobalt: 0.028 grams or 0.006%

Ingredient Statement: Water, calcium chloride, calcium sulfate, magnesium chloride, hydrated magnesium, aluminum silicates, sodium chloride and cobalt sulfate.

Indications: CAL-GEL™ is a specially formulated mineral supplement for use in dairy cows. It is an aid to help maintain normal calcium levels during the critical immediate pre-partum and post-partum period.

Directions: One tube can be administered just before or after calving. If milk fever develops, then one tube is given 2-3 hours after regular IV milk fever treatment and another tube 12-16 hours later.

If condition continues, consult your veterinarian.

Administration: Load cartridge in standard dosing gun and remove protective end cap. Place the nozzle near the back of the oral cavity and empty the tube contents, allowing the cow to swallow.

Caution(s): The cow must have a swallowing reflex and normal ruminal motility for the product to be effective.

Nozzle should be placed near the back of the mouth. Extra care should be taken to not puncture the pharyngeal wall. If puncture occurs, you need to cease administration and contact your veterinarian.

Warning(s): For oral use only. For veterinary use only.

Human Caution: CAL-GEL™ is a strong acidic salt and contact with eyes or open wounds will cause irritation.

Presentation: 447 gm tube, 12/case.

Compendium Code No.: 11520000

CAL-GEL 63

Durvet **Calcium-Oral**

Guaranteed Analysis:

Calcium (Ca), maximum,.......................... 17.40%
Calcium (Ca), minimum,.......................... 14.50%

Ingredients: Calcium chloride and calcium propionate in a special smooth and gentle proprietary base.

Indications: An oral calcium supplement for cattle during parturition.

Directions for Use: Cows: Provide one entire tube (300 mL) per cow within 24 hours prior to calving.

Give another entire tube (300 mL) per cow after calving.

Place tube in gun and remove cap. Hold cow's head in slightly elevated position, and depress contents into mouth, watching for natural swallowing reflex. Use care in regards to wind pipe.

Caution(s): Not for human use. For livestock use only. Contact with eyes or mucous membranes will irritate; flush with cool water if exposed.

Warning(s): Keep out of reach of children.

Presentation: 300 mL (10.14 fl oz) tube.

Compendium Code No.: 10841731 6/00

CALIBER® 3

Boehringer Ingelheim **Toxoid**

Clostridium Perfringens Types C&D Toxoid

U.S. Vet. Lic. No.: 124

Contents: This product contains the antigens listed above.

Indications: Recommended for the vaccination of healthy, susceptible sheep and cattle as an aid in the reduction of enterotoxemia caused by the toxins of *Cl. perfringens* Types B, C, and D.

Dosage and Administration: Using aseptic technique, inject 2 mL subcutaneously. Repeat in 21 to 28 days and once annually.

Precaution(s): Store out of direct sunlight at a temperature between 35-45°F (2-7°C). Avoid freezing. Shake well before using. Use entire contents when first opened.

Caution(s): Anaphylactoid reactions may occur.

Antidote(s): Epinephrine.

Warning(s): Do not vaccinate within 21 days before slaughter.

Presentation: 10 doses (20 mL), 50 doses (100 mL), and 250 doses (500 mL).

Compendium Code No.: 10281350 21501-00 / 21502-00 / 21503-00

CALIBER® 7

Boehringer Ingelheim **Bacterin-Toxoid**

Clostridium Chauvoei-Septicum-Novyi-Sordellii-Perfringens Types C&D Bacterin-Toxoid

U.S. Vet. Lic. No.: 124

Contents: This product contains the antigens listed above.

Indications: Recommended for the vaccination of healthy, susceptible sheep and cattle, including bred and/or lactating beef and dairy cattle, as an aid in the reduction of diseases caused by *Clostridium chauvoei, Cl. septicum, Cl. novyi, Cl. sordellii* and *Cl. perfringens* Types C and D. Although *Cl. perfringens* Type B is not a significant problem in the U.S.A., immunity may be provided against the beta and epsilon toxins elaborated by *Cl. perfringens* Type B. This immunity is derived from the combination of Type C (beta) and Type D (epsilon) fractions.

Dosage and Administration: Using aseptic technique, inject 2 mL subcutaneously. Repeat in 21 to 28 days and once annually.
Precaution(s): Store at 35-45°F (2-7°). Avoid freezing. Shake well before using. Use entire contents when first opened.
Caution(s): Anaphylactoid reactions may occur.
Antidote(s): Epinephrine.
Warning(s): Do not vaccinate within 21 days before slaughter.
Presentation: 10 doses (20 mL), 50 doses (100 mL), and 250 doses (500 mL).
Compendium Code No.: 10280262 33301-01 / 33302-01

CAL M 64 PLUS SE

Butler **Calcium-Combination Therapy**

Ingredient(s): Polyethylene Glycol, Calcium Hydroxide, Calcium Propionate, Magnesium Oxide, Mineral Oil, Vitamin D_3, Cobalt Chloride, Selenium from Selenium Yeast, Thiamine HCl, Niacinamide, d-Pantothenol, Pyridoxine HCl, Vitamin E, Riboflavin, Citric Acid, Cyanocobalamin, Water.

Minimum Contents of 300 mL Tube

Calcium	64 g - 16.2% Minimum
Calcium	76 g - 19.2% Maximum
Magnesium	6.3 g- 1.6%
Cobalt	0.7 g - 0.2%
Vitamin D_3	100,000 IU
Thiamine HCl	100 mg
Niacinamide	100 mg
d-Pantothenol	10 mg
Pyridoxine HCl	10 mg
Vitamin E	5 mg
Riboflavin	5 mg
Citric Acid	5 mg
Selenium	3 mg
Cyanocobalamin	100 mcg

Indications: A nutritional supplement for dairy cattle during calving containing calcium, magnesium, cobalt and selenium.
Directions for Use:
1. Hold head of the cow in a slightly elevated position.
2. Place nozzle near rear of mouth. Use of hook nozzle recommended.
3. Discharge entire contents of the tube.
4. Hold head up and allow animal time to swallow.

Give one tube prior to or after calving and second tube 12 to 24 hours after calving. Do not administer more than one tube in 24 hour period.
Precaution(s): Keep cool.
Presentation: 300 mL tube.
Compendium Code No.: 10820270

CAL-MAG-CO GEL

Durvet **Calcium-Oral**

Active Ingredient(s): Minimum Contents of 300 mL Dose:

Calcium	60.0 g - 14.3% minimum 62.0 g - 14.8% maximum
Magnesium	1.3 g - .33%
Cobalt	0.6 g - 0.1%

Ingredients: Water, calcium chloride, calcium carbonate, dextrose, magnesium chloride, sodium citrate, cobalt sulfate, silicon dioxide.
Indications: A nutritional supplement containing calcium, magnesium, and cobalt for dairy cattle during calving.

Not a drug - No withdrawal time.
Directions for Use:
1. Hold head of the cow in a slightly elevated position.
2. Place nozzle near rear of mouth. Use of hook nozzle is recommended.
3. Discharge entire contents of the tube.
4. Hold head up and allow animal time to swallow.

Give one tube prior to or after calving and second tube 12 to 24 hours after calving.
Precaution(s): Do not freeze.
Caution(s): For animal use only. Not for human use. Keep out of reach of children.
Presentation: 300 mL tubes.
Patent Pending
Compendium Code No.: 10840151 Rev. 6/01

CAL-MAG-SE GEL

Durvet **Calcium-Oral**

Active Ingredient(s): Minimum Contents of 300 mL Dose:

Calcium	64.0 g - 18.3% minimum 67.0 g - 19.1% maximum
Magnesium	6.8 g - 1.7%
Cobalt	0.6 g - 0.1%
Selenium	3.0 mg
Thiamine HCl	100 mg
Niacinamide	100 mg
d-Panthenol	10 mg
Pyridoxine HCl	10 mg
Vitamin E	5 mg
Riboflavin	5 mg
Citric Acid	5 mg
Cyanocobalamin	100 mcg

Ingredients: Polyethylene glycol, calcium propionate, calcium oxide, magnesium chloride, cobalt sulfate, silicon dioxide, thiamine, sodium selenite, niacinamide, calcium pantothenate, riboflavin, pyridoxine, dl-alpha tocopheryl acetate (source of vitamin E), citric acid, vitamin B_{12} (cyanocobalamin).
Indications: A nutritional supplement containing calcium, magnesium, and cobalt for dairy cattle during calving.

Not a drug - No withdrawal time.
Directions for Use:
1. Hold head of cow in a slightly elevated position.
2. Place nozzle near rear of mouth. Use of hook nozzle recommended.
3. Discharge entire contents of the tube.
4. Hold head up and allow animal time to swallow.

Give one tube prior to or after calving and second tube 12 to 24 hours after calving. Never administer more than one tube in 24 hour period.
Precaution(s): Do not freeze.
Caution(s): For animal use only. Not for human use. Keep out of reach of children.
Presentation: 300 mL tubes (NDC 30798-561-15).
Patent Pending
Compendium Code No.: 10840161 Rev. 6/01

CAL-MAG-SV GEL

Butler **Calcium-Oral**

Active Ingredient(s): Contents of 300 mL Dose

Calcium	54 gms (Min.-11.17%) (Max.-16.17%)
Magnesium	6.8 gms (1.56%)
Cobalt	0.6 gms (.14%)
Thiamine HCl	100 mg
Niacinamide	100 mg
d-Panthenol	10 mg
Pyridoxine HCl	10 mg
Vitamin E	5 mg
Riboflavin	5 mg
Citric Acid	5 mg
Sodium Selenite	3 mg
Cyanocobalamin (Vitamin B_{12})	100 mcg

Ingredients: Calcium chloride, water, magnesium chloride, cobalt sulfate, thiamine HCl, niacinamide, d-Panthenol, pyridoxine HCl, vitamin E, riboflavin, citric acid, sodium selenite, cyanocobalamin (Vitamin B_{12}), silicon dioxide, dextrose.
Indications: A nutritional supplement for dairy cattle during and after calving.
Directions for Use:
1. Hold head of the cow in a slightly elevated position.
2. Place nozzle near rear of mouth. Use of hook nozzle recommended.
3. Discharge entire contents of the tube.
4. Hold head up and allow animal time to swallow.

Give one tube prior to or after calving and second tube 12 to 24 hours after calving.

Not a drug-No withdrawal time.
Precaution(s): Store at room temperature.
Caution(s): Follow label directions. Dairy cattle feeding of selenium more than 0.3 PPM is not permitted.
Presentation: 300 mL (435 g) tube (NDC 11695-1735-1).
Compendium Code No.: 10820310

CAL MP-1000 ℞

Butler **Calcium-Combination Therapy**

Active Ingredient(s): Each 500 mL contains:

Dextrose	75.0 g
Calcium (as boryl calcium borogluconate, equiv. to 21.5 g calcium gluconate)	10.0 g
Phosphorus (as sodium hypophosphite)	7.1 g
Magnesium (as magnesium chloride • $6H_2O$)	2.8 g

Indications: For use as an aid in the treatment of hypocalcemia (parturient paresis, milk fever), hypomagnesemia (grass tetany), and other conditions associated with calcium, magnesium, phosphorous and potassium deficiencies in cattle.
Dosage and Administration: Warm the solution to body temperature. The usual intravenous dose in cattle is 500 mL per 800 to 1,000 pounds of body weight.
Contraindication(s): Do not administer the product to animals showing signs of cardiac distress.
Precaution(s): Store at a controlled room temperature between 59°-86°F (15°-30°C). Protect from light.

Administration should be made slowly and with care to avoid adverse effects such as heart block or shock. Perivascular or subcutaneous deposition of hypertonic solutions may result in severe inflammation at the injection site.
Caution(s): Federal law restricts this drug to use by or on the order of a licensed veterinarian.

The product does not contain preservatives. Use the entire contents when first opened. Discard any unused solution.

For veterinary use only.

Keep out of the reach of children.
Presentation: 500 mL bottles.
Compendium Code No.: 10820280

CAL-MP 1700™ ℞

Butler **Calcium-Combination Therapy**

Active Ingredient(s): Each 500 mL of sterile aqueous solution contains:

Dextrose • H_2O	75.0 g
Calcium (as calcium borogluconate, equivalent to 26.7% calcium gluconate)	12.4 g
Phosphorus (as calcium hypophosphite)	7.1 g
Magnesium (as magnesium chloride • $6H_2O$)	2.8 g

Milliequivalents per liter:

Cations:

Calcium	1,698 mEq/L
Magnesium	454 mEq/L

Anions:

Gluconate	1,240 mEq/L
Hypophosphite	458 mEq/L
Chloride	454 mEq/L

Indications: For use as an aid in the treatment of hypocalcemia (parturient paresis, milk fever), hypomagnesemia (grass tetany), and other conditions associated with calcium, phosphorus and magnesium deficiencies in cattle.
Dosage and Administration: Warm the solution to body temperature. The usual intravenous dose in cattle is 500 mL per 800 to 1,000 pounds of body weight.
Contraindication(s): Do not administer the product to animals showing signs of cardiac distress.

Precaution(s): Store at a controlled room temperature between 59°-86°F (15° and 30°C).
Administration should be made slowly and with care to avoid adverse effects such as heart block or shock. Perivascular or subcutaneous disposition of hypertonic solutions may result in severe inflammation at the injection site.
Caution(s): Federal law restricts this drug to use by or on the order of a licensed veterinarian.
The product does not contain preservatives. Use the entire contents when first opened. Discard any unused solution. For veterinary use only. Keep out of the reach of children.
Presentation: 500 mL vials.
Compendium Code No.: 10820320

CAL-MPK™ 1080 INJECTION ℞

Butler **Calcium-Combination Therapy**

Active Ingredient(s): Composition: Each 500 mL of sterile aqueous solution contains:

Calcium	10.8 g
(as calcium borogluconate, equivalent to calcium gluconate 23.2%)	
Potassium	8.0 g
(as potassium chloride)	
Phosphorus	2.5 g
(as sodium hypophosphite • H_2O)	
Magnesium	1.6 g
(as magnesium borogloconate)	
Dextrose • H_2O	75.0 g

Millequivalents per liter

Cations	
Calcium	1,080 mEq/L
Potassium	410 mEq/L
Magnesium	261 mEq/L
Sodium	161 mEq/L
Anions	
Borogluconate	1,341 mEq/L
Chloride	410 mEq/L
Hypophosphite	161 mEq/L

Indications: For use as an aid in the treatment of hypocalcemia (parturient paresis, milk fever), hypomagnesia (grass tetany), and other conditions associated with calcium, magnesium, phosphorous and potassium deficiencies in cattle.
Dosage and Administration: Warm solution to body temperature. The usual intravenous dose in cattle is 500 mL per 800 to 1,000 pounds of body weight.
Contraindication(s): Do not administer this product to animals showing signs of cardiac distress.
Precaution(s): Store between 15°C and 30°C (59°-86°F).
This product contains no preservatives. Use entire contents when first opened. Discard any unused solution.
Caution(s): Federal law restricts this drug to use by or on the order of a licensed veterinarian.
Administration should be made slowly and with care to avoid adverse effects such as heart block or shock. Perivascular or subcutaneous deposition of hypertonic solutions may result in severe inflammation at the injection site.
Warning(s): For animal use only. Keep out of reach of children.
Presentation: 500 mL (NDC 11695-3547-3).
Manufactured by: Phoenix Scientific, Inc., St. Joseph, MO 64506
Compendium Code No.: 10820340 Iss. 3-99

CAL-MPK 1234™ ℞

Butler **Calcium-Combination Therapy**

Active Ingredient(s): Each 500 mL of sterile aqueous solution contains:

Dextrose • H_2O	75.0 g
Calcium (as calcium borogluconate)	10.8 g
Potassium (as potassium chloride)	8.0 g
Phosphorus (as calcium hypophosphite)	2.5 g
Magnesium (as magnesium borogluconate)	1.6 g

Milliequivalents per liter:
Cations:

Calcium	1,234 mEq/L
Potassium	409 mEq/L
Magnesium	259 mEq/L
Anions:	
Borogluconate	1,332 mEq/L
Hypophosphite	161 mEq/L
Chloride	409 mEq/L

Indications: For use as an aid in the treatment of hypocalcemia (parturient paresis, milk fever), hypomagnesemia (grass tetany), and other conditions associated with calcium, magnesium, phosphorous and potassium deficiencies in cattle.
Dosage and Administration: Warm the solution to body temperature. The usual intravenous dose in cattle is 500 mL per 800 to 1,000 pounds of body weight.
Contraindication(s): Do not administer the product to animals showing signs of cardiac distress.
Precaution(s): Store at a controlled room temperature between 59°-86°F (15°-30°C).
Administration should be made slowly and with care to avoid adverse effects such as heart block or shock. Perivascular or subcutaneous deposition of hypertonic solutions may result in severe inflammation at the injection site.
Caution(s): Federal law restricts this drug to use by or on the order of a licensed veterinarian.
The product does not contain preservatives. Use the entire contents when first opened. Discard any unused solution. For veterinary use only. Keep out of the reach of children.
Presentation: 500 mL vials.
Compendium Code No.: 10820330

CAL MPK GEL

Butler **Calcium-Combination Therapy**

Active Ingredient(s): Minimum contents of 300 mL dose:

Calcium	47.3 g (11.5% minimum)
	67.6 g (16.5% maximum)
Phosphorus	6.2 g (1.5%)
Magnesium	2.9 g (1.5%)
Potassium	1.0 g (0.2%)

Ingredients: Calcium chloride, water, phosphoric acid, trisodium phosphate, magnesium hydroxide, glucose, citric acid, potassium chloride, silicon dioxide, sodium citrate, and artificial flavorings.
Indications: A calcium supplement for dairy cattle during calving.
Dosage and Administration:
1. Hold the head of the cow in a slightly elevated position.
2. Place the nozzle near the rear of the mouth. The use of a hook nozzle is recommended.
3. Discharge the entire contents of the tube.
4. Hold the head up and allow the animal time to swallow.

Give one (1) tube prior to calving and a second tube 24 hours after calving.
Precaution(s): Do not freeze. Keep cool.
Presentation: 300 mL tube.
Compendium Code No.: 10820290

CAL-NATE 1069™

Butler **Calcium Therapy**

Active Ingredient(s): Each 500 mL of sterile aqueous solution contains:
Calcium (as calcium borogluconate, equivalent to calcium gluconate 23%) .... 10.7 g
Milliequivalents per liter:
Cations:

Calcium	1,069 mEq/L
Anions:	
Gluconate	1,069 mEq/L

The product does not contain preservatives.
Indications: For use as an aid in the treatment of hypocalcemia (parturient paresis, milk fever) in cattle.
Dosage and Administration: Warm the solution to body temperature before administration. The usual intravenous dose in cattle is 500 mL per 800 to 1,000 pounds of body weight. If given intramuscularly or subcutaneously, divide the dosage among several injection sites and massage to aid in absorption. If improvement does not occur after using the product, consult a veterinarian.
Precaution(s): Store at a controlled room temperature between 15° and 30°C (59°-86°F).
Use the entire contents when first opened. Discard any unused solution.
Caution(s): Follow strict sterile procedures in the use of the product. Intravenous administration should be made slowly to avoid adverse effects such as heart block or shock.
Restricted drug; use only as directed.
For veterinary use only.
Warning(s): Keep out of the reach of children.
Presentation: 500 mL vial.
Compendium Code No.: 10820351

CAL ORAL PLUS™

Butler **Calcium-Oral**

Active Ingredient(s): Contents:

Calcium chloride	400 mg/mL
Vitamin D_3	2,400 I.U.
Water	q.s.

Indications: CAL ORAL PLUS™ is indicated as a supplemental source of calcium in cattle.
Dosage and Administration: Shake well before use.
Administer at a rate of one (1) bottle per day or additionally under the direction of a veterinarian. Administer with care to avoid aspiration.
Caution(s): Overdosage can cause hypercalcemia. At the first sign of hypercalcemia, discontinue use of the product and consult a veterinarian.
For veterinary use only.
Keep out of the reach of children.
Presentation: 12 fl. oz. bottles.
Compendium Code No.: 10820300

CALOX 64 ORAL GEL

Vedco **Calcium-Oral**

Ingredient(s): Polyethylene glycol, calcium propionate, calcium oxide, magnesium chloride, cobalt sulfate, silicon dioxide, thiamine HCl, niacinamide, d-panthenol, pyridoxine, vitamin E, riboflavin, citric acid, cyanocobalamin.
Minimum contents of 300 mL tube:

Calcium	64 g - 18.3% minimum
Calcium	67 g - 19.1% maximum
Magnesium	6.8 g - 17%
Cobalt	0.6 g - 0.1%
Thiamine HCl	100 mg
Niacinamide	100 mg
d-Panthenol	10 mg
Pyridoxine HCl	10 mg
Vitamin E	5 mg
Riboflavin	5 mg
Citric Acid	5 mg
Cyanocobalamin	100 mcg

Indications: A nutritional supplement for dairy cattle during calving containing calcium, magnesium and cobalt.
Dosage and Administration:
1. Hold head of cow in a slightly elevated position.
2. Place nozzle near rear of mouth.
3. Discharge entire contents of the tube.
4. Hold head up and allow animal time to swallow.

Give one tube prior to or after calving and the second tube 12-24 hours after calving.
Precaution(s): Store in a cool place.
Presentation: 300 mL tube.
Compendium Code No.: 10940220

CAL OX 64 PLUS SE

AgriPharm **Calcium-Oral**

A Nutritional Supplement Containing Calcium, Magnesium, and Cobalt

Ingredients: Polyethylene glycol, calcium hydroxide, calcium propionate, magnesium oxide, vitamin D_3, cobalt chloride, sodium selenite, thiamine hydrochloride, niacin, calcium pantothenate, pyridoxine hydrochloride, riboflavin, alpha-tocopherol acetate (source of vitamin E), citric acid, cyanocobalamin (vitamin B_{12}).

Minimum Contents of 300 mL tube:

Calcium	64.0 g - 16.7% minimum
	67.0 g - 17.2% maximum
Magnesium	6.2 g - 1.6%
Cobalt	0.7 g - 0.2%
Thiamine	100 mg
Niacin	100 mg
Pantothenic Acid	10 mg
Pyridoxine	10 mg
Vitamin E	5 mg
Riboflavin	5 mg
Citric Acid	5 mg
Selenium	2.6 mg
Vitamin B_{12}	100 mcg
Vitamin D_3	100,000 IU

Indications: For use as a high calcium nutritional supplement for dairy cattle during calving.

Dosage and Administration: Administer orally on back of tongue.

Prior to calving	1 tube
After calving	1 tube

Give one tube prior to calving and the second tube 12 to 24 hours after calving using the following directions:

1. Hold head of the cow in a slightly elevated position.
2. Place nozzle near rear of mouth. Use of hook nozzle recommended.
3. Discharge entire contents of the tube.
4. Hold up head of cow and allow animal time to swallow.

Precaution(s): Do not freeze. Keep cool.

Warning(s): This product does not require a withdrawal time.

For animal use only.

Keep out of reach of children.

Presentation: 300 mL tube.

Compendium Code No.: 14570170

CALOX 64 SE ORAL GEL

Vedco **Calcium-Oral**

Ingredient(s): Polyethylene glycol, calcium propionate, calcium oxide, magnesium chloride, sodium selenite, cobalt sulfate, silicon dioxide, thiamine HCl, niacinamide, d-panthenol, pyridoxine, vitamin E, riboflavin, citric acid, cyanocobalamin.

Minimum Contents of 300 mL tube:

Calcium	64 g - 18.3% Minimum
Calcium	67 g - 19.1% Maximum
Magnesium	6.8 g - 17%
Cobalt	0.6 g - 0.1%
Selenium	3.0 mg
Thiamine HCl	100 mg
Niacinamide	100 mg
D-Panthenol	10 mg
Pyridoxine HCl	10 mg
Vitamin E	5 mg
Riboflavin	5 mg
Citric Acid	5 mg
Cyanocobalamin	100 mcg

In a special RumiGel base.

Indications: A nutritional supplement for dairy cattle during calving containing calcium, magnesium and cobalt.

Dosage and Administration: Directions for Use:

1. Hold head of the cow in a slightly elevated position.
2. Place nozzle near rear of mouth.
3. Discharge entire contents of the tube.
4. Hold head up and allow animal time to swallow.

Give one tube prior to or after calving and the second tube 12-24 hours after calving.

Precaution(s): Keep cool.

Caution(s): Sold to graduate veterinarians only.

Warning(s): Not a drug. No withdrawal time.

Presentation: 300 mL tube.

Compendium Code No.: 10940230

CAL-PHOS #2 ℞

Vedco **Calcium-Combination Therapy**

Active Ingredient(s): Each 500 mL contains:

Calcium (as calcium borogluconate, equivalent to 26.7% calcium gluconate	12.4 g)
Phosphorus (as sodium hypophosphite • H_2O)	7.1 g
Magnesium (as magnesium chloride • $6H_2O$)	2.8 g
Dextrose • H_2O	750 g
Cations:	
Calcium	1,241 mEq/L
Sodium	459 mEq/L
Magnesium	456 mEq/L
Anions:	
Gluconate	1,241 mEq/L
Hypophosphite	459 mEq/L
Chloride	456 mEq/L

The product does not contain preservatives.

Indications: For use as an aid in the treatment of hypocalcemia (parturient paresis, milk fever), hypomagnesemia (grass tetany), and other conditions associated with calcium, phosphorus and magnesium deficiencies in cattle.

Dosage and Administration: Warm the solution to body temperature. The usual intravenous dose in cattle is 50 mL per 800 to 1,000 pounds of body weight.

Contraindication(s): Do not administer the product to animals showing signs of cardiac distress.

Precaution(s): Store at a controlled room temperature between 59-86°F (15-30°C).

Caution(s): Federal law restricts this drug to use by or on the order of a licensed veterinarian.

Keep out of the reach of children.

Use the entire contents when first opened. Discard any unused solution.

Administration should be made slowly and with care to avoid adverse effects such as heart block or shock. Perivascular or subcutaneous depostion of hypertonic solutions may result in severe inflammation at the injection site.

Presentation: 500 mL containers.

Compendium Code No.: 10940190

C

CAL-PHOS #2 INJECTION ℞

AgriLabs **Calcium-Combination Therapy**

Active Ingredient(s): Each 500 mL contains:

Calcium	10.00 g
(Complexed as boryl esters of gluconic acid)	
Magnesium	2.76 g
(Obtained from 23.07 grams of magnesium chloride hexahydrate)	
Phosphorus	6.03 g
(Obtained from 20.65 grams of sodium hypophosphite • H_2O)	
Dextrose • H_2O	75.00 g
Water for Injection	q.s.

Osmolarity (calc.) 11,760 mOsmol/L.

Indications: For use as an aid in the treatment of hypocalcemia (parturient paresis, milk fever), hypomagnesemia (grass tetany), and other conditions associated with calcium, phosphorous and magnesium deficiencies in cattle.

Dosage and Administration: Warm solution to body temperature. The usual intravenous dose in cattle is 500 mL per 800 to 1,000 pounds of body weight.

Contraindication(s): Do not administer this product to animals showing signs of cardiac distress.

Precaution(s): Store between 15°C and 30°C (59°F-86°F).

This product contains no preservatives. Use entire contents when first opened. Discard any unused solution.

Caution(s): Federal law restricts this drug to use by or on the order of a licensed veterinarian.

Administration should be made slowly and with care to avoid adverse effects such as heart block or shock. Perivascular or subcutaneous deposition of hypertonic solutions may result in severe inflammation of the injection site.

For animal use only.

Keep out of the reach of children.

Presentation: 500 mL vials.

Compendium Code No.: 10581540 Iss. 3-00

CAL-PHOS #2 INJECTION ℞

Phoenix Pharmaceutical **Calcium-Combination Therapy**

Active Ingredient(s): Composition: Each 500 mL contains:

Calcium (complexed as boryl esters of gluconic acid)	10.00 g
Magnesium (obtained from 23.07 g of magnesium chloride hexahydrate)	2.76 g
Phosphorus (obtained from 20.65 g of sodium hypophosphite • H_2O)	6.03 g
Dextrose • H_2O	75.0 g
Water for Injection	q.s.
Osmolarity (calc.)	11,760 mOsmol/L

This product contains no preservatives.

Indications: For use as an aid in the treatment of hypocalcemia (parturient paresis, milk fever), hypomagnesemia (grass tetany), and other conditions associated with calcium, phosphorous, and magnesium deficiencies in cattle.

Dosage and Administration: Warm solution to body temperature. The usual intravenous dose in cattle is 500 mL per 800 to 1,000 pounds of body weight.

Contraindication(s): Do not administer this product to animals showing signs of cardiac distress.

Precaution(s): Store between 15° and 30°C (59°F-86°F).

Use entire contents when first opened. Discard any unused solution.

Caution(s): Federal law restricts this drug to use by or on the order of a licensed veterinarian.

Administration should be made slowly and with care to avoid adverse effects such as heart block or shock. Perivascular or subcutaneous deposition of hypertonic solutions may result in severe inflammation at the injection site.

For animal use only.

Warning(s): Keep out of reach of children.

Presentation: 500 mL vials (NDC 57319-094-07).

Manufactured by: Phoenix Scientific, Inc., St. Joseph, MO 64503.

Compendium Code No.: 12560112 Iss. 2-02

CAL-PHOS #2 WITH POTASSIUM INJECTION ℞

Phoenix Pharmaceutical **Calcium-Combination Therapy**

Active Ingredient(s): Composition: Each 500 mL of sterile aqueous solution contains:

Calcium (as calcium borogluconate, equivalent to calcium gluconate 23.2%)	10.8 g
Potassium (as potassium chloride)	8.0 g
Phosphorus (as sodium hypophosphite • H_2O)	2.5 g
Magnesium (as magnesium borogluconate)	1.6 g
Dextrose • H_2O	75.0 g
Milliequivalents per liter:	
Cations:	
Calcium	1,080 mEq/L
Potassium	410 mEq/L
Magnesium	261 mEq/L
Sodium	161 mEq/L
Anions:	
Borogluconate	1,341 mEq/L
Chloride	410 mEq/L
Hypophosphite	161 mEq/L
Osmolarity (calc.)	11,597 mOsmol/L

This product contains no preservatives.

Indications: For use as an aid in the treatment of hypocalcemia (parturient paresis, milk fever),

hypomagnesemia (grass tetany), and other conditions associated with calcium, magnesium, phosphorous, and potassium deficiencies in cattle.
Dosage and Administration: Warm solution to body temperature. The usual intravenous dose in cattle is 500 mL per 800 to 1,000 pounds of body weight.
Contraindication(s): Do not administer this product to animals showing signs of cardiac distress.
Precaution(s): Store between 15° and 30°C (59°-86°F). Use entire contents when first opened. Discard any unused solution.
Caution(s): Federal law restricts this drug to use by or on the order of a licensed veterinarian.
Administration should be made slowly and with care to avoid adverse effects such as heart block or shock. Perivascular or subcutaneous deposition of hypertonic solutions may result in severe inflammation at the injection site. For animal use only.
Warning(s): Keep out of reach of children.
Presentation: 500 mL vials (NDC 57319-098-07).
Manufactured by: Phoenix Scientific, Inc., St. Joseph, MO 64503.
Compendium Code No.: 12560122 Rev. 4-02

CALPHOSAN® SOLUTION ℞

Glenwood **Calcium Therapy**

Calcium Solution for Injection

Active Ingredient(s): Each 10 mL contains 50 mg calcium glycerophosphate, 50 mg calcium lactate and 0.25% phenol (as preservative), in a physiological solution of sodium chloride.
Indications: For use as an aid in the treatment of canine eclampsia.
Intramuscular or subcutaneous injections of CALPHOSAN® raise blood serum calcium levels, without pain, inflammatory reactions or sloughing.
Dosage and Administration:
Small Dogs: 5 to 10 mL subcutaneously (back of neck) or intramuscularly.
Large Dogs: 10 mL for each 100 lbs of body weight, or as indicated. May also be given by subcutaneous or intravenous injection.
Contraindication(s): As there is a similarity in the actions of calcium and digitalis on the contractility and excitability of the heart muscle, CALPHOSAN® is contraindicated in fully digitalized animals.
Precaution(s): Store in a dark place at room temperature.
Caution(s): Federal law restricts this drug to use by or on the order of a licensed veterinarian.
Presentation: 125 mL vials.
Compendium Code No.: 11330000

CAL-PHOS FORTE ℞

Bimeda **Calcium Therapy**

Parenteral Solution

Active Ingredient(s): Composition: Calcium borogluconate dextrose, magnesium borogluconate, calcium hyposhosphite. pH is adjusted with sodium hydroxide or HCl.

Total calcium chemically equivalent to calcium borogluconate	29.9%
Dextrose	15.0%
Magnesium borogluconate	6.0%
Total phosphorus	0.5%
Total calcium	2.48 g per 100 mL
Milliequivalents per liter:	
Cations:	
Calcium	1240 mEq/L
Magnesium	257 mEq/L
Anions:	
Borogluconate	1336 mEq/L
Hypophosphite	161 mEq/L

Sterile. Contains no preservative.
Indications: For use as an aid in the treatment of milk fever, and other conditions associated with calcium, phosphorus and magnesium deficiencies in cattle.
Dosage and Administration: Cattle: 500 mL. For milk fever prophylaxis, give 200-500 mL at time of calving. Repeat in 2 to 6 hours if needed. Warm solution to body temperature. Administer intravenously.
Precaution(s): Store between 15°-30°C (59°-86°F).
Discard any unused portion.
Caution(s): Federal law restricts this drug to use by or on the order of a licensed veterinarian.
Large doses administered intravenously may have toxic action on heart if the blood level of calcium is raised excessively. Regulate dose carefully according to severity of hypocalcemia and inject slowly so that administration may be stopped if adverse effect becomes evident.
For animal use only.
Warning(s): Keep out of reach of children.
Presentation: 500 mL (NDC# 61133-3398-8).
Manufactured by: Bimeda-MTC Animal Health Inc., Cambridge, Ontario, Canada N3C 2W4.
Compendium Code No.: 13990091 Iss. 6-00

CAL-PHO-SOL ℞

Neogen **Calcium Therapy**

Sterile Solution

Active Ingredient(s): Each 10 mL contains:

Calcium glycerophosphate	50 mg
Calcium Lactate	50 mg
Sodium Chloride	0.9% w/v
Benzyl alcohol (as preservative)	1.5% v/v
Water for injection	q.s.
Milliequivalents per 10 mL	
Calcium	0.9 mEq/10 mL
Sodium	1.54 mEq/10 mL

Indications: As an aid in the treatment of canine eclampsia.
Dosage and Administration: For intramuscular injection. May also be given by subcutaneous or intravenous injection.
Small dogs: 5 to 10 mL.
Large dogs: 10 mL for each 100 lbs body weight or as indicated.
Precaution(s): Store at controlled room temperature between 15°-30°C (59°-86°F).
Caution(s): Federal law restricts this drug to use by or on the order of a licensed veterinarian.
Intravenous administration of this product should be made slowly to avoid adverse effects, such as heart block or shock.
For animal use only.
Warning(s): Keep out of reach of children.
Presentation: 12 x 100 mL amber multi-dose glass vials per carton.
Manufactured by: Omega Laboratories, Montreal, Quebec, H3M 3E4.
Compendium Code No.: 14910042 0201

CAL-PHO-SOL SOLUTION SA ℞

Vedco **Calcium Therapy**

Active Ingredient(s): Each 10 mL contains:

Calcium glycerophosphate	50 mg
Calcium lactate	50 mg
Sodium chloride	0.9% w/v
Benzyl alcohol (as preservative)	1.5% v/v
Water for injection	q.s.
Milliequivalents per 10 mL:	
Calcium	0.9 mEq
Sodium	1.54 mEq

Indications: For use as an aid in the treatment of canine eclampsia.
Dosage and Administration:
Small Dogs: 5 to 10 mL.
Large Dogs: 10 mL for each 100 lbs. of body weight, or as directed.
For intramuscular injection.
May also be given by subcutaneous or intravenous injection.
Precaution(s): Store at temperatures between 2°-30°C (36°-86°F).
Caution(s): Federal law restricts this drug to use by or on the order of a licensed veterinarian.
Intravenous administration of the product should be made slowly to avoid adverse effects, such as heart block or shock.
Sold to veterinarians only.
Keep out of the reach of children.
Presentation: 100 mL vial.
Compendium Code No.: 10940180

CALSORB™

PRN Pharmacal **Calcium-Oral**

A Fast Absorbing Calcium Supplement

Active Ingredient(s): Each milliliter contains:
Calcium .... 170 mg/mL
in a rapidly absorbing gel base.
Indications: A nutritional supplement for canines showing signs of extreme calcium deficiency such as postpartum hypocalcemia.
Dosage and Administration: Initially administer 1 to 3 mL depending on severity of condition. Follow-up doses should be administered as recommended by a veterinarian.
This product may replace I.V. treatment in many cases.
After initially administering CALSORB™, follow up oral calcium supplementation with PSD II Complex chewable tablets through lactation.
References: Available upon request.
Presentation: Available in a 12 mL dosing syringe twelve units per case.
Compendium Code No.: 10900000

CAL SUPREME GEL™

Bimeda **Calcium-Oral**

A nutritional calcium supplement for use pre and post calving.
Guaranteed Analysis: per tube:

Calcium Min	40 g
Calcium Max	42 g

Ingredients: Calcium Propionate, molasses, propylene glycol, xanthan gum.
Description: A dark brown paste containing Calcium Propionate in a palatable molasses base.
Indications: CAL SUPREME GEL™ is designed as a nutritional supplement which can be used to aid in maintaining normal calcium levels in cows during the critical pre-calving period and immediately post calving.
Not a drug. No withdrawal time.
Directions for Use: It is recommended that an initial tube should be given orally prior to calving as close as is practical to the expected calving time. A second tube should be given within the 12 hours following calving.
To administer, place the tube in the dosing gun, remove cap. Introduce the nozzle of the tube at the corner of the animal's mouth directing it backwards so that the paste is delivered at the back of the animal's tongue. Allow the animal to swallow the entire contents of the tube.
The animal should be allowed free access to water after administration.
Take care when administering the product that it does not enter the trachea and lungs. Administer only to cows with swallowing reflex and normal rumen mobility.
Precaution(s): Store at room temperature.
Dispose of empty containers safely.
Caution(s): There will be incidences where oral calcium supplementation alone will not meet the cows demand for calcium, resulting in milk fever. Recumbent/downer cows need immediate veterinary attention.
Keep out of reach of children.
For animal use only.
Presentation: 300 mL (NDC# 61133-03110).
CAL SUPREME GEL is a trademark of Bimeda Animal Health Inc.
Compendium Code No.: 13990070

CALVENZA™ EHV

Boehringer Ingelheim **Vaccine**

Equine Rhinopneumonitis Vaccine, Killed Virus

U.S. Vet. Lic. No.: 124
Contents: This product contains the antigen listed above.
Preservative: Gentamicin.
Indications: For the vaccination of healthy, susceptible horses 6 months of age or older, including pregnant mares, as an aid in the reduction of respiratory disease due to equine herpesvirus type 1 (EHV-1) and type 4 (EHV-4).
Dosage and Administration: Shake well before use. Using aseptic technique, inoculate horses intramuscularly with a 2 mL dose. Administer a second 2 mL dose intramuscularly in 3-4 weeks

using a different injection site. Administer a third 2 mL dose in 3-4 weeks by either the intramuscular or intranasal route.

Revaccinate annually and prior to anticipated exposure, by either the intramuscular or intranasal route.

Precaution(s): Store at a temperature between 35-45°F (2-7°C). Protect from freezing.

Caution(s): Anaphylactoid reactions may occur following use.

This product has been tested under laboratory conditions and safety and efficacy in normal, healthy, immunocompetent animals. This level of performance may be affected by conditions such as stress, weather, nutrition, disease, parasitism, other treatments, individual idiosyncrasies or impaired immunological competency. These factors should be considered by the user when evaluating product performance or freedom from reactions. For veterinary use only.

Antidote(s): Epinephrine.

Warning(s): Do not vaccinate within 21 days before slaughter.

Presentation: 10 x 1 dose (2 mL) and 10 dose (20 mL) syringes.

Compendium Code No.: 10281261 32201-00/32202-00 / 32203-01/32204-00

CALVENZA™ EIV

Boehringer Ingelheim **Vaccine**

Equine Influenza Vaccine, Killed Virus

U.S. Vet. Lic. No.: 124

Contents: This product contains the antigen listed above.

Preservative: Gentamicin.

Indications: For the vaccination of healthy, susceptible horses 6 months of age or older, including pregnant mares, as an aid in the reduction of respiratory disease caused by equine influenza types A1 and A2 viruses.

Dosage and Administration: Shake well before use. Using aseptic technique, inoculate horses intramuscularly with a 2 mL dose. Administer a second 2 mL dose intramuscularly in 3-4 weeks using a different injection site. Administer a third 2 mL dose in 3-4 weeks by either the intramuscular or intranasal route.

Revaccinate annually and prior to anticipated exposure, by either the intramuscular or intranasal route.

Precaution(s): Store at a temperature between 35-45°F (2-7°C). Protect from freezing.

Caution(s): Anaphylactoid reactions may occur following use.

This product has been tested under laboratory conditions and shown to meet all Federal standards for safety and efficacy in normal, healthy, immunocompetent animals. This level of performance may be affected by conditions such as stress, weather, nutrition, disease, parasitism, other treatments, individual idiosyncrasies or impaired immunological competency. These factors should be considered by the user when evaluating product performance or freedom from reactions. For veterinary use only.

Antidote(s): Epinephrine.

Warning(s): Do not vaccinate within 21 days before slaughter.

Presentation: 10 x 1 dose (2 mL) and 10 dose (20 mL) syringes.

Compendium Code No.: 10281271 32101-00/32102-00 / 32103-00/32104-00

CALVENZA™ EIV/EHV

Boehringer Ingelheim **Vaccine**

Equine Rhinopneumonitis-Influenza Vaccine, Killed Virus

U.S. Vet. Lic. No.: 124

Contents: This product contains the antigens listed above.

Preservative: Gentamicin.

Indications: For the vaccination of healthy, susceptible horses 6 months of age or older, including pregnant mares, as an aid in the reduction of respiratory disease caused by equine herpesvirus type 1 (EHV-1) and type 4 (EHV-4) and by equine influenza types A1 and A2 viruses.

Dosage and Administration: Shake well before use. Using aseptic technique, inoculate horses intramuscularly with a 2 mL dose. Administer a second 2 mL dose intramuscularly in 3-4 weeks using a different injection site. Administer a third 2 mL dose in 3-4 weeks by either the intramuscular or intranasal route.

Revaccinate annually and prior to anticipated exposure, by either the intramuscular or intranasal route.

Precaution(s): Store at a temperature between 35-45°F (2-7°C). Protect from freezing.

Caution(s): Anaphylactoid reactions may occur following use.

This product has been tested under laboratory conditions and shown to meet all Federal standards for safety and efficacy in normal, healthy, immunocompetent animals. This level of performance may be affected by conditions such as stress, weather, nutrition, disease, parasitism, other treatments, individual idiosyncrasies or impaired immunological competency. These factors should be considered by the user when evaluating product performance or freedom from reactions. For veterinary use only.

Antidote(s): Epinephrine.

Warning(s): Do not vaccinate within 21 days before slaughter.

Presentation: 10 x 1 dose (2 mL) and 10 dose (20 mL) syringes.

Compendium Code No.: 10281281 32301-00/32302-00 / 32303-00/32304-00

CAMPYLOBACTER FETUS BACTERIN-BOVINE

Colorado Serum **Bacterin**

Campylobacter fetus Bacterin

U.S. Vet. Lic. No.: 188

Contents: A suspension of inactivated cultures of *Campylobacter fetus* subsp. *fetus* in a mineral oil adjuvant.

Contains thimerosal as a preservative.

Indications: For vaccinating healthy female cattle to aid in the control of bovine genital campylobacteriosis (vibriosis) caused by the subspecies named above.

Dosage and Administration: Inject 2 mL subcutaneously in top part of neck, 6" from ear.

Shake well to completely resuspend the organisms. Administer 30 to 60 days prior to exposure or addition to breeding herd. Revaccinate annually.

Precaution(s): Store in dark at 2° to 7°C, but remove from refrigeration and hold at room temperature 10-12 hours before use. Do not freeze.

Use entire contents when bottle is first opened.

Caution(s): Anaphylactoid reaction sometimes follows administration of products of this nature. If noted, administer adrenaline or equivalent.

Warning(s): Do not vaccinate within 60 days before slaughter.

For veterinary use only.

Presentation: 10 dose (20 mL) and 50 dose (100 mL) vials.

Compendium Code No.: 11010070

CAMPYLOBACTER FETUS BACTERIN-OVINE

Colorado Serum **Bacterin**

Campylobacter Fetus Bacterin

U.S. Vet. Lic. No.: 188

Contents: An aqueous suspension of inactivated cultures of *Campylobacter fetus* subsp. *jejuni* and *intestinalis* containing aluminum hydroxide as an adjuvant.

Contains thimerosal as a preservative.

Indications: For vaccination of healthy ewes to aid in the control of ovine genital campylobacteriosis (vibriosis) caused by the subsp. named.

Dosage and Administration: Inject 5 mL subcutaneously in the fold of the skin behind the axillary space, shortly before breeding. Repeat in 60 to 90 days. A booster of 5 mL should be administered annually just prior to breeding or shortly thereafter.

C

Precaution(s): Shake well to assure even distribution of contents. Store in dark at 2° to 7°C.

Use entire contents when bottle is first opened.

Caution(s): Anaphylactic reaction sometimes follows administration of products of this nature. If noted, administer adrenaline or equivalent.

Warning(s): Do not vaccinate within 21 days before slaughter.

For veterinary use only.

Presentation: 10 dose (50 mL) and 50 dose (250 mL) vials.

Compendium Code No.: 11010080

CAMPYLOBACTER FETUS-JEJUNI BACTERIN

Hygieia **Bacterin**

Campylobacter Fetus-Jejuni Bacterin, Inactivated Cultures in Aluminum Hydroxide Adjuvant

U.S. Vet. Lic. No.: 407

Contents: CAMPYLOBACTER FETUS-JEJUNI BACTERIN contains killed cultures of isolates of both bacterial species in an aluminum hydroxide adjuvant.

Indications: CAMPYLOBACTER FETUS-JEJUNI BACTERIN is intended for use in sheep to help prevent losses associated with late-term abortion caused by the vibrio bacteria: *Campylobacter* ("Vibrio") *fetus* or *Campylobacter jejuni.*

Dosage and Administration: The dose is 2.0 cc, administered subcutaneously on the side of the neck just in front of the shoulder. In previously unvaccinated ewes, and all yearling ewes, two doses are recommended: the first dose should be administered immediately prior to breeding, and a second dose should be given at approximately 3-4 months gestation (when animals are tagged). In subsequent years, previously vaccinated animals should receive a booster dose at 3-4 months gestation.

Precaution(s): Keep refrigerated at 35-45°F. Do not freeze. Shake well before using.

Entire contents of this bottle should be used when first opened.

Caution(s): As with any vaccine, anaphylactic or other adverse reactions may occasionally occur. In this event, immediate therapy with epinephrine or other antianaphylactic drugs should be instituted. Any adverse reactions following vaccination should be immediately reported to the manufacturer. This product license is conditional pending the development of an acceptable potency test.

Warning(s): Do not vaccinate within 21 days of slaughter.

Discussion: Abortion due to *Campylobacter* ("Vibrio") bacteria represents a significant economic loss to the sheep industry. The disease is characterized by episodic late-term abortion storms in susceptible pregnant ewes 7-25 days after exposure. Animals are exposed to the bacteria through ingestion, either from licking tissues and fluids aborted from other animals, ingestion of feed and water contaminated with these fluids, or acquiring it from non-symptomatic carriers. Contact with freshly aborted materials during the second half of gestation carries the highest risk of infection and subsequent abortion, stillbirths, or weak lambs.

Vibriosis appears in a in cyclical pattern, both within a lambing season, and from one year to the next. Although exposure to the bacteria (either, by acquiring the infection or by vaccination with a bacterin) usually confers some degree of immunity in the individual animal, both flock and individual immunity are important in determining the extent of abortion losses. In a flock where 90% of the animals are immune, it is unlikely that very many of the remaining 10% will encounter the bacteria and abort. Losses in this flock will, therefore, be limited. However, in a flock where only 10% of the animals are immune, 90% are at risk for abortion, and it is far more likely that several of them will contract the infection and lose their lambs. The level of flock immunity can shift annually as individual immunity varies with time, culling, and replacement practices.

Both *Campylobacter fetus* and *Campylobacter jejuni* are present in the United States. Immunity developed after infection can be incomplete; therefore, flock immunity can be optimized by exposure to the bacteria through vaccination. While commercial bacterins against *C. fetus* have been available, the immunity to one *Campylobacter* species is only weakly cross-protective against infection by the other species. Therefore, the single species vaccines should not be expected to prevent losses caused by a different species.

Trial Data: The performance of the bivalent CAMPYLOBACTER FETUS-JEJUNI BACTERIN was tested in yearling ewes. For this study, vaccinates received one dose of bivalent bacterin at pre-breeding and a second dose at approximately mid-gestation. Pregnancy was confirmed via ultrasound. Fifty-six (twenty-eight vaccinates and twenty-eight controls) pregnant yearlings were challenged at about four months gestation with either virulent *C. fetus* or *C. jejuni* in a prospective cohort-controlled study. The vaccinates experienced no losses attributable to *Campylobacter* infection, while controls experienced 38% abortions due to *C. jejuni* and 29% abortions due to *C. fetus.* This study demonstrated the bivalent bacterin to have a statistically significant effect in protecting ewes from abortion following challenge with either *C. fetus* or *C. jejuni* ($p<0.001$).

Summary of Pregnancy Outcomes in Vaccinated and Non-Vaccinated Yearling Ewes Following Challenge with *C. fetus* or *C. jejuni* Virulent Strains: Pregnancy Outcomes

Vaccination Status	Normal births	*Campylobacter* Losses	Totals*
Vaccinates (n=28)	23	0	23
Controls (n=28)	15	9	24
Totals	38	9	47

*Vaccinates lost 3 due to non-infectious causes (low selenium), and 2 due to unknown cause (animals recorded as pregnant pre-challenge were open three months later without being seen to lamb or abort); controls lost 1 to non-infectious causes, 2 to non-*Campylobacter* infections, and 1 to unknown cause.

Presentation: 125 dose (250 cc) vials.

Compendium Code No.: 15060000

CANIGLIDE™ ℞

Vedco **Amikacin Injection**

(Amikacin Sulfate Injection)

ANADA No.: 200-178

Active Ingredient(s): Each mL of solution contains:

Amikacin (as the sulfate) .... 50 mg
Sodium citrate, USP (as buffer) .... 25.1 mg
Sodium bisulfite .... 6.6 mg
Benzethonium chloride, USP (as preservative) .... 0.1 mg
Water for injection, USP .... q.s.

pH adjusted with sulfuric acid.

C

Indications: CANIGLIDE™ (Amikacin Sulfate Injection) is indicated for the treatment of the following conditions in dogs:

Genitourinary tract infections (cystitis) caused by susceptible strains of *Escherichia coli* and *Proteus* sp.

Skin and soft tissue infections caused by susceptible strains of *Pseudomonas* sp and *Escherichia coli*.

While nearly all strains of *Escherichia coli*, *Pseudomonas* sp, and *Proteus* sp, including those that are resistant to gentamicin, kanamycin or other aminoglycosides, are susceptible to amikacin at levels achieved following treatment, it is recommended that the invading organism be cultured and its susceptibility demonstrated as a guide to therapy. Amikacin susceptibility discs, 30 mcg, should be used for determining *in vitro* susceptibility.

Pharmacology: Description: Amikacin sulfate is a semi-synthetic aminoglycoside antibiotic derived from kanamycin. It is $C_{22}H_{43}N_5O_{13}\bullet 2H_2SO_4$,D-streptamine, 0-3-amino-3-deoxy-α-D-glucopyranosyl-(1→6)-0-[6-amino-6-deoxy-α-D-glucopyranosyl-(1→4)]-N[1]-(4-amino-2-hydroxy-1-oxobutyl)-2-deoxy-,(S)-,sulfate(1:2)(salt).

Action: Amikacin, like other aminoglycoside antibiotics, is a bactericidal agent that exerts its action at the level of the bacterial ribosome. Amikacin has been shown to be effective against many aminoglycoside-resistant strains due to its ability to resist degradation by aminoglycoside inactivating enzymes known to affect gentamicin, tobramycin and kanamycin.[1]

Microbiology: Amikacin has been shown to be effective in the treatment of skin and soft tissue infections caused by *Pseudomonas* sp and *Escherichia coli* and in urinary tract infections caused by *Escherichia coli* and *Proteus* sp. The susceptibility of veterinary isolates to amikacin is summarized in the following table:

Organism (No. of Isolates)	Minimum Inhibitory Concentration (mcg/mL)	
	Range	MIC_{90}*
Escherichia coli (50)	1-32	4
Proteus mirabilis (50)	1-128	6
Enterobacter sp (50)	0.5-128	4
Staphylococcus aureus (50)	1-128	2
Klebsiella pneumoniae (50)	0.5-16	2
Pseudomonas aeruginosa (50)	1-64	8

*Concentration at which 90% of the isolates are susceptible

In addition, the following microorganisms have been shown to be susceptible to amikacin *in vitro*,[2] although the clinical significance of this action has not been demonstrated in animals: *Serratia marcescens*, *Salmonella* sp, *Shigella* sp, *Providencia* sp, *Citrobacter freundii*, *Listeria monocytogenes*.

The aminoglycoside antibiotics in general have limited activity against gram-positive pathogens, although *Staphylococcus aureus* and *Listeria monocytogenes* are susceptible to amikacin as noted above.

Pharmacokinetics: Amikacin is well absorbed following intravenous, subcutaneous, or intramuscular injection but is not appreciably absorbed orally. The serum half-life (T½) averages from 1 to 2 hours in dogs depending on the route of administration.[3] Amikacin is excreted unchanged in urine, concentrations in excess of 1,000 mcg/mL typically being achieved within three hours in dogs. Serum concentration-time profiles in dogs following subcutaneous administration are illustrated graphically in Figure 1.

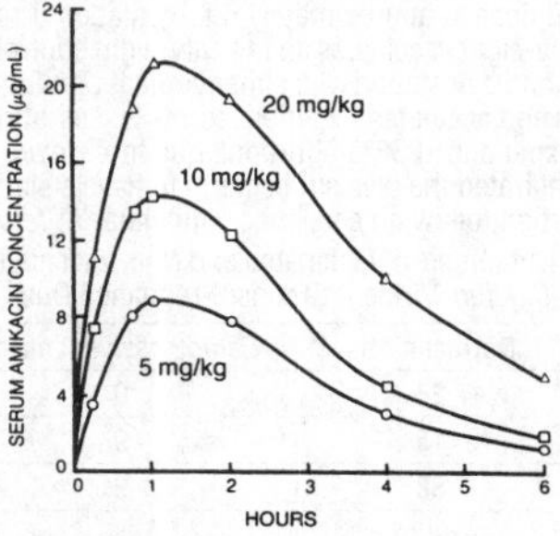

Figure 1: Amikacin Concentration-Time Curves in Dogs (n=6) Following Subcutaneous Injection

Dosage and Administration: CANIGLIDE™ (Amikacin Sulfate Injection) should be administered subcutaneously or intramuscularly at a dosage of 10 mg/kg (5 mg/lb) twice daily. Dogs with skin and soft tissue infections should be treated for a minimum of 7 days and those with genitourinary infections should be treated for 7 to 21 days or until culture negative and asymptomatic. If no response is observed after three days of treatment, therapy should be discontinued and the case re-evaluated. Maximum duration of therapy should not exceed 30 days.

Contraindication(s): Systemic aminoglycoside therapy is contraindicated in dogs with seriously impaired renal function.

Precaution(s): Store vials at controlled room temperature (15°-30°C, 59°-86°F). At times the solution may become pale yellow in color. This does not indicate a decrease in potency.

Caution(s): Federal law restricts this drug to use by or on the order of a licensed veterinarian.

Amikacin should be used with extreme caution in dogs, in which hearing acuity is required for functioning, such as seeing eye, hearing ear or military patrol, as the auditory and vestibular impairment tends not to be reversible.[6]

Aminoglycosides, including amikacin, are not indicated in uncomplicated episodes of cystitis unless the causative agents are susceptible to them and are not susceptible to antibiotics having less potential for toxicity.

Early signs of ototoxicity can include ataxia, nausea and vomiting. Auditory and vestibular impairment may be reversible in the very early stages, but if treatment is continued, the conditions will become irreversible.[6]

The following conditions have been found to contribute to the toxicity of aminoglycosides in dogs:

-Prior renal damage (most commonly found in dogs of advanced age) and dogs infected with heartworm microfilaria.[5]

-Hypovolemic dehydration (dehydrated patients should be rehydrated prior to initiating therapy).

In dogs where decreased renal function is suspected prior to treatment, BUN or serum creatinine levels may not indicate the degree of kidney impairment. A creatinine clearance determination may be more useful.

Monitoring of renal function during treatment is recommended. Although there is not a completely reliable monitoring program for aminoglycoside toxicity, urinalysis may indicate early nephrotoxicity. Unfavorable changes in the urinalysis which may indicate toxicity include:

-Decreased specific gravity in the absence of fluid therapy.

-Appearance in the urine of casts, albumin, glucose or blood.

Continued use of aminoglycosides where any functional renal impairment has occurred may lead to enhanced renal damage as well as increased likelihood of ototoxicity and/or neuromuscular blockade.[6]

Concurrent or sequential use of topically or systemically administered nephrotoxic, ototoxic, or neuromuscular blocking drugs, particularly other aminoglycosides such as streptomycin, gentamicin, kanamycin and neomycin should be avoided because of the potential for additive effects.

Concurrent administration of furosemide with aminoglycosides may enhance nephrotoxicity.[7]

Not for use in breeding dogs as reproductive studies have not been conducted.

Neurotoxic and nephrotoxic antibiotics may be absorbed in significant quantities from body surfaces after local irrigation or application. The potential toxic effect of antibiotics administered in this fashion should be considered.[8]

If hypersensitivity develops, treatment with CANIGLIDE™ (Amikacin Sulfate Injection) should be discontinued and appropriate therapy instituted.

Warning(s): Not for human use. Keep out of reach of children.

For subcutaneous or intramuscular use in the dog only.

Toxicology: The intravenous and intramuscular LD_{50} in dogs is greater than 250 mg/kg. Like other aminoglycosides, amikacin has nephrotoxic, neurotoxic, and ototoxic potential. In dogs, minimal to mild renal changes were detectable histopathologically after amikacin dosage of 45 mg/kg/day for two weeks, and dogs receiving a dosage of 30 mg/kg/day for 90 days had minimal renal alterations which were believed to be entirely reversible. Urinary casts were not observed in dogs receiving a 30 mg/kg dose for 90 days. In efficacy studies involving 80 infected dogs treated with amikacin at the recommended dosage rate of 10 mg/kg b.i.d. for 8-21 consecutive days, no evidence of nephrotoxicity or any other toxicity was encountered. Regarding ototoxicity, studies in cats reveal that amikacin has less potential for ototoxicity than gentamicin.[4]

Adverse Reactions: In clinical studies in dogs, transient pain on injection has been reported as well as rare cases of vomiting or diarrhea following amikacin therapy. In 90 day intramuscular toxicology studies, evidence of muscle damage was detected histologically as well as by elevated creatinine phosphokinase.

References: Available upon request.

Presentation: 50 mL vials.

Manufactured by: Phoenix Scientific, Inc.

Compendium Code No.: 10940240

CANINE ASPIRIN CHEWABLE TABLETS FOR LARGE DOGS ℞

Pala-Tech **Non-Steroidal Anti-Inflammatory**

Microencapsulated, Buffered Aspirin, USP

Active Ingredient(s): Composition: Each tablet contains 450 mg of microencapsulated, buffered aspirin. The recommended dosage of aspirin is 16.5 mg/kg body weight (7.5 mg/lb) every 12 hours.

Indications: Pala-Tech™ CANINE ASPIRIN CHEWABLE TABLETS contain microencapsulated, buffered aspirin in a proprietary, highly palatable roast beef and liver flavor base to ensure dogs readily consume the tablet. Pala-Tech™ CANINE ASPIRIN CHEWABLE TABLETS, a mild analgesic, aids in the temporary relief of pain and inflammation associated with minor muscular aches and joint problems in dogs, and as an antipyretic agent (aid to reduce fever).

Dosage and Administration: Dosage: Consult with your veterinarian. The recommended dosage is one tablet per 60 pounds body weight every 12 hours. This amount may be increased or decreased based on the dog's condition and the recommendation of your veterinarian.

Administration: Each tablet, Pala-Tech™ CANINE ASPIRIN CHEWABLE TABLETS, may be given orally to dogs as a treat, or crumbled over their food. If crumbled over food, consumption should be monitored. Give at or immediately before mealtime.

Precaution(s): Store at room temperature; 15°C-30°C (59°F-86°F). Avoid excessive heat.

Caution(s): Federal law restricts this drug to use by or on the order of a licensed veterinarian.

Not for use in cats. Do not administer to dogs having gastritis, enteritis, or other gastro-intestinal conditions, except as directed by your veterinarian. If vomiting or diarrhea occur, discontinue use or decrease dosage and contact your veterinarian.

Warning(s): Keep out of reach of children.

Presentation: 60 tablets/bottle.

Compendium Code No.: 10680001 8001-0699

CANINE ASPIRIN CHEWABLE TABLETS FOR SMALL AND MEDIUM DOGS ℞

Pala-Tech **Non-Steroidal Anti-Inflammatory**

Microencapsulated, Buffered Aspirin, USP

Active Ingredient(s): Composition: Each tablet contains 150 mg of microencapsulated, buffered aspirin. The recommended dosage of aspirin is 16.5 mg/kg body weight (7.5 mg/lb) every 12 hours.

Indications: Pala-Tech™ CANINE ASPIRIN CHEWABLE TABLETS contain microencapsulated, buffered aspirin in a proprietary, highly palatable roast beef and liver flavor base to ensure dogs readily consume the tablet. Pala-Tech™ CANINE ASPIRIN CHEWABLE TABLETS, a mild analgesic, aids in the temporary relief of pain and inflammation associated with minor muscular aches and joint problems in dogs, and as an antipyretic agent (aid to reduce fever).

Dosage and Administration: Dosage: Consult with your veterinarian. The recommended dosage is one tablet per 20 pounds body weight every 12 hours. This amount may be increased or decreased based on the dog's condition and the recommendation of your veterinarian.

Administration: Each tablet, Pala-Tech™ CANINE ASPIRIN CHEWABLE TABLETS, may be given orally to dogs as a treat, or crumbled over their food. If crumbled over food, consumption should be monitored. Give at or immediately before mealtime.

Precaution(s): Store at room temperature; 15°C-30°C (59°F-86°F). Avoid excessive heat.

Caution(s): Federal law restricts this drug to use by or on the order of a licensed veterinarian.

Not for use in cats. Do not administer to dogs having gastritis, enteritis, or other gastro-intestinal conditions, except as directed by your veterinarian. If vomiting or diarrhea occur, discontinue use or decrease dosage and contact your veterinarian.

Warning(s): Keep out of reach of children.

Presentation: 60 tablets/bottle.

Compendium Code No.: 10680011 8001-0699

CANINE F.A./PLUS CHEWABLE TABLETS FOR LARGE DOGS

Pala-Tech **Small Animal Dietary Supplement**

Omega Fatty Acids, Vitamins and Minerals

Active Ingredient(s): Composition: Each tablet, Pala-Tech™ CANINE F.A./PLUS CHEWABLE TABLETS, contains:

Microencapsulated Fatty Acids

Marine Lipid Concentrates . . . . 400 mg
Flaxseed Oil . . . . 100 mg

Vitamins

Vitamin A . . . . 4,300 I.U.
Vitamin B_1 (thiamine mononitrate) . . . . 2,800 mcg
Vitamin B_2 (riboflavin) . . . . 2,800 mcg
Vitamin B_6 (pyridoxine HCl) . . . . 2,290 mcg
Vitamin B_{12} (cyanocobalamin) . . . . 70 mcg
Vitamin D_3 . . . . 860 I.U.
Vitamin E . . . . 14 I.U.
Vitamin K (menadione) . . . . 710 mcg
Biotin . . . . 28 mcg
Choline . . . . 7 mg
Folic Acid . . . . 86 mcg
Inositol . . . . 21 mg
Niacin . . . . 21 mg
Pantothenic Acid . . . . 3,230 mcg

Minerals

Calcium (from calcium phosphate) . . . . 25.5 mg
Chloride (from sodium chloride) . . . . 5.7 mg
Cobalt (from cobalt sulfate) . . . . 43 mcg
Copper (from copper sulfate) . . . . 500 mcg
Iodine (from potassium iodide) . . . . 105 mcg
Iron (from iron oxide) . . . . 10 mg
Magnesium (from magnesium oxide) . . . . 4.3 mg
Manganese (from manganese sulfate) . . . . 198 mcg
Phosphorus (from calcium phosphate) . . . . 20 mg
Potassium (from potassium iodide) . . . . 42 mcg
Selenium (from sodium selenite) . . . . 8.6 mcg
Sodium (from sodium chloride) . . . . 4.3 mg
Zinc (from zinc oxide) . . . . 7.1 mg

Indications: Pala-Tech™ CANINE F.A./PLUS CHEWABLE TABLETS are a supplemental source of omega fatty acids and other essential vitamins and minerals. For supplementation of the diet to aid in the prophylaxis and treatment of fatty acid, multiple vitamin and mineral deficiencies.

Dosage and Administration: Dosage: The following dosage schedule is recommended for the daily administration of Pala-Tech™ CANINE F.A./PLUS CHEWABLE TABLETS. Consult with your veterinarian to determine the proper dosage level and schedule for each individual animal prescribed this product.

Dogs 20 to 50 pounds . . . . 1 tablet daily
Dogs 50 pounds and over . . . . 1 to 2 tablets daily

Administration: Pala-Tech™ CANINE F.A./PLUS CHEWABLE TABLETS are formulated with a proprietary, highly palatable roast beef and liver flavor base to ensure dogs readily consume the tablet. Administer free choice orally to the dog as a treat, or crumble over the dog's food at mealtime.

Precaution(s): Store at room temperature; (58°F-86°F). Avoid excessive heat.

Warning(s): Keep out of reach of children. For veterinary use only.

Presentation: 60 tablets/bottle.

Compendium Code No.: 10680020 9001-0699

CANINE F.A./PLUS CHEWABLE TABLETS FOR SMALL AND MEDIUM DOGS

Pala-Tech **Small Animal Dietary Supplement**

Omega Fatty Acids, Vitamins and Minerals

Active Ingredient(s): Composition: Each tablet, Pala-Tech™ CANINE F.A./PLUS CHEWABLE TABLETS, contains:

Microencapsulated Fatty Acids

Marine Lipid Concentrates . . . . 280 mg
Flaxseed Oil . . . . 70 mg

Vitamins

Vitamin A . . . . 3,000 I.U.
Vitamin B_1 (thiamine mononitrate) . . . . 2,000 mcg
Vitamin B_2 (riboflavin) . . . . 2,000 mcg
Vitamin B_6 (pyridoxine HCl) . . . . 1,600 mcg
Vitamin B_{12} (cyanocobalamin) . . . . 50 mcg
Vitamin D_3 . . . . 600 I.U.
Vitamin E . . . . 10 I.U.
Vitamin K (menadione) . . . . 500 mcg
Biotin . . . . 20 mcg
Choline . . . . 5 mg
Folic Acid . . . . 60 mcg
Inositol . . . . 15 mg
Niacin . . . . 15 mg
Pantothenic Acid . . . . 2,250 mcg

Minerals

Calcium (from calcium phosphate) . . . . 18 mg
Chloride (from sodium chloride) . . . . 4 mg
Cobalt (from cobalt sulfate) . . . . 30 mcg
Copper (from copper sulfate) . . . . 345 mcg
Iodine (from potassium iodide) . . . . 75 mcg
Iron (from iron oxide) . . . . 7 mg
Magnesium (from magnesium oxide) . . . . 3 mg
Manganese (from manganese sulfate) . . . . 38 mcg
Phosphorus (from calcium phosphate) . . . . 14 mg
Potassium (from potassium iodide) . . . . 30 mcg
Selenium (from sodium selenite) . . . . 6 mcg
Sodium (from sodium chloride) . . . . 3 mg
Zinc (from zinc oxide) . . . . 5 mg

Indications: Pala-Tech™ CANINE F.A./PLUS CHEWABLE TABLETS are a supplemental source of omega fatty acids and other essential vitamins and minerals. For supplementation of the diet to aid in the prophylaxis and treatment of fatty acid, multiple vitamin and mineral deficiencies.

Dosage and Administration: Dosage: The following dosage schedule is recommended for the daily administration of Pala-Tech™ CANINE F.A./PLUS CHEWABLE TABLETS. Consult with your veterinarian to determine the proper dosage level and schedule for each individual animal prescribed this product.

Dogs under 10 pounds . . . . ½ to 1 tablet daily
Dogs 10 pounds and over . . . . 1 to 2 tablets daily

Administration: Pala-Tech™ CANINE F.A./PLUS CHEWABLE TABLETS are formulated with a proprietary, highly palatable roast beef and liver flavor base to ensure dogs readily consume the tablet. Administer free choice orally to the dog as a treat, or crumble over the dog's food at mealtime.

Precaution(s): Store at room temperature; (58°F-86°F). Avoid excessive heat.

Warning(s): Keep out of reach of children.

For veterinary use only.

Presentation: 60 tablets/bottle.

Compendium Code No.: 10680030 9001-0699

CANINE F.A./PLUS GRANULES

Pala-Tech **Small Animal Dietary Supplement**

Omega Fatty Acids, Vitamins and Minerals

Active Ingredient(s): Composition: Each 10 gram scoop of Pala-Tech™ CANINE F.A./PLUS GRANULES (1 scoop) contains:

Microencapsulated Fatty Acids

Marine Lipid Concentrates . . . . 800 mg
Flaxseed Oil . . . . 200 mg

Vitamins

Vitamin A . . . . 1,300 I.U.
Vitamin B_1 (thiamine mononitrate) . . . . 2,800 mcg
Vitamin B_2 (riboflavin) . . . . 810 mcg
Vitamin B_6 (pyridoxine HCl) . . . . 820 mcg
Vitamin B_{12} (cyanocobalamin) . . . . 10 mcg
Vitamin C . . . . 5 mg
Vitamin D_3 . . . . 150 I.U.
Vitamin E . . . . 3 I.U.
Biotin . . . . 10 mcg
Choline . . . . 20 mg
Folic Acid . . . . 40 mcg
Inositol . . . . 5 mg
Niacin . . . . 10 mg
Pantothenic Acid . . . . 2 mg

Minerals

Calcium (from calcium phosphate) . . . . 160 mg
Chloride (from sodium chloride) . . . . 3 mg
Chromium (from chromium chloride) . . . . 1 mcg
Cobalt (from cobalt sulfate) . . . . 14 mcg
Copper (from copper sulfate) . . . . 500 mcg
Fluoride (from sodium fluoride) . . . . 10 mcg
Iodine (from potassium iodide) . . . . 52 mcg
Iron (from ferrous fumarate) . . . . 10 mg
Magnesium (from magnesium oxide) . . . . 1 mg
Manganese (from manganese sulfate) . . . . 60 mcg
Molybdenum (from molybdenum trioxide) . . . . 1 mcg
Nickel (from nickel chloride) . . . . 1 mcg
Phosphorus (from calcium phosphate) . . . . 123 mg
Potassium (from potassium iodide) . . . . 16 mcg
Selenium (from selenium powder) . . . . 4 mcg
Silicon (from silicon dioxide) . . . . 1 mcg
Sodium (from sodium chloride) . . . . 2 mg
Tin (from tin powder) . . . . 1 mcg
Vanadium (from vanadium oxide) . . . . 1 mcg
Zinc (from zinc oxide) . . . . 2.5 mg

Indications: Pala-Tech™ CANINE F.A./PLUS GRANULES is a supplemental source of omega fatty acids and other essential vitamins and minerals. For supplementation of the diet to aid in the prophylaxis and treatment of fatty acid, multiple vitamin and mineral deficiencies.

Dosage and Administration: Dosage: The following dosage schedule is recommended for the daily administration of Pala-Tech™ CANINE F.A./PLUS GRANULES. Consult with your veterinarian to determine the proper dosage level and schedule for each individual animal prescribed this product.

Weight of Dog	Daily Dosage (Scoop Size = 10 grams)
< 20 lbs.	1 scoop/day
21 - 51 lbs.	2 scoops/day
> 51 lbs.	3-4 scoops/day

Administration: A 10 gram precision dosing scoop is enclosed in the container. Measure out the prescribed daily dose and administer over the dog's food. Product may be mixed with food, if necessary, to facilitate complete consumption. Pala-Tech™ CANINE F.A./PLUS GRANULES is formulated with a proprietary, highly palatable roast beef and liver flavor base to ensure dogs readily consume the supplement.

Precaution(s): Store at room temperature; (58°F-86°F). Avoid excessive heat.

Warning(s): Keep out of reach of children.

For veterinary use only.

Presentation: 650 gram container.

Compendium Code No.: 10680040 9002-0699

CANINE FRESH FROZEN PLASMA

P.V.R. **Canine Plasma**

Description: Fresh frozen plasma is the liquid component(s) of whole blood that has been separated by centrifugation and subsequently frozen within 6-8 hours of collection.

Indications: This product is warranted in patients with bleeding disorders involving the loss of platelets, diminished clotting factors, and or diseases which cause prolonged clotting time.

Dosage and Administration:

1. Properly determine if the patient need for blood therapy and which product should be used. Cross match donor and recipient blood (description provided).
2. Utilize a slow intravenous drip for 15-20 minutes while monitoring dog for clinical signs on incompatibility. Without no clinical reaction symptoms, continue steady drip for approximately 2-3 hours.

Type of product	Indications	Hazards
Whole blood	anemia (decreased PCV) with volume deficit	Review adverse reactions section
Red blood cells	anemia without volume deficit. Low PCV only	Review adverse reactions section
Liquid and Frozen Plasma	Deficit of stable coagulations factors and associated proteins (normal PCV)	Review adverse reactions section

3. Never vent infusion bag to outside air.
4. Blood and associated components must be administered through an appropriate blood administration set with a clot filter included.
5. Warm and gently agitate blood components to no more than 37°C prior to administration.
6. Never use blood or blood components as a means to administer other drugs or fluids such as ringers lactate, electrolytes, dextrose, diuretics, etc.
7. During normal handling and shipping, some hemolysis or blood breakdown will occur. This will occasionally appear as a pink supernate. Any cloudy material, clotted fragments, or obvious discoloration of this product should be reported to Professional Veterinary Research, Inc. (812) 358-9078.
8. Gently warm blood by water bath or commercial heater without allowing any water into injection ports. Watertight wraps of bags are suggested prior to emersion into the bath.
9. After warming, administer blood at .10 mL/pound (.05 mL/kilogram body weight) slowly for first 20-30 minutes. During this period, it is essential to clinically monitor these animals for signs of transfusion reactions. Continue to administer blood at slow rate for next 2-4 hours. Please note more rapid infusion of blood can be obtained under emergency situations.
10. Care should be taken in all blood or blood product infusions. Often, medical therapy with proper fluid replacement (ringers lactate, hypotonic saline) can replenish fluid volume loss without the need of blood products.
11. Due to the wide range of infusion rates, in patients always closely monitor animals that receive blood products.

Contraindication(s): Fresh frozen plasma should not be used when other therapeutic treatments can safely replenish the plasma components needed in the recipient.

Caution(s): The safety and efficacy of whole blood administration in dogs has been documented for several years in veterinary literature. If used correctly and as indicated, blood therapy can be extremely beneficial to the recipient. If used incorrectly or haphazardly, an incompatible blood infusion can cause any or all of the listed clinical signs listed below:

1) Fever/chills
2) Urticaria
3) Vomiting, nausea
4) Hemolysis
   A. Hemoglobinemia and hemoglobinuria
   B. Bilirubinemia and bilirubinuria
   C. Recurrent anemia
   D. Acute renal failure
   E. Disseminated intravascular coagulopathy
5) Hypotension
6) Anaphylactic shock
7) Death

Warning(s): Blood products can cause immunologic complications such as reactions caused by incompatible red cells, reactions caused by incompatible white blood cells, and/or reactions caused by incompatible plasma constituents. Nonimmunologic reactions can also occur with improper handling, administration, and/or storage of blood products. To prevent transfusion incompatibility one should: 1) Crossmatch donor and recipient blood prior to transfusion. 2) Use only dog donors: negative for Dea 1.1, Dea 1.2, and Dea 7 canine red cell surface antigens. 3) If a patient has already suffered a serious reaction and does require future transfusions, cross-match blood and administer antihistamines and/or glucocorticoids prior to and during the transfusion. Nonimmunologic reactions can be minimized by: 1) Premix and prewarm blood. 2) Maintain intrinsic warmth by passing blood through gentle waterbaths or commercial warmers. 3) Maintain a continuous but slow rate of infusion except under emergency situations. 4) Use proper filters to remove particulate matter. 5) Maintain sterile technique when placing all in dwelling catheters and setups. 6) Administer appropriate doses based on body weight, need, and blood parameters which should be closely monitored.

Of equal importance, the risk of lateral disease transmission does exist from this product. Professional Veterinary Research, Inc. maintains a closed access colony of universal donor dogs that have been serologically tested for *Brucella canis, Ehrlichia canis, Borrelia burgdorferi*, and *Dirofilaria immitis*. All animals are housed in indoor biosecure kennel runs on plastic flooring and are vaccinated quarterly for Canine Distemper, Adenovirus type 2, Leptospirosis, Parainfluenza, and Canine Parvo Virus. Dogs are also vaccinated yearly for Rabies.

For intravenous use in dogs only.

Adverse Reactions: Hemolytic transfusion reactions either acute or delayed can occur following a blood transfusion with donor/recipient blood incompatibilities. To reduce this risk of hypersensitivity reactions, all donor and recipient blood products should have a major and minor crossmatch prior to every transfusion. Uncommon nonimmunologic complications are listed below:

1. Circulatory overload. All recipient animals must have an absence of overall blood volume prior to infusion. It is strongly recommended to monitor patients hematocrict (PCV), hemoglobin concentration, and all other clinical parameters prior to and during transfusion. Pulmonary edema is generally noted in circulatory overload reactions and can occur when excessive volumes are given. Older geriatric patients, toy breed dogs, and animals with chronic diseases that manifest by reducing red cell mass and increase plasma volume are particularly at risk. If pulmonary edema is noted, stop fluid placements and treat immediately.
2. Air Embolism. Care should be taken to remove excess air from all fluid paths and I.V. lines prior to transfusion.
3. Fever/hypothermia has been noted but usually is benign and transient.
4. Bacterial sepsis generally involving gram negative bacteria. Contamination of this product is rare but can occur with improper handling of the blood. The presence of primarily gram negative bacteria can cause severe endoxic reactions with subsequent fever, hypotension following transfusion which can lead to shock and/or death if left untreated. If the blood has abnormal clumping or discoloration, Professional Veterinary Research Inc. at 812-358-9078 should be contacted.
5. The transmission of infectious agents with blood transfusions are always possible. Donor dogs are tested serologically, and heavily monitored for signs of infection disease but the possibility of subclinical infectious prior to donation blood does exist.
6. Iron overload can occur but is extremely rare in patients receiving repeated transfusions over long periods of time.
7. Depletion or dilution of coagulation proteins can occur rarely after massive transfusion. Treatment with specific blood components may be useful.
8. Metabolic complications following massive transfusions:
   A. Hypothermia from infusing cold blood through a central venous line. Cardiac arrhythmia can occur unless blood is heated and delivered slowly.
   B. Citrate toxicity can occur rarely especially due underlying disease but can generally be treated by discontinuing the transfusion.
   C. Metabolic acidosis or subsequent alkalosis can occur post-transfusion but rarely requires drug intervention.

Presentation: 125 mL and 250 mL.

Compendium Code No.: 10440021

CANINE PACKED RED BLOOD CELLS

P.V.R. **Blood Product**

Description: This product contains concentrated red blood cells without plasmal components.

Indications: This product will increase the circulating red blood cell mass and associated oxygen carrying capabilities of the recipient animal and is warranted in cases of anemia without extensive volume loss. Conditions such as hemolysis, blood loss and/or ineffective red cell production should benefit from packed red blood cells.

Dosage and Administration:

1. Properly determine if the patient need for blood therapy and which product should be used. Cross match donor and recipient blood (description provided).
2. Utilize a slow intravenous drip for 15-20 minutes while monitoring dog for clinical signs on incompatibility. Without no clinical reaction symptoms, continue steady drip for approximately 2-3 hours.

Type of product	Indications	Hazards
Whole blood	anemia (decreased PCV) with volume deficit	Review adverse reactions section
Red blood cells	anemia without volume deficit. Low PCV only	Review adverse reactions section
Liquid and Frozen Plasma	Deficit of stable coagulations factors and associated proteins (normal PCV)	Review adverse reactions section

3. Never vent infusion bag to outside air.
4. Blood and associated components must be administered through an appropriate blood administration set with a clot filter included.
5. Warm and gently agitate blood components to no more than 37°C prior to administration.
6. Never use blood or blood components as a means to administer other drugs or fluids such as ringers lactate, electrolytes, dextrose, diuretics, etc.
7. During normal handling and shipping, some hemolysis or blood breakdown will occur. This will occasionally appear as a pink supernate. Any cloudy material, clotted fragments, or obvious discoloration of this product should be reported to Professional Veterinary Research, Inc. (812) 358-9078.
8. Gently warm blood by water bath or commercial heater without allowing any water into injection ports. Watertight wraps of bags are suggested prior to emersion into the bath.
9. After warming, administer blood at .10 mL/pound (.05 mL/kilogram body weight) slowly for first 20-30 minutes. During this period, it is essential to clinically monitor these animals for signs of transfusion reactions. Continue to administer blood at slow rate for next 2-4 hours. Please note more rapid infusion of blood can be obtained under emergency situations.
10. Care should be taken in all blood or blood product infusions. Often, medical therapy with proper fluid replacement (ringers lactate, hypotonic saline) can replenish fluid volume loss without the need of blood products.
11. Due to the wide range of infusion rates, in patients always closely monitor animals that receive blood products.

Contraindication(s): Red blood cell administration is contraindicated in cases involving advanced cardiac disease, renal impairment, or animals without decreased Hematocrits (PCV). Red blood cells should only be used when other therapeutic treatments can not safely replenish the blood volume and/or oxygen carrying capacity of the circulating red blood cell mass. All blood transfusions are contraindicated in animals with normal packed cell volumes which can result in circulatory overloads.

Caution(s): The safety and efficacy of whole blood administration in dogs has been documented for several years in veterinary literature. If used correctly and as indicated, blood therapy can be extremely beneficial to the recipient. If used incorrectly or haphazardly, an incompatible blood infusion can cause any or all of the listed clinical signs listed below:

1) Fever/chills
2) Urticaria
3) Vomiting, nausea
4) Hemolysis
   A. Hemoglobinemia and hemoglobinuria
   B. Bilirubinemia and bilirubinuria
   C. Recurrent anemia
   D. Acute renal failure
   E. Disseminated intravascular coagulopathy
5) Hypotension
6) Anaphylactic shock
7) Death

Warning(s): Blood products can cause immunologic complications such as reactions caused by incompatible red cells, reactions caused by incompatible white blood cells, and/or reactions caused by incompatible plasma constituents. Nonimmunologic reactions can also occur with improper handling, administration, and/or storage of blood products. To prevent transfusion incompatibility one should: 1) Crossmatch donor and recipient blood prior to transfusion. 2) Use only dog donors: negative for Dea 1.1, Dea 1.2, and Dea 7 canine red cell surface antigens. 3) If a patient has already suffered a serious reaction and does require future transfusions, cross-match blood and administer antihistamines and/or glucocorticoids prior to and during the transfusion. Nonimmunologic reactions can be minimized by: 1) Premix and prewarm blood. 2) Maintain intrinsic warmth by passing blood through gentle waterbaths or commercial warmers. 3) Maintain a continuous but slow rate of infusion except under emergency situations. 4) Use proper filters to remove particulate matter. 5) Maintain sterile technique when placing all in dwelling catheters and setups. 6) Administer appropriate doses based on body weight, need, and blood parameters which should be closely monitored.

Of equal importance, the risk of lateral disease transmission does exist from this product. Professional Veterinary Research, Inc. maintains a closed access colony of universal donor dogs that have been serologically tested for *Brucella canis, Ehrlichia canis, Borrelia burgdorferi*, and *Dirofilaria immitis.* All animals are housed in indoor biosecure kennel runs on plastic flooring and are vaccinated quarterly for Canine Distemper, Adenovirus type 2, Leptospirosis, Parainfluenza, and Canine Parvo Virus. Dogs are also vaccinated yearly for Rabies.

For intravenous use in dogs only.

Adverse Reactions: Hemolytic transfusion reactions either acute or delayed can occur following a blood transfusion with donor/recipient blood incompatibilities. To reduce this risk of hypersensitivity reactions, all donor and recipient blood products should have a major and minor crossmatch prior to every transfusion. Uncommon nonimmunologic complications are listed below:

1. Circulatory overload. All recipient animals must have an absence of overall blood volume prior to infusion. It is strongly recommended to monitor patients hematocrict (PCV), hemoglobin concentration, and all other clinical parameters prior to and during transfusion. Pulmonary edema is generally noted in circulatory overload reactions and can occur when excessive volumes are given. Older geriatric patients, toy breed dogs, and animals with chronic diseases that manifest by reducing red cell mass and increase plasma volume are particularly at risk. If pulmonary edema is noted, stop fluid placements and treat immediately.
2. Air Embolism. Care should be taken to remove excess air from all fluid paths and I.V. lines prior to transfusion.
3. Fever/hypothermia has been noted but usually is benign and transient.
4. Bacterial sepsis generally involving gram negative bacteria. Contamination of this product is rare but can occur with improper handling of the blood. The presence of primarily gram negative bacteria can cause severe endoxic reactions with subsequent fever, hypotension following transfusion which can lead to shock and/or death if left untreated. If the blood has abnormal clumping or discoloration, Professional Veterinary Research Inc. at 812-358-9078 should be contacted.
5. The transmission of infectious agents with blood transfusions are always possible. Donor dogs are tested serologically, and heavily monitored for signs of infection disease but the possibility of subclinical infectious prior to donation blood does exist.
6. Iron overload can occur but is extremely rare in patients receiving repeated transfusions over long periods of time.
7. Depletion or dilution of coagulation proteins can occur rarely after massive transfusion. Treatment with specific blood components may be useful.
8. Metabolic complications following massive transfusions:
   A. Hypothermia from infusing cold blood through a central venous line. Cardiac arrhythmia can occur unless blood is heated and delivered slowly.
   B. Citrate toxicity can occur rarely especially due underlying disease but can generally be treated by discontinuing the transfusion.
   C. Metabolic acidosis or subsequent alkalosis can occur post-transfusion but rarely requires drug intervention.

Presentation: 125 mL and 250 mL.
Compendium Code No.: 10440030

CANINE PLASMA

A.B.B. **Canine Plasma**

CA Vet. Biol. Lic. No.: 83
Active Ingredient(s): Each 10 mL CPDA-1 contains:

Dextrose (hydrous) .... 317 mg USP
Sodium citrate (hydrous) .... 263 mg USP
Citric acid (hydrous) .... 33 mg USP
Monobasic sodium phosphate (monohydrate) .... 22 mg USP
Adenine .... 2.7 mg USP
Water .... q.s. USP

Table of Product Contents:

	Whole Blood	RBC's	Plasma	CPDA-1	Total Fluid Volume	Range
Fresh Frozen (1 unit)	-0-	-0-	approx. 100 mL	approx. 20 mL	approx. 120 mL	105-140 mL
Frozen (1 unit)	-0-	-0-	approx. 100 mL	approx. 20 mL	approx. 120 mL & 50 mL mini-unit	105-140 mL

CANINE PLASMA, Fresh Frozen is a transfusion product aseptically obtained from healthy dogs maintained in an isolated, controlled access colony. Blood is not pooled (ie. each unit of blood is from a single-donor) and euthanasia donors are never used. All colony donors are serologically negative for *Canine brucellosis, Ehrlichia canis, Borrelia burgdorferi* (Lyme Disease), and *Dirofilaria immitis.* The blood type of each donor dog is indicated on the product label. The colony receives intensive onsite veterinary health care, and all animals are current on immunizations, to include: Canine distemper, hepatitis, leptospirosis, parainfluenza, canine parvovirus, and rabies.

The anticoagulant CPDA-1 is present. It consists of citrate, phosphate, dextrose, and adenine.

A unit of CANINE PLASMA, Fresh Frozen is prepared via the centrifugation of canine whole blood, and is produced within six hours of the time of collection of the original whole blood from the donor dog; has a total fluid volume of approximately 120 mL; and a shelf-life of one year.

A unit of CANINE PLASMA, Frozen is distinguished from the fresh frozen plasma in that it may be prepared at any time up to five days after the expiration date applicable to the original unit of whole blood. Clinically, this difference results in reduced amounts of some coagulation factors in the older product, as well as slightly increased levels of potassium and ammonia; however, such plasma is a viable source of the other components of plasma such as albumin, globulins, and electrolytes, as well as replacement fluid volume. A unit of CANINE PLASMA, Frozen has a total fluid volume of approximately 120 mL; and a shelf-life of five years. 50 mL mini-units are also available.

Indications: CANINE PLASMA, Fresh Frozen when properly thawed, is indicated for parenteral replenishment of coagulation factors, albumin, globulins, electrolytes, and fluid volume, as indicated by the clinician's/internist's evaluation of the patient.

CANINE PLASMA, Frozen when properly thawed, is indicated for parenteral replenishment of albumin, globulins, electrolytes, and fluid volume.

Dosage and Administration:

Blood Filter: A blood filter should always be used when administering plasma. When administering over 50 mL of blood to a patient, use the standard blood administration set with its integral 170-230 micron clot screen filter. When administering less than 50 mL of blood to a patient, the standard blood administration set's filter (with a relatively huge surface area) will trap too much blood. Therefore, when transfusing less than 50 mL of blood, the following configuration is recommended:

1. Remove one (1) red cap (white on some models) from the blood bag's diaphragm port, and insert the spike of the drip chamber end of a Venoset 70 Microdrip set into the now uncovered blood bag diaphragm port. The second red cap, found on whole blood bags and red blood cell bags, should remain in place. Technically, non-vented fluid administration sets are safer than using blood bags. This can be simulated by aseptically replacing the Venoset's air filter with the male end of a 3 mL syringe, with its plunger in place. Never leave the Venoset's air filter port uncovered.
2. Attach the needle adaptor end of the Venoset into the female end of a Hemo-Nate neonatal filter, model #HN-179.
3. Then attach the male end of the filter to the female end of a 30 inch IV extension set.
4. Finally, attach the male end of the extension set to an IV catheter pre-positioned in the patient. With the above technique, transfusion can be obtained via a slow continuous drip over several hours (or longer), therefore minimizing volume overload.
5. If the bolus technique is preferred, simply aspirate the blood into a sterile syringe, then aseptically place the Hemo-Nate filter between the syringe and a fresh sterile needle/catheter, before transfusing.

   Plasma bags can readily be adapted for syringe access via Gesco international's Hemo-Tap device, model #HT-180 (2½ inches long, with a spike at one end and a brown hypodermic needle port at the other end).

Route of Administration: The jugular, cephalic, and saphenous veins are common sites for IV catheter placement. The intramedullary cavity of the femur and humerus are alternate sites. Additionally, intraperitoneal transfusions have application in selected patients.

Rate of Infusion:

1. There is virtually no rate of blood infusion that is safe for all canine patients; therefore the following are only general guidelines. The actual rate of infusion of blood must be tailored to each individual patient.
2. If clinical conditions permit, the initial rate should be slow (about 0.11 mL/lb. BW over a 30-minute period), in order to observe the patient for transfusion reactions.
   (0.11 mL/lb. = @ 0.25 mL/kg).
3. If plasma is being administered for hypoproteinemia, a suggested dose is 6 to 10 mL/kg BW (@ 2.7 to 4.5 mL/lb. BW).

Post-Transfusion Patient Care: During and after transfusions, the patient should be closely monitored. In addition to physical examinations and temperature monitoring, measurement of PCV, urine output, body weight, and EKG are recommended. Measurement of CVP may be utilized in some cases. In all cases, infusion rates should be calculated (rather than estimated) and closely monitored.

Contraindication(s): The plasma was frozen in a horizontal position then stored upright. If the frozen plasma bag shows cracks or signs of premature thawing and refreezing (ie. thicker at the bottom than at the top) do not administer.

Do not administer (via the same infusion system) in conjunction with other fluids or drugs, except 0.9% NaCl.

Do not administer to species other than the domestic dog.

Precaution(s):

1. Frozen plasma bags must be carefully handled to avoid cracking the plastic bags and to avoid contamination during thawing. Thawing should be conducted at 86 to 98.6°F (30 to 37°C). Do not exceed 98.6°F at any time. The use of a controlled temperature circulating warm water bath is the preferred thawing method. (Although some clinicians advocate the use of a microwave for thawing frozen plasma, the potential for hot spots prevents the recommendation of this latter technique).
2. Always conduct a minor crossmatch before transfusing plasma.
3. Infusion of plasma should begin within six hours of thawing. Do not re-freeze plasma once it has been thawed.

These units have a shelf-life of one year for Fresh Frozen Plasma and five years for Frozen Plasma from the date of collection of the original unit of whole blood. They should be maintained in a freezer at below 0°F. (chest type freezers work best). Store the frozen plasma bags in a vertical position (to detect thawing, as they were originally frozen in an horizontal position). Caution, the defrost cycle on some freezers allows the temperature to briefly rise above zero. This can be partially compensated for by sandwiching plasma bags between bags of deep frozen artificial ice. (This technique will only work if the artificial ice has been pre-frozen to a temperature of below 0°F).

A method of monitoring freezer and refrigerator temperatures is to install an indoor/outdoor thermometer on the freezer, such that the sensor is inside the freezer, yet the gauge is mounted on its casing so that the temperature can be easily read without opening the door or lid.

It is recommended that one of the hospital technicians view and record, at least twice a day, the internal temperature of the plasma freezer.

Caution(s):

1. During transfusions, fluid flow rates must be carefully calculated and monitored, based on the patient's size, weight, age, and clinical condition. It is recommended that urine output be monitored as well.
2. Gently oscillate each bag before use in order to mix contents.
3. Use gloves when handling the dry ice, which is used when shipping frozen plasma.
4. Do not allow dry ice to contact bare skin.
5. Complications of transfusions are manifest by a variety of clinical signs including jaundice, fever, cardiac arrythmias, erratic respiration, salivation, hemoglobinuria, edema, DIC, hemorrhage, vomiting, and urticaria. If any of these clinical signs develop, immediately stop the transfusion and institute appropriate supportive measures, as determined by the patient's clinical condition and the clinician's medical judgment.
6. For use in domestic dogs only.

Warning(s):

1. Circulatory overload can occur quickly unless all patient parameters are closely monitored.
2. Do not add medications to the blood bags nor via the same infusion system.
3. In spite of serological screening, disease organisms may still be present in these transfusion products.
4. Platelets are not viable in these products.
5. Do not administer any of these blood products without a blood filter.
6. Do not add Lactated Ringer's solution to whole blood or to red blood cells. It is safest to use 0.9% NaCl as the only fluid/drug administered in conjunction with these blood products.
7. Transfusion reactions can still occur in spite of correct blood typing and proper crossmatching.

References: Available upon request.
Presentation: Units of CANINE PLASMA, Fresh Frozen and Frozen are supplied frozen (packed in dry ice), in blood grade plastic bags (with one IV set coupling port, and reference aliquots [tubing segments]).
Compendium Code No.: 13980000

CANINE RED BLOOD CELLS

A.B.B. **Blood Product**

CA Vet. Biol. Lic. No.: 83
Active Ingredient(s): Each 10 mL CPDA-1 contains:

Dextrose (hydrous) .... 317 mg USP
Sodium citrate (hydrous) .... 263 mg USP
Citric acid (hydrous) .... 33 mg USP
Monobasic sodium phosphate (monohydrate) .... 22 mg USP
Adenine .... 2.7 mg USP
Water .... q.s. USP

Table of Product Contents:

	Whole Blood	RBC's	Plasma	CPDA-1	Total Fluid Volume	Range
CANINE RED BLOOD CELLS (packed RBC's) (1 unit)	-0-	approx. 100 mL	approx. 13 mL	approx. 13 mL	approx. 125 mL & 250 mL dbl. unit	115-140 mL

CANINE RED BLOOD CELLS is a transfusion product aseptically obtained from healthy dogs maintained in an isolated, controlled access colony. Blood is not pooled (ie. each unit of blood is from a single-donor) and euthanasia donors are never used. All colony donors are serologically negative for *Canine brucellosis, Ehrlichia canis, Borrelia burgdorferi* (Lyme Disease), and *Dirofilaria immitis*. The blood type of each donor dog is indicated on the product label. The colony receives intensive onsite veterinary health care, and all animals are current on immunizations, to include: Canine distemper, hepatitis, leptospirosis, parainfluenza, canine parvo virus, and rabies.

A unit of CANINE RED BLOOD CELLS, (packed RBC's) is the highly cellular fluid remaining in the primary blood bag, after approximately 80% of the plasma and CPDA-1 have been aseptically moved into the transfer bag; 12 mL of CPDA-1 having then been aseptically added back to the RBC's to retain the 35 day shelf-life of the original unit; for a total fluid volume of approximately 125 mL. Tubing aliquots are present for crossmatching. 250 mL units are also available.
Indications: CANINE RED BLOOD CELLS (packed RBC's) are indicated for parenteral replenishment of RBC's (such as in conditions of chronic anemia) and especially in situations where the patient is additionally at risk of fluid volume overload. May be used in conjunction with crystalloids for treatment of acute blood loss.
Dosage and Administration:
The clinician/surgeon should first determine the PCV of the blood in the donor blood bag by aspirating the contents of an attached numbered tubing segment [reference aliquot] (shake the segment to mix its contents before aspirating), and centrifuging the sample. After ascertaining the microhematocrit of the donor blood, the following formula may be used to calculate the volume of blood to transfuse:

mLs of donor blood needed =

$$\frac{\text{(Recipient wt. [lbs.] x 40 mL/lb.) X (PCV desired – Recipient PCV)}}{\text{PCV of blood in donor bag}}$$

or

mLs of donor blood needed =

$$\frac{\text{(Recipient wt. [lbs.] x 32 mL/lb.) X (Hb desired – Recipent Hb)}}{\text{Hb of blood in donor bag}}$$

Refrigerated blood should be warmed to room temperature before transfusing. Do not exceed 98.6°F (37°C).

Blood Filter: A blood filter should always be used when administering red blood cells (packed RBC's). When administering over 50 mL of blood to a patient, use the standard blood administration set with its integral 170-230 micron clot screen filter. When administering less than 50 mL of blood to a patient, the standard blood administration set's filter (with a relatively huge surface area) will trap too much blood. Therefore, when transfusing less than 50 mL of blood, the following configuration is recommended:

1. Remove one (1) red cap (white on some models) from the blood bag's diaphragm port, and insert the spike of the drip chamber end of a Venoset 70 Microdrip set into the now uncovered blood bag diaphragm port. The second red cap, found on red blood cell bags, should remain in place. This second port is available for piggybacking a second IV system into the primary blood bag; or for attaching a transfer bag to extract plasma. Technically, non-vented fluid administration sets are safer then using blood bags. This can be simulated by aseptically replacing the Venoset's air filter with the male end of a 3 mL syringe, with its plunger in place. Never leave the Venoset's air filter port uncovered.
2. Attach the needle adaptor end of the Venoset into the female end of a Hemo-Nate neonatal filter, model #HN-179.
3. Then attach the male end of the filter to the female end of Abbott's 30 inch IV extension set.
4. Finally, attach the male end of the extension set to an IV catheter pre-positioned in the patient. With the above technique, transfusion can be obtained via a slow continuous drip over several hours (or longer), therefore minimizing volume overload.
5. If the bolus technique is preferred, simply aspirate the blood (from the blood bag's brown hypodermic needle port) into a sterile syringe, then aseptically place the Hemo-Nate filter between the syringe and a fresh sterile needle/catheter, before transfusing. Red blood cell bags have an integral brown hypodermic needle port for syringe access.
6. For puppies and other small patients, adding 0.9% NaCl (not Lactated Ringer's) to the blood will tend to reduce its viscosity and therefore facilitate the use of 22 or 24 gauge needles/catheters.

Route of Administration: The jugular, cephalic, and saphenous veins are common sites for IV catheter placement. The intramedullary cavity of the femur and humerus are alternate sites. Additionally, intraperitoneal transfusions have application in selected patients.

Rate of Infusion:

1. There is virtually no rate of blood infusion that is safe for all canine patients; therefore the following are only general guidelines. The actual rate of infusion of blood must be tailored to each individual patient.
2. If clinical conditions permit, the initial rate should be slow (about 0.11 mL/lb. BW over a 30-minute period), in order to observe the patient for transfusion reactions. (0.11 mL/lb. = @ 0.25 mL/kg).
3. Red blood cells (packed RBC's) can generally be infused at the same rate as whole blood. Transfusion of red blood cells tends to be safer than whole blood in normovolemic patients with chronic anemia.
In treating chronic conditions with red blood cells, the blood may be administered as part of a continuous drip system in conjunction with 0.9% NaCl in a piggyback set or in a secondary set, or in a Y-set.
In using the continuous drip method, the blood products' volume is merely included in the 24 hour IV fluid requirements of the animal; then the drip rate is calculated by converting the 24 hour volume into a certain number of drips per minute, or per second (depending on if an infusion pump is being used or the drip rate is being visually monitored).

Post-Transfusion Patient Care: During and after transfusions, the patient should be closely monitored. In addition to physical examinations and temperature monitoring, measurement of PCV, urine output, body weight, and EKG are recommended. Measurement of CVP may be utilized in some cases. In all cases, infusion rates should be calculated (rather than estimated) and closely monitored.
Contraindication(s): Do not administer if the blood bags are leaking or if the supernatant exhibits brown or purple discoloration or if excessive hemolysis is present.

Do not administer (via the same infusion system) in conjunction with other fluids or drugs, except 0.9% NaCl.

Do not administer to species other than the domestic dog.
Precaution(s): Because these units have 12 mL CPDA-1 added back to them after extracting the plasma, they have a shelf-life of 35 days from the date of collection of the original unit of whole blood. It should be maintained at a temperature of 33.8° to 42.8°F (1 to 6°C), except during shipment, when 33.8 to 50°F (1 to 10°C) is approved. Store the blood bags in a vertical position, with airspace between each bag (ie. avoid a sardine effect - RBC storage survival is apparently enhanced by the plastic bag's ability to breathe - that is one reason why glass is a less desirable storage container for blood).
Caution(s):

1. During transfusions, fluid flow rates must be carefully calculated and monitored, based on the patient's size, weight, age, and clinical condition. It is recommended that urine output be monitored as well.
2. Gently oscillate each bag before use in order to mix contents.
3. Complications of transfusions are manifest by a variety of clinical signs including jaundice, fever, cardiac arrythmias, erratic respiration, salivation, hemoglobinuria, edema, DIC, hemorrhage, vomiting, and urticaria. If any of these clinical signs develop, immediately stop the transfusion and institute appropriate supportive measures, as determined by the patient's clinical condition and the clinician's medical judgment.
4. For use in domestic dogs only.

Warning(s):

1. Circulatory overload can occur quickly unless all patient parameters are closely monitored.
2. Do not add medications to the blood bags nor via the same infusion system.
3. In spite of serological screening, disease organisms may still be present in these transfusion products.
4. Platelets are not viable in these products.
5. Do not administer without a blood filter.
6. Do not add Lactated Ringer's solution to red blood cells. It is safest to use 0.9% NaCl as the only fluid/drug administered in conjunction with this product.
7. Transfusion reactions can still occur in spite of correct blood typing and proper crossmatching.

Discussion: Crossmatching:
Current research divides canine blood types into eight blood groups. Canine blood group A_1 (DEA 1.1 = dog erythrocyte antigen 1.1) has the most clinical significance, followed by Canine blood group A_2 (DEA 1.2). Canine blood group T_r (DEA 7) has apparently limited clinical significance.

For purposes of identifying the blood types of the dog donors, the phrase A negative indicates that the donor does not possess either the DEA 1.1 or 1.2 antigen. Likewise, the phrase A positive is on blood bags to indicate that the donor is positive for DEA 1.1 or 1.2.

It is recommended that A-/A+ blood typing be a routine presurgical procedure and a routine part of each animal's first physical examination (and recorded in its permanent medical record), in order to facilitate subsequent transfusion therapy.

Blood crossmatching is recommended prior to every transfusion (in addition to using donor blood of the same blood type as the recipient). A major and minor crossmatch should be conducted prior to each transfusion involving red blood cells; a minor crossmatch should be conducted prior to every transfusion of plasma.

1. Collect 2 mL of recipient blood in a serum tube and 1 mL of recipient blood in an EDTA or heparin tube.
2. Remove (cut) one or two numbered tubing segments from the bag of donor blood; gently shake this segment(s) in order to mix the contents; then collect 2 mL of this donor blood into an empty tube (the Animal Blood Bank donor blood already has CPDA-1 anticoagulant in it; therefore do not add more anticoagulant).

3. Centrifuge all three glass tubes at 3400 x G for one minute (or allow the cells to sediment down by letting the samples stand for 30 minutes or longer).
4. Decant recipient plasma, retaining recipient packed RBC's. Carefully remove and save the donor plasma, retaining the donor packed RBC's as well. The recipient serum tube may remain as is.
5. Temporarily ignoring the recipient serum tube, wash the two packed RBC tubes as follows: (i) add 2 or 3 mL of 0.9% saline to each RBC tube; (ii) resuspend the cells; (iii) centrifuge as in step (3) above; (iv) discard supernatant, retaining packed RBC's; (v) repeat this wash two more times, ending with two tubes of packed RBC's (donor and recipient).
6. In addition to the donor plasma and recipient serum saved from step (4), prepare new tubes as follows: donor 4% RBC suspension (0.2 mL of packed RBC's plus 4.8 mL of 0.9% saline); and recipient 4% RBC suspension (0.2 mL of recipient packed RBC's plus 4.8 mL of 0.9% saline).
7. Now prepare four more glass tubes as follows:
   Tube G-1: Two drops donor plasma and one drop donor 4% RBC suspension (donor control - should not react).
   Tube G-2: Two drops recipient serum and one drop recipient 4% RBC suspension (recipient control - should not react).
   Tube G-3: Two drops donor plasma and one drop recipient 4% RBC suspension (minor crossmatch).
   Tube G-4: Two drops recipient serum and one drop donor 4% RBC suspension (major crossmatch).
8. If time permits, prepare three sets of the tubes listed in step (7), and incubate one set at 77°F (25°C); one set at 98.6°F (37°C); and the third set at 39.2°F (4°C). If unable to prepare three sets, conduct the crossmatch at 25°C.
9. Now centrifuge all step (8) tubes at 3400 x G for one minute.
10. Examine the supernatant of all step (9) tubes for hemolysis, then gently tap the tubes to resuspend the red cells and observe for agglutination. Compare the control tubes with the major and minor crossmatch tubes.
    If the major or minor crossmatch shows any agglutination or hemolysis, it is strongly recommended that a different donor blood be considered for that particular recipient.
    A crossmatch should still be conducted even if the donor and recipient are known to have the same blood type.

References: Available upon request.
Presentation: Units of CANINE RED BLOOD CELLS are supplied refrigerated, in blood grade plastic bags (with integral hypodermic needle injection port, two IV line coupling ports, and reference aliquots [tubing segments]).
Compendium Code No.: 13980010

CANINE THYROID CHEWABLE TABLETS ℞

Pala-Tech **Thyroid Therapy**

Levothyroxine Sodium, USP

Active Ingredient(s): Composition: Each scored, round chewable tablet contains either 0.1 mg, 0.2 mg, 0.3 mg, 0.4 mg, 0.5 mg, 0.6 mg, 0.7 mg or 0.8 mg of Levothyroxine Sodium, USP in a proprietary, highly palatable roast beef and liver flavor base.
Indications: Provides thyroid replacement therapy in all conditions of inadequate production of thyroid hormones (hypothyroidism) in dogs.
Pharmacology: Each tablet, Pala-Tech™ CANINE THYROID CHEWABLE TABLETS (Levothyroxine Sodium, USP), provides synthetic crystalline levothyroxine sodium (L-thyroxine).
The structural formula for levothyroxine sodium is:

HO–(diiodophenyl)–O–(diiodophenyl)–$CH_2CH(NH_2)COONa \cdot xH_2O$

Levothyroxine Sodium Action: Levothyroxine sodium acts, as does endogenous thyroxine, to stimulate metabolism, growth, development and differentiation of tissues. It increases the rate of energy exchange and increases the maturation rate of the epiphyses. Levothyroxine sodium is absorbed rapidly from the gastrointestinal tract after oral administration. Following absorption, the compound becomes bound to the serum alpha globulin fraction. For purposes of comparison, 0.1 mg of levothyroxine sodium elicits a clinical response approximately equal to that produced by one grain (65 mg) of desiccated thyroid.
Dosage and Administration: Dosage: The initial recommended dose of levothyroxine is 0.1 mg/10 lb (4.5 kg) body weight twice daily. Dosage is then adjusted by monitoring the post-pill blood level of thyroid hormone in the dog every four weeks until an adequate maintenance dosage is established. The usual maintenance dose is 0.1 mg/10 lb (4.5 kg) once daily.
Administration: Each tablet, Pala-Tech™ CANINE THYROID CHEWABLE TABLETS, may be given orally to dogs as a treat, or crumbled over their food at the veterinarian-prescribed dose. If crumbled over food, consumption should be monitored.
Contraindication(s): Levothyroxine sodium therapy is contraindicated in thyrotoxicosis, acute myocardial infarction and uncorrected adrenal insufficiency. Use in pregnant bitches has not been evaluated.
Precaution(s): Store at controlled room temperature; 15°C to 30°C (59°F to 86°F) and protect from light.
Caution(s): Federal law restricts this drug to use by or on the order of a licensed veterinarian.
The effects of levothyroxine sodium therapy are slow to manifest. Overdosage of any thyroid drug may produce the signs and symptoms of thyrotoxicosis including, but not limited to: polydipsia, polyuria, polyphagia, reduced heat tolerance and hyperactivity or personality change. Administer with caution to animals with clinically significant heart disease, hypertension, or other complications for which a sharply increased metabolic rate might prove hazardous.
Adverse Reactions: There are no particular adverse reactions associated with levothyroxine sodium therapy at the recommended dosage levels. Overdosage will result in the signs of thyrotoxicosis listed above under Cautions.
Discussion: Hypothyroidism is the generalized metabolic disease resulting from deficiency of the thyroid hormones levothyroxine (T_4) and liothyronine (T_3). Each tablet, Pala-Tech™ CANINE THYROID CHEWABLE TABLETS (Levothyroxine Sodium, USP), will provide levothyroxine (T_4) as a substrate for the physiologic deiodination to liothyronine (T_3). Administration of levothyroxine sodium alone will result in complete physiologic thyroid replacement.
Canine hypothyroidism is usually primary, i.e. due to the atrophy of the thyroid gland. In the majority of cases the atrophy is associated with lymphocytic thyroiditis and in the remainder it is non-inflammatory and as of yet unknown etiology. Less than 10 percent of cases of hypothyroidism are secondary, i.e. due to deficiency of thyroid stimulating hormone (TSH). TSH deficiency may occur as a component of congenital hypopituitarism or as an acquired disorder in adult dogs, in which case it is invariably due to the growth of a pituitary tumor.
Hypothyroidism in the Dog: Hypothyroidism usually occurs in middle-aged and older dogs although the condition will sometimes be seen in younger dogs of the larger breeds. Neutered animals of either sex are also frequently affected, regardless of age. The following are clinical signs of hypothyroidism in dogs:
Systemic: Lethargy, lack of endurance, increased sleeping; Reduced interest, alertness and excitability; Slow heart rate, weak apex beat and pulse, low voltage on ECG; Preference for warmth, low body temperature, cool skin; Increased body weight.
Musculoskeletal: Stiff and slow movements, dragging of the front feet; Head tilt, disturbed balance, unilateral facial paralysis.
Dermatological: Atrophy of the epidermis, thickening of the dermis; Surface and follicular hyperkeratosis, pigmentation; Puffy face, blepharoptosis, tragic expression; Dry, coarse, sparse haircoat, slow regrowth after clipping; Retarded turnover of hair (carpet coat of boxers).
Reproductive: Shortening or absence of estrus, lack of libido.
Gastrointestinal: Dry feces, occasional diarrhea.
Clinical Pathological: Hypercholesterolemia; Normochromic, normocytic anemia; Elevated serum creatinine phosphokinase.
References: Available upon request.
Presentation: Tablets are bilaterally scored. The tablets are packaged in bottles of 180 tablets (with child-proof caps) and 1,000 tablets.
Compendium Code No.: 10680050 4801-0699

CANINE WHOLE BLOOD

A.B.B. **Blood Product**

CA Vet. Biol. Lic. No.: 83
Active Ingredient(s): Each 10 mL CPDA-1 contains:

Dextrose (hydrous)	317 mg USP
Sodium citrate (hydrous)	263 mg USP
Citric acid (hydrous)	33 mg USP
Monobasic sodium phosphate (monohydrate)	22 mg USP
Adenine	2.7 mg USP
Water	q.s. USP

Table of Product Contents:

	Whole Blood	RBC's	Plasma	CPDA-1	Total Fluid Volume	Range
CANINE WHOLE BLOOD (1 unit)	approx. 112 mL	approx. 50 mL*	approx. 62 mL	approx. 16 mL	approx. 125 mL & 250 mL dbl. unit & 500 mL quad unit	120-130 mL

*Based upon an estimated average donor PCV of 45%.

CANINE WHOLE BLOOD is a transfusion product aseptically obtained from healthy dogs maintained in an isolated, controlled access colony. Blood is not pooled (ie. each unit of blood is from a single-donor) and euthanasia donors are never used. All colony donors are serologically negative for *Canine brucellosis, Ehrlichia canis, Borrelia burgdorferi* (Lyme Disease), and *Dirofilaria immitis*. The blood type of each donor dog is indicated on the product label. The colony receives intensive onsite veterinary health care, and all animals are current on immunizations, to include: Canine distemper, hepatitis, leptospirosis, parainfluenza, canine parvo virus, and rabies.
The anticoagulant CPDA-1 consists of citrate, phosphate, dextrose, and adenine, and provides for a 35 day shelf-life for CANINE WHOLE BLOOD.
Using the single-donor technique, a unit of CANINE WHOLE BLOOD consists of approximately 112 mL whole blood and 16 mL CPDA-1, for a total fluid volume of approximately 125 mL. Each unit (the plastic bag and contents) has blood sequestered in segments of the donor tubing. Crossmatching can be accomplished by means of sampling the contents of these tubing aliquots (without entering the primary bag. 250 mL and 500 mL units are also available.
Indications: CANINE WHOLE BLOOD is indicated for parenteral replenishment of acute blood loss (such as surgical or traumatic hemorrhage) and other anemias as indicated by the clinical condition of the patient and the judgment of the surgeon/clinician.
Dosage and Administration:
The clinician/surgeon should first determine the PCV of the blood in the donor blood bag by aspirating the contents of an attached numbered tubing segment [reference aliquot] (shake the segment to mix its contents before aspirating), and centrifuging the sample. After ascertaining the microhematocrit of the donor blood, the following formula may be used to calculate the volume of blood to transfuse:

$$\text{mLs of donor blood needed} = \frac{(\text{Recipient wt. [lbs.]} \times 40\ \text{mL/lb.}) \times (\text{PCV desired} - \text{Recipient PCV})}{\text{PCV of blood in donor bag}}$$

or

$$\text{mLs of donor blood needed} = \frac{(\text{Recipient wt. [lbs.]} \times 32\ \text{mL/lb.}) \times (\text{Hb desired} - \text{Recipient Hb})}{\text{Hb of blood in donor bag}}$$

Refrigerated blood should be warmed to room temperature before transfusing. Do not exceed 98.6°F (37°C).
Blood Filter: A blood filter should always be used when administering whole blood. When administering over 50 mL of blood to a patient, use the standard blood administration set with its integral 170-230 micron clot screen filter. When administering less than 50 mL of blood to a patient, the standard blood administration set's filter (with a relatively huge surface area) will trap too much blood. Therefore, when transfusing less than 50 mL of blood, the following configuration is recommended:

1. Remove one (1) red cap (white on some models) from the blood bag's diaphragm port, and insert the spike of the drip chamber end of a Venoset 70 Microdrip set into the now uncovered blood bag diaphragm port. The second red cap, found on whole blood bags, should remain in place. This second port is available for piggybacking a second IV system into the primary blood bag; or for attaching a transfer bag to extract plasma. Technically, non-vented fluid administration sets are safer then using blood bags. This can be simulated by aseptically replacing the Venoset's air filter with the male end of a 3 mL syringe, with its plunger in place. Never leave the Venoset's air filter port uncovered.
2. Attach the needle adaptor end of the Venoset into the female end of a Hemo-Nate neonatal filter, model #HN-179.
3. Then attach the male end of the filter to the female end of Abbott's 30 inch IV extension set.
4. Finally, attach the male end of the extension set to an IV catheter pre-positioned in the patient.
   With the above technique, transfusion can be obtained via a slow continuous drip over several hours (or longer), therefore minimizing volume overload.
5. If the bolus technique is preferred, simply aspirate the blood (from the blood bag's brown

hypodermic needle port) into a sterile syringe, then aseptically place the Hemo-Nate filter between the syringe and a fresh sterile needle/catheter, before transfusing.

The whole blood bags have an integral brown hypodermic needle port for syringe access.

6. For puppies and other small patients, adding 0.9% NaCl (not Lactated Ringer's) to the blood will tend to reduce its viscosity and therefore facilitate the use of 22 or 24 gauge needles/catheters.

Route of Administration: The jugular, cephalic, and saphenous veins are common sites for IV catheter placement. The intramedullary cavity of the femur and humerus are alternate sites. Additionally, intraperitoneal transfusions have application in selected patients.

Rate of Infusion:

1. There is virtually no rate of blood infusion that is safe for all canine patients; therefore the following are only general guidelines. The actual rate of infusion of blood must be tailored to each individual patient.
2. If clinical conditions permit, the initial rate should be slow (about 0.11 mL/lb. BW over a 30-minute period), in order to observe the patient for transfusion reactions.
(0.11 mL/lb. = @ 0.25 mL/kg).
3. Following the initial 30 minute trial infusion, in a animal with a normal state of hydration, whole blood may be infused at a rate of 10 mL/lb. BW per 24 hours (22 mL/kg BW per 24 hours). For hypovolemic patients the rate may be increased up to 10 mL/lb. BW per hour; however, given the wide range between those two rates, close monitoring of the patient is essential, with the actual rate being adjusted accordingly.
4. In using the continuous drip method, the blood products' volume is merely included in the 24 hour IV fluid requirements of the animal; then the drip rate is calculated by converting the 24 hour volume into a certain number of drips per minute, or per second (depending on if an infusion pump is being used or the drip rate is being visually monitored).

Post-Transfusion Patient Care: During and after transfusions, the patient should be closely monitored. In addition to physical examinations and temperature monitoring, measurement of PCV, urine output, body weight, and EKG are recommended. Measurement of CVP may be utilized in some cases. In all cases, infusion rates should be calculated (rather than estimated) and closely monitored.

Contraindication(s): Do not administer if the blood bags are leaking or if the supernatant exhibits brown or purple discoloration or if excessive hemolysis is present.

Do not administer (via the same infusion system) in conjunction with other fluids or drugs, except 0.9% NaCl.

Do not administer to species other than the domestic dog.

Precaution(s): The product has a shelf-life of 35 days from the date of collection from the donor dog. It should be maintained at a temperature of 33.8° to 42.8°F (1 to 6°C), except during shipment, when 33.8 to 50°F (1 to 10°C) is approved. Store the blood bags in a vertical position, with airspace between each bag (ie. avoid a sardine effect - RBC storage survival is apparently enhanced by the plastic bag's ability to breathe - that is one reason why glass is a less desirable storage container for blood).

Caution(s):

1. During transfusions, fluid flow rates must be carefully calculated and monitored, based on the patient's size, weight, age, and clinical condition. It is recommended that urine output be monitored as well.
2. Gently oscillate each bag before use in order to mix contents.
3. Complications of transfusions are manifest by a variety of clinical signs including jaundice, fever, cardiac arrythmias, erratic respiration, salivation, hemoglobinuria, edema, DIC, hemorrhage, vomiting, and urticaria. If any of these clinical signs develop, immediately stop the transfusion and institute appropriate supportive measures, as determined by the patient's clinical condition and the clinician's medical judgment.
4. For use in domestic dogs only.

Warning(s):

1. Circulatory overload can occur quickly unless all patient parameters are closely monitored.
2. Do not add medications to the blood bags nor via the same infusion system.
3. In spite of serological screening, disease organisms may still be present in these transfusion products.
4. Platelets are not viable in these products.
5. Do not administer without a blood filter.
6. Do not add Lactated Ringer's solution to whole blood. It is safest to use 0.9% NaCl as the only fluid/drug administered in conjunction with this product.
7. Transfusion reactions can still occur in spite of correct blood typing and proper crossmatching.

Discussion: Crossmatching:

Current research divides canine blood types into eight blood groups. Canine blood group A_1 (DEA 1.1 = dog erythrocyte antigen 1.1) has the most clinical significance, followed by Canine blood group A_2 (DEA 1.2). Canine blood group T_r (DEA 7) has apparently limited clinical significance.

For purposes of identifying the blood types of the dog donors, the phrase A negative indicates that the donor does not possess either the DEA 1.1 or 1.2 antigen. Likewise, the phrase A positive is on blood bags to indicate that the donor is positive for DEA 1.1 or 1.2.

It is recommended that A-/A+ blood typing be a routine presurgical procedure and a routine part of each animal's first physical examination (and recorded in its permanent medical record), in order to facilitate subsequent transfusion therapy.

Blood crossmatching is recommended prior to every transfusion (in addition to using donor blood of the same blood type as the recipient). A major and minor crossmatch should be conducted prior to each transfusion involving whole blood; a minor crossmatch should be conducted prior to every transfusion of plasma.

1. Collect 2 mL of recipient blood in a serum tube and 1 mL of recipient blood in an EDTA or heparin tube.
2. Remove (cut) one or two numbered tubing segments from the bag of donor blood; gently shake this segment(s) in order to mix the contents; then collect 2 mL of this donor blood into an empty tube (the Animal Blood Bank donor blood already has CPDA-1 anticoagulant in it; therefore do not add more anticoagulant).
3. Centrifuge all three glass tubes at 3400 x G for one minute (or allow the cells to sediment down by letting the samples stand for 30 minutes or longer).
4. Decant recipient plasma, retaining recipient packed RBC's. Carefully remove and save the donor plasma, retaining the donor packed RBC's as well. The recipient serum tube may remain as is.
5. Temporarily ignoring the recipient serum tube, wash the two packed RBC tubes as follows: (i) add 2 or 3 mL of 0.9% saline to each RBC tube; (ii) resuspend the cells; (iii) centrifuge as in step (3) above; (iv) discard supernatant, retaining packed RBC's; (v) repeat this wash two more times, ending with two tubes of packed RBC's (donor and recipient).
6. In addition to the donor plasma and recipient serum saved from step (4), prepare new tubes as follows: donor 4% RBC suspension (0.2 mL of packed RBC's plus 4.8 mL of 0.9% saline); and recipient 4% RBC suspension (0.2 mL of recipient packed RBC's plus 4.8 mL of 0.9% saline).
7. Now prepare four more glass tubes as follows:
Tube G-1: Two drops donor plasma and one drop donor 4% RBC suspension (donor control - should not react).
Tube G-2: Two drops recipient serum and one drop recipient 4% RBC suspension (recipient control - should not react).
Tube G-3: Two drops donor plasma and one drop recipient 4% RBC suspension (minor crossmatch).
Tube G-4: Two drops recipient serum and one drop donor 4% RBC suspension (major crossmatch).
8. If time permits, prepare three sets of the tubes listed in step (7), and incubate one set at 77°F (25°C); one set at 98.6°F (37°C); and the third set at 39.2°F (4°C). If unable to prepare three sets, conduct the crossmatch at 25°C.
9. Now centrifuge all step (8) tubes at 3400 x G for one minute.
10. Examine the supernatant of all step (9) tubes for hemolysis, then gently tap the tubes to resuspend the red cells and observe for agglutination. Compare the control tubes with the major and minor crossmatch tubes.
If the major or minor crossmatch shows any agglutination or hemolysis, it is strongly recommended that a different donor blood be considered for that particular recipient.
A crossmatch should still be conducted even if the donor and recipient are known to have the same blood type.

References: Available upon request.

Presentation: Units of CANINE WHOLE BLOOD are supplied refrigerated, in blood grade plastic bags (with integral hypodermic needle injection port, two IV line coupling ports, and reference aliquots [tubing segments]).

Compendium Code No.: 13980020

CANINE WHOLE BLOOD

P.V.R. **Blood Product**

Description: This product contains whole blood which is composed of red blood cells, white blood cells, plasma components, and anticoagulants. Blood is the means by which oxygen and nutritive materials are transported to the tissues and carbon dioxide with other metabolic products are removed for excretion. This product was obtained from universal donor dogs with a packed cell volume (PCV) of 37% to 55%. Actual product packed cell volume (PCV) will range from 35 to 50%.

Indications: Whole blood is indicated for moderate to severe hemostatic defects such as blood loss anemia or any such condition whereas the total blood volume is decreased. Whole blood should not be considered as a provider of viable white blood cells or coagulation factors.

Dosage and Administration:

1. Properly determine if the patient need for blood therapy and which product should be used. Cross match donor and recipient blood (description provided).
2. Utilize a slow intravenous drip for 15-20 minutes while monitoring dog for clinical signs on incompatibility. Without no clinical reaction symptoms, continue steady drip for approximately 2-3 hours.

Type of product	Indications	Hazards
Whole blood	anemia (decreased PCV) with volume deficit	Review adverse reactions section
Packed Red blood cells	anemia without volume deficit. Low PCV only	Review adverse reactions section
Fresh Frozen Plasma	Deficit of stable coagulations factors and associated proteins (normal PCV)	Review adverse reactions section

3. Never vent infusion bag to outside air.
4. Blood and associated components must be administered through an appropriate blood administration set with a clot filter included.
5. Warm and gently agitate blood components to no more than 37°C prior to administration.
6. Never use blood or blood components as a means to administer other drugs or fluids such as ringers lactate, electrolytes, dextrose, diuretics, etc.
7. During normal handling and shipping, some hemolysis or blood breakdown will occur. This will occasionally appear as a pink supernate. Any cloudy material, clotted fragments, or obvious discoloration of this product should be reported to Professional Veterinary Research, Inc. (812) 358-9078.
8. Gently warm blood by water bath or commercial heater without allowing any water into injection ports. Watertight wraps of bags are suggested prior to emersion into the bath.
9. After warming, administer blood at .10 mL/pound (.05 mL/kilogram body weight) slowly for first 20-30 minutes. During this period, it is essential to clinically monitor these animals for signs of transfusion reactions. Continue to administer blood at slow rate for next 2-4 hours. Please note more rapid infusion of blood can be obtained under emergency situations.
10. Care should be taken in all blood or blood product infusions. Often, medical therapy with proper fluid replacement (ringers lactate, hypotonic saline) can replenish fluid volume loss without the need of blood products.
11. Due to the wide range of infusion rates, in patients always closely monitor animals that receive blood products.

Contraindication(s): Whole blood should only be used when other therapeutic treatments can not safely replenish the blood volume and/or oxygen carrying capacity of the circulating red blood cell mass. All blood transfusions are contraindicated in animals with normal to above normal packed cell volumes which can result in circulatory overloads. Whole blood administration is contraindicated in some cases involving advanced cardiac disease or renal impairment.

Caution(s): The safety and efficacy of whole blood administration in dogs has been documented for several years in veterinary literature. If used correctly and as indicated, blood therapy can be extremely beneficial to the recipient. If used incorrectly or haphazardly, an incompatible blood infusion can cause any or all of the listed clinical signs listed below:

1) Fever/chills
2) Urticaria
3) Vomiting, nausea
4) Hemolysis
   A. Hemoglobinemia and hemoglobinuria
   B. Bilirubinemia and bilirubinuria
   C. Recurrent anemia
   D. Acute renal failure

E. Disseminated intravascular coagulopathy
5) Hypotension
6) Anaphylactic shock
7) Death

Warning(s): Blood products can cause immunologic complications such as reactions caused by incompatible red cells, reactions caused by incompatible white blood cells, and/or reactions caused by incompatible plasma constituents. Nonimmunologic reactions can also occur with improper handling, administration, and/or storage of blood products. To prevent transfusion incompatibility one should: 1) Crossmatch donor and recipient blood prior to transfusion. 2) Use only dog donors: negative for Dea 1.1, Dea 1.2, and Dea 7 canine red cell surface antigens. 3) If a patient has already suffered a serious reaction and does require future transfusions, cross-match blood and administer antihistamines and/or glucocorticoids prior to and during the transfusion. Nonimmunologic reactions can be minimized by: 1) Premix and prewarm blood. 2) Maintain intrinsic warmth by passing blood through gentle waterbaths or commercial warmers. 3) Maintain a continuous but slow rate of infusion except under emergency situations. 4) Use proper filters to remove particulate matter. 5) Maintain sterile technique when placing all in dwelling catheters and setups. 6) Administer appropriate doses based on body weight, need, and blood parameters which should be closely monitored.

Of equal importance, the risk of lateral disease transmission does exist from this product. Professional Veterinary Research, Inc. maintains a closed access colony of universal donor dogs that have been serologically tested for *Brucella canis, Ehrlichia canis, Borrelia burgdorferi*, and *Dirofilaria immitis*. All animals are housed in indoor biosecure kennel runs on plastic flooring and are vaccinated quarterly for Canine Distemper, Adenovirus type 2, Leptospirosis, Parainfluenza, and Canine Parvo Virus. Dogs are also vaccinated yearly for Rabies.

For intravenous use in dogs only.

Adverse Reactions: Hemolytic transfusion reactions either acute or delayed can occur following a blood transfusion with donor/recipient blood incompatibilities. To reduce this risk of hypersensitivity reactions, all donor and recipient blood products should have a major and minor crossmatch prior to every transfusion. Uncommon nonimmunologic complications are listed below:

1. Circulatory overload. All recipient animals must have an absence of overall blood volume prior to infusion. It is strongly recommended to monitor patients hematocrict (PCV), hemoglobin concentration, and all other clinical parameters prior to and during transfusion. Pulmonary edema is generally noted in circulatory overload reactions and can occur when excessive volumes are given. Older geriatric patients, toy breed dogs, and animals with chronic diseases that manifest by reducing red cell mass and increase plasma volume are particularly at risk. If pulmonary edema is noted, stop fluid placements and treat immediately.
2. Air Embolism. Care should be taken to remove excess air from all fluid paths and I.V. lines prior to transfusion.
3. Fever/hypothermia has been noted but usually is benign and transient.
4. Bacterial sepsis generally involving gram negative bacteria. Contamination of this product is rare but can occur with improper handling of the blood. The presence of primarily gram negative bacteria can cause severe endoxic reactions with subsequent fever, hypotension following transfusion which can lead to shock and/or death if left untreated. If the blood has abnormal clumping or discoloration, Professional Veterinary Research Inc. at 812-358-9078 should be contacted.
5. The transmission of infectious agents with blood transfusions are always possible. Donor dogs are tested serologically, and heavily monitored for signs of infection disease but the possibility of subclinical infectious prior to donation blood does exist.
6. Iron overload can occur but is extremely rare in patients receiving repeated transfusions over long periods of time.
7. Depletion or dilution of coagulation proteins can occur rarely after massive transfusion. Treatment with specific blood components may be useful.
8. Metabolic complications following massive transfusions:
   A. Hypothermia from infusing cold blood through a central venous line. Cardiac arrhythmia can occur unless blood is heated and delivered slowly.
   B. Citrate toxicity can occur rarely especially due underlying disease but can generally be treated by discontinuing the transfusion.
   C. Metabolic acidosis or subsequent alkalosis can occur post-transfusion but rarely requires drug intervention.

Presentation: 125 mL, 250 mL and 500 mL.
Compendium Code No.: 10440040

CANITEC™

DMS Laboratories **Allergen-Specific IgE Test**

Reagents and Materials:

1. Diluent - Two bottles each containing 125 mL of phosphate buffered saline with protein stabilizers and 0.05% thimerosal as a preservative.
   Mix gently before use. Avoid foaming.
2. Wash Solution Concentrate - Two bottles, each containing 125 mL of phosphate buffered saline with a detergent and 0.05% thimerosal as a preservative.
3. Anti-IgE Conjugate - One vial containing 0.35 mL of affinity purified anti-canine IgE antibody conjugated with horseradish peroxidase, stabilized with protein, in phosphate buffered saline and preserved with 0.05% thimerosal.
4. Substrate Solution - One bottle containing 125 mL of citrate phosphate buffer with urea hydrogen peroxide.
5. Chromogen - Five hermetically sealed packages, each containing a 20 mg tablet of o-Phenylenediamine Dihydrochloride (OPD).
   Warning: Harmful if swallowed, inhaled or absorbed through the skin. May induce contact hypersensitivity.
6. Stop Solution - One bottle containing 60 mL of 1 N sulfuric acid.
   Warning: Avoid contact with skin.
7. Allergen-Coated Wells - Thirty-five strips of allergen-coated wells. Each strip is coated with allergens relevant to either a geographic region or food groups.
8. Calibrator Strips - Five strips of calibrator wells coated with *Poa pratensis*.
9. Calibrator Sera - One set of three calibrators, each vial containing 0.75 mL of canine serum of known reactivity with *Poa pratensis*. Ready to use - Do not dilute. See calibrator label for expected absorbance units. Mix gently before use.
10. Control Sera - Two vials, each containing 0.25 mL, one of High control serum and one of Low control serum, specific for *Poa pratensis*.
11. Black, Uncoated Wells - One package containing three 12-well strips of reusable, black, uncoated wells.
12. Microtiter Well Holder - One reusable microtiter well holder with a 96-well capacity.
13. Microtiter plastic plate cover
14. Sponge
15. Matrix Sheet

Materials Required But Not Provided:
- Micropipettes for dispensing 50-200 μL
- Test tubes
- Microtiter plate washer/aspirator
- Distilled or deionized H_2O
- Microtiter plate reader operable at 490±5 nm
- Assorted glassware for the preparation of reagents and buffer solutions
- Timer
- Vortex mixer
- Absorbent paper toweling
- Microtest plate shaker (500 - 600 rpm) with a uniform horizontally circular movement (3-5 mm)

Indications: Assay for the *in vitro* determination of Allergen-Specific IgE in Canine Serum (CE - 306•SPF).

Intended Use: The IgE canitec-s Test Kit for Canine Allergen-Specific IgE is an enzyme-linked immunosorbent assay (ELISA) for the quantitative determination of allergen-specific IgE antibodies in canine serum. The assay is intended for *in vitro* diagnostic use only.

Test Principles: Principle of the IgE canitec-s Assay: An outline of the principle of the assay is represented in Figure 1. The allergen-specific IgE in the patient's serum binds to the allergen(s)[4] of interest, which have been adsorbed to the surface of polystyrene microtiter wells. After the removal of unbound serum proteins, antibodies specific for canine IgE, labeled with horseradish peroxidase (HRPO) are added, forming complexes with the allergen-bound IgE.

Following additional washing, the enzyme bound to the immunosorbent is assayed by the addition of hydrogen peroxide and o-Phenylenediamine Dihydrochloride (OPD) as the chromogen substrate. The quantity of bound enzyme and thus color varies directly with the concentration of allergen-specific IgE antibodies in the sample. The absorbance, at 490 nm, is a measure of the concentration of allergen-specific IgE in the test sample. The relative serum concentration of allergen-specific IgE antibodies can be expressed by a scoring system based on normalized absorbance (EA) units.

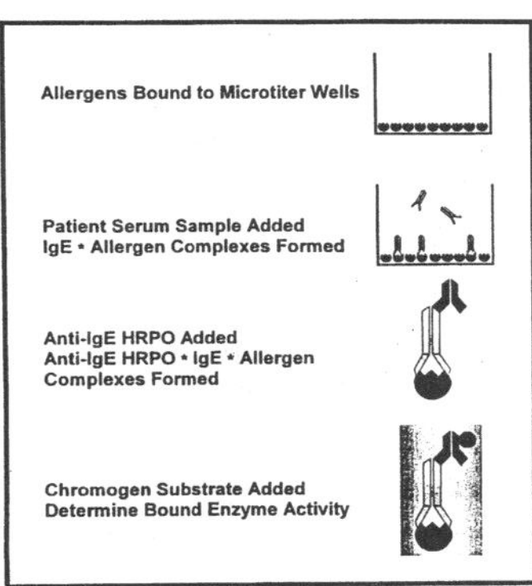

Figure 1

The results of the IgE canitec-s assay are stated in EA units.

These results can then be conveniently organized according to a scoring system which represents a general guideline of the relative likelihood that a particular allergen or group of allergens plays a clinically significant role in a patient already diagnosed as atopic and, as such, are useful when choosing allergens or groups of allergens for incorporation into prescription immunotherapy.

This scoring system also represents a general guideline of the relative likelihood that a particular patient is, in fact, atopic when considering the various factors in a differential diagnosis of atopy. However, the results do not provide a definitive conclusion as to the presence or absence of atopy, as a differential diagnosis of atopy must include clinical signs, patient history, and the results of other diagnostic test procedures as may be appropriate.

One such diagnostic test procedure that may be appropriate is IgG canitec. Allergen-specific IgG antibodies are considered to be "blocking antibodies" in the immune response to the presence of allergens to which the patient may be sensitive. One objective of immunotherapy is to increase the level of these blocking antibodies[5]. The presence of significant levels of such blocking antibodies at the time of initial examination of a patient may indicate that the presence of levels of allergen-specific IgE otherwise likely to be clinically significant may, in fact, be a benign condition in that patient at the time.

Test Procedure: Reagent Preparation:

1. Wash Solution: Add 100 mL of wash solution concentrate to 900 mL of distilled or deionized water to make a total of 1 liter of the working solution. The working solution is stable for one week from the date of preparation when stored at room temperature (20-25°C) or for one month at 2-7°C. Each microtiter well has a fill capacity of 0.4 mL. Mix required amounts in same proportions indicated above.
   Note: Crystal formation in the concentrate is common when storage temperatures are low. Redissolve crystals by warming the concentrate to 30-35°C before dilution.
2. Anti-IgE Conjugate: The working conjugate solution should be diluted immediately prior to use. Add 50 μL of conjugate to 5.0 mL of diluent (1:101 dilution) for each microtiter plate. Mix uniformly but gently. Avoid foaming.
3. Chromogen Substrate Solution: OPD is highly hydroscopic and will react with moisture in the air. Open only one package at a time and use immediately. To prepare the working chromogen substrate, add one 20 mg OPD tablet to 10 mL of substrate solution. Prepare just before use. The chromogen substrate is stable for one hour when kept from excessive heat and light. Mix thoroughly.

Specimen Collection and Handling: Blood should be collected by venipuncture and the serum separated from the cells (after clot formation) by centrifugation. Specimens may be shipped at room temperature and then stored at 2-7°C if testing is to take place within one week after collection. If testing is to take place more than one week after collection, specimens should be stored at -20°C. Avoid repeated freezing and thawing. No additives or preservatives are required for specimen preparation. Avoid sodium azide contamination.

Warning: Handle all specimens as if capable of transmitting disease.

Loading the Microtiter Plate: The microtiter plate is numbered 1-12 for columns, A-H for rows. Figure 2 illustrates a format to test six canine samples for the same panel of 12 allergen groups (wells 1-12).

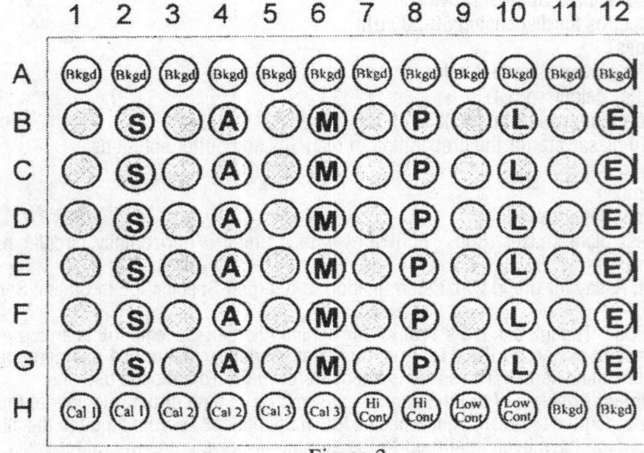

Figure 2

Insert one strip of allergen-coated wells in row A (allergen background), with the marked well positioned in column 12. For each sample to be assayed, insert one strip of allergen-coated wells into subsequent rows with the marked well positioned in column 12.

Insert one calibrator strip for each run for assaying calibrators, controls and the calibrator background. See Figure 2, row H. The calibrator strip is coated with the same allergen in each well, making well positioning unnecessary.

When testing less than six samples, it may be necessary to insert the black wells to fill the microtiter plate when using automated plate washers.

Procedure: Bring reagents to room temperature (20-25°C) before use.

1. Dilute sample and controls 1:26. To assay a single twelve-well panel, add 40 µL of sample to 1.0 mL of diluent, then mix by gentle vortexing. Dilute control sera in the same proportions.
2. Pipette 50 µL of diluted sample into wells B1 through B12. Pipette the next sample into wells C1 through C12. Continue until designated sample wells are filled. The unused portion of the plate can be filled with black, uncoated wells to facilitate plate washing.
3. Pipette 50 µL of Diluent into each of the wells in row A and into designated background wells in row H. See Figure 2.
4. Pipette 50 µL of Calibrator Sera and diluted Control Sera into the designated wells of row H. See Figure 2.
5. Cover the microtiter plate, place upon sponge and secure to the microtest plate shaker. Keeping plate level, shake at room temperature (20-25°C) for 45 minutes at 500-600 rpm.
6. Remove the covered plate from the shaker and aspirate the contents of the wells.
7. Fill each well with Wash Solution, then aspirate. Be sure to keep the plate level during the washing/aspirating procedure. Repeat for a total of four washes. Finally, invert the plate on absorbent paper toweling and wrap the toweling around the plate. Blot excess fluid by striking the plate firmly against a level surface several times.
8. Pipette 50 µL of appropriately diluted Anti-IgE Conjugate into each well. Return and secure the covered plate to the shaker, and shake at room temperature (20-25°C) for 45 minutes at 500-600 rpm.
9. Wash and blot the wells as described in Step 7.
10. Prepare the Chromogen Substrate Solution immediately prior to use. Protect from direct light.
11. Pipette 100 µL of Chromogen Substrate Solution into each well. Return and secure the covered plate to the shaker, and shake at room temperature (20-25°C) for precisely 15 minutes at 500-600 rpm. Protect from direct light.
12. After precisely 15 minutes, pipette 100 µL of Stop Solution into each well.
13. Incubate at room temperature (20-25°C) for 10 minutes.
14. Set the plate reader to 490±5 nm. Use one of the Bkgd wells (H11, H12) to zero the instrument, then read the absorbance of every well.

Stability of the Colorimetric Reaction: The absorbance of the final reaction can be measured up to four hours after the completion of the procedure, provided the plates are stored in a darkened, humidified chamber. However, good laboratory practice dictates that the measurement be made soon after the final incubation period.

Interpretation of Results:

1. Background Correction: To determine the correct absorbance units, each allergen background value must be subtracted from the test values for each corresponding allergen well; e.g., in Figure 2, the absorbance of background well A1 is subtracted from the absorbance values of each of B1, C1, D1, E1, F1, and G1. Subtract the average absorbance of the background wells of the calibrator strip, well H11 and H12, from the other wells in the calibrator strip. Multiply all corrected absorbance values by 1,000 and record.
2. Calculation of Normalization Factor: Review the example in Table 1 to become familiar with the normalization protocol. Determine the ratio of the expected absorbance of each calibrator provided with the observed calibrator values. If more than one set of calibrator wells is assayed, use the averages of the values obtained. Calculate the Normalization Factor using the mean of the ratios of the expected and observed calibrator values.

   The acceptable range of the Normalization Factor is 0.8 to 1.2.

Table 1 - Example: Normalization Factor Calculation

Calibrator	Expected EA Units	Observed EA Units	Ratio Exp/Obs.
1	1150	1197	0.961
2	700	681	1.028
3	250	239	1.046
Normalization Factor (NF) = 1.012			

3. Normalization of Control Values: Multiply the absorbance of high and low controls by the Normalization Factor to obtain the normalized EA units. The normalized EA units must be within ±20% of the expected values for a valid assay. For convenience, the expected range is shown on the label. If the normalized values are not within this range, the assay is invalid and should be repeated.
4. Calculation of Patient Values: Multiply the corrected EA values of the patient's sample by the Normalization Factor to obtain the normalized EA units.

Table 2 - Examples of Normalization:

Sample	Absorbance		NF		EA Units
#1	29	x	1.012	=	29
#2	77	x	1.012	=	78
#3	162	x	1.012	=	164
#4	421	x	1.012	=	426
#5	1250	x	1.012	=	1265

Results (Alternative Method) - Using Computer Software Programs:

1. Background Correction: To obtain corrected absorbance units, the allergen background value must be subtracted from the test values for each allergen, e.g., the absorbance of well A1 is subtracted from the absorbance values of B1, C1, D1, E1, F1 and G1 (see Figure 2). Repeat analogously for other columns (A2 through A12). The allergen background for the calibrator strip (H11, H12) should be averaged and subtracted from wells H1 through H10.
2. Calculation of the Patient and Control Values: Using conventional data reduction computer software programs such as Delta Graph® for IBM®-compatible computers or Cricket Graph® for Macintosh® systems, plot the background corrected observed values for calibrators 1, 2, 3 and the calibrator strip background against the lot-specific calibrator values provided with the kit.

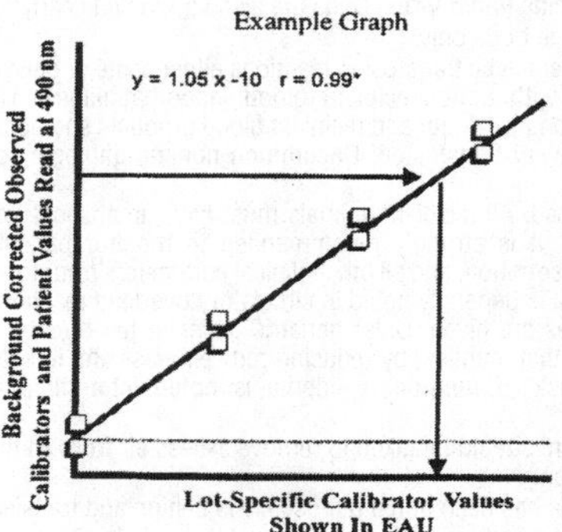

Figure 3

To calculate the corrected EAU (ELISA Absorbant Units) for the control and each sample, use the computer derived slope, $m\left(\frac{dy}{dx}\right)$ and the y intercept, b.

For example: Corrected EAU = $\frac{EAU - b}{m}$

Corrected EAU = $\frac{985 - 10}{1.050}$ = 929 EA units

*The acceptable range for the (r) correlation coefficient is 0.97 to 1.0.

Controls are provided with this kit for validation of procedure. The corrected EA units of each control value must be within ±20% of the expected values in order for the assay to be considered valid. The expected values are provided with each kit and the expected range is shown on the matrix sheet label. If the control values are not within range, the assay is invalid and must be repeated.

5. IgE canitec-s Scoring System: The patient values calculated in EA units can be conveniently organized according to a scoring system which represents a general guideline of the relative likelihood that a particular allergen or group of allergens plays a clinically significant role in a patient already diagnosed as atopic and, as such, are useful when choosing allergens or groups of allergens for incorporation into prescription immunotherapy.

   This scoring system also represents a general guideline of the relative likelihood that a particular patient is, in fact, atopic when considering the various factors in a differential diagnosis of atopy.

Table 3 - canitec Scoring System:

Class 0	EA Units		Class 1	EA Units	
0.1	20	22	1.0	51	54
0.2	23	24	1.1	55	58
0.3	25	27	1.2	59	62
0.4	28	30	1.3	63	67
0.5	31	34	1.4	68	71
0.6	35	37	1.5	72	76
0.7	38	41	1.6	77	82
0.8	42	45	1.7	83	87
0.9	46	50	1.8	88	93
			1.9	94	100
Class 2	EA Units		Class 3	EA Units	
2.0	101	108	3.0	211	232
2.1	109	116	3.1	233	255
2.2	117	126	3.2	256	281
2.3	127	135	3.3	282	310
2.4	136	146	3.4	311	341
2.5	147	157	3.5	342	375
2.6	158	169	3.6	376	413
2.7	170	181	3.7	414	454
2.8	182	195	3.8	455	500
2.9	196	210	3.9	501	550

Class 4	EA Units		Class 5	EA Units	
4.0	551	606	5.0	1451	1560
4.1	607	668	5.1	1561	1677
4.2	669	737	5.2	1678	1804
4.3	738	812	5.3	1805	1940
4.4	813	894	5.4	1941	2086
4.5	895	985	5.5	2087	2244
4.6	986	1085	5.6	2245	2413
4.7	1086	1195	5.7	2414	2594
4.8	1196	1317	5.8	2595	2790
4.9	1318	1450	5.9	2791	3000

Clinical Significance of Results: The EA units shown in Table 3 are expressed in a decimalized scoring system and are directly proportional to the relative level of allergen-specific IgE. The class scores into which the EA units are grouped represent the IgE canitec-s Scoring System.

IgE canitec-s Score 0.0-0.9 (EA units <50): EA units less than 50 are generally obtained from dogs which do not exhibit clinical signs of atopy when exposed to the allergens contained in the regional screen and can be considered negative for allergen-specific IgE.

IgE canitec-s Score 1.0 through 1.9 (EA units 51-100): EA units within this range indicate low levels of allergen-specific IgE and, thus, are unlikely to be clinically significant. These levels will rarely exceed the animal's pruritic threshold.

IgE canitec-s Score 2.0 through 4.9 (EA units 101-1,450): The EA units for each allergen or allergen group within this range are directly proportional to the relative levels of allergen-specific IgE and, therefore, indicate increasing likelihood of clinical significance. However, even these higher levels may not exceed the pruritic threshold of all animals.

In addition, some animals may naturally produce IgG blocking antibodies which, when present in large amounts, may moderate any hypersensitivity reaction. This may be particularly true with respect to dust mites and certain fungi. For these groups, most animals whose assay results are from 101 to 210 EA units (IgE canitec-s Score 2.0 to 2.9) have results on the IgG canitec assay greater than their IgE canitec-s results.

This is also the case for a large percentage of animals whose assay results are from 211 to 550 EA units (IgE canitec-s Score 3.0 to 3.9) and for a significant percentage of animals whose assay results are from 551 to 1,450 EA units (IgE canitec-s Score 4.0 to 4.9). Within each of these groups and in general, the percentage of animals whose IgG canitec results exceed their IgE canitec-s results declines as IgE EA units increase. The actual amount of circulating antibodies associated with canitec IgE EA units and IgG canitec EA units individually has not been established nor has the relationship, if any, between canitec IgE EA units and IgG canitec EA units.

IgE canitec-s Score 5.0 through 5.9 (EA units 1,451 - 3,000): Such a class score indicates extremely high relative levels of allergen-specific IgE and in only rare cases will these levels not exceed the animal's pruritic threshold. Because of differences in physiology and environmental exposure to allergens, diagnosis of atopy must include patient history, clinical signs, and the results of other diagnostic *in vitro* test procedures as may be appropriate, such as IgG canitec Allergen-Specific IgG.

IgE canitec-s Quality Control: In accordance with good laboratory practice, each laboratory should use routine quality control procedures to establish inter- and intra-assay precision and performance characteristics.

Limitations:

1. Proper performance of the IgE canitec-s assay depends upon many factors, including consistent ambient temperature, the quality of distilled or deionized water, and blotting of microtiter wells. Contamination of buffers may result in increasing non-specific background and/or erroneous values.
2. Inconsistent results may occur if there is improper and/or insufficient washing in steps 7 and 9 of the procedure.
3. Inconsistent values may result if the microtiter plate is not kept level during shaking, incubation and washing procedures.
4. The binding capacity of specific IgE from one allergen to another may yield identical results, but this does not necessarily imply clinical equivalence.
5. The assay indicates relative levels of allergen-specific IgE only. It is not intended to provide a definitive diagnosis of atopy. A differential diagnosis must include patient history and clinical signs.

Known Interfering Substances:

Sodium azide is known to interfere with horseradish peroxidase activity.

Chromogen substrate solution is light sensitive and should be protected from direct light and excessive heat.

Performance Characteristics: The precision of the IgE canitec-s assay for the quantitative determination of allergen-specific IgE antibodies in canine serum was evaluated on 6 separate occasions for 12 different allergen groups. The intra-assay and inter-assay coefficients of variation are listed below.

Table 4

EA Units	Intra-Assay C.V. (%)	Inter-Assay C.V. (%)
1478	2.2 to 4.7	4.5
808	4.0 to 5.2	5.1
423	4.5 to 9.7	5.9

Storage and Stability: Each component is stable until the date stated on each reagent label. Store all components at 2-7°C unless otherwise indicated.

Discussion: Summary and Explanation of the Assay: In 1967, Wide, et al[1], introduced the Radioallergosorbent Test (RAST) as an *in vitro* diagnostic method for the detection of IgE-mediated allergic conditions in humans. The canine analog of IgE has been isolated and its physiochemical properties described[2].

An increased understanding of the immunopathological mechanisms of IgE in atopy has resulted in the development of *in vitro* diagnostic procedures for detecting allergen-specific IgE in the canine species[3].

Based on this information, the Iatric Elisarest™ 18-hour assay was developed to determine the relative level of allergen-specific IgE antibodies in canine serum. This work led to the development of the IgE canitec-s, a new sensitive assay taking less than three hours to perform.

References: Available upon request.

Presentation: This test kit contains sufficient materials to test 30 samples when run in 5 batches of 6 samples each.

Elisarest and canitec are trademarks of Vetazyme Corporation.

Manufactured by: Vetazyme Corporation, 1706 West Fourth Street, Tempe, Arizona 85281.

Compendium Code No.: 14810001 PN3020306, 7/31/97

CA-P I.V. THERAPY ℞

RXV **Calcium-Combination Therapy**

Parenteral Solution

Active Ingredient(s): Contains: Calcium borogluconate, dextrose, magnesium borogluconate, calcium hypophosphite and base.

Total calcium chemically equivalent to calcium borogluconate 26.0%
Dextrose 15.0%
Magnesium borogluconate 6.0%
Total phosphorus in amounts chemically equivalent to elemental phosphorus 0.5%

This product contains no preservative.

Indications: For intravenous use in milk fever, and in calcium, phosphorus, magnesium and glucose deficiency in animals.

Dosage and Administration: Dosage: Cattle, 500 mL. For milk fever prophylaxis, give 200-500 mL at time of calving. Horses, 250-500 mL; Sheep 50-125 mL. Repeat in 2 to 6 hours if needed.

Note: Intravenous administration is always preferable. If used subcutaneously, always distribute dose in several places and massage to facilitate absorption.

Precaution(s): Store between 15°C-30°C (59°F-86°F). Unused portion remaining in bottle must be discarded.

Caution(s): Federal law restricts this drug to use by or on the order of a licensed veterinarian.

Large doses administered intravenously may have toxic action on heart if the blood level of calcium is raised excessively. Doses should be carefully regulated according to severity of hypocalcemia and injected slowly so that administration may be stopped if toxic action becomes evident.

For animal use only.

Warning(s): Keep out of reach of children.

Presentation: 12 x 500 mL bottles.

Manufactured by: Nova-Tech, Inc., Grand Island, NE 68801.

Compendium Code No.: 10910400 Iss. 05-01

CAPRINE POSITIVE REAGENT

Allied Monitor **Mycobacterium Test Reagent**

Active Ingredient(s): Serum obtained from adult goats, confirmed paratuberculous by culture and necropsy. It is sterile-filtered and lyophilized.

Indications: For use as a positive control in ELISA and AGID against PPA antigen.

Presentation: 1 mL.

Compendium Code No.: 10800021

CAPRINE SERUM FRACTION, IMMUNOMODULATOR

Professional Biological **Immunostimulant**

U.S. Vet. Lic. No.: 188

Contents: This product is a patented sterile filtered fraction of serum from pre-tested goats. Fraction is purified and standardized to assure uniformity of product.

Contains phenol and thimerosal as preservatives.

Indications: CAPRINE SERUM FRACTION, IMMUNOMODULATOR is recommended for use as an aid in combination with adjunctive therapy in treatment of horses with lower respiratory disease. This problem often occurs in athletic horses involved in racing, rodeo, jumping, endurance and other stressful exercise.

Response in treated horses is of an immunomodulating nature.

Dosage and Administration: Inject one 2 mL dose deep intramuscularly in the neck. Repeat this dose in 7-10 days in the opposite side of the neck.

Contraindication(s): Corticosteroids and other drugs which may cause immunosuppression are not recommended for use with this product.

Precaution(s): Store at 2° to 7°C.

Caution(s): For use by or under the direction of a licensed veterinarian.

Localized reactions - Protein-containing serum origin products may cause local reactions. These can include local swelling with increased heat at the injection site. Studies have demonstrated that these reactions are transient and usually recede within 48-72 hours. Rarely they may last longer. Moderate exercise aids in preventing or reducing local reaction. Discontinue use if a severe local reaction occurs.

Anaphylaxis - A systemic anaphylactic reaction is always possible after administration of a product of this nature. Discontinue use of this product and administer adrenalin or equivalent if such occurs.

Warning(s): Do not vaccinate within 21 days before slaughter.

For veterinary use only.

Discussion: Lower respiratory disease often occurs in athletic horses involved in racing, rodeo, jumping, endurance and other stressful exercise. When horses become ill, performance is reduced and they are usually removed from competition, often for an extended time period.

Trial Data: Efficacy testing included evaluation of recovery as measured by improvement in clinical signs and reduction and/or elimination of exudate of the trachea and lower respiratory tract by bronchoscope exam. These tests demonstrated a significant reduction in recovery time for horses receiving CAPRINE SERUM FRACTION, IMMUNOMODULATOR and adjunctive therapy when compared with horses receiving only adjunctive therapy.

Field safety testing included groups of horses from 6 months to 15 years of age.

Presentation: Packaged only in 10 x 1 dose (10 x 2 mL) containers.

This product license is conditional. Potency test studies are in progress.

Compendium Code No.: 14250050 63321

C

CAPSTAR®

Novartis **Parasiticide Tablets**

(nitenpyram)

NADA No.: 141-175

Active Ingredient(s): CAPSTAR® Tablets contain 11.4 or 57.0 mg of nitenpyram which belongs to the chemical class of neonicotinoids. Nitenpyram kills adult fleas.

Indications: CAPSTAR® Tablets are for the treatment of flea infestations on dogs, puppies, cats and kittens 4 weeks of age and older and 2 pounds of body weight or greater.

Directions: A single dose of CAPSTAR® should kill the adult fleas on your pet. If your pet gets re-infested with fleas, you can safely give another dose as often as once per day.

To give CAPSTAR® Tablets, place the pill directly in your pet's mouth, or hide it in food. If you hide the pill in food, watch closely to make sure your pet swallows the pill. If you are not sure that your pet swallowed the pill, it is safe to give a second pill.

Treat all infested pets in the household. Fleas can reproduce on untreated pets and allow infestations to persist.

Dosage: CAPSTAR® Tablets should be administered according to the following schedule. Weigh your pet prior to administration to ensure proper dosage. Do not administer to pets under 2 pounds.

Recommended Dosage Schedule:

Species	Body Weight	Dose	Nitenpyram per Tablet
Dog or Cat	2-25 lbs.	One tablet	11.4 mg
Dog	25.1-125 lbs.	One tablet	57.0 mg

Precaution(s): Storage Conditions: Store at controlled room temperature, between 59° and 86°F (15-30°C).

Caution(s): Not for human use. Keep this and all drugs out of the reach of children.

Adverse Reactions: Laboratory and clinical studies showed that CAPSTAR® Tablets are safe for use in dogs and cats, puppies and kittens 4 weeks of age and older and 2 pounds of body weight or greater.

Discussion: CAPSTAR® begins working within 30 minutes. In studies, CAPSTAR® achieved greater than 90% effectiveness against adult fleas on dogs within 4 hours and cats within 6 hours.

CAPSTAR® Tablets are safe for pregnant or nursing dogs and cats.

When using this product you may notice that your dog or cat will start scratching itself as fleas begin to die. The scratching behavior is temporary and is a reaction to the fleas, not the drug.

CAPSTAR® Tablets kill adult fleas that cause flea allergy dermatitis (FAD).

CAPSTAR® Tablets may be used together with other products including heartworm preventives, corticosteroids, antibiotics, vaccines, de-worming medications, shampoos, and other flea products.

Flea Infestations on Dogs and Cats: In addition to the common nuisance irritations associated with infestations, fleas can be responsible for skin conditions in your pet such as flea allergy dermatitis (FAD) in the dog and miliary dermatitis in the cat. Also, fleas transmit other parasites, including tapeworms. The control of flea infestations is important to your pet's health and also reduces the problems associated with these parasites.

CAPSTAR® Tablets do not have an effect on fleas in the pet's environment. You may need to treat more than one time because immature fleas in and around the home will continue to develop into adults that can reinfest your pet.

Alternatively, you can treat your pet or environment with an insect growth regulator, or you can treat your pet with an insect development inhibitor. Both insect growth regulators and insect development inhibitors act by preventing the development of immature stages of the flea. This will prevent fleas from reinfesting your pet. Laboratory studies have shown that CAPSTAR® Tablets can be used safely with lufenuron.

The following diagram illustrates the flea's life cycle and where CAPSTAR® Tablets work:

Life Cycle of the Flea:

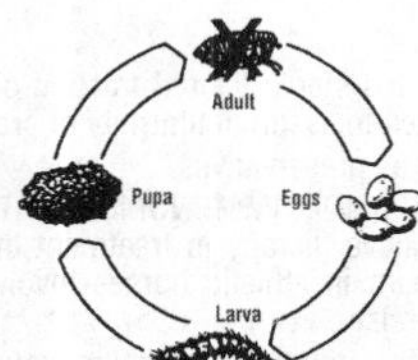

Fleas can be a problem because they reproduce so rapidly. A single female flea may produce up to 2,000 eggs over her lifetime. Eggs hatch and can develop into adults within only three weeks. Adult female fleas feed by ingesting blood from your pet and subsequently lay eggs, which drop off your pet's coat. Within days, larvae hatch from the eggs and live undetected in your pet's surroundings, such as the carpet, bedding and other protected areas. Flea larvae spin a cocoon, and when appropriately stimulated, a young adult flea emerges and jumps onto your pet to continue the life cycle. When these new fleas are seen on your pet, treat with CAPSTAR® Tablets.

Presentation: 6x11.4 mg tablet/package and 6x57.0 mg tablet/package.

U.S. Patent # 5,750,548

CAPSTAR is a registered trademark of Novartis.

Compendium Code No.: 11310102 NAH/CAP-T/PI/1 02/01

CARBOCAINE®-V ℞

Pharmacia & Upjohn **Local Anesthetic**

Mepivacaine hydrochloride USP 2% sterile aqueous solution

NADA No.: 100-703

Active Ingredient(s): Each mL contains 20 mg mepivacaine hydrochloride, 1 mg methylparaben as preservative, and sodium chloride for isotonicity. The pH was adjusted with sodium hydroxide or hydrochloric acid.

Indications: CARBOCAINE®-V Sterile Aqueous Solution is recommended for infiltration, nerve block, intra-articular and epidural anesthesia for horses. It has also been found useful for topical anesthesia of the laryngeal mucosa prior to ventriculectomy. As with other anesthetics, the dosage varies considerably depending upon the anesthetic technic, body area to be desensitized and the surgical procedure.

Pharmacology: Mepivacaine hydrochloride, 1-methyl-2', 6'-pipecoloxylidide monohydrochloride, is a white, crystalline, odorless powder, readily soluble in water, and very stable in aqueous solution. It is available as a 2% sterile aqueous solution containing sodium chloride (for isotonicity) and 0.1% methylparaben (as preservative). The pH is adjusted with sodium hydroxide or hydrochloric acid.

Clinical Pharmacology: Mepivacaine hydrochloride is a potent local anesthetic whose effectiveness and safety have been well established in human medicine and dentistry. Laboratory and clinical studies in animals have confirmed its value in veterinary medicine. Its anesthetic activity is two to two and one half times that of procaine, and it is equal to or better than that of lidocaine. The compound has shown excellent tissue compatibility in laboratory animals and in horses. Moderate transient edema at the site of injection may occur in rare instances.

CARBOCAINE®-V Sterile Aqueous Solution produces rapid and marked local anesthesia lasting for several hours. This enables the veterinarian to proceed with intended manipulations without delay and to complete the work under desensitization which is adequate even for prolonged operations. The innate vasoconstrictive activity of CARBOCAINE®-V Sterile Aqueous Solution may be enhanced by the addition of epinephrine at 1:100,000. The addition should be carried out aseptically for current use and any unused portion should be discarded.

Pharmacological studies in various species of animals, including horses, have shown that the drug produces complete and effective anesthesia at dosages that are no more than half those needed when procaine is used.

Dosage and Administration: The following dosages have generally proved satisfactory in the horse and are therefore suggested as a guide:

For nerve block (diagnosis of lameness, firing, pain relief in osteoarthritis and navicular disease): 3 to 15 mL.

For epidural anesthesia (animal standing): 5 to 20 mL.

For intra-articular anesthesia (removal of fracture chips, bone and bog spavin, arthritis): 10 to 15 mL.

For infiltration (alone or in combination with nerve block or intra-articular anesthesia): as required.

For anesthesia of the laryngeal mucosa prior to ventriculectomy: CARBOCAINE®-V Sterile Aqueous Solution may be administered topically or by infiltration or by a combination of the two. For topical application, a total of 25 to 40 mL applied by spray (3 mL/application) is usually adequate. For infiltration, 20 to 50 mL will suffice.

Precaution(s): Store at controlled room temperature 20° to 25°C (68° to 77°F) [see USP].

When administered by a skilled person, CARBOCAINE®-V Sterile Aqueous Solution may be employed safely for local infiltration, for common nerve blocking procedures, and for intra-articular and epidural anesthesia. The following precautions, which are observed with respect to all local anesthetics, also apply to this anesthetic. (1) Injections should always be made aseptically and with frequent aspirations. If blood is aspirated, the needle should be relocated and the injections continued cautiously. (2) When used for epidural anesthesia, care should be taken to avoid injection into the subarachoid space. The skin should be shaved and sterilized, and the needles used must be sharp and of the proper length. (3) The depth of anesthesia should be checked by pricking the area before manipulations are begun.

Caution: Federal (USA) law restricts this drug to use by or on the order of a licensed veterinarian.

Warning(s): Not for use in horses intended for food. Not for human use. Keep out of reach of children.

Presentation: CARBOCAINE®-V is available as 50 mL multiple-dose vials.

Manufactured by: Abbott Laboratories.

Compendium Code No.: 10490090

CARMILAX® BOLETS®

Pfizer Animal Health **Antacid-Laxative**

Active Ingredient(s): Each CARMILAX® BOLET® contains 27 g of magnesium hydroxide.

Indications: For use in cattle as an antacid and mild laxative.

Directions: Administer 1 bolus per 60 lb of body weight to a maximum of 6 boluses. Carmilax® Powder is recommended as the initial dose for prompt action or in calves less than 200 lb.

Precaution(s): Store at controlled room temperature 15°-30°C (59°-86°F).

Warning(s): Milk taken from dairy animals during treatment and within 12 hours after the latest treatment must not be used for food.

Presentation: 50 boluses per box.

Compendium Code No.: 36900350 20-6152-09

CARMILAX® POWDER

Pfizer Animal Health **Antacid-Laxative**

Active Ingredient(s): Each 1-lb tub contains:

Magnesium hydroxide. . . . . 361.0 grams

Indications: For use in cattle and sheep as an antacid and mild laxative.

Dosage and Administration: Mix 1 lb of CARMILAX® Powder into 1 gallon of water and stir thoroughly. Shake well before administering with a stomach tube.

Cattle, sheep and calves: Administer 1 pint of diluted product per 100 lb of body weight.

Precaution(s): Store at controlled room temperature 15°-30°C (59°-86°F).

Warning(s): Milk that has been taken from animals during treatment and for 12 hours after the latest treatment must not be used for food.

Presentation: 1 lb (454 g) tubs.

Compendium Code No.: 36900360 85-6156-12

CARRASORB™ FREEZE-DRIED GEL (FDG)

V.P.L. **Topical Wound Dressing**

Ingredient(s): (alphabetical order): Acemannan Hydrogel™, Hydroxyethylcellulose, Polyvinylpyrrolidone, Purified Water.

Indications: A topical wound dressing for medium exudating wounds such as pressure ulcers, diabetic ulcers, foot ulcers, stasis ulcers, post-surgical incisions, radiation dermatitis, and abrasions for horses, dogs, cats and other companion animals.

A sterile, preservative-free, freeze-dried pad of Carrasyn® Hydrogel Wound Dressing that absorbs wound exudate, conforms to the contours of the wound and creates the moist wound environment necessary for the natural healing process.

Directions for Use: Flush wound with a suitable wound cleanser. Peel and remove CARRASORB™ in an aseptic manner and apply to wound. Cover with a non-adherent dressing followed by a secondary dressing. Apply as often as necessary, usually daily.

In the case of dry wounds, CARRASORB™ can be moistened with a suitable wound cleanser to provide a moist wound environment.

Caution(s): If condition worsens or does not improve within 10 to 14 days, consult a veterinarian.
For veterinary use only.
Warning(s): Not for use in animals intended for food.
Keep this and all similar products out of reach of children.
Presentation: Fifteen 4" dia. (10 cm) CARRASORB™ Freeze-Dried Gel Pads per box (NDC 053303-013-16).
CARRASORB™ and Acemannan Hydrogel are trademarks of Carrington Laboratories, Inc.
Carrasyn is a registered trademark of Carrington Laboratories, Inc.
Compendium Code No.: 11430420 0B1

CARRAVET™ MULTI PURPOSE CLEANSING FOAM

V.P.L. **Grooming Product**

Ingredient(s): Water, isobutane, propane, ammonium laureth sulfate, methylparaben, fragrance, imidazolidinyl urea potassium sorbate, sodium benzoate, sodium laureth sulfate, sodium metabisulfite, aloe vera gel, extract containing acemannan*, tocopherol (vitamin E).
Contains no chlorofluorocarbons.
Indications: Water free shampoo.
Dosage and Administration: Shake well and direct spray toward area to be cleansed. Wipe away foam. Repeat if necessary. Does not need to be rinsed off.
Precaution(s): Contents under pressure. Do not puncture or incinerate. Do not store at temperatures above 120°F.
Warning(s): For external use only. Avoid spraying in eyes. Keep out of reach of children.
For animal use only.
Presentation: 4 oz (113 g).
* U.S. Patent Nos. 4,735,935 and 4,957,907.
Manufactured by: Carrington Laboratories, Inc.
Compendium Code No.: 11430110

CARRAVET™ SPRAY-GEL WOUND DRESSING

V.P.L. **Topical Wound Dressing**

Ingredient(s): (alphabetical order): Aloe vera gel extract containing Acemannan*, carbomer 940, citric acid, edetate disodium, imidurea, l-glutamic acid, methylparaben, panthenol, polyvinylpyrrolidone, potassium sorbate, purified water, sodium benzoate, sodium chloride, sodium metabisulfite, trolamine.
Indications: This product provides a protective, moist wound environment for the clinical management of 1st and 2nd degree burns, cuts, dermal ulcers, abrasions and other irritations of the skin in horses, dogs, and cats.
Dosage and Administration: Clip excess hair from wound area and thoroughly cleanse and rinse the wound with CARRAVET™ Wound Cleanser. Apply CARRAVET™ Spray Gel Wound Dressing in a quantity sufficient to cover the wound and wound borders. Apply as often as necessary.
Caution(s): For external use on horses, dogs, and cats only. Avoid contact with eyes. Discontinue use if irritation develops.
Warning(s): Not for use in horses intended for food.
Keep out of reach of children. For veterinary use only.
Presentation: 8 oz (226.8 g).
* U.S. Patent Nos. 4,735,935 and 4,957,907
Manufactured by: Carrington Laboratories, Inc.
Compendium Code No.: 11430120

CARRAVET™ WOUND DRESSING

V.P.L. **Topical Wound Dressing**

Ingredient(s): (alphabetical order): Aloe vera gel extract containing Acemannan*, carbomer 940, citric acid, edetate disodium, imidurea, l-glutamic acid, methylparaben, panthenol, polyvinylpyrrolidone, potassium sorbate, purified water, sodium benzoate, sodium chloride, sodium metabisulfite, trolamine.
Indications: This product provides a protective, moist environment for the clinical management of 1st and 2nd degree burns, cuts, dermal ulcers, abrasions and other irritations of the skin in horses, dogs, and cats.
Dosage and Administration: Clip excess hair from wound area and thoroughly cleanse and rinse the wound with CarraVet™ Wound Cleanser. Apply CARRAVET™ Wound Dressing in a quantity sufficient to cover entire wound and wound borders. Apply as often as necessary.
Caution(s): For external use on horses, dogs, and cats only. Avoid contact with eyes. Discontinue use if irritation develops.
Warning(s): Not for use in horses intended for food.
Keep out of reach of children. For veterinary use only.
Presentation: 1 oz (28.4 g) and 3.5 oz (99.2 g).
* U.S. Patent Nos. 4,735,935 and 4,957,907
Manufactured by: Carrington Laboratories, Inc.
Compendium Code No.: 11430130

CASE-BAC™

Colorado Serum **Bacterin-Toxoid**

Corynebacterium pseudotuberculosis Bacterin-Toxoid
U.S. Vet. Lic. No.: 188
Active Ingredient(s): *Corynebacterium pseudotuberculosis* bacterin-toxoid. Contains thimerosal as a preservative.
Indications: The product, when administered to healthy sheep according to label directions, will aid in the prevention and control of caseous lymphadenitis, a disease characterized by localized collections of pus in the tissues of the body.
Dosage and Administration: Shake before using so that the adjuvant, which may precipitate to some extent while the product is held in inventory, is well distributed at the time of use. Thereafter inject 2 mL subcutaneously (axillary space). Repeat the full 2 mL dose four (4) weeks later (axillary space opposite to the first dose). A booster dose of 2 mL should be administered annually.
Slight lameness (soreness) in lambs may be observed, along with lethargy, in a percentage of the mature animals following vaccination. Sheep are inclined to become depressed and may limp after foreign substances are administered or because of the increased exertion and stimulation of vaccination. While noticeable, these symptoms usually disappear within 24-48 hours and can be considered minor vaccination reactions. If suggested care is taken in preparing the vaccination equipment and in administering the product there should not be abscessation at the site of injection.
Precaution(s): Store in the dark at 2° to 7°C.
Caution(s): Handling of the product, filling of syringes, etc., should be done as aseptically as possible. Care has been taken to ensure the purity of the preparation at the time of release for marketing. Reasonable precautions should be taken in the field to maintain this condition.
Anaphylactic reactions sometime follow the use of products of this nature. Adrenalin, or an equivalent drug, should be immediately available for use in these instances. Delayed treatment could result in an irreversible reaction.
Sterilize needles and syringes by boiling in clean water.
Use the entire contents when the bottle is first opened. For veterinary use only.
Warning(s): Do not vaccinate within 21 days before slaughter.
Discussion: Caseous lymphadenitis is a chronic disease of sheep in which clinical signs and lesions may not be observed for several months after the animals become infected. Causative bacteria are likely to be present on the skin of susceptible animals and exposure may occur through wounds resulting from shearing, scratches, splinters or thorns. Abrasions provide access to the organism which thereafter migrates to the lymph nodes of the body. Exposure may also occur by pulmonary transfer so over-crowding of animals should also be avoided. The disease is not usually fatal but condemnations may run as high as 20% when carcasses are inspected following slaughter. Weakness and emaciation may develop in animals that are not held for slaughter, followed by eventual death.
The disease is manifested in two forms: (1) external abscesses in the superficial (mandibular, prescapular, and prefemoral) lymph nodes and (2) internal abscesses in the visceral organs especially in the lung, liver, and kidney and in the mediastinal, bronchial, and lumbar lymph nodes. Both forms may occur simultaneously. The visceral form of the disease is implicated in the thin ewe syndrome and can cause loss of fertility.
Abscesses and lesions formed in caseous lymphadenitis have a cheesy greenish-yellow to off-white odorless pus surrounded by a capsule. These lesions progressively enlarge. In older abscesses the pus becomes somewhat dry and firm and will form concentric layers within the fibrous capsule. *Corynebacterium pseudotuberculosis* is easily isolated from such abscesses and is usually the only organism present.
Once the disease has been introduced into a flock of sheep a relatively large percentage of susceptible animals will be affected. The organism is likely to spread by contamination from ruptured or lanced abscesses or at shearing time. Any infected animals should be shorn last and the shearing equipment thereafter sterilized. It is essential, in the control of caseous lymphadenitis, to exercise strict herd management with careful attention to examination, treatment, separation, and culling of the infected animals.
It has been shown that the product will control caseous lymphadenitis when sheep are vaccinated prior to exposure to the disease. It has also been shown that little or no benefit can be expected when animals with visible signs of the disease are vaccinated. Those showing infection should be immediately culled from the flock and disposed of or held away from those animals that appear to be in good health.
Presentation: Packaged in 10 dose (20 mL) and 50 dose (100 mL) bottles.
Compendium Code No.: 11010091

CASEOUS D-T™

Colorado Serum **Bacterin-Toxoid**

Clostridium tetani-perfringens Type D-Corynebacterium pseudotuberculosis Bacterin-Toxoid
U.S. Vet. Lic. No.: 188
Active Ingredient(s): The product is a combination of three antigenic substances, namely, *Clostridium perfringens* type D, *Cl. tetani* and *Corynebacterium pseudotuberculosis.* Contains thimerosal as a preservative.
Indications: The product is a combination of three antigenic substances adequate, when administered to healthy sheep according to label directions, to protect against (1) enterotoxemia caused by *Cl. perfringens,* type D, (2) toxemia caused by *Cl. tetani,* and (3) to aid in the prevention and control of caseous lymphadenitis, a disease characterized by localized collections of pus in the tissues of the body caused by *C. pseudotuberculosis.*
Dosage and Administration: Shake before using so that the adjuvant, which may precipitate to some extent while the product is held in inventory, is well distributed at the time of use. Thereafter inject 2 mL subcutaneously (axillary space). Repeat the full 2 mL dose four (4) weeks later (axillary space opposite to the first dose). A booster dose of 2 mL should be administered annually.
Slight lameness (soreness) in lambs and lethargy in mature sheep may be observed in a percentage of the animals following vaccination. Sheep are inclined to become depressed or will limp when foreign substances are administered or because of the increased exertion and stimulation of vaccination. While noticeable, these symptoms usually disappear within 24-48 hours and can be considered as minor vaccination reactions. If suggested care is taken in preparing the vaccination equipment and in administering the product there should not be abscessation at the site of injection.
Precaution(s): Store in the dark at 2° to 7°C.
Caution(s): Handling of the product, filling of syringes, etc., should be done as aseptically as possible. Care has been taken to ensure the purity of the preparation at the time of release for marketing. Reasonable precautions should be taken in the field to maintain this condition.
Anaphylactic reactions sometime follow the use of products of this nature. Adrenalin, or an equivalent drug, should be immediately available for use in these instances. Delayed treatment could result in an irreversible reaction.
Sterilize needles and syringes by boiling in clean water.
Use the entire contents when the bottle is first opened. For veterinary use only.
Warning(s): Do not vaccinate within 21 days before slaughter.
Discussion: Caseous lymphadenitis is a chronic disease of sheep, goats, and other small ruminants in which clinical signs and lesions may not be observed for several months after the animals become infected. Causative bacteria are likely to be present on the skin of susceptible animals and exposure may occur through wounds resulting from shearing, scratches, splinters or thorns. Abrasions provide access to the organism which thereafter migrates to the lymph nodes of the body. Exposure may also occur by pulmonary transfer so over-crowding of animals should also be avoided. The disease is not usually fatal but condemnations may run as high as 20% when carcasses are inspected following slaughter. Weakness and emaciation may develop in animals that are not held for slaughter, followed by eventual death.
The disease is manifested in two forms: (1) external abscesses in the superficial (mandibular, prescapular, and prefemoral) lymph nodes and (2) internal abscesses in the visceral organs especially in the lung, liver, and kidney and in the mediastinal, bronchial, and lumbar lymph nodes. Both forms may occur simultaneously. The visceral form of the disease is implicated in the thin ewe syndrome and can cause loss of fertility.
Abscesses and lesions formed in caseous lymphadenitis have a cheesy greenish-yellow to off-white odorless pus surrounded by a capsule. These lesions progressively enlarge. In older abscesses the pus becomes somewhat dry and firm and will form concentric layers within the fibrous capsule. *C. pseudotuberculosis* is easily isolated from such abscesses and is usually the only organism present.
Once the disease has been introduced into a flock of sheep a relatively large percentage of

susceptible animals will be affected. The organism is likely to spread by contamination from ruptured or lanced abscesses or at shearing time. Any infected animals should be shorn last and the shearing equipment thereafter sterilized. It is essential, in the control of caseous lymphadenitis, to exercise strict herd management with careful attention to examination, treatment, separation, and culling of the infected animals.

It has been shown that the product will control caseous lymphadenitis when sheep are vaccinated prior to exposure to the disease. It has also been shown that little or no benefit can be expected when animals with visible signs of the disease are vaccinated. Those showing infection should be immediately culled from the flock and disposed of or held away from those animals that appear to be in good health.

Enterotoxemia is most common in younger sheep and goats being fed a high carbohydrate diet which is a general practice in most feedlots. Animals on grass may also become infected but less frequently. *Cl. tetani* is found in the intestinal tracts of most animals. It is introduced into tissues in much the same manner as the micro-organism that causes caseous lymphadenitis.

Presentation: Packaged in 10 dose (20 mL) and 50 dose (100 mL) bottles.

Compendium Code No.: 11010101

CAT LAX®

Pharmaderm **Laxative**

Active Ingredient(s): Contains: Cod liver oil, caramel, lecithin, malt syrup, white petrolatum, 0.1% sodium benzoate, (preservative), vitamin E (*dl*-alpha-tocopheryl acetate equivalent to 0.033 mg/g *d*-alpha-tocopherol) (antioxidant), purified water.

Indications: A palatable formula for the elimination and prevention of hair balls in cats.

Directions: Many cats will accept CAT LAX® readily. For finicky animals place a small amount on paw - cat will lick his paw and become accustomed to the pleasant taste.

For Hair Ball Removal: For average weight adult cats, administer once daily. Squeeze approximately one inch of CAT LAX® from tube. For smaller cats, vary amount accordingly.

For Prevention of Hair Ball Formation: Administer two or three times per week.

Your veterinarian may give specific directions for treatment, in which case follow veterinarian's instructions.

Precaution(s): Store at room temperature.

Warning(s): For veterinary use only. Keep out of reach of children.

Presentation: 56.70 g (2 oz) tubes.

Compendium Code No.: 10880010

CAT-OFF™

Thornell **Deodorant Product**

Description: Does not contain enzymes, bacteria, nor oxidizers. Non-toxic, non-irritating, biodegradable, non-flammable.

Indications: To eliminate animal odors from urine, tomcat spray, feces and emesis in carpets, upholstery and other porous surfaces. Removes animal originated stains. Unlike enzyme and bacteria based products, CAT-OFF™ remains effective when used with or after most cleaners, shampoo and germicides.

The product penetrates to the source of the odor.

Dosage and Administration: For imbedded odors, apply with a sponge or cloth and soak the area, let dry. CAT-OFF™ must penetrate as deeply as the odor-causing problem. If any odor remains, CAT-OFF™ has not reached the source and the treatment should be repeated. If the odor is recent and not soaked in, CAT-OFF™ may be put in a spray bottle and sprayed on the affected areas.

For stains, rub the area thoroughly with a CAT-OFF™ soaked sponge or cloth. Let dry and vacuum. Although it is a quality stain remover, not all stains can be removed with a single agent.

Precaution(s): CAT-OFF™ has an indefinite shelf life.

Caution(s): For external use only. Always spot test for color fastness before using on fabrics.

Warning(s): Although safe, as with all chemicals, it should be kept out of the reach of children.

Presentation: 16 ounce ready-to-use bottle with applicator cap.

Compendium Code No.: 11210011

CAT-OFF™ CONCENTRATE

Thornell **Deodorant Product**

Carpet Deodorizer

Indications: Fast, permanent, safe elimination of odors from urine, tomcat spray, feces in rugs, upholstery, floors and more.

Directions: Mix up the required amount according to the following:

CAT-OFF™ Concentrate	Water
½ oz	1 pint (16 oz)
1 oz	1 quart (32 oz)
4 oz	1 gallon (128 oz)

Odor, deeply imbedded. In carpeting, upholstery, concrete and other porous materials, thoroughly soak the area, let dry. CAT-OFF™ must penetrate as deeply as the problem odor to be totally effective, If any odor remains repeat treatment. This kind of problem cannot be sprayed away.

Odor, recent. CAT-OFF™ may be used as above or put into a spray bottle and sprayed on the areas affected. Very effective when applied to the surface of litter boxes or tomcat spray.

Stains. Rub area thoroughly with CAT-OFF™ soaked sponge or cloth. Blot with clean cloth. Let dry and vacuum. Although CAT-OFF™ is a quality stain remover, not all stains can be removed by a single agent.

Always spot test before using.

Makes 32 pints (4 gallons).

Warning(s): Nontoxic, however, as with all chemicals, keep out of reach of children.

For external use only.

Presentation: 16 fl oz (474 mL) self measuring bottle.

Compendium Code No.: 11210020

CATRON™ IV

Boehringer Ingelheim **Topical Insecticide**

Permethrin Screwworm and Ear Tick Spray

EPA Reg. No.: 4691-122

Active Ingredient(s):

Permethrin (CAS No. 52645-53-1) 0.50%
Other Ingredients 99.50%
Total 100.00%

Indications: Recommended for use on wounds to kill and repel flies and fly maggots, to control ear ticks on livestock, and to kill and repel flies. For use on beef cattle, dairy cattle, sheep, goats, hogs and horses.

Directions for Use: It is a violation of Federal law to use this product in a manner inconsistent with its labeling.

Shake well before using.

Remove protective cap, hold container upright and spray from a distance of 12 to 15 inches except where stated otherwise. Remove birds and cover fish aquariums before spraying.

Directions for Use on Livestock:

To kill and control screwworms, fleece worms (wool maggots) and other blow fly maggots in and around superficial wounds: Spray wounds thoroughly allowing spray to penetrate into pockets made by maggots. Apply over discharge around wound to prevent reinfestation. Treat at five to seven day intervals until wound is healed.

To protect wounds from flies: For castration, de-horning, docking, branding, wire and shear cut wounds, spray directly onto the wound and on surrounding area. Treat navels of newborn animals. Apply to drainage area below wound to prevent fly infestations. Repeat at five to seven day intervals until wounds are healed. Bacterial infections of wounds should be prevented or treated with supplemental disinfectants or appropriate antibiotic therapy.

To kill ear ticks: For spinose ear ticks: Spray downward directly into animal's ear. Retreat as necessary. For gulf coast ear ticks: Spray directly onto ticks on outer surface of animal's ear. Retreat as necessary.

To protect beef cattle, dairy cattle, goats, sheep, hogs and horses from attacks of stable flies, horse flies, deer flies, face flies, house flies, horn flies, mosquitoes and gnats: Spray about 3 seconds on each side being careful to spray back, withers and forelegs thoroughly. To protect from Face Flies, spray the face and head, but do not spray into eyes. Repeat treatment when flies are troublesome.

To control blood sucking lice: Apply to the infested areas of the animal using a stiff brush to get the spray to the base of the hair. Repeat every 3 weeks if required.

To control poultry lice: Spray roosts, walls and nests or cages thoroughly. This should be followed by spraying over the birds with a fine mist.

Precautionary Statements: Hazards to Humans and Domestic Animals:

Caution: Harmful if swallowed, absorbed through the skin, or inhaled. Causes moderate eye irritation. Avoid breathing vapor or spray mist. Avoid contact with skin, eyes, or clothing. Wash thoroughly with soap and water after handling and before smoking or eating. Remove contaminated clothing and wash before reuse.

Avoid contamination of feed and foodstuffs. Remove pets and birds and cover fish aquaria before space spraying or surface applications. This product is not for use on humans. Vacate room after treatment and ventilate before reoccupying. Do not allow children or pets to contact treated areas until surfaces are dry.

First Aid:

If Swallowed: Call a physician or Poison Control Center. Drink 1 or 2 glasses of water and induce vomiting by touching back of throat with finger. If person is unconscious, do not give anything by mouth and do not induce vomiting.

If on Skin: Wash with plenty of soap and water. Get medical attention if irritation persists.

If in Eyes: Flush eyes with plenty of water. Contact a physician if irritation persists.

If Inhaled: Remove victim to fresh air. If not breathing, give artificial respiration, preferably mouth to mouth. Get medical attention.

Environmental Hazards: This product is toxic to fish. Do not apply directly to water.

Physical Chemical Hazards: Contents under pressure. Do not use or store near heat or open flame. Do not puncture or incinerate container. Exposure to temperatures above 130°F may cause bursting.

Storage and Disposal: Store in a cool, dry area. Do not transport or store below 32°F.

Replace cap, wrap container in several layers of newspaper. Discard in trash. Do not incinerate or puncture.

Warning(s): For swine: Do not ship animals for slaughter within 5 days of last treatment.

Keep out of reach of children.

Disclaimer: Warranty and Limitations of Damages: Seller warrants that this material conforms to its chemical description and is reasonably fit for the purposes stated on the label when used in accordance with directions under normal conditions of use and Buyer assumes the risk of any use contrary to such directions. Seller makes no other express or implied warranty, including any other express or implied warranty of Fitness or of Merchantability, and no agent of Seller is authorized to do so except in writing and with specific reference to this warranty. In no event shall Seller's liability for any breach of warranty exceed the purchase price of the material as to which a claim is made.

Presentation: 10 oz aerosol can.

Compendium Code No.: 10280272 BI 4234-1R-1 7/01

CATTLEMASTER® 4

Pfizer Animal Health **Vaccine**

Bovine Rhinotracheitis-Virus Diarrhea-Parainfluenza$_3$-Respiratory Syncytial Virus Vaccine, Modified Live and Killed Virus

U.S. Vet. Lic. No.: 189

Description: CATTLEMASTER® 4 is a freeze-dried preparation of chemically altered strains of IBR and PI$_3$ viruses and modified live BRSV plus a liquid, adjuvanted preparation of inactivated cytopathic and noncytopathic BVD virus strains. The liquid component is used to rehydrate the freeze-dried component. Viral antigens are propagated on an established cell line. This product is adjuvanted with aluminum hydroxide to enhance immune response.

Contains gentamicin as preservative.

Indications: CATTLEMASTER® 4 is for vaccination of healthy cattle, including pregnant cows, as an aid in preventing infectious bovine rhinotracheitis caused by infectious bovine rhinotracheitis (IBR) virus, bovine viral diarrhea caused by bovine viral diarrhea (BVD) virus, and disease caused by parainfluenza$_3$ (PI$_3$) virus and bovine respiratory syncytial virus (BRSV).

Directions:

1. General Directions: Vaccination of healthy cattle, including pregnant cows, is recommended. Aseptically rehydrate the freeze-dried vaccine with the liquid vaccine provided, shake well, and administer 2 mL intramuscularly. In accordance with Beef Quality Assurance guidelines, this product should be administered in the muscular region of the neck.
2. Primary Vaccination: Healthy cattle should receive 2 doses administered 2-4 weeks apart. To avoid possible maternal antibody interference with active immunization, calves vaccinated before the age of 6 months should be revaccinated after 6 months of age.
3. Revaccination: Annual revaccination with a single dose is recommended.
4. Good animal husbandry and herd health management practices should be employed.

Precaution(s): Store at 2°-7°C. Prolonged exposure to higher temperatures and/or direct sunlight may adversely affect potency. Do not freeze.

Use entire contents when first opened.

Sterilized syringes and needles should be used to administer this vaccine. Do not sterilize with chemicals because traces of disinfectant may inactivate the vaccine.

Burn containers and all unused contents.

Caution(s): As with many vaccines, anaphylaxis may occur after use. Initial antidote of epinephrine is recommended and should be followed with appropriate supportive therapy.

This product has been shown to be efficacious in healthy animals. A protective immune response may not be elicited if animals are persistently infected with BVD virus or incubating an infectious disease, are malnourished or parasitized, are stressed due to shipment or environmental conditions, are otherwise immunocompromised, or the vaccine is not administered in accordance with label directions.

Warning(s): Do not vaccinate within 21 days before slaughter.

For veterinary use only.

Discussion: Disease Description: IBR, BVD, PI_3, and BRSV viruses are commonly associated with respiratory disease and/or reproductive failure in cattle. IBR virus infection is characterized by high temperature, excessive nasal discharge, conjunctivitis and ocular discharge, inflamed nose ("red nose"), increased rate of respiration, coughing, loss of appetite, and depression. Cattle infected during pregnancy may abort.

A characteristic of IBR virus (BHV1) is that it establishes a latent infection in sensory neurons, typically trigeminal ganglia or iliosacral dorsal root ganglia.[1] From these sites of latency, it can be reactivated when an infected animal is stressed or injured. Subsequently, the virus is shed and transmitted by contact to other cattle.

BVD virus may be transmitted in nasal secretions, saliva, blood, feces, and/or urine, and by direct contact with contaminated objects; it invades through the nose and mouth and replicates systemically. Infection during pregnancy may result in abortion, fetal resorption, or congenital malformation of the fetus. Moreover, if susceptible cows are infected with noncytopathic BVD virus during the first trimester of pregnancy, their calves may be born persistently infected with the virus. Exposure of those calves to certain virulent cytopathic BVD virus strains may precipitate BVD-mucosal disease. Clinical signs of BVD include loss of appetite, ulcerations in the mouth, profuse salivation, elevated temperature, diarrhea, dehydration, and lameness.

PI_3 virus usually localizes in the upper respiratory tract, causing elevated temperature and moderate nasal and ocular discharge. Although clinical signs typically are mild, PI_3 infection weakens respiratory tissues. Invasion and replication of other pathogens, particularly *Pasteurella* spp., is thereby facilitated and may result in pneumonia.

BRSV is the etiologic agent of a specific viral respiratory disease of cattle of all ages, including nursing calves. Infection is characterized by rapid breathing, coughing, loss of appetite, discharge from the nose and eyes, fever, and swelling around the throat and neck. In an acute outbreak, deaths may follow within 48 hours after onset of signs. Clinically, BRSV infection may be indistinguishable from other viral infections associated with the bovine respiratory disease complex. BRSV infection, like PI_3, facilitates invasion and replication of other respiratory pathogens. Exacerbation of clinical signs has been documented when concurrent BRSV and BVD or IBR infection exists.

Trial Data: Safety and Efficacy: In safety studies of the fractions of CATTLEMASTER® 4, no adverse reactions to vaccination were observed and vaccinated pregnant cattle delivered normal, healthy calves.

The latency and subsequent excretion of the IBR virus fraction of CATTLEMASTER® 4 was determined in a safety study in which cattle were inoculated intramuscularly with the attenuated, temperature-sensitive IBR virus component and subsequently given corticosteroid to reactivate latent herpesvirus. Vaccination resulted in a characteristic serological response that remained unaltered even after corticosteroid treatment, indicating a lack of viral reactivation. Also, no BHV1 was recovered from mucosal swabs collected postvaccination or postcorticosteroid treatment, nor was it transmitted to nonvaccinated sentinel calves commingled with the vaccinates for the duration of the study. Further, no BHV1 DNA or latency-related RNA was detected in trigeminal or iliosacral spinal dorsal root ganglia collected after the administration of corticosteroid. Both nucleic acids were detected in a single cervical ganglion sample, suggesting a direct or proximate intraneural injection. BHV1 given by IM injection could not be reactivated from trigeminal ganglia, the primary site of BHV1 latency, demonstrating a lack of efficient viral replication in those sensory neurons. Excluding possible injection into nervous tissue (from which reactivation was not observed), the IBR fraction of CATTLEMASTER® 4 given by the IM route showed no propensity to establish latent herpesvirus infections.

Efficacy of each fraction of CATTLEMASTER® 4 was demonstrated in challenge-of-immunity studies. Cattle vaccinated with any fraction of CATTLEMASTER® 4, followed by challenge with a disease-causing strain of that fraction, showed no signs or had significantly fewer clinical signs than nonvaccinated control cattle. Serologic studies also demonstrated no immunologic interference among the fractions of CATTLEMASTER® 4. Antibody response was not significantly different between cattle vaccinated with an individual fraction and cattle vaccinated with the combined fractions.

References: Available upon request.

Presentation: 5 dose, 10 dose and 25 dose vials.

Compendium Code No.: 36900471 75-4135-06

CATTLEMASTER® 4+L5

Pfizer Animal Health **Bacterin-Vaccine**

Bovine Rhinotracheitis-Virus Diarrhea-Parainfluenza$_3$-Respiratory Syncytial Virus Vaccine, Modified Live and Killed Virus-Leptospira Canicola-Grippotyphosa-Hardjo-Icterohaemorrhagiae-Pomona Bacterin

U.S. Vet. Lic. No.: 189

Description: CATTLEMASTER® 4+L5 is a freeze-dried preparation of chemically altered strains of IBR and PI_3 viruses and modified live BRSV plus a liquid, adjuvanted preparation of inactivated cytopathic and noncytopathic BVD virus strains and cultures of the 5 *Leptospira* serovars identified above. The liquid component is used to rehydrate the freeze-dried component. Viral antigens are propagated on an established cell line. This product is adjuvanted with aluminum hydroxide to enhance immune response.

Contains gentamicin as preservative.

Indications: CATTLEMASTER® 4+L5 is for vaccination of healthy cattle, including pregnant cows, as an aid in preventing infectious bovine rhinotracheitis caused by infectious bovine rhinotracheitis (IBR) virus, bovine viral diarrhea caused by bovine viral diarrhea (BVD) virus, disease caused by parainfluenza$_3$ (PI_3) virus and bovine respiratory syncytial virus (BRSV), and leptospirosis caused by *Leptospira canicola, L. grippotyphosa, L. hardjo, L. icterohaemorrhagiae,* and *L. pomona.*

Directions:

1. General Directions: Vaccination of healthy cattle, including pregnant cows, is recommended. Aseptically rehydrate the freeze-dried vaccine with the liquid component provided, shake well, and administer 5 mL intramuscularly. In accordance with Beef Quality Assurance guidelines, this product should be administered in the muscular region of the neck.
2. Primary Vaccination: Healthy cattle should receive 2 doses administered 2-4 weeks apart. To avoid possible maternal antibody interference with active immunization, calves vaccinated before the age of 6 months should be revaccinated after 6 months of age.
3. Revaccination: Annual revaccination with a single dose is recommended.
4. Good animal husbandry and herd health management practices should be employed.

Precaution(s): Store at 2°-7°C. Prolonged exposure to higher temperatures and/or direct sunlight may adversely affect potency. Do not freeze.

Use entire contents when first opened.

Sterilized syringes and needles should be used to administer this vaccine. Do not sterilize with chemicals because traces of disinfectant may inactivate the vaccine.

Burn containers and all unused contents.

Caution(s): As with many vaccines, anaphylaxis may occur after use. Initial antidote of epinephrine is recommended and should be followed with appropriate supportive therapy.

This product has been shown to be efficacious in healthy animals. A protective immune response may not be elicited if animals are persistently infected with BVD virus or incubating an infectious disease, are malnourished or parasitized, are stressed due to shipment or environmental conditions, are otherwise immunocompromised, or the vaccine is not administered in accordance with label directions.

Warning(s): Do not vaccinate within 21 days before slaughter.

For veterinary use only.

Discussion: Disease Description: IBR, BVD, PI_3, and BRSV viruses are commonly associated with respiratory disease and/or reproductive failure in cattle. IBR virus infection is characterized by high temperature, excessive nasal discharge, conjunctivitis and ocular discharge, inflamed nose ("red nose"), increased rate of respiration, coughing, loss of appetite, and depression. Cattle infected during pregnancy may abort.

A characteristic of IBR virus (BHV1) is that it establishes a latent infection in sensory neurons, typically trigeminal ganglia or iliosacral dorsal root ganglia.[1] From these sites of latency, it can be reactivated when an infected animal is stressed or injured. Subsequently, the virus is shed and transmitted by contact to other cattle.

BVD virus may be transmitted in nasal secretions, saliva, blood, feces, and/or urine, and by direct contact with contaminated objects; it invades through the nose and mouth and replicates systemically. Infection during pregnancy may result in abortion, fetal resorption, or congenital malformation of the fetus. Moreover, if susceptible cows are infected with noncytopathic BVD virus during the first trimester of pregnancy, their calves may be born persistently infected with the virus. Exposure of those calves to certain virulent cytopathic BVD virus strains may precipitate BVD-mucosal disease. Clinical signs of BVD include loss of appetite, ulcerations in the mouth, profuse salivation, elevated temperature, diarrhea, dehydration, and lameness.

PI_3 virus usually localizes in the upper respiratory tract, causing elevated temperature and moderate nasal and ocular discharge. Although clinical signs typically are mild, PI_3 infection weakens respiratory tissues. Invasion and replication of other pathogens, particularly *Pasteurella* spp., is thereby facilitated and may result in pneumonia.

BRSV is the etiologic agent of a specific viral respiratory disease of cattle of all ages, including nursing calves. Infection is characterized by rapid breathing, coughing, loss of appetite, discharge from the nose and eyes, fever, and swelling around the throat and neck. In an acute outbreak, deaths may follow within 48 hours after onset of signs. Clinically, BRSV infection may be indistinguishable from other viral infections associated with the bovine respiratory disease complex. BRSV infection, like PI_3, facilitates invasion and replication of other respiratory pathogens. Exacerbation of clinical signs has been documented when concurrent BRSV and BVD or IBR infection exists.

Leptospirosis may be caused by several serovars of *Leptospira,* of which *L. canicola, L. grippotyphosa, L. hardjo, L. icterohaemorrhagiae,* and *L. pomona* are the most common affecting cattle. *Leptospira* localize in the kidneys, are shed in the urine, and cause anemia, bloody urine, fever, loss of appetite, and prostration in calves. Signs are usually subclinical in adult cattle. Infected pregnant cows, however, often abort, and dairy cows may exhibit a marked decrease in milk production. *Leptospira* spp. are known zoonotic pathogens.

Trial Data: Safety and Efficacy: In safety studies of the fractions of CATTLEMASTER® 4+L5, no adverse reactions to vaccination were observed and vaccinated pregnant cattle delivered normal, healthy calves.

The latency and subsequent excretion of the IBR virus fraction of CATTLEMASTER® 4+L5 was determined in a safety study in which cattle were inoculated intramuscularly with the attenuated, temperature-sensitive IBR virus component and subsequently given corticosteroid to reactivate latent herpesvirus. Vaccination resulted in a characteristic serological response that remained unaltered even after corticosteroid treatment, indicating a lack of viral reactivation. Also, no BHV1 was recovered from mucosal swabs collected postvaccination or postcorticosteroid treatment, nor was it transmitted to nonvaccinated sentinel calves commingled with the vaccinates for the duration of the study. Further, no BHV1 DNA or latency-related RNA was detected in trigeminal or iliosacral spinal dorsal root ganglia collected after the administration of corticosteroid. Both nucleic acids were detected in a single cervical ganglion sample, suggesting a direct or proximate intraneural injection. BHV1 given by IM injection could not be reactivated from trigeminal ganglia, the primary site of BHV1 latency, demonstrating a lack of efficient viral replication in those sensory neurons. Excluding possible injection into nervous tissue (from which reactivation was not observed), the IBR fraction of CATTLEMASTER® 4+L5 given by the IM route showed no propensity to establish latent herpesvirus infections.

Efficacy of each fraction of CATTLEMASTER® 4+L5 was demonstrated in challenge-of-immunity studies. Cattle vaccinated with any fraction of CATTLEMASTER® 4+L5, followed by challenge with a disease-causing strain of that fraction, showed no signs or had significantly fewer clinical signs than nonvaccinated control cattle. Serologic studies also demonstrated no immunologic interference among the fractions of CATTLEMASTER® 4+L5. Antibody response was not significantly different between cattle vaccinated with an individual fraction and cattle vaccinated with the combined fractions.

References: Available upon request.

Presentation: 5 dose, 10 dose and 25 dose vials.

Compendium Code No.: 36900481 75-4139-05

CATTLEMASTER® 4+VL5

Pfizer Animal Health **Bacterin-Vaccine**

Bovine Rhinotracheitis-Virus Diarrhea-Parainfluenza$_3$-Respiratory Syncytial Virus Vaccine, Modified Live and Killed Virus-Campylobacter Fetus-Leptospira Canicola-Grippotyphosa-Hardjo-Icterohaemorrhagiae-Pomona Bacterin

U.S. Vet. Lic. No.: 189

Description: CATTLEMASTER® 4+VL5 is a freeze-dried preparation of chemically altered strains of IBR and PI_3 viruses and modified live BRSV plus a liquid, adjuvanted preparation of inactivated cytopathic and noncytopathic BVD virus strains, *C. fetus,* and cultures of the 5 *Leptospira* serovars identified above. The liquid component is used to rehydrate the freeze-dried component. Viral antigens are propagated on an established cell line. This product is adjuvanted with aluminum hydroxide to enhance immune response.

Contains gentamicin as preservative.

Indications: CATTLEMASTER® 4+VL5 is for vaccination of healthy cattle, including pregnant cows, as an aid in preventing infectious bovine rhinotracheitis caused by infectious bovine rhinotracheitis (IBR) virus, bovine viral diarrhea caused by bovine viral diarrhea (BVD) virus, disease caused by parainfluenza$_3$ (PI$_3$) virus and bovine respiratory syncytial virus (BRSV), campylobacteriosis (vibriosis) caused by *Campylobacter fetus*, and leptospirosis caused by *Leptospira canicola, L. grippotyphosa, L. hardjo, L. icterohaemorrhagiae,* and *L. pomona*.

Directions:

1. General Directions: Vaccination of healthy cattle, including pregnant cows, is recommended. Aseptically rehydrate the freeze-dried vaccine with the liquid component provided, shake well, and administer 5 mL intramuscularly. In accordance with Beef Quality Assurance guidelines, this product should be administered in the muscular region of the neck.
2. Primary Vaccination: Healthy cattle should receive 2 doses administered 2-4 weeks apart. To avoid possible maternal antibody interference with active immunization, calves vaccinated before the age of 6 months should be revaccinated after 6 months of age.
3. Revaccination: Annual revaccination with a single dose is recommended.
4. Good animal husbandry and herd health management practices should be employed.

Precaution(s): Store at 2°-7°C. Prolonged exposure to higher temperatures and/or direct sunlight may adversely affect potency. Do not freeze.

Use entire contents when first opened.

Sterilized syringes and needles should be used to administer this vaccine. Do not sterilize with chemicals because traces of disinfectant may inactivate the vaccine.

Burn containers and all unused contents.

Caution(s): Occasional hypersensitivity reactions may occur up to 18 hours postvaccination. Owners should be advised to observe animals during this period. While this event appears to be rare overall, dairy cattle maybe affected more frequently than other cattle. Animals affected may display excessive salivation, incoordination, and/or dyspnea. Animals displaying such signs should be treated immediately with epinephrine or equivalent. In nonresponsive animals, other modes of treatment should be considered.

As with many vaccines, anaphylaxis may occur after use. Initial antidote of epinephrine is recommended and should be followed with appropriate supportive therapy.

This product has been shown to be efficacious in healthy animals. A protective immune response may not be elicited if animals are persistently infected with BVD virus or incubating an infectious disease, are malnourished or parasitized, are stressed due to shipment or environmental conditions, are otherwise immunocompromised, or the vaccine is not administered in accordance with label directions.

Warning(s): Do not vaccinate within 21 days before slaughter.

For veterinary use only.

Discussion: Disease Description: IBR, BVD, PI$_3$, and BRSV viruses are commonly associated with respiratory disease and/or reproductive failure in cattle. IBR virus infection is characterized by high temperature, excessive nasal discharge, conjunctivitis and ocular discharge, inflamed nose ("red nose"), increased rate of respiration, coughing, loss of appetite, and depression. Cattle infected during pregnancy may abort.

A characteristic of IBR virus (BHV1) is that it establishes a latent infection in sensory neurons, typically trigeminal ganglia or iliosacral dorsal root ganglia.[1] From these sites of latency, it can be reactivated when an infected animal is stressed or injured. Subsequently, the virus is shed and transmitted by contact to other cattle.

BVD virus may be transmitted in nasal secretions, saliva, blood, feces, and/or urine, and by direct contact with contaminated objects; it invades through the nose and mouth and replicates systemically. Infection during pregnancy may result in abortion, fetal resorption, or congenital malformation of the fetus. Moreover, if susceptible cows are infected with noncytopathic BVD virus during the first trimester of pregnancy, their calves may be born persistently infected with the virus. Exposure of those calves to certain virulent cytopathic BVD virus strains may precipitate BVD-mucosal disease. Clinical signs of BVD include loss of appetite, ulcerations in the mouth, profuse salivation, elevated temperature, diarrhea, dehydration, and lameness.

PI$_3$ virus usually localizes in the upper respiratory tract, causing elevated temperature and moderate nasal and ocular discharge. Although clinical signs typically are mild, PI$_3$ infection weakens respiratory tissues. Invasion and replication of other pathogens, particularly *Pasteurella* spp., is thereby facilitated and may result in pneumonia.

BRSV is the etiologic agent of a specific viral respiratory disease of cattle of all ages, including nursing calves. Infection is characterized by rapid breathing, coughing, loss of appetite, discharge from the nose and eyes, fever, and swelling around the throat and neck. In an acute outbreak, deaths may follow within 48 hours after onset of signs. Clinically, BRSV infection may be indistinguishable from other viral infections associated with the bovine respiratory disease complex. BRSV infection, like PI$_3$, facilitates invasion and replication of other respiratory pathogens. Exacerbation of clinical signs has been documented when concurrent BRSV and BVD or IBR infection exists.

Campylobacteriosis (vibriosis) is a bovine venereal disease transmitted during breeding, either through coitus or artificial insemination with contaminated semen. Although the disease is often subclinical, in cows it causes temporary infertility, irregular estrus cycles, delayed conception, and occasionally, abortion.

Leptospirosis may be caused by several serovars of *Leptospira*, of which *L. canicola, L. grippotyphosa, L. hardjo, L. icterohaemorrhagiae,* and *L. pomona* are the most common affecting cattle. *Leptospira* localize in the kidneys, are shed in the urine, and cause anemia, bloody urine, fever, loss of appetite, and prostration in calves. Signs are usually subclinical in adult cattle. Infected pregnant cows, however, often abort, and dairy cows may exhibit a marked decrease in milk production. Leptospira spp. are known zoonotic pathogens.

Trial Data: Safety and Efficacy: In safety studies of the fractions of CATTLEMASTER® 4+VL5, no adverse reactions to vaccination were observed and vaccinated pregnant cattle delivered normal, healthy calves.

The latency and subsequent excretion of the IBR virus fraction of CATTLEMASTER® 4+VL5 was determined in a safety study in which cattle were inoculated intramuscularly with the attenuated, temperature-sensitive IBR virus component and subsequently given corticosteroid to reactivate latent herpesvirus. Vaccination resulted in a characteristic serological response that remained unaltered even after corticosteroid treatment, indicating a lack of viral reactivation. Also, no BHV1 was recovered from mucosal swabs collected postvaccination or postcorticosteroid treatment, nor was it transmitted to nonvaccinated sentinel calves commingled with the vaccinates for the duration of the study. Further, no BHV1 DNA or latency-related RNA was detected in trigeminal or iliosacral spinal dorsal root ganglia collected after the administration of corticosteroid. Both nucleic acids were detected in a single cervical ganglion sample, suggesting a direct or proximate intraneural injection. BHV1 given by IM injection could not be reactivated from trigeminal ganglia, the primary site of BHV1 latency, demonstrating a lack of efficient viral replication in those sensory neurons. Excluding possible injection into nervous tissue (from which reactivation was not observed), the IBR fraction of CATTLEMASTER® 4+VL5 given by the IM route showed no propensity to establish latent herpesvirus infections.

Efficacy of each fraction of CATTLEMASTER® 4+VL5 was demonstrated in challenge-of-immunity studies. Cattle vaccinated with any fraction of CATTLEMASTER® 4+VL5, followed by challenge with a disease-causing strain of that fraction, showed no signs or had significantly fewer clinical signs than nonvaccinated control cattle. Serologic studies also demonstrated no immunologic interference among the fractions of CATTLEMASTER® 4+VL5. Antibody response was not significantly different between cattle vaccinated with an individual fraction and cattle vaccinated with the combined fractions.

References: Available upon request.

Presentation: 5 dose, 10 dose and 25 dose vials

Compendium Code No.: 36900462 75-4143-05

CATTLEMASTER® BVD-K

Pfizer Animal Health **Vaccine**

Bovine Virus Diarrhea Vaccine, Killed Virus

U.S. Vet. Lic. No.: 189

Description: CATTLEMASTER® BVD-K is a liquid, adjuvanted preparation of inactivated cytopathic and noncytopathic BVD virus strains, propagated on an established cell line. This product is adjuvanted with aluminum hydroxide to enhance immune response.

Contains gentamicin as preservative.

Indications: CATTLEMASTER® BVD-K is for vaccination of healthy cattle, including pregnant cows, as an aid in preventing bovine viral diarrhea caused by bovine viral diarrhea (BVD) virus.

Directions:

1. General Directions: Vaccination of healthy cattle, including pregnant cows, is recommended. Shake well. Administer 2 mL intramuscularly. In accordance with Beef Quality Assurance guidelines, this product should be administered in the muscular region of the neck.
2. Primary Vaccination: Healthy cattle should receive 2 doses administered 2-4 weeks apart. To avoid possible maternal antibody interference with active immunization, calves vaccinated before the age of 6 months should be revaccinated after 6 months of age.
3. Revaccination: Annual revaccination with a single dose is recommended.
4. Good animal husbandry and herd health management practices should be employed.

Precaution(s): Store at 2°-7°C. Prolonged exposure to higher temperatures and/or direct sunlight may adversely affect potency. Do not freeze.

Use entire contents when first opened.

Caution(s): As with many vaccines, anaphylaxis may occur after use. Initial antidote of epinephrine is recommended and should be followed with appropriate supportive therapy.

This product has been shown to be efficacious in healthy animals. A protective immune response may not be elicited if animals are persistently infected with BVD virus or incubating an infectious disease, are malnourished or parasitized, are stressed due to shipment or environmental conditions, are otherwise immunocompromised, or the vaccine is not administered in accordance with label directions.

Warning(s): Do not vaccinate within 21 days before slaughter.

For veterinary use only.

Discussion: Disease Description: BVD virus is commonly associated with respiratory disease and/or reproductive failure in cattle. BVD virus may be transmitted in nasal secretions, saliva, blood, feces, and/or urine, and by direct contact with contaminated objects; it invades through the nose and mouth and replicates systemically. Infection during pregnancy may result in abortion, fetal resorption, or congenital malformation of the fetus. Moreover, if susceptible cows are infected with noncytopathic BVD virus during the first trimester of pregnancy, their calves may be born persistently infected with the virus. Exposure of those calves to certain virulent cytopathic BVD virus strains may precipitate BVD-mucosal disease. Clinical signs of BVD include loss of appetite, ulcerations in the mouth, profuse salivation, elevated temperature, diarrhea, dehydration, and lameness.

Trial Data: Safety and Efficacy: In safety studies of CATTLEMASTER® BVD-K, no adverse reactions to vaccination were observed and vaccinated pregnant cattle delivered normal, healthy calves. Field reports, however, indicate occasional hypersensitivity reactions may occur up to 6 hours postvaccination. Owners should be advised to observe animals during this period. While this event appears to be rare overall, 500-900 lb dairy heifers may be affected more frequently than other cattle. Animals affected may display excessive salivation, incoordination, and/or dyspnea. Animals displaying such signs should be treated immediately with epinephrine or equivalent. In nonresponsive animals, other modes of treatment should be considered.

Efficacy of CATTLEMASTER® BVD-K was demonstrated in a challenge-of-immunity study. Cattle vaccinated with CATTLEMASTER® BVD-K, followed by challenge with a disease-causing strain of BVD virus, showed no signs or had significantly fewer clinical signs than nonvaccinated control cattle.

Presentation: 10 dose and 50 dose vials.

Compendium Code No.: 36900450 75-4147-03

CATTLE-VAC™ 9-SOMNUS

Durvet **Bacterin-Vaccine**

Bovine Rhinotracheitis-Virus Diarrhea-Parainfluenza 3-Respiratory Syncytial Virus Vaccine, Killed Virus-Haemophilus somnus-Leptospira canicola-grippotyphosa-hardjo-icterohaemorrhagiae-pomona Bacterin

U.S. Vet. Lic. No.: 272

Active Ingredient(s): Bovine rhinotracheitis, bovine virus diarrhea, bovine parainfluenza 3, bovine respiratory syncytial virus vaccine, killed virus, *Haemophilus somnus* and the serovars of *Leptospira canicola, L grippotyphosa, L hardjo, L icterohaemorrhagiae* and *L pomona* bacterin.

The product contains gentamicin and amphotericin B as preservatives.

Indications: CATTLE-VAC™ 9-Somnus is an inactivated, multivalent immunogen recommended for use in the vaccination of healthy cattle against disease caused by the IBR, BVD, PI$_3$ and BRSV viruses, *H somnus* and the serovars of *Leptospira canicola, L grippotyphosa, L hardjo, L icterohaemorrhagiae* and *L pomona.*

Dosage and Administration: Shake well. Administer 5 mL intramuscularly or subcutaneously to healthy cattle. For the initial vaccination, a second dose is required two (2) to four (4) weeks later.

CATTLE-VAC™ 9-Somnus may be used in pregnant cows at any stage of gestation or very young animals nursing pregnant cows. Calves vaccinated before six (6) months of age should be revaccinated at six (6) months of age or older followed by a second dose two (2) to four (4) weeks later.

Annual revaccination with a single 5 mL dose is recommended.

Precaution(s): Store at 35°F-45°F (2°C-7°C). Do not freeze.

Caution(s): Use the entire contents when first opened.
In case of an anaphylactic reaction, epinephrine should be administered immediately.
For veterinary use only.
Warning(s): Do not vaccinate within 21 days before slaughter.
Presentation: 50 mL (10 dose) and 250 mL (50 dose) vials.
Compendium Code No.: 10840220

CATTLE-VAC™ EC

Durvet **Bacterin**
Escherichia Coli Bacterin
U.S. Vet. Lic. No.: 303
Composition: This bacterin contains inactivated cultures of K99 piliated *Escherichia coli* adjuvanted with oil. Contains penicillin, streptomycin and thimerosal as preservatives.
Indications: For use in healthy heifers and cows as an aid in the prevention and control of colibacillosis in calves caused by K99 piliated *Escherichia coli.*
Dosage and Administration: Shake well before using. Administer 1 mL intramuscularly 2 weeks to 12 months prior to calving. Vaccinate dairy cows during the dry off period. Revaccinate annually.
Precaution(s): Store in the dark at 35°-45°F (2°-7°C). Do not freeze. Use entire contents when first opened.
Caution(s): It is essential that calves receive colostrum from the vaccinated dam within 8 hours of birth.
This product causes persistent swelling at the site of injection. Anaphylactic reactions may occur following the use of this biological. Symptomatic treatment: Epinephrine.
Warning(s): Do not vaccinate within 60 days prior to slaughter.
Presentation: 20 dose (20 mL) and 100 dose (100 mL) vials.
Manufactured by: Advance Biologics, Inc., Freeman, SD 57029.
Compendium Code No.: 10840251 8/99

CATTLE VAC™ EC+C

Durvet **Bacterin-Toxoid**
Clostridium Perfringens Type C-Escherichia Coli Bacterin-Toxoid
U.S. Vet. Lic. No.: 303
Composition: This product contains inactivated cultures of *Clostridium perfringens* Type C and K99 piliated *Escherichia coli* adjuvanted with oil. Contains thimerosal as a preservative.
Indications: For use in healthy pregnant cattle as an aid in the prevention and control of enterotoxemia in calves caused by *Clostridium perfringens* Type C and colibacillosis in calves caused by K99 piliated *Escherichia coli.*
Dosage and Administration: Shake well before using. Administer 1 mL intramuscularly 1-3 months prior to calving. Vaccinate dairy cows during the dry off period. Revaccinate prior to each subsequent calving.
Precaution(s): Store in the dark at 35°-45°F (2°-7°). Do not freeze. Use entire contents when first opened.
Caution(s): It is essential that calves receive colostrum from the vaccinated dam. This product may cause persistent swelling at the site of injection. Anaphylactic reactions may occur following use of this biological. Symptomatic treatment: Epinephrine.
Warning(s): Do not vaccinate within 60 days prior to slaughter.
Presentation: 20 dose (20 mL) and 100 dose (100 mL) vials.
Manufactured by: Advance Biologics, Inc., Freeman, SD 57029.
Compendium Code No.: 10841741 10/00

CATTLE-VAC™ E. COLI

Durvet **Antibodies**
Escherichia Coli Antibody, Equine Origin
U.S. Vet. Lic. No.: 303
Composition: This product is prepared from the blood of horses hyperimmunized with K99 piliated *Escherichia coli.* Contains oxytetracycline, phenol, and thimerosal as preservatives.
Indications: For use in newborn calves as an aid in the prevention of colibacillosis caused by K99 piliated *Escherichia coli.*
Dosage and Administration: Directions and Dosage: Shake well before using. Administer 10 mL orally to calves less than 12 hours old. Slowly syringe toward the back of the calf's mouth. Colostrum should be fed to each calf.
Precaution(s): Store in the dark at 35°-45°F (2°-7°C). Do not freeze. Use entire contents when first opened.
Caution(s): Anaphylactic reactions may occur following the use of this biological. Symptomatic treatment: Epinephrine.
Warning(s): Do not administer within 21 days prior to slaughter.
Presentation: 1 dose (10 mL) and 10 dose (100 mL) vials.
Manufactured by: Advance Biologics, Inc., Freeman, SD 57029.
Compendium Code No.: 10840231 8/99

CATTLE-VAC™ E. COLI+C

Durvet **Antibodies-Antitoxin**
Clostridium Perfringens Type C Antitoxin-Escherichia Coli Antibody, Equine Origin
U.S. Vet. Lic. No.: 303
Composition: This product is prepared from the blood of horses hyperimmunized with *Clostridium perfringens* Type C and K99 piliated *Escherichia coli.* Contains oxytetracycline, phenol, and thimerosal as preservatives.
Indications: For use in newborn calves as an aid in the prevention of disease caused by *Clostridium perfringens* Type C and K99 piliated *Escherichia coli.*
Dosage and Administration: Shake well before using. Administer 10 mL orally to calves less than 4 hours old. Slowly syringe toward the back of the calf's mouth. Colostrum should be fed to each calf.
Precaution(s): Store in the dark at 35°-45°F (2°-7°C). Do not freeze. Use entire contents when first opened.
Caution(s): Anaphylactic reactions may occur following the use of this biological. Symptomatic treatment: Epinephrine.
Warning(s): Do not administer within 21 days prior to slaughter.
Presentation: 1 dose (10 mL) and 10 dose (100 mL) vials.
Manufactured by: Advance Biologics, Inc., Freeman, SD 57029.
Compendium Code No.: 10840241 8/99

CATTLE-VAC™ HS

Durvet **Bacterin**
Haemophilus Somnus Bacterin
U.S. Vet. Lic. No.: 303
Composition: This bacterin contains inactivated cultures of *Haemophulus somnus* adjuvanted with aluminum hydroxide. Contains penicillin and streptomycin as preservatives.
Indications: For use in healthy cattle as an aid in the prevention and control of disease caused by *Haemophilus somnus.*
Dosage and Administration: Shake well before using. Administer 2 mL intramuscularly or subcutaneously at 3 months of age or older. Repeat in 2-3 weeks. Revaccinate annually.
Precaution(s): Store in the dark at 35°-45°F (2°-7°C). Do not freeze. Use entire contents when first opened.
Caution(s): Anaphylactic reactions may occur following the use of this biological. Symptomatic treatment: Epinephrine.
Warning(s): Do not vaccinate within 21 days prior to slaughter.
Presentation: 10 dose (20 mL) and 50 dose (100 mL) vials.
Manufactured by: Advance Biologics, Inc., Freeman, SD 57029.
Compendium Code No.: 10840261 8/99

C

CATTLE-VAC™ PINKEYE 4

Durvet **Bacterin**
Moraxella Bovis Bacterin
U.S. Vet. Lic. No.: 303
Composition: This bacterin contains inactivated cultures of *Moraxella bovis* adjuvanted with oil. Contains penicillin, streptomycin, and thimerosal as preservatives.
Indications: For use in healthy cattle as an aid in the prevention and control of ocular lesions caused by *Moraxella bovis.*
Dosage and Administration: Shake well before using. Administer 2 mL intramuscularly. Revaccinate annually.
Precaution(s): Store in the dark at 35°-45°F (2°-7°C). Do not freeze. Use entire contents when first opened.
Caution(s): Transient swelling may occur at the site of injection. Anaphylactic reactions may occur following the use of this biological. Symptomatic treatment: Epinephrine.
Warning(s): Do not vaccinate within 60 days prior to slaughter.
Presentation: 10 dose (20 mL) and 50 dose (100 mL) vials.
Manufactured by: Advance Biologics, Inc., Freeman, SD 57029.
Compendium Code No.: 10840271 8/99

CATTLE-VAC™ SALMO

Durvet **Bacterin**
Salmonella Dublin-Typhimurium Bacterin
U.S. Vet. Lic. No.: 303
Composition: This bacterin contains inactivated cultures of *Salmonella dublin* and *typhimurium* adjuvanted with aluminum hydroxide. Contains penicillin and streptomycin as preservatives.
Indications: For use in healthy cattle as an aid in the prevention and control of disease caused by *Salmonella dublin* and *typhimurium.*
Dosage and Administration: Shake well before using. Administer 2 mL intramuscularly or subcutaneously. Revaccinate in 2-4 weeks. Vaccinate dairy cows during the dry off period. Revaccinate annually.
Precaution(s): Store in the dark at 35°-45°F (2°-7°C). Do not freeze. Use entire contents when first opened.
Caution(s): Transient swelling may occur at the site of injection. Anaphylactic reactions may occur following the use of this biological. Symptomatic treatment: Epinephrine.
Warning(s): Do not vaccinate within 21 days prior to slaughter.
Presentation: 50 dose (100 mL) vials.
Manufactured by: Advance Biologics, Inc., Freeman, SD 57029.
Compendium Code No.: 10840281 8/99

CATTLEVAC™ VIBRIO-PLUS

Durvet **Bacterin**
Campylobacter Fetus Bacterin
U.S. Vet. Lic. No.: 303
Composition: This bacterin contains inactivated cultures of *Campylobacter fetus* subspecies *venerealis* adjuvanted with oil. Contains penicillin, streptomycin, and thimerosal as preservatives.
Indications: For use in healthy cattle as an aid in the prevention and control of vibriosis caused by *Campylobacter fetus.*
Dosage and Administration: Shake well before using. Administer 2 mL intramuscularly into the neck region or the caudal region of the hind legs 2 weeks to 1 year prior to breeding. Vaccinate dairy cows during the dry off period. Revaccinate annually.
Precaution(s): Store in the dark at 35°-45°F (2°-7°C). Do not freeze. Use entire contents when first opened.
Caution(s): This product causes persistent swelling at the site of injection. Anaphylactic reactions may occur following the use of this biological. Symptomatic treatment: Epinephrine.
Warning(s): Do not vaccinate within 60 days prior to slaughter.
Presentation: 10 dose (20 mL) and 50 dose (100 mL) vials.
Manufactured by: Advance Biologics, Inc., Freeman, SD 57029.
Compendium Code No.: 10840291 8/99

CATTLYST® 50

Alpharma **Feed Additive**
Type A Medicated Article-Laidlomycin propionate potassium
NADA No.: 141-025
Active Ingredient(s): Laidlomycin propionate potassium, 50 grams per pound.
Inert Ingredients: Mixed hemicellulose extract, calcium hydroxide, sodium hydroxide, soybean hulls.
Indications: For improved feed efficiency and increased rate of weight gain in cattle fed in confinement for slaughter.
Directions:
Weight Gain and Feed Efficiency: For increased rate of weight gain and improved feed efficiency when incorporated into complete cattle feed at 5 g/ton to provide not less than 30 mg and not more than 75 mg per head per day.

Feed Efficiency: For improved feed efficiency when incorporated into complete cattle feed at 5 to 10 g/ton to provide not less than 30 mg and not more than 150 mg per head per day.

Mixing And Feeding Instructions: Read all directions carefully before mixing and feeding.

Do not feed undiluted.

Type B Medicated Feed: Thoroughly mix the following amounts of CATTLYST® 50 to make one ton of Type B Medicated Feed to provide the concentrations shown in Table 1. With low use levels of CATTLYST® 50 (e.g. under two lb/ton), the use of an intermediate premix is recommended.

Liquid feeds made with CATTLYST® 50 shall have a dry matter content in the range of 62%-75%, pH in the range of 6.0-8.0 and drug level of 100-2000 g/ton. Its label shall carry daily and prior to use recirculating/agitation directions and an expiration of 21 days from date of manufacture. The Type C feed made with this Type B liquid feed shall be fed within seven days from date of manufacture.

Table 1 - Type B Medicated Feed:

Pounds of CATTLYST® 50 per ton of supplement	CATTLYST® concentration in Type B Medicated Feed (Grams per ton)
2.0	100
4.0	200
20.0	1000
40.0	2000

Type C Medicated Feed: Thoroughly mix the following amounts of CATTLYST® 50 to make one ton of Type C Medicated Feed that provides 5-10 grams of laidlomycin propionate potassium per ton of feed on a 90% dry matter basis (Table 2). An intermediate blending step, consistent with mixing equipment specifications, should be performed to ensure adequate mixing. For example, use one part CATTLYST® 50 Type A Medicated Article with nine parts of feed ingredients to prepare an intermediate blend before preparing a Type C Medicated Feed. Feed in the range of 5-10 grams per ton to growing and finishing beef cattle.

Table 2 - Type C Medicated Feed:

Pounds of CATTLYST® 50 per ton of complete feed	Pounds of a 1,000 g/ton Type B Medicated Feed per ton of complete feed	CATTLYST® Concentration in complete feed 90% dry matter basis (grams per ton)
0.1	10	5
0.15	15	7.5
0.2	20	10

Precaution(s): Reseal container immediately after each use.

Avoid excessive heat and moisture. Store below 40°C (104°F).

Caution(s): Do not allow horses or other equines access to feeds containing laidlomycin propionate potassium (CATTLYST® 50). The safety of laidlomycin propionate potassium (CATTLYST® 50) in unapproved species has not been established. Not for use in animals intended for breeding.

Warning(s): Contains sodium hydroxide and calcium hydroxide. Direct contact may be irritating and corrosive to the eye and irritating to the skin. Avoid ingestion, inhalation, skin contact and eye contact. When mixing and handling CATTLYST® 50, use protective clothing, impervious gloves, eye protection and a dust mask. If accidental eye or skin contact occurs, rinse immediately with water. Operators should wash thoroughly with soap and water after handling CATTLYST® 50.

Presentation: 10 lb (4.54 kg) bottle.

Compendium Code No.: 10220252 780310 0104

CAUSTIC DRESSING POWDER

Phoenix Pharmaceutical **Topical Wound Dressing**

Astringent-Antiseptic Topical Powder

Active Ingredient(s):

Copper sulfate • $5H_2O$ . . . . 51.1% w/w

Chloroxylenol . . . . 1.0% w/w

In a free-flowing starch base. Not sterilized.

Indications: For use as an aid in the management of slow-healing surface wounds of horses and mules.

Dosage and Administration: Apply powder freely to wounds twice daily. Repeat as indicated.

Precaution(s): Do not store above 30°C (86°F).

Keep container tightly closed when not in use.

Caution(s): In case of deep or puncture wounds or serious burns, consult a veterinarian. If redness, irritation, or swelling persists or increases, discontinue use and consult a veterinarian.

For external use only.

Warning(s): Not for use on animals intended for food.

Keep out of the reach of children.

Presentation: 5 oz. (142 g) containers (NDC 57319-282-33).

Compendium Code No.: 12560151 Rev. 11-98

CAUSTIC POWDER

Butler **Hemostatic**

Active Ingredient(s):

Copper sulfate • $5H_2O$ . . . . 51.5% w/w

Parachlorometaxylenol . . . . 1.0% w/w

In a free-flowing starch base. Not sterilized.

Indications: For use as an aid in the management of slow-healing wounds of horses and mules.

Dosage and Administration: Apply the powder freely to wounds twice a day. Repeat as indicated. For external use only.

Precaution(s): Do not store above 30°C (86°F). Keep the container tightly closed when not in use.

Caution(s): In case of deep or puncture wounds or serious burns, consult a veterinarian. If redness, irritation or swelling persists or increases, discontinue use of the product and consult a veterinarian. For veterinary use only.

Keep out of the reach of children. Restricted drug; use only as directed.

Warning(s): Not for use on animals intended for food.

Presentation: 6 oz. containers.

Compendium Code No.: 10820360

CAVICIDE®

Metrex **Disinfectant**

EPA Reg. No.: 38526-1

Active Ingredient(s):

Diisobutylphenoxyethoxyethyl dimethyl benzyl ammonium chloride 0.25%

Isopropanol 15.30%

Inert ingredients 84.45%

Contains biodegradable detergent.

Indications: CAVICIDE® is a multipurpose, broad-spectrum, effective cleaner and disinfectant for use on the surfaces of inanimate objects. It is especially useful in hospital operating rooms, emergency departments, isolation areas, neonatal units, and other high risk areas where environmental infection control is important.

Safe for use on delicate medical/dental/surgical equipment and instruments, it can be used to clean and disinfect such items as, infant incubators, oxygen hoods, anesthesia and respiratory therapy equipment, or tables and lights, laboratory equipment and surfaces, and to thoroughly clean and disinfect surgical and dental instruments.

CAVICIDE® is effective against: *Staphylococcus aureus, Pseudomonus aeruginosa, Salmonella choleraesuis, Trichophyton mentagrophytes,* Herpes Simplex 1 and 2 viruses, polio 1 and 2 viruses, coxsackle virus, *Mycobacterium tuberculosis var. bovis* (BCG), mold and mildew.

Deodorizer: Suppresses malodor at its source.

Dosage and Administration: If a violation of U.S. Federal law to use the product in a manner inconsistent with its labeling.

For use on large equipment and surfaces:

1. Apply CAVICIDE® directly to the surface using a spray-type bottle. Allow the surface to remain wet for about 30 seconds. Wipe away solution and debris using a clean paper or cloth towel. Discard the towel.
2. Re-spray the surface thoroughly wetting the pre-cleaned area. Wipe excessive CAVICIDE® from the surface. Allow the remaining CAVICIDE® to air dry.

For use as a manual cleaner/disinfectant for instrumentation:

1. First rinse dirty, contaminated instrumentation under cool running tap water to remove gross debris.
2. Fill an appropriate size container with a sufficient amount of CAVICIDE® to allow complete submersion of the instruments.
3. Place the instruments into the CAVICIDE® solution and allow them to soak for about five (5) minutes before scrubbing surfaces using a stiff bristle brush. Allow the instruments to soak for an additional 10 minutes before removing.
4. Rinse thoroughly.
5. Change the solution as needed.

For use as an ultrasonic cleaner:

1. Thoroughly rinse the instrument under cool running water to remove gross debris.
2. Submerge instruments into CAVICIDE® and activate the ultrasonic unit for 10 minutes.
3. Remove and rinse.
4. Change the solution as needed.

For use as a high-level disinfectant:

1. Thoroughly clean instruments.
2. Rinse under cool tap water and shake excessive water from the surface.
3. Immerse the instruments into CAVICIDE® solution and allow them to remain submerged for 10 minutes at room temperature for tuberculocidal kill.
4. Remove and rinse prior to use.
5. Change the solution as needed.

Mold and mildew: To control mold and mildew on clean hard surfaces, apply and wipe to wet surface thoroughly with CAVICIDE®. Allow to air dry after the application. Repeat the application in seven (7) days or as necessary to maintain control.

Precaution(s): Store in a cool place.

Pesticide Disposal: Dilute with water. Dispose in sanitary sewer.

Container Disposal: Do not re-use the empty container. Wrap the container and put it in the trash.

Caution(s): Precautionary Statements: Harmful to humans and domestic animals. Harmful if swallowed. Keep out of the reach of children. May cause eye and skin irritation. Avoid contamination with food.

In case of eye contact, immediately flush eyes with plenty of water for at least 15 minutes.

Presentation: 2 oz with sprayer, 8 oz spray, 24 oz spray, 1 gallon, and 2.5 gallon.

Compendium Code No.: 13400001

CAV-VAC®

Intervet **Vaccine**

Chicken Anemia Virus Vaccine, Modified Live Virus

U.S. Vet. Lic. No.: 286

Description: CAV-VAC® is a live virus vaccine, prepared from a modified U.S. field isolate. The vaccine is produced using specific pathogen free (SPF) substrates, and contains live chicken anemia vaccine virus suspended in wing web diluent.

This vaccine contains gentamicin and amphotericin B as preservatives.

Quality tested for purity, potency and safety.

Indications: CAV-VAC® is indicated for the immunization of breeder chickens against Chicken Anemia Virus to provide protection of progeny against clinical signs due to chicken infectious anemia. CAV-VAC® should be administered one time to breeder chickens via the wing web stick method from 10 to 12 weeks of age.

Dosage and Administration: Preparation of Vaccine: Do not open the vaccine until ready to begin vaccination. Use vaccine immediately after opening.

1. Shake well.
2. Remove the tear-off seal and stopper from the vaccine vial. Vaccine is now ready for use.

Wing-Web Administration:

For Chickens from 10 to 12 Weeks of Age:

1. Vaccine is applied to the web of the wing. Use the enclosed two-pronged applicator.
2. Vaccinate by dipping the applicator in the vaccine mixture and stabbing the webbed portion of the wing from beneath. Avoid feathered areas of the web.
3. Periodically during use, re-insert stopper and shake vaccine well.

Warning: Use of this product in chickens younger than three weeks of age may cause clinical signs of chicken anemia. Do not vaccinate breeder chickens in lay.

Records: Keep a record of vaccine, quantity, serial number, expiration date, and place of purchase; the date and time of vaccination; the number, age, breed, and locations of chickens; names of operators performing the vaccination and any observed reactions.

Precaution(s): Store vaccine between 2 and 7°C (35 and 45°F).

Do not spill or splash the vaccine.

Use entire contents when first opened.

Burn containers and all unused contents.

This product is non-returnable.

Caution(s): Vaccinate only healthy chickens. Although disease may not be evident, concurrent disease conditions may cause complications or reduce immunity.

All susceptible chickens on the same premises should be vaccinated at the same time.

Efforts should be taken to reduce stress conditions at the time of vaccination.

Do not use less than one dose per bird.

Following vaccination, virus may be shed in the feces. Thus, care should be taken to avoid spread of the vaccine virus to young chickens or to unexposed chickens in lay.

For veterinary use only.

Notice: This vaccine has undergone rigid potency, safety and purity tests, and meets the requirements of Intervet Inc. and the USDA. It is designed to stimulate effective immunity when used as directed, but the user must be advised that the response to the product depends upon many factors, including, but not limited to, conditions of storage and handling by the user, administration of the vaccine, health and responsiveness of the individual chickens, and the degree of field exposure. Therefore, directions should be followed carefully.

This product is not hazardous when used according to directions supplied. A material safety data sheet (MSDS) is available upon request. This and any other consumer information can be obtained by calling Intervet Inc. Customer Service at 1-800-441-8272 or 1-302-934-8051.

The use of this vaccine is subject to applicable local and federal laws and regulations.

Use only as directed.

Warning(s): Do not vaccinate chickens in lay. Do not vaccinate within 21 days of slaughter.

Presentation: 10 x 1,000 doses (10 mL/vial) for wing-web administration.

U.S. Patent No. 5,686,077

24405 AL172

Compendium Code No.: 11060291

C & D ANTITOXIN™

Boehringer Ingelheim **Antitoxin**

Clostridium Perfringens Types C & D Antitoxin, Equine Origin

U.S. Vet. Lic. No.: 124

Composition: Prepared from the blood of horses hyperimmunized with toxins of *Clostridium perfringens* Types C and D. Contains 0.2% cresol as a preservative.

Indications: Recommended for the prevention and treatment of enterotoxemia caused by *Clostridium perfringens* Types C and D in calves, cattle, lambs, sheep, and baby pigs.

Dosage and Administration: (Prophlactic) Using aseptic technique, inject subcutaneously or intravenously: Calves—10 mL; Cattle—30 mL; Suckling lambs—3 mL; All other sheep—10 mL; Baby pigs—2 mL administered orally or injected subcutaneously.

(Therapeutic) Increase dosage 100%.

Precaution(s): Store out of direct sunlight at a temperature between 35-45°F (2-7°C). Avoid freezing. Shake well before using. Use entire contents when first opened.

Caution(s): Anaphylactic reactions may occur.

Antidote(s): Epinephrine.

Warning(s): Do not vaccinate within 21 days before slaughter.

Presentation: 250 mL vial.

Compendium Code No.: 10280252 01801-02

C & D TOXOID

Aspen **Toxoid**

Clostridium perfringens Types C & D Toxoid

U.S. Vet. Lic. No.: 124

Composition: Prepared from cultures of *Clostridium perfringens* types C and D. Alum precipitated.

Indications: Recommended for the immunization of healthy susceptible sheep and cattle against enterotoxemia caused by the toxins of *Clostridium perfringens* type C and D for the immunization of healthy susceptible swine against enterotoxemia caused by the toxins of *Clostridium perfringens* type C.

Dosage and Administration: Sheep 2 mL, cattle and swine 5 mL injected subcutaneously or intramuscularly using aseptic technique. Repeat in 21 to 28 days and annually.

Precaution(s): Store out of direct sunlight at a temperature not over 45°F. Avoid freezing. Shake well. Use entire contents when first opened.

Caution(s): Anaphylactoid reactions may occur.

Antidote(s): Administer epinephrine.

Warning(s): Do not vaccinate within 21 days before slaughter.

Presentation: 50 mL and 250 mL vials.

Compendium Code No.: 14750090

CEFA-DRI®

Fort Dodge **Mastitis Therapy**

Cephapirin Benzathine

NADA No.: 108-114

Active Ingredient(s): Each 10 mL disposable syringe contains 300 mg of cephapirin activity in a stable peanut oil gel. This product was manufactured by a non-sterilizing process.

Indications: For the treatment of mastitis in dairy cows during the dry period.

CEFA-DRI® has been shown by extensive clinical studies to be efficacious in the treatment of mastitis in dry cows, when caused by *Streptococcus agalactiae* and *Staphylococcus aureus*, including penicillin-resistant strains.

Treatment of the dry cow with CEFA-DRI® is indicated in any cow known to harbor any of these organisms in the udder at drying off.

Pharmacology:

Description: CEFA-DRI® (cephapirin benzathine) for intramammary infusion into the dry cow is a product which provides a wide range of bactericidal activity against gram-positive and gram-negative organisms. It is derived biosynthetically from 7-aminocephalosporanic acid.

Action: In the non-lactating mammary gland, CEFA-DRI® (cephapirin benzathine) provides bactericidal levels of the active antibiotic, cephapirin, for a prolonged period of time. This prolonged activity is due to the low solubility of the cephapirin benzathine and to the slow release gel base.

Cephapirin is bactericidal to susceptible organisms; it is known to be highly active against *Streptococcus agalactiae* and *Staphylococcus aureus* including strains resistant to penicillin.

To determine the susceptibility of bacteria to cephapirin in the laboratory, the class disc, Cephalothin Susceptibility Test Discs, 30 mcg, should be used.

Dosage and Administration: CEFA-DRI® (cephapirin benzathine) is for use in dry cows only. Infuse each quarter at the time of drying off with a single 10 mL syringe. Use no later than 30 days prior to calving.

Completely milk out all four quarters. The udder and teats should be thoroughly washed with warm water containing a suitable dairy antiseptic and dried, preferably using individual paper towels. Carefully scrub the teat end and orifice with 70% alcohol, using a separate swab for each teat. Allow to dry.

CEFA-DRI® is packaged with the Opti-Sert® protective cap.

For partial insertion: Twist off upper portion of the Opti-Sert® protective cap to expose 3-4 mm of the syringe tip.

For full insertion: Remove protective cap to expose the full length of the syringe tip.

Insert syringe tip into the teat canal and expel the entire contents of syringe into the quarter. Withdraw the syringe and gently massage the quarter to distribute the medication.

Do not infuse contents of the mastitis syringe into the teat canal if the Opti-Sert® protective cap is broken or damaged.

Precaution(s): Store at controlled room temperature 15° to 30°C (59° to 86°F); avoid excessive heat.

CEFA-DRI® should be administered with caution to subjects which have demonstrated some form of allergy, particularly to penicillin. Such reactions are rare; however, should they occur, consult your veterinarian.

Warning(s):

1. For use in dry cows only. 2. Not to be used within 30 days of calving.
3. Milk from treated cows must not be used for food during the first 72 hours after calving.
4. Any animal infused with this product must not be slaughtered for food until 42 days after the latest infusion.

Presentation: Carton containing 12 x 10 mL syringes (NDC 0856-2726-10)

Opti-Sert® Protective Cap - U.S. Patent No. 4,850,970.

Compendium Code No.: 10030280 4220H

CEFA-DROPS® AND CEFA-TABS® ℞

Fort Dodge **Cefadroxil**

Cefadroxil-Veterinary Powder for Oral Suspension and Tablets

NADA No.: 140-684 (Drops)/119-688 (Tablets)

Active Ingredient(s):

Each 15 mL contains 750 mg cefadroxil.

Each 50 mL contains 2500 mg cefadroxil.

Each scored tablet contains 1 g cefadroxil.

Each film-coated tablet contains 50 mg, 100 mg, or 200 mg cefadroxil.

Indications: CEFA-DROPS® (cefadroxil) and CEFA-TABS® (cefadroxil) are indicated for the treatment of the following conditions:

Dogs: Genitourinary tract infections (cystitis) caused by susceptible strains of *Escherichia coli, Proteus mirabilis* and *Staphylococcus aureus.*

Skin and soft tissue infections including cellulitis, pyoderma, dermatitis, wound infections and abscesses caused by susceptible strains of *Staphylococcus aureus.*

Cats: Skin and soft tissue infections including abscesses, wound infections, cellulitis and dermatitis caused by susceptible strains of *Pasteurella multocida, Staphylococcus aureus, Staphylococcus epidermidis* and *Streptococcus* spp.

Pharmacology: CEFA-DROPS® (cefadroxil) and CEFA-TABS® (cefadroxil) contain a semi-synthetic cephalosporin antibiotic intended for oral administration. CEFA-DROPS® has an orange-pineapple flavor.

Chemistry: Cefadroxil is a member of a group of semi-synthetic derivatives of cephalosporin C, found among the metabolic products of the fungus *Cephalosporium acremonium.* The cephalosporins are structurally related to the penicillins in that both contain a 4-member beta-lactam ring. Cefadroxil is a 7-amino cephalosporanic acid substituted at the 7 position to form a molecule designated chemically as (6R, 7R)-7-[(R)-2-amino-2-(p-hydroxyphenyl) acetamido]-3-methyl-8-oxo-5-thia-1-azabicyclo [4.2.0] oct-2-ene-2-carboxylic acid monohydrate:

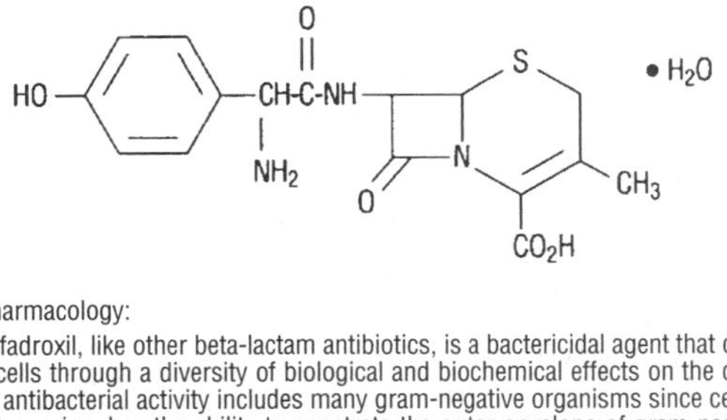

Clinical Pharmacology:

Action: Cefadroxil, like other beta-lactam antibiotics, is a bactericidal agent that causes death of bacterial cells through a diversity of biological and biochemical effects on the cell wall. The spectrum of antibacterial activity includes many gram-negative organisms since cefadroxil, like other cephalosporins, has the ability to penetrate the outer envelope of gram-negative bacilli, thereby gaining access to cell wall target sites. Cefadroxil is generally not broken down by penicillinases such as those produced by penicillin-resistant staphylococci, although cephalosporinases have been identified that can inactivate the molecule.

Microbiology: The effectiveness of CEFA-DROPS® and CEFA-TABS® in skin and soft tissue infections caused by *Staphylococcus aureus*, (including penicillin-resistant strains) and in urinary tract infections caused by *Staphylococcus aureus, Escherichia coli* and *Proteus mirabilis*, has been demonstrated clinically in the dog. In cats, the effectiveness of cefadroxil in skin and soft tissue infections caused by susceptible pathogens such as *Pasteurella multocida, Staphylococcus aureus, Staphylococcus epidermidis* and *Streptococcus* spp. has also been demonstrated. In addition, cefadroxil has a broad spectrum of activity against both gram-positive and gram-negative human isolates. Although the clinical significance of *in vitro* data is unknown in the target species, the following human isolates are generally susceptible to cefadroxil at the indicated concentrations.[1]

Organism (No. of Isolates)	Minimum Inhibitory Concentration (mcg/mL) Range	MIC$_{90}$*
Streptococcus pyogenes (24)	0.063-0.125	0.11
Streptococcus agalactiae (27)	0.25-1	0.92
Streptococcus pneumoniae (29)	0.5-2	1.2
Staphylococcus aureus, penicillin sensitive (16)	2-16	3.2
Staphylococcus aureus, penicillin resistant (63)	1-32	6.2
Staphylococcus epidermidis (28)	0.125-4	2.13
Escherichia coli (59)	4->125	16.0
Proteus mirabilis (62)	4->125	15.6
Klebsiella pneumoniae (61)	4-16	7.85
Salmonella spp. (22)	4-8	7.19
Shigella spp. (12)	2-8	6.98
Pasteurella multocida (2)		1.4

*Concentration at which 90% of the isolates are susceptible.

The susceptibility of organisms to cefadroxil should be determined using the cephalosporin class disc, 30 mcg. Specimens for susceptibility testing should be collected prior to the initiation of antibiotic therapy.

Pharmacokinetics: Cefadroxil is stable in gastric acid and only moderately bound to serum proteins (approximately 20%). Cefadroxil is well absorbed from the gastrointestinal tract even when administered with food. The drug is excreted largely unchanged by the kidney. In humans, high concentrations of cefadroxil activity are found in urine within three hours after oral dosage.[2] The concurrent administration of probenecid retards the elimination rate.

In dogs, oral administration of cefadroxil at a dosage of 10 mg/lb results in mean peak serum concentrations averaging 18.6 mcg/mL within 1 to 2 hours after treatment.[3] The serum half-life (T½) following oral administration is approximately 2 hours. Over 50% of an orally administered dose is excreted unchanged in the urine of dogs within 24 hours. Serum concentration time profiles in dogs following oral administration are illustrated graphically in Figure 1.

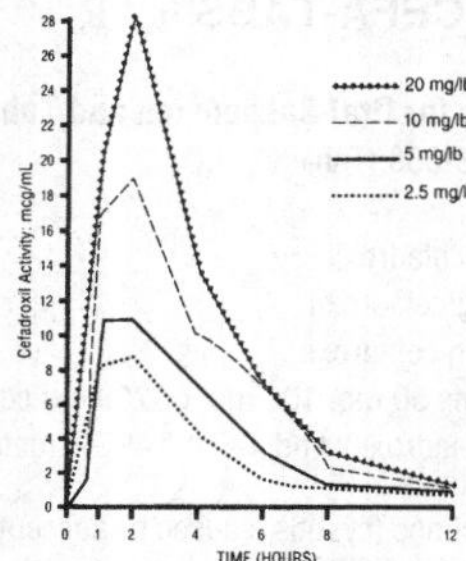

Figure 1: Cefadroxil Serum Concentration Curves in Dogs[3]

In cats, oral administration of cefadroxil at a dosage of 10 mg/lb results in mean peak serum concentrations of 17.4 mcg/mL within 1 to 2 hours after treatment. The serum half-life (T½) following oral administration to cats is 2½ to 3 hours. Serum concentration time profiles in cats following oral administration are illustrated graphically in Figure 2.

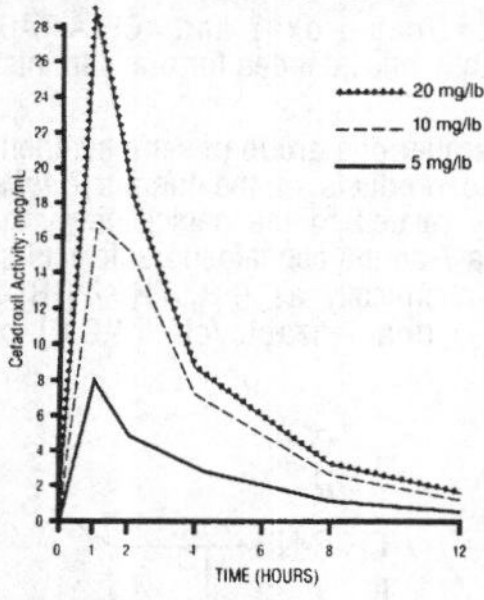

Figure 2: Cefadroxil Serum Concentration Curves in Cats

Dosage and Administration:

Dogs: CEFA-DROPS® and CEFA-TABS® 1 gram, 50 mg, 100 mg and 200 mg should be administered orally at a dosage of 10 mg/lb of body weight twice daily. Dogs with skin or soft tissue infections should be treated for a minimum of three days. Genitourinary tract infections should be treated for a minimum of seven days with cefadroxil. Maximum duration of therapy should not exceed 30 days.

Cats: CEFA-DROPS® and CEFA-TABS® 50 mg and 100 mg should be administered orally at a dosage of 10 mg/lb of body weight once daily. Maximum duration of therapy should not exceed 21 days.

In both species, drug treatment should continue for at least 48 hours after the animal is afebrile or asymptomatic. If no response is observed after three days of treatment, therapy should be discontinued and the case should be re-evaluated.

To Prepare Suspension: Tap bottle lightly to loosen powder. For 15 mL bottle, add 10.4 mL of water in two portions. For 50 mL bottle, add 34 mL of water in two portions. Shake well after each addition. After mixing, store in refrigerator. Shake well before use. Discard unused portion after 14 days.

Droppers supplied with CEFA-DROPS® are calibrated in mL increments. When mixed as directed, each mL contains cefadroxil monohydrate equivalent to 50 mg cefadroxil.

Contraindication(s): CEFA-DROPS® and CEFA-TABS® should not be administered to dogs or cats with a known allergy to cephalosporins. In penicillin-allergic animals, CEFA-DROPS® and CEFA-TABS® should be used with caution.

Precaution(s): Store at controlled room temperature 15° to 30°C (59° to 86°F).

Caution(s): Federal law restricts this drug to use by or on the order of a licensed veterinarian.

The enclosed dose dropper in CEFA-DROPS® contains natural rubber latex which may cause allergic reactions.

Warning(s): For use in dogs and cats only. Not to be used in animals which are raised for food production. Safety for use in pregnant female dogs and cats or in breeding males has not been determined. (See "Toxicology".)

Toxicology: Animal Toxicology: In subacute studies, dogs administered 100, 200 or 400 mg/kg/day for 13 weeks showed no consistent or distinct treatment-related histopathologic changes. In chronic toxicity studies, dogs receiving doses as high as 600 mg/kg/day for six months showed no discernible treatment-related effects, with the exception of emesis in dogs receiving a 400 mg/kg/day dose at one time. No distinct or consistent meaningful drug-related changes in the hematologic, coagulation or urinalysis test results or in histologic examination of tissues were observed when compared to controls.

No teratogenic or antifertility effects were seen in reproductive studies done in mice and rats receiving dosages as high as nine times the maximum recommended canine dosage.

In cats, oral administration of cefadroxil at a dosage of 240 mg/kg/day divided into two equal doses (ten times the recommended daily dosage) for 21 consecutive days produced no clinical chemistry, pathological or other signs of toxicity other than reduced food consumption, vomiting and diarrhea.

Adverse Reactions: Occasional nausea and vomiting have been reported following cefadroxil therapy. Administration with food appears to decrease nausea. Diarrhea and lethargy have been occasionally reported.

References: Available upon request.

Presentation: CEFA-DROPS® (cefadroxil) Veterinary Powder for Oral Suspension equivalent to:
NDC 0856-2365-20 - 750 mg cefadroxil per 15 mL dropper bottle
NDC 0856-2365-50 - 2500 mg cefadroxil per 50 mL dropper bottle
CEFA-TABS® (cefadroxil) Veterinary Tablets:
NDC 0856-2386-30 - 1 gram scored tablets, bottles of 20
CEFA-TABS® Veterinary Film-Coated Tablets:
NDC 0856-2350-80 - 50 mg tablets, bottles of 500
NDC 0856-2351-80 - 100 mg tablets, bottles of 500
NDC 0856-2352-70 - 200 mg tablets, bottles of 250

Manufactured by: Bristol-Myers Barceloneta, Inc., Barceloneta, PR 00708
U.S. Patent No. 4,504,657

Compendium Code No.: 10030291 4230F

CEFA-LAK®

Fort Dodge **Mastitis Therapy**

Cephapirin Sodium

NADA No.: 097-222

Active Ingredient(s): Each 10 mL disposable syringe contains 200 mg of cephapirin activity in a stable peanut oil gel. This product was manufactured by a non-sterilizing process.

Indications: For lactating cows only. For the treatment of bovine mastitis.

CEFA-LAK® (cephapirin sodium) for intramammary infusion should be used at the first signs of inflammation or at the first indication of any alteration in the milk. Treatment is indicated immediately upon determining, by C.M.T. or other tests, that the leucocyte count is elevated, or that a susceptible pathogen has been cultured from the milk.

CEFA-LAK® for intramammary infusion has been shown to be efficacious in the treatment of mastitis in lactating cows caused by susceptible strains of *Streptococcus agalactiae* and *Staphylococcus aureus* including strains resistant to penicillin.

Pharmacology: CEFA-LAK® (cephapirin sodium) is a cephalosporin which possesses a wide range of antimicrobial activity against gram-positive and gram-negative organisms. It is derived biosynthetically from 7-aminocephalosporanic acid.

Action: Cephapirin is bactericidal to susceptible organisms; it is known to be highly active against *Streptococcus agalactiae* and *Staphylococcus aureus* including strains resistant to penicillin.

To determine the susceptibility of bacteria to cephapirin in the laboratory, the class disc, Cephalothin Susceptibility Test Discs, 30 mcg, should be used.

Dosage and Administration:

Infuse the entire contents of one syringe (10 mL) into each infected quarter immediately after the quarter has been completely milked out. Repeat once only in 12 hours. If definite improvement is not noted within 48 hours after treatment, the causal organism should be further investigated. Consult a veterinarian.

Milk out udder completely. Wash the udder and teats thoroughly with warm water containing a suitable dairy antiseptic and dry, preferably using individual paper towels. Carefully scrub the teat end and orifice with 70% alcohol, using a separate swab for each teat. Allow to dry.

CEFA-LAK® (cephapirin sodium) is packaged with the Opti-Sert® protective cap.

For partial insertion: Twist off upper portion of the Opti-Sert® protective cap to expose 3-4 mm of the syringe tip.

For full insertion: Remove protective cap to expose the full length of the syringe tip.

Insert syringe tip into the teat canal and expel the entire contents of one syringe into each infected quarter. Withdraw the syringe and gently massage the quarter to distribute the suspension into the milk cistern. Do not milk out for 12 hours.

Do not infuse contents of the mastitis syringe into the teat canal if the Opti-Sert® protective cap is broken or damaged.

Reinfection - The use of antibiotics, however effective, for the treatment of mastitis will not significantly reduce the incidence of this disease in the herd unless their use is fortified by good herd management, and sanitary and mechanical safety measures are practiced to prevent reinfection.

Precaution(s): Store at controlled room temperature 15° to 30°C (59° to 86°F); avoid excessive heat.

CEFA-LAK® should be administered with caution to subjects which have demonstrated some form of allergy, particularly to penicillin. Such reactions are rare; however, should they occur, discontinue treatment and consult a veterinarian.

Warning(s):

1. Milk that has been taken from animals during treatment and for 96 hours after the last treatment must not be used for food.
2. Treated animals must not be slaughtered for food until four (4) days after the last treatment.
3. Administration of more than the prescribed dose may lead to residue of antibiotic in milk longer than 96 hours.

Presentation: Carton containing 12 x 10 mL syringes (NDC 0856-2723-21).
Opti-Sert® Protective Cap - U.S. Patent No. 4,850, 970.

Compendium Code No.: 10030300 4200I

CENTRINE® ℞

Fort Dodge **Anticholinergic**

(Aminopentamide Hydrogen Sulfate) Injection and Tablets

NADA No.: 043-079 (Injection)/043-078 (Tablets)

Active Ingredient(s):

Injection: Each mL contains 0.5 mg aminopentamide hydrogen sulfate.

Tablets: Each tablet contains 0.2 mg aminopentamide hydrogen sulfate.

Indications: CENTRINE® (aminopentamide hydrogen sulfate) is a potent antispasmodic agent. As a cholinergic blocking agent for smooth muscle, its action is similar to atropine.

CENTRINE® is indicated in the treatment of acute abdominal visceral spasm, pylorospasm or hypertrophic gastritis and associated nausea, vomiting and/or diarrhea.

Pharmacology:

Action: CENTRINE® effectively reduces the tone and amplitude of colonic contractions to a greater degree and for a more extended period than does atropine.

CENTRINE® effects a reduction in gastric secretion, a decrease in gastric acidity and a marked decrease in gastric motility.

The mydriatic and salivary effects of CENTRINE® are less than those produced by atropine at similar dosage, permitting the control of vomiting and diarrhea with less distress to the animal due to dryness of the mouth and blurred vision.

Dosage and Administration: CENTRINE® (aminopentamide hydrogen sulfate) may be administered by subcutaneous or intramuscular injection or by oral tablets according to the following schedule. If the desired effect is not obtained, the dosage may be gradually increased up to a maximum of 5 times the doses listed. When the condition has been brought under control by parenteral medication, treatment can be continued, if desired, with 0.2 mg scored tablets according to the dosage schedule.

Weight of Animal	Amount to be administered every 8 to 12 hours		
	Dosage	Injectable Volume	Oral Tablets
10 lbs or less	0.1 mg	0.2 mL	½ Tab
11 lbs to 20 lbs	0.2 mg	0.4 mL	1 Tab
21 lbs to 50 lbs	0.3 mg	0.6 mL	1½ Tabs
51 lbs to 100 lbs	0.4 mg	0.8 mL	2 Tabs
Over 100 lbs	0.5 mg	1.0 mL	2½ Tabs

Contraindication(s): CENTRINE® should not be used in animals with glaucoma because of the occurrence of mydriasis.

Precaution(s): Dryness of the mouth is the most commonly reported side effect. Blurring of vision may occur and dryness of the eyes may occur if larger (greater than therapeutic) doses are used. CENTRINE® should be used cautiously, if at all, in pyloric obstruction because of its action in delaying gastric emptying. These effects frequently decrease with continued administration of the drug. Disturbances in urination are relatively infrequent. They vary from slightly hesitancy in initiating urination to complete inability to urinate; the latter is an indication for discontinuing the drug. After a day or two, it may be resumed at a lower dosage level.

Caution(s): Federal law restricts this drug to use by or on the order of a licensed veterinarian.

Warning(s): For use in dogs and cats only.

Presentation:

CENTRINE® Injection is supplied in 10 mL vials (NDC 0856-2401-10).

CENTRINE® Tablets are supplied in bottles of 100 (NDC 0856-2400-60).

Compendium Code No.: 10030330 4260F

CEPHALOVAC® EWT

Boehringer Ingelheim **Toxoid-Vaccine**

Encephalomyelitis Vaccine-Eastern and Western Killed Virus, Tetanus Toxoid

U.S. Vet. Lic. No.: 124

Contents: This product contains the antigens listed above.

Contains gentamicin and thimerosal as preservatives.

Indications: For the vaccination of all types and ages of healthy horses against Eastern and Western Equine Encephalomyelitis and tetanus.

Dosage and Administration: Shake well before using. Using aseptic technique, inject 2 mL deep intramuscularly. Administer a second 2 mL dose in 4 to 6 weeks, using a different injection site. Revaccinate annually and prior to anticipated exposure, using a single 2 mL dose. Use a separate, sterile 1½ inch needle for each injection.

Precaution(s): Store at 35-45°F (2-7°C). Protect from freezing. Use entire contents when first opened.

Caution(s): Anaphylactoid reactions may occur following use.

This product has been tested under laboratory conditions and shown to meet all Federal standards for safety and efficacy in normal healthy animals. This level of performance may be affected by conditions such as stress, weather, nutrition, disease, parasitism, other treatments, individual idiosyncrasies, or impaired immunological competency. These factors should be considered by the user when evaluating product performance or freedom from reactions.

For veterinary use only.

Antidote(s): Epinephrine.

Warning(s): Do not vaccinate within 21 days before slaughter.

Presentation: 10 x 1 dose (2 mL) syringes and 10 dose (20 mL) vials.

Compendium Code No.: 10280281 1101-03/31102-03 / 31103-03/31104-03

CEPHALOVAC® VEWT

Boehringer Ingelheim **Toxoid-Vaccine**

Encephalomyelitis Vaccine-Eastern, Western and Venezuelan Killed Virus-Tetanus Toxoid

U.S. Vet. Lic. No.: 124

Contents: This product contains the antigens listed above.

Contains gentamicin and thimerosal as preservatives.

Indications: For vaccination of all types and ages of healthy horses against Eastern, Western, and Venezuelan Equine Encephalomyelitis and tetanus.

Dosage and Administration: Shake well before using. Using aseptic technique, inject 2 mL deep intramuscularly. Administer a second 2 mL dose in 4 to 6 weeks, using a different injection site. Revaccinate annually and prior to anticipated exposure using a single 2 mL dose. Use a separate sterile 1½ inch needle for each injection.

Precaution(s): Store at 35-45°F or (2-7°C. Protect from freezing. Use entire contents when first opened.

Caution(s): Anaphylactoid reactions may occur following use.

This product has been tested under laboratory conditions and shown to meet all Federal standards for safety and ability to immunize normal healthy animals. This level of performance may be affected by conditions of use such as stress, weather, nutrition, disease, parasitism, other treatments, individual idiosyncrasies, or impaired immunological competency. These factors should be considered by the user when evaluating product performance or freedom from reactions.

For veterinary use only.

Antidote(s): Epinephrine.

Warning(s): Do not vaccinate within 21 days before slaughter.

Presentation: 10 x 1 dose (2 mL) syringes and 10 dose (20 mL) vials.

Compendium Code No.: 10280291 31301-03/31302-03 / 31303-02/31304-03

C

CEPHLOPEX®

United **Vaccine**

Fox Encephalitis Vaccine, Killed Virus

U.S. Vet. Lic. No.: 245

Active Ingredient(s): An inactivated vaccine which contains canine hepatitis virus.

Preservatives: Gentamicin and thimerosal.

Indications: CEPHLOPEX® is for use as an aid in the prevention of encephalitis in healthy, susceptible foxes.

Dosage and Administration: Use sharp, sterile needles and sterile syringes. Inject 1 mL into the large muscle of the hind leg of foxes at 10 to 12 weeks of age. For a proper suspension, shake before and occasionally during use. Revaccinate all adults at the time of pup vaccination.

Precaution(s): Store at 35-45°F (2-7°C).

Caution(s): Use the entire contents when the container is first opened.

Consult a veterinarian or United Vaccines Inc. before using the vaccine in foxes on a farm where disease exists or has occurred in the last 18 months, or for an alternate vaccinating schedule.

Presentation: 50 dose, 100 dose, 250 dose, and 500 dose vials.

Compendium Code No.: 11040072

CERULYTIC™

Virbac **Otic Cleanser**

Ear Solution

Active Ingredient(s): Contains: Benzyl alcohol and butylated hydroxytoluene in a propylene glycol dicaprylate/dicaprate base with fragrance.

Indications: CERULYTIC™ has been specifically formulated for conditions where a ceruminolytic (dewaxing) product is of benefit prior to the use of a specific ear treatment. Such conditions may include erythematoceruminous otitis in dogs and otodectic mange in cats. CERULYTIC™ may also be used for dogs and cats known to be prone to hypersecretion of cerumen.

Directions for Use: Turn the nozzle to open and then apply a few drops of CERULYTIC™ into each ear canal. Gently rub the base of the ear and then wipe the interior of the earflap with cotton or cloth. CERULYTIC™ may be administered prior to each use of an ear treatment product, two to three times a week for routine cleansing, or as directed by your veterinarian.

Caution(s): For topical use only. Avoid contact with eyes.

Available through licensed veterinarians only.

Warning(s): Keep out of reach of children.

Presentation: 4 oz (120 mL).

Compendium Code No.: 10230090

CERUMENE™

Evsco **Otic Cleanser**

Active Ingredient(s): Contains cerumene (squalane) 25% in an isopropyl myristate liquid petrolatum base.

Indications: Ear cleaning liquid for dogs and cats.

Dosage and Administration: To help soften and loosen earwax accumulation and to aid in its removal by water flushing, fill the ear canal with CERUMENE™ and gently massage for several minutes. Excess may be removed with cotton or paper towel. Flush gently and thoroughly with clean warm water and dry by blotting. When used routinely (once or twice a month), CERUMENE™ helps prevent earwax accumulation.

CERUMENE™ may be used prior to otic medication or as part of a complete grooming regimen.

Precaution(s): Store at room temperature.

The product is not an ear medication and is intended only for cleaning use as indicated. If pain, redness, rash or irritation develops, or if infection occurs, discontinue use and re-evaluate the condition.

Caution(s): Keep out of the reach of children.

Presentation: 4 fl. oz. and 12 fl. oz. (355 mL) plastic bottles with ear application tip.

Compendium Code No.: 10050031

CERUMITE 3X

Evsco **Otic Parasiticide**

EPA Reg. No.: 2382-116-50414

Active Ingredient(s):

Pyrethrins 0.15%
Technical Piperonyl Butoxide* 1.50%
n-Octyl bicycloheptane Dicarboximide 0.50%
Inert ingredients 97.85%

*Equivalent to 1.2% (butyl-carbityl) (6-propyl-piperonyl) ether and 0.3% related compounds.

Indications: For the treatment of ear mites in dogs, cats, puppies and kittens.

Directions for Use: It is a violation of Federal law to use this product in a manner inconsistent with its labeling.

Read entire label before using.

Use only on dogs, cats, puppies and kittens.

Cleanse ear thoroughly with a low pH ear cleanser. Place sufficient CERUMITE in each ear to wet external ear canal and massage base of ear. Retreat in 7 days. If it is necessary to again clean the ears sooner, retreat with CERUMITE.

Precautionary Statements: Hazards to Human and Domestic Animals:

Caution: Do not use on dogs or cats under 12 weeks of age. Sensitivities may occur after using any pesticide product on pets. If signs of sensitivity occur, consult a veterinarian immediately. Harmful if absorbed through skin. Avoid contact with skin or clothing. Prolonged or frequently repeated skin contact may cause allergic reactions in some individuals. Wash thoroughly with soap and water after handling.

Statement of Practical Treatment:

If on Skin: Wash with plenty of soap and water. Get medical attention if irritation occurs.

Storage and Disposal: Storage: Store in a cool, dry area.

Disposal: Do not reuse empty container. Wrap container and put in trash.

Warning(s): Keep out of reach of children.

Presentation: 0.5 fl oz (14.7 mL).

Sold only by veterinarians.

Compendium Code No.: 10050330 1289 1

CERVIZINE® INJECTABLE ℞

Wildlife **Analgesic-Sedative**

(Xylazine) 100 mg/mL

NADA No.: 139-236

Active Ingredient(s): Each mL contains: Xylazine hydrochloride equivalent to 100 mg of base activity, methylparaben 0.9 mg, propylparaben 0.1 mg, sodium citrate dihydrate 5.0 mg and water for injection. pH adjusted with citric acid and sodium citrate.

Indications: Xylazine should be used in horses and *Cervidae* (Fallow Deer, Mule Deer, Sika Deer, White-Tailed Deer and Elk) when it is desirable to produce a state of sedation accompanied by a shorter period of analgesia. **Horses:** Xylazine has been used successfully as follows:

1. Diagnostic procedures - oral and ophthalmic examinations, abdominal palpation, rectal palpation, vaginal examination, catheterization of the bladder and radiographic examinations.
2. Orthopedic procedures, such as application of casting materials and splints.
3. Dental procedures.
4. Minor surgical procedures of short duration such as debridement, removal of cutaneous neoplasms and suturing of lacerations.
5. To calm and facilitate handling of fractious animals.
6. Major surgical procedures:
   a. When used as a preanesthetic to general anesthesia.
   b. When used in conjunction with local anesthetics

Cervidae: Xylazine may be used for the following:

1. To calm and facilitate handling of fractious animals.
2. Diagnostic procedures.
3. Minor surgical procedures.
4. Therapeutic medication for sedation and relief of pain following injury or surgery.
5. As a preanesthetic to local anesthesia. CERVIZINE® at the recommended dosages can be used in conjunction with local anesthetics, such as procaine or lidocaine.

Pharmacology: Xylazine, a non-narcotic compound, is a sedative and analgesic as well as a muscle relaxant. Its sedative and analgesic activity is related to central nervous system depression. Its muscle-relaxant effect is based on inhibition of the intraneural transmission of impulses in the central nervous system. This principal pharmacological activities develop within 10 to 15 minutes after intramuscular injection in horses and *Cervidae*, and within 3 to 5 minutes following intravenous administration in horses.

A sleeplike state, the depth of which is dose-dependent, is usually maintained for 1 to 2 hours, while analgesia lasts from 15 to 30 minutes. The centrally acting muscle-relaxant effect causes relaxation of the skeletal musculature complementing sedation and analgesia.

In horses and *Cervidae* under the influence of xylazine, the respiratory rate is reduced as in natural sleep. Following treatment with xylazine, the heart rate is decreased and a transient change in the conductivity of the cardiac muscle may occur, as evidenced by a partial atrioventricular block. This resembles the atrioventricular block often observed in normal horses.[1,2,3,4] Although a partial A-V block may occasionally occur following intramuscular injection of xylazine, the incidence is less than when it is administered intravenously. Intravenous administration of xylazine causes a transient rise in blood pressure, followed by a slight decrease.

Xylazine has no effect on blood clotting time or other hematologic parameters.

Dosage and Administration:

1. Dosage

   Horses:

   Intravenous - 0.5 mL/100 lb body weight (0.5 mg/lb or 1.1 mg/kg).

   Intramuscular - 1.0 mL/100 lb body weight (1 mg/lb or 2.2 mg/kg).

   Cervidae:

   Administer intramuscularly, by either hand syringe or syringe dart, in the heavy muscles of the croup or shoulder.

   Fallow Deer *(Dama dama)* - 2.0 to 4.0 mL/100 lbs body weight (2.0 to 4.0 mg/lb or 4.4 to 8.8 mg/kg).

   Mule Deer *(Odocoileus hemionus)* - 1.0 to 2.0 mL/100 lbs body weight (1.0 to 2.0 mg/lb or 2.2 to 4.4 mg/kg).

   Sika Deer *(Cervus nippon)* - 1.0 to 2.0 mL/100 lbs body weight (1.0 to 2.0 mg/lb or 2.2 to 4.4 mg/kg).

   White-Tailed Deer *(Odocoileus virginianus)* - 1.0 to 2.0 mL/100 lbs body weight (1.0 to 2.0 mg/lb or 2.2 to 4.4 mg/kg).

   Elk *(Cervus canadensis)* - 0.25 to 0.5 mL/100 lbs body weight (0.25 to 0.5 mg/lb or 0.55 to 1.1 mg/kg).

   Following injection of xylazine, the animal should be allowed to rest quietly until the full effect has been reached.

   These dosages produce sedation which is usually maintained for 1 to 2 hours, and analgesia which lasts for 15 to 30 minutes.
2. Preanesthetic to Local Anesthesia

   Xylazine at the recommended dosages can be used in conjunction with local anesthetics, such as procaine or lidocaine.
3. Preanesthetic to General Anesthesia

   Xylazine at the recommended dosage rates produces an additive effect to central nervous system depressants such as pentobarbital sodium, thiopental sodium and thiamyl sodium. Therefore, the dosage of such compounds should be reduced and administered to the desired effect. In general, only ⅓ to ½ of the calculated dosage of the barbiturates will be needed to produce a surgical plane of anesthesia. Post-anesthetic or emergence excitement has not been observed in animals pre-anesthetized with xylazine.

   Xylazine has been used successfully as a preanesthetic agent for pentobarbital sodium, thiopental sodium, thiamylal sodium, nitrous oxide, ether, halothane, glyceryl guaiacolate and methoxyflurane anesthesia.

Contraindication(s): Do not use xylazine in conjunction with tranquilizers.

Precaution(s): Protect from heat. Do not store over 30°C (86°F).

Caution(s): Federal law restricts this drug to use by or on the order of a licensed veterinarian.

Careful consideration should be given before administering to horses and *Cervidae* with significantly depressed respiration, severe pathologic heart disease, advanced liver or kidney disease, severe endotoxic or traumatic shock and stress conditions such as extreme heat, cold, high altitude, or fatigue.

Analgesic effect is variable, and depth should be carefully assayed prior to surgical/clinical procedures. Variability of analgesia occurs most frequently at the distal extremities of horses and *Cervidae*. **In spite of sedation, the practitioner and handlers should proceed with caution since defense reactions may not be diminished.**

Intracarotid Arterial Injection Should be Avoided. As with many compounds, including tranquilizers, immediate violent seizures followed by collapse may result from inadvertent administration into the carotid artery. Although the reaction with xylazine is usually transient and recovery may be rapid and complete, special care should be taken to assure that the needle is in the jugular vein rather than the carotid artery.

Horses: Since an additive effect results from the use of xylazine and the barbiturate compounds, it should be used with caution with these central nervous system depressants. Products known to produce respiratory depression or apnea, such as thiamylal sodium should be given at a reduced dosage and, when injected intravenously, should be administered slowly. When intravenous administration is desired, avoid perivascular injection in order to achieve the desired effect. Studies have shown negligible evidence of tissue irritation, however, following perivascular injection of xylazine.

Bradycardia and an arrhythmia in the form of incomplete atrioventricular block have been reported following xylazine administration. Although clinically the importance of this effect is questioned,[1,2,3,4] a standard dose of atropine given prior to or following xylazine will greatly decrease the incidence.

Sedation for transport is most successful if actual transportation is begun after the full effect of the drug has been reached and the animal's stability is maintained while standing. In addition, it should be noted that animals under the influence of xylazine can be aroused by noise or other stimuli and this may increase the risk of injury.

Cervidae: It is preferable to administer CERVIZINE® to fasted *Cervidae*. As in all ruminants, a safeguard against aspiration of food material into the lungs and/or bloat during deep sedation is necessary.

Care should be taken to administer CERVIZINE® in the heavy muscles of the croup or shoulder. Injections given subcutaneously, intraperitoneally or into fat deposits will give unpredictable results.

Cervidae should not be disturbed during induction or until the full effect of the drug has been reached which is usually 10 to 15 minutes following injection.

The usual time to initial effect of the drug is 2 to 5 minutes. The administrator of the drug should be fully cognizant of this interval prior to administration of drug to free-ranging deer or elk, especially at night or in heavily wooded areas.

If the animal has been underdosed (faulty injection or miscalculation on weight), it is advisable to wait one hour before administering a second dose.

Adequate ventilation-especially in cages or crates-is mandatory; keep head and neck in position to ensure patient air passage and to prevent aspiration of stomach contents.

During sedation, *Cervidae* should be prevented from assuming lateral recumbency. A sternal recumbent position is desirable.

While under the effects of xylazine, the animal should be protected from an extremely hot or cold environment.

Efforts should be made to prevent patient from rising until almost complete recovery is attained.

The transportation of *Cervidae* given CERVIZINE® should be carefully monitored to prevent excessive struggling, injury or death.

Hyperthermic reactions may occur, especially if the subject is in a highly excited psychic state when the drug is administered. Hosing the head and entire body with cold water has usually proven to be an effective deterrent.

Data are presently inadequate to recommend CERVIZINE®'s use in pregnant *Cervidae*. Avoid use during breeding season.

Cervidae should be observed closely until all of the sedative effects of CERVIZINE® are gone.

Care should be taken at all times when administering CERVIZINE® to *Cervidae*. This is due to the method of administration (usually darting), the difficulty in estimating body weights and the accepted theory that wild animals are more unpredictable in their response to sedatives and analgesics than the domesticated species.

Warning(s): The drug is for use in horses and *Cervidae* only and should not be administered to food-producing animals.

Avoid accidental administration to humans. Should such exposure occur, notify a physician immediately. Artificial respiration may be indicated.

In *Cervidae*, occasional capture-associated deaths occur. Clinical trials reveal a mortality rate of approximately 3.5% attendant with the administration of xylazine.

Side Effects: Xylazine in horses and *Cervidae* used at recommended dosage levels may occasionally cause slight muscle tremors, bradycardia with partial A-V heart block and a reduced respiratory rate. Movement in response to sharp auditory stimuli may be observed. In horses, sweating, rarely profuse, has been reported following administration. In *Cervidae*, salivation, various vocalizations (bellowing, bleating, groaning, grunting, snoring) on expiration, audible grinding of molar teeth, protruding tongue and elevated temperatures have also been noted in some cases.

Trial Data:

Safety: Xylazine has been tested in horses at 5 times the recommended dose, and at doses above the recommended range in *Cervidae*. However, doses of this magnitude may produce convulsions and long periods of sedation in horses and muscle tremors and long periods of sedation in *Cervidae*.

References: Available upon request.

Presentation: CERVIZINE® is supplied in 50 mL multiple-dose vials.

CERVIZINE® is a registered trademark of Wildlife Pharmaceuticals, Inc.

Compendium Code No.: 10520020

CESTEX® ℞

Pfizer Animal Health **Parasiticide-Oral**

(epsiprantel) Veterinary Tablets

NADA No.: 140-893

Description: CESTEX® tablets are film-coated and contain 12.5 mg, 25 mg, 50 mg or 100 mg of epsiprantel per tablet.

Indications: CESTEX® tablets are indicated for the removal of the following:

Feline cestodes: *Dipylidium caninum* and *Taenia taeniaeformis*.

Canine cestodes: *Dipylidium caninum* and *Taenia pisiformis*.

Pharmacology: Epsiprantel is an anthelmintic that is active as a single dose against the common tapeworms of cats and dogs. Epsiprantel has a molecular weight of 326 and is chemically

2-(cyclohexylcarbonyl)-4-oxo-1,2,3,4,6,7,8,12b-octahydropyrazino[2,1-a][2]benzazepine. It is a stable white solid which is sparingly soluble in water. Its chemical structure is presented below.

Action: Epsiprantel acts directly on the tapeworm. Since it is minimally absorbed following oral administration, epsiprantel remains at the site of action within the gastrointestinal tract. Due to digestive process, tapeworm fragments or proglottids may not be readily visible in the stool.

Dosage and Administration: CESTEX® tablets should be administered orally.

The recommended dosage of epsiprantel is: cats, 1.25 mg/lb of body weight; dogs, 2.5 mg/lb of body weight. The following table may be used as a guide:

Dosage Schedule

Feline

Body Weight	Dose
Seven weeks old	
up to 10 lb	12.5 mg
11-20 lb	25.0 mg

Canine

Body Weight	Dose
Seven weeks old	
up to 5 lb	12.5 mg
6-10 lb	25.0 mg
11-20 lb	50.0 mg
21-40 lb	100.0 mg
41-50 lb	125.0 mg
51-60 lb	150.0 mg
61-80 lb	200.0 mg
81-90 lb	225.0 mg
91-100 lb	250.0 mg
101+ lb	2.5 mg/lb, rounding up to next whole tablet combination

Fasting is not necessary or recommended.

Unless exposure to the infected intermediate hosts is controlled, reinfection is likely and retreatment may be required. In the case of *D. caninum*, an effective flea control program should be instituted.

Contraindication(s): There are no known contraindications to the use of this drug.

Precaution(s): Storage: Store at controlled room temperature 15°-30°C (59°-86°F).

Do not use in kittens or puppies less than 7 weeks of age.

Caution: Federal law restricts this drug to use by or on the order of a licensed veterinarian.

Warning(s): For use in cats and dogs only. Safety of use in pregnant or breeding animals has not been determined. Keep out of reach of children. Not for use in humans.

Trial Data: Safety: Epsiprantel has been evaluated in cats at 5 times the recommended dose given once daily for 3 days with no adverse effects noted. In tolerance studies, epsiprantel produced minimal clinical signs in cats given 40 times the recommended dose once daily for 4 days.

Epsiprantel has been evaluated in 14-day repeat dose studies in dogs at 500 mg/kg (90 times recommended dosage) with no significant adverse results. No side effects were observed during the clinical field studies.

Epsiprantel is not a cholinesterase inhibitor. During the course of clinical field studies, CESTEX® was administered concurrently with diethylcarbamazine citrate (dogs only), anti-inflammatory agents, insecticides, and nematocides with no drug incompatibilities noted.

Presentation: CESTEX® tablets are film-coated and contain 12.5 mg, 25 mg, 50 mg or 100 mg of epsiprantel per tablet. Cestex is supplied as described below:

Concentration	Weight (lbs)		Number Tablets/Bottle
	Cat	Dog	
12.5 mg	10	5	50, 100
25.0 mg	20	10	50, 100
50.0 mg	——	20	25, 50
100.0 mg	——	40	25, 50

Compendium Code No.: 36900881 75-8032-07

C.E.T.® 0.12% CHLORHEXIDINE LAVAGE

Virbac **Dental Preparation**

Active Ingredient(s):

Chlorhexidine gluconate B.P. .... 12% w/v

Ethyl alcohol U.S.P. .... 6% v/v

Also contains purified water, carboxymethylcellulose sodium U.S.P., sorbitol solution 70% U.S.P., mint flavor, FD&C blue #1 and D&C yellow #10.

Indications: For use on dogs, cats and horses between dental visits to help reduce inflammation and bleeding at the gumline. When gingival inflammation and bleeding subside, C.E.T.® 0.12% Chlorhexidine Lavage should be discontinued and a regular home dental care program of brushing with an animal toothpaste should begin.

Dosage and Administration: For the best results, use an applicator such as a soft-bristled toothbrush.

Use with applicators: Place a small amount of C.E.T.® 0.12% Chlorhexidine Lavage in a container. Gently hold the animal's head and dip the toothbrush or other applicator in the C.E.T® 0.12% Chlorhexidine Lavage. Carefully brush the animal's teeth in a gentle, circular motion. Remoisten the applicator as needed.

Use as a rinse: Gently hold the animal's head with one hand, placing the spout inside the corner of the mouth and inserting the nozzle slightly inside the cheek. Gently squeeze the bottle to place a small amount of C.E.T.® 0.12% Chlorhexidine Lavage between the cheek and the gums. Massage the mouth to work C.E.T® 0.12% Chlorhexidine Lavage over the teeth. Repeat on the opposite side of the mouth.

Precaution(s): Store at a controlled room temperature of 59°-86°F (15°-30°C).

Caution(s): Keep all drugs out of the reach of children.

Reversible teeth staining has been reported with the prolonged use of chlorhexidine.

Keep out of the ears and the eyes. For veterinary use only.

Presentation: 8 fl. oz. (237 mL) plastic bottle.

Compendium Code No.: 10230131

C

C.E.T.® CHEWS FOR CATS

Virbac **Dental Preparation**

Enzymatic Oral Hygiene Chews for Cats

Ingredients: Freeze-dried fish, antioxidant (containing tocopherols, ascorbic acid, natural flavor, and citric acid), dextrose, glucose oxidase, lactoperoxidase.

Guaranteed Analysis:

Crude Protein .... 40.0 - 49.2%

Crude Ash .... 2.0 - 2.4%

Crude Fat .... 44.3 - 54.1%

Moisture .... 3.8 - 4.7%

Crude Fiber .... 0.1 - 0.2%

Calories .... 16 per chew

Indications: C.E.T.® Chews for Cats combine the mechanical abrasive action of chewing freeze-dried fish with a dual-enzyme, antibacterial system. The coarse texture of the uniquely-processed, freeze-dried fish cleans the teeth by helping remove plaque and food debris. The dual-enzyme system activates and enhances the cat's naturally-occurring oral defense mechanism.

Dosage and Administration: C.E.T.® Chews should be part of a complete home dental care program which includes toothbrushing. Feed your cat one chew on those days you do not brush. Your veterinarian may give you specific directions. Please follow this professional advice closely.

Caution(s): For veterinary use only.

Presentation: 24 chews.

Compendium Code No.: 10230051

C.E.T.® ENZYMATIC TARTAR CONTROL TOOTHPASTE

Virbac **Dental Preparation**

Active Ingredient(s): Glucose oxidase, lactoperoxidase. Also Contains: Sorbitol USP/NF, purified water USP, hydrated silica, glycerine, dextrose, xanthan gum, flavor, sodium benzoate, potassium thiocyanate.

Indications: Enzymatic dentifrice for dogs.

C.E.T.® Enzymatic Tartar Control Toothpaste is specifically formulated for companion animal use.

Directions: Use a soft-bristled toothbrush such as the C.E.T.® Animal Toothbrush. Apply daily or as directed by your veterinarian. Your veterinarian may give you specific directions; follow this professional advice closely.

Precaution(s): Store at controlled room temperature.

Warning(s): Keep out of reach of children. For veterinary use only.

Presentation: 2.5 oz (70 g) beef and seafood tubes.

Compendium Code No.: 10230061

C.E.T.® ENZYMATIC TOOTHPASTE

Virbac **Dental Preparation**

Active Ingredient(s):

C.E.T.® Malt Flavor: Lactoperoxidase and glucose oxidase.

C.E.T.® Mint Flavor: Lactoperoxidase and glucose oxidase.

C.E.T.® Poultry Flavor: Lactoperoxidase, glucose oxidase and sodium monofluorophosphate.

Indications: An enzymatic dentifrice with fluoride formulated for companion animal use.

Dosage and Administration: Use a soft bristle toothbrush. Apply once a day or as directed by a veterinarian. Follow professional advice closely.

Precaution(s): Store at a controlled room temperature of 59°-86°F (15°-30°C).

Caution(s): Keep out of the reach of children.

Presentation: 2.5 oz. (70 g) tubes.

Compendium Code No.: 10230031

C.E.T.® FIRST•SIGHT

Virbac **Dental Preparation**

Plaque Disclosing Solution-Dry Handle Swabs

Active Ingredient(s): Contains: FD&C red dye #28, potassium sorbate, sorbic acid, methylparaben, propylparaben, glycerin.

Indications: A plaque disclosant that should be used to improve your client's brushing without the mess associated with solutions. Each Dry Handle Swab is an individual package that contains a cotton swab saturated with 0.25 mL of dye to effectively cover and disclose residual plaque.

C.E.T.® Duo-128 is the first product to use this revolutionary packaging to aid in helping your client understand the proper techniques to be employed to achieve better oral hygiene.

Directions:

1. Squeeze applicator where handle and tube join.
2. Gently snap handle to break joint.
3. Pull out. Dab C.E.T.® Duo-128 on area to be examined and allow to remain in place for 10 seconds. Areas of concern will appear dark red and added brushing should be employed.

Precaution(s): Store at room temperature.

Caution(s): For oral use only.

For veterinary use only.

Warning(s): C.E.T.® Duo-128 uses red dye #28 which will permanently stain clothing and other materials if allowed to come in contact with them.

Keep out of the reach of children.

Presentation: 100 x 0.25 mL swabs (NDC 051311-128-01). Patent No. 4,952,204

Compendium Code No.: 10230740

C

C.E.T.® FLURAFOM

Virbac **Dental Preparation**

Active Ingredient(s): C.E.T.® FluraFom contains 1.23% fluoride (from sodium fluoride and hydrogen fluoride) in a phosphoric acid foam at pH 3.0- 3.4.

Indications: Fluoride treatment can be an important adjunct to routine dental prophylaxis. Although dogs and cats are relatively resistant to developing caries, the beneficial uses of fluoride therapy are well documented. These benefits include desensitizing exposed dentin, strengthening tooth enamel, decreasing the rate of plaque re-attachment, and stimulating remineralization of the enamel.[1]

C.E.T.® FluraFom is a fluoride treatment specifically developed for use on animals. C.E.T.® FluraFom's delivery system is more efficient than regular fluoride gels. The dynamic foam provides a continuous supply of fluoride to the tooth surface requiring less fluoride to produce a comparable fluoride uptake.

The reduction of the total amount of fluoride introduced into the oral cavity decreases the danger of ingesting potentially toxic levels of fluoride.

Dosage and Administration: C.E.T.® FluraFom should be used on an intubated and anesthetized patient. After a thorough cleaning, polishing and irrigating, dry the teeth completely using an air syringe.

Shake the applicator vigorously. Gently push down on the nozzle, and apply a ribbon of C.E.T.® FluraFom directly on the upper and lower row of teeth, one (1) side at a time. If necessary, use a soft-bristled toothbrush to evenly distribute the foam over all of the tooth surfaces. Allow one (1) to two (2) minutes for the foam to dissipate and then remove any remaining foam. The fluoride is continuously deposited on the tooth enamel as the foam dissipates. Avoid food and water for 30 minutes after treatment. A fluoride treatment is recommended every four (4) to six (6) months.

Note: Because the nozzle has a tendency to release too much foam, first-time users of C.E.T.® FluraFom may wish to test the application on a smooth surface prior to applying it on the teeth.

Precaution(s): The contents are under pressure. Do not puncture or incinerate. Do not store at temperatures above 120°F.

Caution(s): U.S. federal law prohibits dispensing without a prescription. For veterinary use only.

Discussion:

Fluoride uptake efficiency of C.E.T.® FluraFom: Fluoride gels are available with neutral or acidic pH. The 1.23% acidulated phosphate fluoride gels with a 3-3.5 pH have been shown to have a better capacity to bond with the calcium in the tooth enamel.[2]

The fluoride uptake by teeth exposed to C.E.T.® FluraFom and a commercial gel product (both 1.23% acidulated phosphate fluoride) have been measured under experimental laboratory conditions. Results from one study are summarized, and demonstrate the fluoride uptake achieved by C.E.T.® FluraFom is consistently higher than that provided by the traditional gel-type product.[3]

In addition, since substantially less fluoride is required to produce comparable fluoride uptake, the use of the foam minimizes exposure to systemic fluoride. The foam delivery is also easier to use and requires less cleanup.

References: Available upon request.

Presentation: 2 oz. (56 g) and 6.34 oz. (180 g) bottles.

Note the bottle may look partially empty, but the "empty" portion is the propellent in C.E.T.® FluraFom needed to supply the delivery system. The propellant is a propane/isobutane mixture that is environmentally safe.

Compendium Code No.: 10230301

C.E.T.® ORAL HYGIENE GEL

Virbac **Dental Preparation**

Active Ingredient(s): 0.12% chlorhexidine gluconate. Also contains: Glycerine, safflower oil, food grade carbopol 974P, triethanolamine (TEA) 99, fish oil, barley malt extract, zinc gluconate, vitamin E.

Indications: Long acting oral gel for pets.

Dosage and Administration: Use daily or as directed by your veterinarian.

Precaution(s): Store at room temperature 59°-86°F (15°-30°C).

Caution(s): Reversible teeth staining has been reported with prolonged use of chlorhexidine.

Keep out of ears and eyes.

Warning(s): For veterinary use only.

Keep this and all drugs out of reach of children.

Presentation: 1.1 fl oz (32 mL).

Compendium Code No.: 10230121

C.E.T.® ORAL HYGIENE RINSE

Virbac **Dental Preparation**

0.12% Chlorhexidine Gluconate

Active Ingredient(s): Contains: 0.12% Chlorhexidine gluconate, 0.05 cetylpyridinium chloride, and zinc in a soothing alcohol-free vehicle.

Spherulites: An exclusive & patented encapsulation system which provides slow release of ingredients long after application.

Indications: For use in the prevention of plaque, calculus and gum disease in dogs and cats.

C.E.T.® Oral Hygiene Rinse is a soothing, refreshing and palatable rinse containing chlorhexidine gluconate, cetylpyridinium chloride and zinc. The antimicrobial activity of chlorhexidine and cetylpyridinium chloride, combined with the anti-plaque and anti-calculus properties of zinc, together can aid in the prevention of tooth and gum disease. Encapsulation of chlorhexidine in Spherulites allows for slow release and long-lasting benefit. This alcohol-free formulation will leave your pet with clean breath while providing soothing temporary relief of minor gum irritation.

Directions: Shake well before use. Rinse daily following each meal as directed by your veterinarian. Hold the bottle in the upright position and below your pet's field of vision. Gently elevate the upper lip to expose the teeth and gums. Point and squeeze to apply a gentle stream of C.E.T.® Oral Hygiene Rinse. The foaming formulation of C.E.T.® Oral Hygiene Rinse will allow a quick dispersion and complete coverage of the oral cavity, even in those areas that are difficult to reach. Avoid touching the gum with the nozzle to avoid any injury in case of movement of your pet.

Precaution(s): Store at room temperature.

Caution(s): Keep out of reach of children.

For veterinary use only.

Discussion: Importance of oral hygiene: Plaque is the soft, grayish-white film which is formed continuously on tooth surface by the proliferation of bacteria. Within days, plaque mineralizes into calculus, or tartar, which acts as a framework for further plaque development. If not eliminated, plaque bacteria can infect the gums and structures which support the teeth. The result is gingivitis and eventually periodontal disease, which causes bad breath, pain and tooth loss. Chronic oral infection can also lead to disease in other parts of the body, including the heart, lungs and kidneys.

Good oral hygiene is important to your pet's overall health. Your veterinarian is your best source of advice concerning your pet's oral health. Follow the advice closely.

Presentation: 8 fl oz bottle.

250822-01

Compendium Code No.: 10230341

CGB® OINTMENT ℞

PPC **Otic Preparation Antibiotic-Corticosteroid**

Gentamicin Sulfate Veterinary, Betamethasone Valerate, USP and Clotrimazole, USP-Veterinary

NADA No.: 140-896

Active Ingredient(s): Each gram of CGB® Ointment contains gentamicin sulfate veterinary equivalent to 3 mg gentamicin base; betamethasone valerate, USP equivalent to 1 mg betamethasone; and 10 mg clotrimazole, USP in a mineral oil-based system containing a plasticized hydrocarbon gel.

Indications: CGB® Ointment is indicated for the treatment of canine acute and chronic otitis externa associated with yeast *(Malassezia pachydermatis*, formerly *Pityrosporum canis)* and/or bacteria susceptible to gentamicin.

Pharmacology:

Gentamicin: Gentamicin sulfate is an aminoglycoside antibiotic active against a wide variety of pathogenic gram-negative and gram-positive bacteria. *In vitro* tests have determined that gentamicin is bactericidal and acts by inhibiting normal protein synthesis in susceptible microorganisms. Specifically, gentamicin is active against the following organisms commonly isolated from canine ears: *Staphylococcus aureus*, other *Staphylococcus* spp., *Pseudomonas aeruginosa, Proteus* spp., and *Escherichia coli.*

Betamethasone: Betamethasone valerate is a synthetic adrenocorticoid for dermatologic use. Betamethasone, an analog of prednisolone, has a high degree of corticosteroid activity and a slight degree of mineralocorticosteroid activity. Betamethasone valerate, the 17-valerate ester of betamethasone, has been shown to provide anti-inflammatory and antipruritic activity in the topical management of corticosteroid-responsive otitis externa.

Topical corticosteroids can be absorbed from normal, intact skin. Inflammation can increase percutaneous absorption. Once absorbed through the skin, topical corticosteroids are handled through pharmacokinetic pathways similar to systemically administered corticosteroids.

Clotrimazole: Clotrimazole is a broad-spectrum antifungal agent that is used for the treatment of dermal infections caused by various species of pathogenic dermatophytes and yeasts. The primary action of clotrimazole is against dividing and growing organisms.

In vitro, clotrimazole exhibits fungistatic and fungicidal activity against isolates of *Trichophyton rubrum, Trichophyton mentagrophytes, Epidermophyton floccosum, Microsporum canis, Candida* spp., and *Malassezia pachydermatis (Pityrosporum canis).* Resistance to clotrimazole is very rare among the fungi that cause superficial mycoses.

In an induced otitis externa infected with *Malassezia pachydermatis*, 1% clotrimazole in the CGB® Ointment vehicle was effective both microbiologically and clinically in terms of reduction of exudate odor and swelling.

In studies of the mechanism of action, the minimum fungicidal concentration of clotrimazole caused leakage of intracellular phosphorus compounds into the ambient medium with concomitant breakdown of cellular nucleic acids and accelerated potassium efflux. These events began rapidly and extensively after addition of the drug.

Clotrimazole is very poorly absorbed following dermal application.

Gentamicin-Betamethasone-Clotrimazole: By virtue of its 3 active ingredients, CGB® Ointment has antibacterial, anti-inflammatory, and antifungal activity.

In component efficacy studies, the compatibility and additive effect of each of the components were demonstrated.

In clinical field trials, CGB® Ointment was effective in the treatment of otitis externa associated with bacteria and *Malassezia pachydermatis.* CGB® Ointment reduced discomfort, redness, swelling, exudate, and odor, and exerted a strong antimicrobial effect.

Dosage and Administration: The external ear should be thoroughly cleaned and dried before treatment. Remove foreign material, debris, crusted exudates, etc., with suitable nonirritating solutions. Excessive hair should be clipped from the treatment area. After verifying that the eardrum is intact, instill 4 drops (2 drops from the 215 g bottle) of CGB® Ointment twice daily into the ear canal of dogs weighing less than 30 lbs. Instill 8 drops (4 drops from the 215 g bottle) twice daily into the ear canal of dogs weighing 30 lbs. or more. Therapy should continue for 7 consecutive days.

Contraindication(s): If hypersensitivity to any of the components occurs, treatment should be discontinued and appropriate therapy instituted. Concomitant use of drugs known to induce ototoxicity should be avoided. Do not use in dogs with known perforation of eardrums.

Precaution(s): Store between 2° and 25°C (36° and 77°F).

Caution(s): Federal law restricts this drug to use by or on the order of a licensed veterinarian.

Identification of infecting organisms should be made either by microscopic roll smear evaluation or by culture as appropriate. Antibiotic susceptibility of the pathogenic organism(s) should be determined prior to use of this preparation.

If overgrowth of nonsusceptible bacteria, fungi, or yeasts occurs, or if hypersensitivity develops, treatment should be discontinued and appropriate therapy instituted.

Administration of recommended doses of CGB® Ointment beyond 7 days may result in delayed wound healing.

Avoid ingestion. Adverse systemic reactions have been observed following the oral ingestion of some topical corticosteroid preparations. Patients should be closely observed for the usual signs of adrenocorticoid overdosage which include sodium retention, potassium loss, fluid retention, weight gain, polydipsia, and/or polyuria. Prolonged use or overdosage may produce adverse immunosuppressive effects.

Use of corticosteroids, depending on dose, duration, and specific steroid, may result in endogenous steroid production inhibition following drug withdrawal. In patients presently receiving or recently withdrawn from corticosteroid treatments, therapy with a rapidly acting corticosteroid should be considered in especially stressful situations.

Before instilling any medication into the ear, examine the external ear canal thoroughly to be certain the tympanic membrane is not ruptured in order to avoid the possibility of transmitting infection to the middle ear us well as damaging the cochlea or vestibular apparatus from prolonged contact.

Warning(s): The use of CGB® Ointment has been associated with deafness or partial hearing loss in a small number of sensitive dogs (eg, geriatric). The hearing deficit is usually temporary. If hearing or vestibular dysfunction is noted during the course of treatment, discontinue use of CGB® Ointment immediately and flush the ear canal thoroughly with a nonototoxic solution.

Corticosteroids administered to dogs, rabbits, and rodents during pregnancy have resulted in cleft palate in offspring. Other congenital anomalies including deformed forelegs, phocomelia, and anasarca have been reported in offspring of dogs which received corticosteroids during pregnancy.

Clinical and experimental data have demonstrated that corticosteroids administered orally or parenterally to animals may induce the first stage of parturition if used during the last trimester of pregnancy and may precipitate premature parturition followed by dystocia, fetal death, retained placenta, and metritis.

Keep this and all drugs out of the reach of children.

For otic use in dogs only.

Toxicology: Clinical and safety studies with CGB® Ointment have shown a wide safety margin at the recommended dose level in dogs (see Cautions/Side Effects).

Side Effects:

Gentamicin: While aminoglycosides are absorbed poorly from skin, intoxication may occur when aminoglycosides are applied topically for prolonged periods of time to large wounds, burns, or any denuded skin, particularly if there is renal insufficiency. All aminoglycosides have the potential to produce reversible and irreversible vestibular, cochlear, and renal toxicity.

Betamethasone: Side effects such as SAP and SGPT enzyme elevations, weight loss, anorexia, polydipsia, and polyuria have occurred following the use of parenteral or systemic synthetic corticosteroids in dogs. Vomiting and diarrhea (occasionally bloody) have been observed in dogs and cats.

Cushing's syndrome in dogs has been reported in association with prolonged or repeated steroid therapy.

Clotrimazole: The following have been reported occasionally in humans in connection with the use of clotrimazole: erythema, stinging, blistering, peeling, edema, pruritus, urticaria, and general irritation of the skin not present before therapy.

Presentation: CGB® Ointment is available in 7.5 gram tubes (NDC 61546-6520-6), 15 gram tubes (NDC 61546-6520-7), and 215 gram bottles (NDC 61546-6520-4).

Compendium Code No.: 14870000 January 1998, 81-479242

CHAMPION PROTECTOR™ CANINE 7-WAY VACCINE

AgriLabs **Bacterin-Vaccine**

Canine Distemper-Hepatitis-Parainfluenza-Parvovirus Vaccine, Modified Live Virus-Leptospira Bacterin

U.S. Vet. Lic. No.: 213

Contents: CHAMPION PROTECTOR™ Canine 7-Way Vaccine consists of standardized, lyophilized, attenuated strains of canine distemper virus, infectious canine hepatitis virus (CAV-1), canine parainfluenza virus, and a canine isolate parvovirus; accompanied by liquid, inactivated *Leptospira canicola* and *L. icterohaemorrhagiae* bacterin diluent. All virus fractions are propagated in established cell lines proven free of extraneous agents and are produced under precisely controlled conditions. The vaccine viruses are blended with Bemapar® stabilizer and presented in a lyophilized form. The product has been tested for purity, safety, potency, and efficacy in accordance with regulations of the United States Department of Agriculture.

CHAMPION PROTECTOR™ Canine 7-Way Vaccine contains permissible levels of polymyxin B and neomycin as preservatives.

Indications: For use in healthy dogs for the prevention of canine distemper, hepatitis, parainfluenza, parvovirus, and leptospirosis caused by *Leptospira canicola* and *L. icterohaemorrhagiae.*

Dosage and Administration: Administer two (2) doses (1 mL each) two (2) to three (3) weeks apart. For dogs vaccinated before 14 weeks of age, revaccinate every two (2) to three (3) weeks until at least 14 weeks of age. Revaccinate annually with a single dose to maintain a high level of immunity.

To rehydrate, aseptically add the contents of an accompanying vial of Leptospira bacterin to a vial of lyophilized canine distemper-hepatitis-parainfluenza-parvovirus vaccine. Shake well to rehydrate. After rehydration, the entire contents should be used immediately. For intramuscular or subcutaneous use. Maternal antibodies may interfere with successful immunization with any of the components of the vaccine. It is recommended that a 1 mL dose be administered at approximately nine (9) weeks of age with repeat vaccinations at 2- to 3-week intervals until at least 14 weeks of age.

Precaution(s): Store at 35-45°F (2-7°C).

Use sterile syringes and needles (do not chemically sterilize).

Burn all containers and unused contents.

Caution(s): Anaphylactic reactions may occur following the use of biological products. Symptomatic therapy should be provided, including epinephrine. Occasionally transient corneal opacity may occur following the administration of the product. This is due to the canine hepatitis fraction, however the strain has been used extensively in the field and appears to involve a very low incidence of corneal opacity.

For use in dogs only.

For veterinary use only.

Trial Data: CHAMPION PROTECTOR™ Canine 7-Way Vaccine has been extensively tested in susceptible puppies. Studies conducted have shown that puppies were protected against challenge with virulent canine distemper, canine hepatitis, canine parainfluenza or canine parvo viruses after vaccination with the virus strains used in the CHAMPION PROTECTOR™ Canine 7-Way Vaccine. Protective antibodies against all four viruses were demonstrated following vaccination. Studies also demonstrated that there was no interference between the canine distemper, hepatitis, parainfluenza, parvovirus or the Leptospira fractions. The vaccine proved to be safe and efficacious, and did not cause untoward reactions in vaccinated dogs. The Leptospira bacterin diluent contained with the CHAMPION PROTECTOR™ Canine 7-Way Vaccine has been extensively tested in susceptible dogs. Agglutinating antibodies were present in susceptible dogs in eight days after being vaccinated with a single dose of the *Leptospira canicola* and *L. icterohaemorrhagiae* bacterin. Nonvaccinated dogs showed clinical symptoms such as leptospiremia, leptospiruria, and leptospirae isolation from kidney tissue after challenge with virulent leptospirae. All vaccinated dogs remained healthy and free of clinical symptoms, including renal shedding, after challenge with virulent leptospirae. Studies performed have shown that there is not virucidal activity when the Leptospira bacterin diluent is used to rehydrate the virus vaccine.

Presentation: 1 dose with syringe.

Compendium Code No.: 10581420

CHAMPION PROTECTOR™ FELINE

AgriLabs **Vaccine**

Feline Rhinotracheitis-Calici-Panleukopenia Vaccine, Modified Live Virus

U.S. Vet. Lic. No.: 213

Contents: The Feline Rhinotracheitis portion of this combination package consists of a naturally attenuated strain, designated the AL strain. The Feline Calicivirus portion consists of an attenuated strain of feline calicivirus The vaccines are blended with a special stabilizer and lyophilized. The Feline Panleukopenia portion is a stable liquid vaccine with stabilizer consisting of an attenuated strain of feline panleukopenia (distemper) designated the Alpha-PL strain virus and is used to rehydrate the lyophilized Feline Rhinotracheitis-Calici Vaccine. The Feline Rhinotracheitis-Calici and Feline Panleukopenia Vaccine fractions are all produced in a feline cell line under precisely controlled conditions of a "Frozen Stable Cell Bank™" system.

C

The vaccine contains permissible levels of polymyxin B and neomycin as preservatives.

The vaccine viruses have undergone extensive purification studies ensuring the highest degree of purity. There is no sting or discomfort on administration. The product meets USDA requirements for purity, safety, potency and efficacy.

Indications: For use in healthy cats for the prevention of feline rhinotracheitis, feline calici and feline panleukopenia infections.

Dosage and Administration: To rehydrate, aseptically add the contents of an accompanying vial of Feline Panleukopenia Vaccine to a vial of lyophilized Feline Rhinotracheitis-Calici Vaccine. Shake well to rehydrate. After rehydration, the entire contents should be used immediately. Feline Vaccine is recommended for vaccination of healthy cats. For intramuscular or subcutaneous use. Administer 2 doses (1 mL each) 3 to 4 weeks apart. For cats vaccinated before 9 weeks of age, revaccinate every 3 to 4 weeks until at least 12 weeks of age. Revaccinate annually with a single dose to maintain a high level of immunity.

Vaccination Instructions: (Clean hands, equipment and surroundings will minimize the chance of injection site irritation).

1. Using syringe and needle, withdraw all material from the "liquid" bottle and inject it into the "dry vaccine" bottle.
2. Leave the needle in the vaccine vial and remove the syringe from the needle to ease the vacuum. Replace syringe on the needle.
3. Now you can withdraw the mixed contents of the vaccine vial into the syringe. Gently pumping it between the vial and syringe a few times provides improved mixing.
4. While keeping the animal quiet, gently grasp the loose skin along the back of the neck area with one hand while the other hand rests on the animal's back, with loaded vaccination syringe ready to push forward.
5. Insert and aspirate. (Aspirate means to partially withdraw the plunger to make sure no blood appears in the syringe barrel...in which case the needle should be withdrawn and reinserted.)
6. Pull out needle and gently rub the area. Property dispose of used syringes and bottles. Congratulations! Your pet has just taken a giant step toward good health.

Contraindication(s): Do not vaccinate pregnant cats.

Precaution(s): Store at 35-45°F (2-7°C). Use sterile syringe and needle (do not chemically sterilize). Use the entire contents when the container is first opened. Burn all containers and unused contents.

Caution(s): Anaphylactoid reactions may occur following the use of biological products. Symptomatic treatment should be provided.

For animal use only.

Antidote(s): Epinephrine.

Trial Data:

Purity of the Vaccine Viruses - Studies conducted on the Feline, Rhinotracheitis, Calici, and Panleukopenia Vaccine Master Seed Viruses demonstrated no extraneous viruses, bacteria, fungi, mycoplasma, or other adventitious agents.

Purity of the Cell Cultures - The Master Cell Stock of the feline cell line was prepared and pretested prior to use in vaccine production and demonstrated no bacteria, fungi, mycoplasma or other adventitious agents assuring a vaccine of the highest purity.

Feline Rhinotracheitis Antigenicity (Patency Evaluation in Cats) - Challenge studies were performed in over 100 susceptible cats from a closed colony. The studies showed the vaccine protected cats from virulent challenge. The challenge strain (C27), at 10,000 $TCID_{50}$s caused significant disease and often death in susceptible cats. The cats used in the antigenicity test for licensing were challenged with more than 100 times this concentration.

Feline Calicivirus Antigenicity and Efficacy (Potency Evaluation in Cats) - The vaccine afforded significant protection to felines against the highly virulent FPV-255 challenge strain. A reduction in clinical symptoms ranging from 83% to 97% was demonstrated in vaccinates as compared to challenge controls.

Panleukopenia Antigenicity (Potency Evaluation in Cats) - Serologic studies performed in susceptible seronegative closed colony cats of various ages showed the average serum neutralization antibody titer to be 1:2500 fourteen days after vaccination. Paired sera from clinical field trials were also evaluated and supported the closed colony results which illustrate the high antigenicity in cats. Studies completed and filed USDA illustrate that the Feline Panleukopenia Vaccine provides significant protection when cats were challenged with virulent virus 72 hours after vaccination. This combination product Feline Vaccine was shown to be efficacious and not to cause cross interference with immunity.

Safety Studies in Cats (Feline Rhinotracheitis Fraction) - The vaccine virus when used as directed has been shown to be safe and free from untoward reactions. At exaggerated dosage levels (>100 times the field dose) the virus caused no adverse effects in susceptible animals. Back passages in cats demonstrated no reversion to virulence.

Safety Studies in Cats (Feline Calicivirus Fraction) - The vaccine virus has been shown to be safe in the feline. Back passages substantiate the safety of the vaccine by indicating no reversion to virulence.

Safety studies in Cats (Feline Panleukopenia Fraction) - The vaccine virus has been shown to be safe for use in cats. Ten (10) back passages in susceptible cats prove the virus to be truly attenuated and that it does not revert to virulence. The virus is safe when tested at exaggerated dosage levels (>600 times the field dose). The vaccine virus has been safely used in many cats of various ages. Studies indicate that minimal contact spread of vaccine occurs from cats administered >1000 times the field dose.

Maternal Antibody - Studies determined the decay rate for maternal antibodies to feline rhinotracheitis virus. Felines lose maternal antibodies between eight and nine weeks of age and become susceptible to the disease. Feline calicivirus maternal antibodies also decay within the same approximate period of time. However, animals may be born from nonimmune queens and will be susceptible prior to this age. The level of maternal antibody to Panleukopenia varies greatly depending upon the immune status of the mother, therefore, vaccination at an early age with revaccination as indicated earlier is recommended.

Presentation: 1 dose (1 mL) vial accompanied by 1 mL diluent.

Manufactured by: Diamond Animal Health, Inc.

Compendium Code No.: 10581430

CHAMPION PROTECTOR™ PUPPY PROTECTOR™

AgriLabs **Vaccine**

Canine Distemper-Hepatitis-Parainfluenza-Parvovirus Vaccine, Modified Live Virus

U.S. Vet. Lic. No.: 213

Contents: CHAMPION PROTECTOR™ PUPPY PROTECTOR™ consists of standardized, lyophilized, attenuated strains of canine distemper virus, infectious canine hepatitis virus (CAV-1), canine parainfluenza virus, and a canine isolate parvovirus. All virus fractions are propagated in established cell lines proven free of extraneous agents and are produced under precisely controlled conditions. The vaccine viruses are blended with Bemapar® stabilizer and presented in a lyophilized form. The product has been tested for purity, safety, potency, and efficacy in accordance with regulations of the United States Department of Agriculture. CHAMPION PROTECTOR™ PUPPY PROTECTOR™ is virtually free from foreign serum proteins.

CHAMPION PROTECTOR™ PUPPY PROTECTOR™ contains permissible levels of polymyxin B and neomycin as preservatives.

Indications: For use in healthy dogs for the prevention of canine distemper, hepatitis, parainfluenza and parvovirus.

Dosage and Administration: Administer two (2) doses (1 mL each) two (2) to three (3) weeks apart. For dogs vaccinated before 14 weeks of age, revaccinate every two (2) to three (3) weeks until at least 14 weeks of age. Revaccinate annually with a single dose to maintain a high level of immunity.

To rehydrate, aseptically add the contents of an accompanying vial of sterile diluent to a vial of lyophilized canine distemper-hepatitis-parainfluenza-parvovirus vaccine. Shake well to rehydrate. After rehydration, the entire contents should be used immediately. For intramuscular or subcutaneous use.

Maternal antibodies may interfere with successful immunization with any of the components of the vaccine. It is recommended that a 1 mL dose be administered at approximately nine (9) weeks of age with repeat vaccinations at 2- to 3-week intervals until at least 14 weeks of age.

Precaution(s): Store at 35-45°F (2-7°C).

Use sterile syringes and needles (do not chemically sterilize).

Burn all containers and unused contents.

Caution(s): Anaphylactic reactions may occur following the use of biological products. Symptomatic therapy should be provided, including epinephrine. Occasionally transient corneal opacity may occur following the administration of the product. This is due to the canine hepatitis fraction, however the strain has been used extensively in the field and appears to involve a very low incidence of corneal opacity.

For use in dogs only.

For veterinary use only.

Antidote(s): Epinephrine.

Trial Data: CHAMPION PROTECTOR™ PUPPY PROTECTOR™ has been extensively tested in susceptible puppies. Studies conducted have shown that puppies were protected against challenge with virulent canine distemper, canine hepatitis, canine parainfluenza and canine parvo viruses after vaccination with the virus strains used in the CHAMPION PROTECTOR™ PUPPY PROTECTOR™ vaccine. Protective antibodies against all four viruses were demonstrated following vaccination. Studies also demonstrated that there was not interference between the canine distemper, hepatitis, parainfluenza, or the parvovirus fractions. The vaccine proved to be safe and efficacious, and did not cause untoward reactions in vaccinated dogs.

Presentation: 1 dose with syringe.

Compendium Code No.: 10581440

CHAMPION PROTECTOR™ WORM PROTECTOR™ 2X

AgriLabs **Parasiticide-Oral**

(Pyrantel pamoate) Liquid Wormer

ANADA No.: 200-028

Active Ingredient(s): 4.54 mg of pyrantel base as pyrantel pamoate per mL.

Indications: To prevent reinfestation of *Toxocara canis* in puppies and adult dogs and in lactating bitches after whelping.

For the removal of large roundworms *(Toxocara canis* and *Toxascaris leonina)* and hookworms *(Ancylostoma caninum* and *Uncinaria stenocephala)* in dogs and puppies.

The presence of these parasites should be confirmed by laboratory fecal examination. Consult your veterinarian for assistance in the diagnosis, treatment, and control of parasitism.

Directions for Use: Important: Shake well before use.

For maximum control and prevention of reinfestation, it is recommended that puppies be treated at 2, 3, 4, 6, 8, and 10 weeks of age. Lactating bitches should be treated 2-3 weeks after whelping. Adult dogs kept in heavily contaminated quarters may be treated at monthly intervals to prevent *T. canis* reinfestation. Administer one full teaspoonful (5 mL) for each 10 lb of body weight.

For the removal of large roundworms (ascarids) and hookworms, administer one full teaspoonful (5 mL) for each 10 lb of body weight. It is not necessary to withhold food prior to treatment. If medication is to be dispensed, client can be advised that dogs usually find this wormer very palatable and will lick the dose from the bowl willingly. If there is reluctance to accept the dose, mix in a small quantity of dog food to encourage consumption. It is recommended that dogs maintained under conditions of constant exposure to worm infestation should have a follow-up fecal exam within 2 to 4 weeks after first treatment.

If your dog looks or acts sick, consult your veterinarian before treatment.

Precaution(s): Recommended Storage: Store below 86°F (30°C).

Warning(s): Keep out of reach of children.

Presentation: 2 fl oz (60 mL) and 8 fl oz (240 mL).

Compendium Code No.: 10581450 CT-84262-01

CHAP-GUARD™ PLUS

AgriLabs **Udder Cream**

Active Ingredient(s): Contains stearic acid, homo methyl, silcylate, isopropyl myristate, cetyl alcohol, aloe vera, propylene glycol, silicone, lanolin, mineral oil, triethanolamine, propylparaben, methylparaben, vitamin A, vitamin E, palmitate, vitamin D_3, chloroxylenol and de-ionized water.

Indications: CHAP-GUARD™ Plus with vitamins is for use as an aid in reducing dry, cracked and chapped udders in cattle. Contains humectants which assist in maintaining skin and tissue moisture balance.

The nonsticky, disappearing cream base discourages dirt and manure from sticking to udders.

Dosage and Administration: Apply each day or as needed after milking to aid in reducing dryness, cracking and chapping associated with chapped udders in cattle.

Caution(s): Keep out of the reach of children.

CHAP-GUARD™ Plus is not a substitute for balanced nutrition. Animals with signs of nutritional deficiency in the skin may require injections of therapeutic levels of vitamins. Consult a veterinarian for assistance in the diagnosis and treatment of nutritional deficiency.

If an animal shows signs of uncontrolled generalized infections, consult a veterinarian. Wash the teats and udders thoroughly before milking.

Presentation: 16 oz. (454 g) and 5 lb. (2.27 kg) containers.

Compendium Code No.: 10580290

CHECKMITE+™

Mann Lake

Bee Hive Pest Control Strip

For Control of Varroa Mites in Honeybee Colonies

For Use Only Under Section 18 Authorization

Active Ingredient:	Percent by Weight
0,0-Diethyl 0-(3-chloro-4-methyl-2 oxo-(2H)-1-benzopyran-7-yl) phosphorothioate (coumaphos)	10%
Inert Ingredients:	90%
Total	100%

KEEP OUT OF REACH OF CHILDREN

WARNING

SEE BELOW FOR STATEMENTS OF PRACTICAL TREATMENT AND OTHER PRECAUTIONARY STATEMENTS

READ ENTIRE LABEL FOR DIRECTIONS BEFORE USE

PRECAUTIONARY STATEMENTS

HAZARDS TO HUMANS AND DOMESTIC ANIMALS

WARNING

Do not chew or swallow. Causes moderate eye irritation. Avoid contact with skin, clothing or eyes. Wash thoroughly with soap and warm water after handling. Wash contaminated clothing with soap and hot water before use.

STATEMENTS OF PRACTICAL TREATMENT

If chewed or swallowed: Call a physician or Poison Control Center immediately, If possible, vomiting should be induced under medical supervision. Drink one or two glasses of water and induce vomiting by touching the back of throat with finger. Do not induce vomiting or give anything by mouth to an unconscious person.

If on skin: Remove contaminated clothing and wash affected areas with soap and water. Get medical attention if irritation appears.

If in eyes: Flush eyes with plenty of water. Call a physician immediately.

To Physician: Atropine sulfate by injection is antidotal. Repeat as necessary to the point of tolerance. 2-PAM is also antidotal and may be administered in conjunction with atropine.

ENVIRONMENTAL HAZARDS

This pesticide is toxic to birds, fish and aquatic invertebrates. Do not apply directly to any body of water. Do not contaminate water when disposing of used strips.

SUPPLIED: Code 0511 — 1 X 10 strips 77005110, R.1

EPA Est. No. 4691-KS-1

Distributed exclusively by: Mann Lake Ltd.

Manufactured by: Bayer Corporation, Agriculture Division, Animal Health, Shawnee Mission, Kansas 66201 U.S.A.

Compendium Code No.: 10810001

CHERRYDERM™ GROOMING SHAMPOO

Vetus **Grooming Shampoo**

Ingredient(s): Water, ammonium laureth sulfate, ammonium lauryl sulfate, coconut oil, glycerine, sodium chloride, fragrance, FD&C color.

Indications: Specially formulated to offer quick and easy cleansing while conditioning the animal's coat. Tangles brush out easily and coat smells fresh and clean. Adds body and luster to animal's coat while moisturizing and conditioning the skin. Provides superior cleansing action, and is pH balanced to be gentle enough for everyday use.

For dogs, cats, puppies, kittens, horses, foals.

Directions for Use: Thoroughly wet coat using warm water and apply a small amount of CHERRYDERM™ Grooming Shampoo. Work up a good lather, massaging deep into coat and skin. Rinse thoroughly and dry. May be repeated on extremely dirty animals, and will result in additional conditioning to the animal's coat.

Precaution(s): Avoid storing at excessive heat.

Caution(s): Keep out of reach of children.

Available exclusively through veterinarians.

Presentation: One gallon.

Distributed by: Burns Veterinary Supply, Inc., Westbury, NY 11590

Compendium Code No.: 14440190 ss. 03-00

CHERRY GROOMING SHAMPOO

Butler **Grooming Shampoo**

NDC No.: 11695-2154-5/11695-2154-2

Active Ingredient(s): Water, ammonium laureth sulfate, ammonium lauryl sulfate, coconut oil, glycerine, sodium chloride, fragrance, FD&C color.

Indications: For dogs, cats, puppies, kittens, horses, and foals.

Formulated to cleanse while conditioning the animal's coat. Adds body and luster to the animal's coat while moisturizing and conditioning the skin. Provides a cleansing action and is pH balanced to be gentle enough for everyday use.

Dosage and Administration: Thoroughly wet the coat using warm water and apply a small amount of CHERRY GROOMING SHAMPOO. Work up a good lather, massaging deep into the coat and skin. Rinse thoroughly and dry. The procedure may be repeated on extremely dirty animals, and will result in additional conditioning to the animal's coat.

Caution(s): Keep out of the reach of children.

Presentation: 12 fl. oz. and 2.5 gallon containers.

Compendium Code No.: 10820370

CHERRY GROOMING SHAMPOO

First Priority **Grooming Shampoo**

Ingredient(s): Water, Ammonium Lauryl Sulfate, Sodium Chloride, Cherry Fragrance, Artificial Color, Citric Acid.

Indications: Specially formulated to offer quick and easy cleansing while conditioning the animal's coat. Tangles brush out easily and coat smells fresh and clean. Adds body and luster to animal's coat while moisturizing and conditioning the skin. Provides superior cleansing action, and is pH balanced to be gentle enough for everyday use.

For dogs, cats, puppies, kittens, horses, foals.

Directions for Use: Thoroughly wet coat using warm water and apply a small amount of CHERRY GROOMING SHAMPOO. Work up a good lather, massaging deep into coat and skin. Rinse thoroughly and dry. May be repeated on extremely dirty animals, and will result in additional conditioning to the animal's coat.

Precaution(s): Storage: Store at controlled room temperature between 15°-30°C (59°-86°F). Keep container tightly closed when not in use.

Caution(s): For animal use only.

Warning(s): Keep out of reach of children.

Presentation: 16 fl oz (473 mL) (NDC# 58829-291-16), 1 gallon (3.785 L) (NDC# 58829-291-01), and 2.5 gallon (9.46 L) (NDC# 58829-291-25).

Compendium Code No.: 11390103 Rev. 06-01 / Iss. 05-00 / Rev. 08-01

CHICK ARK BRONC™

L.A.H.I. (New Jersey) **Vaccine**

Bronchitis Vaccine, Mass. and Ark. Types, Live Virus

U.S. Vet. Lic. No.: 196

Active Ingredient(s): This product is a live virus bronchitis vaccine, Massachusetts and Arkansas types. Contains neomycin as a preservative.

This product is manufactured from carefully selected strains of infectious bronchitis virus of Massachusetts and Arkansas types. The viruses are grown in SPF (Specific Pathogen Free) eggs.

The strains of virus in this product were selected to protect against Massachusetts and Arkansas types of infectious bronchitis, yet provide minimum reaction when used as directed.

This vaccine was carefully produced and passed all tests in accordance with the U.S. Government requirements.

Indications: This product is recommended for initial vaccination of chickens at five weeks of age. For drinking water use only.

The older the chicks at the time of administration, the more durable is the immunity produced. Two vaccinations of broilers are usually sufficient. If the birds are to be held as layers, a revaccination must be done at 16 to 20 weeks.

This vaccine will stimulate protective antibodies in susceptible birds. However, if the birds have a high level of antibodies, parental or from a previous vaccination, the vaccine may not be effective.

Parental immunity and immunological incompetence are major factors in preventing young birds from developing immunity. The duration of immunity resulting from vaccination is also directly related to the age of the birds and their susceptibility.

This vaccine will stimulate protective antibodies in susceptible birds. However, the duration of immunity resulting from the use of this vaccine is not permanent, therefore, revaccinations are necessary.

Consult your poultry pathologist for recommendations on revaccination based on conditions existing in your area at any given time.

Dosage and Administration: Preparation of Vaccine for Drinking Water Use: Remove the aluminum overseal and stopper and add clean non-sanitized water. Replace the stopper and shake well. Pour the contents into a quart jar ¾ full of non-sanitized water. Shake well and dilute as outlined in the chart below.

Method of Vaccination: Withhold all medication and disinfectants from the drinking water 24 hours before and 24 hours after vaccinating. Rinse waterers with clean non-sanitized water and remove all water from chicks for at least two hours prior to vaccination. Provide adequate space so that at least two-thirds of the birds can drink at one time.

Add mixture to water as per following chart:

10,000 Doses:

Age of Birds	Heavy	Leghorn
5 Weeks-8 Weeks	80 Gals. of Water	50 Gals. of Water
9 Weeks-15 Weeks	100 Gals. of Water	80 Gals. of Water
16 Weeks-20 Weeks	130 Gals. of Water	100 Gals. of Water

Divide the mixed vaccine into the waterers.

Provide no other drinking water until all vaccine has been consumed.

Precaution(s): Keep vaccine in the dark between 2-7°C (35-45°F).

Use entire contents when first opened. Burn this container and all unused contents.

Caution(s): Distribution in each state shall be limited to authorized recipients designated by proper state officials - under such conditions as these authorities may require.

Recommended use shall be restricted to premises having a history of the disease.

It is imperative that the user of this product comply with the indications for use, contraindication, and method of vaccination stated on the direction sheet. The vaccine must be prepared and administered as directed to obtain best results.

If chicks are to be vaccinated at a very young age, the vaccination must be done at the point of destination to avoid violation of the Postal Laws and Regulations.

Warning(s): Do not vaccinate within 21 days before slaughter.

For veterinary use only.

Presentation: 10,000 doses.

Compendium Code No.: 10080082

CHICK POLY ARK™

L.A.H.I. (New Jersey) **Vaccine**

Newcastle-Bronchitis Vaccine, B_1 Type, B_1 Strain, Mass. and Ark. Type, Live Virus

U.S. Vet. Lic. No.: 196

Active Ingredient(s): This product contains Newcastle disease live virus, B_1 type, B_1 strain, and infectious bronchitis live viruses, Massachusetts and Arkansas types.

Contains neomycin as a preservative.

It is manufactured from carefully selected strains of infectious bronchitis virus of Massachusetts and Arkansas types and the B_1 type, B_1 strain of Newcastle disease virus. The viruses are grown in SPF (Specific Pathogen Free) eggs.

The strains of viruses in this product were selected to protect against Newcastle disease and Massachusetts and Arkansas types of infectious bronchitis, yet provide minimum reaction when used as directed.

This vaccine was carefully produced and passes all tests in accordance with the U.S Government requirements.

Indications: This product is recommended for initial vaccination of chickens at five weeks of age.

The older the chicks at the time of administration, the more durable is the immunity produced. Two vaccinations of broilers are usually sufficient. If the birds are to be held as layers, a revaccination must be done at 16 to 20 weeks.

This vaccine will stimulate protective antibodies in susceptible birds. However, if the birds have a high level of antibodies, either parental or from a previous vaccination, the vaccine may not be effective.

Parental immunity and immunological incompetence are major factors in preventing young birds from developing immunity. The duration of immunity resulting from vaccination is also directly related to the age of the birds and their susceptibility.

This vaccine will stimulate protective antibodies in susceptible birds. However, the duration of immunity resulting from the use of this vaccine is not permanent. Therefore, revaccinations are necessary.

Consult your poultry pathologist for recommendations on revaccination based on conditions existing in your area at any given time.

Dosage and Administration: Preparation of Vaccine: Remove the aluminum overseal and stopper and add clean non-sanitized water. Replace the stopper and shake well. Pour the contents into a quart jar ¾ full of non-sanitized water. Shake well and dilute as outlined in the chart below.

Method of Vaccination: Keep all medication and disinfectants from the drinking water 24 hours before and 24 hours after vaccination. Rinse waterers with clean, non-sanitized water. Water starve the birds for at least two hours prior to vaccination. Provide adequate space so that two-thirds of the birds can drink at the same time.

Add mixture to water as per following chart:

10,000 Doses:

Age of Birds	Heavy	Leghorn
5 Weeks-8 Weeks	80 Gals. of Water	50 Gals. of Water
9 Weeks-15 Weeks	100 Gals. of Water	80 Gals. of Water
16 Weeks-20 Weeks	130 Gals. of Water	100 Gals. of Water

Divide mixed vaccine into the waterers.

Provide no other drinking water until all vaccine has been consumed.

Contraindication(s): Vaccinate healthy chickens only that are free of PPLO and without previous history of a respiratory disease.

If there are susceptible laying birds on the premises there is the possibility that the virus might spread from the vaccinated to the susceptible birds and affect egg production.

Precaution(s): Keep vaccine in the dark between 2-7°C (35-45°F).

Use entire contents when first opened. Burn this container and all unused contents.

Caution(s): Distribution in each state shall be limited to authorized recipients designated by proper state officials - under such conditions as these authorities may require.

Recommended use shall be restricted to premises having a history of the disease.

It is imperative that the user of this product comply with the indications for use, contraindications, and method of vaccination stated on the direction sheet. The vaccine must be prepared and administered as directed to obtain best results.

If chicks are to be vaccinated at a very young age, the vaccination must be done at the point of destination to avoid violation of the Postal Laws and Regulations.

Warning(s): Do not vaccinate within 21 days before slaughter.

Care should be taken to avoid contaminating your hands, eyes and clothing with the vaccine. Newcastle disease virus can cause inflammation of the eyelids in humans.

For veterinary use only.

Presentation: 10,000 doses.

Compendium Code No.: 10080112

CHICK POLY BANCO™

L.A.H.I. (New Jersey) **Vaccine**

Newcastle Bronchitis Vaccine, B_1 Type, B_1 Strain, Mass. and Conn. Type, Live Virus

U.S. Vet. Lic. No.: 196

Description: This product is manufactured from carefully selected strains of Infectious Bronchitis virus of Massachusetts and Connecticut types and the B_1 Type, B_1 strain of Newcastle Disease Virus. The viruses are grown in SPF (Specific Pathogen Free) eggs.

The strains of viruses in this product were selected to protect against Newcastle Disease and Massachusetts and Connecticut Types of Infectious Bronchitis, yet provide minimum reaction when used as directed.

This vaccine was carefully produced and passed all tests in accordance with the U.S. Government requirements.

Contains neomycin as a preservative.

Indications: This product is recommended for initial vaccination of chickens at five weeks of age by the intranasal, intraocular or drinking water method.

The older the chicks at the time of administration, the more durable is the immunity produced. If the chickens are to be held as layers, a revaccination with live virus against both diseases must be done prior to 16 to 20 weeks.

Parental immunity and immunological incompetence are major factors in preventing young chickens from developing immunity. The duration of immunity resulting from the use of this vaccine is also directly related to the age of the chickens and their susceptibility.

This vaccine will stimulate protective antibodies in susceptible chickens. However, the duration of immunity resulting from the use of this vaccine is not permanent. Therefore, revaccinations are necessary. Consult your poultry pathologist for recommendations on revaccination based on conditions existing in your area at any given time.

Dosage and Administration: Read instructions before use.

1,000 Dose - Rehydrate to 30 mL for Intranasal or Intraocular Routes:

Preparation of Vaccine for Intranasal and Intraocular Use: Remove the aluminum tear seal and rubber stopper from the vaccine bottle. Pour some of the diluent provided with the vaccine into the bottle. Replace the rubber stopper and shake vigorously. Pour the mixed vaccine back into the bottle containing the remaining diluent and attach the dropper tip. The vaccine is now ready for intranasal or intraocular use.

Method of Vaccination: The vaccine may be administered by way of the nostril (intranasally) or the eye (intraocularly). When the vaccine is administered by way of the nostril, the chicken's beak is held shut, a finger is placed over one nostril and a drop of vaccine, from the applicator, is dropped into the other nostril.

When used intraocularly, chickens are held on their side and one drop of the mixed vaccine is allowed to fall into the open eye. Hold the chicken until the drop of vaccine disappears. Take care must be taken to prevent injury to the cornea of the eye with the dropper tip.

1,000 Dose, 2,500 Dose and 10,000 Dose - Drinking Water Route:

Preparation of Vaccine for Drinking Water Use: Remove the aluminum overseal and stopper from the vaccine bottle and add clean non-sanitized water. Replace the stopper and shake well. Pour the contents into a quart jar ¾ full of non-sanitized water. Shake well and dilute the vaccine for 1,00 doses, 2,500 doses or 10,000 doses as the case may be as outlined in the chart below. A dried skim milk powder should be used as a vaccine stabilizer at the rate of 8.0 grams per gallon of water. The powdered milk is added prior to the reconstitution of the vaccine.

Method of Vaccination: Keep all medication and disinfectants from the drinking water 24 hours before and 24 hours after vaccinating. Rinse waterers with clean non-sanitized water. Water starve chickens for at least two hours prior to vaccination. Provide adequate space so that at least two-thirds of the chickens can drink at one time.

Add mixture to water as per following chart:

Age of Birds	Water To Use For 1,000 Doses		Water To Use For 2,500 Doses		Water To Use For 10,000 Doses	
	Meat Type	Layers	Meat Type	Layers	Meat Type	Layers
5-8 weeks	30-38 L or 8-10 gal	19-22 L or 5-6 gal	76-95 L or 20-25 gal	45-55 L or 12-15 gal	300-380 L / 80-100 gal	190-220 L or 50-60 gal
9-15 Weeks	38-45 L or 10-12 gal	30-33 L or 8-9 gal	95-113 L or 25-29 gal	76-83 L or 20-21 gal	380-450 L / 100-120 gal	300-330 L / 80-100 gal
16-20 Weeks	49-53 L or 13-14 gal	38-42 L or 10-11 gal	114-133 L or 30-34 gal	95-105 L or 25-27 gal	490-350 L / 130-140 gal	380-420 L / 100-110 gal

Divide the mixed vaccine into the waterers.

Provide no other drinking water until all vaccine has been consumed.

Contraindication(s): Vaccinate healthy chickens only.

If there are susceptible laying chickens on the premises there is the possibility that the virus might spread from the vaccinated to the susceptible chickens and affect egg production.

A mild respiratory reaction can appear three to seven days after vaccination. The development of this reaction is influenced by the level of maternal immunity and/or previous IB vaccinations. Symptoms subside within 10 days post-vaccination.

Precaution(s): Keep refrigerated at 2-7°C (35-45°F).

Use entire contents when first opened. Burn this container and all unused contents.

Caution(s): It is imperative that the user of this product comply with the "Indications", "Contraindications", and "Method of Vaccination" stated on the direction sheet. The vaccine must be prepared and administered as directed to obtain best results.

Warning(s): Do not vaccinate within 21 days before slaughter.

Care should be taken to avoid contaminating hands, eyes and clothing with the vaccine. Newcastle Disease virus can cause inflammation of the eyelids in humans.

For veterinary use only.

Presentation: 1,000 and 10,000 doses.

Compendium Code No.: 10080123 117158-595

CHICK POLY FLORIDA™

L.A.H.I. (New Jersey) **Vaccine**

Newcastle-Bronchitis Vaccine, B_1 Type, B_1 Strain, Mass. and Florida Types, Live Virus

U.S. Vet. Lic. No.: 196

Active Ingredient(s): Description: This product is manufactured from SPF (Specific Pathogen Free) eggs and is a combination live virus vaccine of chicken embryo origin for the prevention of Newcastle Disease and Mass. and Florida types of infectious bronchitis in chickens.

The virus strains in this product are the B_1 type, B_1 strain of Newcastle disease virus and the Mass. and Florida types of bronchitis virus. These viruses were carefully selected to protect against field challenge yet provide minimum reaction when used as directed.

Contains neomycin as a preservative.

This vaccine was carefully produced and passed all tests in accordance with the U.S. government requirements.

Indications: The product is used for the initial vaccination and revaccination of chickens for the prevention of Newcastle disease and Mass. and Florida types of infectious bronchitis. Initial vaccination is administered to birds at 2 weeks of age by the intranasal, intraocular or drinking water routes. If birds are initially vaccinated by these routes under 2 weeks of age, revaccination is required.

The vaccine will stimulate protective antibodies in susceptible birds. However, the duration of immunity resulting from the use of this vaccine is not permanent, therefore, revaccinations are necessary.

Consult your poultry pathologist for recommendations on revaccination based on conditions existing in a designated area at any given time.

Dosage and Administration: Preparation of Vaccine for Intranasal and Intraocular Use: Remove aluminum overseal and stopper from the vaccine bottle and pour part of the diluent into the bottle. Shake well and pour the vaccine back into the remaining diluent and place the dropper tip on the diluent bottle. The vaccine is now ready for intranasal or intraocular use.

Method of Vaccination: The vaccine may be administered by way of the nostril (intranasally) or the eye (intraocularly). When the vaccine is administered by way of the nostril, the chick's beak is held shut, a finger is placed over one nostril and a drop of vaccine, from the special applicator, is dropped into the other nostril.

When used intraocularly, birds should be held on their side and one drop of the mixed vaccine should be allowed to fall into the open eye. Bird should be held until the drop of vaccine disappears. Care must be taken to prevent injury to the cornea of the eye with the dropper tip.

Preparation of Vaccine for Drinking Water Use: Remove the aluminum overseal and stopper and add clean, non-sanitized water. Replace the stopper and shake well. Pour the contents into a quart jar ¾ full of non-sanitized water. Shake well and dilute as outlined in the chart below.

Method of Vaccination: Withhold all medication and disinfectants from the drinking water 24 hours before and 24 hours after vaccinating. Rinse waterers with clean, non-sanitized water and remove all water from chicks for at least two hours prior to vaccination. Provide adequate space so that at least two-thirds of the birds can drink at one time.

Add mixture to water as per the following chart:

Age of Birds	Heavy	Leghorn
2-3 weeks	3 gals. of water	3 gals. of water
4-8 weeks	8 gals. of water	5 gals. of water
9-15 weeks	10 gals. of water	8 gals. of water
16-20 weeks	13 gals. of water	10 gals. of water

Divide the vaccine solution into the waterers.

Provide no other drinking water until all of vaccine has been consumed.

Contraindication(s): Vaccinate healthy chickens only that are free of PPLO and without previous history of respiratory disease.

If there are susceptible laying birds on the premises, there is a possibility that the virus might spread from the vaccinated to the susceptible birds and affect egg production.

Precaution(s): Keep vaccine in the dark between 2-7°C (35-45°F).

Use entire contents when first opened. Burn this container and all unused contents.

Caution(s): It is imperative that the user of this product comply with the indications for use, contraindications, and method of vaccination stated on the direction sheet. The vaccine must be prepared and administered as directed to obtain best results.

If chicks are to be vaccinated at a very young age, the vaccination must be done at the point of destination to avoid violation of the Postal Laws and regulations.

Warning(s): Do not vaccinate within 21 days before slaughter.

Care should be taken to avoid contaminating hands, eyes and clothing with the vaccine since the Newcastle disease virus can cause a mild inflammation of the conjunctiva lasting for 3 to 5 days.

For veterinary use only.

Presentation: 1,000 dose - rehydrate to 30 mL.

Compendium Code No.: 10080132

CHICK SYNO VAC™

L.A.H.I. (New Jersey) **Vaccine**

Tenosynovitis Vaccine, Modified Live Virus

U.S. Vet. Lic. No.: 196

Active Ingredient(s): This product is of chicken tissue culture origin using SPF (Specific Pathogen Free) eggs. The product contains a modified strain of the tenosynovitis virus and is used for the prevention of tenosynovitis (viral arthritis) in young chickens.

The vaccine is made from a live virus that has been modified by a great number of passages through chicken embryos and tissue cultures of chicken embryo origin.

The vaccine contains Gentamicin and a Fungistat as a preservative.

This vaccine was carefully produced and passed all tests in accordance with the U.S. Government requirements.

Indications: The vaccine is recommended for administration by the subcutaneous route in one-day-old chickens. The dosage is 0.2 mL per bird.

Good management practices are recommended to reduce exposure for at least 2 weeks following vaccination.

Dosage and Administration: Sterilize vaccinating equipment by boiling in water for 20 minutes or by autoclaving (15 minutes at 120°C). Do not use chemical disinfectants.

1. Rehydrate one vial of vaccine with one bottle of diluent.
2. Remove the center tab of the aluminum seal from vaccine vial and the diluent bottle. Do not remove rubber stopper. Sanitize the stopper with alcohol and allow to dry.
3. Insert a sterile needle and syringe into the diluent bottle and withdraw 2-3 mL of diluent. Transfer the diluent into the vaccine vial.
4. Shake well to insure that the vaccine is dissolved and withdraw the entire contents into the syringe.
5. Add the rehydrated vaccine to the diluent, shake well and repeat Numbers 3 and 4 above. The repeat step is necessary to insure that all the vaccine is removed from the vial.
6. Fill the automatic syringe according to the manufacturer's recommendations and set the dosage for 0.2 mL.

Method of Vaccination: Subcutaneous Administration

1. Dilute the vaccine as directed above observing all instructions.
2. Hold the chick by the back of the neck just below the head. The loose skin in the area is raised by gently pinching with the thumb and forefinger. Insert the needle beneath the skin in a downward direction away from the head. Inject 0.2 mL per chick. The vaccine should be kept chilled during administration by means of an ice bath.
3. Avoid hitting the muscles and bones in the neck.
4. Entire contents of bottle must be used within 1 hour after mixing, or discarded.

Contraindication(s): Birds to be vaccinated should be healthy and free of all diseases. It is essential that the birds be maintained under good environmental conditions to prevent unnecessary exposure to viral arthritis.

Precaution(s): Burn containers and all unused contents.

Keep vaccine in the dark - between 2-7°C (35-45°F).

Do not use vaccine that has been rehydrated other than immediately before use.

Caution(s): The capacity of this vaccine to produce satisfactory results depends on many factors, including but not limited to conditions of storage and handling by the user, administration of the vaccine, health and responsiveness of individual animals and degree of field exposure. Therefore, directions for use should be followed carefully.

The use of this vaccine is subject to applicable state and federal laws and regulations.

Warning(s): Do not vaccinate within 21 days before slaughter.

Presentation: 1000 doses - rehydrate to 200 mL.

Compendium Code No.: 10080142

CHICK UNI BRONC™

L.A.H.I. (New Jersey) **Vaccine**

Bronchitis Vaccine, Mass. Type, Live Virus

U.S. Vet. Lic. No.: 196

Active Ingredient(s): This product is a live bronchitis vaccine, Massachusetts type. Contains neomycin as a preservative.

It is manufactured from SPF (Specific Pathogen Free) eggs and is a live virus vaccine of chicken embryo origin for the prevention of Massachusetts Type Infectious Bronchitis in chickens.

The strain of virus in this product was carefully selected to protect against field challenges yet provide minimum reaction when used as directed.

This vaccine was carefully produced and passed all tests in accordance with the U.S. Government requirements.

Indications: This product is used for initial vaccination and revaccination of chickens for the prevention of Massachusetts type infectious bronchitis. Initial vaccination is recommended for birds at five weeks of age by the intranasal, intraocular, aerosol spray or water routes. This product is also used in replacement birds before 16 weeks of age that were previously vaccinated.

This vaccine will stimulate protective antibodies in susceptible birds. However, the duration of immunity resulting from the use of this vaccine is not permanent, therefore, revaccinations are necessary.

Consult your poultry pathologist for recommendations on revaccination based on conditions existing in your area at any given time.

Dosage and Administration: 1,000 Dose: Preparation of Vaccine for Intranasal and Intraocular Use: Remove the aluminum tear seal and rubber stopper from the vaccine bottle and pour part of the diluent into the bottle. Shake well and pour the vaccine back into the remaining diluent and place the dropper tip on the diluent bottle. The vaccine is now ready for intranasal or intraocular use.

Method of Vaccination: The vaccine may be administered by way of the nostril (intranasally) or the eye (intraocularly). When the vaccine is administered by way of the nostril, the chick's beak is held shut, a finger is placed over one nostril and a drop of vaccine, from the special applicator, is dropped into the other nostril.

When used intraocularly, birds are held on their side and one drop of the mixed vaccine allowed to fall into the open eye. Hold the bird until the drop of vaccine disappears. Care must be taken to prevent injury to the cornea of the eye with the dropper tip.

Preparation of Vaccine for Aerosol Use: Remove the aluminum overseal and stopper from the vaccine bottle and pour part of the diluent into the bottle. Shake well and pour the vaccine back into the remaining diluent. Pour the entire contents into the reservoir of a sprayer containing 70 mL of deionized water or 5 mL of glycerine and 65 mL of deionized water. Before the vaccination the sprayer should be calibrated so that 100 mL will be delivered in 3 minutes.

Method of Vaccination: Confine the birds to a corner of the house with fences and direct the stream from the sprayer over the heads of the birds. Extreme caution should be taken to prevent birds from smothering during this operation.

1,000 and 2,500 Doses: Preparation of Vaccine for Drinking Water Use: Remove the aluminum overseal and stopper and add clean non-sanitized water. Replace the stopper and shake well. Pour the contents into a quart jar ¾ full of non-sanitized water. Shake well and dilute as outlined in the chart below.

Method of Vaccination: Withhold all medication and disinfectants from the drinking water 24 hours before and 24 hours after vaccinating. Rinse waterers with clean non-sanitized water and remove all water from chicks for at least two hours prior to vaccination. Provide adequate space so that at least two-thirds of the birds can drink at one time.

Add mixture to water as per following chart:

1,000 Doses:

Age of Birds	Heavy per 1,000 birds	Leghorn per 1,000 birds
2 Weeks-3 Weeks	3 Gals. of Water	3 Gals. of Water
4 Weeks-8 Weeks	8 Gals. of Water	5 Gals. of Water
9 Weeks-15 Weeks	10 Gals. of Water	8 Gals. of Water
16 Weeks-20 Weeks	13 Gals. of Water	10 Gals. of Water

2,500 Doses:

Age of Birds	Heavy per 2,500 birds	Leghorn per 2,500 birds
2 Weeks-3 Weeks	7 Gals. of Water	7 Gals. of Water
4 Weeks-8 Weeks	20 Gals. of Water	12 Gals. of Water
9 Weeks-15 Weeks	25 Gals. of Water	20 Gals. of Water
16 Weeks-20 Weeks	30 Gals. of Water	25 Gals. of Water

Divide the mixed vaccine into the waterers.

Provide no other drinking water until all vaccine has been consumed.

Precaution(s): Keep vaccine in the dark between 2-7°C (35-45°F).

Use entire contents when first opened. Burn this container and all unused contents.

Caution(s): It is imperative that the user of this product comply with the indications for use, contraindication, and method of vaccination stated on the direction sheet. The vaccine must be prepared and administered as directed to obtain best results.

If chicks are to be vaccinated at a very young age, the vaccination must be done at the point of destination to avoid violation of the Postal Laws and Regulations.

Warning(s): Do not vaccinate within 21 days before slaughter.

Care should be taken to avoid contaminating hands, eyes, and clothing with the vaccine.

For veterinary use only.

Presentation: 1,000 and 2,500 doses.

Compendium Code No.: 10080152

CHICK UNI HOL™

L.A.H.I. (New Jersey) **Vaccine**

Bronchitis Vaccine, Mass. Type, Live Virus

U.S. Vet. Lic. No.: 196

Description: This product is manufactured from SPF (Specific Pathogen Free) eggs and is a live virus vaccine of chicken embryo origin containing the Massachusetts Type, Holland Strain of bronchitis virus. Contains neomycin as a preservative.

The virus was carefully selected to protect against field challenges yet provide minimum reaction on use.

The vaccine is carefully produced and passes all tests in accordance with the U.S. government requirements.

Indications: This product is used for the initial vaccination and revaccination of chickens for the prevention of Infectious Bronchitis, Massachusetts Type.

Dosage and Administration: Initial vaccination is administered to chickens at two weeks of age by the intranasal, intraocular, drinking water or spray methods.

Parental immunity and immunological incompetence are major factors in preventing young chickens from developing immunity. The duration of immunity resulting from the use of this vaccine is also directly related to the age of the chickens and their susceptibility.

Consult a poultry pathologist for recommendations on revaccination based on conditions existing in a designated area at any given time.

1,000 dose - Rehydrate to 30 mL for Intranasal or Intraocular Routes:

Preparation of Vaccine for Intranasal and Intraocular Use: Remove the aluminum tear seal and rubber stopper from the vaccine bottle. Pour some of the diluent into the bottle. Replace the rubber stopper and shake vigorously. Pour the mixed vaccine back into the bottle containing the remaining diluent and attach the dropper tip. The vaccine is now ready for intranasal or intraocular use.

Method of Vaccination: The vaccine may be administered by way of the nostril (intranasally) or the eye (intraocularly). When the vaccine is administered by way of the nostril, the chicken's beak is held shut, a finger is placed over one nostril and a drop of vaccine, from the applicator, is dropped into the other nostril.

When used intraocularly, chickens are held on their side and one drop of the mixed vaccine is allowed to fall into the open eye. Hold the chickens until the drop of vaccine disappears. Care must be taken to prevent injury to the cornea of the eye with the dropper tip.

1,000, 2,500 and 10,000 dose - for Aerosol Route:

Preparation of Vaccine for Aerosol Use:

Required amount of deionized water or deionized water/glycerine:

1000 Doses:	2500 Doses:	10,000 Doses:
70 mL deionized water or 65 mL deionized water with 5 mL glycerine	175 mL deionized water or 165 mL deionized water with 15 mL glycerine	700 mL deionized water or 650 mL deionized water with 50 mL glycerine

Set aside the required amount of deionized water. Remove the aluminum overseal and rubber stopper from the vaccine bottle. Add a sufficient amount of deionized water, from the required amount set aside, to the vaccine bottle. Replace the rubber stopper and shake well. Pour the remaining deionized water and glycerine (if used) into the reservoir of a sprayer, and add the entire contents of the vaccine bottle. Before the vaccination, the sprayer should be calibrated so that 100 mL will be delivered in 3 minutes.

Method of Vaccination: Confine the chickens to a corner of the house with fences and direct the stream from the sprayer over the heads of the chickens. Extreme caution should be taken to prevent chickens from smothering during this operation.

1,000, 2,500 and 10,000 dose - Drinking Water Route:

Preparation of Vaccine for Drinking Water Use: Remove the aluminum overseal and stopper from the vaccine bottle and add clean, non-sanitized water. Replace the stopper and shake well. Pour the contents into a quart jar ¾ full of non-sanitized water. Shake well and dilute as outlined in the chart below.

Method of Vaccination: Keep all medication and disinfectants from the drinking water for 24 hours before and 24 hours after vaccinating. Rinse the waterers with clean, non-sanitized water. Water starve the chickens for at least two hours prior to vaccination. Provide adequate space so that at least two-thirds of the chickens can drink at one time.

Add mixture to water as per the following chart:

Age of Birds	Water to Use For 1,000 Doses		Water to Use for 2,500 Doses		Water to Use for 10,000 Doses	
	Meat Type	Layers	Meat Type	Layers	Meat Type	Layers
2 weeks 3 weeks	11 - 18 L or 3 - 5 gal	11 - 18 L or 3 - 5 gal	26 - 45 L or 7 - 12 gal	26 - 45 L or 7 - 12 gal	110 - 180 L or 15 - 25 gal	110 - 180 L or 15 - 25 gal
5 weeks 8 weeks	30 - 38 L or 8 - 10 gal	19 - 22 L or 5 - 6 gal	76 - 95 L or 20 - 25 gal	45 - 55 L or 12 - 15 gal	300 - 380 L / 80 - 100 gal	190 - 220 L or 50 - 60 gal
9 weeks 15 weeks	38 - 45 L or 10 - 12 gal	30 - 33 L or 8 - 9 gal	95 - 113 L or 25 - 29 gal	76 - 83 L or 20 - 21 gal	380 - 450 L / 100 - 120 gal	300 - 330 L / 80 - 100 gal
16 weeks 20 weeks	49 - 53 L or 13 - 14 gal	38 - 42 L or 10 - 11 gal	114 - 133 L or 30 - 34 gal	95 - 105 L or 25 - 27 gal	490 - 530 L / 130 - 140 gal	380 - 420 L / 100 - 110 gal

Divide the mixed vaccine into the waterers.

Provide no other drinking water until all of the vaccine has been consumed.

Precaution(s): Use entire contents when first opened.

Keep refrigerated at 2-7°C (35-45° F).

Burn this container and all unused contents.

Caution(s): Vaccinate healthy chickens only.

If there are susceptible laying chickens on the premises, there is a possibility that the virus might spread from the vaccinated to the susceptible chickens and affect egg production.

A mild respiratory reaction can appear three to seven days after vaccination. The development of this reaction is influenced by the level of maternal immunity and/or previous IB vaccinations. Symptoms subside within 10 days post-vaccination.

It is imperative that the user of this product comply with the indications for use, cautions and methods of vaccination stated on the direction sheet. The vaccine must be prepared and administered as directed to obtain the best results.

For veterinary use only.

Warning(s): Do not vaccinate within 21 days before slaughter.

Presentation: 1,000, 2,500, and 10,000 doses.

Compendium Code No.: 10080162

11321-1

CHICK VI BANCO™

L.A.H.I. (New Jersey) **Vaccine**

Newcastle Bronchitis Vaccine, B_1 Type, B_1 Strain, Mass. Type, Live Virus

U.S. Vet. Lic. No.: 196

Description: This product is manufactured from SPF (Specific Pathogen Free) eggs and is a live virus vaccine of chicken embryo origin for the prevention of Newcastle Disease and Massachusetts Type Infectious Bronchitis in chickens.

The virus strains in this product are the Massachusetts Type, Strain 48 of bronchitis virus and the B_1 Type, B_1 Strain of Newcastle Disease virus.

These viruses were carefully selected to protect against field challenges when used as directed.

This vaccine was carefully produced and passed all tests in accordance with the U.S. Government requirements.

Contains neomycin as a preservative.

Indications: This product is used for initial vaccination and revaccination of chickens as an aid for the prevention of Infectious Bronchitis (Massachusetts Type) and Newcastle Disease. Initial vaccination is administered to birds at 5 weeks of age by the intranasal, intraocular, aerosol spray or drinking water routes. This product is also used for vaccination of day old chicks by aerosol method using equipment like Beak-O-Vac machine.

Parental immunity and immunological incompetence are major factors in preventing young

C

birds from developing immunity. The duration of immunity resulting from vaccination is also directly related to the age of the birds and their susceptibility.

Consult your poultry pathologist for recommendations on revaccination based on conditions existing in your area at any given time.

Dosage and Administration: Read instructions before use.

1,000 Dose - Rehydrate to 30 mL:

Preparation of Vaccine for Intranasal and Intraocular Use: Remove aluminum overseal and stopper from the vaccine bottle. Pour some of the diluent into the bottle. Replace the rubber stopper and shake vigorously. Pour the mixed vaccine back into the bottle containing the remaining diluent and attach the dropper tip. The vaccine is now ready for intranasal or intraocular use.

Method of Vaccination: The vaccine may be administered by way of the nostril (intranasally) or the eye (intraocularly). When the vaccine is administered by way of the nostril, the chick's beak is held shut, a finger is placed over one nostril and a drop of vaccine, from the special applicator, is dropped into the other nostril.

When used intraocularly, birds should be held on their side and one drop of the mixed vaccine should be allowed to fall into the open eye. Birds should be held until the drop of vaccine disappears. Care must be taken to prevent injury to the cornea of the eye with the dropper tip.

1000 and 2500 Doses:

Preparation of Vaccine for Aerosol Use: Remove the aluminum overseal and stopper from the vaccine bottle and pour 5 mL of deionized water into the bottle. Shake well. Pour the entire contents into the reservoir of a sprayer containing 70 mL of deionized water or 5 mL of glycerine and 65 mL of deionized water. Before the vaccination, the sprayer should be calibrated so that 100 mL will be delivered in 3 minutes.

Method of Vaccination: Confine the birds to a corner of the house with fences and direct the stream from the sprayer over the heads of the birds. Extreme caution should be taken to prevent birds from smothering during this operation.

Preparation of Vaccine for Drinking Water Use: Remove the aluminum overseal and stopper and add clean non-sanitized water. Replace the stopper and shake well. Pour the contents into a quart jar ¾ full of non-sanitized water. Shake well and dilute the vaccine for 1000 doses or 2500 doses as the case may be as outlined in the chart below. A dried skim milk powder should be used as a vaccine stabilizer at the rate of 8.0 grams per gallon of water. The powdered milk is added prior to the reconstitution of the vaccine.

Method of Vaccination: Withhold all medication and disinfectants from the drinking water 24 hours before and 24 hours after vaccinating. Rinse waterers with clean non-sanitized water and remove all water from chicks for at least two hours prior to vaccination. Provide adequate space so that at least two-thirds of the birds can drink at one time.

Add mixture to water as per following chart:

1000 Doses:

Age of Birds	Heavy per 1,000 birds	Leghorn per 1,000 birds
5-8 Weeks	8 Gals of Water	5 Gals of Water
9-15 Weeks	10 Gals of Water	8 Gals of Water

2,500 Doses:

Age of Birds	Heavy per 2,500 birds	Leghorn per 2,500 birds
5-8 Weeks	20 Gals of Water	12 Gals of Water
9-15 Weeks	25 Gals of Water	20 Gals of Water

Divide the mixed vaccine into the waterers.

Provide no other drinking water until all vaccine has been consumed.

Contraindication(s): Vaccinate healthy chickens only.

If there are susceptible laying birds on the premises there is a possibility that the virus might spread from the vaccinated to the susceptible birds and affect egg production.

Precaution(s): Keep vaccine in the dark - between 2-7°C (35-45°F).

Use entire contents when first opened. Burn this container and all unused contents.

Caution(s): It is imperative that the user of this product comply with the "Indications", "Contraindications" and "Method of Vaccination" stated on the direction sheet. The vaccine must be prepared and administered as directed to obtain best results.

Warning(s): Do not vaccinate within 21 days before slaughter.

Care should be taken to avoid contaminating your hands, eyes and clothing with the vaccine. Newcastle Disease virus can cause inflammation of the eyelids in humans.

For veterinary use only.

Presentation: 1,000, 2,500 and 5,000 doses.

Compendium Code No.: 10080173 R95B

CHICK VI BANCO™ (Drinking Water Use)

L.A.H.I. (New Jersey) **Vaccine**

Newcastle Bronchitis Vaccine, B_1 Type, B_1 Strain, Mass. Type, Live Virus

U.S. Vet. Lic. No.: 196

Description: This product is manufactured with SPF (Specific Pathogen Free) eggs and is a live virus vaccine of chicken embryo origin for the prevention of Newcastle Disease and Massachusetts type infectious bronchitis in chickens.

The strains of viruses in this product was carefully selected to protect against field challenges yet provide minimum reaction when used as directed.

This vaccine was carefully produced and passed all tests in accordance with the U.S. Government requirements.

Contains neomycin as a preservative.

Indications: This product is used for initial vaccination and revaccination of chickens for the prevention of Massachusetts Type Infectious Bronchitis and Newcastle Disease. Initial vaccination is administered to birds at 5 weeks of age. This product is also used in replacement birds before 16 weeks of age that were previously vaccinated.

This vaccine will stimulate protective antibodies in susceptible birds. However, the duration of immunity resulting from the use of this vaccine is not permanent, therefore, revaccinations are necessary.

Consult your poultry pathologist for recommendations on revaccination based conditions existing in your area at any given time.

For drinking water use.

Dosage and Administration: Read instructions before use.

10,000 Dose:

Preparation of Vaccine: Remove the aluminum overseal and stopper and add clean non-sanitized water. Replace the stopper and shake well. Pour the contents into a quart jar ¾ full of non-sanitized water. Shake well and dilute as outlined in the chart below.

Method of Vaccination: Withhold all medication and disinfectants from the drinking water 24 hours before and 24 hours after vaccinating. Rinse waterers with clean non-sanitized water and remove all water from chicks for at least two hours prior to vaccination. Provide adequate space so that at least two-thirds of the birds can drink at one time.

Add mixture to water as per following chart:

Age of Birds	Heavy	Leghorn
5-8 Weeks	80 Gals. of Water	50 Gals. of Water
9-15 Weeks	100 Gals. of Water	80 Gals. of Water
16-20 Weeks	130 Gals. of Water	100 Gals. of Water

Divide the vaccine solution into the waterers.

Provide no other drinking water until all vaccine has been consumed.

Contraindication(s): Vaccinate healthy chickens only that are free of PPLO and without previous history of a respiratory disease.

If there are susceptible laying birds on the premises there is the possibility that the virus might spread from the vaccinated to the susceptible birds and affect egg production.

Precaution(s): Keep vaccine in the dark between 2-7°C (35-45°F).

Use entire contents when first opened.

Burn this container and all unused contents.

Caution(s): It is imperative that the user of this product comply with the "Indications", "Contraindications", and "Method of Vaccination" stated on the direction sheet. The vaccine must be prepared and administered as directed to obtain best results.

If chicks are to be vaccinated at a very young age, the vaccination must be done at the point of destination to avoid violation of the Postal Laws and Regulations.

Warning(s): Do not vaccinate within 21 days before slaughter.

Care should be taken to avoid contaminating hands, eyes and clothing with the vaccine since the Newcastle Disease virus can cause a mild inflammation of the conjunctiva lasting for 3 to 5 days. For veterinary use only.

Presentation: 10,000 dose vial.

Compendium Code No.: 10080651 5860

CHICK VI HANCO™

L.A.H.I. (New Jersey) **Vaccine**

Newcastle-Bronchitis Vaccine, B_1 Type, B_1 Strain, Mass. Type Live Virus

U.S. Vet. Lic. No.: 196

Contents: This product is manufactured from SPF (Specific Pathogen Free) eggs and is a combination live virus vaccine of chicken embryo origin for the prevention of Newcastle Disease and Massachusetts Type Infectious Bronchitis in chickens.

The virus strains in this product are the Massachusetts Type, Holland Strain - high egg passages of bronchitis virus and the B_1 Type, B_1 Strain of Newcastle Disease virus.

These viruses were carefully selected to protect against field challenges yet provide minimum reaction when used as directed.

Contains neomycin as a preservative.

Indications: This product is recommended for initial intranasal or intraocular vaccination of chickens at two weeks of age and initial aerosol or water vaccination of chickens at five weeks of age.

Parental immunity and immunological incompetence are major factors in preventing young birds from developing immunity. The duration of immunity resulting from vaccination is also directly related to the age of the birds and their susceptibility.

Consult your poultry pathologist for recommendations on revaccination based on conditions existing in your area at any given time.

Dosage and Administration: Read instructions before use.

1,000 Doses - Rehydrate to 30 mL:

Preparation of Vaccine for Intranasal and Intraocular Use: Remove the aluminum tear seal and rubber stopper from the vaccine bottle. Pour some of the diluent into the bottle. Replace the rubber stopper and shake vigorously. Pour the mixed vaccine back into the bottle containing the remaining diluent and attach the dropper tip. The vaccine is now ready for use.

Method of Vaccination: The vaccine may be administered by way of the nostril, (intranasally) or the eye, (intraocularly). When the vaccine is administered by way of the nostril, the beak is held shut, a finger is placed over one nostril and a drop of vaccine, from the applicator, is dropped into the other nostril.

When used intraocularly, birds are held on their side and one drop of the mixed vaccine allowed to fall into the open eye. Hold the birds until the drop of vaccine disappears. Take care to prevent injury to the cornea of the eye with the dropper tip.

Preparation of Vaccine for Aerosol Use: Remove the aluminum overseal and stopper from the vaccine bottle and pour 5 mL of deionized water into the bottle. Shake well. Pour the entire contents into the reservoir of a sprayer containing 70 mL of deionized water or 5 mL of glycerine and 65 mL of deionized water. Before the vaccination, the sprayer should be calibrated so that 100 mL will be delivered in 3 minutes.

Method of Vaccination: Confine the birds to a corner of the house with fences and direct the stream from the sprayer over the heads of the birds. Extreme caution should be taken to prevent birds from smothering during this operation.

1000 and 2500 Doses:

Preparation of Vaccine for Drinking Water Use: Remove the aluminum overseal and stopper and add clean non-sanitized water. Replace the stopper and shake well. Pour the contents into a quart jar ¾ full of non-sanitized water. Shake well and dilute the vaccine for 1000 doses or 2500 doses as the case may be as outlined in the chart below. A dried skim milk powder should be used as a vaccine stabilizer at the rate of 8.0 grams per gallon of water. The powdered milk is added prior to the reconstitution of the vaccine.

Method of Vaccination: Withhold all medication and disinfectants from the drinking water 24 hours before and 24 hours after vaccination. Rinse waterers with clean non-sanitized water and remove all water from chicks for at least two hours prior to vaccination. Provide adequate space so that at least two-thirds of the birds can drink at one time.

Add mixture to water as per following chart:

1000 Doses:

Age of birds	Heavy per 1,000 birds	Leghorn per 1,000 birds
5 Weeks-8 weeks	8 Gals of water	5 Gals of water
9 Weeks-15 weeks	10 Gals of water	8 Gals of water

2500 Doses:

Age of birds	Heavy per 2,500 birds	Leghorn per 2,500 birds
5 Weeks-8 weeks	20 Gals of water	12 Gals of water
9 Weeks-15 weeks	25 Gals of water	20 Gals of water

Divide the mixed vaccine into the waterers.
Provide no other drinking water until all vaccine has been consumed.
Contraindication(s): Vaccinate healthy chickens only.
If there are susceptible laying birds on the premises there is the possibility that the virus might spread from the vaccinated to the susceptible birds and affect egg production.
Precaution(s): Keep vaccine in the dark between 2-7°C (35-45°F).
Use entire contents when first opened. Burn this container and all unused contents.
Caution(s): Federal regulations prohibit the repackaging or sale of the contents of the package in fractional units. Do not accept if seal is broken.
Warning(s): Do not vaccinate within 21 days before slaughter.
It is imperative that the user of this product comply with the indications for use, contraindications and method of vaccination stated in the direction sheet. The vaccine must be prepared and administered as directed to obtain best results.
Care should be taken to avoid contaminating your hands, eyes and clothing with the vaccine. Newcastle Disease virus can cause inflammation of the eyelids in humans.
For veterinary use only.
Presentation: 2,500 doses.
Compendium Code No.: 10080182

CHICK VI POX™

L.A.H.I. (New Jersey) **Vaccine**
Fowl Pox Vaccine, Live Virus, Chicken Tissue Culture Origin
U.S. Vet. Lic. No.: 196
Active Ingredient(s): Description: This product is a mild live virus fowlpox vaccine containing a chicken tissue culture propagated fowl pox virus.
Contains gentamicin and a fungistat as preservatives.
This vaccine was carefully produced and passes all tests in accordance with the U.S. Government requirements.
Indications: For the prevention of fowlpox in baby chicks as well as growing birds. For wing web application.
This vaccine is for administration to birds one day of age and older. For meat birds and laying replacements, this product may be administered from 1 day to 10 weeks of age. For replacement chickens, revaccination with Fowl Pox Vaccine (chicken embryo origin) before initiation of lay is necessary.
Dosage and Administration: Preparation of Vaccine: The active agent of the vaccine is supplied in a dried form in the bottle labelled 'Vaccine'. Open the bottle by removing the aluminum tear seal and rubber stopper. Open the diluent and pour a small quantity into the bottle of vaccine, replace the rubber stopper, and shake well. Pour the mixture back into the bottle containing the remainder of the diluent and shake mixture vigorously. Do not open or mix the vaccine until ready for use.
Method of Vaccination: Either a double needle or a single needle can be used. Vaccination is accomplished by dipping the needle in the mixed vaccine and piercing the "web of the wing" from the underside. Do not apply through feathers, muscle or bone. The applicator must be redipped between each application.
Birds from the flock should be examined for evidence of a "take" to ensure that the vaccine was applied properly.
The evidence of a successful vaccination will appear at the point of vaccination in from 7 to 10 days after vaccination. Brownish, black scabs will be found on both the under and upper surfaces of the web of the wing through which the needle vaccinator was thrust.
Contraindication(s): Chickens to be vaccinated should be free of all diseases including the latent form of diseases such as chronic respiratory disease (CRD), coccidiosis, blackhead, parasitic diseases, etc.
Precaution(s): Keep vaccine in the dark, between 2-7°C (35-45°F).
Use entire contents when first opened. Burn this container and all unused contents.
Caution(s): When administered to susceptible birds, a mild form of the disease results which stimulates immunity.
No vaccine confers immediate protection against fowl pox. While immunity begins to develop immediately, it takes 2 to 3 weeks for birds to establish maximum immunity, during which time they should not be placed in contaminated premises nor otherwise exposed to Fowlpox.
All susceptible birds on any farm should be vaccinated at the same time. If this is not possible, individual lots may be vaccinated if strict isolation and separate caretakers are provided for the vaccinated and unvaccinated lots of birds.
It is imperative that the user of this product comply with the indications for use, contraindications, and method of vaccination stated on the direction sheet. The vaccine must be prepared and administered as directed to obtain best results.
Warning(s): Do not vaccinate within 21 days before slaughter.
Care should be taken to avoid contaminating hands, eyes and clothing with the vaccine.
For veterinary use only.
Presentation: 500 doses with a 5 mL diluent
1000 doses with a 10 mL diluent.
Compendium Code No.: 10080192

CHLAMYDIA PSITTACI BACTERIN

Colorado Serum **Bacterin**
Chlamydia psittaci Bacterin
U.S. Vet. Lic. No.: 188
Active Ingredient(s): An aqueous suspension of inactivated cultures of *Chlamydia psittaci* emulsified with a mineral oil adjuvant.
Contains thimerosal as a preservative.
Contains permitted levels of penicillin and streptomycin.
The bacterin is produced from cultures of chlamydia psittaci, a filterable bacteria of the psitticosis-lymphogranuloma-trachoma group of micro-organsims that cause enzootic abortion of ewes. The cultures are formalin killed.
Indications: For use in vaccinating healthy ewes to aid in the control of ovine enzootic abortion.
Dosage and Administration: When to Vaccinate: Two (2) doses are recommended. Administer the first dose at least 60 days before ewes are exposed to rams. The second dose should be administered 30 days later. Revaccinate annually.
Each of the two (2) doses should be 2 mL administered subcutaneously. Injections should be made on top of the neck about four (4) inches from the ear. If small nodules should then appear these will be of little consequence in breeding flocks and will be even less objectionable in the event that an occasional animal must be culled from the flock and sold.
Precaution(s): Store in the dark at 2-7°C. Do not freeze.
Sterile needles and syringes by boiling in clean water.
All biological products should be stored in the refrigerator. Because the product is an emulsion, which is difficult to use when cold, it is suggested that the product be removed from storage 10-12 hours before use so that it will warm slightly. Do not expose to excessive heat or to long periods at room temperature.
Shake the product thoroughly to resuspend any micro-organisms that may have precipitated.
Handling of the product, filling of syringes, etc., should be done as aseptically as possible. Great care has been taken to ensure the purity of the preparation at the time of release for marketing. Reasonable precautions should be taken in the field to maintain this condition.
Caution(s): Anaphylactic reactions sometimes follow administration of products of this nature. If noted, administer adrenaline or an equivalent drug. Use the entire contents when first opened.
For veterinary use only.
Warning(s): Do not vaccinate within 60 days before slaughter.
Discussion: Enzootic abortion of ewes has been an unidentified problem in a vast area of the western and northwestern United States for many years. Isolation of the causative agent, *Chlamydia psittaci*, is fairly recent.
Enzootic abortion in ewes is characterized almost exclusively by the loss of lambs late in pregnancy. Weak or dead lambs may be born at full term. In some instances infected ewes will not show clinical symptoms of any kind and will lamb in a normal manner. Those that do not abort or lamb prematurely are sometimes in poor health showing a rapid deterioration over a short period before lambing. A vaginal discharge is noted after lambing and the placenta may be retained for several days. Generally, the ewes will slowly return to normal condition.
The chlamydia is present in fetal membranes and in the uterine discharge. It is at this time that the disease is spread through the flock, being picked up orally by the ewes, to remain inactive until carried into the developing placenta during the following pregnancy. In Scotland there is evidence that the chlamydia micro-organism can remain in the tissues of a ewe lamb for as long as two years, then cause the animal to abort when she becomes pregnant. It is during the second pregnancy that ewes most often abort or lamb prematurely from the effects of the disease although many are also affected during the first lambing season.
Presentation: 10 dose (20 mL) and 50 dose (100 mL) vials.
Compendium Code No.: 11010110

CHLOR-A-CLENS CLEANSING SOLUTION

Vedco **Topical Wound Dressing**
Ingredient(s): Propylene glycol, malic acid, benzoic acid, salicylic acid, chlorhexidine and glycerin.
Indications: As an aid in the cleansing of superficial skin infections and irrigation of wounds found on dogs and cats. The cleansing creates an ideal environment for healthy tissue to grow.
Dosage and Administration: Apply liberally to infected or wound area and let stand. Repeat application 2-3 times daily or as necessary.
Warning(s): For external use only. Irritating to the eye. Use only as directed by your veterinarian.
Keep out of reach of children.
Presentation: 4 oz (120 mL) bottle.
Compendium Code No.: 10940250

CHLOR-A-CLENS-L CLEANSING SOLUTION

Vedco **Topical Wound Dressing**
Active Ingredient(s): Propylene glycol, malic acid, benzoic acid, lidocaine HCl 0.5%, salicylic acid, chlorhexidine and glycerine.
Indications: As an aid in the cleansing of superficial skin infections and irrigation of wounds found on dogs and cats.
Dosage and Administration: Apply liberally to infected or wound area and let stand. Repeat application 2-3 times daily or as necessary.
Precaution(s): Store at room temperature in dark area.
Warning(s): For external use only. Irritating to the eye. Use only as directed by your veterinarian.
Keep out of reach of children.
Presentation: 4 oz (120 mL) bottle.
Compendium Code No.: 10940260

CHLORADINE SCRUB 4%®

RXV **Surgical Scrub**
Active Ingredient(s):
Chlorhexidine gluconate 4%
Contents: Purified Water, Alkyl Dimethylamineoxide, Diethanolamine, Chlorhexidine Digluconate, Isopropyl Alcohol 99%, Polyoxyethylene-6-Coco Amide, Octylphenoxypolyethoxy-Ethanol, Glycerol, Polyethylene Glycol, Quaternium 33-Ethylhexandiol, Hydroxyethylcellulose, FD&C Red #40 and Fragrance.
Indications: CHLORADINE SCRUB 4%® is a mild scrub that exhibits bactericidal activity against a wide range of micro-organisms.
Directions for Use: Wet hands with water. Pour approximately 5 mL of CHLORADINE SCRUB 4%® in palm of hand. Add enough water to make a lather. Lather thoroughly. Rinse thoroughly under running water.
Caution(s): For animal use only.
Warning(s): Keep out of reach of children.
Presentation: 1 gallon (NDC# 14049-298-01).
Compendium Code No.: 10910331

CHLORA-DIP

First Priority **Teat Dip**
Chapless Teat Dip Concentrate with Chlorhexidine and Glycerin
Active Ingredient(s):
Chlorhexidine Gluconate .... 2.0% w/w
Glycerin .... 23.8% w/w
Inert Ingredients .... 74.2% w/w
Total .... 100.0% w/w
Contains artificial color.
Indications: For use in preparation of 0.5% solution for dipping teats as an aid in controlling mastitis-causing bacteria on teats.
Directions for Use: To prepare a 0.5% solution for dipping teats as an aid in controlling mastitis-causing bacteria on teats, add 48 fluid ounces (3 pints), or 96 fluid ounces (3 quarts) of clean water* or distilled water to 16 fluid ounces (1 pint), or 32 fluid ounces (1 quart) of CHLORA-DIP Teat Dip Concentrate in a clean container.

*Precipitate may occur with certain types of water used for dilution. It is preferable to use distilled water or deionized water.

Directions for use of the 0.5% solution: Dip each teat into the 0.5% solution immediately after milking. Thoroughly wash teats and udder just before the next milking. Dry with a single-use paper towel. Dipping should start at least one week before the cow freshens and should continue until four days or more after drying off.

Precaution(s): Storage: Store at controlled room temperature between 15°-30°C (59°-86°F). Keep container tightly closed when not in use.

Caution(s): Dilute with the proper amount of water before use as a teat dip. Do not use the concentrate as a teat dip.

May be irritating to the eyes and mucous membranes. If contact occurs, flush with copious amounts of water. Call a physician for treatment of eyes. May be harmful if swallowed.

Avoid contamination of feed and foodstuffs. Rinse empty container thoroughly with water and destroy container properly by crushing or burial.

Hazardous - Livestock remedy. Not for human use. For animal use only.

Warning(s): Keep out of reach of children.

Presentation: 16 fl oz (473 mL) (NDC# 58829-245-16) and 1 gallon (3.785 L) (NDC# 58829-245-01).

Compendium Code No.: 11390113 Rev. 7-01 / Rev. 06-01

CHLORASAN ANTISEPTIC OINTMENT

Butler **Topical Wound Dressing**

ANADA No.: 200-301

Active Ingredient(s): 1% chlorhexidine acetate in a hydrophilic ointment base which contains 10% stearyl alcohol.

Indications: Dogs, Cats and Horses - For use as a topical antiseptic ointment for surface wounds.

Dosage and Administration: Suggested Usage:

Dogs, Cats and Horses - Carefully cleanse the wound area and apply daily.

Precaution(s): Storage: Store at controlled room temperature between 15°-30°C (59°-86°F). Keep container tightly closed when not in use. Protect from freezing.

Caution(s): In case of deep or puncture wounds or serious burns, consult veterinarian.

If redness, irritation or swelling persists or increases, discontinue use and consult veterinarian.

Warning(s): Not to be used on horses intended for use as food.

Keep out of reach of children.

Presentation: 7 oz (NDC 11695-2194-7) and 16 oz (NDC 11695-2194-1).

Compendium Code No.: 10822000 Iss. 01-02

CHLORBIOTIC® ℞

Schering-Plough **Ophthalmic Antibiotic**

(Chloramphenicol) 1% Sterile, Ophthalmic Ointment

NADA No.: 065-460

Active Ingredient(s): Each gram contains: Chloramphenicol 10 mg, in a light mineral oil, white petrolatum, polyoxyethylene sorbitan monostearate base.

Indications: Chloramphenicol veterinary ophthalmic ointment 1% is appropriate for use in dogs and cats for the topical treatment of bacterial conjunctivitis caused by pathogens susceptible to chloramphenicol.

Pharmacology: Chloramphenicol is a broad-spectrum antibiotic providing rapid clinical response and having therapeutic activity against susceptible strains of a number of gram-positive and gram-negative organisms including *Escherichia coli*, *Staphylococcus aureus* and *Streptococcus hemolyticus*.

Dosage and Administration: Application of the ointment should be preceded by cleansing to remove discharge and crusts. The ointment is applied every three (3) hours around the clock for 48 hours after which night instillations may be omitted. A small amount of ointment should be placed in the lower conjunctival sac. Treatment should be continued for two (2) days after the eye appears normal. Therapy for cats should not exceed seven (7) days.

Contraindication(s): Chloramphenicol products must not be used in meat, egg, or milk producing animals. The length of time that residues persist in milk or tissues has not been determined.

Precaution(s): Most susceptible bacteria will respond to chloramphenicol therapy in a few days. If improvement is not noted in this period of time, a change of therapy should be considered.

When infection is suspected as the cause of a disease process, especially in purulent or catarrhal conjunctivitis, attempts should be made to determine through susceptibility testing, which antibiotics will be effective prior to applying ophthalmic preparations.

Store at room temperature.

Caution(s): Federal (USA) law restricts this drug to use by or on the order of a licensed veterinarian.

Warning(s): Not for use in animals which are raised for food production. Prolonged use in cats may produce blood dyscrasias.

Presentation: ⅛ oz. sterile, tamper-proof tubes.

Compendium Code No.: 10470270

CHLORHEXIDERM™ 2% SHAMPOO

DVM **Antidermatosis Shampoo**

Antiseptic Cleansing Formulation with Emollients

Active Ingredient(s): Chlorhexidine gluconate 2%.

CHLORHEXIDERM™ is an antiseptic, shampoo combining surface-active penetrating agents and emollients for optimal therapeutic effectiveness.

Indications: For dermatological conditions in dogs, cats and horses where an antiseptic, cleansing and deodorizing formulation may be of benefit.

Directions for Use: Wet coat thoroughly with water. Apply and lather shampoo over the entire body, allowing for 5 to 10 minutes of contact time. Rinse completely with water. Repeat procedure if necessary.

Precaution(s): Store at room temperature.

Caution(s): For topical use only on dogs, cats, and horses. Avoid contact with eyes. Do not use in ears of any animal. If irritation develops, discontinue and consult your veterinarian.

Warning(s): Keep out of reach of children.

Presentation: 8 fl oz (237 mL) (NDC 47203-657-08), 12 fl oz (355 mL) (NDC 47203-657-12), and 1 gallon (3.78 L).

Compendium Code No.: 11420132 Rev 0199

CHLORHEXIDERM™ DISINFECTANT

DVM **Antiseptic**

An Effective Long-Acting Chlorhexidine Disinfectant

Active Ingredient(s): Chlorhexidine gluconate 2%.

Indications: An antiseptic, disinfectant solution for use in areas requiring a broad spectrum agent.

A fragrance-free long acting antiseptic/disinfectant solution providing broad spectrum activity.

For use in dogs, cats and horses.

Directions for Use: Dilute one (1) ounce of CHLORHEXIDERM™ Disinfectant per gallon of water. Apply ample amount of disinfectant solution to area being treated. Remove excess with a sterile gauze or sponge.

Precaution(s): Store at room temperature.

Caution(s): For external use only. Avoid contact with eyes and mucous membranes. Do not use in ears of any animal. If contact occurs, rinse thoroughly with water. Avoid ingestion.

For animal use only (dogs, cats and horses).

Warning(s): This product cannot be used on food-producing animals. Keep out of reach of children.

Presentation: 1 gallon (3.78 L) (NDC 47203-690-28).

Compendium Code No.: 11420061 Rev 0399

CHLORHEXIDERM™ FLUSH

DVM **Topical Wound Dressing**

Topical Antimicrobial Cleansing/Drying Solution

Active Ingredient(s): Water, glycerin, isopropyl alcohol, nonoxynol-12, PPG-12-PEG-50 lanolin, PEG-40 castor oil, chlorhexidine gluconate, fragrance, FD&C blue #1. May contain citric acid to ensure optimal pH. Contains chlorhexidine gluconate in a soothing, solubilizing vehicle.

Indications: CHLORHEXIDERM™ Flush is an astringent, general cleansing, drying formulation for topical use on dogs, cats and horses. For general cleansing of such conditions where an antimicrobial formulation would be of benefit.

Directions: Apply CHLORHEXIDERM™ Flush liberally onto the affected area. Use cotton or an absorbent material to clean the excess solution and debris from the treated area. Repeat the procedure once daily, if necessary, or as directed by a veterinarian.

Precaution(s): Store at room temperature.

Caution(s): For external use on animals only. Do not instill in eyes or on sensitive membranes that are not intact.

Warning(s): Keep out of reach of children.

Presentation: 4 fl oz (118 mL) and 12 fl oz (355 mL).

Compendium Code No.: 11420071 Rev 0597

CHLORHEXIDERM™ MAXIMUM 4% SHAMPOO ℞

DVM **Antidermatosis Shampoo**

Antiseptic Cleansing Formulation with Emollients

Active Ingredient(s): Chlorhexidine gluconate 4%.

CHLORHEXIDERM™ Maximum is a full strength medicated shampoo containing penetrating agents and emollients for optimal therapeutic effectiveness.

Indications: For mild to severe dermatological conditions in dogs, cats and horses where a full strength antiseptic, antimicrobial, cleansing and deodorizing formulation may be of benefit.

Directions for Use: Wet coat thoroughly with water. Apply and lather shampoo over the entire body, allowing for 5 to 10 minutes of contact time. Rinse completely with water. Repeat procedure if necessary.

Precaution(s): Store at room temperature.

Caution(s): Federal law restricts this drug to use by, or on the order of, a licensed veterinarian.

For topical use only on dogs, cats, and horses. Avoid contact with eyes. Not for otic use. If irritation develops, discontinue and consult your veterinarian.

Warning(s): Keep out of reach of children.

Presentation: 8 fl oz (237 mL) (NDC 47203-687-08), 12 fl oz (355 mL) (NDC 47203-687-12) and 1 gallon (3.78 L) (NDC 47203-687-28).

Compendium Code No.: 11420082 Rev 0199

CHLORHEXIDERM™ MAXIMUM 4% SPRAY ℞

DVM **Antidermatosis Spray**

Antiseptic Spray Formulation with Emollients

Active Ingredient(s): Chlorhexidine gluconate 4%.

CHLORHEXIDERM™ Maximum is a full strength antimicrobial spray containing penetrating agents and emollients for optimal therapeutic effectiveness.

Indications: For use in dogs, cats and horses where a full strength antiseptic and deodorizing formulation may be of benefit.

Directions for Use: Shake well before each use. Spray directly onto the affected area(s) 2-3 times daily, or as directed by veterinarian. Distract animal for several minutes following treatment to prevent licking.

Precaution(s): Store at room temperature.

Caution(s): Federal law restricts this drug to use by, or on the order of, a licensed veterinarian.

For topical use only on dogs, cats, and horses. Not for otic use. Avoid contact with eyes. If irritation develops, discontinue and consult your veterinarian.

Warning(s): Keep out of reach of children.

Presentation: 8 fl oz (237 mL) (NDC 47203-647-08).

Compendium Code No.: 11420092 Rev 0199

CHLORHEXIDERM™ PLUS SCRUB

DVM **Surgical Scrub**

Chlorhexidine Gluconate

Active Ingredient(s): Chlorhexidine Gluconate 2%, Isopropyl Alcohol 4%.

Indications: Provides fast-acting activity against a wide range of microorganisms, especially against those commonly found on skin.

Product Description: A broad spectrum antimicrobial surgical scrub and skin/wound cleanser in a dye-free and soap-free surfactant system. Gentle to the skin.

Directions for Use: Surgical Scrub - Apply CHLORHEXIDERM™ Plus liberally to surgical site and swab for at least two minutes. Dry with sterile towel. Repeat procedure for an additional two minutes and dry with a sterile towel.

Skin/Wound Cleanser - Thoroughly rinse the area to be cleansed with water. Apply the minimum amount of CHLORHEXIDERM™ Plus necessary to cover the skin or wound area and wash gently. Rinse again thoroughly.

Precaution(s): Store at room temperature.
Contraindication(s): FDA does not recommend the use of chlorhexidine as a surgical scrub for kittens and cats.
Caution(s): For external and topical use only. Avoid contact with eyes, ears and mucous membranes. If contact occurs, rinse thoroughly with water. Keep out of reach of children.
Presentation: 1 gallon (3.78 L).
Compendium Code No.: 11420100 REV 0699

CHLORHEXIDERM™ S DISINFECTANT

DVM **Antiseptic**

Scented Disinfectant 2% Chlorhexidine
Active Ingredient(s): Chlorhexidine gluconate 2%.
Indications: An antiseptic, disinfectant solution for use on dogs, cats and horses in areas requiring a broad spectrum antimicrobial agent.
A pleasantly-scented antiseptic disinfectant, which provides fasting-acting and long-acting activity against a wide range of micro-organisms, especially those commonly present on skin.
Directions for Use: Dilute one (1) ounce of CHLORHEXIDERM™ S Disinfectant per gallon of water. Apply ample amount of disinfectant solution to area being treated. Remove excess with a sterile gauze or sponge.
Precaution(s): Store at room temperature.
Caution(s): For external use only. Avoid contact with eyes and mucous membranes. Do not use in ears of any animal. If contact occurs, rinse thoroughly with water. Avoid ingestion.
Warning(s): This product cannot be used in food-producing animals. Keep out of reach of children.
Presentation: 1 gallon (3.78 L) (NDC 47203-197-28).
Compendium Code No.: 11420111 Rev 0199

CHLORHEXIDINE DISINFECTANT SOLUTION

AgriLabs **Antiseptic**

Active Ingredient(s):
Chlorhexidine gluconate 2%
Indications: An antiseptic and antimicrobial disinfectant which provides fast-acting activity against a wide range of micro-organisms, especially against those commonly present on the skin.
A non-toxic, non-irritating agent possessing a wide range of antiseptic and antimicrobial activity against organisms which infect the skin, such as bacteria, fungi, ringworm and yeast.
Dosage and Administration: Dilute one (1) ounce (2 tablespoons) of CHLORHEXIDINE DISINFECTANT SOLUTION per gallon of clean water.
Rinse the area to be disinfected with an ample amount of CHLORHEXIDINE DISINFECTANT SOLUTION. Wipe away the excess and pat dry with a sterile gauze or sponge.
Caution(s): Avoid contact with the eyes and mucous membranes. If contact is made, flush immediately and thoroughly with clean water.
For external use only.
For animal use only.
Keep out of the reach of children.
Presentation: 1 gallon containers.
Compendium Code No.: 10580320

CHLORHEXIDINE OINTMENT 1%

Phoenix Pharmaceutical **Topical Wound Dressing**

ANADA No.: 200-301
Active Ingredient(s): 1% chlorhexidine acetate in a hydrophilic ointment base which contains 10% stearyl alcohol.
Indications: Suggested Usage:
Dogs, Cats and Horses - For use as a topical antiseptic ointment for surface wounds.
Dosage and Administration: Dogs, Cats and Horses - Carefully cleanse the wound area and apply daily.
Precaution(s): Storage: Store at controlled room temperature between 15°-30°C (59°-86°F). Keep container tightly closed when not in use. Protect from freezing.
Caution(s): In case of deep or puncture wounds or serious burns, consult veterinarian.
If redness, irritation or swelling persists or increases, discontinue use and consult veterinarian.
For animal use only.
Warning(s): Not to be used on horses intended for use as food.
Keep out of reach of children.
Presentation: 1 lb jar (NDC 57319-470-27).
Manufactured by: First Priority, Inc., Elgin, IL 60123.
Compendium Code No.: 12561170 Iss. 11-01

CHLORHEXIDINE SCRUB

A.A.H. **Surgical Scrub**

Skin and Wound Cleaner
Active Ingredient(s):
Chlorhexidine Gluconate 2.0%
Quaternium-33 . . . . 1.5%
Contents: USP Purified water, Alkyl Dimethylamine oxide, Chlorhexidine Digluconate, Polyoxyethylene-6-Coco Amide, Octylphenoxypolyethoxyethanol, Glycerol, Polyethylene Glycol, Quaternium-33, Hydroxyethylcellulose, and FDC Blue #1.
Indications: Uses: CHLORHEXIDINE SCRUB exhibits a broad range of antimicrobial activity. CHLORHEXIDINE SCRUB is a mild scrub containing Chlorhexidine Digluconate and Quaternium-33 that exhibits bactericidal activity against a wide range of micro-organisms.
Directions: Wet hands with water. Pour approximately 5 mL of CHLORHEXIDINE SCRUB in palm of hand. Add enough water to make a lather. Lather thoroughly. Rinse thoroughly under running water.
Caution(s): For veterinary use only.
Warning(s): Avoid contact of this product with eyes and mucous membranes. If this product inadvertently comes in contact with eyes, immediately flush with cool water for 15 minutes and contact a physician. If this product is inadvertently swallowed, contact a physician and/or poison control center immediately. Keep out of reach of children.
Warning(s): Keep out of reach of children.
Presentation: 4 x 3.78 L (128 fl oz) (1 gal) jugs per case.
Compendium Code No.: 11180200 1101

CHLORHEXIDINE SCRUB 2%

First Priority **Surgical Scrub**

Mild Scrub Containing Chlorhexidine Gluconate
Active Ingredient(s):
Chlorhexidine Gluconate 2%
Indications: CHLORHEXIDINE SCRUB 2% is a mild scrub containing Chlorhexidine Gluconate 2% that exhibits bactericidal activity against a wide range of micro-organisms.
Directions for Use: Wet hands with water. Pour approximately 5 mL of CHLORHEXIDINE SCRUB 2% in palm of hand. Add enough water to make a lather. Lather thoroughly. Rinse thoroughly under running water.
Precaution(s): Storage: Store at controlled room temperature between 15°-30°C (59°-86°F). Keep container tightly closed when not in use.
Caution(s): Avoid contact with eyes and mucous membranes. If in eyes, immediately flush with water for 15 minutes and contact a physician. If swallowed, contact a physician and/or poison control center immediately.
Warning(s): Keep out of reach of children.
Presentation: 1 gallon (3.785 L) (NDC# 58829-140-01).
Compendium Code No.: 11390131 Rev. 07-01

C

CHLORHEXIDINE SCRUB 4%

First Priority **Surgical Scrub**

Maximum Strength-Mild Scrub Containing Chlorhexidine Gluconate
Active Ingredient(s):
Chlorhexidine Gluconate 4%
Indications: CHLORHEXIDINE SCRUB 4% is a mild scrub containing Chlorhexidine Gluconate 4% that exhibits bactericidal activity against a wide range of micro-organisms.
Directions for Use: Wet hands with water. Pour approximately 5 mL of CHLORHEXIDINE SCRUB 4% in palm of hand. Add enough water to make a lather. Lather thoroughly. Rinse thoroughly under running water.
Precaution(s): Storage: Store at controlled room temperature between 15°-30°C (59°-86°F). Keep container tightly closed when not in use.
Caution(s): Avoid contact with eyes and mucous membranes. If in eyes, immediately flush with water for 15 minutes and contact a physician. If swallowed, contact a physician and/or poison control center immediately. For animal use only.
Warning(s): Keep out of reach of children.
Presentation: 1 gallon (3.785 L) (NDC# 58829-298-01).
Compendium Code No.: 11390141 Rev. 07-01

CHLORHEXIDINE SOLUTION

A.A.H. **Antiseptic**

Chlorhexidine Gluconate 2.0%
Active Ingredient(s):
Chlorhexidine gluconate 2.0%
Indications: An antiseptic and antimicrobial disinfectant which provides fast acting activity against a wide range of microorganisms, especially against those commonly present on the skin.
Non-toxic, non-irritating agent possessing a wide range of antiseptic and antimicrobial activity against organisms which infect the skin, such as bacteria, fungi, ringworm and yeast.
Directions for Use: Dilution: One ounce (2 tablespoons) of CHLORHEXIDINE SOLUTION per gallon of water.
Rinse area to be disinfected with an ample amount of diluted CHLORHEXIDINE SOLUTION. Wipe away excess and pat dry with a sterile gauze or sponge.
Caution(s): For external use only. Avoid contact with eyes, ears, and mucous membranes. If contact occurs, immediately flush with water. For animal use only.
Warning(s): Keep out of reach of children. In case of accidental ingestion, seek professional assistance or contact the poison control center immediately.
Presentation: 4 x 3.78 L (128 fl oz) (1 gal) jugs per case.
Compendium Code No.: 11180210 901

CHLORHEXIDINE SOLUTION

Aspen **Antiseptic**

Active Ingredient(s): 2% Chlorhexidine Gluconate.
Indications: A topical aqueous cleaning solution for use on horses and dogs for application to superficial cuts, abrasions or insect stings.
Dosage and Administration: Dilute: 1 ounce (2 tablespoons) of CHLORHEXIDINE SOLUTION per gallon of clean water.
Directions for Use: Rinse skin area to be treated with CHLORHEXIDINE SOLUTION. Wipe away excess and pat dry with a sterile gauze or sponge.
Caution(s): Avoid contact with eyes and mucous membranes. This product is not to be used in ears. If contact is made, flush immediately and thoroughly with clean water. For use on horses and dogs. For animal use only. For external use only.
Warning(s): Keep out of reach of children.
Presentation: 3.785 L (1 gallon).
Compendium Code No.: 14750130

CHLORHEXIDINE SOLUTION

Bimeda **Antiseptic**

2% Chlorhexidine Gluconate
Active Ingredient(s): 2% Chlorhexidine Gluconate.
Indications: Product Description: A topical aqueous cleaning solution for use on horses and dogs for application to superficial cuts, abrasions or insect stings.
Directions for Use: Dilute: 1 ounce (2 tablespoons) of CHLORHEXIDINE SOLUTION per gallon of clean water.
Rinse skin area to be treated with CHLORHEXIDINE SOLUTION. Wipe away excess and pat dry with a sterile gauze or sponge.
Precaution(s): Storage: Store at controlled room temperature between 15°-30°C (59°-86°F). Keep container tightly closed when not in use.
Caution(s): Avoid contact with eyes and mucous membranes. This product is not to be used in ears. If contact is made, flush immediately and thoroughly with clean water. For use on horses and dogs. For external use only. For animal use only.
Warning(s): Keep out of reach of children.
Presentation: 3.785 L (1 gallon) (NDC# 61133-715-05).
Compendium Code No.: 13990530 Iss. 11-98

CHLORHEXIDINE SOLUTION

Butler **Antiseptic**

NDC No.: 11695-2157-1

Active Ingredient(s):

Chlorhexidine gluconate 2%

Indications: A topical aqueous cleaning solution for use on non-food producing animals for application to superficial cuts, abrasions or insect stings.

Dosage and Administration: Dilute one (1) ounce (2 tablespoons) of chlorhexidine solution per gallon of clean water.

Rinse the area to be disinfected with an ample amount of chlorhexidine solution. Wipe away the excess and pat dry with a sterile gauze or sponge.

C

Caution(s): Avoid contact with the eyes and mucous membranes. This product is not to be used in ears. If contact is made, flush immediately and thoroughly with clean water.

Warning(s): Not for use with food producing animals.

For animal use only. For external use only. Keep out of the reach of children.

Presentation: 1 gallon containers.

Compendium Code No.: 10820400

CHLORHEXIDINE SOLUTION

Durvet **Antiseptic**

NDC No.: 30798-624-31/30798-624-35

Active Ingredient(s): 2% Chlorhexidine gluconate.

Indications: A topical aqueous cleaning solution for use on horses and dogs for application to superficial cuts, abrasions or insect stings.

Dosage and Administration: Dilute: 1 ounce (2 tablespoons) of CHLORHEXIDINE SOLUTION per gallon of clean water.

Directions for Use: Rinse skin area to be treated with CHLORHEXIDINE SOLUTION. Wipe away excess and pat dry with a sterile gauze or sponge.

Caution(s): Avoid contact with eyes and mucous membranes. This product is not to be used in ears. If contact is made, flush immediately and thoroughly with clean water. Keep out of reach of children. For use on horses and dogs.

Warning(s): For external use only. For animal use only. Keep out of reach of children.

Presentation: 16 fl oz and 3.785 L (1 gal).

Compendium Code No.: 10840300

CHLORHEXIDINE SOLUTION

First Priority **Antiseptic**

2% Chlorhexidine Gluconate

Active Ingredient(s):

Chlorhexidine Gluconate 2%

Indications: A topical aqueous cleaning solution for use on horses and dogs for application to superficial cuts, abrasions or insect stings.

Directions for Use: Rinse skin area to be treated with CHLORHEXIDINE SOLUTION. Wipe away excess and pat dry with a sterile gauze or sponge.

Dilution: 1 ounce (2 tablespoonfuls) of CHLORHEXIDINE SOLUTION per gallon of clean water.

Precaution(s): Storage: Store at controlled room temperature between 15°-30°C (59°-86°F). Keep container tightly closed when not in use.

Caution(s): Avoid contact with eyes and mucous membranes. This product is not to be used in ears. If contact is made, flush immediately and thoroughly with clean water.

For external use only. For animal use only.

Warning(s): Keep out of reach of children.

Presentation: 16 fl oz (473 mL) (NDC# 58829-141-16) and 1 gallon (3.785 L) (NDC# 58829-141-01).

Compendium Code No.: 11390152 Rev. 06-01 / Rev. 07-01

CHLORHEXIDINE SOLUTION

Phoenix Pharmaceutical **Antiseptic**

2% Chlorhexidine Gluconate

Active Ingredient(s): 2% Chlorhexidine Gluconate.

Indications: A topical aqueous cleaning solution for use on horses and dogs for application to superficial cuts, abrasions or insect stings.

Directions for Use: Dilute: 1 ounce (2 tablespoons) of CHLORHEXIDINE SOLUTION per gallon of clean water.

Rinse skin area to be treated with CHLORHEXIDINE SOLUTION. Wipe away excess and pat dry with a sterile gauze or sponge.

Caution(s): Avoid contact with eyes and mucous membranes. This product is not to be used in ears. If contact is made, flush immediately and thoroughly with clean water. For use on horses and dogs. For external use only. For animal use only.

Warning(s): Keep out of reach of children.

Presentation: 1 gallon (3.785 L) (NDC 57319-421-09).

Manufactured by: Phoenix Scientific, Inc., St. Joseph, MO 64503.

Compendium Code No.: 12560162 Rev. 9-01

CHLORHEXIDINE SOLUTION

Vedco **Antiseptic**

NDC No.: 50989-351-29

Active Ingredient(s): Contains:

Chlorhexidine gluconate 2%

Indications: An antiseptic and antimicrobial disinfectant which provides activity against a wide range of micro-organisms, especially against those commonly present on the skin.

Non-toxic, non-irritating agent possessing a wide range of antiseptic and antimicrobial activity against organisms which infect the skin, such as bacteria, fungi, ringworm and yeast.

Dosage and Administration: Dilute one (1) ounce (2 tablespoons) of CHLORHEXIDINE SOLUTION per gallon of clean water.

Rinse the area to be disinfected with an ample amount of CHLORHEXIDINE SOLUTION. Wipe away the excess and pat dry with a sterile gauze or sponge.

Caution(s): Avoid contact with the eyes and mucous membranes. If contact is made, flush immediately and thoroughly with clean water.

For animal use only. Keep out of the reach of children. For external use only.

Presentation: 1 gallon containers.

Compendium Code No.: 10940290

CHLORHEXIDINE SOLUTION

Vet Solutions **Antiseptic**

2% Chlorhexidine Gluconate-A Concentrated Broad Spectrum Antimicrobial Solution

Active Ingredient(s): Chlorhexidine Gluconate 2%.

Indications: Vet Solutions CHLORHEXIDINE SOLUTION provides rapid antimicrobial activity against a wide range of microorganisms.

Directions: Dilute one (1) ounce (2 tablespoons) per gallon of clean water. Higher concentrations of solution may be used upon veterinarian's discretion. Apply diluted solution liberally to affected area. Remove excess with clean towel or sterile gauze.

Precaution(s): Storage: Store at controlled room temperature.

Caution(s): For external use only. Avoid contact with eyes, ears and mucous membranes. If contact occurs, immediately flush with clean water.

Warning(s): Keep this and all drugs out of the reach of children. In case of accidental ingestion, seek professional assistance or contact the poison control center immediately.

Presentation: 1 gallon (3.79 L).

Compendium Code No.: 10610040 990501

CHLORHEXI-LUBE

Durvet **Lubricant**

Active Ingredient(s): 0.1% Chlorhexidine Gluconate.

Indications: Product Description: A ready to use antiseptic lubricant for topical or intrauterine application. Non-greasy; free from irritating effects; will not injure rubber appliances or surgical instruments.

Directions for Use:

Topical: Remove sufficient amount to cover hand and arm or instruments as required. If desired a small amount of water can be used.

Intrauterine: Add approximately four ounces of CHLORHEXI-LUBE per gallon of warm water and mix well.

Precaution(s): Store at controlled room temperature 15° to 30°C (59° to 86°F). Keep container tightly closed.

Caution(s): For veterinary use only. For animal use only.

Warning(s): Keep out of reach of children.

Presentation: 8 lbs (NDC 30798-632-57).

Compendium Code No.: 10841930 Iss. 07-00

CHLORHEXI-LUBE

First Priority **Lubricant**

Active Ingredient(s):

Chlorhexidine Gluconate 0.1%

Indications: A ready to use antiseptic lubricant for topical or intrauterine application. Non-greasy; free from irritating effects; will not injure rubber appliances or surgical instruments.

Directions for Use:

Topical: Remove sufficient amount to cover hand and arm or instruments as required. If desired a small amount of water can be used.

Intrauterine: Add approximately four ounces of CHLORHEXI-LUBE per gallon of warm water and mix well.

Precaution(s): Storage: Store at controlled room temperature 15° to 30°C (59° to 86°F). Keep container tightly closed when not in use.

Caution(s): For veterinary use only. For animal use only.

Warning(s): Keep out of reach of children.

Presentation: 8 lb (3.785 L) (NDC# 58829-151-01).

Compendium Code No.: 11390122 Rev. 07-01

CHLORHEX SHAMPOO

Vedco **Grooming Shampoo**

Active Ingredient(s): Chlorhexidine 1%. Contains surface-active agents, coat conditioners, and fragrance.

Indications: An antiseptic cleansing shampoo. For use in dogs, cats and horses.

It is recommended for dermatological conditions where antiseptic, antifungal, antimicrobial, cleansing and deodorizing formulation may be of benefit. Also, for routine shampooing of normal animals.

Dosage and Administration: Wet coat thoroughly with water and work sufficient shampoo over as large an area as will allow a mild lather to develop. Then proceed to lather another area. When the entire coat is treated, allow to stand 5 minutes. Rinse thoroughly with water. Repeat procedure if necessary.

Precaution(s): Store product at room temperature.

Caution(s): Avoid contact with eyes.

Warning(s): For veterinary use only. Keep out of reach of children.

Presentation: 8 oz and 1 gallon (3.79 L).

Compendium Code No.: 10940270

CHLORHEX SURGICAL SCRUB

Vedco **Surgical Scrub**

Active Ingredient(s): Contains:

Chlorhexidine citrate . . . . 2% weight to volume

Indications: CHLORHEX SURGICAL SCRUB exhibits a broad range of antimicrobial activity.

CHLORHEX SURGICAL SCRUB is used as a skin and wound cleanser.

Dosage and Administration: Apply 1-5 mL of chlorhexidine surgical scrub to the area to be treated with a clean sponge. Thoroughly scrub the area for three (3) to five (5) minutes. Rinse the area with clean water.

Caution(s): Keep out of the reach of children.

Avoid contact with the eyes and mucous membranes. If in eyes, immediately flush with water for 15 minutes and contact a physician.

If swallowed, contact a physician and/or a poison control center immediately.

Presentation: 128 fl. oz. (1 gallon) containers.

Compendium Code No.: 10940280

CHLORMAX™ 50

Alpharma **Feed Additive**

Chlortetracycline-Type A Medicated Article-Antibacterial

NADA No.: 046-699

Active Ingredient(s):

Chlortetracycline (as hydrochloride). . . . . 50 g/lb

Inert ingredients: Roughage products, silicon dioxide, mineral oil.

Indications: For control and treatment of diseases caused by organisms susceptible to chlortetracycline and for increased feed efficiency and weight gain as indicated.

Directions:

Indications for use	Chlortetracycline mg/lb body wt/day
Cattle	
Calves (up to 250 lbs, in milk replacers or starter feeds): For an increased rate of weight gain and improved feed efficiency.	0.1
Beef cattle (over 700 lbs): Control of active infection of anaplasmosis caused by *Anaplasma marginale* susceptible to chlortetracycline.	0.5
Calves, beef, and non-lactating dairy cattle: Treatment of bacterial enteritis caused by *Escherichia coli* and bacterial pneumonia caused by *Pasteurella multocida* organisms susceptible to chlortetracycline. Treat for not more than 5 days.	10
Swine	
Control of porcine proliferative enteropathies (ileitis) caused by *Lawsonia intracellularis* susceptible to chlortetracycline. Treatment of bacterial enteritis caused by *Escherichia coli* and *Salmonella choleraesuis* and bacterial pneumonia caused by *Pasteurella multocida* organisms susceptible to chlortetracycline. (Note: This dose is equivalent to 400 grams per ton, depending on feed consumption and body weight). Feed for not more than 14 days.	10
Turkeys	
Control of complicating bacterial organisms associated with bluecomb (transmissible enteritis, coronaviral enteritis) susceptible to chlortetracycline. Feed continuously for 7 to 14 days.	25

Indications for use	mg/head/day
Cattle	
Calves (250-400 lbs): For an increased rate of weight gain and improved feed efficiency.	25-70
Growing cattle (over 400 lbs): For an increased rate of weight gain, improved feed efficiency and reduction of liver condemnation due to liver abscesses.	70
Beef cattle: For the control of bacterial pneumonia associated with shipping fever complex caused by *Pasteurella* spp. susceptible to chlortetracycline.	350
Beef cattle (under 700 lbs): Control of active infection of anaplasmosis caused by *Anaplasma marginale* susceptible to chlortetracycline.	350
Sheep	
Breeding sheep: Reducing the incidence of (vibrionic) abortion caused by *Campylobacter fetus* infection susceptible to chlortetracycline.	80

Indications for use	In complete feed Chlortetracycline g/ton
Chickens	
For an increased rate of weight gain and improved feed efficiency.	10-50
Control of infectious synovitis caused by *Mycoplasma synoviae* susceptible to chlortetracycline. Feed continuously for 7 to 14 days.	100-200
Control of chronic respiratory disease (CRD) and air sac infection caused by *Mycoplasma gallisepticum* and *Escherichia coli* susceptible to chlortetracycline. Feed continuously for 7 to 14 days.	200-400
Reduction of mortality due to *Escherichia coli* infections susceptible to chlortetracycline. Feed for 5 days.	500
Turkeys	
Growing turkeys: For an increased rate of weight gain and improved feed efficiency.	10-50
Control of infectious synovitis caused by *Mycoplasma synoviae* susceptible to chlortetracycline. Feed continuously for 7 to 14 days.	200
Control of hexamitiasis caused by *Hexamita meleagrides* susceptible to chlortetracycline. Feed continuously for 7 to 14 days.	400
Turkey poults not over 4 weeks of age: Reduction of mortality due to paratyphoid caused by *Salmonella typhimurium* susceptible to chlortetracycline.	400
Swine	
Growing swine: For an increased rate of weight gain and improved feed efficiency.	10-50
Reducing the incidence of cervical lymphadenitis (jowl abscesses) caused by Group E. *Streptococci* susceptible to chlortetracycline.	50-100
Breeding swine: Control of leptospirosis (reducing the incidence of abortion and shedding of leptospirae) caused by *Leptospira pomona* susceptible to chlortetracycline. Feed continuously for 14 days.	400
Sheep	
Growing sheep: For an increased rate of weight gain and improved feed efficiency.	20-50

Mixing directions: For use in manufacture of complete feeds, mix thoroughly as follows:

Chlortetracycline, g/ton	CHLORMAX™ 50, lb/ton
10-50	0.2-1
20-50	0.4-1
50-100	1-2
100-200	2-4
200-400	4-8
500	10

For use in manufacture of feed supplements to be fed at a rate of 1 lb per head per day, mix thoroughly as follows:

mg/lb body wt/day	If animal wt = 1000 lbs	CHLORMAX™ 50 lb/ton supplement
0.5	500 mg	20
5.0	5,000 mg	200

Precaution(s): Keep container tightly closed to prevent contamination or moisture pick-up.

Caution(s): Observe the limitations of use and withdrawal periods as indicated.

For use in manufacturing medicated feed only.

For animal use only. For use in dry feeds only.

Not for use in liquid type B medicated feeds.

Warning(s): Do not feed to chickens or turkeys producing eggs for human consumption. A withdrawal period has not been established for this product in pre-ruminating calves. Do not use in calves to be processed for veal.

Beef cattle (0.5 mg/lb body wt/day): Withdraw 48 hours prior to slaughter.

Calves, beef, and non-lactating dairy cattle (10 mg/lb body wt/day): Withdraw 24 hours prior to slaughter.

Beef cattle (350 mg/head/day): Withdraw 48 hours prior to slaughter.

Chickens (500 g/ton): Withdraw 24 hours prior to slaughter.

Presentation: 50 lb (22.68 kg) bag.

Compendium Code No.: 10220261 700301 0107

CHLOR-SCRUB 40™

Butler **Surgical Scrub**

NDC No.: 11695-2152-1

Active Ingredient(s): CHLOR-SCRUB 40™ is a mild scrub containing chlorhexidine gluconate 4%. It also contains: Deionized water, alkyl dimethylamineoxide, diethanolamine, chlorhexidine digluconate, isopropyl alcohol 99%, polyoxyethylene-6-coco amide, octylphenoxypolyethoxy-ethanol, glycerol, polyethylene glycol, quaternium 33-ethylhexandiol, hydroxyethylcellulose, and FDC red #40.

Indications: CHLOR-SCRUB 40™ exhibits bactericidal activity against a wide range of micro-organisms.

Dosage and Administration: Wet hands with water. Pour approximately 5 mL of CHLOR-SCRUB 40™ in the palm of the hand. Add enough water to make a lather. Lather thoroughly. Rinse thoroughly under running water.

Caution(s): Keep out of the reach of children.

Presentation: 1 gallon (128 fl. oz.) containers.

Compendium Code No.: 10820380

CHOATE'S® LINIMENT

Hawthorne **Liniment**

Active Ingredient(s): Each 16 U.S. fl oz contains:

Menthol. . . . . 5 g

Camphor . . . . 5 g

Capsicum . . . . 17 g

Acetone base with essential oils.

Indications: For use as an aid in the temporary relief of minor stiffness and soreness caused by over-exertion and as an excellent soothing body brace.

Dosage and Administration: Make sure affected area is clean and free of other medication. Apply sparingly with brush or hand. To use as a body brace after a workout or race, add 2 oz of CHOATE'S® Liniment to 5 gallons of water.

Caution(s): Do not apply to irritated skin or if excessive irritation develops. Avoid contact with eyes or mucous membranes. Keep away from children. For external use only. Keep away from fire and open flame.

Warning(s): Do not use on food animals.

Presentation: 16 U.S. fl oz.

Compendium Code No.: 10670000

CHOLERAMUNE® CU

Biomune **Bacterial Vaccine**

Pasteurella Multocida Vaccine, Avirulent Live Culture, Avian Isolate

U.S. Vet. Lic. No.: 368

Contents: This is a live bacterial vaccine containing the known avirulent isolate of *Pasteurella multocida*, type 3 x 4, Clemson University (CU) strain, in a freeze-dried preparation sealed under vacuum.

The seed culture used to make this vaccine has been laboratory tested for protection against challenge with *P. multocida* strain X-73 (type 1).

Indications: This vaccine is recommended for use in healthy chickens six weeks of age or older as an aid in preventing pasteurellosis (fowl cholera) due to *Pasteurella multocida* type 1.

The CU vaccine strain has been shown to offer protection against naturally occurring field strains of *P. multocida*.

Dosage and Administration: Administer contents of vial to 500 chickens by wing web stab (0.01 mL). Best results are obtained when vaccine is administered initially to chickens 6 to 12 weeks of age and again at 4 to 6 week intervals.

Chickens to be vaccinated should not be given any antibiotic and/or sulfonamide medication for 3 days before and 5 days after vaccination to avoid interference with the immune response.

How To Vaccinate:

1. Keep refrigerated until use. After rehydration, use entire contents within 2 hours.
2. Rehydrate the vaccine vial with the entire contents of the diluent vial provided (5 mL). Mix well.
3. Vaccinate by dipping the applicator needle into the rehydrated vaccine and piercing the

C

webbed portion under the wing. Guard against losing vaccine by touching feathers with applicator. Avoid piercing the wing muscle, bone or large blood vessels.

4. Re-dip the applicator between each vaccination. Remove excess vaccine on applicator by touching to inside of vial.

Contraindication(s): Chickens should be healthy and free of environmental or physical stress at the time of vaccination. Initial vaccination should not be conducted in chickens older than 12 weeks of age, as this may result in larger granulomas at the site of inoculation which may cause possible carcass downgrading at slaughter.

Precaution(s): Store between 35° to 45°F (2°-7°C).

Use entire contents of vial when first opened. Burn this vial and all unused contents

Caution(s): Since this is a live bacterial culture, caution should be used to avoid contact with open wounds or accidental inoculation of personnel. If this occurs, consult a physician immediately.

Warning(s): Do not vaccinate within 21 days before slaughter.

Adverse Reactions: Usually, there is no clinical reaction to this vaccine. However, a small granuloma will develop at the site of inoculation 5 to 10 days after vaccination. The absence of a reaction may indicate that the birds were immune prior to vaccination or that the vaccine was improperly handled or administered.

Presentation: 10 x 500 dose vials of vaccine with 10 vials of diluent (5 mL each) and vaccine applicators/box.

Compendium Code No.: 11290021 122

CHOLERAMUNE® M

Biomune **Vaccine**

Pasteurella Multocida Vaccine, Avirulent Live Culture, Avian Isolate

U.S. Vet. Lic. No.: 368

Contents: This is a live bacterial vaccine containing the known avirulent isolate of *Pasteurella multocida*, M-9 strain in a freeze-dried preparation sealed under vacuum.

The seed culture used to make this vaccine has been laboratory tested for protection against challenge with *P. multocida* strain X-73 (type 1).

Indications: This vaccine is recommended for use in healthy chickens six weeks of age or older as an aid in preventing pasteurellosis (fowl cholera) due to *Pasteurella multocida* type 1.

The M-9 strain has been shown to offer protection against naturally occurring field strains of *P. multocida.*

Dosage and Administration: Administer contents of vial to 1,000 chickens by wing web stab (0.01 mL). Best results are obtained when vaccine is administered initially to chickens 6 to 12 weeks of age and once again at about 18 to 20 weeks of age, prior to start of lay.

Chickens to be vaccinated should not be given any antibiotic and/or sulfonamide medication for 3 days before and 5 days after vaccination to avoid interference with the immune response.

How To Vaccinate:

1. Keep refrigerated until use. After rehydration, use entire contents within 2 hours.
2. Rehydrate the vaccine vial with the entire contents of the diluent vial provided (10 mL). Mix well.
3. Vaccinate by dipping the applicator needle into the rehydrated vaccine and piercing the webbed portion under the wing. Guard against losing vaccine by touching feathers with applicator. Avoid piercing the wing muscle, bone or large blood vessels.
4. Re-dip the applicator between each vaccination. Remove excess vaccine on applicator by touching to inside of vial.

Contraindication(s): Chickens should be healthy and free of environmental or physical stress at the time of vaccination. Initial vaccination should not be conducted in chickens older than 12 weeks of age, as this may result in larger granulomas at the site of inoculation which may cause possible carcass downgrading at slaughter.

Precaution(s): Store between 35° to 45°F (2°-7°C).

Use entire contents of vial when first opened.

Burn this vial and all unused contents.

Caution(s): Since this is a live bacterial culture, caution should be used to avoid contact with open wounds or accidental inoculation of personnel. If this occurs, consult a physician immediately.

Warning(s): Do not vaccinate within 21 days before slaughter

Adverse Reactions: Usually, there is no clinical reaction to this vaccine. However, a small granuloma will develop at the site of inoculation 5 to 10 days after vaccination. The absence of a reaction may indicate that the birds were immune prior to vaccination or that the vaccine was improperly handled or administered.

Presentation: 10 x 1,000 dose vials accompanied by 10 mL diluents and applicators.

Compendium Code No.: 11290032 120

CHOLERVAC-IV™

Intervet **Bacterin**

Pasteurella Multocida Bacterin, Avian Isolates, Types 1, 3, 4 & 3X4

U.S. Vet. Lic. No.: 286

Contents: CHOLERVAC-IV™ is prepared from four inactivated strains of *Pasteurella multocida* belonging to serotypes 1, 3, 4 and 3X4 and suspended in the aqueous phase of an oil adjuvant emulsion.

Indications: CHOLERVAC-IV™ is indicated for the prevention of disease (fowl cholera) in chickens due to *P. multocida* Type 1 infection and in turkeys due to *P. multocida* Types 3, 4 and 3X4. Chickens and turkeys should be in good health when vaccinated. Sick or weak birds will not develop adequate immunity.

Dosage and Administration: Before use, CHOLERVAC-IV™ must reach ambient temperatures 21-27°C (70-80°F) naturally. Shake vigorously before and periodically during use. Inject 0.5 mL subcutaneously in the back of the neck midway between the head and body in a direction away from the head using an 18-gauge needle.

Vaccination Program: CHOLERVAC-IV™ should be used for the initial vaccination of chickens at 10 weeks of age or older or turkeys at 8 weeks of age or older. Revaccination should be performed 5 to 6 weeks later but at least 3 weeks prior to lay.

Vaccination Reaction: Clinical reactions may occur as a result of transient swelling in the neck region following vaccination. These reactions may be aggravated by improper vaccination technique. If shock is observed, this must usually be ascribed to stress by handling.

Records: Keep a record of bacterin, quantity, serial number, expiration date, and place of purchase; the date and time of vaccination; the number, age, breed, and locations of birds; names of operators performing the vaccination and any observed reactions.

Precaution(s): Store in the dark in a refrigerator between 2 and 7°C (35 and 45°F). Do not freeze.

Before use, CHOLERVAC-IV™ must reach ambient temperatures 21-27°C (70-80°F) naturally.

Do not mix this bacterin with any other substances.

Ensure that vaccination equipment is clean and sterile before use.

Do not use vaccination equipment with rubber parts, as the oil emulsion may attack certain types of rubber.

Use entire contents when first opened.

Avoid exposure of this bacterin to sunlight.

Do not expose this bacterin to microwave radiation, boiling water, extensive heat, or any other similar physical processes.

Caution(s): To avoid human injection, extreme caution should be used when injecting any oil emulsion vaccine. Accidental human injection may cause serious local reactions. Contact a physician immediately if accidental human injection occurs.

Vaccinate only healthy birds. Although disease may not be evident, concurrent disease conditions may cause complications and/or reduce immunity.

Do not inject this bacterin by the intramuscular route.

Do not use less than 1 dose per bird per vaccination.

The use of any bacterin may cause false-positive results on Mycoplasma plate tests. Avoid such testing prior to 10 weeks post-vaccination.

For veterinary use only.

Notice: This bacterin has undergone rigid potency, safety and purity tests, and meets Intervet Inc. and USDA requirements. It is designed to stimulate effective immunity when used as directed, but the user must be advised that the response to the product depends upon many factors, including, but not limited to, conditions of storage and handling by the user, administration of the bacterin, health and responsiveness of the individual chickens or turkeys, and the degree of field exposure. Therefore, directions should be followed carefully.

This product is not hazardous when used according to directions supplied. A material safety data sheet (MSDS) is available upon request. This and any other consumer information can be obtained by calling Intervet Customer Service at 1-800-441-8272 or 1-302-934-8051.

The use of this bacterin is subject to applicable local and federal laws and regulations.

Warning(s): Do not administer this bacterin during the critical egg laying period from onset of lay until after peak production. Administration of this product during lay period may result in a drop of egg production.

Do not vaccinate birds within 42 days before slaughter.

Presentation: 500 mL bottle (1000 doses) for subcutaneous injection.

Compendium Code No.: 11060300

CHOLERVAC-PM-1®

Intervet **Vaccine**

Pasteurella Multocida Vaccine, Avirulent Live Culture, Avian Isolate

U.S. Vet. Lic. No.: 286

Description: CHOLERVAC-PM-1® contains the known avirulent isolate of *Pasteurella multocida* designated PM-1, as a freeze-dried preparation sealed under vacuum. The strain has been tested in chickens for protection against challenge with Type 1 (X-73) of *P. multocida.*

This vaccine contains no preservative.

Quality tested for purity, potency, and safety.

Indications: CHOLERVAC-PM-1® is indicated for the prevention of disease due to *P. multocida* Type 1 infection (fowl cholera) in chickens. Chickens should be in good health when vaccinated and not under any environmental, physical or social stress. Sick or weak chickens will not develop adequate immunity. Chickens should be 10 to 12 weeks of age at initial vaccination by the wing-web route. Revaccination should be performed between 6 to 8 weeks following the initial vaccination.

Dosage and Administration: CHOLERVAC-PM-1® should be refrigerated until use and not rehydrated until immediately ready for use. Administer 1,000 doses of vaccine by the wing-web route to 1,000 chickens. Rehydrate the vaccine with the supplied diluent bottle (10 mL). Rehydrate only one bottle at a time and use the entire contents within 2 hours. After mixing the vaccine thoroughly, dip the applicator needle in the vaccine and pierce the webbed portion of the underside of the wing. Avoid contacting feathers as this will wipe the vaccine off the needle. Avoid piercing muscle or bone tissue. Re-dip the applicator needle in the vaccine before each application. Mix the vaccine periodically during the vaccination period.

Records: Keep a record of vaccine, quantity, serial number, expiration date, and place of purchase; the date and time of vaccination; the number, age, breed, and locations of chickens; names of operators performing the vaccination and any observed reactions.

Precaution(s): Storage Conditions: Store in the dark in a refrigerator between 2-7°C (35-45°F). Do not freeze.

Do not spill, splash or mix this vaccine with any other substance.

Use entire contents when first opened.

Burn containers and all unused contents.

Wash hands thoroughly after using the vaccine.

This product is non-returnable.

Caution(s): Vaccinate only healthy chickens. Although disease may not be evident, coccidiosis, respiratory virus infection, infectious bursal disease, avian reovirus disease, Marek's disease, and other disease conditions may cause complications or reduce immunity.

Do not dilute the vaccine or otherwise stretch the dosage.

Do not medicate chickens with antibacterial drugs five days prior to or after vaccination.

Efforts should be taken to reduce stress conditions at the time of vaccination.

All susceptible chickens on the same premises should be vaccinated at the same time.

For veterinary use only.

Notice: This vaccine has undergone rigid potency, safety and purity tests, and meets Intervet Inc. and USDA requirements. It is designed to stimulate effective immunity when used as directed, but the user must be advised that the response to the product depends upon many factors, including, but not limited to, conditions of storage and handling by the user, administration of the vaccine, health and responsiveness of the individual chickens, and the degree of field exposure. Therefore, directions should be followed carefully.

This product is not hazardous when used according to directions supplied. A material safety data sheet (MSDS) is available upon request. This and any other consumer information can be obtained by calling Intervet Customer Service at 1-800-441-8272 or 1-302-934-8051.

The use of the vaccine is subject to applicable local and federal laws and regulations.

Use only as directed.

Warning(s): Do not vaccinate within 21 days before slaughter or 35 days prior to onset of lay or during egg production.

Avoid contact of open wounds or accidental inoculation of vaccination crew personnel. If this occurs, consult a physician immediately.

Presentation: 10 x 1,000 doses for wing web administration with 10 x 10 mL sterile diluent.

U.S. Patent No. 4,999,191

Compendium Code No.: 11060311 Rev. 24206 AL162

CHOLODIN®

MVP **Small Animal Dietary Supplement**

Active Ingredient(s): CHOLODIN® contains: Phosphatidylcholine (from soy lecithin), choline (as chloride), dl-methionine, inositol, zinc (as oxide), niacinamide, vitamin E, thiamine (mononitrate), riboflavin, pyridoxine (HCl), selenium (sodium selenite), vitamin B_{12} (cobalamin concentrate), and dexpanthenol. Formulated with a flavor base.

Indications: A dietary supplement to increase levels of available choline and phosphatidylcholine through dietary loading.

Dosage and Administration: Usual Daily Dose:

Animal	Tablet Form	Powder Form
Cats and Small Dogs	½-1 tablet	¼-½ teaspoonful
Large Dogs	1-2 tablets	½-1 teaspoonful

The tablets may be fed by hand or crumbled and mixed with food.

The powder may be mixed with food.

Caution(s): Keep out of the reach of children.

Side Effects: Infrequently, animals on a choline loading regime will show signs of increased neurological activity such as hyperactivity, social agitation, muscular twitching, etc. If these signs are seen, cessation of tablet or powder administration will quickly result in the disappearance of these signs. After a period of three or four days, the animal may be started again on the same dosage, usually with no adverse reaction.

Presentation: Tablets: 50, 180 and 500-count bottles.
Powder: 1 lb. containers.

Compendium Code No.: 11120011

CHOLODIN®-FEL

MVP **Small Animal Dietary Supplement**

Guaranteed Analysis: Per Tablet - All values are minimum quantities.

Minerals: Zinc 3.6 mg, Selenium 0.01 mg.

Vitamins and other: dl-Methionine 200 mg, Taurine 30 mg, Choline 20 mg, Inositol 20 mg, Vitamin E 2.5 IU, Niacin 2.5 mg, Thiamine 0.75 mg, Riboflavin 0.75 mg, Vitamin B6 0.5 mg, Pantothenic Acid 0.5 mg, Vitamin B12 1.0 mg.

Ingredients: Brewers dried yeast, dl-methionine, cellulose powder, lecithin, bone ash, lactose, starch, animal liver meal (pork), taurine, choline chloride, soy flour, inositol, sodium chloride, dried beans, silicon dioxide, magnesium stearate, torula dried yeast, dl-alpha tocopheryl acetate, zinc oxide, thiamine mononitrate, niacinamide, riboflavin, calcium pantothenate, pyridoxine HCl, sodium selenite, cyanocobalamin.

Indications: A chewable dietary supplement containing choline, amino acids, vitamins, minerals, and taurine for cats.

Directions: 1 tablet per day for each 10 lbs. of body weight. Tablets may be fed by hand or crumbled and mixed with daily diet.

Precaution(s): Store at room temperature.

Caution(s): Infrequently, animals on a choline-loading regime will show signs of increased neurological activity such as hyperactivity, social agitation, muscular twitching, etc. If these responses are noticed, cessation of tablet administrations will quickly result in disappearance of these irregularities. After a period of three or four days the animal may resume the same dosage, usually with no adverse reaction.

Presentation: 50 tablets.

Compendium Code No.: 11120021

CHONDROPROTEC® ℞

Neogen **Topical Wound Dressing**

Polysulfated Glycosaminoglycan

Active Ingredient(s): CHONDROPROTEC® is a sterile 10 mL solution containing 1000 mg of polysulfated glycosaminoglycan. Sodium hydroxide and/or hydrochloric acid is added when necessary to adjust pH to 6.5-6.7.

Indications: For use on partial and full thickness wounds, secreting and bleeding dermal lesions, 1st and 2nd degree burns, pressure ulcers (stages I-IV), surgical incisions, donor sites, venous stasis ulcers.

For use on dogs, cats and horses.

Directions for Use:

1. Irrigate wound site with sterile water or normal saline.
2. Apply CHONDROPROTEC® liberally to wound surface.
3. Cover with gauze or non-stick (Telfa) pad.
4. Redress wound site every 24-48 hours.

Precaution(s): Store at controlled room temperature (15°-30°C). Protect from freezing. Discard unused portion.

Caution(s): Federal Law restricts this device to sale by or on the order of a licensed veterinarian.

Warning(s): Not for food animal use.

Presentation: 10 mL (1000 mg) vial.

Sold to licensed veterinarians only.

Compendium Code No.: 14910211 L145-1097 Rev 0101

CHORIONIC GONADOTROPIN ℞

Butler **Chorionic Gonadotropin**

Chorionic Gonadotropin for Injection, USP (Cryodesiccated)

NADA No.: 047-055

Active Ingredient(s): Chorionic gonadotropin is a gonad-stimulating principle obtained from the urine of pregnant women.

When reconstituted with the diluent provided (bacteriostatic water for injection) each vial of sterile solution contains:

Chorionic gonadotropin . . . . . 10,000 U.S.P. units
Mannitol . . . . . 100 mg
Dibasic sodium phosphate . . . . . 16 mg
Monobasic sodium phosphate . . . . . 14 mg
Benzyl alcohol (as preservative) 0.9%
Water for injection . . . . . q.s.

Sodium hydroxide and/or hydrochloric acid may be used to adjust pH.

Indications: For parenteral use in cows for the treatment of nymphomania (frequent or constant heat) due to cystic ovaries.

Dosage and Administration: The drug is administered at a recommended dose of 10,000 U.S.P. units by deep intramuscular injection, or 2,500 to 5,000 U.S.P. units intravenously, or by intrafollicular injection of 500 to 2,500 units. The dosage may be repeated in 14 days if necessary.

How to use the Monovial® to Prepare the Solution:

1. Remove the protective white plastic cap. Press the upper stopper which dislodges the inner rubber seal down causing the diluent to mix with the solids.
2. Shake the contents in the Monovial® until completely in solution.

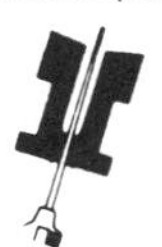

Needle must be inserted directly in center

3. Sterilize the upper stopper. Invert the Monovial®. With the needle of the syringe pierce the center of the rubber seal. Withdraw the desired number of mL or doses.

Precaution(s): Prior to reconstitution, store at a controlled room temperature 15°-30°C (59°-86°F). After reconstitution with bacteriostatic water for injection, refrigerate the solution and use within 30 days. Protect from freezing.

Caution(s): Federal law restricts this drug to use by or on the order of a licensed veterinarian.

Chorionic gonadotropin is a heterologous protein. Due caution against anaphylaxis should be observed.

Antidote(s): Epinephrine hydrochloride and parenteral antihistamine.

Presentation: 10 mL double vial packs containing: 10,000 U.S.P. units per vial with bacteriostatic water for injection.

10 mL multiple dose Monovials® (2-chamber vials containing bacteriostatic water for injection as diluent): 10,000 U.S.P. units per vial.

Compendium Code No.: 10820410

CHORULON® ℞

Intervet **Chorionic Gonadotropin**

NADA No.: 140-927

Active Ingredient(s): CHORULON® is a freeze-dried preparation of chorionic gonadotropin (Human Chorionic Gonadotropin, hCG) for intramuscular administration after reconstitution. When reconstituted with the accompanying sterile diluent, each single dose vial contains 10,000 I.U. chorionic gonadotropin (equivalent to 10,000 USP units chorionic gonadotropin) and 10 mg mannitol, with mono- and disodium phosphate to adjust the pH of the solution.

Indications: CHORULON® is indicated for intramuscular use in cows for the treatment of nymphomania (frequent or constant heat) due to cystic ovaries.

Pharmacology: Action: Chorionic gonadotropin has luteinizing hormone-like activity with little or no follicle stimulating or estrogenic activity.

Dosage and Administration: To reconstitute, transfer the contents of one vial of sterile diluent into one vial of freeze-dried powder. The resulting single dose (10 mL) of CHORULON® contains 10,000 I.U. chorionic gonadotropin.

One dose (10 mL) of reconstituted CHORULON® should be administered as a single deep intramuscular injection. Dosage may be repeated in 14 days if the animal's behavior, or rectal examination of the ovaries, indicates the necessity for retreatment.

Precaution(s): Store at or below room temperature, 77°F (25°C).

Once reconstituted, CHORULON® should be used immediately. Unused solution should be disposed of properly and not stored for future use.

Caution(s): Federal law restricts this drug to use by or on the order of a licensed veterinarian.

For animal use only.

Adverse Reactions: Chorionic gonadotropin is a protein. In the unlikely event of an anaphylactic reaction, epinephrine should be administered. The administration of an antihistamine may also be indicated.

Presentation: CHORULON® is supplied in cartons containing five single dose vials of freeze-dried powder and five 10 mL vials of sterile diluent.

Compendium Code No.: 11060320

CHX+Zn ORAL MIST

Butler **Dental Preparation**

With 0.12% chlorhexidine gluconate and zinc

Active Ingredient(s): Contains: Chlorhexidine gluconate 0.12%, zinc lactate 0.12% and cetylpyridinium chloride 0.05% in a soothing alcohol-free vehicle.

Indications: An oral rinse to be used in pets as an aid in the prevention of plaque, calculus and gum disease.

Directions for Use: Apply CHX+Zn ORAL MIST either as an oral rinse or with a toothbrush. Oral Rinse: Holding the animal's head steady with one hand, spray a small amount of CHX+Zn ORAL MIST between the teeth and gums on one side of the animal's mouth. Massage the mouth over the teeth to work CHX+Zn ORAL MIST over the surface of the teeth. Repeat on the opposite side of the mouth so that the gum surfaces are thoroughly wet on both sides of the mouth. Tooth Brushing: Place a small amount of CHX+Zn ORAL MIST in a clean dish or cup. Holding the animal's head steady with one hand, dip the toothbrush into the solution and carefully brush the teeth with a gentle motion. Re-wet the brush with CHX+Zn ORAL MIST as needed.

Precaution(s): Store at room temperature.

Caution(s): Reversible tooth staining has been reported with prolonged use of chlorhexidine.

Consult your veterinarian at least once a year for a dental heath management program.

Warning(s): For veterinary use only. Keep out of reach of children.

For external use only as oral rinse. Not for use in eye.

Discussion: CHX+Zn ORAL MIST is a soothing, refreshing and highly palatable rinse containing chlorhexidine gluconate, cetylpyridinium chloride and zinc. The antimicrobial activity of chlorhexidine and cetylpyridinium chloride, combined with the anti-plaque and anti-calculus properties of zinc, together can aid in the prevention of tooth and gum disease. This alcohol-free formulation will leave your pet with clean breath while providing soothing, temporary relief of minor gum irritation.

Importance of Oral Hygiene: Plaque results from bacterial proliferation on the tooth surface. Eventually, calculus forms on the tooth and acts as a protective barrier for plaque development. If these are not eliminated, the teeth, sockets and gums can become diseased and lead to such conditions as bad breath, oral pain and loss of teeth. Eventually, dental disease can also lead to severe systemic conditions such as heart, kidney or liver disease.

Presentation: 8 fl oz.

Compendium Code No.: 10820420

C

CIRCOMUNE™

Biomune **Vaccine**

Chicken Anemia Virus Vaccine, Live Virus

U.S. Vet. Lic. No.: 368

Contents: This vaccine contains chicken infectious anemia virus for administration only by wing web inoculation. The virus is stable allowing this vaccine to be presented in a liquid, ready to use preparation.

This vaccine contains gentamicin and amphotericin B as preservatives.

Indications: This vaccine is recommended for use in healthy breeder chickens to provide maternal antibodies to progeny as an aid in the prevention of chicken infectious anemia due to chicken infectious anemia virus. The vaccine is administered only by the wing web route to breeder chickens 9 to 12 weeks of age. Do not vaccinate chickens in lay. Vaccine virus may be shed in the feces and eggs of vaccinated birds. Therefore, avoid spread of vaccine virus to young chickens or unexposed layers. Additionally, avoid vaccinating breeders older than 12 weeks of age to prevent vertical transmission of vaccine virus.

Dosage and Administration: For wing web administration.

Use the enclosed applicator to deliver each dose of 0.01 mL by the wing web stab method.

1. Shake well before opening. Remove the seal and stopper from the vaccine vial. The vaccine is ready to use.
2. Vaccinate by dipping the enclosed two-pronged applicator needle into the vaccine and piercing the webbed portion under the wing. Guard against losing vaccine by touching feathers with applicator. Avoid piercing the wing muscle, bone or large blood vessels.
3. Re-dip the applicator between each vaccination.

Contraindication(s): Carefully follow directions for age of administration. Use of this vaccine in chickens younger than three weeks of age may cause clinical signs of chicken infectious anemia. Use of this vaccine in chickens older than 12 weeks of age may result in vertical transmission to progeny.

Precaution(s): Store between 35 to 45°F (2-7°C).

Use entire contents of vial when first opened. Burn this vial and all unused contents.

Caution(s): Do not dilute the vaccine or administer less than one dose per bird.

All susceptible chickens should be vaccinated at the same time.

Avoid stress conditions during and following vaccination.

Notice: This vaccine has undergone rigid potency, safety and purity tests, and meets the requirements of Biomune Co. The response following vaccination is dependent on many factors, including but not limited to, conditions of vaccine storage and handling by the user, administration of the vaccine, health and responsiveness of the individual chickens, and the degree of field exposure.

This vaccine is not returnable to the manufacturer.

Warning(s): Do not vaccinate within 21 days before slaughter.

Presentation: 10 x 1000 doses.

Patent pending

Compendium Code No.: 11290360 310

CIRCOMUNE™ W

Biomune **Vaccine**

Chicken Anemia Virus Vaccine, Live Virus

U.S. Vet. Lic. No.: 368

Contents: This vaccine contains chicken infectious anemia virus for administration only by drinking water. The virus is stable allowing this vaccine to be presented in a liquid, ready to use preparation.

This vaccine contains gentamicin and amphotericin B as preservatives.

Indications: This vaccine is recommended for use in healthy breeder chickens to provide maternal antibodies to progeny as an aid in the prevention of chicken infectious anemia due to chicken infectious anemia virus. The vaccine is administered only by the drinking water route to breeder chickens 9 to 12 weeks of age. Do not vaccinate chickens in lay. Vaccine virus may be shed in the feces and eggs of vaccinated birds. Therefore, avoid spread of vaccine virus to young chickens or unexposed layers. Additionally, avoid vaccinating breeders older than 12 weeks of age to prevent vertical transmission of vaccine virus.

Dosage and Administration: For drinking water administration.

1. The waterers should be thoroughly cleaned before use. Do not use disinfecting solutions during cleaning as the disinfectant residue may inactivate the virus. Drinking containers must be free of all disinfecting solutions for 48 hours prior to vaccination and for 24 hours after vaccination.
2. Deprive the birds of water two hours prior to vaccination.
3. Shake the vial well before opening. Tear off the aluminum seal from the vial containing the vaccine and remove the stopper.
4. Use clean, cold, nonchlorinated water for diluting the vaccine. Mix a 1,000 dose vial with 2 gallons (7.6 L) of water, and a 2,000 dose vial with 4 gallons (15.2 L) of water.
5. Provide enough waterers so that all birds may have an opportunity to drink the vaccine-treated water.
6. Avoid exposure of the waterers to direct sunlight.
7. Do not resume watering until water containing vaccine has been consumed. Then continue watering with untreated water for 24 hours before resuming the normal watering practice.
8. Vaccinating with less than one dose per bird may fail to protect satisfactorily.

Precaution(s): Store between 35 to 45°F (2-7°C).

Use entire contents of vial when first opened. Burn this vial and all unused contents.

Caution(s): Do not administer less than one dose per bird.

All susceptible chickens should be vaccinated at the same time.

Avoid stress conditions during and following vaccination.

Carefully follow directions for age of administration. Use of this vaccine in chickens younger than three weeks of age may cause clinical signs of chicken infectious anemia.

Notice: This vaccine has undergone rigid potency, safety and purity tests, and meets the requirements of Biomune Co. The response following vaccination is dependent on many factors, including but not limited to, conditions of vaccine storage and handling by the user, administration of the vaccine, health and responsiveness of the individual chickens, and the degree of field exposure.

This vaccine is not returnable to the manufacturer.

Warning(s): Do not vaccinate within 21 days before slaughter.

Presentation: 10 x 1000 doses.

Patent pending

Compendium Code No.: 11290370 215

CITE® BRUCELLA ABORTUS ANTIBODY TEST KIT

Idexx Labs. **Brucella Test**

U.S. Vet. Lic. No.: 313

Description: CITE® *Brucella abortus* Antibody Test Kit is an enzyme immunoassay.

Kit Components:

Item	Reagents	Volume
	B. abortus CITE® Devices	5
A.	5 bottles of Sample Diluent	2 mL
B.	1 bottle of Wash Solution	25 mL
C.	1 vial of Anti-Bovine Alkaline Phosphatase Conjugate	2 mL
D.	1 vial of Substrate Solution	2 mL

Other Components: Transfer pipets.

Indications: For the semi-quantitative measurement of *Brucella abortus (B. abortus)* antibodies in bovine serum or plasma. The test is a supplemental test to be used in the cooperative State/Federal Brucellosis Eradication Program.

Test Principles: CITE® *Brucella abortus* Antibody Test is an enzyme immunoassay designed to detect the presence of antibodies to *B. abortus* in bovine serum or plasma. The test incorporates advanced immunoassay device technology, providing a unique format for a solid phase immunoassay for *B. abortus* antibodies. In the CITE® format, *B. abortus* antigens and bovine immunoglobulin calibrators have been spotted separately onto a fiber membrane in the device. Sample and reagents are applied onto the surface of the membrane and flow through the bioactive spots. Antibodies to *B. abortus*, if present, are captured by the immobilized *B. abortus* antigens on the sample spot. Enzyme conjugated anti-bovine antibodies are then added, and bind to the captured *B. abortus* immunoglobulins forming an antigen-antibody sandwich. After washing away unbound material from the membrane, an enzyme substrate solution is added. Subsequent color development is proportional to the concentration of *B. abortus* antibodies captured.

Color will also develop in the calibration spots. Test interpretation, by comparison of color in the sample and calibration spots, correlates to the Idexx *B. abortus* Particle Concentration Fluorescence Immunoassay (PCFIA) System test results. The low calibration spot is standardized to the PCFIA positive-negative cutoff. The high calibration spot is standardized to the PCFIA reactor cutoff. The mid-range calibration spot has been included to provide an additional comparison for a sample in the suspect category. In addition to their calibration function, these spots indicate that the assay reagents are functional.

Test Procedure:

Specimen Information: Bovine serum or plasma may be used in this test. For serum or plasma, the sample can be either fresh or previously frozen. Hemolyzed samples may be used. Heavily contaminated serum may yield high background color.

Allow reagents and Cite® devices to come to room temperature before starting the test procedure. Then, perform steps below.

1. Dilute Sample: Bovine serum or plasma may be used. Two drops of sample from a transfer pipet (provided in the kit) is required. Remove the cap and dropper tip from one bottle of Solution A (Sample Diluent). Insert one of the transfer pipet into the sample, squeeze bulb end and release to pull sample into the pipet. Wipe excess sample from the outside of the pipet. Add 2 drops of the sample to Solution A by squeezing the bulb end of the pipet. Replace the top and cap of the bottle and mix well.
2. Wet Cite® device: Wet the entire membrane of the Cite® device with Solution B (Wash Solution) by adding 10 to 15 drops onto the membrane. Allow the solution to be completely absorbed before adding sample.
3. Add Diluted Sample: Mix the diluted sample thoroughly by inverting the bottle several times. Add 5 drops of diluted sample directly onto the center of the Cite® device. Wait 3 minutes.
4. Add Conjugate: Add 5 drops of Solution C (Anti-Bovine Alkaline Phosphatase Conjugate) to the Cite® device. Make sure that all four spots are covered with the blue conjugate. Wait 3 minutes.
5. Wash Cite® Device: First, add 10-15 drops of Solution B (Wash Solution) to Cite® device. Most of the blue color should be washed away. Then, fill device (approximately 2 mL) with Solution B up to the line on the inside of the device. Allow Wash Solution to be completely absorbed. All blue color should be washed away.
6. Add Substrate: Add 5 drops of Solution D (Substrate Solution) being careful to cover all four spots. Wait 3 minutes for color development.
7. Stop Reaction: To stop reaction and preserve the result, add 10-15 drops of Solution B (Wash Solution) to Cite® device. Determine the level of *B. abortus* antibodies in the sample by comparing sample spot to the calibration spots. (Note: The addition of Solution B may reduce color intensity of reaction.)

Test Interpretation: The test result is read by first moving the device so that the orientation dot is in the 12 o'clock position (see diagram). In this position, the sample spot is directly below the orientation dot. The low calibration spot is below and to the left of the sample spot; the mid-range calibration spot is directly below the sample spot; and the high calibration spot is below and to the right of the sample spot.

The level of antibody to *B. abortus* is determined by comparing the color intensity of the sample spot to the color intensity of the calibration spots. The presence or absence of antibody to *B. abortus* is determined by comparing the color of the sample spot to that of the low calibration spot. Animals are considered negative if the sample spot has either no color or color less than the low calibration spot.

In addition, a semi-quantitative determination of the level of antibody in a positive sample is made by comparing the color in the sample spot to the level of color in the low, mid and high calibration spots. Animals are considered suspect if the sample spot color is greater than or equal to the low calibration spot but less than the high calibration spot. The animal is considered a reactor if color in the sample spot is greater than or equal to the color in the high calibration spot.

Determination of *B. abortus* antibody level in sample is based upon color development on the Cite® assay device.

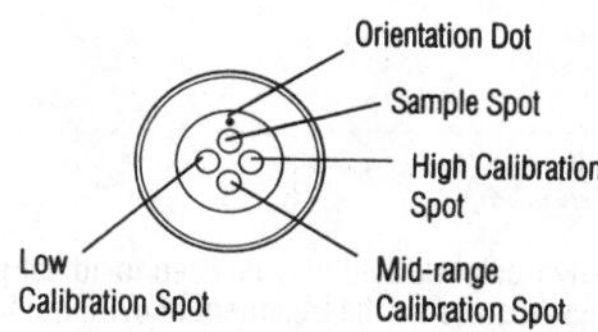

Negative: Sample spot remains white or is lighter than the low calibration spot.

Suspect: Sample spot equal to or darker than the low calibration spot but lighter than the high calibration spot.

Positive: Sample spot equal to or greater than the high calibration spot.

Storage: Store all kit components at 2°-7°C (36°-45°F). Once a device package has been opened, carefully reseal package for storage at 2°-7°C (36°-45°F).

Caution(s): Handle all *B. abortus* biological materials as though capable of transmitting Brucellosis.

No eating, drinking or smoking where specimens or kit reagents are being handled.

Do not use components past expiration date and do not intermix components from kits with different serial numbers.

Use a separate transfer pipet for each sample.

All kit reagents must be at room temperature 15°-30°C (59°-86°F) prior to use.

Dispense reagents into the center of the assay device, taking care to cover the four bioactive spots.

For veterinary use only.

Discussion: Brucellosis in cattle is a disease caused by *B. abortus*, a facultative, intracellular bacterium. The major mode of disease transmission is by ingestion of *B. abortus* organisms that may be present in tissues of aborted fetuses, fetal membranes and uterine fluids. In addition, infection may occur as the result of cattle ingesting *B. abortus* contaminated feed or water. Infection in cows also has occurred through venereal transmission of the organisms by infected bulls.

Abortion is the most outstanding clinical feature of the disease. If a carrier state develops in a majority of infected cows in a herd, the clinical manifestations may be reduced milk production, dead calves at term, and/or a higher frequency of retained placenta. Disease in the bull may produce infections of the seminal vesicles and testicles resulting in the shedding of the organisms in semen.

Diagnosis is based on serological and/or bacteriological procedures. While a positive bacteriological finding is the most definitive diagnosis, several weeks may be required to obtain final culture results. The success of disease eradication is dependent upon the accurate identification and elimination of *B. abortus* reactors in a herd. An assessment of exposure to *B. abortus* via natural infection or vaccine is facilitated by the measurement of specific antibody in the serum.

References: Available upon request.

Presentation: 5 tests.

Compendium Code No.: 11160001

CITRIC ACID

AgriLabs **Water Additive**

Soluble Powder

Active Ingredient(s): U.S.P. anhydrous citric acid in a fine granular, free flowing, soluble powder form.

Indications: Used as a chelating agent, CITRIC ACID may increase the solubility of tetracyclines when used in poultry drinking water. CITRIC ACID may also be used as a waterline cleaner and antimicrobial.

Directions for Use:

Chelating agent or to increase antibiotic solubility: Mix 205 g of CITRIC ACID or half packet of CITRIC ACID 410 with 25.6 g of oxytetracycline, chlortetracycline, or tetracycline soluble antibiotic in a stock solution. Delivery then administered to all label instructions.

Waterline cleaning: Mix 820 g to 1640 g of CITRIC ACID or two to four packets of CITRIC ACID 410 in one gallon of stock solution. Use alone at these levels to clean and reduce microbial growth in waterlines.

Caution(s): Consult MSDS prior to usage.

Warning(s): Not for human use. For animal use only.

Keep out of reach of children.

Presentation: 40 x 410 g packets.

Compendium Code No.: 10580331

CITRIC ACID

Alpharma **Water Acidifier**

Active Ingredient(s): The product contains citric acid.

Indications: For use as an aid in solving solubility problems for a variety of water administered products in poultry, swine and other livestock.

Dosage and Administration: Waterline cleaning instructions: 7.23 oz pack: Use 4 to 8 packs per gallon of stock solution.

14.46 oz or 1 lb packs: Use 2 to 4 packs per gallon of stock solution.

Precaution(s): Store in cool, dry place.

Caution(s): For oral animal use only.

Not for human use.

Keep out of reach of children.

Presentation: 7.23 oz (205 g), 14.46 oz (410 g), 1 lb. (453.6 g) packages.

Compendium Code No.: 10220270 AHF-043 0005, AHF-044 0005, AHF-048 0005

CITRIC ACID SOLUBLE POWDER

AgriPharm **Water Acidifier**

Active Ingredient(s):

U.S.P. citric acid, anhydrous 100%

Indications: Citric Acid increases solubility when used in hard water and is also used as a water line cleaner.

Dosage and Administration: Prepare fresh stock solution daily by mixing:

Solubility Improvement .... 7-14 ounces per gallon
Cleaning Waterlines .... 42-56 ounces per gallon

Use in a proportioner that delivers one ounce of stock solution per gallon.

Precaution(s): Store unopened product in a cool, dry place.

Unused solutions should be refrigerated.

Warning(s): For animal use only.

Keep out of reach of children.

Presentation: 205 g and 410 g.

Compendium Code No.: 14570200

CLAVAMOX® DROPS ℞

Pfizer Animal Health **Amoxicillin Potentiated**

(amoxicillin trihydrate/clavulanate potassium)

NADA No.: 055-101

Active Ingredient(s): Each mL of suspension will contain 50 mg of amoxicillin activity as the trihydrate and 12.5 mg of clavulanic acid activity as the potassium salt.

Indications: CLAVAMOX® Drops are indicated in the treatment of:

Dogs: Skin and soft tissue infections such as wounds, abscesses, cellulitis, superficial/juvenile and deep pyoderma due to susceptible strains of the following organisms: β-lactamase-producing *Staphylococcus aureus,* non-β-lactamase-producing *Staphylococcus aureus, Staphylococcus* spp., *Streptococcus* spp., and *E. coli.*

Periodontal infections due to susceptible strains of both aerobic and anaerobic bacteria. CLAVAMOX® has been shown to be clinically effective for treating cases of canine periodontal disease.

C

Cats: Skin and soft tissue infections such as wounds, abscesses, and cellulitis/dermatitis due to susceptible strains of the following organisms: β-lactamase-producing *Staphylococcus aureus,* non-β-lactamase-producing *Staphylococcus aureus, Staphylococcus* spp., *Streptococcus* spp., *E. coli, Pasteurella multocida,* and *Pasteurella* spp.

Urinary tract infections (cystitis) due to susceptible strains of *E. coli.*

Therapy may be initiated with CLAVAMOX® prior to obtaining results from bacteriological and susceptibility studies. A culture should be obtained prior to treatment to determine susceptibility of the organisms to CLAVAMOX®. Following determination of susceptibility results and clinical response to medication, therapy may be reevaluated.

Pharmacology: Description: CLAVAMOX® (amoxicillin trihydrate/clavulanate potassium) is an orally administered formulation comprised of the broad-spectrum antibiotic Amoxi® (amoxicillin trihydrate) and the β-lactamase inhibitor, clavulanate potassium (the potassium salt of clavulanic acid).

Amoxicillin trihydrate is a semisynthetic antibiotic with a broad spectrum of bactericidal activity against many gram-positive and gram-negative, aerobic and anaerobic microorganisms. It does not resist destruction by β-lactamases; therefore, it is not effective against β-lactamase-producing bacteria. Chemically, it is D(-)-α-amino-p-hydroxybenzyl-penicillin trihydrate.

Clavulanic acid, an inhibitor of β-lactamase enzymes, is produced by the fermentation of *Streptomyces clavuligerus.* Clavulanic acid by itself has only weak antibacterial activity. Chemically, clavulanate potassium is potassium z-(3R,5R)-2-β-hydroxyethylidene clavam-3-carboxylate.

Actions: CLAVAMOX® is stable in the presence of gastric acid and is not significantly influenced by gastric or intestinal contents. The 2 components are rapidly absorbed resulting in amoxicillin and clavulanic acid concentrations in serum, urine, and tissues similar to those produced when each is administered alone.

Amoxicillin and clavulanic acid diffuse readily into most body tissues and fluids with the exception of brain and spinal fluid, which amoxicillin penetrates adequately when meninges are inflamed. Most of the amoxicillin is excreted unchanged in the urine. Clavulanic acid's penetration into spinal fluid is unknown at this time. Approximately 15% of the administered dose of clavulanic acid is excreted in the urine within the first 6 hours.

CLAVAMOX® combines the distinctive properties of a broad-spectrum antibiotic and a β-lactamase inhibitor to effectively extend the antibacterial spectrum of amoxicillin to include β-lactamase as well as non-β-lactamase-producing aerobic and anaerobic organisms.

Microbiology: Amoxicillin is bactericidal in action and acts through the inhibition of biosynthesis of cell wall mucopeptide of susceptible organisms. The action of clavulanic acid extends the antimicrobial spectrum of amoxicillin to include organisms resistant to amoxicillin and other β-lactam antibiotics. Amoxicillin/clavulanate has been shown to have a wide range of activity which includes β-lactamase-producing strains of both gram-positive and gram-negative aerobes, facultative anaerobes, and obligate anaerobes. Many strains of the following organisms, including β-lactamase-producing strains, isolated from veterinary sources, were found to be susceptible to amoxicillin/clavulanate *in vitro* but the clinical significance of this activity has not been demonstrated for some of these organisms in animals.

Aerobic bacteria, including *Staphylococcus aureus**, β-lactamase-producing *Staphylococcus aureus** (penicillin resistant), *Staphylococcus* species*, *Staphylococcus epidermidis, Staphylococcus intermedius, Streptococcus faecalis, Streptococcus* species*, *Corynebacterium pyogenes, Corynebacterium* species, *Erysipelothrix rhusiopathiae, Bordetella bronchiseptica, Escherichia coli**, *Proteus mirabilis, Proteus* species, *Enterobacter* species, *Klebsiella pneumoniae, Salmonella dublin, Salmonella typhimurium, Pasteurella multocida**, *Pasteurella hemolytica, Pasteurella* species*.

* The susceptibility of these organisms has also been demonstrated in *in vivo* studies.

Studies have demonstrated that both aerobic and anaerobic flora are isolated from gingival cultures of dogs with clinical evidence of periodontal disease. Both gram-positive and gram-negative aerobic and anaerobic subgingival isolates indicate sensitivity to amoxicillin/clavulanic acid during antimicrobial susceptibility testing.

Susceptibility Test: The recommended quantitative disc susceptibility method (Federal Register 37:20527-29; Bauer AW, Kirby WMM, Sherris JC, *et al:* Antibiotic susceptibility testing by standardized single disc method. Am J Clin Path 45:493, 1966) utilized 30 μg Augmentin® (AMC) discs for estimating the susceptibility of bacteria to CLAVAMOX® Tablets and Drops.

Dosage and Administration:

Dogs: The recommended dosage is 6.25 mg/lb (1 mL/10 lb) of body weight twice a day. Skin and soft tissue infections such as abscesses, cellulitis, wounds, superficial/juvenile pyoderma, and periodontal infections should be treated for 5-7 days or for 48 hours after all symptoms have subsided. If no response is seen after 5 days of treatment, therapy should be discontinued and the case reevaluated. Deep pyoderma may require treatment for 21 days; the maximum duration of treatment should not exceed 30 days.

Cats: The recommended dosage is 62.5 mg (1 mL) twice a day. Skin and soft tissue infections such as abscesses and cellulitis/dermatitis should be treated for 5-7 days or 48 hours after all symptoms have subsided, not to exceed 30 days. If no response is seen after 3 days of treatment, therapy should be discontinued and the case reevaluated.

Urinary tract infections may require treatment for 10-14 days or longer. The maximum duration of treatment should not exceed 30 days.

Reconstitution Instructions—Oral Suspension: Add 14 mL of water to the 15 mL bottle and shake vigorously.

Note: Any unused portion of the reconstituted suspension must be discarded after 10 days. Refrigeration of the reconstituted suspension is required.

Contraindication(s): The use of this drug is contraindicated in animals with a history of an allergic reaction to any of the penicillins or cephalosporins.

Caution(s): Federal law restricts this drug to use by or on the order of a licensed veterinarian.

Safety of use in pregnant or breeding animals has not been determined.

For veterinary oral suspension.

For use in dogs and cats only.

Adverse Reactions: CLAVAMOX® contains a semisynthetic penicillin (amoxicillin) and has the potential for producing allergic reactions. If an allergic reaction occurs, administer epinephrine and/or steroids.

Presentation: CLAVAMOX® Drops are supplied in 15 mL bottle.

CLAVAMOX and Augmentin are trademarks owned by and used under license from SmithKline Beecham.

Manufactured by: SmithKline Beecham Pharmaceuticals.

Compendium Code No.: 36900890 75-8016-06

CLAVAMOX® TABLETS ℞

Pfizer Animal Health **Amoxicillin Potentiated**

(amoxicillin trihydrate/clavulanate potassium)

NADA No.: 055-099

Active Ingredient(s): CLAVAMOX® Tablets are available in the following strengths:

Each 62.5 mg tablet contains amoxicillin trihydrate equivalent to 50 mg of amoxicillin activity and 12.5 mg of clavulanic acid as the potassium salt.

For use in dogs and cats.

Each 125 mg tablet contains amoxicillin trihydrate equivalent to 100 mg of amoxicillin activity and 25 mg of clavulanic acid as the potassium salt.

For use in dogs only.

Each 250 mg tablet contains amoxicillin trihydrate equivalent to 200 mg of amoxicillin activity and 50 mg of clavulanic acid as the potassium salt.

For use in dogs only.

Each 375 mg tablet contains amoxicillin trihydrate equivalent to 300 mg of amoxicillin activity and 75 mg of clavulanic acid as the potassium salt.

For use in dogs only.

Indications: CLAVAMOX® Tablets are indicated in the treatment of:

Dogs: Skin and soft tissue infections such as wounds, abscesses, cellulitis, superficial/juvenile and deep pyoderma due to susceptible strains of the following organisms: β-lactamase-producing *Staphylococcus aureus*, non-β-lactamase-producing *Staphylococcus aureus, Staphylococcus* spp., *Streptococcus* spp., and *E. coli.*

Periodontal infections due to susceptible strains of both aerobic and anaerobic bacteria. CLAVAMOX® has been shown to be clinically effective for treating cases of canine periodontal disease.

Cats: Skin and soft tissue infections such as wounds, abscesses, and cellulitis/dermatitis due to susceptible strains of the following organisms: β-lactamase-producing *Staphylococcus aureus,* non-β-lactamase-producing *Staphylococcus aureus, Staphylococcus* spp., *Streptococcus* spp., *E. coli,* and *Pasteurella* spp.

Urinary tract infections (cystitis) due to susceptible strains of *E. coli.*

Therapy may be initiated with CLAVAMOX® prior to obtaining results from bacteriological and susceptibility studies. A culture should be obtained prior to treatment to determine susceptibility of the organisms to CLAVAMOX®. Following determination of susceptibility results and clinical response to medication, therapy may be reevaluated.

Pharmacology: Description: CLAVAMOX® (amoxicillin trihydrate/clavulanate potassium) is an orally administered formulation comprised of the broad-spectrum antibiotic Amoxi® (amoxicillin trihydrate) and the β-lactamase inhibitor, clavulanate potassium (the potassium salt of clavulanic acid).

Amoxicillin trihydrate is a semisynthetic antibiotic with a broad spectrum of bactericidal activity against many gram-positive and gram-negative, aerobic and anaerobic microorganisms. It does not resist destruction by β-lactamases; therefore, it is not effective against β-lactamase-producing bacteria. Chemically, it is D(-)-α-amino-p-hydroxybenzyl-penicillin trihydrate.

Clavulanic acid, an inhibitor of β-lactamase enzymes, is produced by the fermentation of *Streptomyces clavuligerus.* Clavulanic acid by itself has only weak antibacterial activity. Chemically, clavulanate potassium is potassium z-(3R,5R)-2-β-hydroxyethylidene clavam-3-carboxylate.

Action: CLAVAMOX® is stable in the presence of gastric acid and is not significantly influenced by gastric or intestinal contents. The 2 components are rapidly absorbed resulting in amoxicillin and clavulanic acid concentrations in serum, urine, and tissues similar to those produced when each is administered alone.

Amoxicillin and clavulanic acid diffuse readily into most body tissues and fluids with the exception of brain and spinal fluid, which amoxicillin penetrates adequately when meninges are inflamed. Most of the amoxicillin is excreted unchanged in the urine. Clavulanic acid's penetration into spinal fluid is unknown at this time. Approximately 15% of the administered dose of clavulanic acid is excreted in the urine within the first 6 hours.

CLAVAMOX® combines the distinctive properties of a broad-spectrum antibiotic and a β-lactamase inhibitor to effectively extend the antibacterial spectrum of amoxicillin to include β-lactamase-producing as well as non-β-lactamase-producing aerobic and anaerobic organisms.

Microbiology: Amoxicillin is bactericidal in action and acts through the inhibition of biosynthesis of cell wall mucopeptide of susceptible organisms. The action of clavulanic acid extends the antimicrobial spectrum of amoxicillin to include organisms resistant to amoxicillin and other β-lactam antibiotics. Amoxicillin/clavulanate has been shown to have a wide range of activity which includes β-lactamase-producing strains of both gram-positive and gram-negative aerobes, facultative anaerobes, and obligate anaerobes. Many strains of the following organisms, including β-lactamase-producing strains, isolated from veterinary sources, were found to be susceptible to amoxicillin/clavulanate *in vitro* but the clinical significance of this activity has not been demonstrated for some of these organisms in animals.

Aerobic bacteria, including *Staphylococcus aureus**, β-lactamase-producing *Staphylococcus aureus** (penicillin resistant), *Staphylococcus* species*, *Staphylococcus epidermidis, Staphylococcus intermedius, Streptococcus faecalis, Streptococcus* species*, *Corynebacterium pyogenes, Corynebacterium* species, *Erysipelothrix rhusiopathiae, Bordetella bronchiseptica, Escherichia coli**, *Proteus mirabilis, Proteus* species, *Enterobacter* species, *Klebsiella pneumoniae, Salmonella dublin, Salmonella typhimurium, Pasteurella multocida**, *Pasteurella hemolytica, Pasteurella* species*.

* The susceptibility of these organisms has also been demonstrated in *in vivo* studies.

Studies have demonstrated that both aerobic and anaerobic flora are isolated from gingival cultures of dogs with clinical evidence of periodontal disease. Both gram-positive and gram-negative aerobic and anaerobic subgingival isolates indicate sensitivity to amoxicillin/clavulanic acid during antimicrobial susceptibility testing.

Susceptibility Test: The recommended quantitative disc susceptibility method (Federal Register 37:20527-29; Bauer AW, Kirby WMM, Sherris JC, *et al:* Antibiotic susceptibility testing by standardized single disc method. Am J Clin Path 45:493, 1966) utilized 30 μg Augmentin® (AMC) discs for estimating the susceptibility of bacteria to CLAVAMOX® Tablets.

Dosage and Administration:

Dogs: The recommended dosage is 6.25 mg/lb of body weight twice a day.

Skin and soft tissue infections such as abscesses, cellulitis, wounds, superficial/juvenile pyoderma, and periodontal infections should be treated for 5-7 days or for 48 hours after all symptoms have subsided. If no response is seen after 5 days of treatment, therapy should be discontinued and the case reevaluated. Deep pyoderma may require treatment for 21 days; the maximum duration of treatment should not exceed 30 days.

Cats: The recommended dosage is 62.5 mg twice a day.

Skin and soft tissue infections such as abscesses and cellulitis/dermatitis should be treated for 5-7 days or for 48 hours after all symptoms have subsided, not to exceed 30 days. If no response is seen after 3 days of treatment, therapy should be discontinued and the case reevaluated.

Urinary tract infections may require treatment for 10-14 days or longer. The maximum duration of treatment should not exceed 30 days.

Contraindication(s): The use of this drug is contraindicated in animals with a history of allergic reaction to any of the penicillins or cephalosporins.

Precaution(s): Store in a dry, cool place at temperatures not above 25°C (77°F). Do not remove from foil strip until ready to use.

Caution(s): Federal law restricts this drug to use by or on the order of a licensed veterinarian.

For use in dogs and cats.

Safety of use in pregnant or breeding animals has not been determined.

Adverse Reactions: CLAVAMOX® contains a semisynthetic penicillin (amoxicillin) and has the potential for producing allergic reactions. If an allergic reaction occurs, administer epinephrine and/or steroids.

Presentation: CLAVAMOX® Tablets are supplied in strip packs of four strengths. Each carton holds 15 strips with 14 tablets per strip (210 tablets per carton).

CLAVAMOX and Augmentin are trademarks owned by and used under license from SmithKline Beecham.

Manufactured by: SmithKline Beecham Pharmaceuticals.

Compendium Code No.: 36900900 75-8012-04

CLEAN AND FRESH™

Butler **Dental Preparation**

Active Ingredient(s): Contains: Chlorhexidine 0.1%, surfactants, ethyl alcohol 6%, FD&C red 40, D&C red 33, peppermint flavored base.

Indications: To assist in the daily maintenance of a healthy and pleasant smelling mouth in dogs and cats through the removal of food particles and other debris from the teeth and gum line.

Dosage and Administration: Apply CLEAN AND FRESH™ either as an oral rinse or with a toothbrush.

Oral rinse: Holding the animal's head steady with one hand, spray a small amount of CLEAN AND FRESH™ between the teeth and gums on one side of the animal's mouth. Massage the mouth over the teeth to work CLEAN AND FRESH™ over the surface of the teeth. Repeat on the opposite side of the mouth so that the gum surfaces are thoroughly wet on both sides of the mouth.

Tooth brushing: Place a small amount of CLEAN AND FRESH™ in a clean dish or cup. Holding the animal's head steady with one hand, dip the toothbrush into the solution and carefully brush the teeth with a gentle motion. Rewet the brush with CLEAN AND FRESH™ as needed.

Caution(s): The use of CLEAN AND FRESH™ should not be considered a substitute for sound veterinary dental treatment. The' product should be used under the direction of a veterinarian who can advise on a complete oral health program.

Published literature has reported some staining of teeth surfaces after the prolonged use of rinses containing chlorhexidine. The build-up of stain can be prevented by applying the solution with a tooth brush.

For veterinary use only. For external use only as an oral rinse. Not for use in eyes.

Warning(s): Keep out of the reach of children.

Presentation: 4 fl. oz. and 8 fl. oz. misters.

Compendium Code No.: 10820431

CLEAN CROP® MALATHION 57EC

Loveland **Premise and Topical Insecticide**

EPA Reg. No.: 2393-280-36208

Active Ingredient(s):

Malathion* 57.0%

Inert Ingredients: 43.0%

Total 100.0%

*O,O-Dimethyl phosphorodithioate of diethyl mercaptosuccinate. This product contains xylene-range aromatic solvents. One gallon contains 5 pounds of Malathion.

Indications:

Cattle (Beef and non-milking) and Horses: To control hornfly, lice, and ticks, and for use with back rubbing devices.

Sheep and Goats: To control keds, lice, and ticks.

Hogs: To control lice and sarcoptic mange.

Poultry (Chicken, Ducks, Geese and Turkeys): To control chiggers, flies, lice, Northern fowl mite, chicken red mite, and ticks.

Domestic Pets: To control fleas, lice, and ticks.

In and Around Homes, Dairies, Food Processing Plants: To control bedbugs.

Directions for Use: It is a violation of Federal Law to use this product in a manner inconsistent with its labeling.

Keep children and pets out of the treated area until sprays have dried.

Livestock:

Insect Controlled	Dosage	Directions for use
Cattle (Beef and non-milking) and Horses		
Hornfly	1-1.5 gal per 100 gal or 6.5-10 oz per 5 gallons	Apply complete coverage spray. Repeat at 2 week intervals, if needed.
Lice	1 gal per 100 gal or 6.5 per 5 gal	Apply complete coverage spray. One treatment may be sufficient. Repeat only if needed.
Ticks	1-2 gal per 100 gal or 6.5-13 oz per 5 gal	Apply complete coverage spray. Repeat at two (2) week intervals if needed.
Back rubbing devices	2% mixture in fuel oil (for example: 1 pt per 4 gal fuel oil)	To reduce lice. May also reduce horn flies. Should be made continuously accessible. One to each 35 to 45 head of cattle and retreated every 2-3 wks.

Insect Controlled	Dosage	Directions for use
Sheep and Goats*		
Keds, Lice, Ticks	1 gal per 100 gal or 6.5-5 oz per 5 gal	Spray animals thoroughly.
*Do not apply to milk goats Repeat application after 2 or 3 weeks if needed. Do not treat animals under one month of age. Residue tolerance: 4 ppm in meat, fat and meat by-products.		
Hogs*		
Lice	1 gal per 100 gal or 6.5-5 oz per 5 gal	Apply complete coverage spray to animals, pens and litter. One treatment may be sufficient. Repeat only if needed.
Sarcoptic mange	1 gal per 100 gal or 6.5-5 oz per 5 gal	Apply complete coverage spray to all animals in herd, bedding and walls. Use extreme care to thoroughly cover all body surfaces of the animal, including inside of ears. One thorough spraying will usually control sarcoptic mange of swine, however, extensive cases will require second treatment about 10 days after first application.
*After spraying, swine should be kept out of sun and wind for a few hours. Residue tolerance: 4 ppm in meat, fat and meat by-products		
Poultry (Chicken, Ducks, Geese and Turkeys)		
Chiggers	1-1.5 pts per acre	Range Treatment: Treat range thoroughly day before placing poultry on range. Repeat every 2-3 weeks.
Flies	4 tbsp. per gal	Premise Treatment: Apply liberally to litter, walls, ceilings, roost nests and adjacent areas. Force spray into cracks and crevices.
Lice, Northern fowl mite	2 tbsp. per gal per 100-150 birds	Direct Application: Repeat application in 4-8 weeks or when necessary.
	8.5 oz per 15 gal per 400 birds	Tail Dipping: Hold bird by wings and dip 3-4 inches of tail into solution. Treat vent and surrounding areas. Repeat in 7-10 days if necessary.
	2-7 oz per gal of water or oil	Roost Paint: Brush on at rate of 1 pint per 150 feet of roost.
	4 tbsp. per gal	Premise Treatment: Apply liberally to litter, walls, ceiling, roost nests and adjacent areas. Force spray into cracks and crevices.
Chicken red mite	2 tbsp. per gal per 100-150 birds	Direct Application: Repeat application in 4-8 weeks or when necessary. Use as a supplement to premise treatment for chicken red mite.
	2-7 oz per gal	Roost Paint: Brush on at rate of 1 pint per 150 feet of roost.
	4 tbsp per gal	Premise Treatment: Apply liberally to walls, ceiling, and adjacent areas. Force spray into cracks and crevices.
Ticks	6-7 oz per gal	Premise Treatment: Apply liberally to walls, ceiling, roost nests and adjacent areas. Force spray into cracks and crevices.
Residue tolerance: 4 ppm in or on meat, fat or meat by-products. 0.1 ppm in eggs (from application to poultry).		

Household Uses:

Insect Controlled	Dosage	Directions for use
Domestic Pets		
Fleas, Lice, Ticks	1 oz per gal	Wet animal thoroughly. Repeat in 2-3 weeks if necessary.
Fleas, Ticks	5 oz per gal	Premise Treatment: Apply per 1,000 sq ft of surface to pet quarters, yards and lawns. Remove manure or debris before treating. Repeat treatment in 3-4 weeks if necessary.
In and Around Homes, Dairies, Food Processing Plants		
Bedbugs	2-4 tbsp. per gal deodorized kerosene	Apply lightly to all mattress surfaces in sufficient quantity to "mist" the fabric and generously to beds and woodwork

Precautionary Statements:

Hazards to Humans: Harmful if swallowed, inhaled or absorbed through skin. Avoid breathing spray mist. Do not get in eyes, on skin or on clothing. Use only with adequate ventilation. After using this product indoors, ventilate thoroughly before occupying enclosed spaces. Do not allow contact with treated surface until sprays have dried.

Personal Protective Equipment: Some materials that are chemical-resistant to this product are listed below. If you want more options, follow the instructions for category F on the EPA chemical resistance category selection chart.

Applicators and other handlers must wear: Long-sleeved shirt and long pants, chemical-resistant gloves, such as barrier laminate, butyl rubber, nitrile rubber or viton, and shoes plus socks. For exposures in enclosed areas, a respirator with either an organic vapor-removing cartridge with a prefilter approved for pesticides (MSHA/NIOSH approval number prefix TC-23C) or a canister approved for pesticides (MSHA/NIOSH approval number prefix TC-14G). For exposures outdoors, a dust/mist filtering respirator (MSHA/NIOSH approval number prefix TC-21C).

Follow manufacturer's instructions for cleaning and maintaining PPE. If no such instructions for washables, use detergent and hot water. Keep and wash PPE separately from other laundry.

Engineering controls statements: When handlers use closed systems, enclosed cabs, or aircraft in a manner that meets with requirements listed in the Worker Protection Standard (WPS) for agricultural pesticides [40 CFR 170 240 (d) (4-6)], the handler PPE requirements may be reduced or modified as specified in the WPS.

Statement of Practical Treatment:

If swallowed: Call a physician or Poison Control Center immediately. Gastric lavage may be indicated if material was taken internally. Do not induce vomiting unless other treatment is not available. Vomiting may cause aspiration pneumonia. If it is necessary to induce vomiting, give victim 1 or 2 glasses of water and insert finger in back of throat. Repeat until vomit fluid is clear. Do not induce vomiting or give anything by mouth to an unconscious person.

If on skin: Wash affected areas with soap and water.

If in eyes: Immediately flush eyes with plenty of water and get medical attention.

If inhaled: Remove victim to fresh air. Assist respiration as needed.

Note to Physician: Empty stomach if material was taken internally. Gastric lavage may be indicated. Xylene-range aromatic solvent is an aspiration hazard. This product may cause cholinesterase inhibition. Atropine is antidotal. 2-PAM may be effective as an adjunct to atropine.

Environmental Hazards: This pesticide is toxic to fish, aquatic invertebrates, and aquatic life stages of amphibians. For terrestrial uses, do not apply directly to water, or to areas where surface water is present or to intertidal areas below the mean high water mark. Do not contaminate water when disposing of equipment washwaters. This pesticide is highly toxic to bees exposed to direct treatment on blooming crops or weeds. Do not apply this product or allow it to drift to blooming crops or weeds if bees are visiting this treatment area.

Physical Hazards: Do not use or store near heat or open flame.

Storage and Disposal: Do not contaminate water, food or feed by storage or disposal.

Storage: Do not use or store near heat or open flame. Keep product in original container, tightly closed and store in a cool, dry place. High temperatures may shorten shelf life of product.

Pesticide Disposal: Pesticide wastes are toxic. Improper disposal of excess pesticide, spray mixture, or rinsate is a violation of Federal law. If these wastes cannot be disposed of by use according to label instructions, contact your State Pesticide or Environmental Control Agency, or the Hazardous Waste representative at the nearest EPA Regional Office for guidance.

Container Disposal: Triple rinse (or equivalent). Then offer for recycling or reconditioning, or puncture and dispose of in a sanitary landfill, or by incineration, or, if allowed by state and local authorities, by burning. If burned, stay out of smoke.

Warning(s): Keep out of reach of children.

Disclaimer: Except as expressly provided herein, neither Loveland nor seller makes any warranties, guarantees, or representations of any kind, either by usage of trade, statutory or otherwise, with regard to the product sold, including, but not limited to merchantability, fitness for a particular purpose, use or eligibility of the product for any particular trade usage.

Unintended consequences may result because of, but not limited to, such factors as presence of other materials, or the manner of use or application, all of which are beyond the control of Loveland Industries, Inc. or seller. In no case shall seller be liable for consequential, special, or indirect damages resulting from the use or handling of this product. All such risks shall be assumed by the buyer or user.

Applicator's or grower's exclusive remedy against Loveland Industries, Inc. or seller for any cause of action relating to the product is a claim for damages, and in no event shall damages or any other recovery exceed the purchase price of the product in respect of which such claim is made.

Presentation: 1 gallon.

Compendium Code No.: 10860321

CLEARCAL 50

Vedco **Calcium-Oral**

Guaranteed Analysis: Each tube contains 300 mL of gel supplying 35% W/W or 47% W/V calcium chloride. Equivalent to 170 mg calcium per mL (127 mg per gram).

Minimum calcium content: 12.00% W/W or 16.08 W/V

Maximum calcium content: 13.27% W/W or 17.78 W/V

Indications: CLEARCAL 50 is an easy to use, high potency oral source of bioactive calcium for nutritionally stabilizing blood calcium levels in cows before and after calving. Aids in maintaining proper blood levels of calcium in the parturient and post-partum cow.

Dosage and Administration: Dosage for Dairy Cows: Give one tube of CLEARCAL 50 Oral Gel 6 to 24 hours prior to calving. Then give one more tube within 24 hours after calving.

Directions for Use: Hold the head of the cow in a normal to slightly elevated position. Remove the cap from the tube of CLEARCAL 50 Oral Gel and place directly over the tongue inside the cow's mouth. Push the entire contents of the tube quickly and carefully into the cow's mouth. Allow the animal to swallow normally. For best results administer the entire contents of the tube and allow access to fresh clean drinking water.

Warning(s): For veterinary use only.

Keep out of reach of children.

Presentation: 300 mL (400 g) tube.

Compendium Code No.: 10940300

CLEAR EYES

Farnam **Ophthalmic Solution**

Active Ingredient(s): Sodium chloride and sodium citrate in a phosphate buffer with benzalkonium chloride 0.01% as a preservative.

Indications: CLEAR EYES is a sterile ophthalmic irrigating solution specially formulated for use on horses and ponies. The ideal preparation for daily use to keep eyes bright. Gently flushes foreign matter from the eyes. Relieves eye irritation due to dust, wind, sun and smog.

Dosage and Administration: Remove top of cap and direct tip of spout toward center of eye. Hold eyelid open with a thumb and forefinger. Squeeze bottle releasing sufficient liquid to flush eye thoroughly. Wipe off any excess with a clean, dry cloth. Repeat treatment daily for best results.

Precaution(s): Do not touch the inside of the cap or the tip of the bottle to any surface, since this may contaminate the solution.

Caution(s): If eye irritation persists or increases, discontinue use of the product and consult a veterinarian.

Warning(s): For animal use only. Not for use on humans. Keep this and other medications out of the reach of children.

Presentation: 3.5 fl. oz. (103 mL) bottle.

Compendium Code No.: 10000090

CLEARx® EAR CLEANSING SOLUTION ℞

DVM **Otic Cleanser**

Active Ingredient(s): Dioctyl sodium sulfosuccinate 6.5%, urea peroxide 6%.

Indications: For use as an initial cleanser in any waxy, dirty or exudative ear that will require an otoscopic exam and treatment. CLEARx® is also an intermittent maintenance cleanser in dogs and cats prone to excessive ear wax formation.

Directions for Use: Shake well before use. Squeeze 1-2 mL into ear canal. Allow to remain for 1-2 minutes. Gently massage outside of ear to help break up accumulated wax and crust. Using a bulb syringe, flush ear canal liberally with water. Repeat once per week or as directed by a veterinarian. Evacuate water and apply an ear drying solution. Change dose proportionately for smaller or larger animals.

Contraindication(s): Do not use in acute inflammatory otitis.

Precaution(s): Store the room temperature.

Caution(s): Federal law restricts this drug to use by, or on the order of, a licensed veterinarian.

Do not use this product if the eardrum is ruptured. If irritation occurs, consult your veterinarian.

Warning(s): Keep out of reach of children.

Presentation: 4 fl oz (118 mL) (NDC 47203-005-04).

Compendium Code No.: 11420141 Rev 0797

CLEAR$_X$® EAR DRYING SOLUTION ℞

DVM **Otic Dryer**

Astringent, Antipruritic, Anti-Inflammatory Drying Formulation.

Active Ingredient(s): Hydrocortisone 1%.

Indications: For otic conditions where an anti-inflammatory formulation may be of benefit.

CLEAR$_X$® Ear Drying Solution is an astringent, antipruritic, anti-inflammatory, drying formulation.

Directions for Use: Shake well before each use. Be sure that ear is free of wax and debris. Fill ear dropper with 0.5 mL CLEAR$_X$® and squeeze into ear canal. Do not remove solution from ear canal. Treatment is completed. Use after cleansing of ears, or up to once daily as directed by a veterinarian. If the ear flap is affected, several drops should be rubbed into the ear flap as well. Change the dose proportionately for smaller or larger animals.

Contraindication(s): Do not use in acute inflammatory otitis.

Precaution(s): Store at room temperature.

Caution(s): Federal law restricts this drug to use by, or on the order of, a licensed veterinarian.

If irritation or pain persists after two days of treatment, consult your veterinarian.

Warning(s): Keep out of reach of children.

Presentation: 1 fl oz (30 mL) (NDC 47203-002-01).

Compendium Code No.: 11420151 Rev 0797

CLEEN SHEEN

Vedco **Grooming Shampoo**

Active Ingredient(s): Water, ammonium laureth sulfate, ammonium lauryl sulfate, coconut oil, glycerine, sodium chloride, fragrance, FD&C color.

Indications: CLEEN SHEEN is a mild, pH balanced grooming shampoo for use on pets. Formulated for cleaning and enriched with coconut oil. CLEEN SHEEN will leave the animal's coat clean and smelling fresh. Gentle enough for every day use. Rinses out easily and completely.

Dosage and Administration: Wet the animal's coat using warm water, and apply enough CLEEN SHEEN shampoo to work up a good lather. Massage deep into the coat. Rinse the animal thoroughly with warm water.

For especially dirty animals, repeat the washing directions. When finished washing, dry the animal.

Caution(s): Keep out of the reach of children.

Presentation: 2.5 gallon containers.

Compendium Code No.: 10940310

CLINACOX™

Schering-Plough **Feed Medication**

(Diclazuril) Anticoccidial Type A Medicated Article

NADA No.: 140-951

Active Ingredient(s): Diclazuril, 0.2%.

Inert Ingredients: Wheat middlings, calcium carbonate, soybean oil with 0.02% TBHQ (preservative), and silicon dioxide.

Indications: Broiler chickens: For the prevention of coccidiosis caused by *Eimeria tenella, E. necatrix, E. acervulina, E. brunetti, E. mitis (mivati),* and *E. maxima.* Because diclazuril is effective against *E. maxima* later in its life cycle, subclinical intestinal lesions may be present for a short time after infection. Diclazuril was shown in studies to reduce lesion scores and improve performance and health of birds challenged with *E. maxima.*

Growing Turkeys: For the prevention of coccidiosis caused by *Eimeria adenoeides, E. gallopavonis,* and *E. meleagrimitis.*

Directions: Important: Must be thoroughly mixed into poultry feeds before use.

Thoroughly mix one pound (1 lb) of CLINACOX™ (0.2% diclazuril) into each ton of complete feed to provide 1 ppm of diclazuril (use level). It is recommended that an intermediate mix containing one part CLINACOX™ Anticoccidial and not less than nine parts appropriate feed ingredient be thoroughly mixed before incorporation into the final feed.

Caution(s): Do not feed to breeding turkeys.

Warning(s): Not for use in hens producing eggs for human food.

Presentation: 50 lb (22.68 kg) bag (NDC 0138-5215-01).

Diclazuril is a licensed product from Janssen Pharmaceutica, Beerse, Belgium.

CLINACOX is a trademark of Johnson & Johnson. U.S. Patent 4,631,278.

Compendium Code No.: 10470281 Rev. 9/01

CLINAFARM® EC

ASL **Disinfectant**

EPA Reg. No.: 773-55-10392

Active Ingredient(s): Each 750 mL tip "N" measure® bottle contains:

Imazalil (enilconazole): 1-(2-(2,4-dichlorophenyl)-2-(2-propenyloxy) ethyl)-1H-imidazole	13.8% w/w
Inert ingredients	86.2%
Total	100.0% w/w

* U.S. Patent No. 3,658,813

Indications: For the control of *Aspergillus* organisms in cleaned poultry and turkey hatchery equipment prior to introduction of the eggs. Equipment would include empty hatcher cabinets, setters, coolers, storerooms, handling equipment, etc. CLINAFARM® EC will dramatically reduce the levels of infectious organisms and spores in treated areas.

Dosage and Administration: It is a violation of federal law to use the product in a manner inconsistent with its labeling.

To make one (1) gallon of a 1:100 dilution, add 1.25 fl. oz. (36 mL) of CLINAFARM® EC to one (1) gallon of clean water to provide an antifungal concentration of 0.15% active ingredient. Do not use the product undiluted.

To ensure proper efficacy, the area or equipment to be treated should be clean and closed off from outside air currents before treatment. Ventilation ducts may be treated, but fans must be shut off.

Fog or spray the area to be treated at the rate of ½ fl. oz. diluted product per 150 cu. ft. (1 mL per 10 cu. ft.). Fog or spray to ensure good contact with surface areas. Do not re-enter the treated areas for two (2) hours.

CLINAFARM® EC is compatible with other commonly used disinfectants such as quaternary ammonium compounds, glutaraldehyde, formaldehyde and phenolic compounds.

Precaution(s):

Storage: Store at room temperature.

Pesticide Disposal: Do not contaminate water, food or feed by storage or disposal. Do not contaminate water when disposing of equipment washwaters. Wastes resulting from the use of the product may be disposed of on site or at an approved waste disposal facility.

Container Disposal: Triple rinse (or equivalent), then offer for recycling or reconditioning, or puncture and dispose of in a sanitary landfill, by incineration or, if allowed by state and local authorities, by burning. If burned, stay out of smoke.

Caution(s): Keep out of the reach of children.

Precautionary Statements:

Hazards to Humans and Domestic Animals: Danger. Corrosive. Causes irreversible eye damage. Harmful or fatal if swallowed. Harmful if absorbed through the skin or inhaled. Avoid breathing spray mist and contact with the skin. Do not get in the eyes. Wear goggles or a face shield. Wash thoroughly with soap and water after handling. Remove contaminated clothing and wash before re-use.

Physical or Chemical Hazards: Do not use or store near heat or an open flame.

Statement of Practical Treatment:

If in eyes: Hold the eyelids open and flush with a steady, gentle stream of water for 15 minutes. Call a physician.

If swallowed: Call a physician or poison control center, drink one or two glasses of water and induce vomiting by touching the back of the throat with a finger. Do not induce vomiting or give anything by mouth to an unconscious person.

If on skin: Wash with plenty of soap and water. Get medical attention.

If inhaled: Remove victim to fresh air. If not breathing, give artificial respiration, preferably mouth to mouth. Get medical attention.

Presentation: 750 mL (1.58 U.S. pints) tip "N" measure® bottles.

CLINAFARM is a registered trademark of Janssen Pharmaceutica N.V.

tip "N" measure is a registered trademark of Container Manufacturing, Inc.

Compendium Code No.: 11020220

CLINAFARM® SG

ASL **Antifungal**

EPA Reg. No.: 773-56-10392

Active Ingredient(s): Each smoke generator will deliver 5 g of the active ingredient imazalil.

Indications: For the control of *Aspergillus* organisms in cleaned poultry and turkey hatchery equipment prior to the introduction of the eggs: such as empty hatcher cabinets, setters, coolers, storerooms, and egg and chick handling equipment. Imazalil will dramatically reduce the levels of infectious organisms and spores in treated areas. Each canister contains sufficient imazalil and smoke generating material to cover an enclosure of 400 to 500 cubic feed.

CLINAFARM® SG is for use in well closed rooms, ventilation systems and hard to reach places between equipment and machines.

Dosage and Administration: Methods of Administration:

Do not remove the canisters from the container except for immediate use. The treatment of the hatchery equipment should be the final step prior to introduction of the eggs. After the equipment has been thoroughly cleaned and disinfected, a smoke canister of imazalil should be placed on a noncombustible surface. Before beginning, the area to be treated should be closed off to prevent air currents from diluting the smoke.

Ventilation ducts may be treated, but all fans must be shut off. The wick of the canister should be ignited and persons should leave the treated area. Within 60 seconds the canister will be through smoking. The smoke should be allowed to settle and contact the surfaces for no less than ½ hour, but preferably for up to 12 hours before the fumigated equipment and areas are used. Delay re-entry into the treatment areas until the smoke has settled or dissipated to avoid possible eye irritation. Do not re-enter the unventilated areas for 12 hours after the treatment. For ventilated areas, do not re-enter the treatment areas until the ventilation ducts and fans have been opened and turned on for at least 30 minutes. For either unventilated or ventilated areas, do not re-enter if treatment smoke is still visible.

Precaution(s): Store in a cool, dry place. The storage temperature should not exceed 100°F.

Container Disposal: Do not reuse the container. Replace the cap and dispose of the container in a sanitary landfill or by incineration, or, if allowed by state or local authorities, by burning. If burned, stay out of smoke.

Pesticide Disposal: Sweep up any spilled powder and place it in a DOT approved container for disposal. Do not contaminate water, food, or feed by storage or disposal. Wastes resulting from the use of the product may be disposed of on site or at an approved waste disposal facility, in accordance with applicable federal, state and local regulations.

Caution(s): Keep out of the reach of children.

Precautionary Statements:

Hazards to Humans and Domestic Animals: Danger. The unignited content of the canister contains a strong oxidizing agent which may cause irreversible eye damage. After ignition of the canister, all persons should leave the treated area immediately. Avoid contact of product with skin, eyes or clothing. Wear goggles. Avoid breathing smoke. Wash thoroughly with soap and water after handling.

Statement of Practical Treatment:

If in Eyes: Hold the eyelids open and flush with a steady, gentle stream of water for 15 minutes. Call a physician.

If Swallowed: Call a physician or poison control center. Promptly drink a large quantity of milk, egg white, gelatin solution, or, if these are not available, drink large quantities of water. Avoid alcohol.

If on Skin: Wash thoroughly using soap and copious amounts of water. Get medical attention.

If Inhaled: Remove to fresh air. If not breathing, give artificial respiration. Get medical attention if respiratory irritation occurs.

Warning(s): The information contained herein is to the best of our knowledge true and accurate. Any recommendations or suggestions are made without warranty or guarantee, since use conditions are beyond our control. Nothing contained herein shall be construed to imply the non-existence of any relevant patents, nor to constitute permission, endorsement or recommendation to produce any inventions covered by any patents owned by American Scientific Laboratories, or by others without authority from the owner of the patent.

Presentation: 24 x 33.4 g canisters.

CLINAFARM® is a registered trademark of Janssen Pharmaceutical N.V.

Compendium Code No.: 11020230

CLINCAPS™ ℞

Vetus **Clindamycin**

Antibiotic-Clindamycin Hydrochloride Capsules

ANADA No.: 200-298

Active Ingredient(s): CLINCAPS™:

25 mg Capsule, each yellow and colorless capsule contains clindamycin hydrochloride equivalent to 25 mg of clindamycin.

75 mg Capsule, each green and colorless capsule contains clindamycin hydrochloride equivalent to 75 mg of clindamycin.

150 mg Capsule, each blue and colorless capsule contains clindamycin hydrochloride equivalent to 150 mg of clindamycin.

Indications: Dogs:

Aerobic bacteria: CLINCAPS™ are indicated for the treatment of soft tissue infections (wounds and abscesses), dental infections and osteomyelitis caused by susceptible strains of *Staphylococcus aureus*.

Anaerobic bacteria: CLINCAPS™ are indicated for the treatment of soft tissue infections (deep wounds and abscesses), dental infections and osteomyelitis caused by or associated with susceptible strains of *Bacteroides fragilis, Bacteroides melaninogenicus, Fusobacterium necrophorum* and *Clostridium perfringens*. (See Microbiology section for additional information.)

Pharmacology: Description: CLINCAPS™ (Clindamycin Hydrochloride Capsules) contain clindamycin hydrochloride which is the hydrated salt of clindamycin. Clindamycin is a semisynthetic antibiotic produced by a 7(S)-chlorosubstitution of the 7(R)-hydroxyl group of a naturally produced antibiotic produced by *Streptomyces lincolnensis var. lincolnensis*.

CLINCAPS™ (Clindamycin Hydrochloride Capsules) is a palatable formulation intended for oral administration to dogs.

Actions:

Site and Mode of Action: Clindamycin is an inhibitor of protein synthesis in the bacterial cell. The site of binding appears to be in the 50S sub-unit of the ribosome.

Binding occurs to the soluble RNA fraction of certain ribosomes, thereby inhibiting the binding of amino acids to those ribosomes. Clindamycin differs from cell wall inhibitors in that it causes irreversible modification of the protein-synthesizing subcellular elements at the ribosomal level.

Microbiology: The following clindamycin *in vitro* data are available but their clinical significance is unknown. Clindamycin has been shown to have *in vitro* activity against the following organisms isolated from animals:

Aerobic gram positive cocci, including: *Staphylococcus aureus* (penicillinase and non-penicillinase producing strains), *Staphylococcus intermedius, Staphylococcus simulans, Staphylococcus epidermidis*, Streptococci (except *Enterococcus faecalis)*.

Anaerobic gram negative bacilli, including: *Bacteroides* species, *Fusobacterium* species.

Anaerobic gram positive nonsporeforming bacilli, including: *Propionibacterium, Eubacterium, Actinomyces* species.

Anaerobic and microaerophilic gram positive cocci, including: *Peptococcus* species, *Peptostreptococcus* species, Microaerophilic streptococci.

Clostridia: Most *C. perfringens* are susceptible, but other species may be resistant to clindamycin.

Overall Susceptibility to Clindamycin of Anaerobes Isolated from Canine Lesions. Data Obtained from Three Veterinary Diagnostic Laboratories.

	Susceptible ≤3.2 μg/mL	Resistant ≥4.0 μg/mL
All Isolates	122/137 (89%)	15/137 (11%)
Clostridium spp.	41/49 (84%)	8/49 (16%)
Bacteroides spp.	42/46 (91%)	4/46 (9%)
Fusobacterium spp.	16/16 (100%)	0/16 (0%)
Peptostreptococcus spp.	15/16 (94%)	1/16 (6%)
Actinomyces spp.	5/6 (83%)	1/6 (17%)
Proprionibacterium spp.	3/4 (75%)	1/4 (25%)

Mycoplasma species: Most mycoplasma species are susceptible to clindamycin.

Clindamycin and erythromycin show parallel resistance. Partial cross resistance has been demonstrated between clindamycin, erythromycin and macrolide antibiotics.

Absorption: Clindamycin hydrochloride is rapidly absorbed from the canine gastrointestinal tract. Dogs orally dosed with therapeutic amounts of clindamycin hydrochloride demonstrated antibacterial serum levels of the drug within 15 minutes post-dosing.

Canine Serum Levels: Therapeutically effective serum levels of clindamycin hydrochloride can be maintained by oral dosing at the rate of 2.5 mg/lb every 12 hours. Dogs orally dosed with clindamycin hydrochloride at 2.5 mg/lb every 12 hours during a 72 hours dosing regimen continuously maintained antibacterial serum levels of the drug. This same study revealed that average peak serum concentrations occurred 1 hour and 15 minutes after dosing. The biological half-life for clindamycin hydrochloride in dog serum was about 5 hours. There was no bioactivity accumulation after a regimen of multiple oral doses.

Metabolism and Excretion: Extensive studies of the metabolism and excretion of clindamycin hydrochloride administered orally in animals and humans have shown that unchanged drug and bioactive and bioinactive metabolites are excreted in urine and feces. Almost all of the bioactivity detected in serum after clindamycin hydrochloride product administration is due to the parent molecule (clindamycin). Urine bioactivity, however, reflects a mixture of clindamycin and active metabolites, especially N-demethyl clindamycin and clindamycin sulfoxide.

Dosage and Administration:

Canine Infected Wounds, Abscesses and Dental Infections:

Oral: 2.5 mg/lb body weight every 12 hours.

Duration: Treatment with CLINCAPS™ may be continued up to a maximum of 28 days if clinical judgment indicates. Treatment of acute infections should not be continued for more than three or four days if no response to therapy is seen.

Dosage Schedule:

Capsules:

CLINCAPS™ 25 mg, administer 1 capsule every 12 hours for each 10 lbs of body weight.

CLINCAPS™ 75 mg, administer 1 capsule every 12 hours for each 30 lbs of body weight.

CLINCAPS™ 150 mg, administer 1 capsule every 12 hours for each 60 lbs of body weight.

Canine Osteomyelitis:

Oral: 5.0 mg/lb body weight every 12 hours.

Duration: Treatment with CLINCAPS™ is recommended for a minimum of 28 days. Treatment should not be continued for longer than 28 days if no response to therapy is seen.

Dosage Schedule:

Capsules:

CLINCAPS™ 25 mg, administer 1 capsule every 12 hours for each 5 lbs of body weight.

CLINCAPS™ 75 mg, administer 1 capsule every 12 hours for each 15 lbs of body weight.

CLINCAPS™ 150 mg, administer 1 capsule every 12 hours for each 30 lbs of body weight.

Contraindication(s): CLINCAPS™ are contraindicated in animals with a history of hypersensitivity to preparations containing clindamycin or lincomycin.

Because of potential adverse gastrointestinal effects, do not administer to rabbits, hamsters, guinea pigs, horses, chinchillas or ruminating animals.

Precaution(s): Store at controlled room temperature 20°-25°C (68°-77°F).

Keep container tightly closed.

Caution(s): Federal law restricts this drug to use by or on the order of a licensed veterinarian.

CLINCAPS™ should be prescribed with caution in atopic animals.

During prolonged therapy of one month or greater, periodic liver and kidney function tests and blood counts should be performed.

The use of clindamycin hydrochloride occasionally results in overgrowth of non-susceptible organisms such as clostridia and yeasts. Therefore, the administration of CLINCAPS™ should be avoided in those species sensitive to the gastrointestinal effects of clindamycin (see Contraindications). Should superinfections occur, appropriate measures should be taken as indicated by the clinical situation.

Patients with very severe renal disease and/or very severe hepatic disease accompanied by severe metabolic aberrations should be dosed with caution, and serum clindamycin levels monitored during high-dose therapy.

Clindamycin hydrochloride has been shown to have neuromuscular blocking properties that may enhance the action of other neuromuscular blocking agents. Therefore, CLINCAPS™ should be used with caution in animals receiving such agents.

Safety in gestating bitches or breeding male dogs has not been established.

For animal use only. Approved for use in canines.

Warning(s): Not for human use. Keep out of reach of children.

Toxicology: Toxicology and Safety:

Rat and Dog Data: One year oral toxicity studies in rats and dogs at doses of 30, 100 and 300 mg/kg/day (13.6, 45.5 and 136.4 mg/lb/day) have shown clindamycin hydrochloride to be well tolerated. Differences did not occur in the parameters evaluated to assess toxicity when comparing groups of treated animals with contemporary controls. Rats administered clindamycin hydrochloride at 600 mg/kg/day (272.7 mg/lb/day) for six months tolerated the drug well; however, dogs orally dosed at 600 mg/kg/day (272.7 mg/lb/day) vomited, had anorexia, and subsequently lost weight.

Safety in gestating bitches or breeding males has not been established.

Side Effects: Side effects occasionally observed in either clinical trials or during clinical use were vomiting and diarrhea.

Discussion: *In Vitro* Susceptibility Testing: Susceptibility tests should be done on samples collected prior to initiation of therapy with CLINCAPS™. Clindamycin susceptibility testing is performed by using Cleocin® Susceptibility Disks (clindamycin 2 mcg) and Cleocin® Susceptibility Powder 20 mg. A standardized disk testing procedure* is recommended for determining susceptibility of aerobic bacteria to clindamycin. A description is contained in the Cleocin® Susceptibility Disk insert. Using this method, the laboratory can designate isolates as resistant, intermediate, or susceptible. Tube or agar dilution methods may be used for aerobic and anaerobic bacteria. When the directions in the Cleocin® Susceptibility Powder insert are followed, a MIC (minimal inhibitory concentration) of 1.6 mcg/mL may be considered susceptible; MICs of 1.6 to 4.8 mcg/mL may be considered intermediate and MICs greater than 4.8 mcg/mL may be considered resistant.

References: *Available upon request.

Presentation: CLINCAPS™ are available as:

25 mg capsules supplied in bottles of 600.
75 mg capsules supplied in bottles of 200 (NDC: 47611-787-02).
150 mg capsules supplied in bottles of 100.

Manufactured by: Phoenix Scientific, Inc., St. Joseph, MO 64503.

Distributed by: Burns Veterinary Supply, Inc., Westbury, NY 11590.

Compendium Code No.: 14441040 T-Iss. 11-01

CLINDACURE™ ℞

Vedco **Clindamycin**

(Clindamycin Hydrochloride Oral Liquid) Antibiotic

ANADA No.: 200-193

Active Ingredient(s): Each mL of CLINDACURE™ (Clindamycin Hydrochloride Oral Liquid) contains clindamycin hydrochloride equivalent to 25 mg clindamycin; and ethyl alcohol, 8.64%.

Indications: Dogs:

Aerobic bacteria: CLINDACURE™ (Clindamycin Hydrochloride Oral Liquid) is indicated for the treatment of soft tissue infections (wounds and abscesses), dental infections and osteomyelitis caused by susceptible strains of *Staphylococcus aureus*.

Anaerobic bacteria: CLINDACURE™ (Clindamycin Hydrochloride Oral Liquid) is indicated for the treatment of soft tissue infections (deep wounds and abscesses), dental infections and osteomyelitis caused by or associated with susceptible strains of *Bacteroides fragilis, Bacteroides melaninogenicus, Fusobacterium necrophorum* and *Clostridium perfringens*. (See Microbiology section for additional information.)

Pharmacology: Description: CLINDACURE™ (Clindamycin Hydrochloride Oral Liquid) contains clindamycin hydrochloride which is the hydrated salt of clindamycin. Clindamycin is a semi-synthetic antibiotic produced by a 7(S)-chlorosubstitution of the 7(R)-hydroxyl group of a naturally produced antibiotic produced by *Streptomyces lincolnensis var. lincolnensis*.

CLINDACURE™ (Clindamycin Hydrochloride Oral Liquid) is a palatable formulation intended for oral administration to dogs.

Actions:

Site and Mode of Action: Clindamycin is an inhibitor of protein synthesis in the bacterial cell. The site of binding appears to be in the 50S sub-unit of the ribosome. Binding occurs to the soluble RNA fraction of certain ribosomes, thereby inhibiting the binding of amino acids to those ribosomes. Clindamycin differs from cell wall inhibitors in that it causes irreversible modification of the protein-synthesizing subcellular elements at the ribosomal level.

Microbiology: The following clindamycin *in vitro* data are available but their clinical significance is unknown. Clindamycin has been shown to have *in vitro* activity against the following organisms isolated from animals:

Aerobic gram positive cocci, including: *Staphylococcus aureus* (penicillinase and non-penicillinase producing strains), *Staphylococcus intermedius, Staphylococcus simulans, Staphylococcus epidermidis*, Streptococci (except *Enterococcus faecalis)*.

Anaerobic gram negative bacilli, including: *Bacteroides* species, *Fusobacterium* species.

Anaerobic gram positive nonsporeforming bacilli, including: *Propionibacterium, Eubacterium, Actinomyces* species.

Anaerobic and microaerophilic gram positive cocci, including: *Peptococcus* species, *Peptostreptococcus* species, Microaerophilic streptococci.

Clostridia: Most *C perfringens* are susceptible, but other species may be resistant to clindamycin.

Overall susceptibility to clindamycin of anaerobes isolated from canine lesions. Data obtained from three veterinary diagnostic laboratories.

	Susceptible ≤3.2 μg/mL	Resistant ≥4.0 μg/mL
All Isolates	122/137 (89%)	15/137 (11%)
Clostridium spp	41/49 (84%)	8/49 (16%)
Bacteroides spp	42/46 (91%)	4/46 (9%)
Fusobacterium spp	16/16 (100%)	0/16 (0%)
Peptostreptococcus spp	15/16 (94%)	1/16 (6%)
Actinomyces spp	5/6 (83%)	1/6 (17%)
Proprionibacterium spp	3/4 (75%)	1/4 (25%)

Mycoplasma species: Most mycoplasma species are susceptible to clindamycin.

Clindamycin and erythromycin show parallel resistance. Partial cross resistance has been demonstrated between clindamycin, erythromycin and macrolide antibiotics.

Absorption: Clindamycin hydrochloride is rapidly absorbed from the canine gastrointestinal tract. Dogs orally dosed with therapeutic amounts of clindamycin hydrochloride demonstrated antibacterial serum levels of the drug within 15 minutes post-dosing.

Canine Serum Levels: Therapeutically effective serum levels of clindamycin hydrochloride can be maintained by oral dosing at the rate of 2.5 mg/lb every 12 hours. Dogs orally dosed with clindamycin hydrochloride at 2.5 mg/lb every 12 hours during a 72 hours dosing regimen continuously maintained antibacterial serum levels of the drug. This same study revealed that average peak serum concentrations occurred 1 hour and 15 minutes after dosing. The biological half-life for clindamycin hydrochloride in dog serum was about 5 hours. There was no bioactivity accumulation after a regimen of multiple oral doses.

Metabolism and Excretion: Extensive studies of the metabolism and excretion of clindamycin hydrochloride administered orally in animals and humans have shown that unchanged drug and bioactive and bioinactive metabolites are excreted in urine and feces. Almost all of the bioactivity detected in serum after clindamycin hydrochloride product administration is due to the parent molecule (clindamycin). Urine bioactivity, however, reflects a mixture of clindamycin and active metabolites, especially N-demethyl clindamycin and clindamycin sulfoxide.

Dosage and Administration:

Canine Infected Wounds, Abscesses and Dental Infections:

Oral: 2.5 mg/lb body weight every 12 hours. Duration: Treatment with clindamycin hydrochloride products may be continued up to a maximum of 28 days if clinical judgment indicates. Treatment of acute infections should not be continued for more than three or four days if no response to therapy is seen.

Dosage Schedule:

CLINDACURE™ (Clindamycin Hydrochloride Oral Liquid): Administer 1 mL/10 lbs body weight every 12 hours.

Canine Osteomyelitis:

Oral: 5.0 mg/lb body weight every 12 hours. Duration: Treatment with CLINDACURE™ (Clindamycin Hydrochloride Oral Liquid) is recommended for a minimum of 28 days. Treatment should not be continued for longer than 28 days if no response to therapy is seen.

Dosage Schedule:

CLINDACURE™ (Clindamycin Hydrochloride Oral Liquid): Administer 2 mL/10 lbs body weight every 12 hours.

Contraindication(s): CLINDACURE™ (Clindamycin Hydrochloride Oral Liquid) is contraindicated in animals with a history of hypersensitivity to preparations containing clindamycin or lincomycin.

Because of potential adverse gastrointestinal effects, do not administer to rabbits, hamsters, guinea pigs, horses, chinchillas or ruminating animals.

Precaution(s): Store at controlled room temperature 15°-30°C (59°-86°F).

Caution(s): Federal (USA) law restricts this drug to use by or on the order of a licensed veterinarian.

CLINDACURE™ (Clindamycin Hydrochloride Oral Liquid) should be prescribed with caution in atopic animals.

During prolonged therapy of one month or greater, periodic liver and kidney function tests and blood counts should be performed.

The use of clindamycin hydrochloride occasionally results in overgrowth of non-susceptible organisms such as clostridia and yeasts. Therefore, the administration of clindamycin hydrochloride should be avoided in those species sensitive to the gastrointestinal effects of clindamycin (see Contraindications). Should superinfections occur, appropriate measures should be taken as indicated by the clinical situation.

Patients with very severe renal disease and/or very severe hepatic disease accompanied by severe metabolic aberrations should be dosed with caution, and serum clindamycin levels monitored during high-dose therapy.

Clindamycin hydrochloride has been shown to have neuromuscular blocking properties that may enhance the action of other neuromuscular blocking agents. Therefore, clindamycin hydrochloride should be used with caution in animals receiving such agents.

Safety in gestating bitches or breeding males has not been established.

Warning(s): Not for human use. For use in animals only.

Toxicology:

Rat and Dog Data: One year oral toxicity studies in rats and dogs at doses of 30, 100 and 300 mg/kg/day (13.6, 45.5 and 136.4 mg/lb/day) have shown clindamycin hydrochloride to be well tolerated. Differences did not occur in the parameters evaluated to assess toxicity when comparing groups of treated animals with contemporary controls. Rats administered clindamycin hydrochloride at 600 mg/kg/day (272.7 mg/lb/day) for six months tolerated the drug well; however, dogs orally dosed at 600 mg/kg/day (272.7 mg/lb/day) vomited, had anorexia, and subsequently lost weight.

Safety in gestating bitches or breeding males has not been established.

Side Effects: Side effects occasionally observed in either clinical trials or during clinical use were vomiting and diarrhea.

Discussion: Susceptibility tests should be done on samples collected prior to initiation of therapy with CLINDACURE™ (Clindamycin Hydrochloride Oral Liquid). Clindamycin susceptibility testing is performed by using Cleocin® Susceptibility Disks (clindamycin 2 mcg) and Cleocin® Susceptibility Powder 20 mg. A standardized disk testing procedure* is recommended for determining susceptibility of aerobic bacteria to clindamycin. A description is contained in the Cleocin® Susceptibility Disk insert. Using this method, the laboratory can designate isolates as resistant, intermediate, or susceptible. Tube or agar dilution methods may be used for aerobic and anaerobic bacteria. When the directions in the Cleocin® Susceptibility Powder insert are followed, a MIC (minimal inhibitory concentration) of 1.6 mcg/mL may be considered susceptible; MICs of 1.6 to 4.8 mcg/mL may be considered intermediate and MICs greater than 4.8 mcg/mL may be considered resistant.

References: Available upon request.

Presentation: CLINDACURE™ (Clindamycin Hydrochloride Oral Liquid) is available as 20 mL filled in 30 mL bottles (25 mg/mL) supplied in packers containing 12 cartoned bottles with direction labels and calibrated dosing droppers.

Manufactured by: Phoenix Scientific, Inc.

Compendium Code No.: 10940320

CLINDA-GUARD™ ℞

RXV **Clindamycin**

(Clindamycin Hydrochloride Oral Liquid) Antibiotic

ANADA No.: 200-193

Active Ingredient(s): Each mL of CLINDA-GUARD™ (Clindamycin Hydrochloride Oral Liquid) contains clindamycin hydrochloride equivalent to 25 mg clindamycin; and ethyl alcohol, 8.64%.

Indications: Dogs:

Aerobic bacteria: CLINDA-GUARD™ (Clindamycin Hydrochloride Oral Liquid) is indicated for the treatment of soft tissue infections (wounds and abscesses), dental infections and osteomyelitis caused by susceptible strains of *Staphylococcus aureus*.

Anaerobic bacteria: CLINDA-GUARD™ (Clindamycin Hydrochloride Oral Liquid) is indicated for the treatment of soft tissue infections (deep wounds and abscesses), dental infections and osteomyelitis caused by or associated with susceptible strains of *Bacteroides fragilis, Bacteroides melaninogenicus, Fusobacterium necrophorum* and *Clostridium perfringens*. (See Microbiology section for additional information.)

Pharmacology: Description: CLINDA-GUARD™ (Clindamycin Hydrochloride Oral Liquid) contains clindamycin hydrochloride which is the hydrated salt of clindamycin. Clindamycin is a semi-synthetic antibiotic produced by a 7(S)-chlorosubstitution of the 7(R)-hydroxyl group of a naturally produced antibiotic produced by *Streptomyces lincolnensis var. lincolnensis*.

CLINDA-GUARD™ (Clindamycin Hydrochloride Oral Liquid) is a palatable formulation intended for oral administration to dogs.

Actions:

Site and Mode of Action: Clindamycin is an inhibitor of protein synthesis in the bacterial cell. The site of binding appears to be in the 50S sub-unit of the ribosome. Binding occurs to the soluble RNA fraction of certain ribosomes, thereby inhibiting the binding of amino acids to those ribosomes. Clindamycin differs from cell wall inhibitors in that it causes irreversible modification of the protein-synthesizing subcellular elements at the ribosomal level.

Microbiology: The following clindamycin *in vitro* data are available but their clinical significance is unknown. Clindamycin has been shown to have *in vitro* activity against the following organisms isolated from animals:

Aerobic gram positive cocci, including: *Staphylococcus aureus* (penicillinase and non-penicillinase producing strains), *Staphylococcus intermedius, Staphylococcus simulans, Staphylococcus epidermidis*, Streptococci (except *Enterococcus faecalis)*.

Anaerobic gram negative bacilli, including: *Bacteroides* species, *Fusobacterium* species.

Anaerobic gram positive nonsporeforming bacilli, including: *Propionibacterium, Eubacterium, Actinomyces* species.

Anaerobic and microaerophilic gram positive cocci, including: *Peptococcus* species, *Peptostreptococcus* species, Microaerophilic streptococci.

Clostridia: Most *C. perfringens* are susceptible, but other species may be resistant to clindamycin.

Overall susceptibility to clindamycin of anaerobes isolated from canine lesions. Data obtained from three veterinary diagnostic laboratories.

	Susceptible ≤3.2 μg/mL	Resistant ≥4.0 μg/mL
All Isolates	122/137 (89%)	15/137 (11%)
Clostridium spp	41/49 (84%)	8/49 (16%)
Bacteroides spp	42/46 (91%)	4/46 (9%)
Fusobacterium spp	16/16 (100%)	0/16 (0%)
Peptostreptococcus spp	15/16 (94%)	1/16 (6%)
Actinomyces spp	5/6 (83%)	1/6 (17%)
Proprionibacterium spp	3/4 (75%)	1/4 (25%)

Mycoplasma species: Most mycoplasma species are susceptible to clindamycin.

Clindamycin and erythromycin show parallel resistance. Partial cross resistance has been demonstrated between clindamycin, erythromycin and macrolide antibiotics.

Absorption: Clindamycin hydrochloride is rapidly absorbed from the canine gastrointestinal tract. Dogs orally dosed with therapeutic amounts of clindamycin hydrochloride demonstrated antibacterial serum levels of the drug within 15 minutes post-dosing.

Canine Serum Levels: Therapeutically effective serum levels of clindamycin hydrochloride can be maintained by oral dosing at the rate of 2.5 mg/lb every 12 hours. Dogs orally dosed with clindamycin hydrochloride at 2.5 mg/lb every 12 hours during a 72 hours dosing regimen continuously maintained antibacterial serum levels of the drug. This same study revealed that average peak serum concentrations occurred 1 hour and 15 minutes after dosing. The biological half-life for clindamycin hydrochloride in dog serum was about 5 hours. There was no bioactivity accumulation after a regimen of multiple oral doses.

Metabolism and Excretion: Extensive studies of the metabolism and excretion of clindamycin hydrochloride administered orally in animals and humans have shown that unchanged drug and bioactive and bioinactive metabolites are excreted in urine and feces. Almost all of the bioactivity detected in serum after clindamycin hydrochloride product administration is due to the parent molecule (clindamycin). Urine bioactivity, however, reflects a mixture of clindamycin and active metabolites, especially N-demethyl clindamycin and clindamycin sulfoxide.

Dosage and Administration:

Canine Infected Wounds, Abscesses and Dental Infections:

Oral: 2.5 mg/lb body weight every 12 hours.

Duration: Treatment with clindamycin hydrochloride products may be continued up to a maximum of 28 days if clinical judgment indicates. Treatment of acute infections should not be continued for more than three or four days if no response to therapy is seen.

Dosage Schedule:

CLINDA-GUARD™ (Clindamycin Hydrochloride Oral Liquid): Administer 1 mL/10 lbs body weight every 12 hours.

Canine Osteomyelitis:

Oral: 5.0 mg/lb body weight every 12 hours.

Duration: Treatment with CLINDA-GUARD™ (Clindamycin Hydrochloride Oral Liquid) is recommended for a minimum of 28 days. Treatment should not be continued for longer than 28 days if no response to therapy is seen.

Dosage Schedule:

CLINDA-GUARD™ (Clindamycin Hydrochloride Oral Liquid): Administer 2 mL/10 lbs body weight every 12 hours.

Contraindication(s): CLINDA-GUARD™ (Clindamycin Hydrochloride Oral Liquid) is contraindicated in animals with a history of hypersensitivity to preparations containing clindamycin or lincomycin.

Because of potential adverse gastrointestinal effects, do not administer to rabbits, hamsters, guinea pigs, horses, chinchillas or ruminating animals.

Precaution(s): Store at controlled room temperature 15°-30°C (59°-86°F).

Caution(s): Federal (USA) law restricts this drug to use by or on the order of a licensed veterinarian.

CLINDA-GUARD™ (Clindamycin Hydrochloride Oral Liquid) should be prescribed with caution in atopic animals.

During prolonged therapy of one month or greater, periodic liver and kidney function tests and blood counts should be performed.

The use of clindamycin hydrochloride occasionally results in overgrowth of non-susceptible organisms such as clostridia and yeasts. Therefore, the administration of clindamycin hydrochloride should be avoided in those species sensitive to the gastrointestinal effects of clindamycin (see Contraindications). Should superinfections occur, appropriate measures should be taken as indicated by the clinical situation.

Patients with very severe renal disease and/or very severe hepatic disease accompanied by severe metabolic aberrations should be dosed with caution, and serum clindamycin levels monitored during high-dose therapy.

Clindamycin hydrochloride has been shown to have neuromuscular blocking properties that may enhance the action of other neuromuscular blocking agents. Therefore, clindamycin hydrochloride should be used with caution in animals receiving such agents.

Safety in gestating bitches or breeding males has not been established.

Warning(s): Not for human use.

For use in animals only.

Toxicology:

Rat and Dog Data: One year oral toxicity studies in rats and dogs at doses of 30, 100 and 300 mg/kg/day (13.6, 45.5 and 136.4 mg/lb/day) have shown clindamycin hydrochloride to be well tolerated. Differences did not occur in the parameters evaluated to assess toxicity when comparing groups of treated animals with contemporary controls. Rats administered clindamycin hydrochloride at 600 mg/kg/day (272.7 mg/lb/day) for six months tolerated the drug well; however, dogs orally dosed at 600 mg/kg/day (272.7 mg/lb/day) vomited, had anorexia, and subsequently lost weight.

Safety in gestating bitches or breeding males has not been established.

Side Effects: Side effects occasionally observed in either clinical trials or during clinical use were vomiting and diarrhea.

Discussion: In Vitro Susceptibility Testing: Susceptibility tests should be done on samples collected prior to initiation of therapy with CLINDA-GUARD™ (Clindamycin Hydrochloride Oral Liquid). Clindamycin susceptibility testing is performed by using Cleocin® Susceptibility Disks (clindamycin 2 mcg) and Cleocin® Susceptibility Powder 20 mg. A standardized disk testing procedure* is recommended for determining susceptibility of aerobic bacteria to clindamycin. A description is contained in the Cleocin® Susceptibility Disk insert. Using this method, the laboratory can designate isolates as resistant, intermediate, or susceptible. Tube or agar dilution methods may be used for aerobic and anaerobic bacteria. When the directions in the Cleocin® Susceptibility Powder insert are followed, a MIC (minimal inhibitory concentration) of 1.6 mcg/mL may be considered susceptible; MICs of 1.6 to 4.8 mcg/mL may be considered intermediate and MICs greater than 4.8 mcg/mL may be considered resistant.

References: Available upon request.

Presentation: CLINDA-GUARD™ (Clindamycin Hydrochloride Oral Liquid) is available as 20 mL filled in 30 mL bottles (25 mg/mL) supplied in packers containing 12 cartoned bottles with direction labels and calibrated dosing droppers.

Manufactured by: Phoenix Scientific, Inc.

Compendium Code No.: 10910020

CLINDAMYCIN HYDROCHLORIDE DROPS ℞

Phoenix Pharmaceutical **Clindamycin**

Antibiotic-25 mg/mL Clindamycin

ANADA No.: 200-193

Active Ingredient(s): Each mL of CLINDAMYCIN HYDROCHLORIDE DROPS contains clindamycin hydrochloride equivalent to 25 mg clindamycin; and ethyl alcohol, 8.64%.

Indications:

Dogs:

Aerobic bacteria: CLINDAMYCIN HYDROCHLORIDE DROPS are indicated for the treatment of soft tissue infections (wounds and abscesses), dental infections and osteomyelitis caused by susceptible strains of *Staphylococcus aureus.*

Anaerobic bacteria: CLINDAMYCIN HYDROCHLORIDE DROPS are indicated for the treatment of soft tissue infections (deep wounds and abscesses), dental infections and osteomyelitis caused by or associated with susceptible strains of *Bacteroides fragilis, Bacteroides melaninogenicus, Fusobacterium necrophorum* and *Clostridium perfringens.* (See Microbiology section for additional information.)

Cats:

Aerobic bacteria: CLINDAMYCIN HYDROCHLORIDE DROPS are indicated for the treatment of soft tissue infections (wounds and abscesses), and dental infections caused by or associated with susceptible strains of *Staphylococcus aureus, Staphylococcus intermedius* and *Streptococcus* spp.

Anaerobic bacteria: CLINDAMYCIN HYDROCHLORIDE DROPS are indicated for the treatment of soft tissue infections (deep wounds and abscesses) and dental infections caused by or associated with susceptible strains of *Clostridium perfringens* and *Bactericides fragilis.* (See Microbiology section for additional information).

Pharmacology: Description: CLINDAMYCIN HYDROCHLORIDE DROPS contain clindamycin hydrochloride which is the hydrated salt of clindamycin. Clindamycin is a semi-synthetic antibiotic produced by a 7(S)-chlorosubstitution of the 7(R)-hydroxyl group of a naturally produced antibiotic produced by *Streptomyces lincolnensis var. lincolnensis.*

CLINDAMYCIN HYDROCHLORIDE DROPS are a palatable formulation intended for oral administration to dogs and cats.

Actions:

Site and Mode of Action: Clindamycin is an inhibitor of protein synthesis in the bacterial cell. The site of binding appears to be in the 50S sub-unit of the ribosome. Binding occurs to the soluble RNA fraction of certain ribosomes, thereby inhibiting the binding of amino acids to those ribosomes. Clindamycin differs from cell wall inhibitors in that it causes irreversible modification of the protein-synthesizing subcellular elements at the ribosomal level.

Microbiology: The following clindamycin *in vitro* data are available but their clinical significance is unknown. Clindamycin has been shown to have *in vitro* activity against the following organisms isolated from animals:

Aerobic gram positive cocci, including: *Staphylococcus aureus* (penicillinase and non-penicillinase producing strains), *Staphylococcus intermedius, Staphylococcus simulans, Staphylococcus epidermidis,* Streptococci (except *Enterococcus faecalis).*

Anaerobic gram negative bacilli, including: *Bacteroides* species, *Fusobacterium* species.

Anaerobic gram positive nonsporeforming bacilli, including: *Propionibacterium, Eubacterium, Actinomyces* species.

Anaerobic and microaerophilic gram positive cocci, including: *Peptococcus* species, *Peptostreptococcus* species, Microaerophilic streptococci.

Clostridia: Most *C. perfringens* are susceptible, but other species may be resistant to clindamycin.

Overall susceptibility to clindamycin of anaerobes isolated from canine lesions. Data obtained from three veterinary diagnostic laboratories.

	Susceptible ≤3.2 µg/mL	Resistant ≥4.0 µg/mL
All Isolates	122/137 (89%)	15/137 (11%)
Clostridium spp	41/49 (84%)	8/49 (16%)
Bacteroides spp	42/46 (91%)	4/46 (9%)
Fusobacterium spp	16/16 (100%)	0/16 (0%)
Peptostreptococcus spp	15/16 (94%)	1/16 (6%)
Actinomyces spp	5/6 (83%)	1/6 (17%)
Proprionibacterium spp	3/4 (75%)	1/4 (25%)

The MIC values for the anaerobes isolated from feline lesions are not different from the MIC values for the anaerobes isolated from canine lesions.

Mycoplasma species: Most mycoplasma species are susceptible to clindamycin.

Clindamycin and erythromycin show parallel resistance. Partial cross resistance has been demonstrated between clindamycin, erythromycin and macrolide antibiotics.

Absorption: Clindamycin hydrochloride is rapidly absorbed from the canine and feline gastrointestinal tract. Dogs and cats orally dosed with therapeutic amounts of clindamycin hydrochloride demonstrated antibacterial serum levels of the drug within 15 minutes post-dosing.

Canine Serum Levels: Therapeutically effective serum levels of clindamycin hydrochloride can be maintained by oral dosing at the rate of 2.5 mg/lb every 12 hours. Dogs orally dosed with clindamycin hydrochloride at 2.5 mg/lb every 12 hours during a 72 hours dosing regimen continuously maintained antibacterial serum levels of the drug. This same study revealed that average peak serum concentrations occurred 1 hour and 15 minutes after dosing. The biological half-life for clindamycin hydrochloride in dog serum was about 5 hours. There was no bioactivity accumulation after a regimen of multiple oral doses.

Feline Serum Levels: Therapeutically effective serum levels of clindamycin can be maintained by oral dosing at the rate of 5 to 10 mg/lb body weight once every 24 hours. The average peak serum concentration of clindamycin occurs about 1 hour after oral administration. The terminal half-life of clindamycin in feline serum is approximately 7.5 hours. Minimal accumulation occurs after multiple oral doses of clindamycin hydrochloride, and steady-state should be achieved by the third dose.

Clindamycin Serum Concentrations 5 mg/lb (11 mg/kg) After Single Oral Dose of Antirobe Aquadrops:

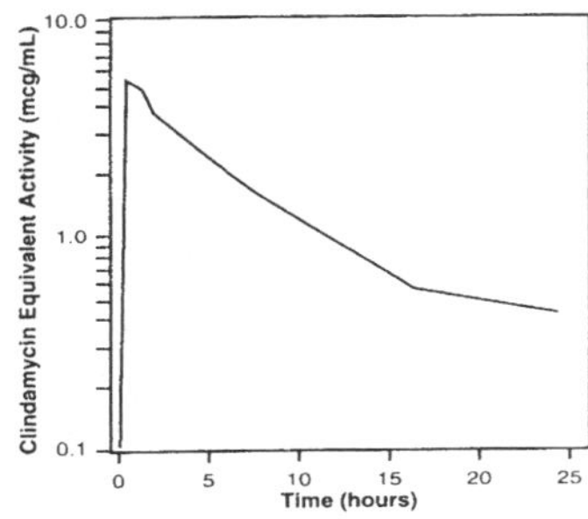

Feline Tissue levels: Tissue concentrations measured at 10 days (µg/g; means) of clindamycin hydrochloride liquid in cats 2 hours after oral administration at 10 mg/lb body weight once every 24 hours for 10 days.

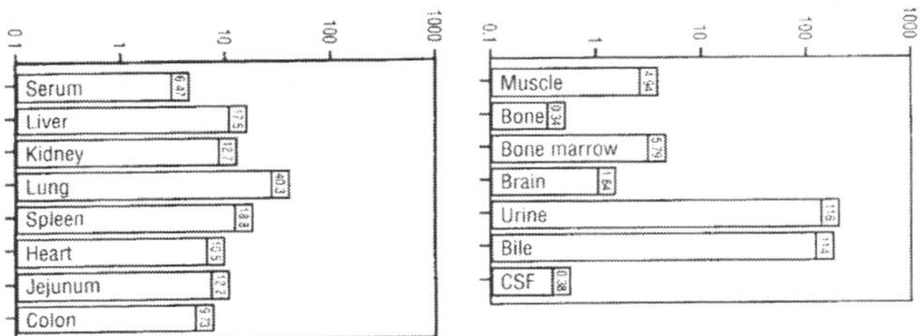

Metabolism and Excretion: Extensive studies of the metabolism and excretion of clindamycin hydrochloride administered orally in animals and humans have shown that unchanged drug and bioactive and bioinactive metabolites are excreted in urine and feces. Almost all of the bioactivity detected in serum after clindamycin hydrochloride product administration is due to the parent molecule (clindamycin). Urine bioactivity, however, reflects a mixture of clindamycin and active metabolites, especially N-demethyl clindamycin and clindamycin sulfoxide.

Dosage and Administration:

Canine Infected Wounds, Abscesses and Dental Infections:

Oral: 2.5 mg/lb body weight every 12 hours.

Duration: Treatment with clindamycin hydrochloride products may be continued up to a maximum of 28 days if clinical judgment indicates. Treatment of acute infections should not be continued for more than three or four days if no response to therapy is seen.

Dosage Schedule:

CLINDAMYCIN HYDROCHLORIDE DROPS: Administer 1 mL/10 lbs body weight every 12 hours.

Canine Osteomyelitis:

Oral: 5.0 mg/lb body weight every 12 hours.

Duration: Treatment with CLINDAMYCIN HYDROCHLORIDE DROPS is recommended for a minimum of 28 days. Treatment should not be continued for longer than 28 days if no response to therapy is seen.

Dosage Schedule:

CLINDAMYCIN HYDROCHLORIDE DROPS: Administer 2 mL/10 lbs body weight every 12 hours.

Feline Infected Wounds, Abscesses and Dental Infections:

Oral: 5.0 to 10.0 mg/lb body weight once every 24 hours depending on the severity of the condition.

Duration: Treatment with CLINDAMYCIN HYDROCHLORIDE DROPS may be continued up to a maximum of 14 days if clinical judgment indicates. Treatment of acute infections should not be continued for more than three to four days if no clinical response to therapy is seen.

Dosage Schedule:

CLINDAMYCIN HYDROCHLORIDE DROPS, to provide 5.0 mg/lb administer 1 mL/5 lb body weight once every 24 hours; to provide 10.0 mg/lb, administer 2 mL/5 lb body weight once every 24 hours.

Contraindication(s): CLINDAMYCIN HYDROCHLORIDE DROPS are contraindicated in animals with a history of hypersensitivity to preparations containing clindamycin or lincomycin.

Because of potential adverse gastrointestinal effects, do not administer to rabbits, hamsters, guinea pigs, horses, chinchillas or ruminating animals.

Precaution(s): Store at controlled room temperature 20°-25°C (68°-77°F).

Caution(s): Federal (USA) law restricts this drug to use by or on the order of a licensed veterinarian.

CLINDAMYCIN HYDROCHLORIDE DROPS should be prescribed with caution in atopic animals.

During prolonged therapy of one month or greater, periodic liver and kidney function tests and blood counts should be performed.

The use of clindamycin hydrochloride occasionally results in overgrowth of non-susceptible organisms such as clostridia and yeasts. Therefore, the administration of clindamycin hydrochloride should be avoided in those species sensitive to the gastrointestinal effects of clindamycin (see Contraindications). Should superinfections occur, appropriate measures should be taken as indicated by the clinical situation.

Patients with very severe renal disease and/or very severe hepatic disease accompanied by severe metabolic aberrations should be dosed with caution, and serum clindamycin levels monitored during high-dose therapy.

Clindamycin hydrochloride has been shown to have neuromuscular blocking properties that may enhance the action of other neuromuscular blocking agents. Therefore, clindamycin hydrochloride should be used with caution in animals receiving such agents.

Safety in gestating bitches and queens or breeding male dogs and cats has not been established.

Warning(s): Not for human use. For use in animals only.

Toxicology: Toxicology and Safety:

Rat and Dog Data: One year oral toxicity studies in rats and dogs at doses of 30, 100 and 300 mg/kg/day (13.6, 45.5 and 136.4 mg/lb/day) have shown clindamycin hydrochloride to be well tolerated. Differences did not occur in the parameters evaluated to assess toxicity when comparing groups of treated animals with contemporary controls. Rats administered clindamycin hydrochloride at 600 mg/kg/day (272.7 mg/lb/day) for six months tolerated the drug well; however, dogs orally dosed at 600 mg/kg/day (272.7 mg/lb/day) vomited, had anorexia, and subsequently lost weight.

Safety in gestating bitches or breeding males has not been established.

Cat Data: The recommended daily therapeutic dose range for CLINDAMYCIN HYDROCHLORIDE DROPS is 11 to 22 mg/kg/day (5 to 10 mg/lb/day) depending on the severity of the condition. CLINDAMYCIN HYDROCHLORIDE DROPS were tolerated with little evidence of toxicity in domestic shorthair cats when administered orally at 10x the minimum recommended therapeutic daily dose (11 mg/kg; 5 mg/lb) for 15 days, and at doses up to 5x the minimum recommended therapeutic dose for 42 days. Gastrointestinal tract upset (soft feces to diarrhea) occurred in control and treated cats with emesis occurring at doses 3x or greater than the minimum recommended therapeutic dose (11 mg/kg/day; 5 mg/lb/day). Lymphocytic inflammation of the gallbladder was noted in a greater number of treated cats at the 110 mg/kg/day (50 mg/lb/day) dose level than for control cats. No other effects were noted. Safety in gestating queens or breeding male cats has not been established.

Side Effects: Side effects occasionally observed in either clinical trials or during clinical use were vomiting and diarrhea.

Discussion: *In Vitro* Susceptibility Testing: Susceptibility tests should be done on samples collected prior to initiation of therapy with CLINDAMYCIN HYDROCHLORIDE DROPS. Clindamycin susceptibility testing is performed by using Cleocin® Susceptibility Disks (clindamycin 2 mcg) and Cleocin® Susceptibility Powder 20 mg. A standardized disk testing procedure* is recommended for determining susceptibility of aerobic bacteria to clindamycin. A description is contained in the Cleocin® Susceptibility Disk insert. Using this method, the laboratory can designate isolates as resistant, intermediate, or susceptible. Tube or agar dilution methods may be used for aerobic and anaerobic bacteria. When the directions in the Cleocin® Susceptibility Powder insert are followed, a MIC (minimal inhibitory concentration) of 1.6 mcg/mL may be considered susceptible; MICs of 1.6 to 4.8 mcg/mL may be considered intermediate and MICs greater than 4.8 mcg/mL may be considered resistant.

References: Available upon request.

Presentation: CLINDAMYCIN HYDROCHLORIDE DROPS are available as 20 mL (0.68 fl oz) filled in 30 mL bottles (25 mg/mL) supplied in packers containing 12 cartoned bottles with direction labels and calibrated dosing droppers (NDC 57319-380-26).

Manufactured by: Phoenix Scientific, Inc., St. Joseph, MO 64503.

Compendium Code No.: 12560172 Rev. 10-01

CLINDROPS™ ℞

Vetus **Clindamycin**

(Clindamycin Hydrochloride Oral Liquid) Antibiotic

ANADA No.: 200-193

Active Ingredient(s): Each mL of CLINDROPS™ (Clindamycin Hydrochloride Oral Liquid) contains clindamycin hydrochloride equivalent to 25 mg clindamycin; and ethyl alcohol, 8.64%.

Indications: Dogs:

Aerobic bacteria: CLINDROPS™ (Clindamycin Hydrochloride Oral Liquid) is indicated for the treatment of soft tissue infections (wounds and abscesses), dental infections and osteomyelitis caused by susceptible strains of *Staphylococcus aureus.*

Anaerobic bacteria: CLINDROPS™ (Clindamycin Hydrochloride Oral Liquid) is indicated for the treatment of soft tissue infections (deep wounds and abscesses), dental infections and osteomyelitis caused by or associated with susceptible strains of *Bacteroides fragilis, Bacteroides melaninogenicus, Fusobacterium necrophorum* and *Clostridium perfringens.* (See Microbiology section for additional information.)

Cats:

Aerobic bacteria: CLINDROPS™ (Clindamycin Hydrochloride Oral Liquid) is indicated for the treatment of soft tissue infections (wounds and abscesses), and dental infections caused by or associated with susceptible strains of *Staphylococcus aureus, Staphylococcus intermedius* and *Streptococcus* spp.

Anaerobic bacteria: CLINDROPS™ (Clindamycin Hydrochloride Oral Liquid) is indicated for the treatment of soft tissue infections (deep wounds and abscesses) and dental infections caused by or associated with susceptible strains of *Clostridium* perfringens and *Bacteroides fragilis.* (See Microbiology section for additional information).

Pharmacology: Description: CLINDROPS™ (Clindamycin Hydrochloride Oral Liquid) contains clindamycin hydrochloride which is the hydrated salt of clindamycin. Clindamycin is a semi-synthetic antibiotic produced by a 7(S)-chlorosubstitution of the 7(R)-hydroxyl group of a naturally produced antibiotic produced by *Streptomyces lincolnensis var. lincolnensis.*

CLINDROPS™ (Clindamycin Hydrochloride Oral Liquid) is a palatable formulation intended for oral administration to dogs and cats.

Actions:

Site and Mode of Action: Clindamycin is an inhibitor of protein synthesis in the bacterial cell. The site of binding appears to be in the 50S sub-unit of the ribosome. Binding occurs to the soluble RNA fraction of certain ribosomes, thereby inhibiting the binding of amino acids to those ribosomes. Clindamycin differs from cell wall inhibitors in that it causes irreversible modification of the protein-synthesizing subcellular elements at the ribosomal level.

Microbiology: The following clindamycin *in vitro* data are available but their clinical significance is unknown. Clindamycin has been shown to have *in vitro* activity against the following organisms isolated from animals:

Aerobic gram positive cocci, including: *Staphylococcus aureus* (penicillinase and non-penicillinase producing strains), *Staphylococcus intermedius, Staphylococcus simulans, Staphylococcus epidermidis,* Streptococci (except *Enterococcus faecalis).*

Anaerobic gram negative bacilli, including: *Bacteroides* species, *Fusobacterium* species.

Anaerobic gram positive nonsporeforming bacilli, including: *Propionibacterium, Eubacterium, Actinomyces* species.

Anaerobic and microaerophilic gram positive cocci, including: *Peptococcus* species, *Peptostreptococcus* species, Microaerophilic streptococci.

Clostridia: Most *C. perfringens* are susceptible, but other species may be resistant to clindamycin.

Overall Susceptibility to Clindamycin of Anaerobes Isolated from Canine Lesions. Data Obtained from Three Veterinary Diagnostic Laboratories.

	Susceptible ≤3.2 µg/mL	Resistant ≥4.0 µg/mL
All Isolates	122/137 (89%)	15/137 (11%)
Clostridium spp.	41/49 (84%)	8/49 (16%)
Bacteroides spp.	42/46 (91%)	4/46 (9%)
Fusobacterium spp.	16/16 (100%)	0/16 (0%)
Peptostreptococcus spp.	15/16 (94%)	1/16 (6%)
Actinomyces spp.	5/6 (83%)	1/6 (17%)
Proprionibacterium spp.	3/4 (75%)	1/4 (25%)

The MIC values for the anaerobes isolated from feline lesions are not different from the MIC values for the anaerobes isolated from canine lesions.

Mycoplasma species: Most mycoplasma species are susceptible to clindamycin.

Clindamycin and erythromycin show parallel resistance. Partial cross resistance has been demonstrated between clindamycin, erythromycin and macrolide antibiotics.

Absorption: Clindamycin hydrochloride is rapidly absorbed from the canine and feline gastrointestinal tract. Dogs and cats orally dosed with therapeutic amounts of clindamycin hydrochloride demonstrated antibacterial serum levels of the drug within 15 minutes post-dosing.

Canine Serum Levels: Therapeutically effective serum levels of clindamycin hydrochloride can be maintained by oral dosing at the rate of 2.5 mg/lb every 12 hours. Dogs orally dosed with clindamycin hydrochloride at 2.5 mg/lb every 12 hours during a 72 hours dosing regimen continuously maintained antibacterial serum levels of the drug. This same study revealed that average peak serum concentrations occurred 1 hour and 15 minutes after dosing. The biological half-life for clindamycin hydrochloride in dog serum was about 5 hours. There was no bioactivity accumulation after a regimen of multiple oral doses.

Feline Serum Levels: Therapeutically effective serum levels of clindamycin can be maintained by oral dosing at the rate of 5 to 10 mg/lb body weight once every 24 hours. The average peak serum concentration of clindamycin occurs about 1 hour after oral administration. The terminal half-life of clindamycin in feline serum is approximately 7.5 hours. Minimal accumulation occurs after multiple oral doses of clindamycin hydrochloride, and steady-state should be achieved by the third dose.

Clindamycin Serum Concentrations 5 mg/lb (11 mg/kg) After Single Oral Dose of Antirobe® Aquadrops®:

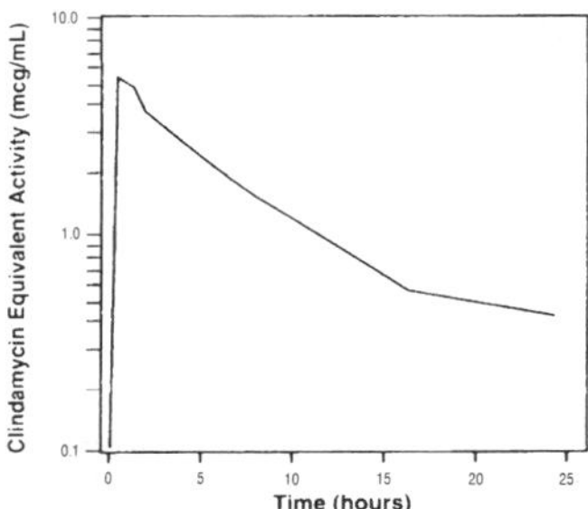

Feline Tissue levels: Tissue concentrations measured at 10 days (μg/g; means) of clindamycin hydrochloride liquid in cats 2 hours after oral administration at 10 mg/lb body weight once every 24 hours for 10 days.

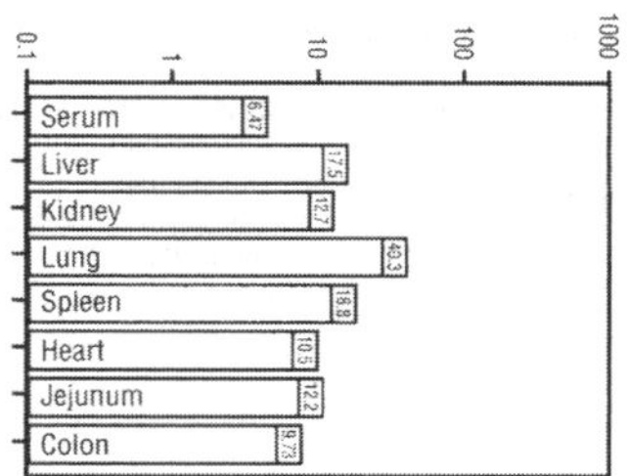

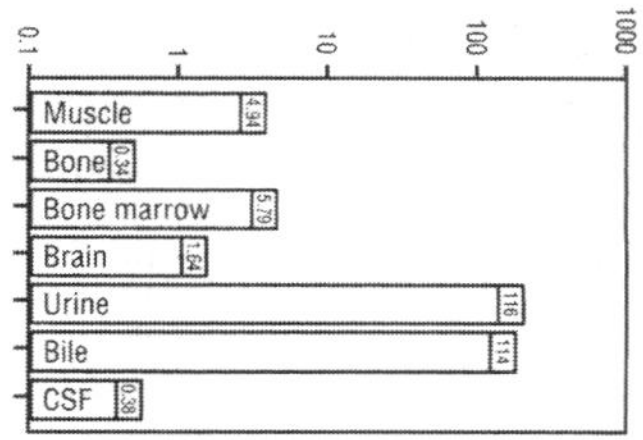

Metabolism and Excretion: Extensive studies of the metabolism and excretion of clindamycin hydrochloride administered orally in animals and humans have shown that unchanged drug and bioactive and bioinactive metabolites are excreted in urine and feces. Almost all of the bioactivity detected in serum after clindamycin hydrochloride product administration is due to the parent molecule (clindamycin). Urine bioactivity, however, reflects a mixture of clindamycin and active metabolites, especially N-demethyl clindamycin and clindamycin sulfoxide.

Dosage and Administration:

Canine Infected Wounds, Abscesses and Dental Infections:

Oral: 2.5 mg/lb body weight every 12 hours.

Duration: Treatment with clindamycin hydrochloride products may be continued up to a maximum of 28 days if clinical judgment indicates. Treatment of acute infections should not be continued for more than three or four days if no response to therapy is seen.

Dosage Schedule:

CLINDROPS™ (Clindamycin Hydrochloride Oral Liquid): Administer 1 mL/10 lbs body weight every 12 hours.

Canine Osteomyelitis:

Oral: 5.0 mg/lb body weight every 12 hours.

Duration: Treatment with CLINDROPS™ (Clindamycin Hydrochloride Oral Liquid) is recommended for a minimum of 28 days. Treatment should not be continued for longer than 28 days if no response to therapy is seen.

Dosage Schedule:

CLINDROPS™ (Clindamycin Hydrochloride Oral Liquid): Administer 2 mL/10 lbs body weight every 12 hours.

Feline Infected Wounds and Abscesses and Dental Infections:

Oral: 5.0 to 10.0 mg/lb body weight once every 24 hours depending on the severity of the condition.

Duration: Treatment with CLINDROPS™ (Clindamycin Hydrochloride Oral Liquid) may be continued up to a maximum of 14 days if clinical judgment indicates. Treatment of acute infections should not be continued for more than three to four days if no clinical response to therapy is seen.

Dosage Schedule: CLINDROPS™ (Clindamycin Hydrochloride Oral Liquid), to provide 5.0 mg/lb, administer 1 mL/5 lb body weight once every 24 hours; to provide 10.0 mg/lb, administer 2 mL/5 lb body weight once every 24 hours.

Contraindication(s): CLINDROPS™ (Clindamycin Hydrochloride Oral Liquid) is contraindicated in animals with a history of hypersensitivity to preparations containing clindamycin or lincomycin.

Because of potential adverse gastrointestinal effects, do not administer to rabbits, hamsters, guinea pigs, horses, chinchillas or ruminating animals.

Precaution(s): Store at controlled room temperature 20°-25°C (68°-77°F).

Caution(s): Federal (USA) law restricts this drug to use by or on the order of a licensed veterinarian.

CLINDROPS™ (Clindamycin Hydrochloride Oral Liquid) should be prescribed with caution in atopic animals.

During prolonged therapy of one month or greater, periodic liver and kidney function tests and blood counts should be performed.

The use of clindamycin hydrochloride occasionally results in overgrowth of non-susceptible organisms such as clostridia and yeasts. Therefore, the administration of clindamycin hydrochloride should be avoided in those species sensitive to the gastrointestinal effects of clindamycin (see Contraindications). Should superinfections occur, appropriate measures should be taken as indicated by the clinical situation.

Patients with very severe renal disease and/or very severe hepatic disease accompanied by severe metabolic aberrations should be dosed with caution, and serum clindamycin levels monitored during high-dose therapy.

Clindamycin hydrochloride has been shown to have neuromuscular blocking properties that may enhance the action of other neuromuscular blocking agents. Therefore, clindamycin hydrochloride should be used with caution in animals receiving such agents.

Safety in gestating bitches and queens or breeding male dogs and cats has not been established.

Warning(s): Not for human use.

Toxicology: Toxicology and Safety:

Rat and Dog Data: One year oral toxicity studies in rats and dogs at doses of 30, 100 and 300 mg/kg/day (13.6, 45.5 and 136.4 mg/lb/day) have shown clindamycin hydrochloride to be well tolerated. Differences did not occur in the parameters evaluated to assess toxicity when comparing groups of treated animals with contemporary controls. Rats administered clindamycin hydrochloride at 600 mg/kg/day (272.7 mg/lb/day) for six months tolerated the drug well; however, dogs orally dosed at 600 mg/kg/day (272.7 mg/lb/day) vomited, had anorexia, and subsequently lost weight.

Safety in gestating bitches or breeding males has not been established.

Cat Data: The recommended daily therapeutic dose range for CLINDROPS™ (Clindamycin Hydrochloride Oral Liquid) is 11 to 22 mg/kg/day (5 to 10 mg/lb/day) depending on the severity of the condition. CLINDROPS™ (Clindamycin Hydrochloride Oral Liquid) was tolerated with little evidence of toxicity in domestic shorthair cats when administered orally at 10x the minimum recommended therapeutic daily dose (11 mg/kg; 5 mg/lb) for 15 days, and at doses up to 5x the minimum recommended therapeutic dose for 42 days. Gastrointestinal tract upset (soft feces to diarrhea) occurred in control and treated cats with emesis occurring at doses 3x or greater than the minimum recommended therapeutic dose (11 mg/kg/day; 5 mg/lb/day). Lymphocytic inflammation of the gallbladder was noted in a greater number of treated cats at the 110 mg/kg/day (50 mg/lb/day) dose level than for control cats. No other effects were noted. Safety in gestating queens or breeding male cats has not been established.

Side Effects: Side effects occasionally observed in either clinical trials or during clinical use were vomiting and diarrhea.

Discussion: *In Vitro* Susceptibility Testing: Susceptibility tests should be done on samples collected prior to initiation of therapy with CLINDROPS™ (Clindamycin Hydrochloride Oral Liquid). Clindamycin susceptibility testing is performed by using Cleocin® Susceptibility Disks (clindamycin 2 mcg) and Cleocin® Susceptibility Powder 20 mg. A standardized disk testing procedure* is recommended for determining susceptibility of aerobic bacteria to clindamycin. A description is contained in the Cleocin® Susceptibility Disk insert. Using this method, the laboratory can designate isolates as resistant, intermediate, or susceptible. Tube or agar dilution methods may be used for aerobic and anaerobic bacteria. When the directions in the Cleocin® Susceptibility Powder insert are followed, a MIC (minimal inhibitory concentration) of 1.6 mcg/mL may be considered susceptible; MICs of 1.6 to 4.8 mcg/mL may be considered intermediate and MICs greater than 4.8 mcg/mL may be considered resistant.

References: *Available upon request.

Presentation: CLINDROPS™ (Clindamycin Hydrochloride Oral Liquid) is available as 20 mL filled in 30 mL bottles (25 mg/mL) supplied in packers containing 12 cartoned bottles with direction labels and calibrated dosing droppers.

Manufactured by: Phoenix Scientific, Inc., St. Joseph, MO 64503.

Distributed by: Burns Veterinary Supply, Inc., Westbury, NY 11590.

Compendium Code No.: 14440211 Rev. 01/01

CLINICARE® CANINE LIQUID DIET

Abbott **Therapeutic Diet**

Guaranteed Analysis:

Crude protein, min 5.4%
Crude fat, min 6.2%
Crude fiber, max 0.05%
Moisture, max. 82.0%
Ash, max. 1.2%
Calcium, min. 0.17%
Phosphorus, min 0.13%
Potassium, min. 0.15%
Sodium, min 0.05%
Chloride, min 0.09%
Magnesium, min 0.01%

Ingredients: Water, maltodextrin (corn), sodium caseinate, soy oil, butter, dried whey protein concentrate, egg yolks, calcium phosphate tribasic, potassium citrate, soy lecithin, calcium carbonate, potassium chloride, potassium phosphate monobasic, choline chloride, magnesium chloride, l-arginine, dl-methionine, potassium phosphate dibasic, carrageenan, ferrous sulfate, taurine, zinc sulfate, calcium phosphate dibasic, ascorbic acid, dl-alpha-tocopherol acetate, manganese sulfate, niacinamide, citric acid, d-calcium pantothenate, copper sulfate, thiamine hydrochloride, vitamin A palmitate, riboflavin, pyridoxine hydrochloride, folic acid, biotin, vitamin D_3 supplement, potassium iodide, sodium molybdate, sodium selenite and vitamin B_{12} supplement.

Calorie Content (ME calculated): 1.0 kcal/mL; 959 kcal/kg.

Calorie Distribution: protein, 20%; fat, 55%; carbohydrate, 25%.

Product Density: 1.04 g/mL.

Indications: CLINICARE® Canine Liquid Diet is a palatable, liquid food designed for the intermittent or supplemental feeding of dogs.

Dosage and Administration:

Suggested daily feeding rates at 1 kcal/mL		
wt (lbs)	wt (kg)	mL
10	4.6	218
20	9.1	366
40	18.2	616
80	36.4	1037

Follow veterinarian's instructions.

Adjust volume and dilution according to animal's condition and tolerance. Avoid contamination during preparation and use.

Precaution(s): Shake well. Store unopened at room temperature. Once opened, cover, refrigerate and use within 48 hours.

Use by date on end of can.

Caution(s): Use only as directed by your veterinarian.

For animal use only.

Not for parenteral use.

Presentation: 8 fl oz (237 mL).

Compendium Code No.: 10240000

CLINICARE® FELINE LIQUID DIET

Abbott **Therapeutic Diet**

Ready to Feed-Veterinary Nutritional Supplement

Guaranteed Analysis:

Crude protein, min 8.2%
Crude fat, min 5.1%
Crude fiber, max. 0.05%
Moisture, max. 81.0%
Ash, max 1.2%
Calcium, min 0.14%
Phosphorus, min 0.12%
Potassium, min 0.13%
Sodium, min 0.05%
Chloride, min 0.10%
Magnesium, min 0.01%

Ingredients: Water, sodium caseinate, malto-dextrin (corn), soy oil, dried whey protein concentrate, butter, egg yolks, calcium phosphate tribasic, potassium citrate, potassium chloride, calcium carbonate, l-arginine, lecithin, magnesium sulfate, choline chloride, taurine, carrageenan, calcium phosphate dibasic, ascorbic acid, ferrous sulfate, zinc sulfate, dl-alpha-tocopherol acetate, niacinamide, manganese sulfate, d-calcium pantothenate, citric acid, thiamine hydrochloride, copper sulfate, riboflavin, pyridoxine hydrochloride, vitamin A palmitate, folic acid, biotin, vitamin D_3 supplement, potassium iodide, sodium molybdate, sodium selenite and vitamin B_{12} supplement.

Calorie Content (ME calculated): 1.0 kcal/mL; 959 kcal/kg.

Calorie Distribution: protein, 30%; fat, 45%; carbohydrate, 25%.

Product Density: 1.04 g/mL.

Indications: CLINICARE® Feline Liquid Diet is a palatable, liquid food designed for the intermittent or supplemental feeding of cats.

Dosage and Administration: Suggested daily feeding rates at 1 kcal/mL:

wt (lbs)	wt (kg)	mL
5	2.3	130
10	4.6	218
15	6.8	295

Follow veterinarian's instructions.

Adjust volume and dilution according to animal's condition and tolerance. Avoid contamination during preparation and use.

Precaution(s): Use by date on end of can. Shake well.

Store unopened at room temperature. Once opened, cover, refrigerate and use within 48 hours.

Caution(s): Use only as directed by your veterinarian.

For animal use only.

Not for parenteral use.

Presentation: 8 fl oz (237 mL).

Compendium Code No.: 10240011 5023 RL-407/2

CLINICARE® RF SPECIALIZED FELINE LIQUID DIET

Abbott **Therapeutic Diet**

Guaranteed Analysis:

Crude protein, min 6.1%
Crude fat, min 6.5%
Crude fiber, max. 0.05%
Moisture, max. 82.0%
Ash, max 1.0%
Calcium, min 0.12%
Phosphorus, min 0.10%
Potassium, min 0.10%
Sodium, min 0.04%
Chloride, min 0.05%
Magnesium, min 0.009%

Ingredients: Water, maltodextrin (corn), sodium caseinate, soy oil, butter, dried whey protein concentrate, calcium phosphate tribasic, potassium citrate, mono- and diglycerides, l-arginine, dl-methionine, citric acid, calcium carbonate, taurine, magnesium chloride, potassium chloride, choline chloride, carrageenan, calcium phosphate dibasic, ascorbic acid, ferrous sulfate, zinc sulfate, niacinamide, dl-alpha-tocopherol acetate, manganese sulfate, d-calcium pantothenate, thiamine hydrochloride, copper sulfate, riboflavin, pyridoxine hydrochloride, vitamin A palmitate, folic acid, biotin, vitamin D_3 supplement, potassium iodide, sodium molybdate, sodium selenite and vitamin B_{12} supplement.

Calorie Content (ME calculated): 1.0 kcal/mL; 971 kcal/kg.

Calorie Distribution: protein, 22%; fat, 57%; carbohydrate, 21%.

Product Density: 1.03 g/mL.

Indications: CLINICARE® RF Specialized Feline Liquid Diet is a palatable, liquid food reduced in protein and electrolytes designed for the intermittent or supplemental feeding of cats.

Dosage and Administration:

Suggested daily feeding rates at 1 kcal/mL		
wt (lbs)	wt (kg)	mL
5	2.3	130
10	4.6	218
15	6.8	295

Follow veterinarian's instructions.

Adjust volume and dilution according to animal's condition and tolerance. Avoid contamination during preparation and use.

Precaution(s): Shake well. Store unopened at room temperature. Once opened, cover, refrigerate and use within 48 hours.

Use by date on end of can.

Caution(s): Use only as directed by your veterinarian.

For animal use only.

Not for parenteral use.

Presentation: 8 fl oz (237 mL).

Compendium Code No.: 10240020

CLOMICALM® ℞

Novartis **Antidepressant**

Clomipramine hydrochloride

NADA No.: 141-120

Active Ingredient(s): CLOMICALM® Tablets are oblong, light brown in color and contain clomipramine hydrochloride formulated together with meat components. CLOMICALM® Tablets are available in 20, 40 and 80 mg tablet strengths in color-coded packaging for oral administration to dogs.

Indications: CLOMICALM® Tablets are to be used as part of a comprehensive behavioral management program to treat separation anxiety in dogs greater than 6 months of age. Inappropriate barking or destructive behavior, as well as inappropriate elimination (urination or defecation) may be alleviated by the use of CLOMICALM® Tablets in conjunction with behavior modification.

Separation anxiety is a complex behavior disorder displayed when the owner (or other attachment figure) leaves the dog. The signs of separation anxiety evaluated in controlled trials were vocalization, destructive behavior, excessive salivation, and inappropriate elimination. In the absence of the owner or attachment figure, dogs with separation anxiety may exhibit one or more of these clinical signs. Although the owner (attachment figure) may inadvertently misinterpret this behavior, which only happens in their absence, as spiteful, it is thought to be the result of anxiety experienced by the dog. Punishment is not considered appropriate for a dog with separation anxiety.

Proper recognition of clinical signs, including a complete patient history and assessment of the patient's household environment, is essential to accurately diagnose and treat separation anxiety.

The use of CLOMICALM® Tablets should not replace appropriate behavioral and environmental management but should be used to facilitate a comprehensive behavior management program.

Pharmacology: Description: CLOMICALM® (clomipramine hydrochloride) Tablets belong to the dibenzazepine class of tricyclic antidepressants. Clomipramine hydrochloride is 3-chloro-5[3-(dimethyl-amino)propyl]-10,11-dihydro-5H-dibenz[b,f]azepine monohydrochloride. The molecular weight of clomipramine hydrochloride is 351.3. The structural formula is:

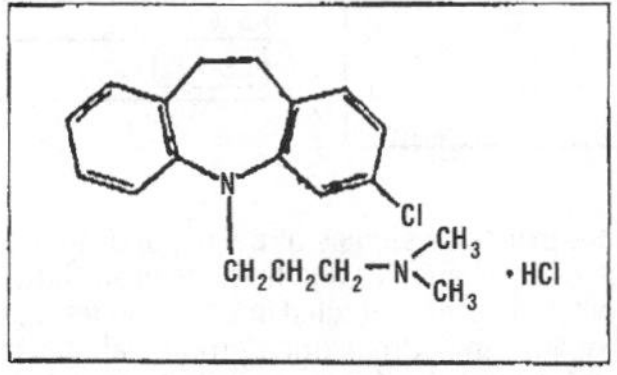

Clinical Pharmacology: Clomipramine hydrochloride reduces the clinical signs of separation anxiety by affecting serotonergic and noradrenergic neuronal transmission in the central nervous system. While clomipramine hydrochloride can cause lethargy in dogs (see Adverse Reactions) its mode of action is not as a sedative. Clomipramine hydrochloride's capacity to inhibit re-uptake of serotonin in the central nervous system is believed to be the primary mechanism of action.

Clomipramine hydrochloride is rapidly absorbed when administered orally. A single-dose crossover study involving 12 dogs evaluated clomipramine hydrochloride bioavailability after IV (2 mg/kg) and oral (4 mg/kg) administration in either a fed or fasted state. The administration of clomipramine hydrochloride in the presence of food resulted in an increase in the rate and extent of drug absorption as shown in the following table (mean ± SD):

	$AUC_{0\text{-inf}}$ (nmol hr/L)	C_{max} (nmol/L)	T_{max} (hr)	Absolute Bioavailability (F)
Fed	1670±575	601±286	1.18±0.32	0.21±0.07
Fasted	1350±447	379±154	1.31±0.32	0.17±0.05

The absolute bioavailability is approximately 25% greater in fed dogs. The apparent terminal plasma half-life ranges from approximately 2 to 9 hours in fed and 3 to 21 hours in fasted dogs. The difference and variability in apparent half-life estimates may be attributable to prolonged drug absorption in the fasted state. The relatively large volume of distribution (3.8 ± 0.8 L/kg) suggests that the drug is widely distributed throughout the body.

Dosage and Administration: The recommended daily dose of CLOMICALM® Tablets is 2 to 4 mg/kg/day (0.9-1.8 mg/lb/day) (see dosing table below). It can be administered as a single daily dose or divided twice daily based on patient response and/or tolerance of the side effects. It may be prudent to initiate treatment in divided doses to minimize side effects by permitting tolerance to side effects to develop or allowing the patient time to adapt if tolerance does not develop. To reduce the incidence of vomiting that may be experienced by some dogs, CLOMICALM® Tablets may be given with a small amount of food.

Dog Weight (lbs)	CLOMICALM® per Day	No. Tablets per Day	Tablet Strength
11-22	20 mg	1	20 mg
22.1-44	40 mg	1	40 mg
44.1-88	80 mg	1	80 mg
88.1-176	160 mg	2	80 mg

The specific methods of behavioral modification used in clinical trials involved desensitization and counterconditioning techniques. Since the manifestation of separation anxiety can vary according to the individual dog, it is advised that a specific behavior modification plan be developed based on a professional assessment of each individual case.

Once the desired clinical effect is achieved and the owners have successfully instituted the appropriate behavioral modification, the dose of CLOMICALM® Tablets may be reduced to maintain the desired effect or discontinued. Withdrawal side effects were not reported in studies with CLOMICALM® Tablets in dogs. However, in clinical practice, it is recommended to taper the individual patient dose while continuing to monitor the dog's behavior and clinical status through the dose reduction or withdrawal period. Continued behavioral modification is recommended to prevent recurrence of the clinical signs.

The effectiveness and clinical safety of CLOMICALM® Tablets for long-term use (i.e., for more than 12 weeks) has not been evaluated.

Professional judgement should be used in monitoring the patient's clinical status, response to therapy and tolerance to side effects to determine the need to continue treatment with CLOMICALM® Tablets and to continue to rule-out physiological disorders which may complicate the diagnosis and treatment of separation anxiety.

Contraindication(s): CLOMICALM® Tablets are contraindicated in dogs with known hypersensitivity to clomipramine or other tricyclic antidepressants.

CLOMICALM® Tablets should not be used in male breeding dogs. Testicular hypoplasia was seen in dogs treated for 1 year at 12.5 times the maximum daily dose.

CLOMICALM® Tablets should not be given in combination, or within 14 days before or after treatment with a monoamine oxidase inhibitor [e.g. selegiline hydrochloride (L-deprenyl), amitraz].

CLOMICALM® Tablets are contraindicated for use in dogs with a history of seizures or concomitantly with drugs which lower the seizure threshold.

Precaution(s): Storage Conditions: Store in a dry place at controlled room temperature, between 59° and 86°F (15-30°C).

Caution(s): Federal (USA) law restricts this drug to use by or on the order of a licensed veterinarian.

General: CLOMICALM® Tablets are not recommended for other behavior problems, such as aggression (see Adverse Reactions). Studies to establish the safety and efficacy of CLOMICALM® Tablets in dogs less than 6 months of age have not been conducted.

Diagnosis: It is critical to conduct a comprehensive physical examination, including appropriate laboratory tests, and to obtain a thorough history and assessment of the patient's household environment, to rule-out causes of inappropriate behavior unrelated to separation anxiety before prescribing CLOMICALM® Tablets.

Veterinarians should be familiar with the risks and benefits of the treatment of behavioral disorders in dogs before initiating therapy. Inappropriate use of CLOMICALM® Tablets, i.e., in the absence of a diagnosis or without concurrent behavioral modification, may expose the animal to unnecessary adverse effects and may not provide any lasting benefit of therapy.

Drug Interactions: Recommendations on the interaction between clomipramine and other medications are extrapolated from data generated in humans. Plasma concentrations of clomipramine have been reported to be increased by the concomitant administration of phenobarbital. Plasma levels of closely related tricyclic antidepressants have been reported to be increased by the concomitant administration of hepatic enzyme inhibitors (e.g., cimetidine, fluoxetine). Plasma levels of closely related tricyclic antidepressants have been reported to be decreased by the concomitant administration of hepatic enzyme inducers (e.g. barbiturates, phenytoin). Caution is advised in using clomipramine with anticholinergic or sympathomimetic drugs or with other CNS-active drugs, including general anesthetics and neuroleptics.

Prior to elective surgery with general anesthetics, clomipramine should be discontinued for as long as clinically feasible.

Use in Concomitant Illness: Use with caution in dogs with cardiovascular disease. At 20 mg/kg/day (5X the maximum recommended dose), bradycardia and arrhythmias (atrioventricular node block and ventricular extrasystole) were observed in dogs. Because of its anticholinergic properties, clomipramine should be used with caution in patients with increased intraocular pressure, a history of narrow angle glaucoma, urinary retention or reduced gastrointestinal motility.

Reproductive Safety: Safety studies to determine the effects of CLOMICALM® Tablets in pregnant or lactating female dogs have not been conducted. CLOMICALM® Tablets should not be used in breeding males (see Contraindications).

Warning(s): Human Warnings: Not for use in humans. Keep out of reach of children. In case of accidental ingestion seek medical attention immediately. In children, accidental ingestion should be regarded as serious. There is no specific antidote for clomipramine. Overdose in humans causes anticholinergic effects including effects on the central nervous (e.g., convulsions) and cardiovascular (e.g., arrhythmia, tachycardia) systems. People with known hypersensitivity to clomipramine should administer the product with caution.

Keep this and all drugs out of reach of children.

To report suspected adverse reactions or in case of accidental human ingestion, call 1-800-637-0281.

Adverse Reactions: Frequency and category of adverse reactions observed in dogs dosed with CLOMICALM® Tablets or placebo were observed in multisite clinical studies as follows.

Adverse Reactions Reported in Placebo-Controlled Clinical Field Trials		
	CLOMICALM® N=180	Placebo N=88
Emesis	36 (20%)	8 (9%)
Lethargy	26 (14%)	7 (8%)
Diarrhea	17 (9%)	4 (5%)
Polydipsia	6 (3%)	0
Decreased Appetite	6 (3%)	3 (3%)
Aggression*	3 (2%)	1 (1%)
Seizure	2 (1%)	0
Dry Mouth	1 (0.5%)	1 (1%)
Tremors	1 (0.5%)	0
Constipation	1 (0.5%)	0
Anisocoria	1 (0.5%)	0
Polyuria	1 (0.5%)	0
Hyperthermia	1 (0.5%)	0

*These dogs displayed growling behavior towards either humans or other dogs.

Trial Data: Efficacy:

Dose Establishment: A 12 week, placebo-controlled, multi-site clinical trial was conducted in the US and Europe to establish an effective dose of CLOMICALM® Tablets in dogs. Treatment with CLOMICALM® Tablets, at 2 - 4 mg/kg/day divided twice daily, in conjunction with behavioral modification (desensitization and counterconditioning) was more effective than behavior modification alone in reducing the signs of separation anxiety in dogs.

Dose Confirmation: In another placebo-controlled, multi-site clinical trial, CLOMICALM® Tablets at 2 - 4 mg/kg/day given either once daily or divided twice daily showed significant improvement in resolving signs of separation anxiety when tested against behavioral modification alone (desensitization and counterconditioning). In this 8 week study, the rate of improvement of the dogs receiving CLOMICALM® Tablets with behavioral modification was significantly faster than the rate of improvement of the dogs receiving behavioral modification alone. After one week on trial, 47% of the dogs receiving CLOMICALM® Tablets once or twice (divided dose) daily in conjunction with behavioral modification showed clinical improvement compared to improvement in 29% of the dogs receiving behavioral modification alone.

Safety: CLOMICALM® Tablets were demonstrated to be well-tolerated in dogs at the recommended label dose of 2-4 mg/kg/day. In a six-month target animal safety study, beagle dogs were dosed daily at 4 (1X), 12 (3X), and 20 (5X) mg/kg/day. Emesis was seen in all groups including the dogs receiving placebo, but occurred more frequently in dogs receiving 12 and 20 mg/kg. Decreased activity was also seen in dogs receiving the 12 and 20 mg/kg. There were no apparent treatment-related alterations in the following: body weights, physical examination findings, electrocardiograph examinations, hematology or biochemistry parameters, ophthalmoscopic examinations, macroscopic or microscopic organ examinations and organ weights. Average food and water consumption over the 26-week period was similar for control and treated groups.

In a one-year study, pure bred dogs were dosed daily at 12.5 (3X), 50 (12.5X), and 100 (25X) mg/kg/day. Emesis and mydriasis were observed within 15 minutes to one hour after dosing in dogs receiving 12.5, 50, and 100 mg/kg/day and lethargy was observed within 1 hour of dosing in dogs receiving 50 and 100 mg/kg. Testicular hypoplasia was seen in dogs receiving 50 mg/kg. At 100 mg/kg/day (25X) convulsions and eventual death occurred in five out of the eight dogs.

Presentation: 25 tablets per bottle.

Compendium Code No.: 11310002

NAH/CLO-T/VI/2 07/00

C

CLONEVAC-30®

Intervet **Vaccine**

Newcastle Disease Vaccine, B_1 Type, LaSota Strain, Live Virus

U.S. Vet. Lic. No.: 286

Description: CLONEVAC-30® is prepared using SPF substrates from the proven Clone 30® strain of Newcastle disease virus. Intervet's Research team cloned several lentogenic ND virus strains to separate possible sub-populations within these strains. These clones were then extensively tested for immunogenicity and reactivity. One clone, designated ND virus Clone 30®, was selected and proven to be of the same order of reactivity as the classical Hitchner B_1, but provided considerably better protection.

The Clone 30® strain has been propagated under exacting standards using SPF substrates. The immunizing capability of this vaccine has also been proven by the Master Seed Immunogenicity Test. This vaccine contains gentamicin as a preservative.

Quality tested for purity, potency, and safety.

Indications: Drinking Water: Vaccination of healthy chickens two weeks of age or older for protection against Newcastle disease.

Coarse Spray: Vaccination of healthy chicken two weeks of age or older for protection against Newcastle disease.

Revaccination at older ages is recommended for optimum protection. Initial vaccination should be by drinking water or intraocular route.

Dosage and Administration: Vaccination Programs: Many factors must be considered in determining a sound vaccination program for a particular farm or poultry complex. To be fully effective, the vaccine must be administered properly to healthy, receptive animals maintained in a proper environment under good management. In addition, the response may be influenced by the age of the animals and their immune status. Seldom does one live virus vaccination under field conditions produce lifetime protection for all individuals in a given flock. The level of immunity required will vary with operational practices and the degree of exposure. Therefore, a program of periodic revaccinations may be necessary.

Preparation of Vaccine:

For Drinking Water or Coarse Spray Use: Do not open and mix the vaccine until ready to begin vaccination. Use the vaccine immediately after mixing.

1. The initial use of the vaccine should be by drinking water or eye drop administration.
2. Remove the tear-off seal and stopper from the vial containing the dried vaccine.
3. Carefully pour clean, cool, non-chlorinated water into the vaccine vial until the vial is approximately two-thirds full.
4. Insert the rubber stopper and shake vigorously until all material is dissolved.
5. The vaccine is now ready for drinking water or coarse spray use in accordance with directions below. For best results, be sure to follow the directions carefully!

Drinking Water Administration:

For Chickens Two Weeks of Age or Older:

1. Do not use any disinfectants in the drinking water for 48 hours before vaccinating and for 24 hours after vaccination.
2. Withhold the drinking water from the chickens until they are thirsty. Withholding periods will vary from 2 to 8 hours according to age of chickens and climatic conditions. Be careful in hot weather.
3. Scrub and rinse waterers thoroughly with fresh, clean water. Do not use disinfectants for cleaning the waterers.
4. Rehydrate the vaccine as directed above.
5. Mix rehydrated vaccine with clean, cool, non-chlorinated water in accordance with the chart below.

Age of Chickens	Water Per 1,000 Doses Vaccine
2-4 weeks	6 gal. (23 liters)
4-8 weeks	10 gal. (38 liters)
8 weeks or older	16 gal. (60 liters)

As an aid in preserving the virus, 3.2 ounces of non-fat powdered milk may be added with each 10 gallons (38 liters) of water used for mixing vaccine. Add the dried milk first and mix until dissolved. Then add the rehydrated vaccine from the vial and again mix thoroughly.

6. Distribute the vaccine solution, as prepared above, among the waterers provided for the chickens. Avoid placing waterers in direct sunlight.
7. Provide no other drinking water until all the vaccine-water solution has been consumed.

Coarse Spray Administration:

For Chickens Two Weeks of Age or Older:

1. Initial spray vaccination should be of coarse spray, i.e., Hardi®.
2. Do not use any disinfectants or skim milk in sprayer.
3. Use sprayer only for administration of vaccines. Clean thoroughly after each use.
4. Shut off all fans while spray vaccinating. Turn on the fan immediately after spraying. Be careful in hot weather.
5. Spray the chickens by walking slowly through the house.
6. Follow the recommendation of the manufacturer of the sprayer regarding water volume and particle size.
7. Use only clean, cool, deionized water.
8. Individual(s) spraying chickens should wear face mask and goggles.

Records: Keep a record of vaccine, quantity, serial number, expiration date, and place of purchase; the date and time of vaccination; the number, age, breed, and location of chickens; names of operators performing the vaccination and any observed reactions.

Precaution(s): Store vaccine between 2 and 7°C (35 and 45°F).

Do not spill or splash the vaccine.
Use entire contents when first opened.
Burn containers and all unused contents.
This product is non-returnable.

Caution(s): Vaccinate only healthy chickens. Although disease may not be evident, coccidiosis, Mycoplasma infection, infectious bursal disease, Avian Reovirus disease, Marek's disease, and other disease conditions may cause complications or reduce immunity.

All susceptible chickens on the same premises should be vaccinated at the same time.

Efforts should be taken to reduce stress conditions at the time of vaccination and during the reaction period.

Do not dilute the vaccine or otherwise stretch the dosage.

For veterinary use only.

Notice: This vaccine has undergone rigid potency, safety and purity tests, and meets Intervet Inc. and USDA requirements. It is designed to stimulate effective immunity when used as directed, but the user must be advised that the response to the product depends upon many factors, including, but not limited to, conditions of storage and handling by the user, administration of the vaccine, health and responsiveness of the individual chickens, and the degree of field exposure. Therefore, directions should be followed carefully!

This product is not hazardous when used according to directions supplied. A material safety data sheet (MSDS) is available upon request. This and any other consumer information can be obtained by calling Intervet Customer Service at 1-800-441-8272 or 1-302-934-8051.

The use of this vaccine is subject to applicable local and federal laws and regulations.

Use only as directed.

Warning(s): Do not vaccinate within 21 days before slaughter.

Newcastle virus occasionally causes conjunctivitis in humans, lasting two or three days. Avoid any contact of vaccine with eyes.

Presentation: 10 x 2,000 doses for drinking water or coarse spray use.
10 x 10,000 doses for drinking water or coarse spray use.

Compendium Code No.: 11060341 IAI 00208 AL 97

CLONEVAC-30®-T

Intervet **Vaccine**

Newcastle Disease Vaccine, B$_1$ Type, LaSota Strain, Live Virus

U.S. Vet. Lic. No.: 286

Description: CLONEVAC-30®-T, a live virus vaccine, is prepared from the proven Clone 30® strain of Newcastle disease virus.

Intervet's Research team cloned several lentogenic ND virus strains to separate possible sub-populations within these strains. These clones were then extensively tested for immunogenicity and reactivity. One clone, designated ND virus Clone 30®, was selected and proven to be of the same order of reactivity as the classical Hitchner B$_1$, but provided considerably better protection.

The Clone 30® strain has been propagated under exacting standards using SPF substrates. The immunizing capability of this vaccine has also been proven by the Master Seed Immunogenicity Test.

This vaccine contains gentamicin as a preservative.

Quality tested for purity, potency, and safety.

Indications: Drinking Water: Vaccination of healthy turkeys two weeks of age or older for protection against Newcastle disease.

If turkeys are vaccinated at two weeks of age, revaccination at later times is recommended for optimum protection for the life of the flock.

Dosage and Administration: Vaccination Program: Many factors must be considered in determining a sound vaccination program for a particular farm or poultry complex. To be fully effective, the vaccine must be administered properly to healthy, receptive animals maintained in a proper environment under good management. In addition, the response may be influenced by the age of the animals and their immune status. Seldom does one live virus vaccination under field conditions produce life-time protection for all individuals in a given flock. The level of immunity required will vary with operational practices and the degree of exposure. Therefore, a program of periodic revaccinations may be necessary.

Preparation of Vaccine:

For Drinking Water Use: Do not open and mix the vaccine until ready to begin vaccination. Use vaccine immediately after mixing.

1. Remove the tear-off seal and stopper from the vial containing the dried vaccine.
2. Carefully pour clean, cool, non-chlorinated tap water into the vaccine vial until the vial is approximately two-thirds full.
3. Insert the rubber stopper and shake vigorously until all material is dissolved.
4. The vaccine is now ready for drinking water use in accordance with directions below. For best results, be sure to follow the directions carefully!

Drinking Water Administration:

For Turkeys Two Weeks of Age or Older:

1. Do not use any disinfectants in the drinking water for 48 hours before vaccinating and for 24 hours after vaccination.
2. Withhold the water from the turkeys until they are thirsty. Withholding periods will vary from 2 to 8 hours according to age of turkeys and climatic conditions. Be careful in hot weather.
3. Scrub and rinse waterers thoroughly with fresh, clean water. Do not use disinfectants for cleaning the waterers.
4. Rehydrate the vaccine as directed above.
5. Mix rehydrated vaccine with clean, cool, non-chlorinated tap water in accordance with the following chart:

Age of Turkeys	Water Per 1,000 Doses Vaccine
2-4 weeks	6 gal. (23 liters)
4-8 weeks	10 gal. (38 liters)
8 weeks or older	16 gal. (60 liters)

As an aid in preserving the virus, 3.2 ounces (100 g) of non-fat powdered milk may be added with each 10 gallons (38 liters) of water used for mixing vaccine. Add the dried milk first and mix until dissolved. Then add the rehydrated vaccine from the vial and mix thoroughly.

6. Distribute the vaccine solution, as prepared above, among the waterers provided for the turkeys. Avoid placing waterers in direct sunlight.
7. Provide no other drinking water until all the vaccine-water solution has been consumed.

Records: Keep a record of vaccine, quantity, serial number, expiration date, and place of purchase; the date and time of vaccination; the number, age, breed, and location of turkeys; names of operators performing the vaccination and any observed reactions.

Precaution(s): Store vaccine between 2 and 7°C (35 and 45°F). Do not freeze.

Do not spill or splash the vaccine.
Use entire contents when first opened.
Burn containers and all unused contents.
This product is non-returnable.

Caution(s): For drinking water use only.

Vaccinate only healthy turkeys. Although disease may not be evident, coccidiosis, Mycoplasma infection, infectious bursal disease, Marek's disease and other disease conditions may cause complications or reduce immunity.

All susceptible turkeys on the same premises should be vaccinated at the same time.

Efforts should be taken to reduce stress conditions at the time of vaccination and during the reaction period.

Do not dilute the vaccine or otherwise stretch the dosage.

For veterinary use only.

Notice: This vaccine has undergone rigid potency, safety and purity tests, and meets Intervet Inc. and USDA requirements. It is designed to stimulate effective immunity when used as directed, but the user must be advised that the response to the product depends upon many factors, including, but not limited to, conditions of storage and handling by the user, administration of the vaccine, health and responsiveness of individual chickens, and the degree of field exposure. Therefore, directions should be followed carefully.

This product is not hazardous when used according to directions supplied. A material safety data sheet (MSDS) is available upon request. This and any other consumer information can be obtained by calling Intervet Customer Service at 1-800-441-8272 or 1-302-934-8051.

The use of this vaccine is subject to applicable federal and local laws and regulations.

Use only as directed.

Warning(s): Do not vaccinate within 21 days before slaughter.

Newcastle virus occasionally causes conjunctivitis in humans, lasting two or three days. Avoid any contact of vaccine with eyes.

Presentation: 10 x 2,000 doses for drinking water use.

Compendium Code No.: 11060361 00256 AL 109.2.0

CLONEVAC D-78®

Intervet **Vaccine**

Bursal Disease Vaccine, Live Virus

U.S. Vet. Lic. No.: 286

Description: CLONEVAC D-78® contains an intermediate strain of infectious bursal disease (IBD) virus propagated in SPF (Specific Pathogen Free) chicken embryos. This strain was developed from a bursal isolate by cloning. The vaccine contains gentamicin as a preservative.

Indications: CLONEVAC D-78®, a live virus vaccine, is indicated for initial vaccination of healthy chickens two weeks of age or older via drinking water or one day or older via coarse spray for the prevention of infectious bursal disease (IBD) - also known as Gumboro Disease. The vaccine may also be used for priming of breeder replacement pullets.

Dosage and Administration: Immune status, general health, and field exposure to IBD virus must be assessed to develop an effective program. Immunological priming of breeder replacement chickens can be accomplished at 10 to 12 weeks of age, followed by the use of an inactivated vaccine at 18-20 weeks of age.

Preparation of Vaccine: For drinking water use or coarse spray use:

Do not open and mix the vaccine until ready to begin vaccination. Use the vaccine immediately after mixing.

1. Remove the tear-off seal and stopper from the vial containing the dried vaccine.
2. Carefully pour clean, cool non-chlorinated tap water into the vaccine vial until the vial is approximately two-thirds (⅔) full.
3. Insert the rubber stopper and shake vigorously until all of the material is dissolved.
4. The vaccine is now ready for use. For the best results, be sure to follow the directions carefully.

Drinking Water Administration: For chickens two (2) weeks of age or older:

1. Do not use any disinfectants in the drinking water for 48 hours before vaccinating and for 24 hours after vaccination.
2. Withhold drinking water from the chickens until they are thirsty. Withholding periods will vary from 2-12 hours according to the age of the chickens and the weather. Be careful in hot weather.
3. Scrub the waterers and rinse thoroughly with fresh, clean water. Do not use disinfectants for cleaning the waterers.
4. Rehydrate the vaccine.
5. Mix the rehydrated vaccine with clean, cool, non-chlorinated tap water.

Age of chickens	Water per 1,000 doses vaccine
2-4 weeks	6 gal. (24 L)
4-8 weeks	10 gal. (40 L)
8 weeks or older	16 gal. (64 L)

As an aid in preserving the virus, 3.2 oz. (85 mL) of non-fat powdered milk may be added with each 10 gallons of water used for mixing the vaccine. Add the dried milk first and mix until dissolved. Then add the rehydrated vaccine from the vial and again mix thoroughly.

6. Distribute the vaccine solution among the waterers provided for the chickens. Avoid placing waterers in direct sunlight.
7. Do not provide any other drinking water until all of the vaccine-water solution has been consumed.

Coarse Spray Administration: For chickens one (1) day of age or older:

1. Use the rehydrated vaccine as indicated for a specific coarse spray vaccination machine. For example, a sprayer which dispenses 20 mL to 100 chickens; - total volume for 2,500 doses is 500 mL., and 10,000 doses is 2,000 mL of deionized water. Mix thoroughly.
2. Add the prepared vaccine solution to the reservoir on the sprayer.
   Prime and adjust the sprayer as instructed in the manual accompanying the specific machine.

If chickens are vaccinated at earlier than two (2) weeks of age, revaccination at four (4) weeks of age may be indicated for optimum protection.

Records: Keep a record of vaccine, quantity, serial number, expiration date, place of purchase; the date and time of vaccination; the number, age, breed, and locations of chickens; names of operators performing the vaccination and any observed reactions.

Precaution(s): Use only as directed. Store the vaccine between 2-7°C (35-45°F). The product is not returnable.

Use the entire contents when first opened.

Burn the containers and all unused contents.

Caution(s): Vaccinate healthy chickens only. Although disease may not be evident, coccidiosis, mycoplasma infection, Marek's disease, and other disease conditions may cause complications or reduce immunity.

All susceptible chickens on the same premises should be vaccinated at the same time.

Efforts should be taken to reduce stress conditions at the time of vaccination and during the reaction period.

Do not spill or splash the vaccine.

Do not dilute the vaccine or otherwise stretch the dosage.

Warning(s): Do not vaccinate within 21 days before slaughter.

Discussion: The vaccine has undergone rigid potency, safety and purity tests, and meets Intervet America Inc. and USDA requirements. It is designed to stimulate effective immunity when used as directed, but the user must be advised that the response to the product depends upon many factors, including, but not limited to, conditions of storage and handling by the user, administration of the vaccine, health and responsiveness of individual chickens, and the degree of field exposure. Therefore, directions should be followed carefully.

The use of the vaccine is subject to applicable local and federal laws and regulations.

Presentation: 10 x 2,000 doses for drinking water or coarse spray use.
10 x 10,000 doses for drinking water or coarse spray use.
10 x 25,000 doses for drinking water or coarse spray use.

* U.S. Patent No. 4,530,831.

Compendium Code No.: 11060331

CLOSTRATOX® BCD

Novartis Animal Vaccines **Antitoxin**

Clostridium perfringens Type C & D Antitoxin

U.S. Vet. Lic. No.: 303

Composition: CLOSTRATOX® BCD is an equine origin serum product containing antibodies against *Clostridium perfringens* types C and D toxins. Contains thimerosal, oxytetracycline, and phenol as preservatives.

Indications: For the use in the prevention and treatment of enterotoxemia caused by *Clostridium perfringens* types C and D. The combination of beta and epsilon antitoxins also provides protection and treatment of enterotoxemia caused by *Clostridium perfringens* type B.

Dosage and Administration: Administer the following doses subcutaneously.

	Prevention	Treatment
Piglets and suckling lambs	3 mL	7 mL
Feeder lambs	5-10 mL	20 mL
Suckling calves	10-15 mL	25 mL
Cattle (mL/100 lbs.)	5 mL	10 mL

Precaution(s): Store in the dark at a temperature between 35°-45°F (2°-7°C). Do not freeze.

Caution(s): All contents of the bottle should be used when first opened. Anaphylactic reactions may occur following the use of biologicals. Symptomatic treatment: Epinephrine.

Warning(s): Do not vaccinate within 21 days prior to slaughter.

Discussion: *Clostridium perfringens* is a common soil inhabitant and is also often found in the intestines of healthy animals. Under favorable conditions, bacteria in the intestines grow rapidly and produce the toxins which cause the various disease symptoms. There are five known types of *Cl. perfringens:* A, B, C, D, and E. Types B, C, and D are the strains which are covered by the product.

Clostridium perfringens type B causes lamb dysentery, but it can also affect calves less than three weeks of age. Symptoms include sudden death, listlessness, recumbency, abdominal pain, and a fetid diarrhea that may be blood tinged. On postmortem, intestines show severe inflammation, ulcers, and necrosis. The mortality rate approaches 100%. *Cl. perfringens* type B is not common in the United States, but is frequently found in England, Europe, South Africa and the near East.

Clostridium perfringens type C causes an acute hemorrhagic enteritis (enterotoxemia) in calves, lambs and piglets less than two weeks of age, and also in older cattle and sheep on full feed. Affected newborn animals are often from dams producing an abundance of milk. Overfeeding can cause changes in the gut environment which enhance growth and toxin production by the organism. Clinical signs include sudden death, abdominal pain, depression, and possible central nervous system involvement (convulsions, coma). The mortality rate is high, and young animals that do survive are often permanently stunted. Post mortem signs are dependent on the relative amounts of alpha and beta toxins produced by the bacteria and on the duration of the disease. If alpha toxin predominates, the guts will be hemorrhagic. If beta toxin predominates, there will be evidence of gut necrosis and peritonitis.

"Overeating disease" is caused by *Clostridium perfringens* type D. The disease is more common in sheep, but is more economically important in cattle. It can affect both young animals and feeders. The disease is often seen in single lambs under three months of age that are nursing high-producing ewes. In feeders, high concentrate rations, especially if introduced suddenly to an animal accustomed to forage, will cause an abrupt pH drop in the rumen. Fermented grain then passes into the small intestine, where the type D organisms multiply and produce alpha and epsilon toxins. The alpha toxin produces hemolytic lesions. The epsilon toxin must be activated by trypsin in the small intestine. It then causes necrosis and increased vascular permeability, which results in hemorrhage and edema. Initially there is central nervous system stimulation, followed by soft foci and liquefaction necrosis in the brain. Clinical signs include sudden death, convulsions, posterior paralysis, coma, and possibly diarrhea. At necropsy, the rumen is full of concentrate feed and may have petechial hemorrhage. There may be excess pericardial fluid, lung fluid, and excess fluid in parts of the small intestines. Often tissues decompose rapidly, which explains why the disease is sometimes called "pulpy kidney" in sheep.

Presentation: Available in 250 mL and 100 mL bottles.

Compendium Code No.: 11140072

CLOSTRATOX® C

Novartis Animal Vaccines **Antitoxin**

Clostridium perfringens Type C Antitoxin

U.S. Vet. Lic. No.: 303

Composition: CLOSTRATOX® C is an equine origin serum product containing antibodies against *Clostridium perfringens* type C toxin. Contains thimerosal, oxytetracycline, and phenol as preservatives.

Indications: For the use in the prevention and treatment of enterotoxemia caused by *Clostridium perfringens* type C.

Dosage and Administration: Administer the following doses subcutaneously.

	Prevention	Treatment
Piglets and suckling lambs	3 mL	7 mL
Feeder lambs	5-10 mL	20 mL
Suckling calves	10-15 mL	25 mL
Cattle (mL/100 lbs.)	5 mL	10 mL

For oral administration to piglets only: Slowly syringe 5 mL into the back of the mouth of suckling pigs within eight (8) hours after birth.

Precaution(s): Store in the dark at a temperature between 35°-45°F (2°-7°C). Do not freeze. All contents of the bottle should be used when first opened.

Caution(s): Anaphylactic reactions may occur following the use of the product. Symptomatic treatment: Epinephrine.

Warning(s): Do not vaccinate within 21 days prior to slaughter.

Discussion: Type C enterotoxemia is caused by an intestinal overgrowth of *Clostridium perfringens* type C which produces primarily beta and some alpha exotoxins. *Clostridium perfringens* type C is widely distributed in the soil and is a common inhabitant of the intestinal tract. It is a gram-positive, spore-forming rod which multiplies rapidly in the small intestine when conditions are right.

Calves, lambs and piglets from one to ten days old may be found dead without previously showing symptoms. Symptoms seen in affected animals include abdominal pain, diarrhea (sometimes blood-tinged), depression, and cessation of nursing.

Engorgement with milk or grain is considered a predisposing factor for enterotoxemia. It is believed that a large intake of milk may slow the digestive processes, allowing the clostridial bacteria time to multiply. In addition, the proteolytic enzyme trypsin, which can inactivate the beta toxin, may not be present in adequate concentrations under these circumstances. It is usually the healthy, vigorous offspring of high-producing mothers which are affected by the disease.

Postmortem lesions vary according to the predominating type of exotoxin. If alpha toxin predominates, there will be extensive hemorrhage in the jejunum and ileum as well as in the mesenteric and intestinal lymph nodes. There will be blood-stained contents in the lower small intestine and the colon. If beta toxin predominates, there will be necrosis of the jejunum and ileum and peritonitis. Petechial hemorrhages will be found on the spleen, heart, thymus, and serosal surfaces.

Older animals may also be affected with type C enterotoxemia. Pigs between 10-20 days old may have a more chronic but still fatal form. Adult sheep changing from dry to lush feed or starting on supplemental grain can show acute symptoms and sudden death. Feedlot cattle which are brought up too rapidly on highly concentrated feeds or adult cattle which accidentally get into the grain bin will show depression, toxemia, and death.

Trial Data: Clostratox® C (5 mL oral administration) *Clostridium perfringens* type C Challenge:

Test Group	% Mortality	
Treatments	13%	2/15
Controls	77%	10/13

Presentation: Available in 250 mL bottles.

Compendium Code No.: 11140083

CLOSTRATOX® ULTRA C 1300

Novartis Animal Vaccines **Antitoxin**

Clostridium perfringens Type C Antitoxin

U.S. Vet. Lic. No.: 303

Composition: CLOSTRATOX® Ultra C 1300 is an equine origin serum product containing 1300 I.A.U.'s of *Clostridium perfringens* type C antitoxin per mL. Contains thimerosal, oxytetracycline, and phenol as preservatives.

Indications: For use as an aid in the prevention and treatment of enterotoxemia caused by *Clostridium perfringens* type C.

Dosage and Administration: Administer the following doses subcutaneously.

	Prevention	Treatment
Piglets and suckling lambs	3 mL	7 mL
Feeder lambs	5-10 mL	20 mL
Suckling calves	10-15 mL	25 mL
Cattle (mL/100 lbs.)	5 mL	10 mL

For oral administration to piglets only: Slowly syringe 5 mL into the back of the mouth of suckling pigs within eight (8) hours after birth.

Precaution(s): Store in the dark at a temperature between 35°-45°F (2°-7°C). Do not freeze. Use the entire contents when first opened.

Caution(s): Anaphylactic reactions may occur following the use of the product. Symptomatic treatment: Epinephrine.

Warning(s): Do not administer within 21 days prior to slaughter.

Discussion: Type C enterotoxemia is caused by an intestinal overgrowth of *Clostridium perfringens* type C which produces primarily beta and some alpha exotoxins. *Clostridium perfringens* type C is widely distributed in the soil and is a common inhabitant of the intestinal tract. It is a gram-positive, spore-forming rod which multiplies rapidly in the small intestine when conditions are suitable.

Calves, lambs and piglets from one to ten days of age may be found dead without previously showing symptoms. Symptoms seen in affected animals include abdominal pain, diarrhea (sometimes blood-tinged), depression, and cessation of nursing.

Engorgement with milk or grain is considered a predisposing factor for enterotoxemia. It is believed that a large intake of milk may slow the digestive processes, allowing the clostridial bacteria time to multiply. In addition, the proteolytic enzyme trypsin, which can inactivate the beta toxin, may not be present in adequate concentrations under these circumstances. It is usually the healthy, vigorous offspring of high-producing mothers which are affected by the disease.

Postmortem lesions vary according to the predominating type of exotoxin. If alpha toxin predominates, there will be extensive hemorrhage in the jejunum and ileum as well as in the mesenteric and intestinal lymph nodes. There will be blood-stained contents in the lower small intestine and the colon. If beta toxin predominates, there will be necrosis of the jejunum and ileum and peritonitis. Petechial hemorrhages will be found on the spleen, heart, thymus, and serosal surfaces.

Older animals may also be affected with type C enterotoxemia. Pigs between 10-20 days of age may have a more chronic, but still fatal form. Adult sheep changing from dry to lush feed or starting on supplemental grain can show acute symptoms and sudden death. Feedlot cattle which are brought up too rapidly on highly concentrated feeds or adult cattle which accidentally get into the grain bin will show depression, toxemia, and death.

Trial Data: Clostratox® C (5 mL oral administration) *Clostridium perfringens* type C Challenge:

Test Group	% Mortality	
Treatments	13%	2/15
Controls	77%	10/13

Presentation: Available in 250 mL bottles.
Compendium Code No.: 11140093

CLOSTRI BOS™ BCD

Novartis Animal Vaccines **Toxoid**
Clostridium Perfringens Types C and D Toxoid
U.S. Vet. Lic. No.: 303

Composition: This toxoid contains inactivated toxins of *Clostridium perfringens* Types C and D adjuvanted with Xtend® III. Contains thimerosal as a preservative.
Indications: For use in healthy cattle as an aid in the prevention and control of enterotoxemia caused by the beta and epsilon toxins of *Clostridium perfringens* Types C and D. Although *Clostridium perfringens* Type B is not a significant problem in the United States, the combination of *Clostridium perfringens* Types C and D fractions may protect against enterotoxemia caused by *Clostridium perfringens* Type B.
Dosage and Administration: Shake well before using. Administer 1 mL intramuscularly or subcutaneously at 3 months of age or older. Calves vaccinated under 3 months of age should be revaccinated at weaning or at 4-6 months of age. Revaccinate annually.
Precaution(s): Store in the dark at 35°-45°F (2°-7°C). Do not freeze. Use entire contents when first opened.
Caution(s): Transient swelling may occur at the site of injection. Anaphylactic reactions may occur following the use of this biological. Symptomatic treatment: Epinephrine.
For veterinary use only.
Warning(s): Do not vaccinate within 60 days prior to slaughter.
Presentation: 20 dose (20 mL) and 100 dose (100 mL) bottles.
Compendium Code No.: 11140730 F268 / F269

CLOSTRIDIAL 7-WAY

AgriLabs **Bacterin-Toxoid**
Clostridium chauvoei-septicum-novyi-sordellii-perfringens Types C & D Bacterin-Toxoid
U.S. Vet. Lic. No.: 272
Active Ingredient(s): *Clostridium chauvoei, Cl. septicum, Cl. novyi, Cl. sordellii, Cl. perfringens* types C and D bacterin-toxoid.
Indications: For the active immunization of healthy cattle and sheep against diseases caused by *Clostridium chauvoei, Cl. septicum, Cl. sordellii, Cl. novyi* and *Cl. perfringens* types C and D.
Dosage and Administration: Shake well.
Dosage for cattle of any age: Using aseptic technique administer 5 mL subcutaneously or intramuscularly.
Revaccinate in two (2) to four (4) weeks for *Cl. sordellii* and *Cl. perfringens* types C and D. For *Cl. novyi*, repeat the dose every five (5) to six (6) months in animals subjected to re-exposure.
Calves vaccinated before three (3) months of age should be revaccinated at weaning or at four (4) to six (6) months of age.
Intramuscular injection: Make intramuscular injections deeply into a large muscle (thigh). Cleanse the area and insert the needle. Needle should be at least ¾" in length.
Subcutaneous injection: Can be made in any area where the skin fits loosely (neck, chest wall, armpit or flank). Cleanse the area and insert the needle through the skin and discharge the dose.
Massage the area to facillitate distribution.
Precaution(s): Store not over 45°F or 7°C.
Caution(s): Use the entire contents when first opened. Anaphylactic reactions may occur following use of this product.
This product has been tested under laboratory conditions and shown to meet all federal standards for safety and ability to immunize normal, healthy animals. The level of performance of this product may be affected by conditions of use such as stress, weather, nutrition, disease, parasitism, other treatments, individual idiosyncrasies or impaired immunological competency. These factors should be considered by the user when evaluating the product performance or freedom from reactions.
Antidote(s): Epinephrine.
Warning(s): Do not vaccinate within 21 days before slaughter.
Presentation: 50 mL (10 dose), 250 mL (50 dose), and 1,000 mL (200 dose) vials.
Compendium Code No.: 10580340

CLOSTRIDIAL 7-WAY PLUS SOMNUMUNE®

AgriLabs **Bacterin-Toxoid**
Clostridium Chauvoei-Septicum-Novyi-Sordellii-Perfringens Types C & D-Haemophilus Somnus Bacterin-Toxoid
U.S. Vet. Lic. No.: 124
Composition: Prepared from cultures of the organisms listed. Alum precipitated.
Although *Clostridium perfringens* Type B is not a significant problem in the U.S.A, immunity may be provided against the beta and epsilon toxins elaborated by *Clostridium perfringens* Type B. This immunity is derived from the combination of Type C (beta) and Type D (epsilon) fractions.
Indications: Recommended for the vaccination of healthy, susceptible cattle against diseases caused by *Clostridium chauvoei, Cl. septicum, Cl. novyi, Cl. sordellii, Cl. perfringens* Types C and D and *Haemophilus somnus.*
Dosage and Administration: Using aseptic technique, inject 5 mL subcutaneously. Repeat in 21 to 28 days and once annually.
Precaution(s): Store out of direct sunlight at a temperature between 35-45°F. Avoid freezing. Shake well before using. Use entire contents when first opened.
Caution(s): Transient swelling at the injection site may occur. Anaphylactoid reactions may occur.
Antidote(s): Epinephrine.
Warning(s): Do not vaccinate within 21 days before slaughter.
Presentation: 10 dose (50 mL), 50 dose (250 mL) and 200 dose (1000 mL) vials.
Manufactured by: Boehringer Ingelheim Vetmedica, Inc., St. Joseph, MO 64506.
Compendium Code No.: 10580351 18731-01

CLOSTRIDIAL 8-WAY

AgriLabs **Bacterin-Toxoid**
Clostridium chauvoei-septicum-haemolyticum-novyi-sordellii-perfringens Types C & D Bacterin-Toxoid
U.S. Vet. Lic. No.: 272
Contents: *Clostridium chauvoei, Cl. septicum, Cl. haemolyticum, Cl. novyi* type B, *Cl. sordellii, Cl. perfringens* types C and D bacterin-toxoid.
Indications: For the active immunization of healthy cattle and sheep against diseases caused by *Clostridium chauvoei, Cl. septicum, Cl. sordellii, Cl. novyi* type B and *Cl. haemolyticum* (known elsewhere as *Cl. novyi* type D), and *Cl. perfringens* types C and D.
Although *Clostridium perfringens* type B is not a significant problem in the U.S.A, immunity may be provided against the beta and epsilon toxins elaborated by *Cl. perfringens* type B. This immunity is derived from the combination of type C (beta) and type D (epsilon) fractions.
Dosage and Administration: Shake well. Using aseptic technique, inject subcutaneously or intramuscularly.
Dosage: 5 mL, repeated in three (3) to four (4) weeks. Revaccinate annually or prior to periods of extreme risk, or parturition. For *Cl. novyi* and *Cl. haemolyticum,* revaccinate every five (5) to six (6) months. Animals vaccinated under three (3) months of age should be revaccinated at weaning or at four (4) to six (6) months of age.
Intramuscular injection: Make intramuscular injections deeply into a large muscle (thigh). Cleanse the area and insert the needle. The needle should be at least ¾" in length.
Subcutaneous injection: Can be made in any area where the skin fits loosely (neck, chest wall, armpit or flank). Lift the skin to facilitate needle entry, insert the needle and discharge the dose. Massage the area to accelerate distribution.
Precaution(s): Store not over 45°F or 7°C.
Caution(s): Use the entire contents when first opened. Anaphylactic reactions may occur following use of this product.
This product has been tested under laboratory conditions and shown to meet all federal standards for safety and ability to immunize normal, healthy animals. The level of performance of this product may be affected by conditions of use such as stress, weather, nutrition, disease, parasitism, other treatments, individual idiosyncrasies or impaired immunological competency. These factors should be considered by the user when evaluating the product performance or freedom from reactions.
Antidote(s): Epinephrine.
Warning(s): Do not vaccinate within 21 days before slaughter.
Presentation: 10 dose (50 mL) and 50 dose (250 mL) vials.
Compendium Code No.: 10580361

CLOSTRIDIAL ANTITOXIN BCD

Durvet **Antitoxin**
Clostridium Perfringens Types C and D Antitoxin, Equine Origin
U.S. Vet. Lic. No.: 303
Composition: This product is prepared from the blood of horses hyperimmunized with *Clostridium perfringens* Types C and D toxins. Contains oxytetracycline, phenol, and thimerosal as preservatives.
Indications: For use as an aid in the prevention and control of enterotoxemia caused by *Clostridium perfringens* Types C and D. Although *Clostridium perfringens* Type B is not a significant problem in the United States, the combination of *Clostridium perfringens* Types C and D antitoxins may protect against enterotoxemia caused by *Clostridium perfringens* Type B.
Dosage and Administration: Shake well before using. Administer the following doses subcutaneously.

	Prophylactic Treatment	Therapeutic Treatment
Feeder lambs	10 mL	20 mL
Suckling calves	15 mL	30 mL
Cattle	30 mL	60 mL

Precaution(s): Store in the dark at 35°-45°F (2°-7°C). Do not freeze. Use entire contents when first opened.
Caution(s): Anaphylactic reactions may occur following the use of this biological. Symptomatic treatment: Epinephrine.
Warning(s): Do not administer within 21 days prior to slaughter.
Presentation: 100 mL and 250 mL vials.
Manufactured by: Advance Biologics, Inc., Freeman, SD 57029.
Compendium Code No.: 10840311 8/99

CLOSTRIDIAL BCD

Durvet **Bacterin-Toxoid**
Clostridium Perfringens Types C and D Bacterin-Toxoid
U.S. Vet. Lic. No.: 303
Composition: This product contains inactivated cultures of *Clostridium perfringens* Types C and D adjuvanted with aluminum hydroxide. Contains penicillin and streptomycin as preservatives.
Indications: For use in healthy cattle and sheep as an aid in the prevention and control of disease caused by *Clostridium perfringens* Types C and D. Although *Clostridium perfringens* Type B is not a significant problem in the United States, the combination of *Clostridium perfringens* Types C and D fractions may protect against enterotoxemia caused by *Clostridium perfringens* Type B.
Dosage and Administration: Shake well before using. Administer 2 mL intramuscularly to cattle and 1 mL intramuscularly to sheep. Repeat in 21 days. Revaccinate annually.
Precaution(s): Store in the dark at 35°-45°F (2°-7°C). Do not freeze. Use entire contents when first opened.
Caution(s): Anaphylactic reactions may occur following the use of this biological. Symptomatic treatment: Epinephrine.
Warning(s): Do not administer within 21 days prior to slaughter.
Presentation: 50 cattle doses and 100 sheep doses (100 mL vials).
Manufactured by: Advance Biologics, Inc., Freeman, SD 57029.
Compendium Code No.: 10840321 8/99

CLOSTRIDIUM BOTULINUM TYPE B ANTITOXIN

V.D.I. **Antitoxin**
Clostridium Botulinum Type B Antitoxin, Equine Origin
U.S. Vet. Lic. No.: 360
Contents: The plasma contains no preservatives, and donors used have been found free of hemolysins and agglutinins against 32 of the main antigens in blood groups A, C, D, K, P, Q and U. Donors have also tested negative for EIA, EVA, dourine, piroplasmosis, brucellosis and glanders.

Indications: This product can be administered in the following situation: For prophylactic administration to foals less than 1 month of age with probable exposure to *Clostridium botulinum* type B toxin or spores.

Dosage and Administration: The plasma should be kept frozen until required. It should be thawed using only warm water and then warmed to body temperature. Plasma can be damaged by thawing in microwaves. Administer directly from the bag by slow filtered intravenous infusion. Do not add anything to the product. Each single dose bag contains approximately 5,000 IU, the recommended dose for a foal, or 20,000 IU, the recommended dose for adult horses. Caution should be taken to avoid volume overload. Complications are very infrequent but may include mild reactions such as tachypnea and trembling. If these symptoms become severe and also include sweating and excessive shaking, it is advisable to slow the rate of administration or to stop and restart in 5-10 minutes. If the symptoms recur or persist, discontinue administration.

Caution(s): This product license is conditional. Efficacy and potency test studies are in progress.

Only for use in horses by a licensed veterinarian.

This product is frozen immediately after collection and is not pasteurized. The transmission of viral disease is possible with the administration of any blood product, as is the development of serum sickness, but these are rare occurrences using plasma in equidae.

Administer through a sterile blood administration set with a 180 micron filter.

Presentation: 5,000 IU single dose for foals under 1 month of age and 20,000 IU single dose for adults.

Compendium Code No.: 11280001

CLOSTRIDIUM CHAUVOEI-SEPTICUM BACTERIN

Colorado Serum **Bacterin**

Clostridium chauvoei-septicum Bacterin

U.S. Vet. Lic. No.: 188

Active Ingredient(s): Formalin killed, aluminum hydroxide adsorbed, cultures of *Clostridium chauvoei* and *Clostridium septicum.*

Contains thimerosal as a preservative.

Indications: For the vaccination of healthy cattle, sheep and goats against blackleg and malignant edema.

Dosage and Administration: Shake well. Inject 2 mL subcutaneously. Calves vaccinated under three (3) months of age should be revaccinated at weaning or at four (4) to six (6) months of age.

Precaution(s): Shake well, each dose must have a proportionate share of the precipitate for a proper response. Store in the dark at 2-7°C. Do not freeze.

Caution(s): Anaphylactic reactions sometimes follow administration of products of this nature. If noted, administer adrenaline or an equivalent drug.

Use the entire contents when the bottle is first opened.

For veterinary use only.

Warning(s): Do not vaccinate within 21 days before slaughter.

Presentation: 10 dose (20 mL) and 50 dose (100 mL) vials.

Compendium Code No.: 11010120

CLOSTRIDIUM CHAUVOEI-SEPTICUM-NOVYI-SORDELLII BACTERIN-TOXOID

Colorado Serum **Bacterin-Toxoid**

Clostridium chauvoei-septicum-novyi-sordellii Bacterin-Toxoid

U.S. Vet. Lic. No.: 188

Active Ingredient(s): Formalin killed, aluminum hydroxide adsorbed, cultures of *Clostridium chauvoei, Clostridium septicum, Clostridium novyi* and *Clostridium sordellii.*

Contains thimerosal as a preservative.

Indications: For the vaccination of healthy cattle, sheep, and goats against blackleg, malignant edema, black disease, and *Clostridium sordellii* infection.

Dosage and Administration: Shake well. Each dose must have a proportionate share of precipitate.

Inject subcutaneously or intramuscularly.

Calves .... 5 mL
Sheep and Goats .... 2½ mL

Revaccination with *Clostridium sordellii* bacterin is recommended in two (2) to four (4) weeks. Calves vaccinated under three (3) months of age should be revaccinated at weaning time or at four (4) to six (6) months of age. For *Clostridium novyi*, repeat the dose every five (5) to six (6) months in animals subject to re-exposure.

Precaution(s): Store in the dark at 2° to 7°C. Do not freeze.

Caution(s): An anaphylactic reaction sometimes follows administration of products of this nature. If noted, administer adrenaline or equivalent.

Use the entire contents when the bottle is first opened.

For veterinary use only.

Warning(s): Do not vaccinate within 21 days before slaughter.

Presentation: 10 dose (50 mL) and 50 dose (250 mL) vials.

Compendium Code No.: 11010130

CLOSTRIDIUM CHAUVOEI-SEPTICUM-PASTEURELLA HAEMOLYTICA-MULTOCIDA BACTERIN

Colorado Serum **Bacterin**

Clostridium chauvoei-septicum-Pasteurella haemolytica-multocida Bacterin

U.S. Vet. Lic. No.: 188

Active Ingredient(s): Formalin killed, aluminum hydroxide adsorbed, cultures of *Clostridium chauvoei, Clostridium septicum, Pasteurella haemolytica* and *Pasteurella multocida,* bovine isolates.

Contains thimerosal as a preservative.

Indications: For the vaccination of healthy cattle, sheep and goats against blackleg, malignant edema and pasteurellosis caused by the micro-organisms named.

Dosage and Administration: Shake well. Each dose must have a proportionate share of the precipitate for a proper response.

Calves: 5 mL injected subcutaneously. Calves vaccinated when less than three (3) months of age should be revaccinated at weaning or at four (4) to six (6) months of age.

Sheep and Goats: 3 mL injected subcutaneously. Revaccination with *Pasteurella haemolytica* and *P. multocida* bacterin is recommended in two (2) to four (4) weeks.

Precaution(s): Store in the dark at 2-7°C. Do not freeze.

Caution(s): Anaphylactic reactions sometimes follow administration of products of this nature. If noted, administer adrenaline or an equivalent drug.

Use the entire contents when the bottle is first opened.

For veterinary use only.

Warning(s): Do not vaccinate within 21 days before slaughter.

Presentation: 10 dose (50 mL) and 50 dose (250 mL) vials.

Compendium Code No.: 11010140

CLOSTRIDIUM HAEMOLYTICUM BACTERIN (RED WATER)

C

Colorado Serum **Bacterin**

Clostridium Haemolyticum Bacterin

U.S. Vet. Lic. No.: 188

Contents: Formalin inactivated *Clostridium haemolyticum*, aluminum hydroxide adsorbed.

Contains thimerosal as a preservative.

Indications: For vaccination of healthy cattle, sheep and goats as an aid in the prevention of "Red Water Disease" (Bacillary Hemoglobinuria).

Dosage and Administration: Inject 2 mL subcutaneously or intramuscularly. In areas where constant exposure is likely revaccinate every 5 to 6 months. Spring vaccination is recommended because disease is most prevalent in Summer months. Initial vaccination for calves should be at 3-4 months of age. Revaccinate yearly.

Precaution(s): Shake well before using to uniformly disperse adjuvant. Use entire contents when bottle is first opened. Store in dark at 2° to 7°C.

Protect from freezing.

Caution(s): Anaphylactoid reaction sometimes follow administration of products of this nature. If noted, administer adrenaline or equivalent.

Warning(s): Do not vaccinate within 21 days before slaughter.

For veterinary use only.

Presentation: 10 dose (20 mL) and 50 dose (100 mL) vials.

Compendium Code No.: 11010150

CLOSTRIDIUM PERFRINGENS TYPES C & D ANTITOXIN, EQUINE ORIGIN

Colorado Serum **Antitoxin**

Clostridium perfringens Types C & D Antitoxin, Equine Origin

U.S. Vet. Lic. No.: 188

Active Ingredient(s): Prepared from the blood of horses hyperimmunized with *Clostridium perfringens* types C and D toxin.

Contains phenol and thimerosal as preservatives.

Indications: A potent multivalent antitoxin specific for the temporary prevention of clostridial enterotoxemia in cattle, sheep and goats caused by types C and D toxin and in swine when caused by type C.

Dosage and Administration: Injections should be made as soon as possible after birth.

CLOSTRIDIUM PERFRINGENS TYPES C & D ANTITOXIN, EQUINE ORIGIN confers a prompt passive immunity lasting about 14-21 days. Administer subcutaneously using aseptic methods. The following doses are recommended:

Suckling lambs, goats and pigs .... 5 mL
Suckling calves .... 10 mL
Feeder lambs and pigs .... 10 mL
Feeder calves and cattle .... 25 mL

Clostridium perfringens type D is not known to cause disease in swine.

Precaution(s): Shake well before withdrawing. Store in the dark at 2-7°C.

Use the entire contents when the bottle is first opened. Sterilize needles and syringes by boiling in clean water.

Caution(s): Anaphylactic reactions sometimes follow the use of products of this nature. The risk of this reaction increases when injections are intravenous. If noted, administer epinephrine or an equivalent drug. Antihistamines injected prior to or simultaneously with intravenous administration may reduce the incidence of shock.

For veterinary use only.

Warning(s): Do not vaccinate within 21 days before slaughter. If the antitoxin must be used under emergency conditions, the animals treated should be withheld from market for 21 days after injection.

Discussion: Type C, sometimes called hemorrhagic enterotoxemia, occurs most often in calves and in swine; type D, occasionally referred to as pulpy kidney disease, most often occurs in sheep and goats. Affected young animals are commonly suckling dams that are heavy milk producers. Because both types of toxin have been identified as the cause of problems in all four species of animals and clinical diagnosis is difficult, more reliable protection is ensured by injection of a multivalent antitoxin.

The essentials for activating *Clostridium perfringens*, rich ingesta and bowel stasis, are likely to be present when animals are on feedlot rations, and digestive problems arise because of excessive grain concentrates. It is for this reason that the infection is also called "overeating" disease. When the disease appears in feeder livestock, the prompt use of antitoxin can often mean the difference between the success of treatment and failure.

Antitoxins contain antibodies formed as a result of hyperimmunization with a specific toxin and which are capable of neutralizing that toxin. An almost immediate response is provided at the time of injection. Antitoxins do not actively stimulate the antibody system of the vaccinated animal and the resulting immunity is passive, lasting only until the injected antibodies are eliminated from the system, a period of approximately 14-21 days.

Clostridium perfringens is a micro-organism that normally exists in the lower intestinal tract of most domestic animals and which lives on decaying organic matter. It is opportunistic and when triggered by proper circumstances becomes highly toxigenic. Fatal intoxication causing a hemorrhagic enteritis and peritonitis follows. Lethal toxins can be grown in nutritive media in the laboratory in just a few hours. As feeds rich in protein and carbohydrates are ingested a suitable medium for the development of the organism is provided in the animals. Progress of the disease is, therefore, almost as rapid as the growth of the organism in the laboratory. Deaths frequently occur without symptoms ever being observed.

Presentation: 250 mL vials.

Compendium Code No.: 11010171

C

CLOSTRIDIUM PERFRINGENS TYPES C&D ANTITOXIN, EQUINE ORIGIN

Professional Biological **Antitoxin**

Clostridium Perfringens Types C&D Antitoxin, Equine Origin

U.S. Vet. Lic. No.: 188

Contents: This product contains the antigens listed above.

Contains phenol and thimerosal as preservatives.

Indications: This is a potent multivalent antitoxin specific for the temporary prevention or treatment of Clostridial enterotoxemia in cattle, sheep and goats caused by types C and D toxin and in swine when caused by type C. Type D is not known to cause disease in swine.

Dosage and Administration: For prevention lasting approximately 3 weeks the following doses should be administered subcutaneously.

Suckling Lambs, Goats and Pigs .... 5 mL
Suckling Calves .... 10 mL
Feeder Lambs and Pigs .... 10 mL
Feeder Calves and Cattle .... 25 mL

For treatment, double the preventative dose. A more rapid effect can be achieved by intravenous administration, with repeat dosages as often as 12 hour intervals.

Precaution(s): Shake well before using. Use entire contents when bottle is first opened. Store in the dark at 2° to 7°C.

Caution(s): Anaphylactoid reaction sometimes follows products of this nature (especially if given intravenously). If noted, administer adrenaline or equivalent. Prior or concurrent administration of antihistamines with intravenous use may reduce the incidence of shock.

For veterinary use only.

Warning(s): Do not administer within 21 days before slaughter.

Presentation: 250 mL vials.

Compendium Code No.: 14250060 63703

CLOSTRIDIUM PERFRINGENS TYPES C & D-TETANUS TOXOID

Colorado Serum **Toxoid**

Clostridium perfringens Types C & D-Tetanus Toxoid

U.S. Vet. Lic. No.: 188

Active Ingredient(s): Purified formalin detoxified filtrates of highly toxic cultures of *Clostridium perfringens* types C and D micro-organisms and of tetanus toxin.

Contains thimerosal as a preservative.

Indications: For the vaccination of healthy cattle, sheep, goats and swine as an aid in the prevention of enterotoxemia caused by *Clostridium perfringens* types C and D and for long-term protection against tetanus.

Dosage and Administration: Inject 2 mL subcutaneously or intramuscularly. Repeat the full dose in three (3) to four (4) weeks.

Precaution(s): Shake well. Store in the dark at 2-7°C. Do not freeze. Each dose must have a proportionate share of the precipitate for a proper response. Use the entire contents when first opened.

Caution(s): Anaphylactic reactions sometimes follow administration of products of this nature. If noted, administer adrenaline or an equivalent drug.

For veterinary use only.

Warning(s): Do not vaccinate with 21 days before slaughter.

Presentation: 10 dose (20 mL) and 50 dose (100 mL) vials.

Compendium Code No.: 11010190

CLOSTRIDIUM PERFRINGENS TYPES C & D-TETANUS TOXOID

Professional Biological **Toxoid**

Clostridium Perfringens Types C & D-Tetanus Toxoid

U.S. Vet. Lic. No.: 188

Contents: Purified formalin detoxified filtrates of highly toxic cultures of *Clostridium perfringens* types C and D micro-organisms and of Tetanus Toxin.

Contains thimerosal as a preservative.

Indications: For the vaccination of healthy cattle, sheep, and goats as an aid in the prevention of enterotoxemia caused by *Clostridium perfringens* types C and D. For the vaccination of healthy swine as an aid in the prevention of enterotoxemia caused by *Clostridium perfringens* type C. For the long-term protection against tetanus.

Dosage and Administration: Inject 2 mL subcutaneously or intramuscularly. Repeat the full dose in 3 to 4 weeks.

Precaution(s): Shake well. Each dose must have a proportionate share of the precipitate for proper responses. Use the entire contents when first opened.

Store in dark at 2° to 7°C. Do not freeze.

Caution(s): Anaphylactoid reaction sometimes follows administration of products of this nature. If noted, administer adrenalin or equivalent.

For veterinary use only.

Warning(s): Do not vaccinate with 21 days before slaughter.

Presentation: 10 dose (20 mL) and 50 dose (100 mL) vials.

Compendium Code No.: 14250070 61302/61304

CLOSTRIDIUM PERFRINGENS TYPES C & D TOXOID

Colorado Serum **Toxoid**

Clostridium perfringens Types C & D Toxoid

U.S. Vet. Lic. No.: 188

Active Ingredient(s): Purified formalin detoxified filtrates of highly toxic cultures of *Clostridium perfringens* types C and D micro-organisms.

Contains thimerosal as a preservative.

Indications: For the vaccination of cattle, sheep, goats and swine as an aid in preventing clostridial enterotoxemia caused by *Clostridium perfringens* types C and D.

Dosage and Administration: Inject 2 mL subcutaneously or intramuscularly. Repeat the full dose in three (3) to four (4) weeks.

Precaution(s): Shake well. Store in the dark at 2-7°C. Do not freeze. Each dose must have a proportionate share of the precipitate for a proper response. Use the entire contents when first opened.

Caution(s): Anaphylactic reactions sometimes follow administration of products of this nature. If noted, administer adrenaline or an equivalent drug.

For veterinary use only.

Warning(s): Do not vaccinate with 21 days before slaughter.

Presentation: 10 dose (20 mL) and 50 dose (100 mL) vials.

Compendium Code No.: 11010180

CLOSTRIDIUM PERFRINGENS TYPES C & D TOXOID

Professional Biological **Toxoid**

Clostridium Perfringens Types C & D Toxoid

U.S. Vet. Lic. No.: 188

Contents: Purified formalin detoxified filtrates of highly toxic cultures of *Clostridium perfringens* types C and D micro-organisms.

Contains thimerosal as a preservative.

Indications: For the vaccination of healthy cattle, sheep, and goats as an aid in the prevention of enterotoxemia caused by *Clostridium perfringens* types C and D. For the vaccination of healthy swine as an aid in the prevention of enterotoxemia caused by *Clostridium perfringens* type C.

Dosage and Administration: Inject 2 mL subcutaneously or intramuscularly. Repeat the full dose in 3 to 4 weeks.

Precaution(s): Shake well. Each dose must have a proportionate share of the precipitate for proper responses. Use entire contents when first opened.

Store in dark at 2° to 7°C. Do not freeze.

Caution(s): Anaphylactoid reaction sometimes follows administration of products of this nature. If noted, administer adrenalin or equivalent.

For veterinary use only.

Warning(s): Do not vaccinate within 21 days before slaughter.

Presentation: 10 dose (20 mL) and 50 dose (100 mL) vials.

Compendium Code No.: 14250080 61312/61314

CLOSTRI SHIELD® BCD

Novartis Animal Vaccines **Bacterin-Toxoid**

Clostridium perfringens Type C & D Bacterin-Toxoid

U.S. Vet. Lic. No.: 303

Composition: This product contains inactivated cultures of *Clostridium perfringens* Type C and D adjuvanted with aluminum hydroxide. Contains penicillin and streptomycin as preservatives.

Indications: For use in healthy cattle and sheep as an aid in the prevention and control of disease caused by *Clostridium perfringens* Types C and D. Although *Clostridium perfringens* Type B is not a significant problem in the United States, the combination of *Clostridium perfringens* Type C and D fractions may protect against enterotoxemia caused by *Clostridium perfringens* Type B.

Dosage and Administration: Shake well before using. Administer 2 mL intramuscularly to cattle and 1 mL intramuscularly to sheep. Repeat in 21 days. Revaccinate annually.

Precautions: Store in the dark at 35°-45°F (2°-7°C). Do not freeze. Use entire contents when first opened.

Caution(s): Anaphylactic reactions may occur following the use of this biological. Symptomatic treatment: Epinephrine.

For veterinary use only.

Warning(s): Do not vaccinate within 21 days prior to slaughter.

Discussion: Disease Information: *Clostridium perfringens* is a common soil inhabitant and is also often found in the intestines of healthy animals. Under favorable conditions, bacteria in the intestines grow rapidly and produce the toxins which cause the various disease symptoms. There are five known types of *Cl perfringens:* A, B, C, D, and E. Types B, C, and D are the strains which are covered by the product.

Clostridium perfringens Type B causes lamb dysentery, but it can also affect calves less than three weeks of age. Symptoms include sudden death, listlessness, recumbency, abdominal pain, and a fetid diarrhea that may be blood tinged. On post-mortem intestines show severe inflammation, ulcers and necrosis. The mortality rate approaches 100%. *Cl perfringens* Type B is not common in the United States but is frequently found in England, Europe, South Africa and the near East.

Clostridium perfringens Type C causes an acute hemorrhagic enteritis (enterotoxemia) in calves and lambs less than two weeks old, and also in older cattle and sheep on full feed. Affected newborn animals are often from dams producing an abundance of milk. Overfeeding can cause changes in the gut environment which enhance growth and toxin production by the organism. Clinical signs include sudden death, abdominal pain, depression and possible central nervous system involvement (such as convulsions and coma). The mortality rate is high and young animals that do survive are often permanently stunted. Post mortem signs are dependent on the relative amounts of alpha and beta toxins produced by the bacteria and on the duration of the disease. If alpha toxin predominates, the intestines will be hemorrhagic. If beta toxin predominates, there will be evidence of stomach and intestinal necrosis and peritonitis.

"Overeating disease" is caused by *Clostridium perfringens* Type D. The disease is more common in sheep, but is more economically important in cattle. It can affect both young animals and feeders. The disease is often seen in single lambs under three months of age that are nursing high-producing ewes. In feeders, high concentrate rations, especially if introduced suddenly to an animal accustomed to forage, will cause an abrupt pH drop in the rumen. Fermented grain then passes into the small intestine, where the Type D organisms multiply and produce alpha and epsilon toxins. The alpha toxin must be activated by trypsin in the small intestine. It then causes necrosis and increased vascular permeability, which results in hemorrhage and edema. Initially there is central nervous system stimulation, followed by soft foci and liquefaction necrosis in the brain. Clinical signs include sudden death, convulsions, posterior paralysis, coma and possibly diarrhea. At necropsy, the rumen is full of concentrate feed and may have petechial hemorrhages. There may be excess pericardial fluid, lung fluid, and excess fluid in parts of the small intestines. Often tissues decompose rapidly, which explains why the disease is sometimes called "pulpy kidney" in sheep.

Vaccination against these diseases is the economical, effective way to combat them, since treatment of affected animals is usually futile, with death the outcome.

Presentation: 50 cattle doses or 100 sheep doses (100 mL bottle).

Compendium Code No.: 11140103

CLOTISOL® LIQUID

BenePet **Hemostatic**

Blood Clotting Suspension-Original Formula

Ingredient(s): Ferric sulfate, aluminum sulfate, collagen protein and chloroxylenol in suspension.

Indications: CLOTISOL® is a blood clotting suspension used as an aid to stop bleeding in animals caused by minor cuts and wounds. It can be used for nail trimming, tail docking and ear cropping.

Directions: Shake well before using. To stop bleeding, apply a liberal amount directly to wound. If bleeding does not stop, consult a veterinarian.
Caution(s): Do not use in deep wounds or on burns.
For external use only.
Presentation: 2 oz (56.8 g) containers.
Compendium Code No.: 14020001

CLOT-IT PLUS™

Evsco **Hemostatic**

Styptic Powder With Benzocaine
Active Ingredient(s): Benzocaine 0.2%, ferric subsulfate, bentonite, diatomaceous earth, aluminum chloride, ammonium chloride, copper sulfate, iodoform.
Indications: CLOT-IT PLUS™ is a specially compounded formula used as an aid to stop minor external bleeding and to temporarily relieve pain caused by clipping nails or dew claws and minor cuts.
Directions: Apply directly to bleeding area. A pressure bandage is sometimes required if claws or nails are cut too short. If bleeding persists, or in the case of deep puncture wounds, consult your veterinarian immediately.
Warning(s): For external animal use only. Keep out of reach of children and pets.
Presentation: 1 oz (28.4 g) bottles.
Compendium Code No.: 10050060

CLOT POWDER

Q.A. Laboratories **Hemostatic**

Active Ingredient(s): Ferric subsulfate, copper sulfate, iodophore complex in an absorptive base.
Indications: CLOT POWDER is for use as an aid to stop bleeding caused by minor cuts and wounds. Useful in nail clips, docking tails and dew claws and trimming beaks. A pressure bandage should be used with CLOT POWDER following tail docking. Do not use in deep wounds, body cavities, or on burns.
Dosage and Administration: Apply with a moistened cotton tipped applicator to the cut nail or other superficial bleeding using moderate, constant pressure for 5-10 seconds. If the bleeding does not stop, consult a veterinarian.
Caution(s): Keep out of the reach of children.
For external veterinary use only on dogs, cats, and birds.
Presentation: ½ oz. and 1½ oz. containers.
Compendium Code No.: 13680010

CLOTRIMAZOLE SOLUTION USP, 1% ℞

Butler **Antifungal**

Antifungal Solution
Active Ingredient(s): Clotrimazole 1%.
Ingredients: Propylene Glycol, SD Alcohol 40, Cocamidopropyl PG-Dimonium Chloride Phosphate, Chloroxylenol (PCMX), Benzyl Alcohol.
Indications: For dermatological conditions associated with infections responsive to Clotrimazole.
Resistance: Resistance to clotrimazole is very rare among the fungi that cause superficial mycoses. Neither natural nor acquired resistance appears to be prevalent.
Directions: Clean and dry affected area. Apply a thin layer morning and evening or as directed by veterinarian. If satisfactory results are not obtained within 2 weeks, consult a veterinarian.
Dosage and Administration: Thoroughly clean and dry the affected area before treatment. Remove foreign material, debris, crusted exudates, etc., with suitable non-irritating solutions. To prevent spreading and reinfection from fungal spores attached to hair shafts, clip the hair in the area of the lesion before and during the treatment period as needed. (Note: Disinfect clipper head before re-use.) Apply a thin layer twice daily. Therapy should continue for 14 consecutive days. Wash hands thoroughly after applying to avoid spread of infection.
Drug Interactions: None.
Contraindication(s): If hypersensitivity to any of the components occurs, treatment should be discontinued and apropriate therapy instituted. Do not use in dogs with known perforation of eardrums.
Precaution(s): Storage: Store at controlled room temperature.
Caution(s): Federal law restricts this drug to use by or on the order of a licensed veterinarian.
Avoid contact with eyes or mucous membranes. If contact occurs, immediately flush with water. If skin irritation occurs, discontinue use and consult a veterinarian.
For veterinary use only.
Warning(s): Keep out of reach of children.
Side Effects: The following have been reported occasionally in connection with the use of clotrimazole: erythema, stinging, blistering, peeling, edema, pruritus, uticaria and general skin irritation not present before therapy.
Presentation: Box of 12 x 30 mL (1 fl oz) plastic bottles with dropper tips and box of 12 x 60 mL (2 fl oz) plastic bottles with pump sprayer.
Sold exclusively through licensed veterinarians.
Compendium Code No.: 10822010

CLOTRIMAZOLE SOLUTION USP, 1% ℞

Vet Solutions **Antifungal**

Antifungal Solution
Active Ingredient(s): Clotrimazole 1%.
Ingredients: Propylene Glycol, SD Alcohol 40, Cocamidopropyl PG-Dimonium Chloride Phosphate, Chloroxylenol (PCMX), Benzyl Alcohol.
Indications: For dermatological conditions associated with infections responsive to Clotrimazole.
Directions: Clean and dry affected area. Apply a thin layer morning and evening or as directed by veterinarian. If satisfactory results are not obtained within 2 weeks, consult a veterinarian.
Precaution(s): Store at controlled room temperature (59-86°F).
Caution(s): Federal Law (USA) restricts this drug to use by or on the order of a licensed veterinarian.
Warning(s): Keep out of the reach of children. Avoid contact with eyes or mucous membranes. If contact occurs, immediately flush with water. If skin irritation occurs, discontinue use and consult a veterinarian.
Presentation: 1 oz., 2 oz., and 237 mL (8 fl. oz.).
Compendium Code No.: 10610050 991001

CLOTRIMAZOLE SOLUTION USP, 1% ℞

Vetus **Antifungal**

Antifungal Solution
Active Ingredient(s):
Clotrimazole 1%
Ingredients: Propylene Glycol, SD Alcohol 40, Cocamidopropyl, Chloroxylenol (PCMX), Benzyl Alcohol.
Indications: For dermatological conditions associated with infections responsive to Clotrimazole.
Directions: Clean and dry affected area. Apply a thin layer morning and evening or as directed by veterinarian. If satisfactory results are not obtained within 2 weeks, consult a veterinarian.
Precaution(s): Storage: Store at controlled room temperature.
Caution(s): Avoid contact with eyes or mucous membranes. If contact occurs, immediately flush with water. If skin irritation occurs, discontinue use and consult a veterinarian.
For veterinary use only.
Warning(s): Keep out of reach of children.
Presentation: 1 fl oz (30 mL) (NDC: 47611-366-95).
Sold exclusively to licensed veterinarians.
Distributed by: Burns Veterinary Supply, Inc., Westbury, NY 11590.
Compendium Code No.: 14441020

C

CLOUT™

All Weather Bait

Bayer

For Indoor And Outdoor Rodent Control
Kills Roof Rats, Norway Rats And House Mice
Roof Rats, Norway Rats and House Mice usually consume a lethal dose in a single day's feeding, but it may take two or more days from time of bait consumption for these rodents to die. Rodents cease feeding after consuming a lethal dose. Clout™ All Weather Bait is effective against anticoagulant-resistant rats and mice.
Contains Bitrex
ACTIVE INGREDIENT:
Bromethalin: N methyl-2,4-dinitro-N-(2,4,6-tribromophenyl)-6-(trifluoromethyl) benzenamine 0.01%
INERT INGREDIENTS 99.99%
100.00%

KEEP OUT OF REACH OF CHILDREN
CAUTION
PRECAUTIONARY STATEMENTS
HAZARD TO HUMANS & DOMESTIC ANIMALS
CAUTION
Keep away from humans, domestic animals and pets. May be harmful or fatal if swallowed. Avoid contact with skin, eyes or clothing. Wash thoroughly with soap and water after handling bait.
NOTE TO PHYSICIAN:
Clout™ All Weather Bait is not an anticoagulant type of rodenticide. If ingested, limit absorption by either emesis or gastric lavage. Sublethal symptoms, if present, would be the result of cerebral edema and should be treated accordingly through administration of an osmotic diuretic and corticosteroid.
ENVIRONMENTAL HAZARDS
This product is toxic to mammals and birds. Do not apply directly to water, or to areas where surface water is present or to intertidal areas below the mean high water mark.
DIRECTIONS FOR USE
It is a violation of Federal Law to use this product in a manner inconsistent with its labeling.
READ THE LABEL: Read the entire label and follow all use directions and use precautions.
IMPORTANT: Do not expose children, pets, or other nontarget animals to rodenticides. To help to prevent accidents:

1. Store product not in use in a location out of reach of children and pets.
2. Apply bait in locations out of reach of children, pets, domestic animals and nontarget wildlife, or in tamper-resistant bait stations. These stations must be resistant to destruction by dogs and by children under six years of age, and must be used in a manner that prevents such children from reaching into bait compartments and obtaining bait. If bait can be shaken from stations when they are lifted, units must be secured or otherwise immobilized. Even stronger bait stations are needed in areas open to hoofed livestock, raccoons, bears, or other potentially destructive animals, or in areas prone to vandalism.
3. Dispose of product container, and unused, spoiled, and unconsumed bait as specified on the label.

USE RESTRICTIONS
This product may be used to control Norway rats, roof rats, and house mice in and around sewers, homes, industrial and agricultural buildings, and similar man-made structures. This product may also be used in alleys located in urban areas, inside transport vehicles (ships, trains, aircraft), and in and around related port or terminal buildings. Do not place this bait in areas where there is a possibility of contaminating food or surfaces that come into contact with food.
SELECTION OF TREATMENT AREAS:
Determine areas where rodents will most likely find and consume the bait. Generally, these areas are along walls, by gnawed openings, in or beside burrows, in corners and concealed places, between floors and walls, or in locations where rodents or their signs have been seen. Remove as much alternative food accessible to rodents as possible.
APPLICATION DIRECTIONS:
RATS: Apply 2 to 12 baits per placement. Space placements at intervals of 20 to 30 feet.
MICE: Apply 1 to 2 baits per placement. Space placements at intervals of 8 to 12 feet.
RATS AND MICE: Adjust the amount of bait applied to the level of rodent feeding expected at each bait placement location. Highest bait consumption is expected to occur on the first day or two after treatment. After several days, inspect the placements and replenish bait at sites where there is heavy feeding, or where there is continued evidence of rodent activity. Maintain bait for at least one week and continue baiting until all signs of rodent activity have ceased or it becomes clear that the remaining rodents are not attracted to the bait.
Collect and properly dispose of all dead rodents and leftover bait. To discourage reinfestation, limit sources of rodent food, water, and harborage as much as possible. If reinfestation does occur, repeat treatment. Where continuous source of infestation is present, establish permanent bait stations and replenish as needed.
STORAGE AND DISPOSAL
Do not contaminate water, food or feed by storage or disposal.
PESTICIDE STORAGE: Store in original container in a cool, dry place inaccessible to children and pets. Keep containers closed and away from other chemicals.

PESTICIDE DISPOSAL: Wastes resulting from the use of this product may be disposed of on site or at an approved waste disposal facility.
CONTAINER DISPOSAL: Do not reuse empty containers. Triple rinse (or equivalent) then offer for recycling or reconditioning, or puncture and dispose of in a sanitary landfill, or by incineration, or, if allowed by state and local authorities, by burning. If burned, stay out of smoke.
EPA Est. No. 67517-MO-1
EPA Reg. No. 67517-66-11556
SUPPLIED: Code 0383—200 x 14 g (0.5 oz) Blocks 0383 R. 1
Manufactured For: Bayer Corporation, Agriculture Division, Animal Health, Shawnee Mission, Kansas 66201 U.S.A.
Compendium Code No.: 10400131

C

CLOUT™
Place Packs
Bayer
Mouse and Rat Poison
For Indoor And Outdoor Rodent Control
Kills House Mice, Norway Rats And Roof Rats
House Mice, Norway Rats and Roof Rats usually consume a lethal dose in a single day's feeding, but it may take two or more days from the time of bait consumption, or pack removal, for these rodents to die. Rodents cease feeding after consuming a lethal dose. Clout™ Place Packs are effective against anticoagulant-resistant mice and rats.
Contains Bitrex
ACTIVE INGREDIENT:
Bromethalin: N methyl-2,4-dinitro-N-(2,4,6-tribromophenyl)-6-(trifluoromethyl) benzenamine.......... 0.01%
INERT INGREDIENTS.......... 99.99%
TOTAL.......... 100.00%
KEEP OUT OF REACH OF CHILDREN
CAUTION
PRECAUTIONARY STATEMENTS
HAZARD TO HUMANS & DOMESTIC ANIMALS
CAUTION
Keep away from humans, domestic animals and pets. May be harmful or fatal if swallowed. Avoid contact with skin, eyes or clothing. Wash thoroughly with soap and water after handling bait.
FIRST AID
IF SWALLOWED: Call a physician or Poison Control Center. Drink 1 or 2 glasses of water and induce vomiting by touching back of the throat with finger. If person is unconscious, do not give anything by mouth and do not induce vomiting.
IF IN EYES: Flush eyes with plenty of water. Call a physician if irritation persists.
IF ON SKIN: Wash with plenty of soap and water. Get medical attention if irritation persists.
NOTE TO PHYSICIAN:
Clout™ Place Packs are not an anticoagulant type of rodenticide. If ingested, limit absorption by either emesis or gastric lavage. Sublethal symptoms, if present, would be the result of cerebral edema and should be treated accordingly through administration of an osmotic diuretic and corticosteroid.
ENVIRONMENTAL HAZARDS
This product is toxic to mammals and birds. Do not apply this product directly to water, or to areas where surface water is present or to intertidal areas below the mean high water mark.
DIRECTIONS FOR USE
It is a violation of Federal Law to use this product in a manner inconsistent with its labeling.
READ THE LABEL: Read the entire label and follow all use directions and use precautions.
IMPORTANT: Do not expose children, pets, or other nontarget animals to rodenticides. To help to prevent accidents:
1. Store product not in use in a location out of reach of children and pets.
2. Apply bait in locations out of reach of children, pets, domestic animals and nontarget wildlife, or in tamper-resistant bait stations. These stations must be resistant to destruction by dogs and by children under six years of age, and must be used in a manner that prevents such children from reaching into bait compartments and obtaining bait. If bait can be shaken from stations when they are lifted, units must be secured or otherwise immobilized. Even stronger bait stations are needed in areas open to hoofed livestock, raccoons, bears, or other potentially destructive animals, or in areas prone to vandalism.
3. Dispose of product container, and unused, spoiled, and unconsumed bait as specified on the label.

USE RESTRICTIONS
For control of Norway rats, roof rats and house mice in and around homes, industrial and agricultural buildings, and similar man-made structures. This product may also be used in alleys located in urban areas, inside transport vehicles (ships, trains, aircraft), and in and around related port or terminal buildings. Do not use Clout™ Place packs in sewers. Do not place this bait in areas where there is a possibility of contaminating food or surfaces that come in contact with food. Do not broadcast placepacks or bait.
SELECTION OF TREATMENT AREAS:
Determine areas where rodents will most likely find and consume the bait. Generally, these are along walls, by gnawed openings, in or beside burrows, in corners and concealed places, between floors and walls, or in locations where rodents or their signs have been seen. Protect bait from rain or snow. Remove as much alternative food as possible.
APPLICATION DIRECTIONS:
The active ingredient in Clout™ Place Packs is different from anticoagulant rodenticides. Individual mice cease feeding after consuming a toxic dose.
RATS: Apply 2 - 12 place packs per placement location. Space placements at intervals of 15 to 30 feet.
MICE: Apply 1 - 2 place packs per placement. Space placements at intervals of 8 to 12 feet. Larger placements up to six place packs, may be needed at points of extremely high mouse activity.
RATS AND MICE: Adjust the amount of bait applied to the level of feeding by target rodents expected at each placement location. Highest bait consumption is expected to occur during the first day or two after treatment. After several days, inspect bait placements and replenish bait at sites where there is heavy feeding or where there is continued evidence of rodent activity. Maintain bait for at least one week and continue baiting until all signs of rodent activity have ceased or it becomes clear that the remaining rodents are not attracted to the bait.
Collect and properly dispose of all dead animals and leftover bait. To discourage reinfestation, limit sources of rodent food, water, and harborage as much as possible. If reinfestation does occur, repeat treatment. Where a continuous source of infestation is present, establish permanent bait stations and replenish as needed.

STORAGE AND DISPOSAL
Do not contaminate water, food or feed by storage or disposal.
PESTICIDE STORAGE: Store in original container in a cool, dry place inaccessible to children and pets. Keep containers closed and away from other chemicals.
PESTICIDE DISPOSAL: Wastes resulting from the use of this product may be disposed of on site or at an approved waste disposal facility.
CONTAINER DISPOSAL: Do not reuse empty containers. Triple rinse (or equivalent) then offer for recycling or reconditioning, or puncture and dispose of in a sanitary landfill, or incineration or, if allowed by state and local authorities, by burning. If burned, stay out of smoke.
EPA Est. No. 67517-MO-1
EPA Reg. No. 67517-72-11556
SUPPLIED: Code 0382—200 x 14 g (0.5 oz) Packets 0382 R. 1
Manufactured For: Bayer Corporation, Agriculture Division, Animal Health, Shawnee Mission, Kansas 66201 U.S.A.
Compendium Code No.: 10400141

CLOVITE® CONDITIONER
Fort Dodge **Vitamins A-B_{12}-D**
Vitamin Supplement for All Species of Animals
Guaranteed Analysis: Minimum Vitamin Guarantee (each pound contains):
Vitamin A .... 110,000 IU (242 IU/g)
Vitamin D .... 50,000 IU (110 IU/g)
Vitamin B_{12} .... 136 mcg (0.3 mcg/g)
Ingredients: Soybean meal, Soy flour, Vitamin A & D oil, Dicalcium phosphate, Vitamin B_{12} supplement, Vitamin A & D_3 supplement, Choline chloride, Vitamin E supplement, Calcium pantothenate, Niacin, Pyridoxine hydrochloride, Thiamine hydrochloride, Riboflavin, Biotin.
Indications: A vitamin supplement for all species of animals.
Dosage and Administration: Suggested Usage:
Young Foals and Weanlings: 1 to 2 tablespoonfuls daily.
Brood Mares: (latter half of pregnancy and lactation) 2 tablespoonfuls twice a day.
Ponies: 1 tablespoonful daily.
Colts, Stallions and Horses in Training: 1 tablespoonful per 400 lb daily.
All Farm Animals: 1 to 3 lb to each 100 lb feed.
Mature Cattle: (milking or on full feed) 1 to 3 lb to each 100 lb feed. Many dairymen prefer adding a handful to each feeding. Feedlot operators simply top off feed with the prescribed amount of CLOVITE®.
Calves: (bucket fed) 1 to 2 tablespoonfuls daily in milk or ground feed.
Range Cattle: Supplemental feeding is simplified by mixing with salt - 1 part to 10 parts salt, or 2½ lb to 25 lb salt. (These calculations are based on normal consumption of ¼ lb of salt per day by a 1,000 lb cow and ⅛ lb. per day by a 400 lb steer.) To prevent the oxidation that tends to destroy all Vitamin A compounds on prolonged exposure, mix only the amount normally consumed in a 3-week period.
Poultry: 1 lb to each 100 lb feed.
Baby Pigs: 3% of the creep-feed.
Dogs and Cats: 1 level teaspoonful per each 10 lb of body weight daily. This dosage should be doubled for growing pups and kittens, lactating animals and animals in the last half of pregnancy. Dosage may be varied as prescribed by the veterinarian.
Mink: 1 level teaspoonful daily.
Presentation: 5 lb (2.2 kg) pail and 25 lb bag.
Compendium Code No.: 10030342 2336H

CLTC® 100 MR
Phibro **Tetracycline-Oral**
NADA No.: 092-287
Active Ingredient(s):
Chlortetracycline 22%
Each pound of CLTC® 100 MR contains 100 g of chlortetracycline hydrochloride, with dextrose monohydrate as an inert ingredient.
Indications: A type A medicated article to be mixed in calf milk replacers and starter feeds to aid in growth promotion and feed efficiency and to aid in the prevention of bacterial diarrhea.
Dosage and Administration: For calves up to 250 lb., in milk replacers or starter feeds:
Growth promotion and feed efficiency: Mix 0.1 mg of chlortetracycline per pound of body weight per day.
Example: To prepare a finished milk replacer or starter feed containing 40 g per ton of chlortetracycline, add 6.4 oz of CLTC® 100 MR.
As an aid in the prevention of bacterial diarrhea: Mix 0.5 mg of chlortetracycline per pound of body weight per day.
Example: To prepare a finished milk replacer or starter feed containing 200 g per ton of chlortetracycline, add 2 lb. of CLTC® 100 MR.
Caution(s): Do not use without diluting.
For further manufacturing use only.
Not for use in liquid feed supplements.
Presentation: 100 lbs. (45.4 kg).
CLTC is a registered trademark of Phibro Animal Health, for chlortetracycline hydrochloride.
Compendium Code No.: 36930051

CMPK ℞
RXV **Calcium-Combination Therapy**
Calcium-Magnesium-Phosphorus-Potassium-Dextrose
Active Ingredient(s): Each 500 mL contains:
Dextrose • H_2O .... 75.0 g
Calcium (as calcium borogluconate) .... 10.8 g
Potassium (as potassium chloride) .... 8.0 g
Phosphorus (as sodium hypophosphite • H_2O) .... 2.5 g
Magnesium (as magnesium borogluconate) .... 1.6 g
Indications: For use in cattle as an aid in the treatment of conditions associated with calcium, magnesium, phosphorus, potassium or glucose deficiencies.
Dosage and Administration:
Cattle .... 500 mL/800-1000 lbs body weight
For intravenous administration only. Solutions should be warmed to room temperature and administered slowly using aseptic precautions, such as using a sterile needle and syringe and disinfecting the site of injection.

Contraindication(s): Do not administer this product to animals showing signs of cardiac distress. Monitor animal's condition closely.
Precaution(s): Store at controlled room temperature between 15°-30°C (59°-86°F).
Caution(s): Federal law restricts this drug to use by or on the order of a licensed veterinarian.
Entire contents should be used when first entered as this product contains no preservatives. Discard any unused portion. For veterinary use only. Keep out of the reach of children.
Presentation: 500 mL vials.
Compendium Code No.: 10910030

CMPK BOLUS

Durvet **Calcium-Oral**

Guaranteed Analysis: Per Bolus (Min):

Calcium (min.)	3.5 g
Calcium (max.)	4.0 g
Phosphorus	2.0 g
Magnesium	1.5 g
Potassium	1.0 g
Sodium	0.5 g
Vitamin D_3	50,000 IU
Vitamin E	300 IU

Ingredients: Dicalcium phosphate, magnesium oxide, sodium chloride, calcium carbonate, potassium chloride, dl-alpha-tocopherol acetate, corn starch, vitamin D_3 supplement, and magnesium stearate.
Indications: Durvet CMPK BOLUS is a nutritional supplement for the additional intake of the minerals calcium, magnesium, phosphorus, and potassium; plus vitamin E and D_3.
Directions for Use:
Cattle/Horses:
1 to 2 boluses per day for daily supplementation.
2 to 3 boluses per day for increased nutrient intake.
Sheep/Swine:
½ to 1 boluses per day for daily supplementation.
1 to 2 boluses per day for increased nutrient intake.
Boluses may be administered orally with a balling gun, crushed and sprinkled in milk or water and given as a drench.
Precaution(s): Store in a cool dry place.
Caution(s): For animal use only.
Warning(s): Not for human use. Keep out of reach of children.
Presentation: 50 boluses 24 g each (NDC 30798-563-69).
Compendium Code No.: 10841940 10-01

CMPK BOLUS

Vets Plus **Calcium-Oral**

Guaranteed Analysis: Per bolus (Min):

Calcium (min)	3.32 g
Calcium (max)	3.68 g
Phosphorus	2.0 g
Magnesium	1.5 g
Potassium	1.0 g
Sodium	0.5 g
Vitamin D_3	50,000 IU
Vitamin E	300 IU

Ingredients: Dicalcium phosphate, magnesium oxide, sodium chloride, calcium carbonate, potassium chloride, dl-alpha-tocopherol acetate, corn starch, vitamin D_3 supplement, and magnesium stearate.
Indications: A source of calcium, magnesium, phosphorus and potassium for cattle, horses, sheep and swine.
Dosage and Administration:
Cattle/Horses:
1 to 2 boluses per day for daily supplementation.
2 to 3 boluses per day for increased nutrient intake.
Sheep/Swine:
½ to 1 boluses per day for daily supplementation.
1 to 2 boluses per day for increased nutrient intake.
Boluses may be administered orally with a balling gun, crushed and sprinkled in milk or water and given as a drench.
Precaution(s): Keep lid tightly closed. Store in a cool, dry place.
Caution(s): Keep out of reach of children. For animal use only.
Presentation: 50 Boluses, 24 g each.
Compendium Code No.: 10730070

CMPK D_3 DRENCH

Durvet **Calcium-Oral**

Guaranteed Analysis: (per 354 mL feeding):
Calcium Chloride ($CaCl_2$) 40%
Ingredients: Water, calcium chloride, magnesium chloride, propylene glycol, potassium chloride, sodium hypophosphite and vitamin D_3.
Indications: CMPK D_3 DRENCH is an oral calcium, magnesium, phosphorus, potassium and vitamin D supplement for use before and after freshening in dairy and beef cattle, sheep and goats as a milk fever preventive. It can also be used after calving as an appetite stimulant. CMPK D_3 DRENCH is also suggested for sheep and goats.
Dosage and Administration:
Cattle: Administer orally one 12 oz bottle pre-birthing and additional feedings post-birthing as needed.
Sheep and Goats: Administer 1-2 oz. orally depending on the body weight, pre-birthing and additional feedings post-birthing or as directed by your veterinarian.
Exercise care in administering to avoid aspiration into the lungs. Do not feed to animals without swallowing reflex.
Precaution(s): Shake well before using. Protect from freezing. Keep in a cool dry place.
Caution(s): For animal use only.
Warning(s): Not for human use. Keep out of reach of children.
Presentation: 354 mL (12 fl oz) bottle.
Compendium Code No.: 10841950 8-01

CMPK-DEX ℞

Vetus **Calcium-Combination Therapy**

Composition: Each 500 mL of aqueous solution contains:

Calcium (as calcium borogluconate, equivalent to calcium gluconate 23.2%)	10.8 g
Potassium (as potassium chloride)	8.0 g
Phosphorus (as sodium hypophosphite•H_2O)	2.5 g
Magnesium (as magnesium borogluconate)	1.6 g
Dextrose•H_2O	75.0 g
Millequivalents per liter - Cations:	
Calcium	1,080 mEq/L
Potassium	410 mEq/L
Magnesium	261 mEq/L
Sodium	161 mEq/L
Millequivalents per liter - Anions:	
Borogluconate	1,341 mEq/L
Chloride	410 mEq/L
Hypophosphite	161 mEq/L
Osmolarity (calc.)	11,597 mOsmol/L

Indications: For use as an aid in the treatment of hypocalcemia (parturient paresis, milk fever), hypomagnesemia (grass tetany), and other conditions associated with calcium, magnesium, phosphorus and potassium deficiencies in cattle.
Dosage and Administration: Warm solution to body temperature. The usual intravenous dose in cattle is 500 mL per 800 to 1,000 pounds of body weight.
Contraindication(s): Do not administer this product to animals showing signs of cardiac distress.
Precaution(s): Store between 15°C and 30°C (59°F-86°F).
Caution(s): Federal law restricts this drug to use by or on the order of a licensed veterinarian.
Administration should be made slowly and with care to avoid adverse effects such as heart block or shock. Perivascular or subcutaneous deposition of hypertonic solutions may result in severe inflammation at the injection site.
This product contains no preservatives. Use entire contents when first opened. Discard any unused solution.
Warning(s): For animal use only.
Keep out of reach of children.
Presentation: 500 mL bottles.
Compendium Code No.: 14440220

C.M.P.K. GEL

AgriLabs **Calcium-Oral**

Active Ingredient(s): Each tube contains:

Calcium (min.)	18%
Calcium (max.)	20% (54 g)
Phosphorous (min.)	10 g
Magnesium (min.)	2.0 g
Potassium (min.)	1 g

Contains calcium chloride, water, sodium hexameta, phosphate, magnesium chloride, potassium chloride, starch and guar gum.
Indications: A nutritional supplement preparation that supplies calcium, magnesium, phosphorus and potassium to ensure normal levels in the blood before, during and after calving.
Dosage and Administration: Give one (1) tube within 6-12 hours prior to calving. Give another tube within 6-12 hours after calving.
Hold the head of the cow in a normal to slightly elevated position. Place the tube in the cow's mouth directly over the tongue. The product is carefully pressed out of the 300 mL tube. Hold the cow's mouth closed and allow time to swallow. Administer the entire 300 mL tube for each dose.
Caution(s): Follow label directions. Keep out of the reach of children. Contact with the eyes or wounds, or prolonged contact with the skin can cause irritation.
Presentation: 14 oz. (400 g) tubes.
Compendium Code No.: 10580240

CMPK GEL

AgriPharm **Calcium-Oral**

Active Ingredient(s): Minimum contents of 300 mL dose:

Calcium	47,250 mg/dose (47.3 g)
Magnesium	2,925 mg/dose (2.9 g)
Phosphorus	6,181 mg/dose (6.2 g)
Potassium	1,010 mg/dose (1.0 g)

Calcium chloride, water, phosphoric acid, trisodium phosphate, magnesium chloride, glucose, citric acid, potassium chloride, silicon dioxide, flavors.
Indications: For use as a high calcium nutritional supplement for dairy cattle during calving.
Dosage and Administration: Administer orally on back of tongue.

Prior to calving	1 tube
After calving	1 tube

Give one tube prior to calving and the second tube 24 hours after calving using the following directions:
1. Hold head of the cow in a slightly elevated position.
2. Place nozzle near rear of mouth. Use of hook nozzle recommended.
3. Discharge entire contents of the tube.
4. Hold up head of cow and allow animal time to swallow.

Precaution(s): Do not freeze. Keep cool.
Warning(s): For animal use only.
Keep out of reach of children.
Presentation: 300 mL.
Compendium Code No.: 14570210

CMPK GEL

Durvet **Calcium-Oral**

Active Ingredient(s): Minimum Contents of 300 mL Dose:

Calcium	47.3 gms - 11.5% minimum 67.6 gms - 16.5% maximum
Phosphorus	6.2 gms - 1.5%
Magnesium	2.9 gms - 0.7%
Potassium	1.0 gms - 0.2%

Ingredients: Calcium chloride, water, phosphorus acid, trisodium phosphate, magnesium hydroxide, glucose, potassium chloride, silicon dioxide, sodium citrate, artificial flavorings.
Indications: A high calcium nutritional supplement for dairy cattle during calving.
Not a drug - No withdrawal time.
Directions for Use:
1. Hold head of the cow in a slightly elevated position.
2. Place nozzle near rear of mouth. Use of hook nozzle recommended.
3. Discharge entire contents of the tube.
4. Hold head up and allow animal time to swallow.

Give one tube prior to or after calving and second tube 12 to 24 hours after calving.
Precaution(s): Do not freeze.
Caution(s): For animal use only. Not for human use. Keep out of reach of children.
Presentation: 300 mL tubes (NDC 30798-560-15).
Patent Pending
Compendium Code No.: 10840331 Rev. 6/01

C

CMPK GEL
Vedco **Calcium-Oral**

Active Ingredient(s): Contents of 375 g dose (mg/dose):
Calcium .... 47,250 - 47.3 g
Magnesium .... 2,925 - 2.9 g
Phosphorus .... 6,181 - 6.2 g
Potassium .... 1,010 - 1.0 g

Ingredients: Calcium chloride, water, phosphoric acid, trisodium phosphate, magnesium chloride, glucose, citric acid, potassium chloride, silicon dioxide, flavors.
Indications: A calcium supplement for dairy cattle during calving.
Dosage and Administration:
1. Hold the head of the cow in a slightly elevated position.
2. Place the nozzle near the rear of the mouth. The use of a hook nozzle is recommended.
3. Discharge the entire contents of the tube.
4. Hold the head up and allow the animal time to swallow.

Give one (1) tube prior to calving and the second tube 24 hours after calving.
Presentation: 375 g tubes.
Compendium Code No.: 10940330

CMPK GEL PLUS™
Vets Plus **Calcium-Oral**

Oral Calcium, Magnesium, Phosphorus, and Potassium Gel
Guaranteed Analysis: (min):

	Per Tube	Per lb.
Calcium	54 g	63 g
Calcium (max)	58 g	68 g
Phosphorus	10 g	11 g
Magnesium	3 g	3 g
Potassium	2 g	2 g

Ingredients: Calcium Chloride, Tri-Calcium Phosphate, Magnesium Chloride, Potassium Chloride, and Xanthan Gum.
Indications: Administer to every fresh cow or heifer before and after calving to lower the incidence of milk fever. CMPK GEL PLUS™ can also be used as a follow up to IV treatment.
Dosage and Administration: Give one tube at the first sign of freshening and give another tube 6 to 12 hours post calving, repeat every 12 hours as needed. If the first dose is missed, a post calving dose is still beneficial. If conditions do not improve, consult your veterinarian.
Feeding Directions: Place the tube in a dosing gun and remove the cap. Hold the head of the cow in a normal to slightly elevated position and place the nozzle on the back of the tongue. Administer the entire contents of the tube slowly, allowing the cow time to swallow. Do not give to cows that are unable to swallow.
Precaution(s): Keep in a cool dry place. Avoid Freezing.
Caution(s): Keep out of the reach of children. Contact with eyes or wounds or prolonged contact with skin can cause irritation. Single dose unit. Properly dispose of unused portion.
Animal use only.
Presentation: 12x300 cc (400 gm) tubes per case.
Compendium Code No.: 10730080

C-M-P-K INJECTION ℞
Vet Tek **Calcium-Combination Therapy**

Calcium-Magnesium-Phosphorus-Potassium-Dextrose Solution
Active Ingredient(s): Composition: Each 500 mL of sterile aqueous solution contains:
Calcium (as calcium borogluconate, equivalent to calcium gluconate 23.2%) .... 10.8 g
Potassium (as potassium chloride) .... 8.0 g
Phosphorus (as sodium hypophosphite • H_2O) .... 2.5 g
Magnesium (as magnesium borogluconate) .... 1.6 g
Dextrose • H_2O .... 75.0 g

Milliequivalents per liter:
Cations:
Calcium .... 1,080 mEq/L
Potassium .... 410 mEq/L
Magnesium .... 261 mEq/L
Sodium .... 161 mEq/L
Anions:
Borogluconate .... 1,341 mEq/L
Chloride .... 410 mEq/L
Hypophosphite .... 161 mEq/L
Osmolarity (calc.) .... 11,597 mOsmol/L

This product contains no preservatives.
Indications: For use as an aid in the treatment of hypocalcemia (parturient paresis, milk fever), hypomagnesemia (grass tetany), and other conditions associated with calcium, magnesium, phosphorous and potassium deficiencies in cattle.
Dosage and Administration: Warm the solution to body temperature. The usual intravenous dose in cattle is 500 mL per 800 to 1,000 pounds of body weight.
Contraindication(s): Do not administer this product to animals showing signs of cardiac distress.
Precaution(s): Store between 15°C and 30°C (59°F-86°F). Use entire contents when first opened. Discard any unused solution.
Caution(s): Federal law restricts this drug to use by or on the order of a licensed veterinarian.
Administration should be made slowly and with care to avoid adverse effects such as heart block or shock. Perivascular or subcutaneous deposition of hypertonic solutions may result in severe inflammation of the injection site.
For animal use only.
Warning(s): Keep out of reach of children.
Presentation: 500 mL vials (NDC No. 60270-026-17).
Manufactured by: Phoenix Scientific, Inc. St. Joseph, MO 64506.
Compendium Code No.: 14200031 Rev. 5-95

CMPK ORAL ℞
AgriPharm **Calcium-Oral**

Active Ingredient(s): Each 500 mL of aqueous solution contains:
Calcium (as calcium borogluconate) .... 10.0 g
Phosphorus (as sodium phosphate monobasic) .... 6.0 g
Magnesium (as magnesium chloride • $6H_2O$) .... 2.8 g
Potassium (as potassium chloride) .... 0.5 g
Dextrose • H_2O .... 75.0 g
Benzyl alcohol .... 1.5% v/v
Indications: For use as a supplemental source of calcium, phosphorus, magnesium, potassium and dextrose in cattle.
Dosage and Administration: Administer orally as a drench. The usual oral dose for adult cattle is 500 mL.
Precaution(s): Store at a controlled room temperature between 59°-86°F (15°-30°C).
Caution(s): Not for human use. Keep out of the reach of children.
Presentation: 500 mL containers.
Compendium Code No.: 14570220

C.M.P.K. ORAL GEL
Phoenix Pharmaceutical **Calcium-Oral**

Nutritional Supplement
Guaranteed Analysis: Per Tube/Dose:
Calcium (Ca), Min. 11.5% .... 47.3 g
Calcium (Ca), Max. 16.5% .... 67.6 g
Phosphorus (P), Min. 1.5% .... 6.2 g
Magnesium (Mg), Min. 0.7% .... 2.9 g
Potassium (K), Min. 0.2% .... 1.0 g

Ingredients: Calcium Chloride, Purified Water, Phosphoric Acid, Tri-Sodium Phosphate, Magnesium Hydroxide, Glucose, Potassium Chloride, Silicon Dioxide, Sodium Citrate, Artificial Flavorings.
Indications: A nutritional supplement for dairy cattle.
Directions for Use: Place the tube in a dosing gun and remove the cap. Hold the head of the cow in a normal to slightly elevated position and carefully place the nozzle into the back of the mouth. Administer the entire contents of one tube per feeding. Do not give to cows or calves that are unable to swallow.
Give one tube within 6 to 12 hours prior to calving. Give another tube within 6 to 12 hours alter calving.
Precaution(s): Store at room temperature.
Caution(s): For animal use only.
Warning(s): Not a drug. No withdrawal time. Keep out of reach of children.
Presentation: 300 mL single dose units (NDC 57319-456-29).
Manufactured by: First Priority, Inc., Elgin, IL 60123-1146.
Compendium Code No.: 12560102 Rev. 03-02

CMPK ORAL SOLUTION 33%
Vedco **Calcium-Oral**

Active Ingredient(s): Each 12 oz. (360 mL) bottle contains:
Calcium chloride .... 118.8 g (33%)
Phosphate 6.2 g (1.7%)
Magnesium 2.9 g (0.8%)
Potassium 1 g (0.3%)
Indications: CMPK ORAL is indicated for use as a supplemental source of calcium, potassium, phosphorus and magnesium in cattle.
Dosage and Administration: Administer at the rate of one (1) bottle each day or additionally upon the direction of a veterinarian. Administer with care to avoid aspiration. Shake well before use.
Caution(s): An overdose can cause hypercalcemia. At the first sign of hypercalcemia, discontinue use and consult a veterinarian.
For use in cattle only. For veterinary use only. Keep out of the reach of children.
Presentation: 12 oz. (360 mL) bottle.
Compendium Code No.: 10940340

CMPK SOLUTION
Aspen **Calcium-Combination Therapy**

Composition: Each 500 mL of aqueous solution contains:
Calcium (As Calcium Borogluconate) .... 10.0 g
Phosphorous (As Sodium Hypophosphite H_2O) .... 6.0 g
Magnesium (As Magnesium Chloride • $6H_2O$) .... 2.8 g
Potassium (As Potassium Chloride) .... 0.5 g
Dextrose • H_2O .... 75.0 g

With methylparaben 0.18%, propylparaben 0.02%, and ethylparaben 0.01% added as preservatives.
Indications: For use as a supplemental nutritive source of calcium, phosphorous, magnesium, potassium and dextrose in cattle.
Dosage and Administration: Administer orally as a drench. The usual dose for adult cattle is 500 mL.
Precaution(s): Store at a controlled room temperature between 15° and 36°C (59°-86°F).
Warning(s): For animal use only. Keep out of reach of children.
Presentation: 500 mL.
Compendium Code No.: 14750140

CMPK SOLUTION ℞

Bimeda **Calcium-Combination Therapy**

Active Ingredient(s): Composition: Each 500 mL of sterile aqueous solution contains:

Dextrose H_2O .... 75.0 g
Calcium (as calcium borogluconate) .... 10.8 g
Potassium (as potassium chloride) .... 8.0 g
Phosphorus (as sodium hypophosphite•H_2O .... 2.5 g
Magnesium (as magnesium borogluconate) .... 1.6 g

Milliequivalents per liter:

Cations:

Calcium .... 1080 mEq/L
Potassium .... 410 mEq/L
Magnesium .... 261 mEq/L
Sodium .... 161 mEq/L

Anions:

Borogluconate .... 1341 mEq/L
Hypophosphite .... 161 mEq/L
Chloride .... 410 mEq/L

This product contains no preservatives.

Indications: For use as an aid in the treatment of hypocalcemia (parturient paresis, milk fever), hypomagnesemia (grass tetany) and other conditions associated with calcium, magnesium, phosphorus, and potassium deficiencies in cattle.

Dosage and Administration: Warm solution to body temperature. The usual intravenous dose in cattle is 500 mL per 800 to 1,000 pounds of body weight.

Contraindication(s): Do not administer this product to animals showing signs of cardiac distress.

Precaution(s): Store at temperature between 15°C-30°C (59°F-86°F).

Use entire contents when first opened. Discard any unused solution.

Caution(s): Federal law restricts this drug to use by or on the order of a licensed veterinarian.

Administration should be made slowly and with care to avoid adverse effects such as heart block or shock. Perivascular or subcutaneous deposition of hypertonic solutions may result in severe inflammation at the injection site.

For animal use only.

Warning(s): Keep out of reach of children.

Presentation: 500 mL bottles (NDC# 61133-2696-9).

Manufactured by: Bimeda-MTC Animal Health Inc., Cambridge, Ontario, Canada N3C 2W4.

Compendium Code No.: 13990081 Iss. 2.99

CMPK SOLUTION ℞

Vedco **Calcium-Combination Therapy**

Active Ingredient(s): Each 100 mL contains:

Calcium Gluconate (provides 2.14 grams Calcium) .... 23.0 g
Magnesium Chloride Hexahydrate .... 4.5 g
Sodium Hypophosphite Monohydrate .... 3.43 g
Potassium Chloride .... 0.2 g
Dextrose Monohydrate .... 25 g
Water for Injection .... q.s.

Contains boric acid as a solubilizing agent.

Electrolytes per 1000 mL; Calcium 1069 mEq; Magnesium 443 mEq; Sodium 324 mEq; Phosphorus 324 mEq; Potassium 27 mEq. Hypertonic.

Indications: To be used as an aid in the treatment of parturient paresis (milk fever) and hypomagnesemic tetany (grass tetany) in cattle.

Dosage and Administration: Cattle: 250 to 500 mL.

For intravenous use only.

Solution should be warmed to body temperature and administered slowly. This product is sterile in unopened container. It contains no preservative. Use entire contents when first opened. It should be handled under aseptic conditions.

Precaution(s): Store between 15 and 30°C.

Caution(s): Federal law restricts this drug to use by or on the order of a licensed veterinarian.

Warning(s): For animal use only. Keep out of reach of children.

Presentation: 500 mL containers.

Compendium Code No.: 10940350

CMPK WITH D_3 DRENCH

Vets Plus **Calcium-Oral**

Guaranteed Analysis: (Per 200 mL):

Calcium, min .... 28.7 g
Calcium, max .... 29.4 g

Ingredients: Water, calcium chloride, magnesium chloride, propylene glycol, potassium chloride, sodium hypophosphite and vitamin D_3.

Indications: An oral nutrient supplement for use on every fresh cow or heifer before and after calving. CMPK drench provides calcium along with phosphorus, magnesium, potassium and vitamin D_3 to lower the incidences of milk fever and propylene glycol for energy. CMPK Drench can also be used as a follow up to IV treatment.

Dosage and Administration: Provide 200 mL at the first sign of freshening and another 200 mL 6 to 12 hours after freshening, repeat as needed. If the first dose is missed, a post calving dose is still beneficial. Shake well before using. If conditions do not improve, consult your veterinarian. 1 gallon provides nineteen 200 mL feedings.

Feeding Directions: Administer orally using a drench gun. Hold the head of the animal in a slightly elevated position and carefully place nozzle into the back of the mouth between the cheek and teeth. Slowly administer recommended dosage. Do not give to cows that are unable to swallow.

Precaution(s): Keep in a cool, dry place. Avoid freezing.

Caution(s): For animal use only.

Warning(s): Keep out of the reach of children. Contact with eyes or wounds or prolonged contact with skin, can cause irritation.

Presentation: 1 gallon (3.8 L), 5 gallons and 15 gallons.

Compendium Code No.: 10730012

CMT (CALIFORNIA MASTITIS TEST)

ImmuCell **Mastitis Test**

Indications: A rapid cow-side test for early detection of bovine mastitis.

ImmuCell's CMT provides the producer with a simple and rapid method for the detection of elevated SCC in mammary glands suspected of having mastitis. This inexpensive cow-side test requires no sophisticated equipment and can be used is often as it is practical. The test is intended in part for use with good mastitis management practices. If ImmuCell's CMT were to detect elevated SCC in specific quarters, actions can quickly be taken to remedy the causes for this increase. The use of antibiotics is frequently the course of therapy to treat mastitic quarters. However, not all antibiotic regimens are successful. Some producers will incorporate microbiological culture and antibiotic sensitivity testing into their mastitis management practices to aid in developing successful treatment strategies. Unfortunately, results from these tests may take days, However, ImmuCell's MASTiK™ Antibiotic Susceptibility Test Kit used in concert with CMT can provide similar results sooner which may enhance your herd's mastitis treatment success by aiding the veterinarian and producer in selecting an effective antibiotic for mastitis therapy. Sensitivity results from the MASTiK™ test can be obtained in as little as 12 hours, saving 24-48 hours compared to the traditional test method.

Test Procedure: Directions:

Collect milk from individual quarters

1. Dilute CMT concentrate. (Makes 1½ gallons of CMT working solution.) See concentrate bottle for directions.
2. Discard first stream of milk.
3. Draw foremilk from each quarter into the corresponding cup of testing paddle.
4. Do not use colostrum, milk from fresh cows (<3 days post-calving) or samples after dry-off.

Pour off excess milk

1. Tilt testing paddle to discharge excess milk until equal volumes remain in each cup.
2. Remaining milk should be level with the outside (largest) circle in the cup.

Add and equal amount of CMT working solution

1. Tilt testing paddle back until milk is halfway between the inner and outer circles.
2. Slowly add CMT working solution into each cup until mixture is even with the inside circle of each cup. This should provide equal parts milk to CMT solution.

Rotary movement of test paddle

1. Gently rotate mixture in a horizontal position.
2. Reaction can be observed almost immediately. Thickening or gel formation indicates high somatic cell counts and likelihood of mastitis.
3. Record results on enclosed chart.
4. Contact your veterinarian with positive CMT results for assistance in adopting a treatment strategy.

Uses and Scoring of the CMT: The CMT could be used regularly (e.g. every 2 weeks) to screen individual quarters within your entire herd for subclinical mastitis, characterized by increases in SCC. Ideally, screening individual quarters can be performed in concert with recent DHIA SCC data to better identity the quarter(s) responsible for elevated SCC. In addition, CMT can also be used to quantify SCC in composite and bulk tank samples. Elevations in SCC in composite samples or the bulk tank can indicate a mastitis problem in individual cows or entire herd, respectively.

Samples tested by CMT should be foremilk samples obtained during the active period of lactation. Milk samples can be stored refrigerated for up to 36 hours prior to testing. CMT should not be used on strippings, milk samples prior to 3 days after calving or after dry-off has started. The CMT reagent reacts with leukocytes (somatic cells) that are elevated during mastitis. The degree of gel formation is proportional to the increasing numbers of leukocytes present during mammary gland inflammation, characteristic of mastitis. Greater gel formation corresponds to a higher CMT score.

Interpretation of Results: Grading CMT Reactions: Defining CMT Scores:

Negative: Mixture remains liquid with no evidence of thickening or formation of a precipitate.

Trace: Slight thickening that tends to disappear with continued movement of the paddle.

1 (Weak): Distinct thickening but no tendency toward gel formation. Thickening may disappear after prolonged rotation of the paddle.

2 (Distinct): Mixture thickens immediately. With continued rotation of paddle, liquid moves towards the center, leaving the bottom of the outer edge of the cup exposed.

3 (Strong): A distinct gel forms which tends to adhere to the bottom of the paddle and during swirling a distinct mass forms.

CMT Scores and Estimates of Corresponding SCC

CMT Score	Est. SCC (cells/mL)	Mastitis Diagnosis
Negative	< 200,000	No mastitis
Trace	150,000 to 500,000	Suspicious
1 (Weak)	400,000 to 1,500,000	Suspicious
2 (Distinct)	800,000 to 5,000,000	Mastitis
3 (Strong)	Over 5,000,000	Mastitis

Positive CMT Results: The CMT is meant to assist the producer in monitoring udder health. Results obtained from the CMT correlate broadly to SCC. Most positive CMT reactions indicate abnormally high SCC. Trace or weak (CMT Score 1) CMT results, indicating a suspicious mastitis diagnosis, may reflect two possible scenarios. First, these results may suggest that the mammary gland is presently recovering from a previous infection. Second, a suspicious diagnosis may suggest early detection of mastitis. In either case, another CMT test should be performed to determine if mastitis is present and any additional actions are needed.

In contrast, distinct and strong positive CMT results (CMT Scores 3 & 4) on milk samples collected from individual quarters or composites indicate an ongoing inflammatory response characterized by elevated SCC. This inflammatory response may be due to the response of the mammary gland to mechanical injury, or most likely the response to mastitis-causing pathogens (bacteria). In order to maintain optimum milk production and high milk quality, producers in cooperation with their veterinarian must decide what appropriate actions should be taken to reduce the SCC.

Interpretation of CMT results from bulk tank samples will be somewhat different. Only a negative CMT response using samples from the bulk tank would indicate low prevalence of mastitis in your milking herd. However, all other positive CMT scores of bulk tank samples tested (including Trace) suggest a prevalence of mastitis that should be addressed. If the producer only checks his bulk tank periodically, any positive CMT response should indicate that an action be taken. At the very least, quarters from all of the cows in the herd should be tested with CMT to identify which cows are contributing the most to the abnormally high SCC in the bulk tank.

Initially, the cause of the mammary inflammation should be determined. The approach to reducing elevated SCC caused by mechanical injury would be different than the approach if caused by microbiological pathogens. If elevated SCC are due to mechanical injury, the root cause of the injury such as stray voltage or milking machine maintenance issues should be identified and corrected immediately. In contrast, high SCC due to mastitis-causing organisms can be reduced by the use of antibiotics indicated to treat intramammary infections. In order to increase the likelihood of successful treatment, two tools are available. Samples from the infected mammary gland can be cultured to identify the organism responsible for the high SCC. Simultaneously, milk samples can be tested using the ImmuCell MASTiK™ Mastitis Antibiotic Susceptibility Test Kit which will aid in selecting FDA approved antibiotics for mastitis therapy.

Whatever actions you choose to correct the cause of the elevated SCC problem, ImmuCell's CMT can then be used to monitor changes in SCC in order to evaluate the effectiveness of the treatment strategy in each infected quarter(s).

Position paddle with handle toward you to record individual quarters.

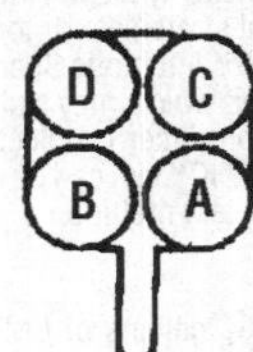

Result codes:

— Negative: Mixture remains liquid with no thickening

T Trace: A slight thickening which disappears with paddle movement

1 Weak: A distinct thickening but no gel formation

2 Distinct: Mixture thickens immediately moving to center of cup

3 Strong: Distinct gel formation which tends to form a mass

Discussion: General Information: Mastitis: Mastitis is responsible for the highest economic losses in the dairy industry with estimates of 1.5-2 billion dollars annually in the United States. These losses are due in part to decreases in milk production and milk quality and the costs associated with veterinarian intervention, treatment(s), milk discard and in extreme cases the need to cull chronically infected animals. Clearly, the easiest way to control these financial losses is to reduce the incidence of mastitis in your herd by improving your dairy farm management practices. There have been steady advances in reducing the incidence of mastitis. Some of these advances include pre- and post teat disinfection, improved dairy hygiene and nutrition, vaccines and antibiotic treatments. However, establishment of on-site protocols to regularly monitor milk quality and udder health, which would aid in identifying the early signs of mastitis, is probably the most practical and cost effective control of the financial losses attributed to mastitis. Specifically, increases in somatic cell counts (SCC) can be used to indicate a decline in milk quality and udder health. The sooner increases in SCC in the bulk tank or individual cows can be detected, the faster actions can be taken to reverse the trend. It is clear that cows diagnosed during early stages of infectious mastitis have a significantly better chance of successful treatment resulting in the return of low SCC and high milk quality.

Mastitis Detection: Clinical cases of mastitis can he easily recognized by the presence of abnormalities of the udder including heat, swelling and sensitivity, as well as changes in the milk including flakes, clots and a watery appearance. However, subclinical mastitis is not as easily identified. Cows with subclinical mastitis have no detectable changes in the udder and no observable abnormalities in the milk. Subclinical cases can often be diagnosed by microbiological culture of milk samples and quantifying SCC. Elevated SCC in milk samples from individual cows indicate the likelihood of subclinical mastitis. Although quantifying SCC are commonplace, few producers have milk samples from their entire herd routinely cultured for mastitis-causing pathogens.

The goal of many well-managed herds is to provide high quality milk by maintaining low SCC in both individual animals and the bulk tank. Early and frequent identification of cows with subclinical mastitis based on increases in SCC will facilitate quick intervention in an attempt to successfully clear the quarter or quarters with the problem. Dairy Herd Improvement Association (DHIA) data provides monthly SCC information on cow-to-cow basis. However, the individual quarters contributing to elevated SCC cannot be determined using this information. In contrast, the CALIFORNIA MASTITIS TEST (CMT) is recognized as the most widely accepted on-farm test for detecting high SCC in individual quarter samples. Interestingly, with all of its advantages, the CMT is also one of the most under-utilized tests available to the producer. Information obtained from the CMT can be used to improve management of udder health problems and maintenance of high milk quality.

Presentation: 525 tests per kit.

Compendium Code No.: 11200050

CMT (CALIFORNIA MASTITIS TEST)

TechniVet **Mastitis Test**

Contents: The Original Schalm CMT Kit Contains:

1. One pint of concentrated reagent—(one pint concentrate = 1 gallon diluted reagent; 1 gallon reagent = approximately 350 tests).
2. Testing paddle—designed for ease in cow-side use and for accurate visual reactions.
3. Dispensing bottle—to apply diluted concentrate. For small quantities of reagent mix directly in dispenser bottles. Add concentrate first, referring to measurement lines on the bottle.

Indications: The Original Schalm CMT is a screening test developed by Dr. O. W. Schalm of the University of California Veterinary School of Medicine. It is a quick and easy cow-side test which immediately detects bovine mastitis in fresh bulk milk or within individual quarters.

The Original Schalm CMT was developed to estimate the leukocyte cell content of fresh milk. It is the finest tool available for the early detection of bovine mastitis.

CMT is a simple, quick, accurate and inexpensive mastitis test applied at cow-side with instant visible reactions, an effective method of monitoring udder health changes.

Using CMT at regular intervals and recording the results makes it possible to detect mastitis in the incipient stages as well as to locate the individual quarters affected.

CMT is a proven procedure which enjoys the respect and endorsement of many of the very top men in the Dairy industry.

Call your veterinarian if tests show a positive mastitis reaction. Your veterinarian will know the extent of the treatment required for your animal's mastitis.

Test Procedure:

A. Collect Milk from Individual Quarters

1. Dilute CMT concentrate (1 pint concentrate = 1 gallon of reagent) or refer to dispenser bottle measuring lines for small quantities.
2. Discard first stream of milk. Do not use colostrum milk or strippings.
3. Draw next milk from each quarter into the respective cup of the testing paddle.

B. Pour off Excess Milk

1. Tilt testing paddle to discharge excess milk.
2. The remaining milk should be level with the outside circle in each cup.

C. Add Equal Amount of Reagent

1. Tilt paddle back until milk is halfway between the circles.
2. Slowly squirt reagent over the milk in each cup. Mixture will be even with the inside circle and the rim of each cup for equal parts.
3. Avoid bubbles!
4. The mixture of milk to reagent must be equal parts.

D. Brief Rotary Movement of Paddle Brings out Reaction

1. Bring paddle down to a horizontal position and gently rotate.
2. Instant reaction occurs between the milk and the reagent during rotation.
3. Results can be graded using the chart below.
4. If test shows positive, call your vet for nature and extent of treatment.

Interpretation of Results:

Paddle position with handle toward you. Record individual quarters.

Acid/Alkaline code
+ Purple color / alkaline milk
y Yellow color / acid milk

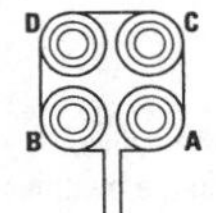

mastitis code symbols

- Negative: Mixture remains fluid, no slime or sediment.

T Trace: Mixture becomes slimy.

1 Weak: Mixture forms distinct sediment.

2 Distinct: Mixture thickens immediately; tends to form a jelly.

3 Strong: Mixture forms jelly peak in center, even after swirling stops.

Original Schalm CMT CALIFORNIA MASTITIS TEST Results

	Negative. Mixture remains liquid. No slime or gel forms.	Suspicious. Mixture becomes slimy or gel like. It's seen to best advantage by tipping the paddle back and forth, while observing mixture as it flows over the bottom of the cup.	Positive. Mixture distinctly forms a gel.	Positive. Mixture thickens immediately, tends to form jelly. Swirling the cup moves mixture in towards the center exposing the outer edges of the cup.
Individual Quarter Sample	No Mastitis	Trace of Mastitis	Mastitis	Mastitis
Bulk Milk Sample	No Mastitis	Mastitis in one or more quarters	Definite Mastitis Check Quarters	Serious Mastitis Check Quarters

Presentation: 350 tests per kit.

Compendium Code No.: 10760000

COBAN® 60

Elanco **Feed Medication**

Monensin Sodium-Type A Medicated Article

NADA No.: 038-878

Active Ingredient(s):

Monensin (as monensin sodium) .... 60 g per lb

Indications:

Chickens: As an aid in the prevention of coccidiosis caused by *Eimeria necatrix, E. tenella, E. acervulina, E. brunetti, E. mivati,* and *E. maxima.*

Turkeys: For the prevention of coccidiosis in turkeys caused by *Eimeria adenoeides, E. meleagrimitis* and *E. gallopavonis.*

Quail: For the prevention of coccidiosis in Bobwhite quail caused by *Eimeria dispersa* and *E. lettyae.*

Directions:

Important: Must be thoroughly mixed in feeds before use.

Mixing Directions (Broiler and Replacement Chickens) - Thoroughly mix the following amounts of COBAN® 60 with a sufficient quantity of unmedicated feed to make one ton of complete chicken feed to provide 90 through 110 grams monensin per ton.

Monensin (Grams Per Ton)	COBAN® 60 (Lbs Per Ton of Type C Feed)
90	1.50
95	1.58
100	1.67
105	1.75
110	1.83

Feeding Directions - Feed continuously as the sole ration.

Mixing Directions (Turkeys) - Thoroughly mix the following amounts of COBAN® 60 with a sufficient quantity of unmedicated feed to make one ton of complete turkey feed to provide 54 through 90 grams monensin per ton.

Monensin (Grams Per Ton)	COBAN® 60 (Lbs Per Ton of Type C Feed)
54	0.90
66	1.10
78	1.30
90	1.50

Feeding Directions - For turkeys, feed continuously as the sole ration. The optimum level depends upon the severity of coccidiosis exposure.

Mixing Directions (Bobwhite Quail) - Thoroughly mix the following amounts of COBAN® 60 with a sufficient quantity of unmedicated feed to make one ton of complete quail feed to provide 73 grams monensin per ton.

Monensin (Grams Per Ton)	COBAN® 60 (Lbs Per Ton of Type C Feed)
73	1.22

Feeding Directions - For Bobwhite quail, feed continuously as the sole ration.

Do not feed undiluted.

Precaution(s): Store in a cool, dry place.

Not to be used after the date printed at top of bag.

When mixing and handling COBAN® 60, use protective clothing, impervious gloves, and a dust mask. Operators should wash thoroughly with soap and water after handling. If accidental eye contact occurs, immediately rinse thoroughly with water.

Caution(s): For replacement chickens intended for use as cage layers only. Do not allow horses, other equines, mature turkeys, or guinea fowl access to feed containing monensin. Ingestion of monensin by horses and guinea fowl has been fatal. Some strains of turkey coccidia may be monensin tolerant or resistant. Monensin may interfere with development of immunity to turkey coccidiosis. In the absence of coccidiosis in broiler chickens the use of monensin with no withdrawal period may limit feed intake resulting in reduced weight gain.

For use in broiler and replacement chicken, growing turkey, and growing bobwhite quail feeds only.

Warning(s): Do not feed to laying chickens. Do not feed to chickens over 16 weeks of age.

Presentation: 50 lbs (22.68 kg)

Compendium Code No.: 10310011 BG 1391 AMB

COCCIVAC®-B

Schering-Plough **Vaccine**

Coccidiosis Vaccine, Live Oocysts, Chicken Isolates

U.S. Vet. Lic. No.: 226

Contents: COCCIVAC®-B contains the oocysts of *Eimeria acervulina, E. maxima, E. mivati* and *E. tenella.*

Indications: COCCIVAC®-B is recommended as an aid in the prevention of coccidiosis caused by 4 species of coccidia: *E. acervulina, E. maxima, E. mivati* and *E. tenella.* This vaccine should be administered in accordance with directions below.

Dosage and Administration: Feed Spray Administration:

1. Do not use any medicated drinking water or water disinfectant 24 hours before and after vaccination or during vaccination.
2. Feed sprinkled on paper under the feed line increases the exposure of chicks to the vaccine.
3. Dilute the vaccine at a ratio of 1000 doses/400 mL of non-chlorinated water. Mix well and place in a clean garden type pressure sprayer.
4. Spray the diluted vaccine over the surface of the feed. Agitate the sprayer during administration.
5. For best results, the vaccine should be sprayed on all of the feed.
6. Avoid wetting the feed. Proper application will only dampen the surface of the feed.
7. Allow the chicks sufficient time to ingest the oocysts on the feed before placing more feed in the pans or on the paper.

Spray Cabinet Administration: For vaccination of chicks at one day of age.

1. Use diluted vaccine as directed for each coarse spray vaccinating machine.
   When using an SPAH-spray cabinet we recommend diluting 1000 doses of vaccine to 210 mL.
2. Add the vaccine solution to pressure reservoir of the spray apparatus. Red dye may be added as a marker.
3. Prime and adjust the machine as indicated on the machine operating instructions.
4. Place boxes holding 100 chickens each on the conveyor belt or in machine. Activate the spray head.
5. Using an SPAH machine, each box of 100 chicks receives 21 mL of vaccine solution.

Eye Spray Administration: For vaccination of chicks at one day of age. For each 1000 doses of vaccine, dilute in 26 mL of non-chlorinated water. Each chick should receive 0.03 mL of this product.

Full directions for use of the Biojector-Immunizer are available from the company.

Using Medicated Feeds: COCCIVAC® vaccine is not ordinarily recommended for use on chicks receiving a feed containing a coccidiostat or high levels of antibiotic. After vaccination, it may become necessary to use high levels of drugs for treatment of disease conditions other than coccidiosis. If such drugs, with coccidiostatic activity, are used during the first or second week post-vaccination with COCCIVAC® vaccine, revaccination with COCCIVAC® vaccine is recommended.

The capacity of this vaccine to produce satisfactory results depends on many factors, including but not limited to conditions of storage and handling by the user, administration of the vaccine, health and responsiveness of individual chickens and degree of field exposure, Therefore, directions for use should be followed carefully.

Precaution(s): Use entire contents of each vial when first opened. Store vaccine in refrigerator under 45°F (7°C).

Do not freeze. Burn container and all unused contents.

Caution(s): Only vaccinate healthy chicks.

Sprayed on the feed at 1-3 days of age; or by eye spray or spray cabinet routes at 1 day of age.

Chicks must have access to their droppings as reinfection is required to give immunity.

Therefore, chicks started on paper, or raised in batteries or on wire, should be put on litter no later than the 4th day post-vaccination.

Moisture is necessary for oocysts to sporulate. If litter conditions are extremely dry during the immunization period, sprinkling or spraying the litter (to slightly damp) with water is recommended.

If there is a noticeable reaction from the vaccine, it usually occurs between the 12th and 14th days post-vaccination. Do not treat coccidiosis unless mortality or severe morbidity is directly attributable to coccidiosis. When positive diagnosis is made, treat with amprolium in the drinking water. Treatment for 48 hours using the manufacturers lowest recommended level, will usually be adequate.

Notice: All Schering Plough Animal Health Corp. vaccines released for sale meet the requirements of the licensing authority (U.S. Department of Agriculture) in regard to safety, purity, potency and the capacity to immunize normal, susceptible chickens.

Federal regulations prohibit the repackaging or sale of the contents of the carton in fractional units. Do not accept if seal is broken.

Warning(s): Do not vaccinate within 21 days before slaughter.

Presentation: 10 x 1,000 dose (NDC-0138-5100-01) and 10 x 10,000 dose (NDC-0138-5100-02) vials.

Compendium Code No.: 10472150 0145R8 / 0158R8

COCCIVAC®-D

Schering-Plough **Vaccine**

Coccidiosis Vaccine, Live Oocysts

U.S. Vet. Lic. No.: 226

Contents: COCCIVAC®-D contains live oocysts of *Eimeria tenella, E. mivati, E. acervulina, E. maxima, E. brunetti, E. hagani, E. necatrix,* and *E. praecox.*

Indications: COCCIVAC®-D is recommended as an aid in the prevention of coccidiosis caused by 8 species of coccidia: *E. tenella, E. mivati, E. acervulina, E. maxima, E. brunetti, E. hagani, E. necatrix,* and *E. praecox.* This vaccine should be administered in accordance with directions below.

Dosage and Administration: Feed Spray Administration:

1. Do not use any medicated drinking water or water disinfectant 24 hours before and after vaccination or during vaccination.
2. Feed sprinkled on paper under the feed line increases the exposure of chicks to the vaccine.
3. Dilute the vaccine at a ratio of 1000 doses/400 mL of non-chlorinated water. Mix well and place in a clean garden type pressure sprayer.
4. Spray the diluted vaccine over the surface of the feed. Agitate the sprayer during administration.
5. For best results, the vaccine should be sprayed on all of the feed.
6. Avoid wetting the feed. Proper application will only dampen the surface of the feed.
7. Allow the chicks sufficient time to ingest the oocysts on the feed before placing more feed in the pans or on the paper.

Spray Cabinet Administration: For vaccination of chicks at one day of age.

1. Use diluted vaccine as directed for each coarse spray vaccinating machine.
   When using an SPAH-spray cabinet we recommend diluting 1000 doses of vaccine to 210 mL.
2. Add the vaccine solution to pressure reservoir of the spray apparatus. Red dye may be added as a marker.
3. Prime and adjust the machine as indicated on the machine operating instructions.
4. Place boxes holding 100 chickens each on the conveyor belt or in machine. Activate the spray head.
5. Using an SPAH machine, each box of 100 chicks receives 21 mL of vaccine solution.

Using Medicated Feeds and COCCIVAC®: COCCIVAC® vaccine is not ordinarily recommended for use on chicks receiving a feed containing a coccidiostat or high levels of antibiotic. After vaccination, it may become necessary to use high levels of drugs for treatment of disease conditions other than coccidiosis. If such drugs, with coccidiostatic activity, are used during the first or second week after vaccination with COCCIVAC® vaccine, revaccination with COCCIVAC® vaccine is recommended.

The capacity of this vaccine to produce satisfactory results depends on many factors, including but not limited to conditions of storage and handling by the user, administration of the vaccine, health and responsiveness of individual chickens and degree of field exposure. Therefore, directions for use should be followed carefully.

Precaution(s): Use entire contents of each vial when first opened. Store vaccine in refrigerator under 45°F (7°C).

Do not freeze. Burn container and all unused contents.

Caution(s): Only vaccinate healthy chicks.

Administer by spray cabinet at one day of age or spray on the feed at 4 days of age.

Chicks may be started on paper, but it should be removed and chicks should be on litter by the 4th day post-vaccination. Chicks must have access to their droppings as reinfection is required to give immunity.

Chicks raised in batteries or on wire, cannot be effectively immunized by COCCIVAC®. Chicks started in batteries, or on wire can be effectively immunized if they are placed on litter not later than the 4th day after vaccination.

Moisture is necessary for oocysts to sporulate. If litter conditions are extremely dry during the immunization period, sprinkling or spraying the litter (to slightly damp) with water is recommended.

If there is a noticeable reaction from COCCIVAC® vaccine, it usually occurs between the 12th and 14th days after vaccination. Do not treat coccidiosis unless mortality or severe morbidity is directly attributable to coccidiosis. When positive diagnosis is made, treat with amprolium in the drinking water. Treatment for 48 hours using the manufacturers lowest recommended level, will usually be adequate.

Notice: All Schering Plough Animal Health Corp. vaccines released for sale meet the requirements of the licensing authority (U.S. Department of Agriculture) in regard to safety, purity, potency and the capacity to immunize normal, susceptible chickens.

Federal regulations prohibit the repackaging or sale of the contents of the carton in fractional units. Do not accept if seal is broken.

Warning(s): Do not vaccinate within 21 days before slaughter.

Presentation: 10 x 1,000 dose (NDC-0318-5102-01) and 10 x 5,000 dose (NDC-0318-5102-02) vials.

Compendium Code No.: 10472160 0116R9 / 0170R5

COCCIVAC®-T

Schering-Plough **Vaccine**

Coccidiosis Vaccine, Live Oocysts

U.S. Vet. Lic. No.: 226

Contents: COCCIVAC®-T contains *Eimeria adenoeides, E. meleagrimitis, E. gallopavonis,* and *E. dispersa.*

Indications: COCCIVAC®-T is recommended as an aid in the prevention of coccidiosis caused by 4 species of coccidia: *E. adenoeides, E. meleagrimitis, E. gallopavonis,* and *E. dispersa.* This vaccine should be administered in accordance with directions below.

Dosage and Administration: Spray Cabinet Administration:

Recommended for vaccination of poults at one day of age.

1. Use diluted vaccine as directed for each coarse spray vaccinating machine.
   When using a SPAH spray cabinet, dilute 1000 doses to 210 mL of non-chlorinated water.
2. Add the vaccine solution to pressure reservoir of the spray apparatus. (Red dye may be added as a marker).
   Do not add water stabilizer to spray solution.
3. Prime and adjust the machine as indicated on the machine operating instructions.
4. Place boxes holding 100 poults on the conveyor belt or in machine. Activate the spray head.
5. Using a SPAH machine, each box of 100 poults receives 21 mL of vaccine solution.

Precaution(s): Store vaccine in refrigerator under 7°C (45°F). Do not freeze.

Use entire contents of each vial when first opened.

Burn container and all unused contents.

C

Caution(s): Only vaccinate healthy poults.

Poults may be started on paper but it should be removed and poults should be on litter by the 5th day after vaccination. Poults must have access to their droppings as reinfection is required to give immunity.

Moisture is necessary for oocysts to sporulate. If litter conditions are extremely dry during vaccination period, sprinkling or spraying the litter (to slightly damp) with water is recommended.

Do not treat for coccidiosis unless mortality or severe morbidity is directly attributable to coccidiosis. When positive diagnosis is made, treat with amprol in the drinking water.

To reduce the incidence of bacterial enteritis, an injectable antibiotic should be administered at day of age followed by an in-feed antibiotic.

The capacity of this vaccine to produce satisfactory results depends on many factors, including but not limited to conditions of storage and handling by the user, administration of the vaccine, health and responsiveness of individual birds and degree of field exposure. Therefore, directions for use should be followed carefully.

C

Warning(s): Do not vaccinate within 21 days before slaughter.
Presentation: 10 x 1,000 dose vials.
Manufactured by: Schering-Plough Animal Health Corp., Millsboro, Delaware 19966 U.S.A.
Compendium Code No.: 10472170 0107R1

COCODERM CONDITIONING SHAMPOO

Vetus **Grooming Shampoo**

NDC No.: 47611-200-98/47611-200-90
Active Ingredient(s): The product contains U.S.P. purified water, sodium lauryl ether sulfate, sodium lauryl sulfate, cocamide DEA, ethoxylated lanolin, sodium chloride, coconut oil, FD&C color.
Indications: A conditioning shampoo for everyday use on dogs, cats and horses.
Dosage and Administration:

General cleansing: Pour a small amount of the shampoo into a large container of water, and agitate to form thick suds. Bathe or sponge onto the animal, and rinse thoroughly.

Maximum conditioning: Wet the animal with water and apply the shampoo full strength to the animal's coat, working into a lather. Rinse thoroughly and remove any excess water.

Presentation: 16 oz. bottles and 1 gallon containers.
Compendium Code No.: 14440230

COLIMUNE®-ORAL

Bioniche Animal Health (formerly Vetrepharm) **Antibodies**

K99 E. coli Antibody for Neonatal Calves

Description: COLIMUNE®-ORAL is an oral preparation of *Escherichia coli* antibody of equine origin.

Contains phenol, thimerosal and oxytetracycline HCl as preservatives.

Indications: It is given to newborn calves as an aid in the reduction of fatal calf scours due to infection with enteropathogenic K99 *E. coli* organisms.
Directions for Use: Administer entire contents of one syringe (10 mL/1 dose), orally to the calf within 12 hours of birth.
Precaution(s): Storage: Store at 2-7°C. (35-45°F.). Do not freeze.

Syringes must be kept sealed until used. Use entire contents when first opened.

Caution(s): If anaphylaxis occurs, administer epinephrine or equivalent.
Presentation: COLIMUNE®-ORAL is available in 10 mL pre-filled, oral syringes, 12 per box.
Compendium Code No.: 11070001

COLLASATE™

PRN Pharmacal **Topical Wound Dressing**

Postoperative Dressing-Medical Hydrolysate of Type I Collagen

Active Ingredient(s): COLLASATE™ contains only a natural medical hydrolysate Type I collagen as its active ingredient. Unlike other collagen products, which are made from native collagen, COLLASATE™ is a patented product manufactured from a proprietary process which creates a product of a specified molecular weight.

Indications: Advanced COLLASATE™ technology provides for topical use in the management of surgical sites, chronic and acute wounds and all partial and full-thickness wounds, including: surgical sites, dental extractions and oral surgery, pressure ulcers (Stages I-IV), venous stasis ulcers, ulcers resulting from arterial insufficiency, traumatic wounds, superficial wounds, first and second degree burns, spays, neutering, de-clawing, foot pad injuries, hot spots, diabetic ulcers, lick granulomas.

COLLASATE™ can be used on many types of animals, including mammals, birds and reptiles, with no known side effects. COLLASATE™ is non-toxic and has no contraindications.

Dosage and Administration: Product Administration:

1. Cleanse the site.
2. Apply COLLASATE™ directly into the wound or incision and onto the surrounding area.
3. Allow gel to dry, then cover with a non-stick dressing (Telfa® pad). Gauze is recommended as the secondary dressing if removing debris from the site. Superficial wounds such as cuts and abrasions may not require a secondary dressing due to the film that COLLASATE™ forms on the wound site after drying.
4. Remove dressing as needed (if secondary dressing sticks to wound, soak in warm water to ease removal) and repeat procedure.

Precaution(s): Storage: Store at controlled room temperature (59-86°F). Protect from freezing. Extreme temperatures may affect viscosity but will not affect product performance.
Caution(s): If condition worsens or does not improve within 10-14 days, contact your veterinarian.
Discussion: COLLASATE™ is a revolutionary scientific breakthrough in the management of surgical and trauma sites. An all-natural gel product, COLLASATE™ interacts with the site to provide a moist healing environment. Collagen also provides a matrix for cellular colonization and tissue regeneration.[1]

COLLASATE™ Characteristics: reduces pain, tissue adhesive properties, protects the site and newly formed granulation tissue, soothes and deodorizes, hemostatic qualities of collagen†, promotes natural autolysis by rehydrating and softening necrotic, tissue and eschar, encouraging autolytic debridement, provides physiologically favorable environment that encourages healing, absorbs exudate, conforms to any site, safe to use, non-toxic, biocompatible, biodegradable.

References: Available upon request.
Presentation: COLLASATE™ is available in a laminate tube containing 7.0 grams of product, 6 tubes to a box.
Compendium Code No.: 10900200 121-73 6-2001

COLOR-GUARD® 500

Alpharma **Feed Additive**

Guaranteed Analysis: Vitamin D_3 500,000 International Chick Units per gram (226,800,000 ICU per pound).

Ingredients: Activated 7-dehydrocholesterol, butylated hydroxytoluene (preservative), vegetable oil, modified edible starch, certified food color.

Indications: Source of cholecalciferol, vitamin D_3.
Dosage and Administration: Use as needed.
Precaution(s): Store in a cool dry location. Keep container closed. Do not accept if container has been opened.
Caution(s): For manufacturing feedstuffs only.
Presentation: 55.1 lb (25 kg).
Compendium Code No.: 10220290

COLOR-GUARD® 1000

Alpharma **Feed Additive**

Guaranteed Analysis: Vitamin D_3 1,000,000 International Chick Units per gram (453,590,000 ICU per pound).

Ingredients: Activated 7-dehydrocholesterol, butylated hydroxytoluene (preservative), vegetable oil, modified edible starch, certified food color.

Indications: Source of cholecalciferol, vitamin D_3.
Dosage and Administration: Use as needed.
Precaution(s): Store in a cool dry location. Keep container closed. Do not accept if container has been opened.
Caution(s): For manufacturing feedstuffs only.
Presentation: 55.1 lb (25 kg).
Compendium Code No.: 10220280

COLOSTRUM BOLUS FORTE

Durvet **Large Animal Dietary Supplement**

Guaranteed Analysis: 7 X 10^8 C.F.U./bolus (equal numbers of each)	mg/bolus
Vitamin A	25000 I.U.
Vitamin D	5000 I.U.
Vitamin E	15 I.U.
Mendione	8 mg
Vitamin B_{12}	50 mcg
Choline Chloride	130 mg
Thiamine	75 mg
Potassium as K	52 mg
Phosphorus as P	54 mg
Magnesium as Mg	48 mg
Sodium as Na	40 mg

Ingredients: Dried Colostrum, Dried Whey, *Lactobacillus acidophilus* fermentation product dehydrated, *Lacillus caseil* fermentation product dehydrated, *Bifidobacterium bifidum* fermentation product dehydrated, *Aspergillus oryzae* fermentation product dehydrated, choline chloride, Vitamin A supplement (stability improved), D-activated animal sterol (source of D), Alpha Tocopherol Acetate (source of Vitamin E), polysaccharide complexes of zinc, manganese, iron, copper, Vitamin B_{12} supplement, anise seed mendione dimenthyl primidinal bisulfite.

Indications: Designed to assist in the replacement of colostrum where calves and sheep may be deficient. Also contains a source of live (viable) naturally occurring microorganisms.
Directions for Use: Calves and Sheep: One bolus following birth. One bolus twice daily as needed.
Precaution(s): Keep cool and dry.
Presentation: 25 x 6.125 g boluses per box (NDC 30798-178-66).
Compendium Code No.: 10840351 2/98

COLOSTRUM BOVINE IgG MIDLAND QUICK TEST KIT™

Midland BioProducts **IgG Test**

Description: A qualitative test to measure the amount of immunoglobulin G (IgG) in bovine colostrum, in a rapid test format.
Contents: Each kit contains: individually pouched cassettes, bag of drop volume sample pipettes, dilution vials, and instruction.
Indications: The COLOSTRUM BOVINE IgG MIDLAND QUICK TEST KIT™, is designed to detect immunoglobulin G (IgG) concentrations in bovine colostrum. The test cassette is a rapid test format and eliminates the need for elaborate laboratory equipment, fragile instruments, or a specific temperature to measure the colostrum IgG. The test will give you a yes/no answer in 20 minutes to the quality of your colostrum in collected milkings.
Test Procedure:

Step 1: Sample Collection: Collection supplies are not included with the kit.

1. Collect colostrum from the first and second milking of fresh cows.[8]
2. Do not use mastitic or abnormal milk.
3. Determine the IgG content of each individual collection.
4. If pooling, use only colostrum that is rated (above 50 mg/mL of IgG) with COLOSTRUM BOVINE IgG MIDLAND QUICK TEST KIT™.

Step 2: Procedure

1. Obtain the colostrum sample (see "Sample Collection").
2. Next, in the foil pouch, remove the Cassette from the foil pouch by tearing at the notched end on the side of the pouch. Discard the Cassette foil pouch and the desiccant inside the pouch.
3. Label or otherwise identify the Cassette so that each colostrum sample can be associated with its Cassette and source.
4. In the kit, take the dilution vial and remove the seal and septum (cap) from the dilution vial.
5. Using a clean pipette provided with the kit, completely depress the bulb, and put the pipette in the colostrum sample. Release the bulb, which will allow the sample to be drawn into the pipette. Note: The pipette will not be completely full. Quickly releasing the bulb increases the likelihood that air will be drawn into the pipette which may effect the accuracy of the test.
6. Transfer one drop of the colostrum sample in the pipette to the dilution vial. Do not add all the contents of the pipette to the dilution vial. Do not rinse the pipette out in the solution of the dilution vial. Discard this pipette.
7. Put the septum (cap) on the dilution vial and invert several times to thoroughly mix the sample. Avoid shaking.
8. Once the sample is thoroughly mixed, remove the septum from the dilution vial. Using a new, clean pipette from the kit. completely depress the bulb and submerge the pipette into

the diluted sample in the dilution vial. Gently release the bulb, which will allow the diluted sample to be drawn into the pipette.

9. Express 3 drops of the diluted sample into the sample well of the Cassette (marked "S"), making sure that the Cassette is on a level surface. Allow the test to proceed for 20 minutes, then read the results. For accuracy, do not read the results before 20 minutes or after 40 minutes.

Test Interpretation: Step 3: Interpretation of Test Results

Example of COLOSTRUM BOVINE IgG MIDLAND QUICK TEST KIT™ cassette results (Control= "C", Test = "T" and Sample = "S"):

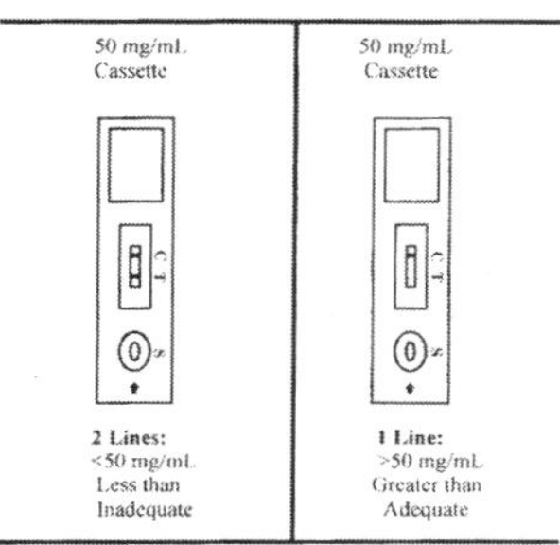

Storage: Avoid prolonged temperature and humidity extremes.

Do not remove the cassette from the foil pouch until ready for use.

Even though the foil pouch includes a desiccant packet, exposure to high humidity conditions should be minimized.

If the buffer in the dilution vial freezes, thaw before using.

Caution(s): Do not use components past expiration date and do not mix components from kits from different lot numbers.

The dilution vial in this kit contains sodium azide. Sodium azide may react with lead or copper plumbing to form highly explosive metal azides. On disposal, flush with a large volume of water to prevent azide build-up. For further information, refer to the manual issued by the Centers for Disease Control.

Do not ingest the desiccant or the buffer solution.

Dispose of all kit components in an appropriate manner.

Discussion: Failure of Passive Transfer (FPT): Calves are born virtually devoid of any detectable level of immunoglobulin G (IgG). The neonatal calf s immunity to infectious agent over the next several weeks relies on the ingestion and absorption of maternal IgG from colostrum in the mother's milk. This process, termed passive transfer, is a critical determinant of a calf s health. Failure of passive transfer (FPT) may occur as a result of inadequate suckling, poor absorption of IgG, low levels of IgG in colostrum, or environmental stress.[2] Because of FPT in calves, the result is a calf at a greater risk of developing severe respiratory illness, diarrhea and other septicemic illnesses.[3,4,5,6]

The calf's ability to absorb IgG is optimal at birth. The highest rate of absorption occurs during the first 6-12 hours. From 12 to 24 hours there is a substantial decline in absorption. Estimated gut closure time for IgG is approximately 24 hours.[3,7] Therefore, the feeding of high quality colostrum is essential in the first hours of life for a healthy calf and body development. Studies have indicated that approximately 100 g of first colostral immunoglobulin must be fed within the first hours after birth in order for the calf to develop an adequate serum IgG level.

Studies have identified the specific concentrations of IgG that indicate adequate passive transfer.[6,7] Serum IgG concentrations above 10 mg/mL (1000 mg/dL) are considered to have an adequate level of immunity.[3]

The rapid identification of IgG in colostrum can be used to assess calf management practices. By eliminating the feeding of poor quality colostrum, the risks of morbidity and mortality will be greatly reduced.

References: Available upon request.

Presentation: Kits are packaged and sold in the following number of tests: Packages of 6, 12 and 24 tests.

Patent Pending

Compendium Code No.: 15010002 — 9020 rev. 2

COLOSTRUM-PLUS

Jorgensen — **Large Animal Dietary Supplement**

Active Ingredient(s): Minimum Guaranteed Analysis:

Bovine origin glycoproteins	32 g
Vitamin A	30,000 I.U.
Vitamin D_3	4,000 I.U.
Vitamin E	200 I.U.
Lactic acid bacteria*	not lessthan, 2,500,000,000 CFU**

**Lactobacillus acidophilus, Lactobacillus lactis, Lactobacillus casei, Streptococcus diacetylactis* and *Bifidobacterium bifidum.*

**CFU (colony-forming units).

Each dose contains: Dehydrated bovine glycoproteins from first and second milking after parturition, viable *Lactobacillus acidophilus*, viable *Lactobacillus lactis*, viable *Lactobacillus casei*, viable *Streptoccoccus diacetylactis*, viable *Bifidobacterium bifidum*, calcium carbonate, vitamin A supplement, vitamin D_3 supplement, vitamin E supplement, dicalcium phosphate, choline chloride, ferrous sulfate, zinc sulfate, magnesium oxide, menadione sodium bisulfite complex (source of vitamin K), manganese sulfate, ascorbic acid, vitamin B_{12} supplement, riboflavin supplement, pyridoxine hydrochloride, niacin supplement, calcium pantothenate, folic acid, thiamine mononitrate, ethylenediamine dihydriodide, cobalt sulfate, sodium selenite, polyethylene mono and dioleates, artificial flavor, silicon dioxide and artificial flavor.

Indications: Bovine origin glycoproteins combined with essential vitamins, minerals and live microbial cultures.

Dosage and Administration:

Newborn Calves: Mix one (1) pack (350 g) of COLOSTRUM-PLUS into one and one-half (1½) quarts of lukewarm water. Administer one (1) dose by bottle, pail or esophageal feeder as soon as possible after birth.

Precaution(s): Keep cool and dry.

Presentation: 350 g packs, 12/box.

Compendium Code No.: 11520010

COLOSTRUM POWDER

Vedco — **Large Animal Dietary Supplement**

Active Ingredient(s): Each ounce contains: *Lactobacillus acidophilus* fermentation product dehydrated, *Lactobacillus casei* fermentation product dehydrated, *Bifido bacterium* fermentation product dehydrated, dried milk colostrum, vitamin A acetate (stability improved), (d-activated animal sterol) source of vitamin D_3 (dl-alpha tocopherol acetate) source of vitamin E, calcium carbonate, rice mill by-product and dextrose.

Guaranteed Minimum Analysis: Each pound contains:

Vitamin A	not less than 1,000,000 U.S.P. units
Vitamin D_3	not less than 500,000 U.S.P. units
Vitamin E	not less than 500 I.U. units

Lactic acid producing micro-organisms - 2.0×10^8 C.F.U. per gram, equal numbers of each micro-organism listed in the ingredients. Antibiotics may affect the viability of the micro-organisms in this product.

Indications: A nutritional product for newborn calves, sheep and goats, which contains a source of live (viable) naturally occurring micro-organisms.

Dosage and Administration: Feeds 30 calves for five (5) days. Administer to newborn calves as soon as possible after birth: One (1) teaspoonful in milk or milk replacer. Continue administration of the product as long as calves are on milk replacer or milk.

Caution(s): For animal use only. Not for human use. Keep out of the reach of children.

Presentation: 18 oz. container.

Compendium Code No.: 10940360

COLOSTRX®

Schering-Plough — **Immunoglobulins**

Escherichia coli Antibody, Bovine Origin

U.S. Vet. Permit No.: 341

Guaranteed Analysis:

Bovine immunoglobulin, minimum	30 grams
Crude Protein, minimum	70.00%

Indications: Failure of Passive Transfer: COLOSTRX® supplies a guaranteed quantity of absorbable immunoglobulins to aid in the treatment of failure of passive transfer in newborn calves less than 24 hours old.

Diarrhea Control: Serves as an aid in the prevention of scours by supplying antibodies that block the K-99 *E coli* process.

Dosage and Administration: First, empty the entire contents of the package into a pail. Second, add approximately 1-1½ quarts of lukewarm water or milk replacer and stir vigorously with a wire whisk until mixed.

For best results, administer with a nipple pail, bottle or esophageal feeder within 10 hours after birth (immediately if practical). Be sure that the calf consumes the entire contents. Follow the normal feeding program after COLOSTRX® is administered.

Precaution(s): Store at temperatures no higher than room temperature (72°F, 23°C) and out of direct sunlight.

Warning(s): For veterinary use only.

Presentation: 1 dose (454 g).

COLOSTRX® is a registered trademark of Protein Technology, Inc., Santa Rosa, CA 95403

Compendium Code No.: 10470290

COMBICILLIN ℞

Anthony — **Penicillin Injection**

Sterile Penicillin G Benzathine and Penicillin G Procaine Aqueous Suspension

NADA No.: 065-506

Active Ingredient(s): Each mL contains:

Penicillin G benzathine	150,000 units
Penicillin G procaine	150,000 units
Lecithin	11.7 mg
Sodium formaldehyde sulfoxylate	1.75 mg
Methylparaben	1.20 mg
Propylparaben	0.14 mg
Tween 40	8.19 mg
Span 40	11.3 mg
Sodium citrate (anhydrous)	3.98 mg
Procaine hydrochloride	20 mg
Sodium carboxymethylcellulose	1.04 mg
Water for injection	q.s.

Indications: COMBICILLIN is indicated for the treatment of the following bacterial infections in dogs, horses, and beef cattle due to penicillin-susceptible micro-organisms that are susceptible to the serum levels common to this particular dosage form, such as:

1. Bacterial pneumonia *(Streptococcus* spp., *Corynebacterium pyogenes, Staphylococcus aureus).*
2. Upper respiratory infections, such as rhinitis or pharyngitis *(Corynebacterium pyogenes).*
3. Equine strangles *(Streptococcus equi).*
4. Blackleg *(Clostridium chauvoei).*

Pharmacology: Penicillin G is an antibiotic which shows a marked bactericidal effect against certain organisms during their growth phase. It is relatively specific in its action against gram-positive bacteria, but is usually ineffective against gram-negative organisms.

When treating an animal for a bacterial infection, it is advisable to isolate and identify the causative organisms and conduct appropriate *in vitro* susceptibility tests. In cases where organisms other than those susceptible to penicillin are present, a re-evaluation of treatment should be made. Organisms normally considered susceptible to penicillin include *Clostridium septicum, Corynebacterium pyogenes, Streptococcus equi, Staphylococcus aureus, Streptococcus canis,* and *Streptococcus pyogenes.*

Dosage and Administration: Shake well before each use.

Dogs: 1 mL per 10 to 25 lbs. of body weight, given intramuscularly or subcutaneously (6,000 to 15,000 units penicillin G procaine and 6,000 to 15,000 units penicillin G benzathine per lb. of body weight). The treatment should be repeated in 48 hours.

Horses: 2 mL per 150 lbs. of body weight, given intramuscularly (2,000 units penicillin G procaine and 2,000 units penicillin G benzathine per lb. of body weight). The treatment should be repeated in 48 hours.

Beef Cattle: 2 mL per 150 lbs. of body weight, given subcutaneously only (2,000 units penicillin G procaine and 2,000 units penicillin G benzathine per lb. of body weight). The treatment should be repeated in 48 hours.

Important: Treatment in beef cattle should be limited to two (2) doses given subcutaneously only.

The product should be given to horses by intramuscular injection. In beef cattle, the recommended dosage should be administered by subcutaneous injection only. Dogs may be injected by either the intramuscular or subcutaneous route.

It is normally recommended that any bacterial infection be treated as early as possible and with a dosage that will give effective blood levels. Although the recommended dosage of the product will give longer detectable penicillin blood levels than penicillin G procaine alone, it is recommended that a second dose be administered at 48 hours when treating a penicillin-susceptible bacterial infection.

If no definite improvement is noted following the second dose of the product, the diagnosis should be re-evaluated and use of another chemotherapeutic agent considered.

Contraindication(s): The product is contraindicated in patients which have shown hypersensitivity to penicillin.

Precaution(s): Store under refrigeration below 59°F (15°C). Protect from freezing.

Caution(s): Federal law restricts this drug to use by or on the order of a licensed veterinarian.

Warning(s): Beef cattle should be withheld from slaughter for food use for 30 days following the last treatment with this drug. Treatment in beef cattle must be limited to two (2) doses.

Not to be used for horses intended for slaughter for food purposes.

Side Effects: Anaphylactic reactions have been reported in cattle given penicillin. Treated animals should be closely observed and if allergic or anaphylactic reactions occur, administer epinephrine or antihistamines immediately.

Presentation: Available in 100 mL and 250 mL vials.

Compendium Code No.: 10250000

COMBICILLIN-AG

Anthony **Penicillin Injection**

(Penicillin G Benzathine & Penicillin G Procaine Injectable Suspension) Injectable Suspension-Antibiotic

NADA No.: 065-506

Active Ingredient(s): Each mL contains 150,000 units penicillin G benzathine, 150,000 units penicillin G procaine, 11.7 mg lecithin, 1.75 mg sodium formaldehyde sulfoxylate, 1.20 mg methylparaben, 0.14 mg propylparaben, 8.19 mg Tween 40, 11.3 mg Span 40, 3.98 mg sodium citrate (anhydrous), 20 mg procaine hydrochloride, 1.04 mg sodium carboxymethylcellulose, Water for injection q.s.

Indications: This product is indicated for the treatment of the following bacterial infections in beef cattle due to penicillin-susceptible microorganisms that are susceptible to the serum levels common to this particular dosage form, such as:

1. Bacterial Pneumonia (shipping fever complex) *(Streptococcus* spp., *Corynebacterium pyogenes, Staphylococcus aureus).*
2. Upper Respiratory Infections such as rhinitis or pharyngitis *(Corynebacterium pyogenes).*
3. Blackleg *(Clostridium chauvoei).*

Pharmacology: Action: Penicillin G is an antibiotic which shows a marked bactericidal effect against certain organisms during their growth phase. It is relatively specific in its action against gram-positive bacteria but is usually ineffective against gram-negative organisms.

It is normally recommended that any bacterial infection be treated as early as possible and with a dosage that will give effective blood levels. Although the recommended dosage of this product will give longer detectable penicillin blood levels than penicillin G procaine alone, it is recommended that a second dose be administered at 48 hours when treating a penicillin-susceptible bacterial infection.

The use of antibiotics in the management of disease is based on an accurate diagnosis and an adequate course of treatment. When properly used in the treatment of diseases caused by penicillin-susceptible organisms, most animals treated with the product will show a noticeable improvement within 24 to 48 hours. If improvement does not occur within this period of time, the diagnosis and course of treatment should be re-evaluated. It is recommended that the diagnosis and treatment of animal diseases be carried out by a veterinarian. Since many diseases look alike but require different types of treatment, the use of professional veterinary and laboratory services can reduce treatment time, costs and needless losses. Good housing, sanitation and nutrition are important in the maintenance of healthy animals and are essential in the treatment of disease.

Dosage and Administration: Administration: The recommended dosage for beef cattle should be administered by subcutaneous injection only. Failure to use the subcutaneous route of administration may result in antibiotic residues in meat beyond the withdrawal time.

Dosage:

Beef cattle: 2 mL per 150 lb body weight given subcutaneously only (2000 units penicillin G procaine and 2000 units penicillin G benzathine per lb body weight). Treatment should be repeated in 48 hours.

Important: Treatment in beef cattle should be limited to two (2) doses given by subcutaneous injection only.

Directions for Use: A thoroughly cleaned, sterile needle and syringe should be used for each injection (needles and syringes may be sterilized by boiling in water for 15 minutes).

Before withdrawing the solution from the bottle, disinfect the rubber cap on the bottle with a suitable disinfectant, such as 70 percent alcohol. The injection site should be similarly cleaned with the disinfectant. Needles of 14 to 16 gauge, and not more than 1 inch long, are adequate for injections.

A subcutaneous injection should be made by pinching up a fold of the skin between the thumb and forefinger. The mid-neck region is the preferred injection site. Insert the needle under the fold in a direction approximately parallel to the surface of the body. When the needle is inserted in this manner, the medication will be delivered underneath the skin between the skin and the muscles. Proper restraint, such as the use of a chute and nose lead is needed for proper administration of the product.

Precaution(s): The product should be stored between 2°-8°C (36°-46°F). Avoid freezing. Shake well before using.

Caution(s): Exceeding the recommended doses and dosage levels may result in antibiotic residues beyond the withdrawal time. Do not inject this product intramuscularly.

Penicillin G is a substance of low toxicity. However, side effects, or so-called allergic or anaphylactic reactions - sometimes fatal, have been known to occur in animals hypersensitive to penicillin and procaine. Such reactions can occur unpredictably with varying intensity. Animals administered penicillin G should be kept under close observation for at least one-half hour. Should allergic or anaphylactic reactions occur, discontinue use of the product and immediately administer epinephrine, following the manufacturer's recommendations, and call a veterinarian.

As with all antibiotic preparations, use of this drug may result in overgrowth of non-susceptible organisms, including fungi. A lack of response by the treated animal, or the development of new signs or symptoms suggests that an overgrowth of non-susceptible organisms has occurred. In such instances, consult your veterinarian.

Since bacterial drugs may interfere with the bacteriostatic action of tetracyclines, it is advisable to avoid giving penicillin in conjunction with tetracyclines.

For animal use only.

For subcutaneous use only.

For use in beef cattle only.

Restricted Drug (under California law); use only as directed.

Warning(s): Beef cattle should be withheld from slaughter for food use for 30 days following the last treatment. Treatment in beef cattle must be limited to two (2) doses, by subcutaneous injection only. Do not inject intramuscularly.

Presentation: Available in 100 mL (NDC 59419-206-11) and 250 mL (NDC 59419-206-12) multiple-dose vials.

Compendium Code No.: 10250030 Rev. 8/99

COMBI-CLENS®

G.C. Hanford **Topical Product**

Sterile Topical Skin Cleanser

Active Ingredient(s): Purified Water, USP containing 20% Poloxamer 155, NF.

Indications: Aids in the cleansing of impurities such as dirt and debris from skin surfaces.

Dosage and Administration: Use as required.

Precaution(s): The bottle is hermetically sealed for your protection. Squeeze bottle prior to use. If bottle leaks do not use.

Caution(s): For external use only.

Presentation: 100 mL (3.4 fl. oz) single unit dose container.

Compendium Code No.: 10340040 10/2000

COMBOVAC-30®

Intervet **Vaccine**

Newcastle-Bronchitis Vaccine, B_1 Type, LaSota Strain, Mass. and Conn. Types, Live Virus

U.S. Vet. Lic. No.: 286

Description: This live virus vaccine is prepared from the proven Clone 30® strain of Newcastle disease virus and the regular Massachusetts and Connecticut bronchitis viruses. The virus strains have been propagated using SPF substrates.

Intervet's research team cloned several lentogenic ND virus strains from separate sub-populations within these strains. These clones were then extensively tested for immunogenicity and reactivity. One clone, designated ND virus Clone 30®, was selected and proven to be of the same order of reactivity as the classical Hitchner B_1, but provided considerably better protection.

This vaccine contains gentamicin as a preservative.

Quality tested for purity, potency, and safety.

Indications: Coarse Spray, or Drinking Water: Vaccination of healthy chickens two weeks of age or older for protection against Newcastle Disease and Massachusetts and Connecticut types of bronchitis. Initial vaccination should be by coarse spray, drinking water.

Dosage and Administration: Vaccination Programs: Many factors must be considered in determining a sound vaccination program for a particular farm or poultry complex. To be fully effective, the vaccine must be administered properly to healthy, receptive birds maintained in a proper environment under good management. In addition, the response may be influenced by the age of the birds and their immune status. Seldom does one live virus vaccination under field conditions produce lifetime protection for all individuals in a given flock. The level of immunity required will vary with operational practices and the degree of exposure. Therefore, a program of periodic revaccinations may be necessary.

Preparation of Vaccine:

For Drinking Water or Coarse Spray Use: Do not open and mix the vaccine until ready to begin vaccination. Use vaccine immediately after mixing.

1. Remove the tear-off seal and stopper from the vial of vaccine.
2. Carefully pour clean, cool non-chlorinated water into the vaccine vial until the vial is approximately two-thirds full.
3. Insert the rubber stopper and shake vigorously until all material is dissolved.
4. Pour the rehydrated vaccine into a container in preparation for drinking water or coarse spray use.

For best results, be sure to follow directions carefully!

Drinking Water Administration:

For Chickens Two Weeks of Age or Older:

1. Do not use any disinfectants in the drinking water for 48 hours before vaccinating and for 24 hours after vaccination.
2. Withhold drinking water from the chickens until they are thirsty. Withholding periods will vary from 2 to 8 hours according to age of chickens and weather conditions.
3. Scrub waterers and rinse thoroughly with fresh, clean water. Do not use disinfectants for cleaning waterers.
4. Mix rehydrated vaccine with clean, cool, non-chlorinated tap water in accordance with the chart below.

Age of Chickens	Water Per 1,000 Doses Vaccine
2-4 weeks	6 gal. (23 liters)
4-8 weeks	10 gal. (38 liters)
8 weeks or older	16 gal. (60 liters)

As an aid in preserving the virus, 3.2 ounces (100 g) of non-fat powdered milk may be added to each 10 U.S. gallons (38 liters) of water used for mixing vaccine. Add the dried milk first and agitate thoroughly. Then add the rehydrated vaccine from the vial and mix thoroughly.

5. Distribute the vaccine solution, as prepared above, to the waterers provided for the chickens. Avoid placing waterers in direct sunlight.
6. Provide no other drinking water until all the vaccine-water solution has been consumed.

Coarse Spray Vaccination:

For Chickens Two Weeks of Age or Older:

1. Initial spray vaccination should be by coarse spray, i.e., Hardi®.
2. Do not use any disinfectants or skim milk in sprayer.
3. Use sprayer for administration of vaccines.
4. Shut off all fans while spray vaccinating. Turn on fan immediately after spraying. Be careful in hot weather.
5. Spray chickens by walking slowly through the house.
6. Follow the recommendation of the manufacturer of the sprayer regarding water volume.
7. Use only clean, cool, deionized water.

8. Individual(s) spraying chickens should wear face mask and goggles.

Records: Keep a record of vaccine, quantity, serial number, expiration date, and place of purchase; the date and time of vaccination; the number, age, breed, and location of chickens; name of operators performing the vaccination and any observed reactions.

Precaution(s): Store vaccine between 2 and 7°C (35 and 45°F).

Do not spill or splash the vaccine.

Use entire contents when first opened.

Burn containers and all unused contents.

This product is non-returnable.

Caution(s): Vaccinate only healthy chickens. Although disease may not be evident, coccidiosis, Mycoplasma infection, infectious bursal disease, Marek's disease, reovirus infection and other disease conditions may cause complications or reduce immunity.

All susceptible chickens on the same premises should be vaccinated at the same time.

The revaccination of laying hens with live Newcastle/Bronchitis vaccine may be detrimental to the flock and cannot be generally recommended. Consult your Intervet representative for more information.

Efforts should be taken to reduce stress conditions at the time of vaccination and during the reaction period.

Do not dilute the vaccine or otherwise stretch the dosage.

For veterinary use only.

Notice: This vaccine has undergone rigid potency, safety and purity tests, and meets Intervet Inc. and USDA requirements and is designed to stimulate effective immunity when used as directed. The user must be advised that the response to the vaccine depends upon many factors, including, but not limited to, conditions of storage and handling by the user, administration of the vaccine, health and responsiveness of individual chickens, and the degree of field exposure. Therefore, directions should be followed carefully.

This product is not hazardous when used according to directions supplied. A material safety data sheet (MSDS) is available upon request. This and any other consumer information can be obtained by calling Intervet Customer Service at 1-800-441-8272 or 1-302-934-8051.

The use of this vaccine is subject to applicable federal and local laws and regulations.

Use only as directed.

Warning(s): Do not vaccinate within 21 days before slaughter.

Newcastle virus occasionally causes conjunctivitis in humans. Avoid any contact of vaccine with eyes.

Presentation: 10 x 2,000 doses for drinking water or coarse spray use.
10 x 10,000 doses for drinking water or coarse spray use.
10 x 25,000 doses for drinking water or coarse spray use.

Compendium Code No.: 11060381 — 20307 AL 90 2.0

COMEBACK™

AgriPharm — **Electrolytes-Oral**

Ingredient(s): Guaranteed Analysis:

Sodium, minimum 3.00%
Potassium, minimum 1.10%

Ingredients: Dextrose, sodium chloride, potassium chloride, glycine, citric acid, and sodium silico aluminate.

Indications: Supplemental nutrients and electrolytes for young calves, lambs, and foals. Designed for oral administration.

Dosage and Administration: Mix and Feed Directions

Feed according to the following schedule:

Calves and Foals:

Mix the entire contents of this packet (5.73 oz) with two (2) quarts of warm water. Stir until dissolved. COMEBACK™ should be prepared just prior to use and can be fed with nursing bottles and pails.

Feed two (2) quarts of this solution twice daily to each calf or foal for the first two days. Discontinue milk or milk replacer feedings for these first two days.

On the third and fourth days, feed one (1) quart of solution mixed with either one (1) quart of milk or one (1) quart of milk replacer twice daily to each calf or foal.

Lambs:

Lambs will require approximately one-fourth (¼) of the above dosage. Follow feeding schedule shown above.

Precaution(s): Store in a cool, dry place.

Warning(s): For animal use only. Keep out of reach of children.

Presentation: 5.73 oz (162.55 g) packet.

Compendium Code No.: 14570230

COMMANDER™ 5

Biocor — **Vaccine**

Canine Distemper-Adenovirus Type 2-Parainfluenza-Parvovirus Vaccine, Modified Live and Killed Virus

U.S. Vet. Lic. No.: 462

Contents: This product contains the antigens listed above.

The Adenovirus fraction is inactivated. The remaining virus fractions are live, and attenuated to assure safety.

This product contains gentamicin and amphotericin B as preservatives.

Indications: COMMANDER™ 5 is recommended for use in the vaccination of healthy dogs against disease caused by Canine Distemper, Infectious Canine Hepatitis, Canine Parvovirus and respiratory disease caused by Canine Adenovirus Type 2 and Parainfluenza.

Directions: Aseptically rehydrate the desiccated product with the accompanying vial of liquid product. Shake well. Administer entire contents (1 mL) intramuscularly or subcutaneously.

Persistence of maternal origin antibody in puppies should receive consideration in determining vaccination programs. Ideally, puppies should be vaccinated at 9 weeks of age with revaccination every 2-4 weeks until at least 18 weeks of age. Dogs vaccinated after 18 weeks of age should receive a 1 mL dose followed by a second dose 2-4 weeks later. Annual revaccination with a single 1 mL dose is recommended.

Precaution(s): Store at 35°F-45°F (2°C-7°C). Do not freeze. Use entire contents when first rehydrated. Burn these containers and all unused contents.

Caution(s): Do not vaccinate pregnant bitches. In case of anaphylactoid reactions, epinephrine should be administered immediately. For use in dogs only. For veterinary use only.

Presentation: Code 75511B - 25 x 1 dose (1 mL) vials with diluent.

Compendium Code No.: 13940042 — BAH11925-999

COMMANDER™ 7 L

Biocor — **Bacterin-Vaccine**

Canine Distemper-Adenovirus Type 2-Parainfluenza-Parvovirus Vaccine, Modified Live and Killed Virus, Leptospira Bacterin

U.S. Vet. Lic. No.: 462

Contents: This product contains the antigens listed above.

The Adenovirus and Leptospira fractions are inactivated. The remaining virus fractions are live, and attenuated to assure safety.

This product contains gentamicin and amphotericin B as preservatives.

Indications: COMMANDER™ 7 L is recommended for use in the vaccination of healthy dogs against disease caused by Canine Distemper, Infectious Canine Hepatitis, Canine Parvovirus, *Leptospira canicola* and *Leptospira icterohaemorrhagiae* and respiratory disease caused by Canine Adenovirus Type 2, and Parainfluenza.

Directions: Aseptically rehydrate the desiccated product with the accompanying vial of liquid product. Shake well. Administer entire contents (1 mL) IM or SC.

Persistence of maternal origin antibody in puppies should receive consideration in determining vaccination programs. Ideally, puppies should be vaccinated at 9 weeks of age with revaccination every 2-4 weeks until at least 18 weeks of age. Dogs vaccinated after 18 weeks of age should receive a 1 mL dose followed by a second dose 2-4 weeks later. Annual revaccination with a single 1 mL dose is recommended.

Precaution(s): Store at 35°F-45°F (2°C-7°C). Do not freeze. Use entire contents when first rehydrated. Burn these containers and all unused contents.

Caution(s): Do not vaccinate pregnant bitches. In case of anaphylactoid reactions, epinephrine should be administered immediately. For use in dogs only For veterinary use only.

Presentation: Code 75311B - 25 x 1 dose (1 mL) vials with diluent.

Compendium Code No.: 13940052 — BAH9525-1098

COMMANDER™ PARVO MLV

Biocor — **Vaccine**

Parvovirus Vaccine, Modified Live Virus

U.S. Vet. Lic. No.: 462

Contents: This product contains the antigen listed above.

This product contains gentamicin, amphotericin B and thimerosal as preservatives.

Indications: COMMANDER™ Parvo MLV is recommended for use in the vaccination of healthy dogs against disease caused by Canine Parvovirus.

Directions: Shake well. Administer entire contents (1 mL) IM or SC. Ideally, puppies should be vaccinated at 9 weeks of age with revaccination every 2-4 weeks until at least 18 weeks of age. Dogs vaccinated after 18 weeks of age should receive a 1 mL dose followed by a second dose 2-4 weeks later. Annual revaccination with a single 1 mL dose is recommended.

Persistence of maternal origin antibodies in puppies should receive consideration in determining vaccination programs.

Precaution(s): Store at 35°F-45°F (2°C-7°C). Do not freeze. Use entire contents when first opened. Burn these containers and all unused contents.

Caution(s): Do not vaccinate pregnant bitches. In case of anaphylactoid reactions, epinephrine should be administered immediately. For use in dogs only. For veterinary use only.

Presentation: Code 75611B - 25 x 1 dose (1 mL) vials.
Code 75654B - 10 dose (10 mL) vials.

Compendium Code No.: 13940062 — BAH11325-1098 / BAH1138-1098

COMMANDO™ INSECTICIDE CATTLE EAR TAG

Boehringer Ingelheim — **Insecticide Ear Tags**

EPA Reg. No.: 4691-157

Active Ingredient: — By Weight

Ethion (CAS #563-12-2) 36.0%
Other Ingredients 64.0%
Total 100.0%

Net Weight: 15 grams per tag minimum.

Tag rivets coated with Infecta-Guard™ - A patented anti-bacterial coating to improve tag retention.

Indications: For use on beef and lactating dairy cattle to control horn flies (including pyrethroid resistant populations), Gulf Coast ticks, Spinose ear ticks, and as an aid to control face flies, lice, stable flies, and house flies.

Directions for Use: It is a violation of Federal law to use this product in a manner inconsistent with its labeling.

For optimum control of horn flies, control of ear ticks, and as an aid in the control of face flies, lice, stable flies and house flies attach one tag to each ear (two tags per animal). Replace as necessary. These tags have been proven to substantially reduce pyrethroid resistant horn flies for up to five months. Apply as indicated. Calves less than 3 months of age should not be tagged as ear damage may result.

Remove tag prior to slaughter.

Figure 1. Disinfect pliers prior to use. Place female tag under clip by depressing lever. Collar on tag must be pointing down.

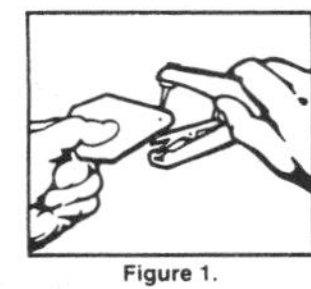

Figure 1.

Figure 2. Slide male rivet on pin. Align tip of male rivet with female portion of tag. Tag and rivet are now ready for application.

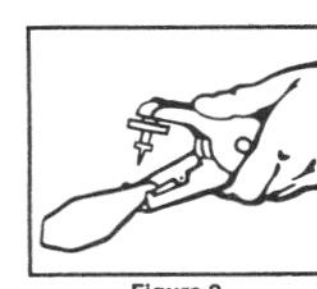

Figure 2.

Figures 3 and 4. Position tag on the inner flat surface in center of ear. Do not allow shaft of the male rivet to penetrate any cartilage rib or blood vessel or ear damage may result. Boehringer

C

Ingelheim Vetmedica, Inc. recommends that tag be rotated at a 90° angle (Fig. 4) for ease of application. Tag may also be extended outward from the plier in a straight manner (Fig. 3).

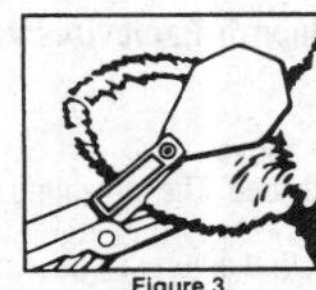
Figure 3.

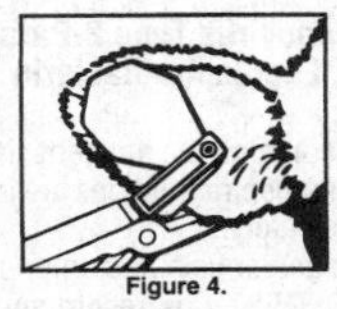
Figure 4.

Figure 5. When properly positioned, the tag should hang as shown.

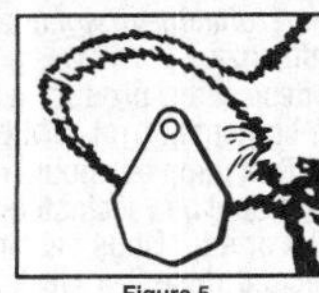
Figure 5.

Precautionary Statements: Hazards to Humans:

Warning: May be fatal if absorbed through skin. Do not get in eyes, on skin or on clothing. Wear protective clothing and rubber gloves. Wash thoroughly with soap and water after handling and before eating, drinking, or using tobacco. Remove contaminated clothing and wash clothing before reuse.

First Aid:

If on Skin: Wash with plenty of soap and water. Get medical attention.

If in Eyes: Flush eyes with plenty of water. Call a physician if irritation persists.

If Swallowed: Call a physician or Poison Control Center immediately. Drink one or two glasses of water and induce vomiting by touching the back of the throat with a finger. Do not induce vomiting or give anything by mouth to an unconscious or convulsing person.

Note to physician: This product is a cholinesterase inhibitor. If symptoms of cholinesterase inhibition are present, atropine sulfate by injection is antidotal. Do not give morphine.

Environmental Hazards: This pesticide is toxic to fish. Do not contaminate water by disposal of used tags.

Storage and Disposal: Store in a cool place in original container.

Opened pouches containing ear tags should be resealed for storage. Do not contaminate water, food, or feed by storage or disposal.

Pesticide Disposal: Waste (spent tags) resulting from the use of this product may be disposed of on site or at an approved waste disposal facility.

Container Disposal: Dispose of empty container in a sanitary landfill or by incineration, or, if allowed by state and local authorities, by burning. If burned, stay out of smoke.

Warning(s): Remove tag prior to slaughter.

Keep out of reach of children.

Disclaimer: Warranty and Limitation of Damages: Seller warrants that this material conforms to its chemical description and is reasonably fit for the purposes stated on the label when used in accordance with direction under normal conditions of use and Buyer assumes the risk of any use contrary to such directions. Seller makes no other express or implied warranty of Fitness or of Merchantability, and no agent of Seller is authorized to do so except in writing and with a specific reference to this warranty. In no event shall Seller's liability for any breach of warranty exceed the purchase price of the material as to which a claim is made.

Presentation: 20's (16 per case) and 120's (6 per case). Boxes contain rivets for use with the AllFlex Applicator.

U.S. Patent No. 5,342,619

Licensed under U.S. Patent No. 4,581,834

Compendium Code No.: 10280301 665009D-01-9808

COMPANIONVAC™ 5

Aspen **Vaccine**

Canine Distemper-Adenovirus Type 2-Parainfluenza-Parvovirus Vaccine, Modified Live and Killed Virus

U.S. Vet. Lic. No.: 462

Contents: This product contains the antigens listed above. The Adenovirus fraction is inactivated. The remaining virus fractions are live, and attenuated to assure safety.

This product contains gentamicin and amphotericin B as preservatives.

Indications: COMPANIONVAC™ 5 is recommended for use in the vaccination of healthy dogs against disease caused by Canine Distemper, Infectious Canine Hepatitis, Canine Parvovirus and respiratory disease caused by Canine Adenovirus Type 2 and Parainfluenza.

Directions: Aseptically rehydrate vial of desiccated antigens by injecting the liquid product into the vial containing the vaccine cake. Shake well. Remove the entire contents back into the syringe. Push out an air trapped in the syringe. Administer entire contents (1 mL) intramuscularly or subcutaneously. To give subcutaneously, vaccinate under loose skin (back of neck). To give intramuscularly, vaccine in large muscle of hind limb. Do not vaccinate into blood vessels. If blood enters the syringe, choose another injection site.

Persistence of maternal origin antibody in puppies should receive consideration in determining vaccination programs. Ideally, puppies should be vaccinated at 9 weeks of age with revaccination every 2-4 weeks until at least 18 weeks of age. Dogs vaccinated after 18 weeks of age should receive a 1 mL dose followed by a second dose 2-4 weeks later. Annual revaccination with a single 1 mL dose is recommended.

Contraindication(s): Do not vaccinate pregnant bitches.

Precaution(s): Store at 35°-45°F (2°-7°C). Do not freeze. Use entire contents when first rehydrated. Burn these containers, including syringe and needle.

Caution(s): In case of anaphylactoid reactions, epinephrine should be administered immediately.

For use in dogs only.

Presentation: One dose (1 mL) vials with syringe.

Manufactured by: Biocor Animal Health Inc., Omaha, NE 68134.

Compendium Code No.: 14750990 AV11901-200

COMPANIONVAC™ 7 L

Aspen **Vaccine**

Canine Distemper-Adenovirus Type 2-Parainfluenza-Parvovirus Vaccine, Modified Live and Killed Virus, Leptospira Bacterin

U.S. Vet. Lic. No.: 462

Contents: This product contains the antigens listed above. The Adenovirus and Leptospira fractions are inactivated. The remaining virus fractions are live, and attenuated to assure safety.

This product contains gentamicin and amphotericin B as preservatives.

Indications: COMPANIONVAC™ 7 L is recommended for use in the vaccination of healthy dogs against disease caused by Canine Distemper, Infectious Canine Hepatitis, Canine Parvovirus, *Leptospira canicola* and *L. icterohaemorrhagiae* and respiratory disease caused by Canine Adenovirus Type 2 and Parainfluenza.

Directions: Aseptically rehydrate vial of desiccated antigens by injecting the liquid product into the vial containing the vaccine cake. Shake well. Remove the entire contents back into the syringe. Push out an air trapped in the syringe. Administer entire contents (1 mL) intramuscularly or subcutaneously. To give subcutaneously, vaccinate under loose skin (back of neck). To give intramuscularly, vaccine in large muscle of hind limb. Do not vaccinate into blood vessels. If blood enters the syringe, choose another injection site.

Persistence of maternal origin antibody in puppies should receive consideration in determining vaccination programs. Ideally, puppies should be vaccinated at 9 weeks of age with revaccination every 2-4 weeks until at least 18 weeks of age. Dogs vaccinated after 18 weeks of age should receive a 1 mL dose followed by a second dose 2-4 weeks later. Annual revaccination with a single 1 mL dose is recommended.

Contraindication(s): Do not vaccinate pregnant bitches.

Precaution(s): Store at 35°-45°F (2°-7°C). Do not freeze. Use entire contents when first rehydrated. Burn these containers, including syringe and needle.

Caution(s): In case of anaphylactoid reactions, epinephrine should be administered immediately.

For use in dogs only.

Presentation: One dose (1 mL) vials with syringe.

Manufactured by: Biocor Animal Health Inc., Omaha, NE 68134.

Compendium Code No.: 14751000 AV9501-200

COMPANIONVAC™ B

Aspen **Bacterin**

Bordetella Bronchiseptica Bacterin, Extracted Cellular Antigens

U.S. Vet. Lic. No.: 462

Contents: COMPANIONVAC™ B is a nonadjuvanted antigenic extract prepared from the cells of *Bordetella bronchiseptica.*

This product contains thimerosal (merthiolate) as a preservative.

Indications: Recommended for use as an aid in the control of Canine Infectious Tracheobronchitis (Kennel Cough) caused by the organism represented.

Directions: Shake well. Aseptically remove entire contents into the syringe. Push out any air trapped in the syringe. Administer entire contents (1 mL) subcutaneously under loose skin (back of neck) to healthy dogs at least 8 weeks of age. Do not vaccinate into blood vessels. If blood enters the syringe, choose another injection site. For initial vaccination, a second dose is required 2-4 weeks later. This product should be administered by subcutaneous injection only. Annual revaccination with a single 1 mL dose is recommended.

Precaution(s): Store at 35°-45°F (2°-7°C). Do not freeze. Use entire contents when first opened. Care should be taken to avoid microbial contamination of the product.

Caution(s): In case of anaphylactoid reactions, epinephrine should be administered immediately. Transient local irritation at the site of injection, though rare, may occur subsequent to use of this product.

Use special caution when vaccinating miniature or small breed dogs.

For use in dogs only.

Discussion: The effect of persisting *B. bronchiseptica* maternal antibody on the immune response in puppies to this bacterin has not been determined. Puppies from bitches immune to the organism usually have low antibody titers that are dissipated by 4-6 weeks of age. Although kennel cough is considered a disease of complex etiology, it can be reproduced by challenge with *B. bronchiseptica* alone. A close association and/or confinement of dogs facilitates spread of the disease syndrome. Antibiotic therapy has been shown to be generally unsuccessful in reducing or eliminating *B. bronchiseptica* in dogs.

Presentation: One dose (1 mL) vials with syringe.

Manufactured by: Biocor Animal Health Inc., Omaha, NE 68134.

Compendium Code No.: 14751010 AV7001-200

COMPANIONVAC™ PARVO MLV

Aspen **Vaccine**

Parvovirus Vaccine, Modified Live Virus

U.S. Vet. Lic. No.: 462

Contents: This product contains the antigen listed above.

This product contains gentamicin, amphotericin B and thimerosal as preservatives.

Indications: COMPANIONVAC™ Parvo MLV is recommended for use in the vaccination of healthy dogs against disease caused by Canine Parvovirus.

Directions: Shake well. Aseptically remove entire contents into the syringe. Push out any air trapped in the syringe. Administer entire contents (1 mL) subcutaneously or intramuscularly. To give subcutaneously, vaccinate under loose skin (back of neck). To give intramuscularly, vaccinate in large muscle of hind limb. Do not vaccinate into blood vessels. If blood enters the syringe, choose another injection site.

Persistence of maternal origin antibody in puppies should receive consideration in determining vaccination programs. Ideally, puppies should be vaccinated at 9 weeks of age with revaccination every 2-4 weeks until at least 18 weeks of age. Dogs vaccinated after 18 weeks of age should receive a 1 mL dose followed by a second dose 2-4 weeks later. Annual revaccination with a single 1 mL dose is recommended.

Contraindication(s): Do not vaccinate pregnant bitches.

Precaution(s): Store at 35°-45°F (2°-7°C). Do not freeze. Use entire contents when first opened. Burn this container, including syringe and needle.

Caution(s): In case of anaphylactoid reactions, epinephrine should be administered immediately.

For use in dogs only.

Presentation: One dose (1 mL) vials with syringe.

Manufactured by: Biocor Animal Health Inc., Omaha, NE, 68134.

Compendium Code No.: 14751020 AV11031-200

COMPANIONVAC™ RCP

Aspen **Vaccine**

Feline Rhinotracheitis-Calici-Panleukopenia Vaccine, Modified Live and Killed Virus

U.S. Vet. Lic. No.: 462

Contents: COMPANIONVAC™ RCP is a combination of modified live Feline Rhinotracheitis and Calici viruses with inactivated Panleukopenia virus vaccine.

All fractions are subjected to tests for potency and safety prior to release for market.

This product contains gentamicin and amphotericin B as preservatives.

Indications: Recommended for use in the vaccination of healthy cats against disease caused by the organisms represented.

Directions: Aseptically rehydrate vial of desiccated antigens by injecting the liquid product into the vial containing the vaccine cake. Shake well. Remove the entire contents back into the syringe. Push out any air trapped in the syringe. Administer entire contents (1 mL) subcutaneously under loose skin (back of neck). Do not vaccinate into blood vessels. If blood enters the syringe, choose another injection site.

Persistence of maternal origin antibody in kittens is known to interfere with development of active immunity following vaccination. Present indications are that Rhinotracheitis and Calicivirus antibodies of maternal origin endure in kittens for approximately 8 weeks. Panleukopenia antibody somewhat longer - up to 13 weeks. Ideally, kittens should be vaccinated at 9 weeks of age with revaccination 3-4 weeks later. Adult cats should receive a 1 mL dose followed by a second dose 3-4 weeks later. Annual revaccination with a single 1 mL dose is recommended.

Contraindication(s): Do not vaccinate pregnant queens.

Precaution(s): Store at 35°-45°F (2°-7°C).

Do not freeze. Use entire contents when first rehydrated.

Burn these containers, including syringe and needle.

Caution(s): An occasional animal may demonstrate a transient fever, and mild arthralgia and/or myalgia within the first week following vaccination. In case of anaphylactoid reactions, epinephrine should be administered immediately.

For use in cats only.

Presentation: One dose vials with accompanying (1 mL) killed virus diluent.

Manufactured by: Biocor Animal Health Inc.

Compendium Code No.: 14750331 AV3301-200

COMPLIANCE™

Metrex **Disinfectant**

Sterilizing and Disinfecting Solution

Active Ingredient(s):

Hydrogen Peroxide 7.35%
Peracetic Acid 0.23%
Inert Ingredients. 92.42%
Total 100.00%

Indications: Intended Use: COMPLIANCE™ solution is a liquid chemical sterilant and a high-level disinfectant when used according to the "Directions for Use".

1. Germicide Level of Activity: COMPLIANCE™ can be used at the following germicide levels of activity:
   High Level Disinfection:
   14 Day Reuse: COMPLIANCE™ is a high-level disinfectant when used or reused, according to the "Directions for Use", at 68°F (20°C) with an immersion time of 15 minutes for a use period not to exceed 14 days.
   Sterilant:
   14 Day Reuse: COMPLIANCE™ is a sterilant when used or reused, according to the "Directions for Use", at 68°F (20°C) with an immersion time of 180 minutes (3 hours) for a use period not to exceed 14 days.
2. Reuse Period: COMPLIANCE™ has demonstrated efficacy in the presence of five percent (5%) organic soil contamination and a simulated amount of microbiological burden under the following temperatures:
   68°F (20°C) - with a contact time of 15 minutes and the product discarded after 14 days for high-level disinfection. For sterilization, a contact time of 180 minutes (3 hours) is required with the product discarded after 14 days.
3. General Sterilization/Disinfection Information: Choose a germicide with the level of microbial activity that is appropriate for the reusable medical device or equipment surface. Follow the reusable device labeling and standard institutional practices. In the absence of complete instructions, use the following guidance:
   First, for patient contacting devices, determine whether the reusable device to be processed is a critical or semi-critical device.
   - A critical device routinely penetrates the skin or mucous membranes during use or is otherwise used in normally sterile tissues of the body.
   - A semi-critical device makes contact with mucous membranes but does not ordinarily penetrate sterile areas of the body.
   Second, determine the level of sterilization/disinfection required:
   - Critical Device - Sterilization is required.
   - Semi-critical Device - Although sterilization is recommended whenever practical, high-level disinfection is acceptable (e.g. GI endoscopes, anesthesia equipment to be used in the airway, diaphragm-fitting rings, etc.)
   Third, determine the time needed to achieve the level of disinfection or sterilization required for the specified medical device as indicated on the COMPLIANCE™ solution label.
4. The germicidal activity of COMPLIANCE™ was demonstrated using stressed solutions* in performance, clinical and simulated use testing using the following organisms:

	20°C 14 Day Reuse*
Spores - *Bacillus subtilis* - *Clostridium sporogenes*	180 minutes
Vegetative Organisms	15 minutes
- *Staphylococcus aureus*	3 minutes
- *Salmonella choleraesuis*	3 minutes
- *Pseudomonas aeruginosa*	3 minutes
- *Mycobacterium bovis*	15 minutes
Fungi - *Trichophyton mentagrophytes*	5 minutes
Non-lipid Small Virus - Polio 2	5 minutes
Lipid Medium Virus - Herpes simplex - HIV 1 (Human Immunodeficiency Virus)	5 minutes

*Testing was performed using COMPLIANCE™ solution which had been stressed in accordance with EPA "Reuse Test Protocol Specifications" and aged 46 days. Due to a lack of a test strip for monitoring concentration of active ingredients the reuse period is limited to 14 days.

5. Device/Material Compatibility: COMPLIANCE™ solution is recommended for usage with medical devices made from the following materials: Black Anodized Aluminum**, 303 Stainless Steel, Teflon*, Polyethylene*, Polyethylene Tubing*, Polyurethane*, Black Rubber*, Cemedine (epoxy)/Liquid Silicone***, Adhesive***, Loctite Impruv-Loctite 330++, Masterbond.
   *Represents 1500 cycles - 20 minute exposure plus rinsing and drying.
   **Some loss of color observed after 48 cycles; complete color loss observed on some specimens from 394 cycle to 657 cycles. (No damage to base metal was observed).
   ***Cemedine epoxy adhesive remained flexible with good adhesion for 72 hours immersed in COMPLIANCE™ at 20°C. Cemedine epoxy adhesive became brittle and failed adhesively at 50°C immersion for 30 hours. Liquid silicone adhesive remained flexible with good adhesion for 72 hours at 20°C. Liquid silicone adhesive maintained shiny appearance with good flexibility, but failed adhesively at 50°C with 30 hours immersion.
   Note: Similar tests were conducted at 50°C in tap water with failure of flexibility and adhesion observed between 20 and 44 hours of immersion. This suggests that adhesive damage and/or failure is likely due to elevated solution temperature rather than due to chemical action.
   ++Loctite Impruv and Loctite 330 adhesive remained optically clear with good adhesion at 63°C with a 24-hour immersion.
   Following sterilization or disinfection, the sterilized or disinfected medical device should be rinsed according to the "Directions for Use", Rinsing (see "Rinsing Instructions"), and dried according to manufacturer's instructions.
6. Pre-cleaning Agent Compatibility: COMPLIANCE™ is compatible with enzymatic detergents which are neutral in pH, low foaming and easily rinsed from equipment. Detergents that are either highly alkaline or acidic are contraindicated as precleaning agents since improper rinsing could effect the efficacy of the COMPLIANCE™ solution by altering its pH.

COMPLIANCE™ Disinfectant/Sterilant Solution Endoscope Reprocessing:

Intended Use: COMPLIANCE™ is a liquid chemical sterilant and high-level disinfectant for medical instruments and devices when used according to the "Directions for Use".

Medical instruments/devices, when expected to penetrate the skin or mucous membranes or are used in otherwise normally sterile tissues of the body during use, are critical devices and are therefore, required to be sterile.

Medical instruments and devices when expected to come in contact without penetration of mucous membranes are semi-critical devices and therefore may be high-level disinfected.

Germicide Level of Activity: COMPLIANCE™ can be used at the following germicide levels of activity:

High-Level Disinfection:

14 Day Reuse: COMPLIANCE™ is a high-level disinfectant when used or reused, according to the "Directions for Use", at 68°F (20°C) with an immersion time of 15 minutes for a use period not to exceed 14 days.

Sterilant:

14 Day Reuse: COMPLIANCE™ is a sterilant when used or reused, according to the "Directions for Use", at 68°F (20°C) with an immersion time of 180 minutes for a use period not to exceed 14 days.

Directions for Use: It is a violation of federal law to use this product in a manner inconsistent with its labeling.

COMPLIANCE™ is a ready to use disinfectant/sterilant solution. COMPLIANCE™ is for use in manual (bucket and tray) systems made from polypropylene, ABS, polyethylene, glass-filled polypropylene or specially molded polycarbonate plastics and stainless steel.

1. Record initial date of use and the expiration date (14 days hence) in a log book or a label affixed to any secondary container used to contain the solution. COMPLIANCE™ must be discarded after 14 days.
2. Cleaning/Decontamination: Blood and other body fluids must be thoroughly cleaned from the surfaces, lumens, and objects before application of the disinfectant/sterilant. Blood and other body fluids should be autoclaved and disposed of according to all applicable federal, state and local regulations for infectious waste disposal.
   For COMPLIANCE™ to be an effective disinfectant or sterilant, thoroughly clean, rinse and rough dry medical instruments and equipment. Clean and rinse the lumens of hollow instruments before filling with COMPLIANCE™ solution. Refer to the reusable device manufacturers labeling for instructions on disassembly, decontamination, cleaning and leak testing of their equipment. Avoid dilution of the COMPLIANCE™ solution.
3. Usage: It is violation of federal law to use this product in a manner inconsistent with its labeling.
   a. Directions for Sterilization (Bucket/Tray Manual System): COMPLIANCE™ is a liquid chemical sterilant for medical instruments and devices when used according to the "Directions for Use".
   14 Day Reuse Solution - at 68°F (20°C).
   Sterilant: COMPLIANCE™ is a sterilant for medical instruments/devices when used or reused, according to the "Directions for Use", at 68°F (20°C) with an immersion time of 180 minutes (3 hours) for a use period not to exceed 14 days.
   Immerse medical equipment/devices completely in COMPLIANCE™ solution for a minimum of 180 minutes (3 hours) at 68°F (20°C) to eliminate all microorganisms including *Clostridium sporogens* and *Bacillus subtilis* spores. Remove equipment from the solution using sterile technique and rinse thoroughly with sterile water following the "Rinsing Instructions" below.
   b. Directions for High-Level Disinfection (Bucket/Tray Manual System): COMPLIANCE™ is a liquid chemical high-level disinfectant for medical instruments and devices when used according to the "Directions for Use". Medical instruments/devices when expected to come in contact without penetration of mucous membranes are semi-critical devices and therefore may be high-level disinfected.
   14 Day Reuse Solution - at 68°F (20°C).
   High-Level Disinfectant: COMPLIANCE™ is a high-level disinfectant for medical instruments/devices when used or reused, according to the "Directions for Use", at 68°F (20°C) with an immersion time of 15 minutes for a use period not to exceed 14 days.
   Immerse medical equipment/devices completely in COMPLIANCE™ solution for a minimum of 15 minutes at 68°F (20°C) to destroy all pathogenic microorganisms, except for large numbers of bacterial endospores, but including *Mycobacterium* strains as represented by *M. bovis* (Quantitative TB Method). Remove equipment/devices from the solution and rinse thoroughly following the rinsing instructions below.
4. Rinsing Instructions: Following immersion in COMPLIANCE™ solution, thoroughly rinse the equipment or medical device by immersing in two gallons of water. Repeat this procedure a second time with a fresh two-gallon volume of water.
   For endoscopic instruments with lumens, a minimum of 500 mL of water should be flushed

through lumens during each separate rinse unless otherwise noted by the device or equipment manufacturer. Use fresh volumes of water for each rinse. Discard the water following each rinse. Do not reuse the water for rinsing or any other purpose as it will become contaminated with hydrogen peroxide.

Refer to the reusable device/equipment manufacturer's labeling for rinsing instructions.

a. Sterile Water Rinse: Critical devices which are sterilized with COMPLIANCE™ must be rinsed with sterile water.

b. Potable Water Rinse: A sterile water rinse is recommended when practical, for all devices. Alternatively, a high quality potable water (one that meets Federal Clean Water Standards at point of use) may be used.

The use of potable water for rinsing, increases the risk of contaminating the device or medical equipment with Pseudomonades and atypical (fast growing) *Mycobacteria* that are often present in potable water supplies. The devices (e.g. colonoscope) need to be completely dried, because any moisture remaining provides an ideal situation for rapid colonization of bacteria. Additionally, mycobacteria are highly resistant to drying, therefore, rapid drying will avoid possible colonization but may not result in a device free from atypical mycobacteria. A final rinse using a 70 percent isopropyl alcohol solution should be used to speed the drying process and reduce the numbers of any organism present as a result of rinsing with potable water.

Reuse: COMPLIANCE™ solution has demonstrated efficacy in the presence of 5 percent (5%) organic soil contamination and a simulated amount of microbiological burden during reuse. The hydrogen peroxide and peracetic acid concentration of this product will remain stable and effective during its use life (14 days). COMPLIANCE™ must be discarded after 14 days.

Due to lack of test strip for monitoring concentration of active ingredients the reuse period is limited to 14 days.

General Procedure for High-Level Disinfection of Flexible Endoscopes (This procedure is recommended in the absence of specific directions from the device manufacturer.):

1. Train Personnel:
   - Personnel involved in the reprocessing of endoscopes should have the ability to read, understand, and implement instructions from manufacturers and regulatory agencies as they relate to endoscopic disinfection.
   - The person(s) to whom the job of reprocessing endoscopes is given should have the opportunity to become completely familiar with the mechanical aspects of the endoscopic equipment.
   - Training should include familiarization with government regulations and in-house policies on how to appropriately and safely handle liquid chemical germicides.
   - Training should also include information on the safe handling of instruments that are contaminated with body fluids after use. This should include familiarization with universal precautions.
2. Cleaning of Flexible Endoscopes:

   a. Cleaning at the Examination Room: Reflux of body fluids from the patient may occur in any of the standard channels. Cleaning of endoscopes and accessories should be performed promptly after removing the endoscope from the patient to prevent drying of secretions.

   1. Don all personal protective equipment.
   2. Prepare an enzyme detergent or one recommended by the scope manufacturer.
   3. Gently wipe all debris from the insertion tube with a moistened gauze or cloth.
   4. Place the distal end of the flexible endoscope into the water and enzyme detergent solution and aspirate through the biopsy/suction channel for 5-10 seconds or until the solution is visibly clean. Alternate aspiration of the detergent solution and air several times. Finish by suctioning air.
   5. Flush or blow out air and water channels in accordance with the endoscope manufacturers instructions.
   6. Transport the endoscope to the reprocessing area.

   b. Cleaning at the Reprocessing Area:

   1. Attach any necessary water-tight caps to the electrical portions of the umbilicus.
   2. Before proceeding with any further cleaning steps, the flexible endoscope should be leak tested. (Refer to manufacturer's leakage test instructions.) Follow the manufacturer's instructions if the instrument appears damaged.
   3. Fill a sink or basin with a freshly made enzyme detergent solution.
   4. Immerse the endoscope. All channels should be irrigated with copious amounts of detergent and tap water to soften, moisten, and dilute the organic debris. All detachable parts (e.g., hoods and suction valves) should be removed and soaked in the detergent solution. The insertion tube should be washed with detergent solution and rinsed.
   5. Use a small soft brush to scrub all detachable parts.
   6. Use a brush to clean under the suction valve, air/water valve and biopsy port openings.
   7. Brush the entire suction/biopsy system including the body, the insertion tube, and the umbilicus of the endoscope in accordance with the manufacturer's instructions.
   8. Accessible channel(s) should be brushed to remove particulate matter, and the detergent solution must be suctioned or pumped through all channels to remove dislodged material. Channel irrigators may be useful for this step. Fill all channels with detergent solution and soak in accordance with the manufacturer's label instructions.
3. Rinse After Cleaning:
   a. Rinse the endoscope and all detachable parts in clean water.
   b. Rinse all channels well with water to remove debris and detergent.
   c. Purge water from all channels and wipe dry the exterior of the endoscope with a soft clean cloth to prevent dilution of the COMPLIANCE™ disinfectant used in subsequent steps.
4. Manual Sterilization/Disinfection:
   a. Attach channel irrigators/adapters and cover the biopsy port in accordance with the manufacturer's instructions.
   b. Pour COMPLIANCE™ into an appropriate sized basin or tray in an amount to completely submerge all surfaces of the endoscope.
   c. Completely immerse the endoscope in the basin of COMPLIANCE™.
   Note: In order to prevent damage to the endoscope, do not soak any other accessory equipment with the endoscope.
   d. Inject the COMPLIANCE™ solution into all channels of the endoscope until it can be seen exiting the opposite end of each channel. Assure that all channels are filled with disinfectant and that no air pockets remain within the channels.
   e. Cover the disinfectant soaking basin with a tight fitting lid to minimize chemical vapor exposure.
   f. Soak the endoscope for the designated use time at the appropriate temperature. Use a timer to ensure adequate soaking time.
   g. Before completely removing the endoscope from the disinfectant, flush all channels with air to remove disinfectant.
5. Rinse After Manual Sterilization or Disinfection:
   a. Rinse 1: Fill a basin with two gallons of water (preferably sterile water). Place the endoscope into the basin and thoroughly rinse the exterior of the scope. Attach channel irrigators/adapters to the endoscope and flush with 500 mL of water through the channel irrigator. Empty basin.
   b. Rinse 2: Fill a basin with two gallons of water (preferably sterile water). Place the endoscope into the basin and thoroughly rinse the exterior of the scope and flush with 500 mL of water through the channel irrigator.
   c. Purge all channels with air.
   d. Flush all channels with 70% isopropyl alcohol until the alcohol can be seen exiting the opposite end of each channel.
   e. Purge all channels with air.
   f. Remove all adapters and devices.
6. Storage:
   a. Dry the exterior of the endoscope with a soft clean cloth. Do not attach detachable parts to the endoscope prior to storage. Storage of endoscopes with the removable parts detached lowers the risk of trapping liquid inside the instrument and facilitates continued drying of the channels and channel openings. To prevent the growth of water borne organisms, the endoscope and all detached parts should be thoroughly dried prior to storage.
   b. Hang the endoscope vertically with the distal tip hanging freely in a well-ventilated, dust-free cabinet.

User Training: The user should be adequately trained in the decontamination and disinfection or sterilization of medical devices and the handling of liquid chemical germicides.

Storage and Disposal: Post Processing Handling and Storage of Reusable Devices: Sterilized or disinfected reusable devices are either to be used immediately or stored in a manner to minimize contamination. Refer to reusable device equipment manufacturer's labeling for additional storage and/or handling instructions.

Storage Conditions and Expiration Date:

1. COMPLIANCE™ solution should be stored in its original sealed container at room temperature 15°-30°C (59°-86°F).
2. The expiration date of COMPLIANCE™ solution will be found on the bottle.
3. Do not allow COMPLIANCE™ solution to freeze. COMPLIANCE™ solution known to have been frozen, cloudy, or exhibit visible precipitants, (i.e. particles) should not be used, but discarded immediately.

Disposal Information:

Container Disposal: Container must be triple rinsed and disposed of in accordance with federal, state and/or local regulations.

Used Solution Disposal: Used solution should be disposed of in accordance with federal, state and/or local regulations.

Caution(s): Material compatibility, adhesive compatibility, tuberculocidal, sporicidal, simulated use, and clinical testing demonstrate that COMPLIANCE™ is compatible with flexible fiberoptic endoscopes used for endoscopic retrograde cholangipancreatography including bronchial scopes, gastrointestinal endoscopes, and colonoscopes. Do not use with devices with labeling contraindicating use with hydrogen peroxide or peracetic acid solutions. Contact the reusable device manufacturer for information on compatibility.

1. Sterilant Usage: Routine biological monitoring is not possible with COMPLIANCE™ solution, and therefore COMPLIANCE™ solution should not be used to sterilize reusable medical devices that are compatible with automated sterilization processes that can be biologically monitored. COMPLIANCE™ solution should not be used for sterilization of critical devices intended for single use (e.g. catheters).
2. High-Level Disinfectant Usage: COMPLIANCE™ should not be used to high-level disinfect a semi-critical device when heat sterilization is practical.
3. Endoscope Usage: COMPLIANCE™ is not the method of choice for sterilization of rigid endoscopes which the device manufacturer indicates are compatible with steam sterilization.
4. Appropriate hand, eye and face protection (goggles, face shield, or safety glasses) as well as liquid proof gowns must be worn when cleaning and sterilizing/disinfecting soiled devices and equipment.
5. Contaminated reusable devices must be thoroughly cleaned prior to disinfection or sterilization, since residual contamination will decrease effectiveness of the germicide.
6. The user must adhere to the "Directions for Use" since any modification will affect the safety and effectiveness of the germicide.
7. The reusable device manufacturer should provide the user with a validated reprocessing procedure for that device using COMPLIANCE™ solution.

Warning(s): COMPLIANCE™ is hazardous to humans and domestic animals.

Danger: Keep out of reach of children. Contains hydrogen peroxide and peracetic acid.

1. Direct contact is corrosive to exposed tissue, causing eye damage and skin irritation/damage. Do not get into eyes, on skin or on clothing.
2. Avoid contamination of food.
3. Use in well-ventilated area in closed containers.

Wash thoroughly with soap and water after handling. Harmful if inhaled. Avoid breathing (vapor or spray mist). Remove contaminated clothing and wash clothing before reuse.

In case of contact, immediately flush eyes or skin with copious amounts of water for at least 15 minutes. For eyes, seek medical attention.

Harmful if swallowed. Drink large quantities of water or milk and call a physician immediately.

Note to Physician: Probable mucosal damage from oral exposure may contraindicate the use of gastric lavage.

Emergency, safety, or technical information about COMPLIANCE™ can be obtained from Metrex Research Corporation Customer Care Department at 1-800-841-1428, or by contacting your local Metrex Research Corporation sales representative.

References: Available upon request.

Presentation: 4 x 1 gallon (3.785 L) bottles per case.

Compendium Code No.: 13400030 2520-3/2522-2

COMPLIANCE™ NEUTRALIZING POWDER

Metrex **Disinfectant Neutralizer**

Indications: Neutralizing Powder for use with sterilizing and disinfecting solution containing Peracetic Acid.

Directions for Use: Pour appropriate amount of neutralizer into tray of used solution.

Use entire contents of the bottle to neutralize 2 gallons.

Use approximately ½ the contents of the bottle to neutralize 1 gallon.

Dissolve powder into solution. Color will change from yellow to brown within 5 minutes. When brown color is achieved, the solution is neutralized.

Storage and Disposal: Dispose of spent neutralized solution in accordance with Federal, State and local regulations.

Avoid storage in heat and moist areas.

Warning(s): Avoid exposure to skin, eyes and clothing.

Presentation: 4 x 220 g bottles.

Compendium Code No.: 13400040 2540-1

COMPONENT® E-C

VetLife **Implant**

Calf Implants

NADA No.: 110-315

Active Ingredient(s): Each dose of pellets contains a total of 100 mg progesterone USP plus 10 mg estradiol benzoate.

Indications: COMPONENT® E-C Implants are indicated for increased rate of weight gain in suckling beef calves up to approximately 400 lbs of body weight.

Dosage and Administration:

General Instructions: Study the instructions which should be followed carefully at all times, avoiding short cuts. Skin infection can be avoided by properly preparing implant site and implanter. During fly season use fly repellent on implant site.

One designated team member should always do the implanting. Cleanliness of hands and instruments is important at all times.

Multi-Dose Implanter Instructions:

Loading the Implanter: Load the Implanter following the instructions supplied with each implanter.

Note: The manufacturer recommends the use of the Component® One Gun™ Implanter**.

Restrain the Animal: Speed of implantation as well as safety of handlers is best achieved by restraining animal in a squeeze chute using head restraint.

Prepare the Implant Site: Scrub the back side of the ear (implant site) with a piece of clean absorbent cotton which has been soaked with topical germicidal solution. Follow manufacturer's directions on germicide for correct strength and preparation of solution. Avoid getting into animal's eyes.

Where to Implant: The full contents (all 4 pellets) should be implanted beneath the skin on the back side of the middle one-third of the ear as illustrated in the drawing.

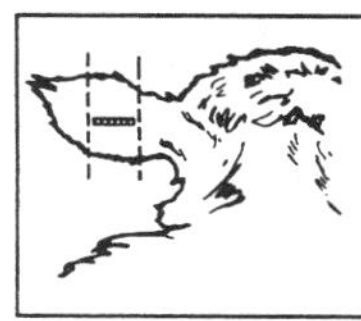

The implant must not be closer to the head than the edge of the auricular cartilage ring farthest from the head. The location for insertion of the needle is a point toward the tip of the ear and at least a needle length away from the intended deposition site. Avoid injuring the large arteries, veins and cartilage of the ear.

Insert the Needle: With one hand firmly grasp the ear. With the other hand insert needle point through the skin and ease forward on a lateral plane until the entire length of the needle is under the skin.

Implant the Pellets: After inserting the needle fully in the correct implant position, squeeze the trigger fully. As the needle is withdrawn from the ear, the controlled-pressure plunger action properly deposits the implant in the needle track. This procedure should prevent breakage or crushing of pellets if otherwise forced into contact with tough fibrous tissue underlying the skin. The length and total contact area of the 4 pellet single dose are designed to permit absorption of the hormones after implantation to stimulate good weight gain. Broken or crushed pellets may interfere with rates of gain and may lead to undesirable side effects such as noted in the Caution.

Clean the Needle: Clean the implanter needle with alcohol or a properly diluted germicidal solution prior to implanting the next animal.

Contraindication(s): Do not use in bull calves intended for reproduction, or in calves less than 45 days old.

Precaution(s): Store at controlled room temperature 15° to 30°C (59° to 86°F).

Do not refrigerate - avoid excessive heat and humidity.

Caution(s): Bulling, rectal prolapse, ventral edema and elevated tail-heads have occasionally been reported in animals implanted with progesterone and estradiol benzoate.

This product is manufactured by a non-sterilizing process.

Warning(s): Implant pellets in ear only. Any other site is in violation of Federal Law. Do not attempt to salvage implant site for animal feed or human use.

Keep this and all other drugs out of reach of children.

Restricted Drug-Use only as directed (California).

For use in animals only.

Presentation: 20 dose Cartridge Belt*.

Manufactured for VetLife by Ivy Laboratories.

*U.S. Patent No. 4,531,938

**U.S. Patent Nos. 4,762,515 and 5,522,797 - Ivy Animal Health, Inc.

COMPONENT and Component One Gun are registered trademarks of Ivy Animal Health, Inc.

Compendium Code No.: 10330000

COMPONENT® E-C WITH TYLAN®

VetLife **Implant**

Calf Implants

NADA No.: 110-315

Active Ingredient(s): Each dose of 5 pellets consists of 4 pellets containing a total of 100 mg progesterone USP and 10 mg estradiol benzoate plus 1 pellet containing 29 mg tylosin tartrate as a local antibacterial.

Manufactured by a non-sterilizing process.

Indications: COMPONENT® E-C Implants are indicated for increased rate of weight gain in suckling beef calves up to approximately 400 lbs of body weight.

Dosage and Administration:

General Instructions: Study the instructions which should be followed carefully at all times, avoiding short cuts. Skin infection can be avoided by properly preparing implant site and implanter. During fly season use fly repellent on implant site. One designated team member should always do the implanting. Cleanliness of hands and instruments is important at all times.

Implanter Instructions:

Loading the Implanter: Load the Implanter following the instructions supplied with each implanter.

For use of the Component® One Gun™**.

Restrain the Animal: Speed of implantation as well as safety of handlers is best achieved by restraining animal in a squeeze chute using head restraint.

Prepare the Implant Site: Scrub the back side of the ear (implant site) with a piece of clean absorbent cotton which has been soaked with topical germicidal solution. Follow manufacturer's directions on germicide for correct strength and preparation of solution. Avoid getting into animal's eyes.

Where to Implant: The full contents should be implanted beneath the skin on the back side of the middle one-third of the ear as illustrated in the drawing.

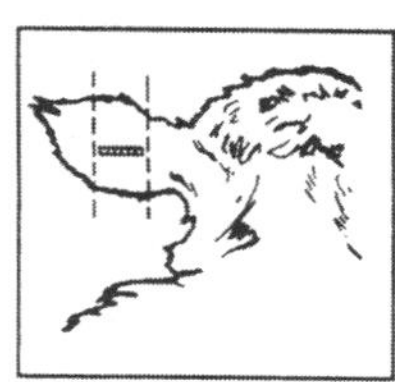

The implant must not be closer to the head than the edge of the auricular cartilage ring farthest from the head. The location for insertion of the needle is a point toward the tip of the ear and at least a needle length away from the intended deposition site. Avoid injuring the large arteries, veins and cartilage of the ear.

Insert the Needle: With one hand firmly grasp the ear. With the other hand insert needle point through the skin and ease forward on a lateral plane until the entire length of the needle is under the skin.

Implant the Pellets: After inserting the needle fully in the correct implant position, squeeze the trigger fully. As the needle is withdrawn from the ear, the controlled-pressure plunger action properly deposits the implant in the needle track. This procedure should prevent breakage or crushing of pellets if otherwise forced into contact with tough fibrous-tissue underlying the skin. The length and total contact area of a single dose are designed to permit absorption of the hormones after implantation to stimulate good weight gain. Broken or crushed pellets may interfere with rates of gain and may lead to undesirable side effects such as noted in the Caution.

Clean the Needle: Clean the implanter needle with alcohol or a properly diluted germicidal solution prior to implanting the next animal.

Contraindication(s): Do not use in bull calves intended for reproduction, or in calves less than 45 days old.

Precaution(s): Store at controlled room temperature 15° to 30°C (59° to 86°F).

Do not refrigerate - avoid excessive heat and humidity.

Caution(s): Bulling, rectal prolapse, ventral edema and elevated tail-heads have occasionally been reported in animals implanted with progesterone and estradiol benzoate.

Warning(s): Implant pellets in ear only. Any other site is in violation of Federal Law. Do not attempt to salvage implant site for animal feed or human use.

Keep this and all other drugs out of reach of children.

Restricted Drug-Use only as directed (California).

For use in animals only.

Presentation: 20 dose Cartridge Belt*.

Manufactured for VetLife by Ivy Laboratories.

*U.S. Patent No. 4,531,938

**U.S. Patent Nos. 4,762,515 and 5,522,797 - Ivy Animal Health, Inc.

COMPONENT E-C WITH TYLAN is covered by U.S. Patent No. 5,874,098

COMPONENT is a registered trademark of Ivy Animal Health, Inc.

TYLAN is a registered trademark of Eli Lilly and Company.

Compendium Code No.: 10330010 01 23 01 00

COMPONENT® E-H

VetLife **Implant**

Heifer Implants

NADA No.: 135-906

Active Ingredient(s): Each dose of 8 pellets contains a total of 200 mg testosterone propionate USP plus 20 mg estradiol benzoate.

Indications: COMPONENT® E-H Implants are recommended for use in heifers weighing 400 lbs or more for improved growth promotion and feed efficiency.

Dosage and Administration:

General Instructions: Study the instructions which should be followed carefully at all times, avoiding short cuts. Skin infection can be avoided by properly preparing implant site and implanter. During fly season use fly repellent on implant site.

One designated team member should always do the implanting. Cleanliness of hands and instruments is important at all times.

Implanting Instructions:

Loading the Implanter: Load the implanter following the instructions supplied with each implanter.

Note: The manufacturer recommends the use of the Component® One Gun™ Implanter**.

Restrain the Animal: Speed of implantation as well as safety of handlers is best achieved by restraining animal in a squeeze chute using head restraint. When implanting horned cattle, better control is obtained with additional use of nose tongs.

Prepare the Implant Site: Scrub the back side of the ear (implant site) with a piece of clean absorbent cotton which has been soaked with a germicidal solution. Follow manufacturer's directions on germicide for correct strength and preparation of solution. Avoid getting into animal's eyes.

Where to Implant: The full contents of the cartridge (all 8 pellets) should be implanted beneath the skin on the back side of the middle one-third of the ear as illustrated in the drawing.

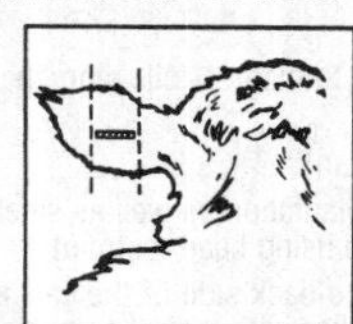

The implant must not be closer to the head than the edge of the auricular cartilage ring farthest from the head. The location for insertion of the needle is a point toward the tip of the ear and at least a needle length away from the intended deposition site.

Avoid injuring the large arteries, veins and cartilage of the ear.

Insert the Needle: With one hand firmly grasp the ear. With other hand insert needle point through the skin and ease forward on a lateral plane until the entire length of the needle is under the skin.

Implant the Pellets: After inserting the needle fully in the correct implant position squeeze the trigger fully. As the needle is withdrawn from the ear, the controlled-pressure plunger action properly deposits the implant in the needle track. This procedure should prevent breakage or crushing of pellets if otherwise forced into contact with tough fibrous tissue underlying the skin. The length and total contact area of the 8 pellet single dose are designed to permit absorption of the hormones after implantation to stimulate good weight gain. Broken or crushed pellets may interfere with rates of gain and may lead to undesirable side effects such as noted in the Caution.

Clean the Needle: Clean the implanter needle with alcohol or a properly diluted germicidal solution prior to implanting the next animal.

Precaution(s): Store at controlled room temperature 15° to 30°C (59° to 86°F).

Do not refrigerate - avoid excessive heat and humidity.

Caution(s): For use in heifers only. Bulling, vaginal and rectal prolapse, udder development, ventral edema and elevated tail-heads have occasionally been reported in animals implanted with testosterone propionate and estradiol benzoate.

This product is manufactured by a non-sterilizing process.

Warning(s): Not for use in dairy or beef replacement heifers.

Implant pellets in ear only. Any other site is in violation of Federal Law. Do not attempt to salvage implant site for animal feed or human use.

Keep this and all other drugs out of reach of children.

Restricted Drug-Use only as directed (California).

For use in animals only.

Presentation: 20 dose Cartridge Belt*.

Manufactured for VetLife by Ivy Laboratories.

*U.S. Patent No. 4,531,938

**U.S. Patent Nos. 4,762,515 and 5,522,797 - Ivy Animal Health, Inc.

COMPONENT and Component One Gun are registered trademarks of Ivy Animal Health, Inc.

Compendium Code No.: 10330020

COMPONENT® E-H WITH TYLAN®

VetLife **Implant**

Heifer Implants

NADA No.: 135-906

Active Ingredient(s): Each dose of 9 pellets consists of 8 pellets containing a total of 200 mg testosterone propionate USP and 20 mg estradiol benzoate plus 1 pellet containing 29 mg tylosin tartrate as a local antibacterial.

Manufactured by a non-sterilizing process.

Indications: COMPONENT® E-H Implants are recommended for use in heifers weighing 400 lbs or more for increased rate of weight gain and improved feed efficiency.

Dosage and Administration:

General Instructions: Study the instructions which should be followed carefully at all times, avoiding short cuts. Skin infection can be avoided by properly preparing implant site and implanter. During fly season use fly repellent on implant site. One designated team member should always do the implanting. Cleanliness of hands and instruments is important at all times.

Implanting Instructions:

Loading the Implanter: Load the Implanter following the instructions supplied with each implanter.

For use with the Component® One Gun™**.

Restrain the Animal: Speed of implantation as well as safety of handlers is best achieved by restraining animal in a squeeze chute using head restraint. When implanting horned cattle, better control is obtained with additional use of nose tongs.

Prepare the Implant Site: Scrub the back side of the ear (implant site) with a piece of clean absorbent cotton which has been soaked with a germicidal solution. Follow manufacturer's directions on germicide for correct strength and preparation of solution. Avoid getting into animal's eyes.

Where to Implant: The full contents of the cartridge should be implanted beneath the skin on the back side of the middle one-third of the ear as illustrated in the drawing.

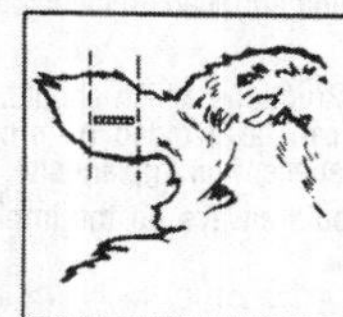

The implant must not be closer to the head than the edge of the auricular cartilage ring farthest from the head. The location for insertion of the needle is a point toward the tip of the ear and at least a needle length away from the intended deposition site.

Avoid injuring the large arteries, veins and cartilage of the ear.

Insert the Needle: With one hand firmly grasp the ear. With other hand insert needle point through the skin and ease forward on a lateral plane until the entire length of the needle is under the skin.

Implant the Pellets: After inserting the needle fully in the correct implant position squeeze the trigger fully. As the needle is withdrawn from the ear, the controlled-pressure plunger action properly deposits the implant in the needle track. This procedure should prevent breakage or crushing of pellets if otherwise forced into contact with tough fibrous-tissue underlying the skin. The length and total contact area of a single dose are designed to permit absorption of the hormones after implantation to stimulate good weight gain. Broken or crushed pellets may interfere with rates of gain and may lead to undesirable side effects such as noted in the Caution.

Clean the Needle: Clean the implanter needle with alcohol or a properly diluted germicidal solution prior to implanting the next animal.

Precaution(s): Store at controlled room temperature 15° to 30°C (59° to 86°F).

Do not refrigerate - avoid excessive heat and humidity.

Caution(s): For use in heifers only. Bulling, vaginal and rectal prolapse, udder development, ventral edema and elevated tail-heads have occasionally been reported in animals implanted with testosterone propionate and estradiol benzoate.

Warning(s): Not for use in dairy or beef replacement heifers. Implant pellets in ear only. Any other site is in violation of Federal Law. Do not attempt to salvage implant site for animal feed or human use.

Keep this and all other drugs out of reach of children.

Restricted Drug-Use only as directed (California).

For use in animals only.

Presentation: 20 dose Cartridge Belt*.

Manufactured for VetLife by Ivy Laboratories.

*U.S. Patent No. 4,531,938

**U.S. Patent Nos. 4,762,515 and 5,522,797 - Ivy Animal Health, Inc.

COMPONENT E-H WITH TYLAN is covered by U.S. Patent No. 5,874,098

COMPONENT is a registered trademark of Ivy Animal Health, Inc.

TYLAN is a registered trademark of Eli Lilly and Company.

Compendium Code No.: 10330030 01 22 01 00

COMPONENT® E-S

VetLife **Implant**

Steer Implants

NADA No.: 110-315

Active Ingredient(s): Each dose of 8 pellets contains a total of 200 mg progesterone USP plus 20 mg estradiol benzoate.

Indications: COMPONENT® E-S Implants are recommended for use in steers weighing 400 lbs or more for improved weight gain and feed efficiency.

Dosage and Administration:

General Instructions: Study the instructions which should be followed carefully at all times, avoiding short cuts. Skin infection can be avoided by properly preparing implant site and implanter. During fly season use fly repellent on implant site. One designated team member should always do the implanting. Cleanliness of hands and instruments is important at all times.

Implanting Instructions:

Loading the Implanter: Load the Implanter following the instructions supplied with each implanter.

Note: The manufacturer recommends the use of the Component® One Gun™ Implanter**.

Restrain the Animal: Speed of implantation as well as safety of handlers is best achieved by restraining animal in a squeeze chute using head restraint. When implanting horned cattle, better control is obtained with additional use of nose tongs.

Prepare the Implant Site: Scrub the back side of the ear (implant site) with a piece of clean absorbent cotton which has been soaked with topical germicidal solution. Follow manufacturer's directions on germicide for correct strength and preparation of solution. Avoid getting into animal's eyes.

Where to Implant: The full contents of the cartridge (all 8 pellets) should be implanted beneath the skin on the back side of the middle one-third of the ear as illustrated in the drawing.

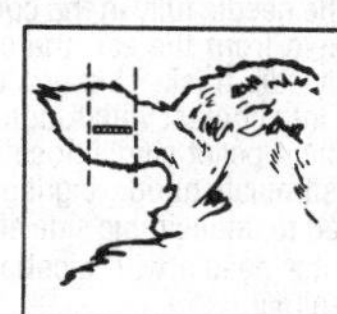

The implant must not be closer to the head than the edge of the auricular cartilage ring farthest from the head. The location for insertion of the needle is a point toward the tip of the ear and at least a needle length away from the intended deposition site.

Avoid injuring the large arteries, veins and cartilage of the ear.

Insert the Needle: With one hand firmly grasp the ear. With the other hand insert needle point through the skin and ease forward on a lateral plane until the entire length of the needle is under the skin.

Implant the Pellets: After inserting the needle fully in the correct implant position squeeze the trigger fully. As the needle is withdrawn from the ear, the controlled-pressure plunger action properly deposits the implant in the needle track. This procedure should prevent breakage or crushing of pellets if otherwise forced into contact with tough fibrous tissue underlying the skin. The length and total contact area of the 8 pellet single dose are designed to permit absorption of the hormones after implantation to stimulate good weight gain. Broken or crushed pellets may interfere with rates of gain and may lead to undesirable side effects such as noted in the Caution.

Clean the Needle: Clean the implanter needle with alcohol or a properly diluted germicidal solution prior to implanting the next animal.

Precaution(s): Store at controlled room temperature 15° to 30°C (59° to 86°F).

Do not refrigerate - avoid excessive heat and humidity.

Caution(s): Bulling, rectal prolapse, ventral edema and elevated tail-heads have occasionally been reported in animals implanted with progesterone and estradiol benzoate.

This product is manufactured by a non-sterilizing process.

Warning(s): Implant pellets in ear only. Any other site is in violation of Federal Law. Do not attempt to salvage implant site for animal feed or human use.

Keep this and all other drugs out of reach of children.

Restricted Drug-Use only as directed (California).

For use in animals only.

Presentation: 20 dose Cartridge Belt*.

Manufactured for VetLife by Ivy Laboratories.

*U.S. Patent No. 4,531,938

**U.S. Patent Nos. 4,762,515 and 5,522,797 - Ivy Animal Health, Inc.

COMPONENT and Component One Gun are registered trademarks of Ivy Animal Health, Inc.

Compendium Code No.: 10330040

COMPONENT® E-S WITH TYLAN®

VetLife **Implant**

Steer Implants

NADA No.: 110-315

Active Ingredient(s): Each dose of 9 pellets consists of 8 pellets containing a total of 200 mg progesterone USP and 20 mg estradiol benzoate plus 1 pellet containing 29 mg tylosin tartrate as a local antibacterial.

Manufactured by a non-sterilizing process.

Indications: COMPONENT® E-S Implants are recommended for use in steers weighing 400 lbs or more for increased rate of weight gain and improved feed efficiency.

Dosage and Administration:

General Instructions: Study the instructions which should be followed carefully at all times, avoiding short cuts. Skin infection can be avoided by properly preparing implant site and implanter. During fly season use fly repellent on implant site. One designated team member should always do the implanting. Cleanliness of hands and instruments is important at all times.

Implanting Instructions:

Loading the Implanter: Load the Implanter following the instructions supplied with each implanter.

For use with the Component® One Gun™**.

Restrain the Animal: Speed of implantation as well as safety of handlers is best achieved by restraining animal in a squeeze chute using head restraint. When implanting horned cattle, better control is obtained with additional use of nose tongs.

Prepare the Implant Site: Scrub the back side of the ear (implant site) with a piece of clean absorbent cotton which has been soaked with topical germicidal solution. Follow manufacturer's directions on germicide for correct strength and preparation of solution. Avoid getting into animal's eyes.

Where to Implant: The full contents of the cartridge should be implanted beneath the skin on the back side of the middle one-third of the ear as illustrated in the drawing.

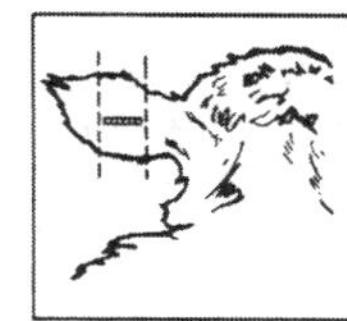

The implant must not be closer to the head than the edge of the auricular cartilage ring farthest from the head. The location for insertion of the needle is a point toward the tip of the ear and at least a needle length away from the intended deposition site.

Avoid injuring the large arteries, veins and cartilage of the ear.

Insert the Needle: With one hand firmly grasp the ear. With the other hand insert needle point through the skin and ease forward on a lateral plane until the entire length of the needle is under the skin.

Implant the Pellets: After inserting the needle fully in the correct implant position squeeze the trigger fully. As the needle is withdrawn from the ear, the controlled-pressure plunger action properly deposits the implant in the needle track. This procedure should prevent breakage or crushing of pellets if otherwise forced into contact with tough fibrous-tissue underlying the skin. The length and total contact area of a single dose are designed to permit absorption of the hormones after implantation to stimulate good weight gain. Broken or crushed pellets may interfere with rates of gain and may lead to undesirable side effects such as noted in the Caution.

Clean the Needle: Clean the implanter needle with alcohol or a properly diluted germicidal solution prior to implanting the next animal.

Precaution(s): Store at controlled room temperature 15° to 30°C (59° to 86°F).

Do not refrigerate - avoid excessive heat and humidity.

Caution(s): Bulling, rectal prolapse, ventral edema and elevated tail-heads have occasionally been reported in animals implanted with progesterone and estradiol benzoate.

Warning(s): Implant pellets in ear only. Any other site is in violation of Federal Law. Do not attempt to salvage implant site for animal feed or human use.

Keep this and all other drugs out of reach of children.

Restricted Drug-Use only as directed (California).

For use in animals only.

Presentation: 20 dose Cartridge Belt*.

Manufactured for VetLife by Ivy Laboratories.

*U.S. Patent No. 4,531,938

**U.S. Patent Nos. 4,762,515 and 5,522,797 - Ivy Animal Health, Inc.

COMPONENT E-S WITH TYLAN is covered by U.S. Patent No. 5,874,098

COMPONENT is a registered trademark of Ivy Animal Health, Inc.

TYLAN is a registered trademark of Eli Lilly and Company.

Compendium Code No.: 10330050 01 21 01 00

COMPONENT® TE-G

VetLife **Implant**

For Pasture Cattle (slaughter, stocker, and feeder steers and heifers)

ANADA No.: 200-221

Active Ingredient(s): Each dose consists of 2 pellets containing a total of 40 mg of trenbolone acetate USP and 8 mg estradiol USP.

Manufactured by a non-sterilizing process.

Indications: This product contains trenbolone acetate and estradiol in a slow-release delivery system which increases rate of weight gain in pasture cattle (slaughter, stocker, and feeder steers and heifers).

Dosage and Administration:

General Instructions: Study the instructions which should be followed carefully at all times, avoiding short cuts. Skin infection can be avoided by properly preparing implant site and implanter. During fly season use fly repellent on implant site. One designated team member should always do the implanting. Cleanliness of hands and instruments is important at all times.

Implanting Instructions:

Loading the Implanter: Load the implanter following the instructions supplied with each implanter.

For use with the Component® One Gun®**.

Restrain the Animal: Speed of implantation as well as safety of handlers is best achieved by restraining animal in a squeeze chute using head restraint. When implanting horned cattle, better control is obtained with additional use of nose tongs.

Prepare the Implant Site: Scrub the back side of the ear (implant site) with a piece of clean absorbent cotton which has been soaked with topical germicidal solution. Follow manufacturer's directions on germicide for correct strength and preparation of solution. Avoid getting disinfectant into animal's eyes.

Where to Implant: The full contents of the cartridge should be implanted beneath the skin on the back side of the middle one-third of the ear as illustrated in the drawing.

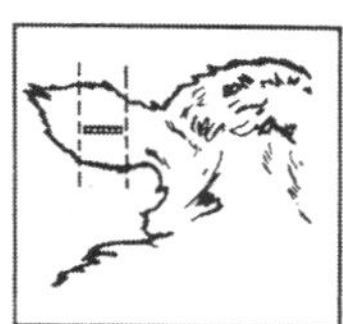

The implant must not be closer to the head than the edge of the auricular cartilage ring farthest from the head. The location for insertion of the needle is a point toward the tip of the ear and at least a needle length away from the intended deposition site. Avoid injuring the large arteries, veins and cartilage of the ear.

Insert the Needle: With one hand firmly grasp the ear. With the other hand insert needle point through the skin and ease forward on a lateral plane until the entire length of the needle is under the skin.

Implant the Pellets: After inserting the needle fully in the correct implant position, squeeze the trigger fully. As the needle is withdrawn from the ear, the controlled-pressure plunger action properly deposits the implant in the needle track. This procedure should prevent breakage or crushing of pellets if otherwise forced into contact with tough fibrous-tissue underlying the skin. The length and total contact area of a single dose are designed to permit absorption of the hormones after implantation to stimulate good weight gain. Broken or crushed pellets may interfere with rates of gain.

Clean the Needle: Clean the implanter needle with alcohol or a properly diluted germicidal solution prior to implanting the next animal.

Precaution(s): Storage Conditions: Store in a refrigerator (2°-8°C; 36°-46°F) and protect from sunlight. Use before the expiration date printed on foil pouch.

Warning(s): Not to be used in animals intended for subsequent breeding, or in dairy animals. For animal treatment only. Not for use in humans. Implant pellets in the ear only. Any other location is in violation of Federal Law. Do not attempt to salvage of implantation site for animal feed or human food.

Keep this and all other drugs out of reach of children.

Restricted Drug-Use only as directed (California).

For use in animals only.

Presentation: 20 dose Cartridge Belt*.

Manufactured for VetLife by Ivy Laboratories.

*U.S. Patent No. 4,531,938

**U.S. Patent Nos. 4,762,515 and 5,522,797 - Ivy Animal Health, Inc.

COMPONENT and Component One Gun are registered trademarks of Ivy Animal Health, Inc.

Compendium Code No.: 10330100

COMPONENT® TE-G WITH TYLAN®

VetLife **Implant**

For Pasture Cattle (slaughter, stocker, feeder steers and heifers)

ANADA No.: 200-221

Active Ingredient(s): Each dose of 3 pellets consists of 2 pellets containing a total of 40 mg of trenbolone acetate and 8 mg estradiol plus 1 pellet containing 29 mg of tylosin tartrate as a local antibacterial.

Manufactured by a non-sterilizing process.

Indications: This product contains trenbolone acetate and estradiol in a slow-release delivery system which increases rate of weight gain in pasture cattle (slaughter, stocker, feeder steers and heifers).

Directions for Use:

General Instructions: Study the instructions which should be followed carefully at all times, avoiding short cuts. Skin infection can be avoided by properly preparing implant site and implanter. During fly season use fly repellent on implant site. One designated team member should always do the implanting. Cleanliness of hands and instruments is important at all times.

Implanting Instructions:

Loading the Implanter: Load the implanter following the instructions supplied with each implanter.

For use with the Component® One Gun®**.

Restrain the Animal: Speed of implantation as well as safety of handlers is best achieved by restraining animal in a squeeze chute using head restraint. When implanting horned cattle, better control is obtained with additional use of nose tongs.

Prepare the Implant Site: Scrub the back side of the ear (implant site) with a piece of clean absorbent cotton which has been soaked with topical germicidal solution. Follow manufacturer's directions on germicide for correct strength and preparation of solution. Avoid getting disinfectant into animal's eyes.

Where to Implant: The full contents of the cartridge should be implanted beneath the skin on the back side of the middle one-third of the ear as illustrated in the drawing.

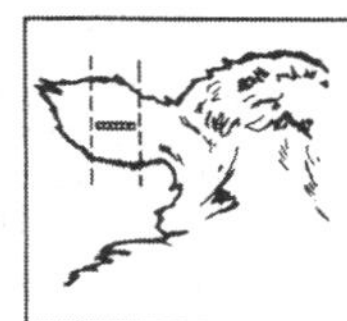

The implant must not be closer to the head than the edge of the auricular cartilage ring farthest from the head. The location for insertion of the needle is a point toward the tip of the ear at least a needle length away from the intended deposition site. Avoid injuring the large arteries, veins and cartilage of the ear.

Insert the Needle: With one hand firmly grasp the ear. With the other hand insert needle point through the skin and ease forward on a lateral plane until the entire length of the needle is under the skin.

Implant the Pellets: After inserting the needle fully in the correct implant position, squeeze the trigger fully. As the needle is withdrawn from the ear, the controlled-pressure plunger action properly deposits the implant in the needle track. This procedure should prevent breakage or crushing of pellets if otherwise forced into contact with tough fibrous-tissue underlying the skin. The length and total contact area of the single dose are designed to permit absorption of the hormones after implantation to stimulate good weight gain. Broken or crushed pellets may interfere with rates of gain.

Clean the Needle: Clean the implanter needle with alcohol or a properly diluted germicidal solution prior to implanting the next animal.

Precaution(s): Storage Conditions: Store in a refrigerator (2°-8°C; 36°-46°F) and protect from sunlight.

Use before the expiration date printed on foil pouch.

Warning(s): Not to be used in animal intended for subsequent breeding, or in dairy animals. For animal treatment only. Not for use in humans. Implant pellets in ear only. Any other location is in violation of Federal Law. Do not attempt to salvage implantation site for animal feed or human food.

Keep this and all other drugs out of reach of children.

Presentation: 20 dose Cartridge Belt*.

Manufactured for VetLife by Ivy Laboratories.

*U.S. Patent No. 4,531,938

**U.S. Patent Nos. 4,762,515 and 5,522,797 — Ivy Animal Health, Inc.

COMPONENT TE-G with TYLAN is covered by U.S. Patent No. 5,874,098

COMPONENT and Component One Gun are registered trademarks of Ivy Animal Health, Inc.

TYLAN is a registered trademark of Eli Lilly and Company.

Compendium Code No.: 10330150 01 28 01 00

COMPONENT® TE-S

VetLife **Implant**

For Feedlot Steers

ANADA No.: 200-221

Active Ingredient(s): Each dose of 6 pellets contains a total of 120 mg of trenbolone acetate and 24 mg estradiol USP.

Indications: COMPONENT® TE-S Implants are recommended for use in feedlot steers for increased rate of weight gain and improved feed efficiency in a slow-release delivery system.

Dosage and Administration:

General Instructions: Study the instructions which should be followed carefully at all times, avoiding short cuts. Skin infection can be avoided by properly preparing implant site and implanter. During fly season use fly repellent on implant site. One designated team member should always do the implanting. Cleanliness of hands and instruments is important at all times.

Implanting Instructions:

Loading the Implanter: Load the Implanter following the instructions supplied with each implanter.

Note: The manufacturer recommends the use of the Component® One Gun™ Implanter**.

Restrain the Animal: Speed of implantation as well as safety of handlers is best achieved by restraining animal in a squeeze chute using head restraint. When implanting horned cattle, better control is obtained with additional use of nose tongs.

Prepare the Implant Site: Scrub the backside of the ear (implant site) with a piece of clean absorbent cotton which has been soaked with topical germicidal solution. Follow manufacturer's directions on germicide for correct strength and preparation of solution. Avoid getting into animal's eyes.

Where to Implant: The full contents of the cartridge (all 6 pellets) should be implanted beneath the skin on the backside of the middle one-third of the ear as illustrated in the drawing.

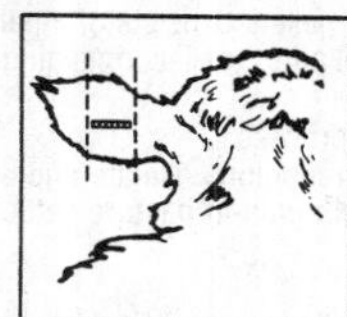

The implant must not be closer to the head than the edge of the auricular cartilage ring farthest from the head. The location for insertion of the needle is a point toward the tip of the ear and at least a needle length away from the intended deposition site.

Avoid injuring the large arteries, veins and cartilage of the ear.

Insert the Needle: With one hand firmly grasp the ear. With other hand insert needle point through the skin and ease forward on a lateral plane until the entire length of the needle is under the skin.

Implant the Pellets: After the needle is completely inserted in the correct implant position squeeze the trigger fully. As the needle is withdrawn from the ear, the controlled-pressure plunger action properly deposits the implant in the needle track. This procedure should prevent breakage or crushing of pellets if otherwise forced into contact with tough fibrous-tissue underlying the skin. The length and total contact area of the 6 pellet single dose are designed to permit absorption of the hormones after implantation to stimulate good weight gain. Broken or crushed pellets may interfere with rates of gain and may lead to undesirable side effects.

Clean the Needle: Clean the implanter needle with alcohol or a properly diluted germicidal solution prior to implanting the next animal.

Precaution(s): Store in a refrigerator (2°-8°C; 36°-46°F) and protect from sunlight. Use before the expiration date printed on the foil pouch.

Caution(s): Studies have demonstrated that the administration of COMPONENT® TE-S can result in decreased marbling scores when compared to non-implanted steers.

This product is manufactured by a non-sterilizing process.

Warning(s): Not to be used in animals intended for subsequent breeding, or in dairy animals. For animal treatment only. Not for use in humans. Implant pellets in the ear only. Any other location is in violation of federal law. Do not attempt salvage of implanted site for human or animal food.

Keep this and all other drugs out of reach of children.

For use in animals only.

Presentation: 20 dose Cartridge Belt*.

Manufactured for VetLife by Ivy Laboratories.

*U.S. Patent No. 4,531,938

**U.S. Patent Nos. 4,762,515 and 5,522,797 - Ivy Animal Health, Inc.

COMPONENT and Component One Gun are registered trademarks of Ivy Animal Health, Inc.

Compendium Code No.: 10330110

COMPONENT® TE-S WITH TYLAN®

VetLife **Implant**

For Feedlot Steers

ANADA No.: 200-221

Active Ingredient(s): Each dose of 7 pellets consists of 6 pellets containing a total of 120 mg of trenbolone acetate USP and 24 mg estradiol USP plus 1 pellet containing 29 mg tylosin tartrate as a local antibacterial.

Manufactured by a non-sterilizing process.

Indications: This product contains trenbolone acetate and estradiol, which increases rate of weight gain and improves feed efficiency in feedlot steers in a slow-release delivery system.

Dosage and Administration:

General Instructions: Study the instructions which should be followed carefully at all times, avoiding short cuts. Skin infection can be avoided by properly preparing implant site and implanter. During fly season use fly repellent on implant site. One designated team member should always do the implanting. Cleanliness of hands and instruments is important at all times.

Implanting Instructions:

Loading the Implanter: Load the Implanter following the instructions supplied with each implanter.

For use with the Component® One Gun™**.

Restrain the Animal: Speed of implantation as well as safety of handlers is best achieved by restraining animal in a squeeze chute using head restraint. When implanting horned cattle, better control is obtained with additional use of nose tongs.

Prepare the Implant Site: Scrub the back side of the ear (implant site) with a piece of clean absorbent cotton which has been soaked with topical germicidal solution. Follow manufacturer's directions on germicide for correct strength and preparation of solution. Avoid getting disinfectant into animal's eyes.

Where to Implant: The full contents of the cartridge should be implanted beneath the skin on the back side of the middle one-third of the ear as illustrated in the drawing.

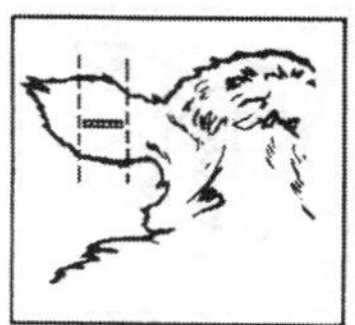

The implant must not be closer to the head than the edge of the auricular cartilage ring farthest from the head. The location for insertion of the needle is a point toward the tip of the ear and at least a needle length away from the intended deposition site. Avoid injuring the large arteries, veins and cartilage of the ear.

Insert the Needle: With one hand firmly grasp the ear. With the other hand insert needle point through the skin and ease forward on a lateral plane until the entire length of the needle is under the skin.

Implant the Pellets: After inserting the needle fully in the correct implant position, squeeze the trigger fully. As the needle is withdrawn from the ear, the controlled-pressure plunger action properly deposits the implant in the needle track. This procedure should prevent breakage or crushing of pellets if otherwise forced into contact with tough fibrous-tissue underlying the skin. The length and total contact area of a single dose are designed to permit absorption of the hormones after implantation to stimulate good weight gain. Broken or crushed pellets may interfere with rates of gain.

Clean the Needle: Clean the implanter needle with alcohol or a properly diluted germicidal solution prior to implanting the next animal.

Precaution(s): Storage Conditions: Store in a refrigerator (2°-8°C; 36°-46°F) and protect from sunlight. Use before the expiration date printed on foil pouch.

Caution(s): Studies have demonstrated that the administration of COMPONENT® TE-S can result in decreased marbling scores when compared to non-implanted steers.

Warning(s): Not to be used in animals intended for subsequent breeding, or in dairy animals. For animal treatment only. Not for use in humans. Implant pellets in ear only. Any other location is in violation of Federal Law. Do not attempt to salvage implantation site for animal feed or human use.

Keep this and all other drugs out of reach of children.

Restricted Drug-Use only as directed (California).

For use in animals only.

Presentation: 20 dose Cartridge Belt*.

Manufactured for VetLife by Ivy Laboratories.

*U.S. Patent No. 4,531,938

**U.S. Patent Nos. 4,762,515 and 5,522,797 - Ivy Animal Health, Inc.

COMPONENT TE-S WITH TYLAN is covered by U.S. Patent No. 5,874,098

COMPONENT is a registered trademark of Ivy Animal Health, Inc.

TYLAN is a registered trademark of Eli Lilly and Company.

Compendium Code No.: 10330120 01 24 01 00

COMPONENT® T-H

VetLife **Implant**

For Feedlot Heifers

ANADA No.: 200-224

Active Ingredient(s): Each dose of 10 pellets contains a total of 200 mg of trenbolone acetate.

Indications: This product is a slow release anabolic agent containing trenbolone acetate which increases rate of weight gain and improves feed efficiency in growing finishing feedlot heifers. This product is to be used in feedlot heifers only during approximately the last 63 days prior to slaughter.

Dosage and Administration:

General Instructions: Study the instructions which should be followed carefully at all times, avoiding short cuts. Skin infection can be avoided by properly preparing implant site and implanter. During fly season use fly repellent on implant site. One designated team member should always do the implanting. Cleanliness of hands and instruments is important at all times.

Implanting Instructions:

Loading the Implanter: Load the Implanter following the instructions supplied with each implanter.

Note: The manufacturer recommends the use of the Component® One Gun™ Implanter**.

Restrain the Animal: Speed of implantation as well as safety of handlers is best achieved by restraining animal in a squeeze chute using head restraint. When implanting horned cattle, better control is obtained with additional use of nose tongs.

Prepare the Implant Site: Scrub the backside of the ear (implant site) with a piece of clean absorbent cotton or gauze which has been soaked with alcohol or topical germicidal solution. Follow manufacturer's directions on germicide for correct strength and preparation of solution. Avoid getting into animal's eyes.

Where to Implant: The full contents of the cartridge (all 10 pellets) should be implanted beneath the skin on the backside of the middle one-third of the ear as illustrated in the drawing.

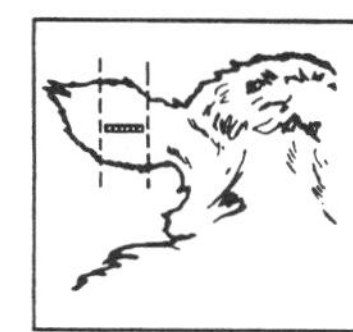

The implant must not be closer to the head than the edge of the auricular cartilage ring farthest from the head. The location for insertion of the needle is a point toward the tip of the ear and at least a needle length away from the intended deposition site. Avoid injuring the large arteries, veins and cartilage of the ear.

Insert the Needle: With one hand firmly grasp the ear. With other hand insert needle point through the skin and ease forward on a lateral plane until the entire length of the needle is under the skin.

Implant the Pellets: After the needle is completely inserted in the correct implant position squeeze the trigger fully. As the needle is withdrawn from the ear, the controlled-pressure plunger action properly deposits the implant in the needle track. This procedure should prevent breakage or crushing of pellets if otherwise forced into contact with tough fibrous-tissue underlying the skin.

Clean the Needle: Clean the implanter needle with alcohol or a properly diluted germicidal solution prior to implanting the next animal.

Precaution(s): Store in a refrigerator (2°-8°C; 36°-46°F) and protect from sunlight. Use before the expiration date printed on the foil pouch.

Caution(s): This product is manufactured by a non-sterilizing process.

Warning(s): Not to be used in animals intended for subsequent breeding, or in dairy animals. Implant one dose 10 pellets (entire contents of one plastic cartridge) in the ear subcutaneously. Any other site is in violation of Federal Law. Do not attempt salvage of implanted site for human or animal food.

Keep this and all other drugs out of reach of children.

For use in animals only.

Presentation: 20 dose Cartridge Belt*.

Manufactured for VetLife by Ivy Laboratories.

*U.S. Patent No. 4,531,938

**U.S. Patent Nos. 4,762,515 and 5,522,797 - Ivy Animal Health, Inc.

COMPONENT and Component One Gun are registered trademarks of Ivy Animal Health, Inc.

Compendium Code No.: 10330060

COMPONENT® T-H WITH TYLAN®

VetLife **Implant**

For Feedlot Heifers

ANADA No.: 200-224

Active Ingredient(s): Each dose of 11 pellets consists of 10 pellets containing a total of 200 mg of trenbolone acetate USP plus 1 pellet containing 29 mg tylosin tartrate as a local antibacterial.

Manufactured by a non-sterilizing process.

Indications: This product is a slow-release anabolic agent containing trenbolone acetate which increases rate of weight gain and improves feed efficiency in growing finishing feedlot heifers. This product is to be used in feedlot heifers only during approximately the last 63 days prior to slaughter.

Dosage and Administration:

General Instructions: Study the instructions which should be followed carefully at all times, avoiding short cuts. Skin infection can be avoided by properly preparing implant site and implanter. During fly season use fly repellent on implant site. One designated team member should always do the implanting. Cleanliness of hands and instruments is important at all times.

Implanting Instructions:

Loading the Implanter: Load the Implanter following the instructions supplied with each implanter.

For use with the Component® One Gun™**.

Restrain the Animal: Speed of implantation as well as safety of handlers is best achieved by restraining animal in a squeeze chute using head restraint. When implanting horned cattle, better control is obtained with additional use of nose tongs.

Prepare the Implant Site: Scrub the back side of the ear (implant site) with a piece of clean absorbent cotton which has been soaked with alcohol or topical germicidal solution. Follow manufacturer's directions on germicide for correct strength and preparation of solution. Avoid getting disinfectant into animal's eyes.

Where to Implant: The full contents should be implanted beneath the skin on the back side of the middle one-third of the ear as illustrated in the drawing.

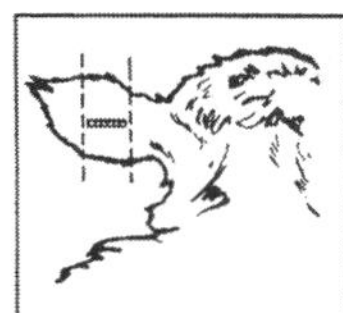

The implant must not be closer to the head than the edge of the auricular cartilage ring farthest from the head. The location for insertion of the needle is a point toward the tip of the ear and at least a needle length away from the intended deposition site. Avoid injuring the large arteries, veins and cartilage of the ear.

Insert the Needle: With one hand firmly grasp the ear. With other hand insert needle point through the skin and ease forward on a lateral plane until the entire length of the needle is under the skin.

Implant the Pellets: After inserting the needle fully in the correct implant position, squeeze the trigger fully. As the needle is withdrawn from the ear, the controlled-pressure plunger action properly deposits the implant in the needle track. This procedure should prevent breakage or crushing of pellets if otherwise forced into contact with tough fibrous-tissue underlying the skin.

Clean the Needle: Clean the implanter needle with alcohol or a properly diluted germicidal solution prior to implanting the next animal.

Precaution(s): Storage Conditions: Store in a refrigerator (2°-8°C; 36°-46°F) and protect from sunlight. Use before the expiration date printed on foil pouch.

Warning(s): Not to be used in animals intended for subsequent breeding, or in dairy animals. For animal treatment only. Not for use in humans. Implant pellets in ear only. Any other location is in violation of Federal Law. Do not attempt to salvage implantation site for animal feed or human use.

Keep this and all other drugs out of reach of children.

Restricted Drug-Use only as directed (California).

For use in animals only.

Presentation: 20 dose Cartridge Belt*.

Manufactured for VetLife by Ivy Laboratories.

*U.S. Patent No. 4,531,938

**U.S. Patent Nos. 4,762,515 and 5,522,797 - Ivy Animal Health, Inc.

COMPONENT T-H WITH TYLAN is covered by U.S. Patent No. 5,874,098

COMPONENT is a registered trademark of Ivy Animal Health, Inc.

TYLAN is a registered trademark of Eli Lilly and Company.

Compendium Code No.: 10330070 01 26 01 00

COMPONENT® T-S

VetLife **Implant**

For Feedlot Steers

ANADA No.: 200-224

Active Ingredient(s): Each dose of 7 pellets contains a total of 140 mg of trenbolone acetate.

Indications: This product is a slow-release anabolic agent containing trenbolone acetate, which improves feed efficiency in growing finishing feedlot steers. For continued effectiveness this product should be reimplanted once after 63 days.

Dosage and Administration:

General Instructions: Study the instructions which should be followed carefully at all times, avoiding short cuts. Skin infection can be avoided by properly preparing implant site and implanter. During fly season use fly repellent on implant site. One designated team member should always do the implanting. Cleanliness of hands and instruments is important at all times.

Implanting Instructions:

Loading the Implanter: Load the Implanter following the instructions supplied with each implanter.

Note: The manufacturer recommends the use of the Component® One Gun™ Implanter**.

Restrain the Animal: Speed of implantation as well as safety of handlers is best achieved by restraining animal in a squeeze chute using head restraint. When implanting horned cattle, better control is obtained with additional use of nose tongs.

Prepare the Implant Site: Scrub the backside of the ear (implant site) with a piece of clean absorbent cotton or gauze which has been soaked with alcohol or a topical germicidal solution. Follow manufacturer's directions on germicide for correct strength and preparation of solution. Avoid getting into animal's eyes.

Where to Implant: The full contents of the cartridge (all 7 pellets) should be implanted beneath the skin on the backside of the middle one-third of the ear as illustrated in the drawing.

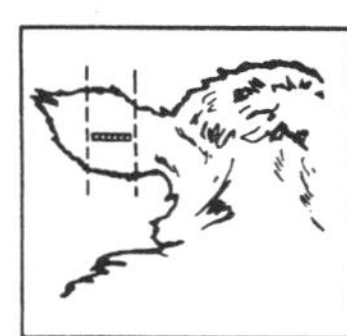

The implant must not be closer to the head than the edge of the auricular cartilage ring farthest from the head. The location for insertion of the needle is a point toward the tip of the ear and at least a needle length away from the intended deposition site. Avoid injuring the large arteries, veins and cartilage of the ear.

Insert the Needle: With one hand firmly grasp the ear. With other hand insert needle point through the skin and ease forward on a lateral plane until the entire length of the needle is under the skin.

Implant the Pellets: After the needle is completely inserted in the correct implant position squeeze the trigger fully. As the needle is withdrawn from the ear, the controlled-pressure plunger action properly deposits the implant in the needle track. This procedure should prevent breakage or crushing of pellets if otherwise forced into contact with tough fibrous-tissue underlying the skin.

Clean the Needle: Clean the implanter needle with alcohol or a properly diluted germicidal solution prior to implanting the next animal.

Precaution(s): Store in a refrigerator (2°-8°C; 36°-46°F) and protect from sunlight. Use before the expiration date printed on the foil pouch.

Caution(s): This product is manufactured by a non-sterilizing process.

Warning(s): Not to be used in animals intended for subsequent breeding, or in dairy animals. For animal treatment only. Not for use in humans. Implant pellets in the ear only. Any other location is in violation of federal law. Do not attempt to salvage implanted site for animal feed or human food.

Keep this and all other drugs out of reach of children.

For use in animals only.

Presentation: 20 dose Cartridge Belt*.

Manufactured for VetLife by Ivy Laboratories.

*U.S. Patent No. 4,531,938

**U.S. Patent Nos. 4,762,515 and 5,522,797 - Ivy Animal Health, Inc.

COMPONENT and Component One Gun are registered trademarks of Ivy Animal Health, Inc.

Compendium Code No.: 10330080

COMPONENT® T-S WITH TYLAN®

VetLife **Implant**

For Feedlot Steers

ANADA No.: 200-224

Active Ingredient(s): Each dose of 8 pellets consists of 7 pellets containing a total of 140 mg of trenbolone acetate USP plus 1 pellet containing 29 mg tylosin tartrate as a local antibacterial.

Manufactured by a non-sterilizing process.

Indications: This product is a slow-release anabolic agent containing trenbolone acetate which improves feed efficiency in growing finishing feedlot steers. For continued effectiveness this product should be reimplanted once after 63 days.

Dosage and Administration:

General Instructions: Study the instructions which should be followed carefully at all times, avoiding short cuts. Skin infection can be avoided by properly preparing implant site and implanter. During fly season use fly repellent on implant site. One designated team member should always do the implanting. Cleanliness of hands and instruments is important at all times.

Implanting Instructions:

Loading the Implanter: Load the Implanter following the instructions supplied with each implanter.

For use with the Component® One Gun™**.

Restrain the Animal: Speed of implantation as well as safety of handlers is best achieved by restraining animal in a squeeze chute using head restraint. When implanting horned cattle, better control is obtained with additional use of nose tongs.

Prepare the Implant Site: Scrub the back side of the ear (implant site) with a piece of clean absorbent cotton which has been soaked with alcohol or topical germicidal solution. Follow manufacturer's directions on germicide for correct strength and preparation of solution. Avoid getting disinfectant into animal's eyes.

Where to Implant: The full contents of the cartridge should be implanted beneath the skin on the back side of the middle one-third of the ear as illustrated in the drawing.

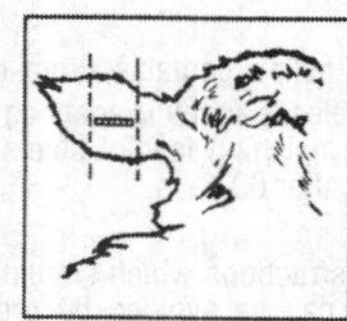

The implant must not be closer to the head than the edge of the auricular cartilage ring farthest from the head. The location for insertion of the needle is a point toward the tip of the ear and at least a needle length away from the intended deposition site. Avoid injuring the large arteries, veins and cartilage of the ear.

Insert the Needle: With one hand firmly grasp the ear. With other hand insert needle point through the skin and ease forward on a lateral plane until the entire length of the needle is under the skin.

Implant the Pellets: After inserting the needle fully in the correct implant position, squeeze the trigger fully. As the needle is withdrawn from the ear, the controlled-pressure plunger action properly deposits the implant in the needle track. This procedure should prevent breakage or crushing of pellets if otherwise forced into contact with tough fibrous-tissue underlying the skin.

Clean the Needle: Clean the implanter needle with alcohol or a properly diluted germicidal solution prior to implanting the next animal.

Precaution(s): Storage Conditions: Store in a refrigerator (2°-8°C; 36°-46°F) and protect from sunlight. Use before the expiration date printed on foil pouch.

Warning(s): Not to be used in animals intended for subsequent breeding, or in dairy animals. For animal treatment only. Not for use in humans. Implant pellets in ear only. Any other location is in violation of Federal Law. Do not attempt to salvage implantation site for animal feed or human food.

Keep this and all other drugs out of reach of children.

Restricted Drug-Use only as directed (California).

For use in animals only.

Presentation: 20 dose Cartridge Belt*.

Manufactured for VetLife by Ivy Laboratories.

*U.S. Patent No. 4,531,938

**U.S. Patent Nos. 4,762,515 and 5,522,797 - Ivy Animal Health, Inc.

COMPONENT T-S WITH TYLAN is covered by U.S. Patent No. 5,874,098

COMPONENT is a registered trademark of Ivy Animal Health, Inc.

TYLAN is a registered trademark of Eli Lilly and Company.

Compendium Code No.: 10330090 01 25 01 00

COMPUDOSE®

VetLife **Implant**

Controlled Release Implants

NADA No.: 118-123

Active Ingredient(s): Each COMPUDOSE® silicone rubber implant contains 25.7 mg estradiol and is coated with not less than 0.5 mg of oxytetracycline powder as a local antibacterial.

Indications: For increased rate of weight gain in suckling and pastured growing steers; for improved feed efficiency and increased rate of weight gain in confined steers and heifers.

COMPUDOSE® Controlled Release Implant will provide an effective daily dose of estradiol for at least 200 days. No additional effectiveness may be expected from reimplanting in less than 200 days.

Dosage and Administration: Insert one implant under the skin of the ear as directed in this leaflet.

When to Implant COMPUDOSE®:

Suckling steers: At castration or later.

Pastured growing steers: At weaning or later.

Finishing steers and heifers: At arrival in feedlot.

Equipment: A COMPUDOSE® Implanter must be used to implant cattle.

Directions for Implantation: Insert one implant under the skin of the ear.

1. Confine animal in a squeeze chute.
2. To reduce the possibility of infection and resulting implant loss, hygienic and antiseptic procedures should be followed during implantation. The ear should be clean and dry. The skin should be cleansed with a suitable antiseptic soap and dried prior to implanting. This is particularly important if the ears are contaminated with urine or feces.
3. To load the COMPUDOSE® Implanter remove the cartridge from the package, release the latch on the magazine, open and insert the cartridge.

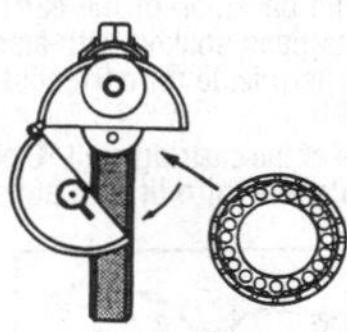

Close the magazine and latch. Advance the cartridge to the next implant by inserting the thumb into the magazine opening and turning the cartridge to the next stop.

Use a sharp needle. The needle should be cleaned and sterilized between each injection by wiping the exterior with a sponge, cloth, or gauze saturated with an appropriate disinfectant. The presence of excessive moisture inside the needle may result in dissolving the oxytetracycline (OTC) from the implant surface and contribute to accumulation of OTC inside the needle.

4. The implant should be deposited under the skin on the back side of the middle third of the ear. It should be placed between the skin and cartilage, avoiding major blood vessels. Grasping the tip of the ear with one hand and the implanter in the other, penetrate the skin in the outer third of the ear.

   Important: Do not penetrate cartilage.
5. Upon penetration. the needle should be fully inserted between the skin and cartilage, avoiding major blood vessels. Full insertion of the needle is important to maximize implant retention.
6. Pull the needle back as the implant is being deposited by squeezing the lever on the implanter grip. The figure below shows the implant in proper position in the middle third of the ear where the skin is tight.

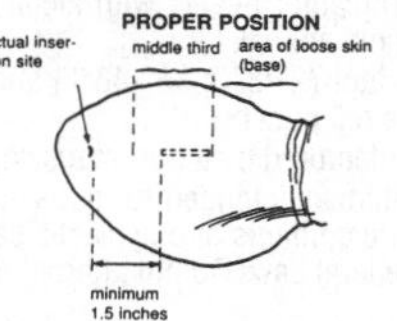

7. After repeated use, sufficient oxytetracycline (OTC) from the implant may accumulate inside the needle to impede implant passage. Periodic removal of the needle from the device and washing it in water will prevent such accumulation. Before reusing, the needle should be disinfected and allowed to dry after shaking vigorously to remove excess water or disinfectant.
8. If reimplantation is desired, it is not necessary to remove the existing COMPUDOSE® implant. Place the second implant at the same level and parallel to, but not in contact with the existing implant or place it in the unimplanted ear in accordance with paragraphs 1-7 of these directions.

To maximize implant retention:

A. Fully insert the needle.

B. Deposit the implant in the middle third of the ear where the skin is tight.

C. Do not deposit the implant where the skin is loose in the third of the ear closest to the head.

The needle has been scientifically designed to maximize retention. When it becomes dull, use a new needle. If the needle is resharpened, sharpen only the point.

Failure to follow antiseptic implanting procedures, particularly when the ears are contaminated with fecal material, may result in infection and excessive implant loss. Implanting cattle during wet weather or just prior to dipping in contaminated solutions may increase infection and implant loss.

Carefully check the ears for implant loss approximately 4 weeks after implantation. If loss occurs, reimplant using recommended procedures.

Caution(s): Increased sexual activity (bulling, riding and excitability) has been reported in animals implanted with COMPUDOSE®. Implanted animals should be observed for such signs particularly during the first few days after implanting and animals being excessively ridden (bullers) should be removed to prevent physical injury. Vaginal and rectal prolapse have been reported in heifers implanted with COMPUDOSE®.

Warning(s): Do not use in animals intended for breeding purposes.

For subcutaneous ear implantation in steers and heifers only.

Keep out of reach of children.

Side Effects: Udder development, swollen or enlarged vulva and high tailheads may be observed in implanted heifers.

Presentation: COMPUDOSE® Implants are supplied in cartridges of 20 implants each.

COMPUDOSE is a registered trademark of Ivy Animal Health, Inc.

Compendium Code No.: 10330131

CONOFITE® CREAM ℞

Schering-Plough **Topical Antifungal**

(Miconazole Nitrate) 2%

NADA No.: 095-183

Active Ingredient(s): Description: CONOFITE® (miconazole nitrate) Cream is a synthetic antifungal agent for use on dogs and cats. Each gram contains 23 mg of miconazole nitrate (equivalent to 20 mg miconazole base) in a base containing: cetyl alcohol, stearyl alcohol, butylated hydroxytoluene, white petrolatum, mineral oil, polyoxyl 40 stearate, butylparaben and purified water.

Indications: CONOFITE® (miconazole nitrate) Cream is indicated for the treatment of fungal infections in dogs and cats caused by *Microsporum canis, Microsporum gypseum* and *Trichophyton mentagrophytes.*

Dosage and Administration: An accurate diagnosis of the infecting organism is essential. Identification should be made either by direct microscopic examination of a mounting of infected tissue in a solution of potassium hydroxide, or by culture on an appropriate medium.

Apply a ¼ inch ribbon of CONOFITE® (miconazole nitrate) Cream once daily per square inch of lesion for 2 to 4 weeks. Rub into infected site and immediate surrounding vicinity. Application is best accomplished using a finger cot or cotton swab. The medication must be continued until the infecting organism is completely eradicated as indicated by appropriate clinical or laboratory examination. If improvement is not noticed within 2 weeks, the diagnosis should be re-evaluated. Difficult cases may require treatment for 6 weeks.

General measures in regard to hygiene should be observed to control sources of infection or re-infection. Clipping of hair around and over the sites of infection should be done at the start of treatment and again as necessary.

Caution(s): Federal law restricts this drug to use by or on the order of a licensed veterinarian.

Avoid contact with the eyes, since irritation may result. Wash hands thoroughly after administration to avoid the spread of fungal infection. Do not allow pet to contact finished wood surfaces until pet is thoroughly dried.

Presentation: 15 g tubes.

Compendium Code No.: 10470301 Rev. 8/97

CONOFITE® SPRAY AND LOTION ℞

Schering-Plough **Topical Antifungal**

(Miconazole Nitrate) 1%

NADA No.: 095-184

Active Ingredient(s): Description: CONOFITE® (miconazole nitrate) Spray or Lotion is a synthetic antifungal agent for use on dogs and cats. It contains 1.15% miconazole nitrate (equivalent to 1% miconazole base by weight), polyethylene glycol 400, and ethyl alcohol 55%.

Indications: CONOFITE® (miconazole nitrate) Spray or Lotion is indicated for the treatment of fungal infections in dogs and cats caused by *Microsporum canis, Microsporum gypseum* and *Trichophyton mentagrophytes.*

Dosage and Administration: An accurate diagnosis of the infecting organism is essential. Identification should be made either by direct microscopic examination of a mounting of infected tissue in a solution of potassium hydroxide, or by culture on an appropriate medium.

Spray: Spray affected areas from a distance of 2 to 4 inches to apply a light covering, once daily for 2 to 4 weeks. Do not allow pet to contact finished wood surfaces until pet is thoroughly dried.

Lotion: Apply a light covering of CONOFITE® (miconazole nitrate) Lotion to affected areas, once daily, for 2 to 4 weeks. Application is best accomplished by using a gauze pad or cotton swab.

Medication must be continued until the infecting organism is completely eradicated as indicated by appropriate clinical or laboratory examination. If no improvement is noticed within 2 weeks, diagnosis should be re-evaluated. Difficult cases may require treatment for 6 weeks.

General measures in regard to hygiene should be observed to control sources of infection or reinfection. Clipping of hair around and over the sites of infection should be done at the start of treatment and again as necessary.

Caution(s): Federal law restricts this drug to use by or on the order of a licensed veterinarian.

In the event of sensitization or irritation due to CONOFITE® Spray or Lotion, treatment should be discontinued. Avoid contact with eyes, since irritation may result. Wash hands thoroughly after administration to avoid spread of fungal infection.

Presentation: Spray: 60 mL containers (NDC 0061-5022-01).
Lotion: 30 mL containers (NDC 0061-5031-01).

Compendium Code No.: 10470311 3/98

CONQUEST™-4K

Aspen **Vaccine**

Bovine Rhinotracheitis-Virus Diarrhea-Parainfluenza$_3$-Respiratory Syncytial Virus Vaccine, Killed Virus

U.S. Vet. Lic. No.: 272

Active Ingredient(s): CONQUEST™-4K is an inactivated virus vaccine containing the Cooper strain of IBR virus and New York plus Singer strains of BVD virus, in addition to PI$_3$ and BRSV.

This product contains gentamicin and amphotericin B as preservatives and is adjuvanted with aluminum hydroxide and *Haemophilus somnus* cultures.

Indications: For use in the vaccination of healthy cattle against disease caused by the organisms represented.

Dosage and Administration: Shake well. Administer 5 mL IM or SC to healthy cattle. For initial vaccination, a second dose is required 2-4 weeks later.

CONQUEST™-4K may be safely used in pregnant cows at any stage of gestation or very young calves nursing pregnant cows. Two doses are required for calves 6 months or older. Calves vaccinated before 6 months of age should be revaccinated at 6 months of age followed by a second dose 2-4 weeks later. Annual revaccination with a single 5 mL dose is recommended.

Precaution(s): Store at 35°F-45°F (2°C-7°C). Do not freeze.

Caution(s): Use entire contents when first opened. In case of anaphylactoid reactions, epinephrine should be administered immediately.

Antidote(s): Epinephrine.

Warning(s): Do not vaccinate within 21 days before slaughter. For veterinary use only.

Presentation: 50 mL (10 dose) and 250 mL (50 dose) vials.

Compendium Code No.: 14750190

CONQUEST™-4K+H.S.

Aspen **Bacterin-Vaccine**

Bovine Rhinotracheitis-Virus Diarrhea-Parainfluenza$_3$-Respiratory Syncytial Virus Vaccine, Killed Virus-Haemophilus somnus Bacterin

U.S. Vet. Lic. No.: 272

Active Ingredient(s): CONQUEST™-4K+H.S. is an inactivated, multivalent immunogen containing the Cooper strain of IBR, New York plus Singer strains of BVD, PI$_3$ and BRSV viruses in combination with *Haemophilus somnus* bacterin.

This product contains gentamicin and amphotericin B as preservatives.

Indications: For use in the vaccination of healthy cattle against diseases caused by the organisms represented.

Dosage and Administration: Shake well. Administer 5 mL IM or SC to healthy cattle. For initial vaccination, a second dose is required 2-4 weeks later.

CONQUEST™-4K+H.S. may be safely used in pregnant cows at any stage of gestation or very young calves nursing pregnant cows. Calves vaccinated before 6 months of age should be revaccinated at 6 months of age followed by a second dose 2-4 weeks later. Annual revaccination with a single 5 mL dose is recommended.

Precaution(s): Store at 35°F-45°F (2°C-7°C). Do not freeze.

Caution(s): Use entire contents when first opened. In case of anaphylactoid reactions, epinephrine should be administered immediately.

Antidote(s): Epinephrine.

Warning(s): Do not vaccinate within 21 days before slaughter. For veterinary use only.

Presentation: 10 dose (50 mL) and 50 dose (250 mL) vials.

Compendium Code No.: 14750200

CONQUEST™-4KW

Aspen **Vaccine**

Bovine Rhinotracheitis-Virus Diarrhea-Parainfluenza$_3$-Respiratory Syncytial Virus Vaccine, Killed Virus

U.S. Vet. Lic. No.: 124

Active Ingredient(s): Bovine rhinotracheitis, virus diarrhea, parainfluenza$_3$ and respiratory syncytial virus vaccine, killed virus.

Neomycin and thimerosal are used as preservatives.

Indications: CONQUEST™-4KW vaccine is recommended for the immunization of healthy, susceptible dairy and beef cattle of all ages including pregnant cattle and veal calves against the diseases caused by bovine rhinotracheitis (IBR) virus, bovine virus diarrhea (BVD) virus, parainfluenza$_3$ (PI$_3$) virus and bovine respiratory syncytial virus (BRSV).

C

Dosage and Administration: Using aseptic technique, inject 5 mL intramuscularly. Repeat in 14-28 days. Calves vaccinated before the age of 6 months should be revaccinated at 6 months of age or weaning. Ideally calves should receive the first dose 2-4 weeks before weaning with a booster dose at weaning. A 5 mL booster dose is recommended annually or prior to time of stress or exposure.

Precaution(s): Store out of direct sunlight. Store at 35-45°F. Do not freeze. Shake well before using.

Caution(s): CONQUEST™-4KW has been shown to be safe and efficacious when used according to label directions. Use entire contents when first opened. Anaphylactic reactions may occur.

Antidote(s): Epinephrine.

Warning(s): Do not vaccinate within 21 days before slaughter.

Toxicology: The efficacy of CONQUEST™-4KW has been demonstrated for each fraction. Pregnant cattle may be vaccinated at any stage of gestation, and lactating dairy cattle may be vaccinated with no post-vaccination milk discard required.

Presentation: 10 dose (50 mL) and 50 dose (250 mL) vials.

Compendium Code No.: 14750210

CONQUEST™-4KW+H.S.

Aspen **Bacterin-Vaccine**

Bovine Rhinotracheitis-Virus Diarrhea-Parainfluenza$_3$-Respiratory Syncytial Virus Vaccine, Killed Virus-Haemophilus somnus Bacterin

U.S. Vet. Lic. No.: 124

Active Ingredient(s): Bovine rhinotracheitis, virus diarrhea, parainfluenza$_3$ and respiratory syncytial virus vaccine, killed virus, plus *Haemophilus somnus* bacterin.

Indications: CONQUEST™-4KW+H.S. is recommended for the immunization of healthy, susceptible dairy and beef cattle of all ages including pregnant cattle and veal calves against the diseases of IBR, BVD, PI$_3$, BRSV and *Haemophilus somnus.*

Dosage and Administration: Shake well before using.

Using aseptic technique, inject 5 mL intramuscularly. Repeat in 14-28 days. Calves vaccinated before the age of 6 months should be revaccinated at 6 months of age or weaning. Ideally calves should receive the first dose 2-4 weeks before weaning with a booster dose at weaning. A 5 mL booster dose is recommended annually or prior to a time of stress or exposure.

Precaution(s): Store out of direct sunlight. Store at 35° to 45°F (2° to 7°C). Do not freeze.

Caution(s): CONQUEST™-4KW+H.S. has been shown to be safe and efficacious when used according to label directions. Use the entire contents when first opened. Anaphylactic reactions may occur.

Antidote(s): Epinephrine.

Warning(s): Do not vaccinate within 21 days before slaughter.

Toxicology: The efficacy of CONQUEST™-4KW+H.S. has been demonstrated for each fraction. Pregnant cattle may be vaccinated at any stage of gestation, and lactating dairy cattle may be vaccinated without post-vaccination milk discard required.

Presentation: 10 dose (50 mL) and 50 dose (250 mL) vials.

Compendium Code No.: 14750220

CONQUEST™ 5K (OIL BASE)

Aspen **Vaccine**

Bovine Rhinotracheitis-Virus Diarrhea-Parainfluenza 3-Respiratory Syncytial Virus Vaccine, Killed Virus

U.S. Vet. Lic. No.: 303

Composition: This vaccine contains an IBR virus, a cytopathic Type 1 BVD virus, a noncytopathic Type 2 BVD virus, a PI$_3$ virus, and a BRS virus propagated on an established bovine cell line. The vaccine is chemically inactivated and adjuvanted with oil. Contains amphotericin B, penicillin, streptomycin, and thimerosal as preservatives.

Indications: For use in healthy cattle as an aid in the prevention of disease caused by infectious bovine rhinotracheitis, bovine virus diarrhea, parainfluenza type 3, and bovine respiratory syncytial viruses.

Dosage and Administration: Shake well before using. Administer 5 mL intramuscularly. Revaccinate in 4-5 weeks. This vaccine may be administered to pregnant animals at any stage of gestation. Vaccinate dairy cows during the dry off period. Revaccinate annually.

Precaution(s): Store in the dark at 35°-45°F (2°-7°C). Do not freeze. Use entire contents when first opened.

Caution(s): Transient swelling may occur at the site of injection. Anaphylactic reactions may occur following the use of this biological. Symptomatic treatment: Epinephrine.

Warning(s): Do not vaccinate within 60 days prior to slaughter.

Presentation: 10 dose (50 mL) and 50 dose (250 mL) vials.

Compendium Code No.: 14750160

CONQUEST™ 5K+HS (OIL BASE)

Aspen **Bacterin-Vaccine**

Bovine Rhinotracheitis-Virus Diarrhea-Parainfluenza 3-Respiratory Syncytial Virus Vaccine, Killed Virus-Haemophilus Somnus Bacterin

U.S. Vet. Lic. No.: 303

Composition: This product contains an IBR virus, a cytopathic Type 1 BVD virus, a noncytopathic Type 2 BVD virus, a PI$_3$ virus, and a BRS virus propagated on an established bovine cell line and cultures of *Haemophilus somnus.* The product is chemically inactivated and adjuvanted with oil. Contains amphotericin B, penicillin, streptomycin, and thimerosal as preservatives.

Indications: For use in healthy cattle as an aid in the prevention of disease caused by infectious bovine rhinotracheitis, bovine virus diarrhea, parainfluenza Type 3, and bovine respiratory syncytial viruses and *Haemophilus somnus.*

Dosage and Administration: Shake well before using. Administer 5 mL intramuscularly at 3

months of age or older. Revaccinate in 4-5 weeks. This vaccine may be administered to pregnant animals at any stage of gestation. Vaccinate dairy cows during the dry off period. Revaccinate annually.
Precaution(s): Store in the dark at 35°-45°F (2°-7°C). Do not freeze. Use entire contents when first opened.
Caution(s): Transient swelling may occur at the site of injection. Anaphylactic reactions may occur following the use of this biological. Symptomatic treatment: Epinephrine.
Warning(s): Do not vaccinate within 60 days prior to slaughter.
Presentation: 10 dose (50 mL) and 50 dose (250 mL) vials.
Produced by: Advance Biologics, Inc.
Compendium Code No.: 14750170

CONQUEST™ 5K+VL5 (OIL BASE)

C

Aspen **Bacterin-Vaccine**

Bovine Rhinotracheitis-Virus Diarrhea-Parainfluenza 3-Respiratory Syncytial Virus Vaccine, Killed Virus-Campylobacter Fetus-Leptospira Canicola-Grippotyphosa-Hardjo-Icterohaemorrhagiae-Pomona Bacterin
U.S. Vet. Lic. No.: 303
Composition: This product contains an IBR virus, a cytopathic Type 1 BVD virus, a noncytopathic Type 2 BVD virus, a PI_3 virus, and a BRS virus propagated on an established bovine cell line and cultures of *Campylobacter fetus, Leptospira canicola, grippotyphosa, hardjo, icterohaemorrhagiae*, and *pomona*. The product is chemically inactivated and adjuvanted with oil. Contains amphotericin B, penicillin, streptomycin, and thimerosal as preservatives.
Indications: For use in healthy cattle as an aid in the prevention of disease caused by infectious bovine rhinotracheitis, bovine virus diarrhea, parainfluenza type 3, and bovine respiratory syncytial viruses and *Campylobacter fetus, Leptospira canicola, grippotyphosa, hardjo, icterohaemorrhagiae*, and *pomona*.
Dosage and Administration: Shake well before using. Administer 5 mL intramuscularly 2-4 weeks prior to breeding. Revaccinate with Conquest™ 5K (oil base) (Bovine Rhinotracheitis-Virus Diarrhea-Parainfluenza 3-Respiratory Syncytial Virus Vaccine) in 4-5 weeks. Revaccinate annually.
Precaution(s): Store in the dark at 35°-45°F (2°-7°C). Do not freeze. Use entire contents when first opened.
Caution(s): Transient swelling may occur at the site of injection. Milk reduction and transient depression may be observed in lactating dairy cows for 3-6 days following vaccination. Anaphylactic reactions may occur following the use of this biological. Symptomatic treatment: Epinephrine.
Warning(s): Do not vaccinate within 60 days prior to slaughter.
Presentation: 10 dose (50 mL) and 50 dose (250 mL) vials.
Compendium Code No.: 14750180

CONQUEST™-8K

Aspen **Bacterin-Vaccine**

Bovine Rhinotracheitis-Virus Diarrhea-Parainfluenza$_3$ Vaccine, Killed Virus-Leptospira canicola-grippotyphosa-hardjo-icterohaemorrhagiae-pomona Bacterin
U.S. Vet. Lic. No.: 272
Active Ingredient(s): CONQUEST™-8K is a multivalent immunogen containing inactivated, adjuvanted strains of IBR, BVD and PI_3 viruses in combination with the Leptospira serovars represented.

This product contains gentamicin and amphotericin B as preservatives and is adjuvanted with aluminum hydroxide and *Haemophilus somnus* cultures.
Indications: For use in the vaccination of healthy cattle against disease caused by the organisms represented.
Dosage and Administration: Shake well. Administer 5 mL IM or SC to healthy cattle. For initial vaccination, a second dose is required 2-4 weeks later.

CONQUEST™-8K may be safely used in pregnant cows at any stage of gestation or very young calves nursing pregnant cows. Calves vaccinated before 6 months of age should be revaccinated at 6 months of age followed by a second dose 2-4 weeks later. Annual revaccination with a single 5 mL dose is recommended.
Precaution(s): Store at 35°F-45°F (2°C-7°C). Do not freeze.
Caution(s): Use entire contents when first opened. In case of anaphylactoid reactions, epinephrine should be administered immediately.
Antidote(s): Epinephrine.
Warning(s): Do not vaccinate within 21 days before slaughter. For veterinary use only.
Presentation: 10 dose (50 mL) and 50 dose (250 mL) vials.
Compendium Code No.: 14750230

CONQUEST™-9K

Aspen **Bacterin-Vaccine**

Bovine Rhinotracheitis-Virus Diarrhea-Parainfluenza$_3$-Respiratory Syncytial Virus Vaccine, Killed Virus-Leptospira canicola-grippotyphosa-hardjo-icterohaemorrhagiae-pomona Bacterin
U.S. Vet. Lic. No.: 272
Active Ingredient(s): Bovine rhinotracheitis (IBR), virus diarrhea (BVD), parainfluenza-3 (PI_3) and respiratory syncytial virus vaccine, killed virus and *Leptospira canicola, L grippotyphosa, L hardjo, L icterohaemorrhagiae, L pomona* bacterin.

This product contains gentamicin and amphotericin B as preservatives and is adjuvanted with aluminum hydroxide and *Haemophilus somnus* cultures.
Indications: CONQUEST™-9K is an inactivated, multivalent immunogen recommended for use in the vaccination of healthy cattle against disease caused by the IBR, BVD, PI_3 and BRSV viruses and the Leptospira serovars represented.
Dosage and Administration: Shake well. Administer 5 mL IM or SC to healthy cattle. For initial vaccination, a second dose is required 2-4 weeks later.

CONQUEST™-9K may be safely used in pregnant cows at any stage of gestation or very young calves nursing pregnant cows. Calves vaccinated before 6 months of age should be revaccinated at 6 months of age or older followed by a second dose 2-4 weeks later. Annual revaccination with a single 5 mL dose is recommended.
Precaution(s): Store at 35°F-45°F (2°C-7°C). Do not freeze.
Caution(s): Use entire contents when first opened. In case of anaphylactoid reactions, epinephrine should be administered immediately.
Antidote(s): Epinephrine.
Warning(s): Do not vaccinate within 21 days before slaughter. For veterinary use only.
Presentation: 10 dose (50 mL) and 50 dose (250 mL) vials.
Compendium Code No.: 14750240

CONQUEST™-9K+H.S.

Aspen **Bacterin-Vaccine**

Bovine Rhinotracheitis-Virus Diarrhea-Parainfluenza$_3$-Respiratory Syncytial Virus Vaccine, Killed Virus-Haemophilus somnus-Leptospira canicola-grippotyphosa-hardjo-icterohaemorrhagiae-pomona Bacterin
U.S. Vet. Lic. No.: 272
Active Ingredient(s): Bovine rhinotracheitis (IBR), virus diarrhea (BVD), parainfluenza-3 (PI_3) and respiratory syncytial virus vaccine, killed virus and *Leptospira canicola, L grippotyphosa, L hardjo, L icterohaemorrhagiae, L pomona* and *Haemophilus somnus* bacterin.

This product contains gentamicin and amphotericin B as preservatives.
Indications: CONQUEST™-9K+H.S. is an inactivated, multivalent immunogen recommended for use in the vaccination of healthy cattle against disease caused by IBR, BVD, PI_3 and BRSV viruses, *H. somnus* and the Leptospira serovars represented.
Dosage and Administration: Shake well. Administer 5 mL IM or SC to healthy cattle. For initial vaccination, a second dose is required 2-4 weeks later.

CONQUEST™-9K+H.S. may be safely used in pregnant cows at any stage of gestation or very young calves nursing pregnant cows. Calves vaccinated before 6 months of age should be revaccinated at 6 months of age followed by a second dose 2-4 weeks later. Annual revaccination with a single 5 mL dose is recommended.
Precaution(s): Store at 35°F-45°F (2°C-7°C). Do not freeze.
Caution(s): Use entire contents when first opened. In case of anaphylactoid reactions, epinephrine should be administered immediately.
Warning(s): Do not vaccinate within 21 days before slaughter.

For veterinary use only.
Presentation: 10 dose (50 mL) and 50 dose (250 mL) vials.
Compendium Code No.: 14750250

CONQUEST™ 10K

Aspen **Bacterin-Vaccine**

Bovine Rhinotracheitis-Virus Diarrhea-Parainfluenza 3-Respiratory Syncytial Virus Vaccine, Killed Virus-Leptospira Canicola-Grippotyphosa-Hardjo-Icterohaemorrhagiae-Pomona Bacterin
U.S. Vet. Lic. No.: 303
Composition: This product contains an IBR virus, a cytopathic Type 1 BVD virus, a noncytopathic Type 2 BVD virus, a PI_3 virus, and a BRS virus propagated on an established bovine cell line and cultures of *Leptospira canicola, grippotyphosa, hardjo, icterohaemorrhagiae*, and *pomona*. The product is chemically inactivated and adjuvanted with oil. Contains amphotericin B, penicillin, streptomycin, and thimerosal as preservatives.
Indications: For use in healthy cattle as an aid in the prevention of disease caused by infectious bovine rhinotracheitis, bovine virus diarrhea, parainfluenza Type 3, and bovine respiratory syncytial viruses and *Leptospira canicola, grippotyphosa, hardjo, icterohaemorrhagiae*, and *pomona*.
Dosage and Administration: Shake well before using. Administer 5 mL intramuscularly. Revaccinate with Conquest™ 5K (oil base) (Bovine Rhinotracheitis-Virus Diarrhea-Parainfluenza 3-Respiratory Syncytial Virus Vaccine) in 4-5 weeks. Vaccinate dairy cows during the dry off period. Revaccinate annually.
Precaution(s): Store in the dark at 35°-45°F (2°-7°C). Do not freeze. Use entire contents when first opened.
Caution(s): Transient swelling may occur at the site of injection. Anaphylactic reactions may occur following the use of this biological. Symptomatic treatment: Epinephrine.
Warning(s): Do not vaccinate within 60 days prior to slaughter.
Presentation: 10 dose (50 mL) and 50 dose (250 mL) vials.
Produced by: Advance Biologics, Inc.
Compendium Code No.: 14750150

CONSEPT® BARRIER SANITIZING TEAT DIP

Westfalia•Surge **Teat Dip**

Active Ingredient(s):

Ambicin N	34 µg/mL
1-Propanol	10%

Contains 10% glycerin plus other emollients.
Indications: CONSEPT® Barrier effectively controls a broad spectrum of organisms that cause mastitis.
Dosage and Administration: Shake well before using. Use at full strength. Do not dilute.

Pre-milking hygiene: Udders and teats must be cleaned and dried before milking. The teats must be treated with a sanitizing solution and wiped dry just prior to milking.

Post dipping: Immediately after milking, thoroughly cover at least the lower one-third (⅓) of each teat with CONSEPT® Barrier Sanitizing Teat Dip. At the end of lactation, apply the product once a day for one (1) week after the last milking. In addition, begin application of the product about one (1) week prior to calving.

Note: A fresh solution of the product should always be used at each milking. The teat dip cup should be emptied, cleaned and rinsed with potable water after each milking session or when the cup becomes contaminated during milking. Do not pour the remaining solution from the dip cup back into the original container.
Precaution(s): Keep away from heat and flame. Avoid storing above 100°F (38°C). Keep from freezing.
Caution(s):

1. Always read label directions completely before using the product.
2. Always exercise caution when handling any chemicals.
3. Avoid contact with the eyes, skin, and clothing.
4. Never dispense any chemical product from its original container into another container for storage or resale.
5. Never mix two or more products together. Mixing of product could result in the release of toxic gases and/or render the product ineffective for the recommended use application.
6. Always use the product in a ventilated area.
7. Avoid the contamination of food.
8. Avoid inhaling vapors or fumes.
9. Always use the product according to recommendations for a particular application.
10. Never exceed the recommended use without consulting trained personnel.
11. Keep out of the reach of children.
12. Harmful if swallowed.
13. Can cause eye damage.

First Aid:

Eyes: In case of contact with the eyes, flush immediately with plenty of water for at least 15 minutes. Get medical attention.

Internal: Do not take internally. If swallowed, promptly rinse the mouth, then give a large quantity of milk or water. Avoid alcohol. Contact a physician immediately. Never give anything by mouth to an unconscious person.

Inhalation of vapors: If inhaled and breathing difficulty occurs, remove to fresh air. If breathing difficulty continues, get medical attention.

Skin: Flush with large amounts of water. If irritation develops, call a physician.

Trial Data: The product has been tested and has been proven effective in reducing the spread of organisms which may cause mastitis. Research data is available upon request.

Presentation: Contact the company for container sizes available.

Compendium Code No.: 10020032

CONSEPT® PRE+POST TEAT DIP

Westfalia•Surge **Teat Dip**

Active Ingredient(s):

Ambicin N, 1-propanol 16.1%
Other ingredients 83.9%

Indications: CONSEPT® Pre+Post Teat Dip has been thoroughly tested using protocols consistent with the National Mastitis Council (NMC) testing protocols and has been proven effective in reducing new intramammary infections caused by major mastitis-causing organisms. CONSEPT® has been proven safe and effective and presents no threat of residue contamination of the milk when used as a pre-dip. Testing has also proven that the most effective method for the use of CONSEPT® is as both a pre-dip and a post-dip.

Dosage and Administration: For the best results, use CONSEPT® Pre+Post Dip to dip teats before milking and again after milking.

Pre dipping: Before milking, dip or spray each teat with CONSEPT®. After 15 to 30 seconds, dry each teat thoroughly with a single service paper towel. If the udder and teats are heavily soiled, wash with a sanitizing solution and dry before the application of CONSEPT®.

Post dipping: Immediately after milking, dip or spray each teat with CONSEPT®. Allow the teats to air dry.

Note: For the best results, CONSEPT® should be applied both before and after milking and the recommended dip cup should be used. A fresh solution of CONSEPT® should always be used at each milking. The teat dip cup should be emptied, cleaned and rinsed with potable water after each milking session or when the cup becomes contaminated during milking. Do not pour the remaining solution from the dip cup back into the original container.

Precaution(s): Avoid storage above 100°F (38°C). Keep from freezing.

Caution(s): Danger. Keep out of the reach of children. Keep away from heat and flame. Shake well before using. Harmful if swallowed. Can cause eye damage.

First Aid:

Eyes: In case of contact with the eyes, flush immediately with plenty of water for at least 15 minutes. Get medical attention.

Internal: Do not take internally. If swallowed, promptly drink a large quantity of milk or water. Avoid alcohol. Contact a physician immediately.

Inhalation of Vapors: If inhaled, and breathing difficulty occurs, remove to fresh air. If breathing difficulty continues, get medical attention.

Skin: Flush with large amounts of water. If irritation develops, call a physician.

Handling Recommendations:

1. Always read the label directions completely before using the product.
2. Always exercise caution when handling any chemicals.
3. Avoid contact with the eyes, skin, and clothing.
4. Never dispense any chemical product from its original container into another container for storage or resale.
5. Never mix two or more products together. Mixing of products could result in the release of toxic gases and/or render the product ineffective for the recommended use application.
6. Always use the product in a ventilated area.
7. Avoid contamination of food.
8. Avoid inhaling vapors or fumes.
9. Always use the product according to the recommendations for a particular application.
10. Never exceed the recommended usage without consulting trained personnel.

Presentation: Contact the company for container sizes available.

Compendium Code No.: 10020042

CONTINUEX™

Farnam **Parasiticide-Oral**

(pyrantel tartrate) Equine Anthelmintic-Daily Dewormer

ANADA No.: 200-282

Active Ingredient(s):

Pyrantel tartrate . . . . . 2.11% (9.6 g/lb)

Guaranteed Analysis:

Crude Protein, not less than 11.5%
Crude Fat, not less than 1.5%
Crude Fiber, not less than 22.0%

Ingredients: Dehydrated alfalfa meal, wheat middlings, cane molasses and preserved with propionic acid.

Indications: For the prevention of *Strongylus vulgaris larval* infections in horses.

For control of the following parasites in horses:

Large Strongyles (adults): *S. vulgaris, S. edentaius, Triodontophorus* spp.

Small Strongyles (adults and fourth stage larvae): *Cyathostomum* spp., *Cylicocyclus* spp., *Cylicodontophorus* spp., *Poteriostomum* spp.

Pinworms (adults and fourth stage larvae): *Oxyuris equi.*

Ascarids (adults and fourth stage larvae): *Parascaris equorum.*

Directions: Mixing and Feeding Directions: CONTINUEX™ (pyrantel tartrate) is to be administered on a continuous basis either as a top-dress or mixed in the horse's daily grain ration at the rate of 1.2 mg pyrantel tartrate per pound of body weight daily. To achieve this dose administer 0.5 oz. of CONTINUEX™ per 250 lb. of body weight. (A CONTINUEX™ measuring cup is enclosed.) CONTINUEX™ should be administered for the entire period that the animal is at risk to internal parasites. Unprotected animals that have grazed may have already established *S. vulgaris* larval infection. Before administering CONTINUEX™, these animals should be treated with a therapeutic dose of a larvicidal product.

Foals may be administered CONTINUEX™ as soon as consistent intake of grain mix is occurring. This is generally between two to three months of age.

CONTINUEX™ may be used in mares at any stage of pregnancy of lactation. Stallion fertility is not affected by the use of CONTINUEX™.

Top-Dress Directions:

Lb Body Weight	Ounces per Day of CONTINUEX™
250	0.5
500	1.0
750	1.5
1000	2.0
1250	2.5

(Measuring cup enclosed)

Medicated Grain Mix Directions:

Lb of Medicated Grain Mix per 100 Lb of Body Weight	Lb of CONTINUEX™	Lb of Non-Medicated Feed	Concentration Grams per Ton
2.0	12.5	1987.5	120
1.5	16.5	1983.5	160
1.0	25.0	1975	240
0.5	50.0	1950	480
0.2	125.0	1875	1200

Precaution(s): Store at controlled room temperature 15-30°C (59-86°F).

Caution(s): Consult your veterinarian before using in severely debilitated animals and for assistance in the diagnosis, treatment and control of parasitism. Do not mix in feeds containing bentonite.

Warning(s): Do not use in horses intended for food.

Presentation: 3.75 lb (1.7 kg), 7.5 lb (3.44 kg), 10 lb (4.54 kg), and 25 lb (11.34 kg) buckets.

CONTINUEX™ is the Farnam, Inc. trademark for pyrantel tartrate.

Compendium Code No.: 10000501 9DD8 / 9DD8 / 9FF8 / 9DD8

CONTROLLED IODINE SPRAY

Durvet **Topical Wound Dressing**

Active Ingredient(s): Contains: %w/w

Polyethoxylated nonylphenyl iodine complex, polyethoxylated fatty alcohol iodine complex (Provides 1.0% minimum titratable iodine) 12.37%
Inert Ingredients 87.63%

Indications: A topical antiseptic for use on horses, cattle, swine and sheep prior to surgical procedures such as castrating and docking. For application to the navel of newborn animals, and for use as an aid in the treatment of minor cuts, bruises and abrasions.

Directions: Remove regular cap from container and replace with spray cap and tube. Hold container approximately 4 to 6 inches from the area to be treated. Point valve at the area to be sprayed. Pull trigger of valve and spray the area once lightly. May be repeated daily when necessary until the abraded area is healed.

Note: When used near the teats or udders, thoroughly wash before the next milking to prevent contamination of milk.

Precaution(s): Store in a cool place.

Caution(s): If redness, irritation, or swelling persists or increases, discontinue use and consult a veterinarian. Not for use on burns or in body cavities or deep wounds.

Hazardous - Livestock remedy. Not for human use. Keep out of the reach of children.

For animal use only.

Presentation: 16 fl oz (473 mL) and 1 gallon containers.

Compendium Code No.: 10840361 0994/0496

COOL-CAST®

Hawthorne **Topical Anti-inflammatory**

Emollient Leg Bandage

Active Ingredient(s): Calamine, zinc oxide, gelatin, glycerin, menthol, water, cab-o-sil, methylparaben and propylparaben.

Indications: For use as an aid to reduce inflammation, swelling and tenderness. Useful for strains and injuries and as a light support following intra-articular injections, and to augment other conventional forms of anti-inflammatory treatment.

Dosage and Administration: Wrap on leg uniformly. Smooth out with palm of hand and let set. Do not use over open sores or where excessive swelling persists.

Precaution(s): Store in a cool place.

Caution(s): Keep away from children.

Presentation: 12 rolls 3" x 10 yds./7.62 cm x 9 m and 12 rolls 4" x 10 yds./10.16 cm x 9 m.

Compendium Code No.: 10670010

COOPER'S® BEST IVERMECTIN PASTE 1.87%

Aspen **Parasiticide-Oral**

Anthelmintic and Boticide

ANADA No.: 200-286

Active Ingredient(s):

Ivermectin 1.87%

Indications: Consult your veterinarian for assistance in the diagnosis, treatment, and control of parasitism. Ivermectin Paste 1.87% provides effective control of the following parasites in horses. Large Strongyles (adults) - *Strongylus vulgaris* (also early forms in blood vessels), *S. edentatus* (also tissue stages), *S. equinus, Triodontophorus* spp.; Small Strongyles including those resistant to some benzimidazole class compounds (adults and fourth-stage larvae) - *Cyathostomum* spp, *Cylicocyclus* spp, *Cylicostephanus* spp, *Cylicodontophorus* spp; Pinworms (adults and fourth-stage larvae) - *Oxyuris equi*; Ascarids (adults and third- and fourth-stage larvae) - *Parascaris equorum;* Hairworms (adults) *Trichostrongylus axei;* Large-mouth Stomach Worms (adults) - *Habronema muscae;* Bots (oral and gastric stages) - *Gasterophilus* spp; Lungworms (adults and fourth-stage larvae) - *Dictyocaulus arnfieldi;* Intestinal Threadworms (adults) - *Strongyloides westeri;* Summer Sores caused by *Habronema* and *Draschia* spp cutaneous third-stage larvae; Dermatitis caused by neck threadworm microfilariae, *Onchocerca* sp.

Dosage and Administration: This syringe contains sufficient paste to treat one 1250 lb horse at the recommended dose rate of 91 mcg ivermectin per lb (200 mcg/kg) body weight. Each weight marking on the syringe plunger delivers enough paste to treat 250 lb body weight. (1) While holding plunger, turn the knurled ring on the plunger to the right so the side nearest the barrel is at the prescribed weight marking. (2) Make sure that the horse's mouth contains no feed.

(3) Remove the cover from the tip of the syringe. (4) Insert the syringe tip into the horse's mouth at the space between the teeth (5) Depress the plunger as far as it will go, depositing paste on the back of the tongue (6) Immediately raise the horse's head for a few seconds after dosing.
Precaution(s): Store at controlled room temperature, 20° to 25°C (68° to 77°F).

Do not contaminate ground or surface water. Dispose of the syringe in an approved landfill or by incineration.
Caution(s): Ivermectin Paste 1.87% has been formulated specifically for use in horses only. This product should not be used in other animal species as severe adverse reactions, including fatalities in dogs, may result. Refrain from smoking and eating when handling. Wash hands after use. Avoid contact with eyes. Keep this and all drugs out of the reach of children. Ivermectin and excreted ivermectin residues may adversely affect aquatic organisms.

Note to User: Swelling and itching reactions after treatment with Ivermectin Paste 1.87% have occurred in horses carrying heavy infections of neck threadworm (*Onchocerca* sp.) microfilariae. These reactions were most likely the result of microfilariae dying in large numbers. Symptomatic treatment may be advisable. Consult your veterinarian should any such reactions occur. Healing of summer sores involving extensive tissue changes may require other appropriate therapy in conjunction with treatment with Ivermectin Paste 1.87%. Reinfection, and measures for its prevention, should also be considered. Consult your veterinarian if the condition does not improve.
Warning(s): Residue Warning: Do not use in horses intended for food purposes.
Side Effects: Safety - Ivermectin Paste 1.87% may be used in horses of all ages, including mares at any stage of pregnancy. Stallions may be treated without adversely affecting their fertility.
Discussion: Parasite Control Program: All horses should be included in a regular parasite control program with particular attention being paid to mares, foals and yearlings. Foals should be treated initially at 6 to 8 weeks of age, and routine treatment repeated as appropriate.

Consult your veterinarian for a control program to meet your specific needs. Ivermectin Paste 1.87% effectively controls gastrointestinal nematodes and bots of horses. Regular treatment will reduce the chances of verminous arteritis caused by *S vulgaris*.
Presentation: 6.08 g (0.21 oz) syringe.
Compendium Code No.: 14751040 Iss. 03-00

COPASURE®-12.5

Butler **Mineral Supplement**

Active Ingredient(s): Each capsule contains 12.5 g copper oxide present as copper wire particles (80% w/w of particles are 0.5 ± 0.1 mm in diameter, and 1 mm to 8 mm in length.
Indications: For use as a copper supplement for calves from 150 to 500 lbs. bodyweight.
Dosage and Administration: Supplementation Directions: Seek the advice of a veterinarian or cattle husbandry specialist to ascertain copper status and the type of supplementation required for cattle under consideration.

Calves from 150 to 500 lbs bodyweight: 1 capsule.

Administer the capsule orally with a suitable balling gun. Regurgitation may be possible with any capsule or bolus if not administered properly. To be effective, capsules must be swallowed. Administer only intact capsules. Do not crush or break.
Contraindication(s): Do not administer to sheep.
Precaution(s): Store in a cool (below 85°F), dry place. Protect from sunlight.
Caution(s): Do not administer to cattle of unknown copper status or those supplemented with other sources of copper.

The COPASURE®-12.5 g bolus should not be administered to newborn calves. Copper toxicity in neonates has been reported. Do not use in cattle suffering from jaundice or any other liver disorder.

Under most conditions, readministration will not be necessary for at least 12 months. Excessive levels of molybdenum, selenium, sulfur, or iron in feed or water may impair copper absorption.

For use in cattle only.
Warning(s): Keep out of reach of children.
Presentation: 25 x 12.5 g capsules per jar (NDC 11695-1251-2).
Manufactured by: Animax Ltd.
Compendium Code No.: 10821940 Issued 9/97

COPASURE®-25

Butler **Mineral Supplement**

Active Ingredient(s): Each capsule contains 25 g copper oxide particles (80% w/w of particles are 0.5 ± 0.1 mm in diameter, and 1 mm to 8 mm in length).
Indications: Copper supplement for cattle over 500 lbs. bodyweight.
Dosage and Administration: Supplementation Directions: Seek the advice of a veterinarian or cattle husbandry specialist to ascertain copper status and the type of supplementation required for cattle under consideration.

Calves over 500 lbs bodyweight: 1 capsule.

Adult cattle in situations of very low copper status: 2 capsules.

Administer the capsule orally with a suitable balling gun. Regurgitation may be possible with any capsule or bolus if not administered properly. To be effective, capsules must be swallowed. Administer only intact capsules. Do not crush or break.
Contraindication(s): Do not administer to sheep.
Precaution(s): Store in a cool (below 85°F), dry place. Protect from sunlight.
Caution(s): Do not administer to cattle of unknown copper status or those supplemented with other sources of copper.

Do not use in cattle suffering from jaundice or any other liver disorder.

Under most conditions, readministration will not be necessary for at least 12 months.

Excessive levels of molybdenum, sulfur, selenium, or iron in feed or water may impair copper absorption.

For use in cattle only.
Warning(s): Keep out of reach of children.
Presentation: 24 x 25 g capsules per box (NDC 11695-1250-1).
Manufactured by: Animax Ltd.
Compendium Code No.: 10821950 Issued 9/97

COPPER BLUE™

AgriLabs **Large Animal Dietary Supplement**

Acidified Copper Sulfate (Soluble Powder)
Guaranteed Analysis:
Copper Sulfate 86.0%
Citric Acid 14.0%

Ingredients: Copper sulfate pentahydrate and citric acid, anhydrous.
Indications: For nutritional supplementation in the feed or drinking water of poultry and livestock.
Dosage and Administration: For drinking water add 1 pound per 256 gallons of drinking water or 1 pound per 2 gallons of stock solution when used in proportioners set to deliver 1 oz per gallon of drinking water. In feed add 2 pounds per ton of complete feed. Pail contains 1 pound volume measure.
Caution(s): Use only with glass or plastic containers in preparing concentrated solutions.
Warning(s): Keep out of reach of children.
Presentation: 40 lb pail.
Compendium Code No.: 10580380

COPRO 25

Zinpro **Feed Additive**

Cobalt Glucoheptonate
Typical Analysis:
Cobalt 2.5%
Protein 2.6%
Fat 0.0%
Fiber 13.5%
Ash 35.0%
Salt 2.5%
Indications: Recommended as a nutritional feed additive for use as a source of cobalt in ruminant animals. When used as a commercial feed ingredient it must be declared as cobalt glucoheptonate.
Physical Description: A brown granular powder. COPRO 25 weighs approximately 30 lbs/cu ft.
Feeding Instructions:

Dairy Cattle: Feed 1 gram per head daily, or 0.5 lb per 200 head daily.
Beef Cattle: Feed 1 gram per head daily, or 0.5 lb per 200 head daily.
Sheep: Feed 0.2 grams per head daily, or 1 gram per 5 head daily.
Swine: Add 0.5 lbs per ton of complete ration.
Horses: Feed 1 grams per head daily.

Toxicology: When correctly used, there is no toxicity hazard in the use of COPRO 25.
Presentation: COPRO 25 is packaged in 50 lb multiwall bags.
Compendium Code No.: 11300110

COP-R-SOL™

Alpharma **Mineral Supplement**

Oral Mineral Supplement
Ingredient(s): Contains: Copper carbonate, ammonium carbonate, ammonium hydroxide, citric acid and water.
Indications: COP-R-SOL™ is a concentrated source of supplemental copper for use in the drinking water of poultry. COP-R-SOL™ is specifically formulated to perform under difficult water conditions and will not react with most metals.
Dosage and Administration: COP-R-SOL™ can be used in either tanks or proportioners.

See table below and administer the correct amount in the drinking water for 3-5 days.

Amount COP-R-SOL™	Treats
1 tablespoon	4 gallons
1 pint	128 gallons
1 quart	256 gallons
½ gallon	512 gallons
1 gallon	1024 gallons

Caution(s): Harmful if swallowed as a concentrate. If ingested, call a physician immediately. The concentrate may cause irritation to the nose, throat and skin.

For animal use only.
Warning(s): Not for human use. Keep out of reach of children.
Presentation: 1 gallon (3785 mL) packages.
COP-R-SOL is a trademark of Alpharma Inc.
Compendium Code No.: 10220301 AHL-453-0109

COR-1™

VacciCel **Vaccine**

Coronavirus Vaccine, Killed Virus
U.S. Vet. Lic. No.: 292
Active Ingredient(s): Contains coronavirus vaccine killed virus.

Contains penicillin and streptomycin as preservatives.
Indications: COR-1™ is a vaccine designed to protect healthy puppies and dogs against disease caused by canine coronavirus.
Dosage and Administration: Shake well before using. Inject 1 mL subcutaneously or intramuscularly using aseptic technique. A second dose two (2) to three (3) weeks later is recommended. Puppies vaccinated at less than 12-16 weeks of age should receive an additional dose at 12-16 weeks of age. Revaccinate annually with one (1) dose.
Precaution(s): Store at less than 45°F or 7°C.
Caution(s): Use the entire contents when first opened. Anaphylactic reactions although rare may occur.
Antidote(s): Epinephrine.
Presentation: 10 dose (10 mL) vials.
Compendium Code No.: 11090000

CO-RAL® 1%

Durvet **Topical Insecticide**

EPA Reg. No.: 67517-21-12281
Active Ingredient(s):
0,0-Diethyl 0-(3-chloro-4-methyl-2-oxo-2H-1-benzopyran-7-yl) phosphorothioate 1%
Inert Ingredients 99%
Total 100%
Indications: For dairy or beef cattle. For control of hornflies and lice. Aids in reducing face flies on cattle.

A ready-to-use insecticide dusting powder for use in the refillable Durvet Co-Ral® 1% Insecticide Bag - a weather-proof bag for use in open or sheltered areas. This product can also be used for hand dusting. Effective in controlling hornflies and lice; aids in controlling face flies.

No withdrawal period required; may be used with dairy cattle in production or beef cattle being fed for slaughter.

Directions for Use: It is a violation of Federal law to use this product in a manner inconsistent with its labeling.

Dust Bag: Empty contents of bag (CO-RAL® 1% Insecticide) into the Co-Ral® 1% Bag through opening along edge of upper side. Close opening. Use 1 lb of CO-RAL® 1% Insecticide per 8 animals every two weeks. Do not exceed 3 lbs of CO-RAL® 1% Insecticide per animal per year.

How to Hang: Hang Co-Ral® 1% Bag by means of rope or chain placed through straps along top edge. For horn fly and lice control, adjust height so that bottom of bag will hang a little below the backline of the animals using it. To aid in reducing face flies, hang bag so that animals will be forced to dust face daily.

Where to Hang: Suspend Co-Ral® 1% Bag in locations where animals will frequently dust themselves on a free-choice basis; or in gateways or lanes through which animals are forced to pass daily for water, feed or mineral.

Dairy Cattle: For lactating dairy cows, hang in the exit of the milking barn.

Restrictions: Do not hang Co-Ral® 1% Bag over feed, mineral or water troughs.

Hand Dusting: Apply not more than 2 oz (6 level tablespoonfuls) evenly into the hair over the head, neck, shoulders, back and tailhead. Repeat as necessary, but not more often than every 14 days. (Maximum Seasonal Application Rate: 26 applications/year).

Precautionary Statements: Hazards to Humans and Domestic Animals:

Caution: Harmful if swallowed, inhaled or absorbed through skin. Avoid breathing dusts. Avoid contact with eyes, skin and clothing. Wash thoroughly with soap and water after handling. Remove contaminated clothing and wash clothing before reuse.

Statement of Practical Treatment:

If Swallowed: Call a physician or Poison Control Center. Drink 1 or 2 glasses of water and induce vomiting by touching the back of throat with finger. Do not induce vomiting or give anything by mouth to an unconscious person.

If Inhaled: Remove victim to fresh air. If not breathing, give artificial respiration, preferably mouth-to-mouth. Get medical attention.

If on Skin: Wash with plenty of soap and water. Get medical attention if irritation persists.

If in Eyes: Flush eyes with plenty of water. Get medical attention if irritation persists.

Note to Physician: Atropine sulfate by injection is antidotal. 2-PAM is also antidotal and may be administered in conjunction with atropine.

Environmental Hazards: This pesticide is toxic to birds, fish, and aquatic invertebrates. Do not apply directly to water. Do not contaminate water when disposing of equipment washwater or rinsate.

Restrictions: For external, insecticidal use on above specified animals only. Avoid contamination of feed, troughs, water and water utensils. Provide thorough ventilation while dusting. Do not apply to sick, stressed or convalescent animals.

Storage and Disposal: Do not contaminate water, food, or feed by storage or disposal.

Pesticide Disposal: Wastes resulting from the use of this product may be disposed of on site or at an approved waste disposal facility.

Container Disposal: Completely empty bag into application equipment. Then dispose of empty bag in a sanitary landfill or by incineration, or, if allowed by State and local authorities, by burning. If burned, stay out of smoke.

Warning(s): Keep out of reach of children.

Disclaimer: Notice of Warranty: Durvet, Inc. makes no warranty of merchantability, fitness for any particular purpose, or otherwise, expressed or implied concerning this product or its uses which extend beyond the use of the product under normal conditions in accord with the statements made on the label.

Presentation: 12.5 lb (5.67 kg).

® A Reg. Trademark of the parent company of Miles, Inc.

U.S. Patent No. 2,748,146.

Compendium Code No.: 10840341 10/97

CO-RAL®

(coumaphos) Emulsifiable Livestock Insecticide

Bayer

RESTRICTED USE PESTICIDE: Due to Acute Oral Hazards-For retail sale to and use only by Certified Applicators or persons under their direct supervision and only for those uses covered by the Certified Applicator's Certification.

For Control of Horn Flies, Face Flies, Lice and Ticks

Active Ingredients:

0,0-Diethyl 0-(3-chloro-4-methyl-2-oxo-(2H)-1-benzopyran-7-yl) phosphorothioate . . . 11.6%

Inert Ingredients:* 88.4%

* Contains aromatic petroleum distillates. 100.0%

This product contains 1.0 lb. 0,0-Diethyl 0-(3-chloro-4-methyl-2-oxo-(2H)-1-benzopyran-7-yl) phosphorothioate per gallon.

STATEMENT OF PRACTICAL TREATMENT: Fatal if swallowed. May be fatal if inhaled. Do not breathe vapors or spray mist. Avoid contact with skin, clothing or eyes. Wash thoroughly w/soap and warm water after handling. Wash contaminated clothing with soap and hot water before reuse. **If swallowed** — Call a physician or Poison Control Center immediately. If possible, vomiting should be induced under medical supervision. Drink one or two glasses of water and induce vomiting by touching the back of throat with finger. Do not induce vomiting or give anything by mouth to an unconscious person. **If inhaled** — Remove victim to fresh air. Apply artificial respiration if indicated. Get medical attention if victim displays signs of poisoning. **If on skin** — Remove contaminated clothing and wash affected areas with soap and water. **If in eyes** — Flush eyes with plenty of water. Call a physician immediately. **To Physician:** Atropine sulfate by injection is antidotal. Repeat as necessary to the point of tolerance. 2-PAM is also antidotal and may be administered in conjunction with atropine.

KEEP OUT OF REACH OF CHILDREN

DANGER POISON

SEE ADDITIONAL PRECAUTIONARY STATEMENTS

HAZARDS TO HUMANS AND DOMESTIC ANIMALS

ENVIRONMENTAL HAZARDS

This pesticide is toxic to fish, birds, and other aquatic invertebrates. Keep out of lakes, streams, or ponds. Coumaphos washed off of wading treated livestock may be hazardous to aquatic organisms. Do not contaminate water when disposing of equipment washwater or rinsate. Apply this product only as specified on this label.

STORAGE AND DISPOSAL

Do not contaminate water, food or feed by storage or disposal.

STORAGE: Do not allow to freeze. Keep from extreme heat.

PESTICIDE DISPOSAL: Pesticide wastes are acutely hazardous. Improper disposal of excess pesticide, spray mixture, or rinsate is a violation of Federal Law. If these wastes cannot be disposed of by use according to label directions, contact your State Pesticide or Environmental Control Agency, or the Hazardous Waste representative at the nearest EPA Regional Office for guidance.

CONTAINER DISPOSAL: Triple rinse (or equivalent). Then offer for recycling or reconditioning, or puncture and dispose of in a sanitary landfill, or by other procedures approved by state and local authorities.

PROTECTIVE CLOTHING STATEMENT

Applicators and handlers exposed to the concentrate or participating in spray operations must wear long sleeve shirt, long pants, chemical-resistant gloves such as barrier laminate or butyl rubber ≥ 14 mils, chemical-resistant footwear plus socks, chemical-resistant apron, face shield or goggles. All other handlers must wear long sleeve shirt, long pants, chemical-resistant gloves such as barrier laminate or butyl rubber ≥ 14 mils, chemical-resistant footwear plus socks.

Users should wash hands before eating, drinking, chewing gum, using tobacco, or using the toilet. Users should remove clothing immediately if pesticide gets inside. Then wash thoroughly and put on clean clothing.

Users should remove personal protective equipment immediately after handling this product. Wash the outside of gloves before removing. As soon as possible, wash thoroughly and change into clean clothing. Follow manufacturer's instructions for cleaning/maintaining personal protective equipment. If no such instructions for washables, use detergent and hot water. Keep and wash personal protective equipment separately from other laundry.

ATTENTION: CONTENTS MUST BE DILUTED BEFORE USE

DIRECTIONS FOR USE

It is a violation of Federal law to use this product in a manner inconsistent with its labeling.

Co-Ral Emulsifiable Livestock Insecticide mixes easily with water to form an emulsion which is easily applied with ordinary spray equipment. One spray treatment is highly effective for control of flies, lice and ticks and provides residual control for several weeks.

Spray Treatment for Specified Ectoparasites: Operate spray equipment so as to thoroughly penetrate the hair coat. Retreatment will be necessary only when insects reappear and constitute a problem.

Backrubber Application for Horn Flies and Face Flies: Co-Ral Emulsifiable Livestock Insecticide has proved to be ideal for backrubber application. When properly mixed and applied, excellent control of horn flies and face flies will be achieved. Best control is obtained when backrubbers are strategically located and properly treated. No. 2 furnace oil (fuel oil) or No. 2 diesel fuel oil is recommended for mixing with Co-Ral Emulsifiable Livestock Insecticide for use in backrubbers. Use of other oils may result in sludge formation that will prevent proper distribution in the reservoir-type backrubber.

Entry Restriction: Do not contact treated animals until their coats are dry.

RECOMMENDED APPLICATIONS

DO NOT APPLY MORE THAN 5 OUNCES OF **Co-Ral** EMULSIFIABLE LIVESTOCK INSECTICIDE PER 4 GALLONS OF WATER. FOR LACTATING DAIRY CATTLE DO NOT APPLY MORE THAN 1 1/4 OUNCES **Co-Ral** EMULSIFIABLE LIVESTOCK INSECTICIDE PER 4 GALLONS OF WATER.

ANIMAL	PARASITE	Fl. oz. Co-Ral	REMARKS
Beef and Non Lactating Dairy Cattle	Horn Flies, Lice	2 1/2	**SPRAY TREATMENT(S):** Apply specified dosage in 4 gallons of water for a complete wetting to run-off. Repeat as necessary.
	Ticks	5	
Beef and Lactating Dairy Cattle	Horn Flies Face Flies	9 3/4	**CATTLE BACKRUBBER(S):** Mix specified dosage in gallon of No. 2 furnace oil or No. 2 diesel fuel. Saturate the fiber portion of the backrubber with this mixture. Place the backrubber where animals congregate or travel regularly. For dairy cattle, suspend at a height that will prevent straddling. Resaturate backrubber as needed. **Note:** For most effective face fly control, the rubber should be constructed so as to permit the animal to rub its face. No interval is required between treatment and slaughter or use of milk.
	Lice	1 1/4	**SPRAY TREATMENT(S):** Apply specified dosage in 4 gallons of water for a complete wetting to run-off. Repeat as necessary. No interval is required between treatment and slaughter or use of milk.
Horses (Not intended for slaughter)	Horn Flies, Lice	2 1/2	**SPRAY TREATMENT(S):** Apply specified dosage in 4 gallons of water for a complete wetting. Treat thoroughly all wounds and injuries. Repeat as necessary.
	Ticks	5	
Swine	Lice	2 1/2	**SPRAY TREATMENT(S):** Apply specified dosage in 4 gallons of water for a complete wetting to run-off. Repeat as necessary.

NOTICE TO VETERINARIANS

If the proper dosage of Co-Ral Emulsifiable Livestock Insecticide has been applied and adverse reactions, such as bloat, excessive salivation and posterior paralysis occur, it is highly probable that a host-parasite reaction exists. Administer symptomatic treatment. Anti-inflammatory agents may be helpful. If necessary, relieve bloat by trocarization, as a stomach tube may traumatize a severely swollen esophagus. Do **not** administer atropine, as it is contraindicated in host-parasite reactions. If toxicity should occur as a result of gross overdosage, atropine is antidotal.

USE RESTRICTIONS

Co-Ral is a cholinesterase inhibitor. Do not use this product on animals simultaneously or within a few days before or after treatment or exposure to cholinesterase-inhibiting drugs or pesticides. Atropine sulfate by injection is antidotal. Consult veterinarian at the first sign of adverse reaction.

Do not apply as a spray at rates above 1 1/4 ounce of Co-Ral Emulsifiable Livestock Insecticide per 4 gallons of water to lactating dairy cattle, or non-lactating dairy cattle within 14 days of freshening. If freshening should occur within this interval after spraying, do not use milk for human food for balance of 14 day interval.

Do not apply to sick, convalescent or stressed livestock, or to animals less than 3 months old.

Do not spray animals for 10 days before or after shipping or weaning, or after exposure to contagious or infectious diseases.

Do not spray in a confined, non-ventilated area.

Do not apply in conjunction with oral drenches or other internal medication such as phenothiazine, nor with natural or synthetic pyrethroids or their synergists or with other organic phosphates.

For external insecticidal use only on specified animals. Do not apply this product in a way that will contact workers or other persons, either directly or through drift. Only protected handlers may be in the area during application.

Individuals must limit the number of animals they treat per day with hand held sprayers to no more than 100, if the animals are treated at the maximum label rate, 200 if they are treated at 1/2 maximum label rate, etc.

Premise

Precautions: Do not spray in a confined, non-ventilated area. Do not treat areas such as drinking cups, mangers, or troughs where livestock feed. Do not contaminate water, food, feedstuffs, food or feed handling equipment, or milk or meat handling equipment.

C

LIMITED WARRANTY AND LIMITATION OF DAMAGES

Bayer Corporation, Agriculture Division warrants that this material conforms to the chemical description on the label. BAYER CORPORATION, MAKES NO OTHER EXPRESS OR IMPLIED WARRANTY, INCLUDING ANY OTHER EXPRESS OR IMPLIED WARRANTY OF FITNESS OR OF MERCHANTABILITY, and no agent of Bayer Corporation, is authorized to do so except in writing with a specific reference to this warranty. Any damages arising from a breach of this warranty shall be limited to direct damages and shall not include consequential commercial damages such as loss of profits or values, etc.

Co-Ral is a Reg. TM of the parent company of Bayer AG, Leverkusen

EPA Reg. No. 11556-23

EPA Est. No. 67517-MO-1

SUPPLIED:

Code 13291 — 3.8L (1 Gallon)

71132911, R.0

Bayer Corporation, Agriculture Division, Animal Health, Shawnee Mission, Kansas 66201 U.S.A.

Compendium Code No.: 10400151

CO-RAL® EQUINE AND LIVESTOCK DUST

AgriLabs **Topical Insecticide**

EPA Reg. No.: 34704-306-53302

Active Ingredient(s):

Coumaphos: 0,0-diethyl 0-(3-chloro-4-methyl-2-oxo-2H-1-benzopyran-7-yl) phosphorothioate 1%

Inert Ingredients: 99%

Total 100%

Indications: For control of horn flies and lice on beef and dairy cattle, lice on swine and horn flies on horses.

Directions for Use: It is a violation of Federal Law to use this product in a manner inconsistent with its labeling.

Important: Read the entire Directions and the Warranty before using this product.

Recommended Applications:

Animal	Insects	Remarks
Cattle (Dairy and Beef)	Horn Flies, Lice	Direct Application: Apply not more than 2 oz.*/animal. Dust evenly into the hair over the head, neck, shoulders, back and tailhead. Repeat as necessary but not more often than every 14 days. No interval is required between treatment and use of meat or milk as food.
Swine	Lice	Direct Application: Apply not more than 1 oz.*/animal as a uniform coat to the shoulders and back. Repeat as necessary, but not more than once every 10 days. No interval is required between treatment and use of meat as food. Bedding Treatment: Apply 2 oz.* uniformly over each 30 square feet of fresh, dry bedding. Repeat as necessary, but not more than once every 10 days. Direct Application and Bedding Treatment: In severe infestations, both individual animals and the bedding may be treated as directed above.
Horses	Horn Flies	Direct Application: Apply not more than 2 oz.*/animal. Dust evenly into the hair over the head, neck, shoulders, back and tailhead. Repeat as necessary.

*Note: 1 oz. of this material equals approximately three level tablespoonsful.

Hold container at a distance from the area to be treated that will permit even distribution of the dust.

Contraindication(s): Use Restrictions: For external insecticidal use only on above specified animals. Do not contaminate feed troughs, water, or water utensils. Provide thorough ventilation while dusting. Use caution when dusting in area of face to avoid exposure to eyes. Do not apply to sick, stressed, or convalescent animals.

Precautionary Statements: Hazards to Humans: Caution: Harmful if swallowed, inhaled, or absorbed through skin. Avoid breathing dusts. Avoid contact with eyes, skin and clothing.

Statement of Practical Treatment:

If swallowed — Call a physician or Poison Control Center immediately. Drink one or two glasses of water and induce vomiting by touching the back of throat with finger. Repeat until vomit fluid is clear. Do not induce vomiting or give anything by mouth to an unconscious person.

If inhaled — Remove victim to fresh air. Apply artificial respiration if indicated. Get medical attention if victim displays signs of poisoning.

If on skin — Remove contaminated clothing and wash affected areas with soap and water.

If in eyes — Flush eyes with plenty of water. Call a physician immediately.

To Physician: Prolonged exposure will result in cholinesterase depression. Atropine sulfate by injection is antidotal. 2-PAM is also antidotal and may be administered in conjunction with atropine.

For a Medical Emergency Involving this Product Call: 1-800-228-5635, ext. 136, or call collect, 612-851-8180, ext. 136.

Environmental Hazards: This pesticide is toxic to birds, fish, and aquatic invertebrates. For terrestrial uses, do not apply directly to water, or to areas where surface water is present, or to intertidal areas below the mean high water mark. Do not contaminate water when disposing of equipment washwater or rinsate.

Storage and Disposal: Do not contaminate water, food, or feed by storage or disposal.

Storage: Store in a cool, dry place.

Pesticide Disposal: Wastes resulting from the use of this product may be disposed of on site or at an approved waste disposal facility.

Container Disposal: Completely empty the container by shaking and tapping sides and bottom to loosen clinging particles, thereby dispensing the entire contents of the can only as directed by the label. Dispose of container in sanitary landfill or by incineration, or, if allowed by state and local authorities, by burning. If burned, stay out of smoke.

Warning(s): Keep out of reach of children.

Disclaimer: Warranty: Manufacturer and Seller warrants that this product conforms to the chemical description on the label thereof and is reasonably fit for the purposes stated on such label only when used in accordance with the directions under normal use conditions. It is impossible to eliminate all risks inherently associated with the use of this product. Livestock injury, ineffectiveness, or other unintended consequences may result because of such factors as weather conditions, presence of other materials, or the manner of use or application, all of which are beyond the control of the Manufacturer or Seller. In no case shall Manufacturer or Seller be liable for consequential, special or indirect damages resulting from the use or handling of this product. All such risks shall be assumed by the Buyer.

Except as expressly provided herein, Manufacturer and Seller makes no warranties, guarantees, or representations of any kind, either expressed or implied, or by usage of trade, statutory or otherwise, with regard to the product sold, including, but not limited to, merchantability, fitness for a particular purpose, use or eligibility of the product for any particular trade usage. Buyer's or User's exclusive remedy, and Manufacturer's or Seller's total liability, shall be for damages not exceeding the cost of the product.

Presentation: 12 x 2 lbs, 2 x 12.5 lbs (5.67 kg) dust bag refills, 4 x 12.5 lbs (5.67 kg) Flip Top dust bag kits and 12.5 lbs (5.67 kg) square dust bag kits.

®CO-RAL is a Registered T.M. of the parent company of Farben Fabriken Bayer GmbH, Leverkusen.

Compendium Code No.: 10580372 3/94

CO-RAL®

(coumaphos) Flowable Insecticide

Bayer

RESTRICTED USE PESTICIDE: Due to Acute Oral Hazard.

For retail sale to and use only by Certified Applicators or persons under their direct supervision and only for those uses covered by the Certified Applicator's Certification.

Use restricted to employees of the U.S. Department of Agriculture Animal and Plant Health Inspection Service (USDA-APHIS) who are enrolled in the USDA-APHIS cholinesterase monitoring program.

For Control Of Scabies On Cattle And For Control Of Horn Flies, Lice, Ticks And Screwworms On Beef And Non-Lactating Dairy Cattle And Horses

ACTIVE INGREDIENTS: 0,0-Diethyl 0-(3-chloro-4-methyl-2-oxo-(2H)-1-benzopyran-7-yl) phosphorothioate 42.0%

INERT INGREDIENTS 58.0%

100.0%

Product contains 4.2 lbs. of coumaphos per gallon.

Shake Well Before Using

EPA Reg. No. 11556-98 EPA Est. No. 3125-MO-1

KEEP OUT OF REACH OF CHILDREN

STATEMENT OF PRACTICAL TREATMENT

Fatal if swallowed or absorbed through the skin. Do not breathe spray mist. Do not get in eyes, on skin, or on clothing. Wash thoroughly with soap and warm water after handling. Wash contaminated clothing with soap and hot water before use.

If swallowed—Call a physician or Poison Control Center immediately. If possible, vomiting should be induced under medical supervision. Drink one or two glasses of water and induce vomiting by touching the back of throat with finger. Do not induce vomiting or give anything by mouth to an unconscious person.

If inhaled—Remove victim to fresh air. Apply artificial respiration if indicated. Get medical attention if victim displays signs of poisoning.

If on skin—Remove contaminated clothing and wash affected areas with soap and water.

If in eyes—Flush eyes with plenty of water. Call a physician immediately.

To Physician: Administer atropine sulfate by injection in therapeutic doses. Repeat as necessary to the point of tolerance. **2-PAM** is also antidotal and may be administered in conjunction with atropine.

SEE ADDITIONAL PRECAUTIONARY STATEMENTS

PRECAUTIONARY STATEMENTS

HAZARDS TO HUMANS AND DOMESTIC ANIMALS

KEEP OUT OF REACH OF CHILDREN

Fatal if swallowed or absorbed through the skin. Do not breathe spray mist. Do not get in eyes, on skin or on clothing. Wash thoroughly with soap and warm water after handling. Wash contaminated clothing with soap and hot water before use.

This material contains a cholinesterase inhibitor. If poisoning should occur, obtain prompt medical aid.

HAZARDS TO DOMESTIC ANIMALS (CATTLE AND HORSES)

Acute symptoms of overdosage in cattle and horses are: Frequent defecation and urination, watering of eyes and muscular twitching. Later the symptoms are: salivation, diarrhea and muscular weakness.

While no claims for control of cattle grubs are made for this product, host parasite reactions such as bloat, salivation, staggering and paralysis may sometimes occur when cattle are treated while the common cattle grub *(Hypoderma lineatum)* is in the gullet, or while the northern grub *(H. bovis)* is in the area of the spinal cord. Cattle should be treated either *before* or *after* these stages of grub development. Consult your veterinarian, extension livestock specialist or extension entomologist regarding the timing of the grub cycle for your cattle based on their origin and history.

Consult veterinarian at the first sign of adverse reaction.

> NOTE: If it is impossible to determine the origin of the cattle, and thus the exact stage of the grubs is unknown, it is recommended that the cattle receive only a maintenance ration of low energy feed during the treatment period. This lessens the likelihood of severe bloat which may occur in cattle on full feed when the common grub is killed while in the gullet.

NOTICE TO VETERINARIANS: If the proper dosage of Co-Ral Flowable has been applied and adverse reactions, such as bloat, excessive salivation and posterior paralysis occur, it is highly probable that a host parasite reaction exists. Administer symptomatic treatment. Anti-inflammatory agents may be helpful. If necessary relieve bloat by trocarization, as a stomach tube may traumatize a severely swollen esophagus. Do not administer atropine, as it is contraindicated in host parasite reactions. If toxicity should occur as a result of gross overdosage, atropine by injection is antidotal.

ENVIRONMENTAL HAZARDS
This pesticide is toxic to birds, fish and aquatic invertebrates. Coumaphos washed off of wading treated livestock may be hazardous to aquatic organisms. Do not contaminate water when disposing of equipment washwater or rinsate.
PROTECTIVE CLOTHING STATEMENT
Applicators and handlers exposed to the concentrate or participating in dip vat operations must wear long sleeve shirt, long pants, chemical-resistant gloves such as barrier laminate or butyl rubber ≥14 mils, chemical-resistant footwear plus socks, chemical-resistant apron, face shield or goggles. All other handlers must wear long sleeve shirt, long pants, chemical-resistant gloves such as barrier laminate or butyl rubber ≥14 mils, chemical-resistant footwear plus socks.
Users should wash hands before eating, drinking, chewing gum, using tobacco, or using the toilet. Users should remove clothing immediately if pesticide gets inside. Then wash thoroughly and put on clean clothing.
Users should remove personal protective equipment immediately after handling this product. Wash the outside of gloves before removing. As soon as possible, wash thoroughly and change into clean clothing. Follow manufacturer's instructions for cleaning/maintaining personal protective equipment. If no such instructions for washables, use detergent and hot water. Keep and wash personal protective equipment separately from other laundry.
DIRECTIONS FOR USE
It is a violation of Federal Law to use this product in a manner inconsistent with its labeling.
AVISO - Al Usuario: Si usted no puede leer o entender ingles, no use este producto hasta que la etiqueta le haya side explicada ampliamente. (To the user: If you cannot read or understand English, do not use this product until the label has been fully explained to you.)
IMPORTANT: Read this entire label including the Limited Warranty and Limitation of Damages provision, before using.
Entry Restriction: Do not contact treated animals until their coats are dry.
Premise Precautions: Do not spray in confined, non-ventilated area. Do not treat areas such as feed bunks, mangers, or troughs where livestock feed or drink. Do not contaminate water, food, feedstuffs, food or feed handling equipment, or milk or meat handling equipment.
FOR USE ON BEEF AND NON-LACTATING DAIRY CATTLE AND ON HORSES.
Co-Ral Flowable has been especially developed to provide a highly concentrated formulation of coumaphos. The physical properties of the formulation allow for quick initial mixing and excellent suspension, as well as ease of resuspension where settling has occurred due to lack of regular use or overwintering.
As a liquid, the difficulties and inconvenience commonly associated with mixing of wettable powders are greatly reduced or eliminated. Because Co-Ral Flowable is a much more concentrated formulation of coumaphos than previously available, a smaller amount is needed to prepare any given volume of spray or dip suspension.
DIP TREATMENT FOR ECTOPARASITES OF CATTLE LISTED BELOW:
Charge dip vats with accurate concentration by using exact quantity of Co-Ral Flowable and volume of water specified. Mix suspension thoroughly before each use. Passage of animals through the vat does not change concentration of remaining suspension. Water lost by evaporation should be replaced. If water is added to the vat due to rainfall or replenishment, an appropriate amount of Co-Ral Flowable should also be added. Continue to use vat until accumulation of debris makes it unsuitable for further use.
NOTE: Be sure cattle have access to drinking water prior to dipping. Do not dip excessively thirsty animals.
SPRAY TREATMENT FOR ECTOPARASITES OF CATTLE AND HORSES LISTED BELOW:
Co-Ral Flowable provides residual control of ectoparasites on livestock. Repeat applications will be necessary only when insects reappear and constitute a problem. Co-Ral Flowable mixes easily with water to form a suspension which is readily usable in spray equipment.
RECOMMENDED APPLICATIONS
Do not apply more than one (1) gallon of Co-Ral Flowable per 165 gallons of water as a dip or more than one (1) gallon of Co-Ral Flowable per 200 gallons of water as a spray.
No withdrawal interval is required between application and use of meat as food.

Parasite	Gallons Co-Ral Flowable	Remarks
Scabies* *(Psoroptes bovis)*	1	**DIP TREATMENT:** Mix specified amount in 165 gallons of water. Agitate dip suspension thoroughly prior to each use. Two treatments, 10 to 14 days apart, are necessary to control scabies. Do not dip more than twice per year.** Submerge each animal to assure complete coverage and thorough wetting of the skin.
Horn Flies Lice	¼ (1 quart)	**SPRAY TREATMENT:** Add specified amount to 200 gallons of water and mix thoroughly. Apply for complete wetting to run-off. Do not spray more than six times per year. Do not make applications less than 10 days apart.
Ticks*	½ - 1	**DIP TREATMENT:** Mix specified quantity of Flowable in 200 gallons of water. Agitate dip thoroughly prior to each use to assure uniform treatment. Do not dip more than twice per year.** Do not make applications less than 10 days apart.
	½ - 1	**SPRAY TREATMENT:** Add specified amount of Flowable to 200 gallons of water and mix thoroughly. Apply for complete wetting to run-off. Do not spray more than six times per year. Do not make applications less than 10 days apart.
Screwworms*	1	**SPRAY TREATMENT:** Mix specified amount in 200 gallons of water and mix thoroughly. Apply as a high pressure spray to wet the skin, not just the hair. Do not spray more than six times per year. Do not make applications less than 10 days apart.

*Approved as a "Permitted Pesticide" by Animal and Plant Health Inspection Service (APHIS) of the U.S. Department of Agriculture for the control of Screwworms, Scabies and Ticks in Federal Eradication Programs when used according to the directions of APHIS Veterinary Service Regulations and/or Memoranda.
**Animals should not be dipped more than twice per year unless additional treatments are required by APHIS Veterinary Services Regulations/Memoranda for Animals included in Federal Eradication Programs.
USE RESTRICTIONS
Co-Ral is a cholinesterase inhibitor. Do not use this product on animals simultaneously or within a few days before or after treatment or exposure to cholinesterase-inhibiting drugs or pesticides. Atropine sulfate by injection is antidotal. Consult veterinarian at the first sign of adverse reaction.
Do not apply this product in a way that will contact workers or other persons, either directly or through drift. Only protected handlers may be in the area during application.
Individuals must limit the number of animals they treat per day with hand held sprayers to no more than 100, if the animals are treated at the maximum label rate, 200 if they are treated at 1/2 maximum label rate, etc.
STORAGE AND DISPOSAL
Do not contaminate water, food or feed by storage or disposal.
Not for storage in or around the home.

Cattle Dip Solution Disposal: Contact your Local and/or State Environmental Control Agency for specific recommendations or details for the geographical area where the dip vat is located. The Agency recommends that spent dip-vat solution be bioremediated in accordance with a method developed by the USDA. The treated solution can then be transferred to lined, shallow evaporation ponds or incorporated into the soil to encourage further degradation. If an evaporation pond is used it should be constructed to prevent overflow or flooding during wet seasons and should be lined with compacted clay, reinforced concrete or flexible membrane liner. Questions concerning the disposal of the spent solution should be directed to the waste representative at the nearest EPA Regional Office. Details are available concerning the bioremediation procedure and ultimate disposition of the remediated solution. Do not apply dried sludge or the bioremediated/treated solution to land for raising crops for human consumption.

Pesticide Disposal: Pesticide wastes are acutely hazardous. Improper disposal of excess pesticide, spray mixture or rinsate is a violation of Federal Law. If these wastes cannot be disposed of by use according to label directions, contact your State Pesticide or Environmental Control Agency or the Hazardous Waste representative at the nearest EPA Regional Office for guidance.

Container Disposal: Triple rinse (or equivalent). Then offer for recycling or reconditioning; or puncture and dispose of in a sanitary landfill or incineration or, if allowed by state and local authorities, by burning. If burned, stay out of smoke.

LIMITED WARRANTY AND LIMITATION OF DAMAGES
We warrant that at the time of manufacture this product was true to label and reasonably fit for the purposes described in its labeling. However, there are numerous factors beyond our control, e.g. storage, diagnosis, dosage, differences among individual animals, etc. which make it impossible to eliminate all risks associated with the use of this product, even if the directions are followed.
This statement is made in lieu of any other warranty, either express or implied, including any warranty of merchantability or fitness: and no representative or agent of this corporation is authorized to vary the terms of this warranty or the contents of the labeling of this product except by printed notice from the corporation's Shawnee Mission, Kansas head office. In the event of damages arising from our breach of this warranty, damages shall be limited to direct damages and shall not include consequential commercial damages such as loss of profit or values, etc.
SUPPLIED:
Code 13265 — 7.6 L (2 Gallons)
71132650, R.10
Co-Ral® is a Reg. TM of the parent company of Bayer Corporation.
Manufactured for Bayer Corporation, Agriculture Division, Animal Health, Shawnee Mission, Kansas 66201 U.S.A.
Compendium Code No.: 10400162

CO-RAL®

(coumaphos) Fly and Tick Spray

Bayer

For Control of Horn Flies, Face Flies, Lice And Ticks
ACTIVE INGREDIENT:
0,0-Diethyl 0-(3-chloro-4-methyl-2-oxo-2H-1-benzopyran-7-yl) phosphorothioate 6.15%
INERT INGREDIENTS* 93.85%
100.0%

*Contains aromatic petroleum distillates.
This product contains 0.25 lb 0,0-Diethyl 0-(3-chloro-4-methyl-2-oxo-2H-1-benzopyran-7-yl) phosphorothioate per half gallon.
EPA Reg. No. 11556-115 EPA Est. No. 67517-MO-1
Keep out of reach of children
WARNING
SEE STATEMENTS OF PRACTICAL TREATMENT AND OTHER PRECAUTIONARY STATEMENTS
DIRECTIONS FOR USE
It is a violation of Federal Law to use this product in a manner inconsistent with its labeling.
Co-Ral Fly and Tick Spray mixes easily with water to form an emulsion which is easily applied with ordinary spray equipment. One spray treatment is highly effective for control of flies, lice and ticks and provides residual control.
SPRAY TREATMENT FOR SPECIFIED ECTOPARASITES: Operate spray equipment so as to thoroughly penetrate the hair coat. Re-treatment will be necessary only when insects reappear and constitute a problem.
BACKRUBBER APPLICATION FOR HORN FLIES AND FACE FLIES: Co-Ral Fly and Tick Spray is ideal for backrubber application. When properly mixed and applied, effective control of horn flies and face flies will be achieved. Best control is obtained when backrubbers are strategically located and properly treated. No. 2 furnace oil (fuel oil) or No. 2 diesel fuel oil is recommended for mixing with Co-Ral Fly and Tick Spray for use in backrubbers. Use of other oils may result in sludge formation that will prevent proper distribution in the reservoir-type backrubber.
Entry Restriction: Do not contact treated animals until their coats are dry.
PROTECTIVE CLOTHING STATEMENT
Applicators and other handlers must wear long sleeve shirt, long pants, chemical-resistant gloves such as barrier laminate or butyl rubber ≥ 14 mils, shoes plus socks.
Users should wash hands before eating, drinking, chewing gum, using tobacco, or using the toilet. Users should remove clothing immediately if pesticide gets inside. Then wash thoroughly and put on clean clothing.
Users should remove personal protective equipment immediately after handling this product. Wash the outside of gloves before removing. As soon as possible, wash thoroughly and change into clean clothing. Follow manufacturer's instructions for cleaning/maintaining personal protective equipment. If no such instructions for washables, use detergent and hot water. Keep and wash personal protective equipment separately from other laundry.
NOTICE TO VETERINARIANS: If the proper dosage of Co-Ral Fly and Tick Spray has been applied and adverse reactions, such as bloat, excessive salivation and posterior paralysis occur, it is highly probable that a host parasite reaction exists. Administer symptomatic treatment. Anti-inflammatory agents may be helpful. If necessary, relieve bloat by trocarization, as a stomach tube may traumatize a severely swollen esophagus. Do not administer atropine, as it is contraindicated in host parasite reactions. If toxicity should occur as a result of gross overdosage, atropine by injection is antidotal.

C

USE RESTRICTIONS

For external insecticidal use only on specified animals. Do not apply as a spray at rates above 1 quart of Co-Ral Fly and Tick Spray per 50 gallons of water to lactating dairy cattle or non-lactating dairy cattle within 14 days of freshening. If freshening should occur within the interval after spraying, do not use milk for human food for balance of 14 day interval. Do not apply to sick, convalescent or stressed livestock or to animals less than 3 months old. Do not spray animals for 10 days before or after shipping or weaning or after exposure to contagious and infecting diseases. Do not spray in a confined, non-ventilated area. Co-Ral is a cholinesterase inhibitor. Do not use this product on animals simultaneously or within a few days before or after treatment or exposure to cholinesterase-inhibiting drugs or pesticides. Atropine by injection is antidotal. Consult veterinarian at the first sign of adverse reaction. Do not apply this product in a way that will contact workers or other persons, either directly or through drift. Only protected handlers may be in the area during application.

Individuals must limit the number of animals they treat per day with hand held sprayers to no more than 100, if the animals are treated at the maximum label rate, 200 if they are treated at 1/2 maximum label rate, etc.

RECOMMENDED APPLICATIONS

DO NOT APPLY MORE THAN 4 QUARTS OF CO-RAL FLY AND TICK SPRAY PER 50 GALLONS OF WATER. FOR LACTATING DAIRY CATTLE DO NOT APPLY MORE THAN 1 QUART OF CO-RAL FLY AND TICK SPRAY PER 50 GALLONS OF WATER.

Animal	Parasite	Quarts Per 50 Gallons of Water	Ounces Per 4 Gallons of Water	Remarks
Beef and Non-Lactating Dairy Cattle	Horn Flies Lice	2	5	SPRAY TREATMENTS: Apply specified dosage for a complete wetting to run-off. Treat no more than six times per year. Do not make applications less than 10 days apart.
	Ticks	4	10	
Lactating Dairy Cattle	Lice	1	2-1/2	SPRAY TREATMENTS: Apply specified dosage for a complete wetting to run-off. Treat no more than six times per year. Do not make applications less than 10 days apart. No interval is required between treatment and slaughter or use of milk.
Backrubber for Beef and Lactating Dairy Cattle	Horn Flies Face Flies	See Remarks	See Remarks	Mix 4 quarts Co-Ral in 13 gallons of No. 2 fuel oil or No. 2 diesel fuel (or 9-3/4 oz Co-Ral per gallon). Saturate the fiber portion of the backrubber with this mixture. Place the backrubber where animals congregate or travel regularly. For dairy cattle suspend at a height that will prevent straddling. Resaturate backrubber as needed. NOTE: For most effective face fly control the rubber should be constructed so as to permit the animal to rub its face. No interval is required between treatment and slaughter or use of milk.
Horses (Not intended for slaughter)	Horn Flies Lice	2	5	SPRAY TREATMENT(S): Apply specified dosage for complete wetting. Treat thoroughly all wounds and injuries. Treat no more than six times per year. Do not make applications less than 10 days apart.
	Ticks	4	10	
Swine	Lice	2	5	SPRAY TREATMENT(S): Apply specified dosage for a complete wetting to run-off. Treat no more than six times per year. Do not make applications less than 10 days apart.

STORAGE AND DISPOSAL

Do not contaminate water, food, or feed by storage or disposal.

STORAGE: Do not allow to freeze. Keep from extreme heat.

PESTICIDE DISPOSAL: Pesticide wastes are acutely hazardous. Improper disposal of excess pesticide, spray mixture, or rinsate is a violation of Federal Law. If these wastes cannot be disposed of by use according to label directions, contact your State Pesticide or Environmental Control Agency or the Hazardous Waste representative at the nearest EPA Regional Office for guidance.

CONTAINER DISPOSAL: Triple rinse (or equivalent). Then offer for recycling or reconditioning, or puncture and dispose of in a sanitary landfill or incineration, or if allowed by state and local authorities, by burning. If burned, stay out of smoke.

PRECAUTIONARY STATEMENTS

HAZARDS TO HUMANS AND DOMESTIC ANIMALS

WARNING

May be fatal if swallowed or inhaled. Do not breathe vapors or spray mist. Causes moderate eye irritation. Avoid contact with skin, clothing or eyes. Wash thoroughly with soap and warm water after handling. Wash contaminated clothing with soap and hot water before use.

STATEMENTS OF PRACTICAL TREATMENT

If swallowed: Call a physician or Poison Control Center immediately. If possible, vomiting should be induced under medical supervision. Drink one or two glasses of water and induce vomiting by touching the back of throat with finger. Do not induce vomiting or give anything by mouth to an unconscious person.

If inhaled: Remove victim to fresh air. Apply artificial respiration if indicated. Get medical attention it victim displays signs of poisoning.

If on skin: Remove contaminated clothing and wash affected areas with soap and water. Get medical attention if irritation appears.

If in eyes: Flush eyes with plenty of water. Call a physician immediately.

To Physician: Atropine sulfate by injection is antidotal. Repeat as necessary to the point of tolerance. 2-PAM is also antidotal and may be administered in conjunction with atropine.

ENVIRONMENTAL HAZARDS

This pesticide is toxic to birds, fish and aquatic invertebrates. Do not contaminate water when disposing of equipment washwater or rinsate. Do not apply directly to any body of water. Coumaphos washed off of wading treated livestock may be hazardous to aquatic organisms. Do not contaminate water when disposing of equipment washwater or rinsate.

Premise Precautions: Do not spray in a confined, non-ventilated area. Do not treat areas such as feed bunks, mangers, or troughs where livestock feed or drink. Do not contaminate water, food, feedstuffs, food or feed handling equipment, or milk or meat handling equipment.

LIMITED WARRANTY AND LIMITATION OF DAMAGES

Bayer Corporation, Agriculture Division, warrants that this material conforms to the chemical description on the label. BAYER CORPORATION MAKES NO OTHER EXPRESS OR IMPLIED WARRANTY, INCLUDING ANY OTHER EXPRESS OR IMPLIED WARRANTY OF FITNESS OR OF MERCHANTABILITY, and no agent of Bayer Corporation is authorized to do so except in writing with a specific reference to this warranty. Any damages arising from a breach of this warranty shall be limited to direct damages and shall not include consequential commercial damages such as loss of profits or values, etc.

Co-Ral is a Reg. TM of the parent company of Bayer Corporation.

SUPPLIED:

Code 13130 — 1.9L (½ gallon)

71131300, R.5

Bayer Corporation, Agriculture Division, Animal Health, Shawnee Mission, Kansas 66201 U.S.A.

Compendium Code No.: 10400171

CO-RAL® PLUS

Insecticide Cattle Ear Tag

Bayer

For Use On Beef And Non-Lactating Dairy Cattle To Control Horn Flies (including pyrethroid-resistant Horn Flies), Gulf Coast Ticks, Spinose Ear Ticks, And As An Aid To Control Face Flies.

Active Ingredients:	Percent By Weight
Coumaphos O, O - diethyl O- (3-chloro-4-methyl-2-oxo-2H-1 benzopyran-7-yl) phosphorothioate	20%
Diazinon O, O - diethyl-O-(2-isopropyl-6-methyl-4-pyrimidinyl)-phosphorothioate	20%
Inert Ingredients	60%
Total	100%

Keep Out of Reach of Children

CAUTION

See Additional Precautionary Statements

PRECAUTIONARY STATEMENTS

HAZARDS TO HUMANS AND DOMESTIC ANIMALS

CAUTION

May be fatal if chewed or swallowed. Harmful if absorbed through skin. Avoid contact with eyes, skin or clothing. Wear nonpermeable protective gloves when applying or removing tags.

User Safety Recommendation: Wash hands before eating, drinking, chewing gum, using tobacco or using the toilet.

FIRST AID

If swallowed: Call poison control center or doctor immediately for treatment advice. Have person sip a glass of water if able to swallow. Do not induce vomiting unless instructed to do so by the poison control center or doctor. Do not give anything by mouth to an unconscious person.

If on skin or clothing: Take off contaminated clothing. Rinse skin immediately with plenty of water for 15-20 minutes. Call poison control center or doctor for treatment advice.

If in eyes: Hold eye open and rinse slowly and gently with water for 15-20 minutes. Remove contact lenses, if present, after the first 5 minutes, then continue rinsing eye. Call a poison control center or doctor for treatment advice.

Note to Physician: This product contains cholinesterase inhibitors. If symptoms of cholinesterase inhibition are present, atropine sulfate, by injection, is antidotal. 2-PAM is also antidotal and may be administered in conjunction with atropine.

Environmental Hazards: This pesticide is toxic to birds, fish and wildlife. Do not apply directly to water. Do not contaminate water when disposing of used tags.

Directions for Use:

It is a violation of Federal law to use this product in a manner inconsistent with its labeling. This labeling must be in the possession of the user at the time of pesticide application.

For the control of Horn Flies (including pyrethroid-resistant Horn Flies), Gulf Coast Ticks and Spinose Ear Ticks on beef and non-lactating dairy cattle and as an aid to control Face Flies.

All mature animals in the herd should be tagged. For adequate control of Horn Flies attach one tag per animal. For optimum control of Horn Flies, Gulf Coast Ticks, and Spinose Ear Ticks, and as an aid in the control of Face Flies, attach one tag to each ear (two per animal). Replace as necessary. Co-Ral® Plus Insecticide Cattle Ear Tags have been proven to be effective against Horn Flies for three to five months.

Apply as indicated (Figures 1-4). Calves less than 3 months of age should not be tagged as ear damage may result. Remove tags at end of fly season or prior to slaughter.

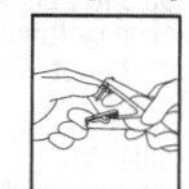

Figure 1

Disinfect pliers prior to use. Place male button onto pin.

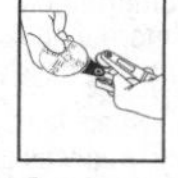

Figure 2

Slide tag under the clip of the pliers by depressing the lever.

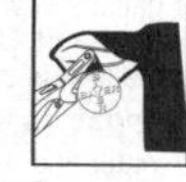

Figure 3

Position tag in the center portion of the front side of the ear.

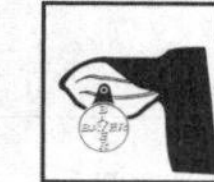

Figure 4

Apply the tag between the second and third rib cartilage.

Continual exposure of Horn Flies to a single class of insecticide (e.g. pyrethroids or organophosphates) may lead to the development of resistance to that class of insecticide. In order to reduce the possibility of Horn Flies developing resistance it is important to rotate the class of insecticide used and/or the method of Horn Fly control on a seasonal basis. Co-Ral® Plus Insecticide Cattle Ear Tags contain the organophosphate insecticides coumaphos and diazinon.

Storage and Disposal:

Do not contaminate water, food or feed by storage or disposal.

Storage: Store in cool place in original container. Opened pouches containing ear tags should be resealed for storage.

Pesticide Disposal: Waste (spent tags) resulting from the use of this product may be disposed of on site or at an approved waste disposal facility.

Container Disposal: Dispose of empty pouch in a sanitary landfill or by incineration, or if allowed by State and local authorities, by burning. If burned stay out of smoke.

LIMITED WARRANTY AND LIMITATION OF DAMAGES

Bayer Corporation, Agriculture Division, Animal Health warrants that this material conforms to the chemical description on the label. BAYER CORPORATION MAKES NO OTHER EXPRESS OR IMPLIED WARRANTY, INCLUDING ANY OTHER EXPRESS OR IMPLIED WARRANTY OF FITNESS OR OF MERCHANTABILITY, and no agent of Bayer Corporation is authorized to do so except in writing with specific reference to this warranty. Any damages arising from a breach of this warranty shall be limited to direct damages and shall not include consequential commercial damages such as loss of profits or values, etc.

EPA Est. No. 4691-KS-01 EPA Reg. No. 11556-123

Supplied: Code 062199—20 tags—13 g Per Tag 77006210, R.0

Manufactured For Bayer Corporation, Agriculture Division, Animal Health, Shawnee Mission, Kansas 66201 U.S.A.

Compendium Code No.: 10400411

CORID® 9.6% ORAL SOLUTION

Merial **Water Medication**

(amprolium) Coccidiostat

NADA No.: 013-149

Active Ingredient(s): CORID® 9.6% Solution contains 9.6% amprolium.

Benzoic acid 0.1% added as preservative.

Indications: An aid in the treatment and prevention of coccidiosis caused by *Eimeria bovis* and *E. zurnii* in calves.

Directions: 1 fl oz = 2 measuring tablespoonfuls; 16 fl oz = 1 pint

In Drinking Water:

Treatment: Add CORID® 9.6% Oral Solution to drinking water at the rate of 16 fl oz/100 gal. At the usual rate of water consumption this will provide an intake of approximately 10 mg amprolium/kg (2.2 lb) body weight. Offer this solution as the only source of water for 5 days.

Use on a herd basis only; when one or more calves show signs of coccidiosis, it is likely that the rest of the group have been exposed, and all calves in the group should be treated.

Prevention: During periods of exposure or when experience indicates that coccidiosis is likely to be a hazard, add CORID® 9.6% Oral Solution to drinking water, at the rate of 8 fl oz/100 gal. At usual rates of water consumption this will provide an intake of approximately 5 mg amprolium/kg (2.2 lb) body weight. Offer this solution as the only source of water for 21 days.

As a Drench:

Treatment: Add 3 fl oz CORID® 9.6% Oral Solution to 1 pt of water and, with a dose syringe, give 1 fl oz of this solution for each 100 lb (45 kg) body weight. This will provide a dose of approximately 10 mg amprolium/kg (2.2 lb) body weight. Give daily for 5 days.

Use on a herd basis only, when one or more calves show signs of coccidiosis, it is likely that the rest of the group have been exposed, and all calves in the group should be treated.

Prevention: During periods of exposure or when experience indicates that coccidiosis is likely to be a hazard, add 1½ fl oz of CORID® 9.6% Oral Solution to 1 pt of water, and with a dose syringe, give 1 fl oz of this solution for each 100 lb (45 kg) body weight. This will provide a dose of approximately 5 mg amprolium/kg (2.2 lb) body weight. Give daily for 21 days.

Note: Make drinking water fresh daily. Drench solutions may be stored in a clean, closed, labeled container for up to 3 days.

Precaution(s): Store at temperatures above 41°F (5°C).

Caution(s): For a satisfactory diagnosis, a microscopic examination of the feces should be done before treatment. When treating outbreaks, drug should be administered promptly after diagnosis is determined.

For oral use in animals only.

Warning(s): Residue Information: Withdraw 24 hours before slaughter. A withdrawal period has not been established for this product in pre-ruminating calves. Do not use in calves to be processed for veal.

Keep this and all drugs out of the reach of children.

May cause eye irritation. For irritation, flush with plenty of water; get medical attention.

Presentation: 4 x 128 fl oz (1 gal) (3.785 L) plastic jugs per case.

CORID is a registered trademark of Merial.

69137601

Compendium Code No.: 11110061

CORID® 20% SOLUBLE POWDER

Merial **Water Medication**

(amprolium) Coccidiostat

NADA No.: 033-165

Active Ingredient(s): CORID® 20% Soluble Powder contains 20% amprolium.

Indications: An aid in the treatment and prevention of bovine coccidiosis caused by *Eimeria bovis* and *E. zurnii* in calves.

Directions: 1 oz = 3½ measuring tablespoonfuls.

In Drinking Water:

Treatment: Add CORID® (amprolium) 20% Soluble Powder to drinking water at the rate of 4 oz/50 gal. For use in automatic water proportioners that meter 1 fl oz of stock solution per gallon of drinking water, add 1 bag (10 oz) in 1 gallon of water to make stock solution. At the usual rate of water consumption this will provide an intake of approximately 10 mg amprolium/kg (2.2 lb) body weight. Offer this solution as the only source of water for 5 days. Use on a herd basis only; when one or more calves show signs of coccidiosis, it is likely that the rest of the group have been exposed, and all calves in the group should be treated.

Prevention: During periods of exposure or when experience indicates that coccidiosis is likely to be a hazard, add CORID® 20% Soluble Powder to drinking water at the rate of 4 oz/100 gal. For use in automatic water proportioners that meter 1 fl oz of stock solution per gallon of drinking water, add ½ bag (5 oz) in 1 gallon of water to make stock solution. At usual rates of water consumption this will provide an intake of approximately 5 mg amprolium/kg (2.2 lb) body weight. Offer this solution as the only source of water for 21 days.

As a Drench:

Treatment: Add 3 oz CORID® 20% Soluble Powder to 1 qt of water and, with a dose syringe, give 1 fl oz of this solution for each 100 lb (45 kg) body weight. This will provide a dose of approximately 10 mg amprolium/kg (2.2 lb) body weight. Give daily for 5 days. Use on a herd basis only; when one or more calves show signs of coccidiosis, it is likely that the rest of the group have been exposed, and all calves in the group should be treated.

Prevention: During periods of exposure or when experience indicates that coccidiosis is likely to be a hazard, add 1½ fl oz of CORID® 20% Soluble Powder to 1 qt of water, and with a dose syringe, give 1 fl oz of this solution for each 100 lb (45 kg) body weight. This will provide a dose of approximately 5 mg amprolium/kg (2.2 lb) body weight. Give daily for 21 days.

Note: Make drinking water fresh daily. Drench solutions or stock solution for proportioners may be stored in a clean, closed, labeled container for up to 3 days.

Caution(s): For a satisfactory diagnosis, a microscopic examination of the feces should be done before treatment. When treating outbreaks, the drug should be administered promptly after diagnosis is determined.

For animal use only.

Warning(s): Withdraw 24 hours before slaughter. A withdrawal period has not been established for this product in pre-ruminating calves. Do not use in calves to be processed for veal.

Keep this and all drugs out of the reach of children.

The Material Safety Data Sheet (MSDS) contains more detailed occupational safety information. To report adverse effects, obtain an MSDS, or for assistance, contact Merial at 1-888-637-4251.

Presentation: 10 oz plastic bags and 24 x 10 oz packets per 15 lb pail.

CORID is a registered trademark of Merial.

(Merial Limited: Registered in England and Wales [Reg. No. 3332751] with registered offices at 27 Knightsbridge, London SW1X 7QT, England and domesticated in Delaware, USA as Merial LLC).

Compendium Code No.: 11110051 668010 / 68413113

CORIUM-20™

Virbac **Otic Cleanser**

Active Ingredient(s): Contains purified water U.S.P., SDA-40B 23%, glycerol triesterfied with fatty acids, glycerine U.S.P., fragrance and B.H.A.

Indications: A nonstinging, nonirritating, alcohol-based cleansing system for use on dogs, cats and horses to remove ear wax and debris.

Dosage and Administration: It is normal for the contents of the bottle to settle. Shake well before using.

Slightly tilt the head and lift the ear flap. Squeeze the bottle to fill the external ear canal. Gently massage the base of the ear. Carefully wipe away any debris in the accessible portion of the ear with a cotton ball or gauze. Allow the pet to shake out any excess liquid and repeat the wiping process. CORIUM-20™ may be used as often as is necessary. Follow professional advice closely.

Precaution(s): Store at room temperature 59°-86°F (15°-30°C).

Caution(s): For external ear canal use only. Do not use if there is a possibility of ear drum damage. Never use instruments like cotton swabs to remove wax from the ear canal.

Keep out of the reach of children. For veterinary use only.

Presentation: 8 fl. oz. (237 mL) and 16 fl.oz. (473 mL) squeezable bottles.

Compendium Code No.: 10230142

CORIUM-Tx™

Virbac **Otic Cleanser**

Anti-Pruritic Ear Cleaner and Treatment with Pramoxine.

Active Ingredient(s): Pramoxine HCl (1%). Also contains: Purified water USP, SDA-40B 23%, glycerol tri-esterfied with fatty acids, glycerine USP, Tween 80, fragrance, B.H.A.

Indications: A non-stinging, non-irritating, alcohol-based cleansing system for use on dogs and cats to remove ear wax and debris

Dosage and Administration: Shake well. Slightly tilt head and lift ear flap. Squeeze bottle to fill the external ear canal. Gently massage the base of the ear. Carefully wipe away any debris in the accessible portion of the ear with a cotton ball or gauze. Allow the pet to shake out any excess liquid and repeat the wiping process. May be used as often as necessary. It is normal for the contents of the bottle to settle.

Caution(s): For external ear canal use only. Do not use if there is a possibility of eardrum damage. Avoid contact with eyes. Keep out of reach of children.

Presentation: 2 fl oz bottle, 12 bottles per inner carton.

Compendium Code No.: 10230150

CORRECTIVE SUSPENSION

Phoenix Pharmaceutical **Antidiarrheal-Adsorbent**

Anti-Diarrheal Suspension

Active Ingredient(s): Contains:

Bismuth Subsalicylate. 1.75%

Indications: For oral administration as an aid in the treatment of noninfectious diarrhea in horses, cattle, dogs and cats.

Dosage and Administration: Shake well before using.

Administration: Oral.

Dosage:

Cattle and Horses: 6-10 oz. every 2 - 3 hours.

Calves and Foals: 3-4 oz. every 2 - 3 hours.

Dogs and Cats: 1-3 tbsp. (½-2 oz.) every 1 - 3 hours.

Precaution(s): Keep from freezing.

Caution(s): If symptoms persist after using the product for 2 to 3 days, consult a veterinarian.

For animal use only.

Not for human use.

Warning(s): Keep this and all medications out of the reach of children.

Presentation: 1 gallon (3.785 L) containers (NDC 57319-393-09).

Compendium Code No.: 12560181 Rev. 4-01

CORTALONE® CREAM ℞

Vedco **Topical Corticosteroid**

Triamcinolone Acetonide Cream USP 0.1%

Active Ingredient(s): CORTALONE® Cream (triamcinoone acetonide cream U.S.P.) provides 1 mg triamcinolone acetonide per gram (0.1%) in a vanishing cream base containing propylene glycol, cetostearyl alcohol (and) ceteareth-20, white petrolatum, sorbitol solution, glyceryl monostearate, polyoxyl 40 stearate, simethicone, sorbic acid and purified water.

Indications: CORTALONE® Cream (triamcinolone acetonide cream U.S.P.) is indicated for topical treatment of allergic dermatitis and summer eczema in dogs.

CORTALONE® Cream is a corticosteroid that provides prompt relief of itching, burning, inflamed skin lesions, by virtue of its anti-inflammatory, antipruritic, and anti-allergic effects.

Dosage and Administration: Apply CORTALONE® Cream (triamcinolone acetonide cream U.S.P.) by rubbing into the affected areas two (2) to four (4) times daily for 4-10 days.

Contraindication(s): CORTALONE® Cream should not be used ophthalmically.

Precaution(s): Store at room temperature; avoid freezing.

Caution(s): Federal law restricts this drug to use by or on the order of a licensed veterinarian.

If local infection exists, suitable concomitant antimicrobial therapy should be administered. If favorable response does not occur promptly, application of CORTALONE® Cream should be discontinued until the infection is adequately controlled by appropriate measures.

CORTALONE® Cream is indicated for use on dogs only. Absorption of triamcinolone acetonide through topical application on the skin and by licking does occur. Therefore, dogs receiving CORTALONE® Cream therapy should be observed closely for signs of polydipsia, polyuria and increased weight gain, particularly when used over large areas or for extended periods of time.

Clinical and experimental data have demonstrated that corticosteroids administered orally or by injection to animals may induce the first stage of parturition if used during the last trimester of pregnancy and may precipitate premature parturition followed by dystocia, fetal death, retained placenta and metritis.

Additionally, corticosteroids administered to dogs, rabbits and rodents during pregnancy have resulted in cleft palate in offspring. Corticosteroids administered to dogs during pregnancy have also resulted in other congenital anomalies including deformed forelegs, phocomelia and anasarca.

For topical use on dogs only.

Warning(s): Do not use CORTALONE® Cream on animals which are raised for food production.

Side Effects: SAP and SGPT (ALT) enzyme elevations, polydipsia and polyuria have occurred following parenteral or systemic use of synthetic corticosteroids in dogs. Vomiting and diarrhea (occasionally bloody) have been observed in dogs.

Cushing's Syndrome in dogs has been reported in association with prolonged or repeated steroid therapy.

Presentation: Available in 7.5 g (NDC 50989-570-66) and 15 g (NDC 50989-570-08) tubes.

Compendium Code No.: 10942190

CORTALONE TABLETS ℞

Vedco — **Corticosteroid-Oral**

Triamcinolone Acetonide

NADA No.: 137-694

Active Ingredient(s): Each tablet contains 0.5 mg or 1.5 mg triamcinolone acetonide.

Indications: Triamcinolone acetonide is a highly potent glucocorticoid effective in the treatment of inflammation and related disorders in dogs and cats. It is indicated in the management and treatment of acute arthritis and allergic and dermatologic disorders.

Dosage and Administration: 0.5 to 1.0 mg per 10 pounds of body weight daily.

Precaution(s): Store at room temperature in a dry place.

Caution(s): Federal law restricts this drug to use by or on the order of a licensed veterinarian.

Warning(s): For oral use in dogs and cats only. For animal use only.

Keep out of reach of children.

For use in animals only.

Presentation: 0.5 mg: 1000 tablets.
1.5 mg: 500 tablets.

Compendium Code No.: 10940380

CORT/ASTRIN SOLUTION

Vedco — **Topical Corticosteroid**

Active Ingredient(s): Each mL contains:

Burow's solution .... 20 mg
Hydrocortisone .... 10 mg

In a water miscible propylene glycol base.

Indications: A topical astringent and anti-inflammatory agent for inflammatory pruritus in small animals.

Dosage and Administration: Apply three (3) to four (4) times a day.

Precaution(s): Store in a cool area.

Caution(s): For topical use only. Not for ophthalmic use.

Not for deep seated infections.

As with any hydrocortisone product, CORT/ASTRIN SOLUTION should not be used in the presence of tuberculosis of the skin.

Presentation: 1 oz. dropper bottles and 16 oz. bottles.

Compendium Code No.: 10940371

CORTICALM™ LOTION ℞

DVM — **Topical Corticosteroid**

Topical Antipruritic Formulation

Active Ingredient(s): Hydrocortisone USP 1%.

Product Description: CORTICALM™ Lotion is a rapidly penetrating topical medication containing 1% hydrocortisone in a clear, non-greasy, non-staining lotion vehicle. Formulated with Lubrasil®, CORTICALM™ Lotion provides enhanced coat manageability, making it ideal for broad area application.

Indications: Reduces itching and further trauma from habitual scratching and biting.

Directions for Use: Apply directly onto affected area(s) 2-3 times daily, or as directed by veterinarian. May also be effectively used following a bath (after towel drying).

Precaution(s): Store at room temperature.

Caution(s): Federal law restricts this drug to use by, or on the order of, a licensed veterinarian.

For external use only. Avoid contact with eyes. If contact occurs, rinse thoroughly with water. Consult veterinarian if swelling, redness and irritation persist after seven (7) days of treatment.

Clinical and experimental data have demonstrated that corticosteroid administered orally or by injection to animals may induce serious adverse reactions. This product should not be used during pregnancy. People handling these medications should wear gloves to prevent exposure and toxic effects.

Warning(s): Not for use in animals intended for food. Keep out of reach of children.

Presentation: 3 fl oz (88 mL) (NDC 47203-810-03) and 6 fl oz (177 mL) (NDC 47203-810-06).

Compendium Code No.: 11420161 — Rev 0199

CORTI-DERM™ CREAM

First Priority — **Topical Corticosteroid**

Zinc Oxide and Hydrocortisone

Active Ingredient(s):

Hydrocortisone 1.0%
Zinc Oxide 40.0%

Other Ingredients: BHA, cod liver oil, lanolin, methylparaben, petrolatum, talc, fragrance.

Indications: Aids in the treatment of minor skin irritations.

Directions for Use: Apply to affected areas as needed.

Precaution(s): Storage: Store at controlled room temperature between 15°-30°C (59°-86°F). Keep container tightly closed when not in use.

Caution(s): Do not use in the eyes or nose. Not for prolonged use. Do not apply to large areas of the body. Do not use where infection is present, since the drug may allow infection to be spread. If redness, irritation or swelling persists or increases, discontinue use and consult a veterinarian.

For animal use only.

Warning(s): Not for use on animals intended as food.

Keep out of reach of children.

Presentation: 1 lb (453.6 g) (NDC# 58829-250-16).

Compendium Code No.: 11390162 — 07-01

CORTI-DERM™ SOLUTION

First Priority — **Topical Corticosteroid**

Topical Treatment

Active Ingredient(s):

Hydrocortisone 1%
Burow's Solution 2%

In a water miscible base containing Propylene Glycol.

Indications: Topical treatment for the relief of discomfort caused by inflammatory pruritis in dogs.

Hydrocortisone is an anti-inflammatory and anti-pruritic agent.

Burow's Solution is used as an astringent for drying of moist dermatitis. It provides cooling relief for discomfort.

Dosage and Administration: Apply 3 to 4 times daily.

Contraindication(s): As with any topical hydrocortisone product CORTI-DERM™ should not be used in the presence of tuberculosis of the skin.

Precaution(s): Storage: Store at controlled room temperature 15° to 30°C (59° to 86°F). Keep container tightly closed when not in use.

Caution(s): For topical use only. Not intended for deep-seated infections. Not for use in the eyes.

For animal use only.

Warning(s): Keep out of reach of children.

Presentation: 1 fl oz (30 mL) (NDC# 58829-160-10), 2 fl oz (60 mL) (NDC# 58829-160-02), 4 fl oz (120 mL) (NDC# 58829-160-04) and 16 fl oz (473 mL) (NDC# 58829-160-16).

Compendium Code No.: 11390173 — Iss. 7-99 / Iss. 4-99 / Iss. 6-98 / Rev. 07-01

CORTISOOTHE™ SHAMPOO ℞

Virbac — **Antidermatosis Shampoo**

NDC No.: 51311-016-06

Active Ingredient(s): Hydrocortisone 1% (10 mg/mL) in a soothing emollient oatmeal shampoo vehicle.

Indications: For the temporary relief of inflammation and pruritus associated with corticosteroid-responsive canine dermatoses.

Dosage and Administration: Shake well before using. Apply to a wet coat. Rub into the skin and coat. Lather well. Wait 5-10 minutes and rinse well. May be used once a day or as directed by a veterinarian.

Caution(s): Federal law (USA) restricts this drug to use by or on the order of a licensed veterinarian.

Keep out of the reach of children.

For external use only on dogs and cats. Avoid contact with the eyes or mucous membranes. Wash hands after using.

Presentation: Available in 8 fl. oz. (237 mL) and 16 fl. oz. (473 mL) containers.

Compendium Code No.: 10230161

CORTISPRAY® ℞

DVM — **Topical Corticosteroid**

Therapeutic Spray-Hydrocortisone-Topical Antipruritic Formulation

Active Ingredient(s): Hydrocortisone 1%.

CORTISPRAY® contains hydrocortisone in an astringent solution. Colorless, non-greasy and non-staining.

Indications: Reduces itching and further trauma from continual biting and scratching.

For topical use only on dogs, cats and horses.

Directions for Use: Spray directly onto affected area(s) 2-3 times daily, or as directed by a veterinarian.

Precaution(s): Store at room temperature.

Caution(s): Federal law restricts this drug to use by, or on the order of, a licensed veterinarian.

Avoid contact with eyes. If contact occurs, rinse thoroughly with water. If irritation develops, discontinue and consult veterinarian.

Clinical and experimental data have demonstrated that corticosteroid administered orally or by injection to animals may induce serious adverse reaction. This product should not be used during pregnancy. People handling these medications should wear gloves to prevent exposure and toxic effects.

Warning(s): Not for use in animals intended for food. Keep out of reach of children.

Presentation: 2 fl oz (60 mL) (NDC 47203-800-02).

Compendium Code No.: 11420171 — Rev 0199

CORVAC-3®

Intervet — **Bacterin**

Haemophilus Paragallinarum Bacterin

U.S. Vet. Lic. No.: 286

Description: CORVAC-3® is prepared from three inactivated strains of *Haemophilus paragallinarum* belonging to serotypes A, B and C (Page classification scheme), and suspended in the aqueous phase of an oil adjuvant emulsion.

Quality tested for purity, potency and safety.

Indications: CORVAC-3® is indicated for the vaccination of chickens against *Haemophilus paragallinarum* infection (coryza). Chickens should be in good health when vaccinated. Sick or weak chickens will not develop adequate immunity.

Dosage and Administration: Before use, CORVAC-3® must reach ambient temperature 21-27°C (70-80°F) naturally. Shake vigorously before and periodically during use. Inject 0.5 mL subcutaneously in the back of the neck midway between the head and the body in a direction away from the head using an 18 gauge needle.

Vaccination Program: CORVAC-3® should be used for the initial vaccination of chickens against *Haemophilus paragallinarum.* The first vaccination should be administered to healthy chickens at least 5 weeks of age. A second vaccination is recommended at least 4 weeks following initial vaccination and 3-4 weeks prior to the onset of lay.

Immunity: Chickens administered two doses of CORVAC-3® with the second dose given a few weeks prior to the onset of lay will achieve a protective level of immunity during the laying period with only small variations between individual chickens.

Vaccination Reaction: Clinical reactions may occur as a result of transient swelling in the neck region following vaccination. These reactions may be aggravated by improper vaccination technique. If shock is observed, this must usually be ascribed to stress by handling.

Records: Keep a record of bacterin, quantity, serial number, expiration date and place of purchase; the date and time of vaccination; the number, age, breed and locations of chickens; names of operators performing the vaccination and any observed reactions.

Precaution(s): Storage Conditions: Store in the dark in a refrigerator between 2 and 7°C (35 and 45°F). Do not freeze.

Before use, the bacterin much reach ambient temperature 21-27°C (70-80°F) naturally.

Do not mix this bacterin with any other substances.

Use entire contents when first opened.

Avoid exposure of this bacterin to sunlight.

Do not expose this bacterin to microwave radiation, boiling water, extensive heat, or any other similar physical processes.

This product is non-returnable.

Caution(s): Vaccinate only healthy birds. Although disease may not be evident, concurrent disease conditions may cause complications and/or reduce immunity.

Ensure that vaccination equipment is clean and sterile before use.

Do not use vaccination equipment with rubber parts, as the oil emulsion may attack certain types of rubber.

Do not inject this bacterin by the intramuscular route.

Do not use less than one dose per bird per vaccination.

The use of any bacterin may cause false-positive results on Mycoplasma plate tests. Avoid such testing prior to 10 weeks post-vaccination.

For veterinary use only.

Notice: This bacterin has undergone rigid potency, safety and purity tests, and meets Intervet Inc. and USDA requirements. It is designed to stimulate effective immunity when used as directed, but the user must be advised that the response to the product depends upon many factors, including, but no limited to, conditions of storage and handling by the user, administration of the bacterin, health and responsiveness of the individual chickens, and the degree of field exposure. Therefore, directions should be followed carefully.

This product is not hazardous when used according to directions supplied. A material safety data sheet (MSDS) is available upon request. This and any other consumer information can be obtained by calling Intervet Customer Service at 1-800-441-8272 or 1-302-934-8051.

The use of this bacterin is subject to applicable local and federal laws and regulations.

Use only as directed.

Warning(s): Do not vaccinate chickens within 42 days of slaughter.

Do not administer this bacterin during the critical egg-laying period from the onset of lay until after peak production. Administration of the product during the laying period may result in a drop in egg production.

To avoid human injection, extreme caution should be used when injecting any oil emulsion vaccine. Accidental human injection may cause serious local reactions. Contact a physician immediately if accidental human injection occurs.

Presentation: 1,000 doses (500 mL).

Compendium Code No.: 11060391 Intervet 12205 AL 146

COTHIVET®

Neogen **Topical Wound Dressing**

89.5% Hydrocotyle Tincture Topical Spray

Active Ingredient(s):

Hydrocotyl tincture 89.5%

Also contains the following ingredients: Horse chestnut tincture, rosemary volatile oil, cypress volatile oil, thyme volatile oil, lavender volatile oil, foenugreek tincture, carlina tincture.

Indications: Aids in healing of sores and wounds in horses, dogs and cats. Helps in keratinization of the hoof in horses.

Directions for Use: Spray COTHIVET® on wounds 3-4 times daily. Repeat until complete healing.

Precaution(s): Product is flammable.

Note: Keep away from open flame or sparks.

Caution(s): Use with extreme care around the head to prevent spraying into the eyes.

For veterinary use only.

Warning(s): Keep out of the reach of children.

Warning(s): The product is not to be administered to horses that are to be slaughtered for use in food.

Presentation: 30 mL containers (NDC: 59051-8888-0).

Manufactured by: Vetoquinol SA.

Compendium Code No.: 14910221

COUGHGUARD® B

Pfizer Animal Health **Bacterin**

Bordetella Bronchiseptica Bacterin

U.S. Vet. Lic. No.: 189

Description: The bacterin contains an inactivated culture of this pathogen.

Indications: COUGHGUARD® B is for vaccination of healthy dogs as an aid in the control of infectious tracheobronchitis ("kennel cough") caused by *Bordetella bronchiseptica*.

Directions:

1. General Directions: Vaccination of healthy dogs is recommended. Shake well. Aseptically administer 1 mL intramuscularly or subcutaneously.
2. Primary Vaccination: Healthy dogs should receive 2 doses administered 2-4 weeks apart. If dogs are vaccinated before the age of 4 months, they should be revaccinated with a single dose upon reaching 4 months of age. (Maternal antibodies may interfere with development of an adequate immune response in puppies less than 4 months old.)
3. Revaccination: Annual revaccination with a single dose is recommended. Where exposure is likely, such as breeding, boarding, and showing situations, additional boosters are indicated or annual revaccination could be timed 2-4 weeks prior to these events.

Precaution(s): Store at 2°-7°C. Prolonged exposure to higher temperatures may adversely affect potency. Do not freeze.

Use entire contents when first opened.

Caution(s): Intramuscular vaccination is recommended to avoid petite nodules which may occur if given subcutaneously.

As with many vaccines, anaphylaxis may occur after use. Initial antidote of epinephrine is recommended and should be followed with appropriate supportive therapy.

This product has been shown to be efficacious in healthy animals. A protective immune response may not be elicited if animals are incubating an infectious disease, are malnourished or parasitized, are stressed due to shipment or environmental conditions, are otherwise immunocompromised, or the vaccine is not administered in accordance with label directions.

For use in dogs only.

For veterinary use only.

Discussion: Disease Description: Although there is no single cause for kennel cough, *B. bronchiseptica* is a primary etiological agent in the kennel cough complex.[1,2] This pathogen predisposes dogs to the influence of other respiratory agents and frequently exists concurrently with them. Kennel cough can be reproduced by challenge with virulent *B. bronchiseptica*. Further, environmental factors such as cold, drafts, and high humidity—often typical conditions in dog kennels—increase susceptibility to the disease.[3] Antibiotics are generally recognized as poor agents to treat the primary disease.[3] In contrast, immunoprophylaxis for *B. bronchiseptica* provides an effective means to aid in the control of disease.

The outstanding sign of *B. bronchiseptica* infection is a harsh, dry cough which is aggravated by activity or excitement. The coughing occurs in paroxysms, followed by retching or gagging in attempts to clear small amounts of mucus from the throat. Body temperature may be elevated as secondary bacterial invasion takes place.

Because kennel cough is highly contagious, the disease can readily be transmitted to susceptible dogs and produce a severe cough. The most severe signs are noted beginning 2-5 days after infection, but can continue for extended periods. Stress, particularly due to adverse environmental conditions, may cause relapse during later stages of the disease.

Trial Data: Safety and Efficacy: COUGHGUARD® B is prepared from a highly antigenic strain of *B. bronchiseptica* which has been inactivated and processed to be nontoxic when administered to dogs. The production method leaves the immunogenic properties of *B. bronchiseptica* intact. Historically, *Bordetella* bacterins have had a tendency toward toxic reactions characterized by lethargy, anorexia, and vomiting 1-6 hours after administration; however, COUGHGUARD® B is safe and effective. In an extensive field trial in which over 1,000 doses of COUGHGUARD® B were administered, no reports of these reactions were received.

In tests conducted with normal, susceptible dogs under controlled conditions, experimental infection with the virulent BC strain of *B. bronchiseptica* consistently resulted in coughing and other respiratory signs typical of kennel cough.

In the usual research model, palpation of the throat is necessary to produce coughing. Due to the severity of the challenge in the test, coughing was spontaneous for extended periods beginning 2-5 days after challenge. (Data on file, Pfizer Animal Health.)

Clinical signs of coughing were significantly ($p \leq 0.05$) reduced when vaccinates were experimentally exposed to the virulent BC strain of *B. bronchiseptica* (Table 1).

Table 1. Reduction in coughing associated with experimental challenge exposure of dogs with the virulent BC strain of *B. bronchiseptica*

Treatment	Total No. of Dogs	Mean Percent (%) Cough Reduction*
Vaccinated	548	77±12**
Nonvaccinated Control	233	—

*Results of 89 efficacy tests ranged from 50% (minimum) to 96% (maximum) cough reduction in vaccinates

**Standard deviation

References: Available upon request.

Presentation: 50 x 1 dose vials.

Compendium Code No.: 36901830 75-4277-05

COUGHGUARD® CPI/B

Pfizer Animal Health **Bacterin-Vaccine**

Canine Parainfluenza Vaccine, Modified Live Virus-Bordetella Bronchiseptica Bacterin

U.S. Vet. Lic. No.: 189

Description: The vaccine component of COUGHGUARD® CPI/B contains an attenuated strain of CPI virus propagated on an established canine cell line. The vaccine is packaged in freeze-dried form with inert gas in place of vacuum. The bacterin component, containing inactivated whole cultures of *B. bronchiseptica*, is supplied as diluent.

Contains penicillin and streptomycin as preservatives.

Indications: COUGHGUARD® CPI/B is for vaccination of healthy dogs as an aid in the prevention and control of canine parainfluenza caused by canine parainfluenza (CPI) virus and infectious tracheobronchitis ("kennel cough") caused by *Bordetella bronchiseptica*.

Directions:

1. General Directions: Vaccination of healthy dogs is recommended. Aseptically rehydrate the freeze-dried vaccine (Vanguard® CPI) with the liquid bacterin provided (Coughguard® B), shake well, and administer 1 mL subcutaneously or intramuscularly.
2. Primary Vaccination: Healthy dogs should receive 2 doses administered 2-4 weeks apart. If dogs are vaccinated before the age of 4 months, they should be revaccinated with a single dose upon reaching 4 months of age. (Maternal antibodies may interfere with development of an adequate immune response in puppies less than 4 months old.) Where *B. bronchiseptica* and canine virus exposure is likely, such as breeding, boarding, and showing situations, an additional booster may be indicated or annual revaccination should be timed 2-4 weeks prior to these events.
3. Revaccination: Annual revaccination with a single dose is recommended.

Precaution(s): Store at 2°-7°C. Prolonged exposure to higher temperatures and/or direct sunlight may adversely affect potency. Do not freeze.

Use entire contents when first opened.

Sterilized syringes and needles should be used to administer this vaccine. Do not sterilize with chemicals because traces of disinfectant may inactivate the vaccine.

Burn containers and all unused contents.

Caution(s): Vaccination of pregnant bitches should be avoided.

Although the *Bordetella* fraction of COUGHGUARD® CPI/B has been specifically designed to be nontoxic, a small, nonirritating, sterile nodule may appear in some puppies after subcutaneous inoculation. For puppies, therefore, intramuscular vaccination may be advisable. Stinging has been reported in up to 10% of dogs vaccinated intramuscularly.

As with many vaccines, anaphylaxis may occur after use. Initial antidote of epinephrine is recommended and should be followed with appropriate supportive therapy.

This product has been shown to be efficacious in healthy animals. A protective immune response may not be elicited if animals are incubating an infectious disease, are malnourished or parasitized, are stressed due to shipment or environmental conditions, are otherwise immunocompromised, or the vaccine is not administered in accordance with label directions.

For use in dogs only

For veterinary use only

Discussion: Disease Description: CPI is a common viral upper respiratory disease. Uncomplicated CPI may be mild or subclinical, with signs becoming more severe if concurrent infection with other respiratory pathogens exists. Although there is no single cause for kennel cough, *B. bronchiseptica* is a primary etiological agent in the kennel cough complex.[1,2] The outstanding sign of *B. bronchiseptica* infection is a harsh, dry cough which is aggravated by activity or excitement. The coughing occurs in paroxysms, followed by retching or gagging in attempts to clear small amounts of mucus from the throat. Body temperature may be elevated as secondary bacterial invasion takes place. Antibiotics are generally recognized as poor agents to treat the primary disease. In contrast, immunoprophylaxis for *B. bronchiseptica* provides an effective means to aid in the control of the disease.[3]

Trial Data: Safety and Efficacy: Laboratory evaluation demonstrated that COUGHGUARD® CPI/B aided in preventing disease caused by CPI and *B. bronchiseptica,* and that no immunologic interference existed between the vaccine fractions.

The *B. bronchiseptica* fraction in COUGHGUARD® CPI/B is prepared from a highly antigenic strain which has been inactivated and processed to be nontoxic when administered to dogs. Historically, *Bordetella* bacterins have had a tendency toward toxic reactions characterized by lethargy, anorexia, and vomiting 1-6 hours after administration; however, the *B. bronchiseptica* fraction is safe and effective. In an extensive field trial in which over 3,268 doses of the *B. bronchiseptica* fraction were administered, no reports of these reactions were received.

When the fractions of COUGHGUARD® CPI/B were administered subcutaneously to adult dogs, serious reactions to the *B. bronchiseptica* fraction were not noted. In puppies, however, petite nodules developed. These were nonirritating, sterile, and transitory in nature. This mild reaction was not observed in puppies when COUGHGUARD® CPI/B was administered by the intramuscular route. A postvaccinal sting has been reported in less than 10% of dogs vaccinated intramuscularly.

In tests conducted with normal, susceptible dogs under controlled conditions, experimental infection with the virulent BC strain of *B. bronchiseptica* resulted in coughing and other respiratory signs typical of kennel cough. In the usual research model, palpation of the throat is necessary to produce coughing. Due to the severity of the challenge in the test, coughing was spontaneous for extended periods beginning 2-5 days after challenge. (Data on file, Pfizer Animal Health.)

Clinical signs of coughing were significantly (p = 0.05) reduced when vaccinates were experimentally exposed to the virulent BC strain of *B. bronchiseptica* (Table 1).

Table 1. Reduction in coughing associated with experimental challenge exposure of dogs with the virulent BC strain of *B. bronchiseptica*.

Treatment	Mean Percent (%)	
	Total No. of Dogs	Cough Reduction*
Vaccinated	548	77±12**
Nonvaccinated control	233	—

*Results of 89 efficacy tests ranged from 50% (minimum) to 96% (maximum) cough reduction in vaccinates

**Standard deviation

References: Available upon request.

Presentation: 25 x 1 dose vials.

U.S. Patent No. 3,616,203

Compendium Code No.: 36901841 75-5311-00

COUGH SYRUP

Life Science **Antitussive**

Active Ingredient(s): Each fluid ounce contains:

Guaifenesin .... 8 g
Ammonium chloride .... 8 g
Sodium citrate .... 8 g
Pyrilamine maleate .... 50 mg
Phenylephrine hydrochloride .... 50 mg

In a flavored syrup base.

Indications: A decongestant, expectorant, and antihistamine for use as an aid in the relief of cough symptoms related to upper respiratory conditions.

Dosage and Administration: Administer orally.

Horses: Two (2) to four (4) ounces.

Dogs and Cats: One (1) to two (2) teaspoonfuls depending on the size of the animal.

Repeat every two (2) hours if necessary.

Caution(s): For animal use only.

Not for human use.

Keep out of the reach of children.

Warning(s): Not for use in food producing animals.

Presentation: 1 pint (16 fl oz), 1 quart (32 fl oz) and 1 gallon (128 fl oz) containers.

Compendium Code No.: 10870001

COUGH TABLETS

Life Science **Antitussive**

Active Ingredient(s):

Guaifenesin .... 100 mg
Dextromethorphan hydrobromide .... 10 mg

Indications: An expectorant, antitussive and cough suppressant for the temporary relief of cough symptoms in dogs and cats.

Dosage and Administration:

Small Dogs and Cats: One-half (½) tablet; repeat in four (4) hours.

Large Dogs: One (1) tablet every four (4) hours.

Caution(s): If the animal's cough is persistent or a chronic cough is accompanied by excessive secretions, prolonged depression or fever, consult a veterinarian.

Keep out of the reach of children.

For animal use only.

Presentation: Bottles of 250 and 1,000 tablets.

Compendium Code No.: 10870010

COVERT™ 5

AgriPharm **Vaccine**

Bovine Rhinotracheitis-Virus Diarrhea-Parinfluenza$_3$-Respiratory Syncytial Virus Vaccine, Modified Live Virus

U.S. Vet. Lic. No.: 124

Contents: This product contains the antigens listed above.

Preservative: Neomycin.

Indications: Recommended for the vaccination of healthy, susceptible cattle as an aid in the reduction of diseases caused by Bovine Rhinotracheitis (IBR) virus, Bovine Virus Diarrhea (BVD) Types 1 and 2, Parainfluenza$_3$ (PI$_3$), and Bovine Respiratory Syncytial Virus (BRSV).

Directions: Rehydrate the modified live virus vaccine by aseptically adding the accompanying liquid diluent to the vaccine vial. Shake well and use immediately.

Dosage: Using aseptic technique, inject 2 mL either intramuscularly or subcutaneously. If using subcutaneous route, inject in front of the shoulder and midway of the neck, away from the suprascapular lymph node. If initial vaccination, repeat the BRSV fraction in 14 to 28 days. Calves vaccinated before 6 months of age should be revaccinated at 6 months. A 2 mL booster dose is recommended annually.

Precaution(s): Store out of direct sunlight at a temperature between 35-45°F (2-7°C). Avoid freezing. Use entire contents when first opened. Burn containers and all unused contents.

Caution(s): Stressed cattle should not be vaccinated. Do not use in pregnant cows or in calves nursing pregnant cows. Injection site swelling may occur. Anaphylactoid reactions may occur.

Note: It is possible that healthy appearing cattle can be persistently infected with or incubating virulent BVD virus at time of vaccination. In view of these findings and suggested causes, BVD vaccine is contraindicated in persistently infected cattle and use should be limited only to healthy, immunocompetent, unstressed, non-pregnant cattle.

Antidote(s): Epinephrine.

Warning(s): Do not vaccinate within 21 days before slaughter.

Animal inoculation only. Accidental injection to humans can cause serious local reactions. Contact a physician immediately if accidental injection occurs.

Presentation: 10 doses (20 mL) and 50 doses (100 mL).

Manufactured by: Boehringer Ingelheim Vetmedica, Inc. St. Joseph, MO 64506, U.S.A.

Compendium Code No.: 14571160 26316-00

COVERT™ 5-HS

AgriPharm **Bacterin-Vaccine**

Bovine Rhinotracheitis-Virus Diarrhea-Parinfluenza$_3$-Respiratory Syncytial Virus Vaccine, Modified Live Virus-Haemophilus Somnus Bacterin

U.S. Vet. Lic. No.: 124

Contents: This product contains the antigens listed above.

Preservative: Neomycin.

Indications: Recommended for the vaccination of healthy, susceptible cattle as an aid in the reduction of diseases caused by Bovine Rhinotracheitis (IBR) virus, Bovine Virus Diarrhea (BVD) Types 1 and 2, Parainfluenza$_3$ (PI$_3$), Bovine Respiratory Syncytial Virus (BRSV), and for the prevention of disease caused by *Haemophilus somnus.*

Directions: Rehydrate the modified live virus vaccine by aseptically adding the accompanying liquid bacterin to the vaccine vial. Shake well and use immediately.

Dosage: Using aseptic technique, inject 2 mL either intramuscularly or subcutaneously. If using subcutaneous route, inject in front of the shoulder and midway of the neck, away from the suprascapular lymph node. If initial vaccination, repeat the BRSV and *H. somnus* fractions in 14 to 28 days. Calves vaccinated before 6 months of age should be revaccinated at 6 months. A 2 mL booster dose is recommended annually.

Precaution(s): Store out of direct sunlight at a temperature between 35-45°F (2-7°C). Avoid freezing. Use entire contents when first opened. Burn containers and all unused contents.

Caution(s): Stressed cattle should not be vaccinated. Do not use in pregnant cows or in calves nursing pregnant cows. Injection site swelling may occur. Anaphylactoid reactions may occur.

Note: It is possible that healthy appearing cattle can be persistently infected with or incubating virulent BVD virus at time of vaccination. In view of these findings and suggested causes, BVD vaccine is contraindicated in persistently infected cattle and use should be limited only to healthy, immunocompetent, unstressed, non-pregnant cattle.

Antidote(s): Epinephrine.

Warning(s): Do not vaccinate within 21 days before slaughter.

Animal inoculation only. Accidental injection to humans can cause serious local reactions. Contact a physician immediately if accidental injection occurs.

Presentation: 10 doses (20 mL) and 50 doses (100 mL).

Manufactured by: Boehringer Ingelheim Vetmedica, Inc. St. Joseph, MO 64506, U.S.A.

Compendium Code No.: 14571170 26408-00

COVERT™ 10

AgriPharm **Bacterin-Vaccine**

Bovine Rhinotracheitis-Virus Diarrhea-Parinfluenza$_3$-Respiratory Syncytial Virus Vaccine, Modified Live Virus-Leptospira Canicola-Grippotyphosa-Hardjo-Icterohaemorrhagiae-Pomona Bacterin

U.S. Vet. Lic. No.: 124

Contents: This product contains the antigens listed above.

Preservatives: The vaccine fraction contains neomycin as a preservative. The bacterin fraction contains gentamicin and Amphotericin B.

Indications: Recommended for the vaccination of healthy, susceptible cattle as an aid in the reduction of diseases caused by Bovine Rhinotracheitis (IBR) virus, Bovine Virus Diarrhea (BVD) Types 1 and 2, Parainfluenza$_3$ (PI$_3$), Bovine Respiratory Syncytial Virus (BRSV), *Leptospira canicola, L. grippotyphosa, L. hardjo, L. icterohaemorrhagiae,* and *L. pomona.*

Directions: Rehydrate the modified live virus vaccine by aseptically adding the accompanying liquid bottle of liquid bacterin to the vaccine vial. Shake well and use immediately.

Dosage: Using aseptic technique, inject 2 mL intramuscularly. Repeat in 14 to 28 days and once annually. Calves vaccinated before 6 months of age should be revaccinated at 6 months. A 2 mL booster dose is recommended prior to time of stress or exposure.

Precaution(s): Store out of direct sunlight at a temperature between 35-45°F (2-7°C). Avoid freezing. Use entire contents when first opened. Burn containers and all unused contents.

Caution(s): Stressed cattle should not be vaccinated. Do not use in pregnant cows or in calves nursing pregnant cows. Injection site swelling may occur. Anaphylactoid reactions may occur.

Note: It is possible that healthy appearing cattle can be persistently infected with or incubating virulent BVD virus at time of vaccination. In view of these findings and suggested causes, BVD vaccine is contraindicated in persistently infected cattle and use should be limited only to healthy, immunocompetent, unstressed, non-pregnant cattle.

Antidote(s): Epinephrine.
Warning(s): Do not vaccinate within 21 days before slaughter.
Animal inoculation only. Accidental injection to humans can cause serious local reactions. Contact a physician immediately if accidental injection occurs.
Presentation: 5 doses (10 mL), 10 doses (20 mL) and 50 doses (100 mL).
Manufactured by: Boehringer Ingelheim Vetmedica, Inc. St. Joseph, MO 64506, U.S.A.
Compendium Code No.: 14571181 27408-00

COVERT™ 10-HS

AgriPharm **Bacterin-Vaccine**

Bovine Rhinotracheitis-Virus Diarrhea-Parinfluenza$_3$-Respiratory Syncytial Virus Vaccine, Modified Live Virus-Haemophilus Somnus-Leptospira Canicola-Grippotyphosa-Hardjo-Icterohaemorrhagiae-Pomona Bacterin
U.S. Vet. Lic. No.: 124
Contents: This product contains the antigens listed above.
Preservative: Neomycin.
Indications: Recommended for the vaccination of healthy, susceptible cattle as an aid in the reduction of diseases caused by Bovine Rhinotracheitis (IBR) virus, Bovine Virus Diarrhea (BVD) Types 1 and 2, Parainfluenza$_3$ (PI$_3$), Bovine Respiratory Syncytial Virus (BRSV), *Leptospira canicola, L. grippotyphosa, L. hardjo, L. icterohaemorrhagiae,* and *L. pomona* and for the prevention of disease caused by *Haemophilus somnus.*
Directions: Rehydrate the modified live virus vaccine by aseptically adding the accompanying liquid bottle of liquid bacterin.
Dosage: Using aseptic technique, inject 2 mL intramuscularly. Repeat in 14 to 28 days and once annually. Calves vaccinated before 6 months of age should be revaccinated at 6 months. A 2 mL booster dose is recommended prior to time of stress or exposure.
Precaution(s): Store out of direct sunlight at a temperature between 35-45°F (2-7°C). Avoid freezing. Shake well before using. Use entire contents when first opened. Burn containers and all unused contents.
Caution(s): Stressed cattle should not be vaccinated. Do not use in pregnant cows or in calves nursing pregnant cows. Injection site swelling may occur. Anaphylactoid reactions may occur.
Note: It is possible that healthy appearing cattle can be persistently infected with or incubating virulent BVD virus at time of vaccination. In view of these findings and suggested causes, BVD vaccine is contraindicated in persistently infected cattle and use should be limited only to healthy, immunocompetent, unstressed, non-pregnant cattle.
Antidote(s): Epinephrine.
Warning(s): Do not vaccinate within 21 days before slaughter.
Animal inoculation only. Accidental injection to humans can cause serious local reactions. Contact a physician immediately if accidental injection occurs.
Presentation: 5 doses (10 mL), 10 doses (20 mL) and 50 doses (100 mL).
Manufactured by: Boehringer Ingelheim Vetmedica, Inc. St. Joseph, MO 64506, U.S.A.
Compendium Code No.: 14571191 27509-00

COVEXIN® 8 VACCINE

Schering-Plough **Bacterin-Toxoid**

Clostridium chauvoei-septicum-haemolyticum-novyi-tetani-perfringens Types C & D Bacterin-Toxoid
U.S. Vet. Lic. No.: 107
Active Ingredient(s): A formalin-inactivated, alum-precipitated bacterin-toxoid prepared from highly toxigenic cultures and culture filtrates of *Clostridium chauvoei, Cl. septicum, Cl. haemolyticum* (known elsewhere as *Cl. novyi* type D), *Cl. novyi, Cl. tetani,* and *Cl. perfringens* types C and D. COVEXIN® 8 is an Electroferm® product produced by an electronically controlled deep culture process.
The specific toxoids and/or cellular antigens required for optimal disease protection are emphasized in the growth of Electroferm® cultures. These cultures are highly concentrated and, when divided for the blending of combination vaccines, make possible the production of the low volume dose. Exacting procedures are employed to ensure that each dose of combination vaccine contains an appropriate amount of each component.
All components of each serial of the final product are tested for potency using USDA-accepted laboratory and/or host animal tests.
Indications: For the active immunization of healthy sheep against diseases caused by *Clostridium chauvoei, Cl. septicum, Cl. haemolyticum* (known elsewhere as *Cl. novyi* type D), *Cl. novyi, Cl. tetani,* and *Cl. perfringens* types C and D.
Although *Cl. perfringens* type B is not a significant problem in the U.S.A., immunity may be provided against the beta and epsilon toxins elaborated by *Cl. perfringens* type B. The immunity is derived from the combination of type C (beta) and type D (epsilon) fractions.
Dosage and Administration: Shake well. Using aseptic technique, inject 5 mL subcutaneously followed by a 2 mL dose in six (6) weeks. Revaccinate annually with 2 mL prior to periods of extreme risk, or parturition. For *Cl. novyi* and *Cl. haemolyticum,* revaccinate every five (5) to six (6) months. Vaccination should be scheduled so that pregnant ewes receive their second vaccination or annual booster two (2) to six (6) weeks before lambing commences in the flock. Lambs should be given their primary course beginning at 10 to 12 weeks of age.
Precaution(s): Store at 35°-45°F (2°-7°C). Protect from freezing.
This product has been tested under laboratory conditions and has met all federal standards for safety and ability to immunize normal healthy animals. The level of performance may be affected by conditions of use such as stress, weather, nutrition, disease, parasitism, other treatments, individual idiosyncrasies or impaired immunological competency. These factors should be considered by the user when evaluating product performance or freedom from reactions.
Caution(s): Use the entire contents when first opened.
Anaphylactic reactions may occur following use.
Antidote(s): Epinephrine.
Warning(s): Do not vaccinate within 21 days before slaughter.
Discussion: The protective value of all components of COVEXIN® 8 has been demonstrated through the most critical test procedures available. Vaccinated sheep withstood the challenge of massive doses of virulent live spores of *Cl. chauvoei, Cl. septicum, Cl. tetani, Cl. novyi* types B and D. *Cl. perfringens* types C and D, for which no host animal direct-challenge test exists, were evaluated by measuring the amount of antitoxin produced by cattle, sheep and laboratory animals.
Presentation: 50 mL and 250 mL vials.
COVEXIN 8 and Electroferm are registered trademarks of Schering-Plough Animal Health Corporation.
Compendium Code No.: 10470330

COW-VAC® 9

Aspen **Bacterin-Vaccine**

Bovine Rhinotracheitis-Virus Diarrhea-Parainfluenza$_3$ Vaccine, Modified Live Virus-Campylobacter fetus-Leptospira canicola-grippotyphosa-hardjo-icterohaemorrhagiae-pomona Bacterin
U.S. Vet. Lic. No.: 272
Active Ingredient(s): Bovine rhinotracheitis, virus diarrhea, parainfluenza-3 modified live virus vaccine, *Campylobacter fetus, Leptospira canicola, L grippotyphosa, L hardjo, L icterohaemorrhagiae* and *L pomona* bacterin.
The viral vaccine contains gentamicin and amphotericin B as preservatives.
Indications: For use in the immunization of healthy cattle against bovine rhinotracheitis, virus diarrhea and parainfluenza-3 infections, *Campylobacter fetus* and leptospirosis caused by *Leptospira canicola, L. grippotyphosa, L. hardjo, L. icterohaemorrhagiae* and *L. pomona.*
Dosage and Administration: Rehydrate the vial of vaccine with the accompanying vial of bacterin. Shake well and administer 5 mL intramuscularly or subcutaneously. Annual revaccination is recommended.
Calves vaccinated under three (3) months of age should be revaccinated at four (4) to six (6) months of age or at weaning because of the possible interfering influence of passive immunity.
In areas where vibriosis is endemic, a second vaccination in 21 days is recommended for primary immunization.
Precaution(s): Store at 35°-45°F (2°-7°C). Protect the vaccine from the direct rays of the sun.
Caution(s): Use the entire contents without delay after rehydration.
Care should be taken to avoid chemical or microbial contamination of the product.
Burn each vaccine container and unused contents.
If an allergic response occurs, epinephrine should be administered immediately.
Scientific evidence demonstrates the inability of some animals to develop antibodies to bovine virus diarrhea after vaccination. The affected animal may exhibit symptoms similar to mucosal disease.
Antidote(s): Epinephrine.
Warning(s): Do not vaccinate pregnant cows or calves nursing pregnant cows.
Do not vaccinate within 21 days before slaughter.
Presentation: 50 mL (10 dose) and 100 mL (20 dose) vials.
Compendium Code No.: 14750260

CPV/LP™

VacciCel **Vaccine**

Parvovirus Vaccine, Modified Live Virus
U.S. Vet. Lic. No.: 292
Active Ingredient(s): Contains modified live virus parvovirus.
Contains penicillin, streptomycin and amphotericin B as preservatives.
Indications: For the active immunization of healthy puppies and dogs against disease caused by canine parvovirus (CPV).
Dosage and Administration: Shake well before using. Inject 1 mL intramuscularly using aseptic technique. Puppies less than 12 weeks of age should receive a second dose at 12-16 weeks of age. Revaccinate annually.
Precaution(s): Store at less than 45°F or 7°C.
Caution(s): Use the entire contents when first opened. Anaphylactic reactions although rare may occur.
Antidote(s): Epinephrine.
Presentation: 10 dose (10 mL) vials.
Compendium Code No.: 11090010

CRF®

Synbiotics **Rheumatoid Test**

U.S. Vet. Lic. No.: 312
Contents: Materials provided:
1. CRF® latex reagent
2. Positive reference serum
3. Negative reference serum
4. Glass reading slide
5. Dropper
6. 10 mcg pipets
7. Stir sticks

Indications: For use in the detection of canine rheumatoid factor.
Test Principle: The latex particles provided as a standardized suspension in the kit are coated with canine IgG specifically altered to react with canine rheumatoid factor (CRF). Serum samples are heated to inactivate complement factors that may interfere with the test. The coated particles agglutinate when mixed with serum containing CRF, present in rheumatoid arthritis, which recognizes and binds to antigen coated on the latex particles. The agglutination reaction is observed visually, without the need for specialized equipment or instruments. Reagent and sample volumes have been specifically optimized to eliminate the need for predilution of patient sample or references. Do not dilute patient samples or references.
Positive and negative reference sera are provided as a comparative aid to the user in identifying positive or negative reactivity.
Test Procedure: Materials required, but not provided:
1. Water bath at 56°C.
2. Light sources - Tensor lamp or similar.
3. Hand magnifier - Useful for weak specimens.

Test procedure (reagents provided):
1. Canine-rheumatoid factor latex slide test reagent, one (1) vial, 5.0 mL. A suspension of polystyrene latex particles coated with treated canine IgG, standardized to provide proper reactivity in the test procedure.
2. RF positive reference serum, one (1) vial, 0.5 mL. Serum demonstrates positive reactivity in the latex slide test.
3. RF negative reference serum, one (1) vial, 0.5 mL. Serum which is nonreactive in the latex slide test.

Procedure: Use clear serum specimens only. The use of plasma is not recommended.
All reagents and serum specimens must be equilibrated to room temperature (18°C-25°C).
1a. Place the serum samples in a 56°C water bath for 30 minutes. Allow the samples to cool to room temperature (70-78°F, 21-25°C) before testing.
b. Using the pipets provided, deposit 10 mcg of the positive reference into well No. 1.
c. Pipet 10 mcg of the negative reference into well No. 2.

d. Pipet 10 mcg of the serum specimens into wells No. 3-6.
2. Mix the CRF® latex-reagent by gently swirling the vial contents for about 10-15 seconds. Do not allow the reagent to foam. Mix the dropper contents by expelling the contents into the bulk reagent a few times.
Place three (3) drops (approximately 120 mcg) of the latex reagent into each well adjacent to the sample of reference serum.
3. Stir the contents of each well with a clean stirring stick. Make sure that the reagent mixes with all of the sample.
4. Rotate the slide evenly in a figure eight pattern for two (2) to three (3) minutes. Examine the slide under a tungsten filament lamp (e.g., tensor or similar) for latex agglutination.
5. Compare the serum samples with the positive and negative reference. Agglutinated reagents indicate positive reactivity, non-agglutinated reagents indicate negative reactivity. The positive reference supplied is adjusted to a mid-range or approximately 2+ reactivity.

Notes on procedure:
1. Use clean serum samples only, do not use plasma samples. After blood clotting, the serum may be separated by centrifugation or by standard serum filter separator tubes.
2. Do not allow the serum to dry before the addition of latex reagent.
3. Use only the proportion of latex reagent and serum specified in the latex slide test procedure. Do not predilute patient sample.
4. After washing the slide in detergent, rinse the slide thoroughly. Residual detergent may affect the test results.

Using the microcapillary pipet provided in the kit:
a. Insert the capillary pipet into the holder provided.
b. Allow the pipet to draw up patient or reference serum by capillary action. The hole at the top of the rubber bulb must be unobstructed.
c. To expel the sample into a well on the glass slide, cover the hole at the top of the black rubber bulb with an index finger and gently squeeze the bulb. The serum will be deposited onto the slide.

It may be helpful to practice the technique a few times with clean water.

If patient or reference serum is accidentally sucked into the glass barrel of the micropipet holder, disassemble, rinse well with water, dry and reassemble before reuse.

Do not reuse capillary pipets.

Other pipeting devices capable of delivering 10 mcg and yielding satisfactory results with the positive and negative reference sera may also be used.

Results: If latex agglutination occurs in the latex slide test, rheumatoid factor is present in the test serum. Lack of reactivity indicates the absence of rheumatoid factor. Occasionally a slight degree of agglutination may be encountered. Such results may indicate the presence of an early stage of progressive disease and the test should be repeated at a later visit. Increased activity provides evidence for progressive disease. Generally, reactions equal to or greater than the positive reference serum indicate the presence of rheumatoid type antibodies. Such findings combined with the criteria "Diagnostic criteria for rheumatoid arthritis" assist in the diagnosis of rheumatoid arthritis in the canine.

Limitations of the procedure:
1. Use clear serum samples only, plasma or lipemic samples may non-specifically agglutinate latex particles.
2. Store the latex slide reagent with the cap tightly closed to prevent evaporation of the buffered liquid.
3. If the glass slide is rotated for more than five (5) minutes, false positive results may occur.

Performance characteristics:
1. Sera from a group of healthy dogs were found to exhibit negative reactivity when tested by the canine rheumatoid factor latex slide test.
2. Sera from a group of dogs exhibiting rheumatoid factor as determined by a qualified clinical laboratory performing veterinary rheumatoid factor determinations were found to exhibit positive reactivity in the canine rheumatoid factor latex slide test.

Utilizing criteria established in humans and accepted by the American Rheumatoid Association the following criteria might be helpful, as quoted from Berkow, et al[1]:
1. Diagnostic criteria for rheumatoid arthritis:
a. Classic rheumatoid arthritis: The diagnosis requires seven (7) of the following criteria. In criteria one (1) through five (5) the joint signs or symptoms must be continuous for at least six (6) weeks.
   1) Morning stiffness.
   2) Pain on motion or tenderness in at least one (1) joint (observed by a physician).
   3) Swelling (soft tissue thickening or fluid, not bony overgrowth alone) in at least one (1) joint (observed by a physician).
   4) Swelling (observed by a physician) of at least one (1) other joint (any interval free of joint symptoms between the two (2) joint involvements may not be more than three (3) months).
   5) Symmetric joint swelling (observed by a physician) with simultaneous involvement of the same joint on both sides of the body (bilateral involvement of proximal interphalangeal, metacarpophalangeal, or metatarsophalangeal joints is acceptable without absolute symmetry). Terminal phalangeal joint involvement will not satisfy this criterion.
   6) Subcutaneous nodules (observed by a physician) over bony prominences, on extensor surfaces, or in juxta-articular regions.
   7) X-ray changes typical of rheumatoid arthritis (which must include at least bony decalcification localized to or greatest around the involved joints and not just degenerative changes). Degenerative changes do not exclude patients from any group classified as rheumatoid arthritis.
   8) Positive agglutination test: Demonstration of the rheumatoid factor by any method which, in two (2) laboratories, has been positive in not >5% of normal controls.
   9) Poor mucin precipitate from synovial fluid (with shreds and cloudy solution).
   10) Characteristic histologic changes in synovial membrane with three (3) or more of the following: Marked villous hypertrophy, proliferation of superficial synovial cells, often with palisading, marked infiltration of chronic inflammatory cells (lymphocytes or plasma cells predominating), with tendency to form "lymphoid nodules", deposition of compact fibrin either on surface or interstitially, foci of cell necrosis.
   11) Characteristic histologic changes in nodules showing granulomatous foci with central zones of cell necrosis, surrounded by a palisade of proliferated macrophages, and peripheral fibrosis and chronic inflammatory cell infiltration, predominantly perivascular.
b. Definite rheumatoid arthritis: The diagnosis requires five (5) of the above criteria. In criteria one (1) through five (5) the joint signs or symptoms must be continuous for at least six (6) weeks.
c. Probable rheumatoid arthritis: The diagnosis requires three (3) of the above criteria. In at least one (1) criteria, one (1) through five (5), the joint signs or symptoms must be continuous for at least six (6) weeks.
d. Possible rheumatoid arthritis: The diagnosis requires two (2) of the following criteria, and the total duration of joint symptoms must be at least three (3) weeks.
   1. Morning stiffness.
   2. Tenderness or pain on motion (observed by a physician) with history of recurrence or persistence for three (3) weeks.
   3. History or observation of joint swelling.
   4. Subcutaneous nodules (observed by a physician).
   5. Elevated ESR or C-reactive protein.
   6. Iritis (of dubious value as a criterion except in the case of juvenile rheumatoid arthritis).

Precaution(s): Store the components at 2-8°C. Do not freeze.

Properly stored reagents are stable until the expiration date.

Warning(s): The toxicological properties of these reagents have not been determined. Do not ingest.

The kit components contain sodium azide. Upon disposal flush with a large volume of water.

For *in vitro* veterinary diagnostic use only.

Discussion: Canine rheumatoid arthritis is an erosive polyarthritis frequently characterized by multi-site lameness and joint swelling.[3] The disease is often progressive in nature and is distinct from osteoarthritis (degenerative joint disease) and septic arthritis.

The diagnosis of canine RA is difficult. Most authors have chosen to adapt the criteria adopted by the American Rheumatism Association[2] for the diagnosis of RA in canines. Among these is the presence of rheumatoid factor (RF), an antibody which binds to altered IgG, and which has been reported to be present in 70% of dogs with RA.[3]

Several methods have been developed for the detection of canine rheumatoid factor (CRF), among these are the latex agglutination, the modified Rose-Waaler, and the bentonite floculation procedures. Of these the latex agglutination procedure has been demonstrated to be a simple, stable and consistent test for the presence of rheumatoid factor in dogs.[4]

References: Available upon request.

Presentation: 12-36 tests/kit (depending on batch size).

Compendium Code No.: 11150040

CTC 50

Durvet **Feed Medication**

Chlortetracycline (Type A Medicated Article)

Active Ingredient(s): Chlortetracycline as Chlortetracycline calcium complex equivalent to 50 grams Chlortetracycline Hydrochloride/lb.

Ingredients: Chlortetracycline, calcium carbonate, roughage products and mineral oil.

Indications:

Chickens:

For Broiler/Fryer Chickens: For an increased rate of weight gain and improved feed efficiency.

For Chickens: Control of infectious synovitis caused by *Mycoplasma synoviae;* susceptible to chlortetracycline.

For Chickens: Control of chronic respiratory disease (CRD) and air sac infection caused by *Mycoplasma gallisepticum* and *Escherichia coli* susceptible to chlortetracycline.

For Chickens: Reduction of mortality due to *Escherichia coli* infections susceptible to chlortetracycline.

Turkeys:

For Growing Turkeys: For an increased rate of weight gain and improved feed efficiency.

For Turkeys: Control of infectious synovitis caused by *Mycoplasma synoviae* susceptible to chlortetracycline.

For Turkeys: Control of hexamitiasis caused by *Hexamita meleagrides* susceptible to chlortetracyline.

For Turkeys: Turkey poults not over 4 weeks of age: Reduction of mortality due to paratyphoid caused by *Salmonella typhimurium* susceptible to chlortetracycline.

For Turkeys: Control of complicating bacterial organisms associated with bluecomb (transmissible enteritis, coronaviral enteritis) susceptible to chlortetracycline.

Sheep:

For Growing Sheep: For an increased rate of weight gain and improved feed efficiency.

For Breeding Sheep: Reducing the incidence of (vibrionic) abortion caused by *Campylobacter fetus* infection susceptible to chlortetracycline.

Swine:

For Growing Swine: For an increased rate of weight gain and improved feed efficiency.

For Swine: Reducing the incidence of cervical lymphadenitis (jowl abscesses) caused by *Group E Streptocci* susceptible to chlortetracycline.

For Breeding Swine: Control of leptospirosis (reducing the instances of abortions and shedding of leptospirae) caused by *Leptospira pomona* susceptible to chlortetracycline.

For Swine: Treatment of bacterial enteritis caused by *Escherichia coli* and *Salmonella choleraesuis* and bacterial pneumonia caused by *Pasteurella multocida* susceptible to chlortetracycline.

Calves, Beef Cattle and Non-Lactating Dairy Cattle:

For Calves (up to 250 lbs): For an increased weight gain and improved feed efficiency.

For Calves (250-400 lbs): For an increased weight gain and improved feed efficiency.

For Growing Cattle (over 400 lbs): For an increased weight gain, improved feed efficiency and reduction of liver condemnation due to liver abscesses.

For Cattle: For the control of bacterial pneumonia associated with shipping fever complex susceptible to chlortetracycline.

For Beef Cattle (under 700 lbs): Control of active infection of anaplasmosis caused by *Anaplasma marginale* susceptible to chlortetracycline.

For Beef Cattle (over 700 lbs): Control of active infection of anaplasmosis caused by *Anaplasma marginale* susceptible to chlortetracycline.

For Calves, Beef and Non-Lactating Dairy Cattle: For treatment of bacterial enteritis caused by *Escherichia coli* and bacterial pneumonia caused by *Pasteurella multocida* susceptible to chlortetracycline.

Directions for Use:

Indications for Use	Use Levels of Chlortetracycline	lbs of CTC 50 per ton
Chickens		
For Broiler/Fryer Chickens: For an increased rate of weight gain and improved feed efficiency.	10-50 g/ton	0.2-1.0
For Chickens: Control of infectious synovitis caused by *Mycoplasma synoviae;* susceptible to chlortetracycline. (Feed continuously for 7-14 days.)	100-200 g/ton	2.0-4.0
For Chickens: Control of chronic respiratory disease (CRD) and air sac infection caused by *Mycoplasma gallisepticum* and *Escherichia coli* susceptible to chlortetracycline. (Feed continuously for 7-14 days.)	200-400 g/ton	4.0-8.0
For Chickens: Reduction of mortality due to *Escherichia coli* infections susceptible to chlortetracycline. (Feed for 5 days.)	500 g/ton	10.0
Turkeys		
For Turkeys: Growing Turkeys: For an increased rate of weight gain and improved feed efficiency.	10-50 g/ton	0.2-1.0
For Turkeys: Control of infectious synovitis caused by *Mycoplasma synoviae* susceptible to chlortetracycline. (Feed continuously for 7-14 days.)	200 g/ton	4.0
For Turkeys: Control of hexamitiasis caused by *Hexamita meleagrides* susceptible to chlortetracyline. (Feed continuously for 7-14 days.)	400 g/ton	8.0
For Turkeys: Turkey poults not over 4 weeks of age: Reduction of mortality due to paratyphoid caused by *Salmonella typhimurium* susceptible to chlortetracycline.	400 g/ton	8.0
For Turkeys: Control of complicating bacterial organisms associated with bluecomb (transmissible enteritis, coronaviral enteritis) susceptible to chlortetracycline. (Feed continuously for 7-14 days.)	25 mg/lb body weight/day	
Sheep		
For Growing Sheep: For an increased rate of weight gain and improved feed efficiency.	20-50 g/ton	0.4-1.0
For Breeding Sheep: Reducing the incidence of (vibrionic) abortion caused by *Campylobacter fetus* infection susceptible to chlortetracycline.	80 mg/head/day	
Swine		
For Growing Swine: For an increased rate of weight gain and improved feed efficiency.	10-50 g/ton	0.20-1.0
For Swine: Reducing the incidence of cervical lymphadenitis (jowl abscesses) caused by *Group E Streptocci* susceptible to chlortetracycline.	50-100 g/ton	1.0-2.0
For Breeding Swine: Control of leptospirosis (reducing the instances of abortions and shedding of leptospirae) caused by *Leptospira pomona* susceptible to chlortetracycline. (Feed continuously for 14 days.)	400 g/ton	8.0
For Swine: Treatment of bacterial enteritis caused by *Escherichia coli* and *Salmonella choleraesuis* and bacterial pneumonia caused by *Pasteurella multocida* susceptible to chlortetracycline. (Feed for not more than 14 days.)	10 mg/lb body weight/day	

Calves, Beef Cattle and Non-Lactating Dairy Cattle	
For Calves (up to 250 lbs): For an increased weight gain and improved feed efficiency.	0.1 mg/lb body weight/day
For Calves (250-400 lbs): For an increased weight gain and improved feed efficiency.	25-70 mg/head/day
For Growing Cattle (over 400 lbs): For an increased weight gain, improved feed efficiency and reduction of liver condemnation due to liver abscesses.	70 mg/head/day
For Cattle: For the control of bacterial pneumonia associated with shipping fever complex susceptible to chlortetracycline.	350 mg/head/day
For Beef Cattle (under 700 lbs): Control of active infection of anaplasmosis caused by *Anaplasma marginale* susceptible to chlortetracycline.	350 mg/head/day
For Beef Cattle (over 700 lbs): Control of active infection of anaplasmosis caused by *Anaplasma marginale* susceptible to chlortetracycline.	0.5 mg/lb body weight/day
For Calves, Beef and Non-Lactating Dairy Cattle: For treatment of bacterial enteritis caused by *Escherichia coli* and bacterial pneumonia caused by *Pasteurella multocida* susceptible to chlortetracycline. (Treat for not more than 5 days.)	10 mg/lb body weight/day

Caution(s): For use in dry feeds only. Not for use in liquid feed supplements.
Restricted Drug (California) — Use only as directed.
For use in the manufacture of medicated feeds.

Warning(s):
Chickens:
Do not feed to chickens producing eggs for human consumption.
When used at levels of up to 400 g/ton: Zero-day withdrawal period.
When used at levels of 500 g/ton: Withdraw 24 hours prior to slaughter.
Turkeys: Do not feed to turkeys producing eggs for human consumption. Zero-day withdrawal period.
Sheep: Zero day withdrawal period.
Swine: Zero day withdrawal period.
Cattle:
A withdrawal period has not been established for this product in pre-ruminating calves. Do not use in calves to be processed for veal.
When used in growing cattle at a level of 70 mg/head/day or less: Zero-day withdrawal period.
When used in beef cattle at a level of 0.5 mg/lb body weight/day: Withdraw 48 hours prior to slaughter.
When used in calves, beef cattle, and non-lactating dairy cattle at levels of 10 mg/lb body weight/day: Withdraw 10 days prior to slaughter.

Presentation: 50 lbs (22.7 kg) (NDC 30798-373-56).
Compendium Code No.: 10840371 4/97

CTC SOLUBLE POWDER

AgriLabs **Water Medication**

Chlortetracycline HCl-Antibiotic
ANADA No.: 200-236
Active Ingredient(s): Each packet contains 102.4 grams of chlortetracycline (64 g/lb).
Indications:
Chickens: Control of infectious synovitis caused by *M. synoviae,* control of chronic respiratory disease (CRD) and air sac infections caused by *M gallisepticum* and *E. coli.*
Turkeys: Control of infectious synovitis caused by *M synoviae,* control of complicating bacterial organisms associated with bluecomb (transmissible enteritis, coronaviral enteritis).
Swine: Control and treatment of bacterial enteritis (scours) caused by *E. coli* and *Salmonella* spp. and bacterial pneumonia associated with *Pasteurella* spp., *Hemophilus* spp., *Klebsiella* spp.
Directions for Use: For use in drinking water of chickens, turkeys and swine.
Dissolve the contents of one packet of CTC SOLUBLE POWDER in four (4) gallons of water to prepare a stock solution, when metered at the rate of 1 oz of stock solution per gallon of drinking water, will deliver 200 mg chlortetracycline HCl per gallon of drinking water. One level measuring teaspoon contains approximately 575 mg chlortetracycline hydrochloride which will treat 57.5 lbs (26 kg) of animal at 10 mg/lb for one day. Not to be used for more than 14 consecutive days in chickens and turkeys and five days in swine. The concentration of drug required in drinking water must be adjusted to provide a correct dosage in order to compensate for variations in the age of the animal, class of poultry, environmental temperature and humidity; each of which affects water consumption.
Chickens and Turkeys: Administer for 7 to 14 days. Medicate continuously at the first clinical signs of disease. The dosage range permitted provides for different levels based on the severity of the infection. Consult a poultry diagnostic laboratory or a poultry pathologist to determine the diagnosis and advice regarding the optimum level of the drug where ranges are permitted. As a generalization, 100 turkeys will drink one gallon of water per day for each week of age. Chickens will consume one half this amount.
Dosage:
Chickens: Control of infectious synovitis caused by *M. synoviae* - 200 to 400 mg chlortetracycline hydrochloride per gallon drinking water (5.0-13.4 mg/lb body weight per day). Control of chronic respiratory disease (CRD) and air sac infections caused by *M. gallisepticum* and *E. coli* - 400 to 800 mg chlortetracycline hydrochloride per gallon drinking water (10.0-26.8 mg/lb body weight per day).
Turkeys: Control of infectious synovitis caused by *M synoviae* - 400 mg chlortetracycline hydrochloride per gallon drinking water (3.2-16.8 mg/lb body weight per day). Control of complicating bacterial organisms associated with bluecomb (transmissible enteritis, coronaviral enteritis)-25 mg chlortetracycline hydrochloride per body weight daily.
Swine: Control and treatment of bacterial enteritis (scours) caused by *E. coli* and *Salmonella* spp. and bacterial pneumonia associated with *Pasteurella* spp., *Hemophilus* spp., *Klebsiella* spp. - 10 mg chlortetracycline hydrochloride per pound body weight daily in divided doses for 3 to 5 days
Precaution(s): Store in cool, dry place.
Caution(s): Prepare a fresh solution daily. When using galvanized waterer, prepare fresh solution every 12 hours. Use only against organisms sensitive to chlortetracycline. Use as the sole source of chlortetracycline. Do not mix in liquid feed supplements, milk or milk replacers. Administer 1 hour before or 2 hours after feeding with milk or milk replacers.
For use in drinking water only.
Use as the sole source of drinking water.
Restricted Drug(s) (California), not for human use.
For animal use only.

Warning(s): Withdraw 24 hours before slaughter of chickens, turkeys and five days for swine. Do not feed to chickens producing eggs for human consumption. For growing turkeys only.

Keep out of reach of children.

Presentation: 30 x 725.8 g (25.6 oz) packets.

Compendium Code No.: 10581350 Iss. 11-01/T-Iss. 9-01

CTC SOLUBLE POWDER CONCENTRATE

Durvet **Water Medication**

Antibiotic

Active Ingredient(s): Each packet contains:

Chlortetracycline hydrochloride .... 25.6 g (64 g/lb.)

The 6.4 oz packet contains 25.6 g Chlortetracycline HCl and will make:

256 gallons containing 100 mg chlortetracycline HCl per gallon.

128 gallons containing 200 mg chlortetracycline HCl per gallon.

64 gallons containing 400 mg chlortetracycline HCl per gallon.

25.6 gallons containing 1000 mg chlortetracycline HCl per gallon.

Indications:

Swine and Calves: For use in the control or treatment of diseases caused by bacterial enteritis (scours) *(Escherichia coli, Salmonella* spp.) and bacterial pneumonia *(Pasteurella* spp., *Hemophilus* spp., *Klebsiella* spp.).

Chickens: For use in the control or treatment of chronic respiratory disease (CRD) and air-sac infection *(Mycoplasma gallisepticum, Escherichia coli),* infectious synovitis *(Mycoplasma synoviae),* and for the control of mortality due to fowl cholera *(Pasteurella multocida)* in growing chickens.

Turkeys: For use in the control or treatment of complicated bluecomb (transmissible enteritis) and infectious synovitis *(Mycoplasma synoviae).*

Dosage and Administration: The dosage in terms of packets per 256 gallons are based on stated dosages per unit of body weight and the average water consumption of the species. Weather conditions and other factors may affect consumption and, except where calves are drenched, the unit dosage should be used as a guide to its effective use in drinking water. The animal must consume enough medicated water to provide the desired therapeutic dose under the conditions that prevail.

Swine (A dose of 10 mg/lb. of body weight per day):

For use in the control or treatment of diseases caused by bacterial enteritis (scours) *(Escherichia coli, Salmonella* spp.), bacterial pneumonia *(Pasteurella* spp., *Hemophilus* spp., *Klebsiella* spp.): 10 packets per 256 gallons will treat 25,600 lbs. of pigs for one day, that is 256-100 lb. pigs providing 10 mg per lb. of body weight. Administer at this rate in the total water consumed over a full 24-hour period. Do not administer for more than 5 days.

Calves (A dose of 10 mg/lb. of body weight per day):

For the control or treatment of diseases caused by bacterial pneumonia *(Pasteurella* spp., *Hemophilus* spp., *Klebsiella* spp.), bacterial enteritis *(Escherichia coli, Salmonella* spp.): One standard measuring teaspoonful of powder contains 500 mg. Administer 4 teaspoonsful in the solution to a 200 lb. calf daily in the total water consumed over a full 24-hour period, or as a drench in divided doses. Do not administer for more than 5 days.

Chickens:

For use in the control or treatment of chronic respiratory disease (CRD) and air-sac infection *(Mycoplasma gallisepticum, Escherichia coli)*: 4-8 packets per 256 gallons.

Infectious synovitis *(Mycoplasma synoviae)*: 2-4 packets per 256 gallons.

For the control of mortality due to fowl cholera *(Pasteurella multocida)* in growing chickens: 10 packets per 256 gallons.

Administer at the indicated rates in the total water consumed over a full 24-hour period.

Turkeys:

For use in the control or treatment of complicated bluecomb (transmissible enteritis): 25 mg/lb. of body wt/day. Administer 1 packet for every 1,024 lbs. of turkeys in the total water consumed over a full 24-hour period.

Infectious synovitis *(Mycoplasma synoviae)*: 4 packets per 256 gallons. Administer at this rate in the total water consumed over a full 24-hour period.

Caution(s): Medicate continuously at the first clinical signs of disease in poultry and continue for 7 to 14 consecutive days. The dosage ranges permitted provide for different levels based on the severity of the infection. Consult a poultry diagnostic laboratory or a poultry pathologist to determine the diagnosis and for advice regarding the optimal level of the drug where ranges are permitted.

When used in plastic or stainless steel waterers or automatic waterers, prepare fresh solutions every 24 hours. When used in galvanized waterers, prepare fresh solutions every 12 hours.

For veterinary use in drinking water.

Warning(s): Use as the sole source of chlortetracycline.

Not to be used for more than 14 consecutive days in chickens and turkeys, 5 days in calves, or 5 days in swine.

Do not use in laying chickens.

For growing turkeys only.

Do not administer to swine and calves within 24 hours of slaughter.

Do not administer to poultry at 1000 mg/gallon of water (1 packet per 25.6 gallons) within 24 hours of slaughter.

Presentation: 6.4 oz and 25.6 oz packets.

Compendium Code No.: 10840381 11/92

CUPLEX 50

Zinpro **Feed Additive**

Copper Lysine

Typical Analysis:

Copper 5.0%
Lysine 22.0%
Protein 25.0%
Fat 0.0%
Fiber 18.0%
Ash 25.0%
Salt 9.0%

Indications: Recommended as a nutritional feed additive for livestock and poultry. When used as a commercial feed ingredient it must be declared as copper lysine.

Physical Description: A green granular powder. CUPLEX 50 weighs approximately 30 lbs/cu ft.

Feeding Instructions:

Swine: Add 1.0 lb (454 grams) per ton of complete ration.

Laying Hens, Broilers and Turkeys: Add 1.0 lb (454 grams) per ton of complete ration.

Dairy Cattle: Feed 2.5 grams per head daily, or 1 ounce per 12 head daily.

Beef Cattle: Feed 2.5 grams per head daily, or 1 ounce per 12 head daily.

Horses: Feed 2.5 grams per head daily.

Contraindication(s): Contains high levels of copper: Do not feed to sheep or related species.

Toxicology: When correctly used, there is no toxicity hazard in the use of CUPLEX 50.

Presentation: CUPLEX 50 is packaged in 50 lb multiwall bags.

Compendium Code No.: 11300130

CUPLEX 100

Zinpro **Feed Additive**

Copper Lysine

Typical Analysis:

Copper 10.0%
Lysine 46.0%
Protein 48.0%
Fat 0.0%
Fiber 0.0%
Ash 30.0%
Salt 19.5%

Indications: Recommended as a nutritional feed additive for livestock and poultry. When used as a commercial feed ingredient it must be declared as copper lysine.

Physical Description: A dark blue fine powder. CUPLEX 100 weighs approximately 35 lbs/cu ft.

Feeding Instructions:

Swine: Add 0.5 lb (227 grams) per ton of complete ration.

Laying Hens, Broilers and Turkeys: Add 0.5 lb (227 grams) per ton of complete ration.

Dairy Cattle: Feed 1.25 grams per head daily, or 1 ounce per 24 head daily.

Beef Cattle: Feed 1.25 grams per head daily, or 1 ounce per 24 head daily.

Horses: Feed 1.25 grams per head daily.

Contraindication(s): Contains high levels of copper: Do not feed to sheep or related species.

Toxicology: When correctly used, there is no toxicity hazard in the use of CUPLEX 100.

Presentation: CUPLEX 100 is packaged in 50 lb multiwall bags.

Compendium Code No.: 11300120

CURATREM®

Merial **Parasiticide-Oral**

(clorsulon) 8.5% Liver Fluke Drench for Cattle (85 mg/mL)

NADA No.: 136-742

Active Ingredient(s): Contains clorsulon 85 mg/mL.

Indications: For the treatment of immature and adult liver fluke *(Fasciola hepatica)* in cattle.

Dosage and Administration: Dose: The recommended dose of CURATREM® Suspension is ¼ fl oz per 200 lb body weight (7½ mL per 200 lb or 91 kg). This equals 7 mg clorsulon per kg of body weight (approximately 3.2 mg per lb).

Administration:

1. Shake container vigorously before using.
2. Use automatic or single-dose drenching equipment.
3. Set equipment gauge at the required dose.
4. Insert the nozzle of the syringe into the corner of the mouth.
5. Deposit the suspension over the back of the tongue.

Timing of retreatment for cattle is based on geographic, climatic, and husbandry considerations.

Consult your veterinarian for assistance in the diagnosis, treatment, and control of parasitism.

Caution(s): For oral use in cattle only.

Warning(s): Residue Information: Because a withdrawal time in milk has not been established, do not use in female dairy cattle of breeding age. Do not treat cattle within 8 days of slaughter.

Keep this and all drugs out of the reach of children.

The Material Safety Data Sheet (MSDS) contains more detailed occupational safety information. To report adverse reactions in users, to obtain more information, or to obtain an MSDS, contact Merial at 1-888-637-4251.

Presentation: 32 fl oz (1 qt) (946.3 mL) and 128 fl oz (1 gal) (3.785 L) jugs.

CURATREM is a registered trademark of Merial.

(Merial Limited: Registered in England and Wales [Reg. No. 3332751] with registered offices at 27 Knightsbridge, London, SW1X 7QT, England and domesticated in Delaware, USA as Merial LLC).

Compendium Code No.: 11110071 8636804 / 8645803

CYDECTIN® POUR-ON

Fort Dodge **Parasiticide-Topical**

Moxidectin-Antiparasitic

NADA No.: 141-099

Active Ingredient(s): Contains 5 mg moxidectin/mL

Indications: CYDECTIN® Pour-On when applied at the recommended dose level of 0.5 mg/2.2 lb (0.5 mg/kg) body weight is effective in the treatment and control of the following internal [adult and fourth-stage larvae (L_4)] and external parasites of cattle:

Gastrointestinal Roundworms:

Ostertagia ostertagi - Adult and L_4 (including inhibited larvae)
Haemonchus placei - Adult
Trichostrongylus axei - Adult and L_4
Trichostrongylus colubriformis - Adult and L_4
Cooperia oncophora - Adult and L_4
Cooperia pectinata - Adult
Cooperia punctata - Adult and L_4
Cooperia spatulata - Adult
Cooperia surnabada - Adult and L_4
Bunostomum phlebotomum - Adult
Nematodirus helvetianus - Adult and L_4
Oesophagostomum radiatum - Adult and L_4

Lungworms:

Dictyocaulus viviparus - Adult and L_4

Cattle Grubs:

Hypoderma bovis
Hypoderma lineatum

Mites:

Chorioptes bovis

Psoroptes ovis (Psoroptes communis var. *bovis)*

Lice:

Linognathus vituli

Haematopinus eurysternus

Solenopotes capillatus

Bovicola (Damalinia) bovis

Horn Flies:

Haematobia irritans

Pharmacology: Mode of Action: Moxidectin is an endectocide in the milbemycin chemical class which shares the distinctive mode of action characteristic of macrocyclic lactones. CYDECTIN® (moxidectin) Pour-On is specially formulated to allow moxidectin to be absorbed through the skin and distributed internally to the areas of the body affected by endo- and/or ectoparasitism. Moxidectin binds selectively and with high affinity to glutamate-gated chloride ion channels which are critical to the function of invertebrate nerve and muscle cells. This interferes with neurotransmission resulting in paralysis and elimination of the parasite.

Persistent Activity: CYDECTIN® Pour-On has been proven to effectively control infections and protect from reinfection with *Haemonchus placei* for 14 days after treatment, *Oesophagostomum radiatum* and *Ostertagia ostertagi* for 28 days after treatment, and *Dictyocaulus viviparus* for 42 days after treatment. Efficacy below 90% was observed in some *Ostertagia ostertagi* persistent activity studies at 21 and 28 days posttreatment.

Dosage and Administration: Dosage: CYDECTIN® (moxidectin) Pour-On is a ready-to-use topical formulation intended for direct application to the hair and skin in a narrow strip extending along the top of the back from the withers to the tailhead (see Figure 1). Due to the angular topline characteristic of most dairy breeds, it is recommended that all pour-on products be applied slowly to dairy cows. Apply to healthy skin avoiding any mange scabs, skin lesions, mud or manure. Treated cattle can be easily recognized by the characteristic purple color, which will remain for a short period of time after treatment. The recommended rate of administration is 1 mL for each 22 lb (10 kg) body weight which provides 0.5 mg moxidectin for each 2.2 lb (0.5 mg/kg) body weight. The table below will assist in the calculation of the appropriate volume of pour-on which must be applied based on the weight of animal being treated.

Body Weight Lb (kg)	Dose mL
88 (40)	4
110 (50)	5
132 (60)	6
154 (70)	7
176 (80)	8
198 (90)	9
220 (100)	10
242 (110)	11
264 (120)	12
286 (130)	13
308 (140)	14
330 (150)	15
440 (200)	20
550 (250)	25
660 (300)	30
770 (350)	35
880 (400)	40
990 (450)	45
1100 (500)	50
1210 (550)	55
1320 (600)	60
1430 (650)	65

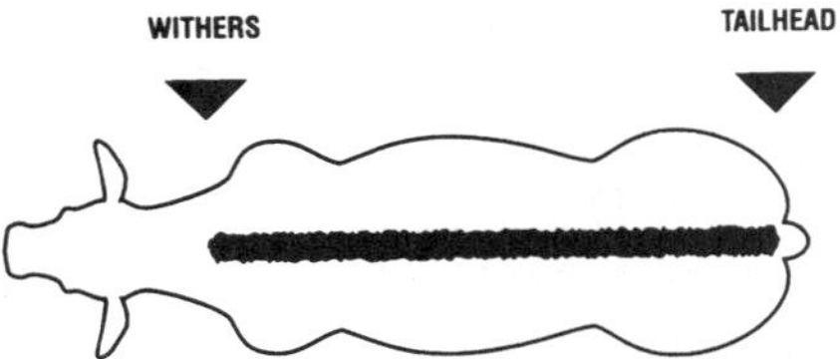

Figure 1. Where to Apply CYDECTIN® Pour-On

Use Conditions: Varying weather conditions, including rainfall do not affect the efficacy of CYDECTIN® Pour-On.

Administration: CYDECTIN® Pour-On is available in three convenient package styles designed for ease of administration and the number of cattle to be treated. Directions for use of each container type follow:

Squeeze-Measure-Pour System (16.91 fl oz/500 mL and 33.81 fl oz/1 L Bottles): Determine the weight of the animal, calculate the recommended volume of CYDECTIN® Pour-On and locate the volume marker equivalent to this dose on the dosing chamber of the bottle. Remove the dosing chamber cap and squeeze the main chamber of bottle until the desired level of solution is present in the dosing chamber. Release pressure on the container to avoid further filling. Holding the dosing chamber as indicated, pour this measured volume of solution evenly along the backline of the animal from the withers to the tailhead (see Figure 1).

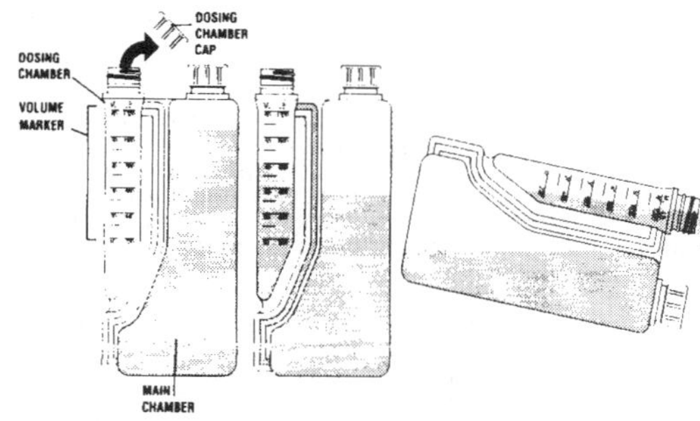

Figure 2. Squeeze-Measure-Pour System (16.91 fl oz/500 mL and 33.81 fl oz/1 L Bottles)

Large Conventional Containers (84.54 fl oz/2.5 L and 169 fl oz/5 L Bottles and 338 fl oz/10 L Cubetainer): These bottles are designed for use with the CYDECTIN® (moxidectin) Pour-On applicators. Simply remove the transient cap and seal and replace with the vented cap. Attach the applicator feeder hose to the vented cap. Invert the container prior to use (2.5 L and 5 L containers only). Apply the recommended volume of CYDECTIN® Pour-On evenly along the backline of the animal from the withers to the tailhead (see Figure 1).

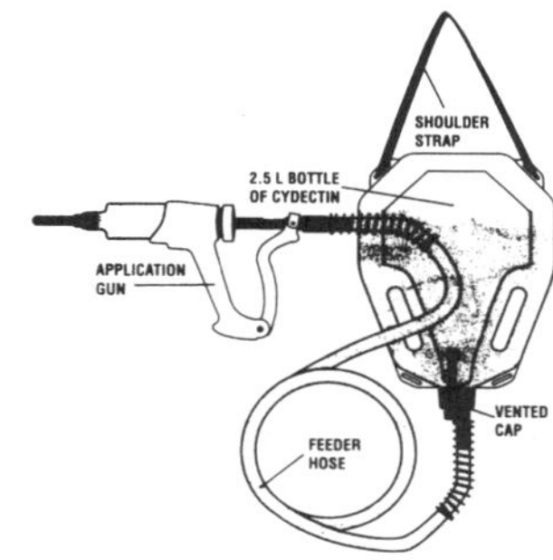

Figure 3. Large Conventional Containers (84.54 fl oz/2.5 L and 169 fl oz/5 L Bottles)

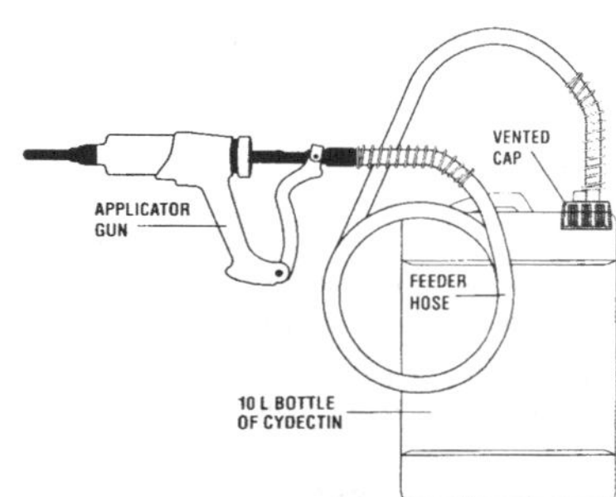

Figure 4. Large Conventional Container (338 fl oz/10 L Cubetainer)

Precaution(s): Storage: Store product at or below room temperature. Avoid prolonged exposure above 25°C (77°F). If product becomes frozen, thaw completely and shake well prior to use.

Disposal: Dispose of containers in an approved landfill or by incineration.

Environmental Safety: Studies indicate that when moxidectin comes in contact with the soil it readily and tightly binds to the soil and becomes inactive. Free moxidectin may adversely affect fish and certain aquatic organisms. Do not contaminate water by direct application or by improper disposal of drug containers.

Caution(s): For external use only. Do not apply to areas of skin with mange scabs, skin lesions, mud or manure. CYDECTIN® Pour-On is not recommended for use in species other than cattle. This product has been formulated specifically for topical use in cattle and should not be used in other animal species or by other routes of administration as adverse reactions may occur.

CYDECTIN® Pour-On is effective against the migrating stage of cattle grubs (*Hypoderma* larvae). Treatment with CYDECTIN® Pour-On during the period when grubs are migrating through vital areas may cause undesirable host-parasite reactions. Killing *H. lineatum* when they are located in peri-esophageal tissues may cause bloat. Killing *H. bovis* when they are in the vertebral canal may cause staggering or hindlimb paralysis. Cattle should be treated as soon as possible after heel fly (warble fly) season to avoid this potential problem. Cattle treated with CYDECTIN® Pour-On at the end of fly season can be re-treated during the winter without danger of grub-related reactions. Consult your veterinarian for more information regarding these secondary grub reactions and the correct time to treat with CYDECTIN® Pour-On.

Consult your veterinarian for assistance in the diagnosis, treatment and control of parasitism. If animals are likely to be reinfected following treatment, a strategic parasite control program should be established.

Warning(s): Not for use in humans. Keep this and all drugs out of the reach of children. This product can cause irritation to skin, eyes, or mucous membranes. In case of accidental skin contact and/or clothing contamination, wash skin thoroughly with soap and water and launder clothing with detergent. In case of accidental eye contact, flush eyes with copious amounts of water. When direct inhalation occurs, cleanse lungs and respiratory passages with fresh air. In case of ingestion do not induce vomiting and seek medical attention immediately. If irritation or any other symptom attributable to exposure to this product persists, consult your physician.

A copy of the material safety data sheet (MSDS) which provides more detailed occupational safety information can be obtained by calling 1-888-339-6761. To report adverse reactions attributable to exposure to this product, call 1-800-477-1365.

Residue Warning: When used according to label directions, neither a pre-slaughter drug withdrawal period nor a milk discard time are required. Meat and milk from cattle treated with CYDECTIN® (moxidectin) Pour-On may be used for human consumption at any time following treatment. A withdrawal period has not been established for this product in pre-ruminating calves. Do not use in calves to be processed for veal.

Toxicology: Animal Safety: Tolerance and toxicity studies have demonstrated an adequate margin of safety to allow treatment of cattle of all ages with CYDECTIN® Pour-On. No toxic signs were seen in cattle given up to 25 times the recommended dose level. Newborn calves similarly showed no toxic signs when treated with up to three times the recommended dose level within 12 hours of birth and nursing from cows concurrently treated with the recommended dose level of CYDECTIN® Pour-On. In breeding animals (bulls and cows in estrous and during early, mid and late pregnancy), treatment with three times the recommended dose level had no effect on breeding performance.

Discussion: Management Considerations for External Parasites: For most effective external parasite control, CYDECTIN® Pour-On should be applied to all cattle in the herd. Cattle entering the herd following this administration should be treated prior to introduction. Consult your veterinarian or a livestock entomologist for the most appropriate time to apply CYDECTIN® Pour-On in your location to effectively control horn flies and external parasites. CYDECTIN® Pour-On provides seven days of persistent activity against horn flies. For optimal control of horn flies, the product should be used as part of an integrated control program utilizing other methods to provide extended control.

Presentation: CYDECTIN® Pour-On is available in five convenient container sizes. The 16.91 fl oz/500 mL (NDC 0856-2680-01) and 33.81 fl oz/1 L (NDC 0856-2680-02) are packaged in specially-designed squeeze-measure-pour polyethylene bottles. When treating larger numbers of cattle, 84.54 fl oz/2.5 L (NDC 0856-2680-03), 169 fl oz/5 L (NDC 0856-2680-04), or 338 fl oz/10 L (NDC 0856-2680-05) conventional polyethylene containers are available for use with most commercially-available topical applicators.

U.S. Patent No. 4,916,154

Compendium Code No.: 10030372 2680G

CYLENCE®

Pour-On Insecticide

Bayer

For Control of Horn Flies, Face Flies, Biting Lice And Sucking Lice On Beef And Dairy Cattle (Including Lactating)

Active Ingredient **% By Weight**

Cyfluthrin; cyano(4-fluoro-3-phenoxyphenyl) methyl-3-(2,2-dichloroethenyl)-2,2-dimethyl-cyclopropanecarboxylate 1%

Inert Ingredients 99%

Total 100%

KEEP OUT OF REACH OF CHILDREN

WARNING

See Statements of Practical Treatment and Other Precautionary Statements

PRECAUTIONARY STATEMENTS

HAZARDS TO HUMANS AND DOMESTIC ANIMALS

WARNING

Causes substantial but temporary eye injury. Harmful if swallowed, or absorbed through the skin. Avoid contact with skin, eyes or clothing.

Wear goggles, face shield or safety glasses. Wash hands thoroughly with soap and warm water after handling.

Keep out of reach of children.

Do not contaminate feed or food.

STATEMENTS OF PRACTICAL TREATMENT

If in eyes: Hold eyelids open and flush with plenty of water. Get medical attention.

If swallowed: Call a physician or Poison Control Center. Do not induce vomiting. Vomiting may cause an aspiration hazard. **If on skin:** Wash with plenty of soap and water. Get medical attention. **If inhaled:** Remove victim to fresh air. Get medical attention if victim displays signs of poisoning.

TO PHYSICIAN: Treat the patient symptomatically.

ENVIRONMENTAL HAZARDS

This pesticide is extremely toxic to fish and aquatic invertebrates. Do not apply directly to water. Do not contaminate water when disposing of equipment washwaters.

Apply this product only as specified on this label.

DIRECTIONS FOR USE

It is a violation of Federal law to use this product in a manner inconsistent with its labeling.

For Control of Horn Flies, Face Flies, Biting Lice and Sucking Lice on Beef and Dairy Cattle (Including Lactating).

How to Apply: CyLence Pour-On Insecticide is a **ready-to-use** solution. To use the package dispenser on the one pint size, hold the container upright, remove the cap from the dosage chamber and gently squeeze the sides of the bottle to fill the chamber to the desired dosage. Apply the required amount of solution directly along the top of the back and top of the head of the animal.

Amount to Use: Apply **CyLence Pour-On Insecticide** at the dosages shown on the following table. Due to the small amount of material required, care must be taken to apply the correct dosage.

Animal Weight	Horn and Face Flies			Biting and Suckling Lice		
	Dosage (mL)	No. of Animals Contents of Container Will Treat		Dosage (mL)	No. of Animals Contents of Container Will Treat	
		1 PT	6 PT		1 PT	6 PT
Less than 400 lbs.	4	118	709	8	59	354
400 - 800 lbs.	8	59	354	16	29	177
Over 800 lbs.	12	39	236	24	19	118

CyLence Pour-On Insecticide can be used on beef and dairy cattle (including lactating) of all ages and sizes. Treatment for flies can be repeated as needed but not more often than once every 3 weeks. For optimal lice control, an initial application followed by a second treatment 3 weeks later is recommended.

CyLence Pour-On Insecticide does not control cattle grubs.

NOTICE TO VETERINARIANS

As with all synthetic pyrethroids, a small percentage of animals may experience a temporary skin sensation known as paresthesia within 24 hours after application. Paresthesia is characterized by one or more of the following signs: head tossing, tail twitching, restlessness, and irritability. Generally, affected animals return to normal within 48 hours without treatment.

STORAGE AND DISPOSAL

Not for Use or Storage In or Around the Home

Do not contaminate water, food or feed by storage or disposal.

Pesticide Disposal:

Pesticide wastes are hazardous. Improper disposal of excess pesticide or rinsate is a violation of Federal law. If these wastes cannot be disposed of by use according to label instructions, contact your State Pesticide or Environmental Control Agency or the Hazardous Waste representative at the nearest EPA Regional Office for guidance.

Container Disposal:

Triple rinse (or equivalent). Then offer for recycling or reconditioning, or puncture and dispose of in a sanitary landfill, or incineration, or, if allowed by state and local authorities, by burning. If burned, stay out of smoke.

Storage:

Store in cool, dry place and in such a manner as to prevent cross contamination with other pesticides, fertilizers, food and feed. Store in original container and out of reach of children, preferably in a locked storage area.

Handle and open container in a manner as to prevent spillage. If the container is leaking, invert to prevent leakage. If the container is leaking or material spilled for any reason or cause, carefully dam up spilled material to prevent runoff. Refer to Precautionary Statements on label for hazards associated with the handling of this material. Do not walk through spilled material. Absorb spilled material with absorbing type compounds and dispose as directed for pesticides above.

Limited Warranty and Limitation of Damages

Bayer Corporation, Animal Health, warrants that this material conforms to the chemical description on this label. BAYER CORPORATION, ANIMAL HEALTH, MAKES NO OTHER EXPRESS OR IMPLIED WARRANTY, INCLUDING ANY OTHER EXPRESS OR IMPLIED WARRANTY OF FITNESS OR OF MERCHANTABILITY, and no agent of Bayer Corporation, Animal Health, is authorized to do so except in writing with a specific reference to this warranty. Any damages arising from a breach of this warranty shall be limited to direct damages and shall not include consequential commercial damages such as loss of profits or values, etc.

EPA EST. No. 67517-MO-1

EPA REG. No. 11556-107

Supplied: Code 13590—473 mL (1 Pint) 71135910, R.4

Code 13596—2.8 L (6 Pints) 71135965, R.4

Bayer Corporation, Agriculture Division, Animal Health, Shawnee Mission, Kansas 66201 U.S.A.

Compendium Code No.: 10400202

CYLENCE® ULTRA

Insecticide Cattle Ear Tag

Bayer

For Use On Beef And Non-Lactating Dairy Cattle To Control Face Flies, Horn Flies, Gulf Coast Ticks And Spinose Ear Ticks

- **Effective Against Face Flies and Pyrethroid Susceptible Horn Flies for up to 5 months.**
- **Kills and Repels Face Flies — mechanical vector of *Moraxella bovis* bacteria causing "pink eye" of cattle.**
- **Synergized for extra performance**

Active Ingredients: Percent By Weight

Beta-cyfluthrin; Cyano (4-fluoro-3-phenyoxyphenyl) methyl 3-(2,2 - dichloroethenyl) 2, 2 - dimethylcyclopropane carboxylate 8%

Piperonyl Butoxide 20%

Other Ingredients 72%

Total 100%

Keep Out of Reach of Children

CAUTION

See Additional Precautionary Statements

PRECAUTIONARY STATEMENTS

HAZARDS TO HUMANS AND DOMESTIC ANIMALS

CAUTION

May cause eye irritation. Harmful if swallowed, inhaled or absorbed through the skin. Avoid contact with eyes, skin, or clothing. Avoid breathing vapors. Wear nonpermeable protective gloves when applying or removing tags. Wash thoroughly with soap and water after use and before eating, drinking, or using tobacco.

FIRST AID

If in Eyes:

- Hold eye open and rinse slowly and gently with water for 15-20 minutes. Remove contact lenses if present after the first 5 minutes, and then continue rinsing eye.
- Call a poison control center or doctor for treatment advice.

If Swallowed:

- Call poison control center or doctor immediately for treatment advice.
- Have person sip a glass of water if able to swallow.
- Do not induce vomiting unless told to do so by a poison control center or doctor.
- Do not give anything to an unconscious person.

If on Skin or Clothing:

- Take off contaminated clothing.
- Rinse skin immediately with plenty of water for 15-20 minutes.
- Call a poison control center or doctor for treatment advice.

If Inhaled:

- Move person to fresh air.
- If person is not breathing call 911 or an ambulance then give artificial respiration, preferably mouth-to-mouth if possible.

HOTLINE NUMBER: Have the product container or label with you when calling a poison control center or doctor, or going for treatment. For emergency medical treatment information, call 1-877-258-2280. For product information, call 1-800-633-3796.

Directions for Use:

It is a violation of Federal law to use this product in a manner inconsistent with its labeling. This labeling must be in the possession of the user at the time of pesticide application.

For the control of horn flies, face flies, gulf coast ticks, and spinose ear ticks on beef and non-lactating dairy cattle.

All mature animals in the herd should be tagged. For adequate control of horn flies attach one tag per animal. For optimum control of face flies, horn flies, gulf coast ticks, and spinose ear ticks, attach one tag to each ear (two per animal). Replace as necessary. CyLence® Ultra

Insecticide Ear Tags have been proven to be effective against face and horn flies for up to five months.

Apply as indicated (Figures 1-4). Calves less than 3 months of age should not be tagged as ear damage may result. Remove tags at end of fly season or prior to slaughter.

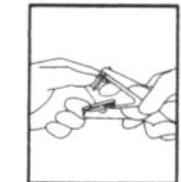

Figure 1

Disinfect pliers prior to use. Place male button onto pin.

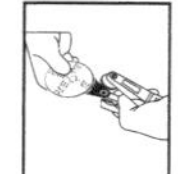

Figure 2

Slide tag under the clip of the pliers by depressing the lever.

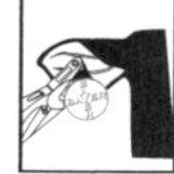

Figure 3

Position tag in the center portion of the front side of the ear.

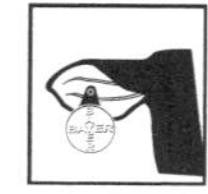

Figure 4

Apply the tag between the second and third rib cartilage.

Continual exposure of horn flies to a single class of insecticide (e.g. pyrethroids or organophosphates) may lead to the development of resistance to that class of insecticide. In order to reduce the possibility of horn flies developing resistance it is important to rotate the class of insecticide used and/or the method of horn fly control on a seasonal basis. CyLence® Ultra Cattle Ear Tag contains the pyrethroid insecticide beta cyfluthrin plus piperonyl butoxide, which is an insecticide synergist.

Storage and Disposal:

Do not contaminate water, food or feed by storage or disposal.

Storage: Store in cool place in original container. Opened pouches containing ear tags should be resealed for storage.

Pesticide Disposal: Waste (spent tags) resulting from the use of this product may be disposed of on site or at an approved waste disposal facility.

Container Disposal: Dispose of empty pouch in a sanitary landfill or by incineration, or if allowed by State and local authorities, by burning. If burned stay out of smoke.

Environmental Hazards: This pesticide is toxic to fish. Do not contaminate water when disposing of used tags. Apply this product only as specified on the label.

LIMITED WARRANTY AND LIMITATION OF DAMAGES

Bayer Corporation, Agriculture Division, Animal Health warrants that this material conforms to the chemical description on the label. BAYER CORPORATION MAKES NO OTHER EXPRESS OR IMPLIED WARRANTY, INCLUDING ANY OTHER EXPRESS OR IMPLIED WARRANTY OF FITNESS OR OF MERCHANTABILITY, and no agent of Bayer Corporation is authorized to do so except in writing with a specific reference to this warranty. Any damages arising from a breach of this warranty shall be limited to direct damages and shall not include consequential commercial damages such as loss of profits or values, etc.

EPA Est. No. 4691-KS-01 EPA Reg. No. 11556-131

Supplied: Code 08712118-062099—20 Tags, 2 Pouches of 10 Tags Each 0.5 oz Per Tag

77006200, R.1

Manufactured For Bayer Corporation, Agriculture Division, Animal Health, Shawnee Mission, Kansas 66201 U.S.A.

Compendium Code No.: 10400421

CYSTORELIN® ℞

Merial **Gonadorelin**

(Gonadorelin Diacetate Tetrahydrate) (50 mcg/mL) Sterile Solution

NADA No.: 098-379

Active Ingredient(s): Each mL of CYSTORELIN® contains:

Gonadorelin diacetate tetrahydrate	50 mcg
Benzyl Alcohol	9 mg
Sodium Chloride	7.47 mg
Water for Injection, U.S.P.	q.s.

pH adjusted with potassium phosphate (monobasic and dibasic).

Indications: For the treatment of cystic ovaries in cattle.

CYSTORELIN® (gonadorelin) is indicated for the treatment of ovarian follicular cysts in dairy cattle. Ovarian cysts are non-ovulated follicles with incomplete luteinization which result in nymphomania or irregular estrus.

Historically, cystic ovaries have responded to an exogenous source of luteinizing hormone (LH) such as human chorionic gonadodotropin. CYSTORELIN® initiates release of endogenous LH to cause ovulation and lutenization.

Pharmacology: Description: CYSTORELIN® is a sterile solution containing 50 micrograms of gonadorelin (GnRH) diacetate tetrahydrate per milliliter suitable for intramuscular or intravenous administration. Gonadorelin is a decapeptide composed of the sequence of amino acids—5-oxoPro-His-Trp-Ser-Tyr-Gly-Leu-Arg-Pro-Gly-NH_2—a molecular weight of 1182.32 and empirical formula $C_{55}H_{75}N_{17}O_{13}$. The diacetate tetrahydrate ester has a molecular weight of 1374.48 and empirical formula $C_{59}H_{91}N_{17}O_{21}$.

Gonadorelin is the hypothalamic releasing factor responsible for the release of gonadotropins (e.g. LH, FSH) from the anterior pituitary. Synthetic gonadorelin is physiologically and chemically identical to the endogenous bovine hypothalamic releasing factor.

Endogenous gonadorelin is synthesized and/or released from the hypothalamus during various stages of the bovine estrus cycle following appropriate neurogenic stimuli. It passes, via the hypophyseal portal vessels, to the anterior pituitary to effect the release of gonadotropins (e.g. LH, FSH). Synthetic gonadorelin administered intravenously or intramuscularly also causes the release of endogenous LH or FSH from the anterior pituitary.

Dosage and Administration: The recommended intravenous or intramuscular dosage of CYSTORELIN® is 100 mcg per cow.

Precaution(s): Keep refrigerated: 2°-8°C (36°-46°F).

Caution(s): Federal (U.S.A.) law restricts this drug to use by or on the order of a licensed veterinarian.

Warning(s): Not for use in humans.

Keep this and all drugs out of reach of children.

The Material Safety Data Sheet (MSDS) contains more detailed occupational safety information. To report adverse effects in users, to obtain an MSDS, or for assistance call 1-888-637-4251.

Toxicology: Gonadorelin diacetate tetrahydrate has been shown to be safe. The LD_{50} for mice and rats is greater than 60 mg/kg, and for dogs, greater than 600 mcg/kg, respectively. No untoward effects were noted among rats or dogs administered 120 mcg/kg/day or 72 mcg/kg/day intravenously for 15 days.

It has no adverse effects on heart rate, blood pressure, or EKG to unanesthetized dogs at 60 mcg/kg. In anesthetized dogs it did not produce depression of myocardial or system hemodynamics or adversely affect coronary oxygen supply or myocardial oxygen requirements.

The intravenous administration of 60 mcg/kg/day of gonadorelin diacetate tetrahydrate to pregnant rats and rabbits during organogenesis did not cause embryotoxic or teratogenic effects.

The intramuscular administration of 1,000 mcg to normally cycling dairy cattle had no effect on hematology or blood chemistry.

Further, CYSTORELIN® does not cause irritation at the site of intramuscular administration in dogs. The dosage administered was 72 mcg/kg/day for seven (7) days.

Presentation: CYSTORELIN® is supplied in multi-dose vials containing 10 mL of sterile solution, 20 per case.

® Registered trademark of Merial.

Merial Limited: Registered in England and Wales [Reg. No. 3332751] with registered offices at 27 Knightsbridge, London, SW1X 7QT, England and domesticated in Delaware, USA as Merial LLC.

Compendium Code No.: 11110081 C-03004-R3

C

Disclaimer
Every effort has been made to ensure the accuracy of the information published. However, it remains the responsibility of the readers to familiarize themselves with the product information contained on the product label or package insert.
Inclusion or omission of products does not imply endorsement or criticism by the Publisher or anyone involved in the publication. Inclusion does not imply product availability and/or product registration. The Publisher, Editorial Team and all those involved in the production of this book cannot be held responsible for publication errors or any consequence that could result from the use of published information.

D

D-128

Vedco **Disinfectant**

Active Ingredient(s): Contains:

Didecyl dimethyl ammonium chloride 4.61%
n-Alkyl (C_{14} 50%, C_{12} 40%, C_{16} 10%) dimethyl benzyl ammonium chloride 3.07%
Inert ingredients 92.32%

Indications: A concentrated, multi-purpose germicidal detergent and deodorant effective in hard waters, up to 400 ppm hard water (calculated as $CaCO_3$) plus 5% organic serum.

Disinfects, cleans and deodorizes in one step.

Recommended for use in veterinary clinics and animal life science laboratories, equine farms, tack shops, pet shops, kennels, poultry and turkey farms, dairy and hog farms, breeding and grooming establishments.

Pharmacology: Bactericidal at 1:28 (1 oz. per gallon of water) against *Pseudomonas aeruginosa, Fusobacterium necrophorum, Staphylococcus aureus* and *Salmonella choleraesuis* according to the current AOAC Use-Dilution Test method, modified in the presence of 400 ppm synthetic hard water (calculated as $CaCO_3$) plus 5% organic serum.

Fungicidal against *Trichophyton interdigitale* and *Candida albicans* according to the AOAC fungicidal test, modified in the presence of 400 ppm hard water (calculated as $CaCO_3$) plus 5% organic serum at a 1:128 dilution (1 oz. per gallon of water).

Virucidal against influenza A/Hong Kong, Herpes simplex type I, Herpes simplex type II, vaccinia, rubella, adenovirus type 4, feline picornavirus, feline leukemia virus, canine distemper virus, rabies virus, porcine parvovirus, pseudorabies virus, infectious bronchitis (avian IBV), canine parvovirus according to the virucidal qualification, modified in the presence of 400 ppm hard water plus 5% organic serum at a 1:128 dilution (1 oz. per gallon of water).

Dosage and Administration: It is a violation of federal law to use the product in a manner inconsistent with its labeling.

General use directions for disinfecting: For use on hard, nonporous surfaces such as floors, walls, metal surfaces, porcelain and plastic surfaces.

Remove gross filth and heavy soil deposits, then thoroughly wet surfaces as recommended and required. Use 1 oz. per gallon of water for a minimum contact time of 10 minutes in a single application. Can be applied with a mop, sponge or cloth, as well as spraying or soaking.

The recommended use solution is prepared fresh for each use, then discarded. Rinsing is not necessary unless floors are to be waxed or polished.

Mildew static instructions: Will effectively inhibit the growth and mildew plus the odors caused by them when applied to hard, nonporous surfaces such as walls, floors and tabletops.

Apply (1 oz. per gallon of water) with a cloth, mop or sponge making sure to wet all surfaces completely. Let air dry. Prepare a fresh solution for each use. Repeat application once a week or when growth reappears.

Precaution(s): Storage and Disposal Prohibitions: Do not contaminate water, food or feed by storage or disposal. Open dumping is prohibited. Do not re-use the empty container.

Pesticide Disposal: Pesticide wastes are acutely hazardous. Improper disposal of excess pesticide, spray mixture or rinsate is a violation of federal law. If these wastes cannot be disposed of according to label instructions, contact a State Pesticide or Environmental Control Agency, or the Hazardous Waste representative at the nearest EPA Regional Office for guidance.

Container Disposal: Plastic containers, triple rinse (or equivalent). Then offer for recycling or reconditioning, or puncture and dispose of in a sanitary landfill, or by incineration, or, if allowed by state and local authorities, by burning. If burned, stay out of smoke.

General: Consult federal, state or local disposal authorities for approved alternative procedures, such as limited open burning.

Caution(s): Hazards to Humans and Domestic Animals: Keep out of the reach of children.

Precautionary Statements:

Corrosive. Causes eye damage and severe skin irritation. Do not get in the eyes, on skin or on clothing. To protect eyes, wear goggles or a face shield and to protect skin, wear rubber gloves when handling. Wash thoroughly with soap and water after handling. Remove contaminated clothing and wash before re-use. Harmful if swallowed.

Statement of Practical Treatment:

In case of contact, immediately flush the eyes or skin with plenty of water for at least 15 minutes. For eyes, call a physician.

If swallowed, drink promptly a large quantity of milk, egg whites, gelatin solution, or if these are not available, drink large quantities of water. Avoid alcohol. Get medical attention.

Note to Physician: Probable mucosal damage may contraindicate the use of gastric lavage. Measures against circulatory shock, respiratory depression and convulsion may be needed.

Presentation: 1 gallon containers.

Compendium Code No.: 10940390

D-256

Vedco **Disinfectant**

EPA Reg. No.: 47371-129-44084

Active Ingredient(s):

Didecyl dimethyl ammonium chloride 9.22%
n-Alkyl (c14 50%, c12 40%, c16 10%) dimethyl benzyl ammonium chloride 6.14%
Inert Ingredients: 84.6%

Dilution: 1:256 (600 ppm quat) ½ ounce per gallon of water.

Indications: One-step, germicidal detergent and deodorant recommended for use in hospitals, nursing homes, schools, colleges, commercial and industrial institutions, office buildings, veterinary clinics, animal life science laboratories, equine farms, dairy farms, hog farms, breeding establishments, grooming establishments, and households. Disinfects, cleans and deodorizes floors, walls, metal surfaces, stainless steel surfaces, glazed porcelain, plastic surfaces (such as polypropylene, polystyrene, etc.), and other hard non-porous surfaces.

This product has disinfectant, pseudomonacidal, staphylocidal, bactericidal, fungicidal-mildewstatic and virucidal action.

Directions for Use: It is a violation of Federal law to use this product in a manner inconsistent with its labeling.

Application: Remove heavy soil deposits from surface. Then thoroughly wet surface with a solution of ½ ounce concentrate per gallon of water. The solution can be applied with a cloth, mop, sponge, or coarse spray, or soaking.

Let solution remain on surface for a minimum of 10 minutes. Rinse or allow to air dry. Rinsing off floors is not necessary unless they are to be waxed or polished. Prepare a fresh solution daily or more often if the solution becomes visibly dirty or dirty.

Mildewstatic Instructions: Will effectively control the growth of mold and mildew plus the odors caused by them when applied to hard non-porous surfaces such as walls, floors, and table tops. Apply solution (½ ounce per gallon of water) with a cloth, mop, sponge, or coarse spray. Make sure to wet all surfaces completely. Let air dry. Repeat application weekly or when growth reappears.

*Kills HIV-1 (AIDS Virus) on precleaned, environmental surfaces/objects previously soiled with blood/body fluids in health care settings or other settings in which there is an expected likelihood of soiling of inanimate surfaces/objects with blood/body fluids, and in which the surface/objects likely to be soiled with blood/body fluids can be associated with the potential for transmission of human immunodeficiency virus Type 1 (HIV-1)(Associated with AIDS).

Special Instructions for Cleaning and Decontamination Against HIV-1 (AIDS Virus) of Surfaces/Objects Soiled with Blood/Body Fluids:

Personal Protection: Disposable latex or vinyl gloves, gowns, face masks, or eye coverings such as appropriate must be worn during all cleaning of blood/body fluids and during decontamination procedures.

Cleaning Procedures: Blood/body fluids must be thoroughly cleaned from surfaces/objects before application of disinfectant.

Contact Time: HIV-1 (AIDS Virus) is inactivated after a contact time of 4 minutes at 25°C (room temperature). Use a 10 minute contact time for other viruses, fungi, and bacteria listed.

Disposal of Infectious Materials: Blood/body fluids should be autoclaved and disposed of according to federal, state and local regulations for infectious waste disposal.

Effective Against the Following Pathogens: *Pseudomonas aeruginosa*[1], *Listeria monocytogenes, Staphylococcus epidermis*[2], *infectious bronchitis; *Staphylococcus aureus*[1], *Pasteurella multocida, Streptococcus faecalis,* *influenza A/Hong Kong; *Salmonella choleraesuis, Proteus mirabilis, Streptococcus pyogenes,* *pseudorabies; *Acinetobacter calcoaceticus, Proteus Vulgaris,* *Adenovirus type 4 *rabies; *Bordetella bronchiseptica, Salmonella enteritidis,* *canine distemper, *respiratory synctial virus; *Chlamydia psittaci, Salmonella typhi,* *feline leukemia, *rubeola (German measles); *Enterobacter aerogenes, Salmonella typhimurium,* *feline picornavirus, *transmissible gastroenteritis virus; *Enterobacter cloacae, Serratia marcescens,* *herpes simplex type 1, *vaccina; *Escherichia coli*[1], *Shigella flexneri,* *herpes simplex type 2, *Aspergillus niger, Fusobacterium necrophorum, Shigella sonnei,* *HIV-1 (AIDS virus), candida albicans; *Klebsiella pneumoniae, Staphylococcus aureus,* *infectious bovine rhinotracheitis; *Trichophyton mentagrophytes,* (methicillin resistant);

* virus

1 ATCC & Antibiotic - resistant strain 2 Antibiotic-resistant strain.

Farm Premise, Livestock, Poultry & Turkey House Disinfectant: Directions for Use:

1. Remove all animals and feeds from premises, trucks, coops, crates and enclosures.
2. Remove all litter and manure from floors, walls and surfaces of barns, pens, stalls, chutes, vehicles, and other facilities and fixtures occupied or traversed by animals.
3. Empty all troughs, racks, and other feeding and watering appliances.
4. Thoroughly clean all surfaces with soap or detergent, and rinse with water.
5. Saturate all surfaces with the recommended disinfecting solution for a period of 10 minutes.
6. Immerse all halters, ropes, and other types of equipment used in handling and restraining animals, as well as forks, shovels and scrapers used for removing litter and manure.
7. Ventilate buildings, coops, cars, boats and other enclosed spaces. Do not house animals or employ equipment until treatment has been absorbed, set or dried.
8. After treatment with disinfectant, thoroughly scrub feed racks, troughs, automatic feeders, fountains, and waterers with soap or detergent, and rinse with potable water before use.

Precautionary Statements: Hazards to Humans and Domestic Animals: Danger: Corrosive: Causes eye damage and severe skin irritation. Harmful if swallowed. Do not get in eyes, on sin or clothing. When handling product, protect eyes by wearing goggles or face shield and protect skin by wearing rubber gloves. Wash thoroughly with soap and water after handling. Remove contaminated clothing and wash before reuse.

Statement of Practical Treatment: In case of contact, immediately flush eyes or skin with plenty of water for at least 15 minutes. For eyes, call a physician. If swallowed, immediately drink a large quantity of water. Avoid alcohol. Get medical attention.

Note to Physician: Probable mucosal damage may contraindicate the use of gastric lavage. Measures against circulatory shock, respiratory depression, and convulsions may be needed.

Storage and Disposal: Keep product under locked storage, inaccessible to children. Do not contaminate water, food, or feed by storage or disposal. Open dumping is prohibited. Do not reuse empty container.

Pesticide Disposal: Pesticide wastes are acutely hazardous. Improper disposal of excess pesticide, spray mixture or rinsate is a violation of Federal law. If these wastes cannot be disposed of by use according to label instructions, contact your state pesticide or Environmental Control Agency, or the Hazardous Waste representatives at the nearest EPA Regional Office for guidance.

Container Disposal: Do not reuse empty container. Rinse thoroughly, securely wrap in several layers of newspaper, and discard empty container in trash.

Warning(s): Keep out of reach of children.

Presentation: 1 gallon and 2.5 gallon.

Compendium Code No.: 10940402

DAIRY BOMB-50

Durvet **Premise and Topical Insecticide**

EPA Reg. No.: 9444-173-12281

Active Ingredient(s):

Pyrethrins 0.50%
Piperonyl Butoxide, technical* 2.50%
Inert Ingredients: 97.00%
Total 100%

*Equivalent to 2.00% (butylcarbityl) (6-propylpiperonyl) ether and 0.5% related compounds.

Contains no CFCs or other ozone depleting substances. Federal regulations prohibit CFC propellants in aerosols.

Indications: Kills house flies, mosquitoes, gnats, wasps, small flying moths, barn flies, deer flies, stable flies and horn flies.

Directions for Use: It is a violation of Federal law to use this product in a manner inconsistent with its labeling.

Dairy Farm Use: Milking Parlor and Milk Room - Close all windows and doors. Direct spray upwards, spraying for 2-3 seconds for 1,000 cubic feet of space. Do not remain in treated areas. Ventilate after treatment. Cover milking utensils and milk to prevent contamination from spray and dead or falling insects.

Animal Use: Thoroughly spray entire animal from approximately 2 feet distance. Do not spray directly toward animal's eyes. Spot treat withers, shoulders and back where saliva accumulates from head tossing.

Beef Cattle Operations: In barns, close all windows and doors. Spray at the rate of 2-3 seconds per 1,000 cubic feet of space. Do not remain in treated area. After 15 minutes, ventilate the area. Repeat application as necessary.

Animal Use: For animal application, thoroughly spray entire animal from approximately 2 feet distance. Do not spray directly toward animal's face or eyes. Repeat application daily or as necessary.

Stanchion Barn Use: Walk behind animals and direct spray over backs, allowing 5 seconds per animal. For most effective results, apply each morning.

Horse Barns or Stables: In horse and pony barns, close all window and doors. Spray at the rate of 2-3 seconds per 1,000 cubic feet of space. Do not remain in treated area. After 15 minutes, ventilate the area. Repeat the application as necessary.

Animal Use: For animal application, lightly mist over backs of horses and ponies from a distance of 2 feet. Do not spray directly toward the animal's face or eyes. Repeat application daily or as necessary.

Hog Operations: In hog houses, close all doors and windows. Spray at the rate of 2-3 seconds per 1,000 cubic feet of space. Do not remain in treated area. After 15 minutes, ventilate the area. Repeat the application as necessary.

Animal Use: For animal application, direct spray over backs of hogs and spray for 5 seconds per hog. Do not spray directly toward the animal's face or eyes. Repeat application daily or as necessary.

Poultry Operations: In poultry houses, close all windows and doors. Spray at the rate of 2-3 seconds per 1,000 cubic feet of space. Do not remain in treated areas. After 15 minutes, ventilate the area. Treat daily or as necessary.

Home Use: To Kill Cockroaches, Spiders, Silverfish, Wasps, Hornets, Crickets - Spray the insect directly when possible, and spray all probable hiding places such as cracks, crevices, baseboards, sinks, cabinets, shelves and under appliances. Repeat as necessary.

Precautionary Statements: Hazards to Humans and Domestic Animals:

Caution: Harmful if swallowed. Avoid breathing of vapor. Avoid contact with skin and eyes. In case of contact, immediately flush eyes with plenty of water. Wash skin with warm water and soap. Get medical attention if irritation persists. Do not contaminate food or foodstuffs. Do not remain in treated areas. Vacate premises for at least 15 minutes after spraying. Ventilate the area after treatment is completed and before re-entering. In medical care facilities, remove all patients prior to treatment. Ventilate area for 2 hours before returning patients.

Volumetric Treatment in Homes: In the home, all food processing surfaces and utensils should be covered during treatment or thoroughly washed before use. Remove pets and birds and cover fish aquariums before spraying.

Physical or Chemical Hazards: Flammable. Contents under pressure. Keep away from heat, sparks and open flame. Do not puncture or incinerate container. Exposure to temperatures above 130°F may cause bursting.

Do not spray on plastic, painted or varnished surfaces or directly into electronic equipment such as radios, TVs, computers, etc.

Storage and Disposal: Do not contaminate water, food or feed by storage or disposal.

Storage: Store in a cool, dry area away from heat or open flame.

Disposal: The container may be recycled in the few but growing number of communities where steel aerosol can recycling is available. Before offering for recycling, empty the can by using the product according to the label. Do not puncture or incinerate! If recycling is not available, wrap the container and discard in the trash.

Warning(s): Keep out of reach of children.

Disclaimer: Buyer assumes all risks of use, storage or handling of this material not in strict accordance with directions given herewith.

Presentation: 25 oz (709 g) aerosol can.

Compendium Code No.: 10840391 2/99

DAIRY BOMB-50Z

Durvet **Premise and Topical Insecticide**

EPA Reg. No.: 9444-210-12281

Active Ingredient(s):

Pyrethrins	0.50%
Piperonyl Butoxide, technical*	4.00%
Inert Ingredients	95.50%
	100.00%

* Equivalent to 3.20% (butylcarbityl) (6-propylpiperonyl) ether and 0.80% related compounds.

Contains no CFCs or other ozone depleting substances. Federal regulations prohibit CFC propellants in aerosols.

Indications: Kills and Repels: Flies, Mosquitoes, Small Flying Moths, Wasps, Hornets, Gnats, Cockroaches, Ants, Fleas, Crickets, Spiders, Barn Flies, Deer Flies, Stable Flies, Horn Flies, Horse Flies, House Flies, Face Flies, Fruit Flies, Lice, Centipedes, Millipedes, Clover Mites, Cluster Flies and Mud Daubers.

For use in Beef Cattle Operations, Dairy Farms (including Milk House, Milk Parlor, Loafing Sheds, and Holding Lot), Hog Operations, Kennels, Barns, Stables, Farms, Animal Quarters, Milkrooms, and Poultry Houses.

Directions for Use: It is a violation of Federal law to use this product in a manner inconsistent with its labeling.

Hold container upright with nozzle away from you. Press valve down and spray as directed. To avoid possible staining of fabrics or surfaces, do not spray at close range.

Note: When using this product in an enclosed area, such as a milkroom, barn or stable, remove animals before spraying.

Dairy Farm Use: Milking Parlor and Milkroom—Close all windows and doors. Direct spray upwards, spraying for 1-3 seconds per 1,000 cubic feet of space. Do not remain in treated areas. Ventilate after treatment. Cover milking utensils and milk to prevent contamination from spray and dead or falling insects.

Animal Use (Do not spray sick animals): Thoroughly spray entire animal from approximately 2 feet distance. Do not spray directly toward animal's eyes. Spot treat withers, shoulders and back where saliva accumulates from head tossing.

Beef Cattle Operations: In barns, close all windows and doors. Spray at the rate of 1-2 seconds per 1,000 cubic feet of space. Do not remain in treated area. After 15 minutes, ventilate the area. Repeat application as necessary.

Animal Use: For animal application, thoroughly spray entire animal from approximately 2 feet distance. Do not spray directly toward animal's face or eyes. Repeat application daily or as necessary.

Stanchion Barn Use: Walk behind animals and direct spray over backs, allowing 1 second per animal. For most effective results, apply each morning.

Horse Barns or Stables: In horse and pony barns, close all windows and doors. Spray at the rate of 1-2 seconds per 1000 cubic feet of space. Do not remain in treated area. After 15 minutes, ventilate the area. Repeat the application as necessary.

Animal Use: For animal application, lightly mist over back of horses and ponies from a distance of 2 feet. Do not spray directly toward the animal's face or eyes. Repeat application daily or as necessary.

Hog Operations: In hog houses, close all doors and windows. Spray at the rate of 1-2 seconds per 1,000 cubic feet of space. Do not remain in treated area. After 15 minutes, ventilate the area. Repeat the application as necessary.

Animal Use: For animal application, direct spray over back of hogs and spray for 1-2 seconds per hog. Do not spray directly toward the animal's face or eyes. Repeat application daily or as necessary.

Poultry Operations: Use only in empty poultry houses (when birds are not present). In poultry houses, close all windows and doors. Spray roosts, walls, nests, and cages thoroughly. Spray at the rate of 1-2 seconds per 1000 cubic feet of space. Do not remain in treated areas. Ventilate after treatment. Treat daily or as necessary.

Mud Dauber and Wasp Nest: Spray mist directly on insects and their nests from approximately 2 ft. distance. Contacted insects will fly away from fog. Applications should be made in late evening when insects are at rest. Spray into hiding and breeding places contacting as many insects as possible.

Fleas: General Volumetric Treatment: Hold aerosol 36" above floor and direct spray toward floor and lower walls at a rate of 10 seconds per 100 sq. ft. making sure that all floor areas are contacted. Change litter before application. Keep area closed for 15 minutes. Remove animals before spraying. Open and ventilate before reoccupying. Repeat treatment after 7 days or as necessary.

Kennels and Catteries: Remove animals before spraying. Ventilate after treatment is completed.

Outdoor Ground Application: Flies, Gnats, and Mosquitoes in open areas near buildings and in campgrounds. Best results are obtained when wind speed is five (5) MPH or less. Apply at a rate of 60-80 seconds per acre. Spray in wide swaths across area to be treated. Allow spray drift to penetrate dense foliage. Repeat treatment as necessary.

Precautionary Statements: Hazards to Humans and Domestic Animals:

Caution: Harmful if absorbed through skin or inhaled. Avoid contact with eyes, skin or clothing. Avoid breathing spray mist. Wash thoroughly with soap and water after handling. Remove contaminated clothing and wash clothing before reuse.

Statement of Practical Treatment:

If Swallowed: Call a physician or Poison Control Center. Do not induce vomiting. Do not give anything by mouth to an unconscious person. Avoid alcohol.

If Inhaled: Remove victim to fresh air. If not breathing, give artificial respiration, preferably mouth-to-mouth. Get medical attention.

If On Skin: Wash with plenty of soap and water. If symptoms persist get medical attention.

May pose an aspiration pneumonia hazard.

Environmental Hazards: This product is toxic to fish, birds, and other wildlife. Do not apply directly to water, or to areas where surface water is present or to intertidal areas below the mean high water mark. Apply this product only as specified on this label.

Physical or Chemical Hazards: Flammable. Contents under pressure. Keep away from heat, sparks and open flame. Do not puncture or incinerate container. Exposure to temperatures above 130°F may cause bursting.

Do not spray on plastic, painted or varnished surfaces or directly into electronic equipment such as radios, TVs, computers, etc.

Storage and Disposal: Do not contaminate water, food or feed by storage or disposal.

Storage: Store in a cool, dry area away from heat or open flame.

Disposal: This container may be recycled in the few but growing number of communities where steel aerosol can recycling is available. Before offering for recycling, empty the can by using the product according to the label. Do not puncture! If recycling is not available, wrap the container and discard in the trash.

Warning(s): Keep out of reach of children.

Presentation: 24 oz / 680 g.

Compendium Code No.: 10840400 38L34-8315DR-57-REV 2/99 (PNT 1/00)

DAIRY BOMB-55

Durvet **Premise and Topical Insecticide**

EPA Reg. No.: 47000-73-12281

Active Ingredient(s): Non-aqueous, low oil pyrethrin and piperonyl butoxide insecticide.

Pyrethrins	0.5%
*Piperonyl Butoxide, Technical	1.0%
N-Octyl Bicycloheptene Dicarboximide	1.0%
Inert Ingredients	97.5%

*Equivalent to 0.8% (butylcarbityl) (6-propylpiperonyl) ether and 0.2% of related compounds.

Indications: For use on cattle, horses, swine, and in homes, restaurants, food handling plants, dairies, milk houses, cattle, horse, poultry, and swine quarters.

Directions for Use: It is a violation of Federal Law to use this product in a manner inconsistent with its labeling.

Remove protective cap. Aim spray opening away from person. Push button to spray.

Dairy Farm Use: Milking parlor and milk room. Close all windows and doors. Spray at the rate of 1 to 2 seconds per 1000 cubic feet. If rooms cannot be closed, double the dosage. Stand in middle of room. Direct spray in all directions. Keep room closed for 15 minutes after treatment. Do not remain in treated area. Ventilate the area after treatment is completed. Cover milking utensils and milk to prevent contamination from spray and dead or falling insects.

Dairy Animal Use: From approximately 2 foot distance thoroughly spray entire animal as it is being released to pasture. Do not spray directly toward animal's eyes. Spot treat withers, shoulders and back where saliva accumulates from head tossing.

Stanchion Barn Use: Walk behind animals and direct spray over backs allowing 1 second per animal. For most effective results, apply each morning.

Poultry Operations: In poultry houses, close all windows and doors. Spray at the rate of 1 to 2 seconds per 1000 cubic feet. Keep area closed for 15 minutes following application. Treat daily or as necessary.

Hog Operations: In hog houses, close all windows and doors. Apply at the rate of 1 to 2 seconds per 1000 cubic feet. Keep area closed for 15 minutes following application. For animal application direct spray over backs and spray for 1 to 2 seconds per hog. Do not spray directly towards animal's face or eyes. Repeat application daily or as necessary.

Horse Barns and Stables: In horse and pony barns close all windows and doors. Spray at the rate of 1 to 2 seconds per 1000 cubic feet. Keep area closed for 15 minutes following application. If area cannot be closed, double the dosage. In animal application, lightly mist over backs of horses and ponies from a distance of at least 2 feet. Do not spray directly toward horses face or eyes. Repeat application daily or as necessary.

Beef Cattle Operations: In barns, close all windows and doors. Apply at the rate of 1 to 2 seconds per 1000 cubic feet. Keep area closed for 15 minutes following application. For animal use, thoroughly spray entire animal as it is being released to pasture. Do not spray directly towards animal's face or eyes. Repeat application daily or as necessary.

Home and Food Processing Area Use: For flies, mosquitoes, small flying moths (millers), and gnats: Close all doors and windows. Point nozzle upward, direct the spray mist to all parts of the room, especially windows and other light sources which attract these insects. Fill the room with mist, then leave the treated areas. Keep the room closed for at least 15 minutes. Ventilate the room when treatment is completed. Roaches, Waterbugs, Sowbugs, Spiders and Centipedes: Spray thoroughly into hiding places such as cracks, crevices, moist areas, openings around pipes and sinks, under refrigerators, baseboards and storage areas. Spray directly on insects where possible. Repeat as necessary. Ants: Spray trails, nests and points of entry. Spray on ants where possible. Repeat as necessary.

Precautionary Statements: Hazards to Humans and Domestic Animals: Caution: Harmful if swallowed. Avoid contact with skin and eyes. Avoid inhalation of spray mist. Avoid contamination of feed and foodstuffs.

When using this product as a space spray in food processing plants, foods must be removed or covered during treatment. Apply only when the facility is not in operation. At home and in food processing establishments, cover or remove food prior to treatment. Cover food contact surfaces, benches, utensils, equipment, etc., during treatment or thoroughly clean prior to use with an effective cleaning compound followed by a potable water rinse.

In hospitals or other medical facilities, remove patients prior to treatment. Ventilate treated area for two hours prior to returning patients.

Do not remain in treated areas and ventilate the area after treatment is completed.

Remove pets, birds and cover fish aquariums before spraying.

Physical or Chemical Hazards: Extremely flammable. Contents under pressure. Keep away from fire, sparks, and heated surfaces. Do not puncture or incinerate container. Exposure to temperatures above 130°F may cause bursting.

Environmental Hazards: This product is toxic to fish, birds, and other wildlife. Keep out of lakes, ponds, or streams. Do not contaminate water when disposing of equipment in washwater. Apply this product only as specified on this label.

Statement of Practical Treatment:

If Swallowed: Call a physician or poison control center immediately. Do not induce vomiting. Vomiting may cause aspiration pneumonia.

If inhaled: Remove patient to fresh air. Apply artificial respiration if indicated.

If on Skin: Remove contaminated clothing and wash affected skin areas with soap and water. Get medical attention if irritation persists.

If in Eyes: Flush eyes with plenty of water. Get medical attention if irritation persists.

Storage and Disposal:

Storage: Store in a cool, dry, secure area.

Disposal: Do not reuse empty container. Wrap container and put in trash collection.

Warning(s): Keep out of reach of children.

Disclaimer: Notice to User: Seller's guarantee shall be limited to the terms of the label, and subject thereto the buyer assumes any risk to persons or property arising out of use or handling and accepts the products on these conditions.

Presentation: 25 oz. container.

Compendium Code No.: 10840412 1/99

DAIRY BOMB-55Z

Durvet **Premise and Topical Insecticide**

EPA Reg. No.: 47000-97-12281

Active Ingredient(s):

Pyrethrins 0.5%
*Piperonyl Butoxide, Technical 5.0%
Other Ingredients 94.50%

*Equivalent to 4.00% (butylcarbityl) (8-Propylpiperonyl) ether and 1.0% related compounds.

Indications: Contains pyrethrum. Kills and repels stable flies, horse flies, face flies, deer flies, house flies, mosquitos and gnats. For use in animal quarters, dairies, milk rooms, milking parlors, calving areas, dairy and hog barns as well as outdoor areas. For use on beef cattle, dairy cattle, horses, hogs, chickens, and other livestock. Quick killing pyrethrin controls crawling and flying insects in the dairies, barns, storage sites and other listed areas. For use in homes for bedbugs, clothes moths, carpet beetles, cockroaches, fleas, ticks, and other listed pests.

Directions for Use: It is a violation of Federal Law to use this product in a manner inconsistent with its labeling.

Read all directions completely before use.

For most effective results, follow directions for specific use areas.

Shake before use and at intervals during prolonged use. Hold container upright with nozzle away from face. Press valve down and spray as directed.

For Use in Animal Quarters, Barns, Dairies, Milking Parlors, Milking Rooms, Poultry Houses and other listed animal areas: For rapid control of Flies, Mosquitos, Gnats, Stable Fly, House Fly, Horse Fly, Lesser House Fly, Deer Fly, Horn Fly, Black Fly: Spray at the rate of 5 to 10 seconds per 1000 cubic feet of space directing the spray toward the ceiling and upper corners and not directly towards the animals or birds. For best results, close doors and windows if possible, before spraying and keep them closed for 10 to 15 minutes. Applicator should vacate the treated area and ventilate it prior to returning. Repeat as necessary.

For Use on Livestock: To protect beef cattle, dairy cattle, horses and other livestock from attacks and to kill and repel Stable Flies, Horse Flies, Deer Flies, House Flies, Horn Flies, Lesser House Flies, Mosquitos and Gnats, spray about 3 seconds on each side being careful to spray back, withers and forelegs thoroughly. Repeat as necessary.

To protect from Face Flies, spray the face and head or spray on a cloth and rub on the face being certain to avoid contact with the eyes. Repeat treatment as necessary when flies are troublesome.

For effective control of biting and suckling lice on cattle, horses, sheep, goats, and hogs, spray to thoroughly wet the hair of the animal including the head and brush of the tail. Repeat treatment in 10 days to kill newly hatched lice.

To control Poultry Lice and exposed stages of Darkling Beetles, spray roosts, walls and nests or cages thoroughly. This should be followed by spraying over the birds with a fine mist. Repeat as necessary.

For control of bedbugs and mites on poultry and in poultry houses, spray crevices of roost poles, cracks in walls and cracks in nests where the Bedbugs and Mites hide. This should be followed by spraying over the birds with a fine mist. Repeat as necessary.

To control sheep "tick" or Ked, thoroughly wet all portions of the body by spraying directly into the wool. Treat at a rate to sufficiently wet the animal. Repeat as necessary.

To kill fleas and ixodid ticks on livestock and to obtain protection against reinfestation, spray to wet animal. Repeat as necessary.

Space Treatment Indoors: For maximum efficacy, close all doors and windows, turn off fans and air conditioner and spray upward into center of room with slow sweeping motion. Spray 5 to 10 seconds for average size room (1,000 cubic feet). Keep room closed for 15 minutes after spraying. Ventilate room for 5 minutes before entry. For use in food areas of food handling establishments: When applying space treatment in food handing areas, the food handling operation should be shut down. In food processing areas, all utensils, shelving, etc., where food will be handled should be covered or removed before treatment or washed with an effective cleaning compound followed by a potable water rinse prior to use.

Flies, Gnats, Mosquitos, Flying Moths, exposed stages of Indian Meal Moth, Angoumois Grain Moth, Tobacco Moth, Clothes Moth, Chocolate Moth, Almond Moth, Miller Moth, and other listed flying insects: Direct spray into all parts of the room, with special attention to hiding places. Sweep up and destroy fallen insects. Repeat as necessary.

Surface Treatment Indoor: For use in Food and Nonfood areas of Food Processing Plants, Industrial Installations, Bakeries, Rice and Wheat Mills, Restaurants, Tobacco Warehouses, Grain Elevators and Warehouses: Spray as directed to control listed flying and crawling insects. The use of this product in food processing or food handling establishments should be confined to time periods when the plant is not in operation. Food should be covered or removed during treatment.

Repeat as necessary.

For use in Storage Sites: This product can be used in warehouse bins and trucks, cargo ships, mills, bin hoppers, elevators and conveying equipment as a clean up prior to using them for storage. In mills and elevators, all grain infested accumulations should be removed from the bin hoppers. All storage and conveying equipment should be thoroughly cleaned by sweeping out the waste grain, cobwebs and other debris from the walls and rafters as well as on the floor and door frames with special attention to material lodged in the cracks and crevices. All of the debris should be removed and burned to kill eggs and insects that might be present.

For Farms, particular attention should be given to cleaning up around the used feed and grain bags, grain residues from wagons, harvesting equipment and feed troughs. Newly harvested grain should not be placed in same bin with carry-over grain and all carry-over grain stocks that are not treated with grain protectant should be fumigated. These cleaning operations should be done within two or three weeks before harvest.

After above sanitation measures have been employed, spray all areas prior to use for storage as directed.

Ants, Foraging Fire Ants, Pharaoh Ants, Carpenter Ants: Treat doors, around window frames, ant trails and hills and other areas of entry. Spray on ants where possible. Repeat as necessary.

Fleas and Ticks: For use in listed pet areas. Remove and either launder or destroy pet's old bedding. To reduce infestation, thoroughly spray the animal's clean bedding, sleeping quarters, kennel, around baseboards, window and door frames, wall cracks, local areas of floors and other resting places until the surface is slightly moist. Treat these areas at the rate of two seconds per linear foot at the distance of 12 to 18 inches. Also spray the entire inside surface of dog houses. Put fresh bedding in pet's quarters after spray has dried. Allow treated areas to dry thoroughly before allowing pets to re-enter. For best results, pets should be treated with an EPA registered flea and tick control product before they return to the treated area. Do not treat pets with this product. Repeat necessary.

Precautionary Statements: Hazards To Humans and Domestic Animals:

Caution: Harmful if absorbed through skin. Avoid contact with skin, eyes, or clothing. Prolonged or frequently repeated skin contact may cause allergic reactions in some individuals. Wash thoroughly with soap and water after handling. Avoid contamination of food or feedstuffs.

Environmental Hazards: For terrestrial uses, do not apply directly to water, or to areas where surface water is present or to intertidal areas below the mean high water mark.

Physical or Chemical Hazards: Contents under pressure. Do not use or store near heat or open flame. Do not puncture or incinerate container. Exposure to temperatures above 130°F may cause BURSTING. Do not use this product in or on electrical equipment due to possibility of shock hazard.

Statement of Practical Treatment:

If Swallowed: Call a physician or Poison Control Center immediately. If in Eyes: Flush with plenty of water. Get medical attention if irritation persists. If on Skin: Wash skin with plenty of soap and water. Get medical attention. If inhaled: Remove victim to fresh air. Apply artificial respiration if indicated.

For information regarding medical emergencies or pesticide incidents call The International Poison Control Center at 1-888-740-8712.

Storage and Disposal: Do not contaminate water, food, or feed by storage or disposal.

Storage: Store in a cool, dry, place away from children, preferably a secure storage area.

Container Disposal: When container is empty, replace cap and offer for recycling. Where recycling is not available, securely wrap container in several layers of newspaper and discard in trash.

Warning(s): Keep out of reach of children.

Disclaimer: Notice To User: Seller's guarantee shall be limited to the terms of the label, and subject thereto the buyer assumes any risk to persons or property arising out of use or handling and accepts the product on these conditions.

Presentation: 25 oz (709 g) can.

Compendium Code No.: 10840420

DAIRYLAND BRAND PRE-POST 5000

Stearns **Teat Dip**

Active Ingredient(s): Contains: Nonylphenoxypolyethoxy ethanol-iodine complex and polyethoxypolypropoxypoly-ethoxyethanol-iodine complex providing 0.5% titratable iodine, equivalent to 5,000 ppm titratable iodine.

Emollient system contains 4% U.S.P. glycerine.

Minimum pH is 4.0.

Indications: The teat dip is an iodophor (a combination of iodine and complexing agents), and when properly used, is effective as an aid in reducing the spread of mastitis-causing organisms. Iodophors are considered relatively non-toxic, but should always be used in accordance with label directions. Consult a veterinarian in case of teat irritation.

Dosage and Administration: Do not dilute. Use full strength.

Important Use Instructions for Pre-Milking:

1. Wash each individual teat with a sanitizing udder wash.
   Note: For the best results, keep the hair around the teat base clipped.
2. Hand strip the teats to initiate let down.
3. Predip the entire teat with PRE-POST 5000 on all four (4) quarters. Repeat the process on the next four (4) to six (6) cows or until the first cow prepped has at least one (1) minute contact time.
4. Wipe each individual teat with a clean paper towel. Utilize a "pulling down" motion which removes iodine solution, germs, and sediment from teat skin. This is very important.

5. Place the machine on the cow and repeat the wiping process on the remaining cows that have been predipped.

For Post-Milking:

Directions for Teat Dipping: Dip the entire teat with undiluted dip solution. Allow to air dry and remain on the teats for a prolonged contact time. Clean, sanitize and thoroughly dry each teat prior to the next milking. Replace the dip solution when visibly cloudy or dirty.

Caution(s): Not for internal use. Avoid contamination of foods. Avoid contact with the eyes.

First Aid:

Eyes: Immediately flush the eyes with plenty of cool running water for at least 15 minutes.

Internal: If swallowed, do not induce vomiting. Drink large quantities of milk, egg whites, and gelatin (or water).

Get medical attention immediately. Keep out of the reach of children.

Presentation: 1 U.S. gallon (3.79 L) containers.

Compendium Code No.: 10170010

D

DAKIL

Davis **Disinfectant**

EPA Reg. No.: 47371-6-50591

Active Ingredient(s):

Didecyl dimethyl ammonium chloride 7.5%

n-Alkyl (C_{14} 50%, C_{12} 40%, C_{16} 10%) dimethyl benzyl ammonium chloride 5.0%

Indications: A concentrated fungicide, virucide, disinfectant, cleaner and deodorant that cleans and deodorizes in one step. Rinsing is not necessary and the product is non-corrosive to stainless steel.

Effective against the following pathogenic organisms: *Pseudomonas aeruginosa, Serratia marcescens, Salmonella choleraesuis, Staphylococcus aureus* phage 80, *Staphylococcus aureus, Trichophyton interdigitale, Aspergillus fumigatus, Aspergillus flavus, Aspergillus glaucus var. tonophilus, Candida albicans,* bovine rhinotracheitis virus, newcastle's disease virus, vaccinia, rubella virus, canine parvovirus, influenza A/Texas, avian influenza, avian infectious bronchitis virus, adenovirus type 3 and herpes simplex.

Dosage and Administration: Use ½ oz. (1 tbsp.) per gallon of water for effectiveness against the following pathogenic organisms: *Pseudomonas aeruginosa, Serratia marcescens, Salmonella choleraesuis, Staphylococcus aureus* phage 80, *Staphylococcus aureus, Trichophyton interdigitale, Aspergillus fumigatus, Aspergillus flavus, Aspergillus glaucus var. tonophilus, Candida albicans,* bovine rhinotracheitis virus, newcastle's disease virus, vaccinia, rubella virus, canine parvovirus, influenza A/Texas, avian influenza, avian infectious bronchitis virus, adenovirus type 3 and herpes simplex.

Presentation: 1 gallon and 5 gallon buckets.

Compendium Code No.: 11410101

D.A.P.™ DOG APPEASING PHEROMONE

V.P.L. **Pheromone**

Composition:

Canine "appeasing pheromone" 2%

Excipients to .... 100 g

Indications: Uses:

D.A.P.™ (Dog Appeasing Pheromone) helps stop or prevent fear and stress-related behavior in puppies and adult dogs that result in: destructive behavior, excessive vocalization (barking, whining, etc.), house soiling, excessive licking, anxiety.

D.A.P.™ helps comfort the puppies and adult dog in stressful situations such as: introduction to visitors or strangers, visits to the veterinarian;, moving to new homes, adoption, novel and unpredictable situations leading to phobic reactions.

Directions: Instructions for Use:

1. Remove the vial cap.
2. Screw the diffuser onto the vial and gently tighten.
3. Plug the diffuser into an electric socket.

Place the D.A.P.™ Diffuser in the room most used by the dog during the day.

Coverage Area: 500-650 sq. ft.

One vial lasts approximately four weeks.

Duration of use may be adapted according to the recommendations of your veterinarian.

Precaution(s): Empty packaging and any remnants of the product should be disposed of in accordance with current regulations covering disposal of waste products.

Caution(s): The physiological effects of this product were not tested by Underwriters Laboratories.

The diffuser is specially designed for this product. The properties of the product cannot be guaranteed if a different device is used.

Do not cover.

Check that the main voltage is the same as indicated on the device. Do not place underneath or behind furniture. When plugged in, do not touch the device with metal objects. When plugged in, do not touch the device with wet hands.

During and immediately after use, do not touch the device with your hands.

The electric device should only be used with this D.A.P.™ diffuser formulation. Use of another substance may increase the toxicity or flammability of the product. The surfaces of the device reach high temperatures to encourage evaporation of active ingredients - these surfaces should not be touched during use of the product.

Warning(s): Keep out of reach of children.

In case of contact with eyes, wash them immediately with water and seek the advice of a physician.

Avoid contact with the skin. In case of contact with the skin, wash thoroughly with soap and water.

If the product is swallowed, consult a doctor immediately and show him/her the packaging.

Discussion: In mammals, lactating females release substances called "appeasing pheromones" the function of which is to reassure the offspring. Canine "appeasing pheromones" are secreted by the sebaceous glands of the intermammary sulcus in the lactating bitch.

These pheromones calm the puppy during times of stress and provide reassurance, particularly in unknown environments and when encountering novel experiences.

Research has shown that the reassuring properties of these pheromones persist even into adult age.

D.A.P.™ (Dog Appeasing Pheromone) reproduces the properties of the natural "appeasing pheromones" of the bitch.

Presentation: Complete Kit Contents: One electric diffuser and 1-48 mL vial.
Refill: 1-48 mL vial only.

D.A.P.™ is a trademark of Ceva Santé Animale.

Compendium Code No.: 11430450 01-2001/01-2003

DARICLOX® ℞

Pfizer Animal Health **Mastitis Therapy**

(sodium cloxacillin) Lactating Cow Formula-Intramammary Infusion

NADA No.: 055-070

Active Ingredient(s): Description: DARICLOX® (sodium cloxacillin) is a stable, nonirritating suspension of sodium cloxacillin containing the equivalent of 200 mg of cloxacillin in saturated vegetable oils per disposable syringe. DARICLOX® is manufactured by a nonsterilizing process.

Indications: DARICLOX® is indicated in the treatment of bovine mastitis in lactating cows due to *Streptococcus agalactiae* and nonpenicillinase-producing *Staphylococcus aureus*.

Clinical experience indicates that antibiotic efficacy in the treatment of mastitis in lactating cows is directly related to the duration of infection. Therefore, treatment should be instituted as early as possible after detection.

Pharmacology: Cloxacillin is a semisynthetic penicillin derived from the penicillin nucleus, 6-amino-penicillanic acid. Sodium cloxacillin is the monohydrate sodium salt of 5-methyl-3-(o-chlorophenyl)-4-isoxazolyl penicillin.

Action: Sodium cloxacillin is bactericidal in action against susceptible organisms during the stage of active multiplication. It acts through the inhibition of biosynthesis of cell wall mucopeptide. It is active against most gram-positive organisms associated with mastitis. It is effective against *Streptococcus agalactiae* and nonpenicillinase-producing *Staphylococcus aureus,* and there is laboratory evidence that indicates cloxacillin is resistant to destruction by penicillinase-producing organisms. Milk cultures and antibiotic susceptibility testing is recommended when using this product.

Susceptibility Test: The Kirby-Bauer* procedure, utilizing antibiotic susceptibility disks, is a quantitative method that may be adapted to determining the sensitivity of bacteria in milk to DARICLOX®.

For testing the effectiveness of DARICLOX® in milk, follow the Kirby-Bauer procedure using the 1 mcg oxacillin susceptibility disk. Zone diameters for interpreting susceptibility are:

Resistant	Intermediate	Susceptible
≤10 mm	11-12 mm	≥13 mm

* Bauer AW, Kirby WMM, Sherris JC, et al: Antibiotic testing by a standardized single disk method, Am J Clin Path 45:493, 1966. Standardized Disk Susceptibility Test, Federal Register 37:20527-29, 1972.

Dosage and Administration: Milk out udder completely. Wash udder and teats thoroughly with warm water containing a suitable dairy antiseptic. Dry thoroughly. Clean and disinfect the teat with alcohol swabs provided in the carton. Remove the syringe tip cover and insert the tip of the syringe into the teat orifice. Express the suspension into the quarter with gentle and continuous pressure. Withdraw the syringe and grasp the end of the teat firmly. Massage the medication up into the milk cistern.

For optimum response the drug should be administered by intra-mammary infusion in each infected quarter as described above. Treatment should be repeated at 12-hour intervals for a total of 3 doses. The treated quarter should be milked out at the next routine milking.

Each carton contains 12 alcohol swabs to facilitate proper cleaning and disinfecting of the teat orifice.

Precaution(s): Do not store above 24°C (75°F).

Caution(s): Federal law restricts this drug to use by or on the order of a licensed veterinarian.

Because it is a derivative of 6-amino-penicillanic acid, DARICLOX® has the potential for producing allergic reactions. Such reactions are rare; however, should they occur, the subject should be treated with the usual agents (antihistamines, pressor amines).

Warning(s): Milk taken from animals during treatment and for 48 hours (4 milkings) after the last treatment must not be used for food. Treated animals must not be slaughtered for food purposes within 10 days after the last treatment.

Presentation: DARICLOX® is supplied in cartons of 12 single-dose syringes with 12 alcohol swabs. Each 10-mL, disposable syringe contains sodium cloxacillin equivalent to 200 mg of cloxacillin.

Manufactured by: G.C. Hanford Mfg. Co., Syracuse, NY 13201

Compendium Code No.: 36900081 75-8162-00

DAVIS BEST LUXURY SHAMPOO

Davis **Grooming Shampoo**

Ingredient(s): Shampoo formula, conditioners and coconut extract.

Indications: A grooming shampoo for dogs, cats, puppies and kittens.

Directions for Use: To use DAVIS BEST as a general grooming and cleansing shampoo, dilute 12 parts water to 1 part shampoo (12:1). For extra dirty pets, dilute 4 parts water to 1 part shampoo (4:1) or apply shampoo undiluted.

Wet pet's coat thoroughly with warm water. Do not get shampoo into eyes. Apply shampoo to head and ears, then lather. Repeat procedure with neck, chest, middle and hind quarter, finishing legs last. Allow pet to stand for 5 to 10 minutes. Rinse pet thoroughly. For best results, repeat procedure.

Warning(s): For external use only.

Keep out of reach of children.

Presentation: 12 fl oz (355 mL) and 1 gallon (3.785 L).

Compendium Code No.: 11410110

DAVIS PYRETHRINS

Davis **Parasiticide Shampoo**

EPA Reg. No.: 50591-2

Active Ingredient(s):

Pyrethrins 7.5%

Piperonyl butoxide, technical* 75.0%

Inert ingredients 17.5%

Total 100.0%

*Equivalent to min. 60% (butylcarbityl) (6-propylpiperonyl) ether and 15% related compounds.

Indications: A concentrate to be added to shampoo for use on cats and dogs to kill fleas and ticks.

Dosage and Administration: It is a violation of federal law to use the product in a manner inconsistent with its labeling.

To shampoo and kill fleas and ticks, follow these steps:

1. Mix 1 oz. of DAVIS PYRETHRINS in one (1) gallon of non-insecticide shampoo.
2. Wet the animal thoroughly.
3. Apply a generous amount of the shampoo mixture to the coat, massaging the lather well into the coat and skin.

4. Allow the lather to remain on the animal for five (5) minutes to permit the pyrethrins to take their full effect.
5. Rinse the animal thoroughly.

Precaution(s): Do not re-use the empty container. Wrap it in newspaper and discard it with the trash. Do not use or store near heat or an open flame.

Caution(s): Keep out of the reach of children. To be applied only by or under the supervision of a licensed veterinarian or pet groomer.

Precautionary Statements:

Hazards to Humans: Harmful if swallowed. Do not get in the eyes. Wash hands thoroughly after each use and before eating or smoking.

Hazards to Domestic Animals: Do not apply directly to or on the eyes, mouth or genitals of pets. Do not treat or cause exposure to kittens or puppies of less than four weeks of age.

Statement of Practical Treatment:

If swallowed: Contact a physician or poison control center immediately. Do not induce vomiting. The product contains petroleum distillate. Vomiting may cause aspiration pneumonia.

If in eyes or on skin: Flush the affected areas with plenty of water. Contact a physician if irritation persists.

Environmental Hazards: The product is toxic to fish. Do not dispose of in lakes, streams or open ponds.

Warning(s): Buyer assumes all risks of use, storage or handling of the material not in strict accordance with directions given on the label.

Presentation: 5 fl. oz. and 16 fl. oz. containers.

Compendium Code No.: 11410121

D-BASIC SHAMPOO

DVM **Grooming Shampoo**

Soap-free Deep-Cleansing Conditioning Formulation

Ingredient(s): Water, ammonium lauryl sulfate, ammonium laureth sulfate, lauramide DEA, cetrimonium chloride, cocamidopropyl betaine, hydroxypropyl methylcellulose, fragrance, kathon CG, citric acid, safflower oil, FD&C yellow #5, FD&C blue #1.

Indications: For general cleansing, grooming and conditioning of dogs and cats. Also to clean skin before using a medicated shampoo for a specific skin disease or before using a topical treatment for ectoparasites.

A concentrated, pH-balanced, deep-cleansing formulation which combines surface-active and penetrating agents with coat conditioners. Leaves coat easy to groom with a silky luster.

Directions for Use: Wet coat thoroughly with water and apply sufficient shampoo to create a rich lather. Rinse well and repeat if necessary. May be used as often as necessary.

Precaution(s): Store at room temperature.

Caution(s): For topical use on dogs and cats. Avoid contact with eyes. If contact occurs, rinse thoroughly with water.

Warning(s): Keep out of reach of children.

Presentation: 12 fl oz (355 mL), 1 gallon (3.78 L) and 2.5 gallons (9.46 L).

Compendium Code No.: 11420181 Rev 0797 / Rev 0597

DC&R® DISINFECTANT

Loveland **Disinfectant**

EPA Reg. No.: 134-65

Active Ingredient(s):

2-(hydroxymethyl)-2-nitro-1,3-propanediol 19.20%
Formaldehyde 2.28%
Alkyl (C_{12}-67%, C_{14}-25%, C_{16}-7%, C_8, C_{10}, C_{18}-1%)
dimethyl benzyl ammonium chloride 3.08%
Inert ingredients........ 75.44%
Total 100.00%

Indications: For use in the disinfection of farm buildings and equipment which are used for poultry and livestock production. Also suitable for equipment which may harbor or spread disease germs within the farm operation or to other farms.

Dosage and Administration: It is a violation of federal law to use the product in a manner inconsistent with its labeling.

Dilute DC&R® Disinfectant in 1 oz. per gallon of water. Use as follows:

Equipment: Empty all the troughs, racks and other feeding and watering appliances. Thoroughly clean all surfaces with soap or detergent and rinse with water. Then thoroughly wet all exposed parts of the cleaned equipment used in the poultry or livestock operation.

All treated feed racks, mangers, troughs, automatic feeders, fountains and waterers must be thoroughly scrubbed with detergents and rinsed with potable water prior to reuse.

Immerse cleaned halters, ropes and other types of equipment used in handling and restraining animals, as well as forks, all shovels and scrapers used for removing litter and manure and allow DC&R® Disinfectant to saturate all surfaces for 10 minutes. Do not spray onto feed to be consumed by the animals.

When disinfecting trucks used for hauling poultry or livestock, rinse the truck cab for a few minutes after the spraying is completed. Do not rinse other parts of the truck. The release of formaldehyde is slight, therefore little odor can be detected. However, allow reasonable ventilation for animals being transported following disinfection.

Buildings: Evacuate all animals from buildings. Remove all litter and manure from floors, walls and surfaces of barns, pens, stalls, chutes and other facilities and fixtures occupied or traversed by the animals. Empty all of the troughs, racks and other feeding and watering appliances. Thoroughly clean all surfaces with soap or detergent and rinse with water. Wet all surfaces by allowing DC&R® Disinfectant to saturate for 10 minutes. The equipment inside the building (cages for laying hens, for example) should be cleaned with soap or detergent first, rinsed with water and then saturated as above with the product.

Ventilate buildings, cars, boats, coops and other closed spaces. Do not house poultry, livestock or employ equipment until the treatment has been absorbed, set or dried. Thoroughly scrub all treated feed racks, troughs, automatic feeders, fountains and waterers with soap or detergent and rinse with potable water before reuse.

Precaution(s): Do not contaminate water, food or feed by storage or disposal.

Keep in an upright position while moving and in storage. The container is equipped with a pressure relief closure. Keep from freezing. Store in the original container only, in a safe place. Do not store under conditions which might adversely affect the container or its ability to function properly. Reduce stacking height where local conditions can affect the package strength. Open the container in a well ventilated area, avoid inhaling vapor. Keep the container tightly closed when not in use.

Spill Control: Soak up the spill in a dry absorbent such as clay. Sweep it up, put it into disposal containers and dispose of it as directed below. Wear protective clothing and equipment consistent with pesticide handling procedures while exposed to the spilled material.

Pesticide Disposal: "Pesticide wastes are toxic. Improper disposal of excess pesticide, spray mixture, or rinsate is a violation of federal law. If these wastes cannot be disposed of according to label instructions, contact the state pesticide or environmental control agency, or the hazardous waste representative at the nearest EPA regional office for guidance."

Container Disposal:

Metal: Triple rinse (or equivalent), then offer for recycling or reconditioning, or puncture and dispose of in a sanitary landfill, or by other procedures approved by state and local authorities.

Plastic: Triple rinse (or equivalent), then offer for recycling or reconditioning, or puncture and dispose of in a sanitary landfill, or by incineration, or if allowed by state and local authorities, by burning. If burned, stay out of smoke.

Caution(s): Keep out of the reach of children.

Precautionary Statements:

Hazards to Humans and Domestic Animals: Causes eye irritation. Do not get into the eyes, on the skin, or on clothing. Harmful if swallowed. Wear rubber gloves when mixing and handling DC&R® Disinfectant. Wear long pants, long sleeve shirts and a plastic or rubber apron when applying the diluted spray mixture. Do not use on animals.

Statement of Practical Treatment:

If swallowed: Induce vomiting (if conscious). Call a physician.

If in the eyes: Flush with water immediately.

If on the skin: Wash thoroughly with soap and water.

Presentation: 55 gallon (208 L) containers.

Compendium Code No.: 10860010

DEALER SELECT HORSE CARE BIOTIN 800

Durvet **Equine Dietary Supplement**

Nutritional Supplement

Active Ingredient(s): Provides a source of d-Biotin, *Yucca Schidigera* (500 mg/oz), d-Calcium Pantothenate, dl-Methionine in a palatable base of Yeast Culture and Distillers Grains with Solubles.

Each level scoop holds approximately one ounce of product and provides the following levels of the above nutrients:

Nutrient	Per Ounce Scoop	Per Pound Equivalency
d-Biotin	50 mg	800 mg
d-Pantothenic Acid	460 mg	7360 mg
dl-Methionine	25 mg	400 mg

Ingredients: Magnesium Mica, d-Biotin, Corn Distillers Dried Grains with Solubles, Yeast Culture, *Yucca Schidigera*, d-Calcium Pantothenate, Mineral Oil and dl-Methionine.

Indications: A very palatable Extra Strength Biotin (800 mg/lb) supplement formulated to optimize the general condition of the hooves, skin and hair coat of horses.

A nutritional supplement for horses of all stages.

Directions for Use:

Horses: Mix one (1) or two (2) scoops with daily feed. Provide daily, or as directed by your veterinarian or nutritionist.

Lactating Mares: Mix two (2) scoops with daily feed. Provide daily, or as directed by your veterinarian or nutritionist.

Foals: Mix one (1) scoop with daily feed. Provide daily, or as directed by your veterinarian or nutritionist.

Can also be top dressed and/or hand fed as desired.

Presentation: 2 lbs (NDC# 30798-180-42) and 20 lbs (9.07 kg).

Compendium Code No.: 10840432 1/00

DEALER SELECT HORSE CARE DURLYTE-A

Durvet **Electrolytes-Oral**

Guaranteed Analysis:

Sodium (minimum)........ 31.0%
Sodium (maximum) 35.0%
Potassium (minimum) 6.5%
Potassium (maximum) 7.5%

Ingredients: Sodium chloride, potassium chloride, magnesium sulfate, calcium lactate, silicon dioxide, dextrose, artificial and natural flavor, FD&C yellow #5 and FD&C blue #1. Apple flavored.

Indications: A nutritional source of electrolytes and minerals for all horses.

Dosage and Administration: Use Directions: DURLYTE-A may be used in the horse's feed as a top dress or mixed with feed at a rate of 2 ounces daily. Alternatively, a drinking water solution may be prepared daily at the rate of 1 ounce per 5 gallons of fresh water. All solutions should be made fresh daily. (Enclosed measuring scoop holds 1 ounce.)

Precaution(s): Close container after use. Store in cool, dry place.

Caution(s): For animal use only.

Warning(s): Keep out of reach of children.

Presentation: 5 lb (2.27 kg) and 25 lb (11.35 kg).

Compendium Code No.: 10840871 11/98

DEALER SELECT HORSE CARE DURLYTE-C

Durvet **Electrolytes-Oral**

Guaranteed Analysis:

Sodium (minimum)........ 31.0%
Sodium (maximum) 35.0%
Potassium (minimum) 6.5%
Potassium (maximum) 8.5%

Ingredients: Sodium chloride, potassium chloride, magnesium sulfate, calcium lactate, silicon dioxide, dextrose, artificial flavorings and FD&C red #3.

Cherry flavored.

Indications: A nutritional source of electrolytes and minerals for all horses.

Dosage and Administration: Use Directions: DURLYTE-C may be used in the horse's feed as a top dress or mixed with feed at a rate of 2 ounces daily. Alternatively, a drinking water solution may be prepared daily at the rate of 1 ounce per 5 gallons of fresh water. All solutions should be made fresh daily. (Enclosed measuring scoop holds 1 ounce.)

Precaution(s): Close container after use. Store in cool, dry place.

Caution(s): For animal use only.

Warning(s): Keep out of reach of children.

Presentation: 5 lb (2.27 kg) and 25 lb (11.35 kg).

Compendium Code No.: 10840881 7/95

DEALER SELECT HORSE CARE DURVIT C POWDER

Durvet **Vitamin C**

Guaranteed Analysis: per pound:
Vitamin C, (minimum) .... 51,000 mg

Ingredients: Roughage products, calcium carbonate, ascorbic acid (vitamin C), mineral oil, saccharin sodium and artificial and natural flavor. Apple flavored.

Indications: A source of ascorbic acid (vitamin C) for horses.

Dosage and Administration: Use Directions: Top feed or hand mix ½ to 1 ounce of DURVIT C POWDER into each horse's daily ration (enclosed measuring scoop holds 1 ounce).

Precaution(s): Close container after use. Store in cool, dry place.

Caution(s): For animal use only.

Warning(s): Keep out of reach of children.

Presentation: 4 lb.

Compendium Code No.: 10840901

D

DEALER SELECT HORSE CARE DURVIT E POWDER

Durvet **Vitamin E**

Guaranteed Analysis: per pound:
Vitamin E, minimum.......... 17,000 I.U.

Ingredients: Roughage products, calcium carbonate, vitamin E supplement, mineral oil, saccharin sodium and artificial and natural flavor. Apple flavored.

Indications: A source of vitamin E for horses.

Dosage and Administration: Use Directions: Top feed or hand mix ½ to 1 ounce of DURVIT E POWDER into each horse's daily ration (enclosed measuring scoop holds 1 ounce).

Precaution(s): Close container after use. Store in cool, dry place.

Caution(s): For animal use only.

Warning(s): Keep out of reach of children.

Presentation: 4 lb.

Compendium Code No.: 10840911 7/95

DEALER SELECT HORSE CARE EPSOM SALT POULTICE

Durvet **Poultice**

Active Ingredient(s): Contains:
Epsom Salt.......... 60%
Methyl Salicylate .... q.s.

In a water soluble base.

Indications: For sprains, strains and bruises. An osmotic agent for external application.

Directions for Use: Apply to painful muscles and joints. Repeat as needed for relief of soreness and to relax muscles.

Caution(s): For veterinary use only.

Warning(s): Keep out of reach of children.

Presentation: 20 oz.

Compendium Code No.: 10840941 5/96

DEALER SELECT HORSE CARE FARRIER'S SELECT

Durvet **Large Animal Dietary Supplement**

Nutritional Supplement

Guaranteed Analysis:
Crude Protein (Min) 17.00%
Crude Fat (Min) 9.00%
Crude Fiber (Max) 20.00%
Ash (Max) 12.00%
Copper (Min) .... 540 ppm
Zinc (Min) .... 1450 ppm

Typical Analysis:

Nutrients	Per 6 oz (170 g)	Percent
DL-Methionine	6188 mg	3.634%
Biotin	5.25 mg	0.003%
Ascorbic Acid	1290 mg	0.758%
Choline	487 mg	0.286%
Inositol	262 mg	0.154%
Glycine	1687 mg	0.991%
Proline	1050 mg	0.617%
Hydroxyproline	750 mg	0.441%
L-Tyrosine	618 mg	0.363%
Iodine (I)	0.8 mg	0.00047%

Ingredients: Dehydrated Alfalfa Meal, Yeast Culture, Lecithin, Gelatin (Porcine Origin), DL-Methionine, Ascorbic Acid, Copper Sulfate, Zinc Oxide, L-Tyrosine, Biotin, Choline Chloride, Inositol, Ethylenediamine dihydriodide, Bentonite and Natural Flavors.

Indications: A nutritional supplement for horses (all classes of horses).

Directions for Use: Daily Feeding Level: Top dress or mix with regular feed.

Adults:
Up to 250 lbs (113 kg).......... 1 scoop
251 - 500 lbs (226 kg) .... 2 scoops
501 - 750 lbs (339 kg) .... 3 scoops
751 - 1000 lbs (452 kg) .... 4 scoops
over 1000 lbs (452 kg).......... 1 scoop for every 250 lbs (113 kg) of body weight.

Weanling to adults: Use above dosage based on expected adult weight.

Foals: 1 scoop (1½ oz or 43 g) per day.

FARRIER'S SELECT contains balanced nutrients designed to be fed for the lifetime of the horse. After feeding the supplement as directed above for 6 to 8 months, the above amounts may usually be reduced by up to one half and still maintain a healthy balance. Resume feeding at the indicated levels during periods of stress for the animal.

Precaution(s): Keep contents dry while in storage. Avoid excessive heat.

Caution(s): For animal consumption only.

Warning(s): Keep out of reach of children.

Presentation: 11 lbs (5 kg), 22 lbs (10 kg) and 44 lbs (20 kg).

Compendium Code No.: 10840442 6/99

DEALER SELECT HORSE CARE GROOM 'N SHOW

Durvet **Grooming Spray**

Active Ingredient(s): Water, amodimethicone, nonxynol-10, tallowtrimonium chloride, cyclomethicone and fragrance.

Indications: A grooming spray that brings out the natural color highlights and conditions horse's hair while leaving a pleasant fragrance.

Directions for Use: For best results, bathe horse and rinse thoroughly. Apply GROOM 'N SHOW in an even mist over the entire hair coat. Work into hair using a soft bristle brush. Use a clean towel to smooth down hair coat, then brush the hair coat into place using a soft bristle brush.

Dry Application: If bathing cannot be done, apply GROOM 'N SHINE in an even mist over the entire hair coat. Work into hair using a soft bristle brush. Use a clean towel to smooth down the hair coat, then brush the hair coat into place using a soft bristle brush.

Mane and Tail: Apply GROOM 'N SHOW to tail and mane and comb with a wide toothed flexible plastic comb.

Caution(s): For animal use only.

Warning(s): Keep out of reach of children.

Presentation: 32 oz (1 qt).

Compendium Code No.: 10840951 7/95

DEALER SELECT HORSE CARE HOOF DRESSING WITH BRUSH

Durvet **Hoof Product**

Ingredient(s): Fish oil, pine tar, linseed oil, wheat germ oil, turpentine, and complexed iodine.

Indications: A hoof dressing for horses.

Directions for Use: Apply HOOF DRESSING with a brush to the walls and frog twice a week. May be used more often if needed.

Caution(s): For animal use only.

Warning(s): Keep out of reach of children.

Presentation: 32 oz container, with brush.

Compendium Code No.: 10840961 7/95

DEALER SELECT HORSE CARE HOOF MOISTURIZER

Durvet **Hoof Product**

Ingredient(s): Water, glycerin, emulsifying wax, petrolatum (and) lanolin (and) beeswax (and) sorbitan sesquioleate (and) polysorbate 81, mineral oil, isopropyl myristrate, glyceryl stearate, cetyl alcohol, hydrolyzed animal protein, stearic acid, panthenol, aloe vera, triethanolamine, methyl and propyl paraben (a preservative), quaternium 15 (a preservative) and FD&C yellow #5 and fragrance.

Indications: A hoof moisturizer and conditioner containing aloe vera, lanolin, protein humectants and essential oils in a moisturizing and conditioning base.

Directions for Use: Apply HOOF MOISTURIZER liberally to the soles, walls, frog and coronary band daily until the dry hooves return to normal condition. Regularly apply to normal hooves twice a week to maintain normal hoof condition.

Caution(s): For animal use only.

Warning(s): Keep out of reach of children.

Presentation: 28 oz (1 pt 12 oz).

Compendium Code No.: 10840971 7/95

DEALER SELECT HORSE CARE HORSE & COLT WORMER

Durvet **Feed Medication**

Medicated Feed Additive

Active Ingredient(s):
Pyrantel tartrate 1.25%
(Equivalent to 5.671 grams per pound)

Ingredients: Wheat middlings, ground yellow corn, dehydrated alfalfa meal, soybean meal, cane molasses.

Indications: A pyrantel tartrate wormer for horses and ponies.

For Removal and Control of Infections of the Following Mature Parasites: Large strongyles *(Strongylus vulgaris, S. endentatus,* and *S. equinus),* small stongyles *(Trichonema* sp. *triodontophorus),* pinworms *(Oxyuris),* large roundworms *(Parascaris).*

Directions: Each horse should be treated individually. Not all horses will consume medicated feed; however, most horses consume HORSE & COLT WORMER readily when mixed in the feed. Mix the required amount of HORSE & COLT WORMER in the feed normally consumed at one feeding. Animals should not be fasted prior to or following treatment. The product may be administered safely to foals and pregnant mares.

Since horses are constantly reinfecting themselves with worms through grazing, periodic worming every two months may be required. Consult your veterinarian for assistance in the diagnosis, treatment, and control of parasitism.

Dosage*

Weight of Horse	Amount of HORSE & COLT WORMER to Mix in Feed
175 lbs	½ cupful** (3 oz)
350 lbs	1 cupful (6 oz)
700 lbs	2 cupfuls (12 oz)
1000 lbs	2⅔ cupfuls (1 lb)

*Provides 12.5 mg of pyrantel tartrate per 2.2 lbs. of body weight.

**One 8 ounce measuring cup holds 6 ounces of Durvet HORSE & COLT WORMER equivalent to 2.126 grams of pyrantel tartrate.

Caution(s): It is recommended that severely debilitated animals not be treated with HORSE & COLT WORMER. Consult a veterinarian at the first sign of adverse reaction such as a marked increase in rate of respiration, profuse sweating or incoordination.

For use only as directed on the label.

Restricted drug - use only as directed.

Warning(s): Do not use in horses or ponies intended for food.

Keep out of reach of children.

Not for human consumption.

Presentation: 16 oz (1 lb) (454 g) (NDC 30798-490-31).

Compendium Code No.: 10840981 7/95

DEALER SELECT HORSE CARE HORSE LINIMENT

Durvet **Liniment**

Ingredient(s): Water, isopropyl alcohol, glycerin, menthol, camphor, methyl salicylate, thymol, wormwood oil and complexed iodine.

Indications: HORSE LINIMENT is a specially formulated leg brace, body wash antiseptic.

Directions for Use:

Liniment: Massage HORSE LINIMENT vigorously and evenly over inflamed area.

Body Wash: Dilute 1 ounce of HORSE LINIMENT to 1 gallon of clean water. Apply to entire horse's body. Keep away from eyes and mucous membranes.

Leg Care: Dilute 1 ounce of HORSE LINIMENT to 16 ounces of water. Vigorously rub solution into legs and wrap if needed.

Precaution(s): Flammable. Keep away from heat or open flame.

Caution(s): For external use only. Discontinue use if excessive irritation develops. Avoid getting into the eyes or mucous membranes.

For animal use only.

Warning(s): Livestock remedy, not for human use. Keep out of reach of children.

Presentation: 16 oz (1 pt) (473 mL).

Compendium Code No.: 10840991

7/95

DEALER SELECT HORSE CARE NUTRIHOOF

Durvet **Equine Dietary Supplement**

Guaranteed Analysis:

Crude Protein (minimum) . . . 11.00%
Lysine (minimum) . . . 0.50%
Methionine (minimum) . . . 0.75%
Crude Fat (minimum) . . . 1.70%
Crude Fiber (maximum) . . . 15.00%
Zinc (Zn) (minimum) . . . 7200 ppm
Biotin (minimum) . . . 250 mg/lb

Ingredients: Forage products, calcium carbonate, animal protein products, dried cane molasses, biotin supplement, calcium lignin sulfonate, grain products, gelatin, brewers yeast, saccharin sodium, zinc oxide, DL-methionine, L-lysine, monohydrochloride, pyridoxine HCl, dicalcium phosphate, sodium propionate (a preservative) and artificial and natural flavor.

Apple flavored.

Indications: A source of biotin, amino acids and minerals for all horses.

Directions for Use: Top feed or hand mix 1 ounce of NUTRIHOOF for every 1,000 lb. of body weight in each horse's daily ration (enclosed measuring scoop holds 1 ounce).

Precaution(s): Close container after each use. Keep in cool, dry place.

Caution(s): For animal use only.

Warning(s): Keep out of reach of children.

Presentation: 5 lb (2.27 kg).

Compendium Code No.: 10841012

7/98

DEALER SELECT HORSE CARE PERMETH 5 FLY SPRAY

Durvet **Parasiticide Spray**

Concentrated Permethrin Stable Emulsion

EPA Reg. No.: 67517-55-12281

Active Ingredients:

*Permethrin . . . 0.50%
Inert Ingredients . . . 99.50%
Total 100.00%

*(3-phenoxyphenyl) methyl (±) cis/trans 3-(2,2-dichloroethenyl) 2,2-dimethylcyclopropane-carboxylate. cis/trans ratio: min. 35% (±) cis and max. 65% (±) trans.

Indications: A concentrated permethrin stable emulsion. To protect horses from horn flies, face flies, house flies, mosquitoes and gnats.

Directions for Use: It is a violation of Federal law to use this product in a manner inconsistent with its labeling.

Shake well before using.

On Horses: To protect horses from horn flies, face flies, house flies, mosquitoes and gnats. Apply a light mist sufficient to wet the surface hair. For face flies, spray face and head, but do not spray into eyes.

To Control Stable Flies, Horse Flies and Deer Flies: Apply at a rate of 2 ounces per adult animal sufficient to wet the hair thoroughly. Repeat treatment daily or at intervals necessary to give continued protection.

Do not use this product in or on electrical equipment due to the possibility of shock hazard.

Do not use in food/feed areas of food/feed handling establishments, restaurants or other areas where food/feed is commercially prepared or processed. Food/feed areas of commercial food/feed handling establishments where the product cannot be used include areas for receiving, serving, storage (dry, cold, frozen, raw), packaging (canning, bottling, wrapping, boxing), preparing (cleaning, slicing, cooking, grinding), edible waste storage, enclosed processing systems (mills, dairies, edible oils, syrups). Do not use in serving areas while food is exposed or facility is in operation. Serving areas are areas where prepared foods are served such as dining rooms but excluding areas where foods may be prepared or held in the home, all food processing surfaces and utensils should be covered during treatment or thoroughly washed before use. Exposed food should be covered or removed.

Non-food areas are areas such as garbage rooms, lavatories, floor drains (to sewers), entries and vestibules, offices, locker rooms, machine rooms, boiler rooms, garages, mop closets and storage (after canning or bottling).

Apply spray with spray/trigger attachment.

Precautionary Statements: Hazards to Humans and Domestic Animals:

Caution: Harmful if swallowed. May be absorbed through skin. Avoid inhalation of spray mist. Avoid contact with skin, eyes, or clothing. Wash thoroughly after handling and before eating or smoking. Avoid contamination of feed and foodstuffs. Do not use on humans. Do not allow children or pets to contact areas until surfaces are dry. Do not apply in classrooms when in use. Do not apply to institutions (including libraries, sports facilities, etc.) when occupants are present in the immediate area. Remove pets and birds and cover fish aquaria before surface applications. Do not use this product on old, sick or debilitated dogs.

Statement of Practical Treatment:

If Swallowed: Drink one or two glasses of water and induce vomiting by touching the back of the throat with finger. Repeat until vomit fluid is clear. Call a physician immediately. Do not induce vomiting or give anything by mouth to an unconscious person.

If on Skin: Remove contaminated clothing and wash affected areas with soap and water.

If in Eyes: Flush eyes with plenty of water. Call a physician if irritation persists.

If Inhaled: Remove affected person to fresh air. Apply artificial respiration if indicated.

Environmental Hazards: This product is extremely toxic to fish. Do not apply directly to water. Do not contaminate water when disposing of equipment wash waters.

Storage and Disposal: Do not contaminate water, food or feed by storage or disposal. Do not reuse container. Wrap container in several layers of newspaper and discard in trash.

Warning(s): Keep out of reach of children.

Disclaimer: Buyer assumes all risks of use, storage or handling of this product in strict accordance with directions given within.

Presentation: 32 oz (946.35 mL).

Compendium Code No.: 10841021

7/95

DECCOX®

Alpharma **Feed Medication**

Decoquinate Type A Medicated Article-Medicated Premix-Coccidiostat

NADA No.: 039-417

Active Ingredient(s):

Decoquinate . . . 6% (27.2 g/lb)

Ingredients: Corn meal, soybean oil, lecithin and silicon dioxide.

Indications:

Cattle: For the prevention of coccidiosis in ruminating and non-ruminating calves (including veal calves) and cattle caused by *Eimeria bovis* and *E. zurnii.*

Sheep: For the prevention of coccidiosis in young sheep caused by *Eimeria ovinoidalis, E. crandallis, E. parva,* and *E. bakuensis.*

Poultry: For the prevention of coccidiosis in broiler chickens - caused by *Eimeria tenella, E. necatrix, E. acervulina, E. mivati, E. maxima,* and *E. burnetti.*

Goats: For the prevention of coccidiosis in young goats caused by *Eimeria christenseni* and *E. ninakohlyakimovae.*

Dosage and Administration: Each pound of DECCOX® contains 27.2 grams of decoquinate.

Cattle: Thoroughly mix DECCOX® into the ration at a rate to provide decoquinate at a daily dose of 22.7 mg/100 lbs (0.5 mg/kg) of body weight. Feed for at least 28 days during periods of coccidiosis exposure or when experience indicates that coccidiosis is likely to be a hazard. Coccidiostats are not indicated for use in adult animals due to continuous previous exposure.

1. For Supplements or Topdress:

a. Dry Supplements - Type C Medicated Product

The table below shows the amount of DECCOX® required per ton of supplement to provide the proper decoquinate levels per head daily.

lbs DECCOX® per ton of Supplement	Decoquinate Levels			Daily Feeding Rate per Head
	g/ton	%	mg/lb	
16.7	454	0.05	227	1⁄10 lb/100 lbs body weight
33.4	908	0.1	454	1⁄10 lb/200 lbs body weight
41.75	1136	0.125	568	1⁄10 lb/250 lbs body weight

b. Dry Supplements - Type B Medicated Product

lbs DECCOX® per ton of Supplement	Decoquinate Levels			Daily Feeding Rate per Head
	g/ton	%	mg/lb	
167.0	4542	0.5	2271	* (See footnote)

* This supplement must be mixed with grain at the rate of 1 part supplement with 9 parts grain. The resulting mixture contains 0.05% decoquinate and is then to be fed at the rate of 1⁄10 lb per 100 lbs body weight daily.

c. Liquid Supplements - Type B Medicated Product

(1) Add the appropriate amount of DECCOX® to liquid supplement to provide the proper decoquinate level per head daily (see table below).

(2) The pH of the supplement must be between 5.0 to 6.5.

(3) Supplements must contain a suspending agent to maintain viscosity of not less than 500 centipoises.

lbs DECCOX® per ton of Liquid Supplement	Decoquinate Levels			Daily Feeding Rate per Head
	g/ton	%	mg/lb	
4.18	139	0.0125	56.8	1⁄10 lb/25 lbs body weight
8.36	277	0.025	113.5	1⁄10 lb/50 lbs body weight
16.7	454	0.05	227.0	1⁄10 lb/100 lbs body weight

2. For Complete Rations - Type C Medicated Product

The table below shows the amount of DECCOX® required per ton of complete feed to provide the proper decoquinate levels daily for animals weighing an average of 600 pounds.

lbs DECCOX® per ton of Feed	Decoquinate Levels			Daily Feeding Rate per Head
	g/ton	%	mg/lb	
0.5	13.6	0.00149	6.8	20 lbs
0.7	19.0	0.00209	9.5	14.5 lbs
1.0	27.2	0.00299	13.6	10 lbs

The following formula can be used to calculate the amount of DECCOX® (6% decoquinate) to be included in one ton of feed to provide the daily dosage of 22.7 mg decoquinate per 100 lbs body weight.

$$\frac{\text{Avg. Weight of Individual Animal to be Medicated} \times 454}{\text{Avg. Pounds of Medicated Feed per Animal, per Day} \times 27{,}200} = \text{lbs DECCOX® to be added per ton feed}$$

Note: Mix DECCOX® in a ratio of 1:9 with ground grain prior to adding it to the mixer.

Sheep: Thoroughly mix DECCOX® into the ration at a rate to provide decoquinate at a daily dose of 22.7 mg/100 lbs (0.5 mg/kg) of body weight. Feed for at least 28 days during periods of coccidiosis exposure or when experience indicates that coccidiosis is likely to be a hazard.

Sheep Body Weight in lbs	lbs DECCOX® per ton of Feed	Decoquinate Levels			Daily Feeding Rate per Head
		g/ton	%	mg/lb	
30	0.5	13.6	0.00149	6.8	1.0 lbs
60	0.5	13.6	0.00149	6.8	2.0 lbs
90	0.5	13.6	0.00149	6.8	3.0 lbs

Poultry: Complete Ration - Type C Medicated Product

Thoroughly mix one (1) pound of DECCOX® in each ton of complete ration and feed continuously.

Goats: Thoroughly mix DECCOX® into the ration at a rate to provide decoquinate at a daily dose of 22.7 mg/100 lbs (0.5 mg/kg) of body weight. Feed for at least 28 days during periods of coccidiosis exposure or when experience indicates that coccidiosis is likely to be a hazard.

Goat Body Weight in lbs	lbs DECCOX® per ton of Feed	Decoquinate Levels			Daily Feeding Rate per Head
		g/ton	%	mg/lb.	
30	0.5	13.6	0.00149	6.8	1.0 lbs

Precaution(s): Store in a cool, dry place. Keep bag tightly closed.

Caution(s): Must be mixed with other ingredients before feeding. Do not use in feeds containing bentonite. Mixing and conveying equipment should be properly grounded.

Restricted Drug - Use only as directed.

Warning(s): Do not feed to cows producing milk for food.

Do not feed to sheep producing milk for food.

Do not feed to laying chickens.

Do not feed to goats producing milk for food.

Presentation: 50 lb (22.68 kg) bag.

Compendium Code No.: 10220311 800306 0110

D

DECCOX®-L

Alpharma **Feed Medication**

Decoquinate-Type B Feed Medicated Supplement

Active Ingredient(s):

Decoquinate . . . . 0.50% (2271 mg/lb)

Inactive ingredients:

Lactose 91.67%

Other (corn meal, soybean oil, lecithin and silicon dioxide) 7.83%

Indications: For the prevention of coccidiosis in ruminating and non-ruminating calves and cattle caused by *E. bovis* and *E. zurnii.*

Directions for Use: Cattle: Each pound of supplement contains 2271 mg of decoquinate. Before feeding mix with feed at the rate of 1 part supplement with 9 parts feed as in the following table:

lbs Supplement	lbs Feed	Total lbs Mixture	Decoquinate mg/lb
10	90	100	227
50	450	500	227
100	900	1000	227
200	1800	2000	227

The resulting mixture should then be top dressed or mixed into the daily ration at the rate of 1⁄10 lb per 100 lbs of body weight - to provide 22.7 mg decoquinate/100 lbs of body weight (0.5 mg/kg) - daily, as in the table below:

lbs Animal Weight	lbs of Mixture per Head per Day	Total lbs Daily for 100 Head
200	0.2	20
400	0.4	40
600	0.6	60
800	0.8	80
1000	1.0	100

Feed for at least 28 days during periods of coccidiosis exposure or when experience indicates that coccidiosis is likely to be a hazard. Coccidiostats are not indicated for use in adult animals due to continuous exposure.

Precaution(s): Storage: Store in a cool, dry place. Keep bag tightly closed.

Warning(s): Do not feed to cows producing milk for food.

Presentation: 50 lbs (22.67 kg) bags.

DECCOX® is a registered trademark of Alpharma Inc.

Compendium Code No.: 10220321 AHG-010 0003

DECCOX®-M

Alpharma **Feed Medication**

Decoquinate-Medicated Powder for Whole Milk

NADA No.: 141-060

Active Ingredient(s):

Decoquinate . . . . (3632 mg/lb) 0.8%

Inactive ingredients:

Lactose 87%

Other (corn meal, soybean oil, lecithin and silicon dioxide) 12.2%

Indications: To be added to whole milk for the prevention of coccidiosis in ruminating and non-ruminating calves, including veal calves caused by *Eimeria bovis* and *E. zuernii.*

Directions for Use: Feed for at least 28 days during periods of coccidiosis exposure or when experience indicates that coccidiosis is likely to be a hazard.

Dosage: Feed at the rate of 22.7 mg per 100 lb (0.5 mg per kg) body weight daily for at least 28 days.

Mixing Directions - Individual Animal: Prepare fresh daily as shown below.

½ teaspoon per 60 lb body weight

1 teaspoon per 120 lb body weight

1½ teaspoons per 180 lb body weight

One level measuring teaspoon contains 28 mg of decoquinate.

Important: Completely stir daily dose of decoquinate powder into whole milk. Feed entire portion immediately.

Mixing Directions - Continuous Agitation: Mix DECCOX®-M into the total amount of whole milk (0.5 to 1.5 gallon per calf daily) needed for the number of calves to be fed, using level measuring cups, teaspoons (tsp) or tablespoons (tbs). Prepare fresh daily and feed each calf an equal portion of the total amount of medicated whole milk prepared as shown below.

If Average Calf Weight (lbs) is:	Amount* of DECCOX®-M for				
	5 Calves	10 Calves	20 Calves	40 Calves	80 Calves
75	1 tbs	2 tbs	¼ cup	½ cup	1 cup
100	4 tsp	8 tsp	⅓ cup	⅔ cup	1⅓ cups
150	2 tbs	¼ cup	½ cup	1 cup	2 cups
200	8 tsp	⅓ cup	⅔ cup	1⅓ cups	2⅔ cups

* This is a measurement of volume not weight (do not convert to ounces).

Important: Stir or agitate continuously.

Feed immediately in containers for individual animals only.

Do not use in bulk feeding containers (i.e., Calf-Bars).

Failure to properly mix and feed this product may result in underdosing or overdosing of some animals due to settling out of the drug.

Caution(s): For animal use only. Not for use in humans.

Restricted drug (CA). Use only as directed.

Presentation: 5 lb (2.27 kg) and 50 lb (22.68 kg).

DECCOX is a registered trademark of Alpharma Inc.

Compendium Code No.: 10220332 800310 0112

DECTOMAX® INJECTABLE SOLUTION

Pfizer Animal Health **Parasiticide Injection**

(doramectin) Antiparasitic 1% (10 mg/mL)

NADA No.: 141-061

Active Ingredient(s): DECTOMAX® Injectable Solution is a ready-to-use, colorless to pale yellow, sterile solution containing 1% w/v doramectin (10 mg/mL).

Indications: Cattle: DECTOMAX® Injectable Solution is indicated for the treatment and control of the following harmful species of gastrointestinal roundworms, lungworms, eyeworms, grubs (see Cautions), sucking lice (see Cautions), and mange mites. Consult your veterinarian for assistance in the diagnosis, treatment, and control of parasitism.

Gastrointestinal Roundworms (adults and fourth stage larvae): *Ostertagia ostertagi* (including inhibited larvae), *O. lyrata, Haemonchus placei, Trichostrongylus axei, T. colubriformis, T. longispicularis*[1], *Cooperia oncophora, C. pectinata*[1], *C. punctata, C. surnabada* (syn. *mcmasteri*), *Bunostomum phlebotomum*[1], *Strongyloides papillosus*[1], *Oesophagostomum radiatum, Trichuris* spp.[1]

[1]adults

Lungworms (adults and fourth stage larvae): *Dictyocaulus viviparus.*

Eyeworms (adults): *Thelazia* spp.

Grubs (parasitic stages): *Hypoderma bovis, H. lineatum.*

Sucking Lice: *Haematopinus eurysternus, Linognathus vituli, Solenopotes capillatus.*

Mange Mites: *Psoroptes bovis, Sarcoptes scabiei.*

DECTOMAX® Injectable Solution has been proved to effectively control infections and to protect cattle from reinfection with *Cooperia oncophora* and *Haemonchus placei* for 14 days, *Ostertagia ostertagi* for 21 days, and *C. punctata, Oesophagostomum radiatum,* and *Dictyocaulus vivapurus* for 28 days after treatment.

Swine: DECTOMAX® Injectable Solution is indicated for the treatment and control of the following species of gastrointestinal roundworms, lungworms, kidney worms, sucking lice (see Cautions), and mange mites. Consult your veterinarian for assistance in the diagnosis, treatment, and control of parasitism.

Gastrointestinal Roundworms (adults and fourth stage larvae): *Ascaris suum, Oesophagostomum dentatum, Oesophagostomum quadrispinulatum*[1], *Strongyloides ransomi*[1], *Hyostrongylus rubidus*[1].

[1]adults

Lungworms (adults): *Metastrongylus* spp.

Kidney Worms (adults): *Stephanurus dentatus.*

Mange Mites (adults and immature stages): *Sarcoptes scabiei var. suis.*

Sucking Lice (adults and immature stages): *Haematopinus suis.*

Pharmacology: Product Characteristics: DECTOMAX® Injectable Solution is a highly active, broad-spectrum parasiticide for parenteral administration to cattle and swine. It contains doramectin, a novel fermentation-derived macrocyclic lactone discovered by Pfizer Inc. Doramectin is isolated from fermentations of selected strains derived from the soil organism *Streptomyces avermitilis.*

A primary mode of action of macrocyclic lactones is to modulate chloride ion channel activity in the nervous system of nematodes and arthropods. Macrocyclic lactones bind to receptors that increase membrane permeability to chloride ions. This inhibits the electrical activity of nerve cells in nematodes and muscle cells in arthropods and causes paralysis and death of the parasites. In mammals, the neuronal receptors to which macrocyclic lactones bind are localized within the central nervous system (CNS), a site reached by only negligible concentrations of doramectin.

Dosage and Administration: In cattle, DECTOMAX® is formulated to deliver the recommended dosage (200 mcg/kg of body weight) when given by subcutaneous (SC) or intramuscular (IM) injection at the rate of 1 mL/110 lb of body weight. In swine, DECTOMAX® is formulated to deliver the recommended dosage (300 mcg/kg of body weight) when given by IM injection at the rate of 1 mL/75 lb of body weight.

Dosage: Cattle: Administer DECTOMAX® Injectable Solution at the recommended dosage of 200 mcg doramectin per kg (91 mcg/lb) of body weight. Each mL contains 10 mg of doramectin, sufficient to treat 110 lb (50 kg) of body weight.

Body Weight (lb)	Dose (mL)
110	1
220	2
330	3
440	4
550	5
660	6
770	7
880	8
990	9
1,100	10

Swine: Administer DECTOMAX® Injectable Solution at the recommended dosage of 300 mcg doramectin per kg (136 mcg/lb) of body weight. Each mL contains 10 mg of doramectin, sufficient to treat 75 lb (34 kg) of body weight.

Body Weight (lb)	Dose (mL)
15	0.2
30	0.4
45	0.6
60	0.8
75	1.0
150	2.0
225	3.0
300	4.0
375	5.0
450	6.0

Recommended treatment program for swine: To effectively initiate control of mange and sucking lice in swine, it is important to treat all animals in the herd. After initial treatment, use DECTOMAX® regularly as follows:

Breeding Animals:

Sows: Treat 7-14 days prior to farrowing to minimize exposure of piglets to mites and sucking lice.

Gilts: Treat 7-14 days prior to breeding. Treat 7-14 days prior to farrowing.

Boars: Treat a minimum of 2 times per year.

Feeder Pigs: Treat any new feeder pigs upon arrival at farm or before placement in clean quarters.

Weaners, Growers, Finishers: Weaners and grow-out/finisher pigs should be treated before placement in clean quarters.

For effective mange elimination, care must be taken to prevent reinfestation from exposure to untreated animals or contaminated facilities.

Administration: Dry, sterile equipment and aseptic procedures should be used when withdrawing and administering DECTOMAX®. For multiple treatments either automatic injection equipment or an aspirating needle should be used.

Cattle: Administer DECTOMAX® Injectable Solution by the SC or IM route. Injections should be made using a 16 gauge needle for adult cattle or an 18 gauge needle for young animals. Needles ½-¾" in length are suggested for SC administration. A 1-½" needle is suggested for IM administration. SC injections should be administered under the loose skin in front of or behind the shoulder. IM injections should be administered into the muscular region of the neck. Beef Quality Assurance guidelines recommend SC administration as the preferred route.

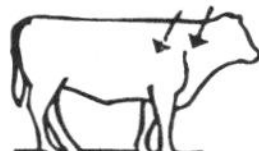

Swine: Administer DECTOMAX® Injectable Solution by the IM route. Inject in the neck region using an 18 gauge x 1" needle for young animals; a 16 gauge x 1-½" needle for sows and boars. To accurately meter doses administered to piglets, use of a tuberculin syringe and 20 gauge x 1" needle is recommended.

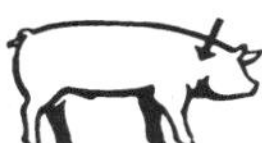

Precaution(s): Store below 30°C (86°F).

Environmental Safety: Studies indicate that when doramectin comes in contact with the soil, it readily and tightly binds to the soil and becomes inactive over time. Free doramectin may adversely affect fish and certain waterborne organisms on which they feed. Do not permit water runoff from feedlots to enter lakes, streams, or groundwater. Do not contaminate water by direct application or by the improper disposal of drug containers. Dispose of containers in an approved landfill.

Caution(s): DECTOMAX® has been developed specifically for use in cattle and swine only. This product should not be used in other animal species as severe adverse reactions, including fatalities in dogs, may result.

For SC injection in cattle only. For IM injection in swine and cattle. This product is approved for the treatment and control of sucking lice. For treatment of biting lice in cattle, use of DECTOMAX® Pour-On is recommended.

DECTOMAX® is highly effective against all stages of cattle grubs. However, proper timing of treatment is important. For most effective results, cattle should be treated as soon as possible after the end of the heel fly (warble) season.

Destruction of *Hypoderma* larvae (cattle grubs) at the period when these grubs are in vital areas may cause undesirable host-parasite reactions including the possibility of fatalities. Killing *H. lineatum* when it is in the tissue surrounding the gullet may cause bloat; killing *H. bovis* when it is in the vertebral canal may cause staggering or paralysis. These reactions are not specific to treatment with DECTOMAX®, but can occur with any successful treatment of grubs. Cattle should be treated either before or after these stages of grub development. Consult your veterinarian concerning the proper time for treatment.

Cattle treated with DECTOMAX® after the end of the heel fly season may be re-treated with DECTOMAX® during the winter for internal parasites, mange mites, or sucking lice, without danger of grub-related reactions. A planned parasite control program is recommended.

Warning(s): Residue Warnings: Cattle: Do not slaughter for human consumption within 35 days of treatment. Not for use in female dairy cattle 20 months of age or older. A withdrawal period has not been established for this product in preruminating calves. Do not use in calves to be processed for veal. Swine: Do not slaughter for human consumption within 24 days of treatment.

Not for human use. Keep out of reach of children. The material safety data sheet (MSDS) contains more detailed occupational safety information. To report adverse effects in users, to obtain more information, or to obtain an MSDS, call 1-800-366-5288.

Trial Data: One dose of DECTOMAX® Injectable Solution effectively treats and controls a wide range of roundworm and arthropod parasites that impair the health and productivity of cattle and swine.

Studies have demonstrated the safety margin of DECTOMAX® injection in cattle and swine. In USA trials, no toxic signs were seen in cattle given up to 25 times the recommended dose, or in swine given up to 10 times the recommended dose. Studies also demonstrated safety in neonatal calves and piglets treated with up to 3 times the recommended dose. In males (bulls and boars) and females (cows and sows during folliculogenesis, implantation, organogenesis, and through gestation), a dose 3 times the recommended dose had no effect on breeding performance.

Presentation: DECTOMAX® is available in 100-mL, 250-mL, and 500-mL multi-dose, rubber-capped glass vials.

U.S. Patent No. 5,089,480

Compendium Code No.: 36900091

79-5199-00-5

DECTOMAX® POUR-ON

Pfizer Animal Health **Parasiticide-Topical**

(doramectin) Antiparasitic 0.5% (5 mg/mL)

NADA No.: 141-095

Active Ingredient(s): DECTOMAX® Pour-On solution is a ready-to-use, systemically active, clear, light blue solution containing 0.5% w/v doramectin (5 mg/mL). It is formulated to deliver the recommended dosage of 500 mcg/kg (227 mcg/lb) of body weight when given by topical administration at the rate of 1 mL/22 lb (10 kg) of body weight.

Indications: DECTOMAX® Pour-On solution is indicated for the treatment and control of the following species of gastrointestinal roundworms, lungworms, eyeworms, grubs (see Cautions), biting and sucking lice, horn flies, and mange mites in cattle. Consult your veterinarian for assistance in the diagnosis, treatment, and control of parasitism.

Gastrointestinal roundworms: *Ostertagia ostertagi* (adults and L_4, including inhibited larvae), *O. lyrata* (adults), *Haemonchus placei* (adults and L_4), *Trichostrongylus axei* (adults), *T. colubriformis* (adults and L_4), *Cooperia oncophora* (adults[1] and L_4), *C. pectinata* (adults), *C. punctata* (adults and L_4), *C. surnabada* (adults), *Bunostomum phlebotomum* (adults), *Oesophagostomum radiatum* (adults and L_4), *Trichuris* spp. (adults).

[1]Efficacy below 90% was observed against adult *C. oncophora* in some clinical studies.

Lungworms (adults and fourth stage larvae): *Dictyocaulus viviparus.*

Eyeworms (adults): *Thelazia gulosa* (adults), *T. skrjabini* (adults).

Grubs: *Hypoderma bovis, H. lineatum.*

Lice:

Biting Lice: *Damalinia bovis.*

Sucking Lice: *Haematopinus eurysternus, Linognathus vituli, Solenopotes capillatus.*

Horn Flies: *Haematobia irritans.*

Mange Mites: *Chorioptes bovis, Sarcoptes scabiei.*

DECTOMAX® Pour-On solution has been proved to effectively control infections and to protect cattle from reinfection with *Cooperia oncophora* and *Dictyocaulus viviparus* for 21 days; *Ostertagia ostertagi, Cooperia punctata,* and *Oesophagostomum radiatum* for 28 days; and *Haemonchus placei* for 35 days after treatment.

Pharmacology: Product Characteristics: DECTOMAX® Pour-On solution is a highly active, broad-spectrum parasiticide for topical administration to cattle. It contains doramectin, a novel fermentation-derived macrocyclic lactone discovered by Pfizer Inc. Doramectin is isolated from fermentations of selected strains derived from the soil organism *Streptomyces avermitilis.*

A primary mode of action of macrocyclic lactones is to modulate chloride ion channel activity in the nervous system of nematodes and arthropods. Macrocyclic lactones bind to receptors that increase membrane permeability to chloride ions. This inhibits the electrical activity of nerve cells in nematodes and muscle cells in arthropods and causes paralysis and death of the parasites. In mammals, the neuronal receptors to which macrocyclic lactones bind are localized within the central nervous system (CNS), a site reached by only negligible concentrations of doramectin.

Dosage and Administration:

Management Considerations for Horn Flies: DECTOMAX® Pour-On solution provides 7 days of persistent activity against horn flies. The product should be used as part of an integrated control program and be combined with other methods for extended horn fly control. For optimal horn fly control, consult with your veterinarian or a livestock entomologist.

Dosage: Administer DECTOMAX® Pour-On solution to cattle topically at a dosage of 500 mcg doramectin per kg (227 mcg/lb) of body weight. Each mL contains 5 mg of doramectin, sufficient to treat 22 lb (10 kg) of body weight.

For the best results, DECTOMAX® Pour-On solution should be a part of a parasite control program for both internal and external parasites based on the epidemiology of these parasites. Consult a veterinarian or an entomologist for information regarding the most effective timing of applications.

Administration: DECTOMAX® Pour-On solution should be applied topically along the mid-line of the back in a narrow strip between the withers and tailhead.

Dosing Cup (250 mL and 1 L bottles): A dosing cup is provided for use with DECTOMAX® Pour-On solution supplied in 250 mL and 1 L bottles. The DECTOMAX® Pour-On solution dosing cup should be installed by rotating the cup on the bottle neck until tight. When installed correctly, the spout is aligned at the mid-point on the wide side of the bottle.

The curved end of the dosing cup tube should be positioned at the bottom of the bottle on the side opposite the spout. When the dosing cup is in the closed position ("zero" at set dosage mark on screw), product does not enter the cup reservoir. Select a dose [1 mL per 22 lb (10 kg) of body weight] by twisting the dosing screw on the top of the dosing cup to the desired position. The first complete turn of the dosing screw will set the dose at 10 mL ("10" shows on the screw at set dose mark). Each additional turn increases the dose in 5 mL increments until a maximum dose of 50 mL ("50" is the bottom number showing on screw at the set dose mark) is reached. When body weight is between weight markings on the dosing cup, use the higher dose volume.

To fill the dosing reservoir, hold the bottle upright and squeeze it until a slight excess has been delivered as indicated by the calibration lines. Release the pressure and excess will automatically drain from the reservoir and return to the bottle.

Tilt the bottle to deliver the dose. DECTOMAX® Pour-On solution should be delivered to cattle on the back in a single pass from the withers to the tailhead.

Applicators (2.5 L and 5 L bottles): Applicators are available for use with DECTOMAX® Pour-On solution supplied in 2.5 and 5 L backpacks. Directions for 2 recommended applicators are provided below. Some applicators may be incompatible with this formulation.

Phillips Pour-on Applicator System:

1. Replace the shipping cap on 2.5 or 5 L backpack with the draw-off cap provided and tighten firmly.
2. Thread the draw-off tubing through the anti-kink spring. Attach the tube to the draw-off cap. Screw the spring counter clockwise over the tubing and draw-off spigot.
3. Invert the backpack.
4. Set the dose to maximum (50 mL). Gently prime the applicator, checking for leaks. To prime, place the nozzle into a clean, dry receptacle and depress lever fully. Pump 3-4 short strokes ensuring that the piston reaches the end of the cylinder, and then release the lever completely to fill the cylinder. A small air bubble may appear within the cylinder. This will not affect the dosing accuracy.
5. Set the required dose and administer.

D

6. To disconnect the system, proceed as follows:
   a) Set backpack in upward position.
   b) Discharge residual material from the applicator and draw-off tubing into a separate, clean, dry receptacle.
7. Follow the manufacturer's recommendation for care and maintenance of the dosing applicator.
8. Remove the draw-off cap. Replace with the original cap and tighten firmly.

Syrvet Pour-on Applicator System:

1. Replace the shipping cap on the 2.5 or 5 L backpack with the draw-off cap provided and tighten firmly.
2. Thread the draw-off tubing through the anti-kink spring. Attach the tube to the draw-off cap. Screw the spring clockwise over the tubing and draw-off spigot.
3. Invert the backpack.
4. Set the dose at the maximum (50 mL) by unscrewing the adjuster at the base of the handle. Gently prime the applicator, checking for leaks. To prime, point the nozzle into a clean, dry receptacle and gently pump the lever back and forth to expel air from the system. When the barrel completely fills after every priming stroke, set the dose.
5. Set the dose as follows:
   a) Use the handle to align the middle of the blue plunger ring with the chosen mark on the barrel. Tighten the adjuster screw against the handle.
   b) Secure the dose with the adjuster screw locknut.

Note: Dose accuracy can be checked by dispensing a known number of set doses into a measuring cylinder. Correct any inaccuracy by adjusting the dose setting screw. Repeat this procedure until desired accuracy is achieved.

6. Administer each dose by fully depressing the handle so that the plunger travels its entire set length. Release the handle and the applicator will automatically refill.
7. To disconnect the system proceed as follows:
   a) Set backpack in upward position.
   b) Discharge residual material from the applicator and draw-off tubing into a separate, dry receptacle.
8. Follow the manufacturer's recommendation for care and maintenance of the dosing applicator.
9. Remove the draw-off cap. Replace with the original cap and tighten firmly.

Use Conditions: Varying weather conditions, including rainfall, do not affect the efficacy of DECTOMAX® Pour-On.

Precaution(s): Store below 30°C (86°F).

Protect from light.

Cloudiness in the formulation may occur when DECTOMAX® Pour-On solution is stored at temperatures below 0°C (32°F). Allowing to warm to room temperature will restore the normal appearance without affecting efficacy.

Environmental Safety: Studies indicate that when doramectin comes in contact with the soil, it readily and tightly binds to the soil and becomes inactive over time. Free doramectin may adversely affect fish or certain water-borne organisms on which they feed. Do not permit cattle to enter lakes, streams or ponds for at least 6 hours after treatment. Do not contaminate water by direct application or by the improper disposal of drug containers. Dispose of containers in an approved landfill or by incineration.

Caution(s): DECTOMAX® Pour-On solution has been developed specifically for use in cattle only. This product should not be used in other animal species as severe adverse reactions, including fatalities in dogs, may result.

This product is to be applied to skin surface only. Do not administer orally or parenterally.

Do not apply to areas of skin which are caked with mud or manure.

Wash hands after use.

Do not smoke or eat while handling the product.

DECTOMAX® Pour-On solution is highly effective against cattle grubs. However, proper timing of treatment is important. For most effective results, cattle should be treated as soon as possible after the end of the heel fly (warble) season.

Destruction of *Hypoderma* larvae (cattle grubs) at the period when these grubs are in vital areas may cause undesirable host-parasite reactions including the possibility of fatalities. Killing *H. lineatum* when it is in the tissue surrounding the gullet may cause bloat; killing *H. bovis* when it is in the vertebral canal may cause staggering or paralysis. These reactions are not specific to treatment with DECTOMAX® Pour-On solution, but can occur with any successful treatment of grubs. Cattle should be treated either before or after the migratory phase of grub development. Consult your veterinarian concerning the proper time for treatment.

Cattle treated with DECTOMAX® Pour-On solution after the end of heel fly season may be re-treated with DECTOMAX® Pour-On during the winter for internal parasites, mange mites, or biting and sucking lice, without danger of grub-related reactions. A planned parasite control program is recommended.

DECTOMAX® Pour-On solution for cattle may be irritating to human skin and eyes, and users should be careful not to apply it to themselves or to other persons. Operators should wear protective clothing including a long-sleeved shirt, rubber gloves, and boots with a waterproof coat when applying the product. Protective clothing should be washed after use. If accidental skin contact occurs, wash the affected area immediately with soap and water. If accidental eye exposure occurs, flush the eyes immediately with water and get medical attention.

Warning(s): Residue Warning: Cattle must not be slaughtered for human consumption within 45 days of treatment. Not for use in female dairy cattle 20 months of age or older. A withdrawal period has not been established for this product in preruminating calves. Do not use in calves to be processed for veal.

Flammable! Keep away from heat, sparks, open flame, and other sources of ignition. Not for human use. Keep out of reach of children. The Material Safety Data Sheet (MSDS) contains more detailed occupational safety information. To report adverse effects in users, to obtain more information, or to obtain an MSDS, call 1-800-366-5288.

Trial Data: One dose of DECTOMAX® Pour-On solution effectively treats and controls a wide range of roundworm and arthropod parasites that impair the health and productivity of cattle.

Studies have demonstrated the safety margin of doramectin. In USA trials, no toxic signs were seen in cattle given up to 25 times the recommended dose of Dectomax® Injectable solution. A study using Dectomax® Injectable solution also demonstrated safety in neonatal calves treated with up to 3 times the recommended dose. In breeding animals (bulls, and cows during folliculogenesis, organogenesis, implantation, and through gestation), a dose 3 times the recommended dose of Dectomax® Injectable solution had no effect on breeding performance. A pharmacokinetic study demonstrated that systemic exposure to doramectin from DECTOMAX® Pour-On was less than systemic exposure to doramectin from Dectomax® Injectable solution.

Presentation: DECTOMAX® Pour-On solution is available in 250 mL, 1 L, 2.5 L, and 5 L multi-dose containers.

Compendium Code No.: 36900321 69-5269-00-4

DEFEND® EXSPOT® TREATMENT FOR DOGS

Schering-Plough **Topical Insecticide**

EPA Reg. No.: 773-73

Active Ingredient(s):

Permethrin (3-phenoxyphenyl) methyl (±)-cis, trans-3-(2,2-dichloroethenyl)-2,2-dimethylcyclopropanecarboxylate**	65%
Inert ingredients	35%
Total	100%

**cis/trans ratio: Max. 56% (±) cis and min. 45% (±) trans

Indications: Kills and repels fleas, deer ticks *(Ixodes dammini)* (vector of lyme disease), and brown dog ticks *(Rhipicephalus sanguineus)* for up to four weeks. It also kills and repels American dog ticks *(Dermacentor variabilis)* for two to three weeks.

Directions for Use: It is a violation of Federal Law to use this product in a manner inconsistent with its labeling.

Read the entire label completely before using. Do not use on cats. May be toxic if applied to or ingested by cats. Do not use the product in or on electrical equipment due to the possibility of a shock hazard.

How to Apply: Hold the card in an upright position, with the cap pointing up and away from user's face and body, then cut along the dotted line. Invert the card over the dog and use the point of the card to part the hair of the dog. Squeeze the tube firmly to apply all of the solution. Wrap the container and put it in the trash.

Dosage for dogs weighing less than 33 lbs.: Apply 1 mL of DEFEND® EXSPOT® insecticide solution to the dog's back between the shoulder blades.

Dosage for dogs weighing more than 33 lbs.: Apply 1 mL of DEFEND® EXSPOT® insecticide solution to the dog's back between the shoulder blades and apply 1 mL of DEFEND® EXSPOT® insecticide solution to the dog's back directly above the tail head area.

DEFEND® EXSPOT® insecticide demonstrates a greater than 92% control of fleas within three (3) days of application. As with all flea and tick control products, DEFEND® EXSPOT® insecticide should be used as part of a control program aimed at reducing flea populations in the dog's environment (bedding, carpets, kennel, yard). Consult a veterinarian or entomologist for program recommendations. If necessary, repeat applications may be made, but do not apply at intervals of less than seven (7) days.

Contraindication(s): Do not use on cats.

Precautionary Statements: Hazards to Humans and Domestic Animals: Caution: Harmful if swallowed or absorbed through the skin. Causes moderate eye irritation. Avoid contact with skin, eyes or clothing. Wash thoroughly with soap and water after handling. Do not use on cats. Cats which actively groom or engage in close physical contact with recently treated dogs may be at risk of toxic exposure. Do not use on sick or debilitated dogs. Consult with a veterinarian before using on dogs with known organ dysfunction.

Statement of Practical Treatment:

If Swallowed: Call a physician or Poison Control Center. Drink 1 or 2 glasses of water and induce vomiting by touching back of throat with finger or, if available, by administration of syrup of Ipecac. Do not induce vomiting or give anything by mouth to an unconscious person. If on Skin: Remove contaminated clothing and wash with plenty of soap and water. Call a physician if irritation persists. If in Eyes: Flush eyes with plenty of water. Call a physician if irritation persists.

Environmental Hazards: This product is toxic to fish. Do not add directly to water. Do not contaminate by cleaning of equipment or disposal of equipment washwaters.

Storage and Disposal: Do not contaminate water, food or feed by storage or disposal.

Storage: Store in a cool, dry place. Protect from freezing. Pesticide Disposal: Securely wrap original container in several layers of newspaper and discard in trash. Container Disposal: Do not reuse empty container. Wrap container and put in trash.

Warning(s): Keep out of reach of children.

Side Effects: Some animals may be sensitive to ingredients in this product. Reported reactions in dogs have included skin sensitivity. Increased itchiness, redness, rash, hair discoloration or hair loss at the application site may occur. Dogs may also show lethargy. Observe the dog following treatment, if sensitivity to for DEFEND® EXSPOT® for Dogs occurs, discontinue use and bathe the dog. Seek veterinary advice.

Disclaimer: Notice of Warranty: Schering-Plough Animal Health Corporation makes no warranty of merchantability, fitness for any particular purpose, or otherwise, expressed or implied concerning the product or its uses which extend beyond the use of the product under normal conditions in accord with the statements made of the label.

Presentation: Each case contains 24 - 2 x 1 mL applicators.

DEFEND is a registered trademark of Schering-Plough Animal Health Corporation.

EXSPOT is a registered trademark of Schering-Plough Animal Health Corporation.

Compendium Code No.: 10470341

DEFENSOR® 1

Pfizer Animal Health **Vaccine**

Rabies Vaccine, Killed Virus

U.S. Vet. Lic. No.: 189

Description: The vaccine is prepared from cell-culture-grown, chemically inactivated rabies virus. The seed virus is a highly immunogenic, fixed strain of rabies virus which originated from Louis Pasteur's original isolate in 1882. The inactivated virus is formulated with a highly purified adjuvant and is packaged in liquid form.

Contains gentamicin as preservative.

Indications: DEFENSOR® 1 is for vaccination of healthy dogs and cats 3 months of age or older as an aid in preventing rabies.

Directions:

1. General Directions: Shake well. Aseptically administer 1 mL subcutaneously. Dogs may be vaccinated intramuscularly or subcutaneously.
2. Primary Vaccination: Healthy dogs and cats should receive a single dose at 3 months of age or older. A repeat dose should be administered 1 year later.
3. Revaccination: Annual revaccination with a single dose is recommended.

Precaution(s): Store at 2°-7°C. Prolonged exposure to higher temperatures may adversely affect potency. Do not freeze.

Use entire contents when first opened.

Sterilized syringes and needles should be used to administer this vaccine.

Caution(s): As with many vaccines, anaphylaxis may occur after use. Initial antidote of epinephrine is recommended and should be followed with appropriate supportive therapy.

This product has been shown to be efficacious in healthy animals. A protective immune response may not be elicited if animals are incubating an infectious disease, are malnourished or parasitized, are stressed due to shipment or environmental conditions, are otherwise immunocompromised, or the vaccine is not administered in accordance with label directions.

Warning(s): For veterinary use only.

Discussion: Disease Description: Rabies is a worldwide, high mortality disease affecting mammalian species. Wild animals are common vectors of the disease and the major source of transmission to humans and domestic animals. Despite successful attempts over the years to reduce the incidence of rabies, recent published reports indicate that in the U.S. more than 30,000 people undergo treatment every year for possible exposure.[1] Domestic animals are the major source of exposure for humans. Since 1980, the most commonly reported rabid domestic animals have been cats, cattle, and dogs. In 1990, a total of 4,881 cases of animal rabies were reported to the Center for Disease Control by all 50 states, the District of Columbia, and Puerto Rico.[2] Susceptibility to rabies varies according to pet species. Rabies is not a treatable disease and suspect pets are usually quarantined until a clinical diagnosis is made, at which time they are destroyed.

The route of infection can be oral, respiratory, or parenteral. Following infection, a paralytic syndrome ensues, emerging as either the "furious" or "dumb" form. "Furious rabies" is characterized by unusual aggression; "dumb rabies" by lethargy and a desire to avoid contact. Respiratory failure is the immediate cause of death.

Trial Data: Safety and Efficacy: Because DEFENSOR® 1 is produced on an established cell line, it has safety advantages over inactivated brain-origin rabies vaccines. Tissue-origin vaccines contain extraneous protein in addition to rabies antigen that can lead to autoimmune disease.

The established cell line used in DEFENSOR® 1 has been extensively tested for freedom from contaminating agents. In addition, use of an established cell line yields a vaccine of consistent potency from serial to serial. DEFENSOR® 1 has proven to be uniformly safe in experimental tests, and no significant adverse reactions were reported in extensive clinical trials of the vaccine.

A duration of immunity study, conducted in accordance with federal regulation and under U.S. Department of Agriculture direction, demonstrated that a 1-mL dose met federal guidelines for protection of dogs and cats against virulent challenge administered more than a year after vaccination.

References: Available upon request.

Presentation: 10-dose vials.

Compendium Code No.: 36900910 75-4654-03

DEFENSOR® 3

Pfizer Animal Health **Vaccine**

Rabies Vaccine, Killed Virus

U.S. Vet. Lic. No.: 189

Description: The vaccine is prepared from cell-culture-grown, chemically inactivated rabies virus. The seed virus is a highly immunogenic, fixed strain of rabies virus which originated from Louis Pasteur's original isolate in 1882. The inactivated virus is formulated with a highly purified adjuvant and is packaged in liquid form.

Contains gentamicin as preservative.

Indications: DEFENSOR® 3 is for vaccination of healthy dogs, cats, cattle, and sheep 3 months of age or older as an aid in preventing rabies.

Directions:

Dogs and Cats:

1. General Directions: Shake well. Aseptically administer 1 mL subcutaneously. Dogs may be vaccinated intramuscularly or subcutaneously.
2. Primary Vaccination: Administer a single 1-mL dose at 3 months of age or older to healthy dogs and cats. A repeat dose should be administered 1 year later.
3. Revaccination: Subsequent revaccination every 3 years with a single dose is recommended.

Cattle and Sheep:

1. General Directions: Shake well. Aseptically administer 2 mL intramuscularly.
2. Primary Vaccination: Administer a single 2-mL dose at 3 months of age or older to healthy cattle and sheep. A repeat dose should be administered 1 year later.
3. Revaccination: Annual revaccination with a single dose is recommended.

Precaution(s): Store at 2°-7°C. Prolonged exposure to higher temperatures may adversely affect potency. Do not freeze.

Use entire contents when first opened.

Sterilized syringes and needles should be used to administer this vaccine.

Caution(s): As with many vaccines, anaphylaxis may occur after use. Initial antidote of epinephrine is recommended and should be followed with appropriate supportive therapy.

This product has been shown to be efficacious in healthy animals. A protective immune response may not be elicited if animals are incubating an infectious disease, are malnourished or parasitized, are stressed due to shipment or environmental conditions, are otherwise immunocompromised, or the vaccine is not administered in accordance with label directions.

Warning(s): Do not vaccinate within 21 days before slaughter.

For use in dogs, cats, cattle, and sheep only. For veterinary use only.

Discussion: Disease Description: Rabies is a worldwide, high mortality disease affecting mammalian species. Wild animals are common vectors of the disease and the major source of transmission to humans and domestic animals. Despite successful attempts over the years to reduce the incidence of rabies, recent published reports indicate that in the U.S. more than 30,000 people undergo treatment every year for possible exposure.[1] Domestic animals are the major source of exposure for humans. Since 1980, the most commonly reported rabid domestic animals have been cats, cattle, and dogs. In 1990, a total of 4,881 cases of animal rabies were reported to the Center for Disease Control by all 50 states, the District of Columbia, and Puerto Rico.[2] Susceptibility to rabies varies according to pet species. Rabies is not a treatable disease and suspect pets are usually quarantined until a clinical diagnosis is made, at which time they are destroyed.

The route of infection can be oral, respiratory, or parenteral. Following infection, a paralytic syndrome ensues, emerging as either the "furious" or "dumb" form. "Furious rabies" is characterized by unusual aggression; "dumb rabies" by lethargy and a desire to avoid contact. Respiratory failure is the immediate cause of death.

Trial Data: Safety and Efficacy: Because DEFENSOR® 3 is produced on an established cell line, it has safety advantages over inactivated brain-origin rabies vaccines. Tissue-origin vaccines contain extraneous protein in addition to rabies antigen that can lead to autoimmune disease.

The established cell line used in DEFENSOR® 3 has been extensively tested for freedom from contaminating agents. In addition, use of an established cell line yields a vaccine of consistent potency from serial to serial. DEFENSOR® 3 has proven to be uniformly safe in experimental tests, and no significant adverse reactions were reported in extensive clinical trials of the vaccine.

A duration of immunity study, conducted in accordance with federal regulation and under U.S. Department of Agriculture direction, demonstrated that a 1-mL dose met federal guidelines for protection of dogs and cats against virulent challenge administered 3 years after vaccination. Cattle and sheep were likewise protected 1 year after receiving a 2-mL dose of DEFENSOR® 3.

References: Available upon request.

Presentation: 1-dose, 10-dose and 25-dose vials.

Compendium Code No.: 36900920 75-4996-01

DEGREASE SHAMPOO

Davis **Antidermatosis Shampoo**

Ingredient(s): Sodium lauryl sulfate, fragrance.

Indications: Davis DEGREASE SHAMPOO is a cleansing agent for oils, grease and dirt to be used on dogs and cats. It can be used on greasy ears, oily coated breeds, motor oil and grease, and oily seborrhea.

Dosage and Administration: Apply full strength directly to coat or wet first and work into a rich lather. Do not get into eyes. Let stand 3-5 minutes, then rinse thoroughly. Repeat if necessary. Can be diluted for a general cleansing and grooming shampoo.

Note: A soft paste when cool, it warms and becomes a thick ivory liquid. Either form performs well.

Warning(s): For external use only. Keep out of reach of children.

Presentation: 16 oz (454 g) and 64 oz.

Compendium Code No.: 11410130

DEHORNING PASTE

AgriPharm **Dehorning Paste**

For Destruction of Horn-Forming Tissue

Active Ingredient(s): Contains:

Calcium and sodium hydroxides 67%
Inert Ingredients: 33%
Total 100%

Indications: For the destruction of horn-forming tissue in baby calves up to 8 weeks of age, preferably 1 to 7 days of age.

Dosage and Administration: Clip hair from horn buttons and roughen the skin from tip to base of buttons (do not draw blood). Protect surrounding tissue with petrolatum. Apply a thin film of DEHORNING PASTE to each horn button by gently squeezing the bottle in an inverted position. Protect hands with rubber gloves. Confine calves for 30 minutes to prevent removal or spreading of paste. Do not expose calves to weather for 12 hours after treatment.

Caution(s): Poison. May be fatal if swallowed.

For animal use only.

Keep out of reach of children.

Antidote(s):

External: Flood with water, then wash with vinegar.

Internal: Give vinegar or citrus juice copiously followed with olive oil.

Eyes: Wash with water for 15 minutes and then with 5% boric acid solution.

Call a physician or Poison Control Center.

Presentation: 85 gm (3 oz).

Compendium Code No.: 14570240

DELIVER® WITH DIALINE™

AgriLabs **Large Animal Dietary Supplement**

Nutritional Supplement

Guaranteed Analysis:

	Percent	App. Grams/Feeding
Salt (NACI)	min. 4.6%; max. 5.5%	3.3-4.0 g
Sodium (Na)	min. 4.5%	3.2 g
Potassium (K)	min. 1.4%	1.0 g
Magnesium (Mg)	min. 0.3%	0.2 g

Contents: Dextrose Monohydrate, Psyllium Seed Husks, Sodium Bicarbonate, Salt, Sodium Citrate, Potassium Chloride, Citric Acid, Magnesium Hydroxide, Guar and Xanthan Gum, Roughage, Silicium Dioxide (anti-caking), Flavor, FD&C Red No. 40-Aluminum Lake.

DIALINE™ is psyllium polysaccharides treated with divalent ions.

Indications: A nutritional supplement for young calves to provide electrolytes, dextrose and fluids when mixed with water.

Directions for Use: After mixing thoroughly with water, DELIVER® may be fed to young calves requiring supplemental electrolytes, dextrose and fluids. DELIVER® may be fed on a short-term basis in place of the usual diet. Since DELIVER® is not a complete source of nutrition, its use should not exceed the following recommended feeding schedule.

0 Hours (1st Feeding): 1 packet (or 2 scoops) DELIVER® in 2 qts. warm water.
12 Hours (2nd Feeding): 1 packet (or 2 scoops) DELIVER® in 2 qts. warm water.
24 Hours (3rd Feeding): 1 packet (or 2 scoops) DELIVER® in 2 qts. warm water.
36 Hours (4th Feeding): 1 qt. milk and ½ packet (or 1 scoop) DELIVER® in 1 qt. warm water.
At 48 hours: Resume usual diet

If desired, the "3rd Feeding" can be omitted, and the "4th Feeding" used in its place, followed in 12 hours with the resumption of the usual diet.

General Guidelines: Mix thoroughly and give immediately or the liquid may become too thick to be ingested by calf.

Precaution(s): Seal bag and replace the bucket lid immediately after use. Store in a cool dry place.

Caution(s): Not for human use.

Presentation: 2.6 oz (74 g) single-feed packet, 1.1 kg and 4.4 kg pails (with scoop).

DELIVER® is a registered trademark of Pharmalett Denmark A/S.

U.S. Patent No. 5,038,396

Compendium Code No.: 10581290

DEL-PHOS® EMULSIFIABLE LIQUID INSECTICIDE

Schering-Plough **Topical Insecticide**

EPA Reg. No.: 773-76

Active Ingredient(s): wt/wt

N-(mercaptomethyl) phthalimide 11.6%
S-(0,0-dimethyl phosphorodithioate) 88.4%
Total 100.0%

Contains ¼ pound active ingredient per quart.

Indications: A beef and non-lactating dairy cattle insecticide for the control of lice, winter ticks, lone star ticks, Gulf Coast ear ticks, horn flies, sarcoptic mange, and a swine insecticide for the control of lice and sarcoptic mange.

For use on cattle and swine only. Not for use on horses, sheep or goats.

Directions for Use: It is a violation of Federal law to use this product in a manner inconsistent with its labeling.

Beef and Non-Lactating Dairy Cattle:

Dilution rate general use 3-day pre-slaughter interval: Do not treat non-lactating dairy cattle within 28 days of freshening.

For the control of lice, spray a 1:150 dilution rate.

For the control of horn flies, spray a 1:200 dilution rate.

For the control of sarcoptic mange, winter ticks, lone star ticks, and Gulf Coast ear ticks, spray a 1:100 dilution rate.

Swine:

Dilution rate general use 1-day pre-slaughter interval: For the control of lice and sarcoptic mange, spray a 1:100 dilution rate.

Spray Method:

Cattle and Swine: At the 1:100 dilution rate, the 1:150 dilution rate or the 1:200 dilution rate, mix one quart of DEL-PHOS® Insecticide with 23, 37.5, or 50 gallons of water respectively, and stir thoroughly. Apply the fresh mixture as a high-pressure spray, taking care to wet the skin, not just the hair. Apply to the point of runoff. For cattle, do not apply within 3 days of slaughter. For swine, do not apply within 1 day of slaughter.

Backrubber Method:

Cattle: To control horn flies on beef cattle, dilute one quart of DEL-PHOS® in 12.5 gallons of fuel oil or other suitable carrier and charge the backrubber device or soak the sack or cloth as required. Retreat with backrubber as needed.

Precautionary Statements: Hazards to Humans and Domestic Animals:

Warning: Causes eye and skin irritation. Do not get in eyes, on skin, or on clothing. Harmful if swallowed. Avoid breathing spray mist. Applicators must wear long-sleeved shirt, long pants, elbow length waterproof gloves, waterproof apron and unlined waterproof boots. Wash all contaminated clothing with soap and hot water before reuse. Wash thoroughly before eating, drinking or using tobacco.

First Aid:

If in Eyes: Rinse immediately with plenty of water. Call a physician immediately.

If on Skin or Clothing: Take off contaminated clothing. Rinse skin immediately with plenty of water for 15-20 minutes. Call a poison control center or doctor for treatment advice.

If Inhaled: Move person to fresh air. If person is not breathing, call 911 or an ambulance, then give artificial respiration, preferably mouth-to-mouth if possible. Call a poison control center or doctor for further treatment advice.

If Swallowed: Call poison control center or doctor immediately for treatment advice. Have person sip a glass of water if able to swallow. Do not induce vomiting unless told to do so by the poison control center or doctor. Do not induce vomiting or give anything by mouth to an unconscious person.

Hotline Number: Have the product container or label with you when calling the poison control center or doctor or going for treatment. You may also contact the Rocky Mountain Poison Center at 1-303-595-4869 for emergency medical treatment information.

Note to Physician and Veterinarian: DEL-PHOS® is an organophosphate insecticide and a cholinesterase inhibitor. If signs of cholinesterase inhibition are present, atropine is antidotal. 2-PAM is also antidotal and may be administered in conjunction with atropine. If ingested, do not induce vomiting as this may cause an aspiration hazard. The usual symptoms of organophosphate poisoning in man include: headache, blurred vision, weakness, nausea, discomfort in the chest, vomiting, abdominal cramps, diarrhea, salivation, sweating and pin-point pupils. The usual symptoms of poisoning in animals include: salivation, labored breathing, loss of balance, staggering and pin-point pupils.

Environmental Hazards: The pesticide is extremely toxic to fish. Do not apply directly to water, to areas where surface water is present, or to intertidal areas below the mean high water mark. Do not contaminate water when disposing of equipment washwaters. Drift or runoff from treated areas may be hazardous to aquatic organisms in neighboring areas.

Physical or Chemical Hazards: Do not use or store near heat or open flame. Protect from temperatures below 20°F.

Storage and Disposal: Do not contaminate water, food or feed by storage or disposal.

Storage: Do not use or store near heat or open flame. Protect from temperatures below 20°F.

Pesticide Disposal: Wastes resulting from the use of this product may be disposed of on site or at an approved waste disposal facility.

Container Disposal: Triple rinse (or equivalent). Then offer for recycling or reconditioning, or puncture and dispose of in a sanitary landfill, or if allowed by State and local authorities, by burning. If burned, stay out of smoke.

Warning(s):

1. DEL-PHOS® Insecticide is a cholinesterase inhibitor. Do not use this product on animals simultaneously or within a few days before or after treatment with or exposure to cholinesterase inhibiting drugs, pesticides or chemicals. Atropine is antidotal. Consult a veterinarian at the first sign of adverse reactions.
2. Cattle treated at a spray rate of 1:100, 1:150 or 1:200 may be slaughtered 3 days after treatment.
3. Swine may be slaughtered 1 day after treatment.
4. In swine, single applications for lice and sarcoptic mange control are usually effective. However, should a second application be necessary, it may be made 14 days following the first treatment.
5. For swine: Do not treat sick, convalescent, or stressed animals. Do not apply directly to suckling pigs.
6. For cattle: Do not treat sick, convalescent, stressed, or animals less than 3 months old. Hand dipping of young animals will prevent swallowing of dip solution.
7. Do not treat non-lactating dairy cattle within 28 days of freshening. If freshening should occur within the 28 day period after treatment, milk must not be used as human food.
8. Important: In cattle, repeat the treatment as necessary, but not more often than every 7 to 10 days. Treatment for lice, ticks, sarcoptic mange and horn flies may be made at any time of the year except when cattle grub larvae are in the gullet or spinal canal. Consult your veterinarian, extension livestock specialist or extension entomologist regarding the timing of treatment.

Presentation: 1 quart (946 mL) (NDC 0061-5150-01) and 1 U.S. gallon (3.785 L) (NDC 0061-5150-02) containers.

Compendium Code No.: 10470412 Rev. 7/01 / Rev. 8/00

DELTA ALBAPLEX® / DELTA ALBAPLEX® 3X ℞

Pharmacia & Upjohn **Antibiotic-Corticosteroid**

brand of tetracycline hydrochloride, novobiocin sodium and prednisolone tablets

NADA No.: 065-090

Active Ingredient(s): DELTA ALBAPLEX® Tablets contain prednisolone, which provides a faster clinical response in the indicated conditions and a combination of two antibiotics—tetracycline hydrochloride and novobiocin sodium—which supplies additive antibacterial effect against certain bacterial pathogens.

Each tablet contains:	DELTA ALBAPLEX®	DELTA ALBAPLEX® 3X
Tetracycline hydrochloride	60 mg	180 mg
Novobiocin sodium equiv. to novobiocin	60 mg	180 mg
Prednisolone anhydrous	1.5 mg	4.5 mg

Indications: DELTA ALBAPLEX® Tablets are indicated in the treatment of acute or chronic upper respiratory conditions, ie, tonsillitis, bronchitis, and tracheobronchitis, when it is necessary to initially reduce the severity of associated clinical signs and when caused by pathogens susceptible to novobiocin sodium and tetracycline hydrochloride such as *Staphylococcus* spp. and *E. coli.*

The product has been shown to be of maximum benefit when used during the first 48 hours of treatment. Subsequent therapy should be continued with ALBAPLEX® Tablets containing novobiocin sodium and tetracycline hydrochloride for an additional 3 days or longer as needed.

As with all antibiotics, appropriate *in vitro* culturing and susceptibility tests should be conducted on samples taken before treatment is started.

Pharmacology: Actions:

Tetracycline Hydrochloride: Tetracycline hydrochloride is an odorless, yellow, fine crystalline powder which is freely soluble in water and gastric juice. It is absorbed readily from the gastrointestinal tract. Following oral administration to dogs, peak blood concentrations are obtained within two to four hours, significant levels are found at twelve hours, and detectable amounts remain in the serum for at least 24 hours. The antibiotic is excreted principally through the kidney.

The *in vitro* spectrum of antimicrobial activity of tetracycline hydrochloride includes a broad range of gram-positive and gram-negative bacteria such as alpha and beta streptococci, some strains of staphylococci, *Klebsiella pneumoniae*, certain clostridia, Shigella, *Aerobacter aerogenes*, and some strains of Salmonella. The clinical significance of this has not been determined.

In an *in vivo* study, it was shown that tetracycline hydrochloride is significantly more effective than novobiocin sodium in eliminating pathogenic streptococci organisms from the throats of dogs suffering from upper respiratory infections. However, it was also shown that tetracycline hydrochloride was significantly less effective than novobiocin sodium in eliminating pathogenic staphylococci.

Studies conducted in laboratory animals show that tetracycline hydrochloride has a low order of toxicity comparable to that of the other tetracyclines.

Novobiocin Sodium: Novobiocin sodium is an antibiotic produced by *Streptomyces niveus* and was developed in the Research Laboratories of The Upjohn Company. The crystalline antibiotic has a light yellow to white color, depending upon the state of subdivision. In contrast to most antibiotics produced by actinomycetes, novobiocin sodium, like penicillin, is acidic in nature and is stable to the degree of acidity or alkalinity present in the gastrointestinal tract. Following oral administration of 10 mg per lb to dogs, peak blood concentrations are obtained within one to two hours and significant levels remain at twelve hours. When an appreciable amount of novobiocin sodium is present in the serum, the drug diffuses into the pleural and ascitic fluids. Novobiocin sodium does not diffuse into the cerebrospinal fluid. The antibiotic is concentrated in the liver and bile and is excreted in the feces and urine. As determined by tests in animals, novobiocin sodium has a relatively low order of toxicity.

In vitro studies show that novobiocin sodium is active against both gram-positive and gram-negative bacteria, including some strains of *Staphylococcus aureus, Streptococcus hemolyticus, Diplococcus pneumoniae*, and some strains of *Proteus vulgaris*. The clinical significance of this has not been determined. Novobiocin sodium shows no cross-resistance with penicillin against resistant strains of *Staphylococcus aureus*. However, *in vitro* studies indicate that *Staphylococcus aureus* may develop resistance to novobiocin sodium as with other antibiotics.

Prednisolone: Prednisolone, a derivative of hydrocortisone, has greater glucocorticoid activity, greater anti-inflammatory activity, less sodium-retaining effect, and less potassium-losing effect than the parent compound. The glucocorticoid activity of prednisolone is approximately three times that of hydrocortisone, and the dose required to produce a given anti-inflammatory effect in dogs is of the order of one-fourth to one-third the required dose of hydrocortisone (or about one-fifth the required dose of cortisone).

Prednisolone exerts an inhibitory influence on the cellular, fibrous, and amorphous components of connective tissue and thereby suppresses the basic processes of inflammation. Vascular permeability is decreased, exudation diminished and migration of inflammatory cells markedly impaired. In infections characterized by stress and/or toxicity, prednisolone therapy, in conjunction with properly indicated antibacterial therapy, is helpful in reducing the clinical signs and in speeding the recovery of the animal being treated.

Combined Antibiotic-Adrenocortical Therapy: DELTA ALBAPLEX® Tablets have been formulated to provide for the use of tetracycline hydrochloride, novobiocin sodium, and prednisolone. It provides a broad antibacterial effect from the combined antibiotics plus the anti-inflammatory effects of prednisolone.

Combined antibiotic therapy offers a wider range of antibacterial activity than therapy with either of the single antibiotics. *In vitro* studies with tetracycline hydrochloride and novobiocin sodium have indicated that this antibiotic combination is effective against such organism as *Staphylococcus aureus, Streptococcus fecalis* and *Proteus rettgeri*. Moreover, *in vitro* studies have shown that the development of resistance by *Staphylococcus aureus* to a combination of tetracycline hydrochloride and novobiocin sodium occurs at a markedly slower rate than to either antibiotic alone. Studies in mice infected with *Staphylococcus aureus* have indicated that tetracycline hydrochloride and novobiocin sodium are compatible *in vivo* against the strains tested.

An *in vivo* clinical study in dogs has shown that the combination of novobiocin sodium and tetracycline hydrochloride is significantly more effective than either single antibiotic in eliminating pathogenic *Staphylococcus* spp. and *E. coli* from the throats of dogs suffering from upper respiratory disease. This study also showed that the incidence of treatment failure is significantly reduced when novobiocin sodium and tetracycline hydrochloride are administered concurrently.

In dogs with upper respiratory infections, the prednisolone component of DELTA ALBAPLEX® results in a significantly faster reduction in the clinical signs of illness in the first 48 hours of treatment than is achievable by therapy with novobiocin sodium and tetracycline hydrochloride, either singly or in combination. After 48 hours, treatment is to be continued for 3 days with ALBAPLEX® Tablets containing tetracycline hydrochloride and novobiocin sodium.

Dosage and Administration: The dosage for dogs is 10 mg of each antibiotic and 0.25 mg prednisolone per lb of body weight repeated at 12 hour intervals for 48 hours. This dose can be given as follows:

DELTA ALBAPLEX® Tablets (one tablet for each 6 lbs of body weight):

Body Weight	DELTA ALBAPLEX® Tablets every 12 Hours
2.5 - 4 lbs	½
5 - 8 lbs	1
9 - 15 lbs	2
16 - 27 lbs	3

DELTA ALBAPLEX® 3X Tablets (one tablet for each 18 lbs of body weight):

Body Weight	DELTA ALBAPLEX® 3X Tablets every 12 Hours
16 - 27 lbs	1
28 - 45 lbs	2
46 - 63 lbs	3
64 - 81 lbs	4

Antibacterial treatment is to be continued with ALBAPLEX® Tablets containing novobiocin sodium and tetracycline hydrochloride at the same dose schedule for an additional 3 days.

Important Note: The prednisolone component of DELTA ALBAPLEX® Tablets containing tetracycline hydrochloride, novobiocin sodium and prednisolone has been shown to contribute to clinical response if administered only for the first 48 hours of treatment. Subsequent antibacterial treatment is to be continued with ALBAPLEX® Tablets containing tetracycline hydrochloride and novobiocin sodium. See Indications and Dosage and Administration sections.

Contraindication(s): As with other adrenocortical steroids, this product is contraindicated in animals with tuberculosis, hyperadrenocorticism and peptic ulcers.

Precaution(s): Store at controlled room temperature 20° to 25°C (65° to 77°F) [see USP].

Caution(s): Federal (USA) law restricts this drug to use by or on the order of a licensed veterinarian.

In the following conditions this product should be used with caution; diabetes mellitus, osteoporosis, predisposition to thrombophlebitis, hypertension, congestive heart failure, and renal insufficiency.

All necessary procedures for establishment of a bacterial diagnosis should be carried out whenever possible before institution of therapy. Combined antibiotic corticosteroid therapy does not obviate the need for indicated surgical procedures.

For use in animals only.

Warning(s): Clinical and experimental data have demonstrated that corticosteroids administered orally or parenterally to animals may induce the first stage of parturition when administered during the last trimester of pregnancy and may precipitate premature parturition followed by dystocia, fetal death, retained placenta, and metritis.

Additionally, corticosteroids administered to dogs, rabbits, and rodents during pregnancy have resulted in cleft palate in offspring. Corticosteroids administered to dogs during pregnancy have also resulted in other congenital anomalies, including deformed forelegs, phocomelia, and anasarca.

Side Effects: Because of the wide antibacterial effect of this antibiotic combination on intestinal flora, a change in the character of the stools may be anticipated in certain animals; however, administration of novobiocin sodium and tetracycline hydrochloride, combined, to dogs at exaggerated doses for six months caused no significant toxicity. If allergic reactions develop during treatment with this product, use of it should be discontinued.

Since the use of any broad spectrum antibiotic may result in overgrowth of nonsusceptible organisms, constant observation of the animal patient is essential. If new infections appear during therapy, appropriate measures should be taken.

Injudicious use of adrenal hormones in animals with infections can be hazardous. It is, therefore, essential that effective antibacterial agents be administered concurrently. Alteration of the inflammatory reaction by corticosteroid therapy may be beneficial; however, it may also mask signs of infection and facilitate spread of micro-organisms. In addition, systemic manifestations, such as fever and signs of toxemia, may be suppressed. A retardant effect on wound healing has not been encountered with prednisolone, but such a possibility should be considered if it is used in conjunction with surgery.

While the use of DELTA ALBAPLEX® Tablets in the recommended doses is not likely to induce the side effects commonly associated with prolonged or intensive adrenocorticoid therapy, overdosage may give rise to the following; hyperglycemia and glycosuria; nitrogen loss; and suppression of endogenous adrenocortical activity. The most commonly observed symptoms of overdosage in the dog are polydipsia and polyuria.

Presentation: DELTA ALBAPLEX® Tablets are available in bottles of 500 (NDC 0009-0593-02).

DELTA ALBAPLEX® 3X Tablets are available in bottles of 250 (NDC 0009-3357-01).

Compendium Code No.: 10490121 811 242 107 / 811 242 207

DEMOTEC® 95

Kane **Hoof Product**

Ingredient(s): Liquid and powder reagents to produce resin. The product is presented in a kit that provides wooden blocks, spatulas and beakers.

Indications: To be used as an adjunct to primary medical care of laming cattle.

Directions for Use: 35 mL of liquid should be measured and poured into a beaker, to which the contents of one sachet (70 g powder) should be added. This should then be thoroughly mixed with the spatula provided. Within seconds, a putty-like malleable mass is produced which is easy to mould and which does not adhese to the hands. Applied directly to both the sole of the claw and wooden block the two are then bonded and the mass moulded round the join.

Discussion: The hooves of cattle are subject to infections and/or inflammation whatever standards of husbandry are employed. Such conditions are not only distressing to see and worthy of attention from an humanitarian aspect, but affect the mobility of the animal and cause pain and stress which can adversely affect both milk yields and weight gains.

It is therefore important to take all steps to treat these conditions in the best possible manner and so limit economic losses that may otherwise occur.

The primary medical treatment of the affected hoof should be undertaken as soon as possible, and as an adjunct to this treatment DEMOTEC® can frequently be employed to great advantage.

Usually it is found that only one claw is affected and so it is possible to bond a wooden block to the sole of the sound claw. This not only raises the affected claw out of the dirt, so making medical and surgical treatment more effective, but more importantly it shifts the weight onto the good claw allowing the affected claw to rest.

Presentation: 2 application sets and 14 application sets with large or small blocks.

Manufactured by: Siegfried Demel, Germany.

Compendium Code No.: 10660011

DEMOTEC® EASY BLOC®

Kane **Hoof Product**

Ingredient(s): A liquid/powder system has been developed, utilizing as resin with a short polymerization time which will cure quickly and effectively.

Indications: EASY BLOC® provides a system which will be applicable to the treatment of most cases of lameness in cattle.

Instructions:

1. The healthy claw is cleaned removing dirt and loose horn with a hoof knife (or grinder if necessary) and thoroughly dried. Special levelling of the sole is not necessary as unevenness is overcome by the resin.
2. Press the perforation on the top of the box, which will allow the insertion of the EASY BLOC® in the correct position to accurately measure the liquid into the BLOC®.
3. Pour the liquid into the BLOC® until it reaches the mark (20 mL).
4. The small hole in the silver foil covering the neck of the powder bottle allows the controlled addition of the powder onto the resin (in volume about twice that of the liquid) until it is nearly to the top of the BLOC®.
5. Remove the EASY BLOC® from the top of the box and quickly mix with the spatula. Immediately take some of the creamy-like resin mix onto the spatula, and spread a thin film around the inside wall of the BLOC®, to guarantee a complete covering glue contact with the claw sole.
6. Next place the EASY BLOC® over the prepared claw, position correctly and exert pressure to ensure the mixed resin spreads evenly. You will find that the BLOC® has been designed to fit securely onto the claw.
7. Any surplus resin mix which exudes must be spread with the spatula into any opening remaining between the top of the EASY BLOC® and the horn. That increases the good adhesion to the claw.
8. After about 4-5 minutes (at a temperature of 21°C) the resin mix will be completely polymerized which will allow the cow to stand on its hoof once more — with the rapid relief of pain and lameness.

Special Note: Temperature has a great influence on the polymerization time of resin. The times quoted relate to a temperature of 21°C. Should the temperature be higher the reaction is accelerated conversely lower temperatures decelerate the reactions. As a rule of thumb it can be said that polymerization time is divided in half for every increase of 10°C i.e. 30°C polymerization time approx. 2½ minutes conversely at 10°C — polymerization 10 minutes.

Logically the resin should be warmed up in winter and cooled in summer. This can be done simply by partially immersing the container of the resin in a bucket of cold or warm water, but care should be taken not to let water come into contact with the resin.

Precaution(s): The synthetic resin in EASY BLOC® should be protected from light and stored in a cool place. All containers should be tightly closed after use — measures should be taken to prevent soiling from a spillage — and all items should be stored out of the reach of children.

Warnings on vessels should be strictly followed. An EC Security Data Sheet with additional information is available on request.

Discussion: The design of the EASY BLOC® was based on the anatomy of the hoof, and its versatility allows claws of any size to be accommodated, without any restriction on their mobility.

The sole of the BLOC® has been made thick enough to ensure that there is no pressure on the affected claw, and the smooth elastic upper cover, is sufficiently flexible to allow claws of very varying sizes to be accommodated.

Presentation: EASY BLOC® is available in kits of 4 applications or 12 applications. Also available in extra length.

Compendium Code No.: 10660022

DENAGARD™ 10

Boehringer Ingelheim **Feed Medication**

(tiamulin) Medicated Premix-Type A Medicated Article

NADA No.: 139-472

Active Ingredient(s):

Tiamulin (as hydrogen fumarate) . . . . 10 g/lb

Ingredients: Roughage products, mineral oil.

Indications: For treatment of swine dysentry associated with *Brachyspira* (formerly *Serpulina* or *Treponema) hyodysenteriae* susceptible to Tiamulin.

For control of porcine proliferative entropathies (ileitis) associated with *Lawsonia intracellularis.*

For control of swine dysentry associated with *Brachyspira* (formerly *Serpulina* or *Treponema) hyodysenteriae* susceptible to Tiamulin.

For increased rate of weight gain and improved feed efficiency.

Dosage and Administration:

Indications	Directions	Amount of DENAGARD™ 10 Per Ton	Tiamulin in Complete Feed Per Ton
For treatment of swine dysentry associated with *Brachyspira* (formerly *Serpulina* or *Treponema) hyodysenteriae* susceptible to Tiamulin	Feed continuously as the sole ration for 14 days	20 lb	200 g
For control of porcine proliferative entropathies (ileitis) associated with *Lawsonia intracellularis*	Feed continuously as the sole ration for not less than 10 days	3.5 lb	35 g
For control of swine dysentry associated with *Brachyspira* (formerly *Serpulina* or *Treponema) hyodysenteriae* susceptible to Tiamulin	Feed continuously as the sole ration	3.5 lb	35 g
For increased rate of weight gain and improved feed efficiency	Feed continuously as the sole ration	1 lb	10 g

Contraindication(s): Swine being treated with DENAGARD™ 10 (tiamulin) should not have access to feeds containing polyether ionophores (e.g., lasalocid, monensin, narasin, salinomycin and semduramicin), as adverse reactions may occur. If signs of toxicity occur, discontinue use.

Precaution(s): Store in a dry place.

Caution(s): Do not feed undiluted. Do not use in feeds for animals other than swine. Not for use in swine weighing over 250 lbs. Do not pellet feeds containing 10 grams tiamulin per ton.

For manufacture of medicated swine feeds only. For use in animals only.

Warning(s): The withdrawal period at the 200 g/ton use level is 7 days.

The withdrawal period at the 35 g/ton use level is 2 days.

There is no withdrawal period at the 10 g/ton use level.

Keep out of reach of children. Avoid contact with skin. Direct contact with skin or mucous membranes may cause irritation.

Presentation: 35 lb (15.9 kg) multi-wall bags.

DENAGARD™ is a Trademark of Boehringer Ingelheim Vetmedica, Inc.

Compendium Code No.: 10280321 634001D-02-0107

DENAGARD™ LIQUID CONCENTRATE

Boehringer Ingelheim **Water Medication**

Tiamulin

NADA No.: 140-916

Active Ingredient(s): DENAGARD™ (tiamulin) Liquid Concentrate is a solution containing 12.3% tiamulin hydrogen fumarate (w/v) in an aqueous base.

Indications: DENAGARD™ Liquid Concentrate is for use only in preparing medicated drinking water for swine.

DENAGARD™ (tiamulin), when administered in the drinking water for five consecutive days, is an effective antibiotic for the treatment of swine dysentery susceptible to tiamulin at a dosage level of 3.5 mg tiamulin per pound of bodyweight daily and for treatment of swine pneumonia susceptible to tiamulin when given at 10.5 mg tiamulin per pound of bodyweight daily.

DENAGARD™ is for treatment of:

- Swine pneumonia *(Actinobacillus pleuropneumoniae)*
- Swine dysentery *(Serpulina hyodysenteriae)*

Pharmacology: The active ingredient, tiamulin, chemically is 14-desoxy-14 [(2-diethylaminoethyl) mercaptoacetoxy] mutilin hydrogen fumarate, a semi-synthetic diterpene antibiotic.

Actions: Tiamulin is active against *Serpulina hyodysenteriae* and *Actinobacillus pleuropneumoniae.* It is readily absorbed from the gut and can be found in the blood within 30 minutes after dosing. Peak blood concentrations occur 2-4 hours after the oral administration of a single dose. At least 85% of a single dose is absorbed, 98% of which is excreted in the urine and feces within 72 hours.

Dosage and Administration:

Use Directions: The concentration of tiamulin hydrogen fumarate in the stock solution and in the drinking water delivered must be adjusted to compensate for variation in the water consumption by pigs due to bodyweight, environmental and other factors. It is important that the pigs receive the proper drug dose of 3.5 mg of tiamulin hydrogen fumarate per pound of bodyweight daily for 5 consecutive days for treatment of swine dysentery or a dose of 10.5 mg per pound bodyweight for 5 consecutive days for treatment of swine pneumonia.

Directions for Preparing DENAGARD™ Medicated Solutions: Determine the amount of DENAGARD™ Liquid Concentrate needed to medicate the desired volume of drinking water at the proper concentration. Carefully measure out this amount, add it to the water and stir to thoroughly mix.

Directions for Using DENAGARD™:

In medicated proportioners: One quart of DENAGARD™ Liquid Concentrate mixed with water to make four gallons of stock solution, and this stock solution, metered at one fluid ounce per gallon will provide 227 mg of tiamulin hydrogen fumarate per gallon to 512 gallons of drinking water for treatment of swine dysentery. Three quarts of DENAGARD™ Liquid Concentrate mixed with water to make four gallons of stock solution, and this stock solution metered at one ounce per gallon will provide 681 mg tiamulin hydrogen fumarate per gallon to a total of 512 gallons of drinking water for treatment of swine pneumonia.

One-half pint (8 fluid ounces) of DENAGARD™ Liquid Concentrate diluted with water to make one gallon of stock solution, and this stock solution metered at one fluid ounce per gallon of drinking water will provide 227 mg of tiamulin hydrogen fumarate per gallon to 128 gallons of drinking water for treatment of swine dysentery. Use one and one-half pints of DENAGARD™ Liquid Concentrate per gallon of stock solution, to be metered at one ounce per gallon, to provide 681 mg per gallon to 128 gallons of drinking water for treatment of swine pneumonia.

In Barrels or Tanks: Three fluid ounces of DENAGARD™ Liquid Concentrate will medicate 48 gallons of drinking water at 227 mg per gallon for treatment of swine dysentery or 16 gallons at 681 mg per gallon for treatment of swine pneumonia.

Measure DENAGARD™ Liquid Concentrate carefully, pour into the proper amount of water and thoroughly mix.

Approximate Daily Water Consumption Per Pig	
Pig Weight/lb	Water Intake/gal
20	0.3-0.5
45	0.4-1.1
75	0.7-1.5
125	1.0-2.0
180	1.2-3.0

Note:

1. Prepare fresh medicated drinking water every day for the 5-day treatment period.
2. Water medicated with DENAGARD™ should be the only source of drinking water during the treatment period.

DENAGARD™ Liquid Concentrate		
One Quart Bottle Net Tiamulin Hydrogen Fumarate Content 116,400 mg		
	Disease to be Treated	
	Swine Dysentery	Swine Pneumonia
Daily Tiamulin Hydrogen Fumarate required per pound bodyweight.	3.5 mg	10.5 mg
Required treatment duration:	5 Days	5 Days
Pig bodyweight this bottle will treat for one day:	33,257 lb	11,086 lb
Number of pigs this bottle will treat for one day:		
Pig Wt. lb		
20	1,663	554
45	739	246
75	443	148
125	266	88
180	185	62

DENAGARD™ Liquid Concentrate		
One Quart Bottle Net Tiamulin Hydrogen Fumarate Content 116,400 mg		
	Disease to be Treated	
	Swine Dysentery	Swine Pneumonia
Suggested final dilution of:*		
1 cup (8 oz)	128 gal	
3 cups (24 oz)		128 gal
1 bottle	512 gal	
3 bottles		512 gal
Tiamulin hydrogen fumarate concentration per gallon at suggested final dilution.*	227 mg (640 ppm)	681 mg (180 ppm)

* Note: Increase or decrease dilution rate as required to obtain proper daily drug dose.

Attention: If no response to treatment is obtained within 5 days, re-establish the diagnosis. Failure of response may be related to the presence of nonsusceptible organisms or other complicating disease conditions. Because of the tendency for the disease to recur on premises with a history of swine dysentery or with swine pneumonia, a control program should be implemented after treatment. Drugs are not substitutes for proper sanitary measures or good management, but should be used in conjunction with such practices.

Contraindication(s): Swine being treated with DENAGARD™ (tiamulin) should not have access to feeds containing polyether ionophores (e.g. monensin, narasin, lasalocid, salinomycin and semduramicin) as adverse reactions may occur.

Caution(s): Avoid contact with skin. Direct contact with skin or mucous membranes may cause irritation.

For use in drinking water of swine only.

Prepare fresh medicated water daily. Not for use in swine over 250 pounds of bodyweight.

For animal use only not for use in humans.

Warning(s): Withdraw medicated water 3 days before slaughter following treatment at 3.5 mg per pound and 7 days before slaughter following treatment at 10.5 mg per pound of bodyweight.

Keep out of reach of children.

Adverse Reactions: Overdoses of DENAGARD™ have sometimes produced transitory salivation, vomiting and an apparent calming effect on the pig.

If signs of toxicity occur, discontinue use of medicated water and replace with clean, fresh water.

In rare cases, redness of the skin primarily over the ham and underline has been observed during medication. If this occurs, discontinue medication immediately. Provide ample clean drinking water. Thoroughly rinse (hose down) the housing to remove urine and feces from animal contact surfaces or move the animals to clean pens. If the condition persists, consult your veterinarian.

Studies to evaluate the safety of the water-soluble form of tiamulin in breeding swine have not been done.

Presentation: 32 oz (946 mL)/6 bottles per case.

Compendium Code No.: 10280331

DEPO-MEDROL® ℞

Pharmacia & Upjohn **Corticosteroid Injection**

Methylprednisolone acetate sterile aqueous suspension

NADA No.: 012-204

Active Ingredient(s): These preparations are recommended for intramuscular and intrasynovial injection in horses and dogs, and intramuscular injection in cats. DEPO-MEDROL® Sterile Aqueous Suspension is available in two concentrations, 20 mg per mL and 40 mg per mL. Each mL of these preparations contains:

	20 mg	40 mg
Methylprednisolone acetate	20 mg	40 mg
Polyethylene glycol 3350	29.6 mg	29 mg
Sodium chloride	8.9 mg	8.7 mg
Myristyl-gamma-picolinium chloride added as preservative	0.198 mg	0.195 mg

When necessary, pH was adjusted with sodium hydroxide and/or hydrochloric acid.

Indications:

Musculoskeletal Conditions: As with other adrenal steroids, DEPO-MEDROL® Sterile Aqueous Suspension has been found useful in alleviating the pain and lameness associated with acute localized arthritic conditions and generalized arthritic conditions. It has been used successfully to treat rheumatoid arthritis, traumatic arthritis, osteoarthritis, periostitis, tendinitis, synovitis, tenosynovitis, bursitis, and myositis of horses; traumatic arthritis, osteoarthritis, and generalized arthritic conditions of dogs. Remission of musculoskeletal conditions may be permanent, or symptoms may recur, depending on the cause and extent of structural degeneration.

Allergic Conditions:. This preparation is especially beneficial in relieving pruritus and inflammation of allergic dermatitis, acute moist dermatitis, dry eczema, urticaria, bronchial asthma, pollen sensitivities and otitis externa in dogs; allergic dermatitis and moist and dry eczema in cats. Onset of relief may begin within a few hours to a few days following injection and may persist for a few days to six weeks. Symptoms may be expected to recur if the cause of the allergic reaction is still present, in which case retreatment may be indicated. In treating acute hypersensitivity reactions, such as anaphylactic shock, intravenous Solu-Delta-Cortef® Sterile Powder containing prednisolone sodium succinate, as well as other appropriate treatments, should be used.

Overwhelming Infections with Severe Toxicity:. In dogs and cats moribund from overwhelmingly severe infections for which antibacterial therapy is available (eg, critical pneumonia, pyometritis), DEPO-MEDROL® may be lifesaving, acting to inhibit the inflammatory reaction, which itself may be lethal; preventing vascular collapse and preserving the integrity of the blood vessels; modifying the patient's reaction to drugs; and preventing or reducing the exudative reaction which often complicates certain infections. As supportive therapy, it improves the general attitude of the animal being treated. All necessary procedures for the establishment of a bacterial diagnosis should be carried out whenever possible before institution of therapy. Corticosteroid therapy in the presence of infection should be administered for the shortest possible time compatible with maintenance of an adequate response, and antibacterial therapy should be continued for at least three days after the hormone has been withdrawn. Combined hormone and antibacterial therapy does not obviate the need for indicated surgical treatment.

Other Conditions: In certain conditions where it is desired to reduce inflammation, vascularization, fibroblastic infiltration, and scar tissue, the use of DEPO-MEDROL® should be considered. Snakebite of dogs also is an indication for the use of this suspension because of its anti-toxemic, anti-shock, and anti-inflammatory activity. It is particularly effective in reducing swelling and preventing sloughing. Its employment in the treatment of such conditions is recommended as a supportive measure to standard procedures and time-honored treatments and will give comfort to the animal and hasten complete recovery.

Pharmacology: Methylprednisolone, an anti-inflammatory steroid synthesized and developed in the Research Laboratories of The Upjohn Company, is the 6-methyl derivative of prednisolone. Exceeding prednisolone in anti-inflammatory potency and having even less tendency than prednisolone to induce sodium and water retention, methylprednisolone offers the advantage over older corticosteroids of affording equally satisfactory anti-inflammatory effect with the use of lower doses and with an enhanced split between anti-inflammatory and mineralocorticoid activities. Estimates of the relative potencies of methylprednisolone and prednisolone range from 1.13 to 2.1, with an average of 1.5. In anti-inflammatory activity, as measured by the granuloma pouch assay, methylprednisolone is twice as active as prednisolone. In mineralocorticoid activity (ie, the capacity to induce retention of sodium and water in the adrenalectomized rat) methylprednisolone is slightly less active than prednisolone. The duration of plasma steroid levels following rapid intravenous injection in intact dogs is appreciably longer for methylprednisolone than for prednisolone, the respective "half-life" value for the two steroids being 80.9 ± 7.5 minutes for methylprednisolone and 71.3 ±1.7 minutes for prednisolone.

While the effect of parenterally administered DEPO-MEDROL® is prolonged, it has the same metabolic and anti-inflammatory actions as orally administered methylprednisolone acetate.

Dosage and Administration:

Intramuscular Administration and Dosage: Following intramuscular injection of methylprednisolone acetate, a prolonged systemic effect results. The dose varies with the size of the animal patient, the severity of the condition under treatment, and the animal's response to therapy.

Dogs and Cats: The average intramuscular dose for dogs is 20 mg. In accordance with the size of the dog and severity of the condition under treatment, the dose may range from 2 mg in miniature breeds to 40 mg in medium breeds, and even as high as 120 mg in extremely large breeds or dogs with severe involvement.

The average intramuscular dose for cats is 10 mg with a range up to 20 mg.

Injections may be made at weekly intervals or in accordance with the severity of the condition and clinical response.

Horses: The usual intramuscular dose for horses is 200 mg repeated as necessary.

For maintenance therapy in chronic conditions, initial doses should be reduced gradually until the smallest effective (ie, individualized) dose is established. Medrol® Tablets containing methylprednisolone may also be used for maintenance in dogs and cats, administered according to the recommended dose.

When treatment is to be withdrawn after prolonged and intensive therapy, the dose should be reduced gradually.

If signs of stress are associated with the condition being treated, the dose should be increased. If a rapid hormonal effect of maximum intensity is required, as in anaphylactic shock, the intravenous administration of highly soluble Solu-Delta-Cortef® Sterile Powder containing prednisolone sodium succinate is indicated.

Intrasynovial Administration and Dosage: Methylprednisolone acetate, a slightly soluble ester of methylprednisolone, is capable of producing a more prolonged local anti-inflammatory effect than equimolar doses of hydrocortisone acetate. Following intrasynovial injection, relief from pain may be experienced within 12 to 24 hours. The duration of relief varies, but averages three to four weeks, with a range of one to five or more weeks. Injections of methylprednisolone acetate have been well tolerated. Intrasynovial (intra-articular) injections may occasionally result in an increased localized inflammatory response.

Intrasynovial injection is recommended as an adjuvant to general therapeutic measures to effect suppression of inflammation in one or a few peripheral structures when (1) the disease is limited to one or a few peripheral structures; (2) the disease is widespread with one or a few peripheral structures actively inflamed; (3) systemic therapy with other corticoids or corticotropin controls all but a few of the more actively involved structures; (4) systemic therapy with cortisone, hydrocortisone, or corticotropin is contraindicated; (5) joints show early but actively progressing deformity (to enhance the effect of physiotherapy and corrective procedures); and (6) surgical or other orthopedic corrective measures are to be or have been done.

The action of DEPO-MEDROL® Sterile Aqueous Suspension injected intrasynovially appears to be well localized since significant metabolic effects characteristic of systemic administration of adrenal steroids have not been observed. In a few instances mild and transient improvement of structures other than those injected have been reported. No other systemic effects have been noted. However, it is possible that mild systemic effects may occur following intrasynovial administration, and this possibility is greater the larger the number of structures injected and the higher the total dose employed.

Procedure for Intrasynovial Injection: The anatomy of the area to be injected should be reviewed in order to assure that the suspension is properly placed and to determine that large blood vessels or nerves are avoided. The injection site is located where the synovial cavity is most superficial. The area is prepared for aseptic injection of the medicament by the removal of hair and cleansing of the skin with alcohol or Mercresin® tincture. A sterile 18- to 21-gauge needle for horses, 20- to 22-gauge needle for dogs, on a dry syringe is quickly inserted into the synovial space and a small amount of synovial fluid withdrawn. If there is an excess of synovia and more than 1 mL of suspension is to be injected, it is well to aspirate a volume of fluid comparable to that which is to be injected. With the needle in place, the aspirating syringe is removed and replaced by a second syringe containing the proper amount of suspension which is then injected. In some animals a transient pain is elicited immediately upon injection into the affected cavity. This pain varies from mild to severe and may last for a few minutes up to 12 hours. After injection, the structure may be moved gently a few times to aid mixing of the synovial fluid and the suspension. The site may be covered with a small sterile dressing.

Areas not suitable for injection are those that are anatomically inaccessible such as spinal joints and those like the sacroiliac joints, which are devoid of synovial space. Treatment failures are most frequently the result of failure to enter the synovial space. If failures occur when injections into the synovial spaces are certain, as determined by aspiration of fluid, repeated injections are usually futile. Local therapy does not alter the underlying disease process, and whenever possible comprehensive therapy including physiotherapy and orthopedic correction should be employed.

The single intrasynovial dose depends on the size of the part, which corresponds to the size of the animal. The interval between repeated injections depends on the duration of relief obtained.

Horses: The average initial dose for a large synovial space in horses is 120 mg with a range from 40 to 240 mg. Smaller spaces will require a correspondingly lesser dose.

Dogs: The average initial dose for a large synovial space in dogs is 20 mg. Smaller spaces will require a correspondingly lesser dose.

Contraindication(s): Systemic therapy with methylprednisolone acetate, as with other corticoids, is contraindicated in animals with arrested tuberculosis, peptic ulcer, and Cushing's syndrome. The presence of active tuberculosis, diabetes mellitus, osteoporosis, renal insufficiency, predisposition to thrombophlebitis, hypertension, or congestive heart failure necessitates carefully controlled use of corticosteroids. Intrasynovial, intratendinous, or other injections of corticosteroids for local effect are contraindicated in the presence of acute infectious conditions. Exacerbation of pain, further loss of joint motion, with fever and malaise following injection may indicate that the condition has become septic. Appropriate antibacterial therapy should be instituted immediately.

Precaution(s): Store at controlled room temperature 20° to 25°C (68° to 77°F) [see USP].

Caution(s): Federal (USA) law restricts this drug to use by or on the order of a licensed veterinarian.

DEPO-MEDROL® Sterile Aqueous Suspension exerts an inhibitory influence on the mechanisms and the tissue changes associated with inflammation. Vascular permeability is decreased, exudation diminished, and migration of the inflammatory cells markedly inhibited. In addition, systemic manifestations such as fever and signs of toxemia may also be suppressed. While certain aspects of this alteration of the inflammatory reaction may be beneficial, the suppression of inflammation may mask the signs of infection and tend to facilitate spread of microorganisms. Hence, all patients receiving this drug should be watched for evidence of intercurrent infection. Should infection occur, it must be brought under control by the use of appropriate antibacterial measures, or administration of this preparation should be discontinued. However, in infections characterized by overwhelming toxicity, methylprednisolone acetate therapy in conjunction with appropriate antibacterial therapy is effective in reducing mortality and morbidity. Without conjoint use of an antibiotic to which the invader-organism is sensitive, injudicious use of the adrenal hormones in animals with infections can be hazardous. As with other corticoids, continued or prolonged use is discouraged.

While no sodium retention or potassium depletion has been observed at the doses recommended, animals receiving methylprednisolone acetate, as with all corticoids, should be under close observation for possible untoward effects. If symptoms of hypopotassemia (hypokalemia) should occur, corticoid therapy should be discontinued and potassium chloride administered by continuous intravenous drip.

Since this drug lacks significant mineralocorticoid activity in usual therapeutic doses, it is not likely to afford adequate support in states of acute adrenocortical insufficiency. For treatment of the latter, the parent adrenocortical steroids, hydrocortisone or cortisone, should be used.

For use in animals only.

Warning(s): Clinical and experimental data have demonstrated that corticosteroids administered orally or parenterally to animals may induce the first stage of parturition when administered during the last trimester of pregnancy and may precipitate premature parturition followed by dystocia, fetal death, retained placenta and metritis.

Additionally, corticosteroids administered to dogs, rabbits, and rodents during pregnancy have resulted in cleft palate in offspring. Corticosteroids administered to dogs during pregnancy have also resulted in other congenital anomalies, including deformed forelegs, phocomelia, and anasarca.

Not for human use.

Presentation: DEPO-MEDROL® Sterile Aqueous Suspension, 20 mg/mL, is available in 10 mL and 20 mL vials, and 40 mg/mL is available in 5 mL vials.

Compendium Code No.: 10490130

DERAMAXX™ CHEWABLE TABLETS ℞

Novartis **Non-Steroidal Anti-Inflammatory**

(deracoxib)

NADA No.: 141-203

Active Ingredient(s): Contains (per tablet) either:

Deracoxib . . . . 25 mg
Deracoxib . . . . 100 mg

Indications: DERAMAXX™ Chewable Tablets are indicated for the control of postoperative pain and inflammation associated with orthopedic surgery in dogs ≥4 lbs (1.8 kg).

Pharmacology: Description: DERAMAXX™ (deracoxib) tablets are a non-narcotic, nonsteroidal anti-inflammatory drug of the coxib class. DERAMAXX™ tablets are round, biconvex, chewable tablets that contain deracoxib formulated with beefy flavoring. The molecular weight of deracoxib is 397.38. The empirical formula is C17-H14-F3-N3-O3-S. Deracoxib is 4-[3-(Difluoromethyl)-5-(3-fluoro-4-methoxyphenyl)-1H-pyrazol-1-yl]benzenesulfonamide, and can be termed a diaryl substituted pyrazole. The structural formula is:

CHF2 F N N O CH3 H2N S O O

Clinical Pharmacology:

Mode of Action: DERAMAXX™ tablets are a member of the coxib class of non-narcotic, non-steroidal, cyclooxygenase-inhibiting antiinflammatory drugs for the control of postoperative pain and inflammation associated with orthopedic surgery.

Data indicate that deracoxib inhibits the production of PGE1 and 6-keto PGF1 by its inhibitory effects on prostaglandin biosynthesis.[1] Deracoxib inhibited COX-2 mediated PGE2 production in LPS-stimulated human whole blood.[2]

Cyclooxygenase-1 (COX-1) is the enzyme responsible for facilitating constitutive physiological processes (e.g., platelet aggregation, gastric mucosal protection, renal perfusion).[3] Cyclooxygenase-2 (COX-2) is responsible for the synthesis of inflammatory mediators.[4] Both COX isoforms are constituitively expressed in the canine kidney.[5] At doses of 2-4 mg/kg/day, DERAMAXX™ tablets do not inhibit COX-1 based on *in vitro* studies using cloned canine cyclooxygenase.[4] The clinical relevance of this *in vitro* data has not been shown.

Although the plasma terminal elimination half-life for DERAMAXX™ tablets is approximately 3 hours, a longer duration of clinical effectiveness is observed.

Summary pharmacokinetics of DERAMAXX™ tablets are listed in Table 1.

Table 1: Pharmacokinetics of Deracoxib:

Parameter	Value
Tmax[a]	2 hours
Oral Bioavailability (F)[a]	>90% at 2 mg/kg
Terminal elimination half-life[b]	3 hours at 2-3 mg/kg 19 hours at 20 mg/kg
Systemic Clearance[b]	~5 mL/kg/min at 2 mg/kg ~1.7 mL/kg/min at 20 mg/kg
Volume of Distribution[c]	~1.5 L/kg
Protein binding[d]	>90%

[a] Values obtained following a single 2.35 mg/kg dose
[b] Estimates following IV administration of deracoxib as an aqueous solution
[c] Based upon a dose of 2 mg/kg of deracoxib
[d] Based upon *in vitro* plasma concentrations of 0.1, 0.3, 1.0, 3.0, 10.0 µg/mL

D

Non-linear elimination kinetics are exhibited at doses above 8 mg/kg/day, at which competitive inhibition of constitutive COX-1 may occur.

Deracoxib is not excreted as parent drug in the urine. The major route of elimination of deracoxib is by hepatic biotransformation producing four major metabolites, two of which are characterized as products of oxidation and o-demethylation. The majority of deracoxib is excreted in feces as parent drug or metabolite.

Large intersubject variability was observed in drug metabolite profiles of urine and feces. No statistically significant differences between genders were observed.

Dosage and Administration: Always provide Client Information Sheet with prescription. The daily dose of DERAMAXX™ tablets for postoperative orthopedic pain is 3 to 4 mg/kg/day (1.4-1.8 mg/lb/day) as a single daily dose, as needed for 7 days. Since DERAMAXX™ tablet bioavailability is greatest when taken with food, postprandial administration is preferable. However, DERAMAXX™ tablets have been shown to be effective under both fed and fasted conditions; therefore, they may be administered in the fasted state if necessary. Administer DERAMAXX™ tablets prior to the procedure. Tablets are scored and dosage should be calculated in half-tablet increments. In clinical practice it is recommended to adjust the individual patient dose while continuing to monitor the dog's status until a minimum effective dose has been reached.

Contraindication(s): Dogs with known hypersensitivity to deracoxib should not receive DERAMAXX™ tablets.

Precaution(s): Storage Conditions: DERAMAXX™ tablets should be stored at room temperature between 59° and 86°F (15-30°C).

Caution(s): U.S. Federal Law restricts the use of this product by or on the order of a licensed veterinarian.

All dogs should undergo a thorough history and physical examination before the initiation of NSAID therapy. Appropriate laboratory tests to establish hematological and serum biochemical baseline data prior to administration of any NSAID is recommended.

For technical assistance or to report suspected adverse events, call 1-800-332-2761.

Plasma levels of deracoxib may increase in a greater than dose-proportional fashion above 8 mg/kg/day. DERAMAXX™ tablets have been safely used during field studies in conjunction with other common medications, including heartworm preventatives, anthelmintics, anesthetics, preanesthetic medications, and antibiotics. If additional pain medication is needed after a daily dose of DERAMAXX™ tablets, a non-NSAID class of analgesic may be necessary. It is not known whether dogs with a history of hypersensitivity to sulfonamide drugs will exhibit hypersensitivity to DERAMAXX™ tablets. The safe use of DERAMAXX™ tablets in dogs younger than 4 months of age, dogs used for breeding, or in pregnant or lactating dogs has not been evaluated.

As a class, cyclooxygenase inhibitory NSAIDs may be associated with gastrointestinal and renal toxicity. Sensitivity to drug-associated adverse events varies with the individual patient. Patients at greatest risk for renal toxicity are those that are dehydrated, on concomitant diuretic therapy, or those with existing renal, cardiovascular, and/or hepatic dysfunction. Concurrent administration of potentially nephrotoxic drugs should be carefully approached. Appropriate monitoring procedures should be employed during all surgical procedures. NSAIDs may inhibit the prostaglandins, which maintain normal homeostatic function. Such anti-prostaglandin effects may result in clinically significant disease in patients with underlying or pre-existing disease that has not been previously diagnosed. The use of parenteral fluids during surgery should be considered to decrease potential renal complications when using NSAIDs perioperatively. Since many NSAIDs possess the potential to produce gastrointestinal ulceration, concomitant use of DERAMAXX™ tablets with other anti-inflammatory drugs, such as NSAIDs or corticosteroids, should be avoided or closely monitored. The use of concomitantly protein-bound drugs with DERAMAXX™ tablets has not been studied in dogs. Commonly used protein-bound drugs include cardiac, anticonvulsant and behavioral medications. The influence of concomitant drugs that may inhibit metabolism of DERAMAXX™ tablets has not been evaluated. Drug compatibility should be monitored in patients requiring adjunctive therapy.

For use in dogs only.

For oral use in dogs only.

Warning(s): Not for use in humans. Keep this and all medications out of reach of children. Consult a physician in case of accidental ingestion by humans.

Adverse Reactions: A total of 207 dogs of forty three (43) different breeds, 1-15 years old, weighing 7-141 lbs were included in the field safety analysis. The following table shows the number of dogs displaying each clinical observation.

Abnormal Health Findings in the Postoperative Orthopedic Pain Field Study*:

Clinical Observation	DERAMAXX™ tablets N=105	Placebo N=102
Vomiting	11	6
Diarrhea	6	7
Hematochezia	4	0
Melena	0	1
Anorexia	0	4
Incision site lesion (drainage, oozing)	11	6
Non-incision Skin Lesions (moist dermatitis, pyoderma)	2	0
Otitis Externa	2	0
Positive joint culture	1	0
Phlebitis	1	0
Hematuria	2	0
Conjunctivitis	1	2
Splenomegaly	1	0
Hepatomegaly	1	0
Death	0	1

*Dogs may have experienced more than one of the observations during the study.

**This table does not include one dog that was dosed at 16.92 mg/kg/day for the study duration. Beginning on the last day of treatment, this dog experienced vomiting, diarrhea, increased water intake and decreased appetite. Hematology and clinical chemistry values were unremarkable. The dog recovered uneventfully within 3 days of cessation of dosing.

Incisional drainage was most prevalent in dogs enrolled at a single study site. There were no statistically significant changes in the mean values for hepatic or renal clinical pathology indices between DERAMAXX™ tablet- and placebo-treated dogs. Four DERAMAXX™ tablet-treated dogs and two placebo-treated dogs exhibited elevated bilirubin during the dosing phase. One DERAMAXX™ tablet-treated dog exhibited elevated ALT, BUN and total bilirubin and a single vomiting event. None of the changes in clinical pathology values were considered clinically significant.

The results of this field study demonstrate that DERAMAXX™ tablets, when administered daily for 7 days to control postoperative orthopedic pain and inflammation in dogs, are well tolerated.

Trial Data: Animal Safety: In a laboratory study, healthy young dogs were dosed with deracoxib tablets once daily, within 30 minutes of feeding, at doses of 0, 4, 6, 8, and 10 mg/kg body weight for 21 consecutive days. No adverse drug events were reported. There were no abnormal findings reported for clinical observations, food and water consumption, body weights, physical examinations, ophthalmic evaluations, organ weights, macroscopic pathologic evaluation, hematology, urinalyses, or buccal mucosal bleeding time. In the clinical chemistry results there was a statistically significant ($p<0.0009$) dose-dependent trend toward increased levels of blood urea nitrogen (BUN). Mean BUN values remained within historical normal limits at the label dose. No effects on other clinical chemistry values associated with renal function were reported. There was no evidence of renal, gastrointestinal, hepatic or biliary lesions noted during gross necropsy. Renal histopathology revealed trace amounts of tubular degeneration/regeneration in all dose groups including placebo, but no clear dose relationship could be determined. There was no histopathologic evidence of gastrointestinal, hepatic or biliary lesions.

In another study, micronized deracoxib in gelatin capsules was administered once daily to healthy young dogs at doses of 10, 25, 50, and 100 mg/kg body weight for periods up to 14 consecutive days. Food was withheld prior to dosing. Non-linear elimination kinetics occurred at all doses. At doses of 25, 50, and 100 mg/kg, reduced body weight, vomiting, and melena occurred. Necropsy revealed gross gastrointestinal lesions in dogs from all dose groups. The frequency and severity of the lesions increased with escalating doses. At 10 mg/kg, moderate diffuse congestion of gut associated lymphoid tissues (GALT) and erosions/ulcers in the jejunum occurred. At 100 mg/kg, all dogs exhibited gastric ulcers and erosions/ulcerations of the small intestines. There were no hepatic or renal lesions reported at any dose in this study.

In a 13-week study, deracoxib in gelatin capsules was administered to healthy dogs at doses of 0, 2, 4, and 8 mg/kg/day. No test-article related changes were identified in clinical observations, physical exams, or any of the other parameters measured. One dog in the 8 mg/kg dose group died from bacterial septicemia secondary to a renal abscess.

The relationship between deracoxib administration and the renal abscess is not clear.

Palatability: DERAMAXX™ tablets were evaluated for palatability in 100 client-owned dogs of a variety of breeds and sizes. Dogs received two doses of DERAMAXX™ tablets, one on each of two consecutive days. DERAMAXX™ tablets were accepted by 94% of dogs on the first day of dosing and by 92% of dogs on the second day of dosing.

Effectiveness: DERAMAXX™ tablets were evaluated in a masked, placebo-controlled multi-site field study involving client-owned animals to determine effectiveness.

Field Study: In this study, 207 dogs admitted to veterinary hospitals for repair of a cranial cruciate injury were randomly administered DERAMAXX™ tablets or a placebo. Drug administration started the evening before surgery and continued once daily for 6 days postoperatively. Effectiveness was evaluated in 119 dogs and safety was evaluated in 207 dogs. Statistically significant differences in favor of DERAMAXX™ tablets were found for lameness at walk and trot, and pain on palpation values at all postsurgical time points. The results of this field study demonstrate that DERAMAXX™ tablets, when administered daily for 7 days are effective for the control of postoperative pain and inflammation associated with orthopedic surgery.

References: Available upon request.

Presentation: DERAMAXX™ tablets are available as 25 mg and 100 mg round, brownish, half-scored tablets in 7, 30 and 90 count bottles.

Manufactured by: G.D. Searle & Co., Caguas, Puerto Rico.

Compendium Code No.: 11310120

NAH/DXB-T/VI/Draft 6/02

DERMACHLOR™ PLUS

Butler **Topical Wound Dressing**

Active Ingredient(s): Contains: Propylene glycol, lidocaine hydrochloride 0.5%, malic acid, benzoic acid, salicylic acid, chlorhexidine 0.2% and glycerin.

Indications: DERMACHLOR™ Plus solution aids in the cleansing of superficial skin infections and irrigation of wounds. The cleaning creates an ideal environment for healthy tissue to grow.

A cleansing and prevention control solution for use on superficial skin infections and irrigation of wounds.

Directions: Apply liberally to infected or wound area and let stand. Repeat application 2-3 times daily or as necessary.

Caution(s): For external use only.

Irritating to the eye.

Use only as directed by your veterinarian.

For veterinary use only.

Keep out of reach of children.

Presentation: 4 oz (NDC #11695-2453-3) and 16 oz (NDC #11695-2453-4).

Compendium Code No.: 10820481

DERMACHLOR™ RINSE

Butler **Topical Wound Dressing**

NDC No.: 11695-113-04/11695-113-16

Active Ingredient(s): Contains propylene glycol, malic acid, benzoic acid, salicylic acid, chlorhexidine and glycerin.

Indications: A cleansing and prevention control solution for use on superficial skin infections and for the irrigation of wounds. The cleaning creates an ideal environment for healthy tissue to grow.

Dosage and Administration: Apply liberally to the infected or wound area and let stand. Repeat the application two (2) to three (3) times a day or as necessary.

Caution(s): For external use only.

Irritating to the eye.

Use only as directed by a veterinarian. For veterinary use only.

Keep out of the reach of children.

Presentation: 4 fl. oz. and 16 fl. oz containers.

Compendium Code No.: 10820490

DERMACIDE™

Butler **Antiseptic**

NDC No.: 11695-2158-6

Active Ingredient(s):

Benzalkonium chloride 0.15%

Other ingredients: Allantoin.

Indications: For use on horses, dogs and cats as an aid in the control of summer itch, girth itch, ringworm and other fungal problems.

Dosage and Administration: Soak the affected area once a day until the hair begins to grow. Leave the treated area uncovered. Rinse the treated area with water prior to re-application. Fresh lesions usually respond within five (5) to seven (7) days. If improvement is not noted within seven (7) days, consult a veterinarian.

Note: Efficiency is neutralized by soap or detergent residues.

Caution(s): Keep out of the reach of children. In case of contact with the eyes or mucous membranes, flush immediately with water. Obtain medical attention for eye inflammation.

For external veterinary use only. For animal use only.

Warning(s): Not for use on animals intended for food.

Presentation: 16 fl. oz. containers.

Compendium Code No.: 10820501

DERMA CIDE™

Westfalia•Surge **Teat Dip**

Pre & Post Sanitizing Teat Conditioner

Active Ingredient(s): 1% caprylic-capric acid.

Inactive Ingredients: 99%*.

*Contains a 10.2% quadruple emollient system.

Indications: This topical liquid product, when used undiluted as a pre and post milking teat dip, effectively aids in reducing the spread of mastitis.

Directions for Use: Use at full strength. Do not dilute.

Pre Dipping: Before milking, dip each teat with DERMA CIDE™. After 15 to 30 seconds, dry each teat thoroughly with a single service paper towel. If the udder and teats are heavily soiled, wash with a sanitizing solution and dry before application of DERMA CIDE™.

Post Dipping: Immediately after milking, dip each teat with DERMA CIDE™. Allow teats to air dry. Do not wipe. If outside temperature is below freezing, allow to air dry on the teat before the cow leaves the parlor to prevent freezing. At the end of lactation, apply this product daily for one week after the last milking. In addition, begin application of this product about one week prior to calving.

If a common teat dip cup is used for application, a fresh solution should always be used at each milking. The teat dip cup should be emptied, cleaned and rinsed with potable water after each milking session or when cup becomes contaminated during milking. Do not pour remaining solution from dip cup back into original container.

Precaution(s): Store this product in a cool dry area away from direct sunlight and heat to avoid deterioration. Keep containers closed to prevent contamination of this product. Keep from freezing.

Warning(s): Danger: Contains materials which may cause eye damage. May be harmful or fatal if swallowed. Individuals with sensitive skin may experience skin irritation. Protect eyes and skin when handling. Do not take internally. Avoid breathing vapors. Do not mix with any other chemical products.

Refer to Material Safety Data Sheet (MSDS).

First Aid:

If in Eyes: Flush with large volumes of water for at least 15 minutes. Call a physician immediately.

If Swallowed: Do not induce vomiting. Rinse mouth promptly then give a small amount/glass of water (4-6 oz child / 10-12 oz adult). Avoid alcohol. Call a physician immediately. Do not give anything by mouth to an unconscious or convulsing person.

If on Skin: While removing contaminated clothing and shoes, flush with large volumes of water for at least 15 minutes. If irritation develops and persists, get medical attention.

Inhalation of Vapors: It breathing difficulty or irritation occurs, remove to fresh air. If symptoms persist, get medical attention.

Keep out of reach of children.

Presentation: Contact the company for container sizes available.

DERMA CIDE is a Trademark of Westfalia•Surge, Inc.

Compendium Code No.: 10020051

DERMA-CLENS®

Pfizer Animal Health **Topical Wound Dressing**

Dermatologic Cream-Vanishing Cream Base

Active Ingredient(s): Contents: Benzoic acid, malic acid, salicylic acid.

Indications: DERMA-CLENS® is an acidic cleansing cream for use on wounds, abrasions, burns and other dermatological conditions.

Directions: Clean affected area and apply an even layer over the entire lesion twice a day. DERMA-CLENS® may also be applied as a dressing when bandaging wounds. Use as required by severity of condition and response.

Precaution(s): Store at room temperature 20°-25°C (68°-77°F).

Caution(s): Avoid contact with eyes.

For external use only.

For veterinary use only.

Presentation: 1 oz tubes and 14 oz (397 g) bottles.

Compendium Code No.: 36900930

85-8021-03

DERMACOOL® HC SPRAY ℞

Virbac **Topical Corticosteroid**

Active Ingredient(s): Hydrocortisone 1% in a cooling astringent vehicle containing hamamelis extract, lactic acid, menthol and propylene glycol.

Indications: For the temporary relief of inflammation and pruritus associated with moist dermatosis, i.e., hot spots.

Dosage and Administration: Spray directly onto the affected areas two (2) to three (3) times a day as needed or as directed by a veterinarian. Wash hands thoroughly after use.

Caution(s): Federal law (USA) restricts this drug to use by or on the order of a licensed veterinarian.

If the condition persists, consult a veterinarian. Avoid contact with the eyes.

Keep out of the reach of children.

Presentation: 2 fl. oz. (59 mL) and 4 fl. oz. (120 mL) containers.

Compendium Code No.: 10230180

DERMACOOL® WITH LIDOCAINE HCL SPRAY

Virbac **Topical Wound Dressing**

NDC No.: 51311-061-04

Active Ingredient(s): Contains hamamelis extract and lidocaine HCl. Also contains purified water, propylene glycol, glycerin, lactic acid, parachlorometaxylenol, menthol, fragrance, FD&C blue no. 1.

Indications: Formulated to provide prompt temporary relief of itching associated with moist weeping lesions, i.e., hot spots. The formulation aids in drying and cleansing. The soothing and cooling effect helps reduce the likelihood of further self-inflicted trauma to the affected area.

Dosage and Administration: Spray directly onto the affected and adjacent areas two (2) to three (3) times a day as needed or as directed by a veterinarian.

Caution(s): For external use only. Avoid contact with the eyes.

Keep out of the reach of children.

Presentation: 4 fl. oz. spray bottles.

Compendium Code No.: 10230190

DERMA-FORM GRANULES F.A.

Vet-A-Mix **Small Animal Dietary Supplement**

Palatable fatty acid granule supplement with vitamins and minerals for dogs and cats

Guaranteed Analysis: per 10 grams:

(All values are minimum quantities unless otherwise stated.)

Minerals:

Calcium (min)	2.0%
Calcium (max)	2.2%
Phosphorus	1.0%
Potassium	1.0%
Zinc	10.0 mg
Iron	6.0 mg
Manganese	1.0 mg
Copper	0.5 mg
Cobalt	0.125 mg
Iodine	0.1 mg
Selenium	0.02 mg

Vitamins:

Vitamin A	1500 IU
Vitamin D_3	150 IU
Choline	30.0 mg
Vitamin E	10.0 IU
Niacin	10.0 mg
Pantothenic acid	0.5 mg
Thiamine	1.0 mg
Riboflavin	1.0 mg
Vitamin B_6	0.1 mg
Folic Acid	0.05 mg
Vitamin B_{12}	3.0 mcg

Fatty acids:

Omega 6 unsaturated	300 mg
Omega 3 unsaturated	50 mg

Ingredients: Brewer's dried yeast, soybean flour, extracted glandular meal (pork), soybean oil, dicalcium phosphate, calcium carbonate, animal liver meal (pork), cellulose powder, fish oil, choline chloride, lactose, DL-methionine, DL-alpha tocopheryl acetate, ferrous fumarate, zinc oxide, dextrose, niacin, lecithin, vitamin A palmitate, sodium selenite, thiamine mononitrate, manganese sulfate, vitamin B_{12} supplement, copper sulfate, povidone, potassium phosphate, riboflavin, calcium pantothenate, cholecalciferol, cobalt sulfate, folic acid, ethylenediamine dihydriodide, pyridoxine hydrochloride; with ethoxyquin, BHT, BHA, and propyl gallate as preservatives.

Indications: Supplementation of diet to aid in prophylaxis and treatment of fatty acid, multiple vitamin and mineral deficiencies. DERMA-FORM GRANULES F.A. may prove beneficial in the improvement and maintenance of healthy skin and coats on dogs and cats.

Dosage and Administration: Dosage: DERMA-FORM GRANULES F.A. are formulated with a special taste appeal for dogs and cats. Administer by mixing with or sprinkling on the food.

For diet supplementation:

Dogs:

Under 10 pounds	½ scoop daily
10 pounds and over	1 to 2 scoops daily

Cats:

All breeds and sizes	1 scoop daily

For sick, convalescing, pregnant or nursing animals:

Dogs:

Under 10 pounds .... 1 scoop daily
10 pounds and over .... 2 scoops daily

Cats:

All breeds and sizes .... 2 scoops daily

One scoop contains approximately 10 grams of product.

Precaution(s): Keep container tightly closed and in a cool, dry place.

Warning(s): Keep out of reach of children.

Presentation: 350 g bottles.

Compendium Code No.: 10500370 0800

DERMA-FORM LIQUID

Vet-A-Mix **Small Animal Dietary Supplement**

Polyunsaturated fatty acid and vitamin supplement

Guaranteed Analysis: per 5 mL:

D

Crude fat .... not less than 90%
Moisture.......... not more than 2%

Nutritional Information per 5 mL:

Vitamin A .... 1,250 IU
Vitamin D_3 .... 250 IU
Vitamin E .... 10 IU
Omega 6, fatty acids .... 2,238 mg
Omega 3 fatty acids .... 370 mg
Other unsaturated fatty acids .... 1,067 mg

Ingredients: Soybean oil, fish oil, sorbitan monooleate, lecithin, DL-alpha tocopheryl acetate, polysorbate 80, vitamin A palmitate, cholecalciferol, with ethoxyquin, BHT, BHA, and propyl gallate as preservatives.

Indications: For improvement of dry skin (Xerodermia) and dry hair (Xerasia) by providing a nutritional source of polyunsaturated fatty acids and vitamins A, D and E in the diet of dogs and cats.

Dosage and Administration: DERMA-FORM LIQUID is a very palatable liquid supplement for oral administration to dogs and cats and contains lecithin and other emulsifiers to facilitate high assimilability.

For diet supplementation:

Dogs and Cats—

Under 5 kg (11 lbs) .... 1 Pump
5 - 10 kg (11 - 22 lbs) .... 2 Pumps
10 - 25 kg (22 - 55 lbs) .... 3 Pumps
Over 25 kg (55 lbs) .... 4 to 5 Pumps

The quantity administered may be adjusted according to the condition and size of the pet.

Three pumps approximate 5 mL (1 teaspoonful).

Warning(s): Keep out of reach of children.

Presentation: 8 oz (236 mL) bottles.

Compendium Code No.: 10500041 0800

DERMA-FORM TABLETS

Vet-A-Mix **Small Animal Dietary Supplement**

Chewable vitamin, mineral and fatty acid supplement for dogs and cats

Guaranteed Analysis: per Tablet:

(All values are minimum quantities unless otherwise stated.)

Minerals:

Zinc .... 11 mg
Iodine.......... 170 mcg
Selenium .... 24 mcg

Vitamins:

Choline.......... 26 mg
Niacin.......... 25 mg
Vitamin E .... 22 IU
Pantothenic acid.......... 11 mg
Riboflavin.......... 4.8 mg
Thiamine .... 22 mg
HCl .... 22 mg
Vitamin A palmitate .... 1100 IU
Folic acid .... 200 mcg
Vitamin B_{12}.......... 50 mcg
Biotin .... 22 mcg
Vitamin D_3 .... 110 IU

Fatty acids:

Omega 6 fatty acids .... 0.3 mg
Omega 3 fatty acids .... 2.1 mg

Ingredients: Brewers dried yeast, extracted glandular meal (pork), DL-methionine, lactose, animal liver meal (pork), starch, soy flour, DL-alpha tocopheryl acetate, choline chloride, vitamin B_{12} supplement, silicon dioxide, niacin, L-lysine, ascorbic acid, cellulose powder, salt, zinc oxide, calcium pantothenate, fish oil, thiamine mononitrate, riboflavin, inositol, menadione sodium bisulfite complex, vitamin A palmitate, povidone, pyridoxine hydrochloride, folic acid, cholecalciferol, ethylenediamine dihydriodide, sodium selenite, biotin with ethoxyquin, BHT and propyl gallate as preservatives.

Indications: For use as a nutritional aid for healthy skin and dietary supplement for mature dogs and cats.

Dosage and Administration: Derma-Form Chewable Tablets may be fed free choice from the hand or crumbled and mixed into the food. For additional flavor release, moisten the tablets before offering to the pet.

For Dietary Supplementation:

Dogs: Small Breeds—one-half tablet.
Medium Breeds—one tablet.
Large Breeds—two tablets.
Extra Large Breeds—3 to 4 tablets.

Cats: All Breeds and Sizes—one-half tablet.

Precaution(s): Store at room temperature.

Warning(s): Keep out of reach of children.

Presentation: Bottles of 50 tablets.

Compendium Code No.: 10500181 0800

DERMAGEN™ CREAM ℞

Butler **Topical Antimicrobial-Antifungal-Corticosteroid**

Nystatin-Neomycin Sulfate-Thiostrepton-Triamcinolone Acetonide Cream Veterinary

ANADA No.: 200-245

Active Ingredient(s): Nystatin-Neomycin Sulfate-Thiostrepton-Triamcinolone Acetonide Cream combines nystatin, neomycin sulfate, thiostrepton, and triamcinolone acetonide.

Each gram contains:

Nystatin.......... 100,000 units
Neomycin sulfate equivalent to neomycin base.......... 2.5 mg
Thiostrepton .... 2500 units
Triamcinolone acetonide .... 1.0 mg

in an aqueous, nonirritating vanishing cream base with cetearyl alcohol (and) ceteareth-20, ethylenediamine hydrochloride, methyl paraben, propyl paraben, propylene glycol, sorbitol solution, titanium dioxide, sodium citrate, citric acid, white petrolatum, glyceryl monostearate, polyethylene glycol monostearate, sorbic acid and simethicone.

Indications: Nystatin-Neomycin Sulfate-Thiostrepton-Triamcinolone Acetonide Cream is indicated in the management of dermatologic disorders in dogs and cats, characterized by inflammation and dry or exudative dermatitis, particularly those caused, complicated or threatened by bacterial or candidal *(Candida albicans)* infections. It is also of value in eczematous dermatitis; contact dermatitis, and seborrheic dermatitis, and as an adjunct in the treatment of dermatitis due to parasitic infestation.

Pharmacology: Actions: By virtue of its four active ingredients, Nystatin-Neomycin Sulfate-Thiostrepton-Triamcinolone Acetonide Cream provides four basic therapeutic effects: antiinflammatory, antipruritic, antifungal and antibacterial. Triamcinolone Acetonide is a potent synthetic corticosteroid providing rapid and prolonged symptomatic relief on topical administration. Inflammation, edema, and pruritus promptly subside, and lesions are permitted to heal. Nystatin is the first well tolerated antifungal agent antibiotic of dependable efficacy for the treatment of cutaneous infections caused by *Candida albicans* (Monilia). Nystatin is fungistatic *in vitro* against a variety of yeast and yeast like fungi including many fungi pathogenic to animals. No appreciable activity is exhibited against bacteria. Thiostrepton has a high order of activity against gram positive organisms, including many which are resistant to other antibiotics; neomycin exerts antimicrobial action against a wide range of gram-positive and gram negative bacteria. Together they provide comprehensive therapy against those organisms responsible for most superficial bacterial infections.

Dosage and Administration: Frequency of administration is dependent on the severity of the condition. For mild inflammation, application may range from once daily to once a week; for severe conditions Nystatin-Neomycin Sulfate-Thiostrepton-Triamcinolone Acetonide Cream may be applied as often as 2 to 3 times daily, if necessary. Frequency of treatment may be decreased as improvement occurs.

Clean affected areas, removing any encrusted discharge or exudate. Apply Nystatin-Neomycin Sulfate-Thiostrepton-Triamcinolone Acetonide Cream sparingly in a thin film.

Contraindication(s): Nystatin-Neomycin Sulfate-Thiostrepton-Triamcinolone Acetonide Cream should not be used ophthalmically.

Precaution(s): Store at room temperature; avoid excessive heat (104°F).

Caution(s): Federal law restricts this drug to use by or on the order of a licensed veterinarian.

Nystatin-Neomycin Sulfate-Thiostrepton-Triamcinolone Acetonide Cream is not intended for the treatment of deep abscesses or deep seated infections such as inflammation of the lymphatic vessels. Parenteral antibiotic therapy is indicated in these infections.

Nystatin-Neomycin Sulfate-Thiostrepton-Triamcinolone Acetonide Cream has been extremely well tolerated. The occurrence of systemic reactions is rarely a problem with topical administration.

Sensitivity to neomycin may occur. If redness, irritation or swelling persists or increases, discontinue use. Do not use if pus is present since the drug may allow the infection to spread.

Avoid ingestion. Oral or parenteral use of corticosteroids, depending on dose, duration and specific steroids, may result in inhibition of endogenous steroid production following drug withdrawal.

For topical use on dogs and cats only.

Warning(s): Nystatin-Neomycin Sulfate-Thiostrepton-Triamcinolone Acetonide Cream is indicated for use in dogs and cats only. Not for use in animals which are raised for food.

Absorption of triamcinolone acetonide through topical application and by licking may occur. Therefore animals should be observed closely for signs of polydipsia, polyuria, and increased weight gain particularly when the preparation is used over large areas or for extended periods of time.

Clinical and experimental data have demonstrated that corticosteroids administered orally or by injection to animals may induce the first stage of parturition if used during the last trimester of pregnancy and may precipitate premature parturition followed by dystocia, fetal death, retained placenta and metritis.

Additionally, corticosteroids administered to dogs, rabbits and rodents during pregnancy have resulted in cleft palate in offspring. Corticosteroids administered to dogs during pregnancy have also resulted in other congenital anomalies including deformed forelegs, phocomelia and anasarca.

Side Effects: SAP and SGPT (ALT) enzyme elevation, polydipsia and polyuria have occurred following parenteral or systemic use of synthetic corticosteroids in dogs. Vomiting and diarrhea (occasionally bloody) have been observed in dogs. Cushing's syndrome in dogs has been reported in association with prolonged or repeated steroid therapy.

Presentation: Nystatin-Neomycin Sulfate-Thiostrepton-Triamcinolone Acetonide Cream is supplied in 7.5 gram and 15 gram tubes.

Manufactured by: Med-Pharmex, Inc.

Compendium Code No.: 10820510

DERMAGEN™ OINTMENT ℞

Butler **Topical Antimicrobial-Antifungal-Corticosteroid**

(Nystatin, Neomycin Sulfate, Thiostrepton and Triamcinolone Acetonide Ointment)

NADA No.: 140-810

Active Ingredient(s): Each mL contains:

Nystatin.......... 100,000 Units
Neomycin sulfate (equivalent to neomycin base) .... 2.5 mg
Thiostrepton .... 2,500 Units
Triamcinolone acetonide.......... 1.0 mg

Vehicle: Polyethylene and mineral oil gel base.

Indications: Recommended for the treatment of acute and chronic otitis of varied etiologies, in interdigital cysts in cats and dogs, and in anal gland infections in dogs. The preparation is also indicated in the management of dermatologic disorders characterized by inflammation and dry or exudative dermatitis, particularly those caused, complicated, or threatened by bacterial or candidal *(Candida albicans)* infections. It is also of value in eczematous dermatitis, contact dermatitis, and seborrheic dermatitis; and as an adjunct in the treatment of dermatitis due to parasitic infestation.

Dosage and Administration: Frequency of administration is dependent on the severity of the condition. For mild inflammations, application may range from once a day to once a week; for severe conditions, the ointment may be applied as often as two to three times daily, if necessary. Frequency of treatment may be decreased as improvement occurs.

Wear gloves during the administration of the ointment or wash hands immediately after application.

Otitis: Clean ear canal of impacted cerumen. Inspect canal and remove any foreign bodies such as grass awns, ticks, etc. Instill three to five drops of ointment.

Preliminary use of a local anesthetic such as proparacaine hydrochloride solution may be advisable.

Infected Anal Glands, Cystic Areas, etc.: Drain gland or cyst and then fill with product.

Other Dermatologic Disorders: Clean affected areas, removing any encrusted discharge or exudate. Apply ointment sparingly in a thin film.

Precaution(s): 240 mL Bottle: Do not store above 86°F. 7.5 mL, 15 mL, 30 mL tubes: Store at room temperature; avoid excessive heat (104°F).

Caution(s): Federal law restricts this drug to use by or on the order of a licensed veterinarian.

This product is not intended for the treatment of deep abscesses or deep-seated infections such as inflammation of the lymphatic vessels. Parenteral antibiotic therapy is indicated in these infections. DERMAGEN™ Ointment (nystatin-neomycin sulfate-thiostrepton- triamcinolone acetonide ointment) has been extremely well tolerated. Cutaneous reactions attributable to its use have been extremely rare. The occurrence of systemic reactions is rarely a problem with topical administration.

There is some evidence that corticosteroids can be absorbed after topical application and cause systemic effects. Therefore, an animal receiving DERMAGEN™ Ointment therapy should be observed closely for signs such as polydipsia, polyuria, and increased weight gain. This product is not generally recommended for the treatment of deep or puncture wounds or serious burns.

Sensitivity to neomycin may occur. If redness, irritation or swelling persists or increases, discontinue use. Do not use if pus is present since the drug may allow the infection to spread.

Avoid ingestion. Oral or parenteral use of corticosteroids (depending on dose, duration of use, and specific steroid) may result in inhibition of endogenous steroid production following drug withdrawal.

Before instilling any medication into the ear, examine the external ear canal thoroughly to be certain the tympanic membrane is not ruptured in order to avoid the possibility of transmitting infection to the middle ear as well as damaging the cochlea or vestibular apparatus from prolonged contact. If hearing or vestibular dysfunction is noted during the course of treatment, discontinue use.

Warning(s): For use in dogs and cats only. Keep this and all medications out of the reach of children.

Side Effects: Clinical and experimental data have demonstrated that corticosteroids administered orally or by injection to animals may induce the first stage of parturition if used during the last trimester of pregnancy and may precipitate premature parturition followed by dystocia, fetal death, retained placenta and metritis.

Additionally, corticosteroids administered to dogs, rabbits, and rodents during pregnancy have resulted in cleft palate in the offspring. In dogs, other congenital anomalies have resulted: Deformed forelegs, phocomelia, and anasarca.

SAP and SGPT (ALT) enzyme elevations, polydipsia/polyuria, vomiting, and diarrhea (occasionally bloody) have been observed following parenteral or systemic use of synthetic corticosteroids in dogs. Cushing's syndrome has been reported in association with prolonged or repeated steroid therapy in dogs. Temporary hearing loss has been reported in conjunction with treatment of otitis with products containing corticosteroids. However, regression usually occurred following withdrawal of the drug. If hearing dysfunction is noted during the course of treatment with this product, discontinue its use.

Discussion: By virtue of its four active ingredients, the ointment provides four basic therapeutic effects: Anti-inflammatory, antipruritic, antifungal and antibacterial. Triamcinolone acetonide is a potent synthetic corticosteroid providing rapid and prolonged symptomatic relief on topical administration. Inflammation, edema and pruritus promptly subside and lesions are permitted to heal. Nystatin is the first well-tolerated antifungal antibiotic of dependable efficacy for the treatment of cutaneous infections caused by *Candida albicans* (monilia). Nystatin is fungistatic *in vitro* against a variety of yeast and yeast-like fungi including many fungi pathogenic to animals. No appreciable activity is exhibited against bacteria.

Thiostrepton has a high order of activity against gram-positive organisms, including many which are resistant to other antibiotics; neomycin exerts antimicrobial action against a wide range of gram-positive and gram-negative bacteria. Together they provide comprehensive therapy against those organisms responsible for most superficial bacterial infections.

Presentation: Tubes of ¼ fl oz (7.5 mL), ½ fl oz (15 mL), and 1 fl oz (30 mL), each with an elongated tip for easy application. Bottles of 8 fl oz (240 mL).

Compendium Code No.: 10820520

DERMA-KOTE™

Westfalia•Surge **Teat Dip**

Iodine Sanitizing Teat Conditioner/Winter Teat Dip

Active Ingredient(s): Contents:

Available Iodine 0.5%
Non-medicinal Ingredients: Emollient. 74%

Indications: This topical liquid product, when used undiluted as a post milking teat dip, effectively aids in reducing the spread of mastitis.

Directions for Use: Use at full strength. Do not dilute.

Pre Dipping: Before milking, dip each teat with a Westfalia•Surge sanitizing teat dip. After 15 to 30 seconds, dry each teat thoroughly with a single service towel. If the udder and teats are heavily soiled, wash with a sanitizing solution and dry before application of a Westfalia•Surge sanitizing teat dip.

Post Dipping: Immediately after milking, dip each teat with DERMA-KOTE™. Allow teats to air dry. Do not wipe. At the end of lactation, apply this product daily for one week after the last milking. In addition, begin application of this product about one week prior to calving. Post dip only. It is not recommended for spraying.

If a common teat dip cup is used for application, a fresh solution should always be used at each milking. The teat dip cup should be emptied, cleaned and rinsed with potable water after each milking session or when cup becomes contaminated during milking. Do not pour remaining solution from dip cup back into original container.

Precaution(s): Storage Instructions: Store this product in a cool dry area away from direct sunlight and heat to avoid deterioration. Keep containers closed to prevent contamination of this product.

Product will not freeze. It may thicken at sub-zero temperatures. If desired, warm to original form.

Precautionary Statements: Danger. Contains materials which may cause eye damage. May be harmful or fatal if swallowed. Individuals with sensitive skin may experience skin irritation. Protect eyes and skin when handling. Do not take internally. Avoid breathing vapors. Do not mix with any other chemical products. Refer to Material Safety Data Sheet (MSDS).

First Aid:

If in Eyes: Flush immediately with large volumes of water for at least 15 minutes. Call a physician immediately.

If Swallowed: Do not induce vomiting. Rinse mouth promptly then give small amount/glass of milk or water (4-6 oz. child/10-12 oz. adult) (120-180 mL child/300-360 mL adult). Avoid alcohol. Call a physician immediately. Do not give anything by mouth to an unconscious or convulsing person.

If on Skin: While removing contaminated clothing and shoes, flush with large volumes of water for at least 15 minutes. If irritation develops and persists, get medical attention.

Inhalation of Vapors: If breathing difficulty or irritation occurs, remove to fresh air. If symptoms persist, get medical attention.

For assistance with medical emergency, call 1-800-451-8346.

For farm, commercial and industrial use only.

Warning(s): Keep out of reach of children.

Presentation: Contact the company for container sizes available.

DERMA-KOTE is a Trademark of Westfalia•Surge, Inc.

Compendium Code No.: 10020230

09-00

DERMALOG® OINTMENT ℞

RXV **Topical Antimicrobial-Corticosteroid**

Nystatin-Neomycin Sulfate-Thiostrepton-Triamcinolone Acetonide Ointment

NADA No.: 140-810

Active Ingredient(s): Each mL contains:

Nystatin. . . . . 100,000 units
Neomycin sulfate (equivalent to neomycin base) . . . . 2.5 mg
Thiostrepton . . . . 2,500 units
Triamcinolone acetonide. . . . . 1.0 mg

Indications: Nystatin, neomycin sulfate, thiostrepton and triamcinolone acetonide ointment is particularly useful in the treatment of acute and chronic otitis of varied etiologies, in interdigital cysts in cats and dogs, and in anal gland infections in dogs. The preparation is also indicated in the management of dermatologic disorders characterized by inflammation and dry or exudative dermatitis, particularly those caused, complicated, or threatened by bacterial or candidal *(Candida albicans)* infections. It is also of value in eczematous dermatitis; contact dermatitis, and seborrheic dermatitis; and as an adjunct in the treatment of dermatitis due to parasitic infestation.

Pharmacology: Description: Nystatin, neomycin sulfate, thiostrepton and triamcinolone acetonide ointment is an ointment in a non-irritating vehicle, a polyethylene and mineral oil gel base.

The preparation is intended for local therapy in a variety of cutaneous disorders of cats and dogs; it is especially useful in disorders caused, complicated or threatened by bacterial and/or candidal (monilial) infections.

Actions: By virtue of its four active ingredients, the ointment provides four basic therapeutic effects: anti-inflammatory, antipruritic, antifungal and antibacterial. Triamcinolone acetonide is a potent synthetic corticosteroid providing rapid and prolonged symptomatic relief on topical administration. Inflammation, edema and pruritus promptly subside and lesions are permitted to heal. Nystatin is the first well tolerated anti-fungal antibiotic of dependable efficacy for the treatment of cutaneous infections caused by *Candida albicans* (monilia). Nystatin is fungistatic in vitro against a variety of yeast and yeast-like fungi including many fungi pathogenic to animals. No appreciable activity is exhibited against bacteria. Thiostrepton has a high order of activity against gram-positive organisms, including many which are resistant to other antibiotics; neomycin exerts antimicrobial action against a wide range of gram-positive and gram-negative bacteria. Together they provide comprehensive therapy against those organisms responsible for most superficial bacterial infections.

Dosage and Administration: Frequency of administration is dependent on the severity of the condition. For mild inflammations, application may range from once daily to once a week; for severe conditions nystatin, neomycin sulfate, thiostrepton and triamcinolone acetonide ointment may be applied as often as two to three times daily, if necessary. Frequency of treatment may be decreased as improvement occurs.

Wear gloves during the administration of the ointment or wash hands immediately after application.

Otitis: Clean ear canal of impacted cerumen. Inspect canal and remove any foreign bodies such as grass awns, ticks, etc. Instill three to five drops of nystatin, neomycin sulfate, thiostrepton and triamcinolone acetonide ointment.

Preliminary use of a local anesthetic such as Proparacaine Hydrochloride Ophthalmic Solution may be advisable.

Infected Anal Glands, Cystic Areas, Etc.: Drain gland or cyst and then fill with nystatin, neomycin sulfate, thiostrepton and triamcinolone acetonide ointment.

Other Dermatologic Disorders: Clean affected areas, removing any encrusted discharge or exudate. Apply nystatin, neomycin sulfate, thiostrepton and triamcinolone acetonide ointment sparingly in a thin film.

Precaution(s): Storage: 240 mL bottle: Do not store above 86°F. 7.5 mL, 15 mL, 30 mL tubes: Store at room temperature; avoid excessive heat (104°F.)

Caution(s): Federal law restricts this drug to use by or on the order of a licensed veterinarian.

Before instilling any medication into the ear, examine the external ear canal thoroughly to be certain the tympanic membrane is not ruptured in order to avoid the possibility of transmitting infection to the middle ear as well as damaging the cochlea or vestibular apparatus from prolonged contact. If hearing or vestibular dysfunction is noted during the course of treatment, discontinue the use of nystatin, neomycin sulfate, thiostrepton and triamcinolone acetonide ointment.

Clinical and experimental data have demonstrated that corticosteroids administered orally or by injection to animals may induce the first stage of parturition if used during the last trimester of pregnancy and may precipitate premature parturition followed by dystocia, fetal death, retained placenta and metritis.

Additionally, corticosteroids administered to dogs, rabbits, and rodents during pregnancy have resulted in cleft palate in the offspring. In dogs, other congenital anomalies have resulted; deformed forelegs, phocomelia, and anasarca.

Nystatin, neomycin sulfate, thiostrepton and triamcinolone acetonide ointment is not intended for the treatment of deep abscesses or deep-seated infections such as inflammation of the lymphatic vessels. Parenteral antibiotic therapy is indicated in these infections. Nystatin, neomycin sulfate, thiostrepton and triamcinolone acetonide ointment has been extremely well tolerated. Cutaneous reactions attributable to its use have been extremely rare. The occurrence of systemic reactions is rarely a problem with topical administration.

There is some evidence that corticosteroids can be absorbed after topical application and cause systemic effects. Therefore, an animal receiving nystatin, neomycin sulfate, thiostrepton and triamcinolone acetonide ointment therapy should be observed closely for signs such as polydipsia, polyuria, and increased weight gain. Nystatin, neomycin sulfate, thiostrepton and triamcinolone acetonide ointment is not generally recommended for the treatment of deep or puncture wounds or serious burns.

Sensitivity to neomycin may occur. If redness, irritation or swelling persists or increases, discontinue use. Do not use if pus is present since the drug may allow the infection to spread.

Avoid ingestion. Oral or parenteral use of corticosteroids (depending on dose, duration of use, and specific steroid) may result in inhibition of endogenous steroid production following drug withdrawal.

D

For use only in dogs and cats.

Warning(s): Keep this and all medications out of the reach of children.

Side Effects: SAP and SGPT (ALT) enzyme elevations, polydipsia/polyuria, vomiting, and diarrhea (occasionally bloody) have been observed following parenteral or systemic use of synthetic corticosteroids in dogs.

Cushing's syndrome has been reported in association with prolonged or repeated steroid therapy in dogs.

Temporary hearing loss has been reported in conjunction with treatment of otitis with products containing corticosteroids. However, regression usually occurred following withdrawal of the drug. If hearing dysfunction is noted during the course of treatment with nystatin, neomycin sulfate, thiostrepton and triamcinolone acetonide ointment, discontinue its use.

Presentation: Nystatin, neomycin sulfate, thiostrepton and triamcinolone acetonide ointment is supplied in tubes of 7.5 mL (¼ fl oz), 15 mL (½ fl oz), and 30 mL (1 fl oz), each with an elongated tip for easy application and in dispensing bottles of 240 mL (8 fl oz).

Manufactured by: Med-Pharmex, Inc.

Compendium Code No.: 10910380 Revised 10/98

DERMALONE™ OINTMENT ℞

Vedco **Topical Antimicrobial-Corticosteroid**

Nystatin-Neomycin Sulfate-Thiostrepton-Triamcinolone Acetonide Ointment

NADA No.: 140-810

Active Ingredient(s): Each mL contains:

Nystatin	100,000 units
Neomycin sulfate (equivalent to neomycin base)	2.5 mg
Thiostrepton	2,500 units
Triamcinolone acetonide	1.0 mg

In a polyethylene and mineral oil gel base.

Indications: DERMALONE™ Ointment is useful in the treatment of acute and chronic otitis of varied etiologies, in interdigital cysts in cats and dogs, and in anal gland infections in dogs. The preparation is also indicated in the management of dermatologic disorders characterized by inflammation and dry or exudative dermatitis, particularly those caused, complicated, or threatened by bacterial or candidal *(Candida albicans)* infections. It is also of value in eczematous dermatitis, contact dermatitis, and seborrheic dermatitis; and as an adjunct in the treatment of dermatitis due to parasitic infestation.

Dosage and Administration: The frequency of administration is dependent upon the severity of the condition. For mild inflammations, application may range from once a day to once a week; for severe conditions DERMALONE™ Ointment may be applied as often as two (2) to three (3) times a day. The frequency of treatment may be decreased as improvement occurs. Wear gloves during the administration of the ointment or wash hands immediately after application.

Otitis: Clean the ear canal of impacted cerumen. Inspect the ear canal and remove any foreign bodies such as grass awns, ticks, etc. Instill three (3) to five (5) drops of DERMALONE™ Ointment. Preliminary use of a local anesthetic such as proparacaine hydrochloride ophthalmic solution may be advisable.

Infected anal glands, cystic areas, etc.: Drain the gland or cyst and then fill with DERMALONE™ Ointment.

Other dermatologic disorders: Clean the affected areas, removing any encrusted discharge of exudate. Apply DERMALONE™ Ointment (nystatin-neomycin sulfate- thiostrepton-triamcinolone acetonide ointment) sparingly in a thin film.

Precaution(s): Store at room temperature; avoid excessive heat (104°F).

Caution(s): Federal law restricts this drug to use by or on the order of a licensed veterinarian.

Keep out of the reach of children.

DERMALONE™ Ointment is not intended for the treatment of deep abscesses or deep-seated infections such as inflammation of the lymphatic vessels. Parenteral antibiotic therapy is indicated in these infections.

DERMALONE™ Ointment has been well tolerated. Cutaneous reactions attributable to its use have been rare. The occurrence of systemic reactions is rarely a problem with topical administration. There is some evidence that corticosteroids can be absorbed after topical application and cause systemic effects. Therefore, an animal receiving DERMALONE™ Ointment therapy should be observed closely for signs such as polydipsia, polyuria, and increased body weight gain.

DERMALONE™ Ointment is not generally recommended for the treatment of deep or puncture wounds or serious burns. Sensitivity to neomycin may occur. If redness, irritation or swelling persists or increases, discontinue use. Do not use if pus is present since the drug may allow the infection to spread. Avoid ingestion. Oral or parenteral use of corticosteroids (depending on dose, duration of use, and specific steroid) may result in the inhibition of endogenous steroid production following drug withdrawal.

Before instilling any medication into the ear, examine the external ear canal thoroughly to be certain that the tympanic membrane is not ruptured in order to avoid the possibility of transmitting infection to the middle ear as well as damaging the cochlea or vestibular apparatus from prolonged contact. If hearing or vestibular dysfunction is noted during the course of treatment, discontinue the use of DERMALONE® Ointment.

Warning(s): For use in dogs and cats only.

Presentation: 7.5 mL, 15 mL, 30 mL and 8 oz tubes.

Compendium Code No.: 10940420

DERMAPET® ALLAY™ OATMEAL SHAMPOO

DermaPet **Grooming Shampoo**

Ingredient(s): 2% solubilized oatmeal, safflower oil (linoleic acid), sodium lactate and glycerine, natural moisturizing factors, and purified water in a hypo-allergenic gentle cleansing system.

Indications: Relief for pets with dry, itchy skin.

Dosage and Administration: Apply to a wet coat. It is best to prime the pet by bathing/cleansing in DermaPet® Conditioning Shampoo. Then rub ALLAY™ Oatmeal Shampoo into skin and/or coat until lightly lathered. Wait 5 to 10 minutes and rinse well. Use as often as necessary or as directed by veterinarian. To help restore natural skin oils and revitalize dry, irritated skin, use DermaPet® Oatmeal Conditioner after bathing and between baths.

Caution(s): Use topically only. Avoid contact with eyes.

Warning(s): Keep out of reach of children.

Presentation: 8 fl oz, 16 fl oz, and 1 gallon.

Compendium Code No.: 14590010

DERMAPET® BENZOYL PEROXIDE PLUS SHAMPOO

DermaPet **Antidermatosis Shampoo**

Active Ingredient(s): Benzoyl peroxide (2.5%) in an all-natural vehicle with moisturizers.

Benzoyl peroxide (2.5%), moisturizing factors, antioxidants, vitamin E and fragrance. All contents are biodegradable.

Indications: Topical treatment of skin infection including pyoderma, seborrhea complex and conditions where a degreasing, antimicrobial, keratolytic shampoo may be beneficial.

Dosage and Administration: Apply to a wet coat. It is to prime the pet by bathing and cleansing in DermaPet® Conditioning Shampoo. Then rub Benzoyl Peroxide into skin and/or coat until lightly lathered. Wait 5 to 10 minutes and rinse well. May be used daily or as directed by veterinarian.

Hot Spots: Clip hair off area, preferably with a #40 clipper blade, apply as directed above.

It is best to use DermaPet® Conditioner/Bath Oil after using Benzoyl Peroxide to relieve associated dryness of skin and coat.

Precaution(s): Store at controlled room temperature (59-86°F).

Warning(s): For external use only on domestic animals. Avoid contact with eyes or mucous membranes. May bleach colored fabric. If irritation develops, discontinue use. Contact hypersensitivity has been seen in humans at a rate of 1-2%, although as yet is unreported in dogs and cats.

Keep out of reach of children.

Presentation: 4 fl oz (118 mL) and 16 fl oz.

Compendium Code No.: 14590020

DERMAPET® DENTACETIC™ WIPES/GEL

DermaPet **Dental Preparation**

Ingredient(s): Contains: 1% acetic acid, sodium hexametaphosphate and cinnamon-clove flavor beads.

Indications: Dental wipes/gel for dogs and cats freshen breath, clean and whiten teeth. The Wipes/Gel also place a protective coating on the teeth to prevent tartar and calculus buildup.

Directions: Brush your pet's teeth daily with DENTACETIC™ Natural Dental Gel.

Presentation: 25-count jar (Wipes) or 2 fl oz bottle (Gel).

Patent Pending

Compendium Code No.: 14590131

DERMAPET® EICOSADERM™

DermaPet **Small Animal Dietary Supplement**

EPA 360 mg/DHA 240 mg

Ingredient(s): Supplement Facts: 1 pump = 2,000 mg Fish Oil; 360 mg EPA (Eicosapentaenoic Acid); 240 mg DHA (Docosahexaenoic Acid); 10 IU Vitamin E; Mercury below lowest level of detection, less than 100 ppb.

Sugar, starch and preservative free.

Indications: Fish oil fortified with 10 IU Vitamin E. For dogs and cats.

Dosage and Administration: Feed directly to pet or apply directly onto pet food.

Current research indicates a dosage of 180 mg of EPA per 10 pounds of weight.

Use the following guide:

1-10 pounds	½ pump
11-20 pounds	1 pump
21-40 pounds	2 pumps
41-60 pounds	3 pumps
61-80 pounds	4 pumps

Servings per container: 120.

Precaution(s): Store in a cool, dark place.

Warning(s): Keep out of reach of children.

Presentation: 8 fl oz (240 mL) container.

Compendium Code No.: 14590150

DERMAPET® HYPOALLERGENIC CONDITIONING SHAMPOO

DermaPet **Grooming Shampoo**

Ingredient(s): Natural coconut oil, safflower oil (linoleic acid), sodium lactate and glycerin as natural moisturizing factors, and purified water in a hypo-allergenic gentle cleansing system.

Indications: For cleansing normal, sensitive and dry skin.

Dosage and Administration: Wet coat, apply shampoo, lather, rinse thoroughly. Repeat. Shampoo may be diluted 4:1 in water. DERMAPET® Shampoo may be used as often as desired. For best results, apply DermaPet® Coat Conditioner/Bath Oil following shampoo.

Discussion: A moisturizing shampoo for cleansing normal, sensitive or dry skin. DERMAPET® Shampoo assists in grooming, aids in restoring natural luster to the coat, is environmentally friendly, biodegradable, non polluting and cruelty free.

Presentation: 8 oz and 1 gallon containers.

Compendium Code No.: 14590040

DERMAPET® MALACETIC™ CONDITIONER FOR DOGS AND CATS

DermaPet **Antidermatosis Conditioner**

Active Ingredient(s): 2% acetic acid (vinegar) and 2% boric acid.

Indications: Aids in the topical treatment of seborrhea complex and as a broad spectrum medicated conditioner for dogs and cats where either acetic and/or boric acid may be beneficial.

Directions: Shake well before using.

For dry application - apply directly. Allow to dry on coat.

For wet application or after shampooing - remove excess moisture and apply directly to skin by parting hairs, then continue grooming as usual.

As a pour on - use 4 caps per quart. Use as often as needed to maintain coat luster and healthy skin.

For best results, use in conjunction with DermaPet® MalAcetic Shampoo.

Warning(s): Use topically only. Avoid contact with eyes. Keep out of reach of children.

Presentation: 12 fl oz (348 mL) and 16 oz container.

U.S. Patent #5,480,658

Compendium Code No.: 14590050

DERMAPET® MALACETIC OTIC (EAR/SKIN CLEANSER FOR PETS)

DermaPet **Otic Cleanser**

(Ear/Skin Cleanser for Pets) Acidifies-pH adjusting-Hypo-allergenic

Active Ingredient(s): Contains: 2% Acetic Acid and 2% Boric Acid with surfactants.

Indications: Description: DERMAPET® MALACETIC OTIC is a unique, all natural, environmentally sensitive solution designed for routine ear cleaning and drying.

For use in pets as an ear cleaning and drying solution.

Directions: Apply liberally to ear. Gently, but firmly massage the base of the ear. Apply a cotton ball to remove any excess solution. Repeat as necessary.

External skin lesions or wounds: Apply liberally 2 to 3 times daily or as directed by veterinarian.

Caution(s): If undue skin irritation develops or increases, discontinue use and consult a veterinarian. Do not use on severely traumatized or irritated skin.

For animal use only.

Presentation: 4 fl oz (118 mL) and 16 fl oz (472 mL) containers.

U.S. Patent Nos. 5,480,658 and 5,853,767

Compendium Code No.: 14590031

DERMAPET® MALACETIC™ SHAMPOO FOR DOGS AND CATS

DermaPet **Antidermatosis Shampoo**

Active Ingredient(s): Acetic acid (2%) and boric acid (2%) in an all natural soapless shampoo vehicle with moisturizers.

Indications: Aids in the topical treatment of seborrhea complex and other conditions where a medicated shampoo may be beneficial.

Directions: Apply to wet coat. Rub MALACETIC™ Shampoo into skin and/or coat until lightly lathered. Wait 5 to 10 minutes, then rinse well. May be used daily or as directed by a veterinarian.

Caution(s): Use topically only. Avoid contact with eyes. Keep out of reach of children.

Presentation: 8 fl. oz. (240 mL), 16 fl. oz. (480 mL) and 1 gallon containers.

U.S. Patent #5,480,658

Compendium Code No.: 14590061

DERMAPET® MALACETIC™ WET WIPES/DRY BATH

DermaPet **Grooming Product**

Active Ingredient(s): Contains: 2% acetic and 2% boric acids pH buffered with surfactants.

Indications: Particularly indicated for cleansing on or around skin folds, perianal, preputial perivulvar, lip, ear, feet, nasal, "hot spots" and other desired areas. For use in dogs and cats.

Directions: Gently cleanse desired areas.

Anal Sacs Expression: Place a MALACETIC™ Wipe over the anal orifice and, with the thumb slightly below and to one side of the anus and the fingers on the other, press forward and together. For further expression, see your veterinarian.

Caution(s): If undue irritation occurs, discontinue and consult veterinarian. Avoid contact with eyes. Keep out of reach of children.

Presentation: Regular size 25 - 4 x 9 inch wet wipes premoistened and unit dosed in dispensing container.

Clinic size strength 100 - 6 x 7 inch wipes per pack.

US Patent #5,480,658

US Patent #5,853,767

Foreign and other patents pending

Compendium Code No.: 14590071

DERMAPET® OATMEAL CONDITIONER

DermaPet **Grooming Rinse**

Active Ingredient(s):

Natural colloidal oatmeal 0.75%

Indications: DERMAPET® Oatmeal Conditioner is a revolutionary soothing, natural dry skin treatment with a pleasant herbal scent and colloidal oatmeal as an active ingredient. Formulated to incorporate natural moisturizing factors and skin nutrients (essential fatty acids) which bind moisture to the skin and restore luster to the hair and coat. Aids in the control of scaling and flaking by stabilizing keratinization.

Dosage and Administration: Shake well before using.

For dry application: Apply directly. Allow to dry on the coat.

For wet application or after shampooing: Remove excess moisture and apply directly to the skin by parting hairs, then continue grooming as usual. Use as often as needed.

As a dip solution: Add two (2) to four (4) caps per gallon of water.

Caution(s): For topical use only.

Avoid contact with the eyes.

Keep out of the reach of children.

Presentation: 8 fl. oz. (230 mL) and 1 gallon (128 fl. oz.) recyclable containers.

Compendium Code No.: 14590100

DERMAPET® O.F.A. PLUS EZ-C CAPS (UP TO 30 LB.)

DermaPet **Small Animal Dietary Supplement**

Nutritional Supplement

Ingredient(s): 87.7 mg Purified marine oil extract, 46 mg borage oil, 10 I.U. natural vitamin E, 5,000 mcg zinc sulfate (2,000 mcg elemental zinc), 50 mg vitamin C, 358 mg safflower oil, garlic oil equivalent to 5,000 mcg of fresh garlic bulb.

Indications: O.F.A. Plus EZ-C Caps is an oral skin supplement with Omega-3 and 6 Fatty Acids and antioxidants. Appropriate fatty acids can reduce chronic itching, excessive shedding, and help dry, lusterless coats. Omega-3/fish oil is the source of eicosapentaenoic, docosahexaenoic, linolenic and oleic acids.

Dosage and Administration: Give one capsule daily orally to pets up to 30 pounds (14 kg) of body weight. Capsules may be punctured and liquid contents squeezed onto food, if desired.

Caution(s): For use in dogs and cats only.

Presentation: Bottles of 60 capsules.

Compendium Code No.: 14590090

D

DERMAPET® O.F.A. PLUS EZ-C CAPS (50-70 LB.)

DermaPet **Small Animal Dietary Supplement**

Nutritional Supplement

Ingredient(s): 263 mg Purified marine oil extract, 138 mg borage oil, 10 I.U. natural vitamin E, 10,000 mcg zinc sulfate (4,000 mcg elemental zinc), 100 mg vitamin C, 358 mg safflower oil, garlic oil equivalent to 100 mcg of fresh garlic bulb.

Indications: O.F.A. Plus EZ-C Caps is an oral skin supplement with Omega-3 and 6 Fatty Acids and antioxidants. Appropriate fatty acids can reduce chronic itching, excessive shedding, and help dry, lusterless coats. Omega-3/fish oil is the source of eicosapentaenoic, docosahexaenoic, linolenic and oleic acids.

Dosage and Administration: Give one capsule daily orally to pets 50 (23 kg) to 70 pounds (32 kg) of body weight. Capsules may be punctured and liquid contents squeezed onto food, if desired.

Caution(s): For use in dogs and cats only.

Presentation: Bottles of 60 capsules.

Compendium Code No.: 14590080

DERMAPET® SEBORRHEIC SHAMPOO

DermaPet **Antidermatosis Shampoo**

Active Ingredient(s): DERMAPET® Seborrheic Shampoo is a clear, golden formulation combining the healing properties of 2% sulfur and 2% salicylic acid with natural coconut oil in a pH balanced, shampoo vehicle.

Does not contain animal protein, dyes or soaps. All the contents are biodegradable.

Indications: For use as an aid in removing scales, crusts and other nonspecific dermatoses. Assists in grooming and aids in restoring natural luster to the coat.

Dosage and Administration: Shake well before using. Apply to the wet coat. Wait for 5-10 minutes and rinse well. Use as often as clinical signs of seborrhea appear, or as directed by a veterinarian.

Caution(s): Use as a topical treatment only.

Avoid contact with the eyes.

Keep out of the reach of children.

Presentation: 8 fl. oz. and 128 fl. oz. (3,792 mL) recyclable containers.

Compendium Code No.: 14590110

DERMAPET® TrizEDTA™ AQUEOUS FLUSH

DermaPet **Otic Cleanser**

Alkalinizing-Ready-to-Use

Active Ingredient(s): Contains: 2,132 mg Tromethamine (Tris) USP, 564 mg Edetate Disodium Dihydrate (EDTA) USP, buffered to pH 8 with Tromethamine HCl and 472 mL of deionized water.

Preservative free.

Indications: A multicleanse TrizEDTA™ flush. For use in dogs and cats as a cleaning and/or alkalinizing and/or pretreatment flush.

Directions: Ear: Apply liberally to ear, gently but firmly massage the base of the ear, apply cotton ball to remove excess flush. Repeat as necessary or as directed by veterinarian.

Caution(s): If undue ear or skin irritation develops or increases, discontinue use and consult a veterinarian.

Use topically only. Avoid contact with eyes.

Warning(s): Keep out of reach of children.

Presentation: 4 fl oz (118 mL) and 16 fl oz (472 mL) bottles.

Patent Pending

Compendium Code No.: 14590140

DERMAPET® TrizEDTA™ CRYSTALS

DermaPet **Otic Cleanser**

Cleanser

Active Ingredient(s): Contains: 533 mg Tromethamine (Tris) USP, 141 mg Edetate Disodium Dihydrate (EDTA) USP, buffered to pH 8 with Tromethamine HCl (after reconstituting with 112 mL distilled water).

Indications: A multicleanse TrizEDTA™ solution. For use in dogs and cats as a cleaning and/or alkalinizing and/or pretreatment solution.

Directions: Shake well before using.

Fill bottle with 112 mL of distilled water and shake well to create a solution with an approximate pH of 8. Ear: Apply liberally to ear, gently but firmly massage the base of the ear, apply cotton ball to remove excess solution. Repeat as necessary or as directed by veterinarian.

Discard after 21 days after reconstituting.

Caution(s): If undue ear or skin irritation develops or increases, discontinue use and consult a veterinarian.

Use topically only.

Avoid contact with eyes.

Warning(s): Keep out of reach of children.

Presentation: 4 fl oz (112 mL) and 16 oz (448 mL) bottles.

Patent Pending

Compendium Code No.: 14590121

DERMA SEPT™

Westfalia•Surge **Teat Dip**

Active Ingredient(s): 1% caprylic-capric acid.

Non-medicinal ingredients: 70% emollient system.

Indications: Sanitizing teat conditioner/winter teat dip.

This product aids in reducing the spread of organisms which may cause mastitis.

Directions for Use: Use at full strength. Do not dilute.

Pre Dipping: Before milking, dip or spray each teat with an approved pre-dip product. After 15 to 30 seconds, dry each teat thoroughly with a single service paper towel. If the udder and teats are heavily soiled, wash with a sanitizing solution and dry before pre-dip application.

Post-Dipping: Immediately after milking, dip each teat with DERMA SEPT™. Allow teats to air dry.

If a common teat cup is used for application, a fresh solution should always be used at each milking. The teat dip cup should be emptied, cleaned and rinsed with potable water after each milking session or when cup becomes contaminated during milking. Do not pour remaining solution from dip cup back into original container.

Precautionary Statements: Contains materials that can cause eye damage. May be harmful if swallowed. Protect eyes and skin when handling. Do not take internally. Refer to Material Safety Data Sheet (MSDS).

First Aid:

If in Eyes: Flush immediately with large volumes of water for at least 15 minutes. Call a physician immediately.

If Swallowed: Do not induce vomiting. Rinse mouth promptly then give a small amount/glass of water. Avoid alcohol. Call a physician immediately. Do not give anything by mouth to an unconscious or convulsing person.

If on Skin: Flush immediately with large volumes of water for at least 15 minutes while removing contaminated clothing and shoes. If irritation develops, get medical attention.

For Assistance with Medical Emergency, Call: 1-800-228-5635 ext. 149 or 1-612-851-8180 ext. 149.

Storage and Disposal: Product will not freeze. It may thicken at sub-zero temperatures. If gelling occurs, warm to original form.

Store this product in a cool dry area away from direct sunlight and heat to avoid deterioration.

Keep containers closed to prevent contamination of this product.

Warning(s): Danger: Keep out of reach of children.

Discussion: Formulated with a fatty acid germicide for broad spectrum kill of mastitis-causing organisms. Germicidal activity evaluations have shown that DERMA SEPT™ possesses superior killing power versus popular 1% iodine products and base and activator products.

Even under extremely cold weather conditions, DERMA SEPT™ will not freeze. This product eliminates the concerns of teat end frostbite by warming skin tissue through increased blood circulation.

Presentation: Contact the company for container sizes available.

Compendium Code No.: 10020061

DERMASOOTHE OATMEAL LEAVE-ON CONDITIONER

Davis **Grooming Product**

Ingredient(s): Conditioners, colloidal oatmeal.

Indications: An aid to relieve irritated, dry and itchy skin in dogs, cats, puppies and kittens.

Directions for Use: Apply Davis DERMASOOTHE LEAVE-ON CONDITIONER full strength on a wet or dry coat after or in-between shampoos. Do not get conditioner into eyes. Start with the head and ears and massage thoroughly. Repeat procedure with neck, chest, middle and hind quarter, finishing legs last. Work well through the coat. To achieve the best results, DERMASOOTHE should remain on the coat until the product is fully absorbed and dry.

Warning(s): For external use only. Keep out of reach of children.

Presentation: 12 fl oz (355 mL) and 1 gallon (3.785 L).

Compendium Code No.: 11410140

DERMA SPRAY

Sungro **Grooming Product**

Active Ingredient(s): Australian Oil of *Maelaleuca alternifolia* which penetrates the skin soothing distress caused by skin irritation.

Indications: Pruritus relief aid for dogs and cats. Gives a glossy coat, cleans, conditions and detangles.

Dosage and Administration: Directions: For relief from stop itch, hot spots, flea bites, tick bites, lick sores, nail infections, fungus and burns.

First bathe your pet with Sungro Fleazy Pet Shampoo. Spray the affected areas, at least 3 times daily or more often if required. Do not spray more than once per hour on any one day. Thereafter, 3 times daily for 7 days.

If the problem persists see your veterinarian.

For detangling, grooming and deodorizing use a little spray while brushing and combing.

Warning(s): Keep out of reach of children.

Presentation: 12 pints/case, 12 quarts/case, and 4x1 gallon.

Compendium Code No.: 10100000

DERMA-TECT KIT

Vetus **Dermatophyte Test**

Active Ingredient(s): Ingredients per liter of demineralized water:

Dermatophyte test medium (base):

Peptone 110	10.0 g
Dextrose	10.0 g
Agar	20.0 g
Phenol red	0.2 g
Cycloheximide	0.5 g

The pH is 5.5 ± 0.2 at 25°C.

Pre-form dermatophyte test medium contains:

Gentamicin	0.1 g
Chlortetracycline	0.1 g

Indications: DERMA-TECT is a formulation for dermatophytes with a yellow to red pH indicator for the growth of dermatophytes and related fungi. Gentamicin and chlortetracycline retard the growth of most bacteria, while cycloheximide inhibits the development of most saprophytic fungi.

Test Procedure: The specimen should be inoculated immediately onto the DERMA-TECT vial. Cutaneous specimens should be implanted by pressing the samples into the agar surface. Incubation at temperatures of 20°-30°C is satisfactory for the growth of most dermatophytes. Optimal growth and indicator change occurs at 29°C. To ensure the presence of an aerobic environment for the best recovery of dermatophytes, do not tighten the tube caps.

After 24 hours the test media may be examined for a color change from yellow to red. Most pathogenic dermatophytes will produce full color changes in three (3) to six (6) days. Other organisms may grow on DERMA-TECT but can be recognized as non-dermatophytes by the absence of color change or by their colonial appearance.

Inoculation onto a conventional cultivation medium is recommended for the identification of species when DERMA-TECT suggests the presence of a dermatophyte.

Test characteristics:

Organisms	Results
Aspergillus flavus	Suppressed
Microsporum audouinil	Growth alkaline (red)
Trichophyton rubeum	Growth, alkaline (red)

Caution(s): For veterinary use only.

Presentation: 10 and 20 vial kits.

Compendium Code No.: 14440240

DERMA-VET™ CREAM ℞

Med-Pharmex **Topical Antimicrobial-Antifungal-Corticosteroid**

Nystatin-Neomycin Sulfate-Thiostrepton-Triamcinolone Acetonide Cream Veterinary

ANADA No.: 200-245

Active Ingredient(s): Nystatin-Neomycin Sulfate-Thiostrepton-Triamcinolone Acetonide Cream combines nystatin, neomycin sulfate, thiostrepton, and triamcinolone acetonide.

Each gram contains:

Nystatin	100,000 units
Neomycin sulfate equivalent to neomycin base	2.5 mg
Thiostrepton	2500 units
Triamcinolone acetonide	1.0 mg

in an aqueous, nonirritating vanishing cream base with cetearyl alcohol (and) ceteareth-20, ethylenediamine hydrochloride, methyl paraben, propyl paraben, propylene glycol, sorbitol solution, titanium dioxide, sodium citrate, citric acid, white petrolatum, glyceryl monostearate, polyethylene glycol monostearate, sorbic acid and simethicone.

Indications: Nystatin-Neomycin Sulfate-Thiostrepton-Triamcinolone Acetonide Cream is indicated in the management of dermatologic disorders in dogs and cats, characterized by inflammation and dry or exudative dermatitis, particularly those caused, complicated or threatened by bacterial or candidal *(Candida albicans)* infections. It is also of value in eczematous dermatitis; contact dermatitis, and seborrheic dermatitis, and as an adjunct in the treatment of dermatitis due to parasitic infestation.

Pharmacology: Actions: By virtue of its four active ingredients, Nystatin-Neomycin Sulfate-Thiostrepton-Triamcinolone Acetonide Cream provides four basic therapeutic effects: antiinflammatory, antipruritic, antifungal and antibacterial. Triamcinolone Acetonide is a potent synthetic corticosteroid providing rapid and prolonged symptomatic relief on topical administration. Inflammation, edema, and pruritus promptly subside, and lesions are permitted to heal. Nystatin is the first well tolerated antifungal agent antibiotic of dependable efficacy for the treatment of cutaneous infections caused by *Candida albicans* (Monilia). Nystatin is fungistatic *in vitro* against a variety of yeast and yeast like fungi including many fungi pathogenic to animals. No appreciable activity is exhibited against bacteria. Thiostrepton has a high order of activity against gram positive organisms, including many which are resistant to other antibiotics; neomycin exerts antimicrobial action against a wide range of gram-positive and gram negative bacteria. Together they provide comprehensive therapy against those organisms responsible for most superficial bacterial infections.

Dosage and Administration: Frequency of administration is dependent on the severity of the condition. For mild inflammation, application may range from once daily to once a week; for severe conditions Nystatin-Neomycin Sulfate-Thiostrepton-Triamcinolone Acetonide Cream may be applied as often as 2 to 3 times daily, if necessary. Frequency of treatment may be decreased as improvement occurs.

Clean affected areas, removing any encrusted discharge or exudate. Apply Nystatin-Neomycin Sulfate-Thiostrepton-Triamcinolone Acetonide Cream sparingly in a thin film.

Contraindication(s): Nystatin-Neomycin Sulfate-Thiostrepton-Triamcinolone Acetonide Cream should not be used ophthalmically.

Precaution(s): Store at room temperature; avoid excessive heat (104°F).

Caution(s): Federal law restricts this drug to use by or on the order of a licensed veterinarian.

Nystatin-Neomycin Sulfate-Thiostrepton-Triamcinolone Acetonide Cream is not intended for the treatment of deep abscesses or deep seated infections such as inflammation of the lymphatic vessels. Parenteral antibiotic therapy is indicated in these infections.

Nystatin-Neomycin Sulfate-Thiostrepton-Triamcinolone Acetonide Cream has been extremely well tolerated. The occurrence of systemic reactions is rarely a problem with topical administration.

Sensitivity to neomycin may occur. If redness, irritation or swelling persists or increases, discontinue use. Do not use if pus is present since the drug may allow the infection to spread.

Avoid ingestion. Oral or parenteral use of corticosteroids, depending on dose, duration and specific steroids, may result in inhibition of endogenous steroid production following drug withdrawal. For topical use on dogs and cats.

Warning(s): Nystatin-Neomycin Sulfate-Thiostrepton-Triamcinolone Acetonide Cream is indicated for use in dogs and cats only. Not for use in animals which are raised for food.

Absorption of triamcinolone acetonide through topical application and by licking may occur. Therefore animals should be observed closely for signs of polydipsia, polyuria, and increased weight gain particularly when the preparation is used over large areas or for extended periods of time.

Clinical and experimental data have demonstrated that corticosteroids administered orally or by injection to animals may induce the first stage of parturition if used during the last trimester of pregnancy and may precipitate premature parturition followed by dystocia, fetal death, retained placenta and metritis.

Additionally, corticosteroids administered to dogs, rabbits and rodents during pregnancy have resulted in cleft palate in offspring. Corticosteroids administered to dogs during pregnancy have also resulted in other congenital anomalies including deformed forelegs, phocomelia and anasarca.

Side Effects: SAP and SGPT (ALT) enzyme elevation, polydipsia and polyuria have occurred following parenteral or systemic use of synthetic corticosteroids in dogs. Vomiting and diarrhea (occasionally bloody) have been observed in dogs. Cushing's syndrome in dogs has been reported in association with prolonged or repeated steroid therapy.

Presentation: Nystatin-Neomycin Sulfate-Thiostrepton-Triamcinolone Acetonide Cream is supplied in 7.5 gram and 15 gram tubes.

Compendium Code No.: 10270020

DERMA-VET™ OINTMENT ℞

Med-Pharmex **Topical Antimicrobial-Antifungal-Corticosteroid**

Nystatin, Neomycin Sulfate, Thiostrepton and Triamcinolone Acetonide Ointment

Active Ingredient(s): DERMA-VET™ Ointment is a combination of nystatin, neomycin sulfate, thiostrepton and triamcinolone acetonide in a non-irritating vehicle, a polyethylene and mineral oil base.

Each mL contains:

Nystatin	100,000 units
Neomycin sulfate (equivalent to neomycin base)	2.5 mg
Thiostrepton	2,500 units
Triamcinolone acetonide	1.0 mg

Indications: DERMA-VET™ Ointment is particularly useful in the treatment of acute and chronic otitis of varied etiologies, in interdigital cysts in cats and dogs, and in anal gland infections in dogs. The preparation is also indicated in the management of dermatologic disorders characterized by inflammation and dry or exudative dermatitis, particularly those caused, complicated, or threatened by bacterial or candidal *(Candida albicans)* infections. It is also of value in eczematous dermatitis, contact dermatitis, seborrheic dermatitis; and as an adjunct in the treatment of dermatitis due to parasitic infestation.

The preparation is intended for local therapy in a variety of cutaneous disorders of cats and dogs; it is especially useful in disorders caused, complicated or threatened by bacterial and/or candidal (monilial) infections.

Pharmacology: By virtue of its four active ingredients, the ointment provides four basic therapeutic effects: anti-inflammatory, antipruritic, antifungal and antibacterial. Triamcinolone acetonide is a potent synthetic corticosteroid providing rapid and prolonged symptomatic relief on topical administration. Inflammation, edema and pruritus promptly subside and lesions are permitted to heal. Nystatin is the first well tolerated anti-fungal antibiotic of dependable efficacy for the treatment of cutaneous infections caused by *Candida albicans* (monillia). Nystatin is fungistatic *in vitro* against a variety of yeast and yeast-like fungi including many fungi pathogenic to animals. No appreciable activity is exhibited against bacteria. Thiostrepton has a high order of activity against gram-positive organisms, including many which are resistant to other antibiotics; neomycin exerts antimicrobial action against a wide range of gram-positive and gram-negative bacteria. Together they provide comprehensive therapy against those organisms responsible for most superficial bacterial infections.

Dosage and Administration: Frequency of administration is dependent on the severity of the condition. For mild inflammations, application may range from once daily to once a week; for severe conditions DERMA-VET™ Ointment may be applied as often as two to three times daily, if necessary. Frequency of treatment may be decreased as improvement occurs.

Wear gloves during the administration of the ointment or wash hands immediately after application.

Otitis: Clean ear canal of impacted cerumen. Inspect canal and remove any foreign bodies such as grass awns, ticks, etc. Instill three to five drops of DERMA-VET™ Ointment.

Preliminary use of a local anesthetic such as Proparacaine Hydrochloride Ophthalmic Solution may be advisable.

Infected anal glands, cystic areas, etc.: Drain gland or cyst and then fill with DERMA-VET™ Ointment.

Other dermatologic disorders: Clean affected areas, removing any encrusted discharge or exudate. Apply DERMA-VET™ Ointment (Nystatin-Neomycin Sulfate-Thiostrepton- Triamcinolone Acetonide Ointment) sparingly in a thin film.

Precaution(s): Bottles: Do not store above 86°F. Tubes: Store at room temperature; avoid excessive heat (104°F).

Caution(s): Federal law restricts this drug to use by or on the order of a licensed veterinarian.

Before instilling any medication into the ear, examine the external ear canal thoroughly to be certain the tympanic membrane is not ruptured in order to avoid the possibility of transmitting infection to the middle ear as well as damaging the cochlea or vestibular apparatus from prolonged contact. If hearing or vestibular dysfunction is noted during the course of treatment, discontinue the use of DERMA-VET™ Ointment.

DERMA-VET™ Ointment is not intended for the treatment of deep abscesses or deep-seated infections such as inflammation of the lymphatic vessels. Parenteral antibiotic therapy is indicated in these infections.

DERMA-VET™ Ointment (Nystatin-Neomycin Sulfate-Thiostrepton-Triamcinolone Acetonide Ointment) has been extremely well tolerated. Cutaneous reactions attributable to its use have been extremely rare. The occurrence of systemic reactions is rarely a problem with topical administration.

There is some evidence that corticosteroids can be absorbed after topical application and cause systemic effects. Therefore, an animal receiving DERMA-VET™ Ointment therapy should be observed closely for signs such as polydipsia, polyuria, and increased weight gain. DERMA-VET™ Ointment is not generally recommended for the treatment of deep or puncture wounds or serious burns.

Sensitivity to neomycin may occur. If redness, irritation or swelling persists or increases, discontinue use. Do not use if pus is present since the drug may allow the infection to spread.

Avoid ingestion. Oral or parenteral use of corticosteroids (depending on dose, duration of use, and specific steroid) may result in inhibition of endogenous steroid production following drug withdrawal.

Warning(s): Keep this and all medications out of the reach of children.

Toxicology: Clinical and experimental data have demonstrated that corticosteroids administered orally or by injection to animals may induce the first stage of parturition if used during the last trimester of pregnancy and may precipitate premature parturition followed by dystocia, fetal death, retained placenta and metritis.

Additionally, corticosteroids administered to dogs, rabbits, and rodents during pregnancy have resulted in cleft palate in the offspring. In dogs, other congenital anomalies have resulted; deformed forelegs, phocomelia, and anasarca.

Side Effects: SAP and SGPT (ALT) enzyme elevations, polydypsia/polyuria, vomiting, and diarrhea (occasionally bloody) have been observed following parenteral or systemic use of synthetic corticosteroids in dogs.

Cushing's syndrome has been reported in association with prolonged or repeated steroid therapy in dogs.

Temporary hearing loss has been reported in conjunction with treatment of otitis with products containing corticosteroids. However, regression usually occurred following withdrawal of the drug. If hearing dysfunction is noted during the course of treatment with DERMA-VET™ Ointment, discontinue its use.

Presentation: DERMA-VET™ Ointment is supplied in tubes of ¼ fl oz (7.5 mL), ½ fl oz (15 mL), and 1 fl oz (30 mL), each with an elongated tip for easy application and in dispensing bottles of 8 fl oz (240 mL).

Compendium Code No.: 10270030

DERMAZOLE™ SHAMPOO ℞

Virbac **Antifungal Shampoo**

Active Ingredient(s): Contains: Miconazole 2% in a conditioning shampoo vehicle consisting of sodium C14-C16 olefin sulfonate, cocamidopropylbetain, lauramide DEA, polyquaternium 7, glycerin, DMDM hydantoin, purified water, fragrance and chlorhexidine 0.5%.

Indications: For the temporary relief of scaling due to dandruff (seborrhea) associated with infections responsive to the ingredients.

Dosage and Administration: Apply to a wet coat. Rub into the skin and coat. Lather freely. Wait 5-10 minutes and rinse well. May be used once a day or as directed by a veterinarian.

Caution(s): Federal law (USA) restricts this drug to use by or on the order of a licensed veterinarian. Keep out of the reach of children.

For external use only on dogs and cats. Avoid contact with the eyes or mucous membranes. Wash hands after using.

Presentation: 6 fl. oz. (170 mL) and 16 fl. oz. (473 mL) containers.

Compendium Code No.: 10230200

DERMCAPS®

DVM **Small Animal Dietary Supplement**

Concentrated Fatty Acid Dietary Supplement

Guaranteed Analysis: Nutritional Information (per capsule):

Crude Protein, not less than	7%
Crude Fat, not less than	90%
Crude Fiber, not more than	1%
Moisture, not more than	2%
Vitamin E	75 IU
Linoleic Acid (LA)	71%
Gamma Linolenic Acid (GLA)*	2%
Eicosapentaenoic Acid (EPA)*	4%
Docosahexaenoic Acid (DHA)*	3%

Ingredients: Safflower oil, fish oil, dl-alpha tocopheryl acetate (vitamin E), borage seed oil, gelatin, water, glycerin.

*Not recognized as an essential nutrient by the AAFCO dog or cat food nutrient profiles.

Indications: A concentrated fatty acid dietary supplement (regular strength) for use in dogs and cats (small and medium breeds).

Dosage and Administration: Recommended Amounts: One capsule per 20 lbs. of body weight per day.

Note: Capsules may be punctured and the liquid contents squeezed onto food if desired.

Precaution(s): Store the container at room temperature.

Caution(s): For animal use only.

Presentation: 645 mg capsules available in bottles of 60, 250 and 1,000.

Compendium Code No.: 11420191 Rev 0299

DERMCAPS® 10 LB.

DVM **Small Animal Dietary Supplement**

Concentrated Fatty Acid Dietary Supplement

Guaranteed Analysis: Nutritional Information (per capsule):

Crude Protein, not less than	7%
Crude Fat, not less than	90%
Crude Fiber, not more than	1%
Moisture, not more than	2%
Vitamin E	75 IU
Linoleic Acid (LA)	57%
Gamma Linolenic Acid (GLA)*	2%
Eicosapentaenoic Acid (EPA)*	4%
Docosahexaenoic Acid (DHA)*	3%

Ingredients: Safflower oil, fish oil, dl-alpha-tocopheryl acetate (vitamin E), borage seed oil, gelatin, water, glycerin.

*Not recognized as an essential nutrient by the AAFCO dog or cat food nutrient profiles.

Indications: A concentrated fatty acid dietary supplement for use in dogs and cats. For petite and miniature breeds.

Dosage and Administration: Recommended Amounts: One capsule per 10 lbs. of body weight per day.

Note: Capsules may be punctured and liquid contents squeezed onto food if desired.

Precaution(s): Store the container at room temperature.

Caution(s): For animal use only.

Presentation: Bottles of 60 (345 mg) capsules.

Compendium Code No.: 11420201 Rev 0299

DERMCAPS® 100 LB.

DVM **Small Animal Dietary Supplement**

Concentrated Fatty Acid Dietary Supplement

Guaranteed Analysis: Nutritional Information (per capsule):

Crude Protein, not less than	7%
Crude Fat, not less than	90%
Crude Fiber, not more than	1%
Moisture, not more than	2%
Vitamin E	75 IU
Linoleic Acid (LA)	36%
Gamma Linolenic Acid (GLA)*	4%
Eicosapentaenoic Acid (EPA)*	10%
Docosahexaenoic Acid (DHA)*	7%

Ingredients: Fish oil, safflower oil, borage seed oil, dl-alpha tocopheryl acetate (vitamin E), gelatin, water, glycerin.

*Not recognized as an essential nutrient by the AAFCO dog or cat food nutrient profiles.

Indications: A concentrated fatty acid dietary supplement for use in dogs and cats. For large and giant breeds.

Dosage and Administration: Recommended Amounts: One capsule per 100 lbs. of body weight per day.

Note: Capsules may be punctured and liquid contents squeezed onto food if desired.

Precaution(s): Store the container at room temperature.

Caution(s): For animal use only.

Presentation: Bottles of 60 (1480 mg) capsules.

Compendium Code No.: 11420211 Rev 0399

DERMCAPS® ECONOMY SIZE LIQUID

DVM **Small Animal Dietary Supplement**

Concentrated Fatty Acid Dietary Supplement

Guaranteed Analysis: Nutritional Information (per 0.75 mL):

Crude Protein, not less than 7%
Crude Fat, not less than 90%
Crude Fiber, not more than 1%
Moisture, not more than 2%
Vitamin E .... 35 IU
Linoleic Acid (LA) 71%
Gamma Linolenic Acid (GLA)* 2%
Eicosapentaenoic Acid (EPA)* 4%
Docosahexaenoic Acid (DHA)* 3%

Ingredients: Safflower oil, fish oil, borage seed oil, dl-alpha-tocopherol acetate (vitamin E).

*Not recognized as an essential nutrient by the AAFCO dog or cat food nutrient profiles.

Indications: A concentrated fatty acid dietary supplement for dogs and cats. Measured strength for all breed sizes.

Dosage and Administration: Recommended Amounts:

Animal Weight	Recommended Daily Amount
1-19 lbs	One-half (½) Pump
20-39 lbs	One (1) Pump**
40-59 lbs	Two (2) Pumps
60-79 lbs	Three (3) Pumps
80-100 lbs	Four (4) Pumps

**Complete depression of the pump delivers 0.75 mL DERMCAPS® Liquid.

Precaution(s): Storage: Store at room temperature.

Caution(s): For use in dogs and cats only.

Presentation: 6 fl oz (177 mL) (694 mg/0.75 mL).

Compendium Code No.: 11420221 Rev. 0399

DERMCAPS® ES

DVM **Small Animal Dietary Supplement**

Concentrated Fatty Acid Dietary Supplement

Guaranteed Analysis: Nutritional Information (per capsule):

Crude Protein, not less than 7%
Crude Fat, not less than 90%
Crude Fiber, not more than 1%
Moisture, not more than 2%
Vitamin E .... 75 IU
Linoleic Acid (LA) 52%
Gamma Linolenic Acid (GLA)* 4%
Eicosapentaenoic Acid (EPA)* 8%
Docosahexaenoic Acid (DHA)* 5%

Ingredients: Fish oil, safflower oil, borage seed oil, dl-alpha-tocopheryl acetate (vitamin E), gelatin, water, glycerin.

*Not recognized as an essential nutrient by the AAFCO dog or cat food nutrient profiles.

Indications: A concentrated fatty acid dietary supplement for dogs and cats. Extra strength for medium and large breeds.

Dosage and Administration: Recommended Amounts: One capsule per 50-70 lbs. of body weight per day.

Note: Capsules may be punctured and liquid contents squeezed onto food if desired.

Precaution(s): Store the container at room temperature.

Caution(s): For animal use only.

Presentation: 945 mg capsules available in bottles of 60, 250 and 500.

Compendium Code No.: 11420231 Rev 0299

DERMCAPS® ES LIQUID

DVM **Small Animal Dietary Supplement**

Concentrated Fatty Acid Dietary Supplement

Guaranteed Analysis:

Crude Protein, not less than 7%
Crude Fat, not less than 90%
Crude Fiber, not more than 1%
Moisture, not more than 2%

Nutritional Information (at 1.0 mL):

Vitamin E .... 46 IU
Linoleic Acid (LA) 52.0%
Gamma Linolenic Acid (GLA) 4.0%
Eicosapentaenoic Acid (EPA) 8.0%
Docosahexaenoic Acid (DHA) 6.0%

Ingredients: Fish oil, safflower oil, borage seed oil, dl-alpha-tocopheryl acetate (vitamin E).

Indications: A concentrated fatty acid dietary supplement for dogs and cats. Extra strength for medium and large breeds.

Dosage and Administration: Recommended Amounts:

Animal Weight	Recommended Daily Amount
30 lbs	0.5 mL
60 lbs	1.0 mL
90 lbs	1.5 mL

Precaution(s): Storage: Store at room temperature.

Caution(s): For animal use only.

Presentation: 2 fl oz (60 mL) (925 mg/1.0 mL) bottles.

Compendium Code No.: 11420241 Rev 0299

DERMCAPS® LIQUID

DVM **Small Animal Dietary Supplement**

Concentrated Fatty Acid Dietary Supplement

Guaranteed Analysis: Nutritional Information (at 1.0 mL):

Crude Protein, not less than 7%
Crude Fat, not less than 90%
Crude Fiber, not more than 1%
Moisture, not more than 2%
Vitamin E .... 46 IU
Linoleic Acid (LA) 71.0%
Gamma Linolenic Acid (GLA)* 2.0%
Eicosapentaenoic Acid (EPA)* 4.0%
Docosahexaenoic Acid (DHA)* 3.0%

Ingredients: Safflower oil, fish oil, borage seed oil, dl-alpha-tocopheryl acetate (vitamin E).

*Not recognized as an essential nutrient by the AAFCO dog or cat food nutrient profiles.

Indications: A concentrated fatty acid dietary supplement for dogs and cats. Regular strength for small and medium breeds.

Dosage and Administration: Recommended Amounts:

Animal Weight	Recommended Daily Amount
10 lbs	0.5 mL
20 lbs	1.0 mL
30 lbs	1.5 mL

Precaution(s): Storage: Store at room temperature.

Presentation: 2 fl oz (60 mL) (925 mg/1.0 mL) bottles.

Compendium Code No.: 11420251 Rev 0399

DESICORT™ CREME

Butler **Topical Corticosteroid**

Active Ingredient(s): Contents:

Hydrocortisone 1.0%
Zinc Oxide 40.0%

Other Ingredients: BHA, Cod Liver Oil, Lanolin, Methylparaben, Petrolatum, Talc, Deionized Water.

Indications: Aids in the treatment of minor skin irritations.

Directions: Apply to affected areas as directed by your veterinarian.

Caution(s): If redness or irritation persists after 72 hours (3 days), consult your veterinarian.

Presentation: 16 oz.

Compendium Code No.: 10820530 Iss. 5-97

DETERGEZYME®

Metrex **Detergent**

Enzymatic Presoak & Cleaning Solution

Ingredient(s): Propylene Glycol, Non-ionic Surfactants, Proteolytic Enzymes, Water and Inerts.

This neutral pH formulated solution containing surfactants, stabilizers, chelating agents and preservatives.

Indications: DETERGEZYME® is a cleaner of surgical instruments, flexible and rigid scopes and other general health care equipment.

It contains a proteolytic enzyme shown to be effective in breaking down a wide range of proteinaceous matter, including hemoglobin.

Directions for Use:

1. Manual Cleaning: One ounce (1 pump) of DETERGEZYME® per gallon of water is recommended for general purpose cleaning. Additional amounts may be required for hard-to-remove matter. DETERGEZYME® is designed to be effective in water temperatures up to 65°C (150°F). The enzyme in DETERGEZYME® may become ineffective in water temperatures exceeding this level. A minimum soak time of 10 minutes is recommended with hard-to-remove matter possibly requiring additional soak time.
2. Automatic Cleaning Units: Follow recommendations under "Manual Cleaning" except that endoscope reprocessors may require less DETERGEZYME®. For endoscope reprocessors, ultrasonic units and washer sterilizers/decontaminators, process instruments according to manufacturer's instructions.
3. Thoroughly rinse DETERGEZYME® from instruments making sure to aspirate rinse water through all channels, box locks, lumens, etc.
4. Once instruments have dried, sterilization or disinfection may follow according to appropriate procedures.
5. Fresh DETERGEZYME® solution should be prepared daily or more frequently if solution is visibly soiled. Used solution may be disposed of into sewage disposal system flushing with large quantities of water and in accordance with federal, state or local regulations.
6. Do not add other chemicals such as bleaches, peroxides or other detergents which could destroy the effectiveness of DETERGEZYME®.

Precautionary Statements: Keep out of reach of children.

Eyes: Eye irritant. Avoid contact with eyes by wearing eye protection. In case of eye contact, flush immediately with plenty of water. Get medical attention.

Skin: Avoid skin contact. Prolonged or repeated contact may cause irritation or skin sensitization. In case of skin contact, flush with water. Get medical attention if irritation occurs.

Ingestion: May be harmful if swallowed. If swallowed, drink large quantities of water or milk. Do not induce vomiting. Get medical attention.

Storage and Disposal: It is recommended that DETERGEZYME® be stored at or below room temperature of 22°C (72°F). Avoid storing at temperatures exceeding 38°C (100°F). Thoroughly rinse container before disposing.

Presentation: 4 x 1 qt bottles, 4 x 1 gallon (128 fl oz) (3.8 L) bottles, 5 gallon bottles, 15 gallon and 30 gallon drums.

Compendium Code No.: 13400050 4500-6

DEXAJECT ℞

Vetus **Corticosteroid Injection**

(Dexamethasone Solution)

ANADA No.: 200-108

Active Ingredient(s): Each mL contains 2 mg dexamethasone, 500 mg polyethylene glycol 400, 9 mg benzyl alcohol, 1.8 mg methylparaben and 0.2 mg propylparaben as preservatives, 4.75% alcohol, HCL to adjust pH to approximately 4.9, water for injection q.s.

Indications: Indicated for the treatment of primary bovine ketosis and as an anti-inflammatory agent in the bovine and equine.

As supportive therapy, dexamethasone may be used in the management of various rheumatic, allergic, dermatologic, and other diseases known to be responsive to anti-inflammatory corticosteroids.

DEXAJECT (Dexamethasone Solution) may be used intravenously as supportive therapy when an immediate hormonal response is required.

Bovine Ketosis: DEXAJECT (Dexamethasone Solution) is offered for the treatment of primary ketosis. The gluconeogenic effects of dexamethasone, when administered intramuscularly, are generally noted within the first 6 to 12 hours.

When Dexamethasone is used intravenously, the effects may be noted sooner. Blood sugar levels rise to normal levels rapidly and generally rise to above normal levels within 12 to 24 hours. Acetone bodies are reduced to normal concentrations usually within 24 hours. The physical attitude of animals treated with dexamethasone brightens and appetite improves, usually within 12 hours. Milk production, which is suppressed as a compensatory reaction in this condition, begins to increase. In some instances, it may even surpass previous peaks. The recovery process usually takes from three to seven days.

Supportive Therapy: Dexamethasone may be used as supportive therapy in mastitis, metritis, traumatic gastritis, and pyelonephritis, while appropriate primary therapy is administered. In these cases, the corticosteroid combats accompanying stress and enhances the feeling of general well-being.

Dexamethasone may also be used as supportive therapy in inflammatory conditions, such as arthritic conditions, snake bite, acute mastitis, shipping fever, pneumonia, laminitis, and retained placenta.

Equine: Dexamethasone is indicated for the treatment of acute musculoskeletal inflammations, such as bursitis, carpitis, osselets, tendonitis, myositis, and sprains. If boney changes exist in any of these conditions, joints, or accessory structures, responses to dexamethasone cannot be expected. In addition, dexamethasone may be used as supportive therapy in fatigue, heat exhaustion, influenza, laminitis, and retained placenta provided that the primary cause is determined and corrected.

Dosage and Administration: For Intravenous or Intramuscular Injection: Therapy with dexamethasone, as with any other potent corticosteroid, should be individualized according to the severity of the condition being treated, anticipated duration of steroid therapy, and the animal's threshold or tolerance for steroid excess. Treatment may be changed over to dexamethasone from any other glucocorticoid with proper reduction or adjustment of dosage.

Bovine:

DEXAJECT (Dexamethasone Solution) - 5 to 20 mg intravenously or intramuscularly.

Equine:

DEXAJECT (Dexamethasone Solution) - 2.5 to 5 mg intravenously or intramuscularly.

Contraindication(s): Except for emergency therapy, do not use in animals with chronic nephritis and hypercorticalism (Cushing's syndrome). Existence of congestive heart failure, diabetes, and osteoporosis are relative contraindications. Do not use in viral infections during the viremic stage.

Precaution(s): Store between 2° and 30°C (36° and 86°F).

Caution(s): Federal law restricts this drug to use by or on the order of a licensed veterinarian.

DEXAJECT (Dexamethasone Solution) is intended for intravenous or intramuscular administration.

Animals receiving dexamethasone should be under close observation. Because of the anti-inflammatory action of corticosteroids, signs of infection may be masked and it may be necessary to stop treatment until a further diagnosis is made. Overdosage of some glucocorticoids may result in sodium retention, fluid retention, potassium loss and weight gain.

Dexamethasone may be administered to animals with acute or chronic bacterial infections providing the infections are controlled with appropriate antibiotic or chemotherapeutic agents.

Doses greater than those recommended in horses may produce as transient drowsiness or lethargy in some horses. The lethargy usually abates in 24 hours.

Use of corticosteroids, depending on dose, duration, and specific steroid, may result in inhibition of endogenous steroid production following drug withdrawal. In patients presently receiving or recently withdrawn from systemic corticosteroid treatments, therapy with a rapidly acting corticosteroid should be considered only in unusually stressful situations.

Warning(s): Not for use in horses intended for food.

A withdrawal period has not been established for this product in pre-ruminal calves. Do not use in calves to be processed for veal.

Toxicology: Clinical and experimental data have demonstrated that corticosteroids administered orally or parenterally to animals may induce the first stage of parturition when administered during the last trimester of pregnancy and may precipitate premature parturition followed by dystocia, fetal death, retained placenta and metritis.

Additionally, corticosteroids administered to dogs, rabbits, and rodents during pregnancy have produced cleft palate. Other congenital anomalies including deformed forelegs, phocomelia, and anascara have been reported in offspring of dogs which received corticosteroids during pregnancy.

Side Effects: Corticosteroids reportedly cause laminitis in horses.

Discussion: Dexamethasone is a synthetic analogue of prednisolone, having similar but more potent anti-inflammatory therapeutic action and diversified hormonal and metabolic effects. Modification of the basic corticoid structure as achieved in dexamethasone offers enhanced anti-inflammatory effect compared to older corticosteroids. The dosage of dexamethasone required is markedly lower than that of prednisone and prednisolone. Dexamethasone is not species-specific; however, the veterinarian should read the sections on Indications, Dosage, Side Effects, Contraindications, Cautions and Toxicology before this drug is used.

Trial Data: Experimental Studies: Experimental animal studies on dexamethasone have revealed it possesses greater anti-inflammatory activity than many steroids. Veterinary clinical evidence indicates dexamethasone has approximately twenty times the anti-inflammatory activity of prednisolone and seventy to eighty times that of hydrocortisone. Thymus involution studies show dexamethasone possesses twenty-five times the activity of prednisolone. In reference to mineralcorticoid activity, dexamethasone does not cause significant sodium or water retention. Metabolic balance studies show that animals on controlled and limited protein intake will exhibit nitrogen losses on exceedingly high dosages.

Presentation: DEXAJECT (Dexamethasone Solution) 2 mg per mL is available in 100 mL multiple dose vial.

Compendium Code No.: 14440250

DEXALYTE ℞

Butler — **Electrolyte Injection**

Active Ingredient(s): Each mL contains:

Dextrose monohydrate	5 g
Sodium chloride	536 mg
Sodium gluconate	510 mg
Sodium acetate	271 mg
Potassium chloride	37 mg
Magnesium chloride $6H_2O$	42 mg

Milliequivalents per 1,000 mL:

Sodium	148 mEq
Potassium	5 mEq
Magnesium	4 mEq
Total Cations	157 mEq
Chloride	101 mEq
Gluconate	23 mEq
Acetate	33 mEq
Total Anions	157 mEq

The osmolar concentration of the solution is approximately 564 mOsm/L. The pH is approximately 6.5.

The product does not contain preservatives.

Indications: For use as an aid in the replacement of fluids and electrolytes lost due to dehydration in cattle, sheep, horses, and swine.

Dosage and Administration: May be injected intravenously, subcutaneously, or intraperitoneally (except horses) using strict aseptic procedures.

Cattle, Horses, Sheep, Swine: 2 mL to 5 mL per pound of body weight. One (1) to three (3) times a day or as required.

If administered by the subcutaneous route, divide the dosage into several sites of injection and massage the points of injection to aid in absorption and to help prevent inflammation and/or sloughing of tissue.

Precaution(s): Store at a controlled temperature between 36°-86°F (2°-30°C).

Discard the unused portion after use.

Caution(s): Federal law (U.S.A.) restricts this drug to use by or on the order of a licensed veterinarian.

For veterinary use only.

The solution should be warmed to body temperature and administered slowly (10 to 30 minutes). It is in a sterile single dose vial.

Do not administer to horses by intraperitoneal injection. Do not administer to animals with inadequate renal function.

Warning(s): Keep out of the reach of children.

Presentation: 500 mL and 1,000 mL vials.

Compendium Code No.: 10820541

DEXALYTE 8X POWDER

Butler — **Electrolytes-Oral**

NDC No.: 11695-4128-4

Active Ingredient(s):

Calcium lactate trihydrate	1.28%
Magnesium citrate soluble purified	0.65%
Potassium chloride	1.27%
Sodium chloride	9.68%
Sodium citrate dihydrate	7.36%
Dextrose monohydrate	79.76%

Indications: For use as a supplemental source of electrolytes and minerals in cattle, horses, sheep and swine.

Dosage and Administration: Mix at the rate of one (1) package (16 oz.) of DEXALYTE 8X POWDER per 40 gallons of drinking water. Prepare the amount of solution that will be consumed in 24 hours and offer free choice to animals. Prepare fresh solutions each day.

Precaution(s): Do not store above 30°C (86°F). Store in a cool, dry place.

Caution(s): The product contains citrate salts which in some cases, may be incompatible with tetracycline antibiotics. For animal use only. Keep out of the reach of children.

Presentation: 454 g (16 oz.) packages.

Compendium Code No.: 10820550

DEXAMETHASONE 2.0 MG INJECTION ℞

Vedco — **Corticosteroid Injection**

NADA No.: 099-607

Active Ingredient(s): Each mL of sterile aqueous solution contains:

Dexamethasone	2 mg
Polyethylene glycol	500 mg
Benzyl alcohol	9 mg
Methylparaben	1.8 mg
Propylparaben	0.2 mg
Alcohol	0.05 mL
Purified water, U.S.P.	q.s.

Indications: Dexamethasone is indicated for use in situations in which a rapid adrenal glucocorticoid and or anti-inflammatory effect is indicated.

Dosage and Administration: For intravenous use in horses only.

Horses: The usual intravenous dosage is 2.5 to 5 mg as the initial dosage in shock and shock-like states followed by equal maintenance doses at 1-, 3-, 6- or 10-hour intervals as determined by the condition of the patient. If a permanent corticosteroid effect is required, oral therapy with dexamethasone tablets may be substituted. When the therapy is to be withdrawn after prolonged corticosteroid administration, the daily dose should be reduced gradually over a number of days, in a stepwise, fashion.

Contraindication(s): Do not use in viral infections.

Caution(s): Federal law restricts this drug to use by or on the order of a licensed veterinarian.

Warning(s): Not for use in horses intended for food.

Presentation: 100 mL sterile, multiple dose vials.

Compendium Code No.: 10940430

DEXAMETHASONE 2 MG/ML INJECTION ℞

RXV — **Corticosteroid Injection**

NADA No.: 099-607

Active Ingredient(s): Each mL contains:

Dexamethasone	2 mg
Polyethylene glycol 400	500 mg
Benzyl alcohol	9 mg
Methylparaben	1.8 mg
Propylparaben	0.2 mg
Alcohol	0.05 mL
Water for injection	U.S.P.

Hydrochloric acid and/or sodium hydroxide used to adjust pH.

DEXAMETHASONE INJECTION

Indications: Dexamethasone is indicated for use in situations in which a rapid adrenal glucocorticoid and or anti-inflammatory effect is indicated.

Dosage and Administration: For intravenous use only.

Horses: The usual intravenous dosage is 2.5 to 5 mg in shock and shock-like states followed by equal maintenance doses at 1-, 3-, 6- or 10-hour intervals as determined by the condition of the patient.

Caution(s): Federal law restricts this drug to use by or on the order of a licensed veterinarian.

Keep out of reach of children.

For animal use only.

Warning(s): Not for use in horses intended for food.

Presentation: 100 mL sterile multiple dose vials.

Compendium Code No.: 10910040

DEXAMETHASONE INJECTION ℞

AgriLabs **Corticosteroid Injection**

Active Ingredient(s): Each mL of sterile aqueous solution contains:

Dexamethasone	2.0 mg
Polyethylene glycol 400	500 mg
Benzyl alcohol	9 mg
Methylparaben	1.8 mg
Propylparaben	0.2 mg
Alcohol	0.05 mL
Purified water, U.S.P.	q.s.

Indications: For use in horses in situations in which a rapid adrenal glucocorticoid and/or anti-inflammatory effect is indicated.

Dosage and Administration: For intravenous use only.

Horses: 2.5 to 5 mg as initial dose, equal maintenance dose 1-, 3-, 6- or 10-hour intervals as determined by the condition of the patient.

Caution(s): Federal law restricts this drug to use by or on the order of a licensed veterinarian.

Not for human use. Keep out of the reach of children.

Warning(s): Not for use in horses intended for food.

Presentation: 100 mL sterile multiple dose vials.

Compendium Code No.: 10581550

DEXAMETHASONE INJECTION ℞

Vet Tek **Corticosteroid Injection**

NADA No.: 128-089

Active Ingredient(s): Each mL of the solution contains 2 mg Dexamethasone; 50% w/v polyethylene glycol 400; 4.75% ethanol; and 0.9% w/v benzyl alcohol; 0.18% methylparaben; 0.02% propylparaben as preservatives, Hydrochloric Acid or Sodium Hydroxide to adjust pH from 4.0 to 6.0, and water for injection q.s.

Indications: Dexamethasone sterile solution is used as an anti-inflammatory agent in horses. Dexamethasone sterile solution may be administered intravenously when an immediate hormonal response is required.

Dexamethasone sterile solution is indicated for use in acute musculoskeletal conditions such as bursitis, carpitis, osselets, tendonitis, myositis and sprains. If boney changes exist in any of the above mentioned inflammatory conditions, responses to dexamethasone cannot be expected. Dexamethasone sterile solution may also be used as supportive therapy pre- and post-operatively to enhance recovery of poor surgical risks, provided that full antibiotic coverage is instituted.

Pharmacology: Description: Dexamethasone is a white or practically white, odorless, crystalline powder. It is stable in air, melts about 250°F with some decomposition. It is practically insoluble in water, sparingly soluble in acetone, in alcohol, in dioxane and in methanol; it is slightly soluble in chloroform, very slightly soluble in ether.

Action: Dexamethasone is a synthetic adrenal steroid derived from prednisolone. It has a similar but more potent anti-inflammatory action than prednisolone by modification of the side groups of the basic corticoid structure. As an anti-inflammatory agent, dexamethasone is about 20 times as potent as prednisolone and about 70 to 80 times as potent as hydrocortisone. With respect to mineralcorticoid activity, dexamethasone is less likely to cause sodium and water retention as the older corticosteroids.

Dosage and Administration: Dexamethasone sterile solution may be used for intramuscular or intravenous injection.

Dexamethasone dosage should be individualized according to the severity of the condition being treated and the animal's threshold or tolerance for steroid excess. Dexamethasone sterile solution is not species specific. The following dosage schedule may be followed.

Equine - 2.5 mg to 5 mg intramuscularly or intravenously. The dose may be repeated for 3 to 5 days.

If condition being treated is of a chronic nature, dexamethasone oral dosage forms may be administered for maintenance therapy. When therapy is to be withdrawn after prolonged corticosteroid administration, the daily dose should be reduced gradually over a number of days in a stepwise fashion.

Contraindication(s): Use of dexamethasone is contraindicated in tuberculosis and peptic ulcers. Except for emergency therapy, do not use in animals with chronic nephritis and hypercorticalism (Cushing syndrome). Existence of congestive heart failure, diabetes and osteoporosis are relative contraindications. Do not use in viral infections.

Overdosage of some glucocorticoids may result in sodium retention, fluid retention, potassium loss and weight gain.

Precaution(s): Store at 2°C-30°C (36°F-86°F).

Caution(s): Federal law restricts this drug to use by or on the order of a licensed veterinarian.

Clinical and experimental data have demonstrated that corticosteroids administered orally or parenterally to animals may induce the first stage of parturition when administered during the last trimester of pregnancy and may precipitate premature parturition followed by dystocia, fetal death, retained placenta, and metritis.

Additionally, corticosteroids administered to dogs, rabbits and rodents during pregnancy have produced cleft palate. Other congenital anomalies including deformed forelegs, phocomelia, and anasarca have been reported in offspring of dogs which received corticosteroids during pregnancy.

Animals receiving dexamethasone should be under close observation. The injudicious use of adrenal hormones in animals can be hazardous. Signs of infection may be masked from anti-inflammatory action of corticosteroids and it may be necessary to stop treatment until a further diagnosis is made.

Dexamethasone sterile solution may be administered to animals with acute or chronic bacterial infection, providing the infections are controlled with the appropriate anti-infective agents.

Horses administered greater than recommended doses may exhibit a transient drowsiness or lethargy. The lethargy usually abates in 24 hours.

Use of corticosteroids, depending on dose, duration, and specific steroid, may result in inhibition of endogenous steroid production following drug withdrawal. In patients presently receiving or recently withdrawn from systemic corticosteroid treatments, therapy with a rapidly acting corticosteroid should be considered in unusually stressful situations.

For animal use only.

Not for human use.

Warning(s): Not for use in horses intended for food use.

Keep out of reach of children.

Side Effects: Use of synthetic corticosteroids may induce such side effects as weight loss, anorexia, diarrhea and polyuria. The intra-articular injection of dexamethasone may lead to osseous metaplasia.

SAP AND SGPT (ALT) enzyme elevations, polydypsia and polyuria have occurred following parenteral or systemic use of synthetic corticosteroids in dogs. Vomiting and diarrhea (occasionally bloody) have been observed in dogs.

Cushing's syndrome in dogs has been reported in association with prolonged or repeated steroid therapy.

Corticosteroids reportedly cause laminitis in horses.

Presentation: 100 mL (3.4 fl oz) multiple dose vials (NDC 60270-309-10).

Manufactured by: Sanofi Animal Health, Inc., a subsidiary of Sanofi, Inc., Overland Park, KS 66210.

Compendium Code No.: 14200051 7/95

DEXAMETHASONE SODIUM PHOSPHATE ℞

Phoenix Pharmaceutical **Corticosteroid Injection**

4 mg/mL Injection

NADA No.: 123-815

Active Ingredient(s): Each mL of sterile aqueous solution contains: Dexamethasone sodium phosphate, 4 mg; sodium citrate, 10 mg; sodium bisulfite, 2 mg; benzyl alcohol, 1.5%; sodium hydroxide and/or hydrochloric acid to adjust pH; water for injection, q.s.

Indications: DEXAMETHASONE SODIUM PHOSPHATE is indicated for use as an anti-inflammatory or glucocorticoid agent in conditions as acute arthritis.

DSP may be used as supportive therapy in non-specific dermatoses such as summer eczema and atopy, provided proper therapy is also instituted to correct the cause of the underlying dermatosis. It may also be used prior to or after surgery to enhance recovery of poor surgical risks, provided that it is used in conjunction with full antibiotic coverage.

Pharmacology: DEXAMETHASONE SODIUM PHOSPHATE (DSP) is a salt of dexamethasone, a synthetic corticosteroid which possesses glucocorticoid activity. DSP is a white or slightly yellow crystalline powder which is particularly suitable for intravenous administration because it is highly water soluble.

Actions: Dexamethasone as a steroid is equivalent in potency to some established steroids and considerably more potent than others. In the case of the dog, dexamethasone is approximately equivalent in dosage to prednisone, but about 30 to 40 times more potent that prednisolone. DSP is especially well suited for intravenous use in situations requiring a rapid and intense glucocorticoid and/or anti-inflammatory effect.

Dosage and Administration: For intravenous use only.

Dogs: 0.25 to 1 mg intravenously as the initial dosage. (Based on 3 mg per mL of dexamethasone). The dose may be repeated for three to five days or until a response is noted.

Horses: 2.5 to 5 mg intravenously. (Based on 3 mg per mL of dexamethasone). If permanent corticosteroid effect is required, oral therapy with dexamethasone may be substituted. When therapy is to be withdrawn after prolonged corticosteroid administration, the daily dose should be reduced gradually over a number of days, in a stepwise fashion.

Contraindication(s): Do not use in viral infections. Except when used for emergency therapy, DSP is contraindicated in animals with tuberculosis, chronic nephritis, Cushing's disease and peptic ulcers. Existence of congestive heart failure, osteoporosis and diabetes are relative contraindications.

When administered in the presence of infections, appropriate antibacterial agents should also be administered and continued for at least 3 days after discontinuance of the steroid.

Precaution(s): Store between 15°C and 30°C (59°F and 86°F).

Caution(s): Federal law restricts this drug to use by or on the order of a licensed veterinarian.

Clinical and experimental data have demonstrated that corticosteroids administered orally or parenterally to animals may induce the first stage of parturition when administered during the last trimester of pregnancy and may precipitate premature parturition followed by dystocia, fetal death, retained placenta and metritis. Additionally, corticosteroids administered in dogs, rabbits, and rodents during pregnancy have resulted in cleft palate in offspring. Corticosteroids administered to dogs during pregnancy have also resulted in other congenital anomalies, including deformed forelegs.

Because of the anti-inflammatory action of corticosteroids, signs of infection may be hidden. It may therefore be necessary to stop treatment until diagnosis is made. Overdosage of some glucocorticoids may result in sodium and fluid retention, potassium loss and weight gains.

In infections characterized by overwhelming toxicity, DSP therapy in conjunction with indicated antibacterial therapy is effective in reducing mortality and morbidity. It is essential that the causative organism be known and an effective anti-bacterial agent be administered concurrently. The injudicious use of adrenal hormones in animals with infections can be hazardous.

Use of corticosteroids, depending on dose, duration and specific steroid, may result in inhibition of endogenous steroid production following drug withdrawal. In patients presently receiving or recently withdrawn from systemic steroid treatments, therapy with a rapid acting corticosteroid should be considered in unusually stressful situations.

Warning(s): Do not use in horses intended for food.

Keep out of reach of children.

Adverse Reactions: The therapeutic use of DSP is unlikely to cause undesired accentuation of metabolic effects. However, if continued corticosteroid therapy is anticipated, a high protein intake should be provided to keep the animal in positive nitrogen balance. A retardant effect on wound healing should be considered when it is used in conjunction with surgery. Euphoria, or an improvement of attitude, and increased appetite are the usual manifestations. The intra-articular injection in leg injuries in the horse may lead to osseous metaplasia.

Side reactions such as glycosuria, hyperglycemia, diarrhea, polydipsia and polyuria have been observed in some species.

- Elevated levels of SGPT and SAP
- Vomiting and diarrhea (occasionally bloody)
- Cushing's syndrome in dogs has been reported in association with prolonged or repeated steroid therapy.
- Corticosteroids reportedly cause laminitis in horses.

Presentation: DEXAMETHASONE SODIUM PHOSPHATE Injection is supplied in 30 mL (NDC 57319-473-03) and 100 mL (NDC 57319-473-05) vials containing 4 mg of dexamethasone sodium phosphate per mL. (Equivalent to 3 mg per mL of dexamethasone).
Manufactured by: Phoenix Scientific, Inc., St. Joseph, MO 64503.
Compendium Code No.: 12561181 Iss. 3-02 / Iss. 2-02

DEXAMETHASONE SODIUM PHOSPHATE INJECTION ℞

Butler **Corticosteroid Injection**

NADA No.: 099-604
Active Ingredient(s): Each mL of sterile aqueous solution contains:

Dexamethasone sodium phosphate .... 4 mg
Sodium citrate .... 10 mg
Sodium bisulfite .... 2.0 mg
Benzyl alcohol 1.5%

Sodium hydroxide is used to adjust the pH to 7.5-8.5. Also contains purified water, U.S.P.
Indications: Dexamethasone sodium phosphate is indicated for use in situations in which a rapid adrenal glucocorticoid and/or anti-inflammatory effect is indicated.
Dosage and Administration: For intravenous use only.
Horses: The usual intravenous dose is 2.5 to 5 mg.
If a permanent corticosteroid effect is required, oral therapy with dexamethasone tablets may be substituted. When therapy is to be withdrawn after prolonged corticosteroid administration, the daily dose should be reduced gradually over a number of days, in a stepwise fashion.
Precaution(s): Do not store above 25°C (77°F).
Caution(s): Federal law restricts this drug to use by or on the order of a licensed veterinarian.
For animal use only.
Because of the anti-inflammatory action of corticosteroid signs of infection may be hidden and it may be necessary to stop treatment until a diagnosis is made. The overdosage of some glucocorticoids may result in sodium retention, fluid retention, potassium loss and weight gains.
In infections characterized by overwhelming toxicity, dexamethasone sodium phosphate therapy in conjunction with indicated antibacterial therapy is effective in reducing mortality and morbidity. It is essential that the causative organism be known and an effective antibacterial agent be administered concurrently. The injudicious use of adrenal hormones in animals with infections can be hazardous.
The use of corticosteroids, depending upon the dose, duration, and specific steroid may result in inhibition of endogenous steroid production following drug withdrawal. In patients presently receiving or recently withdrawn from systemic corticosteroid treatments, therapy with rapidly active corticosteroids should be considered only in unusually stressful situations.
Clinical and experimental data have demonstrated that corticosteroids administered orally or parenterally to animals may induce the first stage of parturition when administered during the last trimester of pregnancy and may precipitate premature parturition followed by dystocia, fetal death, retained placenta and metritis.
Additionally, corticosteroids administered to dogs, rabbits and rodents during pregnancy have resulted in cleft palate in offspring. Corticosteroids administered to dogs during pregnancy have also resulted in other congenital anomalies including deformed forelegs, phocomelia and anasarca.
Warning(s): Not for use in horses intended for food.
Presentation: 100 mL sterile multiple dose vial.
Compendium Code No.: 10820560

DEXAMETHASONE SODIUM PHOSPHATE INJECTION ℞

Vedco **Corticosteroid Injection**

NADA No.: 099-604
Active Ingredient(s): Each mL of sterile aqueous solution contains:

Dexamethasone sodium phosphate .... 4 mg
Sodium citrate .... 10 mg
Sodium bisulfite .... 2.0 mg
Benzyl alcohol 1.5%
Sodium hydroxide to adjust the pH to 7.5-8.5
Purified water, U.S.P. .... q.s.

Indications: Dexamethasone sodium phosphate is indicated for use in situations in which a rapid adrenal glucocorticoid and/or anti-inflammatory effect is indicated. It is suitable for intravenous administration because it is highly water soluble, permitting administration of relatively large doses in a small volume of diluent. It is designed for intravenous use in situations requiring a rapid and intense glucocorticoid and/or anti-inflammatory effect.
Dosage and Administration: For intravenous use only.
Horses: The usual intravenous dosage is 2.5 to 5 mg. If a permanent corticosteroid effect is required, oral therapy with dexamethasone tablets may be substituted. When the therapy is to be withdrawn after prolonged corticosteroid administration, the daily dose should be reduced gradually over a number of days, in a stepwise fashion.
Contraindication(s): Do not use in viral infections. Except when used for emergency therapy, dexamethasone sodium phosphate is contraindicated in animals with tuberculosis and chronic nephritis. Existence of congestive heart failure and osteoporosis are relative contraindications. In the presence of infection, appropriate antibacterial agents should also be administered and should be continued for at least three days after discontinuance of the hormone and the disappearance of all signs of infection.
Precaution(s): Do not store above 25°C (77°F).
Caution(s): Federal law restricts this drug to use by or on the order of a licensed veterinarian.
Clinical and experimental data have demonstrated that corticosteroids administered orally or parenterally to animals may induce the first stage of parturition when administered during the last trimester of pregnancy and may precipitate premature parturition followed by dystocia, fetal death, retained placenta and metritis.
Because of the anti-inflammatory action of corticosteroids, signs of infection may be hidden and it may be necessary to stop treatment until a diagnosis is made. Overdosage of some glucocorticoids may result in sodium retention, fluid retention, potassium loss and weight gains. In infections characterized by overwhelming toxicity, dexamethasone sodium phosphate therapy in conjunction with indicated antibacterial therapy is effective in reducing mortality and morbidity. It is essential that the causative organism be known and an effective antibacterial agent be administered concurrently. The injudicious use of adrenal hormones in animals with infections can be hazardous. The use of corticosteroids, depending upon the dose, duration, and specific steroid, may result in the inhibition of endogenous steroid production following drug withdrawal. In patients presently receiving or recently withdrawn from systemic corticosteroid treatments, therapy with a rapidly acting corticosteroid should be considered only in unusually stressful situations.
Warning(s): Not for use in horses intended for food.
Presentation: 100 mL sterile multiple dose vials.
Compendium Code No.: 10940441

DEXAMETHASONE SOLUTION ℞

Aspen **Corticosteroid Injection**

Dexamethasone Solution (2 mg/mL)
ANADA No.: 200-108
Active Ingredient(s): Each mL contains 2 mg dexamethasone, 500 mg polyethylene glycol 400, 9 mg benzyl alcohol, 1.8 mg methylparaben and 0.2 mg propylparaben as preservatives, 4.75% alcohol, HCl to adjust pH to approximately 4.9, water for injection q.s.
Indications: Dexamethasone Solution is indicated for the treatment of primary bovine ketosis and as an anti-inflammatory agent in the canine, feline, bovine and equine.
As supportive therapy, dexamethasone may be used in the management of various rheumatic, allergic, dermatologic, and other diseases known to be responsive to anti-inflammatory corticosteroids.
Dexamethasone Solution may be used intravenously as supportive therapy when an immediate hormonal response is required.
Dosage and Administration: Therapy with dexamethasone, as with any other potent corticosteroid, should be individualized according to the severity of the condition being treated, anticipated duration of steroid therapy, and the animal's threshold or tolerance for steroid excess.
Treatment may be changed over to dexamethasone from any other glucocorticoid with proper reduction or adjustment of dosage.
Bovine - Dexamethasone Solution - 5 to 20 mg intravenously or intramuscularly.
Equine - Dexamethasone Solution - 2.5 to 5 mg intravenously or intramuscularly.
Canine - Dexamethasone Solution - 0.25 to 1 mg intravenously or intramuscularly. The dose may be repeated for three to five days.
Feline - Dexamethasone Solution - 0.125 to 0.5 mg intravenously or intramuscularly. The dose may be repeated for three to five days.
Contraindication(s): Except for emergency therapy, do not use in animals with chronic nephritis and hypercorticalism (Cushing's syndrome). Existence of congestive heart failure, diabetes, and osteoporosis are relative contraindications. Do not use in viral infections during the viremic stage.
Precaution(s): Store between 2° and 30°C (36° and 86°F).
Caution(s): Federal law restricts this drug to use by or on the order of a licensed veterinarian.
Animals receiving dexamethasone should be under close observation. Because of the anti-inflammatory action of corticosteroids, signs of infection may be masked and it may be necessary to stop treatment until a further diagnosis is made. Overdosage of some glucocorticoids may result in sodium retention, fluid retention, potassium loss, and weight gain.
Dexamethasone may be administered to animals with acute or chronic bacterial infections providing the infections are controlled with appropriate antibiotic or chemotherapeutic agents.
Doses greater than those recommended in horses may produce a transient drowsiness or lethargy in some horses.
Use of corticosteroids, depending on dose, duration, and specific steroid, may result in inhibition of endogenous steroid production following drug withdrawal. In patients presently receiving or recently withdrawn from systemic corticosteroid treatments, therapy with a rapidly acting corticosteroid should be considered in unusually stressful situations.
Warning(s): A withdrawal period has not been established for this product in pre-ruminant calves. Do not use in calves to be processed for veal.
Toxicology: Clinical and experimental data have demonstrated that corticosteroids administered orally or parenterally to animals may induce the first stage of parturition when administered during the last trimester of pregnancy and may precipitate parturition followed by dystocia, fetal death, retained placenta, and metritis.
Additionally, corticosteroids administered to dogs, rabbits, and rodents during pregnancy have produced cleft palate. Other congenital anomalies including deformed forelegs, phocomelia, and anascara have been reported in offspring of dogs which received corticosteroids during pregnancy.
Side Effects: Side effects, such as SAP and SGPT enzyme elevations, weight loss, anorexia, polydipsia, and polyuria have occurred following the use of synthetic corticosteroids in dogs. Vomiting and diarrhea (occasionally bloody) have been observed in dogs and cats.
Cushing's syndrome in dogs has been reported in association with prolonged or repeated steroid therapy.
Corticosteroids reportedly cause laminitis in horses.
Discussion: Dexamethasone is a synthetic analogue of prednisolone, having similar but more potent anti-inflammatory therapeutic action and diversified hormonal and metabolic effects. Modification of the basic corticoid structure as achieved in dexamethasone offers enhanced anti-inflammatory effect compared to older corticosteroids. The dosage of dexamethasone required is markedly lower than that of prednisone and prednisolone.
Dexamethasone is not species-specific; however, the veterinarian should read the information included here before the drug is used.
Dexamethasone Solution is intended for intravenous or intramuscular administration.
Bovine Ketosis
Dexamethasone Solution is offered for the treatment of primary ketosis. The glucogenic effects of dexamethasone, when administered intramuscularly, are generally noted within the first 6 to 12 hours. When Dexamethasone Solution is used intravenously the effects may be noted sooner. Blood sugar levels rise to normal levels rapidly and generally rise to above normal levels within 12 to 24 hours. Acetone bodies are reduced to normal concentrations usually within 24 hours. The physical attitude of animals treated with dexamethasone brightens and appetite improves, usually within 12 hours. Milk production, which is suppressed as a compensatory reaction in this condition, begins to increase. In some instances, it may even surpass previous peaks. The recovery process usually takes from three to seven days.
Supportive Therapy
Dexamethasone may be used as supportive therapy in mastitis, metritis, traumatic gastritis, and pyelonephritis, while appropriate primary therapy is administered. In these cases, the corticosteroid combats accompanying stress and enhances the feeling of general well-being.
Dexamethasone may also be used as supportive therapy in inflammatory conditions, such as arthritic conditions, snake bite, acute mastitis, shipping fever, pneumonia laminitis, and retained placenta.
Equine
Dexamethasone is indicated for the treatment of acute musculoskeletal inflammations, such as bursitis, carpitis, osselets, tendonitis, myositis, and sprains. If boney changes exist in any of

these conditions, joints, or accessory structures, responses to dexamethasone cannot be expected. In addition, dexamethasone may be used as supportive therapy in fatigue, heat exhaustion, influenza, laminitis, and retained placenta provided that the primary cause is determined and corrected.

Canine and Feline

Dexamethasone as supportive therapy may be used in nonspecific dermatosis such as summer eczema and atopy. Primary etiology should be determined and therapy instituted to correct it. The pruritis accompanying these conditions usually subsides within a few hours, followed by regression of inflammatory lesions.

Dexamethasone may be used as supportive therapy and pre-and post-operatively to enhance recovery of poor surgical risks, provided that full antibiotic coverage is instituted.

Dexamethasone, as supportive therapy, may be used in inflammatory conditions such as acute arthritic conditions. If boney changes exist, response to dexamethasone cannot be expected. Dexamethasone may be used as supportive therapy in canine posterior paresis.

D

Trial Data: Experimental animal studies on dexamethasone have revealed it possesses greater anti-inflammatory activity than many steroids. Veterinary clinical evidence indicates dexamethasone has approximately twenty times the anti-inflammatory activity of prednisolone and seventy to eighty times that of hydrocortisone. Thymus involution studies show dexamethasone possesses twenty-five times the activity of prednisolone. In reference to mineralocorticoid activity, dexamethasone does not cause significant sodium or water retention. Metabolic balance studies show that animals on controlled and limited protein intake will exhibit nitrogen losses on exceedingly high dosages.

Presentation: 100 mL multiple dose vial.

Compendium Code No.: 14750270

DEXAMETHASONE SOLUTION ℞

Butler **Corticosteroid Injection**

ANADA No.: 200-108

Active Ingredient(s): Each mL contains: 2 mg dexamethasone, 500 mg polyethylene glycol 400, 9 mg benzyl alcohol, 1.8 mg methyl paraben and 0.2 mg propylparaben, as preservatives, 4.75% alcohol, HCl to adjust pH to approximately 4.9, water for injection.

Indications: For use in situations in which a rapid adrenal glucocorticoid and or anti-inflammatory effect is desirable.

Dosage and Administration:

Bovine: .... 5 to 20 mg

Equine: .... 2.5 to 5 mg

For intravenous or intramuscular injection.

Precaution(s): Store between 2°C and 30°C (36°F-86°F).

Caution(s): Federal law restricts this drug to use by or on the order of a licensed veterinarian.

Warning(s): A withdrawal period has not been established for this product in pre-ruminating calves. Do not use in calves to be processed for veal.

Presentation: 100 mL sterile, multiple dose vials.

Compendium Code No.: 10820570

DEXAMETHASONE SOLUTION ℞

Phoenix Pharmaceutical **Corticosteroid Injection**

2 mg/mL

ANADA No.: 200-108

Active Ingredient(s): Each mL contains 2 mg dexamethasone, 500 mg polyethylene glycol 400, 9 mg benzyl alcohol, 1.8 mg methylparaben and 0.2 mg propylparaben as preservatives, 4.75% alcohol, HCl to adjust pH to approximately 4.9, water for injection q.s.

Indications: DEXAMETHASONE SOLUTION is indicated for the treatment of primary bovine ketosis and as an anti-inflammatory agent in the bovine and equine.

As supportive therapy, dexamethasone may be used in the management of various rheumatic, allergic, dermatologic, and other diseases known to be responsive to anti-inflammatory corticosteroids.

DEXAMETHASONE SOLUTION may be used intravenously as supportive therapy when an immediate hormonal response is required.

Bovine Ketosis: DEXAMETHASONE SOLUTION is offered for the treatment of primary ketosis. The gluconeogenic effects of dexamethasone, when administered intramuscularly, are generally noted within the first 6 to 12 hours. When DEXAMETHASONE SOLUTION is used intravenously, the effects may be noted sooner. Blood sugar levels rise to normal levels rapidly and generally rise to above normal levels within 12 to 24 hours. Acetone bodies are reduced to normal concentrations usually within 24 hours. The physical attitude of animals treated with dexamethasone brightens and appetite improves, usually within 12 hours. Milk production, which is suppressed as a compensatory reaction in this condition, begins to increase. In some instances, it may even surpass previous peaks. The recovery process usually takes from three to seven days.

Supportive Therapy: Dexamethasone may be used as supportive therapy in mastitis, metritis, traumatic gastritis, and pyelonephritis, while appropriate primary therapy is administered. In these cases, the corticosteroid combats accompanying stress and enhances the feeling of general well-being.

Dexamethasone may also be used as supportive therapy in inflammatory conditions, such as arthritic conditions, snake bite, acute mastitis, shipping fever, pneumonia, laminitis, and retained placenta.

Equine: Dexamethasone is indicated for the treatment of acute musculoskeletal inflammations, such as bursitis, carpitis, osselets, tendonitis, myositis, and sprains. If boney changes exist in any of these conditions, joints, or accessory structures, responses to dexamethasone cannot be expected. In addition, dexamethasone may be used as supportive therapy in fatigue, heat exhaustion, influenza, laminitis, and retained placenta provided that the primary cause is determined and corrected.

Pharmacology: Description: Dexamethasone is a synthetic analogue of prednisolone, having similar but more potent anti-inflammatory therapeutic action and diversified hormonal and metabolic effects. Modification of the basic corticoid structure as achieved in dexamethasone offers enhanced anti-inflammatory effect compared to older corticosteroids. The dosage of dexamethasone required is markedly lower than that of prednisone and prednisolone. Dexamethasone is not species-specific; however, the veterinarian should read the sections on Indications, Dosage, Side Effects, Contraindications, Cautions and Toxicology before this drug is used.

Dosage and Administration: DEXAMETHASONE SOLUTION is intended for intravenous or intramuscular administration.

Therapy with dexamethasone as with any other potent corticosteroid, should be individualized according to the severity of the condition being treated, anticipated duration of steroid therapy, and the animal's threshold or tolerance for steroid excess.

Treatment may be changed over to dexamethasone from any other glucocorticoid with proper reduction or adjustment of dosage.

Bovine:

DEXAMETHASONE SOLUTION - 5 to 20 mg intravenously or intramuscularly.

Equine:

DEXAMETHASONE SOLUTION - 2.5 to 5 mg intravenously or intramuscularly.

Contraindication(s): Except for emergency therapy, do not use in animals with chronic nephritis and hypercorticalism (Cushing's syndrome). Existence of congestive heart failure, diabetes, and osteoporosis are relative contraindications. Do not use in viral infections during the viremic stage.

Precaution(s): Store between 2° and 30°C (36° and 86°F).

Caution(s): Federal law restricts this drug to use by or on the order of a licensed veterinarian.

Animals receiving dexamethasone should be under close observation. Because of the anti-inflammatory action of corticosteroids, signs of infection may be masked and it may be necessary to stop treatment until further diagnosis is made. Overdosage of some glucocorticoids may result in sodium retention, fluid retention, potassium loss, and weight gain.

Dexamethasone may be administered to animals with acute or chronic bacterial infections providing the infections are controlled with appropriate antibiotic or chemotherapeutic agents.

Doses greater than those recommended in horses may produce a transient drowsiness or lethargy in some horses. The lethargy usually abates in 24 hours.

Use of corticosteroids, depending on dose, duration, and specific steroid, may result in inhibition of endogenous steroid production following drug withdrawal. In patients presently receiving or recently withdrawn from systemic corticosteroid treatments, therapy with a rapidly acting corticosteroid should be considered in unusually stressful situations.

Warning(s): A withdrawal period has not been established for this product in preruminal calves. Do not use in calves to be processed for veal.

Toxicology: Clinical and experimental data have demonstrated that corticosteroids administered orally or parenterally to animals may induce the first stage of parturition when administered during the last trimester of pregnancy and may precipitate parturition followed by dystocia, fetal death, retained placenta, and metritis.

Additionally, corticosteroids administered to dogs, rabbits, and rodents during pregnancy have produced cleft palate. Other congenital anomalies including deformed forelegs, phocomelia, and anascara have been reported in offspring of dogs which received corticosteroids during pregnancy.

Side Effects: Corticosteroids reportedly cause laminitis in horses.

Trial Data: Experimental Studies: Experimental animal studies on dexamethasone have revealed it possesses greater anti-inflammatory activity than many steroids. Veterinary clinical evidence indicates dexamethasone has approximately twenty times the anti-inflammatory activity of prednisolone and seventy to eighty times that of hydrocortisone. Thymus involution studies show dexamethasone possesses twenty-five times the activity of prednisolone. In reference to mineral-corticoid activity, dexamethasone does not cause significant sodium or water retention. Metabolic balance studies show that animals on controlled and limited protein intake will exhibit nitrogen losses on exceedingly high dosages.

Presentation: DEXAMETHASONE SOLUTION, 2 mg per mL, 100 mL multiple dose vial (NDC 57319-243-05).

Manufactured by: Phoenix Scientific, Inc., St. Joseph, MO 64503.

Compendium Code No.: 12560202 Rev. 10-01

DEXASONE ℞

RXV **Corticosteroid Injection**

Active Ingredient(s): Each mL contains:

Dexamethasone .... 2 mg

Polyethylene glycol 400 .... 500 mg

Benzyl alcohol .... 9 mg

Methylparaben .... 1.8 mg

Propylparaben .... 0.2 mg

Alcohol .... 0.05 mL

Water for injection, U.S.P. .... q.s.

Hydrochloric acid and/or sodium hydroxide used to adjust pH.

Indications: Dexamethasone is indicated for use in situations in which a rapid adrenal glucocorticoid and or anti-inflammatory effect is indicated.

Dosage and Administration: For intravenous use in horses only.

The usual intravenous dosage is 2.5 to 5 mg as the initial dosage in shock and shock-like states followed by equal maintenance doses at 1-, 3-, 6- or 10-hour intervals as determined by the condition of the patient. If a permanent corticosteroid effect is required, oral therapy with dexamethasone tablets may be substituted. When therapy is to be withdrawn after prolonged corticosteroid administration, the daily dose should be reduced gradually over a number of days, in a stepwise fashion.

Contraindication(s): Do not use in viral infections.

Caution(s): Federal law restricts this drug to use by or on the order of a licensed veterinarian.

For animal use only.

Keep out of the reach of children.

Warning(s): Not for use in horses intended for food.

Presentation: 100 mL sterile, multiple dose vials.

Compendium Code No.: 10910050

DEXAZONE™ 2 MG ℞

Bimeda **Corticosteroid Injection**

NADA No.: 099-607

Active Ingredient(s): Each mL of sterile aqueous solution contains:

Dexamethasone .... 2 mg

Polyethylene glycol 400 .... 500 mg

Benzyl alcohol .... 9 mg

Methylparaben .... 1.8 mg

Propylparaben .... 0.2 mg

Alcohol .... 0.05 mL

Water for injection .... q.s.

Hydrochloric acid and/or sodium hydroxide are used to adjust pH.

Indications: Dexamethasone, a synthetic corticosteroid, is indicated for use in situations in which a rapid adrenal glucocorticoid and or anti-inflammatory effect is indicated.

Dosage and Administration: For intravenous use only.

Horses: The usual initial intravenous dose is 2.5 to 5 mg in shock and shock-like states followed by equal maintenance doses at 1-, 3-, 6- or 10-hour intervals as determined by the condition of the patient.

If a permanent corticosteroid effect is required, oral therapy with dexamethasone tablets may be substituted. When therapy is to be withdrawn after prolonged corticosteroid administration, the daily dose should be reduced gradually over a number of days, in a stepwise fashion.

Contraindication(s): Do not use in viral infections. Except when used for emergency therapy, dexamethasone is contraindicated in animals with tuberculosis, and chronic nephritis, Cushing's disease and peptic ulcer. Existence of congestive heart failure, osteoporosis and diabetes are relative contraindications.

In the presence of infection, appropriate antibacterial agents should also be administered and should be continued for at least three days after discontinuance of the hormone and disappearance of all signs of infection.

Caution(s): Because of the anti-inflammatory action of corticosteroids, signs of infection may be hidden and it may be necessary to stop treatment until a diagnosis is made. The overdosage of some glucocorticoids may result in sodium retention, fluid retention, potassium loss and weight gains.

In infections characterized by overwhelming toxicity, dexamethasone therapy in conjunction with indicated antibacterial therapy is effective in reducing mortality and morbidity. It is essential that the causative organism be known and an effective antibacterial agent be administered concurrently. The injudicious use of adrenal hormones in animals with infections can be hazardous. The use of corticosteroids, depending upon the dose, duration, and specific steroid, may result in inhibition of endogenous steroid production following drug withdrawal. In patients presently receiving or recently withdrawn from systemic corticosteroid treatments, therapy with a rapidly acting corticosteroid should be considered only in unusually stressful situations.

Clinical and experimental data have demonstrated that corticosteroids administered orally or parenterally to animals may induce the first stage of parturition when administered during the last trimester of pregnancy and may precipitate premature parturition followed by dystocia, fetal death, retained placenta and metritis.

Additionally, corticosteroids administered to dogs, rabbits, and rodents during pregnancy have resulted in cleft palate in offspring. Corticosteroids administered to dogs during pregnancy have also resulted in other congenital anomalies, including deformed forelegs, phocomelia, and anasarca.

Federal law restricts this drug to use by or on the order of a licensed veterinarian.

Warning(s): Not for use in horses intended for food.

Side Effects: The therapeutic use of dexamethasone is unlikely to cause undesired accentuation of metabolic effects. However, if continued corticosteroid therapy is anticipated, a high protein intake should be provided to keep the animal in positive nitrogen balance. A retardant effect on wound healing has not been encountered, but such a possibility should also be considered when it is used in conjunction with surgery. Euphoria or an improvement in attitude, and increased appetite are usual manifestations.

Side reactions such as glycosuria, hyperglycemia, diarrhea, polydipsia and polyuria have been observed in some species. Corticosteroids reportedly cause laminitis in horses.

Presentation: 100 mL vials.

Compendium Code No.: 13990121

DEXOLYTE SOLUTION ℞

Phoenix Pharmaceutical — **Electrolyte Injection**

Injection-Electrolytes-Dextrose

Active Ingredient(s): Composition: Each 500 mL of sterile aqueous solution contains:

Dextrose • H_2O	12.50 g
Sorbitol	12.50 g
Sodium Lactate	3.95 g
Sodium Chloride	2.40 g
Potassium Chloride	0.37 g
Magnesium Chloride • $6H_2O$	0.21 g
Calcium Chloride • $2H_2O$	0.19 g

Milliequivalents per liter:

Cations:	
Sodium	153 mEq/L
Potassium	9 mEq/L
Calcium	6 mEq/L
Magnesium	4 mEq/L
Anions:	
Chloride	101 mEq/L
Lactate	71 mEq/L
Osmolarity (calc.)	617 mOsmol/L

This product contains no preservatives.

Indications: For use in conditions associated with fluid and electrolyte loss, such as dehydration, shock, vomiting and diarrhea, particularly when an immediate source of energy is also indicated.

Dosage and Administration: Warm solution to body temperature and administer slowly (10 to 30 mL per minute) by intravenous or intraperitoneal injection, using strict aseptic procedures.

Adult Cattle and Horses: 1000 to 2000 mL

Calves, Ponies and Foals: 500 to 1000 mL

Adult Sheep and Swine: 500 to 1000 mL

These are suggested dosages. The actual amount and rate of fluid administration must be judged by the veterinarian in relation to the condition being treated and the clinical response of the animal, being careful to avoid overhydration.

Contraindication(s): Do not administer intraperitoneally to horses.

Precaution(s): Store between 15° and 30°C (59°-86°F). Use entire contents when first opened. Discard any unused solution.

Caution(s): Federal law restricts this drug to use by or on the order of a licensed veterinarian.

For animal use only.

Warning(s): Keep out of reach of children.

Presentation: 500 mL (NDC 57319-075-07) and 1000 mL (NDC 57319-075-08) vials.

Manufactured by: Phoenix Scientific, Inc., St. Joseph, MO 64503.

Compendium Code No.: 12560212 — Rev. 7-01 / Rev. 8-01

DEXSOLYTE POWDER

Neogen — **Electrolytes-Oral**

Ingredient(s): Ascorbic Acid, Calcium Gluconate, Ferrous Sulfate, Magnesium Sulfate, Niacin, Potassium Chloride, Sodium Citrate, Sodium Chloride, Thiamine, Zinc, Sucrose Base.

Indications: A balanced electrolyte powder with vitamins and minerals in a sucrose base for use as a nutritional supplement where a deficiency exists.

Directions: Use 1 tablespoon (½ oz) per bucket of drinking water (10 qt) for individual use; or use 1 lb (16 oz) in approximately 40 gallons of drinking water for herd use; or as directed by veterinarian.

Caution(s): Sold to licensed veterinarians only.

For animal use only.

Warning(s): Keep out of reach of children.

Presentation: 5 lbs.

Compendium Code No.: 14910231 — L105-0997 Rev. 11/01

DEXTROSE 50%

AgriLabs — **Dextrose Therapy**

Active Ingredient(s): Contains:

Dextrose • H_2O	50% w/v
Water	q.s.

Indications: DEXTROSE 50% is indicated for use as an aid in the treatment of uncomplicated primary ketosis in cattle.

Dosage and Administration: The usual dose is 50 mL per 100 lbs. of body weight. It should be administered intravenously only.

Dosage may be repeated in 8-10 hours or on successive days if necessary.

If there is no noticeable improvement in the condition being treated after three (3) to four (4) days of treatment, consult a veterinarian. Aseptic precautions should be observed such as using a sterile needle and syringe. Disinfect the site of injection.

Caution(s): Keep out of the reach of children.

Solution should be warmed to room temperature and administered slowly. Do not use if the solution is cloudy. The entire contents should be used upon entering. Discard any unused portion.

Presentation: 500 mL bottles.

Compendium Code No.: 10580390

DEXTROSE 50%

AgriPharm — **Dextrose Therapy**

Active Ingredient(s): Contains

Dextrose • H_2O	50% w/v
Water for injection	q.s.

Indications: DEXTROSE 50% solution is indicated for use as an aid in the treatment of uncomplicated primary ketosis in cattle.

Dosage and Administration: The usual dose is 50 mL per 100 lbs. of body weight. It should be administered intravenously only. The dosage may be repeated in 8-10 hours or on successive days if necessary.

Precaution(s): Store at a controlled room temperature between 59°-86°F (15°-30°C).

Caution(s): For animal use only.

Keep out of the reach of children.

The solution should be warmed to room temperature and administered slowly. Do not use if the solution is not clear. The product does not contain any preservatives. The entire contents should be used upon entering. Discard any unused portion.

Presentation: 500 mL containers.

Compendium Code No.: 14570250

DEXTROSE 50%

Durvet — **Dextrose Therapy**

NDC No.: 30798-028-17

Active Ingredient(s):

Dextrose • H2O	50% w/v
Water for injection	q.s.

The product does not contain preservatives.

Indications: DEXTROSE 50% is indicated for the treatment of uncomplicated ketosis in cattle.

Dosage and Administration: The usual dose is 50 mL per 100 lbs. of body weight. It may be injected intravenously, intramuscularly, intraperitoneally or subcutaneously. The dose may be repeated in 8-10 hours or on successive days. If administered intramuscularly or subcutaneously, the dose should be divided among several locations and the point of injection massaged to aid in absorption.

If there is not noticeable improvement in the condition being treated after three (3) or four (4) days of treatment, consult a veterinarian. Aseptic precautions should be observed such as using a sterile needle and syringe. Disinfect the site of injection.

Precaution(s): Store at a controlled room temperature between 59°F-86°F (15°-30°C).

Caution(s): The solution should be warmed to room temperature and administered slowly.

The entire contents should be used upon entering. Discard any unused portion.

For animal use only. Livestock drug. Keep out of the reach of children.

Presentation: 500 mL.

Compendium Code No.: 10840450

DEXTROSE 50% SOLUTION ℞

Vedco — **Dextrose Therapy**

Active Ingredient(s): Each mL contains:

Dextrose monohydrate	0.5 g

This product contains no preservatives.

Indications: For use as a fluid and nutrient replenisher. Provides an immediate source of energy in conditions associated with carbohydrate insufficiency. Useful for rapid but temporary symptomatic treatment of ketosis (acetonemia) in cattle, and other hypoglycemic conditions in cattle, and other hypoglycemic conditions in cattle, horses, sheep, swine, dogs and cats.

Dosage and Administration: Warm to body temperature and administer slowly, preferably by intravenous infusion.

Cattle and Horses	100 to 500 mL
Sheep and Swine	30 to 100 mL
Dogs and Cats	10 to 50 mL

If given intramuscularly or subcutaneously dilute with normal saline to 5% dextrose (1 volume DEXTROSE SOLUTION 50% mixed with 9 volumes of normal saline), divided among several injection sites and massaged to aid in absorption.

Contraindication(s): Do not administer intraperitoneally.

Precaution(s): Store at a controlled room temperature between 59-86°F (15-50°C).

Caution(s): Federal law restricts this drug to use by or on the order of a licensed veterinarian.

Keep out of the reach of children.

Use the entire contents when first opened. Discard any unused solution.

Presentation: 500 mL containers.

Compendium Code No.: 10940450

DEXTROSE 50% SOLUTION

Vetus **Dextrose Therapy**

Active Ingredient(s): Each 100 mL contains:

Dextrose • H_2O .... 50 g

Indications: For use as an aid in the treatment of acetonemia (ketosis) in cattle.

Dosage and Administration: For intravenous administration only.

Intravenous administration must be made slowly and under strict aseptic conditions. Solution should be warmed to body temperature prior to administration. Cattle: 100 to 500 mL depending on the size and condition.

The treatment may be repeated in several hours or on successive days as needed.

Precaution(s): Store at 59°-86°F (15°-30°C).

Caution(s): This is a single dose container. This product contains no preservatives. After a quantity has been withdrawn for injection, the remainder should be discarded. Do not administer intraperitoneally.

Warning(s): For animal use only.

Keep out of reach of children.

Presentation: 500 mL single dose container.

Compendium Code No.: 14440270

DEXTROSE SOLUTION

Aspen **Dextrose Therapy**

Active Ingredient(s): Each 100 mL contains:

Dextrose • H_2O .... 50 g

Indications: For use as an aid in the treatment of acetonemia (ketosis) in cattle.

Dosage and Administration: For intravenous administration only.

100 to 500 mL depending on size and condition. Treatment may repeated in several hours or on successive days as needed.

Precaution(s): Store at 15°C-30°C (59°F-86°F).

Caution(s): Intravenous administration must be done slowly and made under strict aseptic conditions.

Solution should be warmed to body temperature prior to administration.

This is a single dose container.

This product contains no preservative. After a quantity has been withdrawn for injection, the remainder should be discarded. Do not administer intraperitoneally.

Warning(s): For animal use only.

Keep out of the reach of children.

Presentation: 500 mL size.

Compendium Code No.: 14750280

DEXTROSE SOLUTION 50% ℞

Butler **Dextrose Therapy**

Active Ingredient(s): Each mL of sterile aqueous solution contains:

Dextrose monohydrate .... 0.5 g

Indications: For use as a fluid and nutrient replenisher. Provides an immediate source of energy in conditions associated with carbohydrate insufficiency. Useful for rapid but temporary symptomatic treatment of ketosis (acetonemia) in cattle, and other hypoglycemic conditions in cattle, horses, sheep, swine, dogs and cats.

Dosage and Administration: Warm to body temperature and administer slowly, preferably by intravenous infusion.

Cattle and Horses .... 100 to 500 mL
Sheep and Swine .... 30 to 100 mL
Dogs and Cats .... 10 to 50 mL

If given intramuscularly or subcutaneously, dilute with normal saline to 5% dextrose (1 volume DEXTROSE SOLUTION 50% mixed with 9 volumes of normal saline), divided among several injection sites, and massage to aid in absorption.

Contraindication(s): Do not administer intraperitoneally.

Precaution(s): Store at a controlled room temperature between 15° and 30°C (59°-86°F).

Caution(s): Federal law restricts this drug to use by or on the order of a licensed veterinarian.

The product does not contain preservatives. Use the entire contents when first opened. Discard any unused solution.

For veterinary use only.

Keep out of the reach of children.

Presentation: 500 mL vials.

Compendium Code No.: 10820580

DEXTROSE SOLUTION 50%

Phoenix Pharmaceutical **Dextrose Therapy**

Active Ingredient(s): Each 100 mL contains:

Dextrose • H_2O .... 50 g

This product contains no preservative.

Indications: For use as an aid in the treatment of acetonemia (Ketosis) in cattle.

Dosage and Administration: For intravenous administration only.

Intravenous administration must be made slowly and under strict aseptic conditions. Solution should be warmed to body temperature prior to administration.

Cattle: 100 to 500 mL depending upon the size and condition.

Treatment may be repeated in several hours or on successive days as needed.

Precaution(s): Store between 15°C and 30°C (59°F and 86°F).

After a quantity has been withdrawn for injection, the remainder should be discarded.

Caution(s): Do not administer intraperitoneally.

For animal use only.

Warning(s): Keep out of reach of children.

Presentation: 500 mL single dose container (NDC 57319-071-07).

Manufactured by: Phoenix Scientific, Inc., St. Joseph, MO 64503.

Compendium Code No.: 12560222 Rev. 10-01

DEXTROSE SOLUTION 50%

Vet Tek **Dextrose Therapy**

NDC No.: 60270-028-17

Active Ingredient(s): Each 100 mL contains:

Dextrose • H_2O .... 50 g

Indications: For use as an aid in the treatment of acetonemia (ketosis) in cattle.

Dosage and Administration: For intravenous administration only.

Intravenous administration must be done slowly and made under strict aseptic conditions. The solution should be warmed to body temperature prior to administration.

Cattle: 100 to 500 mL depending upon the size and condition of the animal.

The treatment may be repeated in several hours or on successive days as needed.

Precaution(s): Store at 59°-86°F (15°-30°C).

Caution(s): Keep out of the reach of children. For animal use only.

After a quantity has been withdrawn for injection, the remainder should be discarded.

Do not administer intraperitoneally.

Presentation: 500 mL single dose container.

Compendium Code No.: 14200060

D-HORN PASTE

Dominion **Dehorning Paste**

Active Ingredient(s):

Sodium Hydroxide .... 46.0% w/w
Calcium Hydroxide .... 18.4% w/w

Indications: To prevent horn growth and remove horn buttons on calves.

Dosage and Administration: Apply a thin film on horn buttons as soon as they can be felt. Isolate calves for 30 minutes to prevent paste removal by rubbing. Protect calves from rain and snow for 6 hours.

Caution(s): First Aid:

External: Flood with water, then wash with vinegar.

Internal: Give citrus juice or vinegar in large amounts, followed by cooking oil.

Eyes: Flood with water or 5% boric acid solution. Call a physician.

The product is extremely corrosive! Keep out of reach of children.

Presentation: 85 gram squeeze bottle; 25 squeeze bottles/carton.
100 gram jar; 12 jars/carton.

Compendium Code No.: 15080020

DIAMINE IODIDE-20 (WITH SALT)

First Priority **Iodine-Oral**

Supplemental Source of Iodine

Active Ingredient(s):

Ethylenediamine Dihydroiodide (EDDI) (equivalent to 21 grams per pound)..... 20 grains/oz

Guaranteed Analysis:

Salt, Min. 89.0%
Max. 94.0%
Iodine, Min. 3.4%

Ingredients: Salt, Ethylenediamine Dihydroiodide, Silicone Dioxide and Artificial Color for identification.

Indications: For use as a supplemental source of iodine.

Directions for Use: Cattle:

Source of Iodine: Feed 10 mg per head per day in feed or salt continuously.

Feed: Thoroughly premix 1 lb with 9 lbs of supplement, ground grain, or another carrier having a particle size similar to DIAMINE IODIDE-20. Then mix 1 lb of the mixture in the feed consumed by 210 head of cattle and feed continuously.

Salt: Thoroughly premix 1 lb with 130 lbs of salt. Then feed 1 oz of the salt mixture per head per day and offer continuously.

Precaution(s): Storage: Store at controlled room temperature between 15°-30°C (59°-86°F). Keep container tightly closed when not in use.

Caution(s): For animal use only.

Warning(s): Not to be fed to dairy cattle in production. Keep out of reach of children.

Presentation: 1 lb (453.6 g) bag (NDC# 58829-253-16) and 25 lb (11.34 kg) pail (NDC# 58829-253-26).

Compendium Code No.: 11390202 Rev. 02-02 / Rev. 08-01

DIAMINE IODIDE-40 (WITH SALT)

First Priority **Iodine-Oral**

Supplemental Source of Iodine

Active Ingredient(s):

Ethylenediamine Dihydroiodide (EDDI) (equivalent to 40 grams per pound)..... 40 grains/oz

Guaranteed Analysis:

Salt, Min. 89.0%
Max. 94.0%
Iodine, Min. 7.6%

Ingredients: Salt, Ethylenediamine Dihydroiodide, Silicone Dioxide.

Indications: For use as a supplemental source of iodine.

Directions for Use: Cattle:

Source of Iodine: Feed 10 mg per head per day in feed or salt continuously.

Feed: Thoroughly premix 1 lb with 9 lbs of supplement, ground grain, or another carrier having a particle size similar to DIAMINE IODIDE-40. Then mix 1 lb of the mixture in the feed consumed by 415 head of cattle and feed continuously.

Salt: Thoroughly premix 1 lb with 260 lbs of salt. Then feed 1 oz of the salt mixture per head per day and offer continuously.

Precaution(s): Storage: Store at controlled room temperature between 15°-30°C (59°-86°F). Keep container tightly closed when not in use.

Caution(s): For animal use only.

Warning(s): Not to be fed to dairy cattle in production. Keep out of reach of children.

Presentation: 1 lb (453.6 g) bag (NDC# 58829-254-16) and 25 lb (11.34 kg) pail (NDC# 58829-254-26).

Compendium Code No.: 11390213 Rev. 02-02 / Rev. 07-01

DIAMINE IODIDE (WITH SUGAR)

First Priority **Iodine-Oral**

Supplemental Source of Iodine

Active Ingredient(s): Each pound (453.6 grams) contains:

Ethylenediamine Dihydroiodide (equivalent to 22 g EDDI/lb) 5.0%

Guaranteed Analysis:

Iodine - Minimum 3.4%

Ingredients: Sucrose, Ethylenediamine Dihydroiodide, Silicone Dioxide and Artificial Color for identification.

Indications: For routine supplementation of iodine in the diet of large animals.

Directions for Use: Mix thoroughly in the ration (protein mix, grain mix or salt) in proportions to provide EDDI at a rate of 10 mg per head per day.

Protein Mix - Add ½ lb per ton of protein mix. Feed at a rate of not more than 2 lb per head per day.

Grain Mix - Add 1 oz per ton of grain mix. Feed at a rate of not more than 15 lb per head per day.

Salt - Add 2 lb per 100 lb of feeding salt.

Precaution(s): Storage: Store at controlled room temperature between 15°-30°C (59°-86°F). Keep container tightly closed when not in use.

Caution(s): For animal use only.

Warning(s): Keep out of reach of children.

Presentation: 1 lb (453.6 g) jar (NDC# 58829-246-16), 1 lb (453.6 g) bag and 25 lb (11.34 kg) pail (NDC# 58829-246-26).

Compendium Code No.: 11390193 Rev. 02-02 / Rev. 07-01

DIARRHEA TABS

Butler **Adsorbent**

Liver Flavored

Active Ingredient(s): Each tablet contains:

Kaolin . . . . . . 8 grains
Aluminum Hydroxide . . . . . . 2 grains
Pectin . . . . . . 1.5 grains
Desiccated Liver

Indications: A soothing and protective aid for simple diarrhea when antibiotics or anticholinergic drugs are not needed. Safe for long term use for dogs and cats with a sensitive digestive system. For dogs, cats, puppies and kittens.

Directions: Give 2 tablets per each 10 lbs. bodyweight, 3 times daily. Withhold food for first 12-24 hours and then feed bland low-fat foods such as boiled rice and low-fat cottage cheese.

Presentation: Contains 500 tablets.

Compendium Code No.: 10820600

DIASYSTEMS® EIA AGID ANTIBODY TEST KIT

Idexx Labs. **EIA Test**

Equine Infectious Anemia Antibody Test Kit

U.S. Vet. Lic. No.: 313

Reagents:

A.	Equine Infectious Anemia Antigen, preserved with sodium azide (Black Cap).	1 bottle-3.9 mL
B.	Equine Infectious Anemia Positive Control Serum, preserved with sodium azide (Red Cap).	1 bottle-11.7 mL

Indications: The purified antigen from equine infectious anemia virus (EIAV) can be used in the agar gel immunodiffusion (AGID) test to detect the presence of antibody against EIAV in the serum of infected horses. Non-specific precipitin lines are virtually eliminated from the AGID test by using highly purified EIAV antigens. These non-specific precipitin lines can interfere with the reading of the test and increase the number of incorrect results.

Test Principles: The movement of antigen and antibody toward one another in an agar gel can result in the formation of precipitin lines. By applying this principle, the AGID test has been shown to reliably detect specific antibody formed after 10 to 30 days of infection with EIAV. Precipitin lines of identity can be visualized in strong positive sera as continuing from the lines between the control serum and center antigen wells. Weakly positive sera are indicated as a bend of the control serum lines towards the antigen well. No precipitin lines of identity form if the serum is negative.

Test Procedure:

Specimen Collection and Preparation for Testing: Use only horse serum for test specimens. Specimens may be stored at 2°-8°C up to five days. If longer storage is desired, store at -20°C (-4°F). The presence of turbidity, hemolysis or visible indications of bacterial growth may interfere with the performance and accuracy of the test. Do not test specimens that exhibit bacterial growth.

Assay Procedure - Preparation of AGID Plates:

1. Prepare 1 liter of buffer by mixing: 2 gm Sodium Hydroxide (NaOH) and 9 gm Boric Acid (H_3BO_3). Add 1 liter distilled water and adjust pH to 8.6 ± 0.1.
2. Prepare a 1.0% solution of Noble agar in the buffer by either method a or b.
   a. Boil the suspension to dissolve the agar and autoclave for seven minutes.
   b. Microwave agar solution for a total of 3 minutes at 30 second intervals or until agar dissolves.
3. Add 15 mL of the liquid agar to a 100 mm diameter petri dish.
4. Plates are cooled for 1 hour at room temperature and then stored at 2°-8°C (if uncut, plates can be stored up to one week).
5. Wells are 5.3 mm diameter and 2.4 mm apart. A seven-well pattern of a center well surrounded by six wells is recommended. Cutting templates may be obtained by approved laboratories from the National Veterinary Services Laboratory, P.O. Box 844, Ames, Iowa 50010.
6. Wells are cut while the agar is cold (from 2°-8°C storage) and just before use. Remove the plugs and any excess moisture in the wells before adding test samples and reagents.

Serum and Antigen Placement in Wells:

1. Completely fill the three alternative outside wells (see pattern I below) with each of the three test sera. Avoid any overflow onto the agar surface.
2. Fill the center well with purified Antigen in the same manner.
3. Fill the three remaining outside wells with Positive Control Serum in the same manner (see pattern I below).
4. Incubate plates for 24-48 hours at room temperature in a moist chamber.

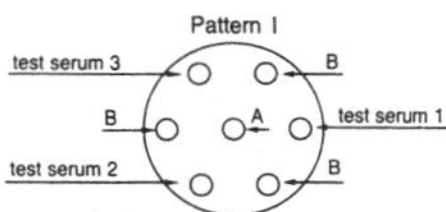

Test Interpretation: Pattern II shows different precipitin patterns in the AGID test:

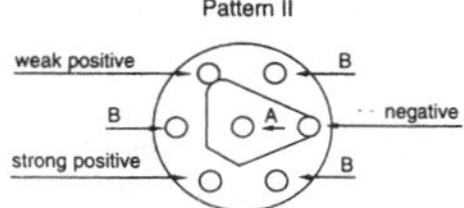

1. Negative serum. Control precipitin lines (B wells) run straight into the negative sample well or bend slightly back towards the B wells.
2. Weakly positive serum. Control precipitin lines (B wells) run into the sample well but bend away from the B wells and towards each other.
3. Strongly positive serum. A precipitin line forms between the sample well and center well A which is continuous with the control precipitin lines between wells B and A.
4. Very strongly positive serum. Control precipitin lines (B wells) bend towards each other before they reach the test serum wells. They may be connected by a broad diffuse precipitin line which will be close to the antigen (A) well. A sharper line can be observed if the serum is two-fold serially diluted and retested.
5. Weak positives may result from:
   a. Serum taken during the incubation period of EIA. Retesting after two to three weeks may show a stronger reaction.
   b. If the horse shows no clinical symptoms and an unchanged AGID reaction, then the horse may be a carrier.
   c. Weak positives may also be characteristic of nursing foals of infected mares. Retest of the foal after six months should show negative AGID results if the foal is uninfected. If the foal's mare (dam) is negative in the AGID test then the foal is probably infected.
6. In the United States, any doubtful samples should be sent to the National Veterinary Services Laboratory.

Quality Control: If the positive control included in the kit does not react, do not use the kit.

Storage: Store the reagents at 2°-8°C. Reagents are stable until expiration date, provided they have been stored properly.

Caution(s):

1. Do not allow reagents to stand at room temperature for extended periods of time.
2. Handle all samples and reagents as if capable of transmitting EIAV. Burn or autoclave unused biological components.
3. Do not use reagents from other kits.
4. Do not use expired reagents.
5. For veterinary use only. In vitro use only.
6. Sale and use in the United States restricted to laboratories approved by State and Federal (USDA) animal health officials.

Presentation: 180 tests.

Compendium Code No.: 11160041

DIASYSTEMS® EIA CELISA ANTIBODY TEST KIT

Idexx Labs. **EIA Test**

U.S. Vet. Lic. No.: 313

Description: Equine infectious anemia antibody test kit.

Components:

Reagents	1 plate kit	5 plate kit
1. Anti-EIAV Coated Wells	1 plate (96 wells)	5 plates (480 wells)
2. Negative Control (Red Band)	1 bottle - 6 mL	1 bottle - 6 mL
3. Positive Control (Blue Band)	1 bottle - 6 mL	1 bottle - 6 mL
4. EIAV Antigen Conjugate (Lavender Band)	1 bottle - 6 mL	1 bottle - 25 mL
5. Substrate Solution (Black Band)	1 bottle - 12 mL	1 bottle - 60 mL

Additional materials required but not provided:

1. Marking pen
2. Wash bottle
3. Pipets and tips
4. 37°C incubator

Indications: It is a rapid, convenient and specific test for the detection of EIA antibody in horse serum. Purified EIA antigen and monoclonal antibodies to p26 are used to reduce non-specific reactions commonly found in ELISA tests. The correlation between the DIASYSTEMS® EIA CELISA and the EIA-AGID assay is greater than 99 percent.

Test Principles: The kit contains plastic wells with monoclonal antibody specific for p26, the major group-specific antigen of Equine Infectious Anemia Virus (EIAV). The p26 antigen has been conjugated to an enzyme. Horse serum is incubated simultaneously with conjugated p26 antigen. Serum antibodies specific for p26 complete with the bound anti-p26 monoclonal antibodies for the enzyme-linked purified p26 antigen.

When antibodies to EIAV p26 antigen are present in the equine serum sample, they prevent the binding of the enzyme-linked antigen to the monoclonal antibody coated on the plastic wells, so little or no color in the positive sample wells results.

If a horse is negative for antibody to EIA, the enzyme-linked antigen will bind to the monoclonal antibody on the plastic wells. The color change of the Substrate Solution to dark blue indicates that EIA specific antibody is not present in the horse serum.

Color in the test sample wells are compared to the color in the Positive Control wells to yield a final assay interpretation.

Test Procedure:

1. Fill wash bottle with distilled or deionized water. Do not use tap water.
2. Run Negative and Positive Controls (included in the kit) each time a test is performed.
3. Use a separate pipet for each serum sample.
4. Washing wells properly is important:
   a. Avoid cross-contamination of wells with reagent during early washes. This is avoided by flicking reagent from wells into sink and blotting dry on clean paper towel. Hold wells at approx. 45° angle facing you. Starting from bottom row of wells and moving side to

side, vigorously flood wells with deionized water from a wash bottle. Make sure no air is trapped in wells.
  b. Improper washing may produce non-specific color development.
  c. The Negative Control will be blue in color and darker than the Positive Control which will show a light-blue color.
  d. Improper washing will result in no color difference between the Negative and Positive Controls (both will be dark blue).

Specimen Collection and Preparation for Testing: Use only horse serum for test. Collect blood by venipuncture into a clean test tube containing no additives. (Serum separator tubes may be used.) Separate serum from blood. Specimens may be stored at 2°-8°C (35°-46°F) up to five days. If longer storage is desired, store at -20°C (-4°F).

Frozen sera may be frozen and thawed only once prior to testing. Mix thawed samples well before use by inverting tube several times. The presence of turbidity or visible indication of bacterial growth (originally clear serum turned cloudy) may interfere with the performance and accuracy of the test.

Assay Procedure:
1. Remove the required number of wells, label and place securely in holder. Use one well per serum sample plus two wells for the two Control samples.
2. Use a separate pipet tip and a separate well for each serum sample. Place 0.10 mL of each serum sample into the appropriately labeled wells. Place 0.10 mL of Negative Control (Red Band) and 0.10 mL of Positive Control (Blue Band) into their respective wells.
3. Place 0.05 mL (50 µl) EIAV Antigen Conjugate (Lavender Band) into all wells.
4. Mix thoroughly by gently tapping well holder 10 times.
5. Incubate uncovered for 30 minutes at 37°C.
6. Flick reagent from wells into sink and blot wells dry on clean paper towel. Tilt the wells at a 45° angle, facing you. Starting from bottom row and moving side to side, vigorously flood wells with deionized water from wash bottle. Make sure each well is filled completely and no air bubbles are trapped. Flick water into sink. Repeat five (5) times. Blot wells dry on paper towel after final rinse.
7. Place two drops of Substrate Solution (black band) into all wells.
8. Mix thoroughly by gently tapping the holder 10 times.
9. Incubate 15 minutes at room temperature. Observe color change.
10. A 650 nm filter is required if reading test wells with a spectrophotometer.

Quality Control: Include Negative and Positive Controls each time a test is performed. In the event that the Negative Control included in the kit does not react (turn dark blue), do not use the kit. Call IDEXX Technical Service at 800-548-9997 or 207-856-0300. In the U.K. call 0800-581786.

Results - Validation:

For the results to be valid, the controls must appear as follows:
1. Negative Control: substrate has turned dark blue.
2. Positive Control: light blue. Improper washing will result in no color difference between the Negative and Positive Controls (both will be dark blue).

Test Interpretation: Sample Evaluation:
1. Little or no color change in test sample indicates the presence of antibodies to EIAV in the serum.
  a. Samples with equal or less color than the light-blue Positive Control are positive.
  b. Many positive samples will be clear (no color).
  c. Positive test results should be verified by DiaSystems™ EIA-AGID.
2. A color change in the test sample of greater intensity than the light blue positive control indicates the absence of antibody to EIAV in the serum.
   Samples with greater color than the light-blue Positive Control are negative.
3. In the United States, doubtful samples should be sent to the National Veterinary Services Laboratory for confirmation.

Limitations:
1. Use only serum. Hemolyzed, lipemic or bacterially contaminated serum may cause erroneous results. (Heparinized or EDTA treated blood may also interfere with test results).
2. Store all reagents in closed containers at refrigerated temperature of 2°-8°C (35°-46°F).
3. Waiting longer than the specified time to read test wells may result in false negatives.

Storage: Store the diagnostic kit at refrigerated temperature of 2°-8°C (35°-46°F). Do not freeze. Do not allow reagents to stand at room temperature for more than 30 minutes. The test may be run at room temperature.

Caution(s):
1. Do not use reagents from other kits.
2. Do not use expired reagents.
3. For veterinary use only. *In vitro* use only.
4. Sale and use restricted to laboratories approved by State and Federal (USDA) animal health officials.

Presentation: 32 to 92 tests.

Compendium Code No.: 11160051

DI-CALCIUM PHOSPHATE

Neogen **Dietary Supplement**

Source of Calcium and Phosphate

Guaranteed Analysis:

Phosphorus
 not more than 21%
 not less than 17%

Calcium
 not more than 26%
 not less than 22%

Indications: As a source of calcium and phosphorus in horses and dogs.

Dosage and Administration:

Horses: 1 to 2 ounces daily in feed.

Dogs: ½ to 2 teaspoons daily in feed.

Precaution(s): Store in a dry place. Keep lid tightly closed.

Caution(s): For animal use only.

Warning(s): Keep out of reach of children.

Presentation: 4 lbs (1.814 kg) (NDC: 59051-9160-6) and 20 lbs (9.072 kg) (NDC: 59051-9161-0).

Compendium Code No.: 14910241 L421-0501 / L433-0501

DICURAL® TABLETS ℞

Fort Dodge **Difloxacin-Oral**

Difloxacin Hydrochloride

NADA No.: 141-096

Active Ingredient(s): Each scored tablet contains either:

Difloxacin hydrochloride . . . . 11.4 mg, 45.5 mg or 136 mg

Indications: DICURAL® (difloxacin hydrochloride) tablets are indicated for the management of diseases in dogs associated with bacteria susceptible to difloxacin.

Pharmacology: Description: Difloxacin hydrochloride [3-quinolinecarboxylic acid, 6-fluoro-1-(4-fluorophenyl)-1,4-dihydro-7-(4-methyl-1-piperazinyl)-4-oxo-, monohydrochloride] is a fluoroquinolone with broad spectrum antimicrobial activity against gram-positive and gram-negative microorganisms.

Difloxacin is poorly water soluble at neutral pH [octanol/water partition coefficient (P) = 8.3 in water, 7.2 at pH 7.0]. Its water solubility is improved under acidic conditions (P = 2.1 at pH 5.0), and difloxacin is highly water soluble under basic conditions (P = 0.33 at pH 9.0). Accordingly, the molecule has two ionizable sites: a carboxylic acid group (pKa=4.33) and a methyl substituted nitrogen group (pKa=9.05).

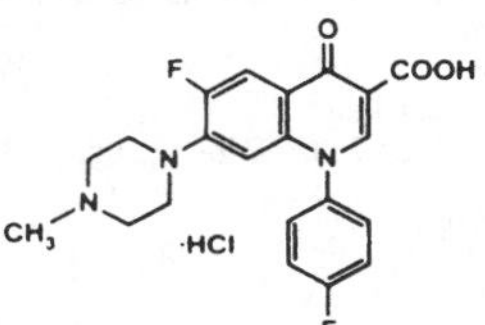

Figure 1. Chemical structure of difloxacin

Efficacy Confirmation: Clinical efficacy was confirmed in skin and soft tissue infections (wounds and abscesses) and urinary tract infections (cystitis). Specific pathogens isolated in clinical field trials are listed in Table 4 in the Microbiology section.

Clinical Pharmacology: Pharmacokinetics in healthy, adult dogs: Difloxacin hydrochloride oral bioavailability exceeds 80% when administered by gavage to fasted dogs. Linear pharmacokinetics have been demonstrated for oral difloxacin up to 60 mg/kg/day. Approximately 90% of the total radioactivity in plasma is attributable to the parent compound following both oral and intravenous administration of ^{14}C-difloxacin.

Difloxacin is associated with two major metabolites: the ester glucuronide and the desmethyl derivative of difloxacin. Difloxacin elimination occurs primarily through glucuronidation with subsequent biliary secretion. However, the glucuronide metabolite may be hydrolyzed in the gastrointestinal tract, and the resulting parent compound reabsorbed. Approximately 80% of an intravenous dose is eliminated in the feces. Renal clearance accounts for less than 5% of difloxacin total body clearance.

Pharmacokinetic estimates for difloxacin tablets following oral administration to fasted dogs are shown in Table 2. No statistically significant gender effects were observed. The effect of food on difloxacin oral bioavailability has not been determined (see Drug Interactions).

Table 2. Plasma pharmacokinetics following administration of difloxacin tablets (5 mg/kg body weight) to dogs (n=20).

Pharmacokinetic Measure	Mean Value
Peak Plasma Concentration (C_{MAX})	1.8 µg/mL
Time to Reach C_{MAX} (T_{MAX})	2.8 hours
Elimination Half-life ($T_{1/2}$)	9.3 hours
Area Under the Plasma Curve (AUC_{0-x})	14.5 µg•hr/mL
Total Body Clearance/F[a] (CL/F)	375 mL/kg/hr
Steady State Volume of Distribution/F[b]	3.8 L/kg
Volume of Distribution (area)/F[c]	4.7 L/kg

[a]Total body clearance/F = Dose/AUC

[b]Steady state volume of distribution/F = Dose•AUMC/AUC^2

[c]Volume of distribution (area)/F = Vd_β = ($T_{1/2}$) (CL/F)/0.693

Blood concentration versus time profiles for difloxacin after a single 5 mg/kg or 10 mg/kg dose of DICURAL® tablets are presented in Figure 2. Negligible accumulation occurs with once daily administration.

Difloxacin Concentrations After a Single Oral Dose

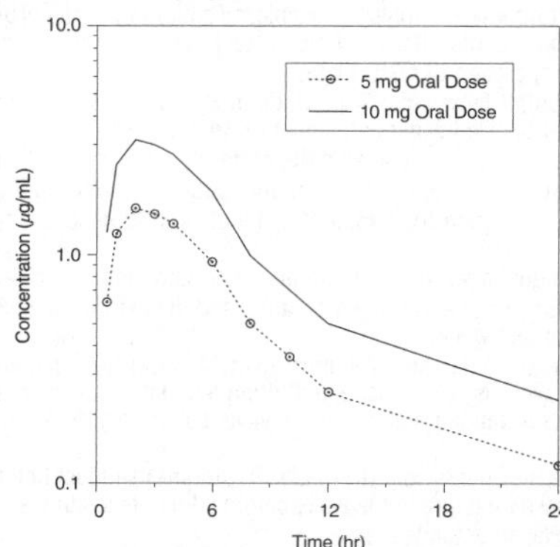

Figure 2: Difloxacin concentration after oral administration of a single DICURAL® tablet. Profile for the 10 mg/kg dose was based upon the mean concentrations observed following a single 5 mg/kg dose.

The affinity of difloxacin for canine plasma proteins is low (plasma protein binding = 46% to 52%). Accordingly, difloxacin readily diffuses into peripheral tissues. This is evidenced by the levels of ^{14}C activity in tissues following oral administration of 10 mg/kg ^{14}C-difloxacin hydrochloride (Table 3). These results are consistent with difloxacin's lipophilic properties and its large volume of distribution.

Table 3. Levels of ^{14}C radioactivity (expressed as µg equivalents of difloxacin per gram or mL) in tissues at 2, 6, and 24 hours following administration of a single oral dose of radiolabeled difloxacin free base at 10 mg/kg.

Body System	2 hours (n=2)	6 hours (n=1)	24 hours (n=1)
Hematopoietic			
Whole Blood	2.3	1.1	0.6
Plasma	2.6	1.2	0.8
Bone	6.5	7.2	6.5
Lymph Node	3.1	2.5	1.7
Liver	10.7	7.8	4.6
Spleen	3.5	1.1	1.1
Urogenital			
Urine*	22.6	21.0	10.7
Kidney	5.0	2.8	1.5
Bladder Wall	3.0	1.8	1.7
Testes	3.1	1.6	0.8
Prostate	3.4	1.5	1.4
Gastrointestinal			
Stomach	66.7	8.5	9.9
Small Intestine	18.3	38.7	16.4
Cardiopulmonary			
Lung	3.2	0.9	0.8
Heart	3.8	1.6	1.1
Other Tissues			
Muscle	4.1	1.2	1.1
Fat	0.7	0.8	0.8

*Based on percent of dose with urine output at 50 mL/kg/day

Considering the comparability of ^{14}C radioactivity in tissues and plasma, AUC, C_{MAX} and the MIC of the targeted pathogen(s) can be used as a guide for clinical dose adjustment.

Microbiology: Difloxacin has broad spectrum activity against gram-negative and gram-positive bacteria. It is bactericidal and exerts its antibacterial effect through interference with the bacterial enzyme DNA gyrase which is needed for the maintenance and synthesis of bacterial DNA. The minimum inhibitory concentrations (MICs) of pathogens isolated in clinical field trials conducted in the United States between 1991 and 1993 were determined using National Committee for Clinical Laboratory Standards (NCCLS). The following table (Table 4) provides the minimum inhibitory concentrations of difloxacin for the bacteria isolated during clinical field trials:

Table 4. MIC values* (µg/mL) of difloxacin for bacterial pathogens isolated from skin and soft tissue infections and urinary tract infections in dogs enrolled in clinical studies conducted during 1991-1993.

Bacteria Name	No. of Isolates	MIC_{50}	MIC_{90}	MIC Range
Enterobacter spp.	9	0.11	3.66	≤0.05-3.66
Escherichia coli	28	≤0.05	0.11	≤0.05-7.3
Klebsiella spp.	8	0.11	0.11	0.11-0.23
Pasteurella spp.	8	≤0.05	≤0.05	≤0.05
Proteus spp.	15	0.92	1.83	0.11-1.83
Pseudomonas spp.	5	0.11	0.92	≤0.05-0.92
Staphylococcus spp.	193	0.23	0.46	≤0.05-1.83
Streptococcus spp.	56	1.83	3.66	0.11-7.3

*The correlation between the *in vitro* susceptibility data (MIC values) and clinical response has not been confirmed. The MIC tests were performed using difloxacin hydrochloride and an adjustment was made to represent the results as difloxacin (free base).

A study was conducted to determine the *in vitro* activity of difloxacin against 300 canine clinical isolates from multiple geographic locations across the United States during 1995-1996. MICs were determined using National Committee for Clinical Laboratory Standards. The study results are summarized in Table 5.

Table 5. MIC values* (µg/mL) of difloxacin for canine bacterial isolates collected during a comprehensive study conducted in the United States during 1995-1996.

Bacteria Name	Number of Isolates	MIC_{50}	MIC_{90}	MIC Range
Escherichia coli	78	0.11	0.23	0.01 - >0.91
Klebsiella pneumoniae	20	0.46	0.46	0.03 - >0.91
Proteus spp.	38	0.91	0.91	0.46 - 1.82
Staphylococcus intermedius	164	0.91	0.91	0.11 - >0.91

*The correlation between the *in vitro* susceptibility data (MIC values) and clinical response has not been confirmed. The MIC tests were performed using difloxacin hydrochloride and an adjustment was made to represent the results as difloxacin (free base).

Dosage and Administration: The dose range of difloxacin in dogs is 5 to 10 mg/kg body weight (2.3 to 4.6 mg/lb) once a day for two to three days beyond the cessation of clinical signs to a maximum of 30 days (see Drug Interactions).

The determination of dosage for any particular patient must take into consideration such factors as the severity and nature of the infection, the susceptibility of the causative organism, and the integrity of the host-defense mechanisms. The dose of 5 mg/kg of body weight administered once daily should be used for the routine treatment of infection caused by susceptible organism(s) in an otherwise healthy dog. The dosage may be increased to the upper limit of the dose range (10 mg/kg), if deemed necessary. Antibiotic susceptibility of the pathogenic organism(s) should be determined prior to use of difloxacin. However, therapy with DICURAL® tablets may be initiated before results of these tests are known. Once test results become available, continue with appropriate therapy.

For the treatment of skin and soft tissue infections, DICURAL® tablets should be given for two (2) to three (3) days beyond the cessation of clinical signs to a maximum of 30 days. For the treatment of urinary tract infections, DICURAL® tablets should be administered for at least 10 consecutive days. If no improvement is noted within five (5) days, the diagnosis should be re-evaluated and a different course of therapy considered.

Table 1. Dose Table for DICURAL® tablets for Dogs

Tablet Color	Tablet Strength (Difloxacin Base)	Daily Dose	
		5 mg/kg	10 mg/kg
Blue	11.4 mg	2.3 kg (5 lb)	1.1 kg (2.5 lb)
White	45.4 mg	9 kg (20 lb)	4.5 kg (10 lb)
Orange	136 mg	27 kg (60 lb)	13.5 kg (30 lb)

Drug Interactions: Compounds (e.g., sucralfate, antacids, and multivitamins) containing divalent and trivalent cations (e.g., iron, aluminum, calcium, magnesium and zinc) may substantially interfere with the absorption of quinolones from the intestinal tract resulting in a decrease in product bioavailability. Therefore, the concomitant oral administration of quinolones with foods, supplements or other preparations containing these compounds should be avoided.

Difloxacin hydrochloride has been administered to dogs concurrently with other animal health products under field conditions with no adverse effects observed. Concurrent therapies included heartworm prevention, thyroid hormone augmentation, ectoparasiticides anesthetics, anti-seizure compounds, topical antibiotics/anti-inflammatory and antihistamine medication.

Contraindication(s): Difloxacin and other quinolones have been shown to cause arthropathy in immature animals of most species tested, the dog being particularly sensitive to this side effect. Difloxacin is contraindicated in immature dogs during the rapid growth phase (between 2 and 8 months of age in small and medium-sized breeds, and up to 18 months of age in large and giant breeds).

Precaution(s):

Storage Conditions: Store DICURAL® tablets between 15°C and 30°C (59°F and 86°F); avoid excessive heat (40°C/104°F).

Caution(s): Federal (U.S.A.) law restricts this drug to use by or on the order of a licensed veterinarian.

Quinolone-class drugs should be used with caution in animals with known or suspected central nervous system (CNS) disorders. In such animals, quinolones have in rare instances, been associated with CNS stimulation which may lead to convulsive seizures. Quinolones have been shown to produce erosions of cartilage of weight-bearing joints and other signs of arthropathy in immature animals of various species.

The safety of DICURAL® tablets in breeding or pregnant dogs has not been determined. DICURAL® tablets should not be used in dogs known to be hypersensitive to quinolones.

Warning(s): For oral use in dogs only.

Federal law prohibits the extra-label use of this drug in food-producing animals.

Human Warnings: For use in animals only. Keep out of the reach of children.

Avoid contact with eyes. In case of contact, immediately flush eyes with copious amounts of water for 15 minutes. In case of dermal contact, wash skin with soap and water. Consult a physician if irritation persists following ocular or dermal exposure. Individuals with a history of hypersensitivity to quinolones should avoid this product. In humans, there is a risk of user photosensitization within a few hours after excessive exposure to quinolones. If excessive accidental exposure occurs, avoid direct sunlight.

Toxicology: Target Animal Safety: Difloxacin administered to 9.5 to 11.5 month-old, 9.5 to 17.6 kg beagles at doses of 5, 15, or 25 mg/kg for 30 consecutive days supports an adequate safety margin for the product. There was no ante or post-mortem evidence of quinolone-induced arthropathy. However, transient erythema/edema on the facial area, diarrhea and decreased appetite and weight loss were observed in some dogs.

In 15 to 16 week-old Beagle puppies dosed at 0, 5, 25, 35, 50 and 125 mg/kg/day for 90 days, lameness and articular cartilage lesions in the femur and proximal tibia were noted in the 50 mg/kg and 125 mg/kg groups. Clinical lameness was not observed in any group below 50 mg/kg. Articular cartilage lesions were also noted in the 5, 25, and 35 mg/kg/day groups (see Contraindications).

Adverse Reactions: Various breeds of dogs, aged 9 months to 16 years, were admitted into the clinical study and received 5 mg/kg/day for up to 10 days. DICURAL® tablets were well tolerated. Potential adverse reactions recorded in clinical cases involved the gastrointestinal tract (e.g., anorexia, emesis, diarrhea, and inappetence), which were self-limiting and did not require additional treatment.

Presentation: DICURAL® tablets are supplied in three strengths: 11.4 mg (100, 250 or 500 single-scored tablets); 45.5 mg (100, 250 or 500 single-scored tablets); and 136 mg (50, 125 or 250 double-scored tablets).

NDC 53501-131-23 — 11.4 mg — 100 tablets
NDC 53501-131-25 — 11.4 mg — 250 tablets
NDC 53501-131-24 — 11.4 mg — 500 tablets
NDC 53501-231-33 — 45.4 mg — 100 tablets
NDC 53501-231-35 — 45.4 mg — 250 tablets
NDC 53501-231-34 — 45.4 mg — 500 tablets
NDC 53501-331-41 — 136 mg — 50 tablets
NDC 53501-331-42 — 136 mg — 125 tablets
NDC 53501-331-44 — 136 mg — 250 tablets

Compendium Code No.: 10030392 13140C

DIGEST AID™

Farnam **Large Animal Dietary Supplement**

Guaranteed Analysis: Each ounce contains:

Crude Protein, not less than 25.5%
Crude Fat, not less than 9.75%
Crude Fiber, not less than 6.7%

Ingredients: Heat treated whole soybeans - ground, yeast culture grown on a medium of ground yellow corn, hominy feed, corn gluten feed, wheat middlings, diastatic malt and corn syrup, dried *Aspergillus oryzae* fermentation extract.

Indications: Recommended as a dietary supplement for horses.

Dosage and Administration: Measuring Cup = One Ounce

Feed DIGEST AID™ at the following daily rates:

Sprinkle the proper amount over feed or mix with the grain ration.

Adult Horses: . . . . 1 ounce per day
Foals, Weanlings, Ponies: . . . . ½ ounce per day
Pregnant and Nursing Mares: . . . . 2 ounces per day

For optimum results, DIGEST AID™ should be fed along with a complete vitamin/mineral supplement such as Farnam's Vita-Plus®.
Caution(s): For oral use in horses.
Warning(s): Keep out of reach of children.
Discussion: Aids in Digestion and Feed Utilization: DIGEST AID™ is a soybean meal base that contains a patented fermentation extract produced by a select sub-strain of *Aspergillus oryzae*. This fermentation extract helps to establish and maintain a balanced microflora in the horse's intestinal tract that will aid in the digestion of protein, fiber, sugars and starches. DIGEST AID™ will help improve the horse's utilization of its feed by increasing the nutrient availability it receives from the hay and grains in its diet. You'll see the difference in your horse's performance, digestion and attitude. Improved feed utilization not only helps with your horse's nutrition, but also helps you as a horseowner to get the most economical use from the feeds you purchase for your home.
Presentation: 3 lbs (1.36 kg) and 7 lbs.
Compendium Code No.: 10000141

D

DI-METHOX® 12.5% ORAL SOLUTION

AgriLabs **Water Medication**
Sulfadimethoxine 12.5%-Antibacterial
ANADA No.: 200-030
Active Ingredient(s): Each fluid ounce contains 3.75 g sulfadimethoxine solubilized with sodium hydroxide.
Indications:
Broiler and Replacement Chickens: Use for the treatment of disease outbreaks of coccidiosis, fowl cholera, and infectious coryza.
Meat Producing Turkeys: Use for the treatment of disease outbreaks of coccidiosis and fowl cholera.
Dairy Calves, Dairy Heifers and Beef Cattle: Use in the treatment of shipping fever complex, bacterial pneumonia, calf diphtheria, and foot rot.
Dosage and Administration:
Chickens: For a 0.05% concentration, add 1 fl oz* to 2 gallons of drinking water, or 25 fl oz to 50 gallons of drinking water.
Turkeys: For a 0.025% concentration, add 1 fl oz* to 4 gallons of drinking water, or 25 fl oz to 100 gallons of drinking water.
Automatic Proportioners** Stock Solution — To make 2 gallons of Stock Solution use:
Chickens: 1 gallon of DI-METHOX® (Sulfadimethoxine) 12.5% Drinking Water Solution Concentrate, plus 1 gallon of water.
Turkeys: 2 qts of DI-METHOX® (Sulfadimethoxine) 12.5% Drinking Water Solution Concentrate, plus 6 qts of water.
Treatment Period — 6 consecutive days.
Dairy Calves, Dairy Heifers and Beef Cattle: 25 mg/lb first day followed by 12.5 mg/lb/day for 4 days.

	Water Consumption	
	(Summer) 1 gallon/† 100 lb b.w.	(Winter) 1 gallon/† 150 lb b.w.
First Day Add:		
1 pint (16 fl oz) to:	25 gallons	16 gallons
1 quart (32 fl oz) to:	50 gallons	33 gallons
1 gallon (128 fl oz) to:	200 gallons	127 gallons
Next 4 Days Add:		
1 pint (16 fl oz) to:	50 gallons	33 gallons
1 quart (32 fl oz) to:	100 gallons	66 gallons
1 gallon (128 fl oz) to:	400 gallons	266 gallons

†This dosage recommendation is based on a water consumption of 1 gallon per 100 lb of body weight per day, the expected water consumption rate for summer. Water consumption during cold months (winter) may drop markedly (30-40%). Accordingly, adjustments in drug concentration in drinking water must be made to ensure proper drug intake.
For individual treatment of cattle, DI-METHOX® (Sulfadimethoxine) 12.5% Drinking Water Solution may be given as a drench. Administer using same mg/lb dosage as outlined above. Four fluid ounces will medicate one-600 lb animal initially, or two-600 lb animals on a maintenance dose.
Treatment Period — 5 consecutive days.
*1 fl oz DI-METHOX® (Sulfadimethoxine) 12.5% Drinking Water Solution = 30 mL or 2 tablespoonfuls.
**Set proportioner to a feed rate of 1 fl oz of DI-METHOX® (Sulfadimethoxine) Stock Solution per gallon of water.
Chickens and Turkeys: If animals show no improvement within 5 days, discontinue treatment and re-evaluate diagnosis. Handle the recommended dilutions (chickens 0.05% and turkeys 0.025%) as regular drinking water. Administer as sole source of drinking water and sulfonamide medication.
Chickens and turkeys that have survived fowl cholera outbreaks should not be kept for replacements or breeders.
Cattle: During treatment period, make certain that animals maintain adequate water intake. If animals show no improvement within 2 or 3 days, re-evaluate diagnosis. Treatment should not be continued beyond 5 days.
Prepare a fresh stock solution daily.
Precaution(s): Store at room temperature; if freezing occurs, thaw before using. Protect from light; direct sunlight may cause discoloration. Freezing or discoloration does not affect potency.
Caution(s): For use in animals only.
Not for human use.
For oral use in chickens, turkeys and cattle.
Warning(s):
Chickens and Turkeys: Withdraw 5 days before slaughter. Do not administer to chickens over 16 weeks (112 days) of age or to turkeys over 24 weeks (168 days) of age.
Cattle: Withdraw 7 days before slaughter. A withdrawal period has not been established for this product in pre-ruminating calves. Do not use in calves to be processed for veal.
Keep out of reach of children.
Presentation: 3.8 L (1 gallon).
® Registered Trademark of Agri Laboratories, Ltd.
Compendium Code No.: 10580401 Iss. 5-00

DI-METHOX® INJECTION-40%

AgriLabs **Sulfadimethoxine**
(Sulfadimethoxine Injection-40%)-Antibacterial
ANADA No.: 200-177
Active Ingredient(s): Composition: Each mL contains 400 mg sulfadimethoxine compounded with 20% propylene glycol, 1% benzyl alcohol (preservative), 0.1 mg disodium edetate, 1 mg sodium formaldehyde sulfoxylate and pH adjusted with sodium hydroxide.
Indications: DI-METHOX® (Sulfadimethoxine Injection 40%) is indicated for the treatment of bovine respiratory disease complex (shipping fever complex) and bacterial pneumonia associated with *Pasteurella* spp. sensitive to sulfadimethoxine, necrotic pododermatitis (foot rot) and calf diphtheria caused by *Fusobacterium necrophorum (Sphaerophorus necrophorus),* sensitive to sulfadimethoxine.
Limitations: Sulfadimethoxine is not effective in viral or rickettsial infections, and as with any antibacterial agent, occasional failures in therapy may occur due to resistant microorganisms. The usual precautions in sulfonamide therapy should be observed.
Pharmacology: Sulfadimethoxine is a white, almost tasteless and odorless compound. Chemically, it is N[1]-(2,6 dimethoxy-4-pyrimidinyl) sulfanilamide. The structural formula is:

$H_2N-C_6H_4-SO_2\cdot NH-C_4HN_2(OCH_3)_2$

Actions: Sulfadimethoxine has been demonstrated clinically or in the laboratory to be effective against a variety of organisms, such as streptococci, klebsiella, proteus, shigella, staphylococci, escherichia, and salmonella.[1,2] The systemic sulfonamides which include sulfadimethoxine are bacteriostatic agents. Sulfonamides competitively inhibit bacterial synthesis of folic acid (pteroylglutamic acid) from para-aminobenzoic acid. Mammalian cells are capable of utilizing folic acid in the presence of sulfonamides.
The tissue distribution of sulfadimethoxine, as with all sulfonamides, is a function of plasma levels, degree of plasma protein binding, and subsequent passive distribution in the tissues of the lipid-soluble unionized form. The relative amounts are determined by both its pKa and by the pH of each tissue. Therefore, levels tend to be higher in less acid tissue and body fluids or those diseased tissues having high concentrations of leucocytes.[2]
Slow renal excretion results from a high degree of tubular reabsorption,[3] and plasma protein binding is very high, providing a blood reservoir of the drug. Thus, sulfadimethoxine maintains higher blood levels than most other long-acting sulfonamides. Single, comparatively low doses of Sulfadimethoxine Injection 40% give rapid and sustained therapeutic blood levels.[1]
To assure successful sulfonamide therapy (1) the drug must be given early in the course of the disease, and it must produce a high sulfonamide level in the body rapidly after administration, (2) therapeutically effective sulfonamide levels must be maintained in the body throughout the treatment period, (3) treatment should continue for a short period of time after the clinical signs have disappeared, and (4) the causative organisms must be sensitive to this class of drugs.
Dosage and Administration: DI-METHOX® (Sulfadimethoxine Injection 40%) must be administered only by the intravenous route in cattle. Cattle should receive 1 mL of DI-METHOX® (Sulfadimethoxine Injection 40%) per 16 pounds of body weight (55 mg/kg) as an initial dose, followed by 0.5 mL per 16 pounds of body weight (27.5 mg/kg) every 24 hours thereafter. Sulfadimethoxine boluses may be utilized for maintenance therapy in cattle. Representative weights and doses are indicated in the following table:

Animal Weight	Initial Dose 25 mg/lb. (55 mg/kg)	Subsequent Daily Doses 12.5 mg/lb. (27.5 mg/kg)
250 lb. (113.6 kg)	15.6 mL	7.8 mL
500 lb. (227.2 kg)	31.2 mL	15.6 mL
750 lb. (340.9 kg)	46.9 mL	23.5 mL
1,000 lb. (454.5 kg)	62.5 mL	31.3 mL

Length of treatment depends on the clinical response. In most cases, treatment for 3 to 5 days is adequate. Treatment should be continued until the animal is asymptomatic for 48 hours.
Directions for Intravenous Injection:
Equipment Needed:
1. A nose lead and/or halter sufficiently strong enough to effectively restrain or hold the animal's head steady so that the intravenous injection can be made with ease.
2. Hypodermic needles, 16 or 18 gauge and 2 inches long. Only new, sharp and sterile hypodermic needles should be used. Dull needles should be discarded. Extra needles should be available in case the needles being used should become clogged.
3. Hypodermic syringes, 40 or 50 mL sterile disposable or reusable glass syringes should be available.
4. Alcohol (70%) or an equally effective antiseptic for disinfecting the skin.

Preparation of equipment: Glass syringes and regular hypodermic needles should be thoroughly cleaned and washed. Following this, the needles and syringes should be immersed in boiling water for 30 minutes prior to each injection. Regular hypodermic needles should not be used more than 3-4 times as repeated skin puncturing and boiling of the needles causes them to become quite dull. Disposable hypodermic needles and syringes should not be used more than once.
Restraint of animal: The cow should preferably be in a stanchion for the maximum restraint. If this is not possible, the animal should be restrained in a manner to prevent excessive movement. A nose lead should be applied and the animal's head turned sidewise to stretch the skin and tense the muscles of the neck region.
Locating the jugular vein: Once animal has been restrained, a long depression of the skin from below the angle of the jaw to just above the shoulder is noticed. This is known as the jugular furrow or jugular groove. The jugular vein is located just under the jugular groove.
Preparation of DI-METHOX® (Sulfadimethoxine Injection 40%) for injection: The rubber cap of the bottle should be thoroughly cleaned with 70% alcohol or other satisfactory antiseptic. The correct amount of DI-METHOX® (Sulfadimethoxine Injection 40%) for treatment should be calculated and that amount withdrawn into a syringe. One or two syringefuls of air should be injected into the bottle first to make withdrawing the drug easier. DI-METHOX® (Sulfadimethoxine Injection 40%) should preferably be at room temperature when filling syringes and when injecting intravenously.
Entering the vein: The skin of the injection area should be clean and free of dirt. Cotton saturated with 70% alcohol (or suitable antiseptic) should be used to wipe the injection site.
Apply pressure over the jugular vein close to the shoulder. This will reduce the flow of blood to the heart and cause the jugular vein to bulge or enlarge. (See Figure 1). When the jugular vein

has been "raised", insert the hypodermic needle at a 45 degree angle through the skin just underneath the jugular vein. The beveled edge of the hypodermic needles should be up.

After the skin has been punctured, the point of the needle should be directed toward the side of the vein and pushed into the center of the vein. (See Figure 2). When the needle is in the center of the vein, there will be a free flow of blood back through the needle. Release external pressure when the needle is within the vein.

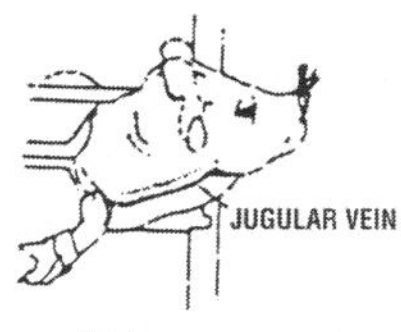

Fig. 1

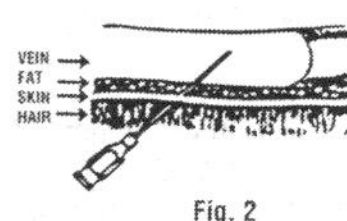

Fig. 2

Injecting the DI-METHOX® (Sulfadimethoxine Injection 40%): After the needle has been accurately inserted into the jugular vein, firmly attach the syringe containing DI-METHOX® (Sulfadimethoxine Injection 40%) to the inserted hypodermic needle. Ensure that the syringe is free of air. Exert firm pressure on the plunger of the syringe to inject the DI-METHOX® (Sulfadimethoxine Injection 40%) while the barrel is held firmly. The injection should be made moderately slow - never rapidly.

If the animal moves, causing resistance in pushing the plunger of the syringe, or if a bubble of the drug is noted under the skin, the needle is no longer within the vein. The needle should be repositioned.

When the injection is completed, quickly withdraw the syringe and needle with a quick pull and apply light pressure over the injection site with alcohol and cotton to minimize bleeding from the puncture site.

Precaution(s): Store at room temperature between 15° and 30°C (59° and 86°F). Should crystallization occur at cold temperatures, crystals will dissolve either by storing at room temperature for several days or by heating the vial in warm water. Crystallization and redissolution do not impair the efficacy of the product.

Caution(s): Restricted drug, use only as directed - Not for human use (California).

For animal use only.

During treatment period, make certain that animals maintain adequate water intake.

If animals show no improvement within 2 or 3 days, consult a veterinarian.

Tissue damage may result from perivascular infiltration.

For intravenous use only in cattle.

Warning(s): Milk taken from animals during treatment and for 60 hours (5 milkings) after the latest treatment must not be used for food. Do not administer within 5 days before slaughter.

A withdrawal period has not been established for this product in pre-ruminating calves. Do not use in calves to be processed for veal.

Keep out of reach of children.

Toxicology: Toxicity and Safety: Data regarding acute (LD_{50}) and chronic toxicities of sulfadimethoxine indicate the drug is very safe. The LD_{50} in mice is greater than 2 g/kg body weight when administered intraperitoneally and greater than 16 g/kg when administered orally. In dogs receiving massive single oral doses of 3.2 g/kg of body weight, diarrhea was the only adverse effect observed. Dogs given 160 mg/kg of body weight orally daily for 13 weeks showed no signs of toxicity.

In cattle sulfadimethoxine has been shown to be safe through extensive clinical use with other dosage forms. In addition, studies with intravenous administration of DI-METHOX® (Sulfadimethoxine Injection 40%) have demonstrated that hemolysis of erythrocytes does not occur by this route of administration. Sulfadimethoxine has a relatively high solubility at the pH normally occurring in the kidney, precluding the possibility of precipitation and crystalluria.

References: Available upon request.

Presentation: 250 mL sterile multiple dose vials.

Compendium Code No.: 10580412 Iss. 10-99

DI-METHOX® SOLUBLE POWDER

AgriLabs **Water Medication**

Sulfadimethoxine Antibacterial Soluble Powder

ANADA No.: 200-031

Active Ingredient(s): Each packet contains 3.34 oz. (94.6 g) Sulfadimethoxine in the form of the soluble sodium salt and disodium edetate.

Indications:

For Broiler and Replacement Chickens Only: Use for the treatment of disease outbreaks of coccidiosis, fowl cholera, and infectious coryza.

For Meat Producing Turkeys Only: Use for the treatment of disease outbreaks of coccidiosis and fowl cholera.

For Dairy Calves, Dairy Heifers and Beef Cattle: Use for the treatment of shipping fever complex, bacterial pneumonia, calf diphtheria, and foot rot.

Dosage and Administration:

Chickens: Concentration - 0.05%. Add the contents of one packet to 50 gallons of water.

Turkeys: Concentration - 0.025%. Add the contents of one packet to 100 gallons of water.

Automatic proportioners: To make a stock solution, add the contents of 5 packets to 2 gallons of water for chickens and to 4 gallons of water for turkeys. Set proportioner to feed at a rate of 1 fl oz of stock solution per gallon of water.

Treatment Period — 6 consecutive days.

Dairy Calves, Dairy Heifers and Beef Cattle: Administer 25 mg/lb first day followed by 12.5 mg/lb/day for 4 days.

	Amount of Stock Solution for Cattle*	DI-METHOX® in Water	
		Water Consumption	
		(Summer) 1 gallon/**100 lb b.w.	(Winter) 1 gallon/**150 lb b.w.
First Day Add:	1 quart	10 gallons	7 gallons
	2 quarts	20 gallons	14 gallons
	1 gallon	40 gallons	28 gallons
Next 4 Days Add:	1 quart	20 gallons	14 gallons
	2 quarts	40 gallons	28 gallons
	1 gallon	80 gallons	56 gallons

*Note: Make a cattle stock solution by adding one packet of DI-METHOX® Soluble Powder to one gallon of water.

**This dosage recommendation is based on a water consumption of one gallon per 100 lb of body weight per day, the expected water consumption rate for summer. Water consumption during the cold months (winter) may drop markedly (30-40%). Accordingly, adjustments must be made in the dilution rates to compensate for this and to ensure proper drug intake.

For treatment of individual cattle, DI-METHOX® Soluble Powder stock solution for cattle may be given as a drench. Administer using the same mg/lb dosage as outlined above.

Twenty fluid ounces of cattle stock solution will medicate one-600 lb animal initially or two-600 lb animals on a maintenance dose. The contents of one packet will medicate six-600 lb animals initially or twelve-600 lb animals on a maintenance dose.

Treatment Period — 5 consecutive days.

Caution(s):

Chickens and Turkeys: If animals show no improvement within 5 days, discontinue treatment and re-evaluate diagnosis. Prepare a fresh stock solution daily. Handle the recommended dilutions (chickens 0.05% and turkeys 0.025%) as regular drinking water. Administer as sole source of drinking water and sulfonamide medication.

Chickens and turkeys that have survived fowl cholera outbreaks should not be kept for replacements or breeders.

Cattle: During treatment period, make certain that animals maintain adequate water intake.

If animals show no improvement within 2 or 3 days, re-evaluate diagnosis. Treatment should not be continued beyond 5 days.

For animal use only.

Not for human use.

Warning(s):

Chickens and Turkeys: Withdraw 5 days before slaughter. Do not administer to chickens over 16 weeks (112 days) of age or to turkeys over 24 weeks (168 days) of age.

Cattle: Withdraw 7 days before slaughter. For dairy calves, dairy heifers and beef cattle only. A withdrawal period has not been established for this product in pre-ruminating calves. Do not use in calves to be processed for veal.

Keep out of reach of children.

Presentation: 107 g (3.77 oz) packets and 25 x 107 g (3.77 oz) packets.

® Registered Trademark of Agri Laboratories, Ltd.

Compendium Code No.: 10580422 8SDM006-101 / 8SDM001-101

DINEOTEX

Stearns **Disinfectant**

EPA Reg. No.: 2495-2-3640

Active Ingredient(s):

a-(P-nonylphenyl)-omega-hydroxypoly (oxyethylene)-iodine complex 18.05%
(providing 1.75% titratable iodine)
Phosphoric acid 16.0%
Inert ingredients 65.95%
Total 100.00%

Indications: Detergent-sanitizer accepted for use on food processing equipment and utensils without rinsing, when used as directed in accordance with federal regulation No. 121.2547.

Dosage and Administration: For milking equipment:

Cleaning operations:

1. Immediately after each milking, thoroughly flush all utensils and milking machines with cold or lukewarm water until all of the milk is washed out. Do not use hot water.
2. Fill the wash tank with lukewarm water (90°F) to which is added one (1) ounce of DINEOTEX for each five (5) gallons of water. (Provides 25 ppm titratable iodine.)
3. Take milking machines apart. Immerse air-hoses, inflations and all parts except pulsator,in DINEOTEX solution before brushing. Wash pails and strainers in the same solution.

Sanitizing operations:

4. In the rinse tank, add one-half (½) ounce of DINEOTEX for each five (5) gallons of lukewarm water to assist in reducing the recontamination of sanitized equipment by contaminated rinse water and by the possible carry-over of organic matter from the wash tank. (Provides 12.5 ppm titratable iodine.)
5. Immerse washed utensils and milking machine parts in the rinse tank solution for at least two (2) minutes. Where local code permits, drain thoroughly, do not rinse.
6. Before each milking, assemble and flush machine parts with a DINEOTEX solution containing one-half (½) ounce of DINEOTEX to five (5) gallons of cold water. (Provides 12.5 ppm titratable iodine.)

Directions for udder washing and sanitizing milking machine cups:

1. Using a clean paper towel for each cow, wash and massage the udder with the above solution approximately one (1) minute before the machine is applied. (If there is excessive dirt, wash away the soil with warm water prior to washing with DINEOTEX.) Udders should be rinsed with potable water prior to milking.
2. Sanitize milking machine cups before applying to each cow. Dip into DINEOTEX solution containing 25 ppm titratable iodine. Drain.

For farm bulk tank:

Cleaning operations:

1. Flush with lukewarm water until all of the milk is washed out.
2. Wash with DINEOTEX solution - One (1) ounce of DINEOTEX to five (5) gallons cold water. (Provides 25 ppm titratable iodine.)
3. Brush thoroughly, drain and rinse for two (2) minutes.

Sanitizing operations: Where code permits, brush or spray the tank with one-quarter (¼) ounce of DINEOTEX to a 10 quart pail of cold water. (Provides 12.5 ppm titratable iodine.)

For udders: Udders should be rinsed with potable water prior to milking. Use a clean paper towel for each cow. Wet in DINEOTEX solution one-half (½) ounce DINEOTEX to a 10 quart pail of lukewarm water (90°F). (Provides 25 ppm titratable iodine.)

For milkstone removal: Should a yellow color show on equipment after the first use of DINEOTEX, milkstone is indicated. Remove it, using a DINEOTEX solution - equal parts of DINEOTEX and lukewarm water. Spread over the surface to be cleaned, wait two (2) to three (3) minutes, then brush and rinse with potable water. The daily use of DINEOTEX will prevent the formation of milkstone.

Note: Use freshly made solutions for each morning and night milking. Where health departments require dismantling twice a day, the same method would be used at night as in the morning. Follow state and health department requirements covering cleaning and sanitizing.

To sanitize previously cleaned food processing equipment and utensils, use one (1) ounce of DINEOTEX to five (5) gallons of water. Drain. Do not rinse.

Important: DINEOTEX is its own indicator of germicidal activity. The amber or yellow color shows the presence of the active ingredient - iodine. When the color fades, prepare a fresh solution. DINEOTEX is not adversely affected by water hardness or cold water. In use dilution, DINEOTEX will not corrode stainless steel, rubber or commonly used plastics. Use only as directed. Formulated from biodegradable detergents.

Precaution(s):

Storage: Keep the container closed when not in use. Do not store below 25°F or above 100°F for extended periods.

Disposal: Do not contaminate water, food, or feed by storage or disposal, or the cleaning of equipment. In case of a spill, flood the area with a large quantity of water, washing into a sewer or collection vessel. Wastes resulting from the use of the product may be disposed of on site or at an approved waste disposal facility. Do not re-use the empty container. Triple rinse, puncture, and dispose of the container in a sanitary landfill or by incineration.

Caution(s): Danger - Keep out of the reach of children.

Use of the product causes damage to the eyes and severe skin irritation. Do not get in eyes or on skin. May be fatal or harmful it swallowed. In case of contact, flush immediately with plenty of water. For eyes, get medical attention. Avoid contamination of food.

First Aid: If swallowed, promptly drink a large quantity of milk, egg whites, gelatin solution or if these are not available, drink large quantities of water. Avoid alcohol. Call a physician immediately.

Note to Physician: Probable mucosal damage may contraindicate the use of gastric lavage. Measures against circulatory shock, respiratory depression and convulsion may be needed.

Presentation: 1 U.S. gallon (3.78 L) containers.

Compendium Code No.: 10170020

DIOCTYNATE

Butler **Enema**

Active Ingredient(s): A 5% water miscible solution of dioctyl sodium sulfosuccinate, which also contains water and propylene glycol.

Indications: For use as an enema in dogs, cats and horses. For use as a laxative in horses. For use as a ceruminolytic agent in dogs and cats.

Dosage and Administration:

Horses: For use as an enema, administer four (4) to six (6) ounces in one (1) gallon of water. For use as a laxative, administer orally eight (8) ounces in one (1) gallon of water or mineral oil.

Dogs and Cats: For use as an enema, administer two (2) to three (3) ounces of a mixture of 5 mL D.S.S. per ounce of water.

For use as a ceruminolytic agent, administer two (2) to three (3) drops in each ear.

Precaution(s): Cooler temperatures will cause the product to become cloudy. Place it in warm water or bring it to room temperature (68°-74°F).

Caution(s): For veterinary use only.

Keep out of the reach of children.

Sold to graduate veterinarians only.

Presentation: 1 gallon (3.785 L) containers.

Compendium Code No.: 10820610

DI-QUAT 10-S™

Butler **Disinfectant**

EPA Reg. No.: 6836-57-6480

Active Ingredient(s):

Alkyl (C_{14}, 60%; C_{16}, 30%; C_{12}, 5%; C_{18}, 5%) dimethyl benzyl ammonium chloride	5.0%
Alkyl (C_{12}, 68%; C_{14}, 32%) dimethyl ethylbenzyl ammonium chloride	5.0%
Inert ingredients	90.0%
Total	100.0%

Indications: A disinfectant, fungicide, and deodorizer for hospital, institutional, industrial, school, dairy and other farm use.

Dosage and Administration:

General classification: It is a violation of federal law to use the product in a manner inconsistent with its labeling.

Apply DI-QUAT 10-S™ with a cloth, mop or mechanical spray device. When applied with a mechanical spray device, the surface must be sprayed until thoroughly wetted. Treated surfaces must remain wet for 10 minutes. Fresh solutions should be prepared daily or when the use solution becomes visibly dirty.

Disinfection of hospitals and other health care institutions: For disinfecting floors, walls, countertops, bathing areas, lavatories, tables, chairs, garbage pails and other hard, nonporous surfaces, add 4.5 oz. DI-QUAT 10-S™ to five (5) gallons of water. Apply to previously cleaned hard surfaces with a mop or cloth.

At this use-level, DI-QUAT 10-S™ is effective against *Pseudomonas aeruginosa*.

Disinfection of institutions, industry and schools: For disinfecting floors, walls, countertops, tables, chairs, garbage pails, bathroom fixtures and other hard, nonporous surfaces, add 3 oz. of DI-QUAT 10-S™ to five (5) gallons of water. Apply to previously cleaned, hard surfaces with a mop or cloth.

At 3 oz./5 gallon use-level, DI-QUAT 10-S™ is effective against *Staphylococcus aureus* and *Salmonella choleraesuis*.

Fungicidal activity: At 8 oz./5 gallons use-level, DI-QUAT 10-S™ is effective against *Trichophyton interdigitale* (athlete's foot fungus) on inanimate, hard surfaces.

Disinfection of poultry equipment, animal quarters and kennels: Poultry brooders, watering founts, feeding equipment and other animal quarters (such as stalls and kennel areas) can be disinfected after thorough cleaning by applying a solution of 4.5 oz. DI-QUAT 10-S™ to five (5) gallons of water with a mop, cloth or brush. Small utensils should be immersed in this solution.

Prior to disinfection, all poultry, other animals and their feeds must be removed from the premises. This includes emptying all troughs, racks and other feeding and watering appliances. Remove all litter and droppings from floors, walls and other surfaces occupied or traversed by poultry or other animals.

After disinfection, ventilate buildings, coops and other closed spaces. Do not house poultry, or other animals, or employ equipment until the treatment has been absorbed, set or dried.

All treated equipment that will contact feed or drinking water must be rinsed with potable water before re-use.

Precaution(s): Storage and Disposal: Do not contaminate water, food, or feed by storage or disposal. Do not store on site. Avoid creasing or impaction of side walls.

Pesticide Disposal: Pesticide wastes are acutely hazardous. Improper disposal of excess pesticide, spray or mixture of rinsate is a violation of federal law. If these wastes cannot be disposed of according to label instructions, contact the State Pesticide or Environmental Control Agency, or the hazardous waste representative at the nearest EPA Regional Office for guidance.

Container Disposal: Do not re-use the empty container (bottle, can, bucket). Wrap the container and put it in the trash.

Caution(s): Precautionary Statements:

Hazardous to Humans and Domestic Animals: Danger. Keep out of the reach of children. Corrosive. Causes eye damage and skin irritation. Do not get in eyes, on skin, or on clothing. Wear goggles or a face shield and rubber gloves when handling. Harmful or fatal if swallowed. Avoid contamination of food.

Statement of Practical Treatment:

In case of contact, immediately flush eyes or skin with plenty of water for at least 15 minutes. For eyes call a physician. Remove and wash contaminated clothing before re-use.

If swallowed, promptly drink a large quantity of milk, egg whites, gelatin solution; or if these are not available, drink large quantities of water. Avoid alcohol. Call a physician immediately.

Note to Physician: Probable mucosal damage may contraindicate the use of gastric lavage. Measures against circulatory shock, respiratory depression, and convulsion may be needed.

Presentation: 1 gallon containers.

Compendium Code No.: 10820590

DiroCHEK®

Synbiotics **Heartworm Test**

Canine Heartworm Antigen Test Kit

U.S. Vet. Lic. No.: 312

Test Description: Canine heartworm antigen test kit.

Contents:

	Regular	Lab Pack
Anti-*D. immitis* Coated Wells	48	144
Tri-Continent Precision pipetter	1	1
Pipette Tips	50	150
Positive Control (Red Cap)	1.0 mL	2.5 mL
Negative Control (Gray Cap)	1.0 mL	2.5 mL
Reagent 1 - HRP Antibody Conjugate (Blue Cap)	2.5 mL	7.0 mL
Reagent 2 - Chromogenic Substrate Buffer (Purple Cap)	7.0 mL	14.0 mL

Materials required but not provided: distilled or deionized water.

Also available: Kilo pack.

Patent No. 4,789,631

Indications: DiroCHEK® is an enzyme-linked immunoassay (ELISA) for the detection of adult *D. immitis* antigen in canine and feline plasma or serum. DiroCHEK® is highly specific, sensitive and simple to use. Test results can be obtained in 15 minutes.

Test Principles: The reaction wells are coated with antibodies directed against *D. immitis* antigen. Another antibody is labeled with the enzyme horseradish peroxidase. Any antigen present in the specimen (plasma or serum) is bound by the antibody coated well and the enzyme-linked antibody to form a specific complex. Any free enzyme-linked antibody is washed away and a chromogenic substrate is added. In the absence of *D. immitis* antigen, no color change will be observed. The development of a blue color specifically indicates the presence of *D. immitis* antigen and heartworms.

Predicting Heartworm Burden: Level of color in sample wells will intensify with increasing level of heartworm antigen. Level of heartworm antigen correlates with the number of heartworms present, although it is more closely related to the actual weight of worms present (a product of both the number and size of worms).

Test Procedure: Sample Information: 50 µL (0.05 mL) of serum or plasma is required. Serum or plasma (not whole blood) may be stored at 2°-7°C (36°-45°F) for 7 days; -20°C or below if stored longer. Hemolyzed and lipemic samples may be used, however, they may produce background color. When in doubt, obtain a better quality sample.

A. Preparation:

1. Calculate required number of wells:
   - 1 well for positive control.
   - 1 well for negative control.
   - 1 well for each sample.

   Remove required number of wells.
   Leave wells attached to each other.
   Place in well holder.

2A. Controls:
   Add 1 drop Positive Control (red cap) into the first well.
   Add 1 drop Negative Control (gray cap) into the second well.

B. Sample(s): Use of the 0.050 mL Precision Pipetter: Place pipette tip firmly onto pipette. Release button slowly to aspirate. Depress button to dispense.
   Draw/aspirate 0.05 mL sample.
   Dispense 0.05 mL sample into the next well following the controls.
   Discard pipette tip.
   Repeat procedure for each sample into subsequent wells.

B. Conjugate:

3. Add 1 drop Reagent 1 - Conjugate (blue cap) into each well.
   Tap well holder (without splashing) for 15 seconds to mix.
   Wait 10 minutes.

C. Blot and Wash:

4. Discard fluid from wells into sink or appropriate container.
   Invert holder and blot firmly onto a paper towel to remove final drops.
5. Wash Wells Vigorously:
   Use liberal amounts of distilled or deionized water.

Direct a forceful stream into each well. (Oversplashing will not contaminate adjacent wells.)
Shake out excess water.
Repeat at least 5 times. (It is impossible to overwash.)
Blot firmly onto a paper towel to remove final drops.

D. Develop:

6. Add 2 drops Reagent 2 (purple cap) to each well.
Tap well holder (without splashing) for 15 seconds to mix.
Wait 5 minutes.
Read results.

Test Interpretation: Controls:

Positive control should be distinctly blue.

Negative control should be completely clear.

Samples:

Positive samples will be blue. Color intensity will vary with level of heartworm antigen present. This may reflect worm burden (see Test Principles).

Negative samples will be clear. Compare directly with the negative control against a white background.

Storage: Storage and Stability: Store the test kit at 2°-7°C (36°-45°F). Do not freeze. Reagents will be stable until expiration date provided they have been stored properly.

Caution(s):

1. Allow kit to come to room temperature (21°-25°C; 70°-78°F) prior to use.
2. Do not expose kit to direct sunlight.
3. Do not use expired reagents or mix from different kit lots.
4. Follow instructions exactly. Improper washing or contamination of reagents may produce nonspecific color development.
5. For veterinary use only.

Discussion: Heartworm Disease: Heartworm disease is caused by *Dirofilaria immitis,* a filarial nematode whose immature stages are transmitted between animals by mosquitoes. The adult heartworms live in the heart and adjacent large blood vessels. Although primarily a disease of dogs, the parasite can also infect cats, ferrets and other mammals, such as the red fox and the coyote.

Presentation: Available in 2 sizes: Lab Pack (48-142) and Kilo Pack (1056 wells).

Licensed under U.S. Patent No. 4,839,275.

DiroCHEK® is a registered trademark of Synbiotics Corporation.

Compendium Code No.: 11150062 03-0024-0100

DISAL® INJECTION ℞

Boehringer Ingelheim **Diuretic**

(furosemide) 50 mg/mL

NADA No.: 131-538

Active Ingredient(s): Each mL contains: 50 mg furosemide as a monoethanolamine salt, myristyl-gamma-picolinium chloride 0.02%, EDTA sodium 0.1%, sodium sulfite 0.1% with sodium chloride 0.2% in water for injection. The pH is adjusted with sodium hydroxide and/or hydrochloric acid.

Indications: Dogs and Horses: DISAL® Injection is an effective diuretic-saluretic for use in the treatment of acute noninflammatory tissue edema in dogs and horses, and for use in the treatment of edema (pulmonary congestion, ascites) associated with cardiac insufficiency in the dog. In cases of edema involving cardiac insufficiency, the continued use of heart stimulants such as digitalis or its glycosides is indicated.

The rationale for the use of diuretic therapy in either dogs or horses is determined by the clinical pathology producing the edema.

Pharmacology: Furosemide is a potent loop diuretic which is a derivative of anthranilic acid. The structure is:

COOH, NH · CH2, NH2SO2, Cl

Chemical name: 4-chloro-N-furfuryl-5-sulfamoylanthranilic acid. Furosemide is pharmacodynamically characterized by the following:

1. Administered intramuscularly, it begins to act in about 30 minutes, and a diuretic response is produced. When administered intravenously, the response is in about 5 minutes.[1,2]
2. DISAL® is a loop diuretic which inhibits the re-absorption of sodium and chloride at the ascending loop of Henle in the kidneys, enhancing water excretion.[3]
3. A dose-response relationship and a ratio of minimum to maximum effective dose range greater than tenfold.[1]
4. A high degree of efficacy, low inherent toxicity and a high therapeutic index.

Actions: The therapeutic efficacy of DISAL® Injection is from the activity of the intact and unaltered molecule throughout the nephron, inhibiting the re-absorption of sodium not only in the proximal and distal tubule but also in the ascending limb of the loop of Henle. The prompt onset of action is a result of the drug's rapid absorption and a poor lipid solubility. The low lipid solubility and a rapid renal excretion minimize the possibility of its accumulation in tissues and organs or crystalluria. Furosemide has no inhibitory effect on carbonic anhydrase or aldosterone activity in the distal tubule. The drug possesses diuretic activity either in the presence of acidosis or alkalosis.[1,3,4,5,6]

Dosage and Administration: Dogs: Administer intravenously or intramuscularly 0.25 to 0.50 mL per 10 pounds of body weight once or twice daily at 6 to 8 hour intervals.

The dosage should be adjusted to the individual's response. In severe edematous or refractory cases, the dose may be doubled or increased by increments of 1.0 mg per pound of body weight. The established effective dose should be administered once or twice daily. Discontinue diuretic therapy with DISAL® Injection, 50 mg/mL after the initiation of acute fluid mobilization or the stabilization of the patient; when necessary Disal® Tablets may be used for maintenance therapy. Do not exceed treatment with DISAL® Injection, 50 mg/mL for more than 3 days. The daily schedule of administration can be timed to control the period of micturition for the convenience of the client or veterinarian. Mobilization of the edema may be most efficiently and safely accomplished by utilizing an intermittent daily dose schedule, i.e., every other day or 2 to 4 consecutive days weekly.

Horses: The usual parenteral dosage of furosemide in horses is approximately 0.5 mg/lb body weight (1.0 mg/kg). See the dosage schedule below. A prompt diuresis usually ensues from the initial treatment. Administer once or twice daily at 6 to 8 hour intervals either intravenously or intramuscularly until the desired results are achieved.

The dosage should be adjusted to the individual's response. In severe edematous or refractory cases, the dose may be doubled or increased by increments of 0.5 mg per pound of body weight. The established effective dose should be administered once or twice daily. The daily schedule of administration can be timed to control the period of micturition for the convenience of the client or veterinarian. Mobilization of the edema may be most efficiently and safely accomplished by utilizing an intermittent daily dose schedule, i.e., every other day or 2 to 4 consecutive days weekly.

Recommended Dosage Schedule:

Horses: Administer I.V. or I.M. once or twice daily at 6 to 8 hour intervals until desired results are achieved.

Body Weight (lbs)	DISAL® Injection (50 mg/mL)
500	4.6 mL
600	5.5 mL
700	6.4 mL
800	7.3 mL
900	8.2 mL
1,000	9.1 mL
1,100	10.0 mL
1,200	10.9 mL

Diuretic therapy for both dogs and horses should be discontinued after reduction of the edema, or maintained after determining a carefully programmed dosage schedule to prevent the recurrence of edema. For long-term treatment, the dose can generally be lowered after the edema has once been reduced. Re-examination and consultations with the client will enhance the establishment of a satisfactorily programmed dosage schedule. Clinical examination and serum BUN, CO_2 and electrolyte determinations should be performed during the early period of therapy and periodically thereafter, especially in refractory cases. Abnormalities should be corrected or the drug temporarily withdrawn.

Contraindication(s): Animal reproductive studies have shown that furosemide may cause fetal abnormality and the drug is contraindicated in pregnant bitches, mares and stallions at stud.

Furosemide is contraindicated in anuria, furosemide hypersensitivity, hepatic coma, or during electrolytic imbalances. Monitor serum electrolytes, BUN and CO_2 frequently. Monitor serum potassium levels and watch for signs of hypocalcemia.

Corticosteroids cause an additive potassium-depletion effect.

Precaution(s): Store at controlled room temperature, 59°-86°F (15°-30°C).

Caution(s): Federal (U.S.A.) law restricts this drug to use by or on the order of a licensed veterinarian.

DISAL® Injection is a highly effective diuretic-saluretic which, if given in excessive amounts, may result in dehydration and have to be adjusted to the patient's needs. The animal should be observed for early signs of electrolyte imbalance, and corrective measures administered. Early signs of electrolyte imbalance are increased thirst, lethargy, drowsiness or restlessness, fatigue, oliguria, gastro-intestinal disturbances and tachycardia. Special attention should be given to potassium levels. DISAL® Injection may lower serum calcium levels and cause tetany in rare cases of animals having an existing hypocalcemic tendency.[7,8,9,10,11]

DISAL® Injection is contraindicated in anuria. Therapy should be discontinued in cases of progressive renal disease if increasing azotemia and oliguria occur during the treatment. Sudden alterations of fluid and electrolyte imbalance in an animal with cirrhosis may precipitate hepatic coma, therefore observation during the period of therapy is necessary. In hepatic coma and in states of electrolyte depletion, therapy should not be instituted until the basic condition is improved or corrected. Potassium supplementation may be necessary in cases routinely treated with potassium-depleting steroids.

Active or latent diabetes melitus may, on rare occasions, be exacerbated by furosemide. Transient loss of auditory capacity has been experimentally produced in cats following intravenous injections of excessive doses of furosemide at a very rapid rate.[12,13,14]

DISAL® Injection is a highly effective diuretic and, if given in excessive amounts, as with any diuretic, may lead to excessive diuresis which could result in electrolyte imbalance, dehydration and reduction of plasma volume, enhancing the risk of circulatory collapse, thrombosis and embolism. Therefore, the animal should be observed for early signs of fluid depletion with electrolyte imbalance, and corrective measures administered. Excessive loss of potassium in patients receiving digitalis or its glycosides may precipitate digitalis toxicity. Caution should be exercised in animals administered potassium-depleting steroids. Correct potassium deficiency with proper dietary supplementation. If an animal needs potassium supplements, use the oral liquid form, do not use enteric-coated potassium tablets.

The concurrent use of furosemide with some antibiotics may be inadvisable. There is evidence that the drug enhances the nephrotoxic potential of aminoglycosides, cephalosporins and polymyxins and increases the ototoxic effects of all aminoglycosides.

Sulfonamide diuretics have been reported to decrease arterial responsiveness to pressor amines and to enhance the effect of tubocurarine. Caution should be exercised in administering curare or its derivatives to patients undergoing therapy with DISAL® Injection and it is advisable to discontinue DISAL® Injection for one day prior to any elective surgery.

For veterinary use only.

Warning(s): Do not use in horses intended for food.

Toxicology: Furosemide demonstrates a very low order of either acute or chronic toxicity. The drug is rapidly absorbed and excreted by both glomerular filtration and tubular secretion. The rates of excretion are of such a magnitude that the cumulation of furosemide does not occur despite repeated administrations.[15]

The main effect observed in clinical toxicity is an abnormality of fluid and electrolyte imbalances. Ototoxicity resulting in transient loss of hearing has been reported with furosemide.[15]

A safety study was performed in dogs to determine the effects of DISAL® Injection at increasing dosages and time elements. The dosage levels were 1.5 mg/lb body weight (recommended dosage), 4.5 mg/lb body weight (3X recommended dosage) and 7.5 mg/lb body weight (5X recommended dosage). The treatment period ranged up to nine days in length. Results demonstrate a very slight tubular nephrosis at the higher dosage levels.

In addition, serum levels of potassium and chloride were slightly lowered in the higher dosage groups. Cumulative evaluation of the data demonstrates that DISAL® Injection is safe when administered at the recommended dosage for a duration of nine consecutive days.

References: Available upon request.

Presentation: Available in 50 mL and 100 mL multi-dose vials.

DISAL® is a Registered Trademark of Boehringer Ingelheim Vetmedica, Inc.

Compendium Code No.: 10280341 BI 673-1 6/00

D

DISCOURAGE TASTE DETERRENT & TRAINING AID

Davis **Topical Product**

Active Ingredient(s): Water, ethanol, denatonium benzoate, artificial flavor.

Indications: An aid to protect wounds and hot spots on dogs.

It also helps save furniture from destructive chewing.

Davis DISCOURAGE leaves an unpleasant taste on surfaces to help stop licking, chewing and biting.

Directions for Use: Shake well before using.

For Pet: To discourage licking, chewing and biting, apply topically on pet. Avoid spraying in eyes. Repeat as often as needed.

For Furniture and Upholstery: Test an inconspicuous area before applying. May stain some surfaces.

Warning(s): For external use only.

Keep out of reach of children.

Presentation: 8 fl oz (236 mL).

Compendium Code No.: 11410150

DISINTEGRATOR®

Phoenix Pharmaceutical **Disinfectant**

One-Step Germicidal Detergent & Deodorant

EPA Reg. No.: 47371-129-58383

Active Ingredient(s):

Didecyl dimethyl ammonium chloride 10.14%
n-Alkyl (C_{14} 50%, C_{12} 40%, C_{16} 10%) dimethyl benzyl ammonium chloride 6.76%
Inert Ingredients: 83.10%
Total 100.00%

Indications: A multi-purpose, neutral pH, germicidal detergent and deodorant effective in hard water up to 400 ppm (calculated as $CaCO_3$) in the presence of a moderate amount of soil (5% organic serum) according to the AOAC Use-dilution Test. Disinfects, cleans, and deodorizes in one step.

Effective against the following pathogens:

Bacteria: *Pseudomonas aeruginosa,*[1] *Staphylococcus aureus,*[1] *Salmonella choleraesuis, Acintobacter calcoaceticus, Bordetella bronchiseptica, Chlamydia psittaci, Enterobacter aerogenes, Enterobacter cloacae, Enterococcus faecalis* - Vancomycin Resistant (VRE), *Escherichia coli,*[1] *Fusobacterium necrophorum, Klebsiella pneumoniae,*[1] *Legionella pneumophila, Listeria monocytogenes, Pasturella multocida, Proteus mirabillis, Proteus vulgaris, Salmonella enteritidis, Salmonella typhi, Salmonella typhimurium, Serratia marcescens, Shigella flexneri, Shigella sonnei, Staphylococcus aureus* - Methicillin resistant (MRSA), *Staphylococcus aureus* - Vancomycin Intermediate Resistant (VISA), *Staphylococcus epidermis,*[2] *Streptococcus faecalis,*[1] *Streptococcus pyogenes.*

Viruses: *Adenovirus type 4, *Hepatitis B Virus (HBV), *Herpes Simplex Type 1, *Herpes Simplex Type 2, *HIV-1 (AIDS virus), *Influenza A/Hong Kong, *Vaccinia, *Rubella (German Measles), *Respiratory Syncytial Virus (RSV).

Animal Viruses: *Avian polyomavirus, *Canine distemper, *Feline leukemia, *Feline picomavirus, *Infectious bovine rhinotracheitis, *Infectious bronchitis (Avian IBV), *Pseudorabies (PRV), *Rabies, *Transmissible gastroenteritis virus (TGE).

Fungi: *Aspergillus niger, Candida albicans, Trichophyton mentagrophytes.*

[1]ATCC and anti antibiotic-resistant strain; [2]antibiotic-resistant strain only; *Kills HIV-1 (AIDS Virus), and HBV (Hepatitis B Virus) on precleaned, environmental surfaces/objects previously soiled with blood/body fluids in health care settings or other settings in which there is an expected likelihood of soiling of inanimate surfaces/objects with bloody/body fluids, and in which the surfaces/objects likely to be soiled with blood/body fluids can be associated with the potential for transmission of Human Immunodeficiency Virus Type 1 (HIV-1) (associated with AIDS) or Hepatitis B Virus (HBV).

Recommended for use in hospitals, nursing homes, schools, colleges, commercial and industrial institutions, office buildings, veterinary clinics, animal life science laboratories, zoos, tack shops, pet shops, airports, kennels, hotels, motels, breeding establishments, grooming establishments, and households. Use to clean and disinfect non-medical (i.e. industrial and fire-fighting) respirators in industrial, commercial and institutional premises. Disinfects, cleans, and deodorizes the following hard, non-porous, inanimate surfaces: floors, walls, (non-medical) metal surfaces, (non-medical) stainless steel surfaces, glazed porcelain, plastic surfaces (such as polypropylene, polystyrene, etc.).

Directions for Use: It is a violation of Federal law to use this product in a manner inconsistent with its labeling.

Dilution: 1:256 .... ½ ounce per gallon of water (600 ppm quat)

Disinfection/Cleaning/Deodorizing Directions: Remove heavy soil deposits from surface. Then thoroughly wet surface with a use-solution of ½ ounce of the concentrate per gallon of water. The use-solution can be applied with a cloth, mop, sponge, or coarse spray, or soaking. Let solution remain on surface for a minimum of 10 minutes. Rinse or allow to air dry. Rinsing of floors is not necessary unless they are to be waxed or polished. Food contact surfaces must be thoroughly rinsed with potable water. This product must not be used to clean the following food contact surfaces: utensils, glassware and dishes. Prepare a fresh solution daily or more often if the solution becomes visibly dirty or diluted.

Toilet Bowls: Swab bowl with brush to remove heavy soil prior to cleaning or disinfecting. Clean by applying use-solution around the bowl and up under the rim. Stubborn stains may require brushing. To disinfect, first remove or expel over the inner trap the residual bowl water. Pour in three ounces of the use-solution. Swab the bowl completely using a scrub brush or mop, making sure to get under rim. Let stand for 10 minutes or overnight, then flush.

Fungicidal Directions: For use in areas such as locker rooms, dressing rooms, shower and bath areas and exercise facilities follow disinfection directions.

Mildewstatic Instructions: Will effectively control the growth of mold and mildew plus the odors caused by them when applied to hard, non-porous surfaces such as walls, floors and table tops. Apply use-solution of ½ ounce per gallon of water with a cloth, mop, sponge, or coarse spray. Make sure to wet all surfaces completely. Let air dry. Repeat application weekly or when growth reappears.

Special Instructions for Cleaning and Decontamination Against HIV-1 (AIDS Virus) or HBV of Surfaces/Objects Soiled with Blood/Body Fluids:

Personal Protection: Disposable latex or vinyl gloves, gowns, face masks, or eye coverings as appropriate must be worn during all cleaning of blood/body fluids and during decontamination procedures.

Cleaning Procedures: Blood/body fluids must be thoroughly cleaned from surfaces/objects before application of disinfectant.

Contact Time: HIV-1 (AIDS virus) is inactivated after a contact time of 4 minutes at 25°C (room temperature). HBV is inactivated after a 10 minute contact time. Use a 10-minute contact time for other viruses, fungi, and bacteria listed.

Disposal of Infectious Materials: Blood/body fluids should be autoclaved and disposed of according to federal, state and local regulations for infectious waste disposal.

Cleaning and Disinfecting Hard Non-Porous Surfaces on Personal Protective Equipment (Respirators): Preclean equipment if heavily soiled to ensure proper surface contact. Add ½ oz of DISINTEGRATOR® to one gallon of water. Gently mix for a uniform solution. Apply solution to hard non-porous surfaces of the respirator with a brush, coarse spray device, sponge, or by immersion. Thoroughly wet all surfaces to be disinfected. Treated surfaces should remain wet for 10 minutes. Remove excess solution from equipment prior to storage. Comply with all OSHA regulations for cleaning respiratory protection (29 CFR Section 1910.134).

Veterinary Practice/Animal Care/Animal Laboratory/Zoos/Pet Shop/Kennels Disinfection Directions: For cleaning and disinfecting the following hard non-porous surfaces: Equipment not used for animal food or water, utensils, instruments, cages, kennels, stables, catteries, etc. Remove all animals and feed from premises, animal transportation vehicles, crates, etc. Remove all litter, droppings and manure from floors, walls and surfaces of facilities occupied or traversed by animals. Thoroughly clean all surfaces with soap or detergent and rinse with water. Saturate surfaces with a use-solution of ½ oz of DISINTEGRATOR® per gallon of water (or equivalent dilution) for a period of 10 minutes. Ventilate buildings and other closed spaces. Do not house animals or employ equipment until treatment has been absorbed, set or dried.

Contraindication(s): This product is not for use on medical device surfaces.

Precautionary Statements: Hazards to Humans and Domestic Animals:

Danger: Corrosive. Causes irreversible eye damage and skin burns. Harmful if swallowed. Do not get in eyes, on skin, or on clothing. When handling product, protect eyes by wearing goggles or face shield and protect skin by wearing rubber gloves. Wash thoroughly with soap and water after handling. Remove contaminated clothing and wash before reuse.

First Aid:

If in Eyes: Hold eye open and rinse slowly and gently with water for 15-20 minutes. Remove contact lenses, if present, after the first 5 minutes, then continue rinsing eye.

If on Skin or Clothing: Take off contaminated clothing. Rinse skin immediately with plenty of water for 15-20 minutes.

If Swallowed: Call a poison control center or doctor immediately for treatment advice. Have person sip a glass of water if able to swallow. Do not induce vomiting unless told to do so by the poison control center or doctor. Do not give anything by mouth to an unconscious person.

Call a poison control center or doctor for treatment advice. Have the product container or label with you when calling a poison control center or doctor or going for treatment.

Note to Physician: Probable mucosal damage may contraindicate the use of gastric lavage. Measures against circulatory shock, respiratory depression, and convulsion may be needed.

Storage and Disposal: Keep product under locked storage, inaccessible to children. Do not reuse empty container. Rinse thoroughly, securely wrap in several layers of newspaper, and discard empty container in trash or recycle.

Warning(s): Keep out of reach of children.

Presentation: 1 U.S. gallon (3.785 L) plastic containers.

Compendium Code No.: 12560252 Rev. 10/01

DISPOSABLE ENEMA ℞

Vedco **Enema**

Active Ingredient(s): Each mL contains: 250 mg of dioctyl sodium sulfosuccinate in glycerine U.S.P.

Indications: For use as an aid in the relief of constipation. For the relief of impaction caused by hard fecal masses in dogs and cats.

Lubricates and softens stool.

Dosage and Administration: Gently insert the flexible nozzle into the rectum and press the plunger to express the contents.

In resistant cases, the treatment may be repeated in one (1) hour.

Caution(s): Federal law restricts this drug to use by or on the order of a licensed veterinarian.

Keep out of the reach of children.

For veterinary use only.

Presentation: 12 mL syringes.

Compendium Code No.: 10940460

DISTEMINK®

United **Vaccine**

Mink Distemper Vaccine, Modified Live Virus

U.S. Vet. Lic. No.: 245

Active Ingredient(s): The vaccine consists of two components: A freeze-dried distemper vaccine consisting of modified live canine distemper virus (DISTEMINK®) and sterile diluent. The diluent is used to dissolve the DISTEMINK®.

Preservative: Gentamicin.

Indications: DISTEMINK® is for use as an aid in the prevention of distemper in healthy, susceptible mink.

Dosage and Administration: Mixing of the Vaccine:

1. Do not mix the vaccine until ready to use.
2. Mix only one pair of vials at a time, and use the entire contents within two (2) hours.
3. Disinfect rubber stoppers with alcohol.
4. Using a sterile transfer needle, transfer the diluent into the bottle of DISTEMINK®.
5. To do this Insert the short end of the double-pointed transfer needle into the diluent and turn the bottle upside down; then, insert the other end of the transfer needle into the DISTEMINK®. The diluent will be drawn into the DISTEMINK® bottle by vacuum.
6. After all the diluent has been transferred, shake gently to suspend evenly.
7. Do not transfer the vaccine to other containers.

Use sharp, sterile needles and sterile syringes. Inject 1 mL under the loose skin of the armpit of mink of at least 10 weeks of age. For a proper suspension,shake before and occasionally during use. Revaccinate all adults at the time of kit vaccination.

Keep a record of brand name, quantity, serial number, expiration date, and place of purchase. Record the date of vaccination, the number, age and location of the mink.

Contact United Vaccines Inc. before mixing with any liquid product other than that provided in the box.

Consult a veterinarian or United Vaccines Inc. for an alternate vaccinating schedule and before using the vaccine on a farm where disease exists or has occurred in the last 18 months or where earlier botulism protection is desired.

Precaution(s): Store at 35-45°F (2-7°C).

Caution(s):
1. Burn the empty containers and any unused portion of the vaccine.
2. Syringes and reusable, stainless steal needles may be sterilized by boiling them in distilled water for 15 to 20 minutes. Do not disinfect them with chemicals as these can destroy the vaccine.
3. Incubating diseases (such as Aleutian disease), parasites, nutritional deficiencies (anemia), maternal antibodies and poor management practices (dehydration, adverse temperatures) will reduce the vaccine's effectiveness.
4. If shock occurs after vaccination, use atropine sulfate or epinephrine.
5. Should disease occur in an unvaccinated herd, the losses may be minimized by promptly vaccinating those animals which are not showing signs of the disease. The best procedure is to first vaccinate the mink located the farthest distance from those showing symptoms. Care should be taken to use a sterile needle for each animal and to disinfect handling gloves as often as is practical. Consult a veterinarian regarding the treatment and handling of sick animals.
6. Animals infected, yet not showing signs of disease at the time of vaccination, will not be protected by the vaccine. Symptoms of the disease may continue to develop for as long as two months after vaccination.

Presentation: 100 dose and 250 dose vials.
Compendium Code No.: 11040081

DISTEM-R TC®

Schering-Plough **Vaccine**

Mink Distemper Vaccine, Modified Live Virus
U.S. Vet. Lic. No.: 165A
Contents: A modified live distemper virus grown in chicken embryo tissue culture and combined with stabilizing agents. Preservative: Gentamicin.
Indications: This vaccine is for use in mink 8 weeks of age or older, as an aid in preventing distemper through vaccination by subcutaneous injection.
Dosage and Administration: Vaccinate eight weeks of age or older. Revaccinate breeders for distemper one month before mating season.

Preparation of the Vaccine:

Do not open and mix the vaccine until ready for use.

Mix only one vial at a time and use entire contents within two hours.

Disinfect exposed rubber stoppers with alcohol or other disinfectants.

Using a sterile transfer needle, or a sterile needle and syringe, transfer the entire contents of the diluent bottle into the bottle of dried vaccine. (Insert transfer needle into diluent first, turn diluent bottle upside down, then insert other end of transfer needle into vaccine bottle. Diluent will be drawn into vaccine bottle by vacuum.)

As soon as all diluent has been transferred, shake the vaccine several times to suspend evenly.

The vaccine is now ready for use.

How to Vaccinate: For all mink, inject 1.0 mL (cc) under the skin, preferably in the region of the armpit (axillary space).

Records: Keep a record of vaccine type, quantity, serial number, expiration date, and place of purchase; the date and time of vaccination; the number, age and location of the mink; names of operators performing the vaccination and any observed reactions.

Contraindication(s): Mink younger than 8 weeks of age and born from vaccinated female breeders may possess strong maternal immunity which can interfere with this vaccine. Thus, vaccination of such mink is not recommended before 8 weeks of age.
Precaution(s): Store at 2° to 7°C (35° to 45°F).

Use only sterile needles and syringes to inject the vaccine. Syringes and needles may be sterilized by boiling for 15 to 20 minutes. Do not disinfect with chemicals since they may destroy the vaccine virus.

Do not transfer vaccine to other containers.

Protect the vaccine from excessive light and heat.

Do not save any unused portion of the vaccine mixture for later use.

Do not spill or splatter the vaccine. Use entire contents of vial when first opened. Burn empty bottles, caps and all unused vaccine and accessories.

Do not dilute the vaccine or otherwise stretch the dosage.

Caution(s): Vaccinate only healthy animals. Although disease may not be evident, Aleutian disease, urinary tract infections, boils or other disease conditions may cause complications or reduce protection.

Do not mix with inactivated products such as botulinum toxoid or enteritis vaccine. Administer distemper vaccine with separate equipment and use separate injection sites.

Warning(s): For veterinary use only.
Discussion: Distemper is a highly contagious disease of mink and dogs which is transmitted through the air, from animal to animal, and on clothing, equipment or supplies. Although the incubation period of distemper is known to be long, the actual time an animal can harbor the disease before visible signs appear has not been determined. Hence, the best insurance a rancher can have against distemper is a routine program of vaccinating kits and breeders.

Outbreak Situations: The best way to avoid distemper is to follow an annual vaccination program. However, when distemper threatens a nonvaccinated herd, losses may be minimized by vaccinating those mink which are not showing signs of the disease. Prompt vaccination will ordinarily protect those mink which do not become infected before protection is developed. Start by vaccinating those mink having the least contact with the infected animals. Vaccination will not cure or arrest the disease in infected animals and because of the long term incubation period of distemper, animals apparently healthy at the time of emergency vaccination may continue to die for several months.

Presentation: 100 dose and 250 dose vials.
Compendium Code No.: 10470420

DISTOX®

Schering-Plough **Bacterin-Toxoid-Vaccine**

Mink Distemper-Enteritis Vaccine, Modified Live and Killed Virus-Clostridium botulinum Type C Bacterin-Toxoid
U.S. Vet. Lic. No.: 165A
Contents: This vaccine is made up of two components: a lyophilized (dried) vaccine containing a modified live virus grown in chicken embryo tissue culture and combined with stabilizing agents; and a liquid fraction containing an inactivated mink enteritis virus grown in feline cell line combined with *Clostridium botulinum* Type C Bacterin-Toxoid with an aluminum adjuvant. The liquid bacterin-toxoid component serves as diluent for rehydrating the dried distemper vaccine and has been processed and tested especially to allow mixing of this triple combination vaccine in the field. Contains gentamicin and amphotericin B as preservatives.
Indications: This vaccine is for use in mink 10 weeks of age or older, as an aid in preventing distemper, virus enteritis and type C botulism through vaccination by subcutaneous injection.
Dosage and Administration: Mink should be vaccinated at 6 weeks of age for mink virus enteritis and then at 10 weeks or older with DISTOX®. Revaccinate breeders one month before mating season for distemper and type C botulism.

Preparation of the Vaccine:

Do not open and mix the vaccine until ready for use.

Mix only one vial at a time and use entire contents within two hours.

Disinfect exposed rubber stoppers with alcohol or other disinfectants.

Shake the liquid bacterin-toxoid component well before use.

Using a sterile transfer needle, or a sterile needle and syringe, transfer the entire contents of the liquid bacterin-toxoid bottle into the bottle of dried distemper vaccine. (Insert transfer needle into bacterin-toxoid diluent first, turn bacterin-toxoid diluent bottle upside down, then insert other end of transfer needle into dried distemper vaccine bottle. Bacterin-toxoid diluent will be drawn into distemper vaccine bottle by vacuum.)

As soon as all bacterin-toxoid diluent has been transferred, shake the completed vaccine well to suspend evenly.

The vaccine is now ready for use.

How to Vaccinate: For all mink, inject 1.0 mL (cc) subcutaneously under the skin, preferably in the region of the armpit (axillary space).

Records: Keep a record of vaccine type, quantity, serial number, expiration date, and place of purchase; the date and time of vaccination; the number, age and location of the mink; names of operators performing the vaccination and any observed reactions.

Contraindication(s): Mink kits younger than 10 weeks of age and born from distemper-vaccinated female breeders may possess strong maternal immunity which can interfere with the distemper fraction of this vaccine. Thus, vaccination of such mink is not recommended before 10 weeks of age.
Precaution(s): Store at 2° to 7°C (35° to 45°F).

Use only sterile needles and syringes to inject the vaccine. Syringes and needles may be sterilized by boiling for 15 to 20 minutes. Do not disinfect with chemicals since they may destroy the distemper vaccine virus.

Do not transfer vaccine to other containers.

Protect the vaccine from excessive light and heat.

Use entire contents of vial when first opened. Do not save any unused portion of the vaccine mixture for later use.

Do not spill or splatter the vaccine. Burn empty bottles, caps and all unused vaccine and accessories.

Do not dilute the vaccine or otherwise stretch the dosage.

Caution(s): Vaccinate only healthy animals. Although disease may not be evident, Aleutian disease, urinary tract infections, boils or other disease conditions may cause complications or reduce protection.

This vaccine has been demonstrated to be safe and efficacious when used according to directions. As with any vaccine, it may not be effective when used in animals with significant levels of maternal immunity.

Warning(s): For veterinary use only.
Presentation: 100 dose and 250 dose vials.
Compendium Code No.: 10470431

DISTOX®-PLUS

Schering-Plough **Bacterin-Toxoid-Vaccine**

Mink Distemper-Enteritis Vaccine, Modified Live and Killed Virus-Clostridium botulinum Type C-Pseudomonas aeruginosa Bacterin-Toxoid
U.S. Vet. Lic. No.: 165A
Contents: This vaccine is made up of two components: a lyophilized (dried) vaccine containing a modified live distemper virus grown in chicken embryo tissue culture and combined with stabilizing agents; and a liquid fraction containing an inactivated mink enteritis virus grown in feline cell line combined with *Clostridium botulinum* Type C-*Pseudomonas aeruginosa* Bacterin-Toxoid with an aluminum adjuvant. The liquid bacterin-toxoid component serves as diluent for rehydrating the dried distemper vaccine and has been processed and tested especially to allow mixing of this triple combination vaccine in the field. Contains gentamicin and amphotericin B as preservatives.
Indications: This vaccine is for use in mink 8 weeks of age or older, as an aid in preventing distemper, virus enteritis and type C botulism and hemorrhagic pneumonia through vaccination by subcutaneous injection.
Dosage and Administration: Eight weeks of age or older. Revaccinate all breeders annually for type C botulism and distemper about one month before mating season.

Preparation of the Vaccine:

Do not open and mix the vaccine until ready for use.

Mix only one vial at a time and use entire contents within two hours.

Disinfect exposed rubber stoppers with alcohol or other disinfectants.

Shake the liquid bacterin-toxoid component well before use.

Using a sterile transfer needle, or a sterile needle and syringe, transfer the entire contents of the liquid bacterin-toxoid bottle into the bottle of dried distemper vaccine. (Insert transfer needle into bacterin-toxoid diluent first, turn bacterin-toxoid diluent bottle upside down, then insert other end of transfer needle into dried distemper vaccine bottle. Bacterin-toxoid diluent will be drawn into distemper vaccine bottle by vacuum.)

As soon as all bacterin-toxoid diluent has been transferred, shake the completed vaccine well to suspend evenly.

The vaccine is now ready for use.

How to Vaccinate: For all mink, inject 1.0 mL (cc) subcutaneously under the skin, preferably in the region of the armpit (axillary space).

Records: Keep a record of vaccine type, quantity, serial number, expiration date, and place of purchase; the date and time of vaccination; the number, age and location of the mink; names of operators performing the vaccination and any observed reactions.

Contraindication(s): Mink kits younger than 8 weeks of age and born from distemper-vaccinated female breeders may possess strong maternal immunity which can interfere with the distemper fraction of this vaccine. Thus, vaccination of such mink is not recommended before 8 weeks of age.
Precaution(s): Store at 2° to 7°C (35° to 45°F).

Use only sterile needles and syringes to inject the vaccine. Syringes and needles may be sterilized by boiling for 15 to 20 minutes. Do not disinfect with chemicals since they may destroy the distemper vaccine virus.

Do not transfer vaccine to other containers.

Protect the vaccine from excessive light and heat.

Use entire contents of vial when first opened. Do not save any unused portion of the vaccine mixture for later use.

Do not spill or splatter the vaccine. Burn empty bottles, caps and all unused vaccine and accessories.

Do not dilute the vaccine or otherwise stretch the dosage.

Caution(s): Vaccinate only healthy animals. Although disease may not be evident, Aleutian disease, urinary tract infections, boils or other disease conditions may cause complications or reduce protection.

Warning(s): For veterinary use only.

Presentation: 100 dose and 250 dose vials.

Compendium Code No.: 10470441

DL-ALPHA TOCOPHEROL ACETATE INJECTION ℞

Vedco **Vitamin E**

Active Ingredient(s): Each mL contains:

dl-alpha tocopherol acetate .... 200 mg
Benzyl alcohol in sesame oil........ 2%

Indications: For use as a supplemental source of dl-alpha tocopherol acetate (vitamin E).

Dosage and Administration:

Lambs and Calves: 100 to 500 mg subcutaneously or intramuscularly.

Larger animals in proportion.

Caution(s): Federal law restricts this drug to use by or on the order of a licensed veterinarian.

For animal use only. For intramuscular or subcutaneous use only.

Presentation: 100 mL sterile multiple dose vials.

Compendium Code No.: 10940470

D'LIMONENE DIP

Davis **Grooming Rinse**

Active Ingredient(s):

D'Limonene 95%

Indications: An insecticide-free product with a citrus ingredient for use on dogs and cats to condition the coat, leaving it lustrous and manageable while leaving a pleasant fragrance.

Dosage and Administration:

To use as a dip: Mix two (2) ounces (4 tbsp.) of D'LIMONENE with one (1) gallon of water. Dip, sponge or spray the animal with the diluted solution until the coat is thoroughly wet. Rub well into the coat, between the toes and on the ears. For the best results, up to seven (7) days, do not rinse, but allow to dry naturally.

To make a citrus shampoo: Mix two (2) ounces (4 tbsp.) of D'LIMONENE in one (1) gallon of shampoo. Mix well.

Caution(s): Do not use on puppies or kittens under four weeks of age.

Presentation: 1 gallon (3.785 L).

Compendium Code No.: 11410081

D'LIMONENE SHAMPOO

Davis **Grooming Shampoo**

Active Ingredient(s): Contains 5% D'Limonene.

Indications: Davis D-LIMONENE SHAMPOO was developed to provide the professional with an all natural, milder citrus shampoo. It is highly concentrated, is a superior cleaning shampoo and has a special agent that keeps the coat cleaner longer.

Davis D'LIMONENE SHAMPOO's citrus ingredient conditions the coat leaving it lustrous and manageable. It eliminates unpleasant pet odor, leaving in its place a pleasing fragrance. It is pH balanced, antistatic and has excellent sudsing action that is easy to rinse.

Effective for dogs on Program®, Advantage™ and Frontline®.

Directions for Use: For use as a general cleansing shampoo, dilute Davis D-LIMONENE SHAMPOO 10 to 20 parts water to 1 part shampoo (10:1 to 20:1). For insecticide-free use, dilute 3 parts water to 1 part shampoo (3:1).

Wet pet's coat thoroughly with warm water. Apply shampoo to head and ears, then lather. Be careful not to get shampoo into eyes. Repeat procedure with neck, chest, middle and hindquarters, finishing legs last. Let the pet stand 5 to 10 minutes (this is an important part of the grooming procedure), then rinse the pet thoroughly. With extremely dirty or scaly animals, the above procedure may be repeated.

Caution(s): For external use only. Keep out of reach of children. Do not use on puppies and kittens under 8 weeks of age. Do not use if human or pet is allergic to this product.

Presentation: 12 fl oz (355 mL) and 1 gallon (3.785 L).

Program® is a registered trademark of Novartis Animal Health US., Inc.
Frontline® is a registered trademark of Merial.

Compendium Code No.: 11410091

d-l-METHIONINE POWDER™

Butler **Urinary Acidifier**

Active Ingredient(s): Each pound contains:

dl methionine........ 100%

Indications: For use as a feed grade nutritional supplement.

Dosage and Administration:

Cats: Administer orally, 250 to 500 mg (⅛ to ¼ level teaspoon) per day, depending upon size.

Dogs: Administer orally, 500 to 1,000 mg (¼ to ½ level teaspoon) per day, depending upon size.

Precaution(s): Do not store above 30°C (86°F).

Caution(s): Keep out of the reach of children. For veterinary use only.

Do not give to animals with severe liver or kidney damage. Gastro-intestinal distress may occur after large doses or when given to animals with empty stomachs.

Presentation: 16 oz. (1 lb., 454 g) containers.

Compendium Code No.: 10820460

DL-METHIONINE POWDER

First Priority **Urinary Acidifier**

Guaranteed Analysis:

(% w/w - DL-Methionine) DL-Methionine .... (min.) 95%

Ingredient: D-L-Methionine.

Indications: For use as a feed grade nutritional supplement.

Directions for Use: Cats: Orally-250 to 500 mg (⅛ to ¼ level teaspoon) daily, depending on size. Dogs: Orally-500 to 1000 mg (¼ to ½ level teaspoon) daily, depending on size.

Precaution(s): Storage: Store at controlled room temperature 15° to 30°C (59° to 86°F). Keep container tightly closed when not in use.

Caution(s): Do not give to animals with severe liver or kidney damage. Gastrointestinal distress may occur after large doses or when given to animals with empty stomachs.

For animal use only.

Warning(s): Keep out of reach of children.

Presentation: 1 lb (453.6 g) (NDC# 58829-186-16).

Compendium Code No.: 11390182 Rev. 07-01

d-l-m TABLETS ℞

Butler **Urinary Acidifier**

Active Ingredient(s): Each tablet contains either:

DL-methionine .... 200 mg or 500 mg

Indications: For use as a urinary acidifier in dogs and cats. May be used as an adjunct to urinary antiseptics and antibiotics in the therapy of bacterial cystitis and to control chronic recurrent bacterial infections of the lower urinary tract; as adjunct therapy in the prophylactic aftercare of urinary salts of calcium and magnesium calculi; prevention and treatment of feline urological syndrome (FUS); and to help reduce ammoniacal urine odor.

Dosage and Administration: Dogs and Cats: The suggested dosage range is 25 to 150 mg per pound of body weight per day, preferably administered in two (2) or three (3) divided doses with meals. Adjust dosage based on the clinical response and by monitoring urine pH.

Contraindication(s): Do not use in animals in a state of metabolic acidosis; with urinary retention from urethral obstruction; or with severe liver or kidney disease.

Precaution(s): Store at a controlled room temperature between 15° and 30°C (59°-86°F).

Caution(s): Federal law restricts this drug to use by or on the order of a licensed veterinarian.

May cause gastric mucosal irritation, particularly if large doses are administered to animals when the stomach is empty.

For veterinary use only.

Keep out of the reach of children.

Presentation: Bottles of 1,000 tablets.

Compendium Code No.: 10820450

DOCUSATE SOLUTION

Life Science **Enema-Cerumenolytic**

A 5% Water Miscible Solution of Dioctyl Sodium Sulfosuccinate

Active Ingredient(s): Each 100 mL contains:

Dioctyl sodium sulfosuccinate (D.S.S.)........ 5 g
Propylene glycol .... 35 g
Deionized water........ q.s.

Indications:

Horses: For use as an enema and a laxative.

Dogs and Cats: For use as an enema and a cerumenolytic agent.

Dosage and Administration: Suggested Use:

Horses: For use as an enema, administer 4-6 fluid ounces per gallon of water. For use as a laxative, administer orally 8 fluid ounces per gallon of water or mineral oil.

Dogs and Cats: For use as an enema, administer 2-3 fluid ounces of a mixture of 5 mL DOCUSATE per fluid ounce of water. For use as a cerumenolytic agent, administer 2 to 3 drops of DOCUSATE in each ear.

Precaution(s): If cold temperatures cause product to become cloudy, place in warm water or store at room temperature (68°-74°F).

Caution(s): For animal use only.

For veterinary use only.

Warning(s): Not for use in horses intended for food use.

Not for human use.

Keep out of reach of children.

Presentation: 1 gallon (3.785 L) containers.

Compendium Code No.: 10870031

DOCU-SOFT™ PET ENEMA

Life Science **Enema**

Active Ingredient(s): Each syringe contains 12 mL concentrated solution of Docusate (DSS) 250 mg in glycerin with sorbic acid as a preservative.

Indications: A ready-to-use disposable enema for dogs and cats.

Dosage and Administration: Gently insert the flexible nozzle into the rectum and press the plunger to express the contents. In resistant cases the treatment may be repeated in one (1) hour.

Caution(s): For rectal use only in animals.

Presentation: 12 mL syringe.

Compendium Code No.: 10870021

DOG-OFF™

Thornell **Deodorant Product**

Description: Does not contain enzymes, bacteria, nor oxidizers. Nontoxic, nonirritating, biodegradable, nonflammable.

Indications: To neutralize dog odors including normal animal body odor, urine, feces and emesis.

For direct application on the dog, accidents, bedding, and cages. Eliminates bathing when odor is the problem.

DOG-OFF™ works chemically through bonding, absorption and counteraction. Unlike enzyme and bacteria based products, DOG-OFF™ remains effective when used with or after most cleaners, shampoo and germicides.

Dosage and Administration: Spray full strength on the source of the odor. Work in if possible. Allow to dry. If the odor persists, DOG-OFF™ has not reached the source of the odor. Re-apply.

Precaution(s): DOG-OFF™ has an indefinite shelf life.

Caution(s): Although not irritating to mucous membranes, spraying directly into the eyes is not recommended. As with all chemicals, keep out of the reach of children. For external use only. Always spot test for color fastness before using on fabrics.

Presentation: 8 oz. pump spray bottle.

Compendium Code No.: 11210030

DOLOREX® CIV

Intervet **Analgesic**

Butorphanol Tartrate

ANADA No.: 200-239

Active Ingredient(s): Each mL of DOLOREX® contains 10 mg butorphanol base (as butorphanol tartrate, USP), 3.3 mg citric acid, Ph. Eur., 6.4 mg sodium citrate, Ph. Eur., 4.7 mg sodium chloride, Ph. Eur., and 0.1 mg benzethonium chloride, Ph. Eur., q.s. with water for injection, Ph. Eur.

Indications: DOLOREX® (butorphanol tartrate) is indicated for the relief of pain associated with colic in adult horses and yearlings. Clinical studies in the horse have shown that butorphanol tartrate alleviates abdominal pain associated with torsion, impaction, intussusception, spasmodic and tympanic colic, and postpartum pain.

Pharmacology: Description: DOLOREX® (butorphanol tartrate) is a totally synthetic, centrally acting, narcotic agonist-antagonist analgesic with potent antitussive activity. It is a member of the phenanthrene series. The chemical name is morphinan-3, 14-diol, 17-(cyclobutylmethyl)-,(-), (S-(R*, R*))-2, 3-dihydroxybutanedioate (1:1) (salt). It is a white crystalline, water soluble substance having a molecular weight of 477.55; its molecular formula is $C_{21}H_{29}NO_2C_4H_6O_6$.

Comparative Pharmacology: In animals, butorphanol has been demonstrated to be 4 to 30 times more potent than morphine and pentazocine (Talwin®-V) respectively.[1] In humans, butorphanol has been shown to have 5 to 7 times the analgesic activity of morphine and 20 times that of pentazocine.[2,3] Butorphanol has 15 to 20 times the oral antitussive activity of codeine or dextromethorphan in dogs and guinea pigs.[4]

As an antagonist, butorphanol is approximately equivalent to nalorphine and 30 times more potent than pentazocine.[1]

Cardiopulmonary depressant effects are minimal after treatment with butorphanol as demonstrated in dogs[5], humans[6,7] and horses.[8] Unlike classical narcotic agonist analgesics which are associated with decreases in blood pressure, reduction in heart rate, and concomitant release of histamine, butorphanol does not cause histamine release.[1] Furthermore, the cardiopulmonary effects of butorphanol are not distinctly dosage related but rather reach a ceiling effect beyond which further dosage increase result in lesser effects.

Reproductive studies performed in mice and rabbits revealed no evidence of impaired fertility or harm to the fetus due to butorphanol tartrate. In the female rat, parenteral administration was associated with increased nervousness and decreased care for newborns, resulting in a decreased survival rate of the new born. This nervousness was seen only in the rat species.

Equine Pharmacology: Following intravenous injection in horses, butorphanol is largely eliminated from the blood within 3 to 4 hours. This drug is extensively metabolized in the liver and excreted in the urine.

In ponies, butorphanol given intramuscularly at a dosage of 0.22 mg/kg was shown to alleviate experimentally induced visceral pain for about 4 hours.[9]

In horses, intravenous dosages of butorphanol ranging from 0.05 to 0.4 mg/kg were shown to be effective in alleviating visceral and superficial pain for at least 4 hours. A definite dosage-response relationship was detected in that butorphanol dosage of 0.1 mg/kg was more effective than 0.05 mg/kg, but not differ from 0.2 mg/kg, in alleviating deep abdominal pain.

Dosage and Administration: The recommended dosage in the horse is 0.1 mg butorphanol per kilogram of body weight (0.05 mg/lb) by intravenous injection. This is equivalent to 5 mL DOLOREX® for each 1000 lb body weight. The dose may be repeated in 3 to 4 hours but treatment should not exceed 48 hours. Preclinical model studies and clinical field trials in horses demonstrated that the analgesic effects of butorphanol are seen within 15 minutes following injection and persist for about 4 hours.

Precaution(s): Store at controlled room temperature 15° to 30°C (59° to 86°F).

Caution(s): Federal Law restricts this drug to use by or on the order of a licensed veterinarian.

DOLOREX®, a potent analgesic, should be used with caution with other sedative or analgesic drugs as these are likely to produce additive effects.

There are no well controlled studies using butorphanol in breeding horses, weanlings, and foals. Therefore the drug should not be used in those groups.

For animal use only.

Warning(s): For use in horses only. Not for use in horses intended for food.

Adverse Reactions: In clinical trials in horses, the most commonly observed side effect was slight ataxia which lasted 3 to 10 minutes. Marked ataxia was reported in 1.5% of the 327 horses treated. Mild sedation was reported in 9% of the horses.

Trial Data: Acute Equine Studies: Rapid intravenous administration of butorphanol at a dosage of 2.0 mg/kg (20 times the recommended dosage) to a previously unmedicated horse resulted in a brief episode of inability to stand, muscle fasciculation, a convulsive seizure of 6 seconds duration, and recovery within 3 minutes. The same dosage administered after 10 successive daily 1.0 mg/kg dosages of butorphanol resulted only in transient sedative effects. During the 10 day course of administration at 1.0 mg/kg (10 times the recommended use level) in 2 horses, the only detectable drug effects were transient behavioral changes typical of narcotic agonist activity. These included muscle fasciculation about the head and neck, dysphoria, lateral nystagmus, ataxia, and salivation. Repeated administration of butorphanol at 1.0 mg/kg (10 times the recommended dosage) every 4 hours for 48 hours caused constipation in one of two horses.

Subacute Equine Studies: Horses were found to tolerate butorphanol given intravenously at dosages of 0.1, 0.3, and 0.5 mg/kg every 4 hours for 48 hours followed by once daily injections for a total of 21 days. The only detectable drug effects were slight transient ataxia observed occasionally in the high dosage group. No clinical, laboratory, or gross or histopathologic evidence of any butorphanol-related toxicity was encountered in the horses.

References: Available upon request.

Presentation: DOLOREX® is supplied in 50 mL vials.

Compendium Code No.: 11060411

DOMINATOR® INSECTICIDE EAR TAGS

Schering-Plough **Insecticide Ear Tags**

EPA Reg. No.: 773-68

Active Ingredient(s):

Pirimiphos-Methyl 0-[2-diethylamino-6-methyl-4-pyrimidinyl] 00-dimethyl phosphorothioate	20%
Other Ingredients	80%
Total	100%

Indications: For up to 5 months' control of Horn flies (including synthetic pyrethroid-resistant Horn flies) and as an aid in the control of Face flies, use two tags per head on beef and non-lactating dairy cattle and calves.

Directions for Use: It is a violation of Federal law to use this product in a manner inconsistent with its labeling. The labeling must be in the possession of the user at the time of pesticide application.

1. Place male button onto pin until it projects through the tip.
2. Dip tag button into disinfectant solution.
3. Press female tag under the clip by depressing lever.
4. Apply through ear between second and third rib, halfway between ear tip and head.

For optimum control and to minimize development of insect resistance, use two tags per animal (one in each ear). All animals in the herd should be tagged. Apply when flies first appear in spring. Replace as necessary. Apply with Allflex®* Tagging System. Tags remain effective up to 5 months. Remove tags in fall.

Continual exposure of Horn flies to a single class of insecticide (e.g., pyrethroids or organophosphates) may lead to the development of resistance to that class of insecticide. In order to reduce the possibility of Horn flies developing resistance, it is important to rotate the class of insecticide used and/or the method of Horn fly control on a seasonal basis. For advice concerning current control practices with relation to specific local conditions, consult resources in resistance management programs such as a veterinarian and/or your Cooperative Agricultural Extension Service.

Precautionary Statements: Hazards to Humans and Domestic Animals:

Caution: Harmful if swallowed or absorbed through the skin. Wear non-permeable protective gloves when applying or removing tags. Wash thoroughly with soap and water after handling and before eating and smoking.

D

First Aid:

If on skin or clothing: Take off contaminated clothing. Rinse skin immediately with plenty of water for 15-20 minutes. Call a poison control center or doctor for treatment advice.

If swallowed: Call a poison control center or doctor immediately for treatment advice. Have person sip a glass of water if able to swallow. Do not induce vomiting unless told to do so by the poison control center or doctor. Do not induce vomiting or give anything by mouth to an unconscious person.

Hotline Number: Have the product container or label with you when calling the poison control center or doctor or going for treatment. You may also contact the Rocky Mountain Poison Center at 1-303-595-4869 for emergency medical treatment information.

Note To Physician: This product is a cholinesterase inhibitor. If symptoms of cholinesterase inhibition are present, atropine sulfate by injection is antidotal.

Environmental Hazards: This pesticide is toxic to fish. Do not add directly to water. Do not contaminate water by disposal of used tags. Use this product only as specified on the label.

Storage and Disposal: Do not contaminate water, food, or feed by storage or disposal.

Storage: Store in cool place away from direct sunlight. Opened pouches containing ear tags should be resealed for storage.

Pesticide Disposal: Remove tags before slaughter. Wastes resulting from the use of this product may be disposed of on site or at an approved waste disposal facility.

Container Disposal: Dispose of empty bag in a sanitary landfill or by incineration, or, if allowed by State and local authorities, by burning. If burned, stay out of smoke.

Warning(s): Remove tags before slaughter.

Keep out of reach of children.

Disclaimer: Notice of Warranty: Schering-Plough Animal Health Corp. makes no warranty of merchantability, fitness for any particular purpose, or otherwise expressed or implied concerning this product or its uses which extend beyond the use of the product under normal conditions in accordance with the statements made on the label.

Presentation: 20 x 9.5 g tags and buttons per case (NDC 0061-5223-01).

*Allflex is a registered trademark of AllFlex USA, Inc.

U.S. Patent No. 4,953,313

Compendium Code No.: 10470451 Rev. 5/01

DOMITOR® ℞

Pfizer Animal Health **Analgesic-Sedative**

(medetomidine hydrochloride) Sterile Injectable Solution—1.0 mg/mL

NADA No.: 140-999

Active Ingredient(s): Each mL of DOMITOR® contains 1.0 mg medetomidine hydrochloride, 1.0 mg methylparaben (NF), 0.2 mg propylparaben (NF), 9.0 mg sodium chloride (USP), and water for injection (USP), q.s.

Indications: DOMITOR® is indicated for use as a sedative and analgesic in dogs over 12 weeks of age to facilitate clinical examinations, clinical procedures, minor surgical procedures not requiring muscle relaxation, and minor dental procedures where intubation is not required. The IV route of administration is more efficacious for dental care.

Pharmacology: DOMITOR® (medetomidine hydrochloride) is a synthetic alpha$_2$-adrenoreceptor agonist with sedative and analgesic properties. The chemical name is (±)-4-[1-(2,3-dimethylphenyl) ethyl]-1H-imidazole monohydrochloride. It is a white, or almost white, crystalline, water soluble substance having a molecular weight of 236.7. The molecular formula is $C_{13}H_{16}N_2 \bullet HCl$ and the structural formula is:

CH3 · N · HCl · CH3 · N H · CH3

Clinical Pharmacology: Medetomidine is a potent non-narcotic alpha$_2$-adrenoreceptor agonist which produces sedation and analgesia. These effects are dose dependent in depth and duration. Profound sedation and recumbency, with reduced sensitivity to environmental stimuli (sounds, etc.), are seen with medetomidine.

The pharmacological restraint and pain relief provided by medetomidine facilitates handling dogs and aids in the conduct of diagnostic or therapeutic procedures. It also facilitates minor surgical procedures (with or without local anesthesia) and dental care where intubation is not required. Spontaneous muscle contractions (twitching) can be expected in some dogs sedated with medetomidine.

With medetomidine administration, blood pressure is initially increased due to peripheral vasoconstriction and thereafter drops to normal or slightly below normal levels. The initial vasopressor response is accompanied by a compensatory marked decrease in heart rate mediated by a vagal baroreceptor mechanism. The bradycardia may be partially prevented by prior (at least 5 minutes before) intravenous administration of an anticholinergic agent (see Cautions). A transient change in the conductivity of the cardiac muscle may occur, as evidenced by atrioventricular blocks. Cardiovascular changes (such as profound bradycardia and second degree heart block) equally affect both heartworm negative and asymptomatic heartworm positive dogs.

Respiratory responses include an initial slowing of respiration within a few seconds to 1-2 minutes after administration, increasing to normal within 120 minutes. An initial decrease in tidal volume is followed by an increase. When medetomidine was given at 3 and 5 times the recommended dose IV, and 5 and 10 times IM, effects were not intensified but were prolonged.

Dosage and Administration: DOMITOR® should be administered at the rate of 750 mcg IV or 1000 mcg IM per square meter of body surface. Use the table below to determine the correct dosage on the basis of body weight.

Body Weight (lb) IV Administration	Injection Volume (mL)	Body Weight (lb) IM Administration
3-4	0.1	
5-7	0.15	4-5
8-11	0.2	6-7
12-15	0.25	8-9
16-21	0.3	10-14
22-31	0.4	15-20
32-43	0.5	21-27
44-55	0.6	28-35
56-68	0.7	36-44
69-82	0.8	45-53
83-97	0.9	54-63
98-121	1.0	64-78
122-156	1.2	79-101
157-194	1.4	102-126
195+	1.6	127-165
	2.0	166+

Following injection of DOMITOR®, the dog should be allowed to rest quietly for 15 minutes.

Contraindication(s): DOMITOR® should not be used in dogs with the following conditions: cardiac disease, respiratory disorders, liver or kidney diseases, dogs in shock, dogs which are severely debilitated, or dogs which are stressed due to extreme heat, cold or fatigue.

Precaution(s): Storage: Store at controlled room temperature 15°-30°C (59°-86°F). Protect from freezing.

Caution(s): Federal law restricts this drug to use by or on the order of a licensed veterinarian.

In extremely nervous or excited dogs, levels of endogenous catecholamines are high due to the animals state of agitation. The pharmacological response elicited by alpha$_2$-agonists (e.g., medetomidine) in such animals is often reduced, with depth and duration of sedative/analgesic effects ranging from slightly diminished to nonexistent. Highly agitated dogs should therefore be put at ease and allowed to rest quietly prior to receiving DOMITOR®. Allowing dogs to rest quietly for 10 to 15 minutes after injection may improve the response to DOMITOR®. In dogs not responding satisfactorily to treatment with DOMITOR®, repeat dosing is not recommended.

DOMITOR® is a potent alpha$_2$-agonist which should be used with caution with other sedative or analgesic drugs. Additive or synergistic effects are likely, possibly resulting in overdose. Although bradycardia may be partially prevented by prior (at least 5 minutes before) intravenous administration of an anticholinergic agent, the administration of anticholinergic agents to treat bradycardia either simultaneously with medetomidine or following sedation with medetomidine could lead to adverse cardiovascular effects.

Special care is recommended when treating very young animals and older animals. Information on the possible reproductive effects of medetomidine is limited; therefore, the drug is not recommended for use in dogs used for breeding purposes or in pregnant dogs.

Warning(s): For intramuscular and intravenous use in dogs only.

Keep out of reach of children. Not for human use.

Medetomidine hydrochloride can be absorbed and may cause irritation following direct exposure to skin, eyes, or mouth. In case of accidental eye exposure, flush with water for 15 minutes. In case of accidental skin exposure, wash with soap and water. Remove contaminated clothing. If irritation or other adverse reaction occurs (e.g., sedation, hypotension, bradycardia), seek medical attention. In case of accidental oral exposure or injection, seek medical attention. Precaution should be used while handling and using filled syringes.

Users with cardiovascular disease (e.g., hypertension or ischemic heart disease) should take special precautions to avoid any exposure to this product.

The material safety data sheet (MSDS) contains more detailed occupational safety information.

To report adverse reactions in users or to obtain a copy of the MSDS for this product call 1-800-366-5288.

Note to Physician: This product contains an alpha-2-adrenergic agonist.

Side Effects: Bradycardia with occasional atrioventricular blocks will occur together with decreased respiratory rates. Body temperature is slightly or moderately decreased. Urination typically occurs during recovery at about 90 to 120 minutes posttreatment. In approximately 10% of treated dogs, occasional episodes of vomiting occur between 5 to 15 minutes posttreatment. An increase in blood glucose concentration is seen due to alpha$_2$-adrenoreceptor-mediated inhibition of insulin secretion.

Adverse Reactions: As with all alpha$_2$-agonists, the potential for isolated cases of hypersensitivity, including paradoxical response (excitation), exists. Incidents of prolonged sedation, bradycardia, cyanosis, vomiting, apnea, death from circulatory failure with severe congestion of lungs, liver, kidney and recurrence of sedation after initial recovery have been reported.

Trial Data: Animal Safety: In target animal safety studies, medetomidine was tolerated in dogs at up to 5 times the recommended IV dose and up to 10 times the recommended IM dose. A single IV administration of 10 times the recommended dose in dogs caused a prolonged anesthesia-like condition accompanied by an increased level of spontaneous muscle contractions (twitching). Repeated IV doses of 3 or 5 times the recommended dose caused a profound sedation, bradycardia and reduced respiratory rates over several hours, accompanied in some animals by occasional spontaneous twitching. Death (approximately 1 in 40,000 treatments) has been noted in clinical use with doses at 2 times the recommended dose of DOMITOR®.

Presentation: DOMITOR® is supplied in 10-mL, multidose vials containing 1.0 mg of medetomidine hydrochloride per mL.

U.S. Patent Nos. 4,544,664 and 4,670,455

DOMITOR® is a trademark of Orion Corporation.

Developed and manufactured by: Orion Corporation, Orion-Farmos, Espoo, Finland

Compendium Code No.: 36900941 75-6294-01

DOMOSO® GEL ℞

Fort Dodge **Topical Anti-inflammatory**

90% Dimethyl Sulfoxide — Medical Grade

NADA No.: 047-925

Active Ingredient(s): DOMOSO® Gel contains 90% dimethyl sulfoxide, carbomer 934, disodium edetate, NaOH and purified water q.s.

Indications: Canine and Equine: DOMOSO® (dimethyl sulfoxide) Gel is recommended as a topical application to reduce acute swelling due to trauma.

Pharmacology: Dimethyl sulfoxide (DMSO), an oxidation product of dimethyl sulfide, is an exceptional solvent possessing a number of commercial uses.

DMSO is the lowest member of the group of alkyl sulfoxides with a general formula of RSOR. Its structural formula is:

$$CH_3-\overset{\overset{\displaystyle O}{\|}}{S}-CH_3$$

It freely mixes with water with the evolution of heat and lowers the freezing point of aqueous solutions. It is soluble in many other compounds including ethanol, acetone, diethyl ether, glycerin, toluene, benzene and chloroform. DMSO is a solvent for many aromatic and unsaturated hydrocarbons as well as inorganic salts and nitrogen-containing compounds. DMSO has a high dielectric constant due to the polarity of the sulphur-oxygen bond. Its basicity is slightly greater than water due to enhanced electron density at the oxygen atom. It forms crystalline salts with strong protic acids and coordinates with Lewis acids. It modifies hydrogen bonding.

DMSO is a hygroscopic stable organic liquid essentially odorless and water white in color. Other physical characteristics include:

Molecular weight.................... 78.13
Melting point.................... 18.45°C
Boiling point.................... 189°C

The original biological applications of DMSO were primarily confined to its use in preserving various tissues and cellular elements including blood[1], blood cells and bone marrow[2], leukocytes[3], lymphocytes[4], platelets[5], spermatozoa[6,7,8], corneal grafts[9,10], skin[11], tissue culture cells[12,13,14,15] and trypanosomes[16], by freezing techniques. DMSO has also been investigated as a radioprotective agent.[17,18]

DMSO has been stated to increase the penetration of low molecular weight allergens such as penicillin G but not large molecular weight allergens such as house dust.[19]

The rate of passage of tritiated water in the presence of DMSO on the epidermis of the hairless mouse was measured *in vitro.* DMSO did not appear to promote the passage of water by its presence, but when concentrated solutions (60% to 100%) were used, permanent changes were produced in the rate of passage of water. It was concluded that the concentration of DMSO used seemed more significant than the time of exposure in establishing the effect on the water barrier.[20]

When the tails of mice were immersed in a 5% solution of various psychoactive drugs in DMSO, the drugs appeared to exert their usual pharmacological effects, indicating drug penetration as judged by the behavioral effects observed in the experimental subjects. Other solvents, including water, also appeared to permit some drug penetration in this study.[21]

Using ten quaternary ammonium salts as test compounds and either water or DMSO as solvents, the oral LD_{50} values were determined in rats and mice. Toxicity changes were obtained in some instances by 50% DMSO and more changes were observed in rats than mice although the results in the two species were not always parallel. When toxicity was altered by DMSO it increased in all instances except one.[22]

When administered systemically in another study, however, various drugs dissolved in DMSO did not differ significantly in their lethality or cellular penetration as compared to the same drugs administered in saline.[23]

When evaluated as a solvent for biologic screening tests, low doses of hormones in DMSO stimulated a response similar to that of the hormone in the control vehicle. Higher doses of hormone, however, failed to give the expected response suggesting a partition coefficient in favor of the solvent.[24] DMSO was also shown to carry physostigmine and phenylbutazone through the skin of the rat.[25]

The absorption of phenylbutazone dissolved in an aqueous solution of DMSO was impaired when administered orally to the rabbit. Absorption of the same drug was not improved using the subcutaneous route simultaneously with DMSO.

However, phenylbutazone could be detected in the rabbit's blood for several hours when an ointment containing DMSO and 5% phenylbutazone was applied to the skin. When the DMSO content of the ointment was increased, the phenylbutazone levels increased. An increase of phenylbutazone in the muscle tissues underlying the site of application over a control ointment containing phenylbutazone without DMSO could be demonstrated in rats.[26]

In a number of other studies in experimental animals[21,25,27] where DMSO has been chiefly administered orally or by injection, no anti-inflammatory or analgesic activity could be established.

Following experimental hypersensitization to human gamma globulin in the horse, antigen challenge resulted in massive erythema, necrosis and slough. This reaction could be markedly reduced by the hourly application of undiluted DMSO to the reaction site, after challenge.[19]

DMSO, by itself, at concentrations of 100%, 66% and 33% has been shown to produce neurolysis following perineural injection in the rat's sciatic nerve.[28]

The conflicting reports cited above for the anti-inflammatory and analgesic properties of DMSO are partially dependent upon the experimental models and methods used to measure these parameters. DMSO fails to show analgesic or anti-inflammatory activity in certain of these situations, particularly when used by the systemic route or when administered topically preceded by an irritant substance. In clinical studies in the horse, it was noted that when iodine, liniments or other strong irritants were present on the skin from previous therapy and DMSO applied, a temporary but marked local reaction would occur. This was due to the ability of DMSO to carry these substances into the underlying skin tissues where their irritant actions could be displayed.

Using the isolated guinea pig heart it was found that DMSO did not influence the amplitude of cardiac contractions, heart rate or coronary flow, although high intravenous doses in the rat and cat resulted in a transient lowering of blood pressure.[25]

Isolated, innervated guinea pig preparations were also used to study the effects of DMSO on skeletal, smooth and cardiac muscles. The compound depressed diaphragm response to both muscle and nerve stimulation and also caused spontaneous skeletal muscle fasciculations. Actual contraction amplitude was augmented although contraction rate appeared unaffected. Vagal threshold was lowered almost 50% by a bath concentration of 6% DMSO. The fasciculations and increased tone of skeletal muscle, and lowering of the vagal threshold by DMSO could be due to cholinesterase inhibition.[29] The *in vitro* oxygen consumption of liver, brain and hemidiaphragm tissues of rats is not affected by the intravenous administration of 75 mg DMSO/100 g body weight during the 7 subsequent days.

Urease, trypsin and chymotrypsin are inhibited by DMSO dependent upon its concentration. The *in vitro* metabolism of corticosterone by rat liver slices is not affected by the intravenous administration of 100 mg DMSO/100 g body weight during 3 subsequent days.[30]

DMSO treatment administered intraperitoneally to rats for 35 days decreased experimentally induced intestinal adhesions by 80% over controls as compared to saline, cortisone acetate or a combination of cortisone and DMSO administered separately.[31]

In rabbits the application of 70% DMSO, adjacent to but not on the wound incision site, appeared to increase the development of wound tensile strength over controls.[32]

Increasing the concentration of DMSO resulted in an increasing inhibition of fibroblast proliferation, *in vitro,* which was reversible.[19]

Dosage and Administration: DOMOSO® Gel is to be administered topically to the skin over the affected area.

Dogs — Liberal application should be administered three to four times daily. Total daily dosage should not exceed 20 g. Total duration of therapy should not exceed 14 days.

Horses — Liberal application should be administered two to three times daily. Total daily dosage should not exceed 100 g. Total duration of therapy should not exceed 30 days.

Contraindication(s): DOMOSO® Gel may mask certain disease signs such as seen in fractures, etc.; this does not obviate the need for specific therapy in such conditions.

Since DOMOSO® Gel effectively alters the biologic membrane, it will in some cases facilitate the systemic absorption of other topically applied drugs and may have a potentiating effect on drugs administered systemically.

DOMOSO® Gel should be judiciously used when administered in conjunction with other pharmaceutical preparations, especially those affecting the cardiovascular and central nervous systems.

DOMOSO® Gel may enhance the absorption of other materials into the skin. The veterinarian should make certain that other medications are not present prior to its application.

DOMOSO® Gel is contraindicated in horses and dogs intended for breeding purposes.

Precaution(s): Store at controlled room temperature 15° to 30°C (59° to 86°F).

Caution(s): Federal law restricts this drug to use by or on the order of a licensed veterinarian.

Contact between DOMOSO® Gel and the skin should be avoided. Rubber gloves should be worn while applying this drug. Forceps and swabs may be used to facilitate application. If absorbed through the skin, DOMOSO® Gel will cause odorous breath and unpleasant mouth taste. Mild sedation or drowsiness, sensations of warmth, burning, irritation, itching and mild erythematous localized or generalized dermatitis have been reported in some persons following exposure to DOMOSO® Gel. Treatment of such side effects is symptomatic. Consult a physician immediately if adverse effects appear.

Keep DOMOSO® Gel out of the reach of children.

DOMOSO® Gel is recommended for topical application only. Do not administer by any other route.

DOMOSO® Gel should not be used under occlusive dressings.

DOMOSO® Gel is a potent solvent and may have a deleterious effect on fabrics, plastics and other materials. Care should be taken to prevent physical contact with DOMOSO® Gel.

Hygroscopic. Close cap tightly after use. Avoid freezing. Due to the rapid penetration ability of DOMOSO® Gel, rubber gloves should be worn when applying this drug.

Warning(s): DOMOSO® Gel should not be administered to horses that are to be slaughtered for food.

For animal use only.

Toxicology: In a study designed to evaluate the effects of Domoso® (dimethyl sulfoxide) Solution at a total daily dose of 100-300 mL administered for a total period of 90 days, no essential or clinically meaningful ophthalmological effects were seen in the horse. There were no significant variations in glucose, sodium, potassium, SGOT or SGPT measurements. There were a few fluctuations in hematologic values but no changes appear to be drug-related or of significance.

Another study was conducted in the dog to determine the effects of Domoso® Solution at a total daily dose of 20-60 mL administered topically for 21 consecutive days. No clinically meaningful ophthalmological effects were noted. No significant variations were observed in blood measurements, including glucose, BUN, SGOT and plasma electrophoresis. Hematologic values were similar to control animals used in this study.

Long-term topical applications of the drug to guinea pigs resulted in histopathologic changes similar to those observed in allergic contact dermatitis. The observed clinical changes were compatible with either an allergic contact dermatitis or a primary irritant effect.[33] DMSO was shown to cause erythema and blistering of human and rat skin resulting in increased permeability of venules and capillaries.[34]

In most cases the local irritation of the skin characterized by erythema, vesicle or blister formation and scurfing abates even with continued treatment. The phenomenon has been described as "accommodation" or "hardening" of the skin, and has been noted with other solvents.

The undiluted compound has low systemic toxicity but a marked local necrotizing and inflammatory effect when it is injected subcutaneously. In rats the subcutaneous injection of 10 g/kg or the intravenous injection of 2.5 g/kg of undiluted DMSO for 2 weeks showed no definite indication of systemic toxicity. The local necrotizing effects produced at these dose levels, however, prevented a longer period of treatment. No significant hematologic or biochemical changes were noted in 3 dogs receiving 0.4 g/kg for 33 days.[24]

Four dogs were administered topical DMSO at 1 g/kg body weight, 5 days weekly for 18 months. Serum glutamic oxaloacetic transaminase (SGOT), serum glutamic pyruvic transaminase (SGPT), prothrombin time, alkaline phosphatase, bilirubin, total protein and albumin globulin (AG) ratio, and blood urea nitrogen (BUN) were determined at the beginning of treatment and at monthly intervals. Significant abnormalities did not occur.[41]

Upon injection of DMSO into the rat pleura, there is an accumulation of fluid, initially appearing as a transudate, but later as a protein-rich exudate. Exudate formation is thought to be due to increased vascular permeability, predominantly in venules, brought about by a delayed release of histamine together with activation of a vaso-active slow contracting substance.[34]

A compilation of the results for a number of acute toxicity (LD_{50}) determinations derived from several published reports[24,40,42,43,44] in several experimental animal species are as follows:

Species	Rt. of Administr.	LD_{50} g/kg
Mouse	SQ	13.9-20.5
Mouse	IV	3.82-10.73
Mouse	Oral	15.0-22
Mouse	IP	20.06
Rat	IV	5.25-5.36
Rat	Oral	16.0-28.3
Rat	IP	6.5-13.621
Dog	IV	2.5
Guinea Pig	IP	6.5
Chicken	Oral	12.5

Hemolysis resulting in hemoglobinuria and methemoglobinuria was noted in anesthetized cats following single intravenous doses of 200 mg/kg DMSO. The intraperitoneal administration of DMSO or the dilution of DMSO with isotonic saline prior to intravenous administration reduced its hemolytic activity.[39]

Tests *in vitro* showed that washed rabbit erythrocytes are hemolyzed in a short time with 40% to 60% DMSO solution. Higher concentrations caused, without hemolysis, an agglutination of the erythrocytes.[40]

Teratology: The intraperitoneal administration of 5.5 g/kg of DMSO as a single dose to pregnant hamsters induced developmental malformations of their embryos.[35] Both dimethyl sulfoxide and diethyl sulfoxide are teratogenic when injected into the chick embryo, the classification of malformations being dependent upon the stage of embryonic development at the time of treatment. The same drugs when administered by various techniques to mice, rats and rabbits in which fertility had been established, did not cause any embryonic malformations.[36]

Ocular Effects: In a variety of experimental animals including rats, dogs, swine, rabbits and primates, following oral or topical administration of DMSO, certain eye changes have been noted. These consist mainly of a change in the refractive index of the lens described as a "lens within a lens". The lens changes are characterized by a decrease in the normal relucency of the lens cortex, causing the normal central zone of the lens to act as a biconvex lens. When viewing the fundus of affected animals, it is necessary to interpose biconcave lenses in order to see the retinal vessels clearly. The functional effect would be a tendency toward myopia.[37]

The lens changes were first observed in dogs receiving 5 g DMSO/kg after 9 weeks of administration. At lower dose levels the change was observed later. In rabbits these changes were seen after 90 days of dermal application, (8 mg 50% DMSO/kg/day and 4 mg 100% DMSO/kg/day and higher). In swine, dermal application of 4.5 g 90% DMSO/kg twice daily caused similar lens changes by 90 days of treatment.[38]

The lens changes appear earlier with oral administration, and also bear a relation to the dosage employed; the higher the dose the more rapid their appearance.

The eye changes are slowly reversible but with a definite species difference, the dog being the slowest to exhibit improvement.

No effects were seen following direct application of aqueous solutions varying from 10% to full strength into the eyes of albino rabbits for a total dosage of DMSO between 0.1 and 0.2 g/kg body weight per day for six months. Rabbits which received daily doses as high as 10 g/kg orally or topically showed lines of discontinuity in their lenses. No cataract was seen after ten weeks of such daily treatment, although discontinuous lens lines could be detected in about two weeks by slit lamp examination. Chemical studies on these lenses revealed reduction in the usual concentrations of urea, glutathione, uric and amino acids.[19]

Side Effects: In general, adverse reactions are local, and while they may prove to be annoying to some patients, they are usually not of a serious nature. Upon topical application, an occasionally animal may develop transient erythema, associated with local "burning" or "smarting". Even when erythema or vesiculation occur, they are self-limiting reversible states, and not necessarily an indication to discontinue medication. Dryness of the skin and an oyster-like breath odor have been reported. These effects are temporary and are not considered to be of serious consequence. Changes in the refractive index of the lens of the eye and nuclear cataracts have been observed in animals, with the use of this drug. This appears to be related to dosage and duration of therapy.

References: Available upon request.

Presentation: DOMOSO® (dimethyl sulfoxide) Gel is supplied in 2.1 oz (60 g) (NDC 0856-0046-50) and 4.2 oz (120 g) (NDC 0856-0046-51) collapsible tubes, and 15 oz (425 g) (NDC 0856-0046-55) containers.

Compendium Code No.: 10030401 0030B

DOMOSO® SOLUTION ℞

Fort Dodge **Topical Anti-inflammatory**

90% Dimethyl Sulfoxide — Medical Grade

NADA No.: 032-168

Active Ingredient(s): Each mL of DOMOSO® (dimethyl sulfoxide) Solution contains 90% dimethyl sulfoxide and 10% water.

Indications: Canine and Equine: DOMOSO® (dimethyl sulfoxide) Solution is recommended as a topical application to reduce acute swelling due to trauma.

Pharmacology: Dimethyl sulfoxide (DMSO), an oxidation product of dimethyl sulfide, is an exceptional solvent possessing a number of commercial uses.

DMSO is the lowest member of the group of alkyl sulfoxides with a general formula of RSOR. Its structural formula is:

$$CH_3-\overset{\overset{\large O}{\|}}{S}-CH_3$$

It freely mixes with water with the evolution of heat and lowers the freezing point of aqueous solutions. It is soluble in many other compounds including ethanol, acetone, diethyl ether, glycerin, toluene, benzene and chloroform. DMSO is a solvent for many aromatic and unsaturated hydrocarbons as well as inorganic salts and nitrogen-containing compounds. DMSO has a high dielectric constant due to the polarity of the sulphur-oxygen bond. Its basicity is slightly greater than water due to enhanced electron density at the oxygen atom. It forms crystalline salts with strong protic acids and coordinates with Lewis acids. It modifies hydrogen bonding.

DMSO is a hygroscopic stable organic liquid essentially odorless and water white in color. Other physical characteristics include:

Molecular weight 78.13
Melting point .... 18.45°C
Boiling point .... 189°C

Metabolism: Dimethyl sulfoxide when administered topically or orally is rapidly absorbed and distributed in living materials.

Using S^{35}-labeled DMSO[1] the maximal blood concentration after cutaneous application was achieved in approximately 10 minutes in rats and less than 1 hour in dogs. In rats and dogs the substance did not accumulate in the organs but the concentration in the treated skin and underlying muscle was increased. The main route of excretion is via the urine partially dependent on the species and route of application. In rats there was no significant difference in the elimination half-time of 6 to 8 hours after intravenous or cutaneous administration; in the dog, the elimination half-time was 1.5 to 2 days after intravenous or oral administration. In the dog, however, after cutaneous application about 55% of the administered material was eliminated within 14 days. The radioactivity eliminated via the lungs, and identified as dimethyl sulfide, was about 3% of the administered dose.

In another S^{35}-labeled study[2] with DMSO, following intravenous or cutaneous administration, the only metabolite detectable in the urine of humans and rats, was dimethyl sulfone ($DMSO_2$).

In another S^{35}-labeled rat study[3], DMSO was administered by the oral, intraperitoneal and dermal routes at a level of 500 mg/kg body weight. Plasma radioactivity after an intraperitoneal dose was highest at 0.5 hours, the half-time being 5 to 6 hours. When applied dermally, levels remained constant for 6 hours. Radioactivity in the urine collected for 22 hours represented 60% to 85% of the intraperitoneal and oral doses and 36% to 50% of the dermal dose. The skin contained 3% to 7% of the labeled dosage in all cases.

A peculiar sweetish odor was noted in the exhaled breath of cats treated with dimethyl sulfoxide.[4] The compound responsible for this was identified as dimethyl sulfide. The same odor has been noted in all species treated with the compound.

In rabbits, dimethyl sulfone was detected in the urine following treatment of DMSO.[5]

It has been shown that dimethyl sulfone is a constituent of normal cow's milk.[6]

The original biological applications of DMSO were primarily confined to its use in preserving various tissues and cellular elements including blood[7], blood cells and bone marrow[8], leukocytes[9], lymphocytes[10], platelets[11], spermatozoa[12,13,14], corneal grafts[15,16], skin[17], tissue culture cells[18,19,20,21] and trypanosomes[22], by freezing techniques. DMSO has also been investigated as a radioprotective agent.[23,24]

In early studies with plants, it was claimed that DMSO exerted a profound effect on the biologic membrane, altering their natural selectivity and enhancing the penetration of antibiotics and fungicides.[25]

In one of the first studies reported in animals, various drugs were added to 15% solution of DMSO instilled into the urinary bladder of intact, anesthetized dogs through which an enhancement of absorption was demonstrated.[25] Utilizing a similar technique the transport of physiologically active insulin across the intact bladder mucosa was demonstrated. Results were judged on a decrease in blood sugar levels over that of controls.[26]

In vivo and *in vitro* methods demonstrated that DMSO enhanced human percutaneous absorption of various compounds including steroids, vasoconstrictors, antiperspirants and dyes, as well as an anthelmintic (thiabendazole) and a skin antiseptic (hexachlorophene).[27,28,29,60,61,62] Enhancement was not due to irreversible damage to the stratum corneum.[28]

DMSO has been stated to increase the penetration of low molecular weight allergens such as penicillin G but not large molecular weight allergens such as house dust.[30]

The rate of passage of tritiated water in the presence of DMSO on the epidermis of the hairless mouse was measured *in vitro.* DMSO did not appear to promote the passage of water by its presence, but when concentrated solutions (60% to 100%) were used, permanent changes were produced in the rate of passage of water. It was concluded that the concentration of DMSO used seemed more significant than the time of exposure in establishing the effect on the water barrier.[31]

When the tails of mice were immersed in a 5% solution of various psychoactive drugs in DMSO, the drugs appeared to exert their usual pharmacological effects, indicating drug penetration as judged by the behavioral effects observed in the experimental subjects. Other solvents, including water, also appeared to permit some drug penetration in this study.[32]

Using ten quaternary ammonium salts as test compounds and either water or DMSO as solvents, the oral LD_{50} values were determined in rats and mice. Toxicity changes were obtained in some instances by 50% DMSO and more changes were observed in rats than mice although the results in the two species were not always parallel. When toxicity was altered by DMSO it increased in all instances except one.[33]

When administered systemically in another study, however, various drugs dissolved in DMSO did not differ significantly in their lethality or cellular penetration as compared to the same drug administered in saline.[34]

When evaluated as a solvent for biologic screening tests, low doses of hormones in DMSO stimulated a response similar to that of the hormone in the control vehicle. Higher doses of hormone, however, failed to give the expected response, suggesting a partition coefficient in favor of the solvent.[35] DMSO was also shown to carry physostigmine and phenylbutazone through the skin of the rat.[36]

The absorption of phenylbutazone dissolved in an aqueous solution of DMSO was impaired when administered orally to the rabbit. Absorption of the same drug was not improved using the subcutaneous route simultaneously with DMSO.

However, phenylbutazone could be detected in the rabbit's blood for several hours when an ointment containing DMSO and 5% phenylbutazone was applied to the skin. When the DMSO content of the ointment was increased, the phenylbutazone levels increased. An increase of phenylbutazone in the muscle tissues underlying the site of application over a control ointment containing phenylbutazone without DMSO could be demonstrated in rats.[37]

When 1% fluorescein was injected intradermally at several different concentrations of DMSO in man, the dermal clearance of this substance was considerably decreased as compared to saline control solutions. This was believed due to reduced diffusion through the dermis.[29]

The addition of 50% DMSO to solutions containing 1% old tuberculin (OT) abolished positive patch test reactions in tuberculin sensitive human subjects, and 50% DMSO also prevented the dermatitis produced by 1% trypsin. A possible explanation of these phenomena is the formation of complexes with proteins causing their denaturation.[28] DMSO has also been reported to alter the Schwartzman reaction.[30] It is believed that, similar to chelating agents, DMSO can form complexes with certain metallic salts.[25,38]

Based on the above evidence as well as gas chromatographic and radio-isotope studies it is established that DMSO can effectively penetrate the stratum corneum of the epidermis and enter the systemic circulation. DMSO also has the ability to allow some substances ordinarily unable to penetrate the skin barrier to be carried through it. The mechanism of penetrant action is not yet understood although some theories have been advanced as explanations.[25,38]

DMSO has been claimed to show anti-inflammatory activity against the baker's yeast granuloma in guinea pigs, and when administered orally, against the carrageenin granuloma in rats. The dose needed to achieve these effects is quite high, requiring 1 to 5 g/kg body weight.[39]

In a number of other studies in experimental animals[32,36,40] where DMSO has been chiefly administered orally or by injection, no anti-inflammatory or analgesic activity could be established.

Following experimental hypersensitization to human gamma globulin in the horse, antigen challenge resulted in massive erythema, necrosis and slough. This reaction could be markedly reduced by the hourly application of undiluted DMSO to the reaction site, after challenge.[30]

In the human, DMSO did not exert any beneficial effects on experimentally induced thermal burns, contact dermatitis or ultraviolet burns. It was noted in this study that the burns were of a non-infected nature.[28,29]

In experimentally induced thermal edema of the legs of rabbits, the leg volume was the same for DMSO treated and untreated groups at 3 and 24 hours, but less at 6 hours for the treated group. The DMSO in this experiment was applied at a site distant to the injury.[30]

Sedative effects have been noted in dogs when 90% DMSO was administered at 10 mg/kg dosage levels and mild reserpine-like actions of the drug have also been described in mice.[30]

DMSO, by itself, at concentrations of 100%, 66% and 33%, has been shown to produce neurolysis following perineural injection in the rat's sciatic nerve.[41]

The conflicting reports cited above for the anti-inflammatory and analgesic properties of DMSO are partially dependent upon the experimental models and methods used to measure these parameters. DMSO fails to show analgesic or anti-inflammatory activity in certain of these situations, particularly when used by the systemic route or when administered topically preceded by an irritant substance. In clinical studies in the horse, it was noted that when iodine, liniments or other strong irritants were present on the skin from previous therapy and DMSO applied, a temporary but marked local reaction would occur. This was due to the ability of DMSO to carry these substances into the underlying skin tissues where their irritant actions could be displayed. When DMSO was used clinically, it was applied topically to the involved area, while in the experimental situation this procedure was seldom used. In clinical situations, a marked reduction of pain and edema has often been noted following topical application. The mechanism of action, although not understood, may be partially related to the heat of dissolution of DMSO. It has been demonstrated that following cutaneous application of DMSO in dogs, the skin, dermis and underlying muscle tissues show a local rise in temperature.[30]

The analgesic and anti-inflammatory activity of DMSO, as observed clinically and the differences noted by classical pharmacological methods, may be partially due to the ability of the compound to alter the underlying pathology of the disease state under treatment.[42]

Using the isolated guinea pig heart it was found that DMSO did not influence the amplitude of cardiac contractions, heart rate or coronary flow, although high intravenous doses in the rat and cat resulted in a transient lowering of blood pressure.[36]

Isolated, innervated guinea pig preparations were also used to study the effects of DMSO on skeletal, smooth and cardiac muscles. The compound depressed diaphragm response to both muscle and nerve stimulation and also caused spontaneous skeletal muscle fasciculations. Actual contraction amplitude was augmented although contraction rate appeared unaffected. Vagal threshold was lowered almost 50% by a bath concentration of 6% DMSO. The fasciculations and increased tone of skeletal muscle, and lowering of the vagal threshold by DMSO could be due to cholinesterase inhibition.[43] Intravenous doses of 50% DMSO in doses as high as 1 g/kg failed to alter the EKG of anesthetized dogs and monkeys.[26]

With single intravenous doses of 200 mg/kg of DMSO to anesthetized cats, apnea and a transient fall in blood pressure were produced. Subsequent doses caused only a transient hypotension and apnea was no longer observed. Vagotomy failed to influence the course of DMSO-induced hypotension and bradycardia but atropine (1 mg/kg) significantly attenuated these effects. Repeated intravenous administration of DMSO where each succeeding dose was doubled, led to a gradually lowered blood pressure until death ensued at about 4 g/kg. Myoneural transmission, ganglionic transmission and force of cardia contraction also deteriorated gradually with repeated doses until death. The transient fall in blood pressure occurred only rarely after intraperitoneal administration. One cat exhibited hypotension following a 1 g/kg dose of DMSO but the remainder received dosages of 4 g/kg without showing this effect.[44]

The *in vitro* oxygen consumption of liver, brain and hemidiaphragm tissues of rats is not affected by the intravenous administration of 75 mg DMSO/100 g body weight during the 7 subsequent days. Urease, trypsin and chymotrypsin are inhibited by DMSO, dependent upon its concentration. The *in vitro* metabolism of corticosterone by rat liver slices is not affected by the intravenous administration of 100 mg DMSO/100 g body weight during 3 subsequent days.[2]

DMSO treatment administered intraperitoneally to rats for 35 days decreased experimentally induced intestinal adhesions by 80% over controls as compared to saline, cortisone acetate or a combination of cortisone and DMSO administered separately.[45]

In rabbits, the application of 70% DMSO, adjacent to but not on the wound incision site, appeared to increase the development of wound tensile strength over controls.[46]

Increasing the concentration of DMSO resulted in an increasing inhibition of fibroblast proliferation *in vitro,* which was reversible.[30]

There is an increase in urinary production following the dermal or systemic administration of DMSO, and a transient doubling of urine volume after the intravenous administration of the drug.[48]

Some studies have indicated that DMSO may potentiate the action of certain compounds including insulin[39], endogenous steroids and others. It was suggested that in the case of steroids it might be due to improved penetration at their sites of action on lysosomal membranes.[30]

The minimal inhibitory concentration (MIC) of DMSO to the nearest 10% was determined for two isolates each of *Staphylococcus aureus, Staphylococcus aureus* var. albus, β-hemolytic Streptococci, *Corynebacterium acnes,* Corynebacterium species, *Alcaligenes faecalis, Escherichia coli* and Proteus species. Twenty percent DMSO was found to be bacteriostatic. For *Staphylococcus aureus,* the bactericidal concentration of 50% was 2.5 times that of the MIC; for the remainder, it ranged from 30% to 40% with the gram negative bacteria being somewhat more susceptible.[29]

No growth of Staphylococci, Pseudomonas or *Escherichia coli* occurred in the presence of 36%, 25%, 33% or greater concentrations, respectively, of DMSO.[49]

The minimal inhibitory concentration of DMSO in Sabouraud's broth to the nearest 10% was determined for three dermatophytes: *Trichophyton mentagrophytes, Microsporum gypseum* and *Microsporum canis.* Ten percent DMSO was inhibitory to all three species. The fungicidal concentrations were 30% for the Microsporum species, while *T. mentagrophytes* survived the highest test concentrations of 50%.[29]

Dosage and Administration: DOMOSO® Solution is to be administered topically to the skin over the affected area. The spray pump should be initially held approximately 6 inches from the animal and the distance adjusted to provide a uniform coverage of the area. The volume delivered by depressing the spray pump is approximately ⅓ mL. Refer to user precautions below under Cautions and Contraindications.

Dogs — Liberal application should be administered three to four times daily. Total daily dosage should not exceed 20 mL. Total duration of therapy should not exceed 14 days.

Horses — Liberal application should be administered two to three times daily. Total daily dosage should not exceed 100 mL. Total duration of therapy should not exceed 30 days.

Contraindication(s): DOMOSO® Solution may mask certain disease signs such as are seen in fractures etc.; this does not obviate the need for specific therapy in such conditions. DOMOSO® should not be used directly prior to racing or other physical stress wherein the drug might mask existing pathology, such as a fracture.

Since DOMOSO® Solution effectively alters the biologic membrane, it will in some cases facilitate the systemic absorption of other topically applied drugs and may have a potentiating effect on drugs administered systemically. Therefore, great care should be exercised in use of other drugs at the DOMOSO® Solution application site because of the demonstrated—if variable—ability of DMSO to carry other chemicals through the dermis into the general circulation. If other topical medications are indicated they should not be applied until DOMOSO® Solution is thoroughly dry. Frequently, due to the heat of resolution, a "smoking" effect following application is noted due to vaporization of the drug.

DOMOSO® Solution should also be judiciously used when administered in conjunction with other pharmaceutical preparations, especially those affecting the cardiovascular and central nervous systems. DMSO may potentiate the activity of atropine, insulin, endogenous steroids and certain other drugs.

DOMOSO® Solution should not be used under occlusive dressings. DOMOSO® Solution is contraindicated in horses and dogs intended for breeding purposes.

Precaution(s): Store at controlled room temperature 15° to 30°C (59° to 86°F).

Caution(s): Federal law restricts this drug to use by or on the order of a licensed veterinarian.

Contact between DOMOSO® Solution and the skin should be avoided. Rubber gloves should be worn while applying this drug. Forceps and swabs may be used to facilitate application. If absorbed through the skin, DOMOSO® Solution will cause odorous breath and unpleasant mouth taste. Mild sedation or drowsiness, sensations of warmth, burning, irritation, itching and mild erythematous localized or generalized dermatitis have been reported in some persons following exposure to DOMOSO® Solution. Treatment of such side effects is symptomatic. Consult a physician immediately if adverse effects appear.

Lowering of the vagal threshold, spontaneous skeletal muscle fasciculation, and increased smooth muscle tone in the stomach following DMSO exposure may be due to cholinesterase inhibition. Therefore, DOMOSO® Solution should not be used on dogs, or horses, simultaneously or within a few days before or after treatment with, or exposure to, cholinesterase-inhibiting pesticides or drugs.

DOMOSO® Solution is recommended for topical application only. The application of DOMOSO® Solution should take place only in well ventilated quarters. Inhalation of the drug should be avoided. Avoid contact of the medication with the eyes.

Keep DOMOSO® Solution out of the reach of children.

Do not administer by any other route.

DOMOSO® Solution is a potent solvent and may have a deleterious effect on fabrics, plastics and other materials. Care should be taken to prevent physical contact with DOMOSO® Solution and these materials, either alone or until drying of the treated skin surface has occurred when applied to an animal.

Extremely hygroscopic! Close bottle cap tightly after use. Avoid freezing. Due to the rapid penetration ability of DOMOSO®, rubber gloves should be worn when applying this drug.

Warning(s): For animal use only.

Toxicology: Absorption of topically applied DMSO results in degranulation of the mast cells at the site of application and a release of histamine followed by characteristic histamine whealing of the overlying skin. Following repeated applications of the compound to the same skin area, the mast cells are eventually depleted and the wheal no longer occurs.[28]

The erythema of the skin following topical application of DMSO is considered to be partially due to the release of histamine. In addition, DMSO has the typical action of most solvents in causing drying and defatting of the skin.

In a study designed to evaluate the effects of DOMOSO® (dimethyl sulfoxide) Solution at a total daily dose of 100-300 mL administered for a total period of 90 days, no essential or clinically meaningful ophthalmological effects were seen in the horse. There were no significant variations in glucose, sodium, potassium, SGOT or SGPT measurements. There were a few fluctuations in hematologic values but no changes appear to be drug-related or of significance.

Another study was conducted in the dog to determine the effects of DOMOSO® Solution at a total daily dose of 20-60 mL administered topically for 21 consecutive days. No clinically meaningful ophthalmological effects were noted. No significant variations were observed in blood measurements, including glucose, BUN, SGOT and plasma electrophoresis. Hematologic values were similar to control animals used in this study.

Long-term topical applications of the drug to guinea pigs resulted in histopathologic changes similar to those observed in allergic contact dermatitis. The observed clinical changes were compatible with either an allergic contact dermatitis or a primary irritant effect.[50] DMSO was shown to cause erythema and blistering of human and rat skin resulting in increased permeability of venules and capillaries.[51]

In most cases the local irritation of the skin characterized by erythema, vesicle or blister formation and scurfing abates even with continued treatment. The phenomenon has been described as "accommodation" or "hardening" of the skin, and has been noted with other solvents.

The undiluted compound has low systemic toxicity but a marked local necrotizing and inflammatory effect when it is injected subcutaneously. In rats the subcutaneous injection of 10 g/kg or the intravenous injection of 2.5 g/kg of undiluted DMSO for 2 weeks showed no definite indication of systemic toxicity. The local necrotizing effects produced at these dose levels, however, prevented a longer period of treatment. No significant hematologic or biochemical changes were noted in 3 dogs receiving 0.4 g/kg for 33 days.[35]

Four dogs were administered topical DMSO at 1 g/kg body weight, 5 days weekly for 18 months. Serum glutamic oxaloacetic transaminase (SGOT), serum glutamic pyruvic transaminase (SGPT), prothrombin time, alkaline phosphatase, bilirubin, total protein and albumin globulin (AG) ratio, and blood urea nitrogen (BUN) were determined at the beginning of treatment and at monthly intervals. Significant abnormalities did not occur.[39]

Upon injection of DMSO into the rat pleura, there is an accumulation of fluid, initially appearing as a transudate, but later as a protein-rich exudate. Exudate formation is thought to be due to increased vascular permeability, predominantly in venules, brought about by a delayed release of histamine together with activation of a vaso-active slow contracting substance.[51]

Rats are orally dosed 5 days a week for 2 weeks at levels of 1, 3.5, 5 and 10 mg/kg of DMSO. The only deaths in this group were due to dosing injuries. No signs of dermal sensitization were noted following a course of intradermal injection of a 10% v/v aqueous solution of DMSO in guinea pigs, nor did the same species show signs of injury following 28 daily applications of the undiluted drug to the clipped skin of the back.[52]

A compilation of the results for a number of acute toxicity (LD_{50}) determinations derived from several published reports[35,52,53,54,55] in several experimental animal species are as follows:

Species	Rt. of Administr.	LD_{50} g/kg
Mouse	SQ	13.9-20.5
Mouse	IV	3.82-10.73
Mouse	Oral	15.0-22
Mouse	IP	20.06
Rat	IV	5.25-5.36
Rat	Oral	16.0-28.3
Rat	IP	6.5-13.621
Dog	IV	2.5
Guinea Pig	IP	6.5
Chicken	Oral	12.5

Hemolysis resulting in hemoglobinuria and methemoglobinuria was noted in anesthetized cats following single intravenous doses of 200 mg/kg DMSO. The intraperitoneal administration of DMSO or the dilution of DMSO with isotonic saline prior to intravenous administration reduced its hemolytic activity.[44]

Tests *in vitro* showed that washed rabbit erythrocytes are hemolyzed in a short time with 40% to 60% DMSO solution. Higher concentrations caused, without hemolysis, an agglutination of the erythrocytes.[55]

Teratology: The intraperitoneal administration of 5.5 g/kg of DMSO as a single dose to pregnant hamsters induced developmental malformations of their embryos.[56] Both dimethyl sulfoxide and diethyl sulfoxide are teratogenic when injected into the chick embryo, the classification of malformations being dependent upon the stage of embryonic development at the time of treatment. The same drugs when administered by various techniques to mice, rats and rabbits in which fertility had been established did not cause any embryonic malformations.[57]

Ocular Effects: In a variety of experimental animals including rats, dogs, swine, rabbits and primates, following oral or topical administration of DMSO, certain eye changes have been noted. These consist mainly of a change in the refractive index of the lens described as a "lens within a lens". The lens changes are characterized by a decrease in the normal relucency of the lens cortex, causing the normal central zone of the lens to act as a biconvex lens. When viewing the fundus of affected animals, it is necessary to interpose biconcave lenses in order to see the retinal vessels clearly. The functional effect would be a tendency toward myopia.[58]

The lens changes were first observed in dogs receiving 5 g DMSO/kg after 9 weeks of administration. At lower dose levels the change was observed later. In rabbits these changes were seen after 90 days of dermal application, (8 mg 50% DMSO/kg/day and 4 mg 100% DMSO/kg/day and higher). In swine, dermal application of 4.5 g 90% DMSO/kg twice daily caused similar lens changes by 90 days of treatment.[59]

The lens changes appear earlier with oral administration, and also bear a relation to the dosage employed; the higher the dose the more rapid their appearance.

The eye changes are slowly reversible but with a definite species difference, the dog being the slowest to exhibit improvement.

No effects were seen following direct application of aqueous solutions varying from 10% to full strength into the eyes of albino rabbits for a total dosage of DMSO between 0.1 and 0.2 g/kg body weight per day for six months. Rabbits which received daily doses as high as 10 g/kg orally or topically showed lines of discontinuity in their lenses. No cataract was seen after ten weeks of such daily treatment, although discontinuous lens lines could be detected in about two weeks by slit lamp examination. Chemical studies on these lenses revealed reduction in the usual concentration of urea, glutathione, uric and amino acids.[30]

Side Effects: In general, adverse reactions are local, and while they may prove to be annoying to some patients, they are usually not of a serious nature. Upon topical application, an occasional animal may develop transient erythema, associated with local "burning" or "smarting". Even when erythema or vesiculation occurs, they are self-limiting reversible states, and not necessarily an indication to discontinue medication. Dryness of the skin and an oyster-like breath odor have been reported. These effects are temporary and are not considered to be of serious consequence. Changes in the refractive index of the lens of the eye and nuclear cataracts have been observed in animals, with the use of this drug. This appears to be related to dosage and duration of therapy.

References: Available upon request.

Presentation: DOMOSO® (dimethyl sulfoxide) Solution is supplied in 1 Pint (473 mL) (NDC 0856-0045-74) and 1 Gallon (3785 mL) (NDC 0856-0045-75) bottles.

Compendium Code No.: 10030411 0020B

DOPRAM®-V INJECTABLE ℞

Fort Dodge **Respiratory Stimulant**

brand of Doxapram Hydrochloride

NADA No.: 034-879

Active Ingredient(s): Each 1 mL contains:

Doxapram hydrochloride. . . . . 20 mg
Benzyl alcohol (as preservative) 0.9%
Water for injection, USP . . . . q.s.

Indications: For Dogs, Cats and Horses:

1. To stimulate respirations during and after general anesthesia.
2. To speed awakening and return of reflexes after anesthesia.

For Neonate Dogs and Cats:

1. Initiate respirations following dystocia or cesarean section.
2. To stimulate respirations following dystocia or cesarean section.

Pharmacology: DOPRAM®-V (doxapram hydrochloride) is a potent respiratory stimulant. It is unique in its ability to stimulate respiration at dosages considerably below those required to evoke cerebral cortical stimulation. In nonanesthetized animals the dose required to produce convulsions is some 70 to 75 times the dose required to produce respiratory stimulation. In anesthetized subjects, doxapram also exerts a marked arousal effect. Thus, by promoting the restoration of normal ventilation and producing early arousal following general anesthesia, doxapram minimizes or prevents the undesirable effects of post-anesthetic respiratory depression or hypoventilation and hastens recovery.

Chemistry[1]: The chemical name of doxapram hydrochloride is 1-ethyl-4-(2-morpholinoethyl)-3,3-diphenyl-2-pyrrolidinone hydrochloride hydrate.

The material is prepared as a clear, colorless, 2% aqueous solution with a pH of 3.5 to 5 and is stable at room temperature. Stability studies of 24 months' duration have shown doxapram to have excellent stability characteristics. The preservative is benzyl alcohol, 0.9% and sterilization is accomplished by aseptic filtration technique. Doxapram is compatible with 5% and 10%

dextrose in water or normal saline, but is physically incompatible with alkaline solutions, such as 2.5% thiopental sodium.

Species Variation[2,5]: The dog responds more dramatically to doxapram than other species. For example, arousal was not observed in the rat, and the cat responded poorly in comparison with the dog. Respiratory stimulation was slight in the rat, moderate in the cat and marked in the dog and horse.

Effect on EEG[3]: Studies show that while the drug acted selectively on respiratory centers of the brain, higher doses stimulated other parts of the neuraxis. The cortex appeared to be the most resistant part of the central nervous system to the action of the drug.

Effect on Cerebral Blood Flow[4]: The effect of doxapram on cerebral blood flow in anesthetized dogs was determined. Initially, the drug caused a transient increase in blood flow concomitant with rising femoral arterial blood pressure. Flow then diminished while the blood pressure remained elevated. The decreased flow appeared to coincide with marked respiratory stimulation; its occurrence, therefore, is consistent with the known vasoconstrictor effect of hypocapnia.

D

Effect on Pituitary-Adrenal Axis[5]: Intravenous administration of doxapram (20 mg/kg) to anesthetized dogs resulted in a marked rise in the adrenal venous blood level of 17-hydroxycorticosteroids. The peak response occurred at 5-7 minutes in most animals. Hypophysectomy prevented this effect of doxapram.

Site and Mechanism of Action[2,3,4,7]: Doxapram appeared to stimulate respirations primarily by an effect on the brain stem, since sectioning of reflex pathways did not abolish its action. The detection of increased electrical activity in both the inspiratory and expiratory centers of the medulla, at doses as low as 0.2 mg/kg, constituted confirmation of this site of action. Only after higher doses were other parts of the brain and spinal cord stimulated. Also, cross circulation experiments have shown that doxapram acts mainly through direct stimulation of central respiratory centers.

The pressor response to doxapram appears to be primarily due to stimulation of brain stem vasomotor areas and it is mediated through the sympathoadrenal system. Adrenalectomy and/or drugs which inhibit transmission at sympathetic ganglia or at sympathetic neuroeffector sites were capable of reducing the pressor response to doxapram. Spinal section at C2 abolished the pressor effect.

Intravenous infusion of doxapram to dogs resulted in a prompt and marked increase in total blood and urinary catecholamines.

Therapeutic Ratio[2]: Doxapram did not produce convulsions as readily as did other respiratory stimulants. In unanesthetized animals the ratios between convulsant and respiratory stimulant doses of several such drugs were as follows: doxapram, 70; ethamivan, 35; bemegride, 15; pentylenetetrazol, 4; and picrotoxin, 2.3. In animals anesthetized with barbiturates, it was not possible to establish this ratio for doxapram because convulsions could not be produced.

Interaction with Other Drugs[2,5,10,11,13]: The respiratory stimulant effects of doxapram in dogs were not blocked by anesthetic doses of the following: phenobarbital sodium, pentobarbital sodium, thiopental sodium, secobarbital sodium, halothane and methoxyflurane. In dogs and cats, doxapram stimulated respiration that was severely depressed with morphine or meperidine. However, convulsions occurred in cats, a species in which morphine is known to be convulsant.

The respiratory stimulant effects of doxapram in horses were not blocked by anesthetic doses of the following: chloral hydrate, chloral hydrate plus magnesium sulfate and pentobarbital sodium.

Nialamide potentiated the respiratory stimulant action of doxapram in dogs and reserpine suppressed this action. In curarized dogs, the respiratory response varied inversely with the degree of muscle relaxation existing at the time doxapram was administered.

Doxapram antagonized the depressant effects of chlorpromazine, mephenesin and methocarbamol on spinal reflexes in unanesthetized cats.

Various combinations of analeptics in acute barbiturate narcosis in dogs have been compared, including metaraminol and phenylephrine, methetharimide and amphetamine, methetharimide and phenylephrine, pentylenetetrazol and phenylephrine, pentylenetetrazol and amphetamine, doxapram and phenylephrine, and doxapram alone. While most combinations improved respiratory minute volume quickly, doxapram gave the best response of all. In a similar study comparing the effects of doxapram and various analeptic combinations in dogs, only doxapram was conspicuously effective in increasing ventilation and in shortening sleeping time.

Absorption, Distribution and Fate[5,8]: Respiratory stimulation was observed in the anesthetized dog after administration by the following routes: intravenous, intramuscular, intraperitoneal, oral, sublingual and subcutaneous.

Spectrophotometric methods were applied to the determination of blood levels and urinary excretion in dogs given doxapram, 10 mg/kg and 20 mg/kg, intravenously. Blood concentrations of doxapram and/or its metabolites were at peak levels immediately after injection and declined rapidly in the first hour. The concentration then further decreased slowly, and an appreciable amount was still present at the end of 24 hours. One dog was given doxapram labeled with radioactive carbon in the 2-position of the pyrrolidinone ring. Blood levels were slightly higher and urinary excretion was slightly lower by isotope assay than by chemical assay. The feces contained 29% of the administered radioactivity after 48 hours and an additional 9% in the following 24 hours.

Dosage and Administration: The action of DOPRAM®-V (doxapram hydrochloride) is rapid, usually beginning in a few seconds. The duration and intensity of response depends upon the dose, the condition of the animal at the time the drug is administered, and depth of anesthesia. Repeated doses should not be given until the effects of the first dose have passed and the condition of the patient requires it.

Dosage of DOPRAM®-V (Doxapram Hydrochloride) for Intravenous Injection

Dogs and Cats

Weight of Animal (lb)	Barbiturate Anesthesia Use 1/8 mL (2.5 mg) to 1/4 mL (5 mg) per lb body weight	Gas Anesthesia Use 1/40 mL (0.5 mg) per lb body weight
10	1 1/4 mL (25 mg) to 2 1/2 mL (50 mg)	1/4 mL (5 mg)
20	2 1/2 mL (50 mg) to 5 mL (100 mg)	1/2 mL (10 mg)
30	3 3/4 mL (75 mg) to 7 1/2 mL (150 mg)	3/4 mL (15 mg)
50	6 1/4 mL (125 mg) to 12 1/2 mL (250 mg)	1 1/4 mL (25 mg)

Dosage should be adjusted for depth of anesthesia, respiratory volume and rate. Dosage can be repeated in 15 to 20 minutes, if necessary.

Horses

Weight of Animal (lb)	Chloral hydrate, chloral hydrate and magnesium sulfate barbiturates, use 0.0125 mL (0.25 mg) per lb body weight	Inhalation anesthesia halothane, methoxyflurane, use 0.01 mL (0.20 mg) per lb body weight
100	1 1/4 mL (25 mg)	1 mL (20 mg)
200	2 1/2 mL (50 mg)	2 mL (40 mg)
500	6 1/4 mL (125 mg)	5 mL (100 mg)
1000	12 1/2 mL (250 mg)	10 mL (200 mg)

Dosage of DOPRAM®-V (Doxapram Hydrochloride) for Neonate Use

Neonate Canine: Doxapram may be administered either subcutaneously, sublingually (topically) or via the umbilical vein in doses of 1-5 drops (1-5 mg) depending on size of neonate and degree of respiratory crisis.

Technique for Umbilical Vein Administration: When the neonate is presented through the incision of the uterus, placental membrane and fluid are removed from mouth and nose. A clamp is placed across the umbilical cord approximately 1-2 inches from abdomen of neonate. The umbilical vein is isolated and the selected dose of doxapram injected directly into the umbilical vein.

Neonate Feline: Doxapram may be administered either subcutaneously or sublingually (topically) in a dose of 1-2 drops (1-2 mg) depending on severity of respiratory crisis.

Precaution(s): Store at controlled room temperature 15° to 30°C (59° to 86°F).

Caution(s): Federal law restricts this drug to use by or on the order of a licensed veterinarian.

For intravenous use only in dogs, cats and horses. May be administered subcutaneously, sublingually (topically) or via umbilical vein in neonatal puppies and either subcutaneously or sublingually (topically) in neonatal kittens. Do not mix with alkaline solutions. DOPRAM®-V (doxapram hydrochloride) is neither an antagonist of muscle relaxant drugs nor a specific narcotic antagonist.

Doses of DOPRAM®-V should be adjusted to meet the requirements of the situation. Excessive doses may produce hyperventilation which may lead to respiratory alkalosis. A patent air passageway is essential. Adequate, but not excessive, doses should be used and the blood pressure and reflexes should be checked periodically.

Toxicology: Animal Toxicology[5,9]: Oral toxicity studies were carried out in nine dogs and sixty rats for 30 days. Dogs were given doxapram orally by capsule at doses of 20, 50 and 125 mg/kg/day, and one group received the drug intravenously at 20 mg/kg/day. Rats received the drug by stomach tube at 40, 80 and 160 mg/kg/day, with one group receiving 20 mg/kg intravenously daily. Four dogs died, three while receiving the high dose of 125 mg/kg and one at 50 mg/kg. At each dosage level signs of tremor, lacrimation, excessive salivation, occasional vomiting, diarrhea, stiffness of the extremities and respiratory stimulation were observed in all dogs. The hemogram, urinalysis and blood chemistry showed no changes which were considered attributable to the drug.

Histologically, the central nervous system in both species showed congestion, perivascular hemorrhages and petechial hemorrhages. These changes were interpreted as resembling hypoxic changes. The experiments were repeated in dogs at 2.5, 5, 10, and 20 mg/kg/day and no such lesions were seen.

The acute LD_{50} of doxapram appears to be in the same dose range for various species of animals including mice, rats, adult dogs, newborn dogs and cats. The intravenous LD_{50} was approximately 75 mg/kg while the oral and subcutaneous LD_{50}'s were three to four times greater and the intraperitoneal LD_{50} about twice as great.

No significant irritation was produced when a saline solution of doxapram at a pH of 4.3 was administered intramuscularly to rabbits at concentrations of 1, 2 and 4%. On the other hand, aqueous solutions of the same concentrations caused tissue irritation in rabbits when given subcutaneously.

Safety Margin for the Various Species[2,9]: The acute LD_{50} of doxapram HCl in unanesthetized animals appears to be in the same dose range for various species of animals including mice, rats, adult and neonatal dogs and cats. Intravenously, the LD_{50} was determined to be approximately 75 mg/kg. The oral and subcutaneous LD_{50} was three to four times the intravenous LD_{50} whereas the intraperitoneal LD_{50} was about twice as great.[2,9]

The maximum tolerated dose (MTD) of doxapram HCl in unanesthetized animals appears to be in the same dose range for various species of animals including mice, rats, adult and neonatal dogs and cats. Intravenously, the highest MTD tested was determined to be approximately 40 mg/kg. The oral and subcutaneous MTD was three or four times the intravenous MTD whereas the intraperitoneal MTD was about twice as great.

The highest dose given intravenously to horses was 66 mg per 100 lbs with chloral hydrate anesthesia, and 60 mg per 100 lbs with gas anesthesia. All animals responded normally and no toxic symptoms were observed.

Trial Data: Clinical Studies[5,12,14]: The clinical use of doxapram in lightly and deeply anesthetized animals has confirmed the respiratory stimulant and arousal effects previously demonstrated in the laboratory. In one study with 48 dogs and 18 cats subjected to various surgical procedures using pentobarbital sodium as the anesthetic, marked increases in ventilation occurred within one minute following a single intravenous injection of 5 mg doxapram per kg of body weight (2.5 mg/lb). The most dramatic improvement occurred in lightly anesthetized dogs pretreated with either promazine or fentanyl-droperidol and atropine. Doxapram accelerated the return of pedal reflexes in all animals.

Doxapram consistently sustained an increased heart rate beginning one minute after injection. A second injection generally failed to further increase heart rate. EKG disturbances of T-wave polarity and magnitude occurred with the use of doxapram but tended to abate with time. Second injections of doxapram generally did not aggravate the EKG distortions.

Ten animals had pre-existing EKG signs of cardiac damage and tolerated doxapram well.

In another study with 73 dogs subjected to various surgical procedures using methoxyflurane or halothane as the anesthetic, the arousal time was materially shortened, and respiratory minute volume and rate were increased following a single intravenous injection ranging from 0.08 to 1.95 mg/lb with an average dose of 0.44 mg/lb.

Doxapram was effective in intravenous dosages of 1 mg/kg or less in increasing ventilation and reducing arousal time, especially following methoxyflurane. Tidal volume and respiratory rates were increased; the response normally occurred in 10-20 seconds following injection. No side effects were observed. There were 35 dogs under halothane and 33 dogs under methoxyflurane anesthesia in this study.

In 20 horses subjected to various surgical procedures using intravenous injections of chloral hydrate, chloral hydrate and magnesium sulfate, or pentobarbital as the anesthetic, marked increases in ventilation occurred within 30 seconds following intravenous injection of doxapram in doses ranging from 0.20 to 0.66 mg/lb with an average of 0.28 mg/lb for chloral hydrate and 0.20 to 0.25 mg/lb for the barbiturate. The arousal time was materially shortened, and respiratory minute volume and rate were increased.

In another study involving 34 horses anesthetized with halothane or methoxyflurane, marked increases in ventilation occurred within 30 seconds following intravenous injection of doxapram in doses ranging from 0.08 to 0.50 mg/lb, with an average dose of 0.21 mg/lb. The average recovery time was shortened by one-third or more.

In a series of clinical studies involving 80 neonatal canine patients, suffering respiratory crisis following dystocia or cesarean section, doxapram administered either subcutaneously, sublingually or via umbilical vein in doses from 1 to 5 drops (1-5 mg) resulted in a marked increase in ventilation and survival of all patients.

In a series of clinical studies involving 16 neonatal feline patients, suffering respiratory crisis following cesarean section or dystocia, doxapram administered either subcutaneously or sublingually (topically) in doses of 1 to 2 drops (1-2 mg) resulted in a marked increase in ventilation and survival of all patients.

References: Available upon request.

Presentation: DOPRAM®-V (doxapram hydrochloride) is available in 20 mL multiple dose vials of the sterile solution (NDC 0856-4851-83).

Manufactured by: Elkins-Sinn, Inc., Cherry Hill, NJ 08003

Compendium Code No.: 10030420

5020C

DORMOSEDAN® ℞

Pfizer Animal Health **Analgesic-Sedative**

(detomidine hydrochloride) Sedative and Analgesic-Sterile Solution 10 mg/mL

NADA No.: 140-862

Active Ingredient(s): Each mL of DORMOSEDAN® contains 10.0 mg detomidine hydrochloride, 1.0 mg methyl paraben, 5.9 mg sodium chloride, and water for injection, q.s.

Indications: DORMOSEDAN® is indicated for use as a sedative and analgesic to facilitate minor surgical and diagnostic procedures in mature horses and yearlings. It has been used successfully for the following: to calm fractious horses, to provide relief from abdominal pain, to facilitate bronchoscopy, bronchoalveolar lavage, nasogastric intubation, nonreproductive rectal palpations, suturing of skin lacerations, and castrations. Additionally, an approved, local infiltration anesthetic is indicated for castration.

Pharmacology: Description: DORMOSEDAN® is a synthetic alpha-2 adrenoreceptor agonist with sedative and analgesic properties. The chemical name is 1H imidazole, 4-[(2,3-dimethylphenyl) methyl]-hydrochloride and the generic name is detomidine hydrochloride. It is a white, crystalline, water-soluble substance having a molecular weight of 222.7. The molecular formula is C12H14N2•HCl.

Chemical Structure:

Clinical Pharmacology: DORMOSEDAN®, a non-narcotic sedative and analgesic, is a potent α2-adrenoreceptor agonist which produces sedation and superficial and visceral analgesia which is dose dependent in its depth and duration. Profound lethargy and a characteristic lowering of the head with reduced sensitivity to environmental stimuli (sounds, etc.) are seen with detomidine. A short period of incoordination is characteristically followed by immobility and a firm stance with front legs well spread. The analgesic effect is most readily seen as an increase in the pain threshold at the body surface. Sensitivity to touch is little affected and in some cases may actually be enhanced.

With detomidine administration, heart rate is markedly decreased, blood pressure is initially elevated, and then a steady decline to normal is seen. A transient change in the conductivity of the cardiac muscle may occur, as evidenced by partial atrioventricular (AV) and sinoauricular (SA) blocks. This change in the conductivity of the cardiac muscle may be prevented by IV administration of atropine at 0.02 mg/kg of body weight.

No effect on blood clotting time or other hematological parameters was encountered at dosages of 20 or 40 mcg/kg of body weight. Respiratory responses include an initial slowing of respiration within a few seconds to 1-2 minutes after administration, increasing to normal within 5 minutes. An initial decrease in tidal volume is followed by an increase.

Dosage and Administration:

For sedation: Administer DORMOSEDAN® IV or IM at the rates of 20 or 40 mcg detomidine hydrochloride per kg of body weight (0.2 or 0.4 mL of DORMOSEDAN® per 100 kg or 220 lb), depending on the depth and duration of sedation required. Onset of sedative effects should be reached within 2-4 minutes after IV administration and 3-5 minutes after IM administration. Twenty mcg/kg will provide 30-90 minutes of sedation and 40 mcg/kg will provide approximately 90 minutes to 2 hours of sedation.

For analgesia: Administer DORMOSEDAN® IV at the rates of 20 or 40 mcg detomidine hydrocloride per kg of body weight (0.2 or 0.4 mL of DORMOSEDAN® per 100 kg or 220 lb), depending on the depth and duration of analgesia required. Twenty mcg/kg will usually begin to take effect in 2-4 minutes and provide 30-45 minutes of analgesia. The 40 mcg/kg dose will also begin to take effect in 2-4 minutes and provide 45-75 minutes of analgesia.

For both sedation and analgesia: Administer DORMOSEDAN® IV at the rates of 20 or 40 mcg detomidine hydrochloride per kg of body weight (0.2 or 0.4 mL of DORMOSEDAN® per 100 kg or 220 lb), depending on the depth and duration of sedation and analgesia required.

Before and after injection, the animal should be allowed to rest quietly.

Contraindication(s): DORMOSEDAN® should not be used in horses with pre-existing AV or SA block, with severe coronary insufficiency, cerebrovascular disease, respiratory disease, or chronic renal failure. Intravenous potentiated sulfonamides should not be used in anesthetized or sedated horses as potentially fatal dysrhythmias may occur.

Information on the possible effects of detomidine hydrochloride in breeding horses is limited to uncontrolled clinical reports; therefore, this drug is not recommended for use in breeding animals.

Precaution(s): Storage: Store at controlled room temperature 15°-30°C (59°-86°F) in the absence of light.

Before administration, careful consideration should be given to administering DORMOSEDAN® to horses approaching or in endotoxic or traumatic shock, to horses with advanced liver or kidney disease, or to horses under stress from extreme heat, cold, fatigue, or high altitude. Protect treated horses from temperature extremes. Some horses, although apparently deeply sedated, may still respond to external stimuli. Routine safety measures should be employed to protect practitioners and handlers. Allowing the horse to stand quietly for 5 minutes before administration and for 10-15 minutes after injection may improve the response to DORMOSEDAN®.

Caution(s): Federal law restricts this drug to use by or on the order of a licensed veterinarian.

DORMOSEDAN® is a potent α2-agonist, and extreme caution should be exercised in its use with other sedative or analgesic drugs for they may produce additive effects.

When using any analgesic to help alleviate abdominal pain, a complete physical examination and diagnostic work-up are necessary to determine the etiology of the pain.

Warning(s): Not for use in horses intended for food. Not for human use. Keep out of reach of children.

Human safety information: Care should be taken to assure that detomidine hydrochloride is not inadvertently ingested as safety studies have indicated that the drug is well absorbed when administered orally. Standard ocular irritation tests in rabbits using the proposed market formulation have shown detomidine hydrochloride to be nonirritating to eyes. Primary dermal irritation tests in guinea pigs using up to 5 times the proposed market concentration of detomidine hydrochloride on intact and abraded skin have demonstrated that the drug is nonirritating to skin and is apparently poorly absorbed dermally. However, in accordance with prudent clinical procedures, exposure of eyes or skin should be avoided and affected areas should be washed immediately if exposure does occur. As with all injectable drugs causing profound physiological effects, routine precautions should be employed by practitioners when handling and using loaded syringes to prevent accidental self-injection.

For use in horses only.

Overdose: Detomidine hydrochloride is tolerated in horses at up to 200 mcg/kg of body weight (10 times the low dosage and 5 times the high dosage). In safety studies in horses, detomidine hydrochloride at 400 mcg/kg of body weight administered daily for 3 consecutive days produced microscopic foci of myocardial necrosis in 1 of 8 horses.

Adverse Reactions: Occasional reports of anaphylactic-like reactions have been received, including 1 or more of the following: urticaria, skin plaques, dyspnea, edema of the upper airways, trembling, recumbency, and death. The use of epinephrine should be avoided since epinephrine may potentiate the effects of α2-agonists. Reports of mild adverse reactions have resolved uneventfully without treatment. Severe adverse reactions should be treated symptomatically. As with all α2-agonists, the potential for isolated cases of hypersensitivity exist, including paradoxical response (excitation).

Side Effects: Horses treated with DORMOSEDAN® exhibit hypertension. Bradycardia routinely occurs 1 minute after injection. The relationship between hypertension and bradycardia is consistent with an adaptive baroreceptor response to the increased pressure and inconsistent with a primary drug-induced bradycardia. Piloerection, sweating, salivation, and slight muscle tremors are frequently seen after administration. Partial transient penis prolapse may be seen. Partial AV and SA blocks may occur with decreased heart and respiratory rates. Urination typically occurs during recovery at about 45-60 minutes posttreatment, depending on dosage. Incoordination or staggering is usually seen only during the first 3-5 minutes after injection, until animals have secured a firm footing.

Because of continued lowering of the head during sedation, mucus discharges from the nose and, occasionally, edema of the head and face may be seen. Holding the head in a slightly elevated position generally prevents these effects.

Presentation: DORMOSEDAN® is supplied in 5- and 20-mL multidose vials.

Manufactured by: Orion Corporation, Espoo, Finland

U.S. Patent Nos. 4,443,466 and 4,584,383

Compendium Code No.: 36900950

75-6290-07

DOUBLE "A" CONCENTRATE

Vedco **Large Animal Dietary Supplement**

Active Ingredient(s): Each 100 mL contains:

Dextrose • H_2O	5 g
Sodium acetate • $3H_2O$	250 mg
Magnesium sulfate • $7H_2O$	200 mg
Potassium chloride	200 mg
Calcium chloride • $2H_2O$	150 mg
Niacinamide	150 mg
Pyridoxine hydrochloride (B_6)	10 mg
Thiamine hydrochloride (B_1)	10 mg
d-panthenol	5 mg
Riboflavin (B_2)	4 mg
Cyanocobalamin (B_{12})	5 mcg
L-leucine	187 mg
L-lysine hydrochloride	170 mg
L-glutamic acid	136 mg
L-valine	136 mg
L-phenylalanine	119 mg
L-arginine hydrochloride	85 mg
L-isoleucine	85 mg
L-threonine	78.2 mg
L-histidine hydrochloride • H_2O	59.5 mg
L-methionine	51 mg
L-cysteine hydrochloride • H_2O	50 mg
L-tryptophan	34 mg
Propylene glycol	2.5%
Sorbitol	2.5%
Lactic acid	0.16%
Citric acid	0.1%
BHA	0.005%
Preservatives:	
Methylparaben	0.18%
Propylparaben	0.02%
Ethylparaben	0.01%

Indications: An oral source of vitamins, amino acids and electrolytes for cattle, swine, sheep and horses when dietary intake is reduced. For use as a supplemental source of concentrated amino acids, electrolytes, B complex vitamins, and dextrose.

Dosage and Administration: For use in drinking water. DOUBLE "A" CONCENTRATE may be used undiluted or diluted with water. Supply fresh drinking water daily. Dosage: Undiluted.

Cattle: Administer 1 oz. DOUBLE "A" CONCENTRATE per 100 pounds of body weight in the drinking water to be consumed in one (1) day.

Horses: Administer 10 oz. DOUBLE "A" CONCENTRATE per 1,000 pounds of body weight in the drinking water to be consumed in one (1) day.

Sheep and Swine: Administer ½ oz. DOUBLE "A" CONCENTRATE per 50 pounds of body weight in the drinking water to be consumed in one (1) day.

Precaution(s): Store at a controlled room temperature between 59-86°F (15-30°C).

Caution(s): Keep out of the reach of children.

Presentation: 500 mL containers.

Compendium Code No.: 10940480

DOUBLE "A" SOLUTION

Vedco **Large Animal Dietary Supplement**

Active Ingredient(s): Each 100 mL contains:

Dextrose • H_2O	5 g
Sodium acetate • 3 H_2O	250 mg
Magnesium sulfate • $7H_2O$	20 mg
Potassium chloride	20 mg
Calcium chloride • $2H_2O$	15 mg
Niacinamide	150 mg
Pyridoxine hydrochloride (B_6)	10 mg
Thiamine hydrochloride (B_1)	10 mg
d-panthenol	5 mg
Riboflavin (B_2)	4 mg
Cyanocobalamin (B_{12})	5 mcg
L-valine	5 mg
L-glutamic acid	4 mg
L-ceucine	4 mg
L-lysine hydrochloride	3 mg
L-phenylalanine	3 mg
L-arginine hydrochloride	2.5 mg
L-isoleucine	2 mg
L-threonine	2 mg
L-histidine hydrochloride • H_2O	1 mg
L-methionine	1 mg
L-cysteine hydrochloride • H_2O	1 mg
L-tryptophan	1 mg
Propylene glycol	2.5%
Sorbitol	2.5%
Lactic acid	0.16%
Citric acid	0.1%
BHA	0.005%
Preservatives:	
Methylparaben	0.18%
Propylparaben	0.02%
Ethylparaben	0.01%

D

Indications: An oral source of vitamins, amino acids and electrolytes for cattle, swine, sheep and horses when dietary intake is reduced. For use as a supplemental source of concentrated amino acids, electrolytes, B complex vitamins, and dextrose in cattle, swine and sheep.

Dosage and Administration: For use in drinking water. Supply fresh drinking water daily.

Cattle: Administer 1 oz. DOUBLE "A" SOLUTION per 10 pounds of body weight in the drinking water to be consumed in one (1) day.

Horses: Administer 10 oz. DOUBLE "A" SOLUTION per 100 pounds of body weight in the drinking water to be consumed in one (1) day.

Sheep and Swine: Administer ½ oz. DOUBLE "A" SOLUTION per five (5) pounds of body weight in the drinking water to be consumed in one (1) day.

Precaution(s): Store at a controlled room temperature between 59-86°F (15-30°C).

Caution(s): Keep out of the reach of children.

Presentation: 500 mL and 1,000 mL containers.

Compendium Code No.: 10940490

DOUBLE BARREL™ VP INSECTICIDE EAR TAGS

Schering-Plough **Insecticide Ear Tags**

EPA Reg. No.: 773-81

Active Ingredient(s):

	%w/w
Lambdacyhalothrin: [1 α(S), 3 α (Z)]-(±)-cyano (3-phenoxyphenyl)-methyl-3-(2-chloro-3,3,3-trifluoro-1-propenyl)-2,2-dimethylcyclopropanecarboxylate	6.8%
Pirimiphos methyl: 0-[2-diethylamino-6-methyl-4-pyrimidinyl] 0,0-dimethylphosphorothioate	14.0%
Other Ingredients	79.2%
Total	100.0%

Indications: For up to 5 months' control of horn flies and face flies, use two tags per head on beef and non-lactating dairy cattle and calves.

Directions for Use: It is a violation of Federal law to use this product in a manner inconsistent with its labeling. The labeling must be in the possession of the user at the time of pesticide application.

1. Place male button onto pin until it projects through the tip.
2. Dip tag button into disinfectant solution.
3. Press female tag under the clip by depressing lever.
4. Apply through ear between second and third rib, halfway between ear tip and head.

For optimum control and to minimize development of insect resistance, use two tags per animal (one in each ear). All animals in the herd should be tagged. Apply when flies first appear in spring. Replace as necessary. Apply with Allflex®* Tagging System. Tags remain effective up to 5 months. Remove tags in fall.

Precautionary Statements: Hazards to Humans and Domestic Animals:

Caution: Harmful if swallowed or absorbed through the skin. Avoid contact with skin, eyes or clothing. Wear rubber or non-permeable protective gloves when applying or removing tags. Wash thoroughly with soap and water after handling and before eating, drinking or using tobacco. Certain individuals are known to have a special sensitivity to some pyrethroid insecticides. Such individuals on contact with the insecticide may experience a "tingling or burning" sensation around the face, arms, armpits and/or groin. If such sensitivity occurs, wash the affected area with mild soap and water. To relieve the sensation apply a thin layer of an oil based ointment. The sensation generally dissipates within 18-24 hours, if not, call a physician.

First Aid:

If on skin or clothing: Take off contaminated clothing. Rinse skin immediately with plenty of water for 15-20 minutes. Call a poison control center or doctor for treatment advice.

If swallowed: Call a poison control center or doctor immediately for treatment advice. Have person sip a glass of water if able to swallow. Do not induce vomiting unless told to do so by the poison control center or doctor. Do not induce vomiting or give anything by mouth to an unconscious person.

Hotline Number: Have the product container or label with you when calling the poison control center or doctor, or going for treatment. You may also contact the Rocky Mountain Poison Center at 1-303-595-4869 for emergency medical treatment information.

Note to Physician: This product contains a cholinesterase inhibitor. If symptoms of cholinesterase inhibition are present, atropine sulfate by injection is antidotal.

Environmental Hazards: This product is toxic to fish. Do not apply directly to water. Do not contaminate water by disposal of used tags. Use the product only as specified on the label.

Storage and Disposal: Do not contaminate water, food or feed by storage or disposal.

Storage: Store in a cool place away from direct sunlight. Opened pouches containing ear tags should be resealed for storage.

Pesticide Disposal: Remove tags before slaughter. Wastes resulting from the use of this product may be disposed of on site or at an approved waste disposal facility.

Container Disposal: Dispose of empty bag in a sanitary landfill or by incineration, or, if allowed by State and local authorities, by burning. If burned, stay out of smoke.

Warning(s): Remove tags before slaughter.

Keep out of reach of children.

Disclaimer: Notice of Warranty: Schering-Plough Animal Health Corp. makes no warranty of merchantability, fitness for any particular purpose or otherwise expressed or implied concerning this product or its uses which extend beyond the use of this product under normal conditions in accord with the statements made on the label.

Presentation: 20 x 9.5 g tags and buttons (NDC 0061-5004-01).

*Allflex is a registered trademark of Allflex USA, Inc.

U.S. Patent No. 4,953,313

Compendium Code No.: 10470461 Rev. 5/01

DOUBLE IMPACT™

AgriLabs **Parasiticide Injection**

(ivermectin) Injection 1% Sterile Solution

Active Ingredient(s): DOUBLE IMPACT™ Injection is a clear, ready-to-use, sterile solution containing 1% ivermectin, 40% glycerol formal, and propylene glycol, q.s. ad 100%.

Indications: A parasiticide for the treatment and control of internal and external parasites in cattle and swine.

Cattle: DOUBLE IMPACT™ Injection is indicated for the effective treatment and control of the following harmful species of gastrointestinal roundworms, lungworms, grubs, sucking lice, and mange mites in cattle:

Gastrointestinal Roundworms (adults and fourth-stage larvae): *Ostertagia ostertagi* (including inhibited *O ostertagi), O lyrata, Haemonchus placei, Trichostrongylus axei, T colubriformis, Cooperia oncophora, C punctata, C pectinata, Oesophagostomum radiatum, Bunostomum phlebotomum, Nematodirus helvetianus* (adults only), *N spathiger* (adults only).

Lungworms (adults and fourth-stage larvae): *Dictyocaulus viviparus.*

Cattle Grubs (parasitic stages): *Hypoderma bovis, H lineatum.*

Sucking Lice: *Linognathus vituli, Haematopinus eurysternus, Solenopotes capillatus.*

Mites (scabies): *Psoroptes ovis* (syn. *P communis* var. *bovis), Sarcoptes scabiei* var. *bovis.*

Further studies have shown that DOUBLE IMPACT™ Injection given at the recommended dosage controls infections of *Dictyocaulus viviparus* and *Ostertagia ostertagi* for 21 days after treatment; *Oesophagostomum radiatum, Haemonchus placei, Trichostrongylus axei, Cooperia punctata* and *Cooperia oncophora* for 14 days after treatment.

Swine: DOUBLE IMPACT™ Injection is indicated for the effective treatment and control of the following harmful species of gastrointestinal roundworms, lungworms, lice, and mange mites in swine:

Gastrointestinal Roundworms:

Large roundworm: *Ascaris suum* (adults and fourth-stage larvae).

Red stomach worm: *Hyostrongylus rubidus* (adults and fourth-stage larvae).

Nodular worm: *Oesophagostomum* spp (adults and fourth-stage larvae).

Threadworm: *Strongyloides ransomi* (adults).

Somatic Roundworm Larvae:

Threadworm: *Strongyloides ransomi* (somatic larvae).

Sows must be treated at least seven days before farrowing to prevent infection in piglets.

Lungworms: *Metastrongylus* spp (adults).

Lice: *Haematopinus suis.*

Mange Mites: *Sarcoptes scabiei* var. *suis.*

Reindeer: For the treatment and control of warbles *(Oedemagena tarandi)* in reindeer (see Special Minor Use section under "Dosage and Administration").

Pharmacology: Product Description: Ivermectin is derived from the avermectins, a family of potent, broad-spectrum antiparasitic agents isolated from fermentation of *Streptomyces avermitilis.*

DOUBLE IMPACT™ Injection is formulated to deliver the recommended dose level of 200 mcg ivermectin/kilogram of body weight in cattle when given subcutaneously at the rate of 1 mL/110 lb (50 kg). In swine, DOUBLE IMPACT™ Injection is formulated to deliver the recommended dose level of 300 mcg ivermectin/kilogram body weight when given in the neck at the rate of 1 mL per 75 lb (33 kg).

Mode of Action: Ivermectin is a member of the macrocyclic lactone class of endectocides which have a unique mode of action. Compounds of the class bind selectively and with high affinity to glutamate-gated chloride ion channels which occur in invertebrate nerve and muscle cells. This leads to an increase in the permeability of the cell membrane to chloride ions with hyperpolarization of the nerve or muscle cell, resulting in paralysis and death of the parasite. Compounds of this class may also interact with other ligand-gated chloride channels, such as those gated by the neurotransmitter gamma-aminobutyric acid (GABA).

The wide margin of safety is attributable to the fact that mammals do not have glutamate-gated chloride channels, the macrocyclic lactones have a low affinity for other mammalian ligand-gated chloride channels and they do not readily cross the blood-brain barrier.

Dosage and Administration:

Dosage:

Cattle: DOUBLE IMPACT™ Injection should be given only by subcutaneous injection under the loose skin in front of or behind the shoulder at the recommended dose level of 200 mcg ivermectin per kilogram of body weight. Each mL of DOUBLE IMPACT™ contains 10 mg of ivermectin, sufficient to treat 110 lb (50 kg) of body weight (maximum 10 mL per injection site).

Body Weight (lb)	Dose Volume (mL)
220	2
330	3
440	4
550	5
660	6
770	7
990	9
1100	10

Swine: DOUBLE IMPACT™ Injection should be given only by subcutaneous injection in the neck of swine at the recommended dose level of 300 mcg of ivermectin per kilogram (2.2 lb) of body weight. Each mL of DOUBLE IMPACT™ contains 10 mg of ivermectin, sufficient to treat 75 lb of body weight.

	Body Weight (lb)	Dose Volume (mL)
Growing Pigs	19	1/4
	38	1/2
	75	1
	150	2
Breeding Animals (Sows, Gilts, and Boars)	225	3
	300	4
	375	5
	450	6

Administration:

Cattle: DOUBLE IMPACT™ Injection is to be given subcutaneously only, to reduce risk of potentially fatal clostridial infection of the injection site. Animals should be appropriately restrained to achieve the proper route of administration. Use of a 16-gauge, ½ to ¾" needle is suggested. Inject under the loose skin in front of or behind the shoulder (see illustration).

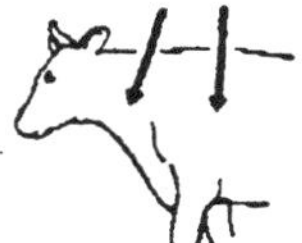

When using the 200 mL and 500 mL pack size, use only automatic syringe equipment.

Use sterile equipment and sanitize the injection site by applying a suitable disinfectant. Clean, properly disinfected needles should be used to reduce the potential for injection site infections. No special handling or protective clothing is necessary.

Swine: DOUBLE IMPACT™ (ivermectin) Injection is to be given subcutaneously in the neck. Animals should be appropriately restrained to achieve the proper route of administration. Use of a 16- or 18-gauge needle is suggested for sows and boars, while an 18- or 20-gauge needle may be appropriate for young animals. Inject under the skin, immediately behind the ear (see illustration).

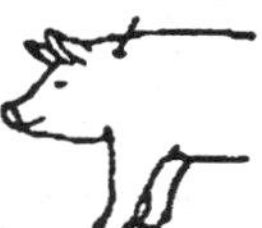

When using the 200 mL and 500 mL pack size, use only automatic syringe equipment. As with any injection, sterile equipment should be used. The injection site should be cleaned and disinfected with alcohol before injection. The rubber stopper should also be disinfected with alcohol to prevent contamination of the contents. Mild and transient pain reactions may be seen in some swine following subcutaneous administration.

Recommended Treatment Program:

Swine: At the time of initiating any parasite control program, it is important to treat all breeding animals in the herd. After the initial treatment, use DOUBLE IMPACT™ Injection regularly as follows:

Breeding Animals:

Sows: Treat prior to farrowing, preferably 7-14 days before, to minimize infection of piglets.

Gilts: Treat 7-14 days prior to breeding.

Treat 7-14 days prior to farrowing.

Boars: Frequency and need for treatments are dependent upon exposure.

Treat at least two times a year.

Feeder Pigs (Weaners/Growers/Finishers): All weaner/feeder pigs should be treated before placement in clean quarters.

Pigs exposed to contaminated soil or pasture may need retreatment if reinfection occurs.

Note:

1. DOUBLE IMPACT™ Injection has a persistent drug level sufficient to control mite infections throughout the egg to adult life cycle. However, since the ivermectin effect is not immediate, care must be taken to prevent reinfestation from exposure to untreated animals or contaminated facilities. Generally, pigs should not be moved to clean quarters or exposed to uninfested pigs for approximately one week after treatment. Sows should be treated at least one week before farrowing to minimize transfer of mites to newborn baby pigs.
2. Louse eggs are unaffected by DOUBLE IMPACT™ Injection and may require up to three weeks to hatch. Louse infestations developing from hatching eggs may require retreatment.
3. Consult a veterinarian for aid in the diagnosis and control of internal parasites of swine.

Special Minor Use:

Reindeer: For the treatment and control of warbles *(Oedemagena tarandi)* in reindeer, inject 200 micrograms ivermectin per kilogram of body weight, subcutaneously. Follow use directions for cattle as described under Administration.

Contraindication(s): DOUBLE IMPACT™ Injection for Cattle and Swine has been developed specifically for use in cattle, swine, and reindeer only. This product should not be used in other animal species as severe adverse reactions, including fatalities in dogs, may result.

Precaution(s): Protect product from light.

Environmental Safety: Studies indicate that when ivermectin comes in contact with the soil, it readily and tightly binds to the soil and becomes inactive over time. Free ivermectin may adversely affect fish and certain water-borne organisms on which they feed. Do not permit water runoff from feedlots or production sites to enter lakes, streams, or ponds. Do not contaminate water by direct application or by the improper disposal of drug containers. Dispose of containers in an approved landfill or by incineration.

Caution(s): Consult your veterinarian for assistance in the diagnosis, treatment and control of parasitism.

Transitory discomfort has been observed in some cattle following subcutaneous administration. A low incidence of soft tissue swelling at the injection site has been observed. These reactions have disappeared without treatment. For cattle, divide doses greater than 10 mL between two injection sites to reduce occasional discomfort or site reaction.

Use sterile equipment and sanitize the injection site by applying a suitable disinfectant. Clean, properly disinfected needles should be used to reduce the potential for injection site infections.

Observe cattle for injection site reactions. Reactions may be due to clostridial infection and should be aggressively treated with appropriate antibiotics. If injection site infections are suspected, consult your veterinarian.

DOUBLE IMPACT™ effectively controls all stages of cattle grubs. However, proper timing of treatment is important. For most effective results, cattle should be treated as soon as possible after the end of the heel fly (warble fly) season.

Cattle treated with DOUBLE IMPACT™ after the end of the heel fly season may be retreated with DOUBLE IMPACT™ during the winter for internal parasites, mange mites, or sucking lice without danger of grub-related reactions. A planned parasite control program is recommended.

This product is not for intravenous or intramuscular use.

Warning(s): Do not treat cattle within 35 days of slaughter. Because a withdrawal time in milk has not been established, do not use in female dairy cattle of breeding age.

Do not treat swine within 18 days of slaughter.

Do not treat reindeer within 8 weeks (56 days) of slaughter.

Keep this and all drugs out of the reach of children.

Adverse Reactions: Destruction of *Hypoderma* larvae (cattle grubs) at the period when these grubs are in vital areas may cause undesirable host-parasite reactions including the possibility of fatalities. Killing *Hypoderma lineatum* when it is in the tissue surrounding the esophagus (gullet) may cause salivation and bloat; killing *H bovis* when it is in the vertebral canal may cause staggering or paralysis. These reactions are not specific to treatment with DOUBLE IMPACT™, but can occur with any successful treatment of grubs. Cattle should be treated either before or after these stages of grub development. Consult your veterinarian concerning the proper time for treatment.

Presentation: DOUBLE IMPACT™ Injection for Cattle and Swine is available in two ready-to-use pack sizes:

The 50 mL pack is a multiple-dose, rubber-capped bottle. Each bottle contains sufficient solution to treat 10 head of 550 lb (250 kg) cattle or 100 head of 38 lb (17.3 kg) swine.

The 200 mL pack is a soft, collapsible pack designed for use with automatic syringe equipment. Each pack contains sufficient solution to treat 40 head of 550 lb (250 kg) cattle or 400 head of 38 lb (17.3 kg) swine.

The 500 mL pack is a soft, collapsible pack designed for use with automatic syringe equipment. Each pack contains sufficient solution to treat 100 head of 550 lb (250 kg) cattle or 1000 head of 38 lb (17.3 kg) swine.

U.S. Pat. 4,199,569

Compendium Code No.: 10580431

DOXIROBE™ ℞

Pharmacia & Upjohn **Doxycycline-Topical**

brand of doxycycline gel

NADA No.: 141-082

Active Ingredient(s): DOXIROBE™ Gel is provided in a 2-syringe system requiring mixing prior to use. Syringe A contains the polymer delivery system (N-methyl-2-pyrrolidone and poly (DL-lactide)) and Syringe B contains the active ingredient (doxycycline). Once mixed, the product is a flowable solution of doxycycline hyclate equivalent to 8.5% doxycycline activity.

Indications: DOXIROBE™ Gel is indicated for the treatment and control of periodontal disease in dogs.

Pharmacology: Clinical Pharmacology: Doxycycline is a semi-synthetic tetracycline derivative. Consistent with the tetracycline class of antibiotics, it has a wide range of antimicrobial activity against microorganisms. Upon contact with the aqueous environment (gingival crevicular fluid) the polymer will coagulate, resulting in the formation of a solid, pliable delivery system within the treated periodontal pocket(s). Doxycycline is released into the gingival crevicular fluid for a local effect on the microorganisms, particularly gram-negative anaerobic bacteria, involved in periodontal disease.

In a clinical trial, the highest plasma doxycycline concentration was observed at 6 hours after treatment administration (2-4 affected teeth in each of 6 dogs). Doxycycline was not detected in plasma samples taken at 24 hours after treatment administration or any time point thereafter. All detectable concentrations of doxycycline were well below levels associated with systemic activity or toxicity.

Dosage and Administration: The formulation is applied subgingivally to the periodontal pocket(s) of affected teeth, and doxycycline is slowly released from the polymer providing a local antimicrobial effect. The product is non-irritating and biodegradable.

Teeth should be cleaned and scaled prior to application of the product. If required, root planing and debridement of affected sites should be performed. The product is applied with the animal under sedation or anesthesia. Use as many units as required to fill the periodontal pockets of affected teeth.

1. Each pouch contains 2 syringes and a blunt cannula. Syringe A contains the polymer delivery system and Syringe B contains doxycycline. Lock the syringes together.
2. Beginning with Syringe A, use the plungers of Syringes A and B to exchange the material between the syringes approximately 100 times to achieve a consistent mixture.
3. Fully deliver the mixture into Syringe A, separate the syringes, and lock the supplied blunt cannula onto Syringe A. The cannula may be bent to the desired angle.
4. Gently place the cannula 1-2 mm below the gingival margin of an affected tooth. Express a small amount of the mixture into each periodontal pocket 4 mm or deeper. Ensure that the pockets are filled approximately to the gingival margin.
5. The formulation will begin to solidify immediately upon application; however, lavage with a few drops of water or saline will facilitate the process. Allow approximately 30-60 seconds for the polymer to harden before beginning to press it into the pocket.
6. The exposed surface of the product may be pressed into the pocket with the edge of a wax spatula or the back of a curette. Pressure may be applied to the gingival margin to avoid

dislodging the polymer inadvertently. As the product is biodegradable, removal at a subsequent visit is not required.

Treatment and control of periodontal disease requires a comprehensive program of routine scaling and cleaning, home care and dental hygiene (e.g., brushing, rinses or the use of chewing devices) in addition to application of this product. Severe cases may require surgical intervention.

Precaution(s): Store in a refrigerator 2° to 8°C (36° to 46°F).

Reconstituted product not used on the day of mixing should be stored in the resealable foil pouch at room temperature (15-25°C or 59-77°F) and used within 3 days of reconstitution. Ten additional exchanges between syringes should be performed if reconstituted product has been stored.

Caution(s): Federal law restricts this drug to use by or on the order of a licensed veterinarian.

Do not use in dogs less than 1 year of age as the use of tetracyclines during tooth development has been associated with permanent discoloration of the teeth. Do not use in pregnant bitches. The use of the product in breeding dogs has not been evaluated.

Clients should be advised to suspend brushing treated teeth for approximately 2 weeks following treatment.

For periodontal use in dogs only.

Adverse Reactions: For Technical Assistance or to report adverse reaction/experience, please call 1-800-253-8600.

Trial Data: Periodontal pocket probing depths ≥ 4 mm are evidence of disease that may be responsive to treatment with the DOXIROBE™ Gel. In clinical trials, use of the product resulted in attachment level gains, periodontal pocket depth reductions and improved gingival health. Noticeable improvements in these parameters should be evident within 2-4 weeks following treatment. The response in individual animals is dependent on the severity of the condition and rigor of adjunctive therapy. This product is not intended for use in oronasal fistulas, periapical abscesses, or severely compromised teeth.

Presentation: Each unit of the DOXIROBE™ Gel contains Syringe A (polymer delivery system) and Syringe B (doxycycline), which when mixed result in approximately 0.5 mL of doxycycline solution. Available as a 3-unit carton (containing 1 additional blunt cannula), NDC 0009-5193-01.

Manufactured by: Atrix Labs, Fort Collins, CO 80525, USA

U.S. Pat. No. B1 4,938,763; U.S. Pat. No. 5,077,049; U.S. Pat. No. 5,278,201; U.S. Pat. No. 5,324,519; Patent Pending

Compendium Code No.: 10490140 818 214 000

D-PANTHENOL INJECTABLE ℞

Vedco **Vitamin Injection**

Active Ingredient(s): Each mL contains:

Dexpanthenol .... 250 mg
Chlorobutanol 0.5%
Water .... q.s.

pH adjusted with acetic acid

Note: The sterility of the product conforms to U.S.P. membrane testing methods.

Indications: For use in intestinal atony, distention, postoperative retention of flatus and feces, paralytic ileus and prophylaxis after abdominal surgery, or trauma resulting in internal injuries, equine colic and any other condition in which there is an impairment of smooth muscle function.

Dosage and Administration:

Dogs and Cats: 25 mg per 5 lbs. of body weight (¼ to 1 mL) intramuscularly. May be repeated in two (2) hours after the initial injection and followed every six (6) to eight (8) hours until the condition is alleviated. The time interval and duration of therapy will depend upon the degree of severity that the animal is exhibiting from the clinical standpoint.

Horses: Initial dose 10 mL intravenously or intramuscularly and repeated every four (4) to six (6) hours until adverse clinical signs have been terminated. The intestinal inhibition elicited by certain parasympatholytic drugs (such as atropine) and adrenergic stimulants (such as adrenaline) is not antagonized. Dexpanthenol does not have a detectable effect on blood coagulation.

Contraindication(s): In therapy of colic resulting from the administration of cholinergic type anthelmintics.

Caution(s): Federal law restricts this drug to use by or on the order of a licensed veterinarian.

Keep out of the reach of children.

Following the administration of succinylcholine chloride, a one-hour waiting period is advisable before initiation of dexpanthenol therapy.

Presentation: 100 mL vials.

Compendium Code No.: 10940411

D-PANTHENOL INJECTION ℞

Butler **Vitamin Injection**

NDC No.: 11695-3525-1

Active Ingredient(s): Each mL contains:

Dexpanthenol .... 250 mg
Benzyl alcohol .... 1% w/v
Water for injection .... q.s.

Indications: For use as a source of d-panthenol.

Dosage and Administration:

Dogs and Cats: 25 mg per 5 lbs. of body weight intramuscularly.

Horses: An initial dose of 10 mL intravenously or intramuscularly.

Contraindication(s): In the therapy of colic resulting from the administration of cholinergic type anthelmintics.

Caution(s): Federal law restricts this drug to use by or on the order of a licensed veterinarian.

Following the administration of succinylcholine chloride, a one-hour waiting period is advisable before the initiation of dexpanthenol therapy.

For animal use only.

Keep out of the reach of children.

Presentation: 100 mL vials.

Compendium Code No.: 10820471

D-PANTHENOL INJECTION ℞

Phoenix Pharmaceutical **Vitamin Injection**

Active Ingredient(s): Each mL contains:

Dexpanthenol .... 250 mg
Benzyl Alcohol .... 1% w/v
Water for Injection .... q.s.
Acetic Acid, Glacial, USP .... to adjust pH

Indications: For use as a nutritional source of d-panthenol.

Dosage and Administration:

Dogs and Cats: 25 mg per 5 lbs. body weight intramuscularly.

Horses: Initial dose 10 cc intravenously or intramuscularly.

Contraindication(s): In therapy of colic resulting from the administration of cholinergic type anthelmintics.

Caution(s): Federal law restricts this drug to use by or on the order of a licensed veterinarian.

Following the administration of succinylcholine chloride, a one-hour waiting period is advisable before the initiation of dexpanthenol therapy.

For animal use only.

Warning(s): Keep out of reach of children.

Presentation: 100 mL vials (NDC 57319-292-05).

Manufactured by: Phoenix Scientific, Inc., St. Joseph, MO 64503.

Compendium Code No.: 12560193 Rev. 11-01

DRAWING SALVE

Neogen **Topical Product**

Ichthammol 20%

Active Ingredient(s): Ichthammol 20%.

Indications: Applied as an ointment in the treatment of weak and brittle hooves and nails of horses and dogs, and chronic skin infections, such as eczema and pruritis. Used as a demulcent, emollient and mild antiseptic alone or in combination with other antiseptics to promote healing in chronic inflammations.

Directions: Apply to affected area once or twice a day. A loose bandage may be applied.

Precaution(s): Avoid prolonged exposure to excessive heat.

Caution(s): External use only.

Warning(s): Keep out of reach of children.

Presentation: 14 oz (400 g) (NDC: 17153-420-16).

Compendium Code No.: 14910251

DR. NAYLOR® BLU-KOTE®

H.W. Naylor **Topical Wound Dressing**

Active Ingredient(s): Sodium propionate, gentian violet, acriflavine, in a special base of water, urea, glycerine, isopropyl alcohol 32% by volume.

Indications: For the effective treatment of fungal infections, surface wounds, cuts, galls, hoof-foot and pad sores, chafes, abrasions, moist lesions, itchy fungus eczema and sores on horses and dogs.

BLU-KOTE® is a germicidal, fungicidal wound dressing and healing aid effective against both bacterial and fungal infections most common in skin lesions of domestic animals. Kills ringworm. Helps to dry up blisters and pox-like sores or lesions.

Dosage and Administration: Clean and dry the affected area thoroughly before spraying. Scrub and remove the scale and scab on ringworm before the first application. Shake well. Remove the protective cap. Hold upright. Point the nozzle opening toward the lesion and spray from a distance of 4-8 inches. Only a light application is needed. Repeat once or twice a day or as indicated until healing occurs.

Precaution(s): Danger: Extremely flammable (aerosol package).

The contents are under pressure. Do not puncture. Do not store or use near heat or an open flame. Exposure to temperatures above 130°F may cause bursting. Never throw the container into a fire or incinerator. BLU-KOTE® stains clothing.

Caution(s): For external veterinary use only. In case of serious burns, deep or puncture wounds, or if redness, irritation or swelling persists or increases, discontinue use and consult a veterinarian. Keep away from the eyes, mouth, nostrils, and mucous membranes. Do not spray in the eyes. Do not inhale. Do not use on cats. Prevent dogs from licking the treated area.

For animal use only.

Keep from the reach of children.

Use only as directed.

Warning(s): Not for use on food producing animals.

Presentation: 4 oz. non-aerosol spray, 4 oz. dauber bottle and 5 oz. aerosol spray.

Compendium Code No.: 10890000

DR. NAYLOR® DEFENDER® TEAT DIP

H.W. Naylor **Teat Dip**

Active Ingredient(s):

N,N'-dimethyldodecanamine 0.4%

In a special emollient base, buffered to neutral pH.

DR. NAYLOR® DEFENDER® Teat Dip has a lotion-like quality with a neural pH. The blue color provides visible evidence that the teats were dipped. Washes off easily at the next milking.

Indications: DR. NAYLOR® DEFENDER® Teat Dip provides a broad-spectrum kill of those micro-organisms on teats that cause mastitis, including coliform and other environmental bacteria.

Dosage and Administration: Make sure to use fresh, full strength DR. NAYLOR® DEFENDER® Teat Dip. Do not mix with any other product. Do not return any dip into the container.

Immediately after milking and upon removal of the milking machine, submerge at least half and preferably all of each teat in DEFENDER® Teat Dip. Allow to air dry. Do not wipe. Discard the used teat dip whenever it becomes dirty. Wash the dip cup thoroughly after each milking.

Precaution(s): Store at room temperature.

The quality of the product is not affected by freezing.

Caution(s): To avoid contamination of milk, thoroughly wash the udder and teats with lukewarm water or an appropriate udder wash and dry with an individual, clean towel before milking.

For animal use only. Keep out of the reach of children. Not for internal use. Protect the eyes from contact with the product.

First Aid: Immediately flush the eyes with cool running water for at least 15 minutes. Seek medical attention.

Presentation: Available in 1 gallon (3.78 L) jugs.

* ® DEFENDER is a registered trademark of H.W. Naylor Company, Inc.

Compendium Code No.: 10890010

DR. NAYLOR® DEHORNING PASTE

H.W. Naylor **Dehorning Paste**

Active Ingredient(s): Calcium hydroxide and sodium hydroxide.

Indications: Prevents horn growth.

Dosage and Administration: Clip off the hair over and around the horn button. With a wood applicator, apply the paste to a spot the size of a quarter once only.

Apply as soon as the horn button can be felt - when the calf or kid is three (3) to seven (7) days old. Keep the animal tied away from others and out of the rain for at least six (6) hours.

Dehorning Older Calves: To dehorn older calves, six (6) to eight (8) weeks of age, where the horn button has started to grow, remove the hair and roughen a ring approximately one-quarter (¼) inch wide around the base of the horn where it joins the skin, with a small scraper or file (do not draw blood). Apply a thin film of paste over the horn button and over the roughened ring around the horn button. Apply once only.

Be particular to apply a thin even coating and only as directed. The reason it is advisable to remove the hair over the horn button before applying the paste is that it is then easier to see that the application is in the right place and in direct contact with the skin.

To further contain the Dehorning Paste, form a ring of udder balm or petroleum jelly around the horn button prior to application.

Caution(s): Poison. Keep from children's reach.

Antidote:

External: Flood with water, then wash with vinegar.

Internal: Give vinegar, or juice of lemon, grapefruit, or orange copiously follow with olive oil.

Eyes: Wash out with 5% boric acid solution.

Call a physician.

For animal use only.

Presentation: 4 oz. jar.

Compendium Code No.: 10890020

DR. NAYLOR® HOOF 'N HEEL®

H.W. Naylor **Topical Wound Dressing**

Active Ingredient(s):

Zinc sulfate equivalent to 20% as the zinc sulfate heptahydrate .... 11.2% (w/v)
Sodium lauryl sulfate .... 2% (w/v)

In a cleansing penetrating aqueous base.

Indications: For use as an aid in the treatment of sheep, goats, cattle and dairy cows with foot rot due to organisms susceptible to zinc sulfate (foot rot, hoof rot, fouls, foot scald).

Dosage and Administration:

1. Clean and trim, when necessary, affected hoofs to expose and remove all dead, loose, undermined tissue. Control any bleeding before treating with DR. NAYLOR® HOOF 'N HEEL®.
2. Slowly squirt DR. NAYLOR® HOOF 'N HEEL® on the lesion, covering and saturating it and surrounding the area thoroughly while holding the hoof inverted. Permit it to penetrate before the releasing the animal. The foot may be wet pack bandaged or soaked to enhance healing. HOOF 'N HEEL® is re-useable and stable.
3. Treat once or twice a day until healing results.
4. Retain the animal in a clean, dry area while it is undergoing treatment. Turn sheep out in a pasture that has been vacant for at least 1-2 weeks. Keep treated animals separate from nontreated animals.

Caution(s): If redness, irritation or swelling persists or increases, consult a veterinarian. Livestock remedy. Not for human use. For external veterinary use only.

Keep out of the reach of children.

Presentation: DR. NAYLOR® HOOF 'N HEEL® is available in a 16 fl. oz. (1 pt.) (474 mL) squeeze bottle, 1 gallon container, and as a 26 lb. powder concentrate to make an antiseptic foot bath for use as a treatment and preventive.

Compendium Code No.: 10890030

DR. NAYLOR® MASTITIS INDICATORS

H.W. Naylor **Mastitis Test**

Active Ingredient(s): Brom thymol.

Indications: A safe and simple cowside test for mastitic milk. The color-change blotter card also reveals flakes and clots.

Dosage and Administration:

Test Procedure: Each quarter section of the blotter is designed to test the milk from the corresponding quarter of the cow's udder. The dark area is for the detection of flakes, and the yellow (round) area is for the determination of alkalinity, either of which conditions, if present, indicates abnormal milk and represents evidence of mastitis infection.

Remove the blotter from the container by grasping it at the place indicated between the thumb and forefinger of left hand. Discard the first stream of milk from the quarter to be tested. Then hold the blotter in a slanting position with the corner downward, so that the milk stream will first cover the dark area and run down over the yellow round area.

If flakes are present they will remain on the surface of the blotter where they will show up clearly against the dark background. If milk is abnormally alkaline the yellow (round) area will change to a greenish blue color. The depth of this color is usually in direct proportion to the degree of mastitis infection.

Many cases of mastitis in the early stages can be successfully treated. For the determination of curable cases and a course of treatment, consult a veterinarian.

Precaution(s): Unused testers should be kept in a clean, dry place away from light and stable odors.

Caution(s): The colormetric test should not be relied upon during a period of two or three weeks after freshening and before drying off.

Reactions will result from long exposure to ammoniated atmosphere.

Presentation: Box of 30 indicator cards.

Compendium Code No.: 10890040

DR. NAYLOR® RED-KOTE®

H.W. Naylor **Topical Wound Dressing**

Active Ingredient(s): Phenol, biebrich scarlet red, isopropyl alcohol 6.2% by volume. In a soothing, softening vegetable oil base.

Indications: For use as an aid in the treatment of superficial wounds, surface and wire cuts, lacerations, slow healing ulcers, abrasions, rope burns and chafes in horses and dogs.

Dosage and Administration: Clean and dry the affected area thoroughly before spraying. Keep the wound clean and dry.

Shake well. Remove the protective cap. Hold the container upright four (4) to six (6) inches from the animal and direct the spray at the site to be treated by pressing down the valve. Only a light coat is needed. Use either as an open wound treatment or under a bandage. Repeat once or twice a day or as indicated until healing takes place.

Thoroughly cleanse and sanitize the dauber after each use.

Precaution(s): Danger: Extremely flammable.

Contents under pressure. Do not use or store near heat or an open flame. Exposure to temperatures above 120°F may cause bursting. Do not puncture or incinerate the can.

Caution(s): Keep out of the reach of children.

For external veterinary use only. Use only as directed. Avoid contact with the eyes and mucous membranes. Do not apply to large areas of broken skin. Do not use on cats. Prevent dogs from licking the treated area. If redness, irritation, or swelling persists or increases, discontinue use and consult a veterinarian. In case of serious burns, deep or puncture wounds, consult a veterinarian. Avoid inhalation.

For external animal use only.

Livestock remedy. Not for human use.

Warning(s): Not for use on food-producing animals.

Presentation: 4 oz. dauber bottle and 5 oz. (142 g) aerosol spray.

Compendium Code No.: 10890050

DR. NAYLOR® STOP-A-LEAK

H.W. Naylor **Udder Product**

Active Ingredient(s): Contains iodine in a base of tannic acid, ethyl acetate, ethylcellulose and isopropyl alcohol 22%.

Indications: Topical liquid for teats that leak milk. Stimulates and tightens the muscle at the end of the teat.

Dosage and Administration: With the applicator attached to the cap, apply Stop-A-Leak over the opening in the teat and over the entire end of the teat. Apply morning and night after milking until the teat stops leaking. Strip the quarter clean and thoroughly dry the end of the teat before applying Stop-A-Leak. In severe cases, milk out the quarter and apply three (3) times a day. Keep the bottle tightly capped.

Caution(s): Treated teats should be thoroughly washed before milking. Do not apply to irritated skin or if excessive irritation develops. Avoid getting into the eyes or on mucous membranes.

Keep out of the reach of children.

Presentation: 1.75 fl. oz. bottle.

Compendium Code No.: 10890060

DR. NAYLOR® TEAT DILATORS

H.W. Naylor **Teat Dilator**

Active Ingredient(s): DR. NAYLOR® Soft Surface Dilators are packed in a special lubricant containing petrolatum, water, lanolin, beeswax, paraffin, isopropyl alcohol 1.2%, methylparaben, propylparaben, sodium borate, oil of clove and color.

Indications: DR. NAYLOR® Dilators keep the teat open in the treatment of cut, bruised, and sore teats.

Assists in preventing scar tissue obstructions while the teat heals.

Dosage and Administration:

1. Thoroughly cleanse the end of the teat with soap and water. Disinfect with a mild antiseptic or dairy disinfectant solution. Insert the DR. NAYLOR® Dilator in the teat and allow it to remain there until the next milking.
2. At the next milking, remove the dilator and discard it. Discard the first few streams of milk in a strip cup, then milk out the quarter. Clean and disinfect the end of the teat each time before inserting the dilator, and use a new DR. NAYLOR® Dilator for each insertion.
3. Keep a DR. NAYLOR® Dilator in the teat between milkings until the teat milks freely by hand.

Precaution(s): Store in a clean, dry, cool place.

Caution(s): Keep out of the reach of children.

Thoroughly clean the udder and teats before milking. Do not remove the cylinder from the box. Keep the lid on.

Presentation: Package of 40 dilators.

Compendium Code No.: 10890070

DR. NAYLOR® UDDER BALM

H.W. Naylor **Udder Product**

NDC No.: 15878-413-13

Active Ingredient(s):

8-hydroxyquinoline 0.14%

Inactive Ingredients: Petrolatum, water, lanolin, wax, oil of clove, sodium borate, color, and isopropyl alcohol 0.2%.

Indications: Chapped teats, minor cuts, scrapes, scratches, chafes, windburn, and sunburn.

Designed to remain in prolonged antiseptic contact, to reduce the danger of external infection by inhibiting bacterial growth.

Dosage and Administration: Apply liberally after each milking or as often as necessary.

Udder Massage: To promote better circulation in a congested udder, apply liberally with a thorough massage, removing milk at each application.

Caution(s): Do not use in case of deep or puncture wounds or serious burns. Consult a veterinarian. If redness, irritation, or swelling persists or increases, discontinue use and consult a veterinarian. Thoroughly wash the udder and teats before each milking.

For animal use only.

Keep from the reach of children.

Presentation: 9 oz. (255 g) tin or 36 oz. pail.

Compendium Code No.: 10890080

DRONCIT® ℞

(praziquantel) Canine Cestocide Tablets

Bayer

Each tablet contains 34 mg praziquantel.

DESCRIPTION: Droncit® (praziquantel) Canine Cestocide Tablets are sized for easy oral administration to either adult dogs or puppies. The tablets may be crumbled and mixed with the feed.

INDICATIONS: Droncit® (praziquantel) Canine Cestocide Tablets are indicated for the removal of the following canine cestodes: *Dipylidium caninum, Taenia pisiformis, Echinococcus granulosus* and for the removal and control of *Echinococcus multilocularis.*

ACTION: Droncit® (praziquantel) is absorbed, metabolized in the liver and excreted in the bile. Upon entering the digestive tract from the bile, cestocidal activity is exhibited.[1] Following exposure to praziquantel, the tapeworm loses its ability to resist digestion by the mammalian host. Because of this, whole tapeworms, including the scolex, are very rarely passed after administration of praziquantel. In many instances only disintegrated and partially digested pieces of tapeworms will be seen in the stool. The majority of tapeworms are digested and are not found in the feces.

USE DIRECTIONS: Droncit® (praziquantel) Canine Cestocide Tablets may be administered directly per os or crumbled and mixed with the feed. The recommended dosage of praziquantel varies according to body weight. Smaller animals require a relatively larger dosage because of their higher metabolic rate. The optimum dose for each individual animal will be achieved by utilizing the following dosage schedule:

Dogs and Puppies*

5 lbs. and under	½ tablet
6-10 lbs.	1 tablet
11-15 lbs.	1½ tablets
16-30 lbs.	2 tablets
31-45 lbs.	3 tablets
46-60 lbs.	4 tablets
Over 60 lbs.	5 tablets max

D

* Not intended for use in puppies less than 4 weeks of age.

FASTING: The recommended dosage of praziquantel is not affected by the presence or absence of food in the gastrointestinal tract, therefore, **FASTING IS NEITHER NECESSARY NOR RECOMMENDED.**

RETREATMENT: For those animals living where reinfections are likely to occur, clients should be instructed in the steps to optimize prevention, otherwise, retreatment may be necessary. This is true in cases of *Dipylidium caninum* where reinfection is almost certain to occur if fleas are not removed from the animal and its environment. In addition, for control of *Echinococcus multilocularis*, a program of regular treatment every 21 to 26 days may be indicated (see *E. multilocularis* section below).

ECHINOCOCCUS MULTILOCULARIS: *Echinococcus multilocularis* is a tapeworm species ordinarily considered to be found in wild canids, including foxes, coyotes and wolves. The parasite has also been identified in domestic dogs and cats and potentially is a serious public health concern by involving humans as accidental intermediate hosts.

The life cycle of the parasite is based on a predator-prey relationship, as depicted below.

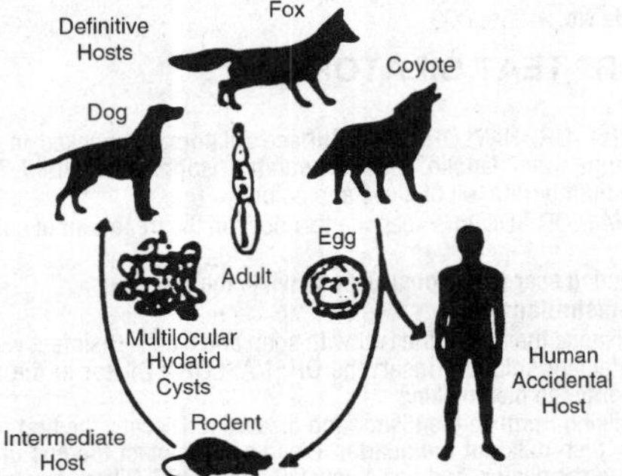

The adult tapeworm is small (1-4mm) and resides in the intestinal tract of the definitive host (wild or domestic canids). Eggs from the adult tapeworm are shed in the feces of the infected canid. Rodents such as mice and voles serve as the intermediate host for *E. multilocularis*. Eggs ingested by rodents develop in the liver, lungs and other organs to form multilocular cysts. The life cycle is completed after a canid consumes a rodent infected with cysts. After ingestion of an infected rodent, larvae contained within the cyst develop into adult tapeworms in the intestinal tract of the canid. Eggs may begin to be passed in the feces of the canid approximately 28 days later.

This parasite poses a serious public health problem because of the possibility for human involvement in the life cycle. If eggs shed by an infected canid are accidentally ingested, a highly pathogenic condition (Alveolar Hydatid Disease) results from development of the cyst stage in humans.

The original geographic distribution of *E. multilocularis* was primarily confined to northern areas of North America. Current evidence indicates migration of the parasite well into the continental United States.[2,3]

Domestic dogs living in *E. multilocularis* endemic areas that roam freely with the opportunity to catch wild rodents are at risk for infection. Pet owners should be advised on how to minimize this risk. Proper restraint of roaming dogs should be encouraged, along with regular treatment with Droncit tablets, following the established dosage schedule (above) and the precautions indicated below.

Additional information on the life cycle and epidemiology of this parasite is available in veterinary parasitology texts.[4,5]

DIAGNOSIS: Diagnosis of *E. multilocularis* in canids is difficult. The adult tapeworm produces no clinical signs of infection. Tapeworm segments (proglottids) are usually not observed in the feces. *E. multilocularis* eggs, observed using microscopic fecal examination procedures, are similar in appearance to the common taeniid species of canids such as *Taenia pisiformis*.

Assistance in the diagnosis of *E. multilocularis* may be available from a state veterinary diagnostic laboratory. Additional information regarding areas where *E. multilocularis* is suspected or has been confirmed may be obtained from area veterinary schools or the Centers for Disease Control in Atlanta, GA.

TREATMENT: Dogs infected with *E. multilocularis* should be treated to prevent exposure of humans to infective eggs and to reduce perpetuation of the parasite's life cycle.

The dosage of Droncit tablets for removal of *E. multilocularis* is the same as that indicated for the removal of the other tapeworm species listed on the label. Laboratory efficacy studies have demonstrated the recommended dosage is 100% efficacious for removal of this tapeworm.

Under condition of continual exposure to wild rodents, retreatment of the dog at 21-26 day intervals is recommended to prevent the shedding of infectious eggs.

PRECAUTIONS: Strict hygienic precautions should be taken when handling dogs or feces suspected of harboring *E. multilocularis*. Infected dogs treated for the first time with Droncit tablets and dogs treated at intervals greater than 28 days may shed eggs in the feces after treatment. The animal should be held in the clinic during this interval and all feces should be incinerated or autoclaved. If these procedures are not possible, the eggs can be destroyed by soaking the feces in a sodium hypochlorite (bleach) solution of 3.75% or greater.[6] All areas where the animal was maintained or in contact with should be thoroughly cleaned with sodium hypochlorite and allowed to dry completely before reuse.

OVERDOSAGE: The safety index has been derived from controlled safety evaluations, clinical trials and prior approved use in foreign countries. Dosages of 5 times the labeled rate at 14 day intervals to dogs as young as 4 weeks did not produce clinical signs of toxicity. No significant clinical chemistry, hematological, cholinesterase, or histopathological changes occurred. Symptoms of gross overdosage include vomition, salivation, diarrhea and depression.

CONTRAINDICATIONS: There are no known contraindications to the use of praziquantel in dogs.

PREGNANCY: Droncit® (praziquantel) has been tested in breeding and pregnant dogs. No adverse effects were noted.

ADVERSE REACTIONS: Seven instances (3.2%) of either vomiting, anorexia, lethargy or diarrhea were reported during the field trials in which 218 dogs were administered Droncit® Canine Cestocide Tablets. The investigators rated these as non-significant.

WARNING: Keep out of the reach of children. Not for human use.

CAUTION: Federal (U.S.A.) law restricts this drug to use by or on the order of a licensed veterinarian.

HOW SUPPLIED: Bottle of 50, and 150 scored tablets. Each scored tablet contains 34 mg praziquantel.

REFERENCES:

1 Andrews, P., Pharmacokinetic Studies with DRONCIT® in Animals Using a Biological Assay. *Veterinary Medical Review*, 2/76, pg. 154-165.

2 Hildreth, M.B., Johnson, M.D. and Kazacos, K.R., 1991. A Zoonosis of Increasing Concern in the United States. *Compendium for Cont Ed*, 13 (5) 727-740.

3 Lieby, P.D., Carney, W.P., and Woods, C.E., 1970. Studies on Sylvatic Echinococcosis. III. Host Occurrence and Geographic Distribution of *Echinococcus multilocularis* in the North Central United States. *J Parasit* 56 (6) 1141-1150.

4 Georgi, J.R. and Georgi, M.E., 1990. *Parasitology for Veterinarians.* W.B. Saunders Co. 118-138.

5 Soulsby, E.J.L., 1982. *Helminths, Arthropods and Protozoa of Domesticated Animals.* 7th Edition. Lea & Febiger. 118-138.

6 Craig, P.S. and McPharson, C.N.L., 1988 Sodium Hypochlorite as an Ovicide for *Echinococcus. Ann Trop Med and Parasit* 82 (2) 211-213.

Droncit is a registered TM of the parent company of Bayer Ag., Leverkusen.

Product Code 1828 — 50 Tablets
July, 1999 71018280, R.11

Code 1860 — 150 Tablets
July, 1999 71018600, R.9

NADA 111-798, Approved by FDA

Bayer Corporation, Agriculture Division, Animal Health, Shawnee Mission, Kansas 66201 U.S.A.

Compendium Code No.: 10400210

DRONCIT® ℞

(praziquantel) Feline Cestocide Tablets

Bayer

Each tablet contains 23 mg praziquantel.

DESCRIPTION: Droncit® Feline Cestocide Tablets are sized for easy oral administration to either adult cats or kittens. The tablets may be crumbled and mixed with the feed.

INDICATIONS: Droncit® Feline Cestocide Tablets are indicated for the removal of the following feline cestodes: *Dipylidium caninum* and *Taenia taeniaeformis*.

ACTION: Droncit® (praziquantel) is absorbed, metabolized in the liver and excreted in the bile. Upon entering the digestive tract from the bile, cestocidal activity is exhibited.[1]

Following exposure to praziquantel, the tapeworm loses its ability to resist digestion by the mammalian host. Because of this, whole tapeworms, including the scolex, are very rarely passed after administration of praziquantel. In many instances only disintegrated and partially digested pieces of tapeworms will be seen in the stool. The majority of tapeworms killed are digested and are not found in the feces.

USE DIRECTIONS: Droncit® Feline Cestocide Tablets may be administered directly per os or crumbled and mixed with the feed. The recommended dosage of praziquantel varies according to body weight. Smaller animals require a relatively larger dosage because of their higher metabolic rate. The optimum dose for each individual animal will be achieved by utilizing the following dosage schedule:

Cats and Kittens*

4 lbs. & under	½ tablet
5-11 lbs.	1 tablet
Over 11 lbs.	1½ tablets

*Not intended for use in kittens less than 6 weeks of age.

FASTING: The recommended dosage of praziquantel is not affected by the presence or absence of food in the gastrointestinal tract, therefore, **FASTING IS NEITHER NECESSARY NOR RECOMMENDED.**

RETREATMENT: For those animals maintained on premises where reinfections are likely to occur, clients should be instructed in the steps necessary to prevent reinfection; otherwise, retreatment may be necessary. This is especially true in cases of *Dipylidium caninum* infections where reinfection is almost certain to occur if fleas are not removed from the animal and its environment.

OVERDOSAGE: The safety index has been derived from controlled safety evaluations, clinical trials and prior approved use in foreign countries. Dosages of 5 times the labeled rate at 14 day intervals to cats as young as 5½ weeks did not produce clinical signs of toxicity. No significant clinical chemistry, hematological, or histopathological changes occurred. Symptoms of gross overdosage include vomition, salivation, diarrhea and depression.

CONTRAINDICATIONS: There are no known contraindications to the use of praziquantel in cats.

PREGNANCY: Droncit® (praziquantel) has been tested in breeding and pregnant cats. No adverse effects were noted.

ADVERSE REACTIONS: One instance of diarrhea and one of salivation (1.5%) were reported during the field trials in which 135 cats were administered Droncit® Feline Cestocide.

WARNING: Keep out of the reach of children. Not for human use.

SOLD TO VETERINARIANS ONLY

CAUTION: Federal (U.S.A.) Law restricts this drug to use by or on the order of a licensed veterinarian.

HOW SUPPLIED: Bottle of 50, and 150 scored tablets. Each scored tablet contains 23 mg praziquantel.

Product Code 1829—50 Tablets 71018290, R.11
Code 1855—150 Tablets 71018550, R.7 July, 1999

REFERENCES

(1) P. Andrews, Pharmacokinetic Studies with DRONCIT in Animals Using a Biological Assay. *Veterinary Medical Review*, 2/76, pg. 154-165.

Droncit is a Reg. TM of the parent company of Bayer AG. Leverkusen.

Bayer Corporation, Agriculture Division, Animal Health, Shawnee Mission, Kansas 66201 U.S.A. Made in U.S.A.

Compendium Code No.: 10400220

DRONCIT® ℞

(praziquantel) Injectable Cestocide for Dogs and Cats

Bayer

56.8 mg/mL Solution

DESCRIPTION:

Droncit Injectable Cestocide is a clear solution containing 56.8 milligrams of praziquantel per mL which has been formulated for subcutaneous or intramuscular use in dogs and cats for removal of cestodes (tapeworms).

INDICATIONS:

Droncit (praziquantel) Injectable Cestocide is indicated for the removal of the following canine and/or feline cestodes: Dogs: *Dipylidium caninum, Taenia pisiformis, Echinococcus granulosus* and for the removal and control of *Echinococcus multilocularis.* Cats: *Taenia taeniaeformis* and *Dipylidium caninum.*

ACTION:

Droncit (praziquantel) is absorbed, metabolized in the liver and excreted via the bile into the digestive tract where its cestocidal activity is exerted.[1] Following exposure to praziquantel, the tapeworm loses its ability to resist digestion by the mammalian host. Because of this, whole tapeworms, including the scolex, are very rarely passed after administration of praziquantel. It is common to see only disintegrated and partially digested pieces of tapeworms in the stool. The majority of tapeworms killed are digested and are not found in the feces.

USE DIRECTIONS:

Droncit (praziquantel) Injectable Cestocide may be administered by either the subcutaneous or intramuscular route to dogs and cats. The recommended dosage of praziquantel varies according to body weight. Smaller animals require a relatively larger dosage. The optimum dosage for each individual animal will be achieved by utilizing the following dosage schedule.

DOGS AND PUPPIES†

Dogs:	
5 lbs. and under	0.3 mL
6-10 lbs.	0.5 mL
11-25 lbs.	1.0 mL
over 25 lbs.	0.2 mL/5 lbs. body weight to a maximum of 3 mL

† Not intended for use in puppies less than four (4) weeks of age.

CATS AND KITTENS††

Cats:	
Under 5 lbs.	0.2 mL
5-10 lbs.	0.4 mL
11 lbs. and over	0.6 mL maximum

†† Not intended for use in kittens less than six (6) weeks of age.

FASTING:

The recommended dosage of praziquantel is not affected by the presence or absence of food in the gastrointestinal tract, therefore, FASTING IS NEITHER NECESSARY NOR RECOMMENDED.

ADMINISTRATION:

Droncit (praziquantel) Injectable Cestocide may be administered by either the subcutaneous or intramuscular route to dogs and cats. The intramuscular route may be preferred in dogs due to a brief period of pain that occasionally follows subcutaneous administration.

Anaphylactoid reactions were not observed in clinical trials. However, as with any drug an anaphylactoid reaction can occur with this product and should be treated symptomatically if it occurs.

RETREATMENT:

For those animals living where reinfections are likely to occur, clients should be instructed in the steps to optimize prevention, otherwise, retreatment may be necessary. This is true in cases of *Dipylidium caninum* where reinfection is almost certain to occur if fleas are not removed from the animal and its environment. In addition, for control of *Echinococcus multilocularis*, a program of regular treatment every 21 to 26 days may be indicated (see *E. multilocularis* section below).

ECHINOCOCCUS MULTILOCULARIS:

Echinococcus multilocularis is a tapeworm species ordinarily considered to be found in wild canids, including foxes, coyotes and wolves. The parasite has also been identified in domestic dogs and cats and potentially is a serious public health concern by involving humans as accidental intermediate hosts.

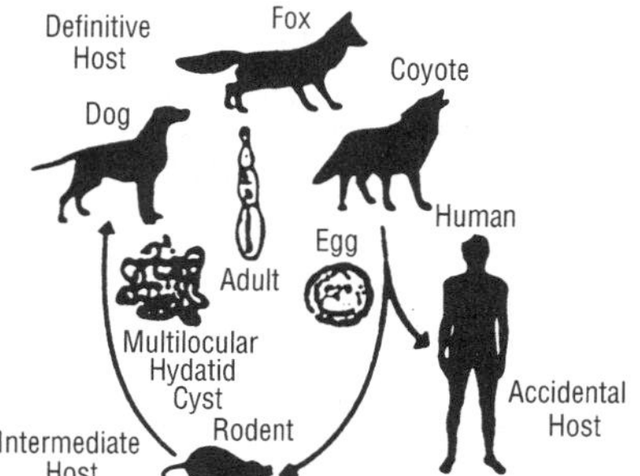

The life cycle of the parasite is based on a predator-prey relationship, as depicted above.

The adult tapeworm is small (1-4mm) and resides in the intestinal tract of the definitive host (wild or domestic canids). Eggs from the adult tapeworm are shed in the feces of the infected canid. Rodents such as mice and voles serve as the intermediate host for *E. multilocularis.* Eggs ingested by rodents develop in the liver, lungs and other organs to form multilocular cysts. The life cycle is completed after a canid consumes a rodent infected with cysts. After ingestion of the infected rodent, larvae within the cyst develop to adult tapeworms in the intestinal tract of the canid. Eggs may begin to be passed in the feces of the canid approximately 28 days later.

This parasite poses a serious public health problem because of the possibility for human involvement in the life cycle. If eggs shed by an infected canid are accidentally ingested, a highly pathogenic condition (Alveolar Hydatid Disease) results from development of the cyst stage in humans.

The original geographic distribution of *E. multilocularis* was primarily confined to northern areas of North America. Current evidence indicates migration of the parasite well into the continental United States.[2,3]

Domestic dogs living in *E. multilocularis* endemic areas that roam freely with the opportunity to catch wild rodents are at risk for infection. Pet owners should be advised on how to minimize this risk. Proper restraint of roaming dogs should be encouraged, along with regular treatment with Droncit Injectable solution, following the dosing schedule aforementioned and precautions indicated below.

Additional information on the life cycle and epidemiology of this parasite is available in veterinary parasitology texts.[4,5]

Diagnosis:

Diagnosis of *E. multilocularis* in canids is difficult. The adult tapeworm produces no clinical signs of infection. Tapeworm segments (proglottids) are usually not observed in the feces. *E. multilocularis* eggs, observed using microscopic fecal examination procedures, are similar in appearance to the common taeniid species of canids such as *Taenia pisiformis.*

Assistance in the diagnosis of *E. multilocularis* may be available from a state veterinary diagnostic laboratory. Additional information regarding areas where *E. multilocularis* is suspected or has been confirmed may be obtained from area veterinary schools or the Centers for Disease Control in Atlanta, GA.

Treatment:

Dogs infected with *E. multilocularis* should be treated to prevent exposure of humans to infective eggs and to reduce perpetuation of the parasite's life cycle.

The dosage of Droncit Injectable solution for removal of *E. multilocularis* is the same as that indicated for the removal of the other tapeworm species listed on the label. Laboratory efficacy studies have demonstrated the recommended dosage is 100% efficacious for removal of this tapeworm.

Under condition of continual exposure to wild rodents, retreatment of the dog at 21-26 day intervals is recommended to prevent the shedding of infectious eggs.

Precautions:

Strict hygienic precautions should be taken when handling dogs or feces suspected of harboring *E. multilocularis.* Infected dogs treated for the first time with Droncit Injectable solution and dogs treated at intervals greater than 28 days may shed eggs in the feces after treatment. The animal should be held in the clinic during this interval and all feces should be incinerated or autoclaved. If these procedures are not possible, the eggs can be destroyed by soaking the feces in a sodium hypochlorite (bleach) solution of 3.75% or greater.[6] All areas where the animal was maintained or in contact with should be thoroughly cleaned with sodium hypochlorite and allowed to dry completely before reuse.

OVERDOSAGE:

The safety index has been derived from controlled safety evaluations, clinical trials and prior approved use in foreign countries. Dosages of 5 times the labeled rate at 14 day intervals to dogs as young as 4 weeks did not produce signs of clinical toxicity following either intramuscular or subcutaneous injections. No significant clinical chemistry, hematological, cholinesterase or histopathological changes occurred. Dosages of 5 times the labeled rate at 14 day intervals to kittens as young as 5 1/2 weeks did not produce signs of clinical toxicity following either intramuscular or subcutaneous injections. Symptoms of overdosage (33.8 to 40 times the labeled dosage rate) in adult dogs included vomition, excessive salivation and depression, but no deaths. Symptoms of overdosage (10 to 20 times the labeled dosage rate) in adult cats included vomition, depression, muscle tremors and incoordination. Deaths occurred in 5 of 8 cats treated subcutaneously and in all 8 injected intramuscularly at doses greater than 20 times the label rate.

CONTRAINDICATIONS:

There are no known contraindications to the use of praziquantel.

PREGNANCY:

Droncit (praziquantel) has been tested in breeding and pregnant dogs and cats. No adverse effects were noted.

ADVERSE REACTION:

Mild side effects were observed in 18 of 189 dogs (9.5%) and 8 of 85 cats (9.4%) administered Droncit Injectable in field trials. For dogs the majority of these were described as brief pain responses following injections to larger dogs (weighing over 50 lbs.). Two dogs exhibited a brief period of mild vomiting and/or drowsy or staggering gait. The eight cats exhibited either diarrhea, weakness, vomition, salivation, sleepiness, burning on injection and/or a temporary lack of appetite. Local irritation or swelling at the site of subcutaneous injections have been reported for cats.

CAUTION:

Federal (U.S.A.) law restricts this drug to use by or on the order of a licensed veterinarian.

HOW SUPPLIED:

Code:	1831	10 mL vial
	1837	50 mL vial

REFERENCES:

1 Andrews, P., Pharmacokinetic Studies with DRONCIT® in Animals Using a Biological Assay. *Veterinary Medical Review*, 2/76, pg. 154-165.

2 Hildreth, M.B., Johnson, M.D. and Kazacos, K.R., 1991. A Zoonosis of Increasing Concern in the United States. *Compendium for Cont Ed*, 13(5) 727-740.

3 Lieby, P.D., Carney, W.P., and Woods, C.E., 1970. Studies on Sylvatic Echinococcosis. III. Host Occurrence and Geographic Distribution of *Echinococcus multilocularis* in the North Central United States. *J Parasit* 56(6) 1141-1150.

4 Georgi, J.R. and Georgi, M.E., 1990. *Parasitology for Veterinarians.* W.B. Saunders Co. 118-138.

5 Soulsby, E.J.L., 1982. *Helminths, Arthropods and Protozoa of Domesticated Animals.* 7th Edition. Lea & Febiger. 118-138.

6 Craig, P.S. and McPharson, C.N.L., 1988 Sodium Hypochlorite as an Ovicide for *Echinococcus. Ann Trop Med and Parasit* 82(2) 211-213.

Droncit is a Registered Trademark of the Parent Company of Bayer AG, Leverkusen.

NADA 111-607, Approved by FDA

December, 1999 79018310, R.12

Bayer Corporation, Agriculture Division, Animal Health, Shawnee Mission, Kansas 66201 U.S.A.

Made in U.S.A.

Compendium Code No.: 10400230

DRONTAL®
(praziquantel/pyrantel pamoate) Tablets
Bayer
Broad Spectrum Dewormer for Cats And Kittens

DESCRIPTION: Drontal® (praziquantel/pyrantel pamoate) Broad Spectrum Dewormer Tablets for Cats and Kittens are scored for easy breakage. Each tablet contains 18.2 mg praziquantel and 72.6 mg pyrantel base as pyrantel pamoate.

DIRECTIONS FOR USE: Drontal® (praziquantel/pyrantel pamoate) tablets will remove Tapeworms *(Dipylidium caninum, Taenia taeniaeformis)*, Hookworms *(Ancylostoma tubaeforme)*, and Large Roundworms *(Toxocara cati)* in cats and kittens.

The presence of tapeworms is indicated by the observance of tapeworm segments passed in the cat's feces. Tapeworm segments are white, pinkish-white or yellow-white in color and are similar in size and shape to flattened grains of rice. The segments are most frequently observed lying on a freshly passed stool. Segments may also be found on the hair around the anus of the animal or on the animal's bedding. Cats become infected with tapeworms after eating fleas or small mammals (rabbits, mice) which may be infected with tapeworm larvae.

D

Hookworms are small whitish or reddish-brown worms less than one inch in length that live in the intestinal tract and feed on blood. Cats can become infected with hookworms by swallowing infected larvae while grooming or when larvae from the environment burrow through the skin. Cats infected with hookworms may have poor physical condition, dull haircoat, and reduced body weight and diarrhea, sometimes with the presence of dark blood.

Large roundworms are white or yellow-white strands 2-7 inches in length (similar in size and color to smooth strings of spaghetti) that may be observed in the cat's vomit or feces. Cats become infected with large roundworms by swallowing infective eggs, particularly while grooming, or by ingestion of mice that may be infected with larval stages.

Large roundworms and hookworms pass eggs in the feces of the cat that can only be observed with the aid of a microscope.

The presence of these parasites should be confirmed through identification of parasite eggs in the feces.

Consult your veterinarian for assistance in the diagnosis, treatment and control of parasites.

Large roundworms and hookworms may be observed in the feces of the cat a day or so after the cat has been treated with Drontal® Tablets. The majority of tapeworms, however, are digested and are not found in the feces after treatment.

DOSAGE AND ADMINISTRATION: To assure proper dosage, weigh the cat prior to treatment. Select the number of whole or partial tablets needed for the cat from the following table.

Body Weight* (lbs.)	Number of Tablets
1.5 - 1.9	¼
2 - 3	½
4 - 8	1
9 - 12	1½
13 - 16	2

*NOT FOR USE IN KITTENS LESS THAN ONE MONTH OF AGE OR WEIGHING LESS THAN 1.5 LBS.

Drontal® Tablets may be given directly by mouth or offered in a small amount of food. Do not withhold food from the cat prior to or after treatment.

EFFICACY: A total of 93 cats with naturally acquired parasite infections were included in two well-controlled laboratory studies to establish the efficacy of Drontal® Tablets. In addition, 85 cats and kittens of various sizes, ages and breeds were included in clinical field studies conducted at six veterinary clinics at different geographic locations throughout the United States. Data indicate 98% of the cats were completely cleared of parasite infections within 7 days of treatment. These studies demonstrated Drontal® Tablets are safe and efficacious for the removal of the parasite species indicated on the label when used as directed.

SAFETY: Cats treated with 10 times the highest recommended Drontal® Tablet dosage during safety studies showed signs of vomition and salivation without other adverse effects. Eighty-three of 85 cats treated with the recommended dosages of Drontal® Tablets in a clinical field study did not exhibit any drug related side effects. A temporary loss of appetite was reported for one cat and transient loose stools were observed in a second cat.

RETREATMENT: *Steps should be taken to prevent parasite infections, otherwise retreatment will be necessary.*

Tapeworms transmitted by fleas will likely recur unless measures are taken to control fleas. Flea control procedures must include insecticide treatment of the cat's environment (i.e. bedding and resting areas) as well as direct treatment of the cat with dips, powders, sprays or other approved insecticides.

Roundworms and hookworms are controlled in cats by maintaining an environment free of infective eggs and larvae. Feces and soiled litter should be removed on a daily basis to prevent build-up of eggs and larvae in the environment.

Certain parasites such as tapeworms and large roundworms are transmitted to the cat after they eat infected rodents. Controlling the predatory habits of cats, i.e., catching and eating rodents, will prevent these parasite infections.

Cats maintained under conditions of constant exposure to parasite infections should have a follow-up fecal exam within 2 to 4 weeks after the first treatment.

If reinfection with tapeworms, hookworms or large roundworms occurs, treatment with Drontal® Tablets may be repeated.

WARNING: KEEP OUT OF REACH OF CHILDREN. Consult your veterinarian before administering to sick or pregnant animals.

HOW SUPPLIED: Drontal® Tablets are available in 50 tablet bottles.

Code 1755—50 tablets/bottle 71017550, R.4

November, 2001

Bayer Corporation, Agriculture Division, Animal Health, Shawnee Mission, Kansas 66201 U.S.A.

NADA 141-008, Approved by FDA

Compendium Code No.: 10400251

DRONTAL® PLUS ℞
(praziquantel/pyrantel pamoate/febantel) Tablets
Bayer
Broad Spectrum Anthelmintic for Dogs

DESCRIPTION: Drontal® Plus (praziquantel/pyrantel pamoate/febantel) Broad Spectrum Anthelmintic Tablets are available in two sizes. Each size is scored for convenient oral administration.

Each Drontal® Plus Tablet for Small Dogs contains 22.7 mg praziquantel, 22.7 mg pyrantel base as pyrantel pamoate and 113.4 mg febantel.

Each Drontal® Plus Tablet for Medium and Large Dogs contains 68.0 mg praziquantel, 68.0 mg pyrantel base as pyrantel pamoate and 340.2 mg febantel.

ACTION: Drontal® Plus Tablets contain three active ingredients having different modes of action and spectra of activity. Praziquantel is active against cestodes (tapeworms). Praziquantel is absorbed, metabolized in the liver and excreted in the bile. Upon entering the digestive tract from the bile, cestocidal activity is exhibited.[1] Following exposure to praziquantel, the tapeworm loses its ability to resist digestion by the mammalian host. Because of this, whole tapeworms, including the scolices, are very rarely passed after administration of praziquantel. In many instances only disintegrated and partially digested pieces of tapeworms will be seen in the stool. The majority of tapeworms are digested and are not found in the feces.

Pyrantel pamoate is active against hookworms and ascarids. Pyrantel pamoate acts on the cholinergic receptors of the nematode resulting in spastic paralysis. Peristaltic action of the intestinal tract then eliminates the parasite.[2]

Febantel is active against nematode parasites including whipworms. Febantel is rapidly absorbed and metabolized in the animal. Available information suggests that the parasite's energy metabolism is blocked, leading to energy exchange breakdown and inhibited glucose uptake.

Laboratory efficacy and clinical studies conducted with Drontal® Plus Tablets demonstrate that each of the three active ingredients act independently without interference. The combined tablet formulation provides a wide spectrum of activity against the indicated species of intestinal helminths.

INDICATIONS: Drontal® Plus (praziquantel/pyrantel pamoate/febantel) Broad Spectrum Anthelmintic Tablets are indicated for removal of Tapeworms *(Dipylidium caninum, Taenia pisiformis, Echinococcus granulosus*, and removal and control of *Echinococcus multilocularis)*. For removal of Hookworms *(Ancylostoma caninum, Uncinaria stenocephala)*, Ascarids *(Toxocara canis, Toxascaris leonina)*, and Whipworms *(Trichuris vulpis)* in dogs.

USE DIRECTIONS

DOSAGE: The presence of parasites should be confirmed by laboratory fecal examination. Weigh the animal before treatment. Administer the proper dosage as specified in the following table as a single oral treatment.

DOSAGE CHARTS

Drontal® Plus Tablets for Small Dogs* (2-25 lbs.)		Drontal® Plus Tablets for Medium & Large Dogs (26 lbs. and over)	
Body Weight (lbs.)	Number of Tablets	Body Weight (lbs.)	Number of Tablets
2 - 4	0.5	26 - 30	1.0
5 - 7	1.0	31 - 44	1.5
8 - 12	1.5	45 - 60	2.0
13 - 18	2.0	61 - 74	2.5
19 - 25	2.5	75 - 90	3.0
		91 - 104	3.5
		105 - 120	4.0

*NOT FOR USE IN DOGS WEIGHING LESS THAN 2 LBS. OR PUPPIES LESS THAN 3 WEEKS OF AGE.

ADMINISTRATION: Drontal® Plus Tablets have been developed for oral administration. Tablets may be given directly by mouth or offered in a small amount of food. Fasting is neither necessary nor recommended prior to or after treatment.

RETREATMENT: For those animals living where reinfections are likely to occur, clients should be instructed in the steps to optimize prevention, otherwise, retreatment may be necessary. This is true in cases of *Dipylidium caninum* where reinfection is almost certain to occur if fleas are not removed from the animal and its environment. In addition, for control of *Echinococcus multilocularis*, a program of regular treatment every 21 to 26 days may be indicated (see *E. multilocularis* section below).

ECHINOCOCCUS MULTILOCULARIS: *Echinococcus multilocularis* is a tapeworm species usually found in wild canids, including foxes, coyotes and wolves. The parasite has also been identified in domestic dogs and cats and is potentially a serious public health concern because it may infect humans.

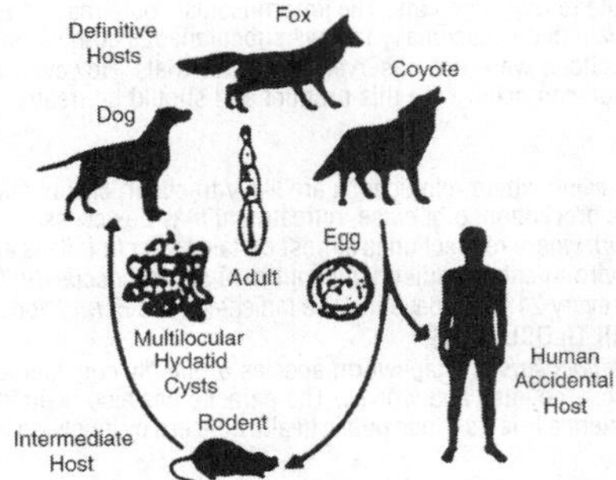

The life cycle of the parasite is based on a predator-prey relationship, as depicted above.

The adult tapeworm is small (1-4 mm) and resides in the intestinal tract of the definitive host (wild or domestic canids). Eggs from the adult tapeworm are shed in the feces. Rodents such as mice and voles serve as the intermediate host. Eggs ingested by rodents develop in the liver, lungs and other organs to form multilocular cysts. The life cycle is completed after a canid consumes a rodent infected with cysts. Larvae within the cyst develop into adult tapeworms in the intestinal tract of the canid. Eggs may be passed in the feces of the canid approximately 28 days later.

This parasite poses a serious public health problem because of the possibility for human involvement in the life cycle. If eggs shed by an infected canid are accidentally ingested, a highly pathogenic condition (Alveolar Hydatid Disease) results from development of the cyst stage in humans.

The original geographic distribution of *E. multilocularis* was primarily confined to northern areas of North America. Current evidence indicates migration of the parasite well into the continental United States.[3,4]

Domestic dogs living in *E. multilocularis* endemic areas that roam freely with the opportunity to catch wild rodents are at risk of infection. Pet owners should be advised on how to minimize this risk. Proper restraint of dogs should be encouraged, along with regular treatment with Drontal® Plus Tablets, following the dosing schedule aforementioned and precautions indicated below.

Additional information on the life cycle and epidemiology of this parasite is available in veterinary parasitology texts.[5,6]

DIAGNOSIS: Diagnosis of *E. multilocularis* in canids is difficult. The adult tapeworm produces no clinical signs of infection. Tapeworm segments (proglottids) are usually not observed in the feces. *E. multilocularis* eggs, observed using microscopic fecal examination procedures, are similar in appearance to those of common species such as *Taenia pisiformis.*

Assistance in the diagnosis of *E. multilocularis* may be available from a state veterinary diagnostic laboratory. Additional information regarding areas where *E. multilocularis* is suspected or has been confirmed may be obtained from area veterinary schools or the Centers for Disease Control in Atlanta, GA.

TREATMENT: Dogs infected with *E. multilocularis* should be treated to prevent exposure of humans to infective eggs and to break the parasite's life cycle.

The dosage of Drontal® Plus Tablets for removal of *E. multilocularis* is the same as that indicated for the removal of the other tapeworm species listed on the label. Laboratory efficacy studies have demonstrated the recommended dosage is 100% effective.

Under condition of continual exposure to wild rodents, retreatment of the dog at 21-26 day intervals is recommended to prevent the shedding of infectious eggs.

PRECAUTIONS: Strict hygienic precautions should be taken when handling dogs or feces suspected of harboring *E. multilocularis.* Infected dogs treated for the first time with Drontal® Plus Tablets and dogs treated at intervals greater than 28 days may shed eggs in the feces after treatment. The animal should be held in the clinic during this interval and all feces should be incinerated or autoclaved. If these procedures are not possible, the eggs can be destroyed by soaking the feces in a sodium hypochlorite (bleach) solution of 3.75% or greater.[7] All areas where the animal was maintained or in contact with should be thoroughly cleaned with sodium hypochlorite and allowed to dry completely before reuse.

CONTRAINDICATIONS: DO NOT USE IN PREGNANT ANIMALS. Dogs treated with elevated levels (6 consecutive days with 3 times the labeled dosage rate) of the combination of febantel and praziquantel in early pregnancy demonstrated an increased incidence of abortion and fetal abnormalities.[8] The effects of Drontal® Plus on pregnant animals have not been determined.

There are no known contraindications against the use of praziquantel or pyrantel pamoate in dogs.

EFFICACY: A total of 176 dogs and puppies with naturally acquired or experimental parasite infections were included in 4 well-controlled laboratory studies to establish the efficacy of Drontal® Plus Tablets. In addition, 103 dogs and puppies were included in clinical field studies conducted in 5 veterinary clinics at different geographic locations throughout the United States to further evaluate safety and efficacy. These studies included dogs of various sizes, ages and breeds. Data from these studies demonstrated Drontal® Plus Tablets are safe and efficacious for the removal of the parasite species indicated on the label when used as directed.

Results obtained in the laboratory and clinical studies indicate small numbers of hookworm or roundworm eggs may be passed in the feces for up to 7 days after treatment although the worms themselves were eliminated. A follow-up fecal examination should be conducted 2 to 4 weeks after treatment to determine the need for retreatment.

SIDE EFFECTS: None of the 103 dogs treated with Drontal® Plus Anthelmintic Tablets in the clinical field studies exhibited drug related side effects.

ANIMAL TOXICOLOGY: Controlled safety evaluations have been conducted in dogs with Drontal® Plus (praziquantel/pyrantel pamoate/febantel) Broad Spectrum Anthelmintic Tablets. Dogs receiving up to 5 times the label dosage (35 mg praziquantel, 35 mg pyrantel pamoate and 179 mg febantel per kg of body weight) for 3 consecutive days (3 times the label duration) showed clinical signs of vomition and non-formed stools. One dog receiving a 3 times labeled dose had elevated SGPT, SGOT, CPK and GGT readings (outside of normal range) at 6 days post-treatment. No additional findings were noted in hematology/clinical chemistry parameters nor were there any treatment related histological lesions. Vomition was the only side effect observed when dogs received a single treatment of 61 mg praziquantel, 61 mg pyrantel pamoate and 305 mg febantel/kg with one dog having an elevated SGPT reading (outside of normal range) at 24 hours post-treatment which had returned to normal by 7 days.

WARNING: KEEP OUT OF REACH OF CHILDREN.

CAUTION: Federal (U.S.A.) law restricts this drug to use by or on the order of a licensed veterinarian.

HOW SUPPLIED: Each tablet size is available in bottles of 50.

Code 1760 — 50 Tablets/Bottle (Small Dogs) 71017600, R.5

Code 1770 — 50 Tablets/Bottle (Medium and Large Dogs) 71017700, R.5

REFERENCES:

1 Andrews, P., 1976. Pharmacokinetic Studies with DRONCIT™ in Animals Using a Biological Assay. *Veterinary Medical Review.* 2:154-165.

2 Campbell, W.C., 1986. The Chemotherapy of Parasitic Infections. *J. Parasit.* 72(1):45-61.

3 Hildreth, M.B., Johnson, M.D. and Kazacos, K.R., 1991. A Zoonosis of Increasing Concern in the United States. *Compendium for Cont. Ed.* 13(5):727-740.

4 Lieby, P.D., Carney, W.P., and Woods, C.E., 1970. Studies on Sylvatic Echinococcosis, III. Host Occurrence and Geographic Distribution of *Echinococcus multilocularis* in the North Central United States. *J. Parasit.* 56(6):1141-1150.

5 Georgi, J.R. and Georgi, M.E., 1990. *Parasitology for Veterinarians.* W.B. Saunders Co. 118-138.

6 Soulsby, E.J.L., 1982. *Helminths, Arthropods and Protozoa of Domesticated Animals.* 7th Edition, Lea & Febiger. 118-138.

7 Craig, P.S. and McPharson, C.N.L., 1988. Sodium Hypochlorite as an Ovicide for *Echinococcus. Ann Trop Med. and Parasit.* 82(2):211-213.

8 Freedom of Information Summary (FOI) NADA 133-953 Vercom Paste (febantel and praziquantel).

November, 2001

Bayer Corporation, Agriculture Division, Animal Health, Shawnee Mission, Kansas 66201 U.S.A.

NADA 141-007, Approved by FDA

Compendium Code No.: 10400241

DRY-CLOX® ℞

Fort Dodge **Mastitis Therapy**

Cloxacillin Benzathine

NADA No.: 055-058

Active Ingredient(s): Each 10 mL disposable syringe contains cloxacillin benzathine equivalent to 500 mg of cloxacillin activity in a stable peanut oil gel. This product was manufactured by a non-sterilizing process.

Indications: For the treatment of mastitis in dairy cows during the dry period.

DRY-CLOX® has been shown by extensive clinical studies to be efficacious in the treatment of mastitis in dry cows, when caused by *Streptococcus agalactiae* and *Staphylococcus aureus* including penicillin-resistant strains.

Treatment of the dry cow with DRY-CLOX® is indicated in any cow known to harbor any of these organisms in the udder at drying off, or which has had repeated attacks of mastitis during the previous lactation, or is affected with mastitis at drying off, if caused by susceptible organisms.

Pharmacology:

Description: DRY-CLOX® (cloxacillin benzathine) for intramammary infusion into the dry cow is a product which provides bactericidal activity against gram-positive bacteria. The active agent, cloxacillin benzathine, is a sparingly soluble salt of the semisynthetic penicillin, cloxacillin. Cloxacillin is a derivative of 6-aminopenicillanic acid, and therefore is chemically related to other penicillins. It has, however, the antibacterial properties described below, which distinguish it from certain other penicillins.

Action: In the non-lactating mammary gland, DRY-CLOX® (cloxacillin benzathine) provides bactericidal levels of the active antibiotic, cloxacillin, for a prolonged period of time. This prolonged activity is due to the low solubility of the cloxacillin benzathine and to the slow-release oil-gel base. This prolonged contact between the antibiotic and the pathogenic organism enhances the probability of a bacteriological cure.

Cloxacillin is not destroyed by the enzyme, penicillinase, and therefore, is active against penicillin-resistant strains of *Staphylococcus aureus.* It is also active against non-penicillinase-producing *Staphylococcus aureus* as well as *Streptococcus agalactiae.*

The class disc, Methicillin 5 mcg, should be used to estimate the *in vitro* susceptibility of bacteria to cloxacillin.

Dosage and Administration:

Dosage for Dry Cows: Infuse the contents of one syringe (10 mL) into each infected quarter following the last milking or early in the dry period. See Directions for Use.

Directions for Use: DRY-CLOX® (cloxacillin benzathine) is for use in dry cows only. Administer immediately after the last milking, or early in the dry period. Use no later than 30 days prior to calving.

Completely milk out all four quarters. The udder and teats should be thoroughly washed with warm water containing a suitable dairy antiseptic and dried, preferably using individual paper towels. Carefully scrub the teat end and orifice with 70% alcohol, using a separate swab for each teat. Allow to dry.

DRY-CLOX® is packaged with the Opti-Sert® protective cap.

For partial insertion: Twist off upper portion of the Opti-Sert® protective cap to expose 3-4 mm of the syringe tip.

For full insertion: Remove protective cap to expose the full length of the syringe tip.

Insert syringe tip into the teat canal and expel the entire contents of syringe into the quarter. Withdraw the syringe and gently massage the quarter to distribute the medication.

Do not infuse contents of the mastitis syringe into the teat canal if the Opti-Sert® protective cap is broken or damaged.

Precaution(s): Store at controlled room temperature 15° to 30°C (59° to 86°F).

Because it is a derivative of 6-aminopenicillanic acid, DRY-CLOX® has the potential for producing allergic reactions. Such reactions are rare; however, should they occur, the subject should be treated with antihistamines or pressor amines, such as epinephrine.

Caution(s): Federal law restricts this drug to use by or on the order of a licensed veterinarian.

Warning(s):

1. For use in dry cows only.
2. Not to be used within 30 days of calving.
3. Any animal infused with this product must not be slaughtered for food until 30 days after the latest infusion.

Presentation: Carton containing 12 x 10 mL syringes (NDC 0856-2722-10).

Opti-Sert® Protective Cap - U.S. Patent No. 4,850,970.

Compendium Code No.: 10030460 4300I

DRY FLOTATION MEDIUM

Butler **Fecal Flotation**

Indications: For fecal flotation analysis.

Directions: Mixed according to directions.

Makes a one gallon flotation solution with a specific gravity of 1.25 to 1.30.

Add 4 lb. pkg. to 1-gallon container. Fill with potable water until brimful. Shake well. When sodium nitrate goes into solution, water level will go down. Do not add more water.

Caution(s): For animal use only.

Keep out of reach of children.

Sold to veterinarians only.

Presentation: Sodium Nitrate 4 lb. (makes 1 gallon) (NDC 11695-1555-02) and Sodium Nitrate 40 lb. (10 4 lb. packages makes 1 gal.) (NDC 11695-1555-06).

Compendium Code No.: 10820630

DRY-IT

Q.A. Laboratories **Topical Wound Dressing**

Active Ingredient(s): Isopropyl alcohol, de-ionized water, sillicon dioxide, boro-tannic acid complex, camphor, polysorbate 60, sallcylic acid, menthol, PEG 75 lanolin oil, sucrose octyl acetate, propylene glycol, acetic acid, FD & C blue #1, FD & C yellow #5.

Indications: DRY-IT is a topical dessicant and antiseptic which aids in the treatment of hot spots, weeping lesions and moist exzemas.

Dosage and Administration: Shake well before using. Apply DRY-IT once or twice a day onto the affected areas according to the directions of a veterinarian or until the lesion is dry. The gel will initially sting when applied to an open wound.

Precaution(s): Flammable: Keep away from heat or open flame.

Caution(s): Keep out of the reach of children.

Harmful if swallowed. If swallowed, call a physician or poison control center. Avoid contact with the eyes and mucous membranes. If in eyes, wash with copious amounts of cool water.

Presentation: 2 oz. containers.

Compendium Code No.: 13680020

DRY-OFF®

Westfalia•Surge **Topical Product**

Teat Protection Sealant for Dry Cows

Indications: DRY-OFF® is a teat protection sealant for dry cows.

Directions for Use: At the end of lactation, apply DRY-OFF® after last milking and about one week prior to calving.

Do not pour unused product back into original container.

After use, immediately discard applicator cup out of reach of children.

Precaution(s): Storage Instructions: Keep container tightly closed when not in use.

Important: Store above 50°F (10°C). Product freezes between 30-35°F (-1 to 2°C). Once frozen, this product is rendered unusable and cannot be reconstituted.

Caution(s): Contains materials which may cause irritation of the eyes, nose, throat, and respiratory system. Individuals with sensitive skin may experience skin irritation. May be harmful if swallowed. Protect eyes and skin when handling. Do not take internally. Avoid breathing vapors. Do not mix with any other chemical products. Refer to Material Safety Data Sheet (MSDS).

If In Eyes: Flush with large volumes of water for at least 15 minutes. Call a physician immediately.

If Swallowed: Do not induce vomiting. Call a physician immediately. If on Skin: Wash thoroughly with soap and water. If irritation develops and persists, get medical attention.

Inhalation: If breathing difficulty or irritation occurs, remove to fresh air. If symptoms persist, get medical attention.

For assistance with medical emergency, call 1-800-451-8346.

Warning(s): Keep out of reach of children.

Presentation: Contact the company for container sizes available.

Compendium Code No.: 10020200 Rev. 01-01

D-TEC® CB

Synbiotics **Brucella Test**

U.S. Vet. Lic. No.: 298

Contents: Kit contains:

Slide cards	13
Pipettes	25
Antigen	2.5 mL
Rubber bulbs	2
Stirring rods	25
2-mercaptoethanol (0.2M solution)	2.5 mL
Anti-serum, sufficient to perform a minimum of 25 tests (procedure one and/or procedure 2)	1.3 mL

Indications: The reagents are used to presumptively diagnose infection with *Brucella canis.*

Test Principles: The rapid slide agglutinagion test (RSAT) for the diagnosis of *Brucella canis* was described by George and Carmichael (Proc. Council Res. Workers in Animal Disease, November 1973). The basis of the test is direct agglutination of the killed stained antigen by *Brucella canis* antibodies.

Test Procedure:

Rapid slide agglutination test (RSAT):

1. Ensure that the reagents are at room temperature: 70°F (21°C).
2. Cut the card on the dotted line. Two (2) circles are used to perform each test.
3. Place one drop of positive control antiserum (white bulb), in one (1) circle of the supplied card.
4. Use a disposable plastic pipette and rubber bulb to place one (1) drop of test serum in another circle. Each test kit contains disposable pipettes to prevent serum cross contamination. Do not dispose of the pipette until the 2ME-RSAT is completed.
5. Thoroughly mix the antigen by shaking the vial and then rapidly squeezing the dropper bulb several times. Add one (1) drop of the *B. canis* agglutination antigen close to each serum drop, being careful not to touch the serum with the dropper tip.
6. Mix each antigen-serum combination with a separate end of an applicator stick, spreading to fill the circular area. Do not allow the positive control test to touch the unknown serum sample.
7. Gently rock the card for 10 to 15 seconds. Place it on a flat surface and observe for agglutination for no longer than two (2) minutes. If the serum is negative (absence of agglutination), no further testing is required and the animal is considered not to be infected with *B. canis.* If the card test is positive, perform the 2ME-RSAT.

2-Mercaptoethanol-rapid slide agglutination test (2ME-RSAT):

1. Add two (2) drops of 2-mercaptoethanol, 0.2M solution to a tube containing two (2) drops of the serum to be tested and mix well.
2. Place one (1) drop of mixture on a card.
3. Add one (1) drop of *B. canis* agglutination antigen as above to the serum solution and mix with the applicator stick.
4. Observe for agglutination for no longer than two (2) minutes.

When the RSAT-positive sample tests positive by 2ME-RSAT, the animal is presumptively diagnosed as being infected with *B. Canus.* Blood should be subjected to a cultural examination for *B. canis.*

When the RSAT-positive tests negative by 2ME-RSAT, the animal may be in the early stage of *B. canis* infection, or alternatively, its serum may contain nonspecific agglutinins to *B. Canis.* To distinguish between these two conditions, a second serum sample should be collected in approximately 30 days and retested by the 2ME-RSAT procedure. Only if the sample tests positive should the animal be presumptively diagnosed as having *B. canis* infection.

A definitive diagnosis of canine brucellosis is based upon the isolation of *B. canis* from the animal.

Precaution(s): Store the components at 35°-45°F (2°-7°C). Do not allow the reagents to stand at room temperature for excessive periods of time. Do not freeze.

Caution(s): The antigen and the accompanying antiserum have been standardized and should be used together.

Discussion: Canine brucellosis is a chronic infection with *Brucella canis* that causes generalized lymphadenitis and mild to severe reproductive symptoms. Prostatitis, epididymitis, scrotal dermatitis, testicular atrophy and impotence can be present in the male. Abortion typically in the final two weeks of gestation, resorption, infertility and vaginal discharge can be present in the female. Its incidence in the continental United states is approximated by current surveys to be between 1% and 10%. *Brucella canis* can infect humans and caution should be exercised when handling the serums to be tested.

The test has been shown to presumptively diagnose infection with *Brucella canis* by detecting specific antibody that is formed one to four weeks after infection.

The basis for serodiagnosis of canine brucellosis is the 2-mercaptoethanol tube agglutination test (2ME-TAT) and the rapid slide agglutination test (RSAT). The 2ME-TAT and RSAT have demonstrated excellent correlation in experimentally infected dogs.

In field situations, it has been recognized that an occasional healthy dog, culturally negative for *Brucella canis,* will react positively in the RSAT, but not in the 2ME-TAT. The 2-mercaptoethanol-rapid slide agglutination test (2ME-RSAT) has been developed in an attempt to eliminate discrepancies between the RSAT and the 2ME-TAT.

Certain nonspecific agglutinins, reported to occur in the sera of normal dogs, are removed from canine sera when 2-mercaptoethanol is employed in the 2ME-TAT. Because of the occurrence, 2-mercaptoethanol is employed in the modified rapid slide agglutination test procedure.

References: Available upon request.

Presentation: 10 tests.

Compendium Code No.: 11150050

D-TROL

DuBois **Disinfectant**

Disinfectant/Sanitizer

EPA Reg. No.: 5736-5

Active Ingredient(s): D-TROL disinfectant/sanitizer is a blend of dual quaternary ammonium chlorides.

Properties:

Appearance: Light yellow

Density: 0.9903 @ 20°C 8.25 lb./gal. Foam Moderate

pH @ 1%: 6.5 to 7.5

Stability: Stable in water up to 750 ppm of hardness

Indications: It is formulated for sanitizing in beverage, dairy, food, meat and poultry operations, and for disinfecting in veterinary operations.

D-TROL disinfectant/sanitizer is authorized for use in federally inspected meat and poultry plants.

D-TROL complies with 21 CFR 178.1010, Sanitizing Solutions Food Additive Law for final sanitizing rinsing of food processing equipment and on food contact surfaces in bars and restaurants.

This product fulfills the criteria of Appendix F of the Grade a Pasteurized Milk Ordinance 1978 Recommendations of the U.S. Public Health Service in waters up to 750 ppm of hardness calculated as calcium carbonate when tested by the A.O.A.C. Germicidal and Detergent Sanitizers Official Method.

Material Safety: D-TROL is safe at recommended use dilutions on stainless steel, steel, aluminum, galvanized, and most soft metals. D-TROL is also safe on painted surfaces and does not attack most plastics when used as directed.

Pharmacology: Microbiological Data: Official A.O.A.C. Procedures 14th Edition, 1984. Hard water tolerance: In the presence of hard water (750 ppm), *Staphylococcus aureus* (ATCC No. 6536), *Escherichia coli* (ATCC No. 11229), and *Listeria monocytogenes* (ATCC No. 15313) are reduced in 30 seconds with ¼ ounce solution of D-TROL disinfectant/sanitizer per gallon of water (200 ppm Quat). This product when used for disinfection on environmental inanimate hard surfaces at ¾ ounce per gallon of water (600 ppm Quat) is effective against influenza A2, Herpes Simplex, Adenovirus Type 5 and Vaccinia viruses. D-TROL disinfectant/sanitizer at this concentration passes the A.O.A.C. Use Dilution Confirmation Test against *Pseudomonas aeruginosa* (ATCC No. 15442), *Salmonella choleraesuis* (ATCC No. 10708), and *Staphylococcus aureus* (ATCC No. 6538). For disinfecting porous surfaces, use 1½ ounces of D-TROL disinfectant/sanitizer per gallon of water (1200 ppm Quat).

D-TROL at 1¾ oz./gal. (1400 ppm Quat.) concentration passes the EPA's Use-Dilution Mildew Fungicidal Test Method (Revised 12/1/70) against *Aspergillus niger* ATCC 6275.

Hand Sanitizing Efficiency Test: In the presence of 408 ppm hard water (24 grain) D-TROL at ¼ ounce per gallon (200 ppm Quat) is more than equivalent for sanitizing than 50 ppm available chlorine using sodium hypochlorite. (Official A.O.A.C. "Available Chlorine Germicidal Equivalent Concentration" as modified by Section 4.4(B) of the "Guidelines for Obtaining Authorization of Compounds to be Used in Meat and Poultry Plants" USDA).

Directions for Use: Using Procedures: For Final Sanitizing Rinsing in Food, Beverage, and Dairy Operations. For Sanitizing Equipment in Meat and Poultry Plants. To Sanitize Utensils and Equipment in Hand Wash, Soak, and Spray Wash Operations.

1. Pre-flush or pre-scrape utensils and equipment to remove gross food particles. Pre-soak if necessary.
2. Wash thoroughly with a DuBois detergent.
3. Rinse with potable water.
4. Sanitize in a solution of 200 ppm Quat (¼ ounce per 1 gallon of water). If spraying, keep surface wet with sanitizer for at least 2 minutes. Immerse all utensils and equipment for at least 2 minutes.
5. Place sanitized utensils on a rack to air dry. Adequately drain all surfaces before contact with food. For hand wash operations, fresh sanitizing solution must be prepared at least daily; prepare more often if the solution becomes diluted or soiled. Solution used in spray operations may be reused for sanitizing. Only one sanitization per solution is allowed. The solution may be used for cleaning or other purposes if it is not soiled.

For Shell Egg Sanitizing: Use D-TROL at use dilution ¼ ounce per gallon of water. Eggs that have been sanitized with D-TROL should be subjected to a thorough potable water rinse only if they are to be immediately broken for use in the manufacture on egg products.

For Hand Sanitizing: The hands must be washed and thoroughly rinsed prior to sanitizing. Sanitize by dipping hands into a solution of ¼ ounce of D-TROL per gallon of water. The hands need not be rinsed with potable water following the use of the compound.

For Disinfecting in Veterinary Operations: Clean equipment with a suitable detergent. For disinfecting hard surfaces such as floors, walls, furnishings, animal cages, pens, or runs, use ¾ ounce per 1 gallon of water (600 ppm Quat). Give cages, pens, or runs a potable water rinse before animals are allowed to enter. Treated surfaces must remain wet for 10 minutes.

For Destroying Mold and Mildew on Hard Surfaces: Clean surfaces with a suitable detergent and rinse. For destroying or killing fungi which cause mold and mildew growth on hard surfaces such as floors and walls in hospitals, meat, poultry, beverage, dairy, food and similar facilities, use 1¾ ounces of D-TROL per 1 gallon of water (1400 ppm Quat).

The concentration of D-TROL will kill on contact. Repeat this application when evidence of mold or mildew appear.

Dispensing: D-TROL disinfectant/sanitizer is most suitably dispensed via the Hose End Sanitizer, Control-A-Matic, and the Crownco Sanitizing System.

Titration: QAC Test Kit: Use the QAC Test Kit (LaMotte Chemical Products Co., Charlestown, MD 21621) for periodically testing the quat concentration in the D-TROL disinfectant/sanitizer use solution. QT-10 Test Paper can also be used.

Acceptability: A Material Safety Data Sheet is available on request.

Precaution(s): Danger: Corrosive. Causes eye damage and skin irritation. Do not get in eyes, on skin, or on clothing. Wear goggles or face shield and rubber gloves when handling. Harmful if swallowed. Avoid contamination of food.

Statement of Practical Treatment: In case of contact, flush eyes or skin with plenty of water for at least 15 minutes. For eyes, call a physician. Remove and wash contaminated clothing before reuse. If swallowed, drink promptly a large quantity of milk, egg whites, gelatin solution or if these are not available, drink large quantities of water. Avoid alcohol. Call a physician immediately.

Note to Physician: Probably mucosal damage may contraindicate the use of gastric lavage. Measures against circulatory shock, respiratory depression, and convulsion may be needed.

Storage: Protect from freezing. If frozen, thaw and mix to make usable. Do not store near heat or open flame.

Warning(s): Keep out of the reach of children.

Disclaimer: The information contained in this bulletin is to our best knowledge, true and accurate, but all recommendations or suggestions are made without guarantee, since the conditions of use are beyond our control. Diversey Corp. disclaims any liability incurred in connection with the use of these data or suggestions.

Presentation: 4x1 gallon case, 55 gallon plastic drum, 330 gallon recyclable tanks, and bulk delivery.

Compendium Code No.: 10070021 8-1477 0193

DUBLVAX®

Schering-Plough **Vaccine**

U.S. Vet. Lic. No.: 165A

Newcastle-Bronchitis Vaccine, B_1 Type, LaSota Strain-Mass. & Conn. Types Live Virus

Active Ingredient(s): DUBLVAX® is a live virus vaccine containing the A.S.L. N-47 (LaSota) strain B_1 type Newcastle virus combined with the mild reaction infectious bronchitis virus strains (Connaught Massachusetts and Connecticut types). The vaccine contains gentamicin as a preservative.

Indications: For the vaccination of chickens four weeks of age or older as an aid in preventing Newcastle disease and Massachusetts and Connecticut types of bronchitis.

Dosage and Administration:

When to Vaccinate:

Initial Vaccination:

Water: Four (4) weeks to 16 weeks of age.

Revaccination:

Spray: Four (4) weeks of age or older.

Water: Four (4) weeks of age or older.

Vaccination Program: The development of a durable, strong protection to both diseases depends upon the use of an effective vaccination program as well as many circumstances such as administration techniques, environment and flock health at the time of vaccination. Also, the immune response to one (1) vaccination under field conditions is seldom complete for all animals within a given flock. Even when vaccination is successful, the protection stimulated in individual animals against different diseases may not be life-long. Therefore, a program of periodic revaccination may be necessary.

Preparation of the Vaccine:

1. Assemble the equipment needed to vaccinate the entire flock at one time.
2. Do not open and mix the vaccine until ready for use.
3. Remove the tear-off aluminum seal from the vaccine vial without disturbing the rubber stopper.
4. Use cool, clean, nonchlorinated tap water to which powdered milk has been added as directed under How to Vaccinate.
5. Hold the vial submerged in a pail of water or under a running stream of water. Lift the lip of the rubber stopper so that the water (milk added) is sucked into the vial.
6. Reseat the stopper and shake to thoroughly dissolve the vaccine.

How to Vaccinate:

1. Drinking Water Method: Do not mix the vaccine into the drinking water until ready for use. Drinking water for vaccination should be mixed with powdered milk to prevent inactivation from chlorine or other water additives and also to stabilize the vaccine virus. The powdered milk should be added to the water at the rate of one (1) heaped teaspoon per three (3) U.S. gallons or 2.5 imperial gallons (3 g per 11 L); or one (1) heaped cupful per 80 U.S. gallons or 66 imperial gallons (90 g per 300 L).

   Withhold water from the birds for several hours before vaccinating so that the birds are thirsty. Thoroughly clean and rinse all watering containers so that no residual disinfectants remain. Dilute the vaccine immediately before use with cool, clean, nonchlorinated water (milk added). Pour the dissolved vaccine material into the following amounts of water and mix thoroughly.

Each 5,000 Birds	U.S. Gallons	Imperial Gallons	Metric Liters
4 weeks to 8 weeks	25	20	100
Over 8 weeks	50	40	200

   Distribute the diluted vaccine so that all of the birds are able to drink within a 1-hour period and do not add any more water until the vaccine is consumed. Avoid placing water in direct sunlight.

2. Spray Method: Use this method for revaccination only. Proper spray application of the vaccine is only accomplished through the use of a clean sprayer emitting a very a fine aerosol (mist) which floats and disseminates easily through the air. Only use the spray method in houses that can be closed during vaccination and for at least 15 minutes thereafter. Cross winds, drafts, or operating ventilation fans prevent effective application.

   Rehydrate the vaccine according to the above instructions. Further dilute each 5,000 doses of vaccine to 500 mL using distilled water. Place the vaccine in the sprayer container and set at the lowest output. Spray droplets of 17 to 20 microns average size and the application of about 700 doses of vaccine per minute are desirable.

   Apply the vaccine over all of the birds at the rate of one (1) dose per square foot, or one (1) dose per bird, whichever is greater.

   Use protective goggles during vaccination to avoid eye contact with Newcastle vaccine.

Records: Keep a record of the vaccine type, quantity, serial number, expiration date, and place of purchase; the date and time of vaccination; the number, age, breed, and location of the birds; the names of operators performing the vaccination; and any observed reactions.

Contraindication(s): As will all bronchitis vaccines, the initial vaccination of layer or breeder replacement stock should be conducted before 16 weeks of age to avoid possible damage to reproductive organs. For the same reason, at least one revaccination with a bronchitis vaccine should be conducted before 16 weeks of age.

Precaution(s): Store at 35° to 45° F (2° to 7°C).

Caution(s): For veterinary use only.

1. Vaccinate healthy birds only. Although disease may not be evident, coccidiosis, chronic respiratory disease, mycoplasma infection, lymphoid leukosis, infectious bursal disease, Marek's disease, or other disease conditions may cause serious complications or reduce protection.
2. All birds within a house should be vaccinated on the same day. Isolate other susceptible birds on the premises from the birds being vaccinated.
3. In outbreak situations, vaccinate healthy birds first, progressing toward outbreak areas in order to vaccinate diseased birds last.
4. Do not spill or spatter the vaccine. Use the entire contents of the vial when first opened. Burn the empty bottles, caps, and all unused vaccine and accessories.
5. Wash hands thoroughly after using the vaccine.
6. Do not dilute the vaccine or otherwise stretch the dosage.
7. Newcastle virus occasionally causes inflammation of the eyelids in humans, lasting two or three days. Avoid contact of the eyes with the vaccine.

The use of the vaccine is subject to state laws wherever applicable.

Warning(s): Do not vaccinate within 21 days before slaughter.

Presentation: Supplied in 10 x 5,000 dose units.

Compendium Code No.: 10470470

DUOCIDE® L.A. SPRAY

Virbac **Parasiticide Spray**

EPA Reg. No.: 46473-5

Active Ingredient(s):

Pyrethrins . . . 0.112%
Permethrin [(3-phenoxyphenyl) methyl (±) cis-trans-3-(2,2-dichloroethenyl) 2,2-dimethylcyclopropane-carboxylate]* . . . 0.100%
Related compounds . . . 0.008%
N-octyl bicycloheptene dicarboxide. . . . 1.000%
Inert ingredients . . . 98.780%

*Cis-trans isomer ratio: min. 35% (±) cis; max. 65% (±) trans.

Indications: Residual insecticide flea and tick spray for dogs and cats.

Directions for Use: It is a violation of federal law to use the product in a manner inconsistent with its labeling. Do not use DUOCIDE® L.A. Spray or any other pesticide on sick, old or debilitated pets.

Shake well before using.

The product will kill fleas for up to 14 days and ticks for up to seven (7) days on dogs and cats.

To operate, hold the container upright and spray the animal from a distance of 8-12 inches. Point the nozzle toward the animal and start spraying at the tail, moving the container rapidly and making sure that the animal's entire body is covered with spray, including the legs and under the body. On long-haired animals, rub the hand against the lay of the hair, spraying into the ruffled hair directly behind the hand so that the spray will penetrate to the skin. The spray should wet ticks thoroughly. Do not spray in the face, eyes or on genitalia. May be sprayed on a brush and applied to the coat and face. Repeat as needed. For cats, apply at the rate of one (1) second per pound of body weight. For dogs, apply at the rate of two (2) seconds per pound of body weight for thin or short-haired dogs, and up to eight (8) seconds per pound of body weight for heavy or long-haired dogs.

Precautionary Statements: Hazards to Humans and Domestic Animals: Harmful if swallowed. Avoid inhaling vapors. Do not spray in eyes, on face or genitalia. Do not use on nursing puppies, or kittens under three months of age.

Statement of Practical Treatment:

If swallowed, call a physician or poison control center immediately. Drink one or two glasses of water and induce vomiting by touching the back of the throat with a finger. Repeat until the vomit fluid is clear. Do not induce vomiting or give anything by mouth to an unconscious person.

If inhaled, remove victim to fresh air. Apply artificial respiration if indicated.

If on skin, remove contaminated clothing and wash the affected areas with soap and water.

If in eyes, flush eyes with plenty of water. Call a physician immediately.

Storage and Disposal:

Storage: Store in a cool area away from heat and open flame.

Disposal: Do not re-use the empty container. Wrap the original container in several layers of newspaper and discard in the trash.

Warning(s): Keep out of the reach of children.

Presentation: 16 fl. oz. (455 mL) and 32 fl. oz. (946 mL) spray bottles.

Compendium Code No.: 10230210

DUOCIDE® SHAMPOO

Virbac **Parasiticide Shampoo**

EPA Reg. No.: 46473-2

Active Ingredient(s):

D-trans allethrin (allyl homolog of cinerin I) . . . 0.080%
Related compounds . . . 0.006%
*3-phenoxybenzyl D-cis and trans**2,2-dimethyl-3-(2-methylpropanyl) cyclopropanecarboxylate . . . 0.024%
*Other isomers . . . 0.001%
N-octyl bicycloheptane dicarboximide*** . . . 0.400%
Petroleum distillate . . . 0.486%
Inert ingredients . . . 99.003%
Total . . . 100.000%

*D-(cis, trans) phenothrin.

**Cis/trans isomer ratio: max. 25% (±) cis; min. 75% (±) trans.

***MGK-264, insecticide synergist.

Indications: Kills fleas on dogs and cats and brown dog ticks on dogs.

Directions for Use: It is a violation of federal law to use the product in a manner inconsistent with its labeling.

To use, wet the coat thoroughly with water. Pour the shampoo into the hand or onto the pet, and rub into coat, starting with the head. Work backwards until the coat is completely covered with a foamy lather. Let the lather stay on for 10 minutes, then rinse and towel dry. Keep away from the eyes. Repeat as necessary.

Precautionary Statements: Hazards to Humans and Domestic Animals: Avoid contact with the eyes. In case of contact, immediately flush eyes with plenty of water. Get medical attention if irritation persists.

Storage and Disposal:

Storage: Store in a cool, dry place.

Product Disposal: Securely wrap the original container in several layers of newspapers and discard in the trash.

Container Disposal: Do not re-use the bottle. Rinse it thoroughly before discarding it in the trash.

Warning(s): Keep out of the reach of children.

Presentation: 8 fl. oz. (237 mL) containers.

Compendium Code No.: 10230221

DUO-PEN®

AgriPharm **Penicillin Injection**

(Sterile Penicillin G Benzathine and Penicillin G Procaine)

NADA No.: 065-506

Active Ingredient(s): Each mL of suspension contains:

Penicillin G benzathine .... 150,000 units
Penicillin G procaine .... 150,000 units
Lecithin .... 11.7 mg
Sodium formaldehyde sulfoxylate .... 1.75 mg
Methylparaben (as preservative) .... 1.20 mg
Propylparaben (as preservative) .... 0.14 mg
Tween 40 .... 8.19 mg
Span 40 .... 11.3 mg
Sodium citrate anhydrous .... 3.98 mg
Procaine hydrochloride .... 20 mg
Sodium carboxymethylcellulose .... 1.04 mg
Water for injection .... q.s.

Dosage and Administration: Given subcutaneously only.
Beef Cattle: 2 mL per 150 lbs. of body weight.

Precaution(s): Store under refrigeration below 59°F (15°C).
Protect from freezing.

Caution(s): For subcutaneous use in beef cattle only.
Shake well before using.
For animal use only.
Restricted drug (California).
Use only as directed.
Keep out of the reach of children.

Warning(s): Do not inject intramuscularly.
Beef cattle should be withheld from slaughter for food use for 30 days following last treatment. Treatment in beef cattle must be limited to two (2) doses.

Presentation: 100 mL and 250 mL multiple dose vials.

Compendium Code No.: 14570320

DURACEPT™

Activon **Hoof Product**

Disinfecting Tablets

Active Ingredient(s): Sodium Dichloro-s-Trizinetrione.

Indications: Helps prevent and treat pathogen based hoof diseases.
Powerful, safe, non-antibiotic.

Directions for Use: Designed for use with DuraCept™ Conditioning Activator.

The DURACEPT™ Cycle:

Control Week		
	Apply	Strength
- First week of use - One week per quarter - One week if flare-up occurs	Daily	8 Tablets/gallon 16 oz Activator/gallon

Herd lesions under 5%:

Apply	Strength
Minimum 2 times per week	4 Tablets/gallon 8 oz Activator/gallon

Herd lesions over 5%:

Apply	Strength
Minimum 2 times per week	8 Tablets/gallon 16 oz Activator/gallon

- Hooves should be rinsed prior to use.
- Spot spray active lesions at higher strength as needed.
- Usage with wrap should be considered for advanced cases (size of quarter or larger).

16 Tablet Size: Makes up to 4 gallons.
64 Tablet Size: Makes up to 16 gallons.

Caution(s): (tablet form) Do not ingest. If swallowed, drink large quantities of water and do not induce vomiting. Avoid contact with eyes. If contact with eyes occurs, flush with water. Call a physician immediately. For emergency information, call 1-800-654-6911.

Presentation: 16 tablets/32 oz Activator Kit or 64 tablets/128 oz Activator Kit.
Also Available: 2 gallon sprayer.

Compendium Code No.: 10600000

DURACREAM

Durvet **Udder Product**

Udder Balm-Emollient and Barrier Cream

Active Ingredient(s): Ingredients: Water, mineral oil, cetearyl alcohol, glycol stearate, stearic acid, propylene glycol, glycerine, sorbitol, lanolin, aloe vera gel, vitamin E, vitamins A and D, ethyl dihydroxypropyl PABA, methylparaben, sodium hydroxide, propylparaben, fragrance, FD&C Yellow #5.

Indications: DURACREAM helps provide a barrier against the effects of weather extremes - low humidity, hot or cold temperatures, wind. Daily application of DURACREAM also aids in soothing and softening chapped and irritated skin.

DURACREAM may be used on teats, udders, hands, and other skin surfaces that are exposed to the effects of weather or to frequent washings.

Aids in frost protection.

Directions:

Udders: Wash and thoroughly dry udder and each teat. Apply DURACREAM liberally and evenly to entire teat and udder area after each milking, being sure to coat teat orifice. Gently massage coated area to work DURACREAM onto skin.

Hands and other skin areas: Wash and thoroughly dry area. Apply DURACREAM and massage onto skin.

Caution(s): To avoid contamination of milk, thoroughly wash entire udder and each teat before milking.

Warning(s): Keep out of reach of children.

Presentation: 4 oz, 1 lb, and 4 lb (1.816 kg).

Compendium Code No.: 10840481 5/97

DURAMUNE® Cv-K

Fort Dodge **Vaccine**

Canine Coronavirus Vaccine, Killed Virus

U.S. Vet. Lic. No.: 112

Contents: This product contains the antigen listed above.
Gentamicin, thimerosal, and amphotericin B added as preservatives.

Indications: For vaccination of healthy dogs six weeks of age or older as an aid in the prevention of disease caused by canine coronavirus.

Dosage and Administration: Dogs, inject one 1 mL subcutaneously or intramuscularly using aseptic technique. All dogs over 12 weeks of age should initially receive one dose of DURAMUNE® Cv-K and a second dose 2 to 3 weeks later. Annual revaccination with one dose is recommended.

A recommended vaccination schedule should start at or about 6 weeks of age. The presence of maternal antibody is known to interfere with the development of active immunity. Puppies should be revaccinated every 2 to 3 weeks until they are at least 12 weeks of age.

InfoVax-ID® System: The InfoVax-ID® System provides a simple and effective method of recording pertinent information on the vaccines administered to animals in a veterinary practice.

For vaccines requiring reconstitution, remove label from both vials and affix both labels to the animal's medical chart.

Using the InfoVax-ID® System:

1. Grasp the lower right hand corner of the tab at the arrow marked "Peel Here" between your thumb and forefinger.
2. Pull steadily at a slight upward angle until the top portion of the label is separated from the vial.
3. Place the label on the animal's medical chart. Press down on the label to ensure adhesion.

Precaution(s): Store in dark at 2° to 7°C (35° to 45°F). Avoid freezing. Shake well.

Caution(s): In the absence of a veterinarian-client-patient relationship, Federal law prohibits the relabeling, repackaging, resale, or redistribution of the individual contents of this package. (9 CFR 112.6)

In case of anaphylactoid reaction, administer epinephrine.
For veterinary use only.

Presentation: 25 doses (25 x 1 mL vials of vaccine) and 100 doses (10 x 10 mL vials of vaccine), featuring the InfoVax-ID® System.

Patent Pending
U.S. Patent Nos. 4,567,042 — 4,567,043 — 4,824,785 — 5,013,663 — 5,047,238
U.S. Pat. No. 5,704,648 (InfoVax-ID® System)

Compendium Code No.: 10030471 1472C

DURAMUNE® LGP

Fort Dodge **Bacterin**

Leptospira Grippotyphosa-Pomona Bacterin

U.S. Vet. Lic. No.: 112

Contents: This product contains the antigens listed above.
Gentamicin and thimerosal added as preservatives.

Indications: For subcutaneous vaccination of healthy dogs six weeks of age or older as an aid in the prevention of disease caused by *Leptospira grippotyphosa* and *Leptospira pomona*.

Dosage and Administration: Dogs, inject one 1 mL dose subcutaneously using aseptic technique. All dogs over 12 weeks of age should initially receive one dose of DURAMUNE® LGP and a second dose 2 to 3 weeks later. Annual revaccination with one dose is recommended.

A recommended vaccination schedule should start at or about 6 weeks of age. Puppies 6 weeks of age or older should be revaccinated every 2 to 3 weeks until they are at least 12 weeks of age.

InfoVax-ID® System: The InfoVax-ID® System provides a simple and effective method of recording pertinent information on the vaccines administered to animals in a veterinary practice.

For vaccines requiring reconstitution, remove label from both vials and affix both labels to the animal's medical chart.

Using the InfoVax-ID® System:

1. Grasp the lower right hand corner of the tab at the arrow marked "Peel Here" between your thumb and forefinger.
2. Pull steadily at a slight upward angle until the top portion of the label is separated from the vial.
3. Place the label on the animal's medical chart. Press down on the label to ensure adhesion.

Precaution(s): Store in dark at 2° to 7°C (35° to 45°F). Avoid freezing. Shake well.

Caution(s): In the absence of a veterinarian-client-patient relationship, Federal law prohibits the relabeling, repackaging, resale, or redistribution of the individual contents of this package. (9 CFR 112.6)

In case of anaphylactoid reaction, administer epinephrine.
Not intended for use as diluent for live vaccines.*

* If the use of these Lepto serovars in combination with modified live vaccines is desired, products containing *Leptospira canicola, Leptospira grippotyphosa, Leptospira icterohaemorrhagiae* and *Leptospira pomona* are specifically designed and available for this purpose.

For veterinary use only.

Presentation: 25 doses (25 x 1 mL vials of vaccine), featuring the InfoVax-ID® System.
U.S. Pat. No. 5,704,648 (InfoVax-ID® System)

Compendium Code No.: 10030521 3455D

DURAMUNE® MAX 5

Fort Dodge **Vaccine**

Canine Distemper-Adenovirus Type 2-Parainfluenza-Parvovirus Vaccine, Modified Live Virus

U.S. Vet. Lic. No.: 112

Contents: This product contains the antigens listed above.
Gentamicin added as preservative.

Indications: For subcutaneous vaccination of healthy dogs 6 weeks of age or older as an aid in the prevention of disease caused by canine distemper, infectious canine hepatitis, canine adenovirus type 2, canine parainfluenza and canine parvovirus.

Directions for Use:

General Directions: Aseptically rehydrate DURAMUNE® Max 5 with Sterile Diluent supplied. Administer one 1 mL dose subcutaneously.

Primary Vaccination: A recommended vaccination schedule should start at or about 6 weeks of age. The presence of maternal antibody is known to interfere with the development of active immunity. Puppies should be revaccinated every 2 to 3 weeks until 12 weeks of age.

All dogs over 12 weeks of age should initially receive one dose of DURAMUNE® Max 5 and a second dose 2 to 3 weeks later.

Annual Vaccination: Annual revaccination with one dose is recommended.

InfoVax-ID® System: The InfoVax-ID® System provides a simple and effective method of recording pertinent information on the vaccines administered to animals in a veterinary practice.

For vaccines requiring reconstitution, remove label from both vials and affix both labels to the animal's medical chart.

Using the InfoVax-ID® System:

1. Grasp the lower right hand corner of the tab at the arrow marked "Peel Here" between your thumb and forefinger.
2. Pull steadily at a slight upward angle until the top portion of the label is separated from the vial.
3. Place the label on the animal's medical chart. Press down on the label to ensure adhesion.

Precaution(s): Store in the dark at 2° to 7°C (35° to 45°F). Avoid freezing. Shake well. Burn container and all unused contents.

Caution(s): In the absence of a veterinarian-client-patient relationship, Federal law prohibits the relabeling, repackaging, resale, or redistribution of the individual contents of this package. (9 CFR Part 112.6)

In case of anaphylactoid reaction, administer epinephrine.

For veterinary use only.

Presentation: 25 doses (25 x 1 mL vials of vaccine plus 25 x 1 mL vials of diluent), featuring the InfoVax-ID® System.

U.S. Pat. No. 5,704,648 (InfoVax-ID® System)

Compendium Code No.: 10030532 1165D

DURAMUNE® MAX 5/4L

Fort Dodge **Bacterin-Vaccine**

Canine Distemper-Adenovirus Type 2-Parainfluenza-Parvovirus Vaccine, Modified Live Virus-Leptospira Bacterin

U.S. Vet. Lic. No.: 112

Contents: This product contains the antigens listed above.

Gentamicin and thimerosal added as preservatives.

Indications: For subcutaneous vaccination of healthy dogs 6 weeks of age or older as an aid in the prevention of disease caused by canine distemper, infectious canine hepatitis, canine adenovirus type 2, canine parainfluenza, canine parvovirus, *Leptospira canicola, Leptospira icterohaemorrhagiae, Leptospira grippotyphosa* and *Leptospira pomona.*

Directions for Use:

General Directions: Aseptically rehydrate Duramune® Max 5 with Leptospira bacterin supplied. Administer one 1 mL dose subcutaneously.

Primary Vaccination: A recommended vaccination schedule should start at or about 6 weeks of age. The presence of maternal antibody is known to interfere with the development of active immunity. Puppies should be revaccinated every 2 to 3 weeks until 12 weeks of age.

All dogs over 12 weeks of age should initially receive one dose of DURAMUNE® Max 5/4L and a second dose 2 to 3 weeks later.

Annual Vaccination: Annual revaccination with one dose is recommended.

InfoVax-ID® System: The InfoVax-ID® System provides a simple and effective method of recording pertinent information on the vaccines administered to animals in a veterinary practice.

For vaccines requiring reconstitution, remove label from both vials and affix both labels to the animal's medical chart.

Using the InfoVax-ID® System:

1. Grasp the lower right hand corner of the tab at the arrow marked "Peel Here" between your thumb and forefinger.
2. Pull steadily at a slight upward angle until the top portion of the label is separated from the vial.
3. Place the label on the animal's medical chart. Press down on the label to ensure adhesion.

Precaution(s): Store in the dark at 2° to 7°C (35° to 45°F). Avoid freezing. Shake well. Burn container and all unused contents.

Caution(s): In the absence of a veterinarian-client-patient relationship, Federal law prohibits the relabeling, repackaging, resale, or redistribution of the individual contents of this package. (9 CFR Part 112.6)

In case of anaphylactoid reaction, administer epinephrine.

For veterinary use only.

Presentation: 25 doses (25 x 1 mL vials of vaccine plus 25 x 1 mL vials of diluent), featuring the InfoVax-ID® System.

U.S. Pat. No. 5,704,648 (InfoVax-ID® System)

Compendium Code No.: 10030562 3595D

DURAMUNE® MAX 5-CvK THE PUPPYSHOT®

Fort Dodge **Bacterin-Vaccine**

Canine Distemper-Adenovirus Type 2-Coronavirus-Parainfluenza-Parvovirus Vaccine, Modified Live and Killed Virus

U.S. Vet. Lic. No.: 112

Contents: This product contains the antigens listed above.

Gentamicin and thimerosal added as preservatives.

Indications: For subcutaneous vaccination of healthy dogs 6 weeks of age or older as an aid in the prevention of disease caused by canine distemper, infectious canine hepatitis, canine adenovirus type 2, canine coronavirus, canine parainfluenza and canine parvovirus.

Directions for Use:

General Directions: Aseptically rehydrate Duramune® Max 5 with Canine Coronavirus vaccine supplied. Administer one 1 mL dose subcutaneously.

Primary Vaccination: A recommended vaccination schedule should start at or about 6 weeks of age. The presence of maternal antibody is known to interfere with the development of active immunity. Puppies should be revaccinated every 2 to 3 weeks until 12 weeks of age.

All dogs over 12 weeks of age should initially receive one dose of DURAMUNE® Max 5-CvK and a second dose 2 to 3 weeks later.

Annual Vaccination: Annual revaccination with one dose is recommended.

InfoVax-ID® System: The InfoVax-ID® System provides a simple and effective method of recording pertinent information on the vaccines administered to animals in a veterinary practice.

For vaccines requiring reconstitution, remove label from both vials and affix both labels to the animal's medical chart.

Using the InfoVax-ID® System:

1. Grasp the lower right hand corner of the tab at the arrow marked "Peel Here" between your thumb and forefinger.
2. Pull steadily at a slight upward angle until the top portion of the label is separated from the vial.
3. Place the label on the animal's medical chart. Press down on the label to ensure adhesion.

Precaution(s): Store in the dark at 2° to 7°C (35° to 45°F). Avoid freezing. Shake well. Burn container and all unused contents.

Caution(s): In the absence of a veterinarian-client-patient relationship, Federal law prohibits the relabeling, repackaging, resale, or redistribution of the individual contents of this package. (9 CFR Part 112.6)

In case of anaphylactoid reaction, administer epinephrine.

For veterinary use only.

Presentation: 25 doses (25 x 1 mL vials of vaccine plus 25 x 1 mL vials of diluent), featuring the InfoVax-ID® System.

U.S. Pat. No. 5,704,648 (InfoVax-ID® System)

Compendium Code No.: 10030542 3545D

DURAMUNE® MAX 5-CvK/4L THE PUPPYSHOT® BOOSTER

Fort Dodge **Bacterin-Vaccine**

Canine Distemper-Adenovirus Type 2-Coronavirus-Parainfluenza-Parvovirus Vaccine, Modified Live and Killed Virus-Leptospira Bacterin

U.S. Vet. Lic. No.: 112

Contents: This product contains the antigens listed above.

Gentamicin and thimerosal added as preservatives.

Indications: For subcutaneous vaccination of healthy dogs 6 weeks of age or older as an aid in the prevention of disease caused by canine distemper, infectious canine hepatitis, canine adenovirus type 2, canine coronavirus, canine parainfluenza, canine parvovirus, *Leptospira canicola, Leptospira icterohaemorrhagiae, Leptospira grippotyphosa* and *Leptospira pomona.*

Directions for Use:

General Directions: Aseptically rehydrate Duramune® Max 5 with Canine Coronavirus vaccine-Leptospira bacterin supplied. Administer one 1 mL dose subcutaneously.

Primary Vaccination: A recommended vaccination schedule should start at or about 6 weeks of age. The presence of maternal antibody is known to interfere with the development of active immunity. Puppies should be revaccinated every 2 to 3 weeks until 12 weeks of age.

All dogs over 12 weeks of age should initially receive one dose of DURAMUNE® Max 5-CvK/4L and a second dose 2 to 3 weeks later.

Annual Vaccination: Annual revaccination with one dose is recommended.

InfoVax-ID® System: The InfoVax-ID® System provides a simple and effective method of recording pertinent information on the vaccines administered to animals in a veterinary practice.

For vaccines requiring reconstitution, remove label from both vials and affix both labels to the animal's medical chart.

Using the InfoVax-ID® System:

1. Grasp the lower right hand corner of the tab at the arrow marked "Peel Here" between your thumb and forefinger.
2. Pull steadily at a slight upward angle until the top portion of the label is separated from the vial.
3. Place the label on the animal's medical chart. Press down on the label to ensure adhesion.

Precaution(s): Store in the dark at 2° to 7°C (35° to 45°F). Avoid freezing. Shake well. Burn container and all unused contents.

Caution(s): In the absence of a veterinarian-client-patient relationship, Federal law prohibits the relabeling, repackaging, resale, or redistribution of the individual contents of this package. (9 CFR Part 112.6)

In case of anaphylactoid reaction, administer epinephrine.

For veterinary use only.

Presentation: 25 doses (25 x 1 mL vials of vaccine plus 25 x 1 mL vials of diluent), featuring the InfoVax-ID® System.

U.S. Pat. No. 5,704,648 (InfoVax-ID® System)

Compendium Code No.: 10030552 2275D

DURAMUNE® MAX PC

Fort Dodge **Vaccine**

Canine Coronavirus-Parvovirus Vaccine, Modified Live and Killed Virus

U.S. Vet. Lic. No.: 112

Contents: This product contains the antigens listed above.

Gentamicin and thimerosal added as preservatives.

Indications: For vaccination of healthy dogs 6 weeks of age or older as an aid in the prevention of disease caused by canine coronavirus and canine parvovirus.

Dosage and Administration: Inject one 1 mL dose subcutaneously using aseptic technique. A recommended vaccination schedule should start at or about 6 weeks of age. The presence of maternal antibody is known to interfere with the development of active immunity. Puppies should be revaccinated every 2 to 3 weeks until they are at least 12 weeks of age. All dogs over 12 weeks of age should initially receive one dose of vaccine and a second dose 2 to 3 weeks later. Annual revaccination with one dose is recommended.

InfoVax-ID® System: The InfoVax-ID® System provides a simple and effective method of recording pertinent information on the vaccines administered to animals in a veterinary practice.

For vaccines requiring reconstitution, remove label from both vials and affix both labels to the animal's medical chart.

Using the InfoVax-ID® System:

1. Grasp the lower right hand corner of the tab at the arrow marked "Peel Here" between your thumb and forefinger.
2. Pull steadily at a slight upward angle until the top portion of the label is separated from the vial.
3. Place the label on the animal's medical chart. Press down on the label to ensure adhesion.

Precaution(s): Store in the dark at 2° to 7°C (35° to 45°F). Avoid freezing. Shake well. Burn container and all unused contents.

Caution(s): In the absence of a veterinarian-client-patient relationship, Federal law prohibits the relabeling, repackaging, resale, or redistribution of the individual contents of this package. (9 CFR Part 112.6)

In case of anaphylactoid reaction, administer epinephrine.

For veterinary use only.

Presentation: 10 doses (10 mL) and 25 doses (25 x 1 mL vials of vaccine), featuring the InfoVax-ID® System.

U.S. Patent Nos. 4,567,042 — 4,567,043 — 4,824,785 — 5,013,663 — 5,047,238

U.S. Pat. No. 5,704,648 (InfoVax-ID® System)

Compendium Code No.: 10030571 3563B / 3565D

DURAMUNE® MAX Pv

Fort Dodge **Vaccine**

Parvovirus Vaccine, Modified Live Virus

U.S. Vet. Lic. No.: 112

Contents: This product contains the antigen listed above.

Gentamicin and thimerosal added as preservatives.

Indications: For vaccination of healthy dogs 6 weeks of age or older as an aid in the prevention of disease caused by canine parvovirus.

Dosage and Administration: Inject one 1 mL dose subcutaneously using aseptic technique. A recommended vaccination schedule should start at or about 6 weeks of age. The presence of maternal antibody is known to interfere with the development of active immunity. Puppies should be revaccinated every 2 to 3 weeks until 12 weeks of age. All dogs over 12 weeks of age should initially receive 1 dose of vaccine and a second dose 2 to 3 weeks later. Annual revaccination with one dose is recommended.

InfoVax-ID® System: The InfoVax-ID® System provides a simple and effective method of recording pertinent information on the vaccines administered to animals in a veterinary practice.

For vaccines requiring reconstitution, remove label from both vials and affix both labels to the animal's medical chart.

Using the InfoVax-ID® System:

1. Grasp the lower right hand corner of the tab at the arrow marked "Peel Here" between your thumb and forefinger.
2. Pull steadily at a slight upward angle until the top portion of the label is separated from the vial.
3. Place the label on the animal's medical chart. Press down on the label to ensure adhesion.

Precaution(s): Store in dark at 2° to 7°C (35° to 45°F). Avoid freezing. Shake well. Burn container.

Caution(s): In the absence of a veterinarian-client-patient relationship, Federal law prohibits the relabeling, repackaging, resale, or redistribution of the individual contents of this package. (9 CFR Part 112.6)

In case of anaphylactoid reaction, administer epinephrine.

For use in dogs only.

For veterinary use only.

Presentation: 10 doses (10 mL) and 25 doses (25 x 1 mL vials of vaccine), featuring the InfoVax-ID® System.

U.S. Pat. No. 5,704,648 (InfoVax-ID® System)

Compendium Code No.: 10030581 1213B / 1215E

DURAMUNE® DA$_2$PP+CvK/LCI+BORRELIA BURGDORFERI BACTERIN THE PUPPYSHOT® BOOSTER+LYMEVAX®

Fort Dodge **Bacterin-Vaccine**

Canine Distemper-Adenovirus Type 2-Coronavirus-Parainfluenza-Parvovirus Vaccine, Modified Live and Killed Virus-Borrelia Burgdorferi-Leptospira Bacterin

U.S. Vet. Lic. No.: 112

Contents: DURAMUNE® DA$_2$PP+CvK/LCI+BORRELIA BURGDORFERI BACTERIN THE PUPPYSHOT® BOOSTER+LYMEVAX® contains the antigens listed above.

Gentamicin, thimerosal and amphotericin B added as preservatives.

Indications: For subcutaneous vaccination of healthy dogs, at least 9 weeks of age, as an aid in the prevention of disease caused by canine distemper, infectious canine hepatitis, respiratory disease caused by adenovirus type 2, canine coronavirus, canine parainfluenza, canine parvovirus, *Leptospira canicola, Leptospira icterohaemorrhagiae* infections and as an aid in the prevention of the disease caused by *Borrelia burgdorferi.*

Directions for Use: Aseptically rehydrate Duramune® DA$_2$P+Pv with Canine Coronavirus Vaccine, Killed Virus, Borrelia Burgdorferi-Leptospira Canicola-Icterohaemorrhagiae Bacterin supplied. Administer one 1 mL dose subcutaneously. A second dose should be administered 2 to 3 weeks later. Annual revaccination with one dose is recommended.

The presence of maternal antibody is known to interfere with the development of active immunity. Puppies should be revaccinated every 2 to 3 weeks until they are at least 16 weeks of age with Duramune® KF-11 or other Duramune® products containing parvovirus.

InfoVax-ID® System: The InfoVax-ID® System provides a simple and effective method of recording pertinent information on the vaccines administered to animals in a veterinary practice.

For vaccines requiring reconstitution, remove label from both vials and affix both labels to the animal's medical chart.

Using the InfoVax-ID® System:

1. Grasp the lower right hand corner of the tab at the arrow marked "Peel Here" between your thumb and forefinger.
2. Pull steadily at a slight upward angle until the top portion of the label is separated from the vial.
3. Place the label on the animal's medical chart. Press down on the label to ensure adhesion.

Precaution(s): Store in dark at 2° to 7°C (35° to 45°F). Avoid freezing. Shake well. Burn container and all unused contents.

Caution(s): In the absence of a veterinarian-client-patient relationship, Federal law prohibits the relabeling, repackaging, resale, or redistribution of the individual contents of this package. (9 CFR 112.6)

In case of anaphylactoid reaction, administer epinephrine.

For veterinary use only.

Presentation: 25 doses (25 x 1 mL vials of vaccine plus 25 x 1 mL vials of diluent), featuring the InfoVax-ID® System.

U.S. Patents Pending

U.S. Patent Nos. 4,567,042 - 4,567,043 - 4,824,785 - 5,013,663 - 5,047,238

Borrelia Burgdorferi Bacterin made under license from MGI Pharma, Inc. U.S. Patents Pending and U.S. Patent No. 4,721,617.

U.S. Pat. No. 5,704,648 (InfoVax-ID® System)

Compendium Code No.: 10030631 2752E

DURAMYCIN 10

Durvet **Water Medication**

Tetracycline Hydrochloride Soluble Powder-Antibiotic

NADA No.: 065-140

Active Ingredient(s): Each pound contains 25 g of tetracycline hydrochloride activity.

The 6.4 oz package contains 10 g of tetracycline hydrochloride activity.

Indications:

Chickens: For use in the control of chronic respiratory disease (CRD air sac disease) caused by *Mycoplasma gallisepticum* and *Escherichia coli,* infectious synovitis caused by *Mycoplasma synoviae* sensitive to tetracycline hydrochloride.

Turkeys: For use in the control of infectious synovitis caused by *Mycoplasma synoviae,* bluecomb (transmissible enteritis, corona viral enteritis) complicated by organisms sensitive to tetracycline hydrochloride.

Swine and Calves: For use in the control and treatment of bacterial enteritis (scours) caused by *Escherichia coli,* bacterial pneumonia associated with *Pasteurella* spp., *Actinobacillus pleuropneumoniae, Klebsiella* spp. sensitive to tetracycline hydrochloride.

Directions for Use: Medicate at the first clinical signs of disease or when experience indicates that the disease may be a problem.

Mixing Instructions(6.4 oz. will make):

100 gal containing 100 mg of tetracycline hydrochloride/gallon.

50 gal containing 200 mg of tetracycline hydrochloride/gallon.

25 gal containing 400 mg of tetracycline hydrochloride/gallon.

12.5 gal containing 800 mg of tetracycline hydrochloride/gallon.

Prepare fresh solutions at least once a day. The solutions are not stable for more than 24 hours. Use as the sole source of tetracycline. Deliver the recommended dosage level in divided doses. The diagnosis should be reconsidered if improvement is not noticed within 3 days. The concentration of the drug required in medicated water must be adequate to compensate for variations in the age and the class of the animals, feed consumption, and environmental temperature and humidity, each of which affects water consumption.

Recommended Dosage Level:

Chickens:

CRD Air Sac Disease: Use the soluble powder in the drinking water at a drug level of 400-800 mg of tetracycline hydrochloride per gallon per day in divided doses.

Infectious synovitis: Use the soluble powder in the drinking water at a drug level of 200-400 mg of tetracycline hydrochloride per gallon per day in divided doses. Administer for 7-14 days.

Turkeys:

Infectious Synovitis: Use the soluble powder in the drinking water at a drug level of 400 mg of tetracycline hydrochloride per gallon per day in divided doses.

Bluecomb: Use the soluble powder in the drinking water at a drug level of tetracycline hydrochloride per gallon to provide 25 mg/pound of body weight per day in divided doses. Administer for 7-14 days.

Swine and Calves:

For use in the control and treatment of bacterial enteritis (scours) caused by *Escherichia coli,* bacterial pneumonia associated with *Pasteurella* spp., *Actinobacillus pleuropneumoniae, Klebsiella* spp. sensitive to tetracycline hydrochloride: Use the soluble powder in the drinking water at a drug level of tetracycline hydrochloride per gallon to provide 10 mg/pound of body weight per day in divided doses. Administer for 3-5 days.

Special directions for baby calves and baby pigs: Administer this product one hour before or two hours after feeding milk or milk replacers. Provide clean (unmedicated) drinking water at all times.

Note: This product is to be administered twice a day in the drinking water of swine, calves and poultry. One-half of the recommended daily dosage level of the antibiotic is to be consumed during each administration period, thus providing the drug in divided doses.

Caution(s): For animal use only.

Restricted Drug (California) — Use only as directed.

Warning(s): Do not slaughter birds or swine for food within 4 days of treatment.

Not for use in turkeys or chickens producing eggs for human consumption. Do not use for more than 14 consecutive days.

A withdrawal period has not been established for this product in pre-ruminating calves. Do not use in calves to be processed for veal.

Do not slaughter animals for food within 5 days of treatment.

Do not use for more than 5 consecutive days.

Presentation: 6.4 oz. (181 g) (NDC: 30798-277-27).

Compendium Code No.: 10840491 4/97

DURAMYCIN 72-200

Durvet **Oxytetracycline Injection**

Oxytetracycline Injection-Antibiotic

ANADA No.: 200-123

Active Ingredient(s): DURAMYCIN 72-200 (oxytetracycline injection) is a sterile, ready-to-use solution for the administration of the broad spectrum antibiotic oxytetracycline by injection. Each mL contains 200 mg of oxytetracycline base as amphoteric oxytetracycline and, on a w/v basis, 40.0% 2-pyrrolidone, 5.0% povidone, 1.8% magnesium oxide, 0.2% sodium formaldehyde sulfoxylate (as a preservative), monoethanolamine and/or hydrochloric acid as required to adjust pH.

Indications: DURAMYCIN 72-200 is intended for use in the treatment of the following diseases in beef cattle, non-lactating dairy cattle; calves, including pre-ruminating (veal) calves; and swine when due to oxytetracycline-susceptible organisms:

Cattle: In cattle, DURAMYCIN 72-200 is indicated in the treatment of pneumonia and shipping fever complex associated with *Pasteurella* spp. and *Hemophilus* spp.; infectious bovine keratoconjunctivitis (pinkeye) caused by *Moraxella bovis;* foot-rot and diphtheria caused by *Fusobacterium necrophorum;* bacterial enteritis (scours) caused by *Escherichia coli;* wooden tongue caused by *Actinobacillus ligniersii;* leptospirosis caused by *Leptospira pomona;* and wound infections and acute metritis caused by strains of staphylococci and streptococci organisms sensitive to oxytetracycline.

Swine: In swine, DURAMYCIN 72-200 (oxytetracycline injection) is indicated in the treatment of bacterial enteritis (scours, colibacillosis) caused by *Escherichia coli;* pneumonia caused by *Pasteurella multocida;* and leptospirosis caused by *Leptospira pomona.*

In sows, DURAMYCIN 72-200 is indicated as an aid in the control of infectious enteritis (baby pig scours, colibacillosis) in suckling pigs caused by *Escherichia coli.*

Dosage and Administration: Dosage:

Cattle: DURAMYCIN 72-200 is to be administered by intramuscular, subcutaneous or intravenous injection to beef cattle and non-lactating dairy cattle and calves, including pre-ruminating (veal) calves.

A single dosage of 9 milligrams of DURAMYCIN 72-200 per pound of body weight administered intramuscularly or subcutaneously is recommended in the treatment of the following conditions: 1) bacterial pneumonia caused by *Pasteurella* spp. (shipping fever) in calves and yearlings, where re-treatment is impractical due to husbandry conditions, such as cattle on range, or where their repeated restraint is inadvisable; 2) infectious bovine keratoconjunctivitis (pinkeye) caused by *Moraxella bovis.*

DURAMYCIN 72-200 can also be administered by intravenous, subcutaneous or intramuscular injection at a level of 3 to 5 milligrams of oxytetracycline per pound of body weight per day. In the treatment of severe foot-rot and advanced cases of other indicated diseases, dosage level of 5 milligrams per pound of body weight per day is recommended. Treatment should be continued 24 to 48 hours following remission of disease signs; however, not to exceed a total of four consecutive days. Consult your veterinarian if improvement is not noted within 24 to 48 hours of the beginning of treatment.

Swine: In swine a single dosage of 9 milligrams of DURAMYCIN 72-200 per pound of body weight administered intramuscularly is recommended in the treatment of bacterial pneumonia caused by *Pasteurella multocida* in swine, where re-treatment is impractical due to husbandry conditions or where repeated restraint is inadvisable.

DURAMYCIN 72-200 can also be administered by intramuscular injection at a level of 3 to 5 milligrams of oxytetracycline per pound of body weight per day. Treatment should be continued 24 to 48 hours following remission of the disease signs; however, not to exceed a total of four consecutive days. Consult your veterinarian if improvement is not noted within 24 to 48 hours of the beginning of treatment.

For sows, administer once intramuscularly 3 milligrams of oxytetracycline per pound of body weight approximately 8 hours before farrowing or immediately after completion of farrowing.

For swine weighing 25 lb of body weight and under, DURAMYCIN 72-200 should be administered undiluted for treatment at 9 mg/lb but should be administered diluted for treatment at 3 to 5 mg/lb body weight.

	9 mg/lb Dosage Volume of Undiluted DURAMYCIN 72-200	3 or 5 mg/lb Dosage Volume of Diluted DURAMYCIN 72-200		
Body Weight	9 mg/lb	3 mg/lb	Dilution*	5 mg/lb
5 lb	0.2 mL	0.6 mL	1:7	1.0 mL
10 lb	0.5 mL	0.9 mL	1:5	1.5 mL
25 lb	1.1 mL	1.5 mL	1:3	2.5 mL

*To prepare dilutions, add one part DURAMYCIN 72-200 to three, five or seven parts of sterile water, or 5 percent dextrose solution as indicated; the diluted product should be used immediately.

Directions for Use: DURAMYCIN 72-200 is intended for use in the treatment of disease due to oxytetracycline-susceptible organisms in beef cattle, non-lactating dairy cattle; calves, including pre-ruminating (veal) calves; and swine. A thoroughly cleaned, sterile needle and syringe should be used for each injection (needles and syringes may be sterilized by boiling in water for 15 minutes). In cold weather, DURAMYCIN 72-200 should be warmed to room temperature before administration to animals. Before withdrawing the solution from the bottle, disinfect the rubber cap on the bottle with suitable disinfectant, such as 70 percent alcohol. The injection site should be similarly cleaned with the disinfectant. Needles of 16 to 18 gauge and 1 to 1½ inches long are adequate for intramuscular and subcutaneous injections. Needles 2 to 3 inches are recommended for intravenous use.

Intramuscular Administration: Intramuscular injections should be made by directing the needle of suitable gauge and length into the fleshy part of a thick muscle such as in the rump, hip, or thigh regions; avoid blood vessels and major nerves. Before injecting the solution, pull back gently on the plunger. If blood appears in the syringe, a blood vessel has been entered; withdraw the needle and select a different site. No more than 10 mL should be injected intramuscularly at any one site in adult beef cattle and non-lactating dairy cattle, and not more than 5 mL per site in adult swine; rotate injection sites for each succeeding treatment. The volume administered per injection site should be reduced according to age and body size so that 1 to 2 mL per site is injected in small calves.

Subcutaneous Administration: Subcutaneous injections in beef cattle, non-lactating dairy cattle, and calves, including pre-ruminating (veal) calves, should be made by directing the needle of suitable gauge and length through the loose folds of the neck skin in front of the shoulder. Care should be taken to ensure that the tip of the needle has penetrated the skin but is not lodged in muscle. Before injecting the solution, pull back gently on the plunger. If blood appears in the syringe, a blood vessel has been entered; withdraw the needle and select a different site. The solution should be injected slowly into the area between the skin and muscles. No more than 10 mL should be injected subcutaneously at any one site in adult beef cattle and non-lactating dairy cattle; rotate injection sites for each succeeding treatment. The volume administered per injection site should be reduced according to age and body size so that 1-2 mL per site is injected in small calves.

Intravenous Administration: DURAMYCIN 72-200 may be administered intravenously to beef cattle and non-lactating dairy cattle. As with all highly concentrated materials, DURAMYCIN 72-200 should be administered slowly by the intravenous route.

Preparation of the Animal for Injection:

1. Approximate location of vein. The jugular vein runs in the jugular groove on each side of the neck from the angle of the jaw to just above the brisket and slightly above and to the side of the windpipe. (See Fig. I)
2. Restraint. A stanchion or chute is ideal for restraining the animal. With a halter, rope, or cattle leader (nose tongs), pull the animal's head around the side of the stanchion, cattle chute, or post in such a manner to form a bow in the neck (See Fig. II), then snub the head securely to prevent movement. By forming the bow in the neck, the outside curvature of the bow tends to expose the jugular vein and make it easily accessible. Caution: Avoid restraining the animal with a tight rope or halter around the throat or upper neck which might impede blood flow. Animals that are down present no problem so far as restraint is concerned.
3. Clip hair in area where injection is to be made (over the vein in the upper third of the neck). Clean and disinfect the skin with alcohol or other suitable antiseptic.

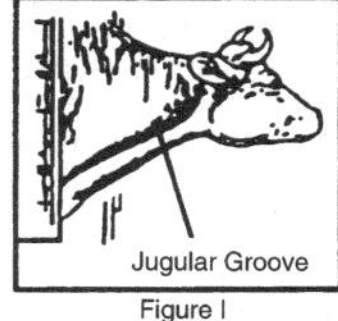

Figure I

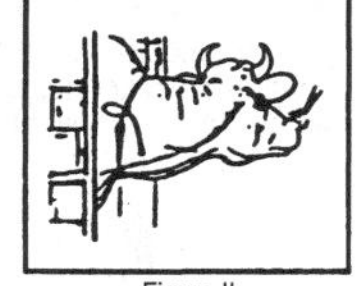
Figure II

Entering the Vein and Making the Injection:

1. Raise the vein. This is accomplished by tying the choke rope tightly around the neck close to the shoulder. The rope should be tied in such a way that it will not come loose and so that it can be untied quickly by pulling the loose end (See Fig. II). In thick-necked animals, a block of wood placed in the jugular groove between the rope and the hide will help considerably in applying the desired pressure at the right point. The vein is a soft flexible tube through which blood flows back to the heart. Under ordinary conditions it cannot be seen or felt with the fingers. When the flow of blood is blocked at the base of the neck by the choke rope, the vein becomes enlarged and rigid because of the back pressure. If the choke rope is sufficiently tight, the vein stands out and can be easily seen and felt in thin-necked animals. As a further check in identifying the vein, tap it with the fingers in front of the choke rope. Pulsations that can be seen or felt with the fingers in front of the point being tapped will confirm the fact that the vein is properly distended. It is impossible to put the needle into the vein unless it is distended. Experienced operators are able to raise the vein simply by hand pressure, but the use of a choke rope is more certain.
2. Inserting the needle. This involves three distinct steps. First, insert the needle through the hide. Second, insert the needle into the vein. This may require two or three attempts before the vein is entered. The vein has a tendency to roll away from the point of the needle, especially if the needle is not sharp. The vein can be steadied with the thumb and finger of one hand. With the other hand, the needle point is placed directly over the vein, slanting it so that its direction is along the length of the vein, either toward the head or toward the heart. Properly positioned this way, a quick thrust of the needle will be followed by a spurt of blood through the needle, which indicates that the vein has been entered. Third, once in the vein, the needle should be inserted along the length of the vein all the way to the hub exercising caution to see that the needle does not penetrate the opposite side of the vein. Continuous steady flow of blood through the needle indicates that the needle is still in the vein. If blood does not flow continuously, the needle is out of the vein (or clogged) and another attempt must be made. If difficulty is encountered, it may be advisable to use the vein on the other side of the neck.
3. While the needle is being placed in proper position in the vein, an assistant should get the medication ready so that the injection can be started without delay after the vein has been entered.
4. Making the injection. With the needle in position as indicated by continuous flow of blood, release the choke rope by a quick pull on the free end. This is essential - the medication cannot flow into the vein while it is blocked. Immediately connect the syringe containing DURAMYCIN 72-200 (oxytetracycline injection) to the needle and slowly depress the plunger. If there is resistance to depression of the plunger, this indicates that the needle has slipped out of the vein (or is clogged) and the procedure will have to be repeated. Watch for any swelling under the skin near the needle which would indicate that the medication is not going into the vein. Should this occur, it is best to try the vein on the opposite side of the neck.
5. Removing the needle. When injection is complete, remove needle with straight pull. Then apply pressure over the area of injection momentarily to control any bleeding through needle puncture, using cotton soaked in alcohol or other suitable antiseptic.

Precaution(s): DURAMYCIN 72-200 does not require refrigeration; however, it is recommended that it be stored at room temperature, 15°-30°C (59°-86°F). The antibiotic activity of oxytetracycline is not appreciably diminished in the presence of body fluids, serum, or exudates. Keep from freezing.

Caution(s): Consult with your veterinarian prior to administering this product in order to determine the proper treatment required in the event of an adverse reaction. At the first sign of any adverse reaction, discontinue use of product and seek the advice of your veterinarian. Some of the reactions may be attributed either to anaphylaxis (an allergic reaction) or to cardiovascular collapse of unknown cause.

Shock may be observed following intravenous administration, especially where highly concentrated materials are involved. To minimize this occurrence, it is recommended that DURAMYCIN 72-200 be administered slowly by this route.

Shortly after injection, treated animals may have transient hemoglobinuria resulting in darkened urine.

As with all antibiotic preparations, use of the drug may result in overgrowth of non-susceptible organisms, including fungi. A lack of response by the treated animal, or the development of new signs, may suggest that an overgrowth of non-susceptible organisms has occurred. If any of these conditions occur, consult your veterinarian.

Since bacteriostatic drugs may interfere with the bactericidal action of penicillin, it is advisable to avoid giving DURAMYCIN 72-200 in conjunction with penicillin.

Livestock drug, not for human use.

Restricted Drug (California), use only as directed.

For animal use only.

Warning(s): Exceeding the highest recommended level of drug per pound of body weight per day, administering more than the recommended number of treatments, and/or exceeding 10 mL intramuscularly or subcutaneously per injection site in adult beef cattle and non-lactating dairy cattle, and 5 mL intramuscularly per injection site in adult swine, may result in antibiotic residues beyond the withdrawal period.

Discontinue treatment at least 28 days prior to slaughter of cattle and swine. Not for use in lactating dairy animals. Rapid intravenous administration may result in animal collapse. Oxytetracycline should be administered intravenously slowly over a period of at least 5 minutes.

Keep out of reach of children.

Adverse Reactions: Reports of adverse reactions associated with oxytetracycline administration include injection site swelling, restlessness, ataxia, trembling, swelling of eyelids, ears, muzzle, anus and vulva (or scrotum and sheath in males), respiratory abnormalities (labored breathing), frothing at the mouth, collapse and possibly death. Some of these reactions may be attributed either to anaphylaxis (an allergic reaction) or to cardiovascular collapse of unknown cause.

Discussion: Care of Sick Animals: The use of antibiotics in the management of diseases is based on an accurate diagnosis and an adequate course of treatment. When properly used in the treatment of diseases caused by oxytetracycline-susceptible organisms, most animals that have been treated with oxytetracycline injection show a noticeable improvement within 24 to 48 hours. It is recommended that the diagnosis and treatment of animal diseases be carried out by a veterinarian. Since many diseases look alike but require different types of treatment, the use of professional veterinary and laboratory services can reduce treatment time, costs and needless losses. Good housing, sanitation and nutrition are important in the maintenance of healthy animals, and are essential in the treatment of diseased animals.

Presentation: 100 mL (NDC 30798-576-10), 250 mL (NDC 30798-576-13) and 500 mL (NDC 30798-576-17).

Compendium Code No.: 10840503

Rev. 9-01

DURAMYCIN-100

Durvet

Oxytetracycline Injection

Oxytetracycline Hydrochloride Injection-Antibiotic

ANADA No.: 200-068

Active Ingredient(s): Each mL contains:

Oxytetracycline base (as HCl) . . . . 100 mg
Magnesium Chloride • $6H_2O$ . . . . 5.76% w/v
Water for Injection . . . . 17% v/v
Propylene Glycol . . . . q.s.

D

with Sodium Formaldehyde Sulfoxylate, 1.3% w/v as a preservative and Monoethanolamine for pH adjustment.

Indications: A great many of the pathogens involved in cattle diseases are known to be susceptible to Oxytetracycline Hydrochloride therapy. Many strains of organisms, however, have shown resistance to Oxytetracycline. In the case of certain coliforms, streptococci and staphylococci, it may be advisable to conduct culture and sensitivity testing to determine susceptibility of the infecting organism to Oxytetracycline. In this manner, the likelihood of successful treatment with DURAMYCIN-100 (Oxytetracycline Hydrochloride Injection) solution can be determined in advance.

Diseases for Which DURAMYCIN-100 (Oxytetracycline Hydrochloride Injection) is Indicated:

The use of DURAMYCIN-100 (Oxytetracycline Hydrochloride Injection) is indicated in beef cattle, beef calves, non-lactating dairy cattle and dairy calves for treatment of the following disease conditions caused by one or more of the Oxytetracycline sensitive pathogens listed as follows:

Disease	Causative Organism(s) Which Show Sensitivity to DURAMYCIN-100 (Oxytetracycline HCl Infection)
Bacterial Pneumonia and Shipping Fever Complex Associated with *Pasteurella* spp	*Pasteurella* spp
Bacterial Enteritis (scours)	*Escherichia coli*
Necrotic Pododermatitis (foot rot)	*Fusobacterium necrophorum*
Calf Diphtheria	*Fusobacterium necrophorum*
Wooden Tongue	*Actinobacillus lignieresii*
Wound Infections; Acute Metritis; Traumatic Injury	Caused by oxytetracycline-susceptible strains of streptococcal and staphylococcal organisms.

Pharmacology: Description: DURAMYCIN-100 (Oxytetracycline Hydrochloride Injection) is a sterile ready-to-use preparation containing 100 mg/mL Oxytetracycline HCl, for administration of the broad spectrum antibiotic, Oxytetracycline, by injection.

Antibiotic Action of Oxytetracycline: Oxytetracycline is effective against a wide range of gram-negative and gram-positive organisms that are pathogenic for cattle. The antibiotic is primarily bacteriostatic in effect, and is believed to exert its antimicrobial action by the inhibition of microbial protein synthesis. The antibiotic activity of Oxytetracycline is not appreciably diminished in the presence of body fluids, serum or exudates. Since the drugs in the tetracycline class have similar antimicrobial spectra, organisms can develop cross resistance among them. Oxytetracycline is concentrated by the liver in the bile and excreted in the urine and feces at high concentrations and in a biologically active form.

Dosage and Administration: Recommended Daily Dosages: Treat at the first clinical signs of disease.

The intravenous injection of 3 to 5 mg of Oxytetracycline Hydrochloride per pound of body weight per day (3 to 5 mL per 100 lbs body weight) is the recommended dosage.

Severe foot-rot and the severe forms of the indicated diseases should be treated with 5 mg per pound of body weight. Surgical procedures may be indicated in some forms of foot-rot or other conditions.

In disease treatment, the daily dose of DURAMYCIN-100 (Oxytetracycline Hydrochloride Injection) should be continued 24 to 48 hours following remission of disease symptoms; however, not to exceed a total of 4 consecutive days.

Directions for Making an Intravenous Injection in Cattle:

Equipment Recommended:

1. Choke rope - a rope or cord about 5 feet long, with a loop in one end, to be used as a tourniquet.
2. Syringe and needles; gravity flow intravenous set.
3. Use new, very sharp hypodermic needles, 16-gauge, 1½ to 2 inches long. Dull needles will not work. Extra needles should be available in case the one being used becomes clogged.
4. Scissors or clippers.
5. 70% rubbing alcohol compound or other equally effective antiseptic for disinfecting the skin.
6. The medication to be given.

Preparation of Equipment: Thoroughly clean the needles, syringe and intravenous set and disinfect them by boiling in water for twenty minutes or by immersing in a suitable chemical disinfectant such as 70% alcohol for a period of not less than 30 minutes. Warm the bottle of medication to approximately body temperature and keep warm until used.

It is recommended that the correct dose be diluted in water for injection, sodium chloride injection or other suitable vehicle immediately prior to administration. Doses up to 50 mL may be diluted in 250 mL. Larger doses may be diluted in 500 mL of one of the diluents. Adverse reactions may be minimized and the drug dose can be better regulated by this method of administration.

Avoid touching the needle with the hands at all times.

In case of the syringe method of administration, disinfect the vial cap by wiping with 70% alcohol or other suitable antiseptic. Touching a sterile needle only by the hub, attach it to the syringe and push the plunger down the barrel to empty it of air. Puncture the rubber cap of the vial and withdraw the plunger upward in the syringe to draw up a volume of DURAMYCIN-100 (Oxytetracycline Hydrochloride Injection), 100 mg/mL of about 5 mL more than is needed for injection. Withdraw from the vial and, pointing the needle upward, remove all air bubbles from the syringe by pushing the plunger upward to the volume required.

If the injection cannot be made immediately, the tip of the needle may be covered with cotton soaked in 70% alcohol to prevent contamination.

Preparation of the Animal for Injection:

1. Approximate location of vein. The jugular vein runs in the jugular groove on each side of the neck from the angle of the jaw to just above the brisket and slightly above and to the side of the windpipe (see Figure 1).

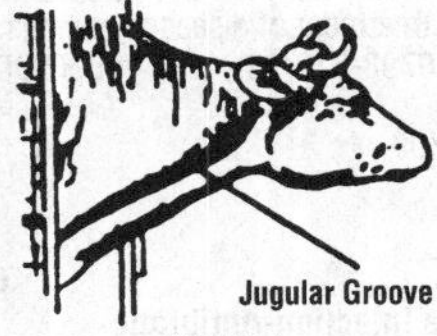

FIGURE 1

2. Method of restraint - A stanchion or chute is ideal for restraining the animal. With a halter, rope or cattle leader (nose tongs), pull the animal's head around the side of the stanchion, cattle chute or post in such a manner to form a bow in the neck, (see Figure 2) then snub the head securely to prevent movement. By forming the bow in the neck, the outside curvature of the bow tends to expose the jugular vein and make it easily accessible. Caution: Avoid a tight rope or halter around the throat or upper neck which might impede blood flow. Animals that are down present no problem so far as restraint is concerned.

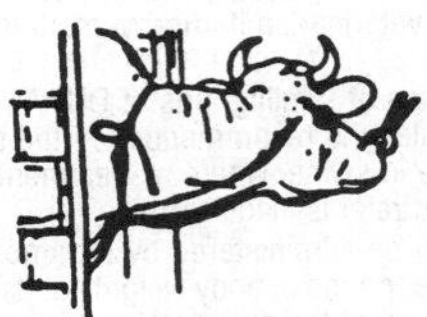

FIGURE 2

3. Clip hair in area where injection is to be made (over the vein in the upper third of the neck). Clean and disinfect the skin with alcohol or other suitable antiseptic.

Dosage for Injection: Refer to the table below for proper dosage according to body weight of the animal.

Weight of Animals, Lbs (Beef Cattle, Beef Calves, Non-Lactating Dairy Cattle, Dairy Calves)	Milligrams of Oxytetracycline Hydrochloride per 100 lbs of Body Weight Per Day	Daily Dosage of DURAMYCIN-100 (Oxytetracycline Hydrochloride Injection) (mL)
50 lbs	300-500 mg	1.5-2.5 mL
100 lbs	300-500 mg	3-5 mL
200 lbs	300-500 mg	6-10 mL
300 lbs	300-500 mg	9-15 mL
400 lbs	300-500 mg	12-20 mL
500 lbs	300-500 mg	15-25 mL
600 lbs	300-500 mg	18-30 mL
800 lbs	300-500 mg	24-40 mL
1000 lbs	300-500 mg	30-50 mL
1200 lbs	300-500 mg	36-60 mL
1400 lbs	300-500 mg	42-70 mL

Caution: If no improvement is noted within 24 to 48 hours consult a veterinarian.

For intravenous use only.

Entering the Vein and Making the Injection:

1. Raise the vein. This is accomplished by tying the choke rope tight around the neck, close to the shoulder. The rope should be tied in such a way that it will not come loose and so that it can be untied quickly by pulling the loose end. In thick-necked animals, a block of wood placed in the jugular groove between the rope and the hide will help considerably in applying the desired pressure at the right point. The vein is a soft flexible tube through which blood flows back to the heart. Under ordinary conditions it cannot be seen or felt with the fingers. When the flow of blood is blocked at the base of the neck by the choke rope, the vein becomes enlarged and rigid because of the back pressure. If the choke rope is sufficiently tight, the vein stands out and can be easily seen and felt in thick-necked animals. As a further check in identifying the vein, tap it with the fingers in front of the choke rope. Pulsations that can be seen or felt with the fingers in front of the point being tapped will confirm the fact that the vein is properly distended. It is impossible to put the needle into the vein unless it is distended. Experienced operators are able to raise the vein simply by hand pressure, but the use of a choke rope is more certain.
2. Inserting the needle. This involves three distinct steps. First, insert the needle through the hide. Second, insert the needle into the vein. This may require two or three attempts before the vein is entered. The vein has a tendency to roll away from the point of the needle, especially if the needle is not sharp. The vein can be steadied with the thumb and finger of one hand. With the other hand, the needle point is placed directly over the vein, slanting it so that its direction is along the length of the vein, either toward the head or toward the heart. Properly positioned this way, a quick thrust of the needle will be followed by a spurt of blood through the needle, which indicates that the vein has been entered. Third, once in the vein, the needle should be inserted along the length of the vein all the way to the hub, exercising caution to see that the needle does not penetrate the opposite side of the vein. Continuous steady flow of blood through the needle indicates that the needle is still in the vein. If blood does not flow continuously, the needle is out of the vein (or clogged) and another attempt must be made. If difficulty is encountered, it may be advisable to use the vein on the other side of the neck.
3. While the needle is being placed in proper position in the vein, an assistant should get the medication ready so that the injection can be started without delay after the vein has been entered. Remove the rubber stopper from the bottle of intravenous solution, connect the intravenous tube to the neck of the bottle, invert the bottle and allow some of the solution to run through the tube to eliminate all air bubbles.
4. Making the injection. With needle in proper position as indicated by continuous flow of blood, release the choke rope by a quick pull on the free end. This is essential - the medication cannot flow into the vein while the vein is blocked. Immediately connect the intravenous tube to the needle, and raise the bottle. The solution will flow by gravity (see Figure 3). Rapid injection may occasionally produce shock. Administer slowly. The animal should be observed at all times during the injection in order not to give the solution too fast. This may be determined by watching the respiration of the animal and feeling or listening to the heart beat. If the heart beat and respiration increase markedly, the rate of injection should be immediately stopped by pinching the tube until the animal recovers approximately to its previous respiration or heart beat rate, when the injection can be resumed at a slower rate. The rate of flow can be controlled by pinching the tube between the thumb and forefinger or by raising and lowering the bottle.

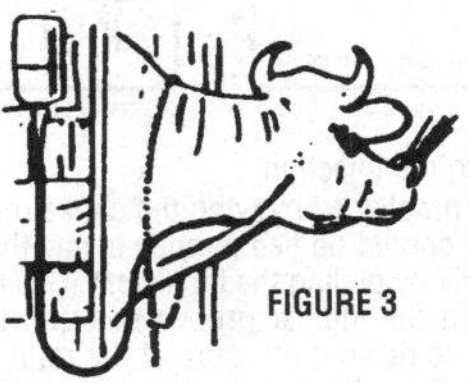

FIGURE 3

Bubbles entering the bottle through the air tube or valve indicate the rate at which the medication is flowing. If the flow should stop, this means the needle has slipped out of the vein (or is clogged) and the operation will have to be repeated. If using the syringe technique, pull back gently on the plunger: if blood flows into the syringe, the needle is in proper position. Depress the plunger slowly. If there is any resistance to the depression of the plunger, stop and repeat insertion procedure. The resistance indicates that either the needle is clogged or it has slipped out of the vein. With either method of administration, syringe or gravity flow, watch for any swelling under the skin near the needle, which would indicate that the medication is not going into the vein. Should this occur, it is best to try the vein on the opposite side of the neck. Sudden movement of the animal, especially twisting of the neck or raising or lowering the head, may sometimes cause the needle to slip out of the vein. To prevent this, tape the needle hub to the skin of the neck to hold the needle in position. Whenever there is any doubt as to the position of the needle, this should be checked in the following manner: Pinch off the intravenous tube to stop flow, disconnect the tube from the needle and re-apply pressure to the vein. Free flow of blood through the needle indicates that it is in proper position and the injection can then be continued. If using the syringe, gently pull back on the plunger. Blood should flow into the syringe.

5. Removing the needle. When the injection is complete, remove needle with a straight pull. Then apply pressure over area of injection momentarily to control any bleeding through needle puncture, using cotton soaked in alcohol or other suitable antiseptic.

Instructions for Care of Sick Animals: The use of antibiotics, as with most medications used in the management of diseases, is based on accurate diagnosis and adequate treatment. When properly used in the treatment of diseases caused by oxytetracycline susceptible organisms, animals usually show a noticeable improvement within 24 to 48 hours. If improvement does not occur within this period of time, the diagnosis and treatment of animal diseases should be carried out by a veterinarian. The use of professional veterinary and laboratory services can reduce treatment costs, time and needless losses. Good management, housing, sanitation and nutrition are essential in the care of animals and in the successful treatment of disease.

Contraindication(s): Because bacteriostatic drugs interfere with the bactericidal action of Penicillin, do not give Oxytetracycline Hydrochloride in conjunction with Penicillin.

Precaution(s): Store between 15° and 30°C (59°-86°F).

Note: Solution may darken on storage but potency remains unaffected.

Caution(s): If no improvement occurs within 24 to 48 hours, consult a veterinarian. Do not use the drug for more than 4 consecutive days. Use beyond 4 days or doses higher than maximum recommended dose may result in antibiotic tissue residues beyond the withdrawal period.

The improper or accidental injection of the drug outside of the vein will cause local tissue irritation manifested by temporary swelling and discoloration at the injection site.

Shortly after injection, treated animals may have a transient hemoglobinuria (darkened urine).

Rapid intravenous administration may result in animal collapse. Oxytetracycline should be administered intravenously slowly over a period of at least 5 minutes.

Consult with your veterinarian prior to administering this product in order to determine the proper treatment required in the event of an adverse reaction. At the first sign of any adverse reaction, discontinue use of product and seek the advice of your veterinarian. Some of the reactions may be attributed either to anaphylaxis (an allergic reaction) or to cardiovascular collapse of unknown cause.

Because bacteriostatic drugs interfere with the bactericidal action of penicillin, do not give oxytetracycline hydrochloride in conjunction with penicillin.

For use in beef cattle, beef calves, non-lactating dairy cattle and dairy calves only.

For use in animals only.

Restricted Drug (California) - Use only as directed.

Warning(s): Discontinue treatment with DURAMYCIN-100 (Oxytetracycline Hydrochloride Injection) at least 22 days prior to slaughter of the animal. Not for use in lactating dairy animals.

A withdrawal period has not been established for this product in pre-ruminating calves. Do not use in calves to be processed for veal.

Keep out of reach of children.

Adverse Reactions: Reports of adverse reactions associated with oxytetracycline administration include injection site swelling, restlessness, ataxia, trembling, swelling of eyelids, ears, muzzle, anus and vulva (or scrotum and sheath in males), respiratory abnormalities (labored breathing), frothing at the mouth, collapse and possibly death. Some of these reactions may be attributed either to anaphylaxis (an allergic reaction) or to cardiovascular collapse of unknown cause.

As with other antibiotics, the use of this drug may result in the over-growth of non-susceptible organisms. If any unusual symptoms occur or in the absence of a favorable response following treatment, discontinue use immediately and call a veterinarian.

Presentation: DURAMYCIN-100 (Oxytetracycline Hydrochloride Injection) is available in 500 mL multidose vials containing 100 mg Oxytetracycline Hydrochloride per mL (NDC 30798-577-17).

Compendium Code No.: 10840513 Rev. 12-00/Rev. 11-00

DURAMYCIN-324

Durvet **Water Medication**

Tetracycline Hydrochloride Soluble Powder 324-Antibiotic

ANADA No.: 200-049

Active Ingredient(s): Each 2.52 oz packet contains 51 g of tetracycline hydrochloride.

Each pound contains 324 g of tetracycline hydrochloride.

Indications: For use in the control and treatment of the following conditions in swine, calves and poultry.

Swine and Calves: Control and treatment of bacterial enteritis (scours) caused by *Escherichia coli* and bacterial pneumonia associated with *Actinobacillus pleuropneumoniae, Pasteurella* spp., *Klebsiella* spp. susceptible to tetracycline.

Chickens: Control of chronic respiratory disease (CRD air sac disease) caused by *Mycoplasma gallisepticum* and *Escherichia coli;* infectious synovitis caused by *Mycoplasma synoviae* sensitive to tetracycline. Recommended Dosage Level: CRD air sac disease; 400-800 mg tetracycline hydrochloride per gallon of drinking water. Infectious synovitis; 200-400 mg tetracycline hydrochloride per gallon of drinking water.

Turkeys: Control of infectious synovitis caused by *Mycoplasma synoviae;* bluecomb (transmissible enteritis, coronaviral enteritis) complicated by organisms sensitive to tetracycline. Recommended Dosage Level: Infectious synovitis; 400 mg tetracycline hydrochloride per gallon of drinking water. Bluecomb; 25 mg/lb body weight of tetracycline hydrochloride per day in divided doses.

Dosage and Administration: Administer DURAMYCIN-324 in the drinking water of swine and calves for 3 to 5 days at a drug level of tetracycline hydrochloride per gallon to provide approximately 10 mg/lb of body weight, per day in divided doses. In turkeys, for bluecomb only, administer in the drinking water for 7-14 days at a drug level of 25 mg/lb of body weight, per day in divided doses.

Mixing Directions for Swine, Calves and Turkeys: Add one packet (2.52 oz) to 500 mL (17 oz), or one level scoop (1.26 oz) to 250 mL (8.5 oz) of warm water and dissolve. This will provide stock solution of 100 mg/mL of tetracycline hydrochloride. For Turkeys Only: This stock solution when metered at approximately 1 oz per gallon, will provide drinking water containing 2957 mg of tetracycline hydrochloride activity per gallon.

Calves: Calves may be treated individually by administering 5 mL (1 measuring teaspoonful) of stock solution twice daily for each 100 lbs body weight as a drench or by dose syringe.

Chickens and Turkeys: To arrive at the recommended dosages, prepare stock solutions as follows and meter into the drinking water at 1 oz per gallon.

200 mg/gallon - dissolve 1 packet (2.52 oz) in 7570 mL (2 gallon), or 1 level scoop (1.26 oz) in 3785 mL warm water (1 gallon). Provides 256 gallons (packet), or 128 gallons (scoop) medicated drinking water.

400 mg/gallon - dissolve 1 packet (2.52 oz) in 3785 mL (1 gallon), or 1 level scoop (1.26 oz) in 1892 mL warm water (0.5 gallon). Provides 128 gallons (packet), or 64 gallons (scoop) medicated drinking water.

800 mg/gallon - dissolve 1 packet (2.52 oz) in 1892 mL (0.5 gallon), or 1 level scoop (1.26 oz) in 946 mL warm water (0.25 gallon). Provides 64 gallons (packet), or 32 gallons (scoop) medicated drinking water.

Note: The concentration of the drug required in medicated water must be adequate to compensate for variation in the age of the animal, feed consumption and the environmental temperature and humidity, each of which affects water consumption.

The contents of each 2.52 oz packet will provide sufficient drug to treat 5,100 total pounds of swine or calves for a single day at the recommended dosage level of 10 mg/lb of body weight in divided doses. The same packet will treat 2,040 lb of turkeys when supplied at 25 mg/lb.

The contents of the 2 lb container will provide sufficient drug to treat 64,800 total pounds of swine or calves for a single day at the recommended dosage level of 10 mg/lb of body weight in divided doses. The same container will treat 25,920 lb of turkeys when supplied at 25 mg/lb.

The contents of the 5 lb container will provide sufficient drug to treat 162,000 total pounds of swine or calves for a single day at the recommended dosage level of 10 mg/lb of body weight in divided doses. The same container will treat 64,800 lb of turkeys when supplied at 25 mg/lb.

Precaution(s): Store at 59-86°F.

Caution(s): Use as sole source of tetracycline. Not to be used in swine or calves for more than 5 days. Not to be used in chickens or turkeys for more than 14 consecutive days. When used in plastic or stainless steel waterers or automatic medicators, prepare fresh solution every 24 hours. When used in galvanized waterers, prepare fresh solution every 12 hours. If condition does not improve within 2 to 3 days, consult your veterinarian.

For use in animals only. Keep out of reach of children.

Warning(s): Do not slaughter swine for food purposes within 4 days of treatment. Do not slaughter cattle for food purposes within 5 days of treatment. Do not slaughter poultry for food within 4 days of treatment. Not for use in poultry producing eggs for human consumption. A withdrawal period has not been established for this product in pre-ruminating calves. Do not use in calves to be processed for veal.

Presentation: 50x2.52 oz (71.4 g) packets (NDC 30798-645-37), 2 lb (907.2 g) (NDC 30798-645-42) and 5 lb (2.27 kg) (NDC 30798-645-44) containers.

Compendium Code No.: 10840521 Rev. 0696

DURA-PEN

Durvet **Penicillin Injection**

Penicillin G Benzathine & Penicillin G Procaine Injectable Suspension-Antibiotic

NADA No.: 065-506

Active Ingredient(s): Description: Each mL of suspension contains:

Penicillin G benzathine	150,000 units
Penicillin G procaine	150,000 units
Lecithin	11.7 mg
Sodium formaldehyde sulfoxylate	1.75 mg
Methylparaben (as preservative)	1.20 mg
Propylparaben (as preservative)	0.14 mg
Tween 40	8.19 mg
Span 40	11.3 mg
Sodium citrate anhydrous	3.98 mg
Procaine hydrochloride	20 mg
Sodium carboxymethylcellulose	1.04 mg
Water for injection	q.s.

Indications: This product is indicated for treatment of the following bacterial infections in beef cattle due to penicillin-susceptible microorganisms that are susceptible to the serum levels common to this particular dosage form, such as:

1. Bacterial Pneumonia (shipping fever complex) *(Streptococcus* spp., *Corynebacterium pyogenes, Staphylococcus aureus).*
2. Upper Respiratory Infections such as rhinitis or pharyngitis *(Corynebacterium pyogenes).*
3. Blackleg *(Clostridium chauvoei).*

Pharmacology: Action: Penicillin G is an antibiotic which shows a marked bactericidal effect against certain organisms during their growth phase. It is relatively specific in its action against gram-positive bacteria but is usually ineffective against gram-negative organisms.

It is normally recommended that any bacterial infection be treated as early as possible and with a dosage that will give effective blood levels. Although the recommended dosage will give longer detectable penicillin blood levels than penicillin G procaine alone, it is recommended that a second dose be administered at 48 hours when treating a penicillin-susceptible bacterial infection.

The use of antibiotics in the management of disease is based on an accurate diagnosis and an adequate course of treatment. When properly used in the treatment of diseases caused by penicillin-susceptible organisms, most animals treated with this product will show a noticeable improvement within 24 to 48 hours. If improvement does not occur within this time period, the diagnosis and course of treatment should be re-evaluated. It is recommended that the diagnosis and treatment of animal diseases be carried out by a veterinarian. Since many diseases look alike but require different types of treatment, the use of professional veterinary and laboratory services can reduce treatment time, costs, and needless losses. Good housing, sanitation and nutrition are important in the maintenance of healthy animals and are essential in the treatment of disease.

Dosage and Administration: Administration: The recommended dosage for beef cattle should be administered by subcutaneous injection only. Failure to use the subcutaneous route of administration may result in antibiotic residues in meat beyond the withdrawal time.

Dosage:

Beef Cattle: 2 mL per 150 pound body weight given subcutaneously only (2,000 units of penicillin G procaine and 2,000 units penicillin G benzathine per pound body weight). Treatment should be repeated in 48 hours. Important: Treatment in beef cattle should be limited to two (2) doses given by subcutaneous injection only.

Directions for Use: A thoroughly cleaned, sterile needle and syringe should be used for each injection (needles and syringes may be sterilized by boiling in water for 15 minutes).

Before withdrawing the solution from the bottle, disinfect the rubber cap on the bottle with a suitable disinfectant, such as 70% alcohol. The injection site should be similarly cleaned with the disinfectant. Needles of 14 to 16 gauge and not more than 1 inch long are adequate for injections.

A subcutaneous injection should be made by pinching up a fold of the skin between the thumb and forefinger. The mid-neck region is the preferred injection site. Insert the needle under the fold in a direction approximately parallel to the surface of the body. When the needle is inserted in this manner the medication will be delivered underneath the skin between the skin and the muscles. Proper restraint, such as the use of a chute and nose lead is needed for proper administration of the product.

Precaution(s): This product should be stored between 2°-8°C (36°-46°F). Avoid freezing. Warm to room temperature, and shake well before using.

Caution(s): Exceeding the recommended doses and dosage levels may result in antibiotic residues beyond the withdrawal time. Do not inject this product intramuscularly.

Penicillin G is a substance of low toxicity. However, side effects, or so-called allergic or anaphylactic reactions-sometimes fatal, have been known to occur in animals hypersensitive to penicillin and procaine. Such reactions can occur unpredictably with varying intensity. Animals administered penicillin G should be kept under close observation for at least one-half hour. Should allergic or anaphylactic reactions occur, discontinue use of the product and immediately administer epinephrine following manufacturer's recommendations and call a veterinarian.

As with all antibiotic preparations, use of this drug may result in overgrowth of non-susceptible organisms, including fungi. A lack of response by the treated animal, or the development of new signs or symptoms suggests that an overgrowth of non-susceptible organisms has occurred. In such instances, consult your veterinarian.

Since bacterial drugs may interfere with the bacteriostatic action of tetracyclines, it is advisable to avoid giving penicillin in conjunction with tetracyclines.

For animal use only.

Restricted drug (California) - Use only as directed.

For subcutaneous use in beef cattle only. Do not inject intramuscularly.

Warning(s): Beef cattle should be withheld from slaughter for food use for thirty (30) days following last treatment. Treatment in beef cattle must be limited to two (2) doses.

Presentation: Available in 100 mL (NDC 30798-231-10) and 250 mL (NDC 30798-231-13) vials.

Manufactured by: Anthony Products Co., Irwindale, CA 91706.

Compendium Code No.: 10840472 Rev. 12/99

DURAPEN™ ℞

Vedco **Penicillin Injection**

Combination Antibiotic (Sterile Penicillin G Benzathine & Penicillin G Procaine) in Aqueous Suspension

NADA No.: 065-500

Active Ingredient(s): Each mL of suspension contains:

Penicillin G benzathine	150,000 units
Penicillin G procaine	150,000 units
Lecithin	11.7 mg
Sodium formaldehyde sulfoxylate	1.75 mg
Methylparaben (as preservative)	1.20 mg
Propylparaben (as preservative)	0.14 mg
Tween 40	8.19 mg
Span 40	11.3 mg
Sodium citrate anhydrous	3.98 mg
Procaine hydrochloride	20.0 mg
Sodium carboxymethylcellulose	1.04 mg
Water for injection	q.s.

Indications: The product is indicated for the treatment of the following bacterial infections in dogs, horses, and beef cattle due to penicillin susceptible micro-organisms that are susceptible to the serum levels common to this particular dosage form, such as bacterial pneumonia *(Streptococcus spp., Corynebacterium pyogenes, Staphylococcus aureus)*, equine strangles *(Streptococcus equi)*, blackleg *(Clostridium chauvoei)*.

Dosage and Administration: Shake well before using.

Sterile penicillin G benzathine and penicillin G procaine in aqueous suspension should be given by intramuscular injection to horses. In beef cattle, the recommended dosage should be administered by subcutaneous injection only. Dogs may be injected by either the intramuscular or subcutaneous route.

Suggested dosage:

Horses: 2 mL per 150 lbs. of body weight given intramuscularly.

Beef Cattle: 2 mL per 150 lbs. of body weight given subcutaneously only.

Dogs: 1 mL per 10-25 lbs. of body weight intramuscularly or subcutaneously.

Precaution(s): Store at a controlled room temperature between 59-86°F (15-30°C).

Caution(s): Federal law restricts this drug to use by or on the order of a licensed veterinarian.

Not for human use. Keep out of the reach of children.

Warning(s): Beef cattle should be withheld from slaughter for food use for 30 days following the last treatment. Treatment in beef cattle must be limited to two (2) doses.

Presentation: 100 mL and 250 mL vials.

Compendium Code No.: 10940510

DURASECT® LONG-ACTING LIVESTOCK POUR-ON

Pfizer Animal Health **Topical Insecticide**

EPA Reg. No.: 1007-90

Active Ingredient(s):

*Permethrin (3-phenoxyphenyl) methyl ± cis, trans-3-(2,2-dichloroethenyl)-2,2-dimethyl-cyclopropanecarboxylate	1.0%
Inert ingredients	99.0%

*cis/trans ratio: Min 35% (±) cis and max 65% (±) trans.

Indications: Ready to use pour-on for beef cattle, lactating and nonlactating dairy cattle, sheep, and goats.

Patented water repellent formulation.

Does not leave an oily residue.

4- to 11-week-control of horn flies†.

Controls face flies for at least 1 month.

Controls lice.

No withdrawal time.

Directions for Use: It is a violation of Federal Law to use this product in a manner inconsistent with its labeling.

Ready to use - No dilution necessary, see below.

Animal Treatments:

Lactating and Nonlactating Dairy Cattle, Beef Cattle, and Calves:

Target Insects: Controls horn flies, face flies, lice, and aids in the control of horse flies, stable flies, and house flies.

Application: **Apply along back and down face. Use ½ fl oz (15 mL) per 100 lb of body weight of animal, up to 5 fl oz for any one animal.

Sheep:

Target Insects: Sheep keds, lice.

Application: **Apply along back. Use ¼ fl oz (7.5 mL) per 50 lb of body weight of animal, up to a maximum of 3 fl oz for any one animal.

Goats:

Target Insects: Lice.

Application: **Apply along back. Use ¼ fl oz (7.5 mL)

per 50 lb of body weight of animal, up to a maximum of 3 fl oz for any one animal.

Repeat treatment as needed, but not more than once every 2 weeks. For optimum lice control, additional treatments at 14 day intervals may be necessary. Do not use more than once every 2 weeks.

†Duration of activity for horn fly control may vary due to pyrethroid resistance, environmental conditions and management factors (i.e., sanitation, animal husbandry, facilities, etc.)

**DURASECT® Long-Acting Livestock Pour-On is to be used in conjunction with the DURASECT® application gun or dipper. Do not use this product as a spray.

Precautionary Statements: Hazards to Humans and Domestic Animals: Caution. Harmful if absorbed through skin. Avoid contact with eyes, skin or clothing. Wash thoroughly with soap and water after handling.

Statement of Practical Treatment:

If on skin: Wash with plenty of soap and water. Get medical attention if irritation persists.

If in eyes: Flush eyes with plenty of water. Get medical attention if irritation persists.

If swallowed: Call a physician immediately.

Environmental Hazards: This pesticide is extremely toxic to fish. Use with care when applying to areas adjacent to any body of water. Do not add directly to water. Do not contaminate water when disposing of equipment washwaters. Apply this product as specified on the label.

Storage and Disposal: Do not contaminate water, food, or feed by storage or disposal.

Storage: Keep container sealed when not in use. Do not store near food or feed.

Disposal: Triple rinse (or equivalent). Then offer for recycling, or puncture and discard in trash. The container is made of High Density Polyethylene (HDPE) #2 and can be offered for recycling.

Caution(s): Keep out of reach of children.

Presentation: 1 gallon.

Compendium Code No.: 36900810 05-9649-35-0

DURASECT® II LONG-ACTING LIVESTOCK POUR-ON

Pfizer Animal Health **Topical Insecticide**

EPA Reg. No.: 1007-91

Active Ingredient(s):

Permethrin (3-phenoxyphenyl) methyl ± cis, trans-3-(2,2-dichlorethyenyl) 2,2-dimethylcyclopropane carboxylate*	5.00%
Pyrethrins	0.10%
Piperonyl butoxide, technical**	1.00%
Inert ingredients	93.90%
Total	100.00%

*cis/trans ratio: Min. 35% (±) cis and max. 65% (±)trans

**Equivalent to 0.80% butylcarbityl (6-propylpiperonyl) ether and 0.20% related compounds

Indications: Ready to use pour-on for beef cattle, lactating and non-lactating dairy cattle, and calves.

Patented water repellent formulation.

Effective in the control of pyrethroid-resistant horn flies.

Up to 6-week control of horn flies†.

Controls face flies for at least 4 weeks.

Controls biting lice.

Treats 60 500-lb cattle or 30 1000-lb cattle.

Directions for Use: It is a violation of Federal Law to use this product in a manner inconsistent with its labeling.

Ready To Use — No dilution necessary, see directions below.

Animal Treatments:

Lactating and Non-Lactating Dairy Cattle, Beef Cattle, and Calves

Target Insects: Horn flies, face flies, and biting lice. Application: Apply along back and down face. Use 0.1 fl oz (3 mL) per 100 lb (45 kg) body wt of animal, up to 1 fl oz (30 mL) for any one animal. If face flies are a particular concern, apply 0.1 fl oz (3 mL) down centerline of forehead and rest of dose along back of animal.

DURASECT® II Long-Acting Livestock Pour-On is to be applied with the squeeze-and pour bottle provided. To use the squeeze-and-pour bottle, remove the cap and inner seal from the calibrated dosing chamber. Estimate the animal's weight and calculate the dose. Squeeze the bottle to fill the dosing chamber to the desired level. Apply product per directions above; do not use product as a spray. Repeat treatment as needed, but not more than once every 2 weeks. For optimum lice control, additional treatments at 14-day intervals may be necessary.

†Duration of activity for horn fly control may vary due to pyrethroid resistance, environmental conditions and management factors (i.e. sanitation, animal husbandry, facilities, etc.).

Precautionary Statements: Hazards to Human and Domestic Animals:

Caution: Harmful if absorbed through skin. Causes moderate eye irritation. Avoid contact with eyes, skin or clothing. Wash thoroughly with soap and water after handling.

Statement of Practical Treatment:

If on Skin: Wash with plenty of soap and water. Get medical attention if irritation persists.

If in Eyes: Flush eyes with plenty of water. Get medical attention if discomfort persists.

If Swallowed: Call a physician immediately.

Environmental Hazards: This pesticide is extremely toxic to fish. Do not contaminate water by cleaning of equipment or disposal of wastes. Apply this product as specified on the label.

Storage and Disposal: Do not contaminate water, food, or feed by storage or disposal.

Storage: Keep container sealed when not in use. Do not store near food or feed.

Disposal: Triple rinse (or equivalent). Then offer for recycling, or puncture and discard in trash. The container is made of High Density Polyethylene (HDPE) #2 and can be offered for recycling.

Warning(s): No withdrawal time. Keep out of reach of children.

Presentation: 450 mL and 900 mL bottles.

Compendium Code No.: 36900101 05-9757-35-0, 07-9757-35-1

DURASOL™

Durvet — **Water Medication**

Liquid Aspirin Concentrate

Active Ingredient(s): Contains 12% Acetylsalicylic Acid (Aspirin).

Indications: A concentrated solution for use in livestock drinking water.

For use in swine, poultry, beef and dairy cattle.

Directions for Use: Open container and add 1 oz of product to 1 gallon of water. Stir stock solution and meter with proportioner at a rate of 1:128 gallons. For seven-day continuous rate, use 4 oz of product to 1 gallon of water on day one and 1 oz of product to 1 gallon of water for the remaining six days.

Precaution(s): Keep container closed when not in use. Store in a cool, dry place.

Flammable - Use with caution.

Caution(s): For animal use only.

Warning(s): Keep out of reach of children.

Presentation: 32 oz (960 mL) (NDC 30798-633-34) containers.

Compendium Code No.: 10840532 — Iss. 09-01

DURAZYME CALF BOLUS

Durvet — **Large Animal Dietary Supplement**

Guaranteed Analysis: Contains 1 x 10^7 CFU/g.

Ingredients: Micro encapsulated *Lactobacillus acidophillus, Bifidobacterium thermophilum, Bifidobacterium longum,* wheat brand, dried whey, limestone cellulose, *Streptococcus faecium,* lactas enzymes, dried egg, maltodextrines.

Indications: DURAZYME CALF BOLUSES are designed to be used on all newborn calves to supplement cow's colostrum. Administer to scouring calves. Calf Boluses enhance appetite, digestion of food, minimizes intestinal infections and aids in fighting diseases.

Directions: Give calf 1 bolus at birth to supplement colostrum. Administer 2 boluses 2 times per day or at first signs of looseness, or first sign of herd health problems. Administer 2 boluses to incoming feedlot cattle and during treatment with antibiotics.

Presentation: Jar of 50 boluses.

Compendium Code No.: 10841751 — 1/01

DURAZYME CALF COLOSTRUM SUPPLEMENT

Durvet — **Large Animal Dietary Supplement**

Guaranteed Analysis: Contains 1 x 10^7 CFU/g.

Ingredients: Dried milk protein, dextrose, dried egg, micro encapsulated *Lactobacilus acidophilus* fermentation product. dried *Bifidobacterium thermophilum* fermentation product, dried *Bifidobacterium longum* fermentation product, dried *Streptococcus faecium* fermentation product. Lactase enzymes, sugar, vegetable oil.

Indications: DURAZYME CALF COLOSTRUM SUPPLEMENT is designed to be used on newborn beef and dairy calves who receive an inadequate supply, or, poor quality colostrum. This special formulation provides nutritional value, energy, and strategic proteins to maintain optimum health coverage. DURAZYME CALF COLOSTRUM SUPPLEMENT is especially formulated for easy mixing and palatability.

Directions: Mix packet with 1 pint to 1 quart of water. Feed or drench the calf within the first 12 hours of life.

Precaution(s): Store package in cool, dry area.

Presentation: 8 oz packet.

Compendium Code No.: 10840541 — 1/01

DURAZYME ENERGY PACK

Durvet — **Large Animal Dietary Supplement**

Guaranteed Analysis: Contains 1 x 10^7 CFU/g.

Ingredients: Malto dextrins, dried whey, dried milk protein, dried egg, micro encapsulated *Lactobacillus acidophilus* fermentation product, dried *Bifidobacterium thermophilum* fermentation product, dried *Bifidobacterium longum* fermentation product, dried *Streptococcus faecium* fermentation product, lactase enzymes.

Indications: Use DURAZYME ENERGY PACK on all chilled and weak calves. DURAZYME ENERGY PACK provides a rapid source of energy which gives calves an immediate energy boost that helps conserve their body reserves. The bacteria, enzymes and strategic proteins (dried egg solids) in DURAZYME ENERGY PACK aid in fighting diseases, minimizing intestinal infections and enhancing the digestion of food. Use when a high energy source is needed.

Directions: Newborn, weak, or chilled calves—Mix packet with 1 pint of warm water. Feed or drench calf immediately. May be administrated as a colostrum supplement or following stress. Repeat dosage as often as needed.

Precaution(s): Store package in cool, dry area.

Presentation: 50 g pack.

Compendium Code No.: 10840551 — 1/01

DURAZYME PASTE FOR CALVES

Durvet — **Large Animal Dietary Supplement**

Guaranteed Analysis: Contains 1 x 10^7 CFU/g.

Ingredients: Corn oil, sodium aluminosilicate, whey dried egg, micro encapsulated *Lactobacillus acidophilus, Bifidobacteriurn longum, Streptococcus faecium,* lactase enzymes, sorbitan monosterate.

Indications: DURAZYME PASTE FOR CALVES aids in fighting diseases, minimizing intestinal infections, and enhancing the digestion of food. Administer DURAZYME PASTE to stressed calves.

Directions:

15 Gram Tube: Give 7-15 grams to calves to supplement colostrum, following stress and at first signs of looseness.

60 Gram Tube: Give 6 to 8 grams to newborn calves to supplement colostrum following stress and at first sign of looseness. Administer 6 to 8 grams to calves and yearlings in feedlots. Give 10 to 15 grams to sick pen cattle.

Precaution(s): Store paste in a cool, dry area.

Presentation: 15 g and 60 g tubes.

Compendium Code No.: 10840561 — 1/01

DURGUARD™ 4

Durvet — **Vaccine**

Bovine Rhinotracheitis-Virus Diarrhea-Parainfluenza 3 Vaccine, Killed Virus

U.S. Vet. Lic. No.: 303

Composition: This vaccine contains an IBR virus, a cytopathic Type 1 BVD virus, a noncytopathic Type 2 BVD virus, and a PI_3 virus propagated on an established bovine cell line. The vaccine is chemically inactivated and adjuvanted with oil. Contains amphotericin B, penicillin, streptomycin, and thimerosal as preservatives.

Indications: For use in healthy cattle as an aid in the prevention of disease caused by infectious bovine rhinotracheitis, bovine virus diarrhea Type 1, bovine virus diarrhea Type 2, and parainfluenza Type 3 viruses.

Dosage and Administration: Shake well before using. Administer 5 mL intramuscularly or subcutaneously. Revaccinate in 4-5 weeks. This vaccine may be administered to pregnant animals at any stage of gestation. Vaccinate dairy cows during the dry off period. Revaccinate annually.

Precaution(s): Store in the dark at 35°-45°F (2°-7°C). Do not freeze. Use entire contents when first opened.

Caution(s): Transient swelling may occur at the site of injection. Anaphylactic reactions may occur following the use of this biological. Symptomatic treatment: Epinephrine.

Warning(s): Do not vaccinate within 60 days prior to slaughter.

Presentation: 10 dose (50 mL), 20 dose (100 mL), and 50 dose (250 mL) vials.

Manufactured by: Advance Biologics, Inc., Freeman, SD 57029

Compendium Code No.: 10841960 — 5/01

DURGUARD™ 5

Durvet — **Vaccine**

Bovine Rhinotracheitis-Virus Diarrhea-Parainfluenza 3-Respiratory Syncytial Virus Vaccine, Killed Virus

U.S. Vet. Lic. No.: 303

Composition: This vaccine contains an IBR virus, a cytopathic Type 1 BVD virus, a non-cytopathic Type 2 BVD virus, a PI_3 virus, and a BRS virus propagated on an established bovine cell line. The vaccine is chemically inactivated and adjuvanted with oil. Contains amphotericin B, penicillin, streptomycin, and thimerosal as preservatives.

Indications: For use in healthy cattle as an aid in the prevention of disease caused by infectious bovine rhinotracheitis, bovine virus diarrhea, parainfluenza Type 3, and bovine respiratory syncytial viruses.

Dosage and Administration: Shake well before using. Administer 5 mL intramuscularly or subcutaneously. Revaccinate in 4-5 weeks. This vaccine may be administered to pregnant animals at any stage of gestation. Vaccinate dairy cows during the dry off period. Revaccinate annually.

Precaution(s): Store in the dark at 35°-45°F (2°-7°C). Do not freeze. Use entire contents when first opened.

Caution(s): Transient swelling may occur at the site of injection. Anaphylactic reactions may occur following the use of this biological. Symptomatic treatment: Epinephrine.

Warning(s): Do not vaccinate within 60 days prior to slaughter.

Presentation: 10 dose (50 mL), 20 dose (100 mL), and 50 dose (250 mL) vials.

Manufactured by: Advance Biologics, Inc., Freeman, SD 57029.

Compendium Code No.: 10840581 — 8/99

DURGUARD™ 5HS

Durvet — **Bacterin-Vaccine**

Bovine Rhinotracheitis-Virus Diarrhea-Parainfluenza 3-Respiratory Syncytial Virus Vaccine, Killed Virus-Haemophilus Somnus Bacterin

U.S. Vet. Lic. No.: 303

Composition: This product contains an IBR virus, a cytopathic Type 1 BVD virus, a non-cytopathic Type 2 BVD virus, a PI_3 virus, and a BRS virus propagated on an established bovine cell line and cultures of *Haemophilus somnus.* The product is chemically inactivated and adjuvanted with oil. Contains amphotericin B, penicillin, streptomycin, and thimerosal as preservatives.

Indications: For use in healthy cattle as an aid in the prevention of disease caused by infectious bovine rhinotracheitis, bovine virus diarrhea, parainfluenza Type 3, and bovine respiratory syncytial viruses and *Haemophilus somnus.*

Dosage and Administration: Shake well before using. Administer 5 mL intramuscularly at 3 months of age or older. Revaccinate in 4-5 weeks. This vaccine may be administered to pregnant animals at any stage of gestation. Vaccinate dairy cows during the dry off period. Revaccinate annually.

Precaution(s): Store in the dark at 35°-45°F (2°-7°C). Do not freeze. Use entire contents when first opened.

Caution(s): Transient swelling may occur at the site of injection. Anaphylactic reactions may occur following the use of this biological. Symptomatic treatment: Epinephrine.

Warning(s): Do not vaccinate within 60 days prior to slaughter.

Presentation: 10 dose (50 mL), 20 dose (100 mL), and 50 dose (250 mL) vials.

Manufactured by: Advance Biologics, Inc., Freeman, SD 57029.

Compendium Code No.: 10840601 — 8/99

DURGUARD™ 5HS+VL5

Durvet — **Bacterin-Vaccine**

Bovine Rhinotracheitis-Virus Diarrhea-Parainfluenza 3-Respiratory Syncytial Virus Vaccine, Killed Virus-Campylobacter Fetus-Haemophilus Somnus-Leptospira Canicola-Grippotyphosa-Hardjo-Icterohaemorrhagiae-Pomona Bacterin

U.S. Vet. Lic. No.: 303

Composition: This product contains an IBR virus, a cytopathic Type 1 BVD virus, a noncytopathic Type 2 BVD virus, a PI_3 virus, and a BRS virus propagated on an established bovine cell line and cultures of *Campylobacter fetus, Haemophilus somnus, Leptospira canicola, grippotyphosa, hardjo, icterohaemorrhagiae,* and *pomona.* The product is chemically inactivated and adjuvanted with oil. Contains amphotericin B, gentamicin, and thimerosal as preservatives.

Indications: For use in healthy breeding cattle as an aid in the prevention of disease caused by infectious bovine rhinotracheitis, bovine virus diarrhea Type 1, bovine virus diarrhea Type 2, parainfluenza Type 3, and bovine respiratory syncytial viruses and *Campylobacter fetus, Haemophilus somnus, Leptospira canicola, grippotyphosa, hardjo, icterohaemorrhagiae,* and *pomona.*

Dosage and Administration: Shake well before using. Administer 5 mL intramuscularly 2-4 weeks prior to breeding. Revaccinate with DurGuard™ 5HS (Bovine Rhinotracheitis-Virus Diarrhea-Parainfluenza 3-Respiratory Syncytial Virus Vaccine-Haemophilus Somnus Bacterin) in 4-5 weeks. Revaccinate annually.
Precaution(s): Store in the dark at 35°-45°F (2°-7°C). Do not freeze. Use entire contents when first opened.
Caution(s): Transient swelling may occur at the site of injection. Milk reduction and transient depression may be observed in lactating dairy cows for 3-6 days following vaccination. Anaphylactic reactions may occur following the use of this biological. Symptomatic treatment: Epinephrine.
Warning(s): Do not vaccinate within 60 days prior to slaughter.
Presentation: 10 dose (50 mL) and 50 dose (250 mL) vials.
Manufactured by: Advance Biologics, Inc., Freeman, SD 57029
Compendium Code No.: 10841970

8/01

D

DURGUARD™ 5+VL5

Durvet **Bacterin-Vaccine**

Bovine Rhinotracheitis-Virus Diarrhea-Parainfluenza 3-Respiratory Syncytial Virus Vaccine, Killed Virus-Campylobacter Fetus-Leptospira Canicola-Grippotyphosa-Hardjo-Icterohaemorrhagiae-Pomona Bacterin

U.S. Vet. Lic. No.: 303
Composition: This product contains an IBR virus, a cytopathic Type 1 BVD virus, a non-cytopathic Type 2 BVD virus, a PI_3 virus, and a BRS virus propagated on an established bovine cell line and cultures of *Campylobacter fetus, Leptospira canicola, grippotyphosa, hardjo, icterohaemorrhagiae*, and *pomona*. The product is chemically inactivated and adjuvanted with oil. Contains amphotericin B, penicillin, streptomycin, and thimerosal as preservatives.
Indications: For use in healthy breeding cattle as an aid in the prevention of disease caused by infectious bovine rhinotracheitis, bovine virus diarrhea, parainfluenza Type 3, and bovine respiratory syncytial viruses and *Campylobacter fetus, Leptospira canicola, grippotyphosa, hardjo, icterohaemorrhagiae*, and *pomona*.
Dosage and Administration: Shake well before using. Administer 5 mL intramuscularly 2-4 weeks prior to breeding. Revaccinate with DurGuard™ 5 (Bovine Rhinotracheitis-Virus Diarrhea-Parainfluenza 3-Respiratory Syncytial Virus Vaccine) in 4-5 weeks. Revaccinate annually.
Precaution(s): Store in the dark at 35°-45°F (2°-7°C). Do not freeze. Use entire contents when first opened.
Caution(s): Transient swelling may occur at the site of injection. Milk reduction and transient depression may be observed in lactating dairy cows for 3-6 days following vaccination. Anaphylactic reactions may occur following the use of this biological. Symptomatic treatment: Epinephrine.
Warning(s): Do not vaccinate within 60 days prior to slaughter.
Presentation: 10 dose (50 mL) and 50 dose (250 mL) vials.
Manufactured by: Advance Biologics, Inc., Freeman, SD 57029.
Compendium Code No.: 10840591

8/99

DURGUARD™ 10

Durvet **Bacterin-Vaccine**

Bovine Rhinotracheitis-Virus Diarrhea-Parainfluenza 3-Respiratory Syncytial Virus Vaccine, Killed Virus-Leptospira Canicola-Grippotyphosa-Hardjo-Icterohaemorrhagiae-Pomona Bacterin

U.S. Vet. Lic. No.: 303
Composition: This product contains an IBR virus, a cytopathic Type 1 BVD virus, a noncytopathic Type 2 BVD virus, a PI_3 virus, and a BRS virus propagated on an established bovine cell line and cultures of *Leptospira canicola, grippotyphosa, hardjo, icterohaemorrhagiae*, and *pomona*. The product is chemically inactivated and adjuvanted with oil. Contains amphotericin B, penicillin, streptomycin, and thimerosal as preservatives.
Indications: For use in healthy cattle as an aid in the prevention of disease caused by infectious bovine rhinotracheitis, bovine virus diarrhea, parainfluenza Type 3, and bovine respiratory syncytial viruses and *Leptospira canicola, grippotyphosa, hardjo, icterohaemorrhagiae*, and *pomona*.
Dosage and Administration: Shake well before using. Administer 5 mL intramuscularly. Revaccinate with DurGuard™ 5 (Bovine Rhinotracheitis-Virus Diarrhea-Parainfluenza 3-Respiratory Syncytial Virus Vaccine) in 4-5 weeks. Revaccinate annually.
Precaution(s): Store in the dark at 35°-45°F (2°-7°C). Do not freeze. Use entire contents when first opened.
Caution(s): Transient swelling may occur at the site of injection. Anaphylactic reactions may occur following the use of this biological. Symptomatic treatment: Epinephrine.
Warning(s): Do not vaccinate within 60 days prior to slaughter.
Presentation: 10 dose (50 mL) and 50 dose (250 mL) vials.
Manufactured by: Advance Biologics, Inc.
Compendium Code No.: 10840570

DURGUARD™ 10HS

Durvet **Bacterin-Vaccine**

Bovine Rhinotracheitis-Virus Diarrhea-Parainfluenza 3-Respiratory Syncytial Virus Vaccine, Killed Virus-Haemophilus Somnus-Leptospira Canicola-Grippotyphosa-Hardjo-Icterohaemorrhagiae-Pomona Bacterin

U.S. Vet. Lic. No.: 303
Composition: This product contains an IBR virus, a cytopathic Type 1 BVD virus, a noncytopathic Type 2 BVD virus, a PI_3 virus, and a BRS virus propagated on an established bovine cell line and cultures of *Haemophilus somnus, Leptospira canicola, grippotyphosa, hardjo, icterohaemorrhagiae*, and *pomona*. The product is chemically inactivated and adjuvanted with oil. Contains amphotericin B, gentamicin, and thimerosal as preservatives.
Indications: For use in healthy breeding cattle as an aid in the prevention of disease caused by infectious bovine rhinotracheitis, bovine virus diarrhea Type 1, bovine virus diarrhea Type 2, parainfluenza Type 3, and bovine respiratory syncytial viruses and *Haemophilus somnus, Leptospira canicola, grippotyphosa, hardjo, icterohaemorrhagiae*, and *pomona*.
Dosage and Administration: Shake well before using. Administer 5 mL intramuscularly. Revaccinate with DurGuard™ 5HS (Bovine Rhinotracheitis-Virus Diarrhea-Parainfluenza 3-Respiratory Syncytial Virus Vaccine-Haemophilus Somnus Bacterin) in 4-5 weeks. Vaccinate dairy cows during the dry off period. Revaccinate annually.
Precaution(s): Store in the dark at 35°-45°F (2°-7°C). Do not freeze. Use entire contents when first opened.
Caution(s): Transient swelling may occur at the site of injection. Anaphylactic reactions may occur following the use of this biological. Symptomatic treatment: Epinephrine.
Warning(s): Do not vaccinate within 60 days prior to slaughter.
Presentation: 10 dose (50 mL) and 50 dose (250 mL) vials.
Manufactured by: Advance Biologics, Inc., Freeman, SD 57029
Compendium Code No.: 10841980

5/01

DURICOL™ CHLORAMPHENICOL CAPSULES U.S.P. ℞

V.P.C. **Chloramphenicol**

NADA No.: 065-150
Active Ingredient(s): Each capsule contains:
Chloramphenicol . . . . . 50 mg
Chloramphenicol . . . . . 100 mg
Chloramphenicol . . . . . 250 mg
Chloramphenicol . . . . . 500 mg
Indications: For oral treatment of the following conditions in dogs caused by susceptible micro-organisms:

Bacterial infections of the urinary tract caused by susceptible micro-organisms: *Escherichia coli, A. aerogenes*, hemolytic staphylococcus, *Streptococcus* spp., *Corynebacterium renalis, Proteus vulgaris*.

Bacterial pulmonary infections caused by susceptible micro-organisms: *Brucella bronchiseptica, Streptococcus pyogenes*, and *Staphylococcus aureus*.

Secondary bacterial infections associated with canine distemper caused by susceptible micro-organisms: *Brucella bronchiseptica, Streptococcus* spp.

Bacterial enteritis caused by susceptible micro-organisms: *E. coli, Proteus* spp., *Salmonella* spp., *Vibrio* spp.

Appropriate supportive therapy should be used when indicated. Most susceptible infectious disease organisms will respond to chloramphenicol therapy in three to five days when the recommended dosage regimen is followed.

Laboratory tests should be conducted including *in vitro* culturing and susceptibility tests on samples collected prior to treatment.

Pharmacology: Chloramphenicol is a broad-spectrum antibiotic providing rapid clinical response and having therapeutic activity against a wide variety of pathogens including many gram-positive and gram-negative bacteria, rickettsiae, and certain of the larger viruses.

In vitro, chloramphenicol exerts its bacteriostatic action by inhibiting protein synthesis in susceptible organisms. When administered orally in dogs, it is rapidly absorbed from the intestinal tract and diffuses readily into all body tissues, but at different concentrations. The highest concentrations are found in the liver and kidney of dogs indicating that these organs are the main routes of inactivation and excretion for the metabolites.

Dosage and Administration: Dogs: 25 mg per pound of body weight every six (6) hours for oral administration.

If a response to chloramphenicol therapy is not obtained within three (3) to five (5) days, discontinue its use and review the diagnosis. Also, a change of therapy should be considered.

Contraindication(s): Because of the potential for antagonism, chloramphenicol should not be administered simultaneously with penicillin or streptomycin.
Caution(s): Federal law restricts this drug to use by or on the order of a licensed veterinarian.

In vitro tissue culture studies using canine bone marrow cells have demonstrated that extremely high concentrations of chloramphenicol inhibit both uptake of iron by the nucleated red cells and incorporation of iron into heme. Considering this, chloramphenicol should be administered cautiously to animals with hematopoietic dysfunction. The drug should be administered cautiously to animals with impaired kidney or liver functions.

Warning(s): Not for use in animals which are raised for food production.

Chloramphenicol products must not be used in meat, egg, or milk producing animals. The length of time that residues persist in milk or tissues has not been determined.

The product is for use in dogs only.

Chloramphenicol products should not be administered in conjunction with or two hours prior to the induction of general anesthesia with pentobarbital.

The safety of chloramphenicol products for use in animals maintained for breeding purposes has not been established.

Side Effects: Certain individual dogs may exhibit transient vomiting or diarrhea after an oral dose of 25 mg per pound of body weight.
Presentation: 50 mg: Bottles of 1,000 capsules
100 mg: Bottles of 1,000 capsules.
250 mg: Bottles of 100 and 1,000 capsules.
500 mg: Bottles of 100, 500 and 1,000 capsules.
Compendium Code No.: 10430001

DURIRON

Durvet **Iron-Oral**

Chelated Oral Supplement

Guaranteed Analysis:

Iron	50 mg/cc	18,000 mg/lb	3.96%
Copper	5 mg/cc	1,800 mg/lb	0.396%

Maximum Moisture 49.1%

Ingredients: Ferrous proteinate, copper proteinate, dried torula yeast, guar gum, artificial flavoring and water.

Indications: DURIRON is designed to raise the piglet's blood iron, and keep it up for up to three weeks. No needle problems with DURIRON.
Pharmacology: The special chelation process bonds iron into easily digestible organic protein molecules. The pig's system absorbs the iron easily.
Directions: Always shake well just before using.

Colostrum: Vital for newborn piglets. It allows the sow to pass on the antibodies to help the piglets ward off infection and disease. The piglets should nurse immediately, within 15 minutes of birth, definitely within 2 hours. Colostrum must be absorbed by the pigs for the first 6-8 hours, and the piglets should be active and nursing well before giving DURIRON. Colostrum helps buffer the harshness of the iron.

Timing: For the best results, give 2 cc (one pump) from 12 hours to 24 hours after farrowing. Before dosing, be sure all piglets are nursing, especially small weak pigs.

For the best efficiency, many do their entire processing routine (clip eye teeth, apply iodine to navel etc.) within the 12 to 24 hour time slot.

If you wait until after 24 hours, the pigs will be less likely to absorb iron due to "gut closure". After this, giving DURIRON is still worthwhile, it is just not quite as efficient.

In most cases, one pump is all they need. The fastest growing piglets may require a second pump at 7-10 days.

Proper Oral Administration: While holding the pig's head parallel to the floor, insert the pump dispenser spout just inside the mouth of the pig, slightly above the center of the tongue. Do not force the product down the throat (inhalation of any foreign matter into the lungs may cause pneumonia or suffocation).

Push the plunger just once for each pig. Each stroke gives 2 cc, including 100 mg of iron and 10 mg of copper.

Housekeeping: The pump will perform best if it is rinsed clean after use, and re-sealed with the cap. The product may thicken due to evaporation. Restore its consistency with distilled water and shake well.

Precaution(s): Store and use at room temperature.
Warning(s): Keep out of reach of children. Not for human use.
Side Effects: Possible Side Effects: DURIRON was designed to make iron easily available to the pig. Unfortunately, as iron becomes more available to the pig, it also becomes more available to bacteria present in the digestive tract.

Certain strains of intestinal bacteria can multiply to a pathological level in the presence of iron and produce toxins. These can cause vomiting, scouring, or even death if left untreated for too long.

The instances are rare, but may occur. Watch the pigs carefully after using the supplement. It may be necessary to follow the iron treatment with an appropriate scours treatment. It is suggested that a veterinarian be consulted.

Presentation: 200 cc (100 pig size).
Compendium Code No.: 10840611 9/93

DURVAC™ APPEAR-HP

Durvet **Bacterin**
Actinobacillus Pleuropneumoniae-Bordetella Bronchiseptica-Erysipelothrix Rhusiopathiae-Haemophilus Parasuis-Pasteurella Multocida Bacterin
U.S. Vet. Lic. No.: 303
Composition: This bacterin contains inactivated cultures of *Actinobacillus pleuropneumoniae* serotypes 1, 5, and 7, *Bordetella bronchiseptica, Erysipelothrix rhusiopathiae, Haemophilus parasuis*, and *Pasteurella multocida* Type A adjuvanted with aluminum hydroxide.
Indications: For use in healthy swine as an aid in the prevention and control of disease caused by *Actinobacillus pleuropneumoniae* serotypes 1, 5, and 7, *Bordetella bronchiseptica, Erysipelothrix rhusiopathiae, Haemophilus parasuis*, and *Pasteurella multocida* Type A.
Dosage and Administration: Shake well before using. This product is designed for use in feeder pigs from sows previously vaccinated with DurVac™ AR-4 (Bordetella Bronchiseptica-Erysipelothrix Rhusiopathiae-Pasteurella Multocida Bacterin). Administer 5 mL intramuscularly at 7 weeks of age or older. Revaccinate in 2-3 weeks.
Precaution(s): Store in the dark at 35°-45°F (2°-7°C). Do not freeze. Use entire contents when first opened.
Caution(s): Anaphylactic reactions may occur following the use of this biological. Symptomatic treatment: Epinephrine.
Warning(s): Do not vaccinate within 21 days prior to slaughter.
Presentation: 20 dose (100 mL) and 50 dose (250 mL) vials.
Manufactured by: Advance Biologics, Inc.
Compendium Code No.: 10840620

DURVAC™ AR

Durvet **Bacterial Vaccine**
Bordetella Bronchiseptica Vaccine, Avirulent Live Culture
U.S. Vet. Lic. No.: 303
Composition: This vaccine contains an avirulent live culture of *Bordetella bronchiseptica.*
Indications: For use in healthy swine as an aid in the prevention and control of atrophic rhinitis caused by *Bordetella bronchiseptica.*
Dosage and Administration: Shake well before using. Administer 2 mL intramuscularly to gilts and sows 5 and 2 weeks prior to farrowing. Administer 1 mL intranasally (½ mL into each nostril) to piglets 1 day of age.
Precaution(s): Store in the dark at 35°-45°F (2°-7°C). Do not freeze. Needles and syringes should not be sterilized with chemicals. Use entire contents when first opened. Burn the container and any unused contents.
Caution(s): Do not use this vaccine in conjunction with antibiotics effective against *Bordetella bronchiseptica.* Anaphylactic reactions may occur following the use of this biological. Symptomatic treatment: Epinephrine.
Warning(s): Do not vaccinate within 21 days prior to slaughter.
Presentation: 30 piglet/15 sow doses (30 mL).
Manufactured by: Advance Biologics, Inc., Freeman, SD 57029.
Compendium Code No.: 10841761 8/99

DURVAC™ AR-4

Durvet **Bacterin-Toxoid**
Bordetella Bronchiseptica-Erysipelothrix Rhusiopathiae-Pasteurella Multocida Bacterin-Toxoid
U.S. Vet. Lic. No.: 303
Composition: This bacterin contains cultures of *Bordetella bronchiseptica, Erysipelothrix rhusiopathiae, Pasteurella multocida* Type A and toxigenic *Pasteurella multocida* Type D adjuvanted with aluminum hydroxide.
Indications: For use in healthy swine as an aid in the prevention and control of atrophic rhinitis caused by *Bordetella bronchiseptica* or the toxin of *Pasteurella multocida* Types A and D, erysipelas caused by *Erysipelothrix rhusiopathiae* and pneumoniae caused by *Pasteurella multocida* Type A.
Dosage and Administration: Shake well before using. Administer intramuscularly or subcutaneously. Four doses must be given (two gilt/sow doses and two piglet doses). Vaccinate gilts and sows with a 5 mL dose at 5 and 2 weeks prior to farrowing. Vaccinate piglets from vaccinated dams with a 1 mL dose at 7-10 days of age and a 2 mL dose 2 weeks later.
Precaution(s): Store in the dark at 35°-45°F (2°-7°C). Do not freeze. Use entire contents when first opened.
Caution(s): Anaphylactic reactions may occur following the use of this biological. Symptomatic treatment: Epinephrine.
Warning(s): Do not vaccinate within 21 days prior to slaughter.
Presentation: 10 gilt/sow doses or 25/50 piglet doses (50 mL vials) and 20 gilt/sow doses or 50/100 piglet doses (100 mL vials).
Manufactured by: Advance Biologics, Inc.
Compendium Code No.: 10840630

DURVAC™ E-AR

Durvet **Vaccine**
Bordetella Bronchiseptica-Erysipelothrix Rhusiopathiae Vaccine, Avirulent Live Culture
U.S. Vet. Lic. No.: 303
Composition: This combination vaccine contains avirulent live cultures of *Bordetella bronchiseptica* and *Erysipelothrix rhusiopathiae.*
Indications: For use in healthy swine as an aid in the prevention and control of disease caused by *Bordetella bronchiseptica* and *Erysipelothrix rhusiopathiae.*
Dosage and Administration: Aseptically rehydrate DurVac™ E with DurVac™ AR supplied. Shake well before using. Administer 2 mL intramuscularly to gilts and sows 5 and 2 weeks prior to farrowing. Administer 1 mL intranasally (½ mL into each nostril) to piglets 1 day of age.
Precaution(s): Store in the dark at 35°-45°F (2°-7°C). Do not freeze. Needles and syringes should not be sterilized with chemicals. Use entire contents when first opened. Burn this container and any unused contents.
Caution(s): Do not use this vaccine in conjunction with antibiotics effective against *Bordetella bronchiseptica* or *Erysipelothrix rhusiopathiae.* Anaphylactic reactions may occur following the use of this biological. Symptomatic treatment: Epinephrine.
Warning(s): Do not vaccinate within 21 days prior to slaughter.
Presentation: 30 piglet doses and 15 gilt/sow doses (30 mL vials).
Manufactured by: Advance Biologics, Inc.
Compendium Code No.: 10840640

DURVAC™ EC

Durvet **Bacterin**
Escherichia Coli Bacterin
U.S. Vet. Lic. No.: 303
Composition: This bacterin contains inactivated cultures of K88, K99, 987P, and F41 piliated *Escherichia coli* adjuvanted with aluminum hydroxide.
Indications: For use in healthy pregnant swine as an aid in the prevention and control of disease in piglets caused by K88, K99, 987P, and F41 piliated *Escherichia coli.*
Dosage and Administration: Shake well before using. Administer 2 mL intramuscularly 5 and 2 weeks prior to farrowing. Revaccinate prior to each subsequent farrowing.
Precaution(s): Store in the dark at 35°-45°F (2°-7°C). Do not freeze. Use entire contents when first opened.
Caution(s): It is essential that newborn pigs receive colostrum from the vaccinated dam. Anaphylactic reactions may occur following the use of this biological. Symptomatic treatment: Epinephrine.
Warning(s): Do not vaccinate within 21 days prior to slaughter.
Presentation: 10 dose (20 mL) and 50 dose (100 mL) vials.
Manufactured by: Advance Biologics, Inc.
Compendium Code No.: 10840670

DURVAC™ EC-C

Durvet **Bacterin-Toxoid**
Clostridium Perfringens Type C-Escherichia Coli Bacterin-Toxoid
U.S. Vet. Lic. No.: 303
Composition: This product contains inactivated cultures of *Clostridium perfringens* Type C and K88, K99, 987P, and F41 piliated *Escherichia coli* adjuvanted with aluminum hydroxide.
Indications: For use in healthy pregnant swine as an aid in the prevention and control of disease in piglets caused by *Clostridium perfringens* Type C and K88, K99, 987P, and F41 piliated *Escherichia coli.*
Dosage and Administration: Shake well before using. Administer 2 mL intramuscularly 5 and 2 weeks prior to farrowing. Revaccinate prior to each subsequent farrowing.
Precaution(s): Store in the dark at 35°-45°F (2°-7°C). Do not freeze. Use entire contents when first opened.
Caution(s): It is essential that newborn pigs receive colostrum from the vaccinated dam. Anaphylactic reactions may occur following the use of this biological. Symptomatic treatment: Epinephrine.
Warning(s): Do not vaccinate within 21 days prior to slaughter.
Presentation: 10 dose (20 mL) and 50 dose (100 mL) vials.
Manufactured by: Advance Biologics, Inc.
Compendium Code No.: 10840680

DURVAC™ E. COLI 3

Durvet **Antibodies**
Escherichia Coli Antibody, Equine Origin
U.S. Vet. Lic. No.: 303
Composition: This product is prepared from the blood of horses hyperimmunized with K88, K99, and 987P piliated *Escherichia coli.* Contains oxytetracycline, phenol, and thimerosal as preservatives.
Indications: For use in newborn piglets as an aid in the prevention of colibacillosis caused by K88, K99, and 987P piliated *Escherichia coli.*
Dosage and Administration: Shake well before using. Insert dispenser into bottle. Place dispenser extender on nozzle. Administer 2 mL (1 pump stroke) orally to piglets less than 12 hours old. Slowly dispense toward the back of the piglet's mouth. Colostrum should be fed to each piglet.
Precaution(s): Store in the dark at 35°-45°F (2°-7°C). Do not freeze. Use entire contents when first opened.

Caution(s): Anaphylactic reactions may occur following the use of this biological. Symptomatic treatment: Epinephrine.
Warning(s): Do not administer within 21 days prior to slaughter.
Presentation: 50 dose (100 mL) and 100 dose (200 mL) vials.
Manufactured by: Advance Biologics, Inc.
Compendium Code No.: 10840650

DURVAC™ E. COLI 3C

Durvet **Antibodies-Antitoxin**

Clostridium Perfringens Type C Antitoxin-Escherichia Coli Antibody, Equine Origin
U.S. Vet. Lic. No.: 303
Composition: This product is prepared from the blood of horses hyperimmunized with *Clostridium perfringens* Type C and K88, K99, and 987P piliated *Escherichia coli.* Contains oxytetracycline, phenol, and thimerosal as preservatives.
Indications: For use in newborn piglets as an aid in the prevention of disease caused by *Clostridium perfringens* Type C and K88, K99, and 987P piliated *Escherichia coli.*
Dosage and Administration: Shake well before using. Insert dispenser into bottle. Place dispenser extender on nozzle. Administer 2 mL (1 pump stroke) orally to piglets less than 6 hours old. Slowly dispense toward the back of the piglet's mouth. Colostrum should be fed to each piglet.
Precaution(s): Store in the dark at 35°-45°F (2°-7°C). Do not freeze. Use entire contents when first opened.
Caution(s): Anaphylactic reactions may occur following the use of this biological. Symptomatic treatment: Epinephrine.
Warning(s): Do not administer within 21 days prior to slaughter.
Presentation: 50 dose (100 mL) and 100 dose (200 mL) vials.
Manufactured by: Advance Biologics, Inc.
Compendium Code No.: 10840660

DURVAC™ ERY

Durvet **Bacterin**

Erysipelothrix Rhusiopathiae Bacterin
U.S. Vet. Lic. No.: 303
Composition: This bacterin contains an inactivated culture of *Erysipelothrix rhusiopathiae* adjuvanted with aluminum hydroxide.
Indications: For use in healthy swine as an aid in the prevention and control of erysipelas caused by *Erysipelothrix rhusiopathiae.*
Dosage and Administration: Shake well before using. Administer 2 mL intramuscularly. Repeat in 21 days. Revaccinate annually.
Precaution(s): Store in the dark at 35°-45°F (2°-7°C). Do not freeze. Use entire contents when first opened.
Caution(s): Anaphylactic reactions may occur following the use of this biological. Symptomatic treatment: Epinephrine.
Warning(s): Do not vaccinate within 21 days prior to slaughter.
Presentation: 50 dose (100 mL), 125 dose (250 mL), and 250 dose (500 mL) vials.
Manufactured by: Advance Biologics, Inc.
Compendium Code No.: 10840690

DURVAC™ MYCO

Durvet **Bacterin**

Mycoplasma Hyopneumoniae Bacterin
U.S. Vet. Lic. No.: 303
Composition: This bacterin contains inactivated culture of *Mycoplasma hyopneumoniae.* Contains penicillin and thimerosal as preservatives.
Indications: For use in healthy swine as an aid in the prevention and control of pneumonia caused by *Mycoplasma hyopneumoniae.*
Dosage and Administration: Shake well before using. Administer 1 mL intramuscularly at 2 weeks of age or older. Revaccinate in 2 weeks.
Precaution(s): Store in the dark at 35°-45°F (2°-7°C). Do not freeze. Use entire contents when first opened.
Caution(s): Anaphylactic reactions may occur following the use of this biological. Symptomatic treatment: Epinephrine.
Warning(s): Do not vaccinate within 21 days prior to slaughter.
Presentation: 100 dose (100 mL) and 250 dose (250 mL) vials.
Manufactured by: Advance Biologics, Inc.
Compendium Code No.: 10840700

DURVAC™ P-E-L

Durvet **Bacterin-Vaccine**

Parvovirus Vaccine, Killed Virus-Erysipelothrix Rhusiopathiae-Leptospira Canicola-Grippotyphosa-Hardjo-Icterohaemorrhagiae-Pomona Bacterin
U.S. Vet. Lic. No.: 303
Composition: This product contains inactivated cultures of porcine parvovirus, *Erysipelothrix rhusiopathiae, Leptospira canicola, grippotyphosa, hardjo, icterohaemorrhagiae,* and *pomona* adjuvanted with aluminum hydroxide. Contains amphotericin B, penicillin, streptomycin, and thimerosal as preservatives.
Indications: For use in healthy swine as an aid in the prevention and control of disease caused by porcine parvovirus, *Erysipelothrix rhusiopathiae, Leptospira canicola, grippotyphosa, hardjo, icterohaemorrhagiae,* and *pomona.*
Dosage and Administration: Shake well before using. Administer 5 mL intramuscularly to gilts and sows 4-6 weeks prior to breeding. Repeat in 3-4 weeks. Revaccinate with a single dose 4-6 weeks prior to each subsequent breeding. Vaccinate boars semiannually.
Precaution(s): Store in the dark at 35°-45°F (2°-7°C). Do not freeze. Use entire contents when first opened.
Caution(s): Anaphylactic reactions may occur following the use of this biological. Symptomatic treatment: Epinephrine.
Warning(s): Do not vaccinate within 21 days prior to slaughter.
Presentation: 10 dose (50 mL), 20 dose (100 mL), and 50 dose (250 mL) vials.
Manufactured by: Advance Biologics, Inc.
Compendium Code No.: 10840710

DURVAC™ STREP

Durvet **Bacterin**

Streptococcus Suis Bacterin
U.S. Vet. Lic. No.: 303
Composition: This bacterin contains an inactivated culture of *Streptococcus suis* adjuvanted with aluminum hydroxide.
Indications: For use In healthy swine as an aid in the prevention and control of disease caused by *Streptococcus suis* serotype 2.
Dosage and Administration: Shake well before using. Administer 2 mL intramuscularly to gilts and sows 5 and 2 weeks prior to each farrowing to provide passive protection in the newborn pigs. Administer 2 mL intramuscularly to piglets at 3 and 5 weeks of age for active immunization.
Precaution(s): Store in the dark at 35°-45°F (2°-7°C). Do not freeze. Use entire contents when first opened.
Caution(s): It is essential that newborn pigs receive colostrum from the vaccinated dam to insure passive immunity. Anaphylactic reactions may occur following the use of this biological. Symptomatic treatment: Epinephrine.
Warning(s): Do not vaccinate within 21 days prior to slaughter.
Presentation: 50 dose (100 mL) and 125 dose (250 mL) vials.
Manufactured by: Advance Biologics, Inc., Freeman, SD 57029.
Compendium Code No.: 10840721 8/99

DVMECTIN™ LIQUID FOR HORSES ℞

DVM **Parasiticide-Oral**

(ivermectin) 10 mg/mL
ANADA No.: 200-292
Active Ingredient(s): DVMECTIN™ (ivermectin) Liquid is a clear, ready-to-use solution with each mL containing 1% ivermectin (10 mg), 0.2 mL propylene glycol, 80 mg polysorbate 80, 9 mg sodium phosphate monobasic monohydrate, 1.3 mg sodium phosphate dibasic anhydrous, 1 mg butylated hydroxytoluene, 0.1 mg disodium edetate, 3% benzyl alcohol and purified water q.s. ad 100%.
Indications: DVMECTIN™ (ivermectin) Liquid is indicated for the effective treatment and control of the following parasites or parasitic conditions in horses:

Large Strongyles: *Strongylus vulgaris* (adults and arterial larval stages), *S. edentatus* (adults and tissue stages), *S. equinus* (adults), *Triodontophorus* spp (adults).

Small Strongyles - including those resistant to some benzimidazole class compounds (adults and fourth-stage larvae): *Cyathostomum* spp, *Cylicocyclus* spp, *Cylicostephanus* spp, *Cylicodontophorus* spp.

Pinworms (adults and fourth-stage larvae): *Oxyuris equi.*
Ascarids (adults and third- and fourth-stage larvae): *Parascaris equorum.*
Hairworms (adults): *Trichostrongylus axei.*
Large-mouth Stomach Worms (adults): *Habronema muscae.*
Bots (oral and gastric stages): *Gastrophilus* spp.
Lungworms (adults and fourth-stage larvae): *Dictyocaulus arnfieldi.*
Intestinal Threadworms (adults): *Strongyloides westeri.*
Summer Sores caused by *Habronema* and *Draschia* spp cutaneous third-stage larvae.
Dermatitis caused by neck threadworm microfilariae, *Onchocerca* sp.

Pharmacology: DVMECTIN™ is derived from the avermectins, a family of potent, broad-spectrum antiparasitic agents, which are isolated from fermentation of *Streptomyces avermitilis.*

Mode of Action: Ivermectin, one of the avermectins, kills certain parasitic roundworms and ectoparasites such as mites and lice. The avermectins are different in their action from other antiparasitic agents. This action involves a chemical that serves as a signal from one nerve cell to another, or from a nerve cell to a muscle cell. This chemical, a neurotransmitter, is called gamma-aminobutyric acid or GABA.

In roundworms, ivermectin stimulates the release of GABA from nerve endings and enhances binding of GABA to special receptors at nerve junctions, thus interrupting nerve impulses-thereby paralyzing and killing the parasite.

The enhancement of the GABA effect in arthropods such as mites and lice resembles that in roundworms except that nerve impulses are interrupted between the nerve ending and the muscle cell. Again, this leads to paralysis and death.

The principal peripheral neurotransmitter in mammals, acetylcholine, is unaffected by ivermectin. Ivermectin does not readily penetrate the central nervous system of mammals where GABA functions as a neurotransmitter.

Dosage and Administration: Dosage: DVMECTIN™ (ivermectin) Liquid for Horses is formulated for administration by stomach tube (nasogastric intubation) or as an oral drench. The recommended dose is 200 mcg of ivermectin per kilogram (91 mcg/lb) of body weight. Each mL contains sufficient ivermectin to treat 110 lb (50 kg) of body weight: 10 mL will treat an 1100 lb (500 kg) horse.

Administration: Use a calibrated dosing syringe inserted into the bottle to measure the appropriate dose, or pour the DVMECTIN™ (ivermectin) Liquid into a graduated cylinder for dose measurement. Use a clean syringe if accessing the bottle to avoid contaminating the remaining product.

Administration by stomach tube (gravity or positive flow): The recommended dose can be used undiluted or diluted up to 40 times with clean tepid water (see Notes to Veterinarian). Use tepid water to flush any drug remaining in the tube into the horse's stomach.

Administration by drench: For administration by this method, an undiluted dose is usually preferred. Clear the horse's mouth of any food material, elevate the horse's head, and using a syringe, deposit the appropriate dose in the back of the mouth. In order to avoid unnecessary coughing or the potential for material to enter the trachea and lungs, do not use excessive pressure (squirting), do not use a large (diluted) dose volume, and do not deposit the dose in the laryngeal area. Increased dose rejection may occur if the dose is deposited in the buccal space. Keep the horse's head elevated and observe the horse to insure the dose is retained.

Suggested Parasite Control Program: All horses should be included in a regular parasite control program with particular attention being paid to mares, foals and yearlings. Foals should be treated initially at 6 to 8 weeks of age, and routine treatment repeated as appropriate. DVMECTIN™ (ivermectin) Liquid effectively controls gastrointestinal nematodes and bots in horses. Regular treatment will reduce the chances of verminous arteritis and colic caused by *S. vulgaris.* With its broad spectrum, DVMECTIN™ (ivermectin) Liquid is well suited to be the major product in a parasite control program.

Precaution(s): Store in a tightly closed container at room temperature. Do not store above 30°C (86°F).

Protect DVMECTIN™ (ivermectin) Liquid (undiluted or diluted) from light.

Environmental Safety: Studies indicate that when ivermectin comes in contact with the soil, it readily and tightly binds to the soil and becomes inactive over time. Free ivermectin may adversely affect fish and certain water-borne organisms on which they feed. Do not contaminate lakes, streams, or ground water by direct application or by improper disposal of drug containers. Dispose of drug container in an approved landfill or by incineration.

Caution(s): Federal (U.S.A.) law restricts this drug to use by or on the order of a licensed veterinarian.

DVMECTIN™ (ivermectin) Liquid has been formulated specifically for use in horses only. This product should not be used in other animal species as severe adverse reactions, including fatalities in dogs, may result.

For veterinary use only.

Warning(s): Residue Warning: Do not use in horses intended for food purposes.

Refrain from smoking and eating when handling. Wash hands after use. Avoid contact with eyes. Keep this and all drugs out of the reach of children.

Toxicology: Safety: DVMECTIN™ (ivermectin) Liquid may be used in horses of all ages including mares at any stage of pregnancy. Stallions may be treated without adversely affecting their fertility. These horses have been treated with no adverse effects other than those noted under Notes to Veterinarian.

Discussion: DVMECTIN™ (ivermectin) Liquid for Horses has been formulated for professional administration by stomach tube or oral drench. One low-volume dose is effective against important internal parasites, including the arterial stages of *Strongylus vulgaris*, and bots.

Notes To Veterinarian: Swelling and itching reactions after treatment with DVMECTIN™ (ivermectin) Liquid have occurred in horses carrying heavy infections of neck threadworm microfilariae, *Onchocerca* sp. These reactions were most likely the result of microfilariae dying in large numbers. Symptomatic treatment may be advisable. Healing of summer sores involving extensive tissue changes may require other therapy in conjunction with DVMECTIN™ (ivermectin) Liquid. Reinfection, and measures for its prevention, should also be considered.

Special consideration should be given to the effects or potential for injury from handling, restraint, and placement of the tube during administration by stomach tube. DVMECTIN™ (ivermectin) Liquid should be administered by drench if the risks associated with tubing are of concern. Due to the consequences of improper administration (also see Dosage and Administration), DVMECTIN™ (ivermectin) Liquid is intended for use by a veterinarian only and is not recommended for dispensing.

DVMECTIN™ (ivermectin) Liquid in 1 to 20 and 1 to 40 dilutions with tap water has been shown to be stable for 72 hours under the conditions recommended for the product (i.e., at room temperature, in a tightly closed container, protected from light). The diluted product does not promote the growth of common organisms. However, prolonged storage of the diluted product cannot be recommended, as the effects of possible contaminants and interactions with untested materials are unknown.

Presentation: DVMECTIN™ (ivermectin) Liquid for Horses is available in 50 mL, 100 mL and 250 mL plastic bottles.

Manufactured by: Med-Pharmex Inc., Pomona, CA 91767.

Compendium Code No.: 11420620 Rev. 1101

DVM HANDSOAP™

DVM **Hand Soap**

Antibacterial Deodorizing Moisturizing Cleansing Formulation-Triclosan

Active Ingredient(s): Triclosan.

Other Ingredients: Water, sodium C14-16 olefin sulfonate, cocamidopropyl betaine, sodium chloride, polysorbate 20, lauramide DEA, PPG-12-PEG-50 lanolin, linoleamide DEA, fragrance, hydroxypropyl methylcellulose, citric acid, D&C red #28.

Indications: DVM HANDSOAP™ is an antibacterial hand cleanser formulated specifically for veterinarians and animal health technicians. The olefin-based surfactant system cleanses and hydrates the skin and prevents chapping. It is formulated for frequent washing between patients. Its germicidal agent, triclosan, eliminates most common pathogens without damaging the natural ecology of the skin. Leaves the hands soft with a pleasant fragrance.

Directions for Use: Apply to wet hands, lather well, then rinse thoroughly.

Precaution(s): Store at room temperature.

Caution(s): For external use only.

Presentation: 12 fl oz (355 mL) and 1 gallon (3.78 L).

Compendium Code No.: 11420261 Rev 0597

DVM TEARLESS™ SHAMPOO

DVM **Grooming Shampoo**

Tearless, Gentle, Soap-free Hypoallergenic Shampoo

Ingredient(s): Water, PEG-80 sorbitan laurate, cocamidopropyl betaine, sodium trideceth sulfate, steareth-10 allyl ether/acrylates copolymer, glycerin, sodium lauroamphoacetate, PEG-150 distearate, sodium laureth-13 carboxylate, polyquaternium-10, fragrance, triethanolimine, quaternium-15, tetrasodium EDTA, and FD&C yellow #5.

Indications: An ultra-sensitive, tearless, soap-free hypoallergenic formulation to reduce eye irritation in routine cleansing and grooming of animals of all ages. May be used in conjunction with other topical therapeutics.

Directions for Use: Wet coat thoroughly with water and apply sufficient amount of DVM TEARLESS™ Shampoo to lather well into haircoat. Rinse thoroughly. May be used as often as necessary, or as directed by your veterinarian.

Precaution(s): Store at room temperature.

Caution(s): For topical use on animals only.

Warning(s): Keep out of reach of children.

Presentation: 12 fl oz (355 mL) and 1 gallon (3.78 L).

Compendium Code No.: 11420271 Rev 0199 / Rev 0797

DVM TEARLESS™ SPRAY-ON SHAMPOO

DVM **Grooming Shampoo**

Ingredient(s): Water, PEG-80 sorbitan laurate, cocamidopropyl betaine, sodium trideceth sulfate, glycerin, sodium lauroamphoacetate, PEG-150 distearate, sodium laureth-13 carboxylate, polyquaternium-10, fragrance, quaternium-15, tetrasodium EDTA, citric acid and FD&C yellow #5.

Indications: Specifically formulated to reduce eye irritation in routine cleansing and grooming of puppies and kittens. May be used in conjunction with other topical therapeutics. May also be used on animals of all ages.

An ultra-sensitive, tearless, soap-free, hypoallergenic formulation to reduce eye irritation. Contains moisturizing agents for conditioning of skin and haircoat in a fresh, pleasant fragrance.

Directions for Use: Wet coat thoroughly. Apply sufficient amount of DVM TEARLESS™ Shampoo to lather well into haircoat. Rinse thoroughly. May be used as often as necessary, or as directed by your veterinarian.

Precaution(s): Store at room temperature.

Caution(s): For topical use on animals only.

Warning(s): Keep out of reach of children.

Presentation: 12 fl oz (355 mL).

Compendium Code No.: 11420281

D-WORM™ 60 LIQUID WORMER

Farnam **Parasiticide-Oral**

(pyrantel pamoate)

ANADA No.: 200-248

Active Ingredient(s): D-WORM™ 60 (pyrantel pamoate suspension 2.27 mg) is a suspension of pyrantel pamoate in a palatable vanilla-flavored vehicle. Each mL contains 2.27 mg of pyrantel base as pyrantel pamoate.

Indications: D-WORM™ 60 suspension is a highly palatable formulation intended as a single treatment for the removal of large roundworms *(Toxocara canis* and *Toxascaris leonina)* and hookworms *(Anclyostoma caninum* and *Uncinaria stenocephala)* in dogs and puppies. D-WORM™ 60 suspension may also be used to prevent reinfection of *Toxocara canis* in puppies and adult dogs and in lactating bitches after whelping. Consult your veterinarian for assistance in the diagnosis, treatment, and control of parasitism.

Pharmacology: Pyrantel pamoate is a compound belonging to a family classified chemically as tetrahydropyrimidines. It is a yellow, water-insoluble crystalline salt of the tetrahydropyrimidine base and pamoic acid containing 34.7% base activity. The chemical structure and name are given below:

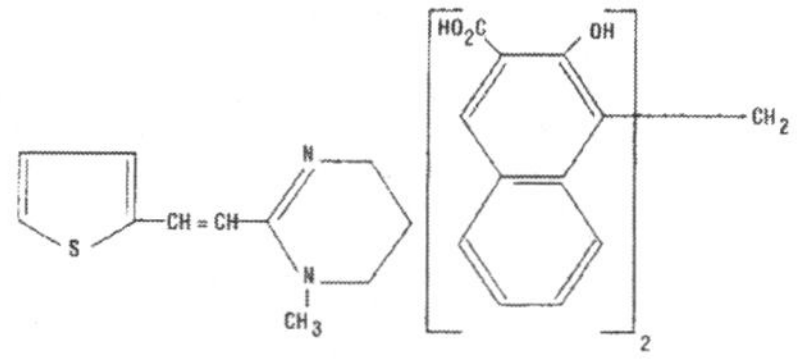

(E)-1,4,5,6-Tetrahydro-1-methyl-2-[2-(2-thienyl) vinyl] pyrimidine 4,4' methylenebis [3-hydroxy-2-naphthoate] (1:1)

Dosage and Administration: Administer one full teaspoon (5 mL) for each 5 lb of body weight (2.27 mg base per lb of body weight). Although most dogs have been observed to find this formulation very palatable and willingly consume it undiluted, it may be necessary to mix a small quantity of formulation in the dog's normal ration to encourage consumption. Fasting prior to or after treatment is not necessary.

For maximum control and prevention of reinfection, it is recommended that puppies be treated at 2, 3, 4, 6, 8 and 10 weeks of age. Lactating bitches should be treated 2-3 weeks after whelping. Adult dogs kept in heavily contaminated quarters may be treated at monthly intervals to prevent *T. canis* reinfection.

Precaution(s): This product is a suspension and as such will separate. To ensure uniform resuspension and to achieve proper dosage, it is extremely important that the product be shaken thoroughly before every use.

Recommended Storage: Store below 86°F (30°C).

Caution(s): For animal use only.

Warning(s): Keep out of reach of children.

Toxicology: Safety: One of the most significant features of D-WORM™ 60 is its wide margin of therapeutic safety in dogs. The acute oral LD_{50} of pyrantel pamoate administered in gelatin capsules to female and male dogs is greater than 314 mg base per lb of body weight, which indicates a therapeutic index in excess of 138 x the recommended dosage. In subacute and chronic studies, no significant morphological abnormalities could be attributed to D-WORM™ 60 when administered to dogs at daily dose rates of up to 94 mg base per lb of body weight (40 x) for periods of 19, 30, and 90 days. Clinical studies conducted in a wide variety of geographic locations using more than 40 different breeds of dogs showed no drug-induced toxic effects. Included in these studies were nursing pups, weaned pups, adults, pregnant bitches, and males at stud. Additional data have demonstrated the safe use of D-WORM™ 60 (pyrantel pamoate) in (1) dogs having heartworm infections and/or receiving medication for heartworm, (2) dogs exposed to organophosphate flea collars or flea/tick dip treatments, and (3) dogs undergoing concurrent treatment or medication at the time of worming such as immunization and antibacterial treatment.

Trial Data: Efficacy: Critical (worm count) studies in dogs demonstrated that D-WORM™ 60 at the recommended dosage is highly efficacious against *T. leonina* (99%), *T. canis* (85%), *A. caninum* (97%), and *U. stenocephala* (94%).

Presentation: 60 mL (2 fl oz) bottle.

Compendium Code No.: 10000621 Iss. 8/98

D-WORM™ 120 LIQUID WORMER

Farnam **Parasiticide-Oral**

(pyrantel pamoate)

ANADA No.: 200-248

Active Ingredient(s): D-WORM™ 120 (pyrantel pamoate suspension 4.54 mg) is a suspension of pyrantel pamoate in a palatable vanilla-flavored vehicle. Each mL contains 4.54 mg of pyrantel base as pyrantel pamoate.

Indications: D-WORM™ 120 suspension is a highly palatable formulation intended as a single treatment for the removal of large roundworms *(Toxocara canis* and *Toxascaris leonina)* and hookworms *(Anclyostoma caninum* and *Uncinaria stenocephala)* in dogs and puppies. D-WORM™ 120 suspension may also be used to prevent reinfection of *Toxocara canis* in puppies and adult dogs and in lactating bitches after whelping. Consult your veterinarian for assistance in the diagnosis, treatment, and control of parasitism.

Pharmacology: Pyrantel pamoate is a compound belonging to a family classified chemically as tetrahydropyrimidines. It is a yellow, water-insoluble crystalline salt of the tetrahydropyrimidine base and pamoic acid containing 34.7% base activity. The chemical structure and name are given below:

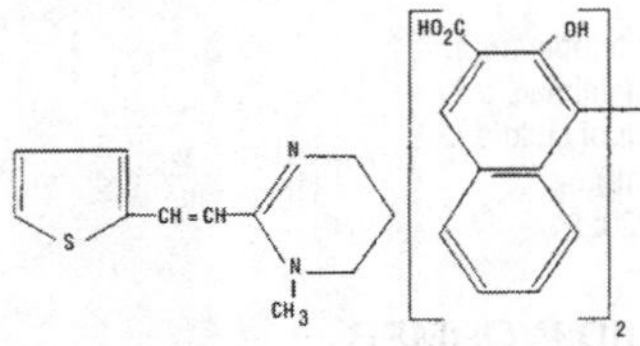

(E)-1,4,5,6-Tetrahydro-1-methyl-2-[2-(2-thienyl) vinyl] pyrimidine 4,4' methylenebis [3-hydroxy-2-naphthoate] (1:1)

Dosage and Administration: Administer one full teaspoon (5 mL) for each 10 lb of body weight (2.27 mg base per lb of body weight). Although most dogs have been observed to find this formulation very palatable and willingly consume it undiluted, it may be necessary to mix a small quantity of formulation in the dog's normal ration to encourage consumption. Fasting prior to or after treatment is not necessary.

For maximum control and prevention of reinfection, it is recommended that puppies be treated at 2, 3, 4, 6, 8 and 10 weeks of age. Lactating bitches should be treated 2-3 weeks after whelping. Adult dogs kept in heavily contaminated quarters may be treated at monthly intervals to prevent *T. canis* reinfection.

Precaution(s): This product is a suspension and as such will separate. To ensure uniform resuspension and to achieve proper dosage, it is extremely important that the product be shaken thoroughly before every use.

Recommended Storage: Store below 86°F (30°C).

Caution(s): For animal use only.

Warning(s): Keep out of reach of children.

Toxicology: Safety: One of the most significant features of D-WORM™ 120 is its wide margin of therapeutic safety in dogs. The acute oral LD_{50} of pyrantel pamoate administered in gelatin capsules to female and male dogs is greater than 314 mg base per lb of body weight, which indicates a therapeutic index in excess of 138 x the recommended dosage. In subacute and chronic studies, no significant morphological abnormalities could be attributed to D-WORM™ 120 when administered to dogs at daily dose rates of up to 94 mg base per lb of body weight (40 x) for periods of 19, 30, and 90 days. Clinical studies conducted in a wide variety of geographic locations using more than 40 different breeds of dogs showed no drug-induced toxic effects. Included in these studies were nursing pups, weaned pups, adults, pregnant bitches, and males at stud. Additional data have demonstrated the safe use of D-WORM™120 (pyrantel pamoate) in (1) dogs having heartworm infections and/or receiving medication for heartworm, (2) dogs exposed to organophosphate flea collars or flea/tick dip treatments, and (3) dogs undergoing concurrent treatment or medication at the time of worming such as immunization and antibacterial treatment.

Trial Data: Efficacy: Critical (worm count) studies in dogs demonstrated that D-WORM™ 120 at the recommended dosage is highly efficacious against *T. leonina* (99%), *T. canis* (85%), *A. caninum* (97%), and *U. stenocephala* (94%).

Presentation: 60 mL (2 fl oz) bottle.

Compendium Code No.: 10000631

Iss. 8/98

D-WORM™ DOG WORMER CHEWABLE TABLETS FOR LARGE DOGS

Farnam **Parasiticide-Oral**

NADA No.: 139-191

Active Ingredient(s): Each tablet contains 113.5 mg pyrantel base as pyrantel pamoate.

Indications: For the removal of large roundworms (ascarids) *(Toxocara canis; Toxascaris leonina)* and hookworms *(Ancylostoma caninum; Uncinaria stenocephala)* in dogs and puppies. To prevent re-infection of *Toxocara canis* in puppies and adult dogs and in lactating bitches after whelping.

For use in animals weighing more than 25 lbs.

Dosage and Administration: For the removal of large roundworms (ascarids) and hookworms in adult dogs or young dogs, weighing more than 25 lbs, administer these tablets according to the weight of the animal.

Weight	Number of Tablets
25 lbs	Give ½ Tablet
26 to 50 lbs	Give 1 Tablet
51 to 75 lbs	Give 1½ Tablets
76 to 100 lbs	Give 2 Tablets

Note: For puppies or small dogs weighing less than 25 lbs, use Farnam Dog Wormer Chewable Tablets For Puppies & Small Dogs.

Offer the proper dosage by hand or in the dog's food container with or without food. Do not withhold food from your dog prior to or after treatment. The presence of these parasites in mature dogs should be confirmed by laboratory fecal examination. A follow-up fecal examination should be conducted in 2 to 4 weeks after first treatment to determine the need for retreatment. Nursing bitches should be treated 2-3 weeks after whelping. Dogs should be routinely treated at monthly intervals to prevent reinfection with large roundworms found in their environment. Retreatment may be necessary at monthly intervals, as determined by laboratory fecal examinations or in animals kept in known contaminated quarters.

Caution(s): Consult your veterinarian for assistance in the diagnosis, treatment and control of parasitism. If your dog looks or acts sick, do not treat with this product.

Warning(s): Not for human consumption.

Keep out of reach of children.

Presentation: 2 tablets and 30 tablets (bulk).

Compendium Code No.: 10000101

D-WORM™ DOG WORMER CHEWABLE TABLETS FOR PUPPIES & SMALL DOGS

Farnam **Parasiticide-Oral**

NADA No.: 139-191

Active Ingredient(s): Each tablet contains 22.7 mg pyrantel base as pyrantel pamoate.

Indications: For the removal of large roundworms (ascarids) *(Toxocara canis; Toxascaris leonina)* and hookworms *(Ancylostoma caninum; Uncinaria stenocephala)* in dogs and puppies. To prevent reinfection of *Toxocara canis* in puppies and adult dogs and in lactating bitches after whelping.

Dosage and Administration: For the removal of large roundworms (ascarids) and hookworms, give 1 tablet for each 10 lbs of body weight. (Dosage is designed to provide at least 2.27 mg per pound of body weight for dogs weighing over 5 lbs, and at least 4.54 mg per pound of body weight for dogs weighing 5 lbs or less). For dogs weighing more than 10 lbs, tablets may be broken in half to provide ½ tablet for each additional 5 lbs body weight. The presence of these parasites should be confirmed by laboratory fecal examination. Do not withhold food from your dog prior to or after treatment.

Offer the proper dosage by hand or in the dog's food container, with or without food. Do not withhold food from your dog prior to or after treatment. A follow-up fecal examination should be conducted in 2 to 4 weeks after first treatment to determine the need for retreatment.

Since anthelmintics cannot be relied upon to prevent reinfection or to remove larvae not present in the intestinal tract at the time of initial treatment, for maximum control, it is recommended that puppies be treated at 2, 3, 4, 6, 8, and 10 weeks of age. Lactating bitches should be treated 2-3 weeks after whelping. Adult dogs should be routinely treated at monthly intervals to protect against environmental *T. canis* reinfection. Retreatment of adult dogs may be necessary at monthly intervals as determined by laboratory fecal examinations or in animals kept in known contaminated quarters.

Caution(s): If your dog looks or acts sick, do not treat with this product. Consult a veterinarian for assistance in the diagnosis, treatment and control of parasitism.

Warning(s): Not for human consumption. Keep out of reach of children.

Presentation: 2 tablets and 30 tablets (bulk).

Compendium Code No.: 10000111

D-WORM™ DOG WORMER TABLETS FOR LARGE DOGS

Farnam **Parasiticide-Oral**

NADA No.: 101-331

Active Ingredient(s): Each tablet contains 113.5 mg pyrantel base as pyrantel pamoate.

Indications: For the removal of ascarids *(Toxocara canis; Toxascaris leonina)* and hookworms *(Ancylostoma caninum; Uncinaria stenocephala)* in dogs and puppies. To prevent reinfection of *Toxocara canis* in puppies and adult dogs and in lactating bitches after whelping.

Dosage and Administration: For the removal of large roundworms (ascarids) and hookworms, give 1 tablet for each 50 lbs of body weight. (Tablets may be broken in half to provide ½ tablet for 25 lbs of body weight. The presence of these parasites should be confirmed by laboratory fecal examination. Do not withhold food from your dog prior to or after treatment.

Place tablet directly into back of mouth or conceal tablet in a small amount of food. A follow-up fecal examination should be conducted in 2 to 4 weeks after first treatment to determine the need for retreatment.

Since anthelmintics cannot be relied upon to prevent reinfection or to remove larvae not present in the intestinal tract at the time of initial treatment, for maximum control, it is recommended that puppies be treated at 2, 3, 4, 6, 8, and 10 weeks of age. Lactating bitches should be treated 2-3 weeks after whelping. Adult dogs should be routinely treated at monthly intervals to protect against environmental *T. canis* reinfection. Retreatment of adult dogs may be necessary at monthly intervals as determined by laboratory fecal examinations or in animals kept in known contaminated quarters..

Caution(s): If your dog looks or acts sick, do not treat with this product. Consult your veterinarian for assistance in the diagnosis, treatment and control of parasitism.

Restricted Drug - Use only as directed.

Warning(s): Not for human consumption. Keep out of reach of children.

Presentation: 2 tablets and 50 tablets (bulk).

Compendium Code No.: 10000121

D-WORM™ DOG WORMER TABLETS FOR PUPPIES & SMALL DOGS

Farnam **Parasiticide-Oral**

NADA No.: 101-331

Active Ingredient(s): Each tablet contains 22.7 mg pyrantel base as pyrantel pamoate.

Indications: For the removal of ascarids *(Toxocara canis; Toxascaris leonina)* and hookworms *(Ancylostoma caninum; Uncinaria stenocephala)* in dogs and puppies. To prevent reinfection of *Toxocara canis* in puppies and adult dogs and in lactating bitches after whelping.

Dosage and Administration: For the removal of large roundworms (ascarids) and hookworms, give 1 tablet for each 10 lbs of body weight. (Dosage is designed to provide at least 2.27 mg per pound body weight for dogs weighing over 5 lbs, and at least 4.54 mg per pound of body weight for dogs weighing less than 5 lbs). For dogs weighing more than 10 lbs, tablets may be broken in half to provide ½ tablet for each additional 5 lbs body weight. The presence of these parasites should be confirmed by laboratory fecal examination. Do not withhold food from your dog prior to or after treatment.

Place tablet directly into back of mouth or conceal tablet in a small amount of food. A follow-up fecal examination should be conducted in 2 to 4 weeks after first treatment to determine the need for retreatment.

Since anthelmintics cannot be relied upon to prevent reinfection or to remove larvae not present in the intestinal tract at the time of initial treatment, for maximum control, it is recommended that puppies be treated at 2, 3, 4, 6, 8, and 10 weeks of age. Lactating bitches should be treated 2-3 weeks after whelping. Adult dogs should be routinely treated at monthly intervals to protect against environmental *T. canis* reinfection. Retreatment of adult dogs may be necessary at monthly intervals as determined by laboratory fecal examinations or in animals kept in known contaminated quarters.

Caution(s): If your dog looks or acts sick, do not treat with this product.

Consult your veterinarian for assistance in the diagnosis, treatment, and control of parasitism.

Restricted Drug - Use only as directed.

Warning(s): Not for human consumption. Keep out of reach of children.

Presentation: 2 tablets and 100 tablets (bulk).

Compendium Code No.: 10000131

D-WORM™ LIQUID WORMER FOR CATS AND DOGS

Farnam **Parasiticide-Oral**

(piperazine)

Active Ingredient(s): Piperazine (Dipiperazine Sulfate)-equivalent to 4.25 grams Piperazine Base per 100 cc.

Indications: Liquid wormer for kittens, cats, puppies and dogs. Removes large roundworms (ascarids) *(Toxocara canis, Toxocara cati, Toxascaris leonina).*

Directions for Use: Mix proper dosage with any amount of palatable feed that will be consumed in one serving. If possible, confine treated pets for a day or two so that the droppings can be collected and destroyed. Heavily infested animals may require a second treatment after two weeks.

Consult your veterinarian for assistance in the diagnosis, treatment and control of parasites.

Dosage Table: (Measure accurately)

Body Weight	Cats	Dogs
2½ lbs. or less	¼ teaspoon	¼ teaspoon
5 lbs.	½ teaspoon	½ teaspoon
7½ lbs.	¾ teaspoon	¾ teaspoon
10 lbs.	1 teaspoon	1 teaspoon
15 lbs.	-	1½ teaspoons
30 lbs.	-	3 teaspoons
60 lbs.	-	6 teaspoons

Precaution(s): Avoid freezing.

Caution(s): Consult veterinarian before using in severely debilitated animals. Do not worm animals more than twice yearly except as advised by a veterinarian. This product is effective for those roundworm stages found in the intestine and does not remove migrating larval stages. Animals should be checked periodically by a veterinarian for the presence of other intestinal parasites.

Warning(s): Keep out of reach of children.

Presentation: 8 fl oz (236 mL).

Distributed by: Farnam Pet Products, Division of Farnam Companies, Inc., P.O. Box 34820, Phoenix, AZ 85067-4820.

Compendium Code No.: 10000640 9CC9

DYNA-LODE® EQUINE SUPPLEMENT

Harlmen **Large Animal Dietary Supplement**

Active Ingredient(s): DYNA-LODE® Equine contains: Lecithin and a typical lipid profile of phospholipids and glycolipids.

Dl-methionine, choline (as choline chloride), inositol, niacinamide, thiamine mononitrate, riboflavin, pantothenic acid, pyridoxine hydrochloride, vitamin B_{12}, zinc, selenium, vitamin E, biotin, formulated with a special flavor base.

Indications: DYNA-LODE® Equine is a dual-phase nutritional supplement. It contains supplements essential for body cell structure. It also contains vitamins needed for cell metabolism.

Dosage and Administration: The powder may be mixed into the diet by pouring over the grain. A leveled scoop contains 30 g.

Usual Dosage: Two (2) level scoops per day (use the scoop provided in the container).

Precaution(s): Store at room temperature and protect from light. Avoid excessive heat and moisture.

Caution(s): For veterinary use only.

Keep out of the reach of children.

Presentation: 5 lb. containers.

Compendium Code No.: 14500010

DYNA-LODE® SUPPLEMENT FOR DOGS & CATS

Harlmen **Small Animal Dietary Supplement**

Active Ingredient(s): Each tablet contains:

Lecithin . . . . 600 mg

Typical Lipid Profile: Phosphatidylcholine, phosphatidylethanolamine, glycolipids, phosphatidylinositol, phosphatidic acid, and phosphatidylserine.

Ingredients: Phosphoric di-calcium carbonate, lecithin, sugar, lumed silica, corn syrup, liver powder, DL methionine, whey, magnesium stearate, zinc sulfate, inositol, vitamin E, niacinamide, riboflavin, thiamine HCl, ubiquinone, pyridoxine, selenium, vitamin B_{12}.

Guarantee per 2 gram tablet:

DL methionine . . . . 55 mg
Zinc. . . . . 10 mg
Selenium. . . . . 20 mcg
Vitamin E . . . . 15 IU
Thiamine. . . . . 2 mg
Pantothenic acid . . . . 1 mg
Riboflavin . . . . 2 mg
Niacinamide . . . . 8 mg
Pyridoxine HCl . . . . 1 mg
Vitamin B_{12}. . . . . 10 mcg
Ubiquinone* . . . . 2 mg
Choline* . . . . 25 mg
Inositol* . . . . 25 mg

*Not recognized as an essential nutrient by the AAFCO Dog food nutrient profile.

Indications: A nutritional supplement which contains choline, phospholipids, and glycolipids to enhance choline loading, and other important ingredients frequently found to be deficient in diets of geriatric animals.

Dosage and Administration: Administration: DYNA-LODE® chewable tablets may be fed free choice, from the hand, or may be crumbled and mixed into food. For additional flavor release, moisten the tablets before offering to the pet.

Usual Dosage:

Cats and small dogs . . . . ½ to 1 tablet a day
Large dogs . . . . 2 to 4 tablets a day

Precaution(s): Store at room temperature and protect from light. Avoid excessive heat (104°F).

Warning(s): Keep out of reach of children.

Presentation: Available in 50 or 150 chewable tablets per container.

Compendium Code No.: 14500001

DYNA-TAURINE™

Harlmen **Small Animal Dietary Supplement**

Ingredient(s): Taurine, enzyme modified soy lecithin, carbomer 934, triethanolamine, methyl p-hydroxybenzoate, propyl p-hydroxybenzoate, water, pH adjusted to 6.0-6.5 with citric acid.

Indications: DYNA-TAURINE™ is a palatable taurine dietary supplement in a liquid lecithin base. To be fed to cats and dogs only.

Dosage and Administration: Dogs: One complete stroke of the pump per 40 pounds of body weight twice daily on the food. Cats: ½ stroke of pump twice daily on the food. (Each stroke of the metered pump is equal to 4 millimeters or 375 mg. of Taurine.)

Warning(s): For oral use only. Keep out of reach of children. Available through licensed veterinarians only.

For veterinary use only. Not for human use.

Presentation: 16 fl oz (473.3 mL).

Compendium Code No.: 14500020

D

Disclaimer

Every effort has been made to ensure the accuracy of the information published. However, it remains the responsibility of the readers to familiarize themselves with the product information contained on the product label or package insert.

Inclusion or omission of products does not imply endorsement or criticism by the Publisher or anyone involved in the publication. Inclusion does not imply product availability and/or product registration. The Publisher, Editorial Team and all those involved in the production of this book cannot be held responsible for publication errors or any consequence that could result from the use of published information.

E

EAR CLEANSING SOLUTION

Butler **Otic Cleanser**

Ingredient(s): Deionized Water, Propylene Glycol, Aloe Vera Gel, SD Alcohol 40-2, Lactic Acid, Glycerin, Dioctyl Sodium Sulfosuccinate, Salicylic Acid, Fragrance, Benzoic Acid, Benzyl Alcohol.
Indications: Butler EAR CLEANSING SOLUTION is specially formulated to deodorize and gently clean, dry and acidify the ear canal. This provides an ideal environment for healthy ears. For dogs and cats.
Directions: Apply liberally into the ear canal. Massage the base of the ear. Allow pet to shake head. Clean excess with a cotton ball. If excessively dirty ears; apply 2-3 times daily over several days. For maintenance of healthy ears; use 1-2 times weekly or as often as recommended by your veterinarian. Always apply after swimming.
Precaution(s): Storage: Store at controlled room temperature.
Caution(s): For topical use only. Avoid contact with eyes. For veterinary use only.
Warning(s): Keep out of reach of children.
Presentation: 8 oz (236.5 mL) (NDC 11695-2470-2), 16 oz (473 mL) (NDC 11695-2470-3). Sold exclusively through veterinarians.
Compendium Code No.: 10822020

EAR CLEANSING SOLUTION

Vet Solutions **Otic Cleanser**

Ingredient(s): Deionized Water, Propylene Glycol, Aloe Vera Gel, SD Alcohol 40-2, Lactic Acid, Glycerin, Dioctyl Sodium Sulfosuccinate, Salicylic Acid, Fragrance, Benzoic Acid, Benzyl Alcohol.
Indications: Vet Solutions EAR CLEANSING SOLUTION is specially formulated to deodorize and gently clean, dry and acidify the ear canal. This provides an ideal environment for healthy ears. For dogs and cats.
Directions: Apply liberally into the ear canal. Massage the base of the ear. Allow pet to shake head. Clean excess with a cotton ball. In excessively dirty ears; apply 2-3 times daily over several days. For maintenance of healthy ears; use 1-2 times weekly or as often as recommended by your veterinarian. Always apply after swimming.
Precaution(s): Storage: Store at controlled room temperature.
Caution(s): For topical use only. Avoid contact with eyes.
Sold exclusively through veterinarians.
Presentation: 8 fl. oz. (237 mL), 16 fl. oz. (474 mL), and 1 gallon.
Compendium Code No.: 10610060 990204

EARMED BORACETIC® FLUSH

Davis **Otic Preparation**

Active Ingredient(s): Boric acid, acetic acid, aloe and deodorants.
Indications: An aid to eliminate ear conditions associated with bacteria and yeast in dogs and cats.
Directions for Use: Apply Davis EARMED BORACETIC® Flush liberally into the ear canal. Gently massage the base of the ear, allowing the solution to come in contact with wax or debris and yeast and bacteria. Use suitable material such as gauze or facial tissue to collect loose wax and debris. Repeat procedure as necessary.
Precaution(s): Store at room temperature.
Caution(s): Use of Davis EARMED BORACETIC® Flush in cats should be limited to once weekly. Not for use in eyes. Do not use if there is suspected damage to the eardrum. Discontinue use if irritation develops.
Warning(s): For external veterinary use only.
Keep out of reach of children. For animal use only.
Presentation: 12 fl oz (355 mL) and 1 gallon (3.785 L).
Compendium Code No.: 114101612 Rev. 5/98

EARMED CLEANSING SOLUTION & WASH

Davis **Otic Cleanser**

Active Ingredient(s): 50A 40B alcohol, propylene glycol, cocamidopropyl phosphatidyl and PE dimonium chloride.
Indications: For use on dogs and cats to remove dirt, wax and dead tissue without harming the pet's ear.
Deodorizing and non-staining, EARMED CLEANSING SOLUTION & WASH can be used routinely to effectively help maintain ear tissue.
Dosage and Administration: Apply liberally into the ear canal. Gently massage the base of the ear, allowing the solution to come into contact with wax and debris. Use suitable material such as gauze or a facial tissue to collect accessible loose wax and debris. Repeat the procedure as necessary.
The use of an ear wash in cats should be limited to once a week.
Presentation: 12 oz.(355 mL) and 1 gallon (3.785 L).
Compendium Code No.: 11410172

EARMED MITE LOTION

Davis **Otic Preparation**

Ingredient(s): Contains: Oil of pennyroyal, oil of lemongrass and oil of lavender.
Contains soothing aloe as a grooming ingredient.
Indications: Davis EARMED MITE LOTION is a an all-natural product for dogs and cats with ear mite problems. It also helps restore a healthy ear environment which promotes the healing process.
Dosage and Administration: Cleanse ear thoroughly.
Cats and Dogs 5-15 lbs - Place 4-5 drops in ear daily.
Dogs 15-30 lbs - Place 5-10 drops in each ear daily.
Dogs over 30 lbs - Place 10-15 drops in each ear daily.
Gently massage base of ear for 3-5 minutes. Leave solution in ear for another few minutes and allow animal to shake its head to remove as much lotion as possible. Wipe the remainder of the lotion from the ear with cotton.
Recommended application, 7-10 days. Repeat application in two weeks, if necessary.
Caution(s): Do not use if there is suspected damage to the eardrum.
If condition persists or if irritation develops, discontinue use and consult a veterinarian.
Presentation: 2 oz (58 mL).
Compendium Code No.: 11410181

EARMED POWDER

Davis **Otic Dryer**

Active Ingredient(s): Micronized silica.
Indications: For use on dogs and cats to help relieve irritated, itching ears of non-parasitic origin, dries wet ears and aids in the inhibition of bacteria growth caused by moist ear environments.
Also helps reduce ear odors and is designed to aid in the removal of excess, unwanted hair from the ear canal.
Dosage and Administration:
To keep ears dry and reduce ear odors: Clean the ears thoroughly with EarMed Cleansing Solution & Wash. Puff the powder into the ear canal. Can be used once a day.
To help remove unwanted hair from the ear canal: Puff the powder into the ear canal and remove unwanted hair with tweezers or forceps. After the hair has been removed, clean the ears with EarMed Cleansing Solution & Wash and re-apply the powder.
Presentation: 16 oz.
Compendium Code No.: 11410192

EAR MITICIDE

Phoenix Pharmaceutical **Otic Parasiticide**

EPA Reg. No.: 28293-42-58383
Active Ingredient(s):

Rotenone	0.12%
Other Associated Resins	0.16%
Inert Ingredients	99.72%
Total:	100.00%

Indications: Use only on dogs, cats, or rabbits to kill ear mites.
Directions for Use: It is a violation of Federal law to use this product in a manner inconsistent with its labeling.
Pets:
Pre-Treatment Directions: Read entire label before each use. Use only on dogs, cats or rabbits to kill ear mites: Do not use on animals under 12 weeks.
Special Animals: Consult a veterinarian or call local Animal Poison Control before using this product on debilitated, aged, pregnant, nursing or medicated animals.
Application Directions: While holding pet firmly, fill each ear canal half full of EAR MITICIDE and massage base of ear to ensure that insecticidal action penetrates ear wax.
Re-Application Directions: Do not reapply product for 1 day. Improvement is usually noted after two applications.
Contraindication(s): Do not use on animals under 12 weeks.
Precautionary Statements: Hazardous to Humans and Domestic Animals:
Warning: Causes substantial, but temporary, eye injury. Wear safety glasses. May be harmful if swallowed, absorbed through the skin, or inhaled. Avoid contact with skin, eyes or clothing. Avoid inhalation of spray. Wash thoroughly with soap and water after handling. Remove contaminated clothing and wash thoroughly before reuse.
Adverse Reaction Information: Sensitivities may occur after using any pesticide product for pets. If signs of sensitivity occur, consult a veterinarian immediately or call local Animal Poison Control.
First Aid: Have label with you when obtaining treatment advice.
If swallowed: Call a poison control center or doctor immediately for treatment advice. Have person sip a glass of water if able to swallow. Do not induce vomiting unless told to do so by the poison control center or doctor.
If on skin or clothing: Take off contaminated clothing. Rinse skin immediately with plenty of water for 15-20 minutes. Call a poison control center or doctor immediately for treatment advice.
If inhaled: Move person to fresh air. If person is not breathing, call an ambulance, then give artificial respiration, preferably mouth-to-mouth, if possible. Call a poison control center or doctor immediately for treatment advice.
If in eyes: Hold eye open and rinse slowly and gently with water for 15-20 minutes. Remove contact lenses, if present, after the first 5 minutes, then continue rinsing eye. Call a poison control center or doctor immediately for treatment advice.
Environmental Hazards: This product is extremely toxic to fish. Do not contaminate water when disposing of product.
Storage and Disposal:
Storage: Store only in original container in a dry place inaccessible to children and pets.
Disposal: Do not reuse empty container. Rinse thoroughly. Securely wrap in newspaper and discard in trash.
Warning(s): Not for use in animals intended for food.
Keep out of reach of children.
Discussion: Diagnosis for Ear Mites: Ear mites usually induce the formation of a dry, dark brown, waxy exudate with crusts in the ears of dogs, cats and rabbits. Ear mites may be detected by placing some of the ear exudate on a dark surface and carefully watching for the movement of tiny white specks away from the exudate. Inflamed, watery, or blocked ear canals indicate a more serious condition which requires the services of a veterinarian.
Presentation: 2 fl oz bottles (NDC 57319-401-18).
Compendium Code No.: 12560292

EAROXIDE™ EAR CLEANSER

Tomlyn **Otic Cleanser**

Active Ingredient(s): Contains carbamide peroxide 6.5% in a stabilized glycerin base.
Indications: Ear cleanser.
Dosage and Administration: The external ear should be clipped and cleaned. Fill the ear canal with EAROXIDE™ and gently massage by pressing on the external ear canal. After a few minutes, the animal may be allowed to shake its head to throw out the dissolved material.
Repeat daily until the canal is free of foreign material.
No cleaning or probing of the ear canal is necessary.
Precaution(s): Store in a cool, dry place. Keep cap tightly closed.
Caution(s): If draining or irritation persists, consult your veterinarian.
For animal use only.
Keep out of reach of children and pets.
Presentation: 2 fl oz (59 mL) and 4 fl oz (118 mL).
Compendium Code No.: 11220031 094-1 5/046-1 4

EAZI-BREED™ CIDR® CATTLE INSERT

Pharmacia & Upjohn **Progesterone**

NADA No.: 141-200

Active Ingredient(s): Each EAZI-BREED™ CIDR® Cattle Insert contains 1.38 grams of progesterone in molded silicone over a flexible nylon spine. Attached to each EAZI-BREED™ CIDR® Cattle Insert is a polyester tail.

Inactive Ingredients: silicone rubber, nylon and polyester.

Indications: Synchronization of estrus in suckled beef cows, and replacement beef and dairy heifers.

Advancement of first postpartum estrus in suckled beef cows.

Advancement of first pubertal estrus in replacement beef heifers.

The EAZI-BREED™ CIDR® Cattle Insert provides an exogenous source of the hormone progesterone during the 7 day administration period. Removal of the EAZI-BREED™ CIDR® Cattle Insert on treatment day 7 results in a rapid fall in plasma progesterone levels which results in synchronization of estrus in those animals responding to treatment.

Directions: Wear latex gloves when handling inserts.

Only use the specially designed EAZI-BREED™ CIDR® Cattle Insert Applicator for administration.

Administer one EAZI-BREED™ CIDR® Cattle Insert per animal for 7 days.

Inject 5 mL of Lutalyse® Sterile Solution (equivalent to 5 mg/mL dinoprost) 1 day prior to EAZI-BREED™ CIDR® Cattle Insert removal, on day 6 of the 7 day administration period.

Observe animals for signs of estrus on days 1 to 3 after removal of EAZI-BREED™ CIDR® Cattle Inserts and inseminate animals about 12 hours after onset of estrus.

Insertion:

1. Restrain cattle appropriately (head catch, squeeze chute, gate, etc.) prior to administration.
2. Wash the EAZI-BREED™ CIDR® Cattle Insert Applicator in a non-irritating antiseptic solution, and then lubricate the front portion of the EAZI-BREED™ CIDR® Cattle Insert Applicator with a veterinary obstetrical lubricant.
3. Push the flexible tail end of the EAZI-BREED™ CIDR® Cattle Insert into the EAZI-BREED™ CIDR® Cattle Insert Applicator taking care to assure the tail is extending upward through the slot of the EAZI-BREED™ CIDR® Cattle Insert Applicator and is pointed toward the handle.
4. Fold the wings of the EAZI-BREED™ CIDR® Cattle Insert to make it longer and continue to advance the EAZI-BREED™ CIDR® Cattle Insert into the applicator until it is fully seated. When fully seated only the tips of the wings should protrude (one half inch) from the end of the EAZI-BREED™ CIDR® Cattle Insert Applicator (see Figure 1).
5. Lubricate the protruding tips of the wings of the EAZI-BREED™ CIDR® Cattle Insert with veterinary obstetrical lubricant.
6. Lift the tail of the animal and clean the exterior of the vulva.
7. Open the lips of the vulva and gently place the loaded EAZI-BREED™ CIDR® Cattle Insert Applicator through the vulva. The slot in the EAZI-BREED™ CIDR® Cattle Insert Applicator should face upwards (see Figure 2).

Figure 1

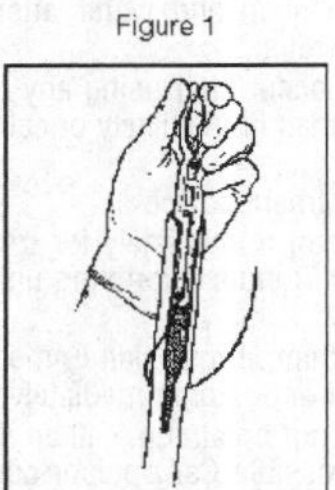

Figure 2

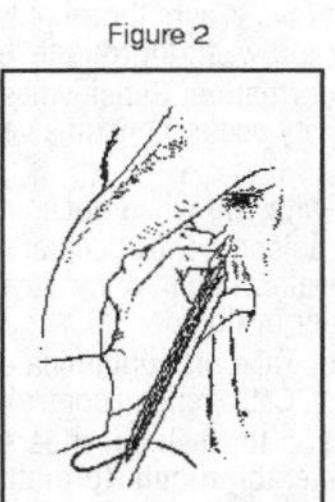

8. Once the loaded EAZI-BREED™ CIDR® Cattle Insert Applicator is past the vulva, slope the EAZI-BREED™ CIDR® Cattle Insert Applicator slightly upwards (35-45° angle) by lowering the handle, and then forward, without forcing, until the EAZI-BREED™ CIDR® Cattle Insert Applicator is fully inserted or resistance is felt (see Figure 3).
9. Squeeze the finger grips within the handle of the EAZI-BREED™ CIDR® Cattle Insert Applicator to deposit the EAZI-BREED™ CIDR® Cattle Insert in the anterior vagina (see Figure 4) and then pull the EAZI-BREED™ CIDR® Cattle Insert Applicator backwards to remove it from the vagina.

Figure 3

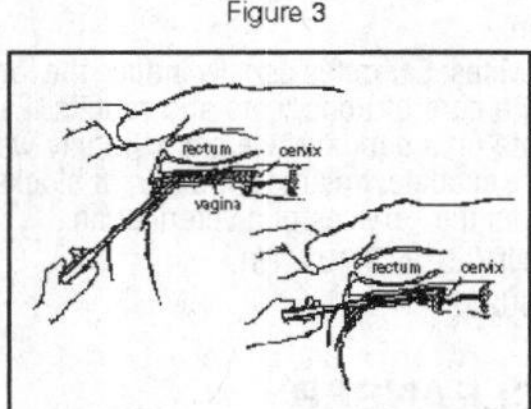

Figure 4

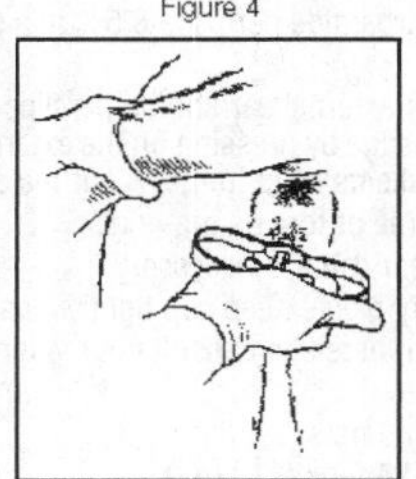

10. With the EAZI-BREED™ CIDR® Cattle Insert correctly placed, with the wings open in the anterior portion of the vagina, the tail of the EAZI-BREED™ CIDR® Cattle Insert should be visible, pointing downward from the vulva of the animal. Tails of EAZI-BREED™ CIDR® Cattle Inserts that protrude more than 2.5 inches from the vulva may be clipped to minimize removal by other animals.

Removal:

1. Remove the EAZI-BREED™ CIDR® Cattle Inserts by pulling, gently but firmly, on the protruding polyester tail.
2. EAZI-BREED™ CIDR® Cattle Inserts have been reported to reverse direction within the vagina; therefore, if the polyester tail of the insert is not visible on the day of removal, check the vagina to determine if an insert is present.

When Using This Product:

- You must use the EAZI-BREED™ CIDR® Cattle Insert concurrently with an injection of 5 mL of Lutalyse® Sterile Solution (equivalent to 5 mg/mL dinoprost) administered on day 6 of the 7 day administration period to assure maximum effectiveness.

- In animals that respond to treatment, the onset of estrus generally occurs within 1 to 3 days after removal of the EAZI-BREED™ CIDR® Cattle Insert.

- Intravaginal administration of EAZI-BREED™ CIDR® Cattle Insert for periods greater than 7 days may result in reduced fertility.

You May Notice:

- Increased loss of EAZI-BREED™ CIDR® Cattle Inserts in animals housed under crowded conditions, especially in heifers. Avoid crowded conditions during treatment as other cattle, particularly heifers, may remove EAZI-BREED™ CIDR® Cattle Inserts by pulling on the tail of the EAZI-BREED™ CIDR® Cattle Insert. If loss rates are high re-evaluate insertion technique and cattle handling facilities.

- Clear, cloudy or bloody mucus on the outside of EAZI-BREED™ CIDR® Cattle Insert when removed from animals. The mucus may have an offensive odor. This is a result of mild irritation to the vaginal lining by the presence of the EAZI-BREED™ CIDR® Cattle Insert, and generally clears between the time of removal and insemination. Such irritation does not affect fertility.

Precaution(s): Store below 86°F (30°C).

Caution(s): Federal law prohibits extra-label use of this drug to enhance food and/or fiber production in animals.

Warning(s): Do Not Use:

- in animals with abnormal, immature or infected genital tracts
- in beef cows that are less than 20 days postpartum
- in beef or dairy heifers of insufficient size or age for breeding
- in lactating dairy cows
- an insert more than once. To prevent the potential transmission of venereal and blood-borne diseases, the EAZI-BREED™ CIDR® Cattle Insert should be disposed after a single use.

Human Warning: Wear latex gloves when handling the inserts. Keep this and all medications out of the reach of children.

Environmental Warning: Store removed EAZI-BREED™ CIDR® Cattle Inserts in a plastic bag or other sealable container until they can be properly disposed in accordance with applicable local, state and Federal regulations.

Presentation: They are packaged in a plastic pouch with 10 inserts to a pouch (NDC 0009-5207-01). The special EAZI-BREED™ CIDR® applicator is packaged separately.

EAZI-BREED is a trademark and CIDR is a registered trademark of DEC International, NZ, Ltd. Lutalyse is a registered trademark of Pharmacia & Upjohn Company.

Made By DEC International, NZ, Ltd., Hamilton, New Zealand

Compendium Code No.: 10490610 819 241 000

E-BAC™

Intervet **Bacterin**

Erysipelothrix Rhusiopathiae Bacterin

U.S. Vet. Lic. No.: 286

Contents: This product contains the antigen listed above. This product is inactivated and adjuvanted to enhance the immune response.

Contains gentamicin as a preservative.

Indications: For the vaccination of healthy swine against infection caused by *Erysipelothrix rhusiopathiae*.

Directions: Administer 2 mL intramuscularly or subcutaneously into pigs at least 3 weeks of age. Repeat in 14-21 days. Semiannual revaccination is recommended.

Precaution(s): Shake well. Use entire contents when first opened. Store at 2° to 7°C (35°-45°F). Do not freeze.

Caution(s): In case of anaphylactoid reactions administer epinephrine.

For veterinary use only.

Warning(s): Do not vaccinate within 21 days before slaughter.

Presentation: 50 dose (100 mL) and 125 dose (250 mL) vials.

Compendium Code No.: 11060450

ECLIPSE® 3

Schering-Plough **Vaccine**

Feline Rhinotracheitis-Calici-Panleukopenia Vaccine, Modified Live Virus

U.S. Vet. Lic. No.: 195A

Active Ingredient(s): Feline rhinotracheitis, calici, panleukopenia vaccine, modified live virus.

The vaccine contains gentamicin and a fungistat as preservatives.

Indications: ECLIPSE® 3 is a modified live virus vaccine for immunization of cats against feline rhinotracheitis, calici, and panleukopenia viruses.

Dosage and Administration: Inject one (1) dose (1 mL) subcutaneously or intramuscularly.

Vaccinate cats at 9-10 weeks of age and repeat in three (3) to four (4) weeks. Cats vaccinated at 12 weeks of age or older require two (2) doses three (3) to four (4) weeks apart. Two (2) doses of feline rhinotracheitis and calici vaccine are required for a prophylactic dose.

Annual revaccination with one (1) dose is recommended. Do not vaccinate pregnant cats. Transfer contents of diluent vial to vaccine vial aseptically.

Do not chemically sterilize needles and syringes.

Precaution(s): Store at 2-7°C. Burn container and all unused contents.

Caution(s): The use of any biological may produce anaphylactic reactions.

Antidote(s): Epinephrine.

Presentation: Box of 25 single doses.

Compendium Code No.: 10470491

ECLIPSE® 3 + FeLV

Schering-Plough **Vaccine**

Feline Leukemia-Rhinotracheitis-Calici-Panleukopenia Vaccine, Modified Live Virus and Killed Virus

U.S. Vet. Lic. No.: 165A

Contents: ECLIPSE® 3 + FeLV is a combination vaccine that unites the benefits of Eclipse®3 and Fevaxyn FeLV® in one vaccination.

Eclipse® 3 is a modified live virus vaccine.

Fevaxyn FeLV® contains a tissue culture derived feline leukemia virus, Subgroups A and B. Viral antigens have been chemically inactivated and combined with an adjuvant designed to enhance the immune response.

Contains gentamicin and amphotericin B as preservatives.

Indications: Eclipse® 3 vaccine is recommended for the vaccination of healthy cats against diseases caused by feline rhinotracheitis, calici, and panleukopenia viruses.

Fevaxyn FeLV® vaccine is recommended for the vaccination of healthy cats as an aid in the prevention of lymphoid tumors caused by and diseases associated with feline leukemia virus (FeLV) infection. Vaccination with this product prevents persistent viremia in cats exposed to virulent feline leukemia virus.

Dosage and Administration: Two doses are required for primary immunization.

Initial vaccination: Inject 1 dose (1 mL) subcutaneously or intramuscularly at 9 weeks of age or older.

Second vaccination: Inject 1 dose (1 mL) subcutaneously or intramuscularly 3 to 4 weeks following the initial vaccination.

Annual revaccination with one dose is recommended.

Prior to use, warm the Fevaxyn FeLV® to room temperature and shake well.

Transfer contents of the Fevaxyn FeLV® vial to the Eclipse® 3 vial aseptically. Mix gently until dissolved. Use entire contents immediately after rehydration.

Contraindication(s): Do not vaccinate pregnant cats.

Precaution(s): Store between 2° and 7°C.

Do not freeze.

Use new, non-chemically sterilized, needles and syringes.

Do not mix with other vaccines.

Burn vaccine container and all unused contents. Dispose of all contents in a proper manner.

Caution(s): The use of a biological product may produce anaphylaxis and/or other inflammatory immune-mediated hypersensitivity reactions.

Some reports suggest that in cats, the administration of certain veterinary biologicals may induce the development of injection-site fibrosarcomas.

Antidote(s): Epinephrine, corticosteroids, and antihistamines may all be indicated depending on the nature of the severity of the reaction.

Warning(s): For use in cats only.

For veterinary use only.

Discussion: It is important to realize that certain conditions and event may cause some cats to be unable to develop or maintain an adequate immune response following FeLV vaccination. Prior exposure to the disease, or disease latency, are conditions in which vaccination may not alter the course of the disease. Therefore, diagnostic testing of all cats for FeLV antigen prior to vaccination is recommended. Also, vaccination with this product will not offer cross-protection against feline immunodeficiency virus (FIV), another feline retrovirus. It is important to advise the cat owner of these situations prior to vaccination.

Presentation: 25 x 1 dose vials of Eclipse® 3.
25 x 1 mL vials of Fevaxyn FeLV®.

Compendium Code No.: 10470501 P20201-10

ECLIPSE® 3 + FeLV/R

Schering-Plough **Vaccine**

Feline Leukemia-Rhinotracheitis-Calici-Panleukopenia-Rabies Vaccine, Modified Live Virus and Killed Virus

U.S. Vet. Lic. No.: 195

Contents: Eclipse® 3 is a modified live virus vaccine for the vaccination of healthy cats against feline rhinotracheitis, calici, and panleukopenia viruses.

Fevaxyn FeLV/R® vaccine diluent is recommended for the vaccination of healthy cats as an aid in the prevention of disease associated with feline leukemia virus infection and rabies. Vaccination with this product prevents persistent viremia in cats exposed to virulent feline leukemia virus. Contains gentamicin and amphotericin B as preservatives.

Fevaxyn FeLV/R® vaccine diluent contains a tissue culture derived feline leukemia virus, Subgroups A and B. Viral antigens have been chemically inactivated and combined with an adjuvant designed to enhance the immune response.

Indications: For the vaccination of healthy cats against the antigens listed above.

Dosage and Administration: Two doses are required for primary immunization of the cat or kitten for feline leukemia, rhinotracheitis, calici, and panleukopenia viruses. Primary immunization of the cat or kitten for rabies requires one dose at 12 weeks of age or older. ECLIPSE® 3 + FeLV/R is recommended for booster vaccination of the cat or kitten 12 weeks of age or older following primary vaccination with feline leukemia, rhinotracheitis, calici and panleukopenia vaccine.

Initial vaccination: Inject 1 dose (1 mL) ECLIPSE® 3 + FeLV/R vaccine subcutaneously or intramuscularly at nine weeks of age or older.

Second vaccination: Inject 1 dose (1 mL) ECLIPSE® 3 + FeLV/R vaccination subcutaneously or intramuscularly three to four weeks following the initial vaccination.

Annual revaccination with one dose of ECLIPSE® 3 + FeLV/R vaccine is recommended.

Prior to use, warm the Fevaxyn FeLV/R® vaccine diluent to room temperature and shake well.

Transfer contents of the Fevaxyn FeLV/R® vaccine diluent vial to the Eclipse® 3 vial aseptically. Mix gently until dissolved. Use entire contents immediately after rehydration.

Contraindication(s): Do not vaccinate pregnant cats.

Precaution(s): Store between 2° and 7°C.

Do not freeze.

Do not chemically sterilize needles and syringes.

Do not mix with other vaccines.

Caution(s): Burn vaccine container and all unused contents. Dispose of all contents in a proper manner.

Antidote(s): The use of any biological product may produce anaphylaxis and/or other inflammatory immune-mediated hypersensitivity reactions. Antidote: Epinephrine, corticosteroids, and antihistamines may all be indicated depending on the nature of the severity of the reaction.*

Warning(s): For veterinary use only.

For use in cats only.

Side Effects: A local reaction may occur at the site following subcutaneous administration.

Some reports suggest that in cats, the administration of certain veterinary biologicals may induce the development of injection-site fibrosarcomas.*

Discussion: It is important to realize that certain conditions and event may cause some cats to be unable to develop or maintain an adequate immune response following FeLV vaccination. Prior exposure to the disease, or disease latency, are conditions in which vaccination may not alter the course of the disease. Therefore, diagnostic testing of all cats for FeLV antigen prior to vaccination is recommended. Also, vaccination with this product will not offer cross-protection against feline immunodeficiency virus (FIV), another feline retrovirus. It is important to advise the cat owner of these situations prior to vaccination.

References: *Available upon request.

Presentation: 25 x 1 dose vials of Eclipse® 3 vaccine.
25 x 1 dose vials of Fevaxyn® FeLV/R vaccine diluent.

Compendium Code No.: 10470510

ECLIPSE® 4

Schering-Plough **Vaccine**

E

Feline Rhinotracheitis-Calici-Panleukopenia-Chlamydia psittaci Vaccine, Modified Live Virus and Chlamydia, Cell Line Origin

U.S. Vet. Lic. No.: 195A

Active Ingredient(s): Feline rhinotracheitis, calici, panleukopenia, *Chlamydia psittaci* vaccine, modified live virus and chlamydia, cell line origin.

The vaccine contains gentamicin and a fungistat as preservatives.

Indications: ECLIPSE® 4 is a modified live virus and chlamydia vaccine for immunization of cats and kittens against feline rhinotracheitis, calici, panleukopenia viruses and chlamydia.

Dosage and Administration: Inject one (1) dose (1 mL) subcutaneously or intramuscularly.

Vaccinate cats at 9-10 weeks of age and repeat in three (3) to four (4) weeks. Cats vaccinated at 12 weeks of age or older require two (2) doses three (3) to four (4) weeks apart. Two (2) doses of feline rhinotracheitis and calici vaccine are required for a prophylactic dose.

Annual revaccination with one (1) dose is recommended. Do not vaccinate pregnant cats.

Transfer contents of diluent vial to vaccine vial aseptically. Do not chemically sterilize needles and syringes.

Precaution(s): Store at 2-7°C. Burn the container and all unused contents.

Caution(s): The use of any biological may produce anaphylactic reactions.

Antidote(s): Epinephrine.

Presentation: Box of 25 single doses.

Compendium Code No.: 10470521

ECLIPSE® 4 + FeLV

Schering-Plough **Vaccine**

Feline Leukemia-Rhinotracheitis-Calici-Panleukopenia-Chlamydia Psittaci Vaccine, Modified Live Virus and Chlamydia and Killed Virus

U.S. Vet. Lic. No.: 165A

Contents: ECLIPSE® 4 + FeLV is a combination vaccine that unites the benefits of Eclipse® 4 and Fevaxyn FeLV® in one vaccination.

Eclipse® 4 is a modified live virus and chlamydia vaccine.

Fevaxyn FeLV® contains a tissue culture derived, feline leukemia virus, Subgroups A and B. Viral antigens have been chemically inactivated and combined with a proprietary adjuvant designed to enhance the immune response.

Contains gentamicin and amphotericin B as preservatives.

Indications: Eclipse® 4 is recommended for the vaccination of healthy cats against diseases caused by feline rhinotracheitis, calici, and panleukopenia viruses and *Chlamydia psittaci*.

Fevaxyn FeLV® is recommended for the vaccination of healthy cats as an aid in the prevention of lymphoid tumors caused by, and diseases associated with feline leukemia virus (FeLV) infection. Vaccination with the product prevents persistent viremia in cats exposed to virulent feline leukemia virus.

Dosage and Administration: Two doses are required for primary immunization.

Initial Vaccination: Inject 1 dose (1 mL) subcutaneously or intramuscularly at 9 weeks of age or older.

Second Vaccination: Inject 1 dose (1 mL) subcutaneously or intramuscularly 3 to 4 weeks following the initial vaccination.

Annual revaccination with one dose is recommended.

Prior to use, warm the Fevaxyn FeLV® to room temperature and shake well.

Transfer the contents of the Fevaxyn FeLV® vial to the Eclipse® 4 vial aseptically. Mix gently until dissolved. Use the entire contents immediately after rehydration.

Contraindication(s): Do not vaccinate pregnant cats.

Precaution(s): Store between 2° and 7°C.

Do not freeze.

Use new, non-chemically sterilized, needles and syringes.

Do not mix with other vaccines.

Burn vaccine container and all unused contents.

Caution(s): The use of any biological product may produce anaphylaxis and/or other inflammatory immune-mediated hypersensitivity reactions.

Some reports suggest that in cats, the administration of certain veterinary biologicals may induce the development of injection-site fibrosarcomas.

Antidote(s): Epinephrine, corticosteroids, and antihistamines may all be indicated depending on the nature of the severity of the reaction.

Warning(s): For use in cats only.

For veterinary use only.

Discussion: It is important to realize that certain conditions and events may cause some cats to be unable to develop or maintain an adequate immune response following vaccination. Prior exposure to the disease, or disease latency, are conditions in which vaccination will not alter the course of the disease. Therefore, diagnostic testing of all cats for FeLV antigen prior to vaccination is recommended. Also, vaccination with the product will not offer cross-protection against feline immunodeficiency virus (FIV), another feline retrovirus. It is important to advise the cat owner of these situations prior to vaccination.

Presentation: 25 x 1 dose vials of Eclipse® 4.
25 x 1 mL vials of Fevaxyn FeLV®.

Compendium Code No.: 10470531 P20601-10

ECLIPSE® 4 + FeLV/R

Schering-Plough **Vaccine**

Feline Leukemia-Rhinotracheitis-Calici-Panleukopenia-Chlamydia psittaci-Rabies Vaccine, Modified Live Virus and Chlamydia and Killed Virus

U.S. Vet. Lic. No.: 195

Contents: Eclipse® 4 is a modified live virus vaccine for the vaccination of healthy cats against feline rhinotracheitis, calici, and panleukopenia viruses and chlamydia.

Fevaxyn FeLV/R® vaccine diluent is recommended for the vaccination of healthy cats as an aid in the prevention of disease associated with feline leukemia virus infection and rabies. Vaccination with this product prevents persistent viremia in cats exposed to virulent feline leukemia virus.

Fevaxyn FeLV/R® vaccine diluent contains a tissue culture derived feline leukemia virus, Subgroups A and B. Viral antigens have been chemically inactivated and combined with an adjuvant designed to enhance the immune response.

Contains gentamicin and amphotericin B as preservatives.

Indications: For the vaccination of healthy cats against the antigens listed above.

Dosage and Administration: Two doses are required for primary immunization of the cat or kitten for feline leukemia, rhinotracheitis, calici, and panleukopenia viruses and chlamydia. Primary immunization of the cat or kitten for rabies requires one dose at 3 months of age or older. ECLIPSE® 4 + FeLV/R is recommended for booster vaccination of the cat or kitten 3 months of age or older following primary vaccination with feline leukemia, rhinotracheitis, calici, panleukopenia, and chlamydia vaccine.

E

Initial vaccination: Inject 1 dose (1 mL) ECLIPSE® 4 + FeLV vaccine subcutaneously or intramuscularly at nine weeks of age or older.

Second vaccination: Inject 1 dose (1 mL) ECLIPSE® 4 + FeLV/R vaccination subcutaneously or intramuscularly three to four weeks following the initial vaccination.

Annual revaccination with one dose of ECLIPSE® 4 + FeLV/R vaccine is recommended.

Prior to use, warm the Fevaxyn FeLV/R® vaccine diluent to room temperature and shake well.

Transfer contents of the Fevaxyn FeLV/R® vaccine diluent vial to the Eclipse® 4 vial aseptically. Mix gently until dissolved. Use entire contents immediately after rehydration.

Contraindication(s): Do not vaccinate pregnant cats.

Precaution(s): Store between 2° and 7°C. Do not freeze.

Use new, non-chemically sterilized needles and syringes.

Do not mix with other vaccines.

Caution(s): Burn vaccine container and all unused contents.

Antidote(s): The use of a biological product may produce anaphylaxis and/or other inflammatory immune-mediated hypersensitivity reactions. Antidote: Epinephrine, corticosteroids, and antihistamines may all be indicated depending on the nature of the severity of the reaction.*

Warning(s): For veterinary use only.

For use in cats only.

Side Effects: A local reaction may occur at the site following subcutaneous administration.

Some reports suggest that in cats, the administration of certain veterinary biologicals may induce the development of injection-site fibrosarcomas.*

Discussion: It is important to realize that certain conditions and event may cause some cats to be unable to develop or maintain an adequate immune response following FeLV vaccination. Prior exposure to the disease, or disease latency, are conditions in which vaccination may not alter the course of the disease. Therefore, diagnostic testing of all cats for FeLV antigen prior to vaccination is recommended. Also, vaccination with this product will not offer cross-protection against feline immunodeficiency virus (FIV), another feline retrovirus. It is important to advise the cat owner of these situations prior to vaccination.

References: *Available upon request.

Presentation: 25 x 1 dose vials of Eclipse® 4 vaccine.
25 x 1 dose vials of Fevaxyn® FeLV/R vaccine diluent.

Compendium Code No.: 10470540

E-COLI + C ANTIBODY

AgriPharm **Antibodies-Antitoxin**

Clostridium Perfringens Type C Antitoxin-Escherichia Coli Antibody, Equine Origin

U.S. Vet. Lic. No.: 303

Composition: This product is prepared from the blood of horses hyperimmunized with *Clostridium perfringens* Type C and K99 piliated *Escherichia coli.* Contains oxytetracycline, phenol, and thimerosal as preservatives.

Indications: For use in newborn calves as an aid in the prevention of disease caused by *Clostridium perfringens* Type C and K99 piliated *Escherichia coli.*

Dosage and Administration: Shake well before using. Administer 10 mL orally to calves less than 4 hours old. Slowly syringe toward the back of the calf's mouth. Colostrum should be fed to each calf.

Precaution(s): Store in the dark at 35°-45°F (2°-7°C). Do not freeze. Use entire contents when first opened.

Caution(s): Anaphylactic reactions may occur following the use of this biological. Symptomatic treatment: Epinephrine.

Warning(s): Do not vaccinate within 21 days prior to slaughter.

For animal use only.

Keep out of reach of children.

Presentation: 1 dose (10 mL) and 10 doses (100 mL).

Produced by: Advance Biologics, Inc.

Compendium Code No.: 14570330

E. COLICIN-B™

AgriLabs **Antiserum**

Escherichia coli Antiserum

U.S. Vet. Lic. No.: 272

Active Ingredient(s): Contains *Escherichia coli* antiserum.

Indications: For use in the prevention of *E. coli* (colibacillosis caused by *Escherichia coli)* both K99 pilus antigens and all of the somatic antigens of whole culture cells.

Dosage and Administration: Administer orally to newborn calves.

Dosage for calves: Administer one (1) 10 mL syringe orally to each calf within 12 hours after birth. Colostrum should be fed to each calf.

How to administer oral dosage: Slowly syringe the contents into the back of the calf's mouth.

How to administer intranasally: To administer intranasally, slowly transfer the entire contents of the diluent vial to the vaccine vial, using aseptic technique and sterile syringes and needles. Use a separate disposable cannula for each animal.

Precaution(s): Store at 35-45°F (2-7°C). Do not freeze.

Warning(s): Do not administer within 21 days of slaughter.

Presentation: 10 mL (1 dose) syringe and 100 mL (10 dose) bottle.

Compendium Code No.: 10580440

E. COLICIN-E®

AgriLabs **Antiserum**

Escherichia Coli Antiserum, Equine Origin

U.S. Vet. Lic. No.: 303

Composition: E. COLICIN-E® is prepared from the blood of horses hyperimmunized with whole cell cultures of *Escherichia coli.* The antiserum contains phenol, thimerosal, and oxytetracycline as preservatives.

Indications: For use as an aid in the prevention and control of endotoxemia and diarrhea caused by *Escherichia coli* in newborn foals.

Dosage and Administration: Shake well before using. Administer entire contents of one syringe (10 mL) orally to each foal within 12 hours after birth. Slowly syringe the contents into the back of the foal's mouth. Colostrum should be fed to each foal.

Precaution(s): Store in the dark at 35°-45°F (2°-7°C). Do not freeze. Use entire contents when first opened.

Caution(s): Anaphylactic reactions may occur following the use of this biological. Symptomatic treatment: Epinephrine.

For veterinary use only.

Presentation: 12 x 10 mL prefilled syringes.

Compendium Code No.: 10581560 AL4400114

E. COLICIN-S$_3$™

AgriLabs **Antiserum**

Escherichia coli Antiserum, Equine Origin

U.S. Vet. Lic. No.: 303

Contents: This product is prepared from the blood of horses hyperimmunized with K88, K99, and 987P, pilated *Escherichia coli.* Contains oxytetracycline, phenol, and thimerosal as preservatives.

Indications: For use in newborn piglets as an aid in the prevention of colibacillosis caused by K88, K99, and 987P pilated *Escherichia coli.*

Dosage and Administration: Shake well before using. Insert dispenser into bottle. Place dispenser extender on nozzle. Administer 2 mL (1 pump stroke) orally to piglets less than 12 hours old. Slowly dispense toward the back of the piglet's mouth. Colostrum should be fed to each piglet.

Precaution(s): Store in the dark at 35°-45° (2°-7°C). Do not freeze. Use entire contents when first opened.

Caution(s): Anaphylactic reactions may occur following the use of this biological.

Antidote(s): Epinephrine (symptomatic treatment).

Warning(s): Do not administer within 21 days prior to slaughter.

For veterinary use only.

Presentation: 50 dose (100 mL) and 100 dose (200 mL) vials.

Compendium Code No.: 10580460

E. COLICIN-S$_3$+C™

AgriLabs **Antiserum-Antitoxin**

Clostridium perfringens Type C Antitoxin-Escherichia coli Antiserum, Equine Origin

U.S. Vet. Lic. No.: 303

Contents: This product contains antibodies against *Clostridium perfringens* Type C and K88, K99, and 987P, pilated *Escherichia coli.* Contains oxytetracycline, phenol, and thimerosal as preservatives.

Indications: For use in newborn piglets as an aid in the prevention of disease caused by *Clostridium perfringens* Type C and K88, K99, and 987P pilated *Escherichia coli.*

Dosage and Administration: Shake well before using. Insert dispenser into bottle. Place dispenser extender on nozzle. Administer 2 mL (1 pump stroke) orally to piglets less than 6 hours old. Slowly dispense toward the back of the piglet's mouth. Colostrum should be fed to each piglet.

Precaution(s): Store in the dark at 35°-45° (2°-7°C). Do not freeze. Use entire contents when first opened.

Caution(s): Anaphylactic reactions may occur following the use of this biological.

Antidote(s): Epinephrine (symptomatic treatment).

Warning(s): Do not administer within 21 days prior to slaughter.

For veterinary use only.

Presentation: 50 dose (100 mL) and 100 dose (200 mL) vials.

Compendium Code No.: 10580450

ECOSECT™ INSECTICIDE

Schering-Plough **Premise and Topical Insecticide**

EPA Reg. No.: 66986-4-45860

Active Ingredient(s):

Potassium salts of fatty acids	49%
Inert Ingredients	51%
Total	100%

Indications: ECOSECT™ is an effective contact insecticide for control of darkling beetles (lesser mealworms) and hide beetles, flies, lice, chicken mites and northern fowl mites found in or on poultry production facilities. The formulation is based on potassium salts of naturally derived fatty acids. For commercial use.

Dosage and Administration: It is a violation of federal law to use this product in a manner inconsistent with its labeling. Do not apply this product in a way that will contact workers or other persons, either directly or through drift. Only protected handlers may be in the area during application. For any requirements specific to your State or Tribe, consult the agency responsible for pesticide regulation.

Application Guidelines: Mix product with water as directed for specific target pests and use a directed spray or mist. Retreat as needed. Obtain through coverage of the pest(s). Ensure that the entire pest population is treated in all areas that the pest is located. Do not apply in thermal foggers. For optimum residual activity, this product may be tank mixed with an approved insecticide and sprayed as directed.

For Direct Application to Poultry:

Pest Target	Gallons per 100 gallons of water	Additional Use Instruction
Lice Northern Fowl Mites Chicken Mites	2-4	Spray thoroughly infested areas of hens or turkeys where mice or lice are located. For Northern Fowl Mites on caged layers: Use one ounce of spray mixture per hen at 100-125 psi to ensure penetration of the feathers. For Northern Fowl Mites on turkeys: Spray enough product to thoroughly wet infested areas. Supplement on bird treatments with treatments to buildings and roosts which are harborages for these pests.

For Control of Pests in Poultry Roosts and Buildings

Pest Target	Gallons per 100 gallons of water	Additional Use Instruction
Lice Flies Northern Fowl Mites Chicken Mites	2-4	When Used Alone: Apply 10-20 gallons of spray mixture per 1000 square feet. When used as a Tank Mix with a Recommended Insecticide: Apply 1-2 gallons of spray mixture per 1000 square feet. Apply spray mixture at the rates listed above to walls, litter or roost surfaces. Force spray into cracks, posts, crevices, around ventilation areas, insulation areas, and areas where insects tend to congregate. For darkling beetles and hide beetles, optimum spray timing is after flock is removed from the house when the beetles are exposed and most active.
Darkling beetles Hide beetles	2-6	

Precaution(s): Storage and Disposal: Do not contaminate water, feed or foodstuff by storage or disposal.

Storage: Keep container tightly sealed when not in use. Store only in original container, in a dry place, inaccessible to children and pets.

Pesticide Disposal: Wastes resulting from the use of this product may be disposed of on site or at an approved waste disposal facility.

Container Disposal: Do not reuse empty container. Triple rinse, then offer for recycling or reconditioning, or puncture and dispose of in a sanitary landfill or by incineration, or, if allowed by state and local authorities, by burning. If burned, stay out of smoke.

Physical or Chemical Hazards: Flammable. Keep away from heat or open flame.

Environmental Hazards: This product may be hazardous to aquatic invertebrates. Do not apply directly to water, areas where surface water is present, or to intertidal areas below the mean high water mark. Do not contaminate water by cleaning of equipment or disposal of water.

Caution(s): Precautionary Statements: Hazards to Humans and Domestic Animals: Causes skin irritation. Causes substantial but temporary eye injury. Do not get in eyes, on skin or on clothing.

Personal Protective Equipment: Some materials that are chemical-resistant to this product are listed below. If you want more options, follow the instructions for category C on an EPA chemical resistance category selection chart.

Handlers who may be exposed to the diluted product through application or other tasks must wear: long-sleeved shirt and long pants, shoes plus socks.

Handlers who may be exposed to the concentrate through mixing, loading, application, or other tasks must wear: Coveralls over short-sleeved shirt and short pants, chemical-resistant gloves such as butyl rubber, nitrile rubber, neoprene rubber or PVC, chemical-resistant footwear plus socks, protective eyewear, chemical-resistant headgear for overhead exposure, and chemical-resistant apron when cleaning equipment, mixing or loading. Discard clothing and other absorbent materials that have been drenched or heavily contaminated with this product's concentrate. Do not reuse them. Follow manufacturer's instructions for cleaning/maintaining PPE. If no such instructions for washables, use detergent and hot water. Keep and wash PPE separately from other laundry.

User Safety Recommendations: Users should wash hands before eating, drinking, chewing gum, using tobacco, or using the toilet. Remove clothing immediately if pesticide gets inside. Then wash thoroughly and put on clean clothing.

Warning(s): First Aid: If in eyes: Hold eyelids open and flush with a steady, gentle stream of water for 15 minutes.

If on skin: Wash with plenty of soap and water. Get medical attention.

If swallowed: Drink promptly a large quantity of milk, egg white, gelatin solution, or, if these are not available, large quantities of water. Avoid alcohol.

Limit of Warranty and Liability: This product conforms to the description on the label and is reasonably fit for the purposes set forth on the label when used according to the label directions and under the specified label conditions. The manufacturer disclaims any and all other express or implied warranties of merchantability and fitness for a particular purpose. Buyer and all users assume all risks and responsibility for loss or damage if this product is used, stored, handled or applied under any condition not reasonably foreseeable or beyond the manufacturer's control, or not as explicitly set forth in the label. The limit of the manufacturer's liability shall be the purchase price for the quantity involved in no event shall the manufacturer be liable for special, incidental or consequential damages.

Keep out of reach of children.

Presentation: 2½ gallons.

Compendium Code No.: 10470550

ECP® STERILE SOLUTION ℞

Pharmacia & Upjohn **Estradiol**

Estradiol cypionate

Active Ingredient(s): The sterile solution contains per mL: 2 mg estradiol cypionate, also 5.4 mg chlorobutanol anhydrous (chloral deriv.) added as preservative in 916 mg cottonseed oil.

Indications: ECP® estradiol cypionate offers all of the functional activity of natural estrogenic substances with the advantage of a prolonged action.

The indications in bovine medicine are[1]:

To correct anestrus (absence of heat period) in the absence of follicular cysts.

To expel purulent material from the uterus in pyometra of cows.

To stimulate uterine expulsion of retained placentas and mummified fetuses.

Pharmacology: Description: This is the oil-soluble 17β-cyclopentylpropionate ester of "alpha" estradiol. It provides estradiol-17β, believed to be most potent of the naturally occurring estrogens, in the form of the cyclopentyl-propionate ester, a highly fat-soluble derivative with profound estrogenic effect.

Actions: Comparative studies have demonstrated that estradiol cypionate produces estrogenic effects which are qualitatively the same as those produced by other estradiol esters.

Dosage and Administration: Sterile Solution ECP® estradiol cypionate is for intramuscular injection only in cattle intended for breeding. The doses should not exceed 4 mg (2 mL). Doses for cows may be repeated, if necessary, in one week. Do not overdose.

The use of ECP® as a supplemental source of estrogen in the bovine has been found beneficial in the following conditions[1]: Anestrus, pyometra, retained placenta, mummified fetus.

Contraindication(s): As with all products of this nature, a complete examination to determine the status of the reproductive tract should be undertaken prior to administration of this drug. Pregnancy may be the prime reason for either anestrus or the persistence of the corpus luteum. Since pregnancy may be terminated by estrogens, ECP® estradiol cypionate is contraindicated where a desired pregnancy exists.

Precaution(s): Store at controlled room temperature 20° to 25°C (68° to 77°F) [see USP].

If this product is exposed to temperature of less than 7°C (45°F), some constituents of the vehicle will solidify. If this should occur, warm the vial to room temperature before using.

Caution(s): Federal (USA) law restricts this drug to use by or on the order of a licensed veterinarian.

Estrogens used in the canine may produce a gradual anemia and a profound leukocytosis which is followed by leukopenia.[2] Thrombocytopenia may result with a concomitant alteration in the clotting mechanisms. First gross signs of alteration of the clotting mechanisms would include petechial and/or ecchymotic hemorrhage of mucus membranes and may result in frank hemorrhage in some animals. The possibility of endometritis and pyometritis following the use of estrogens is always present in the bitch. It has been demonstrated that endometrial hyperplasia is produced more consistently when estrogen and progesterone are given to the bitch.[3] Theoretically then, estrogen given during late estrus or in metestrus in the presence of endogenous progesterone, which is being produced at near maximal rate by the recently developed corpora lutea, could result in endometrial proliferation and pyometra.

ECP® is intended for use only in cattle used for breeding purposes.

Administration of an estrogenic substance to an animal may result in development of follicular cysts.[4]

In the case of prolonged persistence of the corpus luteum in cows, thorough examination should also be made of the uterus to determine the presence of an endometritis or a fetus. Use of appropriate antimicrobial agents, in addition to ECP® estradiol cypionate should be considered if endometritis exists.

In the absence of normally developing follicles on the ovaries, estrus may be produced, but ovulation may not accompany estrus.

Because it is impossible to determine exactly if and when ovulation may occur in treated females during an induced heat period, it may help to breed the female frequently throughout the induced heat periods in order to improve the possibility of conception.

Repeat breeding will improve the chance conception only if ovulation occurs.

For use in animals only.

Warning(s): Not for human use.

Adverse Reactions: Prolonged estrus, precocious development, genital irritation, follicular cysts, and a reduction of milk flow may occur following estrogen therapy, frequently as a result of overdosage. If any of these phenomena are observed, the dosage should be reduced accordingly.

Discussion: Anestrus in Cattle: Reports have suggested that frequently cows with a follicular cyst may be more inclined to be anestrual than nymphomaniac.[5,6] Many cows will recover spontaneously from anestrus (if due to follicular cysts) if less than 60 days postparturient.[6] In cases of anestrus due to follicular cysts, estrogens are not usually indicated.

Frequently, anestrus or follicular cysts have developed in association with a marked loss in body condition due to disease or high milk production.[6]

Anestrus in conjunction with a persistent corpus luteum probably reflects some interference with normal function of the uterine endometrium. Pregnancy must be considered as a cause of the persistence of the corpus luteum. Prolonged maintenance of the corpus luteum has also occurred following hysterectomy or experimental induction of endometritis.[7,8] It is doubtful that corpora lutea are retained indefinitely in cattle with normal uterine function.[6,8] It has been demonstrated that some estrogen esters will cause regression of the corpus luteum in cycling, pregnant, or hysterectomized cattle.[9] The response of the corpus luteum of pregnancy may differ with different estrogen esters. In the absence of a pregnancy or a detectable uterine malfunction, repeated rectal palpations will be required to establish a diagnosis of persistent corpus luteum. Although some estrogen esters may produce luteal regression, consideration of proper uterine treatment should also be given.

The proper diagnosis of anestrus without frequent rectal palpation is difficult since normal ovarian cycles can occur without accompanying estrus. It has been reported that such "silent heat" is more frequent at the first postpartum estrus.[6]

The induced estrus in cows or heifers may not be fertile. Regular cyclic activity may not follow an ECP® estradiol cypionate induced estrus.

References: Available upon request.

Presentation: ECP® estradiol cypionate is available as 2 mg per mL—Supplied in 50 mL vials (NDC 0009-0616-02).

Compendium Code No.: 10490151 811 410 204

ECTIBAN® D

Durvet **Topical Insecticide**

Insecticide-Poultry & Livestock Dust

EPA Reg. No.: 59-212-12281

Active Ingredient(s):

Permethrin-(3-Phenoxyphenyl) methyl (±) cis, trans-3-(2,2-dichloroethenyl)-2,2-dimethyl-cyclopropanecarboxylate*	0.25%
Inert Ingredients	99.75%
Total	100.00%

*cis/trans ratio: Min. 35% (±) cis and max. 65% (±) trans

Indications: For control of horn flies, face flies, lice (dairy, beef and swine) and mites (poultry).

Directions for Use: It is a violation of Federal Law to use this product in a manner inconsistent with its labeling.

Ready-to-use in dust bags or hand dusting equipment. Follow specific use instructions on dust dispensing equipment to be used.

Apply To	Target Insects	Application Instructions
Lactating and Non-Lactating Dairy Cattle and Beef Cattle	Horn Flies, Face Flies, Lice	Dust Bags: Suitable for all refill bags. Place contents of package in dust bag and refill as needed. Results improved by daily forced use. Ready to Use Dustbag: Installation of Cattle Dust Bag. Suspend the dust bags by inserting rope, chain, or wire through the grommets at the top of the bag and attaching to an overhead structure, or by hooking the grommets into hooks fixed to a stationary over-head 2x4 at the heights recommended for louse and horn fly or face fly control. Rope, chain or wire can also be tied or attached to two posts or other fixed points with the dust bag hanging in the center. After the bags are in place, pull the rip cord to allow the insecticide to release from the sifter bottom. Direct Application: Apply up to 2 oz* per animal. For lice, a second treatment at 14 days is recommended and dust should be rubbed well into coat.
Swine	Lice	Apply up to 1 oz* per animal paying particular attention to the ears. A second treatment at 14 days is recommended. Do not ship animals for slaughter within 5 days of last treatment.
Poultry	Mites	Apply at a rate of 1 lb/100 birds. Ensure thorough treatment of vent areas.

*1 oz of this dust equals approximately 2½ level tablespoonsful.

Precautionary Statements: Hazards to Humans and Domestic Animals:

Caution: Avoid contact with skin and eyes. Avoid breathing dust. Food utensils such as teaspoons and measuring cups should not be used for food purposes after use with insecticide.

Statement of Practical Treatment: Harmful if swallowed, inhaled or absorbed through the skin. Causes moderate eye irritation. Avoid breathing dust. Avoid contact with skin, eyes or clothing. Wash thoroughly with soap and water after handling. Remove contaminated clothing and wash clothing before reuse. Prolonged or frequently repeated skin contact may cause allergic reactions in some individuals.

If in Eyes: Flush eyes with plenty of water. Call a physician if irritation persists.

If on Skin: Wash with plenty of soap and water. Get medical attention if irritation persists.

If Inhaled: Move victim to fresh air. If not breathing, give artificial respiration, preferably mouth-to-mouth. Get medical attention.

If Swallowed: Call a physician or Poison Control Center. Drink 1 or 2 glasses of water and induce vomiting by touching back of throat with finger. If person is unconscious, do not give anything by mouth and do not induce vomiting.

Environmental Hazards: This pesticide is extremely toxic to fish. Use with care when applying to areas adjacent to any body of water. Do not apply directly to water. Do not contaminate water by cleaning of equipment or disposal of wastes. Apply this product only as specified on the label.

Physical or Chemical Hazards: Do not use or store near heat or open flame.

Storage and Disposal: Do not contaminate water, food, or feed by storage or disposal.

Storage: Store in cool, dry place.

Pesticide Disposal: Wastes resulting from the use of this product may be disposed of on site or at an approved waste disposal facility.

Container Disposal: Completely empty container into application equipment. Then dispose of empty container in a sanitary landfill or by incineration, or, if allowed by State and local authorities, by burning. If burned, stay out of smoke.

Warning(s): Keep out of reach of children.

Disclaimer: Notice of Warranty: Durvet, Inc., makes no warranty of merchantability, fitness for any particular purpose, or otherwise, expressed or implied concerning this product or its uses which extend beyond the use of the product under normal conditions in accord with the statements made on the label.

Presentation: 2 lbs, 12.5 lbs and 25 lbs.

ECTIBAN® is a registered trademark of Schering-Plough Animal Health.

Compendium Code No.: 10840742 1001

ECTIBAN® DELICE®

Durvet **Topical Insecticide**

Pour-On Insecticide

EPA Reg. No.: 773-66-12281

Active Ingredient(s):

Permethrin: 3-(phenoxyphenyl)methyl (±) cis, trans-3-(2,2-dichloroethenyl)-2,2-dimethylcyclopropanecarboxylate* 1.0%
Inert Ingredients** 99.0%
100.0%

*cis/trans ratio: Min 35% (±) cis and max 65% (±) trans.

**Contains petroleum distillates.

Indications: Controls lice and flies on cattle (beef, lactating and non-lactating dairy); keds and lice on sheep.

Directions for Use: It is a violation of Federal law to use this product in a manner inconsistent with its labeling.

Ready to Use - No dilution necessary.

Apply To	Target Insects	Application Instructions
Lactating and Non-Lactating Dairy Cattle, Beef Cattle and Calves	Lice Horn Flies, Face Flies and Aids in Control of: Horse Flies, Stable Flies, Mosquitoes, Black Flies And Ticks.	Pour along back and down face. Apply ½ fl oz (15 cc) per 100 lbs body wt of animal, up to a maximum of 5 fl oz for any one animal.
Sheep	Sheep Keds Lice	Pour along back. Apply ¼ fl oz (7.5 cc) per 50 lbs body wt of animal, up to a maximum of 3 fl oz for any one animal.

For cattle and sheep, repeat treatment as needed, but not more than once every 2 weeks. For optimum lice control, two treatments at 14 day intervals are recommended.

Special Note: ECTIBAN® DELICE® Pour-On Insecticide is not effective in controlling cattle grubs.

Precautionary Statements: Hazards to Humans and Domestic Animals: Caution: Avoid contact with eyes.

Statement of Practical Treatment:

If in Eyes: Immediately flush eyes with plenty of water. Get medical attention if discomfort persists.

If Swallowed: Call a physician immediately. Do not induce vomiting unless under medical attention.

Note to Physician: Solvent presents aspiration hazard. Gastric lavage is indicated if material was taken internally.

Environmental Hazards: This pesticide is extremely toxic to fish. Use with care when applying to areas adjacent to any body of water. Do not add directly to water. Do not contaminate water by cleaning of equipment or disposal of wastes. Apply this product only as specified on this label.

Physical or Chemical Hazards: Do not use or store near heat or open flame.

Storage and Disposal: Do not contaminate water, food or feed by storage or disposal.

Storage: Keep container sealed when not in use. Do not store near food or feed.

Pesticide Disposal: Wastes resulting from the use of this product may be disposed of on site or at an approved waste disposal facility.

Container Disposal: Triple rinse (or equivalent). Then offer for recycling or reconditioning, or puncture and dispose of in a sanitary landfill or by incineration, or, if allowed by State and local authorities, by burning. If burned, stay out of smoke.

Warning(s): Keep out of reach of children.

Disclaimer: Notice of Warranty: Durvet, Inc. makes no warranty of merchantability, fitness for any particular purpose, or otherwise, expressed or implied concerning this product or its uses which extend beyond the use of the product under normal conditions in accord with the statements made on this label.

Presentation: 1 US gallon (3.785 L) container.

ECTIBAN and DELICE (stylized) are registered trademarks of Schering-Plough Veterinary Corp.

Compendium Code No.: 10840751 9/99

ECTIBAN® EC

Durvet **Premise and Topical Insecticide**

EPA Reg. No.: 59-214-12281

Active Ingredient(s):

Permethrin (3-phenoxyphenyl) methyl (±) cis, trans-3-(2,2-dichloroethenyl)-2,2-dimethyl-cyclopropanecarboxylate* 5.7%
Inert ingredients 94.3%
Total 100.0%

*Cis/trans ratio: Min. 35% (±) cis and max. 65% (±) trans.

Contains 50 g per liter (1.67 oz. active ingredient per quart).

Indications: For the control of horn flies, face flies, stable flies, houseflies, horseflies, black flies, mosquitoes, eye gnats, mange mites, scabies mites, ticks, lice and sheep keds on lactating and nonlactating dairy cattle and goats, beef cattle, horses and sheep.

For the control of lice, northern fowl mites and mange on poultry and swine.

For the control of houseflies, stable flies and little houseflies (*Fannia* spp.) and to aid in the control of cockroaches, ants, spiders, mosquitoes, crickets and face flies in dairies, barns, feedlots, stables, poultry houses, and swine and livestock housing.

For the control of cluster flies on exterior building structures.

Dosage and Administration: It is a violation of federal law to use the product in a manner inconsistent with its labeling.

Apply ECTIBAN® according to the following directions. Retreat as needed, but not more often than once every two (2) weeks. Use as needed on horses not intended for human consumption. Spray lactating dairy cows only after milking is completed.

Lactating and Nonlactating Dairy Cattle and Goats, Beef Cattle, Horses and Sheep:

For horn flies, face flies, stable flies, houseflies, horseflies, black flies, mosquitoes, eye gnats, mange mites, scabies mites, ticks, lice and sheep keds (sprayer): Dilute 1 qt. to 25 gallons of water (2½ tbsp./gallon). Apply 1 to 2 qts. of coarse spray per animal over the whole body surface. For mange, lice, ticks and scabies, be sure to thoroughly wet the animal. Apply a second application at 14 days.

For horn flies only (sprayer): Dilute 1 qt. to 50 gallons of water (1 tbsp./gallon). Apply 1 qt. of coarse spray per animal.

For horn flies, face flies, stable flies, and ear ticks (low pressure sprayer): Dilute 1 qt. to 2½ gallons of water (6 tbsp./qt.). Apply 1 to 2 oz. spray per animal. Spot treat the back, face, legs and ears.

For horn flies, face flies, stable flies, and ear ticks (backrubber/self oiler): Dilute 1 qt. to 10 gallons of diesel oil (6 tbsp./gallon). Keep the rubbing device charged. Results are improved by daily forced use.

Poultry and Swine:

For lice, northern fowl mites, and mange (sprayer): Dilute 1 qt. to 25 gallons of water (2½ tbsp./gallon).

Poultry: Apply one (1) gallon of spray per 100 birds, paying particular attention to the vent.

Swine: Thoroughly soak, including ears. For mange, repeat at 14 days. Spray walls and change bedding.

Premises (dairies, barns, feedlots, stables, poultry houses, swine and livestock housing):

For houseflies, stable flies and little houseflies (*Fannia* spp.), and to aid in the control of cockroaches, ants, spiders, mosquitoes, crickets and face flies (sprayer): Dilute 1 qt. to 10 gallons of water (6 tbsp./gallon). Spray to the point of run-off. As a guide, use one (1) gallon of spray per 750 sq. ft. (400-1,400 sq. ft.).

Mist sprayer: Ready to use. Direct 4 oz. onto 1,000 sq. ft. of surface.

Overhead space spray system: Dilute 1 qt. to 10 gallons of diesel or mineral oil (6 tbsp./gallon). Apply 4 oz. spray per 1,000 cu. ft. of air space.

Exterior building structures:

For cluster flies (mist sprayer): Ready to use. Direct 5 oz. onto 1,000 sq. ft. of surface concentrating on eaves, roof gables and attics.

Spray directly onto walls and ceiling as residue surface treatment only. Do not treat manure or litter. The use of any residual fly spray should be supplemented with proper manure management and general sanitation to reduce or eliminate fly breeding sites.

Precaution(s): Do not contaminate water, food or feed by storage or disposal.

Storage: Keep the container sealed when not in use. Do not store near food or feed.

Pesticide Disposal: Wastes resulting from the use of the product may be disposed of on site or at an approved waste disposal facility.

Container Disposal: Triple rinse (or equivalent). Then offer for recycling or reconditioning, or puncture and dispose of in a sanitary landfill or by incineration, or, if allowed by state and local authorities, by burning. If burned, stay out of smoke.

Physical or Chemical Hazards: Do not use or store near heat or an open flame.

Environmental Hazards: The pesticide is extremely toxic to fish. Use with care when applying to areas adjacent to any body of water. Do not apply directly to water. Do not contaminate water by the cleaning of equipment or the disposal of wastes. Apply the product only as specified on the label.

Caution(s): Precautionary Statements:

Hazards to Humans and Domestic Animals: Avoid contact with the skin and eyes. Avoid inhaling spray mist.

Warning(s): For swine, allow five (5) days between last treatment and slaughter.

Not for use on horses intended for human consumption.

Statement of Practical Treatment:

If swallowed, call a physician. Vomiting should be supervised by a physician or qualified professional medical staff because of the possible pulmonary damage via aspiration of the solvent.

If on skin, wash skin with soap and water.

If in eyes, immediately flush eyes with plenty of water. Get medical attention if discomfort persists.

Notice of Warranty: Durvet, Inc. makes no warranty of merchantability, fitness for any particular purpose, or otherwise, expressed or implied concerning this product or its uses which extend beyond the use of the product under normal conditions in accord with the statements made on the label.

Keep out of the reach of children.

Presentation: 8 oz., 32 oz. and 1 gallon containers.

Compendium Code No.: 10840760

ECTIBAN® SYNERGIZED DELICE® POUR-ON INSECTICIDE

Durvet **Premise and Topical Insecticide**

EPA Reg. No.: 773-72-12281

Active Ingredient(s):

Permethrin: (3-phenoxyphenyl) methyl (±)-cis-trans-3-(2,2-dichloroethenyl)-2,2-dimethylcyclopropanecarboxylate* 1.0%
Piperonyl Butoxide Technical** 1.0%
Inert Ingredients.......... 98.0%
100.0%

*cis/trans ratio: Min 35% (±) cis and max 65% (±) trans

**Equivalent to Min 0.8% (butylcarbityl) (6-propylpiperonyl) ether and 0.2% related compounds.

Indications: Pour-on insecticide for cattle, sheep, and their premises.

Directions for Use: It is a violation of Federal law to use this product in a manner inconsistent with its labeling.

Ready to use — No dilution necessary.

Apply To: Lactating and Non-Lactating Dairy Cattle, Beef Cattle and Calves.

Target Insects: Lice, Horn flies, Face flies. Aids in control of Horse flies, Stable flies, House flies, Mosquitoes, and Black flies.

Application Instructions: Dosage: Apply ½ fl oz (15 cc) per 100 lbs body wt of animal up to a maximum of 5 fl oz for any one animal.

Pour-On: Pour correct dose along back and down face.

Ready-To-Use Spray: Use undiluted in a mist sprayer to apply correct dose. Apply directly to neck, face, back, legs, and ears.

Back Rubber Use: Mix one pint per gallon #2 diesel or mineral oil. Keep rubbing device charged. Results improved by daily forced use.

Apply To: Sheep.

Target Insects: Sheep keds, Lice.

Application Instructions: Pour along back. Apply ¼ fl oz (7.5 cc) per 50 lbs body wt of animal, up to a maximum of 3 fl oz for any one animal. For optimum control, all animals in the flock should be treated after shearing.

Apply To: Premises — In and around Horse, Beef, Dairy, Swine, Sheep, and Poultry premises. Animal Hospital Pens and Kennels and "outside" Meat Processing Premises.

Target Insects: House flies, Stable flies, Face flies, Gnats, Mosquitoes, Black flies, Fleas, Little house flies *(Fannia* spp.). Aid in control of Cockroaches, Ants, Spiders, Crickets.

Application Instructions: For use as a ready-to-use spot spray or premise spray, use undiluted in a mist sprayer. Apply directly to surface to leave a residual insecticidal coating, paying particular attention to areas where insects crawl or alight. One gallon will treat approximately 7300 square feet.

For cattle and sheep, repeat treatment as needed, but not more often than once every 2 weeks. For optimum lice control, two treatments at a 14-day interval are recommended.

Special Note: ECTIBAN® SYNERGIZED DELICE® Insecticide is not effective in controlling cattle grubs. ECTIBAN® SYNERGIZED DELICE® is an oil-based, ready-to-use product, which may leave an oily appearance on the hair coat of some animals. ECTIBAN® SYNERGIZED DELICE® should be used in an integrated pest management system which may involve repeat treatments and the use of other pest control practices.

Precautionary Statements: Hazards to Humans and Domestic Animals:

Caution: Harmful if absorbed through skin. Avoid contact with skin, eyes, and clothing. Prolonged or frequently repeated skin contact may cause allergic reactions in some individuals. Wash thoroughly with soap and water after handling.

Statement of Practical Treatment:

If Swallowed: Call a physician immediately. Do not induce vomiting unless under medical attention. If In Eyes: Immediately flush eyes with plenty of water. Get medical attention if discomfort persists. If On Skin: Wash skin with soap and water. Get medical attention.

Environmental Hazards: This product is extremely toxic to fish and other aquatic invertebrates. Do not add directly to water. Do not contaminate water when disposing of equipment washwaters. Apply this product only as specified on this label.

Physical or Chemical Hazards: Do not use or store near heat or open flame.

Storage and Disposal: Do not contaminate water, food, or feed by storage or disposal.

Storage: Keep container sealed when not in use. Do not store near food or feed. Pesticide Disposal: Wastes resulting from the use of this product may be disposed of on site or at an approved waste disposal facility. Container Disposal: Triple rinse (or equivalent). Then offer for recycling or reconditioning, or puncture and dispose of in a sanitary landfill or incineration, or if allowed by State and local authorities, by burning. If burned, stay out of smoke.

Warning(s): Keep out of reach of children.

Disclaimer: Notice of Warranty: Durvet, Inc. makes no warranty of merchantability, fitness for any particular purpose, or otherwise, expressed or implied, concerning this product or its uses which extend beyond the use of the product under normal conditions in accordance with the statements made on this label.

Presentation: One US gallon.

ECTIBAN and DELICE (stylized) are registered trademarks of Schering-Plough Animal Health Corp.

Compendium Code No.: 10840770 23355507, 23355604 8/99

ECTIBAN® WP

Durvet **Premise Insecticide**

EPA Reg. No.: 773-64-12281

Active Ingredient(s):

Permethrin (3-phenoxyphenyl) methyl (±) cis, trans-3-(2,2-dichloroethenyl)-2,2-dimethylcyclopropanecarboxylate* 25%
Inert Ingredients 75%
Total 100%

*cis/trans ratio: Min 35% (±) cis and max 65% (±) trans

Indications: Long lasting fly killer premise spray.

Directions for Use: For agricultural use only.

Spray directly to walls and ceilings as residual surface treatment only. Do not treat manure or litter. Avoid contamination of feed and water. Do not apply directly to livestock or poultry.

Shake well before measuring.

It is a violation of Federal law to use this product in a manner inconsistent with its labeling.

Apply To	Target Insects	Method of Application	Dilute	Application Rate
Dairies, Barns, Feed lots, Stables, Poultry Houses, Swine and Other Livestock Premises	House Flies, Stable Flies and Other Manure Breeding Flies. Also aids in control of Cockroaches, Mosquitoes, Spiders, Ants, Crickets and Face Flies.	Sprayer	6 oz* to 11 gal water or 8 level tablespoons to 3 gal of water.	Spray to point of runoff. As a guide, use 1 gal spray per 750 sq ft (400-1400 sq ft). Double the concentration for premise application under severe fly pressure.

*1 oz of this powder equals five level tablespoonsful. Shake canister before measuring. Make up only as required.

Apply to surfaces where flies rest. Do not apply as a larvicide. Use proper manure management and sanitation to reduce fly breeding.

Precautionary Statements: Hazards to Humans and Domestic Animals: Warning: May cause eye irritation, harmful if swallowed: Do not get in eyes, on skin or on clothing. Wash thoroughly after handling.

Statement of Practical Treatment: If in Eyes: Flush with water for 15 minutes. Get medical attention if irritation persists.

If Swallowed: Drink 1 or 2 glasses of water and induce vomiting by touching back of throat with finger. Do not induce vomiting or give anything by mouth to an unconscious person.

Environmental Hazards: This pesticide is extremely toxic to fish. Use with care when applying to areas adjacent to any body of water. Do not apply directly to water. Do not contaminate water by cleaning of equipment or disposal of wastes. Apply this product only as specified on this label.

Storage and Disposal: Do not contaminate water, food or feed by storage or disposal. Storage: Mix as needed. Do not store diluted material. Keep container closed when not in use. Do not store near food or feed. Pesticide Disposal: Wastes resulting from the use of this product may be disposed of on site or at an approved waste disposal facility.

In case of spill on floor or paved surfaces, sweep and remove to chemical waste area and dispose of in accordance with State and local regulations.

Container Disposal: Triple rinse (or equivalent). Then offer for recycling or reconditioning, or puncture and dispose of in a sanitary landfill, or incineration, or, if allowed by State and local authorities, by burning. If burned, stay out of smoke.

Warning(s): Keep out of reach of children.

Disclaimer: Notice to Buyer and User: Seller warrants that this product conforms to the chemical description on the label and is reasonably fit for the purpose stated on the label when used in accordance with directions under normal conditions of use. This warranty does not extend to the use of this product contrary to label instructions, or under abnormal use conditions, or under conditions not reasonably foreseeable to Seller and Buyer and User assumes the risk of any such use. Seller disclaims all other warranties expressed or implied, including any other warranty of fitness or merchantability. Seller shall not be liable for consequential, special or indirect damages resulting from the use or handling of this product and Seller's sole liability and Buyer's and User's exclusive remedy shall be limited to the refund of the purchase price.

Presentation: 6 oz (170.1 g).

Compendium Code No.: 10840781 Rev. 10-97

ECTO-FOAM™

Virbac **Parasiticide Foam**

EPA Reg. No.: 499-231-2382

Active Ingredient(s):

Pyrethrins 0.15%
Piperonyl Butoxide Technical* 0.70%
N-Octyl Bicycloheptene Dicarboximide 0.34%
Inert Ingredients 98.81%

*Equivalent to 0.56% (Butylcarbityl) (6-propylpiperonyl) ether and 0.14% related compounds.

Contains no CFCs or other ozone-depleting substances. Federal regulations prohibit CFC propellants in aerosols.

Contains microencapsulated pyrethrins for residual activity and unencapsulated pyrethrins for knockdown.

Indications: Residual flea and tick treatment with knockdown for use on dogs and cats. Also for use on dogs that are sensitive to conventional sprays.

Directions for Use: Shake well before using.

It is a violation of Federal law to use this product in a manner inconsistent with its labeling.

Read entire label before each use.

Use only on dogs, cats, horses and ponies.

Do not use on kittens or puppies under twelve weeks of age. This product is not recommended for use on cats which have been compromised due to previous illness, medication or existing

E

medical condition. Consult a veterinarian before using this product on debilitated, medicated, aged, pregnant or nursing animals.

Fleas: Shake well and invert can to dispense. Foam can be applied directly onto the pet or into the palm of your hand and then applied to the pet. For direct application, apply one-second bursts of ECTO-FOAM™ as hair is back combed. Foam can also be worked from the palm of the hand into the coat. Apply over the entire animal until damp, massaging or brushing the hair until the foam vanishes. Allow pet to dry. Do not apply from can directly to face, rather apply foam by hand around ears and under chin. Ensure that foam contacts and wets ticks thoroughly. Efficacy lasts for up to 8 days. Do not repeat treatment for one week.

Precautionary Statements: Caution:

Statement of Practical Treatment:

If in Eyes: Flush eyes with plenty of water. Call a physician if irritation persists.

Hazards to Humans and Domestic Animals: Caution: Causes moderate eye irritation. Avoid contact with eyes or clothing. Wash thoroughly with soap and water after handling. Sensitivities may occur after using any pesticide product for pets. If signs of sensitivity occur, bathe your pet with mild soap and rinse with large amounts of water. If signs continue, consult a veterinarian immediately.

Environmental Hazards: This product is toxic to fish. Do not apply to water.

Physical or Chemical Hazards: Contents under pressure. Do not puncture or incinerate container. Do not use or store near heat or open flame. Exposure to temperatures above 130°F may cause bursting.

Storage and Disposal: Do not contaminate water, food, or feed by storage and disposal.

Storage: Store in a cool area away from heat or open flame and in an area out of reach of children. Do not store below 32°F.

Disposal: This container may be recycled in aerosol recycling centers. At present there are only a few such centers in the country. Before offering for recycling, empty the can by using the product according to the label. (Do not puncture.) If recycling is not available, wrap the container and discard in the trash.

Warning(s): Keep out of reach of children. Sold only by veterinarians.

Presentation: Available in 9 oz (267 g) cans.

Compendium Code No.: 10230230

ECTOKYL™ 3X FLEA & TICK SHAMPOO

DVM **Parasiticide Shampoo**

EPA Reg. No.: 69061-4-41835

Active Ingredient(s):

Pyrethrins	0.15%
Piperonyl Butoxide, Technical*	1.00%
N-Octyl Bicycloheptene Dicarboximide	0.50%
Di-n-Propyl Isocinchomeronate	0.50%
Inert Ingredients:	97.85%
Total:	100.00%

*Equivalent to 0.80% of (butylcarbityl) (6-propylpiperonyl) ether and 0.20% of related compounds.

Indications: ECTOKYL™ 3X Flea & Tick Shampoo is a 3X pyrethrin formula with oatmeal coat conditioner and natural soothing aloe for dogs and cats.

Directions for Use: It is a violation of Federal Law to use this product in a manner inconsistent with its labeling.

Read entire label before use. Use only on dogs and cats.

To use: Thoroughly soak animal with water. Do not apply shampoo around eyes. Apply shampoo on head, then lather. Repeat procedure with neck, chest, middle and hind quarter, finishing legs last. Allow lather to remain on animal for 3-5 minutes, then rinse thoroughly. In extremely dirty, or scaly animals, the above procedure may be repeated. May be used every 7-10 days. May be used full strength or diluted with two (2) parts water.

Contraindication(s): Do not use on puppies or kittens under 12 weeks.

Precautionary Statements: Hazards to Humans and Domestic Animals:

Humans: Causes eye and skin irritation. Do not get in eyes, on skin or on clothing. Harmful if swallowed. Wash thoroughly with soap and water after handling. Remove contaminated clothing and wash before reuse.

Animals: Do not use on puppies or kittens under 12 weeks. Consult a veterinarian before using this product on debilitated, aged, pregnant, nursing animals or animals on medication. Sensitivities may occur after using any pesticide product for pets. If any signs of sensitivity occur, bathe your pet with mild soap and rinse with large amounts of water. If signs continue, consult a veterinarian immediately.

First Aid:

If in eyes: Flush with plenty of water. Get medical attention.

If swallowed: Drink promptly a large quantity of milk, egg whites, or gelatin solution. If these are not available, drink large quantities of water. Avoid alcohol.

If on skin: Wash with plenty of soap and water. Get medical attention if irritation persists.

Environmental Hazards: This product is toxic to fish. Keep out of lakes, streams, ponds, tidal marshes and estuaries. Do not wash animal where runoff is likely to occur.

Storage and Disposal:

Storage: Store in a cool area. Disposal: Do not reuse container. Wrap and put in trash.

Warning(s): Keep out of reach of children.

Presentation: 8 fl oz (237 mL), 12 fl oz (355 mL) and 1 gallon (3.78 L).

Compendium Code No.: 11420291 Rev 0598

ECTOKYL® IGR EMULSIFIABLE CONCENTRATE

DVM **Premise Insecticide**

EPA Reg. No.: 1021-1620-41835

Active Ingredient(s):

2-[1-Methyl-2-(4-phenoxyphenoxy) ethoxy] pyridine (Nylar®)	1.30%
Inert Ingredients:	98.70%
	100.00%

Indications: For use in apartments, attics, basements, cabinets, cabins, campers, crawl spaces, garages, homes, hotels, kennels, mobile homes, motels, pet bedding, pet carriers, pet grooming parlors, pet sleeping areas, pet stores, pet quarters (enclosed premise treatment), veterinaries and warehouses.

Kills preadult fleas, including eggs. Prevents reinfestation for 7 months (210 days).

Dosage and Administration: It is a violation of Federal Law to use this product in a manner inconsistent with its labeling.

Read all directions completely before use.

For Flea Control: The active ingredient in the container is Nylar®, an insect growth regulator. It terminates the flea life cycle by inhibiting development of the preadult stages (larval and eggs) and preventing growth into the biting adult stage. Treatment lasts for 7 months (210 days). Existing adult fleas and flea pupae are not affected. Application of this product in areas where pets and other animals are known to frequent and where previous infestations have been known to occur, will prevent the emergence of adult fleas. This concentrate can be used prior to the flea season.

Indoors: Prior to treatment, carpets, draperies and upholstered furniture should be vacuumed thoroughly and the vacuum cleaner bag disposed of in an outdoor trash receptacle.

Instructions for Use: This concentrate is intended to be mixed with water and applied with spray equipment such as any low pressure sprayer (tank type sprayer) typically used for indoor application.

Spray Preparation: Prepare a diluted spray solution by adding 1 ounce per gallon of water. Partially fill the mixing container with water, add concentrate, agitate and fill to final volume. Do not allow spray mixture to stand overnight. Mix before each use.

General Surface Application: Apply diluted spray at the rate of 1 gallon per 1,500 square feet of surface area. Treat all areas which may harbor fleas, including carpets, furniture, pet sleeping areas and throw rugs. Treat under cushions of upholstered furniture. Do not allow children or pets to contact treated surfaces until spray has dried. Repeat as necessary.

In Kennels and Doghouses: Using an adjustable hose-end sprayer, tank type sprayer or sprinkling can, prepare a diluted spray solution by adding 1 ounce per gallon of water. Partially fill the sprayer with water, add required amount of concentrate in sprayer, agitate and fill to final volume. Agitate before each spray. Do not allow the spray mixture to stand overnight. Apply at a rate of 1 gallon diluted solution per 1,500 square feet of surface area. Apply to building, resting areas, walls, floor, animal bedding and run areas. Remove animals before spraying and do not return animals to treated areas until spray has dried completely. Pets and their bedding should also be treated with EPA registered flea and tick control products, in conjunction with this application as part of a complete flea control program to prevent the introduction of adult fleas. Repeat as necessary.

In Conjunction with an Adulticide Insecticide: This concentrate may be combined with an insecticide registered for control of adult fleas. The combination would provide immediate control of adult fleas and inhibit the development of the preadult (larval) fleas for 7 months (210 days). This application should conform to accepted use precautions and directions for both products. Use this concentrate at application rates specified above.

Do not use this product in or on electrical equipment due to possibility of shock hazard. Avoid excessive wetting of carpet, draperies and furniture. Always test in an inconspicuous area prior to use, as some natural and synthetic fibers may be adversely affected by any liquid product.

Precaution(s): Storage: Store in a cool, dry place. Keep container closed. Disposal: Do not reuse empty container. Wrap container in several layers of newspaper and discard in trash.

Physical or Chemical Hazards: Do not use or store near heat or open flame.

Caution(s): Precautionary Statements:

Hazards to Humans and Domestic Animals: Harmful if swallowed or absorbed through skin. Do not breathe vapors or spray mist. Avoid contact with skin or eyes. In case of contact, flush with plenty of water. Wash with soap and warm water after use. Obtain medical attention if irritation persists. Avoid contamination of food or feedstuffs.

Warning(s): Statement of Practical Treatment:

If in Eyes: Flush with plenty of water. Get medical attention if irritation persists. If Swallowed: Call a physician or Poison Control Center immediately. Do not induce vomiting. If on Skin or Clothing: Remove contaminated clothing and wash before reuse. Wash skin with soap and warm water. Get medical attention if irritation persists. Keep out of reach of children.

Presentation: 1 fl oz.

Nylar® is a registered trademark of McLaughlin Gormley King Co.

Compendium Code No.: 11420300

ECTOKYL™ IGR PRESSURIZED SPRAY

DVM **Household Insecticide**

EPA Reg. No.: 1021-1622-41835

Active Ingredient(s):

2-[1-Methyl-2-(4-phenoxyphenoxy) ethoxy] pyridine (Nylar®)	0.015%
Tetramethrin [(1-Cyclohexene-1,2-dicarboximido) methyl 2,2-dimethyl-3-(2-methylpropenyl) cyclopropanecarboxylate]	0.400%
3-Phenoxybenzyl-(1RS, 3RS; 1RS, 3SR)-2,2-dimethyl-3-(2-methylprop-1-enyl) cyclopropanecarboxylate	0.300%
Inert Ingredients:	99.285%
	100.000%

Indications: Flea spray for carpets and furniture with Nylar® Insect Growth Regulator.

Kills adult and preadult fleas. Continues to kill fleas for 4 months (120 days). Kills ticks.

Dosage and Administration: It is a violation of Federal Law to use this product in a manner inconsistent with its labeling.

For Indoor Use Only: This spray kills fleas, brown dog ticks and carpet beetles. It contains a unique combination of ingredients that kills both adult and preadult fleas, even fleas before they grow up to bite, Nylar®, a unique ingredient in this product, continues to kill fleas for 4 months (120 days) by preventing development into the adult biting stage. It reaches fleas hidden in carpets, rugs, drapes, upholstery, pet bedding and floor cracks. Protects household from reinfestation and flea build-up, and inhabitants from bites. One treatment with this spray gives continuous flea protection for 120 days. ECTOKYL™ IGR Pressurized Spray leaves no objectionable odor or sticky mess and, used as directed, does not stain furnishings.

For Flea and Tick Control: Shake well. Hold can 2 to 3 feet from surfaces of upholstered to be treated. Using a sweeping motion, apply uniformly to carpets, rugs, drapes and all surfaces of upholstered furniture. Be sure to treat pet bedding as this is a primary hiding place for fleas. No need to remove pet bedding after treatment. Do not treat pets. Use a registered flea control product on your pets in conjunction with this treatment. Retreat as necessary. Avoid wetting furniture and carpeting. A fine mist or spray applied uniformly is all that is necessary to kill fleas and ticks.

Contraindication(s): Do not treat pets.

Precaution(s): Storage: Store in a cool, dry place inaccessible to children. Keep container closed.

Disposal: Do not reuse empty container. Wrap container in several layers of newspaper and discard in trash.

Physical or Chemical Hazards: Contents under pressure. Keep away from heat, sparks, and open flame. Do not puncture or incinerate container. Exposure to temperatures above 130°F may cause bursting.

Caution(s): Precautionary Statements:

Hazards to Humans and Domestic Animals: Harmful if swallowed or absorbed through skin. Contains petroleum distillate. Do not induce vomiting because of aspiration pneumonia hazard. Do not breathe vapors or spray mist. Avoid contact with skin or eyes. In case of contact, flush with plenty of water. Wash with soap and warm water after use. Obtain medical attention if irritation persists. Avoid contamination of food or feedstuffs.

Do not use in commercial food processing, preparation, food storage or serving areas. In the home, all food processing surfaces and utensils should be covered during treatment, or thoroughly washed before use. Exposed food should be covered or removed.

Remove pets, birds, and cover fish aquariums before spraying.

Warning(s): Statement of Practical Treatment:

If Swallowed: Call a physician or Poison Control Center immediately. Do not induce vomiting because of aspiration pneumonia hazard. If in Eyes: Flush with plenty of water. Get medical attention if irritation persists. If on Skin or Clothing: Remove contaminated clothing and wash before reuse. Wash skin with soap and warm water. Get medical attention if irritation persists. If Inhaled: Remove victim to fresh air. Apply artificial respiration if indicated.

Keep out of reach of children.

Presentation: 14 fl oz.

Nylar® is a registered trademark of McLaughlin Gormley King Co.

Compendium Code No.: 11420320

ECTOKYL™ IGR TOTAL RELEASE FOGGER

DVM **Premise Insecticide**

EPA Reg. No.: 1021-1623-41835

Active Ingredient(s):

2-[1-Methyl-2-(4-phenoxyphenoxy) ethoxy] pyridine	0.100%
Pyrethrins	0.050%
N-Octyl bicycloheptene dicarboximide*	0.400%
Permethrin [**(3-Phenoxyphenyl) methyl (±) cis-trans-3-(2,2-dichloroethenyl) 2,2-dimethylcyclopropanecarboxylate]	0.400%
Related Compounds	0.035%
Other Ingredients:	99.015%
Total	100.000%

With Nylar® Insect Growth Regulator.

*MGK® 264, Insecticide Synergist.

**Cis-trans isomers ratio: Min. 45% (±) trans; Max. 55% (±) cis.

Indications: Kills insects such as: Fleas, ticks (that may carry and transmit lyme disease), cockroaches, lice, flies and mosquitoes.

For use in apartments, attics, basements, cabins, campers, food plants, garages, homes, hospitals, hotels, kennels, kitchens, motels, pet grooming parlors, pet sleeping areas, storage areas and warehouses.

Kills adult and preadult fleas. Prevents reinfestation for 7 months (210 days). Treats up to 6,000 cu. ft.

Directions for Use: It is a violation of Federal Law to use this product in a manner inconsistent with its labeling.

Read all directions completely before use.

For use only when building has been vacated by human beings and pets. Ventilate area for 30 minutes before re-entry.

For best results, treat all infested areas. Use one fogger (6 fl oz) for each 6,000 cubic feet of unobstructed area.

Preparation: Do not use more than one fogger per room. Do not use in small, enclosed spaces such as closets, cabinets or under counters or tables. Do not use in a room 5 ft x 5 ft or smaller; instead allow fog to enter from other rooms. Turn off all ignition sources such as pilot lights (shut off gas valves), other open flames or running electrical appliances that cycle off and on (i.e. refrigerators, thermostats, etc.). Call your gas utility or management company if you need assistance with your pilot lights. Remove or cover exposed food, dishes, utensils, surfaces and food-handling equipment. Shut off fans and air conditioners. Close outside doors and windows. Remove pets and birds but leave pets' bedding as this is a primary hiding place for fleas and must be treated for best results. No need to discard pet bedding after treatment. Cover or remove fish tanks and bowls. Leave rugs, draperies and upholstered furniture in place. This product will not harm furniture when used as directed. Open interior closet doors and cabinets of areas to be treated. Cover waxed wood floors and waxed furniture in the immediate area surrounding the fogger. (Newspaper may be used.) For more effective control of storage pests, open all cupboard doors (kitchen, bathrooms, pantry) and drawers for better penetration of fog. For flea and tick control, thoroughly vacuum all carpeting, upholstered furniture, along baseboards, under furniture and in closets. Put vacuum bag into a sack and dispose of in outside trash. Mop all hard floor surfaces.

To Start Fogging: Shake fogger well before using. Hold can at arm's length with top of can pointing away from face and eyes. Push down on finger pad until it locks. This will start fogging action. Set cannister in an upright position on a table, stand, etc. (up to 30 inches in height in the center of the area) and place several thicknesses of newspaper under the canister to prevent marring of the surface. Treat the whole dwelling using multiple units in homes with more than one level and numerous rooms. Leave the building at once.

Do not re-enter building for two hours. After two hours, open all outside doors and windows, turn on air conditioner and/or fans and let treated area air for 30 minutes before reoccupying. If additional units are used for remote rooms or where free flow of fog is not assured, increase airing-out time accordingly.

Precautionary Statements: Hazards to Humans and Domestic Animals:

Caution: Harmful if swallowed. Avoid breathing vapors or spray mist. Avoid contact with skin or eyes. In case of contact, flush with plenty of water. Wash with soap and warm water after use. Obtain medical attention if irritation persists. Avoid contamination of food or feedstuffs.

Do not use in food areas of food handling establishments, restaurants, or other areas where food is commercially prepared or processed. Do not use in serving areas while food is exposed or facility is in operation. Serving areas are areas where prepared foods are served such as dining rooms but excluding areas where foods may be prepared or held. In the home, all food processing surfaces and utensils should be covered during treatment, or thoroughly washed before use. Exposed food should be covered or removed. Non-food areas are areas such as garbage rooms, lavatories, floor drains (to sewers), entries and vestibules, offices, locker rooms, machine rooms, boiler rooms, garages, mop closets and storage (after canning or bottling). Not for use in USDA Meat and Poultry Plants.

Remove pets, birds, and cover fish aquariums before spraying.

Statement of Practical Treatment:

If Swallowed: Call a physician or Poison Control Center immediately.

If in Eyes: Flush with plenty of water. Get medical attention if irritation persists.

If on Skin or Clothing: Remove contaminated clothing and wash before reuse. Wash skin with soap and warm water. Get medical attention if irritation persists.

If Inhaled: Remove victim to fresh air if effects occur, and call a physician.

For more information regarding medical emergencies or pesticide incidents, call the International Poison Center at 1-888-740-8712.

Physical or Chemical Hazards: Contents under pressure. Keep away from heat, sparks, and open flame. Do not puncture or incinerate container. Exposure to temperatures above 130°F may cause bursting. This product contains a highly flammable ingredient. It may cause a fire or explosion if not used properly. Follow the "Directions for Use" on the label very carefully.

Storage and Disposal:

Storage: Store in a cool, dry area away form heat and open flame.

Disposal: Replace cap and discard container in trash. Do not incinerate or puncture.

Warning(s): Keep out of reach of children.

Presentation: 6 fl oz (177 mL).

Nylar® and MGK® are registered trademarks of McLaughlin Gormley King Co.

Compendium Code No.: 11420331 Rev 0799

ECTO-SOOTHE™ SHAMPOO

Virbac **Parasiticide Shampoo**

EPA Reg. No.: 2382-25

Active Ingredient(s):

Pyrethrins	0.05%
Piperonyl butoxide technical*	0.50%
Inert ingredients	99.45%
Total	100.00%

*Equivalent to 0.4% (butylcarbityl) (6-propylpiperonyl) ether and 0.1% related compounds.

Indications: Kills ticks, fleas and lice on dogs, cats, puppies and kittens.

Directions for Use: It is a violation of federal law to use the product in a manner inconsistent with its labeling.

Application: Shake well before using. Wet the animal thoroughly with warm water. Apply the product to the back of the animal and massage well into the skin to obtain a good lathering of the entire body. Allow the lather to remain in contact with the skin for at least 10 minutes. Rinse the animal thoroughly with warm water. For maximum results, repeat the process as directed above. Dry the animal thoroughly and comb. Repeat shampoo as indicated.

Precautionary Statements: Hazards to Humans and Domestic Animals: Harmful if swallowed. Avoid contact with the eyes and mouth of the animal. Do not treat puppies or kittens under six weeks of age. Avoid contamination of feed, foodstuffs, or food handling equipment. Wash thoroughly with soap and water after using.

Statement of Practical Treatment: In case of contact, immediately flush eyes with plenty of water.

Environmental Hazards: The pesticide is toxic to aquatic organisms. Do not apply directly to water. Do not contaminate water by the cleaning of equipment or the disposal of wastes.

Storage and Disposal:

Storage: Store at room temperature in a closed container.

Disposal: Do not re-use the empty container. Wrap the container and put it in the trash.

Warning(s): Keep out of the reach of children.

Presentation: Available in 8 fl. oz. (237 mL), 16 fl. oz. (474 mL) and 1 gallon (3.78 L) containers.

Compendium Code No.: 10230250

ECTO-SOOTHE™ 3X SHAMPOO

Virbac **Parasiticide Shampoo**

EPA Reg. No.: 2382-117

Active Ingredient(s):

Pyrethrins	0.15%
Piperonyl butoxide technical*	1.50%
N-octyl bicycloheptene dicarboximide	0.50%
Inert ingredients	97.85%
Total	100.00%

*Equivalent to 1.2% (butylcarbityl) (6-propylpiperonyl) ether and 0.3% related compounds.

Indications: Kills ticks, fleas and lice on dogs, cats, puppies and kittens.

Directions for Use: It is a violation of federal law to use the product in a manner inconsistent with its labeling.

Application: Shake well before using. Wet the animal thoroughly with warm water. Apply the product to the back of the animal and massage well into the skin to obtain a good lathering of the entire body. Allow the lather to remain in contact with the skin for at least 10 minutes. Rinse the animal thoroughly with warm water. For maximum results, repeat the process as directed above. Dry the animal thoroughly and comb. Repeat shampoo as indicated.

Precautionary Statements: Hazards to Humans and Domestic Animals: Harmful if swallowed. Avoid contact with eyes and mouth of animal. Do not treat puppies or kittens under six weeks of age. Avoid contamination of feed, foodstuffs, or food handling equipment. Wash thoroughly with soap and water after using.

Statement of Practical Treatment: In case of contact, immediately flush eyes with plenty of water and get medical treatment if irritation persists.

Environmental Hazards: The pesticide is toxic to aquatic organisms. Do not apply directly to water. Do not contaminate water by the cleaning of equipment or the disposal of wastes.

Storage and Disposal:

Storage: Store in a closed container in a cool, dry area.

Disposal: Do not re-use the empty container. Wrap the container in newspaper and put it in the trash.

Warning(s): Keep out of the reach of children.

Presentation: Available in 8 fl. oz. (237 mL), 16 fl. oz. (474 mL) and 1 gallon (3.78 L) containers.

Compendium Code No.: 10230240

ECTOZAP™ PLUS POUR-ON INSECTICIDE

Aspen **Premise and Topical Insecticide**

Dual Action Insecticide

EPA Reg. No.: 773-72-40940

Active Ingredient(s):

Permethrin (3-phenoxyphenyl) methyl (±) cis, trans-3-(2,2-dichloroethenyl)-2,2-dimethylcyclopropanecarboxylate*	1.0%
Piperonyl Butoxide Technical**	1.0%
Inert Ingredients**	98.0%
	100.0%

* cis/trans ratio: Min 35% (±) cis and max 65% (±) trans

** Equivalent to Min 0.8% (butylcarbityl) (6-propylpiperonyl) ether and 0.2% related compounds.

Indications: Insecticide for cattle, sheep and their premises. Kills flies and lice.
Directions for Use: It is a violation of Federal law to use this product in a manner inconsistent with its labeling.
Ready to Use No dilution necessary.

Apply To	Target Insects	Application Instruction
Lactating and Non-Lactating, Dairy Cattle, Beef Cattle and Calves	Lice, Horn Flies, Face Flies. Aids in control of Horse Flies, Stable Flies, House Flies, Mosquitoes and Black Flies.	Dosage: Apply ½ fl. oz. (15 cc) per 100 lbs body wt of animal up to a maximum of 5 fl. oz. for any one animal. Pour On: Pour correct dose along back and down face. Ready To Use Spray: Use undiluted in a mist sprayer to apply correct dose. Apply directly to neck, face, back, legs and ears. Back Rubber Use: Mix one pint per gallon #2 diesel or mineral oil. Keep rubbing device charged. Results improved by daily forced use.
Sheep	Sheep Keds, Lice	Pour along back. Apply ¼ fl. oz. (7.5 cc) per 50 lbs body wt of animal, up to a maximum of 3 fl. oz. for any one animal. For optimum control, all animals in the flock should be treated after shearing.
Premises — In and around Horse, Beef, Dairy, Swine, Sheep and Poultry premises. Animal Hospital Pens and Kennels and "outside" Meat Processing Premises.	House Flies, Stable Flies, Face Flies, Gnats, Mosquitoes, Black Flies, Fleas, Little House Flies (*Fannia* app). Aid in control of cockroaches, ants, spiders, crickets.	For use as a ready-to-use spot spray or premise spray, use undiluted in a mist sprayer. Apply directly to surface to leave a residual insecticidal coating, paying particular attention to areas where insects crawl or alight. One gallon will treat approximately 7,300 square feet.

For cattle and sheep, repeat treatment as needed, but not more often than once every two weeks. For optimum lice control, two treatments at a 14-day interval are recommended.

Special Note: ECTOZAP™ Plus Insecticide is not effective in controlling cattle grubs.

ECTOZAP™ Plus is an oil-base, ready-to-use product that may leave an oily appearance on the hair coat of some animals.

ECTOZAP™ Plus should be used in an integrated pest management system which may involve repeat treatments and the use of other pest control practices.

Precautionary Statements: Hazards to Humans and Domestic Animals:

Caution: Harmful if absorbed through skin. Avoid contact with skin, eyes and clothing. Prolonged or frequently repeated skin contact may cause allergic reactions in some individuals. Wash thoroughly with soap and water after handling.

Statement of Practical Treatment:

If Swallowed: Call a physician immediately. Do not induce vomiting unless under medical attention. If in Eyes: Immediately flush eyes with plenty of water. Get medical attention if discomfort persists. If On Skin: Wash skin with soap and water. Get medical attention.

Environmental Hazards: This product is extremely toxic to fish and other aquatic invertebrates. Do not add directly to water. Do not contaminate water when disposing of equipment washwaters. Apply this product only as specified on this label.

Physical or Chemical Hazards: Do not use or store near heat or open flame.

Storage and Disposal: Do not contaminate water, food or feed by storage or disposal.

Storage: Keep container sealed when not in use. Do not store near food or feed. Pesticide Disposal: Wastes resulting from the use of this product may be disposed of on site or at an approved waste disposal facility. Container Disposal: Triple rinse (or equivalent). Then offer for recycling or reconditioning, or puncture and dispose of in a sanitary landfill or incineration, or if allowed by State and local authorities, by burning. If burned, stay out of smoke.

Warning(s): Keep out of reach of children.

Disclaimer: Notice of Warranty: Aspen Veterinary Resources,® Ltd. makes no warranty of merchantability, fitness for any particular purpose, or otherwise, expressed or implied concerning this product or its uses which extend beyond the use of the product under normal conditions in accordance with the statements made on this label.

Presentation: 1 U.S. gallon (3.785 L).

Compendium Code No.: 14750290

ECTOZAP™ POUR-ON INSECTICIDE

Aspen **Topical Insecticide**

EPA Reg. No.: 773-66-40940

Active Ingredient(s):

Permethrin (3-phenoxyphenyl) methyl (±) cis, trans-3-(2,2-dichloroethenyl)-2,2-dimethylcyclopropanecarboxylate* 1.0%
Inert Ingredients** 99.0%
100.0%

* cis/trans ratio: Min 35% (±) cis and max 65% (±) trans
** Contains petroleum distillates.

Indications: Non-systemic pour-on for beef, lactating and non-lactating dairy cattle. Controls lice and flies on cattle. Controls keds and lice on sheep.

Directions for Use: It is a violation of Federal law to use this product in a manner inconsistent with its labeling.

Ready to Use No dilution necessary.

Apply To	Target Insects	Application Instruction
Lactating and Non-Lactating, Dairy Cattle and Beef Cattle and Calves	Lice, Horn Flies, Face Flies and Aids in Control of: Horse Flies, Stable Flies, Mosquitoes, Black Flies and Ticks.	Pour along back and down face. Apply ½ fl. oz. (15 cc) per 100 lbs body wt of animal, up to a maximum of 5 fl. oz. for any one animal.
Sheep	Sheep Keds, Lice	Pour along back. Apply ¼ oz. (7.5 cc) per 50 lbs body wt of animal, up to a maximum of 3 fl oz for any one animal.

For cattle and sheep, repeat treatment as needed, but not more than once every two weeks. For optimum lice control, two treatments at 14 day intervals are recommended.

Special Note: ECTOZAP™ Pour-On Insecticide is not effective in controlling cattle grubs.

Precautionary Statements: Hazards to Humans and Domestic Animals:

Caution: Avoid contact with eyes.

Statement of Practical Treatment:

If in eyes: Immediately flush eyes with plenty of water. Get medical attention if discomfort persists.

If swallowed: Call a physician immediately. Do not induce vomiting unless under medical attention.

Note to Physician: Solvent presents aspiration hazard. Gastric lavage is indicated if material was taken internally.

Environmental Hazards: This pesticide is extremely toxic to fish. Use with care when applying to areas adjacent to any body of water. Do not add directly to water. Do not contaminate water by cleaning of equipment or disposal of wastes. Apply this product only as specified on this label.

Physical or Chemical Hazards: Do not use or store near heat or open flame.

Storage and Disposal: Do not contaminate water, food or feed by storage or disposal.

Storage: Keep container sealed when not in use. Do not store near food or feed.

Pesticide Disposal: Wastes resulting from the use of this product may be disposed of on site or at an approved waste disposal facility.

Container Disposal: Triple rinse (or equivalent). Then offer for recycling or reconditioning, or puncture and dispose of in a sanitary landfill or incineration, or, if allowed by state and local authorities, by burning. If burned, stay out of smoke.

Warning(s): Keep out of reach of children.

Disclaimer: Notice of Warranty: Aspen Veterinary Resources,® Ltd. makes no warranty of merchantability, fitness for any particular purpose, or otherwise, expressed or implied concerning this product or its uses which extend beyond the use of the product under normal conditions in accordance with the statements made on this label.

Presentation: 1 U.S. gallon (3.785 L).

Compendium Code No.: 14750300

ECTRIN® INSECTICIDE CATTLE EAR TAG

Boehringer Ingelheim **Insecticide Ear Tags**

EPA Reg. No.: 4691-125

Active Ingredient(s):

By Weight
Cyano (3-phenoxyphenyl) methyl-4-chloro-alpha-1-methylethyl) benzeneacetate 8.0%
Related compounds 0.6%
Inert ingredients 91.4%
Total 100.0%

The ECTRIN® Insecticide Cattle Ear Tag is a mixture of Ectrin® insecticide (an synthetic pyrethroid), conditioners and a sunlight stablizer all blended with a soft durable plastic which when molded becomes a long acting insecticidal ear tag. A bright yellow color has been added for field visibility. The uniquely shaped tag has more than 12 square inches of active surface although it measures only 2.5 x 2.5 inches. The edges of the tag are insecticidally active.

Indications: For use on dairy cattle (including lactating), beef cattle and calves to control horn flies, face flies, gulf coast ticks, spinose ear ticks and as an aid to control lice, stable flies and houseflies.

Dosage and Administration:

General Classification: It is a violation of federal law to use the product in a manner inconsistent with its labeling.

1. Place the female tag under the clip by depressing the lever. The collar on the tag must be pointing downwards.
2. Disinfect pliers and tags prior to application. Slide the male button on the pin until it projects through the tip. The tag and button are now ready for application.
3. Position the tag on the flat surface in the center of the ear. Do not allow the shaft of the male button to penetrate any cartilage rib or blood vessel. Ear damage may result.
4. When properly positioned, the tag should hang vertically.

For optimum control of flies, ticks and lice, attach one tag to each ear when pests first appear. The tags may remain effective for up to five (5) to six (6) months (horn flies). Replace as necessary. The tags are applied using the Allflex® tagging system.

Precaution(s): Store in a cool place. Remove tags before slaughter. Bury or discard all tags removed from animals in a safe place .

Caution(s): Keep out of the reach of children.

Precautionary Statements:

Hazards to Humans: Wash thoroughly with soap and water after handling and before eating or smoking. Avoid contamination of feed and foodstuffs.

Environmental Hazards: The pesticide is toxic to fish. Keep out of lakes, streams or ponds. Do not contaminate water by the disposal of used tags. Use the product only as specified on the label.

Warning(s): Warranty and limitation of damages: Seller warrants that this material conforms to its chemical description and is reasonably fit for the purposes stated on the label when used in accordance with directions under normal conditions of use and buyer assumes the risk of any use contrary to such directions. Seller makes no other express or implied warranty, including any other express or implied warranty of fitness or of merchantability, and no agent of seller is authorized to do so except in writing and with a specific reference to this warranty. In no event shall seller's liability for any breach of warranty exceed the purchase price of the material as to which a claim is made.

Presentation: 24 tags per box and 96 tags per pail (includes appropriate number of mail buttons for attachment to the ears). Each tag has a net weight of 10 g.

* Allflex is a registered trademark of the Allflex Tag Co.

Compendium Code No.: 10280361

E.D.D.I. 20 GR. (DEXTROSE BASE)

Vedco **Iodine-Oral**

Organic Iodine Dextrose

Guaranteed Analysis:

Iodine (I), minimum 3.65%*

*(Equivalent to 4.6% EDDI; 20 grains/oz of EDDI; 20,880 mg/lb of EDDI or 46 mg/gm of EDDI.)

Ingredients: Ethylenediamine dihydroiodide (EDDI), dextrose, artificial color and silicon dioxide.

Indications: To be used as a nutritional source of iodine.

Directions for Use: Cattle:

Nutritional source of iodine: Feed 217 mg of Vedco EDDI 20 gr per head daily in feed, salt or mineral continuously.

Feed: Thoroughly premix 1 pound of Vedco EDDI 20 gr with 9 pounds of supplement, ground grain or other carrier having a particle size similar to organic iodine. Then mix 1 pound of the mixture in the feed consumed by 210 head of cattle and feed continuously.

Salt: Thoroughly premix 1 pound of Vedco EDDI 20 gr with 130 pounds of salt. Then feed 1 ounce of the salt mixture per head per day and offer continuously.
Caution(s): Do not feed more than 10 mg of EDDI (217 mg of Vedco EDDI 20 gr) per head daily.
Warning(s): For animal use only.
Keep out of reach of children.
Sold to veterinarians only.
Presentation: 1 lb bags and 25 lb containers.
Compendium Code No.: 10940530

E.D.D.I. 20 GR. (ORGANIC IODINE DEXTROSE)

Phoenix Pharmaceutical **Iodine-Oral**

Guaranteed Analysis:
Iodine (I), minimum 3.65%*
*(Equivalent to 4.6% EDDI; 20 grains/oz of EDDI; 20,880 mg/lb of EDDI or 46 mg/g of EDDI.)
Ingredients: Ethylenediamine dihydriodide (EDDI), dextrose, artificial color and silicon dioxide.
Indications: To be used as a nutritional source of iodine in cattle.
Directions for Use: Cattle:
Nutritional source of iodine: Feed 217 mg of Phoenix EDDI 20 GR per head daily in feed, salt or mineral continuously.
Feed: Thoroughly premix 1 pound of Phoenix EDDI 20 GR with 9 pounds of supplement, ground grain or other carrier having a particle size similar to Organic Iodine. Then mix 1 pound of the mixture in the feed consumed by 210 head of cattle and feed continuously.
Premix: Thoroughly premix 1 pound of Phoenix EDDI 20 GR with 130 pounds of salt. Then feed 1 ounce of the salt mixture per head per day and offer continuously.
Caution(s): Do not feed more than 10 mg of EDDI (217 mg of Phoenix EDDI 20 GR) per head daily.
For animal use only.
Warning(s): Keep out of reach of children.
Presentation: 1 lb (0.45 kg) (NDC 57319-367-27).
Sold to veterinarians only.
Manufactured by: Ameri-Pac, Inc., St. Jospeh, MO 64501.
Compendium Code No.: 12560272 Rev. 9-01

E.D.D.I. 20 GR. (ORGANIC IODINE SALT) ℞

Phoenix Pharmaceutical **Iodine-Oral**

Guaranteed Analysis:
Iodine (I), minimum 3.65%*
*(Equivalent to 4.6% EDDI; 20 grains/oz of EDDI; 20,880 mg/lb of EDDI or 46 mg/gm of EDDI.)
Ingredients: Ethylenediamine dihydriodide (EDDI), salt, artificial color and silicon dioxide.
Indications: To be used as a nutritional source of iodine in cattle.
Dosage and Administration: Cattle:
Nutritional source of iodine: Feed 217 mg of Phoenix EDDI 20 GR per head daily in feed, salt or mineral continuously.
Feed: Thoroughly premix 1 pound of Phoenix EDDI 20 GR with 9 pounds of supplement, ground grain or other carrier having a particle size similar to Organic Iodine. Then mix 1 pound of the mixture in the feed consumed by 210 head of cattle and feed continuously.
Premix: Thoroughly premix 1 pound of Phoenix EDDI 20 GR with 130 pounds of salt. Then feed 1 ounce of the salt mixture per head per day and offer continuously.
Caution(s): Federal law restricts this drug to use by or on the order of a licensed veterinarian.
Do not feed more than 10 mg of EDDI (217 mg of Phoenix EDDI 20 GR) per head daily.
For animal use only.
Sold to veterinarians only.
Warning(s): Keep out of reach of children.
Presentation: 1 lb (.45 kg) (NDC 57319-368-27).
Manufactured by: Ameri-Pac, Inc., St. Joseph, MO 64501
Compendium Code No.: 12560281 Rev. 5-01

E.D.D.I. 20 GR. (SALT)

Vedco **Iodine-Oral**

Organic Iodine Salt
Guaranteed Analysis:
Iodine (I), minimum 3.65%*
*(Equivalent to 4.6% EDDI; 20 grains/oz of EDDI; 20,880 mg/lb of EDDI or 46 mg/gm of EDDI.)
Ingredients: Ethylenediamine dihydroiodide (EDDI), salt, artificial color and silicon dioxide.
Indications: To be used as a nutritional source of iodine.
Directions for Use: Cattle:
Nutritional source of iodine: Feed 217 mg of Vedco EDDI 20 gr per head daily in feed, salt or mineral continuously.
Feed: Thoroughly premix 1 pound of Vedco EDDI 20 gr with 9 pounds of supplement, ground grain or other carrier having a particle size similar to organic iodine. Then mix 1 pound of the mixture in the feed consumed by 210 head of cattle and feed continuously.
Salt: Thoroughly premix 1 pound of Vedco EDDI 20 gr with 130 pounds of salt. Then feed 1 ounce of the salt mixture per head per day and offer continuously.
Caution(s): Do not feed more than 10 mg of EDDI (217 mg of Vedco EDDI 20 gr) per head daily.
Warning(s): For animal use only.
Keep out of reach of children.
Sold to veterinarians only.
Presentation: 1 lb (.45 kg) and 25 x 1 lb (.45 kg).
Compendium Code No.: 10940540

E.D.D.I. 40 GR. (SALT)

Vedco **Iodine-Oral**

Organic Iodine Salt
Guaranteed Analysis:
Iodine (I), minimum 7.3%*
*(Equivalent to 9.2% EDDI; 40 grains/oz of EDDI; 41,760 mg/lb of EDDI or 92 mg/gm of EDDI.)
Ingredients: Ethylenediamine dihydroiodide (EDDI), salt, artificial color and silicon dioxide.
Indications: To be used as a nutritional source of iodine.
Directions for Use: Cattle:
Nutritional source of iodine: Feed 109 mg of Vedco EDDI 40 gr per head daily in feed, salt or mineral continuously.
Feed: Thoroughly premix 1 pound of Vedco EDDI 40 gr with 9 pounds of supplement, ground grain or other carrier having a particle size similar to organic iodine. Then mix 1 pound of the mixture in the feed consumed by 415 head of cattle and feed continuously.
Salt: Thoroughly premix 1 pound of Vedco EDDI 40 gr with 260 pounds of salt. Then feed 1 ounce of the salt mixture per head per day and offer continuously.
Caution(s): Do not feed more than 10 mg of EDDI (109 mg of Vedco EDDI 40 gr) per head daily.
Warning(s): For animal use only.
Keep out of reach of children.
Sold to veterinarians only.
Presentation: 1 lb (.45 kg) and 25 x 1 lb (.45 kg).
Compendium Code No.: 10940550

EDDI EQUINE

Butler **Mineral Supplement**

NDC No.: 11695-1744-1
Active Ingredient(s): Each lb contains: Ethylenediamine dihydriodide 320 grains. (Equivalent to 20 grains per ounce) or 1,300 mg EDDI per ounce.
Sugar .... 95.13% w/w
EDDI .... 4.57% w/w
Anticaking Agent .... .3% w/w
Artificial color added.
Indications: An organic iodide feed supplement for oral use as an aid in correcting nutritional deficiencies where the use of supplemental iodine is indicated.
Dosage and Administration: Nutritional source of iodine: Mix 1 oz of EDDI 20 Grain Sugar thoroughly into enough feed for 130 feedings. This provides 10 mg of EDDI per head per day.
Caution(s): Feed animals with caution until tolerance is determined because of variation in susceptibility to iodine.
Warning(s): For animal use only.
Keep out of reach of children.
Presentation: One pound containers.
Compendium Code No.: 10820660

EFFERCEPT®

Activon **Teat Dip & Spray**

Sanitizing Teat Dip & Spray
Active Ingredient(s): Sodium Dichloroisocyanurate 3.0 grams per tablet.
Indications: Kills mastitis causing organisms.
Non-irritating to teats and udder.
Directions for Use:
1. Prepare EFFERCEPT® Vet solutions at least 5 minutes before use.
2. Use dry hands when handling tablets.
3. Fill a clean container with potable water.
4. Add 4-6 tablets per gallon of water (see dilution rates table below).
5. Allow 2-4 minutes for tablets to completely dissolve.
6. If desired, add 2 ounces of SoftGuard™ Conditioning Additive to solution. SoftGuard™ Additives are recommended when using as a post-dip or spray. Follow use instructions on SoftGuard™ label.
7. EFFERCEPT® Vet solutions may be used for up to 7 days after mixing. For best results, store away from direct sunlight.

EFFERCEPT® Vet Dilution Rates:
Teat Dip: Use 5-6 tablets per gallon if milking twice per day, 4-5 tablets per gallon if milking more than twice per day.
Teat Spray: Use 4-5 tablets per gallon if milking twice per day, 4 tablets per gallon if milking more than twice per day.

Dilution Rates	Pre/Post Teat Dip/Spray	Udder Wash
Regular Strength	4 tablets per gal.	3 tablets per 5 gal.
Maximum Strength	6 tablets per gal.	1 tablet per gal.

Container Yields:
50 Tablet Size: Makes up to 12.5 gallons of teat dip or spray.
100 Tablet Size: Makes up to 25 gallons of teat dip or spray.
220 Tablet Size: Makes up to 55 gallons of teat dip or spray.
Caution(s): Keep out of reach of children. Do not take internally. Not for human consumption.
Eye Contact: Flush eyes with clean water. Seek medical advice.
If Swallowed: Drink large quantities of water. Do not induce vomiting. Seek medical advice immediately.
Do not inhale vapors from closed containers of EFFERCEPT® Vet stored solutions or tablets. Open in well ventilated areas.
Do not mix with bleach, acids or ammonia.
Presentation: 50 tablet bottle (10.58 oz), 100 tablet bottle (22.7 oz), and 220 tablet bottle (46.53 oz).
Compendium Code No.: 10600011

EFFERSAN™

Activon **Sanitizer**

EPA Reg. No.: 66750-2-72519
Active Ingredient(s):
Sodium Dichloro-s-Trizinetrione 50%
Inert Ingredients: 50%
Available Chlorine 30%
Total 100%
Indications: Multi-purpose effervescent tablets that sanitize, disinfect and protect against odor.
Directions for Use: It is a violation of Federal law to use this product in a manner inconsistent with its labeling.
Methods of Application of Solutions of this Product: All sanitizing solutions should be freshly prepared. Solutions should be tested during use to make sure the concentration does not drop below the recommended level. Keep in properly labeled containers to protect against contamination. Unused solutions should be discarded.
Method of Sanitizing Equipment: This method is commonly used to sanitize closed systems, such as fluid milk cooling and handling equipment. It is also appropriate for sanitizing weigh tanks, coolers, short-time pasteurizers, pumps, homogenizers, fillers, sanitary piping and fittings, and bottle and can fillers. For mechanical operations, prepared solutions cannot be reused for sanitizing but may be used for other purposes, such as cleaning. For manual operations, fresh

sanitizing solutions must be prepared at least daily or more often if the solution becomes diluted or soiled. First, clean all equipment thoroughly, immediately after use. Remove all gross food particles and soil by a preflush or prescrape and, when necessary, presoak treatment. Wash surfaces or objects with a good detergent or compatible cleaner, followed by a potable water rinse before application of the sanitizing solution. Then place back in operating position. Prepare a solution containing 12 tablets (2 oz) to 40 gallons of water (100 ppm available chlorine) in a volume sufficient to fill the equipment. Allow a 10% excess for waste. Pump the solution through the system until it is filled and air excluded. Close final drain valves and hold under pressure for one minute to ensure proper contact with all surfaces. Then drain the solution and allow to air dry.

Spray Method of Sanitizing Equipment: The spray (or fog) method is generally used to sanitize large, non-porous surfaces that have already been freed of physical soil. It is appropriate for batch pasteurizers, holding tanks, weigh tanks, tank trucks and cars, vats, tile walls, ceilings and floors. Prepare a solution containing 100 ppm available chlorine. If possible, use pressure spraying or fogging equipment designed to resist chlorine-containing solutions (e.g., rubber-coated, plastic or stainless steel). When using any other kind of spraying equipment, be sure to empty and rinse thoroughly with fresh water immediately after treatment. Apply spray or fog heavily to all surfaces the product will touch. All treated surfaces, corners and turns should be thoroughly sprayed. Allow at least a one minute contact time before draining. Allow excess solution to drain off thoroughly and air dry, then place in service.

General Rinse Method: This product containing 100 ppm available chlorine will sanitize plant floors, walls and ceilings, and also control odors in refrigerated areas and drain platforms. Flush or swab surfaces generously with the solution. After one minute contact time allow solution to drain thoroughly and then air dry.

Directions for Sanitizing Hard Non-POROUS Surfaces, Dishes Glasses, Food Processing Equipment and Utensils, Dairy and Brewery Equipment and Utensils: This product is an effective sanitizing agent. Treatment with this product throughout food and beverage processing and food handling operations can help ensure the quality and safety of the final product.

Hand Washing of Items:

1. Remove all gross food particles and soil by a preflush or prescrape and, when necessary, presoak treatment. Wash surfaces or objects with a good detergent or compatible cleaner, followed by a potable water rinse before application of the sanitizing solution.
2. Prepare a sanitizing solution by dissolving 3 tablets of this product in 10 gallons of water. This will give a solution containing 100 ppm free available chlorine (FAC).
3. Place equipment, utensils, dishes, glasses, etc. in the solution or spread the solution over the surface to be sanitized.
4. Allow to stand at least one minute, drain the excess solution from the surface and allow to air dry.
5. Fresh sanitizing solution must be prepared at least daily or more often if the solution becomes diluted or soiled.

Machine Washing of Items:

1. Remove all gross food particles and soil by a preflush or prescrape and, when necessary, presoak treatment. Wash surfaces or objects with a good detergent or compatible cleaner, followed by a potable water rinse before application of the sanitizing solution.
2. Dissolve 3 tablets of this product in 10 gallons of water to obtain a solution having a FAC of 100 ppm.
3. Add the solution to the feed tank of immersion or spray type machines which can provide at least one minute contact time for sanitizing dishes, glasses, food processing equipment or utensils. Allow to drain and air dry before use.
4. The sanitizing solution should be used promptly. Prepared solutions cannot be reused for sanitizing but may be used for other purposes, such as cleaning.

Milk Handling and Processing Equipment: This product can be used on dairy farms and in plants processing milk, cream, ice cream and cheese. Rinse milking machines, utensils and all equipment with cold water to remove excess milk. Clean and rinse prior to sanitizing. To sanitize, spray or rinse all precleaned surfaces with a solution of 3 tablets of this product to 10 gallons of water, to obtain a 100 ppm available chlorine solution. Allow adequate draining before contact with dairy products.

Poultry Houses: The problem of odor control in poultry houses is not completely solved by normal cleaning practices. The regular use of an efficient bactericide and deodorant is strongly recommended and often required by health authorities. Remove all poultry and feed from premises, vehicles and enclosures. Remove all litter and manure from floors, walls and surfaces of barns, pens, stalls, chutes and other facilities occupied or transversed by poultry. Empty all troughs, racks and other feeding and watering appliances. Thoroughly clean all surfaces with soap or detergent and rinse with water. To disinfect, saturate all surfaces with a solution of at least 1,000 ppm available chlorine for a period of two minutes. A 1,000 ppm solution can be made by thoroughly mixing 30 tablets with 10 gallons of water (15 tablets with 5 gallons of water). Immerse all types of equipment used in handling and restraining poultry, as well as the cleaned forks, shovels and scrapers used for removing litter and manure. Ventilate buildings, cars, boats or other closed spaces. Do not house poultry or employ equipment until chlorine has dissipated. All treated feed racks, mangers, troughs, automatic feeders, fountains and waterers must be thoroughly scrubbed with soap or detergent and then rinsed with potable water before reuse.

Egg Processing Plants: To clean egg shells, spray with a solution containing 12 tablets (2 ounces) of this product per 40 gallons of water (100 ppm available chlorine) at 90°F to 120°F. Spray-rinse the cleaned eggs with warm potable water. Only clean, whole eggs can be used for sanitizing. Dirty, cracked or punctured eggs cannot be sanitized.

To destain egg shells, immerse the eggs in a solution containing 100 ppm available chlorine at 90°F to 120°F. After destaining, the eggs must be cleaned by spraying with an acceptable cleaner. Follow with potable water rinse.

To sanitize clean shell eggs intended for food or food products, spray with a solution of 12 tablets (2 oz) per 40 gallons of water (providing 100 ppm available chlorine). The solution must be equal to or warmer than the eggs, but not to exceed 130°F. Wet eggs thoroughly and allow to drain. Eggs that have been sanitized with this chlorine compound may be broken for use in the manufacture of egg products without prior potable water rinse. without prior potable water rinse. Eggs must be reasonably dry before casing or breaking. The solution must not be reused for sanitizing eggs.

All egg cups, breaking knives, trays and other equipment that come into contact with "off" eggs should be thoroughly cleaned and sanitized. First, clean all equipment. Before placing back in use, spray with a solution containing 12 tablets (2 oz) per 40 gallons of water (100 ppm available chlorine). Allow surfaces to drain thoroughly before contact with egg products. To sanitize egg freezers and dryers (tanks, pipelines and pumps), use the spray (or fog) method of treatment. This procedure is generally used to sanitize large, non-porous surfaces that have already been freed of physical soil.

Prepare a solution containing 100 ppm available chlorine. Apply spray heavily to all surfaces the eggs will touch. All treated surfaces, corners and turns should be thoroughly sprayed. Allow at least a one minute contact time before draining. Allow equipment to drain adequately before contact with eggs.

For Use Throughout Food and Beverage Processing and Food Handling Operations: This product is recommended far sanitizing all types of hard-porous equipment and utensils used in food processing and canning plants, bottling plants and breweries, fish processing plants, meat and poultry processing plants, milk handling and processing plants, restaurant and institutional dining establishments and poultry houses. Use 12 tablets of this product to 40 gallons of water (100 ppm available chlorine) to sanitize previously cleaned processing and packaging equipment. Allow at least a one minute contact time before draining. Allow adequate draining before contact with beverages.

To control the growth of bacteria in brewery pasteurizers, badly fouled systems should be cleaned before treatment. When the system is just noticeably fouled, add 50-70 tablets (5-10 oz) of this product per 10,000 gallons of water (17-24 tablets in 343 gallons of water) contained in the system. Repeat this dosage if necessary until a free available chlorine (FAC) level 0.5-1.0 ppm is obtained, as determined by use of a reliable test kit. To maintain a FAC of 0.5-1.0 ppm, add 7-14 tablets (1-2 ounces) of this product per 10,000 gallons of water, daily or as needed. This product should be added to the system at a point where adequate flow is maintained.

Precautionary Statements: Hazards to Humans and Domestic Animals:

Danger: Corrosive. Causes irreversible eye damage. Harmful if swallowed, inhaled or absorbed through skin. Do not get in eyes, on skin or on clothing. Avoid breathing dust. Wear goggles or face shield. Wash thoroughly with soap and water after handling. Remove contaminated clothing and wash before reuse.

Statement of Practical Treatment:

If Swallowed: Drink promptly large quantities of water. Avoid alcohol. Call a physician or poison control center immediately. Do not induce vomiting. Do not give anything by mouth to an unconscious person. If on Skin: Wash with plenty of soap and water. Get medical attention if irritation occurs. If in Eyes: Hold eyelids open and flush with a steady, gentle stream of water for 15 minutes. Get medical attention. If Inhaled: Remove person to fresh air. Get immediate medical attention. Note to Physician: Probable mucosal damage may contraindicate the use of gastric lavage.

Physical or Chemical Hazards: Use only clean, dry utensils. Mix only into water. Contamination with moisture, dirt, organic matter or other chemicals (including other pool chemicals) or any other foreign matter may start a chemical reaction with generation of heat, liberation of hazardous gasses and possible generation of fire and explosion. Avoid any contact with flaming or burning materials such as a lighted cigarette. Do not use this product in any chlorinating device which has been used with any inorganic or unstabilized chlorinating compounds (e.g., calcium hypochlorite). Such use may cause fire or explosion.

Environmental Hazards: This pesticide is toxic to fish and aquatic organisms. Do not discharge effluent containing this product into lakes, streams, ponds, estuaries, oceans or waters unless in accordance with the requirements of a National Pollutant Discharge Elimination System (NPDES) permit and the permitting authority has been notified in writing prior to discharge. Do not discharge effluent containing this product to sewer systems without previously notifying the local sewage treatment plant authority. For guidance contact your State Water Board or Regional Office of the EPA.

Storage and Disposal: Do not contaminate water, food or feed by storage or disposal.

Storage: Keep product dry in tightly closed container when not in use. Store in a cool, dry, well-ventilated area away from heat or open flame. Pesticide Disposal: Pesticide wastes are acutely hazardous. Improper disposal of excess pesticide, spray mixture or rinsate is a violation of Federal law. If these wastes cannot be disposed of by use according to label instructions, contact your state pesticide or environmental control agency, or the hazardous waste representative at the nearest EPA Regional Office for guidance. Container Disposal: Do not reuse empty container. Rinse empty container thoroughly with water to dissolve all material before discarding. Securely wrap container in several layers of newspaper and discard In trash.

Emergency Handling: In case of contamination or decomposition do not reseal container. If possible, isolate container in open and well-ventilated area. Flood with large volumes of water. Dispose of contaminated material in an approved landfill area.

Warning(s): Keep out of reach of children.

Presentation: 24 (0.34 lbs) and 100 (1.42 lbs) tablets. Also available: EFFERSAN™ 32 oz spray bottle.

Compendium Code No.: 10600021

EGT TEST KIT

PRN Pharmacal **Ethylene Glycol Test**

Description: A complete test kit to detect the presence of ethylene glycol in canine or feline blood, plasma or serum.

Components:

Tubes: Each test pack contains several tubes with colored caps. It may be advisable for the first-time user to mark the tubes to correspond with cap color to avoid any possible confusion.

Pipets: Several calibrated (1 mL with 0.25 mL divisions) plastic pipets are included in each test pack that are to be used for transfer operations. Dispose of all pipets when instructed to do so in order to avoid cross-contamination.

Materials required, but not included: Distilled water, centrifuge tubes, centrifuge.

Indications:

Peak blood levels of ethylene glycol are reached in one to four hours post ingestion at which time the early clinical signs of intoxication are apparent (depression, ataxia especially in the rear, polydipsia, polyuria, metabolic acidosis, and serum hyperosmolality). Dogs exhibiting any of these signs of toxicosis should be tested immediately. Additionally, dogs presented up to twelve hours post ingestion may be tested. Beyond twelve hours post ingestion test results will be marginal because most of the ethylene glycol will have been excreted or metabolized. Diagnosis should then be made on the basis of history, metabolic acidosis, and the presence of calcium oxalate and especially hippuric acid crystals in the urine. The determinations of the anion and osmolal gaps as well as serum glycolic acid level are also useful in belated diagnosis of antifreeze poisoning. Unfortunately, these tests often are not readily available.

Test Principles: Blood cells are lysed in water and blood proteins are denatured and precipitated by the addition of sodium tungstate and dilute sulfuric acid. Centrifugation removes precipitated blood components leaving ethylene glycol and other small molecules in solution. Ethylene glycol is oxidized by periodate to formaldehyde which forms a colored complex with 4-Amino-3-hydrazino-5-mercapto-1,2,4-triazole at alkaline pH.[3]

Test Procedure:

1) Draw blood using EDTA or heparin as an anticoagulant. One-half mL of whole blood is required for the test. Serum or plasma may be used if more convenient. (See caution below!)
2) Add 3 mL deionized or distilled water to a centrifuge tube that can hold a total of 5 mL. (If a 5 mL centrifuge tube is not available, use a convenient container such as a small paper cup for steps 2-5 and then distribute contents to two or more centrifuge tubes of any size.)
3) Using one of the plastic transfer pipets provided, add exactly 0.5 mL of whole blood, serum, or plasma to the water and mix completely. Reserve the pipet for use in steps 4 and 5.
4) Carefully open the tube with the white cap, and add the entire contents to the blood-water mixture. Use the plastic pipet saved from step 3 to mix completely.
5) Carefully open the tube with the lavender cap, and add the entire contents to the blood-water mixture. Again use the plastic pipet to mix completely and all the mixture to stand for 5 minutes before proceeding. Dispose of the pipet properly now.
6) Distribute the test sample to appropriate centrifuge tubes (not provided), and spin at blood speed for 5 minutes. A brownish-red pellet of precipitated blood proteins with a water-clear, colorless supernatant should result. Disregard any slight amount of material floating on top of the supernatant. Repeat the test using serum or plasma if a colorless supernatant is not obtained with whole blood.
7) Use a new, clean plastic pipet to transfer exactly 1 mL of the clear test sample supernatant to the yellow-capped reaction tube provided. Avoid any floating material. Dispose of the pipet properly now.
8) Use a new, clean plastic pipet to transfer exactly 0.25 mL of the oxidizer solution (blue-capped tube) to the test sample (yellow-capped tube). Do not allow the pipet to contact the test sample solution. Use the same pipet to transfer exactly 0.25 mL of the oxidizer solution (blue-capped tube) to the control tube (green-capped tube). Securely recap the reaction tube and control tube, shake vigorously, and allow the oxidation reaction to proceed for 10 minutes. Dispose of the pipet properly now.

Important: Be sure that you have added oxidizer solution to both the reaction and control tube.

9) The color reagent is supplied in a pair of red-capped tubes. One tube contains a diluent, the other contains a powder capsule. Activate the color reagent by using a plastic pipet to carefully combine the liquid with the powder. Reserve the pipet for use in step 10.
10) Use the pipet saved from step 9 to transfer 2 mL of the color reagent (red-capped tube mixture) to the yellow-capped reaction tube. Do not allow the pipet to contact the test sample solution. Also transfer 2 mL of the color reagent to the green-capped control tube. Make sure both tubes are recapped securely and shake vigorously. Observe results in 5 minutes. Dispose of the pipet properly now.

Test Interpretation: (See Caution section below!)

A definite reddish-violet (lavender) color should develop in the green-capped control tube within 5 minutes. Color development in the yellow-capped reaction tubs as intense or more so than the control tube is indicative of blood ethylene glycol levels of greater than 0.5 ppt (the standard is 50 μg/mL) and antifreeze poisoning. The color of a strongly positive sample may be very dark. Very faint color may develop in the reaction tube with normal blood due to slight interference from blood aldehydes, but this color should be much less than that of the positive control tube. Commonly, a normal sample will yield a faint yellowish color which may fade to colorless or extremely faint reddish-violet after standing for 30 minutes to an hour.

Please read the caution below concerning false positive reactions due to propylene glycol and glycerol. A false positive test will also result from metaldehyde, a component in some slug baits. If color of a different hue than that of the control tube develops, precipitates form, or no color develops in the control tube, disregard results and contact the manufacturer. If problems should arise, please include the lot number of your test kit in any correspondence.

Caution(s): Draw blood for this test before administration of any preparations containing propylene glycol or glycerol. Failure may result in a false positive test reaction. (Note: Some activated charcoal suspensions and semi-moist diets contain propylene glycol. Propylene glycol may not be listed in ingredients; if in doubt, contact the manufacturer.

Some of the materials in the kit are caustic. No solutions should be allowed to come in contact with the skin or eyes. If contact should occur, flush with copious amounts of water. Use the pipets provided for all operations--do not mouth pipet.

Discussion: A general understanding of the metabolism of ethylene glycol is crucial for accurate diagnosis of poisoning and for choosing a therapy regimen. The metabolic degradation of ethylene glycol takes place in the liver. Alcohol dehydrogenase converts ethylene glycol slowly to glycoaldehyde which is then quickly converted to glycolic acid. Glycolic acid concentration builds because all metabolic pathways that can degrade this compound are slow acting.

Most of the harmful effects of ethylene glycol poisoning are associated with glycolic acid (i.e. severe metabolic acidosis) and metabolites of glycolic acid (i.e. calcium oxalate crystals). Clinical signs and mortality correlate with urinary glycolate concentration. As the ethylene glycol is metabolized, animals often appear to recover from the direct effects of the poisoning only to rapidly deteriorate as glycolic acid concentration builds. Grauer et al.[2] followed the course of toxicosis in fifteen dogs given 9.5 mL of ethylene glycol/kg body weight. Depression, ataxia especially in the rear, polydipsia, polyuria, metabolic acidosis, and serum hyperosmolality were found at one to three hours, whereas calcium oxalate crystalluria was first observed at six hours, and renal function was not obviously impaired until 48 hours.

Most treatment regimens are based on some combination of ethanol, bicarbonate, and fluids.[1] Ethanol competitively inhibits alcohol dehydrogenase thus reducing the metabolism of ethylene glycol into more toxic compounds. [Note: Recently, 4-methylpyrazole has been recommended as an inhibitor of alcohol dehydrogenase that does not cause the undesirable CNS effects of alcohol.[4]] Correction of metabolic acidosis (blood pH < 7.3) is accomplished with sodium bicarbonate in fluid therapy to maintain urine pH at approximately 7.5 to 8.0. Ethanol is not indicated when animals are presented at more than 18 hours because most of the ethylene glycol would already be metabolized by alcohol dehydrogenase and a competitive block of this enzyme would be of no use. Supportive fluid and bicarbonate therapy is appropriate at this time. It should be understood that ethanol treatment will cause blood levels of ethylene glycol to remain elevated for prolonged times (because metabolism by alcohol dehydrogenase is blocked), and treatment periods must be lengthy (up to 72 hours) to allow time for excretion of the ethylene glycol.

Clearly, rapid diagnosis and minimal delay in treatment are positive factors in the prognosis of antifreeze poisoning. The PRN Ethylene Glycol Test Kit is useful in determining toxicosis one to twelve hours after ingestion. An informed diagnosis can be made quickly and the appropriate treatment can be initiated without delay because the test results can be read within 30 minutes. Sequential tests may be made during the course of ethanol treatment to follow blood levels of ethylene glycol.

References: Available upon request.

Presentation: 4 tests per kit.

Compendium Code No.: 10900030

ELECTRAMINE®

Life Science **Electrolytes-Oral**

Electrolyte Amino Acid Solution

Guaranteed Analysis:

Crude Protein, min. 9.0%
Dextrose, min. 65.0%
Salt, max. 14.2%
Salt, min. 13.0%
Potassium, max. 2.1%
Potassium, min. 2.0%

Ingredients: Dextrose, salt (sodium chloride), glycine, dipotassium phosphate, citric acid, ascorbic acid, yeast extract, potassium citrate.

Indications: A supplement providing a source of fluids, essential electrolytes, amino acids, and glucose for oral use in dogs and cats.

Dosage and Administration: Add the contents of one packet to one pint (16 oz/473 mL) of lukewarm tap water. Use one pint of the solution per 5-10 lbs of body weight daily, or as directed by your veterinarian. Refrigerate unused portion. Discard if not used in 24 hours.

Precaution(s): Store in cool, dry place.

Warning(s): Keep out of reach of children.

Presentation: 15 g (0.54 oz) packets; 20 packets/box.

Compendium Code No.: 10870040

ELECTRO DEX®

Horse Health **Electrolytes-Oral**

Oral Electrolyte Feed Supplement for Horses

Guaranteed Analysis:

Calcium, Min. 0.25%
Calcium, Max. 0.75%
Salt (NaCl), Min. 68.00%
Salt (NaCl), Max. 73.00%
Potassium, Min. 11.00%
Magnesium, Min. 0.40%

Ingredients: Salt (Sodium Chloride), Potassium Chloride, Magnesium Sulfate, Calcium Lactate Pentahydrate, Potassium Sulfate, Artificial Cherry Flavor, Artificial Coloring.

Indications: ELECTRO DEX® supplements horses to provide additional electrolyte salts that may be lost by dehydration.

Directions: Dosage: ELECTRO DEX® may be administered in the horse's feed or drinking water at the rate of 2 ounces per 10 gallons of fresh water, or 2 ounces in the horse's daily feed ration in place of regular salt.

Important: When administered in water, allow no other source of drinking water.

Precaution(s): Keep container tightly closed. Store in a cool, dry place.

Caution(s): For animal use only.

Warning(s): Not for use in animals intended for human consumption.

Keep out of reach of children.

Presentation: 5 lb (2.27 kg) and 30 lb.

Compendium Code No.: 15000001

ELECTRO-FLEX™

First Priority **Electrolytes-Oral**

Oral Electrolytes

Active Ingredient(s):

Vitamins	Per Dose	Per Pound
Thiamine HCl (B-1)	25 mg	300 mg
Riboflavin (B-2)	10 mg	120 mg
d Pantothenic Acid	7.5 mg	90 mg
Niacinamide	375 mg	4500 mg
Pyridoxine HCl (B-6)	25 mg	300 mg
Cyanocobalamin (B-12)	7.5 mcg	90 mcg
Minerals		
Sodium Chloride	625 mg	7500 mg
Calcium Chelate	375 mg	4500 mg
Potassium Complex	500 mg	6000 mg
Magnesium Chelate	500 mg	6000 mg
Dextrose	7.5 grams	90 grams
Amino Acids		
Alanine	416 mg	4992 mg
Arginine	212 mg	2544 mg
Aspartic Acid	1100 mg	13,200 mg
Cystine	150 mg	1800 mg
Glutamic Acid	1968 mg	23,616 mg
Glycine	428 mg	5136 mg
Histadine	150 mg	1800 mg
Isoleucine*	212 mg	2544 mg
Leucine*	468 mg	5616 mg
Lysine	425 mg	5100 mg
Methionine*	82 mg	984 mg
Phenylalanine*	267 mg	3564 mg
Proline	472 mg	5664 mg
Serine	436 mg	5232 mg
Theronine*	197 mg	2364 mg
Tryptophan*	101 mg	1212 mg
Tyrosine	332 mg	3984 mg
Valine	340 mg	4080 mg

*Essential Amino Acids

E

Ingredients: Water, Isolated Soy Protein, Dextrose, Propylene Glycol, Sodium Chloride, Potassium Amino Acid Complex, Magnesium Amino Acid Complex, Caramel Color, Niacinamide, Calcium Amino Acid Complex, Sorbic Acid, Xanthan Gum, Apple Flavor, Thiamine HCl, Pyridoxine HCl, Riboflavin, Calcium Pantothenate, Cyanocobalamin.
Indications: To be used after any race or work out to help replace cellular body fluids that are lost due to physical stress.
Directions: Provide ample drinking water. Administer directly from syringe onto back of horse's tongue.
Precaution(s): Store below 86°F.
Caution(s): For equine use only.
Warning(s): Keep out of reach of children.
Presentation: 34 g (NDC# 58829-296-34).
Compendium Code No.: 11390232 Rev. 09-01

ELECTROID® 7 VACCINE

Schering-Plough **Bacterin-Toxoid**
Clostridium chauvoei-septicum-novyi-sordellii-perfringens Types C & D Bacterin-Toxoid
U.S. Vet. Lic. No.: 107
Active Ingredient(s): *Clostridium chauvoei, Cl. septicum, Cl. novyi, Cl. sordellii* and *Cl. perfringens* types C & D bacterin-toxoid.
Indications: For the active immunization of healthy cattle and sheep against diseases caused by *Cl. chauvoei, Cl. septicum, Cl. sordellii, Cl. novyi* type B and *Cl. perfringens* types C and D.
Although *Cl. perfringens* type B is not a significant problem in the U.S.A., immunity may be provided against the beta and epsilon toxins elaborated by *Cl. perfringens* type B. This immunity is derived from the combination of type C (beta) and type D (epsilon) fractions.
Dosage and Administration: Shake well. Using aseptic technique, inject subcutaneously or intramuscularly.
Dosage: 5 mL, repeated in 3-4 weeks. Revaccinate annually prior to periods of extreme risk, or parturition. For *Cl. novyi,* revaccinate every 5-6 months. Animals vaccinated under three (3) months of age should be revaccinated at weaning or at 4-6 months of age.
Precaution(s): Store at 35°-45°F (2°-7°C). Protect from freezing.
The product has been tested under laboratory conditions and has met all federal standards for safety and ability to immunize normal healthy animals. The level of performance may be affected by conditions of use such as stress, weather, nutrition, disease, parasitism, other treatments, individual idiosyncrasies or impaired immunological competency. These factors should be considered by the user when evaluating product performance or freedom from reactions.
Caution(s): Use the entire contents when first opened.
Anaphylactic reactions may occur following use. For veterinary use only.
Antidote(s): Epinephrine.
Warning(s): Do not vaccinate within 21 days before slaughter. @PRS = **Presentation:** 10 dose (50 mL), 50 dose (250 mL), and 200 dose (1,000 mL) vials.
® Registered trademark of Schering-Plough Animal Health Corporation.
Compendium Code No.: 10470560

ELECTROID® D

Schering-Plough **Toxoid**
Clostridium perfringens Type D Toxoid
U.S. Vet. Lic. No.: 311
Contents: *Clostridium perfringens* Type D toxoid.
Indications: For the vaccination of healthy cattle and sheep against disease caused by *Clostridium perfringens* Type D.
Dosage and Administration: Shake well. Using aseptic technique, inject subcutaneously or intramuscularly. Cattle, 4 mL; sheep, 2 mL, repeated in 3 to 4 weeks. Revaccinate annually prior to periods of extreme risk or parturition.
Precaution(s): Store at 35°-45° (2°-7°C). Protect from freezing. Use entire contents when first opened.
Caution(s): Anaphylactoid reactions may occur following use.
This product has been tested under laboratory conditions and shown to meet all Federal standards for safety and efficacy. This level of performance may be affected by conditions of use such as stress, weather, nutrition, disease, parasitism, other treatments, individual idiosyncrasies or impaired immunological competency. These factors should be considered by the user when evaluating product performance or freedom from reactions.
Local reactions may be observed following subcutaneous administration to cattle.
Antidote(s): Epinephrine.
Warning(s): Do not vaccinate within 21 days before slaughter.
For veterinary use only.
Presentation: 500 mL vials (125 cattle doses/250 sheep doses).
Manufactured by: Schering-Plough Animal Health Limited
Compendium Code No.: 10470570

ELECTROLYTE HE WITH VITAMINS

DVM Formula **Electrolytes-Oral**
Guaranteed Analysis: Per Pouch:

Vitamin A	500,000 IU
Vitamin D	240,000 IU
Vitamin E	199 IU
Dextrose	137.2 mEq/L
Sodium	137.0 mEq/L
Chloride	43.2 mEq/L
Potassium	36.1 mEq/L
Glycine	23.6 mEq/L

Ingredients: Dextrose, glycine, sodium bicarbonate, sodium chloride, potassium chloride, citric acid, d-calcium pantothenate, niacinamide, riboflavin, thiamine hydrochloride, vitamin A acetate, d-activated animal sterol (vitamin D_3), DL-alpha-tocopherol acetate (vitamin E), menadione (vitamin K), medium chain triglyceride, and silica.
Indications: Supplement calves during ration change, weaning, disease conditions, shipping, follow up antibiotic treatment, or weather change. DVM Formula ELECTROLYTE HE WITH VITAMINS provides electrolytes, energy, and vitamins to slow fluids loss and assist in more efficient recovery.
Dosage and Administration: Administer one pouch per calf, twice daily for a minimum of two consecutive days or as needed. If conditions do not improve, consult veterinarian.
Feeding Directions: Briskly mix, while slowly adding one pouch of DVM Formula ELECTROLYTE HE WITH VITAMINS into two quarts of warm water, milk, or milk replacer until completely dissolved. Feed DVM Formula ELECTROLYTE HE WITH VITAMINS solution by using an open pail, nipple pail, nursing pail, or esophageal feeder. Discard unused portions; do not store. Provide access to fresh clean drinking water.
Presentation: 3.5 oz (100 gm) pouch.
Compendium Code No.: 15030011

ELECTROLYTE PAK

Alpharma **Electrolytes-Oral**
Ingredient(s): Potassium chloride, sodium chloride, magnesium sulfate, citric acid, natural and/or artificial strawberry flavoring.
Guaranteed analysis per pound:

Sodium	4.0%
Potassium	44.88%
Magnesium	0.05%
Citric acid	Carrier

Indications: An electrolyte supplement for poultry and swine.
Directions:
Poultry and Swine: Mix the contents (16 oz) of this pouch in 256 U.S. gallons (4 oz in 64 gallons) of the drinking water and give at this rate for 3 to 5 days. This dosage may be repeated whenever needed.
Precaution(s): Store in cool, dry place.
Caution(s): For oral animal use only.
Not for human use.
Keep out of reach of children.
Presentation: 1 lb. (453.6 g) pouches.
Compendium Code No.: 10220351 AHF-034A 0004

ELECTROLYTE PAK PLUS STABILIZED VITAMIN C

Alpharma **Electrolytes-Oral**
Guaranteed Analysis: Per Pound:

Sodium	4.0%
Potassium	42.5%
Magnesium	0.05%
Vitamin C Activity as:	
Stabilized Ascorbic Acid	20,000 mg

Ingredients: Potassium chloride, sodium chloride, stabilized ascorbic acid, magnesium sulfate, natural and/or artificial flavoring.
Indications: ELECTROLYTE PAK PLUS STABILIZED VITAMIN C is designed for use during periods of stress such as extremes in temperature (high or low), before and after transportation, or when conditions interfere with normal routine.
Directions: Poultry and Swine: Mix the contents (16 oz) of this pouch in 256 U.S. gallons (4 oz in 64 gallons) of the drinking water and give at this rate for 3 to 5 days. This dosage may be repeated when needed.
Precaution(s): Store in cool, dry place.
Caution(s): For oral animal use only.
Not for human use.
Keep out of reach of children.
Presentation: 1 lb (453.6 g) pouches.
Compendium Code No.: 10220361 AHF-030A 0003

ELECTROLYTE POWDER 8X

Phoenix Pharmaceutical **Electrolytes-Oral**
Active Ingredient(s): Contains:

Calcium lactate trihydrate	1.28%
Magnesium citrate soluble purified	0.65%
Potassium chloride	1.27%
Sodium chloride	9.68%
Sodium citrate dihydrate	7.36%
Dextrose monohydrate	79.76%

Indications: A powdered electrolyte concentrate for use in preparing a balanced electrolyte solution.
Directions for Use: Dissolve one package (16 oz.) in 40 gallons of drinking water.
Precaution(s): Storage: Do not store above 30°C (86°F). Store in a cool, dry place.
Caution(s): This product contains citrate salts which in some cases may be incompatible with tetracycline antibiotics.
For animal use only.
Warning(s): Keep out of reach of children.
Presentation: 16 oz. (1 lb) packages (NDC 57319-241-27).
Manufactured by: Sparhawk Laboratories, Lenexa, KS 66215
Compendium Code No.: 12560302 Rev. 07-01

ELECTROLYTE SOLUTION ℞

AgriLabs **Electrolyte Injection**
Active Ingredient(s): Each liter contains:

Sodium ion	153 mEq
Potassium ion	9 mEq
Calcium ion	6 mEq
Magnesium ion	4 mEq
Chloride ion	101 mEq
Lactate ion	71 mEq
Dextrose • H_2O	25 g
Sorbitol	25 g

It does not contain any preservatives.
Indications: For the correction of electrolyte depletion and dehydration of cattle, calves, horses, sheep and swine.
Dosage and Administration: May be injected intravenously or intraperitoneally (except in horses) using strict aseptic technique.
Cattle, Horses, Swine and Sheep: 2 to 5 mL per pound of body weight depending upon the size and condition of the animal, repeated one (1) to three (3) times a day or as needed.
Precaution(s): Store at 59°-86°F (15°-30°C).

Caution(s): Federal law restricts this drug to use by or on the order of a licensed veterinarian.

The solution should be warmed to body temperature prior to administration and administered at a slow rate. Use the entire contents when first opened, it is a single dose vial.

Not for human use.

Keep out of the reach of children.

Warning(s): Do not administer to horses by intraperitoneal injection. Do not administer to animals with inadequate renal function.

Presentation: 1,000 mL plastic bottles.

Compendium Code No.: 10581570 Rev. 5-89

ELECTROLYTE SOLUTION ℞

Vet Tek **Electrolytes-Injection**

Active Ingredient(s): Composition: Each 500 mL of sterile aqueous solution contains:

Sodium Chloride	2.75 g
Sodium Acetate	1.50 g
Calcium Chloride $2H_2O$	0.20 g
Magnesium Chloride $6H_2O$	0.15 g
Potassium Acetate	0.50 g
Sodium Citrate	0.35 g
Dextrose H_2O	25.00 g

Milliequivalents per liter:

Calcium	5 mEq/L
Sodium	134 mEq/L
Potassium	10 mEq/L
Magnesium	3 mEq/L
Total Cations	152 mEq/L
Chloride	102 mEq/L
Acetate	47 mEq/L
Citrate	3 mEq/L
Total Anions	152 mEq/L
Total Calories	57
Osmolarity (calc.)	approx. 554 mOsmol/L

This product contains no preservatives.

Indications: For use in conditions associated with fluid and electrolyte loss, such as dehydration, shock, vomiting and diarrhea, particularly when an immediate source of energy is also indicated.

Dosage and Administration: Warm solution to body temperature and administer slowly (10 to 30 mL per minute) by intravenous or intraperitoneal injection, using strict aseptic procedures.

Adult Cattle and Horses - 1000 to 2000 mL

Calves, Ponies, and Foals - 500 to 1000 mL

Adult Sheep and Swine - 500 to 1000 mL

These are suggested dosages. The actual amount and rate of fluid administration must be judged by the veterinarian in relation to the condition being treated and clinical response of the animal, being careful to avoid overhydration.

Contraindication(s): Do not administer intraperitoneally to horses.

Precaution(s): Store between 15° and 30°C (59°-86°F).

Use sterile equipment and aseptic procedures. Use entire contents when first opened. Discard any unused solution.

Caution(s): Federal law restricts this drug to use by or on the order of a licensed veterinarian.

Do not use unless solution is clear. Additives may be incompatible. Discontinue infusion if adverse reactions occur.

For animal use only.

Presentation: 1000 mL (NDC 60270-830-20).

Compendium Code No.: 14200071 Iss. 1-99

ELECTROLYTE SOLUTION WITH DEXTROSE ℞

Vedco **Electrolyte Injection**

Active Ingredient(s): Each 500 mL contains:

Dextrose • H_2O	12.50 g
Sorbitol	12.50 g
Sodium lactate	3.95 g
Sodium chloride	2.40 g
Potassium chloride	0.37 g
Magnesium chloride • $6H_2O$	0.21 g
Calcium chloride • $2H_2O$	0.19 g

Cations:

Sodium	153 mEq/L
Potassium	9 mEq/L
Calcium	6 mEq/L
Magnesium	4 mEq/L

Anions:

Chloride	101 mEq/L
Lactate	71 mEq/L

The product does not contain preservatives.

Indications: For use in conditions associated with fluid and electrolyte loss, such as dehydration, shock, vomiting and diarrhea, particularly when an immediate source of energy is also indicated.

Dosage and Administration: Warm the solution to body temperature and administer slowly (10 to 30 mL per minute) by intravenous or interperitoneal injection, using strict aseptic procedures.

Adult Cattle and Horses	1,000 to 2,000 mL
Calves, Ponies and Foals	500 to 1,000 mL
Adult Sheep and Swine	500 to 1,000 mL
Pigs	100 to 500 mL

These are suggested dosages. The actual amount and rate of fluid administration must be judged by the veterinarian in relation to the condition being treated and the clinical response of the animal, being careful to avoid overhydration.

Contraindication(s): Do not administer intraperitoneally to horses.

Precaution(s): Store at a controlled room temperature between 59-86°F (15-30°C).

Caution(s): Federal law restricts this drug to use by or on the order of a licensed veterinarian.

Keep out of the reach of children.

Use the entire contents when first opened. Discard any unused solution.

Presentation: 1,000 mL containers.

Compendium Code No.: 10940570

ELECTROLYTES-PLUS

Alpharma **Electrolytes-Oral**

Ingredient(s): Potassium chloride, sodium chloride, sodium citrate, magnesium sulfate, ferrous sulfate, niacinamide, copper sulfate, vitamin A supplement, menadione sodium bisulfite complex, zinc sulfate, manganese sulfate, d-calcium pantothenic acid, vitamin D_3 supplement, cobalt sulfate, calcium lactate, potassium sulfate, riboflavin, vitamin E supplement, vitamin B_{12} supplement, pyridoxine HCl, thiamine HCl, magnesium carbonate, ethylenediamine dihydriodide, folic acid.

Indications: An oral electrolyte supplement for chickens, turkeys, cattle, sheep and swine.

ELECTROLYTES-PLUS is formulated as a nutritional supplement for use during periods of extreme temperature (high or low), before and after transportation, or when conditions interfere with normal flock or herd routine.

Dosage and Administration: For use in drinking water: Administer to supply essential electrolytes and vitamins. 1 oz. treats 20 gallons of water. One (1) pack treats 256 gallons of water.

Precaution(s): Store in a cool, dry place

Caution(s): For oral animal use only. Not for human use. Keep out of reach of children.

Presentation: 12.5 oz. (354.4 g) packets.

Compendium Code No.: 10220371 AHF-028A 0003

ELECTROLYTE SUPPLEMENT

First Priority **Electrolytes-Oral**

Guaranteed Analysis:

Calcium, Min.	0.32%
Max.	0.40%
Sodium, Min.	3.5%
Max.	4.5%
Potassium, Min.	0.57%
Magnesium, Min.	0.009%

Ingredients: Sucrose, Salt, Potassium Chloride, Calcium Chloride, Silicone Dioxide, Magnesium Sulfate.

Indications: For use as an electrolyte supplement for horses.

Directions for Use: Feed ELECTROLYTE SUPPLEMENT at the rate of 2 ounces per animal daily.

Precaution(s): Storage: Store at controlled room temperature between 15°-30°C (59°-86°F). Keep container tightly closed when not in use.

Caution(s): For animal use only.

Warning(s): Keep out of reach of children.

Presentation: 5 lb (2.67 kg) (NDC# 58829-240-09) and 25 lb (11.34 kg) pails.

Compendium Code No.: 11390243 Rev. 08-01 / Rev. 07-01

ELECTROLYTE W/DEXTROSE INJECTION ℞

Aspen **Electrolyte Injection**

Active Ingredient(s): Each 500 mL of sterile aqueous solution contains:

Dextrose • H_2O	12.50 g
Sorbitol	12.50 g
Sodium lactate	3.95 g
Sodium chloride	2.40 g
Potassium chloride	0.37 g
Magnesium chloride • $6H_2O$	0.21 g
Calcium chloride • $2H_2O$	0.19 g

Milliequivalents per liter:

Cations:

Sodium	153 mEq/L
Potassium	9 mEq/L
Calcium	6 mEq/L
Magnesium	4 mEq/L

Anions:

Chloride	101 mEq/L
Lactate	71 mEq/L
Osmolarity (calc.)	617 mOsmol/L

This product contains no preservatives.

Indications: For use in conditions associated with fluid and electrolyte loss, such as dehydration, shock, vomiting and diarrhea, particularly when an immediate source of energy is also indicated.

Dosage and Administration: Warm the solution to body temperature and administer slowly (10-30 mL per minute) by intravenous or intraperitoneal injection, using strict aseptic procedures.

Adult Cattle and Horses	1000-2000 mL
Calves, Ponies and Foals	500-1000 mL
Adult Sheep and Swine	500-1000 mL

These are suggested dosages. The actual amount and rate of fluid administration must be judged by a veterinarian in relation to the condition being treated and the clinical response of the animal, being careful to avoid overhydration.

Contraindication(s): Do not administer intraperitoneally to horses.

Precaution(s): Store at a controlled room temperature, between 59° and 86° (15°-30°C). Use the entire contents when first opened. Discard any unused solution.

Caution(s): Federal law restricts this drug to use by or on the order of a licensed veterinarian.

Warning(s): Keep out of the reach of children.

Presentation: 1,000 mL vials.

Compendium Code No.: 14750311

ELECTROLYTE WITH THICKENER

DVM Formula **Electrolytes-Oral**

Ingredient(s): Dextrose, glycine, sodium chloride, sodium bicarbonate, potassium chloride, calcium phosphate, citric acid, starch, silica, and guar gum.

Indications: University researched product designed to provide energy, fluids, and electrolytes to re-hydrate calves.

Mix with milk, milk replacer, or water.

Contains an unique amino acid to increase villa size to increase absorption.

Contains starch with pectin to bind to bad bacteria and dispose of via excretion.

Gelling agent to slow loss of fluid and help prevent further dehydration.

Dosage and Administration: Administer one pouch per calf, twice daily for a minimum of two consecutive days or as needed.

Mixing Directions: Mix 1 pouch briskly into two quarts of lukewarm water, milk, or milk replacer.

Presentation: 3.5 oz (100 gm) pouch.

Compendium Code No.: 15030020

ELECTRO R

Alphrama **Electrolytes-Oral**

Ingredient(s): Potassium chloride, sodium chloride, sodium bicarbonate, sodium citrate, magnesium sulfate, niacinamide, vitamin A supplement, menadione sodium bisulfite complex, d-calcium pantothenic acid, vitamin D_3 supplement, riboflavin, vitamin E supplement, vitamin B_{12} supplement, ferrous sulfate, copper sulfate, pyridoxine HCl, thiamine HCl, zinc sulfate, manganese sulfate, cobalt sulfate, calcium lactate, potassium sulfate, ethylenediamine dihydriodide, magnesium carbonate, folic acid.

Indications: Electrolyte supplement for cattle, chickens, hogs, turkeys and sheep.

Dosage and Administration:

For use in drinking water: Administer to supply essential electrolytes and vitamins. 1 oz. treats 20 gallons of water. One (1) pack treats 256 gallons of water.

For use in feed: Replace the salt when using ELECTRO R in feed. Mix thoroughly in the feed and substitute for salt at the following rates.

Percent of electrolytes	Amount of electrolytes/1,000 lbs. feed
0.5%	5 lbs.
1.0%	10 lbs.
1.5%	15 lbs.
2.0%	20 lbs.

Precaution(s): Store in cool, dry place.

Caution(s): For oral animal use only. Not for human use. Keep out of reach of children.

Presentation: 12.5 oz. (354.4 g) packets.

Compendium Code No.: 10220341 AHF-029A 0003

ELECTROSOL-R ℞

Phoenix Pharmaceutical **Fluid Therapy**

Replacement Electrolytes (Sterile Solution-Nonpyrogenic)

Active Ingredient(s): Each 100 mL Contains:

Sodium Chloride	526 mg
Sodium Acetate	222 mg
Sodium Gluconate	502 mg
Potassium Chloride	37 mg
Magnesium Chloride Hexahydrate	30 mg
Water for Injection	q.s.

May contain hydrochloric acid or sodium hydroxide for pH adjustment.

Electrolytes per 1000 mL (not including ions for pH adjustment):

Sodium	140 mEq
Potassium	5 mEq
Magnesium	3 mEq
Chloride	98 mEq
Acetate	27 mEq
Gluconate	23 mEq

295 mOsm/liter (calc.)

pH 5.5-7.5 Isotonic

Contains no preservative.

Indications: ELECTROSOL-R is a sterile, nonpyrogenic solution of balanced electrolytes indicated for replacing acute losses of extracellular fluid and electrolytes, and for correcting moderate to severe acidosis.

Dosage and Administration: Contents or lesser amount as determined by veterinarian as a single dose; usually 3-10% of body weight. In shock, up to 10% of body weight in 1-2 hours. For intravenous or subcutaneous use. Solution should be warmed to body temperature and administered slowly.

Precaution(s): Do not use this product if seal is broken or solution is not clear. If entire contents are not used, discard unused portion.

When introducing additives, use aseptic technique, mix thoroughly and do not store.

Protect from freezing.

Caution(s): Federal law restricts this drug to use by or on the order of a licensed veterinarian.

Additives may be incompatible.

For animal use only.

Not for human use.

Warning(s): Keep out of reach of children.

Presentation: 1000 mL (NDC 57319-365-08).

Compendium Code No.: 12560311 Rev. 10-99

ELIMIN • ODOR® CANINE

Pfizer Animal Health **Deodorant Product**

Indications: Eliminates "doggy-odor" on the dog. Also for use on bedding, rugs, other fabrics.

Body odors of the dog are eliminated by preventing the odor molecule from forming a gas. Without a gas there is no odor. Not just another cover-up.

Directions: Dogs: Spray directly on haircoat, paying special attention to areas such as the ears, anal area, and genitals. Repeat as necessary.

Fabrics: Spot-test on a hidden area to test for color-fastness. May then be sprayed directly on the odoriferous area.

Caution(s): Use externally on specified odor source only.

Nontoxic and nonirritating to skin, eyes, and hair.

Keep out of reach of children.

Presentation: 8 fl oz (236.6 mL).

Compendium Code No.: 36900960 85-8262-03

ELIMIN • ODOR® FELINE

Pfizer Animal Health **Deodorant Product**

Indications: Eliminates cat urine odor in litter boxes, on carpets and upholstery.

Cat urine and stool odors are destroyed—not a cover-up. The odor molecules are prevented from forming a gas; without a gas there is no odor. Safe. May be used as often as required.

Directions: Litter box: Cover entire surface area of litter with spray. For best results, stir in while spraying. Use daily to keep litter fresh and odor-free.

Fabrics: Spray entire area of odor source. Color-fastness should be tested by spraying a small spot in a hidden area of upholstery or carpet. Spray both sides of rugs and carpets whenever practical for best results.

Feline ELIMIN-ODOR® may also be applied to cats as required to eliminate urine odor. Apply only to affected areas.

Caution(s): Use externally on specified odor source only.

Nontoxic and nonirritating to skin and eyes. Keep out of reach of children.

Presentation: 8 fl oz (236.6 mL).

Compendium Code No.: 36900970 85-8264-03

ELIMIN • ODOR® GENERAL PURPOSE

Pfizer Animal Health **Deodorant Product**

Indications: Neutralizes unpleasant pet and household odors—not just a cover-up. General purpose odor eliminator leaves a light, clean, fresh scent. Destroys odors quickly and thoroughly.

Directions: After removing cap, spray the air while holding bottle upright. Spray on, or near, the source of odor for best results.

No need to evacuate premises.

Caution(s): For external use only. Nontoxic and nonirritating to skin and eyes.

Keep out of reach of children.

Presentation: 8 fl oz (236.6 mL).

Compendium Code No.: 36900980 85-8258-03

ELIMIN • ODOR® PET ACCIDENT

Pfizer Animal Health **Deodorant Product**

Ingredient(s): Chemical neutralizers which prevent the odor molecule from forming a gas (without a gas there is no odor).

Indications: Eliminates urine and stool odors from rugs, carpets, upholstery and drapes.

Urine and stool odors of pet accidents are actually destroyed-not a cover-up. Prevents pet from repeatedly returning to the same spot.

Directions for Use: Pull out spout. Spray directly on the entire source of odor by gently squeezing the bottle. If possible spray the bottom as well as the top of rugs and carpets. All fabrics should be spot-tested for color-fastness in a hidden area.

Repeat use as necessary.

Caution(s): Nontoxic and nonirritating to skin and eyes.

Use externally on specified odor source only.

Warning(s): Keep out of reach of children.

Presentation: 8 fl oz (236.6 mL) bottle.

Compendium Code No.: 36900990 85-8255-03

ELIMIN • ODOR® PET STAIN ELIMINATOR

Pfizer Animal Health **Deodorant Product**

Indications: Eliminates pet urine stains. Developed to prevent fresh urine from staining and to help remove stains from carpets, upholstery, drapes, etc. Helps restore original color to fabrics.

Directions for Use: Pull up spout. Squeeze bottle to spray product directly on the area to be treated. Allow product to soak in for a few minutes; then work in thoroughly with a clean damp cloth. Sponge area clean with wet towel; allow to dry naturally. All fabrics should be spot-tested for color-fastness and water spotting in a hidden area.

Repeat use as necessary.

Caution(s): Use on fabric covered surfaces only.

Nontoxic to humans and pets. Keep out of reach of children.

Presentation: 8 fl oz (236.6 mL).

Compendium Code No.: 36901000 85-8269-03

ELITE 4™

Boehringer Ingelheim **Vaccine**

Bovine Rhinotracheitis-Virus Diarrhea-Parainfluenza$_3$-Respiratory Syncytial Virus Vaccine, Killed Virus

U.S. Vet. Lic. No.: 124

Contents: This product contains the antigens listed above.

Neomycin and thimerosal are used as preservatives.

Indications: ELITE 4™ vaccine is recommended for the vaccination of healthy, susceptible dairy and beef cattle of all ages including pregnant cattle and veal calves against diseases caused by bovine rhinotracheitis (IBR) virus, bovine virus diarrhea (BVD) virus, parainfluenza$_3$ (PI_3) virus and bovine respiratory syncytial virus (BRSV).

Dosage and Administration: Using aseptic technique, inject 5 mL intramuscularly. Repeat in 14-28 days. Calves vaccinated before the age of 6 months should be revaccinated at 6 months of age or weaning. Ideally calves should receive the first dose 2-4 weeks before weaning with a booster dose at weaning. A 5 mL booster dose is recommended annually or prior to time of stress or exposure.

Precaution(s): Store out of direct sunlight. Store at 35-45°F (2-7°C). Do not freeze. Shake well before using. Use entire contents when first opened.

Caution(s): ELITE 4™ has been shown to be safe and efficacious when used according to label directions.

Anaphylactoid reactions may occur.

Antidote(s): Administer epinephrine.

Warning(s): Do not vaccinate within 21 days of slaughter.

Toxicology: Safety and Efficacy: The efficacy of ELITE 4™ has been demonstrated for each fraction. Pregnant cattle may be vaccinated at any stage of gestation, and lactating dairy cattle may be vaccinated with no post-vaccination milk discard required.

Presentation: 10 doses (50 mL) and 50 doses (250 mL).

Compendium Code No.: 10280391 23501-03 / 23502-03

ELITE 4-HS™

Boehringer Ingelheim **Bacterin-Vaccine**

Bovine Rhinotracheitis-Virus Diarrhea-Parainfluenza$_3$-Respiratory Syncytial Virus Vaccine, Killed Virus-Haemophilus Somnus Bacterin

U.S. Vet. Lic. No.: 124

Contents: This product contains the antigens listed above.

Neomycin and thimerosal are used as preservatives.

Indications: ELITE 4-HS™ vaccine/bacterin is recommended for the vaccination of healthy, susceptible dairy and beef cattle of all ages including pregnant cattle and veal calves against disease caused by bovine rhinotracheitis (IBR) virus, bovine virus diarrhea (BVD) virus, parainfluenza$_3$ (PI_3) virus, bovine respiratory syncytial virus (BRSV) and *Haemophilus somnus*.

Dosage and Administration: Using aseptic technique, inject 5 mL intramuscularly. Repeat in 14-28 days. Calves vaccinated before the age of 6 months should be revaccinated at 6 months

of age. Ideally calves should receive the first dose 2-4 weeks before weaning with a booster dose at weaning. A 5 mL booster dose is recommended annually or prior to time of stress or exposure.
Precaution(s): Store out of direct sunlight. Store at 35-45°F (2-7°C). Do not freeze. Shake well before using. Use entire contents when first opened.
Caution(s): ELITE 4-HS™ has been shown to be safe and efficacious when used according to label directions.
Anaphylactoid reactions may occur.
Antidote(s): Administer epinephrine.
Warning(s): Do not vaccinate within 21 days of slaughter.
Toxicology: Safety and Efficacy: The efficacy of ELITE 4-HS™ has been demonstrated for each fraction. Pregnant cattle may be vaccinated at any stage of gestation, and lactating dairy cattle may be vaccinated with no post-vaccination milk discard required.
Presentation: 10 doses (50 mL) and 50 doses (250 mL).
Compendium Code No.: 10280381 23601-04 / 23602-04

ELITE 9™

Boehringer Ingelheim **Bacterin-Vaccine**
Bovine Rhinotracheitis-Virus Diarrhea-Parainfluenza$_3$-Respiratory Syncytial Virus Vaccine, Killed Virus-Leptospira Canicola-Grippotyphosa-Hardjo-Icterohaemorrhagiae-Pomona Bacterin
U.S. Vet. Lic. No.: 124
Contents: This product contains the antigens listed above.
Neomycin and thimerosal are used as preservatives.
Indications: ELITE 9™ vaccine/bacterin is recommended for the vaccination of healthy, susceptible dairy and beef cattle of all ages including pregnant cattle and veal calves against the diseases caused by bovine rhinotracheitis (IBR) virus, bovine virus diarrhea (BVD) virus, parainfluenza$_3$ (PI$_3$) virus and bovine respiratory syncytial virus (BRSV), and *Leptospira canicola, L. grippotyphosa, L. hardjo, L. icterohaemorrhagiae* and *L. pomona*.
Dosage and Administration: Using aseptic technique, inject 5 mL intramuscularly. Repeat in 14-28 days. Calves vaccinated before the age of 6 months should be revaccinated at 6 months of age or weaning. Ideally calves should receive the first dose 2-4 weeks before weaning with a booster dose at weaning. A 5 mL booster dose is recommended annually or prior to time of stress or exposure.
Precaution(s): Store out of direct sunlight. Store at 35-45°F (2-7°C). Do not freeze. Shake well before using. Use entire contents when first opened.
Caution(s): ELITE 9™ has been shown to be safe and efficacious when used according to label directions.
Anaphylactoid reactions may occur.
Antidote(s): Administer epinephrine.
Warning(s): Do not vaccinate within 21 days of slaughter.
Toxicology: Safety and Efficacy: The efficacy of ELITE 9™ has been demonstrated for each fraction. Pregnant cattle may be vaccinated at any stage of gestation, and lactating dairy cattle may be vaccinated with no post-vaccination milk discard required.
Presentation: 10 dose (50 mL) and 50 dose (250 mL) vials.
Compendium Code No.: 10280411 26001-02 / 26002-02

ELITE 9-HS™

Boehringer Ingelheim **Bacterin-Vaccine**
Bovine Rhinotracheitis-Virus Diarrhea-Parainfluenza$_3$-Respiratory Syncytial Virus Vaccine, Killed Virus-Haemophilus Somnus-Leptospira Canicola-Grippotyphosa-Hardjo-Icterohaemorrhagiae-Pomona Bacterin
U.S. Vet. Lic. No.: 124
Composition: This product contains inactivated isolates of all the antigens listed above.
Preservatives: Neomycin and thimerosal.
Indications: Recommended for the vaccination of healthy, susceptible dairy and beef cattle of all ages including pregnant cattle and veal calves as an aid in the reduction of diseases caused by the organisms listed above.
Dosage and Administration: Using aseptic technique, inject 5 mL intramuscularly. Repeat in 14-28 days. Calves vaccinated before the age of 6 months should be revaccinated at 6 months. Ideally calves should receive the first dose 2-4 weeks before weaning with a booster dose at weaning. A 5 mL booster dose is recommended annually or prior to time of stress or exposure.
Precaution(s): Store out of direct sunlight. Store at 35-45°F (2-7°C). Do not freeze. Shake well before using. Use entire contents when first opened.
Caution(s): Anaphylactoid reactions may occur.
Antidote(s): Epinephrine.
Warning(s): Do not vaccinate within 21 days of slaughter.
Toxicology: Safety and Efficacy: The efficacy of ELITE 9-HS™ has been demonstrated for each fraction. Pregnant cattle may be vaccinated at any stage of gestation, and lactating dairy cattle may be vaccinated with no post-vaccination milk discard required.
Presentation: 10 doses (50 mL) and 50 doses (250 mL).
Compendium Code No.: 10280401 23401-03 / 23402-03

ELITE™ ELECTROLYTE

Farnam **Electrolytes-Oral**
Electrolyte Salts
Guaranteed Analysis:

Calcium, Minimum	0.25%
Calcium, Maximum	0.75%
Salt (NaCl), Minimum	68.00%
Salt (NaCl), Maximum	73.00%
Potassium, Minimum	11.00%
Magnesium, Minimum	0.40%

Ingredients:
Apple Flavor: Salt (Sodium Chloride), Potassium Chloride, Magnesium Sulfate, Calcium Lactate, Potassium Sulfate, Artificial Apple Flavor, Artificial Coloring.
Cherry Flavor: Salt (Sodium Chloride), Potassium Chloride, Magnesium Sulfate, Calcium Lactate, Potassium Sulfate, Artificial Cherry Flavor, Artificial Coloring.
Orange Flavor: Salt (Sodium Chloride), Potassium Chloride, Magnesium Sulfate, Calcium Lactate Pentahydrate, Potassium Sulfate, Artificial Orange Flavor, Artificial Coloring.
Indications: ELITE™ Electrolyte supplements horses to provide additional electrolyte salts and trace minerals that may be lost by dehydration.
Directions: Dosage: ELITE™ Electrolyte may be administered in the horse's feed or drinking water at the rate of 2 ounces per 10 gallons of fresh water, or 2 ounces in the horse's daily feed ration in place of regular salt. Important: When administered in water allow no other source of drinking water.
Precaution(s): Keep container tightly closed.
Store in a cool, dry place.
Caution(s): For animal use only. For veterinary use only.
Warning(s): Not for use in animals intended for human consumption.
Keep out of reach of children.
Presentation: Apple Flavor: 2.27 kg (5 lbs) and 9.07 kg (20 lbs).
Cherry Flavor: 2.27 kg (5 lbs) and 9.07 kg (20 lbs).
Orange Flavor: 2.27 kg (5 lbs) and 9.07 kg (20 lbs).
Compendium Code No.: 10000151

ELPAK™-G

Vedco **Electrolytes-Oral**
Active Ingredient(s): When ELPAK™-G is diluted with two (2) quarts of water, the solution contains:

Sodium (Na)	180 mEq/liter
Potassium (K)	10 mEq/liter
Bicarbonate (HCO_3)	40 mEq/liter
Chloride (Cl)	70 mEq/liter
Calcium (Ca)	10 mEq/liter
Magnesium (Mg)	5 mEq/liter
Dextrose	55 mM/liter
Glycine	40 mM/liter

Ingredients: Sodium chloride, sodium bicarbonate, sodium citrate, calcium chloride, magnesium sulfate, potassium chloride, dextrose, glycine, sodium alginate (as stabilizer), and sodium propionate and methylparaben as preservatives.
Indications: A concentrated electrolyte product fortified with dextrose, glycine and bicarbonate for oral administration to calves.
Dosage and Administration: Slowly dissolve the contents of one (1) packet in two (2) quarts of warm water. Mix thoroughly until the product is a smooth gel.
Administer two (2) quarts of gel per calf. May be repeated as indicated every four (4) to eight (8) hours.
Mix fresh solutions each day.
Precaution(s): Keep in a cool, dry place.
Caution(s): For animal use only. Not for human use.
Keep out of the reach of children.
Presentation: 80 g packets.
* ELPAK is a trademark of Rhone Merieux, Inc.
Compendium Code No.: 10940580

E-LYTE ℞

Vedco **Fluid Therapy**
Replacement Electrolytes (Sterile Solution-Nonpyrogenic)
Active Ingredient(s): Each 100 mL contains:

Sodium Chloride	526 mg
Sodium Acetate	222 mg
Sodium Gluconate	502 mg
Potassium Chloride	37 mg
Magnesium Chloride Hexahydrate	30 mg
Water for Injection	q.s.

May contain hydrochloric acid or sodium hydroxide for pH adjustment.
Electrolytes per 1000 mL (not including ions for pH adjustment): Sodium 140 mEq; Potassium 5 mEq; Magnesium 3 mEq; Chloride 98 mEq: Acetate 27 mEq; Gluconate 23 mEq.
295 mOsm/Liter (Calc.)
pH 5.5-7.5 Isotonic
Indications: E-LYTE is a sterile, non-pyrogenic solution of balanced electrolytes indicated for replacing acute losses of extracellular fluid and electrolytes, and for correcting moderate to severe acidosis.
Dosage and Administration: Contents or lesser amount as determined by veterinarian as a single dose; usually 3-10% of body weight. In shock, up to 10% of body weight in 1-2 hours. For intravenous or subcutaneous use. Solution should be warmed to body temperature and administered slowly.
Precaution(s): Protect from freezing.
Caution(s): Federal law restricts this drug to use by or on the order of a licensed veterinarian.
Do not use this product if seal is broken or solution is not clear. Contains no preservative. If entire contents are not used, discard unused portion. Additives may be incompatible. When introducing additives, use aseptic technique, mix thoroughly and do not store.
Warning(s): For animal use only.
Not for human use.
Keep out of reach of children.
Presentation: 1000 mL.
Compendium Code No.: 10940520

EMA-SOL™ CONCENTRATE

Alpharma **Mineral Supplement**
Oral Mineral Supplement
Ingredient(s): Contains: Copper sulfate, manganese sulfate, cobalt sulfate, potassium dichromate and hydrochloric acid.
Indications: EMA-SOL™ is a concentrated source of copper, manganese and cobalt for nutritional supplementation in the drinking water or feed of poultry. It is convenient and economical to use in either tanks or proportioners.
Dosage and Administration: Dosage: Consult chart below and administer correct amount as sole source of drinking water for 3 days. When using metal drinking fountains, fill fountain with water first and then add EMA-SOL™ to the water. Do not mix stock concentrate in metal containers.

Amount EMA-SOL™	Treats
1 tablespoon	4 gallons
1 pint	128 gallons
1 quart	256 gallons
½ gallon	512 gallons
1 gallon	1024 gallons

For Feed Use: Mix ½ pint (236 mL) in 4 gallons of water and ribbon on 160 feet of feeder space three times daily for three days.

Caution(s): Harmful if swallowed as a concentrate. If ingested - call a physician immediately. The concentrate may also cause irritation to nose, throat and skin. Wash immediately if spilled on skin, eyes, or clothing.

For oral animal use only.

Warning(s): Not for human use. Keep out of reach of children.

Presentation: 1 gallon (3785 mL).

EMA-SOL is a trademark of Alpharma Inc.

Compendium Code No.: 10220382 AHL-457-0109

E

EMPOWER™

Metrex **Detergent**

Dual Enzymatic Detergent

Ingredient(s): Proteolytic enzymes, low foaming surfactants, corrosion inhibitors and inerts.

Indications: Features: EMPOWER™ is a low-foaming, dual enzymatic detergent that effectively cleans away blood, tissue, mucous and other protein-rich body fluids. EMPOWER™ is designed for use in endoscopy, surgery, central processing, dental or other areas where instruments and equipment may be soiled with organic and inorganic debris. EMPOWER™ contains two different proteolytic enzymes that work in a broad range of temperatures and pH conditions. EMPOWER™ contains low foaming surfactants that efficiently remove lipids, starches, inorganic debris, and prevent debris from redepositing onto instruments. EMPOWER™ also contains corrosion inhibitors to protect a broad range of metals from corrosion.

Directions for Use: Manual Cleaning: Add 1 oz (1 pump yields 1 oz) of concentrate to one gallon of warm water (90°F-145°F). Soak instruments and equipment immediately after use, until soil is dissolved and removed. Soak for a minimum of 1 minute. Soak longer if matter is dried on, until visibly clean. Immerse instruments completely and aspirate solution into any channels and lumens. Use an instrument brush for light mechanical cleaning if necessary. Following soak period, visually inspect for cleanliness and rinse thoroughly with warm water. A power spray unit will assist in thoroughly rinsing the instruments. Rough dry. After cleaning with EMPOWER™, equipment and instruments must be disinfected/sterilized according to appropriate procedures.

Endoscope Reprocessors: Add ½ oz of concentrate per gallon of water to the reprocessor reservoir, or attach container to the reprocessor's automatic dispensing unit.

Ultrasonic Units: Add 1 oz of concentrate per gallon of water. Recommended water temperature is 90°F-145°F (32°C-63°C). A soak time of 2 minutes or more is recommended for ultrasonic cleaners. Process instruments according to manufacturer's directions.

Washer Sterilizers/Decontaminators: Attach concentrate container to the unit's automatic dispensing unit.

Diluted EMPOWER™ solution must be discarded daily, or more frequently if the solution is visibly soiled.

Note: EMPOWER™ is not a sterilant/disinfectant.

A complete line of high-level disinfectants/sterilants is available to complement EMPOWER™ dual enzymatic detergent.

Storage and Disposal: Storage: Keep in a cool area.

Solution Disposal: Flush thoroughly with large quantities of water into sewage disposal system in accordance with federal, state and local regulations.

Container Disposal: Do not reuse empty container. Wrap container and put in trash.

Warning(s): Protective eye gear, gloves and clothing must be worn, especially where exposure to blood and body fluid is expected. If accidental eye contact with EMPOWER™ concentrate occurs, flush immediately with water for 15 minutes and seek medical attention. Temporary redness of the eye may occur.

Discussion: This product is designed for easy one-step pre-cleaning by disintegrating blood and protein from delicate instruments and equipment.

Cleans Fast: In manual, ultrasonic and automatic cleaning systems, EMPOWER™ rapidly dissolves and carries away organic soils.

Safe for Users: EMPOWER™ reduces the need for manual handling and scrubbing, especially in hard-to-reach places like channels, lumens and instrument box locks.

Safe for Instruments and Equipment: EMPOWER™ is a neutral pH formula that provides advanced corrosion protection that is safe for rubber, plastic, stainless steel, carbon steel and soft metals.

Safe for use in evacuation systems.

Presentation: 48 x 2 oz bottles, 4 x 1 qt bottles, 4 x 1 gallon (128 fl oz) (3.8 L) bottles, 5 gallon bottles, 15 gallon, 30 gallon and 55 gallon drums.

Compendium Code No.: 13400060 4050-6

EMULSIBAC® APP

MVP **Bacterin**

Actinobacillus pleuropneumoniae Bacterin, Serotypes 1, 5 and 7

U.S. Vet. Lic. No.: 301

Active Ingredient(s): The bacterin contains inactivated *Actinobacillus pleuropneumoniae* organisms (serotypes 1, 5, and 7). It is adjuvanted with Emulsigen® (brand of emulsified paraffin). Prepared from young cultures of *Actinobacillus pleuropneumoniae* organisms. Chemically inactivated.

Contains polymyxin B sulfate and gentamicin sulfate as preservatives.

Indications: For the vaccination of healthy swine over four weeks of age against pneumonia caused by *Actinobacillus pleuropneumoniae* organisms. The bacterin has been shown to protect susceptible swine against intranasal challenge with virulent serotype(s) 1, 5, and 7 *Actinobacillus pleuropneumoniae* organisms.

Dosage and Administration: Shake before and occasionally during use. Administer 2 mL intramuscularly or subcutaneously in the lower flank or immediately behind the ear. Use sterile syringes and needles. Repeat in 21-28 days. The repeat dose is essential for the maximum immune response. If an outbreak occurs in older swine, administer a third injection at that time.

Annual revaccination of breeding swine is recommended.

Precaution(s): Store at not over 45°F (7°C). Keep from freezing.

Caution(s): Use the entire contents when first opened. Vaccination, especially repeated injections, can result in anaphylaxis.

Antidote(s): Administer epinephrine.

Warning(s): Do not vaccinate within 60 days of slaughter.

Presentation: 100 mL (50 dose) and 250 mL (125 dose) vials.

Compendium Code No.: 11120031

EMULSIBAC® SS

MVP **Bacterin**

Streptococcus suis Bacterin, Porcine Isolates

U.S. Vet. Lic. No.: 301

Active Ingredient(s): The bacterin contains inactivated cultures of *Streptococcus suis* organisms (porcine isolates). It is adjuvanted with Emulsigen® (brand of emulsified paraffin). Prepared from young cultures of *Streptococcus suis* organisms, chemically inactivated. Contains gentamicin sulfate as a preservative.

Indications: For the vaccination of healthy swine against the disease conditions of Streptococcus Suis Syndrome (meningitis, arthritis, pneumonia, pericarditis, endocarditis, and septicemia) associated with *Streptococcus suis* organisms. The bacterin has been shown to protect susceptible swine against challenge with virulent *Streptococcus suis*, serotype 2 organisms, in an efficacy study approved by the USDA.

Dosage and Administration: Read the directions carefully before use. Shake before and occasionally during use. Administer a 1 mL dose intramuscularly to pigs at 10-12 days of age, followed by a 2 mL dose at approximately three (3) to five (5) weeks of age. The repeat dose is essential for the maximum immune response. For the best results, inject into the neck muscules behind the ear. Use sterile syringes and needles. Annual revaccination of breeding swine is recommended.

Precaution(s): Store at not over 45°F (7°C). Keep from freezing.

Caution(s): Use the entire contents when first opened. Vaccination, especially repeated injections, can result in anaphylaxis.

Antidote(s): Administer epinephrine.

Warning(s): Do not vaccinate within 60 days of slaughter.

Trial Data: EMULSIBAC® SS has been shown to be safe in USDA approved field trial studies performed in five states. Each serial of EMULSIBAC® SS has passed rigid quality control testing to ensure the purity, safety and potency standards that are required by the USDA before release.

Presentation: Available in 100 mL vials (100 doses for 10- to 12-day-old pigs or 50 doses for 3- to 5-week-old pigs) and 250 mL vials (250 doses for 10- to 12-day-old pigs or 125 doses for 3- to 5-week-old pigs).

Compendium Code No.: 11120040

EMULSIVIT E-300 ℞

Vedco **Vitamin E**

NDC No.: 50989-335-15

Active Ingredient(s): Each mL contains:

Vitamin E (as d-alpha-tocopherol, a natural source of vitamin E) .... 300 I.U.

Compounded with 2% benzyl alcohol (preservative) in a water emulsifiable base.

EMULSIVIT E-300 is a clear, sterile, nonaqueous solution of d-alpha-tocopherol.

Indications: EMULSIVIT E-300 is for use as an aid in the prevention and treatment of vitamin E deficiencies in swine, cattle, and sheep.

The product is intended as a supplemental source of natural vitamin E.

Dosage and Administration: For intramuscular or subcutaneous administration only. The dose may be repeated. If the dose is greater than 5 mL, equally divide the dose and inject at two (2) different sites.

Suggested Dosage:

Swine:

Sows and Gilts:

2 wks pre-partum .... 4-6 mL (1,200-1,800 I.U.)

2 wks pre-breeding .... 4-6 mL (1,200-1,800 I.U.)

Pigs:

At birth .... 1-2 mL (300-600 I.U.)

Weaning .... 2-3 mL (600-900 I.U.)

Cattle (Dairy and Beef):

Cows and Heifers:

2-3 wks pre-partum .... 8-10 mL (2,400-3,000 I.U.)

At calving .... 8-10 mL (2,400-3,000 I.U.)

Calves:

At birth .... 4-6 mL (1,200-1,800 I.U.)

Weaning .... 4-6 mL (1,200-1,800 I.U.)

Yearlings .... 5-6 mL (1,500-1,800 I.U.)

Sheep:

Ewes:

2-3 wks pre-partum .... 4-5 mL (1,200-1,500 I.U.)

At lambing .... 4-5 mL (1,200-1,500 I.U.)

Lambs:

At birth .... 2-3 mL (600-900 I.U.)

Weaning .... 2-3 mL (600-900 I.U.)

Finishing lambs .... 3-4 mL (900-1,200 I.U.)

Precaution(s): Store between 2° and 30°C (36° and 86°F) in a dark place.

Caution(s): Federal law restricts this drug to use by or on the order of a licensed veterinarian.

Do not exceed the recommended dosage. Occasionally, reactions of an anaphylactic or allergic nature may occur. Should such reactions occur, treat immediately with an injection of epinephrine or antihistamines.

Do not add water to the solution.

Not for human use.

Keep out of the reach of children.

Discussion: Natural tocopherols in feedstuffs can be destroyed through processing, ensiling and storage. A reduced vitamin E intake can result in marginal deficiencies that may not be visible. Intramuscular or subcutaneous injections offer a rapid method to increase the vitamin E status of animals.

Presentation: 250 mL vials.

Compendium Code No.: 10940590

EMULSIVIT E/A&D ℞

Vedco **Vitamins A-D-E**

NDC No.: 50989-344-15

Active Ingredient(s): Each mL contains:

Vitamin E (as d-alpha-tocopherol, a natural source of vitamin E) . . . . . 300 I.U.
Vitamin A propionate . . . . . 100,000 I.U.
Vitamin D_3 . . . . . 10,000 I.U.

Compounded with 2% benzyl alcohol (preservative) in a water emulsifiable base.

EMULSIVIT E/A&D is a clear, sterile nonaqueous solution of vitamin A, vitamin D_3, and vitamin E.

Indications: EMULSIVIT E/A&D is intended as a supplemental source of vitamins A, D, and E.

Dosage and Administration: For intramuscular or subcutaneous administration only. The dose may be repeated as needed. If the dose is greater than 5 mL, equally divide the dose and inject at two (2) different sites.

Suggested Dosage:

Swine:

Sows and Gilts:

1-2 wks pre-breeding	4-6 mL
1-2 wks pre-partum	4-6 mL

Pigs:

At birth	1-2 mL
At weaning	2-3 mL

Cattle (Dairy and Beef):

Cows and Heifers:

2-3 wks pre-partum	8-10 mL
At calving	8-10 mL
End of lactation	8-10 mL

Calves:

At birth	4-6 mL
At weaning	4-6 mL
Yearlings	5-6 mL

Sheep:

Ewes:

2-3 wks pre-partum	4-5 mL
At lambing	4-5 mL

Lambs:

At birth	2-3 mL
At weaning	2-3 mL
Finishing lambs	3-4 mL

Precaution(s): Store between 2° and 30°C (36° and 86°F) in a dark place.

Caution(s): Federal law restricts this drug to use by or on the order of a licensed veterinarian.

Do not exceed the recommended dosage. Occasionally, reactions of an anaphylactic or allergic nature may occur. Should such reactions occur, treat immediately with an injection of epinephrine or antihistamines.

Do not add water to the solution.

Keep out of the reach of children.

Discussion: Natural vitamin A (carotenes), and tocopherols can be destroyed in feedstuffs through processing, ensiling and storage. Due to these losses, reduced intakes of fat-soluble vitamins can occur in animals maintained in continual confinement compared to animals allowed to graze lush pasture. Intramuscular or subcutaneous injections offer a rapid method to increase the vitamin A, vitamin D and vitamin E status of animals.

Presentation: 250 mL vials.

Compendium Code No.: 10940600

ENACARD® TABLETS FOR DOGS ℞

Merial **Cardiac Drug**

(enalapril maleate)

NADA No.: 141-015

Active Ingredient(s): Each ENACARD® tablet contains either:

Enalapril maleate . . . . . 1.0 mg (green)
Enalapril maleate . . . . . 2.5 mg (blue)
Enalapril maleate . . . . . 5.0 mg (pink)
Enalapril maleate . . . . . 10.0 mg (yellow)
Enalapril maleate . . . . . 20.0 mg (white)

Indications: ENACARD® indicated for the treatment of mild, moderate, or severe (modified NYHA Class II[a], III[b], IV[c]) heart failure in dogs. (See Case Management section for etiologies and appropriate conjunctive therapies.)

[a]A dog with modified New York Heart Association Class II heart failure develops fatigue, shortness of breath, coughing, etc., which becomes evident when ordinary exercise is exceeded.

[b]A dog with modified New York Heart Association Class III heart failure is comfortable at rest, but exercise capacity is minimal.

[c]A dog with modified New York Heart Association Class IV heart failure has no capacity for exercise and disabling clinical signs are present at rest.

ENACARD® is indicated for the treatment of dogs in heart failure due to mitral regurgitation (chronic valvular disease) and/or reduced ventricular contractility (dilated cardiomyopathy). Conjunctive therapy which should be used with ENACARD® consists of furosemide and digoxin in the treatment of dilated cardiomyopathy, and furosemide with or without digoxin in the treatment of chronic valvular disease. ENACARD® acts to ameliorate the clinical signs associated with heart failure rather than to reverse the degeneration of the atrioventricular valves or to resolve the underlying myocardial disease in dilated cardiomyopathy. Efficacy against heart failure caused by etiologies other than mitral regurgitation or dilated cardiomyopathy has not been demonstrated.

Pharmacology: Description: ENACARD® contains the maleate salt of enalapril, a derivative of two amino acids, L-alanine and L-proline. Following oral administration, enalapril (a prodrug) is rapidly absorbed and then hydrolyzed to enalaprilat, which is a highly specific, long-acting, non-sulfhydryl angiotensin converting enzyme (ACE) inhibitor. ACE is a dipeptidase that catalyzes the conversion of angiotensin I to angiotensin II. Angiotensin II is a potent vasoconstrictor which stimulates aldosterone secretion by the adrenal cortex. Inhibition of ACE results in decreased plasma angiotensin II levels, which leads to decreased vasopressor activity and to decreased aldosterone secretion. ACE inhibitors are neurohormonal antagonists that are balanced (both arterial and venous) vasodilators resulting in decreased preload and afterload. The overall effect of enalapril treatment is a decrease in the workload of the heart resulting from both arterial and venous dilation and decreased fluid retention.

Chemistry: ENACARD® tablets contain the maleate salt of enalapril, the ethyl ester of the parent diacid, enalaprilat. Enalapril maleate is chemically described as (S)-1(N-(1-(ethoxycarbonyl)-3-phenylpropyl)-L-alanyl)-L-proline, (Z)-2-butenedioate salt (1:1). The empirical formula is $C_{20}H_{28}N_2O_5 \bullet C_4H_4O_4$, and the structural formula is:

CH_3; $-CH_2CH_2CHNHCH-CO-N$; $COOCH_2CH_3$; $COOH$; • CHCOOH ‖ CHCOOH

Dosage and Administration: The recommended starting dose of ENACARD® in dogs is 0.5 mg/kg administered orally s.i.d. (once daily) with or without food. In the absence of an adequate clinical response within 2 weeks, the dosing frequency may be increased to b.i.d. (twice daily) for a total daily dose of 1 mg/kg. The clinical response should be evaluated based upon criteria that include a physical exam, degree of pulmonary congestion/edema demonstrated on chest radiographs, the level of activity displayed by the dog, and exercise tolerance. This dose increase may be initiated earlier if indicated by worsening signs of heart failure such as increased pulmonary congestion/edema, decreased level of activity or decreased exercise tolerance. Dogs should be observed closely for 48 hours following initial dosing or after increasing the dosing frequency for clinical signs consistent with hypotension such as weakness or depression. In addition, renal function should be monitored closely both before and 2 to 7 days after starting treatment with ENACARD®.

Dogs should be receiving standard heart failure therapy including stable doses of furosemide, with or without digoxin. Dogs should be receiving a stable dose of furosemide for at least two days before treatment with ENACARD® and, if included in the treatment regimen, a stable dose of digoxin should be administered for four days prior to the initiation of therapy with ENACARD®.

In the event that clinical signs of hypotension or reduced kidney function occur or that a significant increase in the concentration of blood urea nitrogen (BUN) and/or serum creatinine (CRT) over pretreatment levels is detected, refer to the Cautions section for the appropriate response.

In the clinical studies, dogs with dilated cardiomyopathy generally responded more rapidly than dogs with mitral regurgitation as noted by the higher percentages of dogs demonstrating improved scores on Day 14 for class of heart failure, overall evaluation, mobility, attitude and activity. On Day 28, dogs with dilated cardiomyopathy responded better than dogs with mitral regurgitation as demonstrated by higher percentages of dogs showing improvement for class of heart failure, overall evaluation, mobility, attitude and activity.

Case Management: Because of the complexity of the treatment of dogs with heart failure, it may be necessary to consult with a veterinary cardiologist or internist.

Diagnosis and Monitoring: As the heart failure disease syndrome is complex and usually requires multiple therapies, it is important to establish an accurate diagnosis. Diagnosis is based on procedures such as a complete physical examination, auscultation, electrocardiography, radiography, echocardiography, and pertinent laboratory tests, including hematology, clinical chemistry and urinalysis. In clinical studies, dogs were evaluated by assessing the class of heart failure, severity of pulmonary edema, appetite, level of activity, mobility, and cough prior to initiating treatment and again two (14 days) and four (28 days) weeks after starting treatment (see Efficacy section). Client observations are important in the successful monitoring of treatment. During long-term therapy, dogs were evaluated approximately every three months unless conditions required that individual dogs be monitored more frequently. For dogs receiving digoxin therapy serum digoxin concentrations were also measured at these times or if indicated by inappetence, vomiting or diarrhea.

In addition, pertinent laboratory tests including hematology and clinical chemistry were performed with attention to monitoring BUN and CRT concentrations.

Compatibilities: Concomitant Therapy: As established during clinical studies, ENACARD® may be used concomitantly with other therapy, which may include furosemide, digoxin, antiarrhythmics, beta-blockers, bronchodilators and cough suppressants for the treatment of heart failure in dogs. ENACARD® may be used in combination with sodium restricted diets. The safety of ENACARD® when used concomitantly with other cardiovascular drugs (e.g. vasodilators) has not been established.

Precaution(s): Stability: ENACARD® tablets have been shown to be stable for 24 months at room temperature.

Storage: Protect from moisture. Store below 30°C (86°F) and avoid transient temperatures above 50°C (122°F). When not in use keep container tightly closed. Do not remove desiccant from the container. Subdivision of the product package is not recommended, as the product should be stored in an airtight container.

Caution(s): Federal (U.S.A.) law restricts this drug to use by or on the order of a licensed veterinarian.

Renal Function: The use of diuretics is considered an important part of therapy for heart failure. The result is that some dogs are kept in a volume-depleted (slightly dehydrated) state to control their heart failure. If cardiac function is impaired, the relative volume of blood reaching the kidneys is decreased, leading to prerenal azotemia. If the renal flow, already impaired by heart failure, is further compromised by volume depletion, prerenal azotemia is exacerbated. In normal dogs, prerenal azotemia is confirmed by examination of urine specific gravity; however, administration of diuretics renders this diagnostic test invalid. In clinical trials, the pretreatment serum chemistry profiles showed that the mean BUN was 28.7 mg/dL and the mean serum CRT was 1.27 mg/dL, indicating that dogs in heart failure receiving furosemide therapy may have elevations in BUN and CRT.

Clinical manifestations of the heart failure syndrome may include prerenal azotemia, which is defined as an elevation in BUN and/or CRT with a normal urinalysis. This usually results from decreased renal blood flow induced by impaired cardiovascular performance. Compounds that cause volume depletion, such as diuretics or angiotensin converting enzyme inhibitors, may lower systemic blood pressure, which may further decrease renal perfusion and lead to the development of azotemia. Dogs with no detectable renal disease may develop minor and transient increases in BUN or CRT when ENACARD® is administered concomitantly with furosemide.

1. If clinical signs of hypotension or signs of azotemia develop, the dose of furosemide should be reduced first.
2. If signs of azotemia continue it may be necessary to further reduce the daily dose of furosemide or discontinue administration.

3. If there is still no improvement in clinical signs, dosing with ENACARD® should be decreased in frequency to once daily if being given twice daily, or discontinued.
4. Renal function (BUN and CRT) should be monitored periodically until it returns to pretreatment levels.
5. Appropriate fluid therapy, carefully monitored, should be considered if the above steps do not reverse azotemia.

Use in Breeding Animals: The safety of enalapril in breeding dogs has not been established. Use of enalapril in pregnant bitches is not recommended.

Warning(s): Keep this and all drugs out of the reach of children.

In case of ingestion by humans, clients should be advised to contact a physician immediately.

Toxicology: Safety:

Healthy Dogs: Healthy dogs that received enalapril maleate at a dose rate of 15 mg/kg/day (15X) for up to one year showed no adverse changes. Dogs in acute and subacute toxicity studies also received enalapril maleate at doses including 10, 30, 90, 100 and 200 mg/kg/day for shorter periods. In an acute oral toxicity study, death was observed at 200 mg/kg, but no effect was noted at 100 mg/kg/day. In studies lasting one to three months, death was observed in dogs administered very high doses of 30 and 90 mg/kg/day. Signs observed in these dogs consisted of emesis, anorexia, weight loss, decreased activity, dehydration and tremors. At the highest dose of 90 mg/kg/day, nephrosis, characterized by tubular cell necrosis, tubular casts, crystals and mineralization, tubular cell cytoplasmic vacuolation and diffusely distributed lipids in the tubular cells, was observed. Secondary changes consisted of increased BUN and serum potassium with decreased serum chloride. No drug-induced changes were seen on electrocardiograms.

E

Dogs in heart failure: The safety of ENACARD® was demonstrated in clinical trials when administered at the recommended dose level to dogs in heart failure. In these studies, clinical observations/adverse reactions were reported with similar frequency in both treatment groups (enalapril treated and placebo controls). (See Other Clinical Observations/Adverse Reactions section.)

Adverse Reactions: ENACARD® has been demonstrated to be generally well-tolerated in controlled, open-label field and clinical laboratory studies that involved 414 dogs with mild, moderate, or severe heart failure. In clinical studies, the overall prevalence of adverse effects was no greater in dogs treated with standard therapy (furosemide with or without digoxin) and ENACARD® than in those treated with standard therapy and placebo. Since three therapies (enalapril, furosemide, and digoxin) were used in conjunctive therapy, adverse reactions were difficult to associate with a particular drug. If adverse effects associated with azotemia are observed, refer to the Cautions section for recommended action.

Azotemia: In clinical studies, azotemia was based on the clinical investigator's medical opinion (clinical signs or laboratory values) or defined as a BUN value of ≥50 mg/dL and/or a CRT value of ≥2.5 mg/dL, since dogs in heart failure and dogs receiving furosemide have higher values than normal dogs.

There was no significant difference in the prevalence of azotemia in dogs receiving standard therapy and placebo compared with those receiving standard therapy and ENACARD®. Of 381 dogs in clinical field studies, azotemia as defined above was reported in 25.9% of 116 dogs receiving standard therapy and placebo, and in 28.7% of 265 dogs receiving standard therapy and enalapril. Azotemia was the cause of discontinuation of therapy in 4.3% of the dogs receiving standard therapy and placebo and of 3.0% of the dogs receiving standard therapy and ENACARD® in these clinical studies.

Other Clinical Observations/Adverse Reactions: Some clinical observations are attributable to treatment with furosemide and digoxin, and to the disease process itself. These include polyuria and polydipsia, depression, lethargy, anorexia, and decreased activity. Vomiting and other signs associated with the gastro-intestinal tract may be seen as a result of cardiac glycoside toxicity when digoxin is administered in conjunction with furosemide or furosemide and ENACARD®.

No statistically significant differences in the prevalence of clinical signs were reported between dogs given standard therapy and placebo and those given standard therapy and ENACARD®. Clinical observations/adverse reactions reported in field clinical studies are tabulated as follows.

Prevalence of clinical observations/adverse reactions reported in controlled and open-label field clinical studies involving 381 dogs that were treated for up to 15.5 months.

Observations	ENACARD® % of dogs N=265	Placebo % of dogs N=116
Death:		
Total	6.4	10.3
Heart Failure	1.9	7.8
Sudden	2.6	1.7
Other	1.9	0.9
Gastrointestinal:		
Anorexia or inappetence	18.9	25.0
Vomiting, emesis, gastritis, or gastroenteritis, gastric dilation or upset stomach	17.7	17.2
Diarrhea, loose feces, bloody feces or soft feces	15.5	17.2
Circulatory:		
Hemoptysis	0.0	0.9
Hypotension	1.1	0.0
Collapse	3.4	4.3
Syncope	5.3	3.4
Arrhythmia, atrial fibrillation, cardiac arrest, or ventricular tachycardia	1.1	2.6
Pleural effusion	0.4	0.9
General:		
Lethargy, depression, listlessness, decreased activity or sluggishness	12.1	20.7
Trembling, shaking	1.9	0.0
Weakness, ataxia, immobility, weak hind limb, drowsiness, incoordination or disorientation	7.5	5.2
Dehydration, electrolyte imbalance or hyperkalemia	2.6	0.9
Polyuria, polydipsia	0.0	0.9
Pyrexia	0.4	2.6
Restlessness, anxiety	0.8	0.9
Weight loss	1.1	0.9
Renal:		
Azotemia (clinical signs or BUN ≥50 mg/dL or CRT ≥2.5 mg/dL)	28.7	25.9
Azotemia - Adverse Reaction*	3.0	4.3
Renal Failure	0.4	0.0

*Removed from study

Trial Data: Efficacy: Results of the clinical studies demonstrate that treatment with ENACARD® results in improved exercise tolerance and increased survival time with improved quality of life in dogs with mild, moderate, or severe (modified NYHA Class II, III, IV) heart failure. Efficacy of enalapril tablets was confirmed in studies that included 414 dogs with heart failure due to volume overload caused by chronic valvular disease (mitral regurgitation) or reduced ventricular contractility caused by dilated cardiomyopathy. Efficacy of ENACARD® was evaluated prior to, during, and following the completion of treatment in all studies. Evaluations included physical examination, assessment of clinical variables (class of heart failure, pulmonary edema, activity, attitude, mobility, coughing frequency and appetite), electrocardiographic, hemodynamic (mean blood pressure, pulmonary capillary wedge pressure, cardiac output, pulmonary artery pressure, stroke volume, systemic vascular resistance), echocardiographic (pre-ejection period, left ventricular ejection time, fractional shortening, end diastolic diameter, end systolic diameter, velocity of circumferential fiber shortening) and radiographic examinations, as well as complete blood counts, serum chemistry profiles, urinalyses and serum digoxin concentrations. During these studies furosemide and digoxin dose levels were generally within label directions for each drug when used prior to treatment with enalapril. Following the addition of enalapril, in some cases dosages were increased or decreased beyond label direction as clinical signs indicated.

i. Dose Selection Studies: Two controlled-dose selection studies were conducted using 15 dogs with induced heart failure. Heart failure was induced by surgically removing a section of the mitral valve 1 to 5 months prior to testing ENACARD®. Pulmonary capillary wedge pressure was selected as the primary indicator of efficacy because elevated wedge pressure (≥10 mmHg) is the major cause of pulmonary congestion and edema in dogs with heart failure. A single oral dose of 0.5 mg/kg of ENACARD® significantly ($p<0.05$) decreased mean pulmonary wedge pressure at 8 hours and over the first 24 hours following dosing compared to 0.25 mg/kg. A dose of 0.75 mg/kg did not provide additional benefit over that evident at 0.5 mg/kg.

ii. Dose Confirmation Study: A double-blind study was conducted at six sites and included 47 dogs of various breeds, aged 2.5 to 15 years and weighing 3.2 to 64.1 kg. All dogs received standard therapy [furosemide (range of 1.37-10.91 mg/kg/day) with or without digoxin (range of 4.50-25.00 mcg/kg/day)] for heart failure in addition to the test drug. Dogs were treated with either placebo or enalapril tablets at approximately 0.5 mg/kg b.i.d. (range 0.373-0.646 mg/kg) for approximately 21 days. Over the first 24-hour period after the initiation of treatment, improvement of several hemodynamic variables was observed in the enalapril group. Relative to baseline, mean pulmonary capillary wedge pressure was significantly ($p<0.05$) decreased 8 hours after starting treatment, heart rate decreased significantly ($p<0.01$) at 4 hours and over the first 24 hours following the initiation of treatment, and the scores for class of heart failure and pulmonary edema improved significantly ($p<0.05$) after three weeks of treatment in the enalapril group compared to the placebo group.

iii. Short-Term Efficacy Study: A double-blind study was conducted at 19 sites and included 190 dogs with moderate and severe heart failure. Dogs of various breeds, aged 2.5 to 17 years and weighing 2.4 to 68.6 kg were included in the study. All dogs received standard therapy for heart failure [furosemide (range of 0.70-10.54 mg/kg/day) with or without digoxin (range of 2.03-43.86 mcg/kg/day)] in addition to the test drug. Dogs were treated with either placebo or enalapril tablets at approximately 0.5 mg/kg s.i.d. or b.i.d. (range of 0.383-0.723 mg/kg) for approximately 28 days. Treatment was administered s.i.d. for approximately the first 14 days after which the investigator had the option of increasing the dose to b.i.d. or maintaining the dose s.i.d. for the remaining 14 days.

Significantly ($p<0.05$) more dogs in the placebo group were removed from the study because of an increasing degree of heart failure or death compared to the enalapril group. Two and four weeks after starting treatment, dogs in the enalapril group demonstrated significant ($p<0.05$) improvement relative to baseline in class of heart failure, pulmonary edema score, mobility, overall evaluation, attitude, and activity compared to dogs in the placebo group. During the four-week study, 5 dogs died due to progression of the heart failure in the placebo group whereas none died of heart failure in the enalapril group.

iv. Open-Label Field Efficacy Study: This study was conducted at 17 sites and included 144 dogs with mild, moderate or severe (modified NYHA Class II, III or IV) heart failure. Dogs of various breeds, aged 1.5 to 18 years and weighing 1.9 to 61.0 kg were included in the study. ENACARD® tablets were administered orally s.i.d. or b.i.d. at approximately 0.5 mg/kg (range of 0.225-0.716 mg/kg) for approximately 28 days. All except 11 dogs received standard therapy for heart failure [furosemide (range of 0.52-11.80 mg/kg/day) with or without digoxin (range of 2.42-27.12 mcg/kg/day)]. All scored clinical variables, including class of heart failure, pulmonary edema, activity, mobility, attitude, total cough, appetite, and overall evaluation, showed significant ($p<0.01$) improvement from baseline two and four weeks after starting treatment.

v. Long-Term Efficacy Study: A multicenter study was performed to determine the long-term efficacy of ENACARD® and survival in dogs with moderate and severe heart failure. This study was conducted at 14 sites and included 94 dogs. All dogs received placebo or enalapril tablets at approximately 0.5 mg/kg s.i.d. or b.i.d. (range of 0.363-0.738 mg/kg). In addition, all dogs received standard therapy for heart failure that included [furosemide (range of 1.28-8.67 mg/kg/day) with or without digoxin (range of 2.06-26.04 mcg/kg/day)]. Dogs were evaluated periodically for up to 15.5 months. The primary endpoint in the study was death or removal from the study due to an increase in the degree of heart failure, necessitating unblinding of treatment. Survival was significantly ($p<0.05$) longer in the enalapril group (165.3 days) compared to the placebo group (86.1 days).

vi. Exercise Tolerance and Survival Study: A laboratory study was conducted to determine the effect of ENACARD® on exercise tolerance and survival in 18 dogs with surgically induced heart failure. Heart failure was induced by surgically removing a section of the mitral valve 1 to 5 months prior to testing ENACARD®. Efficacy was assessed by exercising dogs on a treadmill at intervals up to 80 days as well as measuring survival over a period of approximately 1 year. Dogs were treated orally with either ENACARD® at approximately 0.5 mg/kg or an equivalent placebo tablet. Treatment was administered s.i.d. for the first 10 days and b.i.d. thereafter for the remainder of the study. During the entire study no other cardiovascular therapy was administered.

After 80 days of therapy the dogs in the enalapril group ran significantly ($p<0.01$) longer than the dogs in the placebo group. The mean running time was 5.8 minutes in the placebo group and 16.4 minutes in the enalapril group. All dogs in the enalapril group ran longer than they did prior to starting treatment, whereas none of the dogs in the placebo group ran longer than they did prior to starting treatment. In the placebo group 2 out of 9 (22.2%) dogs survived 357 days compared to 6 out of 9 (66.7%) dogs in the enalapril group over the same period. The study results demonstrated that dogs treated with ENACARD® had improved exercise tolerance and survived longer relative to controls.

Results of Clinical Studies:

Study	ENACARD®			Placebo		
Clinical Parameters	All	MR[a]	DCM[b]	All	MR	DCM
i. Dose Selection:						
PCWP (mmHg)[1] Study 1: 0.25 mg/kg	-0.92	-	-	0.22	-	-
0.50 mg/kg	-6.73	-	-	0.22	-	-
Study 2: 0.50 mg/kg	-1.77	-	-	-0.33	-	-
0.75 mg/kg	-4.33	-	-	-0.33	-	-
ii. Dose Confirmation:						
PCWP (mmHg)[1]	-3.22	-1.35	-4.55	0.95	6.0	-1.57
Heart Rate (beats/min)[2]	-10.0	-5.6	-12.9	6.9	12.3	4.1
Class of heart failure[3]	50.0	37.5	57.1	16.7	0.0	23.1
Pulmonary edema[3]	50.0	62.5	42.9	16.7	40.0	7.7
Overall evaluation[3]	63.6	50.0	71.4	27.8	40.0	23.1
iii. Short-term Efficacy:						
Class of heart failure[4]	74.7	67.8	89.3	44.8	45.9	42.3
Pulmonary edema[4]	43.0	42.4	44.4	31.0	32.8	26.9
Overall evaluation[4]	77.0	72.9	85.7	40.2	44.3	30.8
iv. Open-Label:						
Class of heart failure[4]	69.8	72.0	57.1	-	-	-
Pulmonary edema[4]	42.0	39.8	55.0	-	-	-
Overall evaluation[4]	85.6	88.1	71.4	-	-	-
v. Long-term Study:						
Survival (Days to death/failure)	165.3	180.0	141.0	86.1	93.7	66.7
vi. Exercise Tolerance and Survival Study:						
Mean running time (seconds)[5]	988	-	-	389	-	-
Percent surviving to 357 days	67	-	-	22	-	-

[1] Pulmonary capillary wedge pressure, change from baseline at 8 hours after treatment.
[2] Change form baseline at 8 hours after treatment.
[3] Percent improved after three weeks of therapy.
[4] Percent improved after four weeks of therapy.
[5] Running time measured after 80 days of therapy.
[a] Mitral regurgitation
[b] Dilated cardiomyopathy

Presentation: ENACARD® is available in 5 tablet strengths: 1.0 mg (green), 2.5 mg (blue), 5.0 mg (pink), 10.0 mg (yellow) and 20.0 mg (white). Each tablet strength is supplied in bottles containing 30 tablets (with desiccant).

ENACARD is a registered trademark of Merial.

(Merial Limited: Registered in England and Wales [Reg. No. 3332751] with registered offices at 27 Knightsbridge, London, SW1X 7QT, England and domesticated in Delaware, USA as Merial LLC).

U.S. Patent No. 4,374,829

Compendium Code No.: 11110091 8853103 / 8853203 / 8853303 / 8853403 / 8853503

ENCEPHALOID® IM

Fort Dodge **Vaccine**

Encephalomyelitis Vaccine, Eastern and Western, Killed Virus

U.S. Vet. Lic. No.: 112

Contents: This product contains the antigens listed above.

Thimerosal, neomycin, polymyxin B and amphotericin B added as preservatives.

Indications: For vaccination of healthy horses as an aid in the prevention of equine encephalomyelitis caused by Eastern and Western strains.

Dosage and Administration: Horses, inject one 1 mL dose intramuscularly using aseptic technique. Administer a second 1 mL dose 21 days after the first dose. Revaccinate annually using one 1 mL dose.

Precaution(s): Store in dark at 2° to 7°C (35° to 45°F). Avoid freezing. Shake well. Use entire contents when first opened.

Caution(s): In some instances, transient local reactions may occur at the injection site. In case of anaphylactoid reaction, administer epinephrine.

For veterinary use only.

Warning(s): Do not vaccinate within 60 days before slaughter.

Presentation: 10 dose (10 mL) vials.

Compendium Code No.: 10030641 1697H

ENCEPHALOMYELITIS VACCINE EASTERN & WESTERN

Colorado Serum **Vaccine**

Encephalomyelitis Vaccine, Eastern & Western, Killed Virus

U.S. Vet. Lic. No.: 188

Contents: ENCEPHALOMYELITIS VACCINE is prepared from formalin killed cultures of encephalomyelitis viruses propagated in a cell culture system.

Contains thimerosal, penicillin, and streptomycin as preservatives.

Indications: The vaccine is recommended for the vaccination of equines against encephalomyelitis.

Dosage and Administration: Shake well prior to withdrawal from the bottle. Inject 1 mL deep in the muscle. Repeat in 3 to 4 weeks. A booster dose of 1 mL should be administered annually and whenever an epidemic situation develops and exposure is likely.

Precaution(s): Store in dark at 2° to 7°C.

Sterilize syringes and needles by boiling in clean water.

Use entire contents when bottle is first opened.

Caution(s): Transitory local reaction may appear at the site of injection.

Anaphylaxis (shock) may sometimes follow use of products of this nature. Adrenalin, or equivalent should be available for immediate use in these instances.

Shake the product well before withdrawing. Each dose must have proportionate share of precipitate for proper response.

Warning(s): Meat animals should not be vaccinated within 21 days before slaughter.

For veterinary use only.

Discussion: Antigenically different viruses identified as "Eastern" and "Western" types are included in the product. Infections caused by these two types of virus are clinically indistinguishable. Equines vaccinated with a vaccine containing a single virus type are not immune to the other. Similarly, an animal that has recovered from infection caused by one type of virus is not protected from disease that may be caused by the other.

At one time an immunizing program could be planned on the basis of a geographic area but in recent years the "Eastern" type virus has appeared in some of the western states and the "Western" type has been found as far east as the Appalachian mountains.

Encephalomyelitis is often referred to as horse encephalitis (inflammation of the brain), sleeping sickness, blind staggers, and brain fever. It has occurred in nearly all parts of the United States, Canada, Mexico, Central America, and South America.

The first indication of equine encephalomyelitis is fever. Temperature will vary from 102° to 107°F. Sluggishness and drowsiness are early symptoms. Lips are loose and muscles around the head, shoulder or flank may twitch spasmodically. As the disease progresses the affected animal stands dejectedly and will move with an awkward staggering gait, oftentimes stumbling blindly into obstructions. Legs are frequently crossed. Some horses may back up persistently. The sick animal, when aroused, may show interest in food or water only to lapse into a stupor with unchewed food in its mouth. Grinding of the teeth and stretching the head and neck are common.

When to Vaccinate: Encephalomyelitis is spread by mosquitos and perhaps other biting insects so animals should be vaccinated prior to the time insects become prevalent. The incidence of the disease diminishes during cold weather. Annual revaccination of all equines is recommended.

Presentation: 10x1 mL and 10 mL vials.

Compendium Code No.: 11010200

ENCEPHALOMYELITIS VACCINE EASTERN & WESTERN WITH TETANUS TOXOID

Colorado Serum **Toxoid-Vaccine**

Encephalomyelitis Vaccine, Eastern & Western, Killed Virus-Tetanus Toxoid

U.S. Vet. Lic. No.: 188

Contents: This is a combination of three immunizing substances (listed above) that are commonly used in equines.

Contains thimerosal, penicillin, and streptomycin as preservatives.

Indications: When administered as directed this single product provides protection against Eastern and Western types of encephalomyelitis and against tetanus.

Dosage and Administration: Shake well prior to withdrawal from the bottle. Inject 2 mL deep in the muscle. Repeat in 3 to 4 weeks. A booster dose of 2 mL should be administered annually and whenever an epidemic situation develops and exposure is likely.

Precaution(s): Store in dark at 2° to 7°C.

Sterilize needles and syringes before using.

Use entire contents when bottle is first opened.

Caution(s): Transitory local reaction may appear at site of injection.

Anaphylaxis (shock) may sometimes follow use of products of this nature. Adrenalin, or equivalent should be available for immediate use in these instances.

Shake the product well before withdrawing. Each dose must have proportionate share of precipitate for proper response.

Warning(s): Meat animals should not be vaccinated within 21 days before slaughter.

For veterinary use only.

Discussion: Encephalomyelitis is often referred to as horse encephalitis (inflammation of the brain), sleeping sickness, blind staggers, and brain fever. It has occurred in nearly all parts of the United States, Canada, Mexico, Central America, and South America.

The first indication of equine encephalomyelitis is fever. Temperature will vary from 102° to 107°F. Sluggishness and drowsiness are early symptoms. Lips are loose and muscles around the head, shoulder or flank may twitch spasmodically. As the disease progresses the affected animal stands dejectedly and will move with an awkward staggering gait, oftentimes stumbling blindly into obstructions. Legs are frequently crossed. Some horses may back up persistently. When aroused the animal may show interest in food or water only to lapse into a stupor with unchewed food in its mouth. Grinding of the teeth and stretching the head and neck are common.

Tetanus is caused by a toxin (poison) produced by growth of *Clostridium tetani*, an anaerobic (lives without air) micro-organism that may be carried into wounds caused by injury or sites of surgical operations.

Affected animals become stiff, have great difficulty swallowing and the pulse rate is increased. Breathing is labored. Spasmodic contractions of the muscular system occurs, extending muscles of the jaw. Thus, the term "lockjaw" is frequently applied. Legs are often spread, tail stiff with abdominal muscles retracted. Tetanus stricken animals may be unusually sensitive to light and heat. Temperature of the animal generally remains normal, elevating only shortly before death.

The Vaccine fraction of this combination is prepared with formalin inactivated cultures of two antigenically different strains of encephalomyelitis virus which are identified as "Eastern" and "Western". Diseases caused by the two types are clinically indistinguishable. Horses vaccinated with vaccine containing a single virus type are not immune to the other. Similarly, an animal that has recovered from infection caused by one type of virus is not protected from disease that may be caused by the other.

The tetanus toxoid fraction is prepared by detoxifying toxin with formalin and moderate heat in such manner that antigenic properties remain intact. The toxoid is refined to remove most of the nonspecific components and is concentrated to provide a low dose effective product for combination with Encephalomyelitis Vaccine fraction.

When to Vaccinate: Encephalomyelitis is spread by mosquitos and perhaps other biting insects so animals should be vaccinated prior to the time insects become prevalent. The Vaccine-Toxoid may also be used in the event of injury to equines. If a previously immunized animal is injured a booster dose of this combination of Tetanus Toxoid should be administered. If not previously immunized or if the injury occurs within 60 days of primary immunization Tetanus Antitoxin should be used simultaneously with this Vaccine-Toxoid or with Tetanus Toxoid alone.

Presentation: 10x2 mL and 20 mL vials.

Compendium Code No.: 11010210

ENCEVAC® WITH HAVLOGEN®*

Intervet **Vaccine**

Encephalomyelitis Vaccine, Eastern & Western Killed Virus

U.S. Vet. Lic. No.: 286

Description: A formaldehyde inactivated, adjuvanted bivalent equine vaccine consisting of Eastern and Western Equine Encephalomyelitis viruses.

Neomycin, polymyxin B and nystatin added as preservatives.

Indications: For immunization of healthy horses against Eastern and Western Encephalomyelitis.

Dosage and Administration: For primary immunization, aseptically inject 1 mL intramuscularly and repeat the dose in 3 to 4 weeks. A 1 mL dose should be administered annually and at any time epidemic conditions exist or are reported and exposure is imminent.

Precaution(s): Store at 35° to 45° F (2° to 7° C). Shake well before using. Use entire contents when first opened.

Caution(s): Local reactions may occur if this product is given subcutaneously. Inject deep into the muscle only. Anaphylactoid reactions may occur.

For use in animals only.

Antidote(s): Epinephrine.

Warning(s): Do not vaccinate within 21 days before slaughter.

Presentation: 1 dose (1 mL) syringes with separate sterile needles and 10 doses (10 mL).

*Adjuvant—U.S. Patent Nos. 3,790,665 and 3,919,411.

Compendium Code No.: 11060500

ENCEVAC®-T WITH HAVLOGEN®*

Intervet **Toxoid-Vaccine**

Encephalomyelitis Vaccine, Eastern & Western Killed Virus-Tetanus Toxoid

U.S. Vet. Lic. No.: 286

Description: A formaldehyde inactivated, adjuvanted polyvalent equine vaccine-toxoid consisting of Eastern and Western Equine Encephalomyelitis viruses and purified Tetanus Toxoid.

Neomycin, polymyxin B, nystatin and thimerosal added as preservatives.

Indications: For immunization of healthy horses against Eastern and Western Equine Encephalomyelitis and Tetanus.

Dosage and Administration: For primary immunization, aseptically inject 1 mL intramuscularly and repeat the dose in 3 to 4 weeks. A 1 mL dose should be administered annually and at any time epidemic conditions exist or are reported and exposure is imminent.

Precaution(s): Store at 35° to 45°F (2° to 7°C). Shake well before using. Use entire contents when first opened.

Caution(s): Local reactions may occur if this product is given subcutaneously. Inject deep into the muscle only. Injury should be followed by a booster dose of vaccine containing Tetanus Toxoid. Consult your veterinarian regarding indications and precautions for the use of tetanus antitoxin. Anaphylactoid reactions may occur.

For use in animals only.

Antidote(s): Epinephrine.

Warning(s): Do not vaccinate within 21 days before slaughter.

Presentation: 1 dose (1 mL) syringes with separate sterile needles and 10 dose (10 mL) vials.

*Adjuvant—U.S. Patent Nos. 3,790,665 and 3,919,411.

Compendium Code No.: 11060510

ENCEVAC® T + VEE WITH HAVLOGEN®*

Intervet **Toxoid-Vaccine**

Encephalomyelitis Vaccine, Eastern, Western & Venezuelan, Killed Virus-Tetanus Toxoid

U.S. Vet. Lic. No.: 286

Description: A formaldehyde inactivated, adjuvanted polyvalent equine vaccine-toxoid consisting of Eastern, Western and Venezuelan Equine Encephalomyelitis viruses and purified Tetanus Toxoid.

Neomycin, polymyxin B and nystatin added as preservatives.

Indications: For vaccination of healthy horses against Eastern, Western and Venezuelan Equine Encephalomyelitis and Tetanus.

Dosage and Administration: For primary immunization, aseptically inject 1 mL intramuscularly and repeat the dose in 3 to 4 weeks. A 1 mL dose should be administered annually and at any time epidemic conditions exist or are reported and exposure is imminent.

Precaution(s): Store at 35° to 45°F (2° to 7°C). Shake well before using. Use entire contents when first opened.

Caution(s): Local reactions may occur if this product is given subcutaneously. Inject deep into the muscle only. Injury should be followed by a booster dose of vaccine containing Tetanus Toxoid. Consult your veterinarian regarding indications and precautions for the use of Tetanus Antitoxin. Anaphylactoid reactions may occur.

For use in animals only.

Antidote(s): Epinephrine.

Warning(s): Do not vaccinate within 21 days before slaughter.

Presentation: 10 x 1 dose (1 mL) sterile syringes per box, individually printed plastic bag with needle and 10 dose (10 mL) vial.

*Adjuvant—Intervet's proprietary technology.

Compendium Code No.: 11060471

ENCEVAC® TC-4 WITH HAVLOGEN®*

Intervet **Toxoid-Vaccine**

Encephalomyelitis-Influenza Vaccine, Eastern & Western Killed Virus, Tetanus Toxoid

U.S. Vet. Lic. No.: 286

Description: A combination of inactivated, purified, concentrated, adjuvanted, tissue culture origin, Encephalomyelitis Virus, Eastern and Western, Equine Influenza Virus subtypes A1 and A2 including KY 93 strain, and Tetanus Toxoid. Intervet serological data suggest cross protection against certain U.S. and European strains, including Prague 56, KY 63, KY 81 and 87, Fountainbleau 79, and Berlin 84 and 89.**

Neomycin, polymyxin B and nystatin added as preservatives.

Indications: For vaccination of healthy horses against Eastern and Western Equine Encephalomyelitis, Equine Influenza Virus and Tetanus.

Dosage and Administration: For primary immunization, aseptically inject 1 mL intramuscularly and repeat the dose in 3 to 4 weeks. A 1 mL dose should be administered annually and at any time epidemic conditions exist or are reported and exposure is imminent.

Precaution(s): Store at 35° to 45°F (2° to 7°C). Shake well before using. Use entire contents when first opened.

Caution(s): Local reactions may occur if this product is given subcutaneously. Inject deep into the muscle only. Injury should be followed by a booster dose of vaccine containing Tetanus Toxoid. Consult your veterinarian regarding indications and precautions for the use of Tetanus Antitoxin. Anaphylactoid reactions may occur.

For use in animals only.

Antidote(s): Epinephrine.

Warning(s): Do not vaccinate within 21 days before slaughter.

References: **Available upon request.

Presentation: 10 dose (10 x 1 mL) syringes with separate sterile needles (Code 0396), 10 doses (10 mL) and 10 dose (10 x 1 mL) syringes with separate sterile needles (Code 4656).

*Adjuvant—Intervet's Proprietary Technology

Compendium Code No.: 11060490

ENCEVAC® TC-4 + VEE WITH HAVLOGEN®*

Intervet **Toxoid-Vaccine**

Encephalomyelitis-Influenza Vaccine, Eastern, Western & Venezuelan, Killed Virus-Tetanus Toxoid

U.S. Vet. Lic. No.: 286

Description: A combination of inactivated, purified, concentrated, adjuvanted, tissue culture origin, Encephalomyelitis Virus, Eastern, Western and Venezuelan, Equine Influenza Virus subtypes A1 and A2 including KY 93 strain and Tetanus Toxoid. Intervet serological data suggest cross protection against certain U.S. and European strains, including Kentucky 93, 94, 95 and 96, Suffolk 89, Kildare 89 and 92, Austria 92, Switzerland 93, New Market 1/93 and 2/93, Berlin 94, Italy 96 and Meath 96.**

Neomycin, polymyxin B, nystatin and thimerosal added as preservatives.

Indications: For vaccination of healthy horses against Eastern, Western and Venezuelan Equine Encephalomyelitis, Equine Influenza Virus and Tetanus.

Dosage and Administration: For primary immunization, aseptically inject 1 mL intramuscularly and repeat the dose in 3 to 4 weeks. A 1 mL dose should be administered annually and at any time epidemic conditions exist or are reported and exposure is imminent.

Precaution(s): Store at 35° to 45°F (2° to 7°C). Shake well before using. Use entire contents when first opened.

Caution(s): Local reactions may occur if this product is given subcutaneously. Inject deep into the muscle only. Injury should be followed by a booster dose of vaccine containing Tetanus Toxoid. Consult your veterinarian regarding indications and precautions for the use of Tetanus Antitoxin. Anaphylactoid reactions may occur.

For use in animals only.

Antidote(s): Epinephrine.

Warning(s): Do not vaccinate within 21 days before slaughter.

References: **Available upon request.

Presentation: 10 x 1 dose (1 mL) sterile syringes per box, individually printed plastic bag with needle and 10 dose (10 mL) vial.

*Adjuvant—Intervet's proprietary technology.

Compendium Code No.: 11060481

76004860, R.1

ENCORE®

VetLife **Implant**

Estradiol Controlled Release Implants

NADA No.: 118-123

Active Ingredient(s): Each ENCORE® silicone rubber implant contains 43.9 mg estradiol and is coated with not less than 0.5 mg of oxytetracycline powder as a local antibacterial.

Indications: For increased rate of weight gain in suckling and pastured growing steers; for improved feed efficiency and increased rate of weight gain in confined steers and heifers.

An ENCORE® Controlled Release Implant will provide an effective daily dose of estradiol for at least 400 days. No additional effectiveness may be expected from reimplanting in less than 400 days.

Directions for Implantation: Equipment: A Compudose®/ENCORE® Implanter must be used to implant cattle.

Insert one implant under the skin of the ear.

1. Confine animal in a squeeze chute.
2. To reduce the possibility of infection and resulting implant loss, hygienic and antiseptic procedures should be followed during implantation. The ear should be clean and dry. The skin should be cleansed with a suitable antiseptic soap and dried prior to implanting. This is particularly important if the ears are contaminated with urine or feces.
3. To load the Compudose®/ENCORE® Implanter remove the cartridge from the package, release the latch on the magazine, open and insert the cartridge.

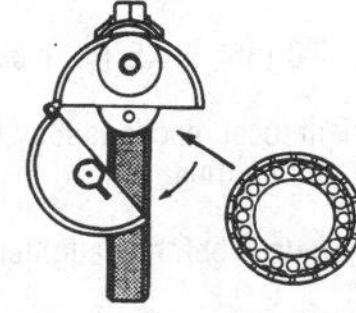

Close the magazine and latch. Advance the cartridge to the next implant by inserting the thumb into the magazine opening and turning the cartridge to the next stop.

Use a sharp needle. The needle should be cleaned and sterilized between each injection by wiping the exterior with a sponge, cloth, or gauze saturated with an appropriate disinfectant. The presence of excessive moisture inside the needle may result in dissolving the oxytetracycline (OTC) from the implant surface and contribute to accumulation of OTC inside the needle.

4. The implant should be deposited under the skin on the back side of the middle third of the ear. It should be placed between the skin and cartilage, avoiding major blood vessels. Grasping the tip of the ear with one hand and the implanter in the other, penetrate the skin in the outer third of the ear.

   Important: Do not penetrate cartilage.
5. Upon penetration. the needle should be fully inserted between the skin and cartilage, avoiding major blood vessels. Full insertion of the needle is important to maximize implant retention.
6. Pull the needle back as the implant is being deposited by squeezing the lever on the implanter

grip. The figure below shows the implant in proper position in the middle third of the ear where the skin is tight.

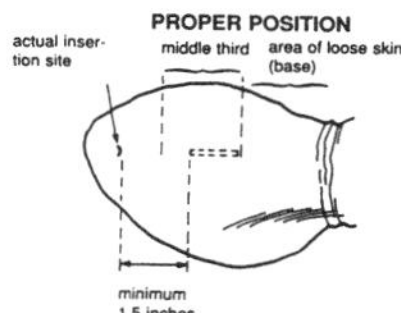

7. After repeated use, sufficient oxytetracycline (OTC) from the implant may accumulate inside the needle to impede implant passage. Periodic removal of the needle from the device and washing it in water will prevent such accumulation. Before reusing, the needle should be disinfected and allowed to dry after shaking vigorously to remove excess water or disinfectant.
8. If reimplantation is desired, it is not necessary to remove the existing ENCORE® implant. Place the second implant at the same level and parallel to, but not in contact with, the existing implant or place it in the unimplanted ear in accordance with paragraphs 1-7 of these directions.

When to Implant ENCORE®:
Suckling steers: At castration or later.
Pastured growing steers: At weaning or later.
Finishing steers and heifers: At arrival in feedlot.

Caution(s): To maximize implant retention:
A. Fully insert the needle.
B. Deposit the implant in the middle third of the ear where the skin is tight.
C. Do not deposit the implant where the skin is loose in the third of the ear closest to the head.

The needle has been scientifically designed to maximize retention. When it becomes dull, use a new needle. If the needle is resharpened, sharpen only the point.

Failure to follow antiseptic implanting procedures, particularly when the ears are contaminated with fecal material, may result in infection and excessive implant loss. Implanting cattle during wet weather or just prior to dipping in contaminated solutions may increase infection and implant loss.

Carefully check the ears for implant loss approximately 4 weeks after implantation. If loss occurs, reimplant using recommended procedures.

Increased sexual activity (bulling, riding and excitability) has been reported in animals implanted with ENCORE®. Implanted animals should be observed for such signs particularly during the first few days after implanting and animals being excessively ridden (bullers) should be removed to prevent physical injury. Vaginal and rectal prolapse have been reported in heifers implanted with ENCORE®.

Do not use in animals intended for breeding purposes.

Warning(s): For subcutaneous ear implantation in steers and heifers only.
Keep out of reach of children.

Side Effects: Udder development, swollen or enlarged vulva and high tailheads may be observed in implanted heifers.

Presentation: ENCORE® Implants are supplied in cartridges of 20 implants each.
ENCORE and Compudose are registered trademarks of Ivy Animal Health, Inc.

Compendium Code No.: 10330141

END-FLUENCE® WITH IMUGEN® II

Intervet **Vaccine**

Swine Influenza Vaccine, Killed Virus

U.S. Vet. Lic. No.: 286

Contents: This product contains the antigen listed above.
Contains gentamicin as a preservative.

Indications: For the vaccination of healthy swine as an aid in the prevention of disease caused by swine influenza virus.

Directions: Inject healthy swine 3 weeks of age or older with 2 mL given intramuscularly. Repeat vaccination 3 weeks later. This product provides protection against clinical signs for three months following vaccination.

Precaution(s): Store at 2°-7°C (35°-45°F). Do not freeze. Shake well. Use entire contents when first opened.

Caution(s): In case of anaphylactoid reaction administer epinephrine.
For veterinary use only.

Warning(s): Do not vaccinate within 21 days before slaughter.

Presentation: 50 dose (100 mL) vial.

Compendium Code No.: 11060001

END-FLUENCE® 2*

Intervet **Vaccine**

Swine Influenza Vaccine, H1N1 & H3N2, Killed Virus

U.S. Vet. Lic. No.: 286

Contents: This product contains an inactivated US Midwest field isolate of subtype H3N2 and an inactivated subtype H1N1 of swine influenza type A virus in Microsol Diluvac Forte® adjuvant.
Contains thimerosal and gentamicin as preservatives.

Indications: For use in healthy swine as an aid in the prevention of influenza caused by serotype A swine influenza (subtypes H1N1 and H3N2).
Duration of immunity study for H3N2 subtype still in progress.

Dosage and Administration: Shake well, aseptically inject intramuscularly (IM). Administer a 2.0 mL dose at 3 weeks of age or older, followed by one 2.0 mL dose 3 weeks later.

Precaution(s): Store in the dark at not over 45°F (7°C). Do not freeze. Do not save partial contents. Burn the container and all unused product.

Caution(s): Use in healthy swine. If allergic reaction occurs, treat with epinephrine.
For veterinary use only.

Warning(s): Do not vaccinate within 21 days of slaughter.

Presentation: 50 dose (100 mL) and 250 dose (500 mL) bottles.

*U.S. Patent Nos. 5,650,155 and 5,667,784

Compendium Code No.: 11062530

ENDOSERUM®

Immvac **Antiserum**

Salmonella typhimurium Antiserum, Equine Origin

U.S. Vet. Lic. No.: 345

Active Ingredient(s): *Salmonella typhimurium* antiserum, equine origin.

Indications: ENDOSERUM® is recommended for attenuating the effects of *Salmonella typhimurium* and *Escherichia coli* in equids when administered prior to challenge. It increases the circulating levels of IgG(t) anti-endotoxin antibodies. It is also recommended for increasing the total IgG levels of FPT foals in properly calculated doses. Contains total IgG levels of 3,000 mg/dl. Prepared from healthy horses negative for equine infectious anemia (EIA), brucellosis, piroplasmosis, dourine, glanders, and anti-red blood cell antibodies.

Dosage and Administration: Shake well before use.

For the treatment of endotoxemia: Administer intravenously 0.7 mL per pound (1.5 mL/kg) of body weight.

For the treatment of foal IgG deficit: For a 70 lb. foal with a 200 mg/dl IgG deficit, administer 500 mL.

Because immunoglobulin may be rapidly depleted during gram-negative diseases, administration should be repeated if signs of endotoxemia recur or persist.

Always dilute with an equal or larger volume of sterile physiological saline or lactated ringer's solution. Warm to room temperature. Administration should not be completed in less than 30 minutes.

Precaution(s): Store at 35°-45°F (2°-7°C). Do not freeze.

Caution(s): Use the entire contents when first opened.
Sales are restricted to licensed veterinarians.
If an allergic reaction occurs, administer epinephrine or its equivalent.

Warning(s): Do not administer within 21 days of slaughter.

Presentation: 250 mL and 500 mL containers.

Compendium Code No.: 11260000

ENDOSORB™ BOLUS

PRN Pharmacal **Antidiarrheal-Adsorbent**

Absorbent Anti-Diarrheal Demulcent

Active Ingredient(s): Each 240 gr. large animal bolus contains activated attapulgite with roasted powdered carob pulp, citrus pectin, magnesium trisilicate, colloidal aluminum silicate (hydrated) with artificial color and base.

Indications: To aid in the supportive treatment of intestinal disturbances in cattle and horses.

Directions: Horses: ½ to 1 bolus; Cattle: 1 to 1½ boluses. Repeat at 4 hour intervals if indicated.

Warning(s): Read and follow label directions carefully. Keep out of reach of children.

Presentation: 50 boluses.

Compendium Code No.: 10900040

ENDOSORB™ SUSPENSION

PRN Pharmacal **Antidiarrheal-Adsorbent**

Active Ingredient(s): Contains activated attapulgite, 750 mg, per 5 mL (teaspoonful) in a base containing pectin, magnesium trisilicate, water, flavors, and sodium saccharin, (an artificial sweetening agent).

Indications: Activated attapulgite is a specially treated mineral clay that adsorbs toxins and toxic materials present in the gut of animals with symptoms of diarrhea. This adsorbent action helps to relieve the irritation, discomfort, and cramping associated with diarrhea.

Dosage and Administration: ENDOSORB™ Suspension is made to help alleviate the symptoms of simple diarrheas in animals. If the diarrhea is caused by, or associated with a bacterial intestinal infection, then appropriate antibiotic therapy should be started as soon as possible. Animals being treated with ENDOSORB™ Suspension should have access to fresh, clean drinking water in liberal portions.

Shake well before using.
Recommended Dosage:
Puppies and Kittens: 1 to 2 tsps every 4 hours.
Dogs and Cats: 1 to 3 tblsps every 4 hours.
Foals and Calves: 2 to 4 fl oz every 2 to 3 hours.
Cattle and Horses: 6 to 8 fl oz every 3 hours.
Pigs: 1 to 2 tsps every 3 to 4 hours.
Hogs: 2 fl oz per 100 lb body weight every 3 to 4 hours.
Note: Dosage should be adjusted as necessary.

Warning(s): If clinical signs persist after 2 or 3 days, diagnosis should be redetermined.
Use only as directed. For veterinary use only. Not for human use.

Presentation: 4 fl oz, 1 pint (16 fl oz) and 1 gallon.

Compendium Code No.: 10900050

ENDOSORB™ TABLETS

PRN Pharmacal **Antidiarrheal-Adsorbent**

Absorbent Anti-Diarrheal Demulcent

Active Ingredient(s): Each 1.5 gram small animal tablet contains activated attapulgite with roasted powdered carob pulp, citrus pectin, magnesium trisilicate, colloidal aluminum silicate (hydrated) with artificial color and base.

Indications: To aid in the supportive treatment of intestinal disturbances in canines.

Directions: Canine: 1 tablet every 4 hours from 5 to 25 lbs of body weight.
2 tablets every 4 hours from 26 lbs to 50 lbs of body weight or as directed by a veterinarian.

Warning(s): Read and follow label directions carefully. Keep out of reach of children.

Presentation: 500 tablets.

Compendium Code No.: 10900060

ENDOVAC-BOVI® WITH IMMUNEPLUS®

Immvac **Bacterin-Toxoid**

Salmonella Typhimurium Bacterin-Toxoid, Re-17 Derived Mutagenically

U.S. Vet. Lic. No.: 345

Contents: This product contains the antigen listed above. This product contains an oil adjuvant.
Preservative: Formaldehyde.

Indications: The Mutant Salmonella Typhimurium Bacterin-Toxoid is for vaccination of healthy cattle to aid in the prevention of clinical mastitis caused by *E. coli* and the effects of endotoxemia in cattle due to *Escherichia coli, Salmonella typhimurium, Pasteurella multocida* and *Pasteurella haemolytica*.

E

ENDOVAC-EQUI® WITH IMMUNEPLUS®

Dosage and Administration: Shake well before use. Inject 2 mL into the musculature of healthy cattle. Repeat in 2 or 3 weeks. Administer a 2 mL booster dose annually. Recommended for vaccination of cows during the dry period and heifers during the third trimester of pregnancy.
Precaution(s): Store at 2°-7°C (35°-45°F). Do not freeze. Use entire contents when opened.
Caution(s): Not recommended for administration to mastic cows or to septicemic cattle. Do not use in horses. Local tenderness at the injection site may occur with the use of this vaccine. If anaphylactoid reaction occurs, administer epinephrine.
Warning(s): Do not use within 60 days of slaughter.
For veterinary use only.
Presentation: 40 mL (20 dose) and 100 mL (50 dose) vials.
U.S. Patent No. 5641492
Compendium Code No.: 11260010

ENDOVAC-EQUI® WITH IMMUNEPLUS®

Immvac **Bacterin-Toxoid**
Salmonella Typhimurium Bacterin-Toxoid, Aluminum Hydroxide Adsorbed
U.S. Vet. Lic. No.: 345
Contents: This product contains the antigen listed above.
Preservative: Merthiolate.
Indications: For the vaccination of healthy equids six months of age or older to aid in the prevention of endotoxin-mediated diseases caused by *Salmonella typhimurium* and *Escherichia coli.*
Dosage and Administration: Shake well before use. Inject 1 mL into the musculature of healthy equids. Repeat in two (2) or three (3) weeks. Administer a 1 mL booster dose annually. Use the entire contents when opened.
Precaution(s): Store at 2°-7°C (35°-45°F). Do not freeze.
Caution(s): Sales are restricted to licensed veterinarians.
Do not vaccinate horses with a history of laminitis or following a recent episode of acute endotoxemia. Do not vaccinate horses recently administered progesterone or steroids. Do not vaccinate horses during active training periods. Horses should be given moderate exercise or turned on pasture following vaccination. Local swelling and tenderness at the injection site may occur with the use of the vaccine. Resolution of these signs usually occurs in 3-5 days, but occasionally in 10 days or more. Lethargy, inappetence and stiffness may occur lasting up to 2-3 days.
If an allergic reaction occurs, administration of epinephrine and other sound medical procedures should be implemented.
Warning(s): Do not vaccinate within 21 days before slaughter.
Presentation: 10 mL (10 dose) vials.
Compendium Code No.: 11260021

ENDOVAC-PORCI® WITH IMMUNEPLUS®

Immvac **Bacterin-Toxoid**
Salmonella Typhimurium Bacterin-Toxoid, Re-17 Derived Mutagenically, Aluminum hydroxide adsorbed, Oil adjuvanted
U.S. Vet. Lic. No.: 345
Contents: This product contains the antigen listed above.
Preservative: Formaldehyde.
Indications: The Mutant Salmonella Typhimurium Bacterin-Toxoid is for vaccination of healthy pigs to aid in the prevention of clinical mastitis caused by *E. coli* and the effects of endotoxin-mediated diseases caused by *Salmonella typhimurium* and *Salmonella choleraesuis.*
Dosage and Administration: Shake well before use. Inject 1 mL into the musculature of healthy pigs. Repeat in 10 to 14 days. Administer a 1 mL booster dose annually.
Precaution(s): Store at 2°-7°C (35°-45°F). Do not freeze. Use entire contents when opened.
Caution(s): Local tenderness at the injection site may occur with the use of this vaccine. If anaphylactoid reaction occurs, administer epinephrine.
Warning(s): Do not use within 60 days of slaughter.
For use in swine only.
For veterinary use only.
Presentation: 100 mL (100 dose) vials.
U.S. Patent No. 5641492
Compendium Code No.: 11260030

ENDURA-LITE™

Creative Science **Electrolytes-Oral**
High Potency Electrolytes-Concentrated Stress Formula
Active Ingredient(s): Contents: Sodium chloride, potassium chloride, calcium acetate, magnesium citrate, in a palatable base (apple flavored).
When dissolved at a rate of 1 oz (scoopful) per 10 gallons of drinking water, resulting solution will contain the following ions: Na^+, K^+, Ca^{++}, Mg^{++}, Cl^-, acetate and citrate.
Indications: As an aid in the replacement of electrolytes and in preventing dehydration due to stress and exercise in horses. Developed for and shown to be especially beneficial when used in endurance horses.
Dosage and Administration:
In drinking water: 1 oz per 10 gallons.
In feed: 1% in place of each 1% salt.
Individually to horses: ½ oz - 1 oz per 800-1,000 pounds or as recommended by a veterinarian.
Caution(s): For animal use only.
Warning(s): For use on horses not intended for food use.
Keep out of reach of children.
Presentation: 1 lb (454 g), 5 lb (2.27 kg) and 25 lb jars.
Compendium Code No.: 13760011

ENDURA-LYTE®

Life Science **Electrolytes-Oral**
Ingredient(s): Sodium chloride, potassium chloride, calcium acetate, magnesium citrate, in a palatable base (apple flavored).
When dissolved at a rate of 1 oz (scoopful) per 10 gallons of drinking water, the resulting solution will contain the following ions (mEq/L): Sodium (Na^+) 5.4, Potassium (K^+) 1.7, Calcium (Ca^{++}) 0.94, Magnesium (Mg^{++}) 0.1, Chloride (Cl^-) 7.1, Acetate 0.94, Citrate 0.1.
Indications: For use as an aid in the replacement of electrolytes and in preventing dehydration due to stress and exercise in horses and large animals. Developed for and shown to be especially beneficial when used in endurance horses.
Dosage and Administration:
In drinking water: 1 oz per 10 gallons.
In feed: 1% in place of each 1% salt.
Individually to horses, cattle, sheep, or swine: ½-1 oz per 800-1,000 pounds of body weight, or as recommended by a veterinarian.
Caution(s): For animal use only.
Warning(s): Keep out of reach of children.
Presentation: 5 lb container.
Compendium Code No.: 10870051

ENDURE™ SWEAT-RESISTANT FLY SPRAY

Farnam **Insect Repellent**
EPA Reg. No.: 270-251
Active Ingredient(s):

Cypermethrin, CAS # 52315-07-8	0.15%
Pyrethrins, CAS # 8003-34-7	0.20%
Piperonyl Butoxide Technical*, CAS # 51-03-6	1.60%
Butoxy Polypropylene Glycol, CAS # 9003-13-8	5.00%
Other Ingredients	93.05%
Total:	100.00%

*Equivalent to 1.28% (butylcarbityl)(6-propylpiperonyl) ether and 0.32% of related compounds.
Indications: Ready-to-use ENDURE™ Sweat-Resistant Fly Spray for Horses insecticide/repellent/sun-screen formula provides repellency, quick knock-down and long lasting protection from flies, gnats, and mosquitoes. Unique formulation stays active and keeps working even in wet conditions and when the horse sweats. The special sun-screening agent in this product protects against both forms of the sun's harmful ultra-violet rays.
Sweat and water resistant fly repellent formula. Up to 14 days fly control. Protects against biting and nuisance flies, gnats, mosquitoes, deer ticks and lice. For horses and ponies.
Directions for Use: It is a violation of Federal law to use this product in a manner inconsistent with its labeling.
Not for use on horses intended for human consumption. Shake well before using. To protect horses from horse flies, house flies, stable flies, face flies, horn flies, deer flies, gnats, mosquitoes, lice, ticks, and deer ticks that may transmit Lyme Disease: Thoroughly brush the horse's coat prior to application to remove loose dirt and debris. For dirty horses, shampoo and rinse thoroughly. Wait until coat is completely dry before applying ENDURE™ Sweat-Resistant Fly Spray for Horses. Its unique water resistant formula contains a special conditioner that binds to the hair shaft so it keeps working even in moist conditions or when the horse sweats.
This product may be applied either as a spray or as a wipe. For horse's face, always apply as a wipe using a piece of clean, absorbent cloth, toweling (Turkish) or sponge. Wear rubber glove or mitt when applying as a wipe. Spray or wipe horse's entire body while brushing against the lay of the coat to ensure adequate coverage. Avoid getting spray into horse's eyes, nose or mouth.
Application should be liberal for best results. Reapply every 5 to 7 days under normal conditions for initial applications. As protection builds, reapply every 10 to 14 days as needed. Also, reapply each time animal is washed or exposed to heavy rain.
Precautionary Statements: Hazards to Humans and Domestic Animals:
Caution:
Humans: For animal use only. Not for use on humans. Harmful if swallowed. Avoid contact with eyes, skin or clothing. Avoid breathing spray mist. Avoid contamination of food. Wash hands with soap and water after use.
Horses: Avoid contact with eyes or mucous membranes. Harmful if swallowed. Avoid breathing spray mist. Avoid contamination of food.
First Aid:
If Swallowed: Call a poison control center or doctor immediately for treatment advice. Have person sip a glass of water if able to swallow. Do not induce vomiting unless told to do so by the poison control center or doctor. Do not give anything by mouth to an unconscious person.
If Inhaled: Move person to fresh air. If person is not breathing, call 911 or an ambulance, then give artificial respiration, preferably by mouth-to-mouth, if possible. Call a poison control center for doctor for further treatment advice.
If on Skin or Clothing: Take off contaminated clothing. Rinse skin immediately with plenty of water for 15-20 minutes. Call a poison control center or doctor for treatment advice.
If in Eyes: Hold eye open and rinse slowly and gently with water for 15-20 minutes. Remove contact lenses, if present, after the first 5 minutes, then continue rinsing eye. Call a poison control center or doctor for treatment advice.
In case of medical emergencies or health and safety inquiries, or in case of fire, leaking or damaged containers or for product use information, call: (602) 285-1660.
Have the product container or label with you when calling a poison control center or doctor, or going for treatment.
Environmental Hazards: This product is toxic to fish. Do not apply to any body of water. Do not contaminate water when disposing of equipment washwaters.
Storage and Disposal:
Storage: Store in a cool, dry place.
Pesticide Disposal: Securely wrap empty original container in several layers of newspaper and discard in trash.
Container Disposal: Do not reuse empty container. Wrap container and put in trash.
Warning(s): Not for use on horses intended for human consumption.
Keep out of reach of children.
Disclaimer: Buyer assumes all risk of use, storage or handling of this product not in strict accordance with directions given herein.
Presentation: 1 qt (.946 L) with sprayer and 1 gallon (3.8 L) containers.
Compendium Code No.: 10000830 0B1 / 01-1362

ENEMA-DSS

Butler **Enema**
Active Ingredient(s): Each syringe contains: 250 mg dioctyl sodium sulfosuccinate in glycerine U.S.P.
Indications: For use as an aid in the relief of all forms of constipation, for pre-operative preparations and for the restoration of bowel habits in post-operative patients.
Dosage and Administration: Gently insert the flexible nozzle into the rectum and press the plunger to express contents. In resistant cases, the treatment may be repeated in one (1) hour.
Caution(s): Keep out of the reach of children.
Presentation: 12 mL syringe.
Compendium Code No.: 10820680

ENEMA SA

Vetus **Enema**

NDC No.: 47611-550-71

Active Ingredient(s): Each mL contains 250 mg of dioctyl sodium sulfosuccinate in glycerin. Sorbic acid is added as a preservative.

Indications: A ready-to-use syringe for rectal use on dogs and cats.

Dosage and Administration: Give a single application to dogs and cats.

Caution(s): For animal use only. For rectal use only.

Presentation: 12 mL syringes.

Compendium Code No.: 14440280

ENERCAL™

Vedco **Small Animal Dietary Supplement**

High Calorie Nutritional Supplement

Ingredient(s): Corn Syrup, Soybean Oil (Source of LA and ALA), Malt Syrup, Cod Liver Oil (Source of EPA and DHA), Cane Molasses, Methylcellulose, Water, Peptones, dl-Alpha Tocopheryl Acetate (Vitamin E), Sodium Benzoate (Preservative), Manganese Sulfate, Iron Peptonate, Thiamine HCl, Nicotinamide, Calcium Pantothenate (Source of Calcium and Pantothenic Acid), Magnesium Sulfate, Pyridoxine HCl, Vitamin A Palmitate, Potassium Iodide (Source of Iodine and Potassium), Riboflavin 5' Phosphate Sodium (Source of Vitamin B2 and Phosphorus), Vitamin A Palmitate and D3 Concentrate, Folic Acid and Cyanocobalamin (Vitamin B12).

Calorie content: 4420 kcal/kg (26.5 kcal/6 g).

Indications: A vitamin and energy supplement for dogs and cats.

ENERCAL™ also acts as an appetite stimulant and added source of energy.

Its highly palatable flavor aids in easy administration.

Directions for Use: To supplement your pet's regular caloric or nutritional intake, give 1½ teaspoons per 10 pounds of body weight daily. For pets that are not eating, give 3 teaspoons (1 tablespoon) per 10 pounds of body weight daily.

To acquaint pet to the flavor of ENERCAL™, place a small amount on your pets nose or paw.

Presentation: 5 oz (141.7 g) tube (NDC 50989-610-22).

Compendium Code No.: 10942200

ENERGEL™ FOR CATS

Pet-Ag **Small Animal Dietary Supplement**

Guaranteed Analysis:

Crude Protein, min.	0.5%
Crude Fat, min.	35.0%
Crude Fiber, max.	3.8%
Moisture, max.	13.0%
Ash, max.	1.1%
Iron, min.	23.0 mg/kg
Manganese, min.	2.9 mg/kg
Pantothenic acid, min.	60.0 mg/kg
Pyridoxine, min.	3.2 mg/kg
Niacin, min.	3.1 mg/kg
Vitamin B12, min.	5.3 mcg/kg
Potassium, min.	5600.0 mg/kg
Vitamin A, min.	11000.0 IU/kg
Vitamin D3, min.	2000.0 IU/kg
Vitamin E, min.	93.0 IU/kg
Riboflavin, min.	12.5 mg/kg
Biotin, min.	0.1 mg/kg

The calorie content (ME) is 4,761 kcal/kg or 21.9 kcal/teaspoon (calculated).

Ingredients: Corn syrup, vegetable oil, malt syrup, molasses, carbohydrate gum, mono and diglycerides, water, lecithin, vitamin E supplement, cod liver oil, vitamin A acetate, vitamin A palmitate, vitamin D3 supplement, vitamin B12 supplement, riboflavin supplement, niacin supplement, calcium pantothenate, menadione dimethylpyrimidinol, folic acid, pyridoxine hydrochloride, thiamine hydrochloride, biotin, potassium sorbate, iron proteinate, polysorbate 80, manganese sulfate, silicon dioxide, ethylenediamine dihydroiodide, and potassium chloride.

Indications: A nutritional supplement for dogs and cats containing essential vitamins, minerals, and trace elements. Helps provide additional energy for working animals, pregnant or lactating females or recovering animals.

Dosage and Administration: Give at the rate of 1-2 teaspoons (4.6 gm-9.2 gm) per 10 lbs. (4.5 kg) of body weight per day. If ENERGEL™ is the principle energy source, double the amount given. Place directly in the animal's mouth or mix in food.

Precaution(s): Store at room temperature.

Presentation: 3.5 oz. (100 g) tube.

Compendium Code No.: 10970061 811

ENERGEL™ FOR DOGS

Pet-Ag **Small Animal Dietary Supplement**

Guaranteed Analysis:

Crude Protein, min.	0.5%
Crude Fat, min.	35.0%
Crude Fiber, max.	3.8%
Moisture, max.	13.0%
Ash, max.	1.1%
Iron, min.	23.0 mg/kg
Manganese, min.	2.9 mg/kg
Pantothenic acid, min.	60.0 mg/kg
Pyridoxine, min.	3.2 mg/kg
Niacin, min.	3.1 mg/kg
Vitamin B12, min.	5.3 mcg/kg
Potassium, min.	5600.0 mg/kg
Vitamin A, min.	11000.0 IU/kg
Vitamin D3, min.	2000.0 IU/kg
Vitamin E, min.	93.0 IU/kg
Riboflavin, min.	12.5 mg/kg
Biotin, min.	0.1 mg/kg

The calorie content (ME) is 4,761 kcal/kg or 21.9 kcal/teaspoon (calculated).

Ingredients: Corn syrup, vegetable oil, malt syrup, molasses, carbohydrate gum, mono and diglycerides, water, lecithin, vitamin E supplement, cod liver oil, vitamin A acetate, vitamin A palmitate, vitamin D3 supplement, vitamin B12 supplement, riboflavin supplement, niacin supplement, calcium pantothenate, menadione dimethylpyrimidinol, folic acid, pyridoxine hydrochloride, thiamine hydrochloride, biotin, potassium sorbate, iron proteinate, polysorbate 80, manganese sulfate, silicon dioxide, ethylenediamine dihydroiodide, and potassium chloride.

Indications: A nutritional supplement for dogs and cats containing essential vitamins, minerals, and trace elements. Helps provide additional energy for working animals, pregnant or lactating females or recovering animals.

Dosage and Administration: Give at the rate of 1-2 teaspoons (4.6 gm-9.2 gm) per 10 lbs. (4.5 kg) of body weight per day. If ENERGEL™ is the principle energy source, double the amount given. Place directly in the animal's mouth or mix in food.

Precaution(s): Store at room temperature.

Presentation: 3.5 oz. (100 g) tube.

Compendium Code No.: 10970071 807

ENERGEL™ POWDER FOR CATS

Pet-Ag **Small Animal Dietary Supplement**

Guaranteed Analysis:

Crude Protein, min.	28.0%
Crude Fat, min.	50.0%
Crude Fiber, max.	0.2%
Moisture, max.	5.0%
Calcium, min.	0.90%
Calcium, max.	1.10%
Phosphorus, min.	0.80%
Vitamin A, min.	66,000 I.U./kg
Vitamin D_3, min.	7,700 I.U./kg
Vitamin E, min.	176 I.U./kg
Vitamin B_{12}, min.	61.6 mcg/kg
Choline, min.	2,860 mg/kg

Ingredients: Animal fat (preserved with BHA, citric acid), casein, dextrose, dicalcium phosphate, dehydrated cheese, potassium chloride, calcium carbonate, choline chloride, lecithin, magnesium sulfate, ascorbic acid, vitamin E supplement, vitamin A supplement, natural and artificial flavors added, zinc methionine, ferrous sulfate, calcium pantothenate, vitamin B_{12} supplement, niacin supplement, manganese sulfate, copper sulfate, vitamin D_3 supplement, riboflavin supplement, thiamine mononitrate, pyridoxine hydrochloride, menadione sodium bisulfite complex, folic acid, biotin, calcium iodate, sodium selenite, mono and diglycerides.

The calorie content (ME) is 5,675 kcal/kg or 12.77 kcal/teaspoon (calculated).

Indications: ENERGEL™ Powdered Formula is a high energy supplement developed especially for cats past weaning age. Natural cheese makes it highly palatable. ENERGEL™ Powdered Formula provides additional calories, protein, vitamins and minerals to maintain weight and energy for:

Active cats—hunting, or just running around.

Show cats—eating irregularly and needing tasty nutrition.

Underweight cats—requiring concentrated protein and calories.

Geriatric cats—needing extra nutrition with taste enhancement.

Breeding/Gestating/Lactating—needing good nutrition for successful reproduction and to maintain weight and milk supply.

Growing—needing extra food palatability and nutrition for good growth.

Directions: Feeding Directions: Top dress or mix into food at the rate of 1 teaspoon per 10 pounds body weight. If condition does not improve in 7 to 10 days gradually increase the amount fed over the next 2 weeks to 3 teaspoons per 10 pounds body weight. For example, a 15 pound pregnant cat would be introduced to 1½ teaspoonfuls of ENERGEL™ Powdered Formula at the beginning of the last trimester of pregnancy. If she does not maintain condition, gradually increase the level to 4½ teaspoonfuls by early lactation.

Since ENERGEL™ Powdered Formula helps to increase food consumption it is recommended that the cat be fed twice per day with half of the daily dose added at each feeding. This will help to equalize meal sizes which will enhance digestibility.

As a guide to how long this container will last, consider that each ounce is equal to approximately 13 level teaspoonfuls. Each teaspoon weighs 2.25 g.

Presentation: 8 oz. (227 g).

Compendium Code No.: 10970080 369

ENERGEL™ POWDER FOR DOGS

Pet-Ag **Small Animal Dietary Supplement**

Guaranteed Analysis:

Crude Protein, min.	28.0%
Crude Fat, min.	50.0%
Crude Fiber, max.	0.2%
Moisture, max.	5.0%
Calcium, min.	0.90%
Calcium, max.	1.10%
Phosphorus, min.	0.80%
Vitamin A, min.	66,000 I.U./kg
Vitamin D_3, min.	7,700 I.U./kg
Vitamin E, min.	176 I.U./kg
Vitamin B_{12}, min.	61.6 mcg/kg
Choline, min.	2,860 mg/kg

Ingredients: Animal fat (preserved with BHA, citric acid), casein, dextrose, dicalcium phosphate, dehydrated cheese, potassium chloride, calcium carbonate, choline chloride, lecithin, magnesium sulfate, ascorbic acid, vitamin E supplement, vitamin A supplement, natural and artificial flavors added, zinc methionine, ferrous sulfate, calcium pantothenate, vitamin B_{12} supplement, niacin supplement, manganese sulfate, copper sulfate, vitamin D_3 supplement, riboflavin supplement, thiamine mononitrate, pyridoxine hydrochloride, menadione sodium bisulfite complex, folic acid, biotin, calcium iodate, sodium selenite, mono and diglycerides.

The calorie content (ME) is 5,675 kcal/kg or 12.77 kcal/teaspoon (calculated).

Indications: ENERGEL™ Powdered Formula is a high energy supplement developed especially for dogs past weaning age. Natural cheese makes it highly palatable. ENERGEL™ Powdered Formula provides additional calories, protein, vitamins and minerals to maintain weight and energy for:

Active dogs—hunting, racing, or just running around.

Show dogs—eating irregularly and needing tasty nutrition.

Underweight dogs—requiring concentrated protein and calories.

Geriatric Dogs—needing extra nutrition with taste enhancement.

Breeding/Gestating/Lactating—needing good nutrition for successful reproduction and to maintain weight and milk supply.

Growing—needing extra food palatability and nutrition for good growth.

Directions: Feeding Directions: Top dress or mix into food at the rate of 1 teaspoon per 10 pounds body weight. If condition does not improve in 7 to 10 days gradually increase the amount fed over the next 2 weeks to 3 teaspoons per 10 pounds body weight, up to 30 teaspoons (10 tablespoons) per day. For example, a 30 pound pregnant bitch would be introduced to 3 teaspoonfuls of ENERGEL™ Powdered Formula at the beginning of the last trimester of pregnancy. If she does not maintain condition, gradually increase the level to 9 teaspoonfuls by early lactation.

Since ENERGEL™ Powdered Formula helps to increase food consumption it is recommended that the dog be fed twice per day with half of the daily dose added at each feeding. This will help to equalize meal sizes which will enhance digestibility.

As a guide to how long this container will last, consider that each ounce is equal to approximately 13 level teaspoonfuls. Each teaspoon weighs 2.25 g.

Presentation: 8 oz. (227 g).

Compendium Code No.: 10970090 364

ENERGY DRENCH

Vedco **Large Animal Dietary Supplement**

Guaranteed Analysis:

Crude Protein, not less than 9.0%
Crude Fat, not less than 0.25%
Crude Fiber, not more than 1.0%
Crude Ash, not more than 4.0%

Ingredients:

Nutrients: Dextrose, dried skimmed milk, dried whey, enzymatic hydrolysates of yeast, sodium caseinate, soy protein, glycine, dl-methionine and corn starch.

Vitamins: Vitamin A (as acetate and palmitate), vitamin D_3, vitamin E, riboflavin (vitamin B_2), d-pantothenic acid, niacin, menadione dimethylpyrimidinol bisulphite (source of vitamin K), folic acid, thiamine mononitrate (vitamin B_1), d-biotin, pyridoxine hydrochloride (vitamin B_6), cyanocobalamin (vitamin B_{12}).

Electrolytes: Sodium chloride, potassium chloride, sodium bicarbonate and potassium phosphate.

Trace Minerals: Proteinates of zinc, cobalt, manganese, iron, and copper.

Indications: ENERGY DRENCH is a source of amino acids, energy, vitamins and electrolytes designed for oral use in cattle and calves.

Dosage and Administration: Give 1 pound per 500-1000 pounds body weight. Suspend product in at least 2 quarts of lukewarm water and administer through a stomach tube or as a drench. Repeat as indicated. Consult your veterinarian concerning correct drenching procedure. Prepare fresh solution daily.

Caution(s): For animal use only. Not for human use.

Warning(s): Keep out of reach of children.

Presentation: 1 lb (454 g) and 20 lb pail.

Compendium Code No.: 10940611

ENERGY+

Butler **Large Animal Dietary Supplement**

Guaranteed Analysis:

Crude Protein, not less than 9.0%
Crude Fat, not less than 0.25%
Crude Fiber, not more than 1.0%
Crude Ash, not more than 4.0%

Ingredients:

Nutrients: Dextrose, dried skimmed milk, dried whey, enzymatic hydrolysates of yeast, sodium caseinate, soy protein, glycine, DL-methionine and corn starch.

Vitamins: Vitamin A (as acetate and palmitate), vitamin D_9, vitamin E, riboflavin (vitamin B_2), d-pantothenic acid (vitamin B_9), niacin (vitamin B_9), menadione dimethylpyrimidinolbisulphite (source of vitamin K), folic acid, thiamine mononitrate (vitamin B_1), d-biotin, pyridoxine hydrochloride (vitamin B_6), cyanocobalamin (vitamin B_{12}).

Electrolytes: Sodium chloride, potassium chloride, sodium bicarbonate and potassium phosphate.

Trace Minerals: Prozeinates of zinc, cobalt, manganese, iron, and copper.

Indications: ENERGY+ is a source of amino acids, energy, vitamins and electrolytes. It is designed for oral use in cattle and calves.

Directions: Give 1 pound per 500-1000 pounds body weight. Suspend product in at least 2 quarts of lukewarm water and administer through a stomach tube or as a drench. Repeat as indicated. Consult your veterinarian concerning correct drenching procedure. Prepare fresh solution daily.

Presentation: 1 lb and 20 lb.

Compendium Code No.: 10820691

ENERGY PLUS

Q.A. Laboratories **Small Animal Dietary Supplement**

Active Ingredient(s): Each 100 g contains:

Vitamin A .... 7,500 I.U.
Vitamin D .... 1,500 I.U.
Vitamin E .... 100 I.U.
Thiamin HCl .... 35 mg
Riboflavin .... 3.5 mg
Pyridoxine .... 17 mg
Cyanocobalamin .... 35 mcg
Nicotinamide .... 35 mg
Calcium panthothenate .... 35 mg
Folic acid .... 3.5 mg

Also contains dextrose, maltose, maltotriose, higher saccharides, palmitic, stearic, oleic, linoleic and linolenic acids, polysorbate 60, xanthan gum, citric acid, potassium sorbate, potassium benzoate, FCD approved flavor and color.

Indications: ENERGY PLUS is a high calorie liquid dietary supplement containing 335 cal. per 100 g. It has been formulated to be palatable and easily digested without straining the animal's digestive system. Useful for stressed animals, pregnancy, lactation, and undernourished newborns.

Dosage and Administration: Suggested dosage: 1 mL per 2 lbs. of body weight, one (1) to three (3) times a day or as indicated.

Precaution(s): Store in a cool, dry place. Shake well. Refrigerate after opening.

Caution(s): Keep out of the reach of children.

Presentation: 2 oz. bottles

Compendium Code No.: 13680030

ENER-LYTE™

Aspen **Large Animal Dietary Supplement**

Suspendable Broth

Guaranteed Analysis:

Vitamin E, minimum .... 122 IU/lb
Sodium (Na), maximum 6.00%
Sodium (Na), minimum 5.50%
Potassium (K), minimum 1.40%
Magnesium (Mg), minimum 0.15%
Lactic Acid Bacteria, minimum *(L acidophilus, L casei, L fermentum, L plantarum, S faecium)*
Total .... 907,200,000 CFU/lb

Ingredients: Glucose, guar gum, sodium chloride, sodium bicarbonate, potassium chloride, lecithin, citric acid, magnesium sulfate, glycine, dried *Lactobacillus acidophilus* fermentation product, dried *Lactobacillus casei* fermentation product, dried *Lactobacillus fermentum* fermentation product, dried *Lactobacillus plantarum* fermentation product, dried *Streptococcus faecium* fermentation product, sodium sulfate, sodium silico aluminate, monocalcium phosphate, corn syrup solids, active yeast *(Saccharomyces cerevisiae)*, vitamin A acetate, d-activated animal sterol (source of vitamin D_3), vitamin E supplement, vitamin B_{12} supplement, riboflavin supplement, niacin supplement, calcium pantothenate, menadione dimethylpyrimidinol bisulphite, folic acid, pyridoxine hydrochloride, thiamine hydrochloride, d-biotin, fumaric acid, dried citrus pulp, ascorbic acid, zinc proteinate, cobalt proteinate, ferrous proteinate, copper proteinate, buttermilk, cellulose gum and manganese proteinate.

Indications: Recommended as a source of electrolytes, nutrients, live microorganisms and sugars for energy in young calves, veal, foals and lambs.

Directions: Mixing: Mix ⅔ cup (100 gm) into 2 quarts warm water/or milk replacer, shake or mix thoroughly.

Calves, Veal and Foals: Feed above mixture per calf twice a day for 2 days. Receiving calves should be given 2 feedings prior to the regular milk program. (Ideal Feeding Directions: Feed 1 qt. milk or milk replacer, followed by 1 qt. ENER-LYTE™ mixture in water or milk replacer. Feed above program 4 times dally for 2 consecutive days.)

Lambs: Feed above mixture at the rate of 4 fluid ounces per 5 pounds body weight, 3 times a day for 2 days.

Precaution(s): Store in a dark, cool, dry place.

Warning(s): Keep out of reach of children.

Presentation: 100 g and 10 lbs (4.536 kg).

Compendium Code No.: 14750320

ENTERISOL® ILEITIS

Boehringer Ingelheim **Bacterial Vaccine**

Lawsonia Intracellularis Vaccine, Avirulent Live Culture

U.S. Vet. Lic. No.: 124

Contents: This product contains the antigens listed above.

Indications: Recommended for the vaccination of healthy, susceptible swine 3 weeks of age or older as an aid in the prevention and control of porcine proliferative enteropathy (Ileitis) caused by *Lawsonia intracellularis.* In clinical studies the vaccine significantly reduced gross and microscopic intestinal lesions of Ileitis. Vaccinated pigs also had significantly reduced colonization by *Lawsonia intracellularis* following challenge with the virulent microorganism. Protective immunity following vaccination has been demonstrated to be at least 7 weeks.

Directions: Vaccine Preparation: Plan vaccination timing to allow thawing of the contents of the vaccine vial in air at controlled room temperature or in a lukewarm water bath (60-70°F) until liquid. Shake well and use entire contents immediately.

Vaccination via the drinking water: Conventional Water Directions (open trough or barrel type [tank] system):

1. Do not thaw vaccine until ready to vaccinate.
2. Remove all medications, sanitizers, and disinfectants from drinking water 72 hours (3 days) prior to vaccination.
3. Flush watering system with nonchlorinated/nontreated clean water to eliminate any antibacterial agents.
4. Thaw vaccine according to directions.
5. Add number of doses of vaccine equal to or more than the number of pigs to vaccinate, to the appropriate amount of clean, nontreated drinking water (see table).
6. Final solution containing vaccine should be consumed within 4 hours after thawing of vaccine.

Directions for Automatic Watering Systems equipped with proportioner: Several types of medicators/proportioners are commercially available.

1. Do not thaw vaccine until ready to vaccinate.
2. Remove all medications, sanitizers, and disinfectants from drinking water 72 hours (3 days) prior to vaccination.
3. Provide sufficient watering space so that all pigs can drink within a 4-hour time frame.
4. Flush watering system with nontreated clean water to eliminate any antibacterial agents.
5. Set proportioner to deliver 1 oz (30 mL) of vaccine solution per 1 gallon (4 liters) of water.
6. See Table to determine how many ounces of stock solution to prepare for pounds of pig to vaccinate.
7. Prepare vaccine concentrate as follows:
   a. Thaw vaccine according to directions.
   b. Add number of doses to the stock solution container equal to or more than the number of pigs to vaccinate.
   c. Add appropriate amount of clean, nontreated water to the container used for the stock solution. d. Mix thoroughly.
8. Insert proportioner hose into vaccine concentrate and start water flow. Continue until all concentrate has been consumed before changing water supply to direct flow. Do not medicate or use disinfectants immediately following vaccination.

Total Weight of Group of Pigs (# of pigs x average pig weight)	Trough/Tank Estimated water[1] consumption in 4-hour vaccination period	Proportioner[2] Oz of stock solution needed. Set proportioner to deliver 1 oz per gal.
100	0.17 gallons	0.17 oz
500	0.85 gallons	0.85 oz
1,000	1.7 gallons	1.7 oz
20,000	34.0 gallons	34 oz
30,000	51.0 gallons	51 oz
40,000	68.0 gallons	68 oz
50,000	85.0 gallons	85 oz

[1] Based on 0.17 gallon consumed (21.8 oz) per 100 pounds body weight in 4 hour period.
[2] Values for pigs 40 pounds or bigger.

Precaution(s): Storage: Store frozen at -70°C. Do not store thawed vaccine. After thawing, shake well and use entire contents immediately.

Disposal: Burn container and all unused contents by a procedure allowed by local, state, and Federal regulations.

Caution(s): Pigs will generally drink 8-12% of their body weight per day, depending on environmental temperatures. The actual amount of water consumed may vary considerably depending on several factors, including environmental temperature.

Incompatibility: All materials used in administration of this vaccine must be free of antibiotic and disinfectant residue to prevent vaccine inactivation and reduced product efficacy.

For use in swine only.

Antidote(s): Epinephrine.

Warning(s): Withdrawal Period: Vaccinated pigs are not to be harvested for human consumption within 21 days after vaccination.

Presentation: 50 doses (100 mL) and 100 doses (100 mL), 250 doses (100 mL) and 500 doses (100 mL).

U.S. Patent Nos. 5,714,375 and 5,885,823

Compendium Code No.: 10281181

BI S129631-RP-12 1/02

ENTERISOL® SC-54

Boehringer Ingelheim **Vaccine**

Salmonella Choleraesuis Vaccine, Avirulent Live Culture

U.S. Vet. Lic. No.: 124

Contents: This product contains the antigen listed above.

Indications: For intranasal or water administration in healthy swine one day of age or older as an aid in the prevention of salmonellosis caused by *Salmonella choleraesuis* var kunzendorf.

Recommended for use only in healthy, susceptible swine, per label directions.

Dosage and Administration: Read entire insert before use.

Read the product label before use.

Rehydrate the vaccine by adding the full contents of the accompanying sterile diluent to the vaccine vial. Shake well and use immediately. Rehydrate only with the diluent provided; do not mix with other materials.

Intranasal Vaccination: Fill syringe with reconstituted vaccine. Place cannula on the syringe tip and administer a single 2 mL dose intranasally to swine one day of age or older. Administer the complete 2 mL dose to each pig vaccinated. Efficacy and safety of the vaccine at other than the dose or routes prescribed on the label is unknown, and therefore, not recommended and not USDA approved.

Vaccination via the drinking water:

Conventional Water Directions (Open Trough or Barrel type (tank) System):

1. Do not open or mix vaccine until ready to vaccinate.
2. Remove all medications, sanitizers and disinfectants from drinking water 72 hours (3 days) prior to vaccination.
3. Flush watering system with nonchlorinated/nontreated clean water to eliminate any antibacterial agents.
4. Rehydrate the vaccine with accompanying diluent.
5. Add 2 mL of rehydrated vaccine to the appropriate amount of clean, nontreated drinking water for each pig to be vaccinated (see table).
6. Final solution containing the vaccine should be consumed within four (4) hours after rehydration of the vaccine.

Directions for Automatic Watering Systems equipped with proportioner: Several types of medicators/proportioners are commercially available.

1. Do not open or mix the vaccine until ready to vaccinate.
2. Remove all medications, sanitizers, and disinfectants from the drinking water 72 hours (3 days) prior to vaccination.
3. Provide sufficient watering space so that all pigs can drink within a 4 hour time frame.
4. Flush the watering system with nontreated clean water to eliminate any antibacterial agents.
5. Set the proportioner to deliver 1 oz (30 mL) of vaccine solution per 1 gallon (4 L) of water.
6. See table to determine how many ounces of stock solution to prepare for pounds of pig to vaccinate.
7. Prepare the vaccine concentrate as follows:
   a. Rehydrate the vaccine with the accompanying diluent.
   b. Add the number of doses to the container for stock solution equal to or more than the number of pigs to vaccinate.
   c. Add the appropriate amount of clean, nontreated water to the container used for the stock solution.
   d. Mix thoroughly.
8. Insert proportioner hose into vaccine concentrate and start water flow. Continue until all the concentrate has been consumed before changing the water supply to direct flow. Do not medicate or use disinfectants immediately following vaccination.

Total Weight of Group of Pigs (# pigs x average pig weight)	Trough/Tank Estimated water* consumption in 4 hour vaccination period	Proportioner** Oz of stock solution needed to vaccinate lbs of pigs in group. When run through proportioner set to deliver 1 oz per gal
100	.17 gallons	.17 oz
200	.34 gallons	.34 oz
300	.51 gallons	.51 oz
400	.68 gallons	.68 oz
500	.85 gallons	.85 oz
600	1.02 gallons	1.02 oz
700	1.19 gallons	1.19 oz
800	1.36 gallons	1.36 oz
900	1.53 gallons	1.53 oz
1,000	1.70 gallons	1.70 oz

*Based on .17 gallon consumed (21.8 oz) per 100 lbs of body weight in 4 hour period.
**Values for pigs 40 lbs or bigger.

Precaution(s): Storage Before Use: Store out of direct sunlight in the outer carton. Store at a temperature between 35°-45°F (2°-7°C). Do not freeze. Use entire contents when first opened. Do not use bottles of damaged product. Do not store reconstituted vaccine.

Disposal: After use, burn containers and all unused contents by a procedure allowed by local, state, and Federal regulations.

Expiration Date: Consult the outer carton for the last date the package of vaccine is acceptable for use.

Caution(s): Incompatibility: All materials used in administering this vaccine must be free of antibiotic and disinfectant residue to prevent inactivation and reduced product efficacy.

Pigs will generally drink 8-12% of their body weight per day depending on environmental temperatures. The actual amount of water consumed may vary considerable depending on several factors including environmental temperature.

Anaphylactoid reactions may occur; Administer epinephrine.

For veterinary use only.

Warning(s): Withdrawal Period: Vaccinated pigs are not to be harvested for human consumption before 21 days after vaccination.

Avoid direct contact. If human exposure occurs, flush area with clean water, administer first aid, and consult physician immediately.

Discussion: Additional Information for Veterinarians: Many factors must be considered in determining a sound *Salmonella choleraesuis* vaccination program for a particular farm. To be most effective, the vaccine must be administered properly to healthy animals maintained in a proper environment under good management. Stressed or immunosuppressed pigs should not be vaccinated as the efficacy of the vaccine in these animals is unknown. The level of individual animal and herd immunity required will vary with management practices, the degree of exposure to salmonella, and the level of susceptibility of each animal. The vaccination program must be carefully planned and implemented in collaboration with the herd veterinarian following label and insert indications and precautions.

Pigs vaccinated intranasally at 3 weeks of age demonstrated a duration of immunity through at least 20 weeks post vaccination. The duration of immunity for pigs vaccinated intranasally at less than 3 weeks of age has not been determined.

Two field studies were conducted representing more than 50,000 total pigs. Non-vaccinated pigs and pigs vaccinated per label instructions via the drinking water when placed in the finishing barn (approximately 60 pounds body weight) were compared for prevalence of salmonella at slaughter. Contrasted with nonvaccinated pigs, vaccinated pigs had a significantly ($p < .05$) lower prevalence of salmonella detected by culture of ileocecal lymph nodes collected at slaughter.

Previous or active Salmonella or other infection: The effect of concurrent or previous infections at or around the time of vaccination on the efficacy of this vaccine in reducing or modifying salmonellosis in pigs is not known.

Presentation: 50 dose (100 mL) amber glass vials.

U.S. Patent No. 5,436,001

Compendium Code No.: 10280431

472303N-00

ENTERISOL® SC-54 FF

Boehringer Ingelheim **Vaccine**

Salmonella Choleraesuis Vaccine, Avirulent Live Culture

U.S. Vet. Lic. No.: 124

Contents: This product contains the antigen listed above.

Indications: For water administration in healthy swine 3 weeks of age or older as an aid in the prevention of salmonellosis caused by *Salmonella choleraesuis* var kunzendorf.

Recommended for use only in healthy, susceptible swine.

Directions: Read entire insert before use.

Read the product label before use.

Vaccine Preparation: Plan vaccination timing to allow thawing of the contents of the vaccine vial in air at controlled room temperature or in a lukewarm water bath (60-75°F) until liquid. Shake well and use immediately.

Vaccination via the drinking water:

Conventional Water Directions (Open Trough or Barrel type (tank) System):

1. Do not thaw vaccine until ready to vaccinate.
2. Remove all medications, sanitizers and disinfectants from drinking water 72 hours (3 days) prior to vaccination.
3. Flush watering system with nonchlorinated/nontreated clean water to eliminate any antibacterial agents.
4. Thaw vaccine according to directions.
5. Add correct number of doses of vaccine to the appropriate amount of clean, nontreated drinking water for each pig to be vaccinated (see table).
6. Final solution containing vaccine should be consumed within 4 hours after rehydration of the vaccine.

Directions for Automatic Watering Systems equipped with proportioner: Several types of medicators/proportioners are commercially available.

1. Do not thaw vaccine until ready to vaccinate.
2. Remove all medications, sanitizers, and disinfectants from the drinking water 72 hours (3 days) prior to vaccination.
3. Provide sufficient watering space so that all pigs can drink within a 4 hour time frame.
4. Flush watering system with nontreated clean water to eliminate any antibacterial agents.
5. Set proportioner to deliver 1 oz (30 mL) of vaccine solution per 1 gallon (4 L) of water.
6. See table to determine how many ounces of stock solution to prepare for pounds of pig to vaccinate.
7. Prepare vaccine concentrate as follows:
   a. Thaw vaccine according to directions.
   b. Add number of doses to container for stock solution equal to or more than number of pigs to vaccinate.
   c. Add appropriate amount of clean, nontreated water to the container used for the stock solution.
   d. Mix thoroughly.
8. Insert proportioner hose into vaccine concentrate and start water flow. Continue until all concentrate has been consumed before changing water supply to direct flow. Do not medicate or use disinfectants immediately following vaccination.

Total Weight of Group of Pigs (# pigs x average pig weight)	Trough/Tank Estimated water* consumption in 4 hour vaccination period	Proportioner** Oz of stock solution needed to vaccinate lbs of pigs in group. When run through proportioner set to deliver 1 oz per gal
100	.17 gallons	.17 oz
500	.85 gallons	.85 oz
1,000	1.7 gallons	1.7 oz
20,000	34.0 gallons	34 oz
30,000	51.0 gallons	51 oz
40,000	68.0 gallons	68 oz
50,000	85.0 gallons	85 oz

*Based on .17 gallon consumed (21.8 oz) per 100 lbs of body weight in 4 hour period.

**Values for pigs 40 lbs or bigger.

Precaution(s): Store frozen at ultra low temperatures below -50°C or with dry ice packs. Can be stored at -20°C for no more than 14 days. Do not re-freeze.

Storage Before Use: Use entire contents when first opened. Do not use bottles of damaged product. Do not store thawed vaccine.

Disposal: After use, burn containers and all unused contents by a procedure allowed by local, state, and Federal regulations.

Expiration Date: Consult the container label for the last date the package of vaccine is acceptable for use.

Caution(s): Incompatibility: All materials used in administration of this vaccine must be free of antibiotic and disinfectant residue to prevent inactivation and reduced product efficacy.

Pigs will generally drink 8-12% of their body weight per day depending on environmental temperatures. The actual amount of water consumed may vary considerable depending on several factors including environmental temperature.

Anaphylactoid reactions may occur. Administer epinephrine.

For veterinary use only.

Warning(s): Withdrawal Period: Vaccinated pigs are not to be harvested for human consumption before 21 days after vaccination.

Avoid contact. If accidental human exposure occurs, flush area with clean water and consult physician immediately.

Discussion: Additional Information for Veterinarians: Many factors must be considered in determining a sound *Salmonella choleraesuis* vaccination program for a particular farm. To be most effective, the vaccine must be administered properly to healthy animals maintained in a proper environment under good management. Stressed or immunosuppressed pigs should not be vaccinated as the efficacy of the vaccine in these animals is unknown. The level of individual animal and herd immunity required will vary with management practices, the degree of exposure to salmonella, and the level of susceptibility of each animal. The vaccination program must be carefully planned and implemented in collaboration with the herd veterinarian following label and insert indications and precautions.

Two field studies were conducted representing more than 50,000 total pigs. Non-vaccinated pigs and pigs vaccinated per label instructions via the drinking water when placed in the finishing barn (approximately 60 pounds body weight) were compared for prevalence of salmonella at slaughter. Contrasted with nonvaccinated pigs, vaccinated pigs had a significantly ($p<.05$) lower prevalence of salmonella detected by culture of ileocecal lymph nodes collected at slaughter.

Previous or active Salmonella or other infection: The effect of concurrent or previous infections at or around the time of vaccination on the efficacy of this vaccine in reducing or modifying salmonellosis in pigs is not known.

Presentation: 250 doses (100 mL) and 500 doses (100 mL).

U.S. Patent No. 5,436,001

Compendium Code No.: 10281360 474201N-00

ENTEROVAX™

Schering-Plough **Vaccine**

Tenosynovitis Vaccine, Modified Live Vaccine

U.S. Vet. Lic. No.: 165A

Active Ingredient(s): ENTEROVAX™ is a modified live vaccine containing an avian reovirus (mild-reacting strain 1,133/C6) in a freeze-dried preparation sealed under vacuum. The vaccine contains gentamicin as a preservative.

Indications: It is recommended for use in healthy chickens two weeks of age or older to aid in the control and prevention of avian reovirus-induced tenosynovitis (viral arthritis) by drinking water administration.

ENTEROVAX™ is a drinking water vaccine developed to prevent viral arthritis (tenosynovitis) which causes serious leg problems and economic loss in broiler, roaster, and breeder flocks. It is for use in flocks where birds are carried to heavier weights. It may be safely administered to birds 14 days of age or older.

Dosage and Administration:

When to Vaccinate: ENTEROVAX™ should be administered to birds two (2) weeks of age or older.

Preparation of the Vaccine:

1. Do not open and mix the vaccine until ready for use.
2. Mix only one (1) vial at a time and use the entire contents within one (1) hour.
3. Remove the tear-off aluminum seal from the vaccine vial without disturbing the rubber stopper.
4. Use cool, clean, nonchlorinated drinking water.
5. Remove the rubber stopper from the vaccine vial and rehydrate the vaccine by filling the vial about half-full with tap water (milk added).
6. Reseat the stopper and shake to thoroughly dissolve the vaccine.

How to Vaccinate: Do not mix the vaccine into the drinking water until ready for use. Drinking water for vaccination should be mixed with powdered milk to prevent possible inactivation from chlorine or other water additives and also to stabilize the vaccine virus. The powdered milk should be added to the water at the rate of one (1) heaped teaspoon per three (3) U.S. gallons or 2.5 imperial gallons (3 g per 11 L); or one (1) heaped cupful per 50 U.S. gallons or 41 imperial gallons (87 g per 190 L).

Use only clean waterers and equipment free of disinfectants or sanitizers. All water must be withheld from the birds for at least two (2) hours prior to vaccination to assure that all chickens drink. Mix the rehydrated vaccine in the quantity of drinking water (milk added) which will be consumed by thirsty chickens in approximately 1-2 hours.

Each 1,000 birds:

Each 1,000 Birds	U.S. Gallons	Imperial Gallons	Liters
2 weeks to 4 weeks	2½	2	10
4 weeks to 8 weeks	5	4	20
Over 8 weeks	10	8	40

Distribute the diluted vaccine so that all of the birds are able to drink within one (1) to two (2) hours. The diluted vaccine should be the sole source of drinking water until it is completely consumed. Avoid placing the water in direct sunlight.

Records: Keep a record of the vaccine type, quantity, serial number, expiration date and place of purchase; the date and time of vaccination; the number, age, breed, and location of the birds; the names of operators performing the vaccination; and any observed reactions.

Precaution(s): Store at 35°-45°F (2°-7°C). Do not freeze.

Caution(s): For veterinary use only.

1. Vaccinate healthy birds only.
2. Do not administer the product by injection. Studies have demonstrated that injection will produce significant mortality in day old birds.
3. Do not administer using an automatic eyedrop vaccinator (e.g. Biojector-Plus) to day old birds.
4. Do not spill or spatter the vaccine. Use the entire contents of the vial when first opened. Burn the empty bottles, caps and all unused vaccine and accessories.
5. Wash hands thoroughly after using the vaccine.
6. All birds within a flock should be vaccinated on the same day.
7. Do not dilute or otherwise stretch the dosage.

Warning(s): Do not vaccinate within 21 days before slaughter.

Do not administer the product to breeders in production. Studies have demonstrated that the vaccine virus may be shed in the eggs.

Presentation: Supplied in 10 x 1,000, 10 x 2,500, and 10 x 5,000 dose units.

Compendium Code No.: 10470580

ENTERVENE™-D

Fort Dodge **Vaccine**

Salmonella Dublin Vaccine, Live Culture

U.S. Vet. Lic. No.: 112

Contents: This product contains the antigen listed above.

Indications: For vaccination of healthy calves, 2 weeks of age or older, as an aid in the prevention of clinical disease due to *Salmonella dublin.*

Dosage and Administration: Dose: Aseptically rehydrate with the accompanying diluent. Calves, inject one 2 mL dose subcutaneously using aseptic technique. A second 2 mL dose should be administered 12 to 16 days following the first vaccination.

Precaution(s): Store in dark at 2° to 7°C (35° to 45°F). Avoid freezing. Shake well after rehydration. Use entire contents when first opened. Burn container and all unused contents.

All material used in administering this vaccine must be free of antibiotic or disinfectant residue. Response to live bacterial vaccination may be affected by concurrent antibiotic administration. Resistance data on the vaccine strain may be obtained from Fort Dodge Animal Health.

Caution(s): In case of anaphylactoid reaction, administer epinephrine.

Warning(s): Do not vaccinate within 21 days of slaughter.

Presentation: 10 dose vial vaccine with 20 mL vial diluent and 50 dose vial vaccine with 100 mL vial diluent.

Compendium Code No.: 10032711 2285B

ENTROLYTE®

Pfizer Animal Health **Electrolytes-Oral**

Oral Nutrient Powder for Calves

Guaranteed Analysis: per 200-gram Twin Pack: Minimum unless otherwise stated.

Crude Protein 13.24%
Glycine 2.81%
Minerals:
Calcium
Minimum 0.31%
Maximum 0.43%
Phosphorus 0.24%
Potassium 1.70%
Salt
Minimum 2.50%
Maximum 3.50%
Sodium
Minimum 4.13%
Maximum 5.13%
Chloride 3.09%
Magnesium 0.14%
Other:
Approximate pH 7.5
Total osmolality . . . . 490 mOsm/liter

Ingredients: Dextrose, dried-meat solubles, sodium bicarbonate, potassium chloride, glycine, salt, dicalcium phosphate, magnesium sulfate.

Indications: ENTROLYTE® is a nutritional supplement formulated to provide a source of electrolytes.

Directions for Use: Mix the contents of 1 packet (both pouches) with 1 gallon (128 oz) of warm water, or mix the contents of ½ packet (1 pouch) with 2 quarts (64 oz) of warm water. Administer ENTROLYTE® solution at body temperature. Allow animal to nurse from a nursing bottle or administer via a stomach tube. Refrigerate if not used immediately. Shake well before using. Discard solution if not used within 24 hours.

Orally administer 1-2 quarts (32-64 oz) to calves 2-3 times per day.

Contraindication(s): Do not use in cases of upper gastrointestinal obstruction or in moribund animals.

Warning(s): Keep out of reach of children. For oral use only. For use in calves only.

For veterinary use only.

Presentation: 7.1 oz (200 g) twin pack.

Compendium Code No.: 36900110 70-8150-06

ENTROLYTE® H.E.

Pfizer Animal Health **Electrolytes-Oral**

A Nutritional Supplement for Young Calves

Guaranteed Analysis: per 178-gram Pouch: Minimum unless otherwise stated.

Crude Protein	19.0%
Glycine	2.3%
Minerals:	
Calcium	
Minimum	0.1%
Maximum	0.6%
Salt	
Minimum	1.2%
Maximum	1.7%
Phosphorus	0.15%
Potassium	0.95%
Sodium	
Minimum	2.2%
Maximum	2.7%
Chloride	1.7%
Magnesium	0.08%

Ingredients: Dextrose, sodium bicarbonate, glycine, potassium chloride, salt, dicalcium phosphate, magnesium sulfate

Indications: ENTROLYTE® H.E. is a nutritional supplement formulated to provide a source of electrolytes and energy.

Directions for Use: ENTROLYTE® H.E. is supplied in twin pouches. Mix the contents of both pouches with ½ gallon (64 oz) of warm water. Allow animal to nurse from a nursing bottle or administer via a stomach tube. Refrigerate if not used immediately. Shake well before using. Discard solution if not used within 24 hours.

Orally administer 1-2 quarts (32-64 oz) to calves 2-3 times per day.

Contraindication(s): Do not use in cases of upper gastrointestinal obstruction or in moribund animals.

Warning(s): Keep out of reach of children. For oral use only. For veterinary use only.

Presentation: 6.3 oz (178 g) pouches.

U.S. Patent No. 4,689,319

Compendium Code No.: 36900121 70-8152-04

ENZYMATIC DETERGENT

Vedco **Detergent**

Dual Enzyme Presoak & Detergent

Active Ingredient(s): Contains Protease #9014-01-0, Amylase #9000-85-5, Surfactant, Propylene Glycol #57-55-6, and water #7732-18-5.

Indications: An extremely effective dual enzyme detergent for the cleaning of flexible and rigid scopes, delicate surgical instruments, and other medical devices. Quickly digests and dissolves blood, fat, mucous, and other soils.

Safe for all surgical instruments and fiberoptic scopes.

Directions for Use: Wear gloves and eye protection.

1. Add 1-2 ounces of Enzymatic to 1 gallon of warm tap water.
2. Soak instruments for 2-3 minutes or longer if required; 15-20 minutes for difficult stains.
3. Solution should be aspirated through lumens and channels of instruments.
4. Lightly scrub scopes and instruments.
5. Rinse thoroughly with warm water aspirating through channels to completely remove all traces of enzymatic solution.
6. If equipment is to be chemically disinfected, dry before immersion into the solution.
7. Discard solution after each use.
8. For ultrasonic washers use ¼ to 1 oz. per gallon water.

Caution(s): HMIS Rating: H-2 F-0 R-0 PPE-B See MSDS for additional information.

Warning(s): Keep out of reach of children.

Presentation: 1 gallon (3.8 L) with pump.

Compendium Code No.: 10942210

EP-1 3X

RXV **Large Animal Dietary Supplement**

Guaranteed Analysis:

Lactobacillus plantarum	7.5 million CFU*/g
Lactobacillus casei	7.5 million CFU*/g
Lactobacillus acidophilus	7.5 million CFU*/g
Enterococcus faecium	7.5 million CFU*/g
*CFU-Colony Forming Units	
Total Lactic Acid Producing Bacteria	30 million CFU*/g

Ingredients: Corn oil, Sodium aluminosilicate, Dried whey, Dextrose, Dried *Lactobacillus plantarum* fermentation product, Dried *Lactobacillus casei* fermentation product, Dried *Lactobacillus acidophilus* fermentation product, Dried *Enterococcus faecium* fermentation product, Sorbitan monostearate, Apple flavoring, FD & C Yellow # 5, FD & C Blue # 1, Potassium sorbate.

Indications: EP-1 3X contains equine host specific lactic acid producing bacteria to provide an oral source of these bacteria.

Directions: Feeding Directions: Administer entire contents orally. Repeat as needed.

Precaution(s): Store product at or below room temperature. Keep unused product dry, cool and out of direct sunlight.

Caution(s): Federal law restricts this drug to use by or on the order of a licensed veterinarian.

For animal use only. Not intended for use as a source of antibody.

Warning(s): Keep out of reach of children.

Presentation: 12 x 30 g tubes.

Compendium Code No.: 10910410 Iss. 12-01

EPIC DAILY FEED SUPPLEMENT FOR HORSES

Bioniche Animal Health (formerly Vetrepharm) **Equine Dietary Supplement**

Pasteurized Spray Dried Whole Egg

Guaranteed Analysis:

Crude Protein (min.)	14%
Crude Fat (min.)	18%
Ash (max.)	9.5%
Moisture (max.)	8%

Ingredients: Rice bran, betaine hydrochloride, pasteurized egg solids, taurine, dried *Lactobacillus acidophilus* fermentation product, dried *Enterococcus faecium* fermentation product, sodium silico aluminate.

Indications: Daily feed supplement for horses.

Egg protein in complexes in a rice bran base, with omega-3 and omega-6 fatty acids.

Dosage and Administration: Recommended use: Top dress and thoroughly mix, 1 scoop with both morning and evening feed.

Presentation: Available in a 2 kg pail with scoop, 6 per case. Supplied scoop holds approximately 25 g of supplement (40 day supply).

Compendium Code No.: 11070060

EPIC NEONATAL FEED SUPPLEMENT FOR FOALS

Bioniche Animal Health (formerly Vetrepharm) **Equine Dietary Supplement**

Guaranteed Analysis: Crude Protein (min.) 43%, Crude Fat (min.) 30%, Ash (max.) 6%, Moisture (max.) 6%.

Ingredients: Pasteurized Spray Dried Whole Egg.

Indications: EPIC is a source of high fat, high protein, readily assimilated complexes for the newborn foal. EPIC mixes easily, is conveniently dispensed for administration by farm staff to help reduce the need for night time emergency calls. It is economical to use.

Directions for Use: EPIC is given immediately after foaling and again in 6-8 hours. EPIC's spray-dried, whole-egg proteins help provide the best start to the foal's performance career. Mix with approximately 40 mL of vegetable oil into a paste consistency. Half of the preparation is given immediately, with the second ½ refrigerated and given 6-8 hours postpartum. One pouch provides both feedings.

Precaution(s): Storage: Store in a cool, dry place.

Presentation: EPIC is packaged in 20 g, foil pouches, 25 per box.

Compendium Code No.: 11070011

EPINEPHRINE ℞

Vedco **Epinephrine**

Active Ingredient(s): Each mL contains:

Epinephrine (prepared with the aid of hydrochloric acid)	1 mg
Sodium bisulfite	1 mg
Sodium chloride	9 mg
Chlorobutanol [chloral derivative (preservative)]	5 mg
Water for injection	q.s.

Indications: Epinephrine injection 1:1,000, sterile.

Dosage and Administration: Parenterally:

Cattle, Horses, Sheep and Swine: 1 mL of 1:1,000 solution per 100 pounds of body weight injected subcutaneously or intramuscularly.

Dogs and Cats: 0.1 to 0.5 mL of 1:1,000 solution injected subcutaneously or intramuscularly.

For veterinary use only. Intravenous injection is not recommended for routine clinical work, but in emergency situations, this route may be desired. When injected intravenously, the dosage should be one-quarter (¼) to one-half (½) of the intramuscular dosages shown above.

Precaution(s): Store at a controlled room temperature between 59-86°F (15-30°C). Do not freeze.

Do not use the product if it is brown in color or if it contains a precipitate.

Caution(s): Federal law restricts this drug to use by or on the order of a licensed veterinarian.

Warning(s): Keep out of reach of children.

Presentation: 30 mL sterile, multiple dose vial.

Compendium Code No.: 10940621

EPINEPHRINE ℞

Vet Tek **Epinephrine**

Injection 1:1000

Active Ingredient(s): Each mL Contains: Epinephrine 1 mg, prepared with the aid of hydrochloric acid, sodium bisulfite 1 mg, sodium chloride 9 mg, chlorobutanol (chloral derivative, preservative) 5 mg. Water for injection q.s.

Indications: For emergency use only in treating anaphylactic shock in cattle, horses, sheep, swine, dogs and cats.

Dosage and Administration: Parenterally:

Cattle, Horses, Sheep, and Swine: 1 mL of 1:1,000 solution per 100 pounds of body weight injected subcutaneously or intramuscularly.

Dogs and Cats: 0.1 to 0.5 mL of 1:1,000 solution injected subcutaneously or intramuscularly.

Intravenous injection is not recommended for routine clinical work, but in emergency situations, this route may be desired.

When injected intravenously, the dosage should be ¼ to ½ of the intramuscular dosages shown above.

Precaution(s): Store in a refrigerator at 2°-8°C (36°-46°F). Do not freeze.

Do not use injection if it is pinkish or darker than slightly yellow or if it contains a precipitate.

Caution(s): Federal law restricts this drug to use by or on the order of a licensed veterinarian.

For veterinary use only.

Warning(s): Keep out of reach of children.

Presentation: 30 mL sterile multiple-dose vial (NDC 30798-009-01).

Compendium Code No.: 14200081 9/93

EPINEPHRINE 1:1000 ℞

AgriPharm **Epinephrine**

Sterile Solution

Active Ingredient(s): Each mL contains:

Epinephrine	1 mg
Sodium Chloride	9 mg
Chlorobutanol (Preservative)	5 mg
Sodium m-Bisulfite	1 mg
Water for Injection	q.s.

Indications: For emergency use only in treating anaphylactic shock.

Dosage and Administration: Cattle, Horses, Sheep and Swine: 1 cubic centimeter per 100 pounds of body weight. Inject subcutaneously.

Precaution(s): Store at temperatures between 2°-15°C (36°-59°F).

Caution(s): Do not use this product if it is brown or contains a precipitate.

Warning(s): For animal use only.
Keep out of reach of children.
Discussion: Symptoms of anaphylactoid shock include glassy eyes, increased salivation, grinding of teeth, rapid breathing, muscular tremors, staggering gait, and collapse with death following. These symptoms may appear shortly after injection of a bacterin, vaccine or antibiotic.
Presentation: 10 mL vials.
Compendium Code No.: 14570340

EPINEPHRINE 1:1000 ℞

Durvet — **Epinephrine**
Sterile Solution
Active Ingredient(s): Each mL contains:
Epinephrine .... 1 mg
Sodium Chloride .... 9 mg
Chlorobutanol (Preservative) .... 5 mg
Sodium m-Bisulfite .... 1 mg
Water for Injection .... q.s.
Indications: For emergency use only in treating anaphylactic shock.
Dosage and Administration: Cattle, horses, sheep, and swine: 1 cubic centimeter per 100 pounds of body weight. Inject subcutaneously.
Precaution(s): Store at temperatures between 2°-15°C (36°-59°F).
Do not use this product if it is brown or contains a precipitate.
Warning(s): For animal use only.
Keep out of reach of children.
Discussion: Symptoms of anaphylactoid shock include glassy eyes, increased salivation, grinding of teeth, rapid breathing, muscular tremors, staggering gait, and collapse with death following. These symptoms may appear shortly after injection of a bacterin, vaccine or antibiotic.
Presentation: 10 mL vials.
Compendium Code No.: 10840790

EPINEPHRINE 1:1000 ℞

Neogen — **Epinephrine**
Sterile Solution
Active Ingredient(s): Each mL contains:
Epinephrine .... 1 mg
Sodium Chloride .... 9 mg
Chlorobutanol (preservative) .... 5 mg
Sodium m-Bisulfite .... 1 mg
Water for injection .... q.s.
Indications: For emergency use only in treating anaphylactoid shock.
Dosage and Administration: Usual Dosage: Cattle, horses, sheep, and swine - 1 cubic centimeter per 100 pounds of body weight. Inject subcutaneously.
Precaution(s): Do not use this product if it is brown or contains a precipitate.
Store at temperature between 2°-15°C (36°-59°F).
Caution(s): Federal law restricts this drug to use by or on the order of a licensed veterinarian.
Symptoms of anaphylactoid shock include glassy eyes, increased salivation, grinding of teeth, rapid breathing, muscular tremors, staggering gait, and collapse with death following. These symptoms may appear shortly after injection of a bacterin, vaccine or antibiotic.
For animal use only.
Warning(s): Keep out of reach of children.
Presentation: 48 x 10 mL amber glass vials (NDC: 59051-9054-1) and 12 x 30 mL amber glass vials (NDC: 59051-9055-3) per carton.
Manufactured by: Omega Laboratories, Montreal, QC H3M 3E4.
Compendium Code No.: 14910052 — L519-0601 / 0201

EPINEPHRINE INJECTION ℞

AgriLabs — **Epinephrine**
Active Ingredient(s): Each mL contains:
Epinephrine (prepared with the aid of hydrochloric acid) .... 1 mg
Sodium bisulfite .... 1 mg
Sodium chloride .... 9 mg
Chlorobutanol [chloral derivative (preservative)] .... 5 mg
Water for injection .... q.s.
Indications: A sterile solution for emergency use only in treating anaphylactic shock.
Dosage and Administration: Parenterally:
Cattle, Horses, Sheep and Swine: 1 mL of 1:1,000 solution per 100 pounds of body weight injected subcutaneously or intramuscularly.
Dogs and Cats: 0.1 to 0.5 mL of 1:1,000 solution injected subcutaneously or intramuscularly.
Intravenous injection is not recommended for routine clinical work, but in emergency situations, this route may be desired. When injected intravenously, the dosage should be one-quarter (¼) to one-half (½) of the intramuscular dosages shown above.
Precaution(s): Store in a refrigerator at 36°-46°F (2°-8°C). Do not freeze.
Caution(s): Federal law restricts this drug to use by or on the order of a licensed veterinarian.
For veterinary use only. Keep out of the reach of children.
Do not use EPINEPHRINE INJECTION if it is brown in color or contains a precipitate.
Presentation: 10 mL multiple dose vials.
Compendium Code No.: 10580470

EPINEPHRINE INJECTION 1:1000 ℞

Bimeda — **Epinephrine**
Active Ingredient(s): Each mL contains:
Epinephrine (prepared with the aid of hydrochloric acid) .... 1 mg
Sodium chloride .... 9 mg
Sodium bisulfite .... 1 mg
Chlorobutanol (as preservative) .... 5 mg
Water for injection U.S.P. .... q.s.
Indications: Epinephrine is a powerful vasoconstrictor for emergency use only in the treatment of anaphylactic shock.
Dosage and Administration: Parenterally:
Cattle, Horses, Sheep, and Swine: Inject subcutaneously 1 mL per 100 lbs. of body weight.
Precaution(s): Protect from light. Store in a refrigerator at 36°-46°F (2°-8°C). Do not freeze.
Caution(s): Federal law restricts this drug to use by or on the order of a licensed veterinarian.
Not for human use. For use in animals only.
Presentation: 10 mL sterile vials.
Compendium Code No.: 13990130

EPINEPHRINE INJECTION 1:1,000 ℞

Butler — **Epinephrine**
Active Ingredient(s): Each mL contains:
Epinephrine (prepared with the aid of hydrochloric acid) .... 1 mg
Sodium bisulfite .... 1 mg
Sodium chloride .... 9 mg
Chlorobutanol [chloral derivative (preservative)] .... 5 mg
Water for injection .... q.s.
Indications: A sterile solution for emergency use only in treating anaphylactic shock.
Dosage and Administration: Parenterally:
Cattle, Horses, Sheep, and Swine: 1 mL of 1:1,000 solution per 100 pounds of body weight injected subcutaneously or intramuscularly.
Dogs and Cats: 0.1 to 0.5 mL of 1:1,000 solution injected subcutaneously or intramuscularly.
Intravenous injection is not recommended for routine clinical work, but in emergency situations, this route may be desired. When injected intravenously, the dosage should be one-quarter (¼) to one-half (½) of the intramuscular dosages shown above.
Precaution(s): Store in a refrigerator at 2-8°C (36-46°F). Do not freeze.
Caution(s): Federal law restricts this drug to use by or on the order of a licensed veterinarian.
Do not use the product if it is brown or contains a precipitate. For veterinary use only.
Presentation: 30 mL sterile multiple dose vials.
Compendium Code No.: 10820700

EPINEPHRINE INJECTION USP 1:1000 ℞

Phoenix Pharmaceutical — **Epinephrine**
Active Ingredient(s): Each mL contains:
Epinephrine .... 1 mg
Sodium Chloride .... 9 mg
Sodium Metabisulfite .... 1 mg
Chlorobutanol (preservative) .... 5 mg
Water For Injection .... q.s.
With Hydrochloric Acid to adjust pH.
Indications: Epinephrine is a powerful, quick-acting vasoconstrictor for emergency use only in the treatment of anaphylactic shock.
Dosage and Administration:
Cattle, Horses, Sheep and Swine - Inject subcutaneously or intramuscularly 1 mL per 100 pounds of body weight.
Intravenous injection is not recommended, but if it is found to be clinically necessary, ¼ to ½ of the intramuscular dose should be used.
Precaution(s): Protect from light. Store in refrigerator at 2°-8°C (36°-46°F). Do not freeze.
Do not use injection if it is pinkish or darker than slightly yellow or if it contains a precipitate.
Caution(s): Federal law restricts this drug to use by or on the order of a licensed veterinarian.
The symptoms of anaphylactoid shock include glassy eyes, increased salivation, grinding of the teeth, rapid breathing, muscular tremors, staggering gait, and collapse with death following. These symptoms may appear after injection of a bacterin, vaccine, or antibiotic.
Hazardous: Not for human use. Use only as directed. For animal use only.
Warning(s): Keep out of reach of children.
Presentation: 30 mL sterile multiple dose vials (NDC 57319-352-03).
Manufactured by: Phoenix Scientific, Inc., St. Joseph, MO 64503
Compendium Code No.: 12560322 — Rev. 8-01

EPINJECT ℞

Vetus — **Epinephrine**
Active Ingredient(s): Each mL contains:
Epinephrine .... 1 mg
Sodium Chloride .... 9 mg
Sodium Metabisulfite .... 1 mg
Chlorobutanol (preservative) .... 5 mg
Water For Injection .... q.s.
With hydrochloric acid to adjust pH.
Indications: Epinephrine is a powerful, quick-acting vasoconstrictor for emergency use only in the treatment of anaphylactoid shock. The symptoms of anaphylactoid shock include glassy eyes, increased salivation, grinding of the teeth, rapid breathing, muscle tremors, staggering gait, and collapse with death following. These symptoms may appear shortly after injection of a bacterin, vaccine or antibiotic.
Dosage and Administration: Cattle, Horses, Sheep and Swine - Inject subcutaneously or intramuscularly 1 mL per 100 pounds of body weight. Intravenous injection is not recommended, but if it is found to be clinically necessary, ¼ to ½ of the intramuscular dose should be used.
Precaution(s): Protect from light. Store in refrigerator at 2°-8°C (38°-46°F). Do not freeze.
Caution(s): Federal law restricts this drug to use by or on the order of a licensed veterinarian.
Do not use injection if it is pinkish or darker than slightly yellow or if it contains precipitate.
Warning(s): Hazardous: Not for human use. For animal use only. Keep out of reach of children.
Presentation: 30 mL sterile multiple-dose vials.
Compendium Code No.: 14440290

EPI-OTIC®

Virbac — **Otic Cleanser**
Ear Solution
Ingredient(s): Contains: Lactic acid and salicylic acid are present in encapsulated (Spherulites®) and free forms. Chitosanide is present in encapsulated form. PCMX, propylene glycol, and sodium docusate are present in free form. Also contains water, fragrance, and FD&C blue #1.
Indications: EPI-OTIC® may be used for routine ear cleansing in healthy ear canal or prior to administration of other ear preparations. It may be used in dogs and cats of any age.
Directions: Shake well before use. Apply product liberally into the ear canal. Gently rub the base of the ear and then wipe the interior of the ear flap with cotton or cloth moistened with EPI-OTIC®.

Frequency of use: From two to three times a week to daily, or as directed by your veterinarian.

Caution(s): For topical use only. Avoid contact with eyes. Do not use in ears with ruptured tympanic membrane.

Available through licensed veterinarians only.

Warning(s): Keep out of reach of children.

Discussion: EPI-OTIC® contains Spherulites®, an exclusive and patented encapsulation system developed by Virbac to provide slow release of ingredients long after product application.

EPI-OTIC® also contains Chitosanide, a natural biopolymer creating a protective film on the skin and hair.

Presentation: 4 oz (120 mL), 8 oz (237 mL), and 16 oz (473 mL) containers.

Compendium Code No.: 10230260

EPI-SOOTHE® CREAM RINSE AND CONDITIONER

Virbac **Grooming Rinse**

Active Ingredient(s): Contains oatmeal in a cream rinse and conditioner base.

Indications: EPI-SOOTHE® Cream Rinse and Conditioner is formulated to help relieve dry, itchy, sensitive skin. The formula also makes the hair coat more manageable and helps prevent tangles, as well as imparting a high sheen.

Dosage and Administration: Shake well before using. EPI-SOOTHE® Cream Rinse and Conditioner should be used after first bathing the dog or cat. Wet the animal's coat thoroughly. Pour EPI-SOOTHE® onto the animal's wetted coat. Gently massage thoroughly into the coat. Allow the cream rinse to remain on the hair coat for five (5) minutes. Lightly rinse with water.

Since many allergic conditions manifest podiatrically, apply EPI-SOOTHE® Rinse with one (1) pint of tepid water and pour over paw areas.

Caution(s): For topical use only. Avoid contact with the eyes. Keep out of the reach of children.

Presentation: 8 oz. (237 mL), 16 oz. (473 mL), and 1 gallon (3.79 L) containers.

Compendium Code No.: 10230270

EPI-SOOTHE® SHAMPOO

Virbac **Grooming Shampoo**

Ingredient(s): Contains: Chitosanide, natural colloidal oatmeal 2%, glycerin 5% and lactic acid in a shampoo base also containing water, sodium C14-16 olefin sulfonate, cocamidopropyl betaine, lauramide DEA, DMDM hydantoin, magnesium aluminum silicate, hydroxypropyl methylcellulose, fragrance, FD & C blue #1. May contain sodium chloride and/or FD & C yellow #5.

Chitosanide, natural colloidal oatmeal and glycerin are present in encapsulated (Spherulites®) and free forms.

Indications: A soothing shampoo aimed to reduce mild itch in dogs and cats of any age.

Directions: Shake well before use. Wet the coat with warm water and apply sufficient shampoo to create a rich lather. Massage EPI-SOOTHE® into wet coat, lather freely. Rinse and repeat. Allow to remain on hair for 5 to 10 minutes, then rinse thoroughly with clean water.

Frequency of use: May be used as often as daily or as directed by your veterinarian.

Caution(s): For topical use only. Avoid contact with eyes. In case of contact, flush eyes with water and seek medical attention if irritation persists.

Available through licensed veterinarians only.

Warning(s): Keep out of reach of children.

Discussion: EPI-SOOTHE® contains Spherulites®, an exclusive and patented encapsulation system developed by Virbac to provide slow release of ingredients long after the shampoo is rinsed off.

EPI-SOOTHE® also contains Chitosanide, a natural biopolymer creating a protective film on the skin and hair.

Presentation: 8 oz (237 mL), 16 oz (473 mL), and 1 gallon (3.79 L) containers.

Compendium Code No.: 10230280

EQSTIM®

Neogen **Immunostimulant**

Propionibacterium Acnes, Immunostimulant

U.S. Vet. Lic. No.: 302

Active Ingredient(s): Description: EQSTIM® is a preparation consisting of 0.4 mg/mL nonviable *Propionibacterium acnes* suspended in 12.5% ethanol in saline.

Indications: EQSTIM® is indicated in the horse as an adjunct to conventional therapy in the treatment of Equine Respiratory Disease Complex (ERDC). The product has been demonstrated to be effective in increasing the rate of recovery when used in conjunction with antibiotic or hyperimmune therapy in the treatment of primary and secondary bacterial and viral infections associated with ERDC.

Dosage and Administration: EQSTIM® must be administered by the intravenous (I.V.) route.

Shake well to obtain uniform suspension.

Dosage:

Foals: 1 mL.

Older horses: 1 mL per 250 lbs body weight.

Repeat the dosage at day 3 (or day 4), at day 7, and weekly as needed.

Contraindication(s): Do not use in conjunction with glucocorticoids or other immune suppressors. Steroid therapy should be withdrawn at least seven days before initiating this therapy.

Precaution(s): Store at room temperature until first used, then store at 2-7°C (35-45°F). Do not freeze.

Caution(s): EQSTIM® is restricted to use by, or under the supervision of, a veterinarian.

The effects of this product have not been studied in pregnant animals. Do not use when pregnancy is known or suspected. There may be a rise in temperature, tremors, temporary loss of appetite, or sluggishness a few hours after injection.

Anaphylactic reactions may occur.

For veterinary use only.

Antidote(s): Epinephrine.

Presentation: 5 mL and 50 mL vials.

Compendium Code No.: 14910261 TC-9/0698 / TC-10/0698

EQU-AID PLUS

Vet-A-Mix **Large Animal Dietary Supplement**

Fortified vitamin-mineral supplement for horses

Guaranteed Analysis:

	Per 2 ounces
Vitamin A, minimum	40,000 I.U.
Vitamin D_3, minimum	5,000 I.U.
Vitamin E, minimum	100 I.U.
Riboflavin, minimum	40 mg
Niacin, minimum	80 mg
Thiamine mononitrate, minimum	20 mg
D-Pantothenic acid, minimum	100 mg
Pyridoxine HCl, minimum	5 mg
D-Biotin, minimum	1 mg
Vitamin B_{12}, minimum	40 mcg
Iodine	2 mg
Iron	100 mg
Copper	20 mg
Cobalt	1 mg
Magnesium	100 mg
Manganese	100 mg
Selenium	1 mg
Zinc	280 mg
Phosphorus, minimum	4,200 mg
Calcium, minimum	4,200 mg
Calcium, maximum	5,000 mg
Salt, minimum	1,125 mg
Salt, maximum	1,418 mg
DL-Methionine	1,000 mg
L-Lysine monohydrate	1,000 mg
Crude fat, minimum	5,670 mg

(Vegetable oils containing not less than 85% unsaturated fatty acids)

Ingredients: Dicalcium phosphate, yeast culture, wheat bran, vegetable oil, sodium tripolyphosphate, salt, L-Lysine monohydrochloride, DL-methionine, linseed meal, zinc oxide, ferrous sulfate, calcium phosphate, vitamin E supplement, magnesium oxide, manganous oxide, calcium pantothenate, biotin supplement, thiamine mononitrate, niacin supplement, copper sulfate, vitamin A supplement, monosodium glutamate, ferric oxide, riboflavin supplement, vitamin B_{12} supplement, corn distiller's dried grain with solubles, mineral oil, vitamin D_3 supplement, pyridoxine HCl, cobalt sulfate, ethylenediamine dihydriodide, sodium selenite, tetrasodium ethylenediaminetetraacetate, with BHT, BHA, ethoxyquin, propyl gallate, and citric acid, preservatives.

Indications: Fortified vitamin-mineral supplement for horses.

Directions: Feed 2 ounces (1 heaping measure) per day to colts and adult horses. Ponies and very small breeds should receive proportional amounts. A ⅓ cup measure is enclosed.

Note: Consider selenium concentrations in the total daily feed intake. The total added selenium should not exceed 0.3 mg/kg (0.3 ppm) in the ration or 3.0 mg selenium per horse per day.

Warning(s): Keep out of the reach of children.

Presentation: 5 lb. (2.268 kg) jars and 40 lb. pails.

Compendium Code No.: 10500051 0799

EQUALIZER™

Evsco **Deodorant Product**

Active Ingredient(s): Contains 2-butoxyethanol and isopropyl alcohol.

Does not contain phosphates or fluorocarbons.

Indications: Formulated for veterinary use to remove organic stains and odors associated with pets, such as those caused by urine, feces, vomit, blood, and food, etc. Recommended for cleaning stains associated with: Puppy and kitten training, sick or debilitated animals, cat litter box aversion, and elimination behavior problems.

Use on carpets, floors, furniture, clothing, auto interiors, litter boxes, cages, pet living and sleeping areas.

Dosage and Administration: Carefully follow the directions to avoid personal injury. The can sprays upside down only. Remove the protective cap. Hold the can upside down. Point the opening in the spray tip towards the spot or stain. Depress the tab on the top of the spray tip to spray. Hold the can at arm's length and avoid spraying toward any part of the body. It is not necessary to bend down to apply the product. To avoid splashback, do not spray at hard surfaces.

Apply in short bursts until the spot or stain is well saturated. Excessive deposits of grease, oil, or ink may require additional applications. Wait until the material is dry before re-applying to see if necessary.

Precaution(s): The contents are under pressure. Do not puncture or incinerate the container. Do not expose to heat or store at temperatures above 120°F.

Caution(s): Keep out of the reach of children.

Check for colorfastness on an inconspicuous area. Do not oversaturate. Not recommended for use on wool.

If the can is cold, the product will foam but this will not impede the product efficacy.

Contact with the skin or eyes can cause irritation and permanent eye damage. The vapor may be harmful. Harmful if swallowed. Use in a well ventilated area.

If sprayed on skin, wash with soap and water. If sprayed in the eyes, flush thoroughly with water for 15 minutes and see a physician.

Presentation: 14 oz. (397 g) aerosol cans.

Compendium Code No.: 10050070

EQUI AID CW®

Equi Aid **Parasiticide-Oral**

(Pyrantel Tartrate) Equine Anthelmintic

Active Ingredient(s):

Pyrantel Tartrate	2.11% (9.6 grams per pound)

Guaranteed Analysis:

Crude Protein (min)	17%
Crude Fat (min)	2%
Crude Fiber (max)	27%
Maximum Moisture	10%

Ingredients: Dehydrated alfalfa meal, brewers dried yeast, brewers dried grains, natural and artificial flavors, and preserved with propionic acid.

Indications: For the prevention of *Strongylus vulgaris* larval infestations in horses.

E

For control of the following parasites in horses:

Large Strongyles (adults): *S. vulgaris, S. edentatus, Triodontophorus* spp.

Small Strongyles (adult and fourth-stage larvae): *Cyathostomum* spp, *Cylicocyclus* spp, *Cylicostephanus* spp, *Cylicodontophorus* spp, *Poteriostomum* spp.

Pinworms (adult and fourth-stage larvae): *Oxyuris equi.*

Ascarids (adult and fourth-stage larvae): *Parascaris equorum.*

Dosage and Administration: EQUI AID CW® (pyrantel tartate) is to be administered on a continuous basis as a top dress on the horse's daily ration. Feed at the rate of 1.2 mg pyrantel tartrate per pound of body weight per day. To achieve this dose administer 0.5 ounces of EQUI AID CW® per 250 lb of body weight (an EQUI AID CW® measuring scoop is enclosed). EQUI AID CW® should be administered for the entire period that the animal is at risk to internal parasites. Unprotected animals that have grazed may already have an established *S vulgaris* larval infestation. Before administering EQUI AID CW®, these animals should be treated with a therapeutic dose of a larvicidal product.

Foals may be fed EQUI AID CW® at such time when consistent intake of grain mix is occurring. This is generally between two and three months of age.

EQUI AID CW® may be used in mares at any stage of pregnancy or lactation. Stallion fertility is not affected by the use of EQUI AID CW®.

Top-Dress Directions:

Pounds Body Weight	Ounces per day of EQUI AID CW®
250	0.5 oz
500	1.0 oz
750	1.5 oz
1,000	2.0 oz
1,250	2.5 oz

(1 oz measuring scoop enclosed - 1 level scoop per 500 lb body weight)

Caution(s): Consult your veterinarian before using in severely debilitated animals and for assistance in the diagnosis, treatment and control of parasitism.

Do not mix in feeds containing Bentonite.

Warning(s): Not for use in horses intended for food.

Presentation: 10 lb (4.5 kg) and 50 lb.

Compendium Code No.: 11130001

EQUICINE® II WITH HAVLOGEN®*

Intervet **Vaccine**

Equine Influenza Vaccine, Killed Virus

U.S. Vet. Lic. No.: 286

Description: A combination of inactivated, purified, concentrated, adjuvanted, tissue culture origin, Equine Influenza virus, subtypes A1 and A2 including KY 93 strain. Intervet serological data suggest cross protection against certain U.S. and European strains, including Prague 56, KY 63, KY 81 and 87, Fountainbleau 79 and Berlin 84 and 89.**

Neomycin, polymyxin B and nystatin added as preservatives.

Indications: For vaccination of healthy horses against Equine Influenza Virus.

Dosage and Administration: For primary immunization, aseptically inject 1 mL intramuscularly and repeat the dose in 3 to 4 weeks. A 1 mL dose should be administered annually and at any time epidemic conditions exist or are reported and exposure is imminent.

Precaution(s): Store at 35° to 45°F (2° to 7°C). Shake well before using. Use entire contents when first opened.

Caution(s): Local reactions may occur if this product is given subcutaneously. Inject deep into the muscle only. Anaphylactoid reactions may occur.

For use in animals only.

Antidote(s): Epinephrine.

Warning(s): Do not vaccinate within 21 days before slaughter.

References: **Available upon request.

Presentation: 10 dose (10 x 1 mL) syringes with separate sterile needles.

*Adjuvant—Intervet's Proprietary Technology

Compendium Code No.: 11060520

EQUI-FLU® EWT

Boehringer Ingelheim **Toxoid-Vaccine**

Encephalomyelitis-Influenza Vaccine, Eastern and Western Killed Virus-Tetanus Toxoid

U.S. Vet. Lic. No.: 124

Contents: This product contains the antigens listed above.

Contains gentamicin and thimerosal as preservatives.

Indications: For the vaccination of all types and ages of healthy horses against Eastern and Western Equine Encephalomyelitis, tetanus and as an aid in the prevention of Equine Influenza due to strains A_1 and A_2 viruses.

Dosage and Administration: Shake well. Using aseptic technique, inject 2 mL deep intramuscularly with a 1½ inch sterile needle preferably in the hind quarters. For primary vaccination administer a second 2 mL dose in 4 to 6 weeks using a different injection site and separate sterile 1½ inch needle for each injection.

Revaccination: Revaccinate annually for protection against tetanus, using a single 2 mL dose. Revaccinate annually and prior to anticipated exposure for maximum benefit against Equine Influenza strains A_1 and A_2 viruses and Eastern and Western Equine Encephalomyelitis. In the event of an outbreak, vaccination should be combined with good hygiene and segregation of affected or newly acquired animals.

Precaution(s): Store at 35-45°F (2-7°C). Protect from freezing. Use entire contents when first opened.

Caution(s): Anaphylactoid reactions may occur following use.

This product has been tested under laboratory conditions and shown to meet all Federal standards for safety and efficacy in normal healthy animals. This level of performance may be affected by conditions of use such as stress, weather, nutrition, disease, parasitism, other treatments, individual idiosyncrasies, or impaired immunological competency. These factors should be considered by the user when evaluating product performance or freedom of reactions.

For veterinary use only.

Antidote(s): Epinephrine.

Warning(s): Do not vaccinate within 21 days before slaughter.

Presentation: 10 x 1 dose (2 mL) syringes and 10 dose (20 mL) vials.

Compendium Code No.: 10280451 31502-03 / 31503-02/31504-03

EQUI-FLU® VEWT

Boehringer Ingelheim **Toxoid-Vaccine**

Encephalomyelitis-Influenza Vaccine, Eastern, Western and Venezuelan Killed Virus-Tetanus Toxoid

U.S. Vet. Lic. No.: 124

Contents: This product contains the antigens listed above.

Contains gentamicin and thimerosal as preservatives.

Indications: For the vaccination of all types and ages of healthy horses against Eastern, Western, and Venezuelan Equine Encephalomyelitis, tetanus and as an aid in the prevention of Equine Influenza due to strains A_1 and A_2 viruses.

Dosage and Administration: Shake well. Using aseptic technique, inject 2 mL deep intramuscularly with a 1½ inch sterile needle preferably in the hind quarters. For primary vaccination administer a second 2 mL dose in 4 to 6 weeks using a different injection site and separate sterile 1½ inch needle for each injection.

Revaccination: Revaccinate annually for protection against tetanus, using a single 2 mL dose. Revaccinate annually and prior to anticipated exposure for maximum benefit against Equine Influenza strains A_1 and A_2 viruses and Eastern, Western, and Venezuelan Equine Encephalomyelitis. In the event of an outbreak, vaccination should be confined with good hygiene and segregation of affected or newly acquired animals.

Precaution(s): Store at 35-45°F (2-7°C). Protect from freezing. Use entire contents when first opened.

Caution(s): Anaphylactoid reactions may occur following use.

This product has been tested under laboratory conditions and shown to meet all Federal standards for safety and efficacy in normal healthy animals. This level of performance may be affected by conditions of use such as stress, weather, nutrition, disease, parasitism, other treatments, individual idiosyncrasies, or impaired immunological competency. These factors should be considered by the user when evaluating product performance or freedom of reactions.

For veterinary use only.

Antidote(s): Epinephrine.

Warning(s): Do not vaccinate within 21 days before slaughter.

Presentation: 10 x 1 dose (2 mL) syringes and 10 dose (20 mL) vials.

Compendium Code No.: 10280461 31601-03/31602-03 / 31603-02/31604/03

EQUILEVE ℞

Vetus **Analgesic-Anti-inflammatory**

Flunixin Meglumine 50 mg/mL

ANADA No.: 200-124

Active Ingredient(s): Each millimeter contains flunixin meglumine equivalent to 50 mg flunixin, 0.1 mg edetate disodium, 2.5 mg sodium formaldehyde sulfoxylate, 4.0 mg diethanolamine, 207.2 mg propylene glycol; 5.0 mg phenol as preservative, hydrochloric acid, water for injection q.s.

Indications: Recommended for the alleviation of inflammation and pain associated with musculoskeletal disorders in the horse.

It is also recommended for the alleviation of visceral pain associated with colic in the horse.

For intravenous or intramuscular use in horses only.

Pharmacology: Flunixin meglumine is a potent, non-narcotic, non-steroidal, analgesic agent with anti-inflammatory and antipyretic activity. It is significantly more potent than pentazocine, meperidine and codeine as an analgesic in the rat yeast paw test. Flunixin is four times as potent on a mg per mg basis as phenylbutazone as measured by the reduction in lameness and swelling in the horse. Plasma half-life in the horse serum is 1.6 hours following a single dose of 1.1 mg/kg. Measurable amounts are detectable in horse plasma at 8 hours post injection.

Dosage and Administration: The recommended dose for musculoskeletal disorders is 0.5 mg per pound (1 mL/100 lbs) of body weight once daily. Treatment may be given by intravenous or intramuscular injection and repeated for up to 5 days. Studies show onset of activity is within 2 hours. Peak response occurs between 12 and 16 hours and duration of activity is 24-36 hours.

The recommended dose for the alleviation of pain associated with equine colic is 0.5 mg per pound of body weight. Intravenous administration is recommended for prompt relief. Clinical studies show pain is alleviated in less than 15 minutes in many cases. Treatment may be repeated when signs of colic recur. During clinical studies approximately 10% of the horses required one or two additional treatments. The cause of colic should be determined and treated with concomitant therapy.

Contraindication(s): There are no known contraindications to this drug when used as directed. Intra-arterial injection should be avoided. Horses inadvertently intra-arterially can show adverse reactions. Signs can be ataxia, incoordination, hyperventilation, hysteria, and muscle weakness. Signs are transient and disappear without antidotal medication within a few minutes. Do not use in horses showing hypersensitivity to flunixin meglumine.

Precaution(s): Store between 2° and 30°C (36° and 86°F).

Caution(s): Federal law restricts this drug to use by or on the order of a licensed veterinarian.

The effect of flunixin meglumine on pregnancy has not been determined. Studies to determine activity of flunixin meglumine when administered concomitantly with other drugs have not been conducted. Drug compatibility should be monitored closely in patients requiring adjunctive therapy.

Isolated reports of local reactions following intramuscular injection, particularly in the neck, have been received. These include localized swelling, sweating, induration, and stiffness.

Warning(s): Not for use in horses intended for food.

Toxicology: Toxicity studies were conducted in horses. A threefold intramuscular dose of 1.5 mg per pound of body weight daily for 10 consecutive days was safe. No changes were observed in hematology, serum chemistry, or urinalysis values. Intravenous dosages of 0.5 mg/lb daily for 15 days; 1.5 mg/lb daily for 10 days; and 2.5 mg/lb daily for 5 days produced no changes in blood or urine parameters. No injection site irritation was observed following intramuscular injection of the 0.5 mg/lb recommended dose. Some irritation was observed following a 3-fold dose administered intramuscularly.

Side Effects: Isolated reports of local reactions following intramuscular injection, particularly in the neck, have been received. These include localized swelling, sweating, induration, and stiffness. In rare instances, fatal or nonfatal clostridial infections or other infections have been reported in association with intramuscular use of flunixin meglumine. In addition, rare instances of anaphylactic-like reactions, some of which have been fatal, have been reported primarily following intravenous use.

Presentation: 100 mL and 250 mL multidose vials.

Compendium Code No.: 14440310

EQUILOID® INNOVATOR

Fort Dodge **Toxoid-Vaccine**

Encephalomyelitis Vaccine-Tetanus Toxoid, Eastern & Western, Killed Virus

U.S. Vet. Lic. No.: 112

Contents: This product contains the antigens listed above.

Thimerosal, neomycin and polymyxin B added as preservatives.

Indications: For vaccination of healthy horses as an aid in the prevention of equine encephalomyelitis due to Eastern and Western viruses, and tetanus.

Dosage and Administration: Horses, inject one 1 mL dose intramuscularly using aseptic technique. Administer a second 1 mL dose 3 to 4 weeks after the first dose. A 1 mL booster should be given annually.

Precaution(s): Store in the dark at 2° to 7°C (35° to 45°F). Avoid freezing. Shake well. Use entire contents when first opened.

Caution(s): In some instances, transient local reactions may occur at the injection site.

In case of anaphylactoid reaction, administer epinephrine.

For veterinary use only.

Warning(s): Do not vaccinate within 21 days before slaughter.

Presentation: 1 dose (1 mL) vial.

Compendium Code No.: 10032740 16611A

EQUIMECTRIN™ PASTE 1.87%

Farnam **Parasiticide-Oral**

Anthelmintic and Boticide

NADA No.: 134-314

Active Ingredient(s): The paste contains:

Ivermectin 1.87%

Indications: EQUIMECTRIN™ (ivermectin) Paste provides effective control of the following parasites in horses. Large strongyles (adults) — *Strongylus vulgaris* (also early forms in blood vessels), *S edentalus* (also tissue stages), *S equinus, Triodontophorus* spp; Small strongyles including those resistant to some benzimidazole class compounds (adults and fourth-stage larvae) — *Cyathostomum* spp, *Cylicocyclus* spp, *Cylicostephanus* spp, *Cylicodontophorus* spp; Pinworms (adults and fourth-stage larvae) — *Oxyuris equi*; Ascarids (adults and third- and fourth-stage larvae) — *Parascaris equorum*; Hairworms (adults) — *Trichostrogylus axei*; Large-mouth Stomach Worms (adults) — *Habronema muscae;* Bots (oral and gastric stages) — *Gasterophilus* spp; Lungworms (adults and forth-stage larvae) — *Dictyocaulus arnfieldi;* Intestinal Threadworms (adults) — *Strongyloides westeri;* Summer Sores caused by *Habronema* and *Draschia* spp cutaneous third-stage larvae; Dermatitis caused by neck threadworm microfilarie, *Onchocerca* sp.

Dosage and Administration: This syringe contains sufficient paste to treat one 1250 lb horse at the recommended dose rate of 91 mcg ivermectin per lb (200 mcg/kg) body weight. Each weight marking on the syringe plunger delivers enough paste to treat 250 lb body weight.

(1) While holding plunger, turn the knurled ring on the plunger ¼ turn to the left and slide it so the side nearest the barrel is at the prescribed weight marking. (2) Lock the ring in place by making a ¼ turn to the right. (3) Make sure that the horse's mouth contains no feed. (4) Remove the cover from the tip of the syringe. (5) Insert the syringe tip into the horse's mouth at the space between the teeth. (6) Depress the plunger as far as it will go, depositing paste on the back of the tongue. (7) Immediately raise the horse's head for a few seconds after dosing.

Contraindication(s): EQUIMECTRIN™ (ivermectin) Paste has been formulated specifically for use in horses only. This product should not be used in other animal species as severe reactions, including fatalities in dogs, may result.

Precaution(s): Ivermectin and excreted ivermectin residues may adversely affect aquatic organisms. Do not contaminate ground or surface water. Dispose of the EQUIMECTRIN™ (ivermectin) Paste syringe in an approved landfill or by incineration.

Caution(s): For oral use in horses only.

Consult your veterinarian for assistance in the diagnosis, treatment, and control of parasitism.

Swelling and itching reactions after treatment with EQUIMECTRIN™ (ivermectin) Paste have occurred in horses carrying heavy infections of neck threadworm (*Onchocerca* sp) microfilariae. These reactions were most likely the result of microfilariae dying in large numbers. Symptomatic treatment may be advisable. Consult your veterinarian should any such reactions occur. Healing of summer sores involving extensive tissue changes may require other appropriate therapy in conjunction with treatment with EQUIMECTRIN™ (ivermectin) Paste. Reinfection, and measures for its prevention, should also be considered. Consult your veterinarian if the condition does not improve.

Warning(s): Do not use on horses intended for food purposes.

Refrain from smoking and eating when handling. Wash hands after use. Avoid contact with eyes. Keep this and all drugs out of the reach of children.

Side Effects: Safety — EQUIMECTRIN™ Paste may be used in horses of all ages, including mares at any stage of pregnancy. Stallions may be treated without adversely affecting their fertility.

Discussion: Parasite Control Program: All horses should be included in a regular parasite control program with particular attention being paid to mares, foals and yearlings. Foals should be treated initially at 6 to 8 weeks of age, and routine treatment repeated as appropriate. Consult your veterinarian for a control program to meet your specific needs. EQUIMECTRIN™ (ivermectin) Paste effectively controls gastrointestinal nematodes and bots of horses. Regular treatment will reduce the chances of verminous arteritis caused by *S vulgaris*.

Product Advantages: Broad-spectrum control, EQUIMECTRIN™ Paste kills important internal parasites, including bots and the arterial stages of *Strongyles vulgaris,* with a single dose. EQUIMECTRIN™ Paste is a potent anti-parasitic agent that is neither a benzimidazole nor an organophosphate.

Presentation: 0.21 oz (6.08 g) tube.

Distributed by: Horse Health.

Compendium Code No.: 10000161

EQUIMECTRIN® PASTE 1.87%

Merial **Parasiticide-Oral**

(ivermectin) Anthelmintic and Boticide

NADA No.: 134-314

Active Ingredient(s): Each syringe contains:

Ivermectin 1.87%

Indications: EQUIMECTRIN® (ivermectin) Paste provides effective control of the following parasites in horses:

Large Strongyles (adults): *Strongylus vulgaris* (also early forms in blood vessels), *S. edentalus* (also tissue stages), *S. equinus, Triodontophorus* spp.

Small Strongyles including those resistant to some benzimidazole class compounds (adults and fourth-stage larvae): *Cyathostomum* spp, *Cylicocyclus* spp, *Cylicostephanus* spp, *Cylicodontophorus* spp.

Pinworms (adults and fourth-stage larvae): *Oxyuris equi.*

Ascarids (adults and third- and fourth-stage larvae): *Parascaris equorum.*

Hairworms (adults): *Trichostrogylus axei.*

Large-mouth Stomach Worms (adults): *Habronema muscae.*

Bots (oral and gastric stages): *Gastrophilus* spp.

Lungworms (adults and forth-stage larvae): *Dictyocaulus arnfieldi.*

Intestinal Threadworms (adults): *Strongyloides westeri.*

Summer Sores caused by *Habronema* and *Draschia* spp cutaneous third-stage larvae.

Dermatitis caused by neck threadworm microfilariae, *Onchocerca* sp.

Dosage and Administration: The syringe contains sufficient paste to treat one 1,250 lb horse at the recommended dose rate of 91 mcg ivermectin per lb (200 mcg/kg) body weight. Each weight marking on the syringe plunger delivers enough paste to treat 250 lb body weight.

(1) While holding plunger, turn the knurled ring on the plunger ¼ turn to the left and slide it so the side nearest the barrel is at the prescribed weight marking. (2) Lock the ring in place by making a ¼ turn to the right. (3) Make sure that the horse's mouth contains no feed. (4) Remove the cover from the tip of the syringe. (5) Insert the syringe tip into the horse's mouth at the space between the teeth. (6) Depress the plunger as far as it will go, depositing paste on the back of the tongue. (7) Immediately raise the horse's head for a few seconds after dosing.

Parasite Control Program: All horses should be included in a regular parasite control program with particular attention being paid to mares, foals and yearlings. Foals should be treated initially at 6 to 8 weeks of age, and routine treatment repeated as appropriate. Consult your veterinarian for a control program to meet your specific needs. EQUIMECTRIN® (ivermectin) Paste effectively controls gastrointestinal nematodes and bots of horses. Regular treatment will reduce the chances of verminous arteritis caused by *Strongylus vulgaris.*

Consult your veterinarian for assistance in the diagnosis, treatment, and control of parasitism.

Precaution(s): Environmental Safety: Ivermectin and excreted ivermectin residues may adversely affect aquatic organisms. Do not contaminate ground or surface water. Dispose of the syringe in an approved landfill or by incineration.

Caution(s): EQUIMECTRIN® Paste has been formulated specifically for use in horses only. This product should not be used in other animal species as severe reactions, including fatalities in dogs, may result.

Note to User: Swelling and itching reactions after treatment with EQUIMECTRIN® (ivermectin) Paste have occurred in horses carrying heavy infections of neck threadworm *(Onchocerca* sp microfilariae). These reactions were most likely the result of microfilariae dying in large numbers. Symptomatic treatment may be advisable. Consult your veterinarian should any such reactions occur. Healing of summer sores involving extensive tissue changes may require other appropriate therapy in conjunction with treatment with EQUIMECTRIN® Paste. Reinfection, and measures for its prevention, should also be considered. Consult your veterinarian if the condition does not improve.

For oral use in horses only.

Warning(s): Do not use on horses intended for food purposes.

Not for use in humans. Keep this and all drugs out of the reach of children. Refrain from smoking and eating when handling. Wash hands after use. Avoid contact with eyes.

The Material Safety Data Sheet (MSDS) contains more detailed occupational safety information. To report adverse reactions in users, to obtain more information, or to obtain an MSDS, contact Merial at 1-888-637-4251.

Discussion: Product Advantages: Broad-spectrum Control — EQUIMECTRIN® Paste kills important internal parasites, including bots and the arterial stages of *S. vulgaris,* with a single dose. EQUIMECTRIN® Paste is a potent anti-parasitic agent that is neither a benzimidazole nor an organophosphate.

Trial Data: Animal Safety: EQUIMECTRIN® (ivermectin) Paste may be used in horses of all ages, including mares at any stage of pregnancy. Stallions may be treated without adversely affecting their fertility.

Presentation: 0.21 oz (6.08 g) syringe.

EQUIMECTRIN is a registered trademark of Merial.

Merial Limited: Registered in England and Wales [Reg. No. 3332751] with registered offices at 27 Knightsbridge, London SW1X 7QT, England and domesticated in Delaware, USA as Merial LLC.

U.S. Patent No. 4,199,569

Compendium Code No.: 11110910 9355600/9355700

EQUIMUNE® I.V.

Bioniche Animal Health (formerly Vetrepharm) **Immunostimulant**

Mycobacterium Cell Wall Fraction Immunostimulant

U.S. Vet. Lic. No.: 289

Active Ingredient(s): Mycobacterium cell wall fraction immunostimulant.

Indications: An immunotherapeutic agent for the treatment of Equine Respiratory Disease Complex, (ERDC). The common causes of ERDC are equine herpesvirus (rhinopneumonitis), influenza A equine 1 and influenza A equine 2.

EQUIMUNE® I.V. is indicated in those conditions where immunotherapy will enhance the immune response to respiratory tract infections. Efficacy of EQUIMUNE® I.V. is not altered by concurrent use of antibiotics.

Pharmacology: Research has shown that mycobacterium cell wall compounds have immunomodulating activity. EQUIMUNE® I.V. is an emulsion of purified mycobacterium cell walls which have been extracted by a process which reduces their toxic and allergic effects, but retains their immunostimulating activity.

EQUIMUNE® I.V. activates antigen presenting cells thereby enhancing the production of the polypeptide cytokine interleukin 1 (IL-1). The IL-1 molecule is one of the body's natural adjuvants, and therefore nonspecifically amplifies the immune response to antigens.[1] This amplification includes both cell-mediated immunity (CMI) and humoral antibody (HA) responses.[1-3,6] IL-1 intensifies the CMI response by inducing the proliferation of cytotoxic lymphocytes (Tc), augmenting the phagocytic abilities of monocytes and macrophages, and by actuating cytokine production.[1] IL-1 also acts directly on the hypothalamus to induce a fever which then enhances the function of T lymphocytes.[1,18] Proliferation of fibroblasts is induced by IL-1 and thus IL-1 production aids in the wound healing processes.[1] Wound healing processes are further augmented by the increased phagocytic action of macrophages and monocytes. This is important in overcoming alveolar cell damage caused by respiratory disease.[17]

Cell mediated immunity plays a major role in resistance to, and recovery from, viral infection[17] such as influenza virus[4,15] and herpesvirus infections[3,11] including equine herpesvirus.[12-15] Immunotherapy trials conducted in Canada and elsewhere have indicated a postive response in horses with viral respiratory tract infections.[15,16] Mycobacterium cell wall preparations have been shown to increase the number of alveolar macrophages in animals[8,9] and to stimulate the release of IL-1 from these cells.[10,14]

In vitro trials demonstrate IL-1 production from equine alveolar macrophages as well as equine peripheral blood monocytes.[16] Mycobacterium cell wall fraction immunostimulant has been shown to cause the transformation of lymphocytes previously sensitized by viruses.[17]

Dosage and Administration: For intravenous use only.

The recommended dose for immunostimulation is 1.5 mL (1 syringe) by intravenous injection into the jugular vein. Treatment may be repeated in one (1) to three (3) weeks.

Contraindication(s): Cortisone reduces the production of IL-1.[1] Horses being treated with corticosteroids or ACTH may not respond to EQUIMUNE® I.V. therapy.

Precaution(s):

1. It is important to ensure that the emulsion remains thoroughly mixed during injections. Shake syringe gently, roll between hands, or heat under 150°F (65°C) water to assist emulsification.
2. Store at 36-45°F (2-7°C). Do not freeze.
3. Use the entire contents when first opened. Discard remaining portions.

Caution(s):

1. Observe aseptic techniques when injecting animals.
2. In the event of an anaphylactic reaction, administer epinephrine.

Warning(s): Keep out of the reach of children.

Toxicology: Safety: EQUIMUNE® I.V. is safe to use in pregnant mares. Other than the contraindications listed above, EQUIMUNE® I.V. is compatible with standard treatment and vaccination regimes.[16]

Side Effects: Mild fever, drowsiness, and an increased catabolic rate leading to decreased appetite may occur for one to two days following an EQUIMUNE® I.V. injection. These are normal responses to the release of IL-1.[1,2,6] An elevated body temperature enhances the immune function by stimulating lymphocyte activity[2,17] and thus is not an adverse side effect.

References: Available upon request.

Presentation: 1.5 mL syringe and 4.5 mL multi-dose vial.

Compendium Code No.: 11070021

EQUINE BENE-BAC™

Pet-Ag **Large Animal Dietary Supplement**

Active Ingredient(s): Guaranteed Analysis:

Total viable lactic acid producing bacteria .... 20 million CFU per gram (min.)

Ingredients: Dried *Lactobacillus acidophilus* fermentation product, dried *L. plantarum* fermentation product, dried *Streptococcus faecium* fermentation product, dried *L. casei* fermentation product, vegetable oil, sugar, silicon dioxide, artificial color, polysorbate 80 preserved with TBHQ, and ethoxyquin.

Indications: EQUINE BENE-BAC™ paste is a blend of naturally occurring viable Lactobacillus bacteria which is administered to the horse to supplement the intestinal microflora. *L. acidophilus* is a normal, desirable inhabitant of the intestine. Adverse conditions, such as stress, upset the natural balance of micro-organisms in the digestive tract by decreasing the number of Lactobacillus. EQUINE BENE-BAC™ provides viable Lactobacillus to help maintain the proper microbial balance.

EQUINE BENE-BAC™ may be used during the following periods of stress:

1. The foal's first week (foal heat scours).
2. At weaning.
3. Loss of appetite, due to fatigue or hot weather.
4. Post worming or antibiotic treatment.
5. Prior to transportation.
6. Ration changes.

Dosage and Administration: Administer orally on the back of the tongue.

Foal:

First week: 10 g at 12 to 24 hours of age. 10 g each on day 4 and day 7.

Weaning: 10 g every other day during the initial week of weaning (three doses total).

Mature equines:

Post worming or antibiotics: 10 g each on day 1, 3 and 7 after the end of treatment.

Training: 10 g every other day for one (1) week (three doses total) when the horse goes off feed due to strenuous training.

Transportation: 10 g each on days 3 and 1 prior to transportation and on the first day after transportation.

Precaution(s): Store in a cool place.

Presentation: 30 g oral syringe (6 syringes per display carton, 6 display cartons per case).

Compendium Code No.: 10970100

EQUINE BLUELITE®

TechMix **Large Animal Dietary Supplement**

Active Ingredient(s): Guaranteed Analysis:

Potassium (K), not less than 5.100%
Sodium (Na), not less than 1.500%
Calcium (Ca), not less than 0.500%
Phosphorus (P), not less than 0.450%
Magnesium (Mg), not less than 0.028%
Iron (Fe), not less than 0.120%
Copper (Cu), not less than 0.088%
Zinc (Zn), not less than 0.040%
Manganese (Mn), not less than 0.032%
Fat, not less than 3.00%

Minimum vitamin content per pound:

Vitamin A .... 1,000,000 I.U. (62.500 I.U./oz.)
Vitamin D_3 .... 200,000 I.U. (12,500 I.U./oz.)
Vitamin E .... 1,000 I.U. (62.5 I.U./oz.)
Choline bitartrate .... 2,000 mg (125.0 mg/oz.)
Niacin .... 400 mg (25.0 mg/oz.)
d-Pantothenic acid .... 167.5 mg (1.00 mg/oz.)
Riboflavin .... 100.0 mg (6.25 mg/oz.)
Thiamin .... 24.0 mg (1.50 mg/oz.)
Pyridoxine .... 22.0 mg (1.30 mg/oz.)
Menadione .... 6,700.0 mg (418.00 mcg/oz.)
Folic acid .... 6,700.0 mg (418.00 mcg/oz.)
d-Biotin .... 2,700.0 mg (168.00 mcg/oz.)

Ingredients: Dextrose, sucrose, lactose, fructose, citric acid, animal fat (preserved with BHA), dipotassium phosphate, potassium chloride, sodium bicarbonate, calcium lactate, magnesium gluconate, glycine, zinc methionine, dl-methionine, l-lysine HCl, cobalt glucoheptonate, aloe vera, vitamin A acetate (stability improved), d-activated animal sterol (source of vitamin D_3), dl-alpha tocopheryl acetate (source of vitamin E activity), choline bitartrate, niacin supplement, ascorbic acid (vitamin C) (1,340 mg/lb.), d-pantothenic acid, riboflavin supplement, pyridoxine HCl, thiamin HCl, folic acid, d-biotin, menadione dimenthylpyrimidinol bisulfite (source of vitamin K activity), vitamin B_{12} supplement, yucca schidigera extract, natural and artificial flavor added, apply and honey, F&DC certified color added.

Indications: EQUINE BLUELITE® is an oral rehydration electrolyte-vitamin-energy supplement specifically designed to rehydrate horses that have lost substantial amounts of body fluid and electrolytes as a result of profuse sweating frequently seen after exercise and during warm weather.

EQUINE BLUELITE® provides a pH regulating action that helps establish and maintain the proper digestive pH, thereby facilitating the absorption of electrolytes and the utilization of nutrients during digestion. EQUINE BLUELITE® can be used in high performance horses, as well as colts, fillies and horses that are stressed from dehydration resulting from digestive upsets such as diarrhea.

EQUINE BLUELITE® contains a broad spectrum of buffered sequestered-chelated electrolytes, thereby reducing the potential of irritating the mucosa of the inflamed intestinal tract.

EQUINE BLUELITE® provides sources of energy in the form of dextrose, sucrose, lactose and fructose in combination with high levels of vitamins. This combination of electrolytes, energy and vitamins makes EQUINE BLUELITE® a nutrient supplement for the horse during competition, training, and trail rides as well as for continued 10-14 day usage for horses stressed from parasites or marginal nutrition.

Dosage and Administration: Top dress EQUINE BLUELITE® on the feed, or add EQUINE BLUELITE® to the drinking water continuously for 10-15 days for horses enduring extensive physical activity, or when horses sweat profusely as a result of hot weather or training, racing, showing, or to horses that may be debilitated as a result of poor nutrition, internal parasites, and for other stresses that may result in the sudden loss of body weight.

I. Feed Administration:

1. Foals and yearlings: Daily top dress 1-2 oz. of EQUINE BLUELITE® on the grain ration.
2. Working and pleasure horses: Top dress EQUINE BLUELITE® on the grain ration according to the degree of dehydration that occurs as a result of energy expended and the amount of fluid lost as sweat during exercise or work based on the following:

	Daily Amount of EQUINE BLUELITE®	
Horse Weight (lbs.)	Routine or Mild Physical Activity	Extensive-Endurance Physical Activity
Ponies and horses 300-600	1-2 oz.	2-3 oz.
600-900	3-4 oz.	4-6 oz.
900-1,200	5-6 oz.	6-10 oz.
1,200 and over	7-8 oz.	8-10 oz.

II. Water Administration: Add 1-2 oz. of EQUINE BLUELITE® to each two (2) gallons of drinking water consumed by the horse each day.

Note: Two (2) heaping tablespoonfuls equal approximately 1 oz. of EQUINE BLUELITE®.

Some horses may occasionally refrain from drinking water with sudden changes in taste. In these situations, EQUINE BLUELITE® should be top dressed or mixed in the feed.

Presentation: 4x6 lb. (2.72 kg) pails (24 lb. case).

Compendium Code No.: 11440060

EQUINE CAPSAICIN GEL

Butler **Analgesic-Topical**

NDC No.: 11695-2174-4

Active Ingredient(s): Capsaicin .020%

Ingredients: Water, carbomer 934, camomile extract (levonemol), cayenne pepper extract (capsaicin .020%), propylene glycol, polysorbate 20, triethanolamine, diazolidinyl urea, methyl paraben, propyl paraben, fragrance.

Indications: For the temporary relief of minor aches and pains associated with arthritis, tendinitis, strains, sprains and simple backaches in horses.

Dosage and Administration: Apply approx. ½-1 oz to the desired area. Rub in until thoroughly absorbed. Clip hair on area to be treated if hair is excessively long. Apply to all sides of a joint where applicable. Do not apply to affected area more than 3-4 times per day. Wash hands after use.

Caution(s): For external use only. Avoid contact with eyes and mucous membranes. Do not apply to open cuts and sores. Discontinue use if excessive irritation occurs. If condition persists or worsens for more than seven days or clears again discontinue use and consult a veterinarian. Do not use other than directed.

Warning(s): For animal use only.

Keep out of reach of children.

Presentation: 8 oz.

Compendium Code No.: 10820720

EQUINE COLI ENDOTOX®

Novartis Animal Vaccines **Antiserum**

Escherichia coli Antiserum

U.S. Vet. Lic. No.: 303

Composition: EQUINE COLI ENDOTOX® is prepared from the blood of horses hyperimmunized with K99 piliated *Escherichia coli*. The antiserum contains phenol, thimerosal, and oxytetracycline as preservatives.

Indications: For use as an aid in the prevention and control of endotoxemia and diarrhea caused by K99 piliated *Escherichia coli*.

Dosage and Administration: Administer 10 mL orally to foals less than 12 hours old. Slowly syringe the contents toward the back of the foal's mouth. Colostrum should be fed to each foal.

Precaution(s): Store in the dark at 35°-45°F (2°-7°C). Do not freeze. Shake well before using. Use the entire contents when first opened.

Caution(s): Anaphylactic reactions may occur following the use of the product. Symptomatic treatment: Epinephrine.

Warning(s): Not for use in horses to be slaughtered for food.

Discussion: Endotoxemia, septicemia and enteric infections are the most severe problems affecting neonatal foals, often culminating in death. Approximately 25% of all septicemias in foals are caused by *Escherichia coli*. Invasive strains of this bacteria enter the foal's bloodstream either through the intestinal tract, the respiratory tract, or the umbilical cord. The bacteria then circulate throughout the body, releasing toxins and causing symptoms such as lethargy, depression, anorexia, and sudden death. Foals that survive the septicemia often wind up with chronic arthritis, since the bacteria tend to take refuge in the joint cavities where they are difficult to reach with antibiotics. Foals with *E. coli* infection may also show diarrhea, but this is less common than in other species such as calves and piglets.

The most common factor predisposing foals to developing *E. coli* septicemia is hypogammaglobulinemia (inadequate levels of passive antibody protection from the mare's colostrum). This is caused by several factors, such as foals failing to nurse adequately, poor quality colostrum in the mare, or the loss of colostrum prior to foaling in mares that leak milk. Up until now, measures to combat this problem were limited to complex procedures such as blood transfusions from mare to foal, or obtaining colostrum from another mare to feed to the foal. Since a foal is often not recognized as being hypogammaglobulinemic until it becomes sick, treatment is seldom effective.

EQUINE COLI ENDOTOX® is not a replacement for colostrum. Colostrum contains components that are necessary for the total health of the foal. Good management practices are necessary to ensure adequate colostral intake by the foal. Since many foals do not receive protective passive immunity and many are born in an environment highly contaminated with *E. coli* organisms, they often lack adequate ability to fight septicemia caused by *E. coli*.

One dose of COLI ENDOTOX™ given orally to the newborn foal provides a safe, easy, effective method of giving the foal specific, passive antibodies it needs to ward off deadly *E. coli* infections.

All donor horses are vaccinated for strangles, tetanus, equine rhinopneumonitis, encephalitis, influenza, potomac horse fever, *Clostridium perfringens* types C & D, *Clostridium chauvoei, Cl. novyi, Cl. sordellii, Cl. septicum,* 5-way lepto and *Salmonella typhimurium,* and have been tested to be free of equine infectious anemia, equine viral arteritis, glanders, and brucellosis.

Trial Data: EQUINE COLI ENDOTOX® Challenge Study:

Group	Mortality	Average Clinical Score
Control	5/7 (71%)	76
Treated	0/9 (0%)	6

All foals were rated for fecal consistency, dehydration, depression, anorexia, and death. Observations were made at 12, 24, 36, 48, 60 and 72 hours post challenge.

Presentation: Available in 1 dose (10 mL) syringes and 10 dose (100 mL) bottles.

Compendium Code No.: 11140122

EQUINE ENTERIC COLLOID

TechMix **Laxative**

Active Ingredient(s): Ground psyllium seed and husks, dried whey, corn distiller's dried grains with solubles, monocalcium phosphate, dicalcium phosphate, live cell yeast, casein, animal fat (preserved with BHA), soy lecithin, dextrose, sucrose, lactose, fructose, citric acid, dipotassium phosphate, potassium chloride, sodium bicarbonate, calcium lactate, magnesium gluconate, glycine, zinc methionine, cobalt glucoheptonate, aloe vera, dried *Lactobacillus acidophilus* fermentation product, dried *Lactobacillus lactis* fermentation product, dried *Lactobacillus plantarum* fermentation product, dried *Streptococcus diacetylactic* fermentation product, dried *Streptococcus faecium* fermentation product, dried *Bacillus subtilis* fermentation product, dried *Bacillus subtilis* fermentation extract, dried *Aspergillus oryzae* fermentation extract, *Yucca schidigera* extract, natural and artificial flavor added, apple and honey, F&DC certified color added.

Indications: EQUINE ENTERIC COLLOID is a laxative for horses for use as an aid in the elimination and expelling of foreign material such as sand and undigested feedstuffs from the digestive tract. EQUINE ENTERIC COLLOID, when administered via a stomach tube, has a lubricating and stool-softening action. It can be used as a top dress following stomach tube administration to help maintain a soft and lubricated stool for horses that habitually eat or consume sand and other undigestible feedstuffs.

Dosage and Administration: Administer EQUINE ENTERIC COLLOID as follows:

1. For lubrication and stool-softening action: Administer EQUINE ENTERIC COLLOID via a stomach tube by preparing a suspension of 8 oz. of EQUINE ENTERIC COLLOID in two (2) to three (3) quarts of water for horses between 600-900 lbs. of body weight. Adjust the dosage depending upon the size of the horse, and administer the suspension immediately after mixing EQUINE ENTERIC COLLOID in water.

   EQUINE ENTERIC COLLOID is dispersible and suspendible in water for short periods of time after mixing in water. Consistency and concentration of EQUINE ENTERIC COLLOID in water can be varied depending upon the preference of the veterinarian administering the suspension. The equipment required for stomach tube administration should be assembled and put in place ready for use prior to mixing EQUINE ENTERIC COLLOID in water.
2. Follow-up therapy: Top dress 8 to 12 oz. of EQUINE ENTERIC COLLOID on the feed each day for horses between 600-900 lbs. of body weight for five (5) to seven (7) days after stomach tube administration. Adjust the dosage depending upon the size of the horse.

   EQUINE ENTERIC COLLOID can be used as follow-up therapy whenever horses are treated with laxatives or lubricants such as mineral oil. Follow-up therapy with EQUINE ENTERIC COLLOID helps maintain desired stool consistency after initial treatments with mineral oil or other laxatives.
3. Prophylactic application: For horses of body weight 600-900 lbs. that habitually eat sand or other undigestible feedstuffs, top dress 4 to 8 oz. of EQUINE ENTERIC COLLOID once a day. Continue administration for as long as horses consume sand, coarse dirt and nondigestible feedstuffs. Adjust the dosage depending upon the size of the horse.

   The viable microbial cultures and yeast-enzyme active ingredients in EQUINE ENTERIC COLLOID help promote and maintain the normal digestive flora in the digestive tract. Horses that habitually or continuously consume sand and other undigestible feedstuffs should be maintained on EQUINE ENTERIC COLLOID for as long as signs of undigested feed or foreign matter persist in the stool or feces. The electrolytes in EQUINE ENTERIC COLLOID are similar to those found in Equine Bluelite™, and the two products may be used together when signs of dehydration are observed.
4. Measure enclosed: Holds approximately 2 oz. of EQUINE ENTERIC COLLOID.

Caution(s): EQUINE ENTERIC COLLOID should be administered via a stomach tube by a veterinarian and prescribed for therapeutic and prophylactic use by the attending veterinarian. EQUINE ENTERIC COLLOID is specifically designed to help provide a stool-softening and lubricating action. Several intestinal impactions or digestive tract disorders may require alternative therapy and additional treatment as determined by the attending veterinarian.

For equine and veterinary use only. Keep out of the reach of children.

Presentation: 4x5 lb. (2.27 kg) pails (20 lb. case).

Compendium Code No.: 11440070

EQUINE EWTF

Merial **Toxoid-Vaccine**

Encephalomyelitis-Influenza Vaccine, Eastern & Western Killed Virus-Tetanus Toxoid

U.S. Vet. Lic. No.: 298

Description: EQUINE EWTF is a combination of inactivated, purified, concentrated and adjuvanted eastern and western equine encephalomyelitis virus, influenza subtypes A1 and A2 and tetanus toxoid. Influenza virus subtypes A1 and A2 confer protection against Kentucky 93, Kentucky 81, Fountainbleau 79, Kentucky 87 and other pertinent U.S. and European strains.

Contains neomycin, polymyxin B and nystatin as preservatives.

Indications: Recommended for vaccination of healthy horses against eastern and western equine encephalomyelitis, influenza and tetanus.

Dosage and Administration: For primary vaccination, aseptically administer 1 mL (1 dose) intramuscularly in healthy horses. Revaccinate with a second 1 mL dose 3 to 4 weeks later. A 1 mL dose should be administered annually and at any time epidemic conditions exist or are reported and exposure is imminent.

Precaution(s): Store at 2-7°C (35-45°F). Shake well before using.

Caution(s): In rare instances, administration of vaccines may cause lethargy, fever, and inflammatory or hypersensitivity types of reactions. Treatment may include antihistamines, anti-inflammatories, and/or epinephrine. A local reaction may occur if given subcutaneously. Injury should be followed by a booster dose of vaccine containing tetanus toxoid.

Sold to veterinarians only. For veterinary use only.

Warning(s): Do not vaccinate within 21 days of slaughter.

Presentation: 5 x 1 dose (1 mL) and 3 x 10 dose (10 mL).

Compendium Code No.: 11110101 RM429RM2 / RM426RM2

EQUINE F.A./PLUS GRANULES

Pala-Tech **Dietary Supplement**

Omega Fatty Acids, Vitamins and Minerals

Active Ingredient(s): Composition: Each 30 gram scoop of Pala-Tech™ EQUINE F.A./PLUS GRANULES (1 scoop) contains:

Microencapsulated Fatty Acids
Flaxseed Oil . . . . . 6,000 mg
Vitamins
Vitamin A . . . . . 4,500 I.U.
Vitamin E . . . . . 30 I.U.
Choline . . . . . 60 mg
Minerals
Zinc (from zinc amino acid chelate) . . . . . 30 mg
Selenium (from selenium amino acid chelate) . . . . . 30 mcg

Indications: Pala-Tech™ EQUINE F.A./PLUS GRANULES is a supplemental source of omega fatty acids and other essential vitamins and minerals. For supplementation of the diet to aid in the maintenance of healthy skin and haircoat in horses.

Dosage and Administration: Dosage: Consult with your veterinarian to determine the proper dosage level and schedule for each individual horse prescribed this product. The recommended dosage schedule for the daily administration of Pala-Tech™ EQUINE F.A./PLUS GRANULES is as follows:

Initial dose (3-4 weeks): 2 scoops/day Maintenance dose: 1 scoop/day

Administration: A 30 gram scoop is enclosed in the container. Measure out the prescribed daily dose and administer over the horse's grain. Product may be mixed with grain, if necessary, to facilitate complete consumption. Pala-Tech™ EQUINE F.A./PLUS GRANULES is formulated with a proprietary, highly palatable molasses and apple flavor base to enhance acceptance by the horse.

Precaution(s): Store at room temperature; (58°F-86°F). Avoid excessive heat.

Warning(s): Keep out of reach of children. For veterinary use only.

Presentation: 1,800 gram container.

Compendium Code No.: 10680060 9901-0699

EQUINE HOOFPRO™ COPPER FORMULATION

SSI Corp. **Hoof Product**

Non-Petroleum Based Ionic Copper Suspension

Active Ingredient(s):

Copper (Cu) 0.67%
Sulfur (S) 2.2%
Inert 99.33%

Indications: Specially formulated as an aid in the treatment and prevention of thrush, seedy toe/white line disease, scratches, heel cracks. Eliminates foul odors. Will not stain, burn, cause hair loss or dry out the hoof. Non-flammable and odor free.

Formulated for horses and ponies.

Directions: Before treatment, clean hoof thoroughly removing debris and dead tissue.

For use as a direct topical application, mix equal parts of EQUINE HOOFPRO™ and water. Spray or drench liberally over the affected area.

As a soak, mix one ounce of EQUINE HOOFPRO™ per one gallon of water. Stand the animal in the solution for at least ten minutes. Environmental conditions may require cleaning and redosing more than once per day.

Precaution(s): Do not allow to freeze.

Caution(s): Eye irritant. In case of eye contact, flush for 15 minutes. If irritation persists, call a physician.

Warning(s): Keep out of the reach of children.

Presentation: 1 and 2.5 gallon containers.

Compendium Code No.: 14930001

EQUINE HOOFPRO™ ZINC FORMULATION

SSI Corp. **Hoof Product**

Non-Petroleum Based Zinc Suspension

Active Ingredient(s):

Zinc (Zn) 1.43%
Sulfur (S) 3.25%
Inert 95.29%

Indications: Specially formulated as an aid in the treatment and prevention of thrush, seedy toe/white line disease, scratches, heel cracks. Eliminates foul odors. Will not stain, burn, cause hair loss or dry out the hoof. Non-flammable and odor free.

Formulated for horses and ponies.
Directions: Before treatment, clean hoof thoroughly removing debris and dead tissue.

For use as a direct topical application, mix equal parts of EQUINE HOOFPRO™ and water. Spray or drench liberally over the affected area.

As a soak, mix one ounce of EQUINE HOOFPRO™ per one gallon of water. Stand the animal in the solution for at least ten minutes. Environmental conditions may require cleaning and redosing more than once per day.
Precaution(s): Do not allow to freeze.
Caution(s): Eye irritant. In case of eye contact, flush for 15 minutes. If irritation persists, call a physician.
Warning(s): Keep out of the reach of children.
Presentation: 1 and 2.5 gallon containers.
Compendium Code No.: 14930011

EQUINE IgG FOALIMMUNE®

Lake Immunogenics — **Plasma**

U.S. Vet. Lic. No.: 318
Active Ingredient(s): Each single bag contains plasma as a source of equine IgG with sodium citrate as an anticoagulant derived from healthy horses with no A or Q r.b.c. factors or no serum r.b.c. antibodies. All donor horses are negative for EIA and EVA. There is no preservative added.
Indications: For intravenous use in the treatment of failure of passive transfer in the equine neonate at the rate of 20 mL/kg body weight.

The diagnosis of failure of passive transfer should be established from a blood sample taken at least 18 hours after birth.
Dosage and Administration: Keep frozen until use. Thaw quickly not exceeding 120°F. Administer by filtered intravenous infusion. Discard the unused portion. In case of a reaction, marked most often by tenesmus and hyperventilation, slow the speed of administration. If this does not abate the signs, stop administration until signs abate, then continue at a slower rate. If signs persist suspend administration and treat with histamine blockers and anti-inflammatory agents. Administration may be attempted again after treatment to relieve the adverse response has been successful.
Caution(s): The possibility of transmission of viral disease is possible with the administration of any blood product. This is a rare occurrence.

For veterinary use only.
Presentation: 950 mL.
Compendium Code No.: 11190000

EQUINE IgG HIGAMM-EQUI™

Lake Immunogenics — **Plasma**

U.S. Vet. Lic. No.: 318
Active Ingredient(s): Each single bag contains plasma as a source of equine IgG with sodium citrate as an anticoagulant derived from healthy horses with no A or Q r.b.c. factors or no serum r.b.c. antibodies. All donor horses are negative for EIA and EVA. There is no preservative added.
Indications: For intravenous use in the treatment of the failure of passive transfer in the equine neonate at the rate of 20 mL/kg body weight.

The diagnosis of failure of passive transfer should be established from a blood sample taken at least 18 hours after birth.
Dosage and Administration: Keep frozen until use. Thaw quickly not exceeding 120°F. Administer by filtered intravenous infusion. Discard the unused portion. In case of a reaction, marked most often by tenesmus and hyperventilation, slow the speed of administration. If this does not abate the signs, stop administration until signs abate, then continue at a slower rate. If signs persist suspend administration and treat with histamine blockers and anti-inflammatory agents. Administration may be attempted again after treatment to relieve the adverse response has been successful.
Caution(s): The possibility of transmission of viral disease is possible with the administration of any blood product. This is a rare occurrence.

For veterinary use only.
Presentation: 500 mL and 950 mL.
Compendium Code No.: 11190010

EQUINE IgG HIGH-GLO

Mg Biologics — **Equine Plasma**

U.S. Vet. Lic. No.: 614
Contents: Each bag contains equine plasma as a source of equine IgG with a minimum level of 2500 mg/dL. It is collected in a sterile closed system from healthy horses whom have tested negative for the antibodies against Aa, Ca, and Qa red cell antigens. Sodium citrate is used as an anticoagulant as part of the manufacturing process. It is frozen immediately after collection and as such does not contain preservatives.
Indications: An intravenous treatment for failure of passive transfer for neonatal foals.
Dosage and Administration: Dose at a rate of 20 mL/kg of body weight.

EQUINE IgG HIGH-GLO requires freezing until used. To thaw, submerge the frozen IgG in warm water (<115°F) for 10 minutes, squeezing the bag periodically to circulate for faster thawing. Warm the liquid plasma to body temperature using the warm water bath. Do not microwave this product. Administer with an IV administration kit with filter. Caution should be observed however, as occasionally intravenous infusion may result in shaking, sweating or hyperventilation. If this occurs, discontinue use for 5 to 10 minutes. Resume at a slower rate of infusion. If adverse reactions persist, discontinue use.
Caution(s): There is always the possibility, while rare, of transmission of viral disease in any blood product.
Presentation: 1,000 mL (other sizes available upon request).
Compendium Code No.: 12600001

EQUINE MEDICATED SHAMPOO

Vet Solutions — **Antidermatosis Shampoo**

Active Ingredient(s): 2% Chloroxylenol, 2% Salicylic Acid, 2% Sodium Thiosulfate (source of soluble sulfur).

Ingredients: Deionized Water, Sodium C14-16 Olefin Sulfonate, Propylene Glycol, Cocamide DEA, Polyquaternium-10, Fragrance, Citric Acid, Methylchloroisothiazolinone, Methylisothiazolinone, FD&C Blue No. 1.
Indications: Vet Solutions EQUINE MEDICATED SHAMPOO may be used as adjunctive therapy for the most common dermatological conditions. For use on horses.

Deep cleansing action, removes scales and crusts, antibacterial, antifungal, deodorizing, gentle for routine use.
Directions: Shake well. With tepid water, thoroughly wet animal's coat. Massage small amounts of shampoo into the coat while continuously adding water to get better dispersion. Continue until a generous lather is generated. Rinse well and repeat procedure. Shampoo may be used weekly or as often as recommended by your veterinarian.
Precaution(s): Storage: Store at controlled room temperature.
Caution(s): Keep out of reach of children. For topical use only. Avoid contact with eyes. If eye contact occurs, immediately flush with water. Sold exclusively through veterinarians.
Presentation: 32 fl. oz. (947 mL) and 1 gallon.
Compendium Code No.: 10610070 — 990902

EQUINE PAIN BLOCK GEL

First Priority — **Analgesic-Topical**

Active Ingredient(s): Contains capsaicin 0.020%.

Ingredients: Water, carbomer 934, camomile extract (levonemol), cayenne pepper extract (capsaicin .020%), propylene glycol, polysorbate 20, triethanolamine, diazolidinyl urea, methyl paraben, propyl paraben, fragrance.
Indications: For the temporary relief of minor aches and pains associated with arthritis, tendinitis, strains, sprains and simple backaches in horses.
Dosage and Administration: Apply Approx: ½-1 oz to the desired area. Rub in until thoroughly absorbed. Clip hair on area to be treated if hair is excessively long. Apply to all sides of a joint where applicable. Do not apply to affected area more than 3-4 times per day. Wash hands after use.
Caution(s): For external use only. Avoid contact with eyes and mucous membranes. Do not apply to open cuts and sores. Discontinue use if excessive irritation occurs. If condition persists or worsens for more than seven days or clears up and occurs again discontinue use and consult a veterinarian. Do not use other than directed.
Warning(s): Keep out of reach of children. For animal use only.
Presentation: 8 oz (227 g) (NDC# 58829-223-08).
Compendium Code No.: 11390261

EQUINE POTOMAVAC®

Merial — **Bacterin**

Ehrlichia Risticii Bacterin
U.S. Vet. Lic. No.: 298
Description: EQUINE POTOMAVAC® is a liquid suspension of inactivated *Ehrlichia risticii*. The efficacy of this combination vaccine has been demonstrated in controlled vaccination challenge tests and the safety in thorough field evaluations.

Contains gentamicin as a preservative.
Indications: Recommended for the vaccination of healthy horses as an aid in the prevention of Potomac Horse Fever (equine monocytic ehrlichiosis) caused by *E. risticii*.
Dosage and Administration: For primary vaccination, acseptically administer 1 mL (1 dose) intramuscularly in healthy horses 3 months of age or older. Revaccinate with 1 dose 3 to 4 weeks later. Revaccinate annually with a single 1 mL dose.
Precaution(s): Store at 2-7°C (35-45°F). Do not freeze. Shake well before using. Use entire contents when first opened.
Caution(s): In rare instances, administration of vaccines may cause lethargy, fever, and inflammatory or hypersensitivity types of reactions. Treatment may include antihistamines, anti-inflammatories, and/or epinephrine. Vaccinating animals whose immune response is compromised by stress, disease, etc. may not product the desired results.

For veterinary use only.
Warning(s): Do not vaccinate within 21 days of slaughter.
Presentation: 5 x 1 dose (1 mL) and 3 x 10 dose (10 mL).
Sold to veterinarians only.
® Trademark of Merial.
Compendium Code No.: 11110482 — RM460RM2 / RM470RM2

EQUINE POTOMAVAC® + IMRAB®

Merial — **Bacterin-Vaccine**

Rabies Vaccine, Killed Virus-Ehrlichia Risticii Bacterin
U.S. Vet. Lic. No.: 298
Description: EQUINE POTOMAVAC® + IMRAB® is a liquid suspension of inactivated rabies virus propagated in a stable cell line, combined with an inactivated suspension of *Ehrlichia risticii*. The efficacy of this combination vaccine has been demonstrated in controlled vaccination challenge tests and the safety in thorough field evaluations.

Contains gentamicin as a preservative.
Indications: Recommended for the vaccination of healthy horses against disease caused by rabies virus and as an aid in the prevention of Potomac Horse Fever (equine monocytic ehrlichiosis) caused by *E. risticii*.
Dosage and Administration: For primary vaccination, aseptically administer 1 mL (1 dose) intramuscularly in healthy horses 3 months of age or older. For *E. risticii*, revaccinate with 1 dose 3 to 4 weeks later using this product or Equine Potomavac®. Revaccinate annually with a single 1 mL dose.
Precaution(s): Store at 2-7°C (35-45°F). Do not freeze. Shake well before using.
Caution(s): In rare instances, administration of vaccines may cause lethargy, fever, and inflammatory or hypersensitivity types of reactions. Treatment may include antihistamines, anti-inflammatories, and/or epinephrine. Vaccinating animals whose immune response is compromised by stress, disease, etc. may not produce the desired results.

For veterinary use only.
Warning(s): Do not vaccinate within 21 days of slaughter.
Presentation: 5 x 1 dose (1 mL) and 3 x 10 dose (10 mL).
Sold to veterinarians only.
® Trademark of Merial.
Compendium Code No.: 11110491 — RM424RM4 / RM425RM4

EQUINE PSYLLIUM

First Priority — **Laxative**

Psyllium Hydrophilic Mucilloid
Guaranteed Analysis:
Crude Fiber . . . . Max. 60.0%

Ingredients: Psyllium Seed Husk, Dextrose, Artificial Flavor.
Indications: A natural fiber product, psyllium is a multi-active fiber that encourages normal elimination without the use of chemical stimulants.
Directions for Use: Add 2 scoops (4 oz) to the feed for 3 days. Discontinue feeding EQUINE

PSYLLIUM for the next 3 days, then repeat with a 3 day feeding. Continue feeding EQUINE PSYLLIUM on 3 days, and off for 3 days for a 30 day period. After 30 days, feed 2 scoops (4 oz) of EQUINE PSYLLIUM once every 7 days or as directed by your veterinarian.

Precaution(s): Storage: Store at controlled room temperature between 15°-30°C (59°-86°F). Keep container tightly closed when not in use.

Caution(s): For animal use only.

Warning(s): Keep out of reach of children.

Presentation: 28 oz (794 g) (NDC# 58829-237-28), 56 oz (1.59 kg), 10 lb (4.5 kg) (NDC# 58829-237-07) and 30 lb (13.6 kg) (NDC# 58829-237-30) pails.

Compendium Code No.: 11390273 Rev. 07-01 / Iss. 03-97 / Rev. 09-99 / Rev. 08-01

EQUINE-RID TEST

V.D.I. **IgG Test**

Active Ingredient(s): An immunodiffusion plate containing antiserum to equine IgG in agarose gel.

Indications: The product is used for the quantification of equine IgG by radial immunodiffusion.

Test Principles: Radial immunodiffusion is based on the diffusion of antigen from a circular well radial into a homogeneous gel containing specific antiserum for each particular antigen. A circle of precipitated antigen and antibody forms, and continues to grow until the equilibrium is reached. The diameters of the rings are a function of antigen concentration. After overnight incubation, the zone diameters of reference sera are plotted against the logarithm (base 10) of the antigen concentration. If equilibrium is reached, the reference sera zone diameters are squared and plotted against their concentration (linear). At intervals in between, a linear relationship does not occur. Unknown concentrations are measured by reference to the standard curve.

Test Procedure: A means of measuring five (5) microliters is required to do the test. Suitable pipettes may be supplied if necessary. The test will work with either plasma or serum.

1. Reagents:

A. Radial immunodiffusion plates contain specific antiserum in agarose gel, 0.1M phosphate buffer pH 7.0, 0.1% sodium azide as a bacteriostatic agent, 1 mcg/mL amphotericin B as an antifungal agent. The plates also contain 0.002M ethylenediaminetetraacetic acid. Store in a refrigerator at temperatures of (2 to 8°C).

B. Equine reference sera - (pooled equine serum at three (3) levels*). Contains sodium azide (0.1%) as a bacteriostatic agent. Store at refrigerator temperature.

2. Specimen Preparation and Handling:

A. Collect whole blood without anticoagulant and allow it to clot at room temperature.

B. Separate the serum by centrifugation at approximately 200 rcf within two (2) to three (3) hours after collection.

C. Plasma may be used, but nonspecific precipitation of fibrin may obscure the precipitation rings. In addition, liquid anticoagulants such as ACD fluid will dilute the specimen.

D. Caution: As noted above, 1B - the unknown specimens should be treated as infectious.

3. Procedure:

A. Materials Provided:

1. Three (3) radial immunodiffusion plates.
2. Reference sera 3 x 0.25 mis.
3. Directions for use.

B. Materials Required:

1. Blood collection tubes.
2. Centrifuge (200 rcf).
3. Microliter dispenser (5 microliters).
4. Reference sera (required if not provided in kit form).
5. Normal control sera (optional) - available separately.
6. Measuring device - calibrated in 0.1 mm increments.
7. Two cycle semi-logarithmic graph paper and/or linear graph paper.

C. General:

1. Do not overfill or underfill the wells. An improperly filled well yields erroneous results and the same specimen should be placed in another well. Overfilling with a five (5) microliter sample indicates that some gel shrinkage has occurred.
2. The reference serum zone diameters should be measured at the same time as the test sera. If a delay in the measurement is anticipated, allow sufficient intervals between filling the wells.
3. The time of filling each plate should be marked on the cover and if more than one (1) plate is filled, they should be read in order of filling.
4. Excess moisture is required to prevent drying. Replace each plate in its plastic bag and reseal it carefully before incubation.
5. The shrinkage of gel or oval shaped wells indicate drying and the plate should not be used.
6. If temperature fluctuations are anticipated, the plates in their bags may be incubated in an insulated container. Fluctuations in temperature may result in multiple precipitin ring formation.
7. The unused sections may be run at a later day if the plate has been stored at 2 to 8°C between incubations in its plastic bag. Check carefully for any evidence of drying.
8. Rough granulation of the gel indicates freezing, therefore the plates should be discarded.

D. Performance of Test:

1. Remove the plates from the refrigerator to room temperature (approximately 30 minutes) before filling the wells. Do not open the bag until it is ready for use.
2. If excess moisture is present, remove the plate from the bag and remove the cover until evaporation has dried the surface and the wells. Replace the cover until it is ready to be used.
3. For the best results, three (3) wells should be filled with reference sera for each plate. The location of each should be noted. Mix each vial of reference serum thoroughly.
4. Deliver the specimen to the well by placing the pipette tip at the bottom of the well. Allow the well to fill to the top of the agar surface. Avoid bubbles to ensure proper volume and diffusion of the sample. Visualization may be aided by placing the plate on a dark background. If practice is required, a used plate may be utilized.
5. More consistent results may be obtained when the wells are filled with a five (5) microliter pipette.
6. Mark the time of the completion on the plate cover and replace the cover.
7. Replace the plate in the bag and reseal it carefully.
8. Incubate the plates in an upright position on a flat surface at room temperature (20-24°C) for 16-20 hours for overnight readings and over 48 hours for end point readings. See C6 above.

E. Calibration:

1. Using the reference sera provided in the kits, determine their ring diameters to the nearest 0.1 mm.
2. Using 2 or 3 cycle semi-logarithmic graph paper, plot the concentration on the Y axis and the zone diameters on the linear or X axis for each protein for overnight readings.
3. Using regular graph paper, plot the concentration on the X axis and the zone diameters squared on the Y axis for each protein for end point readings.
4. Draw a straight line of "best fit" between the three (3) points. A curved line usually indicates that the incubation time and/or temperature should be reduced for overnight values. For valid results, a smooth curve should be fitted to the points and control sera included for additional verification.

F. Quality Control: For consistent results and a comparison of lot to lot, day to day, and week to week variations, a "normal" and abnormal serum should be included each day. The diameters and concentrations obtained can be charted to determine means and standard deviations. For the same specimen, an appropriate series of the wells on the same plate should yield diameters within 0.2 mm of one another. The control sera should be freshly thawed or reconstituted.

G. Reference Sera: All reference sera supplied have been calibrated from two (2) standard sera. The standard sera were calibrated against the appropriate purified proteins.

E

4. Results: Determine the concentration of each unknown of the specimen protein by reading its zone diameter on the reference curve and the corresponding concentration from the X axis. The zone diameter must be squared for end point calibration.

5. Interpretation of Results and Limitation of the Procedure:

A. When an unknown diameter exceeds that of the top standard, the specimen should be diluted with saline and rerun.

B. When an unknown diameter is smaller than that of the lowest standard, its concentration should be reported as "less than" the concentration of the reference serum. If available, "low level" radial immunodiffusion plates may be utilized.

C. Lack of a precipitin ring may be due to:

1. The sample not applied to the well.
2. A concentration too low to be detected by the method.
3. A concentration too high, resulting in the formation of soluble complexes, which are not precipitated.

D. The plates do not measure substitute colostrum sources of IgG from goats, sheep or cows.

6. Expected Values: The incidence of failure of passive transfer (FPT) of immunoglobulins has been estimated to be between 2.9 and 25%.[3,4,5] Partial passive transfer has been defined as immunoglobulin levels of 200 to 400 mg/dl. The total failure of passive transfer has less than 200 mg/dl.

The minimum level of IgG necessary to protect a foal from infection depends upon a number of factors, including the types of bacteria in the environment, management and stress factors and the colostral antibody titer against specific bacteria in the environment. Evidence suggests that foals should have IgG concentrations greater than 800 mg/dl.

The half-life of IgG from colostrum is 20 to 23 days[6,7] therefore serum immunoglobulin levels are at their lowest between one (1) to two (2) months of age.[8,9]

These values are intended as a guideline - each laboratory should establish its own "normal" range. Values vary with age and should be established separately.

7. Performance Characteristics:

A. For investigational use only. The performance characteristics of the product have not been established.

Precaution(s): Store the plate upside down in a refrigerator.

Avoid jarring and freezing temperatures.

Discussion: Single radial immunodiffusion tests have evolved from the work of Fahey and McKelvey[1] and Mancini et al.[2] They are specific for the various proteins in serum or other fluids and depend upon the reaction of each protein with its specific antibody.

Immunoglobulin G (IgG) is one of the first line of defenses against encapsulated bacterial and streptococci. The majority of the newborns IgG is obtained from the dam's colostrum in the first 16 hours after birth, providing the foal nurses. This is called passive transfer. In passive transfer, the IgG from colostrum provides antibodies to infectious agents that the dam has been exposed to, or immunized against. The time it takes IgG to drop to half its original titer in mammals ranges from 20 to 30 days. The foal can start producing its own IgG in sufficient quantities after 30 to 80 days.

References: Available upon request.

Presentation: 24 wells.

Compendium Code No.: 11280020

EQUINE ROTAVIRUS VACCINE

Fort Dodge **Vaccine**

Equine Rotavirus Vaccine, Killed Virus

U.S. Vet. Lic. No.: 112

Contents: This product contains the antigen listed above.

Thimerosal, neomycin, polymixin B and amphotericin B added as preservatives.

Indications: For vaccination of pregnant mares to provide passive transfer of antibodies to foals against equine rotavirus.

Dosage and Administration: Pregnant mares, inject one 1 mL dose intramuscularly at the eighth month of pregnancy using aseptic technique. Administer a second 1 mL dose one month later (i.e., at the ninth month of pregnancy). A third 1 mL dose is then given one month later (i.e., at the tenth month of pregnancy). Each pregnancy requires vaccination with 3 doses.

Precaution(s): Store in dark at 2° to 7°C (35° to 45°F). Avoid freezing. Shake well. Use entire contents when first opened.

Caution(s): This product is conditionally licensed by the USDA while additional efficacy and potency data are being developed.

In case of anaphylactoid reaction, administer epinephrine.

For veterinary use only.

Warning(s): Do not vaccinate within 21 days before slaughter.

Presentation: 10 doses (10 mL vial).

Compendium Code No.: 10030661 2613C

EQUINE THYROID SUPPLEMENT ℞

Pala-Tech **Thyroid Therapy**

Levothyroxine Sodium, USP

Active Ingredient(s): Composition: Each pound (454 grams) contains:

Levothyroxine Sodium, USP .... 0.22% (1.0 g)

One level scoop (approx. 5.5 grams) delivers approximately 12 mg of T4 (Levothyroxine Sodium, USP).

Pala-Tech™ EQUINE THYROID SUPPLEMENT is formulated with a proprietary, highly palatable molasses and apple flavor base to enhance acceptance by the horse.

Indications: For use in horses for correction of conditions associated with low circulating thyroid hormone (hypothyroidism).

Dosage and Administration: Dosage: The suggested initial dosage is 0.5 to 3.0 mg levothyroxine sodium (T-4) per 100 pounds of body weight (1 to 6 mg per 100 kg) once per day or in divided doses. Response to the administration of Pala-Tech™ EQUINE THYROID SUPPLEMENT (Levothyroxine Sodium, USP) should be evaluated clinically until an adequate maintenance dose is established. In most horses, this is usually in the range of 6 to 36 mg total daily dose of T-4. Serum T-3 and T-4 values can vary greatly among individual horses on thyroid supplementation. Dosages should be individualized and animals should be monitored daily for clinical signs of hyperthyroidism or hypersensitivity.

Administration: A 5.5 gram scoop is enclosed in the container. Measure out the prescribed dose and administer by mixing the daily dose in the concentrate or by top dressing on grain, preferably rolled or ground.

Precaution(s): Store at room temperature; 15°C-30°C (59°F-86°F) and protect from light. Avoid excessive heat.

Caution(s): Federal law restricts this drug to use by or on the order of a licensed veterinarian.

Administer with caution to animals with clinically significant heart disease, hypertension or other complications for which a sharply increased metabolic rate might prove hazardous. Use in pregnant mares has not been evaluated.

For use in horses only.

Presentation: Available in two package sizes: 454 gram (1 pound) easy-to-open container and 4,540 gram (10 pound) pail with metal handle.

Compendium Code No.: 10680070 4001-0699

EQUINIME®

Chariton **Large Animal Dietary Supplement**

Active Ingredient(s): Each scoop contains:

Vitamins: A, B_1 (thiamine), B_2 (riboflavin), B_6, K_1, chlorine, biotin and niacin.

Minerals: Calcium, iron, zinc, copper, potassium and magnesium.

Amino acids: Valine, lysine, arginine, isoleucine, methionine, proline, serine and aspartic acid.

Indications: A food supplement for horses in training and breeding.

Dosage and Administration: EQUINIME® can be fed at different times depending on the daily routine:

1. If the horse usually works in the morning, two (2) scoops sprinkled over the morning feed.
2. If the horse usually works in the afternoon, one (1) scoop in the morning feed, one (1) scoop in the afternoon feed. (If the horse is fed only morning and night, combine both in the morning feed.)
3. EQUINIME® can be used two (2) hours prior to any performance.

Feed two (2) to four (4) scoops, depending upon temperament. Two (2) scoops is the average amount. Because of the characteristics of the product, the amount can be increased, if needed, for certain horses. If more information is needed, consult a veterinarian.

Presentation: 2 lb. and 5 lb. sizes.

Compendium Code No.: 13720000

EQUI-PHAR™ ARTHRIBAN

Vedco **Non-Steroidal Anti-Inflammatory**

Microencapsulated Palatable Granules

Active Ingredient(s): Each 39 cc scoop contains 2500 mg/aspirin.

ArthriBan equine granules contain microencapsulated buffered aspirin in a nutritious highly palatable flavor base.

Indications: ArthriBan aids in the temporary relief of pain and inflammation associated with arthritis, laminitis, chronic joint disease and soft tissue pain in horses.

Dosage and Administration: Usual dose for arthritis, lameness and joint pain is one scoop per 1000 lb body weight twice daily. For muscular pain the usual dose is 3 scoops per 1000 lb given twice daily.

Give one level scoop twice daily at or before feeding.

Caution(s): If diarrhea occurs, stop administration and consult a veterinarian. Keep out of reach of children. For horses only.

Presentation: 700 grams.

Compendium Code No.: 10940641

EQUI-PHAR™ BENZAGEL

Vedco **Liniment**

NDC No.: 50989-087-26

Active Ingredient(s): Contains: Benzocaine, camphor, menthol, thymol, witch hazel, isopropyl alcohol in a specially prepared base.

Indications: A topical anesthetic, coolant gel to be used for temporary relief of minor muscle stiffness and soreness due to overexertion.

Dosage and Administration:

For horses in training: Use before and after workouts, under bandages, either wet or dry.

In shipping horses: Apply on legs and use a cotton bandage. BenzaGel will not burn or blister under bandages.

Method of Use: Be certain skin and hair are clean. It is advised that the area to be treated be washed first. Apply by rubbing deeply into hair in the first application, ensuring contact with the skin. Following first application, apply a generous amount for the second application. Use as often as indicated.

For using as a diluted application the indications are: Use after strenuous exercise for any type of performance animal.

Use as a therapeutic bodywash when coolant is indicated.

Directions for Using: Mix 2 tablespoons of BenzaGel into a quart of warm water. Apply with a sponge, covering the horse's entire body. Use a brisk rubbing motion when applying. Guard against creating heat or irritation by overrubbing.

Racetracks: When saliva and urine tests are to be conducted, do not administer before or after racing as horses may pick up components by licking and the ingredients may show up on testing.

Precaution(s): Store in a cool, dry area. Do not store near heat.

Caution(s): Keep out of the reach of children. Avoid contact with eyes and mucous membranes. If the condition for which this preparation is used persists, or if a rash develops, discontinue use and consult your veterinarian.

BenzaGel may be used concentrated or diluted depending on the condition. It will not burn or blister.

Do not apply any other type of external medicants to the same area where BenzaGel has been administered.

It is important to keep the cap on tightly, thereby avoiding evaporation.

Warning(s): Not for use on food producing animals.

Presentation: 1 lb.

Compendium Code No.: 10940650

EQUI-PHAR™ BISMUKOTE PASTE

Vedco **Antidiarrheal-Adsorbent**

Active Ingredient(s): Bismuth subsalicylate, magnesium aluminum silicate, xanthan, benzoic acid, sorbic acid, sucrose, apple flavor, artificial colors, salicylic acid, sodium salicylate, sodium saccharine.

Indications: For horses, as an aid in the treatment and prevention of diarrhea or gastrointestinal inflammation.

Dosage and Administration: Use 5cc per 100 pounds of body weight 3 to 4 times per day, or as directed by a veterinarian. 5cc BISMUKOTE PASTE = 1 g bismuth subsalicylate.

Caution(s): Hospitalization, and oral or intravenous hydration may be necessary in cases of diarrhea or gastrointestinal inflammation. Consult your veterinarian if signs of depression, fever, vomiting, diarrhea, or abdominal discomfort persist. This beneficial medication may cause a temporary and harmless darkening of the tongue and stool.

Presentation: 60cc/60g tube.

Compendium Code No.: 10940660

EQUI-PHAR™ CAUSTIC POWDER

Vedco **Topical Wound Dressing**

Active Ingredient(s):

Copper sulfate • $5H_2O$ .... 51.5% w/w

Chloroxylenol .... 1.0% w/w

In a free-flowing starch base. Not sterilized.

Indications: For use as an aid in the management of slow-healing surface wounds of horses and mules.

Dosage and Administration: Apply the powder freely to wounds twice a day. Repeat as indicated.

Precaution(s): Do not store above 30°C (86°F). Keep the container tightly closed when not in use.

Caution(s): For external use only.

For veterinarian use only.

Keep out of the reach of children.

Restricted drug. Use only as directed.

In case of deep or puncture wounds or serious burns, consult a veterinarian. If redness, irritation, or swelling persists or increases, discontinue use and consult a veterinarian.

Warning(s): Not for use on animals intended for food.

Presentation: 5 oz. (142 g) containers.

Compendium Code No.: 10940670

EQUI-PHAR™ COOLGEL ℞

Vedco **Liniment**

Active Ingredient(s): Contains: Camphor, menthol, thymol, magnesium sulfate, sodium sulfate, sodium chloride, sodium bicarbonate, sodium borate, iodine, potassium iodide, ferrous sulfate, lithium chloride, aluminum sulfate, sodium sesquicarbonate, witch hazel, isopropyl alcohol in a specially prepared base.

Indications: A topical anesthetic, mineral coolant gel to be used for the temporary relief of minor muscle stiffness and soreness due to overexertion.

Dosage and Administration:

For horses in training: Use before and after workouts, under bandages, either wet or dry.

When shipping horses: Apply on the legs and use a cotton bandage.

Method of Use: Be certain that the skin and hair are clean. It is advised that the area to be treated be washed first. Apply by rubbing deeply into the hair in the first application, ensuring contact with the skin. Following the first application, apply a generous amount for the second application. Use as often as indicated.

For using as a diluted application the indications are: Use after strenuous exercise for any type of performance animal.

Use as a therapeutic bodywash when a mineral coolant is indicated.

Directions for Using: Mix two (2) tablespoons of CoolGel into one (1) quart of warm water. When small crystals form, releasing minerals and the medicants, apply with a sponge, covering the horse's entire body. Use a brisk rubbing motion when applying. Guard against creating heat or irritation by overrubbing.

Precaution(s): Store in a cool, dry area. Do not store near heat.

Caution(s): Federal law restricts this drug to use by or on the order of a licensed veterinarian.

Keep out of the reach of children. Avoid contact with the eyes and mucous membranes. If the condition for which the preparation is used persists, or if a rash develops, discontinue use and consult a veterinarian.

CoolGel may be used concentrated or diluted depending upon the condition. It will not burn or blister.

Do not apply any other type of external medicants to the same area where CoolGel has been administered.

It is important to keep the cap on tightly, thereby avoiding evaporation.

Warning(s): Not for use on food producing animals.

Presentation: 1 lb.

Compendium Code No.: 10940680

EQUI-PHAR™ DL-METHIONINE WITH BIOTIN POWDER

Vedco **Large Animal Dietary Supplement**

Ingredient(s): Biotin, methionine, calcium carbonate, alfalfa meal, natural and artificial flavors.
Indications: A palatable nutritional source of biotin and methionine, the essential amino acid for feed supplementation. Intended for intermittent or supplemental feeding only.
Dosage and Administration: Provide the following daily according to body weight:

Under 1000 pounds - 1 tsp
1000 to 1200 pounds - 2 tsp
Over 1200 pounds - 4 tsp

Mix with daily ration. Feed may be moistened with water and top dressed to promote proper adhesion of powder to feed.
Caution(s): For animal use only.
Presentation: 1 lb.
Compendium Code No.: 10940690

EQUI-PHAR™ ELECTRAMINO PASTE

Vedco **Electrolytes-Oral**

Active Ingredient(s): Amino acid chelates with electrolytes:

Calcium	600 mg
Magnesium	600 mg
Potassium	2 g
Sodium chloride	4 g
L-Glutamine	100 mg
Amino acid	22 g

In a molasses base.
Indications: An electrolyte paste for use in athletic horses to help replenish electrolytes lost during times of stress, sweating, or hard exercise.
Dosage and Administration: Insert the paste as far to the rear of the mouth as is practical. Deliver the entire syringe, or give half one (1) hour before the event and half immediately after. After administration, the horse's mouth may be rinsed with a syringe filled with water if desired.
Precaution(s): The manufacturer recommends use at room temperature. Do not freeze.
Caution(s): For veterinary use only.
Presentation: 60 g syringe.
Compendium Code No.: 10940700

EQUI-PHAR™ ELECTROLYTE WITH DEXTROSE ℞

Vedco **Electrolyte Injection**

NDC No.: 50989-128-16
Active Ingredient(s): Each 500 mL of sterile aqueous solution contains:

Dextrose • H_2O	12.50 g
Sorbitol	12.50 g
Sodium lactate	3.95 g
Sodium chloride	2.40 g
Potassium chloride	0.37 g
Magnesium chloride • $6H_2O$	0.21 g
Calcium chloride • $2H_2O$	0.19 g

Milliequivalents per liter:
Cations:

Sodium	153 mEq/L
Potassium	9 mEq/L
Calcium	6 mEq/L
Magnesium	4 mEq/L

Anions:

Chloride	101 mEq/L
Lactate	71 mEq/L

Indications: For use in conditions associated with fluid and electrolyte loss, such as dehydration, shock, vomiting and diarrhea, particularly when an immediate source of energy is also indicated.
Dosage and Administration: Warm the solution to body temperature and administer slowly (10 to 30 mL per minute) by intravenous or interperitoneal injection, using strict aseptic procedures.

Adult Cattle and Horses	1,000 to 2,000 mL
Calves, Ponies, and Foals	500 to 1,000 mL
Adult Sheep and Swine	500 to 1,000 mL
Pigs	100 to 500 mL

These are suggested dosages. The actual amount and rate of fluid administration must be judged by the veterinarian in relation to the condition being treated and the clinical response of the animal, being careful to avoid overhydration.
Contraindication(s): Do not administer intraperitoneally to horses.
Precaution(s): Store at a controlled room temperature between 15° and 30°C (59°-86°F).
Caution(s): Federal law restricts this drug to use by or on the order of a licensed veterinarian.
The product does not contain preservatives. Use the entire contents when first opened. Discard any unused solution.
For animal use only.
Keep out of the reach of children.
Presentation: 500 mL containers.
Compendium Code No.: 10940710

EQUI-PHAR™ EQUIGESIC™ ℞

Vedco **Analgesic-Anti-inflammatory**

Flunixin Meglumine Injection 50 mg/mL
ANADA No.: 200-124
Active Ingredient(s): Each milliliter contains:

Flunixin Meglumine equivalent to Flunixin	50 mg
Edetate Disodium	0.1 mg
Sodium Formaldehyde Sulfoxylate	2.5 mg
Diethanolamine	4.0 mg
Propylene Glycol	207.2 mg
Phenol (as preservative)	5.0 mg
Water for Injection	q.s.

With hydrochloric acid to adjust pH.
Indications: EQUIGESIC™ (flunixin meglumine injection) is recommended for the alleviation of inflammation and pain associated with musculoskeletal disorders in the horse.
It is also recommended for the alleviation of visceral pain associated with colic in the horse.
Pharmacology: Flunixin meglumine is a potent, non-narcotic, nonsteroidal, analgesic agent with anti-inflammatory and antipyretic activity. It is significantly more potent than pentazocine, meperidine, and codeine as an analgesic in the rat yeast paw test. Flunixin is four times as potent on a mg-per-mg basis as phenylbutazone as measured by the reduction in lameness and swelling in the horse. Plasma half-life in horse serum is 1.6 hours following a single dose of 1.1 mg/kg. Measurable amounts are detectable in horse plasma at 8 hours post injection.
Dosage and Administration: The recommended dose for musculoskeletal disorders is 0.5 mg per pound (1 mL/100 lbs) of body weight once daily. Treatment may be given by intravenous or intramuscular injection and repeated for up to 5 days. Studies show onset of activity is within 2 hours. Peak response occurs between 12 and 16 hours and duration of activity is 24-36 hours.
The recommended dose for the alleviation of pain associated with equine colic is 0.5 mg per pound of body weight. Intravenous administration is recommended for prompt relief. Clinical studies show pain is alleviated in less than 15 minutes in many cases. Treatment may be repeated when signs of colic recur. During clinical studies approximately 10% of the horses required one or two additional treatments. The cause of colic should be determined and treated with concomitant therapy.
Contraindication(s): There are no known contraindications to this drug when used as directed. Intra-arterial injection should be avoided. Horses inadvertently injected intra-arterially can show adverse reactions. Signs can be ataxia, incoordination, hyperventilation, hysteria, and muscle weakness. Signs are transient and disappear without antidotal medication within a few minutes. Do not use in horses showing hypersensitivity to flunixin meglumine.
Precaution(s): Store between 2° and 30°C (36° and 86°F).
Caution(s): Federal law restricts this drug to use by or on the order of a licensed veterinarian.
The effect of EQUIGESIC™ (flunixin meglumine injection) on pregnancy has not been determined. Studies to determine activity of EQUIGESIC™ (flunixin meglumine injection) when administered concomitantly with other drugs have not been conducted. Drug compatibility should be monitored closely in patients requiring adjunctive therapy. Isolated reports of local reactions following intramuscular injection, particularly in the neck, have been received. These include localized swelling, sweating, induration, and stiffness.
Warning(s): Not for use in horses intended for food.
For animal use only. Keep out of reach of children.
Toxicology: Toxicity studies were conducted in horses. A 3-fold intramuscular dose of 1.5 mg per pound of body weight daily for 10 consecutive days was safe. No changes were observed in hematology, serum chemistry, or urinalysis values. Intravenous dosages of 0.5 mg/lb daily for 15 days; 1.5 mg/lb daily for 10 days; and 2.5 mg/lb daily for 5 days produced no changes in blood or urine parameters. No injection site irritation was observed following intramuscular injection of the 0.5 mg/lb recommended dose. Some irritation was observed following a 3-fold dose administered intramuscularly.
Adverse Reactions: Isolated reports of local reactions following intramuscular injection, particularly in the neck, have been received. These include localized swelling, sweating, induration, and stiffness. In rare instances, fatal or nonfatal clostridial infections or other infections have been reported in association with intramuscular use of EQUIGESIC™ (flunixin meglumine injection). In addition, rare instances of anaphylactic-like reactions, some of which may have been fatal, have been reported primarily following intravenous use.
Presentation: EQUIGESIC™ (flunixin meglumine injection), 50 mg/mL, is available in 100 mL and 250 mL multi-dose vials.
Manufactured by: Schering-Plough Animal Health Corp.
Compendium Code No.: 10940741

EQUI-PHAR EQUIGLIDE™ ℞

Vedco **Intrauterine Antibiotic**

(Amikacin Sulfate Solution)
ANADA No.: 200-181
Active Ingredient(s): The dosage form supplied is a sterile, colorless to light straw colored solution.
Each mL contains:

Amikacin (as the sulfate)	250 mg
Sodium citrate (as buffer)	25.1 mg
Sodium bisulfite	6.6 mg
Benzethonium chloride (as preservative)	0.1 mg
pH adjusted with sulfuric acid	
Water for injection	q.s.

Indications: EQUIGLIDE™ (Amikacin Sulfate Solution) is indicated for the treatment of uterine infections (endometritis, metritis and pyometra) in mares, when caused by susceptible organisms including *Escherichia coli, Pseudomonas* sp, and *Klebsiella* sp. The use of amikacin sulfate in eliminating infections caused by the above organisms has been shown clinically to improve fertility in infected mares.
While nearly all strains of *Escherichia coli, Pseudomonas* sp and *Klebsiella* sp, including those that are resistant to gentamicin, kanamycin or other aminoglycosides, are susceptible to amikacin at levels achieved following treatment, it is recommended that the invading organism be cultured and its susceptibility demonstrated as a guide to therapy. Amikacin susceptibility discs, 30 mcg, should be used for determining *in vitro* susceptibility.
Pharmacology: Description: Amikacin sulfate is a semisynthetic aminoglycoside antibiotic derived from kanamycin. It is $C_{22}H_{43}N_5O_{13}\bullet 2H_2SO_4$,D-streptamine, 0-3-amino-3-deoxy-α-D-glucopyranosyl-(1→6)-0-[6-amino-6-deoxy-α-D-glucopyranosyl-(1→4)-N[1]-(4-amino-2-hydroxy-1-oxobutyl)-2-deoxy-, (S)-, sulfate (1:2) (salt).

Action:
Antibacterial Activity: The effectiveness of EQUIGLIDE™ (Amikacin Sulfate Solution) in infections caused by *Escherichia coli, Pseudomonas* sp, and *Klebsiella* sp has been demonstrated clinically in the horse. In addition, the following microorganisms have been shown to be susceptible to amikacin *in vitro*,[1] although the clinical significance of this action has not been demonstrated in animals: *Enterobacter* sp, *Proteus mirabilis, Proteus* sp (indole positive),

Serratia marcescens, *Salmonella* sp, *Shigella* sp, *Providencia* sp, *Citrobacter freundii*, *Listeria monocytogenes*, *Staphylococcus aureus* (both penicillin resistant and penicillin sensitive).

The aminoglycoside antibiotics in general have limited activity against gram-positive pathogens, although *Staphylococcus aureus* and *Listeria monocytogenes* are susceptible to amikacin as noted above.

Amikacin has been shown to be effective against many aminoglycoside-resistant strains due to its ability to resist degradation by aminoglycoside inactivating enzymes known to affect gentamicin, tobramycin and kanamycin.[2]

Clinical Pharmacology:

Endometrial Tissue Concentrations: Comparisons of amikacin activity in endometrial biopsy tissue following intrauterine infusion with that following intramuscular injection of amikacin sulfate in mares demonstrate superior endometrial tissue concentrations when the drug is administered by the intrauterine route.

Intrauterine infusion of 2 grams EQUIGLIDE™ (Amikacin Sulfate Solution) daily for three consecutive days in mares results in peak concentrations typically exceeding 40 mcg/g of endometrial biopsy tissue within one hour after infusion. Twenty-four hours after each treatment amikacin activity is still detectable at concentrations averaging 2 to 4 mcg/g. However, the drug is not appreciably absorbed systemically following intrauterine infusion. Endometrial tissue concentrations following intramuscular injection roughly parallel, but are typically somewhat lower than corresponding serum concentrations of amikacin.

E

Safety: EQUIGLIDE™ (Amikacin Sulfate Solution) is non-irritating to equine endometrial tissue when infused into the uterus as directed (see "Dosage and Administration"). In laboratory animals as well as equine studies, the drug was generally found not to be irritating when injected intravenously, subcutaneously or intramuscularly.

Although amikacin, like other aminoglycosides, is potentially nephrotoxic, ototoxic and neurotoxic, parenteral (intravenous) administration of amikacin sulfate twice daily at dosages of up to 10 mg/lb for 15 consecutive days in horses resulted in no clinical, laboratory or histopathologic evidence of toxicity.

Intrauterine infusion of 2 grams of EQUIGLIDE™ (Amikacin Sulfate Solution) 8 hours prior to breeding by natural service did not impair fertility in mares. Therefore, mares should not be bred for at least 8 hours following uterine infusion.

Dosage and Administration: For treatment of uterine infections in mares, 2 grams (8 mL) of EQUIGLIDE™ (Amikacin Sulfate Solution), mixed with 200 mL 0.9% Sodium Chloride Injection, USP and aseptically infused into the uterus daily for three consecutive days, has been found to be the most efficacious dosage.

Contraindication(s): There are no known contraindications for the use of amikacin sulfate in horses other than a history of hypersensitivity to amikacin.

Precaution(s): EQUIGLIDE™ (Amikacin Sulfate Solution) is supplied as a colorless solution which is stable at room temperature. At times the solution may become pale yellow in color. This does not indicate a decrease in potency.

Store at controlled room temperature 15°-30°C (59°-86°F).

Caution(s): Federal law restricts this drug to use by or on the order of a licensed veterinarian.

Although amikacin sulfate is not absorbed to an appreciable extent following intrauterine infusion, concurrent use of other aminoglycosides should be avoided because of the potential additive effects.

In vitro studies have demonstrated that when sperm are exposed to the preservative which is present in the 48 mL vials (250 mg/mL) sperm viability is impaired.

Warning(s): Not to be used in horses intended for food.

For intrauterine use in the horse only.

Not for human use. Keep out of reach of children.

Adverse Reactions: No adverse reactions or other side effects have been reported.

References: Available upon request.

Presentation: 48 mL vial.

Manufactured by: Phoenix Scientific, Inc.

Compendium Code No.: 10940630

EQUI-PHAR EQUI-HIST 1200 GRANULES ℞

Vedco — **Antihistamine**

Active Ingredient(s): Each ounce contains:

Pyrilamine Maleate .... 600 mg
Pseudoephedrine Hydrochloride .... 600 mg

In a palatable base (sucrose).

Indications: For use when a histamine antagonizing preparation is required.

Dosage and Administration: ½ ounce (1 level tablespoon) per 1,000 pounds body weight. Can be mixed with feed and repeated at 12 hour intervals if needed.

Precaution(s): Store at controlled room temperature 15°-30°C (56°-86°F).

Caution(s): Federal law restricts this drug to use by or on the order of a licensed veterinarian.

For animal use only.

Warning(s): Do not use at least 72 hours prior to sporting events. Not for use in horses intended for food.

Keep out of reach of children.

Presentation: 12 x 20 oz jars (NDC 50989-341-96).

Compendium Code No.: 10942220 1098

EQUI-PHAR™ EQUI-LYTE POWDER

Vedco — **Electrolytes-Oral**

Active Ingredient(s): Each lb. contains:

Sodium chloride .... 46.2 g
Potassium chloride .... 5.6 g
Calcium chloride • $2H_2O$ .... 4.8 g
Magnesium sulfate .... 0.4 g

In a palatable dextrose base.

Indications: For use as an oral electrolyte supplement for horses.

Dosage and Administration: Feed Equi-Lyte Powder at the rate of 2 oz. per animal, once a day.

Precaution(s): Keep lid tightly closed when not in use.

Caution(s): Not for human use.

Warning(s): Keep out of reach of children.

Presentation: 5 lb. jars and 25 lb.

Compendium Code No.: 10940721

EQUI-PHAR™ EQUINE 7 HSS ℞

Vedco — **Saline Solution**

NDC No.: 50989-011-17

Active Ingredient(s): Each 100 mL of sterile aqueous solution contains:

Sodium chloride .... 7.0 g

Milliequivalents per liter:

Cations:

Sodium .... 1,198 mEq/L

Anions:

Chloride .... 1,198 mEq/L

Indications: For use in replacement therapy of sodium, chloride and water which may become depleted in many diseases in the horse.

Dosage and Administration: Warm to body temperature and administer slowly by intravenous injection. The amount and rate of administration must be judged by the veterinarian in relation to the condition being treated and the clinical response of the animal, being careful to avoid overhydration.

Precaution(s): Store at a temperature between 15°-30°C (59°-86°F).

Caution(s): Federal law (U.S.A.) restricts this drug to use by or on the order of a licensed veterinarian.

The product does not contain preservatives. Use the entire contents when first opened. Discard any unused solution.

For animal use only.

Keep out of the reach of children.

Presentation: 1,000 mL bottles.

Compendium Code No.: 10940750

EQUI-PHAR™ EQUI-VITA PHOS

Vedco — **Large Animal Dietary Supplement**

Active Ingredient(s): Each lb. contains:

Vitamin A .... 800,000 U.S.P. units
Vitamin E - Int. .... 320 U.S.P. units
Vitamin D_3 .... 40,000 U.S.P. units
Thiamine mononitrate (B_1) .... 800 mg
Riboflavin (B_2) .... 800 mg
Pyridoxine HCL (B_6) .... 128 mg
Vitamin B_{12} .... 2,400 mcg
Niacin .... 1,200 mg
Pantothenic acid .... 480 mg
Calcium .... 40 g
Monosodium phosphate .... 200 g
Iron .... 2,400 mg
Iodine .... 40 mg
Magnesium .... 320 mg
Cobalt .... 16 mg
Copper .... 400 mg
Manganese .... 2,400 mg
Zinc .... 2,400 mg
Selenium .... 4 mg

Indications: An equine nutritional supplement which contains lactobacillus for the prevention or correction of vitamin and/or mineral deficiencies in horses. Effective for horses on a heavy diet of alfalfa hay or legumes.

Dosage and Administration: For the prevention or correction of vitamin and/or mineral deficiencies in the equine, feed Equi-Vita-Phos at the rate of 2 oz. (approximately 1 scoop) per animal once a day, as necessary.

Foals should receive 2 oz. once a day by direct oral administration for six (6) to eight (8) weeks.

Feed mares 2 oz. once a day while nursing.

Precaution(s): Do not store above 86°F (30°C).

Caution(s): Keep out of the reach of children.

Presentation: Packaged in 5 lb. tubs with 2 oz. scoops.

Compendium Code No.: 10940730

EQUI-PHAR™ FOLIC 20 ℞

Vedco — **Large Animal Dietary Supplement**

NDC No.: 50989-009-54

Active Ingredient(s): Each 10 g packet contains:

Folc Acid USP .... 20 mg
Sucrose .... q.s.

Indications: A concentrated vitamin product for oral use, fortified with sucrose for greater palatability.

To stimulate the hemoglobin in horses who have not had access to fresh pasture.

Recommended Use: For horses in competition, brood mares in gestation and foals needing supplemental folic acid.

Dosage and Administration: Empty contents of one packet daily, directly on the horses ration. Prepare fresh ration each day.

Precaution(s): Keep in a cool dry place.

Caution(s): Federal law restricts this drug to use by or on the order of a licensed veterinarian.

For animal use only.

Warning(s): Keep out of reach of children.

Presentation: 40 x 10 g packets per carton.

Compendium Code No.: 10940770

EQUI-PHAR™ FUROSEMIDE INJECTION 5% ℞

Vedco — **Diuretic**

NADA No.: 118-550

Active Ingredient(s): Each mL contains:

Furosemide (as a diethanolamine salt) .... 50 mg
Myristyl-gammapicolinium chloride 0.02%
EDTA sodium 0.1%
Sodium sulfite 0.1%
Sodium chloride 0.2%

Water for injection. The pH is adjusted with sodium hydroxide.

Indications: Furosemide is indicated for the treatment of acute non-inflammatory tissue edema in horses.

Dosage and Administration: Administer 0.5 mg per pound of body weight (approximately 1.0 mg per kg) once or twice a day at 6- to 8-hour intervals either intravenously or intramuscularly.

A prompt diuresis usually ensues from the initial treatment. Diuresis may be initiated by the parenteral administration of Furosemide Injection. The dose should be adjusted according to the individual's response. In severe edematous or refractory cases, the dose may be doubled or increased by increments of 1 mg per pound of body weight. The established effective dose should be administered once or twice a day. The daily schedule of administration can be timed to control the period of micturition for the convenience of the client or veterinarian. Mobilization of the edema may be most efficiently and safely accomplished by utilizing an intermittent daily dosage schedule, i.e., every other day, or two (2) to four (4) consecutive days a week. Diuretic therapy should be discontinued after reduction of the edema or maintained after determining a carefully programmed dosage schedule to prevent recurrence of edema. For long-term treatment, the dose can generally be lowered after the edema has once been reduced. Re-examination and consultations with the client will enhance the establishment of a satisfactorily programmed dosage schedule. Clinical examination and serum BUN, CO2 and electrolyte determination should be performed during the early period of therapy and periodically thereafter, especially in refractory cases. Abnormalities should be corrected or the drug temporarily withdrawn.

Precaution(s): Do not store above 25°C (77°F).

Caution(s): Federal law restricts this drug to use by or on the order of a licensed veterinarian.

Sold to veterinarians only.

For veterinary use only.

Warning(s): Do not use in horses intended for food.

Presentation: 50 mL and 100 mL sterile multiple dose vials.

Compendium Code No.: 10940781

EQUI-PHAR™ HORSE & COLT WORMER

Vedco **Parasiticide-Oral**

NDC No.: 50989-168-26

Active Ingredient(s):

Pyrantel Tartrate 1.25%

(Equivalent to 5.671 grams per pound.)

Ingredients: Wheat middlings, ground yellow corn, dehydrated alfalfa meal, soybean meal, cane molasses.

Indications: A pyrantel tartrate wormer for horses and ponies.

For Removal of Infections of the Following Mature Parasites:

Large Strongyles: *(Strongylus vulgaris, S endentatus,* and *S equinus)*

Small Strongyles: *(Trichonema* sp. *Triodontophorus)*

Pinworms: *(Oxyuris)*

Large Roundworms: *(Parascaris)*

Dosage and Administration: Directions: Each horse should be treated individually. Not all horses will consume medicated feed; however, most horses consume EQUI-PHAR™ Horse & Colt Wormer readily when mixed in the feed. Mix the required amount of EQUI-PHAR™ Horse & Colt Wormer in the feed normally consumed at one feeding. Animals should not be fasted prior to or following treatment. This product may be administered safely to foals and pregnant mares. Since horses are constantly reinfecting themselves with worms through grazing, periodic worming every two months may be required. Consult your veterinarian in the diagnosis, treatment and control of parasitism.

Dosage*

Weight of Horse	Amount of Horse & Colt Wormer to Mix in Feed	Ounces
175 lbs	1/2 cupful**	3 oz
350 lbs	1 cupful	6 oz
700 lbs	2 cupfuls	12 oz
1000 lbs	2 2/3 cupfuls	1 lb

*Provides 12.5 mg of pyrantel tartrate per 2.2 lbs of body weight.

**One 8 ounce measuring cup holds 6 ounces of EQUI-PHAR™ Horse & Colt Wormer equivalent to 2.126 grams of pyrantel tartrate.

Caution(s): It is recommended that severely debilitated animals not be treated with EQUI-PHAR™ Horse & Colt Wormer. Consult a veterinarian at the first sign of adverse reaction such as a marked increase in rate of respiration, profuse sweating or incoordination.

Warning(s): Do not use in horses or ponies intended for food.

Keep out of reach of children.

Restricted Drug. Use only as directed. Not for human consumption.

Presentation: 16 oz (1 lb) (454 g).

Compendium Code No.: 10940790

EQUI-PHAR™ ICHTHAMMOL 20% OINTMENT

Vedco **Topical Wound Dressing**

Active Ingredient(s): Each mL contains:

Ichthammol 20%

Indications: For external use as an emmolient for the skin of horses.

Dosage and Administration: Apply to affected parts once or twice a day. A loose bandage may be applied.

Caution(s): For animal use only.

Keep out of the reach of children.

Presentation: 1 lb. containers.

Compendium Code No.: 10940800

EQUI-PHAR™ LACTOBAC GEL

Vedco **Large Animal Dietary Supplement**

Active Ingredient(s): Each 15 g contains:

Vitamin A .... 100,000 I.U.
Vitamin D_3 .... 20,000 I.U.
Vitamin B_{12} .... 150 mcg
Vitamin E .... 200 I.U.
Calcium pantothenate .... 10 mg
Riboflavin .... 11 mg
Thiamine .... 15.1 mg
Total colony forming units .... 10,000,000,000 C.F.U.

The vitamin base is a formulated U.S.P. grade premix from Hoffman LaRoche.

Indications: A microbial product for foals and horses. Contains a source of live (viable), naturally occurring micro-organisms.

Dosage and Administration: The vitamin premix is formulated for horses. Administer orally on the back of the tongue.

Foals: Administer 10 g on the day of birth, at 12 to 24 hours of age and on day 4.

Adult Horses:

Post worming/antibiotics: At the conclusion of treatment, administer 15 g on days 1, 3 and 7.

Transportation: Before transportation, administer 15 g on days 3 and 1, and on the first day following transportation.

Performance training: For a one (1) week time period, administer 15 g every other day, when the horse is off feed due to training.

Precaution(s): Keep cool, not a drug.

Presentation: 80 g containers.

Compendium Code No.: 10940810

EQUI-PHAR™ LUBOGEL-V™

Vedco **Lubricant**

E

Active Ingredient(s): A solution of sodium carboxy methylcellulose in propylene glycol. Propyl and methyl parahydroxybenzoate are included as preservatives. Nonspermicidal.

Indications: For coating hands, arms, instruments and subject areas in performing gynecological procedures and rectal examinations.

Dosage and Administration: The formula minimizes irritation to the skin of the operator and the delicate mucous membranes of the animal.

Apply liberally immediately before use.

Warning(s): Keep out of reach of children.

Presentation: 8 oz and 1 gallon (3.785 L) (NDC 50989-378-29) containers.

Compendium Code No.: 10940821

EQUI-PHAR™ McKILLIPS POWDER

Vedco **Topical Wound Dressing**

NDC No.: 50989-118-22

Active Ingredient(s): Each ounce contains:

3.5-dimethyl-4-chlorophenol .... 284 mg
Alum .... 2.84 g

Indications: An astringent and antiseptic dressing powder for superficial abrasions, cuts and wounds of horses.

Dosage and Administration: Dust powder on frequently to keep wounds dry. May be applied under a gauze dressing.

Precaution(s): Do not store above 30°C (86°F).

Caution(s): In case of deep puncture wounds or serious burns, consult a veterinarian. If redness, irritation or swelling persists or increases, discontinue use and consult a veterinarian.

Keep out of the reach of children.

For animal use only.

Presentation: 5 oz. containers.

Compendium Code No.: 10940830

EQUI-PHAR™ MIRACLE HEEL

Vedco **Topical Wound Dressing**

Active Ingredient(s): Lanolin, propylene glycol, beeswax, *Symphytum* extract, purified water, vegetable oil, isopropyl alcohol and allantoin.

Indications: Wounds or skin abrasions, dry or cracked hooves, dew poisoning and thrush.

Dosage and Administration: Clean affected area and apply an even layer of Miracle Heel once or twice daily. If used under a bandage, change every 2 to 4 days. For best results, use on wounds before excess granulation begins. To moisturize and promote healthy hooves, apply daily to the coronary band area and hoof.

Precaution(s): Store in a cool place.

Caution(s): This product may cause a burning sensation on an open sore due to its propylene glycol content. Avoid contact with eyes.

Warning(s): For external veterinary use only.

Presentation: 16 oz.

Compendium Code No.: 10940840

EQUI-PHAR™ NITROFURAZONE SOLUBLE DRESSING

Vedco **Topical Antibacterial**

NADA No.: 126-504

Active Ingredient(s): Contains: 0.2% nitrofurazone in a water soluble base of polyethylene glycol.

Indications: An antibacterial preparation for topical application.

For the prevention or treatment of surface bacterial infections of wounds, burns, and cutaneous ulcers, by organisms sensitive to nitrofurazone. For use on dogs, cats, and only on horses not intended for food use.

Dosage and Administration: See Caution statement before applying.

Apply directly on the lesion with a spatula or on a piece of gauze. The application of a bandage is optional. The preparation should be in contact with the lesion for at least 24 hours. The dressing may be changed several times a day or left on the lesion for a longer period of time.

Precaution(s): Keep away from excessive heat or direct sunlight. Avoid exposure to alkaline material and strong fluorescent lighting. Do not freeze.

Caution(s): In case of deep or puncture wounds, or serious burns, consult a veterinarian. If redness, irritation, or swelling persists or increases, discontinue use and consult a veterinarian.

For animal use only.

Not for human use.

Keep out of the reach of children.

Warning(s): Not for use on horses intended for food.

Human Warnings: Carcinogenesis: Nitrofurazone, the active ingredient of Nitrofurazone Soluble Dressing, has been shown to produce mammary tumors in rats and ovarian tumors in mice. Additionally, some people may be hypersensitive to the product. Either wear gloves when applying, or wash hands afterwards.

Presentation: 1 lb. (453.6 g) containers.

Compendium Code No.: 10940850

EQUI-PHAR™ PHENYLBUTAZONE 1 GRAM TABLETS ℞

Vedco **Phenylbutazone-Oral**

NADA No.: 49-187

Active Ingredient(s): Each tablet contains:

Phenylbutazone, U.S.P. .... 1 g

Plus excipients.

Indications: A nonhormonal anti-inflammatory agent for horses only.

Dosage and Administration:

Orally: One (1) to two (2) tablets per 500 lbs. of body weight, but not to exceed 4 g per day. Reduce the dosage as symptoms regress.

The oral dose for horses is two (2) to four (4) tablets (2 to 4 g) per 1,000 lbs. per day. The total daily dose should be limited to four (4) tablets per day. Because of the relatively short half-life of the drug, administration every eight (8) hours is the most satisfactory schedule.

Caution(s): Federal law restricts this drug to use by or on the order of a licensed veterinarian.

Sold to veterinarians only.

Warning(s): Not for use in horses intended for food.

Presentation: 100 tablet containers.

Compendium Code No.: 10940860

E

EQUI-PHAR™ PHENYLBUTAZONE INJECTION 20% ℞

Vedco **Phenylbutazone-Injection**

NADA No.: 46-780

Active Ingredient(s): Each mL of sterile aqueous solution contains:

Phenylbutazone .... 200 mg

Benzyl alcohol 1.5%

Sodium hydroxide used to adjust pH and water for injection U.S.P.

Indications: A nonhormonal anti-inflammatory agent for horses only.

Dosage and Administration: The intravenous dose for horses is 5 to 10 mL (1 to 2 g) per 1,000 lbs. per day. The injection should be administered slowly. Intravenous administration should be limited to five (5) consecutive days. An initial high dose is recommended to obtain a prompt effect. As the symptom regresses, the dose should be reduced.

Precaution(s): Store the product in a cool place (46° to 59°F) or alternatively store in a refrigerator.

Caution(s): Federal law restricts this drug to use by or on the order of a licensed veterinarian.

Sold to veterinarians only.

Warning(s): Not for use in horses intended for food.

Presentation: 100 mL sterile multiple dose vial.

Compendium Code No.: 10940870

EQUI-PHAR PROTAL™ ℞

Vedco **Parasiticide-Oral**

(pyrantel pamoate) Equine Anthelmintic Suspension

ANADA No.: 200-246

Active Ingredient(s): 50 mg of pyrantel base as pyrantel pamoate per mL.

Indications: For the removal and control of mature infections of large strongyles *(Strongylus vulgaris, S. edentatus, S. equinus);* pinworms *(Oxyuris equi);* large roundworms *(Parascaris equorum);* and small strongyles in horses and ponies.

Dosage and Administration: Administer 3 mg pyrantel base per pound of body weight (6 mL PROTAL™ (pyrantel pamoate) per 100 lb body weight). It is recommended that severely debilitated animals not be treated with this preparation.

Directions for Use: PROTAL™ (pyrantel pamoate) may be administered by means of a stomach tube, dose syringe or by mixing into the feed.

Stomach Tube - Measure the appropriate dosage of PROTAL™ and mix in the desired quantity of water. Protect drench from direct sunlight and administer to the animal immediately following mixing. Do not attempt to store diluted suspension. PROTAL™ is inactive against the common horse bot *(Gasterophilus* sp.). However, PROTAL™ may be administered concurrently with carbon disulfide observing the usual precautions with carbon disulfide.

Dose Syringe - Draw the appropriate dosage of PROTAL™ into a dose syringe and administer to the animal. Do not expose PROTAL™ to direct sunlight.

Feed - Mix the appropriate dosage of PROTAL™ in the normal grain ration. Fasting of animals prior to or following treatment is not required.

Precaution(s): Recommended Storage: Store below 86°F (30°C).

This product is a suspension and as such will separate. To insure uniform re-suspension and to achieve proper dosage, it is extremely important that the product be shaken and stirred thoroughly before every use.

Caution(s): Federal law restricts this drug to use by or on the order of a licensed veterinarian.

It is recommended that severely debilitated animals not be treated with this preparation.

Warning(s): Not for horses or ponies intended for food. Keep out of reach of children.

Presentation: 473 mL (1 pt) (NDC 50989-485-26) and 946 mL (1 qt) (NDC 50989-485-27).

Manufactured by: Phoenix Scientific, Inc., St. Joseph, MO 64503.

Compendium Code No.: 10942230 Iss. 11-98

EQUI-PHAR™ SWEET PSYLLIUM ℞

Vedco **Laxative**

Active Ingredient(s): Contains:

Psyllium U.S.P. 99%

Flavoring agents 1%

Indications: Psyllium is a multi-active fiber that encourages normal elimination without the use of chemical stimulants. The product may help prevent sand colic in horses.

Dosage and Administration: For a horse that has been diagnosed as having an accumulation of sand, add two (2) scoops (4 oz.) to the feed for three (3) days. Discontinue feeding Sweet Psyllium for the next three (3) days, then repeat with a three-day feeding. Continue feeding Sweet Psyllium for three (3) days, and then off for three (3) days for a 30-day period. After 30 days, feed two (2) scoops (4 oz.) of Sweet Psyllium once every seven (7) days or as directed by a veterinarian.

If a horse shows symptoms of colic or any other disorders, consult a veterinarian immediately.

Precaution(s): Close the container tightly after each use.

Caution(s): Federal law restricts this drug to use by or on the order of a licensed veterinarian.

Livestock drug. Not for human use.

Warning(s): Keep out of reach of children.

Warning(s): Not for use in horses intended for food.

Presentation: 1 lb. and 3 lb. containers.

Compendium Code No.: 10940891

EQUI-PHAR™ THRUSHGARD

Vedco **Hoof Product**

Active Ingredient(s): 12-Benzene, Di-carboxylic acid, dibutal ester, dibenzoyl peroxide, and melaleuca alternifolia oil.

Indications: To be used for thrush and white line disease (Onychomycosis). ThrushGard contains two powerful antibacterial, antifungal agents in an insoluble base. Ideal for use if chronic thrush persists. ThrushGard is highly effective in cleft of frog and under pads for thrush, under web of shoe for white line disease (Onychomycosis).

Dosage and Administration: For thrush, clean affected area and apply ThrushGard topically every 2 to 3 days until condition clears, then once a week thereafter for maintenance. For white line disease, remove soft debris from white line defect and fill defect with ThushGard, protect with web of shoe or packing.

Precaution(s): Store at room temperature 59-86° Fahrenheit.

Keep away from flame.

Caution(s): For external use only.

Avoid contact with skin, eyes and clothing.

Warning(s): Keep out of reach of children.

Presentation: 30 mL.

Compendium Code No.: 10940900

EQUI-PHAR™ VEDLUBE DRY

Vedco **Lubricant**

Active Ingredient(s): Polyethylene polymer, dispersing agent.

Indications: Powdered hand lubricant concentrate.

Dosage and Administration: Apply to hands as a powdered hand soap. Powder may be stirred into water to make a liquid lubricant for obstetrical use.

This lubricant is easily removed with water. A small amount of table salt added to the hands as a powdered hand soap will facilitate removal of all traces of the lubricant.

Warning(s): For veterinary use only.

Keep out of reach of children.

Presentation: 8 oz (227 g).

Compendium Code No.: 10940910

EQUI-PHAR™ VEDLUBE O.B. LUBRICANT

Vedco **Lubricant**

Ingredient(s): A non-medicated aqueous base lubricant containing methyl and propyl parabens as preservatives. Formulated for use either diluted or as a concentrate.

Indications: For lubrication of the arm or glove for rectal and obstetrical procedures in large or small animals; for lubrication of devices such as stomach tubes, enema nozzles, catheters and obstetrical instruments before insertion into body cavities; as an aid in delivery at dry birth.

Dosage and Administration: Distribute evenly a small mount of lubricant to wet or dry glove, arm or instruments.

To prepare a bulk lubricant to aid in dry birth, add lubricant to two quarts of water until the desired viscosity is reached.

Warning(s): For animal use only.

Not for human use.

Keep out of reach of children.

Presentation: 1 gallon.

Compendium Code No.: 10940920

EQUI-PHAR™ VITA PLEX ORAL HONEY

Vedco **Large Animal Dietary Supplement**

Ingredient(s): Each fluid ounce contains:

Cyanocobalamin .... 10.0 mcg

Pyridoxine HCl .... 5.0 mg

Riboflavin .... 8.0 mg

Thiamine HCl .... 50.0 mg

Niacinamide .... 100.0 mg

Folic Acid .... 30.0 mg

d'Panthenol .... 10.0 mg

Ferrous Sulfate - $7H_2O$ .... 334.0 mg

Citric Acid 0.06%

Cobalt Sulfate - H_2O .... 1.0 mg

Copper Sulfate .... 1.7 mg

Sorbitol Solution .... 10.0% v/v

Compounded with pure honey, apple flavor and preservatives.

Indications: For use as a nutritional supplement for the debilitated horse, competitive horse, pregnant mare, stallion in service or growing foal.

Dosage and Administration: Add to daily rations at following dosage: Horses racing and stallions in service, 2 ounces daily. Yearlings and orphan colts, 1 ounce daily. Foal, ½ ounce daily. Debilitated horses, 3 ounces daily for 15 days, then reduce to 1 ounce daily. Mares in foal, 1 ounce daily for first 6 months, then increase to 2 ounces daily to term.

Precaution(s): Keep container tightly closed and protect from light.

Warning(s): For animal use only.

Presentation: 1 gallon.

Compendium Code No.: 10940930

EQUIPHED ℞

AHC **Antihistamine**

Granules

Active Ingredient(s): Each ounce contains:

Pseudoephedrine HCl, USP .... 600 mg

Pyrilamine Maleate, USP .... 600 mg

in a palatable base.

Indications: Recommended as an oral antihistamine for horses.

Dosage and Administration: ½ ounce (1 level tablespoon) per 1,000 pound body weight, or as recommended by a veterinarian. Can be mixed with feed and repeated at 12 hour intervals as needed.

Shake well before use.

Precaution(s): Keep lid tightly closed and store in a dry place.

Do not store above 3°C (86°F).

Caution(s): Federal (U.S.A.) law restricts this drug to use by or on the order of a licensed veterinarian.

For use in horses only.

For veterinarian use only.

For animal use only.

Keep out of reach of children.

Warning(s): Do not use at least 72 hours prior to sporting event.

Presentation: 20 ounces (NDC 65090-002-15), 5 pounds (NDC 65090-002-30), and 10 pounds (NDC 65090-002-40).

Compendium Code No.: 10770040

EQUIPHEN® PASTE ℞

Luitpold **Phenylbutazone-Oral**

(Phenylbutazone)

NADA No.: 140-958

Active Ingredient(s): Each syringe contains:

Phenylbutazone . . . . 6 g or 12 g

Indications: For the relief of inflammatory conditions associated with the musculoskeletal system in horses.

Pharmacology: EQUIPHEN® Paste (phenylbutazone) is a synthetic, non-hormonal, anti-inflammatory, antipyretic compound useful in the management of inflammatory conditions. The apparent analgesic effect is probably related mainly to the anti-inflammatory properties of the compound.

Chemically, phenylbutazone is 4-butyl-1,2-diphenyl-3,5-pyrazolidine-dione. It is a pyrazolone derivative, entirely unrelated to the steroid hormones, and has the following structural formula:

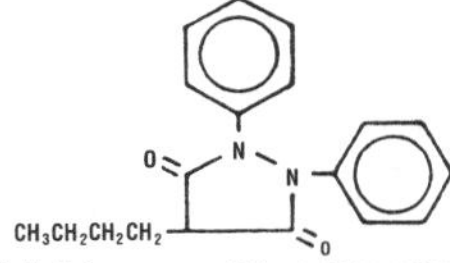

Dosage and Administration: Each increment of the plunger delivers 1 g of phenylbutazone. Administer an oral dose of 1 to 2 g of phenylbutazone per 500 lbs. of body weight, but not to exceed 4 g a day. Use a relatively high dose for the first 48 hours, then reduce it gradually to a maintenance dose. Maintain the lowest dose capable of producing the desired clinical response.

Guidelines To Successful Therapy:

1. Use a relatively high dose for the first 48 hours, then reduce it gradually to a maintenance dose. Maintain the lowest dose capable of producing the desired clinical response.
2. The response to EQUIPHEN® Paste (phenylbutazone) therapy is prompt, usually occurring within 24 hours. If a significant clinical response is not evident after five (5) days, re-evaluate the diagnosis and therapeutic approach.
3. When administering EQUIPHEN® Paste (phenylbutazone), the oral cavity should be empty. Deposit the paste on the back of the tongue by depressing the plunger that has been previously set to deliver the correct dose.
4. Many chronic conditions will respond to EQUIPHEN® Paste (phenylbutazone) therapy, but discontinuance of treatment may result in the recurrence of symptoms.

Contraindication(s): Use with caution in patients who have a history of drug allergy.

Precaution(s): Store at a controlled room temperature of 15°-30°C (59°-86°F).

Stop use of the medication at the first sign of gastro-intestinal upset, jaundice, or blood dyscrasia. Authenticated cases of agranulocytosis associated with the drug have occurred in man; fatal reactions, although rare have been reported in dogs after long-term therapy. To guard against this possibility, conduct routine blood counts at weekly intervals during the early phase of therapy and at intervals of two weeks thereafter. Any significant fall in the total white count, relative decrease in granulocytes, or black or tarry stools, should be regarded as a signal for the immediate cessation of therapy and institution of the appropriate counter measures.

In the treatment of inflammatory conditions associated with infections, specific anti-infective therapy is required.

Caution(s): Federal law restricts this drug to use by or on the order of a licensed veterinarian.

Keep all medication out of the reach of children.

For oral use in horses only.

Warning(s): Not for use in horses intended for food.

Presentation: Syringes containing 12 g of EQUIPHEN® Paste (phenylbutazone).
12 g of phenylbutazone - net wt. 60 g packed in boxes of 12 syringes.

Compendium Code No.: 10390031

EQUI-PLAS™

V.D.I. **Equine Plasma**

Active Ingredient(s): Plasma donors have been tested and are free of agglutinins and hemolysins to the major red cell antigens and are serologically screened for EIA, EVA, dourine, glanders, piroplasmosis and brucellosis.

Indications: Normal equine plasma can be administered in the following situations:

1. Intravenously to horses with hypoproteinemia and/or hypovolemia.
2. Intraperitoneally to horses with hypoproteinemia.
3. Intravenously to horses of any age with a physiologic deficiency of any plasma constituent.

Dosage and Administration: The plasma should be kept frozen until it is required. It should be thawed using warm water only and then warmed to body temperature.

Administer straight from the bag by slow filtered intravenous infusion. Do not mix with anything, and do not dilute. The dose is based on a systemic protein level of the recipient or a clinical assessment of the stage of dehydration.

The recommended dose for a newborn foal is one (1) liter, but care should be taken to avoid a volume overload.

Caution(s): The product is frozen immediately after collection. The transmission of viral diseases is possible with the administration of blood products, as is the development of serum sickness.

For use in horses by a licensed veterinarian only.

Side Effects: Complications are infrequent but may include tachypnea and trembling. If these symptoms become severe, it is advisable to slow the rate of administration, or to stop the administration and repeat in 5-10 minutes. If the symptoms recur or persist, discontinue the administration.

Presentation: 150 mL, 300 mL and 500 mL.

Compendium Code No.: 11280011

EQUIPOISE® Ⓒ III

Fort Dodge **Anabolic Agent**

Boldenone Undecylenate Injection

NADA No.: 034-705

Active Ingredient(s): EQUIPOISE® (boldenone undecylenate injection) is a long-acting injectable anabolic agent for horses, supplied in vials providing 25 or 50 mg boldenone undecylenate per mL in sesame oil with 3% (w/v) benzyl alcohol as a preservative.

Indications: EQUIPOISE® (boldenone undecylenate injection) is recommended as an aid for treating debilitated horses when an improvement in weight, haircoat or general physical condition is desired. Debilitation often follows disease or may occur following overwork and overexertion.

EQUIPOISE® improves the general state of debilitated horses, thus aiding in correcting weight losses and improving appetite. It is not a substitute for a well-balanced diet. Optimal results can be expected only when good management and feeding practices are utilized.

EQUIPOISE® should be considered only as adjunctive therapy to other specific and supportive therapy for diseases, surgical cases and traumatic injuries.

Pharmacology: EQUIPOISE® is a steroid ester possessing marked anabolic properties and a minimal amount of androgenic activity.

Anabolic and androgenic agents have come to be used widely in the treatment of certain pathophysiological or catabolic processes in man and animals. In many instances it is desirable to maintain a constant level of effect over a long period of time. EQUIPOISE® is a long-acting injectable agent which has a rapid onset of action. This is advantageous and is preferred over frequent oral dosing or even repeated injections.

Actions: Anabolic agents are related to the sex hormones, but each varies in its anabolic and androgenic effect. Compounds such as methyltestosterone have anabolic activity, but with prolonged use, animals develop marked androgenic activity which makes these compounds unsuitable for prolonged therapy.

Pharmacological studies conducted in laboratory animals to evaluate the pharmacological activity characterized EQUIPOISE® as having distinct anabolic properties together with a certain degree of androgenic activity. It does not have marked antigonadotrophic properties nor does it produce any clear-cut effects on the endometrium, conditions that are commonly observed when similar substances are used.

In clinical trials, at the recommended dosage, EQUIPOISE® had a marked anabolic effect in debilitated horses; appetite improved, vigor increased, and improvement was noted in musculature and haircoat. This would be expected with an anabolic agent such as EQUIPOISE®, particularly where there had been marked tissue breakdown associated with disease, prolonged anorexia or overwork.

Dosage and Administration: The dosage for horses is 0.5 mg per pound of body weight intramuscularly. Treatment may be repeated at three week intervals.

The condition should be assessed by the veterinarian to determine the duration of treatment; however, most horses will respond with one or two treatments.

Precaution(s): Store at room temperature; avoid freezing.

Caution(s): Federal law restricts this drug to use by or on the order of a licensed veterinarian.

Warning(s): For intramuscular use in horses only. Do not administer to horses intended for use as food. In the absence of data on the effect of boldenone undecylenate on stallions, on pregnant mares and the teratogenicity on the offspring, this drug should not be used in these animals.

Adverse Reactions: With EQUIPOISE® (boldenone undecylenate injection), androgenic (overaggressiveness) effects may be noted in a few animals. If these effects occur, they may persist for up to 6 to 8 weeks. No additional injections of boldenone undecylenate should be administered.

Presentation: EQUIPOISE® is supplied for veterinary use in 10 mL and 50 mL vials.
NDC 53501-414-50 — 25 mg-10 mL vial
NDC 53501-417-10 — 50 mg-10 mL vial
NDC 53501-417-50 — 50 mg-50 mL vial

Compendium Code No.: 10030671 12770C

EQUI-POULTICE

Vetus **Poultice**

Decongestant Poultice

Active Ingredient(s): Composition:

Magnesium Sulphate (epsom salt) 60%

Methyl Salicylate . . . . q.s.

In a water soluble base.

Indications: A poultice paste for use on horses and cattle. For strains, sprains, and bruises. An osmotic agent for external application.

Directions: Apply locally as a poultice (without rubbing) to acute swellings, sprains, contusions, acute mastitis, swollen glands. May be repeated within 24 hours, as indicated.

Precaution(s): Keep container tightly closed. Store in a cool, dry place.

Avoid storing at excessive heat.

Caution(s): Avoid contact with eyes and mucous membranes.

For animal use only.

Keep out of reach of children.

Available exclusively through veterinarians.

Presentation: 20 oz (NDC 47611-209-34).

Distributed by: Burns Veterinary Supply, Inc., Westbury, NY 11590

Compendium Code No.: 14440301 Iss. 03-00

EQUI-PRIN™

First Priority **Non-Steroidal Anti-Inflammatory**

Aspirin Paste

Active Ingredient(s): Each 5 cc marking on the plunger contains:

Aspirin (in paste form) . . . . 2 g

Each syringe contains 24 g aspirin.

Ingredients: Aspirin, mineral oil, silicon dioxide, apple flavor.

Indications: For the temporary relief of pain, inflammation and discomfort associated with musculoskeletal disorders in horses. For use as an antipyretic in horses with respiratory complexes.

Dosage and Administration: 2 g (5 cc) of aspirin per 800 lbs. body weight. Repeat every 4-6 hours if necessary, but not to exceed 15 gms in a 24 hour period. Oral cavity should be empty prior to dispensing. Administer by inserting nozzle of the syringe through the interdental space and depressing plunger that has been previously set to deliver the correct dose onto the back of the tongue.

Contraindication(s): Do not use on horses with gastric ulcers or symptoms related to that

condition, such as intestinal distress or in combination with medication that affects the clotting of blood.
Precaution(s): Store below 86°F.
Caution(s): Do not use on foals under 6 weeks of age.

Use only as directed. If symptoms continue or if irritation develops, discontinue use and consult a veterinarian.

For equine use only.

Keep out of reach of children.
Warning(s): Not for use on animals intended for food.
Presentation: 60 g (NDC 58829-299-60).
Compendium Code No.: 11390252 Iss. 5-00

EQUISIMILIS SHIELD™

Novartis Animal Vaccines **Bacterin**

Streptococcus equisimilis Bacterin
U.S. Vet. Lic. No.: 303
Composition: The bacterin contains whole inactivated cultures of *Streptococcus equisimilis* adjuvanted with aluminum hydroxide.

E

Contains penicillin and streptomycin as preservatives.
Indications: For use in healthy swine as an aid in the prevention and control of diseases caused by *Streptococcus equisimilis.*
Dosage and Administration: Shake well before using. Vaccinate piglets with a 2 mL dose intramuscularly at three (3) and five (5) weeks of age.
Precaution(s): Store at 35°-45°F (2°-7°C). Do not freeze. Use the entire contents when first opened.
Caution(s): Anaphylactic reactions may occur following the use of the product. Symptomatic treatment: Epinephrine.

For veterinary use only.
Warning(s): Do not administer within 21 days of slaughter.
Discussion: *Streptococcus equisimilis,* a member of Lancefield group C, is one of the most common Streps isolated from swine. It causes a variety of disease syndromes, but is most commonly seen in pigs before they are weaned.

Strep. equisimilis is found in nasal, throat, and vaginal secretions, as well as in the tonsils and milk of healthy animals. Newborn pigs are usually infected shortly after birth, and pick up the infection from carrier sows. The organism enters the body through the tonsils, the navel, or wounds and skin abrasions, all of which give the organism direct access to the bloodstream. The disease is more common in herds where teeth are clipped and tails are docked.

Once the organism enters the bloodstream, a septicemia develops and the bacteria circulate throughout the body. They then colonize other parts of the body with some of the more common areas affected being the joints (arthritis), the valves of the heart (valvular endocarditis), and the lining of the brain and spinal cord (meningitis). The bacteria also localize in the bone marrow and may affect bone development. Once the infection enters the joints, it can persist there for up to six months, since antibiotics do not penetrate well into joints and thus have limited effectiveness.

Clinical signs in affected piglets include fever, swollen joints, rough hair coats, and swollen navels. In addition, piglets with meningitis may show lethargy and convulsions. Piglets with endocarditis often have blue, cold skin, since the damaged heart cannot adequately circulate blood to the extremities.

In addition to the problems seen in piglets, *Strep. equisimilis* has been implicated in several diseases of older piglets and sows. It can cause infertility and abortions in sows, as well as mastitis and agalactia (lack of milk). It has been found to cause pneumonia and cutaneous abscesses in feeder pigs, and contributes to the ear necrosis syndrome. It may also cause infections in miscellaneous body organs, since the septicemic phase gives it access to all areas of the body.

Diagnosis of *Strep. equisimilis* infections is best done by necropsy and/or bacteriology, since other infections (i.e. pseudorabies, *Haemophilus parasuis, Pasteurella multocida* and others) produce similar symptoms. Antibiotic treatment may be effective in early cases, but once the bacteria localize in joints or abscesses it is difficult to get antibiotic concentrations into these areas.

Prevention of *Strep. equisimilis* is aimed at limiting the access of bacteria into the bloodstream. This includes taking steps to reduce abrasions, disinfecting navels immediately after birth, and using disinfectants when performing surgical techniques such as tail docking and castration. In addition, vaccination has been shown to be very effective in preventing disease.
Trial Data: EQUISIMILIS SHIELD™ *Streptococcus equisimilis* Challenge Results:

Group	n	Average Clinical Score	Average Number of Colonies Isolated During Necropsy		
			IP[a]	Heart	Lung
Vaccinates	28	156	5	26	25
Controls	30	220	51	143	111
P[b]		0.018	0.062	0.007	0.023

a=intraperitoneal
b=student t test for significance
n=number of animals
Presentation: Available in 50 dose (100 mL) bottles.
Compendium Code No.: 11140132

EQUI-SPOT™ SPOT-ON FLY CONTROL FOR HORSES

Farnam **Parasiticide-Topical**

EPA Reg. No.: 270-279
Active Ingredient(s):
Permethrin*: (CAS #52645-53-1) 45.0%
Other Ingredients 55.0%
Total 100.0%

*cis/trans ratio: Max 55% (+) cis and min 45% (+) trans
Indications: Protects horses from flies, gnats, mosquitoes and ticks. Kills and repels house flies, stable flies, face flies, horn flies, eye gnats, and ticks on horses. Aids in the control of horse flies, deer flies, mosquitoes and black flies on horses.
Directions for Use: It is a violation of Federal law to use this product in a manner inconsistent with its labeling.

Read entire label before each use.

Use only on horses over 12 weeks of age.

Horses: Do not use on horses intended for food use. Do not use on foals under 12 weeks (3 months) of age.

Remove product tubes from package. Fold along perforation between tubes and tear off one tube. Return unused tubes to package. Holding tube with notched end pointing up and away from face and body, snap off narrow end at notches.

Apply one tube (10.0 mL) of product solution as follows:
- 5 mL along the back line starting at the poll (top of head behind the ears), along the base of the mane, down the dorsal midline to the dock (base of the tail).
- 1 mL to the top of the forehead under the forelock.
- 1 mL, as a stripe, to the back of each foreleg, from the ankle up to the knee (2 mL total).
- 1 mL, as a stripe, to the back of each hindleg, from the ankle up to the hock (2 mL total).

Do not allow the product to contact horse's eyes or mucous membranes.

Wrap tube and put in trash.

Do not reapply for 14 days (2 weeks).
Precautionary Statements: Hazards to Humans and Domestic Animals:

Caution:

Hazards to Humans: Harmful if swallowed. Avoid contact with eyes or clothing. Causes moderate eye irritation. Wash thoroughly with soap and water after handling.

Hazards to Domestic Animals: For external use on horses only. Do not use on foals under 12 weeks of age. Consult a veterinarian before using this product on debilitated, aged, medicated, pregnant, or nursing horses. Consult a veterinarian before using on horses with known organ dysfunction. Do not use on animals other than horses. Certain medications can interact with pesticides. It is advisable to consult a veterinarian before using this product with any other pesticide or drug.

First Aid:

If Swallowed: Call a physician or poison control center immediately for treatment advice. Have person sip a glass of water, if able to swallow. Do not induce vomiting unless told to do so by a poison control center or doctor. Do not give anything by mouth to an unconscious person

If in Eyes: Hold eye open and rinse slowly and gently with water for 15 - 20 minutes. Remove contact lenses, if present, after the first 5 minutes, then continue rinsing eye. Call a poison control center or doctor for treatment advice.

In case of medical emergencies or health and safety inquiries, or in case of fire, leaking or damaged containers, or for product use information, call (602) 285-1660.

Have the product container or label with you when calling a poison control center or doctor for treatment.

Adverse Reactions: Some animals may be sensitive to ingredients in this product. Reactions in horses may include skin sensitivity. Horses may show lethargy, increased pruritis (itchiness), erythema (redness), rash and hair discoloration or hair loss at the application site. Observe the horse following treatment. Sensitivity may occur after using any pesticide product on animals. If signs of sensitivity occur, bathe your horse with a mild, non-insecticidal shampoo and rinse with large amounts of water. If signs continue, consult a veterinarian immediately.

Environmental Hazards: This product is extremely toxic to fish. Do not add directly to water. Do not contaminate water when disposing of product or packaging.

Physical or Chemical Hazards: Do not use or store near heat or open flames.

In case of emergency or for product use information, call 602-285-1660 7 AM - 3:45 PM MST M-F.
Storage and Disposal: Do not contaminate water, food or feed by storage or disposal.

Storage: Store in cool, dry place. Protect from freezing.

Disposal: If empty: Do not reuse the container. Place in trash or offer for recycling if available. If partly filled: Call your local solid waste agency or call 1-800-CLEANUP for disposal instructions. Never place unused product down any indoor or outdoor drain.
Warning(s): Do not use on horses intended for food use.

Keep out of reach of children.
Disclaimer: Notice of Warranty: Farnam Companies, Inc. makes no warranty of merchantability, fitness for any particular purpose, or otherwise, expressed or implied concerning this product or its uses which extend beyond the use of the product, under normal conditions, in accordance with the statements made on the label.
Presentation: 3 x 0.34 fl oz (10.0 mL) applicators.
Compendium Code No.: 10000840 01-2031

EQUITEC™

DMS Laboratories **Allergen-Specific IgE Test**

Reagents and Materials:

1. Diluent - Two bottles, each containing 125 mL of phosphate buffered saline with protein stabilizers and 0.05% thimerosal as a preservative.
   Mix gently before use. Avoid foaming.
2. Wash Solution Concentrate - Two bottles, each containing 125 mL of phosphate buffered saline with a detergent and 0.05% thimerosal as a preservative.
3. Anti-IgE Conjugate - One vial containing 0.6 mL of affinity purified anti-equine IgE antibody conjugated with horseradish peroxidase, stabilized with protein, in phosphate buffered saline and preserved with 0.05% thimerosal.
4. Substrate Solution - One bottle containing 125 mL of citrate phosphate buffer with urea hydrogen peroxide.
5. Chromogen - Five hermetically sealed packages, each containing one 20 mg tablet of o-Phenylenediamine Dihydrochloride (OPD).
   Warning: Harmful if swallowed, inhaled or absorbed through the skin. May induce contact hypersensitivity.
6. Stop Solution - One bottle containing 60 mL of 1 N sulfuric acid.
   Warning: Avoid contact with skin.
7. Allergen-Coated Wells - One package containing thirty-five (35) twelve-well strips. Each strip is coated with allergens relevant to either a geographic region or food group.
8. Calibrator Strips - Five twelve-well strips of calibrator wells.
9. Calibrator Sera - One set of three calibrators, each vial containing 1.5 mL of equine serum of different known reactivity on the calibrator strip. Ready to use - Do not dilute. See calibrator label for expected absorbance units. Mix gently before use.
10. Control Sera - Two vials (Control A and B) each containing 0.5 mL of control serum of different known reactivity for use as a batch quality control check.
11. Black, Uncoated Wells - One package containing five 12-well strips of reusable, black, uncoated wells.
12. Microtiter Well Holder - One reusable microtiter well holder with a 96-well capacity.
13. Matrix Sheet
14. Sponge
15. Microtiter plate cover

Materials Required But Not Provided:
- Micropipettes for dispensing 50-200 µL
- Test tubes
- Microtiter plate washer/aspirator
- Distilled or deionized H_2O
- Microtiter plate reader operable at 490±5 nm
- Assorted glassware for the preparation of reagents and buffer solutions
- Timer
- Vortex mixer
- Absorbent paper toweling
- Microtest plate shaker (500 - 600 rpm) with a uniform horizontally circular movement (3-5 mm)

Indications: Assay for the *in vitro* determination of Allergen-Specific IgE in Equine Serum (EE-306•S).

Intended Use: The equitec-s Test Kit for Equine Allergen-Specific IgE consists of an enzyme-linked immunosorbent assay (ELISA) for the semiquantitative determination of allergen-specific IgE antibodies in equine serum. The assay is intended for *in vitro* use only.

The role of allergy in various diseases of the horse has been described[1-5]. Chronic obstructive pulmonary disease (COPD) is a condition of chronic bronchiolitis and/or coughing often associated with molds, dusts and pollens from grasses commonly found in barns and stables[1-2]. Exercise induced pulmonary hemorrhage and exercise intolerance are conditions associated with outdoor allergens such as pollens from grasses, trees and weeds. Urticaria (hives) is a condition that may be insect induced (most frequently by culicoides present in the dorsal cervical mane and tail head) or induced by allergenic components of grass and weeds with which the animal comes in contact in the field[5]. The presence of allergen-specific IgE antibodies in serum represents, in many species, an indicator of some form of allergy involvement in analogous conditions.

The equitec-s Test Kit for Equine Allergen-Specific IgE incorporates a flexible means of testing for IgE antibodies to a wide variety of substances. The choice for each patient should be made by the veterinarian, in consultation with the veterinary clinical pathologist, in light of the medical history, environmental conditions and current clinical signs.

Test Principles: Principle of the IgE equitec-s Assay: The principle of the assay is represented in Figure 1. The allergen-specific IgE in a patient's serum binds to the allergen(s) of interest, which have been adsorbed to the surface of polystyrene microtiter wells. After the removal of unbound serum proteins, antibodies specific for equine IgE, labeled with horseradish peroxidase (HRPO), are added. The enzyme-labeled antibodies form complexes with the allergen-bound IgE.

Following additional washing, the enzyme bound to the immunosorbent is assayed by the addition of hydrogen peroxide and o-Phenylenediamine Dihydrochloride (OPD) as the chromogen substrate. The quantity of bound enzyme varies directly with the concentration of allergen-specific IgE antibodies in the sample. The absorbance, at 490 nm, is a measure of the concentration of allergen-specific IgE in the test sample. The relative serum concentration of allergen-specific IgE antibodies can be expressed according to a scale based on EA absorbance units. The level of sensitivity of the patient to a given allergen or group of allergens is estimated as a multiple of the average expected normal value in normalized absorbance (EA) units.

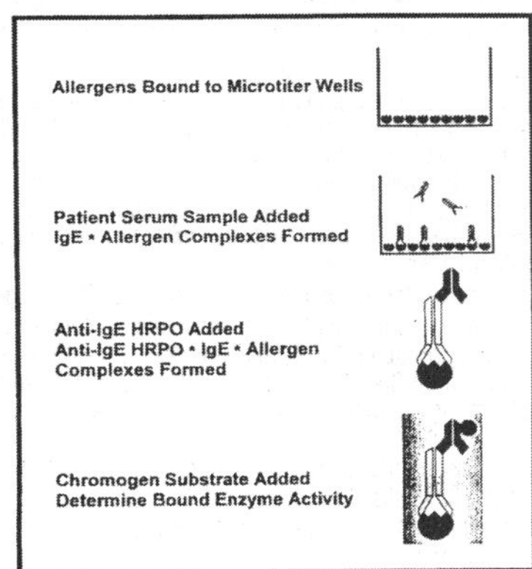

Figure 1

Test Procedure: Reagent Preparation:

1. Wash Solution: Dilute 1:10 by adding 100 mL of wash solution concentrate to 900 mL of distilled or deionized water to make a total of 1 liter of the working solution. The working solution is stable for one week from the date of preparation when stored at room temperature (20-25°C) or for one month at 2-7°C. Each microtiter well has a fill capacity of 0.4 mL. Mix required amounts in same proportions indicated above.

   Note: Crystal formation in the concentrate is common when storage temperatures are low. Redissolve crystals by warming the concentrate to 30-35°C before dilution.
2. Anti-IgE Conjugate: The working conjugate solution should be diluted immediately prior to use. Add 150 µL of conjugate to 10 mL of diluent (1:67 dilution) for each eight-strip microtiter plate (see Figure 2). Mix uniformly but gently. Avoid foaming.
3. Chromogen Substrate Solution: OPD is highly hydroscopic and will react with moisture in the air. Open only one package at a time and use immediately. To prepare the working chromogen substrate, add one 20 mg OPD tablet to 10 mL of substrate solution. Mix thoroughly. This is sufficient for 96 wells. Prepare just before use. The chromogen substrate is stable for one hour when kept from excessive heat and light.

Specimen Collection and Handling: Blood should be collected by venipuncture and the serum separated from the cells (after clot formation) by centrifugation. Specimens may be shipped at room temperature and then stored at 2-7°C if testing is to take place within one week after collection. If testing is to take place more than one week after collection, specimens should be stored at -20°C. Avoid repeated freezing and thawing. No additives or preservatives are required for specimen preparation. Avoid sodium azide contamination.

Warning: Handle all specimens as if capable of transmitting disease.

Loading the Microtiter Plate: The microtiter plate is numbered 1-12 for columns, A-H for rows. Figure 2 illustrates a format to test six equine samples for the same panel of 12 allergen groups (wells 1-12).

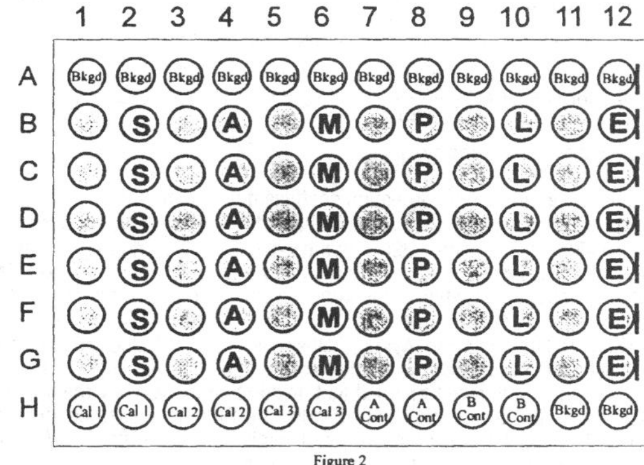

Figure 2

Insert one strip of allergen-coated wells in row A (allergen background), with the marked well positioned in column 12. For each sample to be assayed, insert one strip of allergen-coated wells into subsequent rows with the marked well positioned in column 12.

Insert one calibrator strip for each run for assaying calibrators, controls and the calibrator background. See Figure 2, row H. The calibrator strip is coated with the same allergen in each well, making well positioning unnecessary.

When testing less than six samples, it may be necessary to insert the black wells to fill the microtiter plate when using automated plate washers.

Procedure: Bring reagents to room temperature (20-25°C) before use.

1. Dilute sample and controls 1:26. To assay a single twelve-well panel, add 80 µL of sample to 2.0 mL of diluent, then mix by gentle vortexing. Dilute each control sera in the same proportion.
2. Pipette 100 µL of diluted sample into wells B1 through B12. Pipette the next sample into wells C1 through C12. Continue until designated sample wells are filled.
3. Pipette 100 µL of Diluent into each of the wells in row A and into designated background wells in row H. See Figure 2.
4. Pipette 100 µL of Calibrator Sera and diluted Control Sera into their designated wells of row H. See Figure 2.
5. Cover the microtiter plate, place upon sponge and secure to the microtest plate shaker. Keeping plate level, shake at room temperature (20-25°C) for 45 minutes at 500-600 rpm.
6. Remove the covered plate from the shaker and aspirate the contents of the wells.
7. Fill each well with Wash Solution, then aspirate. Be sure to keep the plate level during the washing/aspirating procedure. Repeat for a total of four washes. Finally, invert the plate on absorbent paper toweling and wrap the toweling around the plate. Blot excess fluid by striking the plate firmly against a level surface several times.
8. Pipette 100 µL of appropriately diluted Anti-IgE Conjugate into each well. Return and secure the covered plate to the shaker, and shake at room temperature (20-25°C) for 45 minutes at 500-600 rpm.
9. Wash and blot the wells as described in Step 7.
10. Prepare the Chromogen Substrate Solution immediately prior to use. Protect from direct light.
11. Pipette 100 µL of Chromogen Substrate Solution into each well. Return and secure the covered plate to the shaker, and shake at room temperature (20-25°C) for precisely 30 minutes at 500-600 rpm. Protect from direct light.
12. After precisely 30 minutes, pipette 100 µL of Stop Solution into each well.
13. Incubate at room temperature (20-25°C) for 10 minutes.
14. Set the plate reader to 490±5 nm. Use one of the Bkgd wells (H11, H12) to zero the instrument, then read the absorbance of every well.

Stability of the Colorimetric Reaction: The absorbance of the final reaction can be measured up to four hours after the completion of the procedure providing the covered plates are stored in a darkened area. However, good laboratory practice dictates that the measurement be made soon after the final incubation period.

Interpretation of Results:

1. Background Correction: To obtain corrected absorbance units, the allergen background value must be subtracted from the test values for each allergen, e.g., the absorbance of well A1 is subtracted from the absorbance values of B1, C1, D1, E1, F1 and G1 (see Figure 2). Repeat analogously for other columns (A2 through A12). The allergen background for the calibrator strip (H11, H12) should be averaged and subtracted from wells H1 through H10.
2. Calculation of the Patient and Control Values: Using conventional data reduction computer software programs such as Delta Graph® for IBM®-compatible computers or Cricket Graph® for Macintosh® systems, plot the background corrected observed values for calibrators 1, 2, 3 and the calibrator strip background against the lot-specific calibrator values provided with the kit.

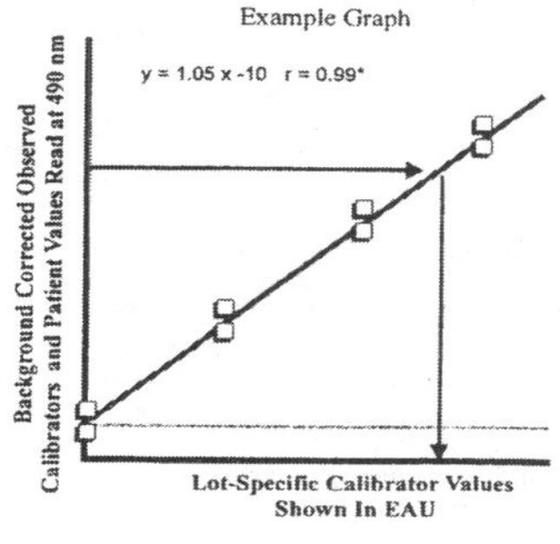

Figure 3

To calculate the corrected EAU (ELISA Absorbant Units) for the control and each sample, use the computer derived slope, $m\left(\frac{dy}{dx}\right)$ and the y intercept, b.

For example: $\text{Corrected EAU} = \frac{\text{EAU} - b}{m}$

$$\text{Corrected EAU} = \frac{985 - 10}{1.050} = 929 \text{ EA units}$$

*The acceptable range for the (r) correlation coefficient is 0.97 to 1.0.

Controls are provided with this kit for validation of procedure. The corrected EA units of each control value must be within ±20% of the expected values in order for the assay to be considered valid. The expected values are provided with each kit and the expected range is shown on the matrix sheet label. If the control values are not within range, the assay is invalid and must be repeated.

3. Calculations of Relationships to Average Observed Normal Values: For convenience in reporting results and discussing the relative likelihood of involvement of seasonal allergy in the underlying signs, it is recommended that, in addition to EA units, the results be stated as a ratio to this value. This is obtained by dividing the EA units measured for each seasonal allergen or group of inhalant allergens for which testing was performed by the equitec Index Divisor (250). The equitec Index Divisor is an approximation of the average results obtained for seasonal allergens in animals showing no signs of atopy. The ratio becomes the equitec Index. It is further recommended the results be categorized according to the equitec Index score presented Table 1.

Table 1. equitec Index

equitec Index	Category
<1.00	N
1.00-1.50	U
1.50-2.00	P
2.00-4.00	L
>4.00	A

"N" Indicates results consistent with those of normal animals.

"U" Indicates results that are unlikely to have clinical significance.

"P" Indicates results consistent with those of animals which exhibit one or more symptoms often associated with allergy.

"L" Indicates results which are sufficiently elevated to be likely to be of clinical significance.

"A" Indicates results that are highly abnormal and would be expected to be exceeded with respect to only a small percentage of animals tested.

Establishment of Normal Ranges: Normal ranges for each regional seasonal allergen panel should be established for this assay based on a Gaussian distribution of test results of approximately thirty (30) horses. Each should have no clinical signs of allergen-associated respiratory diseases such as Chronic Obstructive Pulmonary Disease (COPD) or dermatological disorders such as urticaria. The normal ranges shown in the chart supplied with equitec-s kits were established in this manner. It is provided for reference only. These normal ranges should not be used to define normal ranges for your test subjects unless your test panel is substantially the same.

Clinical Significance of Results: The patient's test results indicate a relative likelihood of clinical significance when considered as an element of a differential diagnosis. The results do not provide a definitive conclusion as to the presence of absence of atopy or COPD. A differential diagnosis must include clinical signs, patient history and the results of diagnostic test procedures as may be appropriate.

In addition to allergen-specific IgE values, the level of allergen-specific IgG "blocking" antibodies may be relevant to the clinical evaluation of patients exhibiting elevated allergen-specific IgE levels. If the allergen-specific IgG is elevated, this will indicate the allergen-specific IgE levels which are normally clinically significant are, in fact, a benign condition.

Limitations:

1. Proper performance of the IgE equitec-s assay depends upon many factors, including consistent ambient temperature, the quality of distilled or deionized water, and blotting of microtiter wells. Contamination of buffers may result in increasing non-specific background and/or erroneous values.
2. Inconsistent results may occur if there is improper and/or insufficient washing in steps 7 and 9 of the procedure.
3. Inconsistent values may result if the microtiter plate is not kept level during shaking, incubation and washing procedures.
4. The binding capacity of specific IgE from one allergen to another may yield identical results, but this does not necessarily imply clinical equivalence.
5. The assay indicates relative levels of allergen-specific IgE only. It is not intended to provide a definitive diagnosis of atopy. A differential diagnosis must include patient history and clinical signs, and other related tests such as allergen-specific IgG.

Known Interfering Substances:

Sodium azide is known to interfere with horseradish peroxidase activity.

Chromogen substrate solution is light sensitive and should be protected from direct light and excessive heat.

Performance Characteristics: The precision of the IgE equitec-s assay for the quantitative determination of allergen-specific IgE antibodies in equine serum was evaluated on 4 separate occasions. The inter-assay coefficients of variation are listed below.

Table 2

EA Units	Inter-Assay C.V. (%)
400	8.0
1400	6.0

Storage and Stability: Each component is stable until the date stated on each reagent label. Store all components at 2-7°C unless otherwise indicated.

Discussion: Summary and Explanation of the Assay: In 1967, Wide, et al[1], introduced the Radioallergosorbent Test (RAST) as an *in vitro* diagnostic method for the detection of IgE-mediated allergic conditions in humans. Recently a team of scientists at the Iatric Research Institute developed an enzyme-linked immunosorbent assay (ELISA) for the semi-quantitative determination of allergen-specific IgE in canine serum[7]. The equine analog of IgE has been isolated and its physiochemical properties described[8].

An increased understanding of the immunopathological mechanisms of IgE in atopy and COPD has resulted in the development of *in vitro* diagnostic procedures for detecting allergen-specific IgE in the equine species[9].

Based on this information, the Iatric equitec-s assay was developed to determine relative levels of allergen-specific IgE antibodies in equine serum.

References: Available upon request.

Presentation: This test kit contains sufficient materials to test 30 samples when run in five batches of six samples each.

equitec is a trademark of Vetazyme Corporation.

Manufactured by: Vetazyme Corporation, 1706 West Fourth Street, Tempe, Arizona 85281.

Compendium Code No.: 14810011 3040306-S/1, 6/18/97

EQUITROL® FEED-THRU FLY CONTROL

Farnam **Larvicide**

EPA Reg. No.: 270-164

Active Ingredient(s):

Tetrachlorvinphos: (Z)-2-chloro-1-(2,4,5-trichlorophenyl) vinyl dimethyl phosphate . 2.468%*
Other Ingredients: 97.532%**
Total 100.00%

*Contains 11.2 grams Rabon® per pound. ** Refers only to ingredients which are not larvicidal.

Feed Ingredients: Wheat Middlings, Dehydrated Alfalfa Meal, Oat By-Product, Calcium Carbonate, Lignin Sulfonate, Sodium Chloride, Propionic and Acetic Acids (preservatives).

Indications: Highly palatable feed additive to prevent the development of stable flies and house flies in the manure of treated horses.

Directions for Use: It is a violation of Federal law to use this product in a manner inconsistent with its labeling.

Feed the recommended dosage to each horse separately to make certain he receives his full portion. This product should be fed top dressed on grain or mixed with the horse's total ration to provide 70 mg of Rabon® per 100 lbs. of body weight. For an occasional finicky eater who does not accept new feeds readily, mix EQUITROL® with sweet feed or grain ration.

Start feeding EQUITROL® early in the spring before flies begin to appear and continue feeding throughout the summer and into the fall until cold weather restricts fly activity.

EQUITROL® Feed-Thru Fly Control prevents the development of house flies and stable flies in the manure of treated horses, but is not effective against existing adult flies.

In some cases, supplemental fly control measures may be needed in and around paddocks and buildings to control adult house flies and stable flies which can breed not only in manure, but in other decaying vegetable matter or silage on premises.

In order to achieve optimum fly control, EQUITROL® should be used in conjunction with other good management and sanitation practices.

Daily Dosages:

300-500 lb. Horse	Feed 2⁄5 oz. (One EQUITROL® measuring cup filled to the blue line) per horse per day.
500-700 lb. Horse	Feed 3⁄5 oz. (One EQUITROL® measuring cup filled to the red line) per horse per day.
700-900 lb. Horse	Feed 4⁄5 oz. (One EQUITROL® measuring cup filled to the green line) per horse per day.
900-1100 lb. Horse	Feed 1 oz. (One full EQUITROL® measuring cup) per horse per day.
For larger horses over 1100 lbs. of body weight, feed 1⁄4 oz for each 250 lbs. of body weight.	

Precautionary Statements: Hazards to Humans:

Caution: Keep out of reach of children. Harmful if swallowed. Avoid breathing dust. Avoid contact with skin or eyes. Wash thoroughly with soap and water after handling and before eating or smoking. This product may cause skin sensitization reactions in certain individuals. If in eyes, wash with plenty of water. If irritation persists, see a physician. Wear long-sleeved shirt and pants; chemical resistant gloves; shoes and socks for protection when handling.

Environmental Hazards: This pesticide is toxic to fish. Do not contaminate water when disposing of equipment washwater.

Storage and Disposal: Do not contaminate water, food, or feed by storage or disposal.

Storage: Store tightly closed in cool, dry place inaccessible to children and pets.

Disposal: Completely empty container. Then, dispose of empty container in a sanitary landfill or by incineration or, if allowed by State or local authorities, by burning. If burned, stay out of smoke. Wastes resulting from the use of this product may be disposed of on site or at an approved waste disposal facility.

Warning(s): Do not use on horses intended for slaughter.

Presentation: 3.75 lbs (1.7 kg), 10 lbs, 20 lbs and 100 lbs.

®Rabon is a registered trademark of Boehringer Ingelheim.

Compendium Code No.: 10000171

EQUIVAC™ EHV-1/4

Fort Dodge **Vaccine**

Equine Rhinopneumonitis Vaccine, Killed Virus

U.S. Vet. Lic. No.: 112

Contents: This product contains the antigen listed above.

Contains thimerosal and gentamicin as preservatives.

Indications: For the vaccination of healthy horses as an aid in the prevention of respiratory disease caused by Equine Herpesvirus type 1 (EHV-1) and type 4 (EHV-4).

Dosage and Administration: Shake well before using. Use entire contents when first opened. Using aseptic technique, vaccinate healthy horses with a 1 mL dose intramuscularly followed by a second 1 mL dose 2 to 4 weeks later. A booster is recommended annually, or in the event of a threatened epizootic. Horses subject to repeated exposure to field virus may benefit from revaccination with a single dose every three months.

Precaution(s): Store at 2° to 7°C (35° to 45°F). Do not freeze. Use new, non-chemically sterilized needles and syringes. Do not mix with other vaccines. Burn vaccine container and all unused contents.

Caution(s): Local reactions are rare. To minimize such reactions, ensure that injections are administered in deep muscle tissue. The use of a biological may produce anaphylaxis and/or other inflammatory immune-mediated hypersensitivity reactions.

Antidote(s): Epinephrine, corticosteroids and antihistamines may all be indicated depending on the nature and severity of the reaction.*

Warning(s): Do not vaccinate within 21 days of slaughter.

For veterinary use only.

References: Available upon request.*

Presentation: 12 x 1 dose (syringe pouch pack) and 10 dose (10 mL) vials.

Compendium Code No.: 10030681 12280B

EQUIVIM™

Butler **Large Animal Dietary Supplement**

Active Ingredient(s): Each fluid ounce contains:

Cyanocobalamin (vitamin B_{12})	10.0 mcg
Pyridoxine HCl (vitamin B_6)	5.0 mg
Riboflavin (vitamin B_2)	8.0 mg
Thiamine HCl	50.0 mg
Niacinamide	100.0 mg
Folic acid	30.0 mcg
d-Panthenol	10.0 mg
Ferrous sulfate • $7H_2O$	334.0 mg
Citric acid	0.06%
Cobalt sulfate • H_2O (Co 340 mcg)	1.0 mg
Copper sulfate (Cu 432 mcg)	1.7 mg
Sorbitol solution U.S.P.	10.0% v/v

Compounded with pure honey, apple flavor and preservatives.

Indications: For use as a nutritional supplement for the debilitated horse, competitive horse, pregnant mare, stallion in service, or growing foal.

A balanced supplemental source of vitamins and minerals.

Dosage and Administration: Add the following doses to the daily rations:

Horses, racing and stallions in service: 2 oz. per day.

Yearlings and orphan colts: 1 oz. per day.

Foals: ½ oz. per day.

Debilitated horses: 3 oz. per day for 15 days then reduce to one (1) ounce per day.

Mares in foal: 1 oz. per day for first six (6) months then increase to 2 oz. per day to term.

Precaution(s): Store in a cool place 8° to 15°C (46°-59°F).

Keep the container tightly closed and protect from light.

Caution(s): For veterinary use only. Keep out of the reach of children.

Presentation: 1 gallon (3.785 L) containers.

Compendium Code No.: 10820730

Equ-SeE

Vet-A-Mix **Vitamin E-Selenium**

Vitamin E and selenium feed supplement for horses

Guaranteed Analysis: per lb:

Selenium 0.02%	90.7 mg
Vitamin E	20,000 IU

Ingredients: Calcium carbonate, Rice hulls, Vitamin E (as DL-alpha tocopheryl acetate), Diatomaceous earth, Sodium bentonite, and Sodium selenite.

One teaspoon contains approximately 5 grams of Equ-SeE providing 1.0 mg selenium and 220 IU of vitamin E.

Indications: For use as a nutritional supplement in horses when a vitamin E and selenium deficiency exists.

Dosage and Administration: Dosage: The normal recommended dosage is 0.1 ppm to 0.3 ppm or ½ to 1½ teaspoons per 10 pounds (4.5 kg) daily feed intake.

Recommended Daily Dosage:

Body Weight	Dose
250 lb (115 kg)	¼-¾ teaspoon
500 lb (225 kg)	½-1½ teaspoons
750 lb (340 kg)	¾-2¼ teaspoons
1000 lb (450 kg)	1-3 teaspoons

Administration: Equ-SeE can be administered by mixing the daily dose in the concentrate or by top dressing on grain, preferably rolled or ground. To facilitate proper adhesion of Equ-SeE to the ration, slightly moisten the grain with water or a liquid supplement.

Caution(s): Follow the label instructions. The addition to feed of higher levels of the premix is not recommended. Do not exceed the recommended dosage.

Consider selenium concentrations in the total daily feed intake. The total added selenium should not exceed 0.3 mg/kg (0.3 ppm) in the ration or 3.0 mg selenium per horse per day.

Warning(s): Keep out of the reach of children.

Presentation: 1 lb. (453.6 g) bottle and 5 lb. jar.

Compendium Code No.: 10500081 0399

Equ-Se5E

Vet-A-Mix **Vitamin E-Selenium**

Guaranteed Analysis:

	per lb
Selenium 0.02%	90.7 mg
Vitamin E	100,000 IU

Ingredients: Sodium selenite, vitamin E (as DL-alpha tocopheryl acetate), sodium bentonite, diatomaceous earth, rice hulls and calcium carbonate.

One teaspoon contains approximately 5 grams of Equ-Se5E to provide 1 mg of selenium and 1,100 IU vitamin E.

Indications: For use as a nutritional supplement in horses when a selenium and vitamin E deficiency exists.

Dosage and Administration: The normal recommended dosage of selenium is 0.1 ppm to 0.3 ppm or ½ to 1½ teaspoons per 10 pounds (4.5 kg) daily feed intake.

Recommended Daily Dosage:

Body Weight	Dose
250 lb (115 kg)	¼-¾ teaspoon
500 lb (225 kg)	½-1½ teaspoons
750 lb (340 kg)	¾-2¼ teaspoons
1000 lb (450 kg)	1-3 teaspoons

Administration: Equ-Se5E can be administered by mixing the daily dose in the concentrate or by top dressing on grain, preferably rolled or ground. To facilitate proper adhesion, slightly moisten the grain with water or liquid supplement.

Caution(s): Consider selenium concentrations in the total daily feed intake. The total added selenium should not exceed 0.3 mg/kg (0.3 ppm) in the ration or 3.0 mg selenium, per horse per day.

Follow label directions. The addition to feed of higher levels of this supplement is not recommended. Do not exceed the recommended dosage.

Warning(s): Keep out of reach of children.

Presentation: One pound (453.6 g) bottle.

Compendium Code No.: 10500070

EQVALAN® LIQUID ℞

Merial **Parasiticide-Oral**

(ivermectin) 10 mg per mL

NADA No.: 140-439

Active Ingredient(s): EQVALAN® Liquid is a clear, ready-to-use solution with each mL containing 1% ivermectin (10 mg), 0.2 mL propylene glycol, 80 mg polysorbate 80, 9 mg sodium phosphate monobasic monohydrate, 1.3 mg sodium phosphate dibasic anhydrous, 1 mg butylated hydroxytoluene, 0.1 mg disodium edetate, 3% benzyl alcohol and purified water q.s. ad 100%.

Indications: EQVALAN® Liquid is indicated for the effective treatment and control of the following parasites or parasitic conditions in horses:

Large Strongyles: *Strongylus vulgaris* (adults and arterial larval stages), *S. edentatus* (adults and tissue stages), *S. equinus* (adults), *Triodontophorus* spp (adults).

Small Strongyles - including those resistant to some benzimidazole class compounds (adults and fourth-stage larvae): *Cyathostomum* spp, *Cylicocyclus* spp, *Cylicostephanus* spp, *Cylicodontophorus* spp.

Pinworms (adults and fourth-stage larvae): *Oxyuris equi.*

Ascarids (adults and third- and fourth-stage larvae): *Parascaris equorum.*

Hairworms (adults): *Trichostrongylus axei.*

Large-mouth Stomach Worms (adults): *Habronema muscae.*

Bots (oral and gastric stages): *Gasterophilus* spp.

Lungworms (adults and fourth-stage larvae): *Dictyocaulus arnfieldi.*

Intestinal Threadworms (adults): *Strongyloides westeri.*

Summer Sores caused by *Habronema* and *Draschia* spp cutaneous third-stage larvae.

Dermatitis caused by neck thread-worm microfilariae, *Onchocerca* sp.

Pharmacology: Product Description: Ivermectin is derived from the avermectins, a family of potent, broad-spectrum antiparasitic agents, which are isolated from fermentation of *Streptomyces avermitilis.*

Mode of Action: Ivermectin, is a member of the macrocyclic lactone class of endectocides which have a unique mode of action. Compounds of the class bind selectively and with high affinity to glutamate-gated chloride ion channels which occur in invertebrate nerve and muscle cells. This leads to an increase in the permeability of the cell membrane to chloride ions with hyperpolarization of the nerve or muscle cell, resulting in paralysis and death of the parasite. Compounds of this class may also interact with other ligand-gated chloride channels, such as those gated by the neurotransmitter gamma-aminobutyric acid (GABA).

The wide margin of safety is attributable to the fact that mammals do not have glutamate-gated chloride channels, the macrocyclic lactones have a low affinity for other mammalian ligand-gated chloride channels and they do not readily cross the blood-brain barrier.

Dosage and Administration: Dosage: EQVALAN® Liquid for Horses is formulated for administration by stomach tube (nasogastric intubation) or as an oral drench. The recommended dose is 200 mcg of ivermectin per kilogram (91 mcg/lb) of body weight. Each mL contains sufficient ivermectin to treat 110 lb (50 kg) of body weight: 10 mL will treat an 1100 lb (500 kg) horse.

Administration: Use a calibrated dosing syringe inserted into the bottle to measure the appropriate dose, or pour the EQVALAN® Liquid into a graduated cylinder for dose measurement. Use a clean syringe if accessing the bottle to avoid contaminating the remaining product.

Administration by stomach tube (gravity or positive flow): The recommended dose can be used undiluted or diluted up to 40 times with clean tepid water (see Notes to Veterinarian). Use tepid water to flush any drug remaining in the tube into the horse's stomach.

Administration by drench: For administration by this method, an undiluted dose is usually preferred. Clear the horse's mouth of any food material, elevate the horse's head, and using a syringe, deposit the appropriate dose in the back of the mouth. In order to avoid unnecessary coughing or the potential for material to enter the trachea and lungs, do not use excessive pressure (squirting), do not use a large (diluted) dose volume, and do not deposit the dose in the laryngeal area. Increased dose rejection may occur if the dose is deposited in the buccal space. Keep the horse's head elevated and observe the horse to insure the dose is retained.

Suggested Parasite Control Program: All horses should be included in a regular parasite control program with particular attention being paid to mares, foals and yearlings. Foals should be treated initially at 6 to 8 weeks of age, and routine treatment repeated as appropriate. EQVALAN® effectively controls gastrointestinal nematodes and bots in horses. Regular treatment will reduce the chances of verminous arteritis and colic caused by *S. vulgaris.* With its broad spectrum, EQVALAN® is well suited to be the major product in a parasite control program.

Precaution(s): Store in a tightly closed container at room temperature. Protect EQVALAN® Liquid (undiluted or diluted) from light.

Environmental Safety: Studies indicate that when ivermectin comes in contact with the soil, it readily and tightly binds to the soil and becomes inactive over time. Free ivermectin may adversely affect fish and certain water-borne organisms on which they feed. Do not contaminate lakes, streams, or ground water by direct application or by improper disposal of drug containers. Dispose of drug container in approved landfill or by incineration.

Caution(s): Federal (U.S.A.) law restricts this drug to use by or on the order of a licensed veterinarian.

EQVALAN® Liquid has been formulated specifically for use in horses only. This product should not be used in other animal species as severe adverse reactions, including fatalities in dogs, may result.

Notes to Veterinarian: Swelling and itching reactions after treatment with EQVALAN® have occurred in horses carrying heavy infections of neck threadworm microfilariae, *Onchocerca* sp. These reactions were most likely the result of microfilariae dying in large numbers. Symptomatic treatment may be advisable.

Healing of summer sores involving extensive tissue changes may require other therapy in conjunction with EQVALAN®. Reinfection, and measures for its prevention, should also be considered.

Special consideration should be given to the effects or potential for injury from handling, restraint, and placement of the tube during administration by stomach tube. EQVALAN® Liquid should be administered by drench if the risks associated with tubing are of concern. Due to the consequences of improper administration (also see Dosage and Administration), EQVALAN® Liquid is intended for use by a veterinarian only and is not recommended for dispensing.

EQVALAN® Liquid in 1 to 20 and 1 to 40 dilutions with tap water has been shown to be stable for 72 hours under the conditions recommended for the product (i.e., at room temperature, in a lightly closed container, protected from light). The diluted product does not promote the growth of common organisms. However, prolonged storage of the diluted product cannot be recommended, as the effects of possible contaminants and interactions with untested materials are unknown.

For veterinary use only.

Warning(s): Do not use in horses intended for food purposes.

Refrain from smoking and eating when handling. Wash hands after use. Avoid contact with eyes.

Keep this and all drugs out of the reach of children.

The Material Safety Data Sheet (MSDS) contains more detailed occupational safety information. To report adverse effects, obtain an MSDS, or for assistance, contact Merial at 1-888-637-4251.

Discussion: EQVALAN® (ivermectin) Liquid for Horses has been formulated for professional administration by stomach tube or oral drench. One low-volume dose is effective against important internal parasites, including the arterial stages of *Strongylus vulgaris,* and bots.

Discovered and developed by scientists from Merck Research Laboratories, ivermectin is a potent antiparasitic agent whose chemical structure is different from those of other antiparasitic agents. Its convenience, broad-spectrum efficacy and safety margin make EQVALAN® Liquid and ideal parasite control product for horses.

Trial Data: Safety: EQVALAN® Liquid may be used in horses of all ages including mares at any stage of pregnancy. Stallions may be treated without adversely affecting their fertility. These horses have been treated with no adverse effects other than those noted under Notes to Veterinarian.

Presentation: EQVALAN® Liquid for Horses is available in a 100 mL plastic bottle. Each bottle contains sufficient ivermectin to treat 10-500 kg (1100 lb) horses. Contents may be poured into a graduated cylinder for dose measurement. Alternatively, a clean syringe may be inserted directly into the bottle to draw off the appropriate dose.

E

EQVALAN is a registered trademark of Merial.

Merial Limited: Registered in England and Wales [Reg. No. 3332751] with registered offices at 27 Knightsbridge, London, SW1X 7QT, England and domesticated in Delaware, USA as Merial LLC.

U.S. Patent No. 4,199,569

Compendium Code No.: 11110112 8688407

EQVALAN® PASTE 1.87%

Merial **Parasiticide-Oral**

(ivermectin) Anthelmintic and Boticide

NADA No.: 134-314

Active Ingredient(s): Each syringe contains:

Ivermectin 1.87%

Indications: EQVALAN® (ivermectin) Paste provides effective control of the following parasites in horses:

Large Strongyles (adults): *Strongylus vulgaris* (also early forms in blood vessels), *S. edentatus* (also tissue stages), *S. equinus, Triodontophorus* spp.

Small Strongyles including those resistant to some benzimidazole class compounds (adults and fourth-stage larvae): *Cyathostomum* spp., *Cylicocyclus* spp., *Cylicostephanus* spp., *Cylicodontophorus* spp.

Pinworms (adults and fourth-stage larvae): *Oxyuris equi.*

Ascarids (adults and third- and fourth-stage larvae): *Parascaris equorum.*

Hairworms (adults): *Trichostrongylus axei.*

Largemouth Stomach Worms: *Habronema muscae.*

Bots (oral and gastric stages): *Gasterophilus* spp.

Lungworms (adults and fourth-stage larvae): *Dictyocaulus arnfieldi.*

Intestinal Threadworms (adults): *Strongyloides westeri.*

Summer sores caused by *Habronema* and *Draschia* spp. cutaneous third-stage larvae.

Dermatitis caused by neck threadworm microfilariae *Onchocerca* spp.

Dosage and Administration: One syringe contains sufficient paste to treat one 1,250 lb horse at the recommended dose rate of 91 mcg ivermectin per lb (200 mcg/kg) body weight. Each weight marking on the syringe plunger delivers enough paste to treat 250 lb body weight.

1. While holding plunger, turn the knurled ring on the plunger ¼ turn to the left and slide it so the side nearest the barrel is at the prescribed weight marking.
2. Lock the ring in place by making a ¼ turn to the right.
3. Make sure that horse's mouth contains no feed.
4. Remove the cover from the tip of the syringe.
5. Insert the syringe tip into the horse's mouth at the space between the teeth.
6. Depress the plunger as far as it will go, depositing paste on the back of the tongue.
7. Immediately raise the horse's head for a few seconds after dosing.

Parasite Control Program: All horses should be included in a regular parasite control program with particular attention being paid to mares, foals and yearlings. Foals should be treated initially at 6 to 8 weeks of age, and routine treatment repeated as appropriate. Consult your veterinarian for a control program to meet your specific needs. EQVALAN® (ivermectin) Paste effectively controls gastrointestinal nematodes and bots of horses. Regular treatment will reduce the chances of verminous arteritis caused by *Strongylus vulgaris.*

Consult your veterinarian for assistance in the diagnosis, treatment, and control of parasitism.

Precaution(s): Environmental Safety: Ivermectin and excreted residues may adversely affect aquatic organisms. Do not contaminate ground or surface water. Dispose of the syringe in an approved landfill or by incineration.

Caution(s): EQVALAN® (ivermectin) Paste has been formulated specifically for use in horses only. This product should not be used in other animal species as severe adverse reactions, including fatalities in dogs, may result.

Note to User: Swelling and itching reactions after treatment with EQVALAN® Paste have occurred in horses carrying heavy infections of neck threadworm microfilariae *(Onchocera* sp microfilariae). These reactions were most likely the result of microfilariae dying in large numbers. Symptomatic treatment may be advisable. Consult your veterinarian should any such reactions occur. Healing of summer sores involving extensive tissue changes may require other appropriate therapy in conjunction with treatment with EQVALAN® (ivermectin) Paste. Reinfection, and measures for its prevention should also be considered. Consult your veterinarian if the condition does not improve.

For oral use in horses only.

Warning(s): Do not use in horses intended for food purposes.

Not for use in humans. Keep this and all drugs out of reach of children. Refrain from smoking and eating when handling. Wash hands after use. Avoid contact with eyes.

The Material Safety Data Sheet (MSDS) contains more detailed occupational safety information. To report adverse reactions in users, to obtain more information, or to obtain a MSDS, contact Merial at 1-888-637-4251.

Discussion: Product Advantages: Broad-spectrum Control — EQVALAN® Paste kills important internal parasites, including bots and the arterial stages of *S. vulgaris,* with a single dose. EQVALAN® Paste is a potent antiparasitic agent that is neither a benzimidazole nor an organophosphate.

Trial Data: Animal Safety: EQVALAN® Paste may be used in horses of all ages, including mares at any stage of pregnancy. Stallions may be treated without adversely affecting their fertility.

Presentation: 0.21 oz (6.08 g) individual syringes.

EQVALAN is a registered trademark of Merial.

Merial Limited: Registered in England and Wales [Reg. No. 3332751] with registered offices at 27 Knightsbridge, London SW1X 7QT, England and domesticated in Delaware, USA as Merial LLC.

U.S. Patent No. 4,199,569

Compendium Code No.: 11110123 8766803

ERADIMITE™

Fort Dodge **Otic Parasiticide**

Ear Mite Treatment

EPA Reg. No.: 15297-19-1117

Active Ingredient(s):

Pyrethrins 0.15%

*Piperonyl butoxide, technical 1.50%

Inert Ingredients 98.35%

100.00%

*Equivalent to 1.2% (butylcarbityl) (6 propylpiperonyl) ether and min. 0.3% related compounds.

Contains aloe vera.

Indications: Kills ear mites and ear ticks, aids in ear wax removal. Use only on dogs, cats and rabbits.

Directions for Use: Read entire labeling before each use.

It is a violation of Federal Law to use this product in a manner inconsistent with its labeling.

To control spinose ear ticks and ear mites and to remove ear wax apply 10 drops to each ear. Massage base of ear a few minutes to assist penetration of the ear wax by the solution. Allow pet to shake its head. Wipe excess solution from the ear with cotton. Repeat every 2 days until condition has cleared up or as directed by your veterinarian. As a preventative treatment, apply this solution every 15 days to reduce ear mite and ear tick infestation and ear wax accumulation. Do not use on dogs, cats or rabbits under 12 weeks of age. Consult a veterinarian before using this product on debilitated, medicated, aged, pregnant or nursing animals.

Precautionary Statements: Hazards to Humans and Domestic Animals:

Caution: Harmful if swallowed or inhaled. Avoid contact with skin, eyes and clothing. Wash thoroughly with soap and water after using. Do not contaminate food or foodstuffs with this solution. Avoid contact with animal's eyes. Sensitivities may occur after using any pesticide product for pets. If signs of sensitivity occur bathe your pets with mild soap and rinse with large amounts of water. If signs continue, consult a veterinarian immediately.

First Aid:

If swallowed: Call poison control center or doctor immediately for treatment advice.

Have person sip a glass of water if able to swallow.

Do not induce vomiting unless told to do so by the poison control center or doctor.

Do not give anything by mouth to an unconscious person.

If inhaled: Move person to fresh air.

If person is not breathing, call 911 or an ambulance, then give artificial respiration, preferably by mouth-to-mouth, if possible.

Call a poison control center or doctor for further treatment advice.

If on skin/clothing: Take off contaminated clothing.

Rinse skin immediately with plenty of water for 15-20 minutes.

Call a poison control center or doctor for treatment advice.

If in eyes: Hold eye open and rinse slowly and gently with water for 15-20 minutes.

Remove contact lenses if present, after the first 5 minutes, then continue rinsing eye.

Call a poison control center or doctor for treatment advice.

Physical or Chemical Hazards: Do not use or store near heat or open flame.

Storage and Disposal:

Storage: Store in original, closed container in a cool, dry place.

Disposal: Do not reuse empty container. Securely wrap original container in several layers of newspaper and discard in trash.

Warning(s): Keep out of reach of children.

Presentation: NDC 0856-1282-10 — 1 fl oz (29 mL).
NDC 0856-1282-12 — 12-1 fl oz (29 mL).

Compendium Code No.: 10030691 12820A

ER BAC®

Pfizer Animal Health **Bacterin**

Erysipelothrix Rhusiopathiae Bacterin, Aluminum Hydroxide Adsorbed

U.S. Vet. Lic. No.: 189

Contents: This product contains the antigen listed above.

Indications: For vaccination of healthy swine as an aid in preventing erysipelas caused by *Erysipelothrix rhusiopathiae.*

Dosage and Administration: Shake well. Aseptically administer 2 mL intramuscularly at 8 weeks of age or older. Animals retained for breeding should receive a second dose at selection. Annual revaccination is recommended.

Precaution(s): Store at 2°-7°C. Do not freeze. Use entire contents when first opened.

Caution(s): As with many vaccines, anaphylaxis may occur after use. Initial antidote of epinephrine is recommended and should be followed with appropriate supportive therapy.

Warning(s): Do not vaccinate within 21 days before slaughter.

For veterinary use only.

Presentation: 50 dose (100 mL) and 250 dose (500 mL) vials.

Compendium Code No.: 36900540 85-4244-06

ER BAC®/LEPTOFERM-5®

Pfizer Animal Health **Bacterin**

Erysipelothrix Rhusiopathiae-Leptospira Canicola-Grippotyphosa-Hardjo-Icterohaemorrhagiae-Pomona Bacterin, Aluminum Hydroxide Adsorbed

U.S. Vet. Lic. No.: 189

Contents: This product contains the antigens listed above.

Indications: For vaccination of healthy swine as an aid in preventing erysipelas caused by *Erysipelothrix rhusiopathiae* and leptospirosis caused by *Leptospira canicola, L. grippotyphosa, L. hardjo, L. icterohaemorrhagiae,* and *L. pomona.*

Dosage and Administration: Shake well. Aseptically administer 5 mL intramuscularly to breeding age swine, followed by a second dose 3-6 weeks later. Annual revaccination is recommended.

Precaution(s): Store 2°-7°C. Do not freeze. Use entire contents when first opened.
Caution(s): As with many vaccines, anaphylaxis may occur after use. Initial antidote of epinephrine is recommended and should be followed with appropriate supportive therapy.
Warning(s): Do not vaccinate within 21 days before slaughter.

For use in swine only.

For veterinary use only.

Presentation: 50 dose (250 mL) vials.
Compendium Code No.: 36901010 85-4233-05

ER BAC® PLUS

Pfizer Animal Health **Bacterin**

Erysipelothrix Rhusiopathiae Bacterin

U.S. Vet. Lic. No.: 189

Description: ER BAC® Plus is a liquid, serum-free, clarified bacterin that has been chemically inactivated and combined with the adjuvant Amphigen® to enhance the immune response.
Indications: ER BAC® Plus is for vaccination of healthy swine 3 weeks of age or older as an aid in preventing disease caused by *Erysipelothrix rhusiopathiae* for a period of 20 weeks following the second dose in the vaccination regimen.
Directions:

1. General Directions: Shake well. Aseptically administer 2 mL intramuscularly.
2. Primary Vaccination: Healthy swine 3 weeks of age or older should receive two 2 mL doses administered 3-4 weeks apart.
3. Revaccination: Semiannual revaccination with single dose is recommended.
4. Good animal husbandry and herd health management practices should be employed.

Precaution(s): Store at 2°-7°C. Prolonged exposure to higher temperatures may adversely affect potency. Do not freeze.

Use entire contents when first opened.

Sterilized syringes and needles should be used to administer this vaccine.

Caution(s): As with many vaccines, anaphylaxis may occur after use. Initial antidote of epinephrine is recommended and should be followed with appropriate supportive therapy.

This product has been shown to be efficacious in healthy animals. A protective immune response may not be elicited if animals are incubating an infectious disease, are malnourished or parasitized, are stressed due to shipment or environmental conditions, are otherwise immunocompromised, or the vaccine is not administered in accordance with label directions.

For use in swine only.

For veterinary use only.

Warning(s): Do not vaccinate within 21 days before slaughter.
Discussion: Disease Description: Erysipelas is caused by the bacterium *E. rhusiopathiae* and has been identified as a pathogen in swine since 1878. The disease is worldwide in distribution and is of economic importance throughout Europe, Asia, Australia, and North and South America. Swine 3 months through 3 years of age are most susceptible to erysipelas; outbreaks are usually more severe in herds on soil and during periods of wet weather. Erysipelas can take one of several forms or a combination of the following forms. Acute erysipelas is a general infection by *E. rhusiopathiae* in the bloodstream. This form often causes sudden death. Abortion may result in sows infected during pregnancy. Skin erysipelas manifests as diamond-shaped patches of swollen, purple skin on a pig's body, especially the belly and thighs. If the tips of the ears and tail are affected, tissues may die and slough. Arthritic erysipelas is a chronic disease occurring in pigs that have survived acute erysipelas. Affected pigs often have swollen and stiff joints. They do not gain weight efficiently, and their carcasses are often trimmed or condemned by inspectors at packing houses. Cardiac erysipelas usually occurs in older pigs raised on farms where the chronic form exists. Cardiac erysipelas may result in growths on the heart valves altering the normal flow of blood.
Trial Data: Safety and Efficacy: In laboratory and field safety studies of ER BAC® Plus, no serious adverse reactions to vaccination were reported. Efficacy of ER BAC® Plus was demonstrated in 2 host animal studies conducted by Pfizer Animal Health; an immunogenicity study and a duration-of-immunity study demonstrating efficacy 20 weeks after second vaccination. Pigs vaccinated with ER BAC® Plus, followed by challenge, had significantly fewer clinical signs of disease, including death, lesions, and fever, than non-vaccinated control pigs in both of the following studies. Host animal immunogenicity study: The purpose of this study was to demonstrate protection against challenge with virulent *E. rhusiopathiae* 2½ weeks after the second vaccination. Pigs were vaccinated at approximately 3 and 6 weeks of age. Pigs were monitored daily for rectal temperature and for clinical signs of disease. Ten of 10 control pigs (100%) were determined to be positive for infection after challenge. Nineteen of 20 vaccinated pigs (95%) were protected. These results indicate that vaccination with ER BAC® Plus with Amphigen® provided significant protection from challenge 2½ weeks after vaccination. (Tables 1 and 2).

Table 1. Results of *E. rhusiopathiae* Challenge in Control Pigs (100% positive).

Control Pigs	2 days*	1 day only	Clinical signs**	Mortality/ Euthanasia	Treated	Organism isolation
10	7	3	8	3	7	3

* Elevation in rectal temperature above 40.9°C (105.6°F) on 2 consecutive days.
** Clinical signs included recumbent, depressed, and/or metastatic skin lesions.

Table 2. Results of *E. rhusiopathiae* Challenge 2½ Weeks Postvaccination (95% protected).

Vaccinated Pigs	2 days*	1 day only	Clinical signs**	Mortality/ Euthanasia	Treated	Organism isolation
20	1	0	0	0	1	Not Sampled

* Elevation in rectal temperature above 40.3°C (104.6°F) on 2 consecutive days.
** Clinical signs included recumbent, depressed, and/or metastatic skin lesions.

Duration-of-immunity study: The purpose of this study was to demonstrate protection against challenge with virulent *E. rhusiopathiae* in a duration-of-immunity study 20 weeks after the second vaccination or at approximately market weight (26 weeks of age). Pigs were vaccinated at approximately 3 and 6 weeks of age. Pigs were monitored daily for rectal temperature and for clinical signs of disease. Nine of 10 control pigs (90%) were determined to be positive for infection after challenge. Fifteen of 20 vaccinated pigs (75%) were protected. These results indicate that vaccination with ER BAC® Plus with Amphigen® provided significant protection from challenge 20 weeks after vaccination. (Tables 3 and 4).

Table 3. Results of *E. rhusiopathiae* Challenge in Control Pigs (90% positive).

Control Pigs	2 days*	1 day only	Clinical signs**	Mortality/ Euthanasia	Treated	Organism isolation
10	3	4	9	7	3	5

* Elevation in rectal temperature above 40.9°C (105.6°F) on 2 consecutive days.
** Clinical signs included recumbent, depressed, and/or metastatic skin lesions.

Table 4. Results of *E. rhusiopathiae* Challenge in 26-week-old Pigs (75% protected).

Vaccinated Pigs	2 days*	1 day only	Clinical signs**	Mortality/ Euthanasia	Treated	Organism isolation
20	3	5	5	1	4	1

* Elevation in rectal temperature above 40.3°C (104.6°F) on 2 consecutive days.
** Clinical signs included recumbent, depressed, and/or metastatic skin lesions.

Presentation: 50 dose (100 mL) and 250 dose (500 mL) vials.
Compendium Code No.: 36900331 75-5040-01

ER BAC® PLUS/LEPTOFERM-5®

Pfizer Animal Health **Bacterin**

Erysipelothrix Rhusiopathiae-Leptospira Canicola-Grippotyphosa-Hardjo-Icterohaemorrhagiae-Pomona Bacterin

U.S. Vet. Lic. No.: 189

Description: ER BAC® Plus/LEPTOFERM-5® is a liquid preparation of a serum-free, clarified *E. rhusiopathiae* culture, and whole cell cultures of the 5 *Leptospira* serovars identified above. The antigens have been chemically inactivated and adjuvanted with 2 adjuvants, including Amphigen®, to enhance the immune response.

Contains gentamicin as preservative.

Indications: ER BAC® Plus/LEPTOFERM-5® is for vaccination of healthy breeding swine as an aid in preventing erysipelas caused by *Erysipelothrix rhusiopathiae* and leptospirosis caused by *Leptospira canicola, L. grippotyphosa, L. hardjo, L. icterohaemorrhagiae* and *L. pomona*. A 26-week duration of immunity following vaccination has been demonstrated against erysipelas.
Directions:

1. General Directions: Shake well. Aseptically administer 5 mL intramuscularly.
2. Primary Vaccination: Healthy swine should receive 2 doses 3-5 weeks apart with the second dose administered 2-4 weeks prior to breeding. Healthy gilts, however, should receive the second dose as near as possible to 14 days prior to breeding.
3. Revaccination: Revaccination with a single dose is recommended prior to subsequent breedings. Boars should be revaccinated semiannually.
4. Good animal husbandry and herd health management practices should be employed.

Precaution(s): Store at 2°-7°C. Prolonged exposure to higher temperatures may adversely affect potency. Do not freeze.

Use entire contents when first opened.

Sterilized syringes and needles should be used to administer this vaccine.

Caution(s): Temporary swelling at the injection site may be observed.

As with many vaccines, anaphylaxis may occur after use. Initial antidote of epinephrine is recommended and should be followed with appropriate supportive therapy.

This product has been shown to be efficacious in healthy animals. A protective immune response may not be elicited if animals are incubating an infectious disease, are malnourished or parasitized, are stressed due to shipment or environmental conditions, are otherwise immunocompromised, or the vaccine is not administered in accordance with label directions.

For use in swine only.

For veterinary use only.

Warning(s): Do not vaccinate within 21 days before slaughter.
Discussion: Disease Description: *Leptospira* are common agents of reproductive loss in swine. While infection with *Leptospira* may produce subclinical disease, infection during the second half of pregnancy may cause abortions and stillbirths; late-term abortions are the most important economic effect of leptospirosis. Leptospirosis caused by any of the serovars represented here cannot be clinically differentiated. Abortions may also occur in sows infected with *E. rhusiopathiae* during pregnancy.
Trial Data: Safety and Efficacy: The safety and efficacy of the fractions in ER BAC® Plus/LEPTOFERM-5® were demonstrated in studies conducted in support of FarrowSure® Plus B.

The safety of FarrowSure® Plus B was demonstrated under both controlled laboratory and field conditions. No serious systemic or allergic reactions were observed following vaccination. In field studies, 1191 sows and gilts were vaccinated with FarrowSure® Plus B. Approximately 10% of the sows and gilts vaccinated exhibited transient local swelling at the site of injection 24 hours after vaccination under field conditions. By 21 days after vaccination, less than 1% of sows and gilts exhibited swelling at the injection site. Efficacy of the fractions of FarrowSure® Plus B was demonstrated in controlled challenge-of-immunity and immunogenicity tests. Serologic responses to all components of FarrowSure® Plus B were compared to those of FarrowSure® B. In all cases FarrowSure® Plus B stimulated higher antibody titers than FarrowSure® B. These results are summarized in Table 1.

Table 1. Comparison of FarrowSure® B and FarrowSure® Plus B Geometric Mean Titers and the Lower 95% Confidence Limit (CL) of the Difference as a Percent of the FarrowSure® B Titer:

Antigen	FarrowSure® B	FarrowSure® Plus B	Lower 95% CL
E. rhusiopathiae	552.8	2305.8	279.9
Porcine Parvovirus	53.2	124.6	145.0
L. bratislava	1024.0	6109.9	384.8
L. canicola	9.6	47.7	242.5
L. grippotyphosa	147.0	1262.2	439.9
L. hardjo	4.2	121.4	1322.0
L. icterohaemorrhagiae	157.6	650.8	256.2
L. pomona	9.0	37.6	195.0

Duration of Immunity: In addition to the above studies, duration-of-immunity studies in pigs were conducted for the *E. rhusiopathiae* fraction. The purpose of these studies was to demonstrate protection against challenge with virulent *E. rhusiopathiae* 20 and 26 weeks after the second vaccination with FarrowSure® Plus B.

20 Week Duration-of-Immunity Study: Four to 5-month-old pigs received 2 doses approximately 3 weeks apart, followed by challenge with virulent *E. rhusiopathiae* 20 weeks after the second vaccination. Following challenge, pigs were monitored daily for rectal temperature and clinical signs of disease. Eight of 10 control pigs (80%) were determined to be positive for infection following challenge. Eighteen of 20 vaccinated pigs (90%) were protected.

26 Week Duration-of-Immunity Study: Four to 5-month-old pigs received 2 doses approximately 3 weeks apart, followed by challenge with virulent *E. rhusiopathiae* 26 weeks after the second vaccination. Following challenge, pigs were monitored daily for rectal temperature and clinical signs of disease. Seven of 10 control pigs (70%) were determined to be positive for infection after challenge. Seventeen of 20 vaccinated pigs (85%) were protected. Results of these studies are illustrated in Tables 2 and 3.

Table 2. Results of *E. rhusiopathiae* Challenge in Control Pigs:

Study	No. of Control pigs	# Positive	# Protected	% Protected
20-week	10	8	2	20%
26-week	10	7	3	30%

Control pigs were considered to be positive for erysipelas if they met one or more of the following criteria: 1) Two consecutive days of temperatures at or above 40.9°C (105.6°F); 2) Sudden death following evidence of systemic erysipelas (including less than 2 consecutive days of elevated temperatures and/or systemic clinical signs); or 3) Recovery of *E. rhusiopathiae* from the spleen or liver.

Table 3. Results of *E. rhusiopathiae* Challenge in Vaccinated Pigs:

Study	No. of Vaccinated Pigs	# Positive	# Protected	% Protected
20-week	20	2	18	90%
26-week	20	3	17	85%

Vaccinated pigs were considered to be protected if they were free of the following criteria: 1) Two consecutive days of temperatures at or above 40.3°C (104.6°F); 2) Sudden death following evidence of systemic erysipelas (including less than 2 consecutive days of elevated temperatures and/or systemic clinical signs); or 3) Recovery of *E. rhusiopathiae* from the spleen or liver.

E

Presentation: 50 doses.

Compendium Code No.: 36902020 75-4234-00

ERMOGEN

Novartis (Aqua Health) **Bacterin**

Yersinia Ruckeri Bacterin

U.S. Vet. Lic. No.: 335

Contents: This bacterin has been shown to be safe and effective for use with 2 grams or larger salmonids. This bacterin contains only formalin inactivated cultures of *Yersinia ruckeri.* No other preservative is used.

Indications: As an aid in the prevention of enteric redmouth disease caused by *Yersinia ruckeri*, serotype I.

Dosage and Administration: Vaccination Program: Vaccination should precede exposure of vaccinates to the disease agent by 14 days if holding water temperatures are 10°-12°C. A longer period of time should be allowed if temperatures are below 10°C. Protection develops in 45 days at 5°C.

Methods of Administration: For immersion and spray delivery dilute entire contents of this bottle with 9 liters of clean hatchery water.

For transport delivery dilute 1:200 with hatchery water.

Immersion Delivery: Measure diluted bacterin in a suitable plastic container. Add fish to attain a density of 500 g per liter of diluted bacterin.

Expose fish for 30 seconds then drain bacterin from fish. Return fish to holding facility. Repeat until a total of 20 groups have been vaccinated in this manner.

Spray Delivery: Pressurize spray unit to 2.1 kg/cm² (30 psi) with compressed gas (O_2, N_2 or air) to deliver 10 liters of diluted bacterin in 12-14 minutes.

Adjust nozzle of unit so that 5 seconds contact time is achieved. Dewater fish from holding facility and place in unit. Expose fish to spray for 5 seconds then return to holding facility. Ten liters of diluted bacterin will vaccinate approximately 250 kg, depending on fish size.

Transport Delivery: Vaccination can be done in hauling tanks using normal loading densities of 2.25 lb rainbow trout per gal. Dilute bacterin to 1:200 with hatchery water and expose fish for a minimum of 20 minutes. A longer exposure interval is beneficial when possible. Oxygen gas must be added to the tank during the exposure period.

Precaution(s): Shake well before using. Store between 2-7°C (35-45°F). Do not freeze. Use entire contents when first opened. The vaccinal solution should be within 2°C of the ambient water temperature.

Caution(s): Vaccinate healthy fish only. Revaccination can be done if immunity is required for longer than 300 days.

For veterinary use only.

Warning(s): Do not vaccinate within 21 days of slaughter.

Presentation: 1000 mL bottles.

Distributed by: Mr. J. Zinn, Buhl, Idaho 83316

Compendium Code No.: 14970002 L-021-2

ERYCELL™

Novartis Animal Vaccines **Vaccine**

Erysipelothrix rhusiopathiae Vaccine, Avirulent Live Culture

U.S. Vet. Lic. No.: 303

Composition: The vaccine contains a highly antigenic, avirulent live culture of *Erysipelothrix rhusiopathiae.*

Indications: For use in healthy swine as an aid in the prevention and control of diseases caused by *Erysipelothrix rhusiopathiae.*

Dosage and Administration: Aseptically rehydrate with the diluent supplied and shake well before using.

Sows and Gilts: It is recommended that adult animals be inoculated intramuscularly (I.M.) with a single 2 mL dose before breeding, however, adverse reactions have not been experienced due to vaccination during the gestation period. Revaccinate annually to maintain high levels of immunity.

Piglets: Administer 1 mL (0.5 mL/nostril) intranasally (I.N.) into piglets one (1) to three (3) days of age.

Feeder pigs: Inject 2 mL intramuscularly or intranasally (1 mL/nostril) at weaning stage.

Precaution(s): Store between 35°-45°F (2°-7°C). Do not freeze. Needles and syringes should be sterilized by boiling. Do not use chemical sterilization as traces of chemicals may inactivate the vaccine. Use the entire contents without delay after rehydration. Burn the container and any unused contents.

Caution(s): Do not use the vaccine in the presence of antibiotics effective against *Erysipelothrix rhusiopathiae.* Anaphylactic reactions may occur with the vaccine. Symptomatic treatment: Epinephrine.

Warning(s): Do not vaccinate within 21 days of slaughter.

Discussion: Swine erysipelas is an infectious disease caused by *Erysipelothrix rhusiopathiae.* The gram positive rod-shaped organism is found worldwide wherever swine are raised. The disease manifests itself in one of three forms: acute, subacute, or chronic. The acute form is most frequently characterized by sudden death or septicemia with fevers up to 108°. The subacute form is less severe and is characterized by diamond-shaped raised skin lesions. The chronic form follows the acute or subacute form and may include arthritis or subclinical infections. Perhaps the major economic losses are in animals infected with the chronic form of the disease because of high treatment costs, retarded growth, arthritic conditions, and poor performance in feeder pigs.

The pathogen is spread via the oral route, and many swine are carriers of the organism. It has been estimated that up to 30% of clinically normal swine have positive tonsils.

Swine of all ages are susceptible to erysipelas. As a group, animals of less than one month of age are less affected due to maternal protection from their immunized dams. However, newborn or young pigs are very susceptible to erysipelas if maternal protection is not in place. Animals older than three years of age are usually resistant to infection because of subclinical exposure or from vaccination programs.

Generally, the most susceptible group of swine to the disease is animals recently weaned. Maternal protection drops off to low levels at about five to eight weeks of age. If the piglets are not actively immunized prior to that time they are very susceptible to erysipelas infection.

Trial Data: ERYCELL™ Challenge Data: Feeder pig protection trial:

Status	Vaccination Route and Dose	Challenge Route and Dose	% Protection (Absence of clinical symptoms)
Feeder pig vaccinates	2 mL I.M.	2 mL I.M.	89%
Feeder pig vaccinates	2 mL I.N.	2 mL I.N.	95%
Feeder pig controls	None	2 mL I.M.	0%

Conclusions:

1. Newborn piglets are susceptible to *E. rhusiopathiae* infection.
2. Immunized dams transfer passive protection against *E. rhusiopathiae* to nursing piglets.
3. Piglets born to immunized dams are actively immunized when vaccinated intranasally at birth with an avirulent *Erysipelothrix rhusiopathiae* vaccine. Maternal antibodies did not interfere with immunity.

Three safety tests were also conducted on this product:

1. Extensive field trial safety testing of the product was completed in swine of mixed breed and various ages with no observations of any untoward or adverse reactions. This study was conducted under the supervision of approved veterinary investigators.
2. Exaggerated dose safety testing of the product was completed in one day old baby piglets. The piglets received six times the concentration of vaccine that they would normally receive and again no untoward or adverse reactions were noted by the independent, qualified veterinarian conducting the study.
3. Reversion to virulence testing (required for all avirulent vaccines) was completed in weaned pigs. The avirulent organism was recovered through each of the five back passages. There were not deaths nor symptoms of erysipelas observed in any pigs through the five consecutive back passages indicating that the vaccine will not revert back to its virulent state. An independent study of the same manner was also conducted in pigeons (animals most susceptible to erysipelas) which also supports the safety of this vaccine.

Data on file with USDA.

Presentation: Available in 30 mL bottles (30 piglet doses, 15 sow and feeder pig doses).

Compendium Code No.: 11140172

ERY SERUM™

Novartis Animal Vaccines **Antiserum**

Erysipelothrix rhusiopathiae Antiserum, Equine Origin

U.S. Vet. Lic. No.: 303

Composition: The antiserum is prepared from the blood of horses hyperimmunized with *Erysipelothrix rhusiopathiae.*

The product contains oxytetracycline, phenol and thimerosal as preservatives.

Indications: For use as an aid in the prevention and treatment of diseases caused by *Erysipelothrix rhusiopathiae* in swine.

Dosage and Administration: Shake well before using. Administer the following doses subcutaneously.

Dosage:	Prevention
Piglets less than 24 hours of age	2 mL
Piglets up to 25 lbs.	3 mL
Pigs 25 to 50 lbs.	5 mL
Pigs 50 to 75 lbs.	10 mL
Pigs 75 to 100 lbs.	15 mL

For treatment: Double the dose and repeat in 24 hours.

Precaution(s): Store in the dark at 35°-45°F (2°-7°C). Do not freeze. Use the entire contents when first opened.

Caution(s): Anaphylactic reactions may occur following the use of the product. Symptomatic treatment: Epinephrine.

Warning(s): Do not administer within 21 days prior to slaughter.

Discussion: Erysipelas in swine is caused by a bacterium, *Erysipelothrix rhusiopathiae.* Pigs become infected most commonly from ingesting the organism, although it may also enter the body through skin wounds. The source of the infection is usually other carrier pigs or wild animals such as rodents and birds.

Clinical signs of erysipelas in swine can be acute, subacute or chronic. In the acute form, animals show signs of systemic disease. They lie around and are reluctant to rise. If forced to rise, they will stand with their legs tucked under their bodies. Affected pigs are off feed and have fevers of 104°-108°F. Pregnant sows may abort. Raised red skin lesions ("diamond skin" lesions) often appear within two to three days, and animals that develop severe skin lesions usually die.

Subacute erysipelas includes many of the same symptoms, but they are less severe, sometimes to the point of being unnoticed.

Chronic erysipelas may follow cases of acute or subacute erysipelas, or it may show up in pigs that have not had any previous signs of illness. Pigs with chronic erysipelas usually show signs of arthritis due to degenerative changes in the joints. The valves of the heart may also be affected, in which case the animals will show signs of heart disease such as shortness of breath. Perhaps the major economic losses are in animals infected with the chronic form of the disease because of high treatment costs, retarded growth, arthritic conditions, and poor performance in feeder pigs.

The pathogen is spread via the oral route, and many swine are carriers of the organism. It has been estimated that up to 30% of clinically normal swine have erysipelas-infected tonsils.

Swine of all ages are susceptible to erysipelas. As a group, animals less than one month of age are less affected due to maternal protection from their immunized dams. However, newborn or young pigs are very susceptible to erysipelas if maternal protection is not in place. Animals older than three years of age are usually resistant to infection because of subclinical exposure or from vaccination programs.

Trial Data: Subcutaneous administration reduces the risk of tissue reaction. ERY SERUM™ is an effective colostrum supplement where colostrum quality and quantity are questionable. 80% survival rates were observed in the treated newborn piglets compared to 0% survival in control piglets when exposed within 24 hours of birth.

Presentation: 250 mL bottles.

Compendium Code No.: 11140142

ERY SHIELD™

Novartis Animal Vaccines **Bacterin**

Erysipelothrix rhusiopathiae Bacterin

U.S. Vet. Lic. No.: 303

Composition: The bacterin contains a chemically inactivated highly antigenic culture of *Erysipelothrix rhusiopathiae* adjuvanted with aluminum hydroxide. Contains penicillin and streptomycin as preservatives.

Indications: For use in healthy swine as an aid in the prevention and control of erysipelas and other diseases caused by *Erysipelothrix rhusiopathiae.*

Dosage and Administration: Shake well before using. Inject 2 mL subcutaneously or intramuscularly. For breeding animals, repeat after 21 days. Revaccinate annually.

Precaution(s): Store between 35°-45°F (2°-7°C). Do not freeze. Use the entire contents when first opened.

Caution(s): Anaphylactic reactions may occur following the use of the product. Symptomatic treatment: Epinephrine.

Warning(s): Do not vaccinate within 21 days prior to slaughter.

Presentation: Available in 50 dose (100 mL), 125 dose (250 mL), and 250 dose (500 mL) bottles.

Compendium Code No.: 11140152

ERY SHIELD™+L5

Novartis Animal Vaccines **Bacterin**

Erysipelothrix Rhusiopathiae-Leptospira Canicola-Grippotyphosa-Hardjo-Icterohaemorrhagiae-Pomona Bacterin

U.S. Vet. Lic. No.: 303

Composition: This bacterin contains inactivated cultures of *Erysipelothrix rhusiopathiae, Leptospira canicola, grippotyphosa, hardjo, icterohaemorrhagiae,* and *pomona* adjuvanted with aluminum hydroxide. Contains penicillin, streptomycin, and thimerosal as preservatives.

Indications: For use in healthy swine as an aid in the prevention and control of disease caused by *Erysipelothrix rhusiopathiae, Leptospira canicola, grippotyphosa, hardjo, icterohaemorrhagiae,* and *pomona.*

Dosage and Administration: Shake well before using. Administer 2 mL intramuscularly. Repeat in 3-4 weeks. Revaccinate annually.

Precaution(s): Store in the dark at 35°-45°F (2°-7°C). Do not freeze. Use entire contents when first opened.

Caution(s): Anaphylactic reactions may occur following the use of this biological. Symptomatic treatment: Epinephrine.

For veterinary use only.

Warning(s): Do not vaccinate within 21 days prior to slaughter.

Discussion: Erysipelas in swine is caused by a bacterium, *Erysipelothrix rhusiopathiae.* Pigs become infected most commonly from ingesting the organism, although it may also enter the body through skin wounds. The source of the infection is usually other carrier pigs or wild animals such as rodents and birds.

Clinical signs of erysipelas in swine can be acute, subacute or chronic. In the acute form, animals show signs of systemic disease. They lie around and are reluctant to rise. If forced to rise, they will stand with their legs tucked under their bodies. Affected pigs are off feed and have fevers of 104°-108°F. Pregnant sows may abort. Raised red skin lesions ("diamond skin" lesions) often appear within 2-3 days, and animals that develop severe skin lesions usually die.

Subacute erysipelas includes many of the same symptoms, but they are less severe, sometimes to the point of being unnoticed.

Chronic erysipelas may follow cases of acute or subacute erysipelas, or it may show up in pigs that have had no previous signs of illness. Pigs with chronic erysipelas usually show signs of arthritis due to degenerative changes in the joints. The valves of the heart may also be affected, in which case the animals will show signs of heart disease such as shortness of breath.

Leptospirosis is a contagious disease of both man and animals and has been estimated to cause losses in excess of 100 million dollars per year to the livestock industry, according to the USDA. This loss is due primarily to abortions and stillbirths in breeding stock and by sickness and death in young animals. The causative organisms belong to a group of pathogens called *Leptospira interrogans,* with five major serovars incriminated: *L grippotyphosa, L hardjo, L pomona, L canicola,* and *L icterohaemorrhagiae.*

This disease is spread to our domestic livestock by the shedding of the organisms in the urine, which contaminates feed or water. These organisms survive well in surface waters. The organism may be found in the udder and be secreted in the milk to suckling piglets, thus infecting them.

In swine, the most common serotypes are *L pomona,* which is shed from pig to pig via the urine, and *L icterohaemorrhagiae* which is spread to pigs from dogs and rats.

The incubation period varies from 1 to 4 days and is followed by a leptospiremia (bacteria in the blood) which lasts for 1-5 days. The organisms may remain in the kidney and multiply in this location, then are shed in the urine for months or years, infecting other farm animals.

Symptoms in swine vary widely. Many of the infections are subclinical and are only recognized by seroconversion, by isolation of the organism from the kidneys and urine, or by cases of leptospirosis in other animals from the swine herd. The most common signs are abortions and stillbirths in pregnant animals, mainly late abortions. Common clinical signs include loss of appetite, intestinal problems and reduced weight gain. Acute or subacute infections are observed in young pigs, with fever and high death loss the primary signs.

Presentation: Available in 50 dose (100 mL) bottles.

Compendium Code No.: 11140162

ERYSIPELAS BACTERIN

AgriLabs **Bacterin**

Erysipelas rhusiopathiae Bacterin

U.S. Vet. Lic. No.: 272

Active Ingredient(s): Contains chemically inactivated cultures of *Erysipelas rhusiopathiae.*

Contains thimerosal as a preservative.

Indications: For the immunization of healthy swine against erysipelas caused by *E. rhusiopathiae.*

Dosage and Administration: Shake well before use.

Administer 2 mL subcutaneously to healthy swine. Pigs vaccinated under six (6) weeks of age should be revaccinated at eight (8) to 12 weeks of age. Breeding animals should be revaccinated in two (2) to four (4) weeks and annually with a single 2 mL dose.

Precaution(s): Refrigerate at 35°-45°F (2°-7°C).

Caution(s): For veterinary use only.

Use the entire contents when first opened. In case of anaphylactic reactions, administer epinephrine.

Warning(s): Do not vaccinate within 21 days before slaughter.

Presentation: 100 mL (50 dose) and 500 mL (250 dose) vials.

Compendium Code No.: 10580480

E

ERYSIPELOTHRIX RHUSIOPATHIAE SERUM ANTIBODIES

Colorado Serum **Antiserum**

Erysipelothrix rhusiopathiae Antiserum

U.S. Vet. Lic. No.: 188

Active Ingredient(s): *Erysipelothrix rhusiopathiae* antiserum, equine origin.

Contains phenol and thimerosal as preservatives.

Prepared from the blood of horses hyperimmunized with *Erysipelothrix rhusiopathiae.*

Indications: An antiserum specific for the treatment and temporary prevention of erysipelas in swine.

Dosage and Administration: ERYSIPELOTHRIX RHUSIOPATHIAE SERUM ANTIBODIES should be used when swine are too young to be actively immunized and during outbreaks when immediate protection is desired. Erysipelas is a bacterial disease, as such, antiserum will provide a significantly helpful response when administered to sick animals in therapeutic doses. Needle punctures and tissue damage may result in condemnation of carcasses.

The following dosage table has been recommended for swine by the U.S. Department of Agriculture.

For Prevention:

Pigs weighing less than 50 lbs.	5 mL
Pigs weighing 50 to 75 lbs.	10 mL
Pigs weighing 75 to 100 lbs.	15 mL
Pigs weighing over 100 lbs.	20 mL

For Treatment:

The dosage shown in the above table should be doubled for treatment of sick animals. Repeat in 24 to 48 hours as indicated.

Injections should be made subcutaneously. Avoid fatty tissue and other areas of poor circulation. Small pigs can be vaccinated in the axillary space (armpit). Larger hogs, sows and boars can be vaccinated in the "pocket" behind the ear.

Precaution(s): Store in the dark at 2-7°C. Sterilize needles and syringes by boiling in clean water. Use the entire contents when the bottle is first opened.

Caution(s): Anaphylaxis (shock) may sometimes follow the use of products of this nature. Epinephrine or an equivalent drug should be available for immediate use in these instances. Artificial respiration is also helpful.

For veterinary use only.

Warning(s): Do not vaccinate within 21 days before slaughter.

Discussion: Antiserums contain antibodies against specific diseases and are beneficial as a means of providing immediate protection to susceptible animals. Antiserums, however, do not actively stimulate the antibody system of the vaccinated animal and the resulting immunity is passive, lasting only until the injected antibodies are eliminated from the system, a period of approximately 14-21 days. The antibody systems of production animals are stimulated by injections of increasingly large doses of *Erysipelothrix rhusiopathiae,* which are repeated until a satisfactory titer can be demonstrated in the recovered serum.

Erysipelas is an infectious disease of swine. Turkeys may also become infected. The disease has been diagnosed in every area of the United States and is a problem in many foreign countries as well. Swine and turkeys of all weights and ages may be affected.

Three forms of erysipelas may be observed in swine:

1. The acute, septicemic form is probably the most common and causes the greatest losses, especially in young pigs. Sudden illness, high temperatures (106-109°) and reddish discoloration of the skin are the most common symptoms. Death follows a few days after the symptoms first appear.
2. The chronic form is characterized by evidence of pain, soreness and stiffness. Affected animals are not easily aroused and when forced will walk on their toes in a stilted fashion. While some death loss will occur, the effect is prolonged with animals developing swollen joints, sloughing skin and general unthriftiness.
3. The mild form of erysipelas usually results in slight skin sloughing or so-called diamond skin eruptions. This form is not as serious as the others, and losses are usually not excessive.

In turkeys acute erysipelas is characterized by multiple diffuse hemorrhages in the large muscles and beneath the serous surfaces of the visceral organs. The liver and spleen are usually congested, enlarged and show hemorrhagic infarcts. Catarrhal exudate may be found in the intestines. Clinical symptoms are anorexia, dull and listless behavior with the development of a greenish-yellow diarrhea. Breathing may be labored with a thick mucous discharge from the nostrils. A red-purple wattle is highly suggestive of erysipelas in turkeys.

Erysipelas in swine resembles hog cholera. Autopsy may not reveal lesions that will permit positive diagnosis and the assistance of a competent laboratory is recommended when erysipelas is suspected. Administration of *Erysipelothrix rhusiopathiae* antiserum may sometimes aid in the diagnosis if two or three typically sick animals are injected with therapeutic doses and significant improvement is noted within 21 hours.

Presentation: 250 mL bottles.

Compendium Code No.: 11010240

ERYSIPELOTHRIX RHUSIOPATHIAE SERUM ANTIBODIES

Professional Biological **Antiserum**

Erysipelothrix rhusiopathiae Antiserum, Equine Origin

U.S. Vet. Lic. No.: 188

Active Ingredient(s): *Erysipelothrix rhusiopathiae* antiserum prepared from the blood of horses hyperimmunized with *Erysipelothrix rhusiopathiae.*

Contains phenol and thimerosal as preservatives.

Indications: For the prevention and treatment of swine erysipelas.

Dosage and Administration: Inject subcutaneously as follows:

For Prevention:

Swine up to 50 lbs. .... 5 mL
Swine 50 to 75 lbs. .... 10 mL
Swine 75 to 100 lbs. .... 15 mL
Swine 100 lbs. and over .... 20 mL

For Treatment:

At least double the preventive dose.

Repeat in 24 to 48 hours as indicated.

E

Precaution(s): Store in the dark at 2° to 7°C.

Caution(s): Anaphylactic reactions sometime follows the administration of products of this nature. If noted, administer adrenalin or equivalent. Use the entire contents when the bottle is first opened.

For veterinary use only.

Warning(s): Do not vaccinate within 21 days before slaughter.

Presentation: 250 mL bottles.

Compendium Code No.: 14250010

ERY VAC 100

Arko **Vaccine**

Erysipelothrix rhusiopathiae Vaccine, Avirulent Live Culture

U.S. Vet. Lic. No.: 337

Contents: *Erysipelothrix rhusiopathiae* vaccine. Avirulent live culture.

Indications: For the oral vaccination of healthy susceptible swine eight weeks of age or older against erysipelas associated with *Erysipelothrix rhusiopathiae.*

Dosage and Administration: Add 20 mL of water, shake well. Combine with 25 oz of water and promptly administer ¼ oz orally per pig.

Precaution(s): Store at not over 45°F (7°C). Use entire contents when first opened. Burn this container and all unused contents.

Caution(s): Anaphylactic reactions occur.

Antidote(s): Administer epinephrine.

Warning(s): Do not vaccinate within 21 days before slaughter.

Presentation: 100 dose vials.

Compendium Code No.: 11230020

ERY VAC 500

Arko **Vaccine**

Erysipelothrix rhusiopathiae Vaccine, Avirulent Live Culture

U.S. Vet. Lic. No.: 337

Contents: *Erysipelothrix rhusiopathiae* vaccine. Avirulent live culture.

Indications: For the oral vaccination of healthy susceptible swine eight weeks of age or older against erysipelas associated with *Erysipelothrix rhusiopathiae.*

Dosage and Administration: Add 20 mL of water, shake well. Combine with 125 oz of water and promptly administer ¼ oz orally per pig.

Precaution(s): Store at not over 45°F (7°C). Use entire contents when first opened. Burn this container and all unused contents.

Caution(s): Anaphylactic reactions occur.

Antidote(s): Administer epinephrine.

Warning(s): Do not vaccinate within 21 days before slaughter.

Presentation: 500 dose vials.

Compendium Code No.: 11230030

ESBILAC® 2ND STEP™ PUPPY WEANING FOOD

Pet-Ag **Weaning Formula**

Guaranteed Analysis:

Crude Protein, min. 26%
Crude Fat, min. 12%
Crude Fiber, max. 1%
Moisture, max 8%
Ash, max. 8.5%

Ingredients: Rice flour, dried milk protein concentrate, dried skimmed milk, animal fat preserved with BHA and BHT, dried meat solubles, condensed whey product, dicalcium phosphate, vegetable oil, potassium chloride, dried whey protein concentrate, calcium carbonate, sodium chloride, lecithin, artificial flavor, sodium silico aluminate, dl-methionine, silicon dioxide, zinc methionine, iron choline citrate, vitamin E supplement, zinc choline citrate, manganese sulfate, calcium pantothenate, niacin supplement, copper choline citrate, vitamin A supplement, ethylenediamine dihydroiodide, cobalt choline citrate, riboflavin supplement, thiamine mononitrate, menadione sodium bisulfite complex, pyridoxine hydrochloride, folic acid, d-biotin supplement, vitamin D_3 supplement, vitamin B_{12} supplement.

Indications: Recommended as the transition diet to take puppies from nursing to solid food.

Directions for Use: 2ND STEP™ Puppy Weaning Food is a complete food for growing puppies. 2ND STEP™ Puppy Weaning Food may be mixed with water, however, for a more gradual change from bitch's milk to a solid diet it is recommended that it be mixed with Esbilac®. 2ND STEP™ Puppy Weaning Food should be fed until puppies are 7 to 8 weeks old when they can be fed commercial puppy or dog food. All changes should be made gradually over a one week period.

Mix 2ND STEP™ Puppy Weaning Food using one of the methods in the table below.

Mixing Directions[1]:

2ND STEP™ Puppy Weaning Food	Esbilac® Powder	Esbilac® Liquid[2]	Water[2]
⅓ cup	2.5 tbls		1 cup
⅓ cup		1 cup	
⅓ cup			1 cup

[1]Amounts given are per pound bodyweight per day. Feed at least 3 times per day. Divide the amount per day by the number of feedings to give amount per feeding.

[2]Reduce to ⅔ cup after 4 days or when puppies are eating well.

Provide fresh, clean water at all times.

Weaning from the Bitch: Introduce 2ND STEP™ Puppy Weaning Food at about 3 weeks of age or as soon as the puppies begin to start eating the bitch's food. Offer only a small quantity at first to reduce waste. Do not leave food with puppies for more than 2 hours. If desired puppies may be weaned entirely to 2ND STEP™ Puppy Weaning Food at 4 weeks of age.

Orphaned Bottle-Reared Puppies: Puppies that are on their feet and are lapping their pre-mixed Esbilac® are ready for introduction to solid food.

Note: Weigh the puppies at least once a week to monitor weight gain and adequacy of feeding. A veterinarian should be consulted about sound puppy care practice. More or less food may be needed by individual puppies to satisfy their food requirements for optimum performance.

Presentation: 14 oz can (12 per case) and 5 lb pail (4 per case).

Compendium Code No.: 10970112

ESBILAC® LIQUID

Pet-Ag **Milk Replacer**

Guaranteed Analysis:

Crude protein, min. 4.5%
Crude fat, min. 6.0%
Crude fiber .... None
Moisture, max. 85.0%
Ash, max. 1.0%

Ingredients: Water, skimmed milk, soy oil, sodium caseinate, butter, egg yolk, calcium caseinate, l-arginine, dl-methionine, calcium carbonate, potassium chloride, potassium phosphate monobasic, lecithin, magnesium sulfate, choline chloride, sodium chloride, carrageenan, potassium phosphate dibasic, ascorbic acid, vitamin A supplement, zinc sulfate, iron sulfate, vitamin E supplement, copper sulfate, niacin supplement, calcium pantothenate, vitamin B_{12} supplement, vitamin D_3 supplement, manganese sulfate, riboflavin, thiamine hydrochloride, pyridoxine hydrochloride, potassium iodide, and folic acid.

Indications: Recommended as a food source for orphaned or rejected puppies or those nursing, but needing supplemental feeding. Also recommended for growing puppies or adult dogs that are stressed and require a source of highly digestible nutrients.

Dosage and Administration:

Orphaned Puppies: All puppies should receive their dam's milk for at least two (2) days, if possible. The colostrum milk gives extra nutrition and temporary immunity against some diseases. ESBILAC® Liquid may be fed at the daily rate of two (2) tablespoons per four (4) ounces (¼ lb) of body weight. The daily feeding rate should be divided into equal portions for each feeding. Puppies' needs will vary and this amount may have to be increased or decreased, depending on the individual. Larger puppies do well when fed ESBILAC® Liquid every eight (8) hours. Small or weak puppies may need to be fed ESBILAC® Liquid every three (3) or four (4) hours. Weigh the puppy three (3) times a week to ensure adequate feeding. Consult a veterinarian for advice. ESBILAC® Liquid should be fed at room temperature.

Food Supplement: ESBILAC® Liquid is a digestible source of nutrients.

When a food supplement is desired, for growing puppies and show dogs or for supplementing large litters, old, or convalescent dogs, mix ESBILAC® Liquid into the daily ration at the rate of one (1) tablespoon per 5 lbs (2.2 kg) of body weight.

Pregnant and Lactating Bitches: Mix ESBILAC® Liquid into the daily ration at the rate of two (2) tablespoons per 5 lbs (2.2 kg) of body weight until two (2) weeks after whelping.

Precaution(s): Shake well before use. Refrigerate after opening. Discard after 72 hours. Do not freeze.

Presentation: 8 oz (24 per case) and 12.5 oz (12 per case) cans.

Compendium Code No.: 10970122

ESBILAC® POWDER

Pet-Ag **Milk Replacer**

Guaranteed Analysis:

Crude Protein, min. 33.0%
Crude Fat, min. 40.0%
Crude Fiber 0.0%
Moisture, max. 5.0%
Ash, max. 7.75%

Ingredients: Vegetable oil, casein, whey protein concentrate, butter fat, dried skimmed milk, egg yolk, monocalcium phosphate, lactose, calcium carbonate, L-arginine, lecithin, DL-methionine, potassium chloride, choline chloride, potassium phosphate monobasic, magnesium carbonate, salt, potassium phosphate dibasic, magnesium sulfate, vitamin E supplement, zinc sulfate, dipotassium phosphate, silico aluminate, ferrous sulfate, vitamin B_{12} supplement, calcium pantothenate, ascorbic acid, copper sulfate, niacin supplement, vitamin A supplement, manganese sulfate, vitamin D_3 supplement, ethylenediamine dihydroiodide, folic acid, riboflavin, thiamine hydrochloride, pyridoxine hydrochloride, biotin, and mono and diglycerides.

Indications: Recommended as a food source for orphaned or rejected puppies or those nursing, but needing supplemental feeding. Also recommended for growing puppies or adult dogs that are stressed and require a source of highly digestible nutrients.

Directions for Use: Gently shake or stir one volume of powdered ESBILAC® into two volumes of warm water. Do not use a blender.

Puppies: All puppies should receive their mother's milk for at least 2 days, if possible. The colostrum milk gives extra nutrition and temporary immunity against some diseases.

Warm reconstituted ESBILAC® to room or body temperature. Feed puppies 2 tablespoons (12 g) per 4 ounces (115 g) of body weight daily. Small and/or weak puppies should be fed every 3 to 4 hours. Larger and/or older puppies can do well being fed every 8 hours. Divide the daily feeding amount into equal portions for each feeding. The amount required should be increased or decreased to meet the individual requirements for each puppy.

Weigh the puppies daily to assure that they are receiving adequate ESBILAC®.

Consult your veterinarian for advice.

The Pet-Ag 4 oz Esbilac® Small Animal Nurser is suited for feeding most puppies. When puppies are old enough to lap, begin offering reconstituted ESBILAC® in a shallow container. During the 3rd week mix reconstituted ESBILAC® with Pet-Ag Puppy Weaning Formula. This will allow the puppy to gradually switch to solid food.

Pregnant and lactating bitches: Feed 2 teaspoons (4 g) ESBILAC® Powder per 5 lbs (2.2 kg) body weight daily until 2 weeks after whelping.

Growing puppies, show dogs, and/or convalescing dogs: Feed 1 teaspoon (2 g) ESBILAC® Powder per 5 lbs (2.2 kg) body weight daily.

Precaution(s): Reconstituted ESBILAC® Powder may be refrigerated up to 24 hours. Opened powder may be refrigerated for 3 months.

Presentation: 12 oz cans (12 per case), 28 oz cans (6 per case), ¾ oz pouch (48 per case), and 5 lb bag (4 per case).

ESBILAC® Emergency Feeding Kit includes: ¾ oz (21 g) ESBILAC® Emergency powder pack, 2 oz nurser bottle and nipple, .035 oz (1 g) Bene-Bac™ "One Shot" and the Guide to Saving Little Lives (12 per case).

Compendium Code No.: 10970132

ESCOGEN

Novartis (Aqua Health) — **Bacterin**

Edwardsiella Ictaluri Bacterin

U.S. Vet. Lic. No.: 335

Contents: This bacterin contains only formalin inactivated cultures of *Edwardsiella ictaluri.* No other preservative is used. This bacterin is safe and effective for use with fingerling or larger ictalurids.

Indications: For the vaccination of healthy ictalurids as an aid in the prevention of Enteric Septicemia of catfish (ESC).

Dosage and Administration:

Instructions for Feed Mills: Feed mills must be FDA registered. During milling process maintain pH between 4.0 and 5.5 and maintain the temperature between 155 and 175°F. Incorporate at the rate of 1%, which is the equivalent of 20 pounds of bacterin per ton of fish feed.

Directions: Administer the pellet feed containing the bacterin at a feeding rate of 4% of body weight/day to fingerling or larger ictalurids.

Vaccination: *Edwardsiella ictaluri* bacterin in fish pellets is given as the only feed for 2 periods of 5 consecutive days with a minimum of 10 days between periods.

Precaution(s): Store at 35-45°F under dry conditions.

Caution(s): Vaccinate only healthy fingerling or larger ictalurids.

Feed containing bacterin should be fed 15 to 30 days prior to an expected ESC outbreak which generally occurs when water temperatures are in the range of 72-82°F.

Warning(s): Do not slaughter within 21 days following final feeding with *Edwardsiella ictaluri* bacterin treated feed.

For veterinary use only.

Presentation: As needed up to 25 kg/bag.

Distributed by: Mr. J. Zinn, Buhl, Idaho 83316

Compendium Code No.: 14970011

E-SE® ℞

Schering-Plough — **Vitamin E-Selenium**

(Selenium, Vitamin E) Injection-Veterinary

NADA No.: 030-315

Active Ingredient(s): Each mL contains: 5.48 mg sodium selenite (equivalent to 2.5 mg selenium), 50 mg (68 IU) vitamin E (as d-alpha tocopheryl acetate), 250 mg polyoxyethylated vegetable oil, 2% benzyl alcohol (preservative), water for injection q.s. Sodium hydroxide and/or hydrochloric acid may be added to adjust pH.

Indications: E-SE® Injection is an emulsion of selenium-tocopherol for the prevention and treatment of myositis (Selenium-Tocopherol Deficiency) syndrome in horses.

E-SE® Injection is recommended for the control of the following clinical signs when associated with myositis (Selenium-Tocopherol Deficiency) syndrome: rapid respiration, profuse sweating, muscle spasms and stiffness, elevated SGOT.

Pharmacology: It has been demonstrated that selenium and tocopherol exert physiological effects and that these effects are intertwined with sulfur metabolism. Additionally, tocopherol appears to have a significant role in the oxidation process, thus suggesting an interrelationship between selenium and tocopherol in overcoming sulfur-induced depletion and restoring normal metabolism. Although oral ingestion of adequate amounts of selenium and tocopherol would seemingly restore normal metabolism, it is apparent that the presence of sulfur and perhaps other factors interfere during the digestive process with proper utilization of selenium and tocopherol. When selenium and tocopherol are injected, they bypass the digestive process and exert their full metabolic effects promptly on cell metabolism. Anti-inflammatory action has been demonstrated by selenium-tocopherol in the Selye Pouch Technique and experimentally induced polyarthritis study in rats.

Dosage and Administration: Administration: Administer by slow intravenous injection (see Cautions), or deep intramuscular injections, in divided doses in two or more sites in the gluteal or cervical muscles.

Dosage: 1 mL per 100 pounds of body weight. May be repeated at 5-10 day intervals.

Precaution(s): Storage: Store between 2° and 30°C (36° and 86°F). Protect from freezing.

Caution(s): Federal law restricts this drug to use by or on the order of a licensed veterinarian.

Selenium-Tocopherol Deficiency (STD) syndrome produces a variety and complexity of symptoms often interfering with a proper diagnosis. Even in selenium deficient areas there are other disease conditions which produce similar clinical signs. It is imperative that all these conditions be carefully considered prior to the treatment of STD syndrome. Serum selenium levels, elevated SGOT, and creatine serum levels may serve as aids in arriving at a diagnosis of STD, when associated with other indices.

Important: Use only the selenium-tocopherol product recommended for each species. Each formulation is designed for the species indicated to produce the maximum efficacy and safety.

Intravenous administration, if elected, should be by slow injection.

Emulsions injected intramuscularly into the horse may produce transitory local muscle soreness and can be prevented to some degree by injecting deeply (2 to 2½ inches), in divided doses, in two or more sites. Do not continue therapy in horses demonstrating such sensitivity.

Selenium is toxic if administered in excess. A fixed dose schedule is therefore important (read the package insert for each selenium-tocopherol product carefully before using).

Anaphylactoid reactions, some of which have been fatal, have been reported in horses administered E-SE® Injection. Signs include excitement, sweating, trembling, ataxia, respiratory distress, and cardiac dysfunction. These reactions have been reported in association with both intravenous and intramuscular injections. It is presently unknown whether the mode of application affects the frequency of such reactions. However, reactions associated with intramuscular injections have been reported to manifest more slowly and hence may give more time to institute treatment for anaphylaxis, such as epinephrine and/or corticosteroid injection.

Medications which have been reported to cause major adverse reactions in horses should be avoided when E-SE® is administered, unless the condition of the animal requires such use.

For veterinary use only.

Warning(s): Not to be used in horses intended for food.

Presentation: 100 mL sterile, multiple dose glass vials (NDC 0061-0709-04).

Compendium Code No.: 10470481 Rev. 10/98

ESTRUMATE® ℞

Schering-Plough — **Prostaglandin**

(cloprostenol sodium) Prostaglandin Analogue for Cattle

NADA No.: 113-645

Active Ingredient(s): Each mL of the colorless aqueous solution contains 263 mcg of cloprostenol sodium (equivalent to 250 mcg of cloprostenol) in a sodium citrate, anhydrous citric acid and sodium chloride buffer containing 0.1% w/v chlorocresol BP as a bactericide. pH is adjusted, as necessary, with sodium hydroxide or citric acid.

Indications: For intramuscular use to induce luteolysis in beef and dairy cattle. The luteolytic action of ESTRUMATE® can be utilized to manipulate the estrous cycle to better fit certain management practices, to terminate pregnancies resulting from mismatings, and to treat certain conditions associated with prolonged luteal function.

Pharmacology: ESTRUMATE® (cloprostenol sodium) is a synthetic prostaglandin analogue structurally related to prostaglandin F2α (PGF2α).

OH COOH OH OH O Cl

Action: ESTRUMATE® causes functional and morphological regression of the *corpus luteum* (luteolysis) in cattle. In normal, nonpregnant cycling animals, this effect on the life span of the corpus luteum usually results in estrus 2 to 5 days after treatment. In animals with prolonged luteal function (pyometra, mummified fetus, and luteal cysts), the induced luteolysis usually results in resolution of the condition and return to cyclicity. Pregnant animals may abort depending on the stage of gestation.

Dosage and Administration: 2 mL of ESTRUMATE® (500 mcg of cloprostenol) should be administered by intramuscular injection for all indications in both beef and dairy cattle.

Recommended Uses:

Unobserved or nondetected estrus: Cows which are not detected in estrus, although ovarian cyclicity continues, can be treated with ESTRUMATE® if a mature corpus luteum is present. Estrus is expected to occur 2 to 5 days following injection, at which time animals may be inseminated. Treated cattle should be inseminated at the usual time following detection of estrus. If estrus detection is not desirable or possible, treated animals may be inseminated twice at about 72 and 96 hours postinjection.

Pyometra or Chronic Endometritis: Damage to the reproductive tract at calving or postpartum retention of the placenta often leads to infection and inflammation of the uterus (endometritis). Under certain circumstances, this may progress into chronic endometritis with the uterus becoming distended with purulent matter. This condition, commonly referred to as pyometra, is characterized by a lack of cyclical estrous behavior and the presence of a persistent corpus luteum. Induction of luteolysis with ESTRUMATE® usually results in evacuation of the uterus and a return to normal cyclical activity within 14 days after treatment. After 14 days posttreatment, recovery rate of treated animals will not be different than that of untreated cattle.

Mummified Fetus: Death of the conceptus during gestation may be followed by its degeneration and dehydration. Induction of luteolysis with ESTRUMATE® usually results in expulsion of the mummified fetus from the uterus. (Manual assistance may be necessary to remove the fetus from the vagina.) Normal cyclical activity usually follows.

Luteal Cysts: A cow may be noncyclic due to the presence of a luteal cyst (a single, anovulatory follicle with a thickened wall which is accompanied by no external signs and by no changes in palpable consistency of the uterus). Treatment with ESTRUMATE® can restore normal ovarian activity by causing regression of the luteal cyst.

Pregnancies from Mismating: Unwanted pregnancies can be safely and efficiently terminated from 1 week after mating until about 5 months of gestation. The induced abortion is normally uncomplicated and the fetus and placenta are usually expelled about four to five days after the injection with the reproductive tract returning to normal soon after the abortion. The ability of ESTRUMATE® to induce abortion decreases beyond the fifth month of gestation while the risk of dystocia and its consequences increases. ESTRUMATE® has not been sufficiently tested under feedlot conditions; therefore, recommendations cannot be made for its use in heifers placed in feedlots.

Controlled Breeding: The luteolytic action of ESTRUMATE® can be utilized to schedule estrus and ovulation for an individual cycling animal or a group of animals. This allows control of the time at which cycling cows or heifers can be bred. ESTRUMATE® can be incorporated into a controlled breeding program by the following methods:

1. Single ESTRUMATE® injection: only animals with a mature *corpus luteum* should be treated to obtain maximum response to the single injection. However, not all cycling cattle should be treated since a mature *corpus luteum* is present for only 11 to 12 days of the 21-day cycle.

   Prior to treatment, cattle should be examined rectally and found to be anatomically normal, be nonpregnant and have a mature *corpus luteum.* If these criteria are met, estrus is expected to occur 2 to 5 days following injection, at which time animals may be inseminated. Treated cattle should be inseminated at the usual time following detection of estrus. If estrus detection is not desirable or possible, treated animals may be inseminated either once at about 72 hours or twice at about 72 and 96 hours post injection.

   With a single injection program, it may be desirable to assess the cyclicity status of the herd before ESTRUMATE® treatment. This can be accomplished by heat detecting and breeding at the usual time following detection of estrus for a 6-day period, all prior to injection. If by the sixth day the cyclicity status appears normal (approximately 25%-30% detected in estrus), all cattle not already inseminated should be palpated for normality, nonpregnancy, and cyclicity, then injected with ESTRUMATE®. Breeding should then be continued at the usual time following signs of estrus on the seventh and eighth day. On the ninth and tenth day breeding may continue at the usual time following detection of estrus or all cattle not already inseminated may be bred either once on the ninth day (at about 72 hours postinjection) or on both the ninth and tenth day (at about 72 and 96 hours postinjection).

2. Double ESTRUMATE® injections: prior to treatment, cattle should be examined rectally and found to be anatomically normal, nonpregnant and cycling (the presence of a mature *corpus*

E

luteum is not necessary when the first injection of a double injection regimen is given). A second injection should be given 11 days after the first injection. In normal, cycling cattle, estrus is expected 2 to 5 days following the second injection. Treated cattle should be inseminated at the usual time following detection of estrus. If estrus detection is not desirable or possible, treated animals may be inseminated either once at about 72 hours or twice at about 72 and 96 hours following the second ESTRUMATE® injection.

Many animals will come into estrus following the first injection; these animals can be inseminated at the usual time following detected estrus. Animals not inseminated should receive a second injection 11 days after the first injection. Animals receiving both injections may be inseminated at the usual time following detection of estrus or may be inseminated either once at about 72 hours or twice at about 72 and 96 hours post second injection.

Any controlled breeding program recommended should be completed by either:

- observing animals (especially during the third week after injection) and inseminating or hand mating any animals returning to estrus,

or

- turning in clean-up bull(s) 5 to 7 days after the last injection of ESTRUMATE® to cover any animals returning to estrus.

Requirements for Controlled Breeding Programs: A variety of programs can be designed to best meet the needs of individual management systems. A controlled breeding program should be selected which is appropriate for the existing circumstances and management practices.

Before a controlled breeding program is planned the producer's objectives must be examined and he must be made aware of the projected results and limitations. The producer and his consulting veterinarian should review the operation's breeding history, herd health and nutritional status, and agree that a controlled breeding program is practical in the producer's specific situation. For any successful controlled breeding program:

- cows and heifers must be normal, nonpregnant, and cycling (rectal palpation should be performed).

- cattle must be in a fit and thrifty breeding condition and on an adequate or increasing plane of nutrition.

- proper program planning and record keeping are essential.

- if artificial insemination is used it must be performed by competent inseminators using high-quality semen.

It is important to understand that ESTRUMATE® is effective only in animals with a mature *corpus luteum* (ovulation must have occurred at least 5 days prior to treatment). This must be considered when breeding is intended following a single ESTRUMATE® injection.

Contraindication(s): ESTRUMATE® should not be administered to a pregnant animal whose calf is not to be aborted.

Precaution(s): Storage Conditions:

1. Protect from light.
2. Store in container.
3. Store at controlled room temperature 59°-86°F. (15°-30°C.).

Caution(s): Federal (USA) law restricts this drug to use by or on the order of a licensed veterinarian.

There is no effect on fertility following the single or double dosage regimen when breeding occurs at induced estrus or at 72 and 96 hours posttreatment. Conception rates may be lower than expected in those fixed time breeding programs which omit the second insemination (i.e., the insemination at or near 96 hours). This is especially true if a fixed time insemination is used following a single ESTRUMATE® injection. As with all parenteral products, careful aseptic techniques should be employed to decrease the possibility of postinjection bacterial infection. Antibiotic therapy should be employed at the first sign of infection.

Warning(s): For veterinary use only.

Women of child-bearing age, asthmatics, and persons with bronchial and other respiratory problems should exercise extreme caution when handling this product. In the early stages, women may be unaware of their pregnancies. ESTRUMATE® is readily absorbed through the skin and may cause abortion and/or bronchospasms; direct contact with the skin should therefore be avoided. Accidental spillage on the skin should be washed off immediately with soap and water.

Toxicology: Safety and Toxicity: At 50 and 100 times the recommended dose, mild side effects may be detected in some cattle. These include increased uneasiness, slight frothing, and milk let-down.

Presentation: 20- mL multidose vials.

Compendium Code No.: 10470670 79005960,R.O.

ETIDERM® SHAMPOO

Virbac **Antidermatosis Shampoo**

Antiseptic Shampoo

Active Ingredient(s): Contains: Chitosanide, ethyl lactate 10%, benzalkonium chloride, lactic acid and propylene glycol in a shampoo base also containing TEA lauryl sulfate, water, diethenolamine, benzyl alcohol, fragrance, hydroxypropyl cellulose, methyl paraben, and propyl paraben. Chitosanide and ethyl lactate are present in encapsulated (Spherulites®) and free forms. Benzalkonium chloride is present in encapsulated form.

Indications: ETIDERM® is a gentle, antiseptic and keratoplastic shampoo for use in dogs and cats of any age.

Directions: Shake well before use. Wet the coat with warm water and apply sufficient shampoo to create a rich lather. Massage ETIDERM® into wet coat, lather freely. Rinse and repeat. Allow to remain on hair for 5 to 10 minutes, then rinse thoroughly with clean water.

Frequency of use: Initially two to three times a week for four weeks, then reducing to once a week, or as directed by your veterinarian.

Caution(s): For topical use only. Avoid contact with eyes. In case of contact, flush eyes with water and seek medical attention if irritation persists.

Available through licensed veterinarians only.

Warning(s): Keep out of reach of children.

Discussion: ETIDERM® contains Spherulites®, an exclusive and patented encapsulation system developed by Virbac to provide slow release of ingredients long after the shampoo is rinsed off.

ETIDERM® also contains Chitosanide, a natural biopolymer creating a protective film on the skin and hair.

Presentation: Available in 8 oz, 16 oz, and 1 gallon containers.

Compendium Code No.: 10230290

ETOGESIC® ℞

Fort Dodge **Non-Steroidal Anti-Inflammatory**

(etodolac) Tablets

NADA No.: 141-108

Active Ingredient(s): Each tablet is biconvex and half-scored and contains either 150 or 300 mg of etodolac.

Indications: ETOGESIC® is recommended for the management of pain and inflammation associated with osteoarthritis in dogs.

Pharmacology: Etodolac is a pyranocarboxylic acid, chemically designated as (±) 1,8-diethyl-1,3,4,9-tetrahydropyrano-[3,4-b] indole-1-acetic acid. The structural formula for etodolac is shown:

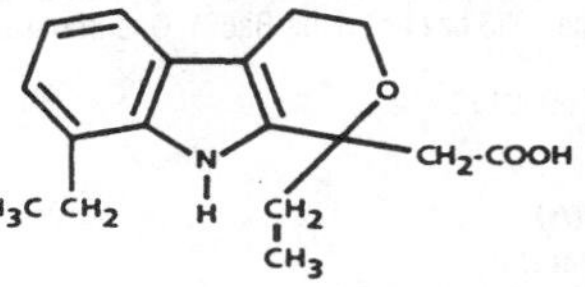

The empirical formula for etodolac is $C_{17}H_{21}NO_3$. The molecular weight of the base is 287.37. It has a pKa of 4.65 and an *n*-octanol:water partition coefficient of 11.4 at pH 7.4. Etodolac is a white crystalline compound, insoluble in water but soluble in alcohols, chloroform, dimethyl sulfoxide, and aqueous polyethylene glycol.

Etodolac is a non-narcotic, nonsteroidal anti-inflammatory drug (NSAID) with anti-inflammatory, anti-pyretic, and analgesic activity. The mechanism of action of etodolac, like that of other NSAIDs, is believed to be associated with the inhibition of cyclooxygenase activity. Two unique cyclooxygenases have been described in mammals[1]. The constitutive cyclooxygenase, COX-1, synthesizes prostaglandins necessary for normal gastrointestinal and renal function. The inducible cyclooxygenase, COX-2, generates prostaglandins involved in inflammation. Inhibition of COX-1 is thought to be associated with gastrointestinal and renal toxicity, while inhibition of COX-2 provides anti-inflammatory activity. In *in vitro* experiments, etodolac demonstrated more selective inhibition of COX-2 than COX-1[2]. Etodolac also inhibits macrophage chemotaxis *in vivo* and *in vitro*.[3] Because of the importance of macrophages in the inflammatory response, the anti-inflammatory effect of etodolac could be partially mediated through inhibition of the chemotactic ability of macrophages.

Pharmacokinetics in healthy beagle dogs: Etodolac is rapidly and almost completely absorbed from the gastrointestinal tract following oral administration. The extent of etodolac absorption (AUC) is not affected by the prandial status of the animal. However, it appears that the peak concentration of the drug decreases in the presence of food. As compared to an oral solution, the relative bioavailability of the tablets when given with or without food is essentially 100%. Peak plasma concentrations are usually attained within 2 hours of administration. Though the terminal half-life increases in a nonfasted state, minimal drug accumulation (less than 30%) is expected after repeated dosing (i.e., steady-state). Pharmacokinetic parameters estimated in a crossover study (fed vs. fasted) in eighteen 5-month-old beagle dogs are summarized in the following table:

Mean Pharmacokinetic Parameters Estimated in 18 Beagle Dogs After Oral Administration of 150 mg of Etodolac (approximately 12-17 mg/kg)

Pharmacokinetic Parameter	Tablet/Fasted	Tablet/Nonfasted
C_{max} (μg/mL)	22.0±6.42	16.9±8.84
T_{max} (hours)	1.69±0.69	1.08±0.46
$AUC_{0-\infty}$ (μg•hours/mL)	64.1±17.9	63.9±28.9
Terminal half-life, $t_{1/2}$ (hrs)	7.66±2.05	11.98±5.52

Pharmacokinetics in dogs with reduced kidney function: In a study involving four beagle dogs with induced acute renal failure, there was no observed change in drug bioavailability after administration of 200 mg single oral etodolac doses. In a study evaluating an additional four beagles, no changes in electrolyte, serum albumin/total protein and creatinine concentrations were observed after single 200 mg doses of etodolac. This was not unexpected since very little etodolac is cleared by the kidneys in normal animals. Most of etodolac and its metabolites are eliminated via the liver and feces. In addition, etodolac is believed to undergo enterohepatic recirculation.[4]

Dosage and Administration: The recommended dose of etodolac in dogs is 10 to 15 mg/kg body weight (4.5 to 6.8 mg/lb) administered once daily. Due to tablet sizes and scoring, dogs weighing less than 5 kg (11 lb) cannot be accurately dosed. The effective dose and duration should be based on clinical judgment of disease condition and patient tolerance of drug treatment. The initial dose level should be adjusted until a satisfactory clinical response is obtained, but should not exceed 15 mg/kg once daily. When a satisfactory clinical response is obtained, the daily dose level should be reduced to the minimum effective dose for longer term administration.

Contraindication(s): ETOGESIC® is contraindicated in animals previously found to be hypersensitive to etodolac.

Precaution(s): Storage Conditions: Store at controlled room temperature, 15-30°C (59-86°F).

Caution(s): Federal (U.S.A.) law restricts this drug to use by or on the order of a licensed veterinarian.

Treatment with ETOGESIC® tablets should be terminated if signs such as inappetence, emesis, fecal abnormalities, or anemia are observed. Dogs treated with nonsteroidal anti-inflammatory drugs, including etodolac, should be evaluated periodically to ensure that the drug is still necessary and well tolerated.

ETOGESIC®, as with other nonsteroidal anti-inflammatory drugs, may exacerbate clinical signs in dogs with pre-existing or occult gastrointestinal, hepatic or cardiovascular abnormalities, blood dyscrasias, or bleeding disorders.

As a class, cyclooxygenase inhibitory NSAIDs may be associated with gastrointestinal and renal toxicity. Sensitivity to drug-associated adverse effects varies with the individual patient. Patients at greatest risk for renal toxicity are those that are dehydrated, on concomitant diuretic therapy, or those with renal, cardiovascular, and/or hepatic dysfunction. Since many NSAIDs possess the potential to induce gastrointestinal ulceration, concomitant use of etodolac with other anti-inflammatory drugs, such as other NSAIDs and corticosteroids, should be avoided or closely monitored.

Studies to determine the activity of ETOGESIC® tablets when administered concomitantly with other protein-bound drugs have not been conducted in dogs. Drug compatibility should be monitored closely in patients requiring adjunctive therapy.

The safety of ETOGESIC® has not been investigated in breeding, pregnant or lactating dogs or in dogs under 12 months of age.

For oral use in dogs only.

Warning(s): Keep out of reach of children. Not for human use. Consult a physician in cases of accidental ingestion by humans. For use in dogs only. Do not use in cats.

All dogs should undergo a thorough history and physical examination before initiation of NSAID therapy. Appropriate laboratory tests to establish hematological and serum biochemical baseline data prior to, and periodically during, administration of any NSAID should be considered. Owners should be advised to observe for signs of potential drug toxicity (see Information for Dog Owners and Adverse Reactions).

Adverse Reactions: In a placebo-controlled clinical field trial involving 116 dogs, where treatment was administered for 8 days, the following adverse reactions were noted:

Adverse Reaction	ETOGESIC® Tablets % of Dogs	Placebo % of Dogs
vomiting	4.3%	1.7%
regurgitation	0.9%	2.6%
lethargy	3.4%	2.6%
diarrhea/loose stool	2.6%	1.7%
hypoproteinemia	2.6%	0
urticaria	0.9%	0
behavioral change, urinating in house	0.9%	0
inappetence	0.9%	1.7%

Following completion of the clinical field trial, 92 dogs continued to receive etodolac. One dog developed diarrhea following 2½ weeks of treatment. Etodolac was discontinued until resolution of clinical signs was observed. When treatment was resumed, the diarrhea returned within 24 hours. One dog experienced vomiting which was attributed to treatment, and etodolac was discontinued. Hypoproteinemia was identified in one dog following 11 months of etodolac therapy. Treatment was discontinued, and serum protein levels subsequently returned to normal.

Post-Approval Experience: As with other drugs in the NSAID class, adverse responses to ETOGESIC® tablets may occur. The adverse drug reactions listed below are based on voluntary post-approval reporting. The categories of adverse event reports are listed below in decreasing order of frequency by body system.

Gastrointestinal: Vomiting, diarrhea, inappetence, gastroenteritis, gastrointestinal bleeding, melena, gastrointestinal ulceration, hypoproteinemia, elevated pancreatic enzymes.

Hepatic: Abnormal liver function test(s), elevated hepatic enzymes, icterus, acute hepatitis.

Hematological: Anemia, hemolytic anemia, thrombocytopenia, prolonged bleeding time.

Neurological/Behavioral/Special Senses: Ataxia, paresis, aggression, sedation, hyperactivity, disorientation, hyperesthesia, seizures, vestibular signs, keratoconjunctivitis sicca.

Renal: Polydipsia, polyuria, urinary incontinence, azotemia, acute renal failure, proteinuria, hematuria.

Dermatological/Immunological: Pruritus, dermatitis, edema, alopecia, urticaria.

Cardiovascular/Respiratory: Tachycardia, dyspnea.

In rare situations, death has been reported as an outcome of some of the adverse responses listed above.

To report suspected adverse reactions, or to obtain technical assistance, call (800) 477-1365.

Discussion: Information for Dog Owners: ETOGESIC®, like other drugs of its class, is not free from adverse reactions. Owners should be advised of the potential for adverse reactions and be informed of the clinical signs associated with drug intolerance. Adverse reactions may include decreased appetite, vomiting, diarrhea, dark or tarry stools, increased water consumption, increased urination, pale gums due to anemia, yellowing of gums, skin or white of the eye due to jaundice, lethargy, incoordination, seizure, or behavioral changes. Serious adverse reactions associated with this drug class can occur without warning and in rare situations result in death (see Adverse Reactions). Owners should be advised to discontinue ETOGESIC® therapy and contact their veterinarian immediately if signs of intolerance are observed. The vast majority of patients with drug related adverse reactions have recovered when the signs are recognized, the drug is withdrawn, and veterinary care, if appropriate, is initiated. Owners should be advised of the importance of periodic follow-up for all dogs during administration of any NSAID.

Trial Data: Efficacy: A placebo-controlled, double-blinded study demonstrated the anti-inflammatory and analgesic efficacy of ETOGESIC® (etodolac) tablets in various breeds of dogs. In this clinical field study, dogs diagnosed with osteoarthritis secondary to hip dysplasia showed objective improvement in mobility as measured by force plate parameters when given ETOGESIC® tablets at the label dosage for 8 days.

Safety: In target animal safety studies, etodolac was well tolerated clinically when given at the label dosage for periods as long as one year (see Cautions).

Oral administration of etodolac at a daily dosage of 10 mg/kg (4.5 mg/lb) for twelve months or 15 mg/kg (6.8 mg/lb) for six months, resulted in some dogs showing a mild weight loss, fecal abnormalities (loose, mucoid, mucosanguineous feces or diarrhea), and hypoproteinemia. Erosions in the small intestine were observed in one of the eight dogs receiving 15 mg/kg following six months of daily dosing.

Elevated dose levels of ETOGESIC® (etodolac), i.e. ≥40 mg/kg/day (18 mg/lb/day, 2.7X the maximum daily dose), caused gastrointestinal ulceration, emesis, fecal occult blood, and weight loss. At a dose of ≥80 mg/kg/day (36 mg/lb/day, 5.3X the maximum daily dose), 6 of 8 treated dogs died or became moribund as a result of gastrointestinal ulceration. One dog died within 3 weeks of treatment initiation while the other 5 died after 3-9 months of daily treatment. Deaths were preceded by clinical signs of emesis, fecal abnormalities, decreased food intake, weight loss, and pale mucous membranes. Renal tubular nephrosis was also found in 1 dog treated with 80 mg/kg for 12 months. Other common abnormalities observed at elevated doses included reductions in red blood cell count, hematocrit, hemoglobin, total protein and albumin concentrations; and increases in fibrinogen concentration and reticulocyte, leukocyte, and platelet counts.

In an additional study which evaluated the effects of etodolac administered to 6 dogs at the labeled dose for approximately 9.5 weeks, the incidence of stool abnormalities (diarrhea, loose stools) was unchanged for dogs in the weeks prior to initiation of etodolac treatment, and during the course of etodolac therapy. Five of the dogs receiving etodolac, versus 2 of the placebo-treated dogs, exhibited excessive bleeding during an experimental surgery. No significant evidence of drug-related toxicity was noted on necropsy.

References: Available upon request.

Presentation: ETOGESIC® is available in 150 and 300 mg single-scored tablets and supplied in bottles containing 7, 30 and 90 tablets.

NDC 0856-5520-03 — 150 mg — bottles of 7
NDC 0856-5520-04 — 150 mg — bottles of 30
NDC 0856-5520-05 — 150 mg — bottles of 90
NDC 0856-5530-03 — 300 mg — bottles of 7
NDC 0856-5530-04 — 300 mg — bottles of 30
NDC 0856-5530-05 — 300 mg — bottles of 90

Compendium Code No.: 10030701 5530D

EUCLENS OTIC CLEANSER

Vetus **Otic Cleanser**

Active Ingredient(s): The product contains propylene glycol, malic acid, benzoic acid, salicylic acid and eucalyptus oil, and is alcohol free.

Indications: EUCLENS OTIC CLEANSER is used to cleanse the ear canal of dogs and cats. Removes dirt and debris from the ears. Reduces ear odor. Contains eucalyptus oil, known for its antiseptic effects in treating inflammation. It is also useful as a wound irrigation solution, in removing necrotic tissue for healthy tissue growth.

Dosage and Administration:

Routine ear cleaning: Fill the ear canal and massage the base of the ear to loosen any dirt or debris. Use a cotton ball to remove any debris and any excess solution. Apply two (2) or three (3) times a week, or as directed by a veterinarian.

Wound cleansing: Apply liberally two (2) or three (3) times a day, or as directed by a veterinarian.

Caution(s): For external use only.

For veterinary use only.

Keep out of the reach of children.

Presentation: 4 oz squeeze bottles with applicator tips and 16 oz twist-to-close Yorker top bottle.

Compendium Code No.: 14440320

EUTHASOL® CIII

Delmarva **Euthanasia Agent**

ANADA No.: 200-071

Active Ingredient(s): Each mL contains:

Pentobarbital sodium (barbituric acid derivative) .... 390 mg
Phenytoin sodium .... 50 mg

Inactive Ingredients:

Ethyl alcohol 10%
Propylene glycol 18%
Rhodamine B .... 0.003688 mg
Benzyl alcohol (preservative) 2%
Water for injection .... q.s.

Sodium hydroxide and/or hydrochloric acid may be added to adjust pH.

A non-sterile solution containing pentobarbital sodium and phenytoin sodium as the active ingredients. Rhodamine B, a bluish-red fluorescent dye, is included in the formulation to help distinguish it from parenteral drugs intended for therapeutic use. Although the solution is not sterile, benzyl alcohol, a bacteriostat, is included to retard the growth of micro-organisms.

Indications: For use in dogs for humane, painless, and rapid euthanasia.

Pharmacology: EUTHASOL® (pentobarbital sodium and phenytoin sodium) contains two active ingredients which are chemically compatible but pharmacologically different. Each ingredient acts in such a manner so as to cause humane, painless, and rapid euthanasia. Euthanasia is due to cerebral death in conjunction with respiratory arrest and circulatory collapse. Cerebral death occurs prior to the cessation of cardiac activity.

When administered intravenously, pentobarbital sodium produces rapid anesthetic action. There is a smooth and rapid onset of unconsciousness. At the lethal dose, there is depression of vital medullary respiratory and vasomotor centers.

When administered intravenously, phenytoin sodium produces toxic signs of cardiovascular collapse and/or central nervous system depression. Hypotension occurs when the drug is administered rapidly.

The sequence of events leading to humane, painless, and rapid euthanasia following the intravenous injection of EUTHASOL® is similar to that following intravenous injection of pentobarbital sodium, or other barbituric acid derivatives. Within seconds, unconsciousness is induced with simultaneous collapse of the dog. This stage rapidly progresses to deep anesthesia with concomitant reduction in the blood pressure. A few seconds later, breathing stops, due to depression of the medullary respiratory center; encephalographic activity becomes isoelectric, indicating cerebral death; and then cardiac activity ceases.

Phenytoin sodium exerts its effect during the deep anesthesia stage caused by the pentobarbital sodium. This ingredient, due to its cardiotoxic properties, hastens the stoppage of electrical activity in the heart.

Dosage and Administration: Dogs, 1 mL for each 10 lbs. of body weight.

Intravenous injection is preferred. Intracardiac injection may be made when intravenous injection is impractical, as in a very small dog, or in a comatose dog with impaired vascular functions. Good injection skill is necessary for intracardiac injection.

The calculated dose should be given in a single bolus injection.

For intravenous injection, a needle of sufficient gauge to ensure intravenous placement of the entire dose should be used.

Precaution(s): Store between 15°C and 30°C (59° and 86°F).

Caution(s): Federal law restricts this drug to use by or on the order of a licensed veterinarian.

For dogs only.

Caution should be exercised to avoid contact of the drug with open wounds or accidental self-inflicted injections. Keep out of the reach of children.

Euthanasia may sometimes be delayed in dogs with severe cardiac or circulatory deficiencies. This may be explained by the impaired movement of the drug to its site of action. An occasional dog may elicit reflex responses manifested by motor movement; however, an unconscious animal does not experience pain, because the cerebral cortex is not functioning.

When restraint may cause the dog pain, injury, or anxiety, or danger to the person making the injection, prior use of tranquilizing or immobilizing drugs may be necessary.

Warning(s): For canine euthanasia only. Must not be used for therapeutic purposes.

Do not use in animals intended for food.

Presentation: EUTHASOL® is available in 100 mL multiple dose vials.

Compendium Code No.: 14260020

E

EWT™

Schering-Plough **Toxoid-Vaccine**

Encephalomyelitis Vaccine, Eastern and Western, Killed Virus, Tetanus Toxoid

U.S. Vet. Lic. No.: 165A

Active Ingredient(s): An encephalomyelitis vaccine, eastern and western, killed virus, tetanus toxoid. Contains gentamicin and amphotericin B as preservatives.

Indications: EWT™ is recommended for the vaccination of healthy equines against eastern and western equine encephalomyelitis and tetanus.

Dosage and Administration: Shake well before using.

Initial vaccination: Using aseptic technique, give 1 mL by deep intramuscular injection with a 20 gauge 1-½" sterile needle. Administer another 1 mL dose in two (2) to four (4) weeks at a different injection site using a separate 20 gauge 1-½" sterile needle for each injection.

Revaccination: A single 1 mL booster should be administered annually. Additional boosters of encephalomyelitis-containing vaccines may be indicated during epidemics or in areas of endemic exposure. In the event of an outbreak, affected or newly acquired animals should be segregated from the unaffected horses.

Precaution(s): Store at 2°-7°C (35°-45°F). Do not freeze.

Caution(s): For veterinary use only.

Vaccinate healthy animals only. Do not vaccinate animals during times of stress.

Inject deep into the muscle tissue only. Transient local reactions may occur if the product is injected subcutaneously. Occasionally, mild stiffness and soreness may occur for two to three days after vaccination in some horses. If an allergic response occurs, administer epinephrine.

Keep a record of the vaccine type, the quantity, the serial number, the expiration date, the place of purchase, and the date and time of vaccination.

Warning(s): Do not vaccinate within 21 days before slaughter.

Presentation: 1 mL (1 dose), 10 mL (10 doses).

Compendium Code No.: 10470680

EWTF™

Schering-Plough **Toxoid-Vaccine**

Encephalomyelitis-Influenza Vaccine, Eastern and Western, Killed Virus, Tetanus Toxoid

U.S. Vet. Lic. No.: 165A

Active Ingredient(s): An encephalomyelitis, influenza vaccine, eastern and western, killed virus, tetanus toxoid. Contains gentamicin and amphotericin B as preservatives.

Indications: EWTF™ is recommended for the vaccination of healthy equines against eastern and western equine encephalomyelitis and tetanus, and as an aid in the prevention of equine influenza due to types A1 and A2.

Dosage and Administration:

Initial vaccination: Shake well before using. Using aseptic technique, give 1 mL by deep intramuscular injection with a 20 gauge 1-½" sterile needle. Administer another 1 mL dose in two (2) to four (4) weeks at a different injection site using a separate 20 gauge 1-½" sterile needle for each injection.

Revaccination: A single 1 mL booster should be administered annually. Additional boosters of encephalomyelitis and/or influenza-containing vaccines may be indicated during epidemics or in areas of endemic exposure. In the event of an outbreak, affected or newly acquired animals should be segregated from the unaffected horses.

Precaution(s): Store at 2°-7°C (35°-45°F). Do not freeze.

Caution(s): For veterinary use only.

Vaccinate healthy animals only. Do not vaccinate animals during times of stress.

Inject deep into the muscle tissue only. Transient local reactions may occur if the product is injected subcutaneously. Occasionally, mild stiffness and soreness may occur for two to three days after vaccination in some horses. If an allergic response occurs, administer epinephrine.

Keep a record of the vaccine type, the quantity, the serial number, the expiration date, the place of purchase, and the date and time of vaccination.

Warning(s): Do not vaccinate within 21 days before slaughter.

Presentation: 1 mL (1 dose), 10 mL (10 doses).

Compendium Code No.: 10470690

EXALT™ 4

AgriPharm **Vaccine**

Bovine Rhinotracheitis-Virus Diarrhea-Parainfluenza 3 Vaccine, Killed Virus

U.S. Vet. Lic. No.: 303

Composition: This vaccine contains an IBR virus, a cytopathic Type 1 BVD virus, a noncytopathic Type 2 BVD virus, and a PI_3 virus propagated on an established bovine cell line. The vaccine is chemically inactivated and adjuvanted with oil. Contains amphotericin B, penicillin, streptomycin, and thimerosal as preservatives.

Indications: For use in healthy cattle as an aid in the prevention of disease caused by infectious bovine rhinotracheitis, bovine virus diarrhea, and parainfluenza Type 3 viruses.

Dosage and Administration: Shake well before using. Administer 5 mL intramuscularly or subcutaneously. Revaccinate in 4-5 weeks. This vaccine may be administered to pregnant animals at any stage of gestation. Vaccinate dairy cows during the dry off period. Revaccinate annually.

Precaution(s): Store in the dark at 35°-45°F (2°-7°C). Do not freeze. Use entire contents when first opened.

Caution(s): Transient swelling may occur at the site of injection. Anaphylactic reactions may occur following the use of this biological. Symptomatic treatment: Epinephrine.

Warning(s): Do not vaccinate within 60 days prior to slaughter.

For animal use only.

Keep out of reach of children.

Presentation: 10 doses (50 mL) and 50 doses (250 mL).

Produced by: Advance Biologics, Inc.

Compendium Code No.: 14570262

EXALT™ 4 + L5

AgriPharm **Bacterin-Vaccine**

Bovine Rhinotracheitis-Virus Diarrhea-Parainfluenza 3 Vaccine, Killed Virus-Leptospira Canicola-Grippotyphosa-Hardjo-Icterohaemorrhagiae-Pomona Bacterin

U.S. Vet. Lic. No.: 303

Composition: This product contains an IBR virus, a cytopathic Type 1 BVD virus, a noncytopathic Type 2 BVD virus, and a PI_3 virus propagated on an established bovine cell line and cultures of *Leptospira canicola, grippotyphosa, hardjo, icterohaemorrhagiae*, and *pomona*. The product is chemically inactivated and adjuvanted with oil. Contains amphotericin B, penicillin, streptomycin, and thimerosal as preservatives.

Indications: For use in healthy cattle as an aid in the prevention of disease caused by infectious bovine rhinotracheitis, bovine virus diarrhea, and parainfluenza Type 3 viruses and *Leptospira canicola, grippotyphosa, hardjo, icterohaemorrhagiae*, and *pomona*.

Dosage and Administration: Shake well before using. Administer 5 mL intramuscularly. Revaccinate with Duo Vac™ 4 (Bovine Rhinotracheitis-Virus Diarrhea-Parainfluenza 3 Vaccine) in 4-5 weeks. Vaccinate dairy cows during the dry off period. Revaccinate annually.

Precaution(s): Store in the dark at 35°-45°F (2°-7°C). Do not freeze. Use entire contents when first opened.

Caution(s): Transient swelling may occur at the site of injection. Anaphylactic reactions may occur following the use of this biological. Symptomatic treatment: Epinephrine.

Warning(s): Do not vaccinate within 60 days prior to slaughter.

For animal use only.

Keep out of reach of children.

Presentation: 10 doses (50 mL) and 50 doses (250 mL).

Produced by: Advance Biologics, Inc.

Compendium Code No.: 14570272

EXALT™ 5

AgriPharm **Vaccine**

Bovine Rhinotracheitis-Virus Diarrhea-Parainfluenza 3-Respiratory Syncytial Virus Vaccine, Killed Virus

U.S. Vet. Lic. No.: 303

Composition: This vaccine contains an IBR virus, a cytopathic Type 1 BVD virus, a noncytopathic Type 2 BVD virus, a PI_3 virus, and a BRS virus propagated on an established bovine cell line. The vaccine is chemically inactivated and adjuvanted with oil. Contains amphotericin B, penicillin, streptomycin, and thimerosal as preservatives.

Indications: For use in healthy cattle as an aid in the prevention of disease caused by infectious bovine rhinotracheitis, bovine virus diarrhea, parainfluenza Type 3 viruses, and bovine respiratory syncytial viruses.

Dosage and Administration: Shake well before using. Administer 5 mL intramuscularly or subcutaneously. Revaccinate in 4-5 weeks. This vaccine may be administered to pregnant animals at any stage of gestation. Vaccinate dairy cows during the dry off period. Revaccinate annually.

Precaution(s): Store in the dark at 35°-45°F (2°-7°C). Do not freeze. Use entire contents when first opened.

Caution(s): Transient swelling may occur at the site of injection. Anaphylactic reactions may occur following the use of this biological. Symptomatic treatment: Epinephrine.

Warning(s): Do not vaccinate within 60 days prior to slaughter.

For animal use only.

Keep out of reach of children.

Presentation: 10 doses (50 mL) and 50 doses (250 mL).

Produced by: Advance Biologics, Inc.

Compendium Code No.: 14570282

EXALT™ 5 + L5

AgriPharm **Bacterin-Vaccine**

Bovine Rhinotracheitis-Virus Diarrhea-Parainfluenza 3-Respiratory Syncytial Virus Vaccine, Killed Virus-Leptospira Canicola-Grippotyphosa-Hardjo-Icterohaemorrhagiae-Pomona Bacterin

U.S. Vet. Lic. No.: 303

Composition: This product contains an IBR virus, a cytopathic Type 1 BVD virus, a noncytopathic Type 2 BVD virus, a PI_3 virus, and a BRS virus propagated on an established bovine cell line and cultures of *Leptospira canicola, grippotyphosa, hardjo, icterohaemorrhagiae*, and *pomona*. The product is chemically inactivated and adjuvanted with oil. Contains amphotericin B, penicillin, streptomycin, and thimerosal as preservatives.

Indications: For use in healthy cattle as an aid in the prevention of disease caused by infectious bovine rhinotracheitis, bovine virus diarrhea, parainfluenza Type 3, and bovine respiratory syncytial viruses and *Leptospira canicola, grippotyphosa, hardjo, icterohaemorrhagiae*, and *pomona*.

Dosage and Administration: Shake well before using. Administer 5 mL intramuscularly. Revaccinate with Exalt™ 5 (Bovine Rhinotracheitis-Virus Diarrhea-Parainfluenza 3-Respiratory Syncytial Virus Vaccine) in 4-5 weeks. Vaccinate dairy cows during the dry off period. Revaccinate annually.

Precaution(s): Store in the dark at 35°-45°F (2°-7°C). Do not freeze. Use entire contents when first opened.

Caution(s): Transient swelling may occur at the site of injection. Anaphylactic reactions may occur following the use of this biological. Symptomatic treatment: Epinephrine.

Warning(s): Do not vaccinate within 60 days prior to slaughter.

For animal use only.

Keep out of reach of children.

Presentation: 10 doses (50 mL) and 50 doses (250 mL).

Produced by: Advance Biologics, Inc.

Compendium Code No.: 14570292

EXALT™ 5 + SOMNUS

AgriPharm **Bacterin-Vaccine**

Bovine Rhinotracheitis-Virus Diarrhea-Parainfluenza 3-Respiratory Syncytial Virus Vaccine, Killed Virus-Haemophilus Somnus Bacterin

U.S. Vet. Lic. No.: 303

Composition: This product contains an IBR virus, a cytopathic Type 1 BVD virus, a noncytopathic Type 2 BVD virus, a PI_3 virus, and a BRS virus propagated on an established bovine cell line and cultures of *Haemophilus somnus*. The product is chemically inactivated and adjuvanted with oil. Contains amphotericin B, penicillin, streptomycin, and thimerosal as preservatives.

Indications: For use in healthy cattle as an aid in the prevention of disease caused by infectious bovine rhinotracheitis, bovine virus diarrhea, parainfluenza Type 3 viruses, and bovine respiratory syncytial viruses and *Haemophilus somnus*.

Dosage and Administration: Shake well before using. Administer 5 mL intramuscularly at 3 months of age or older. Revaccinate in 4-5 weeks. This vaccine may be administered to pregnant animals at any stage of gestation. Vaccinate dairy cows during the dry off period. Revaccinate annually.

Precaution(s): Store in the dark at 35°-45°F (2°-7°C). Do not freeze. Use entire contents when first opened.
Caution(s): Transient swelling may occur at the site of injection. Anaphylactic reactions may occur following the use of this biological. Symptomatic treatment: Epinephrine.
Warning(s): Do not vaccinate within 60 days prior to slaughter.
For animal use only.
Keep out of reach of children.
Presentation: 10 doses (50 mL) and 50 doses (250 mL).
Produced by: Advance Biologics, Inc.
Compendium Code No.: 14570302

EXALT™ 5 + VL5

AgriPharm **Bacterin-Vaccine**

Bovine Rhinotracheitis-Virus Diarrhea-Parainfluenza 3-Respiratory Syncytial Virus Vaccine, Killed Virus-Campylobacter Fetus-Leptospira Canicola-Grippotyphosa-Hardjo-Icterohaemorrhagiae-Pomona Bacterin
U.S. Vet. Lic. No.: 303
Composition: This product contains an IBR virus, a cytopathic Type 1 BVD virus, a noncytopathic Type 2 BVD virus, a PI_3 virus, and a BRS virus propagated on an established bovine cell line and cultures of *Campylobacter fetus, Leptospira canicola, grippotyphosa, hardjo, icterohaemorrhagiae*, and *pomona*. The product is chemically inactivated and adjuvanted with oil. Contains amphotericin B, penicillin, streptomycin, and thimerosal as preservatives.
Indications: For use in healthy cattle as an aid in the prevention of disease caused by infectious bovine rhinotracheitis, bovine virus diarrhea, parainfluenza Type 3, and bovine respiratory syncytial viruses and *Campylobacter fetus, Leptospira canicola, grippotyphosa, hardjo, icterohaemorrhagiae*, and *pomona*.
Dosage and Administration: Shake well before using. Administer 5 mL intramuscularly 2-4 weeks prior to breeding. Revaccinate with Exalt™ 5 (Bovine Rhinotracheitis-Virus Diarrhea-Parainfluenza 3-Respiratory Syncytial Virus Vaccine) in 4-5 weeks. Revaccinate annually.
Precaution(s): Store in the dark at 35°-45°F (2°-7°C). Do not freeze. Use entire contents when first opened.
Caution(s): Transient swelling may occur at the site of injection. Milk reduction and transient depression may be observed in lactating dairy cows for 3-6 days following vaccination. Anaphylactic reactions may occur following the use of this biological. Symptomatic treatment: Epinephrine.
Warning(s): Do not vaccinate within 60 days prior to slaughter.
For animal use only.
Keep out of reach of children.
Presentation: 10 doses (50 mL) and 50 doses (250 mL).
Produced by: Advance Biologics, Inc.
Compendium Code No.: 14570312

EXCALIBUR® SHEATH CLEANER FOR HORSES

Equicare **Grooming Product**

Ingredient(s): Cleaning formula with tea tree oil.
Indications: A gentle cleanser to soften, loosen and remove accumulated body oils, dirt and debris (smegma).
Directions for Use:
Frequency of Use: Most geldings and stallions should have their sheaths cleaned at least every six months. Light-pigmented genital areas, such as in Pintos, tend to develop accumulations more quickly and, therefore, will require more frequent cleaning.
Stallions: A breeding stallion needs to be washed before and after breeding a mare. Washing not only cleanses the penis, but it also helps to stimulate the stallion in preparation for breeding.
Mares: A smegma-like substance occasionally collects between the teats of a mare's udder. This material can cause irritation to the mare resulting in her rubbing her tail. Therefore, mares should be checked periodically for cleanliness.
Directions: For the sake of cleanliness, disposable gloves should be used by the individual performing this cleaning task. Also for the horse's comfort, excessively cold water should be avoided.
Squeeze out a liberal amount of EXCALIBUR® into palm of hand and place up into the horse's sheath. Working the product well into the folds of the sheath. Allow 3-5 minutes for EXCALIBUR® to soften and loosen smegma.
Next, gently pull the horse's penis out of the sheath and, using pieces of cotton batting, gently remove the loose smegma. Occasionally, smegma will accumulate in a mass in the "blind pouch" above the opening of the urethra in the end of the horse's penis. This resulting "bean" may become large enough to interfere with urination if not removed.
After all presence of smegma has been removed, rinse the horse's sheath and penis as thoroughly as possible with clean water. If a horse will accept it, a gently flowing water hose may be used to flush out the sheath.
Warning(s): For external veterinary use only.
Keep out of reach of children.
Presentation: 473 mL (16 fl oz).
Compendium Code No.: 14470010

EXCENEL® RTU ℞

Pharmacia & Upjohn **Cephalosporin(s)**

brand of ceftiofur hydrochloride sterile suspension
NADA No.: 140-890
Active Ingredient(s): Each mL of this ready-to-use sterile suspension contains ceftiofur hydrochloride equivalent to 50 mg ceftiofur, 0.50 mg phospholipon, 1.5 mg sorbitan monooleate, 2.25 mg sterile water for injection, and cottonseed oil.
Indications:
Swine: EXCENEL® RTU Sterile Suspension is indicated for treatment/control of swine bacterial respiratory disease (swine bacterial pneumonia) associated with *Actinobacillus (Haemophilus) pleuropneumoniae, Pasteurella multocida, Salmonella choleraesuis* and *Streptococcus suis* type 2.
Cattle:
EXCENEL® RTU Sterile Suspension is indicated for treatment of the following bacterial diseases:
- Bovine respiratory disease (BRD, shipping fever, pneumonia) associated with *Mannheimia* spp. *(Pasteurella haemolytica), Pasteurella multocida* and *Haemophilus somnus.*
- Acute bovine interdigital necrobacillosis (foot rot, pododermatitis) associated with *Fusobacterium necrophorum* and *Bacteroides melaninogenicus.*
- Acute metritis (0 to 14 days post-partum) associated with bacterial organisms susceptible to ceftiofur.

Pharmacology: EXCENEL® RTU Sterile Suspension is a ready to use formulation that contains the hydrochloride salt of ceftiofur, which is a broad spectrum cephalosporin antibiotic.
Structure:

Figure 1
Chemical Name of Ceftiofur Hydrochloride: 5-Thia-1-azabicyclo[4,2.0]oct-2-ene-2-carboxylic acid, 7-[[(2-amino-4-thiazolyl) (methoxyimino)-acetyl]amino]-3-[[(2-furanylcarbonyl) thio] methyl]-8-oxo-,hydrochloride salt [6R-[6α,7β(Z)]]-
Clinical Pharmacology:
Swine: Ceftiofur administered as either ceftiofur sodium or ceftiofur hydrochloride is metabolized rapidly to desfuroylceftiofur, the primary metabolite. Administration of ceftiofur to swine as either the sodium or hydrochloride salt provides effective concentrations of ceftiofur and desfuroylceftiofur metabolites in plasma above the MIC_{90} for the labeled pathogens: *Actinobacillus pleuropneumoniae, Pasteurella multocida, Streptococcus suis* and *Salmonella choleraesuis* for the 24-hour (h) period between the dosing intervals. The MIC_{90} for *Salmonella choleraesuis* (1.0 μg/mL) is higher than the other three pathogens and plasma concentrations exceed this value for the entire dosing interval only after the 2.27 mg/lb (5.0 mg/kg) body weight (BW) dose.
Comparative Bioavailability Summary: Comparable plasma concentrations of ceftiofur administered as ceftiofur hydrochloride sterile suspension (EXCENEL® RTU Sterile Suspension) or ceftiofur sodium sterile solution (Naxcel® Sterile Powder) were demonstrated after intramuscular administration of 2.27 mg ceftiofur equivalents/lb (5.0 mg/kg) BW. See Table 1 and Figure 2.
Table 1. Swine plasma concentrations and related parameters* of ceftiofur and desfuroylceftiofur metabolites after EXCENEL® RTU Sterile Suspension (ceftiofur hydrochloride sterile suspension, 50 mg/mL) or Naxcel® Sterile Powder (ceftiofur sodium sterile powder, 50 mg/mL) administered at 2.27 mg/lb ceftiofur equivalents/lb (5.0 mg/kg) BW IM.

	Ceftiofur hydrochloride	Ceftiofur sodium
C_{max} μg/mL:	26.1 ± 5.02	29.2 ± 5.01
t_{max} h:	0.66 - 2.0 (range)	0.33 - 2.0 (range)
$AUC_{0\text{-}LOQ}$ μg•h/mL:	321 ± 50.2	314 ± 55.1
$t_{½}$ h:	16.2 ± 1.55	14.0 ± 1.23
C_{24h} μg/mL:	3.45 ± 0.431	3.53 ± 0.791
C_{72h} μg/mL:	0.518 ± 0.126	0.407 ± 0.0675
$t_{>0.2}$ h:	93.8 ± 7.98	85.0 ± 7.71

Definitions:
C_{max} - Maximum plasma concentration in μg/mL
t_{max} - The time after initial injection to when C_{max} occurs, measured in hours
$AUC_{0\text{-}LOQ}$ - the area under the plasma concentration vs. time curve from time of injection to the limit of quantitation of the assay (0.15 μg/mL)
$t_{½}$ - the plasma half life of the drug in hours
$C_{24\,h}$ - the concentration of drug at 24 h after administration
$C_{72\,h}$ - the concentration of drug at 72 h after administration
$t_{>0.2}$ - the time (in hours) plasma concentrations remain above 0.2 μg/mL.
*Due to significant period effect and significant sequence effect in this study, data from period 1 only were used to evaluate these parameters.
Figure 2. Swine plasma concentrations of ceftiofur and desfuroylceftiofur metabolites after EXCENEL® RTU Sterile Suspension (ceftiofur hydrochloride sterile suspension, 50 mg/mL) or Naxcel® Sterile Powder (ceftiofur sodium sterile powder, 50 mg/mL) were administered intramuscularly at 2.27 mg ceftiofur equivalents/lb (5.0 mg/kg) BW.

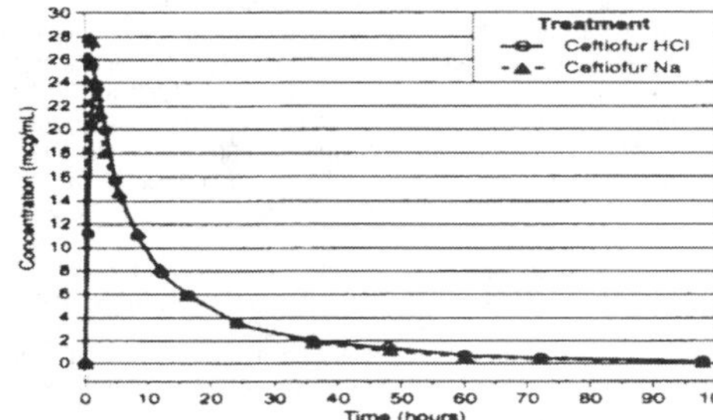

Concentrations of total ceftiofur in the lungs of pigs administered radiolabeled ceftiofur at 2.27 or 3.41 mg ceftiofur equivalents/lb (5.0 or 7.5 mg/kg) BW 12 h after the last of three daily intramuscular injections at 24 h intervals averaged 3.66 and 5.63 μg/g.
Cattle: Ceftiofur administered as either ceftiofur sodium or ceftiofur hydrochloride is metabolized rapidly to desfuroylceftiofur, the primary metabolite. Administration of ceftiofur to cattle as either the sodium or hydrochloride salt provides effective concentrations of ceftiofur and desfuroylceftiofur metabolites in plasma above the MIC_{90} for the bovine respiratory disease (BRD) label pathogens *Mannheimia* spp. *(Pasteurella haemolytica), Pasteurella multocida* and *Haemophilus somnus* for at least 48 h. The relationship between plasma concentrations of ceftiofur and desfuroylceftiofur metabolites above the MIC_{90} in plasma and efficacy has not been

established for the treatment of bovine interdigital necrobacillosis (foot rot) associated with *Fusobacterium necrophorum* and *Bacteroides melaninogenicus*.

Comparative Bioavailability Summary: The comparability of plasma concentrations of ceftiofur following administration of ceftiofur hydrochloride sterile suspension (EXCENEL® RTU Sterile Suspension) or ceftiofur sodium sterile solution (Naxcel® Sterile Powder) was demonstrated after intramuscular or subcutaneous administration of ceftiofur hydrochloride and intramuscular administration of ceftiofur sodium at 1.0 mg ceftiofur equivalents/lb (2.2 mg/kg) BW. See Table 2 and Figure 3.

Table 2. Cattle plasma concentrations and related parameters of ceftiofur and desfuroylceftiofur metabolites after EXCENEL® RTU Sterile Suspension (ceftiofur hydrochloride sterile suspension, 50 mg/mL) administered intramuscularly or subcutaneously at 1.0 mg ceftiofur equivalents/lb (2.2 mg/kg) BW and Naxcel® Sterile Powder (ceftiofur sodium sterile powder, 50 mg/mL) administered intramuscularly at 1.0 mg ceftiofur equivalents/lb (2.2 mg/kg) BW.

	Ceftiofur hydrochloride		Ceftiofur sodium
	IM	SC	IM[1]
C_{max} µg/mL	11.0 ± 1.69	8.56 ± 1.89	14.4 - 16.5
t_{max} h	1 - 4 (range)	1 - 5 (range)	0.33 - 3.0
$t_{>0.2}$ h	60.5 ± 6.27	51.0 ± 6.53	50.7 - 50.9
$AUC_{0\text{-}LOQ}$ µg•h/mL	160 ± 30.7	95.4 ± 17.8	115 - 142
$t_{1/2}$ h	12.0 ± 2.63	11.5 ± 2.57	9.50 - 11.1
C_{24h} µg/mL	1.47 ± 0.380	0.926 ± 0.257	0.86 - 1.16
C_{48h} µg/mL	0.340 ± 0.110	0.271 ± 0.086	0.250 - 0.268

Definitions:

C_{max} - maximum concentration of drug in plasma in µg/mL

t_{max} - The time after initial injection to when C_{max} occurs, measured in hours

$t_{>0.2}$ - the time (in hours) plasma concentrations remain above 0.2 µg/mL

$AUC_{0\text{-}LOQ}$ - the area under the plasma drug concentration vs. time curve from time of injection to the limit of quantitation of the assay (0.15 µg/mL)

$t_{1/2}$ - the drug half life in plasma expressed in hours

$C_{24\,h}$ - the plasma drug concentration 24 h after administration

$C_{48\,h}$ - the plasma drug concentration 48 h after administration

[1] Values represent the separate means from each study.

Figure 3. Cattle plasma concentrations of ceftiofur and desfuroylceftiofur metabolites after administration of 1.0 mg ceftiofur equivalents/lb (2.2 mg/kg) BW of EXCENEL® RTU Sterile Suspension (ceftiofur hydrochloride sterile suspension, 50 mg/mL) by intramuscular or subcutaneous injection or Naxcel® Sterile Powder (ceftiofur sodium sterile powder, 50 mg/mL) by intramuscular injection.

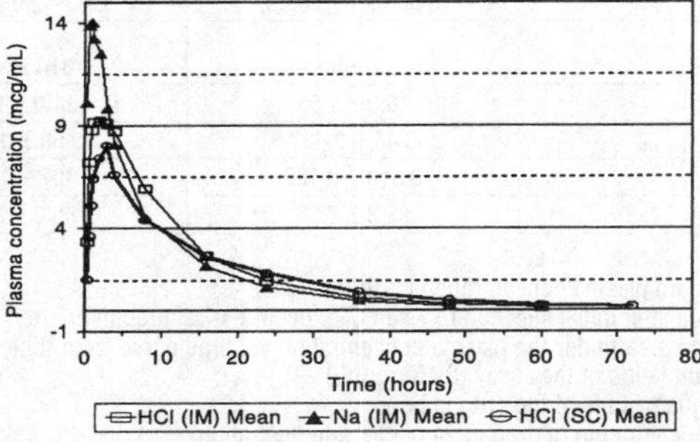

Total residues of ceftiofur were measured in the lungs of cattle administered radiolabeled ceftiofur at 1.0 mg ceftiofur equivalents/lb (2.2 mg/kg) BW at 24 h intervals for five consecutive days. Twelve h after the fifth injection of ceftiofur hydrochloride, total ceftiofur concentrations in the lung averaged 1.15 µg/g, while total ceftiofur concentrations in the lung 8 h after the fifth ceftiofur sodium injection averaged 1.18 µg/g.

Microbiology:

EXCENEL® RTU Sterile Suspension is a ready to use formulation that contains the hydrochloride salt of ceftiofur, which is a broad spectrum cephalosporin antibiotic active against gram-positive and gram-negative bacteria including β-lactamase-producing strains. Like other cephalosporins, ceftiofur is bacteriocidal, *in vitro*, resulting in inhibition of cell wall synthesis.

In vitro activity has been demonstrated for ceftiofur against gram-positive organisms such as *Actinomyces pyogenes*, and other gram-negative organisms, such as *Escherichia coli* and *Salmonella typhimurium*. Ceftiofur was effective when tested in a variety of mouse disease models involving *Escherichia coli, Pasteurella multocida*, and *Salmonella typhimurium*. MIC_{90} values for ceftiofur against other pathogens are as follows: *Salmonella typhimurium* (98 isolates), 2.0 µg/mL; *Escherichia coli* (94 isolates), 1.0 µg/mL. The clinical significance of these findings is not known.

Swine: Studies with ceftiofur have demonstrated *in vitro* and *in vivo* activity against gram-negative pathogens, including *Actinobacillus (Haemophilus) pleuropneumoniae, Pasteurella multocida, Salmonella choleraesuis*, and the gram-positive pathogen *Streptococcus suis* type 2, all of which can be associated with swine bacterial respiratory disease - SRD (swine bacterial pneumonia). A summary of minimum inhibitory concentrations (MIC) for SRD pathogens is provided in Table 3.

Cattle: Studies with ceftiofur have demonstrated *in vitro* and *in vivo* activity against *Mannheimia* spp. *(Pasteurella haemolytica), Pasteurella multocida* and *Haemophilus somnus*, the three major pathogenic bacteria associated with bovine respiratory disease (BRD, pneumonia, shipping fever). A summary of MIC data for BRD pathogens is provided in Table 3.

Studies with ceftiofur have demonstrated *in vitro* and *in vivo* activity against *Fusobacterium necrophorum* and *Bacteroides melaninogenicus*, two of the major pathogenic anaerobic bacteria associated with acute bovine interdigital necrobacillosis (foot rot, pododermatitis).

Antimicrobial Susceptibility: A summary of MIC data for swine (1993-1998) and cattle (1993-1994) pathogens is presented in Table 3. Clinical isolates were obtained in the United States. Testing followed NCCLS Guidelines (National Committee for Clinical Laboratory Standards).

Table 3. Minimum Inhibitory Concentrations for Ceftiofur Against SRD and BRD Clinical Isolates:

Organism (# of strains tested)	MIC µg/mL		
	Range	MIC_{90}	Date Tested
Swine			
Actinobacillus pleuropneumoniae (83)	≤0.03 - 0.06	≤0.03	1993
Pasteurella multocida (74)	≤0.03 - 0.06	≤0.03	1993
Streptococcus suis (94)	≤0.03 - 1.0	0.25	1993
Salmonella choleraesuis (50)	1.0 - 2.0	1.0	1993
beta-hemolytic *Streptococcus* spp. (24)	≤0.03 - 0.06	≤0.03	1993
Actinobacillus suis (77)	0.0019 - 0.0078	0.0078	1998
Haemophilus parasuis (76)	0.0039 - 0.25	0.06	1998
Cattle			
Mannheimia spp. **(Pasteurella haemolytica)* (42)	≤0.003 - 0.03	0.015	1993
**Pasteurella multocida* (48)	≤0.003 - 0.015	≤0.003	1993
**Haemophilus somnus* (59)	no range	≤0.0019	1993
**Fusobacterium necrophorum* (17)	≤0.06	≤0.06	1994
***Bacteroides fragilis* group (29)	≤0.06 - >16.0	16.0	1994
***Bacteroides* spp. non-fragilis group (12)	0.13 - >16.0	16.0	1994
***Peptostreptococcus anaerobius* (12)	0.13 - 2.0	2.0	1994

* Clinical isolates supported by clinical data and indications for use.

** Clinical isolates not supported by clinical data, the clinical significance of these data is not known.

MIC_{90} Minimum inhibitory concentration for 90% of the isolates.

Based on the pharmacokinetic studies of ceftiofur in swine and cattle after a single intramuscular injection of 1.36 to 2.27 mg ceftiofur equivalents/lb (3.0 to 5.0 mg/kg) BW (swine) or 0.5 to 1.0 mg ceftiofur equivalents/lb (1.1 to 2.2 mg/kg) BW (cattle) and the MIC and disk (30 µg) diffusion data, the following breakpoints are recommended by NCCLS.

Zone Diameter (mm)	MIC (µg/mL)	Interpretation
≥ 21	≤ 2.0	(S) Susceptible
18-20	4.0	(I) Intermediate
≤ 17	> 8.0	(R) Resistant

A report of "Susceptible" indicates that the pathogen is likely to be inhibited by generally achievable blood levels. A report of "Intermediate" is a technical buffer zone and isolates falling into this category should be retested. Alternatively the organism may be successfully treated if the infection is in a body site where drug is physiologically concentrated. A report of "Resistant" indicates that the achievable drug concentrations are unlikely to be inhibitory and other therapy should be selected.

Standardized procedures[1] require the use of laboratory control organisms for both standardized diffusion techniques and standardized dilution techniques. The 30 µg ceftiofur sodium disk should give the following zone diameters and the ceftiofur sodium standard reference powder (or disk) should provide the following MIC values for the reference strain. Ceftiofur sodium disks or powder reference standard is appropriate for both ceftiofur salts.

QC Strain	MIC (µg/mL)	Disk Zone Diameter (mm)
E. coli ATCC 25922	0.25-1	24-30

Dosage and Administration:

Swine: Administer intramuscularly at a dosage of 1.36 to 2.27 mg ceftiofur equivalents/lb (3.0 to 5.0 mg/kg) BW (1 mL of sterile suspension per 22 to 37 lb BW). Treatment should be repeated at 24 h intervals for a total of three consecutive days.

Cattle:

- For bovine respiratory disease and acute interdigital necrobacillosis: administer by intramuscular or subcutaneous administration at the dosage of 0.5 to 1.0 mg ceftiofur equivalents/lb (1.1 to 2.2 mg/kg) BW (1 to 2 mL sterile suspension per 100 lb BW). Administer daily at 24 h intervals for a total of three consecutive days. Additional treatments may be administered on Days 4 and 5 for animals which do not show a satisfactory response (not recovered) after the initial three treatments. In addition, for BRD only, administer intramuscularly or subcutaneously 1.0 mg ceftiofur equivalents/lb (2.2 mg/kg) BW every other day on Days 1 and 3 (48 h interval). Do not inject more than 15 mL per injection site.

Selection of dosage level (0.5 to 1.0 mg/lb) and regimen/duration (daily or every other day for BRD only) should be based on an assessment of the severity of disease, pathogen susceptibility and clinical response.

- For acute post-partum metritis: administer by intramuscular or subcutaneous administration at the dosage of 1.0 mg ceftiofur equivalents/lb (2.2 mg/kg) BW (2 mL sterile suspension per 100 lb BW). Administer at 24 h intervals for five consecutive days. Do not inject more than 15 mL per injection site.

Shake well before using.

Contraindication(s): As with all drugs, the use of EXCENEL® RTU Sterile Suspension is contraindicated in animals previously found to be hypersensitive to the drug.

Precaution(s): Storage Conditions: Store at controlled room temperature 20° to 25°C (68° to 77°F) [see USP]. Shake well before using. Protect from freezing.

Caution(s): Federal (USA) law restricts this drug to use by or on the order of a licensed veterinarian.

Swine: Areas of discoloration associated with the injection site at time periods of 11 days or less may result in trim-out of edible tissues at slaughter. The safety of ceftiofur has not been demonstrated for pregnant swine or swine intended for breeding.

Cattle: Following intramuscular or subcutaneous administration in the neck, areas of discoloration at the site may persist beyond 11 days resulting in trim loss of edible tissues at slaughter. Following intramuscular administration in the rear leg, areas of discoloration at the injection site may persist beyond 28 days resulting in trim loss of edible tissues at slaughter.

Warning(s): Residue Warnings: No pre-slaughter drug withdrawal interval is required when this product is used in swine. Treated cattle must not be slaughtered for 48 hours (2 days) following last treatment because unsafe levels of drug remain at the injection sites. No milk discard time is required when this product is used according to label directions. Use of dosages in excess of those indicated or by unapproved routes of administration, such as intramammary, may result in illegal residues in edible tissues and/or in milk. A withdrawal period has not been established in pre-ruminating calves. Do not use in calves to be processed for veal.

Not for human use.

Keep out of reach of children.

Penicillins and cephalosporins can cause allergic reactions in sensitized individuals. Topical exposures to such antimicrobials, including ceftiofur, may elicit mild to severe allergic reactions in some individuals. Repeated or prolonged exposure may lead to sensitization. Avoid direct contact of the product with the skin, eyes, mouth, and clothing.

Persons with a known hypersensitivity to penicillin or cephalosporins should avoid exposure to this product.

In case of accidental eye exposure, flush with water for 15 minutes. In case of accidental skin exposure, wash with soap and water. Remove contaminated clothing. If allergic reaction occurs (e.g., skin rash, hives, difficult breathing), seek medical attention.

The material safety data sheet contains more detailed occupational safety information. To report adverse effects in users, to obtain more information or obtain a material safety data sheet, call 1-800-253-8600.

Trial Data: Clinical Efficacy:

Cattle: In addition to demonstrating comparable plasma concentrations, the following clinical efficacy data are provided.

A clinical study was conducted to evaluate the efficacy of ceftiofur hydrochloride administered subcutaneously for the treatment of the bacterial component of BRD under natural field conditions. When uniform clinical signs of BRD were present, 60 cattle (111 to 207 kg) were randomly assigned to one of the following treatment groups: negative control or ceftiofur hydrochloride at 0.5 or 1.0 ceftiofur equivalents/lb (1.1 or 2.2 mg/kg) BW. Treatments were administered daily for three consecutive days. Cattle were evaluated daily and animals that died or were euthanized were necropsied and the lung lesions scored. On Day 15, all surviving animals were euthanatized and necropsied and the lung lesions scored. Mortality rates were 65%, 10% and 5% for negative controls, 0.5 mg ceftiofur equivalents/lb and 1.0 mg ceftiofur equivalents/lb, (1.1 or 2.2 mg/kg) BW, respectively. Mortality rates for both ceftiofur hydrochloride treatment groups were lower than for negative controls ($P < 0.0001$). Rectal temperatures 24 h after third treatment were 104.0°F, 103.1°F and 102.8°F for negative controls, 0.5 mg/lb and 1.0 mg/lb (1.1 or 2.2 mg/kg) BW, respectively. The temperatures for both ceftiofur hydrochloride treatment groups were lower than the negative controls ($P \leq 0.05$). Ceftiofur hydrochloride administered subcutaneously for three consecutive days at 0.5 or 1.0 mg ceftiofur equivalents/lb (1.1 or 2.2 mg/kg) BW is an effective treatment for the bacterial component of BRD.

A three-location clinical field study was conducted to evaluate the efficacy of ceftiofur hydrochloride administered intramuscularly daily for three days or every other day (Days 1 and 3) for the treatment of the bacterial component of naturally occurring BRD. When uniform signs of BRD were present, 360 beef crossbred cattle were randomly assigned to one of the following treatment groups: negative control, ceftiofur sodium at 0.5 mg ceftiofur equivalents/lb (1.1 mg/kg) BW daily for three days, ceftiofur hydrochloride at 1.0 mg ceftiofur equivalents/lb (2.2 mg/kg) BW daily for three days, or ceftiofur hydrochloride at 1.0 mg ceftiofur equivalents/lb BW on Days 1 and 3 (every other day). All treatments were administered intramuscularly. All ceftiofur treatment groups (hydrochloride and sodium) and treatment regimens (every day and every other day) significantly ($P < 0.05$) reduced Day 4 rectal temperature as compared to the negative control. Clinical success on Days 10 and 28 and mortality to Day 28 were not different for the ceftiofur groups (hydrochloride and sodium) and treatment regimens (every day and every other day). The results of this study demonstrate that daily and every other day (Days 1 and 3) intramuscular administration of ceftiofur hydrochloride are effective treatment regimens for the bacterial component of BRD.

An eight location study was conducted under natural field conditions to evaluate the efficacy of ceftiofur hydrochloride for the treatment of acute post-partum metritis (0 to 14 days post-partum). When clinical signs of acute post-partum metritis (rectal temperature ≥ 103°F and fetid vaginal discharge) were observed, 361 lactating dairy cows were assigned randomly to treatment or negative control. Cattle were dosed either subcutaneously or intramuscularly, daily for five consecutive days. On days 1, 5 and 9 after the last day of dose administration, cows were evaluated for clinical signs of acute post-partum metritis. A cure was defined as rectal temperature < 103°F and lack of fetid discharge. Cure rate for the 1.0 mg ceftiofur equivalents/lb (2.2 mg/kg) BW dose group was significantly improved relative to cure rate of the negative control on day 9. The results of this study demonstrate that ceftiofur hydrochloride administered daily for five consecutive days at a dose of 1.0 mg ceftiofur equivalents/lb (2.2 mg/kg) BW is an effective treatment for acute post-partum metritis.

Animal Safety:

Swine: Results from a five-day tolerance study in normal feeder pigs indicated that ceftiofur sodium was well tolerated when administered at 57 mg ceftiofur equivalents/lb (125 mg/kg) (more than 25 times the highest recommended daily dosage of 2.27 mg/lb (5.0 mg/kg) BW for five consecutive days. Ceftiofur administered intramuscularly to pigs produced no overt adverse signs of toxicity.

To determine the safety margin in swine, a safety-toxicity study was conducted. Five barrows and five gilts per group were administered ceftiofur sodium intramuscularly at 0, 2.27, 6.81 and 11.36 mg ceftiofur equivalents/lb (0, 5, 15, 25 mg/kg) BW for 15 days. This is 0, 1, 3 and 5 times the highest recommended dose of 2.27 mg/lb (5.0 mg/kg) BW/day and 5 times the recommended treatment length of 3 days. There were no adverse systemic effects observed, indicating that ceftiofur has a wide margin of safety when injected intramuscularly into feeder pigs at the highest recommended dose of 2.27 mg ceftiofur equivalents/lb (5.0 mg/kg) BW daily for 3 days or at levels up to 5 times the highest recommended dose for 5 times the recommended length of treatment.

A separate study evaluated the injection site tissue tolerance of EXCENEL® RTU (ceftiofur hydrochloride) in swine when administered intramuscularly in the neck at 1.36 and 2.27 mg ceftiofur equivalents/lb (3.0 to 5.0 mg/kg) BW. Animals were necropsied at intervals to permit evaluations at 12 h, and 3, 5, 7, 9, 11, 15, 20, and 25 days after last injection. Injection sites were evaluated grossly at necropsy. No apparent changes (swelling or inflammation) were observed clinically after 12 h post-injection. Areas of discoloration associated with the injection site were observed at time periods less than 11 days after last injection.

Cattle: Results from a five-day tolerance study in feeder calves indicated that ceftiofur sodium was well tolerated at 25 times (25 mg ceftiofur equivalents/lb {55 mg/kg} BW) the highest recommended dose of 1.0 mg ceftiofur equivalents/lb (2.2 mg/kg) BW for five consecutive days. Ceftiofur administered intramuscularly had no adverse systemic effects.

In a 15-day safety/toxicity study, five steer and five heifer calves per group were administered ceftiofur sodium intramuscularly at 0 (vehicle control), 1, 3, 5 and 10 times the highest recommended dose of 1.0 mg ceftiofur equivalents/lb (2.2 mg/kg) BW to determine the safety factor. There were no adverse systemic effects indicating that ceftiofur sodium has a wide margin of safety when injected intramuscularly into the feeder calves at 10 times (10 mg ceftiofur equivalents/lb {22 mg/kg} BW) the recommended dose for three times (15 days) the recommended length of treatment of three to five days. Local tissue tolerance to intramuscular injection of ceftiofur hydrochloride was evaluated in the following study.

Results from a tissue tolerance study indicated that ceftiofur hydrochloride was well tolerated and produced no systemic toxicity in cattle when administered intramuscularly in the neck and rear leg at a dose of 1.0 mg ceftiofur equivalents/lb (2.2 mg/kg) BW at each injection site. This represents a total dose per animal of 2.0 mg ceftiofur equivalents/lb (4.4 mg/kg) BW. Clinically noted changes (local swelling) at injection sites in the neck were very infrequent (2/48 sites) whereas noted changes in rear leg sites were more frequent (21/48 sites). These changes in the rear leg injection sites were generally evident on the day following injection and lasted from 1 to 11 days. At necropsy, injection sites were recognized by discoloration of the subcutaneous tissues and muscle that resolved in approximately 7 to 15 days in the neck and 19 to 28 days in the rear leg.

Results from another tissue tolerance study indicated that ceftiofur hydrochloride was well tolerated and produced no systemic toxicity to cattle when administered subcutaneously at 0.5 or 1.0 mg ceftiofur equivalents/lb (1.1 or 2.2 mg/kg) BW at 24 h intervals for 5 days. Mild and usually transient, clinically visible or palpable reactions (local swelling) were localized at the injection site. At necropsy, injection sites were routinely recognized by edema, limited increase in thickness and color changes of the subcutaneous tissue and/or facial surface of underlying muscle. The facial surface of the muscle was visibly affected in most cases through 9.5 days after injection. Underlying muscle mass was not involved. There were no apparent differences in tissue response to administration of ceftiofur hydrochloride at 0.5 or 1.0 mg ceftiofur equivalents/lb (1.1 or 2.2 mg/kg) BW.

References: [1] National Committee for Clinical Laboratory Standards. Performance Standards for Antimicrobial Disk and Dilution Susceptibility Tests for Bacteria Isolated from Animals; Proposed Standard. NCCLS Document M31-P (ISBN 1-56238-258-6). NCCLS, 771 East Lancaster Avenue, Villanova, Pennsylvania 19085, 1994.

Presentation: EXCENEL® RTU Sterile Suspension is available in the following package size: 100 mL vial (NDC 0009-3504-03).

U.S. Patent Nos. 4,902,683; 5,736,151

Compendium Code No.: 10490543 816 323 307

EXIT™ INSECTICIDE

AgriPharm **Topical Insecticide**

EPA Reg. No.: 28293-182-10504

Active Ingredient(s):

Permethrin (3-phenoxyphenyl) methyl (±) cis, trans-3-(2,2-dichloroethenyl)-2,2-dimethylcyclopropanecarboxylate* 1.0%

Inert Ingredients** 99.0%

*cis/trans ratio: Min 35% (±) cis and max 65% (±) trans.

**Contains petroleum distillate.

Indications: Kills lice and flies on cattle, and keds on sheep.

Recommended as a pour-on for beef, lactating and non-lactating dairy cattle and sheep.

Directions for Use: It is a violation of Federal law to use this product in a manner inconsistent with its labeling. Ready to use - No dilution necessary.

Application Instructions: Pour along back line and down face. Apply ½ fl oz per 100 lbs body weight of animal, up to a maximum of 5 fl oz for any one animal to kill lice, horn flies and face flies. Aids in the insecticidal control of horse flies, stable flies, mosquitoes, black flies and ticks on lactating and non-lactating dairy cattle, beef cattle, calves and sheep. For keds on sheep, pour along back line over neck, shoulders and rump. Apply ¼ fl oz per 50 lbs body weight of animal, up to a maximum of 3 fl oz for any one animal.

Repeat treatment as needed, but not more than once every two weeks. For optimum insecticidal effectiveness against lice, a double treatment at 14 day intervals is recommended.

Note: This product is not effective for grub control on cattle.

Precautionary Statements: Hazards to Humans and Domestic Animals:

Caution: Avoid contact with eyes.

Statement of Practical Treatment:

If in Eyes: Immediately flush eyes with plenty of water. Get medical attention if discomfort persists.

If Swallowed: Call a physician immediately.

Do not induce vomiting unless advised by a physician.

Note to Physician: Solvent presents aspiration hazard. Gastric lavage is indicated if material was taken internally.

Environmental Hazards: This pesticide is extremely toxic to fish. Use with care when applying to areas adjacent to any body of water. Do not add directly to water. Do not contaminate water by cleaning of equipment or disposal of wastes. Apply this product only as specified on the label.

Physical or Chemical Hazards: Do not use or store near heat or open flame.

Storage and Disposal: Do not contaminate water, food or feed by storage or disposal.

Storage: Keep container sealed when not in use. Do not store near food or feed.

Pesticide Disposal: Wastes resulting from the use of this product may be disposed of on site or at an approved waste disposal facility.

Container Disposal: Triple rinse (or equivalent). Then offer for recycling or reconditioning, or puncture and dispose of in a sanitary landfill or incineration, or if allowed by State and local authorities, by burning. If burned, stay out of smoke.

Containers One Gallon and Under: Do not reuse empty container. Rinse thoroughly, wrap in several layers of newspaper and place in trash.

Warning(s): Keep out of reach of children.

Disclaimer: Notice of Warranty: Agripharm makes no warranty of merchantability, fitness for any particular purpose, or otherwise, expressed or implied concerning this product or its uses which extend beyond the use of the product under normal conditions in accord with the statements made on this label.

Presentation: 1 U.S. gallon (3.785 liters).

Compendium Code No.: 14570410

EXIT™ II SYNERGIZED FORMULA INSECTICIDE

AgriPharm **Premise and Topical Insecticide**

EPA Reg. No.: 28293-259-10504

Active Ingredient(s):

Permethrin (3-phenoxyphenyl) methyl (±) cis, trans 3-(2,2-dichloroethenyl) 2,2-dimethylcyclopropanecarboxylate* 1.0%

Piperonyl Butoxide Technical** 1.0%

Inert Ingredients*** 98.0%

100.0%

*cis/trans ratio: Min. 35% (±) cis max. 65% (±) trans.

**Equivalent to Min. 0.8% (butylcarbityl) (6-propylpiperonyl) ether and 0.2% related compounds.

***Contains petroleum distillate.

Indications: Kills lice and flies on cattle, and keds on sheep.

Recommended as a pour-on for beef, lactating and non-lactating dairy cattle and sheep.

Directions for Use: It is a violation of Federal law to use this product in a manner inconsistent with its labeling. Ready to use - No dilution necessary.

Apply To	Target Insects	Application Instructions
Lactating and Non-Lactating Dairy Cattle, Beef Cattle and Calves	Lice, Horn Flies, Face Flies. Aids in control of Horse Flies, Stable Flies, House Flies, Mosquitoes and Black Flies.	Dosage: Apply ½ fl oz (15 cc) per 100 lbs body wt. of animal up to a maximum of 5 fl oz for any one animal. Pour-On: Pour correct dose along back and down face. Ready-to-Use Spray: Use undiluted in a mist sprayer to apply correct dose. Apply directly to neck, face, back, legs and ears. Back Rubber Use: Mix one pint per gallon of mineral oil. Keep rubbing device charged. Results improved by daily forced use.
Sheep	Sheep Keds, Lice	Pour along back. Apply ¼ fl oz (7.5 cc) per 50 lbs body wt. of animal, up to a maximum of 3 fl oz for any one animal. For optimum control, all animals in the flock should be treated after shearing.
Premises - in and around Horse, Beef, Dairy, Swine, Sheep and Poultry Premises, Animal Hospital Pens and Kennels and "outside" Meat Processing Premises.	House Flies, Stable Flies, Face Flies, Gnats, Mosquitoes, Black Flies, Fleas and Little House Flies. Aids in control of cockroaches, ants, spiders, crickets.	For use as a ready-to-use spot spray or premise spray, use undiluted in a mist sprayer. Apply directly to surface to leave a residual insecticidal coating, paying particular attention to areas where insects crawl or alight. One gallon will treat approximately 7,300 square feet.

For cattle and sheep, repeat treatment as needed, but no more than once every two weeks. For optimum lice control, two treatments at a 14-day interval are recommended.

Special Note: This product is not effective in controlling cattle grubs. This is an oil-base, ready-to-use product that may leave an oily appearance on the hair coat of some animals. This product should be used in an integrated pest management system which may involve repeat treatments and the use of other pest control practices.

Precautionary Statements: Hazards to Humans and Domestic Animals:

Caution: Harmful if absorbed through skin. Avoid contact with skin, eyes and clothing. Prolonged or frequently repeated skin contact may cause allergic reactions in some individuals. Wash thoroughly with soap and water after handling.

Statement of Practical Treatment:

If Swallowed: Call a physician immediately. Do not induce vomiting unless under medical attention.

If in Eyes: Immediately flush eyes with plenty of water. Get medical attention if discomfort persists.

If on Skin: Wash skin with soap and water. Get medical attention.

Environmental Hazards: This product is extremely toxic to fish and other aquatic invertebrates. Do not add directly to water, or to areas where surface waters are present or to intertidal areas below the mean high water mark. Do not contaminate water when disposing of equipment washwaters. Apply this product only as specified on the label.

Physical or Chemical Hazards: Do not use or store near heat or open flame.

Storage and Disposal: Do not contaminate water, food or feed by storage or disposal.

Storage: Keep container sealed when not in use. Do not store near food or feed.

Pesticide Disposal: Wastes resulting from the use of this product may be disposed of on site or at an approved waste disposal facility.

Container Disposal: Triple rinse (or equivalent). Then offer for recycling or reconditioning, or puncture and dispose of in a sanitary landfill or incineration, or, if allowed by State and local authorities, by burning. If burned, stay out of smoke.

Warning(s): Keep out of reach of children.

Disclaimer: Notice of Warranty: Agripharm makes no warranty of merchantability, fitness for any particular purpose, or otherwise, expressed or implied concerning this product or its uses which extend beyond the use of the product under normal conditions in accordance with the statements made on this label.

Presentation: 1 U.S. gallon (3.785 liters).

Compendium Code No.: 14570401

EXODUS™ PASTE

Bimeda **Parasiticide-Oral**

(pyrantel pamoate) Equine Anthelmintic

ANADA No.: 200-350

Active Ingredient(s): EXODUS™ Paste (pyrantel pamoate) is a pale yellow to buff paste containing 43.9% w/w pyrantel pamoate in an inert vehicle. Each 23.6 g syringe contains 3.6 grams pyrantel base in 23.6 grams paste. Each 47.2 g syringe contains 7.2 g pyrantel pamoate base in 47.2 g paste. Each milliliter contains 171 milligrams pyrantel base as pyrantel pamoate.

Apple flavored.

Indications: For the removal and control of mature infections of large strongyles *(Strongylus vulgaris, S. edentatus, S. equinus);* small strongyles, pinworms *(Oxyuris equi),* and large roundworms *(Parascaris equorum)* in horses and ponies.

Consult your veterinarian for assistance in the diagnosis, treatment, and control of parasitism.

Pharmacology: Composition: Pyrantel pamoate is a compound belonging to a family classified chemically as tetrahydropyrimidines. It is a yellow, water-insoluble crystalline salt of the tetrahydropyrimidine base and pamoic acid containing 34.7% base activity. The chemical structure and name are given below.

CH = CH N N CH_3 HO_2C OH CH_2 2

Chemical Name: (E)-1,4,5,6-tetrahydro-1-methyl-2-[2-(2-thienyl)-vinyl]-pyrimidine 4,4' methylenebis [3-hydroxy-2-naphtholate] (1:1).

Dosage and Administration: Dosage and Treatment: EXODUS™ Paste (pyrantel pamoate) is to be administered as a single oral dose of 3 milligrams pyrantel base per pound of body weight. The 23.6 g syringe has four weight mark increments. The 47.2 g syringe has eight weight mark increments. Each weight mark indicates the recommended dose for 300 pounds of body weight. One-half 47.2 g syringe treats a 1200 lb horse.

Dosage for 23.6 g syringe:

Body Weight Range	Quantity	mg Pyrantel Base
Up to 300 lb	¼ syringe	900 mg
301 to 600 lb	½ syringe	1800 mg
601 to 900 lb	¾ syringe	2700 mg
901 to 1200 lb	1 full syringe	3600 mg

Dosage for 47.2 g syringe:

Body Weight Range	Quantity	mg Pyrantel Base
Up to 300 lb	⅛ syringe	900 mg
301 to 600 lb	¼ syringe	1800 mg
601 to 900 lb	⅜ syringe	2700 mg
901 to 1200 lb	½ syringe	3600 mg

Note: Position ring-gauge over appropriate mark on plunger.

For maximum control of parasitism, it is recommended that foals (2-8 months of age) be dosed every 4 weeks. To minimize the potential source of infection that the mare may pose to the foal, the mare should be treated 1 month prior to anticipated foaling date followed by re-treatment 10 days to 2 weeks after birth of foal. Horses and ponies over 8 months of age should be routinely dosed every 6 weeks.

It is recommended that severely debilitated animals not be treated with this preparation.

Administration: After removing the cap, the paste should be deposited on the dorsum of the tongue. Introduce the nozzle end of the syringe at the corner of the mouth. Direct the syringe backwards and depress the plunger to deposit the paste onto the tongue. Given in this manner, it is unlikely that rejection of the paste will occur. Raising the horse's head sometimes assists in the swallowing process. When only part of the paste has been used, replace the cap on the syringe nozzle.

Precaution(s): Storage: Store at 15°-30°C (59°-86°F).

Caution(s): Read entire brochure carefully before using this product.

For oral use only. For animal use only.

Warning(s): Not for use in horses intended for food.

Keep this and all medications out of reach of children.

Trial Data: Efficacy: Critical (worm count) studies in horses demonstrated that pyrantel pamoate administered at the recommended dosage was efficacious against mature infections of *Strongylus vulgaris* (>90%), *S. edentatus* (69%), *S. equinus* (>90%), *Oxyuris equi* (81%), *Parascaris equorum* (>90%), and small strongyles (>90%).

Presentation: 23.6 g (NDC 61133-0141-0) single-dose syringe and 47.2 g (NDC 61133-0141-1) multi-dose syringe.

EXODUS is a trademark of Bimeda, Inc.

Manufactured by: Bimeda-MTC Animal Health, Inc.

Compendium Code No.: 13990630 8PYR003 / 8PYR006

EXPECTADE™ COUGH SYRUP

PRN Pharmacal **Antitussive**

Decongestant-Expectorant-Antihistamine

Active Ingredient(s): Each 5 mL contains:

Guaifenesin .... 100 mg
Sodium Citrate .... 100 mg
Pyrilamine Maleate .... 8 mg
Phenylephrine Hydrochloride .... 8 mg

In a flavored syrup base.

Indications: For effective relief of cough symptoms related to upper respiratory conditions.

Dosage and Administration: Administer orally.

Horses 2 ozs (59.2 mL) to 4 ozs (118.4 mL).

Dogs and Cats 1 tsp (5 mL) to 2 tsp (10 mL) depending on size.

Repeat every two hours if necessary.

Caution(s): If symptoms persist, consult a veterinarian.

Warning(s): Not for use in horses intended for food. For animal use only.

Not for human use. Keep out of reach of children.

Presentation: 4 fl oz and 1 quart (32 fl oz).

Compendium Code No.: 10900070

EXPECTAHIST

Vetus **Antitussive**

Active Ingredient(s): Description: Each fluid ounce contains:

Guaifenesin .... 8 grs.
Ammonium Chloride .... 8 grs.
Sodium Citrate .... 8 grs.
Pyrilamine Maleate .... 50 mg
Phenylephrine Hydrochloride .... 50 mg

In a flavored syrup base.

Indications: A decongestant-expectorant antihistamine for the effective relief of cough symptoms related to upper respiratory conditions.

Dosage and Administration: Administer orally.

Horses: 2 to 4 ounces.

Sheep, Swine and Young Animals: 1 to 2 ounces.

Dogs and Cats: 1 to 2 teaspoonfuls, depending on size.

Repeat every 2 hours if necessary.

Caution(s): For veterinary use only.

Warning(s): Not for human use. Keep out of the reach of children.

Presentation: 1 gallon (128 fl oz, 3,840 mL) containers (NDC#: 47611-551-71).

Distributed by: Burns Veterinary Supply, Inc., Westbury, NY 11590.

Compendium Code No.: 14440960 6-2000

EXPECTORANT POWDER

First Priority **Expectorant**

Active Ingredient(s): Sodium bicarbonate, ammonium chloride, sodium chloride, licorice root, maltrin, dicalcium phosphate, benzoic acid, silicon dioxide.
Indications: For use in horses and cattle as an expectorant to loosen accumulated mucus in the upper respiratory tract.
Directions for Use: For mature horses and cattle, one heaping tablespoon on food three times daily.
Precaution(s): Storage: Store at controlled room temperature between 15°-30°C (59°-86°F). Keep tightly closed when not in use.
Caution(s): For animal use only.
Warning(s): Do not use on animals intended for food.

Keep out of reach of children.

Presentation: 1 lb (453.6 g) (NDC# 58829-281-16).
Compendium Code No.: 11390282 Rev. 06-01

EXPRESS™ 3

Boehringer Ingelheim **Vaccine**

Bovine Rhinotracheitis-Virus Diarrhea Vaccine, Modified Live Virus
U.S. Vet. Lic. No.: 124
Composition: This product contains Bovine Rhinotracheitis (IBR) and Bovine Virus Diarrhea (BVD) Types 1 and 2 modified live viruses.

Preservative: Neomycin.

Indications: Recommended for the vaccination of healthy, susceptible cattle as an aid in the reduction of diseases caused by Bovine Rhinotracheitis (IBR) virus and Bovine Virus Diarrhea (BVD) Types 1 and 2.
Directions: Rehydrate one bottle of modified live virus vaccine by aseptically adding one bottle of liquid diluent. Shake well and use immediately.

Dosage: Using aseptic technique, inject 2 mL subcutaneously. Repeat in 14-28 days and once annually. Calves vaccinated before 6 months of age should be revaccinated at 6 months. A 2 mL booster dose is recommended prior to time of stress or exposure.

Contraindication(s): Note: It is possible that healthy appearing cattle can be persistently infected with or incubating virulent BVD virus at the time of vaccination. In view of these findings and suggested causes, BVD vaccine is contraindicated in persistently infected cattle and use should be limited only to healthy, immunocompetent, unstressed, non-pregnant cattle.
Precaution(s): Storage: Store out of direct sunlight at a temperature between 35-45°F (2-7°C). Avoid freezing.

Use entire contents when first opened.

Disposal: Burn vaccine containers and all unused contents.

Caution(s): Stressed cattle should not be vaccinated. Do not use in pregnant cows or calves nursing pregnant cows. Injection site swelling may occur. Anaphylactoid reactions may occur.

Animal inoculation only. Accidental injection to humans can cause serious local reactions. Contact a physician immediately if accidental injection occurs.

Antidote(s): Epinephrine.
Warning(s): Do not vaccinate within 21 days before slaughter.
Presentation: 5 x 10 doses (20 mL) and 5 x 50 doses (100 mL).
Compendium Code No.: 10281291 BI 1103-1 6/01, 10305-00

EXPRESS™ 3/LP

Boehringer Ingelheim **Bacterin-Vaccine**

Bovine Rhinotracheitis-Virus Diarrhea Vaccine, Modified Live Virus-Leptospira Pomona Bacterin
U.S. Vet. Lic. No.: 124
Composition: This product contains Bovine Rhinotracheitis (IBR) and Bovine Virus Diarrhea (BVD) Types 1 and 2 modified live viruses, and inactivated cultures of *Leptospira pomona.*

Preservatives: The vaccine fraction contains neomycin as a preservative. The bacterin diluent fraction contains gentamicin and Amphotericin B.

Indications: Recommended for the vaccination of healthy, susceptible cattle as an aid in the reduction of diseases caused by Bovine Rhinotracheitis (IBR) virus, Bovine Virus Diarrhea (BVD) Types 1 and 2, and *Leptospira pomona.*
Directions: Rehydrate one bottle of modified live virus vaccine by aseptically adding one bottle of liquid bacterin diluent. Shake well and use immediately.

Dosage: Using aseptic technique, inject 2 mL intramuscularly. Repeat in 14-28 days and once annually. Calves vaccinated before 6 months of age should be revaccinated at 6 months. A 2 mL booster dose is recommended prior to time of stress or exposure.

Precaution(s): Storage: Store out of direct sunlight at a temperature between 35-45°F (2-7°C). Avoid freezing.

Use entire contents when first opened.

Disposal: Burn vaccine containers and all unused contents.

Caution(s): Stressed cattle should not be vaccinated. Do not use in pregnant cows or calves nursing pregnant cows. Injection site swelling may occur. Anaphylactoid reactions may occur.

Animal inoculation only. Accidental injection to humans can cause serious local reactions. Contact a physician immediately if accidental injection occurs.

Note: It is possible that healthy appearing cattle can be persistently infected with or incubating virulent BVD virus at the time of vaccination. In view of these findings and suggested causes, BVD vaccine is contraindicated in persistently infected cattle and use should be limited only to healthy, immunocompetent, unstressed, non-pregnant cattle.

Antidote(s): Antidote: Epinephrine.
Warning(s): Do not vaccinate within 21 days before slaughter.
Presentation: 5 x 10 doses (20 mL) and 5 x 50 doses (100 mL).
Compendium Code No.: 10281300 BI 1095-1 5/01, 09503-01

EXPRESS 4®

Boehringer Ingelheim **Vaccine**

Bovine Rhinotracheitis-Virus Diarrhea-Parainfluenza$_3$-Respiratory Syncytial Virus Vaccine, Modified Live and Killed Virus
U.S. Vet. Lic. No.: 124
Contents: This product contains the antigens listed above.

Contains neomycin as a preservative.

Indications: Recommended for the vaccination of healthy, susceptible cattle against disease caused by bovine rhinotracheitis (IBR) virus, bovine virus diarrhea (BVD) virus, parainfluenza$_3$ (PI$_3$) virus, and bovine respiratory syncytial virus (BRSV).
Directions: Rehydrate the modified live virus vaccine by aseptically adding the accompanying bottle of killed virus vaccine.

Dosage: Using aseptic technique, inject 2 mL intramuscularly. Repeat in 21 days and once annually. Calves vaccinated before 6 months of age should be revaccinated at 6 months. A 2 mL booster dose is recommended annually or prior to time of stress or exposure.

Contraindication(s): It is possible that healthy appearing cattle can be persistently infected with or incubating virulent BVD virus at time of vaccination. In view of these findings and suggested causes, BVD vaccine is contraindicated in persistently infected cattle and use should be limited only to healthy, immunocompetent, unstressed, non-pregnant cattle.
Precaution(s): Store out of direct sunlight at a temperature not over 45°F (7°C). Avoid freezing. Shake well and use entire contents when first opened. Burn containers and all unused contents.
Caution(s): Stressed cattle should not be vaccinated. Do not use in pregnant cows or in calves nursing pregnant cows. Injection site swelling may occur.

Anaphylactoid reactions may occur.

Antidote(s): Epinephrine.
Warning(s): Do not vaccinate within 21 days of slaughter.

Animal inoculation only. Accidental injection to humans can cause serious local reactions. Contact a physician immediately if accidental injection occurs.

Presentation: 10 doses (rehydrate with 20 mL vial of KV vaccine) and 50 doses (rehydrate with 100 mL vial of KV vaccine).
Compendium Code No.: 10280501 26101-02 / 26102-02

E

EXPRESS™ 5

Boehringer Ingelheim **Vaccine**

Bovine Rhinotracheitis-Virus Diarrhea-Parainfluenza$_3$-Respiratory Syncytial Virus Vaccine, Modified Live Virus
U.S. Vet. Lic. No.: 124
Composition: The product in the amber glass vial contains IBR, BVD Types 1 and 2, PI$_3$, and BRSV modified live viruses. The plastic vial contains a unique adjuvant system.

Preservatives: Neomycin and thimerosal.

Indications: Recommended for the vaccination of healthy, susceptible cattle against diseases caused by Bovine Rhinotracheitis (IBR), Bovine Virus Diarrhea (BVD) Types 1 and 2, Parainfluenza$_3$ (PI$_3$), and Bovine Respiratory Syncytial virus (BRSV).
Directions: Rehydrate the vaccine by aseptically adding the accompanying liquid diluent to the vaccine vial.

Dosage: Using aseptic technique, inject 2 mL subcutaneously in front of the shoulder and midway of the neck, away from the suprascapular lymph node. If initial vaccination, repeat the BRSV fraction in 14 to 28 days. Calves vaccinated before 6 months of age should be revaccinated at 6 months. A 2 mL booster dose is recommended annually.

Contraindication(s): It is possible that healthy appearing cattle can be persistently infected with or incubating virulent BVD virus at time of vaccination. In view of these findings and suggested causes, BVD vaccine is contraindicated in persistently infected cattle and use should be limited only to healthy immunocompetent, unstressed, non-pregnant cattle.
Precaution(s): Store out of direct sunlight at a temperature between 35-45°F (2-7°C). Avoid freezing. Shake well before using. Use entire contents when first opened. Burn containers and all unused contents.
Caution(s): Stressed cattle should not be vaccinated. Do not use in pregnant cows or in calves nursing pregnant cows. Injection site swelling may occur. Anaphylactoid reactions may occur.
Antidote(s): Epinephrine.
Warning(s): Do not vaccinate within 21 days of slaughter.

Animal inoculation only. Accidental injection to humans can cause serious local reactions. Contact a physician immediately if accidental injection occurs.

Presentation: 10 dose (20 mL) and 50 dose (100 mL) vials.
Compendium Code No.: 10280531 26304-01 / 26305-01

EXPRESS™ 5-HS

Boehringer Ingelheim **Bacterin-Vaccine**

Bovine Rhinotracheitis-Virus Diarrhea-Parainfluenza$_3$-Respiratory Syncytial Virus Vaccine, Modified Live Virus-Haemophilus Somnus Bacterin
U.S. Vet. Lic. No.: 124
Composition: The product in the amber glass vial contains IBR, BVD Types 1 and 2, PI$_3$, and BRSV modified live viruses. The plastic vial contains *H. somnus* in a unique adjuvant system.

Preservatives: Neomycin.

Indications: Recommended for the vaccination of healthy, susceptible cattle as an aid in the reduction of diseases caused by Bovine Rhinotracheitis (IBR) virus, Bovine Virus Diarrhea (BVD) Types 1 and 2, Parainfluenza$_3$ (PI$_3$) virus, Bovine Respiratory Syncytial virus (BRSV), and *Haemophilus somnus.*
Directions: Rehydrate the modified live virus vaccine by aseptically adding the accompanying bottle of liquid bacterin.

Dosage: Using aseptic technique, inject 2 mL subcutaneously in front of the shoulder and midway of the neck, away from the suprascapular lymph node. If initial vaccination, repeat the BRSV and *H. somnus* fraction in 14 to 28 days. Calves vaccinated before 6 months of age should be revaccinated at 6 months. A 2 mL booster dose is recommended annually.

Contraindication(s): It is possible that healthy appearing cattle can be persistently infected with or incubating virulent BVD virus at time of vaccination. In view of these findings and suggested causes, BVD vaccine is contraindicated in persistently infected cattle and use should be limited only to healthy immunocompetent, unstressed, non-pregnant cattle.
Precaution(s): Store out of direct sunlight at a temperature between 35-45°F (2-7°C). Avoid freezing. Shake well before using. Use entire contents when first opened. Burn containers and all unused contents.
Caution(s): Stressed cattle should not be vaccinated. Do not use in pregnant cows or in calves nursing pregnant cows. Injection site swelling may occur. Anaphylactoid reactions may occur.
Antidote(s): Epinephrine.
Warning(s): Do not vaccinate within 21 days of slaughter.

Animal inoculation only. Accidental injection to humans can cause serious local reactions. Contact a physician immediately if accidental injection occurs.

Presentation: 10 dose (20 mL) and 50 dose (100 mL) vials.
Compendium Code No.: 10280541 26401-01 / 26402-01

EXPRESS™ 5-PHM

Boehringer Ingelheim **Bacterin-Toxoid-Vaccine**

Bovine Rhinotracheitis-Virus Diarrhea-Parainfluenza$_3$-Respiratory Syncytial Virus Vaccine, Modified Live Virus-Pasteurella Haemolytica-Multocida Bacterin-Toxoid

U.S. Vet. Lic. No.: 124

Composition: The amber glass vial contains IBR, BVD Types 1 & 2, PI_3, and BRSV MLV viruses. The plastic vial contains toxoids (leukotoxoids) and cell-associated antigens from multiple isolates of *P. haemolytica* type A-1 fractions, and cell-associated and soluble antigens from *P. multocida*. The antigens are combined in the Life II adjuvant system.

Preservatives: Neomycin and thimerosal.

Indications: Recommended for the vaccination of healthy, susceptible cattle 30 days of age or older as an aid in the reduction of diseases caused by Bovine Rhinotracheitis (IBR) virus, Bovine Virus Diarrhea (BVD) Types 1 and 2, Parainfluenza$_3$ (PI_3) virus, Bovine Respiratory Syncytial virus (BRSV), *Pasteurella haemolytica*, and *P. multocida*.

Directions: Rehydrate the modified live virus vaccine by aseptically adding the accompanying bottle of liquid bacterin.

Dosage: Using aseptic technique, inject 2 mL subcutaneously in front of the shoulder and midway of the neck, away from the suprascapular lymph node. If initial vaccination, repeat the BRSV, *P. haemolytica*, and *P. multocida* fractions in 14-28 days. Calves vaccinated before 6 months age should be revaccinated at 6 months. A 2 mL booster dose is recommended annually.

Contraindication(s): It is possible that healthy appearing cattle can be persistently infected with or incubating virulent BVD virus at time of vaccination. In view of these findings and suggested causes, BVD MLV vaccine is contraindicated in persistently infected cattle and use should be limited only to healthy, immunocompetent, unstressed, non-pregnant cattle.

Precaution(s): Store out of direct sunlight between 35-45°F (2-7°C). Avoid freezing. Shake well before using. Use entire contents when first opened. Burn containers and all unused contents.

Caution(s): Stressed cattle should not be vaccinated. Do not use in pregnant cows or in calves nursing pregnant cows. Injection site swelling may occur, which may be persistent after subcutaneous use. Anaphylactic reactions, including delayed hypersensitivity reactions or death, may occur with a biological product and can cause reduced milk production in lactating dairy cattle.

Antidote(s): Epinephrine.

Warning(s): Do not vaccinate within 60 days before slaughter.

Animal inoculation only. Accidental injection to humans can cause serious local reactions. Contact a physician immediately if accidental injection occurs.

Presentation: 10 doses (20 mL) and 50 doses (100 mL).

Compendium Code No.: 10281191 28301-00 / 28302-00

EXPRESS 10™

Boehringer Ingelheim **Bacterin-Vaccine**

Bovine Rhinotracheitis-Virus Diarrhea-Parainfluenza$_3$-Respiratory Syncytial Virus Vaccine, Modified Live Virus-Leptospira Canicola-Grippotyphosa-Hardjo-Icterohaemorrhagiae-Pomona Bacterin

U.S. Vet. Lic. No.: 124

Contents: This product contains the antigens listed above.

Preservative: Neomycin.

Indications: Recommended for the vaccination of healthy, susceptible cattle against diseases caused by Bovine Rhinotracheitis (IBR) virus, Bovine Virus Diarrhea (BVD) Types 1 and 2, Parainfluenza$_3$ (PI_3) virus, Bovine Respiratory Syncytial virus (BRSV), *Leptospira canicola, L. grippotyphosa, L. hardjo, L. icterohaemorrhagiae*, and *L. pomona*.

Directions: Rehydrate the modified live virus vaccine by aseptically adding the accompanying bottle of liquid bacterin.

Dosage: Using aseptic technique, inject 2 mL intramuscularly. Repeat in 14 to 28 days and once annually. Calves vaccinated before 6 months of age should be revaccinated at 6 months. A 2 mL booster dose is recommended prior to time of stress or exposure.

Contraindication(s): It is possible that healthy appearing cattle can be persistently infected with or incubating virulent BVD virus at time of vaccination. In view of these findings and suggested causes, BVD vaccine is contraindicated in persistently infected cattle and use should be limited only to healthy immunocompetent, unstressed, non-pregnant cattle.

Precaution(s): Store out of direct sunlight at a temperature between 35-45°F (2-7°C). Avoid freezing. Shake well before using. Use entire contents when first opened. Burn containers and all unused contents.

Caution(s): Stressed cattle should not be vaccinated. Do not use in pregnant cows or in calves nursing pregnant cows. Injection site swelling may occur. Anaphylactoid reactions may occur.

Antidote(s): Epinephrine.

Warning(s): Do not vaccinate within 21 days of slaughter.

Animal inoculation only. Accidental injection to humans can cause serious local reactions. Contact a physician immediately if accidental injection occurs.

Presentation: 5 dose (10 mL), 10 dose (20 mL) and 50 dose (100 mL) vials.

Compendium Code No.: 10280512 BI 1274-1R-1 1/02

EXPRESS™ 10-HS

Boehringer Ingelheim **Bacterin-Vaccine**

Bovine Rhinotracheitis-Virus Diarrhea-Parainfluenza$_3$-Respiratory Syncytial Virus Vaccine, Modified Live Virus-Haemophilus Somnus-Leptospira Canicola-Grippotyphosa-Hardjo-Icterohaemorrhagiae-Pomona Bacterin

U.S. Vet. Lic. No.: 124

Description: Bovine Rhinotracheitis-Virus Diarrhea-Parainfluenza$_3$-Respiratory Syncytial Virus Vaccine, Modified Live Virus, Haemophilus Somnus, Leptospira Canicola-Grippotyphosa-Hardjo-Icterohaemorrhagiae-Pomona Bacterin. EXPRESS™ 10-HS contains neomycin as a preservative.

Indications: Recommended for the vaccination of healthy, susceptible cattle against diseases caused by Bovine Rhinotracheitis (IBR) virus, Bovine Virus Diarrhea (BVD) Types 1 and 2, Parainfluenza$_3$ (PI_3) virus, Bovine Respiratory Syncytial virus (BRSV), *Haemophilus somnus, Leptospira canicola, L. grippotyphosa, L. hardjo, L. icterohaemorrhagiae*, and *L. pomona*.

Dosage and Administration: Rehydrate the modified live virus vaccine by aseptically adding the accompanying bottle of liquid bacterin.

Using aseptic technique, inject 2 mL intramuscularly. Repeat in 14 to 28 days and once annually. Calves vaccinated before 6 months of age should be revaccinated at weaning or at 6 months of age. A 2 mL booster dose is recommended annually or prior to time of stress or exposure.

Contraindication(s): It is possible that healthy appearing cattle can be persistently infected with or incubating virulent BVD virus at time of vaccination. In view of these findings and suggested causes, BVD vaccine is contraindicated in persistently infected cattle and use should be limited only to healthy immunocompetent, unstressed, non-pregnant cattle.

Precaution(s): Store out of direct sunlight at a temperature between 35-45°F (2-7°C). Avoid freezing. Shake well before using. Use entire contents when first opened. Burn containers and all unused contents.

Caution(s): Stressed cattle should not be vaccinated. Do not use in pregnant cows or in calves nursing pregnant cows. Injection site swelling may occur. Anaphylactoid reactions may occur.

Antidote(s): Epinephrine.

Warning(s): Do not vaccinate within 21 days of slaughter.

Animal inoculation only. Accidental injection to humans can cause serious local reactions. Contact a physician immediately if accidental injection occurs.

Presentation: 5 doses (10 mL), 10 doses (20 mL) and 50 doses (100 mL) vials.

Compendium Code No.: 10280520

EXPRESS™ I

Boehringer Ingelheim **Vaccine**

Bovine Rhinotracheitis Vaccine, Modified Live Virus

U.S. Vet. Lic. No.: 124

Composition: This product contains Bovine Rhinotracheitis (IBR) modified live virus.

Preservative: Neomycin.

Indications: Recommended for the vaccination of healthy, susceptible cattle as an aid in the reduction of disease caused by Bovine Rhinotracheitis (IBR) virus.

Directions: Rehydrate one bottle of modified live virus vaccine by aseptically adding one bottle of liquid diluent. Shake well and use immediately.

Dosage: Using aseptic technique, inject 2 mL subcutaneously. Calves vaccinated before 6 months of age should be revaccinated at 6 months. A 2 mL booster dose is recommended annually.

Precaution(s): Storage: Store out of direct sunlight at a temperature between 35-45°F (2-7°C). Avoid freezing.

Use entire contents when first opened.

Disposal: Burn vaccine containers and all unused contents.

Caution(s): Do not use in pregnant cows or calves nursing pregnant caws. Anaphylactoid reactions may occur.

Antidote(s): Epinephrine.

Warning(s): Do not vaccinate within 21 days before slaughter.

Presentation: 5 x 10 doses (20 mL) and 5 x 50 doses (100 mL).

Compendium Code No.: 10281311 BI 1125-1 6/01, 12509-00

EXPRESS™ IBP

Boehringer Ingelheim **Vaccine**

Bovine Rhinotracheitis-Virus Diarrhea-Parainfluenza$_3$ Vaccine, Modified Live Virus

U.S. Vet. Lic. No.: 124

Composition: The product in the amber glass vial contains IBR, BVD Type 1 and PI_3 modified live viruses. The plastic vial contains a unique adjuvant system.

Preservative: Neomycin and thimerosal.

Indications: Recommended for the vaccination of healthy, susceptible cattle as an aid in the reduction of diseases caused by bovine rhinotracheitis, virus diarrhea and parainfluenza$_3$ viruses.

Directions: Rehydrate the vaccine by aseptically adding the accompanying liquid diluent to the vaccine vial. Shake well and use immediately.

Dosage: Using aseptic technique, inject 2 mL subcutaneously in front of the shoulder and midway of the neck, away from the suprascapular lymph node. Animals vaccinated before 6 months of age should be revaccinated at 6 months. A 2 mL booster dose is recommended annually.

Contraindication(s): It is possible that healthy appearing cattle can be persistently infected with or incubating virulent BVD virus at time of vaccination. In view of these findings and suggested causes, BVD Vaccine is contraindicated in persistently infected cattle and use should be limited only to healthy, immunocompetent, unstressed, non-pregnant cattle.

Precaution(s): Store out of direct sunlight at a temperature between 35-45°F (2-7°C). Use entire contents when first opened. Burn containers and all unused contents.

Caution(s): Stressed cattle should not be vaccinated. Do not use in pregnant cows or in calves nursing pregnant cows. Anaphylactoid reactions may occur.

Antidote(s): Epinephrine.

Warning(s): Do not vaccinate within 21 days before slaughter.

Presentation: 10 doses (rehydrate with 20 mL vial of diluent) and 50 doses (rehydrate with 100 mL vial of diluent).

Compendium Code No.: 10280551 10205-03 / 10206-03

EXPRESS™ IBP/HS-2P

Boehringer Ingelheim **Bacterin-Vaccine**

Bovine Rhinotracheitis-Virus Diarrhea-Parainfluenza$_3$ Vaccine, Modified Live Virus-Haemophilus Somnus-Pasteurella Haemolytica-Multocida Bacterin

U.S. Vet. Lic. No.: 124

Contents: This product contains the antigens listed above.

Preservative: Neomycin.

Indications: Recommended for the vaccination of healthy, susceptible cattle against disease caused by bovine rhinotracheitis, virus diarrhea and parainfluenza$_3$ viruses and *Haemophilus somnus, Pasteurella haemolytica* and *Pasteurella multocida*.

Dosage and Administration: Rehydrate the vaccine by aseptically adding the accompanying bottle of bacterin. Shake well and use immediately.

Using aseptic technique, inject 2 mL intramuscularly. Repeat bacterin dose in 21 days and once annually. Calves vaccinated before 6 months of age should be revaccinated at 6 months.

Precaution(s): Store out of direct sunlight at a temperature not over 45°F. Avoid freezing. Shake well and use entire contents when first opened. Burn containers and all unused contents.

Caution(s): Stressed cattle should not be vaccinated. Do not use in pregnant cows or in calves nursing pregnant cows. Anaphylactoid reactions may occur.

Antidote(s): Epinephrine.

Warning(s): Do not vaccinate within 21 days before slaughter.

Presentation: 10 doses (20 mL) and 50 doses (100 mL).

Compendium Code No.: 10280560

EXPRESS™ I/LP

Boehringer Ingelheim **Bacterin-Vaccine**

Bovine Rhinotracheitis Vaccine, Modified Live Virus-Leptospira Pomona Bacterin

U.S. Vet. Lic. No.: 124

Composition: This product contains Bovine Rhinotracheitis (IBR) modified live virus and inactivated cultures of *Leptospira pomona*.

Preservatives: The vaccine fraction contains neomycin as a preservative. The bacterin fraction contains gentamicin and Amphotericin B.

Indications: Recommended for the vaccination of healthy, susceptible cattle as an aid in the reduction of disease caused by Bovine Rhinotracheitis (IBR) virus and leptospirosis caused by *Leptospira pomona*.

Directions: Rehydrate one bottle of modified live virus vaccine by aseptically adding one bottle of liquid bacterin diluent. Shake well and use immediately.

Dosage: Using aseptic technique, inject 2 mL intramuscularly. Calves vaccinated before 6 months of age should be revaccinated at 6 months. A 2 mL booster dose is recommended annually.

Precaution(s): Storage: Store out of direct sunlight at a temperature between 35-45°F (2-7°C). Avoid freezing.

Use entire contents when first opened.

Disposal: Burn vaccine containers and all unused contents.

Caution(s): Do not use in pregnant cows or calves nursing pregnant cows. Anaphylactoid reactions may occur.

Antidote(s): Epinephrine.

Warning(s): Do not vaccinate within 21 days before slaughter.

Presentation: 5 x 10 doses (20 mL) and 5 x 50 doses (100 mL).

Compendium Code No.: 10281320 BI 1093-1 5/01, 09305-01

EXPRESS™ IP/HS-2P

Boehringer Ingelheim **Bacterin-Vaccine**

Bovine Rhinotracheitis-Parainfluenza$_3$ Vaccine, Modified Live Virus-Haemophilus Somnus-Pasteurella Haemolytica-Multocida Bacterin

U.S. Vet. Lic. No.: 124

Contents: This product contains the antigens listed above.

Preservative: Neomycin.

Indications: Recommended for the vaccination of healthy, susceptible cattle against disease caused by bovine rhinotracheitis and parainfluenza$_3$ viruses, and *Haemophilus somnus, Pasteurella haemolytica* and *Pasteurella multocida*.

Directions: Rehydrate the vaccine by aseptically adding the accompanying bottle of bacterin.

Dosage: Using aseptic technique, inject 2 mL intramuscularly. Repeat bacterin dose in 21 days and once annually. Calves vaccinated before 6 months of age should be revaccinated at 6 months.

Contraindication(s): It is possible that healthy appearing cattle can be persistently infected with or incubating virulent BVD virus at time of vaccination. In view of these findings and suggested causes, BVD vaccine is contraindicated in persistently infected cattle and use should be limited only to healthy, immunocompetent, unstressed, non-pregnant cattle.

Precaution(s): Store out of direct sunlight at a temperature not over 45°F. Avoid freezing. Shake well. Use entire contents when first opened. Burn containers and all unused contents.

Caution(s): Do not use in pregnant cows or in calves nursing pregnant cows. Anaphylactoid reactions may occur.

Antidote(s): Epinephrine.

Warning(s): Do not vaccinate within 21 days before slaughter.

Presentation: 10 doses (rehydrate with 20 mL) and 50 doses (rehydrate with 100 mL).

Compendium Code No.: 10280571 19401-01 / 19402-01

EYE RINSE

Butler **Ophthalmic Rinse**

Active Ingredient(s): Contents: Water, boric acid, zinc sulfate, glycerin, camphor.

Indications: An aid in cleaning the eye and removing eye stains.

Dosage and Administration: EYE RINSE should be used by applying a few drops to each eye three or four times daily for optimum cleansing. For eye stains, apply a few drops to each eye once daily. Moisten facial tissue or cotton with EYE RINSE and gently rub stained area below the eyes. Repeat daily or as directed by your veterinarian.

Caution(s): For veterinary use only.

Keep out of reach of children.

Presentation: 4 fluid ounces.

Compendium Code No.: 10820750

EYE RINSE

RXV **Ophthalmic Rinse**

Eye Cleaner & Stain Remover

Active Ingredient(s): Contents: Water, Boric acid, Zinc Sulfate, Glycerin, Camphor.

Indications: An aid in cleaning the eye and removing eye stains.

Dosage and Administration: Eye cleaner should be used by applying a few drops to each eye three or four times daily for optimum cleansing.

For eye stains, apply a few drops to each eye once daily. Moisten facial tissue or cotton with Eye Cleaner and gently rub stained area below the eyes.

Repeat daily or as necessary.

Caution(s): For animal use only.

Warning(s): Keep out of reach of children.

Presentation: 4 fl oz.

Compendium Code No.: 10910340

E-Z COPPER™

SSI Corp. **Disinfectant**

Active Ingredient(s):

Copper Sulfate Pentahydrate 20%

Inert Ingredients 80%

Total 100%

*Metallic Copper Equivalent 5%

Indications: For use in footbaths and hoofmats.

Directions:

Footbath Directions: 1 to 150 cows, use one half gallon of E-Z COPPER™ per 50 gallons of water.

If hygienic or environmental conditions are extreme, use one full gallon of E-Z COPPER™ per 50 gallons of water.

Hoofmat Directions: 80 to 100 cows, use 1 pint of E-Z COPPER™ per 8 gallons of water.

If hygienic or environmental conditions are extreme, use 1 quart of E-Z COPPER™ per 8 gallons of water.

Footbaths and hoofmats require careful management. If not properly managed results are reduced significantly.

Precaution(s): Keep from freezing.

Caution(s): Eye irritant. In case of contact, flush for 15 minutes. If irritation persists, call a physician.

Warning(s): Keep out of the reach of children.

Presentation: 5 and 55 gallon containers.

Compendium Code No.: 14930081

F

F-48

Rochester Midland **Disinfectant**

No-Rinse Acid Cleaner Sanitizer

EPA Reg. No.: 527-123

Active Ingredient(s):

Octyl decyl dimethyl ammonium chloride	2.295%
Didecyl dimethyl ammonium chloride	1.377%
Dioctyl dimethyl ammonium chloride	0.918%
Alkyl (C_{14}, 50%; C_{12}, 40%; C_{16}, 10%) dimethyl benzyl ammonium chlorides	3.060%
Inert	92.350%
Total	100.000%

Indications: F-48 is a no-rinse acid cleaner sanitizer for dairy, food processing and farm use and for the removal of milkstone.

Directions for Use: It is a violation of Federal law to use this product in a manner inconsistent with its labeling.

For sale, use and storage by maintenance personnel only.

F-48 is an acid cleaner sanitizer for use on food processing and dairy equipment in water up to 600 ppm hardness (as $CaCO_3$). Do not rinse with water. For heavily soiled equipment, a preliminary cleaning is required. Prepare a fresh solution daily or when the use solution becomes visibly dirty. For mechanical application, use solution may not be reused for sanitizing applications.

Cleaning bulk milk tanks, dairy and food processing:

Sanitizing - To sanitize hard nonporous food contact surfaces, such as milk tanks and milking equipment, clean with a good detergent and rinse thoroughly, dilute 1 oz. of F-48 in 4 gallons of water (150 ppm active quarternary) and apply with a cloth, brush, mechanical spray device (spray surface until thoroughly wetted) or by immersion. Treated surface should remain wet for at least 60 seconds followed by adequate draining and air drying. Do not rinse with water.

Grade A pasteurized milk ordinance: At 1 oz./4 gallons, F-48 fulfills the criteria of Appendix F of the Grade "A" Pasteurized Milk Ordinances 1978 Recommendations of the U.S. Public Health Services in waters up to 600 ppm of hardness calculated as calcium carbonate when evaluated by the AOAC Germicidal and Detergent Sanitizer Method against *Escherichia coli* and *Staphylococcus aureus*.

The udders, flanks and teats of dairy cows can be sanitized by washing with a solution of 1 oz. F-48 in 4 gallons of warm water. A potable water rinse is not required. Use a fresh towel for each cow. Avoid contamination of the sanitizing solution by dirt and soil. Do not dip used towels back into sanitizing solution. When a solution becomes visibly dirty, discard and provide fresh solution.

Precautionary Statements: Hazards to Humans and Domestic Animals:

Danger. Keep out of reach of children. Corrosive. Causes eye damage and skin irritation. Do not get in the eyes, on skin, or on clothing. Wear goggles or a face shield and rubber gloves when handling this product. Harmful if swallowed.

Statement of Practical Treatment: In case of contact, immediately flush eyes or skin with plenty of water for at least 15 minutes. For eyes, call a physician. Remove and wash contaminated clothing before reuse. If swallowed, drink promptly a large quantity of milk, egg whites, gelatin solution; or if these are not available, drink large quantities of water. Avoid alcohol. Call a physician immediately.

Note to Physician: Probable mucosal damage may contraindicate the use of gastric lavage. Measures against circulatory shock, respiratory depression and convulsion may be needed. Medical Emergency Telephone Number: 1-800-535-5053 (U.S.). Outside the U.S. please call 1-352-323-3500.

Environmental Hazards: Do not discharge effluent containing this product into lakes, streams, ponds, estuaries, oceans or other waters unless in accordance with the requirements of a National Pollutant Discharge Elimination System (NPDES) permit and the permitting authority has been notified in writing prior to discharge. Do not discharge effluent containing this product to sewer systems without previously notifying the local sewage treatment plant authority. For guidance contact your State Water Board or Regional Office of the EPA.

Storage and Disposal: Do not contaminate water, food, or feed by storage or disposal. Do not store the container on its side. Avoid creasing or impacting of side walls.

Pesticide Disposal: Pesticide wastes are acutely hazardous. Improper disposal of excess pesticide, spray or mixture of rinsate is a violation of Federal Law. If these wastes cannot be disposed of according to label instructions, contact a State Pesticide or Environmental Control Agency, or the Hazardous Waste representative at the nearest EPA Regional Office for guidance.

Container Disposal: Triple rinse (or equivalent). Then offer for recycling or reconditioning, or puncture and dispose of in a sanitary landfill, or by other procedures approved by state and local authorities.

Presentation: 1 gallon, 4x1 gallon per case, 5 gallon pail, and 55 gallon (208.2 liter) containers.

Compendium Code No.: 13690001 REV. 3/22/99

FACILITATOR™

Idexx Pharm. **Liquid Bandage**

(hydroxyethylated amylopectin)

Description: FACILITATOR™ Liquid Bandage contains hydroxyethylated amylopectin.

Indications: The gel is indicated for management of a variety of wounds in dogs, cats, horses, birds and exotics. Wound management uses: degloving injuries, burns, bite wounds, lick granulomas, hot spots, foot pad injuries, dehisced surgical wounds, cuts and wounds that can't be sutured, where skin grafts may be considered, lacerations and abrasions, hard to bandage areas, open wounds, cat declaws and tail docking. For veterinary use only. For proper wound management, please consult your veterinarian.

Pharmacology: Mode of Action: FACILITATOR™ is a polymeric gel which, upon drying over the wound, forms an adhesive barrier.

Directions for Use: Instructions for Use: Apply FACILITATOR™ as thinly as possible as needed or a minimum of every 3 days. Proper preparation of the wound site is critical for the successful use of FACILITATOR™. The wound should be gently cleansed with water or an antiseptic, e.g. povidone, then rinsed thoroughly. Remove any accumulating blood or moisture from the wound using sterile gauze. Do not use other topical ointments or salves as they may interfere with the formation of the FACILITATOR™ Liquid Bandage. Avoid contaminating the tube by holding the tip of the tube slightly above the wound. Gently apply FACILITATOR™ until the wound is completely covered by a very thin film, allowing it to extend slightly beyond the wound edges. Allow the thin film of FACILITATOR™ to dry completely to assure secure coverage of the wound.

Removal of FACILITATOR™: FACILITATOR™ can be removed from skin or other surfaces with water.

Contraindication(s): FACILITATOR™ is not recommended in the management of infected and deep puncture wounds.

Precaution(s): Storage Conditions: FACILITATOR™ should be stored at room temperature (15°C-30°C).

Warning(s): Avoid contact with eyes.

Presentation: Display cartons of twelve 5 mL dispensing tubes.

FACILITATOR™ is sold only to licensed veterinarians.

FACILITATOR is a trademark of Idexx Pharmaceuticals, Inc. in the United States and/or other countries.

Compendium Code No.: 15070011 BRP/FAC/PI/5-05/00 06-02999-02

FACTREL® ℞

Fort Dodge **Gonadorelin**

Gonadorelin Hydrochloride For Injection

NADA No.: 139-237

Active Ingredient(s): FACTREL® (gonadorelin hydrochloride) is a sterile solution containing 50 mcg of synthetic gonadorelin (as hydrochloride) per mL in aqueous formulation containing 0.6% sodium chloride and 2% benzyl alcohol (as a preservative).

Indications: FACTREL® (gonadorelin hydrochloride) is indicated for the treatment of ovarian follicular cysts in cattle. The treatment effect of FACTREL® when used in cattle with ovarian follicular cysts is a reduction in the number of days to first estrus.

Pharmacology: Gonadorelin is the gonadotropin releasing hormone (GnRH) which is produced by the hypothalamus and causes the release of the gonadotropin luteinizing hormone (LH) and follicle-stimulating hormone (FSH) from the anterior pituitary.

FACTREL® (gonadorelin hydrochloride) has the identical amino acid sequence as endogenous gonadorelin; 5-oxo Pro-His-Trp-Ser-Tyr-Gly-Leu-Arg-Pro-Gly-NH_2 with identical physiological activities. The molecular weight of gonadorelin is 1182 with a molecular formula of $C_{55}H_{75}N_{17}O_{13}$. The corresponding values for gonadorelin hydrochloride are 1219 (1 HCl) expressed as $C_{55}H_{75}N_{17}O_{13}HCl$, or 1255 (2 HCl) expressed as $C_{55}H_{75}N_{17}O_{13}$ 2HCl.

Mechanism of Action: Follicular cysts are enlarged non-ovulatory follicles resulting from a malfunction of the neuroendocrine mechanism controlling follicular maturation and ovulation. Exogenous administration of agents possessing luteinizing hormone (LH) activity, such as pituitary extracts or human chorionic gonadotropin, often causes ovulation or regression of follicular cysts. FACTREL® induces release of endogenous luteinizing hormone (LH) to produce this same effect.

No significant differences have been demonstrated in days from treatment to conception, frequency of cows conceiving at first or subsequent heats, or conception rates among treated or non-treated control animals.

Dosage and Administration: The recommended dosage of FACTREL® is 100 mcg/cow intramuscularly.

Precaution(s): Storage Conditions: Store at refrigerator temperature 2° to 8°C (36° to 46°F).

Caution(s): Federal law restricts this drug to use by or on the order of a licensed veterinarian.

Warning(s): Residue Warning: Because FACTREL® is identical to endogenous GnRH such that both are rapidly metabolized without detectable levels in milk or tissue, no withdrawal period is required.

Toxicology: Safety and Toxicity: In cows the intramuscular administration of up to 25 times recommended dosage (2,500 mcg/day) of FACTREL® for 3 days did not affect any physiological or clinical parameter. Likewise, single intramuscular doses of 5 times recommended dosage (500 mcg) did not interfere with pregnancy. No evidence of irritation at injection site was found in any animal.

Presentation: FACTREL® (gonadorelin hydrochloride) solution 50 mcg/mL is available in single dose vials of 2 mL (box of 25) (NDC 0856-4311-01) and in 20 mL multidose (box of one) (NDC 0856-4311-02).

Compendium Code No.: 10030710 4310G

FARRIER'S HOOF™

Horses Prefer **Antiseptic**

Non-Irritant Topical Spray

Active Ingredient(s):

Ionized Copper (Cu)	0.134%
Ionized Zinc (Zn)	0.700%
Nonionized Surfactant	1.400%
Inert material	97.770%

Indications: FARRIER'S HOOF™ Topical Spray is designed to treat conditions like thrush, while line disease, seed toe abscesses and other related hoof infections in horses. Spraying on a regular basis will help keep infections away during damp weather or whenever conditions are optimal for hoof damage. The unique formula in FARRIER'SHOOF™ Topical works well to prevent bacterial and fungal infection under these conditions.

FARRIER'S HOOF™ will not stain the coat or irritate the skin. It will help eliminate the foul odor common in hoof infections.

For proper and healthy hoof growth, simultaneous feeding of Vets Plus Bio-Hoof™ is recommended.

If conditions do not improve, consult your veterinarian.

Directions: FARRIER'S HOOF™ Topical Spray is a convenient ready-to-use solution designed for direct application to the hoof.

Prevention: For prevention of infections use FARRIER'S HOOF™ Topical whenever the hooves are handled or cleaned. Use of FARRIER'S HOOF™ Topical is especially beneficial after workouts, before and after shoeing, during wet conditions, or anytime cracks or bruises are visible. Spray the hoof liberally with FARRIER'S HOOF™ Topical to help prevent infection.

Treatment: Cleaned the infected hoof as thoroughly as possible and spray FARRIER'S HOOF™ two to three times a day to the point of saturation to achieve maximum exposure. After spraying, contain the horse in a clean, and area if possible. When treating, it is advisable to spray all the hooves to prevent cross contamination.

Continue to use FARRIER'S HOOF™ Topical Spray until the infection subsides. Wrap the hoof if necessary.

Precaution(s): If product freezes, thaw at room temperature. Shake well before using.

Caution(s): Eye irritant. In case of eye contact, flush for 15 minutes. If irritation persists, call a physician.

Presentation: 32 fl oz (946 mL).

Compendium Code No.: 36950022

FARROWSURE®

Pfizer Animal Health **Bacterin-Vaccine**

Parvovirus Vaccine, Killed Virus-Erysipelothrix Rhusiopathiae-Leptospira Canicola-Grippotyphosa-Hardjo-Icterohaemorrhagiae-Pomona Bacterin

U.S. Vet. Lic. No.: 189

Description: FARROWSURE® is a liquid preparation of inactivated PPV, grown on an established porcine cell line; whole cultures of *E. rhusiopathiae;* and the 5 *Leptospira* serovars identified above. The vaccine is combined with a sterile adjuvant to enhance the immune response.

Contains gentamicin as preservative.

Indications: FARROWSURE® is for vaccination of healthy breeding swine as an aid in preventing reproductive failure caused by porcine parvovirus (PPV), erysipelas caused by *Erysipelothrix rhusiopathiae,* and leptospirosis caused by *Leptospira canicola, L. grippotyphosa, L. hardjo, L. icterohaemorrhagiae,* and *L. pomona.*

Directions:

1. General Directions: Shake well. Aseptically administer 5 mL intramuscularly.
2. Primary Vaccination: Administer a single 5 mL dose to healthy sows 14-60 days before breeding. Healthy gilts, however, should receive a single 5 mL dose as near as possible to 14 days before breeding; if gilts are vaccinated sooner, persisting maternal antibodies may interfere with active immunization. Healthy boars should receive a single 5 mL dose at least 14 days prior to introduction into the breeding herd. For protection against leptospirosis, a single dose of Leptoferm-5® is recommended either 3-6 weeks before or 3-6 weeks after administration of FARROWSURE®.
3. Revaccination: Semiannual revaccination with a single dose is recommended before breeding. Boars should be revaccinated semiannually.
4. Good animal husbandry and herd health management practices should be employed.

Precaution(s): Store at 2°-7°C. Prolonged exposure to higher temperatures may adversely affect potency. Do not freeze.

Use entire contents when first opened.

Caution(s): As with many vaccines, anaphylaxis may occur after use. Initial antidote of epinephrine is recommended and should be followed with appropriate supportive therapy.

This product has been shown to be efficacious in healthy animals. A protective immune response may not be elicited if animals are incubating an infectious disease, are malnourished or parasitized, are stressed due to shipment or environmental conditions, are otherwise immunocompromised, or the vaccine is not administered in accordance with label directions.

For veterinary use only.

Warning(s): Do not vaccinate within 21 days before slaughter.

Discussion: Disease Description: PPV and *Leptospira* are common agents of reproductive loss in swine. While infection with any of those pathogens may produce subclinical disease, infection by PPV during pregnancy may result in fetal resorption, stillbirths, and fetal mummification. Infection by *Leptospira* during the second half of pregnancy may cause stillbirths or abortions; late-term abortions are the most important economic effect of leptospirosis. Leptospirosis caused by any of the serovars represented here cannot be clinically differentiated. Abortions may also occur in sows infected with *E. rhusiopathiae* during pregnancy.

Trial Data: Safety and Efficacy: Safety of FARROWSURE® was demonstrated in breeding-age swine. Transient mild swelling and inflammation of the injection site was observed in 3%-10% of vaccinates. No systemic or allergic reactions were observed. Efficacy of the fractions of FARROWSURE® was demonstrated in challenge-of-immunity and immunogenicity tests. After challenge with virulent *E. rhusiopathiae,* vaccinated pigs remained clinically normal while nonvaccinated control pigs developed clinical disease. In addition, vaccinated pigs expressed protective antibody titers to PPV and each of the *Leptospira* serovars, confirming that no significant immunologic interference occurred.

Presentation: 10 dose and 50 dose vials.

Compendium Code No.: 36900661 75-4568-07

FARROWSURE® B

Pfizer Animal Health **Bacterin-Vaccine**

Parvovirus Vaccine, Killed Virus-Erysipelothrix Rhusiopathiae-Leptospira Bratislava-Canicola-Grippotyphosa-Hardjo-Icterohaemorrhagiae-Pomona Bacterin

U.S. Vet. Lic. No.: 189

Description: FARROWSURE® B is a liquid preparation of inactivated PPV, grown on an established porcine cell line; whole cultures of *E. rhusiopathiae;* and the 6 *Leptospira* serovars identified above. The vaccine is combined with a sterile adjuvant to enhance the immune response.

Contains gentamicin as preservative.

Indications: FARROWSURE® B is for vaccination of healthy breeding swine as an aid in preventing reproductive failure caused by porcine parvovirus (PPV), erysipelas caused by *Erysipelothrix rhusiopathiae,* and leptospirosis caused by *Leptospira bratislava, L. canicola, L. grippotyphosa, L. hardjo, L. icterohaemorrhagiae,* and *L. pomona.*

Directions:

1. General Directions: Shake well. Aseptically administer 5 mL intramuscularly.
2. Primary Vaccination: Administer a single 5 mL dose to healthy sows 14-60 days before breeding. Healthy gilts, however, should receive a single 5 mL dose as near as possible to 14 days before breeding; if gilts are vaccinated sooner, persisting maternal antibodies may interfere with active immunization. Healthy boars should receive a single 5 mL dose at least 14 days prior to introduction into the breeding herd. For protection against leptospirosis, a single dose of BratiVac®-6 is recommended either 3-6 weeks before or 3-6 weeks after administration of FARROWSURE® B.
3. Revaccination: Revaccination with a single dose is recommended before breeding. Boars should be revaccinated semiannually.
4. Good animal husbandry and herd health management practices should be employed.

Precaution(s): Store at 2°-7°C. Prolonged exposure to higher temperatures may adversely affect potency. Do not freeze.

Use entire contents when first opened.

Caution(s): As with many vaccines, anaphylaxis may occur after use. Initial antidote of epinephrine is recommended and should be followed with appropriate supportive therapy.

This product has been shown to be efficacious in healthy animals. A protective immune response may not be elicited if animals are incubating an infectious disease, are malnourished or parasitized, are stressed due to shipment or environmental conditions, are otherwise immunocompromised, or the vaccine is not administered in accordance with label directions.

For use in swine only.

For veterinary use only.

Warning(s): Do not vaccinate within 21 days before slaughter.

Discussion: Disease Description: PPV and *Leptospira* are common agents of reproductive loss in swine. While infection with any of these pathogens may produce subclinical disease, infection by PPV during pregnancy may result in fetal resorption, stillbirths, and fetal mummification. Infection by *Leptospira* during the second half of pregnancy may cause stillbirths or abortions; late-term abortions are the most important economic effect of leptospirosis. Leptospirosis caused by any of the serovars represented here cannot be clinically differentiated. Abortions may also occur in sows infected with *E. rhusiopathiae* during pregnancy.

Trial Data: Safety and Efficacy: Safety of vaccine fractions in FARROWSURE® B was demonstrated in breeding-age swine. No significant postvaccination reactions were reported.

Efficacy of the fractions of FARROWSURE® B was demonstrated in challenge-of-immunity and immunogenicity tests. After challenge with virulent *E. rhusiopathiae,* vaccinated pigs remained clinically normal while nonvaccinated control pigs developed clinical disease. Studies conducted to assess immunologic interference based on antibody titers to PPV and all 6 *Leptospira* serovars showed no significant immunologic interference occurred between vaccine fractions.

L. bratislava is fastidious in its growth requirements and has proven difficult to isolate. However, *L. bratislava* has been isolated in aborted pigs and fetuses in European studies; and in 1986, Ellis and Thiermann reported the isolation of *L. bratislava* from the kidney and genital tract of 2 sows in the United States.[1,2] Subsequently, *L. bratislava* was also isolated in the United States from weak pigs, stillborn pigs, and swine placental tissues.[3,4] Recent serological surveys show that infections of swine by *L. bratislava* are prevalent. Antibody to *L. bratislava,* detectable by the microscopic agglutination test (MAT), has been shown to be present in sera from greater than 30% of finishing pigs and 50% of adult pigs.[5,6] Furthermore, controlled vaccination studies conducted in swine herds showing evidence of infection and poor reproductive performance support the conclusion that *L. bratislava* can be controlled through vaccination.[6]

Challenge-of-immunity tests were conducted by scientists at the Veterinary Research Laboratories, Belfast, Northern Ireland to determine the efficacy of the *L. bratislava* fraction of FARROWSURE® B against virulent isolates of *L. bratislava.* Fifteen pigs were divided into 2 groups. Ten pigs were administered 2 doses of the *L. bratislava* bacterin in 2 mL doses given 2 weeks apart, and a group of 5 pigs was used as nonvaccinated controls. Subsequently, all pigs were challenged with virulent strains of *L. bratislava.* After challenge, *L. bratislava* was recovered from the kidneys of all 5 control pigs and from the oviduct of one of them. In contrast, leptospires were not recovered from the kidneys or genital tracts of the 10 vaccinated pigs. Leptospiraemia was demonstrated in the blood of all 5 control pigs beginning on the third postchallenge day. Leptospiraemia was demonstrated in only 2 of the 10 vaccinated pigs on the third postchallenge day. Two controls also experienced a rise in rectal temperature after challenge.

These results are similar to results of previously conducted challenge-of-immunity tests on the other 5 *Leptospira* fractions of FARROWSURE® B. In those studies also, vaccinated animals remained healthy after challenge, while nonvaccinated animals developed clinical signs of leptospirosis.

References: Available upon request.

Presentation: 10 dose and 50 dose vials.

Compendium Code No.: 36900691 75-4560-06

FARROWSURE® B-PRV

Pfizer Animal Health **Bacterin-Vaccine**

Parvovirus-Pseudorabies Vaccine, Modified Live & Killed Virus-Erysipelothrix Rhusiopathiae-Leptospira Bratislava-Canicola-Grippotyphosa-Hardjo-Icterohaemorrhagiae-Pomona Bacterin

U.S. Vet. Lic. No.: 189

Description: FARROWSURE® B-PRV is a freeze-dried preparation of modified live PRV grown on an established porcine cell line, plus a liquid preparation of chemically inactivated PPV, *E. rhusiopathiae,* the 6 Leptospira serovars identified above, and a sterile adjuvant to enhance the immune response. The liquid component is used to rehydrate the freeze-dried component.

Contains gentamicin as preservative.

Indications: FARROWSURE® B-PRV is for vaccination of healthy breeding swine as an aid in preventing pseudorabies caused by pseudorabies virus (PRV), reproductive failure caused by porcine parvovirus (PPV), erysipelas caused by *Erysipelothrix rhusiopathiae,* and leptospirosis caused by *Leptospira bratislava, L. canicola, L. grippotyphosa, L. hardjo, L. icterohaemorrhagiae,* and *L. pomona.*

Directions:

1. General Directions: Vaccination of healthy breeding swine is recommended. Aseptically rehydrate the freeze-dried vaccine with the liquid bacterin provided, shake well, and administer 5 mL intramuscularly.
2. Primary Vaccination: Administer a single 5 mL dose to healthy sows 14-60 days before breeding. Healthy gilts, however, should receive a single 5 mL dose as near as possible to 14 days before breeding; if gilts are vaccinated sooner, persisting maternal antibodies may interfere with active immunization. Healthy boars should receive a single 5 mL dose at least 14 days prior to introduction into the breeding herd. For protection against leptospirosis, a single dose of BratiVac®-6 is recommended either 3-6 weeks before or 3-6 weeks after administration of FARROWSURE® B-PRV.
3. Revaccination: Revaccination with a single dose is recommended before breeding. Boars should be revaccinated semiannually.
4. Good animal husbandry and herd health management practices should be employed.

Precaution(s): Store at 2°-7°C. Prolonged exposure to higher temperatures and/or direct sunlight may adversely affect potency. Do not freeze.

Use entire contents when first opened.

Sterilized syringes and needles should be used to administer this vaccine. Do not sterilize with chemicals because traces of disinfectant may inactivate the vaccine.

Burn containers and all unused contents.

Caution(s): Vaccination with FARROWSURE® B-PRV produces an antibody response to pseudorabies, thereby rendering swine positive to a serum neutralization (SN) test. Vaccinated swine can be differentiated from infected swine using a USDA-approved differential pseudorabies test, Pseudorabies Virus gpI Antibody Test Kit, provided the animals have received a Pfizer Animal Health PRV vaccine. Distribution of this vaccine is limited to authorized recipients designated by proper State Officials and such conditions as these officials may require.

As with many vaccines, anaphylaxis may occur after use. Initial antidote of epinephrine is recommended and should be followed with appropriate supportive therapy.

This product has been shown to be efficacious in healthy animals. A protective immune response may not be elicited if animals are incubating an infectious disease, are malnourished or parasitized, are stressed due to shipment or environmental conditions, are otherwise immunocompromised, or the vaccine is not administered in accordance with label directions.

For use in swine only.

For veterinary use only.

Warning(s): Do not vaccinate within 21 days before slaughter.

Discussion: Disease Description: Pseudorabies is an acute infectious viral disease of swine and many other mammals. Abortions, stillbirths, and mummified fetuses may occur in PRV-infected sows. PPV and *Leptospira* are more common agents of reproductive loss in swine. While infection with any of these pathogens may produce subclinical disease, infection by PPV during pregnancy may result in fetal resorption, stillbirths and fetal mummification. Infection by *Leptospira* during the second half of pregnancy may cause stillbirths or abortions; late-term abortions are the most important economic effect of leptospirosis. Leptospirosis caused by any of the serovars represented here cannot be clinically differentiated. Abortions may also occur in sows infected with *E. rhusiopathiae* during pregnancy.

Trial Data: Safety and Efficacy: Safety of vaccine fractions in FARROWSURE® B-PRV was demonstrated in breeding-age swine. No significant postvaccination reactions were reported.

Efficacy of the fractions of FARROWSURE® B-PRV was demonstrated in challenge-of-immunity and immunogenicity tests. After challenge with virulent *E. rhusiopathiae*, vaccinated pigs remained clinically normal while nonvaccinated control pigs developed clinical disease. Studies conducted to assess immunologic interference based on antibody titers to PRV, PPV, and all 6 *Leptospira* serovars showed no significant immunologic interference occurred between vaccine fractions.

L. bratislava is fastidious in its growth requirements and has proven difficult to isolate. However, *L. bratislava* has been isolated in aborted pigs and fetuses in European studies; and in 1986, Ellis and Thiermann reported the isolation of *L. bratislava* from the kidney and genital tract of 2 sows in the United States.[1,2] Subsequently, *L. bratislava* was also isolated in the United States from weak pigs, stillborn pigs, and swine placental tissues.[3,4] Recent serological surveys show that infections of swine by *L. bratislava* are prevalent. Antibody to *L. bratislava*, detectable by the microscopic agglutination test (MAT), has been shown to be present in sera from greater than 30% of finishing pigs and 50% of adult pigs.[5,6] Furthermore, controlled vaccination studies conducted in swine herds showing evidence of infection and poor reproductive performance support the conclusion that *L. bratislava* can be controlled through vaccination.[6]

Challenge-of-immunity tests were conducted by scientists at the Veterinary Research Laboratories, Belfast, Northern Ireland to determine the efficacy of the *L. bratislava* fraction of FARROWSURE® B-PRV against virulent isolates of *L. bratislava*. Fifteen pigs were divided into 2 groups. Ten pigs were administered 2 doses of the *L. bratislava* bacterin in 2 mL doses given 2 weeks apart, and a group of 5 pigs was used as nonvaccinated controls. Subsequently, all pigs were challenged with virulent strains of *L. bratislava*. After challenge, *L. bratislava* was recovered from the kidneys of all 5 control pigs and from the oviduct of one of them. In contrast, leptospires were not recovered from the kidneys or genital tracts of the 10 vaccinated pigs. Leptospiraemia was demonstrated in the blood of all 5 control pigs beginning on the third postchallenge day. Leptospiraemia was demonstrated in only 2 of the 10 vaccinated pigs on the third postchallenge day. Two controls also experienced a rise in rectal temperature after challenge.

These results are similar to results of previously conducted challenge-of-immunity tests on the other 5 *Leptospira* fractions of FARROWSURE® B-PRV. In those studies also, vaccinated animals remained healthy after challenge, while nonvaccinated animals developed clinical signs of leptospirosis.

References: Available upon request.

Presentation: 10 dose vials.

Compendium Code No.: 36900681 75-4562-07

FARROWSURE® PLUS

Pfizer Animal Health **Bacterin-Vaccine**

Parvovirus Vaccine, Killed Virus-Erysipelothrix Rhusiopathiae-Leptospira Canicola-Grippotyphosa-Hardjo-Icterohaemorrhagiae-Pomona Bacterin

U.S. Vet. Lic. No.: 189

Description: FARROWSURE® Plus is a liquid preparation of porcine parvovirus grown on an established porcine cell line, a serum-free, clarified *E. rhusiopathiae* culture, and whole cell cultures of the 5 *Leptospira* serovars identified above. The antigens have been chemically inactivated and adjuvanted with 2 adjuvants, including Amphigen®, to enhance the immune response.

Contains gentamicin as preservative.

Indications: FARROWSURE® Plus is for vaccination of healthy breeding swine as an aid in preventing reproductive failure caused by porcine parvovirus (PPV), erysipelas caused by *Erysipelothrix rhusiopathiae*, and leptospirosis caused by *Leptospira canicola*, *L. grippotyphosa*, *L. hardjo*, *L. icterohaemorrhagiae* and *L. pomona*. A 26-week duration of immunity following vaccination has been demonstrated against erysipelas.

Directions:

1. General Directions: Shake well. Aseptically administer 5 mL intramuscularly.
2. Primary Vaccination: Healthy swine should receive 2 doses 3-5 weeks apart with the second dose administered 2-4 weeks prior to breeding. Healthy gilts, however, should receive the second dose as near as possible to 14 days prior to breeding.
3. Revaccination: Revaccination with a single dose is recommended prior to subsequent breedings. Boars should be revaccinated semiannually.
4. Good animal husbandry and herd health management practices should be employed.

Precaution(s): Store at 2°-7°C. Prolonged exposure to higher temperatures may adversely affect potency. Do not freeze.

Use entire contents when first opened.

Sterilized syringes and needles should be used to administer this vaccine.

Caution(s): Temporary swelling at the injection site may be observed.

As with many vaccines, anaphylaxis may occur after use. Initial antidote of epinephrine is recommended and should be followed with appropriate supportive therapy.

This product has been shown to be efficacious in healthy animals. A protective immune response may not be elicited if animals are incubating an infectious disease, are malnourished or parasitized, are stressed due to shipment or environmental conditions, are otherwise immunocompromised, or the vaccine is not administered in accordance with label directions.

For use in swine only.

For veterinary use only.

Warning(s): Do not vaccinate within 21 days before slaughter.

Discussion: Disease Description: PPV and *Leptospira* are common agents of reproductive loss in swine. While infection with either of these pathogens may produce subclinical disease, infection with PPV during pregnancy may result in fetal resorption, fetal mummification and stillbirths. Infection by *Leptospira* during the second half of pregnancy may cause abortions and stillbirths; late-term abortions are the most important economic effect of leptospirosis. Leptospirosis caused by any of the serovars represented here cannot be clinically differentiated. Abortions may also occur in sows infected with *E. rhusiopathiae* during pregnancy.

Trial Data: Safety and Efficacy: The safety and efficacy of the fractions in FARROWSURE® Plus were demonstrated in studies conducted in support of FarrowSure® Plus B.

The safety of FarrowSure® Plus B was demonstrated under both controlled laboratory and field conditions. No serious systemic or allergic reactions were observed following vaccination. In field studies, 1191 sows and gilts were vaccinated with FarrowSure® Plus B. Approximately 10% of the sows and gilts vaccinated exhibited transient local swelling at the site of injection 24 hours after vaccination under field conditions. By 21 days after vaccination, less than 1% of sows and gilts exhibited swelling at the injection site. Efficacy of the fractions of FarrowSure® Plus B was demonstrated in controlled challenge-of-immunity and immunogenicity tests. Serologic responses to all components of FarrowSure® Plus B were compared to those of FarrowSure® B. In all cases FarrowSure® Plus B stimulated higher antibody titers than FarrowSure® B. These results are summarized in Table 1.

Table 1. Comparison of FarrowSure® B and FarrowSure® Plus B Geometric Mean Titers and the Lower 95% Confidence Limit (CL) of the Difference as a Percent of the FarrowSure® B Titer:

Antigen	FarrowSure® B	FarrowSure® Plus B	Lower 95% CL
E. rhusiopathiae	552.8	2305.8	279.9
Porcine Parvovirus	53.2	124.6	145.0
L. bratislava	1024.0	6109.9	384.8
L. canicola	9.6	47.7	242.5
L. grippotyphosa	147.0	1262.2	439.9
L. hardjo	4.2	121.4	1322.0
L. icterohaemorrhagiae	157.6	650.8	256.2
L. pomona	9.0	37.6	195.0

Duration of Immunity: In addition to the above studies, duration-of-immunity studies in pigs were conducted for the *E. rhusiopathiae* fraction. The purpose of these studies was to demonstrate protection against challenge with virulent *E. rhusiopathiae* 20 and 26 weeks after the second vaccination with FarrowSure® Plus B.

20 Week Duration-of-Immunity Study: Four to 5-month-old pigs received 2 doses approximately 3 weeks apart, followed by challenge with virulent *E. rhusiopathiae* 20 weeks after the second vaccination. Following challenge, pigs were monitored daily for rectal temperature and clinical signs of disease. Eight of 10 control pigs (80%) were determined to be positive for infection following challenge. Eighteen of 20 vaccinated pigs (90%) were protected.

26 Week Duration-of-Immunity Study: Four to 5-month-old pigs received 2 doses approximately 3 weeks apart, followed by challenge with virulent *E. rhusiopathiae* 26 weeks after the second vaccination. Following challenge, pigs were monitored daily for rectal temperature and clinical signs of disease. Seven of 10 control pigs (70%) were determined to be positive for infection after challenge. Seventeen of 20 vaccinated pigs (85%) were protected. Results of these studies are illustrated in Tables 2 and 3.

Table 2. Results of *E. rhusiopathiae* Challenge in Control Pigs:

Study	No. of Control pigs	# Positive	# Protected	% Protected
20-week	10	8	2	20%
26-week	10	7	3	30%

Control pigs were considered to be positive for erysipelas if they met one or more of the following criteria: 1) Two consecutive days of temperatures at or above 40.9°C (105.6°F); 2) Sudden death following evidence of systemic erysipelas (including less than 2 consecutive days of elevated temperatures and/or systemic clinical signs); or 3) Recovery of *E. rhusiopathiae* from the spleen or liver.

Table 3. Results of *E. rhusiopathiae* Challenge in Vaccinated Pigs:

Study	No. of Vaccinated Pigs	# Positive	# Protected	% Protected
20-week	20	2	18	90%
26-week	20	3	17	85%

Vaccinated pigs were considered to be protected if they were free of the following criteria: 1) Two consecutive days of temperatures at or above 40.3°C (104.6°F); 2) Sudden death following evidence of systemic erysipelas (including less than 2 consecutive days of elevated temperatures and/or systemic clinical signs); or 3) Recovery of *E. rhusiopathiae* from the spleen or liver.

Presentation: 10 doses, 50 doses and 100 doses.

Compendium Code No.: 36902030 75-5138-00

FARROWSURE® PLUS B

Pfizer Animal Health **Bacterin-Vaccine**

Parvovirus Vaccine, Killed Virus-Erysipelothrix Rhusiopathiae-Leptospira-Bratislava-Canicola-Grippotyphosa-Hardjo-Icterohaemorrhagiae-Pomona Bacterin

U.S. Vet. Lic. No.: 189

Description: FARROWSURE® Plus B is a liquid preparation of porcine parvovirus grown on an established porcine cell line, a serum-free, clarified *E. rhusiopathiae* culture, and whole cell cultures of the 6 *Leptospira* serovars identified above. The antigens have been chemically inactivated and adjuvanted with 2 adjuvants, including Amphigen®, to enhance the immune response.

Contains gentamicin as preservative.

Indications: FARROWSURE® Plus B is for vaccination of healthy breeding swine as an aid in preventing reproductive failure caused by porcine parvovirus (PPV), erysipelas caused by *Erysipelothrix rhusiopathiae*, and leptospirosis caused by *Leptospira bratislava*, *L. canicola*, *L. grippotyphosa*, *L. hardjo*, *L. icterohaemorrhagiae* and *L. pomona*. A 26-week duration of immunity following vaccination has been demonstrated against erysipelas.

Directions:

1. General Directions: Shake well. Aseptically administer 5 mL intramuscularly.
2. Primary Vaccination: Healthy swine should receive 2 doses 3-5 weeks apart with the second dose administered 2-4 weeks prior to breeding. Healthy gilts, however, should receive the second dose as near as possible to 14 days prior to breeding.
3. Revaccination: Revaccination with a single dose is recommended prior to subsequent breedings. Boars should be revaccinated semiannually.
4. Good animal husbandry and herd health management practices should be employed.

Precaution(s): Store at 2°-7°C. Prolonged exposure to higher temperatures may adversely affect potency. Do not freeze.

Use entire contents when first opened.

Sterilized syringes and needles should be used to administer this vaccine.

Caution(s): Temporary swelling at the injection site may be observed.

As with many vaccines, anaphylaxis may occur after use. Initial antidote of epinephrine is recommended and should be followed with appropriate supportive therapy.

This product has been shown to be efficacious in healthy animals. A protective immune response may not be elicited if animals are incubating an infectious disease, are malnourished or parasitized, are stressed due to shipment or environmental conditions, are otherwise immunocompromised, or the vaccine is not administered in accordance with label directions.

For use in swine only.

For veterinary use only.
Warning(s): Do not vaccinate within 21 days before slaughter.
Discussion: Disease Description: PPV and *Leptospira* are common agents of reproductive loss in swine. While infection with either of these pathogens may produce subclinical disease, infection with PPV during pregnancy may result in fetal resorption, fetal mummification and stillbirths. Infection by *Leptospira* during the second half of pregnancy may cause abortions and stillbirths; late-term abortions are the most important economic effect of leptospirosis. Leptospirosis caused by any of the serovars represented here cannot be clinically differentiated. Abortions may also occur in sows infected with *E. rhusiopathiae* during pregnancy.
Trial Data: Safety and Efficacy: The safety of FARROWSURE® Plus B was demonstrated under both controlled laboratory and field conditions. No serious systemic or allergic reactions were observed following vaccination. In field studies, 1191 sows and gilts were vaccinated with FARROWSURE® Plus B. Approximately 10% of the sows and gilts vaccinated exhibited transient local swelling at the site of injection 24 hours after vaccination under field conditions. By 21 days after vaccination, less than 1% of sows and gilts exhibited swelling at the injection site. Efficacy of the fractions of FARROWSURE® Plus B was demonstrated in controlled challenge-of-immunity and immunogenicity tests. Serologic responses to all components of FARROWSURE® Plus B were compared to those of FarrowSure® B. In all cases FARROWSURE® Plus B stimulated higher antibody titers than FarrowSure® B. These results are summarized in Table 1.

Table 1. Comparison of FarrowSure® B and FARROWSURE® Plus B Geometric Mean Titers and the Lower 95% Confidence Limit (CL) of the Difference as a Percent of the FarrowSure® B Titer:

Antigen	FarrowSure® B	FARROWSURE® Plus B	Lower 95% CL
E. rhusiopathiae	552.8	2305.8	279.9
Porcine Parvovirus	53.2	124.6	145.0
L. bratislava	1024.0	6109.9	384.8
L. canicola	9.6	47.7	242.5
L. grippotyphosa	147.0	1262.2	439.9
L. hardjo	4.2	121.4	1322.0
L. icterohaemorrhagiae	157.6	650.8	256.2
L. pomona	9.0	37.6	195.0

Duration of Immunity: In addition to the above studies, duration-of-immunity studies in pigs were conducted for the *E. rhusiopathiae* fraction. The purpose of these studies was to demonstrate protection against challenge with virulent *E. rhusiopathiae* 20 and 26 weeks after the second vaccination with FARROWSURE® Plus B.

20 Week Duration-of-Immunity Study: Four to 5-month-old pigs received 2 doses approximately 3 weeks apart, followed by challenge with virulent *E. rhusiopathiae* 20 weeks after the second vaccination. Following challenge, pigs were monitored daily for rectal temperature and clinical signs of disease. Eight of 10 control pigs (80%) were determined to be positive for infection following challenge. Eighteen of 20 vaccinated pigs (90%) were protected.

26 Week Duration-of-Immunity Study: Four to 5-month-old pigs received 2 doses approximately 3 weeks apart, followed by challenge with virulent *E. rhusiopathiae* 26 weeks after the second vaccination. Following challenge, pigs were monitored daily for rectal temperature and clinical signs of disease. Seven of 10 control pigs (70%) were determined to be positive for infection after challenge. Seventeen of 20 vaccinated pigs (85%) were protected. Results of these studies are illustrated in Tables 2 and 3.

Table 2. Results of *E. rhusiopathiae* Challenge in Control Pigs:

Study	No. of Control Pigs	# Positive	# Protected	% Protected
20-week	10	8	2	20%
26-week	10	7	3	30%

Control pigs were considered to be positive for erysipelas if they met one or more of the following criteria: 1) Two consecutive days of temperatures at or above 40.9°C (105.6°F); 2) Sudden death following evidence of systemic erysipelas (including less than 2 consecutive days of elevated temperatures and/or systemic clinical signs); or 3) Recovery of *E. rhusiopathiae* from the spleen or liver.

Table 3. Results of *E. rhusiopathiae* Challenge in Vaccinated Pigs:

Study	No. of Vaccinated Pigs	# Positive	# Protected	% Protected
20-week	20	2	18	90%
26-week	20	3	17	85%

Vaccinated pigs were considered to be protected if they were free of the following criteria: 1) Two consecutive days of temperatures at or above 40.3°C (104.6°F); 2) Sudden death following evidence of systemic erysipelas (including less than 2 consecutive days of elevated temperatures and/or systemic clinical signs); or 3) Recovery of *E. rhusiopathiae* from the spleen or liver.
Presentation: 10 doses, 50 doses and 100 doses.
Compendium Code No.: 36902040 75-5141-00

FARROWSURE® PRV

Pfizer Animal Health **Bacterin-Vaccine**

Parvovirus-Pseudorabies Vaccine, Modified Live & Killed Virus-Erysipelothrix Rhusiopathiae-Leptospira Canicola-Grippotyphosa-Hardjo-Icterohaemorrhagiae-Pomona Bacterin

U.S. Vet. Lic. No.: 189
Description: FARROWSURE® PRV is a freeze-dried preparation of modified live PRV grown on an established porcine cell line, plus a liquid preparation of chemically inactivated PPV, *E. rhusiopathiae*, the 5 *Leptospira* serovars identified above, and a sterile adjuvant to enhance the immune response. The liquid component is used to rehydrate the freeze-dried component.

Contains gentamicin as preservative.
Indications: FARROWSURE® PRV is for vaccination of healthy breeding swine as an aid in preventing pseudorabies caused by pseudorabies virus (PRV), reproductive failure caused by porcine parvovirus (PPV), erysipelas caused by *Erysipelothrix rhusiopathiae*, and leptospirosis caused by *Leptospira canicola, L. grippotyphosa, L. hardjo, L. icterohaemorrhagiae*, and *L. pomona*.
Directions:

1. General Directions: Vaccination of healthy breeding swine is recommended. Aseptically rehydrate the freeze-dried vaccine with the liquid bacterin provided, shake well, and administer 5 mL intramuscularly.
2. Primary Vaccination: Administer a single 5 mL dose to healthy sows 14-60 days before breeding. Healthy gilts, however, should receive a single 5 mL dose as near as possible to 14 days before breeding; if gilts are vaccinated sooner, persisting maternal antibodies may interfere with active immunization. Healthy boars should receive a single 5 mL dose at least 14 days prior to introduction into the breeding herd. For protection against leptospirosis, a single dose of Leptoferm-5® is recommended either 3-6 weeks before or 3-6 weeks after administration of FARROWSURE® PRV.
3. Revaccination: Semiannual revaccination with a single dose is recommended before breeding. Boars should be revaccinated semiannually.
4. Good animal husbandry and herd health management practices should be employed.

Precaution(s): Store at 2°-7°C. Prolonged exposure to higher temperatures and/or direct sunlight may adversely affect potency. Do not freeze.

Use entire contents when first opened.

Sterilized syringes and needles should be used to administer this vaccine. Do not sterilize with chemicals because traces of disinfectant may inactivate the vaccine.

Burn containers and all unused contents.
Caution(s): Vaccination with FARROWSURE® PRV produces an antibody response to pseudorabies, thereby rendering swine positive to a serum neutralization (SN) test. Vaccinated swine can be differentiated from infected swine using a USDA-approved differential pseudorabies test, Pseudorabies Virus gpI Antibody Test Kit, provided the animals have received a Pfizer Animal Health PRV vaccine. Distribution of this vaccine is limited to authorized recipients designated by proper State Officials and under such conditions as these officials may require.

As with many vaccines, anaphylaxis may occur after use. Initial antidote of epinephrine is recommended and should be followed with appropriate supportive therapy.

This product has been shown to be efficacious in healthy animals. A protective immune response may not be elicited if animals are incubating an infectious disease, are malnourished or parasitized, are stressed due to shipment or environmental conditions, are otherwise immunocompromised, or the vaccine is not administered in accordance with label directions.

For veterinary use only.
Warning(s): Do not vaccinate within 21 days before slaughter.
Discussion: Disease Description: Pseudorabies is an acute infectious viral disease of swine and many other mammals. Abortions, stillbirths, and mummified fetuses may occur in PRV-infected sows. PPV and *Leptospira* are more common agents of reproductive loss in swine. While infection with any of those pathogens may produce subclinical disease, infection by PPV during pregnancy may result in fetal resorption, stillbirths, and fetal mummification. Infection by *Leptospira* during the second half of pregnancy may cause stillbirths or abortions; late-term abortions are the most important economic effect of leptospirosis. Leptospirosis caused by any of the serovars represented here cannot be clinically differentiated. Abortions may also occur in sows infected with *E. rhusiopathiae* during pregnancy.
Trial Data: Safety and Efficacy: Safety of FARROWSURE® PRV was demonstrated in breeding-age swine. Transient mild swelling and inflammation of the injection site was observed in 3%-10% of vaccinates. No systemic or allergic reactions were observed. Efficacy of the fractions of FARROWSURE® PRV was demonstrated in challenge-of-immunity and immunogenicity tests. After challenge with virulent *E. rhusiopathiae*, vaccinated pigs remained clinically normal while nonvaccinated control pigs developed clinical disease. In addition, vaccinated pigs expressed protective antibody titers to PRV, PPV, and each of the *Leptospira* serovars, confirming that no significant immunologic interference occurred.
Presentation: 10 dose vials.
Compendium Code No.: 36900651 75-4571-08

FASCURE™

KenVet **Topical Wound Dressing**

Collagen Powder

Ingredient(s): Hydrolyzed collagen powder. Contents are sterile when unopened.
Indications: For topical use in the management of chronic wounds and dermal ulcers, including: Pressure ulcers (stages 1-4), diabetic ulcers, ulcers resulting from arterial insufficiency, venous stasis ulcers, first and second degree burns, surgical wounds, traumatic wounds, and superficial sounds.
Directions for Use: Cleanse the wound site with warm sterile water or normal saline solution, leave the wound moist. Remove cap from bottle and apply FASCURE™ to the wound site by tapping the bottle. Cover wound with a layer of FASCURE™ approx. 6 mm (approx. ¼") thickness. Cover the wound with a non-stick dressing. Change dressing every 24 hours or as needed. With subsequent dressing changes, any remaining FASCURE™ need not be removed.
Precaution(s): Store at room temperature.
Caution(s): To minimize the possibility of cross-contamination, contents of FASCURE™ container should be limited to use in one animal. Wounds often appear larger during the first few days of treatment due to the reduction of edema.
Warning(s): For veterinary use only.
Presentation: 10 grams.
Compendium Code No.: 11340000

FAST ACTING SHAMPOO

Davis **Antidermatosis Shampoo**

Active Ingredient(s): The product contains C_2H_5OH.
Indications: For use on dogs, cats, puppies and kittens with flea problems such as seborrheic dermatitis.
Dosage and Administration: Pour one (1) quart (32 ounces) into a one (1) gallon container. Fill it with water. Shake the mixture before each use. For the best results, do not wet down the pet first with water. Apply generous amounts of the mixture with a sponge or spray bottle. Apply the shampoo on the head and ears, then lather. Repeat the procedure with the neck, chest, middle and hindquarter, finishing with the legs. Rinse the pet thoroughly.
Presentation: 1 gallon (3.785 L).
Compendium Code No.: 11410201

FASTBREAK™ PLUS™

Boehringer Ingelheim **Large Animal Dietary Supplement**

Active Ingredient(s):
Crude fat, minimum 99.50%
Linoleic acid, minimum . . . . . 225,000 mg/lb.
Vitamin A, minimum . . . . . 350,000 I.U./lb.
Vitamin D_3, minimum . . . . . 35,000 I.U./lb.
Vitamin E, minimum . . . . . 600 I.U./lb.

Ingredients: Vegetable oil and fat product, vitamin A supplement, d-activated animal sterol (source of vitamin D_3), vitamin E supplement, ethoxyquin (a preservative) and artificial flavor.
Indications: A nutritional supplement for baby pigs.

Dosage and Administration: Shake before using.

The dispensing system provided with the product uniformly measures 2 mL per pump. Oral dosing is best accomplished by dispensing on the back part of the tongue. This ensures minimizing the possibility of choking and waste of the product.

1. Piglets at processing: 4 mL per pig. Orally dose all piglets by 24 hours of age.
2. Cross-Fosters: Orally dose 4 mL per pig per day.

Precaution(s): Store between 55° and 85°F.
Presentation: 1 pint (480 mL) pump.
Compendium Code No.: 10280580

FASTRACK® CALF BOLUS

Conklin **Large Animal Dietary Supplement**

Guaranteed Analysis: Minimum Guaranteed Analysis Per 7 g (1 bolus): 1 billion colony-forming units (CFU) of total lactic acid-producing bacteria *(Enterococcus faecium* and *Lactobacillus acidophilus);* 200 million live yeast cells *(Saccharomyces cerevisiae);* protease from *Bacillus subtilis* not less than 6,250 PC; amylase from *Bacillus subtilis* and *Aspergillus oryzae* not less than 3,750 BAU; vitamin A, 25,000 IU; vitamin D_3, 5,000 IU; vitamin E, 200 IU; d-pantothenic acid, 30 mg; niacin, 15 mg; riboflavin, 10 mg; thiamine, 5 mg; and vitamin B_{12}, 0.15 mg.

Ingredients: Powdered cellulose, dicalcium phosphate, dried egg yolk, extract from chicory, calcium carbonate, vitamin E supplement, active dry yeast *(Saccharomyces cerevisiae)*, vitamin A supplement, magnesium sterate, D-calcium pantothenate, dried *Enterococcus faecium* fermentation product, sodium carboxymethylcellulose, vitamin B_{12} supplement, niacin, vitamin D_3 supplement, riboflavin, dried *Aspergillus oryzae* fermentation product, dried *Bacillus subtilis* fermentation product, thiamine mononitrate, dried *Lactobacillus acidophilus* fermentation product.

Indications: Contains a source of live (viable) naturally-occurring microorganisms; a source of protease which can hydrolyze proteins; and a source of amylase which can hydrolyze starch.

Directions for Use: FASTRACK® Calf Bolus is provided to the animal using a standard bolus gun (size no. 12). The bolus is formulated for calves under 500 lbs. Use the bolus daily until feed consumption is resumed.

Usage Rates:
Beef Calves under 500 lbs: 1 bolus per day
Dairy Calves under 500 lbs: 1 bolus per day
Sheep and Goats: 1 bolus per day

Precaution(s): Keep Cool: For extended shelf life, store in a refrigerator.
Disclaimer: Limited Guarantee: Conklin Company Inc. warrants that this product conforms to label description. No other warranty is expressed or implied.
Presentation: 0.79 U.S. Pound (350 g). Contains 50 boluses [0.25 oz. (7 g) each].
Compendium Code No.: 10630001

0-000569B

FASTRACK® CANINE GEL

Conklin **Small Animal Dietary Supplement**

Guaranteed Analysis: Minimum Guaranteed Analysis Per 1 cc: Total lactic acid-producing bacteria activity: 750 million colony-forming units *(Enterococcus faecium, Lactobacillus lactis);* live yeast cells: 25 million *(Saccharomyces cerevisiae);* vitamin A, 2,000 IU; vitamin E, 20 IU.

Ingredients: vegetable oil, glucose, dried egg yolk, extract from chicory, silicon dioxide, active dry yeast *(Saccharomyces cerevisiae)*, dl-alpha tocopherol acetate (source of vitamin E activity), vitamin A acetate, dried *Enterococcus faecium* fermentation product and dried *Lactobacillus lactis* fermentation product.

Indications: Contains a source of live (viable) naturally-occurring microorganisms.

Directions for Use: The gel should be placed between the lower teeth and the cheek. This product is intended for intermittent and supplemental feeding only.

Daily Usage Rates:
Puppies and dogs (less than 50 lbs.): 2 cc
Dogs (greater than 50 lbs.): 4 cc

Precaution(s): Keep Cool: For extended shelf life, store in a refrigerator.
Disclaimer: Guarantee: Conklin Company Inc. warrants that this product conforms to label description. No other warranty is expressed or implied.
Presentation: 20 cc (0.70 oz.) tube.
Compendium Code No.: 10630011

0-000523C

FASTRACK® CANINE MICROBIAL SUPPLEMENT

Conklin **Small Animal Dietary Supplement**

FOS Fortified

Guaranteed Analysis: Minimum Guaranteed Analysis Per Gram (¼ teaspoon): Total lactic acid-producing bacteria activity: 400 million colony-forming units *(Enterococcus faecium* and *Lactobacillus acidophilus);* total live yeast cells: 400 million *(Saccharomyces cerevisiae);* protease from *Bacillus subtilis* not less than 1,874 PC; amylase from *Bacillus subtilis* and *Aspergillus oryzae* not less than 1,125 BAU.

Ingredients: Extract of chicory; lactose, whey, active dry yeast *(Saccharomyces cerevisiae)*, dried *Enterococcus faecium* fermentation product; dried *Lactobacillus acidophilus* fermentation product; dried *Aspergillus oryzae* fermentation product; dried *Bacillus subtilis* fermentation product.

Indications: FASTRACK® Canine Microbial Supplement contains a source of live (viable) naturally-occurring microorganisms; a source of protease which can hydrolyze proteins and a source of amylase which can hydrolyze starch.

Directions: Mix FASTRACK® Canine Microbial Supplement with dry or wet dog food at the time of feeding. Sprinkle the appropriate amount over the dog food and then mix. FASTRACK® Canine Microbial Supplement is a daily supplement to complement a complete dog food, and is not a complete dog food. Use Fastrack® Canine Gel for puppies or dogs during times of irregular food intake.

Usage rates:
Puppies or dogs under 20 lbs.: 1 g (¼ teaspoon) per animal daily
Puppies or dogs 20 to 50 lbs.: 2 g (½ teaspoon) per animal daily
Puppies or dogs over 50 lbs.: 4 g (1 teaspoon) per animal daily

Precaution(s): Keep Cool: For extended shelf life, store under refrigeration.
Disclaimer: Limited Guarantee: Conklin Company Inc. warrants that this product conforms to label description. No other warranty is expressed or implied.
Presentation: 0.66 U.S. Pound (300 g).
Compendium Code No.: 10630022

0-000854A

FASTRACK® EQUINE GEL

Conklin **Equine Dietary Supplement**

Guaranteed Analysis: Minimum Guaranteed Analysis Per 1 cc: Total lactic acid-producing bacteria activity, 1.25 billion colony-forming units *(Enterococcus faecium, Lactobacillus acidophilus);* live yeast cells, 25 million *(Saccharomyces cerevisiae);* vitamin A, 10,000 IU; vitamin E, 25 IU.

Ingredients: Vegetable oil, dried egg yolk, extract from chicory, silicon dioxide, active dry yeast *(Saccharomyces cerevisiae)*, dl-alpha tocopherol acetate (source of vitamin E activity), vitamin A acetate, dried *Enterococcus faecium* fermentation product and dried *Lactobacillus acidophilus* fermentation product.

Indications: Contains a source of live (viable) naturally-occurring microorganisms.

Directions for Use: Place between the lower teeth and the cheek.

Daily Usage Rates:
Foals: 2 cc
Adult horses: 4 cc

Precaution(s): Keep Cool: For extended shelf life, store in a refrigerator.
Disclaimer: Limited Guarantee: Conklin Company Inc. warrants that this product conforms to label description. No other warranty is expressed or implied.
Presentation: 20 cc (0.70 oz.) tube.
Compendium Code No.: 10630031

0-000851D

FASTRACK® KICK-OFF

Conklin **Large Animal Dietary Supplement**

Guaranteed Analysis: Minimum Guaranteed Analysis Per 1 g: 1 billion colony-forming units (CFU) of total lactic acid-producing bacteria *(Enterococcus faecium* and *Lactobacillus acidophilus);* 200 million live yeast cells *(Saccharomyces cerevisiae);* protease from *Bacillus subtilis* not less than 2,500 PC; and amylase from *Bacillus subtilis* and *Aspergillus oryzae* not less than 1,500 BAU; vitamin A, 6,000 IU; vitamin D_3, 1,250 IU; vitamin E, 50 IU; d-pantothenic acid, 7.5 mg; niacin, 3 mg; riboflavin, 2.5 mg; thiamine, 1.25 mg; and vitamin B_{12}, 35 mcg.

Ingredients: Dried egg yolk, extract from chicory, lactose, vitamin E supplement, whey, vitamin A supplement, dried *Lactobacillus acidophilus* fermentation product, dried *Aspergillus oryzae* fermentation product, D-calcium pantothenate, dried *Bacillus subtilis* fermentation extract, dried *Enterococcus faecium* fermentation product, vitamin B_{12} supplement, niacin, vitamin D_3 supplement, riboflavin, active dry yeast *(Saccharomyces cerevisiae)*, thiamine mononitrate.

Indications: Contains a source of live (viable) naturally-occurring microorganisms; a source of protease which can hydrolyze proteins and a source of amylase which can hydrolyze starch.

Directions for Use: FASTRACK® Kick-Off is provided to newborn calves and other newborn ruminants for the first five days of life.

Supplement calves and young ruminants with Fastrack® Liquid Dispersible for the remainder of the growing period during regular feed consumption. FASTRACK® Kick-Off is also provided to calves and young ruminants during periods of variable nutrient intake, and until nutrient intake stabilizes.

FASTRACK® Kick-Off is formulated to be mixed with colostrum, whole milk or milk replacer. Agitation is required to assure proper mixing.

Daily Usage Rates:
Beef and dairy calves: 1 g (¼ teaspoon) daily per calf
Lambs and kid goats: 0.5 g (⅛ teaspoon) daily per animal

Precaution(s): Keep Cool: For extended shelf life, store in a refrigerator.
Disclaimer: Limited Guarantee: Conklin Company Inc. warrants that this product conforms to label description. No other warranty is expressed or implied.
Presentation: 1 U.S. Pound (454 g).
Compendium Code No.: 10630041

0-000852A

FASTRACK® LIQUID DISPERSIBLE

Conklin **Large Animal Dietary Supplement**

Guaranteed Analysis:

Minimum Guaranteed Analysis Per Pound (115 teaspoons): Total lactic acid-producing bacteria activity: 400 billion colony-forming units *(Enterococcus faecium* and *Lactobacillus acidophilus);* total live yeast cells: 400 billion *(Saccharomyces cerevisiae)*.

Minimum Guaranteed Analysis Per Gram: Total lactic acid-producing bacteria activity: 880 million colony-forming units *(Enterococcus faecium, Lactobacillus acidophilus);* total live yeast cells: 880 million *(Saccharomyces cerevisiae);* protease from *Bacillus subtilis* not less than 4,225 PC; and amylase from *Bacillus subtilis* and *Aspergillus oryzae* not less than 2,535 BAU.

Ingredients: Lactose, extract from chicory, whey, yeast active dehydrated *(Saccharomyces cerevisiae)*, dried *Enterococcus faecium* fermentation product, dried *Lactobacillus acidophilus* fermentation product, dried *Aspergillus oryzae* fermentation product, dried *Bacillus subtilis* fermentation product.

Indications: Contains a source of live (viable) naturally-occurring microorganisms; a source of protease which can hydrolyze proteins and a source of amylase which can hydrolyze starch.

Directions for Use: FASTRACK® Liquid Dispersible is designed to be mixed with water, cool (body temperature or lower) milk replacers or liquid feeds. Agitation is required to assure proper mixing. Liquid Dispersible can also be mixed in dry feeds.

Poultry: ¼ to ½ pound (in watering system) per each ton of feed consumed.
Calves: Mix with whole milk or milk replacer at the rate of ¼ teaspoon (1 g) per calf per day.
Lactating dairy cattle: 1 oz. per 10 head daily in dry feed.
Growing and mature beef cattle: 1 oz. per 10 head daily in dry feed.
Swine: In liquid feeds (per 10 head per day)
birth to 40 pounds: ¼ teaspoon
40 to 130 pounds: ½ teaspoon
Over 130 pounds: 1 teaspoon
General livestock:
In water system, automated feeders or liquid feeds: ½ pound per each ton of feed consumed.
In dry feeds: 12 pound per ton of feed.

Special note: ½ pound of Liquid Dispersible per ton of feed consumed is equal to 100 million colony-forming units per pound of feed consumed.

For dry mixed feeds, Fastrack® Probiotic Pack is recommended.

Precaution(s): Keep Cool: For extended shelf life, store in a refrigerator.
Disclaimer: Limited Guarantee: Conklin Company Inc. warrants that this product conforms to label description. No other warranty is expressed or implied.
Presentation: 1 U.S. pound (454 g) jar and 22 U.S. pound (10 kg) pail.
Compendium Code No.: 10630051

0-000139D / 0-000845A

FASTRACK® LIQUID DISPERSIBLE-P

Conklin — **Poultry Dietary Supplement**

Guaranteed Analysis: Minimum Guaranteed Analysis Per 1 oz.: 25 billion colony-forming units (CFU) of total lactic acid-producing bacteria *(Enterococcus faecium* and *Lactobacillus acidophilus);* 25 billion live yeast cells *(Saccharomyces cerevisiae)*; protease from *Bacillus subtilis* not less than 120,487 PC; and amylase from *Bacillus subtilis* and *Aspergillus oryzae* not less than 72,292 BAU.

Ingredients: Dried egg yolk, extract from chicory, lactose, active dry yeast *(Saccharomyces cerevisiae)*, whey, dried *Lactobacillus acidophilus* fermentation product, dried *Aspergillus oryzae* fermentation product, dried *Bacillus subtilis* fermentation product, dried *Enterococcus faecium* fermentation extract.

Indications: Contains a source of live (viable) naturally-occurring microorganisms; a source of protease which can hydrolyze proteins and a source of amylase which can hydrolyze starch.

Directions for Use: Provide FASTRACK® Liquid Dispersible-P to poultry the first five days of life. Supplement poultry with Fastrack® Liquid Dispersible for the remainder of the growing period during regular feed consumption. However, FASTRACK® Liquid Dispersible-P should be supplemented to growing and mature poultry during periods of variable nutrient intake, and should be utilized until nutrient intake stabilizes. FASTRACK® Liquid Dispersible-P is formulated to be mixed with water and supplied to poultry via water proportioner systems. Agitation is required to assure proper mixing. The FASTRACK® Liquid Dispersible-P may also be sprinkled over the poultry feed during day one and two of life.

Usage Rates:
Newly-hatched poultry: 1 oz. per 20,000 chicks for each of the first five days of life.
Growing poultry:

Week Of Life	Daily amount of product to be supplemented until teed intake stabilizes	
	Per 20,000 broilers	Per 10,000 turkeys
2	1.5 oz.	1.5 oz.
3 to 4	2.0 oz.	2.0 oz.
5	2.5 oz.	2.5 oz.
6	3.0 oz.	3.0 oz.
7	4.0 oz.	4.0 oz.
8	5.0 oz.	5.0 oz.
9 to 10	6.0 oz.	6.0 oz.
11 to 12	7.0 oz.	8.0 oz.
13 to 14		10.0 oz.
15 to 16		12.0 oz.
17 to 18		14.0 oz.
19 to 20		16.0 oz.

Note: One Fastrack® top-dressing scoop measures 1.5 oz. of FASTRACK® Liquid Dispersible-P.

Precaution(s): Keep Cool: For extended shelf life, store in a refrigerator.

Disclaimer: Limited Guarantee: Conklin Company Inc. warrants that this product conforms to label description. No other warranty is expressed or implied.

Presentation: 1 U.S. pound (454 g).

Compendium Code No.: 10630061 — 0-000853A

FASTRACK® NONRUMINANT MICROBIAL GEL

Conklin — **Dietary Supplement**

Guaranteed Analysis: Minimum Guaranteed Analysis Per 1 cc: Total lactic acid-producing bacteria activity: 50 million colony-forming units *(Enterococcus faecium, Lactobacillus acidophilus)*; live yeast cells: 20 million *(Saccharomyces cerevisiae)*; protease from *Bacillus subtilis* not less than 3,457 PC; amylase from *Bacillus subtilis* and *Aspergillus oryzae* not less than 2,074 BAU; vitamin A, 3,300 IU; vitamin D_3, 900 IU; vitamin E, 11 IU; niacin, 35 mg; d-pantothenic acid, 12 mg; riboflavin, 3.25 mg; thiamine, 1.1 mg; vitamin B_{12}, 15 mcg.

Ingredients: Vegetable oil, extract from chicory, silicon dioxide, dextrose, niacin, dl-alpha tocopheryl acetate (source of vitamin E activity), calcium pantothenate, vitamin B_{12} supplement, active dry yeast *(Saccharomyces cerevisiae)*, vitamin A acetate, riboflavin supplement, thiamine hydrochloride, D-activated animal sterol (source of vitamin D_3), dried *Enterococcus faecium* fermentation product, dried *Lactobacillus acidophilus* fermentation product, dried *Aspergillus oryzae* fermentation product, dried *Bacillus subtilis* fermentation extract.

Indications: Contains a source of live (viable) naturally-occurring microorganisms; a source of protease which can hydrolyze proteins and a source of amylase which can hydrolyze starch.

Directions for Use: Place the FASTRACK® Nonruminant Microbial Gel between the lower teeth and the cheek. Use during periods of irregular nutrient intake. When nutrient intake stabilizes, use the appropriate dry Fastrack® direct-fed microbial product mixed into the feed or top-dressed.

Usage Rates:
New-born pigs: 1 cc at birth
Nursery pigs: 2 cc at weaning
Horses: 5-10 cc
Pets:
Cats and small dogs: ½-1 cc
Large dogs: 1-2 cc

Precaution(s): Keep Cool: For extended shelf life, store in a refrigerator.

Disclaimer: Limited Guarantee: Conklin Company Inc. warrants that this product conforms to label description. No other warranty is expressed or implied.

Presentation: 32 cc and 60 cc tubes.

Compendium Code No.: 10630071 — 0-000846B / 0-000584A

FASTRACK® PROBIOTIC PACK

Conklin — **Large Animal Dietary Supplement**

Guaranteed Analysis: Minimum Guaranteed Analysis Per Ounce: Total lactic acid-producing bacteria activity: 2.5 billion colony-forming units *(Enterococcus faecium, Lactobacillus acidophilus)*; protease from *Bacillus subtilis* not less than 22,125 PC; and amylase from *Bacillus subtilis* and *Aspergillus oryzae* not less than 13,289 BAU.

Ingredients: Yeast culture *(Saccharomyces cerevisiae)*, rice hulls, calcium carbonate, extract from chicory, dried *Enterococcus faecium* fermentation product, dried *Lactobacillus acidophilus* fermentation product, dried *Aspergillus oryzae* fermentation extract, dried *Bacillus subtilis* fermentation extract.

Indications: Contains a source of live (viable) naturally occurring microorganisms; a source of protease which can hydrolyze proteins and a source of amylase which can hydrolyze starch.

Directions for Use:

Growing beef and dairy animals: Supplement at the rate of 0.5 to 1.5 ounces per animal daily.
Lactating dairy cattle: Supplement at the rate of 1 to 2 ounces per animal daily.
Hogs: Mix at the rate of 2.5 to 5 pounds per ton of feed.
Horses: Supplement at the following rates:
Growing horses: 0.5 to 2 ounces per horse daily.
Horses at maintenance: 1 ounce per horse daily.
Horses being trained or strenuously exercised: 1 to 2 ounces per horse daily.
Lactating mares: 1 to 2 ounces per horse daily.
All other horses: 1 to 2 ounces per horse daily.
Poultry: Mix at the rate of 2.5 to 5 pounds per ton of mixed feed.

Precaution(s): Store in a cool, dry place.

Warning(s): For U.S. Health Hazard Information, call (800) 228-5635.

Disclaimer: Limited Guarantee: Conklin Company Inc. warrants that this product conforms to label description. No other warranty is expressed or implied.

Presentation: 5 lb bag, 8 lb (3.6 kg) horse pail and 10 x 5 lb bags per pack.

Compendium Code No.: 10630081 — 0-000842D / 0-000830 / 0-000409C

FASTRACK® RUMINANT BOLUS

Conklin — **Large Animal Dietary Supplement**

Guaranteed Analysis: Minimum Guaranteed Analysis Per 16 g (1 bolus): 3 billion colony-forming units of total lactic acid-producing bacteria *(Enterococcus faecium* and *Lactobacillus acidophilus);* 600 million live yeast cells *(Saccharomyces cerevisiae)*; protease from *Bacillus subtilis* not less than 18,750 PC; amylase from *Bacillus subtilis* and *Aspergillus oryzae* not less than 11,250 BAU; vitamin A, 75,000 IU; vitamin D_3, 15,000 IU; vitamin E, 600 IU; d-pantothenic acid, 90 mg; niacin, 45 mg; riboflavin, 30 mg; thiamine, 15 mg; and vitamin B_{12}.

Ingredients: Powdered cellulose, dicalcium phosphate, extract from chicory, calcium carbonate, vitamin E supplement, active dry yeast *(Saccharomyces cerevisiae)*, vitamin A supplement, magnesium sterate, D-calcium pantothenate, dried *Enterococcus faecium* fermentation product, sodium carboxymethylcellulose, vitamin B_{12} supplement, niacin, vitamin D_3 supplement, riboflavin, dried *Aspergillus oryzae* fermentation extract, dried *Bacillus subtilis* fermentation extract, thiamine mononitrate, dried *Lactobacillus acidophilus* fermentation product.

Indications: FASTRACK® Ruminant Bolus contains a source of live (viable) naturally-occurring microorganisms; a source of protease which can hydrolyze proteins; contains a source of amylase which can hydrolyze starch.

Directions for Use: FASTRACK® Ruminant Bolus is designed to be provided to the animal using a standard bolus gun (size no. 11). Use during periods of irregular nutrient intake. When nutrient intake stabilizes, use the appropriate Fastrack® direct-fed microbial product mixed into the feed or topdressed.

Usage Rates:
Beef Calves
Calves - under 500 lbs.: ½ bolus
Cattle - over 500 lbs.: one bolus
Dairy Calves
Calves - under 500 lbs: ½ bolus
Cattle - over 500 lbs.: one bolus
Lactating cows: one bolus
Sheep and Goats: ½ bolus

Precaution(s): Keep Cool: For extended shelf life, store in a refrigerator.

Disclaimer: Limited Guarantee: Conklin Company Inc. warrants that this product conforms to label description. No other warranty is expressed or implied.

Presentation: 0.88 U.S. pounds (400 g). Contains 25 boluses [0.57 oz. (16 g) each].

Compendium Code No.: 10630091 — 0-000511B

FASTRACK® RUMINANT MICROBIAL GEL

Conklin — **Large Animal Dietary Supplement**

Guaranteed Analysis: Minimum Guaranteed Analysis Per 5 cc: One billion colony-forming units of lactic acid-producing bacteria *(Enterococcus faecium* and *Lactobacillus acidophilus);* 200 million live yeast cells *(Saccharomyces cerevisiae)*; protease from *Bacillus subtilis* not less than 6,250 PC; amylase from *Bacillus subtilis* and *Aspergillus oryzae* not less than 3,750 BAU; 25,000 international units (IU) vitamin A; 5,000 IU vitamin D_3; 200 IU vitamin E; 30 mg d-pantothenic acid; 15 mg niacin; 10 mg riboflavin; 5 mg thiamine and 150 mcg vitamin B_{12}.

Ingredients: Vegetable oil, extract from chicory, silicon dioxide, dl-alpha tocopheryl acetate (source of vitamin E activity), dextrose, vitamin B_{12} supplement, active dry yeast *(Saccharomyces cerevisiae)*, vitamin A acetate, calcium pantothenate, riboflavin supplement, niacin, thiamine hydrochloride, D-activated animal sterol (source of vitamin D_3), dried *Enterococcus faecium* fermentation product, dried *Lactobacillus acidophilus* fermentation product, dried *Aspergillus oryzae* fermentation extract and dried *Bacillus subtilis* fermentation extract.

Indications: Contains a source of live (viable) naturally-occurring microorganisms; a source of protease which can hydrolyze proteins and a source of amylase which can hydrolyze starch.

Directions for Use: Place the FASTRACK® Ruminant Microbial Gel between the lower teeth and the cheek. Use during periods of irregular nutrient intake. When nutrient intake stabilizes, use the appropriate dry Fastrack® direct-fed microbial product mixed into the feed or top-dressed.

Daily Usage Rates:
Calves, birth and up to 500 lbs.: 5 cc
Cattle, 500 to 800 lbs.: 10 cc
Cattle, over 800 lbs.: 15 cc
Lactating cows: 15 cc
Sheep and goats, at birth and pre-weaning: 5 cc
Sheep and goats, weaned and mature: 5 cc

Precaution(s): Keep Cool: For extended shelf life, store in a refrigerator.

Disclaimer: Limited Guarantee: Conklin Company Inc. warrants that this product conforms to label description. No other warranty is expressed or implied.

Presentation: 80 cc and 300 cc tubes.

Compendium Code No.: 10630101 — 0-000585A / 0-000849B

FATAL-PLUS® POWDER Ⓒ

Vortech **Euthanasia Agent**

Active Ingredient(s): When constituted to 250 mL with water, each mL contains:
Pentobarbital Sodium . . . 392 mg/mL

Indications: For fast and humane euthanasia of all animals regardles of species.

Pharmacology: Action: FATAL-PLUS® produces classic euthanasia by sequentially depressing the cerebral cortex, the lungs and the heart. Action on target organs gives humane euthanasia of unparalleled speed, effectiveness and specificity. Instant unconsciousness is induced with simultaneous collapse of the animal. Deep pentobarbital anesthesia ensues with blood pressure fall, stoppage of breathing and cerebral death. Cardiac function stops, quickly and irreversibly.

Dosage and Administration:

Directions for Mixing: Slowly add water (150 mL to 200 mL). Replace cap and shake well until powder is dissolved. Add more water to the 250 mL mark only. Do not exceed the fill line (250 mL).

Intravenous injection is the preferred route. However, intraperitoneal or intracardiac injections may be made where the intravenous injection is impractical, as in the very small dog and cat, or in the comatose animal with depressed vascular function. Inject rapidly 1 mL for every 10 lbs body weight. Minimum 1 mL. The use of tranquilizers is recommended for IP or IC injections.

Precaution(s): FATAL-PLUS® has a shelf life of 2 years.

Once constituted, potency is guaranteed for 35 days.

Caution(s): Federal (USA) law restricts this drug for use by or on the order of a licensed veterinarian.

Euthanasia may sometimes be delayed in animals with severe cardiac or circulatory deficiencies. This may be explained by the impaired movement of the drug to the site of action. When restraint may cause the animal pain, injury or anxiety, or cause danger to the person making the injection, prior use of tranquilizing drugs may be necessary.

Warning(s): For euthanasia only. Must not be used for therapeutic purposes. Do not use in animals intended for food.

Poison. Caution should be exercised to avoid contact of the drug with open wounds or accidental self-inflicted injections. In case of occurrence wash the contact area thoroughly with soap and water. Keep out of reach of children. For additional information consult the FATAL-PLUS® Material Safety Data Sheet. For veterinary use only.

Presentation: Contains 98 g pentobarbital sodium soluble microfine powder in cases of 12 x 250 mL multiple dose screw cap vials ready to be constituted with water (NDC No. 0298-9372-68). DEA Form No. 222 required to purchase.

Compendium Code No.: 10980001

FATAL-PLUS® SOLUTION Ⓒ

Vortech **Euthanasia Agent**

Active Ingredient(s): Contains:
Pentobarbital Sodium . . . 390 mg/mL

Propylene Glycol; Ethyl Alcohol (SDA-3A); Benzyl Alcohol (preservative).

Color added for identification.

Indications: For fast and humane euthanasia of all animals regardless of species.

Pharmacology: Action: FATAL-PLUS® produces classic euthanasia by sequentially depressing the cerebral cortex, the lungs and the heart. Action on target organs gives humane euthanasia of unparalleled speed, effectiveness and specificity. Instant unconsciousness is induced with simultaneous collapse of the animal. Deep pentobarbital anesthesia ensues with blood pressure fall, stoppage of breathing and cerebral death. Cardiac function stops, quickly and irreversibly.

Dosage and Administration: As an average guide, the volume of FATAL-PLUS® required for euthanasia is 1 mL of solution per 10 lbs of body weight of the animal. Intravenous (IV) injection is preferred. The calculated dosage should be given in a single injection. An uninterrupted injection is the most comfortable for the animal. For intravenous injection a needle of suitable gauge to insure intravenous placement of the entire dose should be used. Intraperitoneal (IP) or intracardiac (IC) injection may be made when intravenous injection is impractical, as in very small or comatose animals with impaired vascular functions. Good injection skill is necessary for intracardiac injection. The use of tranquilizers is recommended for IP or IC injections.

Precaution(s): FATAL-PLUS® Solution has a shelf life of 2 years.

Caution(s): Federal (USA) law restricts this drug for use by or on the order of a licensed veterinarian.

Euthanasia may sometimes be delayed in animals with severe cardiac or circulatory deficiencies. This may be explained by the impaired movement of the drug to the site of action. When restraint may cause the animal pain, injury or anxiety, or cause danger to the person making the injection, prior use of tranquilizing drugs may be necessary.

Warning(s): For euthanasia only. Must not be used for therapeutic purposes. Do not use in animals intended for food.

Poison. Caution should be exercised to avoid contact of the drug with open wounds or accidental self-inflicted injections. In case of occurrence wash the contact area thoroughly with soap and water. Keep out of reach of children. For additional information consult the FATAL-PLUS® Material Safety Data Sheet. For veterinary use only.

Presentation: 250 mL multiple dose vial, packed 12 vials per case (NDC No. 0298-9373-68). DEA Form No. 222 required to purchase.

Compendium Code No.: 10980011

FAVOR®

Pfizer Animal Health **Small Animal Dietary Supplement**

Guaranteed Analysis: per tablet: (All values are minimum quantities unless otherwise stated)

Crude Protein (minimum)	19.0%
Crude Fat (minimum)	4.0%
Crude Fiber (maximum)	2.0%
Moisture (maximum)	9.0%
Minerals:	
Calcium (minimum)	2.1%
(maximum)	2.6%
Phosphorus	1.7%
Potassium	0.6%
Salt (minimum)	0.20%
(maximum)	0.70%
Chloride	0.20%
Iron	5.0 mg
Copper	0.2 mg
Manganese	0.2 mg
Zinc	0.3 mg
Iodine	0.1 mg
Vitamins and Others:	
Vitamin A	1,500 IU
Vitamin D	150 IU
Vitamin E	4 IU
Thiamine	0.81 mg
Riboflavin	1.0 mg
Pantothenic Acid	1.0 mg
Niacin	4.0 mg
Pyridoxine	0.41 mg
Choline	40.0 mg
Taurine	2.25%

Ingredients: Brewers dried yeast, malted milk, sucrose, corn syrup, animal digest, dicalcium phosphate, choline chloride, soy flour, spray-dried whey, taurine, nonfat milk powder, wheat flour, dried buttermilk, safflower oil, ferrous fumarate, dl-alpha tocopheryl acetate, inositol, tricalcium phosphate, hydrolyzed vegetable protein, silicon dioxide, vitamin a acetate, niacinamide, zinc gluconate, copper gluconate, potassium iodide, thiamine mononitrate, riboflavin, calcium pantothenate, pyridoxine hydrochloride, manganese sulfate, cobalt sulfate, vitamin D_3 supplement.

Indications: A highly palatable vitamin-mineral supplement for cats.

Directions for Use:

Mature cats—1 tablet daily.

Kittens—¼-1 tablet daily.

FAVOR® tablets are made with a special taste appeal to cats. Administer by hand just prior to feeding, or crumble and mix with food.

Caution(s): Keep out of reach of children.

Keep bottle tightly closed to preserve freshness.

Presentation: 60 tablets.

Compendium Code No.: 36901020

85-8092-07

FC4 GOLD

L.A.H.I. (Maine Biological) **Bacterin**

Pasteurella Multocida Bacterin, Avian Isolates, Types 1, 3, 4 & 3X4

U.S. Vet. Lic. No.: 196

Contents: This product contains the antigens listed above.

Vaccine was carefully produced and passed all tests in accordance with the U.S. Government.

Indications: Recommended for the vaccination of chickens and turkeys against Fowl Cholera caused by *Pasteurella multocida*, type 1 in chickens and types 3, 4 and 3X4 in turkeys.

If fowl cholera is diagnosed before it has spread throughout the flock, it is often possible to check its spread by immediate vaccination of healthy birds.

Directions for Use: Vaccine should be warmed to room temperature before use.

Shake well before and during use.

Inject subcutaneously or intramuscularly using aseptic technique. Use entire contents of bottle when first opened. Vaccinate chickens between 12 and 16 weeks of age. Vaccinate turkeys between 20 and 24 weeks of age. Revaccinate 4 to 6 weeks later. Revaccinate during molt.

Dose - ¼ mL (0.25 mL) per bird. Inject all birds in flock.

Precaution(s): Store at 2°-7°C (35°-45°F). Do not freeze.

Caution(s): For veterinary use only.

Warning(s): Do not vaccinate within 42 days before slaughter.

In case of accidental human injection seek immediate medical attention.

Presentation: 500 doses (125 mL) and 1,000 doses (250 mL).

Compendium Code No.: 11030560

FECA-DRY™ II

Life Science **Fecal Flotation**

Ingredients: Contains zinc sulfate in a pre-measured amount to be reconstituted. This reagent allows the additional detection of *Giardia*.

Indications: For use in fecal flotation analysis.

Directions: Shake well before using.

Fill this container with warm water up to the brim, secure cap and shake well. As the contents go into solution, the water level will drop. Do not add additional water. This procedure will produce a specific gravity of 1.18.

Caution(s): Keep out of reach of children.

Presentation: 1 gallon.

Compendium Code No.: 10870060

FECA-FLOTATION™ READY TO USE

Life Science **Fecal Flotation**

Ingredients: Sodium nitrate solution.

Indications: For use in fecal flotation analysis.

Directions: FECA-FLOTATION™ is a standardized flotation medium with a specific gravity of 1.25 to 1.30 for use in performing fecal analysis.

FECA-FLOTATION™ may be used for all flotation techniques.

Pre-mixed for convenience.

Caution(s): For veterinary use only.

Warning(s): Keep out of reach of children.

Presentation: One gallon (3.785 L).

Compendium Code No.: 10870071

FECAL FLOAT (DRY)

Phoenix Pharmaceutical **Fecal Flotation**

Sodium Nitrate-Fecal Flotation Medium

Indications: Use: Solution to be used for all fecal flotation techniques of fecal analysis.

Directions: Fill the gallon container with water to the top. Screw the cap on and shake vigorously. Slowly the product will go into solution, dropping the water level. Do not add additional water. When the sodium nitrate is completely dissolved, the finished medium will have a specific gravity of 1.25 to 1.30.

Caution(s): For animal use only.

Warning(s): Keep out of reach of children.

Presentation: 3.5 lbs (NDC 57319-461-09).

Manufactured by: Ameri-Pac, Inc., St. Joseph, MO 64502.

Compendium Code No.: 12561030

Rev. 6-01

FECAL FLOAT (READY TO USE)

Phoenix Pharmaceutical **Fecal Flotation**

Sodium Nitrate-Medium Solution

Active Ingredient(s): A saturated solution of Sodium Nitrate to water with specific gravity of 1.25 to 1.30.

Indications: For use in fecal flotation techniques of fecal analysis for veterinary use only.

Directions: Ready to use fecal flotation medium.

Caution(s): For animal use only.

Warning(s): Keep out of reach of children.

Presentation: 1 gallon (3.785 L) (NDC 57319-462-09).

Manufactured by: Ameri-Pac, Inc., St. Joseph, MO 64502.

Compendium Code No.: 12561040 Rev. 7-01

FECALYZER®

Evsco **Fecal Flotation**

Indications: The FECALYZER® disposable diagnostic system is designed so that the odorfree sample collecting device is also the complete apparatus for assaying the fecal sample. Cross-contamination is avoided by using a new FECALYZER® for each sample.

Test Procedure: The client is instructed to remove the insert, press the small end of the insert into the sample, return the insert to the holder, close the lid and return to a veterinarian. To assay the sample, the lid is opened and flotation solution (Fecasol®) is added to the level of the arrows on the vial. The insert is rotated back and forth. Blades at the bottom of the insert and container mix the sample and separate the ova from the fecal matter. The insert is seated firmly and flotation solution is added to form a meniscus. Debris is trapped in the lower section while the ova float to surface where a slide or coverslip has been placed on the meniscus. After 15-20 minutes, the slide is placed on a microscope for examination, FECALYZER® is capped and discarded.

Precaution(s): The attached cap closes tightly for transporting the sample and for disposal after assay.

Presentation: Each box contains 50 individual FECALYZER® test units, instruction card, pad of 50 client instruction sheets, and 50 pressure-sensitive identification labels.

Compendium Code No.: 10050080

FECA-MED

Centaur **Fecal Flotation**

Fecal Analysis Solution

Description: FECA-MED is a standardized flotation medium.

Indications: FECA-MED is a standardized flotation medium with a specific gravity of 1.25-1.30 for use in performing fecal analysis.

Dosage and Administration: Ready to use solution may be used for all flotation techniques.

Caution(s): For veterinary use only.

Warning(s): Keep out of reach of children.

Presentation: 1 gallon (128 fl oz) 3.785 L.

Manufactured by: Unavet, North Kansas City, MO 64116.

Compendium Code No.: 14880140

FECA-MED

First Priority **Fecal Flotation**

Ready to Use Solution

Description: FECA-MED is a standardized solution of sodium nitrate with specific gravity of 1.25 to 1.30.

Indications: For use in all flotation techniques of fecal analysis.

Caution(s): For animal use only.

Warning(s): Keep out of reach of children.

Presentation: 1 gallon (3.785 L) (NDC# 58829-224-01).

Compendium Code No.: 11390291 Rev. 4-01

FECA-MED ℞

Vedco **Fecal Flotation**

Description: FECA-MED is a standardized ready to use solution with specific gravity of 1.25 to 1.30.

Ingredients: Sodium nitrate.

Indications: For use in all flotation techniques of fecal analysis.

Warning(s): For animal use only. Keep out of reach of children.

Caution(s): Federal law restricts this drug to use by or on the order of a licensed veterinarian.

Presentation: 1 gallon.

Compendium Code No.: 10940940

FECA-MIX

Centaur **Fecal Flotation**

Ingredient(s): Sodium nitrate.

Indications: Crystalline sodium nitrate can be used for all flotation techniques of fecal analysis.

Directions: Fill container to the brim. Secure cap on bottle and shake well; this will take repeated periods of agitation. As the contents go into solution, the water level will drop. Do not add additional water. This procedure will produce a specific gravity of 1.25 to 1.30.

Caution(s): For veterinary use only.

Warning(s): Keep out of reach of children.

Presentation: 3.5 lbs.

Manufactured by: Unavet, North Kansas City, MO 64116.

Compendium Code No.: 14880150

FECA-MIX ℞

First Priority **Fecal Flotation**

Fecal Flotation Medium

Description: FECA-MIX is pre-measured dry sodium nitrate crystals. Contains approximately 3.5 lb sodium nitrate.

Indications: Solution can be used for all flotation techniques of fecal analysis.

Directions: Fill container with warm water up to the brim. Secure cap on bottle and shake well; this will take repeated periods of agitation. As the contents go into solution, the water level will drop. Do not add additional water. This procedure will produce a specific gravity of 1.25 to 1.30.

Caution(s): Federal law restricts this drug to use by or on the order of a licensed veterinarian. For veterinarian use only.

Warning(s): Keep out of reach of children.

Presentation: 3.5 lb (1.6 kg) (NDC# 58829-225-01).

Compendium Code No.: 11390302 Rev. 8-98

FECA-MIX ℞

Vedco **Fecal Flotation**

Active Ingredient(s): FECA-MIX is premeasured dry sodium nitrate crystals.

Indications: The solution can be used for all flotation techniques of fecal analysis.

Dosage and Administration: Fill the container with warm water up to the brim. Secure the cap on the bottle and shake well. This will take repeated periods of agitation. As the contents go into solution, the water level will drop. Do not add additional water. The procedure will produce a specific gravity of 1.25 to 1.30.

Caution(s): Federal law restricts this drug to use by or on the order of a licensed veterinarian. Keep out of the reach of children.

For veterinary use only.

Presentation: 3.5 lb. containers.

Compendium Code No.: 10940950

FECASOL®

Evsco **Fecal Flotation**

Active Ingredient(s): Solution of sodium nitrate with a consistent, standardized specific gravity of 1.20 in which parasite eggs preferentially float to the surface.

Indications: Ready-to-use flotation medium with standardized specific gravity for reliable, accurate testing. For the flotation of gastro-intestinal parasite eggs from stool samples of small and large animals.

Discussion: Fecal examination for the presence of parasite eggs can be complicated by plant cells, grains or other extraneous matter that can be mistaken for the parasite eggs. It is important, therefore, to use a method that concentrates the eggs and one in which the final preparation is clearer. FECASOL® Solution's specific gravity and purity allows the eggs to float to the surface where they can be collected and examined without contamination from other sources.

Presentation: 1 gallon (3.785 L) bottle.

Compendium Code No.: 10050090

FECATECT DRY CONCENTRATE

Vetus **Fecal Flotation**

Fecal Floatation Medium

Active Ingredient(s): Zinc Sulfate Heptahydrate.

Indications: FECATECT DRY CONCENTRATE is a pre-measured amount of Zinc Sulfate Heptahydrate to be reconstituted and used for floatation techniques of fecal analysis.

Ideal for identifying ova, including Giardia.

Small Animals: Hookworm *(Ancylostoma)*, Ascarid *(Toxocara)*, Whipworm *(Trichuris)*, Coccidia *(Isopora)*, Giardia *(Protozoa)*.

Horses: Strongyles and Roundworms.

Tapeworm can be detected, however this is primarily identified by "rice packets" around the anal area.

Directions: Fill container with warm water to 1 inch from top, secure cap and shake well. Repeat shaking—do not add additional water. This will produce a specific gravity of 1.18.

Testing Procedure: Thoroughly mix 2 grams of fresh feces with 15 mL of Fecatect Solution into a fecal floatation device. When thoroughly mixed, add enough additional Fecatect Solution until a reverse meniscus forms.

Float a 22 mm cover slip or slide on the meniscus. Allow to stand for at least 15 minutes for ova to float through fecal floatation device screen and adhere to cover slip. Place cover slip on microscope slide and examine under low power to look for ova. Centrifugation can be used if desired to save time. Lugols Iodine can be added to the slide to stain giardia cysts if desired.

Warning(s): Keep out of reach of children.

Presentation: 2.9 lb (1.32 kg) containers.

Distributed by: Burns Veterinary Supply, Inc., Westbury, NY 11590.

Compendium Code No.: 14440351

FELAXIN®

Schering-Plough **Laxative**

Active Ingredient(s): Contains:

White petrolatum	47.4% w/w
Malt syrup	47.4% w/w
Cod liver oil	2% w/w
Lecithin	2% w/w
Sodium benzoate (preservative)	0.1% w/w
Vitamin E (dl-alpha tocopheryl acetate) (antioxidant)	0.036 I.U./g

With caramel and purified water.

Indications: For the removal and prevention of hairballs in cats.

Dosage and Administration: Squeeze from the tube onto the cat's nose or tongue. Many cats will readily accept FELAXIN®. For a finicky animal, place a small amount on a front paw, the cat will lick the paw and become accustomed to the taste.

Dosage: For an adult cat of average weight, a strip approximately one (1) inch (2.54 cm) long. For smaller cats, vary the amount accordingly.

For hairball removal: Administer once a day.

For hairball prevention: Administer two (2) to three (3) times a week.

Presentation: 2 oz. (57 g) tubes.

Compendium Code No.: 10470710

FELINE 3 WAY VACCINE

TradeWinds **Vaccine**

Feline Rhinotracheitis-Calici-Panleukopenia Vaccine, Modified Live Virus

U.S. Vet. Lic. No.: 462

Contents: FELINE 3 WAY VACCINE is a combination of modified live Feline Rhinotracheitis, Calici and Panleukopenia viruses. The live viruses contained have been attenuated to assure safety upon administration.

This product contains gentamicin and amphotericin B as preservatives.

Indications: Recommended for use in the vaccination of healthy cats against disease caused by the organisms represented.

Directions: Aseptically rehydrate vial of desiccated antigens by injecting the liquid product into the vial containing the vaccine cake. Shake well. Remove the entire contents back into the syringe. Push out air trapped in the syringe. Administer entire contents (1 mL) subcutaneously under loose skin (back of neck). Do not vaccinate into blood vessels. If blood enters the syringe, choose another injection site.

Persistence of maternal origin antibody in kittens should receive consideration in determining vaccination programs. Ideally, kittens should be vaccinated at 9 weeks of age with revaccination 3-4 weeks later. Adult cats should receive a 1 mL dose followed by a second dose 3-4 weeks later. Annual revaccination with a single 1 mL dose is recommended.

Precaution(s): Store at 35°F-45°F (2°C-7°C). Do not freeze. Use entire contents when first rehydrated. Burn these containers, including syringe and needle.

Caution(s): Do not vaccinate pregnant queens. An occasional animal may demonstrate a transient fever, and mild arthralgia and/or myalgia within the first week following vaccination. In case of anaphylactoid reactions, epinephrine should be administered immediately.

For veterinary use only.

Presentation: 1 dose (1 mL).

Manufactured by: Biocor Animal Health Inc., Omaha, NE 68134 U.S.A.

Compendium Code No.: 12610010 TW4001-1001

FELINE 4 WAY VACCINE

TradeWinds **Vaccine**

Feline Rhinotracheitis-Calici-Panleukopenia-Chlamydia Psittaci Vaccine, Modified Live Virus and Chlamydia

U.S. Vet. Lic. No.: 462

Contents: FELINE 4 WAY VACCINE is a combination of modified live Feline Rhinotracheitis, Calici and Panleukopenia viruses and *Chlamydia psittaci.*

This product contains gentamicin and amphotericin B as preservatives.

Indications: Recommended for use in the vaccination of healthy cats against disease caused by the organisms represented.

Directions: Aseptically rehydrate vial of desiccated antigens by injecting the liquid product into the vial containing the vaccine cake. Shake well. Remove the entire contents back into the syringe. Push out air trapped in the syringe. Administer entire contents (1 mL) subcutaneously under loose skin (back of neck). Do not vaccinate into blood vessels. If blood enters the syringe, choose another injection site.

Persistence of maternal origin antibody in kittens is known to interfere with development of active immunity following vaccination. Ideally, kittens should be vaccinated at 9 weeks of age with revaccination 3-4 weeks later. Adult cats should receive a 1 mL dose followed by a second dose 3-4 weeks later. Annual revaccination with a single 1 mL dose is recommended.

Precaution(s): Store at 35°F-45°F (2°C-7°C). Do not freeze. Use entire contents when first rehydrated. Burn these containers, including syringe and needle.

Caution(s): Do not vaccinate pregnant queens. An occasional animal may demonstrate a transient fever, and mild arthralgia and/or myalgia within the first week following vaccination. In case of anaphylactoid reactions, epinephrine should be administered immediately.

For veterinary use only.

Presentation: 1 dose (1 mL).

Manufactured by: Biocor Animal Health Inc., Omaha, NE 68134 U.S.A.

Compendium Code No.: 12610020 TW4201-800

FELINE F.A./PLUS CHEWABLE TABLETS

Pala-Tech **Small Animal Dietary Supplement**

Omega Fatty Acids, Vitamins and Minerals

Active Ingredient(s): Composition: Each tablet, Pala-Tech™ FELINE F.A./PLUS CHEWABLE TABLETS, contains:

Microencapsulated Fatty Acids
Marine Lipid Concentrates . . . . . 200 mg
Flaxseed Oil . . . . . 50 mg
Vitamins
Taurine (special nutrient) . . . . . 60 mg
Vitamin A . . . . . 1,500 I.U.
Vitamin B_1 (thiamine mononitrate) . . . . . 900 mcg
Vitamin B_2 (riboflavin) . . . . . 1,000 mcg
Vitamin B_6 (pyridoxine HCl) . . . . . 445 mcg
Vitamin B_{12} (cyanocobalamin) . . . . . 4.9 mcg
Vitamin D_3 . . . . . 150 I.U.
Vitamin E . . . . . 4 I.U.
Biotin . . . . . 4.5 mcg
Choline . . . . . 5 mg
Folic Acid . . . . . 40 mcg
Niacin . . . . . 4 mg
Pantothenic Acid . . . . . 1,500 mcg
Minerals
Calcium (from calcium phosphate) . . . . . 10.5 mg
Chloride (from sodium chloride) . . . . . 2.7 mg
Cobalt (from cobalt sulfate) . . . . . 150 mcg
Copper (from copper sulfate) . . . . . 280 mcg
Iodine (from potassium iodide) . . . . . 270 mcg
Iron (from iron oxide) . . . . . 5.2 mg
Manganese (from manganese sulfate) . . . . . 240 mcg
Phosphorus (from calcium phosphate) . . . . . 9 mg
Potassium (from potassium iodide) . . . . . 75 mcg
Selenium (from sodium selenite) . . . . . 6.5 mcg
Sodium (from sodium chloride) . . . . . 1.7 mg
Zinc (from zinc oxide) . . . . . 3.2 mg

Indications: Pala-Tech™ FELINE F.A./PLUS CHEWABLE TABLETS are a supplemental source of omega fatty acids and other essential vitamins and minerals. For supplementation of the diet to aid in the prophylaxis and treatment of fatty acid, multiple vitamin and mineral deficiencies.

Dosage and Administration: Dosage: The following dosage schedule is recommended for the daily administration of Pala-Tech™ FELINE F.A./PLUS CHEWABLE TABLETS. Consult with your veterinarian to determine the proper dosage level and schedule for each individual animal prescribed this product.

Cats under 10 pounds . . . . . ½ to 1 tablet daily
Cats 10 pounds and over . . . . . 1 to 2 tablets daily

Administration: Pala-Tech™ FELINE F.A./PLUS CHEWABLE TABLETS are formulated with a proprietary, highly palatable roast beef and liver flavor base to ensure cats readily consume the tablet. Administer free choice orally to the cat as a treat, or crumble over the cat's food at mealtime.

Precaution(s): Store at room temperature; (58°F-86°F). Avoid excessive heat.

Warning(s): Keep out of reach of children.

For veterinary use only.

Presentation: 60 tablets/bottle.

Compendium Code No.: 10680080 9003-0699

FELINE PLASMA

A.B.B. **Feline Plasma**

CA Vet. Biol. Lic. No.: 83

Active Ingredient(s): Each 10 mL CPDA-1 contains:

Dextrose (hydrous) . . . . . 317 mg USP
Sodium citrate (hydrous) . . . . . 263 mg USP
Citric acid (hydrous) . . . . . 33 mg USP
Monobasic sodium phosphate (monohydrate) . . . . . 22 mg USP
Adenine . . . . . 2.7 mg USP
Water . . . . . q.s. USP

Table of Product Contents:

	Whole Blood	RBC's	Plasma	CPDA-1	Total Fluid Volume	Range
Frozen (1 unit)	-0-	-0-	approx. 20 mL	approx. 5 mL	approx. 25 mL	23-27 mL

FELINE PLASMA, Frozen is a transfusion product aseptically obtained from healthy cats maintained in an isolated, controlled access colony. Blood is not pooled (i.e. each unit of blood is from a single-donor) and euthanasia donors are never used. All colony donors are serologically negative for *Feline immunodeficiency virus* and *Feline leukemia virus.* The blood type of each donor cat is indicated on the product label. The colony receives intensive on site veterinary health care, and all animals are current on immunizations, to include: Feline rhinotracheiti, calici, panleukopenia, pneumonitis, and rabies.

The anticoagulant CPDA-1 is present. It consists of citrate, phosphate, dextrose, and adenine.

A unit of FELINE PLASMA, Frozen is prepared via the centrifugation or sedimentation of feline whole blood. A unit of FELINE PLASMA, Frozen is prepared at any time up to five days after the expiration date applicable to the original unit of whole blood. Clinically, this results in reduced amounts of some coagulation factors in the older product, as well as slightly increased levels of potassium and ammonia; however, such plasma is a viable source of the other components of plasma such as albumin, globulins, and electrolytes, as well as replacement fluid volume. A unit of FELINE PLASMA, Frozen has a total fluid volume of approximately 25 mL; and a shelf-life of five years.

Indications: FELINE PLASMA, Frozen when properly thawed, is indicated for parenteral replenishment of non-labile coagulation factors, albumin, globulins, electrolytes, and fluid volume, as indicated by the clinician's/internist's evaluation of the patient.

Dosage and Administration:

Blood Filter: A blood filter should always be used when administering plasma. When administering over 50 mL of blood to a patient, use the standard blood administration set with its integral 170-230 micron clot screen filter. When administering less than 50 mL of blood to a patient, the standard blood administration set's filter (with a relatively huge surface area) will trap too much blood. Therefore, when transfusing less than 50 mL of blood, the following configuration is recommended:

1. Remove one (1) cap (or peel back one tab on some bags) from the blood bag's diaphragm port, and insert the spike of the drip chamber end of a Venoset 70 Microdrip set into the now uncovered blood bag diaphragm port. The second port found on the bags should remain in place. Non-vented fluid administration sets should be used when using blood bags. This can be simulated by aseptically replacing the Venoset's air filter with the male end of a 3 mL syringe, with its plunger in place. Never leave the Venoset's air filter port uncovered.
2. Attach the needle adaptor end of the Venoset into the female end of a Hemo-Nate neonatal filter,.
3. Then attach the male end of the filter to the female end of an extension set.
4. Attach the male end of the extension set to an IV catheter pre-positioned in the patient. With the above technique, transfusion can be obtained via a slow continuous drip over several hours (or longer), therefore minimizing volume overload.
5. If the bolus technique is preferred, simply aspirate the plasma from the blood bag's needle port into a sterile syringe, then aseptically place the Hemo-Nate filter between the syringe and a fresh sterile needle/catheter, before transfusing.

A needle port can be added to the plasma bag by inserting a Hemo-Tap port into one of the diaphragm ports.

Route of Administration: The jugular, cephalic, and saphenous veins are common sites for IV catheter placement. The intramedullary cavity of the femur and humerus are alternate sites. Additionally, intraperitoneal transfusions have application in selected patients.

Rate of Infusion:

1. There is virtually no rate of blood infusion that is safe for all feline patients; therefore the following are only general guidelines. The actual rate of infusion of blood must be tailored to each individual patient.
2. If clinical conditions permit, the initial rate should be slow (about 0.11 mL/lb. BW over a 30-minute period), in order to observe the patient for transfusion reactions. (0.11 mL/lb. = @ 0.25 mL/kg).
3. Following the initial 30 minute trial infusion, in a animal with a normal state of hydration, plasma may be infused at a rate of 10 mL/lb. BW per 24 hours (22 mL/kg BW per 24 hours). For hypovolemic patients the rate may be increased up to 10 mL/lb. BW per hour; however, given the wide range between those two rates, close monitoring of the patient is essential, with the actual rate being adjusted accordingly.
4. In using the continuous drip method, the blood products' volume is merely included in the 24 hour IV fluid requirements of the animal; then the drip rate is calculated by converting the 24 hour volume into a certain number of drips per minute, or per second (depending on if an infusion pump is being used or the drip rate is being visually monitored).
5. If plasma is being administered for hypoproteinemia, a suggested dose is 6 to 10 mL/kg BW (@ 2.7 to 4.5 mL/lb. BW).

Post-Transfusion Patient Care: During and after transfusions, the patient should be closely monitored. In addition to physical examinations and temperature monitoring, measurement of PCV, urine output, body weight, and EKG are recommended. Measurement of CVP may be utilized in some cases. In all cases, infusion rates should be calculated (rather than estimated) and closely monitored.

Contraindication(s): The plasma was frozen in a horizontal position then stored upright. If the frozen plasma bag shows cracks or signs of premature thawing and refreezing (ie. thicker at the bottom than at the top) do not administer.

Do not administer (via the same infusion system) in conjunction with other fluids or drugs, except 0.9% NaCl.

Do not administer to species other than the domestic cat.

Precaution(s):

1. Frozen plasma bags must be carefully handled to avoid cracking the plastic bags and to avoid contamination during thawing. Thawing should be conducted at 86 to 98.6°F (30 to 37°C). Do not exceed 98.6°F at any time. The use of a controlled temperature circulating warm water bath is the preferred thawing method. Microwave thawing is not recommended.
2. Always conduct a minor cross match before transfusing plasma.
3. Infusion of plasma should begin within six hours of thawing. Do not re-freeze plasma once it has been warmed above 50 degrees.

Frozen Plasma has a shelf-life of five years from the date of collection of the original unit of whole blood. They should be maintained in a freezer at below 0°F. (chest type freezers work best). Store the frozen plasma bags in a vertical position (to detect thawing, as they were originally frozen in an horizontal position). Caution, the defrost cycle on some freezers allows the temperature to briefly rise above zero. This can be partially compensated for by sandwiching plasma bags between bags of deep frozen artificial ice. (This technique will only work if the artificial ice has been pre-frozen to a temperature of below 0°F).

A method of monitoring freezer and refrigerator temperatures is to install an indoor/outdoor thermometer on the freezer, such that the sensor is inside the freezer, yet the gauge is mounted on its casing so that the temperature can be easily read without opening the door or lid.

It is recommended that one of the hospital technicians view and record, at least twice a day, the internal temperature of the plasma freezer.

Caution(s):

1. During transfusions, fluid flow rates must be carefully calculated and monitored, based on the patient's size, weight, age, and clinical condition. It is recommended that urine output be monitored as well.
2. Gently oscillate each bag before use in order to mix contents.
3. Use gloves when handling the dry ice, which is used when shipping frozen plasma.
4. Do not allow dry ice to contact bare skin.
5. Complications of transfusions are manifest by a variety of clinical signs including jaundice, fever, cardiac arrythmias, erratic respiration, salivation, hemoglobinuria, edema, DIC, hemorrhage, vomiting, and urticaria. If any of these clinical signs develop, immediately stop the transfusion and institute appropriate supportive measures, as determined by the patient's clinical condition and the clinician's medical judgment.
6. For use in domestic cats only.

Warning(s):

1. Circulatory overload can occur quickly unless all patient parameters are closely monitored.
2. Do not add medications to the blood bags nor via the same infusion system.
3. In spite of serological screening, disease organisms may still be present in these transfusion products.
4. Platelets are not viable in these products.
5. Do not administer any of these blood products without a blood filter.
6. Do not add Lactated Ringer's solution to plasma. It is safest to use 0.9% NaCl as the only fluid/drug administered in conjunction with these blood products.
7. Transfusion reactions can still occur in spite of correct blood typing and proper cross matching.

References: Available upon request.

Presentation: Units of FELINE PLASMA, Frozen are supplied frozen (packed in dry ice), in blood grade plastic bags (with one IV set coupling port, and reference aliquots [tubing segments]).

Compendium Code No.: 13980030

FELINE RED BLOOD CELLS

A.B.B. **Blood Product**

CA Vet. Biol. Lic. No.: 83

Active Ingredient(s): Each 10 mL CPDA-1 contains:

Dextrose (hydrous) .... 317 mg USP
Sodium citrate (hydrous) .... 263 mg USP
Citric acid (hydrous) .... 33 mg USP
Monobasic sodium phosphate (monohydrate) .... 22 mg USP
Adenine .... 2.7 mg USP
Water .... q.s. USP

Table of Product Contents:

	Whole Blood	RBC's	Plasma	A-S RBC Nutrient Solution	Total Fluid Volume	Range
FELINE RED BLOOD CELLS (packed RBC's) (1 unit)	-0-	approx. 20 mL	-0-	Approx. 10 mL	approx. 30 mL	28-34 mL

FELINE RED BLOOD CELLS is a transfusion product aseptically obtained from healthy cats maintained in an isolated, controlled access colony. Blood is not pooled (ie. each unit of blood is from a single-donor) and euthanasia donors are never used. All colony donors are serologically negative for *Feline immunodeficiency virus* and *Feline leukemia virus.* The blood type of each donor cat is indicated on the product label. The colony receives intensive on site veterinary health care, and all animals are current on immunizations, to include: Feline rhinotracheiti, calici, panleukopenia, pneumonitis, and rabies.

A unit of FELINE RED BLOOD CELLS, (packed RBC's) is the highly cellular fluid remaining in the primary blood bag, after approximately 95% of the plasma and CPDA-1 have been aseptically moved into the satellite bag; 10 mL of A-S RBC Nutrient Solution having then been aseptically added back to the RBC's to retain the 35 day shelf-life of the original unit; for a total fluid volume of approximately 30 mL. Tubing aliquots are present for cross matching.

Indications: FELINE RED BLOOD CELLS (packed RBC's) are indicated for parenteral replenishment of RBC's (such as in conditions of chronic anemia) and especially in situations where the patient is additionally at risk of fluid volume overload. May be used in conjunction with crystalloids for treatment of acute blood loss.

Dosage and Administration: The clinician/surgeon should first determine the desired PCV of the recipient. The following formula may be used to calculate the volume of blood to transfuse:

1 mL of whole blood / 1 pound of body weight = Approx. 1.5% increase in PCV of recipient. This is only a guide. Actual increase will depend on PCV of whole blood, blood compatibility, disease process, etc.

Refrigerated blood should be warmed to room temperature before transfusing. Do not exceed 98.6°F (37°C).

Blood Filter: A blood filter should always be used when administering RBC's. When administering over 50 mL of blood to a patient, use the standard blood administration set with its integral 170-230 micron clot screen filter. When administering less than 50 mL of blood to a patient, the standard blood administration set's filter (with a relatively huge surface area) will trap too much blood. Therefore, when transfusing less than 50 mL of blood, the following configuration is recommended:

1. Remove one (1) cap (or peel back one tab on some bags) from the blood bag's diaphragm port, and insert the spike of the drip chamber end of a Venoset 70 Microdrip set into the now uncovered blood bag diaphragm port. The second port found on blood bags should remain in place. This second port is available for piggybacking a second IV system into the primary blood bag; or for attaching a transfer bag to extract plasma. Non-vented fluid administration sets should be used when using blood bags. This can be simulated by aseptically replacing the Venoset's air filter with the male end of a 3 mL syringe, with its plunger in place. Never leave the Venoset's air filter port uncovered.
2. Attach the needle adaptor end of the Venoset into the female end of a Hemo-Nate neonatal filter.
3. Then attach the male end of the filter to the female end of an extension set.
4. Attach the male end of the extension set to an IV catheter pre-positioned in the patient. With the above technique, transfusion can be obtained via a slow continuous drip over several hours therefore minimizing volume overload.
5. If the bolus technique is preferred, simply aspirate the blood from the blood bag's needle port into a sterile syringe, then aseptically place the Hemo-Nate filter between the syringe and a fresh sterile needle/catheter, before transfusing. For bags without an integral needle port, access can be obtained by using a Hemo-Tap Spike.
6. For kittens and other small patients, adding 0.9% NaCl (not Lactated Ringer's) to the blood will tend to reduce its viscosity and therefore facilitate the use of 22 or 24 gauge needles/catheters.

Route of Administration: The jugular, cephalic, and saphenous veins are common sites for IV catheter placement. The intramedullary cavity of the femur and humerus are alternate sites. Additionally, intraperitoneal transfusions have application in selected patients.

Rate of Infusion:

1. There is virtually no rate of blood infusion that is safe for all feline patients; therefore the following are only general guidelines. The actual rate of infusion of blood must be tailored to each individual patient.
2. If clinical conditions permit, the initial rate should be slow (about 0.11 mL/lb. BW over a 30-minute period), in order to observe the patient for transfusion reactions. (0.11 mL/lb. = @ 0.25 mL/kg).
3. Following the initial 30 minute trial infusion, in a animal with a normal state of hydration, RBC's may be infused at a rate of 10 mL/lb. BW per 24 hours (22 mL/kg BW per 24 hours). For hypovolemic patients the rate may be increased up to 10 mL/lb. BW per hour; however, given the wide range between those two rates, close monitoring of the patient is essential, with the actual rate being adjusted accordingly.
4. In using the continuous drip method, the blood products' volume is merely included in the 24 hour IV fluid requirements of the animal; then the drip rate is calculated by converting the 24 hour volume into a certain number of drips per minute, or per second (depending on if an infusion pump is being used or the drip rate is being visually monitored).

Post-Transfusion Patient Care: During and after transfusions, the patient should be closely monitored. In addition to physical examinations and temperature monitoring, measurement of PCV, urine output, body weight, and EKG are recommended. Measurement of CVP may be utilized in some cases. In all cases, infusion rates should be calculated (rather than estimated) and closely monitored.

Contraindication(s): Do not administer if the blood bags are leaking or if the supernatant exhibits brown or purple discoloration or if excessive hemolysis is present.

Do not administer (via the same infusion system) in conjunction with other fluids or drugs, except 0.9% NaCl.

Do not administer to species other than the domestic cat.

Precaution(s): The product has a shelf-life of 30 days from the date of collection from the donor cat. It should be maintained at a temperature of 33.8° to 42.8°F (1 to 6°C), except during shipment, when 33.8 to 50°F (1 to 10°C) is approved. Store the blood bags in a vertical position, with airspace between each bag (ie. avoid a sardine effect - RBC storage survival is enhanced by the plastic bag's ability to breathe).

Caution(s):

1. During transfusions, fluid flow rates must be carefully calculated and monitored, based on the patient's size, weight, age, and clinical condition. It is recommended that urine output be monitored as well.
2. Gently oscillate each bag before use in order to mix contents.
3. Complications of transfusions are manifest by a variety of clinical signs including jaundice, fever, cardiac arrythmias, erratic respiration, salivation, hemoglobinuria, edema, DIC, hemorrhage, vomiting, and urticaria. If any of these clinical signs develop, immediately stop the transfusion and institute appropriate supportive measures, as determined by the patient's clinical condition and the clinician's medical judgment.
4. For use in domestic cats only.

Warning(s):

1. Circulatory overload can occur quickly unless all patient parameters are closely monitored.
2. Do not add medications to the blood bags nor via the same infusion system.
3. In spite of serological screening, disease organisms may still be present in these transfusion products.
4. Platelets are not viable in these products.
5. Do not administer without a blood filter.
6. Do not add Lactated Ringer's solution to whole blood. It is safest to use 0.9% NaCl as the only fluid/drug administered in conjunction with this product.
7. Transfusion reactions can still occur in spite of correct blood typing and proper cross matching.

Discussion: Cross matching:

Current research divides feline blood types into three blood groups. Feline blood group A, B, and AB. There is no universal blood type in cats. 95% of the feline population is type A. Unlike dogs, cats are born with antigens against unlike blood types.

It is recommended that blood typing be a routine presurgical procedure and a routine part of each animal's first physical examination (and recorded in its permanent medical record), in order to facilitate subsequent transfusion therapy.

Blood cross matching is recommended prior to every transfusion (in addition to using donor blood of the same blood type as the recipient). A major cross match should be conducted prior to each transfusion involving red blood cells. A minor cross match cannot be run on RBC's as the plasma has been removed.

1. Collect 2 mL of recipient blood in a serum tube.
2. Remove (cut) one or two numbered tubing segments from the bag of donor blood; gently shake this segment(s) in order to mix the contents; then collect 2 mL of this donor blood into an empty tube (the Animal Blood Bank donor blood already has CPDA-1 anticoagulant in it; therefore do not add more anticoagulant).
3. Centrifuge both glass tubes at 3400 x G for one minute (or allow the cells to sediment down by letting the samples stand for 30 minutes or longer).
4. Decant recipient plasma and save. Retain the donor packed RBC's. The recipient serum tube may remain as is.
5. Temporarily ignoring the recipient serum tube, wash the donor packed RBC tube as follows: (i) add 2 or 3 mL of 0.9% saline to each RBC tube; (ii) resuspend the cells; (iii) centrifuge as in step (3) above; (iv) discard supernatant, retaining packed RBC's; (v) repeat this wash two more times, ending with tube of packed RBC's (donor).
6. In addition to the recipient serum saved from step (4), prepare new tube as follows: donor 4% RBC suspension (0.2 mL of packed RBC's plus 4.8 mL of 0.9% saline).
7. Now prepare two more glass tubes as follows:
   Tube 1: Two drops recipient serum and one drop recipient 4% RBC suspension (recipient control - should not react).
   Tube 2: Two drops recipient serum and one drop donor 4% RBC suspension (major cross match).
8. If time permits, prepare three sets of the tubes listed in step (7), and incubate one set at 77°F (25°C); one set at 98.6°F (37°C); and the third set at 39.2°F (4°C). If unable to prepare three sets, conduct the cross match at 25°C.
9. Now centrifuge all step (8) tubes at 3400 x G for one minute.
10. Examine the supernatant of all step (9) tubes for hemolysis, then gently tap the tubes to resuspend the red cells and observe for agglutination. Compare the control tube with the major tube.
    If the major cross match shows any agglutination or hemolysis, it is strongly recommended that a different donor blood be considered for that particular recipient.
    A cross match should still be conducted even if the donor and recipient are known to have the same blood type.

References: Available upon request.
Presentation: Units of FELINE RED BLOOD CELLS are supplied refrigerated, in blood grade plastic bags, with one IV line diaphragm port, and reference aliquots [tubing segments]).
Compendium Code No.: 13980040

FELINE WHOLE BLOOD

A.B.B. **Blood Product**

CA Vet. Biol. Lic. No.: 83
Active Ingredient(s): Each 10 mL CPDA-1 contains:

Dextrose (hydrous) . . . . . 317 mg USP
Sodium citrate (hydrous) . . . . . 263 mg USP
Citric acid (hydrous) . . . . . 33 mg USP
Monobasic sodium phosphate (monohydrate) . . . . . 22 mg USP
Adenine . . . . . 2.7 mg USP
Water . . . . . q.s. USP

Table of Product Contents:

	Whole Blood	RBC's	Plasma	CPDA-1	Total Fluid Volume	Range
FELINE WHOLE BLOOD (1 unit)	approx. 45 mL	approx. 20 mL*	approx. 25 mL	approx. 6 mL	approx. 50 mL	40-50 mL

*Based upon an estimated average donor PCV of 40%.

FELINE WHOLE BLOOD is a transfusion product aseptically obtained from healthy cats maintained in an isolated, controlled access colony. Blood is not pooled (ie. each unit of blood is from a single-donor) and euthanasia donors are never used. All colony donors are serologically negative for *Feline immunodeficiency virus* and *Feline leukemia virus*. The blood type of each donor cat is indicated on the product label. The colony receives intensive on-site veterinary health care, and all animals are current on immunizations, to include: Feline rhinotracheiti, calici, panleukopenia, pneumonitis, and rabies.

The anticoagulant CPDA-1 consists of citrate, phosphate, dextrose, and adenine, and provides for a 30 day shelf-life for FELINE WHOLE BLOOD.

Using the single-donor technique, a unit of FELINE WHOLE BLOOD consists of approximately 45 mL whole blood and 6 mL CPDA-1, for a total fluid volume of approximately 50 mL. Each unit (the plastic bag and contents) has blood sequestered in segments of the donor tubing. Cross matching can be accomplished by means of sampling the contents of these tubing aliquots (without entering the primary bag.

Indications: FELINE WHOLE BLOOD is indicated for parenteral replenishment of acute blood loss (such as surgical or traumatic hemorrhage) and other anemia's as indicated by the clinical condition of the patient and the judgment of the surgeon/clinician.

Dosage and Administration:

The clinician/surgeon should first determine the desired PCV of the recipient. The following formula may be used to calculate the volume of blood to transfuse:

1 mL of whole blood / 1 pound of body weight = 1% increase in PCV of recipient. This is only a guide. Actual increase will depend on PCV of whole blood, blood compatibility, disease process, etc.

Refrigerated blood should be warmed to room temperature before transfusing. Do not exceed 98.6°F (37°C).

Blood Filter: A blood filter should always be used when administering whole blood. When administering over 50 mL of blood to a patient, use the standard blood administration set with its integral 170-230 micron clot screen filter. When administering less than 50 mL of blood to a patient, the standard blood administration set's filter (with a relatively huge surface area) will trap too much blood. Therefore, when transfusing less than 50 mL of blood, the following configuration is recommended:

1. Remove one (1) cap (or peel back one tab on some bags) from the blood bag's diaphragm port, and insert the spike of the drip chamber end of a Venoset 70 Microdrip set into the now uncovered blood bag diaphragm port. The second port found on whole blood bags should remain in place. This second port is available for piggybacking a second IV system into the primary blood bag; or for attaching a transfer bag to extract plasma. Non-vented fluid administration sets should be used when using blood bags. This can be simulated by aseptically replacing the Venoset's air filter with the male end of a 3 mL syringe, with its plunger in place. Never leave the Venoset's air filter port uncovered.
2. Attach the needle adaptor end of the Venoset into the female end of a Hemo-Nate neonatal filter.
3. Then attach the male end of the filter to the female end of an extension set.
4. Attach the male end of the extension set to an IV catheter pre-positioned in the patient.
   With the above technique, transfusion can be obtained via a slow continuous drip over several hours (or longer), therefore minimizing volume overload.
5. If the bolus technique is preferred, simply aspirate the blood from the blood bag's needle port into a sterile syringe, then aseptically place the Hemo-Nate filter between the syringe and a fresh sterile needle/catheter, before transfusing.
   The whole blood blood bags have an integral needle port for syringe access.
6. For kittens and other small patients, adding 0.9% NaCl (not Lactated Ringer's) to the blood will tend to reduce its viscosity and therefore facilitate the use of 22 or 24 gauge needles/catheters.

Route of Administration: The jugular, cephalic, and saphenous veins are common sites for IV catheter placement. The intramedullary cavity of the femur and humerus are alternate sites. Additionally, intraperitoneal transfusions have application in selected patients.

Rate of Infusion:

1. There is virtually no rate of blood infusion that is safe for all feline patients; therefore the following are only general guidelines. The actual rate of infusion of blood must be tailored to each individual patient.
2. If clinical conditions permit, the initial rate should be slow (about 0.11 mL/lb. BW over a 30-minute period), in order to observe the patient for transfusion reactions.
   (0.11 mL/lb. = @ 0.25 mL/kg).
3. Following the initial 30 minute trial infusion, in a animal with a normal state of hydration, whole blood may be infused at a rate of 10 mL/lb. BW per 24 hours (22 mL/kg BW per 24 hours). For hypovolemic patients the rate may be increased up to 10 mL/lb. BW per hour; however, given the wide range between those two rates, close monitoring of the patient is essential, with the actual rate being adjusted accordingly.
4. In using the continuous drip method, the blood products' volume is merely included in the 24 hour IV fluid requirements of the animal; then the drip rate is calculated by converting the 24 hour volume into a certain number of drips per minute, or per second (depending on if an infusion pump is being used or the drip rate is being visually monitored).

Post-Transfusion Patient Care: During and after transfusions, the patient should be closely monitored. In addition to physical examinations and temperature monitoring, measurement of PCV, urine output, body weight, and EKG are recommended. Measurement of CVP may be utilized in some cases. In all cases, infusion rates should be calculated (rather than estimated) and closely monitored.

Contraindication(s): Do not administer if the blood bags are leaking or if the supernatant exhibits brown or purple discoloration or if excessive hemolysis is present.

Do not administer (via the same infusion system) in conjunction with other fluids or drugs, except 0.9% NaCl.

Do not administer to species other than the domestic cat.

Precaution(s): The product has a shelf-life of 30 days from the date of collection from the donor cat. It should be maintained at a temperature of 33.8° to 42.8°F (1 to 6°C), except during shipment, when 33.8 to 50°F (1 to 10°C) is approved. Store the blood bags in a vertical position, with airspace between each bag (ie. avoid a sardine effect - RBC storage survival is enhanced by the plastic bag's ability to breathe).

Caution(s):

1. During transfusions, fluid flow rates must be carefully calculated and monitored, based on the patient's size, weight, age, and clinical condition. It is recommended that urine output be monitored as well.
2. Gently oscillate each bag before use in order to mix contents.
3. Complications of transfusions are manifest by a variety of clinical signs including jaundice, fever, cardiac arrythmias, erratic respiration, salivation, hemoglobinuria, edema, DIC, hemorrhage, vomiting, and urticaria. If any of these clinical signs develop, immediately stop the transfusion and institute appropriate supportive measures, as determined by the patient's clinical condition and the clinician's medical judgment.
4. For use in domestic cats only.

Warning(s):

1. Circulatory overload can occur quickly unless all patient parameters are closely monitored.
2. Do not add medications to the blood bags nor via the same infusion system.
3. In spite of serological screening, disease organisms may still be present in these transfusion products.
4. Platelets are not viable in these products.
5. Do not administer without a blood filter.
6. Do not add Lactated Ringer's solution to whole blood. It is safest to use 0.9% NaCl as the only fluid/drug administered in conjunction with this product.
7. Transfusion reactions can still occur in spite of correct blood typing and proper cross matching.

Discussion: Cross matching:

Current research divides feline blood types into three blood groups. Feline blood group A, B, and AB. There is no universal blood type in cats. 95% of the feline population is type A. Unlike dogs, cats are born with antigens against unlike blood types.

It is recommended that blood typing be a routine presurgical procedure and a routine part of each animal's first physical examination (and recorded in its permanent medical record), in order to facilitate subsequent transfusion therapy.

Blood cross matching is recommended prior to every transfusion (in addition to using donor blood of the same blood type as the recipient). A major and minor cross match should be conducted prior to each transfusion involving whole blood; a minor cross match should be conducted prior to every transfusion of plasma.

1. Collect 2 mL of recipient blood in a serum tube and 1 mL of recipient blood in an EDTA or heparin tube.
2. Remove (cut) one or two numbered tubing segments from the bag of donor blood; gently shake this segment(s) in order to mix the contents; then collect this donor blood into an empty tube (the Animal Blood Bank donor blood already has CPDA-1 anticoagulant in it; therefore do not add more anticoagulant).
3. Centrifuge all three glass tubes at 3400 x G for one minute (or allow the cells to sediment down by letting the samples stand for 30 minutes or longer).
4. Decant recipient plasma, retaining recipient packed RBC's. Carefully remove and save the donor plasma, retaining the donor packed RBC's as well. The recipient serum tube may remain as is.
5. Temporarily ignoring the recipient serum tube, wash the two packed RBC tubes as follows: (i) add 2 or 3 mL of 0.9% saline to each RBC tube; (ii) resuspend the cells; (iii) centrifuge as in step (3) above; (iv) discard supernatant, retaining packed RBC's; (v) repeat this wash two more times, ending with two tubes of packed RBC's (donor and recipient).
6. In addition to the donor plasma and recipient serum saved from step (4), prepare new tubes

F

as follows: donor 4% RBC suspension (0.2 mL of packed RBC's plus 4.8 mL of 0.9% saline); and recipient 4% RBC suspension (0.2 mL of recipient packed RBC's plus 4.8 mL of 0.9% saline).

7. Now prepare four more glass tubes as follows:
Tube G-1: Two drops donor plasma and one drop donor 4% RBC suspension (donor control - should not react).
Tube G-2: Two drops recipient serum and one drop recipient 4% RBC suspension (recipient control - should not react).
Tube G-3: Two drops donor plasma and one drop recipient 4% RBC suspension (minor cross match).
Tube G-4: Two drops recipient serum and one drop donor 4% RBC suspension (major cross match).
8. If time permits, prepare three sets of the tubes listed in step (7), and incubate one set at 77°F (25°C); one set at 98.6°F (37°C); and the third set at 39.2°F (4°C). If unable to prepare three sets, conduct the cross match at 25°C.
9. Now centrifuge all step (8) tubes at 3400 x G for one minute.
10. Examine the supernatant of all step (9) tubes for hemolysis, then gently tap the tubes to resuspend the red cells and observe for agglutination. Compare the control tubes with the major and minor cross match tubes.
If the major or minor cross match shows any agglutination or hemolysis, it is strongly recommended that a different donor blood be considered for that particular recipient.
A cross match should still be conducted even if the donor and recipient are known to have the same blood type.

F

References: Available upon request.
Presentation: Units of FELINE WHOLE BLOOD are supplied refrigerated, in blood grade plastic bags (with integral hypodermic needle injection port, two IV line coupling ports, and reference aliquots [tubing segments]).
Compendium Code No.: 13980050

FELIWAY®

Farnam **Pheromone**

Feline Behavior Modification Spray

Active Ingredient(s): Composition:
Analogue of Feline Facial Pheromones 10%
Ethanol (90%) 77.6%
Excipients to .... 75 mL

Indications: Uses:
To stop or to prevent urinary marking by the cat.
To comfort the cat in an unknown or stressful environment (cage, car, boarding, new house, etc.).
FELIWAY® may be used in other specific cases and we advise you to discuss the use of the product with your veterinarian.

Directions for Use: Do not spray FELIWAY® on animals.
1) To stop urine marking: FELIWAY® should be sprayed directly onto the places soiled by the cat and also on prominent objects that could be attractive to the cat. A single dose (one depression of the nozzle) should be applied daily at about 10 cm (4 in) from site, keeping the bottle vertical. The spray should be applied at a height of about 20 cm (8 in) from the floor.
Maintenance treatment of each site is recommended once weekly after the cat is observed rubbing the site with its head and marking it with its own facial pheromones. Where this is not observed, treatment should be continued for 1 month.
The method of use should be modified in the following circumstances:
Sexually excited cats:
When a male cat is marking in response to the presence of a female in heat (this is usually accompanied by continual calling), it is not necessary to apply FELIWAY® on all prominent objects that could be attractive to the cat. In this case, it is usually sufficient to apply FELIWAY® only to the places marked, which are usually near doors and windows.
Multiple cat households:
The risk of urine marking is greater when several cats are present in a household. The application of FELIWAY® should be increased to two or three times per day on marked sites and once a day on prominent objects that could be attractive to the cat.
Elderly cats:
With elderly cats, FELIWAY® may need to be used for 45 days in the manner described for multiple cat households, then once every 2-3 days for as long as necessary.
Important: The use of many cleaning agents and disinfectants will increase the likelihood of urine marking by the cat. It is essential that the soiled sites are not cleaned with bleaches or detergents or their derivatives.
2) To prevent urine marking: In order to prevent urine marking by a cat (new house, boarding, etc.) FELIWAY® should be sprayed once per day on prominent objects that could be attractive to the cat.
One depression of the nozzle should be used about 10 cm (4 in) from the object at a height of 20 cm (8 in) from the floor.
3) To familiarize a cat in a new environment: For transport in a cage, spray the inside of the cage with FELIWAY® about 20 minutes before introducing the cat.
For transport in a car or other vehicle, spray 3-4 times around the cat's usual place in the vehicle before placing the cat in it.
When boarding, spray each corner of the cattery accommodation before introducing the cat. Repeat the sprays daily until the cat is observed rubbing its head in the areas of the sprays.
4) To prevent or stop scratching: Scratching is part of territory marking in its strictest sense. Like urine marking, scratching deposits both visible and pheromone-based territorial marks. The pheromones are released from the pads under the cat's paws onto the scratched surface.
FELIWAY® should be sprayed once per day on areas or surfaces that could be attractive to the cat (typically surfaces that are fully visible and vertical).
One depression of the nozzle should be used about 10 cm (4 in) from the area at a height of 20 cm (8 in) from the floor.

Precaution(s): Keep container tightly closed. Store at room temperature.
Caution(s): The product will not stain or mark. Nevertheless, owing to the wide variety of materials used in household furnishings, we advise that you should test the product on a sample that is not easily visible prior to using it.
For best results, the product should be allowed to come up to room temperature by leaving it in the room for about 1 hour before using it and it should be shaken prior to use.
Flammable, eye irritant.
Keep away from sources of ignition. Avoid contact with eyes. Avoid breathing vapor or mist.
Warning(s): Keep out of reach of children.
Discussion: Properties: This innovative and patented product has some of the properties of feline facial pheromones. Pheromones are chemical substances secreted by animals to confirm their territory and to communicate with others.
The cat usually uses facial pheromones to familiarize itself with its environment. Surfaces that have been marked with these pheromones are recognized by the cat as familiar and comforting. Facial pheromones are deposited by rubbing the object with the side of the face.
Among other properties, facial pheromones will inhibit urinary marking when applied to an area.
The marking involves a well recognized behavioral sequence where the cat:
- selects a vertical surface
- paws at the ground
- turns its back to the surface
- lifts its tail to a vertical position while remaining standing
- sprays the surface with a horizontal jet of urine
The cat will perform this behavioral sequence of urine marking:
- during a period of sexual activity
- following an event that changes its environment (new arrival: human or animal, new object or new furniture, new house or vacations, or any other event perceived by the cat as stressful).
Urine marks produced in this way are characterized by a strong smell, even though the quantity of urine deposited each time is usually small, and they are found at about 20 cm (8 in) above the floor.
Presentation: Box with 75 mL vial.
FELIWAY® is a registered trademark of Ceva Santé Animale.
Compendium Code No.: 10000850 ODDO/0EE0

FELIWAY® ELECTRIC DIFFUSER

V.P.L. **Pheromone**

Composition:
Synthetic analogue of the F3 fraction of feline facial pheromone 2%
Excipients to .... 100 g

Indications: Uses: FELIWAY® Diffuser enables reactions to stressful situations to be controlled and avoided.
Reactions to Stress Are Expressed As: Urine marking, vertical scratching, loss of appetite, reduced desire to play, reduced desire to interact.
Use FELIWAY® in the Following Stress-Inducing Situations: Moving to a new house, visits to the veterinarian and return from hospitalization, adoption, rearrangement of furniture, vacation homes, introducing new arrivals, overcrowding.
Directions: Instructions for Use:
1. Remove the vial cap.
2. Screw the diffuser onto the vial and gently tighten.
3. Plug the diffuser into an electric socket.
For Urine Marking or Scratching: Place the FELIWAY® Diffuser in the room where marking has taken place. If the cat marks several rooms (with a total surface area of more than 650 sq. ft.), use an additional diffuser in one of the other rooms that have been marked.
For Loss of Appetite or Reduced Desire to Interact and Play: Plug in the FELIWAY® Diffuser in the room most used by the cat.
Area Coverage: 500-650 sq. ft.
One vial lasts approximately four weeks.
Precaution(s): Empty packaging and any remnants of the product should be disposed of in accordance with current regulations covering disposal of waste products.
Caution(s): The physiological effects of this product were not tested by Underwriters Laboratories.
The diffuser is specially designed for this product. The properties of the product cannot be guaranteed if a different device is used.
Do not cover.
Check that the main voltage is the same as indicated on the device. Do not place underneath or behind furniture. When plugged in, do not touch the device with metal objects.
When plugged in, do not touch the device with wet hands.
During and immediately after use, do not touch the device with your hands.
The electric device should only be used with this FELIWAY® Diffuser formulation. Use of another substance may increase the toxicity or flammability of the product. The surfaces of the device reach high temperatures to encourage evaporation of active ingredients - these surfaces should not be touched during use of the product.
Warning(s): Keep out of reach of children.
In case of contact with eyes, wash them immediately with water and seek the advice of a doctor.
Avoid contact with skin. In case of contact with skin, wash thoroughly with soap and water.
If the product is swallowed, consult a doctor immediately and show him/her the packaging.
Discussion: The secret to happy cats: When a cat feels safe in its environment, it rubs its head against the furniture, the corners of walls or the bottom of the curtains, leaving substances called facial pheromones. These pheromones convey a message of well-being, calm and absence of stress.
When there are changes in the cat's environment, (such as visits to the veterinarian, return from hospitalization, moving to a new home, new arrivals, rearrangement of furniture), or if the cat is scared, a state of unrest or stress may develop. This state can be conveyed by changes in behavior, such as urine marking, vertical scratching, loss of appetite, or refusal to play and interact.
In these situations, FELIWAY® Diffuser can be used to restore the natural balance. FELIWAY® Diffuser mimics the cat's facial pheromones, creating a state of well-being and calm.
Presentation: Pack Contents: 1 electric diffuser and 1-48 mL vial.
Refill: 1-48 mL vial.
FELIWAY® is a registered trademark of Ceva Santé Animale.
Compendium Code No.: 11430460 01-1840/01-2005

FELIWAY® PHEROMONE SPRAY

V.P.L. **Pheromone**

Active Ingredient(s): Composition:
Analogue of Feline Facial Pheromones 10%
Ethanol (90%) 77.6%
Excipients to .... 75 mL

Indications: Uses:
To stop or to prevent urinary marking by the cat.
To comfort the cat in an unknown or stressful environment (cage, car, boarding, new house, etc.).

FELIWAY® may be used in other specific cases and we advise you to discuss the use of the product with your veterinarian.

Directions: Instructions for Use: Do not spray FELIWAY® on animals.

1) To stop urine marking: FELIWAY® should be sprayed directly onto the places soiled by the cat and also on prominent objects that could be attractive to the cat. A single dose (one depression of the nozzle) should be applied daily at about 10 cm (4 in) from site, keeping the bottle vertical. The spray should be applied at a height of about 20 cm (8 in) from the floor.

Maintenance treatment of each site is recommended once weekly after the cat is observed rubbing the site with its head and marking it with its own facial pheromones. Where this is not observed, treatment should be continued for 1 month.

The method of use should be modified in the following circumstances:

- Sexually excited cats:

When a male cat is marking in response to the presence of a female in heat (this is usually accompanied by continual calling), it is not necessary to apply FELIWAY® on all prominent objects that could be attractive to the cat. In this case, it is usually sufficient to apply FELIWAY® only to the places marked, which are usually near doors and windows.

- Multiple cat households:

The risk of urine marking is greater when several cats are present in a household. The application of FELIWAY® should be increased to two or three times per day on marked sites and once a day on prominent objects that could be attractive to the cat.

- Elderly cats:

With elderly cats, FELIWAY® may need to be used for 45 days in the manner described for multiple cat households, then once every 2-3 days for as long as necessary.

Important: The use of many cleaning agents and disinfectants will increase the likelihood of urine marking by the cat. It is essential that the soiled sites are not cleaned with bleaches or detergents or their derivatives.

2) To prevent urine marking: In order to prevent urine marking by a cat (new house, boarding, etc.) FELIWAY® should be sprayed once per day on prominent objects that could be attractive to the cat.

One depression of the nozzle should be used about 10 cm (4 in) from the object at a height of 20 cm (8 in) from the floor.

3) To familiarize a cat in a new environment: For transport in a cage, spray the inside of the cage with FELIWAY® 20 minutes before introducing the cat.

For transport in a car or other vehicle, spray 3-4 times around the cat's usual place in the vehicle before placing the cat in it.

When boarding, spray each corner of the cattery accommodation before introducing the cat. Repeat the sprays daily until the cat is observed rubbing its head in the areas of the sprays.

4) To prevent or stop scratching: Scratching is part of territory marking in its strictest sense. Like urine marking, scratching deposits both visible and pheromone-based territorial marks. The pheromones are released from the pads under the cat's paws onto the scratched surface.

FELIWAY® should be sprayed once per day on areas or surfaces that could be attractive to the cat (typically surfaces that are fully visible and vertical).

One depression of the nozzle should be used about 10 cm (4 in) from the area at a height of 20 cm (8 in) from the floor.

Precaution(s): Keep away from sources of ignition.

Keep container tightly closed. Store at room temperature.

Caution(s): Flammable, eye irritant.

Avoid contact with eyes. Avoid breathing vapor or mist.

The product will not stain or mark. Nevertheless, owing to the wide variety of materials used in household furnishings, we advise that you should test the product on a sample that is not easily visible prior to using it.

For best results, the product should be allowed to come up to room temperature by leaving it in the room for about 1 hour before using it and it should be shaken prior to use.

Warning(s): Keep out of reach of children.

Discussion: Properties: This innovative and patented product has some of the properties of feline facial pheromones. Pheromones are chemical substances secreted by animals to confirm their territory and to communicate with others.

The cat usually uses facial pheromones to familiarize itself with its environment. Surfaces that have been marked with these pheromones are recognized by the cat as familiar and comforting. Facial pheromones are deposited by rubbing the object with the side of the face.

Among other properties, facial pheromones will inhibit urinary marking when applied to an area.

The marking involves a well recognized behavioral sequence where the cat:

- selects a vertical surface
- paws at the ground
- turns its back to the surface
- lifts its tail to a vertical position while remaining standing
- sprays the surface with a horizontal jet of urine

The cat will perform this behavioral sequence of urine marking:

- during a period of sexual activity
- following an event that changes its environment (new arrival: human or animal, new object or new furniture, new house or vacations, or any other event perceived by the cat as stressful).

Urine marks produced in this way are characterized by a strong smell, even though the quantity of urine deposited each time is usually small, and they are found at about 20 cm (8 in) above the floor.

Presentation: 75 mL spray bottle.

FELIWAY® is a registered trademark of Ceva Santé Animale.

U.S. Patent No. 5,709,863

Compendium Code No.: 11430412 0AA1

FELOCELL® 3

Pfizer Animal Health **Vaccine**

Feline Rhinotracheitis-Calici-Panleukopenia Vaccine, Modified Live Virus

U.S. Vet. Lic. No.: 189

Description: FELOCELL® 3 contains attenuated strains of feline rhinotracheitis virus, calicivirus, and panleukopenia virus (Johnson Snow Leopard strain), propagated on established cell lines. FELOCELL® 3 is packaged in freeze-dried form with inert gas in place of vacuum.

Contains gentamicin as preservative.

Indications: FELOCELL® 3 is for vaccination of healthy cats as an aid in preventing feline viral rhinotracheitis (FVR) caused by feline herpesvirus-1, feline respiratory disease caused by feline calicivirus (FCV), and feline panleukopenia (FPL) caused by feline parvovirus.

Directions:

1. General Directions: Vaccination of healthy cats is recommended. Aseptically rehydrate the freeze-dried vaccine with the sterile diluent provided, shake well, and administer 1 mL intramuscularly or subcutaneously.
2. Primary Vaccination: Healthy cats 12 weeks of age or older should receive 2 doses administered 3-4 weeks apart. Cats vaccinated at less than 12 weeks of age should be revaccinated at 12 weeks of age.
3. Revaccination: Annual revaccination with a single dose is recommended.

Precaution(s): Store at 2°-7°C. Prolonged exposure to higher temperatures and/or direct sunlight may adversely affect potency. Do not freeze.

Use entire contents when first opened.

Sterilized syringes and needles should be used to administer this vaccine. Do not sterilize with chemicals because traces of disinfectant may inactivate the vaccine.

Burn containers and all unused contents.

Caution(s): Vaccination of pregnant queens should be avoided.

As with many vaccines, anaphylaxis may occur after use. Initial antidote of epinephrine is recommended and should be followed with appropriate supportive therapy.

This product has been shown to be efficacious in healthy animals. A protective immune response may not be elicited if animals are incubating an infectious disease, are malnourished or parasitized, are stressed due to shipment or environmental conditions, are otherwise immunocompromised, or the vaccine is not administered in accordance with label directions.

For use in cats only.

For veterinary use only.

Discussion: Disease Description: FVR, caused by feline herpesvirus-1, is highly contagious, spreading both by horizontal (including aerosol) and vertical transmission from queen to kitten. It accounts for approximately 40-45% of feline respiratory infections.[1] First signs of FVR are sneezing, fever, conjunctivitis, rhinitis, and salivation. An initial serous nasal and ocular discharge which rapidly becomes mucopurulent is typical of the disease. Ulcerative keratitis or lossitis may also occur. As FVR progresses, anorexia, depression, tracheitis, and bronchitis may be observed. Abortion or fetal resorption may occur. The prognosis is guarded if cats remain severely infected for more than 1 week. A carrier state lasting for years with periods of latency alternating with episodes of viral shedding is common. Although few adult cats die from FVR, death rate among affected kittens can range from 50-60%.

FCV infection is believed to account for another 40-45% of feline respiratory infections, and dual FCV-FVR infections are not uncommon.[2] FCV infects oral mucous membranes as well as the respiratory tract. Buccal, nasal, and lingual ulcers are characteristic. Other clinical signs of the infection are similar to FVR: anorexia, depression, fever, salivation, and nasal discharge. A carrier state with persistent shedding occurs. FCV most severely affects kittens and debilitated cats, but overall death loss is generally low.

FPL, also known as feline distemper, was once one of the most widespread and serious diseases of cats but has been well controlled by vaccination programs. Highly contagious, FPL is transmitted both directly by contact with infected animals and indirectly by contact with contaminated objects.

Clinical signs of FPL include fever, anorexia, vomiting, depression, and weakness; diarrhea may also occur, usually 2-4 days after onset of fever. Characteristic hematology includes a dramatic loss of circulating white cells. Particularly among kittens, FPL may result in high death loss. Cats that survive infection often remain debilitated for the remainder of their lives. Kittens infected *in utero* or within a few days after birth may suffer cerebellar damage clinically manifested by ataxia.

Trial Data: Safety and Efficacy: Safety of FELOCELL® 3 was demonstrated in field trials involving 2,288 cats. No serious postvaccination reactions attributable to the vaccine were reported.

Efficacy of FELOCELL® 3 was determined by challenge-of-immunity tests. Vaccinated cats experienced significantly less severe clinical signs than nonvaccinated control cats after challenge with virulent FVR virus, FCV, or FPL virus. Efficacy of the FPL fraction in FELOCELL® 3 was further established in a 3-year repeat antigenicity study. Three years after initial efficacy studies were conducted, FPL challenge tests were repeated. After challenge, all vaccinated cats remained clinically healthy while 80% of control cats developed clinical signs of FPL.

Results of serological studies indicated that no immunologic interference existed among the vaccine fractions. In specific pathogen-free cats, vaccination with FELOCELL® 3 stimulated serum neutralization titers to each of the 3 vaccinal viruses.

References: Available upon request.

Presentation: 25 x 1 dose vials.

Compendium Code No.: 36901870 75-0240-00

FELOCELL® 4

Pfizer Animal Health **Vaccine**

Feline Rhinotracheitis-Calici-Panleukopenia-Chlamydia Psittaci Vaccine, Modified Live Virus & Chlamydia

U.S. Vet. Lic. No.: 189

Description: FELOCELL® 4 contains attenuated strains of feline rhinotracheitis virus, calicivirus, and panleukopenia virus (Johnson Snow Leopard strain), and *Chlamydia psittaci*, propagated on established cell lines. FELOCELL® 4 is packaged in freeze-dried form with inert gas in place of vacuum.

Contains gentamicin as preservative.

Indications: FELOCELL® 4 is for vaccination of healthy cats as an aid in preventing feline viral rhinotracheitis (FVR) caused by feline herpesvirus-1, feline respiratory disease caused by feline calicivirus (FCV), feline panleukopenia (FPL) caused by feline parvovirus, and feline chlamydiosis caused by *C. psittaci*.

Directions:

1. General Directions: Vaccination of healthy cats is recommended. Aseptically rehydrate the freeze-dried vaccine with the sterile diluent provided, shake well, and administer 1 mL intramuscularly or subcutaneously.
2. Primary Vaccination: Healthy cats 12 weeks of age or older should receive 2 doses administered 3-4 weeks apart. Cats vaccinated at less than 12 weeks of age should be revaccinated at 12 weeks of age.
3. Revaccination: Annual revaccination with a single dose is recommended.

Precaution(s): Store at 2°-7°C. Prolonged exposure to higher temperatures and/or direct sunlight may adversely affect potency. Do not freeze.

Use entire contents when first opened.

Sterilized syringes and needles should be used to administer this vaccine. Do not sterilize with chemicals because traces of disinfectant may inactivate the vaccine.

Burn containers and all unused contents.

Caution(s): Vaccination of pregnant queens should be avoided.

The use of this product has been associated with fever, anorexia, and lethargy in 1% of vaccinated cats, often occurring in clusters in association with multiple concurrent vaccinations. The onset is typically delayed 7-21 days after vaccination. Symptoms may persist for 3-30 days with an average of 12 days after onset. Veterinary intervention may be required. When treatment is necessary, supportive care, steroids, and antibiotics have been utilized.

As with many vaccines, anaphylaxis may occur after use. Initial antidote of epinephrine is recommended and should be followed with appropriate supportive therapy.

This product has been shown to be efficacious in healthy animals. A protective immune response may not be elicited if animals are incubating an infectious disease, are malnourished or parasitized, are stressed due to shipment or environmental conditions, are otherwise immunocompromised, or the vaccine is not administered in accordance with label directions.

For use in cats only.

For veterinary use only.

Warning(s): In case of accidental human exposure, consult a physician.

Discussion: Disease Description: FVR, caused by feline herpesvirus-1, is highly contagious, spreading both by horizontal (including aerosol) and vertical transmission from queen to kitten. First signs of FVR are sneezing, fever, conjunctivitis, rhinitis, and salivation. An initial serous nasal and ocular discharge which rapidly becomes mucopurulent is typical of the disease. Ulcerative keratitis or glossitis may also occur. As FVR progresses, anorexia, depression, tracheitis, and bronchitis may be observed. Abortion or fetal resorption may occur. The prognosis is guarded if cats remain severely infected for more than 1 week. A carrier state lasting for years with periods of latency alternating with episodes of viral shedding is common. Although few adult cats die from FVR, death rate among affected kittens can range from 50-60%.

FCV infects oral mucous membranes as well as the respiratory tract. Buccal, nasal, and lingual ulcers are characteristic. Other clinical signs of the infection are similar to FVR: anorexia, depression, fever, salivation, and nasal discharge. A carrier state with persistent shedding occurs. FCV most severely affects kittens and debilitated cats, but overall death loss is generally low.

FPL, also known as feline distemper, was once one of the most widespread and serious diseases of cats but has been well controlled by vaccination programs. Highly contagious, FPL is transmitted both directly by contact with infected animals and indirectly by contact with contaminated objects. Clinical signs of FPL include fever, anorexia, vomiting, depression, and weakness; diarrhea may also occur, usually 2-4 days after onset of fever. Characteristic hematology includes a dramatic loss of circulating white cells. Particularly among kittens, FPL may result in high death loss. Cats that survive infection often remain debilitated for the remainder of their lives. Kittens infected *in utero* or within a few days after birth may suffer cerebellar damage clinically manifested by ataxia.

It is generally agreed that at least 90% of cases of upper respiratory disease are caused by feline herpesvirus-1 or feline calicivirus group. Numerous other agents such as *Chlamydia, Mycoplasma, Bordetella,* and reovirus have also been implicated in feline respiratory disease.

Chlamydia psittaci, an intracellular organism resembling a bacterium, replicates primarily in conjunctival and oronasal epithelium. It accounts for less than 5% of feline respiratory disease overall, although it may be a significant problem in catteries. The disease is typified by chronic conjunctivitis and mild rhinitis. Although the disease was once called "pneumonitis", lower respiratory tract involvement does not appear to be significant. Early conjunctival signs of chlamydiosis usually are unilateral blepharospasm, congestion, and increased lacrimation, which may become bilateral and be accompanied by mucopurulent ocular discharge. Fever, rhinitis, and sneezing are infrequently observed. Anorexia and depression are uncommon. Some cats become carriers with intermittent shedding of organisms from the epithelium of the conjunctiva, gastrointestinal, and lower genital tracts. The course of infection is 2-6 weeks in kittens and up to 2 weeks in older cats, but the disease is rarely fatal.[1-6]

Trial Data: Safety and Efficacy: Safety of FELOCELL® 4 was demonstrated in field trials involving 2,288 cats. The majority of cats exhibited no serious postvaccination reactions attributable to the vaccine. However, approximately 1% of vaccinated cats exhibited lethargy, anorexia, and fever after vaccination. (See Cautions).

Efficacy of FELOCELL® 4 was determined by challenge-of-immunity tests. Vaccinated cats experienced significantly less severe clinical signs than nonvaccinated control cats after challenge with virulent FVR virus, FCV, FPL virus, or *C. psittaci.*

Results of serological studies indicated that no immunologic interference existed among the vaccine fractions. In specific-pathogen-free cats, vaccination with FELOCELL® 4 stimulated serologic titers to each of the 4 vaccine fractions.

References: Available upon request.

Presentation: 1 dose vial and 25 x 1 dose vials.

Compendium Code No.: 36901880 75-0209-00

FELOCELL® FPV

Pfizer Animal Health **Vaccine**

Feline Panleukopenia Vaccine, Modified Live Virus

U.S. Vet. Lic. No.: 189

Description: FELOCELL® FPV contains an attenuated strain of feline panleukopenia virus (Johnson Snow Leopard strain) propagated on an established cell line. FELOCELL® FPV is packaged in freeze-dried form with inert gas in place of vacuum.

Contains gentamicin as preservative.

Indications: FELOCELL® FPV is for vaccination of healthy cats 12 weeks of age or older as an aid in preventing feline panleukopenia (FPL) caused by feline parvovirus (FPV).

Directions:

1. General Directions: Vaccination of healthy cats is recommended. Aseptically rehydrate the freeze-dried vaccine with the sterile diluent provided, shake well, and administer 1 mL intramuscularly or subcutaneously.
2. Primary Vaccination: Healthy cats 12 weeks of age or older should receive 2 doses administered 3-4 weeks apart. Cats vaccinated at less than 12 weeks of age should be revaccinated at 12 weeks of age.
3. Revaccination: Annual revaccination with a single dose is recommended.

Precaution(s): Store at 2°-7°C. Prolonged exposure to higher temperatures and/or direct sunlight may adversely affect potency. Do not freeze.

Use entire contents when first opened.

Sterilized syringes and needles should be used to administer this vaccine. Do not sterilize with chemicals because traces of disinfectant may inactivate the vaccine.

Burn containers and all unused contents.

Caution(s): Vaccination of pregnant queens should be avoided.

As with many vaccines, anaphylaxis may occur after use. Initial antidote of epinephrine is recommended and should be followed with appropriate supportive therapy.

This product has been shown to be efficacious in healthy animals. A protective immune response may not be elicited if animals are incubating an infectious disease, are malnourished or parasitized, are stressed due to shipment or environmental conditions, are otherwise immunocompromised, or the vaccine is not administered in accordance with label directions.

For use in cats only.

For veterinary use only.

Discussion: Disease Description: FPL, also known as feline distemper, was once one of the most widespread and serious diseases of cats but has been well controlled by vaccination programs.

Highly contagious, FPL is transmitted both directly by contact with infected animals and indirectly by contact with contaminated objects. Clinical signs of FPL include fever, anorexia, vomiting, depression, and weakness; diarrhea may also occur, usually 2-4 days after onset of fever. Characteristic hematology includes a dramatic loss of circulating white cells. Particularly among kittens, FPL may result in high death loss. Cats that survive infection often remain debilitated for the remainder of their lives. Kittens infected *in utero* or within a few days after birth may suffer cerebellar damage clinically manifested by ataxia.

Trial Data: Safety and Efficacy: Safety of FELOCELL® FPV was demonstrated in field trials involving 2,288 cats. No serious postvaccination reactions attributable to the vaccine were reported.

Efficacy of FELOCELL® FPV was determined by challenge-of-immunity tests. Vaccinated cats experienced significantly less severe clinical signs than nonvaccinated control cats after challenge with virulent FPL virus. In specific-pathogen-free cats, vaccination with FELOCELL® FPV stimulated serologic titers to the FPL fraction.

Presentation: 25 x 1 dose vials.

Compendium Code No.: 36901890 75-5312-00

FELOCELL® RESP-2

Pfizer Animal Health **Vaccine**

Feline Rhinotracheitis-Calici Vaccine, Modified Live Virus

U.S. Vet. Lic. No.: 189

Description: FELOCELL® RESP-2 contains attenuated strains of feline rhinotracheitis virus and calicivirus propagated on established cell lines. FELOCELL® RESP-2 is packaged in freeze-dried form with inert gas in place of vacuum.

Contains gentamicin as preservative.

Indications: FELOCELL® RESP-2 is for vaccination of healthy cats as an aid in preventing feline viral rhinotracheitis (FVR) caused by feline herpesvirus-1 and feline respiratory disease caused by feline calicivirus (FCV).

Directions:

1. General Directions: Vaccination of healthy cats is recommended. Aseptically rehydrate the freeze-dried vaccine with the sterile diluent provided, shake well, and administer 1 mL intramuscularly or subcutaneously.
2. Primary Vaccination: Healthy cats 12 weeks of age or older should receive 2 doses administered 3-4 weeks apart. Cats vaccinated at less than 12 weeks of age should be revaccinated at 12 weeks of age.
3. Revaccination: Annual revaccination with a single dose is recommended.

Precaution(s): Store at 2°-7°C. Prolonged exposure to higher temperatures and/or direct sunlight may adversely affect potency. Do not freeze.

Use entire contents when first opened.

Sterilized syringes and needles should be used to administer this vaccine. Do not sterilize with chemicals because traces of disinfectant may inactivate the vaccine.

Burn containers and all unused contents.

Caution(s): Vaccination of pregnant queens should be avoided.

As with many vaccines, anaphylaxis may occur after use. Initial antidote of epinephrine is recommended and should be followed with appropriate supportive therapy.

This product has been shown to be efficacious in healthy animals. A protective immune response may not be elicited if animals are incubating an infectious disease, are malnourished or parasitized, are stressed due to shipment or environmental conditions, are otherwise immunocompromised, or the vaccine is not administered in accordance with label directions.

For use in cats only.

For veterinary use only.

Discussion: Disease Description: FVR, caused by feline herpesvirus-1, is highly contagious, spreading both by horizontal (including aerosol) and vertical transmission from queen to kitten. It accounts for approximately 40-45% of feline respiratory infections.[1] First signs of FVR are sneezing, fever, conjunctivitis, rhinitis, and salivation. An initial serous nasal and ocular discharge, which rapidly becomes mucopurulent, is typical of the disease. Ulcerative keratitis or glossitis may also occur. As FVR progresses, anorexia, depression, tracheitis, and bronchitis may be observed. Abortion or fetal resorption may occur. The prognosis is guarded if cats remain severely infected for more than 1 week. A carrier state lasting for years with periods of latency alternating with episodes of viral shedding is common. Although few adult cats die from FVR, death rate among affected kittens can range from 50-60%.

FCV infection is believed to account for another 40-45% of feline respiratory infections, and dual FCV-FVR infections are not uncommon.[2] FCV infects oral mucous membranes as well as the respiratory tract. Buccal, nasal, and lingual ulcers are characteristic. Other clinical signs of the infection are similar to FVR: anorexia, depression, fever, salivation, and nasal discharge. A carrier state with persistent shedding occurs. FCV most severely affects kittens and debilitated cats, but overall death loss is generally low.

Trial Data: Safety and Efficacy: Safety of the fractions contained in FELOCELL® RESP-2 was demonstrated in field trials involving 2,288 cats. No serious postvaccination reactions attributable to the vaccine were reported.

Efficacy of the fractions contained in FELOCELL® RESP-2 was determined by challenge-of-immunity tests. Vaccinated cats experienced significantly less severe clinical signs than nonvaccinated control cats after challenge with virulent FVR virus or FCV.

Results of serological studies indicated that no immunologic interference existed between the vaccine fractions. In specific-pathogen-free cats, vaccination with FELOCELL® RESP-2 antigens stimulated serum neutralization titers to each of the 2 vaccinal viruses.

References: Available upon request.

Presentation: 25 x 1 dose vials.

Compendium Code No.: 36901900 75-5313-01

FELOCELL® RESP-3

Pfizer Animal Health **Vaccine**

Feline Rhinotracheitis-Calici-Chlamydia Psittaci Vaccine, Modified Live Virus & Chlamydia

U.S. Vet. Lic. No.: 189

Description: FELOCELL® RESP-3 contains attenuated strains of feline rhinotracheitis virus, calicivirus, and *Chlamydia psittaci* propagated on established cell lines. FELOCELL® RESP-3 is packaged in freeze-dried form with inert gas in place of vacuum.

Contains gentamicin as preservative.

Indications: FELOCELL® RESP-3 is for vaccination of healthy cats as an aid in preventing feline viral rhinotracheitis (FVR) caused by feline herpesvirus-1, feline respiratory disease caused by feline calicivirus (FCV), and feline chlamydiosis caused by *C. psittaci.*

Directions:

1. General Directions: Vaccination of healthy cats is recommended. Aseptically rehydrate the freeze-dried vaccine with the sterile diluent provided, shake well, and administer 1 mL intramuscularly or subcutaneously.
2. Primary Vaccination: Healthy cats 12 weeks of age or older should receive 2 doses administered 3-4 weeks apart. Cats vaccinated at less than 12 weeks of age should be revaccinated at 12 weeks of age.
3. Revaccination: Annual revaccination with a single dose is recommended.

Precaution(s): Store at 2°-7°C. Prolonged exposure to higher temperatures and/or direct sunlight may adversely affect potency. Do not freeze.

Use entire contents when first opened.

Sterilized syringes and needles should be used to administer this vaccine. Do not sterilize with chemicals because traces of disinfectant may inactivate the vaccine.

Burn containers and all unused contents.

Caution(s): Vaccination of pregnant queens should be avoided.

The use of this product has been associated with fever, anorexia, and lethargy in 1% of vaccinated cats, often occurring in clusters in association with multiple concurrent vaccinations. The onset is typically delayed 7-21 days after vaccination. Symptoms may persist for 3-30 days with an average of 12 days after onset. Veterinary intervention may be required. When treatment is necessary, supportive care, steroids, and antibiotics have been utilized.

As with many vaccines, anaphylaxis may occur after use. Initial antidote of epinephrine is recommended and should be followed with appropriate supportive therapy.

This product has been shown to be efficacious in healthy animals. A protective immune response may not be elicited if animals are incubating an infectious disease, are malnourished or parasitized, are stressed due to shipment or environmental conditions, are otherwise immunocompromised, or the vaccine is not administered in accordance with label directions.

For use in cats only.

For veterinary use only.

Warning(s): In case of accidental human exposure, consult a physician.

Discussion: Disease Description: FVR, caused by feline herpesvirus-1, is highly contagious, spreading both by horizontal (including aerosol) and vertical transmission from queen to kitten. First signs of FVR are sneezing, fever, conjunctivitis, rhinitis, and salivation. An initial serous nasal and ocular discharge which rapidly becomes mucopurulent, is typical of the disease. Ulcerative keratitis or glossitis may also occur. As FVR progresses, anorexia, depression, tracheitis, and bronchitis may be observed. Abortion or fetal resorption may occur. The prognosis is guarded if cats remain severely infected for more than 1 week. A carrier state lasting for years with periods of latency alternating with episodes of viral shedding is common. Although few adult cats die from FVR, death rate among affected kittens can range from 50-60%.

FCV infects oral mucous membranes as well as the respiratory tract. Buccal, nasal, and lingual ulcers are characteristic. Other clinical signs of the infection are similar to FVR: anorexia, depression, fever, salivation, and nasal discharge. A carrier state with persistent shedding occurs. FCV most severely affects kittens and debilitated cats, but overall death loss is generally low.

It is generally agreed that at least 90% of cases of upper respiratory disease are caused by feline herpesvirus-1 or feline calicivirus group. Numerous other agents such as *Chlamydia, Mycoplasma, Bordetella,* and reovirus have also been implicated in feline respiratory disease.

C. psittaci, an intracellular organism resembling a bacterium, replicates primarily in conjunctival and oronasal epithelium. It accounts for less than 5% of feline respiratory disease overall, although it may be a significant problem in catteries. The disease is typified by chronic conjunctivitis and mild rhinitis. Although the disease was once called "pneumonitis", lower respiratory tract involvement does not appear to be significant. Early conjunctival signs of chlamydiosis usually are unilateral blepharospasm, congestion, and increased lacrimation, which may become bilateral and be accompanied by mucopurulent ocular discharge. Fever, rhinitis, and sneezing are infrequently observed. Anorexia and depression are uncommon. Some cats become carriers with intermittent shedding of organisms from the epithelium of the conjunctiva, gastrointestinal, and lower genital tracts. The course of infection is 2-6 weeks in kittens and up to 2 weeks in older cats, but the disease is rarely fatal.[1-6]

Trial Data: Safety and Efficacy: Safety of the fractions contained in FELOCELL® RESP-3 was demonstrated in field trials involving 2,288 cats. The majority of cats exhibited no serious postvaccination reactions attributable to the vaccine. However, approximately 1% of vaccinated cats exhibited lethargy, anorexia, and fever after vaccination. (See Cautions).

Efficacy of the fractions contained in FELOCELL® RESP-3 was determined by challenge-of-immunity tests. Vaccinated cats experienced significantly less severe clinical signs than nonvaccinated control cats after challenge with virulent FVR virus, FCV, or *C. psittaci.*

Results of serological studies indicated that no immunologic interference existed among the vaccine fractions. In specific-pathogen-free cats, vaccination with FELOCELL® RESP-3 stimulated serologic titers to each of the 3 vaccine fractions.

References: Available upon request.

Presentation: 25 x 1 dose vials.

Compendium Code No.: 36901910 75-5314-01

FELO-FORM

Vet-A-Mix **Small Animal Dietary Supplement**

Chewable dietary supplement with taurine and potassium for cats

Guaranteed Analysis: per Tablet:

(All values are minimum quantities unless otherwise stated.)

Minerals:

Calcium (min.)	6.8%
(max.)	8.1%
Phosphorus	3.5%
Potassium	1.4%
Iron	3 mg
Zinc	1.25 mg
Manganese	0.5 mg
Copper	0.18 mg
Cobalt	0.06 mg
Iodine	0.05 mg
Selenium	2 mcg.

Vitamins and Others:

Taurine	60 mg
Choline chloride	10 mg
Niacin	5 mg
Vitamin E	1 IU
Thiamine mononitrate	0.5 mg
Riboflavin	0.5 mg
Vitamin A	750 IU
D-Pantothenic acid	0.25 mg
Pyridoxine hydrochloride	0.05 mg
Folic acid	25 mcg
Vitamin D_3	75 IU
Vitamin B_{12}	1.5 mcg

Ingredients: Extracted glandular meal (pork), Brewer's dried yeast, Dicalcium phosphate, Liver meal (pork), Cellulose powder, Calcium carbonate, Taurine, Glycerin, Potassium chloride, Silicon dioxide, Gelatin, Choline chloride, Soybean oil, DL-methionine, Lactose, Ferrous fumarate, Niacin, D-pantothenic acid, Vitamin A palmitate, Manganese sulfate, DL-alpha tocopheryl acetate, Zinc oxide, Thiamine mononitrate, Povidone, Vitamin B_{12} supplement, Copper sulfate, Potassium phosphate, Riboflavin, Sodium selenite, Cholecalciferol, Cobalt sulfate, Folic acid, Ethylenediamine dihydriodide, Pyridoxine hydrochloride.

Indications: Use as a dietary supplement for cats.

Dosage and Administration: Feed free choice or crumble in food.

Recommended Daily Dosage:

Kittens—½ tablet.

Adult Cats—1 tablet for diet supplementation; 2 tablets for convalescing, pregnant or nursing cats.

Warning(s): Keep out of reach of children.

Presentation: Bottles of 50 and 150 tablets.

Compendium Code No.: 10500091 0399

F

FEL-O-GUARD® PLUS 2

Fort Dodge **Vaccine**

Feline Rhinotracheitis-Calici Vaccine, Modified Live Virus

U.S. Vet. Lic. No.: 112

Contents: This product contains the antigens listed above.

Neomycin and polymyxin B added as preservatives.

Indications: For subcutaneous vaccination of healthy cats, eight weeks of age or older, as an aid in the prevention of disease caused by feline rhinotracheitis and calici viruses.

Directions for Use: Aseptically rehydrate with accompanying diluent. Cats, inject (one) 1 mL dose subcutaneously using aseptic technique. Administer a second 1 mL dose three to four weeks later. Annual revaccination is recommended.

InfoVax-ID® System: The InfoVax-ID® System provides a simple and effective method of recording pertinent information on the vaccines administered to animals in a veterinary practice.

For vaccines requiring reconstitution, remove label from both vials and affix both labels to the animal's medical chart.

Using the InfoVax-ID® System:

1. Grasp the lower right hand corner of the tab at the arrow marked "Peel Here" between your thumb and forefinger.
2. Pull steadily at a slight upward angle until the top portion of the label is separated from the vial.
3. Place the label on the animal's medical chart. Press down on the label to ensure adhesion.

Precaution(s): Store in dark at 2° to 7°C (35° to 45°F). Avoid freezing. Shake well. Burn container and all unused contents.

Caution(s): In the absence of a veterinarian-client-patient relationship, Federal law prohibits the relabeling, repackaging, resale, or redistribution of the individual contents of this package. (9 CFR 112.6)

Do not vaccinate pregnant queens.

In case of anaphylactoid reaction, administer epinephrine.

Warning(s): For use in cats only.

For veterinary use only.

Presentation: 25 doses (25 x 1 mL vials of vaccine plus 25 x 1 mL vials of diluent), featuring the InfoVax-ID® System.

U.S. Pat. No. 5,704,648 (InfoVax-ID® System)

Compendium Code No.: 10030741 1032A

FEL-O-GUARD® PLUS 3

Fort Dodge **Vaccine**

Feline Rhinotracheitis-Calici-Panleukopenia Vaccine, Modified Live Virus

U.S. Vet. Lic. No.: 112

Contents: This product contains the antigens listed above.

Neomycin and polymyxin B added as preservatives.

Indications: For subcutaneous vaccination of healthy cats, eight weeks of age or older, as an aid in the prevention of disease caused by feline rhinotracheitis, calici and panleukopenia viruses.

Directions for Use: Aseptically rehydrate with accompanying diluent. Cats, inject (one) 1 mL dose subcutaneously using aseptic technique. Administer a second 1 mL dose three to four weeks later. Annual revaccination is recommended.

InfoVax-ID® System: The InfoVax-ID® System provides a simple and effective method of recording pertinent information on the vaccines administered to animals in a veterinary practice.

For vaccines requiring reconstitution, remove label from both vials and affix both labels to the animal's medical chart.

Using the InfoVax-ID® System:

1. Grasp the lower right hand corner of the tab at the arrow marked "Peel Here" between your thumb and forefinger.
2. Pull steadily at a slight upward angle until the top portion of the label is separated from the vial.
3. Place the label on the animal's medical chart. Press down on the label to ensure adhesion.

Precaution(s): Store in dark at 2° to 7°C (35° to 45°F). Avoid freezing. Shake well. Burn container and all unused contents.

Caution(s): In the absence of a veterinarian-client-patient relationship, Federal law prohibits the relabeling, repackaging, resale, or redistribution of the individual contents of this package. (9 CFR 112.6)

Do not vaccinate pregnant queens.

In case of anaphylactoid reaction, administer epinephrine.

Warning(s): For veterinary use only.

Presentation: 25 doses (25 x 1 mL vials of vaccine plus 25 x 1 mL vials of diluent), featuring the InfoVax-ID® System.

U.S. Pat. No. 5,704,648 (InfoVax-ID® System)

Compendium Code No.: 10030751 1172A

FEL-O-GUARD® PLUS 3 + Lv-K

Fort Dodge **Vaccine**

Feline Leukemia-Rhinotracheitis-Calici-Panleukopenia Vaccine, Modified Live Virus and Killed Virus

U.S. Vet. Lic. No.: 112

Contents: This product contains the antigens listed above.

Thimerosal, neomycin and polymyxin B added as preservatives.

Indications: For subcutaneous vaccination of healthy cats, eight weeks of age or older, as an aid in the prevention of disease caused by feline leukemia, rhinotracheitis, calici and panleukopenia viruses.

Directions for Use: Aseptically rehydrate with accompanying diluent. Inject (one) 1 mL dose subcutaneously using aseptic technique. Administer a second 1 mL dose three to four weeks later. Annual revaccination is recommended.

InfoVax-ID® System: The InfoVax-ID® System provides a simple and effective method of recording pertinent information on the vaccines administered to animals in a veterinary practice.

For vaccines requiring reconstitution, remove label from both vials and affix both labels to the animal's medical chart.

Using the InfoVax-ID® System:

1. Grasp the lower right hand corner of the tab at the arrow marked "Peel Here" between your thumb and forefinger.
2. Pull steadily at a slight upward angle until the top portion of the label is separated from the vial.
3. Place the label on the animal's medical chart. Press down on the label to ensure adhesion.

F

Precaution(s): Store in dark at 2° to 7°C (35° to 45°F). Avoid freezing. Shake well. Burn container and all unused contents.

Caution(s): In the absence of a veterinarian-client-patient relationship, Federal law prohibits the relabeling, repackaging, resale, or redistribution of the individual contents of this package. (9 CFR 112.6)

Do not vaccinate pregnant queens. In case of anaphylactoid reaction, administer epinephrine.

Warning(s): For veterinary use only.

Presentation: 25 doses (25 x 1 mL vials of vaccine plus 25 x 1 mL vials of diluent), featuring the InfoVax-ID® System.

U.S. Pat. No. 5,704,648 (InfoVax-ID® System)

Compendium Code No.: 10030761 3435A

FEL-O-GUARD® PLUS 4

Fort Dodge **Vaccine**

Feline Rhinotracheitis-Calici-Panleukopenia-Chlamydia Psittaci Vaccine, Modified Live Virus and Killed Chlamydia

U.S. Vet. Lic. No.: 112

Contents: This product contains the antigens listed above.

Neomycin and polymyxin B added as preservatives.

Indications: For subcutaneous vaccination of healthy cats, eight weeks of age or older, as an aid in the prevention of disease caused by feline rhinotracheitis, calici, panleukopenia viruses and feline *Chlamydia psittaci*.

Directions for Use: Aseptically rehydrate with accompanying diluent. Cats, inject (one) 1 mL dose subcutaneously using aseptic technique. Administer a second 1 mL dose three to four weeks later. Annual revaccination is recommended.

InfoVax-ID® System: The InfoVax-ID® System provides a simple and effective method of recording pertinent information on the vaccines administered to animals in a veterinary practice.

For vaccines requiring reconstitution, remove label from both vials and affix both labels to the animal's medical chart.

Using the InfoVax-ID® System:

1. Grasp the lower right hand corner of the tab at the arrow marked "Peel Here" between your thumb and forefinger.
2. Pull steadily at a slight upward angle until the top portion of the label is separated from the vial.
3. Place the label on the animal's medical chart. Press down on the label to ensure adhesion.

Precaution(s): Store in dark at 2° to 7°C (35° to 45°F). Avoid freezing. Shake well. Use entire contents when first opened. Burn container and all unused contents.

Caution(s): In the absence of a veterinarian-client-patient relationship, Federal law prohibits the relabeling, repackaging, resale, or redistribution of the individual contents of this package. (9 CFR 112.6)

Do not vaccinate pregnant queens. In case of anaphylactoid reaction, administer epinephrine.

Warning(s): For veterinary use only.

Presentation: 25 doses (25 x 1 mL vials of vaccine plus 25 x 1 mL vials of diluent), featuring the InfoVax-ID® System.

U.S. Patent Nos. 5,242,686 — 6,004,563

U.S. Pat. No. 5,704,648 (InfoVax-ID® System)

Compendium Code No.: 10030771 1265B

FEL-O-GUARD® PLUS 4 + Lv-K

Fort Dodge **Vaccine**

Feline Leukemia-Rhinotracheitis-Calici-Panleukopenia-Chlamydia Psittaci Vaccine, Modified Live Virus and Killed Virus and Chlamydia

U.S. Vet. Lic. No.: 112

Contents: This product contains the antigens listed above.

Neomycin, thimerosal and polymyxin B added as preservatives.

Indications: For subcutaneous vaccination of healthy cats, eight weeks of age or older, as an aid in the prevention of disease caused by feline leukemia, rhinotracheitis, calici, panleukopenia viruses and feline *Chlamydia psittaci*.

Directions for Use: Aseptically rehydrate with accompanying diluent. Cats, inject (one) 1 mL dose subcutaneously using aseptic technique. Administer a second 1 mL dose three to four weeks later. Annual revaccination is recommended.

InfoVax-ID® System: The InfoVax-ID® System provides a simple and effective method of recording pertinent information on the vaccines administered to animals in a veterinary practice.

For vaccines requiring reconstitution, remove label from both vials and affix both labels to the animal's medical chart.

Using the InfoVax-ID® System:

1. Grasp the lower right hand corner of the tab at the arrow marked "Peel Here" between your thumb and forefinger.
2. Pull steadily at a slight upward angle until the top portion of the label is separated from the vial.
3. Place the label on the animal's medical chart. Press down on the label to ensure adhesion.

Precaution(s): Store in dark at 2° to 7°C (35° to 45°F). Avoid freezing. Shake well. Burn container and all unused contents.

Caution(s): In the absence of a veterinarian-client-patient relationship, Federal law prohibits the relabeling, repackaging, resale, or redistribution of the individual contents of this package. (9 CFR 112.6)

Do not vaccinate pregnant queens.

In case of anaphylactoid reaction, administer epinephrine.

Warning(s): For veterinary use only.

Presentation: 25 doses (25 x 1 mL vials of vaccine plus 25 x 1 mL vials of diluent), featuring the InfoVax-ID® System.

U.S. Patent Nos. 5,242,686 — 6,004,563

U.S. Pat. No. 5,704,648 (InfoVax-ID® System)

Compendium Code No.: 10030781 2822D

FELOMUNE CVR®

Pfizer Animal Health **Vaccine**

Feline Rhinotracheitis-Calici Vaccine, Modified Live Virus

U.S. Vet. Lic. No.: 189

Description: FELOMUNE CVR® contains attenuated strains of feline rhinotracheitis virus and feline calicivirus propagated on an established feline cell line and freeze-dried to preserve stability.

Contains gentamicin as preservative.

Indications: FELOMUNE CVR® is for intranasal vaccination of healthy cats as an aid in preventing feline rhinotracheitis (FVR) caused by feline herpesvirus-1 and feline respiratory disease caused by feline calicivirus (FCV).

Directions:

1. General Directions: Vaccination of healthy cats is recommended. Aseptically rehydrate the freeze-dried vaccine with the sterile diluent provided. Shake well. Using sterile dropper, inoculate nasal passages with entire volume of vaccine. Alternatively, 1 drop of vaccine may be placed in each eye and the remainder placed into nasal passages. Administer vaccine within 30 minutes after rehydration.
2. Primary Vaccination: Healthy cats 12 weeks of age or older should receive one 0.5-mL dose. Cats vaccinated at less than 12 weeks of age should be revaccinated at 12 weeks of age.
3. Revaccination: Annual revaccination with a single dose is recommended.

Precaution(s): Store at 2°-7°C. Prolonged exposure to higher temperatures and/or direct sunlight may adversely affect potency. Do not freeze.

Use entire contents when first opened.

Burn containers and all unused contents.

Caution(s): As with many vaccines, anaphylaxis may occur after use. Initial antidote of epinephrine is recommended and should be followed with appropriate supportive therapy.

This product has been shown to be efficacious in healthy animals. A protective immune response may not be elicited if animals are incubating an infectious disease, are malnourished or parasitized, are stressed due to shipment or environmental conditions, are otherwise immunocompromised, or the vaccine is not administered in accordance with label directions.

Warning(s): Transient sneezing may be observed 4-7 days after vaccination. Oral lesions may be observed postvaccinally, but typically heal without incident. Vaccination of cats incubating or harboring latent infections may result in more pronounced upper respiratory signs, ocular irritation, or febrile response.

For intranasal use in cats only.

For veterinary use only.

Discussion: Disease Description: FVR and FCV infections are considered the two most important forms of feline respiratory disease.[1]

FVR, caused by feline herpesvirus-1, is highly contagious, spreading both by horizontal (including aerosol) and vertical transmission from queen to kitten. It accounts for approximately 40-45% of feline respiratory infections.[2] First signs of FVR are sneezing, fever, conjunctivitis, rhinitis, and salivation. An initial serous nasal and ocular discharge which rapidly becomes mucopurulent is typical of the disease. Ulcerative keratitis or glossitis may also occur. As FVR progresses, anorexia, depression, tracheitis, and bronchitis may be observed. Abortion or fetal resorption may occur. The prognosis is guarded if cats remain severely infected for more than 1 week. A carrier state lasting for years with periods of latency alternating with episodes of viral shedding is common. Although few adult cats die from FVR, death rate among affected kittens can range from 50-60%.

FCV infection is believed to account for another 40-45% of feline respiratory infections, and dual FCV-FVR infections are not uncommon.[3] FCV infects oral mucous membranes as well as the respiratory tract. Buccal, nasal, and lingual ulcers are characteristic. Other clinical signs of the infection are similar to FVR: anorexia, depression, fever, salivation, and nasal discharge. A carrier state with persistent shedding occurs. FCV most severely affects kittens and debilitated cats, but overall death loss is generally low.

Trial Data: Safety and Efficacy: FELOMUNE CVR® was evaluated for safety and efficacy in conventional and specific-pathogen-free cats. Clinical signs of disease or other adverse side effects attributable to vaccination were not observed in any test animals, including pregnant, susceptible cats, which delivered live, healthy litters.

Tests of serologic response to vaccination with FELOMUNE CVR® indicated that no interference existed between the vaccine fractions. Even kittens vaccinated as early as 2 weeks of age developed protective FVR and FCV serum neutralization titers at 3 weeks postvaccination.

In challenge-of-immunity tests, all cats vaccinated intranasally with FELOMUNE CVR® remained clinically normal after challenge with virulent FCV or FVR virus. In contrast, all nonvaccinated control cats showed signs of disease after challenge.[1]

References: Available upon request.

Presentation: Cartons of 25 x 1 dose vials.

Compendium Code No.: 36901060 75-4350-09

FEL-O-VAX® IV

Fort Dodge **Vaccine**

Feline Rhinotracheitis-Calici-Panleukopenia-Chlamydia Psittaci Vaccine, Killed Virus and Chlamydia

U.S. Vet. Lic. No.: 112

Contents: This product contains the antigens listed above.

Thimerosal, neomycin, polymyxin B and amphotericin B added as preservatives.

Indications: For vaccination of healthy cats 8 to 10 weeks of age or older as an aid in the prevention of disease caused by feline rhinotracheitis, calici, panleukopenia viruses and feline *Chlamydia psittaci*.

Dosage and Administration: Inject one 1 mL dose intramuscularly or subcutaneously using aseptic technique. Repeat in 3 to 4 weeks. Annual revaccination with a single dose of vaccine is recommended.

InfoVax-ID® System: The InfoVax-ID® System provides a simple and effective method of recording pertinent information on the vaccines administered to animals in a veterinary practice.

For vaccines requiring reconstitution, remove label from both vials and affix both labels to the animal's medical chart.

Using the InfoVax-ID® System:

1. Grasp the lower right hand corner of the tab at the arrow marked "Peel Here" between your thumb and forefinger.
2. Pull steadily at a slight upward angle until the top portion of the label is separated from the vial.
3. Place the label on the animal's medical chart. Press down on the label to ensure adhesion.

Precaution(s): Store in dark at 2° to 7°C (35° to 45°F). Avoid freezing. Shake well.

Caution(s): In the absence of a veterinarian-client-patient relationship, Federal law prohibits the relabeling, repackaging, resale, or redistribution of the individual contents of this package. (9 CFR 112.6)

In case of anaphylactoid reaction, administer epinephrine.

Warning(s): For veterinary use only.

Presentation: 50 doses (50 x 1 mL vials of vaccine) and 100 doses (10 x 10 mL vials of vaccine), featuring the InfoVax-ID® System.

U.S. Patent Nos. 5,242,686 — 6,004,563

U.S. Pat. No. 5,704,648 (InfoVax-ID® System)

Compendium Code No.: 10030831

2202H

FEL-O-VAX® FIV

Fort Dodge — **Vaccine**

Feline Immunodeficiency Virus Vaccine, Killed Virus

U.S. Vet. Lic. No.: 112

Contents: This product contains the antigen listed above.

Thimerosal, neomycin and polymyxin B added as preservatives.

Indications: For the vaccination of healthy cats 8 weeks of age or older as an aid in the prevention of infection with feline immunodeficiency virus.

Dosage and Administration: Inject one 1 mL dose subcutaneously using aseptic technique. Administer 2 additional doses at intervals of 2 to 3 weeks. Annual revaccination is recommended.

InfoVax-ID® System: The InfoVax-ID® System provides a simple and effective method of recording pertinent information on the vaccines administered to animals in a veterinary practice.

For vaccines requiring reconstitution, remove label from both vials and affix both labels to the animal's medical chart.

Using the InfoVax-ID® System:

1. Grasp the lower right hand corner of the tab at the arrow marked "Peel Here" between your thumb and forefinger.
2. Pull steadily at a slight upward angle until the top portion of the label is separated from the vial.
3. Place the label on the animal's medical chart. Press down on the label to ensure adhesion.

Precaution(s): Store in the dark at 2° to 7°C (35° to 45°F). Avoid freezing. Shake well. Use entire contents when first opened.

Caution(s): In the absence of a veterinarian-client-patient relationship, Federal law prohibits the relabeling, repackaging, resale, or redistribution of the individual contents of this package. (9 CFR Part 112.6)

In case of anaphylactoid reaction, administer epinephrine.

For veterinary use only.

Toxicology: Efficacy was demonstrated in cats that received three doses of vaccine and were challenged one year post vaccination with a heterologous FIV strain. In one study the vaccine protected 67% of the vaccinates against infection (any cat that showed evidence of integration of the viral genome into its white blood cells was considered infected) while 74% of the controls became persistently viremic. In a more recent one year study, the vaccine protected 84% of the vaccinates against infection while 90% of the controls became persistently viremic.

Presentation: 50 doses (50 x 1 mL vials of vaccine) and 100 doses (10 x 10 mL vials of vaccine), featuring the InfoVax-ID® System.

U.S. Pat. No. 6,254,872

U.S. Pat. No. 5,704,648 (InfoVax-ID® System)

Compendium Code No.: 10032820

1296D / 1293D

FEL-O-VAX® GIARDIA

Fort Dodge — **Vaccine**

Giardia Lamblia Vaccine, Killed Protozoa

U.S. Vet. Lic. No.: 112

Contents: This product contains the antigen listed above.

Thimerosal and gentamicin added as preservatives.

Indications: For vaccination of healthy cats, 8 weeks of age or older as an aid in the prevention of disease and shedding caused by *Giardia lamblia* infection.

Dosage and Administration: Cats, inject one 1 mL dose subcutaneously using aseptic technique. A second dose is given two to four weeks after first vaccination. Annual revaccination is recommended.

InfoVax-ID® System: The InfoVax-ID® System provides a simple and effective method of recording pertinent information on the vaccines administered to animals in a veterinary practice.

For vaccines requiring reconstitution, remove label from both vials and affix both labels to the animal's medical chart.

Using the InfoVax-ID® System:

1. Grasp the lower right hand corner of the tab at the arrow marked "Peel Here" between your thumb and forefinger.
2. Pull steadily at a slight upward angle until the top portion of the label is separated from the vial.
3. Place the label on the animal's medical chart. Press down on the label to ensure adhesion.

Precaution(s): Store in the dark at 2° to 7°C (35° to 45°F). Avoid freezing. Shake well. Use entire contents when first opened.

Caution(s): In the absence of a veterinarian-client-patient relationship, Federal law prohibits the relabeling, repackaging, resale, or redistribution of the individual contents of this package. (9 CFR 112.6)

In case of anaphylactoid reaction, administer epinephrine.

Warning(s): For use in cats only.

For veterinary use only.

Discussion: Giardiasis is a health concern for people and cats. While Giardia infection is a recognized zoonotic disease, the role that the cat assumes in human disease is not well established. FEL-O-VAX® Giardia has been proven to prevent clinical disease caused by *Giardia lamblia* infection in cats and to significantly reduce the duration of cyst shedding. Subsequent to *Giardia lamblia* exposure, some vaccinates may shed, therefore, proper hygiene and sanitation practices should be implemented.

Presentation: 25 doses (25 x 1 mL vials of vaccine), featuring the InfoVax-ID® System.

U.S. Patent Nos. 5,512,288 — 5,549,899 — 5,676,953 — 5,935,583 and Patents Pending

U.S. Pat. No. 5,704,648 (InfoVax-ID® System)

Compendium Code No.: 10030821

1335D

FEL-O-VAX Lv-K®

Fort Dodge — **Vaccine**

Feline Leukemia Vaccine, Killed Virus

U.S. Vet. Lic. No.: 112

Contents: This product contains the antigens listed above.

Thimerosal, neomycin, polymyxin B and amphotericin B added as preservatives.

Indications: For vaccination of healthy cats 10 weeks of age or older as an aid in the prevention of disease caused by feline leukemia virus.

Dosage and Administration: Inject one 1 mL dose intramuscularly or subcutaneously using aseptic technique. Repeat in 3 to 4 weeks. Annual revaccination with a single dose of vaccine is recommended.

InfoVax-ID® System: The InfoVax-ID® System provides a simple and effective method of recording pertinent information on the vaccines administered to animals in a veterinary practice.

For vaccines requiring reconstitution, remove label from both vials and affix both labels to the animal's medical chart.

Using the InfoVax-ID® System:

1. Grasp the lower right hand corner of the tab at the arrow marked "Peel Here" between your thumb and forefinger.
2. Pull steadily at a slight upward angle until the top portion of the label is separated from the vial.
3. Place the label on the animal's medical chart. Press down on the label to ensure adhesion.

Precaution(s): Store in dark at 2° to 7°C (35° to 45°F). Avoid freezing. Shake well.

Caution(s): In the absence of a veterinarian-client-patient relationship, Federal law prohibits the relabeling, repackaging, resale, or redistribution of the individual contents of this package. (9 CFR 112.6)

In case of anaphylactoid reaction, administer epinephrine.

Warning(s): For veterinary use only.

Presentation: 50 doses (50 x 1 mL vials of vaccine) and 100 doses (10 x 10 mL vials of vaccine), featuring the InfoVax-ID® System.

Patent Pending

U.S. Pat. No. 5,704,648 (InfoVax-ID® System)

Compendium Code No.: 10030791

1672F

FEL-O-VAX Lv-K® III

Fort Dodge — **Vaccine**

Feline Leukemia-Rhinotracheitis-Calici-Panleukopenia Vaccine, Killed Virus

U.S. Vet. Lic. No.: 112

Contents: This product contains the antigens listed above.

Thimerosal, neomycin, polymyxin B and amphotericin B added as preservatives.

Indications: For vaccination of healthy cats 8 to 10 weeks of age or older, as an aid in the prevention of disease caused by feline leukemia, rhinotracheitis, calici and panleukopenia viruses.

Dosage and Administration: Inject one 1 mL dose intramuscularly or subcutaneously using aseptic technique. Repeat in 3 to 4 weeks. Annual revaccination with a single dose of vaccine is recommended.

InfoVax-ID® System: The InfoVax-ID® System provides a simple and effective method of recording pertinent information on the vaccines administered to animals in a veterinary practice.

For vaccines requiring reconstitution, remove label from both vials and affix both labels to the animal's medical chart.

Using the InfoVax-ID® System:

1. Grasp the lower right hand corner of the tab at the arrow marked "Peel Here" between your thumb and forefinger.
2. Pull steadily at a slight upward angle until the top portion of the label is separated from the vial.
3. Place the label on the animal's medical chart. Press down on the label to ensure adhesion.

Precaution(s): Store in dark at 2° to 7°C (35° to 45°F). Avoid freezing. Shake well.

Caution(s): In the absence of a veterinarian-client-patient relationship, Federal law prohibits the relabeling, repackaging, resale, or redistribution of the individual contents of this package. (9 CFR 112.6)

In case of anaphylactoid reaction, administer epinephrine.

Warning(s): For veterinary use only.

Presentation: 50 doses (50 x 1 mL vials of vaccine), featuring the InfoVax-ID® System.

Patent Pending

U.S. Pat. No. 5,704,648 (InfoVax-ID® System)

Compendium Code No.: 10030801

2192E

FEL-O-VAX Lv-K® IV

Fort Dodge — **Vaccine**

Feline Leukemia-Rhinotracheitis-Calici-Panleukopenia-Chlamydia Psittaci Vaccine, Killed Virus and Chlamydia

U.S. Vet. Lic. No.: 112

Contents: This product contains the antigens listed above.

Thimerosal, neomycin, polymyxin B and amphotericin B added as preservatives.

Indications: For vaccination of healthy cats 8 to 10 weeks of age or older, as an aid in the prevention of disease caused by feline leukemia, rhinotracheitis, calici, panleukopenia viruses and feline *Chlamydia psittaci*.

Dosage and Administration: Inject one 1 mL dose intramuscularly or subcutaneously using aseptic technique. Repeat in 3 to 4 weeks. Annual revaccination with a single dose of vaccine is recommended.

InfoVax-ID® System: The InfoVax-ID® System provides a simple and effective method of recording pertinent information on the vaccines administered to animals in a veterinary practice.

For vaccines requiring reconstitution, remove label from both vials and affix both labels to the animal's medical chart.

Using the InfoVax-ID® System:

1. Grasp the lower right hand corner of the tab at the arrow marked "Peel Here" between your thumb and forefinger.
2. Pull steadily at a slight upward angle until the top portion of the label is separated from the vial.
3. Place the label on the animal's medical chart. Press down on the label to ensure adhesion.

Precaution(s): Store in dark at 2° to 7°C (35° to 45°F). Avoid freezing. Shake well.

Caution(s): In the absence of a veterinarian-client-patient relationship, Federal law prohibits the relabeling, repackaging, resale, or redistribution of the individual contents of this package. (9 CFR 112.6)

In case of anaphylactoid reaction, administer epinephrine.

Warning(s): For veterinary use only.

Presentation: 50 doses (50 x 1 mL vials of vaccine), featuring the InfoVax-ID® System.

U.S. Patent Nos. 5,242,686 — 6,004,563

U.S. Pat. No. 5,704,648 (InfoVax-ID® System)

Compendium Code No.: 10030811 2232H

F

FEL-O-VAX® MC-K

Fort Dodge **Vaccine**

Microsporum Canis Vaccine, Killed Fungus

U.S. Vet. Lic. No.: 112

Composition: FEL-O-VAX® MC-K is an inactivated whole dermatophyte *Microsporum canis* vaccine homogenized for uniformity and adjuvanted with MetaStim®. The dermatophyte is harvested and inactivated using a soft-kill process to preserve immunogenicity.

Formalin, thimerosal, neomycin, polymyxin B and amphotericin B added as preservatives.

Indications: For use in adult cats at least four months of age as an aid in the prevention and treatment of clinical signs of disease caused by *Microsporum canis*. Vaccination has not been demonstrated to eliminate *Microsporum canis* organisms from infected cats.

Dosage and Administration:

Prevention: Vaccinate cats subcutaneously with one 1 mL dose. Administer a second 1 mL dose 12-16 days after the first dose. A third 1 mL dose should be administered 26-30 days following the second dose. Field efficacy studies showed cats remained free of lesions for at least two weeks following the third dose. No further duration of immunity data has been established.

Treatment: Vaccinate cats subcutaneously with one 1 mL dose. Administer a second 1 mL dose 12-16 days after the first dose. A third 1 mL dose should be administered 26-30 days following the second dose, if typical lesions are still present. Field efficacy studies showed cats remained free of lesions for at least two weeks following the third dose. No further duration of immunity data has been established.

InfoVax-ID® System: The InfoVax-ID® System provides a simple and effective method of recording pertinent information on the vaccines administered to animals in a veterinary practice.

For vaccines requiring reconstitution, remove label from both vials and affix both labels to the animal's medical chart.

Using the InfoVax-ID® System:

1. Grasp the lower right hand corner of the tab at the arrow marked "Peel Here" between your thumb and forefinger.
2. Pull steadily at a slight upward angle until the top portion of the label is separated from the vial.
3. Place the label on the animal's medical chart. Press down on the label to ensure adhesion.

Precaution(s): Store in dark at 2° to 7°C (35° to 45°F). Avoid freezing.

Caution(s): In the absence of a veterinarian-client-patient relationship, Federal law prohibits the relabeling, repackaging, resale, or redistribution of the individual contents of this package. (9 CFR 112.6)

This product is intended only for vaccination of adult cats. Please handle carefully and avoid accidental self-inoculation. In case of anaphylactoid reaction, administer epinephrine.

Transient swelling or temporary alopecia may occur at the injection site. Not recommended for use in pregnant queens. Not recommended for use in immune suppressed cats. Vaccination has not been demonstrated to eliminate *Microsporum canis* organisms from infected cats.

Warning(s): For veterinary use only.

Discussion: Ringworm Control Program: The usage of FEL-O-VAX® MC-K is one part of a total ringworm control program. Ringworm can be a frustrating disease to control in cats due to the persistent nature of *Microsporum canis* spores and the presence of carrier cats. The following treatment program is recommended:

1. Obtain a definitive diagnosis via culture to identify the organism present. *Microsporum canis* is the most common of several types of fungus that can affect cats.[1] FEL-O-VAX® MC-K is effective against *Microsporum canis.*
2. Close the environment to new cats during the initial cleanup phase.
3. Treatment of the environment: It is extremely important to clean up the environment for long-term success. Although it is not possible to eliminate all of the fungal spores from the environment, it is possible to significantly reduce the level of *Microsporum canis* contamination by following these steps to minimize exposure.
   a) Clean all non-porous surfaces with an appropriate disinfectant such as Nolvasan® Solution.
   b) For those surfaces difficult to clean (i.e., wooden cages, rusted wire mesh, etc.), consideration should be given to repainting. Walls, ceilings and floors may also be considered for repainting.
   c) Discard items which cannot be properly disinfected (i.e., cat toys, carpet climbers, non-washable pet beds, etc.).
   d) Clean and replace furnace filters. Clean vents and ducts or consider installation of a separate ventilation system.
   e) Clean and disinfect carpets.
4. Adjunctive Therapy:
   a) Efforts should be made to reduce the number of infected particles carried by cats. Prior to vaccination, cats should be bathed and clipped. This will help remove infective particles carried by the hair. Consider bathing the cats every other week following the first FEL-O-VAX® MC-K vaccination to reduce infectious materials above the skin surface. A commercial shampoo such as Nolvasan® Shampoo is recommended.
   b) It is recommended that cats be vaccinated with FEL-O-VAX® MC-K in accordance with label directions.
   c) Immunosuppressed cats are more susceptible to recurring fungal disease.[2] Efforts should be made to protect cats from immunosuppression. Agents such as feline leukemia virus are known to cause immunosuppression. Programs should be implemented to control agents that cause immunosuppression such as feline leukemia virus. If you are not currently vaccinating against feline leukemia, we recommend use of a commercially available vaccine such as Fel-O-Vax Lv-K® or Fel-O-Vax Lv-K® IV. Cats should also be current on vaccinations for other known disease agents.

A small percentage of cats may not adequately respond to vaccination. Due to the nature of fungal disease, these cats should be easily recognizable and should be isolated from healthy cats to prevent continued contamination of the environment. It is important to use a multi-faceted approach to eradicating and preventing ringworm caused by *Microsporum canis* in cats.

The field trials in catteries were supervised by licensed veterinarians who observed the vaccinated cats for untoward reactions. A total of 692 cats received three doses of the vaccine. No untoward reactions were observed in 92.4 percent of the doses. The vaccine induced a small percentage of post-vaccinal reactions. These reactions included swelling or transient nodules, temporary alopecia and soreness at the injection site. Six (6) cats demonstrated additional minor reactions. All post-vaccinal reactions were transient in nature and required no additional care.

Trial Data: Efficacy: The immunogenicity of FEL-O-VAX® MC-K was critically evaluated in catteries in which the disease was endemic using cats of various ages. Each cat was vaccinated three times. Two doses were administered at a 14-day interval and a third dose was administered 28 days after the second dose. A control group was vaccinated with an adjuvanted placebo identical to FEL-O-VAX® MC-K except that it contained no *Microsporum canis* antigen.

A total of 159 cats received FEL-O-VAX® MC-K and 159 cats received the placebo. At the time of the first vaccination, all cats were examined for the presence of ringworm and thereafter were monitored biweekly for fluorescence and ringworm lesions until 14 days after the final vaccination. Cats were considered negative if they showed neither fluorescence nor lesions.

In the therapeutic study, 97.4 percent in the group to be vaccinated showed lesions before vaccination. At 14 days after the third vaccination, 79.1 percent of the vaccinated cats did not have lesions. During the same period, the ringworm positive control cats with lesions slightly decreased from 98.1 percent to 90.2 percent. Ninety-eight (98) percent of the vaccinated cats had some fluorescence prior to vaccination. At 14 days post third vaccination, 72.4 percent of the vaccinated cats did not have fluorescence. During the same period, the ringworm positive control cats with fluorescence decreased from 96.1 percent to 90.9 percent. Clinical scores of the ringworm positive vaccinated cats decreased from an average of 4.12 to 0.79 whereas among the ringworm positive controls, clinical scores rose from 3.85 to 3.96 on a scale of 0 to 10. The results indicate that FEL-O-VAX® MC-K is an effective treatment for clinical signs of feline ringworm caused by *Microsporum canis.*

Six (6) of the catteries contained ringworm negative cats in both the vaccine and control groups at the beginning of the study and a total of 41 such cats were included in the prophylaxis study. During the study, 21 of the 25 ringworm negative vaccinated cats (84 percent) remained free of lesions and/or fluorescence and the remaining 4 vaccinated cats had transient fluorescence or lesions which cleared by the end of the study. By contrast, 12 of 16 ringworm negative control cats (75 percent) developed either lesions and/or fluorescence during the study. The results indicate that FEL-O-VAX® MC-K is effective in preventing clinical signs of feline ringworm caused by *Microsporum canis.*

The environment in the catteries allowed for critical evaluation of the vaccine in that no improvements were made in sanitization or management practices. In addition, no antimycotic therapy was administered during the study. During the vaccination period, control cats mingled constantly with the vaccinates permitting easy transmission of the fungal infection.

References: Available upon request.

Presentation: 25 doses (25 x 1 mL vials of vaccine), featuring the InfoVax-ID® System.

Patent Pending

U.S. Pat. No. 5,704,648 (InfoVax-ID® System)

Compendium Code No.: 10030841 1282E, 1280A

FEL-O-VAX® PCT

Fort Dodge **Vaccine**

Feline Rhinotracheitis-Calici-Panleukopenia Vaccine, Killed Virus

U.S. Vet. Lic. No.: 112

Contents: This product contains the antigens listed above.

Thimerosal, neomycin, polymyxin B and amphotericin B added as preservatives.

Indications: For subcutaneous or intramuscular vaccination of healthy cats and kittens 8 weeks of age or older as an aid in the prevention of disease caused by feline rhinotracheitis, calici and panleukopenia viruses.

Dosage and Administration: Vaccinate healthy cats 8 weeks of age or older with one 1 mL dose, followed by a second 1 mL dose three to four weeks later. Inject intramuscularly or subcutaneously. Cats vaccinated at less than 12 weeks of age should be given an additional 1 mL dose of vaccine at 12 to 16 weeks of age. Annual revaccination with a single dose of vaccine is recommended. Vaccination of pregnant queens has shown no deleterious effects.

InfoVax-ID® System: The InfoVax-ID® System provides a simple and effective method of recording pertinent information on the vaccines administered to animals in a veterinary practice.

For vaccines requiring reconstitution, remove label from both vials and affix both labels to the animal's medical chart.

Using the InfoVax-ID® System:

1. Grasp the lower right hand corner of the tab at the arrow marked "Peel Here" between your thumb and forefinger.
2. Pull steadily at a slight upward angle until the top portion of the label is separated from the vial.
3. Place the label on the animal's medical chart. Press down on the label to ensure adhesion.

Precaution(s): Store in dark at 2° to 7°C (35° to 45°F). Avoid freezing. Shake well.

Caution(s): In the absence of a veterinarian-client-patient relationship, Federal law prohibits the relabeling, repackaging, resale, or redistribution of the individual contents of this package. (9 CFR 112.6)

In case of anaphylactoid reaction, administer epinephrine.

Warning(s): For veterinary use only.

Presentation: 50 doses (50 x 1 mL vials of vaccine) and 100 doses (10 x 10 mL vials of vaccine), featuring the InfoVax-ID® System.

U.S. Pat. No. 5,704,648 (InfoVax-ID® System)

Compendium Code No.: 10030851 1622I

FELOVITE®-II WITH TAURINE

Evsco — **Small Animal Dietary Supplement**

Active Ingredient(s): Guaranteed analysis per teaspoon (6 g):

Calcium (min.)	55 mg (0.9%)
Calcium (max.)	67 mg (1.1%)
Phosphorus	42 mg (0.7%)
Salt (min.)	2.7 mg (0.045%)
Salt (max.)	3.3 mg (0.055%)
Cobalt	0.08 mg (0.0013%)
Copper	0.11 mg (0.0018%)
Iodine	0.28 mg (0.0047%)
Iron	0.75 mg (0.0125%)
Magnesium	4.42 mg (0.0736%)
Manganese	0.24 mg (0.0040%)
Potassium	0.09 mg (0.0015%)
Zinc	0.34 mg (0.0057%)
Vitamin A	1,480 I.U.
Vitamin D_3	148 I.U.
Vitamin E	6 I.U.
Vitamin B_1 (thiamine HCl)	1.5 mg
Vitamin B_2 (riboflavin)	1.5 mg
Vitamin B_6 (pyridoxine HCl)	1.5 mg
Vitamin B_{12}	6 mcg
Vitamin K (menadione)	0.77 mg
Biotin	7.4 mcg
Choline	35 mg
Folic acid	44 mcg
Inositol	1.5 mg
Nicotinamide	7.4 mg
d-pantothenic acid	4 mg
Taurine	100 mg

Ingredients: Corn syrup, malt syrup, soybean oil, dicalcium phosphate (source of calcium and phosphorus), cod liver oil, water, cane molasses, digest of poultry by-products and tuna, methylcellulose, taurine, choline bitartrate, magnesium sulfate, nicotinamide, sodium benzoate (preservative), dl-alpha tocopheryl acetate (vit. E), calcium pantothenate (source of calcium and pantothenic acid), iron peptonate, sodium chloride (salt), riboflavin 5'-phosphate sodium (source of vit. B_2 and phosphorus), potassium iodide (source of iodine and potassium), cobalt sulfate, copper sulfate, folic acid, biotin and cyanocobalamin (vit. B_{12}).

Indications: A palatable vitamin mineral supplement for cats. Tuna flavored.

Dosage and Administration: Place a small amount of FELOVITE®-II with Taurine on the animal's nose or paws to stimulate taste interest. The animal should then freely accept FELOVITE®-II with Taurine.

Adult Cats: One (1) level teaspoon (approx. 6 g) once a day.

Kittens: One-half (½) level teaspoon (approx. 3 g) once a day.

Precaution(s): Store in a cool area.

Presentation: 12 x 2.5 oz. (56.7 g) tubes.

Compendium Code No.: 10050101

FELOVITE® II WITH TAURINE

Tomlyn — **Small Animal Dietary Supplement**

Active Ingredient(s): Minimum guaranteed analysis/teaspoon (6 grams):

Calcium	67.0 mg (1.1167%)
Phosphorus	52.0 mg (0.8667%)
Salt	2.6 mg (0.0433%)
Cobalt	0.07 mg (0.0012%)
Copper	0.10 mg (0.0017%)
Iodine	0.25 mg (0.0042%)
Iron	0.68 mg (0.0113%)
Magnesium	3.98 mg (0.0663%)
Manganese	0.21 mg (0.0035%)
Potassium	0.08 mg (0.0013%)
Zinc	0.31 mg (0.0052%)
Vitamin A	1332 IU
Vitamin D_3	131 IU
Vitamin E	5 IU
Vitamin B_1 (Thiamine)	1.3 mg
Vitamin B_2 (Riboflavin)	1.4 mg
Vitamin B_6 (Pyridoxine)	1.1 mg
Vitamin B_{12}	5.2 mcg
Vitamin K (Menadione)	0.8 mg
Biotin	6.7 mcg
Choline	27.6 mg
Folic Acid	39.6 mcg
Inositol	1.4 mg
Niacin	6.7 mg
d-Pantothenic Acid	1.8 mg
Taurine	90.0 mg

Ingredients: Corn Syrup, Malt Syrup, Soybean Oil, Dicalcium Phosphate (source of Calcium and Phosphorus), Cod Liver Oil, Water, Cane Molasses, Digest of Poultry By-products and Tuna, Methylcellulose, Taurine, Choline Bitartrate, Magnesium Sulfate, Niacin, Sodium Benzoate (Preservative), dl-Alpha Tocopheryl Acetate (Vit. E), Calcium Pantothenate (source of Calcium and Pantothenic Acid), Iron Proteinate, Sodium Chloride (Salt), Riboflavin 5'-Phosphate Sodium (source of Vit. B_2 and Phosphorus), Thiamine HCl, Pyridoxine HCl, Vitamin A Palmitate and D_3 Supplement, Zinc Sulfate, Menadione Sodium Bisulfite, Inositol, Manganese Sulfate, Potassium Iodide (source of Iodine and Potassium), Cobalt Sulfate, Copper Sulfate, Folic Acid, Biotin and Cyanocobalamin (Vit. B_{12}).

Indications: Tuna flavored vitamins and minerals for cats.

Directions: Place a small amount of FELOVITE® II with Taurine on the animal's nose to stimulate taste interest. Animal should then freely accept FELOVITE® II with Taurine. Adult Cats- One level teaspoon (approx. 6 grams) daily. Kittens- One-half level teaspoon (approx. 3 grams) daily.

Precaution(s): Store in a cool area.

Caution(s): For veterinary use only.

Warning(s): Keep out of reach of children.

Presentation: 2.5 oz. (70.9 g) tubes.

Compendium Code No.: 11220260

6780 3

FERRET DROPS™

Tomlyn — **Dietary Supplement**

Guaranteed Analysis: Per dropperful:

Vitamin A	5973 I.U.
Vitamin D_3	812 I.U.
Vitamin E	1.7 I.U.
Thiamine (Vit. B_1)	1.8 mg
Riboflavin (Vit. B_2)	0.54
Pyridoxine (Vit. B_6)	0.9 mg
Cyanocobalamin (Vit. B_{12})	0.42 mcg
Menadione (Vit. K)	5.0 mcg
Nicotinamide	8.1 mg
D-Panthenol	3.4 mg
Iron (0.27%)	2.7 mg
Copper (0.004%)	44.0 mcg

Ingredients: Water sugar, sorbitol, polysorbate 80, liver extract, gelatin by-products, ferric ammonium citrate (source of iron), nicotinamide, vitamin A & D concentrate, d-panthenol, thiamine RCl (Vit. B_1), citric acid (preservative), alpha tocopheryl acetate (Vit. E), saccharin sodium, Vit. A palmitate, pyridoxine HCl (Vit. B_6), sodium benzoate and methylparaben (preservatives), riboflavin 5' phosphate sodium (source of Vit. B_2), copper sulfate, BHA (preservative), menadione sodium bisulfite (source of Vit. K), cyanocobalamin (Vit. B_{12}).

Indications: A vitamin supplement with liver and iron for use In ferrets.

Dosage and Administration: To Supplement Diet: Give ferrets ½ dropperful twice daily. This mixture is water dispersible and may be given by dropping directly on the tongue or mixed with food or milk.

(1 dropperful =1 mL).

Precaution(s): Store at room temperature.

Caution(s): For veterinary use only.

Keep out of reach of children

Presentation: 12 x 1 fl oz (29.6 mL).

Compendium Code No.: 11220040

726-1

FERRET-OFF™

Thornell — **Deodorant Product**

Description: Does not contain enzymes, bacteria, nor oxidizers. Nontoxic, nonirritating, biodegradable, nonflammable.

Indications: To neutralize ferret odors including glandular secretion, urine, feces, emesis and normal animal body odor.

Use directly on the ferret, accidents, bedding, litter boxes, and cages. Eliminates bathing when odor is the problem.

FERRET-OFF™ works chemically through bonding, absorption and counteraction. Unlike enzyme and bacteria based products, FERRET-OFF™ remains effective when used with or after most cleaners, shampoo and germicides.

Dosage and Administration: Spray full strength on the source of the odor. Work in if possible. Allow to dry. If the odor persists, FERRET-OFF™ has not reached the source of the odor. Re-apply.

Precaution(s): FERRET-OFF™ has an indefinite shelf life.

Caution(s): Although not irritating to mucous membranes, spraying directly into the eyes is not recommended. As with all chemicals, keep out of the reach of children. For external use only. Always spot test for color fastness before using on fabrics.

Presentation: 8 oz. pump spray bottle.

Compendium Code No.: 11210040

FERRODEX™ 100

AgriLabs — **Iron Injection**

Iron Hydrogenated Dextran-Hematinic

NADA No.: 134-708

Active Ingredient(s): Each mL of sterile solution contains 100 mg of elemental iron stabilized with a low molecular weight hydrogenated dextran and 0.5% phenol as a preservative.

Indications: For the prevention and treatment of anemia due to iron deficiency in baby pigs.

Dosage and Administration: For intramuscular injection only.

Prevention: 1 mL (100 mg iron) at two (2) to four (4) days of age.

Treatment: 1 mL (100 mg iron). Treatment may be repeated in 10 days.

Notice: Organic iron preparations injected intramuscularly into pigs beyond four (4) weeks of age may cause staining of the muscle tissue.

Precaution(s): Store at a controlled room temperature between 15-30°C (59-86°F). Protect from freezing.

Caution(s): Keep out of the reach of children.

Livestock drug. Use only as directed.

Presentation: 100 mL bottles.

Compendium Code No.: 10580490

FERRODEX™ 200

AgriLabs — **Iron Injection**

Iron Dextran Complex Injection 200 mg/mL-Hematinic

NADA No.: 134-708

Active Ingredient(s): FERRODEX™ 200 is a sterile solution containing a complex of ferric hydroxide with a low molecular weight dextran fraction equivalent to 200 mg elemental iron per mL with 0.5% phenol as a preservative.

Indications: For the prevention or treatment of baby pig anemia due to iron deficiency.

Dosage and Administration: For intramuscular injection only.

Prevention: 1 mL (200 mg iron), intramuscularly, at one (1) to three (3) days of age.

Treatment: 1 mL (200 mg iron) at the first signs of iron deficiency.

Precaution(s): Store at a controlled room temperature between 59-86°F (15-30°C). Protect from freezing.

Caution(s): Keep out of the reach of children.

Use of this product after four weeks of age may cause staining of the ham muscle.

Presentation: 100 mL bottles.

Compendium Code No.: 10580500

FERTAGYL® ℞

Intervet **Gonadorelin**

ANADA No.: 200-134

Active Ingredient(s): FERTAGYL® is a sterile solution containing 43 µg gonadorelin (GnRH; equivalent to 50µg/mL gonadorelin diacetate tetrahydrate) suitable for intramuscular or intravenous administration.

Each mL of FERTAGYL® contains:

Gonadorelin	43 µg
Benzyl Alcohol	9 mg
Sodium Chloride	7.47 mg
Water for Injection PhEur.	q.s.

pH adjusted with sodium phosphate (monobasic and dibasic).

Indications: FERTAGYL® (gonadorelin) is indicated for the treatment of ovarian follicular cysts in dairy cattle. Ovarian cysts are non-ovulated follicles with incomplete luteinization which can result in nymphomania or irregular estrus.

Pharmacology: Gonadorelin is a decapeptide composed of the sequence of amino acids —

5-oxoPro-His-Trp-Ser-Gly-Leu-Arg-Pro-Gly-NH_2

with a molecular weight of 1182.32 and empirical formula $C_{55}H_{75}N_{17}O_{13}$. Gonadorelin is the hypothalamic releasing factor responsible for the release of gonadotropins (e.g., LH, FSH) from the anterior pituitary.

Synthetic gonadorelin is physiologically and chemically identical to the endogenous bovine hypothalamic releasing factor.

Endogenous gonadorelin is synthesized by and/or released from the hypothalamus during various stages of the bovine estrous cycle following appropriate neurogenic stimuli. It passes via the hypophyseal portal vessels, to the anterior pituitary to effect the release of gonadotrophins.

Synthetic gonadorelin administered intramuscularly or intravenously also causes the release of endogenous LH and FSH from the anterior pituitary.

Dosage and Administration: Historically, cystic ovaries have responded to an exogenous source of luteinizing hormone (LH) such as human chorionic gonadotropin.

FERTAGYL® initiates release of endogenous LH to cause ovulation and luteinization. The recommended intramuscular or intravenous dosage of FERTAGYL® is 86 µg/cow (2 mL; equivalent to 100 µg gonadorelin diacetate tertahydrate/cow).

Precaution(s): Keep refrigerated: 2-8°C (36-46°F).

Caution(s): Federal law restricts this drug to use by or on the order of a licensed veterinarian.

Toxicology: Gonadorelin diacetate tetrahydrate has been shown to be safe. The LD_{50} for mice and rats is greater than 60 mg/kg, and for dogs, greater than 600 µg/kg, respectively. No untoward effects were noted among rats or dogs administered 120 µg/kg/day intramuscularly or 72 µg/kg/day intravenously for 15 days. It has no adverse effects on heart rate, blood pressure or EKG, when administered to unanesthetized dogs at 60 µg/kg. In anesthetized dogs it did not produce depression of myocardial or systemic hemodynamics or adversely affect coronary oxygen supply or myocardial oxygen requirements.

The intravenous administration of 60 µg/kg/day gonadorelin diacetate tetrahydrate to pregnant rats and rabbits during organogenesis did not cause embryotoxic or teratogenic effects.

The intramuscular administration of 1000 µg gonadorelin diacetate tetrahydrate to normally cycling dairy cattle had no effect on hematology or blood chemistry.

Further, gonadorelin diacetate tetrahydrate did not cause irritation at the site of intramuscular administration in dogs. The dosage administered was 72 µg/kg/day for 7 days.

Presentation: 10-2 mL single dose vials or 1-20 mL multidose vials of sterile solution.

Compendium Code No.: 11060530

FERVAC®-D

United **Vaccine**

Distemper Vaccine, Modified Live Virus

U.S. Vet. Lic. No.: 245

Active Ingredient(s): FERVAC®-D is a modified live vaccine consisting of a freeze-dried distemper virus and sterile diluent. Contains gentamicin as a preservative.

Indications: The vaccine is for use as an aid in the prevention of distemper in healthy, susceptible ferrets.

Dosage and Administration: Mixing of the Vaccine:

1. Do not mix the vaccine until ready for use.
2. Mix only one (1) pair of vials at a time, and use the entire contents within two (2) hours.
3. Disinfect the rubber stoppers with alcohol.
4. Using a sterile syringe and needle, transfer the diluent into the bottle of freeze-dried vaccine.
5. After all the diluent has been transferred, shake gently to suspend evenly.

Inject 1 mL subcutaneously. The initial dose is given at eight (8) weeks of age. Repeat the dose at 11 weeks of age and give a final dose at 14 weeks of age. Give the booster annually.

Precaution(s): Store at 35° to 45°F (2° to 7°C).

Caution(s):

1. Burn the empty containers and any unused portion of the vaccine.
2. Incubating diseases (such as Aleutian disease), parasites, nutritional deficiencies (anemia), maternal antibodies and poor management practices (dehydration, adverse temperatures) will reduce the effectiveness of the vaccine.
3. Animals infected, yet not showing signs of distemper at the time of vaccination, will not be protected by the vaccine.
4. The use of any biological may produce anaphylactic reactions.
5. For veterinary use only.

Antidote(s): Epinephrine.

Presentation: 10 x 1 dose vials of vaccine and 10 x 1 mL vials of diluent.
50 dose vial of vaccine and diluent.

Compendium Code No.: 11040091

FEVAXYN® FeLV

Schering-Plough **Vaccine**

Feline Leukemia Vaccine, Killed Virus

U.S. Vet. Lic. No.: 165A

Contents: FEVAXYN® FeLV contains a tissue culture derived, feline leukemia virus, Subgroups A and B. Viral antigens have been chemically inactivated and combined with a proprietary adjuvant designed to enhance the immune response.

Contains gentamicin and amphotericin B as preservatives.

Indications: FEVAXYN® FeLV is recommended for the vaccination of healthy cats as an aid in the prevention of lymphoid tumors caused by, and diseases associated with, feline leukemia virus (FeLV) infection. Vaccination with the product prevents persistent viremia in cats exposed to virulent feline leukemia virus.

Dosage and Administration: Two doses are required for primary immunization.

Initial Vaccination: Inject 1 dose (1 mL) subcutaneously or intramuscularly at 9 weeks of age or older.

Second Vaccination: Inject 1 dose (1 mL) subcutaneously or intramuscularly 3 to 4 weeks following the initial vaccination.

Annual revaccination with one dose is recommended.

Allow the vaccine to warm to room temperature prior to use.

Shake well before use.

Contraindication(s): Do not vaccinate pregnant cats.

Precaution(s): Store between 2° and 7°C. Do not freeze.

Use new, non-chemically sterilized, needles and syringes.

Do not mix with other vaccines.

Burn vaccine container and all unused contents.

Caution(s): The use of a biological product may produce anaphylaxis and/or other inflammatory immune-mediated hypersensitivity reactions.

Some reports suggest that in cats, the administration of certain veterinary biologicals may induce the development of injection-site fibrosarcomas.

Antidote(s): Epinephrine, corticosteroids, and antihistamines may all be indicated depending on the nature and severity of the reaction.

Warning(s): For use in cats only.

For veterinary use only.

Discussion: It is important to realize that certain conditions and events may cause some cats to be unable to develop or maintain an adequate immune response following vaccination. Prior exposure to the disease, or disease latency, are conditions in which vaccination will not alter the course of the disease. Therefore, diagnostic testing of all cats for FeLV antigen prior to vaccination is recommended. Also, vaccination with the product will not offer cross-protection against feline immunodeficiency (FIV), another feline retrovirus. It is important to advise the cat owner of these situations prior to vaccination.

Presentation: 25 x 1 dose vials.

Compendium Code No.: 10470721 P20002-10

FIBER FORTE® FELINE

Life Science **Small Animal Dietary Supplement**

Guaranteed Analysis:

Crude Protein, minimum	11.61%
Crude Fat, minimum	1.30%
Crude Fiber, maximum	17.21%
Moisture, maximum	12.41%
Potassium, minimum	0.50%
Iron, minimum	700 ppm
Manganese, minimum	90 ppm
Zinc, minimum	70 ppm
Copper, minimum	45 ppm
Iodine, minimum	10 ppm

Ingredients: Dried beet pulp; dried kelp; dried animal liver meal (beef); psyllium seed husk; extruded canola; extruded rice; ground flax seed; papaya fruit; apple pectin; bentonite; diatomaceous earth; oil of garlic.

Indications: Feline fiber powder supplement with enzymes and minerals.

FIBER FORTE® Feline is 100% natural and safe and may also be used for dogs and rabbits.

Dosage and Administration: For cats shake ½ tsp. (2-3 shakes) on wet or dry food with each meal daily. Mix or moisten if preferred. Increase if needed to 1 tsp. for larger cat.

Discussion: FIBER FORTE® Feline is a unique blend of naturally occurring fibers, minerals and plant enzymes. Taste and protein content have been greatly enhanced by the addition of liver, canola and pure garlic oil. Norwegian kelp is sundried and of the highest quality - a great source of trace minerals. The remaining all-natural ingredients are of the highest quality available working synergistically to form a unique blend which is easily digested. FIBER FORTE® Feline helps support natural body functions without harsh laxatives.

Presentation: 7 oz (198 g).

Compendium Code No.: 10870080

FILARIBITS® ℞

Pfizer Animal Health **Parasiticide-Oral**

(diethylcarbamazine citrate) Chewable Tablets

NADA No.: 104-493

Active Ingredient(s): Composition: Each tablet contains diethylcarbamazine citrate in strengths of 60 mg, 120 mg, or 180 mg.

Indications: FILARIBITS® are indicated for use in the prevention of infection with *Dirofilaria immitis* (heartworm disease), and as an aid in the treatment of ascarid *(Toxocara canis* and *Toxascaris leonina)* infections in dogs. FILARIBITS® may be given to dogs of all ages including bitches throughout the reproductive period and after whelping.

Dosage and Administration: FILARIBITS® tablets are chewable and are palatable to most dogs. Tablets may be fed free choice or crumbled and placed on food. FILARIBITS® tablets are scored for convenient adjustment of dosage.

For the Prevention Of Heartworm Disease in Dogs: FILARIBITS® are given orally (once a day) at a dosage rate of 3 mg diethylcarbamazine citrate per lb of body weight. Young dogs may be started on the preventive program at 2 months of age. Administration of FILARIBITS® in heartworm endemic areas should start 1 month before the beginning of mosquito activity and be continued daily throughout the mosquito season and for approximately 2 months thereafter. Continuous low level administration during the mosquito season effectively prevents the maturation of recently inoculated heartworm larvae into adults *(D. immitis)*.

Recommended Dosage Schedule for Prevention of Heartworms

Body Weight (lb)	FILARIBITS® 60-mg Tablets
5	1/4 Tablet
10	1/2 Tablet
20	1 Tablet
Body Weight (lb)	**FILARIBITS® 120-mg Tablets**
20	1/2 Tablet
40	1 Tablet
Body Weight (lb)	**FILARIBITS® 180-mg Tablets**
15	1/4 Tablet
30	1/2 Tablet
60	1 Tablet

For the Treatment of Ascarid Infection in Dogs: FILARIBITS® are given as a single, oral dose at the dosage rate of 25-50 mg of diethylcarbamazine citrate per lb of body weight (one 180-mg tablet for each 3.6-7.2 lb of body weight, one 120-mg tablet for 2.4-4.8 lb of body weight, or one 60-mg tablet for 1.2-2.4 lb of body weight). Fasting or a laxative after treatment is not necessary. To reduce the possibility of vomiting which occasionally occurs, it is preferable to administer FILARIBITS® with food or directly after feeding. Repeat the dose 10-20 days later to remove immature worms which may enter the intestine from the lungs after the first treatment.

Precaution(s): Store at controlled room temperature 15°-30°C (59°-86°F).

Caution(s): Federal law restricts this drug to use by or on the order of a licensed veterinarian. Do not use in dogs that may be harboring adult heartworms. Keep out of reach of children.

Warning(s): Dogs with established heartworm infection should not receive FILARIBITS® until they have been converted to a negative status by the appropriate use of adulticidal and microfilaricidal drugs. A dog on prophylactic therapy should be examined for the presence of microfilaria every 6 months. For veterinary use only.

Side Effects: The use of diethylcarbamazine citrate is not recommended in dogs with active *D. immitis* infections. Inadvertent administration to heartworm infested dogs may cause adverse reactions due to pulmonary occlusion. Overdosage may cause emesis. The compound causes no cumulative toxic effects.

Presentation: 60-mg (quarter-scored) tablets—bottles of 100 and 200
120-mg (half-scored) tablets—bottles of 100
180-mg (quarter-scored) tablets—bottles of 50, 100, and 200

Compendium Code No.: 36901080

75-6430-11

FILARIBITS PLUS® ℞

Pfizer Animal Health **Parasiticide-Oral**

(diethylcarbamazine citrate/oxibendazole) Chewable Tablets

NADA No.: 136-483

Active Ingredient(s): Composition: Each 60 mg/45 mg FILARIBITS PLUS® tablet contains 60 mg diethylcarbamazine citrate and 45 mg oxibendazole. Each 120 mg/91 mg FILARIBITS PLUS® tablet contains 120 mg diethylcarbamazine citrate and 91 mg oxibendazole. Each 180 mg/136 mg FILARIBITS PLUS® tablet contains 180 mg diethylcarbamazine citrate and 136 mg oxibendazole.

Indications: FILARIBITS PLUS® are indicated for use in the prevention of infection with *Dirofilaria immitis* (heartworm disease) and *Ancylostoma caninum* (hookworm infection) in dogs. FILARIBITS PLUS® are also indicated for removal and control of *Trichuris vulpis* (whipworm infection) and mature and immature stages of intestinal *Toxocara canis* (ascarid infection) in dogs. FILARIBITS PLUS® may be given to dogs of all ages, including bitches, throughout the reproductive period and following whelping.

Dosage and Administration: FILARIBITS PLUS® tablets are chewable and are palatable to most dogs. Tablets may be fed free choice or placed on food. FILARIBITS PLUS® are scored for convenient adjustment of dosage.

For the Prevention of Heartworm Disease, Hookworm Infection and for the Removal and Control of Whipworms and Mature and Immature Stages of Intestinal Ascarids in Dogs: FILARIBITS PLUS® are given orally (once a day) at a dosage rate of 3 mg diethylcarbamazine citrate and 2.27 mg oxibendazole per lb of body weight. Young dogs may be started on the preventive program at 2 months of age. Administration of FILARIBITS PLUS® in heartworm or hookworm endemic areas should start prior to hookworm exposure and at least 1 month before the beginning of the mosquito season. FILARIBITS PLUS® administration should continue daily throughout the entire period of exposure to hookworms and 2 months past the mosquito season since there is little residual effect of the drugs. Continuous low level administration effectively prevents the maturation of hookworms *(A. caninum)*, recently inoculated heartworm larvae *(D. immitis)* into adults, and provides for the removal and control of whipworms *(T. vulpis)* and mature and immature stages of intestinal ascarids *(T. canis)*. If FILARIBITS PLUS® are discontinued because of seasonal heartworm problem, hookworm prevention or therapy and whipworm and ascarid removal and control should be continued.

Recommended Dosage Schedule

Body Weight (lb)	FILARIBITS PLUS® 60 mg/45 mg tablets
1-5	1/4 tablet
6-10	1/2 tablet
11-15	3/4 tablet
16-20	1 tablet
21-25	1 1/4 tablets
26-30	1 1/2 tablets
31-35	1 3/4 tablets
36-40	2 tablets
41-45	2 1/4 tablets
46-50	2 1/2 tablets
Body Weight (lb)	**FILARIBITS PLUS® 120 mg/91 mg tablets**
21-30	3/4 tablet
31-40	1 tablet
41-50	1 1/4 tablets
51-60	1 1/2 tablets
61-70	1 3/4 tablets
71-80	2 tablets
81-90	2 1/4 tablets
91-100	2 1/2 tablets

Body Weight (lb)	FILARIBITS PLUS® 180 mg/136 mg tablets
21-30	1/2 tablet
31-45	3/4 tablet
46-60	1 tablet
61-75	1 1/4 tablets
76-90	1 1/2 tablets
91-105	1 3/4 tablets
106-120	2 tablets
121-135	2 1/4 tablets
136-150	2 1/2 tablets

Precaution(s): Storage: Store at controlled room temperature 15°-30°C (59°-86°F).

Caution(s): Federal law restricts this drug to use by or on the order of a licensed veterinarian.
Do not use in dogs that may be harboring adult heartworms.
Keep out of reach of children

Warning(s): FILARIBITS PLUS® (diethylcarbamazine citrate, oxibendazole) Chewable Tablets have been occasionally associated with hepatic toxicity including several fatalities. Close monitoring of animals receiving this drug may identify early hepatic injury. The hepatic injury has usually been reversible upon discontinuation of FILARIBITS PLUS® administration; thus dogs exhibiting signs of hepatic dysfunction should be removed from treatment immediately. Dogs with a history of liver disease or dogs receiving FILARIBITS PLUS® concurrently with other potentially hepatotoxic drugs should be carefully monitored for clinical or biochemical evidence of hepatic disease.

Dogs with established heartworm infection should not receive FILARIBITS PLUS® until they have been converted to a negative status by the use of appropriate adulticidal and microfilaricidal heartworm therapy. A dog on prophylactic therapy should be examined for the presence of heartworm microfilaria every 6 months. Dogs with established hookworm infection should be treated with an appropriate anthelmintic prior to FILARIBITS PLUS® administration.
For use in dogs only.

Side Effects: Occasionally in dogs, hepatic dysfunction, sometimes fatal, has been reported with the use of FILARIBITS PLUS®.

Clients should be instructed to report any signs and symptoms which may suggest hepatic dysfunction so that appropriate biochemical testing can be done. Signs and symptoms reported as accompanying hepatic dysfunction include anorexia, vomiting, lethargy, jaundice, weight loss, polydipsia, polyuria, ataxia and dark urine.

The use of diethylcarbamazine citrate is not recommended in dogs with active *D. immitis* infections. Inadvertent administration to heartworm infected dogs may cause adverse reactions due to pulmonary occlusion. Overdosage may cause emesis.

Presentation: 60-mg/45-mg tablets—bottles of 100 and 200
120-mg/91-mg tablets—bottles of 100
180-mg/136-mg tablets—bottles of 50, 100, and 200

U.S. Patent Nos. 3,480,642 and 3,574,845

Compendium Code No.: 36901070

75-6423-01

FINAPLIX®-H

Intervet **Implant**

(trenbolone acetate)

NADA No.: 138-612

Active Ingredient(s): FINAPLIX®-H is an implant containing 200 mg of trenbolone acetate.
Manufactured by a non-sterilizing process.

Indications: Increases rate of weight gain and improves feed efficiency in a slow-release delivery system. This product is to be used in feedlot heifers only during approximately the last 63 days prior to slaughter.

Dosage and Administration: Dosage Form: One implant containing 200 mg trenbolone acetate is administered to each animal. The 10 pellets which make up the dosage of FINAPLIX®-H are contained in one division of the multiple cartridge. Ten doses are in each cartridge. The cartridge is designed to be used with a special implant gun.

Route of Administration: The implant is placed under the skin on the posterior aspect of the ear by means of a special implanter available from Intervet Inc. With the animal suitably restrained, the skin on the outer surface of the ear should be cleaned. The implant is then administered by the method shown in the diagram below.

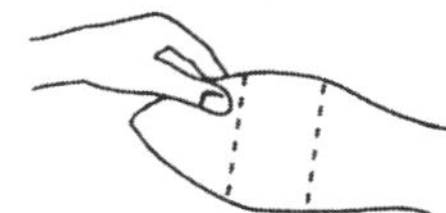

Fig. 1 - Ear of Bovine Ready for Implantation

Site of Implantation: After appropriately restraining the animal to allow access to the ear, cleanse the skin at the implant needle puncture site. It is subcutaneous, between the skin and cartilage on the back side of the ear and below the midline of the ear. The implant must not be placed closer to the head than the edge of the cartilage ring farthest from the head. The location of insertion of the needle is a point toward the tip of the ear and at least a needle length away from the intended deposition site. Care should be taken to avoid injuring the major blood vessels or cartilage of the ear.

Method of Use:

1. Do not remove the cap of the cartridge containing the implants.
2. Place the cartridge (with the capped end to the front) into slot at the top of the implanter magazine.
3. Gently push the cartridge into the slot until it clicks into place.
4. The implanter is then ready to use.
5. Take the ear of the animal firmly with the free hand (in the manner shown in Fig. 1). Then insert the needle into the subcutaneous tissue at the point indicated.
6. After inserting the needle to its full extent, squeeze the trigger gradually. Allow the pellets of the implant will be deposited in a single row.
7. Withdraw the implanter. This will advance the cartridge one groove in the magazine and the next implant is now ready for use.
8. When all the implants have been administered, the cartridge will discharge out of the bottom of the magazine and may be replaced by a new one.
9. To change the needle, loosen the needle locking nut and replace the needle. Tighten the nut finger tight and the implanter is ready for use.

Precaution(s): Storage Conditions: Store in a refrigerator (2-8°C; 36-47°F) and protect from sunlight. Use before the expiration date printed on the box and on the cartridge.
Warning(s): Not to be used in animals intended for subsequent breeding, or in dairy animals. For animal treatment only. Not for use in humans. Implant pellets in the ear only. Any other location may result in violation of Federal Law. Do not attempt salvage of implanted site for human or animal food.
Presentation: Boxes of 10 x 10 cartridge implants. Each implant consists of 10 small yellow pellets. Ten implants are provided in each container.
Compendium Code No.: 11060541

780706-B

FINQUEL®

Argent **Anesthetic-Aquaculture**

Brand of tricaine methanesulfonate
For Anesthesia and Tranquilization of Fishes and Other Cold-Blooded Animals
NADA No.: 042-427
Active Ingredient(s): Contains tricaine methanesulfonate.
Indications: FINQUEL® is intended for the temporary immobilization of fish, amphibians, and other aquatic, cold-blooded animals. It has long been recognized as a valuable tool for the proper handling of these animals during manual spawning (fish stripping), weighing, measuring, marking, surgical operations, transport, photography, and research.
Pharmacology: Tricaine methanesulfonate is the methanesulfonate of meta-amino benzoic acid ethylester, or simply ethyl *m*-amino benzoate. It is thus an isomer of benzocaine have the formula is $C_9H_{11}O_2N + CH_3SO_3H$ and the following structure:

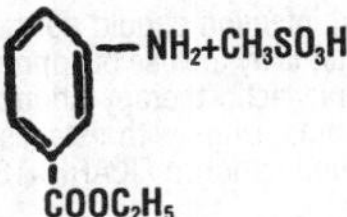

FINQUEL® is a fine white crystalline powder. Its molecular weight is 261.3. Soluble to 11%, it forms clear, colorless, acid solutions in water.
Dosage and Administration: I. Directions for use on fish:

Concentrations: FINQUEL® is effective and safe for the anesthesia of fish when used as directed. Its use is governed by, and can be tailored to, the needs of individual fishery personnel. Sedation and various rates of anesthetization are controlled by the concentration. The versatility of FINQUEL® is demonstrated by the face that it has been used in fisheries at levels ranging from 10 to 1,000 mg/liter.[3] The action of the anesthetic is slowed at cooler temperatures, in extremely soft water (approximately 10 mg/liter of $CaCO_3$, or less), and in larger fish.[4] Also, efficacy may vary with species.[4] Thus, it is imperative that preliminary tests of anesthetic solutions be made against small numbers of fish to determine the desired rates of anesthesia and exposure times for the specific lots of fish under prevailing conditions.

The following tables may be used as guidelines in selecting concentrations of FINQUEL® for the anesthetization of various fishes:

Table 1: Concentrations Required for Rapid Anesthesia (Induction time less than 2-5 minutes; used in spawning, marking, measuring, and some surgical operations).

Fish	Temperature	Concentration (mg/liter)	Max. tolerated exposure time* (min.)	Recovery time in fresh water (min.)
Salmonidae[4]	7-17°C (45-63°F)	80-135	4-12	3-19
(Pacific and Atlantic salmon; trout; chars; etc.)				
Esocidae[5]	8-12°C (46-54°F)	150	8-28	8-31
(Northern pike; muskellunge)				
Cyprinidae[3]	16°C (61°F)	150-200		
(Carp; goldfish)				
Ictaluridae[2]	7-27°C (45-81°F)	140-270	4-11	3-24
(Channel catfish)				
Centrarchidae[6]	10-27°C (50-81°F)	260-330	3-5	7-11
(Bluegill; largemouth bass)				
Percidae[5]	10-16°C (50-61°F)	100-120	7-18	5-40
(Walleye)				
Pet and tropical[7]				
Live-bearers	24-27°C (75-81°F)	85	12 hrs.	
Egg layers	24-27°C (75-81°F)	75	12 hrs.	

* Maximum tolerated exposure time (in minutes) of fish to FINQUEL® solution.

Table 2: Concentrations Required for Moderately Rapid Anesthesia (Induction time less than 15-20 minutes; used in surgical operations and in spawning and marking where longer exposures are more important than rapid immobilization).

Fish	Temperature	Concentration (mg/liter)	Maximum tolerated exposure time* (min.)	Recovery time in fresh water (min.)
Salmonidae[4]	7-17°C (45-63°F)	50-60	30 or >	2-20
(Pacific and Atlantic salmon; trout; chars; etc.)				
Ictaluridae[2]	7-27°C (45-81°F)	70	30 or >	1-10
(Channel catfish)				

* Maximum tolerated exposure time (in minutes) of fish to FINQUEL® solution.

Table 3: Concentrations Required for Sedation (Induction within 15 minutes; used in fish transport).

Fish	Temperature	Concentration (mg/liter)	Maintenance of sedation (hr.)
Salmonidae[4]	7-17°C (45-63°F)	15-30	6
(Pacific and Atlantic salmon; trout; chars; etc.)			
Esocidae[5]		40	
(Chain pickerel)			
Ictaluridae[2]	7-27°C (45-81°F)	20-40	6
(Channel catfish)			
Centrarchidae[6]		25	8-13
(Bluegills)			
Pet and tropical[7]			
[Bettas, Piranhas, etc. (uncrowded)	24-27°C (75-81°F)	66	48
Goldfish]	24-27°C (75-81°F)	37	48

Important: Since, in many cases, relatively rapid rates of anesthesia can be achieved only by exceeding the lethal concentration of FINQUEL®, it is necessary to return anesthetized fish to fresh water before they are overexposed. Excessive exposures are avoided by observing the following sensory and motor responses of the fish which characterize progressively deeper levels of anesthesia:

Sedation: Decreased reactivity to visual and vibrational stimuli; opercular activity reduced.

Total loss of equilibrium: Fish turns over; locomotion ceases; fish swims or extends fins in response to pressure on caudal fin or peduncle.

Total loss of reflex: No response to pressure on caudal fin or peduncle; opercular rate slow and erratic.

Medullary collapse: Opercular activity ceases.

Laboratory and field investigations[3,9] have shown that the action of FINQUEL® is readily reversed when the fish are transferred to fresh water before opercular activity ceases. Additional exposure following medullary collapse may result in mortality. A rough estimate of the safe total exposure can be made by multiplying the time required for anesthesia by a factor of 2 or 3.

Water: Since FINQUEL® is very soluble (1:9) in water, it dissolves with equal readiness in spring water, tap water, or sea water. Do not use distilled or deionized water, or water containing chlorine, heavy metals (copper, zinc, etc.), or other toxic contaminants. The anesthetic solution should be well oxygenated, and its temperature should be similar to that of the water from which the fish are taken. In the field, many water quality problems are eliminated by using natural water to which the fish are acclimated, provided the water does not possess high chemical or biologic oxygen demand.

Methods of Application:

1. General anesthesia: For most situations where rapid or moderately rapid anesthesia is required, FINQUEL® may be applied in a bath, i.e., the fish are immersed in the anesthetic solution. Containers may be of glass, plastic, steel, aluminum, or other suitable material. However, do not use galvanized or brass containers unless treated or sealed to prevent dissolution of zinc. Size of container is determined by individual needs, but the fish should not be overcrowded. Discard anesthetic solutions when a loss in potency is noted, or when the solutions become fouled with mucus or excrement.
2. For surgery and certain physiologic studies, the fish may be anesthetized to loss of reflex, removed from the anesthetic, and then positioned so that the gills are bathed in a sedating concentration of FINQUEL®. Some investigators have developed flowing, recirculating systems for bathing the gills with anesthetic during surgery.
   Large fishes such as sharks and rays are anesthetized within minutes by spraying the gills with a 1 g/liter solution of FINQUEL®.[10] The application is made by means of a water pistol, bulb syringe, hand pump, etc.
3. Transport: FINQUEL® has been used to sedate fish during transport. It is more successful in cold than in warm water, and it is instrumental in reducing injuries because of hyperactivity. Fish are usually transported by means of distribution units (tank trucks), or by air in plastic bags.[11,12] In either case, the fish should be fasted before-hand to reduce metabolic wastes. Also, some workers suggest pretransport sedation for several hours to lower metabolism. With distribution units, the fish may be fasted and sedated prior to loading. The anesthetic solution is prepared in the distribution unit and oxygenated. Then, the fish are added and temperature acclimated.
   In air shipments, the anesthetic solution is placed in a suitable plastic bag, the sedated fish are added, the bag inflated with oxygen, tied securely, and placed in a second bag. This bag is also tied, and then placed on ice in an insulated container.[13] A modification of this method involves complete anesthesia of the fish, and placing them in water bags which contain no anesthetic. In any case, upon arrival, the fish should be acclimated slowly to new environmental temperatures.

Preparation of FINQUEL® Solutions: Prior to use, FINQUEL® may be weighed into amounts which are convenient for the volume of water to be used. A handy unit is 2 g since this quantity in 5 gallons of water yields a concentration of about 100 mg/liter. For rough approximations, one level teaspoonful contains 2.0 to 2.5 g. Thus a level teaspoonful of anesthetic in 5 gallons gives a concentration of about 120 mg/liter.

To convert mg/liter into g/gal: multiply number of mg by 0.00378.
e.g. 80 mg/liter = 80 x 0.00378 = 0.302 g/gal
To convert mg/liter into a ratio of FINQUEL® to water: divide 1,000,000 by the number of mg.
e.g. 80 mg/liter = 1,000,000 ÷ 80 = 1:12,500
Guidelines for Use on Amphibians:
Table 4: Effects of Varying Concentrations of FINQUEL® on Salamanders.

Salamander	Concentration*	Duration of Anesthesia*	Remarks
Embryos	1:10,000 (3b)	2 days	No adverse effects.
Ambystoma opacum	1:3,000 (3c)	to 30 min.	
Larvae	1:10,000 (3b)	2 days	No adverse effects.
	1:12,000 (3f)	10-15 min.	
	1:20,000 (3f)	10-15 min.	
Ambystoma opacum	1:3,000 (3c)	to 30 min.	No adverse effects.
Adults	1:1,000 (3b)	few min.	No adverse effects.
	1:3,000 (3b)	3 days	
Newts	1:1,000 (3b)	few min.	No adverse effects.
	1:10,000 (3b)	2 days	
Triturus sp.	1:1,000 (3k)	20 min.	No adverse effects.
Triturus uridescens	1:3,000 (3g)	1 hour	No adverse effects.

Salamander	Concentration*	Duration of Anesthesia*	Remarks
Mole salamanders			
Ambystoma opacum	1:3,000 (3c)	to 30 min.	No adverse effects.
Ambystoma tigrinum	1:2,000 (3j)	15-30 min.	No adverse effects.
Ambystoma punctatum	1:2,000 (3j)	15-30 min.	No adverse effects.
Mud-puppy			
Necturus maculosus	1:1,500 (3i)	to 6 hours	See below.**

**Remarks: Maintenance dose, 0.1 of induction concentration. At exposure to induction concentration for more than 20-30 min., renal circulation becomes sluggish or stops.

Table 5: Effects of Varying Concentrations of FINQUEL® on Frogs.

Frog	Concentration*	Duration of Anesthesia*	Remarks
Embryos	1:1,000 (3b)	few min.	No adverse effects.
	1:10,000 (3b)	2 days	
	1:15,000 (3h)	3 days	
Tadpoles	1:1,000 (3j)	30 min.	No adverse effects.
	1:3,000 (3f)	10-15 min.	
	1:10,000 (3b)	2 days	
	1:15,000 (3h)	3 days	
Rana sp.	1:5,000 (3k)	5 hours	No adverse effects.
Rana pipiens	1:1,000 (3j)	15-30 min.	
	1:3,333 (3a)	2 min.	
	variable (3d)	1 hour	
Adults	1:1,000 (3e)	30 min.	No adverse effects.
Leopard frog			
Rana pipiens	1:3,000 (3c)	to 30 min.	No adverse effects.
Eastern wood frog			
Rana sylvatica	1:8,000 (3l)	5-10 min.	Only slightly under anesthesia.

* When an individual of any of the species listed is exposed at the designated concentration, the data available suggest that the animal may be safely maintained under anesthesia for the time noted. Prolonging exposure to the anesthetic beyond the time indicated may cause deaths (see Cautions).

Precaution(s): Keep tightly closed. Use only fresh solution. Store at room temperature (approximately 25°C).

Store FINQUEL® solutions in a cool place away from light.*

Discard stock solutions of FINQUEL® after several days.*

* The color of FINQUEL® solutions may change rapidly to yellow or brown when exposed to light. This does not affect activity in any significant way. However, for best results use freshly prepared solutions. A 10 per cent solution stored at room temperature shows no significant loss of potency after three days, but after 10 days, a brownish color and an activity decrease of about 5 per cent is observed.

Caution(s):

1. Avoid inhaling FINQUEL® or getting it into the eyes.
2. Always conduct preliminary tests with FINQUEL® to determine desired rates of anesthesia and optimal length of exposure.
3. Do not overexpose fish to lethal levels of FINQUEL®.
4. Do not anesthetize more fish than can be handled effectively.
5. Do not contaminate eggs or sperm with FINQUEL® when stripping fish.
6. Do not use water containing chlorine, or other toxic agents.
7. Insure adequate oxygen in anesthetic solution.
8. Discard anesthetic solutions when fouled with mucus or metabolic wastes.
9. Do not discard FINQUEL® solutions into water supplies or natural waters.

Warning(s): Keep out of reach of children.

Do not use within 21 days of harvesting fish for food.

When used in food fish, use should be restricted to Ictaluridae, Salmonidae, Esocidae, and Percidae and water temperature should exceed 10°C (50°F).

Limitations in Use: Since FINQUEL® is taken up into the blood of fish, residues of the drug may occur in edible tissues. However, the residues dissipate rapidly after the fish are placed in fresh water.[14] Thus, treated fish which may be used for food must be held in fresh water above 10°C (50°F) for a period of 21 days.

Withdrawal in fresh water is unnecessary for non food fishes such as goldfish, bait fish, and ornamentals. Also, withdrawal is unnecessary for sublegal sizes of the following species of fish because they are not used as food immediately following anesthesia (Table 6).

Table 6: Sublegal Sizes of Fish Species Not Used as Food Immediately after Anesthesia.[15]

Species	Size (in.)
Pink salmon	6
Chum salmon	6
Coho salmon	6
Sockeye salmon	6
Chinook salmon	6
Cutthroat trout	6
Steelhead trout	8
Rainbow trout	6
Atlantic salmon	10
Brown trout	6
Brook trout	6
Lake trout	5
Splake trout	6
Grayling	6
Northern pike	12
Muskellunge	12
Channel catfish	6
Flathead catfish	6
Bluegill	3
Redear sunfish	3
Smallmouth bass	5
Largemouth bass	5
Walleye	6

In other fish and other cold-blooded animals (poikilotherms), FINQUEL® should be limited to hatchery or laboratory use.

Toxicology: Comparative toxicologic studies carried out on fish and frogs gave the following results:

Fish Toxicity Studies: The toxicity[1] of FINQUEL® was measured by standard methods in laboratory bioassays with rainbow trout, brown trout, brook trout, lake trout, northern pike, channel catfish, bluegill, largemouth bass, and walleye. The 24, 48, and 96 hour LC_{50} (lethal concentration for 50 per cent of the animals) values for trout ranged from 52 to 31 mg/liter; for northern pike, from 56 to 48 mg/liter; for catfish, from 66 to 50 mg/liter; for bluegill and largemouth bass, from 61 to 39 mg/liter; and for walleye, the values were 49 to 46 mg/liter.

Safety index: The safety indices for FINQUEL® refer to the margin between concentrations which cause anesthesia and mortality. They are expressed by the quotient of the lethal concentration for 50 per cent of the fish (LC_{50}) and the effective concentration for 50 per cent of the fish (EC_{50}).

Safety Indices for Rainbow Trout and Channel Catfish at 12°C (54°F):

Species	Exposure (min.)	LC_{50} (mg/liter)	EC_{50} (mg/liter)	Index
Rainbow trout[1]	15	65	32	2.0
"	30	57	32	1.8
"	60	56	29	1.9
Channel catfish[2]	15	139	47	3.0
"	30	118	45	2.6
"	60	110	46	2.4

Frog Toxicity Studies[3]: Frogs were put into various concentrations of FINQUEL® for 30 minutes and then transferred to tap water in order to determine the LC_{50}. The LC_{50} was 6.2 per cent FINQUEL®. Therefore, the anesthetic must be used in very high concentrations before it is fatal to frogs.

Trial Data: Comparative Studies: T. Kappanyi and A.G. Karczmar compared tricaine with various aliphatic depressants such as paraldehyde, ethyl alcohol and barbiturates. They showed, using *Ambystoma punctatum* that subanesthetic concentrations of each acted additively with subanesthetic concentrations of tricaine. They stated that tricaine exhibited the property of rapid reversibility of action, i.e., short recovery time.[2]

E. Rothlin concluded that tricaine is three times less toxic than procaine and 10 times less toxic than cocaine.

References: Available upon request.

Presentation: Bottles of 0.18 oz (5 g), 3.5 oz (100 g), and 2.2 lb (1000 grams) of tricaine methanesulfonate).

Compendium Code No.: 10260000

FIRST COMPANION™ CANINE 7-WAY

AgriPharm **Bacterin-Vaccine**

Canine Distemper-Hepatitis-Parainfluenza-Parvovirus Vaccine, Modified Live Virus-Leptospira Bacterin

U.S. Vet. Lic. No.: 124

Contents: Canine 7-Way is a combination of antigenic, attenuated strains of canine distemper, canine parainfluenza, canine hepatitis, and parvovirus propagated in cell line tissue cultures. The liquid diluent is Parvovirus Vaccine-Leptospira canicola-icterohaemorrhagiae Bacterin. The CD virus fraction has been proven safe and non-shedding when injected into susceptible dogs. The infectious canine hepatitis (CAV-1) fraction cross protects against respiratory disease caused by CAV-2.

Preservatives: Gentamicin and a fungistat.

Indications: For the vaccination of healthy susceptible dogs against disease caused by canine distemper, hepatitis (canine adenovirus type 2), parainfluenza, parvovirus, *Leptospira canicola* and *Leptospira icterohaemorrhagiae.*

Dosage and Administration: The dry Distemper-Hepatitis-Parainfluenza Vaccine is rehydrated with 1 mL of liquid Parvovirus Vaccine-Leptospira canicola-icterohaemorrhagiae Bacterin. Shake well and use entire contents when first opened.

Using aseptic technique, inject 1 mL intramuscularly or subcutaneously. Repeat dosage in 3 to 4 weeks. Annual revaccination with a single dose is recommended. Puppies vaccinated before 9 weeks of age should be revaccinated at 3 to 4 week intervals until 14 to 16 weeks of age. Regardless of age, all dogs should receive 2 doses of vaccine in order to insure adequate levels of immunity against canine parainfluenza and parvovirus.

Always use care when handling the dog and provide proper restraint when vaccinating.

Prepare the vaccine by injecting the liquid diluent into the vial containing the vaccine cake.

Shake well. Remove the entire contents back into the syringe. Push out air trapped in the syringe.

To give subcutaneously, inject under loose skin (back of neck or behind front leg) or to give IM, inject into the muscle of the hind limb.

Do not vaccinate into blood vessels. If blood enters the syringe freely or when the plunger is pulled back slightly, choose another injection site.

Precaution(s): Store out of direct sunlight at a temperature not over 45°F. Avoid freezing. Burn containers and all unused contents.

Contraindication(s): Do not vaccinate pregnant animals. Under no circumstances is this product recommended for use in ferrets or mink.

Caution(s): An occasional transitory corneal opacity may occur following administration of the vaccine. This will disappear without untoward effect on the animal. Protective immunity may not be established in all puppies vaccinated at less than 16 weeks of age because of maternal antibody interference. Anaphylactoid reactions may occur.

Antidote(s): Administer epinephrine.

For use in dogs only.

Presentation: This package contains one (1 dose) vial of dry vaccine, one (1 mL) vial of liquid diluent and one disposable syringe.

Manufactured by: Boehringer Ingelheim Animal Health, Inc.

Compendium Code No.: 14570420

FIRST COMPANION™ EQUI-SPIRIN

AgriPharm **Non-Steroidal Anti-Inflammatory**

Microencapsulated Palatable Granules

Active Ingredient(s): Each 39 cc scoop contains 2500 mg of buffered aspirin.

Indications: Equi-Spirin aids in the temporary relief of pain and inflammation associated with arthritis, laminitis, chronic joint disease and soft tissue pain in horses.

Dosage and Administration: Usual dose for arthritis, lameness and joint pain is one scoop per 1000 lb body weight twice daily. For muscular pain the usual dose is 3 scoops per 1000 lb given twice daily. Give one level scoop twice daily at or before feeding.

Caution(s): If diarrhea occurs, stop administration and consult a veterinarian. Keep out of reach of children. For horses only.

Presentation: 700 grams.

Compendium Code No.: 14570431

FIRST DEFENSE®

ImmuCell **Antibodies**

Bovine Coronavirus-Escherichia coli Antibody, Bovine Origin

U.S. Vet. Lic. No.: 327

Active Ingredient(s): The neutralizing antibodies against bovine coronavirus as well as antibodies specific for *Escherichia coli* K99 pilus antigen present in FIRST DEFENSE® are prepared from hyperimmune bovine colostrum.

F

Indications: FIRST DEFENSE® is a capsule containing antibodies which aid in the reduction of morbidity and mortality of neonatal calf scours caused by K99+ *E. coli* and coronavirus. Maximum protection is achieved when the product is administered within the first 12 hours after birth and used in conjunction with colostrum feeding and good calf nutrition programs.

Dosage and Administration: A capsule dose of FIRST DEFENSE® should be given to each calf within the first 12 hours after birth. To administer, remove a FIRST DEFENSE® capsule from its blister pack by tearing off the foil backing and follow the instructions below:

1. Place the large end of the capsule in the dosing gun provided until firmly seated. Similarly sized oral bolus or capsule delivery devices can be used, but avoid guns with undersized openings which may fracture the capsule shell.
2. Restrain the calf and after gently prying open its mouth, place the dosing gun containing the capsule into the back of the throat and administer the capsule into the esophageal opening.
3. To assist the passage of the capsule down the esophagus and to stimulate a swallowing reflex, stroke the surface of the tongue or the outside of the throat.
4. The dosing gun should be cleaned and dried immediately following the administration of a capsule to each calf.

Precaution(s): FIRST DEFENSE® capsules are supplied in individual, moisture resistant blister packs which can be stored at or below room temperature (68° to 72°F or 20° to 23°C). The product is not harmed by freezing. If frozen, allow the blister package capsule to warm to room temperature before removal from the blister and administration. The capsules should remain in their blister packs until administered.

Caution(s): Do not vaccinate calves with oral coronavirus products within five days of administering FIRST DEFENSE®, since the antibodies present in FIRST DEFENSE® may neutralize the vaccine viruses. If an anaphylactic reaction occurs after feeding FIRST DEFENSE®, administer epinephrine, or an equivalent drug.

For veterinary use only.

Side Effects: FIRST DEFENSE® has been tested in a total of 473 beef and dairy calves under both laboratory and field conditions. Allergic or other adverse reactions were not observed.

Discussion: A FIRST DEFENSE® capsule containing dried colostral antibodies dissolves readily upon reaching the calf's stomach and provides protective levels of antibodies to potential sites of intestinal infection. Specific antibodies in FIRST DEFENSE® serve to block enterotoxigenic *E. coli* adherence and interfere with the viral infection of intestinal epithelial cells, thereby reducing scours-related morbidity and mortality.

While diarrhea in newborn calves can result from a variety of nutritional and management-related factors, the most common form of scours in calves during the first week of life is colibacillosis caused by enterotoxigenic K99+ *E. coli* (ETEC). ETEC infections alone cause 30-50% of scour-related deaths in newborn calves.[1,2] Adherence of ETEC to the intestinal epithelial cells via the K99 pili permits colonization and enhances enterotoxin induced hypersecretion of electrolytes and water. The resulting profuse yellowish diarrhea can lead to severe dehydration and death.[3,4]

An additional 15-38% of neonatal scours mortality is associated with infections caused by coronavirus either alone, or in combination with K99+ *E. coli*, rotavirus or cryptosporidium.[2] While coronavirus diarrhea is most common between 7-14 days of age, coronavirus has been isolated in high frequency in calves during the neonatal period and is endemic in many dairy herds.[2,5]

Trial Data: Clinical studies showed that 90% (18 of 20) of the calves treated with FIRST DEFENSE® in the first 12 hours after birth survived without additional treatment following a severe challenge of K99+ *E. coli*. In contrast, only 40% (4 of 10) of the control calves survived the study interval (five days) under the same challenge conditions. Morbidity, as measured by fecal scores and dehydration scores, was also significantly reduced in FIRST DEFENSE® treated calves when compared to the control calves in the K99+ challenge trial.

In a similar challenge study with virulent, calf-passaged coronavirus, animals receiving FIRST DEFENSE® had a significant reduction in mortality (0/18 deaths) when compared to untreated controls (4/10 deaths). FIRST DEFENSE® treated calves also showed a significant reduction in scouring and dehydration compared to the control animals in the study.

References: Available upon request.

Presentation: Capsules packaged in individual, moisture resistant blister packs, five capsules per box.

Compendium Code No.: 11200010

FIRSTDOSE® CPV

Pfizer Animal Health **Vaccine**

Parvovirus Vaccine, Modified Live Virus

U.S. Vet. Lic. No.: 189

Description: FIRSTDOSE® CPV contains a strain of CPV attenuated by low passage on the canine cell line and at that passage level has immunogenic properties capable of overriding maternal antibodies. Some puppies in the field may have higher levels of maternal antibodies than those evaluated in our pivotal efficacy study. FIRSTDOSE® CPV is packaged in liquid form.

Indications: FIRSTDOSE® CPV is for vaccination of healthy dogs as an aid in preventing canine parvoviral enteritis caused by canine parvovirus (CPV).

Directions:

1. General Directions: Vaccination of healthy dogs is recommended. Shake well. Aseptically administer 1 mL subcutaneously or intramuscularly.
2. Primary Vaccination: Administer a single 1-mL dose to healthy dogs. If dogs are vaccinated before the age of 4 months, they should be revaccinated with a single dose upon reaching 4 months of age. (Maternal antibodies may interfere with development of an adequate immune response in puppies less than 4 months old.)
3. Revaccination: Annual revaccination with a single dose is recommended.

Precaution(s): Store at 2°-7°C. Prolonged exposure to higher temperatures and/or direct sunlight may adversely affect potency. Do not freeze.

Use entire contents when first opened.

Sterilized syringes and needles should be used to administer this vaccine. Do not sterilize with chemicals because traces of disinfectant may inactivate the vaccine.

Burn containers and all unused contents.

Caution(s): Vaccination of pregnant bitches should be avoided.

As with many vaccines, anaphylaxis may occur after use. Initial antidote of epinephrine is recommended and should be followed with appropriate supportive therapy.

This product has been shown to be efficacious in healthy animals. A protective immune response may not be elicited if animals are incubating an infectious disease, are malnourished or parasitized, are stressed due to shipment or environmental conditions, are otherwise immunocompromised, or the vaccine is not administered in accordance with label directions.

For use in dogs only.

Warning(s): For veterinary use only.

Discussion: Disease Description: CPV is generally transmitted through direct contact with infectious feces. The virus also can be carried on dogs' hair and feet or other contaminated objects and can remain infective for more than 6 months at room temperature.[1] With an incubation period of 4-14 days, CPV infection results in enteric disease characterized by sudden onset of vomiting and diarrhea, often hemorrhagic.[2,3] Leukopenia commonly accompanies clinical signs.[2] Course of CPV disease may be aggravated by concurrent parasitism or infection with other enteric pathogens.[1,3] Susceptible dogs of any age can be affected, but mortality is greatest in puppies. In puppies 4-12 weeks of age CPV may occasionally cause myocarditis that can result in acute heart failure after a brief and inconspicuous illness. Following infection many dogs are refractory to the disease for a year or more. Similarly, seropositive bitches may transfer to their puppies CPV antibodies which can interfere with active immunization of the puppies through 16 weeks of age.

Trial Data: Safety and Efficacy: FIRSTDOSE® CPV was subjected to comprehensive safety and efficacy testing. It was shown safe and reaction-free in laboratory tests and in clinical trials under field conditions. Product safety was demonstrated by oral administration of multiple doses of the vaccine strain to susceptible dogs, which remained normal. FIRSTDOSE® CPV vaccine virus shares a characteristic with other live CPV vaccine strains in that the vaccinal virus may be present in the feces following administration. Although this CPV vaccinal virus was found occasionally and in low titers in the feces of vaccinated dogs, testing demonstrated that the vaccine strain did not revert to virulence following 6 consecutive backpassages in susceptible dogs.

Susceptible test dogs all developed CPV antibody titers after vaccination and were protected following oral administration of virulent CPV. Conversely, after challenge exposure, nonvaccinated control dogs all developed clinical signs of CPV infection, including vomiting and diarrhea with blood and mucus in the feces. Challenge virus was isolated from the feces of 5/5 control dogs, but only 1/20 vaccinates, and all controls developed marked lymphopenia, while no lymphopenia was demonstrated in vaccinates.

Further research demonstrated a stronger correlation of CPV immunogenicity to number of attenuating virus passages than to antigenic mass; immunogenicity of the vaccinal strain was shown to decline as the number of passages increased. The low-passage vaccinal virus in FIRSTDOSE® CPV is therefore highly immunogenic and capable of stimulating active immunity in the presence of maternal antibodies at the levels shown in Table 1. Studies demonstrating that capability involved forty-one 6- to 8-week-old puppies (32 vaccinates and 9 controls) with the range of maternal antibody titers shown in Table 2. By 14 days after vaccination, 91% of vaccinates' titers were well above the protective threshold. By 21 days, all dogs, including the dog with the initial SN titer of 1:64 seroconverted, giving a group seroconversion rate of 100%. In contrast, seropositive sentinel littermate dogs' CPV antibody titers declined, demonstrating that initial antibody titers were indeed of maternal origin and no adventitious exposure occurred during the study.

Table 1. Pre- and Postvaccination Serum Neutralization (SN) Titers

Number of Dogs	Prevaccination	Postvaccination		
		7 Days	14 Days	21 Days
5	2	39.2	768.0	1433.6
2	4	3.0	36.0	192.0
11	8	45.1	457.5	488.7
9	16	33.8	263.1	739.6
4	32	40.0	450.0	640.0
1	64	32.0	32.0	128.0
Average	13.8	37.3	410.8	696.0

Table 2. Initial Serum Neutralization (SN) Titers of Vaccinates and Controls.

SN Titers	# Vaccinates Included	# Controls Included
1:2	5	0
1:4	2	1
1:8	11	2
1:16	9	4
1:32	4	2
1:64	1	0

References: Available upon request.

Presentation: 10 dose vials.

Compendium Code No.: 36901090

75-4926-05

FIRSTDOSE® CPV/CV

Pfizer Animal Health **Vaccine**

Canine Coronavirus-Parvovirus Vaccine, Modified Live and Killed Virus

U.S. Vet. Lic. No.: 189

Description: The product is a preparation of attenuated CPV and inactivated CCV propagated on established cell lines. The CPV fraction was attenuated by low passage on an established canine cell line and, at that passage level, has immunogenic properties capable of overriding maternal antibodies. Some puppies in the field may have higher levels of maternal antibodies than those evaluated in our pivotal efficacy study. FIRSTDOSE® CPV/CV is packaged in liquid form with an adjuvant.

Contains penicillin and streptomycin as preservatives.

Indications: FIRSTDOSE® CPV/CV is for vaccination of healthy dogs as an aid in preventing canine parvoviral enteritis caused by canine parvovirus (CPV) and canine coronaviral gastroenteritis caused by canine coronavirus (CCV).

Directions:

1. General Directions: Vaccination of healthy dogs is recommended. Shake well. Aseptically administer 1 mL subcutaneously or intramuscularly.
2. Primary Vaccination: Healthy dogs should receive 2 doses administered 2-3 weeks apart. If dogs are vaccinated before the age of 4 months, they should be revaccinated with a single dose upon reaching 4 months of age. (Maternal antibodies may interfere with development of an adequate immune response in puppies less than 4 months old.)
3. Revaccination: Annual revaccination with a single dose is recommended.

Precaution(s): Store at 2°-7°C. Prolonged exposure to higher temperatures and/or direct sunlight may adversely affect potency. Do not freeze.

Use entire contents when first opened.

Sterilized syringes and needles should be used to administer this vaccine. Do not sterilize with chemicals because traces of disinfectant may inactivate the vaccine.

Burn containers and all unused contents.

Caution(s): Vaccination of pregnant bitches should be avoided.

As with many vaccines, anaphylaxis may occur after use. Initial antidote of epinephrine is recommended and should be followed with appropriate supportive therapy.

This product has been shown to be efficacious in healthy animals. A protective immune response may not be elicited if animals are incubating an infectious disease, are malnourished or parasitized, are stressed due to shipment or environmental conditions, are otherwise immunocompromised, or the vaccine is not administered in accordance with label directions.

For use in dogs only.

Warning(s): For veterinary use only.

Discussion: Disease Description: CPV is generally transmitted through direct contact with infectious feces. With an incubation period of 4-14 days, CPV infection results in enteric disease characterized by sudden onset of vomiting and diarrhea, often hemorrhagic. Leukopenia commonly accompanies clinical signs. Susceptible dogs of any age can be affected, but mortality is greatest in puppies.

CCV is also transmitted primarily through direct contact with infectious feces and may cause clinical enteritis within 1-4 days after exposure. Primary signs of CCV infection include depression, anorexia, fever, vomiting, and diarrhea. Leukopenia rarely occurs in uncomplicated cases. Particularly in puppies, potentially life-threatening dehydration may result from severe diarrhea.

Laboratory procedures are frequently employed to differentiate CPV and CCV infections due to their clinical similarities. Laboratory diagnosis based solely on hemagglutination (HA) tests, however, may not distinguish between the 2 agents because HA tests can yield positive results when either CPV or CCV is present, particularly at low levels of HA activity. The result may be a false positive diagnosis for either virus when in fact the other is the agent of disease. Comprehensive protection thus requires vaccination for both CPV and CCV.

Trial Data: Safety and Efficacy: FIRSTDOSE® CPV/CV was subjected to comprehensive safety testing. It was shown safe in laboratory tests and in clinical trials under field conditions.

Safety of the CPV fraction in FIRSTDOSE® CPV/CV was demonstrated by oral administration of multiple doses of the vaccine strain to susceptible dogs, which remained normal. The CPV virus in FIRSTDOSE® CPV/CV shares a characteristic with other live CPV vaccine strains in that the vaccinal virus may be present in the feces following administration. Although this CPV vaccinal virus was found occasionally and in low titers in the feces of vaccinated dogs, testing demonstrated that the vaccine strain did not revert to virulence following 6 consecutive backpassages in susceptible dogs.

Safety of the CCV fraction in FIRSTDOSE® CPV/CV was assessed in a field trial in which 5,999 doses were administered. Postvaccinal reactions occurred in 0.78% of vaccinates. Stinging and pain was observed in 0.08% of vaccinates, transient lameness or swelling was observed in 0.28% of vaccinates, anaphylaxis was observed in 0.12% of vaccinates, and gastroenteritis was observed in 0.30% of vaccinates.

Efficacy of the CPV fraction in FIRSTDOSE® CPV/CV was demonstrated in challenge-of-immunity studies. Susceptible test dogs all developed CPV antibody titers after vaccination and were protected following oral administration of virulent CPV. Conversely, after challenge exposure, nonvaccinated control dogs all developed clinical signs of CPV enteritis, including vomiting and diarrhea with blood and mucus in the feces. Challenge virus was isolated from the feces of 5/5 control dogs, but only 1/20 vaccinates, and all controls developed marked lymphopenia, while no lymphopenia was demonstrated in vaccinates.

Further research demonstrated a stronger correlation of CPV immunogenicity to number of attenuating virus passages than to antigenic mass; immunogenicity of the vaccinal strain was shown to decline as the number of passages increased. The low-passage vaccinal virus in Vanguard 5 is therefore highly immunogenic and capable of stimulating active immunity in the presence of maternal antibodies at the levels shown in Table 1. Studies demonstrating that capability involved forty-one 6- to 8-week-old puppies (32 vaccinates and 9 controls) with the range of maternal antibody titers shown in Table 2. By 14 days after vaccination, 91% of vaccinates' titers were well above the protective threshold. By 21 days, all dogs, including the dog with the initial SN titer of 1:64 seroconverted, giving a group seroconversion rate of 100%. In contrast, seropositive sentinel littermate dogs' CPV antibody titers declined, demonstrating that initial antibody titers were indeed of maternal origin and no adventitious exposure occurred during the study.

Table 1. Pre- and Postvaccination Serum Neutralization (SN) Titers

Number of Dogs	Prevaccination	Postvaccination		
		7 Days	14 Days	21 Days
5	2	39.2	768.0	1433.6
2	4	3.0	36.0	192.0
11	8	45.1	457.5	488.7
9	16	33.8	263.1	739.6
4	32	40.0	450.0	640.0
1	64	32.0	32.0	128.0
Average	13.8	37.3	410.8	696.0

Table 2. Initial Serum Neutralization (SN) Titers of Vaccinates and Controls.

SN Titers	# Vaccinates Included	# Controls Included
1:2	5	0
1:4	2	1
1:8	11	2
1:16	9	4
1:32	4	2
1:64	1	0

Efficacy of the CCV fraction in FirstDose CPV/CV was demonstrated in challenge-of-immunity studies involving 20 vaccinated puppies and 10 controls. Twenty 6- to 7-week-old puppies received 1 dose of vaccine given by the subcutaneous route, followed by a second subcutaneous dose 21 days later. Vaccinates and controls were challenged with virulent CCV 21 days postvaccination. Puppies vaccinated with CCV demonstrated significant differences in reduction of clinical signs, virus shed, and reduction of diarrhea postchallenge when compared to the control group. There was a significant reduction of IFA detectable CCV antigen detected in the intestine at 19 days postchallenge in vaccinates compared to the control group. Serological responses of vaccinates were equal to or higher than the control group.

Presentation: Cartons of 50 x 1 dose vials.

U.S. Patent Nos. 4,567,042; 4,567,043; and 4,824,785

Compendium Code No.: 36901100

75-4930-05

F

FIRSTDOSE® CV

Pfizer Animal Health **Vaccine**

Canine Coronavirus Vaccine, Killed Virus

U.S. Vet. Lic. No.: 189

Description: The product is a liquid preparation of inactivated CCV propagated on an established cell line with an adjuvant to enhance the immune response.

Contains penicillin and streptomycin as preservatives.

Indications: FIRSTDOSE® CV is for vaccination of healthy dogs 6 weeks of age or older as an aid in preventing canine coronaviral gastroenteritis caused by canine coronavirus (CCV).

Directions:

1. General Directions: Vaccination of healthy dogs is recommended. Shake well. Aseptically administer 1 mL subcutaneously or intramuscularly.
2. Primary Vaccination: Healthy dogs 6 weeks of age or older should receive 2 doses administered 2-3 weeks apart. If dogs are vaccinated before the age of 4 months, they should be revaccinated with a single dose upon reaching 4 months of age. (Maternal antibodies may interfere with development of an adequate immune response in puppies less than 4 months old.)
3. Revaccination: Annual revaccination with a single dose is recommended.

Precaution(s): Store at 2°-7°C. Prolonged exposure to higher temperatures may adversely affect potency. Do not freeze.

Use entire contents when first opened.

Caution(s): Vaccination of pregnant bitches should be avoided.

As with many vaccines, anaphylaxis may occur after use. Initial antidote of epinephrine is recommended and should be followed with appropriate supportive therapy.

This product has been shown to be efficacious in healthy animals. A protective immune response may not be elicited if animals are incubating an infectious disease, are malnourished or parasitized, are stressed due to shipment or environmental conditions, are otherwise immunocompromised, or the vaccine is not administered in accordance with label directions.

For use in dogs only.

Warning(s): For veterinary use only.

Discussion: Disease Description: CCV causes enteric disease in susceptible dogs of all ages worldwide. Highly contagious, the virus is transmitted primarily through direct contact with infectious feces and may cause clinical enteritis within 1-4 days after exposure. Severity of disease may be exacerbated by concurrent infection with other agents or by environmental stress.[1] Primary signs of CCV infection include depression, anorexia, fever, vomiting, and diarrhea. Frequency of vomiting usually diminishes within a day or 2 after onset of diarrhea, but diarrhea may linger through the course of infection, and stools occasionally may contain streaks of blood. Particularly in puppies, dehydration is a potentially life-threatening result of severe diarrhea with death loss occasionally occurring within 24-36 hours after onset of disease.[2] With CCV infection most dogs remain afebrile or have subnormal body temperature, and leukopenia is rarely observed in uncomplicated cases.[3]

Laboratory procedures are frequently employed to differentiate CCV and canine parvovirus (CPV) infections due to their clinical similarities. Laboratory diagnosis based solely on hemagglutination (HA) tests, however, may not distinguish between the 2 agents because HA tests can yield positive results when either CCV or CPV is present, particularly at low levels of HA activity. The result may be a false positive diagnosis for either virus when in fact the other is the agent of disease. Initial widespread prevalence of CPV, combined with the ambiguities of the HA test, may have obscured the prevalence of CCV as a source of canine enteritides. Comprehensive protection thus requires vaccination for both CCV and CPV.

Trial Data: Safety and Efficacy: Safety of FIRSTDOSE® CV was assessed in a field trial in which 5,999 doses were administered. Postvaccinal reactions occurred in 0.78% of vaccinates. Stinging and pain was observed in 0.08% of vaccinates, transient lameness or swelling was observed in 0.28% of vaccinates, anaphylaxis was observed in 0.12% of vaccinates, and gastroenteritis was observed in 0.30% of vaccinates.

Efficacy of FIRSTDOSE® CV was demonstrated in a challenge-of-immunity study involving 20 vaccinated puppies and 10 controls. Twenty 6- to 7-week-old puppies received 1 dose of vaccine given by the subcutaneous route, followed by a second subcutaneous dose 21 days later. Vaccinates and controls were challenged with virulent CCV 21 days postvaccination. Puppies vaccinated with CCV demonstrated significant differences in reduction of clinical signs, virus shed, and reduction of diarrhea postchallenge when compared to the control group. There was a significant reduction of IFA detectable CCV antigen detected in the intestine at 19 days postchallenge in vaccinates compared to the control group. Serological responses of vaccinates were equal to or higher than the control group.

References: Available upon request.

Presentation: Cartons of 50 x 1 dose vials of vaccine.

U.S. Patent Nos. 4,567,042; 4,567,043; and 4,824,785

Compendium Code No.: 36901110

75-4928-04

FLAVOMYCIN® 4

Intervet **Feed Additive**

(Bambermycins)-Type A Medicated Article

NADA No.: 44-759

Active Ingredient(s): Bambermycins 4 grams per pound (8.8 grams per kilogram).

Ingredients: Roughage products and/or calcium carbonate, dried bambermycins fermentation product, mineral oil.

Indications: For increased rate of weight gain and improved feed efficiency in broiler chickens, growing-finishing swine and growing turkeys.

Claims: Permitted Claims and Limitations:

Species	Drug	Level/Ton	Claim(s)	Limitations
Broiler Chickens	Bambermycins	1-2 grams*	Increased rate of weight gain; improved feed efficiency	None
Growing-Finishing Swine	Bambermycins	2 grams	Increased rate of weight gain; improved feed efficiency	None
	Bambermycins	2-4 grams*	Increased rate of weight gain	
Growing Turkeys	Bambermycins	2 grams	Increased rate of weight gain; improved feed efficiency	None
	Bambermycins	1-2 grams*	Improved feed efficiency	

*Only a single level of bambermycins (i.e. 4 grams/ton bambermycins) can be indicated on a feed tag. A different tag must be submitted for each level of bambermycins needed for your complete feeding program.

Dosage and Administration:

Mixing Directions: It is recommended that FLAVOMYCIN® 4 be diluted with a suitable grain carrier before addition to the final feed. A dilution of 1 part of FLAVOMYCIN® 4 and 9 parts grain carrier is the suggested working premix. The table below shows premix and working premix addition levels for various commonly used feeds.

Feed	Bambermycins Level	Pounds Premix/Ton FLAVOMYCIN® 4	1-9 Working Premix (Pounds/Ton)
Broiler Chickens	1 gram/ton	.25	2.50
	2 grams/ton	.50	5.00
Growing-Finishing Swine	2 grams/ton	.50	5.00
	3 grams/ton	.75	7.50
	4 grams/ton	1.00	10.00
Growing Turkeys	1 gram/ton	.25	2.50
	2 grams/ton	.50	5.00

Thoroughly mix both working premix and finished feed to ensure complete and uniform distribution of the FLAVOMYCIN®.

Feeding Directions: Feed containing FLAVOMYCIN® should be fed continuously as the sole ration.

Caution(s): For use in manufactured feeds only.

Presentation: 50 pounds (22.68 kg).

Compendium Code No.: 11060560

FLAVORED ASPIRIN POWDER

First Priority **Non-Steroidal Anti-Inflammatory**

Active Ingredient(s):

Acetylsalicylic Acid (Aspirin) .... 226,573 mg
Sucrose .... q.s.
Apple Flavor .... q.s.

Indications: For use as an aid in reducing fever and for mild analgesia.

Directions for Use: Administer orally.

Cattle, Horses: 10-120 g (½-4 oz)
Calves, Foals: 6-12 g (¼-½ oz)
Sheep, Swine: 2-6 g (approx. ¼ oz)
Poultry: 0.30% level in ration
Dogs: 0.30% - 2.0 g
1 level tablespoon is approximately ½ oz.
½ oz contains approximately 7080 mg of Aspirin.

Precaution(s): Storage: Store at controlled room temperature between 15°-30°C (59°-86°F). Keep container tightly closed when not in use.

Caution(s): For animal use only.

Warning(s): Keep out of reach of children.

Presentation: 1 lb (453.6 g) (NDC# 58829-300-16) and 25 lb (11.34 kg) (NDC# 58829-300-26).

Compendium Code No.: 11390313 Rev. 09-01 / Iss. 09-01

FLEA & TICK MIST

Davis **Parasiticide Spray**

EPA Reg. No.: 50591-14

Active Ingredient(s):

Pyrethrins 0.15%
Piperonyl butoxide 1.00%
N-octyl bicycloheptene dicarboximide 0.50%
Di-n-propyl isocinchomeronate 0.50%

Indications: FLEA & TICK MIST with soothing aloe, lanolin and sunscreen is a scented formula for use on dogs, cat, puppies, kittens, horses and foals to kill fleas, ticks and lice on contact and repels mosquitoes, gnats and flies for two or three days.

Dosage and Administration: With a firm stroke to get a proper spray mist, spray the head, ears and chest until damp. With the fingertips, rub into the face around the mouth, nose and eyes. Then spray the neck, middle and hindquarters, finishing with the legs. For the best penetration of spray to the skin, direct the spray against the natural lay of the hair. Repeat the treatment as needed.

Caution(s): Avoid treatment of nursing kittens and puppies under six weeks of age.

Presentation: 16 oz. and 32 oz.

Compendium Code No.: 11410220

FLEA HALT!™ FLEA & TICK REPELLENT TOWELETTES

Farnam **Flea Control & Topical Parasiticide**

EPA Reg. No.: 11715-241-270

Active Ingredient(s):

Pyrethrins 0.116%
Piperonyl Butoxide, Technical* 1.161%
N-Octyl Bicycloheptene Dicarboximide** 0.387%
Inert Ingredients 98.336%
Total 100.000%

*Equivalent to min 0.929% (butylcarbityl) (6-propylpiperonyl) ether and 0.232% related compounds.

**MGK 264 insecticide synergist

Indications: Kills and repels fleas, ticks, lice, deer ticks, mites, and mosquitoes on cats, ferrits, rabbits, guinea pigs, hamsters and gerbils. It also deodorizes and conditions.

Directions for Use: It is a violation of Federal law to use this product in a manner inconsistent with its labeling.

Read entire label before each use.

Use only on cats, ferrits, rabbits, guinea pigs, hamsters or gerbils.

Tear corner of pouch. Remove Towelette and dispose of pouch in trash.

For use on animals: To protect animals from fleas, ticks, deer ticks, mites, and mosquitoes: First brush animal to remove excess dirt and dust. Apply a light coating sufficient to wet the tips of the hair. Reapply every week to give continued protection.

To control lice: Apply wipe lightly to infested areas. Repeat every two to three weeks as required.

Wash hands thoroughly after application.

Precautionary Statements: Hazards to Humans and Domestic Animals:

Caution: Harmful if swallowed. Wash thoroughly with soap and water after handling. Do not use on kittens under 12 weeks of age. Do not use on old, sick or debilitated animals. Consult a veterinarian before using this product on pregnant or nursing animals, or animals on medication. Do not apply to animal's genitalia or get in eyes. Sensitivities may occur after using any pesticide product for pets. If signs of sensitivity occur, bathe your pet with mild soap and rinse with large amounts of water. If signs continue, consult a veterinarian immediately.

First Aid:

If swallowed: Call a physician or Poison Control Center. Drink 1 or 2 glasses of water and induce vomiting by touching back of throat with finger. If person is unconscious, do not give anything by mouth and do not induce vomiting.

If on skin: Wash with plenty of soap and water. Get medical attention if irritation persists.

If in eyes: Flush with plenty of water. Get medical attention if irritation persists.

In case of emergency or for product use information, call (602) 285-1660 M-F 7:00-3:45 MST.

Environmental Hazards: This product is toxic to fish. Keep out of lakes, streams or ponds. Do not contaminate water by disposal of wastes.

Storage and Disposal: Do not contaminate water, food or feed by storage or disposal.

Storage: Store in a cool, dry place away from heat or open flame.

Container Disposal: Securely wrap original container in several layers of newspaper and discard in trash.

Pesticide Disposal: Wastes resulting from use of this product may be disposed of on site or at an approved waste disposal facility.

Warning(s): Keep out of reach of children.

Disclaimer: Buyer assumes all risks of use, storage or handling of this material not in strict accordance with directions given herewith.

Presentation: 2 wipes (0.21 oz) (5.8 g).

Compendium Code No.: 10000181 0AA1

FLEA HALT!™ FLEA & TICK REPELLENT TOWELETTES FOR FERRETS

Farnam **Flea Control & Topical Parasiticide**

EPA Reg. No.: 11715-241-270

Active Ingredient(s):

Pyrethrins 0.116%
Piperonyl Butoxide, Technical* 1.161%
N-Octyl Bicycloheptene Dicarboximide** 0.387%
Inert Ingredients 98.336%
Total 100.000%

*Equivalent to min 0.929% (butylcarbityl) (6-propylpiperonyl) ether and 0.232% related compounds.

**MGK 264 Insecticide Synergist

Indications: Kills and repels fleas, ticks, lice, deer ticks, mites, and mosquitoes on ferrets. Deodorizes and conditions.

Directions for Use: It is a violation of Federal law to use this product in a manner inconsistent with its labeling.

Read entire label before each use.

Tear corner of pouch. Remove Towelette and dispose of pouch in trash.

For use on ferrets: To protect animals from fleas, ticks, deer ticks, mites, and mosquitoes: First brush animal to remove excess dirt and dust. Apply a light coating sufficient to wet the tips of the hair. Reapply every week to give continued protection.

To control lice: Apply wipe lightly to infested areas. Repeat every two to three weeks as required.

Wash hands thoroughly after application.

Precautionary Statements: Hazards to Humans and Domestic Animals:

Caution: Harmful if swallowed. Wash thoroughly with soap and water after handling. Do not use on animals under 12 weeks of age. Do not use on old, sick or debilitated animals. Consult a veterinarian before using this product on pregnant or nursing animals, or animals on medication. Do not apply to animal's genitalia or get in eyes. Sensitivities may occur after using any pesticide product for pets. If signs of sensitivity occur, bathe your pet with mild soap and rinse with large amounts of water. If signs continue, consult a veterinarian immediately.

First Aid:

If swallowed: Call a physician or Poison Control Center. Drink 1 or 2 glasses of water and induce vomiting by touching back of throat with finger. If person is unconscious, do not give anything by mouth and do not induce vomiting.

If on skin: Wash with plenty of soap and water. Get medical attention if irritation persists.

If in eyes: Flush with plenty of water. Get medical attention if irritation persists.

Environmental Hazards: This product is toxic to fish. Keep out of lakes, streams or ponds. Do not contaminate water by disposal of wastes.

In case of emergency, or for product use information, call (602) 285-1660 Monday - Friday 7:00 AM to 3:45 PM, MST.

Storage and Disposal: Do not contaminate water, food or feed by storage or disposal.

Storage: Store in a cool, dry place away from heat or open flame.

Container Disposal: Securely wrap original container in several layers of newspaper and discard in trash.

Pesticide Disposal: Wastes resulting from use of this product may be disposed of on site or at an approved waste disposal facility.

Warning(s): Keep out of reach of children.

Use only on ferrets.

Disclaimer: Buyer assumes all risks of use, storage or handling of this material not in strict accordance with directions given herewith.

Presentation: 2 wipes (0.21 oz) (5.8 g).

Compendium Code No.: 10000191 9EE8

FLEA, TICK AND LICE SHAMPOO

Tomlyn **Parasiticide Shampoo**

EPA Reg. No.: 50414-5

Active Ingredient(s):

Pyrethrins 0.207%
*Piperonyl Butoxide, technical 0.414%
‡N-Octyl bicycloheptene dicarboximide 0.690%
Inert ingredients.......... 98.689%

*Equivalent to .331% butylcarbityl (6-propylpiperonyl) ether and .083% related compounds.

‡MGK 264 insecticide synergist.

With coconut oil and moisturizers for dogs & cats.

Indications: An antiparasitic shampoo to kill fleas, ticks and lice on dogs and cats.

Directions: It is a violation of federal law to use this product in a manner inconsistent with its labeling.

Dilute Tomlyn's FLEA, TICK AND LICE SHAMPOO one part with three parts water. Wet dog or cat with warm water. Apply shampoo liberally beginning at the head and working backward until entire body is covered. For difficult infestations, allow lather to remain on animal for 3-5 minutes. Rinse thoroughly. Keep away from eyes. Repeat as necessary, but do not repeat treatment for 1 week.

Do not use on animals under 12 weeks. Consult a veterinarian before using this product on debilitated, aged, pregnant or nursing animals. Sensitivities may occur after using any pesticide product for pets. If signs of sensitivity occur bathe your pet with mild soap and rinse with large amounts of water. If signs continue, consult a veterinarian immediately. Certain medications can interact with pesticides. Consult a veterinarian before using on medicated animals.

Precautionary Statements: Hazardous to Humans and Domestic Animals.

Caution: Avoid contact with eyes. In case of contact flush eyes thoroughly with water. Obtain medical attention if irritation persists.

Storage and Disposal: Store product in original container in a cool, dry place. Do not reuse container. Wrap empty container and place in trash.

Warning(s): Keep out of reach of children.

Presentation: 8 fl oz (237 mL) -- concentrate makes 1 full quart.
4 x 1 Gallon (128 fl oz - 3.79 liters) -- concentrate makes 4 gallons.

Compendium Code No.: 11220060 087-1

FLOCKCHEK® AE ANTIBODY TEST KIT

Idexx Labs. **Avian Encephalomyelitis Test**

Avian Encephalomyelitis Antibody Test Kit

U.S. Vet. Lic. No.: 313

Components:

Reagent	Volume
1. AE Coated Plates	5
2. AE Positive Control - Diluted chicken Anti-AE, preserved with sodium azide.	1.9 mL
3. Negative Control - Diluted chicken sera non-reactive for Anti-AE, preserved with sodium azide.	1.9 mL
4. (Goat) Anti-Chicken: HRPO Conjugate, preserved with gentamicin.	50 mL
5. Sample Diluent buffer preserved with sodium azide.	235 mL
6. TMB Substrate	60 mL
7. Stop Solution	60 mL

Materials Required but Not Provided: Precision pipets and multiple delivery pipetting device with disposable pipet tips, 96-well plate reader, tubes for diluting samples, distilled or deionized water and device for the delivery and aspiration of wash solution.

Indications: FLOCKCHEK® AE is Idexx's enzyme immunoassay for the detection of antibody to Avian Encephalomyelitis (AE) in chicken serum.

Test Principles: This assay is designed to measure the relative level of antibody to AE in chicken serum. Viral antigen is coated on 96-well plates. Upon incubation of the test sample in the coated well, antibody specific to AE forms a complex with the coated viral antigens. After washing away unbound material from the wells, a conjugate is added which binds to any attached chicken antibody in the wells. Unbound conjugate is washed away and enzyme substrate is added. Subsequent color development is directly related to the amount of antibody to AE present in the test sample.

Test Procedure:

Preparation of Samples: Dilute test samples five hundred fold (1:500) with sample diluent prior to being assayed (e.g., by diluting 1 µL of sample with 500 µL of Sample Diluent). Note: Do not dilute controls. Be sure to change tips for each sample. Samples must be thoroughly mixed prior to dispensing into the coated plate.

Reagents should be allowed to come to room temperature, then mixed by inverting and swirling.

1. Obtain antigen-coated plate(s) and record the sample position on a FlockChek® worksheet.
2. Dispense 100 µL of Undiluted Negative Control into wells A1 and A2.
3. Dispense 100 µL of Undiluted Positive Control into wells A3 and A4.
4. Dispense 100 µL of diluted sample into appropriate wells. All samples should be run in duplicate.
5. Incubate for 30 minutes at room temperature.
6. Wash each well with approximately 350 µL of distilled or deionized water 3-5 times.
7. Dispense 100 µL of (Goat) Anti-Chicken: HRPO Conjugate into each well.
8. Incubate for 30 minutes at room temperature.
9. Repeat step 6.
10. Dispense 100 µL of TMB substrate solution into each well.
11. Incubate for 15 minutes at room temperature.
12. Dispense 100 µL of Stop Solution into each well to stop the reaction.
13. Blank reader with air.
14. Measure and record absorbance at 650nm, A(650).

Test Interpretation:

Results: For the assay to be valid, the difference between the Positive Control mean and the Negative Control mean ($PC\bar{x}-NC\bar{x}$) should be greater than 0.075. The Negative Control mean absorbance should be less than or equal to 0.150. The presence or absence of antibody to AE is determined by relating the A(650) value of the unknown to the Positive Control mean. The Positive Control is standardized and represents significant antibody levels to AE in chicken serum. The relative level of antibody in the unknown is determined by calculating the sample to positive (S/P) ratio. Endpoint titers are calculated using the equation described in the calculations section.

Interpretation of Results: Serum samples with S/P ratios of less than or equal to 0.2 should be considered negative. S/P ratios greater than 0.2 (titers greater than 396) should be considered positive and indicate vaccination or other exposure to AE. Each laboratory should establish its own criterion for immunity with respect to antibody titer based on correlation of FLOCKCHEK® AE to current laboratory test methodologies and on historical antibody responses to specific vaccines and vaccination protocols. The immune status of a flock is best assessed by monitoring and recording antibody titers in representative samples as a function of time. The resulting flock profiles allow an assessment of the distribution of antibody titers and an analysis of changes in titer over time.

Calculations:

1. Negative Control mean ($NC\bar{x}$):
$$\frac{\text{Well A1 A(650)} + \text{Well A2 A(650)}}{2} = NC\bar{x}$$
2. Positive Control mean ($PC\bar{x}$):
$$\frac{\text{Well A3 A(650)} + \text{Well A4 A(650)}}{2} = PC\bar{x}$$
3. S/P Ratio:
$$\frac{\text{Sample Mean} - NC\bar{x}}{PC\bar{x} - NC\bar{x}} = S/P$$
4. Titer - Relates S/P at a 1:500 dilution to an endpoint titer:
$\log_{10}\text{Titer} = 1.09\,(\log_{10} S/P) + 3.36$

Storage: Store all reagents at 2°-7°C (36°-45°F).

Caution(s): Handle all AE biological materials as though capable of transmitting AE. The antigen coated plates may be a source of AE. Prior to coating on the solid phase, the antigen has been inactivated by chemical treatment. Nevertheless, do not assume complete inactivation. Some kit components contain sodium azide as a preservative. Disposal requires flushing plumbing with large volumes of water to prevent formation of copper or lead azide complexes which may explode upon percussion. Do not expose TMB solutions to strong light or any oxidation agents. All wastes should be properly decontaminated prior to disposal. Do not use components past expiration date and do not intermix components from kits with different lot numbers. Careful pipetting and washing throughout this procedure are necessary to maintain precision and accuracy. Optimal results will be obtained by strict adherence to this protocol. For veterinary use only.

Discussion: An assessment of immune status as well as serologic identification of AE requires a measurement of antibody to AE in serum. Enzyme immunoassay systems have proven efficacious in the quantification of antibody levels to AE and facilitate the monitoring of immune status in large flocks.

Presentation: 5 plates per kit.

FLOCKCHEK is a registered trademark of Idexx Laboratories, Inc. in the United States and/or other countries.

Compendium Code No.: 11160092 06-01114-05

FLOCKCHEK® AI VIRUS ANTIBODY TEST KIT

Idexx Labs. **Avian Influenza Test**

Avian Influenza Virus Antibody Test Kit

U.S. Vet. Lic. No.: 313

Components:

Reagent	Volume
1. AI Coated Plates	5
2. AI Positive Control - Diluted chicken Anti-AI, preserved with sodium azide.	1.9 mL
3. Negative Control - Diluted chicken sera non-reactive for Anti-AI, preserved with sodium azide.	1.9 mL
4. (Goat) Anti-Chicken/(Goat) Anti-Turkey: Horseradish Peroxidase Conjugate, preserved with gentamicin.	50 mL
5. Sample Diluent buffer preserved with sodium azide.	235 mL
6. TMB Substrate	60 mL
7. Stop Solution	60 mL

Materials Required but Not Provided: Precision pipets and multiple delivery pipetting device with disposible pipet tips, 96-well plate reader, tubes for diluting samples, distilled or deionized water and device for the delivery and aspiration of wash solution.

Indications: FLOCKCHEK® AI is Idexx's enzyme immunoassay for the detection of antibody to Avian Influenza Virus (AI) in chicken serum.

Test Principles: This assay is designed to measure the relative level of antibody to AI in chicken serum. Viral antigen is coated on 96-well plates. Upon incubation of the test sample in the coated well, antibody specific to AI forms a complex with the coated viral antigens. After washing away unbound material from the wells, a conjugate is added which binds to any attached antibody in the wells. Unbound conjugate is washed away and enzyme substrate is added. Subsequent color development is directly related to the amount of antibody to AI present in the test sample.

Test Procedure:

Preparation of Samples: Dilute test samples five hundred fold (1:500) with sample diluent prior to being assayed (e.g., by diluting 1 µL of sample with 500 µL of Sample Diluent). Note: Do not dilute controls. Be sure to change tips for each sample. Samples must be thoroughly mixed prior to dispensing into the coated plate.

Reagents should be allowed to come to room temperature, then mixed by inverting and swirling.

F

1. Obtain antigen-coated plate(s) and record the sample position on a FlockChek® worksheet.
2. Dispense 100 µL of Undiluted Negative Control into wells A1 and A2.
3. Dispense 100 µL of Undiluted Positive Control into wells A3 and A4.
4. Dispense 100 µL of diluted sample into appropriate wells. All samples should be run in duplicate.
5. Incubate for 30 minutes at room temperature.
6. Wash each well with approximately 350 µL of distilled or deionized water 3-5 times.
7. Dispense 100 µL of (Goat) Anti-Chicken/(Goat) Anti-Turkey: Horseradish Peroxidase Conjugate into each well.
8. Incubate for 30 minutes at room temperature.
9. Repeat step 6.
10. Dispense 100 µL of TMB substrate solution into each well.
11. Incubate for 15 minutes at room temperature.
12. Dispense 100 µL of Stop Solution into each well to stop the reaction.
13. Blank reader with air.
14. Measure and record absorbance values at 650nm, A(650).

Test Interpretation:

Results: For the assay to be valid, the difference between the Positive Control mean and the Negative Control mean ($PC\bar{x}$ - $NC\bar{x}$) should be greater than 0.075. The Negative Control mean absorbance should be less than or equal to 0.150. The presence or absence of antibody to AI is determined by relating the A(650) value of the unknown to the Positive Control mean. The Positive Control is standardized and represents significant antibody levels to AI in chicken serum. The relative level of antibody in the unknown is determined by calculating the sample to positive (S/P) ratio.

F

Interpretation of Results: Serum samples with S/P ratios of less than or equal to 0.5 should be considered negative. S/P ratios greater than 0.5 should be considered positive and indicate exposure to AI. ELISA positive samples should be confirmed by additional serological testing such as Agar Gel Precipitation Test (AGP).

*Note: U.S. Customers must submit all positive samples and/or results to the National Veterinary Services Laboratory for H and N titration.

Calculations:

1. Negative Control mean ($NC\bar{x}$):

$$\frac{\text{Well A1 A(650)} + \text{Well A2 A(650)}}{2} = NC\bar{x}$$

2. Positive Control mean ($PC\bar{x}$):

$$\frac{\text{Well A3 A(650)} + \text{Well A4 A(650)}}{2} = PC\bar{x}$$

3. S/P Ratio:

$$\frac{\text{Sample Mean} - NC\bar{x}}{PC\bar{x} - NC\bar{x}} = S/P$$

Storage: Store all reagents at 2°-7°C (36°-45°F).

Caution(s): Handle all AI biological materials as though capable of transmitting AI. The antigen coated plates may be a source of AI. Prior to coating on the solid phase, the antigen has been inactivated by chemical treatment. Nevertheless, do not assume complete inactivation. Some kit components contain sodium azide as a preservative. Disposal requires flushing plumbing with large volumes of water to prevent formation of copper or lead azide complexes which may explode upon percussion. Do not expose TMB solutions to strong light or any oxidation agents. All wastes should be properly decontaminated prior to disposal. Do not use components past expiration date and do not intermix components from kits with different lot numbers. Careful pipetting and washing throughout this procedure are necessary to maintain precision and accuracy. Optimal results will be obtained by strict adherence to this protocol. For veterinary use only.

Discussion: Domestic and wild avian species are affected by avian influenza viruses. The disease is characterized by a wide range of responses which include virtually no clinical signs to high mortality. Respiratory signs are common, along with drop in egg production, greenish diarrhea, bloodstained nasal and oral discharges, and cyanosis and edema of the head, comb and wattle. Due to the variation and severity of clinical symptoms, serological testing produces significant advantages to detection of infected birds. Monitoring for exposure of a flock to influenza is facilitated by the measurement of antibody to avian influenza in serum.

Presentation: 5 plates per kit.

FLOCKCHEK is a registered trademark of Idexx Laboratories, Inc. in the United States and/or other countries.

Compendium Code No.: 11160521 06-02806-02

FLOCKCHEK® ALV-Ab ANTIBODY TEST KIT

Idexx Labs. **Avian Leukosis Test**

Avian Leukosis Virus Antibody Test Kit

U.S. Vet. Lic. No.: 313

Components:

Reagent	Volume
1. ALV Coated Plates	5
2. ALV Positive Control - Diluted chicken Anti-ALV, preserved with sodium azide.	1.9 mL
3. Negative Control - Diluted chicken sera non-reactive for Anti-ALV, preserved with sodium azide.	1.9 mL
4. (Goat) Anti-Chicken: Horseradish Peroxidase Conjugate, preserved with gentamicin.	50 mL
5. Sample Diluent buffer preserved with sodium azide.	235 mL
6. TMB Substrate	60 mL
7. Stop Solution	60 mL

Materials Required but Not Provided: Precision pipets and multiple delivery pipetting device with disposable pipet tips, 96-well plate reader, tubes for diluting samples, distilled or deionized water and device for the delivery and aspiration of wash solution.

Indications: FLOCKCHEK® ALV Ab is Idexx's enzyme immunoassay for the detection of antibody to Avian Leukosis Virus (ALV-Subgroups A and B) in chicken serum.

Test Principles: This assay is designed to measure the relative level of antibody to ALV subgroups A and B in chicken serum. Antibody to subgroup E viruses, which include the endogenous leukosis viruses, is not detected. Viral antigen is coated on 96-well plates. Upon incubation of the test sample in the coated well, antibody specific to ALV (subgroups A and B) forms a complex with the coated viral antigens. After washing away unbound materials from the wells, a conjugate is added which binds to any attached chicken antibody in the wells. Unbound conjugate is washed away and enzyme substrate is added. Subsequent color development is directly related to the amount of antibody to ALV (subgroups A and B) present in the test sample.

Test Procedure:

Preparation of Samples: Dilute test samples five hundred fold (1:500) with sample diluent (e.g., by diluting 1 µL of sample with 500 µL of Sample Diluent). Note: Do not dilute controls. Be sure to change tips for each sample. Samples must be thoroughly mixed prior to dispensing into the coated plate.

Reagents should be allowed to come to room temperature, then mixed by inverting and swirling.

1. Obtain antigen coated plate(s) and record the sample position on a FlockChek® worksheet.
2. Dispense 100 µL of Undiluted Negative Control into wells A1 and A2.
3. Dispense 100 µL of Undiluted Positive Control into wells A3 and A4.
4. Dispense 100 µL of diluted sample into appropriate wells. All samples should be run in duplicate.
5. Incubate for 30 minutes at room temperature.
6. Wash each well with approximately 350 µL of distilled or deionized water 3-5 times.
7. Dispense 100 µL of (Goat) Anti-Chicken: Horseradish Peroxidase Conjugate into each well.
8. Incubate for 30 minutes at room temperature.
9. Repeat step 6.
10. Dispense 100 µL of TMB substrate solution into each well.
11. Incubate for 15 minutes at room temperature.
12. Dispense 100 µL of Stop Solution into each well to stop the reaction.
13. Blank reader with air.
14. Measure and record absorbance values at 650nm, A(650).

Test Interpretation:

Results: For the assay to be valid, the difference between the Positive Control mean and the Negative Control mean ($PC\bar{x}$-$NC\bar{x}$) should be greater than 0.075. In addition, the Negative Control mean absorbance should be less than or equal to 0.150. The presence or absence of antibody to ALV is determined by relating the A(650) value of the unknown to the Positive Control mean. The Positive Control is standardized and represents significant antibody levels to ALV in chicken serum. The relative level of antibody in the unknown can be determined by calculating the sample to positive (S/P) ratio. Endpoint titers are calculated using the equation described in the calculations section.

Interpretation of Results: Serum samples with S/P ratios of less than or equal to 0.4 should be considered negative. S/P ratios greater than 0.4 (titers greater than 844) should be considered positive and indicate vaccination or other exposure to ALV (Subgroups A and B). Each laboratory should establish its own criterion for the evaluation of a seropositive reaction with respect to antibody titer based on correlation of FLOCKCHEK® ALV to current laboratory test methodologies and on historical antibody responses.

Calculations:

1. Negative Control mean ($NC\bar{x}$):

$$\frac{\text{Well A1 A(650)} + \text{Well A2 A(650)}}{2} = NC\bar{x}$$

2. Positive Control mean ($PC\bar{x}$):

$$\frac{\text{Well A3 A(650)} + \text{Well A4 A(650)}}{2} = PC\bar{x}$$

3. S/P Ratio:

$$\frac{\text{Sample Mean} - NC\bar{x}}{PC\bar{x} - NC\bar{x}} = S/P$$

4. Titer - Relates S/P at a 1:500 dilution to an endpoint titer:

$$\text{Log}_{10}\ \text{Titer} = 1.09\ (\text{Log}_{10}\ S/P) + 3.36$$

Storage: Store all reagents at 2°-7°C (36°-45°F).

Caution(s): Handle all ALV biological materials as though capable of transmitting ALV. The antigen coated plates may be a source of ALV. Prior to coating on the solid phase, the antigen has been inactivated by chemical treatment. Nevertheless, do not assume complete inactivation. Some kit components contain sodium azide as a preservative. Disposal requires flushing plumbing with large volumes of water to prevent formation of copper or lead azide complexes which may explode upon percussion. Do not expose TMB solutions to strong light or any oxidation agents. All wastes should be properly decontaminated prior to disposal. Do not use components past expiration date and do not intermix components from kits with different lot numbers. Careful pipetting and washing throughout this procedure are necessary to maintain precision and accuracy. Optimal results will be obtained by strict adherence to this protocol. For veterinary use only.

Discussion: An assessment of immune status as well as serologic identification of ALV requires a measurement of antibody to ALV in serum. Enzyme immunoassay systems have proven efficacious in the quantification of antibody levels to ALV and facilitate the monitoring of immune status in large flocks.

Presentation: 5 plates per kit.

FLOCKCHEK is a registered trademark of Idexx Laboratories, Inc. in the United States and/or other countries.

Compendium Code No.: 11160102 06-01149-02

FLOCKCHEK® ALV-Ag ANTIGEN TEST KIT

Idexx Labs. **Avian Leukosis Test**

Avian Leukosis Virus Antigen Test Kit, ALV-Ag

U.S. Vet. Lic. No.: 313

Components:

Reagent	Volume
1. Anti-p27 Antibody Coated Plates	5
2. Positive Control: Inactivated virus in buffer with protein stabilizers preserved with sodium azide	1.9 mL
3. Negative Control: Buffer with protein additives nonreactive for p27, preserved with sodium azide	1.9 mL
4. (Rabbit) Anti-p27: Horseradish Peroxidase (HRPO) Conjugate preserved with gentamicin	50 mL
5. Sample Diluent: Buffer with protein stabilizers preserved with sodium azide	235 mL
6. TMB Substrate	60 mL
7. Stop Solution	60 mL
8. 20X Wash Concentrate (for albumin wash protocol)	235 mL

Materials Required but Not Provided: Precision pipets and multiple delivery pipetting device with disposable pipet tips, 96-well plate reader, tubes for diluting samples, distilled or deionized water and device for the delivery and aspiration of wash solution.

Indications: FLOCKCHEK® ALV-Ag is an enzyme immunoassay from Idexx for the detection of Avian Leukosis Virus Antigen p27.

Test Principles: This assay is designed to detect p27, an antigen common to all subgroups of ALV including endogenous viruses. The recommended sample types are light albumin and cloacal swab samples. While serum has been validated for use on the ALV-Ag test, it is not a recommended sample for the detection of exogenous virus because of potential interference from endogenous sequences.[3] A microtitration format has been developed in which anti-p27 antibody is coated onto 96-well plates. Sample p27 forms a complex with the coated antibody. After washing away unbound material, an anti-p27: HRPO Conjugate is added which binds to any attached p27 in the well. In the final step of the assay, unbound conjugate is washed away and enzyme substrate is added to the well. Color development may then be related to the amount of p27 present in the test sample. Because of the viscosity of albumin samples, a modified sample handling/wash protocol is described as a second procedure in this insert.

Test Procedure:

Preparation of Samples:

Albumin - collect light albumin and add directly to the plate without prior dilution. Freeze/thaw the sample to help reduce the viscosity.

Cloacal swabs - place cloacal swab into 1 mL culture media or ample diluent and freeze. Prior to testing, bring the sample to room temperature and allow coarse material to settle. Pipette 100 µL of the supernatant directly onto the ELISA plate.

Serum - for general detection of p27, the sample is added directly to the well without prior dilution. Testing of serum samples for exogenous derived p27 is not recommended because of interference from endogenous virus.

Test Procedure (For Samples other than Albumin):

Reagents should be allowed to come to room temperature, then mixed by inverting and swirling.

1. Obtain antigen coated plate(s) and record the sample positions on a FlockChek® worksheet.
2. Dispense 100 µL of Undiluted Negative Control into wells A1 and A2.
3. Dispense 100 µL of Undiluted Positive Control into wells A3 and A4.
4. Dispense 100 µL of diluted sample into appropriate wells. All samples should be run in duplicate.
5. Incubate for 60 minutes at room temperature.
6. Wash each well with approximately 350 µL of distilled or deionized water 3-5 times.
7. Dispense 100 µL of (Rabbit) Anti-p27: HRPO Conjugate into each well.
8. Incubate for 60 minutes at room temperature.
9. Repeat step 6.
10. Dispense 100 µL of TMB substrate solution into each well.
11. Incubate for 15 minutes at room temperature.
12. Dispense 100 µL of Stop Solution into each well to stop the reaction.
13. Blank reader with air.
14. Measure and record the absorbance values at 650nm, A(650).

Albumin Wash Protocol: Light albumin samples are sometimes difficult to completely wash from the wells with the standard water wash protocol. A 20X Wash Concentrate is provided with the kit for use with albumin samples.

Preparation of 1X Wash Solution: The Wash Concentrate should be brought to room temperature and mixed to ensure dissolution of any precipitated salts. The albumin wash solution is prepared by diluting the concentrate 1 to 20 with distilled/deionized water before use (e.g., 20 mL of concentrate added to 380 mL of water for 1 plate).

Albumin Wash Procedure: The albumin wash procedure is the same as described above with the exception of the wash steps (#6, #9). Aspirator control and test albumin sample wells and wash with approximately 350 µL 1X Wash Solution. Allow wells to soak for 2 minutes; aspirate liquid contents; repeat 4 more times without the 2 minute soak.

Test Interpretation:

Results: For the assay to be valid, the difference between the Positive Control mean and the Negative Control mean ($PC\bar{x}$-$NC\bar{x}$) should be greater than 0.200. The Negative Control mean absorbance should be less than or equal to 0.150.

The presence or absence of p27 antigen is determined by relating the A(650) value of the unknown to the Positive Control mean. The Positive Control has been standardized and represents significant antigen levels (approx. 10ng/mL). The relative level of antigen in the unknown can be determined by calculating the sample to positive (S/P) ratio. If this ratio is less than or equal to 0.2, the sample should be considered negative. S/P ratios greater than 0.2 indicate the presence of p27 antigen.

Calculations:

1. Negative Control mean ($NC\bar{x}$):

$$\frac{\text{Well A1 A(650)} + \text{Well A2 A(650)}}{2} = NC\bar{x}$$

2. Positive Control mean ($PC\bar{x}$):

$$\frac{\text{Well A3 A(650)} + \text{Well A4 A(650)}}{2} = PC\bar{x}$$

3. S/P ratio:

$$\frac{\text{Sample Mean} - NC\bar{x}}{PC\bar{x} - NC\bar{x}} = S/P$$

Storage: Store all reagents at 2°-7°C (36°-45°F).

Caution(s): Handle all biological materials as though capable of transmitting ALV. The Positive Control may be a source of ALV. The Positive Control has been inactivated by chemical treatment. Nevertheless, do not assume complete inactivation. Some kit components contain sodium azide as a preservative. Disposal requires flushing plumbing with large volumes of water to prevent formation of copper or lead azide complexes which may explode upon percussion. Do not expose TMB solutions to strong light or any oxidation agents. All wastes should be properly decontaminated prior to disposal. Do not use components past expiration date and do not intermix components from kits with different lot numbers. Careful pipetting and washing throughout this procedure are necessary to maintain precision and accuracy. Optimal results will be obtained by strict adherence to this protocol. For veterinary use only.

Discussion: Avian leukosis viruses (ALV) produce a variety of neoplastic disease including lymphoid leukosis, erythroblastosis, myeloctomatosis, and others.[1] The major gs antigen, p27, is highly conserved across ALV subgroups (A,B,C,D,E and J) and the detection of this antigen is the basis for the ALV-Ag test. Exogenous ALVs can be transmitted horizontally, from bird to bird by direct or indirect contact, or vertically, from an infected hen to progeny. Viremia in the hen is strongly associated with congenital transmission of the virus through shedding into egg albumen. Endogenous leukosis virus sequences are present in the genome of most normal chicken lines.[2]

References: Available upon request.

Presentation: 5 plates per kit.

FLOCKCHEK is a registered trademark of Idexx Laboratories, Inc. in the United States and/or other countries.

Compendium Code No.: 11160112

06-01154-06

FLOCKCHEK® ALV-J ANTIBODY TEST KIT

Idexx Labs. **Avian Leukosis Test**

Avian Leukosis Virus Antibody Test Kit-Subgroup J

U.S. Vet. Lic. No.: 313

Components:

Reagents	Volume
1. ALV-J gp85 Coated Plates	5
2. ALV-J Positive Control - Diluted chicken anti-ALV-J, preserved with sodium azide.	1.9 mL
3. Negative Control - Diluted chicken sera non-reactive for anti-ALV-J, preserved with sodium azide.	1.9 mL
4. (Goat) Anti-Chicken immunoglobulin: HRPO Conjugate in tris buffer with protein stabilizers preserved with gentamicin.	50 mL
5. Sample Diluent: Buffer with protein stabilizers preserved with sodium azide.	235 mL
6. TMB Substrate	60 mL
7. Stop Solution	60 mL
8. PBS-tween (10X) Wash Concentrate	235 mL

Materials Required But Not Provided: Precision pipets and multiple delivery pipetting device with disposable pipet tips, 96-well plate reader, tubes for diluting samples, distilled or deionized water and device for the delivery and aspiration of wash solution.

Indications: FLOCKCHEK® ALV-J Antibody Test Kit is Idexx's enzyme-linked immunosorbent assay for the detection of antibody to Avian Leukosis Virus - Subgroup J in chicken serum.

Test Principles: The FLOCKCHEK® ALV-J Antibody Test Kit detects antibody produced following horizontal transmission of the ALV-J virus. This assay has been developed in the microtiter format whereby ALV-J gp85 antigen has been coated onto 96-well plates. During incubation of the test sample in the coated well, antibody specific to ALV-J gp85 forms a complex with the coated antigen. After washing unbound materials away from the wells, a (Goat) Anti-Chicken immunoglobulin: Horseradish Peroxidase (HRPO) Conjugate is added which binds to any attached chicken antibodies in the wells. In the final step of the assay, unbound conjugate is washed away and an enzyme substrate, hydrogen peroxide, and a chromogen are added to the wells. Subsequent color development may then be related directly to the amount of Anti-ALV-J present in the test sample.

Test Procedure:

Preparation of Samples: Dilute test samples five hundred fold (1:500) with sample diluent prior to being assayed (e.g., by diluting 1µL of sample with 500 µL of Sample Diluent). Note: Do not dilute controls. Be sure to change tips for each sample. Samples must be thoroughly mixed prior to dispensing into the coated plate.

Preparation of Wash Solution: The 10X Wash Concentrate should be brought to room temperature 22°-27°C (72°-80°F) and mixed to ensure dissolution of any precipitated salts. The Wash Concentrate must be diluted 1:10 with distilled/deionized water before use (e.g. 30 mL of concentrate plus 270 mL of water per plate to be assayed).

Reagents should be allowed to come to room temperature, then mixed by inverting and swirling.

1. Obtain antigen-coated plate(s) and record the sample position on a FlockChek® worksheet.
2. Dispense 100 µL of Undiluted Negative Control into wells A1 and A2.
3. Dispense 100 µL of Undiluted Positive Control into wells A3 and A4.
4. Dispense 100 µL of diluted sample into appropriate wells. All samples should be run in duplicate.
5. Incubate for 30 minutes at room temperature.
6. Wash each well with approximately 350 µL of diluted wash solution 3-5 times.
7. Dispense 100 µL of (Goat) Anti-Chicken: HRPO Conjugate into each well.
8. Incubate for 30 minutes at room temperature.
9. Repeat step 6.
10. Dispense 100 µL of TMB substrate solution into each well.
11. Incubate for 15 minutes at room temperature.
12. Dispense 100 µL of Stop Solution into each well to stop the reaction.
13. Blank reader with air.
14. Measure and record absorbance values at 650nm, A(650).

Test Interpretation:

Results: For the assay to be valid, the difference between the Positive Control mean and the Negative Control mean ($PC\bar{x}$ - $NC\bar{x}$) should be greater than 0.10. In addition, the Negative Control mean absorbance should be less than or equal to 0.150. For invalid tests, technique may be suspect and the assay should be repeated.

The presence of antibody to ALV-J is determined by relating the A(650) value of the unknown to the Positive Control mean. The Positive Control has been standardized and represents significant antibody levels to ALV-J in chicken serum. The relative level of antibody in the unknown can be determined by calculating the sample to positive (S/P) ratio.

If this ratio is less than or equal to 0.6, the sample should be considered negative. S/P ratios greater than 0.6 indicate the presence of antibody to ALV-J.

Interpretation of Results:

1. The ALV-J antibody test kit has been developed as a flock screening tool for monitoring horizontal transmission of the virus. The ALV-J status of individual birds cannot be assessed.
2. ALV-J seroconversion is variable across lines and may depend on endogenous leukosis virus expression.[4] Testing of meat-type birds less than 12-14 weeks of age is not recommended.
3. A positive result on the ALV-J antibody test kit indicates exposure to the ALV-J virus; antibody titer does not indicate whether the virus is being actively shed. A determination of ALV-J flock status should include testing for the virus.
4. Vertical transmission of ALV-J results in seronegative, immune tolerant progeny.

Calculations:

1. Calculation of the Negative Control mean (NC$\bar{x}$):

$$\frac{\text{Well A1 A(650)} + \text{Well A2 A(650)}}{2} = NC\bar{x}$$

2. Calculation of the Positive Control mean (PC$\bar{x}$):

$$\frac{\text{Well A3 A(650)} + \text{Well A4 A(650)}}{2} = PC\bar{x}$$

3. Calculation of the S/P Ratio:

$$\frac{\text{Sample Mean} - NC\bar{x}}{PC\bar{x} - NC\bar{x}} = S/P$$

Storage: Store all reagents at 2°-7°C (36°-45°F).

Caution(s): Handle all ALV-J biological materials as though capable of transmitting ALV-J. Some kit components contain sodium azide as a preservative. Disposal requires flushing plumbing with large volumes of water to prevent formation of copper or lead azide complexes which may explode upon percussion. Do not expose TMB solutions to strong light or any oxidation agents. All wastes should be properly decontaminated prior to disposal. Do not use components past expiration date and do not intermix components from kits with different lot numbers. Careful pipetting and washing throughout this procedure are necessary to maintain precision and accuracy. Optimal results will be obtained by strict adherence to this protocol. For veterinary use only.

Discussion: ALV-J is an avian retrovirus first isolated in meat-type chickens in the late 1980s and designated as a unique subgroup partly based on the envelope glycoprotein (gp85).[1] Clinically, ALV-J causes predominantly myeloid leukosis, with variable tumor frequency across chicken lines.[1,2] As with other avian leukosis viruses, ALV-J is transmitted both vertically (congenital infection of the egg albumen and the chick embryo), and horizontally (through close contact with infected chicks).[2,3]

References: Available upon request.

Presentation: 5 plates per kit.

FLOCKCHEK is a registered trademark of Idexx Laboratories, Inc. in the USA and/or other countries.

U.S. Patent Nos. 4,745,051 and 4,879,236.

Compendium Code No.: 11160531 06-03743-03

FLOCKCHEK® CAV ANTIBODY TEST KIT

Idexx Labs. **CAV Test**

Chicken Anemia Virus Antibody Test Kit

U.S. Vet. Lic. No.: 313

Components:

Reagents	Volume
1. CAV Coated Plates	5
2. Anti-CAV: Horseradish Peroxidase (HRPO) Conjugate in buffer with protein stabilizers	50 mL
3. Negative Control - Chicken serum non-reactive to CAV in buffer with protein stabilizers. Preserved with sodium azide	2 mL
4. CAV Positive Control - Anti-CAV in buffer with protein stabilizers, preserved with sodium azide	2 mL
5. Sample Diluent - buffer with protein stabilizers, preserved with sodium azide	235 mL
6. Wash Concentrate (10X) - Phosphate buffer preserved with gentamicin	235 mL
7. TMB Substrate	60 mL
8. Stop Solution	60 mL

Materials Required but Not Provided: Precision pipets and multiple delivery pipetting device with disposable pipet tips, 96-well plate reader, tubes for diluting samples, distilled or deionized water and device for the delivery and aspiration of wash solution.

Indications: FLOCKCHEK® CAV is Idexx's enzyme immunoassay for the detection of antibody to Chicken Anemia Virus (CAV) in chicken serum.

Test Principles: The FLOCKCHEK® CAV assay is performed in a microtiter well coated with Chicken Anemia Virus antigen. During the first incubation, CAV antibodies present in the sample react with immobilized antigens. After a wash step, an Anti-CAV monoclonal antibody enzyme conjugate is added to the microwell. If no Anti-CAV antibodies are present in the test sample, the anti-CAV conjugate is free to react with the CAV antigen. Conversely, if Anti-CAV antibodies are present in the sample, the enzyme-conjugated monoclonal antibodies are blocked from reacting with the antigen. Following this incubation period, the unreacted conjugate is removed by washing and a substrate/chromogen solution is added. In the presence of enzyme, the substrate is converted to a product which reacts with the chromophore to generate a blue color. The absorbance at 650nm, A(650), is measured using a spectrophotometer. Results are calculated by dividing the A(650) of the sample by the mean A(650) of the negative control, resulting in an S/N value. The quantity of antibodies to CAV is inversely proportional to the A(650) and thus, to the S/N value. The presence of CAV antibodies indicates previous exposure to Chicken Anemia Virus.

Test Procedure:

Preparation of Samples: Dilute test samples ten-fold (1:10) with sample diluent prior to being assayed (e.g., by diluting 10 µl of sample with 90 µl Sample Diluent). Note: Do not dilute controls. Be sure to change tips for each sample and record the position of each sample on the plate using a FlockChek® worksheet. Diluted samples should be mixed prior to dispensing into the antigen coated microtiter plate.

Preparation of Wash Solution: The 10X Wash Concentrate should be brought to room temperature 22°-27°C (72°-80°F) and mixed to ensure dissolution of any precipitated salts. The Wash Concentrate must be diluted 1:10 with distilled/deionized water before use (e.g. 30 mL of concentrate plus 270 mL of water per plate to be assayed).

Reagents should be allowed to come to room temperature, then mixed by inverting and swirling.

1. Obtain antigen coated plate(s) and record the sample position on a FlockChek® worksheet.
2. Dispense 100 µl of Undiluted Negative Control into wells A1 and A2.
3. Dispense 100 µl of Undiluted Positive Control into wells A3 and A4.
4. Dispense 100 µl of diluted sample into appropriate wells. All samples should be run in duplicate.
5. Incubate for 60 minutes at room temperature.
6. Wash each well with approximately 300 µl of wash solution 3-5 times.
7. Dispense 100 µl of Anti-CAV: Horseradish Peroxidase Conjugate into each well.
8. Incubate for 30 minutes at room temperature.
9. Repeat step 6.
10. Dispense 100 µl of TMB substrate solution into each well.
11. Incubate for 15 minutes at room temperature.
12. Dispense 100 µl of Stop Solution into each well to stop the reaction.
13. Blank reader with air.
14. Measure and record absorbance values at 650nm, A(650).

Test Interpretation:

Results: For the assay to be valid, the Negative Control optical density (650 nm) must be greater than or equal to 0.60 and the Positive Control S/N must be less than or equal to 0.50.

For invalid tests, technique may be suspect and the assay should be repeated.

The presence or absence of antibody to CAV is determined by the sample to negative (S/N) ratio for each sample.

Interpretation of Results

1. Samples with S/N ratios greater than 0.6 are considered negative within the limits of the test.
2. Samples with S/N ratios less than or equal to 0.60 are considered positive.

Calculations:

1. Negative Control mean (NC$\bar{x}$):

$$\frac{\text{Well A1 A(650)} + \text{Well A2(650)}}{2} = NC\bar{x}$$

2. Positive Control mean (PC$\bar{x}$):

$$\frac{\text{Well A3 A(650)} + \text{Well A4 A(650)}}{2} = PC\bar{x}$$

3. S/N Ratio:

$$\frac{\text{Sample A(650)}}{NC\bar{x}} = S/N$$

Storage: Store all reagents at 2°-7°C (36°-45°F).

Caution(s): Handle all CAV biological materials as though capable of transmitting CAV. The antigen coated plates may be a source of CAV. Prior to coating on the solid phase, the antigen has been inactivated by chemical treatment. Nevertheless, do not assume complete inactivation. Some kit components contain sodium azide as a preservative. Disposal requires flushing plumbing with large volumes of water to prevent formation of copper or lead azide complexes which may explode upon percussion. Do not expose TMB solutions to strong light or any oxidation agents. All wastes should be properly decontaminated prior to disposal. Do not use components past expiration date and do not intermix components from kits with different lot numbers. Careful pipetting and washing throughout this procedure are necessary to maintain precision and accuracy. Optimal results will be obtained by strict adherence to this protocol. For veterinary use only.

Discussion: Chicken Anemia Virus (CAV) is an important pathogen of poultry and has been found in broilers, breeders and SPF flocks. Virus isolation is difficult and time consuming. Screening for the presence of antibody will indicate exposure to the virus.

The enzyme-linked immunosorbent assay has been utilized to detect antibody against CAV. This method is quite useful in large-scale testing of flocks for exposure to CAV. The FLOCKCHEK® CAV assay can be used as a screen for the presence of Chicken Anemia Virus antibodies.

Presentation: 5 plates per kit.

FLOCKCHEK is a registered trademark of Idexx Laboratories, Inc. in the United States and/or other countries.

Compendium Code No.: 11160062 06-02341-04

FLOCKCHEK® IBD ANTIBODY TEST KIT

Idexx Labs. **Bursal Disease Test**

Infectious Bursal Disease Antibody Test Kit

U.S. Vet. Lic. No.: 313

Components:

Reagent	Volume
1. IBD Coated Plates	5
2. IBD Positive Control - Diluted chicken Anti-IBD, preserved with sodium azide.	1.9 mL
3. Negative Control - Diluted chicken sera non-reactive for Anti-IBD, preserved with sodium azide.	1.9 mL
4. (Goat) Anti-Chicken: Horseradish Peroxidase Conjugate, preserved with gentamicin.	50 mL
5. Sample Diluent buffer preserved with sodium azide.	235 mL
6. TMB Substrate	60 mL
7. Stop Solution	60 mL

Materials Required but Not Provided: Precision pipets and multiple delivery pipetting device with disposable pipet tips, 96-well plate reader, tubes for diluting samples, distilled or deionized water and device for the delivery and aspiration of wash solution.

Indications: FLOCKCHEK® IBD is Idexx's enzyme immunoassay for the detection of antibody to Infectious Bursal Disease (IBD) in chicken serum.

Test Principles: This assay is designed to measure the relative level of antibody to IBD in chicken serum. Viral antigen is coated on 96-well plates. Upon incubation of the test sample in the coated well, antibody specific to IBD forms a complex with the coated viral antigens. After washing away unbound material from the wells, a conjugate is added which binds to any attached chicken antibody in the wells. Unbound conjugate is washed away and enzyme substrate is added. Subsequent color development is directly related to the amount of antibody to IBD present in the test sample.

Test Procedure:

Preparation of Samples: Dilute test samples five hundred fold (1:500) with sample diluent prior to being assayed (e.g., by diluting 1 µL of sample with 500 µL of Sample Diluent). Note: Do not dilute controls. Be sure to change the tips for each sample. Samples must be thoroughly mixed prior to dispensing into the coated plate.

Reagents should be allowed to come to room temperature, then mixed by inverting and swirling.

1. Obtain antigen-coated plate(s) and record the sample position on a FlockChek® worksheet.
2. Dispense 100 µL of Undiluted Negative Control into wells A1 and A2.
3. Dispense 100 µL of Undiluted Positive Control into wells A3 and A4.
4. Dispense 100 µL of diluted sample into appropriate wells. All samples should be run in duplicate.
5. Incubate for 30 minutes at room temperature.

6. Wash each well with approximately 350 μL of distilled or deionized water 3-5 times.
7. Dispense 100 μL of (Goat) Anti-Chicken: Horseradish Peroxidase Conjugate into each well.
8. Incubate for 30 minutes at room temperature.
9. Repeat step 6.
10. Dispense 100 μL of TMB substrate solution into each well.
11. Incubate for 15 minutes at room temperature.
12. Dispense 100 μL of Stop Solution into each well to stop the reaction.
13. Blank reader with air.
14. Measure and record absorbance values at 650nm, A(650).

Test Interpretation:

Results: For the assay to be valid, the difference between the Positive Control mean and the Negative Control mean ($PC\bar{x}$-$NC\bar{x}$) should be greater than 0.075. The Negative Control mean absorbance should be less than or equal to 0.150. The presence or absence of antibody to IBD is determined by relating the A(650) value of the unknown to the Positive Control mean. The Positive Control is standardized and represents significant antibody levels to IBD in chicken serum. The relative level of antibody in the unknown is determined by calculating the sample to positive (S/P) ratio. Endpoint titers are calculated using the equation described in the calculations section.

Interpretation of Results: Serum samples with S/P ratios of less than or equal to 0.2 should be considered negative. S/P ratios greater than 0.2 (titers greater than 396) should be considered positive and indicate vaccination of other exposure to IBD. Each laboratory should establish its own criterion for immunity with respect to antibody titer based on correlation of FLOCKCHEK® IBD to current laboratory test methodologies and on historical antibody responses to specific vaccines and vaccination protocols. The immune status of a flock is best assessed by monitoring and recording antibody titers in representative samples as a function of time. The resulting flock profiles allow an assessment of the distribution of antibody titers and an analysis of changes in titer over time.

Calculations:

1. Negative Control mean ($NC\bar{x}$):
$$\frac{\text{Well A1 A(650)} + \text{Well A2 A(650)}}{2} = NC\bar{x}$$
2. Positive Control mean ($PC\bar{x}$):
$$\frac{\text{Well A3 A(650)} + \text{Well A4 A(650)}}{2} = PC\bar{x}$$
3. S/P Ratio:
$$\frac{\text{Sample Mean} - NC\bar{x}}{PC\bar{x} - NC\bar{x}} = S/P$$
4. Titer - Relates S/P at a 1:500 dilution to an endpoint titer:
$\text{Log}_{10}\text{ Titer} = 1.09\ (\text{Log}_{10}\text{ S/P}) + 3.36$

Storage: Store all reagents at 2°-7°C (36°-45°F).

Caution(s): Handle all IBD biological materials as though capable of transmitting IBD. The antigen coated plates may be a source of IBD. Prior to coating on the solid phase, the antigen has been inactivated by chemical treatment. Nevertheless, do not assume complete inactivation. Some kit components contain sodium azide as a preservative. Disposal requires flushing plumbing with large volumes of water to prevent formation of copper or lead azide complexes which may explode upon percussion. Do not expose TMB solutions to strong light or any oxidation agents. All wastes should be properly decontaminated prior to disposal. Do not use components past expiration date and do not intermix components from kits with different lot numbers. Careful pipetting and washing throughout this procedure are necessary to maintain precision and accuracy. Optimal results will be obtained by strict adherence to this protocol. For veterinary use only.

Discussion: An assessment of immune status as well as serologic identification of IBD requires a measurement of antibody to IBD in serum. Enzyme immunoassay systems have proven efficacious in the quantification of antibody levels to IBD and facilitate the monitoring of immune status in large flocks.

Presentation: 5 plates per kit.

FLOCKCHEK is a registered trademark of Idexx Laboratories, Inc. in the United States and/or other countries.

Compendium Code No.: 11160122 06-01129-05

FLOCKCHEK® IBD-XR ANTIBODY TEST KIT

Idexx Labs. **Bursal Disease Test**

Infectious Bursal Disease Antibody Test Kit

U.S. Vet. Lic. No.: 313

Components:

Reagent	Volume
1. IBD Coated Plates	5
2. IBD Positive Control - Diluted chicken Anti-IBD, preserved with sodium azide.	1.9 mL
3. Negative Control - Diluted chicken sera non-reactive for Anti-IBD, preserved with sodium azide.	1.9 mL
4. (Goat) Anti-Chicken: Horseradish Peroxidase Conjugate, preserved with gentamicin.	50 mL
5. Sample Diluent buffer preserved with sodium azide.	235 mL
6. TMB Substrate	60 mL
7. Stop Solution	60 mL

Materials Required but Not Provided: Precision pipets and multiple delivery pipetting device with disposable pipet tips, 96-well plate reader, tubes for diluting samples, distilled or deionized water and device for the delivery and aspiration of wash solution.

Indications: FLOCKCHEK® IBD-XR is Idexx's immunoassay with enhanced dynamic range for the detection of antibody to Infectious Bursal Disease (IBD) in chicken serum.

Test Principles: This assay is designed to measure the relative level of antibody to IBD in chicken serum. Recombinant IBD antigen is coated on 96-well plates. Upon incubation of the test sample in the coated well, antibody specific to IBD forms a complex with the coated viral antigens. After washing away unbound material from the wells, a conjugate is added which binds to any attached chicken antibody in the wells. Unbound conjugate is washed away and enzyme substrate is added. Subsequent color development is directly related to the amount of antibody to IBD present in the test sample.

Test Procedure:

Preparation of Samples: Dilute test samples five hundred fold (1:500) with sample diluent prior to being assayed (e.g., by diluting 1 μl of sample with 500 μl of Sample Diluent). Note: Do not dilute controls. Be sure to change tips for each sample. Samples must be thoroughly mixed prior to dispensing into the coated plate.

Reagents should be allowed to come to room temperature, then mixed by inverting and swirling.

1. Obtain antigen-coated plate(s) and record the sample position on a FlockChek® worksheet.
2. Dispense 100 μl of undiluted Negative Control into wells A1 and A2.
3. Dispense 100 μl of undiluted Positive Control into wells A3 and A4.
4. Dispense 100 μl of diluted sample into appropriate wells. All samples should be run in duplicate.
5. Incubate for 30 minutes at room temperature.
6. Wash each well with approximately 350 μl of distilled or deionized water 3-5 times.
7. Dispense 100 μl of (Goat) Anti-Chicken: Horseradish Peroxidase Conjugate into each well.
8. Incubate for 30 minutes at room temperature.
9. Repeat step 6.
10. Dispense 100 μl of TMB substrate solution into each well.
11. Incubate for 15 minutes at room temperature.
12. Dispense 100 μl of Stop Solution into each well to stop the reaction.
13. Blank reader with air.
14. Measure and record absorbance values at 650nm, A(650).

Test Interpretation:

Results: For the assay to be valid, the difference between the Positive Control mean and the Negative Control mean ($PC\bar{x}$ - $NC\bar{x}$) should be greater than 0.075. The Negative Control mean absorbance should be less than or equal to 0.150. The presence or absence of antibody to IBD is determined by relating the A(650) value of the unknown to the Positive Control mean. The Positive Control is standardized and represents significant antibody levels to IBD in chicken serum. The relative level of antibody in the unknown is determined by calculating the sample to positive (S/P) ratio. Endpoint titers are calculated using the equation described in the calculations section.

F

Interpretation of Results: Serum samples with S/P ratios of less than or equal to 0.2 should be considered negative. S/P ratios greater than 0.2 (titers greater than 396) should be considered positive and indicate vaccination or other exposure to IBD. Each laboratory should establish its own criterion for immunity with respect to antibody titer based on correlation of FLOCKCHEK® IBD-XR to current laboratory test methodologies and on historical antibody responses to specific vaccines and vaccination protocols. The immune status of a flock is best assessed by monitoring and recording antibody titers in representative samples as a function of time. The resulting flock profiles allow an assessment of the distribution of antibody titers and an analysis of changes in titer over time.

Calculations:

1. Negative Control mean ($NC\bar{x}$):
$$\frac{\text{Well A1 A(650)} + \text{Well A2 A(650)}}{2} = NC\bar{x}$$
2. Positive Control mean ($PC\bar{x}$):
$$\frac{\text{Well A3 A(650)} + \text{Well A4 A(650)}}{2} = PC\bar{x}$$
3. S/P Ratio:
$$\frac{\text{Sample Mean} - NC\bar{x}}{PC\bar{x} - NC\bar{x}} = S/P$$
4. Titer - Relates S/P at a 1:500 dilution to an endpoint titer:
$\text{Log}_{10}\text{ Titer} = 1.09\ (\text{Log}_{10}\text{ S/P}) + 3.36$

Storage: Store all reagents at 2°-7°C (36°-45°F).

Caution(s): Handle all IBD biological materials as though capable of transmitting IBD. Some kit components contain sodium azide as a preservative. Disposal requires flushing plumbing with large volumes of water to prevent formation of copper or lead azide complexes which may explode upon percussion. Do not expose TMB solutions to strong light or any oxidation agents. All wastes should be properly decontaminated prior to disposal. Do not use components past expiration date and do not intermix components from kits with different lot numbers. Careful pipetting and washing throughout this procedure are necessary to maintain precision and accuracy. Optimal results will be obtained by strict adherence to this protocol. For veterinary use only.

Discussion: An assessment of immune status as well as serologic identification of IBD requires a measurement of antibody to IBD in serum. Enzyme immunoassay systems have proven efficacious in the quantitation of antibody levels to IBD and facilitate the monitoring of immune status in large flocks.

Presentation: 5 plates per kit.

FLOCKCHEK is a registered trademark of Idexx Laboratories, Inc. in the United States and/or other countries.

U.S. Patent Nos. 4,745,051; 4,879,236; 5,605,827; 5,605,792.

Compendium Code No.: 11160072 06-02470-03

FLOCKCHEK® IBV ANTIBODY TEST KIT

Idexx Labs. **Bronchitis Test**

Infectious Bronchitis Virus Antibody Test Kit

U.S. Vet. Lic. No.: 313

Components:

Reagent	Volume
1. IBV Coated Plates	5
2. IBV Positive Control - Diluted chicken Anti-IBV, preserved with sodium azide.	1.9 mL
3. Negative Control - Diluted chicken sera non-reactive for Anti-, preserved with sodium azide.	1.9 mL
4. (Goat) Anti-Chicken: HRPO Conjugate, preserved with gentamicin.	50 mL
5. Sample Diluent buffer preserved with sodium azide.	235 mL
6. TMB Substrate	60 mL
7. Stop Solution	60 mL

Materials Required but Not Provided: Precision pipets and multiple delivery pipetting device with disposable pipet tips, 96-well plate reader, tubes for diluting samples, distilled or deionized water and device for the delivery and aspiration of wash solution.

Indications: FLOCKCHEK® IBV is Idexx's enzyme immunoasasy for the detection of antibody to Infectious Bronchitis Virus (IBV) in chicken serum.

Test Principles: This assay is designed to measure the relative level of antibody to IBV in chicken serum. Viral antigen is coated on 96-well plates. Upon incubation of the test sample in the coated well, antibody specific to IBV forms a complex with the coated viral antigens. After washing away unbound material from the wells, a conjugate is added which binds to any attached chicken antibody in the wells. Unbound conjugate is washed away and enzyme substrate is added.

Subsequent color development is directly related to the amount of antibody to IBV present in the test sample.

Test Procedure:

Preparation of Samples: Dilute test samples five hundred fold (1:500) with sample diluent prior to being assayed (e.g., by diluting 1 µL of sample with 500 µL of Sample Diluent). Note: Do not dilute controls. Be sure to change tips for each sample. Samples must be thoroughly mixed prior to dispensing into the coated plate.

Reagents should be allowed to come to room temperature, then mixed by inverting and swirling.

1. Obtain antigen-coated plate(s) and record the sample position on a FlockChek® worksheet.
2. Dispense 100 µL of Undiluted Negative Control into wells A1 and A2.
3. Dispense 100 µL of Undiluted Positive Control into wells A3 and A4.
4. Dispense 100 µL of diluted sample into appropriate wells. All samples should be run in duplicate.
5. Incubate for 30 minutes at room temperature.
6. Wash each well with approximately 350 µL of distilled or deionized water 3-5 times.
7. Dispense 100 µL of (Goat) Anti-Chicken: HRPO Conjugate into each well.
8. Incubate for 30 minutes at room temperature.
9. Repeat step 6.
10. Dispense 100 µL of TMB substrate solution into each well.
11. Incubate for 15 minutes at room temperature.
12. Dispense 100 µL of Stop Solution into each well to stop the reaction.
13. Blank reader with air.
14. Measure and record the absorbance values of 650nm, A(650).

Test Interpretation:

Results: For the assay to be valid, the difference between the Positive Control mean and the Negative Control mean ($PC\bar{x}$-$NC\bar{x}$) should be greater than 0.075. The Negative Control mean absorbance should be less than or equal to 0.150. The presence or absence of antibody to IBV is determined by relating the A(650) value of the unknown to the Positive Control mean. The Positive Control is standardized and represents significant antibody levels to IBV in chicken serum. The relative level of antibody in the unknown is determined by calculating the sample to positive (S/P) ratio. Endpoint titers are calculated using the equation described in the calculations section.

Interpretation of Results: Serum samples with S/P ratios of less than or equal to 0.2 should be considered negative. S/P ratios greater than 0.2 (titers greater than 396) should be considered positive and indicate vaccination or other exposure to IBV. Each laboratory should establish its own criterion for immunity with respect to antibody titer based on correlation of FLOCKCHEK® IBV to current laboratory test methodologies and on historical antibody responses to specific vaccines and vaccination protocols. The immune status of a flock is best assessed by monitoring and recording antibody titers in representative samples as a function of time. The resulting flock profiles allow an assessment of the distribution of antibody titers and an analysis of changes in titer over time.

Calculations:

1. Negative Control mean ($NC\bar{x}$):
$$\frac{\text{Well A1 A(650)} + \text{Well A2 A(650)}}{2} = NC\bar{x}$$
2. Positive Control mean ($PC\bar{x}$):
$$\frac{\text{Well A3 A(650)} + \text{Well A4 A(650)}}{2} = PC\bar{x}$$
3. S/P Ratio:
$$\frac{\text{Sample Mean} - NC\bar{x}}{PC\bar{x} - NC\bar{x}} = S/P$$
4. Titer - Relates S/P at a 1:500 dilution to an endpoint titer:
Log_{10} Titer = 1.09 (Log_{10} S/P) + 3.36

Storage: Store all reagents at 2°-7°C (36°-45°F).

Caution(s): Handle all IBV biological materials as though capable of transmitting IBV. The antigen coated plates may be a source of IBV. Prior to coating on the solid phase, the antigen has been inactivated by chemical treatment. Nevertheless, do not assume complete inactivation. Some kit components contain sodium azide as a preservative. Disposal requires flushing plumbing with large volumes of water to prevent the formation of copper or lead azide complexes which may explode upon percussion. Do not expose TMB solutions to strong light or any oxidation agents. All wastes should be properly decontaminated prior to disposal. Do not use components past expiration date and do not intermix components from kits with different lot numbers. Careful pipetting and washing throughout this procedure are necessary to maintain precision and accuracy. Optimal results will be obtained by strict adherence to this protocol. For veterinary use only.

Discussion: An assessment of immune status as well as serologic identification of IBV requires a measurement of antibody to IBV in serum. Enzyme immunoassay systems have proven efficacious in the quantification of antibody levels to IBV and facilitate the monitoring of immune status in large flocks.

Presentation: 5 plates per kit.

FLOCKCHEK is a registered trademark of Idexx Laboratories Inc. in the United States and/or other countries.

Compendium Code No.: 11160132 06-01102-05

FLOCKCHEK® Mg ANTIBODY TEST KIT

Idexx Labs. **Mycoplasma Test**

Mycoplasma Gallisepticum Antibody Test Kit

U.S. Vet. Lic. No.: 313

Components:

Reagent	Volume
1. Mg Coated Plates	5
2. Mg Positive Control - Diluted chicken Anti-Mg, preserved with sodium azide.	1.9 mL
3. Negative Control - Diluted chicken sera non-reactive for Anti-Mg, preserved with sodium azide.	1.9 mL
4. (Goat) Anti-Chicken/(Goat) Anti-Turkey: HRPO Conjugate, preserved with gentamicin.	50 mL
5. Sample Diluent buffer preserved with sodium azide.	235 mL
6. TMB Substrate	60 mL
7. Stop Solution	60 mL

Materials Required but Not Provided: Precision pipets and multiple delivery pipetting device with disposable pipet tips, 96-well plate reader, tubes for diluting samples, distilled or deionized water and device for the delivery and aspiration of wash solution.

Indications: FLOCKCHEK® Mg is Idexx's enzyme immunoassay for the detection of antibody to *Mycoplasma gallisepticum* (Mg) in chicken and turkey serum.

Test Principles: This assay is designed to measure the relative level of antibody to Mg in chicken and turkey serum. Mg antigen is coated on 96-well plates. Upon incubation of the test sample in the coated well, antibody specific to Mg forms a complex with the coated antigens. After washing away unbound material from the wells, a conjugate is added which binds to any attached antibody in the wells. Unbound conjugate is washed away and enzyme substrate is added. Subsequent color development is directly related to the amount of antibody to Mg present in the test sample.

Test Procedure:

Preparation of Samples: Dilute test samples five hundred fold (1:500) with sample diluent prior to being assayed (e.g., by diluting 1 µL of sample with 500 µL of Sample Diluent). Note: Do not dilute controls. Be sure to change tips for each sample. Samples must be thoroughly mixed prior to dispensing into the coated plate.

Reagents should be allowed to come to room temperature, then mixed by inverting and swirling.

1. Obtain antigen-coated plate(s) and record the sample position on a FlockChek® worksheet.
2. Dispense 100 µL of Undiluted Negative Control into wells A1 and A2.
3. Dispense 100 µL of Undiluted Positive Control into wells A3 and A4.
4. Dispense 100 µL of diluted sample into appropriate wells. All samples should be run in duplicate.
5. Incubate for 30 minutes at room temperature.
6. Wash each well with approximately 350 µL of distilled or deionized water 3-5 times.
7. Dispense 100 µL of (Goat) Anti-Chicken/(Goat) Anti-Turkey: HRPO Conjugate into each well.
8. Incubate for 30 minutes at room temperature.
9. Repeat step 6.
10. Dispense 100 µL of TMB substrate solution into each well.
11. Incubate for 15 minutes at room temperature.
12. Dispense 100 µL of Stop Solution into each well to stop the reaction.
13. Blank reader with air.
14. Measure and record absorbance values at 650nm, A(650).

Test Interpretation:

Results: For the assay to be valid, the difference between the Positive Control mean and the Negative Control mean ($PC\bar{x}$ - $NC\bar{x}$) should be greater than 0.075. The Negative Control mean absorbance should be less than or equal to 0.150. The presence or absence of antibody to Mg is determined by relating the A(650) value of the unknown to the Positive Control mean. The Positive Control is standardized and represents significant antibody levels to Mg in chicken serum. The relative level of antibody in the unknown is determined by calculating the sample to positive (S/P) ratio. Endpoint titers are calculated using the equation described in the calculations section.

Interpretation of Results: Serum samples with S/P ratios of less than or equal to 0.5 should be considered negative. S/P ratios greater than 0.5 (titers greater than 1076) should be considered positive and indicate vaccination or other exposure to Mg. Each laboratory should establish its own criterion for immunity with respect to antibody titer based on correlation of FLOCKCHEK® Mg to current laboratory test methodologies and on historical antibody responses.

Calculations:

1. Negative Control mean ($NC\bar{x}$):
$$\frac{\text{Well A1 A(650)} + \text{Well A2 A(650)}}{2} = NC\bar{x}$$
2. Positive Control mean ($PC\bar{x}$):
$$\frac{\text{Well A3 A(650)} + \text{Well A4 A(650)}}{2} = PC\bar{x}$$
3. S/P ratio:
$$\frac{\text{Sample Mean} - NC\bar{x}}{PC\bar{x} - NC\bar{x}} = S/P$$
4. Titer - Relates S/P at a 1:500 dilution to an endpoint titer:
Log_{10} Titer = 1.09 (Log_{10} S/P) + 3.36

Storage: Store all reagents at 2°-7°C (36°-45°F).

Caution(s): Handle all Mg biological materials as though capable of transmitting Mg. The antigen coated plates may be a source of Mg. Prior to coating on the solid phase, the antigen has been inactivated by chemical treatment. Nevertheless, do not assume complete inactivation. Some kit components contain sodium azide as a preservative. Disposal requires flushing plumbing with large volumes of water to prevent formation of copper or lead azide complexes which may explode upon percussion. Do not expose TMB solutions to strong light or any oxidation agents. All wastes should be properly decontaminated prior to disposal. Do not use components past expiration date and do not intermix components from kits with different lot numbers. Careful pipetting and washing throughout this procedure are necessary to maintain precision and accuracy. Optimal results will be obtained by strict adherence to this protocol. For veterinary use only.

Discussion: An assessment of immune status as well as serologic identification of Mg requires a measurement of antibody to Mg in serum. Enzyme immunoassay systems have proven efficacious in the quantification of antibody levels to Mg and facilitate the monitoring of immune status in large flocks.

Presentation: 5 plates per kit.

FLOCKCHEK is a registered trademark of Idexx Laboratories, Inc. in the United States and/or other countries.

Compendium Code No.: 11160142 06-01144-04

Corporate Index:
For names of manufacturers and distributors,
their addresses and product lists,
see the Manufacturers' Index at the front of this book.

FLOCKCHEK® Mg/Ms ANTIBODY TEST KIT

Idexx Labs. **Mycoplasma Test**

Mycoplasma Gallisepticum-Synoviae Antibody Test Kit

U.S. Vet. Lic. No.: 313

Components:

Reagent	Volume
1. Mg/Ms Coated Plates	5
2. Mg/Ms Positive Control - Diluted chicken Anti-Mg/Ms, preserved with sodium azide.	1.9 mL
3. Negative Control - Diluted chicken sera non-reactive for Anti-Mg/Ms, preserved with sodium azide.	1.9 mL
4. (Goat) Anti-Chicken: Horseradish Peroxidase Conjugate, preserved with gentamicin.	50 mL
5. Sample Diluent buffer preserved with sodium azide.	235 mL
6. TMB Substrate	60 mL
7. Stop Solution	60 mL

Materials Required but Not Provided: Precision pipets and multiple delivery pipetting device with disposable pipet tips, 96-well plate reader, tubes for diluting samples, distilled or deionized water and device for the delivery and aspiration of wash solution.

Indications: FLOCKCHEK® Mg/Ms is Idexx's enzyme immunoassay for the detection of antibody to Mycoplasma gallisepticum-synoviae (Mg/Ms) in chicken serum.

Test Principles: This assay is designed to measure the relative level of antibody to Mg/Ms in chicken serum. Mg/Ms antigen is coated on 96-well plates. Upon incubation of the test sample in the coated well, antibody specific to Mg/Ms forms a complex with the coated antigens. After washing away unbound material from the wells, a conjugate is added which binds to any attached chicken antibody in the wells. Unbound conjugate is washed away and enzyme substrate is added. Subsequent color development is directly related to the amount of antibody to Mg/Ms present in the test sample.

Test Procedure:

Preparation of Samples: Dilute test samples five hundred fold (1:500) with sample diluent prior to being assayed (e.g., by diluting 1 µL of sample with 500 µL of Sample Diluent). Note: Do not dilute controls. Be sure to change tips for each sample. Samples must be thoroughly mixed prior to dispensing into the coated plate.

Reagents should be allowed to come to room temperature, then mixed by inverting and swirling.

1. Obtain antigen-coated plate(s) and record the sample position on a FlockChek® worksheet.
2. Dispense 100 µL of Undiluted Negative Control into wells A1 and A2.
3. Dispense 100 µL of Undiluted Positive Control into wells A3 and A4.
4. Dispense 100 µL of diluted sample into appropriate wells. All samples should be run in duplicate.
5. Incubate for 30 minutes at room temperature.
6. Wash each well with approximately 350 µL of distilled or deionized water 3-5 times.
7. Dispense 100 µL of (Goat) Anti-Chicken: Horseradish Peroxidase Conjugate into each well.
8. Incubate for 30 minutes at room temperature.
9. Repeat step 6.
10. Dispense 100 µL of TMB substrate solution into each well.
11. Incubate for 15 minutes at room temperature.
12. Dispense 100 µL of Stop Solution into each well to stop the reaction.
13. Blank reader with air.
14. Measure and record absorbance values at 650nm, A(650).

Test Interpretation:

Results: For the assay to be valid, the difference between the Positive Control mean and the Negative Control mean ($PC\bar{x}-NC\bar{x}$) should be greater than 0.075. The Negative Control mean absorbance should be less than or equal to 0.150. The presence or absence of antibody to Mg/Ms is determined by relating the A(650) value of the unknown to the Positive Control mean. The Positive Control is standardized and represents significant antibody levels to Mg/Ms in chicken serum. The relative level of antibody in the unknown is determined by calculating the sample to positive (S/P) ratio. Endpoint titers are calculated using the equation described in the calculations section.

Interpretation of Results: Serum samples with S/P ratios of less than or equal to 0.5 should be considered negative. S/P ratios greater than 0.5 (titers greater than 1076) should be considered positive and indicates exposure to Mg/Ms. Each laboratory should establish its own criterion for immunity with respect to antibody titer based on correlation of FLOCKCHEK® Mg/Ms to current laboratory test methodologies and on historical antibody responses.

Calculations:

1. Negative Control mean ($NC\bar{x}$):

$$\frac{\text{Well A1 A(650)} + \text{Well A2 A(650)}}{2} = NC\bar{x}$$

2. Positive Control mean ($PC\bar{x}$):

$$\frac{\text{Well A3 A(650)} + \text{Well A4 A(650)}}{2} = PC\bar{x}$$

3. S/P ratio:

$$\frac{\text{Sample Mean} - NC\bar{x}}{PC\bar{x} - NC\bar{x}} = S/P$$

4. Titer - Relates S/P at a 1:500 dilution to an endpoint titer:

$\text{Log}_{10}\ \text{Titer} = 1.09\ (\text{Log}_{10}\ S/P) + 3.36$

Storage: Store all reagents at 2°-7°C (36°-45°F).

Caution(s): Handle all Mg/Ms biological materials as though capable of transmitting Mg/Ms. The antigen coated plates may be a source of Mg/Ms. Prior to coating on the solid phase, the antigen has been inactivated by chemical treatment. Nevertheless, do not assume complete inactivation. Some kit components contain sodium azide as a preservative. Disposal requires flushing plumbing with large volumes of water to prevent formation of copper or lead azide complexes which may explode upon percussion. Do not expose TMB solutions to strong light or any oxidation agents. All wastes should be properly decontaminated prior to disposal. Do not use components past expiration date and do not intermix components from kits with different lot numbers. Careful pipetting and washing throughout this procedure are necessary to maintain precision and accuracy. Optimal results will be obtained by strict adherence to this protocol. For veterinary use only.

Discussion: An assessment of immune status as well as serologic identification of Mg/Ms requires a measurement of antibody to Mg/Ms in serum. Enzyme immunoassay systems have proven efficacious in the quantification of antibody levels to Mg/Ms and facilitate the monitoring of immune status in large flocks.

Presentation: 5 plates per kit.

FLOCKCHEK is a registered trademark of Idexx Laboratories, Inc. in the United States and/or other countries.

Compendium Code No.: 11160152 06-01139-02

FLOCKCHEK® Mm ANTIBODY TEST KIT

Idexx Labs. **Mycoplasma Test**

Mycoplasma meleagridis Antibody Test Kit

U.S. Vet. Lic. No.: 313

Components:

Reagent	Volume
1. Mm Coated Plates	5
2. Mm Positive Control - Diluted turkey Anti-Mm, preserved with sodium azide.	1.9 mL
3. Negative Control - Diluted sera non-reactive for Anti-Mm, preserved with sodium azide.	1.9 mL
4. (Goat) Anti-Turkey: Horseradish Peroxidase Conjugate (HRPO), preserved with gentamicin.	50 mL
5. Sample Diluent buffer preserved with sodium azide.	235 mL
6. TMB Substrate	60 mL
7. Stop Solution	60 mL

F

Materials Required but Not Provided: Precision pipets and multiple delivery pipetting device with disposable pipet tips, 96-well plate reader, tubes for diluting samples, distilled or deionized water and device for the delivery and aspiration of wash solution.

Indications: FLOCKCHEK® Mm is Idexx's enzyme immunoassay for the detection of antibody to *Mycoplasma meleagridis* (Mm) turkey serum.

Test Principles: This assay is designed to measure the relative level of antibody to Mm in turkey serum. Mm antigen is coated on 96-well plates. Upon incubation of the test sample in the coated well, antibody specific to Mm forms a complex with the coated antigens. After washing away unbound material from the wells, a conjugate is added which binds to any attached antibody in the wells. Unbound conjugate is washed away and enzyme substrate is added. Subsequent color development is directly related to the amount of antibody to Mm present in the test sample.

Test Procedure:

Preparation of Samples: Dilute test samples five hundred fold (1:500) with sample diluent prior to being assayed (e.g., by diluting 1 µL of sample with 500 µL of Sample Diluent). Note: Do not dilute controls. Be sure to change tips for each sample. Samples must be thoroughly mixed prior to dispensing into the coated plate.

Reagents should be allowed to come to room temperature, then mixed by inverting and swirling.

1. Obtain antigen-coated plate(s) and record the sample position on a FlockChek® worksheet.
2. Dispense 100 µL of Undiluted Negative Control into wells A1 and A2.
3. Dispense 100 µL of Undiluted Positive Control into wells A3 and A4.
4. Dispense 100 µL of diluted sample into appropriate wells. All samples should be run in duplicate.
5. Incubate for 30 minutes at room temperature.
6. Wash each well with approximately 350 µL of distilled or deionized water 3-5 times.
7. Dispense 100 µL of (Goat) Anti-Turkey:HRPO Conjugate into each well.
8. Incubate for 30 minutes at room temperature.
9. Repeat step 6.
10. Dispense 100 µL of TMB substrate solution into each well.
11. Incubate for 15 minutes at room temperature.
12. Dispense 100 µL of Stop Solution into each well to stop the reaction.
13. Blank reader with air.
14. Measure and record absorbance values at 650nm, A(650).

Test Interpretation:

Results: For the assay to be valid, the difference between the Positive Control mean and the Negative Control mean ($PC\bar{x} - NC\bar{x}$) should be greater than 0.075. The Negative Control mean absorbance should be less than or equal to 0.150. The presence or absence of antibody to Mm is determined by relating the A(650) value of the unknown to the Positive Control mean. The Positive Control is standardized and represents significant antibody levels to Mm in turkey serum. The relative level of antibody in the unknown is determined by calculating the sample to positive (S/P) ratio. Endpoint titers are calculated using the equation described in the calculations section.

Interpretation of Results: Serum samples with S/P ratios of less than or equal to 0.5 should be considered negative. S/P ratios greater than 0.5 (titers greater than 1076) should be considered positive and indicate vaccination or other exposure to Mm. Each laboratory should establish its own criterion for immunity with respect to antibody titer based on correlation of FLOCKCHEK® Mm to current laboratory test methodologies and on historical antibody responses.

Calculations:

1. Negative Control mean ($NC\bar{x}$):

$$\frac{\text{Well A1 A(650)} + \text{Well A2 A(650)}}{2} = NC\bar{x}$$

2. Positive Control mean ($PC\bar{x}$):

$$\frac{\text{Well A3 A(650)} + \text{Well A4 A(650)}}{2} = PC\bar{x}$$

3. S/P Ratio:

$$\frac{\text{Sample Mean} - NC\bar{x}}{PC\bar{x} - NC\bar{x}} = S/P$$

4. Titer - Relates S/P at a 1:500 dilution to an endpoint titer:

$\text{Log}_{10}\ \text{Titer} = 1.09\ (\text{Log}_{10}\ S/P) + 3.36$

Storage: Store all reagents at 2°-7°C (36°-45°F).

Caution(s): Handle all Mm biological materials as though capable of transmitting Mm. The antigen coated plates may be a source of Mm. Prior to coating on the solid phase, the antigen has been inactivated by chemical treatment. Nevertheless, do not assume complete inactivation. Some kit components contain sodium azide as a preservative. Disposal requires flushing plumbing with large volumes of water to prevent formation of copper or lead azide complexes which may explode upon percussion. Do not expose TMB solutions to strong light or any oxidation agents.

All wastes should be properly decontaminated prior to disposal. Do not use components past expiration date and do not intermix components from kits with different lot numbers. Careful pipetting and washing throughout this procedure are necessary to maintain precision and accuracy. Optimal results will be obtained by strict adherence to this protocol. For veterinary use only.

Discussion: Poultry flocks are susceptible to respiratory infections from a variety of agents. Included in this group are the mycoplasmas. The usual types of infection from mycoplasma are chronic respiratory disease, airsacculitis, sinusitis and synovitis.[1,2] In many cases however, the infection may be identified only through serology, culture or PCR methods. Monitoring for exposure of a flock to mycoplasma is facilitated by the measurement of antibody to mycoplasma in serum.

References: Available upon request.

Presentation: 5 plates per kit.

FLOCKCHEK is a registered trademark of Idexx Laboratories, Inc. in the United States and/or other countries.

Compendium Code No.: 11160551 06-03298-01

F

FLOCKCHEK® Ms ANTIBODY TEST KIT

Idexx Labs. **Mycoplasma Test**

Mycoplasma Synoviae Antibody Test Kit

U.S. Vet. Lic. No.: 313

Components:

Reagent	Volume
1. Ms Coated Plates	5
2. Ms Positive Control - Diluted chicken Anti-Ms, preserved with sodium azide.	1.9 mL
3. Negative Control - Diluted chicken sera non-reactive for Anti-Ms, preserved with sodium azide.	1.9 mL
4. (Goat) Anti-Chicken/(Goat) Anti-Turkey: Horseradish Peroxidase Conjugate (HRPO), preserved with gentamicin.	50 mL
5. Sample Diluent buffer preserved with sodium azide.	235 mL
6. TMB Substrate	60 mL
7. Stop Solution	60 mL

Materials Required but Not Provided: Precision pipets and multiple delivery pipetting device with disposable pipet tips, 96-well plate reader, tubes for diluting samples, distilled or deionized water and device for the delivery and aspiration of wash solution.

Indications: FLOCKCHEK® Ms is Idexx's enzyme immunoassay for the detection of antibody to *Mycoplasma synoviae* (Ms) in chicken and turkey serum.

Test Principles: This assay is designed to measure the relative level of antibody to Ms in chicken and turkey serum. Ms antigen is coated on 96-well plates. Upon incubation of the test sample in the coated well, antibody specific to Ms forms a complex with the coated antigens. After washing away unbound material from the wells, a conjugate is added which binds to any attached chicken antibody in the wells. Unbound conjugate is washed away and enzyme substrate is added. Subsequent color development is directly related to the amount of antibody to Ms present in the test sample.

Test Procedure:

Preparation of Samples: Dilute test samples five hundred fold (1:500) with sample diluent prior to being assayed (e.g., by diluting 1 µL of sample with 500 µL of Sample Diluent). Note: Do not dilute controls. Be sure to change tips for each sample. Samples must be thoroughly mixed prior to dispensing into the coated plate.

Reagents should be allowed to come to room temperature, then mixed by inverting and swirling.

1. Obtain antigen-coated plate(s) and record the sample position on a FlockChek® worksheet.
2. Dispense 100 µL of Undiluted Negative Control into wells A1 and A2.
3. Dispense 100 µL of Undiluted Positive Control into wells A3 and A4.
4. Dispense 100 µL of diluted sample into appropriate wells. All samples should be run in duplicate.
5. Incubate for 30 minutes at room temperature.
6. Wash each well with approximately 350 µL of distilled or deionized water 3-5 times.
7. Dispense 100 µL of (Goat) Anti-Chicken/(Goat) Anti-Turkey: HRPO Conjugate into each well.
8. Incubate for 30 minutes at room temperature.
9. Repeat step 6.
10. Dispense 100 µL of TMB substrate solution into each well.
11. Incubate for 15 minutes at room temperature.
12. Dispense 100 µL of Stop Solution into each well to stop the reaction.
13. Blank reader with air.
14. Measure and record absorbance values at 650nm, A(650).

Test Interpretation:

Results: For the assay to be valid, the difference between the Positive Control mean and the Negative Control mean ($PC\bar{x}$ - $NC\bar{x}$) should be greater than 0.075. The Negative Control mean absorbance should be less than or equal to 0.150. The presence or absence of antibody to Ms is determined by relating the A(650) value of the unknown to the Positive Control mean. The Positive Control is standardized and represents significant antibody levels to Ms in chicken serum. The relative level of antibody in the unknown is determined by calculating the sample to positive (S/P) ratio. Endpoint titers are calculated using the equation described in the calculations section.

Interpretation of Results: Serum samples with S/P ratios of less than or equal to 0.5 should be considered negative. S/P ratios greater than 0.5 (titers greater than 1076) should be considered positive and indicate vaccination or other exposure to Ms. Each laboratory should establish its own criterion for immunity with respect to antibody titer based on correlation of FLOCKCHEK® Ms to current laboratory test methodologies and on historical antibody responses.

Calculations:

1. Negative Control mean ($NC\bar{x}$):
$$\frac{\text{Well A1 A(650)} + \text{Well A2 A(650)}}{2} = NC\bar{x}$$
2. Positive Control mean ($PC\bar{x}$):
$$\frac{\text{Well A3 A(650)} + \text{Well A4 A(650)}}{2} = PC\bar{x}$$
3. S/P ratio:
$$\frac{\text{Sample Mean} - NC\bar{x}}{PC\bar{x} - NC\bar{x}} = S/P$$
4. Titer - Relates S/P at a 1:500 dilution to an endpoint titer:
$\text{Log}_{10}\text{ Titer} = 1.09 (\text{Log}_{10}\text{ S/P}) + 3.36$

Storage: Store all reagents at 2°-7°C (36°-45°F).

Caution(s): Handle all Ms biological materials as though capable of transmitting Ms. The antigen coated plates may be a source of Ms. Prior to coating on the solid phase, the antigen has been inactivated by chemical treatment. Nevertheless, do not assume complete inactivation. Some kit components contain sodium azide as a preservative. Disposal requires flushing plumbing with large volumes of water to prevent formation of copper or lead azide complexes which may explode upon percussion. Do not expose TMB solutions to strong light or any oxidation agents. All wastes should be properly decontaminated prior to disposal. Do not use components past expiration date and do not intermix components from kits with different lot numbers. Careful pipetting and washing throughout this procedure are necessary to maintain precision and accuracy. Optimal results will be obtained by strict adherence to this protocol. For veterinary use only.

Discussion: An assessment of immune status as well as serologic identification of Ms requires a measurement of antibody to Ms in serum. Enzyme immunoassay systems have proven efficacious in the quantification of antibody levels to Ms and facilitate the monitoring of immune status in large flocks.

Presentation: 5 plates per kit.

FLOCKCHEK is a registered trademark of Idexx Laboratories. Inc. in the United States and/or other countries

Compendium Code No.: 11160162 06-02003-03

FLOCKCHEK® NDV ANTIBODY TEST KIT

Idexx Labs. **Newcastle Disease Test**

Newcastle Disease Antibody Test Kit

U.S. Vet. Lic. No.: 313

Components:

Reagent	Volume
1. NDV Coated Plates	5
2. NDV Positive Control - Diluted chicken Anti-NDV, preserved with sodium azide.	1.9 mL
3. Negative Control - Diluted chicken sera non-reactive for Anti-NDV, preserved with sodium azide.	1.9 mL
4. (Goat) Anti-Chicken: Horseradish Peroxidase Conjugate, preserved with gentamicin.	50 mL
5. Sample Diluent buffer preserved with sodium azide.	235 mL
6. TMB Substrate	60 mL
7. Stop Solution	60 mL

Materials Required but Not Provided: Precision pipets and multiple delivery pipetting device with disposable pipet tips, 96-well plate reader, tubes for diluting samples, distilled or deionized water and device for the delivery and aspiration of wash solution.

Indications: FLOCKCHEK® NDV is Idexx's enzyme immunoassay for the detection of antibody to Newcastle Disease (NDV) in chicken serum.

Test Principles: This assay is designed to measure the relative level of antibody to NDV in chicken serum. Viral antigen is coated on 96-well plates. Upon incubation of the test sample in the coated well, antibody specific to NDV forms a complex with the coated viral antigens. After washing away unbound material from the wells, a conjugate is added which binds to any attached chicken antibody in the wells. Unbound conjugate is washed away and enzyme substrate is added. Subsequent color development is directly related to the amount of antibody to NDV present in the test sample.

Test Procedure:

Preparation of Samples: Dilute test samples five hundred fold (1:500) with sample diluent prior to being assayed (e.g., by diluting 1 µL of sample with 500 µL of Sample Diluent). Note: Do not dilute controls. Be sure to change tips for each sample. Samples must be thoroughly mixed prior to dispensing into the coated plate.

Reagents should be allowed to come to room temperature, then mixed by gentle inverting and swirling.

1. Obtain antigen-coated plate(s) and record the sample position on a FlockChek® worksheet.
2. Dispense 100 µL of Undiluted Negative Control into wells A1 and A2.
3. Dispense 100 µL of Undiluted Positive Control into wells A3 and A4.
4. Dispense 100 µL of diluted sample into appropriate wells. All samples should be run in duplicate.
5. Incubate for 30 minutes at room temperature.
6. Wash each well with approximately 350 µL of distilled or deionized water 3-5 times.
7. Dispense 100 µL of (Goat) Anti-Chicken: Horseradish Peroxidase Conjugate into each well.
8. Incubate for 30 minutes at room temperature.
9. Repeat step 6.
10. Dispense 100 µL of TMB substrate solution into each well.
11. Incubate for 15 minutes at room temperature.
12. Dispense 100 µL of Stop Solution into each well to stop the reaction.
13. Blank reader with air.
14. Measure and record absorbance values at 650 nm, A(650).

Test Interpretation:

Results: For the assay to be valid, the difference between the Positive Control mean and the Negative Control mean ($PC\bar{x}$ - $NC\bar{x}$) should be greater than 0.075. The Negative Control mean absorbance should be less than or equal to 0.150. The presence or absence of antibody to NDV is determined by relating the A(650) value of the unknown to the Positive Control mean. The Positive Control is standardized and represents significant antibody levels to NDV in chicken serum. The relative level of antibody in the unknown is determined by calculating the sample to positive (S/P) ratio. Endpoint titers are calculated using the equation described in the calculations section.

Interpretation of Results: Serum samples with S/P ratios of less than or equal to 0.2 should be considered negative. S/P ratios greater than 0.2 (titers greater than 396) should be considered positive and indicate vaccination or other exposure to NDV. Each laboratory should establish its own criterion for immunity with respect to antibody titer based on correlation of FLOCKCHEK® NDV to current laboratory test methodologies and on historical antibody responses to specific vaccines and vaccination protocols. The immune status of a flock is best assessed by monitoring and recording antibody titers in representative samples as a function of time. The resulting flock profiles allow an assessment of the distribution of antibody titers and an analysis of changes in titer over time.

Calculations:

1. Negative Control mean ($NC\bar{x}$):

$$\frac{\text{Well A1 A(650)} + \text{Well A2 A(650)}}{2} = NC\bar{x}$$

2. Positive Control mean ($PC\bar{x}$):

$$\frac{\text{Well A3 A(650)} + \text{Well A4 A(650)}}{2} = PC\bar{x}$$

3. S/P Ratio:

$$\frac{\text{Sample Mean} - NC\bar{x}}{PC\bar{x} - NC\bar{x}} = S/P$$

4. Titer - Relates S/P at a 1:500 dilution to an endpoint titer:

$$\text{Log}_{10}\text{ Titer} = 1.09 (\text{Log}_{10}\text{ S/P}) + 3.36$$

Storage: Store all reagents at 2°-7°C (36°-45°F).

Caution(s): Handle all NDV biological materials as though capable of transmitting NDV. The antigen coated plates may be a source of NDV. Prior to coating on the solid phase, the antigen has been inactivated by chemical treatment. Nevertheless, do not assume complete inactivation. Some kit components contain sodium azide as a preservative. Disposal requires flushing plumbing with large volumes of water to prevent the formation of copper or lead azide complexes which may explode upon percussion. Do not expose TMB solutions to strong light or any oxidation agents. All wastes should be properly decontaminated prior to disposal. Do not use components past expiration date and do not intermix components from kits with different lot numbers. Careful pipetting and washing throughout this procedure are necessary to maintain precision and accuracy. Optimal results will be obtained by strict adherence to this protocol. For veterinary use only.

Discussion: An assessment of immune status as well as serologic identification of NDV requires a measurement of antibody to NDV in serum. Enzyme immunoassay systems have proven efficacious in the quantification of antibody levels to NDV and facilitate the monitoring of immune status in large flocks.

Presentation: 5 plates per kit.

FLOCKCHEK is a registered trademark of Idexx Laboratories, Inc. in the United States and/or other countries.

Compendium Code No.: 11160182 06-01096-04

FLOCKCHEK® NDV (T) ANTIBODY TEST KIT

Idexx Labs. **Newcastle Disease Test**

Newcastle Disease Antibody Test Kit (For use in Turkeys)

U.S. Vet. Lic. No.: 313

Components:

Reagent	Volume
1. NDV Coated Plates	5
2. NDV Positive Control - Diluted avian NDV anti-sera, preserved with sodium azide.	1.9 mL
3. Negative Control - Diluted avian sera non-reactive for Anti-NDV, preserved with sodium azide.	1.9 mL
4. (Goat) Anti-Turkey: Horseradish Peroxidase Conjugate, preserved with gentamicin.	50 mL
5. Sample Diluent buffer preserved with sodium azide.	235 mL
6. TMB Substrate	60 mL
7. Stop Solution	60 mL

Materials Required but Not Provided: Precision pipets and multiple delivery pipetting device with disposible pipet tips, 96-well plate reader, tubes far diluting samples, distilled or deionized water and device for the delivery and aspiration of wash solution.

Indications: FLOCKCHEK® NDV (T) is Idexx's enzyme immunoassay for the detection of antibody to Newcastle Disease (NDV) in turkey serum.

Test Principles: This assay is designed to measure the relative level of antibody to NDV in turkey serum. Viral antigen is coated on 96-well plates. Upon incubation of the test sample in the coated well, antibody specific to NDV forms a complex with the coated viral antigens. After washing away unbound material from the wells, a conjugate is added which binds to any attached turkey antibody in the wells. Unbound conjugate is washed away and enzyme substrate is added. Subsequent color development is directly related to the amount of antibody to NDV present in the test sample.

Test Procedure:

Preparation of Samples: Dilute test samples five hundred fold (1:500) with sample diluent prior to being assayed (e.g., by diluting 1 µL of sample with 500 µL of Sample Diluent). Note: Do not dilute controls. Be sure to change tips for each sample. Samples must be thoroughly mixed prior to dispensing into the coated plate.

Reagents should be allowed to come to room temperature, then mixed by inverting and swirling.

1. Obtain antigen-coated plate(s) and record the sample position on a FlockChek® worksheet.
2. Dispense 100 µL of Undiluted Negative Control into wells A1 and A2.
3. Dispense 100 µL of Undiluted Positive Control into wells A3 and A4.
4. Dispense 100 µL of diluted sample into appropriate wells. All samples should be run in duplicate.
5. Incubate for 30 minutes at room temperature.
6. Wash each well with approximately 350 µL of distilled or deionized water 3-5 times.
7. Dispense 100 µL of (Goat) Anti-Turkey: Horseradish Peroxidase Conjugate into each well.
8. Incubate for 30 minutes at room temperature.
9. Repeat step 6.
10. Dispense 100 µL of TMB substrate solution into each well.
11. Incubate for 15 minutes at room temperature.
12. Dispense 100 µL of Stop Solution into each well to stop the reaction.
13. Blank reader with air.
14. Measure and record absorbance values at 650nm, A(650).

Test Interpretation:

Results: For the assay to be valid, the difference between the Positive Control mean and the Negative Control mean ($PC\bar{x}$ - $NC\bar{x}$) should be greater than 0.075. The Negative Control mean absorbance should be less than or equal to 0.150. The presence or absence of antibody to NDV is determined by relating the A(650) value of the unknown to the Positive Control mean. The Positive Control is standardized and represents significant antibody levels to NDV in serum. The relative level of antibody in the unknown is determined by calculating the sample to positive (S/P) ratio. Endpoint titers are calculated using the equation described in the calculations section.

Interpretation of Results: Serum samples with S/P ratios of less than or equal to 0.2 should be considered negative. S/P ratios greater than 0.2 (titers greater than 396) should be considered positive and indicate vaccination or other exposure to NDV. Each laboratory should establish its own criterion for immunity with respect to antibody titer based on correlation of FLOCKCHEK® NDV (T) to current laboratory test methodologies and on historical antibody responses to specific vaccines and vaccination protocols. The immune status of a flock is best assessed by monitoring and recording antibody titers in representative samples as a function of time. The resulting flock profiles allow an assessment of the distribution of antibody titers and an analysis of changes in titer over time.

Calculations:

1. Negative Control mean ($NC\bar{x}$):

$$\frac{\text{Well A1 A(650)} + \text{Well A2 A(650)}}{2} = NC\bar{x}$$

2. Positive Control mean ($PC\bar{x}$):

$$\frac{\text{Well A3 A(650)} + \text{Well A4 A(650)}}{2} = PC\bar{x}$$

3. S/P Ratio:

$$\frac{\text{Sample Mean} - NC\bar{x}}{PC\bar{x} - NC\bar{x}} = S/P$$

4. Titer - Relates S/P at a 1:500 dilution to an endpoint titer:

$$\text{Log}_{10}\text{ Titer} = 1.09 (\text{Log}_{10}\text{ S/P}) + 3.36$$

Storage: Store all reagents at 2°-7°C (36°-45°F).

Caution(s): Handle all NDV biological materials as though capable of transmitting NDV. The antigen coated plates may be a source of NDV. Prior to coating on the solid phase, the antigen has been inactivated by chemical treatment. Nevertheless, do not assume complete inactivation. Some kit components contain sodium azide as a preservative. Disposal requires flushing plumbing with large volumes of water to prevent formation of copper or lead azide complexes which may explode upon percussion. Do not expose TMB solutions to strong light or any oxidation agents. All wastes should be properly decontaminated prior to disposal. Do not use components past expiration date and do not intermix components from kits with different lot numbers. Careful pipetting and washing throughout this procedure are necessary to maintain precision and accuracy. Optimal results will be obtained by strict adherence to this protocol. For veterinary use only.

Discussion: An assessment of immune status as well as serologic identification of NDV requires a measurement of antibody to NDV in turkey serum. Enzyme immunoassay systems have proven efficacious in the quantification of antibody levels to NDV and facilitate the monitoring of immune status in large flocks.

Presentation: 5 plates per kit.

FLOCKCHEK is a registered trademark of Idexx Laboratories, Inc. in the United States and/or other countries.

Compendium Code No.: 11160172 06-01134-02

FLOCKCHEK® Pm ANTIBODY TEST KIT

Idexx Labs. **Pasteurella Test**

Pasteurella Multocida Antibody Test Kit (For use with Chickens)

U.S. Vet. Lic. No.: 313

Components:

Reagent	Volume
1. Pm Coated Plates	5
2. Pm Positive Control - Diluted chicken Anti-Pm, preserved with sodium azide.	1.9 mL
3. Negative Control - Diluted chicken sera non-reactive for Anti-Pm, preserved with sodium azide.	1.9 mL
4. (Goat) Anti-Chicken: Horseradish Peroxidase Conjugate, preserved with gentamicin.	50 mL
5. Sample Diluent buffer preserved with sodium azide.	235 mL
6. TMB Substrate	60 mL
7. Stop Solution	60 mL

Materials Required but Not Provided: Precision pipets and multiple delivery pipetting device with disposible pipet tips, 96-well plate reader, tubes for diluting samples, distilled or deionized water and device for the delivery and aspiration of wash solution.

Indications: FLOCKCHEK® Pm is Idexx's enzyme immunoassay for the detection of antibody to *Pasteurella multocida* (Pm) in chicken serum.

Test Principles: This assay is designed to measure the relative level of antibody to Pm in chicken serum. Viral antigen is coated on 96-well plates. Upon incubation of the test sample in the coated well, antibody specific to Pm forms a complex with the coated viral antigens. After washing away unbound material from the wells, a conjugate is added which binds to any attached chicken antibody in the wells. Unbound conjugate is washed away and enzyme substrate is added. Subsequent color development is directly related to the amount of antibody to Pm present in the test sample.

Test Procedure:

Preparation of Samples: Dilute test samples five hundred fold (1:500) with sample diluent prior to being assayed (e.g., by diluting 1 µL of sample with 500 µL of Sample Diluent). Note: Do not dilute controls. Be sure to change tips for each sample. Samples must be thoroughly mixed prior to dispensing into the coated plate.

Reagents should be allowed to come to room temperature, then mixed by inverting and swirling.

1. Obtain antigen-coated plate(s) and record the sample position on a FlockChek® worksheet.
2. Dispense 100 µL of Undiluted Negative Control into wells A1 and A2.
3. Dispense 100 µL of Undiluted Positive Control into wells A3 and A4.
4. Dispense 100 µL of diluted sample into appropriate wells. All samples should be run in duplicate.

5. Incubate for 30 minutes at room temperature.
6. Wash each well with approximately 350 µL of distilled or deionized water 3-5 times.
7. Dispense 100 µL of (Goat) Anti-Chicken: Horseradish Peroxidase Conjugate into each well.
8. Incubate for 30 minutes at room temperature.
9. Repeat step 6.
10. Dispense 100 µL of TMB substrate solution into each well.
11. Incubate for 15 minutes at room temperature.
12. Dispense 100 µL of Stop Solution into each well to stop the reaction.
13. Blank reader with air.
14. Measure and record absorbance values at 650nm, A(650).

Test Interpretation:

Results: For the assay to be valid, the difference between the Positive Control mean and the Negative Control mean (PC$\bar{x}$ - NC$\bar{x}$) should be greater than 0.075. The Negative Control mean absorbance should be less than or equal to 0.150. The presence or absence of antibody to Pm is determined by relating the A(650) value of the unknown to the Positive Control mean. The Positive Control is standardized and represents significant antibody levels to Pm in chicken serum. The relative level of antibody in the unknown is determined by calculating the sample to positive (S/P) ratio. Endpoint titers are calculated using the equation described in the calculations section.

Interpretation of Results: Serum samples with S/P ratios of less than or equal to 0.2 should be considered negative. S/P ratios greater than 0.2 (titers greater than 396) should be considered positive and indicate vaccination or other exposure to Pm. Each laboratory should establish its own criterion for immunity with respect to antibody titer based on correlation of FLOCKCHEK® Pm to current laboratory test methodologies and on historical antibody responses to specific vaccines and vaccination protocols. The immune status of a flock is best assessed by monitoring and recording antibody titers in representative samples as a function of time. The resulting flock profiles allow an assessment of the distribution of antibody titers and an analysis of changes in titer over time.

Calculations:

1. Negative Control mean (NC$\bar{x}$):

$$\frac{\text{Well A1 A(650)} + \text{Well A2 A(650)}}{2} = NC\bar{x}$$

2. Positive Control mean (PC$\bar{x}$):

$$\frac{\text{Well A3 A(650)} + \text{Well A4 A(650)}}{2} = PC\bar{x}$$

3. S/P Ratio:

$$\frac{\text{Sample Mean} - NC\bar{x}}{PC\bar{x} - NC\bar{x}} = S/P$$

4. Titer - Relates S/P at a 1:500 dilution to an endpoint titer:

$\text{Log}_{10}\ \text{Titer} = 1.09\ (\text{Log}_{10}\ S/P) + 3.36$

Storage: Store all reagents at 2°-7°C (36°-45°F).

Caution(s): Handle all Pm biological materials as though capable of transmitting Pm. The antigen coated plates may be a source of Pm. Prior to coating on the solid phase. the antigen has been inactivated by chemical treatment. Nevertheless, do not assume complete inactivation. Some kit components contain sodium azide as a preservative. Disposal requires flushing plumbing with large volumes of water to prevent formation of copper or lead azide complexes which may explode upon percussion. Do not expose TMB solutions to strong light or any oxidation agents. All wastes should be properly decontaminated prior to disposal. Do not use components past expiration date and do not intermix components from kits with different lot numbers. Careful pipetting and washing throughout this procedure are necessary to maintain precision and accuracy. Optimal results will be obtained by strict adherence to this protocol. For veterinary use only.

Discussion: An assessment of immune status as well as serologic identification of Pm requires a measurement of antibody to Pm in serum. Enzyme immunoassay systems have proven efficacious in the quantification of antibody levels to Pm and facilitate the monitoring of immune status in large flocks.

Presentation: 5 plates per kit.

FLOCKCHEK is a registered trademark of Idexx Laboratories, Inc. in the United States and/or other countries.

Compendium Code No.: 11160202 06-01160-02

FLOCKCHEK® Pm (T) ANTIBODY TEST KIT

Idexx Labs. **Pasteurella Test**

Pasteurella Multocida Antibody Test Kit (For use in Turkeys)

U.S. Vet. Lic. No.: 313

Components:

Reagent	Volume
1. Pm Coated Plates	5
2. Pm Positive Control - Diluted avian Anti-Pm, preserved with sodium azide.	1.9 mL
3. Negative Control - Diluted avian sera non-reactive for Anti-Pm, preserved with sodium azide.	1.9 mL
4. (Goat) Anti-Turkey: Horseradish Peroxidase Conjugate, preserved with gentamicin.	50 mL
5. Sample Diluent buffer preserved with sodium azide.	235 mL
6. TMB Substrate	60 mL
7. Stop Solution	60 mL

Materials Required but Not Provided: Precision pipets and multiple delivery pipetting device with disposable pipet tips, 96-well plate reader, tubes for diluting samples, distilled or deionized water and device for the delivery and aspiration of wash solution.

Indications: FLOCKCHEK® Pm (T) is Idexx's enzyme immunoassay for the detection of antibody to *Pasteurella multocida* (Pm) in turkey serum.

Test Principles: This assay is designed to measure the relative level of antibody to Pm in turkey serum. Pm antigen is coated on 96-well plates. Upon incubation of the test sample in the coated well, antibody specific to Pm forms a complex with the coated antigen. After washing away unbound material from the wells, a conjugate is added which binds to any attached turkey antibody in the wells. Unbound conjugate is washed away and enzyme substrate is added. Subsequent color development is directly related to the amount of antibody to Pm present in the test sample.

Test Procedure:

Preparation of Samples: Dilute test samples five hundred fold (1:500) with sample diluent prior to being assayed (e.g., by diluting 1 µL of sample with 500 µL of Sample Diluent). Note: Do not dilute controls. Be sure to change tips for each sample. Samples must be thoroughly mixed prior to dispensing into the coated plate.

Reagents should be allowed to come to room temperature, then mixed by inverting and swirling.

1. Obtain antigen-coated plate(s) and record the sample position on a FlockChek® worksheet.
2. Dispense 100 µL of Undiluted Negative Control into wells A1 and A2.
3. Dispense 100 µL of Undiluted Positive Control into wells A3 and A4
4. Dispense 100 µL of diluted sample into appropriate wells. All samples should be run in duplicate.
5. Incubate for 30 minutes at room temperature.
6. Wash each well with approximately 350 µL of distilled or deionized water 3-5 times.
7. Dispense 100 µL of (Goat) Anti-Turkey: Horseradish Peroxidase Conjugate into each well.
8. Incubate for 30 minutes at room temperature.
9. Repeat step 6.
10. Dispense 100 µL of TMB substrate solution into each well.
11. Incubate for 15 minutes at room temperature.
12. Dispense 100 µL of Stop Solution into each well to stop the reaction.
13. Blank reader with air.
14. Measure and record absorbance values at 650nm, A(650).

Test Interpretation:

Results: For the assay to be valid, the difference between the Positive Control mean and the Negative Control mean (PC$\bar{x}$ - NC$\bar{x}$) should be greater than 0.075. The Negative Control mean absorbance should be less than or equal to 0.150. The presence or absence of antibody to Pm is determined by relating the A(650) value of the unknown to the Positive Control mean. The Positive Control is standardized and represents significant antibody levels to Pm in turkey serum. The relative level of antibody in the unknown is determined by calculating the sample to positive (S/P) ratio. Endpoint titers are calculated using the equation described in the calculations section.

Interpretation of Results: Serum samples with S/P ratios of less than or equal to 0.2 should be considered negative. S/P ratios greater than 0.2 (titers greater than 396) should be considered positive and indicate vaccination or other exposure to Pm. Each laboratory should establish its own criterion for immunity with respect to antibody titer based on correlation of FLOCKCHEK® Pm (T) to current laboratory test methodologies and on historical antibody responses to specific vaccines and vaccination protocols. The immune status of a flock is best assessed by monitoring and recording antibody titers in representative samples as a function of time. The resulting flock profiles allow an assessment of the distribution of antibody titers and an analysis of changes in titer over time.

Calculations:

1. Negative Control mean (NC$\bar{x}$):

$$\frac{\text{Well A1 A(650)} + \text{Well A2 A(650)}}{2} = NC\bar{x}$$

2. Positive Control mean (PC$\bar{x}$):

$$\frac{\text{Well A3 A(650)} + \text{Well A4 A(650)}}{2} = PC\bar{x}$$

3. S/P Ratio:

$$\frac{\text{Sample Mean} - NC\bar{x}}{PC\bar{x} - NC\bar{x}} = S/P$$

4. Titer - Relates S/P at a 1:500 dilution to an endpoint titer:

$\text{Log}_{10}\ \text{Titer} = 1.09\ (\text{Log}_{10}\ S/P) + 3.36$

Storage: Store all reagents at 2°-7°C (36°-45°F).

Caution(s): Handle all Pm biological materials as though capable of transmitting Pm. The antigen coated plates may be a source of Pm. Prior to coating on the solid phase, the antigen has been inactivated by chemical treatment. Nevertheless, do not assume complete inactivation. Some kit components contain sodium azide as a preservative. Disposal requires flushing plumbing with large volumes of water to prevent formation of copper or lead azide complexes which may explode upon percussion. Do not expose TMB solutions to strong light or any oxidation agents. All wastes should be properly decontaminated prior to disposal. Do not use components past expiration date and do not intermix components from kits with different lot numbers. Careful pipetting and washing throughout this procedure are necessary to maintain precision and accuracy. Optimal results will be obtained by strict adherence to this protocol. For veterinary use only.

Discussion: An assessment of immune status as well as serologic identification of Pm requires a measurement of antibody to Pm in serum. Enzyme immunoassay systems have proven efficacious in the quantification of antibody levels to Pm and facilitate the monitoring of immune status in large flocks.

Presentation: 5 plates per kit.

FLOCKCHEK is a registered trademark of Idexx Laboratories, Inc. in the United States and/or other countries.

Compendium Code No.: 11160192 06-01170-02

FLOCKCHEK® PROBE® MYCOPLASMA GALLISEPTICUM DNA TEST KIT

Idexx Labs. **Mycoplasma Test**

Mycoplasma Gallisepticum DNA Test Kit

U.S. Vet. Lic. No.: 313

Components: Reagents:

1. Nylon Membrane
2. Blocking Solution
3. 6X Blot Wash Solution 1
4. 6X Blot Wash Solution 2
5. 6X Substrate Buffer

6a. *M. gallisepticum* Vir/F Conjugate Concentrate

7. *M. gallisepticum* PCR Mix 1
8. *M. gallisepticum* PCR Mix 2
9. *M. gallisepticum* Positive Control
10. Sample Wash Solution

A. Substrate A

B. Substrate B

Materials Required But Not Provided:

1. IDEXX DNAmplifier™
2. Mineral oil (light)
3. Rotating platform
4. Heat block (120°C)

5. Analytical reagent grade 10N NaOH
6. Ethanol
7. Water baths (37°C and 55°C)
8. Latex gloves
9. 1-20 µL and 10-200 µL precision pipets and tips with aerosol filters
10. 1 mL disposable transfer pipets graduated to 0.25 mL
11. 25 µL positive displacement pipet with tips
12. Heat sealer and heat-sealable pouches
13. 1.5 mL screw cap microcentrifuge tubes
14. 0.5 mL microcentrifuge tubes with caps
15. 15 mL and 50 mL sterile conical tubes with caps
16. Flat-bottomed containers
17. Heavy filter paper or blotting pad
18. 1% glacial acetic acid
19. Sterile HPLC Grade water, or sterile water for injection

Indications: The FLOCKCHEK® PROBE® Mycoplasma Gallisepticum DNA Test Kit is a nonradioactive probe based test utilizing PCR amplification for the specific detection of *Mycoplasma gallisepticum* genomic DNA from chicken and turkey tracheal swab samples.

Test Principles: Tracheal swab samples are processed to effect the removal of interfering sample components.

The Polymerase Chain Reaction® (PCR®)* DNA amplification procedure utilizes two synthetic DNA molecules whose properties are based on a DNA sequence specific to *M. gallisepticum*. These DNA molecules are used in conjunction with AmpliTaq® DNA polymerase to amplify small amounts of *M. gallisepticum* target DNA to provide enhancement of sensitivity.

A third synthetic DNA molecule, labeled with an enzyme is used as sequence specific hybridization probe to provide colorimetric detection of the amplified target DNA.

Test Procedure: Specimen Information: Obtain tracheal sample by swabbing the trachea of a chicken or turkey. Place the swab in a tube containing 1.0 to 1.5 mL of transport medium. The sample should be stored on ice and delivered to the laboratory within 24 hours.

For pooled samples, place three swabs in a tube containing 2.0 to 2.5 mL of transport medium. The sample should be stored on ice and delivered to the laboratory within 24 hours.

There are three stages required for implementation of the *M. gallisepticum* DNA Test Kit from a tracheal swab sample:

Stage 1 - Sample Preparation Procedure
Stage 2 - DNA Amplification Procedure
Stage 3 - DNA Detection Procedure

Note: Set up the IDEXX DNAmplifier as outlined in the *M. gallisepticum* instructions of the FlockChek® DNA Probe Manual.

Stage 1: Sample Preparation Procedure - For Single Tracheal Swab Sample:

1. Remove swab from transport medium and gently squeeze excess liquid from the swab by rolling the swab against the wall of tube. Discard the swab.
2. Using a disposable transfer pipet, transfer 1 mL of the transport medium to a 1.5 mL screw cap tube.
3. Centrifuge the sample for 10 minutes at 16,000xg in a microcentrifuge.
4. Decant the supernatant, invert the tube and gently tap on a clean paper towel to remove excess fluid.
5. Transfer 21 mL of Sample Wash Solution (10) from stock bottle to a sterile disposable tube. This amount is sufficient for 10 samples.
6. Using a disposable transfer pipet, transfer 1 mL of Sample Wash Solution to the sample tube. Gently resuspend the sample pellet using the transfer pipet.
7. Centrifuge the sample for 10 minutes at 16,000xg.
8. Decant the supernatant and gently tap the tube on a clean paper towel to remove excess fluid. Transfer 1 mL of Sample Wash Solution to the sample tube. Gently resuspend the sample pellet using the transfer pipet.
   Centrifuge the sample for 10 minutes at 16,000xg.
9. Decant supernatant, invert the tube and gently tap on a clean paper towel to remove excess liquid. There should be no more than 10-20 µL of wash solution remaining in the tube.
10. To each sample add 25 µL of Sample Wash Solution. Gently resuspend the sample pellet using the pipettor.
11. Heat the sample for 10 minutes in a 120°C heating block.
12. Place the samples on ice for 10 minutes then centrifuge the sample for 2 minutes at 16,000xg and return to ice.
13. Transfer 20µL of sample solution to a labeled sterile tube, then place on ice.

Sample Preparation Procedure - For a Pool of 3 Tracheal Swabs:

1. Remove swabs from transport medium and gently squeeze excess liquid from the swab by rolling the swab against the wall of tube. Discard the swabs.
2. Using a disposable transfer pipet, transfer 1 mL of the transport medium to a 1.5 mL screw cap tube.
3. Centrifuge the sample for 10 minutes at 16,000xg in a microcentrifuge.
4. Decant the supernatant, invert the tube and gently tap on a clean paper towel to remove excess fluid.
5. Transfer 21 mL of Sample Wash Solution (10) from stock bottle to a sterile disposable tube. This amount is sufficient for 10 samples.
6. Using a disposable transfer pipet, transfer 1 mL of Sample Wash Solution to the sample tube. Gently resuspend the sample pellet using the transfer pipet.
7. Centrifuge the sample for 10 minutes at 16,000xg.
8. Decant the supernatant and gently tap the tube on a clean paper towel to remove excess fluid. Transfer 1 mL of Sample Wash Solution to the sample tube. Gently resuspend the sample pellet using the transfer pipet.
   Centrifuge the sample for 10 minutes at 16,000xg.
9. Decant supernatant, invert the tube and gently tap on a clean paper towel to remove excess liquid. There should be no more than 10-20 µL of wash solution remaining in the tube.
10. To each sample add 25 µL of Sample Wash Solution. Gently resuspend the sample pellet using the pipettor.
11. Heat the sample for 10 minutes in a 120°C heating block.
12. Place the samples on ice for 10 minutes then centrifuge the sample for 2 minutes at 16,000xg and return to ice.
13. Transfer 20µL of sample solution to a labeled sterile tube, then place on ice.

Sample Preparation Procedure - For a Pool of 9 Tracheal Swabs:

1. Follow steps 1-12 of Sample Preparation Procedure - For a pool of 3 tracheal swabs.
2. Transfer 3-20 µL aliquots of sample solution (each represents a pool of 3 tracheal swabs) to a labeled sterile screw cap tube.
3. Add 150 µL of cold absolute ethanol to the sample. Gently invert the tube to mix.
4. Place the sample at -20°C for 1 hour.
5. Centrifuge the sample for 10 minutes at 16,000xg.
6. Decant the supernatant, gently tap the tube on a clean paper towel to remove excess fluid.
7. Resuspend the sample pellet with 20 µL of Sample Wash Solution.
   Place the sample on ice.

Stage 2 - DNA Amplification Procedure:

Note: Use of a 1-20 µL precision pipet and sterile tips with aerosol filters is strongly recommended to minimize the possibility of DNA contamination of the PCR Mixes during sample inoculation. Turn on the IDEXX DNAmplifier 10 to 15 minutes before use to allow the instrument to warm up.

1. Label tops of 0.5 mL microcentrifuge tubes to maintain sample identification during the process.
   One 0.5 mL microcentrifuge tube is required for each sample and two additional tubes are required, one for the positive control and one for the negative control.
2. Add 25 µL of *M. gallisepticum* PCR Mix 1 (7) and 25 µL of *M. gallisepticum* PCR Mix 2 (8) to each labeled 0.5 mL tube with a positive displacement pipet.
3. Add 1 drop of mineral oil to each microcentrifuge tube.
4. Using a 1-20 µL precision pipet, transfer 3 µL of each sample to the appropriately labeled 0.5 mL microcentrifuge tube. Cap each tube. Clean end of pipet plunger by wiping with a disposable tissue dampened with 70% ethanol between samples.

Figure 1. DNA Detection Procedure

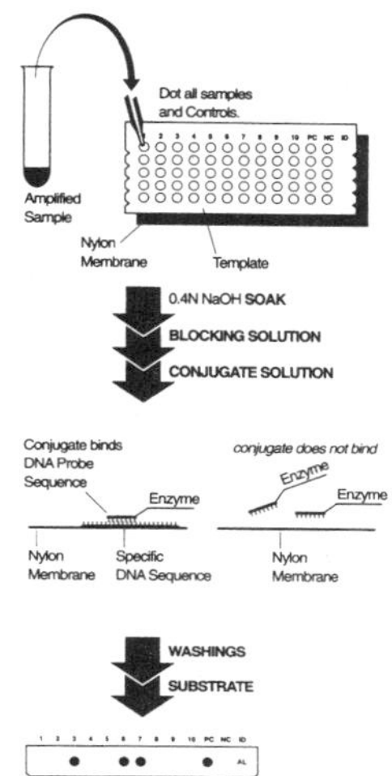

5. Transfer 3 µL of the *M. gallisepticum* Positive Control (9) to the appropriately labeled 0.5 mL microcentrifuge tube. For the negative control, transfer 3 µL of the Sample Wash Solution (10) from the aliquot (Stage 1, Step 5) used during sample preparation to the appropriate tube. Cap each tube.
6. Place the capped tubes into the IDEXX DNAmplifier and close the cover of the instrument.
7. Activate the PCR program.
8. When the PCR program is complete, remove the samples from the IDEXX DNAmplifier and proceed to the DNA detection procedure.

Stage 3. DNA Detection Procedure:

Note: When handling the nylon membrane, always wear gloves and use forceps. Do not allow membranes to come in contact with each other after samples have been added. This contact may result in the transfer of sample nucleic acids or proteins from one membrane to the other. The nylon membrane may be cut with scissors to facilitate analysis of less than 30 samples. A sufficient quantity of reagents have been supplied to perform the DNA detection procedure on 5 separate strips of nylon membrane.

The following procedure gives the appropriate volumes for running 10 samples on a 1 X 11 cm strip of nylon membrane.

1. Preheat the Blocking Solution (2) and the 6X Blot Wash Solutions 1 (3) and 2 (4) by placing the unopened containers into a 55°C water bath. Be certain these items are in solution before use.
2. Prepare 1X stocks of each Blot Wash Solution by mixing 40 mL of the 6X Wash Solutions with 200 mL of sterile, distilled, deionized water. Keep the 1X solutions in the 55°C water bath until Step 15 is completed.
   Prepare a 1X stock of Substrate Buffer by mixing 40 mL of 6X Substrate Buffer (5) with 200 mL sterile, distilled, deionized water. Store the solution at room temperature.
3. Using a pencil, mark the righthand end of the membrane strip with a reference number/name. Using a 1-20 µL pipet, dot 3 µL of each PCR amplificate onto the membrane (a dotting template will be provided if needed). Wipe mineral oil off the pipet tip with a disposable tissue before dotting. Record positions of samples.
4. In a flat-bottomed container, lay membrane sample-side up on heavy filter paper which has been soaked with a solution of 0.4 N NaOH. Allow the membrane to set for 5 minutes.
5. Place the membrane in a heat sealable pouch. Add 5 mL of Blocking Solution per 1X11 cm strip of membrane.
6. Place the pouch onto absorbent paper, and gently pass an object (such as 10 mL pipet) upward from the bottom of the pouch to facilitate removal of air bubbles. Some liquid may be allowed to run out onto the absorbent paper. Heat seal the pouch and incubate for 30 minutes in a 55°C water bath.
7. Prepare conjugate solution by adding 50 µL of *M. gallisepticum* Vir/F Conjugate Concentrate (6a) to 5 mL of Blocking Solution per membrane strip. Mix thoroughly by inverting the tube several times.
   Note: Prepare conjugate solution no more than 5 minutes before use.
8. Cut a corner of the pouch and pour off all of the Blocking Solution.
9. Add the Conjugate Solution prepared in Step 7 and remove the air bubbles as described in Step 6. Heat seal the pouch and incubate for 30 minutes in a 55°C water bath.
10. Cut open the pouch, pour off the Conjugate Solution.
11. Remove the membrane and place sample side down, into a flat-bottomed container.

12. Add 120 mL of prewarmed 1X Blot Wash Solution 1 per membrane strip. Agitate on a rotating platform for 5 minutes. Pour off wash.
13. Repeat step 12.
14. Add 120 mL of prewarmed 1X Blot Wash Solution 2 per membrane strip. Agitate on a rotating platform for 5 minutes. Pour off wash.
15. Repeat step 14.
16. Add 120 mL of 1X Substrate Buffer per membrane strip. Agitate on a rotating platform for 5 minutes. Pour off buffer.
17. Repeat step 16.
18. Prepare Substrate Solution, about 5 minutes before use, by adding 25 µL of Substrate A (A) and 25 µL of Substrate B (B) to 5 mL of 1X Substrate Buffer per membrane strip.
19. Place each membrane into a fresh, heat-sealable pouch. Add the substrate solution prepared in Step 18, removing air bubbles as described in Step 6. Heat seal the pouch and incubate the membrane for 30 minutes at 37°C, protected from the light.
20. Remove the membrane from the pouch and rinse with 1% glacial acetic acid. Place it on absorbent paper to dry, with the sample-side up.

Test Interpretation:

Results: The presence or absence of *M. gallisepticum* DNA is based upon the presence of a colored spot on the nylon membrane. Any sample producing a color reaction is positive for *M. gallisepticum.* Limits of detection for the procedure have been determined to be 100 organisms per tracheal sampling. The DNA detection procedure should be repeated if the negative control spot develops any color or if the positive control spot does not develop color.

F

The results of the *M. gallisepticum* DNA Test may depend on proper timing and technique of specimen collection, proper handling of specimens and proper assay technique. The results of the test therefore, do not necessarily indicate the absence of infection or the presence of disease. Results of this test should be used in conjunction with information available from clinical evaluation and other diagnostic procedures.

Note: A further differentiation of the *M. gallisepticum* F Strain from other *M. gallisepticum* strains can be performed using the PCR amplificates produced by the PCR reagents in this kit. These amplificates are tested using the FLOCKCHEK® PROBE® *Mycoplasma gallisepticum* DNA Test Kit, Accessory F Strain Kit which contains two separate probes specific for the strain type.

Storage: Store all components as designated on labels.

Caution(s): Because of the enormous amplification of DNA possible with this procedure; small levels of DNA contamination, from previous PCR runs, can cause a positive result even in the absence of intentionally added DNA.

The use of pipets, vessels and solutions specifically designated for sample preparation, amplification and analysis will minimize cross contamination.

If possible, perform the DNA detection procedure in an area separate from that used for sample preparation.

Handle all tracheal samples as though capable of transmitting disease.

No eating, drinking or smoking in area where specimens or kit reagents are handled.

Reagents contain sodium azide as a preservative. Flush waste reagents with large volumes of water upon disposal.

All kit reagents must be brought to room temperature prior to use.

When preparing reagents (NaOH, Membrane Wash Solutions, Substrate Buffer), use only sterile, distilled water.

When preparing NaOH, use only analytical reagent grade 10N NaOH. (See manual for order information.) Prepare NaOH fresh the day of use.

Always disinfect work areas using a 70% ethanol solution before and after use.

Discussion: *Mycoplasma gallisepticum (M. gallisepticum)* is associated with chronic respiratory disease in chickens and infectious sinusitis in turkeys. The symptoms generally seen are coryza, coughing, nasal exudate and respiratory rales. Economic losses due to *M. gallisepticum* infection include reduced egg production, lowered hatchability of chicks and downgraded meat quality.

Presentation: 30 test kit.

*The Polymerase Chain Reaction (PCR) process is covered by patents owned by Hoffman-LaRoche. GeneAmp and AmpliTaq are trademarks owned by Hoffman-LaRoche.

Compendium Code No.: 11160541 06-01911-00

FLOCKCHEK® PROBE® MYCOPLASMA SYNOVIAE DNA TEST KIT

Idexx Labs. **Mycoplasma Test**

Mycoplasma Synoviae DNA Test Kit

U.S. Vet. Lic. No.: 313

Components: Reagents:
1. Nylon Membrane
2. Blocking Solution
3. 6X Blot Wash Solution 1
4. 6X Blot Wash Solution 2
5. 6X Substrate Buffer
6. *M. synoviae* Conjugate Concentrate
7. *M. synoviae* PCR Mix 1
8. *M. synoviae* PCR Mix 2
9. *M. synoviae* Positive Control
10. Sample Wash Solution
A. Substrate A
B. Substrate B

Materials Required But Not Provided:
1. IDEXX DNAmplifier™
2. Mineral oil (light)
3. Rotating platform
4. Heat block (120°C)
5. Analytical reagent grade 10N NaOH
6. Ethanol
7. Water baths (37°C and 55°C)
8. Latex gloves
9. 1-20 µL and 10-200 µL precision pipets and tips with aerosol filters
10. 1 mL disposable transfer pipets graduated to 0.25 mL
11. 25 µL positive displacement pipet with tips
12. Heat sealer and heat-sealable pouches
13. 1.5 mL screw cap microcentrifuge tubes
14. 0.5 mL microcentrifuge tubes with caps
15. 15 mL and 50 mL sterile conical tubes with caps
16. Flat-bottomed containers
17. Heavy filter paper or blotting pad
18. 1% glacial acetic acid
19. Sterile HPLC Grade water, or sterile water for injection

Indications: The FLOCKCHEK® PROBE® Mycoplasma Synoviae DNA Test Kit is a nonradioactive probe based test utilizing PCR amplification for the specific detection of *Mycoplasma synoviae* genomic DNA from chicken and turkey tracheal swab samples.

Test Principles: Tracheal swab samples are processed to effect the removal of interfering sample components.

The Polymerase Chain Reaction® (PCR®)* DNA amplification procedure utilizes two synthetic DNA molecules whose properties are based on a DNA sequence specific to *M. synoviae.* These DNA molecules are used in conjunction with AmpliTaq® DNA polymerase to amplify small amounts of *M. synoviae* target DNA to provide enhancement of sensitivity.

A third synthetic DNA molecule, labeled with an enzyme is used as sequence specific hybridization probe to provide colorimetric detection of the amplified target DNA.

Test Procedure: Specimen Information: Obtain tracheal sample by swabbing the trachea of a chicken or turkey. Place the swab in a tube containing 1.0 to 1.5 mL of transport medium. The sample should be stored on ice and delivered to the laboratory within 24 hours.

For pooled samples, place three swabs in a tube containing 2.0 to 2.5 mL of transport medium. The sample should be stored on ice and delivered to the laboratory within 24 hours.

There are three stages required for implementation of the *M. synoviae* DNA Test Kit from a tracheal swab sample:

Stage 1 - Sample Preparation Procedure
Stage 2 - DNA Amplification Procedure
Stage 3 - DNA Detection Procedure

Note: Set up the IDEXX DNAmplifier as outlined in the *M. synoviae* instructions of the FlockChek® DNA Probe Manual.

Stage 1: Sample Preparation Procedure - For Single Tracheal Swab Sample:
1. Remove swab from transport medium and gently squeeze excess liquid from the swab by rolling the swab against the wall of tube. Discard the swab.
2. Using a disposable transfer pipet, transfer 1 mL of the transport medium to a 1.5 mL screw cap tube.
3. Centrifuge the sample for 10 minutes at 16,000xg in a microcentrifuge.
4. Decant the supernatant, invert the tube and gently tap on a clean paper towel to remove excess fluid.
5. Transfer 21 mL of Sample Wash Solution (10) from stock bottle to a sterile disposable tube. This amount is sufficient for 10 samples.
6. Using a disposable transfer pipet, transfer 1 mL of Sample Wash Solution to the sample tube. Gently resuspend the sample pellet using the transfer pipet.
7. Centrifuge the sample for 10 minutes at 16,000xg.
8. Decant the supernatant and gently tap the tube on a clean paper towel to remove excess fluid. Transfer 1 mL of Sample Wash Solution to the sample tube. Gently resuspend the sample pellet using the transfer pipet. Centrifuge the sample for 10 minutes at 16,000xg.
9. Decant supernatant, invert the tube and gently tap on a clean paper towel to remove excess liquid. There should be no more than 10-20 µL of wash solution remaining in the tube.
10. To each sample add 25 µL of Sample Wash Solution. Gently resuspend the sample pellet using the pipettor.
11. Heat the sample for 10 minutes in a 120°C heating block.
12. Place the samples on ice for 10 minutes then centrifuge the sample for 2 minutes at 16,000xg and return to ice.
13. Transfer 20µL of sample solution to a labeled sterile tube, then place on ice.

Sample Preparation Procedure - For a Pool of 3 Tracheal Swabs
1. Remove swabs from transport medium and gently squeeze excess liquid from the swab by rolling the swab against the wall of tube. Discard the swabs.
2. Using a disposable transfer pipet, transfer 1 mL of the transport medium to a 1.5 mL screw cap tube.
3. Centrifuge the sample for 10 minutes at 16,000xg in a microcentrifuge.
4. Decant the supernatant, invert the tube and gently tap on a clean paper towel to remove excess fluid.
5. Transfer 21 mL of Sample Wash Solution (10) from stock bottle to a sterile disposable tube. This amount is sufficient for 10 samples.
6. Using a disposable transfer pipet, transfer 1 mL of Sample Wash Solution to the sample tube. Gently resuspend the sample pellet using the transfer pipet.
7. Centrifuge the sample for 10 minutes at 16,000xg.
8. Decant the supernatant and gently tap the tube on a clean paper towel to remove excess fluid. Transfer 1 mL of Sample Wash Solution to the sample tube. Gently resuspend the sample pellet using the transfer pipet. Centrifuge the sample for 10 minutes at 16,000xg.
9. Decant supernatant, invert the tube and gently tap on a clean paper towel to remove excess liquid. There should be no more than 10-20 µL of wash solution remaining in the tube.
10. To each sample add 25 µL of Sample Wash Solution. Gently resuspend the sample pellet using the pipettor.
11. Heat the sample for 10 minutes in a 120°C heating block.
12. Place the samples on ice for 10 minutes then centrifuge the sample for 2 minutes at 16,000xg and return to ice.
13. Transfer 20µL of sample solution to a labeled sterile tube, then place on ice.

Sample Preparation Procedure - For a Pool of 9 Tracheal Swabs:
1. Follow steps 1-12 of Sample Preparation Procedure - For a pool of 3 tracheal swabs.
2. Transfer 3-20 µL aliquots of sample solution (each represents a Pool of 3 Tracheal Swabs) to a labeled sterile screw cap tube.
3. Add 150 µL of cold absolute ethanol to the sample. Gently invert the tube to mix.
4. Place the sample at -20°C for 1 hour.
5. Centrifuge the sample for 10 minutes at 16,000xg.
6. Decant the supernatant, gently tap the tube on a clean paper towel to remove excess fluid.
7. Resuspend the sample pellet with 20 µL of Sample Wash Solution. Place the sample on ice.

Stage 2 - DNA Amplification Procedure:

Note: Use of a 1-20 µL precision pipet and sterile tips with aerosol filters is strongly recommended to minimize the possibility of DNA contamination of the PCR Mixes during sample inoculation. Turn on the IDEXX DNAmplifier 10 to 15 minutes before use to allow the instrument to warm up.
1. Label tops of 0.5 mL microcentrifuge tubes to maintain sample identification during the process. One 0.5 mL microcentrifuge tube is required for each sample and two additional tubes are required, one for the positive control and one for the negative control.

2. Add 25 µL of *M. synoviae* PCR Mix 1 (7) and 25 µL of *M. synoviae* PCR Mix 2 (8) to each labeled 0.5 mL tube with a positive displacement pipet.
3. Add 1 drop of mineral oil to each microcentrifuge tube.
4. Using a 1-20 µL precision pipet, transfer 3 µL of each sample to the appropriately labeled 0.5 mL microcentrifuge tube. Cap each tube. Clean end of pipet plunger by wiping with a disposable tissue dampened with 70% ethanol between samples.

Figure 1. DNA Detection Procedure

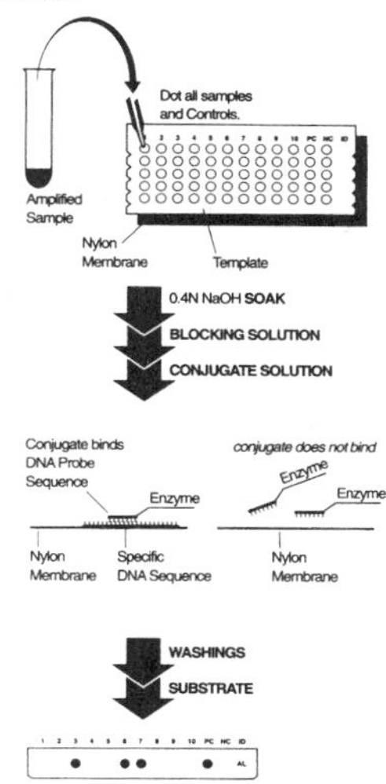

5. Transfer 3 µL of the *M. synoviae* Positive Control (9) to the appropriately labeled 0.5 mL microcentrifuge tube. For the negative control, transfer 3 µL of the Sample Wash Solution (10) from the aliquot (Stage 1, Step 5) used during sample preparation to the appropriate tube. Cap each tube.
6. Place the capped tubes into the IDEXX DNAmplifier and close the cover of the instrument.
7. Activate the PCR program.
8. When the PCR program is complete, remove the samples from the IDEXX DNAmplifier and proceed to the DNA detection procedure.

Stage 3. DNA Detection Procedure:

Note: When handling the nylon membrane, always wear gloves and use forceps. Do not allow membranes to come in contact with each other after samples have been added. This contact may result in the transfer of sample nucleic acids or proteins from membrane to the other. The nylon membrane may be cut with scissors to facilitate analysis of less than 30 samples. A sufficient quantity of reagents have been supplied to perform the DNA detection procedure on 5 separate strips of nylon membrane.

The following procedure gives the appropriate volumes for running 10 samples on a 1 X 11 cm strip of nylon membrane.

1. Preheat the Blocking Solution (2) and the 6X Blot Wash Solutions 1 (3) and 2 (4) by placing the unopened containers into a 55°C water bath. Be certain these items are in solution before use.
2. Prepare 1X stocks of each Blot Wash Solution by mixing 40 mL of the 6X Wash Solutions with 200 mL of sterile, distilled, deionized water. Keep the 1X solutions in the 55°C water bath until Step 15 is completed.
   Prepare a 1X stock of Substrate Buffer by mixing 41 mL of 6X Substrate Buffer (5) with 205 mL sterile, distilled, deionized water. Store the solution at room temperature.
3. Using a pencil, mark the righthand end of the membrane strip with a reference number/name. Using a 1-20 µL pipet, dot 3 µL of each PCR amplificate onto the membrane (a dotting template will be provided if needed). Wipe mineral oil off the pipet tip with a disposable tissue before dotting. Record positions of samples.
4. In a flat-bottomed container, lay membrane sample-side up on heavy filter paper which has been soaked with a solution of 0.4 N NaOH. Allow the membrane to set for 5 minutes.
5. Place the membrane in a heat sealable pouch. Add 5 mL of Blocking Solution per 1X11 cm strip of membrane.
6. Place the pouch onto absorbent paper, and gently pass an object (such as 10 mL pipet) upward from the bottom of the pouch to facilitate removal of air bubbles. Some liquid may be allowed to run out onto the absorbent paper. Heat seal the pouch and incubate for 30 minutes in a 55°C water bath.
7. Prepare conjugate solution by adding 50 µL of *M. synoviae* Conjugate Concentrate (6) to 5 mL of Blocking Solution per membrane strip. Mix thoroughly by inverting the tube several times.
   Note: Prepare conjugate solution no more than 5 minutes before use.
8. Cut a corner of the pouch and pour off all of the Blocking Solution.
9. Add the Conjugate Solution prepared in Step 7 and remove the air bubbles as described in Step 6.
   Heat seal the pouch and incubate for 30 minutes in a 55°C water bath.
10. Cut open the pouch, pour off the Conjugate Solution.
11. Remove the membrane and place sample side down, into a flat-bottomed container.
12. Add 120 mL of prewarmed 1X Blot Wash Solution 1 per membrane strip. Agitate on a rotating platform for 5 minutes. Pour off wash.
13. Repeat step 12.
14. Add 120 mL of prewarmed 1X Blot Wash Solution 2 per membrane strip. Agitate on a rotating platform for 5 minutes. Pour off wash.
15. Repeat step 14.
16. Add 120 mL of 1X Substrate Buffer per membrane strip. Agitate on a rotating platform for 5 minutes. Pour off buffer.
17. Repeat step 16.
18. Prepare Substrate Solution, about 5 minutes before use, by adding 25 µL of Substrate A (A) and 25 µL of Substrate B (B) to 5 mL of 1X Substrate Buffer per membrane strip.
19. Place each membrane into a fresh, heat-sealable pouch. Add the substrate solution prepared in Step 18, removing air bubbles as described in Step 6. Heat seal the pouch and incubate the membrane for 30 minutes at 37°C, protected from the light.
20. Remove the membrane from the pouch and rinse with 1% glacial acetic acid. Place it on absorbent paper to dry, with the sample-side up.

Test Interpretation: Results: The presence or absence of *M. synoviae* DNA is based upon the presence of a colored spot on the nylon membrane. Any sample producing a color reaction is positive for *M. synoviae.* Limits of detection for the procedure have been determined to be 100 organisms per tracheal sampling. The DNA detection procedure should be repeated if the negative control spot develops any color or if the positive control spot does not develop color.

The results of the *M. synoviae* DNA Test may depend on proper timing and technique of specimen collection, proper handling of specimens and proper assay technique. The results of the test therefore, do not necessarily indicate the absence of infection or the presence of disease. Results of this test should be used in conjunction with information available from clinical evaluation and other diagnostic procedures.

Storage: Store all components as designated on labels.

Caution(s): Because of the enormous amplification of DNA possible with this procedure; small levels of DNA contamination, from previous PCR runs, can cause a positive result even in the absence of intentionally added DNA.

The use of pipets, vessels and solutions specifically designated for sample preparation, amplification and analysis will minimize cross contamination.

If possible, perform the DNA detection procedure in an area separate from that used for sample preparation.

Handle all tracheal samples as though capable of transmitting disease.

No eating, drinking or smoking in area where specimens or kit reagents are handled.

Reagents contain sodium azide as a preservative. Flush waste reagents with large volumes of water upon disposal.

All kit reagents must be brought to room temperature prior to use.

When preparing reagents (NaOH, Membrane Wash Solutions, Substrate Buffer), use only sterile, distilled water.

When preparing NaOH, use only analytical reagent grade 10N NaOH. (See manual for order information.) Prepare NaOH fresh the day of use.

Always disinfect work areas using a 70% ethanol solution before and after use.

Discussion: *Mycoplasma synoviae (M. synoviae)* is a known pathogen associated with the development of synovitis and chronic respiratory disease in chickens and turkeys. Clinical symptoms include joint swelling, coryza and respiratory rales. Economic losses due to *M. synoviae* infection include reduced egg production, lowered hatchability of chicks and downgraded meat quality.

Presentation: Kit contains enough reagents to test 50 samples.

*The Polymerase Chain Reaction (PCR) process is covered by patents owned by Hoffman-La Roche. GeneAmp and AmpliTaq are trademarks owned by Hoffman-La Roche.

Compendium Code No.: 11160561 06-01373-02

FLOCKCHEK® REO ANTIBODY TEST KIT

Idexx Labs. **Reovirus Test**

Avian Reovirus Antibody Test Kit

U.S. Vet. Lic. No.: 313

Components:

Reagent	Volume
1. REO Coated Plates	5
2. REO Positive Control - Diluted chicken Anti-REO, preserved with sodium azide.	1.9 mL
3. Negative Control - Diluted chicken sera non-reactive for Anti-REO, preserved with sodium azide.	1.9 mL
4. (Goat) Anti-Chicken: Horseradish Peroxidase Conjugate, preserved with gentamicin.	50 mL
5. Sample Diluent buffer preserved with sodium azide.	235 mL
6. TMB Substrate	60 mL
7. Stop Solution	60 mL

Materials Required but Not Provided: Precision pipets and multiple delivery pipetting device with disposable pipet tips, 96-well plate reader, tubes for diluting samples, distilled or deionized water and device for the delivery and aspiration of wash solution.

Indications: FLOCKCHEK® REO is Idexx's enzyme immunoassay for the detection of antibody to Avian Reovirus (REO) in chicken serum.

Test Principles: This assay is designed to measure the relative level of antibody to REO in chicken serum. Viral antigen is coated on 96-well plates. Upon incubation of the test sample in the coated well, antibody specific to REO forms a complex with the coated viral antigens. After washing away unbound material from the wells, a conjugate is added which binds to any attached chicken antibody in the wells. Unbound conjugate is washed away and enzyme substrate is added. Subsequent color development is directly related to the amount of antibody to REO present in the test sample.

Test Procedure:

Preparation of Samples: Dilute test samples five hundred fold (1:500) with sample diluent prior to being assayed (e.g., by diluting 1 µL of sample with 500 µL of Sample Diluent). Note: Do not dilute controls. Be sure to change tips for each sample. Samples must be thoroughly mixed prior to dispensing into the coated plate.

Reagents should be allowed to come to room temperature, then mixed by inverting and swirling.

1. Obtain antigen-coated plate(s) and record the sample position on a FlockChek® worksheet.
2. Dispense 100 µL of Undiluted Negative Control into wells A1 and A2.
3. Dispense 100 µL of Undiluted Positive Control into wells A3 and A4.
4. Dispense 100 µL of diluted sample into appropriate wells. All samples should be run in duplicate.
5. Incubate for 30 minutes at room temperature.
6. Wash each well with approximately 350 µL of distilled or deionized water 3-5 times.
7. Dispense 100 µL of (Goat) Anti-Chicken: Horseradish Peroxidase Conjugate into each well.
8. Incubate for 30 minutes at room temperature.
9. Repeat step 6.
10. Dispense 100 µL of TMB substrate solution into each well.
11. Incubate for 15 minutes at room temperature.
12. Dispense 100 µL of Stop Solution into each well to stop the reaction.
13. Blank reader with air.
14. Measure and record absorbance values at 650nm, A(650).

Test Interpretation:

Results: For the assay to be valid, the difference between the Positive Control mean and the Negative Control mean (PC$\bar{x}$ - NC$\bar{x}$) should be greater than 0.075. The Negative Control mean absorbance should be less than or equal to 0.150. The presence or absence of antibody to REO is determined by relating the A(650) value of the unknown to the Positive Control mean. The Positive Control is standardized and represents significant antibody levels to REO in chicken serum. The relative level of antibody in the unknown is determined by calculating the sample to positive (S/P) ratio. Endpoint titers are calculated using the equation described in the calculations section.

Interpretation of Results: Serum samples with S/P ratios of less than or equal to 0.2 should be considered negative. S/P ratios greater than 0.2 (titers greater than 396) should be considered positive and indicate vaccination or other exposure to REO. Each laboratory should establish its own criterion for immunity with respect to antibody titer based on correlation of FLOCKCHEK® REO to current laboratory test methodologies and on historical antibody responses to specific vaccines and vaccination protocols. The immune status of a flock is best assessed by monitoring and recording antibody titers in representative samples as a function of time. The resulting flock profiles allow an assessment of the distribution of antibody titers and an analysis of changes in titer over time.

Calculations:

1. Negative Control mean (NC$\bar{x}$):
$$\frac{\text{Well A1 A(650)} + \text{Well A2 A(650)}}{2} = NC\bar{x}$$
2. Positive Control mean (PC$\bar{x}$):
$$\frac{\text{Well A3 A(650)} + \text{Well A4 A(650)}}{2} = PC\bar{x}$$
3. S/P Ratio:
$$\frac{\text{Sample Mean} - NC\bar{x}}{PC\bar{x} - NC\bar{x}} = S/P$$
4. Titer - Relates S/P at a 1:500 dilution to an endpoint titer:
$\text{Log}_{10}\ \text{Titer} = 1.09\ (\text{Log}_{10}\ S/P) + 3.36$

Storage: Store all reagents at 2°-7°C (36°-45°F).

Caution(s): Handle all REO biological materials as though capable of transmitting REO. The antigen coated plates may be a source of REO. Prior to coating on the solid phase, the antigen has been inactivated by chemical treatment. Nevertheless, do not assume complete inactivation. Some kit components contain sodium azide as a preservative. Disposal requires flushing plumbing with large volumes of water to prevent formation of copper or lead azide complexes which may explode upon percussion. Do not expose TMB solutions to strong light or any oxidation agents. All wastes should be properly decontaminated prior to disposal. Do not use components past expiration date and do not intermix components from kits with different lot numbers. Careful pipetting and washing throughout this procedure are necessary to maintain precision and accuracy. Optimal results will be obtained by strict adherence to this protocol. For veterinary use only.

Discussion: An assessment of immune status as well as serologic identification of REO requires a measurement of antibody to REO in serum. Enzyme immunoassay systems have proven efficacious in the quantification of antibody levels to REO and facilitate the monitoring of immune status in large flocks.

Presentation: 5 plates per kit.

FLOCKCHEK® is a registered trademark of Idexx Laboratories, Inc. in the United States and/or other countries.

Compendium Code No.: 11160212 06-01108-04

FLOCKCHEK® REV ANTIBODY TEST KIT

Idexx Labs. **REV Test**

Reticuloendotheliosis Virus Antibody Test Kit

U.S. Vet. Lic. No.: 313

Components:

Reagent	Volume
1. REV Coated Plates	5
2. REV Positive Control - Diluted chicken Anti-REV, preserved with sodium azide.	1.9 mL
3. Negative Control - Diluted chicken sera non-reactive for Anti-REV, preserved with sodium azide.	1.9 mL
4. (Goat) Anti-Chicken: Horseradish Peroxidase Conjugate, preserved with gentamicin.	50 mL
5. Sample Diluent buffer preserved with sodium azide.	235 mL
6. TMB Substrate	60 mL
7. Stop Solution	60 mL

Materials Required but Not Provided: Precision pipets and multiple delivery pipetting device with disposable pipet tips, 96-well plate reader, tubes for diluting samples, distilled or deionized water and device for the delivery and aspiration of wash solution.

Indications: FLOCKCHEK® REV is Idexx's enzyme immunoassay for the detection of antibody to Reticuloendotheliosis (REV) in chicken serum.

Test Principles: This assay is designed to measure the relative level of antibody to REV in chicken serum. Viral antigen is coated on 96-well plates. Upon incubation of the test sample in the coated well, antibody specific to REV forms a complex with the coated viral antigens. After washing away unbound material from the wells, a conjugate is added which binds to any attached chicken antibody in the wells. Unbound conjugate is washed away and enzyme substrate is added. Subsequent color development is directly related to the amount of antibody to REV present in the test sample.

Test Procedure:

Preparation of Samples: Dilute test samples five hundred fold (1:500) with sample diluent prior to being assayed (e.g., by diluting 1 µL of sample with 500 µL of Sample Diluent). Note: Do not dilute controls. Be sure to change tips for each sample. Samples must be thoroughly mixed prior to dispensing into the coated plate.

Reagents should be allowed to come to room temperature, then mixed by inverting and swirling.

1. Obtain antigen-coated plate(s) and record the sample position on a FlockChek® worksheet.
2. Dispense 100 µL of Undiluted Negative Control into wells A1 and A2.
3. Dispense 100 µL of Undiluted Positive Control into wells A3 and A4.
4. Dispense 100 µL of diluted sample into appropriate wells. All samples should be run in duplicate.
5. Incubate for 30 minutes at room temperature.
6. Wash each well with approximately 350 µL of distilled or deionized water 3-5 times.
7. Dispense 100 µL of (Goat) Anti-Chicken: Horseradish Peroxidase Conjugate into each well.
8. Incubate for 30 minutes at room temperature.
9. Repeat step 6.
10. Dispense 100 µL of TMB substrate solution into each well.
11. Incubate for 15 minutes at room temperature.
12. Dispense 100 µL of Stop Solution into each well to stop the reaction.
13. Blank reader with air.
14. Measure and record absorbance values at 650nm, A(650).

Test Interpretation:

Results: For the assay to be valid, the difference between the Positive Control mean and the Negative Control mean (PC$\bar{x}$ - NC$\bar{x}$) should be greater than 0.075. The Negative Control mean absorbance should be less than or equal to 0.150. The presence or absence of antibody to REV is determined by relating the A(650) value of the unknown to the Positive Control mean. The Positive Control is standardized and represents significant antibody levels to REV in chicken serum. The relative level of antibody in the unknown is determined by calculating the sample to positive (S/P) ratio. Endpoint titers are calculated using the equation described in the calculations section.

Interpretation of Results: Serum samples with S/P ratios of less than or equal to 0.5 should be considered negative. S/P ratios greater than 0.5 (titers greater than 1076) should be considered positive and indicate vaccination or other exposure to REV. Each laboratory should establish its own criterion for immunity with respect to antibody titer based on correlation of FLOCKCHEK® REV to current laboratory test methodologies and on historical antibody responses.

Calculations:

1. Negative Control mean (NC$\bar{x}$):
$$\frac{\text{Well A1 A(650)} + \text{Well A2 A(650)}}{2} = NC\bar{x}$$
2. Positive Control mean (PC$\bar{x}$):
$$\frac{\text{Well A3 A(650)} + \text{Well A4 A(650)}}{2} = PC\bar{x}$$
3. S/P Ratio:
$$\frac{\text{Sample Mean} - NC\bar{x}}{PC\bar{x} - NC\bar{x}} = S/P$$
4. Titer - Relates S/P at a 1:500 dilution to an endpoint titer:
$\text{Log}_{10}\ \text{Titer} = 1.09\ (\text{Log}_{10}\ S/P) + 3.36$

Storage: Store all reagents at 2°-7°C (36°-45°F).

Caution(s): Handle all REV biological materials as though capable of transmitting REV. The antigen coated plates may be a source of REV. Prior to coating on the solid phase, the antigen has been inactivated by chemical treatment. Nevertheless, do not assume complete inactivation. Some kit components contain sodium azide as a preservative. Disposal requires flushing plumbing with large volumes of water to prevent formation of copper or lead azide complexes which may explode upon percussion. Do not expose TMB solutions to strong light or any oxidation agents. All wastes should be properly decontaminated prior to disposal. Do not use components past expiration date and do not intermix components from kits with different lot numbers. Careful pipetting and washing throughout this procedure are necessary to maintain precision and accuracy. Optimal results will be obtained by strict adherence to this protocol. For veterinary use only.

Discussion: An assessment of immune status as well as serologic identification of REV requires a measurement of antibody to REV in serum. Enzyme immunoassay systems have proven efficacious in the quantification of antibody levels to REV and facilitate the monitoring of immune status in large flocks.

Presentation: 5 plates per kit.

FLOCKCHEK is a registered trademark of Idexx Laboratories, Inc. in the United States and/or other countries.

Compendium Code No.: 11160222 06-01165-02

FLOCKCHEK® Se ANTIBODY TEST KIT

Idexx Labs. **Salmonella Test**

Salmonella Enteritidis Antibody Test Kit

U.S. Vet. Lic. No.: 313

Components:

Reagents	Volume
1. Se Coated Plates	5
2. Anti-Se: Horseradish Peroxidase (HRPO) Conjugate Concentrate in buffer with protein stabilizers	0.1 mL
2a. HRPO Conjugate Diluent Buffer with Protein Stabilizers	60 mL
3. Negative Control - Chicken serum non-reactive to Se in buffer with protein stabilizers. Preserved with Sodium Azide	2 mL
4. Se Positive Control-Anti-Se in buffer with protein stabilizers, preserved with Sodium Azide	2 mL
5. Sample Diluent - buffer with protein stabilizers, preserved with Sodium Azide	235 mL
6. Wash Concentrate (10X) Phosphate buffer preserved with gentamicin	235 mL
7. TMB Substrate	60 mL
8. Stop Solution	60 mL

Materials Required but Not Provided: Precision pipets and multiple delivery pipetting device with disposable pipet tips, 96-well plate reader, tubes for diluting samples, distilled or deionized water and device for the delivery and aspiration of wash solution.

Indications: FLOCKCHECK® Se is Idexx's enzyme immunoassay for the detection of antibody to *Salmonella enteritidis* (Se) in chicken serum or egg yolk.

Test Principles: The FLOCKCHEK® Se assay is performed in microtiter well coated with purified *Salmonella enteritidis* antigen. During the first incubation, Se antibodies present in the sample react with immobilized antigens. After a wash step, an Anti-Se monoclonal antibody enzyme conjugate is added to the microwell. If no Anti-Se antibodies are present in the test sample, the anti-Se conjugate if free to react with the Se antigen. Conversely, if Anti-Se antibodies are present in the sample, the enzyme-conjugated monoclonal antibodies are blocked from reacting with the antigen. Following this incubation period, the unreacted conjugate is removed by washing and a substrate/chromogen solution is added. In the presence of the enzyme, the substrate is converted to a product which reacts with the chromophore to generate a blue color. The absorbance at 650 nm, A(650), is measured using a spectrophotometer. Results are calculated by dividing the A(650) of the sample by the mean A(650) of the negative control, resulting in an S/N value. The quantity of antibodies to Se is inversely proportional to the A(650) and thus, to the S/N value. The presence of Se antibodies indicates previous exposure to *Salmonella enteritidis* either by natural infection or vaccination.

Test Procedure: Preparation of Samples:

Note: Dilution of serum samples may be made in microdilution tubes or directly in the microtiter plate by adding the appropriate amount of serum to previously pipetted Sample Diluent.

A. Field Exposure: Dilute serum samples two-fold (1:2) with Sample Diluent prior to being assayed (e.g., by diluting 100 µL of serum with 100 µL of Sample Diluent).

B. Vaccination: For the detection of antibody subsequent to vaccination, dilute serum samples 1:250 or 1:500. These dilutions will afford adequate differentiation of responses from samples within a vaccinated flock.
These dilution factors should serve as guidelines only. Responses to vaccination will depend upon dose, route of administration, age of flock, etc. Individual laboratories should establish their own parameters with which to monitor vaccine response and efficacy.

C. Egg Yolks: Dilute egg yolks two-fold (1:2) with Sample Diluent prior to being assayed (e.g., by diluting 100 µL of egg yolk with 100 µL of Sample Diluent). Mix sample thoroughly before pipetting into microtiter well.
Note: Do not dilute controls.

Preparation of Conjugate: Anti-Se: HRPO Concentrate must be diluted in Conjugate Diluent before use. The diluted Conjugate should be used on the same day it is prepared. Dilute the HRPO Concentrate according to the instructions on the label and keep the HRPO Concentrate at 2°-7°C (36°-45°F) when not in use.

Preparation of Wash Solution: The 10X Wash Concentrate should be brought to room temperature 22°-27°C (72°-80°F) and mixed to ensure dissolution of any precipitated salts. The Wash Concentrate must be diluted 1:10 with distilled/deionized water before use (e.g. 30 mL of concentrate plus 270 mL of water per plate to be assayed).

Reagents should be allowed to come to room temperature, then mixed by inverting and swirling.

1. Obtain antigen coated plate(s) and record the sample positions on a FlockChek® worksheet.
2. Dispense 100 µL of Undiluted Negative Control into wells A1 and A2.
3. Dispense 100 µL of Undiluted Positive Control into wells A3 and A4.
4. Dispense 100 µL of diluted sample into the appropriate wells. All samples should be run in duplicate.
5. Incubate for 60 minutes.
6. Wash each well with approximately 350 µL of wash solution 3-5 times.
7. Dispense 100 µL of diluted Anti-Se: Horseradish Peroxidase Conjugate into each well.
8. Incubate for 30 minutes at room temperature.
9. Repeat step 6.
10. Dispense 100 µL of TMB substrate solution into each well.
11. Incubate for 15 minutes at room temperature.
12. Dispense 100 µL of Stop Solution into each well to stop the reaction.
13. Blank reader with air.
14. Measure and record absorbance values at 650nm, A(650).

Test Interpretation:

Results: For the assay to be valid, the Negative Control optical density (650 nm) must be greater than or equal to 0.80 and the Positive Control S/N must be less than or equal to 0.50. For invalid tests, technique may be suspect and the assay should be repeated. The presence or absence of antibody to Se is determined by the sample to negative (S/N) ratio for each sample.

Interpretation of Results:

1. Samples with S/N ratios greater than or equal to 0.75 are considered negative within the limits of the test.
2. If the S/N ratio is between 0.74 and 0.60, the sample should be retested. If the test result repeats, the animal should be sampled and tested at a later date.
3. Samples with S/N ratios less than or equal to 0.59 are considered positive and should be confirmed by culture.
4. The immune status of a flock is best assessed by monitoring and recording antibody levels in representative samples as a function of time. The resulting flock profiles allow an assessment of the distribution of antibody levels and an analysis of changes in status over time.

Calculations:

1. Negative Control mean ($NC\bar{x}$):
$$\frac{\text{Well A1 A(650)} + \text{Well A2(650)}}{2} = NC\bar{x}$$
2. Positive Control mean ($PC\bar{x}$):
$$\frac{\text{Well A3 A(650)} + \text{Well A4 A(650)}}{2} = PC\bar{x}$$
3. S/N Ratio:
$$\frac{\text{Sample A(650)}}{NC\bar{x}} = S/N$$

Storage: Store all reagents at 2°-7°C (36°-45°F).

Caution(s): Handle all Se biological materials as though capable of transmitting Se. The antigen coated plates may be a source of Se. Prior to coating on the solid phase, the antigen has been inactivated by chemical treatment. Nevertheless, do not assume complete inactivation. Some kit components contain sodium azide as a preservative. Disposal requires flushing plumbing with large volumes of water to prevent the formation of copper or lead azide complexes which may explode upon percussion. Do not expose TMB solutions to strong light or any oxidation agents. All wastes should be properly decontaminated prior to disposal. Do not use components past expiration date and do not intermix components from kits with different lot numbers. Careful pipetting and washing throughout the procedure is necessary to maintain precision and accuracy. Optimal results will be obtained by strict adherence to the protocol. For veterinary use only.

Discussion: *Salmonella enteritidis* is an important pathogen of poultry and has been isolated from broilers, breeders, and commercial egg laying flocks. Bacteriological identification of positive birds is difficult due to the intermittent excretion of the organism. The presence of antibody does not always signify infection but will indicate previous exposure.

The enzyme-linked immunoabsorbent assay has shown utility in the detection of antibody to *Salmonella* in poultry, and is particularly useful in large-scale monitoring of flocks for *Salmonella enteritidis* infection. The FLOCKCHECK® Se Assay can be used as an initial screening method for the presence of *S. enteritidis* antibodies. However, since the Se ELISA is g,m flagellin based, other *salmonella* serotypes that share the epitopes of g,m flagellin can potentially yield positive results. Therefore, positive screening results must always be confirmed by standard bacteriological methods.

Presentation: 5 plates per kit.

FLOCKCHEK is a registered trademark of Idexx Laboratories, Inc. in the United States and/or other countries.

Compendium Code No.: 11160082 06-01381-09

FLU AVERT™ I.N. VACCINE

Intervet **Vaccine**

Equine Influenza Vaccine, Modified Live Virus

U.S. Vet. Lic. No.: 213

Composition: This vaccine is a lyophilized preparation containing an attenuated, cold adapted, viable A equine-2 influenza virus. Contains no preservatives.

Indications: For the vaccination of healthy horses, 11 months of age or older, as an aid in the reduction of clinical disease caused by equine influenza viruses of both the American and Eurasian lineages.

Dosage and Administration: Single Dose Vial: Administer a single one (1) mL dose intranasally in one (1) nostril.

Step 1: Securely attach a nasal applicator to a 3-cc luer lock syringe.

Step 2: Remove the cap and rubber stopper from one vial of diluent and one vial of vaccine.

Step 3: Using the nasal applicator with the attached syringe, draw 1 mL of the sterile diluent into the nasal applicator. The applicator should be nearly full, no diluent should be drawn into the syringe. Transfer the sterile diluent to the lyophilized vaccine vial.

Step 4: Mix the vaccine and diluent in the vial with a gentle swirling motion, Once dissolved, immediately withdraw the full amount of rehydrated vaccine into the nasal applicator. Take caution to do draw vaccine into the syringe.

Step 5: Place the full length of the applicator into the nasal passage. The syringe should still be in full view outside the nostril. Once in place, depress the plunger to administer the vaccine over approximately a 1-second interval. Withdraw and discard the applicator and syringe.

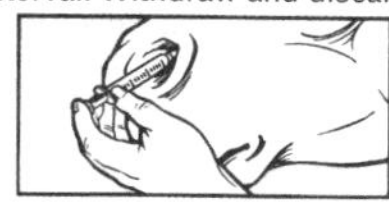

Step 6: After vaccination, there may be some residual vaccine in the applicator and a small amount may drip out of the nostril. This is normal, vaccination has been completed successfully.

Five Dose Vial: Administer a single one (1) mL dose intranasally in one (1) nostril.

Step 1: Use a syringe and needle to transfer the entire amount of the sterile diluent to the lyophilized vaccine vial. Mix the vaccine and diluent in the vial with a gentle swirling motion.

Step 2: Once dissolved, remove the seal and rubber stopper from the vial.

Step 3: Securely attach a nasal applicator to a 3-cc luer lock syringe.

Step 4: Place the tip of the applicator into the vaccine and draw vaccine into the applicator up to the mark. Take caution not to draw vaccine into the syringe.

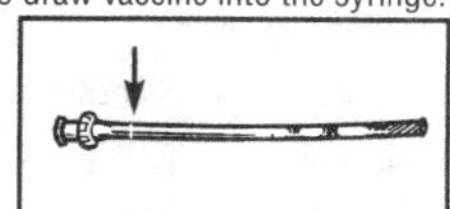

Step 5: Place the full length of the applicator into the nasal passage. The syringe should still be in full view outside the nostril. Once in place, depress the plunger to administer the vaccine over approximately a 1-second interval. Withdraw and discard the applicator and syringe.

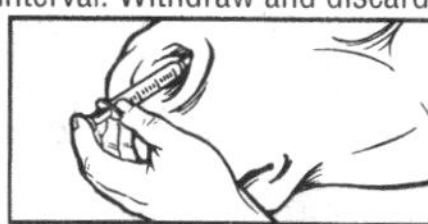

Step 6: After vaccination, there may be some residual vaccine in the applicator and a small amount may drip out of the nostril. This is normal, vaccination has been completed successfully.

Note: A new applicator should be used to vaccinate each horse. This vaccine is not intended for intramuscular or subcutaneous injection. For primary immunization, a single dose is required in horses 11 months of age or older. Horses vaccinated at less than 11 months of age should be given a dose of the vaccine at age 11 months. Revaccination every six months is recommended. Horses at high risk of exposure may benefit from revaccination every three months.

Precaution(s): Keep refrigerated at a temperature between 35° and 45°F (2-7°C). Store out of direct sunlight. Use the entire contents of the vaccine after reconstitution. Burn containers after use.

Caution(s): Do not vaccinate pregnant animals. In rare instances, reactions may occur due to unusual sensitivity following the administration of vaccines. In such cases, administer epinephrine as an antidote. The manufacturer recommends that the vaccine be administered by a veterinarian or a trained technician. A small number of horses may experience mild post-vaccination side effects including slight nasal discharge. These signs should clear in a few days without additional treatment.

For intranasal use only.

For veterinary use only.

Discussion: Description: FLU AVERT™ I.N. vaccine is a unique, proprietary, intranasal, modified-live equine influenza vaccine proven by challenge studies to be safe and effective against North American and Eurasian strains of the equine influenza virus. It is the only intranasal equine influenza vaccine commercially available in the U.S. that has been proven effective against equine influenza viral infection in a challenge model. FLU AVERT™ I.N. vaccine showed significant protection from severe viral exposure and was efficacious against one of the most recent respiratory isolates of equine influenza (KY98).

Presentation: Package contains either: 10 vials (1 dose each) of lyophilized vaccine, 10 vials (1.0 mL) of sterile diluent and 10 nasal applicators, or 6 vials (5 dose each) of lyophilized vaccine, 6 vials (5 mL) of sterile diluent and 30 nasal applicators.

Manufactured by: Heska Corporation, Fort Collins, CO 80525.

Compendium Code No.: 11062811 50148-MAG 08/02

FLUCORT® SOLUTION ℞

Fort Dodge **Steroidal-Anti-inflammatory**

Flumethasone 0.5 mg/mL

NADA No.: 030-414

Active Ingredient(s): Each mL of the injectable preparation contains 0.5 mg flumethasone, 420 mg polyethylene glycol 400, 9 mg benzyl alcohol as a preservative, 8 mg sodium chloride, 0.1 mg citric acid, sodium hydroxide and/or hydrochloric acid for pH adjustment when necessary, and water for injection USP, q.s.

Indications: FLUCORT® (flumethasone) Solution is recommended for the various rheumatic, allergic, dermatologic and other disease states which are known to be responsive to the anti-inflammatory corticoids.

Equine Indications

1. Musculoskeletal conditions due to inflammation, where permanent structural changes do not exist, such as bursitis, carpitis, osselets and myositis. Following therapy an appropriate period of rest should be instituted to allow a more normal return to function of the affected part.
2. In allergic states such as hives, urticaria and insect bites.

Canine Indications

1. Musculoskeletal conditions due to inflammation of muscles or joints and accessory structures, where permanent structural changes do not exist, such as arthritis, osteoarthritis, the disc syndrome and myositis. In septic arthritis appropriate antibacterial therapy should be concurrently administered.
2. In certain acute and chronic dermatoses of varying etiology to help control the pruritus, irritation and inflammation associated with these conditions. The drug has proven useful in otitis externa in conjunction with topical medication for similar reasons.
3. In allergic states such as hives, urticaria and insect bites.
4. Shock and shock-like states,[4] by intravenous administration.

Feline Indications

1. In certain acute and chronic dermatoses of varying etiology to help control the pruritus, irritation and inflammation associated with these conditions.

Pharmacology: General: FLUCORT® is a chemical modification of prednisolone which possesses greater anti-inflammatory and gluconeogenic properties than the parent compound when compared on an equivalent basis. Due to the potency of FLUCORT® Solution, dosage recommendations should be consulted prior to drug administration. Chemically, it is 6α, 9α-difluoro-16α methylprednisolone. The structural formula is as follows:

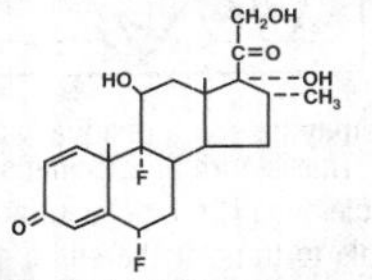

The active ingredient of FLUCORT® Solution is flumethasone which occurs as a white to creamy white, odorless, crystalline powder. The appearance of FLUCORT® Solution is a clear colorless to slightly yellowish mobile liquid.

Clinical Pharmacology: Flumethasone has been reported[1] to possess 700 times the glucocorticoid activity of cortisol (hydrocortisone) as measured in the liver glycogen deposition assay in the rat; 120 times that of cortisol in the cotton pellet assay in the rat; and also in the same animal, shows a net excretion of sodium.

In similar tests in rats, another report[2] showed flumethasone 730 times more potent than cortisol in the granuloma inhibition assay and 165 times the activity of cortisol in the glycogen deposition assay. The same report showed that in man, the compound possessed 7.8 times the potency of prednisolone.

An additional report[3] indicated that flumethasone possessed 677 times the potency of cortisol in the liver glycogen deposition test in the rat, and 30, 25, and 31 times respectively, the eosinopenic, hyperglycemic and antirheumatic potency of cortisol, as measured in man.

Veterinary experimental studies utilizing the eosinophil depression test in normal dogs and blood glucose elevation and eosinophil depression in normal cattle as parameters of drug activity, in comparison tests involving prednisone and dexamethasone, indicate that flumethasone possesses greater anti-inflammatory and gluconeogenic activity than these compounds, on an equivalent basis.

Clinical evidence of drug potency obtained during evaluation of the compound and based upon effective drug dosage levels further substantiates the above experimental findings.

General Effects of Adrenocorticoids: The adrenocorticoids are divided into two main classes: mineralocorticoids and glucocorticoids, based on their major physiologic and pharmacologic actions.

Mineralocorticoids such as the naturally occurring desoxycorticosterone and aldosterone are mainly concerned with hydration, sodium and potassium regulation and the normal renal glomerular filtration of these two electrolytes. The mineralocorticoids have little if any effect as anti-inflammatory agents, and are not widely used in medicine.

Glucocorticoids include the naturally occurring compounds, cortisone and hydrocortisone. Their major effects are as follows:

1. Increase protein catabolism and gluconeogenesis.
2. Depression of lymphoid tissue, fibroblasts and eosinophils.
3. Increase the sense of well being and tolerance to pain.
4. Depress thyroid function and anterior pituitary function through reciprocal influences.
5. Influence vasoconstrictive response of the circulatory system to norepinephrine, helping to maintain blood pressure.
6. Increase renal flow.
7. Influence gastric HCl and pepsin production.
8. Reduces the secretion of mucus from respiratory and enteric mucosa.
9. Affect to some degree sodium retention and potassium excretion.
10. Stimulate erythropoiesis and myelopoiesis.

Synthetic analogues of cortisone and hydrocortisone containing a double bond between carbon 1 and 2 of the corticosteroid nucleus, resulted in compounds with a greatly decreased effect on electrolyte metabolism. Additional molecular changes present in other synthetic corticoids presently used in medicine such as methylation at carbons 6 or 16 and hydroxylation at carbon 16, have led to a further decrease in electrolyte imbalance noted with the naturally occurring glucocorticoids. Fluorination at carbon 6 and/or 9 have led to a marked increase in anti-inflammatory activity.

The synthetic glucocorticoids exhibit a marked increase in potency in that a smaller amount of drug is required to elicit the same effects seen only with larger amounts of the natural glucocorticoids. It is also noted that the synthetic analogues persist for a longer period of time in the body which is believed due to their slower metabolism and excretion.

Dosage and Administration: FLUCORT® (flumethasone) Solution is recommended for administration by injection using various routes depending on the animal species and conditions under treatment. Injection should be accomplished slowly, with the drug at or near body temperature.

The following recommended dosages should be used as therapeutic guides. Each animal should be treated on an individual basis and dosage adjusted according to the response noted.

Dosage of FLUCORT® Solution:

Equine: 1.25 to 2.5 mg daily by intravenous, intramuscular or intra-articular injection. If necessary, the dose may be repeated.

Canine: 0.0625 to 0.25 mg daily by intravenous, intramuscular or subcutaneous injection. If necessary, the dose may be repeated. With chronic conditions, the preceding doses may be used and oral maintenance therapy with FLUCORT® Tablets instituted at a daily dose of 0.0625 to 0.25 mg.

Intralesional dosages in the dog have ranged from 0.125 to 1 mg depending on the size and location of the lesion under treatment.

Intra-articular dosages in the dog have ranged from 0.166 to 1 mg depending on the severity of the condition under treatment and the size of the involved joint.

Feline: 0.03125 to 0.125 mg by intravenous, intramuscular or subcutaneous injection. If necessary, the dose may be repeated. With chronic conditions, the preceding injectable doses may be used and oral maintenance therapy with FLUCORT® Tablets instituted at a daily dose of 0.03125 to 0.125 mg.

Note: The use of a microsyringe or standard tuberculin syringe may facilitate the accurate administration of small amounts of the drug.

If desired, therapy with FLUCORT® Solution may be substituted for other corticoids by the appropriate adjustment of dose levels.

Contraindication(s): Do not use in viral infections. Except for emergency therapy, do not use in animals with tuberculosis, chronic nephritis, cushingoid syndrome and peptic ulcers. Existence of congestive heart failure, diabetes and osteoporosis are relative contraindications.

Precaution(s): Store at room temperature. Avoid freezing.

Caution(s): Federal law restricts this drug to use by or on the order of a licensed veterinarian.

The usual precautions and contraindications for adrenocorticoid hormones are applicable with this compound. The close observation of animals under treatment with this drug is necessary, since the usual signs of adrenocorticoid overdosage which include sodium retention, potassium loss, fluid retention, weight gain, etc., may not be readily observed.

Use of corticosteroids depending on dose duration and specific steroid may result in inhibition of endogenous steroid production following drug withdrawal. In patients presently receiving or recently withdrawn from systemic steroid treatments, therapy with a rapidly acting corticosteroid should be considered in unusually stressful situations.

Experimentally, it has been demonstrated that corticosteroids especially at high dose levels may result in delayed wound healing. An increase in the incidence of osteoporosis may be noted, mainly in the elderly, with the prolonged use of these compounds. Their use in older dogs and cats, during the healing stages of a bone fracture is not indicated for this reason. The intra-articular injection in leg injuries of the horse may produce osseous metaplasia.

If side effects occur, the veterinarian should be prepared to take the necessary steps to correct them, which consist of temporarily discontinuing therapy with the drug until the side effects disappear, when therapy may be resumed at a lower dose level.

When long-term therapy with corticosteroids is used, as is necessary on occasion in the dog and cat, the dose should be individually adjusted so that the minimum maintenance dose (which will keep the condition being treated under control) is desirable. In dogs and cats on long-term therapy with these drugs, a protein-rich diet is useful to counteract nitrogen loss, if it should occur.

Similarly, a small amount of potassium chloride daily in the diet will counteract excessive potassium loss if this is present. Some natural dietary sources of potassium include dry nonfat milk solids, citrus juice, bran flakes, meat, fish and light cane molasses.

FLUCORT® (flumethasone) Solution may be administered to animals with bacterial diseases provided that specific and appropriate antibacterial therapy with antibiotic is administered simultaneously. In the absence of specific concomitant antimicrobial therapy, the prolonged use of corticosteroids is likely to lead to the spread of pathogenic microorganisms. The use of corticosteroids in such situations is not indicated. It should be borne in mind that flumethasone, like cortisone, through its anti-inflammatory action, may mask the usual signs of an infection such as pyrexia, inappetence, lassitude, etc. In the course of therapy with FLUCORT® Solution, should the question of determining the presence of an infectious disease arise, the drug should be withheld temporarily until a diagnosis or rediagnosis establishes the facts.

For animal use only.

Warning(s): Clinical and experimental data have demonstrated that corticosteroids administered orally or by injection to animals may induce the first stage of parturition when administered during the last trimester of pregnancy and may precipitate premature parturition followed by dystocia, fetal death, retained placenta and metritis.

Additionally, corticosteroids administered to dogs, rabbits, and rodents during pregnancy have resulted in cleft palate in offspring. Corticosteroids administered to dogs during pregnancy have also resulted in other congenital anomalies, including deformed forelegs, phocomelia and anasarca.

Side Effects: Side effects such as SAP and SGPT (ALT) enzyme elevations, weight loss, anorexia, polydypsia and polyuria have occurred following parenteral or systemic use of synthetic corticosteroids. In dogs, vomiting and diarrhea, and Cushing's syndrome have been reported in association with prolonged or repeated steroid therapy.

Corticosteroids reportedly cause laminitis in horses.

References: Available upon request.

Presentation: FLUCORT® (flumethasone) Solution is supplied in 100 mL vials (NDC 0856-0820-20). U.S. Pat. No. 3,499,016

Compendium Code No.: 10030861 0050B

FLUMEGLUMINE® ℞

Phoenix Pharmaceutical **Analgesic-Anti-inflammatory**

(flunixin meglumine injection) 50 mg/mL

ANADA No.: 200-124

Active Ingredient(s): Each millimeter of FLUMEGLUMINE® (flunixin meglumine injection 50 mg/mL) contains:

Flunixin Meglumine equivalent to Flunixin	50 mg
Edetate Disodium	0.1 mg
Sodium Formaldehyde Sulfoxylate	2.5 mg
Diethanolamine	4.0 mg
Propylene Glycol	207.2 mg
Phenol (as preservative)	5.0 mg
Water For Injection	q.s.

With hydrochloric acid to adjust pH.

Indications: Horse: FLUMEGLUMINE® (flunixin meglumine injection 50 mg/mL) is recommended for the alleviation of inflammation and pain associated with musculoskeletal disorders in the horse. It is also recommended for the alleviation of visceral pain associated with colic in the horse.

Cattle: FLUMEGLUMINE® (flunixin meglumine injection 50 mg/mL) is indicated for the control of pyrexia associated with bovine respiratory disease and endotoxemia. Flunixin Meglumine Injection is also indicated for the control of inflammation in endotoxemia.

Pharmacology: Flunixin meglumine is a potent, non-narcotic, nonsteroidal, analgesic agent with anti-inflammatory and antipyretic activity. It is significantly more potent than pentazocine, meperidine and codeine as an analgesic in the rat yeast paw test.

Horse: Flunixin is four times as potent on a mg-per-mg basis as phenylbutazone as measured by the reduction in lameness and swelling in the horse. Plasma half-life in horse serum is 1.6 hours following a single dose of 1.1 mg/kg. Measurable amounts are detectable in horse plasma at 8 hours post injection.

Cattle: Flunixin meglumine is a weak acid (pKa=5.82)[1] which exhibits a high degree of plasma protein binding (approximately 99%).[2] However, free (unbound) drug appears to readily partition into body tissues (V_{ss}predictions range from 297 to 782 mL/kg.[2-5] Total body water is approximately equal to 570 mL/kg.[6] In cattle, elimination occurs primarily through biliary excretion.[7] This may, at least in part, explain the presence of multiple peaks in the blood concentration/time profile following IV administration.[2]

In healthy cattle, total body clearance has been reported to range from 90 to 151 mL/kg/hr.[2-5] These studies also report a large discrepancy between the volume of distribution at a steady state (V_{ss}) and the volume of distribution associated with the terminal elimination phase (V_{β}). This discrepancy appears to be attributable to extended drug elimination from a deep compartment.[8] The terminal half-life has been shown to vary from 3.14 to 8.12 hours.[2-5]

Flunixin persists in inflammatory tissues[9] and is associated with anti-flammatory properties which extend well beyond the period associated with detectable plasma drug concentrations.[4,9] These observations account for the counterclockwise hysteresis associated with flunixin's pharmacokinetic/pharmacodynamic relationships.[10] Therefore, prediction of drug concentrations based upon the estimated plasma terminal elimination half-life will likely underestimate both the duration of drug action and the concentration of drug remaining at the site of activity.

Dosage and Administration: Horse: The recommended dose for musculoskeletal disorders is 0.5 mg per pound (1 mL/100 lbs) of body weight once daily. Treatment may be given by intravenous or intramuscular injection and repeated for up to 5 days. Studies show onset of activity is within 2 hours. Peak response occurs between 12 and 16 hours and duration of activity is 24-36 hours.

The recommended dose for the alleviation of pain associated with equine colic is 0.5 mg per pound of body weight. Intravenous administration is recommended for prompt relief. Clinical studies show pain is alleviated in less than 15 minutes in many cases. Treatment may be repeated when signs of colic recur. During clinical studies approximately 10% of the horses required one or two additional treatments. The cause of colic should be determined and treated with concomitant therapy.

Cattle: The recommended dose for cattle is 1.1 to 2.2 mg/kg (0.5 to 1 mg/lb; 1 to 2 mL per 100 lbs) given by slow intravenous administration either once a day as a single dose or divided into two doses administered at 12-hour intervals for up to 3 days. The total daily dose should not exceed 2.2 mg/kg (1.0 mg/lb) of body weight. Avoid rapid intravenous administration of the drug.

Contraindication(s): Horse: There are no known contraindications to this drug when used as directed. Intra-arterial injection should be avoided. Horses inadvertently injected intra-arterially can show adverse reactions. Signs can be ataxia, incoordination, hyperventilation, hysteria, and muscle weakness. Signs are transient and disappear without antidotal medication within a few minutes. Do not use in horses showing hypersensitivity to flunixin meglumine.

Cattle: There are no known contraindications to this drug in cattle when used as directed. Do not use in animals showing hypersensitivity to flunixin meglumine. Use judiciously when renal impairment or gastric ulceration are suspected.

Precaution(s): Store between 2° and 30°C (36° and 86°F).

Caution(s): Federal law restricts this drug to use by or on the order of a licensed veterinarian.

As a class, cyclo-oxygenase inhibitory NSAIDs may be associated with gastrointestinal and renal toxicity. Sensitivity to drug-associated adverse effects varies with the individual patient. Patients at greatest risk for renal toxicity are those that are dehydrated, on concomitant diuretic therapy, or those with renal, cardiovascular, and/or hepatic dysfunction.

Since many NSAIDs possess the potential to induce gastrointestinal ulceration, concomitant use of FLUMEGLUMINE® with other anti-inflammatory drugs, such as other NSAIDs and corticosteroids, should be avoided or closely monitored.

Horse: The effect of FLUMEGLUMINE® (flunixin meglumine injection 50 mg/mL) on pregnancy has not been determined. Studies to determine activity of FLUMEGLUMINE® when administered concomitantly with other drugs have not been conducted. Drug compatibility should be monitored closely in patients requiring adjunctive therapy.

Cattle: Do not use in bulls intended for breeding, as reproductive effects of FLUMEGLUMINE® in these classes of cattle have not been investigated. NSAIDS are known to have potential effects on both parturition and the estrous cycle. There may be a delay in the onset of estrus if flunixin is administered during the prostaglandin phase of the estrous cycle. The effects of flunixin on imminent parturition have not been evaluated in a controlled study. NSAIDs are known to have the potential to delay parturition through a tocolytic effect. Do not exceed the recommended dose.

For intravenous or intramuscular use in horses and for intravenous use in beef and nonlactating dairy cattle only. Not for use in lactating and dry dairy cows. Not for use in veal calves.

For animal use only.

Warning(s): Residue Warnings: Cattle must not be slaughtered for human consumption within 4 days of the last treatment. Not for use in lactating or dry dairy cows. A withdrawal period has not been established for this product in preruminating calves. Do not use in calves to be processed for veal. Not for use in horses intended for food.

Keep out of reach of children.

Toxicology: Safety:

Horse: A 3-fold intramuscular dose of 1.5 mg/lb of body weight daily for 10 consecutive days was safe. No changes were observed in hematology, serum chemistry, or urinalysis values. Intravenous dosages of 0.5 mg/lb daily for 15 days; 1.5 mg/lb daily for 10 days; and 2.5 mg/lb daily for 5 days produced no changes in blood or urine parameters. No injection site irritation was observed following intramuscular injection of the 0.5 mg/lb recommended dose. Some irritation was observed following a 3-fold dose administered intramuscularly.

Cattle: No flunixin-related changes (adverse reactions) were noted in cattle administered a 1X (22 mg/kg; 1.0 mg/lb) dose for 9 days (three times the maximum clinical duration). Minimal toxicity manifested itself at moderately elevated doses (3X and 5X) when flunixin was administered daily for 9 days, with occasional findings of blood in the feces and/or urine. Discontinue use if hematuria or fecal blood are observed.

Adverse Reactions: In horses, isolated reports of local reactions following intramuscular injection, particularly in the neck, have been received. These include localized swelling, sweating, induration, and stiffness. In rare instances in horses, fatal or nonfatal clostridial infections or other infections have been reported in association with intramuscular use of FLUMEGLUMINE® (flunixin meglumine injection 50 mg/mL) Solution. In horses and cattle, rare instances of anaphylactic-like reactions, some of which have been fatal, have been reported primarily following intravenous use.

References: Available upon request.

Presentation: FLUMEGLUMINE® (flunixin meglumine injection 50 mg/mL), is available in 100 mL (NDC 57319-303-05) and 250 mL (NDC 57319-303-06) multidose vials.

Manufactured by: Phoenix Scientific, Inc., St. Joseph, MO 64503

Compendium Code No.: 12560332 Rev. 10-01 / Rev. 8-01

FLUMUNE®

Pfizer Animal Health **Vaccine**

Equine Influenza Vaccine, Killed Virus

U.S. Vet. Lic. No.: 189

Description: FLUMUNE® is a liquid preparation of inactivated equine influenza virus combined with an adjuvant to enhance the immune response.

Contains gentamicin as preservative.

Indications: FLUMUNE® is for vaccination of healthy horses 3 months of age or older as an aid in preventing respiratory disease caused by equine influenza virus subtypes A1 and A2.

Directions:

1. General Directions: Vaccination of all horses on the premises is recommended to enhance herd immunity. Shake well. Aseptically administer 1 mL intramuscularly.
2. Primary Vaccination: Healthy horses 3 months of age or older should receive 2 doses administered 3 weeks apart.
3. Revaccination: Annual revaccination with a single dose is recommended. However, a booster dose should be given whenever epizootic conditions exist or exposure is likely.
4. Good animal husbandry and herd health management practices should be employed.

Precaution(s): Store at 2°-7°C. Prolonged exposure to higher temperatures may adversely affect potency. Do not freeze.

Use entire contents when first opened.

Sterilized syringes and needles should be used to administer this vaccine.

Caution(s): As with many vaccines, anaphylaxis may occur after use. Initial antidote of epinephrine is recommended and should be followed with appropriate supportive therapy.

This product has been shown to be efficacious in healthy animals. A protective immune response may not be elicited if animals are incubating an infectious disease, are malnourished or parasitized, are stressed due to shipment or environmental conditions, are otherwise immunocompromised, or the vaccine is not administered in accordance with label directions.

Warning(s): Do not vaccinate within 21 days before slaughter.

For veterinary use only.

Discussion: Disease Description: Equine influenza is an acute disease, primarily of the lower respiratory tract, that affects horses of all ages. Subtype A2 is more virulent than A1 and produces more pronounced pneumotrophic effects, especially elevated fever and a persistent, harsh cough that is particularly severe 2-3 days after the onset of the disease. These symptoms diminish and disappear after 1-3 weeks. Nasal discharge, at first serous and then mucoid, is also common. Infection is usually accompanied by distinct lymphopenia, which can last from several hours to 3-4 days. The incubation period for the disease is 1-3 days, with 95%-98% morbidity and low mortality in cases without complications. Foals, however, are extremely susceptible to the disease and frequently succumb to pneumonia within a few days after clinical signs appear. In foals infected with subtype A2, encephalopathy can occur. Infected horses shed the virus from the respiratory tract for several days. The disease spreads rapidly because of its short incubation period and because the harsh, violent coughing of infected animals facilitates aerosol transmission of the virus.

Trial Data: Safety and Efficacy: Efficacy of FLUMUNE® was measured by the seroconversion of vaccinates to both subtypes A1 and A2. A total of 35 susceptible test animals (30 vaccinates and 5 nonvaccinated controls) were used. Two vaccinations were given 3 weeks apart. At 2 weeks after administration of the second dose, contact controls showed no significant titer increases, while vaccinates seroconverted to subtypes A1 and A2. Mean titer increases in vaccinates were 13-fold for A1 and 44-fold for A2.

FLUMUNE® produced no postvaccinal lesions in any test animals, demonstrating the safety of the vaccine's unique adjuvant.

Presentation: 1 dose and 10 dose vials.

Compendium Code No.: 36901130 75-4342-04

FLU-NIX™ ℞

AgriLabs **Analgesic-Anti-inflammatory**

(Flunixin Meglumine) Injectable Solution-50 mg/mL

NADA No.: 101-479

Active Ingredient(s): Description: Each milliliter of FLU-NIX™ Injectable Solution contains flunixin meglumine equivalent to 50 mg flunixin, 0.1 mg edetate disodium, 2.5 mg sodium formaldehyde sulfoxylate, 4.0 mg diethanolamine, 207.2 mg propylene glycol; 5.0 mg phenol as preservative, hydrochloric acid, water for injection q.s.

Indications:

Horse: FLU-NIX™ Injectable Solution is recommended for the alleviation of inflammation and pain associated with musculoskeletal disorders in the horse. It is also recommended for the alleviation of visceral pain associated with colic in the horse.

Cattle: FLU-NIX™ Injectable Solution is indicated for the control of pyrexia associated with bovine respiratory disease and endotoxemia. FLU-NIX™ Injectable Solution is also indicated for the control of inflammation in endotoxemia.

Pharmacology: Flunixin meglumine is a potent, nonnarcotic, nonsteroidal, analgesic agent with anti-inflammatory and antipyretic activity. It is significantly more potent than pentazocine, meperidine, and codeine as an analgesic in the rat yeast paw test.

Horse: Flunixin is four times as potent on a mg-per-mg basis as phenylbutazone as measured by the reduction in lameness and swelling in the horse. Plasma half-life in horse serum is 1.6 hours following a single dose of 1.1 mg/kg. Measurable amounts are detectable in horse plasma at 8 hours postinjection.

Cattle: Flunixin meglumine is a weak acid (pKa=5.82)[1] which exhibits a high degree of plasma protein binding (approximately 99%).[2] However, free (unbound) drug appears to readily partition into body issues (V_{SS} predictions range from 297 to 782 mL/kg.[2-5] Total body water is approximately equal to 570 mL/kg).[6] In cattle, elimination occurs primarily through biliary excretion.[7] This may, at least in part, explain the presence of multiple peaks in the blood concentration/time profile following IV administration.[2]

In healthy cattle, total body clearance has been reported to range from 90 to 151 mL/kg/hr.[2-5] These studies also report a large discrepancy between the volume of distribution at steady state (V_{SS}) and the volume of distribution associated with the terminal elimination phase (V_{β}). This discrepancy appears to be attributable to extended drug elimination from a deep compartment.[8] The terminal half-life has been shown to vary from 3.14 to 8.12 hours.[2-5]

Flunixin persists in inflammatory tissues[9] and is associated with anti-inflammatory properties which extend well beyond the period associated with detectable plasma drug concentrations.[4,9] These observations account for the counterclockwise hysteresis associated with flunixin's pharmacokinetic/pharmacodynamic relationships.[10] Therefore, prediction of drug concentrations based upon the estimated plasma terminal elimination half-life will likely underestimate both the duration of drug action and the concentration of drug remaining at the site of activity.

Dosage and Administration:

Horse: The recommended dose for musculoskeletal disorders is 0.5 mg per pound (1 mL/100 lbs) of body weight once daily. Treatment may be given by intravenous or intramuscular injection and repeated for up to 5 days. Studies show onset of activity is within 2 hours. Peak response occurs between 12 and 16 hours and duration of activity is 24-36 hours.

F

The recommended dose for the alleviation of pain associated with equine colic is 0.5 mg per pound of body weight. Intravenous administration is recommended for prompt relief. Clinical studies show pain is alleviated in less than 15 minutes in many cases. Treatment may be repeated when signs of colic recur. During clinical studies approximately 10% of the horses required one or two additional treatments. The cause of colic should be determined and treated with concomitant therapy.

Cattle: The recommended dose for cattle is 1.1 to 2.2 mg/kg (0.5 to 1 mg/lb; 1 to 2 mL per 100 lbs) given by slow intravenous administration either once a day as a single dose or divided into two doses administered at 12-hour intervals for up to 3 days. The total daily dose should not exceed 2.2 mg/kg (1.0 mg/lb) of body weight. Avoid rapid intravenous administration of the drug.

Contraindication(s):

Horse: There are no known contraindications to this drug when used as directed. Intra-arterial injection should be avoided. Horses inadvertently injected intra-arterially can show adverse reactions. Signs can be ataxia, incoordination, hyperventilation, hysteria, and muscle weakness. Signs are transient and disappear without antidotal medication within a few minutes. Do not use in horses showing hypersensitivity to flunixin meglumine.

Cattle: There are no known contraindications to this drug in cattle when used as directed. Do not use in animals showing hypersensitivity to flunixin meglumine. Use judiciously when renal impairment or gastric ulceration are suspected.

Precaution(s): Store between 2° and 30°C (36° and 86°F).

Caution(s): Federal law restricts this drug to use by or on the order of a licensed veterinarian.

As a class, cyclo-oxygenase inhibitory NSAIDs may be associated with gastrointestinal and renal toxicity. Sensitivity to drug-associated adverse effects varies with the individual patient. Patients at greatest risk for renal toxicity are those that are dehydrated, on concomitant diuretic therapy, or those with renal, cardiovascular, and/or hepatic dysfunction.

Since many NSAIDs possess the potential to induce gastrointestinal ulceration, concomitant use of FLU-NIX™ Injectable Solution with other anti-inflammatory drugs, such as other NSAIDs and corticosteroids, should be avoided or closely monitored.

Horse: The effect of FLU-NIX™ Injectable Solution on pregnancy has not been determined. Studies to determine the activity of FLU-NIX™ Injectable Solution when administered concomitantly with other drugs have not been conducted. Drug compatibility should be monitored closely in patients requiring adjunctive therapy.

Cattle: Do not use in bulls intended for breeding, as reproductive effects of FLU-NIX™ Injectable Solution in these classes of cattle have not been investigated. NSAIDs are known to have potential effects on both parturition and the estrous cycle. There may be a delay in the onset of estrus if flunixin is administered during the prostaglandin phase of the estrous cycle. The effects of flunixin on imminent parturition have not been evaluated in a controlled study. NSAIDs are known to have the potential to delay parturition through a tocolytic effect. Do not exceed the recommended dose.

Warning(s): Residue Warnings: Cattle must not be slaughtered for human consumption within 4 days of the last treatment. Not for use in lactating or dry dairy cows. A withdrawal period has not been established for this product in preruminating calves. Do not use in calves to be processed for veal. Not for use in horses intended for food.

For intravenous or intramuscular use in horses and for intravenous use in beef and nonlactating dairy cattle only.

Adverse Reactions: In horses, isolated reports of local reactions following intramuscular injection, particularly in the neck, have been received. These include localized swelling, sweating, induration, and stiffness. In rare instances in horses, fatal or nonfatal clostridial infections or other infections have been reported in association with intramuscular use of FLU-NIX™ Injectable Solution. In horses and cattle, rare instances of anaphylactic-like reactions, some of which have been fatal, have been reported, primarily following intravenous use.

Toxicology: Safety:

Horse: A three-fold intramuscular dose of 1.5 mg/lb of body weight daily for 10 consecutive days was safe. No changes were observed in hematology, serum chemistry, or urinalysis values. Intravenous dosages of 0.5 mg/lb daily for 15 days; 1.5 mg/lb daily for 10 days; and 2.5 mg/lb daily for 5 days produced no changes in blood or urine parameters. No injection site irritation was observed following intramuscular injection of the 0.5 mg/lb recommended dose. Some irritation was observed following a three-fold dose administered intramuscularly.

Cattle: No flunixin-related changes (adverse reactions) were noted in cattle administered a 1X (2.2 mg/kg; 1.0 mg/lb) dose for 9 days (three times the maximum clinical duration). Minimal toxicity manifested itself at moderately elevated doses (3X and 5X) when flunixin was administered daily for 9 days, with occasional findings of blood in the feces and/or urine. Discontinue use if hematuria or fecal blood are observed.

References: Available upon request.

Presentation: FLU-NIX™ Injectable Solution, 50 mg/mL, is available in 50 mL (NDC 0061-0851-02), 100 mL (NDC 0061-0851-03), and 250 mL (NDC 0061-0851-04) multi-dose vials.

Compendium Code No.: 10581580 Oct 2000

FLUNIXAMINE™ ℞

Fort Dodge **Analgesic-Anti-inflammatory**

Flunixin Meglumine Injection-50 mg/mL

ANADA No.: 200-124

Active Ingredient(s): Description: Each milliliter of FLUNIXAMINE™ (flunixin meglumine injection 50 mg/mL) contains flunixin meglumine equivalent to 50 mg flunixin, 0.1 mg edetate disodium, 2.5 mg sodium formaldehyde sulfoxylate, 4.0 mg diethanolamine, 207.2 mg propylene glycol; 5.0 mg phenol as preservative, hydrochloric acid, water for injection q.s.

Indications:

Horse: FLUNIXAMINE™ is recommended for the alleviation of inflammation and pain associated with musculoskeletal disorders in the horse. It is also recommended for the alleviation of visceral pain associated with colic in the horse.

Cattle: FLUNIXAMINE™ is indicated for the control of pyrexia associated with bovine respiratory disease and endotoxemia. FLUNIXAMINE™ is also indicated for the control of inflammation in endotoxemia.

Pharmacology: Flunixin meglumine is a potent, non-narcotic, non-steroidal, analgesic agent with anti-inflammatory and antipyretic activity. It is significantly more potent than pentazocine, meperidine and codeine as an analgesic in the rat yeast paw test.

Horse: Flunixin is four times as potent on a mg per mg basis as phenylbutazone as measured by the reduction in lameness and swelling in the horse. Plasma half-life in horse serum is 1.6 hours following a single dose of 1.1 mg/kg. Measurable amounts are detectable in horse plasma at 8 hours post injection.

Cattle: Flunixin meglumine is a weak acid (pKa=5.82)[1] which exhibits a high degree of plasma protein binding (approximately 99%).[2] However, free (unbound) drug appears to readily partition into body tissues (V_{SS}predictions range from 297 to 782 mL/kg.[2-5] Total body water is approximately equal to 570 mL/kg).[6] In cattle, elimination occurs primarily through biliary excretion.[7] This may, at least in part, explain the presence of multiple peaks in the blood concentration/time profile following IV administration.[2]

In healthy cattle, total body clearance has been reported to range from 90 to 151 mL/kg/hr.[2-5] These studies also report a large discrepancy between the volume of distribution at a steady state (V_{SS}) and the volume of distribution associated with the terminal elimination phase (V_{β}). This discrepancy appears to be attributable to extended drug elimination from a deep compartment.[8] The terminal half-life has been shown to vary from 3.14 to 8.12 hours.[2-5]

Flunixin persists in inflammatory tissues[9] and is associated with anti-inflammatory properties which extend well beyond the period associated with detectable plasma drug concentrations.[4,9] These observations account for the counterclockwise hysteresis associated with flunixin's pharmacokinetic/pharmacodynamic relationships.[10] Therefore, prediction of drug concentrations based upon the estimated plasma terminal elimination half-life will likely underestimate both the duration of drug action and the concentration of drug remaining at the site of activity.

Dosage and Administration:

Horse: The recommended dose for musculoskeletal disorders is 0.5 mg per pound (1 mL/100 lbs) of body weight once daily. Treatment may be given by intravenous or intramuscular injection and repeated for up to 5 days. Studies show onset of activity is within 2 hours. Peak response occurs between 12 and 16 hours and duration of activity is 24-36 hours.

The recommended dose for the alleviation of pain associated with equine colic is 0.5 mg per pound of body weight. Intravenous administration is recommended for prompt relief. Clinical studies show pain is alleviated in less than 15 minutes in many cases. Treatment may be repeated when signs of colic recur. During clinical studies approximately 10% of the horses required one or two additional treatments. The cause of colic should be determined and treated with concomitant therapy.

Cattle: The recommended dose for cattle is 1.1 to 2.2 mg/kg (0.5 to 1 mg/lb; 1 to 2 mL per 100 lbs) given by slow intravenous administration either once a day as a single dose or divided into two doses administered at 12-hour intervals for up to 3 days. The total daily dose should not exceed 2.2 mg/kg (1.0 mg/lb) of body weight. Avoid rapid intravenous administration of the drug.

Contraindication(s):

Horse: There are no known contraindications to this drug when used as directed. Intra-arterial injection should be avoided. Horses inadvertently injected intra-arterially can show adverse reactions. Signs can be ataxia, incoordination, hyperventilation, hysteria, and muscle weakness. Signs are transient and disappear without antidotal medication within a few minutes. Do not use in horses showing hypersensitivity to flunixin meglumine.

Cattle: There are no known contraindications to this drug in cattle when used as directed. Do not use in animals showing hypersensitivity to flunixin meglumine. Use judiciously when renal impairment or gastric ulceration are suspected.

Precaution(s): Store between 2° and 30°C (36° and 86°F).

Caution(s): Federal law restricts this drug to use by or on the order of a licensed veterinarian.

As a class, cyclo-oxygenase inhibitory NSAIDs may be associated with gastrointestinal and renal toxicity. Sensitivity to drug-associated adverse effects varies with the individual patient. Patients at greatest risk for renal toxicity are those that are dehydrated, on concomitant diuretic therapy, or those with renal, cardiovascular, and/or hepatic dysfunction.

Since many NSAIDs possess the potential to induce gastrointestinal ulceration, concomitant use of FLUNIXAMINE™ (flunixin meglumine injection 50 mg/mL) with other anti-inflammatory drugs, such as other NSAIDs and corticosteroids, should be avoided or closely monitored.

Horse: The effect of FLUNIXAMINE™ on pregnancy has not been determined. Studies to determine activity of FLUNIXAMINE™ when administered concomitantly with other drugs have not been conducted. Drug compatibility should be monitored closely in patients requiring adjunctive therapy.

Cattle: Do not use in bulls intended for breeding, as reproductive effects of FLUNIXAMINE™ in these classes of cattle have not been investigated. NSAIDs are known to have potential effects on both parturition and the estrous cycle. There may be a delay in the onset of estrous if flunixin is administered during the prostaglandin phase of the estrous cycle. The effects of flunixin on imminent parturition have not been evaluated in a controlled study. NSAIDs are known to have the potential to delay parturition through a tocolytic effect. Do not exceed the recommended dose.

Warning(s): Residue Warnings: Cattle must not be slaughtered for human consumption within 4 days of the last treatment. Not for use in lactating or dry dairy cows. A withdrawal period has not been established for this product in pre-ruminating calves. Do not use in calves to be processed for veal. Not for use in horses intended for food.

For intravenous or intramuscular use in horses and for intravenous use in beef and non-lactating dairy cattle only.

Toxicology: Safety:

Horse: A 3-fold intramuscular dose of 1.5 mg/lb of body weight daily for 10 consecutive days was safe. No changes were observed in hematology, serum chemistry, or urinalysis values.

Intravenous dosages of 0.5 mg/lb daily for 15 days; 1.5 mg/lb daily for 10 days; and 2.5 mg/lb daily for 5 days produced no changes in blood or urine parameters. No injection site irritation was observed following intramuscular injection of the 0.5 mg/lb recommended dose. Some irritation was observed following a 3-fold dose administered intramuscularly.

Cattle: No flunixin-related changes (adverse reactions) were noted in cattle administered a 1X (2.2 mg/kg; 1.0 mg/lb) dose for 9 days (three times the maximum clinical duration). Minimal toxicity manifested itself at moderately elevated doses (3X and 5X) when flunixin was administered daily for 9 days, with occasional findings of blood in the feces and/or urine. Discontinue use if hematuria or fecal blood are observed.

Adverse Reactions: In horses, isolated reports of local reactions following intramuscular injection, particularly in the neck, have been received. These include localized swelling, sweating, induration, and stiffness. In rare instances in horses, fatal or nonfatal clostridial infections or other infections have been reported in association with intramuscular use of FLUNIXAMINE™. In horses and cattle, rare instances of anaphylactic-like reactions, some of which have been fatal, have been reported primarily following intravenous use.

References: Available upon request.

Presentation: FLUNIXAMINE™ (flunixin meglumine injection 50 mg/mL) is available in 100 mL and 250 mL multidose vials.

NDC 0856-0851-10 — 50 mg/mL — 100 mL vials
NDC 0856-0851-20 — 50 mg/mL — 250 mL vials

Manufactured by: Phoenix Scientific, Inc., St. Joseph, MO 64503.

Compendium Code No.: 10030871 5600C

FLUNIXIN MEGLUMINE ℞

Vet Tek **Analgesic-Anti-inflammatory**

Flunixin Meglumine Injection 50 mg/mL

ANADA No.: 200-124

Active Ingredient(s): Description: Each milliliter of Flunixin Meglumine Injection contains flunixin meglumine equivalent to 50 mg flunixin, 0.1 mg edetate disodium, 2.5 mg sodium formaldehyde sulfoxylate, 4.0 mg diethanolamine, 207.2 mg propylene glycol; 5.0 mg phenol as preservative, hydrochloric acid, water for injection q.s.

Indications: Horse: Flunixin Meglumine Injection is recommended for the alleviation of inflammation and pain associated with musculoskeletal disorders in the horse. It is also recommended for the alleviation of visceral pain associated with colic in the horse.

Cattle: Flunixin Meglumine Injection is indicated for the control of pyrexia associated with bovine respiratory disease and endotoxemia. Flunixin Meglumine Injection is also indicated for the control of inflammation in endotoxemia.

Pharmacology: Flunixin meglumine is a potent non-narcotic, nonsteroidal analgesic agent with anti-inflammatory and antipyretic activity. It is significantly more potent than pentazocine, meperidine and codeine as an analgesic in the rat yeast paw test.

Horse: Flunixin is four times as potent on a mg per mg basis as phenylbutazone as measured by the reduction in lameness and swelling in the horse. Plasma half-life in horse serum is 1.6 hours following a single dose of 1.1 mg/kg. Measurable amounts are detectable in horse plasma at 8 hours post injection.

Cattle: Flunixin meglumine is a weak acid (pKa=5.82)[1] which exhibits a high degree of plasma protein binding (approximately 99%).[2] However, free (unbound) drug appears to readily partition into body tissues (V_{ss}predictions range from 297 to 782 mL/kg.[2-5] Total body water is approximately equal to 570 mL/kg.[6] In cattle, elimination occurs primarily through biliary excretion.[7] This may, at least in part, explain the presence of multiple peaks in the blood concentration/time profile following IV administration.[2]

In healthy cattle, total body clearance has been reported to range from 90 to 151 mL/kg/hr.[2-5] These studies also report a large discrepancy between the volume of distribution at a steady state (V_{ss}) and the volume of distribution associated with the terminal elimination phase (V_β). This discrepancy appears to be attributable to extended drug elimination from a deep compartment.[8] The terminal half-life has been shown to vary from 3.14 to 8.12 hours.[2-5]

Flunixin persists in inflammatory tissues[9] and is associated with anti-flammatory properties which extend well beyond the period associated with detectable plasma drug concentrations.[4,9] These observations account for the counterclockwise hysteresis associated with flunixin's pharmacokinetic/pharmacodynamic relationships.[10] Therefore, prediction of drug concentrations based upon the estimated plasma terminal elimination half-life will likely underestimate both the duration of drug action and the concentration of drug remaining at the site of activity.

Dosage and Administration: Horse: The recommended dose for musculoskeletal disorders is 0.5 mg per pound (1 mL/100 lbs) of body weight once daily. Treatment may be given by intravenous or intramuscular injection and repeated for up to 5 days. Studies show onset of activity is within 2 hours. Peak response occurs between 12 and 16 hours and duration of activity is 24-36 hours.

The recommended dose for the alleviation of pain associated with equine colic is 0.5 mg per pound of body weight. Intravenous administration is recommended for prompt relief. Clinical studies show pain is alleviated in less than 15 minutes in many cases. Treatment may be repeated when signs of colic recur. During clinical studies approximately 10% of the horses required one or two additional treatments. The cause of colic should be determined and treated with concomitant therapy.

Cattle: The recommended dose for cattle is 1.1 to 2.2 mg/kg (0.5 to 1 mg/lb; 1 to 2 mL per 100 lbs) given by slow intravenous administration either once a day as a single dose or divided into two doses administered at 12-hour intervals for up to 3 days. The total daily dose should not exceed 2.2 mg/kg (1.0 mg/lb) of body weight. Avoid rapid intravenous administration of the drug.

Contraindication(s): Horse: There are no known contraindications to this drug when used as directed. Intra-arterial injection should be avoided. Horses inadvertently injected intra-arterially can show adverse reactions. Signs can be ataxia, incoordination, hyperventilation, hysteria, and muscle weakness. Signs are transient and disappear without antidotal medication within a few minutes. Do not use in horses showing hypersensitivity to flunixin meglumine.

Cattle: There are no known contraindications to this drug in cattle when used as directed. Do not use in animals showing hypersensitivity to flunixin meglumine. Use judiciously when renal impairment or gastric ulceration are suspected.

Precaution(s): Store between 2° and 30°C (36° and 86°F).

Caution(s): Federal law restricts this drug to use by or on the order of a licensed veterinarian.

As a class, cyclo-oxygenase inhibitory NSAIDs may be associated with gastrointestinal and renal toxicity. Sensitivity to drug-associated adverse effects varies with the individual patient. Patients at greatest risk for renal toxicity are those that are dehydrated, on concomitant diuretic therapy, or those with renal, cardiovascular, and/or hepatic dysfunction.

Since many NSAIDs possess the potential to induce gastrointestinal ulceration, concomitant use of Flunixin Meglumine Injection with other anti-inflammatory drugs, such as other NSAIDs and corticosteroids, should be avoided or closely monitored.

Horse: The effect of Flunixin Meglumine Injection on pregnancy has not been determined. Studies to determine activity of Flunixin Meglumine Injection when administered concomitantly with other drugs have not been conducted. Drug compatibility should be monitored closely in patients requiring adjunctive therapy.

Cattle: Do not use in bulls intended for breeding, as reproductive effects of Flunixin Meglumine Injection in these classes of cattle have not been investigated. NSAIDS are known to have potential effects on both parturition and the estrous cycle. There may be a delay in the onset of estrus if flunixin is administered during the prostaglandin phase of the estrous cycle. The effects of flunixin on imminent parturition have not been evaluated in a controlled study. NSAIDs are known to have the potential to delay parturition through a tocolytic effect. Do not exceed the recommended dose.

For intravenous or intramuscular use in horses and for intravenous use in beef and nonlactating dairy cattle only. Not for use in lactating and dry dairy cows. Not for use in veal calves.

Warning(s): Residue warnings: Cattle must not be slaughtered for human consumption within 4 days of the last treatment. Not for use in lactating or dry dairy cows. A withdrawal period has not been established for this product in preruminating calves. Do not use in calves to be processed for veal. Not for use in horses intended for food.

Toxicology: Safety:

Horse: A 3-fold intramuscular dose of 1.5 mg/lb of body weight daily for 10 consecutive days was safe. No changes were observed in hematology, serum chemistry, or urinalysis values. Intravenous dosages of 0.5 mg/lb daily for 15 days; 1.5 mg/lb daily for 10 days; and 2.5 mg/lb daily for 5 days produced no changes in blood or urine parameters. No injection site irritation was observed following intramuscular injection of the 0.5 mg/lb recommended dose. Some irritation was observed following a 3-fold dose administered intramuscularly.

Cattle: No flunixin-related changes (adverse reactions) were noted in cattle administered a 1X (22 mg/kg; 1.0 mg/lb) dose for 9 days (three times the maximum clinical duration). Minimal toxicity manifested itself at moderately elevated doses (3X and 5X) when flunixin was administered daily for 9 days, with occasional findings of blood in the feces and/or urine. Discontinue use if hematuria or fecal blood are observed.

Adverse Reactions: In horses, isolated reports of local reactions following intramuscular injection, particularly in the neck, have been received. These include localized swelling, sweating, induration, and stiffness. In rare instances in horses, fatal or nonfatal clostridial infections or other infections have been reported in association with intramuscular use of Flunixin Meglumine Injectable Solution. In horses and cattle, rare instances of anaphylactic-like reactions, some of which have been fatal, have been reported primarily following intravenous use.

References: Available upon request.

Presentation: Flunixin Meglumine Injection, 50 mg/mL, is available in 100 mL (NDC 60270-580-10) and 250 mL (NDC 60270-580-13) multidose vials.

Manufactured by: Phoenix Scientific Inc., St. Joseph, MO 64503.

Compendium Code No.: 14200091 Rev. 11-01

FLUNIXIN MEGLUMINE INJECTION ℞

Butler **Analgesic-Anti-inflammatory**

Flunixin Meglumine Injection 50 mg/mL

ANADA No.: 200-124

Active Ingredient(s): Each millimeter contains:

Flunixin Meglumine equivalent to Flunixin	50 mg
Edetate Disodium	0.1 mg
Sodium Formaldehyde Sulfoxylate	2.5 mg
Diethanolamine	4.0 mg
Propylene Glycol	207.2 mg
Phenol (as preservative)	5.0 mg
Water For Injection	q.s.

with hydrochloric acid to adjust pH.

Indications: FLUNIXIN MEGLUMINE INJECTION is recommended for the alleviation of inflammation and pain associated with musculoskeletal disorders in the horse.

It is also recommended for the alleviation of visceral pain associated with colic in the horse.

Pharmacology: Activity: Flunixin meglumine is a potent, nonnarcotic, nonsteroidal, analgesic agent with anti-inflammatory and antipyretic activity. It is significantly more potent than pentazocine, meperidine and codeine as an analgesic in the rat yeast paw test. Flunixin is four times as potent on a mg per mg basis as phenylbutazone as measured by the reduction in lameness and swelling in the horse. Plasma half-life in horse serum is 1.6 hours following a single dose of 1.1 mg/kg. Measurable amounts are detectable in horse plasma at 8 hours post injection.

Dosage and Administration: The recommended dose for musculoskeletal disorders is 0.5 mg per pound (1 mL/100 lbs) of body weight once daily. Treatment may be given by intravenous or intramuscular injection and repeated for up to 5 days. Studies show onset of activity is within 2 hours. Peak response occurs between 12 and 16 hours and duration of activity is 24-36 hours.

The recommended dose for the alleviation of pain associated with equine colic is 0.5 mg per pound of body weight. Intravenous administration is recommended for prompt relief. Clinical studies show pain is alleviated in less than 15 minutes in many cases.

Treatment may be repeated when signs of colic recur.

The cause of colic should be determined and treated with concomitant therapy.

Precaution(s): Store between 2° and 30°C (36° and 86°F).

Caution(s): Federal law restricts this drug to use by or on the written order of a licensed veterinarian.

For intravenous or intramuscular use in horses only.

For animal use only.

Keep out of reach of children.

Warning(s): Not for use in horses intended for food.

Toxicology: Toxicity: Toxicity studies were conducted in horses. A threefold intramuscular dose of 1.5 mg per pound of body weight daily for 10 consecutive days was safe. No changes were observed in hematology, serum chemistry, or urinalysis values. Intravenous dosages of 0.5 mg/lb daily for 15 days; 1.5 mg/lb daily for 10 days; and 2.5 mg/lb daily for 5 days produced no changes in blood or urine parameters. No injection site irritation was observed following intramuscular injection of the 0.5 mg/lb recommended dose. Some irritation was observed following a 3-fold dose administered intramuscularly.

Presentation: 100 mL (NDC 11695-3539-1).

Manufactured by: Phoenix Scientific, Inc., St. Joseph, MO 64506

Compendium Code No.: 10820760 Iss. 3-97

FLUSURE™

Pfizer Animal Health **Vaccine**

Swine Influenza Vaccine, H1N1 & H3N2, Killed Virus

U.S. Vet. Lic. No.: 189

Description: FLUSURE™ is a freeze-dried preparation containing 2 type A field isolates, subtypes H1N1 and H3N2, of inactivated swine influenza viruses grown on an established cell line. A sterile diluent containing Amphigen®, a unique oil-in-water adjuvant to enhance the immune response, is used to rehydrate the freeze-dried vaccine.

Indications: FLUSURE™ is for vaccination of healthy swine 3 weeks of age or older as an aid in preventing respiratory disease caused by swine influenza virus (SIV) subtypes H1N1 and H3N2.

Directions:

1. General Directions: Vaccination of all pigs on the premises is recommended to enhance herd immunity. Shake diluent before use. Aseptically rehydrate the freeze-dried vaccine with the accompanying adjuvant-containing sterile diluent, shake well, and administer 2 mL intramuscularly.
2. Primary Vaccination: Healthy swine 3 weeks of age or older should receive two 2 mL doses administered approximately 3 weeks apart. In young pigs, vaccinate after maternally derived antibodies to SIV have declined.
3. Revaccination: Semiannual revaccination with a single dose is recommended.
4. Good animal husbandry and herd health management practices should be employed.

Precaution(s): Store at 2-7°C. Prolonged exposure to higher temperatures may adversely affect potency. Do not freeze.

Use entire contents when first opened or rehydrated.

Sterilized syringes and needles should be used to administer this vaccine.

Caution(s): As with many vaccines, anaphylaxis may occur after use. Initial antidote of epinephrine is recommended and should be followed with appropriate supportive therapy.

This product has been shown to be efficacious in healthy animals. A protective immune response may not be elicited if animals are incubating an infectious disease, are malnourished or parasitized, are stressed due to shipment or environmental conditions, are otherwise immunocompromised, or the vaccine is not administered in accordance with label directions.

For use in swine only. For veterinary use only.

Warning(s): Do not vaccinate within 21 days before slaughter.

Discussion: Disease Description: Swine influenza (SI) is an acute respiratory disease caused by Type A influenza viruses. In the USA, 2 subtypes of SIV (H1N1 and H3N2) have emerged as the major disease-causing agents. SIV is a common component of the porcine respiratory disease complex (PRDC). A typical outbreak of respiratory disease caused by SIV is characterized by sudden onset and rapid spread within herds.

Clinical signs include depression, anorexia, coughing, fever (105-107°F/40.5-41.7°C) and serous discharge from the eyes and nose. The duration of the disease is usually 5-7 days. While clinical signs can be severe, recovery is generally rapid and death loss is usually less than 1%. However, SIV does predispose animals to secondary infections. The virus multiplies in the epithelial cells lining the bronchi and bronchioles causing necrosis of these cells.[1] Gross lung lesions appear firm and purple and are indistinguishable in many cases from *Mycoplasma hyopneumoniae* lesions. Laboratory testing is required for definitive diagnosis.

Nose-to-nose contact is the primary mode of transmission. Inhalation of contaminated aerosol particles is another possible means of transmission. Tentative diagnosis of SI may be based on clinical signs, gross lesions at necropsy, and the widespread prevalence of respiratory disease in the herd. Confirmation of infection may be based on either antibody presence or viral isolation. Good herd hygiene and proper facility maintenance are important in managing SI. There is no specific treatment for SI, but supportive care may be helpful.

Trial Data: Safety and Efficacy: The safety of FLUSURE™ was demonstrated in 3 field safety studies conducted in 3 different geographic locations. Nine hundred and six pigs were vaccinated at approximately 3 and 6 weeks of age. No injection site reactions or serious systemic reactions were observed following vaccination.

Efficacy of FLUSURE™ was demonstrated in 2 host animal challenge studies. Pigs were vaccinated at 3-15 days of age and again 14 days later. Sixteen days following the second vaccination, the pigs were challenged with a heterologous isolate of either SIV H1N1 or H3N2. Pigs were necropsied 5 days postchallenge and lung damage evaluated. As compared to nonvaccinated controls, pigs vaccinated with FLUSURE™ had significantly lower rectal temperatures, clinical signs, and lung lesion scores following challenge with either SIV H1N1 or H3N2. Study results are presented in Tables 1-4.

H1N1 Challenge Study:

Table 1. H1N1 serum hemagglutination inhibition geometric mean titers:

	Day 0*	Day 14	Day 28	Day 35
Controls	5.0**	5.0	5.0[a]	11.7[a]
Vaccinates	5.2	5.7	49.5[b]	49.4[b]

* Day 0 = Day of first vaccination

** Titers of < 10 were factored as 5.0 in calculation of geometric mean titers.

a,b Geometric mean titers within the same column with different lower-case superscripts are significantly different.

Table 2. Mean percent lung damage and frequency of clinical signs:

	Mean percent lung damage*	Frequency of animals with at least 1 clinical sign** postchallenge
Controls	23.41[a]	9/18[a]
Vaccinates	5.04[b]	0/19[b]

* Back-transformed least-squares means

** Depression and/or rapid breathing and/or persistent coughing

a,b Geometric mean titers within the same column with different lower-case superscripts are significantly different.

H3N2 Challenge Study:

Table 3. H3N2 serum hemagglutination inhibition geometric mean titers:

	Day 0*	Day 14	Day 28	Day 35
Controls	5.0**	5.0[a]	5.9[a]	9.7[a]
Vaccinates	5.0	7.5[b]	267.2[b]	166.3[b]

* Day 0 = Day of first vaccination

** Titers of < 10 were factored as 5.0 in calculation of geometric mean titers.

a,b Geometric mean titers within the same column with different lower-case superscripts are significantly different.

Table 4. Mean percent lung damage and frequency of clinical signs:

	Mean percent lung damage*	Frequency of animals with at least 1 clinical sign** postchallenge
Controls	33.43[a]	13/20[a]
Vaccinates	0.65[b]	0/19[b]

* Back-transformed least-squares means

** Depression and/or rapid breathing and/or persistent coughing

a,b Geometric mean titers within the same column with different lower-case superscripts are significantly different.

A study evaluating the duration of immunity of the H3N2 component of FLUSURE™ is in progress.

References: Available upon request.

Presentation: 50 dose (100 mL) and 250 dose (500 mL) vials.

Compendium Code No.: 36901940 75-0228-00

FLUSURE™/ER BAC PLUS®

Pfizer Animal Health **Bacterin-Vaccine**

Swine Influenza Vaccine, H1N1 & H3N2, Killed Virus-Erysipelothrix Rhusiopathiae Bacterin

U.S. Vet. Lic. No.: 189

Description: FLUSURE™/ER BAC PLUS® is a freeze-dried preparation containing 2 type A field isolates, subtypes H1N1 and H3N2, of inactivated swine influenza viruses grown on an established cell line, plus a liquid preparation of a serum-free, clarified *Erysipelothrix rhusiopathiae* culture. The liquid component contains Amphigen®, a unique oil-in-water adjuvant to enhance the immune response, and is used to rehydrate the freeze-dried vaccine.

Indications: FLUSURE™/ER BAC PLUS® is for vaccination of healthy swine 3 weeks of age or older as an aid in preventing respiratory disease caused by swine influenza virus (SIV) subtypes H1N1 and H3N2 and erysipelas caused by *E. rhusiopathiae* for a period of 20 weeks.

Directions:

1. General Directions: Vaccination of all pigs on the premises is recommended to enhance herd immunity. Shake diluent before use. Aseptically rehydrate the freeze-dried vaccine with the liquid bacterin provided, shake well, and administer 2 mL intramuscularly.
2. Primary Vaccination: Healthy swine 3 weeks of age or older should receive two 2 mL doses administered approximately 3 weeks apart. In young pigs, vaccinate after maternally derived antibodies have declined.
3. Revaccination: Semiannual revaccination with a single dose is recommended.
4. Good animal husbandry and herd health management practices should be employed.

Precaution(s): Store at 2°-7°C. Prolonged exposure to higher temperatures may adversely affect potency. Do not freeze.

Use entire contents when first opened or rehydrated.

Sterilized syringes and needles should be used to administer this vaccine.

Caution(s): As with many vaccines, anaphylaxis may occur after use. Initial antidote of epinephrine is recommended and should be followed with appropriate supportive therapy.

This product has been shown to be efficacious in healthy animals. A protective immune response may not be elicited if animals are incubating an infectious disease, are malnourished or parasitized, are stressed due to shipment or environmental conditions, are otherwise immunocompromised, or the vaccine is not administered in accordance with label directions.

For use in swine only.

For veterinary use only.

Warning(s): Do not vaccinate within 21 days before slaughter.

Discussion: Disease Description: Swine influenza (SI) is an acute respiratory disease caused by Type A influenza viruses. In the USA, 2 subtypes of SIV (H1N1 and H3N2) have emerged as the major disease-causing agents. SIV is a common component of porcine respiratory disease complex (PRDC). A typical outbreak of SI is characterized by sudden onset and rapid spread within herds. Clinical signs include depression, anorexia, coughing, fever (105-107°F/40.5-41.7°C) and serous discharge from the eyes and nose. The duration of the disease is usually 5-7 days. While clinical signs can be severe, recovery is generally rapid and death loss is usually less than 1%. However, SIV does predispose animals to secondary infections. The virus multiplies in the epithelial cells lining the bronchi and bronchioles causing necrosis of these cells.[1] Gross lung lesions appear firm and purple and are indistinguishable in many cases from *Mycoplasma hyopneumoniae* lesions. Laboratory testing is required for definitive diagnosis.

Erysipelas is caused by the bacterium *E. rhusiopathiae* and has been identified as a pathogen in swine since 1878. The disease is worldwide in distribution and is of economic importance throughout Europe, Asia, Australia, and North and South America. Swine 3 months through 3 years of age are most susceptible to erysipelas; outbreaks are usually more severe in herds on soil and during periods of wet weather. Erysipelas can take one of several forms or a combination of the following forms. Acute erysipelas is a general infection by *E. rhusiopathiae* in the bloodstream. This form often causes sudden death. Abortion may result in sows infected during pregnancy. Skin erysipelas manifests as diamond-shaped patches of swollen, purple skin on a pig's body, especially the belly and thighs. If the tips of the ears and tail are affected, tissues may die and slough. Arthritic erysipelas is a chronic disease occurring in pigs that have survived acute erysipelas. Affected pigs often have swollen and stiff joints. They do not gain weight efficiently, and their carcasses are often trimmed or condemned by inspectors at packing houses. Cardiac erysipelas usually occurs in older pigs raised on farms where the chronic form exists. Cardiac erysipelas may result in growths on the heart valves altering the normal flow of blood.[2]

Trial Data: Safety and Efficacy: The safety of FLUSURE™/ER BAC PLUS® was demonstrated in 3 field safety studies conducted in 3 different geographic locations. Nine hundred and six pigs were vaccinated at approximately 3 and 6 weeks of age. No injection site reactions or serious systemic reactions were observed following vaccination.

Efficacy of FLUSURE™/ER BAC PLUS® was demonstrated in 2 host animal challenge studies. Pigs were vaccinated at 3-15 days of age and again 14 days later. Sixteen days following the second vaccination, the pigs were challenged with a heterologous isolate of either SIV H1N1 or H3N2. Pigs were necropsied 5 days postchallenge and lung damage evaluated. As compared to nonvaccinated controls, pigs vaccinated with FLUSURE™/ER BAC PLUS® had significantly lower rectal temperatures, clinical signs, and lung lesion scores following challenge with either SIV H1N1 or H3N2. Study results are presented in Tables 1-4.

H1N1 Challenge Study:

Table 1. H1N1 serum hemagglutination inhibition geometric mean titers:

	Day 0*	Day 14	Day 28	Day 35
Controls	5.0**	5.0	5.0[a]	11.7[a]
Vaccinates	5.2	5.7	49.5[b]	49.4[b]

* Day 0 = Day of first vaccination

** Titers of < 10 were factored as 5.0 in calculation of geometric mean titers.

a,b Geometric mean titers within the same column with different lower-case superscripts are significantly different.

Table 2. Mean percent lung damage and frequency of clinical signs:

	Mean percent lung damage*	Frequency of animals with at least 1 clinical sign** postchallenge
Controls	23.41[a]	9/18[a]
Vaccinates	5.04[b]	0/19[b]

* Back-transformed least-squares means

** Depression and/or rapid breathing and/or persistent coughing

a,b Geometric mean titers within the same column with different lower-case superscripts are significantly different.

H3N2 Challenge Study:

Table 3. H3N2 serum hemagglutination inhibition geometric mean titers:

	Day 0*	Day 14	Day 28	Day 35
Controls	5.0**	5.0[a]	5.9[a]	9.7[a]
Vaccinates	5.0	7.5[b]	267.2[b]	166.3[b]

* Day 0 = Day of first vaccination

** Titers of < 10 were factored as 5.0 in calculation of geometric mean titers.

a,b Geometric mean titers within the same column with different lower-case superscripts are significantly different.

Table 4. Mean percent lung damage and frequency of clinical signs:

	Mean percent lung damage*	Frequency of animals with at least 1 clinical sign** postchallenge
Controls	33.43[a]	13/20[a]
Vaccinates	0.65[b]	0/19[b]

* Back-transformed least-squares means

** Depression and/or rapid breathing and/or persistent coughing

a,b Geometric mean titers within the same column with different lower-case superscripts are significantly different.

A study evaluating the duration of immunity of the H3N2 component of FLUSURE™/ER BAC PLUS® is in progress.

References: Available upon request.

Presentation: 50 dose (100 mL) and 250 dose (500 mL) vials.

Compendium Code No.: 36901950 75-0237-00

FLUSURE™/RESPISURE®

Pfizer Animal Health **Bacterin-Vaccine**

Swine Influenza Vaccine, H1N1 & H3N2, Killed Virus-Mycoplasma Hyopneumoniae Bacterin

U.S. Vet. Lic. No.: 189

Description: FLUSURE™/RESPISURE® is a freeze-dried preparation containing 2 type A field isolates, subtypes H1N1 and H3N2, of inactivated swine influenza viruses grown on an established cell line, plus a liquid preparation of a chemically inactivated whole cell culture of *Mycoplasma hyopneumoniae*. The liquid component contains Amphigen®, a unique oil-in-water adjuvant to enhance the immune response, and is used to rehydrate the freeze-dried vaccine.

Indications: FLUSURE™/RESPISURE® is for vaccination of healthy swine 3 weeks of age or older as an aid in preventing respiratory disease caused by swine influenza virus (SIV) subtypes H1N1 and H3N2 and *M. hyopneumoniae*.

Directions:

1. General Directions: Vaccination of all pigs on the premises is recommended to enhance herd immunity. Shake diluent before use. Aseptically rehydrate the freeze-dried vaccine with the liquid bacterin provided, shake well, and administer 2 mL intramuscularly.
2. Primary Vaccination: Healthy swine 3 weeks of age or older should receive two 2 mL doses administered approximately 3 weeks apart. In young pigs, vaccinate after maternally derived antibodies to SIV have declined.
3. Revaccination: Semiannual revaccination with a single dose is recommended.
4. Good animal husbandry and herd health management practices should be employed.

Precaution(s): Store at 2°-7°C. Prolonged exposure to higher temperatures may adversely affect potency. Do not freeze.

Use entire contents when first opened or rehydrated.

Sterilized syringes and needles should be used to administer this vaccine.

Caution(s): As with many vaccines, anaphylaxis may occur after use. Initial antidote of epinephrine is recommended and should be followed with appropriate supportive therapy.

This product has been shown to be efficacious in healthy animals. A protective immune response may not be elicited if animals are incubating an infectious disease, are malnourished or parasitized, are stressed due to shipment or environmental conditions, are otherwise immunocompromised, or the vaccine is not administered in accordance with label directions.

For use in swine only.

For veterinary use only.

Warning(s): Do not vaccinate within 21 days before slaughter.

Discussion: Disease Description: Swine influenza (SI) is an acute respiratory disease caused by Type A influenza viruses. In the USA, 2 subtypes of SIV (H1N1 and H3N2) have emerged as the major disease-causing agents. SIV and *M. hyopneumoniae* are both common components of porcine respiratory disease complex (PRDC). A typical outbreak of SI is characterized by sudden onset and rapid spread within herds. Clinical signs include depression, anorexia, coughing, fever (105-107°F/40.5-41.7°C) and serous discharge from the eyes and nose. The duration of the disease is usually 5-7 days. While clinical signs can be severe, recovery is generally rapid and death loss is usually less than 1%. However, SIV does predispose animals to secondary infections. The virus multiplies in the epithelial cells lining the bronchi and bronchioles causing necrosis of these cells.[1] Gross lung lesions appear firm and purple and are indistinguishable in many cases from *M. hyopneumoniae* lesions. Laboratory testing is required for definitive diagnosis.

Mycoplasmal pneumonia of swine (MPS), or enzootic pneumonia, is a widespread, chronic disease characterized by coughing, growth retardation, and reduced feed efficiency. The etiologic agent is *M. hyopneumoniae;* however, the naturally occurring disease often results from a combination of bacterial and mycoplasmal infections.

MPS causes considerable economic loss in all areas where swine are raised. Surveys conducted at various locations throughout the world indicate that lesions typical of those seen with MPS occur in 30%-80% of slaughter-weight swine. Because mycoplasmal lesions may resolve before hogs reach slaughter weight, the actual incidence may be higher. The prevalence of *M. hyopneumoniae* infection in chronic swine pneumonia has been reported to range from 25%[2]-93%.[3] Pigs of all ages are susceptible to MPS, but the disease is most common in growing and finishing swine. Current evidence indicates that *M. hyopneumoniae* is transmitted by aerosol or direct contact with respiratory tract secretions from infected swine. Transmission from sow to pig during lactation is possible.[4] Once established, MPS occurs year after year in infected herds, varying in severity with such environmental factors as season, ventilation, and concentration of swine.

Clinical signs of MPS include a chronic, nonproductive cough continuing for weeks or months, unthrifty appearance, and retarded growth, even though the appetites of infected swine remain normal. Stunting may occur, resulting in considerable variation in size among affected pigs. Death loss associated with secondary bacterial infection and stress may occur.

M. hyopneumoniae causes a loss of ciliary motility in the bronchial passages. Eventually the cilia are destroyed, resulting in reduction in natural defense in the upper respiratory tract and increased susceptibility to secondary infection with bacterial agents such as *Pasteurella multocida, Haemophilus parasuis, Actinobacillus pleuropneumoniae,* and *Bordetella bronchiseptica.* Swine lungworm and roundworm larvae infections may also increase the severity of MPS.

Trial Data: Safety and Efficacy: The safety of FLUSURE™/RESPISURE® was demonstrated in 3 field safety studies conducted in 3 different geographic locations. Nine hundred and six pigs were vaccinated at approximately 3 and 6 weeks of age. No injection site reactions or serious systemic reactions were observed following vaccination.

Efficacy of FLUSURE™/RESPISURE® was demonstrated in 2 host animal challenge studies. Pigs were vaccinated at 3-15 days of age and again 14 days later. Sixteen days following the second vaccination, the pigs were challenged with a heterologous isolate of either SIV H1N1 or H3N2. Pigs were necropsied 5 days postchallenge and lung damage evaluated. As compared to nonvaccinated controls, pigs vaccinated with FLUSURE™/RESPISURE® had significantly lower rectal temperatures, clinical signs, and lung lesion scores following challenge with either SIV H1N1 or H3N2. Study results are presented in Tables 1-4.

H1N1 Challenge Study:

Table 1. H1N1 serum hemagglutination inhibition geometric mean titers:

	Day 0*	Day 14	Day 28	Day 35
Controls	5.0**	5.0	5.0[a]	11.7[a]
Vaccinates	5.2	5.7	49.5[b]	49.4[b]

* Day 0 = Day of first vaccination

** Titers of < 10 were factored as 5.0 in calculation of geometric mean titers.

a,b Geometric mean titers within the same column with different lower-case superscripts are significantly different.

Table 2. Mean percent lung damage and frequency of clinical signs:

	Mean percent lung damage*	Frequency of animals with at least 1 clinical sign** postchallenge
Controls	23.41[a]	9/18[a]
Vaccinates	5.04[b]	0/19[b]

* Back-transformed least-squares means

** Depression and/or rapid breathing and/or persistent coughing

a,b Geometric mean titers within the same column with different lower-case superscripts are significantly different.

H3N2 Challenge Study:

Table 3. H3N2 serum hemagglutination inhibition geometric mean titers:

	Day 0*	Day 14	Day 28	Day 35
Controls	5.0**	5.0[a]	5.9[a]	9.7[a]
Vaccinates	5.0	7.5[b]	267.2[b]	166.3[b]

* Day 0 = Day of first vaccination

** Titers of < 10 were factored as 5.0 in calculation of geometric mean titers.

a,b Geometric mean titers within the same column with different lower-case superscripts are significantly different.

Table 4. Mean percent lung damage and frequency of clinical signs:

	Mean percent lung damage*	Frequency of animals with at least 1 clinical sign** postchallenge
Controls	33.43[a]	13/20[a]
Vaccinates	0.65[b]	0/19[b]

* Back-transformed least-squares means

** Depression and/or rapid breathing and/or persistent coughing

a,b Geometric mean titers within the same column with different lower-case superscripts are significantly different.

A study evaluating the duration of immunity of the H3N2 component of FLUSURE™/RESPISURE® is in progress.

References: Available upon request.

Presentation: 50 dose (100 mL) and 250 dose (500 mL) vials.

Compendium Code No.: 36901960 75-0235-00

FLUSURE™/RESPISURE 1 ONE®

Pfizer Animal Health **Bacterin-Vaccine**

Swine Influenza Vaccine, H1N1 & H3N2, Killed Virus-Mycoplasma Hyopneumoniae Bacterin

U.S. Vet. Lic. No.: 189

Description: FLUSURE™/RESPISURE-ONE® is a freeze-dried preparation containing 2 type A field isolates, subtypes H1N1 and H3N2, of inactivated swine influenza viruses grown on an established cell line, plus a liquid preparation of a chemically inactivated whole cell culture of *Mycoplasma hyopneumoniae*. The liquid component contains Amphigen®, a unique oil-in-water adjuvant to enhance the immune response, and is used to rehydrate the freeze-dried vaccine.

Indications: FLUSURE™/RESPISURE-ONE® is for vaccination of healthy swine 3 weeks of age or older as an aid in preventing respiratory disease caused by swine influenza virus (SIV) subtypes H1N1 and H3N2 and respiratory disease caused by *M. hyopneumoniae* for a period of 23 weeks.

Directions:

1. General Directions: Vaccination of all pigs on the premises is recommended to enhance herd immunity. Shake diluent before use. Aseptically rehydrate the freeze-dried vaccine with the liquid bacterin provided, shake well, and administer 2 mL intramuscularly.

F

2. Primary Vaccination: Administer a single 2 mL dose to healthy swine 3 weeks of age or older, followed by a single dose of Flusure™ approximately 3 weeks later. In young pigs, vaccinate after maternally derived antibodies to SIV have declined.
3. Revaccination: Semiannual revaccination with a single dose is recommended.
4. Good animal husbandry and herd health management practices should be employed.

Precaution(s): Store at 2°-7°C. Prolonged exposure to higher temperatures may adversely affect potency. Do not freeze.

Use entire contents when first opened or rehydrated.

Sterilized syringes and needles should be used to administer this vaccine.

Caution(s): As with many vaccines, anaphylaxis may occur after use. Initial antidote of epinephrine is recommended and should be followed with appropriate supportive therapy.

This product has been shown to be efficacious in healthy animals. A protective immune response may not be elicited if animals are incubating an infectious disease, are malnourished or parasitized, are stressed due to shipment or environmental conditions, are otherwise immunocompromised, or the vaccine is not administered in accordance with label directions.

For use in swine only.

For veterinary use only.

Warning(s): Do not vaccinate within 21 days before slaughter.

Discussion: Disease Description: Swine influenza (SI) is an acute respiratory disease caused by Type A influenza viruses. In the USA, 2 subtypes of SIV (H1N1 and H3N2) have emerged as the major disease-causing agents. SIV and *M. hyopneumoniae* are both common components of porcine respiratory disease complex (PRDC). A typical outbreak of SI is characterized by sudden onset and rapid spread within herds. Clinical signs include depression, anorexia, coughing, fever (105-107°F/40.5-41.7°C) and serous discharge from the eyes and nose. The duration of the disease is usually 5-7 days. While clinical signs can be severe, recovery is generally rapid and death loss is usually less than 1%. However, SIV does predispose animals to secondary infections. The virus multiplies in the epithelial cells lining the bronchi and bronchioles causing necrosis of these cells.[1] Gross lung lesions appear firm and purple and are indistinguishable in many cases from *M. hyopneumoniae* lesions. Laboratory testing is required for definitive diagnosis.

F

Mycoplasmal pneumonia of swine (MPS), or enzootic pneumonia, is a widespread, chronic disease characterized by coughing, growth retardation, and reduced feed efficiency. The etiologic agent is *M. hyopneumoniae;* however, the naturally occurring disease often results from a combination of bacterial and mycoplasmal infections.

MPS causes considerable economic loss in all areas where swine are raised. Surveys conducted at various locations throughout the world indicate that lesions typical of those seen with MPS occur in 30%-80% of slaughter-weight swine. Because mycoplasmal lesions may resolve before hogs reach slaughter weight, the actual incidence may be higher. The prevalence of *M. hyopneumoniae* infection in chronic swine pneumonia has been reported to range from 25%[2]-93%.[3] Pigs of all ages are susceptible to MPS, but the disease is most common in growing and finishing swine. Current evidence indicates that *M. hyopneumoniae* is transmitted by aerosol or direct contact with respiratory tract secretions from infected swine. Transmission from sow to pig during lactation is possible.[4] Once established, MPS occurs year after year in infected herds, varying in severity with such environmental factors as season, ventilation, and concentration of swine.

Clinical signs of MPS include a chronic, nonproductive cough continuing for weeks or months, unthrifty appearance, and retarded growth, even though the appetites of infected swine remain normal. Stunting may occur, resulting in considerable variation in size among affected pigs. Death loss associated with secondary bacterial infection and stress may occur.

M. hyopneumoniae causes a loss of ciliary motility in the bronchial passages. Eventually the cilia are destroyed, resulting in reduction in natural defense in the upper respiratory tract and increased susceptibility to secondary infection with bacterial agents such as *Pasteurella multocida, Haemophilus parasuis, Actinobacillus pleuropneumoniae,* and *Bordetella bronchiseptica.* Swine lungworm and roundworm larvae infections may also increase the severity of MPS.

Trial Data: Safety and Efficacy: The safety of FLUSURE™/RESPISURE-ONE® was demonstrated in 3 field safety studies conducted in 3 different geographic locations. Nine hundred and six pigs were vaccinated at approximately 3 and 6 weeks of age. No injection site reactions or serious systemic reactions were observed following vaccination.

Efficacy of FLUSURE™/RESPISURE-ONE® was demonstrated in 2 host animal challenge studies. Pigs were vaccinated at 3-15 days of age and again 14 days later. Sixteen days following the second vaccination, the pigs were challenged with a heterologous isolate of either SIV H1N1 or H3N2. Pigs were necropsied 5 days postchallenge and lung damage evaluated. As compared to nonvaccinated controls, pigs vaccinated with FLUSURE™/RESPISURE-ONE® had significantly lower rectal temperatures, clinical signs, and lung lesion scores following challenge with either SIV H1N1 or H3N2. Study results are presented in Tables 1-4.

H1N1 Challenge Study:

Table 1. H1N1 serum hemagglutination inhibition geometric mean titers:

	Day 0*	Day 14	Day 28	Day 35
Controls	5.0**	5.0	5.0[a]	11.7[a]
Vaccinates	5.2	5.7	49.5[b]	49.4[b]

* Day 0 = Day of first vaccination

** Titers of < 10 were factored as 5.0 in calculation of geometric mean titers.

a,b Geometric mean titers within the same column with different lower-case superscripts are significantly different.

Table 2. Mean percent lung damage and frequency of clinical signs:

	Mean percent lung damage*	Frequency of animals with at least 1 clinical sign** postchallenge
Controls	23.41[a]	9/18[a]
Vaccinates	5.04[b]	0/19b

* Back-transformed least-squares means

** Depression and/or rapid breathing and/or persistent coughing

a,b Geometric mean titers within the same column with different lower-case superscripts are significantly different.

H3N2 Challenge Study:

Table 3. H3N2 serum hemagglutination inhibition geometric mean titers:

	Day 0*	Day 14	Day 28	Day 35
Controls	5.0**	5.0[a]	5.9[a]	9.7[a]
Vaccinates	5.0	7.5[b]	267.2[b]	166.3[b]

* Day 0 = Day of first vaccination

** Titers of < 10 were factored as 5.0 in calculation of geometric mean titers.

a,b Geometric mean titers within the same column with different lower-case superscripts are significantly different.

Table 4. Mean percent lung damage and frequency of clinical signs:

	Mean percent lung damage*	Frequency of animals with at least 1 clinical sign** postchallenge
Controls	33.43[a]	13/20[a]
Vaccinates	0.65[b]	0/19[b]

* Back-transformed least-squares means

** Depression and/or rapid breathing and/or persistent coughing

a,b Geometric mean titers within the same column with different lower-case superscripts are significantly different.

A study evaluating the duration of immunity of the H3N2 component of FLUSURE™/RESPISURE-ONE® is in progress.

References: Available upon request.

Presentation: 50 dose (100 mL) and 250 dose (500 mL) vials.

Compendium Code No.: 36901970 75-0233-00

FLUSURE™/RESPISURE 1 ONE®/ER BAC PLUS®

Pfizer Animal Health **Bacterin-Vaccine**

Swine Influenza Vaccine, H1N1 & H3N2, Killed Virus-Erysipelothrix Rhusiopathiae-Mycoplasma Hyopneumoniae Bacterin

U.S. Vet. Lic. No.: 189

Description: FLUSURE™/RESPISURE-ONE®/ER BAC PLUS® is a freeze-dried preparation containing 2 type A field isolates, subtypes H1N1 and H3N2, of inactivated swine influenza viruses grown on an established cell line, plus a liquid preparation of a chemically inactivated whole cell culture of *Mycoplasma hyopneumoniae* and a serum-free, clarified *Erysipelothrix rhusiopathiae* culture. The liquid component contains Amphigen®, a unique oil-in-water adjuvant to enhance the immune response, and is used to rehydrate the freeze-dried vaccine.

Indications:

FLUSURE™/RESPISURE-ONE®/ER BAC PLUS® is for vaccination of healthy swine 3 weeks of age or older as an aid in preventing respiratory disease caused by swine influenza virus (SIV) subtypes H1N1 and H3N2, erysipelas caused by *E. rhusiopathiae* for a period of 20 weeks, and respiratory disease caused by *M. hyopneumoniae* for a period of 23 weeks.

Directions:

1. General Directions: Vaccination of all pigs on the premises is recommended to enhance herd immunity. Shake diluent before use. Aseptically rehydrate the freeze-dried vaccine with the liquid bacterin provided, shake well, and administer 2 mL intramuscularly.
2. Primary Vaccination: Administer a single 2 mL dose to healthy swine 3 weeks of age or older, followed by a single dose of Flusure™/ER Bac Plus® approximately 3 weeks later. In young pigs, vaccinate after maternally derived antibodies to SIV and *E. rhusiopathiae* have declined.
3. Revaccination: Semiannual revaccination with a single dose is recommended.
4. Good animal husbandry and herd health management practices should be employed.

Precaution(s): Store at 2°-7°C. Prolonged exposure to higher temperatures may adversely affect potency. Do not freeze.

Use entire contents when first opened or rehydrated.

Sterilized syringes and needles should be used to administer this vaccine.

Caution(s): As with many vaccines, anaphylaxis may occur after use. Initial antidote of epinephrine is recommended and should be followed with appropriate supportive therapy.

This product has been shown to be efficacious in healthy animals. A protective immune response may not be elicited if animals are incubating an infectious disease, are malnourished or parasitized, are stressed due to shipment or environmental conditions, are otherwise immunocompromised, or the vaccine is not administered in accordance with label directions.

For use in swine only.

For veterinary use only.

Warning(s): Do not vaccinate within 21 days before slaughter.

Discussion: Disease Description: Swine influenza (SI) is an acute respiratory disease caused by Type A influenza viruses. In the USA, 2 subtypes of SIV (H1N1 and H3N2) have emerged as the major disease-causing agents. SIV and *M. hyopneumoniae* are both common components of porcine respiratory disease complex (PRDC). A typical outbreak of SI is characterized by sudden onset and rapid spread within herds. Clinical signs include depression, anorexia, coughing, fever (105-107°F/40.5-41.7°C) and serous discharge from the eyes and nose. The duration of the disease is usually 5-7 days. While clinical signs can be severe, recovery is generally rapid and death loss is usually less than 1%. However, SIV does predispose animals to secondary infections. The virus multiplies in the epithelial cells lining the bronchi and bronchioles causing necrosis of these cells.[1] Gross lung lesions appear firm and purple and are indistinguishable in many cases from *M. hyopneumoniae* lesions. Laboratory testing is required for definitive diagnosis.

Mycoplasmal pneumonia of swine (MPS), or enzootic pneumonia, is a widespread, chronic disease characterized by coughing, growth retardation, and reduced feed efficiency. The etiologic agent is *M. hyopneumoniae;* however, the naturally occurring disease often results from a combination of bacterial and mycoplasmal infections.

MPS causes considerable economic loss in all areas where swine are raised. Surveys conducted at various locations throughout the world indicate that lesions typical of those seen with MPS occur in 30%-80% of slaughter-weight swine. Because mycoplasmal lesions may resolve before hogs reach slaughter weight, the actual incidence may be higher. The prevalence of *M. hyopneumoniae* infection in chronic swine pneumonia has been reported to range from 25%[2]-93%.[3] Pigs of all ages are susceptible to MPS, but the disease is most common in growing and finishing swine. Current evidence indicates that *M. hyopneumoniae* is transmitted by aerosol or direct contact with respiratory tract secretions from infected swine. Transmission from sow to pig during lactation is possible.[4] Once established, MPS occurs year after year in infected herds, varying in severity with such environmental factors as season, ventilation, and concentration of swine.

Clinical signs of MPS include a chronic, nonproductive cough continuing for weeks or months, unthrifty appearance, and retarded growth, even though the appetites of infected swine remain normal. Stunting may occur, resulting in considerable variation in size among affected pigs. Death loss associated with secondary bacterial infection and stress may occur.

M. hyopneumoniae causes a loss of ciliary motility in the bronchial passages. Eventually the cilia are destroyed, resulting in reduction in natural defense in the upper respiratory tract and increased susceptibility to secondary infection with bacterial agents such as *Pasteurella multocida, Haemophilus parasuis, Actinobacillus pleuropneumoniae,* and *Bordetella bronchiseptica.* Swine lungworm and roundworm larvae infections may also increase the severity of MPS.

Erysipelas is caused by the bacterium *E. rhusiopathiae* and has been identified as a pathogen in swine since 1878. The disease is worldwide in distribution and is of economic importance throughout Europe, Asia, Australia, and North and South America. Swine 3 months through 3 years of age are most susceptible to erysipelas; outbreaks are usually more severe in herds on soil and during periods of wet weather. Erysipelas can take one of several forms or a combination of the following forms. Acute erysipelas is a general infection by *E. rhusiopathiae* in the bloodstream. This form often causes sudden death. Abortion may result in sows infected during pregnancy. Skin erysipelas manifests as diamond-shaped patches of swollen, purple skin on a pig's body, especially the belly and thighs. If the tips of the ears and tail are affected, tissues may die and slough. Arthritic erysipelas is a chronic disease occurring in pigs that have survived acute erysipelas. Affected pigs often have swollen and stiff joints. They do not gain weight efficiently, and their carcasses are often trimmed or condemned by inspectors at packing houses. Cardiac erysipelas usually occurs in older pigs raised on farms where the chronic form exists. Cardiac erysipelas may result in growths on the heart valves altering the normal flow of blood.[5]

Trial Data: Safety and Efficacy: The safety of FLUSURE™/RESPISURE-ONE®/ER BAC PLUS® was demonstrated in 3 field safety studies conducted in 3 different geographic locations. Nine hundred and six pigs were vaccinated at approximately 3 and 6 weeks of age. No injection site reactions or serious systemic reactions were observed following vaccination.

Efficacy of FLUSURE™/RESPISURE-ONE®/ER BAC PLUS® was demonstrated in 2 host animal challenge studies. Pigs were vaccinated at 3-15 days of age and again 14 days later. Sixteen days following the second vaccination, the pigs were challenged with a heterologous isolate of either SIV H1N1 or H3N2. Pigs were necropsied 5 days postchallenge and lung damage evaluated. As compared to nonvaccinated controls, pigs vaccinated with FLUSURE™/RESPISURE-ONE®/ER BAC PLUS® had significantly lower rectal temperatures, clinical signs, and lung lesion scores following challenge with either SIV H1N1 or H3N2. Study results are presented in Tables 1-4.

H1N1 Challenge Study:

Table 1. H1N1 serum hemagglutination inhibition geometric mean titers:

	Day 0*	Day 14	Day 28	Day 35
Controls	5.0**	5.0	5.0[a]	11.7[a]
Vaccinates	5.2	5.7	49.5[b]	49.4[b]

* Day 0 = Day of first vaccination

** Titers of < 10 were factored as 5.0 in calculation of geometric mean titers.

[a,b] Geometric mean titers within the same column with different lower-case superscripts are significantly different.

Table 2. Mean percent lung damage and frequency of clinical signs:

	Mean percent lung damage*	Frequency of animals with at least 1 clinical sign** postchallenge
Controls	23.41[a]	9/18[a]
Vaccinates	5.04[b]	0/19[b]

* Back-transformed least-squares means

** Depression and/or rapid breathing and/or persistent coughing

[a,b] Geometric mean titers within the same column with different lower-case superscripts are significantly different.

H3N2 Challenge Study:

Table 3. H3N2 serum hemagglutination inhibition geometric mean titers:

	Day 0*	Day 14	Day 28	Day 35
Controls	5.0**	5.0[a]	5.9[a]	9.7[a]
Vaccinates	5.0	7.5[b]	267.2[b]	166.3[b]

* Day 0 = Day of first vaccination

** Titers of < 10 were factored as 5.0 in calculation of geometric mean titers.

[a,b] Geometric mean titers within the same column with different lower-case superscripts are significantly different.

Table 4. Mean percent lung damage and frequency of clinical signs:

	Mean percent lung damage*	Frequency of animals with at least 1 clinical sign** postchallenge
Controls	33.43[a]	13/20[a]
Vaccinates	0.65[b]	0/19[b]

* Back-transformed least-squares means

** Depression and/or rapid breathing and/or persistent coughing

[a,b] Geometric mean titers within the same column with different lower-case superscripts are significantly different.

A study evaluating the duration of immunity of the H3N2 component of FLUSURE™/RESPISURE-ONE®/ER BAC PLUS® is in progress.

References: Available upon request.

Presentation: 50 dose (100 mL) and 250 dose (500 mL) vials.

Compendium Code No.: 36901980 75-0229-00

FLUSURE™/RESPISURE® RTU

Pfizer Animal Health **Bacterin-Vaccine**

Swine Influenza Vaccine, H1N1 & H3N2, Killed Virus-Mycoplasma Hyopneumoniae Bacterin

U.S. Vet. Lic. No.: 189

Description: FLUSURE™/RESPISURE® RTU is a liquid preparation containing 2 type A field isolates, subtypes H1N1 and H3N2, of inactivated swine influenza viruses grown on an established cell line, plus a chemically inactivated whole cell culture of *Mycoplasma hyopneumoniae*. FLUSURE™/RESPISURE® RTU contains Amphigen®, a unique oil-in-water adjuvant, to enhance the immune response.

Indications: FLUSURE™/RESPISURE® RTU is for vaccination of healthy swine 3 weeks of age or older as an aid in preventing respiratory disease caused by swine influenza virus (SIV) subtypes H1N1 and H3N2 and *M. hyopneumoniae*.

Directions:

1. General Directions: Vaccination of all pigs on the premises is recommended to enhance herd immunity. Shake well. Aseptically administer 2 mL intramuscularly.
2. Primary Vaccination: Healthy swine 3 weeks of age or older should receive two 2 mL doses administered approximately 3 weeks apart. In young pigs, vaccinate after maternally derived antibodies to SIV have declined.
3. Revaccination: Semiannual revaccination with a single dose is recommended.
4. Good animal husbandry and herd health management practices should be employed.

Precaution(s): Store at 2°-7°C. Prolonged exposure to higher temperatures may adversely affect potency. Do not freeze.

Use entire contents when first opened.

Sterilized syringes and needles should be used to administer this vaccine.

Caution(s): As with many vaccines, anaphylaxis may occur after use. Initial antidote of epinephrine is recommended and should be followed with appropriate supportive therapy.

This product has been shown to be efficacious in healthy animals. A protective immune response may not be elicited if animals are incubating an infectious disease, are malnourished or parasitized, are stressed due to shipment or environmental conditions, are otherwise immunocompromised, or the vaccine is not administered in accordance with label directions.

For use in swine only.

For veterinary use only.

Warning(s): Do not vaccinate within 21 days before slaughter.

Discussion: Disease Description: Swine influenza (SI) is an acute respiratory disease caused by Type A influenza viruses. In the USA, 2 subtypes of SIV (H1N1 and H3N2) have emerged as the major disease-causing agents. SIV and *M. hyopneumoniae* are both common components of porcine respiratory disease complex (PRDC). A typical outbreak of SI is characterized by sudden onset and rapid spread within herds. Clinical signs include depression, anorexia, coughing, fever (105-107°F/40.5-41.7°C) and serous discharge from the eyes and nose. The duration of the disease is usually 5-7 days. While clinical signs can be severe, recovery is generally rapid and death loss is usually less than 1%. However, SIV does predispose animals to secondary infections. The virus multiplies in the epithelial cells lining the bronchi and bronchioles causing necrosis of these cells.[1] Gross lung lesions appear firm and purple and are indistinguishable in many cases from *M. hyopneumoniae* lesions. Laboratory testing is required for definitive diagnosis.

Mycoplasmal pneumonia of swine (MPS), or enzootic pneumonia, is a widespread, chronic disease characterized by coughing, growth retardation, and reduced feed efficiency. The etiologic agent is *M. hyopneumoniae;* however, the naturally occurring disease often results from a combination of bacterial and mycoplasmal infections.

MPS causes considerable economic loss in all areas where swine are raised. Surveys conducted at various locations throughout the world indicate that lesions typical of those seen with MPS occur in 30%-80% of slaughter-weight swine. Because mycoplasmal lesions may resolve before hogs reach slaughter weight, the actual incidence may be higher. The prevalence of *M. hyopneumoniae* infection in chronic swine pneumonia has been reported to range from 25%[2]-93%.[3] Pigs of all ages are susceptible to MPS, but the disease is most common in growing and finishing swine. Current evidence indicates that *M. hyopneumoniae* is transmitted by aerosol or direct contact with respiratory tract secretions from infected swine. Transmission from sow to pig during lactation is possible.[4] Once established, MPS occurs year after year in infected herds, varying in severity with such environmental factors as season, ventilation, and concentration of swine.

Clinical signs of MPS include a chronic, nonproductive cough continuing for weeks or months, unthrifty appearance, and retarded growth, even though the appetites of infected swine remain normal. Stunting may occur, resulting in considerable variation in size among affected pigs. Death loss associated with secondary bacterial infection and stress may occur.

M. hyopneumoniae causes a loss of ciliary motility in the bronchial passages. Eventually the cilia are destroyed, resulting in reduction in natural defense in the upper respiratory tract and increased susceptibility to secondary infection with bacterial agents such as *Pasteurella multocida, Haemophilus parasuis, Actinobacillus pleuropneumoniae,* and *Bordetella bronchiseptica*. Swine lungworm and roundworm larvae infections may also increase the severity of MPS.

Trial Data: Safety and Efficacy: The safety of FLUSURE™/RESPISURE® RTU was demonstrated in 3 field safety studies conducted in 3 different geographic locations. Nine hundred and six pigs were vaccinated at approximately 3 and 6 weeks of age. No injection site reactions or serious systemic reactions were observed following vaccination.

Efficacy of FLUSURE™/RESPISURE® RTU was demonstrated in 2 host animal challenge studies. Pigs were vaccinated at 3-15 days of age and again 14 days later. Sixteen days following the second vaccination, the pigs were challenged with a heterologous isolate of either SIV H1N1 or H3N2. Pigs were necropsied 5 days postchallenge and lung damage evaluated. As compared to nonvaccinated controls, vaccinated pigs had significantly lower rectal temperatures, clinical signs, and lung lesion scores following challenge with either SIV H1N1 or H3N2. Study results are presented in Tables 1-4.

H1N1 Challenge Study:

Table 1. H1N1 serum hemagglutination inhibition geometric mean titers:

	Day 0*	Day 14	Day 28	Day 35
Controls	5.0**	5.0	5.0[a]	11.7[a]
Vaccinates	5.2	5.7	49.5[b]	49.4[b]

* Day 0 = Day of first vaccination

** Titers of < 10 were factored as 5.0 in calculation of geometric mean titers.

[a,b] Geometric mean titers within the same column with different lower-case superscripts are significantly different.

Table 2. Mean percent lung damage and frequency of clinical signs:

	Mean percent lung damage*	Frequency of animals with at least 1 clinical sign** postchallenge
Controls	23.41[a]	9/18[a]
Vaccinates	5.04[b]	0/19[b]

* Back-transformed least-squares means

** Depression and/or rapid breathing and/or persistent coughing

[a,b] Geometric mean titers within the same column with different lower-case superscripts are significantly different.

H3N2 Challenge Study:

Table 3. H3N2 serum hemagglutination inhibition geometric mean titers:

	Day 0*	Day 14	Day 28	Day 35
Controls	5.0**	5.0[a]	5.9[a]	9.7[a]
Vaccinates	5.0	7.5[b]	267.2[b]	166.3[b]

* Day 0 = Day of first vaccination

** Titers of < 10 were factored as 5.0 in calculation of geometric mean titers.

[a,b] Geometric mean titers within the same column with different lower-case superscripts are significantly different.

Table 4. Mean percent lung damage and frequency of clinical signs:

	Mean percent lung damage*	Frequency of animals with at least 1 clinical sign** postchallenge
Controls	33.43[a]	13/20[a]
Vaccinates	0.65[b]	0/19[b]

* Back-transformed least-squares means

** Depression and/or rapid breathing and/or persistent coughing

a,b Geometric mean titers within the same column with different lower-case superscripts are significantly different.

A study evaluating the duration of immunity of the H3N2 component of FLUSURE™/RESPISURE® RTU is in progress.

References: Available upon request.

Presentation: 50 dose (100 mL) and 250 dose (500 mL) vials.

Compendium Code No.: 36901990 75-0281-00

FLUSURE™ RTU

Pfizer Animal Health **Vaccine**

Swine Influenza Vaccine, H1N1 & H3N2, Killed Virus

U.S. Vet. Lic. No.: 189

Description: FLUSURE™ RTU is a liquid preparation containing 2 type A field isolates, subtypes H1N1 and H3N2, of inactivated swine influenza viruses grown on an established cell line. FLUSURE™ RTU contains Amphigen®, a unique oil-in-water adjuvant, to enhance the immune response.

Indications: FLUSURE™ RTU is for vaccination of healthy swine 3 weeks of age or older as an aid in preventing respiratory disease caused by swine influenza virus (SIV) subtypes H1N1 and H3N2.

F

Directions:

1. General Directions: Vaccination of all pigs on the premises is recommended to enhance herd immunity. Shake well. Aseptically administer 2 mL intramuscularly.
2. Primary Vaccination: Healthy swine 3 weeks of age or older should receive two 2 mL doses administered approximately 3 weeks apart. In young pigs, vaccinate after maternally derived antibodies to SIV have declined.
3. Revaccination: Semiannual revaccination with a single dose is recommended.
4. Good animal husbandry and herd health management practices should be employed.

Precaution(s): Store at 2°-7°C. Prolonged exposure to higher temperatures may adversely affect potency. Do not freeze.

Use entire contents when first opened.

Sterilized syringes and needles should be used to administer this vaccine.

Caution(s): As with many vaccines, anaphylaxis may occur after use. Initial antidote of epinephrine is recommended and should be followed with appropriate supportive therapy.

This product has been shown to be efficacious in healthy animals. A protective immune response may not be elicited if animals are incubating an infectious disease, are malnourished or parasitized, are stressed due to shipment or environmental conditions, are otherwise immunocompromised, or the vaccine is not administered in accordance with label directions.

For use in swine only.

For veterinary use only.

Warning(s): Do not vaccinate within 21 days before slaughter.

Discussion: Disease Description: Swine influenza (SI) is an acute respiratory disease caused by Type A influenza viruses. In the USA, 2 subtypes of SIV (H1N1 and H3N2) have emerged as the major disease-causing agents. SIV is a common component of the porcine respiratory disease complex (PRDC). A typical outbreak of respiratory disease caused by SIV is characterized by sudden onset and rapid spread within herds.

Clinical signs include depression, anorexia, coughing, fever (105-107°F/40.5-41.7°C) and serous discharge from the eyes and nose. The duration of the disease is usually 5-7 days. While clinical signs can be severe, recovery is generally rapid and death loss is usually less than 1%. However, SIV does predispose animals to secondary infections. The virus multiplies in the epithelial cells lining the bronchi and bronchioles causing necrosis of these cells.[1] Gross lung lesions appear firm and purple and are indistinguishable in many cases from *Mycoplasma hyopneumoniae* lesions. Laboratory testing is required for definitive diagnosis.

Nose-to-nose contact is the primary mode of transmission. Inhalation of contaminated aerosol particles is another possible means of transmission. Tentative diagnosis of SI may be based on clinical signs, gross lesions at necropsy, and the widespread prevalence of respiratory disease in the herd. Confirmation of infection may be based on either antibody presence or viral isolation. Good herd hygiene and proper facility maintenance are important in managing SI. There is no specific treatment for SI, but supportive care may be helpful.

Trial Data: Safety and Efficacy: The safety of FLUSURE™ RTU was demonstrated in 3 field safety studies conducted in 3 different geographic locations. Nine hundred and six pigs were vaccinated at approximately 3 and 6 weeks of age. No injection site reactions or serious systemic reactions were observed following vaccination.

Efficacy of FLUSURE™ RTU was demonstrated in 2 host animal challenge studies. Pigs were vaccinated at 3-15 days of age and again 14 days later. Sixteen days following the second vaccination, the pigs were challenged with a heterologous isolate of either SIV H1N1 or H3N2. Pigs were necropsied 5 days postchallenge and lung damage evaluated. As compared to nonvaccinated controls, vaccinated pigs had significantly lower rectal temperatures, clinical signs, and lung lesion scores following challenge with either SIV H1N1 or H3N2. Study results are presented in Tables 1-4.

H1N1 Challenge Study:

Table 1. H1N1 serum hemagglutination inhibition geometric mean titers:

	Day 0*	Day 14	Day 28	Day 35
Controls	5.0**	5.0	5.0[a]	11.7[a]
Vaccinates	5.2	5.7	49.5[b]	49.4[b]

* Day 0 = Day of first vaccination

** Titers of < 10 were factored as 5.0 in calculation of geometric mean titers.

a,b Geometric mean titers within the same column with different lower-case superscripts are significantly different.

Table 2. Mean percent lung damage and frequency of clinical signs:

	Mean percent lung damage*	Frequency of animals with at least 1 clinical sign** postchallenge
Controls	23.41[a]	9/18[a]
Vaccinates	5.04[b]	0/19[b]

* Back-transformed least-squares means

** Depression and/or rapid breathing and/or persistent coughing

a,b Geometric mean titers within the same column with different lower-case superscripts are significantly different.

H3N2 Challenge Study:

Table 3. H3N2 serum hemagglutination inhibition geometric mean titers:

	Day 0*	Day 14	Day 28	Day 35
Controls	5.0**	5.0[a]	5.9[a]	9.7[a]
Vaccinates	5.0	7.5[b]	267.2[b]	166.3[b]

* Day 0 = Day of first vaccination

** Titers of < 10 were factored as 5.0 in calculation of geometric mean titers.

a,b Geometric mean titers within the same column with different lower-case superscripts are significantly different.

Table 4. Mean percent lung damage and frequency of clinical signs:

	Mean percent lung damage*	Frequency of animals with at least 1 clinical sign** postchallenge
Controls	33.43[a]	13/20[a]
Vaccinates	0.65[b]	0/19[b]

* Back-transformed least-squares means

** Depression and/or rapid breathing and/or persistent coughing

a,b Geometric mean titers within the same column with different lower-case superscripts are significantly different.

A study evaluating the duration of immunity of the H3N2 component of FLUSURE™ RTU is in progress.

References: Available upon request.

Presentation: 50 dose (100 mL) and 250 dose (500 mL) vials.

Compendium Code No.: 36902000 75-0268-00

FLUVAC® INNOVATOR

Fort Dodge **Vaccine**

Equine Influenza Vaccine, Killed Virus

U.S. Vet. Lic. No.: 112

Contents: This product contains the antigen listed above.

Thimerosal, neomycin and polymyxin B added as preservatives.

Indications: For vaccination of healthy horses as an aid in the prevention of equine influenza due to types A_1 and A_2 viruses.

Dosage and Administration: Horses, inject one 1 mL dose intramuscularly using aseptic technique. Administer a second 1 mL dose 3 to 4 weeks after the first dose. A 1 mL booster dose should be given annually.

Precaution(s): Store in the dark at 2° to 7°C (35° to 45°F). Avoid freezing. Shake well. Use entire contents when first opened.

Caution(s): In some instances, transient local reactions may occur at the injection site.

In case of anaphylactoid reaction, administer epinephrine.

For veterinary use only.

Warning(s): Do not vaccinate within 21 days before slaughter.

Presentation: 1 dose (1 mL) vial.

Compendium Code No.: 10032750 16651B

FLUVAC® INNOVATOR DOUBLE-E FT®

Fort Dodge **Toxoid-Vaccine**

Encephalomyelitis-Influenza Vaccine-Tetanus Toxoid, Eastern & Western, Killed Virus

U.S. Vet. Lic. No.: 112

Contents: This product contains the antigens listed above.

Thimerosal, neomycin and polymyxin B added as preservatives.

Indications: For vaccination of healthy horses as an aid in the prevention of equine encephalomyelitis due to Eastern and Western viruses, equine influenza due to types A_1 and A_2 viruses, and tetanus.

Dosage and Administration: Horses, inject one 1 mL dose intramuscularly using aseptic technique. Administer a second 1 mL dose 3 to 4 weeks after the first dose. A 1 mL booster dose should be given annually.

Precaution(s): Store in the dark at 2° to 7°C (35° to 45°F). Avoid freezing. Shake well. Use entire contents when first opened.

Caution(s): In some instances, transient local reactions may occur at the injection site.

In case of anaphylactoid reaction, administer epinephrine.

For veterinary use only.

Warning(s): Do not vaccinate within 21 days before slaughter.

Presentation: 1 dose (1 mL) vial.

Compendium Code No.: 10032760 16631A

FLUVAC® INNOVATOR DOUBLE-E FT®+EHV

Fort Dodge **Toxoid-Vaccine**

Encephalomyelitis-Rhinopneumonitis-Influenza Vaccine, Eastern & Western, Killed Virus-Tetanus Toxoid

U.S. Vet. Lic. No.: 112

Contents: This product contains the antigens listed above.

Thimerosal, neomycin and polymyxin B added as preservatives.

Indications: For vaccination of healthy horses as an aid in the prevention of equine encephalomyelitis due to Eastern and Western viruses, equine rhinopneumonitis due to type 1 and 4 viruses, equine influenza due to types A_1 and A_2 viruses and tetanus.

Dosage and Administration: Horses, inject one 1 mL dose intramuscularly using aseptic technique. Administer a second 1 mL dose 3 to 4 weeks after the first dose. A 1 mL booster dose should be given annually.

Precaution(s): Store in the dark at 2° to 7°C (35° to 45°F). Avoid freezing. Shake well. Use entire contents when first opened.

Caution(s): In some instances, transient local reactions may occur at the injection site.

In case of anaphylactoid reaction, administer epinephrine.

For veterinary use only.

Warning(s): Do not vaccinate within 21 days before slaughter.

Presentation: 1 dose (1 mL) vial.

Compendium Code No.: 10032770 16601A

FLUVAC® INNOVATOR EHV-4/1

Fort Dodge **Vaccine**

Equine Rhinopneumonitis-Influenza Vaccine, Killed Virus

U.S. Vet. Lic. No.: 112

Contents: This product contains the antigens listed above.

Thimerosal, neomycin and polymyxin B added as preservatives.

Indications: For vaccination of healthy horses as an aid in the prevention of equine rhinopneumonitis due to types 1 and 4 viruses, and equine influenza due to types A_1 and A_2 viruses.

Dosage and Administration: Horses, inject one 1 mL dose intramuscularly using aseptic technique. Administer a second 1 mL dose 3 to 4 weeks after the first dose. A 1 mL booster dose should be given annually.

Precaution(s): Store in the dark at 2° to 7°C (35° to 45°F). Avoid freezing. Shake well. Use entire contents when first opened.

Caution(s): In some instances, transient local reactions may occur at the injection site.

In case of anaphylactoid reaction, administer epinephrine.

For veterinary use only.

Warning(s): Do not vaccinate within 21 days before slaughter.

Presentation: 1 dose (1 mL) vial.

Compendium Code No.: 10032780

16641A

FLUVAC® INNOVATOR TRIPLE-E® FT

Fort Dodge **Toxoid-Vaccine**

Encephalomyelitis-Influenza Vaccine-Tetanus Toxoid, Eastern, Western & Venezuelan, Killed Virus

U.S. Vet. Lic. No.: 112

Contents: This product contains the antigens listed above.

Thimerosal, neomycin and polymyxin B added as preservatives.

Indications: For vaccination of healthy horses as an aid in the prevention of equine encephalomyelitis due to Eastern, Western and Venezuelan viruses, equine influenza due to types A_1 and A_2 viruses and tetanus.

Dosage and Administration: Horses, inject one 1 mL dose intramuscularly using aseptic technique. Administer a second 1 mL dose 3 to 4 weeks after the first dose. A 1 mL booster dose should be given annually.

Precaution(s): Store in the dark at 2° to 7°C (35° to 45°F). Avoid freezing. Shake well. Use entire contents when first opened.

Caution(s): In some instances, transient local reactions may occur at the injection site.

In case of anaphylactoid reaction, administer epinephrine.

For veterinary use only.

Warning(s): Do not vaccinate within 21 days before slaughter.

Presentation: 1 dose (1 mL) vial.

Compendium Code No.: 10032790

16621A

FLUVAC® INNOVATOR TRIPLE-E® FT+EHV

Fort Dodge **Toxoid-Vaccine**

Encephalomyelitis-Rhinopneumonitis-Influenza Vaccine-Tetanus Toxoid, Eastern, Western & Venezuelan, Killed Virus

U.S. Vet. Lic. No.: 112

Contents: This product contains the antigens listed above.

Thimerosal, neomycin and polymyxin B added as preservatives.

Indications: For vaccination of healthy horses as an aid in the prevention of equine encephalomyelitis due to Eastern, Western and Venezuelan viruses, equine rhinopneumonitis due to type 1 and 4 viruses, equine influenza due to types A_1 and A_2 viruses and tetanus.

Dosage and Administration: Horses, inject one 1 mL dose intramuscularly using aseptic technique. Administer a second 1 mL dose 3 to 4 weeks after the first dose. A 1 mL booster dose should be given annually.

Precaution(s): Store in the dark at 2° to 7°C (35° to 45°F). Avoid freezing. Shake well. Use entire contents when first opened.

Caution(s): In some instances, transient local reactions may occur at the injection site.

In case of anaphylactoid reaction, administer epinephrine.

For veterinary use only.

Warning(s): Do not vaccinate within 21 days before slaughter.

Presentation: 1 dose (1 mL) vial.

Compendium Code No.: 10032800

16351B

FLY GUARD™ COLLAR/BROW BAND

Farnam **Parasiticide Collar**

EPA Reg. No.: 4691-140-270

Active Ingredient(s):

Cyano (3-phenoxyphenyl) methyl-4-chloro-alpha-(1-methylethyl) benzeneacetate 8.0%
Other Ingredients 92.0%
Total 100.0%

This product contains the toxic inert ingredient Di-(2-ethylhexyl) adipate.

Indications: For control of face flies and horn flies and to aid in control of house flies and stable flies on horses and ponies.

FLY GUARD™ Collar/Brow Band utilizes a breakaway feature providing assurance that if the collar becomes snagged, it will automatically release with the tension of the horse pulling.

Directions for Use: It is a violation of Federal law to use this product in a manner inconsistent with its labeling.

For control of face flies, horn flies, and as an aid in the control of house flies and stable flies, the collar/brow band should be placed on your horse when pests first appear in spring. The bands may remain effective up to 4-5 months. Place collar/brow band around horse's throat with closure on left side of horse's head and fasten. Make sure fit is snug so that neck band does not slide down neck. Cut off excess strap extending more than one inch beyond fastener. When effectiveness diminishes, replace with a new FLY GUARD™ Collar/Brow Band.

Precautionary Statements: Hazards to Humans: Caution: Wash thoroughly with soap and water after handling and before eating or smoking. Avoid contamination of feed and food stuffs.

Environmental Hazards: This pesticide is toxic to fish. Do not contaminate water by disposal of used product. Use this product only as specified on the label.

Storage and Disposal: Store in a cool place. Wrap removed bands and put in trash collection.

Warning(s): Keep out of reach of children.

Presentation: One 45 g FLY GUARD™ collar/brow band.

This product contains Ectrin® Insecticide. Ectrin is a registered trademark of Boehringer Ingelheim.

Licensed under U.S. Patent No. 4,062,968 to Sumitomo Chemical Co. and U.S. Patent No. 4,196,075 to Shell Oil Company.

Compendium Code No.: 10000200

FLYPEL® INSECTICIDE SPRAY FOR HORSES

Virbac **Topical Insecticide**

EPA Reg. No.: 2382-132

Active Ingredient(s):

Permethrin: [(3-phenoxyphenyl)methyl(±)cis-trans-3-(2,2-dichloroethenyl) 2,2-dimethylcyclopropanecarboxylate]* 2.0%
Inert Ingredients 98.0%
Total 100.0%

*cis-trans isomer ratio: Min. 35% (±)cis, Max. 65%(±)trans

Indications: FLYPEL® Insecticide Spray provides hours of continuing protection from biting and nuisance insects, ticks, mosquitoes and gnats. Contains sunscreen. Dries quickly. Silicone confers a high gloss to the coat.

Directions for Use: It is a violation of Federal law to use this product in a manner inconsistent with its labeling. Shake Well. Spray in a well ventilated area. Spray areas of hide that are subject to attack by nuisance and biting flies. Wet hair thoroughly. Avoid spraying onto horse's face and eyes, treating these areas by wiping with a spray-moistened cloth or sponge. Control ticks by spraying around the ears and areas on which ticks attach. Repeat treatment as necessary.

Precautionary Statements: Hazards to Humans and Domestic Animals:

Hazards to Humans: May cause eye irritation. Do not get in eyes or on skin or clothing. Avoid breathing spray mist. Avoid contamination of food. Wash hands after using. Remove contaminated clothing and wash before reuse.

Statement of Practical Treatment: If in Eyes: Flush with plenty of water. Call a physician if irritation persists.

Storage and Disposal: Storage: Store in a cool dry area, away from heat and open flame. Disposal: Do not reuse empty container. Wrap in several layers of newspaper and discard in trash.

Physical and Chemical Hazards: Do not store or use near heat or open flame.

Warning(s): Do not apply to horses to be slaughtered for food.

Keep out of reach of children.

Presentation: 16 fl oz (474 mL) and 1 gallon.

Compendium Code No.: 10230311

FLY-RID PLUS

Durvet **Premise and Topical Insecticide**

Multi-Purpose Insect Control Spray

EPA Reg. No.: 1021-1740-12281

Active Ingredient(s):

Permethrin [(3-Phenoxyphenyl) methyl (±)cis-trans-3-2 (2,2-dichloroethenyl) 2,2-dimethylcyoclopropanecarboxylate)] 0.50%
Other Ingredients 99.50%
Total 100.00%

Indications: For indoor/outdoor and on-animal use. Kills and repels flies (6 types), mosquitoes and gnats. 35 day control of fleas and ticks on dogs. 60 day control of cockroaches, spiders and ants.

Directions for Use: It is a violation of Federal law to use this product in a manner inconsistent with its labeling.

Read entire label before each use. Shake well before using. For pet use, use only on dogs.

Indoor Application: For spot application only. Do not use as a space spray indoors. Do not apply to classrooms while in use. In the home, all food processing surfaces and utensils should be covered during treatment or thoroughly washed before use. Exposed food/feed should be covered or removed.

Surface Spraying: For 60 day (two months) control of cockroaches, scorpions, millipedes, centipedes, ants, spiders and crickets. Spray into hiding places, cracks and crevices and behind shelves and drawers.

To Control Fleas (Adults and Larvae) and Ticks, including ticks which may carry Lyme Disease (Adults and Larvae): Thoroughly spray infested areas, pet beds, resting quarters, nearby cracks and crevices, along and behind baseboards, moldings, window and door frames, and entire areas of floor and floor covering. Fresh bedding should be placed in animal quarters following treatment. Repeat treatment as needed. Allow to dry thoroughly before allowing pets to contact treated areas.

On Livestock:

To Protect Cattle (Beef and Dairy), Goats, Sheep, Hogs and Horses from Horn Flies, Face Flies, House Flies, Mosquitoes and Gnats: Apply a light mist sufficient to wet the surface of the hair. For face flies, spray face and head, but do not spray into eyes.

To Control Stable Flies, Horse Flies and Deer Flies: Apply at a rate of 2 ounces per adult animal sufficient to wet the hair thoroughly. Repeat treatment daily or at intervals necessary to give continued protection.

To Control Blood Sucking Lice: Apply to the infested areas of the animal using a stiff brush to get the spray to the base of the hair. Repeat every 3 weeks if required.

To Control Poultry Lice: Spray roosts, walls and nests or cages thoroughly. This should be followed by spraying over the birds with a fine mist.

On Dogs: Consult a veterinarian before using this product on debilitated, medicated, aged, pregnant or nursing dogs. Sensitivities may occur after using any pesticide product for pets. If signs of sensitivity occur bathe your pet with mild soap and rinse with large amounts of water. If signs continue, consult a veterinarian immediately.

To Control Fleas, Ticks and Lice: Start spraying at the tail, moving the dispenser rapidly and making sure that the animal's entire body is covered, including the legs and under body. While spraying, fluff the hair so that the spray will penetrate to the skin. Make sure spray wets thoroughly but do not saturate animal. Do not spray into eyes or face. Avoid contact with genitalia. Use protective gloves or mitts when applying product. Repeat monthly as necessary for control.

Note: Not recommended for use on puppies less that 12 weeks old. Do not use on cats or kittens.

Outdoor Application:

To Control Ticks, including ticks which may carry Lyme Disease (Perimeter Treatment): Use as a residual treatment to control ticks, including Deer Tick, Lone Star Tick, Brown Dog Tick, American Dog Tick and Western Black Legged Tick. Treat around windows and doors, porches, screens, eaves, patios, garages, under stairways and in crawl spaces where these pests may enter. Treat a band of vegetation and leaf litter 6 to 10 feet wide around and the outside of buildings to help control ticks occurring there. To help control ticks in outdoor activity areas, treat a band of vegetation and leaf litter 6 to 10 feet wide and adjacent to activity areas, especially where dense vegetation occurs.

Precautionary Statements: Hazards to Humans and Domestic Animals:

Caution: Wash thoroughly after handling and before smoking or eating. Avoid contamination of feed and foodstuffs. Remove pets and birds and cover fish aquariums before surface applications. Do not use on humans. Do not allow children or pets to contact treated areas until surfaces are dry.

First Aid:

If Inhaled: Remove affected person to fresh air. If person is not breathing, call 911 or an ambulance, then give artificial respiration, preferably mouth-to-mouth, if possible.

If in Eyes: Hold eye open and rinse slowly and gently with water for 15-20 minutes. Remove contact lenses, if present, after the first 5 minutes, then continue rinsing eye. Call a poison control center or doctor for treatment advice.

If on Skin: Rinse skin immediately with plenty of soap and water for 15-20 minutes. Call a poison control center or doctor for treatment advice. Have the product container or label with you when calling a poison control center or doctor or going for treatment.

F

For information regarding medical emergencies or pesticide incidents, call the International Poison Center at 1-888-740-8712.

Environmental Hazards: This product is toxic to fish. Do not apply directly to water, to areas where surface water is present or to intertidal areas below the high water mark. Do not contaminate water by disposing of equipment washwaters.

Storage and Disposal: Do not contaminate water, food or feed by storage or disposal.

Container Disposal: Do not reuse container. Wrap container in several layers of newspaper and discard in trash.

Warning(s): Keep out of reach of children.

Presentation: 32 oz (946 mL).

Compendium Code No.: 10842050 Iss. 3/02

FLYSECT® CITRONELLA SPRAY

Equicare **Topical Insecticide**

EPA Reg. No.: 4816-366-11787

Active Ingredient(s):

Pyrethrins 0.1%
Piperonyl butoxide, technical* 1.0%
Butoxypolypropylene glycol 15.0%
Inert ingredients:**
Oil of citronella 1.0%
Other inerts 82.9%

*Equivalent to 0.8% of (butylcarbityl) (6-propylpiperonyl) ether and 0.2% related compounds.

**Contains petroleum distillate.

Indications: FLYSECT® Citronella Spray provides protection against flies while imparting a high sheen to the hair when brushed out. For use on horses to kill and repel stable flies, house flies, face flies, horse flies, deer flies, mosquitoes and gnats. Also can be used as a grooming aid and coat conditioner.

Dosage and Administration: It is a violation of federal law to use the product in a manner inconsistent with its labeling.

One (1) to two (2) ounces per head per day gives adequate protection. Apply by either a soft cloth or a fine mist spray.

Wipe on: First, brush the animal to remove excess dirt and dust. Moisten (but do not wet to the point of dripping) a soft cloth and rub over the hair. It is best to apply by rubbing against hair growth. Give special attention to the legs, shoulders, shanks, neck and facial areas where flies are most often seen. Only a light application is required. Avoid using an excessive amount. Do not wet the skin. After application, brush out thoroughly. Repeat once a day or as required.

Spray: May be applied as a fine mist spray to the stable area and over and around stabled horses for fast paralysis and killing of flies. Do not wet the horse's skin or exceed two (2) ounces per application.

Precaution(s):

Storage: Store in the original container inaccessible to children and pets.

Disposal: Do not re-use the container. Wrap the container in several layers of newspaper and discard it in the trash.

Caution(s): Keep out of the reach of children.

Precautionary Statements:

Hazards to Humans and Domestic Animals: Harmful if swallowed. Remove or cover exposed foods before spraying.

Statement of Practical Treatment:

If swallowed, do not induce vomiting unless directed by a physician. Petroleum distillate may cause aspiration. Contact a physician immediately.

If in eyes, flush eyes with plenty of water. Contact a physician if irritation persists.

If inhaled, remove victim to fresh air. Apply artificial respiration if indicated.

If on skin, remove contaminated clothing and wash the affected areas with plenty of soap and water.

Environmental Hazards: This product is toxic to fish. Do not apply directly to water. Do not apply where runoff is likely to occur. Do not contaminate water by the cleaning of equipment or the disposal of wastes. Apply this product only as specified on the label.

Physical or Chemical Hazards: Do not use or store near heat or open flame.

Warning(s): Do not apply to dairy animals.

Seller makes no warranty, express or implied, concerning the use of this product other than indicated on the label. Buyer assumes all risk of use and handling of this material when such use and handling are contrary to label instructions.

Presentation: 32 oz. with sprayer and 128 oz. refills.

* FLYSECT and Equicare are trademarks of Sandoz Ltd.

Compendium Code No.: 14470020

FLYSECT® REPELLENT SPRAY

Equicare **Topical Insecticide**

EPA Reg. No.: 51793-154-11787

Active Ingredient(s):

Pyrethrins 0.15%
Piperonyl butoxide, technical* 1.00%
N-octyl bicycloheptene dicarboximide 0.50%
Di-n-propyl isocinchomeronate 0.50%
Inert ingredients 97.85%

*Equivalent to 0.80% (butylcarbityl) (6-propylpiperonyl) ether and 0.20% related compounds.

Indications: FLYSECT® Repellent Spray provides effective control of stable flies, horse flies, deer flies, face flies, gnats and mosquitoes for horses.

Directions for Use: It is a violation of Federal law to use this product in a manner inconsistent with its labeling.

Use only in well-ventilated area. Hold the bottle in an upright position when spraying.

Use full strength to control stable flies, horse flies, deer flies, face flies, gnats and mosquitoes. Apply to the face, legs, flanks, top line and other body areas commonly attacked by these flies. Do not wet the horse's skin with excessive spray. After the application, brush thoroughly. Repeat the treatment as needed.

Precautionary Statements: Hazards to Humans and Domestic Animals:

Humans: Harmful if swallowed or inhaled. Avoid inhaling mist. Keep out of the eyes. Avoid contamination of food. Wash hands with soap and water after using.

Animals: Avoid treatment of foals under six weeks of age. If treatment is necessary, spray on the tips of the fingers and rub the coat.

Environmental Hazards: This product is toxic to fish. Keep out of lakes, streams, ponds, tidal marshes and estuaries. Do not apply where runoff is likely to occur.

Physical or Chemical Hazards: Flammable. Keep away from heat and open flame.

Storage and Disposal:

Storage: Do not use or store near heat or open flame.

Disposal: Do not reuse the empty container. Wrap the container and put it in the trash collection.

Warning(s): Keep out of the reach of children.

Disclaimer: Seller makes no warranty, express or implied, concerning the use of this product other than indicated on the label. Buyer assumes all risk of use and handling of this material when such use and handling are contrary to label instructions.

Presentation: 32 oz with sprayer.

* FLYSECT and Equicare are trademarks of Sandoz Ltd.

Compendium Code No.: 14470041

FLYSECT® ROLL-ON FLY REPELLENT FACE LOTION

Equicare **Insect Repellent**

EPA Reg. No.: 270-107

Active Ingredient(s):

Pyrethrins 0.40%
Piperonyl Butoxide Technical* 1.00%
Di-n-propyl isocinchomeronate 1.00%
N-octyl bicycloheptene dicarboximide 0.40%
Other Ingredients: 97.20%

*Equivalent to 0.80% (butylcarbityl)(6-propylpiperonyl) ether and 0.20% related compounds.

Indications: Fly repellent for horses, ponies and dogs. Repels house flies, stable flies, face flies, and horn flies from sensitive areas of the face and head and also from wounds. Kills on contact.

Directions for Use: It is a violation of Federal law to use this product in a manner inconsistent with its labeling.

Read entire label before each use.

Use only on horses, ponies or dogs.

Shake well before using. Remove cap from bottle. Apply around animal's nose, eyes, ears, mouth; also around wounds and other surface lesions. Do not put solution directly in animal's eyes, mouth or wounds. Reapply everyday. Replace cap after use. Do not use on horses intended for human consumption.

Precautionary Statements: Hazards to Humans and Domestic Animals:

Caution: Harmful if swallowed. For animal use only. Do not use on animals under 12 weeks. Consult a veterinarian before using this product on debilitated, aged, medicated, pregnant or nursing animals. Not for human use. Wash hands after using. Sensitivities may occur after using any pesticide product for pets. If signs of sensitivity occur, bathe your pet with mild soap and rinse with large amounts of water.

If signs continue, consult a veterinarian immediately.

First Aid: If swallowed do not induce vomiting. Call a physician or Poison Control Center immediately.

Environmental Hazards: This product is toxic to fish. Keep out of lakes, streams or ponds. Do not apply where runoff is likely to occur. Do not contaminate water by cleaning of equipment or disposal of wastes. Apply this product only as specified on the label.

Storage and Disposal:

Storage: Store in original container in a cool place inaccessible to children and pets.

Disposal: Dispose of container by wrapping in several layers of newspaper and discard in trash.

Warning(s): Do not use on horses intended for human consumption.

Keep out of reach of children.

Presentation: 2 fl oz (59 mL) roll-on applicator.

Compendium Code No.: 14470250 0B0

FLYSECT® SUPER-7

Equicare **External Parasiticide**

EPA Reg. No.: 51793-91-11787

Active Ingredient(s):

Permethrin [(3-phenoxyphenyl) methyl (±) cis-trans-3-(2,2-dichloroethenyl)-2,2-dimethylcyclopropanecarboxylate] 0.20%
Pyrethrins 0.20%
Piperonyl butoxide, technical* 0.50%
N-octyl bicycloheptene dicarboximide 2.00%
Di-n-propyl isocinchomeronate 1.00%
Butoxypolypropylene glycol 5.00%
Inert ingredients 91.10%

*Equivalent to 0.40% (butylcarbityl) (6-propylpiperonyl) ether and 0.10% related compounds.

Indications: FLYSECT® Super-7 Repellent Spray for horses and dogs combines oil of aloe with other repellents to moisturize the skin and produce a show condition coat. It contains two insecticide systems and three repellents for use on horses and dogs for the immediate and residual control of face flies, stable flies, house flies, mosquitoes, gnats, mites, chiggers and lice.

Dosage and Administration: It is a violation of federal law to use the product in a manner inconsistent with its labeling.

For initial treatment, apply once a day for 2-3 days. As the infestation subsides, repeat the treatment every 5-10 days or as prescribed by a veterinarian. Also, re-apply every time the animal is washed or exposed to a heavy rain. Use only in a well ventilated area. Hold the bottle in an upright position when spraying.

Horses: Thoroughly brush the horse's coat prior to application, to remove loose dirt and debris. For dirty horses, and as a preparation for show grooming, clean the coat with a shampoo. Wait until the coat is completely dry before applying. Cover the entire surface of the animal with the spray, but avoid getting the product into the horse's eyes or other sensitive areas such as the mouth or nose. Brush the coat against the grain while spraying to ensure adequate penetration of the product. As a wipe, apply liberally with a clean cloth or sponge. Make sure the spray has completely dried before covering with any tack.

Dogs: Cover the animal's eyes with a hand. With a firm stroke to get a proper spray mist, spray the head, ears and chest until damp. With fingertips, rub into the face around the mouth, nose and eyes. Then spray the neck, middle and hind quarters, finishing with the legs. For the best penetration of the spray to the skin, direct the spray against the natural lay of the hair. On long-haired dogs, rub a hand against the lay of the hair, spraying the ruffled hair directly behind the hand. Make sure the spray thoroughly wets the ticks. Repeat the treatment as needed.

Precaution(s):

Storage: Do not use or store near heat or open flame.

Disposal: Do not re-use the empty container. Wrap the container and put it in the trash collection.

Caution(s): Keep out of the reach of children.

Precautionary Statements: Hazards to Humans and Domestic Animals:

Humans: Do not get on eyes, skin or clothing. Wear protective gloves or a mitt when applying the product. May cause eye injury. Wear safety glasses or other appropriate eye protection. Harmful if swallowed. Avoid inhaling vapors. Wash hands with soap and water after using. Do not contaminate foodstuffs. Remove contaminated clothing and wash before re-use. Do not smoke while using. If accidental contact occurs, see Statement of Practical Treatment.

Animals: Avoid contact with eyes, or mucous membranes. Avoid the treatment of nursing puppies and foals under six weeks of age unless prescribed by a veterinarian.

Environmental Hazards: This product is toxic to fish. Do not apply directly to water. Do not apply where runoff is likely to occur.

Physical or Chemical Hazards: Flammable. Keep away from heat and open flame. Contains alcohol. Do not apply to painted or finished wood surfaces.

Statement of Practical Treatment:

If swallowed, call a physician or poison control center. Drink one or two glasses of water and induce vomiting by touching the back of the throat with a finger. Do not induce vomiting or give anything by mouth to an unconscious person.

If in eyes, flush with plenty of water. Get medical attention if irritation persists.

If on skin, wash with plenty of soap and water. Get medical attention if irritation persists.

Presentation: 32 oz. with sprayer, 32 oz. and 128 oz. refills.

* FLYSECT and Equicare are trademarks of Sandoz Ltd.

Compendium Code No.: 14470050

FLYSECT® SUPER-C

Equicare **Topical Insecticide**

EPA Reg. No.: 51793-107-11787

Active Ingredient(s):

Permethrin [(3-phenoxyphenyl) methyl (±) cis-trans-3-(2,2-dichloroethenyl)-2,2-dimethylcyclopropanecarboxylate]*	1.00%
Pyrethrins	0.50%
Piperonyl butoxide, technical**	1.85%
N-octyl bicycloheptene dicarboximide	3.10%
Di-n-propyl isocinchomeronate	2.50%
Inert ingredients	91.05%

*Cis-trans isomer ratio: Min. 35% (±) cis Max. 65% (±) trans.

**Equivalent to 1.48% (butylcarbityl) (6-propylpiperonyl) ether and 0.37% related compounds.

Indications: FLYSECT® Super-C Repellent Concentrate contains two insecticide systems and one repellent for use on horses for the immediate and temporary control of face flies, stable flies, horse flies, deer flies, mosquitoes, gnats, mites, chiggers, lice and house flies.

Dosage and Administration: It is a violation of federal law to use the product in a manner inconsistent with its labeling.

Thoroughly brush the horse's coat prior to application to remove loose dirt and debris. For dirty horses, and as a preparation for show grooming, clean the coat with a shampoo. Use at a one (1) to four (4) ratio with water. Put the required amount of concentrate into a sprayer or mixing container and add the appropriate amount of water (1 qt. of concentrate makes 5 qts. of spray). Cover the entire surface of the animal with the spray, but avoid getting the product into the horse's eyes, or other sensitive areas such as the mouth or nose. Spray the horse's coat especially around the shoulders, flanks, neck and legs. Brush the coat against the grain while spraying to ensure adequate penetration of the product. Make sure the application has completely dried on the hair coat before covering with tack. As a wipe, apply liberally with a clean cloth or sponge. For initial treatment, apply FLYSECT® Super-C once a day. As the infestation subsides and protection builds, re-apply every 2-3 days as needed. Also, re-apply every time the animal is washed or exposed to a heavy rain.

Precaution(s):

Storage: Store in a cool, dry area. Do not contaminate water, food or feed by storage or disposal.

Disposal: Do not re-use the container. Wrap and put it in the trash.

Caution(s): Keep out of the reach of children.

Precautionary Statements: Hazards to Humans and Domestic Animals:

Humans: May cause eye injury. Harmful if swallowed or inhaled. Avoid inhaling mist. Avoid contact with the skin, eyes or clothing. Remove contaminated clothing and wash before re-use. Wash hands with soap and water after using. If accidental contact occurs, see Statement of Practical Treatment.

Animals: Avoid contact with eyes or mucous membranes. Do not treat foals under six weeks of age. Do not use this or any other pesticide on sick, old, or debilitated animals.

Physical or Chemical Hazards: Keep away from heat and open flame. Do not apply to painted or finished wood surfaces.

Environmental Hazards: This product is toxic to fish. Do not apply directly to water. Do not apply where runoff is likely to occur. Do not contaminate water when disposing of equipment washwaters.

Statement of Practical Treatment:

If swallowed, call a physician or poison control center. Drink one or two glasses of water and induce vomiting by touching the back of the throat with a finger. Never give anything by mouth to an unconscious person.

If inhaled, remove the victim to fresh air. Get medical attention.

If on skin, wash with plenty of soap and water. Get medical attention if irritation persists.

If in eyes, flush with plenty of water. Get medical attention if irritation persists.

Warning(s): Do not use on animals intended for food.

Seller makes no warranty, express or implied, concerning the use of this product other than indicated on the label. Buyer assumes all risk of use and handling of this material when such use and handling are contrary to label instructions.

Presentation: 16 oz. and 32 oz. spray bottles.

* FLYSECT and Equicare are trademarks of Sandoz Ltd.

Compendium Code No.: 14470060

FLYSECT® WATER-BASED REPELLENT SPRAY

Equicare **Premise and Topical Insecticide**

EPA Reg. No.: 21165-34-270

Active Ingredient(s):

Permethrin [(3-Phenoxyphenyl)methyl (±) cis-trans**-3-(2,2-dichloroethenyl)2,2-dimethylcyclopropanecarboxylate]	0.150%
Pyrethrins	0.075%
Piperonyl butoxide, technical*	0.750%
Inert Ingredients:	99.025%
	100.000%

*Equivalent to 0.60% (Butylcarbityl)(6-Propylpiperonyl) ether and to 0.15% related compounds.

**cis/trans ratio min. 35% (±) cis and max. 65% (±) trans

Indications: FLYSECT® Water-Based Repellent Spray kills and repels stable flies, horse flies, face flies, deer flies, bot flies, house flies, horn flies, mosquitoes, gnats, ticks, fleas, and chiggers. For use on horses and animal quarters.

Directions for Use: It is a violation of Federal law to use this product in a manner inconsistent with its labeling.

For use on horses. Use full strength. This non-oily insecticide/repellent may be applied with a trigger spray applicator, or as a wipe.

Directions for Trigger Spray Use: Remove excess dirt and dust. Apply light spray mist to coat while brushing lightly against lay of the hair. Avoid spray in eyes and mucous membranes. Apply with sponge or soft cloth to those areas.

Directions For Wipe-On Use: Thoroughly brush horse to remove excess dirt and dust. Extremely dirty horses should be shampooed, rinsed, and allowed to dry before applying wipe. Use a sponge or clean soft cloth or mitt. Apply FLYSECT® Water-Based Repellent Spray liberally over areas to be protected. Pay special attention to legs, belly, shoulders, neck, and facial areas. Avoid eyes and mucous membranes.

To kill and repel flying insects in animal quarters: Spray in areas where insects congregate. Direct spray to contact insects for rapid knockdown and kill. Spray around outside of door facings, screens to render area unattractive to insects. This helps to repel insects and prevent entrance into building.

Precautionary Statements: Hazards to Humans and Domestic Animals:

Caution: For animal use only. Not for use on humans. Harmful if swallowed. Avoid breathing spray mist. Avoid contact with eyes, skin or clothing. Wash hands with soap and water after using. Avoid contamination of food and foodstuffs.

Environmental Hazards: This product is extremely toxic to fish. Do not apply directly to any body of water. Do not contaminate water when disposing of equipment washwaters.

Physical and Chemical Hazard: Do not use or store near heat or open flame.

Statement of Practical Treatment: If in eyes, flush eyes with plenty of water. Call a physician if irritation persists. If swallowed, call a physician or poison control center immediately. Drink 1 or 2 glasses of water and induce vomiting by touching back of throat with finger. Do not induce vomiting or give anything by mouth to an unconscious person. If on skin, remove contaminated clothing and wash affected areas with soap and water. It inhaled, remove victim to fresh air. Apply artificial respiration if indicated.

Storage and Disposal: Storage - Store in a cool, dry place. Do not store near heat or open flame. Disposal - Securely wrap original container in several layers of newspaper and discard in trash. Container Disposal - Do not reuse empty container. Wrap container and put in trash.

Warning(s): Not for use on horses intended for human consumption.

Keep out of reach of children.

Disclaimer: Buyer assumes all risks of use, storage or handling of this material not in strict accordance with label directions and usage. In no event shall Seller's liability exceed the purchase price of this product.

Presentation: 32 fl oz (1 qt) 946 mL.

Compendium Code No.: 14470070

FLYS-OFF® FLY REPELLENT OINTMENT

Farnam **Topical Insecticide**

EPA Reg. No.: 270-103

Active Ingredient(s):

Piperonyl Butoxide, Technical*	0.5%
Pyrethrins I and II	0.2%
Di-n-propyl isocinchomeronate	1.0%
Other Ingredients	98.3%

*Equivalent to 0.4% (butylcarbityl) (6-propylpiperonyl) ether and 0.1% of related compounds.

Indications: Repels house flies, stable flies, face flies and horn flies from wounds and open sores. Also kills them on contact. Effective for hours. For use on dogs, ponies and horses.

Directions for Use: It is a violation of Federal law to use this product in a manner inconsistent with its labeling.

Read entire label before each use.

Use only on dogs, ponies or horses.

To treat superficial wounds, abrasions, sores and scratches, apply enough ointment to cover the wound. Apply directly to the wound. Repeat every day.

Do not use on animals under 12 weeks. Consult a veterinarian before using this product on debilitated, aged, pregnant, nursing or medicated animals. Sensitivities may occur after using any pesticide product for pets. If signs of sensitivity occur, bathe your pet with mild soap and rinse with large amounts of water. If signs continue, consult a veterinarian immediately.

Precautionary Statements: Caution: Not for human use. Wash hands after using.

Environmental Hazards: This product is toxic to fish. Keep out of lakes, streams or ponds. Do not apply where runoff is likely to occur.

Storage and Disposal:

Storage: Store tightly in a cool, dry place.

Disposal: Do not reuse empty container. Wrap container and put in trash.

Warning(s): Do not use on animals that are to be used for human consumption.

Keep out of reach of children.

Presentation: 2 oz (56.7 g) and 5 oz (141.8 g) jars.

Compendium Code No.: 10000670 0A1 / 9DD7

FLYS-OFF® INSECT REPELLENT FOR DOGS

Farnam **External Parasiticide**

EPA Reg. No.: 270-218

Active Ingredient(s):

Butoxypolypropylene Glycol 17.589%
Technical Piperonyl Butoxide* 0.375%
Pyrethrins 0.136%
Other Ingredients:** 81.900%

*Equivalent to 0.3% (butylcarbityl) (6-propylpiperonyl) ether and 0.075% related compounds.

**Contains petroleum distillates.

Contains no CFC's or other ozone depleting substances.

Indications: Use only on dogs and non-food/non-feed surfaces to repel flies, gnats and mosquitoes.

Directions for Use: It is a violation of Federal law to use this product in a manner inconsistent with its labeling.

Read the entire label before each use.

Use Restrictions: Use only on dogs and non-food/non-feed surfaces to repel flies, gnats and mosquitoes. Do not use on puppies less than 12 weeks old or on cats.

Consult a veterinarian before using this product on debilitated, aged, pregnant, nursing or medicated animals.

Sensitivities may occur after using any pesticide product for pets. If signs of sensitivity occur, bathe your pet with mild soap and rinse with large amounts of water. If signs continue, consult a veterinarian immediately.

Application Directions for Dogs: Hold container 8 to 10 inches from dog and lightly spray on back, underside, legs, back of neck, base of tail, and inside and outside ears. Do not get in eyes, nose or mouth. Avoid any contact with sores. If hissing noise disturbs dog during ear application, mist cotton swab and rub product on ear surfaces. Repeat every day.

Application Directions for Surfaces: Hold container 8 to 10 inches from non-food/non-feed surfaces such as pet bedding where insects rest. Do not spray this product when there is food present or when there are pets present. Remove any pets from the area before spraying. Repeat application when needed.

Precautionary Statements: Hazards to Humans and Domestic Animals:

Warning: Causes substantial but temporary eye injury. Do not get in eyes, on skin or on clothing. Wear safety glasses. Harmful if swallowed. Wash hands thoroughly with soap and water after handling. Remove contaminated clothing and wash before reuse. Do not spray food, feed, serving or cooking utensils.

First Aid:

If in Eyes: Hold eyelids open and flush with a steady, gentle stream of water for 15 minutes. Get medical attention.

If on Skin: Wash with plenty of soap and water. Get medical attention if irritation persists.

If Swallowed: Call a physician or Poison Control Center. Drink 1 or 2 glasses of water and induce vomiting by touching finger to back of throat. Do not induce vomiting or give anything by mouth to an unconscious person.

Environmental Hazards: This product is extremely toxic to fish. Do not apply directly to water. Do not contaminate water when disposing of equipment washwaters.

Physical or Chemical Hazards: Extremely flammable. Do not use or store near fire, sparks, or heated surfaces. Turn off pilot lights in gas appliances and unplug or turn off electrical equipment in the use area. After airing out phase is completed, relight pilot lights and reconnect electrical current. Do not smoke in the use area. Contents under pressure. Do not puncture or incinerate container. Exposure to temperatures above 130°F may cause bursting. Incineration of container may cause explosion.

Storage and Disposal:

Storage: Store only in a cool, dry place away from heat and sunlight and inaccessible to children and pets.

Disposal: When empty, replace cap, securely wrap in newspaper, and discard in trash. Do not incinerate or puncture.

Warning(s): Keep out of reach of children.

Presentation: 6 oz. (170 g) and 9 oz (255 g) aerosol spray cans.

Compendium Code No.: 10000650 9DD9 / 0C1

FLYS-OFF® LOTION INSECT REPELLENT FOR DOGS

Farnam **External Parasiticide**

EPA Reg. No.: 270-225

Active Ingredient(s):

Butoxypolypropylene Glycol 17.589%
Pyrethrins 0.136%
Piperonyl Butoxide* 0.375%
Inert Ingredients:** 81.900%

*Equivalent to 0.3% (butylcarbityl) (6-propylpiperonyl) ether and 0.075% related compounds.

**Contains petroleum distillates.

Indications: Use only on dogs and non-food/non-feed surfaces to repel flies, gnats and mosquitoes.

Directions for Use: It is a violation of Federal law to use this product in a manner inconsistent with its labeling.

Read the entire label before each use.

Use Restrictions: Use only on dogs and non-food/non-feed surfaces to repel flies, gnats and mosquitoes.

Do not use on puppies less than 12 weeks old or on cats. Consult a veterinarian before using this product on debilitated, aged, pregnant, nursing or medicated animals. Sensitivities may occur after using any pesticide product for pets. If signs of sensitivity occur, bathe your pet with mild soap and rinse with large amounts of water. If signs continue, consult a veterinarian immediately.

Application Directions: Spray lightly, or moisten cloth or sponge with FLYS-OFF® Lotion and rub on lightly. Use in and around ears, base of tail, and underside. Avoid any sores. Also apply a thin film to dog's coat. Do not get in eyes, nose or mouth. Repeat every day.

Precautionary Statements: Hazards to Humans and Domestic Animals:

Warning: Causes substantial but temporary eye injury. Do not get in eyes or on clothing. Wear safety glasses. Harmful if swallowed, inhaled, or absorbed through the skin. Avoid breathing vapor. Wash hands thoroughly with soap and water after handling. Remove contaminated clothing and wash before reuse.

First Aid:

If Swallowed: Do not induce vomiting. Contact a physician immediately. Product contains aromatic solvents.

If in Eyes: Flush with water for 15 minutes, contact a physician.

If on Skin: Wash with plenty of soap and water. Get medical attention if irritation persists.

If Inhaled: Remove victim to fresh air. Contact a physician if irritation persists.

Environmental Hazards: This product is extremely toxic to fish. Do not apply directly to water. Do not contaminate water when disposing of equipment washwaters.

Physical or Chemical Hazards: Flammable. Keep away from heat and open flame.

Storage and Disposal:

Storage: Store tightly closed in a cool, dry place inaccessible to children and pets, and away from heat and sunlight.

Disposal: Do not reuse empty container. Rinse bottle. Wrap and put in trash.

Warning(s): Keep out of reach of children.

Presentation: 6 fl oz (177 mL) pump spray bottle.

Compendium Code No.: 10000660 9EE8

FLY-ZAP™ FLY BAIT

Aspen **Premise Insecticide**

EPA Reg. No.: 53871-3-40940

Active Ingredient(s):

(Z)-9-tricosene 0.025%
Methomyl (S-Methyl-N-[(Methylcarbamoyl)oxy]thioacetimidate) 1.000%
Inert Ingredients: 98.975%

Indications: Fly bait for outdoor use.

Dosage and Administration: It is a violation of Federal Law to use this product in a manner inconsistent with its labeling. FLY-ZAP™ Fly Bait is an improved fly bait formula containing a sex attractant and feeding synergists which encourages both male and female flies to remain in the treated area and stimulates vigorous feeding on the bait. Bait should be scattered over specified fly feeding surfaces daily or as needed to provide initial knockdown and reduction of fly populations. Distribute bait from container or other device to avoid handling bait.

Personal Protective Clothing: Use only when wearing the following personal protective clothing during loading, applications, repairing and cleaning of application equipment, and disposal of the pesticide: long-sleeve shirt; long-legged pants; shoes and socks; gloves.

Important! If pesticide comes in contact with skin, wash off with soap and water.

Always wash hands, face and arms with soap and water before using tobacco products, eating, drinking, or toileting.

Use FLY-ZAP™ Fly Bait only around the outside of feedlots, broiler houses, livestock barns, kennels, fast food establishments, canneries, beverage plants, meat and poultry processing plants, commissaries, bakeries, supermarkets, refuse dumpsters, food processing plants, and restaurants. Bait may be used on walkways in caged layer houses. Scatter bait (do not put in piles) at the rate of approximately ¼ lb per sq ft of fly feeding area, keeping 1 to 2 inch intervals between particles. Do not treat areas where animals can feed on bait.

Precaution(s): Do not contaminate water, food or feed by storage or disposal. Pesticide Disposal: Pesticide and rinsate that cannot be used according to label instructions must be disposed of according to applicable Federal, State, or local governmental procedures. Waste Disposal: Waste resulting from the use of this product may be disposed of on site or at an approved waste disposal facility. Container Disposal: Triple rinse and dispose of according to local governmental procedures.

Do not contaminate feed and foodstuffs. Do not apply where poultry or animals, especially dogs and young calves, can pick it up or lick it. Do not use in homes or where milk is processed or stored. Do not feed treated garbage. Use only in areas inaccessible to food producing animals.

Do not use in edible product areas of food processing plants, restaurants or other areas where food is commercially prepared, or processed. Do not use in serving areas while food is exposed. Do not apply to floors or other surfaces likely to be contacted by children or pets.

Environmental Hazards: Accessible areas treated with this bait are hazardous to birds and other wildlife. Use with care when applying in areas frequented by wildlife or adjacent to any body of water. Collect, cover or incorporate granules spilled on the soil surface. This pesticide is toxic to birds. Do not apply directly to water, or to areas when surface water is present or to intertidal areas below the mean high water mark. Do not contaminate water by cleaning of equipment and when disposing of equipment washwaters. Do not contaminate water by disposal of wastes.

Caution(s): Precautionary Statement: Hazards to humans and domestic animals - Caution:

Harmful if swallowed, inhaled or absorbed through skin. Avoid breathing dust. Avoid contact with skin, eyes or clothing. Wash thoroughly after handling.

Antidote(s): Atropine.

Warning(s): Statement of Practical Treatment: In case of poisoning call a physician immediately.

If in eyes: Flush eyes with water for 15 minutes. Get medical assistance if irritation persists.

If on skin: Remove contaminated clothing and wash skin immediately with soap and water. Wash contaminated clothing before reuse.

If swallowed: Drink 1 or 2 glasses of water and induce vomiting by touching back of throat with finger. Never induce vomiting or give anything by mouth to an unconscious person.

Note to Physician: Methomyl is a cholinesterase inhibitor. Atropine is an antidote.

Warranty - Limitation of Damages: Aspen Veterinary Resources, Ltd. warrants that this material conforms to the chemical description and guaranteed limits of active ingredients as stated on the label. Aspen Veterinary Resources, Ltd. makes no other express or implied warranty of fitness or merchantability of any kind. Aspen Veterinary Resources, Ltd.'s maximum liability for breach of this warranty shall not exceed the purchase price of this product. In no event shall Aspen Veterinary Resources, Ltd. be liable for indirect or consequential damages. This warranty shall not be changed by oral or written agreement unless signed by a duly authorized officer of Aspen Veterinary Resources, Ltd. Buyer assumes all risk of use or handling whether in accordance with directions or not.

Keep out of reach of children.

Presentation: 1 lb, 5 lb and 65 lb containers.

Compendium Code No.: 14750340

FOALCHECK®

Centaur

Equine IgG Test Kit — **IgG Test**

Description: FOALCHECK® is a highly sensitive latex agglutination test for IgG in foals. The test can be conducted on either blood or serum with results obtainable within minutes of collecting a blood sample.

Components:

24 Pack: 24 glass bottles of diluent, 3 plastic squeeze bottles of latex, 1 vial containing fifty 5-microliter heparinized capillary pipettes, 1 plastic mixing stick, 24 disposable plastic Pasteur pipettes, 1 agglutination slide (black with 3 test rings).

10 Pack: 10 glass bottles of diluent, 1 plastic squeeze bottle of latex, 1 vial containing twenty 5-microliter heparinized capillary pipettes, 1 plastic mixing stick, 10 disposable plastic Pasteur pipettes, 1 agglutination slide (black with 3 test rings.)

Indications: A diagnostic test for determination of IgG levels in foals.

The FOALCHECK® test is recommended as a routine part of neonatal health care to screen foals for passive transfer of colostral immunoglobulins from mares to foals. Immunoglobulin levels should be determined after allowing time for absorption. Although sampling between two and three days of age is optimal, twelve to fifteen hours after the first nursing is usually adequate.[2,6] If a low test result is obtained before 24 hrs. of age, the test should be repeated 12-24 hrs. later.

Test Procedure: Specimen Requirements: Either whole blood or serum may be used for the test.

Serum - collect blood specimen without anticoagulant and allow to clot. After retraction of the clot draw off 5 microliters of serum from the layer above the clot using a single 5 microliter capillary pipette. Touch the pipette to the serum, holding the pipette almost horizontal and allow it to fill. The capillary pipette must be completely filled from tip to tip. Care must be taken to assure that the capillary pipette does not contain air bubbles. Wipe excess serum from the outside of the pipette being careful not to draw any serum out of the pipette (fingers work best for this). Hemolysis does not interfere with the test.

Blood - whole blood may be collected directly into the capillary pipettes or first placed into an anti-coagulant tube (heparin or EDTA may be used). Either one or two capillary pipettes filled with whole blood are required for the test. (See Test Procedures) The capillary pipettes are filled in the same manner as with serum. The same care must be taken to insure the pipettes are completely filled and excess blood is removed from the exterior.

A: To Test >400 mg/dl: Drop the filled 5 microliter pipette(s) into the diluent vial (one pipette if serum is used and two pipettes if whole blood is used).

B: To Test >800 mg/dl: Drop one 5 microliter pipette of whole blood into the diluent vial.

1. Allow 5 minutes for the specimen to disperse throughout the diluent. Shake well to insure mixing before removing a sample for testing.
2. Use a plastic Pasteur pipette to draw a small amount of the specimen-diluent mixture, making sure that excess is removed from outside of the pipette. Deliver 2 drops inside the first ceramic ring, 3 drops inside the second ring and 4 drops inside the third ring of the glass slide. Take care to hold the pipette vertically to insure accurate dispensing of proper size drops.
3. Shake latex bottle to insure mixing. Remove cap and add 2 drops of latex to each ceramic ring. Hold dropper bottle vertically to insure accurate dispensing of proper size drops.
4. Use the provided mixing stick to stir the drops and spread them over the entire area inside the rings.
5. Gently tilt and rotate the slide to maintain suspension of the reactants.
6. Observe for agglutination after rotating for approximately 15 seconds. If agglutination does not occur in all 3 rings, continue to rotate for an additional 45 seconds. Read slide and record findings at this time.*

*Some samples that are truly negative will appear to have glossy type patches floating on top. This is not to be considered a positive agglutination. The glossy sheen and patches on top are almost always linked with a negative sample.

Test Interpretation: Timing is important. Specimens with high IgG levels will agglutinate in all three rings within 15 seconds. When agglutination has not occurred in all 3 rings by 15 seconds, the slide should be rotated an additional 45 seconds, then read. The following table should be used to interpret the results at this time.

Agglutination	Procedure A IgG mg/dl	Procedure B IgG mg/dl
all 3 rings+	>400	>800
- + +	200-400	400-800
- - +	<200	200-400
- - -	<100	<200

Important: If one or more rings have a questionable or very weak agglutination reaction, these rings should be considered negative.

Storage: Store latex between 35°F and 45°F. Latex can degrade at extremes of low and/or high temperatures.

Caution(s): The accuracy of this test is dependent upon delivery of consistent-size drops of both latex and serum diluent. It is, therefore, extremely important that care be taken to hold the dropper bottle and Pasteur pipette vertically while dispensing drops. Also, care must be taken to avoid delivering air bubbles with the drops of liquid. The agglutination slide should be rinsed with water and dried between tests.

Latex: If latex is difficult to squeeze from vial, or if it has a stringy appearance, do not use.

Diluent: The diluent can become contaminated if opened prior to use. If diluent has a cloudy appearance, do not use.

Discussion: In equine species, young are born without significant amounts of circulating protective antibody. Normally, maternal antibodies are transmitted to the foal in the colostrum ingested during the first 24 hours after birth. These maternal antibodies provide protection against a variety of pathogens common to the animals' environment until the foal matures sufficiently to produce its own immunoglobulins.

It has been reported that 10-12 percent of foals fail to acquire even partially effective antibody levels from their dam's colostrum, and an additional 12% acquire only partially protective levels.[1-3] These foals are prone to infection which may result in serious illness or death. The survival rate of these animals, if diagnosed, may be improved by various treatments, particularly serum transfusion.[2,4-6]

McGuire and co-workers have suggested the following immunoglobulin levels as meaningful indicators of passive transfer.[3] <200 mg/dl - failure of passive transfer; 200 mg-400 mg/dl - partial failure of passive transfer; >400 mg/dl - adequate transfer

Current trends indicate a number of veterinarians prefer to measure an IgG level >800 mg/dl. Either of these IgG levels can be measured with the FOALCHECK® test kit. (See Test Procedures)

References: Available upon request.

Presentation: 10 and 24 tests.

Compendium Code No.: 14880040

FOAL-LAC® PELLETS

Pet-Ag

Large Animal Dietary Supplement

Active Ingredient(s):

Guaranteed Analysis	Equine System	Formula V™
Crude protein, min.	19.50%	19.50%
Crude fat, min.	14.00%	14.00%
Crude fiber, max.	0.50%	0.50%
Ash, max.	8.50%	8.50%
Calcium, min.	0.90%	0.90%
Calcium, max.	1.20%	1.20%
Phosphorus, min.	0.75%	0.75%
Vitamin A, min.	15,000 I.U./lb.	15,000 I.U./lb.
Vitamin D_3, min.	1,500 I.U./lb.	1,500 I.U./lb.
Vitamin E, min.	36 I.U./lb.	36 I.U./lb.

Ingredients:

Equine System and Formula V™: Dried whey, soy flour, animal fat and vegetable fat (preserved with BHA), dried skimmed milk, dried whey protein concentrate, dried corn syrup, dicalcium phosphate, calcium carbonate, l-lysine, potassium chloride, dl methionine, natural and artificial flavors added, vitamin E supplement, magnesium sulfate, ferrous sulfate, manganese sulfate, vitamin A supplement, vitamin D_3 supplement, copper sulfate, zinc sulfate, vitamin B_{12} supplement, calcium pantothenate, niacin supplement, riboflavin supplement, thiamine mononitrate, folic acid, pyridoxine hydrochloride, menadione sodium bisulfite complex, ethylenediamine dihydroiodide, biotin, sodium selenite.

Indications: FOAL-LAC® Pellets provides milk protein and other essential nutrients to older orphaned and early weaned foals to maintain growth rate through weaning. It is also an excellent supplement for broodmares, breeding stallions and all growing horses.

Dosage and Administration: Feeding Directions:

Orphaned/Early Weaned Foals:

Age of Foal	Reconstituted Foal-Lac® Powder	Daily	
		FOAL-LAC® Pellets	16% Protein Foal Feed
1-14 days	According to directions on the Foal-Lac® Powder container		½ lb
2-3 weeks			
3-4 weeks		1 cup	½ lb
4-5 weeks	Reconstituted FOAL-LAC® is gradually decreased for weaning at 8 weeks	2 cups	¾ lb
5-6 weeks		3 cups	1 lb
6-7 weeks		4 cups	1 lb
7-8 weeks		5 cups	1½ lbs
2-3 months	weaned from liquid FOAL-LAC®	6 cups	2 lbs
3-4 months		6 cups	3 lbs
4-5 months		3 cups	4 lbs
5-6 months		3 cups	5 lbs

Good quality tender hay, salt and water should be provided free choice starting at 10 days of age.

Consult your veterinarian for immunization, parasite control programs and for any sign of illness.

Weanlings/Yearlings: Feed a 14% protein roughage/grain ration. If extra condition is desired, feed 1 to 3 cups of FOAL-LAC® Pellets daily.

Broodmares:

Gestation: Depending on condition of mare, supplement the mare's ration with 1 to 3 cups of FOAL-LAC® Pellets daily during the last 3 months of gestation. Most of the fetal development occurs at this time, and the mare's nutrient requirement increases accordingly. Do not allow the mare to become fat.

Lactation: To help ensure adequate milk production, supplement the ration with 3 cups of Pellets daily. If the mare begins to lose weight, gradually increase to a maximum of 6 cups daily.

Breeding Stallions: During breeding season supplement the stallions ration with 1 to 3 cups of Pellets daily to maintain condition.

Performance Horses: Supplement the ration with 1 to 3 cups of Pellets daily to maintain condition.

Precaution(s): Store in cool dry place.

Presentation: Equine System: 8 lb. and 25 lb. pails, and 40 lb. bags.
Formula V™: 25 lb. pails.

Compendium Code No.: 10970140

FOAL-LAC® POWDER

Pet-Ag

Milk Replacer

Guaranteed Analysis:

	Equine System	Formula V™
Crude protein, min.	19.50%	19.50%
Crude fat, min.	14.00%	14.00%
Crude fiber, max.	0.10%	0.10%
Ash, max.	8.50%	8.50%
Calcium, min.	0.90%	0.90%
Calcium, max.	1.20%	1.20%
Phosphorus, min.	0.75%	0.75%
Vitamin A, min.	15,000 I.U./lb.	15,000 I.U./lb.
Vitamin D_3, min.	1,500 I.U./lb.	1,500 I.U./lb.
Vitamin E, min.	36 I.U./lb.	36 I.U./lb.

Ingredients:

Equine System and Formula V™: Dried whey, dried skimmed milk, animal and vegetable fat (preserved with BHA), dried whey protein concentrate, malto dextrins, dried corn syrup, dried milk protein, lecithin, calcium carbonate, dicalcium phosphate, natural and artificial flavors added, vitamin E supplement, magnesium sulfate, ferrous sulfate, dried *Lactobacillus casei* fermentation product, dried *Lactobacillus fermentum* fermentation product, dried *Streptococcus faecium* fermentation product, dried *Lactobacillus plantarum* fermentation product, manganese

F

sulfate, vitamin A supplement, vitamin D_3 supplement, copper sulfate, zinc sulfate, vitamin B_{12} supplement, calcium pantothenate, niacin supplement, riboflavin supplement, thiamin mononitrate, folic acid, pyridoxine hydrochloride, menadione sodium bisulfite complex, ethylenediamine dihydroiodide, biotin, and sodium selenite.

Indications: FOAL-LAC® milk replacer is a nutritionally complete powder that is reconstituted with water for feeding to orphaned or early weaned foals. Formulated specifically for foals, FOAL-LAC® simulates the nutritional composition of mare's milk. FOAL-LAC® Powder may be used in young orphaned foals, foals weaned prior to two months of age, foals nursing dams with an inadequate milk supply, and for mixing into the foals first feed to enhance palatability.

Dosage and Administration: Mix one (1) cup (8 oz. cup enclosed) of FOAL-LAC® Powder with three (3) cups of warm water. This yields approximately one and one-half (1½) pints of milk replacer.

Orphaned Foals:

1. The foal should receive colostrum during the first 24 hours after foaling. A physical examination of the foal by a veterinarian is recommended at this time.
2. Administer Bene-Bac™ Lactobacillus paste between 12 and 24 hours of age and on days 4 and 7.
3. The following schedule for feeding FOAL-LAC® milk replacer is a guideline for foals that will mature to about 1,100 lbs. of body weight. Since each foal is an individual, more or less milk replacer can be fed, depending upon appetite. Pony foals should be fed about half these quantities. Draft breed foals will require up to twice these quantities.
4. Feeding Schedule:

Age of Foal	FOAL-LAC® (pts./feeding)	No. of feedings/day	Foal-Lac® Pellets & 16% foal creep fed (amount/day)
1-14 days	1½	8	—
2-3 weeks	2	8	Provide ½ lb. foal feed
3-4 weeks	3	6	Feed 1 cup Pellets + ½ lb. foal feed
4-5 weeks	3	6	Feed 2 cups Pellets + ¾ lb. foal feed
5-6 weeks	3	4	Feed 3 cups Pellets + 1 lb. foal feed
6-7 weeks	3	4	Feed 4 cups Pellets + 1 lb. foal feed
7-8 weeks	3	2	Feed 5 cups Pellets + 1½ lbs. foal feed
2-3 months	—	—	Wean from liquid milk replacer. Feed 6 cups Pellets + 2 lbs. foal feed
3-4 months	—	—	Feed 6 cups Pellets + 3 lbs. foal feed daily
4-5 months	—	—	Feed 3 cups Pellets + 4 lbs. foal feed daily
5-6 months	—	—	Feed 3 cups Pellets + 5 lbs. foal feed daily
6-12 months	—	—	Change to a 14% protein weanling ration of grain and hay/pasture. If extra condition is required, supplement with 1 to 3 cups of Foal-Lac® Pellets daily.

5. Reconstituted FOAL-LAC® Powder can be fed in an open bucket. Any milk left by the foal after three (3) hours should be discarded. Always wash the feeding utensils with hot, soapy water and rinse well after each feeding.
6. Good quality tender, hay, salt, and water should be provided free choice starting at 10 days of age.
7. The foal should receive exercise each day to stimulate appetite and to develop bone and muscle.
8. Consult a veterinarian for parasite control, necessary immunizations and signs of illness.

Early Weaned and Nursing Foals: Early weaned foals can be placed on the orphan foal feeding schedule. The age of the foal will determine the place to start in the feeding schedule. Nursing foals receiving an inadequate amount of milk from the mare can be placed on the orphan foal schedule. Start with half the amount of FOAL-LAC® recommended for orphans, then adjust up or down according to the foal's appetite.

Precaution(s): Store in a cool, dry place.

Presentation: Equine System: 5 lb. (4 per case) and 25 lb. pails, and 40 lb. bags.
Formula V™: 4 lb. (4 per case) and 25 lb. pails.

Compendium Code No.: 10970151

FOALWATCH™

Chemetrics **Foaling Test**

Titrets® for Daytime Foaling Management

Components: Each kit includes: 3 mL syringe, 10 mL syringe, distilled water, A-1700 indicator solution, valve assembly, Titret® ampoules, Titrettor device.

Indications: This kit is designed to assist in determining when a mare is likely to foal.

Test Principles: The test is based on changes in the pre-foaling milk calcium level.

Test Procedure:

When to Begin Testing: Begin sampling and testing approximately 10 to 14 days in advance of the mare's expected foaling date (calculated as 335 to 340 days from her last known breeding date). In mares with an unknown breading date, testing should begin as soon as there is some udder enlargement, and secretions can be obtained from the teats without undue effort. It is best to keep a close check on udder development an a daily basis and practice massage of the mare's udder and teats to allow her to get used to your presence in this area. Once a day sampling is sufficient until you begin to get test results that exceed 100 ppm. Then twice daily sampling is recommended. The more accurate assessment of the mare's readiness to foal will be a late afternoon or an evening sampling each day (as most mares foal at night). Since a few mares do foal in the daytime, a morning sampling should not be neglected and is highly advisable when test results first exceed 125 ppm.

Sample Collection: Some mares are resentful of being milked, especially if they are maiden (first-time foaling) mares. Standing to the left side of the mare and facing her tail, press your shoulder firmly against her chest, reach with your right hand first to her belly near the umbilicus and rub gently and progressively toward the udder. Several attempts may need to be made to reassure the mare that you mean no harm. Try to make this a pleasurable experience for the mare by offering her some grain while collecting the sample. The more comfortable she is while collecting her milk, the easier it will be for her to accept her new foal attempting the same procedure.

It is not unusual for maiden mares to fail to develop much of an udder prior to foaling, in which case, the ability to obtain a sample for testing will be greatly hampered. The 'first milk' (colostrum) is typically a very thick, honey-colored, sticky secretion. This is an appropriate sample to recover as calcium levels will be detectable just as with more 'normal' appearing milk.

Since calcium contributes to the hardness of water, all precaution should be used to rinse all re-usable items exceptionally well with distilled water prior to drying. Use only distilled water (supplied or purchased) for all sample dilutions in the testing procedure.

Testing Procedure:

1. Wipe the udder with a clean, dry, soft paper towel.
   Note: This will reduce contamination in the sample and is most critical if the mare has been out in the weather and is wet. Your hands should also be clean and dry.
2. Obtain a 2 to 5 mL sample of mammary secretion by gently stripping a small amount from each teat. (using thumb and index or middle finger) into the small 5 mL sample cup.
   Note: The collected sample may be transported to a clean, dry, warm area to perform the remainder of the test procedure.
3. Using the 3 mL syringe, draw up exactly 1.5 mL (cc) of the mammary secretion sample.
   Note: Be sure that there are no air bubbles in the syringe barrel.
4. Dispense the 1.5 mL sample into the 25 mL sample cup.
5. Using the 10 mL syringe, draw up exactly 9 mL (cc) of distilled water.
   Note: Be sure that there are no air bubbles in the syringe barrel.
6. Dispense the 9 mL of distilled water into the 25 mL sample cup.
7. Cap the sample cup. Mix the contents gently.
8. Add 1 drop of A-1700 indicator Solution and once again mix the contents of the cap gently.
9. Push the valve assembly onto the Titret® ampoule tip until it fits snugly.
   Note: The valve assembly should reach the reference line on the neck of the ampoule.
10. Gently snap the tip of the ampoule at the score mark.
11. Lift the control bar and insert the Titret® assembly into the body of the Titrettor.
12. Hold the Titrettor with the sample pipe in the sample and press the control bar firmly, but briefly, to pull in a small amount of sample. The contents will turn bright orange.
13. Press the control bar again briefly to allow another small amount of sample to be drawn into the Titret® ampoule.
    Caution: Do not press the control bar unless the sample pipe is in the liquid.
14. After each addition, rock the entire assembly to mix the contents of the ampoule. Watch for a color change from orange to bright blue.
    Note: The endpoint color may appear in flashes, but the endpoint is reached only when the blue color is permanent (lasts for at least 30 seconds).
15. Repeat steps 13 and 14 until a permanent color change occurs.
16. When the color of the liquid in the Titret® ampoule changes to blue, remove the ampoule from the Titrettor. Hold the Titret® ampoule in a vertical position and carefully read the test result on the scale opposite the liquid level to obtain test results in ppm (mg/liter) calcium carbonate.
17. Rinse both syringes and sample cups thoroughly with distilled water, then allow them to air dry.

Test Interpretation: In mares that have been evaluated by this test, there was a 54% probability that foaling would occur within 24 hours when the pre-foaling mammary secretion calcium first meets or exceeds 200 ppm. There was an 84% probability that foaling would occur within 48 hours when pre-foaling mammary secretion calcium first meets or exceeds 200 ppm, and a 98% probability that foaling would within 72 hours when pre-foaling mammary secretion calcium first meets or exceeds 200 ppm. The majority of mares foal within a short period of time when a value of 300 to 500 ppm is obtained. But not all mares can be expected to reach these high values. For mares that had not yet reached or exceeded 200 ppm, there was a 98% probability that foaling would not occur within the next 24 hour period.

It is not unusual for some mares to reach 100 to 175 ppm and remain at that level for several days at a time before proceeding up the scale to 200 ppm (or above). Variations occur between mares, and even within the same mare from year to year. Patience and careful monitoring on a once to twice daily schedule are a must. A dramatic rise, or significant in value, over a 12- to 24-hour interval indicates that the mare is advancing towards her actual delivery.

Occasionally a value will drop from the previous day's sampling; this is not cause for alarm. You may want to repeat the test procedure using care to follow the directions exactly.

Initial color of the diluted sample once the Indicator Solution has been added to it will vary from early in the mare's testing period to later when she is closer to foaling. Early samples will appear more orange in color, later samples will appear a rose-pink to reddish purple. This is a normal variation we have observed will is not a cause for concern in accuracy of the result.

Interferences: Mares that have been exposed to fescue grass pastures (specifically the Kentucky 31 variety) contaminated by the fungus *Acremonium coephenophialum* during the last 60-90 days of gestation may suffer from the toxins that are produced within the grass. Such mares very often fail to undergo normal udder development prior to foaling (and often even after), a problem referred to as agalactia. Without a sample for testing, this kit will be of little help to your management of such mares. Consult your veterinarian for prevention of this problem.

Caution(s): This test does not claim to be 100% accurate in all mares. As with any biological system, exceptions are encountered, and no test can be expected to provide completely accurate and reliable results all of the time, in all situations. This is an aid to the foaling management program, and is not intended to guarantee a successful outcome in all mares.

The procedure of pre-foaling mammary secretion sampling slightly increases the risk of mastitis development (infection of the milk and mammary tissue or udder). This is true for any animal when milking is performed manually, especially if precautions are not taken to wipe the skin and teat surfaces clean, and dry them prior to obtaining the sample. If you note clumps of debris, or pink to red discoloration in the milk sample obtained from your mare, this may indicate an infection. Consult the veterinarian for proper treatment.

Obtaining the small sample volume that is required for testing on a once to twice daily basis, for 10 to 14 days prior to foaling, does not deprive the foal of any significant amount of colostrum (or its antibody content) once it is born and begins to nurse. Many foals have been monitored during the research and development of this procedure, and in no case was a failure of passive transfer (inadequate colostrum consumption and passing of antibodies from the mare's milk to the foal) attributable to the sampling of pre-foaling mammary secretions. Also, the quality of the mare's colostrum (its content of antibodies) is not affected. Mares that are prone to 'running milk' prior to foaling will do so whether they have been sampled for testing or not. Such mares are still at risk of losing too much colostrum prior to foaling and should be managed accordingly regardless of testing. Consult your veterinarian if you are not familiar with this problem.

Discussion: Normal pregnancy length can vary widely in the mare. Thus many nights can be spent waiting up for the mare to foal. Physical signs of the mare's approaching readiness for foaling include an appropriate gestation length of greater then 320 days, udder enlargement with the presence of colostrum (milk) in the teats, waxing on teat ends and relaxation around the tail head, buttocks and lips of the vulva. While helpful, none of these signs are extremely accurate as a means of predicting when the mare will foal. Recent studies of pre-foaling milk (mammary secretion) electrolyte changes have demonstrated an increased ability to predict foaling time. These electrolyte changes (especially with regard to calcium level) have also been shown to be related to the development of maturity of the foal in the uterus and its subsequent survivability (viability) following a normal delivery.

This kit has been developed from years of extensive research and testing. The intent is to assist you in determining when the mare is likely to foal based upon changes in the pre-foaling milk calcium level. It is a tool that can allow the operator to attend the mare's foaling without an excessive number of sleepless nights.

The advantages of this kit include its accuracy and repeatability compared with other test kits on the market, its ease of use, its quantitative determination of the calcium carbonate level in each sample tested and its economy.

References: Available upon request.

Presentation: 20 individual tests per kit.

Titrets® is a registered trademark of CHEMetrics, Inc. U.S. Patent No. 4,332,769

Compendium Code No.: 14890000

FOAMING DISINFECTANT CLEANER

Davis **Disinfectant**

EPA Reg. No.: 10807-21-50591

Active Ingredient(s):

n-Alkyl (C_{14} 60%, C_{16} 30%, C_{12} 5%, C_{18} 5%) dimethyl benzyl ammonium chlorides . . . 0.10%
n-Alkyl (C_{12} 68%, C_{14} 32%) dimethyl ethylbenzyl ammonium chlorides . . . 0.10%
Inert Ingredients . . . 99.80%
Total . . . 100.00%

Indications: This is a concentrated general purpose cleaner which cleans, disinfects and deodorizes. It kills Staph, Salmonella, Pseudomonas and HIV-1 (AIDS Virus)* on hard surfaces when used as directed. This is a foaming cleaner that should be used on tile, porcelain, ceramics, metal, stainless steel, bathtubs, hampers, tables, chairs, and walls. For use in hospitals, schools, hotels, motels, offices, restaurants, lockers and rest rooms. Surfaces should be cleaned and disinfected on a regular basis. All food contact surfaces must be rinsed with potable water before reuse.

This product is not to be used as a terminal sterilant/high level disinfectant on any surface or instrument that (1) is introduced directly into the human body, either into or in contact with the bloodstream or normally sterile areas of the body, or (2) contacts intact mucous membranes but which does not ordinarily penetrate the blood barrier or otherwise enter normally sterile areas of the body. This product may be used to preclean or decontaminate critical or semi-critical medical devices prior to sterilization or high level disinfection.

Directions for Use: It is a violation of Federal law to use this product in a manner inconsistent with its labeling. To disinfect hard non-porous surfaces (such as those listed above), proceed as indicated below. (1) Shake can before using. (2) Hold six to eight inches from surface to be treated. (3) Spray area until it is covered with a white foam. Allow foam to penetrate and remain wet for 10 minutes. No scrubbing necessary. (4) Wipe off with a clean cloth, mop or sponge. The product will not leave grit or soap scum. For heavy soiled area, remove gross soil before treatment.

*Kills HIV-1 on precleaned environmental surfaces/objects previously soiled with blood/body fluids in health care settings or other settings in which there is an expected likelihood of soiling on inanimate surfaces/objects with blood or body fluids, and in which the surfaces/objects likely to be soiled with blood or body fluids can be associated with the potential for transmission of human immunodeficiency virus Type 1 (HIV-1) (associated with AIDS) Contact Time: Leave surfaces wet for 10 minutes at 25°C.

Special Instructions for Cleaning and Decontamination Against HIV of Surfaces/Objects Soiled with Blood/Body Fluids: Personal Protection: Specific barrier protection items to be used when handling items soiled with blood or body fluids are disposable latex gloves, gowns, masks, or eye coverings. Cleaning Procedures: Blood and other body fluids must be thoroughly cleaned from surfaces and objects before application of this disinfectant. Disposal of Infectious Materials: Blood and other body fluids should be autoclaved and disposed of according to federal, state and local regulations for infectious waste disposal. Contact Time: Leave surfaces wet for 10 minutes at 25°C.

Precautionary Statements: Hazards to Humans and Domestic Animals:

Warning: Keep out of reach of children. Causes eye and skin irritation. Do not get into eyes, skin or clothing. Harmful if swallowed.

Statement of Practical Treatment: In case of contact, immediately flush eyes or skin with plenty of water for at least 15 minutes. For eyes, call a physician. Remove and wash all contaminated clothing before reuse. If swallowed, drink promptly a large quantity of water. Call a physician. Note to physician: Probable mucosal damage may contraindicate the use of gastric lavage.

Physical or Chemical Hazards: This product contains an extremely flammable propellant. Do not use or store near fire, sparks, or heated surfaces. Turn off pilot lights in gas appliance and unplug or turn off electrical equipment in the use area. After airing out phase is completed, relight pilot lights and reconnect electrical current. Do not smoke in use area. Contents under pressure. Do not puncture or incinerate container. Exposure to temperatures above 130°F may cause bursting. Incineration of container may cause explosion.

Storage and Disposal: Storage: Store in a cool area away from heat and open flame. Disposal: Do not reuse empty container. Wrap container and put in trash collection.

Presentation: 19 oz (1 lb 3 oz) (539 g).

Compendium Code No.: 11410450 Rev. 9/98

FOAM-KOTE 5™

Westfalia•Surge **Teat Dip**

0.5% Iodine Foaming Teat Dip

Active Ingredient(s): Contents:

Titratable iodine . . . 0.5%
Inactive Ingredients: . . . 99.5%*

*Contains 5% glycerin

Indications: This topical liquid product, when used undiluted as a pre milking teat dip, effectively aids in reducing the spread of mastics.

Directions for Use: Use at full strength. Do not dilute.

Pre Foam: Before milking, foam each teat with FOAM-KOTE 5™ Iodine Foaming Teat Dip using the proper teat foamer system. After 15 to 30 seconds, dry each teat thoroughly with a single service towel. If the udder and teats are heavily soiled, wash with a sanitizing solution and dry before application of FOAM-KOTE 5™.

Post Dipping: Immediately after milking, dip each teat with a Westfalia•Surge Sanitizing teat dip. Allow teats to air dry. Do not wipe. If outside temperature is below freezing, allow to air dry on the teat before the cow leaves the parlor to prevent freezing. At the end of lactation, apply this product daily for one week after the last milking. In addition, begin application of this product about one week prior to calving.

At each milking, make sure to have a clean teat foamer applicator. The applicator should be emptied, cleaned and rinsed with potable water after each milking session or when it becomes contaminated during milking. Do not pour remaining solution from teat foamer applicator back into original container.

Precaution(s): Storage Instructions: Store this product in a cool dry area away from direct sunlight and heat to avoid deterioration. Keep containers closed to prevent contamination of this product. Keep from freezing.

Precautionary Statements: Danger. Contains materials which may cause eye damage. May be harmful or fatal if swallowed. Individuals with sensitive skin may experience skin irritation. Protect eyes and skin when handling. Do not take internally. Avoid breathing vapors. Do not mix with any other chemical products. Refer to Material Safety Data Sheet (MSDS).

First Aid:

If in Eyes: Flush with large volumes of water for at least 15 minutes. Call a physician immediately.

If Swallowed: Do not induce vomiting. Rinse mouth promptly then give small amount/glass of milk or water (4-6 oz. child/10-12 oz adult) (120-180 mL child/300-360 mL adult). Avoid alcohol. Call a physician immediately. Do not give anything by mouth to an unconscious or convulsing person.

If on Skin: While removing contaminated clothing and shoes, flush with large volumes of water for at least 15 minutes.

If irritation develops and persists, get medical attention.

Inhalation of Vapors: If breathing difficulty or irritation occurs, remove to fresh air. If symptoms persist, get medical attention.

For assistance with medical emergency, call 1-800-451-8346.

For farm, commercial and industrial use only.

Warning(s): Keep out of reach of children.

Presentation: Contact the company for container sizes available.

FOAM-KOTE 5 is a Trademark of Westfalia•Surge, Inc.

Compendium Code No.: 10020240 01-01

FOAM-KOTE 10™

Westfalia•Surge **Teat Dip**

1% Iodine Foaming Teat Dip

Active Ingredient(s): Contents:

Titratable iodine . . . 1%
Inactive Ingredients: . . . 99%*

*Contains a proprietary emollient system.

Indications: This topical liquid product, when used undiluted as a pre milking teat dip, effectively aids in reducing the spread of mastitis.

Directions for Use: Use at full strength. Do not dilute.

Pre Foam: Before milking, foam each teat with FOAM-KOTE 10™ Foaming Teat Dip using the proper teat foamer system. After 15 to 30 seconds, dry each teat thoroughly with a single service towel. If the udder and teats are heavily soiled, wash with a sanitizing solution and dry before application of FOAM-KOTE 10™.

Post Dipping: Immediately after milking, dip each teat with a Westfalia•Surge Sanitizing teat dip. Allow teats to air dry. Do not wipe. If outside temperature is below freezing, allow to air dry on the teat before the cow leaves the parlor to prevent freezing. At the end of lactation, apply this product daily for one week after the last milking. In addition, begin application of this product about one week prior to calving. At each milking, make sure to have a clean teat foamer applicator. The applicator should be emptied, cleaned and rinsed with potable water after each milking session or when it becomes contaminated during milking. Do not pour remaining solution from teat foamer applicator back into original container.

Precaution(s): Storage Instructions: Store this product in a cool dry area away from direct sunlight and heat to avoid deterioration. Keep containers closed to prevent contamination of this product. Keep from freezing.

Precautionary Statements: Danger. Contains materials which may cause eye damage. May be harmful or fatal if swallowed. Individuals with sensitive skin may experience skin irritation. Protect eyes and skin when handling. Do not take internally. Avoid breathing vapors. Do not mix with any other chemical products. Refer to Material Safety Data Sheet (MSDS).

First Aid:

If in Eyes: Flush with large volumes of water for at least 15 minutes. Call a physician immediately.

If Swallowed: Do not induce vomiting. Rinse mouth promptly then give small amount/glass of milk or water (4-6 oz. child/10-12 oz. adult) (120-160 mL child/300-360 mL adult). Avoid alcohol. Call a physician immediately. Do not give anything by mouth to an unconscious or convulsing person.

If on Skin: While removing contaminated clothing and shoes, flush with large volumes of water for at least 15 minutes. If irritation develops and persists, get medical attention.

Inhalation of Vapors: If breathing difficulty or irritation occurs, remove to fresh air. If symptoms persist, get medical attention.

For assistance with medical emergency, call 1-800-451-8346.

For farm, commercial and industrial use only.

Warning(s): Keep out of reach of children.

Presentation: Contact the company for container sizes available.

FOAM-KOTE 10 is a Trademark of Westfalia•Surge, Inc.

Compendium Code No.: 10020250 01-01

FOAM QUAT

Vet Solutions **Disinfectant**

One-Step Disinfectant, Cleaner and Deodorant

EPA Reg. No.: 47371-89-72896

Active Ingredient(s):

n-Alkyl (C_{14} 60%, C_{16} 30%, C_{12} 5%, C_{18} 5%) dimethyl benzyl ammonium chloride 0.09%
n-Alkyl (C_{12} 50%, C_{14} 30%, C_{16} 17%, C_{18} 3%)
dimethyl ethylbenzyl ammonium chloride . . . 0.09%
Inert Ingredients: . . . 99.82%

Indications: A ready-to-use, multi-purpose formula effective in the presence of a moderate amount of soil (5% organic serum) against *Pseudomonas aeruginosa, Staphylococcus aureus, Salmonella choleraesuis, Trichophyton mentagrophytes*, *Herpes simplex type 2, and *HIV-1 (AIDS virus).

Bactericidal, Fungicidal, *Virucidal.

Directions for Use: It is a violation of Federal law to use this product in a manner inconsistent with its labeling.

Shake before using.

General Use Directions: Recommended for use in households, hospitals, nursing homes, schools, colleges, airports, hotels, motels, greenhouses, and kennels. Disinfects, cleans, and deodorizes non-porous, inanimate surfaces such as floors, walls, metal surfaces, stainless steel surfaces, plastic surfaces (such as polypropylene, polystyrene, etc.), plastic/vinyl chairs, porcelain, garbage cans, laundry chutes, bathroom fixtures, shower stalls, exterior bowl surfaces, empty basins, knobs, handles, railings, vehicles (ships, trains, and airplanes), and many other similar public and residential surfaces which could harbor and transmit dangerous microorganisms.

To Clean: Shake can. Spray evenly over surface, allowing sufficient time for the foam to penetrate heavy soil deposits. Wipe off. Chrome fixtures may be rinsed for high shine.

To Disinfect: Clean surface thoroughly as instructed above. Then apply a thin coat of foam, making sure to cover entire surface to be disinfected. Allow foam to remain for at least 10 minutes, then wipe off or allow to air dry.

Mildewstatic Instructions: Follow the disinfection instructions above. Repeat application weekly or when growth reappears.

*Kills HIV-1 (AIDS virus) on precleaned, environmental surfaces/objects previously soiled with blood/body fluids in health care settings or other settings in which there is an expected likelihood of soiling of inanimate surfaces/objects with blood/body fluids, and in which the surfaces/objects likely to be soiled with blood/body fluids can be associated with the potential for transmission of human immunodeficiency virus type 1 (HIV-1) (associated with AIDS).

Special Instructions For Cleaning and Decontamination Against HIV-1 (AIDS Virus) of Surfaces/Objects Soiled with Blood/Body Fluids.

Personal Protection: Disposable latex or vinyl gloves, gowns, face masks, or eye coverings as appropriate, must be worn during all cleaning of body fluids, blood, and during decontamination procedures.

Cleaning Procedures: Blood/body fluids must be thoroughly cleaned from surfaces/objects before application of disinfectant.

Contact Time: HIV-1 (AIDS virus) is inactivated after a contact time of 5 minutes at 25°C (room temperature). Use a 10 minute contact time for disinfection against all other viruses, fungi, and bacteria listed.

Disposal of Infectious Materials: Blood/body fluids should be autoclaved and disposed of according to federal, state, and local regulations for infectious waste disposal.

Precautionary Statements: Hazards to Humans and Domestic Animals:

Physical and Chemical Hazards. Caution: Contents under pressure. Do not use or store near heat or open flame. Do not puncture or incinerate container. Exposure to temperatures above 130°F may cause bursting.

Storage and Disposal: Keep product under locked storage, inaccessible to children. Do not contaminate water, food, or feed by storage or disposal. Open dumping is prohibited. Do not reuse empty container.

Container Disposal: This container may be recycled in aerosol recycling centers. At present, there are only a few such centers in the country. Before offering for recycling, empty the can by using the product according to the label (Do not puncture!). If recycling is not available, replace cap and discard container in trash.

Warning(s): Keep out of reach of children.

Presentation: 19 oz. (532 grams).

Compendium Code No.: 10610080 000301

FOLIC ACID & VITAMIN E POWDER

AHC **Equine Dietary Supplement**

Feed Supplement

Guaranteed Analysis: Each pound contains not less than:

D alpha-tocopherol (Vitamin E) .... 128,000 IU
Folic Acid .... 640.00 mg

Blended into a yeast culture base.

Ingredients: brewers yeast (source of calcium, iron, magnesium, phosphorus, potassium, sodium, copper, thiamine, riboflavin, B-6, biotin, choline, niacin, pantothenic acid), alpha-tocopherol acetate (vitamin E), silica, folic acid, calcium carbonate, roughage products and mineral oil.

Indications: A nutritional supplement to provide Folic Acid and Vitamin E and B-complex vitamins. Research has shown that Vitamin E is beneficial in neuromuscular function and treatment. B-complex vitamins are beneficial for horses under stress

Dosage and Administration: Recommended Dosage: Feeding 1 ounce per day will provide 8,000 IU Vitamin E and 40 mg of Folic Acid.

Caution(s): For animal use only. Keep out of reach of children.

Presentation: 16 oz jar, 2.5 lb jar and 5 lb pail.

Compendium Code No.: 10770050

FOOT ROT & RINGWORM SPRAY

AgriLabs **Hoof Product**

Active Ingredient(s):

Benzalkonium Chloride 0.15%

Other ingredients Allantoin

Indications: For use on cattle, sheep, horses, dogs and cats as an aid in the control of summer itch, girth itch, foot rot, ringworm and other fungal problems.

Dosage and Administration: Soak affected area liberally with FOOT ROT & RINGWORM SPRAY solution. Apply daily until hair begins to grow. Leave treated areas uncovered. Rinse treated areas with clear water before reapplying. Results should be apparent in a matter of days. If no improvement is noted within seven days, consult veterinarian.

Note: Efficiency is neutralized by soap or detergent residues.

Warning(s): In case of contact with eyes or mucous membranes, flush immediately with water. Obtain medical attention for eye inflammation.

For external veterinary use only. Not for human use.

Presentation: 16 oz and 32 oz.

Compendium Code No.: 10580511

FOOTVAX® 10 STRAIN

Schering-Plough **Bacterin**

Bacteroides nodosus Bacterin

U.S. Vet. Lic. No.: 311

Contents: The FOOTVAX® product contains 10 strains of killed *Bacteroides nodosus* organisms suspended in a water-in-oil emulsion.

Indications: A multi-strain ovine footrot bacterin for the prevention and treatment of footrot in sheep.

Dosage and Administration: Aseptically administer 1 mL under the skin in the anterior half of the neck.

Primary Vaccination: The primary course of treatment should be initiated prior to the anticipated outbreak period as dictated by local conditions. Following the first (sensitizing) dose, a second vaccination should be administered not sooner than six (6) weeks and not later than six (6) months following the initial dose.

Booster Vaccination: Following the original two dose course of treatment, booster vaccinations should be given bi-annually or just prior to an anticipated outbreak. Protection after vaccination is usually longer than four (4) months but local conditions are known to be very important in affecting this period. Booster inoculations at 4 to 6 month intervals may be beneficial in cases of severe challenge.

Administration: The FOOTVAX® product is very viscous because it contains an oil adjuvant. A considerable excess is included in each Flexipack since some of the product adheres to the sides of the container and cannot be withdrawn. Before use it should be thoroughly shaken. In very cold weather the Flexipack should be immersed in lukewarm water to make the product flow more readily. The use of an 18 gauge x 1 inch needle is recommended, except in cold weather when a 16 gauge x 1 inch needle is recommended. The product can be given through standard automatic syringes that can be accurately set to 1 mL. Sterilize all injection equipment by boiling in water for at least 10 minutes prior to use. Maintain maximum cleanliness at all times. Use aseptic technique and change needles frequently.

Precaution(s): Store away from light at not over 45°F or 7°C. Do not freeze. Use entire contents when first opened.

Caution(s): Avoid injection of dirty or wet sheep. To reduce injection site contamination use only sharp sterile disposable needles. Inject only under the skin, and not into the muscle.

The FOOTVAX® product contains an oil adjuvant which is likely to cause a localized reaction at the site of injection. The reaction can take the form of either a lump, a plaquelike swelling or occasionally a sterile abscess may occur. These reactions will normally disappear over a period of 10 weeks. However, some reactions may remain. Some evidence of localized reactions may be present for longer periods of time. Anaphylactoid reactions may occur following use.

Antidote(s): Epinephrine.

Warning(s): Do not vaccinate within 60 days before slaughter.

Accidental Human Exposure: This product does not represent an etiological hazard to humans. Accidental self-injection of the product can cause serious local reactions due to the oil emulsion. If accidental injection occurs seek medical attention at once. Inform the physician that the product contains an oil emulsion.

To the doctor: Accidental self-injection with this oil-based product can cause intense vascular spasm which may, for example, result in the loss of a digit. Expert prompt surgical attention is required and may necessitate early incision and irrigation of the injected area, especially where there is involvement of muscle, tendon sheaths or joint capsules.

For veterinary use only.

Discussion: FOOTVAX® is designed to stimulate a strong immunological response for the protection from new infection, and treatment of infection already present. It forms an essential part of the recommended footrot control program. Owing to the large differences in flock susceptibility, prevalence of the disease, and seasonal climatic factors in different parts of the United States, a specific control program incorporating FOOTVAX® should be designed in consultation with your local veterinarian.

Footrot in sheep is common in many areas of the United States and is principally caused by the bacterium *Bacteroides nodosus*, also known as *Dichelobacter nodosus*. The development of footrot is aided by wet conditions when mud and feces may accumulate on the feet, resulting in inflammation between the claws (scald). This inflammatory response facilitates invasion of the hoof by *B. nodosus* organisms. The disease is characterized by a progressive separation of the horny tissues from the soft tissues of the foot due to necrosis of the sensitive laminae. This usually starts to the rear of the inside of the claw proceeding to the sole and eventually progresses to the outside wall of the claw. In severe cases, there can be almost complete separation of the wall from the underlying structures. Where underrunning is severe the foot may be carried and if both front feet are severely affected the sheep may move about on its knees. There is a characteristic foul odor present.

Bacteroides nodosus, the organism responsible for footrot in sheep, is separated into groups by the differences in the hairlike structures (or pili) on the surfaces of the bacteria.

The differences between strains can only be identified by laboratory tests. Not all strains are equally pathogenic and the least destructive of them often cause only minor clinical signs. "Scald" for instance is now thought to be caused by relatively non-proteolytic (non-tissue-destructive) strains of *B. nodosus*. Lameness in a small portion of the flock is usually the first indication of the presence of footrot. The interdigital skin is moist with some erosion and some minor underrunning may occur. Death of the underlying tissues does not occur although the usual footrot odor is present. In most cases of "scald" there is natural regression and healing. "Scald" of this nature should be referred to as benign footrot. In fact, any infection of the interdigital skin by bacteria such as with *Fusobacterium necrophorum* will present symptoms of "scald" and it is suggested that this term be used only to describe the early non-specific signs of foot disease of indeterminate origin.

Presentation: 50 dose (50 mL) and 100 dose (100 mL) vials.

Manufactured by: Schering-Plough Animal Health Limited.

Compendium Code No.: 10470730

FORMALDEHYDE

Centaur **Reagent**

Active Ingredient(s):

Formaldehyde 37%

Inactive Ingredients:

Water and Methanol (Methanol 11.5 to 12.5%) 63%

Solution: 40% by volume U.S.P. analysis by weight.

Indications: For use as an aid in preserving tissue samples.

Precaution(s): Store above 50°F.

Caution(s): For veterinary use only.

Warning(s): Poison. Causes irritation to skin, eyes, nose and throat. Avoid prolonged or repeated contact with skin. Avoid breathing vapor. Use with adequate ventilation.

First Aid Treatment-Antidote:

If Swallowed: Give a tablespoon of salt in a glass of warm water and repeat until vomit fluid is clear. Give milk, or white of egg beaten with water.

Keep out of reach of children.

Presentation: 1 gallon (128 fl oz) 3.785 L.

Manufactured by: Unavet, North Kansas City, MO 64116.

Compendium Code No.: 14880160 Rev. 4-97

FORMALDEHYDE SOLUTION

Vedco

Reagent

Active Ingredient(s):

Formaldehyde 37%

Inactive ingredients:

Water and methanol........ 63%

(Methanol 11.5 to 12.5%).

Indications: FORMALDEHYDE SOLUTION 40% by volume U.S.P.

Dosage and Administration: The product is a reagent only.

Caution(s): Rinse formaldehyde bottles with water before making them available for disposal.

Strong sensitizer. Causes irritation of skin, eyes, nose, and throat. Do not inhale vapor. Avoid contact with skin and clothing.

Warning(s): Poison. Keep out of the reach of children. Causes irritation to skin, eyes, nose, and throat. Avoid prolonged or repeated contact with skin. Avoid inhaling vapor. Use with adequate ventilation.

First Aid Treatment - Antidote:

If swallowed: Give a tablespoonful of salt in a glass of warm water and repeat until vomit fluid is clear. Give milk, or white of egg beaten with water.

If inhaled: Remove to fresh air. Flush eyes and skin with plenty of water for at least 15 minutes. Call a physician. If not breathing, give artificial respiration, preferably mouth to mouth. If breathing is difficult, give oxygen. Induce vomiting. Never administer anything by mouth to an unconscious person.

Presentation: 1 gallon container.

Compendium Code No.: 10940960

FORMALDEHYDE SOLUTION 37%

Butler

Disinfectant

Active Ingredient(s):

Formaldehyde 37.0%

Inert ingredient:

Water........ 63.0%

Total........ 100.0%

Indications: For use as a disinfectant or preservative.

Dosage and Administration: It is a violation of federal law to use the product in a manner inconsistent with its labeling.

Formaldehyde can be used successfully when eggs are in the incubator without injury to the eggs. However, eggs should not be fumigated for the first five (5) days of their incubating period. If a separate hatching unit is maintained, the ideal procedure is to fumigate the eggs as soon as they are transferred from the incubating to the hatching unit. To be effective, formaldehyde fumigation should not be used in temperatures below 60°F and the relative humidity should be high.

For fumigation of hatching eggs: For each 100 cu. ft. of space to be fumigated, use ½ oz. Vinco® Potassium Permanganate and 1 oz. Formaldehyde Solution.

Precaution(s): Rinse FORMALDEHYDE bottles with water before making them available for disposal.

Caution(s): Poison. Keep out of the reach of children.

Sold to graduate veterinarians only.

Strong sensitizer. Causes irritation of the skin, eyes, nose, and throat. Do not inhale vapor. Avoid contact with skin and clothing.

If inhaled, remove to fresh air. Flush eyes and skin with plenty of water for at least 15 minutes. Call a physician. If not breathing, give artificial respiration, preferably mouth to mouth. If breathing is difficult, give oxygen. Induce vomiting. Never administer anything by mouth to an unconscious person.

Rinse formaldehyde bottles with water before making them available for disposal.

Presentation: 1 gallon.

Compendium Code No.: 10820770

FORMALDEHYDE SOLUTION 37%

First Priority

Reagent

Active Ingredient(s):

Formaldehyde 37%

Inactive Ingredients:

Water and Methanol (Methanol 11.5 to 12.5%)........ 63%

Indications: For laboratory use.

Precaution(s): Storage: Store at controlled room temperature between 15°-30°C (59°-86°F). Keep container tightly closed when not in use.

Rinse formaldehyde bottles with water before making them available for disposal.

Caution(s): Poison. Strong sensitizer that can cause irritation of skin, eyes, nose and throat. Do not breathe vapor. Avoid contact with skin and clothing.

First Aid: If inhaled, remove to fresh air. Flush eyes and skin with plenty of water for at least 15 minutes. Call a physician. If not breathing, give artificial respiration, preferably mouth to mouth. If breathing is difficult, give oxygen. Induce vomiting. Never administer anything by mouth to an unconscious person.

Antidote(s): Treatment-Antidote: If Swallowed: Give a tablespoonful of salt in a glass of warm water and repeat until vomit fluid is clear. Give milk, or white of egg beaten with water.

Warning(s): Keep out of reach of children.

Presentation: 1 gallon (3.785 L) (NDC# 58829-226-01).

Compendium Code No.: 11390321

Rev. 07-01

FORMALDEHYDE SOLUTION 37%

Phoenix Pharmaceutical

Reagent

Active Ingredient(s):

Formaldehyde 37%

Inactive Ingredients:

Water and Methanol (Methanol 11.5 to 12.5%)........ 63%

Indications: For laboratory use.

Precaution(s): Rinse formaldehyde bottles with water before making them available for disposal.

Caution(s): Strong sensitizer. Causes irritation of skin, eyes, nose and throat. Do not breathe vapor. Avoid contact with skin and clothing.

Antidote(s): If inhaled, remove to fresh air. Flush eyes and skin with plenty of water for at least 15 minutes. Call a physician. If not breathing, give artificial respiration, preferably mouth to mouth. If breathing is difficult, give oxygen. Induce vomiting. Never administer anything by mouth to an unconscious person.

First Aid Treatment-Antidote:

If Swallowed: Give a tablespoonful of salt in a glass of warm water and repeat until vomit fluid is clear. Give milk, or white of egg beaten with water.

Warning(s): Keep out of reach of children.

Presentation: 1 gallon (3.785 L) (NDC 57319-436-09).

Sold to veterinarians only.

Manufactured by: Ameri-Pac, St. Joseph, MO 64502.

Compendium Code No.: 12561151

Rev. 8-01

FORMULA F-500

Aire-Mate

Premise Insecticide

EPA Reg. No.: 5011-128

Active Ingredient(s):

*Resmethrin 0.50%

**Inert Ingredients 99.50%

Total:........ 100.00%

*Cis/trans isomers ratio: max. 30% (±) cis and min. 70% (±) trans.

**Contains petroleum distillates.

Indications: A fogging and contact insecticide containing Resmethrin.

Directions for Use: It is a violation of Federal Law to use this product in a manner inconsistent with its labeling.

An insecticide for use in horse stables and kennels. See caution limitations. For fogging control of flies, mosquitoes, and gnats and direct contact spraying control of roaches, ants, spiders, water bugs and house centipedes. Recommended for use in thermal fogging applicators and can also be applied by ULV and other power and hand operated sprayers. Fogging application indoors for control of flies, mosquitoes and gnats: After closing off all air currents, direct fog upwards at walls and ceilings so that as many insects as possible can be contacted with a direct fog. When application is made with foggers, use 1 oz of GH-60 per 1000 cubic feet of space. Keep premises closed for at least 10 minutes after fogging. Sweep up and destroy all dead and dying insects. Repeat when necessary. Direct contact spray application for control of roaches, ants, spiders, water bugs and house centipedes: Direct a wet spray toward infested areas, floors, cracks and crevices to hit the insects. Apply GH-60 with an efficient electric or other power or hand operated sprayer that will deliver a coarse spray. Thorough application should be made with repeated treatment whenever reinfestation occurs.

Precautionary Statements: Hazards to Humans (and Domestic Animals):

Caution: Harmful if swallowed. Do not breathe spray mist, vapor or fog. Avoid contact with skin, and clothing. Remove pets before using.

Personal Protective Equipment: Some materials that are chemical-resistant to this product are listed below. If you want more options, follow the instructions for category E an the EPA resistance category selection chart.

Applicators and other handlers must wear:

A. Long-sleeved shirt and long pants.

B. Chemical-resistant gloves, such as nitrile rubber ≥ 14 mils or barrier laminate ≥ 14 mils or neoprene rubber ≥ 14 mils or viton ≥ 14 mils.

C. Shoes plus socks.

D. Protective eyewear.

E. A respirator with either an organic vapor-removing cartridge with prefilter approved for pesticides (MSHA/NIOSH approval number prefix TC-23C), or a canister approved for pesticides (MSHA/NIOSH approval number prefix TC-14G).

Follow manufacturer's instructions for cleaning/maintaining PPE. If no such instructions for washables, use detergent and hot water. Keep and wash PPE separately from other laundry.

User Safety Recommendations: Users should:

Wash hands before eating, drinking, chewing gum, using tobacco or using the toilet.

Remove clothing immediately if pesticide gets inside. Then wash thoroughly and put on clean clothing.

Remove PPE immediately after handling this product. Wash the outside of gloves before removing. As soon as possible, wash thoroughly and change into clean clothing.

Environmental Hazards: This product is highly toxic to fish. Do not apply directly to water or wetlands (swamps, bogs, marshes, and potholes). Drift and runoff from treated sites may be hazardous to fish in adjacent waters. Do not contaminate water when disposing of equipment washwaters.

Physical or Chemical Hazards: Do not use or store near open flame or heat.

Do not apply this product in a way that will contact workers or other persons, either directly or through drift. Only protected handlers may be in the area during application. For any requirements specific to your State or Tribe, consult the agency responsible for pesticide regulation.

Agricultural Use Requirements:

Use this product only in accordance with its labeling and with the Worker Protection Standard, 40 CFR part 170. This Standard contains requirements for the protection of agricultural workers on farms, forests, nurseries, and greenhouses, and handlers of agricultural pesticides. It contains requirements for training, decontamination, notification, and emergency assistance. It also contains specific instructions and exceptions pertaining to the statements on this label about personal protective equipment (PPE), notification to workers and restricted-entry interval. The requirements in this box only apply to uses of this product that are covered by the Worker Protection Standard.

Do not enter or allow worker entry into treated areas during the restricted entry interval (REI) of 24 hours.

PPE required for early entry to treated areas that is permitted under the Worker Protection Standard and that involves contact with anything that has been treated, such as plants, soil, or water, is: (A) Coveralls (B) Chemical-resistant gloves, such as nitrile rubber ≥ 14 mils or viton ≥ 14 mils, or neoprene rubber ≥ 14 mils or barrier laminate ≥ 14 mils (C) Shoes plus socks (D) Protective eyewear.

Non-Agricultural Use Requirements:

The requirements in this box apply to uses of this product that are not within the scope of the Worker Protection Standard for agricultural pesticides (40 CFR Part 170). The WPS applies when this product is used to produce agricultural plants on farms, forests, nurseries or greenhouses.

Use this product in food processing plants only when plant is not in operation. Foods should be removed or covered during treatment. All processing surfaces should be covered or thoroughly cleaned before using. All food handling surfaces, utensils, and equipment must be covered or removed during treatment or thoroughly washed with an effective cleaning compound followed by a potable water rinse prior to use. In hospitals, remove patients prior to treatment. Ventilate 2 hours after treatment before returning patients. In horse stables, not for application

F

if horses will be used for food. Do not remain in treated area and ventilate after treatment is completed. Observe usual caution as should be followed with any insecticide. Remove pet birds and cover fish aquariums before spraying.

Statement of Practical Treatment:

If Swallowed: Call a physician or Poison Control Center immediately. Do not induce vomiting because of aspiration of pneumonia hazard.

If in Eyes: Flush with plenty of water. Get medical attention it irritation persists.

If on Skin or Clothing: Remove contaminated clothing and wash before reuse. Wash skin with soap and warm water. Get medical attention if irritation persists.

If Inhaled: Remove victim to fresh air. Apply artificial respiration if indicated.

Storage and Disposal:

Prohibitions: Do not contaminate water, food or feed by storage or disposal. Open dumping is prohibited.

Pesticide Storage: Do not use, pour, spill or store near heat or open flame. Do not store with food, feed, drugs or clothing. Store securely. Store to prevent cross contamination of other pesticides and fertilizer. Store in original, tightly closed container. Store above 35°F.

Pesticide Disposal: Pesticide wastes are toxic. Improper disposal of excess pesticide, spray mixture or rinsate is a violation of Federal Law. If these wastes cannot be disposed of by use according to label instructions, contact your State Pesticide or Environmental Control Agency, or the Hazardous Waste representative at the nearest EPA Regional Office for guidance. Container Disposal—Plastic: Triple rinse (or equivalent). Then offer for recycling or reconditioning, or puncture and dispose of in a sanitary landfill, or incineration, or if allowed by state and local authorities, by burning. If burned, stay out of smoke. Container Disposal—Metal: Triple rinse (or equivalent). Then offer for recycling or reconditioning, or puncture and dispose of in a sanitary landfill, or by other procedures approved by state and local authorities. If subjected to temperatures below 32°F, move container to warm storage until reaching average room temperature and thoroughly mix before use.

Warning(s): Keep out of reach of children.

Disclaimer: Seller makes no warranty other than specified on this label. The buyer agrees that the seller shall not be responsible or liable for injury to crop, soil, person or property arising from careless or improper use or handling of the product. Please use in accordance with seller's directions.

Presentation: 1 gallon.

Compendium Code No.: 13970010

FORMULA V™ TAURINE TABLETS

Pet-Ag — **Small Animal Dietary Supplement**

Guaranteed Analysis: Each tablet contains:

Taurine .... 250 mg

In a protein chewable base.

Indications: Recommended for use as a supplement for cats of all ages with a taurine deficiency determined by blood analysis or clinical manifestations of taurine deficiency. Cats and especially growing kittens have a very limited ability to produce taurine through metabolic pathways. Consequently preformed taurine is required from dietary sources. A taurine deficiency may result in dilated cardiomyopathy (DCM), feline central retinal degeneration (FCRD) and reproductive problems characterized by poor growth, survival and other abnormalities of kittens born to taurine deficient queens.

Dosage and Administration: Taurine tablets can be hand fed or crumbled and offered with the cat's food.

One-half (½) tablet per day meets the daily requirement of cats for maintenance and growth. One (1) tablet per day meets the daily requirement of cats for gestation and lactation.

Precaution(s): Store in cool, dry conditions.

Caution(s): For animal use only - not for human use. Use only as directed by a veterinarian.

Presentation: 100 count, tamper evident bottles (12 bottles per case).

Compendium Code No.: 10970161

FORSHNER'S® MEDICATED HOOF PACKING

Equicare — **Hoof Product**

Active Ingredient(s): Per ounce:

Petrolatum .... 7.5 g
Pine tar .... 2.4 g

Indications: FORSHNER'S® Medicated Hoof Packing is useful in preventing drying of the horny tissues, in case of contracted heels and hardening frog; and as an aid in keeping them pliable.

Dosage and Administration: No mixing required.

Make sure that the hoof is thoroughly clean and dry. Pack in and around the frog. Spread a layer over the sole and cover with paper. Apply two (2) or three (3) times a week. For easier application in cold weather keep where warm.

Presentation: 4 lbs (1.814 g), 14 lbs (6.35 kg), 24 lbs and 35 lbs.

Compendium Code No.: 14470091

FORTE V1

Novartis (Aqua Health) — **Bacterin-Vaccine**

Infectious Salmon Anaemia Virus Vaccine, Killed Virus-Aeromonas salmonicida, Vibrio anguillarum-ordalii-salmonicida Bacterin

U.S. Vet. Lic. No.: 335

Contents: Contains formalin inactivated cultures of Infectious Salmon Anaemia Virus, *Aeromonas salmonicida, Vibrio anguillarum* Types I and II, *Vibrio ordalli*, and *Vibrio salmonicida* Types I and II in liquid emulsion with oil based adjuvants. No other preservatives are used.

Indications: Uses: As an aid to the prevention of infectious salmon anaemia, furunculosis, vibriosis, and cold water vibriosis by injection of healthy salmonids.

Dosage and Administration: Vaccination Program: This vaccine has been shown to be safe and effective when administered by manual intraperitoneal injection to salmonids 30 grams or larger. It is recommended that vaccination should precede exposure of vaccinates to the disease agents by 800 degree-days (number of days multiplied by the mean water temperature (°C) during period). This product should be used as part of a comprehensive fish health program in consultation with a licensed veterinarian.

Fish are anaesthetized to immobilize and administered a 0.15 mL injection intraperitoneally one fin length ahead of the pelvic fins along the midline. Warming of the vaccine to room temperature (15-20°C) overnight may facilitate injection.

Precaution(s): Shake well before using.

Store between 2-7°C (35-45°F). Do not freeze.

Use entire contents when first opened.

Any unused product should be disposed of according to local waste disposal regulations and/or requirements.

Caution(s): Vaccinate healthy fish only.

If accidental injection of the operator occurs, the operator should discontinue activity and seek medical attention immediately.

For veterinary use only.

Warning(s): Do not vaccinate within 60 days of slaughter.

Presentation: 1,000 mL bag.

Produced for: J. Zinn, Aqua Health USA, Inc., Buhl, ID 83316.

Compendium Code No.: 14970101 L-35-0

FORTIFIED VITAMIN B COMPLEX

AgriLabs — **Vitamin B-Complex**

Active Ingredient(s): Each mL contains:

Thiamine HCl .... 100 mg
Riboflavin (as 5' phosphate sodium) .... 5 mg
Niacinamide .... 100 mg
d-panthenol .... 10 mg
Pyridoxine HCl .... 10 mg
Cyanocobalamin (cryst.) .... 100 mcg
Benzyl alcohol (preservative) 1.5%
Water .... q.s.

Indications: A sterile aqueous solution of B-complex vitamins to provide a supplementation of these vitamins to cattle, horses, sheep, swine and small animals (dogs and cats).

Dosage and Administration: Administer intramuscularly or subcutaneously.

Dogs and Cats .... ½ to 2 mL
Sheep and Swine .... 5 to 10 mL
Cattle and Horses .... 10 to 20 mL

Repeat daily as indicated.

Precaution(s): Store at a controlled room temperature between 59-86°F (15-30°C).

Caution(s): Keep out of the reach of children.

Anaphylactic reactions to parenteral thiamine HCl have been reported. Administer slowly and with caution in doses over 50 mg.

Presentation: 100 mL, 250 mL and 500 mL bottles.

Compendium Code No.: 10580520

FORTIFIED VITAMIN B-COMPLEX

AgriPharm — **Vitamin B-Complex**

Active Ingredient(s): Each mL contains:

Thiamine HCl .... 100 mg
Riboflavin (as 5'phosphate sodium) .... 5 mg
Niacinamide .... 100 mg
d-Panthenol .... 10 mg
Pyridoxine HCl .... 10 mg
Cobalt (as cyanocobalamin) .... 4.0 ppm
Benzyl alcohol (preservative) .... 1.5% v/v
Citric acid .... 5 mg
Water for injection .... q.s.

Indications: An aqueous solution of B complex vitamins for use as a supplemental source of these vitamins and complexed cobalt for cattle, sheep, and swine.

Dosage and Administration: Administer intramuscularly. The dosage may be repeated once a day as needed.

Cattle .... 10 to 20 mL
Sheep and Swine .... 5 to 10 mL

Precaution(s): Store at a controlled room temperature between 59°-86°F (15°-30°C).

Keep from freezing.

Caution(s): Keep out of the reach of children.

For animal use only.

Not for intravenous use. Parenteral administration of thiamine has resulted in anphylactic shock. Administer slowly and with caution in doses over 0.5 mL (50 mg thiamine).

Presentation: 100 mL, 250 mL and 500 mL containers.

Compendium Code No.: 14570440

FORTRESS® 7

Pfizer Animal Health — **Bacterin-Toxoid**

Clostridium Chauvoei-Septicum-Novyi-Sordellii-Perfringens Types C & D Bacterin-Toxoid

U.S. Vet. Lic. No.: 189

Contents: This product consists of killed, standardized cultures of *Clostridium chauvoei, Cl. septicum, Cl. novyi, Cl. sordellii*, and *Cl. perfringens* types C and D, with a special, water-soluble adjuvant (Stimugen™). Contains formalin as preservative.

Indications: For use in healthy cattle as an aid in preventing blackleg caused by *Cl. chauvoei;* malignant edema caused by *Cl. septicum;* black disease caused by *Cl. novyi;* gas-gangrene caused by *Cl. sordellii;* and enterotoxemia and enteritis caused by *Cl. perfringens* types B, C, and D. Although *Cl. perfringens* type B is not a significant problem in North America, immunity is provided by the beta toxoid of type C and the epsilon toxoid of type D.

Directions: Shake well. Aseptically administer 5 mL subcutaneously. Healthy cattle should receive 2 doses administered 4-6 weeks apart. Annual revaccination with a single dose is recommended.

Precaution(s): Store at 2°-7°C. Do not freeze. Use entire contents when first opened. Not for use in sheep. Transient local swelling at injection site may occur following administration. As with many vaccine, anaphylaxis may occur after use. Initial antidote of epinephrine is recommended and should be followed with appropriate supportive therapy.

Warning(s): Do not vaccinate within 21 days before slaughter.

For veterinary use only.

Presentation: 10 dose (50 mL), 50 dose (250 mL) and 200 dose (1,000 mL) vials.

Compendium Code No.: 36900130 974 85-4419-04

FORTRESS® 8

Pfizer Animal Health **Bacterin-Toxoid**

Clostridium Chauvoei-Septicum-Haemolyticum-Novyi-Sordellii-Perfringens Types C & D Bacterin-Toxoid

U.S. Vet. Lic. No.: 189

Contents: This product consists of killed, standardized cultures of *Clostridium chauvoei, Cl. septicum, Cl. haemolyticum, Cl. novyi, Cl. sordellii,* and *Cl. perfringens* types C and D, with a special, water-soluble adjuvant (Stimugen™). Contains formalin as preservative.

Indications: For use in healthy cattle as an aid in preventing blackleg caused by *Cl. chauvoei;* malignant edema caused by *Cl. septicum;* bacillary hemoglobinuria caused by *Cl. haemolyticum;* black disease caused by *Cl. novyi;* gas-gangrene caused by *Cl. sordellii;* and enterotoxemia and enteritis caused by *Cl. perfringens* types B, C, and D. Although *Cl. perfringens* type B is not a significant problem in North America, immunity is provided by the beta toxoid of type C and the epsilon toxoid of type D.

Directions: Shake well. Aseptically administer 5 mL subcutaneously. Healthy cattle should receive 2 doses administered 4-6 weeks apart. For *Cl. haemolyticum* repeat the dose every 6 months in animals subject to reexposure. Annual revaccination with a single dose is recommended.

Precaution(s): Store at 2°-7°C. Do not freeze. Use entire contents when first opened.

Caution(s): Not for use in sheep. Transient local swelling at injection site may occur following administration. As with many vaccines, anaphylaxis may occur after use. Initial antidote of epinephrine is recommended and should be followed with appropriate supportive therapy.

For veterinary use only.

Warning(s): Do not vaccinate within 21 days before slaughter.

For veterinary use only.

Presentation: 10 dose (50 mL), 50 dose (250 mL) and 200 dose (1,000 mL) vials.

Compendium Code No.: 36900140 974 85-4425-04

FORTRESS® CD

Pfizer Animal Health **Bacterin-Toxoid**

Clostridium Perfringens Types C & D Bacterin-Toxoid

U.S. Vet. Lic. No.: 189

Contents: This product consists of killed, standardized cultures of *Clostridium perfringens* types C and D, with a special, water-soluble adjuvant (Stimugen™). Contains formalin as preservative.

Indications: For use in healthy cattle as an aid in preventing enterotoxemia and enteritis caused by *Cl. perfringens* types B, C, and D. Although *Cl. perfringens* type B is not a significant problem in North America, immunity is provided by the beta toxoid of type C and the epsilon toxoid of type D.

Dosage and Administration: Shake well. Aseptically administer 2 mL subcutaneously. Healthy cattle should receive 2 doses administered 4-6 weeks apart. Annual revaccination with a single dose is recommended.

Precaution(s): Store at 2°-7°C. Do not freeze. Use entire contents when first opened.

Caution(s): Not for use in sheep. Transient local swelling at injection site may occur following administration. As with many vaccines, anaphylaxis may occur after use. Initial antidote of epinephrine is recommended and should be followed with appropriate supportive therapy.

Warning(s): Do not vaccinate within 21 days before slaughter.

For veterinary use only.

Presentation: 10 dose (50 mL), 50 dose (100 mL) and 50 dose (250 mL) vials.

Compendium Code No.: 36900150 975 85-4413-05

FOWL LARYNGOTRACHEITIS VACCINE

L.A.H.I. (New Jersey) **Vaccine**

Fowl Laryngotracheitis Vaccine, Live Virus

U.S. Vet. Lic. No.: 196

Active Ingredient(s): This product is a live virus fowl laryngotracheitis vaccine of chicken embryo origin manufactured from SPF (Specific Pathogen Free) eggs.

Contains streptomycin and penicillin as preservatives.

This vaccine was carefully produced and passed all tests in accordance with the U.S. Government requirements.

Indications: For administration to chickens for the prevention of Laryngotracheitis.

For intranasal, intraocular, or aerosol use.

It is recommended that birds be at least 5 weeks of age when vaccinated. The older the birds at time of vaccination, the more effective will be the immunization using this product. Vaccinate younger birds only if absolutely necessary. Revaccinate birds if they are under 5 weeks of age when first given vaccine if they are to be held for layers.

In the event of a natural outbreak of Laryngotracheitis on a farm, this vaccine should be used immediately to help stop the outbreak. Unaffected birds should be vaccinated first, followed by the pens of birds in which the outbreak occurred.

Dosage and Administration: Preparation of Vaccine for Intranasal and Intraocular Use: Remove the aluminum tear seal and rubber stopper from the vaccine bottle. Pour some of the diluent into the bottle. Replace the rubber stopper and shake vigorously. Pour the mixed vaccine back into the bottle containing the remaining diluent and attach the dropper tip. The vaccine is now ready for use.

Method of Vaccination: The vaccine may be administered by way of the nostril (intranasally) or the eye (intraocularly). When the vaccine is administered by way of the nostril, the beak is held shut, a finger is placed over one nostril and a drop of vaccine, from the applicator, is dropped into the other nostril.

When used intraocularly, birds are held on their side and one drop of the mixed vaccine allowed to fall into the open eye. Hold the bird until the drop of vaccine disappears. Take care to prevent injury to the cornea of the eye with the dropper tip.

Preparation of Vaccine for Aerosol Use: Remove the aluminum overseal and stopper from the vaccine bottle and pour part of the diluent into the bottle. Shake well and pour the vaccine back into the remaining diluent. Pour the entire contents into the reservoir of a sprayer containing 70 mL of deionized water or 5 mL of glycerine and 65 mL of deionized water. Before the vaccination the sprayer should be calibrated so that 100 mL will be delivered in 3 minutes.

Method of Vaccination: Confine the birds to a corner of the house with fences and direct the stream from the sprayer over the heads of the birds. Extreme caution should be taken to prevent birds from smothering during this operation.

Contraindication(s): Birds to be vaccinated should be free of disease, including the latent form of diseases such as Chronic Respiratory Disease (CRD), coccidiosis, blackhead, parasitic disease, etc.

If there are susceptible laying birds on the premises there is the possibility that the virus might spread from the vaccinated to the susceptible birds and affect egg production.

Precaution(s): Keep vaccine in the dark, between 2-7°C (35-45°F).

Use the entire contents when first opened. Burn this container and all unused contents.

Caution(s): When administered to susceptible birds, a mild form of the disease results which stimulates immunity.

Parental immunity and immunological incompetence is a major factor in preventing young birds from developing immunity. When this vaccine is administered, the duration of immunity resulting from vaccination is directly related to the age of the birds and their susceptibility at the time this vaccine is administered.

The duration of immunity resulting from the use of this vaccine is not permanent; therefore, revaccinations are necessary.

It is imperative that the user of this product comply with the indications for use, contraindications, and method of vaccination stated on the direction sheet. The vaccine must be prepared and administered as directed to obtain best results.

No vaccine confers immediate protection. While immunity begins to develop immediately, it takes 9 days to two weeks for birds to establish immunity, during which time they should not be placed in contaminated premises nor otherwise exposed to Laryngotracheitis.

All susceptible birds on any farm should be vaccinated at the same time.

Warning(s): Do not vaccinate within 21 days before slaughter.

Care should be taken to avoid contaminating hands, eyes and clothing with the vaccine.

For veterinary use only.

Presentation: 1,000 and 5,000 doses.

Compendium Code No.: 10080212

FOWL POX VACCINE

L.A.H.I. (New Jersey) **Vaccine**

Fowl Pox Vaccine, Live Virus

U.S. Vet. Lic. No.: 196

Active Ingredient(s): This product is a live virus fowlpox vaccine of chicken embryo origin manufactured from SPF (Specific Pathogen Free) eggs.

Contains neomycin as a preservative.

This vaccine was carefully produced and passed all tests in accordance with the U.S. Government requirements.

Indications: For the prevention of Fowlpox in chickens. For wing web application.

This vaccine is for administration to chickens 5 weeks of age and older. For laying replacements, the ideal time for administration is when birds are 8 to 20 weeks of age. If administered to birds under 5 weeks of age, revaccination is necessary.

The older the birds at the time of administration, the more durable is the immunity produced.

Dosage and Administration: Preparation of Vaccine: The active agent of the vaccine is supplied in a dried form in the bottle labelled 'Vaccine'. Open the bottle by removing the aluminum tear seal and the rubber stopper. Open the diluent and pour a small quantity into the bottle of vaccine, replace the rubber stopper, and shake well. Pour the mixture back into the bottle of diluent and shake mixture vigorously. Do not open or mix the vaccine until ready for use.

Method of Vaccination: Vaccination is accomplished by dipping the double needle in the mixed vaccine and piercing the "web of the wing" from the underside. Do not apply through feathers, muscle or bone. The applicator must be redipped between each application.

Birds from the flock should be examined for evidence of a "take" to ensure that the vaccine was applied properly.

The evidence of a successful vaccination will appear at the point of vaccination in from 7 to 10 days after vaccination. Brownish, black scabs will be found on both the under and upper surfaces of the web of the wing through which the needle vaccinator was thrust.

Contraindication(s): Birds to be vaccinated should be free of all diseases, including the latent form of diseases such as chronic respiratory disease (CRD), coccidiosis, blackhead, parasitic disease, etc.

Precaution(s): Keep vaccine in the dark, between 2-7°C (35-45°F).

Use entire contents when first opened. Burn this container and all unused contents.

Caution(s): When administered to susceptible birds, a mild form of the disease results which stimulates immunity. No vaccine confers immediate protection against fowl pox. While immunity begins to develop immediately, it takes 2 to 3 weeks for birds to establish maximum immunity to fowlpox following vaccination, during which time they should not be placed in contaminated premises nor otherwise exposed to fowlpox.

All susceptible birds on any farm should be vaccinated at the same time. If this is not possible, individual lots may be vaccinated if strict isolation and separate caretakers are provided for the vaccinated and unvaccinated lots of birds.

It is imperative that the user of this product comply with the indications for use, contraindications, and method of vaccination stated on the direction sheet. The vaccine must be prepared and administered as directed to obtain best results.

Warning(s): Do not vaccinate within 21 days before slaughter.

Care should be taken to avoid contaminating hands, eyes and clothing with the vaccine.

For veterinary use only.

Presentation: 500 dose - rehydrate to 5 mL.

Compendium Code No.: 10080222

FOWL POX VACCINE

Merial Select **Vaccine**

Fowl Pox Vaccine, Live Virus

U.S. Vet. Lic. No.: 279

Active Ingredient(s): The vaccine contains a live strain of fowl pox virus.

Penicillin and streptomycin sulfate are added as bacteriostatic agents.

Contains fungizone as a fungistat.

Notice: The vaccine meets the requirements of the U.S. Department of Agriculture in regards to safety, potency and the ability to immunize normal, susceptible chickens.

Indications: The vaccine is recommended for subcutaneous injection of one day old chickens to aid in the prevention of fowl pox.

Chickens to be vaccinated must be healthy and free of all diseases. It is essential that the birds be maintained under good environmental conditions, and that the exposure to disease viruses be reduced as much as possible in the field.

Dosage and Administration: Frozen Vaccine:

Preparation of the Vaccine for Use:

Important: Sterilize the vaccinating equipment by autoclaving for a minimum 15 minutes at 121°C or by boiling in water for at least 20 minutes. Never allow chemical disinfectants to come into contact with the vaccinating equipment.

1. Use 200 mL of sterile diluent for each 1,000 doses of vaccine indicated on the ampule.
2. When the fowl pox vaccine is used in combination with Merial Select's turkey herpesvirus

vaccine, add the contents of two (2) ampules of HVT and one (1) ampule of fowl pox vaccine to 400 mL of diluent.

3. Remove only one (1) ampule of vaccine at a time from the liquid nitrogen container. Thaw and use immediately. Carefully observe all liquid nitrogen precautions, including wearing eye protection and gloves. Caution: Do not hold the ampule toward the face when removing it from a nitrogen container. Never refreeze a vaccine ampule after thawing.
4. The contents of the ampule are thawed rapidly by immersing it in water at room temperature (15-25°C). Gently mix the ampule to disperse the contents. Break the ampule at its neck and quickly proceed as described below.
5. Remove the cover from the diluent container. Draw the contents of the ampule into a sterile 10 mL syringe fitted with an 18 to 20 gauge needle. Slowly add the contents of the vaccine ampule to the appropriate volume of diluent. Withdraw a small amount of the diluent, rinse the ampule once and add this to the vaccine-diluent mixture. Mix the contents of the bottle thoroughly by swirling and inverting the bottle, but do not shake vigorously.
6. Use the vaccine-diluent mixture immediately as described below.

Method of Vaccination: Give subcutaneously only.

1. Use a sterile, automatic syringe with a 20-22 gauge, ⅜"-½" needle which is accurately set to deliver 0.2 mL per dose. Check the accuracy of delivery several times during the vaccination procedure.
2. Dilute the vaccine only as directed, observing all precautions and warnings for handling.
3. Keep the bottle of diluted vaccine in an ice bath and agitate continuously.
4. Inject chickens under the loose skin at the back of the neck (subcutaneously), holding the chicken by the back of the neck just below the head. The loose skin in this area is raised by gently pinching the thumb and forefinger. Insert the needle beneath the skin in a direction away from the head. Inject 0.2 mL per chicken. Avoid hitting the muscles and bones in the neck.
5. Use the entire contents of the bottle within one (1) hour after mixing.
6. Be careful not to touch any part of the bird with the vaccine except the area to be inoculated.

Precaution(s):

Ampules: Store in a liquid nitrogen container.

Diluent: Store at room temperature.

Liquid nitrogen container: Store in a cool, well-ventilated area. Check the liquid nitrogen level once a day. Keep the container away from incubator intakes and chicken boxes.

Liquid Nitrogen Precautions: The liquid nitrogen containers and vaccine should be handled by properly trained personnel only. These persons should be familiar with the Union Carbide publication "Precautions and Safe Practices - Liquified Atmospheric Gases", form #9888. Liquid nitrogen is extremely cold. Accidental contact with the skin or eyes can cause serious frostbite. Protect the eyes with goggles or a face shield, wear gloves and long sleeves when removing and handling frozen ampules, or when adding liquid nitrogen to the container. Storage and handling of liquid nitrogen containers should be in a well-ventilated area. Excessive amounts of nitrogen reduces the concentration of oxygen in the air of an unventilated space and can cause asphyxiation. If drowsiness occurs, get fresh air quickly and ventilate the entire area. If a person seems to become groggy or loses consciousness while working with liquid nitrogen, get the person to a well-ventilated area immediately. If breathing has stopped, apply artificial respiration. If difficulties persist, or there is a loss of consciousness, summon a physician immediately.

Caution(s): Use the entire contents when first opened.

Burn the container and all unused contents.

The ability of the vaccine to produce satisfactory results may depend on many factors, including, but not limited to, conditions of storage and handling by the user, administration of the vaccine, health and the responsiveness of individual chickens and the degree of field exposure. Therefore, directions for use should be followed carefully.

The use of the vaccine is subject to applicable state and federal laws and regulations.

Warning(s): Do not vaccinate within 21 days before slaughter.

Presentation: 5 x 2,000 dose vials, with 200 mL of sterile diluent included per 1,000 doses.

Compendium Code No.: 11050191

FOWL POX VACCINE

Schering-Plough **Vaccine**

Fowl Pox Vaccine, Live Virus

U.S. Vet. Lic. No.: 165A

Active Ingredient(s): FOWL POX VACCINE is a live virus vaccine of chicken embryo origin containing a fowl pox virus selected for its ability to stimulate strong protection against a wide variety of fowl pox strains. The vaccine contains gentamicin as a preservative.

Indications: For the vaccination of healthy chickens and turkeys six weeks of age or older, as an aid in preventing fowl pox through immunization by the wing-web method (for chickens) and the thigh-stab method (for turkeys).

Dosage and Administration: When to Vaccinate:

Chickens: Six (6) weeks of age or older.

Turkeys: Six (6) weeks of age or older.

Vaccination Program: The development of a durable, strong protection depends upon the use of an effective vaccination program as well as many circumstances such as administration techniques, environment and flock health at the time of vaccination. Also, the immune response to one (1) vaccination under field conditions is seldom complete for all animals within a given flock. Even when vaccination is successful, the protection stimulated in individual animals against different diseases may not be life-long. Therefore, under certain circumstances revaccination may be necessary.

Preparation of the Vaccine:

1. Do not open and mix the vaccine until ready for use.
2. Mix only one (1) vial at a time and use the entire contents within two (2) hours.
3. Remove the tear-off aluminum seal and stopper from the vial containing the dried vaccine.
4. Remove the tear-off aluminum seal and stopper from the bottle containing the diluent.
5. Hold the diluent bottle firmly in an upright position and insert the vaccine vial on the adapter of the diluent bottle. The neck of the vaccine vial should snap into position and should be seated securely on the adapter on the diluent bottle.
6. Invert the two (2) containers so that the vaccine vial is on the bottom and allow the diluent to flow into the vaccine vial. If the diluent does not flow freely, squeeze the bottle gently and the diluent will flow into the vaccine vial. The vaccine vial should be completely filled with diluent to prevent excess foaming.
7. Hold the joined containers by the ends and shake vigorously until the vaccine plug is completely dissolved.
8. Return the joined containers to their original position (diluent bottle on the bottom). Allow the vaccine to flow into the diluent bottle. If the vaccine does not flow into the diluent bottle, tap or squeeze the diluent bottle gently and release to draw the vaccine into the diluent bottle. Be sure that all of the product is removed from the vaccine vial.
9. Remove the vaccine vial and adapter from the neck of the diluent bottle.
10. The vaccine is now ready for use.

How to Vaccinate:

Chickens: Vaccination is accomplished by dipping the needle applicator into the mixed vaccine and piercing the webbed portion of the underside of the wing. Avoid piercing through feathers which may wipe off the vaccine, and avoid hitting the wing muscle or bone to minimize reaction. The applicator is designed to pick up the proper amount of vaccine on the needle, which is deposited in the tissues when the wing is pierced. Redip the applicator in the vaccine before each application. Excess vaccine adhering to the applicator should be removed by touching the applicator to the side of the vaccine vial.

Turkeys: Vaccination may be successfully accomplished by the thigh-stab method as follows: The helper grasps the legs of the turkey with one hand as it is handed to him, and holds the bird head downward with its back toward him. He then passes his other hand downward on the outside of one thigh, turning the feathers back and exposing a bare spot about midway. With the freshly dipped applicator, the vaccinator stabs into the thigh muscle going only deep enough to break the skin and deliver the vaccine, but taking care to avoid piercing the tendons or injuring the bone.

Be careful not to touch any part of the bird with the vaccine except the area to be inoculated.

Examine for Takes: Examine the birds for takes six (6) to eight (8) days following vaccination. A positive take, showing that the vaccination was successful, is indicated by swelling of the skin or a scab formation at the point of inoculation. The absence of takes may mean that the birds were immune before vaccination or that improper vaccination methods were used. Protection will normally develop within about 10 to 14 days after vaccination. Swelling and scabs will disappear two (2) to three (3) weeks following vaccination.

Records: Keep a record of the vaccine type, quantity, serial number, expiration date, and place of purchase; the date and time of vaccination; the number, age, breed, and location of the birds; the names of operators performing the vaccination; and any observed reactions.

Precaution(s): Store at 35° to 45° F (2° to 7°C).

Caution(s): For veterinary use only.

1. Vaccinate healthy birds only. Although disease may not be evident, coccidiosis, chronic respiratory disease, mycoplasma infection, lymphoid leukosis, infectious bursal disease, Marek's disease, or other disease conditions may cause serious complications or reduce protection.
2. All birds within a house should be vaccinated on the same day. Isolate other susceptible birds on the premises from the birds being vaccinated.
3. In outbreak situations, vaccinate healthy birds first, progressing toward outbreak areas in order to vaccinate diseased birds last.
4. Do not spill or spatter the vaccine. Use the entire contents of the vial when first opened. Burn the empty bottles, caps, and all unused vaccine and accessories.
5. Wash hands thoroughly after using the vaccine.
6. Do not dilute the vaccine or otherwise stretch the dosage.

Warning(s): Do not vaccinate within 21 days before slaughter.

Presentation: Supplied in 10 x 1,000 dose units with diluent.

Compendium Code No.: 10470740

FP BLEN®

Merial Select **Vaccine**

Fowl Pox Vaccine Live Virus

U.S. Vet. Lic. No.: 279

Contents: This vaccine contains live fowl pox virus.

Contains Gentamicin as a bacteriostatic agent.

Notice: Merial Select's vaccines have met the requirements of the USDA in regard to safety, purity, potency, and the capability to protect susceptible chickens. This vaccine has been tested by the Master Seed immunogenicity test for efficacy.

Indications: This vaccine is for the vaccination of healthy chickens between four and sixteen weeks of age, but no later than four weeks before egg production by wing web stab as an aid in the prevention of fowl pox. Fowl pox vaccine will cause a drop in production if birds are vaccinated while they are in production.

This vaccine is recommended for the protection of healthy chickens. It is essential that the chickens be maintained under good environmental conditions and that exposure to disease viruses be reduced as much as possible.

Dosage and Administration: Wing Web Method: Ten (10) mL of diluent is supplied for each 1,000 doses of vaccine.

1. Pull up on the plastic tear-flip-up top to remove the aluminum seal from the bottle containing the lyophilized vaccine. Carefully pry up one edge of the rubber stopper to permit air to replace the vacuum in the bottle, then remove the stopper.
2. Pull up on the plastic tear-flip-up top to remove the aluminum seal from the bottle containing the diluent and transfer the entire contents to the bottle containing the lyophilized vaccine. Replace the stopper and shake the contents vigorously a few times until the vaccine is evenly suspended. The vaccine is now ready for use. Wash hands thoroughly after mixing the vaccine.
3. The vaccine is applied to the web of the wing using the two-pronged applicator supplied in the package. Avoid stabbing through feathers which may wipe off the vaccine.
4. The applicator is designed to carry the proper amount of vaccine in the grooves of the needles. The needle should be touched briefly to the inner lip of the bottle before withdrawing to avoid waste of the vaccine which may drop from the needles. Dip the applicator before each application.

Check for Takes: At about seven to ten days after vaccination, the birds may be examined for takes. A good take reaction, indicating that a satisfactory vaccination job was done, shows swelling of the skin at the point of vaccination with scab formation. The scabs will fall off about two to three weeks following vaccination. Good immunity to fowl pox is established two to three weeks after vaccination.

If good takes are not seen, it may mean that the birds were immune to fowl pox, that the vaccination was poor or that the vaccine used had lost its potency through extended storage or mishandling.

Precaution(s): Improper storage or handling of the vaccine may result in loss of potency. Store vaccine at 35-45°F (2-7°C). Do not freeze. Use entire vial contents when first opened. Burn this container and all unused contents.

Do not spill or splatter the vaccine. Burn all vaccine containers, used applicators, and unused vaccine when the vaccination is completed.

This vaccine is non-returnable.

Caution(s): All birds on a farm should be vaccinated at one time, or if not, the vaccinated groups should be segregated from the non-vaccinated birds.

Mix the vaccine outside the poultry pens to avoid dangers involved in accidental spilling.

Mix only one vial of vaccine at a time and use promptly. Use all at one time and do not stretch the dosage.

This vaccine is prepared for the vaccination of healthy birds. Improper handling or administration may result in variable responses.

The capability of this vaccine to produce satisfactory results depends upon many factors, including — but not limited to — conditions of storage and handling by the user, administration of the vaccine, health and responsiveness of individual chickens, and degree of field exposure. Therefore, directions for use should be followed carefully. The use of this vaccine is subject to applicable state and federal laws and regulations.

Warning(s): Do not vaccinate within 21 days of slaughter.

Presentation: 25 x 1,000 doses.

Compendium Code No.: 11050202 PE-1M 0699

FPV-1

Biocor **Vaccine**

Feline Panleukopenia Vaccine, Killed Virus-Non-adjuvanted

U.S. Vet. Lic. No.: 462

Contents: FPV-1 is an inactivated Panleukopenia virus vaccine.

This product contains gentamicin and amphotericin B as preservatives.

Indications: Recommended for use in the vaccination of healthy cats and kittens against disease caused by Feline Panleukopenia virus.

Directions: Shake well. Vaccinate healthy cats with one 1 mL dose, followed by a second 1 mL dose 3-4 weeks later. Inject subcutaneously. Kittens vaccinated at less than 12 weeks of age should be given an additional 1 mL dose of vaccine at 12-13 weeks of age with revaccination 3-4 weeks later. Annual revaccination with a single 1 mL dose is recommended.

Precaution(s): Store at 35°F-45°F (2°C-7°C). Do not freeze. Use entire contents when first opened. In case of anaphylactoid reactions, epinephrine should be administered immediately.

Caution(s): May be safely used in pregnant queens. Persistence of maternal origin antibody in kittens is known to interfere with development of active immunity following vaccination. Present indications are that antibodies of maternal origin may endure in kittens up to 13 weeks.

For use in cats only.

Presentation: Code 62411B - 25 x 1 dose (1 mL) vials.

Compendium Code No.: 13940250 BAH5125-900

FP-VAC®

Intervet **Vaccine**

Fowl Pox Vaccine, Live Virus

U.S. Vet. Lic. No.: 286

Active Ingredient(s): FP-VAC®, a live virus vaccine, is prepared from a proven strain of fowl pox virus which was back passaged through specific pathogen free (SPF) chickens to assure its full potential. The virus has been propagated in fertile eggs from (SPF) specific pathogen free flocks. The immunizing capability of this vaccine has also been proven by the Master Seed Immunogenicity Test.

The vaccine contains gentamicin as a preservative.

Indications: FP-VAC® is indicated for immunization of commercial layers, commercial layer breeders, broiler breeders and turkey breeder replacements against fowl pox via wing-web stick method. The vaccine is recommended for use via wing-web stick method in chickens of 8-17 weeks of age and in turkeys of 10-22 weeks of age.

Dosage and Administration: Preparation of Vaccine:

Do not open and mix the vaccine until ready to begin vaccination. Use the vaccine immediately after mixing.

1. Remove the tear-off seal and stopper from the vial containing the vaccine and the vial containing the diluent.
2. Pour the diluent into the vial containing the vaccine. Replace the stopper and shake the bottle thoroughly. The vaccine is ready for use.

Wing-Web Administration: For chickens 8-17 weeks of age and turkeys 10-22 weeks of age:

1. The vaccine is applied to the web of the wing. Use the enclosed two-pronged applicator.
2. Vaccinate by dipping the applicator into the vaccine mixture and stabbing the webbed portion of the wing from beneath. Avoid feathered areas of the web.
3. At about 7-10 days after vaccination, a few birds should be examined for takes. A good take reaction, indicating that a satisfactory vaccination job was done, shows swelling of the skin at the point of vaccination with scab formation. The scabs will fall off in about two (2) to three (3) weeks following vaccination. Good immunity is established two (2) to three (3) weeks after vaccination.

Records: Keep a record of vaccine, quantity, serial number, expiration date and place of purchase; the date and time of vaccination; the number, age, breed and locations of birds; names of operators performing the vaccination and any observed reactions.

Precaution(s): Use only as directed. Store the vaccine between 2-7°C (35-45°F). The product is not returnable.

Caution(s):

1. Vaccinate healthy birds only. Although disease may not be evident, concurrent disease conditions may cause complications or reduce immunity.
2. All susceptible birds on the same premises should be vaccinated at the same time.
3. Efforts should be taken to reduce stress conditions at the time of vaccination.
4. Do not spill or splash the vaccine.
5. Do not use less than one dose per bird.
6. Use the entire contents when first opened.
7. Burn the containers and all unused contents.

Warning(s): Do not vaccinate within 21 days of slaughter or 28 days prior to the onset and during egg production.

Discussion: The vaccine has undergone rigid potency, safety and purity tests, and meets Intervet America Inc. and USDA requirements. It is designed to stimulate effective immunity when used as directed, but the user must be advised that the response to the product depends upon many factors, including, but not limited to, conditions of storage and handling by the user, administration of the vaccine, health and responsiveness of individual birds and the degree of field exposure. Therefore, directions should be followed carefully.

The use of the vaccine is subject to applicable Federal and local laws and regulations.

Presentation: 10 x 500 doses for wing-web administration with 10 x 5 mL vials of sterile diluent.

Compendium Code No.: 11060570

FREEZEX® FREEZE

Hawthorne **Liniment**

Active Ingredient(s): Each 16 U.S. fl oz contains:

Menthol . . . . . 17.1 g

Indications: Deep, penetrating aid for the temporary relief of aches, pains, stiffness and soreness in horses' legs before and after racing or riding.

Dosage and Administration: Thoroughly clean leg with soap and warm water, rinse and dry. Apply FREEZEX® 4 to 6 hours before racing, workouts or eventing. During this time, apply FREEZEX® two or three times, using hot applications the first hour. Then apply cold, wet bandages and use ice tub or ice boots. Exercise only according to severity of ailment. To treat soreness and stiffness, apply FREEZEX® liberally, rub in, then bandage. Repeat for one to three days, according to severity. Discontinue for one or two days and repeat treatment if necessary.

Precaution(s): Keep in a cool, dry place.

Caution(s): Keep away from children. Consult veterinarian if condition persists.

Warning(s): Do not use on food animals.

Presentation: 4 U.S. oz and 16 U.S. fl oz.

Compendium Code No.: 10670020

FREEZEX® HOOF FREEZE

Hawthorne **Hoof Product**

Active Ingredient(s): Each 8 U.S. fl oz contains:

Iodine . . . . . 42 g
Alcohol . . . . . 45 mL
Potassium iodide . . . . . 22 g
Tannic acid

Acetone base with essential oils.

Indications: For use on tender-footed horses, as an aid in the temporary relief of soreness caused by concussion, or as an aid in the treatment of thrush. Do not apply to heel or hair.

Dosage and Administration: Horse must be in dry area. Beginning two hours prior to race or workout, apply to entire bottom of clean, dry hoof every 15 to 20 minutes. To treat thrush, place cotton on frog and saturate with Hoof Freeze. Press cotton into crevices with hoof pick. Repeat process three times during week.

Precaution(s): Keep in cool, dry place. Keep away from fire, flame or excessive heat.

Caution(s): Do not apply to heel or hair. Keep away from children.

Warning(s): Do not use on food animals.

Presentation: 8 U.S. fl oz.

Compendium Code No.: 10670030

F

FRESH COW YMCP PLUS

TechMix **Calcium-Oral**

Guaranteed Analysis:

Calcium (Ca), minimum 12.00%
Calcium (Ca), maximum 13.00%
Potassium (K), minimum 12.00%
Magnesium (Mg), minimum 5.00%
Sodium (Na), minimum 1.45%
Zinc (Zn), minimum . . . . . 100 ppm
Vitamin A, minimum . . . . . 500,000 I. Units/lb
Vitamin D, minimum . . . . . 100,000 I. Units/lb
Vitamin E, minimum . . . . . 500 I. Units/lb
Niacin, minimum . . . . . 3,00 mg/lb

Ingredients: Calcium carbonate, calcium lactate, calcium propionate, propylene glycol, betaine, dextrose, magnesium oxide, salt, potassium chloride, dried whey, sucrose, dried skimmed milk, lactose, fructose, sodium bicarbonate, dipotassium phosphate, citric acid, magnesium gluconate, glycine, zinc methionine complex, choline chloride, vitamin A acetate, d-activated animal sterol (source of vitamin D_3), dl-alpha tocopheryl acetate (source of vitamin E activity), ascorbic acid, folic acid, niacin supplement, vitamin B_{12} supplement, d-biotin, d-calcium pantothenate, menadione sodium bisulfite complex (source of vitamin K activity), riboflavin supplement, pyridoxine hydrochloride, thiamine mononitrate, dried *Saccharomyces cervisiae* fermentation product, dried *Aspergillus oryzae* fermentation extract, dried *Lactobacillus acidophilus* fermentation product, dried *Lactobacillus lactis* fermentation product, dried *Lactobacillus plantarum* fermentation product, dried *Enterococcus faecium* fermentation product, dried *Bacillus subtilus* fermentation product, dried *Bacillus subtilus* fermentation extract, ethoxyquin (a preservative), sodium silico aluminate, silicon dioxide, natural and artificial flavors added.

Indications: For use in high-producing dairy cows immediately after calving to prepare the animals for the demands of lactation.

Directions for Use:

At Calving Time: Administer one pound of FRESH COW YMCP PLUS as soon as possible or feasible immediately after calving. Administer another one pound of FRESH COW YMCP PLUS within 12-18 hours after calving or an additional two-one half pound doses of FRESH COW YMCP PLUS during the first 24 hours after calving to total two pounds administered within 24 hours after calving.

Drench Administration: FRESH COW YMCP PLUS is convenient to administer as a drench suspension by mixing one pound of FRESH COW YMCP PLUS with one pint of warm water Drench suspension slowly to permit swallowing. Do not drench cows that are down or struggle excessively with fluids or gels as their swallowing reflexes may be impaired.

Water Administration: Many cows will consume the initial one pound dose of FRESH COW YMCP PLUS when mixed with warm drinking water. The quicker the offering of FRESH COW YMCP PLUS in the drinking water after calving the better the consumption. When added to the drinking water, mix one half pound of FRESH COW YMCP PLUS with 5 gallons of warm water and repeat it again to provide an initial intake of one pound of FRESH COW YMCP PLUS.

Feed Mixing and Top Dressing: When feed mixing or top dressing, mix sufficient FRESH COW YMCP PLUS in the total ration or grain ration to provide a daily intake of one pound of FRESH COW YMCP PLUS the first three days after calving. When top dressing, hand mix or disperse FRESH COW YMCP PLUS throughout the grain or total ration.

Discussion: Yeast — Specially selected strains of yeast help establish optimum rumen fermentation. By administering immediately after calving and enhancing rumen fermentation action, the cow can utilize and maximize dry matter or feed intake in preparation for lactation.

Magnesium — Complements the utilization of calcium immediately after and through lactation. Many biochemists and animal scientists recommend magnesium to stimulate parathyroid activity essential for calcium mobilization after calving.

Calcium — FRESH COW YMCP PLUS provides three readily available noncaustic forms of calcium in water dispersible form. This dispersibility and solubility enhances absorption and utilization. The three sources of calcium are absorbed independently to provide a higher combination of metabolizable calcium essential to cows with a history of hypocalcemia. The calcium sources in this product are not irritating compared to chloride forms used in many oral drenches and as such, they can be administered with less danger when used as a drench.

Potassium — During the dry period, most cows consume an excess or more than an adequate supply of potassium. Once cows freshen, the demands of recovery from calving and lactation quickly use up supplies of potassium. Potassium is the primary electrolyte responsible for intracellular energy mobilization and utilization.

Betaine — Is an active energy preserving osmolyte that helps maintain normal fluid and energy reserves within the cells during potential stresses of dehydration.

Niacin — A field tested and university proven ketosis preventative. When administered as directed, FRESH COW YMCP PLUS provides an essential preventive level immediately after calving when feed intake by the fresh cow is often depressed or less than desired.

Presentation: FRESH COW YMCP PLUS is available in 4x2 lb bags (8 lb case), 25 lb pails and 40 lb bags.

Compendium Code No.: 11440080

FRESH-EAR

Q.A. Laboratories **Otic Cleanser**

Active Ingredient(s): De-ionized water, isopropyl alcohol, propylene glycol, glycerine, fragrance, salicylic acid, PEG 75 lanolin oil, lidocaine hydrochloride, boric acid, acetic acid, FD & C blue #1.

Indications: FRESH-EAR is used on dogs and cats for the routine cleaning and odor control of the ear canal.

Dosage and Administration: Fill the ear canal with FRESH-EAR and gently massage. Ear debris and excess solution should be wiped from the inner ear surface. For dirty ears, repeat the process. To keep ears clean and fresh-smelling, use on the direction of a veterinarian. May be used before and after bathing or swimming.

Precaution(s): Flammable: Keep away from heat or an open flame.

Caution(s): Harmful if swallowed. If swallowed, call a physician or the nearest poison control center. Avoid contact with the eyes and mucous membranes. If in eyes, wash with copious amounts of cool water.

Keep out of the reach of children.

Presentation: 4 oz. and 1 gallon containers.

Compendium Code No.: 13680040

FRESH EXPRESS® SEMEN EXTENDER

Synbiotics **Semen Extender**

Indications: Extender for use in canine semen collection. This product is a component of FRESH EXPRESS® kits for artificial insemination.

Directions for Use: The extender must be brought to room temperature before use. Dilute one part sperm rich fraction to two parts of extender. It is important to add the extender slowly to avoid osmotic shock to the sperm cells.

Precaution(s): Keep in refrigeration for up to 30 days. If longer storage is required, it can be stored in the freezer for up to six months. Do not refreeze.

Presentation: 10 mL vials.

Compendium Code No.: 11150080

FRESH® IODINE TEAT DIP (.50%)

Metz **Teat Dip**

Pre & Post Milking Teat Dip (0.5% Iodine)

Active Ingredient(s):

Iodine .... .50% w/w

(Provides 50% titratable iodine. Equivalent to 5,000 parts per million titratable iodine.)

Glycerine 5.0%

Minimum pH 4.0

Indications: An aid in controlling the spread of bacteria that may cause mastitis.

Directions for Use:

As a Pre-Dip: Remove all visible dirt by washing the teats and the base of the udder, using a minimal amount of an approved udder wash solution and a clean single service towel. Dry the teats and the udder completely with a clean single service paper towel. Dip or spray the teats. Allow 30 seconds contact time. Before attaching milker, remove the teat dip by drying thoroughly with a clean single service paper towel.

As a Post-Dip: Immediately after milker is removed, dip or spray the teats with undiluted product. If the cow will be returned to a below freezing temperature environment allow the teat dip to dry before discharging her from the milking area. Immediately before the next milking wash and/or pre-dip the teats and udder.

Caution(s): Do not use for cleaning or sanitizing milking equipment.

Warning(s): Harmful if swallowed. If swallowed, drink large quantities of milk or water and induce vomiting. Call a physician immediately. Will irritate eyes and mucous membranes. Flush gently with large amounts of water and see a physician immediately.

Avoid contact with food.

Keep out of the reach of children.

Presentation: 5 gallon, 15 gallon, 30 gallon, and 55 gallon.

Patent No 5 534,266 and patent pending

Patent No. 5720984

Compendium Code No.: 10190000

FRESH® IODINE TEAT DIP (1.00%)

Metz **Teat Dip**

Post Milking Teat Dip (1% Iodine)

Active Ingredient(s):

Iodine .... 1.00% w/w

(Provides 1.00% titratable iodine. Equivalent to 10,000 parts per million titratable iodine.)

Glycerine 10.0%

Minimum pH 4.0

Indications: An aid in controlling the spread of bacteria that may cause mastitis.

Directions for Use:

As a Post-Dip: Immediately after milker is removed, dip or spray the teats with undiluted product. If the cow will be returned to a below freezing temperature environment allow the teat dip to dry before discharging her from the milking area. Immediately before the next milking wash and/or pre-dip the teats and udder.

Caution(s): Do not use for cleaning or sanitizing milking equipment.

Warning(s): Harmful if swallowed. If swallowed, drink large quantities of milk or water and induce vomiting. Call a physician immediately. Will irritate eyes and mucous membranes. Flush gently with large amounts of water and see a physician immediately.

Avoid contact with food.

Keep out of the reach of children.

Presentation: 5 gallon, 15 gallon, 30 gallon, and 55 gallon.

Patent No 5 534,266 and patent pending

Patent No. 5720984

Compendium Code No.: 10190010

FRESH MOUTH ORAL SPRAY

Vedco **Dental Preparation**

Active Ingredient(s): Contains: Chlorhexidine 0.1%, surfactants, ethyl alcohol 6%, FD&C red 40, D&C red 33, peppermint flavored base.

Indications: To assist in the daily maintenance of a healthy and pleasant smelling mouth in dogs and cats through the removal of food particles and other debris from the teeth and gum line.

Dosage and Administration: Apply FRESH MOUTH either as an oral rinse or with a toothbrush.

Oral Rinse: Holding the animal's head steady with one (1) hand, spray a small amount of FRESH MOUTH between the teeth and gums on one side of the animal's mouth. Massage the mouth over the teeth to work FRESH MOUTH over the surface of the teeth. Repeat on the opposite side of the mouth so that the gum surfaces are thoroughly wet on both sides of the mouth.

Tooth Brushing: Place a small amount of FRESH MOUTH in a clean dish or cup. Holding the animal's head steady with one (1) hand, dip the toothbrush into the solution and carefully brush the teeth with a gentle motion. Rewet the brush with FRESH MOUTH as needed.

Caution(s): The use of FRESH MOUTH should not be considered a substitute for sound veterinary dental treatment. The product should be used under the direction of a veterinarian who can advise on a complete oral health program.

Published literature has reported some staining of teeth surfaces after the prolonged use of rinses containing chlorhexidine. The build up of stain can be prevented by applying the solution with a toothbrush.

For veterinary use only.

Keep out of the reach of children.

Presentation: 8 oz. (240 mL) container.

Compendium Code No.: 10940970

FRONTLINE® PLUS FOR CATS & KITTENS

Merial **Flea Control & Topical Parasiticide**

EPA Reg. No.: 65331-4

Active Ingredient(s):

fipronil: 9.8%

(S)-methoprene 11.8%

Inert Ingredients 78.4%

Total 100.0%

Indications: FRONTLINE® Plus for Cats provides fast, effective and convenient treatment and control of fleas and ticks for cats and kittens 8 weeks or older.

Directions for Use: It is a violation of Federal Law to use this product in a manner inconsistent with its labeling. Do not allow children to apply product. To prevent harm to you and your pet, read entire label and directions before each use. Follow all directions and precautionary statements carefully. Use on cats only. Do not use on rabbits. Do not use on other animals.

To kill fleas and all stages of brown dog ticks, American dog ticks, lone star ticks, and deer ticks (which may carry Lyme disease), apply to cats and kittens (8 weeks or older) as follows: Remove applicator from child-resistant package. Hold applicator upright and snap applicator tip away from face and body. Place applicator tip through animal's hair to the skin level between the shoulder blades. Squeeze applicator, applying entire contents in a single spot to the animal's skin. Avoid superficial application to the animal's hair. Only one applicator per treatment is needed.

Frequency of Application: When used monthly, FRONTLINE® Plus for Cats completely breaks the flea life cycle and controls tick infestations. Research demonstrates that FRONTLINE® Plus kills adult fleas, flea eggs, and flea larvae for up to six weeks. FRONTLINE® Plus also prevents development of all flea stages for up to six weeks. FRONTLINE® Plus kills ticks for at least one month. A once monthly application is recommended where tick control is needed. Although FRONTLINE® Plus can control fleas for up to six weeks, if there is a high risk of reinfestation or if the pet has fleas which may cause flea allergy dermatitis, a once monthly application may be needed.

FRONTLINE® Plus for Cats remains effective even after bathing, water immersion, or exposure to sunlight. Avoid contact with treated area until dry. Do not reapply FRONTLINE® Plus for 30 days.

Precautionary Statements: Hazards to Humans: Caution.

Harmful if swallowed. Causes eye irritation. Avoid contact with skin, eyes or clothing. Wash thoroughly with soap and water after handling.

Hazards to Domestic Animals: For external use only. Do not use on kittens under 8 weeks of age. Individual sensitivities, while rare, may occur after using any pesticide product. Pets may experience some temporary irritation at the site of product application. If signs persist, or become more severe within a few days of application, consult a veterinarian immediately. Certain medications can interact with pesticides. Consult a veterinarian before using on medicated, debilitated, aged, pregnant, or nursing animals. Call 1-800-660-1842 for 24-hour assistance.

First Aid: Have the product container or label with you when calling a poison control center or doctor, or going for treatment.

If Swallowed: Call a poison control center or doctor immediately for treatment advice. Have person sip a glass of water if able to swallow. Do not induce vomiting unless told to do so by a poison control center or doctor. Do not give anything by mouth to an unconscious person.

If in Eyes: Flush eyes with plenty of water. Call a doctor if irritation persists.

If on Skin: Wash with plenty of soap and water. Get medical attention if irritation persists.

Physical or Chemical Hazards: Combustible: Do not use or store near heat or open flame.

Storage and Disposal: Do not contaminate water, food, or feed by storage and disposal.

Storage: Store unused product in original container only, out of reach of children and animals.

Pesticide Disposal: Waste resulting from use of this product may be disposed of on-site or at an approved waste disposal facility.

Container Disposal: Securely wrap original container in several layers of newspaper and discard in trash.

Warning(s): Keep out of reach of children.

Disclaimer: Warranty: Seller makes no warranty, expressed or implied, concerning the use of this product other than indicated on the label. Buyer assumes all risk of use and handling of this material when such use and handling are contrary to label instructions.

Discussion: Stops and prevents infestations. Kills adult fleas, flea eggs, and flea larvae. Prevents all flea stages (eggs, larvae, pupae) from developing. Kills fleas which may cause flea allergy dermatitis. Kills all stages of deer ticks (which may carry Lyme disease), brown dog ticks, American dog ticks, and lone star ticks. Prevents and controls reinfestations. Fast-acting. Long-lasting. Waterproof. Convenient to use.

FRONTLINE® Plus For Cats contains fipronil and the insect growth regulator (IGR) (S)-methoprene. FRONTLINE® Plus effectively targets all stages of fleas. Fipronil collects in the oils of the skin and hair follicles, and continues to be released from hair follicles onto the skin and coat, resulting in long-lasting activity against fleas and ticks.

Presentation: Available in cartons of 3 x 0.017 fl oz (0.50 mL) and 6 x 0.017 fl oz (0.50 mL) applicators.

® FRONTLINE is a registered trademark of Merial.

Compendium Code No.: 11110131 037 811633

FRONTLINE® PLUS FOR DOGS & PUPPIES

Merial **Flea Control & Topical Parasiticide**

EPA Reg. No.: 65331-5

Active Ingredient(s):

fipronil:	9.8%
(S)-methoprene	8.8%
Inert Ingredients	81.4%
Total	100.0%

Indications: FRONTLINE® Plus for Dogs provides fast, effective and convenient treatment and control of fleas and ticks for dogs and puppies 8 weeks or older.

Directions for Use: It is a violation of Federal Law to use this product in a manner inconsistent with its labeling. Do not allow children to apply product. To prevent harm to you and your pet, read entire label and directions before each use. Follow all directions and precautionary statements carefully. Use on dogs only. Do not use on rabbits. Do not use on other animals.

To kill fleas and all stages of brown dog ticks, American dog ticks, lone star ticks, and deer ticks (which may carry Lyme disease), apply to dogs or puppies (8 weeks or older) as follows: Remove applicator from child-resistant package. Hold applicator upright and snap applicator tip away from face and body. Place applicator tip through animal's hair to the skin level between the shoulder blades. Squeeze applicator, applying entire contents in a single spot to the animal's skin. Avoid superficial application to the animal's hair. Only one applicator per treatment is needed.

Frequency of Application: When used monthly, FRONTLINE® Plus for Dogs completely breaks the flea life cycle and controls tick infestations. Research demonstrates that FRONTLINE® Plus kills adult fleas, flea eggs, and flea larvae for up to three months. FRONTLINE® Plus also prevents development of all flea stages for up to three months. FRONTLINE® Plus kills ticks for at least one month. A once monthly application is recommended where tick control is needed. Although FRONTLINE® Plus can control fleas for up to three months, if there is a high risk of reinfestation or if the pet has fleas which may cause flea allergy dermatitis, a once monthly application may be needed.

FRONTLINE® Plus for Dogs remains effective even after bathing, water immersion, or exposure to sunlight. Avoid contact with treated area until dry. Do not reapply FRONTLINE® Plus for 30 days.

Precautionary Statements: Hazards to Humans: Caution.

Harmful if swallowed. Causes eye irritation. Avoid contact with skin, eyes or clothing. Wash thoroughly with soap and water after handling.

Hazards to Domestic Animals: For external use only. Do not use on puppies under 8 weeks of age. Individual sensitivities, while rare, may occur after using any pesticide product. Pets may experience some temporary irritation at the site of product application. If signs persist, or become more severe within a few days of application, consult a veterinarian immediately. Certain medications can interact with pesticides. Consult a veterinarian before using on medicated, debilitated, aged, pregnant, or nursing animals. Call 1-800-660-1842 for 24-hour assistance.

First Aid: Have the product container or label with you when calling a poison control center or doctor, or going for treatment.

If Swallowed: Call a poison control center or doctor immediately for treatment advice. Have person sip a glass of water if able to swallow. Do not induce vomiting unless told to do so by a poison control center or doctor. Do not give anything by mouth to an unconscious person.

If in Eyes: Flush eyes with plenty of water. Call a doctor if irritation persists.

If on Skin: Wash with plenty of soap and water. Get medical attention if irritation persists.

Physical or Chemical Hazards: Combustible: Do not use or store near heat or open flame.

Storage and Disposal: Do not contaminate water, food, or feed by storage and disposal.

Storage: Store unused product in original container only, out of reach of children and animals.

Pesticide Disposal: Waste resulting from use of this product may be disposed of on-site or at an approved waste disposal facility.

Container Disposal: Securely wrap original container in several layers of newspaper and discard in trash.

Warning(s): Keep out of reach of children.

Disclaimer: Warranty: Seller makes no warranty, expressed or implied, concerning the use of this product other than indicated on the label. Buyer assumes all risk of use and handling of this material when such use and handling are contrary to label instructions.

Discussion: Stops and prevents infestations. Kills adult fleas, flea eggs, and flea larvae. Prevents all flea stages (eggs, larvae, pupae) from developing. Kills fleas which may cause flea allergy dermatitis. Kills all stages of deer ticks (which may carry Lyme disease), brown dog ticks, American dog ticks, and lone star ticks. Prevents and controls reinfestations. Fast-acting. Long-lasting. Waterproof. Convenient to use.

FRONTLINE® Plus For Dogs contains fipronil and the insect growth regulator (IGR) (S)-methoprene. FRONTLINE® Plus effectively targets all stages of fleas. Fipronil collects in the oils of the skin and hair follicles, and continues to be released from hair follicles onto the skin and coat, resulting in long-lasting activity against fleas and ticks.

Presentation: For small dogs and puppies 11-22 lbs, cartons of three or six 0.023 fl oz (0.67 mL) applicators.
For medium dogs 23-44 lbs, cartons of three or six 0.045 fl oz (1.34 mL) applicators.
For large dogs 45-88 lbs, cartons of three or six 0.091 fl oz (2.68 mL) applicators.
For extra large dogs 89-132 lbs, cartons of three or six 0.136 fl oz (4.02 mL) applicators.

® FRONTLINE is a registered trademark of Merial.

Compendium Code No.: 11110141 037 811634

FRONTLINE® SPRAY TREATMENT FOR CATS & DOGS

Merial **Parasiticide Spray**

EPA Reg. No.: 65331-1

Active Ingredient(s):

fipronil:	0.29%
Inert Ingredients	99.71%
Total	100.00%

Indications: FRONTLINE® Spray Treatment provides effective flea and tick control for adult dogs and cats and for puppies and kittens 8 weeks of age or older.

Directions for Use: It is a violation of Federal law to use this product in a manner inconsistent with its labeling. To prevent harm to you and your pets, read entire label and attached directions before each use. Follow all directions and precautionary statements carefully. Use only on dogs and cats. Do not use on rabbits. Do not use on any other animals.

To kill fleas and all stages of brown dog ticks, American dog ticks, lone star ticks, and deer ticks (which may carry Lyme Disease), apply to dogs, cats, puppies or kittens as follows:

How to unlock the trigger pump: Press down on lock button located at the top of the trigger pump. At the same time, rotate the nozzle counterclockwise one full turn so that the tab on the lock button aligns with the notch in the nozzle. To lock the trigger pump, reverse the process. The trigger pump should be left in the locked position when not in use.

Wear household latex gloves. Hold bottle in upright position. Ruffle the animal's coat with one hand while applying spray mist to the animal's back, sides, stomach, legs, shoulders, and neck. For head and eye area, spray FRONTLINE® on a gloved hand and rub gently into animal's hair. Do not get this product in your pet's eyes or mouth.

Apply spray mist until animal's hair is damp to thoroughly wet.

Approximately 1 to 2 pumps per pound of the animal's body weight will be required. Pets with long or dense coats will require the higher rate.

As with any flea control product wash hands and exposed skin thoroughly with soap and water after use.

To prevent flea build-up or reinfestation, use FRONTLINE® prior to the onset of flea season and monthly thereafter. Ticks do not need to receive spray directly upon their body for complete control. Do not reapply FRONTLINE® for 30 days.

Product performance is unaffected by exposure to moderate rainfall or by bathing with most brands of pet shampoo.

Precautionary Statements: Hazards to Humans. Caution.

Harmful if swallowed or absorbed through the skin. May cause severe eye irritation. Avoid breathing spray. Avoid contact with skin, eyes or clothing. Wash thoroughly with soap and water after handling. Persons applying this product must wear household latex gloves.

Hazards to Domestic Animals: For external use only. May cause severe eye irritation. Take care not to spray in the animal's eye or facial area. Do not use on kittens and puppies under 8 weeks. Individual sensitivities, while rare, may occur after using any pesticide product for pets. If signs persist, or become more severe, consult a veterinarian immediately. Consult a veterinarian before using with any other pesticides. Certain medications can interact with pesticides. Consult a veterinarian before using this product on medicated animals. This product may be harmful to debilitated, aged, pregnant or nursing animals. Consult a veterinarian before using. Call 1-800-660-1842 for 24 hr. assistance.

First Aid: Have the product container or label with you when calling a poison control center or doctor, or going for treatment.

If in Eyes: Hold eye open and rinse slowly and gently with water for 15-20 minutes. Remove contact lenses, if present, after the first 5 minutes, then continue rinsing eye. Call a poison control center or doctor for treatment advice.

If on Skin or Clothing: Take off contaminated clothing. Rinse skin immediately with plenty of water for 15-20 minutes. Call a poison control center or doctor for treatment advice.

If Swallowed: Call a poison control center or doctor immediately for treatment advice. Have person sip a glass of water if able to swallow. Do not induce vomiting unless told to do so by a poison control center or doctor. Do not give anything by mouth to an unconscious person.

If Inhaled: Move person to fresh air. If person is not breathing, call 911 or an ambulance, then give artificial respiration, preferably mouth-to-mouth if possible. Call a poison control center or doctor for further treatment advice.

Physical or Chemical Hazards: Flammable. Keep away from heat and open flame.

Storage and Disposal: Do not contaminate water, food, or feed by storage and disposal.

Storage: Store unused product in original container only, out of reach of children and animals.

Pesticide Disposal: Waste resulting from use of this product may be disposed of on site or at an approved waste disposal facility.

Container Disposal: Securely wrap original container in several layers of newspaper and discard in trash.

Warning(s): Keep out of reach of children.

Disclaimer: Warranty: Seller makes no warranty, expressed or implied, concerning the use of this product other than indicated on the label. Buyer assumes all risk of use and handling of this material when such use and handling are contrary to label instructions.

Discussion: Fast-acting control. Prevents reinfestation. Kills adult fleas before they lay eggs. Kills fleas which may cause flea allergy dermatitis. Kills fleas and ticks for a minimum of 30 days.

FRONTLINE® is the only flea control product that contains fipronil, a patented GABA inhibitor. FRONTLINE® rapidly controls flea infestation by killing adult fleas.

FRONTLINE® residual activity prevents reinfestation by killing fleas and ticks for at least 30 days. Studies have shown FRONTLINE® may protect dogs against fleas for up to 90 days.

Presentation: 8.5 fl oz (250 mL) and 17 fl oz (500 mL) bottles.

® FRONTLINE is a registered trademark of Merial.

Compendium Code No.: 11110152 037 812687

FRONTLINE® TOP SPOT® FOR CATS & KITTENS

Merial **Topical Insecticide**

EPA Reg. No.: 65331-2

Active Ingredient(s):

fipronil:	9.7%
Inert Ingredients	90.3%
Total	100.0%

Indications: FRONTLINE® provides convenient and effective flea and tick control for cats and kittens.

Directions for Use: It is a violation of Federal Law to use this product in a manner inconsistent with its labeling. Do not allow children to apply product. To prevent harm to you and your pet, read entire label and directions before each use. Follow all directions and precautionary statements carefully. Use on cats only. Do not use on rabbits. Do not use on other animals.

To kill fleas and all stages of brown dog ticks, American dog ticks, lone star ticks, and deer ticks (which may carry Lyme disease), apply to cats and kittens (12 weeks or older) as follows:

Remove applicator from child-resistant package. Hold applicator upright and snap applicator tip away from face and body. Place applicator tip through animal's hair to the skin level between the shoulder blades. Squeeze applicator, applying entire contents in a single spot to the animal's skin. Avoid superficial application to the animal's hair. Only one applicator per treatment is needed.

Frequency of Application: When used monthly, FRONTLINE® TOP SPOT® for Cats completely controls both flea and tick infestations. Research demonstrates that FRONTLINE® kills adult fleas for up to six weeks. FRONTLINE® kills ticks for at least one month. A once monthly application is recommended where tick control is needed. Although FRONTLINE® can control fleas for up to six weeks, if there is a high risk of reinfestation or if the pet has fleas which may cause flea allergy dermatitis, a once monthly application may be needed.

FRONTLINE® remains effective even after bathing, water immersion, or exposure to sunlight. Avoid contact with treated area until dry. Do not reapply FRONTLINE® for 30 days.

Precautionary Statements: Hazards to Humans: Caution.

Harmful if swallowed. Causes eye irritation. Avoid contact with skin, eyes or clothing. Wash thoroughly with soap and water after handling.

Hazards to Domestic Animals: For external use only. Do not use on kittens under 12 weeks of age. Individual sensitivities, while rare, may occur after using any pesticide product for pets. Pets may experience some temporary irritation at the site of product application. If signs persist, or become more severe within a few days of application, consult a veterinarian immediately. Certain medications can interact with pesticides. Consult a veterinarian before using on medicated animals. Consult a veterinarian before using this product with other pesticides. This product may be harmful to debilitated, aged, pregnant, or nursing animals; consult a veterinarian before using. Call 1-800-660-1842 for 24-hour assistance.

F

First Aid: Have the product container or label with you when calling a poison control center or doctor or going for treatment.

If Swallowed: Call a poison control center or doctor immediately for treatment advice. Have person sip a glass of water if able to swallow. Do not induce vomiting unless told to do so by a poison control center or doctor. Do not give anything by mouth to an unconscious person.

If in Eyes: Hold eye open and rinse slowly and gently with water for 15-20 minutes. Remove contact lenses, if present, after the first 5 minutes, then continue rinsing eye. Call a poison control center or doctor for treatment advice.

If on Skin: Wash with plenty of soap and water. Get medical attention if irritation persists.

Physical or Chemical Hazards: Flammable: Keep away from heat and open flame.

Storage and Disposal: Do not contaminate water, food, or feed by storage and disposal.

Storage: Store unused product in original container only, out of reach of children and animals.

Pesticide Disposal: Waste resulting from use of this product may be disposed of on-site or at an approved waste disposal facility.

Container Disposal: Securely wrap original container in several layers of newspaper and discard in trash.

Warning(s): Keep out of reach of children.

Disclaimer: Warranty: Seller makes no warranty, expressed or implied, concerning the use of this product other than indicated on the label. Buyer assumes all risk of use and handling of this material when such use and handling are contrary to label instructions.

Discussion: Fast-acting and long-lasting. Prevents reinfestation. Convenient to use. Kills newly emerged adult fleas before they lay eggs. Controls fleas which may cause flea allergy dermatitis. Kills all stages of brown dog ticks, American dog ticks, lone star ticks, and deer ticks (which may carry Lyme disease).

FRONTLINE® contains the active ingredient fipronil which has a unique mode of action that effectively targets fleas and ticks. Fipronil collects in the oils of the skin and hair follicles, and continues to be released from hair follicles onto the skin and coat, resulting in long-lasting activity.

Presentation: Available in cartons of 3 x 0.017 fl oz (0.50 mL) and 6 x 0.017 fl oz (0.50 mL) applicators.

® FRONTLINE and TOP SPOT are registered trademarks of Merial.

Compendium Code No.: 11110161 037 812248

FRONTLINE® TOP SPOT® FOR DOGS & PUPPIES

Merial **Topical Insecticide**

EPA Reg. No.: 65331-3

Active Ingredient(s):

fipronil:.......... 9.7%
Inert Ingredients.......... 90.3%
Total.......... 100.0%

Indications: FRONTLINE® provides convenient and effective flea and tick control for dogs and puppies 10 weeks or older.

Directions for Use: It is a violation of Federal Law to use this product in a manner inconsistent with its labeling. Do not allow children to apply product. To prevent harm to you and your pet, read entire label and directions before each use. Follow all directions and precautionary statements carefully. Use on dogs only. Do not use on rabbits. Do not use on other animals.

To kill fleas and all stages of brown dog ticks, American dog ticks, lone star ticks, and deer ticks (which may carry Lyme disease), apply to dogs and puppies (10 weeks or older) as follows: Remove applicator from child-resistant package. Hold applicator upright and snap applicator tip away from face and body. Place applicator tip through animal's hair to the skin level between the shoulder blades. Squeeze applicator, applying entire contents in a single spot to the animal's skin. Avoid superficial application to the animal's hair. Only one applicator per treatment is needed.

Frequency of Application: When used monthly, FRONTLINE® TOP SPOT® for Dogs completely controls both flea and tick infestations. Research demonstrates that FRONTLINE® kills adult fleas up to three months. FRONTLINE® kills ticks for at least one month. A once monthly application is recommended where tick control is needed. Although FRONTLINE® can control fleas for up to 3 months, if there is a high risk of reinfestation or if the pet has fleas which may cause flea allergy dermatitis, a once monthly application may be needed.

FRONTLINE® remains effective even after bathing, water immersion, or exposure to sunlight. Avoid contact with treated area until dry. Do not reapply FRONTLINE® for 30 days.

Precautionary Statements: Hazards to Humans: Caution.

Harmful if swallowed. Causes eye irritation. Avoid contact with skin, eyes or clothing. Wash thoroughly with soap and water after handling.

Hazards to Domestic Animals: For external use only. Do not use on puppies under 10 weeks of age. Individual sensitivities, while rare, may occur after using any pesticide product for pets. Pets may experience some temporary irritation at the site of product application. If signs persist, or become more severe within a few days of application, consult a veterinarian immediately. Certain medications can interact with pesticides. Consult a veterinarian before using on medicated animals. Consult a veterinarian before using this product with other pesticides. This product may be harmful to debilitated, aged, pregnant, or nursing animals; consult a veterinarian before using. Call 1-800-660-1842 for 24-hour assistance.

First Aid: Have the product container or label with you when calling a poison control center or doctor or going for treatment.

If Swallowed: Call a poison control center or doctor immediately for treatment advice. Have person sip a glass of water if able to swallow. Do not induce vomiting unless told to do so by a poison control center or doctor. Do not give anything by mouth to an unconscious person.

If in Eyes: Hold eye open and rinse slowly and gently with water for 15-20 minutes. Remove contact lenses, if present, after the first 5 minutes, then continue rinsing eye. Call a poison control center or doctor for treatment advice.

If on Skin: Wash with plenty of soap and water. Get medical attention if irritation persists.

Physical or Chemical Hazards: Flammable. Keep away from heat and open flame.

Storage and Disposal: Do not contaminate water, food, or feed by storage and disposal.

Storage: Store unused product in original container only, out of reach of children and animals.

Pesticide Disposal: Waste resulting from use of this product may be disposed of on site or at an approved waste disposal facility.

Container Disposal: Securely wrap original container in several layers of newspaper and discard in trash.

Warning(s): Keep out of reach of children.

Disclaimer: Warranty: Seller makes no warranty, expressed or implied, concerning the use of this product other than indicated on the label. Buyer assumes all risk of use and handling of this material when such use and handling are contrary to label instructions.

Discussion: Fast acting and long lasting. Prevents reinfestation. Convenient to use. Kills newly emerged adult fleas before they lay eggs. Controls fleas which may cause flea allergy dermatitis. Kills all stages of brown dog ticks, American dog ticks, lone star ticks, and deer ticks (which may carry Lyme disease).

FRONTLINE® contains the active ingredient fipronil which has a unique mode of action that effectively targets fleas and ticks. Fipronil collects in the oils of the skin and hair follicles, and continues to be released from hair follicles onto the skin and coat, resulting in long lasting activity.

Presentation: For small dogs and puppies up to 22 lbs, carton of three or six 0.023 fl oz (0.67 mL) applicators.
For medium dogs 23-44 lbs, carton of three or six 0.045 fl oz (1.3 mL) applicators.
For large dogs 45-88 lbs, carton of three or six 0.091 fl oz (2.68 mL) applicators.
For extra large dogs 89-132 lbs, carton of three or six 0.136 fl oz (4.02 mL) applicators.

® FRONTLINE and TOP SPOT are registered trademarks of Merial.

Compendium Code No.: 11110171 037 812249

FROSTSHIELD

Durvet **Udder Product**

All Season Teat & Udder Balm

Ingredient(s): Water, Mineral Oil, Cetearyl Alcohol, Glycol Stearate, Glycerol Stearate, Stearic Acid, Phenoxyethanol, Propylene Glycol, Glycerin, Sorbitol, Lanolin, Aloe Vera, PABA, Folic Acid, Calcium Pantothenate, Niacinamide, Thiamine, Pyridoxine, Methionine, Chloroxylenol, Methyl Paraben, Propyl Paraben, Sodium Hydroxide, Fragrance, FD&C Blue #1.

Indications: An easy to apply, non-stick cream base formulation with vitamins, chloroxylenol germicide, PABA, lanolin. Aids in frost protection.

Use on chapped, scraped, cracked, bruised and irritated teats and udders.

Use on tissues subjected to windburn, sunburn, minor abrasions and inflammations.

Non sticky cream-base formulation for easy application, washing and cleaning.

Excellent cream for use on exposed tissues to frequent washings, warm-cold weather, low humidity, wet conditions, below freezing temperatures.

Directions: Thoroughly dry the udder and each teat before application of FROSTSHIELD with Aloe Vera. Apply FROSTSHIELD liberally to entire teat and udder area after each milking. Be sure to coat teat orifice.

Caution(s): Before milking, thoroughly wash the entire udder and teat area to avoid contamination of milk.

For animal use only.

Warning(s): Keep out of reach of children.

Presentation: 1 lb (16 oz) 454 g, 4 lb (64 oz) 1816 g, and 8 lb (128 oz) 3632 g.

Compendium Code No.: 10840822 Rev. 10-01

FRYVACC 1

Novartis (Aqua Health) **Bacterin**

Flavobacterium Columnare Bacterin

U.S. Vet. Lic. No.: 335

Contents: FRYVACC 1 contains only formalin inactivated cultures of *Flavobacterium columnare (Flexibacter columnaris)*. No other preservative is used.

Indications: For the vaccination of healthy salmonids against Columnaris Disease by mucoid strains of *Flavobacterium columnare (Flexibacter columnaris)*.

Dosage and Administration: Shake well before using.

Vaccination Program: Vaccination should precede exposure of vaccinates to the disease agent by 250 degree-days (number of days multiplied by the mean water temperature (°C) during period). The bacterin is recommended for immunization of salmonids that are 3 grams or more in size.

Method of Administration:

Immersion Delivery: For immersion delivery, dilute entire contents of this container with 9 litres of clean hatchery water. Measure diluted bacterin in a suitable plastic container. Add fish to attain a density of 500 g per litre of diluted bacterin. Expose fish for 30 seconds then drain bacterin from fish. Return fish to holding facility. Repeat until a total of 20 groups have been vaccinated in this manner.

Precaution(s): Store between 2-7°C (35-45°F). Do not freeze.

Caution(s): Use entire contents when first opened.

Vaccinate healthy fish only.

Warning(s): Do not vaccinate within 21 days of slaughter.

For veterinary use only.

Presentation: 1000 mL bottles.

Distributed by: Mr. J. Zinn, Buhl, Idaho 83316

Compendium Code No.: 14970021

FULVICIN-U/F® POWDER ℞

Schering-Plough **Antifungal**

(Griseofulvin)

NADA No.: 039-792

Active Ingredient(s): FULVICIN-U/F® Powder is available in 15 g packets, each containing 2.5 g of griseofulvin (microsize).

Indications: FULVICIN-U/F® is recommended for ringworm infection caused by *Trichophyton equinum* and *Microsporum gypseum.*

FULVICIN-U/F® is an orally effective antifungal antibiotic specifically active against superficial fungi which cause tinea (ringworm) of the skin and hair.

Pharmacology: The microsize form of griseofulvin differs from regular FULVICIN® in that its finer particle size results in a much greater surface area for absorbtion. An increased blood level has been obtained in experimental studies in man using the fine particle size griseofulvin, indicating better absorption and a greater amount of the drug available for fungistatic action in the skin and hair.

General Considerations: In human medicine, FULVICIN-U/F® is indicated in the treatment of infections caused by dermatophytic fungi of the skin, hair and nails. Of those organisms which cause these conditions, the following are responsive to oral therapy with FULVICIN-U/F®: *Trichophyton mentagrophytes, Trichophyton rubrum, Trichophyton schoenleini, Trichophyton sulphureum, Trichophyton verrucosum, Trichophyton interdigitale, Epidermophyton floccosum, Microsporum gypseum, Microsporum canis, Microsporum audouini.* FULVICIN-U/F® is inactive against bacteria and yeasts including monilia, actinomycetes, nocardia, blastomyces, coccidiodes, histoplasma, cryptococcus, sporotrichum and aspergillus.

FULVICIN-U/F® is administered orally until the fungi have been eliminated from the skin and hair. The length of therapy will vary with the severity of the infection. The time necessary for the newly formed fungal-resistant keratin to reach the surface varies greatly with different structures, such as hair and thin body skin. Experimental and clinical work indicates that animals showing involvement of skin and hair may only require treatment for three to four weeks. Cure is considered complete when repeated cultures are negative for the presence of fungi. In the absence of these tests, therapy should be continued until the lesions are clinically improved and there is evidence of resumed hair growth.

The infected skin in many cases shows a remarkably rapid improvement with decreased itching and inflammation occurring in a few days. In some cases, the skin may appear clinically normal in as little as 10 days. Viable fungi in the outer layers may persist, however, and the possibility of re-infection is not known with certainty. The optimal period of treatment has not yet been determined. Clipping of the hair to help remove any remaining viable fungi is indicated. Hair clipped from the infected lesion should be burned.

Dosage and Administration:

Equine (adults): One (1) packet per day (2.5 g).

Yearlings: One-half (½) to one (1) packet per day (1.25-2.5 g).

Foals: One-half (½) packet per day.

Cases of ringworm in horses caused by *T. equinum* should be treated with FULVICIN-U/F® POWDER for a period of not less than 10 days. Responsive cases may show clinical signs of recovery in five (5) to seven (7) days after griseofulvin therapy is initiated. In responsive cases, the treatment should be continued until all the infected areas are negative by appropriate culture.

If cases do not respond to therapy in three (3) weeks, it is recommended that the diagnosis be re-evaluated.

The powder may be given on a small amount of feed or in a drench.

General Measures: Clearing of dermatophytic infections with oral griseofulvin therapy is a great advance. However, it is necessary to maintain general hygienic precautions. The possibility of recurrence is not known. Destruction of old bedding, disinfection of the stall, a close clipping of hair just before termination of therapy, etc., are measures which should reduce the incidence of re-infection.

Precaution(s): Store between 2-30°C (36-86°F).

Caution(s): Federal law restricts this drug to use by or on the order of a licensed veterinarian.

Patients on prolonged therapy with any potent medication should be under close observation. Periodic monitoring of organ system function, including renal, hepatic and hemopotetic, should be done.

The antibiotic is derived from a species of penicillium griseofulvin. A number of known penicillin-sensitive humans have been treated with griseofulvin without difficulty. In veterinary medicine, the drug apparently does not have allergenic properties, however, considerably more experience in this area must be obtained before definite conclusions may be drawn.

Griseofulvin administered to animals intraperitoneally or intravenously in massive doses will produce damage to the seminal epithelium, however, these effects have not been observed following oral administration of usual clinical doses to dogs and cats.

Studies to date indicate that the usual clinical doses of FULVICIN-U/F® administered orally do not have an effect on spermatogenesis. More evidence is needed, but it appears likely that such effects noted are related to the massive doss administered by the parenteral routes. The effects of griseofulvin on stallion spermatogenesis are not known.

Warning(s): The safety and efficacy of the prophylactic use of griseofulvin, has not been established. The drug should not be used to treat minor or trivial infections.

Not for use in horses intended for food.

The safety of griseofulvin for use in pregnant animals has not been established. It has been reported in the Soviet literature (N.N. Slonitskaya, Teratogenic Effect of Griseofulvin-Forte on the Rat Fetus/Antibiotiki 14 (1): 44-48, 1969) that a griseofulvin preparation was found to be embryotoxic on oral administration to pregnant Wistar rats. In addition, pups and kittens with either cleft palates or other abnormalities have been reported in litters of bitches and queens treated with griseofulvin during gestation.

Side Effects: Close observation of human and animal patients receiving therapeutic doses thus far, does not reveal any effect on body weight, fasting blood sugar, blood electrolytes, total or differential counts, thymol turbidity tests, urinalyses or sternal marrow counts.

In the human, heartburn, nausea, epigastric discomfort and diarrhea have occasionally been reported. In a few instances, urticaria or drug rashes have developed and in these instances the drug should be withdrawn. Generally the incidence of side effects has been quite low and the drug seems to be well tolerated when given orally.

The veterinarian is alerted to the following griseofulvin-associated side effects which have been reported in either human or veterinary literature: irritability, dizziness, memory loss, visual disturbances, antagonism to barbituates and other drugs metabolized by the liver, such as warfarin-type anticoagulants.

It has also been reported that griseofulvin affects disturbances in porphyrin metabolism, formation of hepatomala and cocarcinogenicity with methylcholanthrene, also, a higher fat diet increases absorption of the antibiotic.

Presentation: 15 g packets in cartons of 50 packets.

Compendium Code No.: 10470750

FULVICIN-U/F® TABLETS ℞

Schering-Plough **Antifungal**

(Griseofulvin)

NADA No.: 012-227

Active Ingredient(s): Each bolus contains 250 mg and 500 mg of griseofulvin (microsize).

Indications: FULVICIN-U/F® is recommended in the treatment of infections caused by dermatophytic fungi of the skin, hair and claws. Of those organisms which cause these conditions, the following are responsive to oral therapy with FULVICIN-U/F®: *Trichophyton mentagrophytes, Trichophyton rubrum, Trichophyton schoenleini, Trichophyton sulphureum, Trichophyton verrucosum, Trichophyton interdigitale, Epidermophyton floccosum, Microsporum gypseum, Microsporum canis, Microsporum audouini.* FULVICIN-U/F® is inactive against bacteria and yeasts including monilia, actinomycetes, nocardia, blastomyces, coccidiodes, histoplasma, cryptococcus, sporotrichum and aspergillus.

FULVICIN-U/F® is an orally effective antifungal antibiotic specifically active against superficial fungi which cause tinea (ringworm) of the skin and hair.

Pharmacology: The microsize form of griseofulvin differs from regular FULVICIN® in that its finer particle size results in a much greater surface area for absorption. An increased blood level has been obtained in experimental studies in man using the fine particle size griseofulvin, indicating better absorption and a greater amount of the drug available for fungistatic action in the skin, hair and nails.

Dosage and Administration: FULVICIN-U/F® is administered orally until the fungi have been eliminated from the skin, hair or claws. The length of therapy will vary with the site and severity of the infection. The time necessary for the newly formed fungal-resistant keratin to reach the surface varies greatly with different structures, such as thin body skin, hair and nails. Experimental and clinical work indicates that animals showing involvement of skin and hair only may require treatment for three (3) to four (4) weeks. Since nails or claws grow more slowly than hair, onychomycotic lesions may require three (3) to four (4) months continuous therapy. Cure is considered complete when repeated cultures and potassium hydroxide scrapings are negative for the presence of fungi. In the absence of these tests, therapy should be continued at least one (1) week after the patient is clinically free from infection.

The infected skin in many cases shows a remarkably rapid improvement with decreased itching and inflammation occurring in a few days. In some cases, the skin may appear normal clinically in as short as 10 days. Viable fungi in the outer layers may persist, however, and the possibility of re-infection is not known with certainty. The optimal period of treatment has not yet been determined. Clipping of the hair to help remove any remaining viable fungi is indicated. Surgical removal of nails with simultaneous oral FULVICIN-U/F® thereby should shorten the period of therapy for onychomycosis.

When nails and skin or hair are involved, response will be noted first in skin or hair. Treatment, however, should be continued until the nail is cured to prevent re-infection of skin or hair from this source.

Two (2) dosage regimens are offered to the veterinarian the daily oral dose and a weekly dose.

The following daily doses of FULVICIN-U/F® are recommended and may be given singly or in divided doses.

Dogs and Cats:

Body Weight	Oral Dosage
Up to 6 lbs.	62.5 mg daily
6 to 18 lbs.	125 mg daily
18 to 36 lbs.	250 mg daily
36 to 48 lbs.	375 mg daily
48 to 75 lbs.	500 mg daily

Weekly Dosage: Clinical experience indicates that many animals respond to FULVICIN-U/F® when the drug is given at intervals of 7-10 days. The dosage used when this method is employed has varied from approximately 5 to 10 mg of FULVICIN-U/F® per pound of body weight multiplied by a factor of 7-10 (the interval in days). For example, a 25 pound animal being treated at weekly intervals at a dosage of 10 mg per pound of body weight would receive 25 x 10 x 7 = 1,750 mg of FULVICIN-U/F®. The entire computed dose is given at one time. Some animals may require a higher dosage either initially or throughout therapy to achieve beneficial results. The veterinarian should adjust dosage according to the response noted. It is recommended that one additional weekly dose be administered after the patient is clinically free from infection.

General Measures: Clearing of dermatophytic infections with oral griseofulvin therapy is a great advance. However, it is necessary to maintain general hygienic precautions. The possibility of recurrence is not known. Destruction of old bedding, disinfection of stall, a close clipping of hair just before termination of therapy, etc., are measures which should reduce incidence of re-infection.

Precaution(s): Store between 2-30°C (36-86°F).

Caution(s): Federal law restricts this drug to use by or on the order of a licensed veterinarian.

Patients on prolonged therapy with any potent medication should be under close observation. Periodic monitoring of organ system function, including renal, hepatic and hemopotetic, should be done.

The antibiotic is derived from a species of penicillium griseofulvin. A number of known penicillin-sensitive humans have been treated with griseofulvin without difficulty. In veterinary medicine, the drug apparently does not have allergenic properties, however, considerably more experience in this area must be obtained before definite conclusions may be drawn.

Griseofulvin administered to animals intraperitoneally or intravenously in massive doses will produce damage to the seminal epithelium, however, these effects have not been observed following oral administration of usual clinical doses to dogs and cats.

Studies to date indicate that the usual clinical doses of FLUVICIN-U/F® Tablets administered orally do not have an effect on spermatogenesis. More evidence is needed, but it appears likely that such effects noted are related to the massive doses administered by the parenteral routes.

Warning(s): The safety and efficacy of the prophylactic use of griseofulvin, has not been established. The drug should not be used to treat minor or trivial infections.

The safety of griseofulvin for use in pregnant animals has not been established. It has been reported in the Soviet literature (N.N. Slonitskaya, Teratogenic Effect of Griseofulvin-Forte on the Rat Fetus/Antibiotiki 14 (1): 44-48, 1969) that a griseofulvin preparation was found to be embryotoxic on oral administration to pregnant Wistar rats. In addition, pups and kittens with either cleft palates or other abnormalities have been reported in litters of bitches and queens treated with griseofulvin during gestation.

Side Effects: Close observation of human and animal patients receiving therapeutic doses thus far, does not reveals any effect on body weight, fasting blood sugar, blood electrolytes, total or differential counts, thymol turbidity tests, urinalyses or sternal marrow counts.

In the human, heartburn, nausea, epigastric discomfort and diarrhea have occasionally been reported. In a few instances, urticiaria or drug rashes have developed and in these instances the drug should be withdrawn. Generally the incidence of side effects has been quite low and the drug seems to be well tolerated when given orally.

The veterinarian is alerted to the following griseofulvin-associated side effects which have been

F

reported in either human or veterinary literature: irritability, dizziness, memory loss, visual disturbances, antagonism to barbiturates and other drugs metabolized by the liver, such as warfarin-type anticoagulants.

It has also been reported that griseofulvin affects disturbances in porphyrin metabolism, formation of hepatomala and cocarcinogenicity with methylcholanthrene; also, higher fat diet increases absorption of the antibiotic.

Presentation: 250 mg and 500 mg scored tablets in bottles of 100.

Compendium Code No.: 10470760

FUNGASSAY®

Synbiotics **Dermatophyte Test**

Dermatophyte Test Medium

U.S. Vet. Lic. No.: 312

Indications: FUNGASSAY® Dermatophyte Test Medium is a culture medium that provides a simple, rapid and practical method for confirming diagnosis of dermatophyte infections.

Test Principle: The test is based on a color change within the medium from amber to red[1], caused by the growth of pathogenic fungi, such as *Microsporum* and *Trichophyton* species. These fungi cause most of the dermatomycoses in veterinary medicine.

Test Procedure: For optimum results, it is necessary to follow the directions given below.

1. Washing is indicated only in cases of heavy contamination or encrustation.[2,3] If the site is washed prior to sampling, a non-medicated, non-fungicidal soap is recommended, followed by drying with an absorptive material. These steps remove saprophytic organisms which could overgrow the culture, thus masking the growth of pathogenic fungi.
2. Select hair and scales for culture from both the periphery and the center of the lesion. Broken, frayed or distorted hairs, and those that fluoresce with Wood's light, are the best specimens.
3. Remove only a small portion of hair and scales from the lesion with a hemostat or thumb forcep. Avoid placing large amounts of hair and scales on the medium, which will produce useless overgrowth of the contaminants.
4. When removing the cap from the FUNGASSAY® Dermatophyte Test Medium bottle, take care to avoid contamination.
5. Press the hair and scales on the culture medium to ensure good contact, but do not bury the specimen in the medium.
6. When replacing the cap, make certain that it remains loose so that air exchange can occur in the bottle during incubation. When the cap is too tight, the color change will not develop.
7. Identify the bottle with the patient and the date.
8. Incubate at room temperature (72°-86°F) so that suitable growth will occur.
9. Evaluation of the test results can begin as early as 48 hours after inoculation. A pinkish color will appear in the amber medium under the specimen and developing colony. The color will intensify as growth proceeds and is due to alkaline metabolites produced by the dermatophytes. When a positive dermatophyte infection is present, the entire medium will turn red by the seventh to fourteenth day. If there is no growth within ten days, redistribute the sample on the medium. Occasionally growth does not occur because of improper inoculation.
10. A color change may occasionally be produced by a specimen heavily contaminated with saprophytic fungi or bacteria.[1] However, it is not a problem because differentiation from dermatophytes can be made as follows:
    Dermatophyte: A color change appears in the medium with colony growth. The colony pigments are usually light colored.
    Saprophyte fungi: Colony growth is well established before any color change appears in the medium. The colony pigments are usually dark colored.
    Bacteria: The morphology of bacterial colonies differs from the morphology of fungal colonies.

Precaution(s): Refrigerate the FUNGASSAY® Dermatophyte Test Medium for optimum storage. Warming to room temperature before using is not necessary.

Destroy the used FUNGASSAY® Dermatophyte Test Medium bottle by incineration to eliminate the spread of all organisms.

Caution(s): For veterinary use only.

Warning(s): Keep out of reach of children.

References: Available upon request.

Presentation: FUNGASSAY® Dermatophyte Test Medium is supplied in a package containing 10 individual bottles (10 tests).

Compendium Code No.: 11150091 03-0150-0299

FUNGI-DRY-EAR

Q.A. Laboratories **Otic Dryer**

Active Ingredient(s): Isopropyl alcohol, de-ionized water, silicon dioxide, zinc undecylenate (undecylenic acid), methyl salicylate, PEG 75 lanolin oil, sucrose octyl acetate, polysorbate 60, propylene glycol, acetic acid, FD & C blue #1.

Indications: FUNGI-DRY-EAR is a gel with antifungal properties for soothing dessication of the ear canal in dogs and cats.

Dosage and Administration: Shake well before using. Clean ears with an ear cleaning solution. Do not probe into the ear. Apply a few drops of FUNGI-DRY-EAR into the ear canal. Massage the base of the ear allowing FUNGI-DRY-EAR to contact the entire ear canal. Apply on the direction of a veterinarian. May be used before and after bathing or swimming. Accumulated powder may be cleaned out with an ear cleaning solution.

Precaution(s): Flammable: Keep away from heat or an open flame.

Caution(s): Keep out of the reach of children.

Harmful if swallowed. If swallowed, call a physician or the nearest poison control center. Avoid contact with the eyes and mucous membranes. If in eyes, wash with copious amounts of cool water.

Presentation: 2 oz. dropper bottles.

Compendium Code No.: 13680050

FUNGISAN™

Tomlyn **Antiseptic**

Antiseptic Germicidal Solution with Allantoin

Active Ingredient(s):

Benzalkonium Chloride 0.13%

Indications: First aid to help prevent skin infection.

Painless, penetrating, non-staining formula is recommended for use on horses, dogs or cats.

Directions: Clean the affected area. Apply a small amount of FUNGISAN™ solution to the affected area 1 to 3 times daily until hair begins to grow. Leave treated area uncovered. Rinse treated areas with clear water before reapplying. Results in a matter of days. If no improvement is noted within 7 days, consult your veterinarian.

Note: Efficiency, is neutralized by soap or detergent residues.

Caution(s): In case of contact with eyes or other mucous membranes, flush immediately with water. Obtain medical attention for eye inflammation.

For external animal use only.

Warning(s): Not for use on animals intended for food.

Keep out of the reach of children.

Presentation: 4 fl oz (118 mL) (dogs); 4 fl oz (118 mL) (cats and kittens); 12 fl oz (335 mL) (horses and dogs).

Compendium Code No.: 11220270 673-2 5/673-1 4/620-1 7

FURALL™ (FURAZOLIDONE)

Farnam **Topical Antibacterial**

Aerosol Powder

NADA No.: 111-104

Active Ingredient(s):

Furazolidone 4%

Inert Ingredients: 96%

Indications: A topical application for use on horses and ponies. For prevention or treatment of bacterial infections of superficial wounds, abrasions and lacerations due to *Staphylococcus aureus, Streptococcus* spp, and *Proteus* spp, sensitive to furazolidone.

Directions: Shake well before using. Cleanse affected area thoroughly prior to application of FURALL™. Apply lightly once or twice daily. Repeat treatment as necessary.

Holding container approximately six to twelve inches from the affected area, apply FURALL™ lightly. Use only that amount of powder necessary to impart a light yellow color to the affected area. Heavy application may cause caking and retard healing process.

Precaution(s): Contents under pressure. Avoid prolonged exposure to sunlight or heat from radiators, stoves, hot water and other heat sources that may cause bursting. Do not puncture, incinerate, burn or store above 120°F. Do not discard empty can in home garbage compactor.

Caution(s): Use only as recommended by a veterinarian in the treatment of puncture wounds, wounds requiring surgical debridement or suturing, those of a chronic nature involving proud flesh, generalized and chronic infections of the skin, and those skin conditions associated with intense itching. If redness, irritation, or swelling persists or increases, discontinue use and reconsult veterinarian.

Warning(s): Not for use on animals intended for food.

Federal law prohibits the use of this product in food producing animals.

Human Warnings: This product contains chemicals known to the State of California to cause cancer. Carcinogenesis: Furazolidone, the active ingredient of FURALL™, has been shown to produce mammary tumors in rats and ovarian tumors in mice. Additionally, some people may be hypersensitive to this product. Either wear gloves when applying, or wash hands afterwards. Avoid contact with eyes.

Flammable! Do not spray near sparks, heat or open flames. Vapors will accumulate readily and may ignite explosively. Keep area ventilated during use and until vapors are gone. Do not smoke - extinguish all flames, pilot lights and heaters - Turn off stoves, electric tools and appliances, and any other sources of ignition.

Vapor Harmful: Use with adequate ventilation. Avoid continuous breathing of vapor and spray mist by standing up-wind or using a dust mask. Keep away from children.

Use only as directed. Intentional misuse by deliberately concentrating and inhaling the contents can be harmful or fatal.

Keep out of reach of children.

Not for human use.

Presentation: 198 g (7 oz) can.

Compendium Code No.: 10000220

FURA-OINTMENT®

Farnam **Topical Antibacterial**

Nitrofurazone Soluble Dressing

NADA No.: 122-447

Active Ingredient(s): 0.2% nitrofurazone in a water soluble base of polyethylene glycols.

Indications: For the prevention or treatment of surface bacterial infections of wounds, burns, cutaneous ulcers. For use only on horses, dogs and cats.

Dosage and Administration: Apply directly on the lesion with a spatula or first place on a piece of gauze. Application of a bandage is optional.

The preparation should be in contact with the lesion for at least 24 hours. The dressing may be changed several times daily or left on the lesion for a longer period.

Precaution(s): Avoid exposure to excessive heat or direct sunlight and strong fluorescent lighting.

Caution(s): In case of deep or puncture wounds or serious burns, consult veterinarian. If redness, irritation, or swelling persists or increases, discontinue use of the product and consult a veterinarian.

Warning(s): This product contains a chemical known to the State of California to cause cancer.

Carcinogenesis: Nitrofurazone, the active ingredient of FURA-OINTMENT®, has been shown to produce mammary tumors in rats and ovarian tumors in mice. Additionally, some people may be hypersensitive to the product. Either wear gloves when applying, or wash hands afterwards.

For use only on horses, dogs, and cats.

Not to be used on animals intended for food purposes.

Keep out of reach of children.

Presentation: 8 oz and 454 g (16 oz) containers.

Compendium Code No.: 10000211

FURA-SEPTIN

Anthony **Topical Antibacterial**

Brand of Nitrofurazone Soluble Dressing

NADA No.: 132-427

Active Ingredient(s): Contents: 0.2% Nitrofurazone in a water soluble base of polyethylene glycols.

Indications: An antibacterial preparation for topical application. For the prevention or treatment of surface bacterial infections of wounds, burns, and cutaneous ulcers. For use in horses only.

Dosage and Administration: Apply directly on the lesion with a spatula or first place on a piece of gauze. Application of a bandage is optional.

This preparation should be in contact with the lesion for at least 24 hours. The dressing may be changed several times daily or left on the lesion for a longer period of time.

Precaution(s): Avoid exposure to alkaline material and fluorescent lighting. Keep away from excessive heat or direct sunlight.

Caution(s): In case of deep or puncture wounds or serious burns, use only as recommended by a veterinarian. If redness, irritation, or swelling persists or increases, discontinue use and reconsult veterinarian.

Warning(s): Federal law prohibits the use of this product in food-producing animals.

Not for use on horses intended for food.

Human Warnings:

Carcinogenesis: Nitrofurazone, the active ingredient of FURA-SEPTIN ointment, has been shown to produce mammary tumors in rats and ovarian tumors in mice.

Some people may be hypersensitive to this product.

Either wear gloves when applying, or wash hands afterwards.

Keep out of reach of children.

Presentation: 1 pound containers.

Manufactured by: Squire Laboratories, Inc., Revere, MA 02151.

Compendium Code No.: 10250011 C/N 01-3001.0

FURAZOLIDONE AEROSOL POWDER

V.P.L. **Topical Antibacterial**

Topical Antibacterial For Wounds And Sores

NADA No.: 111-104

Active Ingredient(s):

Furazolidone.......... 4%
Inert Ingredients:.......... 96%

Indications: A topical application for use on horses and ponies. For prevention or treatment of bacterial infections of superficial wounds, abrasions and lacerations due to *Staphylococcus aureus, Streptococcus* spp. and *Proteus* spp. sensitive to furazolidone.

Directions: Shake well before using. Cleanse affected area thoroughly prior to application of FURAZOLIDONE AEROSOL POWDER. Apply lightly once or twice daily. Repeat treatment as necessary.

Holding the container approximately six to twelve inches from the affected area, apply FURAZOLIDONE AEROSOL POWDER lightly. Use only that amount of powder necessary to impart a light yellow color to the affected area. Heavy application may cause caking and retard healing process.

Precaution(s): Flammable! Do not spray near sparks, heat or open flames. Vapors will accumulate readily and may ignite explosively. Keep area ventilated during use and until all vapors are gone. Do not smoke - extinguish all flames, pilot lights and heaters - Turn off stoves, electric tools and appliances, and any other sources of ignition. Contents under pressure. Avoid prolonged exposure to sunlight or heat from radiators, stoves, hot water and other heat sources that may cause bursting. Do not puncture, incinerate, burn or store above 120°F. Do not discard empty can in home garbage compactor.

Caution(s): Use only as recommended by a veterinarian in the treatment of puncture wounds, wounds requiring surgical debridement or suturing, those of a chronic nature involving proud flesh, generalized and chronic infections of the skin and those skin conditions associated with intense itching. If redness, irritation or swelling persist or increase, discontinue use and reconsult veterinarian.

Vapor harmful. Use with adequate ventilation. Avoid continuous breathing of vapor and spray mist by standing up-wind or using a dust mask. Keep away from children.

Use only as directed. Intentional misuse by deliberately concentrating and inhaling the contents can be harmful or fatal.

Warning(s): Federal law prohibits the use of this product in food-producing animals.

Not for use on animals intended for food.

Human Warnings: This product contains chemicals known to the state of California to cause cancer. Carcinogenesis: Furazolidone, the active ingredient of FURAZOLIDONE AEROSOL POWDER, has been shown to produce mammary tumors in rats and ovarian tumors in mice. Additionally, some people may be hypersensitive to this product. Either wear gloves when applying or wash hands afterwards. Avoid contact with eyes.

Keep out of reach of children.

Not for human use.

Presentation: Available in 7 oz (198 g) can.

Compendium Code No.: 11430160

FURA-ZONE

Neogen **Topical Antibacterial**

Brand of Nitrofurazone Soluble Dressing

NADA No.: 132-427

Active Ingredient(s): Contains: 0.2% Nitrofurazone, in a water soluble base of Polyethylene Glycols.

Indications: An antibacterial preparation for topical application for the prevention or treatment of surface bacterial infections of wounds, burns, and cutaneous ulcers.

Dosage and Administration: Apply directly on the lesion with a spatula or first place on a piece of gauze. The application of a bandage is optional. The preparation should be in contact with the lesion for at least 24 hours. The dressing may be changed several times a day or left on the lesion for a longer period.

Precaution(s): Keep away from excessive heat or direct sunlight.

Caution(s): In case of deep or puncture wounds or serious burns, use only as recommended by a veterinarian. If redness, irritation, or swelling persists or increases, discontinue use; reconsult veterinarian. Avoid exposure to alkaline material and fluorescent lighting.

For use in horses only.

Warning(s): Not for use on horses intended for food.

Federal law prohibits the use of this product in food-producing animals.

Human Warning:

Carcinogenesis: Nitrofurazone, the active ingredient of furazone ointment has been shown to produce mammary tumors in rats and ovarian tumors in mice. Some people may be hypersensitive to this product. Either wear gloves when applying, or wash hands afterwards.

Keep out of reach of children.

Presentation: 1 lb. (454 g) containers (NDC - 1753-340-16).

Compendium Code No.: 14910281

FUROGEN™

Novartis (Aqua Health) **Bacterin**

Aeromonas Salmonicida Bacterin

U.S. Vet. Lic. No.: 335

Contents: FUROGEN™, produced by Aqua Health Ltd., contains inactivated cultures of *Aeromonas salmonicida*. It has been shown to be safe and effective for use with 5 g or larger salmonids.

Indications: For the immunization of healthy salmonids against furunculosis caused by typical isolates of *Aeromonas salmonicida*.

Dosage and Administration: Vaccination Program: Vaccination should precede exposure of vaccinates to the disease agent by 40 days if holding water temperatures are 10°-12°C. A longer period of time should be allowed if temperatures are below 10°C.

Injection Administration: Fish are anesthetized until immobilized and given 0.1 mL of bacterin intraperitoneally in the area of the pelvic fins.

Precaution(s): Shake well before using. Store between 2-7°C (35-45°F). Do not freeze. Use entire contents when first opened. Temperature of anesthetic solution should be within 2°C of hatchery water ambient temperature.

Caution(s): Vaccinate healthy fish only. Allow at least 40 days following vaccination before fish are exposed to the disease agent, longer at water temperature below 10°C. Vaccinate salmonids when 5 g or larger in size. For injection use. For veterinary use only.

Warning(s): Do not vaccinate within 21 days of slaughter.

Presentation: 5 mL vials and 500 mL bottles.

Distributed by: Mr. J. Zinn, Buhl, Idaho 83316

Compendium Code No.: 14970052 L-32-0 / L-24-1

F

FUROGEN 2

Novartis (Aqua Health) **Bacterin**

Aeromonas Salmonicida Bacterin

U.S. Vet. Lic. No.: 335

Contents: A formalin inactivated liquid emulsion containing *Aeromonas salmonicida* in an oil based adjuvant.

Indications: Uses: As an aid in the prevention of Furunculosis caused by *Aeromonas salmonicida* in healthy salmonids.

Dosage and Administration: Vaccination Program: This bacterin has been shown to be safe and effective when administered by intraperitoneal injection to salmonids 10 g or larger. Vaccination should precede exposure of vaccinates to the disease agent by 400 degree-days (number of days multiplied by the mean water temperature (°C) during period).

Injection Administration: Fish are anaesthetized until immobilized and given a 0.1 mL injection of bacterin intraperitoneally one fin length ahead of the pelvic fins along the midline.

Warming of the vaccine to 15-20°C may facilitate injection.

Precaution(s): Shake well before using. Store between 2-7°C (35-45°F). Do not freeze. Use entire contents when first opened. Empty bags must be destroyed in a safe way.

Caution(s): Vaccinate healthy fish only. If accidental injection occurs, the operator should discontinue and seek medical advice immediately. For veterinary use only.

Warning(s): Do not vaccinate within 60 days of slaughter. Keep away from children.

Presentation: 1000 mL bags.

Distributed by: Mr. J. Zinn, Buhl, Idaho 83316

Compendium Code No.: 14970032 L-31-0

FUROGEN B

Novartis (Aqua Health) **Bacterin**

Aeromonas Salmonicida Bacterin

U.S. Vet. Lic. No.: 335

Contents: This bacterin contains only formalin inactivated culture of *Aeromonas salmonicida* and has been shown to be safe and effective when administered by immersion to Koi carp *(Cyprinus carpio)* greater than or equal to 3.0 grams.

Indications: For the vaccination of healthy Koi carp *(Cyprinus carpio)* as an aid to the prevention of carp erythrodermatitis (ulcer disease) caused by atypical *Aeromonas salmonicida* sub-species *nova*.

Dosage and Administration: Vaccination Program: First vaccination should precede exposure of vaccinates to the disease agent by 800 degree days (number of days multiplied by the mean water temperature (°C) during period). A booster immersion vaccination is administered at not less than 14 days and not greater than 30 days following the first vaccination. Revaccination is also recommended biannually for long term holding of Koi carp. Shake well before using. To vaccinate fish, dilute entire contents of the container with 38 oz. (1,125 mL) of clean rearing water. Measure diluted bacterin in a suitable plastic container. Add fish to attain a density of 500 grams per litre of diluted bacterin. Expose fish for 60 seconds, then remove fish from bacterin solution. Return fish to holding facility. Diluted bacterin may be used up to 20 dips before discarding.

Precaution(s): Shake well before using.

Store between 35-45°F (2-7°C). Do not freeze. Use entire contents when first opened.

The vaccinal solution should be within 2°C of the ambient water temperature.

Caution(s): Vaccinate healthy fish only. For veterinary use only.

Presentation: 125 mL, 500 mL and 1,000 mL bottles.

Produced for: J. Zinn, Buhl, ID 83316.

Compendium Code No.: 14970111 L-28-0 / L-28.1-0 / L-28.2-1

FUROGEN DIP

Novartis (Aqua Health) **Bacterin**

Aeromonas Salmonicida Bacterin

U.S. Vet. Lic. No.: 335

Contents: This bacterin contains only formalin inactivated cultures of *Aeromonas salmonicida*. No other preservative is used.

Indications: For the vaccination of healthy salmonids as an aid in the prevention of furunculosis caused by *Aeromonas salmonicida*.

Dosage and Administration: Vaccination Program: Vaccination should precede exposure of vaccinates to the disease agent by 400 degree days (number of days multiplied by the mean water temperature (°C) during period). Not recommended for use in fish under 2.0 grams for immersion use.

Method of Administration:

Immersion Delivery: For immersion delivery, dilute entire contents of this container with 9 liters of clean hatchery water. Measure diluted bacterin in a suitable plastic container. Add fish to attain a density of 500 g per liter of diluted bacterin. Expose fish for 60 seconds, then drain bacterin from fish. Return fish to holding facility. Repeat until a total of 20 groups have been vaccinated in this manner.

Precaution(s): Shake well before using. Store between 35-45°F (2-7°C). Do not freeze. Use entire contents when first opened. The vaccinal solution should be within 2°C of the ambient water temperature. Any unused bacterin should be disposed of according to local waste disposal regulations and/or requirements.

Caution(s): Vaccinate healthy fish only. For veterinary use only.

Warning(s): Do not vaccinate within 21 days of slaughter

Presentation: 500 mL and 1000 mL bottles.

Distributed by: Mr. J. Zinn, Buhl, Idaho 83316

Compendium Code No.: 14970042 L-26-1 / L-27-0

FUROJECT ℞

Vetus **Diuretic**

(furosemide) 50 mg/mL-Diuretic-Saluretic

NADA No.: 131-538

Active Ingredient(s): Each mL contains: 50 mg furosemide as a monoethanolamine salt, myristyl-gamma-picolinium chloride 0.02%, EDTA sodium 0.1%, sodium sulfite 0.1% with sodium chloride 0.2% in water for injection, pH adjusted with sodium hydroxide and/or hydrochloric acid.

Indications: Dogs and Horses: FUROJECT Injection is an effective diuretic-saluretic for use in the treatment of acute noninflammatory tissue edema in dogs and horses, and for use in the treatment of edema (pulmonary congestion, ascites) associated with cardiac insufficiency in the dog. In cases of edema involving cardiac insufficiency, the continued use of heart stimulants such as digitalis or its glycosides is indicated.

The rationale for efficacious use of diuretic therapy in either dogs or horses is determined by the clinical pathology producing the edema.

Pharmacology: Description: Furosemide is a potent loop diuretic which is a derivative of anthranilic acid. The structure is:

COOH
NH - CH2
NH_2SO_2
Cl

Chemical Name: 4-Chloro-N-furfuryl-5-sulfamoylanthranilic acid. Furosemide is pharmacodynamically characterized by the following:

1) Administered intramuscularly, it begins to act in about 30 minutes, and diuretic response is produced. When administered intravenously, the response is in about 5 minutes.[1,2]
2) Is a loop diuretic which inhibits reabsorption of sodium and chloride at the ascending loop of Henle in the kidneys, enhancing water excretion.[3]
3) A dose-response relationship and a ratio of minimum to maximum effective dose range greater than tenfold.[1]
4) A high degree of efficacy, low inherent toxicity and a high therapeutic index.

Actions: The therapeutic efficacy of FUROJECT Injection is from the activity of the intact and unaltered molecule throughout the nephron, inhibiting the re-absorption of sodium not only in the proximal and distal tubule but also in the ascending limb of the loop of Henle. The prompt onset of action is a result of the drug's rapid absorption and a poor lipid solubility. The low lipid solubility and a rapid renal excretion minimize the possibility of its accumulation in tissues and organs or crystalluria. FUROJECT Injection has no inhibitory effect on carbonic anhydrase or aldosterone activity in the distal tubule. The drug possesses diuretic activity either in the presence of acidosis or alkosis.[1,3,4,5,6]

Dosage and Administration: Dogs: Administer intravenously or intramuscularly 0.25 to 0.50 mL per 10 pounds body weight once or twice daily at 6 to 8 hour intervals.

The dosage should be adjusted to the individual's response. In severe edematous or refractory cases, the dose may be doubled or increased by increments of 1.0 mg per pound of body weight. The established effective dose should be administered once or twice daily. Discontinue diuretic therapy with FUROJECT Injection, 50 mg/mL after initiation of acute fluid mobilization or stabilization of patient; when necessary Furotabs (furosemide) Tablets may be used for maintenance therapy (see Furotabs (furosemide) Tablets for details). Do not exceed treatment with FUROJECT Injection, 50 mg/mL for more than 3 days. The daily schedule of administration can be timed to control the period of micturition for the convenience of the client or veterinarian. Mobilization of the edema may be efficiently and safely accomplished by utilizing an intermittent daily dose schedule, i.e., every other day or 2 to 4 consecutive days weekly.

Horses: The usual parenteral dosage of furosemide in horses is approximately 0.5 mg/lb body weight (1.0 mg/kg). See dosage schedule below. A prompt diuresis usually ensues from the initial treatment. Administer once or twice daily at 6 to 8 hour intervals either intravenously or intramuscularly until desired results are achieved.

The dosage should be adjusted to the individual's response. In severe edematous or refractory cases, the dose may be doubled or increased by increments of 0.5 mg per pound of body weight. The established effective dose should be administered once or twice daily. The daily schedule of administration can be timed to control the period of micturition for the convenience of the client or veterinarian. Mobilization of the edema may be most efficiently and safely accomplished by utilizing an intermittent daily dose schedule, i.e., every other day or 2 to 4 consecutive days weekly.

Recommended Dosage Schedule:

Horses: Administer IV or IM once or twice daily at 6-8 hour intervals until desired results are achieved.

Body Weight (lbs)	FUROJECT Injection (50 mg/mL)
500	4.6 mL
600	5.5 mL
700	6.4 mL
800	7.3 mL
900	8.2 mL
1000	9.1 mL
1100	10.0 mL
1200	10.9 mL

Diuretic therapy for both dogs and horses should be discontinued after reduction of the edema, or maintained after determining a carefully programmed dosage schedule to prevent recurrence of edema. For long-term treatment, the dose can generally be lowered after the edema has been reduced. Re-examination and consultations with the client will enhance the establishment of a satisfactorily programmed dosage schedule. Clinical examination and serum BUN, CO_2 and electrolyte determinations should be performed during the early period of therapy and periodically thereafter, especially in refractory cases. Abnormalities should be corrected or the drug temporarily withdrawn.

Contraindication(s): Animal reproductive studies have shown that furosemide may cause fetal abnormality and the drug is contraindicated in pregnant bitches, mares and stallions at stud. Furosemide is contraindicated in anuria, furosemide hypersensitivity, hepatic coma, or during electrolytic imbalances. Monitor serum electrolytes, BUN and CO_2 frequently. Monitor serum potassium levels and watch for signs of hypocalcemia.

Corticosteroids cause an additive potassium-depletion effect.

Precaution(s): Store at controlled room temperature 59°-86°F (15°-30°C).

Caution(s): Federal law restricts this drug to use by or on the order of a licensed veterinarian.

For use in animals only.

FUROJECT Injection is a highly effective diuretic-saluretic which, if given in excessive amounts, may result in dehydration and have to be adjusted to the patient's needs. The animal should be observed for early signs of electrolyte imbalance, and corrective measures administered. Early signs of electrolyte imbalance are increased thirst, lethargy, drowsiness or restlessness, fatigue, oliguria, gastrointestinal disturbances and tachycardia. Special attention should be given to potassium levels. FUROJECT Injection may lower serum calcium levels and cause tetany in rare cases of animals having an existing hypocalcemic tendency.[7,8,9,10,11]

FUROJECT Injection is contraindicated in anuria. Therapy should be discontinued in case of progressive renal disease if increasing azotemia and oliguria occur during the treatment. Sudden alterations of fluid and electrolyte imbalance in an animal with cirrhosis may precipitate hepatic coma, therefore observation during the period of therapy is necessary. In hepatic coma and in states of electrolyte depletion, therapy should not be instituted until the basic condition is improved or corrected. Potassium supplementation may be necessary in cases routinely treated with potassium-depleting steroids.

Active or latent diabetes mellitis may, on rare occasions, be exacerbated by furosemide. Transient loss of auditory capacity has been experimentally produced in cats following intravenous injections of excessive doses of furosemide at a very rapid rate.[12,13,14]

FUROJECT Injection is a highly effective diuretic and, if given in excessive amounts, as with any diuretic, may lead to excessive diuresis which could result in electrolyte imbalance, dehydration and reduction of plasma volume, enhancing the risk of circulatory collapse, thrombosis and embolism. Therefore, the animal should be observed for early signs of fluid depletion with electrolyte imbalance, and corrective measures administered. Excessive loss of potassium in patients receiving digitalis or its glycosides may precipitate digitalis toxicity. Caution should be exercised in animals administered potassium-depleting steroids. Correct potassium deficiency with a proper dietary supplementation. If the animal needs potassium supplements, use an oral liquid form; do not use enteric-coated potassium tablets.

The concurrent use of furosemide with some antibiotics may be inadvisable. There is evidence that the drug enhances the nephrotoxic potential of aminoglycosides, cephalosporins and polymixins and increases the ototoxic effects of all aminoglycosides.

Sulfonamide diuretics have been reported to decrease arterial responsiveness to pressor amines and to enhance the effect of tubocurarine. Caution should be exercised in administering curare or its derivatives to patients undergoing therapy with FUROJECT Injection, and it is advisable to discontinue FUROJECT Injection for one day prior to elective surgery.

Warning(s): Do not use in horses intended for food.

Toxicology: Furosemide demonstrates a very low order of either acute or chronic toxicity. The drug is rapidly absorbed and excreted by both glomerular filtration and tubular secretion. The rates of excretion are of such magnitude that accumulation of furosemide does not occur despite repeated administrations.[15]

The main effect observed in clinical toxicity is an abnormality of fluid and electrolyte imbalances. Ototoxicity resulting in transient loss of hearing has been reported with furosemide.[15]

A safety study was performed in dogs to determine the effects of FUROJECT Injection at increasing dosages and time elements. The dosage levels were 1.5 mg/lb body weight (recommended dosage), 4.5 mg/lb body weight (3X recommended dosage) and 7.5 mg/lb body weight (5X recommended dosage). The treatment period ranged up to nine days in length. Results demonstrate very slight tubular nephrosis at the higher dosage levels.

In addition, serum levels of potassium and chloride were slightly lowered in the higher dosage groups. Cumulative evaluation of the data demonstrates that FUROJECT Injection is safe when administered at the recommended dosage for a duration of nine consecutive days.

References: Available upon request.

Presentation: 100 mL multi dose vials (NDC 47611-255-82).

Distributed by: Burns Veterinary Supply, Rockville Centre, NY 11570.

Compendium Code No.: 14440361 ECL-1835 9608

FUROSEMIDE INJECTABLE 5% ℞

AgriLabs **Diuretic**

Diuretic-Saluretic

ANADA No.: 200-293

Active Ingredient(s): Each mL contains 50 mg furosemide as a diethanolamine salt preserved and stabilized with myristyl-gamma-picolinium chloride 0.02%, EDTA sodium 0.1%, sodium metasulfite 0.1% with sodium chloride 0.2% in Water For Injection, USP, pH adjusted with sodium hydroxide.

Indications:

Dogs, Cats & Horses: FUROSEMIDE INJECTABLE 5% is an effective diuretic possessing a wide therapeutic range. Pharmacologically it promotes the rapid removal of abnormally retained extracellular fluids. The rationale for the efficacious use of diuretic therapy is determined by the clinical pathology producing the edema. FUROSEMIDE INJECTABLE 5% is indicated for the treatment of edema, (pulmonary congestion, ascites) associated with cardiac insufficiency and acute noninflammatory tissue edema.

The continued use of heart stimulants, such as digitalis or its glycosides is indicated in cases of edema involving cardiac insufficiency.

Cattle: FUROSEMIDE INJECTABLE 5% is indicated for the treatment of physiological parturient edema of the mammary gland and associated structures.

Pharmacology: Description: FUROSEMIDE INJECTABLE 5% is a chemically distinct diuretic and saluretic pharmacodynamically characterized by the following:

1) A high degree of efficacy, low-inherent toxicity and a high therapeutic index.
2) A rapid onset of action of comparatively short duration.
3) A pharmacological action in the functional area of the nephron, i.e., proximal and distal tubules and the ascending limb of the loop of Henle.
4) A dose-response relationship and a ratio of minimum to maximum effective dose range greater than tenfold.

The intravenous route produces the most rapid diuretic response.

The CAS Registry Number is 54-31-9.

FUROSEMIDE INJECTABLE 5%, a diuretic, is an anthranilic acid derivative with the following structural formula:

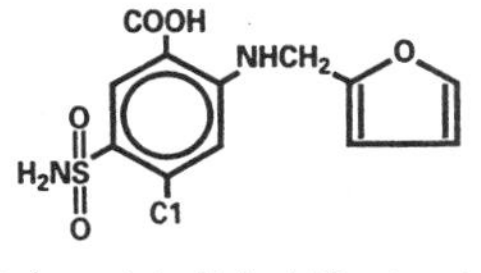

Generic name: Furosemide (except in United Kingdom-furosemide). Chemical name: 4-chloro-N-furfuryl-5-sulfamoylanthranilic acid.

Actions: The therapeutic efficacy of FUROSEMIDE INJECTABLE 5% is from the activity of the intact and unaltered molecule throughout the nephron, inhibiting the reabsorption of sodium not only in the proximal and distal tubule but also in the ascending limb of the loop of Henle. The prompt onset of action is a result of the drug's rapid absorption and a poor lipid solubility. The low lipid solubility and a rapid renal excretion minimize the possibility of its accumulation in tissues and organs or crystalluria. FUROSEMIDE INJECTABLE 5% has no inhibitory effect on carbonic anhydrase or aldosterone activity in the distal tubule. The drug possesses diuretic activity either in the presence of acidosis or alkalosis.

Dosage and Administration: The usual dosage of FUROSEMIDE INJECTABLE 5% is 1 to 2 mg/lb. body weight (approximately 2.5 to 5 mg/kg). The lower dose is suggested for cats. Administer once or twice daily at 6- to 8-hour intervals either intravenously or intramuscularly. A prompt diuresis usually ensues from the initial treatment. Diuresis may be initiated by the parenteral administration of FUROSEMIDE INJECTABLE 5%.

The dosage should be adjusted to the individual's response. In severe edematous or refractory cases, the dose may be doubled or increased by increments of 1 mg per pound body weight. The established effective dose should be administered once or twice daily. The daily schedule of administration can be timed to control the period of micturition for the convenience of the client or veterinarian. Mobilization of the edema may be most efficiently and safely accomplished by utilizing an intermittent daily dosage schedule, i.e., every other day or 2 to 4 consecutive days weekly.

Diuretic therapy should be discontinued after reduction of the edema, or maintained after determining a carefully programmed dosage schedule to prevent recurrence of edema. For long-term treatment, the dose can generally be lowered after the edema has once been reduced. Re-examination and consultations with client will enhance the establishment of a satisfactorily programmed dosage schedule. Clinical examination and serum BUN, CO_2 and electrolyte determinations should be performed during the early period of therapy and periodically thereafter, especially in refractory cases. Abnormalities should be corrected or the drug temporarily withdrawn.

Dosage: Parenteral:

Dogs & Cats: Administer intramuscularly or intravenously ¼ to ½ mL per 10 pounds body weight. Administer one or twice daily, permitting a 6- to 8-hour interval between treatments. In refractory or severe edematous cases the dosage may be doubled or increased by increments of 1 mg per pound body weight as recommended in preceding paragraphs. "Dosage and Administration".

Horse: The individual dose is 250 to 500 mg (5 to 10 mL) administered intramuscularly or intravenously once or twice daily at 6- to 8-hour intervals until desired results are achieved. The veterinarian should evaluate the degree of edema present and adjust dosage schedule accordingly.

Cattle: The individual dose administered intramuscularly or intravenously is 500 mg (10 mL) once daily or 250 g (5 mL) twice daily at 12-hour intervals. Treatment not to exceed 48 hours postparturition.

Contraindication(s): FUROSEMIDE INJECTABLE 5% is a highly effective diuretic-saluretic which if given in excessive amounts may result in dehydration and electrolyte imbalance. Therefore, the dosage and schedule may have to be adjusted to the patient's needs. The animal should be observed for early signs of electrolyte imbalance, and corrective measures administered. Early signs of electrolyte imbalance are: increased thirst, lethargy, drowsiness or restlessness, fatigue, oliguria, gastro-intestinal disturbances and tachycardia. Special attention should be given to potassium levels. FUROSEMIDE INJECTABLE 5% may lower serum calcium levels and cause tetany in rare cases of animals having an existing hypocalcemic tendency.

Although diabetes mellitus is a rarely reported disease in animals, active or latent diabetes mellitus may on rare occasions be exacerbated by FUROSEMIDE INJECTABLE 5%. While it has not been reported in animals the use of high doses of salicylates, as in rheumatic diseases, in conjunction with FUROSEMIDE INJECTABLE 5% may result in salicylate toxicity because of competition for renal excretory sites.

Transient loss of auditory capacity has been experimentally produced in cats following intravenous injection of excessive doses of FUROSEMIDE INJECTABLE 5% at a very rapid rate.

Electrolyte balance should be monitored prior to surgery in patients receiving FUROSEMIDE INJECTABLE 5%. Imbalances must be corrected by administration of suitable fluid therapy.

FUROSEMIDE INJECTABLE 5% is contraindicated in anuria. Therapy should be discontinued in cases of progressive renal disease if increasing azotemia and oliguria occur during the treatment. Sudden alterations of fluid and electrolyte imbalance in an animal with cirrhosis may precipitate hepatic coma, therefore observation during period of therapy is necessary. In hepatic coma and in states of electrolyte depletion, therapy should not be instituted until the basic condition is improved or corrected. Potassium supplementation may be necessary in cases routinely treated with potassium-depleting steroids.

Precaution(s): Store between 15°C and 30°C (59°-86°F).

Caution(s): Federal law restricts this drug to use by or on the order of a licensed veterinarian.

FUROSEMIDE INJECTABLE 5% is a highly effective diuretic and if given in excessive amounts as with any diuretic may lead to excessive diuresis which could result in electrolyte imbalance, dehydration and reduction of plasma volume enhancing the risk of circulatory collapse, thrombosis, and embolism. Therefore, the animal should be observed for early signs of fluid depletion with electrolyte imbalance, and corrective measures administered. Excessive loss of potassium in patients receiving digitalis or its glycosides may precipitate digitalis toxicity. Caution should be exercised in animals administered potassium-depleting steroids.

It is important to correct potassium deficiency with dietary supplementation. Caution should be exercised in prescribing enteric-coated potassium tablets.

There have been several reports in human literature, published and unpublished, concerning nonspecific small-bowel lesions consisting of stenosis, with or without ulceration, associated with the administration of enteric-coated thiazides with potassium salts. These lesions may occur with enteric-coated potassium tablets alone or when they are used with nonenteric-coated thiazides, or certain other oral diuretics. These small-bowel lesions may have caused obstruction, hemorrhage, and perforation. Surgery was frequently required, and deaths have occurred. Available information tends to implicate enteric-coated potassium salts, although lesions of this type also occur spontaneously. Therefore, coated potassium-containing formulations should be administered only when indicated and should be discontinued immediately if abdominal pain, distension, nausea, vomiting, or gastro-intestinal bleeding occurs.

Human patients with known sulfonamide sensitivity may show allergic reactions to FUROSEMIDE INJECTABLE 5%, however, these reactions have not been reported in animals.

Sulfonamide diuretics have been reported to decrease arterial responsiveness to pressor amines and to enhance the effect of tubocurarine. Caution should be exercised in administering curare or its derivatives to patients undergoing therapy with FUROSEMIDE INJECTABLE 5% and it is advisable to discontinue FUROSEMIDE INJECTABLE 5% for one day prior to any elective surgery.

For animal use only.

Warning(s):

Cattle: Milk taken from animals during treatment and for 48 hours (four milkings) after the last treatment must not be used for food. Cattle must not be slaughtered for food within 48 hours following last treatment.

Horses: Do not use in horses intended for food.

Keep out of reach of children.

Toxicology: Acute Toxicity: The following table illustrates low acute toxicity of FUROSEMIDE INJECTABLE 5% in three different species. (Two values indicate two different studies.)

LD50 of FUROSEMIDE INJECTABLE 5% in mg/kg body weight:

Species	Oral	Intravenous
Mouse	1050-1500	308
Rat	2650-4600*	680
Dog	>1000 and >4640	>300 and >464

*Note: The lower value for the rat oral LD50 was obtained in a group of fasted animals; the higher figure is from a study performed in fed rats.

Toxic doses lead to convulsions, ataxia, paralysis and collapse. Animals surviving toxic dosages may become dehydrated and depleted of electrolytes due to the massive diuresis and saluresis.

Chronic Toxicity: Chronic toxicity studies with FUROSEMIDE INJECTABLE 5% were done in a one-year study in rats and dogs. In a one-year study in rats, renal tubular degeneration occurred with all doses higher than 50 mg/kg. A six-month study in dogs revealed calcification and scarring of the renal parenchyma at all doses above 10 mg/kg.

Reproductive Studies: Reproductive studies were conducted in mice, rats and rabbits. Only in rabbits administered high doses (equivalent to 10 to 25 times the recommended average dose of 2 mg/kg for dogs, cats, horses, and cattle) of furosemide during the second trimester period did unexplained maternal deaths and abortions occur. The administration of FUROSEMIDE INJECTABLE 5% is not recommended during the second trimester of pregnancy.

Presentation: Available in 50 mL multidose vials for dogs, cats, horses and cattle and 100 mL multidose vials for horses and cattle.

Compendium Code No.: 10581590

Iss. 12-01

FUROSEMIDE INJECTION ℞

AgriLabs

Diuretic

NADA No.: 131-538

Active Ingredient(s): Each mL Contains: 50 mg furosemide as a monoethanolamine salt, myristyl-gamma-picolinium chloride 0.02%, EDTA sodium 0.1%, sodium sulfite 0.1% with sodium chloride 0.2% in water for injection, pH adjusted with sodium hydroxide and/or hydrochloric acid.

Indications: Dogs and Horses—FUROSEMIDE INJECTION is an effective diuretic-saluretic for use in the treatment of acute noninflammatory tissue edema in dogs and horses, and for use in the treatment of edema (pulmonary congestion, ascites) associated with cardiac insufficiency in the dog. In cases of edema involving cardiac insufficiency, the continued use of heart stimulants such as digitalis or its glycosides is indicated. The rationale for efficacious use of diuretic therapy in either dogs or horses is determined by the clinical pathology producing the edema.

Pharmacology: Description: Furosemide is a potent loop diuretic which is a derivative of anthranilic acid. The structure is:

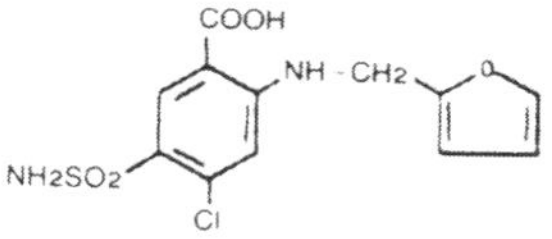

Chemical Name: 4-Chloro-N-furfuryl-5-sulfamoylanthranilic acid. Furosemide is pharmacodynamically characterized by the following:

1) Administered intramuscularly, it begins to act in about 30 minutes, and diuretic response is produced. When administered intravenously, the response is in about 5 minutes.[1,2]
2) Is a loop diuretic which inhibits reabsorption of sodium and chloride at the ascending loop of Henle in the kidneys, enhancing water excretion.[3]
3) A dose-response relationship and a ratio of minimum to maximum effective dose range greater than tenfold.[1]
4) A high degree of efficacy, low inherent toxicity and a high therapeutic index.

Actions: The therapeutic efficacy of FUROSEMIDE INJECTION is from the activity of the intact and unaltered molecule throughout the nephron, inhibiting the reabsorption of sodium not only in the proximal and distal tubule but also in the ascending limb of the loop of Henle. The prompt onset of action is a result of the drug's rapid absorption and a poor lipid solubility. The low lipid solubility and a rapid renal excretion minimize the possibility of its accumulation in tissues and organs or crystalluria. Furosemide has no inhibitory effect on carbonic anhydrase or aldosterone activity in the distal tubule. The drug possesses diuretic activity either in the presence of acidosis or alkosis.[1,3,4,5,6]

Dosage and Administration: Dogs—Administer intravenously or intramuscularly 0.25 to 0.50 mL per 10 pounds body weight once or twice daily at 6 to 8 hour intervals.

The dosage should be adjusted to the individual's response. In severe edematous or refractory cases, the dose may be doubled or increased by increments of 1.0 mg per pound of body weight. The established effective dose should be administered once or twice daily. Discontinue diuretic therapy with FUROSEMIDE INJECTION, 50 mg/mL after initiation of acute fluid mobilization or stabilization of patient; when necessary Furosemide Tablets may be used for maintenance therapy (see Furosemide Tablets insert for details). Do not exceed treatment with FUROSEMIDE INJECTION, 50 mg/mL for more than 3 days. The daily schedule of administration can be timed to control the period of micturition for the convenience of the client or veterinarian. Mobilization of the edema may be efficiently and safely accomplished by utilizing an intermittent daily dose schedule, i.e., every other day or 2 to 4 consecutive days weekly.

Horses—The usual parenteral dosage of furosemide in horses is approximately 0.5 mg/lb body weight (1.0 mg/kg). See dosage schedule below. A prompt diuresis usually ensues from the initial treatment. Administer once or twice daily at 6 to 8 hour intervals either intravenously or intramuscularly until desired results are achieved.

The dosage should be adjusted to the individual's response. In severe edematous or refractory cases, the dose may be doubled or increased by increments of 0.5 mg per pound of body weight. The established effective dose should be administered once or twice daily. The daily schedule of administration can be timed to control the period of micturition for the convenience of the client or veterinarian. Mobilization of the edema may be most efficiently and safely accomplished by utilizing an intermittent daily dose schedule, i.e., every other day or 2 to 4 consecutive days weekly.

Recommended Dosage Schedule: Horses: Administer IV or IM once or twice daily at 6-8 hour intervals until desired results are achieved.

Body Weight (lbs)	FUROSEMIDE INJECTION (50 mg/mL)
500	4.6 mL
600	5.5 mL
700	6.4 mL
800	7.3 mL
900	8.2 mL
1000	9.1 mL
1100	10.0 mL
1200	10.9 mL

F

Diuretic therapy for both dogs and horses should be discontinued after reduction of the edema, or maintained after determining a carefully programmed dosage schedule to prevent recurrence of edema. For long-term treatment, the dose can generally be lowered after the edema has been reduced. Re-examination and consultations with the client will enhance the establishment of a satisfactory programmed dosage schedule. Clinical examination and serum BUN, CO_2 and electrolyte determinations should be performed during the early period of therapy and periodically thereafter, especially in refractory cases. Abnormalities should be corrected or the drug temporarily withdrawn.

Contraindication(s): Animal reproductive studies have shown that furosemide may cause fetal abnormality and the drug is contraindicated in pregnant bitches, mares and stallions at stud.

Furosemide is contraindicated in anuria, furosemide hypersensitivity, hepatic coma, or during electrolytic imbalances. Monitor serum electrolytes, BUN and CO_2 frequently. Monitor serum potassium levels and watch for signs of hypocalcemia.

Corticosteroids cause an additive potassium-depletion effect.

Precaution(s): Store at controlled room temperature, 59°-86°F (15°-30°C).

Caution(s): Federal (U.S.A.) law restricts this drug to use by or on the order of a licensed veterinarian.

FUROSEMIDE INJECTION is a highly effective diuretic-saluretic which, if given in excessive amounts, may result in dehydration and have to be adjusted to the patient's needs. The animal should be observed for early signs of electrolyte imbalance, and corrective measures administered. Early signs of electrolyte imbalance are increased thirst, lethargy, drowsiness or restlessness, fatigue, oliguria, gastro-intestinal disturbances and tachycardia. Special attention should be given to potassium levels. FUROSEMIDE INJECTION may lower serum calcium levels and cause tetany in rare cases of animals having an existing hypocalcemic tendency.[7,8,9,10,11]

FUROSEMIDE INJECTION is contraindicated in anuria. Therapy should be discontinued in case of progressive renal disease if increasing azotemia and oliguria occur during the treatment. Sudden alterations of fluid and electrolyte imbalance in an animal with cirrhosis may precipitate hepatic coma, therefore, observation during period of therapy is necessary. In hepatic coma and in states of electrolyte depletion, therapy should not be instituted until the basic condition is improved or corrected. Potassium supplementation may be necessary in cases routinely treated with potassium-depleting steroids.

Active or latent diabetes mellitis may on rare occasions be exacerbated by furosemide. Transient loss of auditory capacity has been experimentally produced in cats following intravenous injections of excessive doses of furosemide at a very rapid rate.[12,13,14]

FUROSEMIDE INJECTION is a highly effective diuretic and, if given in excessive amounts, as with any diuretic, may lead to excessive diuresis which could result in electrolyte imbalance, dehydration and reduction of plasma volume, enhancing the risk of circulatory collapse, thrombosis and embolism. Therefore, the animal should be observed for early signs of fluid depletion with electrolyte imbalance, and corrective measures administered. Excessive loss of potassium in patients receiving digitalis or its glycosides may precipitate digitalis toxicity. Caution should be exercised in animals administered potassium-depleting steroids. Correct potassium deficiency with proper dietary supplementation. If animal needs potassium supplements, use an oral liquid form; do not use enteric-coated potassium tablets.

The concurrent use of furosemide with some antibiotics may be inadvisable. There is evidence that the drug enhances the nephrotoxic potential of aminoglycosides, cephalosporins and polymixins and increases the ototoxic effects of all aminoglycosides.

Sulfonamide diuretics have been reported to decrease arterial responsiveness to pressor amines and to enhance the effect of tubocurarine. Caution should be exercised in administering curare or its derivatives to patients undergoing therapy with FUROSEMIDE INJECTION and it is advisable to discontinue FUROSEMIDE INJECTION for one day prior to elective surgery.

For use in animals only.

Warning(s): Do not use in horses intended for food.

Keep out of reach of children.

Toxicology: Furosemide demonstrates a very low order of either acute or chronic toxicity. The drug is rapidly absorbed and excreted by both glomerular filtration and tubular secretion. The rates of excretion are of such magnitude that cumulation of furosemide does not occur despite repeated administrations.[15]

The main effect observed in clinical toxicity is an abnormality of fluid and electrolyte imbalances. Ototoxicity resulting in transient loss of hearing has been reported with furosemide.[15]

A safety study was performed in dogs to determine the effects of FUROSEMIDE INJECTION at increasing dosages and time elements. The dosage levels were 1.5 mg/lb body weight (recommended dosage), 4.5 mg/lb body weight (3X recommended dosage) and 7.5 mg/lb body weight (5X recommended dosage). The treatment period ranged up to nine days in length. Results demonstrate very slight tubular nephrosis at the higher dosage levels.

In addition, serum levels of potassium and chloride were slightly lowered in the higher dosage groups.

Cumulative evaluation of the data demonstrates that FUROSEMIDE INJECTION is safe when administered at the recommended dosage for a duration of nine consecutive days.

References: Available upon request.

Presentation: Available in 50 and 100 mL multi dose vials.

Compendium Code No.: 10581600 673719L-00-0002 / 673717L-00-9909

FUROSEMIDE INJECTION 5% ℞

Butler **Diuretic**

NADA No.: 118-550

Active Ingredient(s): Each mL contains:

Furosemide (as a diethanolamine salt)	50 mg
Myristyl-gamma-picolinium chloride	0.02%
EDTA sodium	0.1%
Sodium sulfite	0.1%
Sodium chloride	0.2%
Water for injection	q.s.

The pH is adjusted with sodium hydroxide.

Indications: Horses: FUROSEMIDE is indicated for the treatment of acute noninflammatory tissue edema.

Pharmacology: Furosemide is a chemically distinct diuretic and saluretic pharmacodynamically characterized by the following:

1. A high degree of efficacy, low-inherent toxicity and a high therapeutic index.
2. A rapid onset of action and of comparatively short duration.[1]
3. A pharmacological action in the functional area of the nephron, i.e., proximal and distal tubules and the ascending limb of the loop of Henle.[3,4]
4. A dose-response relationship and a ratio of minimum to maximum effective dose range greater than tenfold.[1]
5. It is administered parenterally. The intravenous route produces the most rapid diuretic response.

Furosemide, a diuretic, is an anthranilic acid derivative with the following structural formula:

Cl N H-CH$_2$ O H_2NO_2S COOH

Generic name: Furosemide (except in United Kingdom - frusemide).

Chemical name: 4-chloro-N-furfuryl-5-sulfamoylanthranilic acid.

The therapeutic efficacy of furosemide is from the activity of the intact and unaltered molecule throughout the nephron, inhibiting the re-absorption of sodium not only in the proximal and distal tubule but also in the ascending limb of the loop of Henle. The prompt onset of action is a result of the drug's rapid absorption and poor lipid solubility. The low lipid solubility and a rapid renal excretion minimize the possibility of its accumulation in tissues and organs or crystalluria. Furosemide does not have an inhibitory effect on carbonic anhydrase activity in the distal tubule.[2,3,4,5]

Dosage and Administration: Administer 0.5 mg per pound of body weight (approximately 1.0 mg per kg) once or twice a day at 6- to 8-hour intervals either intravenously or intramuscularly.

A prompt diuresis usually ensues from the initial treatment. Diuresis may be initiated by the parenteral administration of furosemide injection. The dosage should be adjusted to the individual's response. In severe edematous or refractory cases, the dose may be doubled or increased by increments of 1 mg per pound of body weight. The established effective dose should be administered once or twice a day. The daily schedule of administration can be timed to control the period of micturition for the convenience of the client or veterinarian. Mobilization of the edema may be most efficiently and safely accomplished by utilizing an intermittent daily dosage schedule, i.e., every other day or two (2) to four (4) consecutive days a week.

Diuretic therapy should be discontinued after reduction of the edema, or maintained after determining a carefully programmed dosage schedule to prevent recurrence of edema. For long-term treatment, the dose can generally be lowered after the edema has once been reduced. Re-examination and consultations with the client will enhance the establishment of a satisfactory dosage schedule. Clinical examination and serum BUN, CO_2 and electrolyte determination should be performed during the early period of therapy and periodically thereafter, especially in refractory cases. Abnormalities should be corrected or the drug temporarily withdrawn.

Contraindication(s): Furosemide is contraindicated in anuria. Therapy should be discontinued in cases of progressive renal disease if increasing azotemia and oliguria occur during the treatment. Sudden alterations of fluid and electrolyte imbalance in an animal with cirrhosis may precipitate hepatic coma, therefore observation during the period of therapy is necessary. In hepatic coma and in states of electrolyte depletion, therapy should not be instituted until the basic condition is improved or corrected. Potassium supplementation may be necessary in cases routinely treated with potassium-depleting steroids.

Although diabetes mellitus is a rarely reported disease in animals, active or latent diabetes mellitus may on rare occasions be exacerbated by furosemide. While it has not been reported in animals, the use of high doses of salicylates, as in rheumatic diseases, in conjunction with furosemide may result in salicylate toxicity because of competition for renal excretory sites.

Precaution(s): Concurrent therapy for the treatment of systemic conditions causing edema (pulmonary congestion, ascites, cardiac insufficiency) should be instituted.

The continued use of heart stimulants, such as digitalis or its glycosides is indicated in cases of edema involving cardiac insufficiency.

Furosemide is a highly effective diuretic-saluretic which if given in excessive amounts may result in dehydration and electrolyte imbalance. Therefore, the dosage and schedule may have to be adjusted to the patient's needs. The animal should be observed for early signs of electrolyte imbalance and corrective measures administered. Early signs of electrolyte imbalance are: Increased thirst, lethargy, drowsiness or restlessness, fatigue, oliguria, gastro-intestinal disturbances and tachycardia. Special attention should be given to potassium levels. Furosemide may lower serum calcium levels and cause tetany in rare cases of animals having an existing hypocalcemic tendency.[6,7,8,9,10]

Electrolyte balance should be monitored prior to surgery in patients receiving furosemide. Imbalances must be corrected by the administration of suitable fluid therapy.

Caution(s): Federal law restricts this drug to use by or on the order of a licensed veterinarian.

Furosemide is a highly effective diuretic and if given in excessive amounts, as with any diuretic, may lead to excessive diuresis which could result in electrolyte imbalance, dehydration and the reduction of plasma volume enhancing the risk of circulatory collapse, thrombosis and embolism. Therefore, the animal should be observed for early signs of fluid depletion with electrolyte imbalance, and corrective measures administered. Excessive loss of potassium in patients receiving digitalis or its glycosides may precipitate digitalis toxicity. Caution should be exercised in animals administered potassium-depleting steroids.

It is important to correct potassium deficiency with dietary supplementation. Caution should be exercised in prescribing enteric-coated potassium tablets.

There have been several reports in human literature, published and unpublished, concerning nonspecific small-bowel lesions consisting of stenosis, with or without ulceration, associated with the administration of enteric-coated thiazides with potassium salts. These lesions may occur with enteric-coated potassium tablets alone or when they are used with nonenteric-coated thiazides, or certain other oral diuretics. These small-bowel lesions may have caused obstruction, hemorrhage, and perforation. Surgery was frequently required and deaths have occurred. Available information tends to implicate enteric-coated potassium salts, although lesions of this type also occur spontaneously. Therefore, coated potassium- containing formulations should be administered only when indicated and should be discontinued immediately if abdominal pain, distention, nausea, vomiting or gastro-intestinal bleeding occurs.

Human patients with known sulfonamide sensitivity may show allergic reactions to furosemide, however, these reactions have not been reported in animals. Sulfonamide diuretics have been reported to decrease arterial responsiveness to pressor amines and to enhance the effect of tubocurarine. Caution should be exercised in administering curare or its derivatives to patients undergoing therapy with furosemide and it is advisable to discontinue furosemide for one (1) day prior to any elective surgery.

Warning(s): Do not use in horses intended for food.

Toxicology: The following table illustrates the low acute toxicity of furosemide in three different species. (Two values indicate two different studies) LD_{50} of furosemide in mg/kg of body weight.

Species	Intravenous
Mouse	308
Rat	680
Dog	>300 and >464

Toxic doses lead to convulsions, ataxia, paralysis and collapse. Animals surviving toxic dosages may become dehydrated and depleted of electrolytes due to the massive diuresis and saluresis.

Chronic toxicity studies with furosemide were done in a one-year study in rats and dogs. In a one-year study in rats, renal tubular degeneration occurred with all doses higher than 50 mg/kg. A six-month study in dogs revealed calcification and scarring of the renal parenchyma at all doses above 10 mg/kg.

Reproductive studies were conducted in mice, rats and rabbits. Only in rabbits administered high doses (equivalent to 10 to 25 times the recommended average dose of 2 mg/kg) of furosemide during the second trimester period did unexplained maternal deaths and abortions occur.

The safety of furosemide in breeding animals or in pregnant mares has not been investigated. Therefore, do not use in stallions at stud or in pregnant mares.

References: Available upon request.

Presentation: Available in 50 mL and 100 mL multiple dose vials.

Compendium Code No.: 10820781

FUROSEMIDE INJECTION 5% ℞

Phoenix Pharmaceutical **Diuretic**

Diuretic-Saluretic

ANADA No.: 200-293

Active Ingredient(s): Each mL contains 50 mg furosemide as a diethanolamine salt preserved and stabilized with myristyl-gamma-picolinium chloride 0.02%, EDTA sodium 0.1%, sodium metasulfite 0.1% with sodium chloride 0.2% in water for injection, USP, pH adjusted with sodium hydroxide.

Indications: Horses: FUROSEMIDE INJECTION 5% is an effective diuretic possessing a wide therapeutic range. Pharmacologically it promotes the rapid removal of abnormally retained extracellular fluids. The rationale for the efficacious use of diuretic therapy is determined by the clinical pathology producing the edema. FUROSEMIDE INJECTION 5% is indicated for the treatment of edema (pulmonary congestion, ascites) associated with cardiac insufficiency and acute noninflammatory tissue edema.

The continued use of heart stimulants, such as digitalis or its glycosides, is indicated in cases of edema involving cardiac insufficiency.

Cattle: FUROSEMIDE INJECTION 5% is indicated for the treatment of physiological parturient edema of the mammary gland and associated structures.

Pharmacology: Description: FUROSEMIDE INJECTION 5% is a chemically distinct diuretic and saluretic pharmacodynamically characterized by the following:

1) A high degree of efficacy, low-inherent toxicity and a high therapeutic index.
2) A rapid onset of action of comparatively short duration.
3) A pharmacological action in the functional area of the nephron, i.e., proximal and distal tubules and the ascending limb of the loop of Henle.
4) A dose-response relationship and a ratio of minimum to maximum effective dose range greater than tenfold.

The intravenous route produces the most rapid diuretic response.

The CAS Registry Number is 54-31-9.

FUROSEMIDE INJECTION 5%, a diuretic, is an anthranilic acid derivative with the following structural formula:

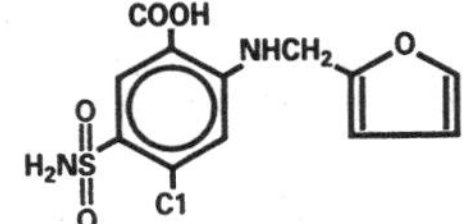

Generic name: Furosemide (except in United Kingdom-furosemide). Chemical name: 4-chloro-N-furfuryl-5-sulfamoylanthranilic acid.

Actions: The therapeutic efficacy of FUROSEMIDE INJECTION 5% is from the activity of the intact and unaltered molecule throughout the nephron, inhibiting the reabsorption of sodium not only in the proximal and distal tubule but also in the ascending limb of the loop of Henle. The prompt onset of action is a result of the drug's rapid absorption and a poor lipid solubility. The low lipid solubility and a rapid renal excretion minimize the possibility of its accumulation in tissues and organs or crystalluria. FUROSEMIDE INJECTION 5% has no inhibitory effect on carbonic anhydrase or aldosterone activity in the distal tubule. The drug possesses diuretic activity either in the presence of acidosis or alkalosis.

Dosage and Administration: The usual dosage of FUROSEMIDE INJECTION 5% is 1 to 2 mg/lb. body weight (approximately 2.5 to 5 mg/kg). Administer once or twice daily at 6- to 8-hour intervals either intravenously or intramuscularly. A prompt diuresis usually ensues from the initial treatment. Diuresis may be initiated by the parenteral administration of FUROSEMIDE INJECTION 5%.

The dosage should be adjusted to the individual's response. In severe edematous or refractory cases, the dose may be doubled or increased by increments of 1 mg per pound body weight. The established effective dose should be administered once or twice daily. The daily schedule of administration can be timed to control the period of micturition for the convenience of the client or veterinarian. Mobilization of the edema may be most efficiently and safely accomplished by utilizing an intermittent daily dosage schedule, i.e., every other day or 2 to 4 consecutive days weekly.

Diuretic therapy should be discontinued after reduction of the edema, or maintained after determining a carefully programmed dosage schedule to prevent recurrence of edema. For long-term treatment, the dose can generally be lowered after the edema has once been reduced. Re-examination and consultations with client will enhance the establishment of a satisfactorily programmed dosage schedule. Clinical examination and serum BUN, CO_2 and electrolyte determinations should be performed during the early period of therapy and periodically thereafter, especially in refractory cases. Abnormalities should be corrected or the drug temporarily withdrawn.

Dosage: Parenteral:

Horse: The individual dose is 250 to 500 mg (5 to 10 mL) administered intramuscularly or intravenously once or twice daily at 6- to 8-hour intervals until desired results are achieved. The veterinarian should evaluate the degree of edema present and adjust dosage schedule accordingly.

Cattle: The individual dose administered intramuscularly or intravenously is 500 mg (10 mL) once a day or 250 g (5 mL) twice daily at 12-hour intervals. Treatment not to exceed 48 hours postparturition.

Contraindication(s): FUROSEMIDE INJECTION 5% is a highly effective diuretic-saluretic which if given in excessive amounts may result in dehydration and electrolyte imbalance. Therefore, the dosage and schedule may have to be adjusted to the patient's needs. The animal should be observed for early signs of electrolyte imbalance, and corrective measures administered. Early signs of electrolyte imbalance are: increased thirst, lethargy, drowsiness or restlessness, fatigue, oliguria, gastro-intestinal disturbances and tachycardia. Special attention should be given to potassium levels. FUROSEMIDE INJECTION 5% may lower serum calcium levels and cause tetany in rare cases of animals having an existing hypocalcemic tendency.

Although diabetes mellitus is a rarely reported disease in animals, active or latent diabetes mellitus may on rare occasions be exacerbated by FUROSEMIDE INJECTION 5%. While it has not been reported in animals the use of high doses of salicylates, as in rheumatic diseases, in conjunction with FUROSEMIDE INJECTION 5% may result in salicylate toxicity because of competition for renal excretory sites.

Transient loss of auditory capacity has been experimentally produced in cats following intravenous injection of excessive doses of FUROSEMIDE INJECTION 5% at a very rapid rate.

Electrolyte balance should be monitored prior to surgery in patients receiving FUROSEMIDE INJECTION 5%. Imbalances must be corrected by administration of suitable fluid therapy.

FUROSEMIDE INJECTION 5% is contraindicated in anuria. Therapy should be discontinued in cases of progressive renal disease if increasing azotemia and oliguria occur during the treatment. Sudden alterations of fluid and electrolyte imbalance in an animal with cirrhosis may precipitate hepatic coma, therefore observation during period of therapy is necessary. In hepatic coma and in states of electrolyte depletion, therapy should not be instituted until the basic condition is improved or corrected. Potassium supplementation may be necessary in cases routinely treated with potassium-depleting steroids.

Precaution(s): Store between 15°C and 30°C (59°-86°F).

Caution(s): Federal law restricts this drug to use by or on the order of a licensed veterinarian.

FUROSEMIDE INJECTION 5% is a highly effective diuretic and if given in excessive amounts as with any diuretic may lead to excessive diuresis which could result in electrolyte imbalance, dehydration and reduction of plasma volume enhancing the risk of circulatory collapse, thrombosis, and embolism. Therefore, the animal should be observed for early signs of fluid depletion with electrolyte imbalance, and corrective measures administered. Excessive loss of potassium in patients receiving digitalis or its glycosides may precipitate digitalis toxicity. Caution should be exercised in animals administered potassium-depleting steroids.

It is important to correct potassium deficiency with dietary supplementation. Caution should be exercised in prescribing enteric-coated potassium tablets.

There have been several reports in human literature, published and unpublished, concerning nonspecific small-bowel lesions consisting of stenosis, with or without ulceration, associated with the administration of enteric-coated thiazides with potassium salts. These lesions may occur with enteric-coated potassium tablets alone or when they are used with nonenteric-coated thiazides, or certain other oral diuretics. These small-bowel lesions may have caused obstruction, hemorrhage, and perforation. Surgery was frequently required, and deaths have occurred. Available information tends to implicate enteric-coated potassium salts, although lesions of this type also occur spontaneously. Therefore, coated potassium-containing formulations should be administered only when indicated and should be discontinued immediately if abdominal pain, distension, nausea, vomiting, or gastro-intestinal bleeding occurs.

Human patients with known sulfonamide sensitivity may show allergic reactions to FUROSEMIDE INJECTION 5%, however, these reactions have not been reported in animals.

Sulfonamide diuretics have been reported to decrease arterial responsiveness to pressor amines and to enhance the effect of tubocurarine. Caution should be exercised in administering curare or its derivatives to patients undergoing therapy with FUROSEMIDE INJECTION 5% and it is advisable to discontinue FUROSEMIDE INJECTION 5% for one day prior to any elective surgery.

For animal use only.

Warning(s):

Cattle: Milk taken from animals during treatment and for 48 hours (four milkings) after the last treatment must not be used for food. Cattle must not be slaughtered for food within 48 hours following the last treatment.

Horses: Do not use in horses intended for food.

Keep out of reach of children.

Toxicology: Acute Toxicity: The following table illustrates low acute toxicity of FUROSEMIDE INJECTION 5% in three different species. (Two values indicate two different studies.)

LD50 of FUROSEMIDE INJECTION 5% in mg/kg body weight:

Species	Oral	Intravenous
Mouse	1050-1500	308
Rat	2650-4600*	680
Dog	>1000 and >4640	>300 and >464

*Note: The lower value for the rat oral LD50 was obtained in a group of fasted animals; the higher figure is from a study performed in fed rats.

Toxic doses lead to convulsions, ataxia, paralysis and collapse. Animals surviving toxic dosages may become dehydrated and depleted of electrolytes due to the massive diuresis and saluresis.

Chronic Toxicity: Chronic toxicity studies with FUROSEMIDE INJECTION 5% were done in a one-year study in rats and dogs. In a one-year study in rats, renal tubular degeneration occurred with all doses higher than 50 mg/kg. A six-month study in dogs revealed calcification and scarring of the renal parenchyma at all doses above 10 mg/kg.

Reproductive Studies: Reproductive studies were conducted in mice, rats and rabbits. Only in rabbits administered high doses (equivalent to 10 to 25 times the recommended average dose of 2 mg/kg for dogs, cats, horses, and cattle) of furosemide during the second trimester period did unexplained maternal deaths and abortions occur. The administration of FUROSEMIDE INJECTION 5% is not recommended during the second trimester of pregnancy.

Presentation: Available in 100 mL multi dose vials for horses and cattle (NDC 57319-471-05).

Manufactured by: Phoenix Scientific, Inc., St. Joseph, MO 64503

Compendium Code No.: 12560341 Iss. 12-01

FUROSEMIDE TABLETS ℞

Butler **Diuretic**

NADA No.: 131-806

Active Ingredient(s): Each tablet contains:

Furosemide .... 12.5 mg or 50.0 mg

Indications: A diuretic-saluretic for oral use in the treatment of edema (pulmonary congestion, ascites) associated with cardiac insufficiency and acute noninflammatory tissue edema in dogs.

Dosage and Administration: One (1) 12.5 mg scored tablet per 5 to 10 lbs. of body weight or one (1) 50 mg scored tablet per 25 to 50 lbs. of body weight. Administer once or twice a day at 6- to 8-hour intervals. The dose may be doubled or increased by increments of 1 mg per pound of body weight in refractory or severe edema cases.

Contraindication(s): Because animal reproductive studies have shown that furosemide may cause fetal abnormality, the drug is contraindicated in pregnant animals.

Precaution(s): Store at a controlled room temperature 15°-30°C (59°-86°F).

Caution(s): Federal law restricts this drug to use by or on the order of a licensed veterinarian.

Keep out of the reach of children.

Presentation: Bottles of 100 and 500 tablets.

Compendium Code No.: 10820790

FUROSEMIDE TABLETS ℞

Vedco **Diuretic**

A diuretic saluretic for relief of edema.

NADA No.: 129-034

Active Ingredient(s): Each tablet contains 12.5 mg or 50.0 mg furosemide: 4-chloro-N-furfuryl-5-sulfamoylanthranilic acid.

Indications: Dogs - FUROSEMIDE is an effective diuretic-saluretic for oral use in the treatment of edema (pulmonary congestion, ascites) associated with cardiac insufficiency and acute noninflammatory tissue edema.

Dosage and Administration: Dogs: One 12.5 mg tablet per 5 to 10 pounds body weight; one 50 mg scored tablet per 25 to 50 pounds body weight. Administer once or twice daily at 6-8-hour intervals. The dosage may be doubled or increased by increments of 1 mg per pound of body weight in refractory or severe edematous cases.

Contraindication(s): Because animal reproductive studies have shown that furosemide may cause fetal abnormality, the drug is contraindicated in pregnant animals.

Precaution(s): Store at controlled room temperature (59°-86°F).

Caution(s): Federal law restricts this drug to use by or on the order of a licensed veterinarian.

For use in dogs only.

Keep out of reach of children.

Warning(s): FUROSEMIDE is a highly effective diuretic and if given in excessive amounts as with any diuretic may lead to excessive diuresis which could result in electrolyte imbalance, dehydration and reduction of plasma volume enhancing the risk of circulatory collapse, thrombosis and embolism. Observe animal for early signs of fluid depletion with electrolyte imbalance and if necessary take corrective action. The concurrent use of furosemide with some antibiotics may be inadvisable. There is evidence that the drug enhances the nephrotoxic potential of aminoglycosides, cephalosporins, and polymyxins and increases the ototoxic effects of aminoglycosides. Not for animals intended for food.

Presentation: 12.5 mg - Bottles of 100 and 500 tablets.
50.0 mg - Bottles of 100 and 500 tablets.

Compendium Code No.: 10940980

FUROTABS ℞

Vetus **Diuretic**

NDC No.: 47611-252-01/47611-252-05/47611-253-01/47611-253-05

Active Ingredient(s): Each tablet contains:

Furosemide .... 12.5 mg or 50 mg

Indications: Furosemide is indicated for use in dogs for the treatment of edema (pulmonary congestion, ascites) associated with cardiac insufficiency and acute noninflammatory tissue edema. In cases of edema involving cardiac insufficiency, the continued use of heart stimulants such as digitalis or its glycosides is indicated. The rationale for the efficacious use of diuretic therapy is determined by the clinical pathology producing the edema.

Pharmacology: Furosemide is a loop diuretic derivative of anthranillic acid. The chemical name is 4-chloro-N-furfuryl-5-sulfamoylanthranilic acid. Furosemide is pharmacodynamically characterized by the following:

1. It is administered orally. It is absorbed from the intestinal tract and begins to act in 30 to 60 minutes after oral administration.
2. Is a loop diuretic which inhibits the re-absorption of sodium and chloride at the ascending loop of Henle in the kidneys, enhancing water excretion.
3. A dose-response relationship and a ratio of a minimum to maximum effective dose range that is greater than tenfold.
4. A high degree of efficacy, low inherent toxicity and a high therapeutic index.

The therapeutic efficacy of furosemide is from the activity of the intact and unaltered molecule throughout the nephron, inhibiting the re-absorption of sodium not only in the proximal and distal tubule but also in the ascending limb of the loop of Henle. The prompt onset of action is a result of the drug's rapid absorption and a poor lipid solubility. The low lipid solubility and a rapid renal excretion minimize the possibility of its accumulation in tissues and organs or crystalluria.

Furosemide does not have an inhibitory effect on carbonic anhydrase or aldosterone activity in the distal tubule. The drug possesses diuretic activity in the presence of acidosis or alkalosis.

Dosage and Administration: The usual oral dose of furosemide is 1-2 mg/lb. of body weight (approximately 2.5-5 mg/kg). A prompt diuresis usually ensues from the initial treatment.

Administer orally once or twice a day at six (6) to eight (8) hour intervals. The dose should be adjusted to the individual's response. In severe edematous or refractory cases, the dose may be doubled or increased by increments of 1.0 mg per lb. of body weight. The established effective dose should be administered once or twice a day.

The daily schedule of administration can be timed to control the period of micturition for the convenience of the client or veterinarian.

Mobilization of the edema may be efficiently and safely accomplished by utilizing an intermittent daily dose schedule, every other day or two (2) to four (4) consecutive days a week.

Diuretic therapy should be discontinued after reduction of the edema, or maintained after determining a carefully programmed dosage schedule to prevent recurrence of the edema. For long-term treatment, the dose can be lowered after the edema has been reduced. Re-examination and consultations with the client will enhance the establishment of a satisfactory programmed dosage schedule. Clinical examination and serum BUN, CO_2 and electrolyte determinations should be performed during the early period of therapy and periodically thereafter, especially in refractory cases. Abnormalities should be corrected or the drug temporarily withdrawn.

Dogs: Give one-half (½) to one (1) 50 mg scored tablet per 25 lbs. of body weight, or one (1) 12.5 mg tablet per 5-10 lbs. of body weight.

Administer once or twice a day, permitting a six (6) to eight (8) hour interval between treatments.

In refractory or severe edematous cases, the dose may be doubled or increased by increments of 1 mg per lb. of body weight.

Contraindication(s): Animal reproductive studies have shown that furosemide may cause fetal abnormality and use of the drug is contraindicated in pregnant animals.

Furosemide is contraindicated in anuria, furosemide hypersensitivity, hepatic coma, or during electrolytic imbalances. Monitor serum electrolytes, BUN and CO_2 frequently. Monitor serum potassium levels and watch for signs of hypocalcemia. Corticosteroids cause an additive potassium-depletion effect.

Caution(s): Federal law restricts this drug to use by or on the order of a licensed veterinarian.

For use in dogs only.

Furosemide is a highly effective diuretic-saluretic which, if given in excessive amounts, may result in dehydration and have to be adjusted to the patient's needs. The animal should be observed for early signs of electrolyte imbalance, and corrective measures administered. Early signs of electrolyte imbalance are increased thirst, lethargy, drowsiness or restlessness, fatigue, oliguria, gastrointestinal disturbances and tachycardia. Special attention should be given to potassium levels. Furosemide may lower serum calcium levels and cause tetany in rare cases of animals having an existing hypocalcemic tendency.

Furosemide is contraindicated in anuria. Therapy should be discontinued in case of progressive renal disease if increasing azotemia and oliguria occur during the treatment. Sudden alterations of fluid and electrolyte imbalance in an animal with cirrhosis may precipitate hepatic coma, therefore observation during the period of therapy is necessary. In hepatic coma and in states of electrolyte depletion, therapy should not be instituted until the basic condition is improved or corrected.

Potassium supplementation may be necessary in cases routinely treated with potassium-depleting steroids. Active or latent diabetes may, on rare occasions, be exacerbated by furosemide.

A transient loss of auditory capacity has been experimentally produced in cats following intravenous injections of excessive doses of furosemide at a rapid rate.

Furosemide is a highly effective diuretic and, if given in excessive amounts, as with any diuretic, may lead to excessive diuresis which could result in electrolyte imbalance, dehydration and a reduction of plasma volume, enhancing the risk of circulatory collapse, thrombosis and embolism. Therefore, the animal should be observed for early signs of fluid depletion with electrolyte imbalance, and corrective measures administered.

Excessive loss of potassium in patients receiving digitalis or its glycosides may precipitate digitalis toxicity. Caution should be exercised in animals administered potassium-depleting steroids.

Correct potassium deficiency with a proper dietary supplementation. If the animal needs potassium supplements, use an oral liquid form, do not use enteric-coated potassium tablets.

The concurrent use of furosemide with some antibiotics may be inadvisable. There is evidence that the drug enhances the nephrotoxic potential of aminoglycosides, cephalosporins and polymyxins and increases the ototoxic effects of aminoglycosides.

Sulfonamide diuretics have been reported to decrease arterial responsiveness to pressor amines and to enhance the effect of tubocurarine. Caution should be exercised in administering curare or its derivatives to patients undergoing therapy with furosemide, and it is advisable to discontinue furosemide for one day prior to elective surgery.

Toxicology: Furosemide demonstrates a low order of either acute or chronic toxicity. The drug is rapidly absorbed and excreted by both glomerular filtration and tubular secretion. Due to the high rates of excretion, the cumulation of furosemide does not occur despite repeated administrations.

The main effect observed in clinical toxicity is an abnormality of fluid and electrolyte imbalances. Ototoxicity resulting in a transient loss of hearing has been reported with furosemide.

A safety study was performed in dogs to determine the effects of FUROTABS at increasing doses and time elements. The dose levels were 2 mg/lb. of body weight (upper recommended dose), 6 mg/lb. of body weight (3X upper recommended dose) and 10 mg/lb. of body weight (5X upper recommended dose). The treatment period ranged up to nine days. The results demonstrated a mild dehydration at the 5X level with a slight elevation of hemoglobin and dosage groups. Cumulative evaluation of the data demonstrates that FUROTABS are safe when administered at the upper level of the recommended dose for a duration of nine consecutive days.

Presentation: Bottles of 100 and 500 tablets.

Compendium Code No.: 14440370

FUSION® 4

Merial **Vaccine**

Bovine Rhinotracheitis-Virus Diarrhea-Parainfluenza 3-Respiratory Syncytial Virus Vaccine, Modified Live & Killed Virus

U.S. Vet. Lic. No.: 298

Contents: FUSION® 4 contains modified-live and killed forms of the IBR virus as well as modified-live PI3 and killed BVD and BRSV.

Contains gentamicin and a fungistat as preservatives.

Indications: For the vaccination of healthy cattle against infectious bovine rhinotracheitis, bovine virus diarrhea, parainfluenza 3, and respiratory syncytial virus.

Dosage and Administration: Aseptically rehydrate the lyophilized vaccine with the accompanying liquid diluent and inject 2 mL (1 dose) intramuscularly; for primary vaccination, revaccinate with a second 2 mL dose 2 to 4 weeks later. Calves vaccinated under 3 months of age should be revaccinated at 4 to 6 months or weaning. Revaccinate with a single 2 mL dose annually or prior to the time of stress or exposure.

Precaution(s): Store at 2-7°C (35-45°F). Use entire contents when first opened. Burn this container and all unused contents.

Caution(s): In case of anaphylaxis, administer epinephrine.

Warning(s): Do not vaccinate pregnant cows or calves nursing pregnant cows.

Do not vaccinate within 21 days of slaughter.

Presentation: 10 dose (20 mL) and 50 dose (100 mL) vials.

® FUSION is a registered trademark of Merial.

Compendium Code No.: 11110191 RM171RM5 / RM175RM5

FUSOGARD™

Novartis Animal Vaccines **Bacterin**

Fusobacterium Necrophorum Bacterin

U.S. Vet. Lic. No.: 303

Contents: Contains chemically inactivated culture of *Fusobacterium necrophorum* and SuprImm® adjuvant.

Indications: For the vaccination of healthy cattle six months of age or older as an aid in the reduction of clinical signs of footrot and the number and size of liver abscesses caused by *Fusobacterium necrophorum.*

Dosage and Administration: For footrot, inject 2 mL subcutaneously with a second dose 21 days later. For liver abscesses, inject 2 mL subcutaneously with a second dose 60 days later.

Precaution(s): Refrigerate at 2-7°C. Shake thoroughly before use. Use entire contents when first opened.

Caution(s): In case of anaphylactoid reaction, administer epinephrine.

For veterinary use only.

Warning(s): Do not vaccinate within 60 days of slaughter.

Presentation: 10 dose (20 mL), 50 dose (100 mL), 125 dose (250 mL), and 300 dose (600 mL) bottles.

Compendium Code No.: 11140710

FUS-SOL™ DROPS

PPI **Urinary Acidifier**

Active Ingredient(s): Each 0.5 mL contains: 100 mg of Ammonium Chloride, in aqueous solution with dl-Methionine and multiple B-complex vitamins and flavors. pH balanced, flavored.

Indications: Oral urinary acidifier for dogs and cats.

Dosage and Administration: Dosage for dogs and cats: Administer 0.5 mL per 10 lb. of bodyweight, twice a day. Or at a dosage schedule recommended by the veterinarian.

Administer orally directly from dropper or mix into a small amount of food.

Caution(s): Keep this and all other medications out of the reach of children.

Presentation: 60 mL bottle with convenient calibrated dropper.

Distributed by: The Triton Group, St. Louis, MO 63103, U.S.A.

Compendium Code No.: 12270020

F VAX-MG®

Schering-Plough **Vaccine**

Mycoplasma gallisepticum Vaccine, Live Culture, Avian Isolate

U.S. Vet. Lic. No.: 165A

Contents: Live vaccine containing the F strain of *Mycoplasma gallisepticum* in a freeze-dried preparation sealed under vacuum. Preservative: Penicillin.

Indications: It is recommended for use in healthy chickens 9 weeks of age or older by spray administration to aid in the prevention of clinical signs associated with *Mycoplasma gallisepticum* infection.

Dosage and Administration: F VAX-MG® should be administered to birds 9 weeks of age or older prior to field exposure and prior to the onset of egg production.

Preparation of the Vaccine:

Do not open and mix the vaccine until ready for use.

Mix only one vial at a time and use the entire contents within one hour.

Remove the tear-off aluminum seal from the vaccine vial without disturbing the rubber stopper.

Use cool, clean, non-chlorinated drinking water to which evaporated milk has been added at a rate of one ounce per quart (30 mL per liter).

Holding the vial submerged in water, lift the lip of the rubber stopper so that the water is sucked into the vial.

Reseat the stopper and shake to thoroughly dissolve the vaccine. The vaccine is now ready for use.

Proper spray application of the vaccine is accomplished only through the use of a clean sprayer emitting a coarse spray. Use the spray method only in houses that can be closed during vaccination and for at least 15 minutes thereafter. Cross winds, drafts, or operation ventilation fans may prevent effective application.

After rehydrating the vaccine, further dilute each 1000 doses to 100 mL using the water with milk. Place the vaccine in a sprayer container. Spray droplets of 40-50 microns (coarse) average size are desirable.

Apply the vaccine over all birds at the rate of one dose per square foot, or one dose per bird, whichever is greater.

Records: Keep a record of the vaccine type, quantity, serial number, expiration date and place of purchase; the date and time of vaccination; the number, age, breed, and location of the birds, names of operators performing the vaccination; and any observed reactions.

Contraindication(s): F VAX-MG® should not be administered within 1 week before or after vaccination with live Newcastle, bronchitis, or laryngotracheitis vaccines, or within 3 days before to 7 days after treatment with oxytetracycline or chlortetracycline.

Precaution(s): Store at 35°-45°F (2°-7°C). Do not freeze.

Do not dilute the vaccine or otherwise stretch the dosage.

Do not spill or spatter the vaccine. Use the entire contents of the vial when first opened. Burn the empty bottles, caps and all unused vaccine and accessories.

Caution(s): Use only in states where permitted.

Vaccinate healthy birds only. To avoid interference with the development of protection, chickens to be vaccinated should not be given oxytetracycline or chlortetracycline and/or sulfonamide medication for 3 days before and 7 days after vaccination.

All birds within a flock should be vaccinated on the same day. Isolate other susceptible birds on the premises from the birds being vaccinated.

Mycoplasma gallisepticum F strain is known to produce clinical disease in turkeys. Do not allow turkeys to come in contact with the vaccine or vaccinated chickens.

For veterinary use only.

Warning(s): Do not vaccinate within 21 days before slaughter.

Wash hands thoroughly after using the vaccine.

Presentation: 1000 dose vials.

Compendium Code No.: 10470701

F

FVR® C-P VACCINE

Schering-Plough **Vaccine**

Feline Rhinotracheitis-Calici-Panleukopenia Vaccine, Modified Live and Killed Virus

U.S. Vet. Lic. No.: 264

Active Ingredient(s): The feline rhinotracheitis-calici component is a lyophilized suspension of modified live virus propagated in a stable cell line of feline origin and backfilled with an inert gas. The panleukopenia vaccine is propagated in a stable cell line of feline origin, and has been chemically inactivated and processed to be nonviricidal when used as a diluent to rehydrate the feline rhinotracheitis-calici vaccine. The safety and immunogenicity of each virus strain have been demonstrated by vaccination and challenge tests in healthy susceptible cats. Contains neomycin, polymyxin B, and a fungistat as preservatives.

Indications: For the immunization of healthy cats of any age against disease caused by feline rhinotracheitis, feline calici and feline panleukopenia viruses.

Dosage and Administration: Aseptically rehydrate the vaccine with the accompanying diluent (feline panleukopenia vaccine) and vaccinate intramuscularly or subcutaneously. Administer two (2) 1 mL doses three (3) to (4) four weeks apart to healthy cats of any age, but if the animal is less than 12 weeks of age, it should be revaccinated at 3- to 4-week intervals until it is 12 to 16 weeks of age. Annual revaccination with a single dose is recommended.

Precaution(s): Store at 35°-45°F (2°-7°C).

Caution(s): Use the entire contents when first opened. Do not use chemicals to sterilize syringes and needles. Burn the container and all unused contents. It is generally recommended to avoid the vaccination of pregnant cats. In case of an anaphylactic reaction, administer epinephrine.

The product is tested before release for sale and meets all tests required by the United States government as well as the laboratories of Pitman-Moore, Inc.

For veterinary use only.

Presentation: 25 x 1 dose vials.

* ® Registered trademark of Schering-Plough Animal Health Corporation.

Compendium Code No.: 10470780

FVR® C VACCINE

Schering-Plough **Vaccine**

Feline Rhinotracheitis-Calici Vaccine, Modified Live Virus

U.S. Vet. Lic. No.: 165A

Contents: This product contains the antigens listed above.

Contains gentamicin as a preservative.

Indications: FVR® C vaccine is a modified live virus vaccine for the vaccination of healthy cats 8 to 9 weeks of age or older against diseases caused by feline rhinotracheitis and calici viruses.

Dosage and Administration: Inject one dose (1 mL) subcutaneously or intramuscularly at 8 to 9 weeks of age or older and repeat with a second dose 3 to 4 weeks later. If the animal is less than 12 weeks of age, it should be revaccinated every three to four weeks until 12 to 16 weeks of age.

Annual revaccination with one dose is recommended.

Transfer the contents of the diluent vial to the FVR® C vial aseptically. Use entire contents immediately after rehydration.

Contraindication(s): Do not vaccinate pregnant cats.

Precaution(s): Store between 2° and 7°C. Do not freeze. Do not chemically sterilize needles and syringes. Do not mix with other vaccines. Burn vaccine container and all unused contents.

Caution(s): The use of a biological product may produce anaphylaxis and/or other inflammatory immune-mediated hypersensitivity reactions.

Some reports suggest that in cats, the administration of certain veterinary biologicals may induce the development of injection-site fibrosarcomas.

For veterinary use only.

Antidote(s): Epinephrine, corticosteroids, and antihistamines may all be indicated depending on the nature and severity of the reaction.

Presentation: 25 x 1 dose vials (NDC 0061-5285-01).

Compendium Code No.: 10472180 P18706-10

F

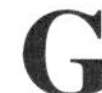

GAINPRO®-10

Intervet **Feed Additive**

Bambermycins-Type A Medicated Article

NADA No.: 141-034

Active Ingredient(s): Bambermycins 10 grams per pound (22 grams per kilogram).

Ingredients: Roughage products and/or calcium carbonate, dried bambermycins fermentation product, mineral oil.

Indications: For increased rate of weight gain and improved feed efficiency in cattle fed in confinement for slaughter. For increased rate of weight gain in pasture cattle (slaughter, stocker and feeder cattle, and dairy and beef replacement heifers) when fed daily in at least one pound and not more than 10 pounds of supplemental feed.

Claims: Permitted Claims and Limitations:

Species	Drug	Level	Claim(s)	Limitations
Cattle Fed in Confinement for Slaughter*	Bambermycins	10 to 20 mg/hd/day**	Increased rate of weight gain, improved feed efficiency	None
Pasture Cattle*	Bambermycins	10 to 20 mg/hd/day***	Increased rate of weight gain	None

*Only a single level of bambermycins (i.e. 2 grams bambermycins/ton) can be indicated on a feed tag. A different tag must be submitted for each level of bambermycins needed for your complete feeding program.

Dosage and Administration:

Cattle Fed in Confinement for Slaughter: **The approved dosage in cattle fed in confinement for slaughter is 10 to 20 mg of bambermycins/hd/day. The amount of bambermycins will range between 1 and 4 grams per ton of feed depending upon the daily feed consumption of the cattle fed in confinement for slaughter. The amount of Type A Medicated Article added to the complete ration (Type C Medicated Feed) must be based on daily feed consumption, the number of animals in the pen and the level (10-20 mg/hd/day) of bambermycins being fed. From this information the grams of bambermycins per ton of feed can be calculated in order to fulfill feed assay requirements. No Type C Medicated Feed should be manufactured with less than 1 g bambermycins/ton. Feed assays for bambermycins with expected levels below 1 g/t may not be accurate. See the following table for conversions from mg/head/day to g/t.

Example of Converting the Bambermycins Cattle Dosage from mg/head/day to grams/ton*:

Cattle Weight		Average Feed Consumption/Head/Day	Grams Bambermycins/Ton of Feed		Mg Bambermycins Fed Daily to each Animal	
Lbs	kg	Lbs[1]	Low	High	Low	High
400	181.4	10.0	2.00	4.00	10.0	20.0
500	226.8	14.0	1.50	2.80	10.5	19.6
600	272.2	17.0	1.25	2.30	10.6	19.6
700	317.5	20.0	1.00	2.00	10.0	20.0
800	362.9	22.0	1.00	1.80	11.0	19.8
900	406.2	23.0	1.00	1.70	11.5	19.6
1000	453.6	24.0	1.00	1.60	12.0	19.2
1100	499.0	25.0	1.00	1.60	12.5	20.0
1200	544.3	26.0	1.00	1.50	13.0	19.5
1300	589.7	27.0	1.00	1.40	13.5	18.9

*Dosage range is 10 to 20 mg/head/day consumption and average daily gain of 2.0 to 3.0 lbs/day

[1]Assumes as fed *ad libitum*

Example Calculation - Amount of GAINPRO®-10 premix added to feed for a pen of cattle.

Given: Average Weight - 800 lbs; Number in pen - 100 hd; Dosage - 20 mg/hd/day; Daily Feed Consumption - 22 lbs/day.

- 100 hd x 20 mg = 2,000 mg or 2 grams bambermycins.
- GAINPRO®-10 contains 10 grams bambermycins/lb, therefore add 0.2 pounds of GAINPRO®-10 premix to the daily feed for this pen of 100 animals.
- 22 lbs/day x 100 hd = 2,200 lbs total feed consumption.
- 2 grams bambermycins ÷ 2,200 lbs = .000909 g/lb.
- .000909 x 2,000 lbs = 1.82 g bambermycins/ton of feed.

Mixing Directions: It is recommended that GAINPRO®-10 be diluted with a suitable grain carrier before addition to the final feed. A dilution of 1 part of GAINPRO®-10 and 9 parts grain carrier is the suggested working premix. The table below shows premix and working premix addition levels for various commonly used feeds.

Feed	Bambermycins Level	Pounds Premix To Be Added Per Ton	
		GAINPRO® 10	1-9 Working Premix
Cattle Fed in Confinement for Slaughter	1 gram/ton	0.1	1
	2 grams/ton	0.2	2
	3 grams/ton	0.3	3
	4 grams/ton	0.4	4

Thoroughly mix both working premix and finished feed to ensure complete and uniform distribution of the GAINPRO®-10.

Feeding Directions: Feeds containing GAINPRO®-10 should be fed continuously in a complete feed. Complete feed for cattle fed in confinement for slaughter must be fed continuously at a rate of 10-20 mg bambermycins/hd/day from Type C Medicated Feed containing 1-4 g bambermycins/ton.

Type B Liquid Feeds Intended for Addition to Dry Feeds for Confinement Cattle:

- Type B Liquid Feeds should be in a pH range of 3.8 to 7.5 and should have a moisture content between 30 and 45%.
- Type B Liquid Feeds must be mixed into the dry feed within 8 weeks of manufacture.
- Type B Liquid Feeds can be manufactured containing 40.0 to 800.0 g of bambermycins/ton.

Mixing directions into dry feed are as follows: Before feeding, the Type B Medicated Liquid feed must be thoroughly mixed with other feed materials to make a complete feed (Type C Medicated Feed).

Examples of addition rates to complete feeds are shown in the following table.

Bambermycins (g/ton) in Type B Liquid Feed	Addition Rate of Type B Liquid Feed (pounds/ton) to Complete Feed	Bambermycins (g/ton) in Final Complete Feed (Type C Medicated Feed)
40.0	50.0	1.0
40.0	200.0	4.0
100.0	20.0	1.0
100.0	80.0	4.0
400.0	5.0	1.0
400.0	20.0	4.0
800.0	2.5	1.0
800.0	10.0	4.0

The complete dry feed (Type C Medicated Feed) may only be fed to cattle in confinement for slaughter and must be fed within one week after mixing.

Pasture Cattle: ***The approved dosage in pasture cattle is 10 to 20 mg of bambermycins/hd/day. Blend 0.2 pounds of GAINPRO®-10 with 999.8 pounds of suitable grain carrier. This supplemental feed will contain 2 mg bambermycins per pound (4 g/ton). This supplemental feed can be fed at a rate of 5 to 10 pounds per head per day to achieve a daily intake of 10 to 20 mg bambermycins/head/day. See the following table for additional examples of conversion from mg/hd/day to g/t.

Mixing Directions: It is recommended that GAINPRO®-10 be diluted with a suitable grain carrier to provide a supplemental feed. The table below shows examples of premix addition levels.

Feed	Bambermycins Level	Pounds GAINPRO®-10g To Be Added Per Ton	Feeding Rate
Pasture Cattle	2 grams/ton	0.2	10.0 lb/hd/day
	4 grams/ton	0.4	5.0-10.0 lb/hd/day
	8 grams/ton	0.8	2.5-5.0 lb/hd/day
	20 grams/ton	2.0	1.0-2.0 lb/hd/day
	40 grams/ton	4.0	1.0 lb/hd/day

Thoroughly mix both working premix and supplemental feed to ensure complete and uniform distribution of the GAINPRO®-10.

Feeding Directions: Feed for Pasture Cattle must be fed continuously at a rate of 10-20 mg bambermycins/hd/day in at least one pound and not more than 10 pounds of Type C Medicated Feed containing 2-40 g bambermycins/ton.

Free-Choice (Self-Fed) Supplement: Free-choice supplements must be formulated to provide not less than 10 mg nor more than 20 mg bambermycins per head per day. (Only a licensed feed mill may manufacture medicated self-fed supplements according to an FDA approved formula.)

Caution(s): For use in manufactured feeds only.

Presentation: 50 lb (22.68 kg).

Compendium Code No.: 11060641

G

GALAXY® Cv

Schering-Plough **Vaccine**

Canine Coronavirus Vaccine, Killed Virus

U.S. Vet. Lic. No.: 165A

Contents: GALAXY® Cv (feline enteric coronavirus) is a killed virus vaccine.

Viral antigens have been chemically inactivated and combined with an adjuvant designed to enhance the immune response.

Contains gentamicin as a preservative.

Indications: GALAXY® Cv is recommended for the vaccination of healthy dogs against disease caused by canine coronavirus infection.

Dosage and Administration: Inject one dose (1 mL) subcutaneously or intramuscularly. The initial dose may be given at 6 weeks of age. A second dose is given 2 to 4 weeks later. A minimum of two doses are required for primary immunization. Annual revaccination with one dose is recommended. Use entire contents immediately.

Contraindication(s): Do not vaccinate pregnant bitches.

Precaution(s): Store between 2° and 7°C. Do not freeze.

Use new, non-chemically sterilized, needles and syringes.

Do not mix with other vaccines.

Burn vaccine container and all unused contents.

Caution(s): Vaccinate only healthy, non-parasitized dogs.

The use of a biological product may produce anaphylaxis and/or other inflammatory immune-mediated hypersensitivity reactions.

Antidote(s): Epinephrine, corticosteroids, and antihistamines may all be indicated depending on the nature and severity of the reaction.

Warning(s): For use in dogs only.

For veterinary use only.

Presentation: 25 x 1 dose vials of GALAXY® Cv.

Patent Pending (feline enteric coronavirus)

Compendium Code No.: 10470801 P23002-10

GALAXY® D

Schering-Plough **Vaccine**

Canine Distemper Vaccine, Modified Live Virus

U.S. Vet. Lic. No.: 195

Active Ingredient(s): Canine distemper vaccine, modified live virus.

The vaccine contains gentamicin as a preservative.

Indications: For use in the vaccination of healthy dogs nine weeks of age or older against canine distemper.

Dosage and Administration: Transfer the contents of the sterile diluent vial to the GALAXY® D vial aseptically. Mix gently until dissolved. Use the entire contents immediately after rehydration.

Inject one (1) dose (1 mL) subcutaneously or intramuscularly and repeat at two (2) to three (3) week intervals until the dog is 18 weeks of age. A minimum of two (2) doses are required for primary immunization.

Annual revaccination with one (1) dose is recommended.

Precaution(s): Store between 2° and 7°C.

Caution(s):

1. Do not chemically sterilize needles and syringes.
2. Do not mix with other vaccines.

3. The use of any biologic may produce an anaphylactic reaction.
4. Burn the vaccine container and all the unused contents. Dispose of all the contents in a proper manner.
5. For use in dogs only.
6. For veterinary use only.

Antidote(s): Epinephrine.
Presentation: 25 - 1 dose vials of GALAXY® D, and 25 - 1 dose vials of sterile diluent.
Compendium Code No.: 10470810

GALAXY® DA2PPv

Schering-Plough **Vaccine**

Canine Distemper-Adenovirus Type 2-Parainfluenza-Parvovirus Vaccine, Modified Live Virus

U.S. Vet. Lic. No.: 165A

Contents: Canine distemper, adenovirus type 2, parainfluenza, and parvovirus vaccine, modified live virus.

Contains gentamicin as a preservative.

Indications: GALAXY® DA2PPv is for the vaccination of healthy dogs against diseases caused by canine distemper virus, adenovirus type 1 (hepatitis) and adenovirus type 2 (respiratory disease), canine parainfluenza virus, and canine parvovirus.

Dosage and Administration: Inject one dose (1 mL) subcutaneously or intramuscularly. The initial dose may be given at 6 weeks of age or older. Repeat at 2 to 4 week intervals until the dog is 12 weeks of age. A minimum of two doses is required for primary immunization. Annual revaccination with one dose is recommended.

Transfer contents of the sterile diluent vial to the GALAXY® DA2PPv vial aseptically. Mix gently until dissolved. Use entire contents immediately after rehydration.

Contraindication(s): Do not vaccinate pregnant bitches.

Precaution(s): Store between 2° and 7°C. Do not freeze.

Use new, non-chemically sterilized, needles and syringes.

Do not mix with other vaccines.

Burn vaccine container and all unused contents.

Caution(s): Vaccinate only healthy, non-parasitized dogs.

The use of a biological product may produce anaphylaxis and/or other inflammatory immune-mediated hypersensitivity reactions.

The age at which maternal antibodies for canine parvovirus no longer interferes with the development of active immunity and varies according to the bitch's titer and quantity of colostral antibodies absorbed by the puppy.

Antidote(s): Epinephrine, corticosteroids, and antihistamines may all be indicated depending on the nature and severity of the reaction.

Warning(s): For veterinary use only.

For use in dogs only.

Trial Data: Data indicate the development of corneal opacity is not associated with the use of this product.

Presentation: 25 x 1 dose vials of GALAXY® DA2PPv.
25 x 1 dose vials of sterile diluent.

Patent pending (feline enteric coronavirus)

Compendium Code No.: 10470821 P25001-10

GALAXY® DA2PPv+Cv

Schering-Plough **Vaccine**

Canine Distemper-Adenovirus Type 2-Coronavirus-Parainfluenza-Parvovirus Vaccine, Modified Live and Killed Virus

U.S. Vet. Lic. No.: 195

Contents: Canine distemper, adenovirus type 2, parainfluenza, and parvovirus vaccine modified live virus vaccine combined with feline enteric coronavirus (killed virus vaccine).

Feline enteric coronavirus antigens have been chemically inactivated and combined with an adjuvant designed to enhance the immune response.

Contains gentamicin as a preservative.

Indications: GALAXY® DA2PPv+Cv is a combination vaccine that unites the benefits of Galaxy® DA2PPv and Galaxy® Cv in one vaccination.

Galaxy® DA2PPv is a modified live virus vaccine for the vaccination of healthy dogs against canine distemper, adenovirus type 2, hepatitis, parainfluenza and parvovirus.

Galaxy® Cv (feline enteric coronavirus) is a killed virus vaccine for the vaccination of healthy dogs against disease caused by canine coronavirus infection.

Dosage and Administration: Inject one dose (1 mL) subcutaneously or intramuscularly. The initial dose may be given at 6 weeks of age or older. Repeat at 2 to 4 week intervals until the dog is 12 weeks of age. A minimum of two doses are required for primary immunization. Annual revaccination with one dose is recommended.

Shake the Galaxy® Cv vial and transfer its contents to the Galaxy® DA2PPv vial aseptically. Mix gently until dissolved. Use entire contents immediately after rehydration.

Contraindication(s): Do not vaccinate pregnant bitches.

Precaution(s): Store between 2° and 7°C. Do not freeze.

Use new, non-chemically sterilized, needles and syringes.

Do not mix with other vaccines.

Caution(s): Vaccinate only healthy, non-parasitized dogs.

The age at which maternal antibody for canine parvovirus no longer interferes with the development of the active immunity varies according to the bitch's titer and quantity of colostral antibodies absorbed by the puppy.*

Burn vaccine container and all unused contents.

Antidote(s): The use of a biological may produce anaphylaxis and/or other inflammatory immune-mediated hypersensitivity reactions. Antidote: Epinephrine, corticosteroids, and antihistamines may all be indicated depending on the nature and severity of the reaction.*

Warning(s): For veterinary use only.

For use in dogs only.

Trial Data: Data indicate the development of corneal opacity is not associated with the use of this product.

References: *Available upon request.

Presentation: 25 x 1 dose vials of Galaxy® DA2PPv.
25 x 1 dose vials of Galaxy® Cv.

Compendium Code No.: 10470831

GALAXY® DA2PPvL

Schering-Plough **Bacterin-Vaccine**

Canine Distemper-Adenovirus Type 2-Parainfluenza-Parvovirus Vaccine, Modified Live Virus-Leptospira Bacterin

U.S. Vet. Lic. No.: 165A

Contents: GALAXY® DA2PPvL is a modified live virus vaccine which is combined with inactivated *Leptospira canicola* and *L. icterohaemorrhagiae* bacterin.

Contains gentamicin as a preservative.

Indications: GALAXY® DA2PPvL is for the vaccination of healthy dogs against diseases caused by canine distemper virus, adenovirus type 1 (hepatitis) and adenovirus type 2 (respiratory disease), canine parainfluenza virus, canine parvovirus and leptospirosis.

Dosage and Administration: Inject one dose (1 mL) subcutaneously or intramuscularly. The initial dose may be given at 6 weeks of age or older. Repeat at 2 to 4 week intervals until the dog is 12 weeks of age. A minimum of two doses is required for primary immunization. Annual revaccination with one dose is recommended.

Transfer contents of the sterile diluent vial to the GALAXY® DA2PPvL vial aseptically. Mix gently until dissolved. Use entire contents immediately after rehydration.

Contraindication(s): Do not vaccinate pregnant bitches.

Precaution(s): Store between 2° and 7°C. Do not freeze.

Use new, non-chemically sterilized, needles and syringes.

Do not mix with other vaccines.

Burn vaccine container and all unused contents.

Caution(s): Vaccinate only healthy, non-parasitized dogs.

The use of a biological product may produce anaphylaxis and/or other inflammatory immune-mediated hypersensitivity reactions.

The age at which maternal antibodies for canine parvovirus no longer interferes with the development of active immunity and varies according to the bitch's titer and quantity of colostral antibodies absorbed by the puppy.

Antidote(s): Epinephrine, corticosteroids, and antihistamines may all be indicated depending on the nature and severity of the reaction.

Warning(s): For veterinary use only.

For use in dogs only.

Trial Data: Data indicate the development of corneal opacity is not associated with the use of this product.

Presentation: 25 x 1 dose vials of GALAXY® DA2PPvL.
25 x 1 mL vials of sterile diluent.

Pat. Pending (feline enteric coronavirus)

Compendium Code No.: 10470841 P26001-10

GALAXY® DA2PPvL+Cv

Schering-Plough **Bacterin-Vaccine**

Canine Distemper-Adenovirus Type 2-Coronavirus-Parainfluenza-Parvovirus Vaccine, Modified Live and Killed Virus-Leptospira Bacterin

U.S. Vet. Lic. No.: 165A

Contents: GALAXY® DA2PPvL+Cv is a combination vaccine that unites the benefits of Galaxy® DA2PPvL and Galaxy® Cv in one vaccination.

Galaxy® DA2PPvL is a modified live virus vaccine which is combined with inactivated *Leptospira canicola* and *Leptospira icterohaemorrhagiae* bacterin.

Galaxy® Cv (feline enteric coronavirus) is a killed virus vaccine.

Coronavirus antigen has been chemically inactivated and combined with an adjuvant designed to enhance the immune response.

Contains gentamicin as a preservative.

Indications: Galaxy® DA2PPvL is for the vaccination of healthy dogs against diseases caused by canine distemper virus, adenovirus type 1 (hepatitis) adenovirus type 2 (respiratory disease), canine parainfluenza virus, canine parvovirus and leptospirosis.

Galaxy® Cv is for the vaccination of healthy dogs against disease caused by canine coronavirus infection.

Dosage and Administration: Inject one dose (1 mL) subcutaneously or intramuscularly. The initial dose may be given at 6 weeks of age. Repeat at 2 to 4 week intervals until the dog is 12 weeks of age. A minimum of two doses are required for primary immunization. Annual revaccination with one dose is recommended.

Shake the Galaxy® Cv vial and transfer its contents to the Galaxy® DA2PPvL vial aseptically. Mix gently until dissolved. Use entire contents immediately after rehydration.

Contraindication(s): Do not vaccinate pregnant bitches.

Precaution(s): Store between 2° and 7°C. Do not freeze.

Use new, non-chemically sterilized, needles and syringes.

Do not mix with other vaccines.

Burn vaccine container and all unused contents.

Caution(s): Vaccinate only healthy, non-parasitized dogs.

The use of a biological product may produce anaphylaxis and/or other inflammatory immune-mediated hypersensitivity reactions.

The age at which maternal antibody for canine parvovirus no longer interferes with the development of the active immunity varies according to the bitch's titer and quantity of colostral antibodies absorbed by the puppy.

Antidote(s): Epinephrine, corticosteroids, and antihistamines may all be indicated depending on the nature and severity of the reaction.

Warning(s): For veterinary use only.

For use in dogs only.

Trial Data: Data indicate the development of corneal opacity is not associated with the use of Galaxy® DA2PPvL.

Presentation: 25 x 1 dose vials of Galaxy® DA2PPvL.
25 x 1 dose vials of Galaxy® Cv.

Pat. Pending (feline enteric coronavirus)

Compendium Code No.: 10470851 P28000-10

GALAXY® LYME

Schering-Plough **Bacterin**

Borrelia Burgdorferi Bacterin

U.S. Vet. Lic. No.: 165A

Contents: GALAXY® Lyme is an inactivated bacterin containing two isolates of *Borrelia burgdorferi.*

Contains gentamicin and nystatin as preservatives.

Indications: This bacterin is for the vaccination of healthy dogs against disease caused by *Borrelia burgdorferi.*

Dosage and Administration: Inject one dose (1 mL) intramuscularly.

Dogs require an initial dose at 12 weeks of age or older. A second dose is needed 2 to 4 weeks after the initial vaccination. Two doses are required for primary immunization.

Annual revaccination with one dose is recommended.

Precaution(s): Store between 2° and 7°C.

Do not freeze.

Use new, non-chemically sterilized, needles and syringes.

Do not mix with other vaccines.

Caution(s): The use of a biological product may produce anaphylaxis and/or other inflammatory immune-mediated hypersensitivity reactions.

Antidote(s): Epinephrine, corticosteroids, and antihistamines may all be indicated depending on the nature and severity of the reaction.

Warning(s): For veterinary use only.

For use in dogs only.

Presentation: 25 x 1 dose and 50 x 1 dose vials.

Pat. Pending

Compendium Code No.: 10470861 P24002-10

GALAXY® Pv

Schering-Plough **Vaccine**

Parvovirus Vaccine, Modified Live Virus

U.S. Vet. Lic. No.: 195

Contents: GALAXY® Pv vaccine is a modified live virus containing a CPV Type 2b strain.

Contains gentamicin as a preservative.

Indications: GALAXY® Pv is for the vaccination of healthy dogs against canine parvovirus.

Dosage and Administration: Inject one dose (1 mL) subcutaneously or intramuscularly. The initial dose may be given at 6 weeks of age or older. Repeat at 2 to 4 week intervals until the dog is 12 weeks of age. Annual revaccination with one dose is recommended. Use entire contents immediately.

Contraindication(s): Do not vaccinate pregnant bitches.

Precaution(s): Store between 2° and 7°C.

Use new, non-chemically sterilized, needles and syringes.

Do not mix with other vaccines.

Burn vaccine container and all unused contents.

Caution(s): Vaccinate only healthy, non-parasitized dogs.

The use of a biological product may produce anaphylaxis and/or other inflammatory immune-mediated hypersensitivity reactions.

The age at which maternal antibody for canine parvovirus no longer interferes with the development of the active immunity varies according to the bitch's titer and quantity of colostral antibodies absorbed by the puppy.

Antidote(s): Epinephrine, corticosteroids, and antihistamines may all be indicated depending on the nature and severity of the reaction.

Warning(s): For veterinary use only.

For use in dogs only.

Presentation: 25 x 1 dose (1 mL) and 5 x 10 dose (10 mL) vials of vaccine.

Compendium Code No.: 10470871 P21005-10

GALLIMUNE™ NC-BR

Merial Select **Vaccine**

Newcastle-Bronchitis Vaccine, Mass. and Ark. Types, Killed Virus

U.S. Vet. Lic. No.: 279

Composition: This product is a suspension of Newcastle disease and bronchitis viruses emulsified in oil. The following strains are utilized:

Newcastle - LaSota

Bronchitis - Mass. and Ark.

Newcastle, bronchitis origin: Chick embryo 100%

Indications: Use in chicken pullet/hens to protect them against Newcastle disease and bronchitis.

Directions: Warm vaccine to room temperature. Shake well. Inject 0.5 mL subcutaneously using aseptic technique. Vaccinate at 12 to 13 weeks of age and repeat at 20 to 21 weeks of age. Birds should be primed with live bronchitis vaccine at least four weeks prior to the first use of this product.

Precaution(s): Store in the dark between 36 and 45°F (2 and 7°C). Do not freeze. Use entire contents when first opened.

Caution(s): For veterinary use only.

Warning(s): Do not vaccinate within 42 days before slaughter.

Humans injected with this vaccine should seek immediate medical attention. Advise medical personnel that the vaccine is an oil emulsion type.

Presentation: 10 x 1,000 dose (500 mL) bottles.

Compendium Code No.: 11050470

GALLIMUNE™ REOGUARD™

Merial Select **Vaccine**

Reovirus Vaccine, Killed Virus

U.S. Vet. Lic. No.: 279

Composition: This product is a suspension of 1133, 2408, and MSB reoviruses emulsified in oil.

Indications: Use in chickens to protect their progeny against tenosynovitis or malabsorption caused by avian reoviruses.

Directions: Warm vaccine to room temperature. Shake well. Inject 0.5 mL subcutaneously using aseptic technique. Vaccinate at 12-13 weeks of age and repeat at 20-21 weeks of age. Birds should be primed with live reovirus vaccine at least four weeks prior to the first use of this product.

Precaution(s): Store in the dark between 36°-45°F (2°-7°C). Do not freeze. Use entire contents when first opened.

For veterinary use only.

Warning(s): Do not vaccinate within 42 days before slaughter.

Humans injected with this vaccine should seek immediate medical attention. Advise medical personnel that the vaccine is an oil emulsion type.

Presentation: 1000 doses (500 mL).

Compendium Code No.: 11050413 1200

GALLIMYCIN®-36

AgriLabs **Mastitis Therapy**

NADA No.: 035-456

Active Ingredient(s): Each mL contains:

Erythromycin . . . . 50 mg

Indications: A mastitis syringe for lactating cows that is effective against the leading mastitis-causing organisms: *Staphylococcus aureus, Streptococcus agalactiae, Streptococcus dysgalactiae,* and *Streptococcus uberis.*

Works against both acute and chronic causes.

Dosage and Administration: Infuse the entire contents of the 6 mL syringe into each infected quarter. Repeat after each milking for a total of three (3) consecutive infusions.

Precaution(s): Store at a controlled room temperature between 59-86°F (15-30°C).

Caution(s): Discard the empty container. Do not re-use.

Not for human use. Keep out of the reach of children.

For the treatment of bovine mastitis in lactating cows only.

Restricted drug, use only as directed.

Warning(s): Discard milk for 36 hours (3 milkings) following the last treatment with this drug. Animals must not be slaughtered for food within 14 days from the time of the last infusion with this drug.

Presentation: 12 x 6 mL tubes per carton, 144 per case.

Compendium Code No.: 10580530

GALLIMYCIN®-36

Bimeda **Mastitis Therapy**

(Erythromycin)

NADA No.: 035-455

Active Ingredient(s): Each 6 mL single dose syringe contains:

Erythromycin (GALLIMYCIN®) . . . . 300 mg

Manufactured by a non-sterilizing process.

Indications: For the treatment of bovine mastitis in lactating cows.

GALLIMYCIN®-36 is recommended for treatment of mastitis in lactating cows caused by the following organisms: *Staphylococcus aureus, Streptococcus agalactiae, Streptococcus dysgalactiae, Streptococcus uberis.*

Dosage and Administration: Thoroughly milk out each infected quarter. Clean the udder and teats by washing carefully. Disinfect the teat orifice(s) with cotton soaked in alcohol or another suitable disinfectant (starting with the teats opposite the operator first). Infuse the entire contents of one (1) syringe into each infected quarter starting with the teats nearest the operator if more than one (1) quarter is to be treated. Close the teat orifice with gentle pressure and massage the udder to distribute the medication.

Lactating Cows: Infuse the entire contents of one GALLIMYCIN®-36 syringe into each infected quarter. Repeat after each milking for a total of three consecutive infusions. Discard milk for 36 hours (3 milkings) following the last treatment.

Precaution(s): Protect from freezing.

Store at controlled room temperature, 15°C-30°C (59°F-86°F).

Discard empty container. Do not reuse.

Caution(s): For the treatment of bovine mastitis in lactating cows only.

Restricted drug (California), use only as directed.

For animal use only.

Not for human use.

Warning(s): Milk taken from animals during treatment and for 36 hours (3 milkings) after the latest treatment must not be used for food. Animals treated with this drug must not be slaughtered for food within 14 days from the time of infusion.

Keep out of the reach of children.

Presentation: 12 syringes, 6 mL (0.2 fl oz) each.

® Registered Trademark of Bimeda, Inc.

Compendium Code No.: 13990171 8GAL016-301

GALLIMYCIN®-100 INJECTION

Bimeda **Erythromycin**

Erythromycin Injectable-100 mg per mL

NADA No.: 012-123

Active Ingredient(s):

GALLIMYCIN® (Erythromycin) . . . . 100 mg
Butesin® (Butyl aminobenzoate) 2%
Ethyl alcohol 10%
Benzyl alcohol as preservative. 0.9%
Polyethylene glycol . . . . q.s.

GALLIMYCIN® Injectable is a specially prepared solution in a polyethylene glycol vehicle with Butesin® 2% (Butyl Aminobenzoate) as a local anesthetic. It contains 100 mg of erythromycin activity per mL.

Indications: A large animal anti-infective for cattle, sheep and swine.

When to Use:

Beef Cattle: Shipping fever, pneumonia (or pneumonia-enteritis complex), foot rot, stress (handling, transporting to feedlot, vaccination, dehorning, etc.), metritis.

Dairy Cattle: Pneumonia, foot rot, metritis, shipping fever, stress (handling, transporting to and from pasture, etc.).

Swine:

Swine (Hogs): Pneumonia, rhinitis, bronchitis.

Sows: Metritis, leptospirosis* (at farrowing time).

Baby Pigs (one week of age or older): "Scours".

Sheep: Prevention of "dysentery"** in newborn lambs, upper respiratory infections.

* In most states, leptospirosis is a reportable disease because of its public health significance. When this disease is suspected, professional advice should be sought.

** Where organisms susceptible to erythromycin may be the infective agent.

Dosage and Administration: How to Use: GALLIMYCIN® is designed for deep injection into the heavy muscles of the neck or legs. Where more than one treatment is needed, change the site of injection. Use a 16 or 18 gauge needle.

How to Inject GALLIMYCIN®:

Important: Always inject deep into muscle tissue, not fat. Swine, Cattle or Sheep can be injected in either the "round" or heavy neck muscles. Young Pigs should be injected only deep in the ham muscles. Inject ½ mL for each 5 lbs of body weight. Use ¾- to 1-inch needles — 18 or 19 gauge for best results.

	When to Use	How Much to Use	How Often to Use	Where to Use
Beef Cattle	Shipping Fever, Pneumonia (or pneumonia-enteritis complex, Foot Rot, Stress (handling, transporting to feedlot, vaccination, dehorning, etc.), Metritis	Inject 0.5-1.0 mL per 100 lbs. For example... 100 lb calves} 0.5-1.0 mL 300 lb calves} 1.5-3.0 mL 500 lb calves} 2.5-5.0 mL 1000 lb steers} 5.0-10.0 mL	1 dose daily as needed.	Inject deep into neck or "round" muscle tissue. Use 2-inch needles — 16 or 18 gauge
Dairy Cattle	Pneumonia, Foot Rot, Metritis, Shipping Fever, Stress (handling, transporting to and from pasture, etc.)	Inject 0.5-1.0 mL per 100 lbs. For example... 50 lb calf} 0.25-0.50 mL 100 lb calves} 0.50-1.0 mL 800 lb calves} 4.0-8.0 mL Each additional 100 lbs} 0.50-1.0 mL	1 dose daily as needed.	Inject deep into neck or "round" muscle tissue. Use 2-inch needles — 16 or 18 gauge.
Swine	Swine (Hogs): Pneumonia, Rhinitis, Bronchitis Sows: Metritis, Leptospirosis* (at farrowing time)	Inject 0.5-1.5 mL per 100 lb pig.	1 dose daily as needed.	Inject deep into muscle tissue — not fat. Use 2-inch needles — 18 gauge for best results.
	Baby Pigs (one week of age or older): "Scours"	Inject 0.25 mL per 5 lbs of body weight.	1 dose daily as needed.	Inject deep into ham muscle. Use ¾ to 1-inch needles — 18 or 19 gauge for best results.
Sheep	Prevention of "dystentry"** in newborn lambs, Upper Respiratory Infections	Inject 0.25 mL per 10 lbs of body weight. Older Animals — Inject 0.50 mL per 100 lbs of weight.	1 dose daily as needed.	Inject deep into muscle tissue. Use 1- or 2-inch needles — 16 or 18 gauge for best results.

* In most states, leptospirosis is a reportable disease because of its public health significance. When this disease is suspected, professional advice should be sought.

** Where organisms susceptible to erythromycin may be the infective agent.

Precaution(s): Store at room temperature 15-30°C (59-86°F). Extreme temperatures will vary the viscosity. If very cold weather causes solidification, GALLIMYCIN® Injectable can be returned to its normal fluid consistency by placing the bottle in warm water for 15 to 20 minutes before use. The antibiotic remains fully effective.

Protect from freezing.

Caution(s): During extensive clinical investigation of GALLIMYCIN® Injectable no significant side effects were reported. Since there may be a transient swelling or soreness at the site of injection, it is advisable, where more than one treatment is required, to vary the site of injection, alternating legs or alternating between the leg and the neck muscle. Swelling or soreness encountered at the site of injection is usually mild, transient and disappears in one or two days. Deep intramuscular injections will minimize the incidence of local soreness and swelling.

Special Note: It is imperative that you do not wash syringes with water. The manufacturer recommends flushing syringes clean with isopropyl alcohol, rubbing alcohol, ethyl alcohol, or acetone.

Restricted Drug (California), use only as directed.

For animal use only.

Warning(s): Milk taken from animals during treatment and for 72 hours (6 milkings) after the latest treatment must not be used for food.

Cattle must not be treated within 14 days of slaughter for food.

Swine must not be treated within 7 days of slaughter for food.

Sheep must not be treated within 3 days of slaughter for food.

Not for human use.

Keep out of reach of children.

Presentation: Supplied in sterile 100 mL (3.4 fl oz) multiple dose rubber-stoppered vials. The rubber stopper facilitates convenient withdrawal when using a single syringe and needle.

GALLIMYCIN is a Registered Trademark of Bimeda, Inc.

Butesin is a Registered Trademark of Abbott Laboratories.

Compendium Code No.: 13990161

GALLIMYCIN®-100P

Bimeda **Feed Medication**

(Erythromycin) Medicated Premix Antibiotic (Type A medicated article)

NADA No.: 035-157

Active Ingredient(s): Each pound contains 100 grams of erythromycin thiocyanate (equivalent to 92.5 grams of erythromycin). Inert ingredients are corn germ meal and soybean oil.

Indications: For use in manufacturing non-pelletized registered feeds for chickens and turkeys.

Chickens and Turkeys: As an aid in the prevention and reduction of lesions and in lowering severity of chronic respiratory disease.

Chickens: As an aid in the prevention of infectious coryza.

Chickens and Turkeys: As an aid in the prevention of chronic respiratory disease during periods of stress.

Directions for Use: To assure effectiveness, treated birds must consume enough medicated feed to provide a therapeutic dosage.

Species	Purpose	Level of Erythromycin
Chickens and Turkeys	As an aid in the prevention and reduction of lesions and in lowering severity of chronic respiratory disease.	185 g erythromycin per ton of feed for 5 to 8 days.
Chickens	As an aid in the prevention of infectious coryza.	92.5 g erythromycin per ton of feed for 7 to 14 days.
Chickens and Turkeys	As an aid in the prevention of chronic respiratory disease during periods of stress.	92.5 g erythromycin per ton of feed for 2 days before stress and 3 to 6 days after stress.

Mixing Directions — Complete Feeds (Type C medicated product)

Erythromycin Thiocyanate (g/ton)	Erythromycin Activity (g/ton)	GALLIMYCIN™-100P Premix (lbs/ton)
100	92.5	1.0
200	185.0	2.0

Precaution(s): Medicated feeds prepared with this product should be consumed within approximately two weeks of preparation. Do not store for future use.

Caution(s): For use in manufacturing non-pelletized registered feeds.

Restricted drug, use only as directed. Not for human use.

Warning(s): Do not use in birds producing eggs for food purposes at the 185 g erythromycin per ton level.

Chickens: Withdraw feed containing 185 g erythromycin per ton 48 hours before slaughter. Withdraw feed containing 92.5 g erythromycin per ton 24 hours before slaughter.

Presentation: 50 lb bag.

GALLIMYCIN® is a registered trademark of The Cross Vetpharm Group, Ltd. DBA Bimeda Inc.

Use of this product is covered by U.S. Patent No. 2,855,321.

Compendium Code No.: 13990141

GALLIMYCIN®-200 INJECTION

Bimeda **Erythromycin Injection**

Erythromycin Injectable 200 mg per mL-Sterile-Antibacterial

NADA No.: 012-123

Active Ingredient(s): Description: GALLIMYCIN® Injection is an erythromycin preparation formulated in a sterile solution for intramuscular administration only.

Each mL contains:

Erythromycin Base .... 200 mg

In a non-aqueous, buffered, alcohol base sterile solution.

Indications: GALLIMYCIN® Injection is indicated for the treatment of bovine respiratory disease (shipping fever complex and bacterial pneumonia) associated with *Pasteurella multocida* organisms susceptible to erythromycin.

Dosage and Administration: Deep intramuscular injection into the heavy neck muscles, or if necessary for alternating injection sites, into the heavy muscular portion of the leg muscle (round). In calves under 200 lbs, deep intramuscular injection into the heavy muscles of the leg only. Administer 2 mL/100 lbs body weight (4 mg/lb body weight) once daily for up to 5 days as needed. Use a 1-inch to 2-inch, 16- or 18-gauge needle depending on the animal's size.

Thoroughly clean and sterilize syringes and needles before using (needles and syringes may be sterilized by boiling in water for 15 minutes) or use prepackaged sterile syringes and needles.

Use all precautions to prevent contamination of contents of the bottle.

Disinfect the injection site with a suitable disinfectant such as 70% isopropyl alcohol just prior to injection.

Precaution(s): Storage: Store at room temperature (15°-30°C, 59°-86°F).

Caution(s): In animals weighing over 200 lbs, the neck region is the preferred site for deep intramuscular injection. Since there may be a transient swelling or soreness at the site of injection, it is advisable, when more than one treatment is required, to vary the site of the injection. This is achieved by alternating sides of the neck or if necessary, alternating between the leg and neck muscles. No more than 10 mL should be injected at any one site (in small calves under 200 lbs no more than 4 mL should be injected per site and then only in the heavy muscles of the leg). Swelling or soreness encountered at the site of injection is usually mild, transient and disappears in 2 to 4 days. Deep intramuscular injections will minimize the incidence of local soreness and swelling.

Restricted Drug (California), use only as directed.

For animal use only.

Warning(s): Treated animals should not be slaughtered for food within 6 days of the last injection. Temporary tissue irritation follows injection. To avoid excessive trim do not slaughter cattle within 21 days of the last injection. Do not use in female dairy cattle greater than 20 months of age.

Not for human use.

Keep out of reach of children.

Presentation: GALLIMYCIN® is supplied in sterile 100 mL (3.4 fl oz) and 250 mL (8.5 fl oz) multiple-dose, rubber-stoppered vials.

® Registered Trademark of Bimeda, Inc.

Compendium Code No.: 13990151

GALLIMYCIN®-DRY COW

AgriLabs **Mastitis Therapy**

NADA No.: 035-455

Active Ingredient(s): Each mL contains:

Erythromycin .... 50 mg

Indications: A mastitis syringe for nonlactating cows that is effective against the following major mastitis-causing organisms.

Organisms	Treated Qtrs./Responding Qtrs.	Response Rate
Staphylococcus aureus	160/99	62%
Staphylococcus agalactiae	81/79	97%
Staphylococcus nonagalactiae	13/13	100%

Dosage and Administration: Infuse the entire contents of the 12 mL syringe into each infected quarter at the time of drying off.

Precaution(s): Store at a controlled room temperature between 59-86°F (15-30°C).

Caution(s): Discard the empty container. Do not re-use.

Not for human use. Keep out of the reach of children.

For the treatment of bovine mastitis in dry cows only.

Restricted drug, use only as directed.

Warning(s): Not for use in lactating dairy cattle. Animals must not be slaughtered for food within 14 days from the time of the last infusion with this drug.

Milk taken from animals during treatment and for 36 hours (3 milkings) after the last treatment with this drug must not be used for food.

Calves born to treated cows must not be slaughtered for food at less than 10 days of age.

Presentation: 12 x 12 mL tubes per carton, 144 per case.

Compendium Code No.: 10580541

GALLIMYCIN®-DRY COW

Bimeda **Mastitis Therapy**

NADA No.: 035-455

Active Ingredient(s): Each 12 mL single dose syringe contains a clear solution of:

Erythromycin .... 600 mg

Indications: GALLIMYCIN®-DRY COW is a clear solution of erythromycin which provides antibacterial activity in the presence of common mastitis-causing micro-organsims.

GALLIMYCIN®-DRY COW is recommended for the treatment of mastitis due to *Staphylococcus aureus, Streptococcus agalactiae, Streptococcus dysgalactiae,* and *Streptococcus uberis.* GALLIMYCIN®-DRY COW is generally effective in eliminating the signs of mastitis caused by the above organisms.

Dosage and Administration: Thoroughly milk out each infected quarter. Clean the udder and teats by washing carefully. Disinfect the teat orifice(s) with cotton soaked in alcohol or another suitable disinfectant (starting with the teats opposite the operator first). Infuse the entire contents of one (1) syringe into each infected quarter starting with the teats nearest the operator if more than one (1) quarter is to be treated. Close the teat orifice with gentle pressure and massage the udder to distribute the medication.

Dosage (one treatment): Dry cows only. Infuse the entire contents of one (1) GALLIMYCIN®-DRY COW syringe into each infected quarter at the time of drying-off.

Precaution(s): Protect from freezing.

Store at a controlled room temperature 59°-86°F (15°-30°C).

Discard the empty container. Do not re-use.

Caution(s): Not for human use. Keep out of the reach of children.

For the treatment of bovine mastitis in dry cows only.

Restricted drug, use only as directed.

Warning(s): Milk taken from animals during treatment and for 36 hours (3 milkings) after the last treatment with this drug must not be used for food.

Animals treated with this drug must not be slaughtered for food within 14 days from the time of infusion nor within 96 hours after calving.

Calves born to treated cows must not be slaughtered for food at less than 10 days of age.

Presentation: 12 mL single dose disposable syringes, 12 syringes per carton.

Compendium Code No.: 13990180

GALLIMYCIN® PFC

Bimeda **Water Medication**

(Erythromycin) Poultry Formula Concentrated-Water Soluble-Anti-Infective

NADA No.: 035-157

Active Ingredient(s): Each 250 g package contains 65 g erythromycin phosphate (Equivalent to 57.8 g erythromycin).

Indications: In Broilers and Replacement Chickens:

Chronic Respiratory Disease: As an aid in the control of Chronic Respiratory Disease due to *Mycoplasma gallisepticum* susceptible to erythromycin.

In Replacement Chickens and Chicken Breeders:

Infectious Coryza: As an aid in the control of Infectious Coryza due to *Haemophilus gallinarum* susceptible to erythromycin.

In Growing Turkeys:

Bluecomb: As an aid in the control Bluecomb (Non-specific Infectious Enteritis) caused by organisms susceptible to erythromycin.

Directions for Use: To assure effectiveness, treated birds must consume enough medicated water to provide a therapeutic dosage.

Indications	Dosage of Erythromycin Phosphate
Chronic Respiratory Disease	½ g/gal of drinking water for 5 days
Infectious Coryza	½ g/gal of drinking water for 7 days
Bluecomb (Non-specific Infectious Enteritis)	½ g/gal of drinking water for 7 days

Mixing Instructions for Drinking Water: Add one (1) package (250 g) per 130 gallons and mix thoroughly.

For proportioners which meter 1 oz/gal, add one (1) package (250 g) to each gallon of stock solution.

In chickens, this dosage provides 5.0 to 17.9 mg/lb and, in turkeys, 3.1 to 34.2 mg/lb body weight per bird per day of erythromycin activity depending upon age, class of chicken (or turkey), feed consumption, environmental temperature, and relative humidity during medication period.

Caution(s): Important: Solutions older than 3 days should not be used.

Restricted drug (California), use only as directed.

For animal use only.

Warning(s): Do not use in chickens or turkeys producing eggs for human consumption.

Do not use in replacement pullets over 16 weeks of age.

Withdraw one (1) day before slaughter.

Not for human use.

Keep out of reach of children.

Presentation: 250 g (8.8 oz) package.

The use of this product in poultry is covered by U.S. Pat. No. 3,276,956.

GALLIMYCIN® is a Registered Trademark of Bimeda, Inc.

Compendium Code No.: 13990540 8GAL001-600

GAMMA-CHECK-B™

V.D.I. **IgG Test**

Indications: The product is used for the semiquantitative detection of bovine gammaglobulin levels in blood and serum.

Test Principle: The test is based on the principal that glutaraldehyde reacts with certain blood proteins (gammaglobulin and fibrinogen) to form a solid gel. The time taken for the gel to form is inversely proportional to the concentration of these proteins. There have been reports on the application of this reaction as a means of detecting gammaglobulin levels in foals, calves, puppies and nondomestic neonatal ruminants.[1-7] Many of these papers have reported excellent results when using serum. The GAMMA-CHECK-B™ test is available as a means of semi-quantitatively measuring IgG in whole blood or serum.

Through new production methods, the glutaraldehyde used in the test is available in a pure, stable form. This allows a long shelf life and avoids some of the pitfalls found by earlier researchers.[8] Because glutaraldehyde is potentially toxic, it has been sealed into a tube so that operator exposure does not occur.

Test Procedure:

When to Test: GAMMA-CHECK-B™ can be used to screen calves at any age for gammaglobulin levels.

Recent research has shown that most neonates that ingest good quality colostrum will have a high (>800 mg/dl) IgG level by eight (8) hours of age.[9,10] Using the test at eight (8) hours still allows the oral route to be used for additional supplementation of colostrum or plasma (absorption can occur via this route for up to 24 hours).[11]

When used on calves of more than 24 hours of age, supplementation of IgG, if required, must occur parenterally.

a. Whole Blood:

1. The GAMMA-CHECK tube should be filled to the red line on the label with whole blood. The vacuum in the tube is sufficient to fill the tube to this line. The filling can be done either directly from the vein, as in the routine collection of blood samples, or by introducing previously drawn blood (with EDTA - lavender top - anticoagulant) into the tube. The reason for the latter alternative is because when the blood is mixed with the stabilized glut, the reaction time must begin. The practitioner may not be in a position to do that when drawing the blood straight from the animal - it may be inconvenient.
2. As soon as the whole blood enters the GAMMA-CHECK tube, the time must be noted. The end point is the formation of a firm clot/gel. Every minute or so, the tube should be gently tilted to approximately 45 degrees. Tilting too far may obscure the contents of the tube because the thickening blood sticks to the side. Blood will no longer run along the sides of the tube when the end-point is reached. Note the time taken when this occurs and calculate the length of time to form the solid gel.

If a solid clot forms in less than five (5) minutes, the IgG level is above 800 mg/dl.

A solid clot formation in less than three (3) minutes indicates a level of >1,500 mg/dl.

Occasionally a soft jelly-like clot will form. In the majority of such cases, this can be interpreted as a firm clot. However, the test should be repeated with another sample or using a different type of test.

b. Serum:

1. Whole blood is first collected into a plain 5 mL or larger red-top tube. When clotting and clot retraction is complete (approximately 1 to 2 hours), the tube should be centrifuged.
2. Using a hypodermic syringe and needle, 1.5 mL of the serum is removed from the collection tube and inserted into the GAMMA-CHECK-B™ tube. The time is noted and the contents are observed by occasionally tilting the tube until a solid gel forms. The time taken for this to occur is noted.

Solid clot formation in less than five (5) minutes indicates an IgG level of >500 mg/dl.

Precaution(s): The kit should be kept in the refrigerator at 4°C.

Caution(s): Using the test with whole blood in calves that may be septic (with elevated fibrinogen levels), dehydrated or hemolyzed may give a false-positive result. If any of these conditions are present, the test should be repeated with serum (see Test Procedure) or another type of test.

Glutaraldehyde is caustic to the skin and eyes. If a tube breaks and skin or eye contact occurs, wash with copious quantities of cold water and consult a physician.

References: Available upon request.

Presentation: 10 and 25 tests per kit.

Compendium Code No.: 11280032

GAMMA-CHECK-C™

V.D.I. **IgG Test**

Indications: The product is used for the semi-quantitative estimation of gammaglobulin levels in equine colostrum.

Test Principle: The test is based on the principal that glutaraldehyde reacts with gammaglobulin to form a solid gel. The time taken for the gel to form is inversely proportional to the concentration of these proteins. There have been reports on the application of this reaction as a means of detecting gammaglobulin levels in foals, calves, puppies and nondomestic neonatal ruminants.[1-7] Many of these papers have reported excellent results when using serum. The GAMMA-CHECK-C™ test is available as a means of semi-quantitatively measuring gammaglobulin in colostrum.[8]

Through new production methods, the glutaraldehyde used in the test is available in a pure, stable form. This allows a long shelf life and avoids some of the pitfalls experienced by earlier researchers.[9] Because glutaraldehyde is potentially toxic, it has been sealed into a tube so that operator exposure does not occur.

Test Procedure:

When to Test: GAMMA-CHECK-C™ can be used to assess the quality of colostrum either just prior to, or just after foaling but before the foal nurses. If the mare drips colostrum prior to foaling, the test will show if adequate gammaglobulin remains. The colostrum quality can also be evaluated prior to freezing. The test will also work on thawed colostrum.

A means of measuring a 1.5 mL liquid is needed, such as a 3 mL syringe.

1. Gently clean the mare's udder with warm water and collect a small quantity (1 teaspoon) of the colostrum into a cup or in the syringe case cap.
2. Draw 0.5 mL of the colostrum into the plastic disposable pipette provided (the 0.5 mL mark is half-way up the stem). Remove the stopper from one (1) of the red top tubes and add the colostrum to the diluent and mix.
3. Draw up 1.5 mL of the diluted colostrum into a 3 mL syringe and add it to the GAMMA-CHECK tube using a hypodermic needle. Do not remove the stopper from the tube. This should fill the GAMMA-CHECK tube to the red line. As soon as the sample is added, note the time. By gently tilting the tube every minute or so, determine the time for a solid gel to appear.

If the solid gel forms in less than 10 minutes, the IgG level is above 4,000 mg/dl.

A solid clot formation in less than three (3) minutes indicates a level of >6,000 mg/dl.

Research indicates that a foal requires 1-1.25 g IgG per kilogram orally to achieve a circulating level of >800 mg/dl.[10] This translates to the average foal requiring 50-60 g IgG, or 1 to 1½ L of colostrum with an IgG of >4,000 mg/dl.

Precaution(s): The kit should be kept in the refrigerator at 4°C.

Caution(s): Glutaraldehyde can be irritating to the skin and eyes. If a tube breaks and the enclosed liquid contacts the skin, wash with copious quantities of cold water, etc.

References: Available upon request.

Presentation: 10 tests per kit.

Compendium Code No.: 11280041

GAMMA-CHECK-E™

V.D.I. **IgG Test**

Indications: The product is used for the semi-quantitative estimation of gammaglobulin levels in foals.

Test Principle: The test is based on the principal that glutaraldehyde reacts with certain blood proteins (gammaglobulin and fibrinogen) to form a solid gel. The time taken for the gel to form is inversely proportional to the concentration of these proteins. There have been reports on the application of this reaction as a means of detecting gammaglobulin levels in foals, calves, puppies and nondomestic neonatal ruminants.[1-7] Many of these papers have reported excellent results when using serum. The GAMMA-CHECK-E™ test is available as a means of semi-quantitatively measuring IgG in whole blood or serum.

Through new production methods, the glutaraldehyde used in the test is available in a pure, stable form. This allows a long shelf life and avoids some of the pitfalls found by earlier researchers.[8] Because glutaraldehyde is potentially toxic, it has been sealed into a tube so that operator exposure does not occur.

Test Procedure:

When to Test: GAMMA-CHECK-E™ can be used to screen foals for IgG levels at any age.

Recent research has shown that most foals that ingest good quality colostrum will have a high (>800 mg/dl) IgG level by eight (8) hours of age.[9,10] Using the test at eight (8) hours still allows the oral route to be used for additional supplementation of colostrum or plasma (absorption can occur via this route for up to 24 hours).[11]

When used on foals of more than 24 hours of age, supplementation of IgG, if required, must occur parenterally.

a. Whole Blood:

1. The GAMMA-CHECK tube should be filled to the red line on the label with whole blood. The vacuum in the tube is sufficient to fill the tube to this line. The filling can be done either directly from the vein, as in the routine collection of blood samples, or by introducing previously drawn blood (with EDTA - lavender top - anticoagulant) into the tube. The reason for the latter alternative is because when the blood is mixed with the stabilized glut, the reaction time must begin. The practitioner may not be in a position to do that when drawing the blood straight from the animal - it may be inconvenient.
2. As soon as the whole blood enters the GAMMA-CHECK tube, the time must be noted. The end point is the formation of a firm clot/gel. Every minute or so, the tube should be gently tilted to approximately 45 degrees. Tilting too far may obscure the contents of the tube because the thickening blood sticks to the side. Blood will no longer run along the sides of the tube when the end-point is reached. Note the time taken when this occurs and calculate the length of time to form the solid gel.

If a solid clot forms in less than 10 minutes, the IgG level is above 800 mg/dl.

A solid clot formation in less than three (3) minutes indicates a level of >1,500 mg/dl.

On rare occasions a false-negative result can occur, i.e. the blood does not clot even in the presence of adequate IgG. If there is not an apparent problem, i.e. the foal nursed normally and the colostrum was of high quality, retest any foal whose blood does not clot in less than 10 minutes using serum or another type of test. In foals over 24 hours of age, this is not the only test recommended when deciding if a foal needs a plasma transfusion. If is advisable to repeat the test on negative samples using the Equine-RID Test.

Occasionally a soft jelly-like clot will form. In the majority of such cases, this can be interpreted as a firm clot. However, the test should be repeated with another sample or using a different type of test.

b. Serum:

1. Whole blood is first collected into a plain 5 mL or larger red-top tube. When clotting and clot retraction is complete (approximately 1 to 2 hours), the tube should be centrifuged.
2. Using a hypodermic syringe and needle, 1.5 mL of the serum is removed from the collection tube and inserted into the GAMMA-CHECK-E™ tube. The time is noted and the contents are observed by occasionally tilting the tube until a solid gel forms. The time taken for this to occur is noted.

Solid clot formation in less than five (5) minutes indicates an IgG level of >400 mg/dl.

Precaution(s): The kit should be kept in the refrigerator at 4°C.

Caution(s): Using the test with whole blood in foals that may be septic (with elevated fibrinogen levels), dehydrated or hemolyzed may give a false-positive result. If any of these conditions are present, the test should be repeated with serum (see Test Procedure) or another type of test.

Glutaraldehyde is caustic to the skin and eyes. If a tube breaks and skin or eye contact occurs, wash with copious quantities of cold water.

References: Available upon request.

Presentation: 10 tests per kit and 25 tests per kit.

Compendium Code No.: 11280051

GARACIN® PIGLET INJECTION

Schering-Plough **Gentamicin**

(Gentamicin Sulfate)

NADA No.: 103-037

Active Ingredient(s): GARACIN® Piglet Injection is a sterile preparation for intramuscular administration in piglets up to three (3) days of age. Each milliliter contains:

Gentamicin sulfate veterinary (equivalent to gentamicin base)	5 mg
Sodium bisulfate	2 mg
Edetate disodium	0.1 mg
Sodium acetate	7.46 mg
Glacial acetic acid	3 mg
Methylparaben (preservative)	1.3 mg
Propylparaben (preservative)	0.2 mg
Water for injection	q.s.

Indications: GARACIN® Piglet Injection is recommended for the treatment of porcine colibacillus caused by strains of *E. coli* sensitive to gentamicin.

Pharmacology: Gentamicin is a mixture of aminoglycoside antibiotics derived from the fermentation of *Micromonospora purpurea.* Gentamicin sulfate veterinary is a mixture of sulfate salts of the antibiotics produced in this fermentation. The salts are weakly acidic and freely soluble in water. Gentamicin sulfate veterinary is stable in solution for the period of time indicated by the expiration date.

Dosage and Administration: The recommended dose is 1 mL (5 mg) administered intramuscularly. GARACIN® Piglet Injection is not to be used more than once in each piglet. If the piglets do not respond to treatment with GARACIN® Piglet Injection, the diagnosis should be re-evaluated.

Clean and sterilize the needles and syringes by boiling in water for 15 minutes prior to use. Prior to injection, disinfect the injection site and the top of the vial with a suitable disinfectant, such as 70% alcohol.

Use all precautions to prevent contamination of the vial contents.

Contraindication(s): There are not any known contraindications to this drug when used as directed.

Precaution(s): Store between 2° and 30°C (36° and 86°F).

Warning(s): For use in piglets up to three (3) days of age only. Piglets injected with GARACIN® Piglet Injection must not be slaughtered for food for a least 40 days following treatment. Use of more than the recommended dose will result in gentamicin tissue residues beyond 40 days.

Presentation: 5 mg/mL available in 250 mL multiple dose vials.

Compendium Code No.: 10470900

GARACIN® PIG PUMP

Schering-Plough **Gentamicin**

(Gentamicin sulfate) Oral Solution—4.35 mg/mL

NADA No.: 130-464

Active Ingredient(s): Each mL of GARACIN® Pig Pump contains gentamicin sulfate veterinary, equivalent to 4.35 mg gentamicin base.

Indications: GARACIN® Pig Pump is recommended for the control and treatment of colibacillosis in neonatal pigs one to three days of age, caused by strains of *E. coli* sensitive to gentamicin.

Pharmacology: Gentamicin is a mixture of aminoglycoside antibiotics derived from the fermentation of *Micromonospora purpurea.* Gentamicin sulfate veterinary is a mixture of sulfate salts of the antibiotics produced in this fermentation. The salts are weakly acidic and freely soluble in water. Gentamicin sulfate veterinary is stable in the subject solution under usual storage conditions for the periods indicated by the expiration date.

Dosage and Administration: Administer orally to baby pigs. Recommended dose is one (1) full pump per pig one (1) time at the first sign of disease. One (1) pump delivers 1.15 mL of gentamicin pig pump solution (5 mg gentamicin).

Unlock the pump with a counterclockwise turn, and press the plunger down two (2) times to fill the delivery unit. A separate extension tube is enclosed for administration convenience. Administer one (1) full pump (plunger depression) directly into the mouth of each affected pig.

Contraindication(s): There are not any known contraindications to the drug when used as directed.

Precaution(s): Store between 2-30°C (36-86°F).

Warning(s): For use in neonatal swine only. Pigs treated with the recommended dose of GARACIN® Pig Pump must not be slaughtered for food for at least 14 days following the last treatment.

Presentation: 4.35 mg/mL available in 115 mL bottles, carton of 1 or 12.

Compendium Code No.: 10470890

GARACIN® SOLUBLE POWDER

Schering-Plough **Gentamicin**

(Gentamicin sulfate veterinary) 2 g gentamicin/30 g powder

NADA No.: 133-836

Active Ingredient(s): Each gram of GARACIN® Soluble Powder contains gentamicin sulfate veterinary, equivalent to 66.7 mg gentamicin base.

Indications: GARACIN® Soluble Powder is recommended for the control and treatment of colibacillosis in weanling swine caused by strains of *E. coli* sensitive to gentamicin, and for the treatment of swine dysentery associated with *Treponema hyodysenteriae.*

Dosage and Administration:

For control and treatment of colibacillosis: Administer GARACIN® Soluble Powder in drinking water at the recommended level of 25 mg per gallon (30 g per 80 gallons) for three (3) consecutive days.

For control and treatment of swine dysentery: Administer GARACIN® Soluble Powder in drinking water at the recommended level of 50 mg per gallon (30 g per 40 gallons) for three (3) consecutive days.

The concentration of the medication should be adjusted in extremely hot or cold weather to ensure a gentamicin dosage of approximately 0.5 mg/lb./day for three (3) days for colibacillosis or 1.0 mg/lb./day for three (3) days for swine dysentery. A 50 lb. pig, under average conditions, will consume 0.9 gallons of water per day.

For swine dysentery, if the condition recurs the medication may be repeated. Because of the tendency for the disease to recur on a premise with a history of swine dysentery, a control program should be used following treatment.

To prepare medicated water, mix GARACIN® Soluble Powder and drinking water according to the following tables:

Mixing chart:

For control and treatment of colibacillosis:

A. For proportioner use: Add 30 g GARACIN® (approximately 1 level scoop) to ⅔ gallon water (80 oz.) to make a stock solution and dispense at the rate of one (1) ounce per gallon of drinking water. This will result in drinking water that contains 25 mg/gallon.

B. Bulk preparation:

Scoops of GARACIN® Soluble Powder (30 g)	Gallons of Water	Gentamicin (mg/gallon)
1	80	25
2	160	25
4	320	25

For control and treatment of swine dysentery:

A. For proportioner use: Add 30 g GARACIN® (approximately 1 level scoop) to ⅓ gallon water (40 oz.) to make a stock solution and dispense at the rate of one (1) ounce per gallon of drinking water. This will result in drinking water that contains 50 mg/gallon.

B. Bulk preparation:

Scoops of GARACIN® Soluble Powder (30 g)	Gallons of Water	Gentamicin (mg/gallon)
1	40	50
2	80	50
4	160	50

Medicated drinking water should not be stored or offered in rusty containers since the drug is quickly destroyed in such containers.

Medicated water should be prepared daily and be the sole source of drinking water for three (3) consecutive days.

The daily water consumption figures shown below are approximations for mild temperatures and are presented as a guide only. Actual water consumption varies with environmental temperature, humidity and diet.

Approximate Daily Water Consumption:

Weight of Pig (lbs.)	Gallons for 5 pigs	Gallons for 10 pigs
25	3.0	6.0
50	4.5	9.0
75	6.0	12.0
100	7.5	15.0

Contraindication(s): There are not any known contraindications to the drug when used as directed.
Precaution(s): Store between 2-30°C (36-86°F).
Warning(s): For use in swine drinking water only. Swine treated with the recommended dose of GARACIN® Soluble Powder must not be slaughtered for food for at least 10 days following the last treatment.
Side Effects: There have not been side effects reported following the recommended use of GARACIN® Soluble Powder in swine.
Presentation: GARACIN® Soluble Powder is available in a 360 g jar with a 30 g scoop in a shelf display box of six and 6 x 18 g packets.
Compendium Code No.: 10470911

GARAGEN™ OPHTHALMIC SOLUTION AND OINTMENT ℞

PPC **Ophthalmic Antibiotic**

Gentamicin Sulfate-Sterile-Veterinary
NADA No.: 099-008 (Solution) / 098-989 (Ointment)
Active Ingredient(s): GARAGEN™ Ophthalmic Solution is a sterile aqueous solution buffered to approximately pH 7 for use in the eye. Each mL contains gentamicin sulfate equivalent to 3 mg gentamicin, 2.9 mg disodium phosphate, 0.1 mg monosodium phosphate, 7.4 mg sodium chloride, 0.1 mg benzalkonium chloride as preservative, and purified water q.s.

GARAGEN™ Ophthalmic Ointment is a sterile ointment, each gram containing gentamicin sulfate equivalent to 3 mg gentamicin with 0.5 mg methylparaben and 0.1 mg propylparaben as preservatives in a bland base of white petrolatum.
Indications: GARAGEN™ Ophthalmic Solution and Ointment are indicated for topical treatment of conjunctivitis caused by susceptible bacteria in dogs and cats.
Pharmacology: Gentamicin sulfate is a water soluble antibiotic of the aminoglycoside group active against a wide variety of pathogenic gram-negative and gram-positive bacteria.

Chemistry: Gentamicin is an aminoglycoside antibiotic mixture derived from *Micromonospora purpurea* of the Actinomycetes group. It is a powder, white to buff in color, readily soluble in water, and heat stable.

Action: Gentamicin sulfate, a broad-spectrum antibiotic, is a highly effective topical treatment in primary and secondary bacterial infections of the eye and surrounding tissues. Gentamicin is bactericidal *in vitro* against a wide variety of gram-positive and gram-negative bacteria. Concentrations of gentamicin sulfate required to inhibit growth of gram-positive and gram-negative clinical and laboratory strains of bacteria tested were less than those of neomycin in most instances.[1,2] Gentamicin is active against most gram-negative bacteria including *Pseudomonas aeruginosa*, indole positive and negative *Proteus* species, *Escherichia coli, Klebsiella* sp. and *Enterobacter* sp. Gentamicin is also active against strains of gram-positive bacteria including *Staphylococcus* species and *Streptococcus* species.
Dosage and Administration: GARAGEN™ Ophthalmic Solution—1 or 2 drops instilled into the conjuctival sac 2 to 4 times a day. GARAGEN™ Ophthalmic Ointment—apply approximately ½-inch strip to the affected eye 2 to 4 times a day.
Precaution(s): Store Solution and Ointment between 2° and 30°C (36° and 86°F).
Caution(s): Federal law restricts this drug to use by or on the order of a licensed veterinarian.

Antibiotic susceptibility of infecting organisms should be determined prior to the use of these preparations. Prolonged use of topical antibiotics may give rise to overgrowth of nonsusceptible organisms such as fungi. Should this occur or if irritation or hypersensitivity to any component develops, discontinue use of the preparation and institute appropriate therapy. Ophthalmic ointments may retard corneal healing.
References: Available upon request.
Presentation: GARAGEN™ Ophthalmic Solution—Sterile—5 mL plastic dropper bottle, box of 12, NDC 61546-6521-2.

GARAGEN™ Ophthalmic Ointment—Sterile—⅛-oz. tube, box of 12, NDC 61546-6527-2.
Compendium Code No.: 14870020 January 1998, 21298700

GARAGEN™ OTIC SOLUTION ℞

PPC **Otic Preparation Antibiotic-Corticosteroid**

Gentamicin Sulfate with Betamethasone Valerate-Veterinary
NADA No.: 046-821
Active Ingredient(s): GARAGEN™ Otic Solution is packaged in a convenient plastic squeeze bottle for easy application. Each mL of GARAGEN™ Otic Solution contains gentamicin sulfate equivalent to 3 mg gentamicin base, betamethasone valerate equivalent to 1 mg betamethasone, 1.0 mg hydroxyethylcellulose, 2.5 mg glacial acetic acid, 200 mg purified water, 19% ethanol, 9.4 mg benzyl alcohol as preservative, 300 mg glycerin, and propylene glycol q.s.
Indications: GARAGEN™ Otic Solution is indicated for the treatment of acute and chronic canine otitis externa and canine and feline superficial infected lesions caused by bacteria sensitive to gentamicin.
Pharmacology: Chemistry: Gentamicin is a bactericidal antibiotic of the aminoglycoside group derived from *Micromonospora purpurea* of the *Actinomyces* group. It is a powder, white to buff in color, basic in nature, readily soluble in water, and highly stable in solution.

Betamethasone valerate is a synthetic corticosteroid derivative of prednisolone.

Action: GARAGEN™ Otic Solution combines the broad-spectrum activity of gentamicin sulfate with the anti-inflammatory and antipruritic activity of betamethasone valerate. *In vitro* antibacterial activity[1] has shown that gentamicin is active against most gram-negative bacteria including *Pseudomonas aeruginosa*, indole-positive and -negative *Proteus* species, *Escherichia coli, Klebsiella pneumoniae, Aerobacter aerogenes*, and *Neisseria*. Gentamicin is also active against strains of gram-positive bacteria including *Staphylococcus* species and some *Streptococcus* species.

Betamethasone valerate has emerged from intensive research as the most promising of some 50 newly synthesized corticosteroids in the experimental model described by McKenzie[2] et al. This human bioassay technique has been found reliable for evaluating the vasoconstrictor properties of new topical corticosteroids and is useful in predicting clinical efficacy.

Betamethasone valerate in human medicine has been shown to provide anti-inflammatory and antipruritic activity in the topical management of corticosteroid-responsive dermatoses. In the responsive cases, the local anti-inflammatory activity is sustained by the vasoconstrictor properties of the steroid.

Dosage and Administration: Duration of treatment will depend upon the severity of the condition and the response obtained. The duration of treatment and/or frequency of the dosage may be reduced, but care should be taken not to discontinue therapy prematurely.

Otitis externa—The external ear and ear canal should be properly cleaned and dried before treatment. Remove foreign material, debris, crusted exudates, etc., with suitable nonirritating solutions. Excessive hair should be clipped from the treatment area of the external ear. Instill 3 to 8 drops of GARAGEN™ Otic Solution (approximately room temperature) into the ear canal twice daily for 7 to 14 days.

Superficial infected lesions—The lesion and adjacent area should be properly cleaned before treatment. Excessive hair should be removed. Apply a sufficient amount of GARAGEN™ to cover the treatment area twice daily for 7 to 14 days.
Contraindication(s): If hypersensitivity to any of the components occurs, treatment with this product should be discontinued and appropriate therapy instituted.

Concomitant use of drugs known to induce ototoxicity should be avoided.

This preparation should not be used in conditions where corticosteroids are contraindicated.

Do not administer parenteral corticosteroids during treatment with GARAGEN™ Otic Solution.
Precaution(s): Store between 2° and 25°C (36° and 77°F).
Caution(s): Federal law restricts this drug to use by or on the order of a licensed veterinarian.

Before instilling any medication into the ear, examine the external ear canal thoroughly to be certain the tympanic membrane is not ruptured in order to avoid the possibility of transmitting infection to the middle ear as well as damaging the cochlea or vestibular apparatus from prolonged contact. If hearing or vestibular dysfunction is noted during the course of treatment, discontinue use of GARAGEN™ Otic Solution.

The antibiotic sensitivity of the pathogenic organism should be determined prior to the use of this preparation. Use of topical antibiotics occasionally allows overgrowth of nonsusceptible bacteria, fungi, or yeasts. In these cases, treatment should be instituted with other appropriate agents as indicated.

Adverse systemic reactions have been observed following the oral ingestion of some topical corticosteroid preparations. Patients should be closely observed for the usual signs of adrenocorticosteroid overdosage which include sodium retention, potassium loss, fluid retention, weight gain, polydipsia, and/or polyuria. Prolonged use or overdosage may produce adverse immunosuppressive effects.

Experimentally it has been demonstrated that corticosteroids, especially at high dosage levels, may result in delayed wound healing. An increase in the incidence of osteoporosis may be noted, mainly in the elderly, with prolonged use of these compounds. Their use in older dogs during the healing stages of bone fracture is not indicated for the reason listed above.

Use of corticosteroids, depending on dose, duration, and specific steroid, may result in inhibition of endogenous steroid production following drug withdrawal. In patients presently receiving or recently withdrawn from systemic corticosteroid treatments, therapy with a rapidly acting corticosteroid should be considered in unusually stressful situations.
Warning(s): Clinical and experimental data have demonstrated that corticosteroids administered orally or parenterally to animals may induce the first stage of parturition when administered during the last trimester of pregnancy and may precipitate premature parturition followed by dystocia, fetal death, retained placenta, and metritis. Additionally, corticosteroids can induce cleft palates in offspring when given to pregnant animals during the period of palate closure of the embryos. Other congenital anomalies, including deformed forelegs, phocomelia, and anasarca have been reported in the offspring of dogs which received corticosteroids during pregnancy.

Avoid ingestion.

For use in dogs and cats only.
Toxicology: Toxicity Studies: Parenterally, no toxic effects were observed in rats given gentamicin sulfate 20 mg/kg/day for 24 days; in cats given 10 mg/kg/day for 40 days. Gentamicin sulfate given to dogs at 6 mg/lb/day, 6 days weekly for 3 weeks, caused no detectable kidney damage. At higher doses, impairment of equilibrium and of renal function were observed in these species.

Subacute otic toxicity study in dogs showed GARAGEN™ Otic Solution to be well tolerated locally with no adverse systemic effects when administered 5 drops twice a day for 21 consecutive days.

GARAGEN™ Otic Solution in a 21-day subacute dermal toxicity study in dogs was shown to be well tolerated when applied topically to abraded skin. There were no meaningful findings except a reduction in eosinophil count attributable to absorption of the corticosteroid component.
Side Effects: Side effects, such as SAP and SGPT enzyme elevations, weight loss, anorexia, polydipsia, and polyuria have occurred following the use of parenteral or systemic synthetic corticosteroids in dogs. Vomiting and diarrhea (occasionally bloody) have been observed in dogs and cats.

Cushing's syndrome in dogs has been reported in association with prolonged or repeated steroid therapy.
References: Available upon request.
Presentation: GARAGEN™ Otic Solution, squeeze bottles of 7.5 mL, 15 mL, and 240 mL (8 fl. oz.).
Compendium Code No.: 14870040 January 1998, F-21296104/B-21296104

GARAGEN™ TOPICAL SPRAY ℞

PPC **Antibiotic-Corticosteroid**

Gentamicin Sulfate Veterinary with Betamethasone Valerate
NADA No.: 132-338
Active Ingredient(s): Each mL of GARAGEN™ contains: gentamicin sulfate veterinary equivalent to 0.57 mg gentamicin base, betamethasone valerate equivalent to 0.284 mg betamethasone, 163 mg isopropyl alcohol, propylene glycol, methylparaben and propylparaben as preservatives, and purified water q.s. Hydrochloric acid may be added to adjust pH.
Indications: For the treatment of infected superficial lesions in dogs caused by bacteria susceptible to gentamicin.
Pharmacology: Chemistry: Gentamicin is a mixture of aminoglycoside antibiotics derived from the fermentation of *Micromonospora purpurea*. Gentamicin sulfate veterinary is a mixture of salts of the antibiotics produced in this fermentation. The salts are weakly acidic and freely soluble in water.

Gentamicin sulfate veterinary contains not less than 500 micrograms of gentamicin base per milligram.

Betamethasone valerate is a synthetic glucocorticoid.

Pharmacology: Gentamicin, a broad-spectrum antibiotic, is a highly effective topical treatment for bacterial infections of the skin. *In vitro*, gentamicin is bactericidal against a wide variety of gram-positive and gram-negative bacteria isolated from domestic animals.[1,2] Specifically, gentamicin is active against the following organisms isolated from canine skin: *Alcaligenes* sp., *Citrobacter* sp., *Klebsiella* sp., *Pseudomonas aeruginosa*, indole-positive and -negative *Proteus* sp., *Escherichia coli, Enterobacter* sp., *Staphylococcus* sp., and *Streptococcus* sp.

Betamethasone valerate emerged from intensive research as the most promising of some 50

G

newly synthesized corticosteroids in the experimental model described by McKenzie,[3] et al. This human bioassay technique has been found reliable for evaluating vasoconstrictor properties of new topical corticosteroids and is useful in predicting clinical efficacy.

Betamethasone valerate in veterinary medicine has been shown to provide anti-inflammatory and antipruritic activity in the topical management of corticosteroid-responsive infected superficial lesions in dogs.

Dosage and Administration: Prior to treatment, remove excessive hair and clean the lesion and adjacent area. Hold bottle upright 3 to 6 inches from the lesion and depress the sprayer head twice.

Administer 2 to 4 times daily for 7 days.

Each depression of the sprayer head delivers 0.7 mL of GARAGEN™ Topical Spray.

Contraindication(s): If hypersensitivity to any of the components occurs, discontinue treatment and institute appropriate therapy.

Precaution(s): Store upright between 2° and 30°C (36° and 86°F).

Caution(s): Federal law restricts this drug to use by or on the order of a licensed veterinarian.

Antibiotic susceptibility of the pathogenic organism(s) should be determined prior to use of this preparation. Use of topical antibiotics may permit overgrowth of nonsusceptible bacteria, fungi, or yeasts. If this occurs, treatment should be instituted with other appropriate agents as indicated.

Administration of recommended dose beyond 7 days may result in delayed wound healing. Animals treated longer than 7 days should be monitored closely.

Avoid ingestion. Oral or parenteral use of corticosteroids, depending on dose, duration, and specific steroid may result in inhibition of endogenous steroid production following drug withdrawal.

In patients presently receiving or recently withdrawn from systemic corticosteroid treatments, therapy with a rapidly acting corticosteroid should be considered in especially stressful situations.

If ingestion should occur, patients should be closely observed for the usual signs of adrenocorticoid overdosage which include sodium retention, potassium loss, fluid retention, weight gain, polydipsia, and/or polyuria. Prolonged use or overdosage may produce adverse immunosuppressive effects.

Warning(s): Clinical and experimental data have demonstrated that corticosteroids administered orally or parenterally to animals may induce the first stage of parturition when administered during the last trimester of pregnancy and may precipitate premature parturition followed by dystocia, fetal death, retained placenta, and metritis.

Additionally, corticosteroids administered to dogs, rabbits, and rodents during pregnancy have produced cleft palate. Other congenital anomalies, including deformed forelegs, phocomelia, and anasarca have been reported in the offspring of dogs which received corticosteroids during pregnancy.

For topical use in dogs only.

Toxicology: Toxicity Study: GARAGEN™ Topical Spray was well tolerated in an abraded skin study in dogs. No treatment-related toxicological changes in the skin were observed.

Systemic effects directly related to treatment were confined to histological changes in the adrenals, liver, and kidney and to organ-to-body weight ratios of adrenals. All were dose related, were typical for or not unexpected with corticosteroid therapy, and were considered reversible with cessation of treatment.

Side Effects: Side effects, such as SAP and SGPT enzyme elevations, weight loss, anorexia, polydipsia, and polyuria have occurred following parenteral or systemic use of synthetic corticosteroids in dogs. Vomiting and diarrhea (occasionally bloody) have been observed in dogs.

Cushing's syndrome in dogs has been reported in association with prolonged or repeated steroid therapy.

References: Available upon request.

Presentation: Plastic spray bottle containing 72 mL of GARAGEN™ Topical Spray.

Compendium Code No.: 14870050 November 1998, F-21297127/B-21297127

GARASOL® INJECTION (100 mg/mL)

Schering-Plough **Gentamicin**

(Gentamicin Sulfate Veterinary)

NADA No.: 101-862

Active Ingredient(s): Description: Each milliliter contains gentamicin sulfate veterinary, equivalent to 100 mg gentamicin base; 3.2 mg sodium bisulfite; 0.1 mg edetate disodium; 4.5 mg sodium acetate, anhydrous; 3.0 mg glacial acetic acid; 0.8 mg methylparaben and 0.1 mg propylparaben as preservatives; water for injection q.s.

Indications: Day-old chickens — GARASOL® is recommended for the prevention of early mortality associated with *Escherichia coli, Salmonella typhimurium* and *Pseudomonas aeruginosa* susceptible to gentamicin sulfate. Turkeys — As an aid in the prevention of early mortality of 1- to 3-day-old turkeys associated with *Arizona paracolon* infections susceptible to gentamicin sulfate.

Pharmacology: Chemistry: Gentamicin sulfate is a bactericidal aminoglycoside antibiotic derived from *Micromonospora purpurea* of the actinomycetes group. It is a powder, readily soluble in water and basic in nature. Gentamicin aqueous solutions do not require refrigeration and are stable over a wide range of temperatures and pH.

Dosage and Administration: Chickens: Each day-old chicken should be aseptically injected subcutaneously in the neck with GARASOL® Injection diluted with sterile, physiological saline solution to provide 0.2 mg gentamicin in a 0.2 mL dose. This concentration can be provided by diluting as follows:

GARASOL® mL	Sterile Saline mL	# Doses	Dose/Chicken mL
1	99	500	0.2
2	198	1000	0.2
4	396	2000	0.2
10	990	5000	0.2
80 (1 bottle)	7920	40000	0.2

Turkeys: Each 1-to 3-day old turkey should be aseptically injected subcutaneously in the neck with GARASOL® Injection diluted with sterile, physiologic saline solution to provide 1 mg gentamicin in a 0.2 mL dose. The dose should be injected under the loose skin on top of the neck, halfway between the head and the base of the neck. This concentration can be provided by diluting GARASOL® as follows:

GARASOL® mL	Sterile Saline mL	# Doses	Dose/Turkey mL
1	19	100	0.2
2	38	200	0.2
4	76	400	0.2
10	190	1000	0.2
80 (1 bottle)	1520	8000	0.2

Clean and sterilize needles and syringes by boiling in water for 15 minutes prior to use. Disinfect the injection site and top of the bottle with a suitable disinfectant, such as 70% isopropyl alcohol. Use all precautions to prevent contamination of vial contents.

Precaution(s): Store between 2° and 30°C (36° and 86°F).

Caution(s): For use in day-old chickens and 1- to 3-day old turkeys only.

Warning(s): Chickens injected with GARASOL® Injection must not be slaughtered for food for a least five (5) weeks following treatment. Turkeys injected with GARASOL® Injection must not be slaughtered for food for at least nine (9) weeks following treatment.

Presentation: GARASOL® Injection, 100 mg/mL, is available in 80 mL multiple-dose vials, NDC 0138-0134-02.

Compendium Code No.: 10470921 February 1996

GARAVAX®-T

Schering-Plough **Vaccine**

Escherichia coli Vaccine, Avirulent Live Culture, Avian Isolate

U.S. Vet. Lic. No.: 165A

Contents: GARAVAX™ is a live bacterial vaccine containing an avirulent temperature sensitive mutant of *Escherichia coli* in a freeze-dried preparation sealed under vacuum. The seed culture used to make this vaccine has been demonstrated in laboratory tests to protect turkeys against challenge with *E coli* serotype 078.

Indications: GARAVAX®-T is recommended for use in healthy turkeys to aid in the prevention of colibacillosis associated with infection by *Escherichia coli* serotype 078.

Dosage and Administration: Vaccinate by spray at day-of-age. Revaccinate at 3 weeks of age by drinking water and again 3-5 weeks thereafter as necessary according to exposure conditions.

Preparation of the Vaccine:

For Spray Use:

Do not open and rehydrate the vaccine until ready for use.

Assemble the vaccine and equipment needed to vaccinate the entire flock at one time.

Remove the tear-off aluminum seal from the vaccine without disturbing the rubber stopper.

Remove the rubber stopper from the vaccine vial and rehydrate the vaccine by filling the vial about half-full with distilled water.

Reseat the stopper and shake to thoroughly dissolve the vaccine.

For Drinking Water Use:

Do not open and rehydrate the vaccine until ready for use.

Assemble the vaccine and equipment needed to vaccinate the entire flock at one time.

Remove the tear-off aluminum seal from the vaccine without disturbing the rubber stopper.

Remove the rubber stopper from the vaccine vial and rehydrate the vaccine by filling the vial about half-full with clean, cool, non-chlorinated water to which powdered milk has been added as directed under How To Vaccinate.

Reseat the stopper and shake to thoroughly dissolve the vaccine.

How to Vaccinate:

By Spray: Use this method for day-of-age vaccination. Proper spray application of this vaccine is best accomplished through use of a clean spray cabinet which delivers 7 mL per second.

Rehydrate each 1000 dose vial to 140 mL or each 5000 dose vial to 700 mL using non-chlorinated water or distilled water. Spray each poult box twice for a total of 14 mL of vaccine per 100 poults.

By Drinking Water: Do not mix the vaccine into the drinking water until ready for use. Drinking water for vaccination should be mixed with powdered milk to prevent possible inactivation from chlorine or other water additives and also to stabilize the vaccine bacteria. The powdered milk should be added to the water at the rate of 3 grams per 11 liters (one heaped teaspoon per 3 U.S. gallons or 2.5 Imp. gallons); or 90 grams per 300 liters (one heaped cupful per 80 U.S. gallons or 66 Imp. gallons).

Use only clean waterers and equipment free of disinfectants or sanitizers. All water must be withheld for at least 2 hours prior to vaccination to assure that all poults drink. This is best done early in the morning to prevent heat stress or dehydration in the birds during hot weather. Mix the rehydrated vaccine in the quantity of drinking water (milk added) which will be consumed by thirsty poults in approximately 1-2 hours.

The following schedule is a general guideline for the amount of water to use with the vaccine. These amounts will vary depending upon the individual management conditions, climate, age and sex of the birds.

Each 1000 birds:

Age	Liters	U.S. Gal	Imp. Gal
3 weeks	45	12	10
4 weeks	61	16	14
5 weeks	76	20	17
6 weeks	99	26	22
7 weeks	121	32	27
8 weeks	152	40	34
9 weeks	182	48	41

Another helpful guideline for daily water consumption is 3.8 liters (one U.S. gallon or 0.8 Imp. gallon) of water per week of age per 1000 poults; figure 40% of this amount. This 40% is about a three-hour supply for the flock.

Distribute 1,000 doses of vaccine in water as used by 1,000 turkeys or 5000 doses of vaccine in water as used by 5000 turkeys. Provide ample water space so that all turkeys can drink easily. Do not administer through water lines with a proportioner or medication tank.

Records: Keep a record of vaccine type, quantity, serial number, expiration date, and place of purchase; the date and time of vaccination; the number, age, breed, and location of the birds; names of operators performing the vaccination and any observed reactions.

Contraindication(s): Turkeys must be healthy and free of environmental or physical stress at the time of vaccination. To avoid interference with development of protection, turkeys to be vaccinated should not be given any antibiotic and/or sulfonamide medication for 3 days before and 5 days after vaccination.

Precaution(s): Store at 2° to 7°C (35° to 45°F).

Do not dilute the vaccine or otherwise stretch the dosage.

Do not spill or splatter the vaccine. Use entire contents of vial when first opened. Burn empty bottles, caps and all unused vaccine and accessories.

Caution(s): Vaccinate only healthy birds. Although disease may not be evident, coccidiosis, respiratory disease, mycoplasma infection, or other disease conditions may cause complications or reduce protection.

All birds within a flock should be vaccinated on the same day.

Vaccination in the face of an acute outbreak is not recommended. Under these conditions, use an effective colibacillosis treatment, wait at least 5 days or until the outbreak subsides and then vaccinate.

Birds infected with *E coli* at time of hatch require treatment with an effective day of age antibiotic injection. This vaccine is not a replacement for day of age antibiotic treatment but should be considered as a part of an effective *E coli* prevention program.

For veterinary use only.

Warning(s): Do not vaccinate within 21 days before slaughter.

Wash hands thoroughly after using the vaccine.

Discussion: Vaccination Program: The development of a durable, strong protection against this disease depends upon the use of an effective vaccination program as well as many circumstances such as administration techniques, environment and flock health at time of vaccination. Also, the immune response to one vaccination under field conditions is seldom compete for all birds within a given flock. Even when vaccination is successful, the protection stimulated in individual birds against different diseases may not be life long. Therefore, a program of periodic revaccination may be necessary.

Presentation: 1000 dose and 5000 dose vials.

Compendium Code No.: 10470941

GASTRO-COTE

Butler **Adsorbent**

Active Ingredient(s): Contains:

Bismuth subsalicylate 1.75%

Indications: A palatable oral solution for use as an aid in the control of nonspecific diarrhea by protecting the intestinal mucosa thus lessening the irritation and hyperperistalsis; also acts as an adsorbent to counter the effects of toxins in the gastro-intestinal tract of cattle, horses, dogs and cats.

Dosage and Administration: Shake well before using. The dose may be repeated until the condition improves.

Horses and Cattle: 6-10 ounces every two (2) to three (3) hours.

Foals and Calves: 3-4 ounces every two (2) to three (3) hours.

Dogs and Cats: 1-3 tablespoons every one (1) to three (3) hours.

Administration: Oral.

Precaution(s): Store at 2° to 30°C (36°-86°F). Keep from freezing.

Caution(s): For veterinary use only.

Keep out of the reach of children.

If symptoms persist after using the product for two to three days, consult a veterinarian.

Presentation: 1 gallon (3.79 L) containers.

Compendium Code No.: 10820800

GASTROGARD® ℞

Merial **Anti-ulcer**

(omeprazole) Oral Paste for Equine Ulcers

NADA No.: 141-123

Active Ingredient(s): GASTROGARD® Paste for horses contains 37% w/w omeprazole. Each syringe contains 2.28 g of omeprazole.

Indications: For treatment and prevention of recurrence of gastric ulcers in horses and foals 4 weeks of age and older.

Pharmacology: Description:

Chemical name: 5-Methoxy-2-[[(4-methoxy-3,5-dimethyl-2-pyridinyl) methyl]sulfinyl]-1-*H*-benzimidazole. Empirical formula: $C_{17}H_{19}N_3O_3S$. Molecular weight: 345.42.

Structural formula:

Clinical Pharmacology:

Mechanism of Action: Omeprazole is a gastric acid pump inhibitor that regulates the final step in hydrogen ion production and blocks gastric acid secretion regardless of the stimulus. Omeprazole irreversibly binds to the gastric parietal cell's H+, K+ ATPase enzyme which pumps hydrogen ions into the lumen of the stomach in exchange for potassium ions. Since omeprazole accumulates in the cell cannaliculi and is irreversibly bound to the effect site, the plasma concentration at steady state is not directly related to the amount that is bound to the enzyme. The relationship between omeprazole action and plasma concentration is a function of the rate-limiting process of H+, K+ ATPase activity/turnover. Once all of the enzyme becomes bound, acid secretion resumes only after new H+, K+ ATPase is synthesized in the parietal cell (i.e., the rate of new enzyme synthesis exceeds the rate of inhibition).

Pharmacodynamics: In a study of pharmacodynamic effects using horses with gastric cannulae, secretion of gastric acid was inhibited in horses given 4 mg omeprazole/kg/day. After the expected maximum suppression of gastric acid secretion was reached (5 days), the actual secretion of gastric acid was reduced by 99%, 95% and 90% at 8, 16, and 24 hours, respectively.

Pharmacokinetics: In a pharmacokinetic study involving thirteen healthy, mixed breed horses (8 female, 5 male) receiving multiple doses of omeprazole paste (1.8 mg/lb once daily for fifteen days) in either a fed or fasted state, there was no evidence of drug accumulation in the plasma when comparing the extent of systemic exposure ($AUC_{0-\infty}$). When comparing the individual bioavailability data ($AUC_{0-\infty}$, C_{max}, and T_{max} measurements) across the study days, there was great inter- and intrasubject variability in the rate and extent of product absorption. Also, the extent of omeprazole absorption in horses was reduced by approximately 67% in the presence of food. This is evidenced by the observation that the mean ($AUC_{0-\infty}$) values measured during the fifth day of omeprazole therapy when the animals were fasted for 24 hours was approximately three times greater than the AUC estimated after the first and fifteenth doses when the horses were fed hay ad libitum and sweet feed (grain) twice daily. Prandial status did not affect the rate of drug elimination. The terminal half-life estimates (N=38) ranged from approximately one-half to eight hours.

Dosage and Administration: Dosage Regimen: For treatment of gastric ulcers, GASTROGARD® Paste should be administered orally once-a-day for 4 weeks at the recommended dosage of 1.8 mg omeprazole/lb body weight (4 mg/kg). For the prevention of recurrence of ulcers, continue treatment for at least an additional 4 weeks by administering GASTROGARD® Paste at the recommended daily maintenance dose of 0.9 mg/lb (2 mg/kg).

Directions for Use: GASTROGARD® Paste for horses is recommended for use in horses and foals 4 weeks of age and older. The contents of one syringe will dose a 1250 lb (568 kg) horse at the rate of 1.8 mg omeprazole/lb body weight (4 mg/kg). For treatment of gastric ulcers, each weight marking on the syringe plunger will deliver sufficient omeprazole to treat 250 lb (114 kg) body weight. For prevention of recurrence of gastric ulcers, each weight marking will deliver sufficient omeprazole to dose 500 lb (227 kg) body weight.

To deliver GASTROGARD® Paste at the treatment dose rate of 1.8 mg omeprazole/lb body weight (4 mg/kg), set the syringe plunger to the appropriate weight marking according to the horse's weight in pounds.

To deliver GASTROGARD® Paste at the dose rate of 0.9 mg/lb (2 mg/kg) to prevent recurrence of ulcers, set the syringe plunger to the weight marking corresponding to half of the horse's weight in pounds.

To set the syringe plunger, unlock the knurled ring by rotating it ¼ turn. Slide the knurled ring along the plunger shaft so that the side nearest the barrel is at the appropriate notch. Rotate the plunger ring ¼ turn to lock it in place and ensure it is locked. Make sure the horse's mouth contains no feed. Remove the cover from the tip of the syringe, and insert the syringe into the horse's mouth at the interdental space. Depress the plunger until stopped by the knurled ring. The dose should be deposited on the back of the tongue or deep into the cheek pouch. Care should be taken to ensure that the horse consumes the complete dose. Treated animals should be observed briefly after administration to ensure that part of the dose is not lost or rejected. If any of the dose is lost, redosing is recommended.

If, after dosing, the syringe is not completely empty, it may be reused on following days until emptied. Replace the cap after each use.

Precaution(s): Store below 86°F (30°C). Transient exposure to temperatures up to 104°F (40°C) is permitted.

Caution(s): Federal (USA) law restricts this drug to use by or on the order of a licensed veterinarian.

The safety of GASTROGARD® Paste has not been determined in pregnant or lactating mares.

Warning(s): Do not use in horses intended for human consumption. Keep this and all drugs out of the reach of children. In case of ingestion, contact a physician. Physicians may contact a poison control center for advice concerning accidental ingestion.

Adverse Reactions: In efficacy trials, when the drug was administered at 1.8 mg omeprazole/lb (4 mg/kg) body weight daily for 28 days and 0.9 mg omeprazole/lb (2 mg/kg) body weight daily for 30 additional days, no adverse reactions were observed.

Trial Data: Efficacy:

Dose Confirmation: GASTROGARD® Paste, administered to provide omeprazole at 1.8 mg/lb (4 mg/kg) daily for 28 days, effectively healed or reduced the severity of gastric ulcers in 92% of omeprazole-treated horses. In comparison, 32% of controls exhibited healed or less severe ulcers. Horses enrolled in this study were healthy animals confirmed to have gastric ulcers by gastroscopy. Subsequent daily administration of GASTROGARD® Paste to provide omeprazole at 0.9 mg/lb (2 mg/kg) for 30 days prevented recurrence of gastric ulcers in 84% of treated horses, whereas ulcers recurred or became more severe were in horses removed from omeprazole treatment.

Clinical Field Trials: GASTROGARD® Paste administered at 1.8 mg/lb (4 mg/kg) daily for 28 days healed or reduced severity of gastric ulcers in 99% of omeprazole-treated horses. In comparison, 32.4% of control horses had healed ulcers or ulcers which were reduced in severity. These trials included horses of various breeds and under different management conditions, and included horses in race or show training, pleasure horses, and foals as young as one month. Horses enrolled in the efficacy trials were healthy animals confirmed to have gastric ulcers by gastroscopy. In these field trials, horses readily accepted GASTROGARD® Paste. There were no drug related adverse reactions. In the clinical trials, GASTROGARD® Paste was used concomitantly with other therapies, which included: anthelmintics, antibiotics, non-steroidal and steroidal anti-inflammatory agents, diuretics, tranquilizers and vaccines.

Diagnostic and Management Considerations: The following clinical signs may be associated with gastric ulceration in adult horses: inappetence or decreased appetite, recurrent colic, intermittent loose stools or chronic diarrhea, poor hair coat, poor body condition, or poor performance. Clinical signs in foals may include: bruxism (grinding of teeth), excess salivation, colic, cranial abdominal tenderness, anorexia, diarrhea, sternal recumbency or weakness. A more accurate diagnosis of gastric ulceration in horses and foals may be made if ulcers are visualized directly by endoscopic examination of the gastric mucosa.

Gastric ulcers may recur in horses if therapy to prevent recurrence is not administered after the initial treatment is completed. Use GASTROGARD® Paste at 0.9 mg omeprazole/lb body weight (2 mg/kg) for control of gastric ulcers following treatment. The safety of administration of GASTROGARD® Paste for longer than 91 days has not been determined.

Maximal acid suppression occurs after three to five days of treatment with omeprazole.

Safety: GASTROGARD® Paste was well tolerated in the following controlled efficacy and safety studies.

In field trials involving 139 horses, including foals as young as one month of age, no adverse reactions attributable to omeprazole treatment were noted.

In a placebo controlled adult horse safety study, horses received 20 mg/kg/day omeprazole (5X the recommended dose) for 90 days. No treatment related adverse effects were observed.

In a placebo controlled tolerance study, adult horses were treated with GASTROGARD® Paste at a dosage of 40 mg/kg/day (10X the recommended dose) for 21 days. No treatment related adverse effects were observed.

A placebo controlled foal safety study evaluated the safety of omeprazole at doses of 4, 12 or 20 mg/kg (1, 3, or 5X) once daily for 91 days. Foals ranged in age from 66 to 110 days at study initiation. Gamma glutamyltransferase (GGT) levels were significantly elevated in horses treated at exaggerated doses of 20 mg/kg (5X the recommended dose). Mean stomach to body weight ratio was higher for foals in the 3X and 5X groups than for controls; however, no abnormalities of the stomach were evident on histological examination.

Reproductive Safety: In a male reproductive safety study, 10 stallions received GASTROGARD® Paste at 12 mg/kg/day (3X the recommended dose) for 70 days. No treatment related adverse effects on semen quality or breeding behavior were observed. A safety study in breeding mares has not been conducted.

Presentation: GASTROGARD® Paste for horses is available in an adjustable-dose syringe. Syringes are calibrated according to body weight and are available in boxes of 7 or 72 units.
GASTROGARD is a registered trademark of the AstraZeneca Group of Companies.
(Merial Limited: Registered in England and Wales [Reg. No. 3332751] with registered offices at 27 Knightsbridge, London, SW1X 7QT, England and domesticated in Delaware, USA as Merial LLC).
U.S. Patent Nos. 4,255,431 and 5,708,017
9201103
Compendium Code No.: 11110201

GASTRO-SORB™ BOLUS

Butler **Adsorbent**

NDC No.: 11695-4114-3
Active Ingredient(s): Each bolus contains: Activated attapulgite, carob flour, pectin, and magnesium trisilicate, in a suitable base.
Indications: For use as an aid in relief of simple noninfectious diarrhea in horses and cattle.
Dosage and Administration: Administer orally. Give two (2) boluses to adult cattle and horses. Give one (1) bolus to calves and foals.

Repeat the treatment at 4- to 6-hour intervals as needed. Discontinue use of the product after three (3) days. If symptoms persist after using the preparation for three (3) days, consult a veterinarian.
Precaution(s): Store a room temperature between 15° and 30°C (59°-86°F).
Caution(s): For animal use only.

Keep out of the reach of children.
Presentation: 50 boluses.
Compendium Code No.: 10820810

GASTRO-SORB™ CALF BOLUS

Butler **Antidiarrheal-Adsorbent**

NDC No.: 11695-4130-3
Active Ingredient(s): Each bolus contains: Activated attapulgite, carob flour, pectin, and magnesium trisilicate, in a suitable base.
Indications: An antidiarrheal and demulcent for use as an aid in relief of simple noninfectious diarrhea in colts and calves.
Dosage and Administration: Administer orally. Give two (2) boluses to calves and foals.

Repeat treatment at 4 to 6 hour intervals as needed. Discontinue use of product after 3 days. If symptoms persist after using the preparation for 3 days, consult a veterinarian.
Precaution(s): Store a room temperature between 15°C and 30°C (59°F-86°F).
Warning(s): For animal use only.

Keep out of the reach of children.
Presentation: 50 boluses.
Compendium Code No.: 10820820

GAUGE™ C&D

AgriPharm **Toxoid**

Clostridium Perfringens Types C & D Bacterin-Toxoid
U.S. Vet. Lic. No.: 124
Description: *Clostridium Perfringens* Types C & D Toxoid. GAUGE™ C&D toxoid is prepared from chemically inactivated cultures of the above organisms.
Indications: Uses: GAUGE™ C&D is recommended for vaccination of healthy, susceptible cattle and sheep as an aid in the reduction of enterotoxemia caused by the toxins of *Cl. perfringens* types B, C, D.
Dosage and Administration: Using aseptic technique inject a 2 mL dose. Repeat in 21 to 28 days. A 2 mL booster dose is recommended annually.
Precaution(s): Store at 35°-45°F (2°-7°C). Avoid freezing. Shake well before using. Use entire contents when first opened.
Caution(s): Anaphylactoid reactions may occur.
Antidote(s): Epinephrine.
Warning(s): Do not vaccinate within 21 days of slaughter.

Animals inoculation only. Accidental injection in humans can cause serious local reactions. Contact a physician immediately if accidental injection occurs.
Presentation: 50 dose (100 mL) and 250 dose (500 mL) bottles.
Compendium Code No.: 14571290

GELMATE

V.D.I. **Inflammation Test**

Active Ingredient(s): Each tube contains stabilized glutaraldehyde, EDTA, a wetting agent and a partial vacuum.
Indications: GELMATE is used for the detection of acute or chronic inflammation in horses and farm animals.
Test Principle: The GELMATE test is for the detection of acute and chronic inflammation in horses and farm animals. The test works on the principle that glutaraldehyde reacts with gammaglobulin (GG) and fibrinogen in whole blood to form a solid gel. The higher the concentrations of these proteins, the quicker the reaction occurs. Each tube contains stabilized glutaraldehyde, EDTA, a wetting agent and a partial vacuum.
Test Procedure: To perform the test, collect a blood sample by attaching a needle to a standard blood collection tube holder. Insert the GELMATE tube into the holder and, via venipuncture, draw whole blood into the tube to the level of the blue line. The vacuum is adjusted so that the correct amount of blood will be drawn in. If this does not occur, discard the tube.

As soon as the blood enters the tube, note the time. Periodically (every minute or so) tilt the tube and observe for gel formation (the sample will turn solid). Note the time and calculate the amount of time it takes to clot.

Interpretation:
1. Solid clot formation in less than five (5) minutes indicates severe inflammation.
2. Clot formation in 5-10 minutes indicates moderate inflammation.
3. Clot formation in 10-15 minutes indicates mild inflammation.
4. Clot formation in >15 minutes represents essentially normal conditions.

Typical Gammaglobulin and Fibrinogen Levels:
1. A clot time in less than five (5) minutes will usually be caused by fibrinogen over 700 mg/dl and gammaglobulin over 3,000 mg/dl.
2. A clot time of 5-10 minutes would have a fibrinogen of 500-700 mg/dl and a GG of 2,500 mg/dl.
3. A clot time of 10-15 minutes will have a fibrinogen of 300-500 mg/dl and a gammaglobulin level of 2,000-2,500 mg/dl.

Conditions which could cause these gammaglobulin and fibrinogen levels:
Cattle:
1. Traumatic reticuloperitonitis
2. Pleurisy
3. Purulent bronchopneumonia
4. Tuberculosis
5. Peritonitis
6. Purulent mastitis
7. Fibrinous pneumonia

Horses:
1. Pleurisy
2. Peritonitis
3. *Corynebacterium pseudotuberculosis* infections
4. Pelvic, liver and kidney abscesses

Pigs:
1. Abscesses
2. Infected joints

Other species: Feedback on the use of the test in other species is welcome and where possible back-up laboratory analysis on blood samples showing a rapid gel time will be provided. Call (800) 654-9743 for details. Because the test is not species specific, it will be helpful in any animal.
Precaution(s): Store at 4°C.
Caution(s): False readings can occur in cases of severe anaemia (excessive plasma) or severe dehydration (abnormally low level of plasma).

A cow with a normal appetite will sometimes show a rapid gel time if there is an internal problem which is completely walled off. These cows are not likely to perform at optimal levels if expected to produce milk. These animals will often show normal temperatures and white cell counts.
References: Available upon request.
Presentation: 10 and 25 tests per kit.
Compendium Code No.: 11280061

GENERAL LUBE

A.A.H. **Lubricant**

Non-Sterile Lubricating Jelly
Ingredient(s): Deionized water, sodium carboxy methylcellulose, propylene glycol, propyl and methyl parahydroxybenzoate.
Indications: A non-greasy, ready to use lubricant to aid in minimizing irritation to skin and membranes. This product has not been tested for spermicidal activity.
Directions: To be used when performing gynecological procedures and rectal exams. Apply liberally to hands and arms. Maybe used as a lubricant for catheters, instruments, etc.
Precaution(s): Keep from freezing.
Caution(s): For animal use only.
Warning(s): Keep out of reach of children.
Presentation: 4 x 3.78 L (128 fl oz) (1 gal) jugs per case.
Compendium Code No.: 11180220 901

GENERAL LUBE

Aspen **Lubricant**

All Purpose Non-Spermicidal Lubricating Jelly
Ingredient(s): Deionized water, propylene glycol, sodium carboxymethocellulose, methyl and propyl para-hydroxybenzoate.
Indications: A non-sterile, non-spermicidal all purpose lubricating jelly for use when performing gynecological procedures and rectal exams.

The bland lubricating qualities aid in minimizing irritation to both the operator's skin and membranes of the animal.
Dosage and Administration: Apply liberally as needed.
Precaution(s): Store and use at room temperature.
Warning(s): For animal use only.

Keep out of reach of children.
Presentation: 1 gallon (3.785 L).
Compendium Code No.: 14750350

GENERAL LUBE

First Priority **Lubricant**

All Purpose Non-Spermicidal Lubricating Jelly
Ingredient(s): Purified water, propylene glycol, sodium carboxymethocellulose, methyl and propyl parahydroxybenzoate.
Indications: A non-sterile, non-spermicidal all purpose lubricating jelly for use when performing gynecological procedures and rectal exams.

The bland lubricating qualities aid in minimizing irritation to both the operator's skin and the membranes of the animal.
Directions for Use: Apply liberally as needed.
Precaution(s): Store and use at room temperature.
Caution(s): For animal use only.
Warning(s): Keep out of reach of children.
Presentation: 8 fl oz (240 mL), 1 gallon (3.785 L) (NDC# 58829-150-01) and 2.5 gallons (9.46 L).
Compendium Code No.: 11390332 Rev. 4-01

GEN-GARD™ SOLUBLE POWDER

AgriLabs **Water Medication**

Gentamicin Sulfate Soluble Powder-Antibacterial
ANADA No.: 200-185
Active Ingredient(s): Each g Contains: Gentamicin sulfate equivalent to 333.33 mg gentamicin base.
Indications: GEN-GARD™ Soluble Powder is recommended for the control and treatment of colibacillosis in weanling swine caused by strains of *E. coli* sensitive to gentamicin, and for the control and treatment of swine dysentery associated with *Treponema hyodysenteriae.*
Dosage and Administration:

Colibacillosis - 1 level scoop per 240 gallons of drinking water for 3 consecutive days,

0.5 mg/lb/day. For proportioner use, add 1 level scoop to 2 gallons stock solution and dispense at the rate of 1 oz/gal drinking water (25 mg/gal).

Swine Dysentery - 1 level scoop per 120 gallons of drinking water for 3 consecutive days, 1.0 mg/lb/day. For proportioner use, add 1 level scoop to 1 gallon stock solution and dispense at the rate of 1 oz/gal drinking water (50 mg/gal).

Precaution(s): Do not store or offer medicated water in rusty metal containers.

Store between 2° and 30°C (36° and 86°F).

Caution(s): For use in swine drinking water only.

Restricted Drug (California).

Use only as directed.

For use in animals only.

Warning(s): Residue Warning: Swine treated with the recommended dose of GEN-GARD™ Soluble Powder must not be slaughtered for food for at least ten (10) days following the last treatment.

Keep out of reach of children.

Presentation: 360 g (12.7 oz) jar.

Compendium Code No.: 10580551 Issue Date 4/97

GENOTIC B-C™ ℞

Butler **Otic Antifungal-Antimicrobial-Corticosteroid**

(Gentamicin Sulfate, Betamethasone Valerate, USP and Clotrimazole, USP Ointment)

ANADA No.: 200-229

Active Ingredient(s): Each gram contains: gentamicin sulfate equivalent to 3 mg gentamicin base, betamethasone valerate, USP equivalent to 1 mg betamethasone; and 10 mg clotrimazole, USP in a mineral oil-based system containing a plasticized hydrocarbon gel.

Indications: GENOTIC B-C™ is indicated for the treatment of canine acute and chronic Otitis externa associated with yeast *(Malassezia pachydermatis*, formerly *Pityrosporum canis)* and/or bacteria susceptible to gentamicin.

Pharmacology:

Gentamicin: Gentamicin sulfate is an aminoglycoside antibiotic active against a wide variety of pathogenic gram-negative and gram-positive bacteria. *In vitro* tests have determined that gentamicin is bactericidal and acts by inhibiting normal protein synthesis in susceptible microorganisms. Specifically, gentamicin is active against the following organisms commonly isolated from canine ears: *Staphylococcus aureus*, other *Staphylococcus* spp., *Pseudomonas aeruginosa*, *Proteus* spp., and *Escherichia coli*.

Betamethasone: Betamethasone valerate is a synthetic adrenocorticoid for dermatologic use. Betamethasone, an analog of prednisolone, has a high degree of corticosteroid activity and a slight degree of mineralocorticosteroid activity. Betamethasone valerate, the 17-valerate ester of betamethasone, has been shown to provide anti-inflammatory and anti-pruritic activity in the topical management of corticosteroid-responsive otitis externa. Topical corticosteroids can be absorbed from normal, intact skin. Inflammation can increase percutaneous absorption. Once absorbed through the skin, topical corticosteroids are handled through pharmacokinetic pathways similar to systemically administered corticosteroids.

Clotrimazole: Clotrimazole is a broad-spectrum antifungal agent that is used for the treatment of dermal infections caused by various species of pathogenic dermatophytes and yeasts. The primary action of clotrimazole is against dividing and growing organisms.

In vitro, clotrimazole exhibits fungistatic and fungicidal activity against isolates of *Trichophyton rubrum, Trichophyton mentagrophytes, Epidermophyton floccosum, Microsporum canis, Candida* spp. and *Malassezia pachydermatis (Pityrosporum canis)*. Resistance to clotrimazole is very rare among the fungi that cause superficial mycoses.

In an induced otitis externa infected with *Malassezia pachydermatis*, 1% clotrimazole in the gentamicin-betamethasone-clotrimazole ointment vehicle was effective both microbiologically and clinically in terms of reduction of exudate odor and swelling.

In studies of the mechanism of action, the minimum fungicidal concentration of clotrimazole caused leakage of intracellular phosphorus compounds into the ambient medium with concomitant breakdown of cellular nucleic acids and accelerated potassium efflux. These events began rapidly and extensively after addition of the drug. Clotrimazole is very poorly absorbed following dermal application.

Gentamicin-Betamethasone-Clotrimazole: By virtue of its three active ingredients, gentamicin-betamethasone-clotrimazole ointment has antibacterial, anti-inflammatory, and antifungal activity.

In component efficacy studies, the compatibility and additive effect of each of the components were demonstrated. In clinical field trials, gentamicin-betamethasone-clotrimazole was effective in the treatment of otitis externa associated with bacteria and *Malassezia pachydermatis*. Gentamicin sulfate USP, betamethasone valerate, USP and clotrimazole, USP ointment reduced discomfort, redness, swelling, exudate, and odor, and exerted a strong antimicrobial effect.

Dosage and Administration: The external ear should be thoroughly cleaned and dried before treatment. Remove foreign material, debris, crusted exudates, etc., with suitable non-irritating solutions. Excessive hair should be clipped from the treatment area. After verifying that the eardrum is intact, instill 4 drops (2 drops from the 215 g bottle) of gentamicin-betamethasone-clotrimazole ointment twice daily into the ear canal of dogs weighing less than 30 lbs. Instill 8 drops (4 drops from the 215 g bottle) twice daily into the ear canal of dogs weighing 30 lbs or more. Massage external ear canal carefully after instillation to ensure appropriate distribution of medication. Therapy should continue for 7 consecutive days.

Contraindication(s): If hypersensitivity to any of the components occurs, treatment should be discontinued and appropriate therapy instituted. Concomitant use of drugs known to induce ototoxicity should be avoided. Do not use in dogs with known perforation of eardrums.

Precaution(s): Store between 2°C and 25°C (36°F and 77°F).

Shake well before use.

Caution(s): Federal law restricts this drug to use by or on the order of a licensed veterinarian.

The use of gentamicin-betamethasone-clotrimazole ointment has been associated with deafness or partial hearing loss in a small number of sensitive dogs (eg. geriatric). The hearing deficit is usually temporary. If hearing or vestibular dysfunction is noted during the course of treatment, discontinue use of gentamicin-betamethasone-clotrimazole ointment immediately and flush the ear canal thoroughly with a non-ototoxic solution. Corticosteroids administered to dogs, rabbits, and rodents during pregnancy have resulted in cleft palate in offspring. Other congenital anomalies including deformed forelegs, phocomelia, and anasarca have been reported in offspring of dogs which received corticosteroids during pregnancy.

Clinical and experimental data have demonstrated that corticosteroids administered orally or parenterally to animals may induce the first stage of parturition if used during the last trimester of pregnancy and may precipitate premature parturition followed by dystocia, fetal death, retained placenta and metritis.

Identification of infecting organisms should be made either by microscopic roll smear evaluation or by culture as appropriate. Antibiotic susceptibility of the pathogenic organism(s) should be determined prior to use of this preparation.

If overgrowth of nonsusceptible bacteria, fungi or yeasts occur, or if hypersensitivity develops, treatment should be discontinued and appropriate therapy instituted.

Administration of recommended doses of gentamicin-betamethasone-clotrimazole ointment beyond 7 days may result in delayed wound healing.

Avoid ingestion. Adverse systemic reactions have been observed following the oral ingestion of some topical corticosteroid preparations. Patients should be closely observed for the usual signs of adrenocorticoid overdosage which include sodium retention, potassium loss, fluid retention, weight gain, polydipsia and/or polyuria. Prolonged use or overdosage may produce adverse immunosuppressive effects.

Use of corticosteroids, depending on dose, duration, and specific steroid, may result in endogenous steroid production inhibition following drug withdrawal. In patients presently receiving or recently withdrawn from corticosteroid treatments, therapy with a rapidly acting corticosteroid should be considered in especially stressful situations.

Before instilling any medication into the ear, examine the external ear canal thoroughly to be certain the tympanic membrane is not ruptured in order to avoid the possibility of transmitting infection to the middle ear as well as damaging the cochlea or vestibular apparatus from prolonged contact.

For otic use in dogs only.

Keep out of reach of children.

Toxicology: Clinical and safety studies with gentamicin sulfate USP, betamethasone valerate, USP and clotrimazole, USP ointment have shown a wide safety margin at the recommended dose level in dogs (see Cautions/Side Effects).

Side Effects:

Gentamicin: While aminoglycosides are absorbed poorly from skin, intoxication may occur when aminoglycosides are applied topically for prolonged periods of time to large wounds, burns, or any denuded skin, particularly if there is renal insufficiency. All aminoglycosides have the potential to produce reversible and irreversible vestibular, cochlear and renal toxicity.

Betamethasone: Side effects such as SAP and SGPT enzyme elevations, weight loss, anorexia, polydipsia, and polyuria have occurred following the use of parenteral or systemic synthetic corticosteroids in dogs. Vomiting and diarrhea (occasionally bloody) have been observed in dogs and cats.

Cushing's syndrome in dogs has been reported in association with prolonged or repeated steroid therapy.

Clotrimazole: The following have been reported occasionally in humans in connection with the use of clotrimazole: erythema, stinging, blistering, peeling, edema, pruritus, urticaria, and general irritation of the skin not present before therapy.

Presentation: 12x7.5 g, 12x15 g and 215 g tubes.

Manufactured by: Med-Pharmex Inc., Pomona, California

Compendium Code No.: 10820830

GENTADIP

Med-Pharmex **Egg Dip Concentrate**

(Gentamicin Sulfate Solution) 50 mg/mL-For Turkey Egg Dipping

ANADA No.: 200-191

Active Ingredient(s): Each milliliter of Gentamicin Sulfate Solution for Turkey Egg Dipping contains gentamicin sulfate equivalent to 50 mg gentamicin base, 3.2 mg sodium bisulfite, 0.1 mg edetate disodium, 7.46 mg sodium acetate, 3.0 mg glacial acetic acid; 1.8 mg methylparaben and 0.2 mg propylparaben as preservatives, purified water q.s.

Indications: Gentamicin Sulfate for Turkey Egg Dipping is recommended as an aid in the reduction or elimination of the following microorganisms from turkey hatching eggs: *Arizona hinshawii* (paracolon), *Salmonella st. paul, Mycoplasma meleagridis*.

Pharmacology: Chemistry: Gentamicin Sulfate is a bactericidal aminoglycoside antibiotic derived from *Micromonospora purpurea* of the Actinomycetes group. It is a powder, readily soluble in water and basic in nature. Gentamicin aqueous solutions do not require refrigeration and are stable over a wide range of temperatures and pH.

Directions for Use: Gentamicin Sulfate Solution should be added to clean water to provide a dip solution with a gentamicin concentration of 250 to 1000 ppm. A gentamicin concentration of 500 ppm is recommended.

To make a solution of approximately 500 ppm gentamicin activity, mix one bottle of Gentamicin Sulfate Solution for Turkey Egg Dipping to each 2 gallons of water.

Mixing Chart:

Gentamicin ppm	Water Gallons	Grams Gentamicin Needed	Bottles Gentamicin Sol. to be added
250	4	4	1
	40	40	10
	80	80	20
500	2	4	1
	40	80	20
	80	160	40
1000	1	4	1
	40	160	40
	80	320	80

Egg dipping procedures - These are general suggestions and will vary with equipment and operator.

Temperature differential method - clean eggs should be warmed 3 to 6 hours at approximately 100°F, then immediately dipped in gentamicin solution maintained at about 40°F and held completely submerged for 10-15 minutes.

Pressure differential method - clean eggs should be held completely submerged in a gentamicin solution under a vacuum of about 27.5-38 cm mercury for 5 minutes, followed by additional soaking in gentamicin solution for approximately 10 minutes at atmospheric pressure.

Egg dipping solutions should be maintained free of dirt and organic contamination. Gentamicin is stable in aqueous solution with the exception of action from microorganisms.

It is recommended that periodically, samples of egg dig solution be sent to a laboratory, such as a State Laboratory, using standard culture techniques to monitor for bacterial, mold or yeast contamination not sensitive to gentamicin.

Since gentamicin sulfate is stable at autoclaving temperatures and pressures, the egg dip solutions may undergo pasteurization procedures to eliminate possible microbial contamination.

Contraindication(s): There are no known contraindications for Gentamicin Sulfate Solution for Turkey Egg Dipping when used as directed.

Precaution(s): Store between 15° and 30°C (59°F and 86°F).
Caution(s): Filters composed of cellulose, diatomaceous earth or asbestos may remove significant amounts of gentamicin from the dipping solution during filtration.

It is recommended that egg dip solutions be analyzed for antibiotic concentration to establish whether the filtering system is removing a significant amount of antibiotic.
Warning(s): For use in the dipping treatment of turkey hatching eggs only. Eggs which have been dipped in Gentamicin Sulphate solution should not be used for food.
Presentation: Gentamicin Sulfate Solution for Turkey Egg Dipping, 50 mg/ml, is available in 2⅔ fl oz (80 mL) screw top bottles.
Compendium Code No.: 10270041

GENTA-FUSE ℞

Vetus **Gentamicin**

Gentamicin Sulfate 100 mg/mL
ANADA No.: 200-115
Active Ingredient(s): Each mL of GENTA-FUSE (Gentamicin sulfate) contains: gentamicin sulfate equivalent to 100 mg gentamicin base; 2.4 mg sodium metabisulfite; 0.8 mg sodium sulfite, anhydrous; 0.1 mg edetate disodium; 10 mg benzyl alcohol as preservative; water for injection q.s.
Indications: For use in horses only. GENTA-FUSE is recommended for the control of bacterial infections of the uterus (metritis) in horses and as an aid in improving conception in mares with uterine infections caused by bacteria sensitive to gentamicin.

Bacteriologic studies should be conducted to identify the causative organism and to determine its sensitivity to gentamicin sulfate.
Pharmacology: Chemistry: Gentamicin is a mixture of aminoglycoside antibiotics derived from the fermentation of *Micromonospora purpurea.* Gentamicin sulfate is a mixture of sulfate salts of the antibiotics produced in this fermentation. The salts are weakly acidic, freely soluble in water, and stable in solution.

Antibacterial Activity: *In vitro* activity has shown that gentamicin is active against most gram-negative and gram-positive bacterial isolated from domestic animals. Gentamicin is active against *Pseudomonas aeruginosa,* indole-positive and -negative *Proteus* species, *Escherichia coli, Klebsiella* species, *Enterobacter* species, *Alcaligenes* species, *Staphylococcus* species, and *Streptococcus* species.

Studies in man indicate that recommended doses of gentamicin produce serum concentrations bactericidal for most bacteria sensitive to gentamicin within an hour after intramuscular injection; these concentrations last for 6 to 12 hours. Some 30% of the administered dose of gentamicin is bound by serum proteins and released as the drug is excreted.

Gentamicin is excreted almost entirely by glomerular filtration. High concentrations of the active form are found in the urine. Fifty to 100% of the gentamicin injected can be recovered unchanged within 24 hours from the urine of patients with normal renal function. A small amount is excreted into the bile.
Dosage and Administration: The recommended dose is 20 to 25 mL (2.0 - 2.5 grams) GENTA-FUSE (Gentamicin Sulfate) per day for 3 to 5 days during estrus. Each dose should be diluted with 200-500 mL of sterile physiological saline before aseptic uterine infusion.
Contraindication(s): There are no known contraindications to this drug when used as directed.
Precaution(s): Store between 2° and 30°C (36° and 86°F).

Protect from freezing.
Caution(s): Federal law restricts this drug to use by or on the order of a licensed veterinarian.

If hypersensitivity to any of the components develops, or if overgrowth of non-susceptible bacteria, fungi, or yeasts occurs, treatment with GENTA-FUSE (Gentamicin sulfate) should be discontinued and appropriate therapy instituted. Although gentamicin sulfate is not spermicidal, treatment should not be given the day of breeding.
Warning(s): Not for use in horses intended for food.
Toxicology: No toxic effects were observed in rats given gentamicin sulfate 20 mg/kg/day for 24 days; in cats given 10 mg/kg/day for forty days. Gentamicin sulfate given to dogs at 6 mg/kg/day, 6 days weekly for 3 weeks, caused no detectable kidney damage. At higher doses, impairment of equilibrium and renal function were observed in these species.
Side Effects: There have been no reports of drug hypersensitivity or adverse side effects following the recommended intra-uterine infusion of gentamicin sulfate combined with sterile physiological saline in mares.
References: Available upon request.
Presentation: 100 mL multiple-dose vials.
Compendium Code No.: 14440380

GENTAMAX™ 100 ℞

Phoenix Pharmaceutical **Gentamicin**

(Gentamicin Sulfate Solution) 100 mg per mL
ANADA No.: 200-137
Active Ingredient(s): Each mL of GENTAMAX™ 100 (Gentamicin Sulfate Solution) contains: Gentamicin sulfate equivalent to 100 mg gentamicin base; 3.2 mg sodium metabisulfite; 0.1 mg edetate disodium; 1.8 mg methylparaben and 0.2 mg propylparaben as preservatives; water for injection q.s.
Indications: GENTAMAX™ 100 (Gentamicin Sulfate Solution) is recommended for the control of bacterial infections of the uterus (metritis) in horses and as an aid in improving conception in mares with uterine infections caused by bacteria sensitive to gentamicin.

Bacteriologic studies should be conducted to identify the causative organism and to determine its sensitivity to gentamicin sulfate. Sensitivity discs of the drug are available for this purpose.
Pharmacology: Chemistry: Gentamicin is a mixture of aminoglycoside antibiotics derived from the fermentation of *Micromonospora purpurea.* Gentamicin sulfate is a mixture of sulfate salts of the antibiotics produced in this fermentation. The salts are weakly acidic, freely soluble in water, and stable in solution.

Antibacterial Activity: *In vitro* antibacterial activity has shown that gentamicin is active against most gram-negative and gram-positive bacteria isolated from domestic animals.[1] Gentamicin is active against *Pseudomonas aeruginosa,* indole-positive and -negative *Proteus* species, *Escherichia coli, Klebsiella* species, *Enterobacter* species, *Alcaligenes* species, *Staphylococcus* species, and *Streptococcus* species.

Studies in man indicate that recommended doses of gentamicin produce serum concentrations bactericidal for most bacteria sensitive to gentamicin within an hour after intramuscular injection; these concentrations last for 6 to 12 hours.[2] Some 30% of the administered dose of gentamicin is bound by serum proteins and released as the drug is excreted.

Gentamicin is excreted almost entirely by glomerular filtration. High concentrations of the active form are found in the urine. Fifty to 100% of the gentamicin injected can be recovered unchanged within 24 hours from the urine of patients with normal renal function. A small amount is excreted into the bile.
Dosage and Administration: The recommended dose is 20 to 25 mL (2.0-2.5 grams) gentamicin sulfate solution per day for 3 to 5 days during estrus. Each dose should be diluted with 200-500 mL of sterile physiological saline before aseptic uterine infusion.
Contraindication(s): There are no known contraindications to this drug when used as directed.
Precaution(s): Store between 2° and 30°C (36° and 86°F). Protect from freezing.
Caution(s): Federal law restricts this drug to use by or on the order of a licensed veterinarian.

If hypersensitivity to any of the components develops, or if an overgrowth of nonsusceptible bacteria, fungi, or yeasts occurs, treatment with GENTAMAX™ 100 (Gentamicin Sulfate Solution) should be discontinued and appropriate therapy instituted.

Although GENTAMAX™ 100 (Gentamicin Sulfate Solution) is not spermicidal, treatment should not be given the day of breeding. For intra-uterine use in horses only.
Warning(s): Not for use in horses intended for food.
Toxicology: Toxicity Studies: No toxic effects were observed in rats given gentamicin sulfate 20 mg/kg/day for 24 days; in cats given 10 mg/kg/day for 40 days. Gentamicin sulfate given to dogs at 6 mg/lb/day, 6 days weekly for 3 weeks, caused no detectable kidney damage. At higher doses, impairment of equilibrium and renal function were observed in these species.
Side Effects: There have been no reports of drug hypersensitivity or adverse side effects following the recommended intrauterine infusion of gentamicin sulfate solution combined with sterile physiological saline in mares.
References: Available upon request.
Presentation: GENTAMAX™ 100 (Gentamicin Sulfate Solution), 100 mg per mL for intrauterine use, is available in 100 mL (NDC 57319-286-05) and 250 mL (NDC 57319-286-06) multiple dose vials.
Manufactured by: Phoenix Scientific, Inc., St. Joseph, MO 64503
Compendium Code No.: 12560362 Rev. 09-01 / Rev. 01-01

GENTAMICIN OTIC SOLUTION ℞

Butler **Otic Antimicrobial-Corticosteroid**

(Gentamicin Sulfate with Betamethasone Valerate)
ANADA No.: 200-183
Active Ingredient(s): Each mL of GENTAMICIN OTIC SOLUTION contains gentamicin sulfate equivalent to 3 mg gentamicin base, betamethasone valerate equivalent to 1 mg betamethasone, 1.0 mg hydroxyethylcellulose, 2.5 mg glacial acetic acid, 200 mg purified water, 19% ethanol, 9.4 mg benzyl alcohol as preservative, 300 mg glycerin and propylene glycol q.s.
Indications: GENTAMICIN OTIC SOLUTION is indicated for the treatment of acute and chronic canine otitis externa and canine and feline superficial infected lesions caused by bacteria sensitive to gentamicin.
Pharmacology: Chemistry: Gentamicin is a bactericidal antibiotic of the aminoglycoside group derived from *Micromonospora purpurea* of the *Actinomyces* group. It is a powder, white to buff in color, basic in nature, readily soluble in water and highly stable in solution.

Betamethasone valerate is a synthetic corticosteroid derivative of prednisolone.

Action: GENTAMICIN OTIC SOLUTION combines the broad-spectrum activity of gentamicin sulfate with the anti-inflammatory and antipruritic activity of betamethasone valerate. *In vitro* antibacterial activity[1] has shown that gentamicin is active against most gram-negative bacteria including *Pseudomonas aeruginosa,* indole-positive and negative *Proteus* sp., *Escherichia coli, Klebsiella pneumoniae, Aerobacter aerogenes,* and *Neisseria.* Gentamicin is also active against strains of gram-positive bacteria including *Staphylococcus* species and some *Streptococcus* species.

Betamethasone valerate has emerged from intensive research as the most promising of some 50 newly synthesized corticosteroids in the experimental model described by McKenzie[2] *et al.* This human bioassay technique has been found reliable for evaluating the vasoconstrictor properties of new topical corticosteroids and is useful in predicting clinical efficacy.

Betamethasone valerate in human medicine has been shown to provide anti-inflammatory and antipruritic activity in the topical management of corticosteroid-responsive dermatoses. In the responsive cases, the local anti-inflammatory activity is sustained by the vasoconstrictor properties of the steroid.
Dosage and Administration: Duration of treatment will depend upon the severity of the condition and the response obtained. The duration of treatment and/or frequency of the dosage may be reduced, but care should be taken not to discontinue therapy prematurely.

Otitis externa-The external ear and ear canal should be properly cleaned and dried before treatment. Remove foreign material, debris, crusted exudates, etc., with suitable nonirritating solutions. Excessive hair should be clipped from the treatment area of the external ear. Instill 3 to 8 drops of GENTAMICIN OTIC SOLUTION (approximately room temperature) into the ear canal twice daily for seven to fourteen days.

Superficial infected lesions-The lesion and adjacent area should be properly cleaned before treatment. Excessive hair should be removed. Apply a sufficient amount of GENTAMICIN OTIC SOLUTION to cover the treatment area twice daily for seven to fourteen days.
Contraindication(s): If hypersensitivity to any of the components occurs, treatment with this product should be discontinued and appropriate therapy instituted.

Concomitant use of drugs known to induce ototoxicity should be avoided.

This preparation should not be used in conditions where corticosteroids are contraindicated.

Do not administer parenteral corticosteroids during treatment with GENTAMICIN OTIC SOLUTION.
Precaution(s): Store between 2°C and 25°C (36°F and 77°F).
Caution(s): Federal law restricts this drug to use by or on the order of a licensed veterinarian.

Clinical and experimental data have demonstrated that corticosteroids administered orally or parenterally to animals may induce the first stage of parturition when administered during the last trimester of pregnancy and may precipitate premature parturition followed by dystocia, fetal death, retained placenta, and metritis. Additionally, corticosteroids can induce cleft palates in offspring when given to pregnant animals during the period of palate closure of the embryos. Other congenital anomalies including deformed forelegs, phocomelia, and anasarca have been reported in offspring of dogs which received corticosteroids during pregnancy.

Avoid ingestion.

Before instilling any medication into the ear, examine the external ear canal thoroughly to be certain the tympanic membrane is not ruptured in order to avoid the possibility of transmitting infection to the middle ear as well as damaging the cochlea or vestibular apparatus from prolonged contact. If hearing or vestibular dysfunction is noted during the course of treatment, discontinue use of GENTAMICIN OTIC SOLUTION.

The antibiotic sensitivity of the pathogenic organism should be determined prior to the use of this preparation. Use of topical antibiotics occasionally allows overgrowth of non-susceptible bacteria, fungi, or yeasts. In these cases, treatment should be instituted with other appropriate agents as indicated.

Adverse systemic reactions have been observed following the oral ingestion of some topical corticosteroid preparations. Patients should be closely observed for the usual signs of adrenocorticosteroid overdosage which include sodium retention, potassium loss, fluid retention, weight gains, polydipsia and/or polyuria. Prolonged use or overdosage may produce adverse immunosuppressive effects.

Experimentally it has been demonstrated that corticosteroids, especially at high dosage levels, may result in delayed wound healing, An increase in the incidence of osteoporosis may be noted, mainly in the elderly, with prolonged use of these compounds. Their use in older dogs during the healing stages of bone fracture is not indicated for the reason listed above.

Use of corticosteroids, depending on dose, duration, and specific steroid, may result in inhibition of endogenous steroid production following drug withdrawal. In patients presently receiving or recently withdrawn from systemic corticosteroid treatments, therapy with a rapidly acting corticosteroid should be considered in unusually stressful situations.

For use in dogs and cats only.

Toxicology: Toxicity Studies: Parenterally, no toxic effects were observed in rats given gentamicin sulfate 20 mg/kg/day for twenty-four days; in cats given 10 mg/kg/day for forty days. Gentamicin sulfate given to dogs at 6 mg/lb/day, 6 days weekly for three weeks, caused no detectable kidney damage. At higher doses, impairment of equilibrium and of renal function were observed in these species.

Subacute otic toxicity study in dogs showed gentamicin sulfate with betamethasone valerate solution to be well tolerated locally with no adverse systemic effects when administered 5 drops twice a day for 21 consecutive days.

Gentamicin sulfate solution in a 21-day subacute dermal toxicity study in dogs was shown to be well tolerated when applied topically to abraded skin. There were no meaningful findings except a reduction in eosinophil count attributable to absorption of the corticosteroid component.

Side Effects: Side, effects such as SAP and SGPT enzyme elevations, weight loss, anorexia, polydipsia, and polyuria have occurred following the use of parenteral or systemic synthetic corticosteroids in dogs. Vomiting and diarrhea (occasionally bloody) have been observed in dogs and cats.

Cushing's Syndrome in dogs has been reported in association with prolonged or repeated steroid therapy.

References: Available upon request.

Presentation: GENTAMICIN OTIC SOLUTION, squeeze bottles of 7.5 mL, 15 mL, and 240 mL (8 fl oz).

Compendium Code No.: 10820840

GENTAMICIN SULFATE SOLUTION ℞

Aspen **Gentamicin**

100 mg/mL Gentamicin

ANADA No.: 200-037

Active Ingredient(s): Each mL contains: Gentamicin sulfate equivalent to 100 mg gentamicin base, 2.4 mg sodium metabisulfite, 0.8 mg sodium sulfite, anhydrous, 0.1 mg edetate disodium, 10 mg benzyl alcohol as preservative, water for injection q.s.

Indications: Gentamicin Sulfate Solution is recommended for the control of bacterial infections of the uterus (metritis) in horses and as an aid in improving conception in mares with uterine infections caused by bacteria sensitive to gentamicin. For intra-uterine use in horses only.

Dosage and Administration: The recommended dose is 20 to 25 mL (2.0-2.5 grams) Gentamicin Sulfate Solution per day for 3 to 5 days during estrus. Each dose should be diluted with 200-500 mL of sterile physiological saline before aseptic uterine infusion.

Precaution(s): Store between 2°C-30°C (36°F-86°F). Protect from freezing.

Caution(s): Federal law restricts this drug to use by or on the order of a licensed veterinarian.

Warning(s): Not for use in horses intended for food.

For animal use only. Not for human use. Keep out of reach of children.

Presentation: 100 mL sterile multiple dose vial.

Compendium Code No.: 14750360

GENTAMICIN SULFATE SOLUTION ℞

Butler **Gentamicin**

100 mg per mL

ANADA No.: 200-137

Active Ingredient(s): Each mL of GENTAMICIN SULFATE SOLUTION contains: gentamicin sulfate equivalent to 100 mg gentamicin base; 3.2 mg sodium metabisulfite; 0.1 mg edetate disodium; 1.8 mg methylparaben and 0.2 mg propylparaben as preservatives; water for injection q.s.

Indications: GENTAMICIN SULFATE SOLUTION is recommended for the control of bacterial infections of the uterus (metritis) in horses and as an aid in improving conception in mares with uterine infections caused by bacteria sensitive to gentamicin.

Bacteriologic studies should be conducted to identify the causative organism and to determine its sensitivity to gentamicin sulfate. Sensitivity discs of the drug are available for this purpose.

Pharmacology: Chemistry: Gentamicin is a mixture of aminoglycoside antibiotics derived from the fermentation of *Micromonospora purpurea.* Gentamicin sulfate is a mixture of sulfate salts of the antibiotics produced in this fermentation. The salts are weakly acidic, freely soluble in water, and stable in solution.

Antibacterial Activity: *In vitro* antibacterial activity has shown that gentamicin is active against most gram-negative and gram-positive bacteria isolated from domestic animals.[1] Gentamicin is active against *Pseudomonas aeruginosa,* indole-positive and -negative *Proteus* species, *Escherichia coli, Klebsiella* species, *Enterobacter* species, *Alcaligenes* species, *Staphylococcus* species, and *Streptococcus* species.

Studies in man indicate that recommended doses of gentamicin produce serum concentrations bactericidal for most bacteria sensitive to gentamicin within an hour after intramuscular injection; these concentrations last for 6 to 12 hours.[2] Some 30% of the administered dose of gentamicin is bound by serum proteins and released as the drug is excreted.

Gentamicin is excreted almost entirely by glomerular filtration. High concentrations of the active form are found in the urine. Fifty to 100% of the gentamicin injected can be recovered unchanged within 24 hours from the urine of patients with normal renal function. A small amount is excreted into the bile.

Dosage and Administration: The recommended dose is 20 to 25 mL (2.0-2.5 grams) gentamicin sulfate solution per day for 3 to 5 days during estrus. Each dose should be diluted with 200-500 mL of sterile physiological saline before aseptic uterine infusion.

Contraindication(s): There are no known contraindications to this drug when used as directed.

Precaution(s): Store between 2° and 30°C (36° and 86°F).

Protect from freezing.

Caution(s): Federal law restricts this drug to use by or on the order of a licensed veterinarian.

If hypersensitivity to any of the components develops, or if an overgrowth of nonsusceptible bacteria, fungi, or yeasts occurs, treatment with GENTAMICIN SULFATE SOLUTION should be discontinued and appropriate therapy instituted.

Although GENTAMICIN SULFATE SOLUTION is not spermicidal, treatment should not be given the day of breeding. For intra-uterine use in horses only.

Warning(s): Not for use in horses intended for food.

Toxicity Studies: No toxic effects were observed in rats given gentamicin sulfate 20 mg/kg/day for 24 days; in cats given 10 mg/kg/day for 40 days. Gentamicin sulfate given to dogs at 6 mg/lb/day, 6 days weekly for 3 weeks, caused no detectable kidney damage. At higher doses, impairment of equilibrium and renal function were observed in these species.

Side Effects: There have been no reports of drug hypersensitivity or adverse side effects following the recommended intrauterine infusion of gentamicin sulfate solution combined with sterile physiological saline in mares.

References: Available upon request.

Presentation: GENTAMICIN SULFATE SOLUTION, 100 mg per mL for intrauterine use, is available in 250 mL multiple dose vials.

Manufactured by: Phoenix Scientific, Inc.

Compendium Code No.: 10820850

GENTAMICIN SULFATE SOLUTION ℞

RXV **Gentamicin**

100 mg per mL

ANADA No.: 200-137

Active Ingredient(s): Each mL contains: Gentamicin sulfate equivalent to 100 mg gentamicin base; 3.2 mg sodium metabisulfite; 0.1 mg edetate disodium; 1.8 mg methylparaben and 0.2 mg propylparaben as preservatives; water for injection q.s.

Indications: GENTAMICIN SULFATE SOLUTION is recommended for the control of bacterial infections of the uterus (metritis) in horses and as an aid in improving conception in mares with uterine infections caused by bacteria sensitive to gentamicin.

Dosage and Administration: The recommended dose is 20 to 25 mL (2.0-2.5 grams) of GENTAMICIN SULFATE SOLUTION per day for 3 to 5 days during estrus. Each dose should be diluted with 200-500 mL of sterile physiological saline before aseptic uterine infusion.

Precaution(s): Store between 36°-86°F (2°-30°C).

Protect from freezing.

Caution(s): Federal law restricts this drug to use by or on the order of a licensed veterinarian.

Warning(s): Not for use in horses intended for food. For intra-uterine use in horses only.

Presentation: 250 mL vials.

Manufactured by: Phoenix Scientific, Inc.

Compendium Code No.: 10910060

GENTAMICIN SULFATE SOLUTION ℞

Vet Tek **Gentamicin**

100 mg/mL

ANADA No.: 200-137

Active Ingredient(s): Description: Each mL of GENTAMICIN SULFATE SOLUTION contains: gentamicin sulfate equivalent to 100 mg gentamicin base; 3.2 mg sodium metabisulfite; 0.1 mg edetate disodium; 1.8 mg methylparaben and 0.2 mg propylparaben as preservatives; water for injection q.s.

Indications: GENTAMICIN SULFATE SOLUTION is recommended for the control of bacterial infections of the uterus (metritis) in horses and as an aid in improving conception in mares with uterine infections caused by bacteria sensitive to gentamicin.

Bacteriologic studies should be conducted to identify the causative organism and to determine its sensitivity to gentamicin sulfate. Sensitivity discs of the drug are available for this purpose.

Pharmacology: Chemistry: Gentamicin is a mixture of aminoglycoside antibiotics derived from the fermentation of *Micromonospora purpurea.* Gentamicin sulfate is a mixture of sulfate salts of the antibiotics produced in this fermentation. The salts are weakly acidic, freely soluble in water, and stable in solution.

Antibacterial Activity: *In vitro* antibacterial activity has shown that gentamicin is active against most gram-negative and gram-positive bacteria isolated from domestic animals.[1] Gentamicin is active against *Pseudomonas aeruginosa,* indole-positive and -negative *Proteus* species, *Escherichia coli, Klebsiella* species, *Enterobacter* species, *Alcaligenes* species, *Staphylococcus* species, and *Streptococcus* species.

Pharmacology: Studies in man indicate that recommended doses of gentamicin produce serum concentrations bactericidal for most bacteria sensitive to gentamicin within an hour after intramuscular injection; these concentrations last for 6 to 12 hours.[2] Some 30% of the administered dose of gentamicin is bound by serum proteins and released as the drug is excreted.

Gentamicin is excreted almost entirely by glomerular filtration. High concentrations of the active form are found in the urine. Fifty to 100% of the gentamicin injected can be recovered unchanged within 24 hours from the urine of patients with normal renal function. A small amount is excreted into the bile.

Dosage and Administration: The recommended dose is 20 to 25 mL (2.0-2.5 grams) GENTAMICIN SULFATE SOLUTION per day for 3 to 5 days during estrus. Each dose should be diluted with 200-500 mL of sterile physiological saline before aseptic uterine infusion.

Contraindication(s): There are no known contraindications to this drug when used as directed.

Precaution(s): Store between 2° and 30°C (36° and 86°F). Protect from freezing.

Caution(s): Federal law restricts this drug to use by or on the order of a licensed veterinarian.

If hypersensitivity to any of the components develops, or if overgrowth of nonsusceptible bacteria, fungi, or yeast occurs, treatment with GENTAMICIN SULFATE SOLUTION should be discontinued and appropriate therapy instituted.

Although GENTAMICIN SULFATE SOLUTION is not spermicidal, treatment should not be given the day of breeding.

For intrauterine use in horses only.

For use in horses only.

Warning(s): Not for use in horses intended for food.

Toxicology: Toxicity Studies: No toxic effects were observed in rats given gentamicin sulfate 20 mg/kg/day for 24 days; in cats given 10 mg/kg/day for 40 days. Gentamicin sulfate given to dogs at 6 mg/lb/day, 6 days weekly for 3 weeks, caused no detectable kidney damage. At higher doses, impairment of equilibrium and renal function were observed in these species.

Side Effects: There have been no reports of drug hypersensitivity or adverse side effects following the recommended intrauterine infusion of GENTAMICIN SULFATE SOLUTION combined with sterile physiological saline in mares.

References: Available upon request.

Presentation: 100 mL (NDC 60270-584-10) and 250 mL (NDC 60270-584-13) multiple dose vials.

Manufactured by: Phoenix Scientific, Inc. St. Joseph, MO 64503.

Compendium Code No.: 14200101 Rev. 01-00

GENTAMICIN TOPICAL SPRAY ℞

Butler **Topical Antimicrobial-Corticosteroid**

Gentamicin Sulfate with Betamethasone Valerate

Active Ingredient(s): Each mL contains: gentamicin sulfate equivalent to 0.57 mg gentamicin base, betamethasone valerate equivalent to 0.284 mg betamethasone, 163 mg isopropyl alcohol, propylene glycol, methylparaben and propylparaben as preservatives, purified water q.s. Hydrochloric acid may be added to adjust pH.

Indications: For the treatment of infected superficial lesions in dogs caused by bacteria sensitive to gentamicin.

Pharmacology: Chemistry: Gentamicin is a mixture of aminoglycoside antibiotics derived from the fermentation of *Micromonospora purpurea*. Gentamicin sulfate is a mixture of sulfate salts of the antibiotics produced in this fermentation. The salts are weakly acidic and freely soluble in water.

Gentamicin sulfate contains not less than 500 micrograms of gentamicin base per milligram.

Betamethasone valerate is a synthetic glucocorticoid.

Gentamicin, a broad-spectrum antibiotic, is a highly effective topical treatment for bacterial infections of the skin. *In vitro*, gentamicin is bactericidal against a wide variety of gram-positive and gram-negative bacteria isolated from domestic animals.[1,2] Specifically, gentamicin is active against the following organisms isolated from canine skin: *Alcaligenes* sp., *Citrobacter* sp., *Klebsiella* sp., *Pseudomonas aeruginosa*, indole-positive and negative *Proteus* sp., *Escherichia coli*, *Enterobacter* sp., *Staphylococcus* sp., and *Streptococcus* sp.

Betamethasone valerate emerged from intensive research as the most promising of some 50 newly synthesized corticosteroids in the experimental model described by McKenzie[3], *et al.* This human bioassay technique has been found reliable for evaluating the vasoconstrictor properties of new topical corticosteroids and is useful in predicting clinical efficacy.

Betamethasone valerate in veterinary medicine has been shown to provide anti-inflammatory and antipruritic activity in the topical management of corticosteroid responsive infected superficial lesions in dogs.

Dosage and Administration: Prior to treatment, remove excessive hair and clean the lesion and adjacent area. Hold bottle upright 3 to 6 inches from the lesion and depress the sprayer head twice. Administer 2 to 4 times daily for 7 days.

Each depression of the sprayer head delivers 0.7 mL of GENTAMICIN TOPICAL SPRAY.

Contraindication(s): If hypersensitivity to any of the components occurs, treatment with this product should be discontinued and appropriate therapy instituted.

Precaution(s): Store upright between 2°C and 30°C (36°F and 86°F).

Caution(s): Federal law restricts this drug to use by or on the order of a licensed veterinarian.

Clinical and experimental data have demonstrated that corticosteroids administered orally or parenterally to animals may induce the first stage of parturition when administered during the last trimester of pregnancy and may precipitate premature parturition followed by dystocia, fetal death, retained placenta, and metritis.

Additionally, corticosteroids administered to dogs, rabbits and rodents during pregnancy have produced cleft palate. Other congenital anomalies including deformed forelegs, phocomelia, and anasarca have been reported in offspring of dogs which received corticosteroids during pregnancy.

Antibiotic susceptibility of the pathogenic organism(s) should be determined prior to the use of this preparation. Use of topical antibiotics may permit overgrowth of non-susceptible bacteria, fungi, or yeasts. If this occurs, treatment should be instituted with other appropriate agents as indicated.

Administration of recommended dose beyond 7 days may result in delayed wound healing. Animals treated longer than 7 days should be monitored closely.

Avoid ingestion. Oral or parenteral use of corticosteroids, depending on dose, duration, and specific steroid may result in inhibition of endogenous steroid production following drug withdrawal.

In patients presently receiving or recently withdrawn from systemic corticosteroid treatments, therapy with a rapidly acting corticosteroid should be considered in especially stressful situations.

If ingestion should occur, patients should be closely observed for the usual signs of adrenocorticoid overdosage which include sodium retention, potassium loss, fluid retention, weight gains, polydipsia, and/or polyuria. Prolonged use or overdosage may produce adverse immunosuppressive effects.

For topical use in dogs only.

Toxicology: Gentamicin sulfate with betamethasone valerate topical spray was well tolerated in an abraded skin study in dogs. No treatment-related toxicological changes in the skin were observed.

Systemic effects directly related to treatment were confined to histological changes in the adrenals, liver, and kidney and to organ-to-body weight ratios of adrenals. All were dose related, were typical for or not unexpected with corticosteroid therapy, and were considered reversible with cessation of treatment.

Side Effects: Side effects such as SAP and SGPT enzyme elevations, weight loss, anorexia, polydipsia, and polyuria have occurred following parenteral or systemic use of synthetic corticosteroids in dogs. Vomiting and diarrhea (occasionally bloody) have been observed in dogs.

Cushings syndrome in dogs has been reported in association with prolonged or repeated steroid therapy.

References: Available upon request.

Presentation: Plastic spray bottle containing 60 mL, 120 mL or 240 mL of GENTAMICIN TOPICAL SPRAY.

Manufactured by: Med-Pharmex, Inc.

Compendium Code No.: 10820861

GENTAMICIN TOPICAL SPRAY ℞

RXV **Topical Antimicrobial-Corticosteroid**

Gentamicin Sulfate with Betamethasone Valerate

ANADA No.: 200-188

Active Ingredient(s): Description: Each mL Contains: gentamicin sulfate equivalent to 0.57 mg gentamicin base, betamethasone valerate equivalent to 0.284 mg betamethasone, 163 mg isopropyl alcohol, propylene glycol, methylparaben and propylparaben as preservatives, purified water q.s. Hydrochloric acid may be added to adjust pH.

Indications: For the treatment of infected superficial lesions in dogs caused by bacteria sensitive to gentamicin.

Pharmacology: Chemistry: Gentamicin is a mixture of aminoglycoside antibiotics derived from the fermentation of *Micromonospora purpurea*. Gentamicin sulfate is a mixture of sulfate salts of the antibiotics produced in this fermentation. The salts are weakly acidic and freely soluble in water.

Gentamicin sulfate contains not less than 500 micrograms of gentamicin base per milligram.

Betamethasone valerate is a synthetic glucocorticoid.

Gentamicin, a broad-spectrum antibiotic, is a highly effective topical treatment for bacterial infections of the skin. *In vitro*, gentamicin is bactericidal against a wide variety of gram-positive and gram-negative bacteria isolated from domestic animals.[1,2] Specifically, gentamicin is active against the following organisms isolated from canine skin: *Alcaligenes* sp., *Citrobacter* sp., *Klebsiella* sp., *Pseudomonas aeruginosa*, indole-positive and negative *Proteus* sp., *Escherichia coli*, *Enterobacter* sp., *Staphylococcus* sp., and *Streptococcus* sp.

Betamethasone valerate emerged from intensive research as the most promising of some 50 newly synthesized corticosteroids in the experimental model described by McKenzie[3], *et al.* This human bioassay technique has been found reliable for evaluating the vasoconstrictor properties of new topical corticosteroids and is useful in predicting clinical efficacy.

Betamethasone valerate in veterinary medicine has been shown to provide anti-inflammatory and antipruritic activity in the topical management of corticosteroid responsive infected superficial lesions in dogs.

Dosage and Administration: Prior to treatment, remove excessive hair and clean the lesion and adjacent area. Hold bottle upright 3 to 6 inches from the lesion and depress the sprayer head twice. Administer 2 to 4 times daily for 7 days.

Each depression of the sprayer head delivers 0.7 mL of Gentamicin Sulfate with Betamethasone Valerate Topical Spray.

Contraindication(s): If hypersensitivity to any of the components occurs, treatment with this product should be discontinued and appropriate therapy instituted.

Precaution(s): Store upright between 2°C and 30°C (36°F and 86°F).

Caution(s): Federal law restricts this drug to use by or on the order of a licensed veterinarian.

Clinical and experimental data have demonstrated that corticosteroids administered orally or parenterally to animals may induce the first stage of parturition when administered during the last trimester of pregnancy and may precipitate premature parturition followed by dystocia, fetal death, retained placenta, and metritis.

Additionally, corticosteroids administered to dogs, rabbits and rodents during pregnancy have produced cleft palate. Other congenital anomalies including deformed forelegs, phocomelia, and anasarca have been reported in offspring of dogs which received corticosteroids during pregnancy.

Antibiotic susceptibility of the pathogenic organism(s) should be determined prior to the use of this preparation. Use of topical antibiotics may permit overgrowth of non-susceptible bacteria, fungi, or yeasts. If this occurs, treatment should be instituted with other appropriate agents as indicated.

Administration of recommended dose beyond 7 days may result in delayed wound healing. Animals treated longer than 7 days should be monitored closely.

Avoid ingestion. Oral or parenteral use of corticosteroids, depending on dose, duration, and specific steroid may result in inhibition of endogenous steroid production following drug withdrawal.

In patients presently receiving or recently withdrawn from systemic corticosteroid treatments, therapy with a rapidly acting corticosteroid should be considered in especially stressful situations.

If ingestion should occur, patients should be closely observed for the usual signs of adrenocorticoid overdosage which include sodium retention, potassium loss, fluid retention, weight gains, polydipsia, and/or polyuria. Prolonged use or overdosage may produce adverse immunosuppressive effects.

For topical use in dogs only.

Toxicology: Gentamicin sulfate with betamethasone valerate topical spray was well tolerated in an abraded skin study in dogs. No treatment-related toxicological changes in the skin were observed.

Systemic effects directly related to treatment were confined to histological changes in the adrenals, liver, and kidney and to organ-to-body weight ratios of adrenals. All were dose related, were typical for or not unexpected with corticosteroid therapy, and were considered reversible with cessation of treatment.

Side Effects: Side effects such as SAP and SGPT enzyme elevations, weight loss, anorexia, polydipsia, and polyuria have occurred following parenteral or systemic use of synthetic corticosteroids in dogs. Vomiting and diarrhea (occasionally bloody) have been observed in dogs.

Cushings syndrome in dogs has been reported in association with prolonged or repeated steroid therapy.

References: Available upon request.

Presentation: 60 mL and 120 mL plastic spray bottles.

Manufactured by: Med-Pharmex, Inc.

Compendium Code No.: 10910350

April 1999

GENTA-OTIC ℞

Vetus **Otic Antimicrobial-Corticosteroid**

(Gentamicin Sulfate with Betamethasone Valerate)

ANADA No.: 200-183

Active Ingredient(s): Each mL of GENTA-OTIC Otic Solution contains gentamicin sulfate equivalent to 3 mg gentamicin base, betamethasone valerate equivalent to 1 mg betamethasone, 1.0 mg hydroxyethylcellulose, 2.5 mg glacial acetic acid, 200 mg purified water, 19% ethanol, 9.4 mg benzyl alcohol as preservative, 300 mg glycerin and propylene glycol q.s.

Indications: GENTA-OTIC Otic Solution is indicated for the treatment of acute and chronic canine otitis externa and canine and feline superficial infected lesions caused by bacteria sensitive to gentamicin.

Pharmacology: Chemistry: Gentamicin is a bactericidal antibiotic of the aminoglycoside group derived from *Micromonospora purpurea* of the *Actinomyces* group. It is a powder, white to buff in color, basic in nature, readily soluble in water and highly stable in solution.

Betamethasone valerate is a synthetic corticosteroid derivative of prednisolone.

Action: GENTA-OTIC Otic Solution combines the broad-spectrum activity of gentamicin sulfate with the anti-inflammatory and antipruritic activity of betamethasone valerate. *In vitro* antibacterial activity has shown that gentamicin is active against most gram-negative bacteria including *Pseudomonas aeruginosa*, indole-positive and negative *Proteus* sp., *Escherichia coli*, *Klebsiella pneumoniae*, *Aerobacter aerogenes*, and *Neisseria*. Gentamicin is also active against strains of gram-positive bacteria including *Staphylococcus* species and some *Streptococcus* species.

Betamethasone valerate has emerged from intensive research as the most promising of some 50 newly synthesized corticosteroids in the experimental model described by McKenzie *et al.* This human bioassay technique has been found reliable for evaluating the vasoconstrictor properties of new topical corticosteroids and is useful in predicting clinical efficacy.

Betamethasone valerate in human medicine had been shown to provide anti-inflammatory and antipruritic activity in the topical management of corticosteroid-responsive dermatoses. In the responsive cases, the local anti-inflammatory activity is sustained by the vasoconstrictor properties of the steroid.

Dosage and Administration: Duration of treatment will depend upon the severity of the condition and the response obtained. The duration of treatment and/or frequency of the dosage may be reduced, but care should be taken not to discontinue therapy prematurely.

Otitis externa: The external ear and ear canal should be properly cleaned and dried before treatment. Remove foreign material, debris, crusted exudates, etc., with suitable non-irritating solutions. Excessive hair should be clipped from the treatment area of the external ear. Instill 3 to 8 drops of GENTA-OTIC Otic Solution (approximately room temperature) into the ear canal twice daily for seven to fourteen days.

Superficial infected lesions: The lesion and adjacent area should be properly cleaned before treatment. Excessive hair should be removed. Apply a sufficient amount of GENTA-OTIC Otic Solution to cover the treatment area twice daily for seven to fourteen days.

Contraindication(s): If hypersensitivity to any of the components occurs, treatment with this product should be discontinued and appropriate therapy instituted. Concomitant use of drugs known to induce ototoxicity should be avoided. This preparation should not be used in conditions where corticosteroids are contraindicated. Do not administer parenteral corticosteroids during treatment with GENTA-OTIC Otic Solution.

Precaution(s): Store between 2°C and 25°C (36°F and 77°F).

Caution(s): Federal law restricts this drug to use by or on the order of a licensed veterinarian.

For use in dogs and cats only.

The antibiotic sensitivity of the pathogenic organism should be determined prior to the use of this preparation. Use of topical antibiotics occasionally allows overgrowth of non-susceptible bacteria, fungi, or yeasts. In these cases, treatment should be instituted with other appropriate agents as indicated.

Adverse systemic reactions have been observed following the oral ingestion of some topical corticosteroid preparations. Patients should be closely observed for the usual signs of adrenocorticoid overdosage which includes sodium retention, potassium loss, fluid retention, weight gains, polydipsia and/or polyuria. Prolonged use or overdosage may produce adverse immunosuppressive effects.

Experimentally it has been demonstrated that corticosteroids, especially at high dosage levels, may result in delayed wound healing. An increase in the incidence of osteoporosis may be noted, mainly in the elderly, with prolonged use of these compounds. Their use in older dogs during the healing stages of bone fracture is not indicated for the reason listed above.

Use of corticosteroids depending on dose, duration, and specific steroid, may result in inhibition of endogenous steroid production following drug withdrawal. In patients presently receiving or recently withdrawn from systemic corticosteroid treatments, therapy with a rapidly acting corticosteroid should be considered in unusually stressful situations.

Before instilling any medication into the ear, examine the external ear canal thoroughly to be certain the tympanic membrane is not ruptured in order to avoid the possibility of transmitting infection to the middle ear as well as damaging the cochlea or vestibular apparatus from prolonged contact. If hearing or vestibular dysfunction in noted during the course of treatment, discontinue use of GENTA-OTIC Otic Solution.

Toxicology: Parenterally, no toxic effects were observed in rats given gentamicin sulfate 20 mg/kg/day for twenty-four days; in cats given 10 mg/kg/day for forty days. Gentamicin sulfate given to dogs at 6 mg/lb/day, 6 days weekly for three weeks, caused no detectable kidney damage. At higher doses, impairment of equilibrium and renal function were observed in these species.

Subacute otic toxicity in dogs showed gentamicin sulfate with betamethasone valerate solution to be well tolerated locally with no adverse systemic effects when administered at 5 drops twice a day for 21 consecutive days.

Gentamicin sulfate in a 21-day subacute dermal toxicity study in dogs was shown to be well tolerated when applied topically to abraded skin. There were no meaningful findings except a reduction in eosinophil count attributable to absorption of the corticosteroid component.

Clinical and experimental data have demonstrated that corticosteroids administered orally or parenterally to animals may induce the first stage of parturition when administered during the last trimester of pregnancy and may precipitate premature parturition followed by dystocia, fetal death, retained placenta, and metritis. Additionally, corticosteroids may induce cleft palates in offspring when given to pregnant animals during the period of palate closure of the embryos. Other congenital anomalies including deformed forelegs, phocomelia, and anasarca have been reported in offspring of dogs which received corticosteroids during pregnancy. Avoid ingestion.

Side Effects: Side effects such as SAP and SGPT enzyme elevations, weight loss, anorexia, polydipsia, and polyuria have occurred following the use of parenteral or systemic synthetic corticosteroids in dogs. Vomiting and diarrhea (occasionally bloody) have been observed in dogs and cats.

Cushing's Syndrome in dogs has been reported in association with prolonged or repeated steroid therapy.

Presentation: GENTA-OTIC Otic Solution, squeeze bottles of 7.5 mL, 15 mL, and 240 mL (8 fl oz).

Compendium Code No.: 14440390

GENTA-SPRAY ℞

Vetus **Topical Antimicrobial-Corticosteroid**

(Gentamicin Sulfate with Betamethasone Valerate)

ANADA No.: 200-188

Active Ingredient(s): Each mL contains: gentamicin sulfate equivalent to 0.57 mg gentamicin base, betamethasone valerate equivalent to 0.284 mg betamethasone, 163 mg isopropyl alcohol, propylene glycol, methylparaben and propylparaben as preservatives, purified water q.s. Hydrochloric acid may be added to adjust pH.

Indications: For the treatment of infected superficial lesions in dogs caused by bacteria sensitive to gentamicin.

Pharmacology: Chemistry: Gentamicin is a mixture of aminoglycoside antibiotics derived from the fermentation of *Micromonospora purpurea*. Gentamicin sulfate is a mixture of sulfate salts of the antibiotics produced in this fermentation. The salts are weakly acidic and freely soluble in water.

Gentamicin sulfate veterinary contains not less than 500 micrograms of gentamicin base per milligram.

Betamethasone valerate is a synthetic glucocorticoid.

Gentamicin, a broad-spectrum antibiotic, is a highly effective topical treatment for bacterial infections of the skin. *In vitro* gentamicin is bactericidal against a wide variety of gram-positive and gram-negative bacteria isolated from domestic animals. Specifically, gentamicin is active against the following organisms isolated from canine skin: *Alcaligenes* sp., *Citrobacter* sp., *Klebsiella* sp., *Pseudomonas aeruginosa*, indole-positive and negative *Proteus* sp, *Escherichia coli*, *Enterobacter* sp., *Staphylococcus* sp., and *Streptococcus* sp.

Betamethasone valerate emerged from intensive research as the most promising of some 50 newly synthesized corticosteroids in the experimental model described by McKenzie, *et al.* This human bioassay technique has been found reliable for evaluating the vasoconstriction properties of new topical corticosteroids and is useful in predicting clinical efficacy.

Betamethasone valerate in veterinary medicine has been shown to provide anti-inflammatory and antipruritic activity in the topical management of corticosteroid-responsive infected superficial lesions in dogs.

Dosage and Administration: Prior to treatment, remove excessive hair and clean the lesion and adjacent area. Hold the bottle upright 3 to 6 inches from the lesion and depress the sprayer head twice. Administer 2 to 4 times daily for 7 days.

Each depression of the sprayer head delivers 0.7 mL of GENTA-SPRAY.

Contraindication(s): If hypersensitivity to any of the components occurs, treatment with this product should be discontinued and appropriate therapy instituted.

Precaution(s): Store upright between 2°C and 30°C (36°F and 86°F).

Caution(s): Federal law restricts this drug to use by or on the order of a licensed veterinarian.

Antibiotic susceptibility of the pathogenic organism(s) should be determined prior to the use of this preparation. The use of topical antibiotics may permit overgrowth of non-susceptible bacteria, fungi, or yeasts. If this occurs, treatment should be instituted with other appropriate agents as indicated.

Administration of recommended dose beyond 7 days may result in delayed wound healing. Animals treated longer than 7 days should be monitored closely.

Avoid ingestion. Oral or parenteral use of corticosteroids, depending on dose, duration, and specific steroid, may result in the inhibition of endogenous steroid production following drug withdrawal.

In patients presently receiving or recently withdrawn from systemic corticosteroid treatments, therapy with a rapidly acting corticosteroid should be considered in especially stressful situations.

If ingestion should occur, patients should be closely observed for the usual signs of adrenocorticoid overdosage which include sodium retention, potassium loss, fluid retention, weight gains, polydipsia and/or polyuria. Prolonged use or overdosage may produce adverse immunosuppressive effects.

Toxicology: Gentamicin sulfate with betamethasone valerate topical spray was well tolerated in an abraded skin study in dogs. No treatment-related toxicological changes in the skin were observed.

Systemic effects directly related to treatment were confined to histological changes in the adrenals, liver and kidney and to organ-to-body weight ratios of adrenals. All were dose-related, were typical for or not unexpected with corticosteroid therapy, and were considered reversible with cessation of treatment.

Clinical and experimental data have demonstrated that corticosteroids administered orally or parenterally to animals may induce the first stage of parturition when administered during the last trimester of pregnancy and may precipitate premature parturition followed by dystocia, fetal death, retained placenta, and metritis.

Additionally, corticosteroids administered to dogs, rabbits, and rodents during pregnancy have produced cleft palate in offspring. Other congenital anomalies including deformed forelegs, phocomelia, and anasarca have been reported in offspring of dogs which received corticosteroids during pregnancy.

Side Effects: Side effects such as SAP and SGPT enzyme elevations, weight loss, anorexia, polydipsia and polyuria have occurred following parenteral or systemic use of synthetic corticosteroids in dogs. Vomiting and diarrhea (occasionally bloody) have been observed in dogs.

Cushing's syndrome in dogs has been reported in association with prolonged or repeated steroid therapy.

References: Available upon request.

Presentation: Plastic spray bottle containing 60 mL, 120 mL, or 240 mL of GENTA-SPRAY Topical Spray.

Compendium Code No.: 14440400

GENTAVED™ 50 ℞

Vedco **Gentamicin**

50 mg/mL Gentamicin Base

NADA No.: 137-310

Active Ingredient(s): Each mL contains: Gentamicin sulfate equivalent to 50 mg gentamicin base, 3.2 mg sodium bisulfite, 0.1 mg disodium edetate, 1.8 mg methylparaben and 0.2 mg propylparaben as preservatives, water for injection q.s., and glacial acetic acid and/or sodium hydroxide for pH adjustment.

Indications: Indicated for use in the treatment of urinary tract infections (cystitis) in dogs caused by susceptible strains of *Proteus mirabilis, Escherichia coli* and *Staphylococcus aureus*. As with all antibiotics, pretreatment cultures and sensitivity testing should be done on samples collected prior to treatment to determine the susceptibility of the microorganism to gentamicin.

Dosage and Administration: The recommended dosage for cystitis in dogs is 2 mg per pound of body weight twice the first day, then once per day thereafter to be administered by intramuscular or subcutaneous injection. Treatment should not exceed 7 days.

If no improvement is seen after 3 days, treatment should be discontinued and the diagnosis re-evaluated.

Warning(s): Keep out of reach of children.

Caution(s): Federal law restricts this drug to use by or on the order of a licensed veterinarian.

Presentation: 50 mL.

Compendium Code No.: 10941020

GENTAVED™ 100 ℞

Vedco **Gentamicin**

Gentamicin Sulfate Solution

100 mg/mL Gentamicin

ANADA No.: 200-037

Active Ingredient(s): Each mL of GENTAVED™ 100 contains:

Gentamicin sulfate equivalent to gentamicin base	100 mg
Sodium metabisulfite	2.4 mg
Sodium sulfite, anhydrous	0.8 mg
Edetate disodium	0.1 mg
Benzyl alcohol as preservative	10 mg
Water for injection	q.s.

Indications: GENTAVED™ 100 is recommended for the control of bacterial infections of the uterus (metritis) in horses and as an aid in improving conception in mares with uterine infections caused by bacteria sensitive to gentamicin.

Bacteriologic studies should be conducted to identify the causative organism and to determine its sensitivity to gentamicin sulfate. Sensitivity discs of the drug are available for this purpose.

Pharmacology: Gentamicin is a mixture of aminoglycoside antibiotics derived from the fermentation of *Micromonospora purpurea*. Gentamicin sulfate is a mixture of sulfate salts of the antibiotics produced in this fermentation. The salts are weakly acidic, freely soluble in water, and stable in solution.

Antibacterial Activity: *In vitro* antibacterial activity has shown that gentamicin is active against

G

most gram-negative and gram-positive bacteria isolated from domestic animals.[1] Gentamicin is active against *Pseudomonas aeruginosa*, indole-positive and -negative *Proteus* species, *Escherichia coli, Klebsiella* species, *Enterobacter* species, *Alcaligenes* species, *Staphylococcus* species, and *Streptococcus* species.

Studies in man indicate that the recommended doses of gentamicin produce serum concentrations bactericidal for most bacteria sensitive to gentamicin within an hour after intramuscular injection; these concentrations last for 6 to 12 hours.[2] Some 30% of the administered dose of gentamicin is bound by serum proteins and released as the drug is excreted.

Gentamicin is excreted almost entirely by glomerular filtration. High concentrations of the active form are found in the urine. Fifty to 100% of the gentamicin injected can be recovered unchanged within 24 hours from the urine of patients with normal renal function. A small amount is excreted into the bile.

Dosage and Administration: The recommended dose is 20 to 25 mL (2.0-2.5 g) of GENTAVED™ 100 per day for three (3) to five (5) days during estrus. Each dose should be diluted with 200-500 mL of sterile physiological saline before aseptic uterine infusion.

Contraindication(s): There are not any known contraindications to this drug when used as directed.

Precaution(s): Store between 2°-30°C (36°-86°F). Protect from freezing.

If hypersensitivity to any of the components develops, or if an overgrowth of nonsusceptible bacteria, fungi, or yeasts occurs, treatment with GENTAVED™ 100 should be discontinued and appropriate therapy instituted. Although GENTAVED™ 100 is not spermicidal, treatment should not be given on the day of breeding.

Caution(s): Federal law restricts this drug to use by or on the order of a licensed veterinarian.

For intra-uterine use in horses only. For animal use only.

Not for human use. Keep out of the reach of children.

Warning(s): Not for use in horses intended for food.

G

Toxicology: Toxic effects were not observed in rats given gentamicin sulfate 20 mg/kg/day for 24 days; nor in cats given 10 mg/kg/day for 40 days. Gentamicin sulfate given to dogs at 6 mg/lb./day, six days a week for three weeks, did not cause detectable kidney damage. At higher doses, impairment of equilibrium and renal function were observed in these species.

Side Effects: There have not been reports of drug hypersensitivity nor other adverse side effects following the recommended intra-uterine infusion of GENTAVED™ 100 combined with sterile physiological saline in mares.

References: Available upon request.

Presentation: GENTAVED™ 100 is available in 100 mL and 250 mL multiple dose vials.

Compendium Code No.: 10941010

GENTAVED® OTIC SOLUTION ℞

Vedco **Otic Antimicrobial-Corticosteroid**

(Gentamicin Sulfate with Betamethasone Valerate)

ANADA No.: 200-183

Active Ingredient(s): Each mL of GENTAVED® Otic Solution contains gentamicin sulfate equivalent to 3 mg gentamicin base, betamethasone valerate equivalent to 1 mg betamethasone, 1.0 mg hydroxyethylcellulose, 2.5 mg glacial acetic acid, 200 mg purified water, 19% ethanol, 9.4 mg benzyl alcohol as preservative, 300 mg glycerin and propylene glycol q.s.

Indications: GENTAVED® Otic Solution is indicated for the treatment of acute and chronic canine otitis externa and canine and feline superficial infected lesions caused by bacteria sensitive to gentamicin.

Pharmacology: Gentamicin is a bactericidal antibiotic of the aminoglycoside group derived from *Micromonospora purpurea* of the *Actinomyces* group. It is a powder, white to buff in color, basic in nature, readily soluble in water and highly stable in solution.

Betamethasone valerate is a synthetic corticosteroid derivative of prednisolone.

GENTAVED® Otic Solution combines the broad-spectrum activity of gentamicin sulfate with the anti-inflammatory and antipruritic activity of betamethasone valerate. *In vitro* antibacterial activity[1] has shown that gentamicin is active against most gram-negative bacteria including *Pseudomonas aeruginosa*, indole-positive and negative *Proteus* sp., *Escherichia coli, Klebsiella pneumoniae, Aerobacter aerogenes* and *Neisseria*. Gentamicin is also active against strains of gram-positive bacteria including *Staphylococcus* species and some *Streptococcus* species.

Betamethasone valerate has emerged from intensive research as the most promising of some 50 newly synthesized corticosteroids in the experimental model described by McKenzie[2] *et al.* This human bioassay technique has been found reliable for evaluating the vasoconstrictor properties of new topical corticosteroids and is useful in predicting clinical efficacy.

Betamethasone valerate in human medicine has been shown to provide anti-inflammatory and antipruritic activity in the topical management of corticosteroid-responsive dermatoses. In the response cases, the local anti-inflammatory activity is sustained by the vasoconstrictor properties of the steroid.

Dosage and Administration: Duration of treatment will depend upon the severity of the condition and the response obtained. The duration of treatment and/or frequency of the dosage may be reduced, but care should be taken not to discontinue therapy prematurely.

Otitis externa: The external ear and ear canal should be properly cleaned and dried before treatment. Remove foreign material, debris, crusted exudates, etc., with suitable nonirritating solutions. Excessive hair should be clipped from the treatment area of the external ear. Instill 3 to 8 drops of GENTAVED® Otic Solution (approximately room temperature) into the ear canal twice daily for seven to fourteen days.

Superficial infected lesions: The lesion and adjacent area should be properly cleaned before treatment. Excessive hair should be removed. Apply a sufficient amount of GENTAVED® Otic Solution to cover the treatment area twice daily for seven to fourteen days.

Contraindication(s): If hypersensitivity to any of the components occurs, treatment with this product should be discontinued and appropriate therapy instituted.

Concomitant use of drugs known to induce ototoxicity should be avoided.

This preparation should not be used in conditions where corticosteroids are contraindicated.

Do not administer parenteral corticosteroids during treatment with GENTAVED® Otic Solution.

Precaution(s): Store between 2°C and 25°C (36°F and 77°F).

Caution(s): Federal law restricts this drug to use by or on the order of a licensed veterinarian.

The antibiotic sensitivity of the pathogenic organism should be determined prior to the use of this preparation. Use of topical antibiotics occasionally allows overgrowth of non-susceptible bacteria, fungi, or yeasts. In these cases, treatment should be instituted with other appropriate agents as indicated.

Adverse systemic reactions have been observed following the oral ingestion of some topical corticosteroid preparations. Patients should be closely observed for the usual signs of adrenocorticoid overdosage which include sodium retention, potassium loss, fluid retention, weight gains, polydipsia and/or polyuria. Prolonged use or overdosage may produce adverse immunosuppressive effects.

Experimentally it has been demonstrated that corticosteroids, especially at high dosage levels, may result in delayed wound healing. An increase in the incidence of osteoporosis may be noted, mainly in the elderly, with prolonged use of these compounds. Their use in older dogs during the healing stages of bone fracture is not indicated for the reason listed above.

Use of corticosteroids, depending on dose, duration, and specific steroid, may result in inhibition of endogenous steroid production following drug withdrawal. In patients presently receiving or recently withdrawn from systemic corticosteroid treatments, therapy with a rapidly acting corticosteroid should be considered in unusually stressful situations.

Before instilling any medication into the ear, examine the external ear canal thoroughly to be certain the tympanic membrane is not ruptured in order to avoid the possibility of transmitting infection to the middle ear as well as damaging the cochlea or vestibular apparatus from prolonged contact. If hearing or vestibular dysfunction in noted during the course of treatment, discontinue use of GENTAVED® Otic Solution.

Warning(s): Clinical and experimental data have demonstrated that corticosteroids administered orally or parenterally to animals may induce the first stage of parturition when administered during the last trimester of pregnancy and may precipitate premature parturition followed by dystocia, fetal death, retained placenta, and metritis. Additionally, corticosteroids can induce cleft palates in offspring when given to pregnant animals during the period of palate closure of the embryos. Other congenital anomalies including deformed forelegs, phocomelia, and anasarca have been reported in offspring of dogs which received corticosteroids during pregnancy.

Avoid ingestion.

For use in dogs and cats only.

Toxicology: Parenterally, no toxic effects were observed in rats given gentamicin sulfate 20 mg/kg/day for twenty-four days; in cats given 10 mg/kg/day for forty days. Gentamicin sulfate given to dogs at 6 mg/lb/day, 6 days weekly for three weeks, caused no detectable kidney damage. At higher doses, impairment of equilibrium and of renal function were observed in these species.

Subacute otic toxicity in dogs showed gentamicin sulfate with betamethasone valerate solution to be well tolerated locally with no adverse systemic effects when administered at 5 drops twice a day for 21 consecutive days.

Gentamicin sulfate in a 21-day subacute dermal toxicity study in dogs was shown to be well tolerated when applied topically to abraded skin. There were no meaningful findings except a reduction in eosinophil count attributable to absorption of the corticosteroid component.

Side Effects: Side effects such as SAP and SGPT enzyme elevations, weight loss, anorexia, polydipsia, and polyuria have occurred following the use of parenteral or systemic synthetic corticosteroids in dogs. Vomiting and diarrhea (occasionally bloody) have been observed in cats and dogs.

Cushing's Syndrome in dogs has been reported in association with prolonged or repeated steroid therapy.

References: Available upon request.

Presentation: GENTAVED® Otic Solution, squeeze bottles of 7.5 mL, 15 mL, and 240 mL (8 fl oz).

Compendium Code No.: 10940990

GENTAVED® TOPICAL SPRAY ℞

Vedco **Topical Antimicrobial-Corticosteroid**

(Gentamicin Sulfate with Betamethasone Valerate)

ANADA No.: 200-188

Active Ingredient(s): Each mL contains: gentamicin sulfate equivalent to 0.57 mg gentamicin base, betamethasone valerate equivalent to 0.284 mg betamethasone, 163 mg isopropyl alcohol, propylene glycol, methylparaben and propylparaben as preservatives, purified water q.s. Hydrochloric acid may be added to adjust pH.

Indications: For the treatment of infected superficial lesions in dogs caused by bacteria sensitive to gentamicin.

Pharmacology: Chemistry: Gentamicin is a mixture of aminoglycoside antibiotics derived from the fermentation of *Micromonospora purpurea*. Gentamicin sulfate is a mixture of sulfate salts of the antibiotics produced in this fermentation. The salts are weakly acidic and freely soluble in water.

Gentamicin sulfate contains not less than 500 micrograms of gentamicin base per milligram.

Betamethasone valerate is a synthetic glucocorticoid.

Gentamicin, a broad-spectrum antibiotic, is a highly effective topical treatment for bacterial infections of the skin. *In vitro*, gentamicin is bactericidal against a wide variety of gram-positive and gram-negative bacteria isolated from domestic animals.[1,2] Specifically, gentamicin is active against the following organisms isolated from canine skin: *Alcaligenes* sp., *Citrobacter* sp., *Klebsiella* sp., *Pseudomonas aeruginosa*, indole-positive and negative *Proteus* sp, *Escherichia coli, Enterobacter* sp., *Staphylococcus* sp., and *Streptococcus* sp.

Betamethasone valerate emerged from intensive research as the most promising of some 50 newly synthesized corticosteroids in the experimental model described by McKenzie[3], *et al.* This human bioassay technique has been found reliable for evaluating the vasoconstrictor properties of new topical corticosteroids and is useful in predicting clinical efficacy.

Betamethasone valerate in veterinary medicine has been shown to provide anti-inflammatory and antipruritic activity in the topical management of corticosteroid responsive infected superficial lesions in dogs.

Dosage and Administration: Prior to treatment, remove excessive hair and clean the lesion and adjacent area. Hold bottle upright 3 to 6 inches from the lesion and depress the sprayer head twice. Administer 2 to 4 times daily for 7 days.

Each depression of the sprayer head delivers 0.7 mL of GENTAVED® Topical Spray.

Contraindication(s): If hypersensitivity to any of the components occurs, treatment with this product should be discontinued and appropriate therapy instituted.

Precaution(s): Store upright between 2°C and 30°C (36°F and 86°F).

Caution(s): Federal law restricts this drug to use by or on the order of a licensed veterinarian.

Antibiotic susceptibility of the pathogenic organism(s) should be determined prior to the use of this preparation. Use of topical antibiotics may permit overgrowth of non-susceptible bacteria, fungi, or yeasts. If this occurs, treatment should be instituted with other appropriate agents as indicated.

Administration of recommended dose beyond 7 days may result in delayed wound healing. Animals treated longer than 7 days should be monitored closely.

Avoid ingestion. Oral or parenteral use of corticosteroids, depending on dose, duration, and specific steroid may result in inhibition of endogenous steroid production following drug withdrawal.

In patients presently receiving or recently withdrawn from systemic corticosteroid treatments, therapy with a rapidly acting corticosteroid should be considered in especially stressful situations.

If ingestion should occur, patients should be closely observed for the usual signs of adrenocorticoid overdosage which include sodium retention, potassium loss, fluid retention, weight gains, polydipsia, and/or polyuria. Prolonged use or overdosage may produce adverse immunosuppressive effects.

Warning(s): Clinical and experimental data have demonstrated that corticosteroids administered orally or parenterally to animals may induce the first stage of parturition when administered during the last trimester of pregnancy and may precipitate premature parturition followed by dystocia, fetal death, retained placenta, and metritis.

Additionally, corticosteroids administered to dogs, rabbits and rodents during pregnancy have produced cleft palate. Other congenital anomalies including deformed forelegs, phocomelia, and anasarca have been reported in offspring of dogs which received corticosteroids during pregnancy.

For topical use in dogs only.

Toxicology: Gentamicin sulfate with betamethasone valerate topical spray was well tolerated in an abraded skin study in dogs. No treatment-related toxicological changes in the skin were observed.

Systemic effects directly related to treatment were confined to histological changes in the adrenals, liver, and kidney and to organ-to-body weight ratios of adrenals. All were dose related, were typical for or not unexpected with corticosteroid therapy, and were considered reversible with cessation of treatment.

Side Effects: Side effects such as SAP and SGPT enzyme elevations, weight loss, anorexia, polydipsia, and polyuria have occurred following parenteral or systemic use of synthetic corticosteroids in dogs. Vomiting and diarrhea (occasionally bloody) have been observed in dogs.

Cushings syndrome in dogs has been reported in association with prolonged or repeated steroid therapy.

References: Available upon request.

Presentation: Plastic spray bottle containing 60 mL, 120 mL or 240 mL of GENTAVED® Topical Spray.

Compendium Code No.: 10941000

GENT-L-CLENS™

Schering-Plough **Otic Cleanser**

NDC No.: 0061-0108-01

Active Ingredient(s): GENT-L-CLENS™ contains lactic acid and salicylic acid in a propylene glycol surface-acting vehicle preserved with PCMX.

Indications: For cleansing prior to the treatment of otic conditions.

Presentation: 4 fl. oz. (120 mL) squeeze bottles.

Compendium Code No.: 10470970

GENTLE IODINE 1%

Aspen **Topical Wound Dressing**

Active Ingredient(s):

Alpha-(P-Nonylphenyl Omega-Hydroxypoly (Oxyethylene)-Iodine Complex
(Equivalent to 1.0% Titratable Iodine) 5.0%
Isopropyl Alcohol 30.0%
Inert Ingredients 65.0%
Total 100.0%

Indications: A topical antiseptic for use prior to surgical procedures such as castrating and docking, for application to the navel of newborn animals, and for teat sores, minor cuts, bruises and abrasions.

Dosage and Administration: For use as a refill for the 16 oz spray bottle. Hold the container approximately six (6) inches from the area to be treated. Point the valve at the area to be sprayed. Pull the trigger of the valve and spray the area once, lightly. The product may also be applied directly with a swab, if desired. May be treated once a day, if necessary, until the area is healed.

Contraindication(s): Not for use on burns or in body cavities or deep wounds.

Precaution(s): Store in a cool place. Do not expose to heat or store at a temperature above 120°F.

Caution(s): Flammable. Do not use near an open flame. Keep out of the reach of children.

In case of deep or puncture wounds or serious burns, consult a veterinarian. If redness, irritation, or swelling persists or increases, discontinue use and consult a veterinarian.

Harmful if swallowed. Do not apply to the eyes, mucous membranes or large areas of abraded skin. Avoid inhaling mist.

Note: When used on or near the teats or udders of dairy animals, the teats and udders should be thoroughly washed before the next milking to prevent the contamination of milk.

Presentation: 16 fl oz (1 pint) spray bottle and 1 gallon (3.785 L) container.

Compendium Code No.: 14750370

"GENTLE" IODINE WOUND SPRAY

Centaur **Topical Wound Dressing**

Topical Antiseptic

Active Ingredient(s):

Alpha (P-Nonylphenyl) Omega-Hydroxypoly (Oxyethylene) Iodine Complex
(providing 2.44% Minimum Titratable Iodine) 8.7%
Isopropanol 52.8%
Inert Ingredients 38.5%

Indications: A topical antiseptic for use on large and small animals prior to surgical procedures such as castrating and docking. For application to the navel of newborn animals, and for aid in treatment of minor cuts, bruises and abrasions.

Directions for Use: Apply freely to infected area. When spraying hold container approximately 4 to 6 inches from the area to be treated. Point valve and spray area once lightly. May be repeated daily, when necessary, until abraded skin is healed.

Contraindication(s): Not for use on burns or in body cavities or deep wounds.

Precaution(s): Store in a cool place. Flammable. Do not expose to heat or store at a temperature above 120°F. Do not use near an open flame.

Caution(s): If redness, irritation, or swelling persists or increases, discontinue use and consult a veterinarian.

Harmful if swallowed. Do not apply to the eyes, mucous membranes or large areas of abraded skin. Avoid inhalation of mist.

Note: When used on or near the teats or udders of dairy animals, the teats and udders should be thoroughly washed before the next milking to prevent the contamination of milk.

Hazardous: Livestock remedy.

For animal use only.

Warning(s): Keep out of reach of children.

Not for human use.

Presentation: 1 pint (16 fl oz) 473 mL and 1 gallon (128 fl oz) 3.785 L containers.

Manufactured by: Unavet, North Kansas City, MO 64116.

Compendium Code No.: 14880170 Iss. 5-91 / Rev. 4/97

GENTLE IODINE WOUND SPRAY

First Priority **Disinfectant**

Active Ingredient(s):

Titratable Iodine 1%

Indications: In cattle, horses and swine as a topical antiseptic for use prior to surgical procedures such as castrating and docking; for ringworm and foot rot; for application to the navel of newborn animals; and for minor cuts, teat sores, bruises and abrasions.

Directions for Use: Remove spray cap from 16 oz container and refill from gallon container. Replace spray cap tightly. Hold container approximately 4 to 6 inches from the area to be sprayed. Pull trigger of valve and spray area once lightly. May be repeated daily, if necessary, until the area is healed.

Contraindication(s): Not for use on burns or in body cavities or deep wounds.

Precaution(s): Storage: Store at controlled room temperature between 15°-30°C (59°-86°F). Keep tightly closed when not in use.

Store in a cool place.

Caution(s): If redness, irritation or swelling persists or increases, discontinue use and consult a veterinarian.

Note: When used on or near the teats or udders of dairy animals, the teats and udders should be thoroughly washed before the next milking to prevent contamination of milk.

Harmful or fatal if swallowed. Do not apply to the eyes, mucous membranes or large areas of abraded skin. Avoid inhalation of mist.

For animal use only.

Warning(s): Keep out of reach of children.

Presentation: 16 fl oz (473 mL) with trigger sprayer (NDC# 58829-227-16) and 1 gallon (3.785 L) (NDC# 58829-227-01).

Compendium Code No.: 11390342 Rev. 06-01 / Rev. 07-01

G

GENTLE IODINE WOUND SPRAY

Vedco **Topical Wound Dressing**

Active Ingredient(s):

Alpha-(P-nonylphenyl)-omega-hyhphenyl)-omega-hydroxypoly-
(oxyethylene) iodine-complete, v/v; (equivalent to 2.4% titratable iodine) 8.7%
Isopropanol 52.8%
Inert ingredients 38.5%

Indications: For skin disinfections, superficial wounds, navel cords, sores. A topical antiseptic for use on horses, cattle, swine and sheep prior to surgical procedures such as castrating and docking; for application to the navel of newborn animals, and for aid in the treatment of footrot, sores, minor cuts, bruises, and abrasions.

Dosage and Administration: Hold the container approximately four (4) to six (6) inches from the area to be treated. Point the valve at the area to be sprayed. Pull the trigger of the valve and spray the area once lightly. May be repeated once a day, when necessary, until the abraded area is healed. If redness, irritation, or swelling persists or increases, discontinue use and consult a veterinarian.

Note: When used on or near the teats or udders of dairy animals, the teat and udders should be thoroughly washed before the next milking to prevent the contamination of milk.

Contraindication(s): Not for use on burns or in body cavities or deep wounds.

Precaution(s): Store in a cool place. Do not expose to heat or store at a temperature above 120°F.

Warning(s): Flammable. Do not use near an open flame.

Keep out of the reach of children.

Hazardous: Livestock remedy. Not for human use. For external animal use only.

Harmful if swallowed. Do not apply to the eyes, mucous membranes, or large areas of abraded skin. Avoid inhalation of mist.

Presentation: 16 fl. oz. (1 pt.) and 1 gallon containers.

Compendium Code No.: 10941030

GENTOCIN® DURAFILM® SOLUTION ℞

Schering-Plough **Ophthalmic Antimicrobial-Corticosteroid**

(Gentamicin sulfate) Ophthalmic Solution with Betamethasone

NADA No.: 034-267

Active Ingredient(s): GENTOCIN® DURAFILM® Ophthalmic Solution is a sterile preparation for topical application. Each mL of buffered solution (pH approximately 6.5) contains gentamicin base, 1 mg betamethasone acetate equivalent to 0.89 mg betamethasone alcohol, polyoxyl 40 stearate, polyoxyethylated vegetable oil, edetate disodium, 0.02 mg phenylmercuric nitrate as preservative and purified water q.s.

Indications: GENTOCIN® DURAFILM® Ophthalmic Solution is indicated for the treatment of external bacterial infections of the eye (conjunctiva and cornea) in dogs.

Clinical reports indicate it is useful for the management of some cases of pigmentary keratitis and pannus. Temporary remission of some of the pathological lesions of the aforementioned conditions, have been noted following therapy with GENTOCIN® DURAFILM® Ophthalmic Solution.

Pharmacology: Gentamicin is a bacterial antibiotic of the aminoglycoside group derived from *Micromonospora purpurea* of the Actinomycetes group. It is a powder, white to buff in color, basic in nature, readily soluble in water and highly stable in solution.

Betamethasone, a synthetic derivative of prednisolone, is 9-alpha- fluoro-16-betamethylprednisolone.

GENTOCIN® DURAFILM® Ophthalmic Solution incorporates polyoxyl 40 stearate and polyoxyethylated vegetable oil which provide a colloidal dispersion of active ingredients. This aqueous colloidal solution offers specific advantages in treating eye conditions. DURAFILM® covers the conjunctiva with a thin, clear, quickly spreading film which carries therapeutic components to accessible structures and maintains prolonged contact.

GENTOCIN® DURAFILM® Ophthalmic Solution provides the antibacterial properties of gentamicin sulfate plus the anti-inflammatory action of betamethasone acetate.

Gentamicin sulfate, a wide-spectrum antibiotic, is a highly effective topical treatment in primary and secondary bacterial infections of the eye and surrounding tissues. Gentamicin is bactericidal *in vitro* against a wide variety of gram-positive and gram-negative bacteria. Concentrations of gentamicin sulfate required to inhibit growth of gram-positive and gram-negative clinical and laboratory strains of bacteria tested were less than those of neomycin in most instances.[1] Gentamicin is active against most gram-negative bacteria including *Pseudomonas aeruginosa* indole-positive and -negative *Proteus* species, *Escherichia, coli, Klebsiella pneumoniae, Aerobacter aerogens* and Neisseria. Gentamicin is also active against strains of gram-positive bacteria including *Staphylococcus* species and Group A Beta-Hemolytic Streptococci.

Betamethasone produces hormonal and metabolic effects common to all adrenocortical steroids, and in low dosage affords anti-inflammatory, anti-allergic and anti-rheumatic effects.

Studies in man show the glucocorticoid activity of betamethasone to be 10 to 15 times greater than prednisone. Betamethasone helps to control excessive tissue reaction to infections, allergens and trauma. The corticoids control the inflammatory and exudate phases of eye conditions, particularly those affecting the anterior chamber and external structure of the eye. However, they do not curtail the growth of the causative organisms. Betamethasone therapy may reduce the damaging sequelae in certain eye diseases and injuries as well as scarring and vascularization, and appear to alter the usual tissue response to injury. In the initial acute phases of inflammation, the local application of betamethasone provides prompt, symptomatic relief, accomplishing temporary control of the exudative phase whether of bacterial, allergic or traumatic origin. Betamethasone also inhibits fibroblast formation during tissue repair.

Dosage and Administration: The topical application of GENTOCIN® DURAFILM® Ophthalmic Solution should, in each instance, be administered to meet the specific needs of the individual case. One (1) or two (2) drops of the solution may be instilled into the conjunctival sac three (3) or four (4) times a day. Thereafter, the frequency of the dosage may be reduced but care should be taken not to discontinue therapy prematurely. In chronic conditions, withdrawal of treatment should be carried out by gradually decreasing the frequency of application.

Contraindication(s): Corticosteroids are contraindicated in the initial treatment of conrneal ulcers.

GENTOCIN® DURAFILM® Ophthalmic Solution is contraindicated in ocular conditions where there is deep ulceration without vascularization and in conditions of viral origin before healing has commenced.

Precaution(s): Store between 2-30°C (36-86°F).

Caution(s): Federal law restricts this drug to use by or on the order of a licensed veterinarian.

The antibiotic sensitivity of the infective organism in bacterial conjunctivitis should be determined prior to the use of the preparation. The preparation is contraindicated in the case of nonsusceptible micro-organisms. In deep-seated infections or when systemic infection threatens, specific antibiotic or sulfonamide therapy should be employed.

G

The extended use of topical corticosteroids may cause increased intra-ocular pressure in susceptible patients. In prolonged therapy, it is advisable to measure intra-ocular pressure. In human medicine, in diseases that cause thinning of the cornea, perforation has been known to have occurred with the use of topical steroids.

The use of corticosteroids, depending upon dose, duration, and specific steroid, may result in the inhibition of endogenous steroid production following drug withdrawal. In patients presently receiving or recently withdrawn from systemic corticosteroid treatment, therapy with a rapidly acting corticosteroid should be considered only in especially stressful situations.

Warning(s): Clinical and experimental data have demonstrated that corticosteroids administered orally or parenterally to animals may induce the first stage of parturition when administered during the last trimester of pregnancy and may precipitate premature parturition followed by dystocia, fetal death, retained placenta and metritis.

Additionally, corticosteroids administered to dogs, rabbits, and rodents during pregnancy have produced cleft palate. Other congenital anomalies including deformed forelegs, phocomelia, and anasarca have been reported in offspring of dogs which received corticosteroids during pregnancy.

Side Effects: Side effects such as SAP and SGPT enzyme elevations, weight loss, anorexia, polydipsia, and polyuria have occurred following the use of synthetic corticosteroids in dogs. Vomiting and diarrhea (occasionally bloody) have been observed in cats and dogs.

Cushing's syndrome in dogs has been reported in association with prolonged or repeated steroid therapy.

A transient stinging sensation usually expressed as some form of resentment by the animal, following topical application of the drug, has been noted in a small number of cases. Usually this does not require discontinuance of therapy.

References: Available upon request.

Presentation: 5 mL squeeze dropper bottle, box of 12.

Compendium Code No.: 10470980

GENTOCIN® INJECTION (Cats and Dogs) ℞

Schering-Plough **Gentamicin**

(Gentamicin Sulfate)

NADA No.: 038-292

Active Ingredient(s): Each mL of GENTOCIN® Injection contains gentamicin sulfate veterinary equivalent to 50 mg gentamicin base, 3.2 mg sodium bisulfite, 0.1 mg edetate disodium; 1.8 mg methylparaben and 0.2 mg propylparaben as preservatives, water for injection q.s.

Indications: GENTOCIN® Injection is indicated for the treatment of the following canine, feline, and equine bacterial infections due to organisms susceptible to gentamicin.

Canine:

Urinary tract infections: cystitis and nephritis.

Respiratory tract infections: tonsillitis, pneumonia, and tracheobronchitis.

Skin and soft tissue: pyodermatitis, wounds, lacerations, and peritonitis.

Feline:

Urinary tract infections: cystitis and nephritis.

Respiratory tract infections: pneumonitis, pneumonia, and upper respiratory tract infections.

Skin and soft tissue: wounds, lacerations, and peritonitis.

Supportive therapy for secondary bacterial infections associated with panleukopenia.

Bacteriologic studies should be conducted to identify the causative organism and to determine its sensitivity to gentamicin sulfate. Sensitivity discs of the drug are available for this purpose.

Pharmacology: Gentamicin is a mixture of aminoglycoside antibiotics derived from the fermentation of *Micromonospora purpurea*. Gentamicin sulfate veterinary is a mixture of sulfate salts of the antibiotics produced in this fermentation. The salts are weakly acidic, freely soluble in water, and stable in solution.

Antibacterial Activity: *In vitro* antibacterial activity has shown that gentamicin is active against most gram-negative and gram-positive bacteria isolated from domestic animals.[1] Gentamicin is active against *Pseudomonas aeruginosa*, indole-positive and -negative *Proteus* species, *Escherichia coli*, *Klebsiella* species, *Aerobacter* species, *Alcaligenes* species, *Staphylococcus* species and *Streptococcus* species.

Studies in man indicate that recommended doses of gentamicin produce serum concentrations bactericidal for most bacteria sensitive to gentamicin within an hour after intramuscular injection; these concentrations last for 6 to 12 hours.[2] Some 30% of the administered dose of gentamicin is bound by serum proteins and released as the drug is excreted.

Gentamicin is excreted almost entirely by glomerular filtration. High concentrations of the active form are found in the urine. Fifty to 100% of the gentamicin injected can be recovered unchanged within 24 hours from the urine of patients with normal renal function. A small amount is excreted into the bile.

Dosage and Administration: GENTOCIN® Injection may be given by intramuscular or subcutaneous injection to dogs and cats.

Canine and Feline: The recommended dose is 2 mg/lb. of body weight twice the first day, then once a day thereafter. Duration of treatment depends on the response obtained and the condition being treated.

Treatment should not exceed seven (7) days.

In clinical studies response was evident in most of the treated dogs and cats after four (4) to six (6) days of therapy. If response is not noted after seven (7) days, the antibiotic sensitivity of the infecting organism should be retested.

Results of *in vivo* and *in vitro* studies indicate that alkalinization of the urine may be a useful therapeutic adjunct.

Contraindication(s): Gentamicin and other aminoglycosides are contraindicated in animals with renal azotemia.

Precaution(s): Store between 15° and 30° (59° and 86°F).

Protect from freezing.

Caution(s): Federal law restricts this drug to use by or on the order of a licensed veterinarian.

The following conditions have been found to contribute to the toxicity of gentamicin:

1. Prior renal damage, most commonly found in dogs of advanced age and dogs with heartworm microfilariae.[4]
2. Hypovolemic dehydration (dehydrated dogs and cats should be rehydrated prior to initiating therapy).[5,6]

The monitoring of renal function during treatment is recommended. Although there is not a completely reliable monitoring program for gentamicin toxicity, urinalysis may indicate early nephrotoxicity.[7] Unfavorable changes in the urinalysis which may indicate toxicity include:

1. Decreased specific gravity in the absence of fluid therapy.
2. Appearance of casts, albumin, glucose, or blood, in the urine in the absence of pyuria and bacteria.[7]

In animals where decreased renal function is suspected prior to treatment, BUN or serum creatinine levels may not indicate the degree of kidney impairment. A creatinine clearance determination may be more useful.

Once there is an indication of toxicosis, the gentamicin should be discontinued and the patient should be closely monitored and treated appropriately.[7]

Continued use of gentamicin where any functional renal impairment has occurred may lead to enhanced renal damage as well as the increased likelihood of ototoxicity and/or neuromuscular blockade.[3]

Animals receiving a full course of gentamicin therapy may not develop signs of nephrotoxicity until 1-3 weeks after therapy has terminated. Observations of animals and/or tests to determine renal function may be considered post treatment.[7]

Gentamicin sulfate should be used with caution in conjunction with drugs having nephrotoxic, ototoxic, or neuromuscular blocking characteristics.[8]

Neurotoxic and nephrotoxic antibiotics may be absorbed in significant quantities from body surfaces after local irrigation or application. The potential toxic effect of antibiotics administered in this fashion should be considered.[8]

Concurrent administration of furosemide and/or aminoglycosides may enhance nephrotoxicity in the dog. The co-administration of cephalosporins and gentamicin has been associated with increased prevalence of nephrotoxicosis in man.[5]

Reproductive studies have not been conducted in breeding dogs and cats.

If an overgrowth of nonsusceptible bacteria, fungi, or yeasts occur, treatment with gentamicin solution should be discontinued and appropriate therapy instituted.

If hypersensitivity develops, treatment with GENTOCIN® Injection should be discontinued and appropriate therapy instituted.

Warning(s): Gentamicin should be used with extreme caution in dogs in which hearing acuity is required for functioning, ie, seeing eye, hearing ear, or military patrol.[3]

To maintain the integrity of the septum and ensure the sterility of the product, no more than 50 entries should be made into a single vial.

Toxicology: Toxic effects were not observed in rats given gentamicin sulfate 20 mg/kg/day for 24 days; nor in cats given 10 mg/kg/day for 40 days. Gentamicin sulfate given to dogs at 6 mg/lb./day, six days a week for three weeks, did not cause detectable kidney damage. At higher doses, impairment of equilibrium and renal function were observed in these species.

Side Effects: There have not been reports of blood dyscrasia in dogs or cats treated with gentamicin. Injection site irritation has been reported in dogs and cats.

Neurotoxicity: Accumulation of ototoxicity can include ataxia, nausea, and vomiting. Auditory and vestibular impairment may be reversible in the very early stages, but if treatment is continued the conditions may become irreversible.[3,9]

Aminoglycoside auditory damage is dose related. Initial effects are associated with high frequency hearing loss. Total hearing loss can follow.

Nephrotoxicity: Accumulation of gentamicin in the kidney proximal tubule cells can lead to acute renal failure.[10] Renal toxicity has been accompanied by decreased urine specific gravity, proteinuria, casts in the urine, hematuria, increased BUN, and serum creatinine. Toxicity occurred more frequently in animals treated for longer periods or with larger doses than recommended.

Based on adverse drug reactions received by FDA, in many of the dogs in which nonfatal nephrotoxicity was associated with gentamicin therapy, drug withdrawal was followed by a decrease in the level of the BUN indicating that the nephrotoxicosis may be reversible when the drug is withdrawn.

References: Available upon request.

Presentation: GENTOCIN® Injection, 50 mg per mL, is packaged in 50 mL multiple dose vials, boxes of 1.

Compendium Code No.: 10470991

GENTOCIN® OPHTHALMIC ℞

Schering-Plough **Ophthalmic Antibiotic**

(Gentamicin sulfate) Solution and Ointment

NADA No.: 099-989/099-008

Active Ingredient(s): GENTOCIN® Ophthalmic Ointment is a sterile ointment containing gentamicin sulfate equivalent to 3 mg gentamicin with 0.5 mg methylparaben and 0.05 mg propylparaben as preservatives in a bland base of white petrolatum.

GENTOCIN® Ophthalmic Solution is a sterile aqueous solution buffered to approximately pH 7 for use in the eye. Each mL contains gentamicin sulfate equivalent to 3 mg gentamicin, 2.9 mg disodium phosphate, 0.1 mg monosodium phosphate, 7.4 mg sodium chloride and 0.1 mg benzalkonium chloride as preservative, and purified water q.s.

Indications: GENTOCIN® Ophthalmic is indicated for the topical treatment of conjunctivitis caused by susceptible bacteria in dogs and cats.

Pharmacology: Gentamicin sulfate is a water soluble antibiotic of the aminoglycoside group active against a wide variety of pathogenic gram-negative and gram-positive bacteria.

Gentamicin is an aminoglycoside antibiotic mixture derived from *Micromonospora purpurea* of the actinomycetes group. It is a powder, white to buff in color, readily soluble in water and heat stable.

Gentamicin sulfate, a broad spectrum antibiotic is a highly effective topical treatment in primary and secondary bacterial infections of the eye and surrounding tissues. Gentamicin is bactericidal *in vitro* against a wide variety of gram-positive and gram-negative bacteria. The concentrations of gentamicin sulfate required to inhibit growth of gram-positive and gram-negative clinical and laboratory strains of bacteria tested were less than those of neomycin in most instances.[1,2] Gentamicin is active against most gram-negative bacteria including *Pseudomonas aeruginosa*, indole-positive and -negative *Proteus* species, *Escherichia coli, Klebsiella* sp. and *Enterobacter* sp. Gentamicin is also active against strains of gram-positive bacteria including *Staphylococcus* species and *Streptococcus* species.

Dosage and Administration: GENTOCIN® Ophthalmic Ointment: Apply approximately one-half (½) inch strip to the affected eye two (2) to four (4) times a day.

GENTOCIN® Ophthalmic Solution: One (1) or two (2) drops instilled into the conjunctival sac two (2) to four (4) times a day.

Precaution(s): Store the solution and ointment between 2-30°C (36-86°F).

Caution(s): Federal law restricts this drug to use by or on the order of a licensed veterinarian.

The antibiotic susceptibility of infecting organisms should be determined prior to the use of the preparation. Prolonged use of topical antibiotics may give rise to the overgrowth of nonsusceptible organisms such as fungi. Should this occur or if irritation or hypersensitivity to any component develops, discontinue use of the preparation and institute appropriate therapy. Ophthalmic ointments may retard corneal healing.

References: Available upon request.

Presentation: GENTOCIN® Ophthalmic Ointment: ⅛ oz. tube, box of 12.
GENTOCIN® Ophthalmic Solution: 5 mL plastic sterile dropper bottle, box of 12.

Compendium Code No.: 10471000

GENTOCIN® OTIC SOLUTION ℞

Schering-Plough **Otic Antimicrobial-Corticosteroid**

(Gentamicin sulfate with betamethasone valerate)

NADA No.: 046-821

Active Ingredient(s): Each mL of GENTOCIN® Otic Solution contains gentamicin sulfate equivalent to 3 mg gentamicin base, betamethasone valerate equivalent to 1 mg betamethasone, 1.0 mg hydroxyethylcellulose, 2.5 mg glacial acetic acid, 200 mg purified water, 19% ethanol, 9.4 mg benzyl alcohol as preservative, 300 mg glycerin and propylene glycol q.s.

Indications: GENTOCIN® Otic Solution is indicated for the treatment of acute and chronic canine otitis externa and canine and feline superficial infected lesions caused by bacteria sensitive to gentamicin.

Pharmacology: Gentamicin is a bacterial antibiotic of the aminoglycoside group derived from *Micromonospora purpurea* of the Actinomycetes group. It is a powder, white to buff in color, basic in nature, readily soluble in water and highly stable in solution.

Betamethasone valerate is a synthetic corticosteroid derivative of prednisolone.

GENTOCIN® Otic Solution combines the broad spectrum activity of gentamicin sulfate with the anti-inflammatory and antipruritic activity of betamethasone valerate. *In vitro* antibacterial activity[1] has shown that gentamicin is active against most gram-negative bacteria including *Pseudomonas aeruginosa*, indole-positive and -negative *Proteus* sp., *Escherichia coli, Klebsiella pneumoniae, Aerobacter aerogenes* and *Neisseria*. Gentamicin is also active against strains of gram-positive bacteria including *Staphylococcus* species and some *Streptococcus* species.

Betamethasone valerate has emerged from intensive research as the most promising of some 50 newly synthesized corticosteroids in the experimental model described by Mckenzie[2] et al. This human bio-assay technique has been found reliable for evaluating the vasoconstrictor properties of new topical corticosteroids and is useful in predicting clinical efficacy.

Betamethasone valerate in human medicine has been shown to provide anti-inflammatory and antipruritic activity in the topical management of corticosteroid-responsive dermatoses. In the response cases, the local anti-inflammatory activity is sustained by the vasoconstrictor properties of the steroid.

Dosage and Administration: The duration of treatment will depend upon the severity of the condition and the response obtained. The duration of treatment and/or frequency of the dosage may be reduced, but care should be taken not to discontinue therapy prematurely.

Otitis externa: The external ear and ear canal should be properly cleaned and dried before treatment. Remove foreign material, debris, crusted exudates, etc., with suitable non-irritating solutions. Excessive hair should be clipped from the treatment area of the external ear. Instill three (3) to eight (8) drops of GENTOCIN® Otic Solution (approximately room temperature) into the ear canal twice a day for 7-14 days.

Superficial infected lesions: The lesion and adjacent area should be properly cleaned before treatment. Excessive hair should be removed. Apply a sufficient amount of GENTOCIN® Otic Solution to cover the treatment area twice a day for 7-14 days.

Contraindication(s): If hypersensitivity to any of the components occurs, treatment with the product should be discontinued and appropriate therapy instituted.

Concomitant use of drugs known to induce ototoxicity should be avoided.

The preparation should not be used in conditions where corticosteroids are contraindicated.

Do not administer parenteral corticosteroids during treatment with GENTOCIN® Otic Solution.

Precaution(s): Store between 2-30°C (36-86°F).

Caution(s): Federal law restricts this drug to use by or on the order of a licensed veterinarian.

The antibiotic sensitivity of the pathogenic organism should be determined prior to the use of the preparation. The use of antibiotics occasionally allows overgrowth of non-susceptible bacteria, fungi or yeasts. In these cases, treatment should be instituted with other appropriate agents as indicated.

Adverse systemic reactions have been observed following the oral ingestion of some topical corticosteroid preparations. Patients should be closely observed for the usual signs of adrenocorticoid overdosage which include sodium retention, potassium loss, fluid retention, weight gains, polydipsia and/or polyuria. Prolonged use or overdosage may produce adverse immunosuppressive effects.

Experimentally it has been demonstrated that corticosteroids especially at high dosage levels, may result in delayed wound healing. An increase in the incidence of osteoporosis may be noted, mainly in the elderly, with the prolonged use of these compounds. Their use in older dogs during the healing stages of bone fracture are not indicated for the reason listed above.

The use of corticosteroids, depending upon dose, duration, and specific steroid may result in the inhibition of endogenous steroid production following drug withdrawal. In patients receiving or recently withdrawn from systemic corticosteroid treatments, therapy with a rapidly acting corticosteroid should be considered only in unusually stressful situations.

Warning(s): Clinical and experimental data have demonstrated that corticosteroids administered orally or parenterally to animals may induce the first stage of parturition when administered during the last trimester of pregnancy and may precipitate premature parturition followed by dystocia, fetal death, retained placenta and metritis.

Additionally, corticosteroids can induce cleft palate in offspring when given to pregnant animals during the period of palate closure of the embryos. Other congenital anomalies including deformed forelegs, phocomelia, and anasarca have been reported in offspring of dogs which received corticosteroids during pregnancy.

Avoid ingestion.

Toxicology: Parenterally, toxic effects were not observed in rats given gentamicin sulfate 20 mg/kg/day for 24 days, or in cats given 10 mg/kg/day for 40 days. Gentamicin sulfate given to dogs at 6 mg/lb./day, six days weekly for three weeks, did not cause detectable kidney damage. At higher doses, impairment of equilibrium and of renal function were observed in these species.

Subacute otic toxicity in dogs showed GENTOCIN® Otic Solution to be well tolerated locally without adverse systemic effects when administered at five drops twice a day for 21 consecutive days.

GENTOCIN® Otic Solution in a 21 day subacute dermal toxicity study in dogs was shown to be well tolerated when applied topically to abraded skin. There were not meaningful findings except a reduction in eosinophil count attributable to absorption of the corticosteroid component.

Side Effects: Side effects such as SAP and SGPT enzyme elevations, weight loss, anorexia, polydipsia, and polyuria have occurred following the use of synthetic corticosteroids in dogs. Vomiting and diarrhea (occasionally bloody) have been observed in cats and dogs.

Cushing's syndrome in dogs has been reported in association with prolonged or repeated steroid therapy.

References: Available upon request.

Presentation: Squeeze bottles of 7.5 mL, 15 mL and 240 mL (8 fl. oz.).

Compendium Code No.: 10471020

GENTOCIN® PINKEYE SPRAY

Schering-Plough **Ophthalmic Antibacterial**

Gentamicin Sulfate, USP-1.07 mg/mL-Antibacterial

NADA No.: 130-952

Active Ingredient(s): GENTOCIN® Pinkeye Spray is a sterile aqueous solution, buffered to approximately pH 7 for topical use in the bovine eye. Each mL contains gentamicin sulfate, USP equivalent to 1.07 mg gentamicin base, 0.1 mg sodium phosphate monobasic, 2.9 mg sodium phosphate dibasic, 7.4 mg sodium chloride, 0.1 mg benzalkonium chloride as preservative, and purified water q.s.

Indications: GENTOCIN® Pinkeye Spray is indicated for the treatment of pinkeye in cattle (infectious bovine keratoconjunctivitis) caused by *Moraxella bovis.*

Pharmacology: Chemistry: Gentamicin is a mixture of aminoglycoside antibiotics derived from the fermentation of *Micromonospora purpurea*. Gentamicin sulfate veterinary is a mixture of sulfate salts of the antibiotics produced in this fermentation. The salts are weakly acidic and freely soluble in water. Gentamicin sulfate, USP is stable in solution for the period of time indicated on the label by the expiration date.

Dosage and Administration: One actuation of the sprayer delivers 0.7 mL containing 0.75 mg gentamicin. The sprayer should be held 3 to 6 inches from the affected eye and pumped once. It is advisable to treat the affected eye once a day for up to 3 days. In mild acute cases, recovery may occur with fewer treatments.

Contraindication(s): There are no known contraindications to this drug when used as directed.

Precaution(s): Store between 2° and 30°C (36° and 86°F).

Caution(s): Other conditions of the bovine eye may produce clinical signs similar to infectious bovine keratoconjunctivitis caused by *Moraxella bovis*. If clinical signs persist or worsen, diagnosis should be reevaluated. If condition persists or increases, discontinue use and consult a veterinarian.

For use in cattle only.

Restricted Drug (CA) - Use only as directed.

Presentation: GENTOCIN® Pinkeye Spray-Sterile-70 mL sealed plastic bottle with separate sterile packaged pump, boxes of 12.

Compendium Code No.: 10472130 22268007 Rev. 10/98

GENTOCIN® SOLUTION (Equine) ℞

Schering-Plough **Gentamicin**

(Gentamicin Sulfate)

NADA No.: 046-724

Active Ingredient(s):

50 mg/mL: Each mL of GENTOCIN® Solution contains gentamicin sulfate veterinary equivalent to 50 mg gentamicin base, 3.2 mg sodium bisulfite, 0.1 mg edetate disodium, 1.8 mg methylparaben and 0.2 mg propylparaben as preservatives, water for injection q.s.

100 mg/mL: Each mL of GENTOCIN® Solution contains gentamicin sulfate veterinary equivalent to 100 mg gentamicin base, 2.4 mg sodium metabisulfite, 0.8 mg sodium sulfite, anhydrous, 0.1 mg edetate disodium, 10 mg benzyl alcohol as preservative, water for injection q.s.

Indications: GENTOCIN® Solution is recommended for the control of bacterial infections of the uterus (metritis) in horses and as an aid in improving conception in mares with uterine infections caused by bacteria sensitive to gentamicin.

Bacteriologic studies should be conducted to identify the causative organism and to determine its sensitivity to gentamicin sulfate. Sensitivity discs of the drug are available for this purpose.

Pharmacology: Gentamicin is a mixture of aminoglycoside antibiotics derived from the fermentation of *Micromonospora purpurea*. Gentamicin sulfate veterinary is a mixture of sulfate salts of the antibiotics produced in this fermentation. The salts are weakly acidic, freely soluble in water, and stable in solution.

Antibacterial Activity: *In vitro* antibacterial activity has shown that gentamicin is active against most gram-negative and gram-positive bacteria isolated from domestic animals.[1] Gentamicin is active against *Pseudomonas aeruginosa*, indole-positive and -negative *Proteus* species, *Escherichia coli, Klebsiella* species, *Aerobacter* species, *Alcaligenes* species, *Staphylococcus* species, and *Streptococcus* species.

Studies in man indicate that recommended doses of gentamicin produce serum concentrations bactericidal for most bacteria sensitive to gentamicin within an hour after intramuscular injection; these concentrations last for 6 to 12 hours.[2] Some 30% of the administered dose of gentamicin is bound by serum proteins and released as the drug is excreted.

Gentamicin is excreted almost entirely by glomerular filtration. High concentrations of the active form are found in the urine. Fifty to 100% of the gentamicin injected can be recovered unchanged within 24 hours from the urine of patients with normal renal function. A small amount is excreted into the bile.

Dosage and Administration:

50 mg/mL: The recommended dose is 40 to 50 mL (2.0-2.5 g) GENTOCIN® Solution per day

for three (3) to five (5) days during estrus. Each dose should be diluted with 200-500 mL of sterile physiological saline before aseptic uterine infusion.

100 mg/mL: The recommended dose is 20 to 25 mL (2.0-2.5 g) GENTOCIN® Solution per day for three (3) to five (5) days during estrus. Each dose should be diluted with 200-500 mL of sterile physiological saline before aseptic uterine infusion.

Contraindication(s): There are not any known contraindications to this drug when used as directed.

Precaution(s): Store between 2° and 30°C (36° and 86°F).

If hypersensitivity to any of the components develops, or if an overgrowth of nonsusceptible bacteria, fungi, or yeasts occurs, treatment with GENTOCIN® Solution should be discontinued and appropriate therapy instituted.

Although GENTOCIN® Solution is not spermicidal, treatment should not be given the day of breeding.

Caution(s): Federal law restricts this drug to use by or on the order of a licensed veterinarian.

Warning(s): Not for use in horses intended for food.

Toxicology: Toxic effects were not observed in rats given gentamicin sulfate 20 mg/kg/day for 24 days; nor in cats given 10 mg/kg/day for 40 days. Gentamicin sulfate given to dogs at 6 mg/lb./day, six days a week for three weeks, did not cause detectable kidney damage. At higher doses, impairment of equilibrium and renal function were observed in these species.

Side Effects: There have not been reports of drug hypersensitivity nor other adverse side effects following the recommended intra-uterine infusion of GENTOCIN® Solution combined with sterile physiological saline in mares.

References: Available upon request.

Presentation: 50 mg/mL available in 100 mL multiple dose vials.
100 mg/mL available in 100 mL and 250 mL multiple dose vials.

Compendium Code No.: 10471030

GENTOCIN® TOPICAL SPRAY ℞

Schering-Plough **Topical Antimicrobial-Corticosteroid**

(Gentamicin sulfate with betamethasone valerate)

NADA No.: 132-338

Active Ingredient(s): Each mL contains: Gentamicin sulfate equivalent to 0.57 mg gentamicin base, betamethasone valerate equivalent to 0.284 mg betamethasone, 163 mg isopropyl alcohol, propylene glycol, methylparaben and propylparaben as preservatives, and purified water q.s. Hydrochloric acid may be added to adjust pH.

Indications: For the treatment of infected superficial lesions in dogs caused by bacteria susceptible to gentamicin.

Pharmacology: Gentamicin is a mixture of glycoside antibiotics derived from the fermentation of *Micromonospora purpurea.* Gentamicin sulfate veterinary is a mixture of sulfate salts of the antibiotics produced in this fermentation. The salts are weakly acidic, freely soluble in water and stable in solution.

Gentamicin sulfate veterinary contains not less than 500 micrograms of gentamicin base per mg.

Betamethasone valerate is a synthetic glucocorticoid.

Gentamicin, a broad-spectrum antibiotic is a highly effective topical treatment for bacterial infections of the skin. *In vitro* gentamicin is bactericidal against a wide variety of gram-positive and gram-negative bacteria isolated from domestic animals.[1,2] Specifically, gentamicin is active against the following organisms isolated from canine skin: *Alcaligenes* sp., *Citrobacter* sp., *Klebsiella* sp., *Pseudomonas aeruginosa*, indole-positive and -negative *Proteus* sp., *Escherichia coli*, *Enterobacter* sp., and *Staphylococcus* sp., and *Streptococcus* sp.

Betamethasone valerate emerged from intensive research as the most promising of some 50 newly synthesized corticosteroids in the experimental model described by McKenzie,[3] *et al.* This human bio-assay technique has been found reliable for evaluating vasoconstriction properties of new topical corticosteroids and is useful in predicting clinical efficacy.

Betamethasone valerate in veterinary medicine has been shown to provide anti-inflammatory and anti-pruritic activity in the topical management of corticosteroid responsive infected superficial lesions in dogs.

Dosage and Administration: Prior to treatment, remove excessive hair and clean the lesion and adjacent area. Hold the bottle upright three (3) to six (6) inches from the lesion and depress the sprayer head twice. Administer two (2) to four (4) times a day for seven (7) days.

Each depression of the sprayer head delivers 0.7 mL of GENTOCIN® Topical Spray.

Contraindication(s): If hypersensitivity to any of the components occurs, discontinue treatment and institute appropriate therapy.

Precaution(s): Store upright between 2-30°C (36-86°F).

Caution(s): Federal law restricts this drug to use by or on the order of a licensed veterinarian.

Antibiotic susceptibility fo the pathogenic organisms should be determined prior to the use of GENTOCIN® TOPICAL SPRAY. The use of topical antibiotics may permit the overgrowth of non-susceptible bacteria, fungi, or yeasts. If this occurs, treatment should be instituted with other appropriate agents as indicated.

Administration of the recommended dose beyond seven days may result in delayed wound healing. Animals treated for longer than seven days should be monitored closely.

Avoid ingestion. Oral or parenteral use of corticosteroids, depending upon dose, duration and specific steroid, may result in the inhibition of endogenous steroid production following drug withdrawal.

In patients presently receiving or recently withdrawn from systemic corticosteroid treatments, therapy with a rapidly acting corticosteroid should be considered in especially stressful situations.

If ingestion should occur, patients should be closely observed for the usual signs of adrenocorticoid overdosage which include sodium retention, potassium loss, fluid retention, weight gains, polydipsia and/or polyuria.

Prolonged use or overdosage may produce adverse immunosuppressive effects.

Warning(s): Clinical and experimental data have demonstrated that corticosteroids administered orally or parenterally to animals may induce the first stage of parturition when administered during the last trimester of pregnancy and may precipitate premature parturition followed by dystocia, fetal death, retained placenta and metritis.

Additionally, corticosteroids administered to dogs, rabbits, and rodents during pregnancy have produced cleft palate in offspring. Other congenital anomalies including deformed forelegs, phocomelia, and anasarca have been reported in offspring of dogs which received corticosteroids during pregnancy.

Toxicology: GENTOCIN® Topical Spray was well tolerated in an abraded skin study in dogs. Treatment related toxicological changes in the skin were not observed.

Systemic effects directly related to treatment were confined to histological changes in the adrenals, liver and kidney and to organ-to-body weight ratios of adrenals. All were dose-related, were typical for or not unexpected with corticosteroid therapy, and were considered reversible with cessation of treatment.

Side Effects: Side effects such as SAP and SGPT enzyme elevations, weight loss, anorexia, polydipsia, and polyuria have occurred following the use of synthetic corticosteroids in dogs. Vomiting and diarrhea (occasionally bloody) have been observed in cats and dogs.

Cushing's syndrome in dogs has been reported in association with prolonged or repeated steroid therapy.

References: Available upon request.

Presentation: Plastic spray bottle containing 72 mL of GENTOCIN® Topical Spray.

Compendium Code No.: 10471040

GERI-FORM

Vet-A-Mix **Small Animal Dietary Supplement**

Chewable, high-potency supplement for older dogs

Guaranteed Analysis: per Tablet:

(All values are minimum quantities unless otherwise stated.)

Minerals:

Zinc	10 mg
Selenium	20 mcg

Vitamins and Others:

Choline	40 mg
Inositol	25 mg
Vitamin E	15 IU
Niacinamide	10 mg
D-Pantothenic Acid	10 mg
Thiamine mononitrate	2 mg
Riboflavin	2 mg
Pyridoxine hydrochloride	1 mg
Vitamin A acetate	1,000 IU
Vitamin K	0.3 mg
Vitamin B_{12}	10 mcg
Vitamin D_3	80 IU

Ingredients: Lactose, Lecithin, Cellulose powder, Silicon dioxide, Choline chloride, DL-Methionine, DL-Alpha tocopheryl acetate, Animal liver meal (pork), Inositol, Magnesium stearate, Torula dried yeast, Calcium pantothenate, Zinc oxide, Niacinamide, Thiamine mononitrate, Riboflavin, Vitamin A acetate, Pyridoxine hydrochloride, Menadione sodium bisulfite complex, Cholecalciferol, Sodium selenite, Vitamin B_{12} supplement. Lipids: Acetone fractionated soy lecithin 600 mg, (Typical lipid profile: Phosphatidylcholine, Phosphatidylethanolamine, Glycolipids, Phosphatidylinositol, Phosphatidic acid, Phosphatidylserine).

Indications: For use as a dietary supplement in nutritional programs to increase levels of phospholipids and glycolipids, plus choline (acetylcholine precursor) and other important nutrients. Designed for older pets.

Dosage and Administration: Feed free choice, from the hand or crumble and mix into the food.

Dosage: Cats and small dogs - ½ to 1 tablet daily. Large dogs - 1 to 2 tablets daily.

Precaution(s): Store at room temperature. Protect from light. Avoid excessive heat (40°C or 104°F).

Warning(s): Keep out of reach of children.

Presentation: Bottles of 50 and 150 tablets.

Compendium Code No.: 10500101 1099

GERMICIDAL DETERGENT AND DEODORANT

Aire-Mate **Disinfectant**

EPA Reg. No.: 47371-131-5011

Active Ingredient(s):

Didecyl dimethyl ammonium chloride	2.31%
n-Alkyl (C_{14} 50%, C_{12} 40%, C_{16} 10%) dimethyl benzyl ammonium chloride	1.54%
Inert ingredients	96.15%
Total	100.00%

Indications: A germicidal detergent and deodorant that kills canine parvovirus. A concentrated, multi-purpose germicidal detergent and deodorant effective in hard waters up to 400 ppm (calculated as $CaCO_3$) plus 5% organic serum. Disinfects, cleans, and deodorizes in one step. Recommended for use in hospitals, schools and colleges, veterinary clinics and animal life science laboratories and the household.

Kills canine parvovirus.

Pharmacology: Bactericidal at 1:64 dilution (two ounces per gallon of water) against the following pathogenic bacteria according to the current AOAC use-dilution test method, modified in the presence of 400 ppm synthetic hard water (calculated as $CaCO_3$) plus 5% organic serum: *Pseudomonas aeruginosa, Staphylococcus aureus, Salmonella choleraesuis, Enterobacter cloacae, Streptococcus pyogenes, Streptococcus facaelis, Enterobacter aerogenes, Salmonella typhimurium, Klebsiella pneumoniae, Proteus vulgaris, Serratia marcescens, Shigella flexneri, Shigella sonnei, Salmonella typhi, Proteus mirabilis, E. coli, Staphylococcus aureus* (antibiotic resistant), *Streptococcus facaelis* (antibiotic resistant), *E. coli* (antibiotic resistant), *Klebsiella pneumoniae* (antibiotic resistant), *Staphylococcus epidermidis* (antibiotic resistant), *Pseudomonas aeruginosa* (antibiotic resistant).

Kills canine parvovirus.

Fungicidal against *Trichophyton interdigitale* and *Candida albicans* according to the AOAC fungicidal test, modified in the presence of 400 ppm hard water (calculated as $CaCO_3$) plus 5% organic serum at a 1:64 dilution.

Virucidal against influenza A/Hong Kong, herpes simplex type I, herpes simplex type II, vaccinia, rubella, adenovirus type 4, canine parvovirus, canine distemper virus, rabies virus, pseudorabies virus, porcine parvovirus, feline picorna virus, feline leukemia virus, infectious bronchitis virus (avian IBV) according to the virucidal qualification, modified in the presence of 400 ppm hard water plus 5% serum at a 1:64 dilution.

Virucidal also against HIV-1 (AIDS virus).

Dosage and Administration: It is a violation of federal law to use the product in a manner inconsistent with its labeling.

General use directions for disinfecting: For use on hard, nonporous surfaces such as floors, walls, metal surfaces, porcelain, and plastic surfaces. Remove gross filth and heavy soil deposits then thoroughly wet surfaces. Use two (2) ounces or one-quarter (¼) cup per gallon of water for a minimum contact time of 10 minutes in a single application. Can be applied with a mop, sponge, or cloth as well as spraying or soaking. The recommended use solution is prepared fresh for each use then discarded. Rinsing is not necessary unless floors are to be waxed or polished.

Mildewstatic instructions: Will effectively inhibit the growth and mildew plus the odors caused by them when applied to hard, non-porous surfaces such as walls, floors, and tabletops. Apply two (2) ounces per gallon of water with cloth, mop, or sponge, making sure to wet all surfaces completely. Let air dry. Prepare a fresh solution for each use. Repeat application once a week or when growth reappears.

For use in federally inspected meat and poultry plants: As a general cleaning agent on all surfaces, or for use with steam or mechanical cleaning device in all departments (dilute 2 oz. per gallon of water). Before use of this compound, food products and packaging materials must be removed from the room or carefully protected. After use of this compound, all surfaces in the area must be thoroughly rinsed with potable water.

Precaution(s):

Prohibitions: Do not contaminate water, food or feed by storage or disposal. Open dumping is prohibited. Do not re-use the empty container.

Pesticide Disposal: Wastes resulting from the use of this product may be disposed of on site or at an approved waste disposal facility.

Container Disposal:

Plastic containers: Triple rinse (or equivalent). Then offer for recycling or reconditioning, or puncture and dispose of in a sanitary landfill, or by incineration, or, if allowed by state and local authorities, by burning. If burned, stay out of smoke.

Fiber drums with liners: Completely empty the liner by shaking and tapping the sides and bottom to loosen clinging particles. Empty the residue into application equipment. Then dispose of the liner in a sanitary landfill or by incineration if allowed by state and local authorities. If the drum is contaminated and cannot be re-used, dispose of in the same manner.

Metal containers: Triple rinse (or equivalent). Then offer for recycling or reconditioning, or puncture and dispose of in a sanitary landfill, or by another procedure approved by state and local authorities.

General: Consult federal, state, or local disposal authorities for approved alternative procedures such as limited open burning.

Caution(s): Keep out of the reach of children.

Precautionary Statements:

Hazards to Humans and Domestic Animals: Causes eye irritation. Avoid contact with the eyes. Wash thoroughly after handling.

Statement of Practical Treatment: In case of contact, immediately flush eyes or skin with plenty of water for at least 15 minutes. For eyes call a physician.

Presentation: 1 gallon, 5 gallon, 30 gallon, and 55 gallon containers.

Compendium Code No.: 13970020

GERMICIDE SOLUTION

Phoenix Pharmaceutical **Disinfectant**

One Step Cleaner, Disinfectant & Deodorizer

EPA Reg. No.: 1130-15-58383

Active Ingredient(s):

N-Alkyl (68%C_{12}, 32%C_{14}) dimethyl ethylbenzyl ammonium chloride	0.154%
N-Alkyl (60%C_{14}, 30%C_{16}, 5%C_{12}, 5%C_{18}) dimethyl benzyl ammonium chloride	0.154%
Isopropanol	21.000%
Inert Ingredients	78.692%

Indications: A novel way to effectively clean, deodorize and sanitize against odor-causing organisms and disinfect hard surfaces. Kills dangerous germs such as *Salmonella choleraesuis, Staphylococcus aureus, Pseudomonas aeruginosa* and *Klebsiella pneumoniae* in 10 minutes. Kills dangerous viruses such as Influenza A2/HK and Herpes Simplex Type II in 30 seconds. Kills *Mycobacterium bovis* BCG (Tuberculosis) in 6 minutes at 20°C. Kills Polio I Virus and Rhinovirus (associated with common colds) in 3 minutes.

Kills HIV-1 (AIDS Virus) on pre-cleaned environmental surfaces or objects previously soiled with blood or body fluids in 30 seconds at room temperature (20-25°C) in health care settings or other settings in which there is an expected likelihood of soiling of inanimate surfaces/objects with blood or body fluids and in which the surfaces/objects likely to be soiled with blood or body fluids can be associated with the potential for transmission of human immunodeficiency virus Type 1 (HIV-1) associated with AIDS.

Kills *Trichophyron mentagrophytes, Aspergillus niger* and *Candida albicans* in 5 minutes at 20°C. Kills pathogenic fungi in 5 minutes at 20°C.

Bactericidal, Tuberculocidal, Fungicidal and Virucidal.

For use in hospitals and other critical care areas where control of hazards of cross-contamination is required. Use on surfaces and equipment surfaces such as tables, carts, baskets, counters, cabinets, telephones in operating rooms, intensive care and emergency units. Use on stainless steel, Formica, glass and other hard, non-porous surfaces. For use in households; in hospitals veterinary clinics; in laundromats in washers and dryers; on folding tables; on toilet seats and bathroom fixtures; hampers and bedpans; sickrooms; offices; on telephones; and hardhats and headphones. For use in dairies, food processing plants, food establishments, restaurants, taverns and commercial kitchens (disinfected food contact surfaces must be rinsed with potable water before reuse); in hotels, in public restrooms accommodations and commercial laundries; on stainless steel, chrome, porcelain, glass, Formica, vinyl, plastic and other hard, nonporous surfaces of respirators and respirator facepieces and CPR training mannequins.

Some areas of use: Hard surfaces in: Surgery, Recovery, Anesthesia, X-Ray Cat. Lab, E.R., Orthopedics, Newborn Nursery, Respiratory Therapy, Radiology, Central Supply.

Directions for Use: It is a violation of Federal law to use this product in a manner inconsistent with its labeling.

To Disinfect Non-Food Contact Surfaces: This product is not to be used as a terminal sterilant/high-level disinfectant on any surface or instrument that (1) is introduced directly into the human body, either into or in contact with the bloodstream or normally sterile areas of the body, or (2) contacts intact mucous membranes but which does not ordinarily penetrate the blood barrier or otherwise enter normally sterile areas of the body. This product may be used to preclean or decontaminate critical or semi-critical medical devices prior to sterilization or high-level disinfection. Remove gross filth. Use solution as is. Do not dilute. Soak items to be disinfected or apply solution with cloth or sponge so as to thoroughly wet surface. Allow to remain wet for 10 minutes, let air dry.

For Surgical Instrument Presoak: Remove gross filth. Presoak surgical instruments in undiluted solution for 10 minutes or more. Proceed with normal decontamination procedure.

Special Instructions for Cleaning and Decontamination Against HIV 1 (AIDS Virus) for Surfaces or Objects Soiled With Blood or Body Fluids.

Personal Protection: When using GERMICIDE SOLUTION, wear disposable latex gloves, protective gown, face masks, or eye coverings as appropriate when handling HIV 1 infected blood or body fluids.

Cleaning Procedure: All blood and other body fluids must be thoroughly cleaned from surfaces and objects before application of the GERMICIDE SOLUTION.

Contact Time: Thoroughly wet surface. Allow to remain wet 30 seconds; let air dry. Although efficacy at a 30-second contact time has been shown to be adequate against HIV 1 (AIDS Virus), this contact time would not be sufficient for other organisms. Use a 10-minute contact time for disinfection against all of the organisms claimed.

Precautionary Statements: Hazards to humans and domestic animals.

Caution: Harmful if absorbed through skin. Causes moderate eye irritation. Avoid contact with eyes, skin, or clothing. Wash thoroughly with soap and water after handling.

Statement of Practical Treatment:

If on skin: Wash with plenty of soap and water.

If in eyes: Flush eyes with plenty of water. Call a physician if irritation persists.

Physical or Chemical Hazards: Do not store near heat or open flame.

Storage and Disposal: Store in cool, well-ventilated area.

Disposal: Wastes resulting from the use of this product may be discarded by pouring down drain and flushing with large quantity of water.

Container Disposal: Do not reuse empty container. Wrap container and put in trash.

Disposal of Infectious Materials: Dispose of used solution in accordance with local regulations for infectious waste disposal.

Warning(s): Keep out of reach of children.

Presentation: 1 gallon (3.8 L).

Compendium Code No.: 12561050

GIARDIAVAX®

Fort Dodge **Protozoal Vaccine**

Giardia Lamblia Vaccine, Killed Protozoa

U.S. Vet. Lic. No.: 112

Contents: This product contains the antigen listed above.

Thimerosal and gentamicin added as preservatives.

Indications: For vaccination of healthy dogs, 8 weeks of age or older, as an aid in the prevention of disease and shedding caused by *Giardia lamblia* infections.

Dosage and Administration: Dogs, inject one 1 mL dose subcutaneously using aseptic technique. A second dose is given two to four weeks after first vaccination. Annual revaccination is recommended.

InfoVax-ID® System: The InfoVax-ID® System provides a simple and effective method of recording pertinent information on the vaccines administered to animals in a veterinary practice.

For vaccines requiring reconstitution, remove label from both vials and affix both labels to the animal's medical chart.

Using the InfoVax-ID® System:

1. Grasp the lower right hand corner of the tab at the arrow marked "Peel Here" between your thumb and forefinger.
2. Pull steadily at a slight upward angle until the top portion of the label is separated from the vial.
3. Place the label on the animal's medical chart. Press down on the label to ensure adhesion.

Precaution(s): Store in the dark at 2° to 7°C (35° to 45°F). Avoid freezing. Shake well. Use entire contents when first opened.

Caution(s): In the absence of a veterinarian-client-patient relationship, Federal law prohibits the relabeling, repackaging, resale, or redistribution of the individual contents of this package. (9 CFR 112.6)

In case of anaphylactoid reaction, administer epinephrine.

Warning(s): For use in dogs only.

For veterinary use only.

Discussion: Giardiasis is a health concern for people and dogs. While Giardia infection is a recognized zoonotic disease, the role that the dog assumes in human disease is not well established. GIARDIAVAX® has been proven to prevent clinical disease caused by *Giardia lamblia* infection in dogs and to significantly reduce the incidence, severity and duration of cyst shedding. Subsequent to *Giardia lamblia* exposure, some vaccinates may shed, therefore, proper hygiene and sanitation practices should be implemented.

Presentation: 25 doses (25 x 1 mL vials of vaccine), featuring the InfoVax-ID® System.

U.S. Patent Nos. 5,512,288 - 5,549,899 - 5,676,953 - 5,935,583 and Patents Pending

U.S. Pat. No. 5,704,648 (InfoVax-ID® System)

Compendium Code No.: 10030922 2795B

GLUCAMINOLYTE FORTE

AgriPharm **Electrolytes-Oral**

Oral Solution

Active Ingredient(s): Each 1000 mL of aqueous solution contains:

Dextrose - H_2O	300.0 g
Sodium Chloride	5.4 g
Sodium Acetate, Anhydrous	3.0 g
Potassium Acetate	1.0 g
Calcium Chloride - $2H_2O$	330.0 mg
Magnesium Chloride - $6H_2O$	260.0 mg
L-Glutamic acid	560.0 mg
L-Arginine Hydrochloride	450.0 mg
L-Proline	400.0 mg
L-Lysine Hydrochloride	240.0 mg
L-Leucine	160.0 mg
L-Phenylalanine	110.0 mg
L-Valine	110.0 mg
L-Threonine	100.0 mg
L-Isoleucine	70.0 mg
L-Histidine Hydrochloride	40.0 mg
L-Methionine	40.0 mg
L-Tyrosine	24.0 mg
Methylparaben (preservative)	0.18%
Propylparaben (preservative)	0.02%

Indications: For use as a supplemental nutritive source of dextrose, electrolytes, and amino acids in cattle.

Dosage and Administration: Administer orally as a drench or by use of a stomach tube. The usual recommended dose in adult cattle is 500 to 1000 mL, depending on size and condition.

Precaution(s): Store at controlled room temperature between 15°C and 30°C (59°F-86°F).

Caution(s): For animal use only.

Warning(s): Keep out of reach of children.

Presentation: 1000 mL.

Compendium Code No.: 14571200

GLUCAMINOLYTE FORTE

Vedco **Electrolytes-Oral**

Active Ingredient(s): Each 1,000 mL of aqueous solution contains:

Dextrose • H_2O .... 300.0 g
Sodium chloride........ 5.4 g
Sodium acetate anhydrous........ 3.0 g
Potassium acetate .... 1.0 g
Calcium chloride • $2H_2O$ .... 330.0 mg
Magnesium chloride • $6H_2O$ .... 260.0 mg
L-glutamic acid .... 560.0 mg
L-arginine hydrochloride .... 450.0 mg
L-proline .... 400.0 mg
L-lysine hydrochloride........ 240.0 mg
L-leucine .... 160.0 mg
L-phenylalanine .... 110.0 mg
L-valine .... 110.0 mg
L-threonine .... 100.0 mg
L-isoleucine........ 70.0 mg
L-histidine hydrochloride........ 40.0 mg
L-methionine .... 40.0 mg
L-tyrosine........ 240.0 mg
Methylparaben (preservative)........ 0.09%
Propylparben (preservative)........ 0.01%

Indications: For use as a supplemental source of electrolytes, dextrose, and amino acids in cattle.

Dosage and Administration: Administer orally as a drench or by the use of a stomach tube. The usual recommended dose in adult cattle is 500 to 1,000 mL, depending upon the size and the condition of the animal.

G

Precaution(s): Store at a controlled room temperature between 59-86°F (15-30°C).

Caution(s): Keep out of the reach of children. Not for human use.

Presentation: 1,000 mL containers.

Compendium Code No.: 10941041

GLUCO-AMINO-FORTE ORAL SOLUTION

Phoenix Pharmaceutical **Electrolytes-Oral**

Dextrose-Electrolytes-Amino Acids

Active Ingredient(s): Composition: Each 1000 mL of aqueous solution contains:

Dextrose • H_2O .... 300.0 g
Sodium Chloride .... 5.4 g
Sodium Acetate, Anhydrous........ 3.0 g
Potassium Acetate .... 1.0 g
Calcium Chloride • $2H_2O$ .... 330.0 mg
Magnesium Chloride • $6H_2O$ .... 260.0 mg
Total Protein .... 2.3 g

Containing Amino Acids: L-glutamic acid, L-arginine hydrochloride, L-proline, L-lysine hydrochloride, L-leucine, L-phenylalanine, L-valine, L-threonine, L-isoleucine, L-histidine hydrochloride, L-methionine, L-tyrosine.

Methylparaben (preservative)........ 0.09%
Propylparaben (preservative)........ 0.01%

Indications: For use as a supplemental nutritive source of dextrose, electrolytes, and amino acids in cattle.

Dosage and Administration: Administer orally as a drench. The usual recommended dose in adult cattle is 500 to 1000 mL, depending on size and condition.

Precaution(s): Store between 15° and 30°C (59°-86°F).

Caution(s): For animal use only.

Warning(s): Keep out of reach of children.

Presentation: 1000 mL bottles (NDC 57319-102-08).

Manufactured by: Phoenix Scientific, Inc., St. Joseph, MO 64503

Compendium Code No.: 12560373 Rev. 1-02

GLUCO AMINO FORTE ORAL SOLUTION

Vetus **Electrolytes-Oral**

Dextrose-Electrolytes-Amino Acids

Composition: Each 1000 mL of aqueous solution contains:

Dextrose•H_2O .... 300.0 g
Sodium Chloride .... 5.4 g
Sodium Acetate, Anhydrous........ 3.0 g
Potassium Acetate........ 1.0 g
Calcium Chloride•$2H_2O$........ 330.0 mg
Magnesium Chloride•$6H_2O$ .... 260.0 mg
Total Protein .... 2.3 g

Containing Amino Acids: L-Glutamic Acid, L-Arginine Hydrochloride, L-Proline, L-Lysine Hydrochloride, L-Leucine, L-Phenylalanine, L-Valine, L-Threonine, L-Isoleucine, L-Histidine Hydrochloride, L-Methionine, L-Tyrosine.

Methylparaben (preservative)........ 0.09%
Propylparaben (preservative)........ 0.01%

Indications: For use as a supplemental nutritive source of dextrose, electrolytes, and amino acids in cattle.

Dosage and Administration: Administer orally as a drench. The usual recommended dose in adult cattle is 500 to 1000 mL, depending on size and condition.

Precaution(s): Store between 15° and 30°C (59°-86°F).

Caution(s): For animal use only.

Warning(s): Keep out of reach of children.

Presentation: 1000 mL (NDC 47611-784-10).

Manufactured by: Phoenix Scientific, Inc.

Distributed by: Burns Veterinary Supply, Inc.

Compendium Code No.: 14440890 Iss. 08-00

GLUCOSE

Fort Dodge **Dextrose Therapy**

50% Sterile Solution

Active Ingredient(s): Each mL contains:

Dextrose, USP........ 500 mg

With 0.2% sodium biphosphate, water for injection, USP, q.s.

Indications: GLUCOSE (dextrose) solution for veterinary use in cattle (including lactating dairy cows) for treatment of Acetonemia (ketosis).

Dosage and Administration: Cattle — 25 mL to 50 mL/100 lb body weight. May be repeated after 3 to 5 hours if necessary. Administer intravenously, intraperitoneally or subcutaneously.

To Open Container: Wipe cap, top and neck of bottle with 70% alcohol. Screw down cap until a snap is heard indicating bottle top seal is broken. Carefully unscrew cap removing top of bottle. Attach sterile IV administration unit.

Precaution(s): Unused portion remaining in bottle should be discarded. Store at controlled room temperature 15° to 30°C (59° to 86°F). Protect from freezing.

Caution(s): Keep out of reach of children.

Presentation: 500 mL bottles, package of 12 (NDC 0856-0808-01).

Compendium Code No.: 10030930 2305D

GLYCERIN U.S.P.

First Priority **Lubricant**

Active Ingredient(s): Glycerin U.S.P.

Indications: For use as a solvent, humectant, emollient or lubricant.

Dosage and Administration: As required.

Precaution(s): Storage: Store at controlled room temperature between 15°-30°C (59°-86°F).

Keep container tightly closed when not in use.

Caution(s): For animal use only.

Warning(s): Keep out of reach of children.

Presentation: 32 fl oz (960 mL) (NDC# 58829-228-32) and 1 gallon (3.785 L) (NDC# 58829-228-01).

Compendium Code No.: 11390352 Rev. 07-01 / Rev. 06-01

GLYCERIN U.S.P.

Vedco **Lubricant**

Active Ingredient(s): Glycerin U.S.P.

Indications: For use as a solvent, humectant, emollient or lubricant.

Dosage and Administration: As required.

Precaution(s): Store at a controlled room temperature between 15° and 30°C (59° and 86°F).

Caution(s): Keep tightly closed when not in use.

Not for human use.

Keep out of the reach of children.

Presentation: 1 gallon (3.785 L) container.

Compendium Code No.: 10941050

GME™ POWDER AND LIQUID (GOAT'S MILK ESBILAC®)

Pet-Ag **Milk Replacer**

Guaranteed Analysis:

	Powder	Liquid
Crude Protein, min.	33.0%	4.5%
Crude Fat, min.	40.0%	6.0%
Crude Fiber, max.	0.0%	0.0%
Moisture, max.	5.0%	85.0%
Ash, max.	7.75%	1.0%

Ingredients:

Powder: Dried whole goat milk, vegetable oil, calcium sodium caseinate, soy oil, whey protein concentrate, dicalcium phosphate, L-arginine, DL-methionine, choline chloride, potassium chloride, calcium carbonate, potassium phosphate monobasic, magnesium carbonate, sodium chloride, potassium phosphate dibasic, magnesium sulfate, zinc sulfate, vitamin A supplement, iron sulfate, vitamin B_{12} supplement, calcium pantothenate, copper sulfate, ascorbic acid, niacin supplement, manganese sulfate, folic acid, riboflavin, vitamin D_3 supplement, thiamine hydrochloride, potassium iodide, pyridoxine hydrochloride, potassium citrate, vitamin E supplement, biotin.

Liquid: Water, goat's milk powder, soy oil, sodium caseinate, butter, egg yolk, calcium caseinate, lactose, L-methionine, L-arginine, calcium carbonate, choline chloride, potassium chloride, lecithin, magnesium sulfate, mono-potassium phosphate, sodium chloride, tri-calcium phosphate, carrageenan, di-potassium phosphate, di-calcium phosphate, ascorbic acid, ferrous sulfate, zinc sulfate, vitamin A supplement, vitamin E supplement, niacin supplement, d-calcium pantothenate, copper sulfate, thiamine hydrochloride, riboflavin, pyridoxine hydrochloride, manganese sulfate, vitamin D_3 supplement, potassium citrate, potassium iodide, folic acid, D-biotin, vitamin K_1 supplement, vitamin B_{12} supplement.

Indications: Milk formula for puppies with sensitive digestive systems and food supplement for adult dogs.

Dosage and Administration:

Directions for Mixing GME™ Powder: Shake one volume of powdered GME™ into two volumes of cold water. Do not mix more GME™ than can be consumed in 24 hours. Use teaspoons, tablespoons, or cups as measures. This reconstituted GME™ should be kept refrigerated. Feed at room temperature.

Directions for Feeding GOAT'S MILK ESBILAC® (GME™):

Puppies: All puppies should drink their mother's milk for at least 2 days, if possible. This colostrum milk gives extra nutrition and temporary immunity against some diseases.

Warm GME™ to room or body temperature. Reconstituted GME™ should be fed at the daily rate of 1 tablespoon per 2 ounces body weight. The daily feeding rate should be divided into equal portions for each feeding. Puppies' needs will vary and this amount may have to be increased or decreased, depending on the individual. Older puppies do well when fed reconstituted GME™ every 8 hours. Young, small or weak puppies may need to be fed reconstituted GME™ every 3 to 4 hours. Weigh the puppy 3 times a week to assure adequate feeding. Reconstituted GME™ should be fed slightly below body temperature (96°F).

Some nursing puppies that are not receiving adequate milk from the bitch may need to receive supplemental feedings. Nursing puppies supplemented with GME™ will require less milk replacer depending on the bitch's milk supply. Weigh the puppies daily to assure that they are receiving adequate GME™.

Consult your veterinarian for advice.

Use of a nurser bottle is recommended. The PetAg Small Animal Nurser is suited for feeding most puppies. When puppies are old enough to lap, begin offering GME™ in a shallow container. During the 3rd or 4th week mix GME™ with PetAg 2nd Step™ Puppy Weaning Food. Use of the GME™ and Weaning Food will allow the puppy to be gradually switched to solid food.

GME™ as a Food Supplement for Growing Puppies, Show Dogs, or Convalescent Dogs: GME™ is a highly digestible source of protein and energy. Mix powdered GME™ into the daily ration at a rate of 1 teaspoon per 5 lbs (2.2 kg) body weight, or feed 1 tablespoon of GME™ Liquid per 5 lbs (2.2 kg) body weight.

Pregnant and Lactating Bitches: Mix powdered GME™ into the daily ration at the rate of 2 teaspoons per 5 lbs (2.2 kg) body weight or feed 2 tablespoons GME™ Liquid formula per 5 lbs (2.2 kg) body weight until 2 weeks after whelping.

Precaution(s): Storage:

Powder: Refrigerate reconstituted liquid. To assure freshness, discard or freeze unused portion within 24 hours. Powdered packages can be resealed and refrigerated up to 1 month, or frozen up to 6 months.

Liquid: Shake well. Refrigerate after opening. To assure freshness, discard or freeze within 3 days. Do not freeze in original container.

Caution(s): Your veterinarian should be consulted for advice about the care and feeding of puppies.

Presentation: Powder: 5 lb (2.27 kg) (4 per case).
Liquid: 12.5 fl. oz. (370 mL) (12 per case).

Compendium Code No.: 10970172 20644-01

GO-DRY™

G.C. Hanford **Mastitis Therapy**

Dry Cow Mastitis Treatment

NADA No.: 065-081

Active Ingredient(s): Each 10 mL single dose syringe contains:

Penicillin G procaine in sesame oil: .... 100,000 units

Indications: This product is intended for the treatment of bovine mastitis in dry cows. This product is effective against udder infections caused by the following susceptible microorganism: *Streptococcus agalactiae.*

Dosage and Administration: Administer at the time of drying-off by infusing all four quarters, one time only, with a single 10 mL syringe.

Shake well before using.

At the time of drying-off, milk the udder dry. Wash the teats and udder thoroughly with warm water containing a suitable dairy disinfectant. Dry thoroughly. Saturate a small piece of cotton with a suitable antiseptic such as 70 percent alcohol and wipe off teat, using a separate piece of cotton for each teat. The hands of the operator should be washed and dried before administration of each treatment.

When using this product, remove plastic cover from tip of syringe and, while holding teat firmly, insert tip into streak canal, then push plunger and inject entire contents. After injection, grasp the end of the teat firmly, then gently massage the medication up the teat canal into the udder. It is recommended to use a suitable teat dip on all teats following treatment.

Precaution(s): Discard empty container. Do not reuse.

Store at room temperature: 15°-30°C (59°-86°F).

This product was manufactured by a non-sterilizing process.

Warning(s): Discard all milk for 72 hours (6 milkings) following calving or later as indicated by the marketable quality of the milk.

Animals should not be slaughtered for food within fourteen (14) days after treatment.

For use in dry cows only.

Not for human use.

Restricted drug (California) - Use only as directed.

Keep this and all medications out of the reach of children.

Presentation: 12x10 mL single dose syringe with 12 alcohol pads.

Compendium Code No.: 10340001

GO MAX™ LIQUID

Farnam **Equine Dietary Supplement**

Vitamin-Iron-Mineral Liquid Supplement

Guaranteed Analysis:

	Contains not Less Than:	Per Fluid Oz.	Per Pound
Cobalt	157 ppm	5 mg	71 mg
Copper	939 ppm	30 mg	426 mg
Iron	9,393 ppm	300 mg	4,261 mg
Magnesium	0.4%	15 mg	213 mg
Manganese	626 ppm	20 mg	284 mg
Potassium	0.31%	100 mg	1,420 mg
Selenium	8 ppm	250 mcg	3,551 mcg
Zinc	3,131 ppm	100 mg	1,491 mg
Vitamin A		25,000 IU	348,460 IU
Vitamin D_3		3,500 IU	48,785 IU
Vitamin E		35 IU	487 IU
Vitamin B_{12}		120 mcg	1,704 mcg
Riboflavin		28 mg	398 mg
d-Pantothenic Acid		50 mg	710 mg
Thiamine (Vitamin B_1)		30 mg	426 mg
Niacin		200 mcg	3 mg
Vitamin B_6		10 mg	142 mg
Folic Acid		10 mg	142 mg
Choline		179 mg	2,542 mg
Biotin		0.025 mg	0.36 mg

Ingredients: Purified Water, Cane Molasses, Ferrous Sulfate, Choline Chloride, Zinc Sulfate, Potassium Chloride, Magnesium Sulfate, Copper Sulfate, Guar Gum, Vitamin A Supplement, Vitamin D_3 Supplement, Vitamin E Supplement, Natural Cherry Flavor, Manganese Sulfate, Calcium Pantothenate, Thiamine Hydrochloride, Saccharin Sodium, Riboflavin Supplement, Xanthan Gum, Cobalt Sulfate, Ferric Ammonium Citrate, Methylparaben and Sodium Benzoate (as preservatives), Folic Acid, Pyridoxine Hydrochloride, Biotin, Ferronyl Iron, Yucca Schidigera Extract, Sodium Selenite, Niacin Supplement, and Vitamin B_{12} Supplement.

Super palatable. Yucca flavored. Selenium fortified.

Contains no beef product ingredients.

Indications: GO MAX™ Liquid is a highly palatable vitamin-iron-mineral feed supplement for horses.

Directions: Feeding Directions: Apply to the top of the grain as top dressing.

Pleasure Horses: Normal Use — 2 ounces daily. Light Use — 1 ounce daily.

Racing and Training Horses: 2 ounces daily.

Horses in Poor Condition: 2 ounces daily for two weeks or until the horse returns to full feed, then 1 to 2 ounces daily.

Idle Horses: 1 ounce daily.

Mares in Foal: 2 ounces daily.

Barren Mares: 2 ounces daily.

Stallions in Breeding Service: 2 ounces daily.

Foals: ½ ounce daily.

One gallon equals 2 month supply for 1 horse in training.

Precaution(s): Important:

1. Shake product before each use.
2. Store in a cool, clean place.
3. Keep container tightly closed when not in use.
4. Keep container away from direct sunlight and heat.
5. Keep from freezing.

Caution(s): Follow label directions. The addition to feed of higher levels of this premix containing selenium is not permitted. Overdosing product may be toxic.

For veterinary use only.

Warning(s): Keep out of reach of children.

Presentation: 3.78 L (one gallon/128 fl oz).

Compendium Code No.: 10000231 0CC1

GOOD START CALF BOLUS

AgriPharm **Large Animal Dietary Supplement**

Guaranteed Analysis:

	Amount per Gram	Amount per Bolus
Lactobacillus acidopholus	4.28×10^7 cfu	3×10^8 (3 billion)
Streptococcus faecium	4.28×10^7 cfu	3×10^8 (3 billion)
Bifidobacterium thermophilum	4.28×10^7 cfu	3×10^8 (3 billion)
Bifidobacterium longum	4.28×10^7 cfu	3×10^8 (3 billion)
Bacillus subtilus	4.28×10^7 cfu	3×10^8 (3 billion)
Lactase enzyme	106 units	750 units
Vitamin A	1,412 iu	10,000 iu
Vitamin E	71 iu	500 iu

This total colony forming units (cfu's) is 1.5×10^9 or 15 billion cfu's per bolus.

Ingredients: Limestone, dried egg, dried colostrum, cellulose, polyglycol, lactase enzyme, vitamin A, vitamin E, *Lactobacillus acidopholus, Streptococcus faecium, Bifidobacterium thermophilum, Bifidobacterium longum, Bacillus subtilus.*

Indications: GOOD START CALF BOLUS contains bovine host specific lactic acid producing bacteria to provide an oral source of these bacterias. GOOD START CALF BOLUS also contains lactase enzymes and a nutritional source of vitamin A and vitamin E.

Dosage and Administration: 1-2 boluses per calf at birth or at receiving. Repeat dosage as necessary.

Caution(s): For animal use only.

Not intended for use as a source of antibody.

Keep out of reach of children.

Presentation: 50 - 7.087 g (¼ oz.) boluses per jar, 12 per case.

Compendium Code No.: 14570450

GOOD START CALF PASTE

AgriPharm **Large Animal Dietary Supplement**

Active Ingredient(s):

Guaranteed Analysis:	Amount per Gram	Amount per Tube
Lactobacillus acidopholus	5×10^7 cfu	7.5×10^8 (7.5 billion)
Bifidobacterium thermophilum	5×10^7 cfu	7.5×10^8 (7.5 billion)
Bifidobacterium longum	5×10^7 cfu	7.5×10^8 (7.5 billion)
Streptococcus faecium	5×10^7 cfu	7.5×10^8 (7.5 billion)
Lactase, not less than	100 units	1,500 units
Vitamin A	1,333 iu	20,000 iu
Vitamin E	66 iu	1,000 iu

This total colony forming units (cfu's) is 3.0×10^9 or 30 billion cfu's per tube.

Ingredients: Vegetable oil, sodium aluminium silicate, dried egg, dried whey, colostrum, dextrose, sorbitan monostearate, potassium sorbate, vitamin A, vitamin E, lactase enzymes, *Lactobacillus acidopholus, Streptococcus faecium, Bifidobacterium thermophilum, Bifidobacterium longum, Bacillus subtilus.*

Indications: GOOD START CALF PASTE contains bovine host specific lactic acid producing bacteria to provide an oral source of these bacterias. GOOD START CALF PASTE also contains lactase enzymes and a nutritional source of vitamin A and vitamin E.

Dosage and Administration: One (1) tube per newborn calf or at receiving. Repeat as needed. No withdrawal required.

Precaution(s): Store product at or below room temperature. Keep unused product dry, cool and out of direct sunlight.

Caution(s): For animal use only – Keep out of reach of children.

Not intended for use as a source of antibody.

Presentation: 15 g tube, 25 per case.

Compendium Code No.: 14570460

GOODWINOL OINTMENT

Goodwinol **Parasiticide-Topical**

Active Ingredient(s): Contains benzocaine, rotenone and lanolin.

Indications: An ointment for the treatment of demodectic and follicular mange of dogs.

Dosage and Administration: Apply once every 24 hours, massaging thoroughly until absorbed.

Caution(s): Exercise care in treatment to avoid getting ointment into the eyes.

Presentation: Available in 1 oz. jars and 1 lb. containers.

Compendium Code No.: 14380000

GRADE A™

Intercon **Disinfectant**

EPA Reg. No.: 48211-4

Active Ingredient(s):

Octyl decyl dimethyl ammonium chloride	2.250%
Dioctyl dimethyl ammonium chloride	1.125%
Didecyl dimethyl ammonium chloride	1.125%
Alkyl (C_{14}, 50%; C_{12}, 40%; C_{16}, 10%) dimethyl benzyl ammonium chloride	3.000%
Inert ingredients	92.500%
Total	100.000%

Indications: Disinfectant, sanitizer, fungicide, virucide, deodorizer with organic soil tolerance for hospital, institutional, industrial, school, dairy and other farm use.

Virucidal performance: At a 3.5 oz./4.5 gallon use level this product was evaluated in the presence of 5% serum and found to be effective against the following viruses: Herpes simplex, vaccina, and influenza A_2 (Hong Kong) on inanimate environmental surfaces.

Fungicidal performance: At 0.5 oz. to 2.25 gallons of water use level, this product is an effective fungicide against *Trichophyton mentagrophytes* (the athlete's foot fungus) when used on surfaces in areas such as locker rooms, dressing rooms, shower and bath areas and exercise facilities, utilizing the AOAC fungicidal test.

Dosage and Administration:

General Classification: It is a violation of federal law to use the product in a manner inconsistent with its labeling.

Apply this disinfectant with a cloth, mop or mechanical spray device. When applied with a mechanical spray device, surface must be sprayed until thoroughly wetted. Treated surfaces must remain wet for 10 minutes. Fresh solution should be prepared daily or when the use solution becomes visibly dirty.

Disinfection in hospitals, nursing homes and other health care institutions. For disinfecting floors, walls, countertops, bathing areas, lavatories, tables, chairs, garbage pails and other hard nonporous surfaces.

Add 3.5 oz. of this disinfectant to 4.5 gallons of water. Apply to previously cleaned hard surfaces. At this use level, this product is effective against *Pseudomonas aeruginosa, Staphylococcus aureus* and *Salmonella choleraesuis* in the presence of 5% blood serum when evaluated by the AOAC use-dilution test.

Disinfection of poultry equipment, animal quarters and kennels: Poultry brooders, watering founts, feeding equipment and other animal quarters (such as stalls and kennel areas) can be disinfected after thorough cleaning by applying a solution of 2 oz. of this product to 4.5 gallons of water. Small utensils should be immersed in this solution. Prior to disinfection, all poultry, other animals and their feeds must be removed from the premises. This includes emptying all troughs, racks and other feeding and watering appliances. Remove all litter and droppings from floors, walls and other surfaces occupied or traversed by poultry or other animals.

After disinfection, ventilate buildings, coops and other closed spaces. Do not house poultry, or other animals or employ equipment until treatment has been absorbed, set or dried.

All treated equipment that will contact feed or drinking water must be rinsed with potable water before re-use.

Sanitizing of food processing equipment and other hard surfaces in food contact locations: For sanitizing food processing equipment, dairy equipment, food utensils, dishes, silverware, glasses, sinktops, countertops, refrigerated storage and display equipment and other hard nonporous surfaces. No potable water rinse is required.

Wash and rinse all articles thoroughly, then apply a solution of 1 oz. of this sanitizer in four (4) gallons of water. (150 ppm active). Surfaces should remain wet for at least one (1) minute followed by adequate draining and air drying. Fresh solutions should be prepared daily or when use solution becomes visibly dirty. For mechanical application, use solution may not be re-used for sanitizing applications.

Apply to sinktops, countertops, refrigerated storage and display equipment and other stationary hard surfaces by cloth or brush or mechanical spray device. No potable water rinse is required.

Dishes, silverware, glasses, cooking utensils and other similar size food processing equipment can be sanitized by immersion in a 1 oz./4 gallon solution of this product. No potable water rinse is required.

At 1 oz./4 gallon this sanitizer fulfills the criteria of appendix F of the GRADE A™ pasteurized milk ordinances 1978 recommendations of the U.S. public health services in waters up to 800 ppm of hardness calculated as $CaCo_3$ when evaluated by the AOAC germicidal and detergent sanitizer method against *Escherichia coli* and *Staphylococcus aureus.*

The udders, flanks and teats of dairy cows can be sanitized by washing with a solution of 1 oz. of this product in for (4) gallons of warm water. No potable rinse is required. Use a fresh towel for each cow. Avoid contamination of sanitizing solution by dirt and soil. Do not dip used towel back into sanitizing solution. When solution becomes visibly dirty, discard and provide fresh solution

Precaution(s): Do not contaminate water, food or feed by storage or disposal.

Do not store container on its side.

Avoid creasing or impacting of container side walls.

Pesticide wastes are acutely hazardous. Improper disposal of excess pesticide, spray mixture, or rinsate is a violation of federal law. If these wastes cannot be disposed of by use according to label instructions, contact the nearest State Pesticide or Environmental Control Agency, or the Hazardous Waste representative at the nearest EPA Regional Office for guidance.

Do not re-use empty container. Triple rinse empty container with water. Return metal drums to reconditioner or puncture and dispose of in a sanitary landfill or by other procedures approved by state and local authorities. Plastic containers may be disposed of in a sanitary landfill, incinerated or, if allowed by local authorities, by burning. If burned, stay out of smoke.

If container is one gallon or less, use this container disposal statement: Do not re-use empty container. Rinse thoroughly before discarding in trash.

Caution(s): Keep out of the reach of children.

Corrosive. Causes eye and skin irritation. Do not get in eyes, on skin, or on clothing. Wear goggles or face shield and rubber gloves when handling. Harmful if swallowed. Do not breathe spray mist. Avoid contamination of food.

Precautionary Statements:

Hazards to Humans and Domestic Animals:

Statement of Practical Treatment: In case of contact, immediately flush eyes or skin with plenty of water for at least 15 minutes. For eyes, call a physician. Remove and wash contaminated clothing before re-use.

If swallowed, drink promptly a large quantity of milk, egg whites, gelatin solution, or if these are not available, drink large quantities of water. Avoid alcohol. Call a physician immediately.

Note to Physician: Probable mucosal damage may contraindicate the use of gastric lavage. Measures against circulatory shock, respiratory depression and convulsion may be needed.

Presentation: 4x1 gallon, 5 gallon containers, and 55 gallon drums.

Compendium Code No.: 10130011

GRAND CHAMPION® DRI-KLEEN™

Farnam **Grooming Shampoo**

Indications: For use on horses or ponies as a shampoo in winter when weather conditions prevent the use of water and in summer if no water is available. An all-season shampoo that cleans deep down without water. DRI-KLEEN™ removes stains and dirt. Does not contain oils or soap to leave a filmy residue. Leaves horse's hair clean, smooth, shiny and stain resistant.

Directions: Shake well.

Spray DRI-KLEEN™ on one section of the horse at a time. Rub each section with a heavy towel, stroking with and against the grain of the hair. After applying DRI-KLEEN™ to the whole horse, allow to air dry completely. Brush thoroughly until all dirt is removed. Repeat if necessary to eliminate resistant stains. DRI-KLEEN™ is mild and non-irritating.

Caution(s): Avoid excessive inhalation of spray mist. Do not use in subfreezing weather.

Warning(s): Keep DRI-KLEEN™ out of reach of children.

Presentation: 32 fl oz (0.946 L) with sprayer.

Compendium Code No.: 10000760 9D7

GRAND CHAMPION® FLY REPELLENT FORMULA

Farnam **Insect Repellent**

Instant Coat Brightener & Conditioner

EPA Reg. No.: 43591-3-270

Active Ingredient(s):

Pyrethrins	0.10%
Piperonyl Butoxide, Technical*	1.00%
Inert Ingredients	98.90%
Total	100.00%

* Equivalent to min. 0.8% (butylcarbityl) (6-propylpiperonyl) ether and 0.2% related compounds.

Indications: GRAND CHAMPION® gives you the perfect show combination - a high-tech silicone shine and a pyrethrin fly repellent in one product. All the advantages of a silicone polish - detangles manes and tails quickly; a lustrous, healthy looking coat that shines like a winner; repels dust and dirt and prevents stains from grass, urine, manure and latigo - plus protection from annoying flies.

Directions for Use: It is a violation of Federal law to use this product in a manner inconsistent with its labeling.

Read entire label before each use.

Use only on horses or ponies.

Do not use on horses intended for slaughter.

To protect horses from horn flies, house flies, mosquitoes and gnats, apply a light mist sufficient to wet the surface of the hair. To control stable flies, horse flies and deer flies, apply at a rate of 2 ounces per adult animal, sufficient to wet the hair thoroughly. Repeat treatment daily or at intervals necessary to give continued protection.

To control blood-sucking lice, apply to the infested areas of the animal using a stiff brush to get the spray to the base of the hair. Repeat every 2 to 3 weeks if required.

Precautionary Statements: Hazards to Humans and Domestic Animals:

Caution: Harmful if swallowed or absorbed through skin. Avoid breathing vapors or spray mist. Avoid contact with skin and eyes. Remove pets, birds and cover fish aquaria before space spraying or surface application. Do not use on animals under 12 weeks. Consult a veterinarian before using this product on debilitated, aged, medicated, pregnant or nursing animals. Sensitivities may occur after using any pesticide product for pets. If signs of sensitivity occur, bathe your pet with mild soap and rinse with large amounts of water. If signs continue, consult a veterinarian immediately. Avoid contamination of feed and foodstuffs.

First Aid:

If Swallowed: Drink one or two glasses of water and induce vomiting by touching the back of the throat with finger. Repeat until vomit fluid is clear. Do not induce vomiting or give anything by mouth to an unconscious person. Call a physician or Poison Control Center immediately.

If on Skin: Remove contaminated clothing and wash affected areas with soap and water. Seek medical attention if irritation persists.

If in Eyes: Flush eyes with plenty of water. Seek medical attention if irritation persists.

If Inhaled: Remove victim to fresh air. Apply artificial respiration if indicated. Seek medical attention if indicated.

Environmental Hazards: This product is toxic to fish. Do not apply directly to lakes, ponds, streams, tidal marshes or estuaries. Do not contaminate water by cleaning of equipment or disposal of waste.

Physical or Chemical Hazards: Flammable. Contents under pressure. Keep away from heat, sparks, and open flame. Do not puncture or incinerate container. Exposure to temperatures above 130°F may cause bursting.

Storage and Disposal: Do not transport or store under 32°F.

Storage: Store in a cool dry area away from heat and open flame. Store above 32°F in a place inaccessible to children and pets.

Disposal: Securely wrap container in several layers of newspaper and discard in trash. Do not puncture or incinerate.

Warning(s): Do not use on horses intended for slaughter.

Keep out of reach of children.

Disclaimer: Buyer assumes all risks of use, storage, or handling of this product not in strict accordance with directions given herein.

Presentation: 0.414 L (14 fl oz) spray can.

Compendium Code No.: 10000860 9D7

GRANULEX® V AEROSOL SPRAY

Pfizer Animal Health **Topical Wound Dressing**

NADA No.: 039-583

Active Ingredient(s): Each gram delivered to the wound site contains:

Trypsin, crystalline, N.F.. . . . . 0.12 mg
Balsam Peru, N.F. . . . . 87.0 mg
Castor Oil, USP . . . . . 788.0 mg

With a water-dispersible emulsifier and propellants.

Inert propellant 25% of total content.

Indications: GRANULEX® is an aid in the treatment of external wounds such as wire cuts, rope burns, abrasions, and lacerations in dogs, cats, horses, and cattle; and assists healing by facilitating the removal of necrotic tissue, exudate, and organic debris.

Directions: Shake well. Hold can upright approximately 12 inches from the area to be treated. Press valve and coat rapidly. Wound may be left unbandaged or apply a wet dressing. Apply twice daily or as often as necessary. To remove, wash gently with warm water. When applied to sensitive areas, a temporary stinging sensation may be noted.

Precaution(s): Flammable—Do not use near fire or open flame. Contents under pressure, do not puncture or incinerate. Do not expose to temperatures above 120°F.

Caution(s): Do not use on fresh arterial clots. Avoid spraying in eyes and nostrils. Keep out of reach of children. Use only as directed. Intentional misuse by deliberately concentrating and inhaling the contents can be harmful or fatal.

Warning(s): For veterinary use only.

Presentation: 4 oz (113.4 g).

Manufactured by: Bertek Pharmaceuticals Inc., Sugar Land, Texas 77487

Compendium Code No.: 36901140 90-8252-01

GRANULEX® V LIQUID

Pfizer Animal Health **Topical Wound Dressing**

NADA No.: 039-583

Active Ingredient(s): Each gram of medication contains:

Trypsin, crystalline, N.F.. . . . . 0.12 mg
Balsam Peru, N.F. . . . . 87.0 mg
Castor Oil, USP . . . . . 788.0 mg

With a water-dispersible emulsifier.

Indications: GRANULEX® is an aid in treatment of external wounds such as wire cuts, rope burns, abrasions, and lacerations in dogs, cats, horses, and cattle; and assists healing by facilitating the removal of necrotic tissue, exudate, and organic debris.

Directions: Shake well. Apply twice daily or as often as necessary. When applied to sensitive areas, a temporary stinging sensation may be noted.

Caution(s): Do not use on fresh arterial clots. Do not apply to eyes. Keep out of reach of children. Use only as directed.

Warning(s): For veterinary use only.

Presentation: 1 oz (28.35 g).

Manufactured by: Bertek Pharmaceuticals Inc., Sugar Land, TX 77487

Compendium Code No.: 36901150 50-8253-01

GREENLYTE®

Bimeda **Feed & Water Additive**

Guaranteed Analysis:

Calcium (Ca) not less than. 0.50%
Calcium (Ca) not more than. 1.00%
Phosphorus (P) not less than 0.25%
Salt (NaCl) not less than 18.00%
Salt (NaCl) not more than 21.60%
Sodium (Na) not lass than. 7.50%
Potassium (K) not less than. 30.00%
Magnesium (Mg) not less than 0.60%
Sulfur (S) not less than 0.06%
Zinc (Zn) not less than. 0.15%
Methionine not less than 0.30%

Bacillus subtilis, Bacillus licheniformis - not less than 9.9 billion CFU units per kilo (45 billion CFU units per pound).

Ingredients: Potassium chloride, salt, citric acid, calcium lactate, magnesium gluconate, monosodium phosphate, zinc methionine, dextrose, sodium bicarbonate, dried bacillus subtilis fermentation product, dried bacillus licheniformis fermentation product, natural and artificial flavors, artificial colors.

Indications: A supplemental source of buffered, soluble mineral electrolytes and acidifiers to be added to the drinking water or feed. For use in beef cattle, dairy cattle, veal calves, sheep, swine, horses, poultry, ostriches, emus, and rheas.

Directions for Use:

Beef, Dairy and Adult Sheep: *Use 1 pound per 128 gallons of drinking water. *Use 1 pound per gallon of stock solution; use 2 ounces stock solutions per gallon drinking water. *Use 6 pounds per ton of feed.

Veal, Replacement Calves & Lambs: *Use 1 pound per 128 gallons of drinking water. *Use 1 tsp. per gallon of water, milk or milk replacer. *Use 1 ounce per quart of water per 25 pounds of body weight for drenching solution. *Use 6 pounds per ton of feed.

Swine: *Use 1 pound per 128 gallons of drinking water. *Use 1 pound per gallon of stock solution and use 1 ounce per gallon of drinking water. *Use 6 pounds per ton of feed.

Equine (Horse, Foals and Colts): *Use 1 pound per 50 to 100 gallons of drinking water *Use 1-2 ounces per 10 gallons of drinking water per day. *Use 1 ounce top dressing in a grain ration for mature horses; ½ ounce for foals and colts.

Poultry & Ratites (Ostrich, Emu & Rhea): *Use 1 pound per 256 gallons of drinking water. *Use ½ pound per 1 gallon of stock solution and use 1 ounce stock solution per gallon of water. *Use 2 pounds per ton of feed.

Companion and Fur-bearing animals: Use 1 tbsp. per gallon of drinking water.

There are 2½ level tablespoons per ounce.

Caution(s): For animal use only.

Keep out of reach of children.

Presentation: 1 lb., 3 lb. and 25 lb.

GREENLYTE® is a registered trademark of Ameri-Pac Inc.

Compendium Code No.: 13990190

GRENADE® ER PREMISE INSECTICIDE

Schering-Plough **Premise Insecticide**

EPA No.: 10182-361-773

Active Ingredient(s):

Lambda-cyhalothrin[1] [1α(S*),3α(Z)]-(±)-cyano-(3-phenoxyphenyl)-methyl-3-(2-chloro-3,3,3-trifluoro-1-propenyl)-2,2-dimethylcyclopropanecarboxylate 9.7%
Inert Ingredients: 90.3%
Total 100.0%

[1]Synthetic pyrethroid

Indications: A premise insecticide for use in and around livestock housing, poultry housing and pet kennels.

Directions for Use: It is a violation of Federal law to use this product in a manner inconsistent with its labeling.

For agricultural use only.

For use as a general surface (non-food/non-feed areas), crack and crevice or spot treatment in, on and around buildings and structures and their immediate surroundings, and on modes of transport. Permitted areas of use include, but are not limited to, livestock/poultry housing structures, pet kennels, railcars, trucks and trailers. GRENADE® ER insecticide can be reapplied at 21-day intervals if necessary.

GRENADE® ER insecticide is intended for dilution with water for application using hand held or power operated application equipment as a coarse spray for crack and crevice or spot and general surface treatments. Application equipment that delivers low volume treatments, such as the Microgen® or Actisol® applicator, may also be used to make crack and crevice or spot and general surface treatments. Fill applicator tank with the desired volume of water and add GRENADE® ER insecticide. Close and shake before use in order to ensure proper mixing. Shake or reagitate applicator tank before use if application is interrupted. Make up only amount of treatment volume as required.

Pests	Concentration of Active Ingredient	Dilution Rate
Ants Bees Confused Flour Beetles Fleas* Flies Lesser Grain Borers Red Flour Beetles Saw-toothed Grain Beetles Wasps	0.015% - 0.03%	0.015%: 0.2 fl oz (6 mL)/gal water 0.03%: 0.4 fl oz (12 mL)/gal water
Crickets Litter Beetles** (adults/immature stages such as Darkling, Hide and Carrion) Mosquitoes Pill Bugs Scorpions Sow Bugs Spiders Ticks	0.06%	0.8 fl oz (24 mL)/gal water

*For outdoor use only and use 0.03% rate.

**For control of light beetle infestations, use 0.03% rate.

1. Flies, Mosquitoes, Bees and Wasps: Apply directly to walls, ceilings, window screens, and other resting areas as a residual surface treatment. May be used in and around carports, garages, and storage sheds; also see Outdoor Surfaces Use.
2. Ants: Apply to any trails around doors and windows and other places where ants may be found. Apply barrier treatments to prevent infestation as directed below; also see Outdoor Surfaces Use.
3. Spiders and Crickets: Apply as a coarse, low-pressure spray to areas where these pests hide, such as corners, storage areas, closets, around water pipes, doors and windows, attics and eaves, baseboards, behind and under sinks, furnaces, and stoves, the underside of shelves, drawers and similar areas. Pay particular attention to cracks and crevices; also see Outdoor Surfaces Use.
4. Confused Flour Beetle, Lesser Grain Borer, Red Flour Beetle and Saw-Toothed Grain Beetle: Apply to cupboards, shelving, and storage areas. Remove all uncovered foodstuffs (or any having original package opened). Allow treated surfaces to dry before replacing any foodstuff or other items. Any foodstuff accidentally contaminated with treatment solution should be destroyed.
5. Sow Bugs and Pill Bugs: Apply around doors and windows and other places where these pests may be found or where they may enter premises. Treat storage areas and other locations. Apply barrier treatments to prevent infestation as described below; also see Outdoor Surfaces Use.
6. Litter Beetles (Darkling, Hide and Carrion Beetles) in Animal Housing (such as Poultry Housing): To control adult litter beetles, apply GRENADE® ER to walls and floors at cleanout, before reintroduction of animals. This will suppress beetles that escaped earlier treatment and will help delay onset of future infestations. Pay attention to areas where beetles frequently occur, such as walls, supports, cages, stalls, and around feeders; also see Livestock/Poultry Housing Structures and Pet Kennels.

Livestock/Poultry Housing Structures and Pet Kennels: Apply as a general surface and/or crack and crevice treatment. Control is enhanced when interior and exterior perimeter applications are made in and around the livestock, poultry, and pet housing structures. Normal cleaning practices of the structure also must be followed along with applications of GRENADE® ER insecticide to effectively control the crawling and flying insect pests listed in the table.

For poultry houses, apply to floor area (birds grown on litter) or to walls, posts, and cage framing (birds grown in cages). Application should also be made into cracks and crevices around insulation. Reapply after each growout or sanitization procedure. Indoor control can be enhanced by making perimeter treatments around the outside of the building foundations to prevent immigrating beetles. Apply in a uniform band at least one foot up and one foot out from foundation. Maintaining a year-round treatment program will prevent background populations from reaching problem levels.

Do not make applications of GRENADE® ER insecticide in areas where animals are present in the facility. Allow treated surfaces to completely dry before restocking the facility. Do not make applications to any animal feedstuffs, water, or watering equipment. Do not contaminate any animal food, feed, or water in and around livestock, poultry, or pet housing when making applications.

Outdoor Surfaces Use: For control of flies, fleas, mosquitoes, ants, bees, wasps, crickets, pill bugs, scorpions, sow bugs, spiders, ticks, and other similar perimeter insect pests. Apply with either hand or power application equipment as a residual treatment to surfaces of buildings, screens, window frames, eaves, patios, garages, and other similar areas. Also may be applied to lawn areas around non-residential buildings, refuse dumps and similar areas where these insect pests are active.

Barrier Treatments: To help prevent infestation of building, apply to a band 6 to 10 feet wide around and adjacent to the building. Also, treat the building foundation to a height of 2 to 3 feet where pests are active and may find entrance. Apply as a coarse spray to thoroughly and uniformly wet the foundation and/or band area, using 1-5 gallons of treatment solution applied to 800-1600 square feet.

Note: Do not use water base sprays of GRENADE® ER insecticide in conduits, motor housings, junction boxes, switch boxes, or other electrical equipment because of possible shock hazard. For best results thoroughly wash out sprayer and screen with water and detergent before using GRENADE® ER insecticide. GRENADE® ER insecticide has not stained or caused damage to painted or varnished surfaces, plastics, fabrics, or other surfaces where water applied alone causes no damage.

Let treated surfaces dry before allowing humans and pets to contact surfaces.

Do not use this product with oil.

Do not allow applications to contact water inhabited by fish, such as in aquariums and ornamental fish ponds that are located in/around structures being treated.

Precautionary Statements: Hazards to Humans and Domestic Animals:

Caution: Harmful if absorbed through skin. Prolonged or frequently repeated skin contact may cause allergic skin reactions in some individuals. Avoid contact with skin, eyes, or clothing. Avoid breathing spray mist or vapors. Wash thoroughly with soap and water after handling. Remove contaminated clothing and wash before reuse.

Statement of Practical Treatment:

If on Skin: Wash with plenty of soap and water. Get medical attention if irritation persists.

If Swallowed: If victim is alert and not convulsing, rinse mouth out and give 200 to 300 mL (1 cup) of water to dilute material. Immediately contact local Poison Control Center. Vomiting should only be induced under the direction of a physician or a Poison Control Center. If spontaneous vomiting occurs, have victim lean forward with head down to avoid breathing in of vomitus, rinse mouth and administer more water. Immediately transport victim to an emergency facility.

If in Eyes: Flush with plenty of water for at least 15 minutes. Get medical attention if irritation persists.

For 24-hour emergency medical assistance, call 1-800-228-5635.

For Chemical Emergency: Spill, leak, fire, exposure, or accident call CHEMTREC, 1-800-424-9300.

Environmental Hazards: This product is extremely toxic to fish. Do not contaminate water when cleaning equipment or disposing of equipment washwaters. Do not apply directly to any body of water. Apply this product only as specified on the label. Care should be used when making applications to avoid household pets, particularly fish and reptile pets.

Physical and Chemical Hazards: Do not use this product in or on electrical equipment due to the possibility of shock hazard.

Storage and Disposal:

Prohibitions: Do not contaminate water, food or feed by storage or disposal. Open dumping is prohibited. Do not reuse empty container.

Storage: Keep container closed when not in use. Do not store near food or feed. Shake well before use. Protect from freezing. In case of spill or leak on floor or paved surfaces, soak up with sand, earth or synthetic absorbent. Remove to chemical waste storage area until proper disposal can be made.

Pesticide Disposal: Pesticide wastes are toxic. Improper disposal of excess pesticide, spray mixture or rinsate is a violation of Federal law. If these wastes cannot be disposed of by use according to label instructions, contact your State Pesticide or Environmental Control Agency, or the Hazardous Waste representative of the nearest EPA Regional Office guidance.

Container Disposal: Triple rinse (or equivalent). Completely empty container into application equipment, then offer for recycling or reconditioning, or puncture and dispose of empty container in a sanitary landfill, by incineration, or by other procedures approved by state and local authorities.

Warning(s): Keep out of reach of children.

Disclaimer: In no event shall Schering-Plough Animal Health Corp. or Seller be liable for any incidental, consequential, or special damages resulting from the use or handling of this product. The exclusive remedy of the User or Buyer, and the exclusive liability of Schering-Plough Animal Health Corp. and Seller for any and all claims, losses, injuries or damages (including claims based on breach of warranty, contract, negligence, tort, strict liability or otherwise) resulting from the use or handling of this product, shall be the return of the purchase price of the product or, at the election of Schering-Plough Animal Health Corp. or Seller, the replacement of the product.

Schering-Plough Animal Health Corp. and Seller offer this product, and Buyer and User accept it, subject to the foregoing conditions of sale and limitations of warranty and liability, which may not be modified except by written agreement signed by a duly authorized representative of Schering-Plough Animal Health Corp.

Conditions of Sale and Limitation of Warranty and Liability:

Notice: Read the entire Directions for Use and Conditions of Sale and Limitation of Warranty and Liability before buying or using this product. If the terms are not acceptable, return the product at once, unopened, and the purchase price will be refunded.

The Directions for Use of this product should be followed carefully. It is impossible to eliminate all risks inherently associated with the use of this product. Ineffectiveness or other unintended consequences may result because such factors as manner of use or application, weather, presence of other materials or other influencing factors in the use of the product, which are beyond the control of Schering-Plough Animal Health Corp. or Seller. All such risks shall be assumed by Buyer and User, and Buyer and User agree to hold Schering-Plough Animal Health Corp. and Seller harmless for any claims relating to such factors.

Schering-Plough Animal Health Corp. warrants that this product conforms to the chemical description on the label and is reasonably fit for the purposes stated in the Directions for Use, subject to the inherent risks referred to above, when used in accordance with directions under normal use conditions. This warranty does not extend to the use of this product contrary to label instructions, or under abnormal conditions or under conditions not reasonably foreseeable to or beyond the control of Seller or Schering-Plough Animal Health Corp., and Buyer and User assume the risk of any such use.

Schering-Plough Animal Health Corp. makes no warranties of merchantability or of fitness for a particular purpose nor any other expressed or implied warranty except as stated above.

Presentation: 8 x 8 fl oz (0.24 L) plastic containers (NDC 0061-5211-01).

GRENADE is a registered trademark of Schering-Plough Veterinary Corp.

Compendium Code No.: 10471051 Rev 11/00

GROOM-AID® 35X

Evsco **Grooming Shampoo**

Contents: Lanolin.

Indications: A concentrated grooming, tearless shampoo for use on dogs, cats, puppies, kittens and horses.

Directions: Add 1 gallon of water to about 3.5 fluid ounces of GROOM-AID® 35x. 1 gallon of concentrate will make 35 gallons of shampoo. Wet coat thoroughly before applying shampoo. Work into coat until a lather is produced. Rinse thoroughly. Keep pet in a warm area until dry.

Caution(s): For topical use only on dogs, cats and horses. Do not use on animals under 4 weeks of age. Discontinue use if skin becomes irritated or inflamed.

Keep out of reach of children.

For animal use only.

Presentation: 4 x 1 gallon (128 fl oz - 3.79 L).

Compendium Code No.: 10050110

GROOM-AID® SPRAY

Evsco **Grooming Product**

Active Ingredient(s): The product contains isopropyl alcohol and mineral spirits, and an absorbable lanolin derivative in a scented deodorant.

Indications: A deodorizing, detangling and moisturizing spray for damp, musty odors absorbed by dog's and cat's coats during kennel stays.

Dosage and Administration: To operate, remove the protective cap from the top of the can. Hold the can in a upright position, approximately 8-12 inches from the pet's hair. Point the opening on the side of the valve in the desired direction for spray. To release the spray, place a finger on top of the valve and press down. Move the bomb over the entire animal, using a "zig-zag" motion, until the coat is slightly damp. It may be advantageous, especially on long haired animals, to rub the hand against the lay of the hair, spraying into the ruffled hair directly behind the hand.

Precaution(s): Flammable. Contents under pressure.

Do not use or store near heat, sparks or an open flame.

Do not puncture or incinerate the container.

Do not store at temperatures above 120°F.

Caution(s): Avoid spraying into the animal's eyes.

For veterinary use only.

Keep out of the reach of children.

Presentation: 7.3 oz. (207 g) containers.

Compendium Code No.: 10050120

GROOMING SHAMPOO

First Priority **Grooming Shampoo**

Ingredient(s): Water, ammonium laureth sulfate, ammonium lauryl sulfate, coconut oil, glycerine, sodium chloride, fragrance, FD&C color.

Indications: A mild, pH balanced shampoo. Enriched with coconut oil. GROOMING SHAMPOO will leave the animal's coat clean and smelling fresh. Gentle enough for every day use on pets. Rinses out easily and completely.

Directions for Use: Wet the animal's coat using warm water, and apply enough shampoo to work up a good lather. Massage deep into coat. Rinse animal thoroughly with warm water. For especially dirty animals, repeat washing directions. When finished washing, dry the animal.

Presentation: 16 fl oz (473 mL) (NDC# 58829-243-16), 1 gallon (3.785 L) (NDC# 58829-243-01) and 2.5 gallon (9.46 L).

Compendium Code No.: 11390362 Rev. 05-00 / Rev. 4-99

GROW COLT®

Farnam **Large Animal Dietary Supplement**

Guaranteed Analysis: Each pound contains not less than:

Calcium (Min.)	7.0500%
Calcium (Max.)	8.0500%
Phosphorus (Min.)	5.2800%
Salt (Min.)	1.6500%
Salt (Max.)	2.1500%
Potassium	0.9300%
Magnesium	0.2200%
Manganese	2200 ppm
Iron	1800 ppm
Copper	100 ppm
Zinc	100 ppm
Iodine	400 ppm
Cobalt	30 ppm
Selenium	4 ppm
Vitamin A	480,000 I.U.
Vitamin D_3	100,000 I.U.
Vitamin E	320 I.U.
Vitamin B_{12}	3.2 mg
Riboflavin	400 mg
d-Pantothenic Acid	360 mg
Thiamine	120 mg
Niacin	2400 mg
Vitamin B_6	60 mg
Folic Acid	10 mg
Choline	3600 mg
Biotin	6 mcg
P-Amino Benzoic Acid	90 mg
Ascorbic Acid	10 mg

Ingredients: Corn, Dicalcium Phosphate, Wheat middlings, Calcium Carbonate, dehydrated alfalfa meal, Sodium Chloride, vitamin A acetate, cholecalciferol (source of Vitamin D_3), choline chloride, niacinamide, riboflavin supplement, dl-alpha tocopherol acetate (source of Vitamin E), calcium pantothenate, para-aminobenzoic acid, thiamine hydrochloride, pyridoxine hydrochloride (source of Vitamin B_6), folic acid, ascorbic acid, biotin, cyanocobalamin (source of Vitamin B_{12}), magnesium oxide, manganous oxide, ferrous carbonate, copper oxide, potassium iodide, cobalt carbonate, sodium selenite and cane molasses.

Indications: GROW COLT® aids in growth and development under appropriate conditions of use. GROW COLT® provides 27 important vitamin and mineral nutrients. Prepared specifically for colts in their first year of development.

Dosage and Administration: General: To aid in maximum growth and development, add 2 ounces (four (4) heaping tablespoons) of GROW COLT® to grain daily for each foal. Continue feeding daily throughout the foal's first year of development. Provides 27 important vitamin and mineral nutrients.

Feeding Before Weaning: To avoid set-backs resulting from weaning and to speed early development, the foal should be given some supplementary feed while still nursing the mare. Usually the foal can start eating small amounts of feed when he is two to three weeks old. Creep feeding - in which the newborn foal can feed on grain and hay separately from the mare - is highly recommended. Several good starting rations are outlined below:

Recommended Grain Formulas for Suckling Foals
(Ingredients for 12-Pound Batch)

Ration No. 1		Ration No. 2		Ration No. 3	
Rolled Oats	6 lbs.	Rolled Oats	4 lbs.	Rolled Oats	9 lbs.
Wheat Bran	4 lbs.	Rolled Barley	3 lbs.	Wheat Bran	2 lbs.
Linseed Meal	1 lb.	Wheat Bran	3 lbs.	GROW COLT®	1-3/4 lbs.
GROW COLT®	1-3/4 lbs.	Linseed Meal	1 lb.		12-3/4 lbs.
	12-3/4 lbs.	GROW COLT®	1-3/4 lbs.		
			12-3/4 lbs.		

Feed 3/4 to 1 lb. of grain daily with fresh legume hay.

Feeding After Weaning: Foals are usually weaned at four to six months of age. At weaning, separate the foal from the mare and feed him 1 to 1-½ lbs. of hay per 100 lbs. of body weight. Also feed 2 ounces of GROW COLT® daily. The weaning period is the most critical time for feeding the growth supplement. Similarly the grain ration is quite critical. Three suggested grain rations for the weanling foal are outlined below:

Recommended Grain Formulas For Weanling Foals To One Year
(Ingredients for 40-Pound Batch)

Ration No. 1		Ration No. 2		Ration No. 3	
Oats	12 lbs.	Oats	27 lbs.	Oats	31 lbs.
Barley	12 lbs.	Wheat Bran	6 lbs.	Linseed Meal	8 lbs.
Wheat Bran	11 lbs.	Linseed Meal	6 lbs.	GROW COLT®	2 lbs.
Linseed Meal	4 lbs.	GROW COLT®	2 lbs.		41 lbs.
GROW COLT®	2 lbs.		41 lbs.		
	41 lbs.				

Feed 3 lbs. of grain daily with grass or legume hay.

You can also add brown sugar to each of these rations to encourage the foal to start eating grain as early as possible. Your choice of rations will, of course, depend on the cost an availability of various grains.

Presentation: 3 lb (1.361 kg), 7 lb, 20 lb, and 100 lb containers.
Compendium Code No.: 10000251

GUAIFENESIN INJECTION ℞

Butler **General Anesthetic**

50 mg per mL

ANADA No.: 200-230

Active Ingredient(s): Each mL of the injection contains: 50 mg guaifenesin, 50 mg dextrose (anhydrous), 20 mg propylene glycol, 50 mg dimethylacetamide (parenteral grade), 0.75 mg edetate disodium, water for injection q.s.

Indications: For intravenous use as a skeletal muscle relaxant for horses.

Pharmacology: Description: Guaifenesin, 3 - (o-Methoxyphenoxy) 1,2-propanediol, is a white to slightly gray, crystalline powder having a bitter taste. It may have a slight characteristic odor.

Actions: Guaifenesin is a guaiacol derivative closely related to mephenesin. The propanediol derivatives are central-acting skeletal muscle relaxants which selectively depress transmission of nerve impulses at the internuncial neurons of the spinal cord, brainstem, and subcortical regions of the brain.

Propanediol derivatives have a wide margin of safety, the toxic dose is three times greater than the recommended dose. Respiration is not severely depressed, and the function of the diaphragm is uninterrupted.[1,2] Tidal volume is slightly decreased and minute volume remains normal. In addition to skeletal muscle, the pharyngeal and laryngeal muscles are sufficiently relaxed for easier surgical intubation procedures. At the beginning of relaxation, there is a slight fall in blood pressure, however, throughout the relaxation period the heart function is unchanged. There is a slight increase in gastrointestinal activity. There is no apparent impairment of lung and kidney functions.

With the recommended administration and dosage of GUAIFENESIN INJECTION, induction is usually smooth and rapid (two to four minutes) providing a duration of action between 15 to 25 minutes. A slightly transient hemolysis occurs at a 5% concentration.[3,4] Higher concentrations cause intravascular hemolysis.[3,5]

The 5% dextrose minimizes the hemolytic action of guaifenesin alone and reduces the tendency to form thrombi at the intravenous injection site.[6] Guaifenesin appears safe when administered to pregnant mares[7] and in human studies did not pass the placental barrier.[2]

Metabolism and excretion of guaifenesin is not well understood. Oxidation products are excreted in the urine as a glycuronimide.

Dosage and Administration: For intravenous use only. Administer rapidly with a positive pressure system or gravity flow using a 12 to 14 gauge needle at the dose rate of 1 mL/pound of body weight. From a standing position the patient will begin to relax and gradually fall when approximately ½ the total dose has been given. Continue the remaining calculated dose for complete relaxation. Average duration of muscle relaxation is 10-25 minutes. For continued relaxation time, additional GUAIFENESIN INJECTION may be administered as determined by the veterinarian at a rate necessary to achieve the desired plane of relaxation. Recovery is usually smooth and uneventful with the horse regaining an upright position usually within 45 minutes after the medication is discontinued.

Contraindication(s): Do not administer physostigmire to horses receiving GUAIFENESIN INJECTION.

Precaution(s): Store between 2° and 30°C (36° and 86°F). Do not freeze.

Destroy partially used vials.

Caution(s): Federal law restricts this drug to use by or on the order of a licensed veterinarian.

Avoid perivascular leakage to prevent local tissue irritation.

If used for prolonged periods, such as in tetanus, serum hemoglobin levels should be monitored.

Oxygen or sustained artificial respiration facilities should be available when the drug is employed.

Additional care should be employed when administering the drug to anemic or hypovolemic animals with cardiac or respiratory problems.

Extreme care should be exercised at all times in handling this product to prevent the introduction of microbial contamination.

Warning(s): Not to be used in horses intended for food.
References: Available upon request.
Presentation: 1,000 mL sterile, single dose plastic vial.
Manufactured by: Phoenix Scientific, Inc.
Compendium Code No.: 10820880

GUAIFENESIN INJECTION ℞

Phoenix Pharmaceutical **General Anesthetic**

50 mg/mL-Sterile

ANADA No.: 200-230

Active Ingredient(s): Each mL of the injection contains:

Guaifenesin	50 mg
Dextrose (anhydrous)	50 mg
Propylene Glycol	20 mg
Dimethylacetamide (parenteral grade)	50 mg
Edetate Disodium	0.75 mg
Water for Injection	q.s.

Indications: For intravenous use as a skeletal muscle relaxant for horses.

Pharmacology: Description: Guaifenesin, 3 - (o-Methoxyphenoxy) 1,2-propanediol, is a white to slightly gray, crystalline powder having a bitter taste. It may have a slight characteristic odor.

Actions: Guaifenesin is a guaiacol derivative closely related to mephenesin. The propanediol derivatives are central-acting skeletal muscle relaxants which selectively depress transmission of nerve impulses at the internuncial neurons of the spinal cord, brainstem, and subcortical regions of the brain.

Propanediol derivatives have a wide margin of safety, the toxic dose is three times greater than the recommended dose. Respiration is not severely depressed, and the function of the diaphragm is uninterrupted.[1,2] Tidal volume is slightly decreased and minute volume remains normal. In addition to skeletal muscle, the pharyngeal and laryngeal muscles are sufficiently relaxed for easier surgical intubation procedures. At the beginning of relaxation, there is a slight fall in blood pressure, however, throughout the relaxation period the heart function is unchanged. There is a slight increase in gastrointestinal activity. There is no apparent impairment of lung and kidney functions.

With the recommended administration and dosage of GUAIFENESIN INJECTION, induction is usually smooth and rapid (two to four minutes) providing a duration of action between 15 to 25 minutes. A slightly transient hemolysis occurs at a 5% concentration.[3,4] Higher concentrations cause intravascular hemolysis.[3,5]

The 5% dextrose minimizes the hemolytic action of guaifenesin alone and reduces the tendency to form thrombi at the intravenous injection site.[6] Guaifenesin appears safe when administered to pregnant mares[7] and in human studies did not pass the placental barrier.[2]

Metabolism and excretion of guaifenesin is not well understood. Oxidation products are excreted in the urine as a glycuronimide.

Dosage and Administration: For intravenous use only. Administer rapidly with a positive pressure system or gravity flow using a 12 to 14 gauge needle at the dose rate of 1 mL/pound of body weight. From a standing position the patient will begin to relax and gradually fall when approximately ½ the total dose has been given. Continue the remaining calculated dose for complete relaxation. Average duration of muscle relaxation is 10-25 minutes. For continued relaxation time, additional GUAIFENESIN INJECTION may be administered as determined by the veterinarian at a rate necessary to achieve the desired plane of relaxation. Recovery is usually smooth and uneventful with the horse regaining an upright position usually within 45 minutes after the medication is discontinued.

Contraindication(s): Do not administer physostigmine to horses receiving GUAIFENESIN INJECTION.

Precaution(s): Store between 2° and 30°C (36° and 86°F). Do not freeze.

This is a single dose vial, containing no preservative. Destroy partially used vials.

Caution(s): Federal law restricts this drug to use by or on the order of a licensed veterinarian.

Avoid perivascular leakage to prevent local tissue irritation.

If used for prolonged periods, such as in tetanus, serum hemoglobin levels should be monitored.

Oxygen or sustained artificial respiration facilities should be available when the drug is employed.

Additional care should be employed when administering the drug to anemic or hypovolemic animals with cardiac or respiratory problems.

Extreme care should be exercised at all times in handling this product to prevent the introduction of microbial contamination.

For intravenous use in horses only.

For animal use only.

Not for human use.

Warning(s): Not to be used in horses intended for food.

Keep out of the reach of children.

References: Available upon request.
Presentation: 1,000 mL sterile, single dose plastic vial (NDC 57319-397-08).
Manufactured by: Phoenix Scientific, Inc., St. Joseph, MO 64503
Compendium Code No.: 12560382

Rev. 12-01

GUAILAXIN® ℞

Fort Dodge **General Anesthetic**

Guaifenesin for Injection, USP-Sterile Powder

NADA No.: 136-651

Active Ingredient(s): Each mL of reconstituted solution contains 50 mg of guaifenesin USP.

Indications: GUAILAXIN® is indicated for intravenous administration for muscle relaxation in horses.

Pharmacology: Description: GUAILAXIN® (Guaifenesin for Injection, USP) is 3-(0-methoxyphenoxy)-1,2-propanediol, an intravenous muscle relaxant with the following structural formula:

G

$$CH_3-O-C_6H_4-O-CH_2-CH(OH)-CH_2(OH)$$

Actions and Uses: Guaifenesin (formerly termed glyceryl guaiacolate) is an intravenous, central-acting skeletal muscle relaxant of the myanesin group that selectively depresses or blocks nerve impulse transmission at the internuncial neuron level of the spinal cord, brainstem and subcortical areas of the brain.[1] In therapeutic amounts guaifenesin produces relaxation of skeletal muscles but the diaphragm continues to function unaffected so that no respiratory paralysis occurs and respiratory activity usually remains normal. Relaxation of the pharyngeal and laryngeal muscles is sufficient to facilitate intubation.[2] These muscle relaxing properties make it an excellent drug for use in induction of general anesthesia with both injectable and inhalant anesthetics.

In addition to its muscle relaxant properties, guaifenesin appears to produce some analgesia and sedation due to its action on the brainstem and subcortical areas of the brain.[3]

Inductions are usually smooth and quiet with duration of action lasting from 10-20 minutes.[2,3] In a study in ponies a significant sex difference in the duration of action was observed with guaifenesin use, the stallions requiring a longer period to recover.[7] Changes in ventilation are small with the usual effect being an increase in respiratory rate associated with a decrease in tidal volume.[4] At increased doses (160 mg/kg) guaifenesin produced only minor changes in heart and respiratory rates and a slight fall in mean arterial blood pressure and in arterial blood PO_2 values.[4] Administration of guaifenesin at 134 mg/kg caused insignificant changes in heart rate, respiratory rate, right atrial pressure, pulmonary arterial pressure and cardiac output.[5] At recommended doses liver and kidney function are unimpaired while gastrointestinal activity is slightly increased.[2] The activity of guaifenesin can be shortened by conventional central analeptic agents.[6]

G

The liver is the main site of degradation of guaifenesin, where it undergoes dealkylation to form catechol that is then conjugated to more polar substances.[7] Following degradation and conjugation in the liver the metabolites are excreted largely in the urine.[6,8] The drug has been administered to pregnant mares without ill effects.[3]

Dosage and Administration: Preparation of GUAILAXIN® Solutions: The sterile powder contained in the 4-ounce container should be transferred to a sterile 1-liter administration bottle using a pre-sterilized funnel prior to preparing. The sterile powder contained in the 32-ounce bottle may be reconstituted in its marketed container. To reconstitute, dissolve 50 g of sterile powder in 954 mL warm [not to exceed 37°C (100°F)] Sterile Water for Injection, USP to make 1 liter of solution. Add the water in two equal portions and shake well after each water addition. GUAILAXIN® solutions should be used within 24 hours following preparation.

If thiamylal sodium is to be added, 2 g of the barbiturate should be added to the 50 g of GUAILAXIN® sterile powder prior to dissolving in USP sterile water for injection to make 1 liter of solution. This provides 2 mg thiamylal sodium and 50 mg guaifenesin USP per 1 mL of solution.

GUAILAXIN® should be administered only by the intravenous route. If preanesthetic agents are to be used for chemical restraint, the horse should remain quiet for the recommended period of time. The 5% GUAILAXIN® solution should be administered by rapid intravenous infusion through a 12-gauge needle at a dose of 1 mL/lb of body weight. When administered in this way the dose of guaifenesin is 50 mg/lb of body weight. The horse will fall gently, usually after receiving ⅓ to ½ the dose; however, the entire dose should be given unless adverse respiratory or cardiovascular effects are observed. The duration of action of a single dose is usually from 10-20 minutes.

Recovery from GUAILAXIN® effects is normally smooth with very little incoordination or struggling observed. The horse will usually rest quietly until adequate muscle tonus returns and it can assume a standing position.[3] After standing, some weakness occurs initially, but maximum stability is regained in a short period of time with slow exercise.[3,9]

When thiamylal sodium is added to the guaifenesin as described, the resulting solution should also be administered by rapid intravenous infusion through a 12-gauge needle at a dose of 1 mL/lb of body weight. This provides a dose of 50 mg/lb of guaifenesin and 2 mg/lb of thiamylal sodium. Anesthesia obtained with this procedure is adequate for short surgical operations and the complete muscle relaxation which results is an aid in performing other procedures. If it becomes necessary to prolong anesthesia additional doses of the solution should be given. Use of additional doses requires the person administering the solution to be familiar with the planes of anesthesia as they relate to ocular reflexes, analgesia and respiratory and cardiac rates.[3] A longer period of surgical anesthesia generally requires a longer period for recovery.

Contraindication(s): Administration of physostigmine is contraindicated in horses receiving GUAILAXIN®.

Caution(s): Federal law restricts this drug to use by or on the order of a licensed veterinarian.

Perivascular leakage should be avoided as this may result in irritation to surrounding tissues. Hemolysis may be induced when guaifenesin is used in concentrations in excess of 5%. This effect is related to concentration of guaifenesin rather than to total dosage administered.[1] As is true with use of any drugs incorporated in anesthetic regimens, care should be taken when anesthetizing anemic or hypovolemic animals with cardiac or respiratory problems. Oxygen should be available when guaifenesin is used in conjunction with barbiturates and/or tranquilizers.

GUAILAXIN® is supplied as a sterile powder but contains no bacteriostatic agent and, therefore, GUAILAXIN® (Guaifenesin for Injection, USP) solutions should be prepared aseptically. Sterilization by heating should not be employed. GUAILAXIN® solutions should be used within 24 hours following preparation. If a solution of GUAILAXIN® precipitates slightly within the 24-hour period, it should be warmed (not to exceed 100°F) until in solution once again.

For use in horses.

Warning(s): Not to be used in horses intended for food.

Toxicology: In a toxicity study using GUAILAXIN® the margin of safety was determined to be at least 2 times the recommended dose. Clinical signs of toxicity observed included extensor rigidity in 4 horses, apnea in 1 horse, and nystagmus in 1 horse all of which occurred at 100 mg/lb of body weight or 2 times the recommended dose of GUAILAXIN®.

References: Available upon request.

Presentation: GUAILAXIN® (Guaifenesin for Injection, USP) Sterile Powder is supplied 50 g per container in 4-oz containers and 32-oz containers.

NDC 0856-5320-12 — 4 oz — bottle

NDC 0856-5320-77 — 32 oz — bottle

Compendium Code No.: 10030941

5040E

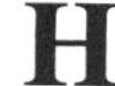

H

HAEMOPHILUS PARAGALLINARUM BACTERIN

L.A.H.I. (New Jersey) **Bacterin**

Infectious Coryza Bacterin

U.S. Vet. Lic. No.: 196

Active Ingredient(s): The infectious coryza bacterin is prepared from concentrated cultures of three antigenic strains of *Haemophilus paragallinarum.*

The vaccine was carefully produced and passed all tests in accordance with the U.S. government requirements.

Indications: The product is used as an aid in the prevention of infectious coryza due to *H. paragallinarum.*

Dosage and Administration: The pullets can be vaccinated when they are three weeks of age or older. Revaccination can be done at least three weeks after first vaccination and at least four weeks prior to onset of lay.

Shake for two (2) minutes before use.

Preparation of Vaccine: Remove the aluminum overseal, the vaccine is ready to use. Should greater than four (4) hours elapse between the first and last use of the vaccine from any one container, it is recommended that the vaccine be shaken again before continuing with the vaccinations.

Dosage: Inject each bird with a 0.5 mL dose intramuscularly in the breast or leg muscle.

Precaution(s): Keep the vaccine in the dark between 35-45°F (2-7°C). Do not freeze.

Caution(s): For veterinary use only.

Use aseptic precautions. Sterilize needles, syringes and stopper.

Vaccinate healthy birds only. Consult a poultry pathologist before vaccinating.

Burn the vaccine containers and all unused contents.

Use the entire contents when first opened.

It is imperative that the user of this product comply with the instructions stated in the direction sheet packed with each product. The vaccine must be prepared and administered as directed to obtain the best results.

The use of nonsterile needles under field vaccination may result in abscess formation and condemnation of the birds.

Warning(s): Do not market birds for at least six (6) weeks after vaccinating. Make sure that the birds marketed do not have swellings at the site of vaccine administration since this may result in condemnations of the birds.

Presentation: 1,000 dose bottles.

Compendium Code No.: 10080232

HAEMO SHIELD® P

Novartis Animal Vaccines **Bacterin**

Haemophilus pleuropneumoniae-Pasteurella multocida Bacterin

U.S. Vet. Lic. No.: 303

Composition: The bacterin contains inactivated cultures of *Haemophilus pleuropneumoniae* serotypes 1, 5 and 7 and *Pasteurella multocida* adjuvanted with aluminum hydroxide. Contains penicillin and streptomycin as preservatives.

Indications: For use in healthy swine as an aid in the prevention and control of diseases caused by *Haemophilus pleuropneumoniae* and *Pasteurella multocida.*

Dosage and Administration: Shake well before and during use. Administer 1 mL intramuscularly or subcutaneously to pigs under 30 pounds and 2 mL to pigs over 30 pounds. Revaccinate two (2) to three (3) weeks later. Sows and gilts should receive two (2) doses prior to farrowing. The first dose should be given approximately five (5) weeks prior to farrowing and a second dose should be given two (2) to three (3) weeks later.

Precaution(s): Store at 35°-45°F (2°-7°C). Do not freeze. Use the entire contents when first opened.

Caution(s): Anaphylactic reactions can occur following the use of the product. Symptomatic treatment: Epinephrine.

Warning(s): Do not vaccinate within 21 days of slaughter.

Discussion: *Haemophilus pleuropneumoniae* is a major cause of pleuropneumonia in hogs. It is distributed throughout the world, but different serovars of the bacteria are more prevalent in certain areas. In the United States, serovars 1 and 5 are most common with serovar 7 causing problems in some areas. Animals of all ages are susceptible, but the majority of cases occur during the growing and finishing stages of production. In acute outbreaks, the morbidity rate is usually high and may approach 100%. The mortality rate in untreated animals may also approach 100%.

Pleuropneumonia is spread by aerosol and through direct pig to pig contact. Animals may carry the organism without showing symptoms, and movement of these carrier animals spreads the disease to other herds. There is not evidence to indicate that other animals, such as rodents and birds, play any role in transmission. There is a slight possibility that the disease could spread by clothing and equipment moved from a herd experiencing an acute outbreak to a clean herd, since the bacteria can survive for a few days in the environment.

H. pleuropneumoniae is a very virulent organism, with as few as 100 organisms needed to cause disease in experimental animals. The disease can also progress very rapidly. Animals experimentally infected with high doses of the bacteria often die within six hours. Much of this can be attributed to the actions of a potent toxin produced by the bacteria as they grow.[1]

In natural infections, producers may find a dead pig as their first clue that something is wrong. On closer inspection, they may notice pigs that seem lethargic, and fevers of 107°F are not uncommon. Pigs rapidly progress to show very labored breathing, and there may be a bloody discharge from the mouth and nose. The disease rapidly progresses through the herd. Animals that recover often become chronic poor-doers.

At necropsy, lesions are confined mainly to the lungs and chest cavity. The lining of the chest cavity is inflamed, and the lungs are often tightly attached to it by adhesions. The lungs themselves show evidence of severe pneumonia.

Definite diagnosis can often be made on the basis of these characteristic signs and lesions. If there is doubt, culturing can be done to detect the organism responsible, since other bacterial infections may mimic *H. pleuropneumoniae.*

The response to treatment is variable. If the disease is detected early and is aggressively treated, animals can fully recover. Other animals may become permanently stunted. Penicillin or ampicillin are often the first drugs of choice, since many strains are sensitive to them. However, it is a good idea to test each strain for its antibiotic resistance pattern, since there are many exceptions to this rule.

Pasteurella multocida is another important cause of pneumonia in swine. It is found worldwide, and it is a common inhabitant of the respiratory tract of healthy animals. It can affect animals of any age.

P. multocida alone causes either no disease or a mild pneumonia. Its importance is as a secondary invader. When lungs are damaged due to some other cause, such as poor air quality, larval ascarid migrations, or other bacterial or mycoplasmal infections, Pasteurella will begin to invade and cause further lung damage, culminating in a severe pneumonia.

Animals infected by *P. multocida* show the typical signs associated with pneumonia - coughing, shortness of breath, "thumping" and high fevers (up to 107°F). If pigs are not treated, the disease tends to linger on, and many of the animals become chronic cases. Death loss is typically fairly low, but can be high in individual cases.

At necropsy, lung lesions are typical of a bronchopneumonia, and the lungs may adhere to the chest cavity. Lung cultures should be done to determine the exact causes, since most are mixed infections.

Treatment can be effective if the proper antibiotic is used. Antibacterial sensitivity of different strains of *P. multocida* varies greatly, which is another important reason culturing should be done. Sulfas, penicillin, tetracycline, and tylosin are commonly used drugs, and all are effective if used properly against sensitive strains.

Prevention is the alternative to the expense of dealing with outbreaks of *Haemophilus pleuropneumoniae* or *Pasteurella multocida,* two of the major causes of pneumonia in swine.

References: Available upon request.

Presentation: Available in 100 mL bottles.

Compendium Code No.: 11140183

HAIRBALL PREPARATION

Vet Solutions **Laxative**

Active Ingredient(s):

White petrolatum, USP .... 214 mg/g
Light mineral oil, NF .... 20 mg/g

Other Ingredients: Malt syrup, refined soya bean oil, cane molasses, water, polypro 5000 hydrolyzed collagen, sorbic acid (a preservative), potassium sorbate (a preservative).

Indications: A laxative and lubricant for hairball removal, for cats and kittens.

Directions for Use: For hairball removal, administer orally daily for three days, then repeat once or twice a week to prevent recurrence. Place a small amount of Vet Solutions® HAIRBALL PREPARATION on cat's nose to stimulate taste interest.

Daily Dosage:

Adult cats: ¼-½ teaspoonful.

Kittens over four weeks old: ¼ teaspoon.

Precaution(s): Store at controlled room temperature.

Caution(s): Sold exclusively through veterinarians.

Presentation: 3.0 oz. (85.0 grams).

Compendium Code No.: 10610090

HAIRBALL SOLUTION

Pet-Ag **Laxative**

Guaranteed Analysis:

Moisture, max. 13.0%
Vitamin A, min .... 50,000 IU/kg
Vitamin E, min .... 500 IU/kg
Vitamin B_6, min .... 820 IU/kg
d-Biotin, min .... 2.2 mg/kg
Zinc, min .... 1,000 ppm
Taurine, min .... 500 mg/kg

Ingredients: Malt Syrup, Mineral Oil, Glycerin, Vegetable Fats, Lecithin, Chicken Digest, Vegetable Gums, Zinc Sulfate, Vitamin A, Vitamin D_3, Vitamin E, Vitamin B_{12}, Riboflavin, Niacin, Calcium Pantothenate, Vitamin K_3, Folic Acid, Vitamin B_6, Thiamine, Taurine and d-Biotin.

Plus Mirra-Coat® Skin and Coat Conditioner.

3,149 Kcal (ME)/kg or 16 Kcal/tsp (calculated).

Chicken flavored.

Indications: HAIRBALL SOLUTION is a highly palatable gel effective in eliminating and preventing hairballs in cats. Mirra-Coat® Skin and Coat conditioner with Zinc and Biotin and essential fatty acids reduces off season shedding and creates a shiny skin and coat. Taurine is an essential amino acid necessary for eye development and muscle health. HAIRBALL SOLUTION is an excellent source of vitamins A, E and K.

Dosage and Administration: Feeding Instructions:

To eliminate hairballs:

Kittens older than six weeks: Feed 1 tsp (5.6 g) daily.

Adult cats: Feed 1-2 tsp (5.2 - 10.4 g) daily.

For hairball prevention: Feed above amounts 3 times weekly. Consult your veterinarian regularly.

Precaution(s): Store at room temperature.

Caution(s): This product is intended for intermittent or supplemental feeding only.

Warning(s): Not for human consumption.

Presentation: 3.5 oz (100 g).

Compendium Code No.: 10970350

HALOTHANE, USP ℞

Halocarbon **Inhalation Anesthetic**

ANADA No.: 200-200

Active Ingredient(s): HALOTHANE, USP stabilized with 0.01% thymol (w/w).

Indications: HALOTHANE, USP is indicated for the induction and maintenance of general anesthesia for dogs, cats and other non-food animals.

Pharmacology: Description: HALOTHANE, USP (2-bromo-2-chloro-1,1,1-trifluoroethane) has the following structural formula:

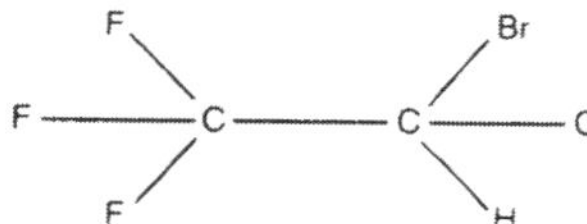

The specific gravity is 1.872-1.877 at 20°C, and the boiling point (range) is 49° to 51°C at 760 mm Hg. The vapor pressure is 243 mm Hg at 20°C. The blood/gas coefficient is 2.5 at 37°C, and the olive oil/water coefficient is 220 at 37°C. Vapor concentrations within the anesthetic range have a pleasant and nonirritating odor. HALOTHANE, USP is nonflammable and its vapors mixed with oxygen in proportions from 0.5% to 50% (v/v) are not explosive. HALOTHANE, USP is twice as potent as chloroform and four times as potent as ether.

HALOTHANE, USP does not decompose in contact with warm soda lime. When moisture is present, the vapor attacks aluminum, brass and lead, but not copper. Rubber, some plastics and similar materials are soluble in HALOTHANE, USP; such materials will deteriorate rapidly in contact with HALOTHANE, USP vapor or liquid.

Actions: HALOTHANE, USP is an inhalation anesthetic. Induction and recovery are rapid, and depth of anesthesia can be rapidly altered.

HALOTHANE, USP acts first by depressing the higher centers of the brain, then the motor and sensory nerves, and finally, in high concentrations, the vital medullary centers. It is an exceptionally potent anesthetic with rapidly, easily reversible action.[1-5,8,11,12]

HALOTHANE, USP progressively depresses respiration.[1,5-7] There may be tachypnea with reduced tidal volume and alveolar ventilation. HALOTHANE, USP is not an irritant to the respiratory tract, and minimal increase in salivary or bronchial secretions ordinarily occurs.[1,6] Pharyngeal and laryngeal reflexes are rapidly diminished. It causes bronchodilation. Hypoxia, acidosis or apnea may develop during deep anesthesia.[11]

HALOTHANE, USP reduces the blood pressure, and frequently results in bradycardia (decreased pulse rate).[1,5,8,9] The greater the concentration of the drug, the more evident these changes become. In those instances where bradycardia is not caused by HALOTHANE, USP administration, but is the result of vagal stimulation, it can be effectively reversed by the use of atropine. HALOTHANE, USP also causes dilation of the vessels of the skin and skeletal muscles.

Cardiac arrhythmias may occur during HALOTHANE, USP anesthesia.[7] HALOTHANE, USP sensitizes the myocardial conduction system to the action of epinephrine and norepinephrine. HALOTHANE, USP ordinarily produces a satisfactory degree of muscular relaxation for most surgical procedures including abdominal surgery and bone-pinning operations.[3,4,10,11]

HALOTHANE, USP is a potent uterine relaxant.

Dosage and Administration: Caution: This product should be used in a manner which will effectively reduce the accumulation of waste anesthetic gases. To aid in this process, reduce the amount of anesthetic gas that is discharged into areas where this product is used (i.e., induction or operating rooms) or where patients are housed during recovery from anesthesia and use an anesthetic gas scavenging system in conjunction with a nonrecirculating ventilation system.

HALOTHANE, USP may be administered by the non-rebreathing technique, partial rebreathing or closed technique. Because of the high potency and other physical and pharmacological properties, these methods all have their advantages and disadvantages. Use of an open or semi-open method using non-rebreathing technique is possible, but is wasteful, costly and permits anesthetic gas to be discharged into the atmosphere.

Because of these disadvantages the closed and semi-closed rebreathing methods employing a carbon dioxide absorber have been developed which are preferable to the non-rebreathing technique. HALOTHANE, USP should be used in vaporizers that provide accurate concentrations which can be adjusted in percentage fractions over the entire clinical range of 0.5 to 5% (v/v). It is important that the anesthetic equipment be in good condition, and that the operator be familiar with inhalation anesthesiology techniques.

It is absolutely necessary that the vaporizer be placed between the gas supply and breathing bag. If between the bag and the patient, overdosage may result.

The concentration of HALOTHANE, USP required to induce anesthesia will vary from patient to patient, but will usually be between 2% to 5%. Maintenance dose of HALOTHANE, USP usually will vary between 0.5% and 2% in the inhaled atmosphere.

As with all inhalation anesthetics the required concentration of HALOTHANE, USP will depend on the technique of the operator, the depth of anesthesia desired and also the additional effect that can be observed if the inhaled atmosphere is composed of a mixture of oxygen and nitrous oxide, if a preanesthetic agent is used; or if a short-acting barbiturate is used to facilitate intubation of the animal.

HALOTHANE, USP may be administered in an atmosphere of oxygen or a mixture of oxygen and nitrous oxide.[8,12] Use of the oxygen/nitrous oxide mixture will normally require a slightly lower concentration of HALOTHANE, USP to achieve the same plane of anesthesia as opposed to use of oxygen alone.[13] Use of a tranquilizer as a pre-anesthetic agent will also normally require a slightly lower concentration of HALOTHANE, USP.

Induction should not be hurried, and the concentration of vapor should not be suddenly increased. As with any anesthetic the operator must monitor the patient to achieve the desired degree of anesthesia.

When endotracheal intubation is desired, the intubation may be accomplished by using an anesthetic dose of one of the short-acting barbiturates.[2,3,5,7,10,11,14] Maintenance anesthesia using HALOTHANE, USP should be administered as soon as the intravenous administration is completed. In these cases care should be taken to control the concentration of HALOTHANE, USP. While under the effects of the barbiturates the required maintenance concentration of HALOTHANE, USP will normally be lower than after the effect of the barbiturate has terminated.

Contraindication(s): HALOTHANE, USP is not recommended for obstetrical anesthesia except when uterine relaxation is required.

HALOTHANE, USP should not be used in pregnant animals, since the safe use of HALOTHANE, USP has not been established with respect to possible adverse effects upon fetal development.

A condition known as malignant hyperthermia has, on rare occasion, been reported with the use of HALOTHANE, USP in dogs, cats, pigs and horses.

HALOTHANE, USP should be used only in vaporizers that permit a reasonable approximation of output, and preferably of the calibrated type.

It is absolutely necessary that the vaporizer be placed between the gas supply and breathing bag. If between the bag and the patient, overdosage may result.

The patient should be closely observed for signs of overdosage, i.e., depression of blood pressure, pulse rate and ventilation, particularly during assisted or controlled ventilation.

Precaution(s): Stability of HALOTHANE, USP is maintained by the addition of 0.01% thymol (w/w) and storage is in amber colored bottles.

HALOTHANE, USP should not be kept indefinitely in vaporizer bottles not specifically designed for its use. Thymol does not volatilize along with HALOTHANE, USP and, therefore, accumulates in the vaporizer, and may, in time, impart a yellow color to the remaining liquid or to wicks in vaporizers. The development of such discoloration may be used as an indicator that the vaporizer should be drained and cleaned, and the discolored HALOTHANE, USP discarded. Accumulation of thymol may be removed by washing with a small amount of fresh Halothane, USP.

Keep bottle securely closed.

Store in a cool, dry place and protect from undue exposure to light. Avoid excessive heat.

Caution(s): Federal law restricts this drug to use by or on the order of a licensed veterinarian.

HALOTHANE, USP increases cerebrospinal fluid pressure. Therefore, in patients with markedly increased intracranial pressure, HALOTHANE, USP administration should be preceded by measures ordinarily used to reduce cerebrospinal fluid pressure.

Ganglionic blocking agents (muscle relaxants) should be administered cautiously, since their hypotensive effect may be augmented by HALOTHANE, USP. Epinephrine or norepinephrine should be employed cautiously, if at all, during HALOTHANE, USP anesthesia, since their simultaneous use may induce cardiac arrhythmias.

HALOTHANE, USP should be administered cautiously to patients in shock, in those with minimal cardiac reserve, and in those with grossly distributed cardiac rhythm.

Aminoglycoside antibiotics should be employed cautiously, if at all, in patients who are in shock and receiving HALOTHANE, USP since there is moderate circulatory depression that is attributed to these antibiotics.

After cessation of the HALOTHANE, USP anesthesia, reflexes are evident within one to two minutes, and sometimes slight muscular tremors occur. Horses, when recovering and semiconscious, do attempt to rise to their feet prematurely. If they are quietly restrained for about one hour, it will help prevent self-injury to the patient.[2,11] Cattle often voluntarily assume breast recumbancy within 15 minutes and rise to their feet unaided in approximately one hour. They show no excitement during recovery and no inhibition of salivation.

The uterine relaxation caused by HALOTHANE, USP anesthesia may fail to respond to oxytocin. HALOTHANE, USP produces marked relaxation of the anus during anesthesia, which may result in voiding of feces.[4]

The use of inhalation anesthetic agents, like halothane, will normally result in waste anesthetic gases being released into the room environment. This results in the potential for exposure of personnel to these agents. Hepatic dysfunction has been reported secondary to occupational exposure to waste anesthetic agents. In addition, adverse reproductive effects in pregnant women have been reported. The role that anesthetic agents plays in the etiology of these events remains controversial. Nevertheless, it is prudent to reduce to the lowest possible level the exposure of all personnel to environmental anesthetic gases. This product should be used in such a manner to prevent the accumulation of waste anesthetic gases.

Operating rooms should be provided with adequate ventilation to prevent the accumulation of anesthetic gases and vapors.

Warning(s): HALOTHANE, USP should not be used in animals intended for use as food.

Adverse Reactions: The following adverse reactions have been reported: mild hepatic dysfunction, cardiac arrest, hypotension, hypothermia, respiratory arrest, cardiac arrhythmias, hyperpyrexia and shivering.[6,8] Nausea and vomiting are relatively uncommon complications observed with HALOTHANE, USP anesthesia.[1,3,9]

References: Available upon request.

Presentation: Bottles of 250 mL (NDC 12164-004-25).

Compendium Code No.: 10700001

HAPPY JACK® COD LIVER OIL

Happy Jack — **Small Animal Dietary Supplement**

Active Ingredient(s): Certified to contain not less than 1,000 vitamin A and 300 vitamin D units per gram U.S.P.

Indications: A supplement that provides a source of vitamin A and vitamin D to growing pups and brood females.

Dosage and Administration: For general use, one (1) teaspoonful each day to dogs of smaller breeds such as Cocker spaniels and Beagles. Comparative doses for larger breeds. Double the dosage in special instances for sickness and winter weather.

Mink: 8 oz. each day per 100 animals.

Foxes: 24 oz. each day per 100 animals.

Precaution(s): Keep in a cool place away from light.

Presentation: 16 fl. oz. (1 pint) and 1 gallon containers.

Compendium Code No.: 10350020

HAPPY JACK® DD-33™ FLEA & TICK MIST

Happy Jack — **Parasiticide Spray**

EPA Reg. No.: 2781-41

Active Ingredient(s):

Pyrethrins	0.112%
Permethrin [*(3-phenoxyphenyl) methyl (±) cis-trans-3-(2,2-dichloroethenyl) 2,2-dimethylcyclopropanecarboxylate]	0.101%
Other related compounds	0.009%
Inert ingredients	99.778%
Total	100.000%

* cis-trans isomer ratio: Min. 35% (±) and cis: Max. 65% (±) trans.

Indications: The product will kill fleas for up to 14 days on dogs and cats and will kill ticks for four days on dogs and nine days on cats.

Dosage and Administration: It is a violation of federal law to use the product in a manner inconsistent with its labeling.

Hold the container upright. Shake well before using.

Spray the animal from a distance of 8-12 inches. Start spraying at the tail, moving the dispenser rapidly and making sure that the animal's entire body is covered, including the legs and under the body. Fluff the hair while spraying so that the spray will penetrate to the skin. The spray should wet the ticks thoroughly. Do not spray in the face, eyes, or genitalia. Repeat as needed.

For cats, apply at the rate of one (1) second per pound of body weight. For dogs, apply at the rate of two (2) seconds per pound of body weight for thin or short-haired dogs and up to eight (8) seconds per pound of body weight for heavy or long-haired dogs.

Precaution(s):

Storage: Store in a cool, dry area away from heat or open flame.

Disposal: Securely wrap the original container in several layers of newspaper and discard it in the trash. Do not re-use the empty container.

Caution(s): Keep out of the reach of children.

Precautionary Statements:

Hazards to Humans and Domestic Animals: Do not spray into the pet's eyes, face, or on genitalia. Do not use on nursing puppies or kittens, or animals under three months of age.

Do not use this or any other pesticide on sick, old, or debilitated animals.

Environmental Hazards: The product is toxic to fish and other aquatic animals. Do not apply directly to any body of water. Do not contaminate water by the cleaning of equipment or the disposal of wastes.

Physical or Chemical Hazards: Do not use or store near heat or open flame.

Statement of Practical Treatment:

If swallowed: Call a physician or poison control center immediately. Drink one or two glasses of water and induce vomiting by touching the back of the throat with a finger. Repeat until vomit fluid is clear.

If in eyes: Flush with plenty of water. Get medical attention if irritation persists.

If on skin or clothing: Remove contaminated clothing and wash before re-use. Wash skin with soap and warm water. Get medical attention if irritation persists.

If inhaled: Remove victim to fresh air. Apply artificial respiration if indicated.

Presentation: 16 fl. oz. (1 pint) containers.

Compendium Code No.: 10350030

HAPPY JACK® DERMAPLEX™

Happy Jack **Small Animal Dietary Supplement**

Active Ingredient(s): Guaranteed analysis:

Vitamin A	50,000 units/lb. (116.3 I.U./g)
Vitamin B_6	22.7 mg/lb. (46.5 mcg/g)
Vitamin E	200 units/lb. (441 I.U./g)
d-Pantothenic acid	4 mg/lb. (8.81 mcg/g)
Zinc (Zn)	minimum 0.01% (100 mcg/g)
Polyunsaturated fatty acids	62.2 g/lb.

Ingredients: Soybean oil, safflower oil, corn oil, soybean flour, sugar sodium silico aluminate, vitamin A palmitate, d-alpha-tocopherol acetate (vitamin E), pyridoxine hydrochloride, calcium pantothenate, zinc proteinate, BHA and BHT (preservatives), flavoring.

Indications: A supplement especially designed to aid in the maintenance of healthy skin and coat of dogs and cats.

Dosage and Administration: Add DERMAPLEX™ to the daily ration according to the following proportions:

Weight of Dog	Add DERMAPLEX™
10 lbs. or less	1 rounded tsp.
10 to 20 lbs.	2 rounded tsp.
20 to 50 lbs.	1 rounded tbsp.
50 lbs. or more	2 rounded tbsp.

Presentation: 14 oz. (397 g) and 5 lb. container.

Compendium Code No.: 10350040

HAPPY JACK® EAR CANKER POWDER

Happy Jack **Otic Dryer**

Active Ingredient(s): Zinc oxide and iodoform.

Indications: A healing aid for ear canker and other sores and rashes on dogs and horses.

Dosage and Administration: If necessary, snip the top of the container for easier flow. Clean the area to be treated. Apply the powder once a day.

Caution(s): Not for human use. Keep out of the reach of children.

If redness, irritation, or swelling persist or increase, discontinue use and consult a veterinarian.

Presentation: ½ oz. (14 g) containers.

Compendium Code No.: 10350050

HAPPY JACK® ENDURACIDE® DIP II

Happy Jack **Parasiticide Dip**

EPA Reg. No.: 2781-19

Active Ingredient(s):

Chlorpyrifos [0,0-diethyl-0-(3,5,6-trichloro-2-pyridyl) phosphorothioate]	4.85%
Inert ingredients	95.15%

Contains petroleum distillates.

Indications: Kills fleas, ticks and sarcoptic mange mites (sarcoptic) on dogs.

Directions for Use: It is a violation of federal law to use the product in a manner inconsistent with its labeling.

To kill fleas, ticks and mange mites on dogs (for medium to large dogs, 25 lbs. or more. For dogs less than 25 lbs. use at ½ strength): Mix two (2) fluid ounces (4 tablespoons) of HAPPY JACK® ENDURACIDE® Dip II to a gallon of water (1 gallon to 64 gallons). Measure accurately and stir well. First wet the animal and then dip the animal in the solution or pour, sponge, or spray on the animal until the hair coat is thoroughly wet to the skin. Do not rinse. Allow the solution to dry on the animal. The initial kill of fleas, mites, and nonengorged ticks is rapid, but 24 to 48 hours may be required to completely kill engorged ticks. Do not repeat more often than once every four (4) weeks. Remove and destroy infested bedding. Do not use the product on animals simultaneously or within 30 days before or after treatment with or exposure to cholinesterase inhibiting drugs, pesticides, or chemicals.

Precautionary Statements: Hazards to Humans and Domestic Animals:

Animal Caution: Do not use the product undiluted. Must be mixed as directed before use. Do not treat nursing animals or animals under four months of age. Do not treat sick or debilitated animals. Do not get into the pets eyes. Do not use on cats or toy breeds.

Human Caution: Harmful if swallowed, inhaled or absorbed through the skin. Avoid contact with the skin, eyes, or clothes. Wear gloves when using the product to bathe dogs. Excessive or prolonged contact of the dip solution with the skin should be avoided. Contaminated utensils should not be used for food purposes after use with insecticides.

Physical and Chemical Hazards: Do not use, pour or store near heat or an open flame.

Statement of Practical Treatment:

If swallowed, call a physician or poison control center. Drink milk and water. Do not induce vomiting because of a possible aspiration hazard.

If in eyes, flush eyes with plenty of water. Get medical attention if irritation persists.

If on skin, wash off with soap and water. Get medical attention if irritation persists.

Note to Physician: Atropine sulfate by injection is antidotal only if signs of cholinesterase inhibition are present.

Storage and Disposal: Do not re-use the empty container. Wrap the container and put it in the trash collection.

Warning(s): Keep out of the reach of children.

Do not use full strength - Mix as directed.

Presentation: 8 oz containers.

Compendium Code No.: 10350060

HAPPY JACK® FLEA FLOGGER PLUS

Happy Jack **Premise Insecticide**

EPA Reg. No.: 1021-1623-2781

Active Ingredient(s):

2-[1 Methyl-2-(4-phenoxyphenoxy) ethoxyl] pyridine*	0.100%
Pyrethrins	0.050%
N-Octyl bicycloheptene dicarboximide	0.400%
Permethrin (3-Phenoxyphenyl) methyl (+ or -) Cis-trans-3-(2,2-dichlorethenyl)-(2,2 dimethyl cyclopropanecarboxylate)	0.400%
Related Compounds	0.035%
Inert Ingredients	99.015%

Nylar® (Insect Growth Regulator) Trademark of *MGK

Indications: Kills fleas, flea eggs and larva, roaches, ants, ticks, spiders and other insects.

7 month total release fogger.

For use in: Apartments, attics, basements, boats, cabins, campers, closed porches, condominiums, dormitories, drive-ins, drug stores, factories, food plants, garages, homes, hospitals, hotels, institutions, kennels, kitchens, motels, nursing homes, office buildings, other public buildings, pet grooming parlors, pet sleeping areas, railroad cars, restaurants, rooms, schools, ships, storage areas, supermarkets, theatres, trailers, treehouses, trucks, verandas, warehouses, and zoos.

Directions for Use: It is a violation of Federal Law to use this product in a manner inconsistent with its labeling.

Read all directions completely before use.

For use only when building has been vacated by humans and pets. Ventilate area for 30 minutes before re-entry. For best results, treat all infested areas (sites). Use one fogger for each 6,000 cubic feet (approximately 27 ft. x 27 ft. x 8 ft. ceiling) of unobstructed area. Use additional units for remote rooms or where the free flow of fog is not assured.

Note: Do not use more than one unit per average size room. Do not use this unit in a cabinet or under a counter or table. Do not use this unit in an area less than 100 cubic feet.

Preparation: Remove or cover exposed food, dishes, utensils, surfaces and floor-handling equipment. Shut off fans and air conditioners. Put out all flames and pilot lights. Close outside doors and windows. Remove pets and birds but leave pets bedding as this is a primary hiding place for fleas and must be treated for best results. No need to discard pet bedding after treatment. Cover or remove fish tanks or bowls. Leave rugs, draperies and upholstered furniture in place. This product will not harm furniture when used as directed. Open interior closed doors and cabinets are areas to be treated. (Cover waxed wood floors and waxed wood furniture in the immediate area surrounding the fogger). (Newspapers may be used).

For more effective control of storage pests open all cupboard doors, (kitchen, bathrooms, pantry), and drawers for better penetration of fog. Remove all infested foodstuffs and dispose of in outside trash.

For flea and tick control, thoroughly vacuum all carpeting, upholstered furniture, along baseboards, under furniture and in closets. Put vacuum bag into a sack and dispose of in outside trash. Mop all hard floor surfaces.

To Start Fogging: Shake Fogger Well Before Using: Hold can at arms length and top pointing away from face and eyes. Push down on finger pad until it locks. This will start fogging action. Set canister in an upright position on a table, stand, etc. (up to 30 inches in height in the center of the area) and place several thicknesses of newspaper under the cannister to prevent marring of the surface. Treat the whole dwelling using multiple units in homes with more than one level and numerous rooms. Leave the building at once.

Do Not Re-Enter Building For Two Hours: After two hours, open all outside doors and windows, turn on air conditioner and/or fans and let treated area air for 30 minutes before reoccupying. If additional units are used for remote rooms or where free flow of fog is not assured. Increase airing out time accordingly.

Precautionary Statements: Hazards to Humans and Domestic Animals:

Harmful if swallowed. Avoid breathing vapors or spray mist. Avoid contact with skin or eyes. In case of contact, flush with plenty of water. Wash with soap and warm water after use. Obtain medical attention if irritation persists. Avoid contamination of food and feedstuffs.

Do not use in food areas or food handling establishments, restaurants or other areas where food is commercially prepared or processed. Do not use in serving areas where prepared foods are served such as dining rooms but excluding areas where foods may be prepared or held. In the home, all food processing surfaces and utensils should be covered during treatment, or thoroughly washed before use. Exposed food should be covered or removed. Non-food areas are areas such as garbage rooms, lavatories, floor drains (to sewers), entries and vestibules, offices, locker rooms, machine rooms, boiler rooms, garages, mop closets and storage (after canning or bottling). Not for use in USDA Meat and Poultry Plants.

Remove pets, birds, and cover fish aquariums before spraying.

Physical or Chemical Hazards: Contents under pressure. Keep away from heat, sparks, and open flame. Do not puncture or incinerate container. Exposure to temperatures above 130°F may cause bursting.

Statement Of Practical Treatment:

If swallowed: Call physician or Poison Control Center immediately. Do not induce vomiting because of aspiration pneumonia hazard.

If inhaled: Remove victim to fresh air if effects occur and call physician.

If on skin or clothing: Remove contaminated clothing and wash before reuse. Wash skin with soap and warm water. Get medical attention if irritation persists.

If in eyes: Flush eyes with plenty of water. Obtain medical attention if irritation persists.

Storage and Disposal:

Storage: Store in a cool, dry area away from heat or open flame.

Disposal: Replace cap and discard container in trash. Do not incinerate or puncture.

Warning(s): Keep out of reach of children.

Presentation: 6 oz canister.

Compendium Code No.: 10350071

HAPPY JACK® FLEA-TICK POWDER II

Happy Jack **Parasiticide Powder**

EPA Reg. No.: 2781-25

Active Ingredient(s):

Carbaryl (1-naphthyl N-methyl carbamate)	5%
Inert ingredients	95%

Indications: Kills fleas, ticks and lice on dogs and cats.

Dosage and Administration: It is a violation of federal law to use the product in a manner inconsistent with its labeling.

For dogs and cats: To kill ticks, fleas and lice, dust liberally all over the animal and rub down to the skin. Apply to the feet, between the toes, and legs. Repeat once a week if needed. Allow a

H

few hours to kill large engorged ticks. Dust sleeping quarters liberally to kill brown dog ticks and fleas. Do not use on pregnant dogs.

Precaution(s): Do not re-use the empty container. Wrap the container and put it in the trash collection.

Caution(s): Keep out of the reach of children.

Precautionary Statements: Hazards to Humans and Domestic Animals:

Humans: May be harmful if swallowed. Avoid inhaling dust. Avoid contact with the eyes, skin or clothing. Wash thoroughly after handling.

Animals: Sensitive cats may exhibit temporary but harmless salivation. Avoid treatment of kittens or puppies of less than four weeks of age.

Note to Physician: Carbaryl is a moderate reversible cholinesterase inhibitor. Atropine sulfate is antidotal.

Environmental Hazard: The product is extremely toxic to aquatic invertebrates. Do not apply directly to water or wetlands. Do not contaminate water by the cleaning of equipment or the disposal of wastes.

Presentation: 5 oz. (141 g) and 1 lb. bottles.

Compendium Code No.: 10350090

HAPPY JACK® FLEA ZINGER PLUS

Happy Jack **Premise Insecticide**

EPA Reg. No.: 1021-1622-2781

Active Ingredient(s):

2-[1 Methyl-2-(4-phenoxyphenoxy) ethoxyl] pyridine* 0.015%

Tetramethrin [(Cyclohexene-1,2-dicarboximide) methyl 2, 2-dimethyl-3-(2-methylpropenyl) cyclopropanecarboxylate] 0.400%

3-Phenoxbenzyl -(1 RS, 3RS, 3SR)-2,2-dimethyl-3-(2-methylprop-1-enyl) cyclopropanecarboxylate.......... 0.300%

Inert Ingredients.......... 99.285%

Nylar® (Insect Growth Regulator) Trademark of *MGK

H

Indications: 120 day flea and flea egg spray for carpets and furniture.

Kills fleas, flea eggs and larva, kills ticks.

Dosage and Administration:

Directions for Use: It is a violation of Federal Law to use this product in a manner inconsistent with its labeling. For indoor use only.

Flea Zinger Plus kills fleas and ticks. It contains a unique combination of ingredients that kills both adult and pre-adult fleas. Even kills fleas before they grow up to bite. Nylar®, a unique ingredient in this flea spray, continues to kill fleas for 120 days (4 months) by preventing their development into the adult biting stage. It reaches fleas hidden in carpets, rugs, drapes, upholstery, pet bedding, floor cracks. Protects your home from reinfestation and fleas buildup, your pets and family from bites. One treatment with this spray gives continuous flea protection for 120 days. Leaves no objectionable odor or sticky mess, and used as directed, does not stain furnishings.

Fleas and Ticks: Shake Well. Hold can 2 or 3 feet from surfaces to be treated. Be sure to apply uniformly using a sweeping motion to carpets, rugs, drapes and all surfaces of upholstered furniture. Be sure to treat pet bedding as this is a primary hiding place for fleas. No need to remove pet bedding after treatment. Do Not Treat Pets. Use a registered flea control product on your pet in conjunction with this treatment. Repeat as necessary. Avoid wetting furniture and carpeting. A fine mist or spray applied is all that is necessary to kill fleas and ticks.

Precaution(s):

Storage: Store in a cool, dry place inaccessible to children. Keep container closed.

Disposal: Do not reuse empty container. Wrap container in several layers of newspaper and discard in trash.

Physical or Chemical Hazards: Contents under pressure. Keep away from heat, sparks, and open flame. Do not puncture or incinerate container. Exposure to temperatures above 130°F may cause bursting.

Caution(s): Precautionary Statements:

Hazards to Humans and Domestic Animals:

Harmful if swallowed or absorbed through skin. Contains petroleum distillate. Do not induce vomiting because of aspiration hazard. Do not breathe vapors or spray mist. Avoid contact with skin or eyes. In case of contact, flush with plenty of water. Wash with soap and warm water after use. Obtain medical attention if irritation persists. Avoid contamination of food and feedstuffs. Do not use in commercial food processing, preparation, food storage or serving areas. In the home, all food processing surfaces and utensils should be covered during treatment or thoroughly washed before use. Exposed food should be covered or removed.

Remove pets, birds, and cover fish aquariums before spraying.

Warning(s): Statement of Practical Treatment:

If swallowed: Call physician or Poison Control Center immediately. Do not induce vomiting because of aspiration pneumonia hazard.

If inhaled: Remove victim to fresh air. Apply artificial respiration if indicated.

If on skin or clothing: Remove contaminated clothing and wash before reuse. Wash skin with soap and warm water. Get medical attention if irritation persists.

If in eyes: Flush eyes with plenty of water. Obtain medical attention if irritation persists.

Keep out of reach of children.

Presentation: 10 oz canister.

Compendium Code No.: 10350080

HAPPY JACK® KENNEL DIP II

Happy Jack **Parasiticide-Topical**

Broad Spectrum Insecticide/Acaricide

EPA Reg. No.: 2781-52

Active Ingredient(s):

Permethrin* (CAS No.: 52645-53-1) 17.00%

Piperonyl Butoxide Technical (CAS No.: 51-03-6) 4.25%

Other Inerts:.......... 78.75%

Total 100.00%

*Cis/trans ratio: Max. 65% (±) trans and min. 35% (±) cis.

Contains: 43.44 g permethrin and 10.86 g piperonyl butoxide technical per 8 oz.

Water based.

Indications: A water base, synergized, concentrate insecticide with up to 30 days residual effects.

For use on dogs and their premises to kill fleas, mange mites, and ticks including deer ticks (carrier of Lyme Disease).

Directions for Use: It is a violation of Federal law to use this product in a manner inconsistent with its labeling.

Read entire label before each use.

Shake well before use. Protect from freezing. Add the required amount of concentrate to water and blend thoroughly. Do not hold dilutions for more than 24 hours. Use only on dogs. Do not use on cats. Do not treat puppies under 12 weeks of age. Do not get this product in your dog's eyes or mouth. Retreat dogs as needed but not more often than once every fourteen days. Mix the product and apply the use-diluted material to dogs and/or their premises at the rates shown. These dilutions and rates will provide the most efficient pest control under conditions of heavy pressure (infestation) when good contact is achieved.

For use on Dogs to control Fleas, Ticks (including Deer Ticks, carrier of Lyme Disease), Mange Mites, Lice and Stable Flies:

Spray, Dip or Sponge On: Mix 1 part concentrate in 256 parts water (1 fl oz in 2 gal or 30 mL in 2 gal or 8 fl oz in 16 gal). Spray, dip or pour diluted product on the dog until the dog's hair and skin are thoroughly wet (saturated), making sure the dog's entire body is treated. Do not treat dog's face. Let drip dry on dog and do not rinse off.

Low Volume Spray: Mix 1 part concentrate in 32 parts water (1 fl oz or 30 mL in 1 quart). Spray 1-2 fl oz per dog. Starting at the tail, stroke against lay of the hair, spraying the parted hair with a fine mist directly behind the hand to insure penetrating the hair coat. Spray entire dog until the hair coat is damp.

For use on Dog Premises to control Fleas and Ticks:

Indoor Premise Spray: Mix 1 to 2 parts concentrate in 80 parts water (8 oz in 2.5 to 5 gal or 1 pt in 5 to 10 gal or 48 mL to 96 mL in 1 gal). Thoroughly spray infested areas, pet beds, resting quarters, nearby cracks and crevices, along baseboards, moldings, windows, door frames, and localized areas of floor and floor covering. Fresh bedding should be placed in animals quarters following treatment.

Outdoor Premise Spray: Mix 2 fl oz (60 mL) concentrate in 10.5 gal water or 14 mL in 2.5 gal water. Use enough finish spray to penetrate foliage, usually 50-100 gal per acre (1-2 gal per 1000 sq ft). To prevent infestation of buildings, treat a band of vegetation 6-10 feet adjacent to the structure.

Conversion Equivalents: 1 fl oz = 30 mL = 2 Tablespoons = 6 Teaspoons

Precautionary Statements: Hazards to Humans and Domestic Animals: Caution:

Hazards to Humans: Causes moderate eye irritation. Harmful if swallowed or absorbed through the skin. Avoid contact with eyes, skin or clothing. Wash thoroughly with soap and water after handling. Remove contaminated clothing and wash clothing before reuse. Groomers or other persons applying the product frequently must wear chemically resistant gloves.

Hazards to Domestic Animals: For external use on dogs only. Do not use on cats. Do not use on puppies under 12 weeks of age. Consult a veterinarian before using this product on debilitated, aged, pregnant, or nursing dogs. Sensitivities may occur after using any pesticide product for pets. If signs of sensitivity occur, bathe your pet with mild soap and rinse with large amounts of water. If signs continue, consult a veterinarian immediately. Certain medications can interact with pesticides. Consult a veterinarian before using on medicated dogs.

First Aid:

If Swallowed: Call poison control center or doctor immediately for treatment advice. Have person sip a glass of water if able to swallow. Do not induce vomiting unless told to do so by a poison control center or doctor. Do not give anything by mouth to an unconscious person.

If on Skin or Clothing: Take off contaminated clothing. Rinse skin immediately with plenty of water for 15-20 minutes. Call a poison control center or doctor for treatment advice.

If in Eyes: Hold eyes open and rinse slowly and gently with water for 15-20 minutes. Remove contact lenses, if present, after the first 5 minutes, then continue rinsing eyes. Call a poison control center or doctor for treatment advice.

Hot Line Number: Have the product container or label with you when calling a poison control center or doctor for treatment. You may also contact 1-800-345-4735 for emergency medical treatment information.

Environmental Hazards: This product is highly toxic to fish, and other aquatic organisms. Do not apply directly to any body of water. Do not contaminate water when disposing of dip or equipment washwaters.

Physical or Chemical Hazards: Do not use this product in or on electrical equipment due to the possibility of shock hazard.

Storage and Disposal: Pesticide Storage: Store in original container in a cool dry place inaccessible to children and pets. Protect from freezing.

Disposal: Do not reuse empty container. Securely wrap original container in several layers of newspaper and discard in trash.

Warning(s): Keep out of the reach of children.

Disclaimer: Notice of Warranty: Happy Jack, Inc makes no warranty of merchantability, fitness for any particular purpose, or otherwise, expressed or implied concerning this product or its uses which extend beyond the use of the product under normal conditions in accord with the statements made on the label.

Presentation: 8 fl oz (236 mL).

Compendium Code No.: 10350260

HAPPY JACK® KENNELSPOT™ FOR DOGS (UNDER 33 LBS)

Happy Jack **Parasiticide-Topical**

EPA Reg. No.: 69332-1-2781

Active Ingredient(s):

Permethrin (CAS# 52645-53-1) 45%

Other Ingredients:.......... 55%

Indications: One easy application for effective control. Kills and repels fleas and ticks quickly. Protects for up to 4 weeks.

What the drops do: One drop KENNELSPOT™ kills and repels fleas and ticks on your dog for up to 4 weeks. It is recommended that you also use a product labeled to treat your dog's basket and favorite sleeping areas.

Directions for Use: It is a violation of Federal Law to use this product in a manner inconsistent with its labeling.

Read entire label before each use. Use only on dogs.

How to use the drops:

For dogs weighing up to 33 lb (15 kg):

1. Only open the tube, immediately prior to use by holding upright and twisting the cap off, taking care not to squeeze the tube.
2. Part the dog's coat to expose the skin between the shoulder blades, at the nape of the neck.
3. Squeeze the entire contents of the tube onto the exposed skin.

If the dog's coat is subsequently wetted, such as when shampooing, the 4 week period of protection may be reduced.

Additional precautions to protect your dog:

1. Do not massage the drops into the dog's skin. Avoid applying to the dog's fur.

2. Do not administer any other flea control product to your dog during the 4 week period of protection.
3. Retreat after 28 days if reinfestation is apparent.

Additional precautions to protect your family: Do not allow children to play with tubes. A pet treated with this product should not sleep with people, particularly children, for the 8 hours immediately following treatment. Do not handle the area of application for 3 to 6 hours following treatment.

What else you must do: Treating your dog's basket and favorite sleeping areas with a suitable insecticidal product labeled for this use and vacuuming these areas regularly will also help to remove dead fleas and ticks. Consult your veterinarian for product recommendations.

Precautionary Statements: Hazards to Humans and Domestic Animals:

Hazards to Humans: Harmful if swallowed or absorbed through the skin. Causes moderate eye irritation. Avoid contact with skin, eyes, or clothing. Wash thoroughly with soap and water after handling.

Hazards to Domestic Animals: For external use only. Do not apply to dogs less than 6 months of age. Repeat applications may be made as necessary, but do not apply at intervals less than 7 days. Do not use on cats. Cats which actively groom or engage in close physical contact with recently treated dogs may be at risk of toxic exposure. Consult a veterinarian before using this product on debilitated, aged, or medicated animals. Consult a veterinarian before using this product on dogs with known organ dysfunction. Sensitivities may occur after using any pesticide product for pets. If signs of sensitivity occur, bathe your pet with a mild soap and rinse with large amounts of water. If signs continue, consult a veterinarian immediately. Signs of sensitivity to this product include skin sensitivity, increased itchiness, redness, rash, hair discoloration or hair loss at the application site. Dogs may also show "lethargy".

First Aid:

If swallowed: Call a physician or Poison Control Center. Drink 1 or 2 glasses of water and induce vomiting by touching back of threat with finger or, if available, administer syrup of ipecac. Do not induce vomiting or give anything by mouth to an unconscious person.

If in eyes: Flush with plenty of water. Get medical attention if irritation persists.

If on skin: Remove contaminated clothing and wash with plenty of soap and water. Get medical attention if symptoms or irritation develops.

To Physician: Treat patient symptomatically.

Environmental Hazards: This product is extremely toxic to fish and aquatic organisms. Do not apply directly to any body of water. Treated dogs should not be allowed to go swimming for 12 hours following treatment.

Physical or Chemical Hazards: Do not use or store near heat or open flame.

In case of emergency, call 1-877-767-4943, 24 hours a day.

Storage and Disposal: Storage: Do not remove tube from the pack until ready to use. Store in a cool (below 25°C) dry place, out of the reach of children. Do not refrigerate. Protect from direct sunlight.

Disposal: Do not reuse empty container. Wrap and put in trash.

Warning(s): Keep out of reach of children.

Disclaimer: Notice: Buyer assumes all responsibility for safety and use not in accordance with directions.

Presentation: 1.5 mL tube (one month supply) and 3 x 1.5 mL tubes (three month supply).

Compendium Code No.: 10350270

P006151

HAPPY JACK® KENNELSPOT™ FOR DOGS (OVER 33 LBS)

Happy Jack **Parasiticide-Topical**

EPA Reg. No.: 69332-1-2781

Active Ingredient(s):

Permethrin (CAS# 52645-53-1)	45%
Other Ingredients:	55%

Indications: One easy application for effective control. Kills and repels fleas and ticks quickly. Protects for up to 4 weeks.

What the drops do: One drop KENNELSPOT™ kills and repels fleas and ticks on your dog for up to 4 weeks. It is recommended that you also use a product labeled to treat your dog's basket and favorite sleeping areas.

Directions for Use: It is a violation of Federal Law to use this product in a manner inconsistent with its labeling.

Read entire label before each use. Use only on dogs.

How to use the drops:

For dogs weighing over 33 lb (15 kg):

1. Only open the tube, immediately prior to use by holding upright and twisting the cap off, taking care not to squeeze the tube.
2. Part the dog's coat to expose the skin between the shoulder blades, at the nape of the neck, then squeeze approximately one-half the contents of one tube onto the exposed skin.
3. Next, part the dog's coat at the base of the tail, then squeeze the remaining contents of the tube onto the exposed skin.

If the dog's coat is subsequently wetted, such as when shampooing, the 4 week period of protection may be reduced.

Additional precautions to protect your dog:

1. Do not massage the drops into the dog's skin. Avoid applying to the dog's fur.
2. Do not administer any other flea control product to your dog during the 4 week period of protection.
3. Retreat after 28 days if reinfestation is apparent.

Additional precautions to protect your family: Do not allow children to play with tubes. A pet treated with this product should not sleep with people, particularly children, for the 8 hours immediately following treatment. Do not handle the area of application for 3 to 6 hours following treatment.

What else you must do: Treating your dog's basket and favorite sleeping areas with a suitable insecticidal product labeled for this use and vacuuming these areas regularly will also help to remove dead fleas and ticks. Consult your veterinarian for product recommendations.

Precautionary Statements: Hazards to Humans and Domestic Animals:

Hazards to Humans: Harmful if swallowed or absorbed through the skin. Causes moderate eye irritation. Avoid contact with skin, eyes, or clothing. Wash thoroughly with soap and water after handling.

Hazards to Domestic Animals: For external use only. Do not apply to dogs less than 6 months of age. Repeat applications may be made as necessary, but do not apply at intervals less than 7 days. Do not use on cats. Cats which actively groom or engage in close physical contact with recently treated dogs may be at risk of toxic exposure. Consult a veterinarian before using this product on debilitated, aged, or medicated animals. Consult a veterinarian before using this product on dogs with known organ dysfunction. Sensitivities may occur after using any pesticide product for pets. If signs of sensitivity occur, bathe your pet with a mild soap and rinse with large amounts of water. If signs continue, consult a veterinarian immediately. Signs of sensitivity to this product include skin sensitivity, increased itchiness, redness, rash, hair discoloration or hair loss at the application site. Dogs may also show "lethargy".

First Aid:

If swallowed: Call a physician or Poison Control Center. Drink 1 or 2 glasses of water and induce vomiting by touching back of threat with finger or, if available, administer syrup of ipecac. Do not induce vomiting or give anything by mouth to an unconscious person.

If in eyes: Flush with plenty of water. Get medical attention if irritation persists.

If on skin: Remove contaminated clothing and wash with plenty of soap and water. Get medical attention if symptoms or irritation develops.

To Physician: Treat patient symptomatically.

Environmental Hazards: This product is extremely toxic to fish and aquatic organisms. Do not apply directly to any body of water. Treated dogs should not be allowed to go swimming for 12 hours following treatment.

Physical or Chemical Hazards: Do not use or store near heat or open flame.

In case of emergency, call 1-877-767-4943, 24 hours a day.

Storage and Disposal: Storage: Do not remove tube from the pack until ready to use. Store in a cool (below 25°C) dry place, out of the reach of children. Do not refrigerate. Protect from direct sunlight.

Disposal: Do not reuse empty container. Wrap and put in trash.

Warning(s): Keep out of reach of children.

Disclaimer: Notice: Buyer assumes all responsibility for safety and use not in accordance with directions.

Presentation: 3 mL tube (one month supply) and 3 x 3 mL tubes (three month supply).

Compendium Code No.: 10350280

P006161

HAPPY JACK® LIQUI-VICT 2X™

Happy Jack **Parasiticide-Oral**

(pyrantel pamoate) Canine Anthelmintic Suspension

ANADA No.: 200-007

Active Ingredient(s): 4.54 mg of pyrantel base as pyrantel pamoate per mL.

Indications: To prevent reinfestation of *Toxacara canis* in puppies and adult dogs and in lactating bitches after whelping.

For the removal of large roundworms (*Toxacara canis* and *Toxacara leonina)* and hookworms (*Ancylostoma caninum* and *Uncinaria stenocephala)* in dogs and puppies.

Consult your veterinarian for assistance in the diagnosis, treatment and control of parasitism.

Dosage and Administration: Shake well before use.

For maximum control and prevention of reinfestation, it is recommended that puppies be treated at 2, 3, 4, 6 8, and 10 weeks of age. Lactating bitches should be treated 2-3 weeks after whelping. Adult dogs kept in heavily contaminated quarters may be treated at monthly intervals to prevent *T canis* reinfestation. Administer one full teaspoonful (5 mL) for each 5 lb of body weight.

For the removal of large roundworms (ascarids) and hookworms. Administer one full teaspoonful (5 mL) for each 5 lb of dog's body weight. It is not necessary to withhold food from your dog prior to treatment. If medication is to be dispensed, client can be advised that dogs usually find this wormer very palatable and will lick the dose from the bowl willingly. If there is a reluctance to accept the dose, mix in a small quantity of dog food to encourage consumption.

The presence of large roundworms (ascarids) and hookworms should be confirmed by lab fecal examination. It is recommended that dogs maintained under conditions of constant exposure to worm infestation should have a follow-up fecal exam within 2 to 4 weeks after first treatment.

Precaution(s): Store below 30°C (86°F).

Warning(s): For animal use only.

Keep out of reach of children.

Presentation: 2 oz (56.4 g) (60 mL) liquid.

Compendium Code No.: 10350120

HAPPY JACK® MANGE MEDICINE

Happy Jack **Parasiticide Dip**

EPA Reg. No.: 2781-1

Active Ingredient(s):

Sulfur	28%
Inert ingredients*	72%
Total	100%

*Linseed oil, turpentine, pine tar oil, cod liver oil, lanolin, and tar acid oil

Indications: A sarcoptic mange medicine for dogs and horses.

Dosage and Administration: It is a violation of federal law to use the product in a manner inconsistent with its labeling.

Shake well before using.

For sarcoptic mange, apply once a day for several days. Wear rubber gloves and work well into the skin with a slow, firm finger massage. On areas that respond slowly, use twice a day until healed. After applying, tie the dog up for at least 20 to 30 minutes.

Important: For the best results, disinfect the animal's environment. Accompany the treatment with a periodic check of the infection and sound a nutritional program. If dermatitis persists, consult a veterinarian. If stiff sediment is found, turn bottle upside down overnight.

Precaution(s): Do not re-use the empty container. Wrap the container and put it in the trash collection.

Caution(s): Keep out of the reach of children.

Precautionary Statements: Hazards to Humans and Domestic Animals:

Humans: May cause eye and skin irritation. Do not get in eyes, on skin or clothing. Harmful if swallowed or absorbed through the skin. Wash thoroughly after handling.

Animals: Do not use on cats.

Statement of Practical Treatment:

If swallowed, call a physician or poison control center immediately. Drink one or two glasses of water and induce vomiting by touching the back of the throat with a finger. Do not induce vomiting or give anything by mouth to an unconscious or convulsing person.

If inhaled, remove the victim to fresh air. Apply artificial respiration if indicated.

If on skin, remove contaminated clothing and wash the affected areas with soap and water.

If in eyes, flush eyes with plenty of water. Call a physician if irritation persists.

Presentation: 8 oz, 16 oz and 1 gallon containers.

Compendium Code No.: 10350130

HAPPY JACK® MILKADE

Happy Jack — **Small Animal Dietary Supplement**

Active Ingredient(s): Salts of sodium, potassium, calcium, and thiamine hydrochloride (3%).

Indications: For use as an aid to the female dog in producing a healthy quantity of milk for her puppies.

Dosage and Administration: Mix the full contents of one (1) bottle with one (1) pint of water. Stir until dissolved. A small sediment on the bottom is normal.

Give one (1) tablespoon twice a day in the food or by mouth, beginning four (4) or five (5) days before whelping and for about 10 days thereafter. Then decrease the dosage gradually until the pups are weaned.

A large dosage is permissible when faster action is desired or where excessively acid milk is encountered.

Important: Some setting and caking can be expected.

Do not mix until ready to use and refrigerate after mixing.

Caution(s): Not for human use. Keep out of the reach of children.

Presentation: 2 oz. (57 g) bottles.

Compendium Code No.: 10350140

HAPPY JACK® MITEX™

Happy Jack — **Otic Parasiticide**

EPA Reg. No.: 2382-54-2781

Active Ingredient(s):

Pyrethrins	0.05%
Piperonyl butoxide, technical*	0.50%
Inert ingredients	99.45%

*Equivalent to 0.4% (butylcarbityl) (6-propylpiperonyl) ether and 0.1% related compounds.

Indications: For the treatment of ear mites in dogs and cats.

Dosage and Administration: It is a violation of federal law to use the product in a manner inconsistent with its labeling.

Cats or Dogs: Clean the ear thoroughly. Place the recommended number of drops in each ear once a day for 7-10 days. Repeat the treatment in two (2) weeks if necessary.

Body Weight	Dosage
5 to 15 lbs.	4 to 5 drops
15 to 30 lbs.	5 to 10 drops
30 lbs. or over	10 to 15 drops

Precaution(s):

Storage: Keep away from heat.

Disposal: Do not re-use the empty container. Wrap the container and put it in the trash collection.

Caution(s): Keep out of the reach of children.

Precautionary Statements:

Hazards to Humans and Domestic Animals: Harmful if swallowed.

Presentation: ½ fl. oz. (14.5 mL) and 1 fl. oz. containers.

Compendium Code No.: 10350150

HAPPY JACK® NO-HOP FLEA-TICK SPRAY

Happy Jack — **Parasiticide Spray**

EPA Reg. No.: 11715-191-2781

Active Ingredient(s):

Pyrethrins	0.056%
Permethrin [*(3-Phenoxyphenyl) methyl (±) cis trans-3-(2,2-dichloroethenyl) 2,2-dimethylcyclopropanecarboxylate]	0.050%
Related reaction products	0.004%
Inert Ingredients	99.890%
Total	100.000%

*cis-trans isomer ratio: Min 35% (±) cis. Max 65% (±) trans

Indications: Residually kills fleas and ticks on dogs and cats.

Directions for Use: It is a violation of Federal Law to use this product in a manner inconsistent with its labeling.

Hold container upright. Shake well before using. This product will kill fleas for up to 14 days on dogs and cats and will kill ticks for 4 days on dogs and 9 days on cats.

Spray animal from a distance of 8-12 inches. Start spraying at the tail, moving the dispenser rapidly and making sure the animal's entire body is covered, including the legs and under the body. Fluff the hair as you spray so the spray will penetrate to the skin. The spray should wet the ticks thoroughly. Do not spray in the face, eyes or on genitalia. Repeat as needed.

For cats, apply at the rate of 1 second per pound of body weight. For dogs, apply at the rate of 2 seconds per pound of body weight for thin or short-haired dogs and up to eight seconds per pound of body weight for heavy or long-haired dogs.

Precautionary Statements: Hazards to Humans and Domestic Animals:

Caution: Do not spray in pet's eyes, face or on genitalia. Do not use on nursing puppies or kittens or animals under 3 months of age. Do not use this or any pesticide on sick, old, or debilitated animals. Causes moderate eye irritation. Harmful if absorbed through skin. Avoid contact with skin, eyes, or clothing. Wash thoroughly with soap and water after handling.

Statement of Practical Treatment:

If swallowed: Call a physician or Poison Control Center immediately.

If in eyes: Flush with plenty of water. Get medical attention if irritation persists.

If on skin or clothing: Remove contaminated clothing and wash before re-use. Wash skin with soap and warm water. Get medical attention if irritation persists.

If inhaled: Remove victim to fresh air. Apply artificial respiration if indicated.

Environmental Hazards: This product is toxic to fish and other aquatic animals. Do not apply directly to any body of water. Do not contaminate water by cleaning of equipment or disposal of wastes.

Physical or Chemical Hazards: Contents under pressure. Do not use or store near heat or open flame. Do not puncture or incinerate container. Exposure to temperatures above 130°F may cause bursting.

Storage and Disposal: Storage: Store in a cool, dry area away from heat or open flame.

Disposal: Replace the cap and discard container in trash. Do not incinerate or puncture.

Warning(s): Keep out of reach of children.

Presentation: 7 oz containers.

Compendium Code No.: 10350290

HAPPY JACK® NOVATION™ FLEA & TICK COLLAR FOR DOGS

Happy Jack — **Parasiticide Collar**

EPA Reg. No.: 68451-1-2781

Active Ingredient(s):

	Percentage by Weight
Deltamethrin	4.0%
Inert Ingredients:	96.0%
Total	100.00%

Indications: Kills fleas and ticks (including Brown and American ticks, and Deer ticks, which may cause Lyme disease). Provides full-season protection against fleas and ticks. Effective for up to 6 months. Water resistant.

Directions for Use: It is a violation of Federal law to use this product in a manner inconsistent with its labeling.

Read entire label before each use. Use only on dogs.

HAPPY JACK® NOVATION™ Collar, containing deltamethrin insecticide, has been specially formulated using patented insecticide-release technology. Maximum effectiveness may not occur for 2-3 weeks after collar placement. Fleas *(Ctenocephalides* sp.) on the dog will be killed and ones which are present in the dog's environment that may appear on your pet will be killed. Collar will kill ticks including Brown dog tick *(Rhipicephalus sanguineus)*, American dog tick *(Dermacentor variabilis)* and deer ticks *(Ixodes scapularis* and *I. pacificus)* which may carry the Lyme disease. This collar should be worn continuously. Reapply a new collar every 6 months.

Place the collar around the dog's neck, buckle and adjust for proper fit. Cut off approximately 2 inches from the buckle and dispose of excess length by wrapping in newspaper and placing in trash. The collar must be worn loosely so that two fingers may be placed between collar and dog's neck. Living and rest areas of pet must also be treated with appropriate pest control measures to ensure control of pests. Wetting will not impair the collar's effectiveness or the pet's protection. If the dog goes swimming or is out in the rain, it is not necessary to remove the collar. HAPPY JACK® NOVATION™ Collar may be used in addition to a lead or constraint collar. Use only one HAPPY JACK® NOVATION™ Collar at a time.

Precautionary Statements: Hazards to Humans and Domestic Animals:

Caution: Do not open protective pouch until ready to use. Do not let children play with this collar. Harmful if swallowed or absorbed through skin. Causes moderate eye irritation. Avoid contact with skin, eyes, or clothing. Wash thoroughly with soap and water after handling. Do not use on puppies under 12 weeks. Consult a veterinarian before using this product on debilitated, aged, pregnant, medicated, or nursing animals. Sensitivities may occur after using any pesticide product for pets. If signs of sensitivity occur, remove collar and bathe your pet with mild soap and rinse with large amounts of water. If signs continue, consult a veterinarian immediately.

First Aid:

If swallowed: Call a physician or poison control center. Do not induce vomiting or give anything by mouth to an unconscious person.

If on skin: Wash with plenty of soap and water. Get medical attention.

If in eyes: Flush eyes with plenty of water. Call a physician if irritation persists.

Emergency Phone Numbers:

For human, fire and environmental: 1-800-228-5635, ext. 132.

For animals: 1-800-4735, ext. 104.

Collar is intended for use only as an insecticide generator and is not to be taken internally by man or animals. Applying other pesticides on the dog may not be necessary while the collar is being worn.

Storage and Disposal: Store in original, unopened container, away from children. Do not reuse container or used collar. Wrap in a newspaper and put in trash.

Warning(s): Do not let children play with this collar.

Disclaimer: Important Notice: Disclaimer: Read "Important Notice: Disclaimer" before buying or using. If terms are not acceptable, return at once unopened. Happy Jack, Inc., warrants only that the product conforms to the chemical description on the label and is reasonably fit for the purpose stated on the label when used in accordance with the directions under normal conditions of use. This warranty does not extend to the use of this product contrary to label instructions or under abnormal conditions, or under conditions not reasonably foreseeable to Happy Jack, Inc., and user assumes the risk of any such use. Happy Jack, Inc., makes no other warranty, expressed or implied, including any implied warranty of fitness for a particular purpose or of merchantability. In no case shall Happy Jack, Inc., be liable for consequential, special, indirect or incidental damages resulting from the use of handling of this product. The foregoing conditions of sale and warranty can be varied only by an agreement in writing signed by a duly authorized representative of Happy Jack, Inc.

Presentation: 1 x 1.1 oz (26") collar.

The Happy Jack name is a registered trademark of Happy Jack, Inc.

Compendium Code No.: 10350300

HAPPY JACK® ONEX

Happy Jack — **External Parasiticide**

EPA Reg. No.: 2781-9

Active Ingredient(s):

Pyrethrins I & II	0.2%
Piperonyl butoxide, technical*	0.5%
Di-n-propyl isocinchomeronate	1.0%
Inert ingredients	98.3%

*Equivalent to 0.4% (butylcarbityl) (6-propylpiperonyl) ether and 0.1% related compounds.

Indications: Repels house flies, stable flies, face flies, and horn flies from wounds and open sores. Also kills on contact. For use on dogs and horses.

Dosage and Administration: It is a violation of federal law to use the product in a manner inconsistent with its labeling.

To treat superficial wounds, abrasions, sores and scratches apply enough ointment to completely cover the affected area. Use once a day.

Precaution(s): Do not re-use the empty container. Wrap the container and put it in the trash collection.

Caution(s): Precautionary Statements:

Hazards to Humans and Domestic Animals: Not for human use. Wash hands after using.

Environmental Hazards: The product is toxic to fish. Keep out of lakes, streams, or ponds. Do not apply where runoff is likely to occur. Do not contaminate water by the cleaning of equipment or the disposal of wastes.

Warning(s): Do not use on horses to be used for human consumption.

Presentation: 4 oz. (113 g) containers.

Compendium Code No.: 10350160

HAPPY JACK® PAD KOTE

Happy Jack **Topical Wound Dressing**

Active Ingredient(s): Cod liver oil, cade oil, balsam peru, tannic acid, turpentine, gentian violet, brilliant green, isopropyl alcohol (50%).

Indications: Developed for conditions of the feet and pads of dogs due to wear or minor skin eczemas. PAD KOTE is a healing aid for moist, weeping spots due to minor skin eczemas, galls, saddle sores and other minor abrasions of the skin of dogs and horses. It aids in the healing and toughening of all types of wounds and sores and relieves itching.

Dosage and Administration: Shake well. Apply once or twice a day. Allow to dry before releasing the dog. Use alcohol to remove stains from the hands.

Caution(s): Not for human use. Keep out of the reach of children.

Presentation: 2 fl. oz. (58 mL) containers.

Compendium Code No.: 10350170

HAPPY JACK® PARACIDE II SHAMPOO

Happy Jack **Parasiticide Shampoo**

EPA Reg. No.: 2781-17

Active Ingredient(s):

Chlorpyrifos* [0,0-diethyl-0-(3,5,6-trichloro-2-pyridyl) phosphorothioate] 0.125%
Inert ingredients. 99.875%

Indications: A residual, insecticidal shampoo with conditioners that add luster to the hair. Kills fleas, ticks, and sarcoptic mange mites on dogs.

Dosage and Administration: It is a violation of federal law to use the product in a manner inconsistent with its labeling.

Wet the dog and apply approximately 2 oz. of shampoo for every 15 lbs. of body weight, working it well into the hair. For the best results, the dog should be left in a lathered state for one (1) to two (2) minutes before rinsing.

Do not use the product on animals simultaneously or within 30 days before or after treatment with or exposure to cholinesterase-inhibiting drugs, pesticides, or chemicals.

Do not treat dogs more than once every four (4) weeks.

Precaution(s): Do not re-use the empty container. Wrap the container and put it in the trash collection.

Caution(s): Keep out of the reach of children.

Precautionary Statements:

Hazards to Humans and Domestic Animals: Not for human use. Harmful if swallowed. Avoid eye contact. Avoid excessive contact with skin or clothing. Wash hands thoroughly with soap and warm water after treating animals. Contaminated utensils should not be used for food purposes after use with insecticides. Chlorpyrifos is a cholinesterase inhibitor.

Use rubber gloves when using this product to bathe dogs.

Statement of Practical Treatment:

If swallowed, call a physician. Atropine by injection is antidotal.

If in eyes, flush eyes immediately with plenty of water and get medical attention if irritation persists.

If on skin, remove contaminated clothing and wash skin with soap and warm water.

Antidote(s): Atropine by injection is antidotal only if symptoms of cholinesterase inhibition are present.

Presentation: 8 fl. oz. (314 mL) containers.

* U.S. Patent 3,244,586

Compendium Code No.: 10350180

HAPPY JACK® SARDEX II®

Happy Jack **Parasiticide Spray**

Dog Mange Remedy

EPA Reg. No.: 2781-51

Active Ingredient(s):

Benzyl benzoate 29.00%
Inert Ingredients. 71.00%
Total 100.00%

Indications: An effective treatment for sarcoptic mange. For dogs only. Stainless. Low odor.

Directions for Use: It is a violation of Federal law to use this product in a manner inconsistent with its labeling.

Read entire label before each use. Use only on dogs. Shake well before using.

Directions: Clip hair around all affected areas, if necessary clip entire body. Then wash animal thoroughly with soap and water, rinse and allow animal to dry or wipe dry before application. Spray product on the affected areas, rub in slightly, allow to dry, then apply a second time. Repeat applications at 7-day intervals until the condition clears up.

Do not spray in or towards the eyes, affected areas around the eyes should be treated with care to avoid getting the product into the eyes. Do not use on puppies less than 12 weeks, nor on pregnant or nursing bitches. Consult a veterinarian before using this product on debilitated, aged or medicated dogs. Sensitivities may occur after using any pesticide product for pets. If signs of sensitivity occur, bathe the dog with mild soap and rinse with large amounts of water. If signs continue, consult a veterinarian immediately.

Dogs under treatment should be fed an adequate diet containing all essential vitamins and minerals. To prevent reinfestation, change bedding daily. Wash bedding thoroughly after use.

Precautionary Statements: Hazards to Humans and Domestic Animals:

For use on dogs only.

Caution: Harmful if swallowed, absorbed through the skin or inhaled. Avoid contact with skin, eyes or clothing. Avoid breathing spray mist. Wash thoroughly with soap and water after handling. Remove contaminated clothing and wash clothing before reuse.

Physical Hazards: Contents under pressure. Do not use or store near heat or open flame. Do not puncture or incinerate container. Exposure to temperatures above 130°F may cause the container to burst.

To receive information concerning the proper use of the product and/or specific actions to be taken in case of emergencies, call 1-800-326-5225.

Storage and Disposal: Do not contaminate water, food or feed by storage and disposal.

Pesticide Storage: Store in a cool, dry area away from heat or flame.

Container Disposal: This container may be recycled in aerosol recycling centers. Before offering for recycling, empty the can by using the product according to the label - Do not puncture! If recycling is not available, wrap container in several layers of newspaper and discard in the trash.

Warning(s): Keep out of reach of children.

Presentation: 9.5 oz containers.

Compendium Code No.: 10350310

HAPPY JACK® SKIN BALM

Happy Jack **Topical Wound Dressing**

Active Ingredient(s):

Mercaptobenzothiazole 1.4%
Inert ingredients 98.6%

Indications: SKIN BALM® affords relief to certain minor, external skin problems of dogs, cats and horses such as summer eczema or kennel itch. In early stages, intense itching and scratching normally occur followed by the skin becoming rough and scaly with some loss of hair. Raw areas may appear.

Dosage and Administration: Apply well to affected areas once or twice a day. Rub into the skin with a finger massage. If the condition persists, consult a veterinarian.

Caution(s): For external use only. Not for human use. Keep out of the reach of children.

Presentation: 4 fl. oz. (117 mL) liquid and 6 oz. aerosol.

Compendium Code No.: 10350200

HAPPY JACK® TAPEWORM TABLETS

Happy Jack **Parasiticide-Oral**

(Dichlorophene)

NADA No.: 007-829

Active Ingredient(s): Each tablet contains:

2,2'methylenebis (4 chlorophenol) (dichlorophene) . . . . 1.0 g

Indications: For use as an aid in the removal of tapeworms *(Taenia pisiformis* and *Dipylidium caninum)* from dogs.

Dosage and Administration: One (1) tablet for each 10 lbs. of body weight. Withhold solid foods and milk (broth may be given) for at least 12 hours prior to medication and for four (4) hours afterward.

Consult a veterinarian for assistance in the diagnosis, treatment and control of parasitism.

Precaution(s): Store in a cool, dry place, not over 70°F.

Caution(s): For oral animal use only.

Consult a veterinarian before administering to weak or debilitated animals.

Side Effects: Vomiting and diarrhea may occur in dogs one to three days post-treatment.

Presentation: Bottles of 30 tablets.

Compendium Code No.: 10350220

HAPPY JACK® TONEKOTE®

Happy Jack **Small Animal Dietary Supplement**

Active Ingredient(s): Guaranteed analysis and statement of ingredients: Each pound of TONEKOTE® food supplement contains:

Linoleic acid . . . . 230,000 mg
Linolenic acid . . . . 30,000 mg
Vitamin A (palmitate) . . . . 100,000 I.U.
Vitamin D_3 (d-activated animal sterol). . . . . 10,000 I.U.
Vitamin E (dl-alpha tocopherol) . . . . 210 I.U.

Other ingredients: Choline (from lecithin), inositol (from lecithin), BHA and BHT (preservatives).

Indications: TONEKOTE® contains essential fatty acids the lack of which may result in shedding, itching, dull coat and dry skin.

Dosage and Administration:

Adult Dogs: One (1) teaspoonful for each 10 lbs. of body weight each day.

Puppies, Pregnant and Nursing Dogs: One (1) teaspoonful for each 10 lbs. of body weight each day.

Double the directions for daily use for the first five (5) days if the skin is very dry or dull.

TONEKOTE® can be mixed in food or may be fed directly. TONEKOTE® contains linoleic acid, an essential fatty acid, that cannot be synthesized by the body. It is a necessary nutrient for normal healthy skin and lustrous hair condition.

When used as directed, TONEKOTE® food supplement provides 170% of the daily adult's and 115% of the daily puppy's requirement for vitamin D and 115% of the daily requirement for vitamin A (Source: National Research Council).

Presentation: 16 fl. oz. and 1 gallon container.

Compendium Code No.: 10350230

HAPPY JACK® VITA TABS

Happy Jack **Small Animal Dietary Supplement**

Active Ingredient(s): Each tablet contains:

Vitamin A (as acetate). . . . . 1,000 I.U.
Vitamin D (cholecalciferol) . . . . 100 I.U.
Niacinamide . . . . 10 mg
Thiamine mononitrate. . . . . 810 mcg
Riboflavin . . . . 1 mg
Pyridoxine hydrochloride . . . . 82 mcg
Vitamin B_{12} (cyanocobalamin) . . . . 0.2 mcg
Vitamin E (dl-alpha-tocopheryl) . . . . 2 I.U.
Iron (from ferric ammonium citrate). . . . . 6 mg
Zinc (as gluconate) 1.5 mg
Cobalt (as gluconate) 0.001%
Potassium (as iodide) 0.001%
Iodine (from potassium iodide). 0.003%
Copper (as sulfate) 0.003%
Magnesium (as oxide) 0.015%
Manganese (as sulfate). 0.004%
Linoleic acid . . . . 30 mg
Calcium (from di-calcium phosphate). . . . . 100 mg
Phosphorus . . . . 77 mg

Indications: A chewable vitamin and mineral tablet for dogs and cats in a palatable protein base.

Dosage and Administration: Administer by hand just prior to feeding or crumble and mix with food.

For diet supplement:

Dogs under 10 lbs.: One-half (½) tablet each day.

Dogs over 10 lbs.: One (1) tablet each day.

Growing Pups: One (1) to two (2) tablets each day.

For sick, convalescing, pregnant or nursing dogs: Two (2) tablets each day.

Cats: One-half (½) to one (1) tablet each day, depending upon the size and condition.

Presentation: 50 and 100 tablets.

Compendium Code No.: 10350250

HAROLD WHITE'S® LEG PAINT

Hawthorne **Counterirritant**

Active Ingredient(s): Each 16 U.S. fl oz contains:

Isopropyl alcohol . . . . . 107.0 g
Ether . . . . . 83.4 g

Turpentine, oil of peppermint, iodine, gum camphor, oil of cedarwood.

Indications: Promotes heavy scurfing.

Aids in preventing and treating bog spavin, bucked shins, curbs, osselets, pop-knee, ringbone, and splints.

Dosage and Administration: Leg must be clean and free of medication. Using a soft brush, apply with hair. Dilute for light-skinned horses. Leave open or wrap with bandage for maximum counter-irritant results. Check daily for desired irritation.

Caution(s): Keep away from children. Flammable - keep away from fire or flame.

For external use only.

Warning(s): Do not use on food animals.

Presentation: 16 U.S. fl oz.

Compendium Code No.: 10670040

HARTZ® 2 IN 1® FLEA & TICK COLLAR FOR CATS AND KITTENS

Hartz Mountain **Parasiticide Collar**

EPA Reg. No.: 2596-63

Active Ingredient(s): By Weight (Nom.):

Tetrachlorvinphos (CAS# 22248-79-9) 14.55%
Other Ingredients: 85.45%
Total 100.00%

Contains Rabon®*.

Indications: For use only on cats. The 2 IN 1® collar will kill ticks, including the Deer Tick, which may carry Lyme Disease, for five months under normal conditions.

Directions for Use: It is a violation of Federal law to use this product in a manner inconsistent with its labeling.

Read entire label before each use.

Remove collar from package, unroll and stretch to activate insecticide generator.

Do not use on kittens under 12 weeks of age. Do not unroll collar until ready to use. Place the HARTZ® 2 IN 1® Flea & Tick Collar around the cat's neck, adjust to proper fit, and buckle in place. The collar must be worn loosely to allow for growth of the cat and to permit the collar to move about the neck. Generally, a properly fitted collar is one that when fastened will snugly slide over the cat's head. Leave 2 or 3 inches on the collar for extra adjustment and cut off and dispose of the extra length. Consult a veterinarian before using this product on debilitated, aged, medicated, pregnant or nursing animals. Sensitivities may occur after using any pesticide product for pets. Some animals may become irritated by any collar if its applied too tightly. If this occurs, loosen the collar. If irritation continues, remove the collar from the animal. If signs of sensitivity occur, remove the collar and bathe your pet with mild soap and rinse with large amounts of water. If signs continue, consult a veterinarian immediately. Do not use this product on animals simultaneously or within 30 days before or after treatment with or exposure to cholinesterase inhibiting drugs, pesticides, or chemicals. However flea & tick collars may be immediately replaced. This collar is intended for use only as an insecticide generator. For continuous flea and tick protection under normal conditions replace the collar every five months. Under conditions when cats are exposed to severe flea & tick infestations, it may be necessary to replace the collar every 4 months. Ticks, which may be an occasional problem for cats, are harder to kill. The collar's full protection against ticks will be built up within a few days after being placed on the animal. The cat should be examined from time to time and the collar replaced when mature tick or flea populations begin to appear. Wetting will not impair the collar's effectiveness or the pet's protection. If the cat is out in the rain it is not necessary to remove the collar. The HARTZ® 2 IN 1® collar may be worn with a regular collar.

Disposal: Do not use empty pouch. Dispose in trash collection.

Warning(s): Do not let children play with this collar.

Presentation: 1 Bright Blue Collar, 0.53 oz (15 g).
1 Pink Collar, 0.53 oz (15 g).
1 Purple Collar, 0.53 oz (15 g).
1 White Collar, 0.53 oz (15 g).
1 White Collar with Safety Snap, 0.53 oz (15 g).
1 White Collar, (for kittens) 0.42 oz (12 g).

* Rabon™ is the Hartz trademark for Tetrachlorvinphos.

Compendium Code No.: 10360010

HARTZ® 2 IN 1® FLEA & TICK COLLAR FOR DOGS AND PUPPIES

Hartz Mountain **Parasiticide Collar**

EPA Reg. No.: 2596-62

Active Ingredient(s): By Weight (Nom.):

Tetrachlorvinphos (CAS# 22248-79-9) 14.55%
Other Ingredients: 85.45%
Total 100.00%

Contains Rabon®*.

Indications: Kills fleas and ticks common to dogs for five months, including Rocky Mountain Wood Tick, carrier of Rocky Mountain Spotted Fever, and the Deer Tick, which may carry Lyme Disease.

Directions for Use: It is a violation of Federal law to use this product in a manner inconsistent with its labeling.

Read entire label before each use.

Remove collar from package, unroll and stretch to activate insecticide generator.

Do not use on puppies under 6 weeks of age. Do not unroll collar until ready to use. Place the HARTZ® 2 IN 1® Flea and Tick Collar around the dog's neck, adjust to proper fit, and buckle in place. The collar must be worn loosely to allow for growth of the dog and to permit the collar to move about the neck. Generally, a properly fitted collar is one that when fastened will snugly slide over the dog's head. Leave 2 or 3 inches of the collar for extra adjustment and cut off and dispose of the extra length. Consult a veterinarian before using this product on debilitated, aged or medicated animals. If used on pregnant or nursing dogs, do not replace collar until the puppies are at least 6 weeks old. Sensitivities may occur after using any pesticide product for pets. Some animals may become irritated by any collar if its applied too tightly. If this occurs, loosen the collar. If irritation continues, remove the collar from the animal. If signs of sensitivity occur, remove the collar and bathe your pet with mild soap and rinse with large amounts of water. If signs continue, consult a veterinarian immediately. Do not use this product on animals simultaneously or within 30 days before or after treatment with or exposure to cholinesterase inhibiting drugs, pesticides, or chemicals. However, flea and tick collars may be immediately replaced. This collar is intended for use only as an insecticide generator. The collar will begin to kill fleas and ticks immediately. Its full protection against harder to kill ticks will be built up within a few days after being placed on the pet. For continuous flea and tick protection under normal conditions replace the collar every five months. Under conditions where dogs are exposed to severe flea and tick infestations it may be necessary to replace the collar more frequently. Wetting will not impair the collar's effectiveness or the pet's protection. If the dog goes swimming or is out in the rain it is not necessary to remove the collar. The HARTZ® 2 IN 1® collar may be worn with a regular collar.

Disposal: Do not use empty pouch. Dispose in trash collection.

Warning(s): Do not let children play with this collar.

Use only on dogs.

Presentation:

1 Bright White Collar, 0.68 oz (19 g) - for puppies with necks to 15".
1 Bright White Collar, 0.85 oz (24 g) - for dogs with necks to 20".
1 Bright White Collar, 1.15 oz (32 g) - for large dogs with necks to 26".
1 Bright Blue Collar, 1.0 oz (28 g) - for dogs with necks to 23".
1 Bright Purple Collar, 1.0 oz (28 g) - for dogs with necks to 23".
1 Bright Red Collar, 1.0 oz (28 g) - for dogs with necks to 23".

* Rabon® is the Hartz® trademark for Tetrachlorvinphos.

Compendium Code No.: 10360020

HARTZ® 2 IN 1® FLEA & TICK DIP FOR DOGS AND CATS

Hartz Mountain **Parasiticide Dip**

EPA Reg. No.: 2596-86

Active Ingredient(s):

Pyrethrins (CAS# 121-29-9) 0.33%
Piperonyl Butoxide, Technical* (CAS# 51-03-6) 0.67%
N-Octyl Bicycloheptene Dicarboximide (CAS# 113-48-4) 1.11%
Other Ingredients: 97.89%

* Equivalent to 0.54% (butylcarbityl) (6-propylpiperonyl) ether and 0.13% related compounds.

Contains Petroleum Distillate.

Indications: For use only on dogs and cats. Kills fleas and ticks, including the Deer Tick which may carry Lyme Disease.

Directions for Use: It is a violation of Federal law to use this product in a manner inconsistent with its labeling.

Read entire label before each use.

For control of fleas, lice and ticks on dogs and cats, dilute 4 ounces of HARTZ® 2 IN 1® Flea & Tick Dip with 1 gallon of water. Dip animal into solution, making sure hair is thoroughly wet to the skin. The area around the ears should be sponged thoroughly. Avoid contact of material with eyes and mouth of animal. Do not rinse. Towel dry. Repeat weekly (if necessary) for control. Consult a veterinarian before using this product on debilitated, aged, pregnant or nursing or medicated animals. Sensitivity may occur after using any pesticide product for pets. If signs of sensitivity occur bathe your pet with mild soap and rinse with large amounts of water. If signs continue, consult a veterinarian immediately.

Precautionary Statements: Hazards to Humans and Domestic Animals: Caution: Harmful if swallowed. Avoid contact with skin or eyes. Do not contaminate food or feedstuffs with this concentrate or dip. Toxic to fish. Do not use on puppies or kittens less than 12 weeks of age.

Physical Hazards: Do not use, pour, spill or store near heat or open flames. Do not contaminate any body of water with this concentrate or dip.

Storage and Disposal: Store in cool place, away from heat or open flame. Do not reuse empty container. Wrap container and put in trash collection.

Warning(s): Keep out of reach of children.

Presentation: 12 fl oz (355 mL). Concentrated - Makes three gallons.

Compendium Code No.: 10360031

HARTZ® 2 IN 1® FLEA & TICK KILLER FOR DOGS

Hartz Mountain **Parasiticide Spray**

EPA Reg. No.: 2596-94

Active Ingredient(s):

Pyrethrins (CAS# 121-29-9) 0.060%
Piperonyl Butoxide Technical* (CAS# 51-03-6) 0.120%
N-Octyl Bicycloheptene Dicarboximide (CAS# 113-48-4) 0.200%
Other Ingredients: 99.620%

*Equivalent to 0.096% (butylcarbityl) (6-propylpiperonyl) ether and 0.024% related compounds.

Indications: For use only on dogs. Kills fleas, ticks and flies.

Directions for Use: It is a violation of Federal law to use this product in a manner inconsistent with its labeling.

Read entire label before each use.

1. Hold bottle upright 6 inches from pet. Direct spray toward pat and spray entire coat, pressing dispenser with quick, short strokes. Move bottle to get even coverage of coat (until tips of hair are moist).
2. Apply lightly and rub into animal's coat. For long haired dogs, ruffle hair for spray to reach skin.
3. After 10 minutes, dry dog with towel.
4. Comb and brush coat.
5. Repeat once a week for fresh, glossy coat. Use on bedding and other areas as needed.
6. Kills fleas in 5 to 10 minutes. Ticks are tough - spray directly.

Precautionary Statements: Hazards to Humans and Domestic Animals: Caution: Do not use near birds, fish or foodstuffs. Do not spray in eyes or face of dog. Do not use on puppies under 12 weeks old. Consult a veterinarian before using this product on debilitated, aged, pregnant or nursing or medicated animals. Sensitivities may occur after using any pesticide product for pets. If signs of sensitivity occur, bathe your pet with mild soap and rinse with large amounts of water. If signs continue, consult a veterinarian immediately. Wash hands thoroughly after use.

Storage and Disposal: Do not re-use empty container. Wrap container and put in trash collection.

Warning(s): Keep out of reach of children.

Presentation: 20 fl oz (591 mL).

Compendium Code No.: 10360040

RM139143 554453, RM139886 555148

HARTZ® 2 IN 1® FLEA & TICK POWDER FOR CATS

Hartz Mountain **Parasiticide Powder**

EPA Reg. No.: 2596-78

Active Ingredient(s):

Tetrachlorvinphos: (CAS# 22248-79-9) 3.3%
Other Ingredients: 96.7%
Total 100.0%
Contains Rabon®*.

Indications: For use only on cats. Kills fleas and ticks, including the Deer Tick, which may carry Lyme Disease.

Directions: It is a violation of Federal law to use this product in a manner inconsistent with its labeling.

Read entire label before each use.

To kill fleas, ticks and lice, and to reduce itching and scratching due to insect bites, dust entire cat beginning at head and working back. Make sure that the powder gets down to the skin. Take care to treat feet and legs. Dust cat's bedding and living quarters. Repeat at weekly intervals if necessary.

Precautionary Statements: Hazards to Humans & Domestic Animals: Caution: Wash hands and exposed skin after use. Avoid contact with eyes. In case of contact, flush with water. If irritation persists, seek medical attention. Do not use on kittens under 12 weeks of age. Consult a veterinarian before using this product on debilitated, aged, medicated, pregnant or nursing animals. Sensitivities may occur after using any pesticide product for pets. If signs of sensitivity occur, bathe your pet with mild soap and rinse with large amounts of water. If signs continue, consult a veterinarian immediately. Do not use this product on animals simultaneously or within 30 days before or after treatment with or exposure to cholinesterase inhibiting drugs, pesticides, or chemicals. However, flea & tick collars may be immediately replaced.

Disposal: Do not re-use empty container. Wrap container and put in trash collection. Do not contaminate water by disposal of waste.

Warning(s): Keep out of reach of children.

Presentation: 4 oz (113 g).

*Rabon® is a registered trademark for Tetrachlorvinphos.

Compendium Code No.: 10360050

554338

HARTZ® 2 IN 1® FLEA & TICK POWDER FOR DOGS

Hartz Mountain **Parasiticide Powder**

EPA Reg. No.: 2596-79

Active Ingredient(s):

Tetrachlorvinphos: (CAS# 22248-79-9) 3.3%
Other Ingredients: 96.7%
Total 100.0%
Contains Rabon®*.

Indications: For use only on dogs. Kills fleas and ticks, including the Deer Tick, which may carry Lyme Disease, and controls sarcoptic mange.

Directions: It is a violation of Federal law to use this product in a manner inconsistent with its labeling.

Read entire label before each use.

To kill fleas, ticks and lice and to reduce itching and scratching due to insect bites, dust entire dog beginning at head and working back. Make sure that the powder gets down to the skin. Take care to treat feet and legs. Dust dog's bedding and living quarters. Repeat at weekly intervals if necessary.

To Control Sarcoptic Mange - a problem often encountered by dogs: Lesions which form are usually characterized by loss of hair, redness and possible open sores. HARTZ® 2 IN 1® Flea and Tick Powder will kill the mite which causes this problem. To treat the dog, apply the powder as directed above making sure that all sores and lesions are covered. Repeat application weekly for at least 3 treatments. More advanced lesions may require further weekly treatments. The area will begin to heal immediately but complete healing, including hair growth may take several weeks. If irritation persists, consult your veterinarian.

Precautionary Statements: Hazards to Humans & Domestic Animals: Caution: Wash hands and exposed skin after use. Avoid contact with eyes. In case of contact, flush with water. If irritation persists, seek medical attention. Do not use on puppies under 6 weeks of age. Consult a veterinarian before using this product on debilitated, aged or medicated animals. If used on pregnant or nursing dogs, do not retreat until the puppies are at least 6 weeks old. Sensitivities may occur after using any pesticide product for pets. If signs of sensitivity occur, bathe your pet with mild soap and rinse with large amounts of water. If signs continue, consult a veterinarian immediately. Do not use this product on animals simultaneously or within 30 days before or after treatment with or exposure to cholinesterase inhibiting drugs, pesticides, or chemicals. However, flea & tick collars may be immediately replaced.

Disposal: Do not re-use empty container. Wrap container and put in trash collection.

Warning(s): Keep out of reach of children.

Presentation: 4 oz (113 g).

* Rabon® is a registered trademark for Tetrachlorvinphos.

Compendium Code No.: 10360060

554337

HARTZ® 2 IN 1® FLEA & TICK SPRAY FOR CATS

Hartz Mountain **Parasiticide Spray**

EPA Reg. No.: 2596-123

Active Ingredient(s): By Weight (Nom.):

Tetrachlorvinphos (CAS# 22248-79-9) 1.08%
Other Ingredients: 98.92%
Contains Rabon®*.

Contains no CFC's or other ozone depleting substances. Federal regulations prohibit CFC propellants in aerosols.

Indications: For use only on cats. Kills fleas and ticks, including the Deer Tick, which may carry Lyme Disease.

Directions for Use: It is a violation of Federal law to use this product in a manner inconsistent with its labeling.

Read entire label before each use.

Shake Well Before Use: To kill fleas, ticks and lice, thereby reducing incidence of itching and scratching, hold container 6 to 10 inches from the animal and spray lightly over the entire body. Do not spray in eyes. For best penetration of spray to the skin, direct spray against the natural lay of the hair to cause fluffing of the coat. In addition to controlling fleas and ticks, this product leaves your pet's coat soft, glossy and manageable.

Under normal circumstances, repeat spray once a week until infestation is brought under control. For more prolonged flea and tick control, the animals bedding, quarters, and surrounding area should also be sprayed lightly until damp to help prevent reinfestation.

Precautionary Statements: Hazards to Humans and Domestic Animals: Caution: Causes moderate eye irritation. Avoid contact with eyes or clothing. Wash hands and exposed skin thoroughly with soap and water after handling. Do not use on kittens under 12 weeks of age. Consult a veterinarian before using this product on debilitated, aged, medicated, pregnant or nursing animals. Sensitivity may occur after using any pesticide product for pets. If signs of sensitivity occur, bathe your pet with mild soap and rinse with large amounts of water. If signs continue, consult a veterinarian immediately. Do not use this product on animals simultaneously or within 30 days before or after treatment with or exposure to cholinesterase inhibiting drugs, pesticides, or chemicals. However, flea and tick collars may be immediately replaced.

Physical or Chemical Hazards: Contents under pressure. Do not use or store near heat or open flame. Do not puncture or incinerate container. Exposure to temperatures above 130° F may cause bursting.

First Aid: If in Eyes: Rinse eyes with plenty of water. Call a physician if irritation persists.

Storage and Disposal: Do not contaminate water, food or feed by storage and disposal. Wrap empty container and put in trash collection.

Warning(s): Keep out of reach of children.

Presentation: 7 oz (198 g).

* Rabon® is a registered trademark for Tetrachlorvinphos.

Compendium Code No.: 10360072

555828

HARTZ® 2 IN 1® FLEA & TICK SPRAY FOR DOGS

Hartz Mountain **Parasiticide Spray**

EPA Reg. No.: 2596-122

Active Ingredient(s): By Weight (Nom.):

Tetrachlorvinphos (CAS# 22248-79-9) 1.08%
Other Ingredients: 98.92%
Contains Rabon®*.

Contains no CFC's or other ozone depleting substances. Federal regulations prohibit CFC propellants in aerosols.

Indications: For use only on dogs. Kills fleas and ticks, including the Deer Tick, which may carry Lyme Disease.

Directions for Use: It is a violation of Federal law to use this product in a manner inconsistent with its labeling.

Read entire label before each use.

Shake Well Before Use: To kill fleas, ticks and lice, thereby reducing incidence of itching and scratching, hold container 6 to 10 inches from the animal and spray lightly over the entire body. Do not spray in eyes. For best penetration of spray to the skin, direct spray against the natural lay of the hair to cause fluffing of the coat. In addition to controlling fleas and ticks, this product leaves your pet's coat soft, glossy and manageable.

Under normal circumstances, repeat spray once a week until infestation is brought under control. For more prolonged flea and tick control, the animals bedding, quarters, and surrounding area should also be sprayed lightly until damp to help prevent reinfestation.

Precautionary Statements: Hazards to Humans and Domestic Animals: Caution: Causes moderate eye irritation. Avoid contact with eyes or clothing. Wash hands and exposed skin thoroughly with soap and water after handling. Do not use on puppies under 6 weeks of age. Consult a veterinarian before using this product on debilitated, aged or medicated animals. If used on pregnant or nursing dogs, do not retreat until the puppies are at least 6 weeks old. Sensitivity may occur after using any pesticide product for pets. If signs of sensitivity occur, bathe your pet with mild soap and rinse with large amounts of water. If signs continue, consult a veterinarian immediately. Do not use this product on animals simultaneously or within 30 days before or after treatment with or exposure to cholinesterase inhibiting drugs, pesticides, or chemicals. However, flea and tick collars may be immediately replaced.

Physical or Chemical Hazards: Contents under pressure. Do not use or store near heat or open flame. Do not puncture or incinerate container. Exposure to temperatures above 130° F may cause bursting.

First Aid: If in Eyes: Rinse eyes with plenty of water. Call a physician if irritation persists.

Storage and Disposal: Do not contaminate water, food or feed by storage and disposal. Wrap empty container and put in trash collection.

Warning(s): Keep out of reach of children.

Presentation: 7 oz (198 g). * Rabon® is a registered trademark for Tetrachlorvinphos.

Compendium Code No.: 10360082

555827

HARTZ® 2 IN 1® LUSTER BATH FOR CATS

Hartz Mountain **Parasiticide-Topical**

EPA Reg. No.: 2596-23

Active Ingredient(s):

Pyrethrins (CAS # 121-29-9) 0.050%
Piperonyl Butoxide, Technical* (CAS# 51-03-6) 0.100%
N-Octyl Bicycloheptene Dicarboximide (CAS# 113-48-4) 0.168%
Other Ingredients: 99.682%

*Equivalent to 0.080% (butylcarbityl) (6-propylpiperonyl) ether and 0.020% related compounds.

Contains Lanolin.

Indications: 2 IN 1® Luster Bath for Cats brings together in one formula the scientific knowledge to clean, groom, freshen and protect against infestation of fleas, lice and ticks, including the Deer Tick, which may carry Lyme Disease. 2 IN 1® Luster Bath kills fleas, lice and ticks within 24 hours under normal conditions and protects against reinfestation if used as frequently as needed. 2 IN 1® Luster Bath grooms the coat, gives it a lustrous shine and kills cat odors leaving your cat bath-fresh.

Directions for Use: It is a violation of Federal law to use this product in a manner inconsistent with its labeling.

Read entire label before each use.

Do not use on kittens less than 12 weeks of age. Shake well. Add no water. Apply with sponge or cloth first to ears and head to prevent fleas from crawling inside ears and nose in an effort to escape. Keep away from eyes. Apply to rest of body, including feet. Rub in. To kill ticks, apply directly. Leave on a few minutes, then wipe off with coarse towel. Swab out ears. Repeat weekly (if necessary). Consult a veterinarian before using this product on debilitated, aged, pregnant or nursing or medicated animals. Sensitivities may occur after using any pesticide product for pets. If signs of sensitivity occur, bathe your pet with mild soap and rinse with large amounts of water. If signs continue, consult a veterinarian immediately.

Storage and Disposal: Do not reuse empty container. Wrap and put in trash

Warning(s): Keep out of reach of children.

Presentation: 12 fl oz (355 mL).

Compendium Code No.: 10360091

HARTZ® 2 IN 1® RID FLEA™ DOG SHAMPOO WITH ALLETHRIN

Hartz Mountain

EPA Reg. No.: 2596-71

Active Ingredient(s):

d-trans Allethrin (CAS# 584-79-2) 0.108%
N-Octyl Bicycloheptene Dicarboximide (CAS# 113-48-4) 0.135%
Other Ingredients: 99.757%

Indications: For use only on dogs. Kills fleas and ticks, including the Deer Tick, which may carry Lyme Disease.

Directions for Use: It is a violation of Federal law to use this product in a manner inconsistent with its labeling.

Read entire label before each use.

Wet dog's coat thoroughly with water. Rub shampoo into coat, starting with head. Work backward until coat is completely covered with foamy lather. Let lather stay on 5 minutes, then rinse and towel dry. Keep away from eyes. Repeat weekly (if necessary). It is recommended that the pet's bedding or sleeping quarters be treated for flea and tick control with a product registered for this use, such as Hartz® Home Flea and Tick Killer.

Precautionary Statements: Hazards to Humans & Domestic Animals: Caution: Avoid contact with eyes. In case of contact, immediately flush eyes with plenty of water. Get medical attention if irritation persists. It is not advisable to use this product or similar pesticides on puppies less than 12 weeks of age. Consult a veterinarian before using this product on debilitated, aged, pregnant or nursing or medicated animals. Sensitivities may occur after using any pesticide product for pets. If signs of sensitivity occur, bathe your pet with mild soap and rinse with large amounts of water. If signs continue, consult a veterinarian immediately.

Environmental Hazards: Do not contaminate lakes or streams by disposal of waste water.

Disposal: Do not reuse empty container. Wrap container and put in trash collection.

Warning(s): Keep out of reach of children.

Presentation: 12 fl oz (355 mL).

Compendium Code No.: 10360100 RM000000 550000, RM130000 550000

H

HARTZ® 2 IN 1® RID FLEA™ DOG SHAMPOO WITH PYRETHRIN

Hartz Mountain **Parasiticide Shampoo**

EPA Reg. No.: 2596-22

Active Ingredient(s):

Pyrethrins (CAS# 121-29-9) 0.040%
Piperonyl Butoxide, Technical* (CAS# 51-03-6) 0.080%
N-Octyl Bicycloheptene Dicarboximide (CAS# 113-48-4) 0.135%
Other Ingredients: 99.745%

*Equivalent to 0.064% (butylcarbityl) (6-propylpiperonyl) ether and 0.016% related compounds.

Indications: For use only on dogs. Kills fleas and ticks, including the Deer Tick, which may carry Lyme Disease.

Directions for Use: It is a violation of Federal law to use this product in a manner inconsistent with its labeling.

Read entire label before each use.

Do not use on puppies under 12 weeks of age. Wet dog's coat thoroughly with water. Rub shampoo into coat, starting with head. Work backward until coat is completely covered with foamy lather. Let lather stay on 5 minutes, then rinse and towel dry. Keep away from eyes. Repeat weekly (if necessary). Consult a veterinarian before using this product on debilitated, aged, pregnant or nursing or medicated animals. Sensitivities may occur after using any pesticide product for pets. If signs of sensitivity occur, bathe your pet with mild soap and rinse with large amounts of water. If signs continue, consult a veterinarian immediately.

Storage and Disposal: Do not reuse empty container. Wrap container and put in trash collection.

Warning(s): Keep out of reach of children.

Presentation: 18 fl oz (532 mL).

Compendium Code No.: 10360110 RM142139 555627, RM142352 555841

HARTZ® ADVANCED CARE™ BRAND FLEA & TICK DROPS PLUS+ FOR CATS AND KITTENS (10 LBS. & UNDER)

Hartz Mountain **Parasiticide-Topical**

EPA Reg. No.: 2596-148

Active Ingredient(s):

Phenothrin (CAS# 26002-80-2) 85.7%
(S)-Methoprene (CAS# 65733-16-6) 2.9%
Other Ingredients: 11.4%

Indications: HARTZ® ADVANCED CARE™ Brand Flea and Tick Drops Plus+ for Cats and Kittens is the monthly treatment that effectively controls flea and tick infestations. This gentle formula kills and prevents adult fleas, ticks and mosquitos, plus flea eggs and larvae thereby breaking the flea life cycle. It is also waterproof.

Kills 95% of fleas and repels 96% of ticks within 24 hours.

Directions for Use: It is a violation Federal Law to use this product in a manner inconsistent with its labeling.

Read entire label before each use.

1. Use only on cats or kittens over 12 weeks of age.
2. Remove one applicator tube from package and hold in an upright position (pointed away from your face).
3. Hold bottom of tube with one hand. With other hand, snap cap off.
4. Position tip of tube on the cat's back between the shoulder blades. Use the tip of the tube to part the cat's hair so that the product will be applied at skin level. Begin squeezing out the contents of the tube to form a stripe as you move from the shoulder blades along the cat's back to the base of the tail.
5. Repeat every month.
6. Hartz recommends that you visit your veterinarian twice a year.

Precautionary Statements: Hazards to Humans - Caution: May cause eye irritation. Avoid contact with eyes and clothing. Wash thoroughly with soap and water after handling.

Hazards to Domestic Animals: Do not use on kittens less than 12 weeks old. Consult a veterinarian before using this product on debilitated, aged, medicated, pregnant, or nursing animals. Sensitivity, such as slight transitory redness of the skin at the site of application may occur after using any pesticide product for pets. If signs of sensitivity occur, bathe your pet with mild soap and rinse with large amounts of water. If signs continue, consult a veterinarian immediately.

Environmental Hazards: This product is toxic to fish.

First Aid: If in eyes: Flush eyes with plenty of water. Call a physician if irritation persists.

Storage and Disposal: Do not contaminate water, food, or feed by storage and disposal. Store in a cool, dry place. Do not reuse empty tube. Wrap and discard in trash.

Warning(s): Keep out of reach of children.

Presentation: 3 Tubes, 1 cc (0.03 fl oz.) each, 3 cc (0.09 fl oz.) total (3 month supply).

Compendium Code No.: 10360121 RM142783 556309

HARTZ® ADVANCED CARE™ BRAND FLEA & TICK DROPS PLUS+ FOR CATS AND KITTENS (OVER 10 LBS.)

Hartz Mountain **Flea Control & Topical Parasiticide**

EPA Reg. No.: 2596-148

Active Ingredient(s):

Phenothrin (CAS#26002-80-2) 85.7%
(S)-Methoprene (CAS#65733-16-6) 2.9%
Other Ingredients: 11.4%

Indications: HARTZ® ADVANCED CARE™ Brand Flea and Tick Drops Plus+ for Cats is the monthly treatment that effectively controls flea and tick infestations. This gentle formula kills and prevents adult fleas, ticks and mosquitoes, plus flea eggs and larvae thereby breaking the flea life cycle. It is also waterproof.

Kills 95% of fleas and repels 96% of ticks within 24 hours.

Directions for Use: It is a violation of Federal Law to use this product in a manner, inconsistent with its labeling.

Read entire label before each use.

1. Use only on cats or kittens over 12 weeks of age.
2. Remove one applicator tube from package and hold in an upright position (pointed away from your face).
3. Hold bottom of tube with one hand. With other hand, snap cap off.
4. Position tip of tube on the cat's back between the shoulder blades. Use the tip of the tube to part the cat's hair so that the product will be applied at skin level. Begin squeezing out the contents of the tube to form a stripe as you move from the shoulder blades along the cat's back to the base of the tail.
5. Repeat every month.

Precautionary Statements: Hazards to Humans - Caution: May cause eye irritation. Avoid contact with eyes and clothing. Wash thoroughly with soap and water after handling.

Hazards to Domestic Animals: Do not use on kittens less than 12 weeks old. Consult a veterinarian before using this product on debilitated, aged, medicated, pregnant, or nursing animals. Sensitivity, such as slight transitory redness of the skin at the site of application may occur after using any pesticide product for pets. It signs of sensitivity occur, bathe your pet with mild soap and rinse with large amounts of water. If signs continue, consult a veterinarian immediately.

Environmental Hazards: This product is toxic to fish.

First Aid: If in eyes: Flush eyes with plenty of water. Call a physician if irritation persists.

Storage and Disposal: Do not contaminate water, food, or feed by storage and disposal. Store in a cool, dry place. Do not reuse empty tube. Wrap and discard in trash.

Warning(s): Keep out of reach of children.

Presentation: 3 tubes, 1.3 cc 0.04 fl oz each, 3.9 cc 0.13 fl oz total (3 month supply).

Compendium Code No.: 10360670 RM142785 556316

HARTZ® ADVANCED CARE™ BRAND FLEA & TICK DROPS PLUS+ FOR DOGS AND PUPPIES (4 TO 15 LBS.)

Hartz Mountain **Parasiticide-Topical**

EPA Reg. No.: 2596-150

Active Ingredient(s):

Phenothrin (CAS# 26002-80-2) 85.7%
(S)-Methoprene (CAS# 65733-16-6) 2.3%
Other Ingredients: 12.0%

Indications: HARTZ® ADVANCED CARE™ Brand Flea and Tick Drops Plus+ for Dogs and Puppies is the monthly treatment that effectively controls flea and tick infestations. This gentle formula kills and prevents adult fleas, ticks and mosquitoes, plus flea eggs and larvae thereby breaking the flea life cycle. It is also waterproof.

Kills 95% of fleas and repels 96% of ticks within 24 hours.

Directions for Use: It is a violation Federal law to use this product in a manner inconsistent with its labeling.

Read entire label before each use.

1. Use only on dogs or puppies over 12 weeks of age.
2. Remove one applicator tube from package and hold in an upright position (pointed away from your face).
3. Hold bottom of tube with one hand. With other hand, snap cap off.
4. Position tip of tube on the dog's back between the shoulder blades. Use the tip of the tube to part the dog's hair so that the product will be applied at skin level. Begin squeezing out the contents of the tube to form a stripe as you move from the shoulder blades along the dog's back to the base of the tail.
5. Repeat every month.

Precautionary Statements: Hazards to Humans - Caution: May cause eye irritation. Avoid contact with eyes or clothing. Wash thoroughly with soap and water after handling.

Hazards to Domestic Animals: Do not use on puppies less than 12 weeks old. Consult a veterinarian before using this product on debilitated, aged, medicated, pregnant, or nursing animals. Sensitivity, such as slight transitory redness of the skin at the site of application may occur after using any pesticide product for pets. If signs of sensitivity occur, bathe your pet with mild soap and rinse with large amounts of water. If signs continue, consult a veterinarian immediately.

Environmental Hazards: This product is toxic to fish.

First Aid: If in eyes: Flush eyes with plenty of water. Call a physician if irritation persists.

Storage and Disposal: Do not contaminate water, food, or feed by storage and disposal. Store in a cool, dry place. Do not reuse empty tube. Wrap and discard in trash.

Warning(s): Keep out of reach of children.

Presentation: 3 Tubes, 1.1 cc (0.04 fl oz.) each, 3.3 cc (0.11 fl oz.) total (3 month supply).

Compendium Code No.: 10360152 RM142789 556311/RM142788 556321

HARTZ® ADVANCED CARE™ BRAND FLEA & TICK DROPS PLUS+ FOR DOGS AND PUPPIES (16 TO 30 LBS.)

Hartz Mountain **Parasiticide-Topical**

EPA Reg. No.: 2596-150

Active Ingredient(s):

Phenothrin (CAS# 26002-80-2) 85.7%
(S)-Methoprene (CAS# 65733-16-6) 2.3%
Other Ingredients: 12.0%

Indications: HARTZ® ADVANCED CARE™ Brand Flea and Tick Drops Plus+ for Dogs and Puppies is the monthly treatment that effectively controls flea and tick infestations. This gentle formula kills and prevents adult fleas, ticks and mosquitoes, plus flea eggs and larvae thereby breaking the flea life cycle. It is also waterproof.

Kills 95% of fleas and repels 96% of ticks within 24 hours.

Directions for Use: It is a violation Federal law to use this product in a manner inconsistent with its labeling.

Read entire label before each use.

1. Use only on dogs or puppies over 12 weeks of age.
2. Remove one applicator tube from package and hold in an upright position (pointed away from your face).
3. Hold bottom of tube with one hand. With other hand, snap cap off.
4. Position tip of tube on the dog's back between the shoulder blades. Use the tip of the tube to part the dog's hair so that the product will be applied at skin level. Begin squeezing out the contents of the tube to form a stripe as you move from the shoulder blades along the dog's back to the base of the tail.
5. Repeat every month.

Precautionary Statements: Hazards to Humans - Caution: May cause eye irritation. Avoid contact with eyes or clothing. Wash thoroughly with soap and water after handling.

Hazards to Domestic Animals: Do not use on puppies less than 12 weeks old. Consult a veterinarian before using this product on debilitated, aged, medicated, pregnant, or nursing animals. Sensitivity, such as slight transitory redness of the skin at the site of application may occur after using any pesticide product for pets. If signs of sensitivity occur, bathe your pet with mild soap and rinse with large amounts of water. If signs continue, consult a veterinarian immediately.

Environmental Hazards: This product is toxic to fish.

First Aid: If in eyes: Flush eyes with plenty of water. Call a physician if irritation persists.

Storage and Disposal: Do not contaminate water, food, or feed by storage and disposal. Store in a cool, dry place. Do not reuse empty tube. Wrap and discard in trash.

Warning(s): Keep out of reach of children.

Presentation: 3 Tubes, 1.3 cc (0.04 fl oz.) each, 3.9 cc (0.13 fl oz.) total (3 month supply).

Compendium Code No.: 10360132 RM142792 556312, RM142791 555322

HARTZ® ADVANCED CARE™ BRAND FLEA & TICK DROPS PLUS+ FOR DOGS AND PUPPIES (31 TO 45 LBS.)

Hartz Mountain **Parasiticide-Topical**

EPA Reg. No.: 2596-150

Active Ingredient(s):

Phenothrin (CAS# 26002-80-2) 85.7%
(S)-Methoprene (CAS# 65733-16-6) 2.3%
Other Ingredients: 12.0%

Indications: HARTZ® ADVANCED CARE™ Brand Flea and Tick Drops Plus+ for Dogs and Puppies is the monthly treatment that effectively controls flea and tick infestations. This gentle formula kills and prevents adult fleas, ticks and mosquitoes, plus flea eggs and larvae thereby breaking the flea life cycle. It is also waterproof.

Kills 95% of fleas and repels 96% of ticks within 24 hours.

Directions for Use: It is a violation Federal law to use this product in a manner inconsistent with its labeling.

Read entire label before each use.

1. Use only on dogs or puppies over 12 weeks of age.
2. Remove one applicator tube from package and hold in an upright position (pointed away from your face).
3. Hold bottom of tube with one hand. With other hand, snap cap off.
4. Position tip of tube on the dog's back between the shoulder blades. Use the tip of the tube to part the dog's hair so that the product will be applied at skin level. Begin squeezing out the contents of the tube to form a stripe as you move from the shoulder blades along the dog's back to the base of the tail.
5. Repeat every month.

Precautionary Statements: Hazards to Humans - Caution: May cause eye irritation. Avoid contact with eyes or clothing. Wash thoroughly with soap and water after handling.

Hazards to Domestic Animals: Do not use on puppies less than 12 weeks old. Consult a veterinarian before using this product on debilitated, aged, medicated, pregnant, or nursing animals. Sensitivity, such as slight transitory redness of the skin at the site of application may occur after using any pesticide product for pets. If signs of sensitivity occur, bathe your pet with mild soap and rinse with large amounts of water. If signs continue, consult a veterinarian immediately.

Environmental Hazards: This product is toxic to fish.

First Aid: If in eyes: Flush eyes with plenty of water. Call a physician if irritation persists.

Storage and Disposal: Do not contaminate water, food, or feed by storage and disposal. Store in a cool, dry place. Do not reuse empty tube. Wrap and discard in trash.

Warning(s): Keep out of reach of children.

Presentation: 3 Tubes, 2.6 cc (0.09 fl oz.) each, 7.8 cc (0.26 fl oz.) total (3 month supply).

Compendium Code No.: 10360142 RM142794 556313/RM142793 556323

HARTZ® ADVANCED CARE™ BRAND FLEA & TICK DROPS PLUS+ FOR DOGS AND PUPPIES (46 TO 60 LBS.)

Hartz Mountain **Parasiticide-Topical**

EPA Reg. No.: 2596-150

Active Ingredient(s):

Phenothrin (CAS# 26002-80-2) 85.7%
(S)-Methoprene (CAS# 65733-16-6) 2.3%
Other Ingredients: 12.0%

Indications: HARTZ® ADVANCED CARE™ Brand Flea and Tick Drops Plus+ for Dogs and Puppies is the monthly treatment that effectively controls flea and tick infestations. This gentle formula kills and prevents adult fleas, ticks and mosquitoes, plus flea eggs and larvae thereby breaking the flea life cycle. It is also waterproof.

Kills 95% of fleas and repels 96% of ticks within 24 hours.

Directions for Use: It is a violation Federal law to use this product in a manner inconsistent with its labeling.

Read entire label before each use.

1. Use only on dogs or puppies over 12 weeks of age.
2. Remove one applicator tube from package and hold in an upright position (pointed away from your face).
3. Hold bottom of tube with one hand. With other hand, snap cap off.
4. Position tip of tube on the dog's back between the shoulder blades. Use the tip of the tube to part the dog's hair so that the product will be applied at skin level. Begin squeezing out the contents of the tube to form a stripe as you move from the shoulder blades along the dog's back to the base of the tail.
5. Repeat every month.

Precautionary Statements: Hazards to Humans - Caution: May cause eye irritation. Avoid contact with eyes or clothing. Wash thoroughly with soap and water after handling.

Hazards to Domestic Animals: Do not use on puppies less than 12 weeks old. Consult a veterinarian before using this product on debilitated, aged, medicated, pregnant, or nursing animals. Sensitivity, such as slight transitory redness of the skin at the site of application may occur after using any pesticide product for pets. If signs of sensitivity occur, bathe your pet with mild soap and rinse with large amounts of water. If signs continue, consult a veterinarian immediately.

Environmental Hazards: This product is toxic to fish.

First Aid: If in eyes: Flush eyes with plenty of water. Call a physician if irritation persists.

Storage and Disposal: Do not contaminate water, food, or feed by storage and disposal. Store in a cool, dry place. Do not reuse empty tube. Wrap and discard in trash.

Warning(s): Keep out of reach of children.

Presentation: 3 Tubes, 4.1 cc (0.14 fl oz.) each, 12.3 cc (0.42 fl oz.) total (3 month supply).

Compendium Code No.: 10360162 RM142956 556314/RM142955 556319

HARTZ® ADVANCED CARE™ BRAND FLEA & TICK DROPS PLUS+ FOR DOGS AND PUPPIES (61 TO 90 LBS.)

Hartz Mountain **Parasiticide-Topical**

EPA Reg. No.: 2596-150

Active Ingredient(s):

Phenothrin (CAS# 26002-80-2) 85.7%
(S)-Methoprene (CAS# 65733-16-6) 2.3%
Other Ingredients: 12.0%

Indications: HARTZ® ADVANCED CARE™ Brand Flea and Tick Drops Plus+ for Dogs and Puppies is the monthly treatment that effectively controls flea and tick infestations. This gentle formula kills and prevents adult fleas, ticks and mosquitoes, plus flea eggs and larvae thereby breaking the flea life cycle. It is also waterproof.

Kills 95% of fleas and repels 96% of ticks within 24 hours.

Directions for Use: It is a violation Federal law to use this product in a manner inconsistent with its labeling.

Read entire label before each use.

1. Use only on dogs or puppies over 12 weeks of age.
2. Remove one applicator tube from package and hold in an upright position (pointed away from your face).
3. Hold bottom of tube with one hand. With other hand, snap cap off.
4. Position tip of tube on the dog's back between the shoulder blades. Use the tip of the tube to part the dog's hair so that the product will be applied at skin level. Begin squeezing out the contents of the tube to form a stripe as you move from the shoulder blades along the dog's back to the base of the tail.
5. Repeat every month.

Precautionary Statements: Hazards to Humans - Caution: May cause eye irritation. Avoid contact with eyes or clothing. Wash thoroughly with soap and water after handling.

Hazards to Domestic Animals: Do not use on puppies less than 12 weeks old. Consult a veterinarian before using this product on debilitated, aged, medicated, pregnant, or nursing animals. Sensitivity, such as slight transitory redness of the skin at the site of application may occur after using any pesticide product for pets. If signs of sensitivity occur, bathe your pet with mild soap and rinse with large amounts of water. If signs continue, consult a veterinarian immediately.

Environmental Hazards: This product is toxic to fish.

First Aid: If in eyes: Flush eyes with plenty of water. Call a physician if irritation persists.

Storage and Disposal: Do not contaminate water, food, or feed by storage and disposal. Store in a cool, dry place. Do not reuse empty tube. Wrap and discard in trash.

Warning(s): Keep out of reach of children.

Presentation: 3 Tubes, 4.6 cc (0.16 fl oz.) each, 13.8 cc (0.47 fl oz.) total (3 month supply).

Compendium Code No.: 10360172 RM142796 556315/RM142795 556324

HARTZ® ADVANCED CARE™ BRAND FLEA & TICK DROPS PLUS+ FOR DOGS AND PUPPIES (OVER 90 LBS.)

Hartz Mountain **Parasiticide-Topical**

EPA Reg. No.: 2596-150

Active Ingredient(s):

Phenothrin (CAS# 26002-80-2) 85.7%
(S)-Methoprene (CAS# 65733-16-6) 2.3%
Other Ingredients: 12.0%

Indications: HARTZ® ADVANCED CARE™ Brand Flea and Tick Drops Plus+ for Dogs and Puppies is the monthly treatment that effectively controls flea and tick infestations. This gentle formula kills and prevents adult fleas, ticks and mosquitoes, plus flea eggs and larvae thereby breaking the flea life cycle. It is also waterproof.

Kills 95% of fleas and repels 96% of ticks within 24 hours.

Directions for Use: It is a violation Federal law to use this product in a manner inconsistent with its labeling.

Read entire label before each use.

1. Use only on dogs or puppies over 12 weeks of age.
2. Remove one applicator tube from package and hold in an upright position (pointed away from your face).
3. Hold bottom of tube with one hand. With other hand, snap cap off.

4. Position tip of tube on the dog's back between the shoulder blades. Use the tip of the tube to part the dog's hair so that the product will be applied at skin level. Begin squeezing out the contents of the tube to form a stripe as you move from the shoulder blades along the dog's back to the base of the tail.
5. Repeat every month.

Precautionary Statements: Hazards to Humans - Caution: May cause eye irritation. Avoid contact with eyes or clothing. Wash thoroughly with soap and water after handling.

Hazards to Domestic Animals: Do not use on puppies less than 12 weeks old. Consult a veterinarian before using this product on debilitated, aged, medicated, pregnant, or nursing animals. Sensitivity, such as slight transitory redness of the skin at the site of application may occur after using any pesticide product for pets. If signs of sensitivity occur, bathe your pet with mild soap and rinse with large amounts of water. If signs continue, consult a veterinarian immediately.

Environmental Hazards: This product is toxic to fish.

First Aid: If in eyes: Flush eyes with plenty of water. Call a physician if irritation persists.

Storage and Disposal: Do not contaminate water, food, or feed by storage and disposal. Store in a cool, dry place. Do not reuse empty tube. Wrap and discard in trash.

Warning(s): Keep out of reach of children.

Presentation: 3 Tubes, 5.9 cc (0.19 fl oz.) each, 17.7 cc (0.59 fl oz.) total (3 month supply).

Compendium Code No.: 10360680 RM142456 556288/RM142455 556287

HARTZ® ADVANCED CARE® BRAND™ FLEA CONTROL CAPSULES™ FOR DOGS

Hartz Mountain **Flea Control**

((S)-Methoprene)

NADA No.: 141-162

Active Ingredient(s): Each capsule contains either:

(S)-Methoprene . . . . 154 mg
(S)-Methoprene . . . . 308 mg
(S)-Methoprene . . . . 462 mg

H

Indications: HARTZ® ADVANCED CARE® BRAND™ FLEA CONTROL CAPSULES™ are indicated for use in dogs, 9 weeks of age and older and 11 pounds body weight or greater, for the prevention and control of flea populations. (S)-Methoprene prevents and controls flea populations by preventing the development of flea eggs and does not kill adult fleas. Concurrent use of insecticides may be necessary for adequate control of adult fleas.

HARTZ® ADVANCED CARE® BRAND™ FLEA CONTROL CAPSULES™ is a weekly medication that works by preventing flea eggs from hatching and developing into biting adults that can harm your dog.

Each capsule is formulated to provide a minimum of 10 mg per pound (22 mg/kg) body weight of (S)-Methoprene.

Pharmacology: The active ingredient of HARTZ® ADVANCED CARE® BRAND™ FLEA CONTROL CAPSULES™ is (S)-Methoprene with the following chemical composition: isopropyl (2E,4E,7S)-11-methoxy-3,7,11-trimethyl-2,4-doderadienoate). (S)-Methoprene is an Insect Growth Regulator (IGR) which does not kill the adult flea but controls flea populations by breaking the life cycle at the egg stage.

Dosage and Administration: Dosage: HARTZ® ADVANCED CARE® BRAND™ FLEA CONTROL CAPSULES™ are administered orally, once a week, at the recommended minimum dosage of 10 mg (S)-Methoprene per pound (22 mg/kg) of body weight. This product is dosed according to your dog's weight. Be sure to weigh your dog before treatment to ensure proper dosage:

Recommended Dosage Schedule:

Body Weight	Dosage and Capsule Color	(S)-Methoprene per Capsule
11 to 15 lbs	1 Green Capsule	154 mg
16 to 30 lbs	1 Red Capsule	308 mg
31 to 45 lbs	1 Lavender Capsule	462 mg
46 to 60 lbs	2 Blue Capsules	308 mg
61 to 90 lbs	2 Brown Capsules	462 mg
91 to 135 lbs	3 Brown Capsules	462 mg
136 to 180 lbs	4 Brown Capsules	462 mg

Administration: HARTZ® ADVANCED CARE® BRAND™ FLEA CONTROL CAPSULES™ can be offered to your dog a variety of ways. Place the entire unopened capsule securely inside a treat. You may also administer HARTZ® ADVANCED CARE® BRAND™ FLEA CONTROL CAPSULES™ without using a treat. Open your pet's mouth wide and place the capsule as far back into the center of the tongue as possible. Gently close your pet's mouth and encourage swallowing through praise and petting underneath the jaw line.

Another alternative is to place a small amount of moist food into your dog's bowl, gently pull apart the capsule to open it and pour the contents directly onto the food. Mix well and serve to your dog. If you use this method, make sure that your dog consumes all of the food that you have mixed with the medication. If you have multiple dogs or puppies, make sure that each pet is fed separately to ensure they each receive the proper dosage. You may notice a change in the color of your dog's feces due to the coloring in the capsules. This has no effect on the safety and efficacy of the product.

HARTZ® ADVANCED CARE® BRAND™ FLEA CONTROL CAPSULES™ must be administered weekly, preferably on the same day each week, to maximize benefits. If you miss a weekly dose, administer HARTZ® ADVANCED CARE® BRAND™ FLEA CONTROL CAPSULES™ immediately and resume your weekly schedule. To maximize results, it is important to treat all dogs and/or puppies in the household. Untreated animals may develop fleas, which reduce the overall flea control within a given household.

Precaution(s): Storage Conditions: Store at room temperature; avoid excessive heat (40°C; 104°F).

Caution(s): Do not give to dogs and puppies under 9 weeks of age and under 11 lbs. Be sure to weigh your dog or puppy to ensure proper dosage. Do not overdose.

Warning(s): Human Warnings: Not for human use. Keep this and all other medications out of reach of children.

Adverse Reactions: The following adverse reactions have been reported after giving HARTZ® ADVANCED CARE® BRAND™ FLEA CONTROL CAPSULES™: lethargy/depression, loss of balance, vomiting, nervousness, trembling, hyperactivity, and diarrhea.

Discussion: HARTZ® ADVANCED CARE® BRAND™ FLEA CONTROL CAPSULES™ have no effect on adult fleas but act to break the flea life cycle by preventing eggs from developing into adults. However, pre-existing fleas in the dog's environment may continue to develop and emerge as adults after treatment with HARTZ® ADVANCED CARE® BRAND™ FLEA CONTROL CAPSULES™. Based on results of clinical studies, this emergence generally occurs during the first 30-60 days. Therefore, noticeable control may not be observed until several weeks after dosing when a pre-existing infestation is present. In cooler climates, immature fleas may take longer to complete the life cycle and emerge as adults.

If a HARTZ® ADVANCED CARE® BRAND™ FLEA CONTROL CAPSULES™ treated dog comes in contact with a flea-infested environment, adult fleas may infest the treated animal. These adult fleas are unable to produce viable offspring. Depending on the severity of infestation, the concurrent use of insecticidal products that kill adult fleas is recommended.

Fleas on Your Dog: Fleas can live on your dog and develop in your home and in your yard. They feed on your dog's blood, mate with other fleas, and lay thousands of eggs that fall off your dog and survive in their surroundings. The eggs hatch and grow into biting adults within just a few weeks. The bite of the flea may cause intense itching that causes your dog to scratch incessantly. Flea allergy dermatitis can develop from flea bites and can cause darkening and crusting of the skin and lead to hair loss and skin abrasions. Additionally, fleas transmit tapeworms and severe cases of fleas can lead to life-threatening anemia.

The Flea Life Cycle: It is important to understand the life stages of the flea life cycle in order to control and prevent flea populations on your dog. One of the most difficult aspects to controlling fleas is the flea's capacity to reproduce. A single female flea may lay over a thousand eggs in a lifetime. Here is how (S)-Methoprene breaks the flea life cycle:

Adult Fleas: After biting a HARTZ® ADVANCED CARE® BRAND™ FLEA CONTROL CAPSULES™ treated dog, the female adult flea ingests a blood meal containing (S)-Methoprene which is deposited in her eggs.

Flea Eggs: (S)-Methoprene prevents those flea eggs from hatching.

Flea Larvae: By preventing flea eggs from hatching, larvae production is stopped.

Flea Pupae: By preventing flea eggs from hatching, pupae production is stopped. Over a period of time, you will find that flea populations in your home are controlled.

When a dog or puppy that is being treated with HARTZ® ADVANCED CARE® BRAND™ FLEA CONTROL CAPSULES™ enters a flea-infested area, the dog may become temporarily reinfested. You may need to treat your dog and home with other flea control products to kill existing adult flea populations.

How do you know if your dog has a flea problem?

Adult fleas are about the size of a dark brown sesame seed and flattened from side to side. Their hind legs are extremely powerful and they use this jumping ability to leap onto a passing dog.

The "Flea Dirt" Test: You can easily check your dog for fleas:

1. Put white paper towels on the floor, under your pet. Have your dog sit or lay down.
2. Vigorousy scruff up the hair on the neck, stomach area and the rump just above the tail.
3. Remove your dog and look for what appears to be "black pepper".
4. Dampen the paper towel containing the "black pepper". If it turns to a dark red color, your dog probably has fleas. This black pepper-like substance is "flea dirt" (which is actually dried blood), left by fleas biting your dog. Live fleas can often be spotted on the inside fold of the back legs where the body temperature is warmest.

Presentation: HARTZ® ADVANCED CARE® BRAND™ FLEA CONTROL CAPSULES™ are available in five packages (see Dosage section), formulated and color-coded according to weight of the dog. Each dose is available in color-coded packages of 8 or 16 capsules each.

HARTZ®, HARTZ® ADVANCED CARE® and other trademarks are the trademarks of The Hartz Mountain Corporation.

Compendium Code No.: 10360371 RM144132

HARTZ® ADVANCED CARE™ BRAND ONCE-A-MONTH™ FLEA & TICK DROPS FOR CATS AND KITTENS (10 LBS. & UNDER)

Hartz Mountain **External Parasiticide**

EPA Reg. No.: 2596-151

Active Ingredient(s): By Weight (Nom):

Phenothrin (CAS#26002-80-2) 85.7%
Other Ingredients 14.3%

Indications: Kills and repels fleas, ticks and mosquitoes on cats and kittens (10 lbs. and under), including the Deer Tick, which may carry Lyme Disease.

Kills 95% of fleas and repels 96% of ticks within 24 hours.

Directions for Use: It is a violation of Federal Law to use this product in a manner inconsistent with its labeling.

Read entire label before each use.

1. Use only on cats or kittens over 12 weeks of age.
2. Remove one applicator tube from package and hold in on upright position (pointed away from your face).
3. Pull off cap. Turn the cap around and place on top of tube.
4. Simply press cap down to break the seal of tube.
5. Remove cap carefully. Position the tip of the tube on the cat's back between the shoulder blades. Use the tip of the tube to part the cat's hair so that the product will be applied at skin level. Begin squeezing out the contents of the tube to form a stripe as you move from the shoulder blades along the cat's back to the base of the tail.
6. Repeat every month.

Precautionary Statements: Hazards To Humans: Caution: May cause eye irritation. Avoid contact with eyes or clothing. Wash thoroughly with soap and water after handling.

Hazards to Domestic Animals: Do not use on kittens less than 12 weeks old. Consult a veterinarian before using this product on debilitated, aged, medicated, pregnant or nursing animals. Sensitivity, such as slight transitory redness of the skin at the site of application, may occur after using any pesticide product for pets. If signs of sensitivity occur, bathe your pet with mild soap and rinse with large amounts of water. If signs continue, consult a veterinarian immediately.

Environmental Hazards: This product is toxic to fish.

First Aid: If in eyes:

1. Hold eyes open and rinse slowly and gently with water for 15-20 minutes.
2. Remove contact lenses, if present, after 5 minutes, then continue rinsing eye.
3. Call a Poison Control Center or doctor for treatment advice if irritation persists. Have the product container or label with you when calling for advice or going for treatment.

Storage and Disposal: Do not contaminate water, food or feed by storage and disposal. Store in a cool, dry place. Do not reuse empty tube. Wrap and discard in trash.

Warning(s): Keep out of reach of children.

Presentation: 3 tubes, 1 cc 0.03 fl oz each, 3 cc 0.09 fl oz total (3 month supply).

Compendium Code No.: 10360600 RM142416 556326

HARTZ® ADVANCED CARE™ BRAND ONCE-A-MONTH™ FLEA & TICK DROPS FOR CATS AND KITTENS (OVER 10 LBS.)

Hartz Mountain **External Parasiticide**

EPA Reg. No.: 2596-151

Active Ingredient(s): By Weight (Nom):

Phenothrin (CAS#26002-80-2) 85.7%
Other Ingredients 14.3%

Indications: Kills and repels fleas, ticks and mosquitoes on cats and kittens (over 10 lbs.), including the Deer Tick, which may carry Lyme Disease.

Kills 95% of fleas and repels 96% of ticks within 24 hours.

Directions for Use: It is a violation of Federal Law to use this product in a manner inconsistent with its labeling.

Read entire label before each use.

1. Use only on cats or kittens over 12 weeks of age.
2. Remove one applicator tube from package and hold in an upright position (pointed away from your face).
3. Pull off cap. Turn the cap around and place on top of tube.
4. Simply press cap down to break the seal of tube.
5. Remove cap carefully. Position the tip of the tube on the cat's back between the shoulder blades. Use the tip of the tube to part the cat's hair so that the product will be applied at skin level. Begin squeezing out the contents of the tube to form a stripe as you move from the shoulder blades along the cat's back to the base of the tail.
6. Repeat every month.

Precautionary Statements: Hazards to Humans: Caution: May cause eye irritation. Avoid contact with eyes or clothing. Wash thoroughly with soap and water after handling.

Hazards to Domestic Animals: Do not use on kittens less than 12 weeks old. Consult a veterinarian before using this product on debilitated, aged, medicated, pregnant or nursing animals. Sensitivity, such as slight transitory redness of the skin at the site of application, may occur after using any pesticide product for pets. If signs of sensitivity occur, bathe your pet with mild soap and rinse with large amounts of water. If signs continue, consult a veterinarian immediately.

Environmental Hazards: This product is toxic to fish.

First Aid: If in eyes:

1. Hold eyes open and rinse slowly and gently with water for 15-20 minutes.
2. Remove contact lenses, if present, after 5 minutes, then continue rinsing eye.
3. Call a Poison Control Center or doctor for treatment advice if irritation persists. Have the product container or label with you when calling for advice or going for treatment.

Storage and Disposal: Do not contaminate water, food or feed by storage and disposal. Store in a cool, dry place. Do not reuse empty tube. Wrap and discard in trash.

Warning(s): Keep out of reach of children.

Presentation: 3 tubes, 1.3 cc 0.04 fl oz each, 3.9 cc 0.13 fl oz total (3 month supply).

Compendium Code No.: 10360610 RM142406 556333

HARTZ® ADVANCED CARE™ BRAND ONCE-A-MONTH™ FLEA & TICK DROPS FOR DOGS AND PUPPIES (16 TO 30 LBS.)

Hartz Mountain **External Parasiticide**

EPA Reg. No.: 2596-151

Active Ingredient(s): By Weight (Nom):

Phenothrin (CAS#26002-80-2) 85.7%
Other Ingredients: 14.3%

Indications: Kills and repels fleas, ticks and mosquitoes on dogs and puppies (16 to 30 lbs.), including the Deer Tick, which may carry Lyme Disease.

Kills 95% of fleas and repels 96% of ticks within 24 hours.

Directions for Use: It is a violation of Federal Law to use this product in a manner inconsistent with its labeling.

Read entire label before each use.

1. Use only on dogs or puppies over 12 weeks of age.
2. Remove one applicator tube from package and fold in an upright position (pointed away from your face).
3. Pull off cap. Turn the cap around and place on top of tube.
4. Simply press cap down to break the seal of tube.
5. Remove cap carefully. Position the tip of the tube on the dog's back between the shoulder blades. Use the tip of the tube to part the dog's hair so that the product will be applied at skin level. Begin squeezing out the contents of the tube to form a stripe as you move from the shoulder blades along the dog's back to the base of the tail.
6. Repeat every month.

Precautionary Statements: Hazards to Humans: Caution: May cause eye irritation. Avoid contact with eyes or clothing. Wash thoroughly with soap and water after handling.

Hazards to Domestic Animals: Do not use on puppies less than 12 weeks old. Consult a veterinarian before using this product on debilitated, aged, medicated, pregnant or nursing animals. Sensitivity, such as slight transitory redness of the skin at the site of application, may occur alter using any pesticide product for pets. If signs of sensitivity occur, bathe your pet with mild soap and rinse with large amounts of water. It signs continue, consult a veterinarian immediately.

Environmental Hazards: This product is toxic to fish.

First Aid: If in eyes:

1. Hold eyes open and rinse slowly and gently with water for 15-20 minutes.
2. Remove contact lenses, if present, after 5 minutes, then continue rinsing eye.
3. Call a Prison Control Center a doctor for treatment advice if irritation persists. Have the product container or label with you when calling for advice or going for treatment.

Storage and Disposal: Do not contaminate water, food or feed by storage and disposal. Store in a cool, dry place. Do not reuse empty tube. Wrap and discard in trash.

Warning(s): Keep out of reach of children.

Presentation: 3 tubes, 1.3 cc 0.04 fl oz each, 3.9 cc 0.13 fl oz total (3 month supply).

Compendium Code No.: 10360630 RM142591 556328

HARTZ® ADVANCED CARE™ BRAND ONCE-A-MONTH™ FLEA & TICK DROPS FOR DOGS AND PUPPIES (15 LBS. & UNDER)

Hartz Mountain **External Parasiticide**

EPA Reg. No.: 2596-151

Active Ingredient(s): By Weight (Nom):

Phenothrin (CAS#26002-80-2) 85 7%
Other Ingredients: 14 3%

Indications: Kills and repels fleas, ticks and mosquitoes on dogs and puppies (15 lbs. and under), including the Deer Tick, which may carry Lyme Disease.

Kills 95% of fleas and repels 96% of ticks within 24 hours.

Directions for Use: It is a violation of Federal Law to use this product in a manner inconsistent with its labeling.

Read entire label before each use.

1. Use only on dogs or puppies over 12 weeks of age.
2. Remove one applicator tube from package and hold in an upright position (pointed away from your face).
3. Pull off cap. Turn the cap around and place on top of tube.
4. Simply press cap down to break the seal of tube.
5. Remove cap carefully. Position the tip of the tube on the dog's back between the shoulder blades. Use the tip of the tube to part the dog's hair so that the product will be applied at skin level. Begin squeezing out the contents of the tube to form a stripe as you move from the shoulder blades along the dog's back to the base of the tail.
6. Repeat every month.

Precautionary Statements: Hazards to Humans: Caution: May cause eye irritation. Avoid contact with eyes or clothing. Wash thoroughly with soap and water after handling.

Hazards to Domestic Animals: Do not use on puppies less than 12 weeks old. Consult a veterinarian before using this product on debilitated, aged, medicated, pregnant or nursing animals. Sensitivity, such as slight transitory redness of the skin at the site of application, may occur after using any pesticide product for pets. If signs of sensitivity occur, bathe your pet with mild soap and rinse with large amounts of water. If signs continue, consult a veterinarian immediately.

Environmental Hazards: This product is toxic to fish.

First Aid: If in eyes:

1. Hold eyes open and rinse slowly and gently with water for 15-20 minutes.
2. Remove contact lenses, if present, after 5 minutes, then continue rinsing eye.
3. Call a Poison Control Center or doctor for treatment advice if irritation persists. Have the product container or label with you when calling for advice or going for treatment.

Storage and Disposal: Do not contaminate water, food or feed by storage and disposal. Store in a cool, dry place. Do not reuse empty tube. Wrap and discard in trash.

Warning(s): Keep out of reach of children.

Presentation: 3 tubes, 1.1 cc 0.04 fl oz each, 3.3 cc 0.11 fl oz total (3 month supply).

Compendium Code No.: 10360620 RM142597 556331

HARTZ® ADVANCED CARE™ BRAND ONCE-A-MONTH™ FLEA & TICK DROPS FOR DOGS AND PUPPIES (31 TO 60 LBS.)

Hartz Mountain **External Parasiticide**

EPA Reg. No.: 2596-151

Active Ingredient(s): By Weight (Nom):

Phenothrin (CAS#26002-80-2) 85.7%
Other Ingredients 14.3%

Indications: Kills and repels fleas, ticks and mosquitoes on dogs and puppies (31 to 60 lbs.), including the Deer Tick, which may carry Lyme Disease.

Kills 95% of fleas and repels 96% of ticks within 24 hours.

Directions for Use: It is a violation of Federal Law to use this product in a manner inconsistent with its labeling.

Read entire label before each use.

1. Use only on dogs or puppies over 12 weeks of age.
2. Remove one applicator tube from package and hold in an upright position (pointed away from your face).
3. Pull off cap. Turn the cap around and place on top of tube.
4. Simply press cap down to break the seal of tube.
5. Remove cap carefully. Position the tip of the tube on the dog's back between the shoulder blades. Use the tip of the tube to part the dog's hair so that the product will be applied at skin level. Begin squeezing out the contents of the tube to form a stripe as you move from the shoulder blades along the dog's back to the base of the tail.
6. Repeat every month.

Precautionary Statements: Hazards to Humans: Caution: May cause eye irritation. Avoid contact with eyes or clothing. Wash thoroughly with soap and water after handling.

Hazards to Domestic Animals: Do not use on puppies less than 12 weeks old. Consult a veterinarian before using this product on debilitated, aged, medicated, pregnant or nursing animals. Sensitivity, such as slight transitory redness of the skin at the site of application, may occur after using any pesticide product for pets. If signs of sensitivity occur, bathe your pet with mild soap and rinse with large amounts of water. If signs continue, consult a veterinarian immediately.

Environmental Hazards: This product is toxic to fish.

First Aid: If in eyes:

1. Hold eyes open and rinse slowly and gently with water for 15-20 minutes.
2. Remove contact lenses, if present, after 5 minutes, then continue rinsing eye.
3. Call a Poison Control Center or doctor for treatment advice if irritation persists. Have the product container or label with you when calling for advice or going for treatment.

Storage and Disposal: Do not contaminate water, food or teed by storage and disposal. Store in a cool, dry place. Do not reuse empty tube. Wrap and discard in trash.

Warning(s): Keep out of reach of children.

Presentation: 3 tubes, 2.6 cc 0.09 fl oz each, 7.8 cc 0.26 fl oz total (3 month supply).

Compendium Code No.: 10360640 RM142594 556329

HARTZ® ADVANCED CARE™ BRAND ONCE-A-MONTH™ FLEA & TICK DROPS FOR DOGS AND PUPPIES (61 TO 90 LBS.)

Hartz Mountain — **External Parasiticide**

EPA Reg. No.: 2596-151

Active Ingredient(s): By Weight (Nom):

Phenothrin (CAS#26002-80-2) 85.7%
Other Ingredients: 14.3%

Indications: Kills and repels fleas, ticks and mosquitoes on dogs and puppies (61 to 90 lbs.), including the Deer Tick, which may carry Lyme Disease.

Kills 95% of fleas and repels 96% of ticks within 24 hours.

Directions for Use: It is a violation of Federal Law to use this product in a manner inconsistent with its labeling.

Read entire label before each use.

1. Use only on dogs or puppies over 12 weeks of age.
2. Remove one applicator tube from package and hold in an upright position (pointed away from your face).
3. Pull off cap. Turn the cap around and place on top of tube.
4. Simply press cup down to break the seal of tube.
5. Remove cap carefully. Position the tip of the tube on the dog's back between the shoulder blades. Use the tip of the tube to part the dog's hair so that the product will be applied at skin level. Begin squeezing out the contents of the tube to form a stripe as you move from the shoulder blades along the dog's back to the base of the tail.
6. Repeat every month.

Precautionary Statements: Hazards to Humans: Caution: May cause eye irritation. Avoid contact with eyes or clothing. Wash thoroughly with soap and water after handling.

Hazards to Domestic Animals: Do not use on puppies less than 12 weeks old. Consult a veterinarian before using this product on debilitated, aged, medicated, pregnant or nursing animals. Sensitivity, such as slight transitory redness of the skin at the site of application, may occur after using any pesticide product for pets. If signs of sensitivity occur, bathe your pet with mild soap and rinse with large amounts of water. If signs continue, consult a veterinarian immediately.

Environmental Hazards: This product is toxic to fish.

First Aid: If in eyes:

1. Hold eyes open and rinse slowly and gently with water for 15-20 minutes.
2. Remove contact lenses, if present, after 5 minutes, then continue rinsing eye.
3. Call a Poison Control Center or doctor for treatment advice if irritation persists. Have the product container or label with you when calling for advice or going for treatment.

Storage and Disposal: Do not contaminate water, food or feed by storage and disposal. Store in a cool, dry place. Do not reuse empty tube. Wrap and discard in trash.

Warning(s): Keep out of reach of children.

Presentation: 3 tubes, 4.6 cc 0.16 fl oz each, 13.8 cc 0.47 fl oz total (3 month supply).

Compendium Code No.: 10360650 RM142601 556332

HARTZ® ADVANCED CARE™ BRAND ONCE-A-MONTH™ FLEA & TICK DROPS FOR DOGS AND PUPPIES (OVER 90 LBS.)

Hartz Mountain — **External Parasiticide**

EPA Reg. No.: 2596-151

Active Ingredient(s): By Weight (Nom):

Phenothrin (CAS#26002-80-2) 85.7%
Other Ingredients: 14.3%

Indications: Kills and repels fleas, ticks and mosquitoes on dogs and puppies (over 90 lbs.), including the Deer Tick, which may carry Lyme Disease.

Kills 95% of fleas and repels 96% of ticks within 24 hours.

Directions for Use: It is a violation of Federal Law to use this product in a manner inconsistent with its labeling.

Read entire label before each use.

1. Use only on dogs or puppies over 12 weeks of age.
2. Remove one applicator tube from package and hold in an upright position (pointed away from your face).
3. Pull off cap. Turn the cap around and place on top of tube.
4. Simply press cap down to break the seal of tube.
5. Remove cap carefully. Position the tip of the tube on the dog's back between the shoulder blades. Use the tip of the tube to part the dog's hair so that the product will be applied at skin level. Begin squeezing out the contents of the tube to form a stripe as you move from the shoulder blades along the dog's back to the base of the tail.
6. Repeat every month.

Precautionary Statements: Hazards to Humans: Caution: May cause eye irritation. Avoid contact with eyes or clothing. Wash thoroughly with soap and water after handling.

Hazards to Domestic Animals: Do not use on puppies less than 12 weeks old. Consult a veterinarian before using this product on debilitated, aged, medicated, pregnant or nursing animals. Sensitivity, such as slight transitory redness of the skin at the site of application, may occur after using any pesticide product for pets. If signs of sensitivity occur, bathe your pet with mild soap and rinse with large amounts of water. If signs continue, consult a veterinarian immediately.

Environmental Hazards: This product is toxic to fish.

First Aid: If in eyes:

1. Hold eyes open and rinse slowly and gently with water for 15-20 minutes.
2. Remove contact lenses, if present, after 5 minutes, then continue rinsing eye.
3. Call a Poison Control Center or doctor for treatment advice if irritation persists. Have the product container or label with you when calling for advice or going for treatment.

Storage and Disposal: Do not contaminate water, food or feed by storage and disposal. Store in a cool, dry place. Do not reuse empty tube. Wrap and discard in trash.

Warning(s): Keep out of reach of children.

Presentation: 3 tubes, 5.9 cc 0.19 fl oz each, 17.7 cc 0.59 fl oz total (3 month supply).

Compendium Code No.: 10360660 RM142487 556327

HARTZ® ADVANCED CARE® BRAND TICK DABBER™ APPLICATOR

Hartz Mountain — **Parasiticide-Topical**

EPA Reg. No.: 2596-152

Active Ingredient(s):

Phenothrin: (CAS# 26002-80-2) 85.7%
Other Ingredients: 14.3%

Indications: A spot treatment designed to help you effectively kill ticks that have landed on your dog or cat.

This is not a preventative treatment.

Directions for Use: It is in violation of Federal law to use this product in a manner inconsistent with its labeling.

Read entire label before each use.

Place HARTZ® ADVANCED CARE® BRAND TICK DABBER™ Applicator on tick and hold for 30 seconds.

Remove HARTZ® ADVANCED CARE® BRAND TICK DABBER™ Applicator and allow tick to die. Some ticks have harder shells and may take longer to die.

Consult your veterinarian if redness and itching occur near bite area.

Precautionary Statements: Hazards to Humans:

Caution: May cause eye irritation. Avoid contact with eyes and clothing. Wash thoroughly with soap and water after handling.

Hazards to Domestic Animals: Do not use on puppies and kittens less than 12 weeks old. Consult a veterinarian before using this product on debilitated, aged, medicated, pregnant or nursing animals. Sensitivity, such as slight transitory redness of the skin at the site of application, may occur after using any pesticide product. If signs of sensitivity occur, bathe your pet with mild soap and rinse with large amounts of water.

If signs continue, consult a veterinarian immediately.

First Aid:

If in eye: Hold eye open and rinse slowly and gently with water for 15-20 minutes. Remove contact lenses, if present, after 5 minutes, then continue rinsing eye. Call a Poison Control Center or doctor for treatment advice if irritation persists. Have the product container or label with you when calling for advice or going for treatment.

Environmental Hazards: This product is toxic to fish.

Storage and Disposal: Do not contaminate water, food or feed by storage and disposal. Store in a cool, dry place.

If empty: Do not reuse empty HARTZ® ADVANCED CARE® BRAND TICK DABBER™ Applicator. Place in trash or offer for recycling if available.

If partly filled: Call your local solid waste agency or 1-800-CLEANUP for disposal instructions. Never place unused product down any indoor or outdoor drain.

Warning(s): Keep out of reach of children.

Do not use on humans.

Presentation: 1 x 0.068 fl oz tick dabber per kit.

HARTZ® and other trademarks are trademarks of The Hartz Mountain Corporation.

Compendium Code No.: 10360690 557107/557106

HARTZ® CONTROL PET CARE SYSTEM® FLEA & FLEA EGG KILLER FOR DOGS

Hartz Mountain — **Flea Control & Topical Parasiticide**

EPA Reg. No.: 2596-140

Active Ingredient(s): By Weight (Nom.)

Tetrachlorvinphos: (CAS# 22248-79-9) 1.08%
(S)-Methoprene: (CAS# 65733-16-6) 0.07%
Other Ingredients: 98.85%

Indications: HARTZ® CONTROL PET CARE SYSTEM® Flea & Flea Egg Killer for Dogs and Puppies contains Rabon®, an insecticide which kills and repels adult fleas and ticks. Kills flea eggs for one month. Waterproof-works even after bathing or swimming.

Directions for Use: It is a violation of Federal law to use this product In a manner inconsistent with its labeling.

Read entire label before each use.

Use only on dogs.

Shake Well Before Use: To kill and repel adult fleas, ticks and lice for 1 week and to kill flea eggs and prevent their hatching for 4 weeks, hold container upright 6 inches from the animal and spray lightly over the entire body, pressing dispenser with quick short strokes. Move bottle to get even coverage of coat until tips of hair are moist. Do not spray in eyes. Apply lightly and rub into coat. Ruffle hair for spray to reach skin. Once sprayed, fleas will be killed within 5 to 10 minutes. Ticks are tough - spray directly. After 10 minutes, dry animal with towel. Comb and brush coat. In addition to controlling fleas and ticks, this product leaves your pet's coat soft, glossy and manageable.

Under normal circumstances, to kill adult fleas and ticks, repeat spray once every few days until infestation is brought under control, then repeat as necessary. For more prolonged flea and tick control, the animal's bedding, quarters and surrounding area should also be sprayed lightly until damp to help prevent reinfestation.

Precautionary Statements: Hazards to Humans - Caution: Causes moderate eye irritation. Avoid contact with eyes or clothing. Wash thoroughly with soap and water after handling. To prevent harm to you and your pet, read entire label before use.

Hazards to Domestic Animals - Do not use on puppies less than 12 weeks of age. Consult a veterinarian before using this product on debilitated, aged or medicated animals. Sensitivity may occur after using any pesticide product for pets. If signs of sensitivity occur, bathe your pet with mild soap and rinse with large amounts of water. If signs continue, consult a veterinarian immediately.

First Aid:

If in Eyes: Rinse eyes with plenty of water. Call a physician if irritation persists.

Storage and Disposal: Do not contaminate water, food or feed by storage and disposal. Do not reuse empty container. Wrap empty container and put in trash collection.

Warning(s): Keep out of reach of children.

Presentation: 10 fl oz (295 mL).

Rabon® is a registered trademark for Tetrachlorvinphos.

Compendium Code No.: 10360181 555609

HARTZ® CONTROL PET CARE SYSTEM® FLEA & TICK CONDITIONING SHAMPOO FOR CATS

Hartz Mountain **Parasiticide Shampoo**

EPA Reg. No.: 2596-124

Active Ingredient(s):

d-trans Allethrin (CAS# 584-79-2) 0.109%
N-Octyl Bicycloheptene Dicarboximide (CAS# 113-48-4) 0.151%
Other Ingredients: 99.740%

Indications: For use only on cats. Kills fleas, lice and ticks, including the Deer Tick which may carry Lyme Disease.

Directions: It is a violation of Federal Law to use this product in a manner inconsistent with its labeling.

Read entire label before each use.

Do not use on kittens less than 12 weeks of age. To kill fleas, lice and ticks, including the Deer Tick, which may carry Lyme Disease, wet cat's coat thoroughly with water and rub shampoo into coat starting with head. Work backward until coat is completely covered with foamy lather. Let lather stay on 5 minutes, then rinse and towel dry. Repeat weekly (if necessary). It is recommended that the pet's bedding or sleeping quarters be treated for flea and tick control with a product registered for this use, such as Control Pet Care System® Home Flea & Tick Killer.

Precautionary Statements: Hazards to Humans and Domestic Animals: Caution: Do not let children or pets play with this product. Consult a veterinarian before using this product on debilitated, aged, pregnant or nursing or medicated animals. Sensitivity may occur after using any pesticide product for pets. If signs of sensitivity occur, bathe your pet with mild soap and rinse with large amounts of water. If signs continue, consult a veterinarian immediately.

Environmental Hazards: Do not contaminate lakes or streams by disposal of waste water.

Disposal: Do not reuse empty container. Wrap container and put in trash collection.

Warning(s): Keep out of reach of children.

Presentation: 12 fl oz (354 mL).

Compendium Code No.: 10360191 RM142443 555996

HARTZ® CONTROL PET CARE SYSTEM® FLEA & TICK CONDITIONING SHAMPOO FOR DOGS

Hartz Mountain **Parasiticide Shampoo**

EPA Reg. No.: 2596-124

Active Ingredient(s):

d-trans Allethrin (CAS# 584-79-2) 0.109%
N-Octyl Bicycloheptene Dicarboximide (CAS# 113-48-4) 0.151%
Other Ingredients: 99.740%

Indications: For use only on dogs. Kills fleas, lice and ticks, including the Deer Tick which may carry Lyme Disease.

Directions: It is a violation of Federal Law to use this product in a manner inconsistent with its labeling.

Read entire label before each use.

Do not use on puppies less than 12 weeks of age. To kill fleas, lice and ticks, including the Deer Tick, which may carry Lyme Disease, wet dog's coat thoroughly with water and rub shampoo into coat starting with head. Work backward until coat is completely covered with foamy lather. Let lather stay on 5 minutes, then rinse and towel dry. Repeat weekly (if necessary). It is recommended that the pet's bedding or sleeping quarters be treated for flea and tick control with a product registered for this use, such as Control Pet Care System® Home Flea & Tick Killer.

Precautionary Statements: Hazards to Humans and Domestic Animals: Caution: Do not let children or pets play with this product. Consult a veterinarian before using this product on debilitated, aged, pregnant or nursing or medicated animals. Sensitivity may occur after using any pesticide product for pets. If signs of sensitivity occur, bathe your pet with mild soap and rinse with large amounts of water. If signs continue, consult a veterinarian immediately.

Environmental Hazards: Do not contaminate lakes or streams by disposal of waste water.

Disposal: Do not reuse empty container. Wrap container and put in trash collection.

Warning(s): Keep out of reach of children.

Presentation: 16 fl oz (473 mL).

Compendium Code No.: 10360201 RM143483 555997

HARTZ® CONTROL PET CARE SYSTEM® FLEA & TICK DIP FOR DOGS

Hartz Mountain **Parasiticide Dip**

EPA Reg. No.: 2596-119

Active Ingredient(s): By Weight (Nom.):

Tetrachlorvinphos: (CAS# 22248-79-9) 2.8%
Other Ingredients: 97.2%

Indications: For use only on dogs to control fleas, ticks, and lice including the Deer Tick which may carry Lyme Disease.

Directions for Use: It is a violation of Federal law to use this product in a manner inconsistent with its labeling.

Read entire label before each use.

For dogs, to control fleas, ticks, and lice including the Deer Tick which may carry Lyme Disease, dilute 2 ounces of CONTROL PET CARE SYSTEM® Dip with each 1 gallon of water. Dip animal into solution, or sponge solution on, making sure hair is thoroughly wet to the skin. The area around the ears should be sponged thoroughly. Avoid contact of material with eyes and mouth of animal. Do not rinse. Towel dry. Repeat once a week if necessary.

Precautionary Statements: Hazards to Humans and Domestic Animals: Caution: Avoid contact with eyes. It is good practice to wash thoroughly with soap and water after handling any pesticide. Do not use on puppies under 6 weeks of age. Consult a veterinarian before using this product on debilitated, aged or medicated animals. If used on pregnant or nursing dogs, do not retreat until the puppies are at least 6 weeks old. Sensitivities may occur after using any pesticide product for pets. If signs of sensitivity occur, bathe your pet with mild soap and rinse with large amounts of water. If signs continue, consult a veterinarian immediately. Do not use this product on animals simultaneously or within 30 days before or after treatment with or exposure to cholinesterase inhibiting drugs, pesticides, or chemicals. However, flea & tick collars may be immediately replaced.

Environmental Hazards: Toxic to fish. Do not contaminate water when disposing of dip solution.

Storage and Disposal: Storage: Store in a cool place, away from heat or open flame.

Disposal: Do not reuse empty container. Wrap container and put in trash collection. Do not contaminate water, food or feed stuffs by storage or disposal of this concentrate or dip.

Warning(s): Keep out of reach of children.

Presentation: 8 fl oz (236 mL). Concentrated - Makes 4 Gallons.

Compendium Code No.: 10360210 RM139156 554707

HARTZ® CONTROL PET CARE SYSTEM® FLEA & TICK REPELLENT FOR CATS

Hartz Mountain **Parasiticide Spray**

EPA Reg. No.: 2596-126

Active Ingredient(s): By Weight (Nom.):

Tetrachlorvinphos: (CAS# 22248-79-9) 1.08%
Other Ingredients: 98.92%

Indications: CONTROL PET CARE SYSTEM® Flea & Tick Repellent for Cats kills and repels fleas and ticks, and kills the Deer Tick which may carry Lyme Disease.

Once sprayed, fleas will be killed within 5 to 10 minutes. In addition to controlling fleas and ticks, this product leaves your pet's coat soft, glossy, and manageable.

Directions for Use: It is a violation of Federal Law to use this product in a manner inconsistent with its labeling.

Read entire label before each use. Shake well before using.

1. Hold bottle upright 6 inches from pet. Direct spray toward pet and spray entire coat, pressing dispenser with quick short strokes. Move bottle to get even coverage of coat (until tips of hair are moist).
2. Apply lightly and rub into coat, ruffle hair for spray to reach skin.
3. Ticks are tough - spray directly.
4. After 10 minutes, dry cat with towel.
5. Comb and brush coat.
6. Repeat once a week.

Precautionary Statements: Hazards to Humans and Domestic Animals: Caution: Causes moderate eye irritation. Avoid contact with eyes or clothing. Wash hands and exposed skin thoroughly with soap and water after handling. Consult a veterinarian before using this product on debilitated, aged, medicated, pregnant or nursing animals. Sensitivities may occur after using any pesticide product for pets. If signs of sensitivity occur, bathe your pet with mild soap and rinse with large amounts of water. If signs continue, consult a veterinarian immediately. Do not use near birds, fish or foodstuffs. Do not use on kittens under 12 weeks old. Do not use this product on animals simultaneously or within 30 days before or after treatment with or exposure to cholinesterase inhibiting drugs, pesticides, or chemicals. However, flea and tick collars may be immediately replaced.

First Aid: If in Eyes: Flush with plenty of water. Call a physician if irritation persists.

Storage and Disposal: Do not re-use empty container. Wrap container and put in trash collection. Do not contaminate water, food or feed by storage and disposal.

Warning(s): Keep out of reach of children. Use only on cats.

Presentation: 8 fl oz (236 mL).

U.S. Patent No. 5,595,749

Compendium Code No.: 10360220 RM139008 554462, RM139009 554463

HARTZ® CONTROL PET CARE SYSTEM® FLEA & TICK REPELLENT FOR DOGS

Hartz Mountain **Parasiticide Spray**

EPA Reg. No.: 2596-125

Active Ingredient(s): By Weight (Nom.):

Tetrachlorvinphos: (CAS# 22248-79-9) 1.08%
Other Ingredients: 98.92%

Indications: CONTROL PET CARE SYSTEM® Flea & Tick Repellent for Dogs kills and repels fleas and ticks, and kills the Deer Tick which may carry Lyme Disease.

Once sprayed, fleas will be killed within 5 to 10 minutes. In addition to controlling fleas and ticks, this product leaves your pet's coat soft, glossy, and manageable.

Directions for Use: It is a violation of Federal Law to use this product in a manner inconsistent with its labeling.

Read entire label before each use. Shake well before using.

1. Hold bottle upright 6 inches from pet. Direct spray toward pet and spray entire coat, pressing dispenser with quick short strokes. Move bottle to get even coverage of coat (until tips of hair are moist).
2. Apply lightly and rub into animal's coat. For long haired dogs, ruffle hair for spray to reach skin.
3. Ticks are tough - spray directly.
4. After 10 minutes, dry dog with towel.
5. Comb and brush coat.
6. Repeat once a week.

Precautionary Statements: Hazards to Humans and Domestic Animals: Caution: Causes moderate eye irritation. Avoid contact with eyes or clothing. Wash hands and exposed skin thoroughly with soap and water after handling. Consult a veterinarian before using this product on debilitated, aged or medicated animals. If used on pregnant or nursing dogs, do not retreat until the puppies are at least 6 weeks old. Sensitivities may occur after using any pesticide product for pets. If signs of sensitivity occur, bathe your pet with mild soap and rinse with large amounts of water. If signs continue, consult a veterinarian immediately. Do not use near birds, fish or foodstuffs. Do not use on puppies under 6 weeks of age. Do not use this product on animals simultaneously or within 30 days before or after treatment with or exposure to cholinesterase inhibiting drugs, pesticides or chemicals. However, flea & tick collars may be immediately replaced.

First Aid: If in Eyes: Flush with plenty of water. Call a physician if irritation persists.

Storage and Disposal: Do not re-use empty container. Wrap container and put in trash collection. Do not contaminate water, food or feed by storage and disposal.

Warning(s): Keep out of reach of children. Use only on dogs.

Presentation: 14.5 fl oz (428 mL).

U.S. Patent No. 5,595,749

Compendium Code No.: 10360230 RM138979 554459, RM138981 554461

HARTZ® CONTROL PET CARE SYSTEM® MOUSSE FOR CATS AND KITTENS

Hartz Mountain **Flea Control & Topical Parasiticide**

EPA Reg. No.: 2724-467-2596

Active Ingredient(s):

(S)-Methoprene (CAS# 65733-16-6) 0.26%
Pyrethrin (CAS# 121-29-9) 0.21%
Piperonyl Butoxide (CAS# 113-48-4) . . . . 2.11 %
Other Ingredients: 97.42%

Contains vIGRen®.

H

Indications: CONTROL PET CARE SYSTEM® Mousse for Cat and Kittens contains natural pyrethrins which kill adult and immature fleas and ticks on your pet. CONTROL PET CARE SYSTEM® Mousse for Cats and Kittens takes flea control a step further by utilizing vIGRen®, an insect growth regulator. vIGRen® breaks the flea life cycle by killing flea eggs, a major source of reinfestation for 21 days. For complete flea and tick control, use CONTROL PET CARE SYSTEM® Mousse for Cats and Kittens in conjunction with the Control Pet Care System® Home Flea & Tick Killer.

Directions for Use: It is a violation of Federal law to use this product in a manner inconsistent with its labeling.

Read entire label before each use. Shake can well before using.

Apply mousse based on pet's bodyweight. Dispense 1 second of spray per 2 pounds of body weight (1 second of spray equals a portion the size of a golf ball. For example, a 3 pound cat needs 4 golf ball size portions for proper treatment) into the palm of your hand and work into the pet's fur starting with the head and working towards the tail. Rub the foam thoroughly into the pet's coat with fingertips. Brush when dry for a better coat appearance. Do not repeat treatment for 1 week (if necessary). Do not treat face, eyes or genitals. Do not use on kittens less than 12 weeks old. Consult a veterinarian before using this product on pregnant or nursing animals, aged, debilitated animals, or animals on medication.

Precautionary Statements: Hazards to Humans - Caution: Harmful if swallowed. Avoid contact with eyes, After using, wash hands with soap and water.

Hazards to Animals: Some cats may be sensitive to products containing pyrethrins. Excessive salivation and paw flicking may occur, however, these effects are temporary and not harmful. Sensitivities may occur after using any pesticide product for pets. If signs of sensitivity occur, bathe your pet with mild soap and rinse with large amounts of water. If signs continue, consult a veterinarian immediately.

Physical Hazards: Flammable. Contents under pressure. Keep away from heat, sparks and open flame. Do not puncture or incinerate container. Exposure to temperatures above 130° F may cause bursting.

First Aid in Humans: If swallowed, call physician or Poison Control Center. Drink 1 or 2 glasses of water and induce vomiting by touching the back of the throat with finger. Do not induce vomiting or give anything by mouth to an unconscious person. If in eyes, flush with plenty of water. Get medical attention if irritation persists.

H

Storage and Disposal: Do not store near heat or open flame. Store away from children and pets. Do not reuse empty container. Wrap can and put in trash.

Warning(s): Keep out of reach of children. Use only on cats.

Presentation: 5.29 oz (150 g).

vIGRen® is a registered trademark of Wellmark Intl.

Compendium Code No.: 10360240 554451

HARTZ® CONTROL PET CARE SYSTEM® ONESPOT® FOR CATS AND KITTENS

Hartz Mountain **Flea Control**

Flea Egg and Larvae Treatment

EPA Reg. No.: 2596-147

Active Ingredient(s):

(S)-Methoprene (CAS# 65733-16-6) 2.9%
Other Ingredients: 97.1%

Indications: ONESPOT® provides relief from flea populations on cats and kittens by controlling and preventing flea eggs and larvae. Adult fleas can live on your pet while also producing vast numbers of eggs which drop off your pet and develop in the surrounding environment. ONESPOT® kills flea eggs and larvae for 1 month, thereby breaking the flea life cycle.

Directions for Use: It is a violation of Federal Law to use this product in a manner inconsistent with its labeling.

Read entire label before each use.

1. Use only on cats or kittens over 12 weeks of age. Do not use on other animals.
2. Remove one applicator tube from package and hold in an upright position (pointed away from your face).
3. Hold bottom of tube with one hand. With other hand, snap cap off.
4. Position tip of tube on the cat's back between the shoulder blades. Use the tip of the tube to part the cat's hair so that the product will be applied at skin level. Begin squeezing out the contents of the tube to form a stripe as you move from the shoulder blades along the cat's back to the base of the tail.
5. Repeat every mouth.

After application, the treated area may appear wet or oily for up to 24 hours. Through its natural movement, your cat's skin and hair oils carry ONESPOT® over the cat's body for protection against flea eggs and larvae. To kill existing eggs and larvae and kill adult flea populations, you may need to treat your pet, home, pet's bed and yard with traditional flea products approved for use on pets around the home or in the yard. ONESPOT® can be used in conjunction with the entire Control Pet Care System® product line.

Precautionary Statements: Hazards to Humans: Causes eye irritation. Avoid contact with eyes or clothing. Wash thoroughly with soap and water after handling.

Hazards to Domestic Animals - Do not use on kittens less than 12 weeks old. Consult a veterinarian before using this product on debilitated, aged, medicated, pregnant, or nursing animals. Sensitivities may occur alter using any pesticide product for pets. If signs of sensitivity occur, bathe your pet with mild soap and rinse with large amounts of water. If signs continue, consult a veterinarian.

Environmental Hazards: This product is toxic to fish.

First Aid: If in eyes, flush eyes with plenty of water. Call a physician if irritation persists.

Storage and Disposal: Do not contaminate water, food or feed by storage and disposal. Store in a cool, dry place. Do not reuse empty tube. Wrap and discard in trash.

Warning(s): Keep out of reach of children.

Presentation: 3 tubes, 1 cc (0.03 fl. oz.) each, 3 cc (0.09 fl. oz.) total (3 month supply).

Compendium Code No.: 10360301 RM139857 555128

HARTZ® CONTROL PET CARE SYSTEM® ULTIMATE FLEA COLLAR® FOR CATS

Hartz Mountain **Flea Control & Topical Parasiticide**

EPA Reg. No.: 2596-139

Active Ingredient(s): By Weight (Nom.):

Tetrachlorvinphos (CAS# 22248-79-9) 14.55%
(S)-Methoprene (CAS# 65733-16-6) 1.02%
Other Ingredients: 84.43%

Indications: The HARTZ® CONTROL PET CARE SYSTEM® ULTIMATE FLEA COLLAR® contains an insecticide (Rabon®) to kill adult fleas and ticks.

This collar is intended for use only as an insecticide/IGR generator. Use only on cats.

Directions for Use: It is a violation of Federal law to use this product in a manner inconsistent with its labeling.

Read entire label before each use.

Remove collar from package, unroll and stretch to activate insecticide generator. As the collar begins to work, a fine white powder will appear on the surface.

Do not use on kittens under 12 weeks old. Do not unroll collar until ready to use. Place the HARTZ® CONTROL PET CARE SYSTEM® ULTIMATE FLEA COLLAR® around the cat's neck, adjust for proper fit, and buckle in place. The collar must be worn loosely to allow for growth of the animal and to permit the collar to move around the neck. A properly fitted collar is one that, when fastened, will snugly slide over the pet's head. Leave 2 or 3 inches on the collar for extra adjustment and cut off and dispose of the extra length. Consult a veterinarian before using this product on debilitated, aged, medicated, pregnant or nursing animals. Sensitivity may occur after using any pesticide product for pets. Some animals may become irritated by any collar if it is applied too tightly. If this occurs, loosen the collar. If irritation continues, remove the collar from the animal. If signs of sensitivity occur bathe your pet with mild soap and rinse with large amounts of water. If signs continue, consult a veterinarian immediately.

The collar will begin to kill fleas, ticks, flea eggs and larvae immediately. Its full protection against harder-to-kill ticks will be built up within a few days after being placed on the pet. For continuous protection under normal conditions replace the collar every 7 months. Under conditions where pets are exposed to severe flea and tick infestations, it may be necessary to replace the collar more frequently. Wetting will not impart the collar's effectiveness or the pet's protection. If the pet goes swimming or is out in the rain, it is not necessary to remove the collar. The HARTZ® CONTROL PET CARE SYSTEM® ULTIMATE FLEA COLLAR® may be worn with a regular collar. This collar is intended for use only as an insecticide/IGR generator.

Do not use this collar on animals simultaneously or within 30 days before or after treatment with or exposure to cholinesterase inhibiting drugs, pesticides or chemicals. However, flea and tick collars may be replaced immediately.

Storage: Store at room temperature.

Disposal: Do not reuse empty pouch. Dispose in trash collection.

Warning(s): Do not let children play with this collar.

Presentation: 1 Purple Collar, 0.6 oz (17 g) or 1 White & Purple Collar, 0.6 oz (17 g) with safety snap buckle. Fits up to 11" necks (27 cm).

Rabon® is a registered trademark for Tetrachlorvinphos.

Compendium Code No.: 10360341 RM139172 555623 / RM139173 555588

HARTZ® CONTROL PET CARE SYSTEM® ULTIMATE FLEA COLLAR® FOR DOGS AND PUPPIES

Hartz Mountain **Flea Control & Topical Parasiticide**

EPA Reg. No.: 2596-139

Active Ingredient(s): By Weight (Nom.):

Tetrachlorvinphos (CAS# 22248-79-9) 14.55%
(S)-Methoprene (CAS# 65733-16-6) 1.02%
Other Ingredients: 84.43%

Indications: The HARTZ® CONTROL PET CARE SYSTEM® ULTIMATE FLEA COLLAR® contains an insecticide (Rabon®) to kill adult fleas and ticks.

This collar is intended for use only as an insecticide/IGR generator. Use only on dogs.

Directions for Use: It is a violation of Federal law to use this product in a manner inconsistent with its labeling.

Read entire label before each use.

Remove collar from package, unroll and stretch to activate insecticide generator. As the collar begins to work, a fine white powder will appear on the surface.

Do not use on puppies under 6 weeks old. Do not unroll collar until ready to use. Place the HARTZ® CONTROL PET CARE SYSTEM® ULTIMATE FLEA COLLAR® around the dog's neck, adjust for proper fit, and buckle in place. The collar must be worn loosely to allow for growth of the animal and to permit the collar to move around the neck. A properly fitted collar is one that, when fastened, will snugly slide over the pet's head. Leave 2 or 3 inches on the collar for extra adjustment and cut off and dispose of the extra length. Consult a veterinarian before using this product on debilitated, aged, medicated, pregnant or nursing animals. Sensitivity may occur after using any pesticide product for pets. Some animals may become irritated by any collar if it is applied too tightly. If this occurs, loosen the collar. If irritation continues, remove the collar from the animal. If signs of sensitivity occur bathe your pet with mild soap and rinse with large amounts of water. If signs continue, consult a veterinarian immediately.

The collar will begin to kill fleas, ticks, flea eggs and larvae immediately. Its full protection against harder-to-kill ticks will be built up within a few days after being placed on the pet. For continuous protection under normal conditions replace the collar every 7 months. Under conditions where pets are exposed to severe flea and tick infestations, it may be necessary to replace the collar more frequently. Wetting will not impart the collar's effectiveness or the pet's protection. If the pet goes swimming or is out in the rain, it is not necessary to remove the collar. The HARTZ® CONTROL PET CARE SYSTEM® ULTIMATE FLEA COLLAR® may be worn with a regular collar. This collar is intended for use only as an insecticide/IGR generator.

Do not use this collar on animals simultaneously or within 30 days before or after treatment with or exposure to cholinesterase inhibiting drugs, pesticides or chemicals. However, flea and tick collars may be replaced immediately.

Storage: Store at room temperature.

Disposal: Do not reuse empty pouch. Dispose in trash collection.

Warning(s): Do not let children play with this collar.

Presentation:

For Dogs: 1 White & Blue Collar, 1.16 oz (33 g). Fits up to 23" necks (58 cm).

For Puppies: 1 White & Blue Collar, 0.77 oz (22 g). Fits up to 15" necks (38 cm).

Rabon® is a registered trademark for Tetrachlorvinphos.

Compendium Code No.: 10360351 RM139174 555587 / RM139171 555588

HARTZ® EASY WASH™ FLEA & TICK SHAMPOO FOR DOGS

Hartz Mountain **Parasiticide Shampoo**

EPA Reg. No.: 2596-22

Active Ingredient(s):

Pyrethrins (CAS# 121-29-9) 0.040%
Piperonyl Butoxide, technical* (CAS# 51-03-6) 0.080%
N-Octyl Bicycloheptene Dicarboximide (CAS# 113-48-4) 0.135%
Other Ingredients: 99.745%

*Equivalent to 0.064% (butylcarbityl) (6-propylpiperonyl) ether and 0.016% related compounds.

Indications: For use only on dogs. Kills fleas, lice and ticks, including the Deer Tick, which may carry Lyme Disease.

Directions for Use: It Is a violation of Federal Law to use this product in a manner inconsistent with its labeling.

Read entire label before each use.

1. Make sure that water control knob on hose sprayer is in the "off" position.
2. Hold the product by handle and shake gently, turning bottle as you shake it.
3. Attach hose to spray nozzle.
4. Bend safety tab down and turn control to "water" position.
5. Slowly turn on the water supply to any appropriate flow rate and pre-dampen file entire dog.
6. Turn the control knob to the "on" position (shampoo will automatically begin to mix with the water).
7. Apply shampoo starting with the head (be careful not to spray in the dog's eyes) and work backwards until the coat is completely covered in shampoo.
8. Turn the sprayer to the "off" position and rub the shampoo into the coat with your hands so that a foamy lather is produced.
9. Turn the spray nozzle to the "water" position and thoroughly rinse the dog.
10. Turn the spray nozzle to tile "off" position and disconnect from the hose for storage. Repeat weekly (if necessary).

Do not use on puppies less than 12 weeks of age. Consult a veterinarian before using this product on debilitated, aged, pregnant or nursing or medicated animals. Sensitivities may occur after using any pesticide product for pets. If signs of sensitivity occur, bathe your pet with mild soap and rinse with large amounts of water. If signs continue, consult a veterinarian immediately.

Disposal: Do not reuse empty container. Wrap container and put in trash collection.

Warning(s): Keep out of reach of children.

Presentation: 35 fl oz (1 qt. 3 fl oz) 1035 mL.

Compendium Code No.: 10360361

HARTZ® GROOMER'S BEST™ CONDITIONING SHAMPOO

Hartz Mountain — **Grooming Shampoo**

Indications: HARTZ® GROOMER'S BEST™ Conditioning Shampoo is specially formulated for long haired breeds of dogs. HARTZ® GROOMER'S BEST™ Conditioning Shampoo formula softens and rehydrates the dog's coat for a clean, healthy shine and leaves the coat with a refreshing scent.

HARTZ® GROOMER'S BEST™ Conditioning Shampoo is safe and gentle and can be used on all breeds of dogs.

Directions:

1. Before shampooing, thoroughly and gently brush out pet's coat to remove knots, tangles and mats.
2. Saturate dog's coat with lukewarm water to remove all dirt and debris. Pay special attention to the inside area of the hind legs and the stomach.
3. Dispense a small amount of shampoo into the palm of your hand. Rub hands together to evenly distribute shampoo.
4. Work shampoo into coat by starting behind the dog's head and working back towards the tail. Use a scrunching motion to thoroughly clean the coat. When shampooing the head, avoid getting shampoo into pet's eyes and ears.
5. Remove all shampoo from pet's head by rinsing thoroughly with lukewarm water several times. To avoid getting rinse water in your dog's eyes, place one hand gently over the pet's eyes when rinsing the area. Avoid getting water in pet's ears. Hold the ear flap down over the ear canal with thumb and rinse.
6. To remove all shampoo from coat and groin area, rinse several times with lukewarm water. Be sure to thoroughly rinse within the folds of the hind legs. Leaving a shampoo residue can irritate the coat and other sensitive areas.
7. Towel dry and gently comb or brush coat. Hartz® provides a full line of Grooming Tools for your pet.

Caution(s): Use only as directed. Biodegradable. Keep shampoo out of the reach of children and pets.

Presentation: 12 fl oz (355 mL).

Compendium Code No.: 10360420 RM139153 554477

HARTZ® GROOMER'S BEST™ MEDICATED SHAMPOO

Hartz Mountain — **Antidermatosis Shampoo**

Active Ingredient(s): Coal tar-U.S.P.

Indications: Specially formulated to remove scales, excess oil and grease, HARTZ® GROOMER'S BEST™ Medicated Shampoo also controls seborrhea and non-specific dermatitis on dogs.

Directions:

1. Before shampooing, thoroughly and gently brush out dog's coat to remove knots, tangles and mats.
2. Saturate pet's coat with lukewarm water to remove all dirt and debris. Pay special attention to the inside area of the hind legs and the stomach.
3. Dispense a small amount of shampoo into the palm of your hand. Rub hands together to evenly distribute shampoo.
4. Work shampoo into coat by starting behind the head and working back towards the tail. Use a scrunching motion to thoroughly clean the coat. When shampooing the dog's head, avoid getting shampoo into their eyes and ear canals.
5. Remove all shampoo by rinsing thoroughly with lukewarm water several times. To avoid getting rinse water in your pet's eyes, place one hand gently over the dog's eyes when rinsing the head. Avoid getting water in pet's ear canal. Hold the ear flap down over the ear canal with thumb and rinse.
6. To remove all shampoo from coat and groin area, rinse several times with lukewarm water. Be sure to thoroughly rinse within the folds of the hind legs. Leaving a shampoo residue can irritate the dog's coat and other sensitive areas.
7. Remove all shampoo from head and body by rinsing thoroughly with lukewarm water. Repeat shampooing and leave lather on for approximately five minutes. Repeat rinse method previously mentioned.
8. Towel dry and gently comb or brush coat. Hartz® provides a full line of Grooming Tools for your pet.

Caution(s): HARTZ® GROOMER'S BEST™ Medicated Shampoo is safe for all dogs when used as directed. Keep shampoo out of the reach of children and pets. For external use only; avoid contact with eyes. Not recommended for cats or kittens.

Presentation: 12 fl oz (355 mL).

Compendium Code No.: 10360430 85833 2 RM138907 554393, RM138908 554394

HARTZ® GROOMER'S BEST™ OATMEAL SHAMPOO

Hartz Mountain — **Grooming Shampoo**

Active Ingredient(s): Oatmeal.

Indications: HARTZ® GROOMER'S BEST™ Oatmeal Shampoo's pH-balanced formula cleans the coat and soothes irritated skin.

HARTZ® GROOMER'S BEST™ Oatmeal Shampoo is safe and gentle and can be used on all breeds of dogs.

Directions:

1. Before shampooing, thoroughly and gently brush out pet's coat to remove knots, tangles and mats.
2. Saturate dog's coat with lukewarm water to remove all dirt and debris. Pay special attention to the inside area of the hind legs and the stomach.
3. Dispense a small amount of shampoo into the palm of your hand. Rub hands together to evenly distribute shampoo.
4. Work shampoo into coat by starting behind the dog's head and working back towards the tail. Use a scrunching motion to thoroughly clean the coat. When shampooing the head, avoid getting shampoo into pet's eyes and ears.
5. Remove all shampoo from pet's head by rinsing thoroughly with lukewarm water several times. To avoid getting rinse water in your dog's eyes, place one hand gently over the pet's eyes when rinsing the area. Avoid getting water in pet's ears. Hold the ear flap down over the ear canal with thumb and rinse.
6. To remove all shampoo from coat and groin area, rinse several times with lukewarm water. Be sure to thoroughly rinse within the folds of the hind legs. Leaving a shampoo residue can irritate the coat and other sensitive areas.
7. Towel dry and gently comb or brush coat. Hartz® provides a full line of Grooming Tools for your pet.

Caution(s): Use only as directed. Biodegradable. Keep shampoo out of the reach of children and pets.

Presentation: 12 fl oz (355 mL).

Compendium Code No.: 10360440 91481 2 RM138916 554399, RM138917 554401

HARTZ® HEALTH MEASURES™ ANTI-ITCH HYDROCORTISONE SHAMPOO

Hartz Mountain — **Antidermatosis Shampoo**

Active Ingredient(s): Hydrocortisone USP (0.5%), aloe.

Indications: Use for temporary relief of itching or minor skin irritations, inflammation and rashes due to flea and tick bites, eczema, scrapes, abrasions and allergies. For use on dogs, cats and horses.

Directions: Wet coat thoroughly. Apply a liberal amount of shampoo into the entire coat and massage into a lather. For best results, leave on coat for 3-5 minutes. Rinse thoroughly, then reapply shampoo to specific areas where pet has itching or visible skin irritation. Lather and leave on for another 3-5 minutes. Rinse thoroughly and dry gently with a towel. For continued relief between shampooing, apply Health measures™ Anti-Itch Hydrocortisone Spray to affected areas.

Caution(s): For external use only. Avoid contact with eyes. Do not use where infection (pus) is present, since the drug may allow infection to spread. If symptoms persist or if irritation develops or worsens, discontinue use of product and consult a veterinarian. In case of accidental ingestion, seek professional assistance or contact a Poison Control Center immediately. Keep out of reach of children.

Presentation: 8 fl oz (236 mL).

Compendium Code No.: 10360450 94751 5, RM136178 553078

HARTZ® HEALTH MEASURES™ ANTI-ITCH HYDROCORTISONE SPRAY

Hartz Mountain — **Topical Corticosteroid**

Active Ingredient(s): Hydrocortisone USP (0.5%), Aloe.

Indications: Use for temporary relief of itching or minor skin irritations, inflammation and rashes due to flea and tick bites, eczema, scrapes, abrasions and allergies. For use on dogs, cats and horses.

Directions: Hold sprayer 4 to 6 inches from affected area and apply directly. Apply 2-3 times daily to irritated area until relief is achieved. For best results, cleanse affected area with Health measures™ Anti-Itch Hydrocortisone Shampoo prior to use.

Caution(s): For external use only. Avoid contact with eyes. Do not use where infection (pus) is present, since the drug may allow infection to spread. If symptoms persist or if irritation develops or worsens, discontinue use of product and consult a veterinarian. In case of accidental ingestion, seek professional assistance or contact a Poison Control Center immediately. Keep out of reach of children.

Presentation: 5 fl oz (147 mL).

Compendium Code No.: 10360460 94752 3, RM136179 553079

HARTZ® HEALTH MEASURES™ EAR MITE TREATMENT FOR CATS

Hartz Mountain — **Otic Parasiticide**

EPA Reg. No.: 68688-41-2596

Active Ingredient(s):

Pyrethrins (CAS# 121-29-9)	0.05%
*Piperonyl Butoxide, Technical (CAS# 51-03-6)	0.50%
Other Ingredients:	99.45%
	100.00%

*Equivalent to 0.40% of Butylcarbityl 6-propylpiperonyl ether and 0.10% of related compound.

Indications: HARTZ® HEALTH MEASURES™ Ear Mite Treatment with Aloe from Hartz® offers relief for cats suffering from ear mites. Cats that have ear mites will typically shake their heads and scratch their ears frequently. Ear mites live in the ear canal of the animal and cause a brownish, waxy debris to be formed. Ear mites may be detected by placing some of the waxy debris on a dark surface and carefully watching for the movement of tiny white specks away from the debris. Inflamed, watery or blocked ear canals indicate a more serious condition which requires the services of a veterinarian.

Directions for Use: It is a violation of Federal law to use this product in a manner inconsistent with its labeling.

Read entire label before each use.

To Kill Ear Mites:

1. Remove one applicator tube from package and hold in an upright position.

2. Pull off cap. Turn the cap around and place on top of tube. Simply press cap down to break the seal of tube and remove cap carefully.
3. Position the tip of the tube at the base of the pet's ear. Firmly holding pet, fill each ear canal with recommended number of drops.
4. Massage base of ear to insure insecticidal action penetrates ear wax.
5. Gently dry with a cotton ball, soft cloth or cotton swab.
6. After application simply invert the cap of the tube and snap back on the tube for easy closure.

Body Weight	Dosage
Under 15 lbs	4-5 drops a day per ear
Over 15 lbs	5-10 drops a day per ear

If conditions for which this preparation is used persist or if an irritation develops, discontinue use and consult a veterinarian.

This product may be applied daily for 7 to 10 days.

Repeat treatment in two weeks if necessary. Do not use on kittens less than 12 weeks.

Consult a veterinarian before using this product on debilitated, aged, pregnant or nursing animals or animals on medications.

Precautionary Statements: Hazards to Humans and Domestic Animals: Caution

Humans: Harmful if swallowed. Avoid breathing vapors. Avoid contact with eyes. In case of contact, immediately flush eyes with plenty of water. Obtain medical attention if irritation persists. If swallowed, do not induce vomiting. Wash hands with soap and water after using.

Animals: Avoid contact with eyes. If in eyes, flush with water. Do not use on any meat or milk producing animals. Sensitivities may occur after using any pesticide product for pets. If signs of sensitivity occur, bathe your pet with mild soap and rinse with large amounts of water. If signs continue, consult a veterinarian immediately.

First Aid:

If Swallowed: Call a physician or Poison Control Center. Do not induce vomiting because of aspiration hazard.

If on Skin: Wash immediately with soap and water.

If in Eyes: Flush with plenty of water. See a physician if irritation persists.

If Inhaled: Remove victim to fresh air.

Storage and Disposal: Storage: Store in a cool, dry area away from heat or open flame.

Disposal: Do not reuse empty container. Wrap and put in trash.

Warning(s): Keep out of reach of children.

Use only on cats.

Presentation: 3 Tubes, 3 cc (0.06 fl. oz.) each, 9 cc (0.18 fl. oz.) total. Each tube contains 100 drops.

Compendium Code No.: 10360471 RM139846 555071

HARTZ® HEALTH MEASURES™ EAR MITE TREATMENT FOR DOGS

Hartz Mountain **Otic Parasiticide**

EPA Reg. No.: 68688-41-2596

Active Ingredient(s):

Pyrethrins (CAS# 121-29-9)	0.05%
*Piperonyl Butoxide, Technical (CAS# 51-03-6)	0.50%
Other Ingredients:	99.45%
	100.00%

*Equivalent to 0.40% of Butylcarbityl 6-propylpiperonyl ether and 0.10% of related compound.

Indications: HARTZ® HEALTH MEASURES™ Ear Mite Treatment with Aloe from Hartz® offers relief for dogs suffering from ear mites. Dogs that have ear mites will typically shake their heads and scratch their ears frequently. Ear mites live in the ear canal of the animal and cause a brownish, waxy debris to be formed. Ear mites may be detected by placing some of the waxy debris on a dark surface and carefully watching for the movement of tiny white specks away from the debris. Inflamed, watery or blocked ear canals indicate a more serious condition which requires the services of a veterinarian.

Directions for Use: It is a violation of Federal law to use this product in a manner inconsistent with its labeling.

Read entire label before each use.

To Kill Ear Mites:

1. Remove one applicator tube from package and hold in an upright position.
2. Pull off cap. Turn the cap around and place on top of tube. Simply press cap down to break the seal of tube and remove cap carefully.
3. Position the tip of the tube at the base of the pet's ear. Firmly holding pet, fill each ear canal with recommended number of drops.
4. Massage base of ear to insure insecticidal action penetrates ear wax.
5. Gently dry with a cotton ball, soft cloth or cotton swab.
6. After application simply invert the cap of the tube and snap back on the tube for easy closure.

Body Weight	Dosage
Under 15 lbs	4-5 drops a day per ear
16-30 lbs	5-10 drops a day per ear
Over 30 lbs	10-15 drops a day per ear

Each tube contains 100 drops.

If conditions for which this preparation is used persist or if an irritation develops, discontinue use and consult a veterinarian.

This product may be applied daily for 7 to 10 days.

Repeat treatment in two weeks if necessary. Do not use on kittens less than 12 weeks.

Consult a veterinarian before using this product on debilitated, aged, pregnant or nursing animals or animals on medications.

Precautionary Statements: Hazards to Humans and Domestic Animals: Caution

Humans: Harmful if swallowed. Avoid breathing vapors. Avoid contact with eyes. In case of contact, immediately flush eyes with plenty of water. Obtain medical attention if irritation persists. If swallowed, do not induce vomiting. Wash hands with soap and water after using.

Animals: Avoid contact with eyes. If in eyes, flush with water. Do not use on any meat or milk producing animals. Sensitivities may occur after using any pesticide product for pets. If signs of sensitivity occur, bathe your pet with mild soap and rinse with large amounts of water. If signs continue, consult a veterinarian immediately.

First Aid:

If Swallowed: Call a physician or Poison Control Center. Do not induce vomiting because of aspiration hazard.

If on Skin: Wash immediately with soap and water.

If in Eyes: Flush with plenty of water. See a physician if irritation persists.

If Inhaled: Remove victim to fresh air.

Storage and Disposal: Storage: Store in a cool, dry area away from heat or open flame.

Disposal: Do not reuse empty container. Wrap and put in trash.

Warning(s): Keep out of reach of children.

Use only on dogs.

Presentation: 3 Tubes, 3 cc (0.06 fl. oz.) each, 9 cc (0.18 fl. oz.) total.

Compendium Code No.: 10360481 RM139748 555072

HARTZ® HEALTH MEASURES™ ENTERIC-COATED ASPIRIN FOR DOGS

Hartz Mountain **Non-Steroidal Anti-Inflammatory Analgesic**

Active Ingredient(s): Each tablet contains 81 mg aspirin.

Indications: HARTZ® HEALTH MEASURES™ Enteric-Coated Aspirin for Dogs can be used in the temporary relief of everyday aches and pains and inflammation associated with arthritis and joint problems in dogs. The special enteric-coating allows the aspirin to pass through the dog's stomach and to be dissolved in the intestine thus reducing stomach upset.

Dosage and Administration: Recommended Dosage: Give 1 tablet per each 15 lbs of body weight 2 times a day. Whole tablet should not be chewed, but be swallowed intact, either directly or wrapped in a treat. Do not give to dogs under 15 lbs of body weight.

Contraindication(s): Not for use in cats.

Precaution(s): Store in a cool dry place below 86°F (30°C). Keep container closed after each use.

Do not use this product if imprinted foil seal under bottle cap is cut, torn, broken or missing.

Caution(s): If vomiting or diarrhea occurs in your dog, stop administration and consult your veterinarian. Do not give this product to your dog if your pet is allergic to aspirin, has gastrointestinal problems or if your dog has ulcers or bleeding problems, unless directed by a veterinarian. If your dog is pregnant or nursing, seek advice of a veterinarian before using this product. If symptoms for use persist for more than 7 days, stop administration and consult your veterinarian. Do not give this product if your pet is taking prescription drugs for arthritis, anticoagulation (thinning the blood), diabetes or gout unless directed by a veterinarian. Do not use this product for dogs 7 days prior to surgery.

For use only with dogs.

Warning(s): Do not use for food animals intended for human consumption.

Keep this and all medicines out of reach of children and pets. In case of accidental overdose, contact a veterinarian/physician or Poison Control Center. Not for human consumption.

Presentation: Bottles of 120 tablets.

HARTZ® and other trademarks are trademarks of The Hartz Mountain Corporation.

Compendium Code No.: 10360492

HARTZ® HEALTH MEASURES™ EVERYDAY CHEWABLE VITAMINS FOR CATS AND KITTENS

Hartz Mountain **Small Animal Dietary Supplement**

Active Ingredient(s): Each tablet supplies:

Vitamin A	250.0 I.U.
Vitamin D	25.0 I.U.
Vitamin E	2.5 I.U.
Thiamine (B_1)	0.25 mg
Riboflavin (B_2)	0.2 mg
Vitamin B_6	0.2 mg
Vitamin B_{12}	1.0 mcg
Niacinamide	3.0 mg
Brewers Dried Yeast	650.0 mg
Protein	50.0 mg
Choline (from brewers dried yeast and lecithin)	2.5 mg
Inositol (from brewers dried yeast and lecithin)	2.0 mg
Folic Acid	40.0 mcg
Taurine	50.0 mg
Pantothenic Acid	0.25 mg

Ingredients: Brewers Dried Yeast, Dried Whey, Taurine, Desiccated Liver, Lecithin, Vitamin A Supplement, Vitamin D_3 Supplement, Vitamin E Supplement, Vitamin B_{12} Supplement, Riboflavin Supplement, Niacin Supplement, Calcium Pantothenate, Folic acid, Pyridoxine Hydrochloride, Thiamine Mononitrate.

Indications: A highly palatable liver flavored vitamin and mineral supplement specially formulated for all cats and kittens.

They help maintain your cat and kitten's healthy skin and shiny coat.

Dosage and Administration: HEALTH MEASURES™ Everyday Chewable Vitamins can be hand fed as a treat, just prior to feeding or crumbled and mixed with food. For pregnant, lactating or convalescing pets, increase dosage by 50% or as directed by your veterinarian.

Kittens: ½ to 1 tablet daily.

Cats: 1 to 2 tablets daily.

Precaution(s): Protect from heat and moisture.

Caution(s): Keep out of reach of children.

Presentation: Bottles of 100 tablets.

Compendium Code No.: 10360500 97701 6, 554031

HARTZ® HEALTH MEASURES™ EVERYDAY CHEWABLE VITAMINS FOR DOGS AND PUPPIES

Hartz Mountain **Small Animal Dietary Supplement**

Active Ingredient(s): Each tablet supplies:

Vitamin A	1000.0 I.U.
Vitamin D_3	100.0 I.U.
Vitamin E	2.0 I.U.
Thiamine (B_1)	810.0 mcg
Riboflavin (B_2)	1.0 mg
Pyridoxine (B_6)	82.0 mcg
Vitamin B_{12}	0.2 mcg
Niacin	10.0 mg
Choline (from Brewers Dried Yeast and Lecithin)	7.0 mg
Inositol (from Brewers Dried Yeast and Lecithin)	6.0 mg

Calcium . . . 100.0 mg
Phosphorus . . . 77.0 mg
Potassium (from Brewers Dried Yeast) . . . 10.0 mg
Iron . . . 1.0 mg
Iodine . . . 16.0 mcg
Copper . . . 55.0 mcg
Manganese . . . 60.0 mcg
Zinc . . . 1.5 mg
Cobalt . . . 14.0 mcg
Linoleic Acid . . . 30.0 mg
Glutathione . . . 4.0 mg

Ingredients: Brewers Dried Yeast, Dried Whey, Dicalcium Phosphate, Desiccated Liver, Lecithin, Zinc Proteinate, Iron Proteinate, Manganese Proteinate, Copper Proteinate, Potassium Iodide, Cobalt Sulfate, Vitamin A Acetate, Cholecalciferol (Vitamin D_3), d-Alpha Tocopheryl Acetate (Vitamin E), Niacin, Riboflavin, Thiamine Mononitrate, Pyridoxine Hydrochloride, Vitamin B_{12} Supplement.

Indications: A highly palatable liver flavored vitamin and mineral supplement specially formulated for all dogs and puppies.

They help maintain your dogs and puppy's healthy skin and shiny coat.

Dosage and Administration: HEALTH MEASURES™ Everyday Chewable Vitamins can be hand fed as a treat, just prior to feeding or crumbled and mixed with food.

Puppies and dogs under 10 lbs: ½ tablet daily.

Dogs over 10 lbs: 1 tablet daily.

For sick, convalescing, pregnant or nursing dogs: 2 tablets daily.

Precaution(s): Protect from heat and moisture.

Caution(s): Keep out of reach of children.

Presentation: Bottles of 100 tablets.

Compendium Code No.: 10360510 97699 3, 553779

HARTZ® HEALTH MEASURES™ HAIRBALL REMEDY

Hartz Mountain **Laxative**

Active Ingredient(s):

Malt Flavor: HEALTH MEASURES™ Hairball Remedy is an emulsion of malt extract, liquid petrolatum, glycerine, acacia and vitamin B_1 (thiamine HCl).

Salmon Flavor: HEALTH MEASURES™ Hairball Remedy is an emulsion of malt extract, liquid petrolatum, glycerine, natural salmon flavor, acacia and vitamin B_1 (thiamine HCl).

Indications: Aids in the elimination of swallowed hair and prevention of hairballs for cats, kittens and rabbits.

Directions for Use:

To eliminate hairballs: For adult cats and rabbits, feed a one-inch ribbon of HEALTH MEASURES™ Hairball Remedy daily until symptoms disappear. Give between meals, either from your finger or by placing on the pet's front paws where it can be licked off readily.

To prevent hairballs: Feed adult cats and rabbits a one-inch ribbon of HEALTH MEASURES™ Hairball Remedy once or twice a week and brush frequently. For young rabbits and kittens over four weeks of age, give a half-inch ribbon once or twice a week.

Precaution(s): Store at room temperature.

Caution(s): Keep out of reach of children.

Presentation: 3 oz (88 g).

Malt Flavor (95118 6, RM132767 551203); Salmon Flavor (95009 1, RM132766 551204)

Compendium Code No.: 10360520

HARTZ® HEALTH MEASURES™ HYDROCORTISONE SPOT

Hartz Mountain **Topical Corticosteroid**

Ingredient(s): Hydrocortisone USP (0.5%), Aloe.

Indications: HARTZ® HEALTH MEASURES™ Hydrocortisone Spot with aloe is the easy-to-apply formula that provides your pet with soothing, effective relief of itching or skin irritation with the proven healing powers of hydrocortisone and aloe.

Use for the temporary relief of itching or minor skin irritations, inflammation and rashes due to flea and tick bites, eczema, scrapes, abrasions and allergies.

For dogs and cats.

Directions for Use:

1. Remove one applicator tube from package and hold in an upright position.
2. Pull off cap. Turn the cap around and place on top of tube. Simply press cap down to break the seal of tube and remove cap carefully.
3. Position the tip of the tube at the irritated area and dispense contents of the tube.
4. Repeat daily until relief is achieved.

Caution(s): For external use only. Avoid contact with eyes. Do not use where infection (pus) is present, since the drug may allow infection to spread. If symptoms persist or if irritation develops or worsens, discontinue use of product and consult a veterinarian.

Warning(s): In case of accidental ingestion, seek professional assistance or contact a Poison Control Center immediately.

Keep out of reach of children.

Presentation: 3 tubes, 3 cc 0.10 fl oz each, 9 cc 0.30 fl oz total.

Compendium Code No.: 10360700 RM142465/556034

HARTZ® HEALTH MEASURES™ LIQUID WORMER

Hartz Mountain **Parasiticide-Oral**

Active Ingredient(s): Each teaspoon (5 mL) contains 250 mg piperazine base as piperazine citrate.

Indications: Use for removal of large roundworms, *Toxocara canis* in dogs and *Toxascaris leonina* in cats.

Directions: Dogs and puppies (6 weeks or older): 1 teaspoon per 10 lbs of body weight. Repeat dosage the following day. At 30 day intervals, repeat 2-day dosage to prevent further infestation.

Cats and kittens (6 weeks or older): ½ teaspoon per 5 lbs of body weight. Repeat dosage the following day. At 30 day intervals, repeat 2-day dosage to prevent further infestation.

Caution(s): Do not worm puppies or kittens that are sick, under 6 weeks of age, or those with known liver or kidney insufficiencies. Consult your veterinarian for assistance in the diagnosis, treatment and control of parasitism.

Keep this and all other medications out of reach of children.

Presentation: 5 fl oz (147 mL). Convenient dosage cup enclosed.

Compendium Code No.: 10360530 95122 8, RM133062 551307

HARTZ® HEALTH MEASURES™ ONCE-A-MONTH® WORMER FOR CATS AND KITTENS

Hartz Mountain **Parasiticide-Oral**

Piperazine Adipate

Active Ingredient(s): Each capsule contains 80 mg piperazine base.

Indications: Use for removal of the large roundworms *(Toxascaris leonina)* in cats and kittens.

Directions: For kittens 8 weeks and older use one capsule. Twist and pull to open capsule. Sprinkle directly into pet's food. Repeat dosage the following day. For older cats use one capsule for each 2 lbs of body weight. Repeat dosage the following day. At 30 day intervals, repeat 2-day dosage to prevent further infestation.

Caution(s): Do not worm a sick kitten or cat or those with known liver or kidney insufficiencies. Consult your veterinarian for assistance in the diagnosis, treatment and control of parasitism.

Keep this and all other medications out of reach of children.

Presentation: 24 capsules (0.3 oz 8 g).

Compendium Code No.: 10360540 84347 4, RM131005 551165

HARTZ® HEALTH MEASURES™ ONCE-A-MONTH® WORMER FOR DOGS

Hartz Mountain **Parasiticide-Oral**

Piperazine Adipate

Active Ingredient(s): Each capsule contains 80 mg piperazine base.

Indications: Use for removal of the large roundworms *(Toxascaris canis)* in dogs.

Directions: Use two capsules for each 5 lbs of body weight. Twist and pull to open capsule. Sprinkle directly into pet's food. Repeat dosage the following day. At 30-day intervals, repeat 2-day dosage to prevent further infestation.

Caution(s): Do not worm puppies or dogs that are sick, under 6 weeks of age, or those with known liver or kidney insufficiencies. Consult your veterinarian for assistance in the diagnosis, treatment and control of parasitism.

Keep this and all other medications out of reach of children.

Presentation: 24 capsules (0.3 oz 8 g).

Compendium Code No.: 10360550 84345 8, RM131007 551163

H

HARTZ® HEALTH MEASURES™ ONCE-A-MONTH® WORMER FOR LARGE DOGS

Hartz Mountain **Parasiticide-Oral**

Piperazine Adipate

Active Ingredient(s): Each capsule contains 303 mg piperazine base.

Indications: Use for removal of the large roundworms *(Toxascaris canis)* in large dogs.

Directions: Use one capsule for each 10 lbs of body weight. Twist and pull to open capsule. Sprinkle directly into pet's food. Repeat dosage the following day. At 30-day intervals, repeat 2-day dosage to prevent further infestation.

Caution(s): Do not worm puppies or dogs that are sick, under 6 weeks of age, or those with known liver or kidney insufficiencies. Consult your veterinarian for assistance in the diagnosis, treatment and control of parasitism.

Keep this and all other medications out of reach of children.

Presentation: 10 capsules (0.45 oz 12 g).

Compendium Code No.: 10360560 84348 2, RM131006 551166

HARTZ® HEALTH MEASURES™ ONCE-A-MONTH® WORMER FOR PUPPIES

Hartz Mountain **Parasiticide-Oral**

Piperazine Adipate

Active Ingredient(s): Each capsule contains 80 mg piperazine base.

Indications: Use for removal of the large roundworms *(Toxascaris canis)* in dogs.

Directions: Use one capsule for each 2 lbs of body weight. Twist and pull to open capsule. Sprinkle directly into pet's food. Repeat dosage the following day. At 30-day intervals, repeat 2-day dosage to prevent further infestation.

Caution(s): Do not worm puppies or dogs that are sick, under 6 weeks of age, or those with known liver or kidney insufficiencies. Consult your veterinarian for assistance in the diagnosis, treatment and control of parasitism.

Keep this and all other medications out of reach of children.

Presentation: 24 capsules (0.3 oz 8 g).

Compendium Code No.: 10360570 84346 6, RM131004 551164

HATCHGARD-3™

Intervet **Vaccine**

Newcastle-Bronchitis Vaccine, B_1 Type, B_1 Strain, Mass. and Conn. Types, Live Virus

U.S. Vet. Lic. No.: 286

Description: HATCHGARD-3™ is prepared from the proven B_1 strain of Newcastle disease virus and the mild Massachusetts and Connecticut types of infectious bronchitis virus. The viruses have been propagated using SPF substrates.

This vaccine contains gentamicin as a preservative.

Quality tested for purity, potency, and safety.

Indications: Coarse Spray: Vaccination of healthy chickens one day of age or older (spray) for protection against Newcastle disease and Massachusetts and Connecticut types bronchitis.

If chickens are vaccinated earlier than two weeks of age, revaccination is recommended for optimum protection.

Dosage and Administration: Vaccination Programs: Many factors must be considered in determining a sound vaccination program for a particular farm or poultry complex. To be fully effective, the vaccine must be administered properly to healthy, receptive birds maintained in a proper environment under good management. In addition, the response may be influenced by the age of the birds and their immune status. Seldom does one live virus vaccination under field conditions produce lifetime protection for all individuals in a given flock. The level of immunity required will vary with operational practices and the degree of exposure. Therefore, a program of periodic revaccinations may be necessary.

Preparation of Vaccine:

Coarse Spray Use: Do not open and mix the vaccine until ready to begin vaccination. Use vaccine immediately after mixing.

Caution: Read the "Safety Precautions" advice on handling vaccine ampule.

1. Before withdrawing the vaccine from the liquid nitrogen canister, protect hands with gloves, wear long sleeves and use a face mask or goggles. It is possible an accident could occur with either the liquid nitrogen or the ampules from the cane, hold palm of gloved hand away from body and face.
2. When withdrawing a can of ampules from the canister in the liquid nitrogen refrigerator, expose only the ampule to be used immediately. We recommend handling only one ampule at a time. After removing the ampule from the cane, the remaining ampules should be replaced immediately in the canister of the liquid nitrogen refrigerator.
3. The contents of the ampule are thawed rapidly by immersing in water at room temperature. Shake ampule to dispense contents. Then break ampule at its neck and immediately proceed as below. Caution: Ampules have been known to explode on sudden temperature changes. Do not thaw in hot or ice cold water.
4. Draw contents of ampule into a sterile 5 or 10 mL syringe, mounted with an 18-guage needle.
5. The contents of the filled syringe are then added to diluent (room temperature distilled water). It is important that this be done slowly. Slowly empty the syringe, allowing the vaccine to run down the side of the bottle. Gently shake the bottle as the vaccine is being mixed. Withdraw a portion of the diluent with the syringe to flush ampule. Inject the washing back into the diluent bottle. Remove the syringe.
6. The vaccine is now ready for use.

Coarse Spray Administration - For Chickens One Day of Age:

1. Use prepared vaccine as indicated for specific coarse spray vaccination machine. For example, a machine which dispenses 10 mL to a box of chickens - total volume for 10,000 doses is 1,000 mL. Mix thoroughly.
2. Add the vaccine solution to reservoir on machine.
3. Prime and adjust machine as instructed in manual accompanying specific machine.
4. Place boxes holding 100 chickens each on the conveyor belt or in machine. Activate spray head.

Records: Keep a record of vaccine, quantity, serial number, expiration date and place of purchase; the date and time of vaccination; the number, age, breed and location of chickens; names of operators performing the vaccination and any observed reactions.

Precaution(s): Safety Precautions: Liquid nitrogen container and vaccine should be handled only by properly trained personnel who are thoroughly conversant with the Union Carbide publication and instruction booklet regarding the use of precautions and safe practice for liquified atmospheric gases (particularly liquid nitrogen).

When removing the ampule cane, handling frozen ampules, or adding liquid nitrogen, wear long sleeves, a plastic face shield and gloves to protect the skin from contact with the liquid nitrogen. All storage and handling of the liquid nitrogen container must be in a dry, ventilated area. Do not inhale liquid nitrogen vapors. If drowsiness occurs, get fresh air quickly; then ventilate the entire area. If breathing difficulty occurs, apply artificial respiration. If any of these difficulties persist or there is a loss of consciousness, summon a physician immediately. Care should be exercised to prevent contaminating your hands, eyes and clothing with the vaccine.

Do not spill or splash the vaccine.

Use entire contents when first opened.

Burn containers and all unused contents.

Once prepared, the vaccine should be used with 2 hours and unused vaccine should be discarded into disinfectant or burned.

Once thawed, the product should not be refrozen.

Store in liquid nitrogen.

This product is non-returnable.

Caution(s): Vaccinate only healthy chickens. Although disease may not be evident, coccidiosis, Mycoplasma infection, infectious bursal disease, Marek's disease, reovirus infection and other disease conditions may cause complications or reduce immunity.

Efforts should be taken to reduce stress conditions at the time of vaccination and during the reaction period.

Do not dilute the vaccine or otherwise stretch the dosage.

For veterinary use only.

Notice: This vaccine has undergone rigid potency, safety and purity tests, and meets Intervet Inc. and USDA requirements and is designed to stimulate effective immunity when used as directed. The user must be advised that the response to the vaccine depends on many factors, including, but not limited to, conditions of storage and handling by the user, administration of the vaccine, health and responsiveness of the individual chickens, and the degree of field exposure. Therefore, directions should be followed carefully!

This product is not hazardous when used according to directions supplied. A material safety data sheet (MSDS) is available upon request. This and any other consumer information can be obtained by calling Intervet Customer Service at 1-800-441-8272 or 1-302-934-8051.

The use of this vaccine is subject to applicable federal and local laws and regulations.

Use only as directed.

Warning(s): Do not vaccinate within 21 days before slaughter.

Newcastle virus occasionally causes conjunctivitis in humans. Avoid any contact of vaccine with eyes.

Presentation: 1 x 10,000 doses for coarse spray use.

Compendium Code No.: 11060661 22601 AL 149

H.B. 15™

Farnam **Equine Dietary Supplement**

Biotin Supplement

Guaranteed Analysis: Each pound contains not less than:

	Per Pound
Crude Protein, min.	11%
Lysine, min.	0.44%
Methionine	0.265%
Crude Fat, min.	2.5%
Crude Fiber, max.	12%
Calcium, min.	3.5%
Calcium, max.	4%
Vitamin B_6	320 mg
Biotin	320 mg

Ingredients: Wheat Middlings, Oat By-Product, Calcium Carbonate, Dehydrated Alfalfa Meal, Sodium Chloride, Biotin, DL-Methionine, L-Lysine, Pyridoxine Hydrochloride (Source of Vitamin B_6, Molasses, and Propionic and Acetic Acids (Preservatives).

Directions: Measuring Cup = One Ounce

Feed H.B. 15™ at the following daily rates:

Adult Horses: 1 ounce per day

Foals, Weanlings, Ponies: ½ ounce per day

Pregnant and Nursing Mares: 2 ounces per day

Sprinkle the proper amount over feed or mix with the grain ration.

Precaution(s): Close container after each use. Store in cool, dry place.

Caution(s): For oral use in horses.

Warning(s): Keep out of reach of children.

Discussion: Proteins are one of the most important at all nutrients, vital to life and health. H.B. 15™ has been specially formulated to contain biotin and the amino acids lysine and methionine. Amino acids are the "building blocks" of the body and enable a horse to make the best possible use of the vegetable proteins present in hay and grains. Lysine and methionine are recognized as especially vital for horses for this reason. H.B. 15™ also contains Vitamin B_6, which aids in the metabolism of these amino acids.

Presentation: 3 lbs (1.36 kg) and 7 lbs.

Compendium Code No.: 10000261

H-BALM UDDER CREAM

Centaur **Udder Cream**

Ingredient(s): Stearic acid, homo menthyl, salicylate, isopropyl myristate, cetyl alcohol, aloe vera, propylene glycol, silicone, lanolin, mineral oil, triethanolamine, propyl paraben, methyl paraben, vitamin A, vitamin E, vitamin D, chloroxylenol, in a specially prepared base.

Indications: H-BALM with multi vitamins for use as an aid in reducing dry, cracked and chapped udders in cattle. Contains humectants which assist in maintaining skin and tissue moisture balance.

The non-sticky, disappearing cream base discourages dirt and manure from sticking to udders.

Directions: Apply daily or as needed after milking to aid in reducing dryness, cracking and chapping associated with chapped udders in cattle.

Caution(s): H-BALM is not a substitute for balanced nutrition. Animals with signs of nutritional deficiency in the skin may require injections of therapeutic levels of vitamins. Consult your veterinarian for assistance in the diagnosis and treatment of nutritional deficiency.

If animal shows signs of uncontrolled generalized infections, consult your veterinarian. Wash the teats and udders thoroughly before milking.

For veterinary use only.

Warning(s): Keep out of reach of children.

Discussion: Milking machines, inclement weather and other factors strip natural moisture from the udders, leaving them dry and chapped. H-BALM is a unique blend of vitamins which are naturally present in healthy skin. Helps promote natural moisture balance of chapped udders in cattle.

Presentation: 16 oz (454 g) and 5 lb (2.27 kg) containers.

Compendium Code No.: 14880180

HEALTHY FOOT™

SSI Corp. **Hoof Product**

Super Concentrated Formula

Indications: For use in footbaths and footmats.

Aids in the treatment and prevention of footwarts.

Directions: Footbath Directions:

Treatment Rate: 1 to 150 cows, begin with one gallon of HEALTHY FOOT™ per 50 gallons of water daily for 1 week. After the initial treatment period, the control rate may be used.

Control Rate: 1 to 150 cows, use one half gallon of HEALTHY FOOT™ per 50 gallons of water.

Footmat Directions:

Treatment Rate: 1 to 80 cows, use 1 quart of HEALTHY FOOT™ per 8 gallons of water.

Control Rate: 1 to 80 cows, use 1 pint of HEALTHY FOOT™ per 8 gallons of water.

If hygienic or environmental conditions are extreme or an increase in foot problems occurs, return to treatment rate. If footbath/footmat is not changed according to label directions, results are reduced significantly.

Precaution(s): Keep from freezing.

Caution(s): Eye irritant. In case of contact, flush for 15 minutes. If irritation persists, call a physician.

Warning(s): Keep out of the reach of children.

Presentation: 2.5 gallon, 5 gallon and 30 gallon containers.

Compendium Code No.: 14930100

HEARTGARD® CHEWABLES FOR CATS ℞

Merial **Parasiticide-Oral**

(ivermectin)

NADA No.: 141-078

Active Ingredient(s): Each chewable tablet contains either:

Ivermectin .... 55 mcg (red)

Ivermectin .... 165 mcg (purple)

Indications: For use in cats to prevent feline heartworm disease by eliminating the tissue stage of heartworm larvae *(Dirofilaria immitis)* for a month (30 days) after infection, and for the removal and control of adult and immature hookworms *(Ancylostoma tubaeforme* and *A. braziliense)*.

Dosage and Administration: Dosage: HEARTGARD® for Cats should be administered orally at monthly intervals at the recommended minimum dose level of 24 mcg of ivermectin per kg (10.9 mcg/lb) of body weight. The recommended dosage schedule for prevention of feline heartworm disease and control of hookworms is as follows:

Cat Weight	HEARTGARD® for Cats Chewables per month	Ivermectin content
Up to 5 lb	1	55 mcg
5 to 15 lb	1	165 mcg

For cats over 15 lb, use the appropriate combination of chewables.

HEARTGARD® for Cats is recommended for use in cats 6 weeks of age and older.

Administration: Remove only one chewable at a time from the foil-backed blister card. Return the card with the remaining chewables to its box to protect the product from light. HEARTGARD® for Cats can be offered to the cat by hand or may be added to a small amount of cat food. If manual dosing is required, the chewable should be broken into pieces for administration. Food should be routinely available during the day of treatment administration. If cats are fasted, or if the chewable is not broken into pieces for manual dosing, then reduced absorption may result. A relationship between reduced absorption and reduced efficacy has not been established.

Care should be taken to see that the cat consumes the complete dose. Treated animals should be observed for a few minutes after administration to ensure that part of the dose is not lost or rejected. If it is suspected that any of the dose has been lost, redosing with a new chewable is recommended. Fragments of chewables have occasionally been observed in the feces of some cats; efficacy of the product was not adversely affected.

HEARTGARD® for Cats should be given at monthly intervals when mosquitoes potentially carrying infective heartworm larvae are active. The initial dose must be given within a month (30 days) after the cat's first exposure to mosquitoes. The final dose must be given within a month (30 days) after the cat's last exposure to mosquitoes. For optimal performance, HEARTGARD® for Cats must be given once a month on or about the same date. If treatment is delayed, whether by a few days or many, immediate treatment with HEARTGARD® for Cats and resumption of the recommended dosing regimen will minimize the opportunity for development of adult heartworm.

It is recommended that cats should be tested for existing heartworm infection prior to starting treatment with HEARTGARD® for Cats. Cats already infected with adult heartworms can safely be given HEARTGARD® for Cats monthly to prevent further infections.

Monthly treatment with HEARTGARD® (ivermectin) for Cats also provides effective removal and control of adult and immature hookworms *(A. tubaeforme* and *A. braziliense)*.

Precaution(s): Stability: HEARTGARD® Chewables for Cats are stable for 2 years when stored below 77°F (25°C) and protected from light. Store at controlled room temperature of 68°F-77°F (20°C-25°C). Excursions between 59°F-86°F (15°C-30°C) are permitted.

Caution(s): Federal (U.S.A.) law restricts this drug to use by or on the order of a licensed veterinarian.

Warning(s): Keep this and all drugs out of the reach of children. In case of ingestion by humans, clients should be advised to contact a physician immediately.

Trial Data: Safety: In the clinical studies involving more that 3000 doses of HEARTGARD® for Cats, observations reported with 24 hours of treatment included vomition in $\leq$0.3% and diarrhea in $\leq$0.2% of the doses administered. There were no statistical differences between HEARTGARD® for Cats and the product vehicle (control) for these observations.

A wide margin of safety was demonstrated in clinical trials at the recommended dose level in cats and kittens 6 weeks of age and older and in laboratory studies in cats with circulating microfilariae of *D. immitis*. A wide margin of safety has also been demonstrated at 3 times the recommended dose in pregnant or breeding queens and breeding toms. No adverse effects were observed in either male or female cats or their offspring in breeding studies. A 30-fold safety margin over the minimum recommended dosage was established in a single dose tolerance study. In growing kittens dosed monthly for 8 consecutive doses, one cat given 5 times the market dose vomited and a second cat in this group experienced diarrhea within 24 hours of the initial treatment. In clinical trials, many commonly used flea control products, anthelmintics, vaccines, antibiotics and steroid preparations were administered with HEARTGARD® for Cats without incident.

Presentation: HEARTGARD® for Cats is available in two dosage strengths (see Dosage section) for cats of different weights. Each strength comes in a convenient carton of 6 chewables, packed 10 cartons per tray.

HEARTGARD is a registered trademark of Merial.

(Merial Limited: Registered in England and Wales [Reg. No. 3332751] with registered offices at 27 Knightsbridge, London, SW1X 7QT, England and domesticated in Delaware, USA as Merial LLC).

U.S. Patent No. 4,199,569

8924303

Compendium Code No.: 11110221

HEARTGARD® CHEWABLES FOR DOGS ℞

Merial **Parasiticide-Oral**

(ivermectin)

NADA No.: 140-886

Active Ingredient(s): Each chewable tablet contains either:

Ivermectin . . . . . 68 mcg (blue)
Ivermectin . . . . . 136 mcg (green)
Ivermectin . . . . . 272 mcg (brown)

Indications: For use in dogs to prevent canine heartworm disease by eliminating the tissue stage of heartworm larvae *(Dirofilaria immitis)* for a month (30 days) after infection.

Dosage and Administration: Dosage: HEARTGARD® Chewables should be administered orally at monthly intervals at the recommended minimum dose level of 6.0 mcg ivermectin per kilogram (2.72 mcg/lb) of body weight (See Administration). The recommended dosage schedule for prevention of canine heartworm disease is as follows:

Dog Weight	Chewables Per Month	Ivermectin Content	Color Coding on Foil Backing and Carton
Up to 25 lb	1	68 mcg	Blue
26 to 50 lb	1	136 mcg	Green
51 to 100 lb	1	272 mcg	Brown

Give dogs over 100 lb the appropriate combination of these chewables.

HEARTGARD® Chewables are recommended for use in dogs 6 weeks of age and older.

Administration: Remove only one chewable at a time from the foil-backed blister package. Return the card with the remaining chewables to the box to protect the product from light. Because most dogs find HEARTGARD® Chewables palatable, the product can be offered to the dog by hand. Alternatively, it may be added to a small amount of dog food. The chewable should be administered in a manner that encourages the dog to chew, rather than to swallow without chewing. Chewables may be broken into pieces and fed to dogs that normally swallow treats whole.

Care should be taken to see that the dog consumes the complete dose, and treated animals should be observed for a few minutes after administration to ensure that part of the dose is not lost or rejected. If it is suspected that any of the dose has been lost, redosing is recommended.

HEARTGARD® Chewables should be given at monthly intervals during the period of the year when mosquitoes (vectors), potentially carrying infective heartworm larvae, are active. The initial dose must be given within a month (30 days) after the dog's first exposure to mosquitoes. The final dose must be given within a month (30 days) after the dog's last exposure to mosquitoes.

When replacing another heartworm preventive in a heartworm disease preventive program, the first dose of HEARTGARD® must be given within a month (30 days) after the last dose of the former medication.

If the interval between doses exceeds a month (30 days), the efficacy of ivermectin can be reduced. For optimal performance, the chewable must be given once a month on or about the same day of the month. If treatment is delayed, whether by a few days or many, immediate treatment with HEARTGARD® and resumption of the recommended dosing regimen minimizes the opportunity for the development of adult heartworms.

Precaution(s): Store at controlled room temperature of 59°-86°F (15°-30°C). Protect product from light.

Caution(s): Federal (U.S.A.) law restricts this drug to use by or on the order of a licensed veterinarian.

All dogs should be tested for existing heartworm infection before starting treatment with HEARTGARD® which is not effective against adult *D. immitis*. Infected dogs must be treated to remove adult heartworms and microfilariae prior to initiating a program with HEARTGARD®.

While some microfilariae may be killed by the ivermectin in HEARTGARD® at the recommended dose level, HEARTGARD® is not effective for microfilariae clearance. A mild hypersensitivity-type reaction, presumably due to dead or dying microfilariae and particularly involving a transient diarrhea, has been observed in clinical trials with ivermectin after treatment of some dogs that have circulating microfilariae.

Warning(s): Keep this and all drugs out of the reach of children. In case of ingestion by humans, clients should be advised to contact a physician immediately. Physicians may contact a Poison Control Center for advice concerning cases of ingestion by humans.

Adverse Reactions: The following adverse reactions have been reported following the use of HEARTGARD®: Depression/lethargy, vomiting, anorexia, diarrhea, mydriasis, ataxia, staggering, convulsions and hypersalivation.

Trial Data: Efficacy: HEARTGARD® (ivermectin) Chewables, given orally using the recommended dose and regimen, are effective against the tissue larval stage of *Dirofilaria immitis* for a month (30 days) after infection and, as a result, prevent the development of the adult stage.

Acceptability: In acceptability and field trials, HEARTGARD® Chewables were shown to be an acceptable oral dosage that was consumed at the first offering by the majority of dogs.

Safety: HEARTGARD® has shown a wide margin of safety at the recommended dose level in dogs (See Cautions for exceptions) including pregnant or breeding bitches, stud dogs and puppies aged 6 or more weeks. In clinical trials, many commonly used flea collars, dips, shampoos, anthelmintics, antibiotics, vaccines, and steroid preparations have been administered with HEARTGARD® Chewables in a heartworm disease preventive program.

Studies with ivermectin indicate that certain dogs of the Collie breed are more sensitive to the effects of ivermectin administered at elevated dose levels (more than 16 times the target use level) than dogs of other breeds. At elevated doses, sensitive dogs showed adverse reactions which included mydriasis, depression, ataxia, tremors, drooling, paresis, recumbency, excitability, stupor, coma and death. HEARTGARD® demonstrated no signs of toxicity at 10 times the recommended dose (60 mcg/kg) in sensitive Collies. Results of these trials support the safety of HEARTGARD® products in dogs, including Collies, when used as recommended.

Presentation: HEARTGARD® Chewables are available in three dosage strengths (see Dosage section) for dogs of different weights. Each strength comes in convenient cartons of 6 chewables, packed 10 cartons per tray.

HEARTGARD is a registered trademark of Merial.

(Merial Limited: Registered in England and Wales [Reg. No. 3332751] with registered offices at 27 Knightsbridge, London, SW1X 7QT, England and domesticated in Delaware, USA as Merial LLC).

U.S. Patent No. 4, 199,569

8828106

Compendium Code No.: 11110211

HEARTGARD® PLUS CHEWABLES FOR DOGS ℞

Merial **Parasiticide-Oral**

(ivermectin/pyrantel)

NADA No.: 140-971

Active Ingredient(s): Each chewable tablet contains:

Color Coding	Ivermectin Content	Pyrantel Content
Blue	68 mcg	57 mg
Green	136 mcg	114 mg
Brown	272 mcg	227 mg

Indications: For use in dogs to prevent canine heartworm disease by eliminating the tissue stage of heartworm larvae *(Dirofilaria immitis)* for a month (30 days) after infection and for the treatment and control of ascarids *(Toxocara canis, Toxascaris leonina)* and hookworms *(Ancylostoma caninum, Uncinaria stenocephala, Ancylostoma braziliense)*.

Dosage and Administration: Dosage: HEARTGARD® Plus should be administered orally at monthly intervals at the recommended minimum dose level of 6 mcg of ivermectin per kilogram (2.72 mcg/lb) and 5 mg of pyrantel (as pamoate salt) per kg (2.27 mg/lb) of body weight. The recommended dosing schedule for prevention of canine heartworm disease and for the treatment and control of ascarids and hookworms is as follows:

Dog Weight	Chewables Per Month	Ivermectin Content	Pyrantel Content	Color Coding on Foil-Backing and Carton
Up to 25 lb	1	68 mcg	57 mg	Blue
26 - 50 lb	1	136 mcg	114 mg	Green
51 - 100 lb	1	272 mcg	227 mg	Brown

HEARTGARD® Plus is recommended for dogs 6 weeks of age and older.

For dogs over 100 lb use the appropriate combination of these chewables.

Administration: Remove only one chewable at a time from the foil-backed blister card. Return the card with the remaining chewables to its box to protect the product from light. Because most dogs find HEARTGARD® Plus palatable, the product can be offered to the dog by hand. Alternatively, it may be added intact to a small amount of dog food. The chewable should be administered in a manner that encourages the dog to chew, rather than to swallow without chewing. Chewables may be broken into pieces and fed to dogs that normally swallow treats whole.

Care should be taken that the dog consumes the complete dose, and treated animals should be observed for a few minutes after administration to ensure that part of the dose is not lost or rejected. If it is suspected that any of the dose has been lost, redosing is recommended.

HEARTGARD® Plus should be given at monthly intervals during the period of the year when mosquitoes (vectors), potentially carrying infective heartworm larvae, are active. The initial dose must be given within a month (30 days) after the dog's first exposure to mosquitoes. The final dose must be given within a month (30 days) after the dog's last exposure to mosquitoes.

When replacing another heartworm preventive product in a heartworm disease prevention program, the first dose of HEARTGARD® Plus must be given within a month (30 days) of the last dose of the former medication.

If the interval between doses exceeds a month (30 days), the efficacy of ivermectin can be reduced. Therefore, for optimal performance, the chewable must be given once a month on or about the same day of the month. If treatment is delayed, whether by a few days or many, immediate treatment with HEARTGARD® Plus and resumption of the recommended dosing regimen minimizes the opportunity for the development of adult heartworms.

Monthly treatment with HEARTGARD® Plus also provides effective treatment and control of ascarids *(T. canis, T. leonina)* and hookworms *(A. caninum, U. stenocephala, A. braziliense)*. Clients should be advised of measures to be taken to prevent reinfection with intestinal parasites.

Precaution(s): Store at controlled room temperature of 59°-86°F (15°-30°C). Protect product from light.

Caution(s): Federal (U.S.A.) law restricts this drug to use by or on the order of a licensed veterinarian.

All dogs should be tested for existing heartworm infection before starting treatment with HEARTGARD® Plus which is not effective against adult *D. immitis*. Infected dogs must be treated to remove adult heartworms and microfilariae before initiating a program with HEARTGARD® Plus.

While some microfilariae may be killed by the ivermectin in HEARTGARD® Plus at the recommended dose level, HEARTGARD® Plus is not effective for microfilariae clearance. A mild hypersensitivity-type reaction, presumably due to dead or dying microfilariae and particularly involving a transient diarrhea, has been observed in clinical trials with ivermectin alone after treatment of some dogs that have circulating microfilariae.

Warning(s): Keep this and all drugs out of the reach of children. In case of ingestion by humans, clients should be advised to contact a physician immediately. Physicians may contact a Poison Control Center for advice concerning cases of ingestion by humans.

Adverse Reactions: In clinical field trials with HEARTGARD® Plus, vomiting or diarrhea within 24 hours of dosing was rarely observed (1.1% of administered doses). The following adverse reactions have been reported following the use of Heartgard®: Depression/lethargy, vomiting, anorexia, diarrhea, mydriasis, ataxia, staggering, convulsions and hypersalivation.

Trial Data: Efficacy: HEARTGARD® Plus (ivermectin/pyrantel) Chewables, given orally using the recommended dose and regimen, are effective against the tissue larval stage of *D. immitis* for a month (30 days) after infection and, as a result, prevent the development of the adult stage. HEARTGARD® Plus Chewables are also effective against canine ascarids *(T. canis, T. leonina)* and hookworms *(A. caninum, U. stenocephala, A. braziliense)*.

Acceptability: In acceptability and field trials, HEARTGARD® Plus was shown to be an acceptable oral dosage form that was consumed at first offering by the majority of dogs.

H

Safety: HEARTGARD® Plus has been shown to be bioequivalent to Heartgard®, with respect to the bioavailability of ivermectin. The dose regimens of HEARTGARD® Plus and Heartgard® are the same with regard to ivermectin (6 mcg/kg). Studies with ivermectin indicate that certain dogs of the Collie breed are more sensitive to the effects of ivermectin administered at elevated dose levels (more than 16 times the target use level) than dogs of other breeds. At elevated doses, sensitive dogs showed adverse reactions which included mydriasis, depression, ataxia, tremors, drooling, paresis, recumbency, excitability, stupor, coma and death. Heartgard® demonstrated no signs of toxicity at 10 times the recommended dose (60 mcg/kg) in sensitive Collies. Results of these trials and bioequivalency studies, support the safety of Heartgard® products in dogs, including Collies, when used as recommended.

HEARTGARD® Plus has shown a wide margin of safety at the recommended dose level in dogs, including pregnant or breeding bitches, stud dogs and puppies aged 6 or more weeks. In clinical trials, many commonly used flea collars, dips, shampoos, anthelmintics, antibiotics, vaccines and steroid preparations have been administered with HEARTGARD® Plus in a heartworm disease prevention program.

In one trial, where some pups had parvovirus, there was a marginal reduction in efficacy against intestinal nematodes, possibly due to a change in intestinal transit time.

Presentation: HEARTGARD® Plus is available in three dosage strengths (see Dosage section) for dogs of different weights. Each strength comes in convenient cartons of 6 and 12 chewables.

HEARTGARD is a registered trademark of Merial.

(Merial Limited: Registered in England and Wales [Reg. No. 3332751] with registered offices at 27 Knightsbridge, London, SW1X 7QT, England and domesticated in Delaware, USA as Merial LLC).

U.S. Patent No. 4,199,569

8823112

Compendium Code No.: 11110231

HEARTGARD® TABLETS FOR DOGS ℞

Merial **Parasiticide-Oral**

(ivermectin)

NADA No.: 138-412

Active Ingredient(s): Each tablet contains either:

Ivermectin .... 68 mcg (blue)
Ivermectin .... 136 mcg (green)
Ivermectin .... 272 mcg (brown)

Indications: For use in dogs to prevent canine heartworm disease. HEARTGARD® prevents heartworm disease by eliminating the tissue stage of heartworm larvae *(Dirofilaria immitis)* for a month (30 days) after infection.

Dosage and Administration: Dosage: HEARTGARD® Tablets should be administered orally at monthly intervals at the recommended minimum dose level of 6 mcg of ivermectin per kilogram (2.72 mcg/lb) of body weight (See Administration). The recommended dosage schedule for prevention of canine heartworm disease is as follows:

Dog Weight	Tablets Per Month	Ivermectin Per Tablet	Color on Carton
Up to 25 lb	1	68 mcg	Blue
26 to 50 lb	1	136 mcg	Green
51 to 100 lb	1	272 mcg	Brown

Give dogs over 100 lb the appropriate combination of tablets.

HEARTGARD® is recommended for use in dogs 6 weeks of age and older.

Administration: The HEARTGARD® tablet should be given so that dogs swallow the whole tablet. (The tablet may be wrapped in food to encourage consumption.) Care should be taken to see that the dog consumes the complete dose, and treated animals should be observed for a few minutes after administration to ensure that part of the dose is not lost or rejected. If it is suspected that any of the dose has been lost, redosing is recommended. HEARTGARD® Tablets should be given at monthly intervals during the period of the year when mosquitoes (vectors), potentially carrying infective heartworm larvae, are active. The initial dose must be given within a month (30 days) after the first exposure to mosquitoes. The final dose must be given within a month (30 days) after the last exposure to mosquitoes.

When replacing another heartworm preventive in a heartworm disease prevention program, the first dose of HEARTGARD® must be given within a month (30 days) after the last dose of the former medication.

If the interval between doses exceeds a month (30 days), the efficacy of ivermectin can be reduced. For optimum performance, the tablet must be given once a month on or about the same day of the month. If treatment is delayed, whether by a few days or many, immediate treatment with HEARTGARD® and resumption of the recommended dosing regimen minimizes the opportunity for the development of adult heartworms.

Caution(s): Federal (U.S.A.) law restricts this drug to use by or on the order of a licensed veterinarian.

All dogs should be tested for existing heartworm infection before starting treatment with HEARTGARD® (ivermectin) Tablets which is not effective against adult *D. immitis*. Infected dogs must be treated to remove adult heartworms and microfilariae prior to initiating a program with HEARTGARD®.

While some microfilariae may be killed by the ivermectin in HEARTGARD® at the recommended dose level, HEARTGARD® is not effective for microfilariae clearance. A mild hypersensitivity-type reaction, presumably due to dead or dying microfilariae and particularly involving a transient diarrhea, has been observed in clinical trials with ivermectin after the treatment of some dogs that have circulating microfilariae.

Warning(s): Keep this and all drugs out of the reach of children. In case of ingestion by human, clients should be advised to contact a physician immediately. Physicians may contact a Poison Control Center for advice concerning cases of ingestion by humans.

Adverse Reactions: The following adverse reactions have been reported following the use of HEARTGARD®: Depression/lethargy, vomiting, anorexia, diarrhea, mydriasis, ataxia, staggering, convulsions and hypersalivation.

Trial Data: Efficacy: HEARTGARD® Tablets, given orally using the recommended dose and regimen, are effective against the tissue larval stage of *Dirofilaria immitis* for up to a month (30 days) after infection and, as a result, prevent the development of the adult stage.

Safety: HEARTGARD® has shown a wide margin of safety at the recommended dose level in dogs (See Cautions for exceptions) including pregnant or breeding bitches, stud dogs and puppies aged 6 or more weeks. In clinical trials, many commonly used flea collars, dips, shampoos, anthelmintics, antibiotics, vaccines, and steroid preparations have been administered with HEARTGARD® in a heartworm disease preventive program.

Studies with ivermectin indicate that certain dogs of the Collie breed are more sensitive to the effects of ivermectin administered at elevated dose levels (more than 16 times the target use level) than dogs of other breeds. At elevated doses, sensitive dogs showed adverse reactions which included mydriasis, depression, ataxia, tremors, drooling, paresis, recumbency, excitability, stupor, coma and death. HEARTGARD® demonstrated no signs of toxicity at 10 times the recommended dose (60 mcg/kg) in sensitive Collies. Results of these trials support the safety of HEARTGARD® products in dogs, including Collies, when used as recommended.

Presentation: HEARTGARD® is available in three dosage strengths (see Dosage section) for dogs of different weights. Each strength comes in a convenient carton of 6 or 9 tablets, packed 10 cartons per tray.

HEARTGARD is a registered trademark of Merial.

(Merial Limited: Registered in England and Wales [Reg. No. 3332751] with registered offices at 27 Knightsbridge, London, SW1X 7QT, England and domesticated in Delaware, USA as Merial LLC).

U.S. Patent No. 4,199,569

8828307

Compendium Code No.: 11110241

HEARTWORM TEST STAIN

Vedco **Heartworm Test**

Indications: For use in the detection of heartworm microfilariae.

Dosage and Administration: Diagnostic reagent for *in vitro* use only.

Precaution(s): Store at room temperature.

Caution(s): For veterinary use only.

Presentation: 15 mL.

Compendium Code No.: 10941060

HEMABLOCK™

Abbott **Hemostatic**

Description: Description and Function: HEMABLOCK™ is composed of microporous particles that have been naturally synthesized from a plant based polysaccharide source. Upon contact with blood or other wound exudates, the particles act as a hydrophilic molecular sieve and accelerate natural hemostasis by concentrating blood solids such as platelets, red blood cells, and blood proteins such as albumin, thrombin and fibrinogen to form a tenacious gel around the beads on contact.

HEMABLOCK™ has been demonstrated to be useful to control bleeding.

Indications: When used by a medical professional, HEMABLOCK™ is intended for the management of bleeding.

Directions: Application of HEMABLOCK™:

1. To open, twist the cap and pull off.
2. Remove excess blood by blotting with sterile gauze pad.
3. Apply liberally to a cleansed wound site directly to the source of bleeding, covering the entire wound surface. Provide light pressure to the applicator tube or simply pour directly on the area of bleeding. Do not apply HEMABLOCK™ over a pool of blood or fluid. This will result in incomplete hemostasis and the HEMABLOCK™ will be washed away.
4. Immediately apply gentle pressure with a sterile gauze pad to ensure contact of beads with both blood and tissue.
5. Remove pressure. Observe the wound for re-bleeding. Repeat the previous steps if bleeding continues.
6. After several minutes, remove excess powder by gently washing with water.
7. Cover the wound site with traditional dressing to promote healing.

Contraindication(s): Not for intravenous application.

Precaution(s): Storage: Protect from extreme heat.

To prevent product or applicator contamination, follow aseptic techniques.

Do not use if the foil package has been damaged or opened prior to use.

Caution(s): To be used by or under the supervision of a licensed veterinarian.

Do not inject into blood vessels. Do not resterilize.

Warning(s): Do not use in animals intended for food.

This device is not intended for human application.

Presentation: HEMABLOCK™ is supplied as ten individually sterilized packages and a package insert, list number 5123, with each package containing a 0.5 g tube and an applicator.

Manufactured by: Medafor, Inc., Minneapolis, MN 55421, under Patent #6,060,461.

Compendium Code No.: 10240130 04-3631/R1

HEMAJECT 200

Vedco **Iron Injection**

(Iron Dextran Injection) Hematinic 200 mg/mL

ANADA No.: 200-256

Active Ingredient(s): Description: HEMAJECT 200 is a sterile solution containing ferric hydroxide in complex with a low molecular weight dextran fraction equivalent to 200 mg elemental iron per mL with 0.5% phenol as a preservative.

Indications: HEMAJECT 200 is intended for the prevention or treatment of anemia in baby pigs due to iron deficiency.

Dosage and Administration: For intramuscular injection only.

For the prevention of anemia due to iron deficiency, administer an intramuscular injection of 200 milligrams of elemental iron (1 mL) at 1 to 3 days of age. For the treatment of anemia due to iron deficiency, administer an intramuscular injection of 200 milligrams of elemental iron (1 mL) at the first signs of anemia.

Directions for Use: Disinfect rubber stopper of vial as well as site of injection. Use small needle (20 gauge, 5/8 inch) that has been sterilized (boiled in water for 20 minutes). Injection should be intramuscular into the back of the ham. Place tension on the skin over the rear of the ham and inject to a depth of 1/2" or slightly more.

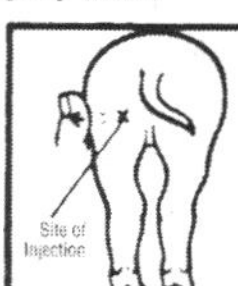

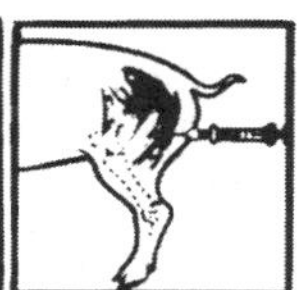

HEMAJECT 200 cannot be considered a substitute for sound animal husbandry. If disease is present in the litter, consult a veterinarian.

Precaution(s): Store at controlled room temperature 59°-86°F (15°-30°C).

Caution(s): For animal use only.

Warning(s): Keep out of reach of children.

Side Effects: Occasionally pigs may show a reaction to injectable iron, clinically characterized by prostration with muscular weakness. In extreme cases, death may result.

Notice: Organic iron preparation injected intramuscularly into pigs beyond 4 weeks of age may cause staining of the ham muscle.

Discussion: Actions: HEMAJECT 200 is easy and economical to use. Injection into the ham is rapid, safe, effective, quickly absorbed by the blood and goes to work immediately. With HEMAJECT 200, the right dosage can be given to every animal with assurance that it will be utilized. Iron deficiency anemia occurs commonly in the suckling pig, often within the first few days following birth. As body size and blood volume increase rapidly from the first few days following birth, hemoglobin levels in the blood fall due to diminishing iron reserves which cannot be replaced adequately from iron in the sow's milk. This natural deficiency lowers the resistance of the pig and scours, pneumonia or other infections may develop and lead to death of the animal. Pigs not hampered by iron deficiency anemia are more likely to experience normal growth and to maintain their normal level of resistance to disease. Adequate iron is necessary for normal, healthy, vigorous growth.

Presentation: HEMAJECT 200, 200 mg/mL is available in 100 mL multidose vials (NDC 50989-488-12).

Manufactured by: Phoenix Scientific, Inc., St. Joseph, MO 64503

Compendium Code No.: 10942460 Iss. 9-98

HEMOSTATIC POWDER

Butler **Hemostatic**

Active Ingredient(s):

Ferrous sulfate $7H_2O$	84%
Chloroxylenol	1%
Diphenyl amine	1%

In a free-flowing absorbent base. Not sterilized.

Indications: For use as an aid in controlling capillary hemorrhage from superficial cuts and wounds and after dehorning.

Dosage and Administration: Apply the powder freely to the bleeding surface. Repeat as needed. Bandage if necessary.

Precaution(s): Store at a controlled room temperature between 59°-86°F (15° and 30°C). Keep the container tightly closed when not in use.

Caution(s): In case of deep or puncture wounds or serious burns consult a veterinarian. If redness, irritation, or swelling persists or increases, discontinue use and consult veterinarian.

For external use only. For animal use only. Keep out of the reach of children.

Restricted drug, use only as directed.

Presentation: 6 oz. and 16 oz. (1 lb., 454 g) containers.

Compendium Code No.: 10820890

HEMOSTAT POWDER

Phoenix Pharmaceutical **Hemostatic**

Active Ingredient(s): Composition:

Ferrous Sulfate • $7H_2O$	84%
Ammonium Alum	5%
Chloroxylenol	1%
Tannic Acid	1%

In a free-flowing absorbent base.

Not sterilized.

Indications: For use as an aid in controlling minor bleeding of superficial cuts and wounds and after dehorning.

Dosage and Administration: Apply powder freely to bleeding surface. Repeat as needed. Bandage if necessary.

Precaution(s): Store at a controlled room temperature between 15° and 30°C (59°-86°F).

Keep container tightly closed.

Caution(s): In case of deep or puncture wounds or serious burns, consult a veterinarian. If redness, irritation or swelling persists or increases, discontinue use and consult a veterinarian.

For animal use only. For external use only.

Warning(s): Keep out of reach of children.

Presentation: 16 oz. (454 g) containers (NDC 57319-392-12).

Compendium Code No.: 12560391 Iss. 11-97

HERDCHECK®: ANTI-PRV-gpX ANTIBODY TEST KIT

Idexx Labs. **Pseudorabies Test**

U.S. Vet. Lic. No.: 313

Description: This pseudorabies virus gpX antibody test kit is an enzyme immunoassay.

Components: Reagents:

1. PRV Coated Plates.
2. Anti-PRV-gpX: Horseradish Peroxidase (HRPO) Conjugate in buffer with protein stabilizers, preserved with gentamicin.
3. Porcine Negative Control, porcine serum non-reactive to PRV-gpX in buffer with protein stabilizers, preserved with sodium azide.
4. PRV-gpX Positive Control, porcine Anti-gpX in buffer with protein stabilizers, preserved with sodium azide.
5. Sample Diluent, buffer with protein stabilizers, preserved with sodium azide.
6. TMB Concentrate.
7. TMB Diluent, citrate-phosphate buffer containing hydrogen peroxide.
8. Wash Concentrate (10X concentrate), phosphate buffer, preserved with gentamicin.

Materials Required but Not Provided:

1. 0.12% Hydrofluoric Acid (HF): Prepared by diluting 1 mL of concentrated HF (48%) in 400 mL with distilled/deionized water. Note: Always add concentrated acids to water. Take precautions to prevent accidental skin contact (i.e., safety glasses and gloves). Use only plasticware for storage and handling HF.
2. Precision Pipet: Suitable for delivering 0.100 and 0.200 mL or multiple delivery pipetting devices.
3. Disposable pipet tips.
4. Graduated cylinders: 500 mL for HF and wash solution; 5 to 50 mL for TMB Diluent and Concentrate.
5. 96-Well Plate Reader.
6. Glass or plastic tubes for diluting samples.
7. Distilled or deionized water.
8. Device for the delivery and aspiration of wash solution.
9. A vacuum source and a trap for retaining the aspirate.

Indications: For the detection of antibodies in swine serum to gpX antigen of pseudorabies virus (PRV). The presence of antibodies to gpX indicates exposure to field strains of PRV and/or vaccines containing gpX antigens. It is intended for use in herd management and pseudorabies eradication applications. When used with SyntroVet's™ gpX-deleted PRV Marker® or SyntroVet's gpX/gI-deleted PRV/Marker Gold vaccines and when performed at approved laboratories, it is an approved differential pseudorabies test for use in the Cooperative State/Federal Pseudorabies Eradication Program. This product should be used in strict accordance with state and federal regulations regarding pseudorabies testing and the movement of swine based on pseudorabies test results.

Test Principles: The Anti-gpX assay is performed in a PRV antigen coated microwell using a two-fold (1:2) serum dilution. During the first incubation, PRV antibodies present in the serum, including those produced against gpX, react with antigens on the plastic. Subsequent to a wash step, an Anti-gpX monoclonal antibody conjugate is added to the microwell and is allowed to compete for the gpX viral antigen during a second incubation. If no gpX antibodies are present in the test serums, the conjugated gpX antibodies are free to react with the gpX antigen. Conversely, if gpX antibodies are present in the test serum, the enzyme-conjugated monoclonal antibodies are blocked from reacting with the antigen. Following this incubation period, the unreacted conjugate is removed by washing and a substrate/chromogen solution is added. In the presence of enzyme, the substrate is converted to a product which reacts with the chromophore to generate a blue color. The absorbance at 650 nm, A(650), is measured using a spectrophotometer. Results are calculated by dividing the A(650) of the sample by the mean A(650) of the negative control, resulting in a S/N value. The quantity of antibodies to gpX is inversely proportional to the A(650) and, thus, to the S/N value. The presence of PRV antibodies, including Anti-gpX, indicates a previous exposure to a field strain of PRV, or application of conventionally modified live, killed virus, or non-gpX deleted vaccines. The presence of PRV antibodies detected by the Anti-PRV Screen and/or Verification assays but absence of antibodies to gpX antigen as assessed by the Anti-gpX assay indicates a response to a gpX deleted vaccine.

Test Procedure:

Preparation of Samples: Dilute test samples two-fold (1:2) with Sample Diluent (e.g., by diluting 200 µL of sample with 200 µL of Sample Diluent).

Note: Do not dilute controls.

Be sure to change tips for each sample and record the position of each sample on the plate using an HerdChek® worksheet. Samples should be mixed prior to dispensing into the PRV Coated Plate and assayed in duplicate.

Preparation of TMB Substrate Solution: The TMB Concentrate must be added to the TMB Diluent before use (5 mL TMB Concentrate plus 5 mL of TMB Diluent; 100 µL required per well). The TMB substrate solution must be stored at room temperature and used within 60 minutes after preparation. The TMB Diluent should not be exposed to any metal during the preparation.

Preparation of Wash Solution: The Wash Concentrate should be brought to room temperature and mixed to ensure dissolution of any precipitated salts. The Wash Concentrate must be diluted 1 to 10 with distilled/deionized water before use (e.g. 30 mL of concentrate plus 270 mL of water per plate to be assayed).

All reagents should be allowed to come to room temperature before use. Reagents should be mixed by gentle swirling or vortexing.

1. Obtain antigen coated plate(s) and record the sample position on an HerdChek® worksheet.
2. Dispense 100 µL of Undiluted Negative Control into wells A1, A2 and A3.
3. Dispense 100 µL of Undiluted Positive Control into wells A4 and A5.
4. Dispense 100 µL of diluted sample into appropriate wells.
5. Incubate for 2 hours at room temperature.
6. Wash each well with approximately 300 µL of wash solution three to five times. Aspirate liquid contents of all wells after each wash. Avoid plate drying between plate washings and prior to the addition of conjugate. Following the final wash fluid aspiration, gently, but firmly tap residual wash fluid from each plate onto absorbent material.
7. Dispense 100 µL of Anti-PRV-gpX: HRPO Conjugate into each well.
8. Incubate for 20 minutes at room temperature. TMB substrate solution should be prepared at this point.
9. Repeat Step 6.
10. Dispense 100 µL of TMB substrate solution into each test well.
11. Incubate for 15 minutes at room temperature.
12. Dispense 100 µL of 1:400 HF into each well to stop the reaction.
13. Blank the spectrophotometer on air.
14. Measure and record the A(650) for samples and controls.

H

15. Calculate results.

Results: For the assay to be valid, negative control A(650) mean minus the positive control A(650) mean must be greater than or equal to 0.3. For invalid assays, technique may be suspect and the assay should be repeated following a thorough review of the product insert. The presence or absence of antibody to the gpX antigen is determined by first calculating the S/N value for each sample. See Calculations for examples.

Note: Idexx Laboratories, Inc. has instrument and software systems available which calculate means, S/N values and provide data summaries.

Test Interpretation:

1. If the S/N is less than or equal to 0.70, the test is classified as positive for antibodies to the gpX antigen of PRV.
2. If the S/N is greater than 0.70, the test is classified as negative for antibodies to the gpX antigen of PRV.

Calculations:

1. Calculation of Negative Control Mean ($NC\overline{x}$):

$$NC\overline{x} = \frac{A1\ A(650) + A2\ A(650) + A3\ A(650)}{3}$$

2. Calculation of Positive Control mean ($PC\overline{x}$):

$$PC\overline{x} = \frac{A4\ A(650) + A5\ A(650)}{2}$$

3. Calculation of Sample/Negative (S/N) Ratio:

$$S/N = \frac{Sample\ \overline{x}\ A(650)}{NC\overline{x}}$$

Storage: Store all reagents at 2°-7°C (36°-45°F). Bring to room temperature prior to use, and return to 2°-7°C (36°-45°F) following use.

Caution(s): Handle all PRV biological materials as though capable of transmitting PRV. Although the virus has been chemically treated, the antigen coated microwell plate may be a source of PRV.

Do not pipet by mouth.

No eating, drinking or smoking where specimens or kit reagents are being handled.

TMB Concentrate, Diluent and acid solutions may be irritating to the skin. Use only plasticware for storage or handling of HF solutions. Safety glasses should be worn while pouring concentrated acids.

Some kit components contain sodium azide as a preservative. Disposal requires flushing plumbing with large volumes of water to prevent formation of copper or lead azide complexes which may explode upon percussion. Care should be taken to prevent the contamination of the Anti-PRV-gpX: HRPO Conjugate with this preservative.

Do not expose TMB solutions to strong light or any oxidizing agents. Handle all TMB substrate solutions with clean glass or plasticware.

All wastes should be properly decontaminated prior to disposal.

Care should be taken to prevent contamination of kit components.

Do not use the components past expiration date and do not intermix components from different serials.

Avoid using heavily hemolyzed or contaminated samples. False positives may result from using sera of this type in the assay.

Optimal results will be obtained by strict adherence to this protocol. Careful pipetting, timing and washing throughout this procedure are necessary to maintain precision and accuracy.

Discussion: Strategies traditionally used to provide protection for swine from the effects of pseudorabies infection have included the administration of conventional and genetically engineered, USDA licensed PRV vaccines.[1] Standard serologic procedures used to assess PRV exposure following vaccination are of limited value since they cannot distinguish naturally infected from vaccinated swine.

Safe and efficacious genetically engineered PRV vaccines have been developed by SyntroVet that allows for serologic differentiation. The virus used in these vaccines was modified such that the synthesis of virulence factors was eliminated without compromising the immunogenicity of the virus. In addition, a mechanism for serologic differentiation was provided by deleting the DNA sequences that code for gpX, an apparently non-essential viral glycoprotein. Thus, the HERDCHECK® Anti-PRV-GPX assay being specific for antibodies to gpX, ignores antibody titers in animals vaccinated with the SyntroVet's gpX-deleted vaccines, but detects Anti-gpX in animals infected with field strains or vaccinated with strains that contain the gpX antigen. The assay utilizes monoclonal antibodies that are specific for gpX.

Prior to vaccination with SyntroVet's products, swine should be tested using the HerdChek® Anti-PRV screening and/or Verification assays to determine their immune status. Subsequent to vaccination the swine should be routinely monitored at least semi-annually for exposure to field strains of PRV using the Anti-gpX assay.

References:

1. Gustafson, D.P., Pseudorabies in Disease of Swine, 5th edition. Eds. Leman, A.D., Glock, R.D., Mengeling, W.L., Penny, R.H., Scholl, E., and Straw, B., pp. 209-223, 1984.

Presentation: 2 plates per kit.

HERDCHECK®: Anti-PRV-gpX is an Idexx registered trademark.

Compendium Code No.: 11160351

HERDCHEK® BLV ANTIBODY TEST KIT

Idexx Labs. **Leukemia Test**

Bovine Leukemia Virus Antibody Test Kit (Serum/Verification)

U.S. Vet. Lic. No.: 313

Components:

Reagent	No. / Volume
A. Bovine Leukemia Virus Antigen/Normal Host Cell Antigen (BLV/NHC) Coated Strips	6
B. BLV Anti-Bovine IgG: Horseradish Peroxidase (HRPO) Conjugate in Tris buffer with protein stabilizers	60 mL
C. BLV Positive Control - Bovine anti-BLV in buffer with protein stabilizers	8 mL
D. BLV Negative Control (Serum) - Bovine serum non-reactive to BLV in buffer with protein stabilizers	8 mL
E. BLV Sample Diluent (Serum) - Buffer with protein stabilizers	235 mL
F. Wash Concentrate (10X) phosphate/Tween wash, preserved with gentamicin	235 mL
G. TMB Substrate - 3,3', 5,5' Tetramethylbenzidine	60 mL
H. Stop Solution	60 mL

Materials Required But Not Provided:

1. Precision pipets or multiple delivery pipetting devices suitable for delivering 10, 100, 200 and 240 µL.
2. Disposable pipet tips.
3. 500 mL graduated cylinder for wash solution.
4. 96-well plate reader.
5. Glass or plastic tubes for sample dilution.
6. Distilled or deionized water.
7. Device for the delivery and aspiration of wash solution.
8. A vacuum source, and a trap for retaining aspirate and disinfectant.

Indications: HERDCHEK® Anti-BLV is Idexx's enzyme immunoassay for the detection and verification of antibody to Bovine Leukemia Virus (BLV), the causative agent of enzootic bovine leukosis. The antibody is detected in bovine serum using BLV and normal host cell (NHC) antigens.

Test Principles: HERDCHEK® Anti-BLV is an enzyme immunoassay designed to detect the presence of antibody to BLV in bovine serum. A microtitration format has been configured using BLV and normal host cell antigens (NHC) that are bound on alternate columns of the microtiter plate. The NHC antigens are used to determine if non-specific immunoglobulins are contributing to positive test results. The extent of host cell contribution to the total signal is assessed by relating the reactivity of specific BLV wells and NHC antigen wells. Upon incubation of the test sample in the BLV antigen wells, antibodies specific for BLV (if present) form a complex with the bound viral antigens. Following a wash step to remove unbound components, an anti-bovine IgG: Horseradish Peroxidase Conjugate is added which binds to bovine antibody attached in the wells. Next, unbound conjugate is removed by washing and enzyme substrate (hydrogen peroxide) and a chromogen (3,3', 5,5' tetramethylbenzidine, TMB) are added. The absorbance at a wavelength between 620 and 650 nm [A(650)] is measured using a spectrophotometer. This absorbance is proportional to the amount of specific antibody in the test sample.

Test Procedure: Test Protocol:

Preparation of Samples: Dilute serum samples twenty-five fold (1:25) with Sample Diluent (e.g., by diluting 20 µL of serum with 480 µL of Sample Diluent).

Note: Do not dilute controls.

Be sure to change tips for each sample and record the position of each sample on the plate using a HerdChek® worksheet. Diluted samples should be mixed prior to dispensing into the antigen coated microtiter plate.

Preparation of Wash Solution: The 10X Wash Concentrate should be brought to room temperature (20°-25°C) and mixed to ensure dissolution of any precipitated salts. The Wash Concentrate must be diluted 1:10 with distilled/deionized water before use (e.g., 30 mL of concentrate plus 270 mL of water per plate to be assayed).

	BLV	NHC	BLV	NHC	BLV	NHC	BLV	NHC	BLV	NHC	BLV	NHC
A	N	N	5	5								
B	N	N	6	6								
C	P	P										
D	P	P										
E	1	1										
F	2	2										
G	3	3										
H	4	4										
	1	2	3	4	5	6	7	8	9	10	11	12

N = Negative Control
P = Positive Control
1, 2, 3, etc. = Sample #
Columns 1, 3, 5, 7, 9, 11 coated with BLV antigen
Columns 2, 4, 6, 8, 10, 12 coated with NHC antigen

1. Obtain BLV and NHC strips and record sample position on a HerdChek® worksheet.
2. Dispense 200 µL of Negative Control into BLV wells A1 and B1 and NHC wells A2 and B2. Note: No dilution required.
3. Dispense 200 µL of Positive Control into BLV wells C1 and D1 and NHC wells C2 and D2. Note: No dilution required.
4. Dispense 200 µL diluted samples into adjacent BLV and NHC wells.
5. Incubate for 90 minutes at room temperature (20°-25°C). Samples may be incubated overnight, 12-18 hours, (2°-7°C). If the latter option is chosen, place plate(s) in a tightly sealed plastic bag.
6. Aspirate liquid contents of all wells into an appropriate waste reservoir.
7. Wash each well four times with approximately 300 µL of wash solution. Aspirate liquid contents of all wells after each wash. Avoid plate drying between plate washings and prior to the addition of conjugate. Following the final aspiration, firmly tap residual wash fluid from each plate onto absorbent material.
8. Dispense 100 µL of Anti-Bovine IgG:HRPO Conjugate into each well.
9. Incubate for 30 minutes at room temperature (20°-25°C).
10. Repeat steps 6 and 7.
11. Dispense 100 µL of TMB Substrate Solution into each well.
12. Incubate 15 minutes at room temperature (20°-25°C).
13. Dispense 100 µL of Stop Solution into each well.
14. Blank spectrophotometer with air.
15. Measure and record the A650 for samples and controls.
16. Calculate results.

Test Interpretation:

Results: For the assay to be valid, the negative control mean ($NC\overline{x}$) for the BLV wells and the NHC wells must be less than or equal to 0.200 (for overnight assays, (0.25). The difference ($PC\overline{x}$ minus $NC\overline{x}$) between the positive control mean ($PC\overline{x}$) for the BLV wells and the negative control mean ($NC\overline{x}$) for the BLV wells must be greater than or equal to 0.075.

For invalid assays, technique may be suspect and the assay should be repeated following a thorough review of the package insert.

The presence or absence of antibody to BLV is determined by the sample to positive (S/P) ratio of the BLV antigen well for each sample. The positive control has been standardized and contains a significant level of antibody to BLV. The normal host cell antigen provides a measure of the NHC contribution to the total BLV signal. The verification of samples reactive for antibody to BLV is determined by calculating the sample to NHC ratio.

See Calculations for examples.

Note: Idexx Laboratories, Inc. has instrument and software systems available which calculate means and S/P ratios and provide data summaries.

Interpretation of Results:

1. Serum samples with BLV well S/P ratios less than 0.500 are classified as negative for BLV antibodies.
2. If the BLV well S/P ratio is greater than or equal to 0.500, the sample is classified as reactive for BLV antibodies. Reactive samples can be confirmed by calculating the S/NHC ratio.
   a. If the S/NHC ratio is less than 1.80, then the sample is classified as negative for antibodies to BLV.
   b. It the S/NHC ratio is greater than or equal to 1.80, then the sample is classified as positive for BLV antibodies.

Calculations:

1. Calculation of negative control mean ($NC\bar{x}$):

$$NC\bar{x} = \frac{A1\ A(650) + B1\ A(650)}{2}$$

Example:

$$\frac{0.67 + 0.073}{2} = 0.070$$

2. Calculation of positive control mean ($PC\bar{x}$):

$$PC\bar{x} = \frac{C1\ A(650) + D1\ A(650)}{2}$$

Example:

$$\frac{0.333 + 0.347}{2} = 0.340$$

3. Calculation of S/P ratio:

$$S/P = \frac{\text{Sample } A(650) - NC\bar{x}}{PC\bar{x} - NC\bar{x}}$$

Example: Sample A(650) = 1.230

$$S/P = \frac{1.230 - 0.070}{0.340 - 0.070} = \frac{1.160}{0.270} = 4.300$$

4. Calculation of sample to normal host cell (S/NHC) ratio:

$$S/NHC = \frac{A(650):BLV}{A(650):NHC}$$

Example:

If A(650): BLV = 0.500, and the A(650): NHC = 0.100, then:

$$S/NHC = \frac{0.500}{0.100} = 5$$

Storage: Store all reagents at 2°-7°C (36°-45°F).

Caution(s):

1. Handle all BLV biological materials as though capable of transmitting BLV.
2. Do not pipet by mouth.
3. There should be no eating, drinking, or smoking where specimens or kit reagents are being handled.
4. TMB and stop solutions may be irritating to the skin.
5. Do not expose TMB Substrate to strong light or any oxidizing agents. Handle the TMB Substrate with clean glass or plasticware.
6. Bring to room temperature (20°-25°C) prior to use, and return to 2°-7°C following use.
7. All wastes should be properly decontaminated prior to disposal.
8. Care should be taken to prevent contamination of kit components.
9. Do not use components past expiration dates and do not intermix components from different serials.
10. Optimal results will be obtained by strict adherence to this protocol. Careful pipetting, timing and washing throughout this procedure are necessary to maintain precision and accuracy.

For veterinary use only.

Discussion: The bovine leukemia virus (BLV) is the causative agent of enzootic bovine leukosis in cattle. This is a highly fatal neoplasia of cattle characterized by the aggregation of neoplastic lymphocytes in lymph nodes. Clinical signs most commonly associated with infection include weight loss, decreased milk production, lymphadenopathy and posterior paresis.[1] Diagnosis of BLV infection based on clinical signs alone is often difficult because of the wide range of symptoms. Once acquired, viral infection is lifelong and is spread by contact between animals. An assessment of exposure to BLV via natural infection can be made by measurement of specific antibody titer to BLV using an enzyme immunoassay system. A positive antibody titer to BLV indicates that the animal has been exposed to BLV and may be persistently and chronically infected.

References: Available upon request.

Presentation: 6 strips per kit.

HERDCHEK is a registered trademark of Idexx Laboratories, Inc., in the United States and/or other countries.

Compendium Code No.: 11160571 06-03560-01

HERDCHEK® BLV ANTIBODY TEST KIT (SERUM)

Idexx Labs. **Leukemia Test**

Bovine Leukemia Virus Antibody Test Kit (Serum) (Screening/Verification)

U.S. Vet. Lic. No.: 313

Components:

Reagent	Volume
A. Bovine Leukemia Virus (BLV) Antigen Coated Plates	5
B. Bovine Leukemia Virus Antigen/Normal Host Cell Antigen (BLV/NHC) Coated Strips	1
C. BLV Anti-Bovine IgG: Horseradish Peroxidase (HRPO) Conjugate in Tris buffer with protein stabilizers	60 mL
D. BLV Positive Control - Bovine anti-BLV in buffer with protein stabilizers	8 mL
E. BLV Negative Control (Serum) - Bovine serum non-reactive to BLV in buffer with protein stabilizers	8 mL
F. BLV Sample Diluent (Serum) - Buffer with protein stabilizers	235 mL
G. Wash Concentrate (10X) phosphate/Tween wash, preserved with gentamicin	235 mL
H. TMB Substrate-3,3', 5,5' Tetramethylbenzidine	60 mL
I. Stop Solution	60 mL

Materials Required But Not Provided:

1. Precision pipets or multiple delivery pipetting devices suitable for delivering 10, 100, 200 and 240 μL.
2. Disposable pipet tips.
3. 500 mL graduated cylinder for wash solution.
4. 96-well plate reader.
5. Glass or plastic tubes for sample dilution.
6. Distilled or deionized water.
7. Device for the delivery and aspiration of wash solution.
8. A vacuum source, and a trap for retaining aspirate and disinfectant.

Indications: HERDCHEK® Anti-BLV is Idexx's enzyme immunoassay for the detection and verification of antibody to Bovine Leukemia Virus (BLV), the causative agent of enzootic bovine leukosis. The antibody is detected in bovine serum using BLV and normal host cell (NHC) antigens.

Test Principles: Description and Principles: HERDCHEK® Anti-BLV is an enzyme immunoassay designed to detect the presence of antibody to BLV in bovine serum. A microtitration format has been configured using specifically captured BLV antigens in individual microassay wells. Upon incubation of the test sample in the well, antibodies specific to BLV (if present) form a complex with the bound viral antigens. Following a wash step to remove unbound components, an anti-bovine IgG:Horseradish Peroxidase Conjugate is added which binds to bovine antibody attached in the wells. Next, unbound conjugate is removed by washing and enzyme substrate (hydrogen peroxide) and a chromogen (3,3',5,5' tetramethylbenzidine, TMB) are added. The absorbance at a wavelength between 620 and 650 nm [A(650)] is measured using a spectrophotometer. This absorbance is proportional to the amount of specific antibody in the test sample.

A verification plate has been included to confirm positive results. In this format, BLV and normal host cell antigens (NHC) are bound on alternate columns of the microtiter plate. The NHC antigens are used to determine if non-specific immunoglobulins are contributing to positive test results. The extent of host cell contribution to the total signal is assessed by relating the reactivity of specific BLV wells and NHC antigen wells.

Test Procedure:

Preparation of Samples: Dilute Serum samples twenty-five-fold (1:25) with Sample Diluent (e.g., by diluting 10 μL of serum with 240 μL of Sample Diluent).

In order to standardize incubation periods and to permit proper mixing and timely transfer of the diluted samples to the coated plates, the 1:25 dilution should be made in microtubes according to the following procedure:

1. Using a 96-tube rack, deliver respectively:

   Screening Protocol:

   -240 μL of Sample Diluent per microtube using a multi-channel pipet;

   -10 μL of undiluted sample per microtube in accordance with the already established plate worksheet

   Verification Protocol:

   -480 μL of Sample Diluent per microtube using a multichannel pipet;

   -20 μL of undiluted sample per microtube in accordance with the already established plate worksheet
2. Mix dilutions by aspiration and delivery (3 times) using the multichannel pipet.
3. Transfer 200 μL of diluted sample row by row into each well of the coated plate using the multichannel pipet.

Note: Do not dilute controls.

Be sure to change tips for each sample and record the position of each sample on the plate using a HerdChek® worksheet. Diluted samples should be mixed prior to dispensing into the antigen coated microtiter plate.

Preparation of Wash Solution: The 10X Wash Concentrate should be brought to room temperature (20°-25°C) and mixed to ensure dissolution of any precipitated salts. The Wash Concentrate must be diluted 1:10 with distilled/deionized water before use (e.g., 30 mL of concentrate plus 270 mL of water per plate to be assayed).

Test Protocol (Screening): All reagents must be allowed to come to room temperature before use. Reagents should be mixed by gentle swirling or vortexing.

1. Obtain BLV antigen plate(s) and record the sample position on a HerdChek® worksheet.
2. Dispense 200 μL of Negative Control into wells A1 and A2. Note: No dilution required.
3. Dispense 200 μL of Positive Control into wells A3 and A4. Note: No dilution required.
4. Dispense 200 μL diluted samples into remaining wells.
5. Incubate for 90 minutes at room temperature (20°-25°C) or overnight, 12-18 hours, (2°-7°C). If the latter option is chosen, place plate(s) in a tightly sealed plastic bag.
6. Aspirate liquid contents of all wells into an appropriate waste reservoir.
7. Wash each well four times with approximately 300 μL of wash solution. Aspirate liquid contents of all wells after each wash. Avoid plate drying between plate washings and prior to the addition of conjugate. Following the final aspiration, firmly tap residual wash fluid from each plate onto absorbent material.
8. Dispense 100 μL of Anti-Bovine IgG:HRPO Conjugate into each well.
9. Incubate for 30 minutes at room temperature (20°-25°C).
10. Repeat steps 6 and 7.
11. Dispense 100 μL of TMB Substrate Solution into each well.
12. Incubate 15 minutes at room temperature.
13. Dispense 100 μL of Stop Solution into each well to stop the reaction.
14. Blank spectrophotometer with air.
15. Measure and record the A650 for samples and controls.
16. Calculate results.

Test Protocol (Verification):

Preparation of Samples: Dilute reactive Serum samples twenty-five fold (1:25) with Sample Diluent (e.g., by diluting 20 μL of serum with 480 μL of Sample Diluent).

Note: Do not dilute controls.

Be sure to change tips for each sample and record the position of each sample on the plate using a HerdChek® worksheet. Diluted samples should be mixed prior to dispensing into the antigen coated microtiter plate.

Note: The same sample dilutions prepared for screening may be used to verify reactive results. (See diagram for verification plate format).

	BLV	NHC	BLV	NHC	BLV	NHC	BLV	NHC	BLV	NHC	BLV	NHC
A	N	N	5	5								
B	N	N	6	6								
C	P	P										
D	P	P										
E	1	1										
F	2	2										
G	3	3										
H	4	4										
	1	2	3	4	5	6	7	8	9	10	11	12

N = Negative Control
P = Positive Control
1, 2, 3, etc. = Sample #
Columns 1, 3, 5, 7, 9, 11 coated with BLV antigen
Columns 2, 4, 6, 8, 10, 12 coated with NHC antigen

1. Obtain BLV and NHC strips and record sample position on a HerdChek® worksheet.
2. Dispense 200 µL of Negative Control into BLV wells A1 and B1 and NHC wells A2 and B2. Note: No dilution required.
3. Dispense 200 µL of Positive Control into BLV wells C1 and D1 and NHC wells C2 and D2. Note: No dilution required.
4. Dispense 200 µL diluted samples into adjacent BLV and NHC wells.
5. Incubate for 90 minutes at room temperature (20°-25°C). Samples may be incubated overnight, 12-18 hours, (2°-7°C). If the latter option is chosen, place plate(s) in a tightly sealed plastic bag.
6. Aspirate liquid contents of all wells into an appropriate waste reservoir.
7. Wash each well four times with approximately 300 µL of wash solution. Aspirate liquid contents of all wells after each wash. Avoid plate drying between plate washings and prior to the addition of conjugate. Following the final aspiration, firmly tap residual wash fluid from each plate onto absorbent material.
8. Dispense 100 µL of Anti-Bovine IgG:HRPO Conjugate into each well.
9. Incubate for 30 minutes at room temperature (20°-25°C).
10. Repeat steps 6 and 7.
11. Dispense 100 µL of TMB Substrate Solution into each well.
12. Incubate 15 minutes at room temperature (20-25°C).
13. Dispense 100 µL of Stop Solution into each well.
14. Blank spectrophotometer with air.
15. Measure and record the A650 for samples and controls.
16. Calculate results.

Test Interpretation:

Results (Screening): For the assay to be valid, the $NC\bar{x}$ must be less than or equal to 0.200 Optical Density (OD). In addition, the difference (P-N) between the positive control mean ($PC\bar{x}$) and the negative control mean ($NC\bar{x}$) must be greater than or equal to 0.075 OD.

For invalid assays, technique may be suspect and the assay should be repeated following a thorough review of the package insert.

The presence or absence of antibody to BLV is determined by the sample to positive (S/P) ratio for each sample. The Positive Control has been standardized and contains a significant level of antibody to BLV.

See Calculations for examples.

Note: Idexx Laboratories, Inc. has instrument and software systems available which calculate means and S/P ratios and provide data summaries.

Interpretation of Results (Screening):

1. Serum samples with S/P ratios less than 0.500 are classified as negative for BLV antibodies.
2. If the S/P ratio is greater than or equal to 0.500, the sample is classified as reactive for BLV antibodies. When samples are classified reactive on the screening test, they should be retested using the verification protocol.

Calculations: (Screening):

1. Calculation of Negative Control mean ($NC\bar{x}$):

$$NC\bar{x} = \frac{A1\ A(650) + A2\ A(650)}{2}$$

Example:

$$\frac{0.67 + 0.073}{2} = 0.070$$

2. Calculation of Positive Control mean ($PC\bar{x}$):

$$PC\bar{x} = \frac{A3\ A(650) + A4\ A(650)}{2}$$

Example:

$$\frac{0.333 + 0.347}{2} = 0.340$$

3. Calculation of S/P ratio:

$$S/P = \frac{\text{Sample } A(650) - NC\bar{x}}{PC\bar{x} - NC\bar{x}}$$

Example: Sample A(650) = 1.230

$$S/P = \frac{1.230 - 0.070}{0.340 - 0.070} = \frac{1.160}{0.270} = 4.300$$

Results (Verification): For the assay to be valid, the negative control mean ($NC\bar{x}$) for the BLV wells and the NHC wells must be less than or equal to 0.200. The difference ($PC\bar{x}$ minus $NC\bar{x}$) between the positive control mean for the BLV wells ($PC\bar{x}$) and the negative control mean for the BLV wells ($NC\bar{x}$) must be greater than or equal to 0.075.

The Positive Control has been standardized and contains a significant level of antibody to BLV. The normal host cell antigen provides a measure of the NHC contribution to the total BLV signal. The verification of samples reactive for antibody to BLV is determined by calculating the sample to NHC (S/NHC) ratio.

Interpretation of Results (Verification): Calculate S/P ratios as previously described.

Samples with S/P values less than 0.500 are negative.

Samples with S/P ratios greater than or equal to 0.500 on both the screening and verification assays can be confirmed by calculating the S/NHC ratio.

a. If the S/NHC ratio is less than 1.80, then the sample is classified as negative for antibodies to BLV.
b. If the S/NHC ratio is greater than or equal to 1.80, then the sample is classified as positive for BLV antibodies.

Calculations (Verification): Calculate the sample to normal host cell (S/NHC) ratio.

$$S/NHC = \frac{A(650){:}BLV}{A(650){:}NHC}$$

Example:

If A(650): BLV = 0.500, and the A(650): NHC = 0.100, then:

$$S/NHC = \frac{0.500}{0.100} = 5$$

Storage: Store all reagents at 2°-7°C (36°-45°F).

Caution(s):

1. Handle all BLV biological materials as though capable of transmitting BLV.
2. Do not pipet by mouth.
3. There should be no eating, drinking or smoking where specimens or kit reagents are being handled.
4. TMB and stop solutions may be irritating to the skin.
5. Do not expose TMB Substrate to strong light or any oxidizing agents. Handle the TMB Substrate with clean glass or plasticware.
6. Bring to room temperature (20°-25°C) prior to use, and return to 2°-7°C following use.
7. All wastes should be properly decontaminated prior to disposal.
8. Care should be taken to prevent the contamination of kit components.
9. Do not use components past expiration dates and do not intermix components from different serials.
10. Optimal results will be obtained by strict adherence to this protocol. Careful pipetting, timing and washing throughout this procedure are necessary to maintain precision and accuracy.

For veterinary use only.

Discussion: The bovine leukemia virus (BLV) is the causative agent of enzootic bovine leukosis in cattle. This is a highly fatal neoplasia of cattle characterized by the aggregation of neoplastic lymphocytes in lymph nodes. Clinical signs most commonly associated with infection include weight loss, decreased milk production, lymphadenopathy and posterior paresis. Diagnosis of BLV infection based on clinical signs alone is often difficult because of the wide range of symptoms. Once acquired, viral infection is lifelong and is spread by contact between animals. An assessment of exposure to BLV via natural infection can be made by measurement of specific antibody titer to BLV using an enzyme immunoassay system. A positive antibody titer to BLV indicates that the animal has been exposed to BLV and may be persistently and chronically infected.

References: Available upon request.

Presentation: 5 plates per kit.

HERDCHEK is a registered trademark of Idexx Laboratories, Inc. in the United States and/or other countries.

Compendium Code No.: 11160312 06-03600-01

HERDCHEK® BRUCELLA ABORTUS ANTIBODY TEST KIT

Idexx Labs. **Brucella Test**

Brucella abortus Antibody Test Kit

U.S. Vet. Lic. No.: 313

Components:

Reagents	Volume	
	6 Plate	30 Plate
A. *B. abortus* LPS Coated Plates		
B. Anti-Bovine IgG:Horseradish Peroxidase (HRPO) Conjugate in buffer with protein stabilizers	60	315 mL
C. *B. abortus* Positive Control Bovine anti-*B. abortus* in buffer with protein stabilizers, preserved with sodium azide	14	14 mL
D. *B. abortus* Negative Control - Milk-based control non-reactive to *B. abortus* in buffer with protein stabilizers, preserved with sodium azide	14	14 mL
E. Sample Diluent- Buffer with protein stabilizers, preserved with sodium azide	235	700 mL
F. Wash Concentrate - 10x phosphate/Tween wash, preserved with gentamicin	235	960 mL
G. TMB Substrate 3, 3', 5, 5', Tetramethylbenzidine	60	315 mL
H. Stop Solution	60	315 mL

Materials Required But Not Provided:

1. Precision Pipets or multiple delivery pipetting devices suitable for delivering 10, 100, 200 and 400 µL
2. Disposable pipet tips
3. 500 mL graduated cylinder for wash solution
4. 96-well plate reader
5. Glass or plastic tubes for sample dilution
6. Distilled or deionized water
7. Device for the delivery and aspiration of wash solution
8. A vacuum source, a trap for retaining aspirate and disinfectant

Indications: HERDCHEK® Anti-*Brucella abortus* is Idexx's enzyme immunoassay for the detection of antibody to *Brucella abortus* in bovine milk using *Brucella abortus* LPS antigens. This test has been validated on herds up to 1000 animals. Larger herds will require multiple samples.

Test Principles: HERDCHEK® Anti-*B. abortus* is an enzyme immunoassay designed to detect the presence of antibody to *B. abortus* in bovine milk. A microtitration format has been configured by immobilizing *B. abortus* LPS antigens on the plate. *B. abortus* is propagated in standard microbiological media. Upon incubation of the test sample in the antigen coated well, antibody specific to *B. abortus* forms a complex with the immobilized antigens. After washing away unbound materials from the wells, an anti-bovine IgG:Horseradish Peroxidase conjugate is added which binds to any bovine antibody attached in the wells. Next, unbound conjugate is washed away and a substrate/chromogen solution is added. In the presence of enzyme, substrate is converted into a product which reacts with the chromogen to generate a blue color. The absorbance at a wavelength between 620 and 650 nm [A(650)] is measured using a spectrophotometer. This absorbance is proportional to the amount of specific antibody in the test sample.

Test Procedure:

Preparation of Samples: Dilute Milk samples (individual and bulk tank samples) two-fold (1:2) with Sample Diluent (e.g., by diluting 200 µL of milk with 200 µL Sample Diluent).

In order to standardize incubation times, samples should be prepared in dilution tubes. Then, it is possible to rapidly transfer (column by column) samples using a multi-channel pipet.

Subsequent additions of conjugate, substrate and stop solutions should also be pipetted in this manner.

Whole milk may be used as a sample although centrifugation to separate the cream will aid in sample pipetting.

Note: Do not dilute controls.

Be sure to change tips for each sample and record the position of each sample on the plate using a HerdChek® worksheet. Diluted samples should be mixed prior to dispensing into the antigen coated microtiter plate.

Preparation of Wash Solution: The 10x Wash Concentrate should be brought to room temperature and mixed to ensure dissolution of any precipitated salts. The Wash Concentrate must be diluted 1 to 10 with distilled/deionized water before use (e.g., 30 mL of concentrate plus 270 mL of water per plate to be assayed).

Note: When running milk samples, wash solution can be warmed to 37°C (98.6°F) to aid in removal of cream from the microtiter wells.

Test Protocol: All reagents must be allowed to come to room temperature before use. Reagents should be mixed by gentle swirling or vortexing.

1. Obtain antigen coated plate(s) and record the sample position on a HerdChek® worksheet.
2. Dispense 100 µL Negative Control into wells A1 and A2. Note: No dilution required.
3. Dispense 100 µL Positive Control into wells A3 and A4. Note: No dilution required.
4. Dispense 100 µL diluted samples into remaining wells.
5. Incubate for 90 minutes at 25°-30°C (77°-86°F). If desired, the use of a temperature controlled chamber may be utilized for sample incubations.
6. Aspirate liquid contents of all wells into an appropriate waste reservoir.
7. Wash each well with approximately 300 µL of wash solution four times. Aspirate liquid contents of all wells after each wash. Avoid plate drying between washes and prior to the addition of conjugate. Following the final aspiration, firmly tap residual wash fluid from each plate onto absorbent material.
8. Dispense 100 µL of Anti-Bovine IgG:HRPO Conjugate into each well.
9. Incubate for 30 minutes at 25°-30°C (77°-86°F).
10. Repeat steps 6 and 7.
11. Dispense 100 µL of TMB Substrate Solution into each well.
12. Incubate 15 minutes at 25°-30°C (77°-86°F).
13. Dispense 100 µL of Stop Solution into each well to stop the reaction.
14. Blank spectrophotometer on air.
15. Measure and record the A650 for samples and controls.
16. Calculate results.

Test Interpretation:

Results: For the assay to be valid, the difference (P-N) between the positive control mean ($PC\bar{x}$) and the negative control mean ($NC\bar{x}$) must be greater than or equal to 0.150 Optical Density (OD). In addition, the $NC\bar{x}$ must be less than or equal to 0.20 OD.

For invalid assays, technique may be suspect and the assay should be repeated following a thorough review of the package insert.

The presence or absence of antibody to *B. abortus* is determined by the sample to positive (S/P) ratio for each sample. The Positive Control has been standardized and represents a significant level of antibody to *B. abortus*.

See Calculations for examples.

Note: Idexx Laboratories, Inc. has instrument and software systems available which calculate means and S/P ratios and provide data summaries.

Interpretation of Results:

I. United States:

A. Individual Milk Samples:

Individual milk samples with S/P values less than 1.0 are considered negative for *B. abortus* antibodies.

Individual milk samples with S/P values between 1.0 and 1.49 are considered suspect and should be re-tested.

Individual milk samples with S/P values greater than or equal to 1.50 are considered positive for *B. abortus* antibodies.

B. Pooled or Bulk Tank:

Pooled or bulk tank samples with S/P values less than 0.75 are considered negative for *B. abortus* antibodies.

Pooled or bulk tank samples with S/P values between 0.75 and 1.49 are considered suspect and should be re-tested.

Pooled or bulk tank samples with S/P values greater than or equal to 1.50 are considered positive for *B. abortus* antibodies.

II. International:

The international cutoffs have been established so that they conform to sensitivity requirements dictated by European Community (EC) directives.

The positive control has been standardized to the 2nd International Brucellosis Standard Serum produced by the Central Veterinary Laboratory, Weybridge, England.

Milk samples with S/P ratios less than 0.25 are classified as negative for *B. abortus* antibodies.

Milk samples with S/P ratios greater than or equal to 0.25 but less than 0.50 are considered suspect and must be retested.

Milk samples with S/P ratios of 0.50 and greater are considered positive for *B. abortus* antibodies.

Calculations:

1. Calculation of negative control mean ($NC\bar{x}$):

$$NC\bar{x} = \frac{A1\ A(650) + A2\ A(650)}{2}$$

Example:

$$\frac{0.67 + 0.073}{2} = 0.070$$

2. Calculation of positive control mean ($PC\bar{x}$):

$$PC\bar{x} = \frac{A3\ A(650) + A4\ A(650)}{2}$$

Example:

$$\frac{0.333 + 0.347}{2} = 0.340$$

3. Calculation of S/P ratio:

$$S/P = \frac{\text{Sample } A(650) - NC\bar{x}}{PC\bar{x} - NC\bar{x}}$$

Example: Sample mean = 0.347

$$S/P = \frac{0.347 - 0.070}{0.340 - 0.070} = \frac{0.277}{0.270} = 1.03$$

4. Calculation of cutoff level; OD(650).

$S/P = ((PC\bar{x} - NC\bar{x}) \times 0.5) + NC\bar{x}$

Example: $((0.340 - 0.070) \times 0.5) + 0.070 = 0.205$

Storage: Store all reagents at 2°-7°C (36°-45°F).

Caution(s):

1. Handle all *B. abortus* biological material as though capable of transmitting *B. abortus*.
2. Do not pipet by mouth.
3. There should be no eating, drinking, or smoking where specimens or kit reagents are being handled.
4. TMB and stop solutions may be irritating to the skin.
5. Some kit components contain sodium azide as a preservative. Disposal requires flushing plumbing with large volumes of water to prevent formation of copper or lead azide complexes which may explode upon percussion.
6. Do not expose TMB solutions to strong light or any oxidizing agents. Handle all TMB solutions with clean glass or plasticware.
7. Bring to room temperature 21°-26°C (70°-79°F) prior to use and return to 2°-7°C (36°-45°F) following use.
8. All wastes should be properly decontaminated prior to disposal.
9. Care should be taken to prevent contamination of kit components.
10. Do not use components past expiration dates and do not intermix components from different serials.
11. Optimal results will be obtained by strict adherence to this protocol. Careful pipetting, timing and washing throughout this procedure are necessary to maintain precision and accuracy.

For veterinary use only.

Discussion: Brucellosis in cattle is a disease caused by *Brucella abortus (B. abortus)*, a facultative, intracellular bacterium. The major mode of disease transmission is by ingestion of *B. abortus* organisms that may be present in tissues of aborted fetuses, fetal membranes and uterine fluids. In addition, infection may occur as the result of cattle ingesting *B. abortus* contaminated feed or water. Infection in cows also has occurred through venereal transmission of the organisms by infected bulls.[1]

Abortion is the most outstanding clinical feature of the disease. If a carrier state develops in a majority of infected cows in a herd, the clinical manifestations may be reduced milk production, dead calves at term, and/or a higher frequency of retained placenta. Disease in the bull may produce infections of the seminal vesicles and testicles resulting in shedding of the organisms in semen.

Diagnosis is based on serological (serum/milk) and/or bacteriological procedures. While a positive bacteriological finding is the most definite diagnosis, several weeks may be required to obtain final culture results. The success of disease eradication is dependent upon the accurate identification and elimination of *B. abortus* reactors in a herd.[1] Reliable serological techniques for *B. abortus* provide rapid and accurate assessments of antibody to *B. abortus* in milk samples.

References: Available upon request.

Presentation: 6 plate and 30 plate kits.

HERDCHEK is a registered trademark of Idexx Laboratories, Inc. in the United States and/or other countries.

Compendium Code No.: 11160232 06-01077-06

HERDCHEK® IBR ANTIBODY TEST KIT

Idexx Labs. **IBR Test**

Bovine Rhinotracheitis Virus Antibody Test Kit (Screening/Verification)

U.S. Vet. Lic. No.: 313

Components:

Reagents	Volume	
	6 Plate	30 Plate
A. Infectious Bovine Rhinotracheitis (IBR) Viral Antigen Coated Plates/Strips		
B. Infectious Bovine Rhinotracheitis Antigen/Normal Host Cell Antigen (IBR/NHC) Coated Strips		
C. IBR Anti-Bovine IgG:Horseradish Peroxidase (HRPO) Conjugate in buffer with protein stabilizers	60	315 mL
D. IBR Positive Control Bovine anti-IBR in buffer with protein stabilizers, preserved with sodium azide	14	14 mL
E. IBR Negative Control - Bovine serum non-reactive to IBR in buffer with protein stabilizers preserved with sodium azide	14	14 mL
F. IBR Sample Diluent Buffer with protein stabilizers preserved with sodium azide	235	350 mL
G. Wash Concentrate (10X) 10x phosphate/Tween wash preserved with gentamicin	235	480 mL
H. TMB Substrate-3,3', 5,5' Tetramethylbenzidine	60	315 mL
I. Stop Solution	60	315 mL

Materials Required But Not Provided:

1. Precision pipettes or multiple delivery pipetting devices suitable for delivering 10, 100, 200 and 240 µL.
2. Disposable pipet tips.
3. 500 mL graduated cylinder for wash solution.
4. 96-well plate reader.
5. Glass or plastic tubes for sample dilution.
6. Distilled or deionized water.
7. Device for the delivery and aspiration of wash solution.
8. A vacuum source, and a trap for retaining aspirate and disinfectant.

Indications: HERDCHEK® Anti-IBR is Idexx's enzyme immunoassay for the detection and verification of antibody to Infectious Bovine Rhinotracheitis Virus (IBR) in bovine serum or milk using IBR and normal host cell (NHC) antigens.

Test Principles: Description and Principles: HERDCHEK® Anti-IBR is an enzyme immunoassay designed to detect the presence of antibody to IBR in bovine serum or milk. A microtitration format has been configured by immobilizing IBR viral antigens on the plate. Upon incubation of the test sample in the antigen-coated well, antibody specific to IBR forms a complex with the immobilized viral antigens. After washing away unbound materials from the wells, an anti-bovine IgG:Horseradish Peroxidase conjugate is added which binds to bovine antibody attached in the wells. Next, unbound conjugate is washed away and a substrate/chromogen solution is added. In the presence of enzyme, substrate is converted into a product which reacts with the chromogen to generate a blue color. The absorbance at a wavelength between 620 and 650 nm [A(650)] is measured using a spectrophotometer. This absorbance is proportional to the amount of specific antibody in the test sample.

A verification plate has been included to verify positive results. In this format, IBR and NHC antigens are immobilized in alternate columns. The immobilized NHC antigens are used to determine if immunoglobulins against tissue culture components present in vaccines are contributing to test results. The extent of host cell contribution to the total signal is assessed by relating IBR reactivity to NHC activity.

Test Procedure:

Preparation of Samples: Dilute Serum samples twenty-five-fold (1:25) with Sample Diluent (e.g., by diluting 10 µL of serum with 240 µL of Sample Diluent).

In order to standardize incubation times, samples should be prepared in dilution tubes. Then it is possible to rapidly transfer (column by column) samples using a multi-channel pipet.

Subsequent additions of Conjugate, Substrate and Stop Solutions should also be pipetted in this manner.

Whole milk may be used as a sample although centrifugation to separate the cream will aid in sample pipetting.

Dilute Milk samples (including pooled milk) two-fold (1:2) with Sample Diluent (e.g., by diluting 200 µL of milk with 200 µL Sample Diluent).

Note: Do not dilute controls.

Be sure to change tips for each sample and record the position of each sample on the plate using a HerdChek® worksheet. Diluted samples should be mixed prior to dispensing into the antigen coated microtiter plate.

Preparation of Wash Solution: The 10X Wash Concentrate should be brought to room temperature and mixed to ensure dissolution of any precipitated salts. The Wash Concentrate must be diluted 1 to 10 with distilled/deionized water before use (e.g., 30 mL of concentrate plus 270 mL of water per plate to be assayed.

Test Protocol (Screening): All reagents must be allowed to come to room temperature before use. Reagents should be mixed by gentle swirling or vortexing.

1. Obtain antigen coated plate(s) and record the sample position on a HerdChek® worksheet.
2. Dispense 100 µL of Negative Control into wells A1 and A2. Note: No dilution required.
3. Dispense 100 µL of Positive Control into wells A3 and A4. Note: No dilution required.
4. Dispense 100 µL diluted samples into remaining wells.
5. Incubate for 90 minutes at room temperature (20-25°C). If desired, the use of a temperature controlled chamber may be utilized for sample incubations. Samples may be incubated overnight at 2-7°C (12-18 hours). If this option is chosen, tightly seal plates to avoid any evaporation.
6. Aspirate liquid contents of all wells into an appropriate waste reservoir.
7. Wash each well with approximately 300 µL of wash solution four times. Aspirate liquid contents of all wells after each wash. Avoid plate drying between plate washings and prior to the addition of conjugate. Following the final aspiration, firmly tap residual wash fluid from each plate onto absorbent material.
8. Dispense 100 µL of Anti-Bovine IgG:HRPO Conjugate into each well.
9. Incubate for 30 minutes at room temperature (20-25°C).
10. Repeat steps 6 and 7.
11. Dispense 100 µL of TMB Substrate Solution into each well.
12. Incubate 15 minutes at room temperature (20-25°C).
13. Dispense 100 µL of Stop Solution into each well to stop the reaction.
14. Blank spectrophotometer on air.
15. Measure and record the A650 for samples and controls.
16. Calculate results.

Test Protocol (Verification):

Preparation of Samples: Dilute Serum samples twenty-five-fold (1:25) with Sample Diluent (e.g., by diluting 10 µL of serum with 240 µL of Sample Diluent).

Whole milk may be used as a sample although centrifugation to separate the cream will aid in sample pipetting.

Dilute Milk (including pooled milk), two-fold (1:2) with Sample Diluent (e.g., by diluting 200 µL of milk with 200 µL of Sample Diluent).

Note: Do not dilute controls.

Be sure to change tips for each sample and record the position of each sample on the plate using a HerdChek® worksheet. Diluted samples should be mixed prior to dispensing into the antigen coated microtiter plate.

	IBR	NHC	IBR	NHC	IBR	NHC	IBR	NHC	IBR	NHC	IBR	NHC
A	N	N	5	5								
B	N	N	6	6								
C	P	P										
D	P	P										
E	1	1										
F	2	2										
G	3	3										
H	4	4										
	1	2	3	4	5	6	7	8	9	10	11	12

N = Negative Control
P = Positive Control
1, 2, 3, etc. = Sample #
Columns 1, 3, 5, 7, 9, 11 coated with IBR antigen
Columns 2, 4, 6, 8, 10, 12 coated with NHC antigen

1. Obtain IBR and NHC coated strips and record sample position on a HerdChek® worksheet.
2. Dispense 100 µL Negative Control into IBR wells A1, B1 and NHC wells A2 and B2. Note: No dilution required.
3. Dispense 100 µL Positive Control into IBR wells C1, D1 and NHC wells C2 and D2. Note: No dilution required.
4. Dispense 100 µL diluted samples into adjacent IBR and NHC wells.
5. Incubate for 90 minutes at room temperature (20°-25°C). If desired, the use of a temperature controlled chamber may be utilized for sample incubations. Sample may be incubated overnight at 2°-7°C (12-18 hours). If this option is chosen, tightly seal plates to avoid any evaporation.
6. Aspirate liquid contents of all wells into an appropriate waste reservoir.
7. Wash each well with approximately 300 µL of wash solution four times. Aspirate liquid contents of all wells after each wash. Avoid plate drying between plate washings and prior to the addition of conjugate. Following the final aspiration, firmly tap residual wash fluid from each plate onto absorbent material.
8. Dispense 100 µL of Anti-Bovine IgG:HRPO Conjugate into each well.
9. Incubate for 30 minutes at room temperature (20-25°C).
10. Repeat steps 6 and 7.
11. Dispense 100 µL of TMB Substrate Solution into each well.
12. Incubate 15 minutes at room temperature (20°-25°C).
13. Dispense 100 µL of Stop Solution into each well to stop the reaction.
14. Blank spectrophotometer on air.
15. Measure and record the A650 for samples and controls.
16. Calculate results.

Test Interpretation:

Results (Screening): For the assay to be valid, the difference (P-N) between the positive control mean ($PC\bar{x}$) and the negative control mean ($NC\bar{x}$) must be greater than or equal to 0.200 Optical Density (OD). In addition, the $NC\bar{x}$ must be less than or equal to 0.25 OD.

For invalid assays, technique may be suspect and the assay should be repeated following a thorough review of the package insert.

The presence or absence of antibody to IBR is determined by the sample to positive (S/P) ratio for each sample. The Positive Control has been standardized and contains a significant level of antibody to IBR.

See Calculations for examples.

Note: Idexx Laboratories, Inc. has instrument and software systems available which calculate means and S/P ratios and provide data summaries.

Interpretation of Results (Screening):

1. Milk and serum samples with S/P ratios less than 0.250 are classified as negative for IBR antibodies.
2. Milks and serum samples with S/P ratios greater than or equal to 0.250 but less than 0.500 are considered suspect and must be confirmed using the verification format.
3. Milk and serum samples with S/P ratios of 0.500 and greater are considered positive for IBR antibodies and do not require verification.

Calculations: (Screening):

1. Calculation of negative control mean ($NC\bar{x}$):

$$NC\bar{x} = \frac{A1\ A(650) + A2\ A(650)}{2}$$

Example:

$$\frac{0.67 + 0.073}{2} = 0.070$$

2. Calculation of positive control mean ($PC\bar{x}$):

$$PC\bar{x} = \frac{A3\ A(650) + A4\ A(650)}{2}$$

Example:

$$\frac{0.333 + 0.347}{2} = 0.340$$

3. Calculation of S/P ratio:

$$S/P = \frac{\text{Sample } A(650) - NC\bar{x}}{PC\bar{x} - NC\bar{x}}$$

Example: Sample mean = 0.347

$$S/P = \frac{0.347 - 0.070}{0.340 - 0.070} = \frac{0.277}{0.270} = 1.03$$

4. Calculation of cutoff level; OD(650).

$OD = ((PC\bar{x} - NC\bar{x}) \times 0.25) + NC\bar{x}$

Example: $((0.340 - 0.070) \times 0.25) + 0.070 = 0.138$

Results (Verification): For the assay to be valid the following specifications must be met.

The mean negative control absorbance value for the IBR wells (NC:IBR) must be less than or equal to 0.25 OD. The difference between the positive control for the IBR well (PC:IBR) and the NC:IBR must be greater than or equal to 0.200 OD. The mean negative control for the NHC well (NC:NHC) must be less than or equal to 0.25 OD.

The Positive Control has been standardized and represents a significant level of antibody to IBR. The normal host cell antigen provides a measure of the NHC contribution to the total IBR signal. The verification of samples reactive for antibody to IBR is determined by calculating the sample to NHC (S/NHC) ratio for each sample.

Interpretation of Results (Verification): Calculate S/P ratios as previously described, ignoring NHC values.

Samples with S/P values less than 0.250 are negative.

Samples that give S/P values greater than or equal to 0.250 can be verified by calculating the S/NHC ratio.

a. If the S/NHC ratio is less than 1.80, then the sample is classified as a negative, non-confirming sample.
b. If the S/NHC ratio is greater than or equal to 1.80, then the sample is classified as a verified positive for IBR antibodies.

Calculations (Verification): Calculate the sample to normal host cell (S/NHC) ratio. This ratio should be calculated only when the S/P ratio for the sample was ≥0.250 and less than 0.500.

$$\text{Sample S/NHC} = \frac{\text{Sample } A(650)\text{:IBR}}{\text{Sample } A(650)\text{:NHC}}$$

Example:

If Sample A(650):IBR = 0.500, and sample A(650):NHC = 0.100, then:

$$S/NHC = \frac{0.500}{0.100} = 5$$

Storage: Store all reagents at 2°-7°C (36°-45°F). For veterinary use only.

Caution(s):

1. Handle all IBR biological material as though capable of transmitting IBR.

2. Do not pipette by mouth.
3. No eating, drinking or smoking where specimens or kit reagents are being handled.
4. TMB and Stop solutions may be irritating to the skin.
5. Some kit components contain sodium azide as a preservative. Disposal requires flushing plumbing with large volumes of water to prevent formation of copper or lead azide complexes which may explode upon percussion.
6. Do not expose TMB solutions to strong light or any oxidizing agents. Handle the TMB Substrate with clean glass or plasticware.
7. Bring to room temperature (20°-25°C) prior to use, and return to 2°-7°C following use.
8. All wastes should be properly decontaminated prior to disposal.
9. Care should be taken to prevent the contamination of kit components.
10. Do not use components past expiration dates and do not intermix components from different serials.
11. Optimal results will be obtained by strict adherence to this protocol. Careful pipetting and washing throughout the procedure is necessary to maintain precision and accuracy.

Discussion: Infectious Bovine Rhinotracheitis is a highly contagious, infectious disease that is caused by Bovine Herpesvirus-1 (BHV-1). In addition to causing respiratory disease, this virus can cause conjunctivitis, vulvovaginitis, abortions, encephalitis and generalized systemic infections.[1] Although clinical findings may be highly suggestive of IBR, no real pathopneumonic signs are restricted to IBR. Therefore, laboratory confirmation is necessary in order to definitely identify BHV-1 infection.[2] Confirmation of exposure to BHV-1 via natural infection is facilitated by a measurement of antibody in serum or milk.

The enzyme-linked immunoabsorbent assay (ELISA) for the detection of antibodies against BHV-1 in cattle has been shown to correlate with the virus neutralization test (VN), although it can be more sensitive.[3,4,5]

References: Available upon request.

Presentation: 6 plate kits and 30 plate kits.

HERDCHEK is a registered trademark of Idexx Laboratories, Inc. in the United States and/or other countries.

Compendium Code No.: 11160322 06-01021-06

HERDCHEK® M HYO ANTIBODY TEST KIT

Idexx Labs. **Mycoplasma Test**

Mycoplasma Hyopneumoniae Antibody Test Kit

U.S. Vet. Lic. No.: 313

Components:

Reagent	Volume
A. M hyo Coated Plates	5
B. Anti-porcine: Horseradish Peroxidase (HRPO) Conjugate. Contains gentamicin as a preservative.	60 mL
C. M hyo Positive Control - Anti-M hyo in buffer with protein stabilizers, preserved with sodium azide	4 mL
D. Negative Control - Porcine serum non-reactive to M hyo in buffer with protein stabilizers. Preserved with sodium azide	4 mL
E. Sample Diluent - buffer with protein stabilizers, preserved with sodium azide	235 mL
F. Wash Concentrate (10X) Phosphate buffer preserved with gentamicin	235 mL
G. TMB Substrate	60 mL
H. Stop Solution	60 mL

Materials Required but Not Provided: Precision pipets and multiple delivery pipetting device with disposable pipet tips, 96-well plate reader, tubes for diluting samples, distilled or deionized water and device for the delivery and aspiration of wash solution.

Indications: HERDCHEK® M live, is Idexx's enzyme immunoassay for the detection of antibody to *Mycoplasma hyopneumoniae* (M hyo) in porcine serum and plasma.

Test Principles: This assay is designed to measure the relative level of antibody to M hyo in swine serum and plasma. Antigen is coated on 96-well plates. Upon incubation of the test sample in the coated well, antibody specific to M hyo forms a complex with the coated antigens. After washing away unbound material from the wells, a conjugate is added which binds to any attached porcine antibody in the wells. Unbound conjugate is washed away and enzyme substrate is added. Subsequent color development is directly related to the amount of antibody to M hyo present in the test sample.

Test Procedure:

Preparation of Samples: Dilute test samples forty fold (1:40) with sample diluent prior to being assayed (e.g., by diluting 10 µL of sample with 390 µL of Sample Diluent). Note: Do not dilute controls. Be sure to change tips for each sample. Diluted samples must be thoroughly mixed prior to dispensing into the coated plate. Record the position of each sample on the plate using a worksheet.

Preparation of Wash Solution: The 10X Wash Concentrate should be brought to room temperature 20°-27°C (68°-80°F) and mixed to ensure dissolution of any precipitated salts. The Wash Concentrate must be diluted 1:10 with distilled/deionized water before use (e.g. 30 mL of concentrate plus 270 mL of water per plate to be assayed).

Allow the reagents to come to room temperature, then mix gently by inverting and swirling.
1. Obtain antigen-coated plate(s) and record the sample position on a worksheet.
2. Dispense 100 µL of Undiluted Negative Control into wells A1 and B1.
3. Dispense 100 µL of Undiluted Positive Control into wells C1 and D1.
4. Dispense 100 µL of diluted sample into appropriate wells.
5. Incubate for 30 minutes at room temperature.
6. Aspirate liquid contents of all wells into appropriate waste reservoir.
7. Wash each well with approximately 350 µL of wash solution 3-5 times. Aspirate completely.
8. Dispense 100 µL of Anti-Porcine: Horseradish Peroxidase Conjugate into each well.
9. Incubate for 30 minutes at room temperature.
10. Repeat steps 6 and 7.
11. Dispense 100 µL of TMB substrate solution into each well.
12. Incubate for 15 minutes at room temperature.
13. Dispense 100 µL of Stop Solution into each well to stop the reaction.
14. Blank reader with air.
15. Measure and record absorbance values at 650nm, A(650).

Test Interpretation:

Results: For the assay to be valid, the difference between the Positive Control mean and the Negative Control mean ($PC\bar{x}$ - $NC\bar{x}$) should be greater than or equal to 0.150. The Negative Control mean absorbance should be less than or equal to 0.150. The presence or absence of antibody to M hyo is determined by relating the A(650) value of the unknown to the Positive Control mean. The Positive Control is standardized and represents significant antibody levels to M hyo in swine serum and plasma. The relative level of antibody in the unknown is determined by calculating the sample to positive (S/P) ratio.

Interpretation of Results:
1. Samples with S/P ratios less than 0.3 are considered negative within the limits of the test.
2. Samples with S/P ratios from 0.3 to 0.4 are classified as suspect for M hyo antibodies.
3. Samples with S/P ratios greater than 0.4 are considered positive.

Calculations:
1. Negative Control mean ($NC\bar{x}$):

$$\frac{\text{Well A1 A(650)} + \text{Well B1 A(650)}}{2} = NC\bar{x}$$

2. Positive Control mean ($PC\bar{x}$):

$$\frac{\text{Well C1 A(650)} + \text{Well D1 A(650)}}{2} = PC\bar{x}$$

3. S/P Ratio:

$$\frac{\text{Sample A(650)} - NC\bar{x}}{PC\bar{x} - NC\bar{x}} = S/P$$

4. Titer - relates S/P at a 1:40 dilution to an endpoint titer:

$\log_{10}$ Titer = 1.09 ($\log_{10}$ S/P) + 3.36

Storage: Do not expose TMB solution to strong light or any oxidation agents. Store all reagents at 2°-7°C (36°-45°F).

Caution(s): Handle all M hyo biological materials as though capable of transmitting M hyo. The antigen coated plates may be a source of M hyo. Prior to coating on the solid phase, the antigen has been inactivated by chemical treatment. Nevertheless, do not assume complete inactivation. Some kit components contain sodium azide as a preservative. Disposal requires flushing plumbing with large volumes of water to prevent formation of copper or lead azide complexes which may explode upon percussion.

All wastes should be properly decontaminated prior to disposal. Do not use components past expiration date and do not intermix components from kits with different lot numbers. Careful pipetting and washing throughout this procedure are necessary to maintain precision and accuracy. Optimal results will be obtained by strict adherence to this protocol. For veterinary use only.

Discussion: Enzootic pneumonia or Mycoplasmal Pneumonia of Swine (MPS), a chronic disease with a high morbidity and a low mortality, is caused by *Mycoplasma hyopneumoniae*. The clinical signs include a chronic non-productive cough, retarded growth, slow onset and spread, and repeated occurrence of the disease.[1] The M hyo antibody ELISA allows rapid screening for the presence of antibodies to *Mycoplasma hyopneumoniae*, which can be an indicator of exposure to the agent. Monitoring the immune status of a herd with regard to M hyo can play an important role in the control of this disease.

References: Available upon request.

Presentation: 5 plates per kit.

HERDCHEK is a registered trademark of Idexx Laboratories, Inc. in the United States and/or other countries.

Compendium Code No.: 11160591 06-04174-00

HERDCHEK® M.pt. ANTIBODY TEST KIT

Idexx Labs. **Mycobacterium Test**

Mycobacterium paratuberculosis Antibody Test Kit

U.S. Vet. Lic. No.: 313

Components:

Reagents	Volume
A. *M.pt.* Coated Strips/Plates	5
B. HRPO Conjugate	60 mL
C. Positive Control - Bovine anti-*M.pt.* in buffer with protein stabilizers. Preserved with Sodium Azide.	3 mL
D. Negative Control - Bovine serum non-reactive to *M.pt.* in buffer with protein stabilizers. Preserved with Sodium Azide.	3 mL
E. Sample Diluent - Buffer with protein stabilizers. Preserved with Sodium Azide.	235 mL
F. Wash Concentrate (10X) - contains gentamicin sulfate	235 mL
G. TMB Substrate	60 mL
H. Stop Solution	60 mL

Materials Required But Not Provided:
1. Precision Pipets. Suitable for delivering 0.005, 0.100 mL and 0.500 mL or multiple delivery pipetting devices.
2. Disposable pipet tips.
3. Graduated cylinder: 500 mL for wash solution.
4. 96 Well Plate Reader.
5. Glass or plastic tubes for diluting samples.
6. Distilled or deionized water.
7. Device for the delivery and aspiration of wash solution.
8. A vacuum source and a trap for retaining the aspirate.

Indications: The Idexx *Mycobacterium paratuberculosis* Antibody Test Kit is an enzyme-linked immunoassay for the detection of antibody to *Mycobacterium paratuberculosis (M.pt.)* in bovine serum or plasma. This test is to be used as an initial screening method.

Test Principles: The Idexx *Mycobacterium paratuberculosis* Antibody Test Kit is designed to detect the presence of antibody to *M.pt.* in bovine serum or plasma. A microtitration format has been developed in which *M.pt.* antigens are coated on 96-well plates, or strips. Samples are diluted in Sample Diluent containing *M.phlei* to remove crossreacting antibodies. Upon incubation of the diluted sample in the coated well, antibody specific to *M.pt.* forms a complex with the coated antigens. After washing away unbound materials from the wells, a horseradish peroxidase (HRPO) conjugate is added which binds to immunoglobulins bound to the solid-phase antigen. In the final step of the assay, unbound conjugate is washed away, and enzyme substrate is added to the wells. The rate of conversion of substrate is proportional to the amount of bound immunoglobulin. Subsequent color, measured spectrophotometrically, is proportional to the amount of antibody present in the test sample.

Test Procedure:

Preparation of Samples: Dilute test samples twenty-fold (1:20) with Sample Diluent (e.g., by diluting 25 µL of sample with 475 µL of Sample Diluent). Note: Do not dilute controls.

Be sure to change tips for each sample and record the position of each sample on the plate using a HerdChek® worksheet. Samples should be mixed prior to dispensing into the *M.pt.* coated plate.

Preparation of Wash Solution: The Wash Concentrate should be brought to room temperature and mixed to assure dissolution of any precipitated salts. The Wash Concentrate must be diluted 1 to 10 with distilled/deionized water before use (e.g., 30 mL of concentrate plus 270 mL of water per plate to be assayed).

All reagents and serum samples must be allowed to come to room temperature before use. Reagents should be mixed by gentle swirling or vortexing.

1. Obtain antigen coated plate(s) and record the sample position on a HerdChek® worksheet.
2. Dilute samples in Sample Diluent at the recommended dilution factor and allow to incubate for 30 minutes.
3. Dispense 100 µL of Undiluted Negative Control into wells A1 and A2.
4. Dispense 100 µL of Undiluted Positive Control into wells A3 and A4.
5. Dispense 100 µL of Diluted samples into appropriate wells. It is recommended that serum samples be run in duplicate but a single well test is acceptable.
6. Incubate for 30 minutes at room temperature.
7. Aspirate liquid contents of all wells into appropriate waste reservoir.
8. Wash each well with approximately 300 µL of phosphate buffered wash solution four times. Aspirate liquid contents of all wells after each wash. Avoid plate drying between plate washings and prior to the addition of conjugate. Following the final wash fluid aspiration, gently, but firmly tap residual wash fluid from each plate onto absorbent material.
9. Dispense 100 µL of HRPO Conjugate into each well.
10. Incubate for 30 minutes at room temperature.
11. Repeat steps 7 and 8.
12. Dispense 100 µL of TMB Substrate Solution into each well.
    Note: All wells should be observed for color development during the first 1-3 minutes of incubation with substrate. Abnormal color development includes variation within areas or "spots" in the well. If this occurs, the results for those samples should be considered invalid and the samples should be re-tested in duplicate using a fresh dilution. However, the other results on the plate may be considered valid.
13. Incubate for 15 minutes at room temperature.
14. Dispense 100 µL of Stop Solution into each well of the test plate to stop the reaction.
15. Blank on air.
16. Measure and record the absorbance at 620 nm, 630 nm or 650 nm.
17. Calculate results.

Test Interpretation:

Assay Validity: The parameters listed below should be confirmed for validation of each plate assayed.

-The optical density (OD) of the negative control should be less than 0.12 (using a 650 nm filter).

-The difference between the mean positive control OD ($PC\bar{x}$) and the mean negative control OD ($NC\bar{x}$) should be greater than 0.15.

If either value is outside of the described limits, the results from the plate are considered invalid. The assay should be repeated following a thorough review of the package insert.

As a guideline, the difference in OD values between positive control wells should not deviate more than 20%. This is derived by: dividing the difference between the positive controls (A3, A4) by the mean of the positive control (A3, A4), then multiplying the answer by 100.

Note: The Idexx *M.pt.* Antibody Test Kit is optimized using a plate reader equipped with a 650 nm filter. Other filters may be used, as noted in step 16, but will yield somewhat lower optical density values. The use of 630 nm or 620 nm filters will lower the optical densities by approximately 12% and 25%, respectively. The use of alternative filters will not affect test results.

Results: The presence or absence of antibody to *M.pt.* is determined by the sample to positive (S/P) ratio for each sample. The positive control has been standardized and represents a significant level of antibody to *M.pt.* in bovine serum.

See Calculations for examples.

Note: Idexx Laboratories, Inc., has instrument and software systems available which calculate means and S/P ratios and provide data summaries.

Interpretation of Results:

1. Serum samples with S/P ratios of less than 0.25 are classified as Negative for *M.pt.* antibodies.
2. If the S/P ratio is greater than or equal to 0.25, the sample is classified Positive for *M.pt.* antibodies.

Calculations:

1. Calculation of Negative Control Mean ($NC\bar{x}$):

$$NC\bar{x} = \frac{A1\ A(650) + A2\ A(650)}{2}$$

Example:

$$\frac{0.080 + 0.090}{2} = 0.085$$

2. Calculation of Positive Control Mean ($PC\bar{x}$):

$$PC\bar{x} = \frac{A3\ A(650) + A4\ A(650)}{2}$$

Example:

$$\frac{0.510 + 0.500}{2} = 0.505$$

3. Calculation of S/P Ratio:

$$S/P = \frac{\text{Sample A} - NC\bar{x}}{PC\bar{x} - NC\bar{x}}$$

Example: Sample Mean = 0.450

$$S/P = \frac{0.450 - 0.085}{0.505 - 0.085} = \frac{0.365}{0.420} = 0.87$$

Storage: Store all reagents at 2°-7°C.

Caution(s):

1. Handle all *M.pt.* biological materials as though capable of transmitting *M.pt.* although the organism has been disrupted.
2. Do not pipet by mouth.
3. There should be no eating, drinking or smoking where specimens or kit reagents are being handled.
4. TMB Substrate and stop solutions may be irritating to the skin.
5. Some kit components contain sodium azide as a preservative. Care should be taken to prevent the contamination of the HRPO Conjugate with this preservative.
6. Do not expose TMB Solution to strong light or any oxidizing agents. Handle TMB substrate Solution with clean glass or plasticware.
7. The HRPO conjugate may be adversely affected by very small amounts of immunoglobulins, which can come from serum samples. This can cause low sample or positive control optical densities and questionable or invalid assays. Take steps to prevent this by handling samples away from conjugate solutions. It is recommended to use sterile, disposable weigh boats or reservoirs for the conjugate solutions. Do not pour any unused conjugate solution back into the original container.
8. Bring to room temperature prior to use, and return to 2°-7°C following use.
9. All wastes should be properly decontaminated prior to disposal.
10. Care should be taken to prevent contamination of kit components.
11. Do not use components past expiration date and do not intermix components from different serials.
12. Optimal results will be obtained by strict adherence to this protocol. Careful pipetting, timing and washing throughout this procedure are necessary to maintain precision and accuracy.

For veterinary use only.

Discussion: Johne's disease is a chronic, debilitating enteritis of ruminants caused by infection with *M.pt.* During the active stage of infection and prior to onset of clinical disease, cattle generally develop antibodies to *M.pt.* antigens. Uninfected cattle lack specific antibodies to *M.pt.* but may have cross-reacting antibodies to other mycobacteria. These crossreacting antibodies can be removed by absorption of the serum or plasma sample with *M.phlei* antigens prior to commencement of the enzyme-linked immunosorbent assay.[1,2]

This test is a solid phase, enzyme-linked immunosorbent assay (ELISA) and may be used as a specific test for Johne's disease in cattle. In this test, cross-reacting antibodies are removed in a rapid absorption step where *M.phlei* antigens are included in the Sample Diluent. This test shows a sensitivity in excess of 50% and a specificity above 99%.[3,4] This is similar to performance characteristics of fecal culture in a single herd test.

References: Available upon request.

Presentation: 5 plates per kit (strips).

HERDCHEK is a registered trademark of Idexx Laboratories, Inc in the United States and/or other countries.

Compendium Code No.: 11160252 06-03120-02

HERDCHEK® MYCOBACTERIUM PARATUBERCULOSIS DNA TEST KIT

Idexx Labs. **Mycobacterium Test**

Mycobacterium Paratuberculosis DNA Test Kit

U.S. Vet. Lic. No.: 313

Components:

Reagents	
Stage 1: Sample Preparation	
1. Polycarbonate Beads	1500
2. Extraction Detergent	2.75 mL
Stage 2: Sample Lysis	
3. Sample Lysis Buffer 1†	40 mL
4. Sample Lysis Buffer 2†	20 mL
5. Sample Lysis Buffer 3	10 mL
6. Lysing Matrix Tubes†	100
Stage 3: DNA Purification	
7. Matrix Binding Solution†	70 mL
8. Matrix Wash Buffer† (user must add 100 mL of 100% ethanol)	12 mL
9. Matrix Elution Buffer†	10 mL
10. DNA Purification Columns	2 X 50
11. DNA Column Buffer A	2 X 25 mL
12. DNA Column Buffer B (user must add 40 mL of 100% ethanol per bottle)	2 X 10 mL
13. DNA Column Buffer C	10 mL
14. DNA Precipitation Solution	3 mL
15. DNA Suspension Solution	10 mL
Stage 4: DNA Amplification	
16. PCR Reagent 1	2 X 1.5 mL
17. PCR Reagent 2	2 X 1.5 mL
18. PCR Positive Control	0.05 mL
19. PCR Negative Control	0.05 mL
Stage 5: DNA Detection	
20. Blocking Solution	100 mL
21. Conjugate Concentrate	0.02 mL
22. Blot Wash Concentrate 1 (contains sodium azide as a preservative)	200 mL
23. Blot Wash Concentrate 2 (contains sodium azide as a preservative)	200 mL
24. Substrate Buffer Concentrate	200 mL
25. Substrate	40 mL
Materials	
26. Nylon Membrane	

Materials Required But Not Provided:

1. Thermal cycler

2. Microcentrifuge
3. Cell-disrupter (Qbiogene "FastPrep" system, Model FP120 or equivalent)
4. Two water baths: 37°C and 60°C
5. Rotating platform
6. Rotating Wheel/Test Tube Rotator
7. Precision micropipettors capable of delivering the following suggested volumes: 1 - 10 μL, 20 - 200 μL, and 200 - 1000 μL
8. Aerosol resistant micropipettor tips
9. Heat sealer and heat-sealable pouches
10. Latex (or similar) gloves, powder-free
11. Ten and twenty-five mL disposable pipets
12. Fifty mL disposable conical tubes with caps
13. PCR tubes
14. 1.5 mL microcentrifuge tubes with caps
15. 2.0 mL microcentrifuge tubes without caps
16. Flat-bottom containers
17. Blotting paper (e.g. Whatman 3M paper)
18. Glacial acetic acid
19. Sterile distilled water
20. Molecular Biology grade ethanol
21. Analytical reagent grade 10N NaOH
22. Mineral oil for GeneAmp® PCR Cycler 480 user
23. Table-top Centrifuge (50 mL)
24. UV Radiation Source

Indications: The HERDCHEK® Mycobacterium Paratuberculosis DNA Test Kit from Idexx is an assay designed to specifically detect genomic DNA of *Mycobacterium paratuberculosis* (M. pt.), present in bovine feces. It is intended for veterinary use only.

Test Principles: The HERDCHEK® M. pt. DNA Test Kit is designed for the purification and detection of M. pt. genomic DNA from fecal specimens. Five stages are required for the procedure:

Stage 1: Sample Preparation
Stage 2: Sample Lysis
Stage 3: DNA Purification
Stage 4: DNA Amplification
Stage 5: DNA Detection

Fecal samples are suspended in a solution to lyse non-*Mycobacterium* organisms. The particulate materials are allowed to settle and *Mycobacterium paratuberculosis* organisms in the supernatant are pelleted. DNA is isolated from the pellet, and purified using silica matrices. The DNA is then amplified using the polymerase chain reaction with a set of synthetic DNA molecules whose properties are based on repetitive DNA sequence specific to M. pt. Amplified DNA is detected using dot-blot hybridization with an enzyme-labeled synthetic DNA molecule specific for *Mycobacterium paratuberculosis*.

Test Procedure: Before starting, kit users must add ethanol to two solutions. Add 100 mL of 100% ethanol to the bottle containing Matrix Wash Buffer and 40 mL of 100% ethanol to each bottle containing DNA Column Buffer B. These solutions are stable at room temperature for one year.

Specimen Information: Obtain bovine fecal sample by rectal examination using a gloved hand. Standard lubricant (mineral oil) will not interfere with the analysis. Place the sample in an airtight bag. Samples can be stored frozen at -20°C.

Sample Preparation - Stage 1:

Fecal Specimens:

1. Prepare fresh sample suspension solution the day of use. For each fecal sample, 25 mL of sample suspension solution is needed. For 10 samples, prepare sample suspension solution by adding 5.5 mL of 10 N NaOH (use only analytical reagent grade) and 275 μL of Extraction Detergent to 270 mL of sterile, distilled water. Mix solution well.
2. Transfer 1.0 (± 0.1) g of fecal sample to a 50 mL conical tube. Aseptically transfer 10-15 Polycarbonate Beads and add 25 mL of prepared sample suspension solution. Cap tube and vortex for 2 minutes to completely disperse fecal sample.
3. Allow sample to stand undisturbed for 30 minutes at room temperature.
4. Transfer the M. pt. containing-supernatant to a clean 50 mL conical tube using a 25 mL pipet; avoid transferring particulate matter.
5. Cap tube and centrifuge the supernatant at 1,750 X g for 30 minutes.
6. Remove and discard the supernatant via pipetting; leave 1-2 mL of solution above the pellet. Be careful to retain the flocculent sludge-like material on top of the bacterial pellet. The M. pt. organisms are in both fractions.
7. Add 25 mL of sterile distilled water, cap tube and vortex for 15 seconds.
8. Centrifuge the washed pellet at 1,750 X g for 30 minutes. Carefully remove all the supernatant using a 25 mL pipet. Do not remove the flocculent sludge-like material. The pellet can be stored for up to 2 hours at 2-7°C; do not freeze.
9. Add 400 microliters (μL) of Sample Lysis Buffer 1, 200 μL of Sample Lysis Buffer 2 and 100 μL of Sample Lysis Buffer 3 to the pellet. Cap tube and vortex for 15-25 seconds or until fully suspended.
10. Carefully pour the bacterial lysate into a labeled Lysing Matrix Tube. Fill the tube between the marks illustrated in Figure 1. If the sample volume is low, add water to increase the volume.

Figure 1

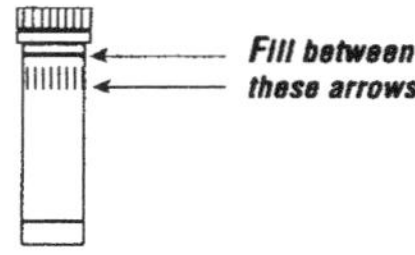

Sample Lysis - Stage 2:

1. Tightly screw the cap on each tube and place in the cell-disrupter device making sure each tube is counter balanced.
2. Disrupt the sample at 5.5 meters/second for 30 seconds.
3. Place tube on ice for 10 minutes.
4. Centrifuge the tube at 8,000 X g for 5 minutes.
5. Pipet the supernatant into a microcentrifuge tube. Cap and centrifuge the tube at 16,000 X g for 10 minutes.
6. Transfer 700 μL of the supernatants to a new microcentrifuge tube. Samples can be stored for up to 2 hours at 2-7°C or at -20°C until needed.

DNA Purification - Stage 3:

Note: Vortex the Matrix Binding Solution to generate a homogeneous solution, just prior to use.

1. Add 700 μL of Matrix Binding Solution to each tube; cap and gently mix by inversion for 10 minutes.
2. Centrifuge the mixture at 16,000 X g for 1 minute.
3. Gently remove and discard the supernatant.
4. Add 500 μL of prepared Matrix Wash Buffer (containing ethanol) to each tube. Cap and suspend completely by gentle vortexing.
5. Centrifuge the mixture at 16,000 X g for 1 minute.
6. Remove and discard the wash buffer.
7. Cap and recentrifuge the Matrix Binding Solution at 16,000 X g for 30 sec and discard the wash solution via pipetting.
8. Add 100 μL of the Matrix Elution Buffer. Cap and vigorously vortex the mixture to ensure total suspension of the Matrix Binding Solution.
9. Incubate at 37°C for 10 minutes.
10. Centrifuge at 16,000 X g for 2 minutes.
11. Carefully remove the top aqueous solution to a new microcentrifuge tube.
12. Add 500 μL of DNA Column Buffer A to each tube and mix via pipetting 1-3 times.
13. Ensure that the DNA Purification Column is in a 2 mL capless microcentrifuge tube.
14. Apply the sample mixture to the DNA Purification Column and centrifuge at 16,000 X g for 1 minute.
15. Place the DNA Purification Column into a new 2 mL capless microcentrifuge tube and discard the tube containing the flow-through.
16. Add 750 μL of DNA Column Buffer B to the DNA Purification Column and centrifuge at 16,000 X g for 1 minute.
17. Place the DNA Purification Column into a new 2 mL capless microcentrifuge tube and discard the tube containing the Buffer.
18. Centrifuge the DNA Purification Column at 16,000 X g for an additional minute to ensure total removal of the Buffer.
19. Place the DNA Purification Column into a new 2 mL sterile capless microcentrifuge tube and discard the tube containing the Buffer.
20. Add 100 μL of DNA Column Buffer C to column. Allow the DNA Purification Column to stand at 20-24°C for 2 minutes.
21. Centrifuge the tube at 16,000 X g for 1 minute.
22. Transfer the DNA-containing solution to a sterile-capped microcentrifuge tube.
23. Sequentially add 30 μL of DNA Precipitation Solution and 300 μL of 100% ethanol and cap tube.
24. Mix by inversion and incubate at < -60°C for at least 20 minutes. The DNA can also be precipitated by incubation at -20°C for greater than 5 hours.
25. Pellet the DNA by centrifugation at 16,000 X g for 10 minutes. Pour off the solution.
26. Wash the DNA pellets with 500 μL of ice cold 70% ethanol. Gently mix and centrifuge at 16,000 X g for 5 minutes.
27. Pour off the ethanol and dry the DNA pellets overnight by laying the tubes onto absorbent paper.
28. Dissolve the DNA in 100 μL of DNA Suspension Solution. Cap tube and incubate at 37°C for 30 minutes or overnight at 4°C. Store the DNA solution at-20°C until needed.

DNA Amplification - Stage 4: Refer to Figure 2 for a diagram of thermal cycler parameters.

Figure 2 - Thermal cycling parameters for the M. pt. DNA Test Kit.

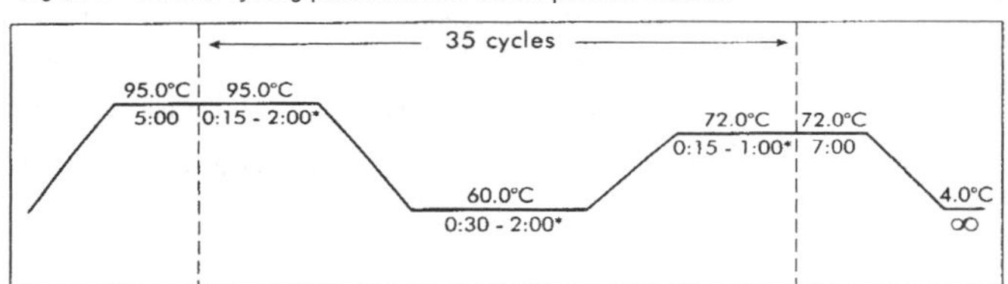

* refer to the technical manual for guidance of thermal cycler specific times.

Use of sterile aerosol resistant lips and three micropipettors: one for master mix preparation (200-1000 μL), a second for aliquoting the master mix into amplification tubes (20-100 μL) and a third for DNA addition (1-10 μL) are mandatory for the amplification procedure to minimize the possibility of DNA contamination.

1. Label tops of PCR tubes to maintain sample identification during the process. One PCR tube is required for each sample and two additional tubes are required for the Positive and Negative Controls.
2. For 12 PCR amplifications (10 samples and two controls) prepare a master mix by adding 300 μL of PCR Reagent 1 and 300 μL for PCR Reagent 2 to a clean, dry, graduate PCR reagent tube. Cap the PCR reagent tube and mix thoroughly by inverting. Transfer 45 μL of the master mix to each PCR tube.
3. Centrifuge the DNA samples at 16,000 X g for approximately 15 seconds.
4. For each reaction, transfer 5 μL of the DNA sample to the appropriately labeled PCR tube. Clean the micropipettor shaft by wiping with a disposable tissue dampened with ethanol between samples. Cap each tube.
5. Place the capped tubes into the thermal cycler and activate the PCR program.
6. When the PCR program is complete, remove the samples from the thermal cycler and proceed to the DNA detection procedure. Refer to the technical manual for specific instructions. Amplified samples can be stored frozen at-20°C.

DNA Detection - Stage 5:

Note: Use gloves and forceps when handling the nylon membrane. The membrane may be cut with scissors to facilitate analysis of less than 100 samples. Do not allow membranes to come in contact with each other after samples have been added.

The following procedure gives appropriate volumes for running 12 samples on a 10 cm X 1 cm membrane strip.

1. Preheat Blocking Solution and Blot Wash Concentrate 1 and 2 by placing the unopened containers into a 60°C water bath. Mix periodically and be certain they are in solution before use.
2. Prepare 1X stocks from 4x concentrates (Blot Wash Concentrate 1, Blot Wash Concentrate 2, and Substrate Buffer Concentrate) by mixing 20 mL of Concentrate with 60 mL of distilled, deionized water. The 1x solutions should remain in the 60°C water bath. Leave the 1 x Substrate Buffer at room temperature.
3. Heat the tubes containing PCR products at 99-100°C for 5 minutes.

H

4. Immediately after heating, place the tubes on ice/water bath for 5 minutes.
5. Centrifuge the tubes at 10,000 X g for 10 seconds
6. Using a pencil, mark the upper left-hand corner of the membrane strip as a reference and mark a grid on the membrane strip to indicate dot placement. Using a micropipettor and aerosol resistant tips, dot 3 µL of each PCR product onto the membrane strip. Record the position of each sample using the M. pt. DNA Test Kit Worksheet.
7. Allow the membrane strip to dry for 10 minutes at room temperature.
8. Cross-link the DNA by placing the membrane strip, sample-side up, under a UV radiation source for two minutes.
9. Place each membrane strip into a heat sealable pouch. Add 5 mL of Blocking Solution per membrane strip.
10. Place the pouch onto absorbent paper and remove any air bubbles. Heat-seal the pouch. Check to make sure the pouch is sealed by inverting and wiping with paper towel.
11. Incubate the sealed membrane strip for 30 minutes in a 60°C water bath.
12. Prepare Conjugate Solution by adding 1.3 µL of Conjugate Concentrate to 5 mL of Blocking Solution per membrane strip. Mix thoroughly by inverting the tube several times.

Note: Prepare conjugate solution no more than 5 minutes before use.

13. Cut open pouch, and pour off Blocking Solution.
14. Add the conjugate solution prepared in step 12 and repeat steps number 10 and 11.
15. Cut open pouch, pour off conjugate solution, and remove membrane strip.
16. Place the membrane strip, sample-side up, into a flat-bottomed container.
17. Add 40 mL of 1x Blot Wash Solution 1 (60°C) per membrane strip. Rapidly agitate on a rotating platform for 10 minutes at room temperature. Pour off solution.
18. Repeat step 17 with 1x Blot Wash Solution 1 (60°C).
19. Repeat steps 17 and 18 using 1x Blot Wash Solution 2 (60°C).
20. Add 40 mL of 1x Substrate Buffer per membrane strip. Agitate for 5 minutes on a rotating platform at room temperature. Pour off solution.
21. Repeat step 20 with 1x substrate buffer.
22. Place each membrane strip into a fresh, heat-sealable pouch. Add 4 mL of substrate solution per membrane strip. Heat-seal the pouch. Incubate substrate solution with membrane strip for 45 minutes at 37°C, protected from the light.
23. Remove the membrane strip and rinse with 1.0% glacial acetic acid for 2 minutes. Discard the acetic acid and rinse three times with distilled water. Place it on absorbent paper to dry, with the sample-side up.

Test Interpretation:

Results: The presence or absence of M. pt. DNA is based upon the presence of a colored spot on the membrane. Any sample producing a color reaction greater than the negative control is positive for *Mycobacterium paratuberculosis*.

If the negative control spot develops color or if the positive control spot does not develop color, the test is invalid. Please refer to the trouble shooting section of the technical manual for suggestions.

Storage: Store all components as designated on labels.

Caution(s): To eliminate potential sources of contaminating DNA,[3] perform the DNA extraction, amplification and detection procedures in three different rooms. Dedicate a set of micropipettors for each phase (extraction, amplification and detection) to minimize cross contamination. Refer to technical manual for detailed instructions on how to prevent DNA contamination.

Handle all samples as though capable of transmitting disease.

No eating, drinking or smoking in area where specimens or kit reagents are handled.

The Matrix Binding Solution and DNA Column Buffer A contain chaotropic salts, which are irritants. Wear gloves when handling. These reagents are incompatible with disinfecting agents that contain bleach.

Reagents may contain sodium azide as a preservative. Wear gloves when handling and flush waste reagents with large volumes of water upon disposal.

When preparing reagents (Sample Suspension Solution, NaOH, Blot Wash Solutions, and Substrate Buffer) use only sterile, distilled, deionized water.

Always disinfect work areas by wiping with 10% bleach and then 70% ethanol solution before and after use.

Note: Use disposable serological pipets and aerosol resistant micropipettor tips for manipulations in stages 1-5.

Discussion: Johne's disease is a chronic, debilitating enteritis of cattle and other ruminants caused by the organism M. pt., a slow growing aerobic bacterium.[1]

Calves less than 6 months of age are most susceptible and are usually infected by ingestion of contaminated feces. In an infected herd, approximately 5% of the animals develop obvious clinical disease. Subclinical infection can also cause economic losses.[2]

References: Available upon request.

This kit is manufactured under one or more of the following U.S. patents: 4,683,195; 4,683,202; and 5,225,324. Other U.S. and/or foreign patents issued or pending.

† Manufactured by Qbiogene, Inc. under one or more of the following U.S. patent numbers: 5,567,050; 5,643,767; and 6,027,750.

Compendium Code No.: 11160581 06-01394-02

HERDCHEK® NEOSPORA CANINUM ANTIBODY TEST KIT

Idexx Labs. **N caninum Test**

Neospora caninum Antibody Test Kit

U.S. Vet. Lic. No.: 313

Components:

Reagents	Volume
A. *Neospora* Antigen Coated Plates. Burn container and all unused contents.	2
B. Anti-Bovine: HRPO conjugate.	30 mL
C. *Neospora* Positive Control. Bovine Anti-*Neospora* in Buffer with protein stabilizers. Preserved with sodium azide.	3 mL
D. *Neospora* Negative Control. Bovine serum non-reactive to *Neospora* in Phosphate Buffer with protein stabilizers. Preserved with sodium azide.	3 mL
E. Sample Diluent. Buffers with protein stabilizers. Preserved with sodium azide.	235 mL
F. Wash Concentrate. 10x phosphate/Tween wash. Contains gentamicin as a preservative.	235 mL
G. TMB Substrate	60 mL
H. Stop Solution	60 mL

Materials Required But Not Provided:

1. Precision Pipets. Suitable for delivering 0.005, 0.100 mL and 0.500 mL or multiple delivery pipetting devices.
2. Disposable pipet tips.
3. Graduated cylinder: 500 mL for wash solution.
4. 96 Well Plate Reader.
5. Glass or plastic tubes for diluting samples.
6. Distilled or deionized water.
7. Device for the delivery and aspiration of wash solution.
8. A vacuum source and a trap for retaining the aspirate.

Indications: HERDCHEK® Anti-*Neospora* is Idexx's enzyme immunoassay for the detection of antibody to *Neospora caninum* in bovine serum.

Test Principles: HERDCHEK® Anti-*Neospora* is an enzyme immunoassay designed to detect the presence of antibody to *Neospora* in bovine serum. A microtitration format has been developed in which *Neospora* antigens are coated on 96 well plates. Upon incubation of the test sample in the coated well, antibody to *Neospora* forms a complex with the coated antigens. After washing away unbound material from the wells, an anti-bovine: horseradish peroxidase conjugate is added which binds to any bovine antibody attached in the wells. In the final step of the assay, unbound conjugate is washed away, and enzyme substrate (hydrogen peroxide) and a chromogen, 3,3',5,5' tetramethylbenzidine, are added to the wells. Subsequent color is proportional to the amount of antibody present in the test sample.

Test Procedure:

Preparation of Samples: Dilute test samples one hundred-fold (1:100) with Sample Diluent (e.g., by diluting 5 µL of sample with 500 µL of Sample Diluent). Note: Do not dilute controls.

Be sure to change tips for each sample and record the position of each sample on the plate using a HerdChek® worksheet. Samples should be mixed prior to dispensing into the *Neospora*-coated plate.

Preparation of Wash Solution: The Wash Concentrate should be brought to room temperature and mixed to assure dissolution of any precipitated salts. The Wash Concentrate must be diluted 1 to 10 with distilled/deionized water before use (e.g., 30 mL of concentrate plus 270 mL of water per plate to be assayed).

All reagents must be allowed to come to room temperature before use. Reagents should be mixed by gentle swirling or vortexing.

1. Obtain antigen coated plate(s) and record the sample position on a HerdChek® worksheet.
2. Dispense 100 µL of Undiluted Negative Control into wells A1 and A2.
3. Dispense 100 µL of Undiluted Positive Control into wells A3 and A4.
4. Dispense 100 µL of Diluted sample into appropriate wells. All samples should be run in duplicates.
5. Incubate for 30 minutes at room temperature.
6. Aspirate liquid contents of all wells into appropriate waste reservoir.
7. Wash each well with approximately 300 µL of phosphate buffered wash solution four times. Aspirate liquid contents of all wells after each wash. Avoid plate drying between plate washings and prior to the addition of conjugate. Following the final wash fluid aspiration, gently, but firmly tap residual wash fluid from each plate onto absorbent material.
8. Dispense 100 µL of Anti-Bovine: HRPO Conjugate into each well.
9. Incubate for 30 minutes at room temperature.
10. Repeat steps 6 and 7.
11. Dispense 100 µL of TMB Substrate Solution into each test plate well.
12. Incubate for 15 minutes at room temperature.
13. Dispense 100 µL of Stop Solution into each well of the test plate to stop the reaction.
14. Blank on air.
15. Measure and record the absorbance at (620 nm, 630 nm or 650 nm).
16. Calculate results.

Test Interpretation:

Results: For the assay to be valid the difference (P-N) between the positive control mean ($PC\bar{x}$), and the negative control mean ($NC\bar{x}$) must be greater than or equal to 0.150. In addition, the $NC\bar{x}$ must be less than or equal to 0.20.

For invalid assays, technique may be suspect and the assay should be repeated following a thorough review of the product insert.

The presence or absence of antibody to *Neospora* is determined by sample to positive (S/P) ratio for each sample. The positive control has been standardized and represents a significant level of antibody to *Neospora* in bovine serum.

See Calculations for examples.

Note: Idexx Laboratories, Inc., has instrument and software systems available which calculate means and S/P ratios and provide data summaries.

Interpretation of Results:

1. Serum samples with S/P ratios of less than 0.50 are classified as Negative for *Neospora* antibodies.
2. If the S/P ratio is greater than or equal to 0.50, the sample is classified Positive for *Neospora* antibodies.

Calculations:

1. Calculation of Negative Control Mean ($NC\bar{x}$):

$$NC\bar{x} = \frac{A1\ A(650) + A2\ A(650)}{2}$$

Example:

$$\frac{0.080 + 0.090}{2} = 0.085$$

2. Calculation of Positive Control Mean ($PC\bar{x}$):

$$PC\bar{x} = \frac{A3\ A(650) + A4\ A(650)}{2}$$

Example:

$$\frac{0.510 + 0.500}{2} = 0.505$$

3. Calculation of the (S/P) ratio:

$$S/P = \frac{\text{Sample A(650)} - NC\bar{x}}{PC\bar{x} - NC\bar{x}}$$

Example: Sample Mean = 0.450

$$S/P = \frac{0.450 - 0.085}{0.505 - 0.085} = \frac{0.365}{0.420} = 0.87$$

Storage: Store all reagents at 2°-7°C.

Caution(s):

1. Handle all *Neospora* biological materials as though capable of transmitting *Neospora*, although the organism has been disrupted.
2. Do not pipet by mouth.
3. There should be no eating, drinking or smoking where specimens or kit reagents are being handled.
4. TMB Substrate and acid solutions may be irritating to the skin.
5. Some kit components contain sodium azide as a preservative. Care should be taken to prevent the contamination of the Anti-Bovine:HRPO Conjugate with this preservative.
6. Do not expose TMB Solution to strong light or any oxidizing agents. Handle TMB substrate Solution with clean glass or plasticware.
7. All wastes should be properly decontaminated prior to disposal.
8. Bring to room temperature 15-30°C before use, and return to 2°-7°C following use.
9. Care should be taken to prevent contamination of kit components.
10. Do not use components past expiration date and do not intermix components from different serials.
11. Optimal results will be obtained by strict adherence to this protocol. Careful pipetting, timing and washing throughout this procedure are necessary to maintain precision and accuracy.

For veterinary use only.

Discussion: *Neospora caninum* is a recently discovered protozoal (Apicomplexan) parasite which can cause abortion and neonatal morbidity and mortality in cattle, sheep, goats and horses.[1] It has been reported in California (U.S.A.) that infection with *Neospora* is the most important diagnosed cause of abortion in dairy cattle.[2,3,4] Neosporosis has been reported as a cause of abortion in other countries as well.[5,6,7] Currently, it is not known how the organism is introduced into herds or whether there are means of transmitting the organism between cattle other than by congenital transmission.[8]

An ELISA has been developed for the serological diagnosis of *Neospora* infection in cattle which may be useful in epidemiological studies or in management and control measures for reducing *Neospora* infection within a herd. Since definitive diagnosis is made only by isolation of the organism, the serological status of an animal is only one of many criteria to be considered in overall herd management.

References: Available upon request.

Presentation: 2 plates per kit (strips).

HERDCHEK is a registered trademark of Idexx Laboratories, Inc., in the United States and/or other countries.

Compendium Code No.: 11160262 06-02995-03

HERDCHEK® PRRS VIRUS ANTIBODY TEST KIT

Idexx Labs. **PRRS Test**

Porcine Reproductive and Respiratory Syndrome Virus Antibody Test Kit

U.S. Vet. Lic. No.: 313

Components:

Reagents	Volume
A. Porcine reproductive and respiratory syndrome Viral Antigens/Normal Host Cell Antigens. PRRS/NHC Coated Strips/Plates. Burn container and all unused contents.	5 Plates
B. Anti-Porcine: HRPO conjugate. Contains gentamicin as a preservative.	60 mL
C. PRRS Positive Control. Porcine Anti-PRRS in phosphate buffer with protein stabilizers. Preserved with sodium azide.	4 mL
D. Porcine Negative Control. Porcine Serum nonreactive to PRRS in phosphate buffer with protein stabilizers.	4 mL
E. Sample Diluent. Phosphate Buffers with protein stabilizers. Contains azide as a preservative.	150 mL
F. Wash Concentrate. 10x phosphate/Tween wash. Contains gentamicin as a preservative.	235 mL
G. TMB Substrate. 3,3', 5,5' Tetramethylbenzidine (TMB)	60 mL
H. Stop Solution.	60 mL

Materials Required But Not Provided:

1. Precision Pipettes. Suitable for delivering 0.010, 0.100 mL and 0.400 mL or multiple delivery pipetting devices.
2. Disposable pipette tips.
3. Graduated cylinders: 500 mL for wash solution.
4. 96 Well Plate Reader.
5. Glass or plastic tubed for diluting samples.
6. Distilled or deionized water.
7. Device for the delivery and aspiration of wash solution.
8. A vacuum source and a trap for retaining the aspirate.

Indications: HERDCHEK® PRRS Virus Antibody Test Kit is Idexx's product for an enzyme immunoassay for the detection of antibody to porcine reproductive and respiratory syndrome (PRRS) in swine serum using PRRS and normal host cell (NHC) antigens.

Test Principles: HERDCHEK® PRRS is an enzyme immunoassay designed to detect the presence of antibody to PRRS in swine serum. A microtitration format has been configured by coating PRRS and NHC antigens in alternating columns on the plate. Upon incubation of the test sample in the coated well, antibody specific to PRRS forms a complex with the coated viral antigens. The NHC antigens coated on the plate are used to assess whether immunoglobulins against tissue culture components present in vaccine are contributing to test results. After washing away unbound material from the wells, an anti-porcine: horseradish peroxidase conjugate is added which binds to any porcine antibody attached in the wells. In the final step of the assay, unbound conjugate is washed away, and enzyme substrate (hydrogen peroxide) and a chromogen 3,3',5,5' Tetramethylbenzidine (TMB), are added to the wells. The extent of host cell contribution to the total signal is assessed by relating PRRS activity to NHC reactivity.

Test Procedure:

Preparation of Samples: Dilute test samples forty-fold (1:40) with Sample Diluent (e.g., by diluting 10 µL of sample with 390 µL of Sample Diluent). Note: Do not dilute controls.

Be sure to change tips for each sample and record the position of each sample on the plate using a HerdChek® worksheet. Samples should be mixed prior to dispensing into the PRRS/NHC coated plate.

	PRRS	NHC	PRRS	NHC	PRRS	NHC	PRRS	NHC	PRRS	NHC	PRRS	NHC
A	P	P	5	5								
B	P	P	6	6								
C	N	N										
D	N	N										
E	1	1										
F	2	2										
G	3	3										
H	4	4										
	1	2	3	4	5	6	7	8	9	10	11	12

N = Negative Control
P = Positive Control
1, 2, 3, etc, = Sample #
Columns 1, 3, 5, 7, 9, 11 coated with PRRS antigen
Columns 2, 4, 6, 8, 10, 12 coated with NHC antigen

Preparation of Wash Solution: The Wash Concentrate should be brought to room temperature and mixed to ensure dissolution of any precipitated salts. The Wash Concentrate must be diluted 1 to 10 with distilled/deionized water before use (e.g., 30 mL of concentrate plus 270 mL of water per plate to be assayed).

All reagents must be allowed to come to room temperature before use. Reagents should be mixed by gentle swirling or vortexing.

1. Obtain antigen coated plate(s) and record the sample position on a HerdChek® worksheet.
2. Dispense 100 µL of Undiluted Negative Control into PRRS wells and C1 and D1 and NHC wells C2 and D2.
3. Dispense 100 µL of Undiluted Positive Control into PRRS wells A1 and B1 and NHC wells A2 and B2.
4. Dispense 100 µL of Diluted sample into adjacent PRRS and NHC wells. All samples should be run in duplicate.
5. Incubate for 30 minutes at room temperature.
6. Aspirate liquid contents of all wells into appropriate waste reservoir.
7. Wash each well with approximately 300 µL of phosphate buffered wash solution three to five times. Aspirate liquid contents of all wells after each wash. Avoid plate drying between plate washings and prior to the addition of conjugate. Following the initial final wash fluid aspiration, gently, but firmly tap residual wash fluid from each plate onto absorbent material.
8. Dispense 100 µL of Anti-Porcine: HRPO Conjugate into each well.
9. Incubate for 30 minutes at room temperature.
   TMB Substrate Solution should be prepared at this point.
10. Repeat steps 6 and 7.
11. Dispense 100 µL of TMB Substrate Solution into each test plate well.
12. Incubate for 15 minutes at room temperature.
13. Dispense 100 µL of Stop Solution into each well of the test plate to stop the reaction.
14. Measure and record the A(650) for samples and controls. If a reference filter is available with the reader, the operating manual should be consulted to determine the method of reference filter selection.
15. Calculate results.

Test Interpretation: For the assay to be valid the following specifications must be met:

The positive control mean for the PRRS side (PC:PRRS) minus the NC:PRRS must be greater than or equal to 0.150. For invalid assays, technique may be suspect and the assay should be repeated following a thorough review of the product insert. The Positive Control has been standardized and represents a significant level of antibody to PRRS in swine serum. The normal host cell antigen provides a measure of the NHC contribution to the total PRRS antigen signal. The presence or absence of antibody to PRRS is determined by calculating the sample to positive (S/P) ratio.

Interpretation of Results: The presence or absence of antibody to PRRS is determined by calculating the S/P ratio for each sample.

1. If the S/P ratio is less than 0.4, the sample is classified as Negative for PRRS antibodies.
2. If the S/P ratio is greater than or equal to 0.4, then the sample is classified as Positive for PRRS antibodies.

Calculations:

1. Calculation of Negative Control Mean (NC:PRRS)

PRRS Antigen (wells C1, D1)

$$NC{:}PRRS = \frac{C1\ A(650) + D1\ A(650)}{2}$$

Example:

$$\frac{0.11 + 0.13}{2} = 0.12$$

2. Calculation of Positive Control Mean (PC:PRRS), PC(NHC)

PRRS Antigen (wells A1, B1)

$$PC{:}PRRS = \frac{A1\ A(650) + B1\ A(650)}{2}$$

Example:

$$\frac{0.360 + 0.384}{2} = 0.372$$

NHC (wells A2, B2)

$$PC{:}NHC = \frac{A2\ A(650) + B2\ A(650)}{2}$$

Example:

$$\frac{0.060 + 0.070}{2} = 0.065$$

3. Calculation of the sample to positive (S/P) ratio:

$$S/P = \frac{\text{Sample A(650):PRRS} - \text{(Sample A(650):NHC)}}{\text{(PC:PRRS)} - \text{(PC:NHC)}}$$

Example: if sample A(650) = 0.750, and A(650) NHC = 0.15, then

$$S/P = \frac{0.750 - 0.15}{0.372 - 0.065} = \frac{0.60}{0.307} = 1.95$$

Note: IDEXX Laboratories, Inc. has instrument and software systems available which calculate means, and S/P ratios and provide data summaries.

Storage: Store all reagents at 2°-7°C (36°-45°F).

Caution(s):

1. Handle all PRRS biological materials as though capable of transmitting PRRS.
2. Do not pipette by mouth.
3. There should be no eating, drinking or smoking where specimens or kit reagents are being handled.
4. TMB Concentrate, Diluent, and acid solutions may be irritating to the skin and eyes. Use only plasticware for storage or handling stop solutions. Safety glasses should be worn while pouring acids.
5. Some kit components contain sodium azide as a preservative. Care should be taken to prevent the contamination of the Anti-Porcine: HRPO Conjugate with this preservative.
6. Do not expose TMB Solutions to strong light or any oxidizing agents. Handle all TMB Substrate Solutions with clean glass or plasticware.
7. Store all reagents at 2°-7°C. Bring to room temperature prior to use, and return to 2°-7°C following use.
8. All wastes should be properly decontaminated prior to disposal.
9. Care should be taken to prevent contamination of kit components.
10. Do not use components past expiration date and do not intermix components from different serials.
11. Optimal results will be obtained by strict adherence to this protocol. Careful pipetting, timing and washing throughout this procedure are necessary to maintain precision and accuracy.

Warning(s): For veterinary use only.

Discussion: A new swine disease causing reproductive problems, respiratory disease and mild neurologic signs was first reported in 1987. Due to the general clinical symptoms presented in most cases, diagnosis was often confused with swine influenza, pseudorabies, hog cholera, parvovirus, encephalomyocarditis, chlamydia and mycoplasma. A major component of the syndrome is reproductive failure resulting in premature births, late term abortions, pigs born weak, increased stillbirths, mummified fetuses, decreased farrowing rates and delayed return to estrus. These aspects of the syndrome have been observed to last 1 to 3 months. Respiratory disease is another significant feature of the disease that most affects pigs less than 3 to 4 weeks of age. Respiratory signs can occur in most stages of the production cycle.

Due to the many confusing features of the disease, it was first called mystery swine disease (MSD) and later, swine infertility and respiratory syndrome (SIRS). During 1990, Europeans reported a disease with almost identical characteristics to MSD/SIRS. Outbreaks were described in Germany, The Netherlands, Spain, France, England and Canada under the names of New Pig Disease, porcine epidemic abortion and respiratory syndrome (PEARS), blue ear disease and porcine reproductive and respiratory syndrome (PRRS).[4-9] The globally accepted designation for this emerging swine disease has become PRRS.

European and North American scientists have successfully isolated and characterized the agent responsible for this disease.[4,10,11] The disease was also reproduced experimentally by both research groups. Researchers have demonstrated that the European and US isolates producing nearly identical clinical symptoms represent strains of the virus responsible for PRRS.[10,11,15] The etiologic agent has been described as a virus similar to equine arteritis virus (EAV) and the lactate dehydrogenase-elevating virus (LDV). Researchers in The Netherlands have proposed that these viruses be grouped in a new family, *Arteriviridae,* based on genomic sequencing information.[13] These viruses were originally assigned to the *Togaviridae* family as unclassified viruses.

Current infection rates remain to be accurately determined in most areas of the world. Estimates in some countries have been as high as 80% while other countries claim to be free of the disease. Two pertinent features of the PRRS virus described in several of the studies have been (A) strain variability among different isolates of the virus[14] and (B) persistent infection apparently present at different times during recovery.[15] Both of these characteristics of the PRRS virus strains can confound the diagnosis of the disease.

An assessment of exposure to the PRRS virus as a result of natural infection is facilitated by a measurement of antibodies in the serum. It is extremely important that the immunodiagnostic assay measuring the antibodies be sensitive to the several strains of the virus.

References: Available upon request.

Presentation: 5 plates per kit (strips).

HERDCHEK is a registered trademark of Idexx Laboratories, Inc. in the United States and/or other countries.

Compendium Code No.: 11160362 06-01553-09

HERDCHEK® PRV gpI ANTIBODY TEST KIT

Idexx Labs. **Pseudorabies Test**

Pseudorabies Virus gpI Antibody Test Kit

U.S. Vet. Lic. No.: 313

Components:

Reagents	Volume	
	6	30
1. PRV Coated Plates	6	30
2. Anti-PRV-gpI: Horseradish Peroxidase (HRPO) Conjugate in buffer with protein stabilizers. Preserved with gentamicin.	60 mL	350 mL
3. Porcine Negative Control - Porcine serum non-reactive to PRV-gpI. Preserved with sodium azide.	5 mL	5 mL
4. PRV-gpI Positive Control - Anti-PRV gpI. Preserved with sodium azide.	5 mL	5 mL
5. Sample Diluent - Buffer with protein stabilizers. Preserved with sodium azide.	120 mL	300 mL
6. Wash Concentrate - (10X concentrate)-Phosphate buffer. Preserved with gentamicin.	235 mL	1440 mL
7. TMB Substrate	60 mL	315 mL
8. Stop Solution	60 mL	315 mL

Materials Required but not Provided:

1. Precision pipets suitable for delivering 50 and 100 µL multiple delivery pipetting devices.
2. Disposable pipet tips.
3. Graduated cylinders: 500 mL for wash solution.
4. 96 well plate reader.
5. Glass or plastic tubes for diluting samples.
6. Distilled or deionized water.
7. Device for the delivery and aspiration of wash solution.
8. A vacuum source and a trap for retaining the aspirate.

Indications: HERDCHEK® Anti-PRV gpI is Idexx's enzyme immunoassay for the detection of antibodies in swine serum to the gpI antigen of pseudorabies virus (PRV/Aujeszky's disease). The presence of antibodies to gpI indicates exposure to field strains of PRV and/or vaccines containing gpI antigen. In the United States, it is intended for use in management and pseudorabies eradication applications. When used with gpI-deleted PRV vaccines manufactured by Boehringer Ingelheim Inc., Norden Laboratories, Syntrovet Inc., and Solvay Animal Health, Inc., and when performed at approved laboratories, it is an official differential pseudorabies test for use in the Cooperative State/Federal Pseudorabies Eradication Program.

Test Principles: The HERDCHEK® Anti-PRV-gpI assay is performed in a PRV antigen-coated microwell using a two-fold (1:2) serum dilution. During the first incubation, PRV antibodies present in the serum, including those produced against gpI, react with antigens on the plastic. Subsequent to a wash step, an Anti-PRV-gpI monoclonal antibody conjugate is added to the microwell and is allowed to compete for the gpI viral antigen during a second incubation. If no gpI antibodies are present in the test serum, the conjugated gpI antibodies are free to react with the gpI antigen. Conversely, if gpI antibodies are present in the test serum, the enzyme-conjugated monoclonal antibodies are blocked from reacting with the antigen. Following the incubation period, the unreacted conjugate is removed by washing, and a substrate/chromogen solution is added. In the presence of enzyme, the substrate is converted to a product which reacts with the chromophore to generate a blue color. The absorbance at 650 nm, A(650), is measured using a spectrophotometer. The results are calculated by dividing the A(650) of the sample by the mean A(650) of the negative control, resulting in an S/N value. The quantity of antibodies to gpI is inversely proportional to the A(650) and, thus, to the S/N value. The presence of PRV antibodies, including anti-gpI, indicates a previous exposure to a field strain of PRV or application of conventional modified-live or killed virus vaccines. The presence of PRV antibodies detected by the HERDCHEK® Anti-PRV Screening and/or Verification assays, but absence of antibodies to gpI antigen as assessed by the HERDCHEK® Anti-PRV-gpI assay, indicates a response to a gpI-deleted vaccine.

Test Procedure:

Preparation of Samples: Dilute test samples two-fold (1:2) with Sample Diluent.

Be sure to change the tips for each sample and record the position of each sample on the plate using a HerdChek® worksheet. The samples should be mixed prior to dispensing into the PRV-coated plate.

Preparation of the Wash Solution: The Wash Concentrate should be brought to room temperature and mixed to ensure dissolution of any precipitated salts. The Wash Concentrate must be diluted 1 to 10 with distilled/deionized water before use (e.g. 30 mL of Concentrate plus 270 mL of water per plate to be assayed).

All reagents must be allowed to come to room temperature before use. Reagents should be mixed by gentle swirling or vortexing.

1. Obtain antigen coated plate(s) and record the sample position on a HerdChek® worksheet.
2. Dispense 100 µL of Negative Control (Diluted 1:2) into wells A1, A2 and A3.
3. Dispense 100 µL of Positive Control (Diluted 1:2) into wells A4 and A5.
4. Dispense 100 µL of diluted sample into the appropriate wells.
5. Incubate for 1 hour at room temperature or overnight at 2°-7°C.
6. Wash each well with approximately 300 µL of wash solution 3 to 5 times. Aspirate the liquid contents of all the wells after each wash. Avoid plate drying between plate washings and prior to the addition of conjugate. Following the final wash fluid aspiration, gently but firmly tap residual wash fluid from each plate into absorbent material.
7. Dispense 100 µL of Anti-PRV-gpI: HRPO Conjugate into each well.
8. Incubate for 20 minutes at room temperature.
9. Repeat step 6.
10. Dispense 100 µL of TMB substrate solution into each test well.
11. Incubate for 15 minutes at room temperature.
12. Dispense 50 µL of Stop Solution into each well to stop the reaction.
13. Blank the spectrophotometer on air.
14. Measure and record the A(650) for the samples and controls.
15. Calculate results.

Test Interpretation:

Results: For the assay to be valid, negative control mean A(650) minus the positive control mean A(650) must be greater than or equal to 0.3. For invalid assays, technique may be suspect and the assay should be repeated following a thorough review of the product insert. The presence or absence of antibody to the gpI antigen is determined by first calculating the S/N value for each sample.

See Calculations for examples.

Note: Idexx Laboratories, Inc. has instruments and software systems available which calculate means, and S/N values and provide data summaries.

Interpretation of Results:

1. If the S/N is less than or equal to 0.60, the sample is classified as positive for antibodies to the gpI antigen of PRV.
2. If the S/N is less than or equal to 0.7 but greater than 0.6, the sample should be retested. If the test result repeats, the animal should be sampled and tested at a later date.
3. If the S/N is greater than 0.7, the sample is classified as negative for antibodies to the gpI antigen of PRV.

Note: Confirm all positives in duplicate.

Calculations:

1. Calculation of Negative Control Mean ($NC\bar{x}$):

$$NC\bar{x} = \frac{A1\ A(650) + A2\ A(650) + A3\ A(650)}{3}$$

2. Calculation of Positive Control Mean ($PC\bar{x}$):

$$PC\bar{x} = \frac{A4\ A(650) + A5\ A(650)}{2}$$

3. Calculation of Sample/Negative (S/N) Ratio:

$$S/N = \frac{\text{Sample A(650)}}{NC\bar{x}}$$

Storage: Store all reagents at 2°-7°C (36°-45°F).

Caution(s):

1. Handle all PRV biological materials as though capable of transmitting PRV. Although the virus has been chemically treated, the antigen-coated microwell plate may be a source of PRV.
2. Do not pipet by mouth.
3. No eating, drinking or smoking where specimens or kit reagents are being handled.
4. TMB Substrate and Stop Solution may be irritating to the skin.
5. Some kit components contain sodium azide as a preservative. Disposal requires flushing plumbing with large volumes of water to prevent the formation of copper or lead azide complexes which may explode upon percussion. Care should be taken to prevent the contamination of the Anti-PRV-gpI: HRPO Conjugate with the preservative.
5. Do not expose TMB solutions to strong light or any oxidizing agents. Handle all TMB substrate solutions with clean glass or plasticware.
7. Bring to room temperature prior to use and return to 2°-7°C (36°-45°F) following use.
8. All wastes should be properly decontaminated prior to disposal.
9. Care should be taken to prevent the contamination of kit components.
10. Do not use components past expiration date and do not intermix components from different serials.
11. Optimal results will be obtained by strict adherence to this protocol. Careful pipetting, timing and washing throughout this procedure are necessary to maintain precision and accuracy.

Discussion: Strategies traditionally used to provide protection for swine from the effects of pseudorabies infection have included the administration of conventional and gene deleted, USDA licensed PRV vaccines.[1] Standard serologic procedures used to assess PRV exposure following vaccination are of limited value as they cannot distinguish naturally infected from vaccinated swine.

Safe and efficacious gpI-deleted PRV vaccines which allow for serologic differentiation have been developed by the manufacturers listed above. The virus used in these vaccines was selected such that the synthesis of virulence factors were eliminated without compromising the immunogenicity of the virus. In addition, a mechanism for serologic differentiation is provided by the natural deletion of the DNA sequences that code for gpI, and apparently non-essential viral protein. Thus, the HERDCHEK® Anti-PRV-gpI assay, being specific for antibodies to gpI, ignores antibody titers in animals vaccinated with gpI-deleted PRV vaccines by approved manufacturers, but detects animals infected with field strains or vaccinated with strains that contain the gpI antigen. The assay uses monoclonal antibodies specific for gpI.

Prior to vaccination with gpI-deleted products, swine should be tested using either this assay or the HERDCHEK® Anti-PRV Screening and/or Verification assays to determine immune status. Subsequent to vaccination the swine should be routinely monitored at least semiannually for exposure to field strains of PRV using the Anti-PRV-gpI assay.

References: Available upon request.

Presentation: 6 plate kits and 30 plate kits.

Licensed under U.S. Patent Nos. 4,810,634 and 5,352,575.

Compendium Code No.: 11160342 06-01040-09

HERDCHEK® PRV-PCFIA ANTIBODY TEST KIT

Idexx Labs. **Pseudorabies Test**

Pseudorabies Virus Antibody Test Kit-Particle Concentration Fluorescence Immunoassay

U.S. Vet. Lic. No.: 313

Components:

1. PRV Coated Particles - Antigen coated polystyrene particles in phosphate buffered saline with protein stabilizers.
2. Anti-PRV: Fluorescent Conjugate; Fluorescently labeled monoclonal antibody to PRV lyophilized in phosphate buffered saline with protein stabilizers.
3. Conjugate Diluent - Deionized Water.
4. PRV Strong Positive Control - Porcine anti-PRV serum.
5. PRV Weak Positive Control - Porcine anti-PRV serum diluted in Negative Control.
6. Negative Control - Porcine serum nonreactive to PRV.
7. Wash Solution - Phosphate buffered saline
8. Sample Diluent

Materials Required But Not Provided:

1. IDEXX® Screen Machine or FCA.
2. 96-well IDEXX PCFIA assay plates.
3. Precision pipet, suitable for delivery of 5 µL and 20 µL.

Indications: HERDCHEK® PRV-PCFIA is Idexx's trademark for a Particle Concentration Fluorescence Immunoassay (PCFIA) for the detection of antibody to Porcine Pseudorabies Virus (PRV) in swine serum. It is intended for use in management and Pseudorabies eradication applications. This is an official test to be used in the Cooperative State/Federal Pseudorabies Program.

Test Principles: PCFIA is a fluorescence immunoassay technique which utilizes polystyrene particles as the solid phase onto which PRV antigens are attached. The conjugate is comprised of fluorescently labeled monoclonal antibody to PRV.

In the assay, the test sample and coated polystyrene particles are initially mixed and incubated in a specially designed 96-well plate. After this initial incubation period, conjugate is added, allowed to react and the reaction mixture is then filtered through the membrane at the bottom of each well. The polystyrene particles, being too large to pass through the membrane, are retained on the surface of the membrane. Each well is washed to remove unbound conjugate and antibody, and then moved into position below a front-surface fluorimetric read system. The amount of particle-bound fluorescence is measured as counts from the membrane surface. The system reads fluorescence in two channels; a sample channel (C) and a reference channel (B). The ratio of counts in each channel normalizes any variation due to pipeting.

The PRV-PCFIA test is a competitive immunoassay to detect antibodies specific for PRV. During the reaction, specific antibodies in the sample compete with the conjugate for antigen binding sites on the polystyrene particles. The system provides an inverse measurement of specific antibody - i.e. the amount of conjugate bound to the polystyrene particles will decrease as the specific antibody concentration in the sample increases. Binding of a non-specific antibody to the polystyrene particles does not affect the competition between specific antibody in the sample and the conjugate, and thus does not affect the resulting signal.

Test Procedure:

Sample Preparation: Controls and serum samples must be diluted 1:5 with Sample Diluent (see Step 3 of the test procedure).

Serum samples should be of good quality, with no flocculation or precipitation. If clogged wells occur frequently, then samples can be centrifuged prior to testing.

If you have questions regarding sample quality, please contact IDEXX Customer Service at 1-800-548-6733.

Test Procedure: The PRV-PCFIA antibody test is performed using the IDEXX PCFIA System. (Refer to the IDEXX PCFIA Operation Manual for complete instructions on maintenance and operation of the instrument and use of the data management program.)

Conjugate Reconstitution: Transfer the contents of one bottle of Conjugate Diluent (25 mL) into one bottle of lyophilized Anti-PRV: Fluorescent Conjugate. Allow to sit undisturbed for 10 minutes, then mix by gently swirling. Store reconstituted Conjugate at 2°-7°C (36°-45°F).

1. Allow all reagents to come to room temperature prior to use.
2. Mix particles gently by inversion; avoid foaming.
3. Add 20 µL sample diluent to each well.
4. Add controls and test sera to the appropriate wells of each plate.
   a. Create a layout to indicate sample position in the assay plate(s).
   b. Add 5 µL of Undiluted Negative control to wells A1, A2, A3, A10, A11, A12.
   c. Add 5 µL of Undiluted PRV Weak Positive Control to wells A4, A5, A8, A9.
   d. Add 5 µL of Undiluted PRV Strong Positive Control to wells A6 and A7.
   e. Add 5 µL of each serum sample to the appropriate remaining wells using the layout created in Step 4a as a guide.
5. Running the Assay
   a. To Reagent Tray, add the following reagents:
   - Wash Solution to Wash Compartment (or fill external reservoir if applicable).
   - Wash Solution to Aux Compartment (or fill external reservoir if applicable).
   - Particles to Compartment A. Mix particles by inversion before adding to tray.
   - Conjugate to Compartment B. (Refer to Volume Chart in the IDEXX PCFIA Operation Manual for appropriate volumes of particles and conjugate).

   b. Load Reagent Tray. Insert plates containing samples in numerical plate order.
   c. Press Process Plates.
   d. Press PRV.
   e. Press Identify Wells.
   f. The total number of plates to the processed must be indicated. To do this, press Plate 1 until the plate number displayed on the screen equals the total number of plates in your batch.
   g. Press Check Reagents. At this point, the instrument will verify if sufficient reagent volumes are present to process the indicated number of plates. Insufficient volumes will be highlighted on the screen. If this occurs, remove the reagent tray and add additional reagents as appropriate.
   h. Press Check Data Link to begin assay. (If applicable, press Configure Output, then press Personal Computer, then press Save to begin assay.)
6. Follow the instructions in the IDEXX PCFIA Operation Manual to generate a computer printout of results upon assay completion.

Test Interpretation:

Results: Results are expressed as a sample to negative ratio (S/N) which is the ratio of sample or positive control signal to the negative control signal. For the assay to be valid, the PRV Strong Positive Control must have an S/N value less than 0.40 and the Weak Positive Control must have an S/N value equal to or less than 0.90. The system automatically checks for these parameters to validate or invalidate the assay. (Refer to "Calculations Section" for a definition of the S/N value.)

The presence or absence of antibody to PRV is determined by comparison of test sample S/N to the Weak Positive S/N. Serum samples with an S/N value greater than the Weak Positive Control are considered negative for PRV antibody; samples with an S/N value less than or equal to the Weak Positive Control are considered positive.

Interpretation of the Results:

1. Serum samples with S/N ratios greater than the Weak Positive Control are classified as Negative for PRV antibodies.
2. If the S/N ratio is equal to or less than the Weak Positive Control, the sample is classified as Positive for PRV antibodies.

Calculations:

1. Calculations of Negative Control ($\bar{x}$NC) Mean:

$$\bar{x}NC = \frac{\text{Sum of } C/B^{*} \text{ ratios for wells A1, A2, A3, A10, A11, A12}}{6}$$

2. Calculation of S/N for PRV Weak Positive Control ($\bar{x}$WPC) Mean:

$$\bar{x}WPC\ S/N = \frac{\dfrac{\text{Sum of } C/B \text{ ratios for wells A4, A5, A8 and A9}}{4}}{\bar{x}NC}$$

3. Calculation of S/N for PRV Strong Positive Control ($\bar{x}$SPC) Mean:

$$\bar{x}SPC\ S/N = \frac{\dfrac{\text{Sum of } C/B \text{ ratios for wells A6 and A7}}{2}}{\bar{x}NC}$$

4. Calculation of S/N for serum sample:

$$S/N = \frac{C/B \text{ ratio of sample well}}{\bar{x}NC}$$

$$^{*}C/B \text{ ratio} = \frac{\text{channel C counts}}{\text{channel B counts}}$$

Storage: Store all reagents at 2°-7°C (36°-45°F).

Store PRV Coated Particles and Anti-PRV Conjugate protected from light.

Caution(s): Thoroughly read all directions prior to starting test procedure.

Handle all PRV biological materials as though capable of transmitting PRV.

Use the dropper top to dispense particles. Do not return unused particles or conjugate to stock bottles.

Do not eat, drink or smoke where specimens or kit reagents are being handled.

All wastes should be properly decontaminated prior to disposal.

Do not use kit past expiration date and do not intermix components from different serial lots.

Discussion: Pseudorabies, Aujesky's Disease, is caused by a type 1 porcine herpesvirus. The highest mortality rates occur in suckling pigs born to a susceptible sow. Baby pigs in the fatal course of the disease exhibit difficulty in breathing, fever, hypersalivation, anorexia, vomiting, diarrhea, trembling, and depression. Within this age group, the final stages of infection are commonly characterized by ataxia, nystagmus, running fits, intermittent convulsions, coma, and death. Death usually occurs within 24 to 48 hours following apparent clinical symptoms. The clinical events of the disease in weanling and fattening pigs are essentially the same except the course of the disease is usually protracted from 4 to 8 days. The mortality rate in mature pigs may reach 2%, however, losses do not usually occur.[1,2] While the clinical course in pregnant swine is virtually the same as described in mature pigs, there is a variation due to transplacental infection of the fetuses. Transplacental infection with PRV can occur, and depending upon the stage of gestation, may result in one of the following sequelae: resorption, premature expulsion of fetuses, birth of macerated fetuses, stillbirth, or birth of weak, infected pigs. Gustafson reported that as many as 20% of the sows in a recently recovered herd will not conceive at the next breeding.[1]

An assessment of exposure to PRV via natural infection or whole virus vaccine is facilitated by a measurement of antibody in the serum.

References: Available upon request.

Presentation: Kit of reagents to run 4,880 tests.

Compendium Code No.: 11160282 06-01001-05

HERDCHEK® PRV (S) ANTIBODY TEST KIT

Idexx Labs. **Pseudorabies Test**

Pseudorabies Virus Antibody Test Kit (For Screening)

U.S. Vet. Lic. No.: 313

Components:

Reagents	Volume
A. PRV Coated Plates. Burn container and all unused contents.	5
B. Anti-Porcine:HRPO conjugate. Contains gentamicin as a preservative.	60 mL
C. PRV Positive Control. Porcine Anti-PRV in Phosphate Buffer with protein stabilizers. Preserved with sodium azide.	4 mL
D. Porcine Negative Control. Porcine Serum nonreactive to PRV in Phosphate Buffer with protein stabilizers. Preserved with Sodium Azide	4 mL
E. Sample Diluent. Phosphate Buffers with protein stabilizers. Contains sodium azide as a preservative.	175 mL
F. Wash Concentrate. 10x phosphate/Tween wash. Contains gentamicin as a preservative.	235 mL
G. TMB Substrate	60 mL
H. Stop Solution	60 mL

Materials Required But Not Provided:

1. Precision Pipettes. Suitable for delivering 0.020, 0.100 mL and 0.380 mL or multiple delivery pipetting devices.
2. Disposable pipette tips.
3. Graduated cylinders: 500 mL for wash solution.
4. 96 Well Plate Reader.
5. Glass or plastic tubes for diluting samples.
6. Distilled or deionized water.
7. Device for the delivery and aspiration of wash solution.
8. A vacuum source and a trap for retaining the aspirate.

Indications: HERDCHEK® Anti-PRV (S) is Idexx's enzyme immunoassay for the detection of antibody to porcine pseudorabies virus (PRV) in swine serum.

Test Principles: HERDCHEK® Anti-PRV (S) is an enzyme immunoassay designed to detect the presence of antibody to PRV in swine serum. A microtitration format has been developed in which PRV antigens are coated on 96 well plates. Upon incubation of the test sample in the coated well, antibody specific to PRV forms a complex with the coated viral antigens. After washing away unbound material from the wells, an anti-porcine:horseradish peroxidase conjugate is added which binds to any porcine antibody attached in the wells. In the final step of the assay, unbound conjugate is washed away, and enzyme substrate (hydrogen peroxide) and a chromogen, 3,3', 5,5' tetramethylbenzidine, are added to the wells. Subsequent color is proportional to the amount of specific antibody present in the test sample.

Test Procedure:

Preparation of Samples: Dilute test samples twenty-fold (1:20) with Sample Diluent (e.g., by diluting 20 μL of sample with 380 μL of Sample Diluent). Note: Do not dilute controls.

Be sure to change tips for each sample and record the position of each sample on the plate using a HerdChek® worksheet. Samples should be mixed prior to dispensing into the PRV coated plate.

Preparation of Wash Solution: The Wash Concentrate should be brought to room temperature and mixed to assure dissolution of any precipitated salts. The Wash Concentrate must be diluted 1 to 10 with distilled/deionized water before use (e.g., 30 mL of concentrate plus 270 mL of water per plate to be assayed).

Test Procedure: All reagents should be allowed to come to room temperature before use. Reagents should be mixed by gentle swirling or vortexing.

1. Obtain antigen coated plate(s) and record the sample positions on a HerdChek® worksheet.
2. Dispense 100 μL of Undiluted Negative Control into wells A1, A2 and A3.
3. Dispense 100 μL of Undiluted Positive Control into wells A4, A5 and A6.
4. Dispense 100 μL of Diluted sample into appropriate wells. All samples should be run in duplicate.
5. Incubate for 30 minutes at room temperature.
6. Aspirate liquid contents of all wells into appropriate waste reservoir.
7. Wash each well with approximately 300 μL of phosphate buffered wash solution three to five times. Aspirate liquid contents of all wells after each wash. Avoid plate drying between plate washings and prior to the addition of conjugate. Following the final wash fluid aspiration, gently, but firmly tap residual wash fluid from each plate onto absorbent material.
8. Dispense 100 μL of Anti-Porcine:HRPO Conjugate into each well.
9. Incubate for 30 minutes at room temperature.
10. Repeat steps 6 and 7.
11. Dispense 100 μL of TMB Substrate Solution into each test plate well.
12. Incubate for 15 minutes at room temperature.
13. Dispense 100 μL of Stop Solution into each well of the test plate to stop the reaction.
14. Blank on air.
15. Measure and record the A(620 nm, 630 nm, 650 nm) for samples and controls. If a reference filter is available with the reader, the operating manual should be consulted to determine the method of reference filter selection.
16. Calculate results.

Test Interpretation:

Results: For the assay to be valid the difference (P-N) between the positive control mean ($PC\overline{x}$), and the negative control mean ($NC\overline{x}$) must be greater than or equal to 0.150. In addition, the $NC\overline{x}$ must be less than or equal to 0.150.

For invalid assays, technique may be suspect and the assay should be repeated following a thorough review of the product insert.

The presence or absence of antibody to PRV is determined by sample to weak positive (S/P) ratio for each sample. The positive control has been standardized and represents a significant level of antibody to PRV in swine serum.

See Calculations for examples.

Note: Idexx Laboratories, Inc., has instrument and software systems available which calculate means and S/P ratios and provide data summaries.

Interpretation of Results:

1. Serum samples with S/P ratios of less than 0.4 are classified as Negative for PRV antibodies.
2. If the S/P ratio is greater than or equal to 0.4, the sample is classified as Positive for PRV antibodies. When samples are classified positive in a screening test, they should be retested using the "Pseudorabies Virus Antibody Test Kit (Verification)".

Calculations:

1. Calculation of Negative Control Mean ($NC\overline{x}$):

$$NC\overline{x} = \frac{A1\ A(410) + A2\ A(410) + A3\ A(410)}{3}$$

Example:

$$\frac{0.060 + 0.063 + 0.069}{3} = 0.064$$

2. Calculation of Positive Control Mean ($PC\overline{x}$):

$$PC\overline{x} = \frac{A4\ A(650) + A5\ A(650) + A6\ A(650)}{3}$$

Example:

$$\frac{0.313 + 0.299 + 0.330}{3} = 0.314$$

3. Calculation of (S/P) Ratio:

$$S/P = \frac{\text{Sample } A(650) - NC\overline{x}}{PC\overline{x} - NC\overline{x}}$$

Example: Sample Mean = 0.350

$$S/P = \frac{0.350 - 0.064}{0.314 - 0.064} = \frac{0.286}{0.250} = 1.14$$

Storage: Store all reagents at 2°-7°C (36°-45°F).

Caution(s):

1. Handle all PRV biological materials as though capable of transmitting PRV, although the virus has been chemically treated.
2. Do not pipette by mouth.
3. There should be no eating, drinking or smoking where specimens or kit reagents are being handled.
4. TMB Substrate and Stop Solutions may be irritating to the skin.
5. Some kit components contain sodium azide as a preservative. Care should be taken to prevent the contamination of the Anti-Porcine:HRPO Conjugate with this preservative.
6. Do not expose TMB Solution to strong light or any oxidizing agents. Handle all TMB substrate Solution with clean glass or plasticware.
7. Bring to room temperature prior to use, and return to 2-7°C following use.
8. All wastes should be properly decontaminated prior to disposal.
9. Care should be taken to prevent contamination of kit components.
10. Do not use components past expiration date and do not intermix components from different serials.
11. Optimal results will be obtained by strict adherence to this protocol. Careful pipetting, timing and washing throughout this procedure are necessary to maintain precision and accuracy.

For veterinary use only.

Discussion: Pseudorabies, or Aujeszky's Disease, is caused by a type 1 porcine herpesvirus. Infections with the highest mortality rate are those affecting suckling pigs born to a susceptible sow. Baby pigs in the fatal course of the disease exhibit difficulty in breathing, fever, hypersalivation, anorexia, vomition, diarrhea, trembling, and depression. Within this age group, the final stages of infection are commonly characterized by ataxia, nystagmus, running fits, intermittent convulsions, coma, and death. Death usually occurs within 24 to 48 hours following apparent clinical symptoms. The clinical events of the disease in weanling and fattening pigs are essentially the same except the course of the disease is usually protracted from 4 to 8 days. The mortality rate in mature pigs may reach 2%, however, losses do not usually occur.[1,2] While the clinical course in pregnant swine is virtually the same as described in mature pigs, there is a variation due to transplacental infection of the fetuses. Transplacental infection with PRV can occur, and depending upon the stage of gestation, one of the following sequelae may occur: resorption, premature expulsion, birth of macerated fetuses, stillbirth, or birth of weak, infected pigs. Gustafson reported that as many as 20% of the sows in a recently recovered herd will not conceive at the next breeding.[1]

An assessment of exposure to pseudorabies virus via natural infection or vaccine is facilitated by a measurement of antibody in the serum.

References: Available upon request.

Presentation: 5 plates per kit.

HERDCHEK is a registered trademark of Idexx Laboratories, Inc. in the United States and/or other countries.

Compendium Code No.: 11160332 06-01449-07

HERDCHEK® PRV (V) ANTIBODY TEST KIT

Idexx Labs. **Pseudorabies Test**

Pseudorabies Virus Antibody Test Kit (For Verification)

U.S. Vet. Lic. No.: 313

Components:

Reagents	Volume
A. Pseudorabies Viral Antigens/Normal Host Cell Antigens, PRV/NHC, Coated Plates. Burn container and all unused contents.	2
B. Anti-Porcine: HRPO conjugate. Contains gentamicin as a preservative.	60 mL

Reagents	Volume
C. PRV Positive Control. Porcine Anti-PRV in phosphate buffer with protein stabilizers. Preserved with sodium azide.	4 mL
D. Porcine Negative Control. Porcine Serum nonreactive to PRV in phosphate buffer with protein stabilizers. Preserved with sodium azide.	4 mL
E. Sample Diluent. Phosphate Buffers with protein stabilizers. Contains azide as a preservative.	175 mL
F. Wash Concentrate. 10x phosphate/Tween wash. Contains gentamicin as a preservative.	235 mL
G. TMB Substrate	60 mL
H. Stop Solution	60 mL

Materials Required But Not Provided:

1. Precision Pipettes. Suitable for delivering 0.020, 0.100 mL and 0.380 mL or multiple delivery pipetting devices.
2. Disposable pipette tips.
3. Graduated cylinder: 500 mL for wash solution.
4. 96 Well Plate Reader.
5. Glass or plastic tubes for diluting samples.
6. Distilled or deionized water.
7. Device for the delivery and aspiration of wash solution.
8. A vacuum source and a trap for retaining the aspirate.

Indications: HERDCHEK® Anti-PRV (V) is Idexx's enzyme immunoassay for the detection of antibody to porcine pseudorabies virus (PRV) in swine serum using PRV and normal host cell (NHC) antigens.

Test Principles: HERDCHEK® Anti-PRV (V) is an enzyme immunoassay designed to detect the presence of antibody to PRV in swine serum. A microtitration format has been configured by coating PRV and NHC antigens and alternating rows on the plate. Upon incubation of the test sample in the coated well, antibody specific to PRV forms a complex with the coated viral antigens. The NHC antigens coated on the plate are used to assess whether immunoglobulins against tissue culture components present in vaccine are contributing to test results. After washing away unbound material from the wells, an anti-porcine:horseradish peroxidase conjugate is added which binds to any porcine antibody attached in the wells. In the final step of the assay, unbound conjugate is washed away, and enzyme substrate (hydrogen peroxide) and a chromogen, 3,3', 5,5' tetramethylbenzidine, are added to the wells. The extent of host cell contribution to the total signal is assessed by relating PRV activity to NHC reactivity.

Test Procedure:

Preparation of Samples: Dilute test samples twenty-fold (1:20) with Sample Diluent (e.g., by diluting 20 µL of sample with 380 µL of Sample Diluent). Note: Do not dilute controls.

Be sure to change tips for each sample and record the position of each sample on the plate using a HerdChek® worksheet. Samples should be mixed prior to dispensing into the PRV/NHC coated plate.

Preparation of Wash Solution: The Wash Concentrate should be brought to room temperature and mixed to insure dissolution of any precipitated salts. The Wash Concentrate must be diluted 1 to 10 with distilled/deionized water before use (e.g., 30 mL of concentrate plus 270 mL of water per plate to be assayed).

All reagents must be allowed to come to room temperature before use. Reagents should be mixed by gentle swirling or vortexing.

1. Obtain antigen coated plate(s) and record the sample position on a HerdChek® worksheet.
2. Dispense 100 µL of Undiluted Negative Control into PRV wells A1, A2 and A3 and NHC wells B1, B2 and B3.
3. Dispense 100 µL of Undiluted Positive Control into PRV wells A4, A5, and A6 and NHC wells B4, B5, and B6.
4. Dispense 100 µL of Diluted sample into adjacent PRV and NHC wells. All samples should be run in duplicate.
5. Incubate for 30 minutes at room temperature.
6. Aspirate liquid contents of all wells into appropriate waste reservoir.
7. Wash each well with approximately 300 µL of phosphate buffered wash solution three to five times. Aspirate liquid contents of all wells after each wash. Avoid plate drying between plate washings and prior to the addition of conjugate. Following the final wash fluid aspiration, gently, but firmly tap residual wash fluid from each plate onto absorbent material.
8. Dispense 100 µL of Anti-Porcine:HRPO Conjugate into each well.
9. Incubate for 30 minutes at room temperature.
10. Repeat steps 6 and 7.
11. Dispense 100 µL of TMB Substrate Solution into each test plate well.
12. Incubate for 15 minutes at room temperature.
13. Dispense 100 µL of Stop Solution into each well of the test plate to stop the reaction.
14. Blank on air.
15. Measure and record the A(620 nm, 630 nm, 650 nm) for samples and controls. If a reference filter is available with the reader, the operating manual should be consulted to determine the method of reference filter selection.
16. Calculate results.

Test Interpretation:

Results: For the assay to be valid the following specifications must be met.

The negative control mean for the PRV side (NC:PRV) must be less than or equal to 0.150. The positive control mean for the PRV side (PC:PRV) minus the NC:PRV must be greater than or equal to 0.150. The negative control mean for the NHC side (NC:NHC) must be less than or equal to 0.150.

For invalid assays, technique may be suspect and the assay should be repeated following a thorough review of the product insert. The Positive Control has been standardized and represents a significant level of antibody to PRV in swine serum. The normal host cell antigen provides a measure of the NHC contribution to the total PRV antigen signal. The presence or absence of antibody to PRV is determined by first calculating the sample to positive (S/P) ratio and when appropriate the sample to NHC (S/NHC) ratio for each sample.

See Calculations for examples.

Note: Idexx Laboratories, Inc. has instrument and software systems available which calculate means, S/NHC and S/P ratios and provide data summaries.

Interpretation of Results: The presence or absence of antibody to PRV is determined by first calculating the S/P ratio for each sample.

1. If the S/P ratio is less than 0.4, the sample is classified as Negative for PRV antibodies.
2. If the S/P ratio is greater than or equal to 0.4, then calculate the S/NHC ratio for each sample.
   a. If the S/NHC ratio is less than 1.8, then the sample is classified as Negative, non-confirming sample.
   b. If the S/NHC ratio is greater than or equal to 1.8, then the sample is classified as a verified Positive for PRV antibodies.

Calculations:

1. Calculation of Negative Control Mean (NCx) for both antigens (NCx:PRV and NCx:NHC).

PRV Antigen wells (A1, A2, A3)

$$\text{NCx:PRV} = \frac{\text{A1 A(650)} + \text{A2 A(650)} + \text{A3 A(650)}}{3}$$

NHC Antigen wells (B1, B2, B3)

$$\text{NCx:NHC} = \frac{\text{B1 A(650)} + \text{B2 A(650)} + \text{B3 A(650)}}{3}$$

2. Calculation of Positive Control Mean (PCx) for wells containing PRV antigens.

PRV Antigen wells (A4, A5, A6)

$$\text{PCx:PRV} = \frac{\text{A4 A(650)} + \text{A5 A(650)} + \text{A6 A(650)}}{3}$$

Example:

$$\frac{0.310 + 0.330 + 0.320}{3} = 0.320$$

3. Calculation of the sample to positive (S/P) ratio:

$$\text{S/P} = \frac{\text{(Sample A(650):PRV)} - \text{(NCx:PRV)}}{\text{(PCx:PRV)} - \text{(NCx:PRV)}}$$

Example: If sample A(650) = 0.750, then

$$\text{S/P} = \frac{0.750 - 0.065}{0.320 - 0.065} = \frac{0.685}{0.255} = 2.69$$

4. Calculation of the sample to normal host cell (S/NHC) ratio.

This ratio should be calculated only when the S/P ratio for the sample is greater than or equal to 0.4.

$$\text{Sample S/NHC} = \frac{\text{(Sample A(650):PRV)}}{\text{(Sample A(650):NHC)}}$$

Example:

If sample A(650):PRV = 0.750, and sample A(650):NHC = 0.100, then

$$\text{S/NHC} = \frac{0.750}{0.100} = 7.50$$

Storage: Store all reagents at 2-7°C (36-45°F).

Caution(s):

1. Handle all PRV biological materials as though capable of transmitting PRV, although the virus has been chemically treated.
2. Do not pipette by mouth.
3. There should be no eating, drinking or smoking where specimens or kit reagents are being handled.
4. TMB substrate, and stop solutions may be irritating to the skin.
5. Some kit components contain sodium azide as a preservative. Care should be taken lo prevent the contamination of the Anti-Porcine:HRPO Conjugate with this preservative.
6. Do not expose TMB Solution to strong light or any oxidizing agents. Handle TMB Substrate Solution with clean glass or plasticware.
7. Bring to room temperature prior to use, and return to 2-7°C following use.
8. All wastes should be properly decontaminated prior to disposal.
9. Care should be taken to prevent contamination of kit components.
10. Do not use components past expiration date and do not intermix components from different serials.
11. Optimal results will be obtained by strict adherence to this protocol. Careful pipetting. timing and washing throughout this procedure are necessary to maintain precision and accuracy.

For veterinary use only.

Discussion: Pseudorabies, or Aujeszky's Disease, is caused by a type 1 porcine herpesvirus. Infections with the highest mortality rate are those affecting suckling pigs born to a susceptible sow. Baby pigs in the fatal course of the disease exhibit difficulty in breathing, fever, hypersalivation, anorexia, vomition, diarrhea, trembling, and depression. Within this age group, the final stages of infection are commonly characterized by ataxia, nystagmus, running fits, intermittent convulsions, coma, and death. Death usually occurs within 24 to 48 hours following apparent clinical symptoms. The clinical events of the disease in weanling and fattening pigs are essentially the same except the course of the disease is usually protracted from 4 to 8 days. The mortality rate in mature pigs may reach 2%, however, losses do not usually occur.[1,2] While the clinical course in pregnant swine is virtually the same as described in mature pigs, there is a variation due to transplacental infection of the fetuses. Transplacental infection with PRV can occur, and depending upon the stage of gestation, one of the following sequelae may occur: resorption, premature expulsion, birth of macerated fetuses, stillbirth, or birth of weak, infected pigs. Gustafson reported that as many as 20% of the sows in a recently recovered herd will not conceive at the next breeding.[1]

An assessment of exposure to pseudorabies virus via natural infection or vaccine is facilitated by a measurement of antibody in the serum.

References: Available upon request.

Presentation: 2 plates per kit.

HERDCHEK is a registered trademark of Idexx Laboratories, Inc. in the United States and/or other countries.

Compendium Code No.: 11160292

06-01450-07

H

HERDCHEK® SWINE INFLUENZA VIRUS ANTIBODY TEST KIT (H1N1)

Idexx Labs. **Swine Influenza Test**

Swine Influenza Virus Antibody Test Kit-H1N1

U.S. Vet. Lic. No.: 313

Components:

Reagents	Volume
A. SI Antigen Coated Strips/Plates.	5 Plates
B. Anti-Porcine: HRPO conjugate. Contains gentamicin as a preservative.	60 mL
C. SI Positive Control. Porcine Anti-SI in phosphate buffer with protein stabilizers. Contains sodium azide as a preservative.	4 mL
D. Porcine Negative Control. Porcine Serum nonreactive to SI in phosphate buffer with protein stabilizers. Contains sodium azide as a preservative.	4 mL
E. Sample Diluent. Phosphate Buffer with protein stabilizers. Contains sodium azide as a preservative.	235 mL
F. Wash Concentrate. 10X phosphate/Tween wash. Contains gentamicin as a preservative.	235 mL
G. TMB Substrate	60 mL
H. Stop Solution	60 mL

H

Materials Required But Not Provided: Precision pipets and multiple delivery pipetting device with disposable pipet tips, 96-well plate reader, tubes for diluting samples, distilled or deionized water and device for the delivery and aspiration of wash solution.

Indications: HERDCHEK® Swine Influenza Virus Antibody Test Kit - H1N1 is an enzyme-linked immunosorbant assay (ELISA) for the detection of antibodies to swine influenza, subtype H1N1 in porcine serum. This SI-H1N1 ELISA is not intended for use in distinguishing between SIV subtype exposure (vaccine application or field infection) because of some low level cross reactivity with antibody to other SIV subtypes.

Test Principles: HERDCHEK® SI is an enzyme immunoassay designed to detect the presence of antibody to swine influenza virus subtype H1N1 in swine serum. To a limited extent, the SI ELISA may detect antibody against other swine influenza subtypes. The SI assay is performed in a microtiter well coated with swine influenza virus antigen. Upon incubation of the test sample in the coated well, antibody specific to SI forms a complex with the coated viral antigens. After washing away unbound material from the wells, an anti-porcine:horseradish peroxidase conjugate is added which binds to any porcine antibody attached in the wells. In the final step of the assay, unbound conjugate is washed away, and an enzyme substrate/chromogen solution is added to the wells. Subsequent color development may then be related directly to the amount of anti-SI antibody present in the test sample.

Test Procedure:

Preparation of Samples: Dilute test samples forty-fold (1:40) with Sample Diluent (e.g., by diluting 10 µL of sample with 390 µL of Sample Diluent). Note: Do not dilute controls.

Be sure to change tips for each sample and record the position of each sample on the plate using a HerdChek® worksheet. Samples should be mixed prior to dispensing into the SI coated plate.

Preparation of Wash Solution: The Wash Concentrate should be brought to room temperature and mixed to ensure dissolution of any precipitated salts. The Wash Concentrate must be diluted 1 to 10 with distilled/deionized water before use (e.g., 30 mL of concentrate plus 270 mL of water per plate to be assayed).

All reagents must be allowed to come to room temperature before use. Reagents should be mixed by gentle swirling or vortexing.

1. Obtain SI antigen coated plate(s) and record the sample position on a HerdChek® worksheet.
2. Dispense 100 µL of Undiluted Negative Control into SI wells A1 and B1.
3. Dispense 100 µL of Undiluted Positive Control into SI wells C1 and D1.
4. Dispense 100 µL of diluted sample into appropriate wells. It is recommended that samples should be run in duplicate.
5. Incubate for 30 minutes at room temperature.
6. Aspirate liquid contents of all wells into appropriate waste reservoir.
7. Wash each well with approximately 350 µL of phosphate buffered Wash Solution three to five times. Aspirate liquid contents of all wells after each wash. Avoid plate drying between plate washings and prior to the addition of conjugate. Following the final wash fluid aspiration, gently, but firmly tap residual wash fluid from each plate onto absorbent material.
8. Dispense 100 µL of Anti-Porcine:HRPO Conjugate into each well.
9. Incubate for 30 minutes at room temperature.
10. Repeat steps 6 and 7.
11. Dispense 100 µL of TMB Substrate Solution into each test plate well.
12. Incubate for 15 minutes at room temperature.
13. Dispense 100 µL of Stop Solution into each well of the test plate to stop the reaction.
14. Measure and record the absorbance values at 650nm, A(650).
15. Calculate results.

Test Interpretation:

Results: For the assay to be valid the difference between the Positive Control mean and the Negative Control mean ($PC\bar{x}$ - $NC\bar{x}$) should be greater than 0.150. In addition, the Negative Control mean absorbance should be less than or equal to 0.150. The presence of antibody to SI is determined by relating the A(650) value of the sample to the Positive Control mean. The Positive Control has been standardized and represents a significant level of antibody to SI in swine serum. The relative level of antibody to SI in the unknown sample is determined by calculating the sample to positive (S/P) ratio.

Interpretation of Results: The presence or absence of antibody to SI subtype H1N1 is determined by calculating the S/P ratio for each sample.

1. If the S/P ratio is less than 0.4, the sample is classified as Negative for SI H1N1 antibodies.
2. If the S/P ratio is greater than or equal to 0.4, then the sample is classified as Positive for SI antibodies.

Calculations:

1. Calculation of the Negative Control mean ($NC\bar{x}$):
$$\frac{\text{Well A1 A(650)} + \text{Well B1 A(650)}}{2} = NC\bar{x}$$
2. Calculation of the Positive Control mean ($PC\bar{x}$):
$$\frac{\text{Well C1 A(650)} + \text{Well D1 A(650)}}{2} = PC\bar{x}$$
3. Calculation of the S/P Ratio:
$$\frac{\text{Sample Mean} - NC\bar{x}}{PC\bar{x} - NC\bar{x}} = S/P$$

Note: Idexx Laboratories, Inc. has instrument and software systems available, which calculate means, and S/P ratios and provide data summaries.

Storage: Store all reagents at 2°-7°C (36°-45°F.)

Caution(s): Handle all SI biological materials as though capable of transmitting SI. The antigen-coated plates may be a source of SI. Prior to coating on the solid phase, the antigen has been inactivated by chemical treatment. Nevertheless, do not assume complete inactivation. Some kit components contain sodium aside as a preservative. Disposal requires flushing plumbing with large volumes of water to prevent formation of copper or lead azide complexes, which may explode upon percussion. Do not expose TMB solution to strong light or any oxidation agents.

All wastes should be properly decontaminated prior to disposal. Do not use components past expiration date and do not intermix components from kits with different lot numbers. Careful pipetting and washing throughout this procedure are necessary to maintain precision and accuracy. Optimal results will be obtained by strict adherence to this protocol. For veterinary use only.

Discussion: Swine influenza is an acute infectious respiratory disease of swine caused by type A influenza viruses. The disease is characterized by a sudden onset, coughing, dyspnea, fever, and prostration, followed by rapid recovery.[1] The Idexx SI antibody ELISA allows rapid screening for the presence of antibodies to H1N1 swine influenza, which can be an indicator of exposure to the virus. Monitoring the immune status of a herd with regard to SI can play an important role in the control of swine influenza virus.

References: Available upon request.

Presentation: 5 plates per kit (strips).

HERDCHEK is a registered trademark of Idexx Laboratories, Inc. in the United States and/or other countries.

Compendium Code No.: 11160601 06-04220-01

HERD-VAC™ 3

Biocor **Vaccine**

Bovine Rhinotracheitis-Virus Diarrhea-Parainfluenza 3 Vaccine, Modified Live Virus

U.S. Vet. Lic. No.: 462

Contents: This product contains the antigens listed above.

This product contains gentamicin and amphotericin B as preservatives.

Indications: HERD-VAC™ 3 is recommended for use in the vaccination of healthy cattle against disease caused by the organisms represented.

Directions: Aseptically rehydrate vial of desiccated virus with the accompanying vial of diluent. Shake well. Administer 2 mL intramuscularly or subcutaneously to healthy cattle.

Persistence of maternal antibody in calves may interfere with development of active immunity following vaccination Calves vaccinated before 3 months of age should be revaccinated at 4-6 months of age or at weaning. Annual revaccination with a single 2 mL dose is recommended.

Precaution(s): Store at 35°F-45°F (2°C-7°C). Do not freeze. Protect the vaccine from direct rays of the sun. Care should be taken to avoid chemical or microbial contamination of the product. Use entire contents when first rehydrated. Burn these containers and all unused contents.

Caution(s): In case of anaphylactoid reactions, epinephrine should be administered immediately. Do not use in pregnant cows or calves nursing pregnant cows.

Scientific evidence demonstrates the inability of some animals of an occasional herd to develop antibodies to Bovine Virus Diarrhea after vaccination. The affected animal may exhibit symptoms similar to mucosal disease.

For use in cattle only.

Warning(s): Do not vaccinate within 21 days before slaughter.

Presentation: Code 63854 - 10 dose (20 mL) vials with diluent.
Code 63864 - 50 dose (100 mL) vials with diluent.

™ Trademark of Biocor Animal Health Inc.

Compendium Code No.: 13940072 BAH5638-1000 / BAH5688-1000

HERD-VAC™ 3 S

Biocor **Bacterin-Vaccine**

Bovine Rhinotracheitis-Virus Diarrhea-Parainfluenza 3 Vaccine, Modified Live Virus-Haemophilus Somnus Bacterin

U.S. Vet. Lic. No.: 462

Contents: This product contains the antigens listed above.

This product contains gentamicin and amphotericin B as preservatives.

Indications: HERD-VAC™ 3 S is recommended for use in the vaccination of healthy cattle against disease caused by the organisms represented.

Directions: Aseptically rehydrate the vial of desiccated virus with the accompanying vial of bacterin. Shake well. Administer 2 mL intramuscularly or subcutaneously to healthy cattle. Two doses are required for calves vaccinated 4-6 months of age or before placement on full feed.

Calves vaccinated before 4 months of age should be revaccinated at 6 months of age followed by a second dose 2-4 weeks later because of the persistence of maternal antibody that may interfere with development of active immunity. Annual revaccination with a single 2 mL dose is recommended.

Precaution(s): Store at 35°F-45°F (2°C-7°C). Do not freeze. Use entire contents when first rehydrated. Care should be taken to avoid chemical or microbial contamination of the product. Burn these containers and all unused contents.

Caution(s): In case of anaphylactoid reactions, epinephrine should be administered immediately. Do not use in pregnant cows or calves nursing pregnant cows.

Scientific evidence demonstrates the inability of some animals of an occasional herd to develop antibodies to Bovine Virus Diarrhea after vaccination. The affected animal may exhibit symptoms similar to mucosal disease.

For use in cattle only.

Warning(s): Do not vaccinate within 21 days before slaughter.

Presentation: Code 64454 - 10 dose (20 mL) vials with diluent.
Code 64464 - 50 dose (100 mL) vials with diluent.

™ Trademark of Biocor Animal Health Inc.

Compendium Code No.: 13940082 BAH 8638-1000 / BAH8688-1000

HERD-VAC™ 8

Biocor **Bacterin-Vaccine**

Bovine Rhinotracheitis-Virus Diarrhea-Parainfluenza 3 Vaccine, Modified Live Virus-Leptospira Canicola-Grippotyphosa-Hardjo-Icterohaemorrhagiae-Pomona Bacterin

U.S. Vet. Lic. No.: 462

Contents: This product contains the antigens listed above.

This product contains gentamicin and amphotericin B as preservatives.

Indications: HERD-VAC™ 8 is recommended for use in the vaccination of healthy cattle against disease caused by the viral and bacterial fractions represented.

Directions: Aseptically rehydrate vial of desiccated virus with accompanying vial of bacterin. Shake well. Administer 2 mL intramuscularly or subcutaneously to healthy cattle.

Calves vaccinated before 3 months of age should be revaccinated at 4-6 months of age or at weaning because of the persistence of maternal antibody that may interfere with the development of active immunity. Annual revaccination with a single 2 mL dose is recommended.

Precaution(s): Store at 35°F-45°F (2°C-7°C). Do not freeze. Use entire contents when first rehydrated. Protect the vaccine from the direct rays of the sun. Care should be taken to avoid chemical or microbial contamination of the product. Burn these containers and all unused contents.

Caution(s): In case of anaphylactoid reactions, epinephrine should be administered immediately. Do not vaccinate pregnant cows or calves nursing pregnant cows.

Scientific evidence demonstrates the inability of some animals of an occasional herd to develop antibodies to Bovine Virus Diarrhea after vaccination. The affected animal may exhibit symptoms similar to mucosal disease.

For use in cattle only.

Warning(s): Do not vaccinate within 21 days before slaughter.

Presentation: Code 64254 - 10 dose (20 mL) vials with diluent.
Code 64264 - 50 dose (100 mL) vials with diluent.

™ Trademark of Biocor Animal Health Inc.

Compendium Code No.: 13940102 BAH6938-1000 / BAH6988-1000

HERD-VAC™ 9

Biocor **Bacterin-Vaccine**

Bovine Rhinotracheitis-Virus Diarrhea-Parainfluenza 3 Vaccine, Modified Live Virus-Campylobacter Fetus-Leptospira Canicola-Grippotyphosa-Hardjo-Icterohaemorrhagiae-Pomona Bacterin

U.S. Vet. Lic. No.: 462

Contents: This product contains the antigens listed above.

This product contains gentamicin and amphotericin B as preservatives.

Indications: HERD-VAC™ 9 is recommended for use in the vaccination of healthy cattle against disease caused by the viral and bacterial fractions represented.

Directions: Aseptically rehydrate vial of desiccated virus with the accompanying vial of bacterin. Shake well. Administer 5 mL intramuscularly or subcutaneously to healthy cattle. In *Campylobacter fetus* infected herds or endemic areas, a second vaccination in 21 days is required.

Persistence of maternal antibody in calves may interfere with development of active immunity following vaccination. Calves vaccinated before 3 months of age should be revaccinated at 4-6 months of age or at weaning. Annual revaccination with a single 5 mL dose is recommended.

Precaution(s): Store at 35°F-45°F (2°C-7°C). Do not freeze. Protect the vaccine from the direct rays of the sun. Use entire contents when first rehydrated. Care should be taken to avoid chemical or microbial contamination of the product. Burn these containers and all unused contents.

Caution(s): In case of anaphylactoid reactions, epinephrine should be administered immediately. Do not use in pregnant cows or calves nursing pregnant cows.

Scientific evidence demonstrates the inability of some animals of an occasional herd to develop antibodies to Bovine Virus Diarrhea after vaccination. The affected animal may exhibit symptoms similar to mucosal disease.

For use in cattle only.

Warning(s): Do not vaccinate within 21 days before slaughter.

Presentation: Code 63055 - 10 dose (50 mL) vials with diluent.
Code 63058 - 20 dose (100 mL) vials with diluent.

™ Trademark of Biocor Animal Health Inc.

Compendium Code No.: 13940112 BAH 7438-1000 / BAH7448-1000

HESKA® ALLERCEPT™ E-SCREEN™ IgE TEST

Heska **Allergen-Specific IgE Test**

Canine IgE Antibody Detection Kit

Test Description: The ALLERCEPT™ E-SCREEN™ test is a rapid immunoassay for the detection of allergen-specific IgE antibodies in canine serum or plasma. The test is specific, sensitive and simple to use. Results are read immediately upon completion of the final step.

Components: Required Materials:

1. Canine Serum or Plasma (do not use whole blood)
2. Test Device (provided)
3. Wash Buffer and Reagents (provided)
   - Wash Buffer: white cap and label
   - Reagent A: green cap and label
   - Reagent B: black cap and label
   - Reagent C: purple cap and label
4. Pipette (provided)
5. Timing Device

Indications: When a clinical diagnosis of atopic dermatitis has been made, a positive E-SCREEN™ test result supports the diagnosis by detecting allergen-specific IgE antibodies in the canine patient's serum or plasma. The ALLERCEPT™ E-SCREEN™ test is intended to determine whether more comprehensive allergen-specific IgE testing is warranted. Heska® Allercept™ Definitive Allergen Panels or intra-dermal skin test results can then be used to formulate customized immunotherapy.

Sample Collection: Sample Collection and Storage:

Plasma: Collect an anticoagulated (EDTA, heparin or citrate) blood sample using standard clinical laboratory procedures. Separate plasma by centrifugation. Plasma samples may be stored refrigerated at 2°-7°C (36°-45°F) for up to 72 hours. For longer storage, freeze at or below -20°C (-4°F) in vials with air-tight seals.

Serum: Collect and prepare serum samples using standard clinical laboratory procedures. Serum samples may be stored refrigerated at 2°-7°C (36°-45°F) for up to 72 hours. For longer storage, freeze at or below -20°C (-4°F) in vials with air-tight seals.

Test Procedure: Directions for Use: Allow test devices, samples and reagents to come to room temperature (15°-30°C [59°-86°F]) before use.

The entire test can be performed within 5 minutes according to the following procedure:

- Open the test kit.
- Open one foil pouch for each sample to be tested. Remove the test device from the pouch by the edges. Avoid touching the center of the device where the test window is located.

Place the test device on a solid, flat surface with the letter "C" (control) positioned on the left side and the letter "T" (test) on the right side of the sample well.

- Perform test following these easy steps:

Note: Do not touch the test membrane with the pipette or bottle tips at any time during the test procedure.

Step 1:

Add two drops of Wash Buffer (bottle with white cap and label) to the test window. Let drops absorb before proceeding.

Step 2:

Using a new pipette for each serum or plasma sample, draw up the patient's sample into the stem portion of the pipette. Avoid air bubbles and do not fill the bulb. Add two drops of sample to the test window. Let drops absorb before proceeding.

Add two drops of Wash Buffer (bottle with white cap and label). Let drops absorb before proceeding.

Step 3:

Add two drops of Reagent A (bottle with green cap and label). Let drops absorb before proceeding.

Add two drops of Wash Buffer (bottle with white cap and label). Let drops absorb before proceeding.

Step 4:

Add two drops of Reagent B (bottle with black cap and label). Let drops absorb before proceeding.

Add two drops of Wash Buffer (bottle with white cap and label). Let drops absorb before proceeding.

Step 5:

Add two drops of Reagent C (bottle with purple cap and label). Wait 30 - 40 seconds.

Add four drops of Wash Buffer.

Note: Results can be read immediately and will remain stable for at least 30 minutes.

Interpretation of Results: Procedural Control Spot (C): You must see a purple spot on the test membrane by the letter "C" within 30 - 40 seconds of completion of Step 5 for the test to be valid. If the control spot does not develop within 30 - 40 seconds, the test is invalid and should be repeated. Repeat the test with a new test device.

Negative Results: If the control spot "C" is the only visible spot within 30 - 40 seconds of test completion, the test is negative.

A negative test result indicates:

1. The dog does not have detectable serum or plasma levels of allergen-specific IgE to the allergens in the test spot.
2. Re-testing with the ALLERCEPT™ E-SCREEN™ test at a later date (e.g. after further allergen exposure or after a longer steroid withdrawal time), may be necessary.
3. Definitive serum testing at this time is unlikely to yield useful information.

Positive Results: If control "C" and test "T" spots both appear within 30 - 40 seconds of test completion, the test is positive. The ALLERCEPT™ E-SCREEN™ test is not a quantitative test and even faint color in the test spot is considered significant.

A positive E-SCREEN™ test result indicates:

1. The dog has readily detectable allergen-specific IgE to one or more of the allergens contained in the test spot.
2. The dog has a high probability of testing positive to individual clinically relevant allergens when evaluated by Heska® Allercept™ Definitive Allergen Panels.

Heska Corporation provides comprehensive allergen-specific IgE *in vitro* testing with Allercept™ Definitive Allergen Panels.

Allercept™ regional panels are tailored to the predominant climatic and botanic regions of North America. Call 1-800-GO HESKA (1-800-464-3752) for more details. Allercept™ Definitive Allergen Panel results come with a free case consultation and an immunotherapy recommendation from Heska's Medical and Technical Consultation Group.

Storage: Storage and Stability: Store the complete test kit in the refrigerator at 2°-7°C (36°-45°F). See package for expiration date.

Caution(s):

1. Do not use lipemic samples of plasma or serum. Lipemic samples may cause background color that could interfere with interpretation of the test.
2. Let liquid absorb fully into the membrane before proceeding to the next step:
   - Inadequate absorption between steps may cause background color that could interfere with interpretation of the test.
   - Sample or reagent overflowing the test window invalidates the test result.
3. Do not expose a test device to direct sunlight or extreme heat.
4. Do not use a test device or pipette more than once.
5. A test device must be used within two hours after opening the foil pouch. Discard any opened unused test devices.

Discussion: Allergen-Specific IgE Test for Dogs: The ALLERCEPT™ E-SCREEN™ test is a rapid immunoassay that detects allergen-specific IgE antibodies in canine serum or plasma. It is intended to be used, after a clinical diagnosis of atopy has been made, to determine whether more comprehensive testing for allergen-specific IgE is indicated at this time.

Canine atopic dermatitis, also referred to as canine allergic dermatitis, is a relatively common disease accounting for approximately 10 - 15% of the dermatological disorders seen in general practice. Atopic dermatitis occurs in susceptible animals upon exposure to a wide range of allergens such as house dust mites and pollens. In the majority of animals allergic to environmental allergens, the initial event is believed to be the formation of IgE antibodies specific for the offending allergen. These antibodies may be detected in serum or plasma by *in vitro* assays using antibodies or other detection reagents specific for canine IgE and in the skin by intradermal skin testing.

Under certain circumstances, clinically normal dogs may produce allergen-specific IgE antibodies. Therefore, the diagnosis of allergy should be based on patient history, clinical signs and a differential diagnostic plan ruling out other causes of pruritic dermatitis.

The presence of allergen-specific IgE in the context of appropriate clinical signs, known allergen exposure and the absence of other causes of pruritus supports a diagnosis of allergy.

The ALLERCEPT™ E-SCREEN™ test detects serum or plasma IgE antibodies specific for one or more of a carefully chosen panel of common allergens, combined in a single test spot within the device test window. A positive E-SCREEN™ test result indicates a high probability that more comprehensive testing for allergen-specific IgE by a proven serum assay (such as Heska® Allercept™ Definitive Allergen Panels) or intradermal skin test will define the relevant allergens for the patient's disease.

Tips for Using the ALLERCEPT™ E-SCREEN™ Test:

1. When using test devices from the box, use only those reagents included in that box.
2. Centrifuge the blood sample, or let it stand so that plasma/serum separates.
3. Have 1 pipette for each sample ready.
4. Have a timing device ready.
5. Use only after the following clinical conditions have been ruled out or treated appropriately: Pyoderma, malassezia, flea infestation, scabies, other parasite infection/infestation.

Presentation: Available in cartons of 10 tests.

U.S. Patent Nos. 5,646,115; 5,795,862; 5,840,695 and Patents Pending

Compendium Code No.: 14820070 02224-1

HESKA® BIVALENT INTRANASAL/INTRAOCULAR VACCINE

Heska **Vaccine**

Feline Rhinotracheitis-Calici Vaccine, Modified Live Virus

U.S. Vet. Lic. No.: 124

Contents: This product contains the antigens listed above (feline cell line origin).

Contains gentamicin and fungistat as preservatives.

H

Indications: Recommended for the vaccination of healthy, susceptible cats against feline rhinotracheitis (herpesvirus) and feline calicivirus.

Dosage and Administration: Cats can be vaccinated with a single dose at 12 weeks of age. If cats are vaccinated at less than 12 weeks of age, a second vaccination should be administered at 12-16 weeks of age. Annual revaccination is recommended.

Remove the ring and rubber stopper from the vials. Using the dropper, rehydrate the lyophilized vaccine with the accompanying bottle of 0.5 mL sterile diluent. Immediately withdraw the rehydrated vaccine into the dropper. Place one drop of vaccine in the corner of each eye. The remaining vaccine is administered by placing the vaccine equally in each nostril as the animal inhales. Use a new dropper for each cat vaccinated.

Precaution(s): Store out of direct sunlight at a temperature not over 45°F. Use the entire contents of the vaccine when first opened. Burn containers and all unused contents.

Caution(s): The vaccine is not to be injected.

Do not vaccinate pregnant animals.

In rare instances, reactions can occur due to unusual sensitivity following use of this product. In such cases, administer epinephrine as an antidote.

The vaccine will not protect against disease in the face of incubating feline rhinotracheitis or feline calicivirus infection. Therefore, only healthy cats should be considered as candidates for vaccination.

In some cats, a slight watery discharge and occasional sneezing may occur four to seven days after vaccination. Oral lesions may be observed after vaccination but heal without incident.

For use in cats only.

Presentation: The package contains 20 (1 dose) vials of dry vaccine, 20 (0.5 mL) vials of sterile diluent and 20 droppers.

Manufactured by: Boehringer Ingelheim Animal Health, Inc.

Compendium Code No.: 14820001 16204-00

HESKA® E.R.D.-SCREEN™ URINE TEST

Heska **Renal Disease Test**

Canine Microalbuminuria Detection Kit

Test Description: The E.R.D.-SCREEN™ test is a rapid immunoassay for the detection of low levels of albumin in canine urine. The test is specific, sensitive and simple to use. Results are read upon completion of the final step.

Components: Required Materials:

1. A sample of canine urine (2 mL)
2. Refractometer
3. Distilled water (for dilution of sample if indicated)
4. Sample dilution tube (provided)
5. Test device (provided)
6. Timing device

Indications: The E.R.D.-SCREEN™ test is a tool developed specifically to assist veterinarians in the detection of ongoing nephron damage in dogs, to help monitor the progression of early renal disease, and to help monitor the success of treatment programs.

Sample Collection: Sample Collection and Storage:

Collect a urine sample (2 mL minimum volume) using standard clinical procedures (free catch, catheterization, cystocentesis). Urine samples may be stored refrigerated at 2°-7°C (36°-45°F) for up to 24 hours. For longer storage, freeze at or below -20°C (-4°F) in vials with airtight seals. Stored samples must be warmed to room temperature prior to testing.

Test Procedure: The entire test can be performed within 5 minutes according to the following procedure:

1. Using a refractometer, measure the specific gravity of the urine sample. If the upper limit of the refractometer's range is 1.040, and the sample's specific gravity is greater than 1.040, dilute 1 mL of the urine sample with 1 mL of distilled water, measure the specific gravity of the diluted sample, and proceed using the diluted sample.
2. Add urine to the sample dilution tube to the line marked "Sample" (= 1 mL). If the sample's specific gravity is less than 1.020, add undiluted sample to the 1.020 mark.
3. Add distilled water to the mark that corresponds to the sample's specific gravity.
4. Cap the tube and mix the sample by inverting the tube 3 times.
5. Open one foil pouch and place the test device into the prepared sample. Move the test device up and down twice to assure proper liquid flow.
6. Leave the device in the sample for at least 3 minutes and not more than 1 hour.
7. Remove device and read by comparing the relative intensities of the 2 bands (refer to Interpretation of Results card).

Interpretation of Results: The relative intensity of the two bands is used to classify the sample into one of two categories: negative or positive. The sample is negative if the bottom band is darker than the top band. The sample is positive if the 2 bands are equal in intensity (low positive), if the top band is slightly darker than the bottom band (medium positive), or if the top band is very dark and the bottom band is very faint or absent (high positive).

If no bands are present, if only the bottom band is present, or if the bands appear broken or blotched, the test is invalid and should be repeated.

A negative E.R.D.-SCREEN™ test result indicates the dog does not have detectable microalbuminuria.

A positive E.R.D.-SCREEN™ test result indicates the dog has readily detectable microalbuminuria.

The presence of persistent microalbuminuria (positive on at least 2 out of 3 urine samples acquired 2 weeks apart) is indicative of nephron damage and in the absence of azotemia supports a diagnosis of early renal disease.

Heska Corporation provides a quantitative microalbuminuria *in vitro* test for determining the level of microalbuminuria as an adjunct diagnostic for monitoring the progression of early renal disease, and to help monitor the success of treatment. Call 1-800-GO HESKA (800-464-3752) for more details.

Storage: Storage and Stability: Store test kit at room temperature (15°-30°C [59°-86°F]). See package for expiration date.

Caution(s):

1. Do not use grossly hematuric samples. Urine samples that are visibly pink or red will be positive due to contamination with serum albumin.
2. Do not use a sample tube or test device more than once.
3. A test device must be used within 1 hour after opening the foil pouch. Discard any opened, unused test devices.

Discussion: Early Renal Disease Test for Dogs: The E.R.D.-SCREEN™ test is a rapid immunoassay that detects low levels of albumin in canine urine. This test is intended to be used to determine whether more comprehensive evaluation for early renal disease is indicated.

Renal Disease in Dogs: Chronic renal disease in dogs is routinely diagnosed by the presence of azotemia, (elevated blood urea nitrogen [BUN] and serum creatinine) which occurs after approximately 75% of nephrons become non-functional. While the underlying etiology of nephron damage and subsequent loss is frequently not determined, glomerulonephritis is considered to be a common cause of chronic renal disease in dogs. Experimental models of glomerulonephritis in dogs have demonstrated that detectable abnormalities in kidney structure and function occur prior to the onset of azotemia. The consequence of these structural changes is an increase in glomerular permeability that results in a continuous low level of albumin being excreted in the urine. The E.R.D.-SCREEN™ test detects this low level of albumin (~1.0 mg/dL).

Trial Data: Accuracy of Conventional Urine Dipsticks for the Detection of Proteinuria: Sensitivity of conventional urine dipsticks for detection of proteinuria is approximately 10.0 - 30.0 mg/dL. However, urine pH has been demonstrated to affect the detection of protein using urine dipsticks, producing false positive results. To determine the accuracy of urine protein dipsticks for the detection of albumin, urine protein dipstick results were compared with the normalized urine albumin concentrations for 246 samples (Table 1). Of the 50 trace positive urine samples, 33 (66%) were negative for microalbuminuria.

Of the 17 +1 positive urine samples, 5 (29%) were negative for microalbuminuria. We interpreted these discrepant results (38/67 = 57%) to be false positive urine protein dipstick results.

Table 1. Urine protein dipstick result versus normalized urine albumin concentration.

Normalized Urine Albumin Concentration	Urine Protein Dipstick Result			
	negative	trace	+1	+2-4
< 1.0 mg/dL	109	33	5	1
>1.0 and < 30.0 mg/dL	57	16	3	2
> 30.0 mg/dL	1	1	9	9

Presentation: Available in cartons of 10 tests.

Patents Pending

Compendium Code No.: 14820080

HESKA® F.A. GRANULES

Heska **Small Animal Dietary Supplement**

Omega-3 and Omega-6 Fatty Acid Supplement

Active Ingredient(s): Each 5 gram scoop of HESKA® F.A. Granules contains:

Ingredient	Nutrient	Amount
Flaxseed oil	Alpha Linolenic Acid (Omega-3)	500 mg
Flaxseed oil	Linoleic Acid (Omega-6)	125 mg
Vitamin E acetate	Vitamin E	5 IU
Vitamin A acetate	Vitamin A	750 IU
Choline chloride	Choline	10 mg
Zinc amino acid chelate	Zinc	5 mg
Selenium amino acid chelate	Selenium	5 mcg

The fatty acids are microencapsulated to enhance bioavailability and usefulness.

Flaxseed oil, which is derived from the flax plant, is a safe and natural source of high levels of omega fatty acids. Flaxseed oil provides Omega-3 and Omega-6 essential fatty acids in the preferred ratio to maximize the benefit to the skin and haircoat.

Indications: A supplemental source of omega fatty acids to aid in dry skin relief and benefit the improvement and maintenance of healthy skin and haircoat of dogs.

Dosage and Administration: Dosage Schedule: The following dosage schedule is recommended for daily administration of HESKA® F.A. Granules. Consult your veterinarian to determine the proper dosage level and schedule for each individual animal prescribed this product.

Weight of Dog	Induction Dosage (6 - 8 weeks)	Maintenance Dosage
	Scoop size = 5 grams	
5 lbs.	¼ scoop/day	⅛ scoop/day
10 lbs.	½ scoop/day	⅛ - ¼ scoop/day
20 lbs.	1 scoop/day	¼ - ½ scoop/day
40 lbs.	2 scoops/day	½ - 1 scoop/day
60 lbs.	3 scoops/day	¾ - 1½ scoops/day
80 lbs.	4 scoops/day	1 - 2 scoops/day
100 lbs.	5 scoops/day	1¼ - 2½ scoops/day

Each 5 gram scoop delivers a total of 500 mg Omega-3 fatty acids and 125 mg Omega-6 fatty acids.

Administration: A 5 gram scoop is enclosed in the container. Measure out the prescribed daily dose and administer over the dog's food. Product may be mixed with food, if necessary, to facilitate complete consumption.

Precaution(s): Store at room temperature (59°F-86°F). Avoid excessive heat.

Caution(s): For veterinary use only.

Warning(s): Keep out of reach of children.

Presentation: 450 g containers.

Compendium Code No.: 14820021

HESKA® SOLO STEP® CH

Heska **Heartworm Test**

Canine Heartworm Antigen Test Kit

U.S. Vet. Lic. No.: 213

Indications: HESKA® SOLO STEP® CH is a diagnostic tool which has been developed to assist veterinarians in detecting *D. immitis* infections in dogs and to help monitor the success of canine heartworm prevention and treatment programs.

Test Principles: HESKA® SOLO STEP® CH is a one-step, lateral flow immunoassay for the detection of antigens produced by adult, *Dirofilaria immitis* in canine serum, plasma and anticoagulated whole blood. This test is highly specific and sensitive, very simple to use, and results are read within 5-10 minutes.

Diagnosis of the infection is based on the detection of circulating antigens produced by adult heartworms. Antigen detection is possible beginning approximately 6 months post-infection.

Test Procedure: The test cassette is for use in detecting antigens produced by *D. immitis* in serum, plasma or anticoagulated whole blood from dogs.

Required Materials:
1. A sample of canine serum, plasma or anticoagulated whole blood
2. Test cassette (provided)
3. Pipette (provided)
4. Timer or clock

Procedure:
1. Open the foil package and place the test cassette on a flat solid surface (Figure 1).

Figure 1

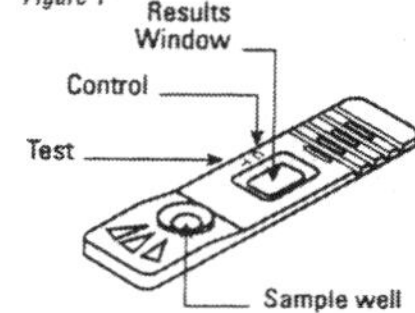

2. Using the pipette, draw up the patient sample into the stem portion of the pipette. Do not fill the bulb.
3. Holding the pipette vertically, dispense 3 drops of the sample into the round sample well of the test cassette.
4. Allow the test cassette to sit undisturbed for 5-10 minutes.
5. Read the results in the rectangular Results Window 5 minutes after applying serum or plasma. For anticoagulated whole blood, read results 10 minutes after application. A blue line (Procedural Control Line) must appear on all samples, and a red line (Test Line) may or may not appear (Figure 2).

Figure 2

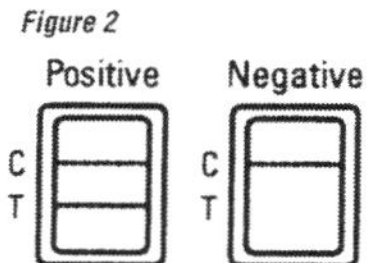

Sample Collection: Anticoagulated Whole Blood: Collect an anticoagulated blood sample in EDTA, heparin or citrate using standard clinical laboratory procedures. Anticoagulated whole blood samples should be tested within 24 hours of drawing. If delays are expected between sample collection and testing, anticoagulated whole blood samples should be stored either on ice or refrigerated (2-7°C), but should not be frozen. If anticoagulated whole blood samples cannot be tested within this period of time, separate plasma by centrifugation and store as described below.

Plasma: Collect an anticoagulated blood sample using standard clinical laboratory procedures. Separate plasma by centrifugation. Plasma samples may be stored refrigerated (2-7°C) for up to 72 hours; for longer storage, freeze at or below -20°C in vials with air-tight seals.

Serum: Collect and prepare serum samples using standard clinical laboratory procedures. Serum samples may be stored refrigerated (2-7°C) for up to 72 hours; for longer storage, freeze at or below -20°C in vials with air-tight seals.

Interpretation of Test Results: Procedural Control Line (C): You must see a blue line within 5 minutes of adding serum or plasma, or within 10 minutes of adding anticoagulated whole blood, for the test to be valid. This blue procedural control line indicates proper flow of the sample through the test cassette. If the blue line does not develop, the test is invalid and should be repeated. Discard the cassette, and repeat the test with a new cassette.

Test Line (T): Any visible red line within 5 minutes of adding serum or plasma, or within 10 minutes of adding anticoagulated whole blood, indicates a positive result. Antigens from adult *D. immitis* are present.

No red line within 5 minutes of adding serum or plasma, or within 10 minutes of adding anticoagulated whole blood, indicates a negative test result. There are no antigens present.

Storage:
1. Store at room temperature (15-30°C [59-86°F]).
2. See package for expiration date.

Caution(s):
1. Do not expose the test cassette to direct sunlight.
2. Do not use the test cassette more than once.
3. Use the test cassette immediately after opening the foil pouch.

Discussion: Heartworm in Dogs: Although heartworms infect a wide variety of mammals, the definitive host is the dog. Adult heartworms live in the right ventricle and pulmonary arteries where, as adults, they produce microfilariae which can be found circulating in the blood of an infected dog. Transmission of the infection occurs when a mosquito ingests circulating microfilariae while feeding on an infected dog. The microfilariae develop within the mosquito to the infective 3rd stage larvae after which they can be transmitted to another animal when the mosquito feeds again. Once infective larvae have been transmitted, they continue to develop and migrate until they reach the heart and pulmonary arteries as young adult worms. Heartworms can interfere with heart function and cause serious damage to the heart, pulmonary vasculature and other organ systems.

Serologic diagnosis of canine heartworm infection is based on detection of circulating antigens or microfilariae, each of which are detectable beginning at about 6 months post-infection. However, even in areas where the prevalence of heartworm infection is high, many heartworm-infected dogs do not have a detectable microfilaremia; therefore antigen testing is considered the primary diagnostic method. In addition, most heartworm-infected dogs that receive regular monthly doses of macrolide heartworm preventives will become amicrofilaremic, further reinforcing the role of antigen testing as the primary tool for the diagnosis of canine heartworm infection.

Presentation: HESKA® SOLO STEP® CH is available in kits containing 10 or 25 test cassettes.

HESKA® SOLO STEP® CH Batch Test Results — An integrated results card which allows you to run as few as 10 tests at a time. Available in packs of 10x10's.

US 4,839,275; US 4,943,522; CA 1,232,849; AU 582,129 and Patents Pending

Compendium Code No.: 14820041

HESKA® SOLO STEP® FH

Heska **Heartworm Test**

Feline Heartworm Antibody Test Kit

U.S. Vet. Lic. No.: 213

Contents: Required Materials:
1. A sample of feline serum, plasma or anticoagulated whole blood
2. Test cassette (provided)
3. Pipette (provided)
4. Timer or clock

Indications: HESKA® SOLO STEP® FH is a diagnostic tool developed specifically to assist veterinarians in detecting *D. immitis* infections in cats. This test will also aid in determining prevalence rates of *D. immitis* infection in the cat population.

Test Principles: Product Description: HESKA® SOLO STEP® FH is a one-step, lateral flow immunoassay for the detection of antibodies to *D. immitis* in feline serum, plasma or anticoagulated whole blood. This test is highly specific and sensitive, and is the first single-step test kit designed specifically for the diagnosis of feline heartworm infection. The test kit is very simple to use, and results are read within 10 minutes.

Diagnosis of the infection is based on the detection of circulating IgG antibodies to a specific heartworm antigen. The antigen, which is expressed by a single *D. immitis* gene isolated and cloned by Heska scientists, is present in male and female heartworms. Antibodies to the antigen are first detected in some cats at 50-60 days post-infection (corresponding to the late fourth larval stage (L4) to early adult stage of *D. immitis* development). HESKA® SOLO STEP® FH was developed to detect these antibodies and will detect antibodies resulting from heartworm infections commonly seen in cats, including immature worms, adult male and female heartworms, and single-sex male or female heartworm infections.

Sample Collection: Sample Collection and Storage:

Anticoagulated Whole Blood: Collect an anticoagulated blood sample in EDTA, heparin or citrate using standard clinical laboratory procedures. Anticoagulated whole blood samples should be tested within 24 hours of drawing. If delays are expected between sample collection and testing, anticoagulated whole blood samples should be stored either on ice or refrigerated (2-7°C) but should not be frozen. If anticoagulated whole blood samples cannot be tested within this period of time, separate plasma by centrifugation and store as described below.

Plasma: Collect an anticoagulated blood sample using standard clinical laboratory procedures. Separate plasma by centrifugation. Plasma samples may be stored refrigerated (2-7°C) for up to 72 hours; for longer storage, freeze at or below -20°C in vials with air-tight seals.

Serum: Collect and prepare serum samples using standard clinical laboratory procedures. Serum samples may be stored refrigerated (2-7°C) for up to 72 hours; for longer storage, freeze at or below -20°C in vials with air-tight seals.

Test Procedure: Directions for Use: The test cassette is for use in detecting IgG antibodies against *D. immitis* in serum, plasma or anticoagulated whole blood from cats.

Procedure:
1. Open the foil package and place the test cassette on a flat solid surface (Figure 1).

Figure 1

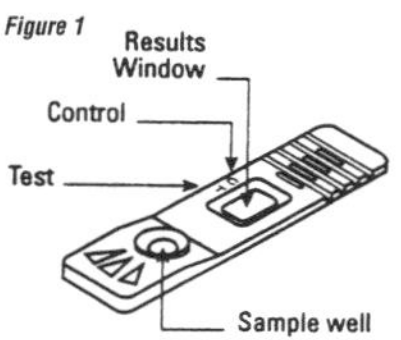

2. Using the pipette, draw up the patient sample into the stem portion of the pipette. Do not fill the bulb.
3. Holding the pipette vertically, dispense 3 drops of the sample into the round sample well of the test cassette.
4. Allow the test cassette to sit undisturbed for 5-10 minutes.
5. Read the results in the rectangular Results Window 5 minutes after applying plasma or serum. For anticoagulated whole blood, read results 10 minutes after application. A blue line (Procedural Control Line) must appear on all samples, and a red line (Test Line) may or may not appear (Figure 2).

Figure 2

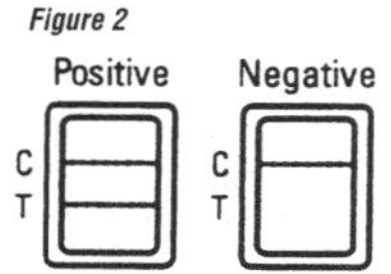

Interpretation of Results:

Procedural Control Line (C): You must see a blue line within 5 minutes of adding serum or plasma, or within 10 minutes of adding anticoagulated whole blood, for the test to be valid. This blue procedural control line indicates proper flow of the sample through the test cassette. If the

H

blue line does not develop, the test is invalid and should be repeated. Discard the test cassette, and repeat the test with a new test cassette.

Test Line (T): Any visible red line within 5 minutes of adding serum or plasma, or within 10 minutes of adding anticoagulated whole blood, indicates a positive result. Antibodies to *D. immitis* are present. This means one or more of the following:

- Adult heartworms are present in the heart and/or pulmonary arteries.
- The cat is infected with late L4 or adult worm(s).
- Heartworm infection has been cleared, but antibodies are still present.
- Ectopic heartworm infection may be present.

In the presence of suggestive clinical signs and other supportive diagnostic data (e.g., radiographic findings, echocardiographic findings, etc.), a positive result will help confirm cardiovascular heartworm disease.

No red line within 5 minutes of adding serum or plasma, or within 10 minutes of adding anticoagulated whole blood, indicates a negative test result. There are no antibodies to *D. immitis* present. This means one of the following:

- The cat is not infected with *D. immitis*.
- The cat was infected less than 60 days prior to collection of the sample.

If a negative result is obtained and clinical signs are present, a retest within 2-3 months is recommended. Additional diagnostic tests should be employed to rule out other causes of the clinical signs.

Storage: Storage and Stability:

1. Store at room temperature (15-30°C [59-86°]).
2. See package for expiration date.

Caution(s):

1. Do not expose the test cassette to direct sunlight.
2. Do not use to test species other than cats.
3. After 10 minutes, a very faint red line may appear in the Results Window with samples from some cats which are negative for heartworm infection.
4. Do not use the test cassette more than once.
5. Use the test cassette immediately after opening the foil pouch.

Discussion: Heartworm in Cats: Feline heartworm infection *(Dirofilaria immitis)* is seen wherever canine heartworm infection is present. Heartworm infections in cats are frequently characterized by single-sex infections (approximately ⅓ of infections) with small numbers of worms (1 to 3 worms per cat on average). For these reasons, antigen tests commonly used for heartworm diagnosis in dogs will not detect a large percentage of heartworm infections in cats.

Heartworms live approximately 1 to 2 years in cats and ectopic infections are not uncommon. Clinical signs of feline heartworm disease include, among others, vomiting, coughing, respiratory distress, central nervous system abnormalities and acute death.

Presentation: Available in kits containing 10 or 25 test cassettes.

US 4,943,522 and Patents Pending

Compendium Code No.: 14820051 01666 / 01533 ; 02213-1

HESKA® TRIVALENT INTRANASAL/INTRAOCULAR VACCINE

Heska **Vaccine**

Feline Rhinotracheitis-Calici-Panleukopenia Vaccine, Modified Live Virus

U.S. Vet. Lic. No.: 213

Contents: This product contains the antigens listed above.

Contains gentamicin, amphotericin B, neomycin and thimerosal as preservatives.

Indications: Recommended for the vaccination of healthy, susceptible cats against feline rhinotracheitis (herpesvirus), feline calicivirus, and feline panleukopenia.

Dosage and Administration: Cats can be vaccinated with a single dose at 12 weeks of age. If cats are vaccinated at less than 12 weeks of age, a second vaccination should be administered at 12-16 weeks of age. Annual revaccination is recommended.

Remove the ring and rubber stopper from the vials. Using the dropper, rehydrate the lyophilized vaccine with the accompanying bottle of 0.5 mL liquid vaccine. Immediately withdraw the rehydrated vaccine into the dropper. Place one drop of vaccine in the corner of each eye. The remaining vaccine is administered by placing the vaccine equally in each nostril as the animal inhales. Use a new dropper for each cat vaccinated.

Precaution(s): Store out of direct sunlight at a temperature not over 45°F. Use the entire contents of the vaccine when first opened. Burn containers and all unused contents.

Caution(s): The vaccine is not to be injected.

Do not vaccinate pregnant animals.

In rare instances, reactions can occur due to unusual sensitivity following use of this product. In such cases, administer epinephrine as an antidote.

The vaccine will not protect against disease in the face of incubating feline rhinotracheitis (herpesvirus), feline calicivirus or feline panleukopenia virus infection. Therefore, only healthy cats should be considered as candidates for vaccination.

In some cats, a slight watery discharge and occasional sneezing may occur four to seven days after vaccination. A transient drop in the white blood cell count has been noted at times five to six days after vaccination. Oral lesions may be observed after vaccination but heal without incident.

For intranasal/intraocular use in cats only.

For veterinary use only.

Discussion: Performance Characteristics of the Vaccine: Based on extensive laboratory and field studies, the HESKA® Trivalent Intranasal/Intraocular Vaccine was shown to provide rapid and effective protection against feline rhinotracheitis virus, calicivirus and panleukopenia virus. A single 0.5 mL dose, administered to kittens as young as three weeks of age, provided protective immunity against feline rhinotracheitis and calicivirus. Kittens vaccinated at less than 12 weeks of age should receive a second vaccination at or after 12 weeks of age to maximize protection against panleukopenia.

For rhinotracheitis, significant protection against virulent virus challenge was observed as early as two days post-vaccination and protection was complete by four days post-vaccination.[1] Data generated in another study suggested vaccination of previously uninfected cats via the intranasal route may prevent the subsequent development of a rhinotracheitis virus carrier state following challenge with virulent field virus, at least in the short term.[2]

The safety of the vaccine was also extensively evaluated.[3] One thousand seventy-seven cats, ranging in age from 1 month to 19 years, were given the rhinotracheitis-calicivirus components with only 17 cats (1.6%) demonstrating mild post-vaccinal reactions. In 747 cats (ages 1 month to 18 years) given the rhinotracheitis, calici and panleukopenia components, vaccine-associated adverse signs were observed in 18 cats (2.4%). The most common clinical sign observed after vaccination was transient sneezing and all vaccinated cats recovered without incident.

References: Available upon request.

Presentation: The package contains 20 (1 dose) vials of dry vaccine, 20 (0.5 mL) vials of liquid vaccine and 20 droppers.

Compendium Code No.: 14820061

HETACIN-K® INTRAMAMMARY INFUSION ℞

Fort Dodge **Mastitis Therapy**

Hetacillin Potassium

NADA No.: 055-054

Active Ingredient(s): Each 10 mL disposable syringe contains hetacillin potassium equivalent to 62.5 mg ampicillin activity in a stable peanut oil gel. This product was manufactured by a non-sterilizing process.

Indications: For lactating cows only.

For the treatment of acute, chronic or subclinical bovine mastitis. HETACIN-K® (hetacillin potassium) for intramammary infusion should be used at the first signs of inflammation or at the first indication of any alteration in the milk. Subclinical infections should be treated immediately upon determining, by C.M.T. or other tests, that the leucocyte count is elevated, or that a susceptible pathogen has been cultured from the milk.

HETACIN-K® for intramammary infusion has been shown to be efficacious in the treatment of mastitis in lactating cows caused by susceptible strains of *Streptococcus agalactiae, Streptococcus dysgalactiae, Staphylococcus aureus* and *Escherichia coli*.

Polycillin® (ampicillin) Susceptibility Test Discs, 10 mcg, should be used to estimate the *in vitro* susceptibility of bacteria to hetacillin.

Pharmacology:

Description: HETACIN-K® (hetacillin potassium) is a broad-spectrum agent which provides bactericidal activity against a wide range of common gram-positive and gram-negative bacteria. It is derived from 6-aminopenicillanic acid and is chemically related to ampicillin.

Action: Hetacillin provides bactericidal levels of the active antibiotic, ampicillin. *In vitro* studies have demonstrated susceptibility of the following organisms to ampicillin: *Streptococcus agalactiae, Streptococcus dysgalactiae, Staphylococcus aureus* and *Escherichia coli*.

Dosage and Administration: Infuse the entire contents of one syringe (10 mL) into each infected quarter. Repeat at 24-hour intervals until a maximum of three treatments has been given.

If definite improvement is not noted within 48 hours after treatment, the causal organism should be further investigated.

Wash the udder and teats thoroughly with warm water containing a suitable dairy antiseptic and dry, preferably using individual paper towels. Carefully scrub the teat end and orifice with 70% alcohol, using a separate swab for each teat. Allow to dry.

HETACIN-K® (hetacillin potassium) is packaged with the Opti-Sert® protective cap.

For partial insertion: Twist off upper portion of the Opti-Sert® protective cap to expose 3-4 mm of the syringe tip.

For full insertion: Remove protective cap to expose the full length of the syringe tip.

Insert syringe tip into the teat canal and expel the entire contents of one syringe into each infected quarter. Withdraw the syringe and gently massage the quarter to distribute the medication.

Do not infuse contents of the mastitis syringe into the teat canal if the Opti-Sert® protective cap is broken or damaged.

Precaution(s): Store at controlled room temperature 15° to 30°C (59° to 86°F).

Because it is a derivative of 6-aminopenicillanic acid, HETACIN-K® has the potential for producing allergic reactions. Such reactions are rare; however, should they occur, treatment should be discontinued and the subject treated with antihistamines, pressor amines, such as epinephrine or corticosteroids.

The drug does not resist destruction by penicillinase and, hence, is not effective against strains of staphylococcus resistant to penicillin G.

Caution(s): Federal law restricts this drug to use by or on the order of a licensed veterinarian.

Warning(s): Milk that has been taken from animals during treatment and for 72 hours (6 milkings) after the latest treatment must not be used for food. Treated animals must not be slaughtered for food until 10 days after the latest treatment.

Presentation: Carton containing 12 x 10 mL syringes (NDC 0856-2713-10).

Opti-Sert® Protective Cap - U.S. Patent No. 4,850,970.

Compendium Code No.: 10030951 43401

H.E. VAC

Arko **Vaccine**

Hemorrhagic Enteritis Vaccine, Live Virus

U.S. Vet. Lic. No.: 337

Active Ingredient(s): This turkey hemorrhagic enteritis virus vaccine is prepared from an apathogenic isolate of an avian adenovirus that is cytopathic in tissue culture and immunogenic in susceptible turkeys. The type II avian adenovirus is propagated in a lymphoblastoid cell line (MDTC-RP 19) of turkey origin. The tissue culture fluids are harvested, stabilized and refrigerated to provide the maximum concentration of viable vaccine virus at the time of use. The vaccine is pink in color and contains a minimal amount of particulate material which consists of ruptured, virus-laden cells.

Contains gentamicin sulfate and an antifungal agent as preservatives.

Indications: H.E. VAC is recommended for use in reducing losses due to hemorrhagic enteritis.

The vaccine is recommended for oral immunization of healthy susceptible turkeys at 30 days of age. The vaccine provides for protection against morbidity and mortality losses due to the effects of field strain hemorrhagic enteritis virus.

This vaccine will produce effective immunity. It has passed potency, safety and purity tests meeting all the requirements set forth by Arko Laboratories Ltd. and the USDA. The response to the product, the stimulation of antibodies within the turkey and the resultant level of immunity may be affected by other factors: Management conditions, concurrent infections and stress levels at vaccination.

Dosage and Administration: The vaccine should be administered to turkeys via the drinking water at 30 days of age or older. Repeat annually. Birds vaccinated at a younger age may not develop adequate immunity due to maternal antibody interferance.

1. Medications and disinfecting products in the drinking water are not compatible with the H.E. Vaccine. Discontinue their use at least 24 hours before vaccinating and do not resume their use for 24 hours after vaccination.
2. Do not use chlorinated water for vaccination. Scrub and clean all waterers before vaccination with nonchlorinated water.

3. Flush the water lines with one (1) pound of powdered milk per 100 gallons of water prior to vaccinating.
4. Shake each vial of vaccine before removing the aluminum seal.
5. The vaccine is to be administered to 30 day old turkeys based on one (1) vial of vaccine for every 1,000 birds. Using the information that four (4) week old turkeys drink 40 gallons of water per 1,000 birds per day, a stock solution would be prepared as follows. One (1) vial of vaccine would go to each 20 gallons of drinking water. For a proportioner that delivers 1 oz. per gallon or one (1) gallon per 128 gallons, six (6) vials of vaccine would be added to each gallon of stock solution. This should provide vaccine to the flock for about 12 hours which should allow for adequate vaccine coverage.
6. Never administer less than one (1) dose of vaccine per bird.
7. Always distribute the vaccine evenly among clean waterers. Do not place the waterers in direct sunlight. Resume regular water administration only after all the vaccine water has been consumed.

Precaution(s): Store this vaccine at less than 45°F (7°C). Protect from sunlight.

It is advised to record the vaccine serial number, the expiration date, the date of vaccination and any reactions observed. This product should be stored, transported and administered in accordance with the instructions and directions.

Caution(s): Use the entire contents when first opened. Burn the vaccine container and all unused contents.

Warning(s): Do not vaccinate within 21 days before slaughter.

Discussion: Hemorrhagic enteritis is an acute disease of young growing turkeys caused by an avian adenovirus. It is characterized by depression, bloody droppings and sudden death. It generally affects poults between seven and 12 weeks of age, but some outbreaks have occurred as early as three weeks and as late as 20 weeks. Although mortality diminishes with increasing age, depending on the concentration of exposure virus, susceptible turkeys suffer a severe to moderate retardation in growth and weight gains.

Presentation: 1,000 and 5,000 dose vials.

Compendium Code No.: 11230040

HEXA-CAINE

PRN Pharmacal — **Topical Antipruritic**

Anti-Itch Spray

Active Ingredient(s): Lidocaine HCl, 2.46%. Contains benzethonium chloride, allantoin, together with denatonium benzoate (Bitrex®), aloe vera, and lanolin in a non-stinging, non-sticky liquid base with normal skin pH.

HEXA-CAINE contains Bitrex® to stop fur and wound biting.

Indications: Helps relieve itching and pain. Aids in the treatment of minor skin problems.

Safe for puppies and kittens 6 weeks or older.

Directions: Shake well before using. Spray liberally on affected areas. Gently wipe away excess around wound with sterile gauze or cotton. Repeat as often as necessary for continued relief.

Precaution(s): Store at room temperature.

Caution(s): Avoid contact with eyes. Do not use on severely traumatized or irritated skin. If undue skin irritation develops or increases, discontinue use and consult a veterinarian.

Warning(s): Keep out of reach of children. For external use only.

Presentation: 4 fl oz, 8 fl oz and 16 fl oz.

Compendium Code No.: 10900080

HEXACLENS 1 ANTISEPTIC SHAMPOO

Vetus — **Antidermatosis Shampoo**

Active Ingredient(s):

Chlorhexidine 1.0%

In a fragrant, lathering shampoo, combining surface-active and penetrating agents and coat conditioners.

Indications: An antiseptic, antimicrobial, antifungal cleansing shampoo for use in the treatment and prevention of dermatological conditions of dogs, cats and horses. May also be used for routine shampooing and deodorizing of animals without skin conditions.

Dosage and Administration: Wet the coat thoroughly with water. Apply enough shampoo to one (1) area to allow a mild lather to develop when worked into the coat. Continue to lather additional areas until the entire coat is treated. Allow to stand on the coat for five (5) minutes before rinsing thoroughly with water. Repeat if necessary.

Precaution(s): Store the product at room temperature.

Caution(s): For topical use on dogs, cats and horses.

Avoid contact with the eyes.

For veterinary use only.

Warning(s): Keep out of the reach of children.

Presentation: 8 oz applicator bottles.

Compendium Code No.: 14440421

HEXACLENS 2% ANTISEPTIC SHAMPOO

Vetus — **Antidermatosis Shampoo**

Chlorhexidine 2%-Antiseptic, Cleansing and Deodorizing Formula

Active Ingredient(s): Contents: Chlorhexidine 2%, in a fragrant, lathering shampoo, which combines surface-active and penetrating agents and coat conditioners.

Indications: For dermatological conditions of dogs, cats and horses where an antifungal and cleansing formulation would be beneficial. May also be used for routine shampooing and deodorizing of animals without dermatological conditions.

Directions: Wet the coat thoroughly with water. Apply enough shampoo to one area to allow a mild lather to develop when worked into the coat.

Continue to lather additional areas until the entire coat is treated. Allow to stand on the coat for 5 minutes before rinsing thoroughly with water. Repeat if necessary.

Precaution(s): Store product at room temperature.

Caution(s): For topical use only on dogs, cats and horses. Avoid contact with the eyes and rinse thoroughly from ears.

For veterinary use only.

Warning(s): Keep out of reach of children.

Presentation: 8 oz bottle and 1 gallon (3.84 L) jug (NDC: 47611-360-90).

Distributed by: Burns Veterinary Supply, Inc., Rockville Centre, NY 11570.

Compendium Code No.: 14440970

HEXADENE® FLUSH

Virbac — **Antiseptic**

Chlorhexidine and Triclosan

Active Ingredient(s): Contains: Chlorhexidine 0.25% (as chlorhexidine digluconate) in water, propylene glycol, triclosan, FD&C blue 11, fragrance. May also contain lactic acid or sodium hydroxide to adjust pH.

Indications: HEXADENE® Flush has been specifically formulated for dermatologic conditions where an antiseptic flush may be beneficial.

Directions for Use: Turn the nozzle to open and then apply HEXADENE® Flush onto the affected area once a day or as directed by your veterinarian. Continue for 2 to 3 days after apparent resolution of clinical signs. If necessary, remove excess solution or debris after use with cotton or absorbent material.

Caution(s): For external use on dogs and cats only. Avoid contact with eyes and mucous membranes. Consult a veterinarian before using on a debilitated animal. If condition does not show improvement after one week, discontinue use of the product and consult with your veterinarian. Wash hands and exposed skin after using.

Available through licensed veterinarians only.

Warning(s): Keep out of reach of children.

Presentation: 4 oz (120 mL) and 8 oz (237 mL).

Compendium Code No.: 10230320

HEXADENE® SHAMPOO ℞

Virbac — **Antidermatosis Shampoo**

Medicated Shampoo Antiseptic with Spherulites®

Ingredient(s): Contains: Chlorhexidine gluconate 3% in a shampoo base containing water, lauryl glucoside, cocamidopropyl betaine, Spherulites, chitosanide and lactic acid. Chitosanide, chlorhexidine gluconate and lactic acid are present in free forms. Chlorhexidine acetate is present in encapsulated (Spherulites) form. May contain sodium hydroxide and sodium chloride.

Indications: HEXADENE® is a gentle, antimicrobial and antiseptic shampoo for use on dogs and cats of any age.

Directions: Shake well before use. Wet the coat with warm water and apply sufficient shampoo to create a rich lather. Massage HEXADENE® into wet coat, lather freely. Rinse and repeat. Allow to remain on hair for 5 to 10 minutes, then rinse thoroughly with clean water.

Frequency of use: initially two to three times a week for four weeks, then reducing to once a week, or as directed by your veterinarian.

Caution(s): Federal Law (USA) restricts this drug to use by or on the order of a licensed veterinarian. For external use only on dogs and cats. Avoid contact with eyes or mucous membranes. If undue skin irritation develops or increases, discontinue use and consult a veterinarian.

Available through licensed veterinarians only.

Warning(s): Keep out of reach of children.

Discussion: HEXADENE® contains Spherulites, an exclusive and patented encapsulation system developed by Virbac to provide slow release of ingredients long after the shampoo is rinsed off.

HEXADENE® also contains Chitosanide, a natural biopolymer creating a protective film on the skin and hair.

Presentation: 8 fl oz (237 mL), 16 oz (474 mL) and 1 gallon (3.79 L).

Compendium Code No.: 10230330

HEXASCRUB MEDICAL SCRUB 2%

Vetus — **Surgical Scrub**

Active Ingredient(s): The product contains USP purified water, surfactants, chlorhexidine gluconate 2%, fragrance, FD&C color.

Indications: HEXASCRUB MEDICAL SCRUB 2% is used for pre-surgical and post-surgical skin cleaning on dogs, horses, cattle and swine.

For use as a surgical or examination scrub for veterinarian use.

Dosage and Administration: Wet the animal's coat with water and apply a sufficient amount of the scrub to work into a lather. Allow the lather to remain on the animal for three (3) or five (5) minutes. Rinse thoroughly. Repeat once a day, or as needed.

Precaution(s): Avoid storing at excessive heat.

Caution(s): For external use only.

Do not use on cats.

May be harmful if swallowed. Not for use in the ears. Avoid contact with the eyes. If irritation develops, discontinue use.

For veterinary use only.

Keep out of the reach of children.

Presentation: 1 gallon containers.

Compendium Code No.: 14440430

HEXASCRUB MEDICAL SCRUB 4%

Vetus — **Hand Cleanser**

A Mild Scrub Containing Chlorhexidine Gluconate

Active Ingredient(s): Contents: Purified water, Alkyl Dimethylamineoxide, Diethanolamine, Chlorhexidine Digluconate, Isopropyl Alcohol 99%, Polyoxyethylene-6-Coco Amide, Octylphenoxypolyethoxy-Ethanol, Glycerol, Polyethylene Glycol, Quaternium 33-Ethylhexandiol, Hydroxyethylcellulose, and FD&C Red #40.

Indications: HEXASCRUB 4 is a mild scrub containing Chlorhexidine Gluconate 4% that exhibits bactericidal activity against a wide range of microorganisms.

Directions: Wet hands with water. Pour approximately 5 mL of HEXASCRUB 4 in palm of hand. Add enough water to make a lather. Lather thoroughly. Rinse thoroughly under running water.

Precaution(s): Avoid storing at excessive heat.

Caution(s): For animal use only.

Keep out of reach of children.

Available exclusively through veterinarians.

Presentation: One gallon (NDC 47611-208-90).

Distributed by: Burns Veterinary Supply, Inc., Westbury, NY 11590

Compendium Code No.: 14440440

Iss. 03-00

HEXASEPTIC FLUSH

Vetus **Topical Wound Dressing**

Active Ingredient(s): The product contains chlorhexidine 0.2% and propylene glycol, malic acid, benzoic acid, salicylic acid, chlorhexidine, glycerin and eucalyptus oil.

Indications: A topical antiseptic containing eucalyptus oil, known for its antiseptic effects in skin inflammation, aids in the cleaning and healing of superficial skin infections in dogs and cats, and is useful for the irrigation of wounds.

Dosage and Administration: Apply liberally to the infected area. Use a cotton ball to remove any debris or excess solution and allow to dry. Repeat the application two (2) or three (3) times a day, or as recommended by a veterinarian.

Caution(s): For external use only. Irritating to the eye. Use only as directed by a veterinarian.

For veterinary use only. Keep out of the reach of children.

Presentation: 4 oz squeeze bottles with a Yorker applicator tip and safety seal and 16 oz twist-to-close Yorker top bottle.

Compendium Code No.: 14440450

HEXASEPTIC FLUSH PLUS

Vetus **Topical Wound Dressing**

Ingredient(s): Propylene glycol, lidocaine, hydrochloride 0.5%, malic acid, benzoic acid, salicylic acid, chlorhexidine 0.2%, glycerin, eucalyptus oil, and denatonium benzoate NF (Bitrex®).

Indications: A general cleansing solution with chlorhexidine as a topical antiseptic. It aids in the healing of superficial skin infections in dogs and cats, therefore creating an ideal environment for healthy tissue growth. Also contains Bitrex®, a non-toxic substance that is so bitter tasting that it discourages biting and licking of the wound.

Dosage and Administration: Apply an amount sufficient to cover the wound, and use a cotton ball to gently remove any debris or excess solution, and allow to dry. Repeat application 2-3 times daily, or as recommended by your veterinarian. Avoid excessive application.

Caution(s): Do not apply to large areas of broken skin. As with any chlorhexidine product, avoid use in the inner ear canal. For external use only. Irritating to the eye.

Use only as directed by your veterinarian.

Warning(s): Keep out of reach of children.

Presentation: 4 oz squeeze bottle with a Yorker applicator tip and safety seal.

Compendium Code No.: 14440460

HEXASOL SOLUTION

Vetus **Topical Wound Dressing**

Active Ingredient(s): The product contains USP purified water, surfactants, chlorhexidine gluconate 2%, fragrance, FD&C color.

Indications: A topical drying agent for use on dogs, horses, cattle and swine for use in conditions where an antimicrobial would be of benefit.

Dosage and Administration: Rinse the subject area with a sufficient amount of the solution. Wipe away any excess solution. Repeat as needed.

Precaution(s): Avoid storing at excessive heat.

Caution(s): For external use only. Do not use on cats.

May be harmful if swallowed. Not for use in the ears. Avoid contact with the eyes. If irritation develops, discontinue use. For veterinary use only. Keep out of the reach of children.

Presentation: 1 gallon containers.

Compendium Code No.: 14440470

HEXORAL RINSE

Vetus **Dental Preparation**

NDC No.: 47611-352-59

Active Ingredient(s):

Chlorhexidine 0.1%
Ethyl alcohol 6%

Surfactants, FD&C red 40, D&C red 33, in a peppermint flavored base.

Indications: An oral cleansing solution for dogs and cats to assist in the daily maintenance of oral health and fresh breath. Also removes food particles from the teeth and the gum line.

Dosage and Administration: Apply HEXORAL RINSE either as an oral rinse or with a toothbrush.

Oral rinse: Use one (1) hand to gently spread the animal's lips on one side to expose the teeth and gum line. Spray a small amount between the teeth and the gums, so that the gum surfaces are thoroughly wet. After closing the animal's mouth, gently rub the animal's lips over the teeth to work the rinse over the surface of the teeth. Repeat on the other side of the animal's mouth.

Toothbrushing: Place a small amount in a small dish. While gently spreading the animal's lips on one side, dip the toothbrush into the solution and carefully brush the teeth with a gentle motion. Re-wet the brush as needed. Repeat on the other side of the animal's mouth.

Caution(s): The use of HEXORAL RINSE should not be considered as a substitute for veterinary dental treatment.

The product should be used as part of a complete oral health program.

Some staining of the teeth surfaces have been reported after the prolonged use of rinses containing chlorhexidine. The accumulation of stain can be prevented by applying the solution with a toothbrush.

Not for use in the eyes. Keep out of the reach of children. For veterinary use only.

Presentation: 8 oz. bottles with a pump spray applicator.

Compendium Code No.: 14440480

HEXORAL Zn RINSE

Vetus **Dental Preparation**

Oral Rinse-0.12% Chlorhexidine and 0.12% Zinc Chloride

Active Ingredient(s): Contains: Chlorhexidine 0.12%, Zinc Chloride 0.12% and Cetylpyridinium Chloride 0.05%, Glycerine, Peppermint flavor, Cherry flavor, FD&C Red 40, FD&C Blue #1, in a non-alcohol base.

Indications: HEXORAL Zn RINSE is a soothing, refreshing and highly palatable rinse containing chlorhexidine gluconate, cetylpyridinium chloride and zinc. The antimicrobial activity of chlorhexidine and cetylpyridinium chloride, combined with the anti-plaque and anti-calculus properties of zinc, together can aid in the prevention of tooth and gum disease. This formulation will leave your pet with clean breath while providing soothing, temporary relief of minor gum irritation.

Directions: Apply HEXORAL Zn RINSE either as an oral rinse or with a toothbrush.

Oral Rinse: Holding the animal's head steady with one hand, spray a small amount of HEXORAL Zn RINSE between the teeth and gums on one side of the animal's mouth. Massage the mouth over the teeth to work HEXORAL Zn RINSE over the side of the mouth so that the gum surfaces are thoroughly wet on both sides of the mouth.

Tooth Brushing: Place a small amount of HEXORAL Zn RINSE in a clean dish or cup. Holding the animal's head steady with one hand, dip the toothbrush into the solution and carefully brush the teeth with a gentle motion. Re-wet the brush with HEXORAL Zn RINSE as needed.

Precaution(s): Store at room temperature.

Caution(s): Reversible tooth staining has been reported with prolonged use of chlorhexidine.

For use only as an oral rinse or a toothbrushing solution.

Warning(s): Keep out of reach of children.

Discussion: Importance of Oral Hygiene: Plaque results from bacterial proliferation on the tooth surface. Eventually, calculus forms on the tooth and acts as a protective barrier for plaque development. If these are not eliminated, the teeth, sockets and gums can become diseased and lead to such conditions as bad breath, oral pain and loss of teeth. Eventually, dental disease can also lead to severe systemic conditions such as heart, kidney or liver disease.

Dental care plays an important role in your pet's overall health. A veterinarian is your best source of advice for the care of your pet's teeth and gums. Consult a veterinarian at least once a year for a dental health management program adapted to your pet's specific needs.

Presentation: 8 fl oz (240 mL) bottles with a pump spray applicator (NDC: 47611-362-59).

Distributed by: Burns Veterinary Supply, Inc.

Compendium Code No.: 14440980

HI-BOOT® ETHYLENEDIAMINE DIHYDRIODIDE

WestAgro **Iodine-Oral**

(EDDI)

Active Ingredient(s): This product is formulated in white, free flowing crystals, consisting of essentially pure ethylenediamine dihydriodide.

Generally recognized as safe.

Ethylenediamine Dihydriodide 99.0%
Elemental Iodine 79.5%
Moisture .... <0.2%
pH of 50% Aqueous Solution .... 4.0 to 4.6
Bulk Density .... 92.4#/cubic foot

Indications: A nutritional source of iodine for livestock and poultry. Recommended for use in animal feed.

Dosage and Administration: Use the following table for recommended rates:

EDDI: As a recommended daily source of iodine in feed.

Species:	Recommended Range:
Cattle	0.1 mg/kg to 0.6 mg/kg
Horses	0.2 mg/kg to 0.4 mg/kg
Sheep	0.6 mg/kg to 0.9 mg/kg
Goats	0.1 mg/kg to 0.9 mg/kg
Poultry	0.4 mg/kg to 0.6 mg/kg
Fish	0.7 mg/kg to 1.5 mg/kg

Presentation: 100 lb polyethylene lined fiber drum.

® HI-BOOT is a registered trademark of WestAgro, Inc.

Compendium Code No.: 10180000

HI-CAL SUSPENSION

Vedco **Dietary Supplement**

Guaranteed Analysis:

	per ounce	per pound
Crude protein not less than	3.0%	3.0%
Crude fat not less than	50.0%	50.0%
Vitamin A	500 IU	8000 IU
Vitamin D_3	40 IU	640 IU
Vitamin E	3 IU	48 IU
Thiamine	0.15 mg	2.4 mg
Riboflavin	0.17 mg	2.72 mg
Pyridoxine	0.20 mg	3.2 mg
Ascorbic Acid	6 mg	96 mg
Niacin	2 mg	32 mg
d-Pantothenic Acid	1 mg	16 mg
Folic Acid	0.04 mg	0.64 mg
Omega 3 Fatty Acids	1200 mg	19200 mg

Ingredients: Vegetable oil, sucrose, fructose, malto dextrins, non fat dry milk solids, vegetable gums, egg white solids, glycerine, citrus pectin, sodium benzoate, vitamin A palmitate, cholecalciferol (vitamin D_3), dl-alpha tocopheryl acetate (vitamin E), ascorbic acid (vitamin C), niacinamide, calcium pantothenate, pyridoxine hydrochloride, riboflavin, thiamine mononitrate, folic acid.

Indications: A high calorie liquid diet and vitamin supplement for dogs, cats, pigs and calves.

Dosage and Administration:

Dogs and Cats:

Maintenance:

5-10 lbs body weight .... One tsp daily
10-30 lbs body weight .... Two tsp daily
30 lbs or more - One tbsp daily

Show and working conditions:

5-10 lbs body weight .... One tsp 3 times daily
10-30 lbs or more .... One tbsp twice a day
30 lbs or more .... Two tbsp 3 times daily

Pigs and Calves: Mix 1 oz of HI-CAL SUSPENSION with 10 oz of water.

Then dose as follows:

Calf Dosage .... 4 tbsp per calf three times daily
Pig Dosage .... 1 tsp per pig 3 times daily

Warning(s): For animal use only. Keep out of reach of children.

Presentation: 16 fl oz (473 mL) containers.

Compendium Code No.: 10941070

HIGH-CAL

Vet Solutions **Small Animal Dietary Supplement**

Guaranteed Analysis: Per teaspoon (6 grams):

Crude Protein (Min)	0.7%
Crude Fat (Min)	34.5%
Crude Fiber (Max)	3.8%
Moisture (Max)	14%
Calcium (Min) (0.0026%)	0.16 mg
Calcium (Max) (0.0033%)	0.20 mg
Phosphorus (0.0006%)	0.03 mg
Iron (0.0088%)	0.53 mg
Iodine (0.0088%)	0.53 mg
Magnesium (0.0067%)	0.42 mg
Manganese (0.0176%)	1 mg
Potassium (0.0027%)	0.16 mg
Vitamin A	1045 IU
Vitamin D_3	60 IU
Vitamin E	6 IU
Vitamin B_1 (Thiamine HCl)	2 mg
Vitamin B_2 (Riboflavin)	0.2 mg
Vitamin B_6 (Pyridoxine HCl)	1 mg
Vitamin B_{12}	2 mcg
Folic Acid	0.2 mg
Nicotinamide	2 mg
Pantothenic Acid	1 mg
Linoleic Acid (LA)	990 mg
Linolenic Acid (ALA)	138 mg
Eicosapentaenoic Acid (EPA)	32 mg
Docosahexaenoic Acid (DHA)	21 mg

Ingredients: Malt syrup, corn syrup, refined soybean oil (source of LA and ALA), methylcellulose USP, cane molasses, cod liver oil USP (source of EPA and DHA), water, polypro 5000 hydrolyzed collagen, dl-alpha tocopheryl acetate (Vit. E), sodium benzoate (preservative), manganese sulfate, iron peptonized, thiamine HCl, nicotinamide USP, calcium pantothenate USP (source of calcium and pantothenic acid), magnesium sulfate, pyridoxine HCl USP, Vitamin A palmitate & D_3 concentrate, potassium iodide USP (source of iodine and potassium), riboflavin 5' phosphate sodium (source of Vitamin B_2 and phosphorus), folic acid, Vitamin A palmitate and cyanocobalamin USP (Vit. B_{12}).

Indications: A high calorie, palatable dietary supplement in a low volume form for dogs, cats, puppies & kittens.

Directions: When the animal's caloric or nutritional intake is to be supplemented, give 1½ teaspoons per 10 pounds of body weight daily. When animal is not consuming full feed ration, give 3 teaspoons (1 tablespoon) per 10 pounds of body weight daily.

Calorie content: 4420 kcal/kg (26.5 kcal/6g).

Precaution(s): Store at controlled room temperature.

Caution(s): Sold exclusively through veterinarians.

Presentation: 5.0 oz. (141.6 grams).

Compendium Code No.: 10610100

HIGH-D 2X DISPERSIBLE

Alpharma **Vitamin D_3**

Vitamin D_3 Liquid Concentrate

Active Ingredient(s): Guaranteed to Contain: 4,000,000 IU Vitamin D_3 per ounce.

Ingredients: Vitamin D_3, polysorbate 80, potassium sorbate, n-propyl alcohol, BHT, propylene glycol, polyethylene glycol monooleate.

Indications: A supplementary nutrition for hogs, chickens, turkeys, calves, and beef cattle.

Directions for Use: Mix ¼ oz (½ tablespoon) in 128 gallons of drinking water or ¼ oz per gallon of stock solution for water proportioners that meter at the rate of 1 oz per gallon of drinking water. Double concentration to ½ oz (1 tablespoon) during periods of stress.

Mix fresh solutions daily.

Precaution(s): Store in a cool, dry place.

Caution(s): For oral animal use only.

Warning(s): Not for human consumption. Keep out of reach of children.

Presentation: 16 oz.

Compendium Code No.: 10221310 AHL-449 0104

HIGH LEVEL VITAMIN-B COMPLEX

Durvet **Vitamin B-Complex**

Injectable Sterile Solution

Active Ingredient(s): Each mL contains:

Thiamine HCl	100 mg
Riboflavin 5' Phosphate Sodium	5 mg
Niacinamide	100 mg
d-Panthenol	10 mg
Pyridoxine HCl	10 mg
Cobalt (As Cyanocobalamin)	4.0 ppm
Benzyl Alcohol (preservative)	1.5%
Citric Acid	5 mg
Water For Injection	q.s.

Indications: A sterile aqueous solution of B Complex vitamins to provide a supplemental nutritional supply of these vitamins and complexed cobalt to cattle, sheep and swine.

Dosage and Administration: Administer intramuscularly or subcutaneously. Sheep and Swine: 5 to 10 mL; Cattle: 10 to 20 mL. Repeat daily as indicated.

Precaution(s): Store between 15°C-30°C (59°F-86°F). Keep from freezing.

Caution(s): Anaphylactogenesis to parenteral Thiamine HCl has been reported. Administer slowly and with caution in doses over 50 mg.

For animal use only.

Warning(s): Keep out of reach of children.

Presentation: 250 mL (NDC 30798-041-13) and 500 mL (NDC 30798-041-17).

Compendium Code No.: 10840841 Rev. 10-95/1-97

HIGH PERFORMANCE POULTRY PAK

Durvet **Water Additive**

Guaranteed Analysis: per pound:

Vitamin A	16,500,000 IU
Vitamin D3	6,400,000 IU
Vitamin E	11,000 IU
Niacin	66,000 mg
d-Pantothenic Acid	28,000 mg
Ascorbic Acid	20,000 mg
Riboflavin	6,600 mg
MSBC	6,000 mg
Thiamine	4,050 mg
Pyridoxine	2,000 mg
Folic Acid	840 mg
Biotin	150 mg
Vitamin B12	20 mg

Ingredients: Vitamin A supplement, Vitamin D3 supplement, Vitamin E supplement, Vitamin B12 supplement, Riboflavin, D-Calcium Pantothenate, Niacin supplement, Menadione Sodium Bisulfite Complex, Pyridoxine Hydrochloride, Thiamine Mononitrate, Folic Acid, D-Biotin, Ascorbic Acid, Potassium Chloride, Sodium Chloride, Magnesium Sulfate, Iron Sulfate, Zinc Methionine Complex, Manganese Amino Acid Chelate, Copper Sulfate, Sodium Saccharin, and artificial flavoring.

Indications: A water-soluble vitamin and electrolytes mix for use in starting poultry during periods of reduced feed intake.

Directions: Use Directions/Dosage: Mix fresh solution daily. Automatic Watering System - add the following amount to two gallons of stock solution when proportioner is set to meter at the rate of one ounce per gallon. Reduced feed intake: one-4 oz. packet. Extreme Conditions: two-4 oz. packets.

Precaution(s): Storage: Store in a cool dry place.

Warning(s): Keep out of reach of children.

Presentation: Net wt. 12.5 lb (5.67 kg) (contains 50 x 4 oz packets).

Compendium Code No.: 10841990 6/01

HI-PO B COMPLEX™

Butler **Vitamin B-Complex**

Active Ingredient(s): Each mL of sterile aqueous solution contains:

Thiamine hydrochloride (B_1)	100 mg
Riboflavin (B_2) (as riboflavin 5[1]-phosphate sodium)	5 mg
Niacinamide	100 mg
Pyridoxine hydrochloride (B_6)	10 mg
d-Panthenol	10 mg
Cyanocobalamin (B_{12})	100 mcg

Preservatives:

Sorbitol	32.5%
Glycerin	6.34%
Lactic acid	0.32%
Citric acid	0.24%
Sodium citrate	0.15%
Benzyl alcohol	1.59%
BHA	0.005%

Indications: For use as a supplement of B-complex vitamins.

Dosage and Administration: Administer intramuscularly.

Adult Cattle and Calves: 1 to 5 mL per 100 pounds of body weight, depending upon the size and condition of the animal.

Horses: 1 to 2 mL per 100 pounds of body weight.

Swine and Sheep: 5 mL per 100 pounds of body weight.

Dogs and Cats: 0.5 to 2 mL, depending upon the size and condition of the animal.

May be repeated each day, as indicated.

Precaution(s): Store in a cool place between 36°-46°F (2°-8°C).

Protect from light.

Caution(s): Hypersensitivity reactions to the parenteral administration of thiamine have been reported. Administer with caution and keep animals under close observation.

For veterinary use only.

Keep out of the reach of children.

Presentation: 100 mL and 250 mL vials.

Compendium Code No.: 10820900

HISTACALM® SHAMPOO ℞

Virbac **Antidermatosis Shampoo**

NDC No.: 51311-023-08/51311-023-16/51311-023-10

Active Ingredient(s): Diphenhydramine hydrochloride, U.S.P. 2%, in a colloidal oatmeal shampoo vehicle containing omega-6 fatty acids.

Indications: HISTACALM® antihistaminic emollient anti-itch shampoo provides temporary relief of itching associated with sensitive skin. HISTACALM® Shampoo contains both diphenhydramine hydrochloride, an antihistamine that stops the itch, and colloidal oatmeal, to cleanse and soothe irritated skin.

Dosage and Administration: Shake well before using. Wet the hair coat and gently massage in HISTACALM®. Lather freely and rinse. Repeat and allow the lather to remain on the hair and skin for 5-10 minutes; then rinse. May be used once a day or as directed by a veterinarian. If the condition persists, discontinue use of the product and consult a veterinarian.

Caution(s): Federal law (USA) restricts this drug to use by or on the order of a licensed veterinarian.

Keep out of the reach of children.

For external use only on dogs and cats. Avoid contact with the eyes or mucous membranes. Wash hands after using.

Presentation: Available in 8 fl. oz. (237 mL), 16 fl. oz. (473 mL) and 1 gallon (3.79 L) containers.

Compendium Code No.: 10230350

HISTACALM® SPRAY ℞

Virbac **Topical Antihistamine**

NDC No.: 51311-023-02

Active Ingredient(s): Diphenhydramine hydrochloride, U.S.P. 2%, in a water-based vehicle containing omega-3 and omega-6 essential fatty acids.

Indications: HISTACALM® antihistaminic/analgesic spray provides temporary relief of the pain and itching associated with allergic reactions in sensitive skin. Application as a spray avoids the allergic flare caused by rubbing on a cream or ointment. HISTACALM® Shampoo contains diphenhydramine hydrochloride, an antihistamine that stops the itch, and essential fatty acids, omega-3 and omega-6, to help moisturize the skin.

Dosage and Administration: Shake well before using. Spray directly onto the affected area two (2) to three (3) times a day or as directed by a veterinarian. If the condition persists, discontinue use of the product and consult a veterinarian.

Caution(s): Federal law (USA) restricts this drug to use by or on the order of a licensed veterinarian.

Keep out of the reach of children.

For external use only on dogs and cats. Avoid contact with the eyes or mucous membranes. Wash hands after using.

Presentation: Available 2 fl. oz. (59 mL) spray bottles.

Compendium Code No.: 10230360

HIST-EQ POWDER

Butler **Expectorant**

Active Ingredient(s): Each ounce contains:

Guaifenesin, USP . . . . 2400 mg
Pyrilamine Maleate, USP . . . . 600 mg

Indications: For use as an antihistamine and expectorant.

Directions for Use: ½ ounce (1 level tablespoon) per 1,000 lb body weight, or as recommended by a veterinarian.

Can be mixed with feed and repeated at 12 hour intervals as needed.

Precaution(s): Keep lid tightly closed and store in a dry place. Do not store above 30°C (86°F).

Shake well before use.

Caution(s): For use in animals only.

For use in horses only.

For veterinary use only.

Warning(s): Do not use at least 72 hours prior to sporting events.

Keep out of reach of children.

Presentation: 20 oz (NDC 11695-1300-2) and 5 lb (NDC 11695-1300-4).

Compendium Code No.: 10820911

HISTOSTAT® 50

Alpharma **Feed Medication**

Nitarsone-Type A Medicated Article

NADA No.: 007-616

Active Ingredient(s):

Nitarsone (4-nitrophenylarsonic acid) 50%
(equivalent to 226.8 grams nitarsone per pound of product)
in a carrier suitable for incorporation in feed.

Indications: An aid in the prevention of blackhead in turkeys and chickens.

Dosage and Administration: Must be mixed thoroughly in feed before use.

Turkeys: Mix in feed so that 2,000 lbs (909 kg) of complete ration contain 12 oz. (340.2 g) of HISTOSTAT® 50 equivalent to 0.01875% nitarsone. Start HISTOSTAT® 50 medication depending on such factors as record of blackhead occurrence on the farm or in the area; climate and weather; and soil or litter condition. Continue as long as prevention is desired.

Chickens: Mix in feed so that 2,000 lbs (909 kg) of complete ration contain 12 oz. (340.2 g) of HISTOSTAT® 50 equivalent to 0.01875% nitarsone. Give continuously for at least 3 weeks during periods of stress. Long-term medication is not necessary for chickens because of their natural resistance except at times of undue stress. Reduced feed consumption, onset of production, and errors in management may produce stresses which lower the resistance of chickens to blackhead.

Mixing directions: To secure an even distribution, mix HISTOSTAT® 50 with a small amount of feed ingredients, then add the remainder of the ingredients and mix thoroughly.

Caution(s): Early medication is essential to prevent spread of the disease. Adequate drinking water must be provided near feeders at all times. The drug is not effective in preventing blackhead in birds infected more than 4 or 5 days. Symptoms of blackhead do not appear until 10 to 15 days after birds become infected.

Use as the sole source of arsenic.

Keep out of reach of children. Overdosage or lack of water may result in leg weakness or paralysis. In mixing, avoid inhaling dust. Avoid contact of product with skin, eyes and clothing. Wash thoroughly after handling. Dangerous for ducks, geese and dogs.

Poison-Arsenic. Antidote: If swallowed, call a physician, poison control center, or hospital immediately. Induce vomiting by giving Ipecac Syrup as directed.

Warning(s): Discontinue use 5 days before slaughtering for human consumption to allow for elimination of the drug from edible tissue.

Presentation: 50 lb (22.68 kg) bag.

Compendium Code No.: 10220401

560310 0106

HI-VITE™ DROPS

Evsco **Small Animal Dietary Supplement**

Active Ingredient(s): Guaranteed analysis per fl. oz.:

Vitamin A . . . . 150,000 I.U.
Vitamin D_3 . . . . 24,000 I.U.
Vitamin E . . . . 50 I.U.
Vitamin B_1 . . . . 60 mg
Vitamin B_2 . . . . 16 mg
Vitamin B_6 . . . . 32 mg
Nicotinamide . . . . 240 mg
D-panthenol . . . . 100 mg
Iron . . . . 52 mg (0.18%)

Ingredients: Water, sugar, sorbitol, liver extract, polysorbate 80, propylene glycol, peptones, ferric ammonium citrate (source of iron), nicotinamide, vitamin A and D_3 concentrate, d-panthenol, thiamine HCl (vit. B_1), citric acid (preservative), alpha tocopheryl acetate (vit. E), saccharin sodium, vit. A palmitate, pyridoxine HCl (vit. B_6), sodium benzoate and methylparaben (preservatives), riboflavin 5'-phosphate sodium (source of vit. B_2), BHA (preservative).

Indications: A vitamin supplement with liver and iron.

Dosage and Administration: To supplement the diet, give puppies and kittens one-half (½) of a dropperful twice a day. Give dogs and cats one (1) dropperful two (2) to three (3) times a day. The mixture is water dispersible and may be given by dropping directly on the tongue or by mixing with food or milk. (1 dropperful = 1 mL.)

Precaution(s): Store at room temperature.

Presentation: 12 x 1 fl. oz. (29.57 mL) bottles with plastic droppers.

Compendium Code No.: 10050130

HOG & CATTLE VITAMINS AND ELECTROLYTES

Fort Dodge **Electrolytes-Oral**

Nutritional Supplement

Active Ingredient(s):

Guaranteed Minimum Analysis	Per Pound	Per Kilo
Salt (Min.) %	0.40	0.40
Salt (Max.) %	0.60	0.60
Potassium, (K) %	1.300	1.300
Vitamin A, I.U	5,000,000	11,023,000
Vitamin D_3, I.U	500,000	1,102,300
Vitamin E, I.U	1,000	2,205
Riboflavin, mg	500	1,102
Niacin, mg	12,500	27,558
d-Pantothenic Acid, mg	6,000	13,228
(Calcium d-Pantothenate, mg)	(6,521)	(14,376)

Ingredients: Dextrose, vitamin A supplement, D-activated animal sterol (source of vitamin D_3), vitamin E supplement, riboflavin supplement, niacin supplement, calcium pantothenate, menadione sodium bisulfite complex, thiamine mononitrate, potassium chloride, salt.

Indications: A supplementary nutritional product, HOG & CATTLE VITAMINS AND ELECTROLYTES is indicated for both healthy animals and sick or convalescent animals eating less feed than normal.

Directions:

For drinking-water use: Mix the contents of 1 pouch in 128 gallons (486 liters) of drinking water and give for 3 to 5 days. This dosage may be repeated whenever needed.

For use in automatic proportioners: To make a stock solution, mix the contents of 1 pouch in U.S. gallon (3.8 liters) of water. Set the proportioner to deliver 1 fluid ounce (30 mL) per gallon (3.8 liters) of drinking water. Prepare fresh stock solutions daily.

For feed use: Mix the contents of 1 pouch in 500 pounds (227 kg) of complete feed. Give for 3 to 5 days. This dosage may be repeated whenever needed.

Caution(s): Keep out of reach of children.

For animal oral use only.

Not for human use.

Presentation: 8 oz (227 g) foil pouches.

Compendium Code No.: 10030960

12682B

HOOF CONDITIONER

First Priority **Hoof Product**

Active Ingredient(s): Composition: Lanolin Oil, Acetate Ester, Stearic Acid, Sorbitan Stearate, Lanolin Quaternary, Propylene Glycol, Diisostearate, Triethanolamine, Deionized Water.

Indications: Deep, penetrating formula promotes healthy hooves. Supports proper moisture balance that helps prevent and treat dry, cracked, or brittle hooves in an easy-to-apply, pleasantly-fragranced vanishing cream base. Normal, pliable hooves result from proper nutrition, moisture content, and shoeing. A regular program using HOOF CONDITIONER and Hoof Supplement will help maintain healthy hooves. Safe for use in all racing, shows, and events.

Dosage and Administration: Thoroughly clean coronary band, hoof wall, sole, and frog. Apply HOOF CONDITIONER directly to the coronary band, the entire hoof wall, and the frog and sole. Repeat daily to help maintain healthy hooves.

Precaution(s): Store at a controlled room temperature between 32°F and 90°F.

Caution(s): For severe or persisting conditions, consult your farrier or veterinarian.

For animal use only.

Warning(s): Keep out of reach of children.

Presentation: 1 lb (453.6 g) (NDC# 58829-283-16) and 4 lb (1.8 kg) (NDC# 58829-283-18).

Compendium Code No.: 11390373

Iss. 12-98 / Rev. 06-99

HOOF PACKING

Fiebing **Hoof Product**

Active Ingredient(s): Bentonite.

Indications: For use as an aid in the treatment of acute inflammatory conditions of the frog and sole of horses' hoofs.

Dosage and Administration: For every two (2) quarts of water, add one (1) pound of rock. Add approximately four (4) ounces of rock at a time while stirring. When the rock becomes a jelly-like mass it is ready for use. Pack the hoof level with the shoe and wrap.

Caution(s): Not intended for use in thrush. Keep out of the reach of children.

Presentation: Packaged in 5 lb. cartons and 25 lb. pails.

Compendium Code No.: 10590001

HOOFPRO+®

SSI Corp. **Hoof Product**

Active Ingredient(s):

Copper (Cu) 0.67%
Sulfur (S) 2.2%
Inert 97.15%

Indications: Aids in the treatment and prevention of foot warts in dairy cattle.

Directions:

Using Spray for Treatment: As an aid in treatment, use HOOFPRO+® in a spray bottle as a topical application. Mix three parts water to one part HOOFPRO+®. Clean feet thoroughly beforehand. Spray lesion(s) to the point of run-off twice daily. Improvement should be noticed in three to four days. If problem animal does not respond to the 1:3 dilution, wrapping may be necessary.

Using Spray for Prevention: For use as a preventative, spray all animals, all feet, or at least the back two feed, with the 1:3 dilution four to six milkings per week.

Using Footbaths for Prevention: In the footbath mix one half gallon of HOOFPRO+® per 50 gallons of water (two liters per 200 liters of water). Clean hooves as thoroughly as possible before entry into the footbath. Footbath should be cleaned and redosed after every 150 animals. Environmental and hygiene conditions may require cleaning and redosing more often. Use four to six milkings per week. Footbaths require careful management. If footbath is not properly managed results are reduced significantly.

Precaution(s): Do not allow to freeze.

Caution(s): Eye irritant. In case of eye contact, flush for 15 minutes. If irritation persists, call a physician.

Warning(s): Keep out of the reach of children.

Presentation: 2.5, 5, 30 and 55 gallon drums.

Compendium Code No.: 14930021

HOOF SUPPLEMENT

First Priority **Large Animal Dietary Supplement**

Biotin-Methionine-Thiamine-Zinc Supplement

Ingredient(s): Composition: Each 60 g contains:

DL-Methionine	10 g
Zinc (as Zinc Oxide)	300 mg
Thiamine Hydrochloride (B_1)	100 mg
Biotin	15 mg

In a palatable soybean meal base.

Indications: For use as a supplemental source of the nutrients methionine, zinc, thiamine, and biotin in horses.

Dosage and Administration: 60 g (2 oz) mixed with grain or sweet feed for 15 days, then 30 g (1 oz) daily for maintenance. A plastic measuring scoop is provided for convenience. One (1) scoopful contains 60 g (2 oz) of HOOF SUPPLEMENT.

Precaution(s): Store at controlled room temperature between 15° and 30°C (59°-86°F).

Warning(s): For veterinary use only.

Keep out of reach of children.

Presentation: 4 lb (1.8 kg) pail (NDC# 58829-244-18) and 22 lb (10 kg) pail (NDC# 58829-244-22).

Compendium Code No.: 11390382 Rev. 10-99 / Rev. 06-01

HORSE CARE BIOTIN CRUMBLES

Durvet **Equine Dietary Supplement**

Guaranteed Analysis:

Biotin	110 mg/lb
Crude Protein (minimum)	13%
Crude Fat (minimum)	2%
Crude Fiber (maximum)	15%

Ingredients: Forage products, processed grain by products, calcium carbonate, grain products, dried cane molasses, calcium lignin sulfonate, biotin, roughage products, sodium propionate (a preservative), ethoxyquin (a preservative) and artificial and natural flavor.

Apple flavored.

Indications: A source of biotin for horses.

Dosage and Administration: Top feed or hand mix ½ to 1 ounce of BIOTIN CRUMBLES into each horse's daily ration (enclosed measuring scoop holds 1 ounce).

Precaution(s): Close container after use. Store in cool, dry place.

Warning(s): For animal use only.

Keep out of reach of children.

Presentation: 40 oz (2 lb 8 oz) and 18 lb.

Compendium Code No.: 10840851

HORSE CARE IVERMECTIN PASTE 1.87%

Durvet **Parasiticide-Oral**

Anthelmintic and Boticide

ANADA No.: 200-286

Active Ingredient(s):

Ivermectin	1.87%

Indications: Consult your veterinarian for assistance in the diagnosis, treatment, and control of parasitism. IVERMECTIN PASTE 1.87% provides effective control of the following parasites in horses. Large Strongyles (adults) - *Strongylus vulgaris* (also early forms in blood vessels), *S. edentatus* (also tissue stages), *S. equinus, Triodontophorus* spp.; Small Strongyles including those resistant to some benzimidazole class compounds (adults and fourth-stage larvae) - *Cyathostomum* spp, *Cylicocyclus* spp, *Cylicostephanus* spp, *Cylicodontophorus* spp; Pinworms (adults and fourth-stage larvae) - *Oxyuris equi*; Ascarids (adults and third- and fourth-stage larvae) - *Parascaris equorum;* Hairworms (adults) *Trichostrongylus axei;* Large-mouth Stomach Worms (adults) - *Habronema muscae;* Bots (oral and gastric stages) - *Gasterophilus* spp; Lungworms (adults and fourth-stage larvae) - *Dictyocaulus arnfieldi;* Intestinal Threadworms (adults) - *Strongyloides westeri;* Summer Sores caused by *Habronema* and *Draschia* spp cutaneous third-stage larvae; Dermatitis caused by neck threadworm microfilariae, *Onchocerca* sp.

Dosage and Administration: This syringe contains sufficient paste to treat one 1250 lb horse at the recommended dose rate of 91 mcg ivermectin per lb (200 mcg/kg) body weight. Each weight marking on the syringe plunger delivers enough paste to treat 250 lb body weight. (1) While holding plunger, turn the knurled ring on the plunger to the right so the side nearest the barrel is at the prescribed weight marking. (2) Make sure that the horse's mouth contains no feed. (3) Remove the cover from the tip of the syringe. (4) Insert the syringe tip into the horse's mouth at the space between the teeth (5) Depress the plunger as far as it will go, depositing paste on the back of the tongue (6) Immediately raise the horse's head for a few seconds after dosing.

Precaution(s): Store at controlled room temperature, 20° to 25°C (68° to 77°F).

Do not contaminate ground or surface water. Dispose of the syringe in an approved landfill or by incineration.

Caution(s): IVERMECTIN PASTE 1.87% has been formulated specifically for use in horses only. This product should not be used in other animal species as severe adverse reactions, including fatalities in dogs, may result. Refrain from smoking and eating when handling. Wash hands after use. Avoid contact with eyes. Keep this and all drugs out of the reach of children. Ivermectin and excreted ivermectin residues may adversely affect aquatic organisms.

Note to User: Swelling and itching reactions after treatment with IVERMECTIN PASTE 1.87% have occurred in horses carrying heavy infections of neck threadworm (*Onchocerca* sp.) microfilariae. These reactions were most likely the result of microfilariae dying in large numbers. Symptomatic treatment may be advisable. Consult your veterinarian should any such reactions occur. Healing of summer sores involving extensive tissue changes may require other appropriate therapy in conjunction with treatment with IVERMECTIN PASTE 1.87%. Reinfection, and measures for its prevention, should also be considered. Consult your veterinarian if the condition does not improve.

Warning(s): Residue Warning: Do not use in horses intended for food purposes.

Side Effects: Safety - IVERMECTIN PASTE 1.87% may be used in horses of all ages, including mares at any stage of pregnancy. Stallions may be treated without adversely affecting their fertility.

Discussion: Parasite Control Program: All horses should be included in a regular parasite control program with particular attention being paid to mares, foals and yearlings. Foals should be treated initially at 6 to 8 weeks of age, and routine treatment repeated as appropriate.

Consult your veterinarian for a control program to meet your specific needs. IVERMECTIN PASTE 1.87% effectively controls gastrointestinal nematodes and bots of horses. Regular treatment will reduce the chances of verminous arteritis caused by *S vulgaris.*

Presentation: 6.08 g (0.21 oz) syringe (NDC 30798-898-81).

Compendium Code No.: 10841770 Iss. 01-00

HORSE CARE STALL POWDER

Durvet **Deodorant Product**

Indications: An aid to eliminate manure and ammonia odors in barn stall.

Directions For Use: Spread stall powder evenly on any type of bedding to extend the life of its use.

Use approximately one pound per stall every ten (10) days.

This container will help to deodorize stall for approximately three months.

Presentation: 10 lb and 50 lb.

Compendium Code No.: 10841031

H

HORSE LICE DUSTER™ III

Farnam **Parasiticide Powder**

EPA Reg. No.: 270-309

Active Ingredient(s):

Permethrin*	0.25%
Inert Ingredients:	99.75%
	100.0%

*(3-phenoxyphenyl) methyl(±) cis, trans-3-(2,2 dichloro-ethenyl)-2, 2-dimethylcyclopropane-carboxylate

cis/trans ratio: min. 35% (±) cis, max. 65% (±) trans

Indications: For use on horses, cattle and swine. Also for dogs and cats to control fleas, ticks, and lice up to 10 days.

Use only on horses, beef and dairy cattle, swine, dogs and cats.

Directions for Use: It is a violation of Federal law to use this product in a manner inconsistent with its labeling.

Read entire label before each use.

Horses, Beef and Dairy Cattle: For use in dust bags, shaker can and mechanical dust applicator.

Horn Flies, Lice, Face Flies: Place contents of the package in any commercially available dust bag. Suspend bag in areas frequented by cattle or in gateways or lanes through which the animals must pass daily for water, feed, or minerals. Bags may also be placed in loafing sheds or in front of mineral feeders.

For dairy cows, bags may be suspended in the exit through which the cows leave the milking barn. The bags should hang 4 to 6 inches below the back line of the cattle.

For reduction of Face Flies, bags must be located so animals will be forced to use them daily and hung at a height so that the face is dusted.

Direct Application: Apply 2 oz. of dust per animal by shaker can or dust glove over the head, neck shoulders, back, legs and tailhead. Repeat as necessary.

Swine:

Direct application for lice: Apply only 1 ounce per head as a uniform coat to the head, shoulder and back by use of a shaker can or suitable mechanical dust applicator. Repeat as necessary but not more often than once every 10 days. In severe infestation, both animals and the bedding may be treated.

Pets:

To control Fleas, Ticks and Lice on Dogs and Cats: Apply powder liberally over the entire body. Work dust into hair and around the feet, pads and between the toes by rubbing against the lay of the hair until dust penetrates to skin. Contact ticks with powder. Take care not to get the powder in pet's eyes, nose or mouth. Dust bedding, kennel, sleeping areas, carpeting and furniture used by infested animals regularly, applying at a rate of 3 to 6 ounces per 100 square feet. Repeat as needed, but not more often than once weekly. Do not use on dogs or cats less than 12 weeks of age.

Consult a veterinarian before using this product on debilitated, aged, pregnant, nursing or medicated animals. Sensitivities may occur after using any pesticide product for pets. If signs of sensitivity occur, bathe your pet with mild soap and rinse with large amounts of water. If signs continue, consult a veterinarian immediately.

Precautionary Statements: Hazards to Humans and Domestic Animals:

Caution: Harmful if swallowed or inhaled. Avoid breathing dust. Avoid contact with eyes and skin. Wash thoroughly with soap and water after handling. Avoid contamination of feed and foodstuffs.

First Aid:

If in Eyes: Flush with plenty of water. Get medical attention if irritation persists.

If on Skin: Wash with plenty of soap and water. Get medical attention if irritation persists.

If Inhaled: Remove victim to fresh air. Apply artificial respiration it indicated. Get medical attention.

Physical and Chemical Hazards: Do not use or store near heat or open flame.

Environmental Hazards: This product is extremely toxic to fish and aquatic invertebrates. Do not apply directly to water. Do not contaminate water by cleaning of equipment or disposal of equipment wash waters.

Storage and Disposal: Do not contaminate feed or foodstuffs by storage or disposal.

Storage: Store in cool, dry area away from children.

Pesticide Disposal: Wastes resulting from the use of this product may be disposed of on site or at an approved waste disposal facility.

Container Disposal: Do not reuse container. Wrap and discard in trash.

Warning(s): Do not ship swine for slaughter within 5 days of treatment.

Keep out of reach of children.

Disclaimer: This container is sold by weight, not by volume. You can be assured of the proper weight even though some settling of contents normally occurs during transportation and handling.

Buyer assumes all risks of use, storage or handling of this product not in strict accordance with the label.

Presentation: 6 oz (170 g).

Compendium Code No.: 10000270

HOSPITAL HAND SOAP

Vedco **Hand Soap**

Active Ingredient(s): Water, sodium lauryl sulfate, cocamide DEA, ethylene glycol monoslearate, glycerin, tetrasodium EDTA, methylparaben, aloe vera, phosphoric acid, sodium chloride, fragrance, FD&C red #40.

Indications: HOSPITAL HAND SOAP not only is an excellent cleanser, but it is formulated to help prevent skin from drying and cracking by adding lotion moisturizers.

Dosage and Administration: Use as a liquid handsoap.

Presentation: 1 gallon.

Compendium Code No.: 10941081

H. SOMNUS BACTERIN

Aspen **Bacterin**

Haemophilus Somnus Bacterin

Contents: H. SOMNUS BACTERIN is an inactivated bacterin.

Indications: Recommended for use in the vaccination of healthy cattle against disease caused by the *Haemophilus somnus* organisms.

Directions: Shake well. Administer 2 mL IM or SC to healthy cattle. For initial vaccination, a second dose is required 2-4 weeks later. Ideally calves should be 4 months of age or older when vaccination procedures are instituted. Annual revaccination with a single 2 mL dose is recommended.

Precaution(s): Store at 35°F-45°F (2°C-7°C). Do not freeze. Use entire contents when first opened.

Caution(s): In case of anaphylactoid reactions, epinephrine should be administered immediately.

For veterinary use only.

Warning(s): Do not vaccinate within 21 days before slaughter.

Presentation: 10 dose (20 mL) and 50 dose (100 mL) vials.

Manufactured by: BioCor®, Inc.

Compendium Code No.: 14750721 AV469-694

HUMILAC® SPRAY

Virbac **Grooming Product**

Active Ingredient(s): Contains purified water, propylene glycol, urea, lactic acid, glycerin, benzalkonium chloride, fragrance.

Indications: HUMILAC® is a soothing dry skin treatment incorporating an oil free humectant. Formulated to aid in moisturizing dry skin and in restoring luster to the hair coat without leaving a greasy or oily film.

Dosage and Administration: While parting the hair, thoroughly spray the entire coat. Groom as usual. Use once a day or as recommended by a veterinarian.

May be used as an after shampoo rinse. Add five (5) capfuls of HUMILAC® to one (1) quart of warm water. Pour the solution over the animal, avoiding the eyes and the ears.

Presentation: 8 fl. oz. (237 mL) and 32 fl. oz. (1 quart) containers.

Compendium Code No.: 10230370

HVT

Intervet **Vaccine**

Monovalent Marek's Disease Vaccine, Serotype 3, Live Virus (HVT, strain FC 126)

U.S. Vet. Lic. No.: 286

Contents: HVT monovalent Marek's disease vaccine is derived from the serotype 3 Marek's disease virus, turkey herpesvirus (East Lansing strain FC 126).

The vaccine contains gentamicin and amphotericin B as preservatives.

Notice: This vaccine has undergone rigid safety, purity and potency tests to meet USDA and Intervet Inc. standards. The use of this vaccine is subject to state laws, where applicable.

Indications: Marek's disease vaccines are recommended for vaccination of healthy one-day-old chicks through subcutaneous route.

Dosage and Administration: Read the instructions fully. Instructions must be followed exactly for best results. Prevent exposure to Marek's disease for at least two weeks.

1. Know and follow all precautions and safety practices for handling liquid nitrogen.
2. Before withdrawing vaccine from liquid nitrogen, protect hands with gloves, wear long sleeves and protect face with a plastic face shield or wear protective goggles.
3. Remove from the liquid nitrogen only the ampules that are going to be used immediately. Match the dosage size of the vaccine ampules and diluent bottle. Move quickly but carefully.

1000 doses of vaccine - 200 mL diluent

2000 to 9000 doses of vaccine - 400 mL to 1800 mL diluent

4. Place the ampule(s) in a clean large container of lukewarm water (75-85°F) to thaw ampule(s) quickly. Gentle agitation promotes rapid thawing and evenly distributes the vaccine in the ampule. Thaw the entire contents.
5. Mix vaccine with the room temperature diluent immediately after thawing. Remove closure from top of diluent bottle. Draw vaccine from the ampule into the sterile disposable mixing syringe.
6. Gently agitate syringe and expel contents into the diluent bottle. Rinse the ampule once with the diluted vaccine.
7. Place the diluted vaccine into an ice bath. Agitate as needed to ensure uniform suspension of the cells.
8. For subcutaneous vaccination, set sterilized automatic syringe to 0.2 mL per dose. Syringe, needles and accessory equipment should be sterilized by autoclaving or boiling.
9. For administering the vaccine subcutaneously, use a short (3/8" or 1/2"), 20 gauge needle to prevent injury to chicks. @NUM2 = 10. Vaccinate only healthy chicks at one day of age. Inject 0.2 mL (two-tenths of a milliliter) subcutaneously into the back of the neck.
11. Keep accurate records of chicks or eggs, vaccine serial numbers, vaccinator and doses used. Be sure to note unusual circumstances that occur before, during, or after vaccinating which may affect the level of immunity.

Precaution(s): Marek's disease vaccines, produced by Intervet, Inc. contain cell associated virus in live chicken cells. The cells and virus particles are very fragile and require careful handling to prevent damage and to preserve them intact to be used as a vaccine in chicks.

This product should be stored, transported and administered in accordance with the instructions and directions.

Make all preparations in advance and follow directions carefully.

Thaw vaccine immediately before use.

Make sure all personnel handling and/or using vaccine understand the importance of following these instructions completely.

Storage Conditions:

Vaccine Ampule - Store in liquid nitrogen.

Diluent - Store at room temperature. Chill after concentrated vaccine has been added as well as during use.

Burn all discarded containers and unused contents.

Caution(s): Combining this product with other biological products is not recommended.

For subcutaneous injection in one-day old chicks only.

Warning(s): Do not vaccinate within 21 days before slaughter.

Presentation: HVT is available for use in frozen form and comes packaged in 2,000 dose size units.

Compendium Code No.: 11060751

HVT + SB-1

Intervet **Vaccine**

Marek's Disease Vaccine, Live Chicken and Turkey Herpesvirus

U.S. Vet. Lic. No.: 286

Contents: Bivalent Marek's disease vaccine contains a cell associated virus in live chicken cells. Live chicken and turkey herpesvirus strains SB-1 and FC 126 (HVT) in one ampule. The cells and virus particles are fragile and require careful handling to prevent damage and to preserve them intact to be used as a vaccine in chicks.

Indications: The vaccine is recommended for use in healthy one-day old chicks for protection against Marek's disease, live chicken and turkey herpesvirus strains SB-1 and FC 126 (HVT). Good management practices are recommended to reduce exposure for at least two weeks following vaccination.

Dosage and Administration: Read fully. Instructions must be followed exactly for the best results. Guard against exposure to Marek's disease for at least two (2) weeks.

Preparation and Administration:

1. Know and follow all precautions and safety practices for the handling of liquid nitrogen.
2. Before withdrawing the vaccine from the liquid nitrogen, protect hands with gloves, wear long sleeves and protect face with a plastic face shield or wear protective goggles.
3. Remove from the liquid nitrogen only the ampules that are going to be used immediately. Match the dosage size of the vaccine ampules and diluent bottle. Move quickly but carefully.
4. Place the ampule(s) in a clean large container of lukewarm water (75°-85°F) to thaw the ampule quickly. Gentle agitation promotes rapid thawing and evenly distributes the vaccine in the ampule. Thaw the entire contents.
5. Mix the vaccine with room temperature diluent immediately after thawing. Mix the contents of one (1) ampule containing 1,000 doses of vaccine to 200 mL of sterile diluent. Remove the closure from the top of the diluent bottle. Draw the vaccine from the ampule into the sterile disposable mixing syringe included with each delivery.
6. Gently agitate the syringe and expel the contents into the diluent bottle. Rinse the ampule once with the diluted vaccine.
7. Place the diluted vaccine into an ice bath. Agitate as needed to ensure a uniform suspension of the cells. Set sterilized automatic syringe to 0.2 mL per dose. Syringe, needles and accessory equipment should be sterilized by autoclaving or boiling. Never sterilize with chemical disinfectants any equipment which comes in contact with the vaccine.
8. Use a short (3/8) or (1/2 inch), 20 to 24 gauge needle to prevent injury to chicks.
9. Vaccinate only healthy chicks at one (1) day of age. Inject 0.2 mL subcutaneously into the back of the neck.
10. Use all the diluted vaccine within one (1) hour of mixing . Do not refreeze or store unused vaccine for later use. Refreezing and thawing destroys the vaccine virus.

This vaccine can also be administered *in ovo,* using the Inovoject® system of Embrex, Inc.

Precaution(s): Vaccine Ampule - Store in a liquid nitrogen container.

Diluent - Store at room temperature. Chill after the concentrated vaccine has been added and during use.

Thaw the vaccine immediately before use.

Make sure all personnel handling and/or using the vaccine understand the importance of following directions completely.

Use all of the diluted vaccine within one hour of mixing. Do not refreeze or store unused vaccine for later use. Refreezing and thawing destroys the vaccine virus.

Burn all of the discarded containers and unused contents.

The vaccine is not returnable.

Caution(s): The product should be stored, transported and administered in accordance with the instructions and directions.

Make all preparations in advance and follow the directions carefully.

The recommended dose is 0.2 mL.

Keep accurate records of chicks, vaccine serial numbers, vaccinator and doses used. Be sure to note unusual circumstances that occur before, during or after vaccinating which may affect the level of immunity.

Warning(s): Do not vaccinate within 21 days before slaughter.

Presentation: One ampule containing 2,000 doses of vaccine with 200 mL of sterile diluent.

Compendium Code No.: 11060781

HYALOVET® ℞

Fort Dodge **Hyaluronate**

Hyaluronic Sodium Veterinary Injection

NADA No.: 140-806

Active Ingredient(s): Each filled 2 mL glass syringe or 2 mL glass vial contains:

Hyaluronate sodium	20.0 mg
Sodium chloride	17.0 mg
Monobasic sodium phosphate	0.1 mg
Dibasic sodium phosphate	1.2 mg
Water for injection	q.s., 2 mL

HYALOVET® (hyaluronate sodium) is a clear, colorless, viscous solution of a specific fraction of highly purified hyaluronic acid obtained by a molecular filtration procedure from biological material (rooster combs). The specific hyaluronic acid fraction from which HYALOVET® is made

H

has a high degree of molecular definition with an average molecular weight of 500,000-730,000 D.

Indications: HYALOVET® (hyaluronate sodium) is indicated for the intra-articular treatment of carpal or fetlock joint dysfunction in horses due to acute or chronic, non-infectious synovitis associated with equine osteoarthritis.

Pharmacology: Hyaluronic acid is the prototype of a wide range of saccharide biopolymers (glycosaminoglycans or mucopolysaccharides) consisting of repeating disaccharide units of N-acetyl-D-glucosamine and D-glucuronic acid linked by beta 1-3 and beta 1-4 glycosidic bonds. A component of all mammalian connective tissue, hyaluronic acid confers viscoelastic and lubricating properties to synovial fluid[1] and structural integrity to cartilage matrix.[2] As a therapeutic agent, hyaluronic acid injected into arthritic joints has been shown, in a variety of animal model systems including horses[3], to improve joint function and to activate tissue repair processes in articular cartilage.

Dosage and Administration: The recommended dose of HYALOVET® (hyaluronate sodium) is 2 mL (20 mg hyaluronate sodium) in small or medium sized joints (carpus, fetlock) given by intra-articular injection. More than one joint may be treated at the same time. If necessary, the injection may be repeated after one or more weeks, but do not exceed 2 injections per week for a total of 4 weeks.

HYALOVET® should be injected using strict aseptic technique. Excess synovial fluid should be removed prior to injection.

For best results, horses should be given two days of rest or limited exercise before resuming normal training.

Contraindication(s): There are no known contraindications.

Precaution(s): Storage Conditions: Store at or below 25°C (77°F).

Used or partially used syringes should be crushed and disposed of in an approved landfill.

Caution(s): Federal law restricts this drug to use by or on the order of a licensed veterinarian.

Warning(s): Not for use in horses intended for food. Not for human use. HYALOVET® Injection must not be administered intravascularly.

Toxicology: In subacute toxicity studies, in horses, intra-articular injection of HYALOVET® at the recommended dosage (20 mg/joint) and at 3X and 5X multiples of that dosage, daily for four days followed by twice weekly injections for four additional weeks, resulted in no evidence of toxicity either locally within the joint or systemically in the horses. Slight increases in synovial fluid leucocytes and protein were attributed to the trauma associated with frequent joint injections.

Results of skin testing in horses following repeated intra-articular injections of 40 mg HYALOVET® into tibiotarsal joints indicated that the product is nonantigenic in horses; no sensitization was detected.

Side Effects: As with any intra-articular injection, a mild inflammatory response (tenderness, heat and swelling) may be seen in the joint following HYALOVET® injection. The response is self limiting but may last from two to five days after treatment. If inflammation is excessive or severe, the possibility of infection should be considered and appropriate antibiotic therapy instituted.

Trial Data: Results of gel chromatography studies demonstrate that HYALOVET® (hyaluronate sodium) induces aggregation of cartilage proteoglycans sub-units as previously described for other fractions of hyaluronic acid.[2]

In equine model studies of acute synovitis of the carpal joint, a single, intra-articular injection of HYALOVET® (hyaluronate sodium) resulted in statistically significant ($p<0.05$) functional improvement with regard to lameness, swelling, pain, heat, and joint flexion in a dosage dependent fashion. In chronic osteoarthritis secondary to carpal fracture in horses, a single intra-articular injection of 20 mg HYALOVET® (hyaluronate sodium) resulted in statistically significant ($p<0.05$) reduction in radiopharmaceutical uptake in subchondral bone, as compared to saline injected controls, a finding consistent with reduced inflammation.

In controlled clinical trials in horses with lameness due to arthroses of the carpal or fetlock joints, intra-articular injection of 20 mg HYALOVET® (hyaluronate sodium) resulted in marked reduction in clinical lameness, pain on palpation, pain on flexion, and facilitated return to training. A measurable and statistically significant ($p<0.005$) decrease in joint circumference was detected in the horses.

References: Available upon request.

Presentation: HYALOVET® (hyaluronate sodium) Veterinary Injection
NDC 0856-2096-01 — 2 mL filled syringe (20 mg/2 mL)
NDC 0856-2096-11 — 12 X 2 mL filled syringes (20 mg/2 mL)
NDC 0856-2096-02 — 2 mL vial (20 mg/2 mL)
NDC 0856-2096-12 — 24 X 2 mL vials (20 mg/2 mL)

HYALOVET is a registered trademark of Trans Bussan s.a., Geneva, Switzerland.

Compendium Code No.: 10030971 4450C

HYCOAT® ℞

Neogen **Topical Wound Dressing**

Hyaluronate Sodium Sterile Solution

Active Ingredient(s): HYCOAT® is either a sterile 6 mL solution containing 30 mg of sodium hyaluronate or a sterile 10 mL solution containing 50 mg of sodium hyaluronate.

Avg Rel MW > 1.0 mm daltons.

Indications: For use in surgical procedures on dogs, cats and horses as a protective tissue coating.

Directions for Use:

1. Apply HYCOAT® liberally to the surgical field during and after the surgical procedure.
2. Introduce the contents of the vial to the bursa, joint, or body cavity, and exposed tissue surfaces.

Precaution(s): Store at controlled room temperature (15°-30°C). Protect from freezing.

Caution(s): Federal law restricts this device to sale by or on the order or a licensed veterinarian.

Warning(s): Not for food animal use.

Presentation: 6 mL and 10 mL vials.

Patent pending.

Compendium Code No.: 14910292 Rev 0501

HYDRA-LYTE

Vet-A-Mix **Electrolytes-Oral**

Ingredient(s): Contents per Package:

Sodium chloride	1.65 g
Sodium citrate	1.85 g
Glycine	2.2 g
Potassium chloride	4.2 g
Sodium acetate	15.4 g
Dextrose	138.0 g

Indications: For use as a buffered nutritional supplement in young calves, lambs and foals.

Dosage and Administration: HYDRA-LYTE readily dissolves in water and is easily absorbed. Prepare the solution by dissolving the contents of both compartments of the package in two quarts of warm water. Prepare the solution just prior to use and administer with an esophageal probe, nursing bottle or pail. Milk or milk replacer should be discontinued for the first two days of therapy.

Administer two quarts of HYDRA-LYTE solution to each calf or foal twice a day for the first two days. Important: Milk or milk replacer should not be used during this period. On the third and fourth day, administer one quart HYDRA-LYTE solution mixed with either one quart of milk or milk replacer to each calf or foal two times each day. Lambs will require about one-fourth of the above dosage.

Most treated animals can be returned to normal feeding on the fifth day, but treatment can be continued on the fifth through seventh day.

Note: In cases of severe dehydration or large neonatal animals, two quarts of HYDRA-LYTE solution should be administered to each calf or foal four times each day for the first two days. One-fourth this dosage is required for lambs. Use the same dosage regimen for the third and fourth days as recommended above.

Precaution(s): Store in a cool dry place.

Warning(s): Keep out of reach of children.

Presentation: Available in 5.76 oz. (163.4 g) two compartment foil packets - packed 48 packets per case.

Compendium Code No.: 10500110

HYDRO-B 1020™ ℞

Butler **Topical Corticosteroid**

Active Ingredient(s): Each mL contains:

Hydrocortisone	10 mg
Burow's Solution	20 mg

In a water miscible base containing propylene glycol.

Indications: Topical treatment for the relief of discomfort caused by inflammatory pruritis in dogs.

Hydrocortisone provides anti-inflammatory and anti-pruritic activity. Burow's solution is an astringent for drying moist dermatitis and provides cooling for relief of discomfort.

Dosage and Administration: Apply 3 to 4 times daily.

Contraindication(s): As with any topical hydrocortisone product, HYDRO-B 1020™ should not be used in the presence of tuberculosis of the skin.

Precaution(s): Store in a cool area. Protect from freezing.

Caution(s): Federal law restricts this drug to use by or on the order of a licensed veterinarian.

For topical use only. Not intended for deep-seated infections. Not for use in the eyes.

For veterinary use only.

Keep out of reach of children.

Presentation: 1 fl. oz. bottle (12 per box), 2 fl. oz. bottle (12 per box) and 16 fl. oz. bottle.

Compendium Code No.: 10820930

H

HYDROCORTISONE SOLUTION USP, 1% ℞

Vet Solutions **Steroidal Anti-inflammatory**

Anti-inflammatory-Antipruritic Solution

Active Ingredient(s): Hydrocortisone 1%, Pramoxine HCl 1%.

Ingredients: Propylene Glycol, SD Alcohol 40, Cocamidopropyl PG-Dimonium Chloride Phosphate, Deionized Water, Chloroxylenol (PCMX), Lactic Acid, Methylchloroisothiazolinone, Methylisothiazolinone.

Indications: For dermatological conditions associated with infections responsive to Hydrocortisone and Pramoxine HCl.

Directions: Clean and dry affected area. Apply a thin layer morning and evening or as directed by veterinarian. If satisfactory results are not obtained within 2 weeks, consult a veterinarian.

Precaution(s): Store at controlled room temperature (59-86°F).

Caution(s): Federal Law (USA) restricts this drug to use by or on the order of a licensed veterinarian.

Warning(s): Keep out of the reach of children. Avoid contact with eyes or mucous membranes. If contact occurs, immediately flush with water. If skin irritation occurs, discontinue use and consult a veterinarian.

Presentation: 29.5 mL (1 fl. oz.) and 59 mL (2 fl. oz.).

Compendium Code No.: 10610110 991101

HYDROGEN PEROXIDE

Butler **Antiseptic**

Antiseptic Solution U.S.P. 3%

Active Ingredient(s): Hydrogen Peroxide 3%.

Inert Ingredients: Water, Stabilizer q.s.

Indications: Recommended for first aid prophylaxis and treatment of minor cuts and abrasions apply to affected area.

Dosage and Administration: Use as required.

Precaution(s): Store in a cool area.

Caution(s): If irritation, swelling persists or increases or infection occurs discontinue use and get medical assistance.

For animal use only.

Keep out of reach of children.

Sold to veterinarians only.

Presentation: 16 fl. oz. (1 pt.) (NDC 11695-1557-01) and 1 gallon (NDC 11695-1557-02).

Compendium Code No.: 10820940

HYDROGEN PEROXIDE 3% SOLUTION

First Priority **Antiseptic**

Topical Antiseptic-Cleansing Agent

Active Ingredient(s): An aqueous solution of 3% hydrogen peroxide.

Indications: For use as a topical antiseptic and cleansing agent for minor cuts, abrasions and wounds.

Directions for Use: Apply freely to cleanse cuts, abrasions and wounds. In addition to its germicidal activity, the effervescence of hydrogen peroxide is beneficial to mechanically remove pus and debris from wounds.

Precaution(s): Storage: Store at controlled room temperature between 15°-30°C (59°-86°F). Keep tightly closed when not in use. Protect from light.

Caution(s): In case of deep or puncture wounds or serious burns consult veterinarian. If redness, irritation, or swelling persists or increases, discontinue use and consult veterinarian.

For animal use only.

Warning(s): Keep out of reach of children.

Presentation: 16 fl oz (473 mL) (NDC# 58829-229-16) and 1 gallon (3.785 L) (NDC# 58829-229-01).

Compendium Code No.: 11390393 Rev. 06-01 / Rev. 07-01

HYDROGEN PEROXIDE 3% SOLUTION

Phoenix Pharmaceutical **Antiseptic**

Topical Antiseptic-Cleansing Agent

Active Ingredient(s): Composition: Each mL of aqueous solution contains:

Hydrogen Peroxide. 3%

Indications: For use as a topical antiseptic and cleansing agent for minor cuts, abrasions and wounds in cattle, horses, sheep, swine, dogs and cats.

Directions for Use: Apply freely to cleanse cuts, abrasions and wounds. In addition to its germicidal activity, the effervescence of hydrogen peroxide is beneficial to mechanically remove pus and debris from wounds.

Precaution(s): Store at controlled room temperature between 15°-30°C (59°-86°F). Protect from light. Keep tightly closed when not in use.

Caution(s): In case of deep or puncture wounds or serious burns consult veterinarian. If redness, irritation, or swelling persists or increases, discontinue use and consult veterinarian.

For external animal use only.

For animal use only.

Warning(s): Keep out of reach of children.

Presentation: 1 gallon (3.785 L) (NDC 57319-428-09).

Manufactured by: Sparhawk Laboratories, Lenexa, KS 66215.

Compendium Code No.: 12561132 Rev. 7-01

H

HYDROGEN PEROXIDE U.S.P.

Vedco **Antiseptic**

Active Ingredient(s): Contains:

Hydrogen peroxide. 3%

Inert ingredients. 97%

Indications: For antiseptic use.

Dosage and Administration: Use full strength as an antiseptic cleanser. Apply locally on minor cuts, boils and abrasions. For mouthwash or gargle, dilute with three (3) parts of water. Preserve in a tightly closed container at room temperature and away from direct sunlight. Avoid contamination of the product.

Caution(s): Keep out of the reach of children.

In case of deep puncture wounds, consult a physician. If redness, irritation, swelling or pain develops, persists or increases, or if infection occurs, discontinue use and consult a physician.

Avoid swallowing. In case of accidental ingestion seek professional assistance.

For veterinary use only.

Presentation: 1 pint and 1 gallon containers.

Compendium Code No.: 10941091

HYDRO-PLUS ℞

Phoenix Pharmaceutical **Topical Corticosteroid**

Active Ingredient(s): Each mL contains:

Hydrocortisone . . . . 10 mg

Burrow's Solution . . . . 20 mg

In a water miscible base containing Propylene Glycol.

Indications: Topical treatment for the relief of discomfort caused by inflammatory pruritis in dogs.

Pharmacology: Hydrocortisone: Anti-inflammatory and antipruritic.

Burrow's Solution: Astringent for the drying of moist dermatitis and it provides cooling for the relief of discomfort.

Dosage and Administration: Apply 3 to 4 times daily.

Contraindication(s): As with any topical hydrocortisone product HYDRO-PLUS should not be used in the presence of tuberculosis of the skin.

Precaution(s): Store in a cool area. Protect from freezing.

Caution(s): Federal law restricts this drug to use by or on the order of a licensed veterinarian.

For topical use only. Not intended for deep-seated infections. Not for use in the eyes.

Warning(s): Keep out of reach of children.

Presentation: 1 fl. oz. (NDC 57319-054-17), 2 fl. oz with pump (NDC 57319-054-18) and 16 fl. oz. (NDC 57319-054-21) containers.

Compendium Code No.: 12560401

HYGROMIX® 8

Elanco **Feed Medication**

Hygromycin B-Type A Medicated Article-Anthelmintic

NADA No.: 010-948 (Chickens) / 010-918 (Swine)

Active Ingredient(s):

Hygromycin B . . . . 8 g/lb

Ingredient—Soybean mill run.

Indications:

Swine: As an aid in the control of infestation of the following intestinal parasites: Large Roundworms *(Ascaris)*, Nodular Worms *(Oesophagostomum)*, Whipworms *(Trichuris)*.

Chickens: As an aid in the control of infestation of the following intestinal parasites: Large Roundworms *(Ascaridia galli)*, Cecal Worms *(Heterakis gallinarum)*, Capillaria Worms *(Capillaria obsignata)*.

Directions:

Important: Must be mixed in feeds before use. Follow mixing directions carefully.

Mixing Directions for Swine Feeds:

Lbs of HYGROMIX® 8 per Ton of Feed Concentrate	g of Hygromycin B per Ton of Concentrate	Lbs of Concentrate to Lbs of Grain
3	24 g	1 lb to 1 lb
7.5	60 g	1 lb to 4 lbs
10.5	84 g	1 lb to 6 lbs
13.5	108 g	1 lb to 8 lbs
16.5	132 g	1 lb to 10 lbs

Complete Ration—Thoroughly mix 1.5 pounds of HYGROMIX® 8 in one ton of feed. This will give 12 g of Hygromycin B per ton.

Feed Concentrates—See table above. Amount of HYGROMIX® 8 in a concentrate must not exceed 16.5 pounds per ton (132 g of Hygromycin B per ton). All concentrate tags must have mixing directions which provide for a complete ration containing 12 g of Hygromycin B per ton. Rations fed to swine must contain 12 g of Hygromycin B per ton.

Use Programs:

In Market Hogs: Use HYGROMIX® for 8 weeks during the growing period.

In Gilts to be Used as Breeding Stock: Do not use HYGROMIX® because of hearing and vision impairment side effects.

In Sows: Consideration should be given to hearing and vision impairment side effects. If fed, use for no longer than 8 weeks during gestation and lactation.

Mixing Directions for Chicken Feeds:

Lbs of HYGROMIX® 8 per Ton of Feed Concentration	g of Hygromycin B per Ton of Concentrate	Lbs of Concentrate to Lbs of Grain to provide the following levels of Hygromycin B per Lb of Complete Ration	
		0.004 g	0.006 g
3	24 g	1 lb to 2 lbs	1 lb to 1 lb
4	32 g	1 lb to 3 lbs	1 lb to 1.67 lbs

Complete Ration—Thoroughly mix 1 or 1.5 pounds of HYGROMIX® 8 in one ton of feed. This will give 8 g or 12 g of Hygromycin B per ton. Rations fed to chickens must contain at least 8 g and not more than 12 g of Hygromycin B per ton.

Feed Concentrates—See table above. Amount of HYGROMIX® 8 in a concentrate must not exceed 4 pounds per ton (32 g of Hygromycin B per ton). All concentrate tags must have mixing directions which provide for a complete ration containing 8 g and not to exceed 12 g of Hygromycin B per ton.

Precaution(s): Avoid moisture and excessive heat.

Not to be used after the date printed on bottom of bag.

When mixing and handling HYGROMIX® 8 Premix, use protective clothing, impervious gloves and a dust mask.

Operators should wash thoroughly with soap and water after handling. Do not breathe dust. Since it may cause severe and potentially permanent eye damage, do not get on skin or in eyes. In case of eye contact, flush with water and obtain prompt medical aid. For skin exposure, wash with soap and water. In case of ingestion, induce vomiting.

Caution(s): Livestock Remedy—Not for human use.

To prevent cross-contamination, equipment must be thoroughly cleaned before and after the manufacture of medicated feeds. Avoid contact with skin surfaces.

Consult your veterinarian for assistance in the diagnosis, treatment and control of parasitism.

For use in swine and chicken feeds only.

Warning(s): Discontinue swine feeds containing Hygromycin B 15 days before slaughter.

Discontinue chicken feeds containing Hygromycin B 3 days before slaughter.

Side Effects: A reduced response to sound and vision has been noticed in some swine fed Hygromycin B. This impairment of hearing and vision is not an important problem in the market hog. It should, however, be carefully evaluated for breeding stock. Should sows be affected, they will become less responsive to the squeal of baby pigs, possibly resulting in crushed pigs.

Presentation: 50 lbs (22.68 kg).

Compendium Code No.: 10310022 BG 3128 AMB

HYLARTIN® V ℞

Pharmacia & Upjohn **Hyaluronate**

Sodium hyaluronate injection 10 mg/mL

NADA No.: 112-048

Active Ingredient(s): HYLARTIN® V is a sterile pyrogen-free solution of a highly purified, specific fraction of the sodium salt of hyaluronic acid extracted from rooster combs.

Each mL contains: Sodium hyaluronate 10.0 mg, sodium chloride 8.5 mg, disodium hydrogen phosphate dihydrate 0.28 mg, sodium dihydrogen phosphate hydrate 0.04 mg, water for injection U.S.P. q.s.

Indications: HYLARTIN® V is indicated in the treatment of joint dysfunction in horses due to non-infectious synovitis associated with equine osteoarthritis.

Pharmacology: Sodium hyaluronate is a natural, physiological substance which occurs extracellularly in connective tissue in both animals and man and is chemically identical in different species. High concentrations (>0.2 mg/mL) of hyaluronate are found in the synovial fluid, the vitreous of the eye and the umbilical cord.

Sodium hyaluronate is a normal component of connective tissue matrix and it is injected therapeutically only in compartments where it constitutes a normal component, specifically the joint cavity.

Chemistry: Sodium hyaluronate is a high molecular weight polymer made up of repeating disaccharide units of N-acetylglucosamine and sodium glucuronate linked by beta 1-3 and beta 1-4 glycosidic bonds. HYLARTIN® V contains only traces of protein.

Dosage and Administration: 2 mL (20 mg) of HYLARTIN® V given to horses intra-articularly in small and medium size joints (carpal, fetlock). In the treatment of larger joints (hock), the dosage is 4 mL (40 mg). The treatment may be repeated at weekly intervals for a total of three treatments.

HYLARTIN® V should be injected in horses intra-articularly under strict aseptic conditions. Effusion should be removed prior to injection. When performing the injections, care should be taken not to scratch the cartilage surface as this may result in diffuse swelling lasting for 24 to 48 hours. This transient swelling, however, will not have an effect on the ultimate clinical result. For the best results, the horse should be given two days stall rest before gradually resuming normal activity.

Contraindication(s): None known.

Precaution(s): Store at 2° to 8°C. The expiration date is stated on the package. Protect from freezing. Protect from light.

Caution(s): Federal law restricts this drug to use by or on the order of a licensed veterinarian.

Used or partially used syringes should be crushed and disposed of in an approved landfill.

Do not use if numerous small air bubbles are present throughout the solution.

Warning(s): Not for use in horses intended for food.

HYLARTIN® V must not be administered intra-vascularly.

Toxicology: Acute, sub-acute and chronic toxicity studies in mice, rats, rabbits, dogs, monkeys and horses have not demonstrated any significant adverse reactions or sensitization.

In an acute toxicity study in horses, HYLARTIN® V was injected intra-articularly at dosages corresponding to five times the recommended dose per animal (200 mg total). In a sub-acute study, horses were injected intra-articularly with the recommended dose per joint (20 mg) at weekly intervals for nine weeks. The results of both investigations showed that hematological and blood chemistry values remained within normal ranges. In mice, the intravenous LD_{100} was found to be of the order of 50 mg/kg of body weight.

There is always a potential immunological risk with repeated parenteral administration of biological material. However, as shown by Richter (1974), sodium hyaluronate, of both human and avian origin, did not produce any antibodies after repeated immunization, nor did intense stimulation of the immunization process by coupling of protein to the hyaluronate and simultaneous administration of Freund's adjuvant give rise to antibodies.

Side Effects: The side effects observed in clinical trials were heat (15%), transient edema (12%), and pain (9%) around the treated joint. These side effects have been observed after intra-articular injection. Most of these reactions were of mild nature and in no case did they require the discontinuance of treatment. These reactions subsided in 24 to 48 hours.

Trial Data: Clinical field trials with thoroughbred and standard-bred race horses were undertaken at four separate clinics. A total of 252 joints were injected with HYLARTIN® V in these investigations. In one study, only horses which were conventional treatment failures were included and the overall improvement rate following HYLARTIN® V treatment approached 90%. In the other studies, the improvement rate surpassed this figure.

In another case, electrogoniometry was used to objectively show that HYLARTIN® V can improve the function of arthritic carpal and fetlock joints. HYLARTIN® V brought return to symmetry with respect to the timing and duration of various angular motions of the joints. In cases where HYLARTIN® V was not able to achieve contralateral symmetry of the joint motion pattern, blocking of the joint with anesthetic also had no effect, indicating that most probably mechanical damage was responsible for the joint dysfunction.

References: Available upon request.

Presentation: HYLARTIN® V is supplied sterile in disposable glass syringes, each containing 20 mg (10 mg/mL) of sodium hyaluronate in 2.0 mL physiological sodium chloride-phosphate buffer with a pH of 7.0-7.5.

Compendium Code No.: 10490180

HYLYT*EFA® BATH OIL/COAT CONDITIONER

DVM — **Grooming Rinse**

Ingredient(s): Water, sodium lactate, mineral oil, PVP, polysorbate 60, safflower oil, diazolidinyl urea, lanolin oil, methylparaben, PEG-4 dilaurate, oleth-2, propylparaben, fragrance, sodium dehydroacetate.

Indications: After bath, rinse for improved luster and sheen of haircoat. Aids in control of flaking and scaling by normalizing keratin.

A gentle, hypoallergenic formulation to replenish skin following or in between bathing. Natural moisturizing factors and essential fatty acids for conditioning of haircoat and renourishment of skin.

Directions for Use: Shake well before use. Use HYLYT® Bath Oil as a spray or rinse to restore proper moisture balance to skin immediately following medicated or routine shampooing.

As a Spray: Be sure to push down on sprayer with sufficient pressure to obtain a fine mist. Mist entire haircoat or areas of dry skin. Part hair so that spray makes direct contact with skin. Rub in well and groom with a brush.

As a Rinse: Add 5 capfuls to one-half gallon of warm water, mix thoroughly and pour mixture evenly over haircoat. Gently rub into haircoat, then towel dry.

May be used daily, or as directed by a veterinarian.

Precaution(s): Store at room temperature.

Caution(s): For topical use on animals only. Avoid contact with eyes.

Warning(s): Keep out of reach of children.

Presentation: 8 fl oz (237 mL) sprayers.

* Essential Fatty Acids

Compendium Code No.: 11420341 — Rev 0597

HYLYT*EFA® HYPOALLERGENIC CREME RINSE

DVM — **Grooming Rinse**

Ingredient(s): Water, quaternium-18, cetearyl alcohol and polysorbate 60, stearamidopropyl dimethylamine lactate, sodium lactate, safflower oil, hydrolyzed collagen, PEG-8 stearate, glycerin, polyquaternium-7, fragrance, methylchloroisothiazolinone and methylisothiazolinone.

Indications: After bath creme rinse for improved luster and sheen of haircoat. Reduces static electricity, tangles and snarls.

A gentle, hypoallergenic, soap-free formulation with optimal pH balance. Contains emollients for moisturizing and protein for conditioning. Natural moisturizing factors promote hydration of skin and coat, while essential fatty acids nourish skin and aid in the control of flaking and scaling.

Directions for Use: After shampooing, apply HYLYT® Creme Rinse evenly and thoroughly into haircoat. Allow to stand for 5-10 minutes, then rinse well with water. May be used as often as necessary.

Precaution(s): Store at room temperature.

Caution(s): For topical use on animals only. Avoid contact with eyes.

Warning(s): Keep out of reach of children.

Presentation: 8 fl oz (237 mL) and 1 gallon (3.78 L).

Compendium Code No.: 11420351 — Rev 0597

HYLYT*EFA® HYPOALLERGENIC SHAMPOO

DVM — **Grooming Shampoo**

Soap-Free Hypoallergenic Shampoo

Ingredient(s): Water, sodium C14-16 olefin sulfonate, cocamidopropyl betaine, sodium lactate, PEG-120 methyl glucose dioleate, glycerin, hydrolyzed collagen, PEG-75 lanolin, sodium chloride, fragrance, methylchloroisothiazolinone and methylisothiazolinone, safflower oil, and FD&C yellow #5. May contain citric acid to ensure optimal pH.

Indications: For routine cleansing and grooming. May be used in conjunction with topical therapeutics.

A gentle, hypoallergenic, soap-free formulation with optimal pH balance. Contains emollients for moisturizing and protein for conditioning. Natural moisturizing factors promote hydration of skin and coat, while essential fatty acids nourish skin and aid in the control of flaking and scaling.

Directions for Use: Wet coat thoroughly. Apply sufficient HYLYT® Shampoo to lather well into haircoat. Rinse thoroughly. May be used as often as necessary.

Precaution(s): Store at room temperature.

Caution(s): For topical use on animals only. Avoid contact with eyes.

Warning(s): Keep out of reach of children.

Presentation: 8 fl oz (273 mL), 12 fl oz (355 mL) and 1 gallon (3.78 L).

*Essential Fatty Acids

Compendium Code No.: 11420361 — Rev 0597

HYLYT*EFA® SPRAY-ON SHAMPOO

DVM — **Grooming Shampoo**

Soap-Free Hypoallergenic Conditioning Shampoo

Ingredient(s): Water, sodium C14-16 olefin sulfonate, cocamidopropyl betaine, sodium lactate, glycerin, hydrolyzed collagen, PEG-75 lanolin, PEG-120 methyl glucose dioleate, fragrance, methylchloroisothiazolinone and methylisothiazolinone, safflower oil, FD&C yellow #5, and may contain citric acid.

Indications: For routine cleansing and grooming of dogs and cats. May be used in conjunction with topical therapeutics.

A gentle, hypoallergenic, soap-free formulation with an optimal pH balance. Contains emollients for moisturizing and protein for conditioning. Natural moisturizing factors promote hydration of skin and coat, while essential fatty acids nourish skin and aid in the control of flaking and scaling.

Directions for Use: Wet coat thoroughly. Apply sufficient HYLYT® Spray-On Shampoo to lather well into haircoat. Rinse thoroughly. May be used as often as necessary, or as directed by your veterinarian.

Storage: Store at room temperature.

Caution(s): For topical use on animals only. Avoid contact with eyes.

Warning(s): Keep out of reach of children.

Presentation: 12 fl oz (355 mL).

*Essential Fatty Acids

Compendium Code No.: 11420371 — Rev 0598

HYPERSALINE E ℞

Vetus — **Saline Solution**

Composition: Each 100 mL of sterile aqueous solution contains:

Sodium Chloride . . . . . 7.2 g

Millequivalents per liter:

Cations:

Sodium . . . . . 1232 mEq/L

Anions:

Chloride . . . . . 1232 mEq/L

Total osmolarity is 2464 milliosmoles per liter.

Indications: For use in replacement therapy of sodium, chloride and water which may become depleted in many diseases.

Dosage and Administration: Warm to body temperature and administer slowly by intravenous or subcutaneous injection. The amount and rate of administration must be judged by the veterinarian in relation to the condition being treated and the clinical response of the animal, being careful to avoid overhydration.

Precaution(s): Store between 15°C and 30°C (59°F-86°F).

This product contains no preservatives. Use entire contents when fist opened. Discard any unused solution.

Caution(s): Federal law restricts this drug to use by or on the order of a licensed veterinarian.

Warning(s): For animal use only. Keep out of reach of children.

Presentation: 1000 mL single dose container.

Compendium Code No.: 14440490

HYPER SALINE SOLUTION 8X ℞

Butler — **Saline Solution**

Active Ingredient(s): Each 100 mL of sterile aqueous solution contains:

Sodium chloride . . . . . 7.2 g

Milliequivalents per liter:

Cations:

Sodium . . . . . 1,232 mEq/L

Anions:

Chloride . . . . . 1,232 mEq/L

Total osmolarity is 2,464 milliosmoles per liter.

This product contains no preservatives.

Indications: For use in replacement therapy of sodium, chloride and water which may become depleted in many diseases.

Dosage and Administration: Warm to body temperature and administer slowly by intravenous or subcutaneous injection. The amount and rate of administration must be judged by the veterinarian in relation to the condition being treated and the clinical response of the animal, being careful to avoid overhydration.

Precaution(s): Store at a controlled room temperature between 15° and 30°C (59°-86°F).

Use the entire contents when first opened. Discard any unused solution.

Caution(s): Federal law restricts this drug to use by or on the order of a licensed veterinarian.

For animal use only.

Warning(s): Keep out of the reach of children.

Presentation: 1,000 mL bottle (NDC 11695-628-04).

Compendium Code No.: 10820961

HYPERTONIC SALINE SOLUTION 7.2% ℞

AgriLabs — **Saline Solution**

Sterile-Preservative Free

Active Ingredient(s): Composition: Each 100 mL of sterile aqueous solution contains:

Sodium Chloride . . . . . 7.2 g

Milliequivalents per liter:

Cations:

Sodium . . . . . 1232 mEq/L

Anions:

Chloride . . . . . 1232 mEq/L

Total osmolarity is 2464 milliosmoles per liter.

This product contains no preservatives.
Indications: For use in replacement therapy of sodium, chloride and water which may become depleted in many diseases.
Dosage and Administration: Warm to body temperature and administer slowly by intravenous or subcutaneous injection. The amount and rate of administration must be judged in relation to the condition being treated and the clinical response of the animal, being careful to avoid overhydration.
Precaution(s): Store between 15°C-30°C (59°F-86°F). Use entire contents when first opened. Discard any unused solution.
Caution(s): Federal law restricts this drug to use by or on the order of a licensed veterinarian.
For animal use only.
Warning(s): Keep out of reach of children.
Presentation: 1000 mL bottle.
Compendium Code No.: 10581610 Iss. 1-97

HYPERTONIC SALINE SOLUTION 7.2%

Aspen **Saline Solution**

Composition: Each 100 mL of sterile aqueous solution contains:
Sodium Chloride .... 7.2 g
Milliequivalents per liter:
Cations:
Sodium .... 1232 mEq/L
Anions:
Chloride .... 1,32 mEq/L
Total osmolarity is 2,464 milliosmoles per liter.
Indications: For use in replacement therapy of sodium, chloride and water which may become depleted in many diseases.
Dosage and Administration: Warm to body temperature and administer slowly by intravenous or subcutaneous injection. The amount and rate of administration must be judged in relation to the condition being treated and the clinical response of the animal, being careful to avoid overhydration.
Precaution(s): Store between 15°C-30°C (59°F-86°F).
Caution(s): This product contains no preservatives. Use entire contents when first opened. Discard any unused solution.
Warning(s): For animal use only.
Keep out of reach of children.
Presentation: 1000 mL.
Compendium Code No.: 14750380

HYPERTONIC SALINE SOLUTION 7.2% ℞

Bimeda **Saline Solution**

Active Ingredient(s): Composition: Each 100 mL of sterile aqueous solution contains:
Sodium Chloride .... 7.2 g
Milliequivalents per liter:
Cations:
Sodium .... 1232 mEq/L
Anions:
Chloride .... 1232 mEq/L
Total osmolarity is 2464 milliosmoles per liter.
This product contains no preservatives.
Indications: For use in replacement therapy of sodium, chloride and water which may become depleted in many diseases.
Dosage and Administration: Horses/Cattle: 50 to 100 mL per 100 lb body weight. Warm to body temperature and administer slowly by intravenous or subcutaneous injection. The amount and rate of administration must be judged by the veterinarian in relation to the condition being treated and the clinical response of the animal, being careful to avoid overhydration.
Precaution(s): Store at controlled room temperature between 15°-30°C (59°-86°F). Use entire contents when first opened. Discard any unused solution.
Caution(s): Federal law restricts this drug to use by or on the order of a licensed veterinarian.
For animal use only.
Warning(s): Keep out of reach of children.
Presentation: 1000 mL (NDC# 61133-0264-9).
Manufactured by: Bimeda-MTC Animal Health Inc., Cambridge, Ontario, Canada N3C 2W4.
Compendium Code No.: 13990550 8111B

HYPERTONIC SALINE SOLUTION 7.2% ℞

Phoenix Pharmaceutical **Saline Solution**

Active Ingredient(s): Composition: Each 100 mL of sterile aqueous solution contains:
Sodium Chloride .... 7.2 g
Milliequivalents per liter:
Cations:
Sodium .... 1232 mEq/L
Anions:
Chloride .... 1232 mEq/L
Total osmolarity is 2464 milliosmoles per liter.
This product contains no preservatives.
Indications: For use in replacement therapy of sodium, chloride and water which may become depleted in many diseases.
Dosage and Administration: Warm to body temperature and administer slowly by intravenous or subcutaneous injection. The amount and rate of administration must be judged by the veterinarian in relation to the condition being treated and the clinical response of the animal, being careful to avoid overhydration.
Precaution(s): Store between 15° and 30°C (59°-86°F).
Use the entire contents when first opened. Discard any unused solution.
Caution(s): Federal law restricts this drug to use by or on the order of a licensed veterinarian.
For animal use only.
Warning(s): Keep out of reach of children.
Presentation: 1000 mL bottles (NDC 57319-104-08).
Compendium Code No.: 12560411 Rev. 6-01

HYPERTONIC SALINE SOLUTION 7.2%

RXV **Saline Solution**

Active Ingredient(s): Each 100 mL of sterile aqueous solution contains:
Sodium chloride .... 7.2 g
Milliequivalents per liter:
Cations:
Sodium .... 1,232 mEq/L
Anions:
Chloride .... 1,232 mEq/L
Total osmolarity is 2,464 milliosmoles per liter.
Sterile-Preservative free.
Indications: For use in replacement therapy of sodium, chloride and water which may become depleted in many diseases.
Dosage and Administration: Warm to body temperature and administer slowly by intravenous or subcutaneous injection. The amount and rate of administration must be judged by the veterinarian in relation to the condition being treated and the clinical response of the animal, being careful to avoid overhydration.
Precaution(s): Store between 15°C-30°C (59°F-86°F).
Caution(s): This product contains no preservatives. Use entire contents when first opened. Discard any unused solution.
For animal use only. Keep out of reach of children.
Presentation: 1,000 mL, 12 per case.
Compendium Code No.: 10910070

HYPERTONIC SALINE SOLUTION 7.2% ℞

Vet Tek **Saline Solution**

Active Ingredient(s): Composition: Each 100 mL of sterile aqueous solution contains:
Sodium chloride .... 7.2 g
Milliequivalents per liter:
Cations:
Sodium .... 1,232 mEq/L
Anions:
Chloride .... 1,232 mEq/L
Total osmolarity is 2464 milliosmoles per liter.
Indications: For use in replacement therapy of sodium, chloride and water which may become depleted in many diseases.
Dosage and Administration: Warm to body temperature and administer slowly by intravenous or subcutaneous injection. The amount and rate of administration must be judged by the veterinarian in relation to the condition being treated and the clinical response of the animal, being careful to avoid overhydration.
Precaution(s): Store between 15°-30°C (59°-86°F).
This product contains no preservatives. Use entire contents when first opened. Discard any unused solution.
Caution(s): Federal law restricts this drug to use by or on the order of a licensed veterinarian.
For animal use only.
Warning(s): Keep out of reach of children.
Presentation: 1,000 mL bottles (NDC 60270-813-20).
Manufactured by: Phoenix Scientific, Inc., St. Joseph, MO 64503
Compendium Code No.: 14200280 Iss. 8-99

HYPO-CHLOR FORMULA 6.40

Stearns **Sanitizer**

EPA Reg. No.: 3640-64
Active Ingredient(s):
Sodium hypochlorite 6.4%
Inert ingredients:
Water 93.6%
Indications: Deodorant for dairy plants and farms.
Dosage and Administration: It is a violation of federal law to use the product in a manner inconsistent with its labeling.

Note: The product degrades with age. Use a chrome test kit and increase the dosage as necessary to obtain the required level of available chlorine.

Sanitation Note: All surfaces to be sanitized with HYPO-CHLOR FORMULA 6.40 should be thoroughly cleaned. In addition, the solution should be applied immediately before using the equipment.

General sanitation: For emergency drinking water, chlorinate water supplies with 0.1 to 0.5 ppm and check for residual chlorine level with chlorine test kits acceptable to local health authorities. Add ½ oz. to 400 gallons of water for 0.5 ppm.

Canning, federally inspected meat and poultry plants, institutional and egg sanitation: Spray or circulate a 200 ppm solution on all processing equipment for at least a two (2) minute exposure period after a thorough cleaning. Open water cooling troughs in canning factories should maintain 5 ppm solution.

Milk and cheese plant sanitation: General applications - After all surfaces have been thoroughly cleaned and just before use, all equipment should be sanitized with a 200 ppm solution of HYPO-CHLOR FORMULA 6.40. The solution should be in contact with the surface for at least two (2) minutes. Do not rinse with potable water after sanitizing.

Butter producing equipment: Just prior to using and after thorough cleaning, all vats, churns, coolers, separators, holding tanks and pipelines should be sanitized with 200 ppm solution of HYPO-CHLOR FORMULA 6.40 for at least two (2) minutes. Butter wash water should contain 10 ppm available chlorine. Do not rinse with potable water.

Milk bottles: The bottles should be sanitized with a solution of 50 ppm available chlorine just before being filled. Do not rinse with potable water.

Dairy farm sanitation: Milking machines - Immediately prior to each milking, sanitize all inflations, utensils and milking machines with a 200 ppm available chlorine solution for at least two (2) minutes. The hoses and inflations may be stored in a 200 ppm available chlorine solution when not in use.

Milking room: A 500 ppm available chlorine solution may be used to wash all equipment, walls, and floors. (To aid in controlling harmful bacteria and promoting quality milk production.)

Dilution Table:

Available Chlorine	Preparation HYPO-CHLOR/Water	Applications
500 ppm	5 oz./4 gals.	Bathhouse, milking room.
200 ppm	1 oz./2 gals.	For sanitizing dairy equipment.
100 ppm	1 oz./4 gals.	To meet minimum sanitizing requirements for two-minute contact.
50 ppm	1 oz./8 gals.	For sanitizing milk bottles.
1 ppm	1 oz./400 gals.	For swimming pool disinfection.
1%	1 gal./5 gals.	Commercial laundry stock bleach.
5¼%	1 gal./1 gal.	Standard household bleach.

Five Step Procedure:

1. Equipment and utensils shall be preflushed or prescraped and when necessary, presoaked to remove gross food particles and soil.
2. Utensils and equipment shall be washed in water having a minimum temperature of 110°F (43°C) and containing an adequate amount of an effective soap or detergent. Water shall be kept clean by changing it frequently.
3. Equipment and utensils shall then be rinsed free of detergent and abrasives with clean water; and
4. Following washing and rinsing, all utensils and equipment shall be sanitized by immersion in a solution of 1 oz. of Quatamine™ to four (4) gallons of water (200 ppm), for at least two (2) minutes or for another contact time observed by the governing sanitation code. A minimum of 100 ppm concentration must be continuously maintained. Check the concentration frequently with an approved chlorine test kit.
5. After sanitization, all equipment and utensils shall be air-dried. A potable water rinse is not required.

Caution(s): Danger - Keep out of the reach of children.

Avoid contact with the eyes. The concentrate may irritate eyes, skin, and lungs. Harmful if swallowed. Do not use with acid containing bowl cleaners.

First Aid:

External: Flood with water for at least 15 minutes. In case of eye contact consult a physician immediately.

Internal: Drink raw egg, milk or rice gruel. Induce vomiting (use a teaspoonful of mustard in a glass of warm water for an emetic). Contact a physician immediately.

Presentation: 1 gallon containers.

Compendium Code No.: 10170031

HY-SORB™

Bimeda **Electrolytes-Oral**

Active Ingredient(s): A concentrated electrolyte product containing: Sodium Chloride 5.52 g; Sodium Bicarbonate 6.36 g; Sodium Citrate, Anhydrous 4.88 g; Calcium Chloride, Anhydrous 1.05 g; Magnesium Sulfate, Dried 0.81 g; Potassium Chloride 1.41 g; Dextrose, Anhydrous 19.11 g; Glycine 5.68 g; Maltrin q.s. to 60 g.

When HY-SORB™ is diluted with two quarts water, the solution contains: Sodium 120 mEq/Liter; Potassium 10 mEq/Liter; Bicarbonate 40 mEq/Liter; Chloride 70 mEq/Liter; Calcium 10 mEq/Liter; Magnesium 5 mEq/Liter; Sulfate 5 mEq/Liter; Dextrose 56 mM/Liter; Glycine 40 mM/Liter.

Indications: A concentrated electrolyte product fortified with dextrose, glycine and bicarbonate for oral administration to calves.

Directions for Use: Dissolve contents of one packet in two quarts of warm water. Administer two quarts of solution per calf via oral administration 2 to 3 times a day. Prepare fresh solution daily.

When mixed as directed, the resulting solution containing electrolytes, dextrose and glycine is approximately 360 mOsm/L.

Precaution(s): Keep in a cool, dry place.

Caution(s): For animal use only.

Warning(s): Not for human use.

Keep out of reach of children.

Presentation: 60 g (2 oz) pouch.

™ Trademark of Bimeda, Inc.

Manufactured by: Bimeda, Inc., LaSueur, MN 56058.

Compendium Code No.: 13990201 8HYS003-700

HYVISC® ℞

Boehringer Ingelheim **Hyaluronate**

Hyaluronate sodium 11 mg/mL sterile injection

NADA No.: 122-578

Active Ingredient(s): Each mL of HYVISC® Injection contains 11 mg of hyaluronate sodium and 8.47 mg of sodium chloride, U.S.P., in sterile water for injection, U.S.P., q.s.

Indications: HYVISC® (hyaluronate sodium) Injection is recommended for the treatment of joint dysfunction in horses due to non-infectious synovitis associated with equine osteoarthritis.

Pharmacology: HYVISC® (hyaluronate sodium) is a clear, colorless, viscous fluid contained in a 5 mL disposable syringe, as a single 2 mL dose. Chemically, hyaluronate acid is a high molecular weight mucopolysaccharide composed of repeating di-saccharide units, each unit consisting of D-glucuronic acid and N-acetyl-D-glucosamine.

Actions: Hyaluronate sodium is a natural constituent of connective tissue and synovial fluid in both man and animals. In synovial fluid, hyaluronate sodium confers viscoelastic as well as lubricating properties.[1-2] In connective tissue, hyaluronate sodium specifically interacts with cartilage proteoglycans to form stable aggregates.[3-5] The mechanism of action by which exogenous hyaluronate sodium exerts its therapeutic effect in arthritic joints is not known at this time.

Dosage and Administration: The recommended dose of HYVISC® (hyaluronate sodium) Injection is 2 mL (22 mg) given to horses intra-articularly in small or medium-sized joints (carpal, fetlock). In larger joints (hock), the dosage is 4 mL (44 mg). Treatment may be repeated at weekly intervals for a total of three treatments. As with any intra-articular injection, aseptic technique is used. The following are suggested use directions regardless of the type of joint to be treated.

1. Carefully diagnose each case using routine methods. The origin of lameness should be pinpointed to be within a specific joint or joints (e.g., lameness is localized to a specific joint using intra-articular anesthesia). Radiographs or other diagnostic aids should not reveal recent fractures or other serious abnormalities which would suggest a poor prognosis.
2. Aseptically remove as much synovial fluid from the afflicted joint as can be easily withdrawn.
3. Remove tip cap from the HYVISC® syringe and inject through a sterile needle, 20 gauge or larger.
4. Inject a single 2 mL dose (one syringe) of HYVISC® into each joint to be treated; if the joint being treated is the hock joint, inject 4 mL (two syringes). Since HYVISC® is a viscous fluid, care should be exercised on injection so as not to dislodge the needle from the syringe.
5. Two or four days of rest or light exercise is recommended before resumption of normal activity. Improvement of joint function should be seen within one to two weeks after HYVISC® Injection.

As with any intra-articular injection, a mild inflammatory response (tenderness, heat and swelling) may be seen in the joint following the HYVISC® Injection. This response is self-limiting, but may last from two to five days after treatment. If inflammation is excessive or severe, the possibility of infection should be considered and appropriate antibiotic therapy instituted.

Contraindication(s): There are no known contraindications to the use of HYVISC® (hyaluronate sodium) Injection.

Precaution(s): Used or partially used syringes should be crushed and disposed of in an appropriate landfill.

Do not use if numerous small air bubbles are present throughout the solution.

Store under refrigerated conditions. Protect from freezing and avoid excessive heat.

Caution(s): Federal Law restricts this drug to use by or on the order of a licensed veterinarian.

Warning(s): Not for use in horses intended for food. HYVISC® (hyaluronate sodium) Injection must not be administered intravascularly.

For intra-articular injection in horses only.

Toxicology: Safety Margin in Horses: In toxicity studies of HYVISC® (hyaluronate sodium) Injection in horses, intra-articular doses at one, three, and five times the recommended dose once weekly for three consecutive weeks did not result in any drug related local or systemic toxic effects. The mild transient post-injection inflammatory response observed within the joints of some horses was qualitatively and quantitatively similar to that detected in the physiologic saline injected controls. In a reproductive study in mares, 16 mL of HYVISC® (10 mg/mL) injected intramuscularly or subcutaneously once or twice during the second or third stage of pregnancy resulted in no adverse effects on the mares or newborn foals.

Adverse Reactions: In the clinical trial with HYVISC® (hyaluronate sodium) Injection, a mild, transient post-injection inflammatory response in the joint was reported in 12% of the cases treated. There were no other side effects.

References: Available upon request.

Presentation: HYVISC® (hyaluronate sodium) Injection, 11 mg/mL, is available in 2 mL prefilled, disposable syringes individually packaged.

HYVISC® is a registered trademark of Anika Therapeutics, Inc.

Manufactured by: Anika Therapeutics, Inc.

Compendium Code No.: 10280610

H

I

IBD BLEN®

Merial Select **Vaccine**

Bursal Disease Vaccine, Live Virus

U.S. Vet. Lic. No.: 279

Contents: This vaccine contains live bursal disease virus.

Contains Gentamicin as a bacteriostatic agent.

Notice: Merial Select's vaccines have met the requirements of the USDA in regard to safety, purity, potency, and the capability to protect susceptible chickens. This vaccine has been tested by the Master Seed immunogenicity test for efficacy.

Indications: This vaccine is for the initial vaccination of healthy meat-type chickens seven to fourteen days of age by drinking water as an aid in the prevention of infectious bursal disease.

This vaccine is recommended for the protection of healthy chickens. It is essential that the chickens be maintained under good environmental conditions and that exposure to disease viruses be reduced as much as possible.

Dosage and Administration: Drinking Water Vaccination Using Pouring Application: Drinking water vaccination is recommended for healthy chickens seven to fourteen days of age.

1. Remove all medications, sanitizers and disinfectants from the drinking water 72 hours (three days) prior to vaccination.
2. Provide sufficient waterers so that all the chickens can drink at one time. Shut off water supply and allow chickens to consume all the water in the lines.
3. Raise water lines above the chickens' heads. Clean and rinse the waterers thoroughly.
4. Withhold all water from the chickens for a minimum of two hours in warm weather to four hours in cool weather prior to vaccination to stimulate thirst. Withdrawal time should be reduced if half-house brooding is in process.
5. Do not open or mix vaccine until ready to vaccinate.
6. Drinking water for vaccine delivery should contain one ounce (29 gram) of non-fat dry milk per gallon (3.8 liters) of non-chlorinated water, or should contain milk product based stabilizer prepared according to the manufacturer's instructions.
7. Reconstitute the vaccine in 3 gallons (11 liters) of milk-water during cool weather or 4 gallons (15 liters) of milk-water during warm weather for each 1,000 doses.
8. Distribute vaccine solution among waterers. Avoid direct sunlight.
9. Lower waterers and allow the chickens to drink freely. Add the remaining vaccine solution to the water lines as the chickens drink.
10. Do not provide additional drinking water until all the vaccine is consumed.

Drinking Water Vaccination Using Proportioner Application: Drinking water vaccination is recommended for healthy chickens seven to fourteen days of age. Several types of medicator/proportioners are commercially available. Set proportioner to deliver one ounce (30 mL) of vaccine concentrate per one gallon (3.8 liters) of water.

1. Remove all medications. sanitizers and disinfectants from the drinking water 72 hours (three days) prior to vaccination.
2. Clean all containers, hoses and waterers prior to vaccination.
3. Withhold all water from the chickens for a minimum of two hours in warm weather to four hours in cool weather prior to vaccination to stimulate thirst. Withdrawal time should be reduced if halfhouse brooding is in process.
4. Do not open or mix vaccine until ready to vaccinate.
5. Calculate to supply vaccine solution at a rate of 3 gallons (11 liters) per 1,000 chickens in cool weather and 4 gallons (15 liters) per 1,000 chickens in warm weather. The age of the chickens should be considered when calculating water supply. Always use non-chlorinated water when vaccinating chickens.
   Example:
   1,000 chickens in cool weather x 3 gallons (11 liters) = 3 gallons (11 liters).
   1,000 chickens in warm weather x 4 gallons (15 liters) = 4 gallons (15 liters).
6. Prepare vaccine stock solution as follows:
   a. Determine the quantity of vaccine concentrate required by multiplying one ounce (30 mL) x gallons of water needed for vaccine/drinking water.
   Example:
   For 1,000 chickens: 3 gallons x 1 ounce (30 mL) = 3 ounces (90 mL).
   b. Add 3 ounces (85 gm) of non-fat dry milk per 16 ounces (480 mL) of cool water, or use a commercial milk product based stabilizer according to the manufacturer's instructions. For 1,000 chickens add 0.5 ounces (16 gm) non-fat dry milk to the 3 ounces (90 mL) of water.
   c. Reconstitute the dried vaccine with the milk solution. Rinse the vaccine vial to remove all the vaccine.
7. Insert proportioner hose into the vaccine stock solution and start water flow. Continue until all solution has been consumed before changing water supply to direct flow.
8. Do not medicate or use disinfectants for 24 hours after vaccination.

Precaution(s): Store vaccine at 35-45°F (2-7°C). Do not freeze. Use entire vial contents when first opened. Burn the container and all unused contents.

This vaccine is non-returnable.

Caution(s): Do not vaccinate diseased chickens.

Vaccinate all chickens on the premises at one time.

Administer a minimum of one dose per chicken.

Avoid stress conditions during and following vaccination.

Do not place chickens in contaminated facilities.

Exposure to disease must be minimized as much as possible.

For veterinary use only.

The capability of this vaccine to produce satisfactory results depends upon many factors, including — but not limited to — conditions of storage and handling by the user, administration of the vaccine, health and responsiveness of individual chickens, and degree of field exposure. Therefore, directions for use should be followed carefully. The use of this vaccine is subject to applicable state and federal laws and regulations.

Warning(s): Do not vaccinate within 21 days of slaughter.

Presentation: IBD BLEN® is supplied without a diluent for water administration only (25 x 2,000 and 15 x 10,000 doses).

Compendium Code No.: 11050213 LM-1M/LN-2M/LO-2.5M/LP-10M 0699

IBL VACCINE

Aspen **Bacterin-Vaccine**

Bovine Rhinotracheitis-Virus Diarrhea Vaccine, Modified Live Virus-Leptospira pomona Bacterin

U.S. Vet. Lic. No.: 213

Contents: Bovine rhinotracheitis (IBR) and bovine viral diarrhea (BVD) modified live virus, and *Leptospira pomona* bacterin.

Virus vial contains neomycin as a preservative.

Indications: For the immunization of healthy cattle against disease caused by bovine rhinotracheitis, bovine virus diarrhea, and *L pomona* infections in cattle.

Leptospira pomona diluent can also be used as an aid in the prevention of leptospirosis in cattle and swine.

Dosage and Administration: Rehydrate with accompanying diluent and inject 2 mL intramuscularly using aseptic techniques. Calves vaccinated before weaning should be revaccinated 30 days after weaning when maternal antibodies will not interfere with development of a durable immunity.

For swine, inject 2 mL of L pomona bacterin intramuscularly, a second dose should be given 3-4 weeks after the first dose. Annual revaccination is recommended.

Precaution(s): Store at 35° to 45°F (2° to 7°C). Do not freeze. Use entire contents when first opened. Burn container and all unused contents.

Caution(s): Allergic reactions may follow the use of vaccines. Do not use in pregnant animals or in calves nursing pregnant animals. Abortions may result.

Antidote(s): Epinephrine.

Warning(s): Do not vaccinate within 21 days before slaughter.

For use in animals only.

Presentation: 10 dose vial, with 10 dose (20 mL) bacterin diluent.
50 dose vial, with 50 dose (100 mL) bacterin diluent.

Compendium Code No.: 14750391

IBP-L5 VACCINE

Aspen **Bacterin-Vaccine**

Bovine Rhinotracheitis-Virus Diarrhea-Parainfluenza$_3$ Vaccine, Modified Live Virus-Leptospira canicola-grippotyphosa-hardjo-icterohaemorrhagia-pomona Bacterin

U.S. Vet. Lic. No.: 272

Contents: Bovine rhinotracheitis, virus diarrhea, and parainfluenza$_3$ vaccine (modified live virus), and *Leptospira canicola, L grippotyphosa, L hardjo, L icterohaemorrhagia, L pomona* bacterin.

This product contains gentamicin and amphotericin B as preservatives.

Indications: IBP-L5 is recommended for use in the vaccination of healthy cattle against disease caused by the viral and bacterial fractions represented.

Dosage and Administration: Aseptically rehydrate vial of desiccated virus with the accompanying vial of bacterin. Shake well. Administer 2 mL IM or SC to healthy cattle. Calves vaccinated under 3 months of age should be revaccinated at 4-6 months of age or at weaning because of the persistence of maternal antibody that may interfere with the development of active immunity. Annual revaccination with a single 2 mL dose is recommended.

Precaution(s): Store at 35°F-45°F (2°C-7°C). Do not freeze. Protect the vaccine from the direct rays of the sun. Use entire contents when first rehydrated. Care should be taken to avoid microbial contamination of the product.

Caution(s): Do not use in pregnant cows or calves nursing pregnant cows. Burn these containers and all unused contents. In case of anaphylactoid reactions, epinephrine should be administered immediately.

Scientific evidence demonstrates the inability of some animals of an occasional herd to develop antibodies to bovine virus diarrhea after vaccination. The affected animal may exhibit symptoms similar to mucosal disease.

Antidote(s): Epinephrine.

Warning(s): Do not vaccinate within 21 days before slaughter.

For veterinary use only.

Presentation: 50 dose vial, with 100 mL diluent.

Compendium Code No.: 14750410

IBP-SOMNUMUNE® VACCINE

Aspen **Bacterin-Vaccine**

Bovine Rhinotracheitis-Virus Diarrhea-Parainfluenza$_3$ Vaccine, Modified Live Virus-Haemophilus somnus Bacterin

U.S. Vet. Lic. No.: 272

Contents: Bovine rhinotracheitis, virus diarrhea, and parainfluenza$_3$ vaccine (modified live virus), and *Haemophilus somnus* bacterin.

This product contains gentamicin and amphotericin B as preservatives.

Indications: IBP-*H somnus* is recommended for use in the vaccination of healthy cattle against disease caused by the organisms represented.

Dosage and Administration: Aseptically rehydrate vial of desiccated virus with the accompanying vial of diluent. Shake well. Administer 2 mL IM or SC to healthy cattle.

Persistence of maternal antibody in calves may interfere with development of active immunity following vaccination. Calves vaccinated before 3 months of age should be revaccinated at 4-6 months of age or at weaning. Annual revaccination with a single 2 mL dose is recommended.

Precaution(s): Store at 35°F-45°F (2°C-7°C). Do not freeze. Use entire contents when first rehydrated. Care should be taken to avoid microbial contamination of the product. Burn these containers and all unused contents.

Caution(s): Do not use in pregnant cows or calves nursing pregnant cows. In case of anaphylactoid reactions, epinephrine should be administered immediately.

Scientific evidence demonstrates the inability of some animals of an occasional herd to develop antibodies to bovine virus diarrhea after vaccination. The affected animal may exhibit symptoms similar to mucosal disease.

Antidote(s): Epinephrine.

Warning(s): Do not vaccinate within 21 days before slaughter.

For veterinary use only.

Presentation: 10 and 50 doses.

Compendium Code No.: 14750420

IBP VACCINE

Aspen **Vaccine**

Bovine Rhinotracheitis-Virus Diarrhea-Parainfluenza$_3$ Vaccine, Modified Live Virus

U.S. Vet. Lic. No.: 272

Contents: Bovine rhinotracheitis, virus diarrhea, and parainfluenza$_3$ vaccine (modified live virus).

This product contains gentamicin and amphotericin B as preservatives.

Indications: IBP is recommended for use in the vaccination of healthy cattle against disease caused by the organisms represented.

Dosage and Administration: Aseptically rehydrate vial of desiccated virus with the accompanying vial of diluent. Shake well. Administer 2 mL IM or SC to healthy cattle.

Persistence of maternal antibody in calves may interfere with development of active immunity following vaccination. Calves vaccinated before 3 months of age should be revaccinated at 4-6 months of age or at weaning. Annual revaccination with a single 2 mL dose is recommended.

Precaution(s): Store at 35°F-45°F (2°C-7°C). Do not freeze. Protect the vaccine from the direct rays of the sun. Use entire contents when first rehydrated. Care should be taken to avoid microbial contamination of the product. Burn these containers and all unused contents.

Caution(s): Do not use in pregnant cows or calves nursing pregnant cows. In case of anaphylactoid reactions, epinephrine should be administered immediately.

Scientific evidence demonstrates the inability of some animals of an occasional herd to develop antibodies to bovine virus diarrhea after vaccination. The affected animal may exhibit symptoms similar to mucosal disease.

Antidote(s): Epinephrine.

Warning(s): Do not vaccinate within 21 days before slaughter.

For veterinary use only.

Presentation: 50 dose vial, with 100 mL sterile diluent.

Compendium Code No.: 14750400

IB-VAC-H®

Intervet **Vaccine**

Bronchitis Vaccine, Massachusetts Type, Live Virus

U.S. Vet. Lic. No.: 286

Active Ingredient(s): IB-VAC-H®, a live virus vaccine, is prepared from the proven Holland strain of infectious bronchitis virus. The virus has been propagated using SPF (Specific Pathogen Free) substrates. The immunizing capability of this vaccine has also been proven by the Master Seed Immunogenicity Test. The vaccine contains gentamicin as a preservative.

Indications: Coarse spray or drinking water: Vaccination of healthy chickens four weeks of age or older for protection against Mass. type bronchitis after vaccination with milder bronchitis vaccines.

Dosage and Administration: Many factors must be considered in determining a sound vaccination program for a particular farm or poultry complex. To be fully effective, the vaccine must be administered properly to healthy, receptive birds maintained in a proper environment under good management. In addition, the response may be influenced by the age of the birds and their immune status. Seldom does one live virus vaccination under field conditions produce lifetime protection for all individuals in a given flock. The level of immunity required will vary with operational practices and the degree of exposure. Therefore, a program of periodic revaccination may be necessary.

Preparation of Vaccine: For drinking water use:

Do not open and mix the vaccine until ready to begin vaccination. Use the vaccine immediately after mixing.

1. Remove the tear-off seal and stopper from the vial containing the dried vaccine.
2. Carefully pour clean, cool, non-chlorinated water into the vaccine vial until the vial is approximately two-thirds (⅔) full.
3. Insert the rubber stopper and shake vigorously until all of the material is dissolved.
4. The vaccine is now ready for drinking water use. For the best results, be sure to follow the directions carefully.

Drinking Water Administration: For chickens four (4) weeks of age or older:

1. Do not use any disinfectants in the drinking water for 48 hours before vaccinating and for 24 hours after vaccination.
2. Withhold drinking water from the chickens until they are thirsty. Withholding periods will vary from two (2) to eight (8) hours according to the age of the chickens and the weather. Be careful in hot weather.
3. Scrub the waterers and rinse thoroughly with fresh, clean water. Do not use disinfectants for cleaning the waterers.
4. Rehydrate the vaccine.
5. Mix the rehydrated vaccine with clean, cool, non-chlorinated tap water.

Age of chickens	Water per 1,000 doses vaccine
2-4 weeks	6 gal. (23 L)
4-8 weeks	10 gal. (38 L)
8 weeks or older	16 gal. (60 L)

As an aid in preserving the virus, 3.2 oz. (100 g) of non-fat powdered milk may be added with each 10 gallons (38 L) of water used for mixing the vaccine. Add the dried milk first and mix until dissolved. Then add the rehydrated vaccine from the vial and again mix thoroughly.

6. Distribute the vaccine solution among the waterers provided for the chickens. Avoid placing the waterers in direct sunlight.
7. Do not provide any other drinking water until all of the vaccine-water solution has been consumed.

Coarse Spray Administration: For chickens four (4) weeks of age or older:

1. Do not use any disinfectants or skim milk in the sprayer.
2. Use the sprayer for administration of the vaccines only.
3. Shut off all fans while spray vaccinating. Turn on the fan immediately after spraying.
4. Be careful in hot weather.
5. Spray the chickens by walking slowly through the house.
6. Follow the manufacturer's directions regarding water volume.
7. Use only clean, cool, deionized water.
8. Individual(s) spraying chickens should wear a face mask and goggles.

Records: Keep a record of vaccine, quantity, serial number, expiration date, and place of purchase; the date and time of vaccination; the number, age, breed, and locations of chickens; names of operators performing the vaccination and any observed reactions.

Precaution(s): Use only as directed. Store the vaccine between 2-7°C (35-45°F). The product is not returnable.

Caution(s):

1. The vaccine should not be used for initial bronchitis vaccination or initial spray bronchitis vaccination.
2. Vaccinate healthy chickens only. Although disease may not be evident, coccidiosis, mycoplasma infection, infectious bursal disease, Marek's disease, and other disease conditions may cause complications or reduce immunity.
3. All susceptible chickens on the same premises should be vaccinated at the same time.
4. The revaccination of laying hens against bronchitis may be detrimental to the flock and cannot be generally recommended. Consult an Intervet representative for more information.
5. Efforts should be taken to reduce stress conditions at the time of vaccination and during the reaction period.
6. Do not spill or splash the vaccine.
7. Do not dilute the vaccine or otherwise stretch the dosage.
8. Use the entire contents when first opened.
9. Burn the containers and all unused contents.

Warning(s): Do not vaccinate within 21 days before slaughter.

Discussion: The vaccine has undergone rigid potency, safety and purity tests, and meets Intervet America Inc. and USDA requirements. It is designed to stimulate effective immunity when used as directed, but the user must be advised that the response to the product depends upon many factors, including, but not limited to, conditions of storage and handling by the user, administration of the vaccine, health and responsiveness of individual chickens, and the degree of field exposure. Therefore, directions should be followed carefully.

The use of the vaccine is subject to applicable local and federal laws and regulations.

Presentation: 10 x 2,000 doses for drinking water or coarse spray use.

Compendium Code No.: 11060800

ICE-O-GEL®

Hawthorne **Liniment**

Tightener/Freeze

Active Ingredient(s): Each 16 U.S. oz contains:

Alcohol	150 g
Menthol	6 g
Camphor	6 g

Indications: For aid in the temporary relief of minor stiffness and soreness caused by overexertion. ICE-O-GEL® cools the leg and tightens at the same time.

Dosage and Administration: Apply freely to leg first rubbing against hair and then apply more with the hair. Wrap with paper towel and bandage, leaving the treatment on the leg for 48 to 72 hours. Repeat if necessary. Leave ICE-O-GEL® on leg while working or walking. Remove with warm water. To freeze horse before racing, apply ICE-O-GEL® 24 to 36 hours prior. Before post time, reapply ICE-O-GEL® using wet, cold water bandages. Place leg in ice tub or ice boots.

Precaution(s): Store at room temperature. Stir well before using if ingredients are separated.

Caution(s): Keep away from children. For veterinary use only.

Warning(s): Do not use on food animals.

Presentation: 16 U.S. oz., 48 U.S. oz. and 1 gallon.

Compendium Code No.: 10670050

ICE-O-POULTICE®

Hawthorne **Cataplasm**

Non-irritating

Active Ingredient(s): Aluminum sillicate (derived from earth montmoullonite), zinc oxide, acetic acid, and aromic oils.

Indications: For temporary relief of soreness and stiffness due to swollen legs and muscles in horses. ICE-O-POULTICE® cools the legs and tightens at the same time. ICE-O-POULTICE® is also recommended for packing sore, tender feet, and as an aid to reduce swelling of healed incisions.

Directions: Cleanse leg and moisten area of application with water. Work small amount of ICE-O-POULTICE® into hair. Then apply to desired thickness. Can be left uncovered or wrapped with paper. For a more penetrating effect, wrap with plastic and cover with stall bandage. For feet, pack around frog and sole. Cover with paper.

Caution(s): Keep away from children.

Presentation: 5.21 kg (10 lb), 10.43 kg (23 lb), and 22.68 kg (50 lb).

Compendium Code No.: 10670060

ICETIGHT®

Horse Health **Poultice**

Ingredient(s): Kaolin, water, bentonite, glycerine, boric acid, ferrous sulfate, and aloe vera with artificial peppermint fragrance added.

Indications: A topical poultice for use on horse's knees, tendons and ankles.

Directions for Use: Clean all medication, chemicals and foreign matter from the area to be treated. Apply a layer of ICETIGHT® up to ¼ inch thick over the area to be treated. Wrap the preparation with plastic or moist brown paper. Cover with cotton bandage. ICETIGHT® is easily removed with water.

Notice: Due to varying temperature changes and ICETIGHT®'s high moisture content, occasional liquid may accumulate on the surface. This in no way affects the quality of the product. Use this liquid as a starter to moisturize the horse's leg or pour it off.

Precaution(s): Close container after each use. Protect from freezing.

Caution(s): For animal use only.

Warning(s): Keep out of reach of children.

Presentation: 7.5 lb, 25 lb (11.34 kg) and 46 lb.

Compendium Code No.: 15000021

ICG STATUS-LH®

Synbiotics **Ovulation Test**

Canine Ovulation Timing Test

U.S. Vet. Lic. No.: 312

Description: The ICG STATUS-LH® test provides an accurate, semi-quantitative measurement of canine luteinizing hormone (LH). The test is simple to perform and rapidly provides information for the veterinary clinician. This assay, when used in conjunction with in-hospital progesterone testing, identifies the pre-ovulatory LH surge, and thus, the time of ovulation.

Indications: For the detection of canine serum luteinizing hormone.

Identification of the LH surge provides the most accurate means of ovulation timing. It may be used for routine breeding situations and is especially recommended in those instances where there are factors present that could adversely affect conception rates. These include:

- chilled/extended semen breedings
- frozen semen breedings
- bitches with a history of infertility

- breedings with stud dogs with low semen quality
- limited access to the stud dog

Test Principles: ICG STATUS-LH® is a luteinizing hormone assay that provides a convenient semi-quantitative measurement of luteinizing hormone levels without special equipment. The test is an immunochromatographic assay that uses gold-conjugated antibodies to give a visual line in the presence of luteinizing hormone. Use of this assay, as directed, will allow identification of the bitch's fertile period.

One test device is used for each serum sample to be tested. A control line is included on each test device. Color development of the control line is indicative of proper testing technique.

The ICG STATUS-LH® luteinizing hormone assay allows you to identify the occurrence of the LH surge. A positive result occurs when a line appears in the test area which is of similar or greater intensity than the control line. When this occurs, the LH level in the serum sample is greater than 1 nanogram per milliliter. The first time that a positive result is observed is the day of the LH peak. This day is counted as day 0.

Test Procedure: Sample Information: ICG STATUS-LH® requires only four drops of serum to run each test. Collect the blood sample in a plain (red top) vacutainer or serum separator tube. Allow the blood to clot and separate the serum by centrifugation. The sample should not be hemolyzed or lipemic. Testing should be performed the same day as sample collection. If this is not possible, refrigerate the serum. Do not freeze the serum.

Note: Only use serum as a sample.

Prior to use, allow sample to come to room temperature (68°-77°F; 20°25°C).

A. Sample Collection and Preparation:

1. Collect the blood sample into a plain (red top) vacutainer or serum separator tube.
   Allow to clot and spin the cells down.
   Transfer serum to a clean glass or polypropylene tube. Serum must be free of red cells, clots and visible debris.
   Do not use severely hemolyzed or grossly lipemic samples. When in doubt, collect a better quality sample.
   If sample will not be tested immediately, store in refrigerator, do not freeze the serum.

Remember: Sample must be at room temperature prior to testing.

B. Test Procedure: The ICG STATUS-LH® test includes a pipet and a test device. The device has a serum well "S" and a window with a control area "C" and a test area "T".

2. Remove test device and pipet from foil pouch by tearing at the notch. Place the device on a flat level surface at room temperature.
3. Draw some serum up into the provided pipet. Hold the pipet perpendicular to the device and add 4 drops of serum to the Serum Well (S).
4. Allow the test device is sit undisturbed for 20 minutes.

Do not use lipemic or grossly hemolyzed samples. Such samples may interfere with the rate at which the sample flows in the device or create a background color which will make interpretation of the results difficult.

Store the kit at room temperature. Do not freeze.

Do not freeze samples. If samples cannot be tested the same day, refrigerate.

Do not use the kit beyond its expiration date.

Do not open the foil pouch until ready to perform the test.

Do not touch any of the surfaces in the windows of the device.

Keep device flat during testing. Do not disturb while test is being conducted.

Test Interpretation: Control: At the end of the test, a pink line should always appear in the area marked C. This is your assurance that the test is complete.

Negative Result: If no line appears in the area marked T or if the line is less intense than the control line C, the LH value is less than 1 nanogram per milliliter.

You should continue LH testing on a daily basis.

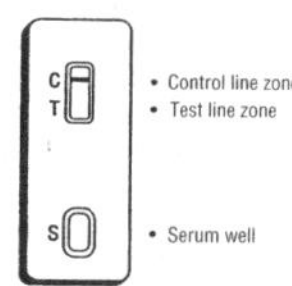

Positive Result: If a line appears at the area marked T which is of similar or greater intensity than the control line C, the LH value is greater than 1 nanogram per milliliter.

The first time a positive result is observed is the day of the LH peak. This day is counted as day 0.

Follow the instructions under "When to Conduct Inseminations".

Note: It is recommended that you perform a progesterone test in 3 to 4 days to confirm a rise in progesterone.

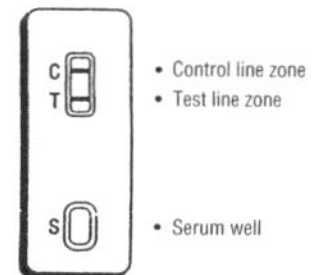

Storage: Store kit at room temperature. Do not freeze. The foil pouch containing the test device and pipette should not be opened prior to running the test. ICG STATUS-LH® will remain stable until expiration date provided that the kit has been stored properly.

For Technical Assistance: 1-800-228-4305

Discussion: When to Test: Since the LH surge may occur within a 24-hour period, it is crucial that daily serum samples are tested. Blood should be drawn every day at approximately the same time beginning the 4th or 5th day of proestrus, or when vaginal cytology approaches 50% cornification (Cornification is defined as cells with a roughened, angulated border with or without a nucleus). A progesterone test should also be performed on the first day of testing to confirm a baseline progesterone level. If testing is started after the onset of estrus, it is likely that the LH surge will have already occurred and cannot be identified in retrospect.

Once an increase in LH is identified, Synbiotics recommends that daily serum samples should be tested for progesterone levels. If the detected increase in LH was indeed the actual pre-ovulatory surge, progesterone levels should rise, usually reaching a value above 2 ng/mL within 3 days, and then stay elevated. If progesterone remains low, it indicates that a proestrus fluctuation in LH was identified. Continue daily LH testing until the true LH surge occurs.

Note: the ICG STATUS-LH® test and test interpretation is referenced against the ICG Status-Pro® Progesterone Test. Use of other progesterone tests may require different interpretations to explain test results.

Reproductive Physiology: Unsuccessful breedings result more often from improper ovulation timing than any other cause. While the estrous cycle of the bitch typically lasts for several weeks, the true fertile period is short (48-72 hours) and is difficult to identify without the use of hormonal assays.

The common indicators of estrus and breeding time, such as vaginal cytology and receptive behavior, are primarily controlled by changes in the hormone estrogen. Unfortunately, these changes are only an approximation of ovulation. Using only these parameters, ovulation could be "missed" by more than a week. Precise identification of the fertile period is made by measurement of the LH surge which actually triggers ovulation. This surge, which consists of rapid increase in LH level, occurs in many cases within a 24-hour period. Ovulation occurs 2 days after the LH surge; the oocytes then require an additional 2-3 days to mature, and will live for about 48-72 hours. Thus, the fertile period of the bitch falls between days 4-7 after the LH surge with the most fertile days being on days 5 and 6 post-LH surge.

Progesterone assays are useful for ovulation timing. Before the LH surge, serum progesterone remains low, generally between 0 and 1.0 ng/mL. At about the time of the LH surge, progesterone levels will begin to rise, usually changing from a baseline of 0-1.0 ng/mL into a range of 1.5-2.0 ng/mL. Progesterone will then continue to rise as the cycle progresses and will remain elevated for 2-3 months in non-pregnant as well as pregnant bitches. It is important to appreciate that the absolute progesterone values discussed above may vary by individual. The key event progesterone assays seek to identity is the initial rise of progesterone above the particular individual's baseline level. Once identified, this initial rise in progesterone may be used as an estimate of the LH surge. However, this first rise in progesterone may vary from the day of the actual LH surge in many bitches. While progesterone is elevated during the fertile period, the rate of rise varies from bitch to bitch, as does the absolute value of progesterone which coincides with the LH surge or with the optimal time to breed. As a result, progesterone measurements alone are, at best, only an approximation of the LH surge. Given the fact that good breeding management often plans for multiple breedings over a period of several days, relying on the information provided by progesterone assays alone may be sufficient. Some breedings, however, will benefit from a more exact identification of the bitch's fertile period. Identification of the LH surge itself allows the most precise ovulation timing.

During proestrus, small, pulsatile fluctuations in LH may occur, while progesterone remains at low, baseline levels. Progesterone rises, however, after the pre-ovulatory surge in LH. By the third day post LH peak, the majority of bitches will evidence a rise in progesterone levels above the 2 ng/mL level. Daily progesterone testing after a positive ICG STATUS-LH® test result allows simple differentiation between small fluctuating increases in LH during proestrus and the true, pre-ovulatory LH surge. If there is no confirmation of progesterone rise within 3 days of a positive ICG STATUS-LH® test, it may be assumed that the positive test result was due to a baseline LH fluctuation.

When to Conduct Inseminations: The positive ICG STATUS-LH® test identifies the day of the LH surge. This day is designated as day 0. Count forward to determine the fertile period. Days 4-7 post-LH surge encompass the true fertile period, with peak fertility on days 5 and 6. By properly planned breedings or inseminations coinciding with this window of fertility, you will optimize the probability of success.

Natural Breeding or Fresh Artificial Insemination: Fresh semen of a normal healthy stud may live up to 5 or more days in the bitch. Therefore, semen inseminated a day of two before the fertile period should be viable at the time of peak fertility. Synbiotics recommends breeding on days 2, 4 and 6 post-LH surge to completely cover the fertile period, and to maximize viable sperm numbers on the bitch's most fertile days. If only two breedings are being performed, they should be accomplished between days 3 and 7 post-LH surge.

Natural Breeding with Compromised Semen Quality: At times, stud dogs produce semen of compromised quality due to age, stress or disease. Breeding during the true fertile period will increase the likelihood of limited sperm numbers encountering mature eggs and will increase the chance of conception. Synbiotics recommends breeding on days 4, 5, 6, and 7.

Surgical Insemination with Fresh Semen: Occasionally, it is desirable to perform surgical inseminations with fresh semen due to low fertility of either the stud dog or the bitch. Synbiotics recommends that this procedure be performed on either days 5 or 6 post-LH surge.

Chilled Extended Semen Breeding: Chilled extended semen will usually live for 2 to 4 days post collection. One day of this time is typically used in shipping. This reduced survival time requires the breeding to be conducted closer to the short fertile period of the bitch. Synbiotics recommends that 2 inseminations be conducted on days 4 and 6 or 3 and 5 post-LH surge. If a surgical insemination is desired, it should be performed on day 5 or 6 post-LH surge.

Frozen Semen Breeding: Frozen semen survives less than 24 hours after thawing, so timing is crucial. Inseminations must be performed during the true fertile period. If one surgical insemination is planned, it should be performed on day 5 or 6 post-LH surge. If multiple vaginal or trans-cervical inseminations are to be conducted, they are recommended on days 4, 5 and 6.

Presentation: 6 test kits.

Compendium Code No.: 11150101

ICG STATUS-PRO®

Synbiotics **Ovulation Test**

Canine Ovulation Timing Test

U.S. Vet. Lic. No.: 312

Test Description: Canine ovulation timing test.

Contents:

ICG STATUS-PRO® Test Cups 6
Bottle 1 - Pretreatment Solution (Yellow Cap) . . . . . 1 vial
Bottle 2 - Conjugate (Red Cap) . . . . . 1 vial
Bottle 3 - Wash Solution (White Cap) . . . . . 1 bottle
Bottle 4 - Substrate (Blue Cap) . . . . . 1 vial
Box 5 - Substrate Activator . . . . . 6 vials
Disposable Transfer Pipets (12)
Direction Insert

Materials required but not provided: Blood collection/separation tubes, marking pen, timer, test tubes.

Indications: For the detection of canine serum progesterone.

Test Principles: ICG STATUS-PRO® is a progesterone assay that provides a convenient semi-quantitative measurement of progesterone levels without special equipment. The test uses monoclonal antibodies that react with enzyme-labeled progesterone to indicate high or low levels of progesterone by color development. Use of this assay, as directed, will allow identification of a bitch's fertile period.

One cup will be used for each serum sample to be tested. A control spot is included on each test cup. Color development of this spot is indicative of proper testing technique and of reagent integrity.

Test Procedure: Sample Information: 1 mL of canine serum is required to run each test. Collect the blood sample into a plain (red top) vacutainer or serum separator tube. Allow to clot and spin the cells down within 20 minutes of collection. Transfer serum to a clean glass or polypropylene tube. Serum must be free of red cells, clots or any visible debris and should not be severely hemolyzed or grossly lipemic. If the sample is to be run immediately, it may remain at room temperature; otherwise store in the refrigerator (up to 8 hours) or freezer (overnight or longer). If the sample is cold, warm it to room temperature for 2 hours prior to testing.

A. Sample Collection:

1. Collect the blood sample into a plain (red top) vacutainer or serum separator tube.
   Allow to clot. Spin the cells down within 20 minutes of collection.
   Transfer serum to a clean glass or polypropylene tube. Serum must be free of red cells, clots and visible debris.
   Do not use severely hemolyzed or grossly lipemic samples. When in doubt, collect a better quality sample.
   If sample will not be tested immediately, store in refrigerator (up to 8 hours) or in the freezer (overnight or longer).
   Remember: Prior to testing, allow sample to warm to room temperature.

B. Test Preparation:

2. For each sample to be tested, prepare 1 vial of Activated Substrate. Using a clean transfer piper, draw Substrate (Bottle 4 - White Cap) up to the 1 mL mark.
   Add the 1 mL of Substrate to a vial of Substrate Activator (Box 5) by placing the tip of the transfer pipet into the vial and squeezing the pipet bulb until all of the Substrate has been added.
   Remove the empty pipet from the vial. Save the pipet for Step 8. Replace cap, tighten and mix the Activated Substrate by inverting several times.
   Allow Activated Substrate to stabilize for 15 minutes prior to use.
   Note: Activated Substrate should be used the same day it is prepared.
3. For each sample to be tested, remove 1 test cup from the foil pouch. Label each test cup with the sample ID.

4a. Using a clean transfer piper, draw serum up to the 1 mL mark. Transfer the 1 mL of serum to a clean tube. Save the pipet for Step 5.

4b. Add 1 drop Bottle 1 Pretreatment Solution (Yellow Cap) to the tube. Tap gently to mix.

C. Sample Addition:

5. Draw the pretreated serum up into the pipet saved from Step 4a.
   Hold the pipet vertically about 1 inch above the surface of the test cup.
   Dispense 6 drops of the pretreated serum onto the surface of the test cup.
   Be sure the sample completely covers the testing surface.
   Wait exactly 2 minutes.

D. Conjugate:

6. Add 6 drops Bottle 2 - Conjugate (Red Cap) to the center of the cup.
   Wait exactly 1 minute.

E. Wash:

7. Fill the well of the test cup to the top of the inner lip with Bottle 3 - Wash Solution (White Cap). Do not overfill.
   Wait for the liquid to completely soak into the test surface.

F. Develop:

8. Using piper saved from Step 2, draw up approximately 0.5 mL of Activated Substrate.
   Squeezing bulb gently. add 6 drops of Activated Substrate to the center of the cup.
   Wait exactly 15 minutes.

Test Interpretation: Read results at exactly 15 minutes.
Test results correlate with level of progesterone:

Result	Progesterone Level
3 Blue Spots	less than 2.0 ng/mL
2 Blue Spots	approx. 2.0 to 5.0 ng/mL
1 Blue Spot	5.0 ng/mL or greater

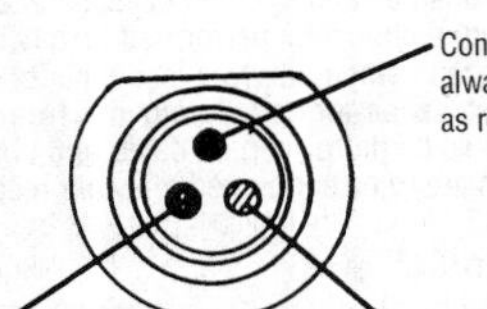
Control Spot: Color always present as reagent control.
High Spot: Color intensity fades as progesterone concentration rises. Not detectable above 5.0 ng/mL.
Low Spot: Color visible at baseline progesterone levels. Key spot in determination of LH surge and timings. Color intensity fades as progesterone rises. Not detectable above 2.0 ng/mL.

To ensure accurate results:
Kit components and sample must be at room temperature before running the test.
Spin down whole blood within 20 minutes of sample collection.
Do not use severely hemolyzed or grossly lipemic samples.
Do not use the kit past expiration date and do not mix components from different kit serials.
Good technique in Test Preparation is critical.
When adding sample to the test cup, be sure to cover the entire testing surface.
Hold dropper bottles vertically when adding reagents to the test cup.
Read the results of the test exactly 15 minutes after addition of the Activated Substrate. Any result read after 15 minutes is not considered to be accurate.

Storage: Storage and Stability: Store kit at 2° to 7°C (35° to 45°F). Do not freeze. The foil pouch containing the unused test cups and the desiccant pack must remain sealed. Reagents are stable until expiration date provided they have been stored properly.

Caution(s):

1. Allow components to come to room temperature (20°-25°C; 68°-77°F) prior to use.
2. Do not use expired reagents or mix from different kit lots.
3. Allow sample to clot; centrifuge promptly. Warm sample to room temperature prior to testing.
4. Do not use grossly hemolyzed or lipemic samples.
5. Follow instructions exactly. Improper washing or contamination of reagents may produce non-specific color development.
6. Allow Activated Substrate Reagent to stabilize for at least 15 minutes before use. Activated Substrate should be used the same day it is prepared.
7. Open foil pouch containing test cups above zip lock closure. Do not remove desiccant. Reseal pouch immediately after removing one test cup for each sample to be run.
8. Failure to completely cover test cup surface with serum may result in an incomplete reaction which may appear as a partial spot (crescent) located on the outer edge of the spot.
9. For veterinary use only.

Discussion: Detection of Canine Progesterone: The ICG STATUS-PRO® Test is designed to be a rapid and simple method of determining the level of progesterone in canine serum. During anestrus and proestrus, the progesterone level is very low (0 to 1.0 ng/mL). Prior to the luteinizing hormone (LH) surge, the progesterone level begins to increase, reaching a level of 2.0 ng/mL (or greater) 1 to 4 days after the LH surge. To identify the bitch's fertile period, count the spots that develop on the test cup. The first day the change from 3 spots to 2 spots is detected indicates that progesterone has risen above 2.0 ng/mL and that the LH surge has occurred. Breeding should begin at that time. It is recommended that an additional sample be tested 2 to 4 days later to ensure that progesterone levels continue to rise, confirming that ovulation has occurred.

When to Start Testing: At least 1 serum sample should be run during the first 5 days of the cycle, during proestrus, to determine the bitch's baseline progesterone level. This varies in individual dogs but will usually range between 0 and 1.0 ng/mL — giving a test result of 3 blue spots.

If you are not comfortable performing and interpreting vaginal smears and the breeding is extremely important, or if the bitch has had trouble conceiving, begin testing early — e.g. day 3 or 4 — and continue testing until you are certain of the progesterone rise indicating the LH peak. Sampling every other day is usually adequate.

If you are comfortable performing and interpreting vaginal smears, you may want to use vaginal cytology as a guideline for continued progesterone testing. Once vaginal cytology shows 50% to 60% cornification, run progesterone levels every other day. (Cornification is defined as cells with roughened, angulated borders with or without a nuclei).

Timing of the Fertile Period: Unsuccessful breeding results more often from improper timing than any other cause. Proper timing of breedings can be achieved conveniently with the use of hormonal assays. The outward signs of heat (flagging and vaginal smears) are primarily controlled by changes in the hormone estrogen. Unfortunately, these changes are only an approximation of ovulation and can vary by more than a week. A much more precise measure is the LH surge which actually triggers ovulation. Ovulation occurs 2 days after the LH surge. The oocytes then require an additional 2 to 3 days to mature and will live for about 48 to 72 hours. Thus, the fertile period of the bitch falls between days 4 to 7 after the LH peak with the most fertile days beginning on days 5 and 6 post-LH peak.

The ICG STATUS-PRO® progesterone assay allows you to identify the occurrence of the LH surge. On the day of the LH surge, progesterone levels will begin to rise to the 1.5-2.0 ng/mL level. Progesterone will continue to rise as the cycle progresses and remain elevated for 2 to 3 months in non-pregnant as well as pregnant bitches.

When to Conduct Inseminations: By properly planned multiple breedings or inseminations, you will optimize the probability of success.

Natural Breeding or Fresh Artificial Insemination: Fresh semen of a normal healthy stud often lives up to 5 or more days in the bitch. Therefore, semen inseminated a day or two before the fertile period will usually be viable at the time of peak fertility.

Synbiotics recommends that breeding begin when the progesterone level has risen above 2 ng/mL. To most effectively cover the fertile period, breeding should be repeated every 2 to 3 days for a total of 2 to 3 breedings.

Fresh Chilled Semen Breeding: Fresh chilled semen will usually live for 2 to 4 days, post collection — one day of this time is used in shipping. The reduced survival time of the sperm requires the breeding to be conducted closer to the short fertile period of the bitch. The LH surge can be most accurately identified using the ICG Status-LH® assay kit; Synbiotics recommends that 2 inseminations, using separate ejaculates, be conducted on days 3 and 5 or days 4 and 6 post-LH peak.

Frozen Semen Breeding: Frozen semen survives less than 24 hours once it is thawed, so timing is even more crucial than with fresh chilled semen breedings. It is critical that the LH surge be identified using the ICG Status-LH® assay. Frozen semen breedings should be conducted on days 4, 5 and 6 post-LH peak with multiple vaginal inseminations. If one surgical insemination is planned, it should be performed on day 5 or 6 post-LH peak.

Presentation: 6 test kits.

ICG STATUS-PRO is a registered trademark of Synbiotics Corporation.

Compendium Code No.: 11150113 03-2000-0901

ICHTHAMMOL 20%

Butler **Topical Wound Dressing**

Active Ingredient(s):
Ichthammol. 20%

Indications: For external use as an emollient for the skin.

Dosage and Administration: Apply to the affected parts once or twice a day.
A loose bandage may be applied.

Presentation: 1 lb. containers.

Compendium Code No.: 10820970

ICHTHAMMOL 20% OINTMENT

Phoenix Pharmaceutical **Topical Wound Dressing**

Active Ingredient(s): Contains:
Ichthammol. 20%
Emollient Base 80%

Indications: A soothing external application for horses with minor skin wounds or irritations.

Directions: For external use as an emollient for the skin. Apply to affected lesions once or twice daily. A loose bandage may be applied.

Precaution(s): Store at 15°C-30°C (59°F-86°F).

Caution(s): Use only as directed. Avoid contact with the eyes and mucous membranes. If redness, irritation, or swelling persists or increases, discontinue use and consult veterinarian.
For animal use only.
Livestock drug.

Warning(s): Keep out of reach of children.

Presentation: 16 oz. (1 lb.) jars (NDC 57319-390-27).

Manufactured by: First Priority, Inc., Elgin, IL 60123

Compendium Code No.: 12560422 Rev. 10-01

ICHTHAMMOL OINTMENT 20%

Aspen **Topical Wound Dressing**

Active Ingredient(s):

Ichthammol 20%

Indications: For external use as an emollient for the skin of horses.

Directions for Use: Apply to affected areas once or twice daily. A loose bandage may be applied.

Warning(s): For animal use only.

Keep out of reach of children.

Presentation: 1 lb (16 oz).

Compendium Code No.: 14750440

ICHTHAMMOL OINTMENT 20%

First Priority **Topical Product**

Active Ingredient(s): Each mL contains:

Ichthammol 20%

Indications: For external use as an emollient for the skin.

Directions: Apply to affected areas once or twice daily. A loose bandage may be applied.

Caution(s): For animal use only.

Warning(s): Keep out of reach of children.

Presentation: 4 oz (113.3 g) (NDC# 58829-15-04), 1 lb (453.6 g) (NDC# 58829-215-16) and 4 lb (1.8 kg) (NDC# 58829-215-18).

Compendium Code No.: 11390402 Rev. 4-99 / Rev. 06-01 / Iss. 10-98

I-DEAL™ BARRIER TEAT DIP

Ecolab Food & Bev. Div. **Teat Dip**

1% Iodine Barrier Teat Dip

Active Ingredient(s):

Iodine 1.0%

Formula ingredients contain no phosphorus.

Contains glycerine plus other emollients.

Indications: I-DEAL™ is a unique germicidal 10,000 ppm iodine teat dip that forms a protective barrier on the teat. Helps control common bacterial organisms known to cause mastitis by providing broad spectrum antimicrobial protection after dipping.

Equally effective against both infectious mastitis organisms and environmental types, such as *Escherichia coli*.

Use a post-milking teat dip on each teat as an aid in a complete cow-care program to help reduce the spread of organisms which may cause mastitis.

Pharmacology: Properties:

Form . . . . . liquid
Color . . . . . dark brown
Odor . . . . . mild
Wetting ability . . . . . excellent
Specific gravity @ 68°F 1.045
Pounds per gallon . . . . . 8.70 (3.94 kg)

Directions for Use: Immediately after milking, use I-DEAL™ at full strength. Submerge entire teat in I-DEAL™ solution. Allow to air dry. Do not wipe. Always use fresh, full strength I-DEAL™. If product in dip cup becomes visibly dirty, discard contents and replenish with undiluted product. Do not reuse or return unused product to the original container. Do not turn cows out in freezing weather until I-DEAL™ is completely dry.

Wash teats thoroughly just prior to next milking with appropriate udder wash solution or pre-milking teat dip. Teats should then be dried with a single-service towel. Use proper procedures for washing or pre-dipping.

Note: I-DEAL™ is not intended to cure to help the healing of chapped or irritated teats. In case of teat irritation or chapping, have the condition examined and, if necessary, treated by a veterinarian.

For cautionary and first aid information, consult the Material Safety Data Sheet (MSDS) or product label.

Precaution(s): Transport and store between 40°F (4°C) and 100°F (37.8°C). Do not freeze. Product damaged if frozen. Product that has been frozen and thawed may appear watery with clumps of material and will not produce a uniform film on the teat.

Caution(s): Important: Do not mix I-DEAL™ with any other teat dip or other products. If transferred from product container to any other, make sure that other container is thoroughly precleaned and bears the proper container labeling for I-DEAL™.

Presentation: 5 gallons, 15 gallons, and 55 gallons.

Compendium Code No.: 14490170 29644/0300/1099

IDEXX® BRUCELLA ABORTUS ANTIBODY TEST KIT PCFIA SYSTEM

Idexx Labs. **Brucella Test**

U.S. Vet. Lic. No.: 313

Description: *Brucella abortus* Antibody Test Kit is a Particle Concentration Fluorescence Immunoassay (PCFIA).

Components: Reagents:

1. *B. abortus* Coated Particles - antigen coated particles in phosphate buffered saline with protein stabilizers, contains a preservative.
2. Anti-*B. abortus:* FITC Conjugate - Fluorescein isothiocyanate labelled antibody to *B. abortus* in phosphate buffered saline with protein stabilizers, contains a preservative.
3. *B. abortus* Strong Positive Control - Bovine Anti-*B. abortus* serum, diluted in Sample Diluent, contains a preservative.
4. *B. abortus* Weak Positive Control - Bovine anti-*B. abortus* serum, diluted in Sample Diluent, contains a preservative.
5. Negative Control - Bovine serum nonreactive to *B. abortus*, diluted in Sample Diluent, contains a preservative.
6. Sample Diluent - phosphate buffered saline with protein stabilizers, contains a preservative.
7. Wash Concentrate (10X) - phosphate buffered saline - contains a preservative.

Materials Required but Not Provided:

1. Idexx Screen Machine™.
2. Special 96-well IDEXX® PCFIA System assay plates.
3. 500 mL graduated cylinder for preparing wash solution.
4. Precision pipets: Suitable for delivering 2 µL and 50 µL.
5. Distilled or deionized water.

Indications: For the detection of antibody to *B. abortus* in bovine serum. This is an official test to be used in the cooperative State/Federal Brucellosis Eradication Program.

Test Principles: PCFIA is a fluorescence immunoassay technique which utilizes submicron polystyrene particles as the solid phase onto which *B. abortus* antigens are attached. The Conjugate is comprised of fluorescein labelled *B. abortus* antibodies.

In the assay, the test sample and coated particles are initially mixed and incubated in a specially designed 96 well plate. After the initial incubation period, Conjugate is added, allowed to react, and the reaction mixture is then filtered through the membrane at the bottom of each well. The particles, being too large to pass through the membrane, are retained on the surface of the membrane. Each well is washed to remove unbound Conjugate and antibody, and then moved into position below a front surface fluorimetric read system. The amount of particle-bound fluorescence is measured as counts from the membrane surface. The system reads fluorescence in two channels, a sample channel (A) and a reference channel (B). The ratio of these counts in each channel normalizes any variation due to pipetting.

Anti-*B. abortus* PCFIA is a competitive immunoassay for antigen-specific antibodies. During the reaction, specific antibodies in the sample compete with the Conjugate for antigen binding sites on the solid phase. The amount of Conjugate bound to the solid phase will decrease as the specific antibody concentration in the sample increases, thus providing an inverse measurement of specific antibody. Binding of a non-specific antibody to the solid phase does not affect the competition between specific antibody in the sample and the Conjugate, and thus, does not affect the resulting signal. Non-specific binding to the antigen on the solid phase is displaced by either the higher affinity Conjugate or specific antibody in the sample, and again, does not affect the resulting signal.

Test Procedure:

Preparation of Wash Solution: The Wash Concentrate (10X) should be brought to room temperature, and must be diluted 1 to 10 with distilled or deionized water before use (e.g. add 100 mL of Wash Concentrate to 900 mL of water). Store the diluted (1X) wash solution at room temperature.

Sample Preparation: Serum samples must be diluted 1:25 with Sample Diluent (e.g. by adding 2 µL of serum to 50 µL of Sample Diluent). Note: Do not dilute controls. Some hemolyzed samples may cause clogging of the membrane in the well, resulting in an invalid test for that sample. Treatment of these serums with kaolin (hydrated aluminum silicate) has been shown to effectively reduce clogging without detrimental effect on the specific reaction. A recognized kaolin treatment for this type of sample is as follows:

Mix approximately 20 mg of dry kaolin with 0.3 mL of serum. Vortex and allow to stand at room temperature for 30 minutes. Centrifuge at 650xg for 30 minutes. Dilute the supernatant 1:25 for testing.

The *B. abortus* Antibody Test is performed using the IDEXX® PCFIA System. (Refer to the IDEXX® PCFIA System, Operation Manual for complete instructions on maintenance and operation of the instrument and use of the data management program.)

1. Allow all reagents to come to room temperature prior to use.
2. Mix particles gently by inversion; avoid foaming.
3. Add Sample Diluent to the assay plates using the following procedure:
   a. Leave row A, wells 1-12 and row B, wells 1-4 of plate 1, empty so that the controls can be added directly to the assay plate. Pipette 50 µL of Sample Diluent into assay plate #1 beginning with the wells in row B column 5 and continuing through other rows C-H.
   b. Continue pipetting 50 µL of Sample Diluent into each well of the remaining plates to be processed, all rows and columns.
4. Add controls and serum to the appropriate wells.
   a. Create a layout with the PCFIA software program to indicate sample position in the assay plate(s). Note: Refer to the IDEXX® PCFIA Software Manual for instructions.
   b. Add 50 µL of undiluted Negative Control to row A, all wells.
   c. Add 50 µL of undiluted *B. abortus* Weak Positive Control to wells B1 and B2 of plate 1.
   d. Add 50 µL of undiluted *B. abortus* Strong Positive Control to wells B3 and B4 of plate 1.
   e. Add 2 µL of each serum sample to the appropriate remaining wells using the layout created in step 4a as a guide.
5. Running the Assay:
   a. To Reagent Tray, add the following reagents: 1X wash solution to WASH Compartment (or fill external reservoir if applicable). 1X wash solution to AUX Compartment (or fill external reservoir if applicable). Particles to compartment A. Conjugate to compartment B. (Refer to Volume chart in the IDEXX® PCFIA System Operation Manual for appropriate volumes).
   b. Load Reagent Tray. Insert plates with diluted samples in numerical plate order.
   c. Press PROCESS PLATES.
   d. Press BRUCELLA.
   e. Press IDENTIFY WELLS.
   f. The total number of plates to be processed must be indicated. To do this, press PLATE 1 until the plate number displayed on the screen equals the total number of plates in your batch.
   g. Press CHECK REAGENTS. At this point, the instrument will verify if sufficient reagent volumes are present to process the indicated number of plates. Insufficient volumes will be highlighted on the screen. If this occurs, remove the reagent tray and add additional reagents as appropriate.
   h. Press CHECK DATE LINK to begin the assay. (If applicable, press CONFIGURE OUTPUT, then press PERSONAL COMPUTER, then press SAVE to begin assay.)
6. Follow the instructions in the IDEXX® PCFIA Software Manual to generate a computer printout of results upon assay completion.

Results: Results are expressed as an S/N value which is the ratio of sample or Positive Control signal to the Negative Control signal. For the assay to be valid, the *B. abortus* Weak Positive Control must have an S/N value less than 0.700, and the *B. abortus* Strong Positive Control must have a value less than 0.300. The system automatically checks for these parameters to validate or invalidate the assay. (Refer to "Calculation Section" for a definition of the S/N value.)

The presence or absence of antibody to *B. abortus* is determined on the basis of the S/N value. Serum samples with an S/N value greater than 0.700 are considered negative for *B. abortus* antibody; samples with S/N less than or equal to 0.700 are considered positive.

Test Interpretation: Animals are considered reactors when the S/N value is less than or equal to 0.250, an S/N value greater than 0.250, and less than or equal to 0.700 indicates suspect status; an S/N value greater than 0.700 is considered negative. Expected results on a 30 day retest of a test eligible vaccinate typically show an increase in the S/N value.

Calculations:

1. Calculation of Negative Control (NC) mean:

$$\overline{NCx} = \frac{\text{Sum of A/B ratios for row A, all wells}}{12}$$

$$\text{A/B ratio} = \frac{\text{channel A counts}}{\text{channel B counts}}$$

2. Calculation of S/N for *B. abortus* Weak Positive Control (WPC) mean:

$$\text{S/N} = \frac{\frac{\text{Sum of A/B ratios for wells B1 and B2}}{2}}{\text{NC (A/B ratio)}}$$

3. Calculation of S/N for *B. abortus* Strong Positive Control (SPC) mean:

$$\text{S/N} = \frac{\frac{\text{Sum of A/B ratios for wells B3 and B4}}{2}}{\text{NC (A/B ratio)}}$$

4. Calculation of S/N for serum sample:

$$\text{S/N} = \frac{\text{A/B ratio of sample well}}{\text{NC (A/B ratio)}}$$

Storage: Store all reagents at 2°-7°C (36°-45°F).

Store *B. abortus* Coated Particles and Anti-*B. abortus:* FTIC Conjugate protected from light. Use the dropper tops to dispense the reagents; Do not return unused reagent to stock bottles.

Caution(s): Handle all *B. abortus* biological materials as though capable of transmitting Brucellosis.

No eating, drinking or smoking where specimens or kit reagents are being handled.

All wastes should be properly decontaminated prior to disposal.

Do not use kit past expiration date and do not intermix components from kits with different lot numbers.

Discussion: Brucellosis in cattle is a disease caused by *Brucella abortus*, a facilitative, intracellular bacterium. The primary mode of disease transmission is by ingestion of *B. abortus* organisms that may be present in tissues of aborted fetuses, fetal membranes and uterine fluids. In addition, infection may occur as the result of cattle ingesting *B. abortus* contaminated feed or water. Infection in cows also has occurred through venereal transmission of the organisms by infected bulls.

Abortion is the most outstanding clinical feature of the disease. If a carrier state develops in a majority of infected cows in a herd, the clinical manifestations may be reduced milk production, dead calves at term, and/or a higher frequency of retained placenta. Disease in the bull may produce infections of the seminal vesicles and testicles resulting in shedding of the organisms in semen.

Diagnosis is based on serological and/or bacteriological procedures. While a positive bacteriological finding is the most definite diagnosis, several weeks may be required to obtain final culture results. The success of disease eradication is dependent upon the accurate identification and elimination of *B. abortus* reactors in a herd. Reliable serological techniques for *B. abortus* provide a rapid and accurate assessment of natural infection or response to vaccine by a measurement of antibodies to *B. abortus* in the serum.

References: Available upon request.

Presentation: 10,560 wells.

Screen Machine™ is a trademark of Baxter Diagnostics, Inc.

Compendium Code No.: 11160372

IGR HOUSE & AREA FOGGER

Durvet **Household Insecticide**

EPA Reg. No.:1021-1623-12281

Active Ingredient(s):

2-[1-Methyl-2-(4-phenoxyphenoxy) ethoxy] pyridine	0.100%
Pyrethrins	0.050%
*N-Octyl bicycloheptene dicarboximide	0.400%
Permethrin [**(3-Phenoxyphenyl) methyl (+ or -) cis-trans-3-(2,2-dichloroethenyl) 2,2-dimethylcyclopropanecarboxylate)	0.400%
Related compounds	0.035%
Inert Ingredients:	99.015%
	100.000%

*MGK® 264, Insecticide Synergist

**Cis-trans isomers ratio: Min. 35% (+ or -) cis and Max. 65% (+ or -) trans.

Indications: Kills adult and preadult fleas. Inhibits reinfestation for 7 months. Also kills cochroaches, spiders, ants, flies, mosquitos, gnats, lice, millipedes, Boxelder bugs, flying moths, hornets, carpenter bees, wasps, yellowjackets and ticks, including deer ticks, brown dog ticks, Golf Coast ticks and other ixodid species that may carry and transmit Lyme Disease.

Pharmacology: IGR HOUSE & AREA FOGGER contains a combination of three insecticides that stops the flea life cycle in three ways and controls other insects. The first insecticide is Nylar®, an insect growth regulator, that will not allow the flea to reproduce thereby providing long term control. The second insecticide is the botanical Pyrethrum, which provides effective, quick kill of insects upon direct contact and an added benefit of flushing the insects from their hiding place to aid in a more complete control. Permethrin, the third active insecticide, provides activity until the Nylar® takes effect.

IGR HOUSE & AREA FOGGER contains a combination of ingredients that kills both adult and hatching fleas. Nylar®, the insect growth regulator in this fogger, continues to kill hatching fleas for 7 months by preventing their development into adults. The fogger reaches fleas (and other listed insects) hidden in carpets, rugs, drapes upholstery, pet bedding, floor cracks and open cabinets. Occasionally adult fleas may be present in treated areas when reintroduced from infested animals.

Directions for Use: It is a violation of Federal Law to use this product in a manner inconsistent with its labeling.

Read all instructions completely before use.

For use only when building has been vacated by human beings and pets. Ventilate area for 30 minutes before re-entry. For best results, treat all infested areas. Use one fogger for each 6,000 cubic feet (approx. 27' x 27' x 8' ceiling) of unobstructed area. Use additional units for remote rooms or where the free flow of fog is not assured. Preparation: Do not use more than one fogger per room. Do not use in small, enclosed spaces such as closets, cabinets or under counters or tables. Do not use in a room 5 ft x 5 ft or smaller; instead allow fog to enter from other rooms. Turn off all ignition sources such as pilot lights (shut off gas valves), other open flames or running electrical appliances that cycle off and on (i.e., refrigerators, thermostats, etc.). Call your gas utility or management company if you need assistance with your pilot lights.

Preparation: Remove or cover exposed food, dishes, utensils, surfaces and food-handling equipment. Shut off fans and air conditioners. Close outside doors and windows. Remove pets and birds but leave pets' bedding as this is a primary hiding place for fleas and must be treated for best results. No need to discard pet bedding after treatment. Cover or remove fish tanks and bowls. Leave rugs, draperies and upholstered furniture in place. This product will not harm furniture when used as directed. Open interior closet doors and cabinets or areas to be treated. Cover waxed furniture and waxed wood floors in the immediate area surrounding the fogger.

For more effective control of storage pests and cockroaches, open all cupboard doors and drawers for better penetration of fog. Remove all infested foodstuffs and dispose of in outdoor trash.

For flea and tick control, thoroughly vacuum all carpeting, upholstered furniture, along baseboards, under furniture and in closets. Put vacuum bag into a sack and dispose of in outside trash. Mop all hard floor surfaces.

Read all directions and cautions before using.

To Start Fogging: Shake fogger well before using: Hold can at arm's length with top of can pointing away from face and eyes. Push down on finger pad until it locks. This will start fogging action. Set canister in an upright position on a table, stand, etc. (up to 30" inches in height in the center of the area) and place several thicknesses of newspaper under the canister to prevent marring of the surface. Treat the whole dwelling using multiple units in homes with more than one level and numerous rooms. Leave the building at once.

Do Not Re-Enter Building for Two Hours: After two hours, open all outside doors and windows, turn on air conditioner and/or fans and let treated area air for 30 minutes before reoccupying. If additional units are used for remote rooms or where free flow of fog is not assured, increase airing-out time accordingly.

Storage and Disposal:

Storage: Store in a cool, dry area away from heat or open flame.

Disposal: Replace cap and discard container in trash. Do not incinerate or puncture.

Precautionary Statements: Hazards to Humans and Domestic Animals: Caution: Harmful if swallowed. Avoid breathing vapors or spray mist. Avoid contact with skin or eyes. In case of contact, flush with plenty of water. Wash with soap and warm water after use. Obtain medical attention if irritation persists. Avoid contamination of food or feedstuffs.

Do not use in food areas of food handling establishments, restaurants or other areas where food is commercially prepared or processed. Do not use in serving areas while food is exposed or facility is in operation. Serving areas are areas where prepared foods are served such as dining rooms but excluding areas where foods may be prepared or held. In the home, all food processing surfaces and utensils should be covered during treatment or thoroughly washed before use. Exposed food should be covered or removed. Non-food areas are areas such as garbage rooms, lavatories, floor drains (to sewers), entries and vestibules, offices, locker rooms, machine rooms, boiler rooms, garages, mop closets and storage (after canning or bottling). Not for use in USDA Meat and Poultry Plants.

Remove pets, birds, and cover fish aquariums before spraying.

First Aid:

If Swallowed: Call a physician or Poison Control Center immediately.

If In Eyes: Flush with plenty of water. Get medical attention if irritation persists.

If On Skin Or Clothing: Remove contaminated clothing and wash before reuse. Wash skin with soap and warm water. Get medical attention if irritation persists.

If Inhaled: Remove victim to fresh air if effects occur, and call a physician. For more information regarding medical emergencies or pesticide incidents, call thte International Poison Center at 1-888-740-8712.

Physical or Chemical Hazards: Contents under pressure. Keep away from heat, sparks, and open flame. Do not puncture or incinerate container. Exposure to temperatures above 130F may cause bursting. This product contains a highly flammable ingredient.

Warning(s): Keep out of reach of children.

Presentation: 6 fl. oz. (170 gm) can.

One unit treats a room for up to 6,000 cubic feet of unobstructed space (27x27x8).

Nylar®, MGK® Registered trademark of McLaughlin Gormley King Co.

Compendium Code No.: 10841361 8/01

IL VACCINE

Aspen **Bacterin-Vaccine**

Bovine Rhinotracheitis Vaccine, Modified Live Virus-Leptospira pomona Bacterin

U.S. Vet. Lic. No.: 213

Active Ingredient(s): Bovine rhinotracheitis (IBR) vaccine, modified live virus and *Leptospira pomona* bacterin.

Contains neomycin as a preservative.

Indications: For the vaccination of healthy cattle against disease caused by IBR virus and *Leptospira pomona.*

Diluent may be used for the immunization of swine against *L pomona* only.

Dosage and Administration: Rehydrate with the accompanying diluent and inject 2 mL intramuscularly using aseptic techniques.

Calves vaccinated before weaning should be revaccinated 30 days after weaning when the possible influence of maternal antibodies is decreased.

When only diluent is being used: Shake well before using. Inject 2 mL subcutaneously or intramuscularly into cattle using aseptic techniques. Inject 2 mL intramuscularly into swine using aseptic techniques. For swine, a second dose should be given 3-4 weeks after the first dose. Annual revaccination is recommended.

Precaution(s): Store at 35° to 45°F (2° to 7°C). Do not freeze.

Caution(s): Use the entire contents when first opened. Burn the container and all unused contents.

Do not use in pregnant animals or in calves nursing pregnant animals. Abortions may result.

For use in animals only.

Allergic reactions may follow the use of the vaccine.

Antidote(s): Epinephrine.

Warning(s): Do not vaccinate within 21 days before slaughter.

Presentation: 10 dose (20 mL) and 50 dose (100 mL) vials.

Compendium Code No.: 14750450

IMIZOL® ℞

Schering-Plough **Parasiticide Injection**

(Imidocarb Dipropionate)

NADA No.: 141-071

Active Ingredient(s): Each mL contains 120 mg of imidocarb dipropionate.

Indications: For the treatment of dogs with clinical signs of babesiosis and/or demonstrated *Babesia* organisms in the blood.

Pharmacology: Description: IMIZOL® (imidocarb dipropionate) is a sterile solution containing

120 mg/mL of imidocarb dipropionate suitable for intramuscular or subcutaneous administration. Imidocarb is chemically described as *N,N'*-bis[3-(4,5-dihydro-1*H*-imidazol-2-yl)-phenyl]urea dipropionate and has a molecular weight of 496.6. In addition to the active component, imidocarb dipropionate, the formulation also contains propionic acid (22.34 mg/mL), and water for injection.

Pharmacodynamics: The pharmacodynamics of imidocarb were studied in various species as described by Rao et al (1980)[2]. The study suggests that there is a potential for adverse reactions mediated by the autonomic nervous system and especially through anticholinesterase mechanisms. Clinical experience in dogs at therapeutic dosages of less than 10 mg/kg body weight given intramuscularly or subcutaneously has established a pattern of adverse reactions. These reactions in descending order of frequency are: salivation, vomiting, and occasionally diarrhea.

Dosage and Administration: Use intramuscularly or subcutaneously at a rate of 6.6 mg/kg (3 mg/lb) body weight. Repeat the dose in two (2) weeks, for a total of two (2) treatments.

IMIZOL® Dosing Guide 6.6 mg/kg Body Weight

Animal Weight	IMIZOL® Dosage
10 lb (4.5 kg)	0.25 mL
20 lb (9.1 kg)	0.50 mL
30 lb (13.6 kg)	0.75 mL
40 lb (18.2 kg)	1.00 mL
60 lb (27.3 kg)	1.50 mL
80 lb (36.4 kg)	2.00 mL
100 lb (45.5 kg)	2.50 mL

Contraindication(s): Do not use this product simultaneously with exposure to cholinesterase-inhibiting drugs, pesticides, or chemicals.

Precaution(s): Store between 2° and 25°C (36° and 77°F). Protect from light.

Caution(s): Federal (USA) law restricts this drug to use by or on the order of a licensed veterinarian.

Must not be administered intravenously. The safety and effectiveness of imidocarb have not been determined in puppies or in breeding, lactating or pregnant animals. Risk versus benefit should be considered before using this drug in dogs with impaired lung, liver or kidney function.

Warning(s): Not for human use. Keep out of reach of children. In the event of human exposure, immediately contact the manufacturer for medical advice for humans.

Oncogenesis: Increased incidence of tumors was observed in rats given imidocarb. Refer to Material Safety Data Sheet (MSDS) for more detailed occupational safety information.

Toxicology: IMIZOL® solution was administered subcutaneously to four groups of five dogs at 2.2, 5.5, 7.7, or 9.9 mg/kg. The treatment was repeated 2 weeks later. There were no effects attributed to IMIZOL® on body temperature, body weight, hematology, most clinical chemistries or gross pathology. At 9.9 mg/kg there was a slight increase in serum alanine aminotransferase (ALT, SGPT) and arginine aminotransferase (AST, SGOT) indicative of mild liver injury. Other effects noted were pain on injection, injection site swelling, and vomiting. Two of the injection sites ulcerated but healed readily without complication.

In a 90-day toxicity study, imidocarb was given orally to three groups of eight dogs at the rate of 5, 20, or 80 mg/kg/day. The target organs of toxicity were liver and intestines. These results may have been influenced by the oral dosing route. In a pharmacokinetic study by Abdullah et al (1984)[1], imidocarb was administered to dogs intravenously at a dose of 4 mg/kg. One of 13 dogs died. The target organs of toxicity in this dog were lungs and kidneys, and some changes were noted in the liver and spleen.

The toxic syndrome involves lethargy, weakness and anorexia, with possible signs of gastrointestinal, liver, kidney, and lung dysfunction.

Adverse Reactions: Adverse effects commonly seen are pain during injection and mild cholinergic signs such as salivation, nasal drip or brief episodes of vomiting. Other effects seen less frequently are panting, restlessness, diarrhea , and mild injection site inflammation lasting one to several days. Rarely, injection site ulceration occurs, but the lesion is not resistant to healing.

If severe cholinergic signs occur, they may be reversed with atropine sulfate. To report an adverse reaction, call 1-800-932-0473.

References:

[1] A.S. Abdullah et al, Veterinary Research Communications. 1984; (8):55-59.

[2] K.S. Rao, Indian Veterinary Journal. 1980; 57(4):283-287.

Presentation: IMIZOL® solution is packaged in 10 mL glass, sterile, multiple-dose vials.

Compendium Code No.: 10471110

IMMITICIDE® ℞

Merial **Parasiticide Injection**

(melarsomine dihydrochloride) Sterile Powder-Canine Heartworm Treatment

NADA No.: 141-042

Active Ingredient(s): IMMITICIDE® Sterile Powder contains 50.0 mg melarsomine dihydrochloride and 33.75 mg glycine USP.

1 vial: when reconstituted with 2 mL of sterile water for injection (provided) contains 25 mg/mL of active ingredient.

Indications: IMMITICIDE® Sterile Powder is indicated for the treatment of stabilized Class 1[a], 2[b], and 3[c] heartworm disease caused by immature (4-month old, stage L_5) to mature adult infections of *Dirofilaria immitis* in dogs.

Heartworm Disease Classification: The following parameters were used to classify the dogs in the clinical field trials for IMMITICIDE®. Other parameters may be considered. As a general rule, conservative treatment should be employed since heartworm disease is serious and potentially fatal. If there is evidence of a high worm burden patients should be categorized as Class 3.

[a]Class 1: Patients in this category are characterized as having asymptomatic to mild heartworm disease. No radiographic signs or signs of anemia are evident. Patients with mild disease may have subjective signs such as a general loss of condition, fatigue on exercise, or occasional cough; however, no objective radiographic or other abnormal laboratory parameters will be present.

[b]Class 2: Patients in this category are characterized as having moderate heartworm disease. Radiographic signs or signs of anemia [Packed Cell Volume (PCV) less than 30% but greater than 20%, or other hematologic parameters below normal] are evident. Mild proteinuria (2+) may be present. Radiographic signs may include right ventricular enlargement, slight pulmonary artery enlargement, or circumscribed perivascular densities plus mixed alveolar/interstitial lesions. Patients may be free of subjective clinical signs or may have a general loss of condition, fatigue on exercise, or occasional cough. If necessary, patients should be stabilized prior to treatment.

[c]Class 3: Patients in this category are characterized as having severe heartworm disease. These patients have a guarded prognosis. Subjective signs of disease may include cardiac cachexia (wasting), constant fatigue, persistent cough, dyspnea, or other signs associated with right heart failure such as ascites and/or jugular pulse. Radiographic signs may include right ventricular enlargement or right ventricular plus right atrial enlargement, severe pulmonary artery enlargement, circumscribed to chronic mixed patterns and diffuse patterns of pulmonary densities or radiographic signs of thromboembolism. Signs of significant anemia (PCV <20% or other hematologic abnormalities) may be present. Proteinuria (>2+) may be present. Patients may have only moderate clinical signs and significant laboratory or radiographic alterations or they may have significant clinical signs with only moderate laboratory and radiographic signs and be categorized as Class 3. Patients in Class 3 should be stabilized prior to treatment and then administered the alternate dosing regime (See Cautions and Dosage and Administration).

Pharmacology: Melarsomine dihydrochloride is an organic arsenical chemotherapeutic agent. Melarsomine has a molecular weight of 501.34 and is chemically designated as 4 - [(4, 6-diamino-1, 3, 5-triazon-2-yl) amino] phenyl-dithioarsenite of di (2-aminoethyl), dihydrochloride. It is freely soluble in water. When injected intramuscularly, it is rapidly absorbed. The exact mode of action on *D. immitis* is unknown.

Dosage and Administration: IMMITICIDE® should be administered only by deep intramuscular injection in the epaxial (lumbar) muscles in the third through fifth lumbar region (see graphic). Do not administer at any other site. Avoid superficial injection or leakage. Use a 23 gauge 1 inch needle for dogs equal to or less than 10 kg (22 lb) in weight. Use a 22 gauge 1½ inch needle for dogs greater than 10 kg (22 lb). Use alternating sides with each administration. If repeated administrations are warranted avoid injecting at the same lumbar location. Record the location of the first injection(s) in the patient's medical record for future reference.

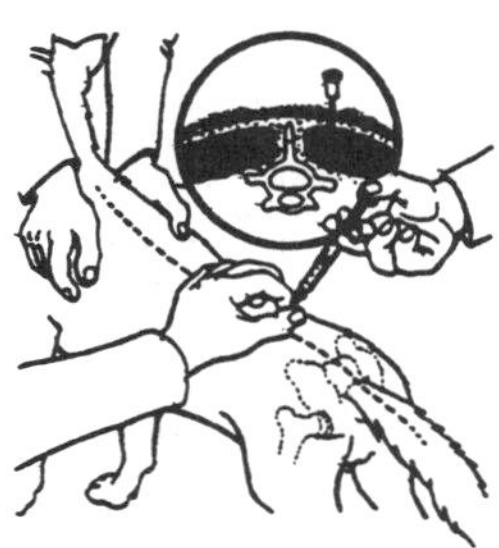

Disease Classification: It is vital to classify the severity of heartworm disease to apply the appropriate dosage regime for IMMITICIDE® (See Indications).

Class 1 and 2: If necessary, dogs should be stabilized prior to treatment. IMMITICIDE® should be administered intramuscularly in the lumbar (L_3-L_5) muscles at a dose of 2.5 mg/kg twice, 24 hours apart (See Dosing Table). Four months following treatment, a second treatment series (2.5 mg/kg twice, 24 hours apart) can be elected taking into consideration the response to the first IMMITICIDE® treatment and the condition, age, and use of the dog. Worms that were too young to be killed by the first treatment series, i.e., < 4 months, may be killed by a second treatment series.

Class 3: Alternate Dosing Regime: Dogs with severe (Class 3) heartworm disease should be stabilized prior to treatment and then dosed intramuscularly in the lumbar (L_3-L_5) muscles with a single injection of 2.5 mg/kg then approximately 1 month later with 2.5 mg/kg administered twice 24 hours apart (See Dosing Table).

Dosing Table: Care must be taken to administer the proper dose. Accurately weigh the dog and calculate the volume to be injected based on the dose of 2.5 mg/kg (1.1 mg/lb). This is equivalent to 0.1 mL/kg (0.045 mL/lb). The following table should be used as a guide to ensure that the proper volume has been calculated.

Weight (lb)	Weight (kg)	Volume per Injection (mL)
2.2	1	0.1
4.4	2	0.2
6.6	3	0.3
8.8	4	0.4
11.0	5	0.5
13.2	6	0.6
15.4	7	0.7
17.6	8	0.8
19.8	9	0.9
22.0	10	1.0
44.0	20	2.0
66.0	30	3.0
88.0	40	4.0
110.0	50	5.0*

*Limited data were collected on the administration > 5.0 mL at a single injection site.

Preparation: IMMITICIDE® should be aseptically reconstituted only with 2.0 mL of sterile water for injection (provided as 2.0 mL sterile water for injection U.S.P.). This provides 2.5 mg melarsomine dihydrochloride per 0.1 mL of injectable solution. Two 50 mg vials will be required for dogs weighing > 20 kg and ≤ 40 kg and 3 vials will be required for dogs > 40 kg and ≤ 60 kg. Use immediately. Reconstituted solution may be used within 24 hours if refrigerated and kept from light.

Treatment Response: A baseline can be established pre-treatment by using commercially available in-office heartworm antigen testing kits prior to treatment. Treatment response can be assessed best by heartworm antigen testing applied 4 months after treatment. A successful treatment is determined to be conversion from an antigen positive to an antigen negative status. In dogs with signs of heartworm disease, gradual improvement should be observed as the long-term effects of the heartworm infection resolve. Some dogs may have chronic effects that will not totally resolve.

Concomitant Therapy: During the course of clinical field trials, IMMITICIDE® was administered concurrently with anti-inflammatories, antibiotics, insecticides, heartworm prophylactics, and various other drugs commonly used to stabilize and support dogs with heartworm disease with no adverse interactions noted.

Routine Prophylaxis: If the dog is not currently receiving commercially available heartworm preventatives, they may be administered consistent with label recommendations and re-exposure risk.

Contraindication(s): IMMITICIDE® is contraindicated in dogs with very severe (Class 4) heartworm disease. Patients in this category have Caval Syndrome (*D. immitis* present in the venae cavae and right atrium).

Precaution(s): Storage Conditions: Store upright at room temperature. After reconstitution, solutions should be stored under refrigeration and kept from light in the original packaging for 24 hours. Do not freeze reconstituted solution.

Caution(s): Federal law restricts this drug to use by or on the order of a licensed veterinarian.

IMMITICIDE® should be administered by deep intramuscular injection in the lumbar (epaxial) muscles (L_3-L_5) only.

Do not use in any other muscle group.

Do not use intravenously.

Care should be taken to avoid superficial injection or leakage. (See Safety).

For use in dogs only. Safety for use in breeding animals and lactating or pregnant bitches has not been determined.

General: All dogs with heartworm disease are at risk for post-treatment pulmonary thromboembolism (death of worms which may result in fever, weakness, and coughing), though dogs with severe pulmonary arterial disease have an increased risk and may exhibit more severe signs (dyspnea, hemoptysis, right heart failure and possibly death). Dogs should be restricted from light to heavy exercise post-treatment depending on the severity of their heartworm disease.

Studies in healthy (heartworm negative) dogs indicate that adverse reactions may occur after the second injection in the series even if no problems were encountered with the first injection. All patients should be closely monitored during treatment and for up to 24 hours after the last injection.

Special Considerations for Class 3 dogs: Following stabilization, severely ill (Class 3) dogs should be treated according to the alternate dosing regime in an attempt to decrease post-treatment mortality associated with thromboembolism (See Dosage and Administration). Post-treatment mortality due to thromboembolism and/or progression of the underlying disease may occur in 10 to 20% of the Class 3 patients treated with IMMITICIDE® (see Mortality). Hospitalization post-treatment and strict exercise restriction are recommended. Other supportive therapies should be considered on a case-by-case basis.

If the alternate dosing regime is used, expect increased injection site reactions on the side receiving the second injection since the skeletal muscles at the first injection site may not have fully recovered or healed. If persistent swelling is present at 1 month, the second injections may be delayed for several weeks up to 1 month.

Special Considerations for Older Dogs: In clinical field trials, dogs 8 years or older experienced more post-treatment depression/lethargy, anorexia/inappetence, and vomiting than younger dogs.

Antidote(s): BAL in Oil Ampules (Dimercaprol Injection, USP) [Akorn, San Clemente, California, at 1-800-223-9851] is reported in the literature to be an antidote for arsenic toxicity and was shown in one study to reduce the signs of toxicity associated with overdosage of IMMITICIDE®. The efficacy of IMMITICIDE® may be reduced with co-administration of BAL.

Warning(s): Human Warnings: Keep this and all medications out of the reach of children. Avoid human exposure. Wash hands thoroughly after use or wear gloves. Potentially irritating to eyes. Rinse eyes with copious amounts of water if exposed. Consult a physician in cases of accidental exposure by any route (dermal, oral, or by injection).

The Material Safety Data Sheet (MSDS) contains more detailed occupational safety information. To report adverse effects, obtain an MSDS, or for assistance, contact Merial at 1-888-637-4251, option 3.

Overdose: Three dogs were inadvertently overdosed with IMMITICIDE® in the clinical field trials when the dose was calculated on a mg/lb basis rather than a mg/kg basis (2X overdosage). Within 30 minutes of injection, one dog showed excessive salivation, panting, restlessness, and fever with all signs resolving within 4 hours. Vomiting and diarrhea were seen in the second dog within 24 hours of injection. The dog vomited once and the diarrhea resolved within 24 hours. The third dog showed no systemic reaction to the overdosage. Clinical observations in healthy beagle dogs after receiving up to 3X the recommended dose included tremors, lethargy, unsteadiness/ataxia, restlessness, panting, shallow and labored respiration, rales, severe salivation, and vomiting which progressed to respiratory distress, collapse, cyanosis, stupor, and death (See Safety).

Adverse Reactions: (Side Effects):

Injection Sites: At the recommended dosage in clinical field trials, significant irritation was observed at the intramuscular injection sites, accompanied by pain, swelling, tenderness, and reluctance to move. Approximately 30% of treated dogs experienced some kind of reaction at the injection site(s). Though injection site reactions were generally mild to moderate in severity and recovery occurred in 1 week to 1 month, severe reactions did occur (< 1.0%), so care should be taken to avoid superficial or subcutaneous injection and leakage. Firm nodules can persist indefinitely.

Other Reactions: Coughing/gagging, depression/lethargy, anorexia/inappetence, fever, lung congestion, and vomiting were the most common reactions observed in IMMITICIDE®-treated dogs. Hypersalivation and panting occurred rarely in clinical trials (1.9% and 1.6%, respectively); however, when seen, they generally occurred within 30 minutes of injection and may be severe. One dog vomited after each injection of IMMITICIDE®, despite pretreatment with anti-emetics. All adverse reactions resolved with time or treatment with the exception of a limited number of injection site reactions [persistent nodules, (See Table: Average Onset Time and Duration (with ranges) of the Most Common Reactions in Clinical Trials)] and a low number of post-treatment deaths (See Mortality).

Prevalence of Clinical Observations/Adverse Reactions Reported in Clinical Field Trials: The following table enumerates adverse events that occurred in 1.5% or more of dogs with Class 1, 2, and 3 heartworm disease treated with IMMITICIDE® in clinical field trials. Comparison is made with the same adverse events reported in dogs treated with placebo. Some of the following clinical observations/adverse reactions seen in dogs treated with IMMITICIDE® may be directly attributable to the drug or they may be secondary to worm death and/or the underlying heartworm disease process.

Prevalence of Clinical Observation/Adverse Reactions Reported in Clinical Field Trials:

Clinical Observation/ Adverse Reaction	IMMITICIDE® % of dogs n=311	Placebo % of dogs n=63
Injection Site Reactions	32.8	3.2
Coughing/Gagging	22.2	14.3
Depression/Lethargy	15.4	4.8
Anorexia/Inappetence	13.2	3.2
Pyrexia (fever)	7.4	0.0
Lung Congestion/Sounds	5.5	1.6
Emesis	5.1	1.6
Diarrhea	2.6	0.0
Dyspnea	2.6	1.6
Hypersalivation	1.9	0.0
Panting	1.6	0.0
Hemoptysis	1.6	0.0

Clinical observations/adverse reactions occurring in less than 1.5% of the dogs treated with IMMITICIDE® include: abdominal hemorrhage, abdominal pain, bloody stool/diarrhea, colitis, gingivitis, pancreatitis, anemia, DIC, hemoglobinemia, icterus (mucous membranes), discolored urine, hematuria, inappropriate urination, low specific gravity, polyuria, pyuria, bronchitis, miscellaneous respiratory problem, pneumonia, tachypnea, tracheobronchitis, wheezing, alopecia, hair color and coat character change, miscellaneous skin problem, ataxia, disorientation, fatigue/tires easily, miscellaneous eye problem, weight loss, convulsion/seizure, leukocytosis, polydipsia, and restlessness.

Onset and Duration of Clinical Observations/Adverse Reactions: The following table is provided to show the average onset time post-treatment for the most common reactions and the average duration of each event, as calculated from the 311 dogs treated with IMMITICIDE® in the clinical field trials.

Average Onset Time and Duration (with Ranges) of the Most Common Reactions in Clinical Trials:

Clinical Observation/ Adverse Reaction	Ave. Onset Time in Days (range*)	Ave. Duration in Days (range*)
Injection Site		
Swelling/Edema/Seroma	6 (0*-77)	18 (< 1-210)
Pain/Discomfort/Irritation/Inflammation/Heat	1 (0-6)	3 (< 1-30)
Generalized/Local Myalgia with Tenderness and Stiffness	3 (1-8)	9 (< 1-30)
Persistent (lumps, knots, nodules, masses)	22 (0-99)	47 (1-152)
Abscess (sterile and septic)	24 (10-42)	21 (5-36)
Coughing/Gagging	10 (0-103)	13 (< 1-134)
Depression/Lethargy	5 (0-46)	6 (< 1-48)
Anorexia/Inappetence	5 (0-63)	5 (< 1-30)

*A zero indicates that the reaction first occurred on the day of treatment.

Mortality: Death is a possible sequelae of heartworm disease in dogs with or without treatment, especially in the Class 3 dogs. The following table shows the percentage of dogs that died in clinical trials with IMMITICIDE® and the causes of death, if known.

Mortality in Dogs with Class 1,2, and 3 Heartworm Disease Treated with IMMITICIDE® in Clinical Field Trials:

	Class 1, 2 % of Dogs n=267	Class 3 % of Dogs n=44
Total Deaths	5.2	18.2
Cause:		
Trauma	2.3	2.3
Thromboembolism	0.0	4.6
Euthanasia (unrelated to treatment or underlying disease)	1.1	0.0
Euthanasia (related to treatment or underlying disease)	0.0	2.3
Underlying Disease	0.8	2.3
Undetermined	1.1	6.8

In one small (n=15), uncontrolled field study in severely ill (Class 3) dogs, 5 dogs died following treatment. Pulmonary thromboembolism was the cause of one death. The remaining dogs were not necropsied. All 5 dogs were in right heart failure at the time of treatment. Clinical signs seen in this study which were not seen in the larger studies include atrial fibrillation, collapse, hypothermia, and weakness.

Post Approval Experience: In addition to the aforementioned adverse reactions reported in pre-approval clinical studies, there have also been rare reports of paresis and paralysis in dogs following administration of IMMITICIDE®. To report a suspected adverse reaction, contact Merial at 1-888-637-4251, option 3.

Trial Data: Safety: IMMITICIDE® has a low margin of safety. A single dose of 7.5 mg/kg (3X the recommended dose) can result in pulmonary inflammation, edema, and death. Daily administration of 2X and 3X the recommended dose for 6 days caused no renal injury; however, daily administration of these doses for 14 days caused renal damage in healthy dogs. Adverse reactions, primarily at the injection sites, were seen at the recommended dose in clinical trials (see Adverse Reactions).

Studies in Healthy (Heartworm Negative) Dogs: The safety of IMMITICIDE® was studied in 24 healthy beagle dogs. Drug was administered at 0, 2.5, 5.0, and 7.5 mg/kg for 6 consecutive days (0, 1, 2, and 3 times the recommended dosage). Clinical observations included tremors, lethargy, unsteadiness/ataxia, restlessness, panting, shallow and labored respiration, and/or rales. These signs were seen in all groups treated with IMMITICIDE® with frequency and intensity increasing with increasing dosage. Death or euthanasia in a moribund state occurred in 3/6 dogs in the 7.5 mg/kg (3X) group. The signs exhibited by these dogs, in addition to the signs described above, including collapse, severe salivation, vomiting, respiratory distress, cyanosis, stupor, and death within 4 hours of the first dose in two dogs and within 20 hours of the second dose in one dog.

Body weights, water consumption, hematology and urine parameters were compatible to controls. Decreased food consumption occurred sporadically in the two high dose groups. Elevations, up to 25-fold, in creatinine kinase (CK) and elevations, up to 7-fold, in aspartate aminotransferase (AST) were observed and related grossly and histologically to muscle damage at the injection sites. Up to 2-fold elevations in alanine aminotransferase (ALT) were also noted. Gross and microscopic pathology revealed no organ-related toxicity other than edema and acute inflammation in the lungs and pleural effusion in the 3 dogs that died at the 7.5 mg/kg dose. Injection site irritation was observed in the skeletal muscles at all dose levels. At 5.0 mg/kg an injection site abscess was observed in one dog.

A separate study was conducted to examine the intensity and duration of injection site reactions. The dogs were dosed at 2.5 and 5.0 mg/kg (1X and 2X the recommended dose) twice

24 hours apart. This treatment series was repeated 4 months later. One group received the second treatment series after 1 month to mimic the alternate dosing regime. Swelling, which occurred within 7 days of injection and persisted from 1 to 72 days (average 30 days), was the most common clinical observation. A small, firm nodule in the lumbar region of one dog in the 1X group appeared during the first month of the study and persisted for 41 days. Pain at or following injection was not observed in this study. Elevations of the same magnitude as in the previous study and again related to muscle damage were observed in CK and AST within 8 hours of injection. The values approached pretest levels by 72 hours and were within the normal range established by control animals by 1 month post-injection.

Gross and microscopic evidence of injection site irritation (cellular infiltrate, fibrosis, necrosis, and hemorrhage) was still evident in the muscles 1 month post-injection in dogs at both dose levels. By 3 months post-injection, resolution (healing) was evident microscopically in the skeletal muscles at the 2.5 mg/kg dose level. One dog treated at the 2X dose had extension of treatment-related injection site inflammation into deeper tissues (i.e., abdominal cavity) as evidenced by an adhesion between the spleen and mesentery.

Efficacy: Results of the laboratory and clinical filed trials demonstrate that treatment with IMMITICIDE® results in reduction and/or clearance of *D. immitis* infection in dogs with Class 1, 2, and 3 heartworm disease. Evaluations for efficacy were determined by post-mortem worm counts in the laboratory studies and detection of antigen in the blood and subjective clinical assessments in the clinical trials. Physical exams, assessments of clinical variables, class of heartworm disease, radiographic examinations, as well as complete blood counts, serum chemistry profiles, and urinalysis were evaluated in the field trials.

Laboratory Studies: In placebo-controlled studies, IMMITICIDE®, administered at 2.5 mg/kg twice, 24 hours apart, was 90.7% effective against transplanted adult heartworms and 90.8% effective against induced infections of 4 month old (L_5) immature heartworms. To evaluate the effectiveness of the alternate dosing regimen, dogs with transplanted heartworms were treated with either 2.5 mg/kg once or 2.5 mg/kg once followed 1 month later with 2.5 mg/kg administered twice 24 hours apart. A single injection of IMMITICIDE® at 2.5 mg/kg reduced male worms 87.7% and female worms 16.9% (total 51.7%). When the full regime was used 100% of male worms and 98% of female worms were killed (total 99%). Dogs with natural *D. immitis* infections were treated with IMMITICIDE® at 2.5 mg/kg twice, 24 hours apart. This dose was repeated 4 months later. Antigen tests performed at month 4 showed a 90% conversion from antigen positive to negative status. Worm counts at month 9 showed a 98.7% reduction in worm numbers as compared to placebo controls.

Clinical Field Studies: In two well-controlled field studies, 169 client-owned dogs, 1 to 12 years old and weighing 3.0 to 59.0 kg, with Class 1 or stabilized Class 2 heartworm disease were treated with the recommended dose of IMMITICIDE®. In-office blood antigen tests were used pretreatment to diagnose the *D. immitis* infection and 4 months after drug administration to assess treatment response. At month 4, 76.2 to 81% of the dogs had converted from antigen positive to antigen negative status. The conversion rate ranged from 89.7 to 98.2% after two treatment series. In an open-label study in 102 dogs, 1 to 18 years old and weighing 4.4 to 40.8 kg, with Class 1 or stabilized Class 2 heartworm disease, the conversion rate was 84% 4 months after one series of treatments. When a second series was given 4 months later, the conversion rate was 94%.

An open-label clinical field study was conducted in 44 dogs, 1.5 to 14 years and weighing 3.2 to 50.0 kg, with stabilized, Class 3 heartworm disease. Dogs received the alternate dosing regime (2.5 mg/kg once followed 1 month later by 2.5 mg/kg twice 24 hours apart). The conversion rate was 89.2% 4 months after the final treatment. In a small, uncontrolled field trial (n=10) in Class 3 dogs the conversion rate was 100% 4 months after treatment.

Presentation: IMMITICIDE® is provided as: 5 x 50 mg vials of lyophilized melarsomine dihydrochloride with accompanying 5 x 2 mL vials of sterile water for injection U.S.P.

®IMMITICIDE is a Registered trademark of Merial.

Merial Limited, a company limited by shares registered in England and Wales (registered number 3332751) with a registered office at PO Box 327, Sandringham House, Sandringham Avenue, Harlow Business Park, Harlow, Essex CM19 5TG, England, and domesticated in Delaware, USA as Merial LLC).

Compendium Code No.: 11110263 1050-0065-00

IMMULITE® CANINE TOTAL T4

DPC **T_4 Determination Test**

Test Description: Summary and Explanation of the Test: Thyroid hormone assays have also proved of value in veterinary medicine.[1,5,14] However, most commercially available T4 RIAs have been designed for measurements in human serum. The reference range for dogs is much lower (approximately 0.73-2.9 μg/dL), with hyperthyroidism characterized by increased levels of circulating T4, hypothyroidism by decreased levels.[17] The differential diagnosis of hypothyroidism is of primary concern, since hyperthyroidism is a rare condition in dogs. The kit is supplied with adjustors prepared in T4-free canine serum, to avoid the systematic inaccuracies which can occur due to matrix differences.[3,8,16]

Components: Materials Supplied: Components are a matched set. The barcode labels are needed for the assay.

Canine Total T4 Test Units (LCT1): Each barcode-labeled unit contains one bead coated with monoclonal murine anti-T4 antibody. Stable at 2-8°C until expiration date.

LKCT1: 100 units.

Allow the Test Unit bags to come to room temperature before opening. Open by cutting along the top edge, leaving the ziplock ridge intact. Reseal the bags to protect from moisture.

Canine Total T4 Reagent Wedge (LCT2): With barcode. 6.5 mL alkaline phosphatase (bovine calf intestine) conjugated to T4 in buffer, with preservative. Store capped and refrigerated: Stable at 2-8°C until expiration date. Recommended usage is within 30 days after opening when stored as indicated.

LKCT1: 2 wedges.

Canine Total T4 Adjustors (LCTL, LCTH): Two vials (Low and High) of lyophilized T4 in processed canine serum, with preservative. At least 30 minutes before use, reconstitute each vial with 2.0 mL distilled or deionized water. Stable at 2-8°C for 30 days after opening, or for 6 months (aliquotted) at -20°C.

Kit Components Supplied Separately:

LSUBX: Chemiluminescent Substrate

LPWS2: Probe Wash

LKPM: Probe Cleaning Kit

LCHx-y: Sample Cup Holders (barcoded)

LSCP: Sample Cups (disposable)

LSCC: Sample Cup Caps (optional)

K9CON: A bi-level, canine serum-based control, containing canine T4 as one of multiple assayed constituents.

LK9TCM: A bi-level, canine serum-based control module, containing canine T4 as one of 3 assayed constituents.

Also Required: Sample transfer pipets, distilled or deionized water, controls.

Indications: Intended Use: For *in vitro* use with the IMMULITE® Analyzer - for the quantitative measurement of total circulating thyroxine (T4) in canine serum. It is intended strictly for *in vitro* veterinary use as an aid in the clinical assessment of thyroid status.

Test Principles: Principle of the Procedure: IMMULITE® Canine Total T4 is a solid-phase, chemiluminescent competitive immunoassay.

Incubation Cycles: 1 x 30 minutes.

Sample Collection: Specimen Collection: The animal need not be fasting, and no special preparations are necessary. Collect blood by venipuncture into plain tubes (without anticoagulant), and separate the serum from the cells.

The use of an ultracentrifuge is recommended to clear lipemic samples.

Centrifuging serum samples before a complete clot forms may result in the presence of fibrin. To prevent erroneous results due to the presence of fibrin, ensure that complete clot formation has taken place prior to centrifugation of samples. Some samples, particularly those from patients receiving anticoagulant therapy, may require increased clotting time.

Volume Required: 30 μL serum. (Sample cup must contain at least 100 μL more than the total volume required.)

Test Procedure: Assay Procedure: See the IMMULITE® Operator's Manual for: Preparation, setup, dilutions, adjustment, assay and quality control procedures.

Adjustment Interval: 2 weeks.

Quality Control Samples: Use controls or sample pools with at least two levels (low and high) of T4.

Interpretation of Results: Expected Values: A reference range study performed with the IMMULITE® Canine Total T4 kit on a total of 46 apparently healthy dogs yielded a median of 2.2 μg/dL (28 nmol/L) and a range of 1.3 to 2.9 μg/dL (17 to 37 nmol/L).

Consider these limits as guidelines only. Each laboratory should establish its own reference ranges.

Storage: 7 days at 2-8°C or 1 month at -20°C.[18] Before assay, allow the samples to come to room temperature (15-28°C) and mix by gentle swirling or inversion. Aliquot, if necessary, to avoid repeated thawing and freezing. Do not attempt to thaw frozen specimens by heating them in a waterbath.

Reagents: Store at 2-8°C. Dispose of in accordance with applicable laws.

Follow universal precautions, and handle all components as if capable of transmitting infectious agents.

Sodium azide, at concentrations less than 0.1 g/dL, has been added as a preservative. On disposal, flush with large volumes of water to prevent the buildup of potentially explosive metal azides in lead and copper plumbing.

Chemiluminescent Substrate: Avoid contamination and exposure to direct sunlight.

Water: Use distilled or deionized water.

Caution(s): For *in vitro* veterinary use only.

Trial Data: Performance Data: Results are expressed in μg/dL. (Unless otherwise specified, all results were generated on canine samples collected in tubes without anticoagulants, gel barriers, or clot-promoting additives.)

Conversion Factor:

μg/dL x 12.87 → nmol/L

Calibration Range: 0.5-15 μg/dL (6.4-193 nmol/L).

Sensitivity: 0.12 μg/dL (1.5 nmol/L).

Precision: Samples were assayed in duplicate over the course of 20 days, two runs per day, for a total of 40 runs and 80 replicates (μg/dL).

		Within-Run		Total	
	Mean	SD	CV	SD	CV
1	0.65	0.07	10.8%	0.09	13.8%
2	0.83	0.08	9.6%	0.11	13.2%
3	1.95	0.1	5.1%	0.16	8.2%
4	3.84	0.17	4.4%	0.26	6.8%
5	6.11	0.29	4.7%	0.35	5.7%
6	11.9	0.47	3.9%	0.62	5.2%

Linearity: Samples were assayed under various dilutions.

	Dilution	Observed μg/dL	Expected μg/dL	%O/E
1	4 in 4	1.8	—	—
	2 in 4	0.95	0.90	106%
	1 in 4	0.52	0.45	116%
2	4 in 4	2.2	—	—
	2 in 4	1.2	1.1	109%
	1 in 4	0.59	0.55	107%
3	4 in 4	2.8	—	—
	2 in 4	1.5	1.4	107%
	1 in 4	0.64	0.70	91%
4	4 in 4	6.2	—	—
	2 in 4	3.2	3.1	103%
	1 in 4	1.6	1.6	100%

Recovery: Samples spiked 1 to 19 with three T4 solutions (17, 32 and 62 μg/dL) were assayed.

	Solution[1]	Observed μg/dL	Expected μg/dL	%O/E
1	—	0.57	—	—
	A	1.5	1.4	107%
	B	2.4	2.1	114%
	C	4.1	3.6	114%
2	—	1.1	—	—
	A	1.9	1.9	100%
	B	2.8	2.6	108%
	C	4.6	4.1	112%

	Solution[1]	Observed µg/dL	Expected µg/dL	%O/E
3	—	1.2	—	—
	A	2.1	2.0	105%
	B	2.8	2.7	104%
	C	4.6	4.2	110%
4	—	1.8	—	—
	A	2.5	2.6	96%
	B	3.3	3.3	100%
	C	4.9	4.8	102%

Specificity: The antibody used in the IMMULITE® Canine Total T4 procedure is highly specific for T4, with low crossreactivity to other compounds and therapeutic drugs that may be present in canine samples.

Compound	µg/dL Added	Apparent µg/dL	% Cross-reactivity
L-Thyroxine (T4)	—	—	100%
D-Thyroxine	10	5.5	55%
Tetraiodothyroacetic acid	10	1.6	16%
Triiodo-L-thyronine	100	3.2	3.2%
	25	1.1	4.4%
Triiodo-D-thyronine	1	ND	ND
Triiodothyroacetic acid	1,000	6.3	0.63%
	10	ND	ND
	1,000	1.6	0.16%
Monoiodotyrosine	10	ND	ND
Diiodo-L-tyrosine	1,000	ND	ND
Methimazole	1,000	ND	ND
5,5'-Diphenylhydantoin	1,000	ND	ND
Phenylbutazone	1,000	ND	ND
6-*n*-Propyl-2-thiouracil	1,000	ND	ND

ND: Not detectable.

Effect of Gel Barrier Tubes: Blood was collected from 8 dogs into plain and Becton Dickinson SST® vacutainer tubes. The samples were processed by the IMMULITE® Canine Total T4 procedure, with the following results.

(SST) = 0.92 (Plain Tubes) + 0.06 µg/dL

r = 0.985

Means:

0.59 µg/dL (Plain Tubes)

0.60 µg/dL (SST Tubes)

Method Comparison: The assay was compared to DPC's Coat-A-Count Canine T4 assay on 154 canine samples. (Concentration range: approximately 0.53 to 5.6 µg/dL. See graph.) By linear regression:

(IMMULITE®) = 0.88 (CAC) + 0.01 µg/dL

r = 0.942

Means:

1.9 µg/dL (IMMULITE®)

2.1 µg/dL (CAC)

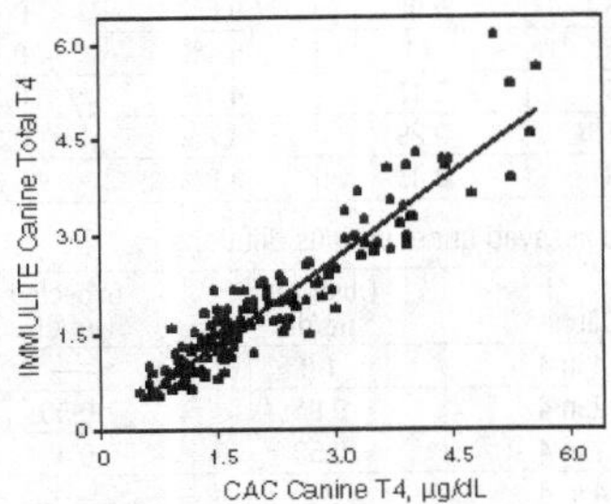

References: Available upon request.

Presentation: 100 test kit.

Compendium Code No.: 12620000

PILKCT-1

IMMULITE® CANINE TSH

DPC **TSH Determination Test**

Test Description: Summary and Explanation of the Test: Thyroid stimulating hormone (TSH, thyrotropin) in dogs is similar in function and structure to TSH found in other mammalian species, including humans. TSH is a glycoprotein produced by the anterior pituitary gland. Through its action on the thyroid gland, it plays a major role in maintaining normal circulating levels of the iodothyronines, T4 and T3. The production and secretion of TSH is controlled by negative feedback from circulating T4 and T3, and by the hypothalamic hormone TRH (thyrotropin releasing hormone.) The TSH molecule is composed of two nonidentical subunits, α and β, that are bound together in a noncovalent manner. Within a species, the TSH α subunit is structurally identical to the α subunits of the related glycoprotein hormones (luteinizing hormone, follicle stimulating hormone and chorionic gonadotropin.) The β subunit of TSH and the β subunits of the related hormones are structurally hormone-specific, and confer upon them their unique biological activities.

Hypothyroidism is considered to be a common endocrine disorder in dogs, whereas hyperthyroidism in this species is relatively unknown. Most cases of canine hypothyroidism are primary in nature, involving impaired production of the thyroid hormones, T4 and T3. In this condition, elevated TSH levels are expected. Secondary or tertiary hypothyroidism, where thyroid hormone production is low as a consequence of hypothalamic or pituitary disease, is believed to account for less than 5% of canine hypothyroidism cases. In the latter conditions, lowered levels of TSH would be expected. Usually, hypothyroidism in dogs is suspected on the basis of clinical history and the presence of lowered levels of thyroid hormones. However, suppressed thyroid hormone levels are nonspecific indicators of the disease, since they are often observed in nonthyroidal illnesses. The evaluation of thyroid function and the diagnosis of hypothyroidism in dogs can be greatly improved through the use of a valid assay for the determination of canine TSH.

Components: Materials Supplied: Components are a matched set. The barcode labels are needed for the assay.

Canine TSH Test Units (LKT1): Each barcode-labeled unit contains one bead coated with monoclonal murine anti-cTSH antibody. Stable at 2-8°C until expiration date.

LKKT1: 100 units.

Allow the Test Unit bags to come to room temperature before opening. Open by cutting along the top edge, leaving the ziplock ridge intact. Reseal the bags to protect from moisture.

Canine TSH Reagent Wedge (LKT2): With barcode. 6.5 mL alkaline phosphatase (bovine calf intestine) conjugated to polyclonal rabbit anti-cTSH antibody in buffer, with preservative. Store capped and refrigerated: Stable at 2-8°C until expiration date. Recommended usage is within 30 days after opening when stored as indicated.

LKKT1: 1 wedge.

Canine TSH Adjustors (LKTL, LKTH): Two vials (Low and High) of lyophilized canine TSH in cTSH-free canine serum/buffer matrix, with preservative. Reconstitute each vial with 4.0 mL distilled or deionized water, and mix by gentle inversion. Stable at 2-8°C for 7 days after reconstitution, or for 6 months (aliquotted) at -20°C.

LKKT1: 1 set. LKKT5: 2 sets.

Kit Components Supplied Separately:

Canine TSH Sample Diluent (LKTZ): For the manual dilution of canine samples. 25 mL of a cTSH-free canine serum/buffer matrix, with preservative. Stable at 2-8°C for 30 days after opening, or for 6 months (aliquotted) at -20°C.

LSUBX: Chemiluminescent Substrate

LPWS2: Probe Wash

LKPM: Probe Cleaning Kit

LCHx-y: Sample Cup Holders (barcoded)

LSCP: Sample Cups (disposable)

LSCC: Sample Cup Caps (optional)

K9CON: A bi-level, canine serum-based control, containing canine TSH as one of multiple assayed constituents.

LK9TCM: A bi-level, canine serum-based control module, containing canine TSH as one of three assayed constituents.

Also Required: Sample transfer pipets; distilled or deionized water; controls.

Indications: Intended Use: For *in vitro* veterinary use with the IMMULITE® Analyzer - for the quantitative measurement of canine thyroid stimulating hormone (canine thyrotropin, cTSH) in serum. It is intended strictly for *in vitro* veterinary use as an aid in the assessment of thyroid status in dogs.

Test Principles: Principle of the Procedure: IMMULITE® Canine TSH is a solid-phase, two-site chemiluminescent immunometric assay.

Incubation Cycles: 1 x 60 minutes.

Sample Collection: Specimen Collection: The animal need not be fasting, and no special preparations are necessary. Collect blood by venipuncture into plain tubes and separate the serum from the cells.

Hemolyzed samples may indicate mistreatment of a specimen before receipt by the laboratory; hence the results should be interpreted with caution.

The use of an ultracentrifuge is recommended to clear lipemic samples.

Centrifuging serum samples before a complete clot forms may result in the presence of fibrin. To prevent erroneous results due to the presence of fibrin, ensure that complete clot formation has taken place prior to centrifugation of samples. Some samples, particularly those from patients receiving anticoagulant therapy, may require increased clotting time.

Volume Required: 25 µL serum. (Sample cup should contain at least 100 µL more than the total volume required.)

Test Procedure: Assay Procedure: Note that for optimal performance, it is important to perform all routine maintenance procedures as defined in the IMMULITE® Operator's Manual.

See the IMMULITE® Operator's Manual for: Preparation, setup, dilutions, adjustment, assay and quality control procedures.

Visually inspect each Test Unit for the presence of a bead before loading it onto the system.

Adjustment Interval: 2 Weeks.

Quality Control Samples: Use controls or sample pools with at least two levels (low and high) of canine TSH.

Test Interpretation: Expected Values: Based on its relation to DPC's Coat-a-Count Canine TSH assay (see the Method Comparison section), the IMMULITE® Canine TSH assay can be expected to have the following approximate reference ranges: Nondetectable to 0.5 ng/mL.

Consider these limits as guidelines only.

Each laboratory should establish its own reference ranges for the diagnostic evaluation of canine results.

Storage: 1 week at 2-8°C or 2 months (aliquotted) at -20°C.

Reagents: Store at 2-8°C. Dispose of in accordance with applicable laws.

Follow universal precautions, and handle all components as if capable of transmitting infectious agents.

Sodium azide, at concentrations less than 0.1 g/dL, has been added as a preservative. On disposal, flush with large volumes of water to prevent the buildup of potentially explosive metal azides in lead and copper plumbing.

Chemiluminescent Substrate: Avoid contamination and exposure to direct sunlight.

Water: Use distilled or deionized water.

Caution(s): For *in vitro* veterinary use.

Trial Data: Performance Data: Results are expressed in ng/mL. (Unless otherwise specified, all results were generated on canine samples collected in tubes without anticoagulants, gel barriers, or clot-promoting additives.)

Calibration Range: Up to 12 ng/mL

Analytical Sensitivity: 0.01 ng/mL

High-dose Hook Effect: None up to 5,000 ng/mL.

Intraassay Precision (Within-Run): Statistics were calculated for samples from the results of 20 replicates in a single run. (See "Intraassay Precision" table.)

Intraassay Precision (ng/mL):

	Mean	SD	CV
1	0.20	0.01	5.0%
2	0.50	0.02	4.0%
3	1.6	0.05	3.1%
4	2.6	0.10	3.8%

Interassay Precision (Run-to-Run): Statistics were calculated for samples assayed in 10 different runs. (See "Interassay Precision" table.)

Interassay Precision (ng/mL):

	Mean	SD	CV
1	0.16	0.01	6.3%
2	0.27	0.02	7.4%
3	2.8	0.23	8.2%

Linearity: Samples were assayed under various dilutions. (See "Linearity" table for representative data.)

Linearity (ng/mL):

	Dilution	Observed	Expected	%O/E
1	16 in 16	5.1	—	—
	8 in 16	2.3	2.6	93%
	4 in 16	1.2	1.3	93%
	2 in 16	0.6	0.6	97%
	1 in 16	0.3	0.3	94%
2	16 in 16	5.96	—	—
	8 in 16	2.9	3.0	97%
	4 in 16	1.5	1.5	101%
	2 in 16	0.8	0.8	102%
	1 in 16	0.4	0.4	102%
3	16 in 16	8.12	—	—
	8 in 16	3.6	4.1	88%
	4 in 16	1.8	2.0	89%
	2 in 16	0.9	1.0	94%
	1 in 16	0.5	0.5	95%

Recovery: Samples spiked 1 to 19 with three TSH solutions (4.3, 8.5 and 18 ng/mL) were assayed. (See "Recovery" table for representative data.)

Recovery (ng/mL):

	Solution	Observed	Expected	%O/E
1	—	0.46	—	—
	A	0.64	0.65	98%
	B	0.75	0.86	87%
	C	1.1	1.3	85%
2	—	2.8	—	—
	A	2.8	2.9	97%
	B	3.0	3.1	97%
	C	3.4	3.6	94%
3	—	5.2	—	—
	A	5.4	5.2	104%
	B	5.5	5.4	102%
	C	5.6	5.8	97%

Specificity: The antibodies used in the IMMULITE® Canine TSH procedure are highly specific for canine TSH, with negligible crossreactivity to related canine pituitary glycoprotein hormones such as FSH, HCG and LH.

Hemolysis: Presence of packed red blood cells in concentrations up to 25 µL/mL has no effect on results, within the precision of the assay.

Lipemia: Presence of lipemia in concentrations up to 5,000 mg/dL has no effect on results, within the precision of the assay.

Method Comparison: The assay was compared to DPC's Coat-A-Count Canine TSH IRMA on 61 canine samples.

(Concentration range: Approximately 0.04 to 9.0 ng/mL. See graph.) By linear regression:

(IML) = 1.00 (CAC IRMA) + 0.02 ng/mL

r = 0.996

Means:

1.39 ng/mL (IMMULITE®)

1.37 ng/mL (CAC IRMA)

Method Comparison:

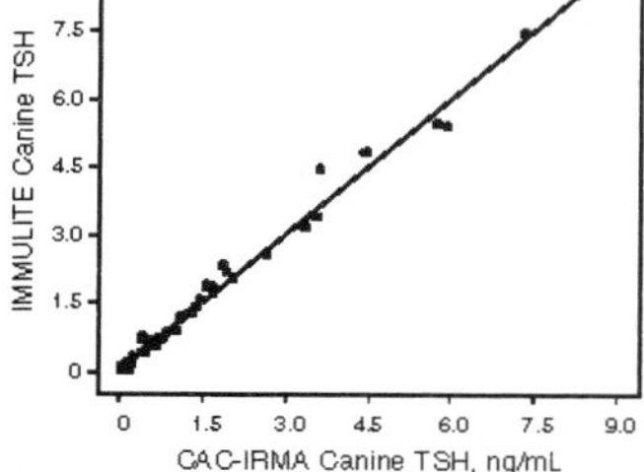

(IML) = 1.00 (CAC IRMA) + 0.02 ng/mL r = 0.996

References: Available upon request.

Presentation: 100 test kit.

Compendium Code No.: 12620010 PILKKT-2

IMMUNOBOOST®

Bioniche Animal Health (formerly Vetrepharm) **Immunostimulant**

Mycobacterium Cell Wall Fraction Immunostimulant

U.S. Vet. Lic. No.: 289

Contents: This product contains the antigen listed above.

Contains gentamicin as a preservative.

Indications: For use in calves, 1 to 5 days of age, as a one-time immunotherapeutic treatment for reduction of mortality and clinical signs associated with calf scours caused by *E. coli* (K99).

Dosage and Administration: Aseptically administer 1 mL intravenously.

Precaution(s): Store at 2-7°C (35-45°F). Use entire contents when first opened.

Caution(s): In case of anaphylaxis, administer epinephrine.

For use by or under the direction of a licensed veterinarian.

Warning(s): Do not inoculate within 21 days of slaughter.

Presentation: 5 dose (5 mL) and 20 dose (20 mL) multi-vials.

U.S. Patent No. 4,744,984

Compendium Code No.: 11070031

IMMUNO-GLO NEP

Mg Biologics **Equine Plasma**

Normal Equine Plasma

Contents: IMMUNO-GLO NEP is collected in a sterile closed system from healthy horses testing negative for the antibodies against Aa, Ca, and Qa red cell antigens. Sodium citrate is used as an anticoagulant as part of the manufacturing process. It is frozen immediately after collection and as such does not contain preservatives.

Indications: IMMUNO-GLO NEP is for IV administration in situations requiring fluid replacement or protein supplementation.

Dosage and Administration: IMMUNO-GLO NEP requires freezing until used. To thaw submerge the frozen plasma in warm water (<115°F) for 10 minutes, squeezing the bag periodically to circulate for faster thawing. Warm the liquid plasma to body temperature using the warm water bath. Do not microwave this product. Administer with an IV administration kit with filter. Dose at a rate of 20 mL/kg of body weight (approximately 10 mL/lb). Caution should be observed however, as occasionally intravenous infusion may result in shaking, sweating or hyperventilation. If this occurs, discontinue use for 5 to 10 minutes. Resume at a slower rate of infusion. If adverse reactions persist, discontinue use.

Caution(s): Each serial is tested for endotoxin and sold after clearance through Quality Assurance. While this plasma has been reviewed and found to be safe, there is always the possibility, while rare, of transmission of viral disease. Every reasonable precaution has been take to safeguard this product.

Presentation: 1,000 mL (other sizes available upon request).

Compendium Code No.: 12600011

IMMUNOREGULIN®

Neogen **Immunostimulant**

Propionibacterium Acnes, Immunostimulant

U.S. Vet. Lic. No.: 302

Active Ingredient(s): IMMUNOREGULIN® is a preparation consisting of 0.4 mg/mL non-viable *Propionibacterium acnes* suspended in 12.5% ethanol in saline.

Indications: For use as an adjunct to antibiotic therapy in controlling and reducing the lesions of chronic recurrent pyoderma in the dog.

Dosage and Administration: Administration: IMMUNOREGULIN® must be administered by the intravenous (IV) route. Shake well to obtain the uniform suspension.

Dosage: Two injections per week for the first two weeks followed by one injection per week until the 12th week; thereafter, once a month until symptoms abate or stabilize.

Recommended Dosage:

Weight Range	Dose
Up to 15 lbs.	0.25 mL
15 to 45 lbs.	0.50 mL
45 to 75 lbs.	1.00 mL
75 lbs. or greater	2.00 mL

Contraindication(s): The therapeutic effect of the immunostimulant may be compromised if used with glucocorticoids. Steroid therapy should be withdrawn at least seven days before initiating the immunostimulant therapy.

Precaution(s): Store at room temperature until first used then store at 2-7°C (35-45°F). Do not freeze.

Caution(s): The effects of this product have not been studied in pregnant animals. Do not use when pregnancy is suspected or a suspected cardiac condition exists. There may be a minor rise in temperature, chills, temporary inappetance, or sluggishness a few hours after injection.

Anaphylactic reactions may occur.

IMMUNOREGULIN® is restricted to use by, or under the supervision of, a veterinarian.

For veterinary use only.

Antidote(s): Epinephrine.

Presentation: 5 mL vials.

Compendium Code No.: 14910301 TC-11/0898

IMPROVED HOOF DRESSING

Fiebing **Hoof Product**

Active Ingredient(s): Mineral oil, soyoil, gilsonite, and less than 1% cresol complex added as a preservative.

Indications: For use as an aid in the treatment of split hoofs, corns, quarter cracks, hard, dry, brittle, tender and contracted feet.

Dosage and Administration: Wash the hoof thoroughly. Apply the dressing with a brush and work well into the edge of the hair (coronet) and frog. For the best results, use two (2) or three (3) times a week.

Caution(s): Keep out of the reach of children.

Presentation: 32 fl. oz. (1 qt.) and 1 gallon with or without applicator.

Compendium Code No.: 10590012

IMRAB® 1

Merial **Vaccine**
Rabies Vaccine, Killed Virus-(Rabies 1 Year)
U.S. Vet. Lic. No.: 298
Description: IMRAB® 1 contains the same virus strain that is used in the Pasteur Merieux Connaught human vaccine. The virus is grown in a stable cell line, inactivated, and mixed with a safe and potent adjuvant. Safety and immunogenicity of this product have been demonstrated by vaccination and challenge tests in susceptible animals.
Contains gentamicin as a preservative.
Indications: IMRAB® 1 is recommended for the vaccination of healthy dogs and cats 12 weeks of age and older for prevention of disease due to rabies virus.
Dosage and Administration: Aseptically inject 1 mL (1 dose) subcutaneously into healthy dogs and cats. Revaccinate annually.
Precaution(s): Store at 2-7°C (35-45°F). Do not freeze. Shake well before using. Use entire contents when first opened. Do not use chemicals to sterilize syringes and needles.
Caution(s): A transient local reaction may occur at the injection site following subcutaneous administration.
Some reports suggest that in cats, the administration of certain veterinary biologicals may induce the development of injection site fibrosarcomas. In rare instances, administration of vaccines may cause lethargy, fever, and inflammatory or hypersensitivity types of reactions. Treatment may include antihistamines, anti-inflammatories, and/or epinephrine.
For veterinary use only.
Presentation: 5 x 10 doses (10 mL).
Sold to veterinarians only.
IMRAB is a registered trademark of Merial.
Compendium Code No.: 11110271 RM384R6

IMRAB® 3

Merial **Vaccine**
Rabies Vaccine, Killed Virus-(Rabies 3 Year)
U.S. Vet. Lic. No.: 298
Description: IMRAB® 3 contains the same virus strain that is used in the Pasteur Merieux Connaught human vaccine. The virus is grown in a stable cell line, inactivated, and mixed with a safe and potent adjuvant. Safety and immunogenicity of this product have been demonstrated by vaccination and challenge tests in susceptible animals.
Contains gentamicin as a preservative.
Indications: IMRAB® 3 is recommended for the vaccination of healthy cats, dogs, sheep, cattle, horses, and ferrets 12 weeks of age and older for prevention of disease due to rabies virus.
Dosage and Administration: Aseptically inject 1 mL (1 dose) subcutaneously or intramuscularly into healthy cats or dogs; 2 mL into healthy sheep, cattle, and horses. Inject 1 mL subcutaneously into healthy ferrets. Revaccinate ferrets, cattle, and horses annually; cats, dogs, and sheep 1 year after first vaccination, then every 3 years.
Precaution(s): Store at 2-7°C (35-45°F). Do not freeze. Shake well before using. Use entire contents when first opened. Do not use chemicals to sterilize syringes and needles.
Caution(s): A transient local reaction may occur at the injection site following subcutaneous administration. Some reports suggest that in cats, the administration of certain veterinary biologicals may induce the development of injection site fibrosarcomas. In rare instances, administration of vaccines may cause lethargy, fever, and inflammatory or hypersensitivity types of reactions. Treatment may include antihistamines, anti-inflammatories, and/or epinephrine.
For veterinary use only.
Warning(s): Do not vaccinate food producing animals within 21 days prior to slaughter.
Presentation: 50 x 1 dose (1 mL) vials (for cats, dogs, and ferrets only).
5 x 10 dose (10 mL) vials.
Sold to veterinarians only.
IMRAB is a registered trademark of Merial.
Compendium Code No.: 11110281 RM949R6 / RM959R5

IMRAB® LARGE ANIMAL

Merial **Vaccine**
Rabies Vaccine, Killed Virus
U.S. Vet. Lic. No.: 298
Contents: This product contains the antigen listed above.
Contains gentamicin as a preservative.
Indications: IMRAB® Bovine Plus is recommended for the vaccination of healthy cattle, horses and sheep against rabies viruses.
Dosage and Administration: Aseptically inject 2 mL subcutaneously or intramuscularly into healthy sheep, cattle or horses when 3 months of age or older. Revaccinate cattle and horses annually and sheep one year after the first vaccination, then every 3 years.
Precaution(s): Store at 2-7°C (35-45°F). Shake well before using. Do not freeze. Use entire contents when first opened.
Caution(s): In case of anaphylactic reaction, administer epinephrine.
For veterinary use only.
Warning(s): Do not vaccinate within 21 days of slaughter.
Presentation: 25 dose (50 mL) vials.
IMRAB is a registered trademark of Merial.
Compendium Code No.: 11110292 RM569R6

INACTI/VAC® AE

L.A.H.I. (Maine Biological) **Vaccine**
Avian Encephalomyelitis Vaccine, Killed Virus, Oil Emulsion
U.S. Vet. Lic. No.: 196
Active Ingredient(s): INACTI/VAC® AE is produced with a high titering strain of avian encephalomyelitis (AE) virus, suspended in a stable oil emulsion.
Indications: Recommended for the immunization of chickens and turkeys against avian encephalomyelitis.
Dosage and Administration: The vaccine should be warmed to room temperature before use. Shake well before using. Inject subcutaneously in the lower neck region using aseptic technique.
Inject all of the birds in the flock with ½ mL (0.5 mL) per bird.
Vaccinate between 16 and 24 weeks of age, but the vaccine can safely be given after birds are in production if necessary. Do not vaccinate before 12 weeks of age. Revaccinate during molt.
This is a killed virus vaccine. There is no danger of spread to susceptible birds, or of egg transmission of the virus.
Precaution(s): Store below 45°F (7°C). Do not freeze.
Caution(s): Use the entire contents of the bottle when first opened.
Warning(s): Do not vaccinate within 42 days before slaughter.
Presentation: 1,000 dose (500 mL) bottles.
Compendium Code No.: 11030132

INACTI/VAC® BD

L.A.H.I. (Maine Biological) **Vaccine**
Bursal Disease Vaccine, Killed Virus, Oil Emulsion
U.S. Vet. Lic. No.: 196
Active Ingredient(s): INACTI/VAC® BD is produced with a high titering strain of infectious bursal disease (IBD) virus, suspended in a stable oil emulsion. It contains the type 1 IBD virus.
Indications: Recommended for the immunization of breeder hens and replacements against infectious bursal disease.
Dosage and Administration: The vaccine should be warmed to room temperature before use. Shake well before using. Inject subcutaneously in the lower neck region using aseptic technique.
Inject all of the birds in the flock with ½ mL (0.5 mL) per bird.
Vaccinate with live virus bursal disease vaccine at least 4 weeks prior to the use of this vaccine. Vaccinate between 16 and 20 weeks of age. Revaccinate during molt.
This is a killed virus vaccine. There is no danger of spread to susceptible birds, or of egg transmission of the virus.
Precaution(s): Store below 45°F (7°C). Do not freeze.
Caution(s): Use the entire contents of the bottle when first opened.
Warning(s): Do not vaccinate within 42 days before slaughter.
Presentation: 1,000 dose (500 mL) bottles.
Compendium Code No.: 11030142

INACTI/VAC® BD-ND

L.A.H.I. (Maine Biological) **Vaccine**
Bursal Disease-Newcastle Disease Vaccine, Killed Virus, Oil Emulsion
U.S. Vet. Lic. No.: 196
Active Ingredient(s): INACTI/VAC® BD-ND is produced with high titering strains of Newcastle disease and infectious bursal disease (IBD) viruses, suspended in a stable oil emulsion.
Indications: Recommended for the immunization of breeder hens and replacements against infectious bursal disease and Newcastle disease.
Dosage and Administration: The vaccine should be warmed to room temperature before use. Shake well before using. Inject subcutaneously in the lower neck region using aseptic technique.
Inject all of the birds in the flock with ½ mL (0.5 mL) per bird.
Vaccinate with live virus bursal disease vaccine and Newcastle disease vaccine at least 4 weeks prior to the use of this vaccine. Vaccinate between 16 and 20 weeks of age. Revaccinate during molt.
This is a killed virus vaccine. There is no danger of spread to susceptible birds, or of egg transmission of the virus.
Precaution(s): Store below 45°F (7°C). Do not freeze.
Caution(s): Use the entire contents of the bottle when first opened.
Warning(s): Do not vaccinate within 42 days before slaughter.
Presentation: 1,000 dose (500 mL) bottles.
Compendium Code No.: 11030152

INACTI/VAC® BD-ND-FC3

L.A.H.I. (Maine Biological) **Bacterin-Vaccine**
Bursal Disease-Newcastle Disease Vaccine, Killed Virus-Pasteurella Multocida Bacterin, Avian Isolates, Types 1, 3 & 4
U.S. Vet. Lic. No.: 196
Contents: This product contains the antigens listed above.
Indications: Recommended for the vaccination of chickens against infectious bursal disease, and for the vaccination of chickens and turkeys against Newcastle disease and fowl cholera caused by *Pasteurella multocida*, Type 1 in chickens and Types 3 and 4 in turkeys.
Directions for Use: The vaccine should be warmed to room temperature before use.
Shake well before using.
Inject subcutaneously in the lower neck region using aseptic technique.
Dose—½ mL (0.5 mL) per bird.
Inject all birds in flock.
Vaccinate chickens (prime) with live virus vaccines for bursal disease, and chickens and turkeys against Newcastle disease and with *Pasteurella multocida* bacterin at least 4 weeks prior to use of this vaccine. Vaccinate chickens between 16 and 20 weeks of age. Vaccinate turkeys between 24 and 30 weeks of age. Revaccinate during molt.
Precaution(s): Store below 45°F (7°C). Do not freeze. Use entire contents of bottle when first opened.
Caution(s): In case of accidental human injection seek immediate medical attention.
Warning(s): Do not vaccinate within 42 days before slaughter.
Presentation: 1000 dose (500 mL) bottles.
Compendium Code No.: 11030163

INACTI/VAC® BD3

L.A.H.I. (Maine Biological) **Vaccine**
Bursal Disease Vaccine, Killed Virus, Standard & Variant, Oil Emulsion
U.S. Vet. Lic. No.: 196
Active Ingredient(s): INACTI/VAC® BD3 is produced with high titering strains of infectious bursal disease (IBD) viruses, suspended in a stable oil emulsion. It is a quadrivalent vaccine containing the Delaware variant A and E, and the Maryland isolates, all three of which are variant IBD strains, in addition to the standard type 1 IBD virus. Variant E is of bursal tissue origin.
Indications: Recommended for the immunization of breeder hens and replacements against infectious bursal disease, type 1 standard, and variant strains.
Dosage and Administration: The vaccine should be warmed to room temperature before use. Shake well before using. Inject subcutaneously in the lower neck region using aseptic technique.
Inject all of the birds in the flock with ½ mL (0.5 mL) per bird.
Vaccinate with live virus bursal disease vaccine at least 4 weeks prior to the use of this vaccine. Vaccinate between 16 and 20 weeks of age. Revaccinate during molt.

This is a killed virus vaccine. There is no danger of spread to susceptible birds, or of egg transmission of the virus.
Precaution(s): Store below 45°F (7°C). Do not freeze.
Caution(s): Use the entire contents of the bottle when first opened.
Warning(s): Do not vaccinate within 42 days before slaughter.
Presentation: 1,000 dose (500 mL) bottles.
Compendium Code No.: 11030172

INACTI/VAC® BD3-IB2-REO

L.A.H.I. (Maine Biological) **Vaccine**
Bronchitis-Bursal Disease-Reovirus Vaccine, Mass. & Ark. Types, Standard & Variant, Killed Virus
U.S. Vet. Lic. No.: 196
Contents: This product contains the antigens listed above.
Indications: Recommended for the vaccination of breeder hens and replacement pullets against infectious bronchitis (Mass. and Ark. Types) and to passively protect the progeny of vaccinated hens against infectious bursal disease (standard and variant strains) and reovirus malabsorption syndrome.
Dosage and Administration: Vaccine should be warmed to room temperature before use.
Shake well before using.
Inject subcutaneously in the lower neck region using aseptic technique.
Dose - ½ mL (0.5 mL) per bird.
Inject all birds in flock.
Vaccinate (prime) with live virus vaccines for bursal disease, bronchitis and tenosynovitis at least 4 weeks prior to the use of this vaccine. Vaccinate between 16 and 20 weeks of age. Revaccinate during molt.
Precaution(s): Store below 45°F (7°C). Do not freeze.
Caution(s): Use entire contents of bottle when first opened.
Warning(s): Do not vaccinate within 42 days before slaughter.
In case of accidental human injection seek immediate medical attention.
Presentation: 1,000 dose (500 mL) bottles.
Compendium Code No.: 11030412

INACTI/VAC® BD3-ND

L.A.H.I. (Maine Biological) **Vaccine**
Bursal Disease-Newcastle Disease Vaccine, Killed Virus, Standard & Variant, Oil Emulsion
U.S. Vet. Lic. No.: 196
Active Ingredient(s): INACTI/VAC® BD3-ND is produced with high titering strains of Newcastle disease and infectious bursal disease (IBD) viruses, suspended in a stable oil emulsion. It is a quadrivalent IBD vaccine containing the Delaware variants A and E, and the Maryland isolate, all of which are variant IBD strains, in addition to the standard type 1 IBD virus.
Indications: Recommended for the immunization of breeder hens and replacements against infectious bursal disease (type 1 standard and variant strains), and Newcastle disease.
Dosage and Administration: The vaccine should be warmed to room temperature before use. Shake well before using. Inject subcutaneously in the lower neck region using aseptic technique.
Inject all of the birds in the flock with ½ mL (0.5 mL) per bird.
Vaccinate with live virus bursal disease vaccine and Newcastle disease vaccine at least 4 weeks prior to the use of this vaccine. Vaccinate between 16 and 20 weeks of age. Revaccinate during molt.
This is a killed virus vaccine. There is no danger of spread to susceptible birds, or of egg transmission of the virus.
Precaution(s): Store below 45°F (7°C). Do not freeze.
Caution(s): Use the entire contents of the bottle when first opened.
Warning(s): Do not vaccinate within 42 days before slaughter.
Presentation: 1,000 dose (500 mL) bottles.
Compendium Code No.: 11030182

INACTI/VAC® BD3-ND-IB1-REO

L.A.H.I. (Maine Biological) **Vaccine**
Bursal Disease-Newcastle Disease-Bronchitis-Reovirus Vaccine, Standard & Variant, Mass. Type, Killed Virus
U.S. Vet. Lic. No.: 196
Contents: This product contains the antigens listed above.
Indications: Recommended for the vaccination of breeder hens and replacement pullets against Newcastle disease and infectious bronchitis (Mass. Type) and to provide maternal antibodies for the early protection of progeny against reovirus related malabsorption syndrome and tenosynovitis and to type 1, infectious bursal disease, standard and variant strains.
Directions for Use: Vaccine should be warmed to room temperature before use.
Shake well before using.
Inject subcutaneously in the lower neck region using aseptic technique.
Dose - ½ mL (0.5 mL) per bird. Inject all birds in flock.
Vaccinate (prime) with live virus vaccines for bursal disease, Newcastle disease, bronchitis and tenosynovitis at least 4 weeks prior to the use of this vaccine. Vaccinate between 16 and 20 weeks of age. Revaccinate during molt.
Precaution(s): Store below 45°F (7°C). Do not freeze.
Use entire contents of bottle when first opened.
Warning(s): Do not vaccinate within 42 days before slaughter.
In case of accidental human injection seek immediate medical attention.
Presentation: 1000 dose (500 mL) bottles.
Compendium Code No.: 11030192

INACTI/VAC® BD3-ND-IB2

L.A.H.I. (Maine Biological) **Vaccine**
Bursal Disease-Newcastle Disease-Bronchitis Vaccine, Killed Virus, Standard & Variant, Mass.-Ark. Type, Oil Emulsion
U.S. Vet. Lic. No.: 196
Active Ingredient(s): INACTI/VAC® BD3-ND-IB2 is produced with a high titering strain of Newcastle disease and two strains of infectious bronchitis virus. Whereas there is very poor cross protection between the different bronchitis strains, this vaccine contains the Massachusetts and Arkansas strains of IB virus, the Massachusetts and Arkansas strains of IB virus. These are the two most serious and common strains that infect flocks in the U.S. It also contains four IBD strains; the standard type 1 strain and the Delaware variants A and E, and Maryland strain, the three of which are variant IBD strains.
Indications: Recommended for the immunization of breeder hens and replacement pullets to give broad protection against Newcastle disease, and infectious bronchitis (Mass. and Ark. types) and to provide maternal antibodies for the early protection of their progeny against Type 1 infectious bursal disease (Gumboro disease) standard and variant strains.
Dosage and Administration: The vaccine should be warmed to room temperature before use. Shake well before using. Inject subcutaneously in the lower neck region using aseptic technique.
Inject all of the birds in the flock with ½ mL (0.5 mL) per bird.
Birds should be primed with live virus Newcastle-Bronchitis vaccine at 10 to 14 days and at 12 weeks of age and with mild or intermediate strains of live virus IBD vaccine at 21 days and 12 weeks of age. Vaccinate with INACTI/VAC® BD3-ND-IB2 between 16 and 20 weeks of age.
Revaccinate during molt.
This is a killed virus vaccine. There is no danger of spread to susceptible birds.
Precaution(s): Store below 45°F (7°C). Do not freeze.
Caution(s): Use the entire contents of the bottle when first opened.
Warning(s): Do not vaccinate within 42 days before slaughter.
Presentation: 1,000 dose (500 mL) bottles.
Compendium Code No.: 11030202

INACTI/VAC® BD3-ND-IB2-REO

L.A.H.I. (Maine Biological) **Vaccine**
Bursal Disease-Newcastle-Bronchitis-Reovirus Vaccine, Standard & Variant, Mass. & Ark. Types, Killed Virus
U.S. Vet. Lic. No.: 196
Active Ingredient(s): INACTI/VAC® BD3-ND-IB2-REO is produced with a high titering strain of Newcastle disease virus. Whereas there is very poor cross protection between the different bronchitis strains, this vaccine contains the Massachusetts and Arkansas strains of IB virus. These are the two most serious and common strains that infect flocks in the U.S.
It contains two reovirus strains; the S1133 (a tenosynovitis pathotype) and the 1733 strain (a malabsorption syndrome pathotype). It also contains four IBD strains; the standard type 1 strain and the Delaware variants A and E, and Maryland strain, the last three of which are variant IBD strains.
Indications: Recommended for the immunization of breeder hens and replacement pullets to give broad protection against Newcastle disease and infectious bronchitis (Mass. and Ark. types) and to provide maternal antibodies for the early protection of progeny against reovirus related malabsorption syndrome and tenosynovitis and to Type 1 infectious bursal disease (Gumboro disease) standard and variant strains.
Dosage and Administration: The vaccine should be warmed to room temperature before use. Shake well before using. Inject subcutaneously in the lower neck region using aseptic technique.
Inject all of the birds in the flock with ½ mL (0.5 mL) per bird.
Birds should be primed with live virus Newcastle-Bronchitis vaccine at 10 to 14 days and 12 weeks of age. Prime with attenuated live virus tenosynovitis vaccine at 7 days and at 12 weeks of age. Prime with mild or intermediate strains of live virus IBD vaccine at 21 days and 12 weeks of age. Vaccination with INACTI/VAC® BD3-ND-IB2-REO between 16 and 20 weeks of age.
Revaccinate during molt.
Precaution(s): Store below 45°F (7°C). Do not freeze.
Caution(s): Use the entire contents of the bottle when first opened.
Warning(s): Do not vaccinate within 42 days before slaughter.
Presentation: 1,000 dose (500 mL) bottles.
Compendium Code No.: 11030212

INACTI/VAC® BD3-ND-REO

L.A.H.I. (Maine Biological) **Vaccine**
Bursal Disease-Newcastle Disease-Reovirus Vaccine, Killed Virus, Standard & Variant, Oil Emulsion
U.S. Vet. Lic. No.: 196
Active Ingredient(s): INACTI/VAC® BD3-ND-REO is produced with a high titering strain of Newcastle disease virus. It contains two reovirus strains; the S1133 strain (a tenosynovitis pathotype) and the 1733 strain (a malabsorption syndrome pathotype). It also contains four IBD strains; the standard type 1 strain and the Delaware variants A and E, and Maryland strain, the last three of which are variant IBD strains.
Indications: Recommended for the immunization of breeder hens and replacement pullets to give broad protection against Newcastle disease and to provide maternal antibodies for the early protection of progeny against reovirus related malabsorption syndrome and tenosynovitis and to Type a infectious bursal disease (Gumboro disease), standard and variant strains.
Dosage and Administration: The vaccine should be warmed to room temperature before use. Shake well before using. Inject subcutaneously in the lower neck region using aseptic technique.
Birds should be primed with live virus Newcastle vaccine at 10 to 14 days and at 12 weeks of age. Prime with attenuated live virus tenosynovitis vaccine at 7 days and at 12 weeks of age. Prime with mild or intermediate strains of live virus IBD vaccine at 21 days and 12 weeks of age. Vaccinate with INACTI/VAC® BD3-ND-REO between 16 and 20 weeks of age. Revaccinate during molt.
This is a killed virus vaccine. There is no danger of spread to susceptible birds.
Precaution(s): Store below 45°F (7°C). Do not freeze.
Caution(s): Use the entire contents of the bottle when first opened.
Warning(s): Do not vaccinate within 42 days before slaughter.
Presentation: 1,000 dose (500 mL) bottles.
Compendium Code No.: 11030222

INACTI/VAC® BD3-REO

L.A.H.I. (Maine Biological) **Vaccine**
Avian Reovirus-Bursal Disease Vaccine, Killed Virus, Standard & Variant, Oil Emulsion
U.S. Vet. Lic. No.: 196
Active Ingredient(s): Produced with high titering strains of avian reovirus and infectious bursal disease (IBD) viruses, suspended in a stable oil emulsion. It contains two reovirus strains: the S1133 strain (a tenosynovitis pathotype) and the 1733 strain (a malabsorption syndrome pathotype), as well as BTO Variant E IBD.
Indications: Recommended for the immunization of breeder hens and replacement pullets to give broad protection against avian reovirus and Type 1 infectious bursal disease (Gumboro disease), standard and variant strains.

Dosage and Administration: The vaccine should be warmed to room temperature before use. Shake well before using. Inject subcutaneously in the lower neck region using aseptic technique.

Inject all of the birds in the flock with ½ mL (0.5 mL) per bird.

Birds should be primed with attenuated live virus vaccines for tenosynovitis and with mild or intermediate strains of bursal disease at least 4 weeks prior to the use of this vaccine. Vaccinate with INACTI/VAC® BD3-REO between 16 and 20 weeks of age.

Revaccinate during molt.

Precaution(s): Store below 45°F (7°C). Do not freeze.

Caution(s): Use the entire contents of the bottle when first opened.

Warning(s): Do not vaccinate within 42 days before slaughter.

Presentation: 1,000 dose (500 mL) bottles.

Compendium Code No.: 11030232

INACTI/VAC® BTO1

L.A.H.I. (Maine Biological) **Vaccine**

Bursal Disease Vaccine, Killed Virus

U.S. Vet. Lic. No.: 196

Contents: This product contains the antigen listed above.

Indications: Recommended for the vaccination of breeder hens and replacement pullets to provide maternal antibodies for the early protection of the progeny against type 1 infectious bursal disease, standard strain.

Directions for Use: Vaccine should be warmed to room temperature before use.

Shake well before using.

Inject subcutaneously in the lower neck region using aseptic technique.

Dose - ½ mL (0.5 mL) per bird. Inject all birds in flock.

Vaccinate (prime) with live virus vaccines for bursal disease at least 4 weeks prior to the use of this vaccine. Vaccinate between 12 and 20 weeks of age. Revaccinate during molt.

Precaution(s): Store below 45°F (7°C). Do not freeze.

Use entire contents of bottle when first opened.

Warning(s): Do not vaccinate within 42 days before slaughter.

In case of accidental human injection seek immediate medical attention.

Presentation: 1000 dose (500 mL) bottles.

Compendium Code No.: 11030242

INACTI/VAC® BTO1-ND-IB

L.A.H.I. (Maine Biological) **Vaccine**

Bursal Disease-Newcastle Disease-Bronchitis Vaccine, Mass. Type, Killed Virus

U.S. Vet. Lic. No.: 196

Contents: This product contains the antigens listed above.

Indications: Recommended for the vaccination of breeder hens and replacement pullets against Newcastle disease and infectious bronchitis (Mass. Type) and to provide maternal antibodies for the early protection of progeny against type 1, infectious bursal disease, standard strain.

Directions for Use: Vaccine should be warmed to room temperature before use.

Shake well before using.

Inject subcutaneously in the lower neck region using aseptic technique.

Dose - ½ mL (0.5 mL) per bird. Inject all birds in flock.

Vaccinate (prime) with live virus vaccines for bursal disease, Newcastle disease and bronchitis at least 4 weeks prior to the use of this vaccine. Vaccinate between 12 and 20 weeks of age. Revaccinate during molt.

Precaution(s): Store below 45°F (7°C). Do not freeze.

Use entire contents of bottle when first opened.

Warning(s): Do not vaccinate within 42 days before slaughter.

In case of accidental human injection seek immediate medical attention.

Presentation: 1000 dose (500 mL) bottles.

Compendium Code No.: 11030252

INACTI/VAC® BTO1-ND-IB-REO

L.A.H.I. (Maine Biological) **Vaccine**

Bursal Disease-Newcastle Disease-Bronchitis-Reovirus Vaccine, Mass. Type, Killed Virus

U.S. Vet. Lic. No.: 196

Contents: This product contains the antigens listed above.

Indications: Recommended for the vaccination of breeder hens and replacement pullets against Newcastle disease and infectious bronchitis (Mass. Type) and to provide maternal antibodies for the early protection of progeny against reovirus related malabsorption syndrome and tenosynovitis and to type 1, infectious bursal disease, standard strain.

Directions for Use: Vaccine should be warmed to room temperature before use.

Shake well before using.

Inject subcutaneously in the lower neck region using aseptic technique.

Dose - ½ mL (0.5 mL) per bird. Inject all birds in flock.

Vaccinate (prime) with live virus vaccines for bursal disease, Newcastle disease, bronchitis and tenosynovitis at least 4 weeks prior to the use of this vaccine. Vaccinate between 12 and 20 weeks of age. Revaccinate during molt.

Precaution(s): Store below 45°F (7°C). Do not freeze.

Use entire contents of bottle when first opened.

Warning(s): Do not vaccinate within 42 days before slaughter.

In case of accidental human injection seek immediate medical attention.

Presentation: 1000 dose (500 mL) bottles.

Compendium Code No.: 11030262

INACTI/VAC® BTO1-ND-REO

L.A.H.I. (Maine Biological) **Vaccine**

Bursal Disease-Newcastle Disease-Reovirus Vaccine, Killed Virus

U.S. Vet. Lic. No.: 196

Contents: This product contains the antigens listed above.

Indications: Recommended for the vaccination of breeder hens and replacement pullets against Newcastle disease and to provide maternal antibodies for the early protection of progeny against reovirus related malabsorption syndrome and tenosynovitis and to type 1, infectious bursal disease, standard strain.

Directions for Use: Vaccine should be warmed to room temperature before use.

Shake well before using.

Inject subcutaneously in the lower neck region using aseptic technique.

Dose - ½ mL (0.5 mL) per bird. Inject all birds in flock.

Vaccinate (prime) with live virus vaccines for bursal disease, Newcastle disease, and tenosynovitis at least 4 weeks prior to the use of this vaccine. Vaccinate between 12 and 20 weeks of age. Revaccinate during molt.

Precaution(s): Store below 45°F (7°C). Do not freeze.

Use entire contents of bottle when first opened.

Warning(s): Do not vaccinate within 42 days before slaughter.

In case of accidental human injection seek immediate medical attention.

Presentation: 1000 dose (500 mL) bottles.

Compendium Code No.: 11030272

INACTI/VAC® BTO1-REO

L.A.H.I. (Maine Biological) **Vaccine**

Bursal Disease-Reovirus Vaccine, Killed Virus

U.S. Vet. Lic. No.: 196

Contents: This product contains the antigens listed above.

Indications: Recommended for the vaccination of breeder hens and replacement pullets to provide maternal antibodies for the early protection of progeny against reovirus related malabsorption syndrome and tenosynovitis and type 1 infectious bursal disease, standard strain.

Directions for Use: Vaccine should be warmed to room temperature before use.

Shake well before using.

Inject subcutaneously in the lower neck region using aseptic technique.

Dose - ½ mL (0.5 mL) per bird. Inject all birds in flock.

Vaccinate (prime) with live virus tenosynovitis and bursal disease vaccines at least 4 weeks prior to the use of this vaccine. Vaccinate between 12 and 20 weeks of age. Revaccinate during molt.

Precaution(s): Store below 45°F (7°C). Do not freeze.

Use entire contents of bottle when first opened.

Warning(s): Do not vaccinate within 42 days before slaughter.

In case of accidental human injection seek immediate medical attention.

Presentation: 1000 dose (500 mL) bottles.

Compendium Code No.: 11030282

INACTI/VAC® BTO2

L.A.H.I. (Maine Biological) **Vaccine**

Bursal Disease Vaccine, BTO Standard and Variant, Killed Virus, Oil Emulsion

U.S. Vet. Lic. No.: 196

Contents: Bursal disease vaccine, BTO standard and variant, killed virus in an oil emulsion.

Indications: For use in breeder hens and replacement pullets to give broad protection against Type 1, infectious bursal disease (Gumboro disease), standard and variant strains. When injected, the vaccine produces high levels of circulating antibodies (humoral immunity) which are maintained throughout the production cycle. This provides high levels of parental immunity in the progeny, which provides protection during the critical first few days of life. Early infection with IBD causes permanent damage to the immune system, leaving the flock susceptible to many other diseases.

Dosage and Administration: Birds should be "primed" with mild or intermediate strains of live virus IBD vaccine at least 4 weeks prior to the use of this vaccine. Vaccinate with INACTI/VAC® BTO2 between 12 and 20 weeks of age. If birds are being held for a second year, revaccinate during molt. Dosage is ½ mL (0.5 mL) per bird. INACTI/VAC® BTO2 is also available, upon request, in a concentrated form. The same amount of antigen per dose is provided in a ¼ mL (0.25 mL) dose size. The vaccine should be warmed to room temperature before using. Inject subcutaneously in the lower neck region using aseptic technique. Inject all birds in flock.

Precaution(s): Store below 45°F (7°C). Do not freeze. Use the entire contents of the bottle when first opened.

Warning(s): Do not vaccinate within 42 days before slaughter.

Discussion: INACTI/VAC® BTO2 is produced with high titering strains of infectious bursal disease (IBD) viruses, suspended in a stable oil emulsion. The vaccine contains bursal tissue origin (BTO) Delaware variant E and BTO standard strain IBD viruses. Large amounts of all antigens are provided in a ½ mL dose. When injected, the oil emulsion controls the absorption of the virus and greatly enhances the development of high levels of long lasting immunity.

INACTI/VAC® BTO2 is completely safe because it contains no living virus and it can be safely administered at any age. It cannot spread from vaccinated to susceptible flocks. It provides high and persistent levels of antibody in the breeder hens to provide parental immunity to the progeny. IBD immunity is delivered to the farm with the chicks.

Presentation: 1000 dose (500 mL) polypropylene bottles.

Compendium Code No.: 11030292

INACTI/VAC® BTO2-ND-IB2-REO

L.A.H.I. (Maine Biological) **Vaccine**

Bursal Disease-Newcastle Disease-Bronchitis-Reovirus Vaccine, Standard & Variant, Mass. & Ark. Types, Killed Virus

U.S. Vet. Lic. No.: 196

Contents: This product contains the antigens listed above.

Indications: Recommended for the vaccination of breeder hens and replacement pullets against Newcastle disease and infectious bronchitis (Mass. and Ark. Types) and to provide maternal antibodies for the early protection of progeny against reovirus related malabsorption syndrome and tenosynovitis and to type 1, infectious bursal disease, standard and variant strains.

Dosage and Administration: Vaccine should be warmed to room temperature before use.

Shake well before using.

Inject subcutaneously in the lower neck region using aseptic technique.

Dose - ½ mL (0.5 mL) per bird.

Inject all birds in flock.

Vaccinate (prime) with live virus vaccines for bursal disease, Newcastle disease, bronchitis and tenosynovitis at least 4 weeks prior to the use of this vaccine. Vaccinate between 16 and 20 weeks of age. Revaccinate during molt.

Precaution(s): Store below 45°F (7°C). Do not freeze.

Caution(s): Use entire contents of bottle when first opened.

Warning(s): Do not vaccinate within 42 days before slaughter.

In case of accidental human injection seek immediate medical attention.

Presentation: 1,000 dose (500 mL) bottles.

Compendium Code No.: 11030302

INACTI/VAC® BTO2-ND-REO

L.A.H.I. (Maine Biological) **Vaccine**

Bursal Disease-Newcastle Disease-Reovirus Vaccine, Standard & Variant, Killed Virus

U.S. Vet. Lic. No.: 196

Contents: This product contains the antigens listed above.

Indications: Recommended for the vaccination of breeder hens and replacement pullets against Newcastle disease and to provide maternal antibodies for the early protection of the progeny against reovirus related malabsorption syndrome and tenosynovitis and to type 1, infectious bursal disease, standard and variant strains.

Dosage and Administration: Vaccine should be warmed to room temperature before use.

Shake well before using.

Inject subcutaneously in the lower neck region using aseptic technique.

Dose - ½ mL (0.5 mL) per bird.

Inject all birds in flock.

Vaccinate (prime) with live virus vaccines for bursal disease, Newcastle disease, and tenosynovitis at least 4 weeks prior to the use of this vaccine. Vaccinate between 16 and 20 weeks of age. Revaccinate during molt.

Precaution(s): Store below 45°F (7°C). Do not freeze.

Caution(s): Use entire contents of bottle when first opened.

Warning(s): Do not vaccinate within 42 days before slaughter.

In case of accidental human injection seek immediate medical attention.

Presentation: 1,000 dose (500 mL) bottles.

Compendium Code No.: 11030312

INACTI/VAC® BTO2-REO

L.A.H.I. (Maine Biological) **Vaccine**

Bursal Disease-Reovirus Vaccine, Standard & Variant, Killed Virus

U.S. Vet. Lic. No.: 196

Contents: This product contains the antigens listed above.

Indications: Recommended for the vaccination of breeder hens and replacement pullets to provide maternal antibodies for the early protection of the progeny against reovirus related malabsorption syndrome and tenosynovitis and type 1 infectious bursal disease, standard and variant strains.

Directions for Use: Vaccine should be warmed to room temperature before use.

Shake well before using.

Inject subcutaneously in the lower neck region using aseptic technique.

Dose - ½ mL (0.5 mL) per bird. Inject all birds in flock.

Vaccinate (prime) with live virus tenosynovitis and bursal disease vaccines at least 4 weeks prior to the use of this vaccine. Vaccinate between 12 and 20 weeks of age. Revaccinate during molt.

Precaution(s): Store below 45°F (7°C). Do not freeze.

Use entire contents of bottle when first opened.

Warning(s): Do not vaccinate within 42 days before slaughter.

In case of accidental human injection seek immediate medical attention.

Presentation: 1000 dose (500 mL) bottles.

Compendium Code No.: 11030322

INACTI-VAC® BTO2-REOC

L.A.H.I. (Maine Biological) **Vaccine**

Bursal Disease-Reovirus Vaccine, Standard & Variant, Killed Virus

U.S. Vet. Lic. No.: 196

Contents: This product contains the antigens listed above.

Indications: Recommended for the vaccination of breeder hens and replacement pullets to provide maternal antibodies for the early protection of the progeny reovirus related malabsorption syndrome tenosynovitis and type 1 infectious bursal disease, standard and variant strains.

Dosage and Administration: Vaccine should be warmed to room temperature before use.

Shake well before using.

Inject subcutaneously in the lower neck region using aseptic technique

Dose - ¼ mL (0.25 mL) per bird.

Inject all birds in flock.

Vaccinate (prime) with live virus tenosynovitis and bursal disease vaccines at least 4 weeks prior to the use of this vaccine. Vaccinate between 12 and 20 weeks of age. Revaccinate during molt.

Precaution(s): Store below 45°F (7°C). Do not freeze.

Use entire contents of bottle when first opened.

Caution(s): In case of accidental human injection seek immediate medical attention.

Warning(s): Do not vaccinate within 42 days before slaughter.

Presentation: 1000 dose (250 mL) bottle.

Compendium Code No.: 11030551

INACTI/VAC® CHICK-ND

L.A.H.I. (Maine Biological) **Vaccine**

Newcastle Disease Vaccine, Killed Virus, Oil Emulsion

U.S. Vet. Lic. No.: 196

Active Ingredient(s): INACTI/VAC® CHICK-ND is produced with a high concentration of a high titering strain of Newcastle disease virus suspended in a stable oil emulsion. When injected, the oil emulsion controls the absorption of the virus and enhances the development of high levels of immunity.

Indications: INACTI/VAC® CHICK-ND has been developed specifically for use in young chicks in geographical areas where highly pathogenic Newcastle disease is endemic. It is recommended that it be injected subcutaneously into one day old chicks and that it be used in conjunction with the Hitchner B1 strain of live virus Newcastle disease vaccine. Depending on the prevalence of Newcastle disease, this vaccination program may be used as late as 10 days of age.

Dosage and Administration: The vaccine should be warmed to room temperature before using. Shake well before using. Inject subcutaneously in the lower neck region using aseptic technique.

Inject all of the birds in the flock with ⅒ mL (0.1 mL) per chick.

When given at 1-10 days of age in conjunction with live virus Newcastle disease vaccine, it neutralizes the parental antibody that is present in the chicks and enables the live virus vaccine to replicate and provide rapid immunity to the chick. This protects the chick until the immune system responds to the killed virus oil emulsion vaccine to provide higher and longer lasting levels of active immunity.

This is a killed virus vaccine. There is no danger of spread to susceptible birds.

Precaution(s): Store below 45°F (7°C). Do not freeze.

Caution(s): Use the entire contents of the bottle when first opened.

Warning(s): Do not vaccinate within 42 days before slaughter.

Presentation: 5,000 dose (500 mL) bottles.

Compendium Code No.: 11030332

INACTI/VAC® FC2

L.A.H.I. (Maine Biological) **Bacterin**

Pasteurella Multocida Bacterin, Avian Isolates, Types 1 & 3x4

U.S. Vet. Lic. No.: 196

Contents: This product contains the antigens listed above.

Indications: Recommended for the vaccination of chickens and turkeys against Fowl Cholera caused by *Pasteurella multocida*, Type 1 in chickens and Type 3x4 in turkeys.

Dosage and Administration: Vaccine should be warmed to room temperature before use.

Shake well before using.

Inject subcutaneously in the lower neck region using aseptic technique.

Dose - ½ mL (0.5 mL) per bird.

Inject all birds in flock.

Vaccinate chickens between 12 and 16 weeks of age. Vaccinate turkeys between 20 and 24 weeks of age. Revaccinate 4 to 6 weeks later. Revaccinate during molt.

If fowl cholera is diagnosed before it has spread throughout the flock, it is often possible to check its spread by immediate vaccination of healthy birds.

Precaution(s): Store below 45°F (7°C). Do not freeze.

Caution(s): Use entire contents of bottle when first opened.

Warning(s): Do not vaccinate within 42 days before slaughter.

In case of accidental human injection seek immediate medical attention.

Presentation: 1,000 dose (500 mL) bottles.

Compendium Code No.: 11030342

INACTI/VAC® FC2C

L.A.H.I. (Maine Biological) **Bacterin**

Pasteurella Multocida Bacterin, Avian Isolates, Types 1 & 3x4

U.S. Vet. Lic. No.: 196

Contents: This product contains the antigens listed above.

Indications: Recommended for the vaccination of chickens and turkeys against Fowl Cholera caused by *Pasteurella multocida*, Type 1 in chickens and Type 3x4 in turkeys.

Dosage and Administration: Vaccine should be warmed to room temperature before use.

Shake well before using.

Inject subcutaneously in the lower neck region using aseptic technique.

Dose - 0.3 mL per bird.

Inject all birds in flock.

Vaccinate chickens between 12 and 16 weeks of age. Vaccinate turkeys between 20 and 24 weeks of age. Revaccinate 4 to 6 weeks later. Revaccinate during molt.

If fowl cholera is diagnosed before it has spread throughout the flock, it is often possible to check its spread by immediate vaccination of healthy birds.

Precaution(s): Store below 45°F (7°C). Do not freeze.

Caution(s): Use entire contents of bottle when first opened.

Warning(s): Do not vaccinate within 42 days before slaughter.

In case of accidental human injection seek immediate medical attention.

Presentation: 1,000 dose (300 mL) bottles.

Compendium Code No.: 11030352

INACTI/VAC® FC3

L.A.H.I. (Maine Biological) **Bacterin**

Pasteurella multocida Bacterin, Avian Isolates, Types 1, 3 & 4, Oil Emulsion

U.S. Vet. Lic. No.: 196

Active Ingredient(s): Produced with three serotypes of *Pasteurella multocida*, Types 1, 3 and 4 that most commonly infect chicken and turkey flocks. High concentrations of these strains are suspended in a stable oil emulsion.

Indications: Recommended for the immunization of chickens and turkeys against fowl cholera caused by *Pasteurella multocida*, Types 1, 3 and 4.

Dosage and Administration: The vaccine should be warmed to room temperature before use. Shake well before using. Inject subcutaneously in the lower neck region using aseptic technique.

Inject all of the birds in the flock with ½ mL (0.5 mL) per bird.

Breeder Hens and Commercial Layers: Vaccinate between 12 and 16 weeks of age. Revaccinate four (4) to six (6) weeks later.

Turkeys: Vaccinate between 20 and 24 weeks of age. Revaccinate 4 to 6 weeks later.

Precaution(s): Store below 45°F (7°C). Do not freeze.

Caution(s): Use the entire contents of the bottle when first opened.

Warning(s): Do not vaccinate within 42 days before slaughter.

Presentation: 1,000 dose (500 mL) bottles.

Compendium Code No.: 11030362

INACTI/VAC® FC3-C

L.A.H.I. (Maine Biological) **Bacterin**

Pasteurella multocida Bacterin, Avian Isolates, Types 1, 3 & 4, Oil Emulsion

U.S. Vet. Lic. No.: 196

Active Ingredient(s): INACTI/VAC® FC3-C is produced with three serotypes of *Pasteurella multocida*, types 1, 3 and 4. These are the serotypes that most commonly infect chicken and turkey flocks. High concentrations of these strains are suspended in a stable oil emulsion. When injected, the oil emulsion concentrate controls the absorption of the antigen and enhances the production of high levels of immunity.

INACTI/VAC® FC3-C has been developed specifically for use in conjunction with autogenous *Pasteurella multocida* bacterin. The same amount of antigen that is used in 1,000 doses (500 mL) of regular Inacti/Vac® FC3 is concentrated into 300 mL of bacterin which is filled into 500 mL bottles. The autogenous bacterin is also produced in a concentrated form with 1,000 doses in 200 mL and filled into 250 mL bottles.

Indications: Recommended for the immunization of chickens and turkeys against fowl cholera caused by *Pasteurella multocida*, types 1, 3 and 4. Two inoculations, given in the late growing period, produce high levels of immunity during the critical early period of production when acute fowl cholera usually occurs.

Dosage and Administration: The vaccine should be warmed to room temperature before use. Shake well before using. Inject subcutaneously in the lower neck region using aseptic technique.

Dose: 0.3 mL per bird. Inject all of the birds in the flock.

Vaccination Recommendation:

Breeder Hens and Commercial Layers: Vaccinate between 12 and 16 weeks of age. Revaccinate 4 to 6 weeks later.

Turkeys: Vaccinate between 20 and 24 weeks of age. Revaccinate 4 to 6 weeks later.

This is a killed bacterin. There is no danger of spread to susceptible birds.

Precaution(s): Store below 45°F (7°C). Do not freeze.

Caution(s): Use the entire contents of the bottle when first opened.

Warning(s): Do not vaccinate within 42 days before slaughter.

Presentation: 1,000 dose bottles with a 300 mL fill of bacterin.

Compendium Code No.: 11030372

INACTI/VAC® FC4

L.A.H.I. (Maine Biological) **Bacterin**

Pasteurella Multocida Bacterin, Avian Isolates, Types 1,3,4 & 3x4

U.S. Vet. Lic. No.: 196

Contents: This product contains the antigens listed above.

Indications: Recommended for the vaccination of chickens and turkeys against Fowl Cholera caused by *Pasteurella multocida*, Type 1 in chickens and Types 3, 4 and 3x4 in turkeys.

Dosage and Administration: Vaccine should be warmed to room temperature before use.

Shake well before using.

Inject subcutaneously in the lower neck region using aseptic technique.

Dose - ½ mL (0.5 mL) per bird.

Inject all birds in flock.

Vaccinate chickens between 12 and 16 weeks of age. Vaccinate turkeys between 20 and 24 weeks of age. Revaccinate 4 to 6 weeks later. Revaccinate during molt.

If fowl cholera is diagnosed before it has spread throughout the flock, it is often possible to check its spread by immediate vaccination of healthy birds.

Precaution(s): Store below 45°F (7°C). Do not freeze.

Caution(s): Use entire contents of bottle when first opened.

Warning(s): Do not vaccinate within 42 days before slaughter.

In case of accidental human injection seek immediate medical attention.

Presentation: 1,000 dose (500 mL) bottles.

Compendium Code No.: 11030382

INACTI/VAC® FC4C

L.A.H.I. (Maine Biological) **Bacterin**

Pasteurella Multocida Bacterin, Avian Isolates, Types 1,3,4 & 3x4

U.S. Vet. Lic. No.: 196

Contents: This product contains the antigens listed above.

Indications: Recommended for the vaccination of chickens and turkeys against Fowl Cholera caused by *Pasteurella multocida*, Type 1 in chickens and Types 3, 4 and 3x4 in turkeys.

Dosage and Administration: Vaccine should be warmed to room temperature before use.

Shake well before using.

Inject subcutaneously in the lower neck region using aseptic technique.

Dose - 0.3 mL per bird.

Inject all birds in flock.

Vaccinate chickens between 12 and 16 weeks of age. Vaccinate turkeys between 20 and 24 weeks of age. Revaccinate 4 to 6 weeks later. Revaccinate during molt.

If fowl cholera is diagnosed before it has spread throughout the flock, it is often possible to check its spread by immediate vaccination of healthy birds.

Precaution(s): Store below 45°F (7°C). Do not freeze.

Caution(s): Use entire contents of bottle when first opened.

Warning(s): Do not vaccinate within 42 days before slaughter.

In case of accidental human injection seek immediate medical attention.

Presentation: 1,000 dose (300 mL) bottles.

Compendium Code No.: 11030392

INACTI/VAC® IB2

L.A.H.I. (Maine Biological) **Vaccine**

Bronchitis Vaccine, Mass. & Ark. Types, Killed Virus

U.S. Vet. Lic. No.: 196

Contents: This product contains the antigens listed above.

Indications: Recommended for the vaccination of chickens and turkeys against infectious bronchitis (Mass. and Ark. types).

Directions for Use: Vaccine should be warmed to room temperature before use.

Shake well before using.

Inject subcutaneously in the lower neck region using aseptic technique.

Dose—½ mL (0.5 mL) per bird.

Inject all birds in flock.

Vaccinate (prime) with live virus bronchitis vaccine at least 4 weeks prior to the use of this vaccine. Vaccinate between 16 and 20 weeks of age. Revaccinate during molt.

Precaution(s): Store below 45°F (7°C). Do not freeze. Use entire contents of bottle when first opened.

Caution(s): In case of accidental human injection seek immediate medical attention.

Warning(s): Do not vaccinate within 42 days before slaughter.

Presentation: 1000 dose (500 mL) bottles.

Compendium Code No.: 11030403

INACTI/VAC® ND

L.A.H.I. (Maine Biological) **Vaccine**

Newcastle Disease Vaccine, Killed Virus, Oil Emulsion

U.S. Vet. Lic. No.: 196

Active Ingredient(s): Produced with a high titering strain of Newcastle disease virus, suspended in a stable oil emulsion.

Indications: Recommended for the immunization of chickens and turkeys against Newcastle disease.

Dosage and Administration: The vaccine should be warmed to room temperature before use. Shake well before using. Inject subcutaneously in the lower neck region using aseptic technique.

Inject all of the birds in the flock with ½ mL (0.5 mL) per bird.

Vaccinate (prime) with live virus vaccine for Newcastle disease at least 4 weeks prior to the use of this vaccine. Vaccinate between 16 and 20 weeks of age. Revaccinate during molt.

This is a killed virus vaccine. There is no danger of spread to susceptible birds.

Precaution(s): Store below 45°F (7°C). Do not freeze.

Caution(s): Use the entire contents of the bottle when first opened.

Warning(s): Do not vaccinate within 42 days before slaughter.

Presentation: 1,000 dose (500 mL) bottles.

Compendium Code No.: 11030422

INACTI/VAC® ND-AE

L.A.H.I. (Maine Biological) **Vaccine**

Newcastle Disease-Avian Encephalomyelitis Vaccine, Killed Virus, Oil Emulsion

U.S. Vet. Lic. No.: 196

Active Ingredient(s): Produced with high titering strains of Newcastle disease and avian encephalomyelitis (AE) viruses, suspended in a stable oil emulsion.

Indications: Recommended for the immunization of breeder hens to give broad protection against Newcastle disease and avian encephalomyelitis.

Dosage and Administration: The vaccine should be warmed to room temperature before use. Inject subcutaneously in the lower neck region using aseptic technique.

Inject all of the birds in the flock with ½ mL (0.5 mL) per bird.

Birds should be primed with live virus Newcastle disease vaccine at seven (7) days and at 12 weeks of age. Vaccinate with INACTI/VAC® ND-AE between 16 and 20 weeks of age. If birds are being held for a second year, revaccinate during molt.

This is a killed virus vaccine. There is no danger of spread to susceptible birds, or of egg transmission of the virus.

Precaution(s): Store below 45°F (7°C). Do not freeze.

Caution(s): Use the entire contents of the bottle when first opened.

Warning(s): Do not vaccinate within 42 days before slaughter.

Presentation: 1,000 dose (500 mL) bottles.

Compendium Code No.: 11030432

INACTI/VAC® ND-IB1

L.A.H.I. (Maine Biological) **Vaccine**

Newcastle-Bronchitis Vaccine, Mass. Type, Killed Virus

U.S. Vet. Lic. No.: 196

Contents: This product contains the antigens listed above.

Indications: Recommended for the vaccination of breeder hens and replacement pullets against Newcastle disease and infectious bronchitis (Mass. Type).

Directions for Use: Vaccine should be warmed to room temperature before use.

Shake well before using.

Inject subcutaneously in the lower neck region using aseptic technique.

Dose - ½ mL (0.5 mL) per bird. Inject all birds in flock.

Vaccinate (prime) with live virus vaccines for Newcastle disease and bronchitis at least 4 weeks prior to the use of this vaccine. Vaccinate between 16 and 20 weeks of age. Revaccinate during molt.

Precaution(s): Store below 45°F (7°C). Do not freeze.

Use entire contents of bottle when first opened.

Warning(s): Do not vaccinate within 42 days before slaughter.

In case of accidental human injection seek immediate medical attention.

Presentation: 1000 dose (500 mL) bottles.

Compendium Code No.: 11030442

INACTI/VAC® ND-IB1C

L.A.H.I (Maine Biological) **Vaccine**

Newcastle-Bronchitis Vaccine, Mass. Type, Killed Virus

U.S. Vet. Lic. No.: 196

Contents: This product contains the antigens listed above.

Indications: Recommended for the vaccination of breeder hens and replacement pullets against Newcastle disease and infectious bronchitis (Mass. Type).

Directions for Use: Vaccine should be warmed to room temperature before use.

Shake well before using.

Inject subcutaneously in the lower neck region using aseptic technique.

Dose - ¼ mL (0.25 mL) per bird. Inject all birds in flock.

Vaccinate (prime) with live virus vaccines for Newcastle disease and bronchitis at least 4 weeks prior to the use of this vaccine. Vaccinate between 16 and 20 weeks of age. Revaccinate during molt.

Precaution(s): Store below 45°F (7°C). Do not freeze.

Use entire contents of bottle when first opened.

Warning(s): Do not vaccinate within 42 days before slaughter.

In case of accidental human injection seek immediate medical attention.

Presentation: 500 dose (125 mL) and 1000 dose (250 mL) bottles.

Compendium Code No.: 11030452

INACTI/VAC® ND-IB2

L.A.H.I. (Maine Biological) **Vaccine**

Newcastle-Bronchitis Vaccine, Mass.-Ark. Types, Killed Virus

U.S. Vet. Lic. No.: 196

Active Ingredient(s): Produced with a high titering strain of Newcastle disease and two strains of infectious bronchitis virus. This vaccine also contains the Massachusetts and Arkansas types of IB virus. These are the two most serious and common strains that infect flocks.

Indications: Recommended for the immunization of breeder hens and commercial layers to give broad protection against Newcastle disease and infectious bronchitis.

Dosage and Administration: The vaccine should be warmed to room temperature before use. Shake well before using. Inject subcutaneously in the lower neck region using aseptic technique.

Inject all of the birds in the flock with ½ mL (0.5 mL) per bird.

Birds should be primed with live virus vaccines for Newcastle disease and bronchitis at least 4 weeks prior to the use of this vaccine. Vaccinate with INACTI/VAC® ND-IB2 between 16 and 20 weeks of age.

Revaccinate during molt.

Precaution(s): Store below 45°F (7°C). Do not freeze.
Caution(s): Use the entire contents of the bottle when first opened.
Warning(s): Do not vaccinate within 42 days before slaughter.
In case of accidental human injection seek immediate medical attention.
Presentation: 1,000 dose (500 mL) bottles.
Compendium Code No.: 11030462

INACTI/VAC® ND-PMV3

L.A.H.I. (Maine Biological) **Vaccine**
Newcastle-Paramyxovirus Vaccine, Type 3, Killed Virus
U.S. Vet. Lic. No.: 196
Contents: INACTI/VAC ND-PMV3 is produced with high titering strains of Newcastle disease and Avian Paramyxovirus, Type 3 viruses, suspended in a stable oil emulsion.
Indications: Recommended for use in turkey breeder hens to give broad protection against Newcastle disease and Avian Paramyxovirus - Type 3 (PMV3).
Dosage and Administration: The vaccine should be warmed to room temperature before use. Shake well before using. Inject subcutaneously in the lower neck region using aseptic technique. Inject all of the birds in the flock with ½ mL (0.5 mL) per bird.
Vaccinate between 16 and 24 weeks of age. Revaccinate 4 to 6 weeks later. Do not vaccinate before 12 weeks of age. This is a killed virus vaccine. There is no danger of spread to susceptible birds, or of egg transmission of the virus.
Precaution(s): Store below 45°F (7°C). Do not freeze.
Caution(s): Use entire contents of bottle when first opened.
Warning(s): Do not vaccinate within 42 days before slaughter.
Presentation: 1000 dose (500 mL) bottle.
Compendium Code No.: 11030472

INACTI/VAC® PMV3

L.A.H.I. (Maine Biological) **Vaccine**
Avian Paramyxovirus Vaccine, Type 3, Killed Virus, Oil Emulsion
U.S. Vet. Lic. No.: 196
Active Ingredient(s): A high titering strain of avian paramyxovirus, type 3 vaccine, killed virus, in an oil emulsion.
Indications: Recommended for the immunization of turkeys against avian paramyxovirus, type 3.
Dosage and Administration: The vaccine should be warmed to room temperature before use. Shake well before using. Inject subcutaneously in the lower neck region using aseptic technique.
Inject all of the birds in the flock with ½ mL (0.5 mL) per bird.
Vaccinate between 20 and 24 weeks of age. Revaccinate four (4) to six (6) weeks later.
This is a killed virus vaccine. There is no danger of spread to susceptible birds, or of egg transmission of the virus.
Precaution(s): Store below 45°F (7°C). Do not freeze.
Caution(s): Use the entire contents of the bottle when first opened.
Warning(s): Do not vaccinate within 42 days before slaughter.
Presentation: 1,000 dose (500 mL) bottles.
Compendium Code No.: 11030482

INACTI/VAC® PULLET-ND

L.A.H.I. (Maine Biological) **Vaccine**
Newcastle Disease Vaccine, Killed Virus
U.S. Vet. Lic. No.: 196
Contents: This product contains the antigen listed above.
Indications: Recommended for the vaccination of mature chickens against Newcastle disease.
Directions for Use: Vaccine should be warmed to room temperature before use.
Shake well before using.
Inject subcutaneously in the lower neck region using aseptic technique.
Dose - ¼ mL (0.25 mL) per bird. Inject all birds in flock.
Vaccinate (prime) with live virus vaccine for Newcastle disease at least 4 weeks prior to the use of this vaccine. Vaccinate between 16 and 20 weeks of age. Revaccinate during molt.
Precaution(s): Store below 45°F (7°C). Do not freeze.
Use entire contents of bottle when first opened.
Warning(s): Do not vaccinate within 42 days before slaughter.
In case of accidental human injection seek immediate medical attention.
Presentation: 2000 dose (500 mL) bottles.
Compendium Code No.: 11030492

INACTI/VAC® REO

L.A.H.I. (Maine Biological) **Vaccine**
Avian Reovirus Vaccine, Killed Virus, Oil Emulsion
U.S. Vet. Lic. No.: 196
Active Ingredient(s): Produced with high titering strains of avian reovirus suspended in a stable oil emulsion. It contains two reovirus stains: the S1133 strain (a tenosynovitis pathotype) and the 1733 strain (a malabsorption syndrome pathotype).
Indications: Recommended for the immunization of breeder hens to give broad protection against avian reovirus infection.
Dosage and Administration: The vaccine should be warmed to room temperature before use. Shake well before using. Inject subcutaneously in the lower neck region using aseptic technique.
Inject all of the birds in the flock with ½ mL (0.5 mL) per bird.
Birds should be primed with live virus tenosynovitis vaccine at least four (4) weeks prior to the use of this vaccine. Vaccinate between 16 and 20 weeks of age and revaccinate four (4) to six (6) weeks later. Revaccinate during molt.
Precaution(s): Store below 45°F (7°C). Do not freeze.
Caution(s): Use the entire contents of the bottle when first opened.
Warning(s): Do not vaccinate within 42 days before slaughter.
Presentation: 1,000 dose (500 mL) bottles.
Compendium Code No.: 11030502

INACTI/VAC® SE4

L.A.H.I. (Maine Biological) **Bacterin**
Salmonella enteritidis Bacterin
U.S. Vet. Lic. No.: 196
Contents: INACTI/VAC SE4 is produced with four phage types of *Salmonella enteritidis.* These four phage types are the most common types isolated from poultry houses. High concentrations of these strains are suspended in a stable oil emulsion.
Indications: Developed for use in commercial layers and breeder hens to aid in the reduction of *Salmonella enteritidis* colonization of internal organs, including the reproductive tract.
Dosage and Administration: The vaccine should be warmed to room temperature before use. Shake well before using. Inject subcutaneously in the lower neck region using aseptic technique. Inject all of the birds in the flock with ½ mL (0.5 mL) per bird. Commercial layers and breeder hens should be vaccinated between 12 and 16 weeks of age. Revaccinate 4 weeks later. INACTI/VAC SE4 is completely safe because it contains no living bacteria.
Precaution(s): Do not store below 45°F (7°C). Do not freeze.
Caution(s): Use entire contents of bottle when first opened.
Warning(s): Do not vaccinate within 42 days before slaughter.
Presentation: 1000 dose (500 mL) bottle.
Compendium Code No.: 11030512

INACTI/VAC® SE4-C

L.A.H.I. (Maine Biological) **Bacterin**
Salmonella enteritidis Bacterin - Concentrate, Oil Emulsion
U.S. Vet. Lic. No.: 196
Contents: *Salmonella enteritidis* bacterin (concentrate) in an oil emulsion.
Indications: Recommended for commercial layers and breeder hens.
Dosage and Administration: Commercial layers and breeder hens should be vaccinated between 12 and 16 weeks of age. Revaccinate 4 weeks later. dosage is ⅕ mL (0.2 mL) per bird. The vaccine should be warmed to room temperature before using. Inject subcutaneously in the lower neck region using aseptic technique. Inject all birds in flock.
Precaution(s): Store below 45°F (7°C). Do not freeze. Use entire contents of bottle when first opened.
Warning(s): Do not vaccinate within 42 days before slaughter.
Discussion: INACTI/VAC® SE4-C Concentrate is produced with four phage types of *Salmonella enteritidis.* These four phage types are the most common isolates from poultry houses. The combination of these four phage types provides a high level of protection. High concentrations of these strains are suspended in a stable oil emulsion. It is recommended for use in commercial layers and breeder hens. A dose of bacterin contains a large amount of inactivated *Salmonella enteritidis.* Two injections, given in the late growing period, produce a high level of immunity to aid in the reduction of *Salmonella enteritidis* colonization of internal organs, including the reproductive tract. This helps decrease the chance of *Salmonella enteritidis* egg contamination. Although the infection in layers does not usually cause health problems in a flock, contaminated eggs are a serious human health risk.
INACTI/VAC® SE4-C has been produced with the same amount of antigen per dose as the regular Inacti/Vac SE4. The concentrate dose size is ¼ mL (0.25 mL) compared to ½ mL (0.5 mL) in the regular product. The bottle is filled to 500 mL containing 2000 doses per bottle. When injected, the oil emulsion releases the antigen over time and greatly enhances the development of high levels of immunity.
INACTI/VAC® SE4-C is completely safe because it contains no living bacteria. Vaccination with INACTI/VAC® SE4-C decreases *Salmonella enteritidis* cecal colonization. The immunity developed also significantly reduces the incidence of internal organ and reproductive tract infections with *Salmonella enteritidis.*
Presentation: 2000 dose (500 mL) polypropylene bottles.
Compendium Code No.: 11030522

INACTI/VAC® SE4-ND-IB2

L.A.H.I. (Maine Biological) **Bacterin-Vaccine**
Newcastle Disease-Bronchitis Vaccine, Mass. & Ark. Types, Killed Virus, Salmonella Enteritidis Bacterin
U.S. Vet. Lic. No.: 196
Contents: This product contains the antigens listed above.
Indications: Recommended for the vaccination of chickens against Newcastle disease and infectious bronchitis (Mass. and Ark. Types) and as an aid to reduce the colonization of the internal organs, including the reproductive tract, by *Salmonella enteritidis.*
Dosage and Administration: Vaccine should be warmed to room temperature before use.
Shake well before using.
Inject subcutaneously in the lower neck region using aseptic technique.
Dose - ½ mL (0.5 mL) per chicken. Inject all birds in flock.
Vaccinate (prime) with live virus vaccines for Newcastle disease and bronchitis at least 4 weeks prior to the use of this vaccine. Vaccinate between 12 and 16 weeks of age. Revaccinate with monovalent Salmonella Enteritidis Bacterin 4 weeks later. Revaccinate during molt.
Precaution(s): Store below 45°F (7°C). Do not freeze.
Caution(s): Use entire contents of bottle when first opened.
Warning(s): Do not vaccinate within 42 days before slaughter.
In case of accidental human injection seek immediate medical attention.
Presentation: 1,000 dose (500 mL) bottles.
Compendium Code No.: 11030532

INACTI/VAC® TURKEY-ND

L.A.H.I. (Maine Biological) **Vaccine**
Newcastle Disease Vaccine, Killed Virus, Oil Emulsion
U.S. Vet. Lic. No.: 196
Active Ingredient(s): INACTI/VAC® TURKEY-ND is produced with a high concentration of a high titering strain of Newcastle disease virus suspended in a stable oil emulsion. When injected, the oil emulsion controls the absorption of the virus and greatly enhances the development of high levels of immunity.
Indications: INACTI/VAC® TURKEY-ND has been developed for use in turkey breeder hens to give broad protection against Newcastle disease.
When injected, the vaccine produces high levels of circulating antibody (humoral immunity) which is maintained throughout the production cycle. This provides high levels of parental immunity in the progeny. This is the only way to provide protection during the critical first days of life. Early infection with Newcastle disease causes high mortality.

INACTI/VAC® TURKEY-ND is a specialty vaccine designed for use in turkeys. The immune system of the turkey is not as responsive as that of a chicken. The high potency vaccine was developed to overcome this deficiency.

Dosage and Administration: The vaccine should be warmed to room temperature before using. Shake well before using. Inject subcutaneously in the lower neck region using aseptic technique.

Inject all of the birds in the flock with ½ mL (0.5 mL) per bird.

Birds should be primed with live virus Newcastle disease vaccine during the growing period. Vaccinate with INACTI/VAC® TURKEY-ND at 28 to 30 weeks of age. If birds are being held for a second year, revaccinate during molt.

This is a killed virus vaccine. There is no danger of spread to susceptible birds.

Precaution(s): Store below 45°F (7°C). Do not freeze.

Caution(s): Use the entire contents of the bottle when first opened.

Warning(s): Do not vaccinate within 42 days before slaughter.

Presentation: 1,000 dose (500 mL) bottles.

Compendium Code No.: 11030542

INDICATORx*

Idexx Labs. **Urinary Microbiology Test**

Test Kit for Canine/Feline Urinary Tract Infection

Components: Each INDICATORx* Test Kit contains the materials necessary to perform 10 tests.

- 10 INDICATORx* tests (each foil bag contains 1 test device and 1 sample pipette)
- 10 sample diluent bottles (5 mLs/bottle)
- 10 sterile wrapped device pipettes for dispensing diluted sample into device
- 10 sealable plastic bags for storing devices during the incubation step

Other Equipment Required for Testing

- 6 watt 365 nm UV Lamp
- Laboratory Incubator set @ 35°C

Indications: The INDICATORx* Test Kit, developed by Idexx Laboratories, Inc., screens for a variety of bacterial infections in canine and feline urine specimens and provides early indication of whether an effective antibiotic is being used to treat an infection.

Test Principles: INDICATORx* is a 24 hour test that:

1) Defects the presence of bacteria in canine or feline urine samples.
2) Identifies bacteria as one of the primary gram-negative uropathogens (i.e., *Escherichia coli, Klebsiella, Enterobacter* spp., and *Proteus* spp.) that are responsible for feline and canine urinary tract infections (UTI).
3) Predicts the antibiotic resistance pattern for the UTI-related gram-negative bacteria found in canine and feline urine samples.

The INDICATORx* test device is composed of 5 test wells, labeled "BAC", "GM(-)", "FQ", "AMO", "CEP" and 2 control wells labeled "NC" and "PC". Each test well contains a specific medium coupled with a fluorogenic enzyme substrate for the detection of target bacteria and their respective antibiotic resistance patterns. Fluorescence in the BAC well is indicative of viable bacteria in the urine sample, but does not differentiate the type of bacteria present. Fluorescence in the GM(-) well identifies the viable bacteria as one of the common gram-negative uropathogens (i.e., *E. coli, Klebsiella, Enterobacter* spp., and *Proteus* spp.). The FQ, AMO, and CEP wells each contain reagent mixtures with a different indicator antibiotic that serves as a predictor for a specific class of antibiotics. FQ is the predictor for the fluoroquinolones (i.e., ciprofloxacin, enrofloxacin and marbofloxacin). AMO is the predictor for some beta-lactams (i.e., amoxicillin, ampicillin and Clavamox). CEP is the predictor for the cephalosporins (i.e., cephalothin, cephalexin and cephadroxil). Fluorescence in the antibiotic wells indicates that the bacterium is resistant to the corresponding antibiotic. Non-fluorescence in the antibiotic wells indicates that the bacterium is susceptible to the antibiotic in that well.

Note: The antibiotic wells do not predict the susceptibility for the BAG well, only the GM(-). Therefore, in cases where only the BAC well is fluorescent, indicative of gram positive bacteria, the clinician should not assume that these bacteria are susceptible to all three antibiotics.

Limitations: INDICATORx* is recommended for use as a screening method for detection of bacteria in feline or canine urine specimens. It is intended for use in detecting the most common gram negative uropathogens (*E. coli, Klebsiella, Enterobacter* spp., and *Proteus* spp.) and in determining their antibiotic resistance patterns. The antibiotic resistance patterns of other bacteria e.g., *Staphylococcus aureus, Enterococcus* spp., and some strains of *Pseudomonas*, should be determined by a reference laboratory. The INDICATORx* test is not intended for use as a method of quantitative antimicrobial susceptibility testing. If the quantitative antimicrobial susceptibility information is desired, an approved antimicrobial susceptibility test should be used.

The INDICATORx* test is intended to assist veterinary practitioners in confirming or selecting an antibiotic treatment regimen for feline and canine bacterial urinary tract infections. As with any diagnosis or treatment decision, however, the practitioner should use clinical discretion with each patient based on a complete evaluation of the patient, including physical presentation and other relevant data.

Sample Collection: Sample Information: For best results, fresh urine specimens should be tested as soon as possible. If it is not possible to test within 4 hours, urine specimens may be stored at 2°-7°C (36°-45°F) for no more than 48 hours prior to testing. Samples collected either by catheterization, by cystocentesis, or as clean-catch specimens must be tested according to the protocol outlined in the test instructions of the insert (4 drops of urine).

Test Procedure:

1. For each specimen to be tested, remove one foil package, one sample diluent bottle, one sterile wrapped device pipette and one sealable plastic bag from kit box. Remove the INDICATORx* test device from the foil package. Leave the sample pipette in the foil bag until ready to transfer urine specimen. Label the device and sample diluent bottle with the patient identification.
2. Loosen cap on the diluent bottle for easier handling during the sample transfer step.
3. Using the sample pipette provided in the foil bag, carefully transfer 4 drops of the urine specimen into the sample diluent bottle. Hold the sample pipette vertically while dispensing urine sample into bottle. Be careful not to contaminate the bottle cap by setting it down on a non-sterile surface.
4. Tightly cap the sample diluent bottle and mix thoroughly by inverting several times.
5. Place the test device on a flat surface. Verify that the device windows are in the open position (blue button of the device should be set at position "o"). Care must be taken not to touch or contaminate the open wells with fingers, etc., prior to running the test.
6. Uncap the sample diluent bottle. Open the sterile wrapped device pipette and draw sample/diluent mixture up into the pipette. Holding device pipette vertically over the center of the BAC well, add 2 drops of the sample/diluent mixture into the BAC well of the device. Repeat this procedure for each of the other 6 wells, refilling the device pipette if necessary.
7. Slide the blue button of the device (from position "o" to position "x") to close the test well windows.
8. Insert each device into a separate sealable plastic bag (included with the kit). Seal bag tightly to prevent dehydration during the incubation step.
9. Incubate the sealed device at 35°C for 24 hours. Note: Results are valid for up to 28 hours of total incubation.
10. Do not remove device from sealable plastic bag. Read the test results by placing a 6 watt 365 nm UV lamp 6 to 8 inches above the test device. The INDICATORx* device contains examples of positive (PC) and negative (NC) test results that can be visualized using a UV lamp. Fluorescent wells produce a bright blue color that can be distinguished from the dull blue color in negative wells. Wells that develop a fluorescent color more intense than the negative control are positive. Use the PC and NC wells as guides to determine the test distance of the lamp from the device while reading test results. A fluorescent BAC or GM(-) well signifies a positive result indicative of bacterial growth. A non-fluorescent BAG or GM(-) well signifies a negative result indicative of no bacterial growth. Fluorescent and non-fluorescent FQ, AMO and CEP wells signify the results indicated in the table below. Be careful not to look directly at the UV source while reading the test results.

Interpretation of Results:

BAC	GM-	FQ	AMO	CEP	Result interpretation	Recommendations
-	-	-	-	-	No bacterial growth	Confirm by a reference laboratory.[1] This is indicative of bacteria other than the common gram-negative uropathogens (e.g., *Staphylococcus* spp. or *Enterococcus* spp. or some strains of *Pseudomonas*).[2]
+	-	-	-	-	Positive bacterial growth; no common gram negative uropathogens detected. Antibiotic wells do not apply.	
+	+	-	-	-	Common gram negative uropathogens detected. The detected uropathogens are susceptible to all three classes of antibiotics.[3]	+
+	+	-	+	-	Common gram negative uropathogens detected. The detected uropathogens are susceptible to the fluoroquinolones and cephalosporins, but are resistant to the beta-lactams.	
+	+	-	-	+	Common gram negative uropathogens detected. The detected uropathogens are susceptible to the fluoroquinolones and beta-lactams, but are resistant to the cephalosporins.	
+	+	+	+	-	Common gram negative uropathogens detected. The detected uropathogens are susceptible to the cephalosporins, but are resistant to the fluoroquinolones and beta-lactams.	
+	+	+	-	+	Common gram negative uropathogens detected. The detected uropathogens are susceptible to the beta-lactams, but are resistant to fluoroquinolones and cephalosporins.	
+	+	-	+	+	Common gram negative uropathogens detected. The detected uropathogens are susceptible to the fluoroquinolones, but are resistant to the beta-lactams and cephalosporins.	
+	+	+	+	+	Common gram negative uropathogens detected. The detected uropathogens are resistant to all three antibiotic classes (fluoroquinolone, beta-lactam and cephalosporin).	Confirm by a reference laboratory.[1] This may be indicative of a resistant strain or a mixed culture containing several different bacteria.

Test Result Patterns other than those reported in this table are invalid. Repeat testing is recommended.

[1] If this result pattern is obtained, it is recommended that a fresh urine sample be collected and analyzed by a reference laboratory for confirmatory testing, e.g., standard microbial identification and antimicrobial susceptibility assays. Alternatively, you may call Idexx Customer Support at the number listed at the end of the insert to inquire about confirmatory testing using the sealed INDICATORx* device.

[2] Aucoin, DVM, David, 1998. Target The Antimicrobial Reference Guide to Effective Treatment, 1998 Edition. North American Compendiums, Inc., pp. 1-2.

[3] Correlation of INDICATORx* to Kirby-Bauer Standard Method of Susceptibility/Resistance prediction for a population of 138 canine/feline urine samples:

FQ Well - CIP 5: 95%, ENO 5: 95%

AMO Well - AM 10: 92%

CEP Well - CF 30: 84%

Storage: The INDICATORx* devices and test reagents are stable until expiration date when stored at 2°-7°C (36°-45°F). Alternatively, the INDICATORx* test kit may be stored at room temperature 15°-30°C (59°-86°F) for 90 days. Once INDICATORx* reagents and devices are removed from 2°-7°C (36°-45°F) for more than 24 hours, the expiration date is 90 days or the printed expiration

date whichever occurs first. If the 90 day expiration date would occur prior to the printed expiration, record the new date in the space provided on the outer box.
Caution(s): For *in vitro* veterinary diagnostic use only.

After use, the INDICATORx* device and test reagents may contain viable microorganisms. Handle and discard all waste by following Good Laboratory Practice for decontamination prior to disposal.

The expiration date applies to the product in its intact container when stored as directed. Do not use test components past the expiration date.

A separate test device, sample pipette, device pipette and sample dilution bottle should be used for each sample. Do not reuse the test device, sample pipette, device pipette or sample dilution bottle once the urine sample has been introduced.
Presentation: 10 tests per kit.
*INDICATORx is either a trademark or a registered trademark of Idexx Laboratories, Inc. in the United States and/or other countries.
Compendium Code No.: 11160610 06-04283-01

INGELVAC® APP-ALC

Boehringer Ingelheim **Vaccine**
Actinobacillus Pleuropneumoniae Vaccine, Live Culture
U.S. Vet. Lic. No.: 124
Contents: This product contains the antigen listed above.
Indications: Recommended for use in healthy swine 6 weeks of age or older as an aid in the prevention of disease associated with *Actinobacillus pleuropneumoniae.*
Dosage and Administration: Vaccinate intramuscularly with a 2 mL dose. Revaccinate 3 to 4 weeks later.

Directions: Plan vaccination timing to allow thawing of the contents of the vaccine vial in air at controlled room temperature or in a lukewarm water bath (60-75°F) until liquid. Shake well and use immediately.
Precaution(s): Store frozen at ultralow temperatures below -50°C or with dry ice packs. Product must not be stored in conventional freezer (-20°C) for more than 2 weeks. Promptly use entire contents when thawed (within 6 hours or less when stored at 35-70°F). To maintain maximum vaccine potency, keep each bottle of thawed vaccine chilled in a cooler until transfer to a syringe for immediate use. All materials used in administering this vaccine must be free of antimicrobial or disinfectant residue to prevent inactivation. Avoid contact. If accidental human exposure occurs, flush area with clean water and consult physician. Burn this container and all unused contents.
Caution(s): For veterinary use only. In case of anaphylactoid reactions epinephrine is symptomatic treatment. Administration of this product has been associated with lethargy (100%), fever and vomiting (20%), and visible injection site swelling in up to 11% of vaccinated pigs. Do not vaccinate pregnant swine or breeding age boars. This vaccine may be shed by vaccinates and transmitted to swine which are in contact with vaccinates.
Warning(s): Do not vaccinate within 21 days of animal harvest for human consumption.
Presentation: 50 dose (100 mL) vials.
Compendium Code No.: 10280621

INGELVAC® AR4

Boehringer Ingelheim **Bacterin-Toxoid**
Bordetella Bronchiseptica-Pasteurella Multocida Bacterin-Toxoid
U.S. Vet. Lic. No.: 124
Contents: This product contains the antigens listed above.

Preservative: Gentamicin.
Indications: Recommended for the vaccination of healthy, susceptible swine against atrophic rhinitis caused by toxigenic *Bordetella bronchiseptica* and *Pasteurella multocida* toxigenic Type D and protects against toxin produced by *Pasteurella multocida* toxigenic Type A.
Dosage and Administration:

Sows and Gilts: Using aseptic technique, inject 2 mL intramuscularly 5 weeks prior to farrowing. Repeat with a second 2 mL dose 2 to 3 weeks prior to farrowing. Administer one 2 mL dose 2 to 3 weeks prior to each subsequent farrowing.

Pigs: Using aseptic technique, vaccinate intramuscularly or subcutaneously with 1 mL prior to weaning. Recommended revaccination of pigs in 2 to 3 weeks.
Precaution(s): Store out of direct sunlight at a temperature between 35-45°F (2-7°C). Avoid freezing. Shake well. Use entire contents when first opened.
Caution(s): Anaphylactoid reactions may occur.
Antidote(s): Epinephrine.
Warning(s): Do not vaccinate within 21 days before slaughter.
Discussion: Protection in the piglet is provided by the maternal antibodies in colostrum. Therefore, piglets should receive colostrum from the vaccinated sow as soon as possible after birth. Vaccination of the piglet is also necessary for protection.
Presentation: 50 sow doses or 100 pig doses (100 mL).
Compendium Code No.: 10280630

INGELVAC® ERY-ALC

Boehringer Ingelheim **Bacterial Vaccine**
Erysipelothrix Rhusiopathiae Vaccine, Avirulent Live Culture
U.S. Vet. Lic. No.: 124
Description: *Erysipelothrix Rhusiopathiae* Vaccine, Avirulent Live Culture is a desiccated vaccine prepared from a specially selected strain of *Erysipelothrix rhusiopathiae.* The strain is not virulent when injected parenterally in mice or pigeons (the most susceptible animals to erysipelas organisms). Immunizing characteristics of the strain have been fully maintained.
Indications: Recommended for the subcutaneous or intramuscular vaccination of healthy, susceptible swine four weeks of age or older or for the oral administration to healthy, susceptible swine eight weeks of age or older against disease caused by *Erysipelothrix rhusiopathiae* (erysipelas). Accumulated experimental and field trial data show over 90% protection with one dose of vaccine in susceptible swine. Where the possibility of maternal antibody interference exists, or if some pigs did not drink the vaccine-treated water, a second dose is recommended 3 to 5 weeks later. Sows or gilts should be revaccinated prior to breeding.
Directions: Directions for Rehydration for Subcutaneous or Intramuscular Injection: Add the contents of the vial of Sterile Diluent to the dry vaccine vial. Shake well and use at once.

Directions for Rehydration for Oral Use: For each dose of vaccine in the vial, add 2 mL of clean water (or use 2 mL per dose of Sterile Diluent) to rehydrate the dry vaccine. Shake well and use at once.

Dosage and Administration:

There are two possible routes of administration: 2 mL injected subcutaneously or intramuscularly or 2 mL per pig administered orally to each pig by squirting in the mouth or pouring in the drinking water.

For Oral Administration: Withhold water from pigs to be vaccinated until they are thirsty. Depending upon the size of pigs and environmental temperature, a thirsty pig will drink 500 to 1000 mL (1 to 2 pints) of water in approximately 3-4 hours. Observation of water intake is recommended to assure vaccine consumption by all pigs.

Open trough method of vaccination: Withhold water from pigs 5 to 12 hours. Add 2 mL of rehydrated vaccine per pig to the appropriate quantity of drinking water and mix thoroughly. Eight linear inches of trough space are recommended for each 50 lb pig. The addition of small amounts of ground feed to the water may stimulate rapid consumption.

Barrel-type watering systems: To prevent pigs from fighting for water, a shorter withdrawal time than for open trough method is recommended. Add 2 mL of rehydrated vaccine per pig to the drinking water and mix thoroughly.

Automatic watering systems equipped with proportioner: To prevent pigs from fighting for water, a shorter withdrawal time than for open trough method is recommended. Adjust the proportioner to deliver ½ oz of stock solution in the drinking water. Use the rehydrated vaccine as the proportioner stock solution as follows:

a) For proportioner adjusted to deliver ½ oz of stock solution per gallon of drinking water, use the rehydrated vaccine as the stock solution.
b) For proportioner adjusted to deliver 1 oz stock solution per gallon of drinking water, further dilute the rehydrated vaccine by adding an equal amount of clean water.

Two gallons of water proportioned by either of these methods will contain 15 doses of vaccine.
Quick Reference Oral Dosage Table:

No. of Pigs	Total Dosage (mL)	Trough Space Approx. (inches)	Average Volume Water Required			
			Minimum		Maximum	
			qts App.	mL	qts App.	mL
1	2	8	0.5	500	1.0	1,000
2	4	16	1.0	1,000	2.0	2,000
3	6	24	1.5	1,500	3.0	3,000
4	8	32	2.0	2,000	4.0	4,000
5	10	40	2.5	2,500	5.0	5,000
6	12	48	3.0	3,000	6.0	6,000
7	14	56	3.5	3,500	7.0	7,000
8	16	64	4.0	4,000	8.0	8,000
9	18	72	4.5	4,500	9.0	9,000
10	20	80	5.0	5,000	10.0	10,000

General Recommendations: If swine erysipelas antiserum has been used recently on the pigs, interference with erysipelas vaccination may occur. A period of two weeks after swine erysipelas antiserum usage is generally considered an adequate interval before vaccination. It is recommended that animals being treated with parenteral antibiotics not be vaccinated with this vaccine or similar modified live vaccines.
Precaution(s): Store out of direct sunlight at a temperature between 35-45°F (2°-7°C). Use entire contents when first opened. Burn the container and all unused contents.
Caution(s): All instruments, watering equipment and proportioners used for antibiotics or other medications or which have been recently disinfected should be thoroughly washed and rinsed with clean water before use.

Anaphylactoid reactions may occur.
Antidote(s): Administer epinephrine.
Warning(s): Do not vaccinate within 21 days before slaughter.
Presentation: 125 doses (250 mL).
Compendium Code No.: 10281201 BI S174331-PI-2 2/00

INGELVAC® HP-1

Boehringer Ingelheim **Bacterin**
Haemophilus Parasuis Bacterin
U.S. Vet. Lic. No.: 124
Contents: This product contains the antigen listed above.
Indications: This product is intended to aid in the prevention and control of Glasser's Disease caused by *Haemophilus parasuis* in swine. The duration of immunity is at least 132 days.
Directions: Shake well. Recommended as a single 2 mL intramuscular dose in healthy swine 3 weeks of age or older. Repeat vaccination of breeding swine every six months.
Precaution(s): Store at 35-45°F (2-7°C). Do not freeze. Use entire contents when first opened.
Caution(s): In case of anaphylactoid reaction, epinephrine is symptomatic treatment.

Do not use as a diluent for live vaccines.

For veterinary use only.
Warning(s): Do not vaccinate within 60 days of slaughter.
Presentation: 50 doses (100 mL) and 250 doses (500 mL).
Compendium Code No.: 10281370 BI S174621-RP-1 12/01

INGELVAC® M. HYO

Boehringer Ingelheim **Bacterin**
Mycoplasma Hyopneumoniae Bacterin
U.S. Vet. Lic. No.: 124
Contents: Prepared from chemically inactivated cultures of *M. hyopneumoniae*, emulsified with a special adjuvant to maximize immune response.
Indications: Recommended for the vaccination of healthy, susceptible swine 3 weeks of age or older as an aid in the prevention of pneumonia caused by *Mycoplasma hyopneumoniae.*
Dosage and Administration: Using aseptic technique, inject a single 2 mL dose intramuscularly. The duration of immunity is 120 days.

Semi-annual revaccination is recommended for breeding swine.
Precaution(s): Store at 35-45°F (2-7°C). Do not freeze. Shake well before using. Use entire contents when first opened.
Caution(s): Anaphylactoid reactions may occur.
Antidote(s): Epinephrine.
Warning(s): Do not vaccinate within 60 days of slaughter.

Accidental injection to humans can cause serious local reactions. Contact a physician immediately if accidental injection occurs.
Presentation: 50 doses (100 mL) and 500 doses (1000 mL).
Compendium Code No.: 10280660

INGELVAC® PRRS ATP

Boehringer Ingelheim **Vaccine**

Porcine Reproductive and Respiratory Syndrome Vaccine, Respiratory Form, Modified Live Virus, Atypical Virus

U.S. Vet. Lic. No.: 124

Contents: This product contains the antigen listed above.

Preservative: Neomycin.

Indications: Recommended for the vaccination of healthy, susceptible swine 3 weeks of age or older, up to 18 weeks of age, as an aid in the reduction of disease associated with atypical Porcine Reproductive and Respiratory Syndrome Virus, respiratory form. The duration of immunity is throughout the finishing period, or up to 4 months post-vaccination. Studies to demonstrate protection against typical isolates of PRRS have not been conducted.

Recommended for use in healthy, susceptible swine in PRRS virus positive herds only, per label directions.

Dosage and Administration: Read entire insert before use.

Rehydrate the vaccine by adding the full contents of the accompanying liquid diluent to the vaccine vial. Shake well and use immediately. Rehydrate only with the diluent provided; do not mix with other materials.

Using aseptic technique, administer a single 2 mL dose intramuscularly to swine 3 weeks of age or older, up to 18 weeks of age. Administer only to healthy pigs in PRRS virus positive herds, and only by intramuscular injection. Administer the complete 2 mL dose to each pig vaccinated. Efficacy and safety of the vaccine at other than the dose or route prescribed on the label is unknown and, therefore, not recommended and not USDA approved.

Contraindication(s): Do not vaccinate adult sows, gilts, or boars of breeding age. Do not vaccinate pregnant sows.

Precaution(s): Store out of direct sunlight in the outer carton. Store at a temperature between 35-45°F (2-7°C). Do not freeze. Use entire contents when first opened. Do not use bottles of damaged product. Do not store reconstituted vaccine.

Disposal: After use, burn containers and all unused contents by a procedure allowed by local, state, and Federal regulations.

Caution(s): Anaphylactoid reactions may occur.

Expiration Date: Consult the outer carton for the last date this package of vaccine is acceptable for use.

Antidote(s): Epinephrine.

Warning(s): Vaccinated pigs are not to be harvested for human consumption before 21 days after vaccination.

For veterinary use only; for use only in swine in PRRS virus positive herds as directed.

If human exposure occurs, administer first aid and consult physician immediately.

Discussion: Many factors must be considered in determining a sound PRRS vaccination program for a particular farm. To be most effective, the vaccine must be administered properly to healthy animals maintained in a proper environment under good management. Stressed or immunosuppressed pigs should not be vaccinated, as the efficacy of the vaccine in these animals is unknown. The level of individual animal and herd immunity required will vary with management practices, the degree of exposure to PRRS virus, and the level of susceptibility of each animal. The benefits and risks from vaccination will vary in part with the levels of PRRS virus in the herd, and the need for the herd or individual animals to maintain a particular status for virus isolation, serological, or other diagnostic tests. Therefore, the vaccination program must be carefully planned and implemented in collaboration with the herd veterinarian following label and insert indications and precautions.

Previous or active PRRS virus or other infection: The effect of concurrent or previous infections at or around the time of vaccination on the efficacy of this vaccine in reducing or modifying PRRS virus disease in pigs is not known.

Shedding and transmission of vaccine virus by vaccinates: Vaccine virus may be shed and transmitted to other populations of swine which are in contact, with vaccinated swine. The duration of potential vaccine virus transmission may vary.

Vaccine virus is found at varying times post-vaccination at locations (tonsil, nasal mucosa, urine, feces) from which the potential for shedding exists. The chances of vaccine virus shedding may be increased when animals are treated with glucocorticoids and possibly by disease or environmental conditions which stress pigs and elevate levels of endogenous glucocorticoids.

Non-vaccinated pigs in contact with INGELVAC® PRRS ATP vaccinated pigs may seroconvert to vaccine virus. Use of the vaccine on farms or transport of pigs from the farms where vaccine has been used to farms wanting to remain PRRS virus seronegative is contraindicated.

Vaccination of Breeding Animals: Do not vaccinate adult boars, sows, or gilts. Do not vaccinate pregnant sows.

Vaccination during the latter part of gestation of pregnant sows or gilts which are PRRS virus naive and previously unvaccinated can result in piglets born vaccine viremic. The impact of vaccine viremia in the newborn pig is not known.

Vaccination of adult boars may result in the shedding of vaccine virus in the semen. Because the impact of shedding is not known, do not use in boars of breeding age.

This vaccine is not USDA licensed for use in pregnant swine or breeding boars.

Presentation: INGELVAC® PRRS ATP is supplied in 10 dose and 50 dose amber glass vials, together with either 20 mL or 100 mL of sterile diluent in plastic or clear glass vials, contained in an outer carton.

Compendium Code No.: 10280670

INGELVAC® PRRS-HP

Boehringer Ingelheim **Bacterin-Vaccine**

Porcine Reproductive and Respiratory Syndrome Vaccine, Respiratory Form-Haemophilus Parasuis Bacterin, Modified Live Virus

U.S. Vet. Lic. No.: 319

Contents: This product contains the antigens described above in lyophilized form (for the modified live virus) and in a bacterin diluent.

Contains amphotericin B, gentamicin, and neomycin as preservatives.

Indications: Recommended for the vaccination of healthy, susceptible swine 3 weeks of age or older as an aid in the reduction of disease associated with Porcine Reproductive and Respiratory Syndrome Virus, Respiratory Form and as an aid in the prevention and control of Glasser's disease caused by *Haemophilus parasuis*.

Recommended for use in healthy, susceptible swine in PRRS virus positive herds only, per label directions.

Dosage and Administration: Read entire insert before use.

Read the product label before use.

Rehydrate the vaccine by adding the full contents of the accompanying bacterin diluent to the vaccine vial. Shake well and use immediately. Rehydrate only with the bacterin diluent provided; do not mix with other materials. Other diluents may be virucidal.

Using aseptic technique, administer a single 2 mL dose, intramuscularly to swine 3 weeks of age or older. Administer only to healthy pigs in PRRS virus positive herds, and only by intramuscular injection. Administer the complete 2 mL dose to each pig vaccinated. Efficacy and safety of the vaccine at other than the dose or route prescribed on the label is unknown, and therefore, not recommended and not USDA approved.

Revaccination of pigs in 2 to 3 weeks with a Boehringer Ingelheim Haemophilus Parasuis Bacterin is recommended. Repeat vaccination of breeding swine every six months with a Boehringer Ingelheim Haemophilus Parasuis Bacterin is recommended.

Contraindication(s): Do not vaccinate pregnant sows or gilts, or boars of breeding age.

Precaution(s): Store out of direct sunlight in the outer carton. Store at a temperature between 35-45°F (2-7°C). Do not freeze. Use entire contents when first opened. Do not use bottles of damaged product. Do not store reconstituted vaccine.

Disposal: After use, burn containers and all unused contents by a procedure allowed by local, state, and federal regulations.

Caution(s): Anaphylactoid reactions may occur.

Expiration Date: Consult the outer carton for the last date this package of vaccine is acceptable for use.

Antidote(s): Administer epinephrine.

Warning(s): Vaccinated pigs are not to be harvested for human consumption before 21 days after vaccination.

For veterinary use only; for use only in swine in PRRS virus positive herds as directed.

If human exposure occurs, administer first aid and consult physician immediately.

Discussion: Many factors must be considered in determining a sound PRRS vaccination program for a particular farm. To be most effective, the vaccine must be administered properly to healthy animals maintained in a proper environment under good management. Stressed or immunosuppressed pigs should not be vaccinated as the efficacy of the vaccine in these animals is unknown. The level of individual animal and herd immunity required will vary with management practices, the degree of exposure to PRRS virus, and the level of susceptibility of each animal. The benefits and risks from vaccination will vary in part with the levels of PRRS virus in the herd, and the need for the herd or individual animals to maintain a particular status for virus isolation, serological or other diagnostic tests. Therefore, the vaccination program must be carefully planned and implemented in collaboration with the herd veterinarian following label and insert indications and precautions.

Previous or Active PRRS Virus or Other Infection: The effect of concurrent or previous infections at or around the time of vaccination on the efficacy of this vaccine in reducing or modifying PRRS virus disease in pigs is not known.

Shedding and Transmission of Vaccine Virus by Vaccinates: Vaccine virus may be shed and transmitted to other populations of swine which are in contact with vaccinated swine. The duration of potential vaccine virus transmission may vary.

Research (Gorcyca et. al., unpublished) indicates that vaccine virus is found at varying times post vaccination at locations (tonsil, nasal mucosa, urine, feces) from which the potential for shedding exists. The chances of vaccine virus shedding may be increased when animals are treated with glucocorticoids, and possibly by disease or environmental conditions which stress pigs and elevate levels of endogenous glucocorticoids.

One field study (Torrison, 1996) indicated that non-vaccinated pigs in contact with RespPRRS/Pig™ vaccinated pigs, may seroconvert to vaccine virus. Use of the vaccine on farms or transport of pigs from the farms where vaccine has been used to farms wanting to remain PRRS virus seronegative is contraindicated.

Vaccination of Breeding Animals: Do not vaccinate pregnant sows or gilts, or boars of breeding age.

Vaccination during the latter part of gestation of pregnant sows or gilts, either intramuscularly (Gorcyca et. al., 1995b) or oronasally (Mengeling et. al., 1995), which are PRRS virus naive and previously unvaccinated can result in piglets born vaccine viremic. The impact of vaccine viremia in the newborn pig is not known.

Vaccination of PRRS negative herds prior to breeding may result in a transient reduction of reproductive performance.

Vaccination of adult boars may result in the shedding of vaccine virus in the semen (Molitor et. al., 1995; Nielsen et. al., 1995; Christoper-Hennings et. al., 1995). Because the impact of shedding is not known, do not use in boars of breeding age.

This vaccine is not USDA licensed for use in pregnant swine or breeding boars.

References: Available upon request.

Presentation: Porcine Reproductive and Respiratory Syndrome Vaccine, Respiratory Form—Haemophilus Parasuis Bacterin, modified live virus is supplied in 10 dose and 50 dose cartons containing the lyophilized modified live virus in amber glass vials together with either 20 mL or 100 mL of bacterin diluent in plastic vials.

Compendium Code No.: 10280690

INGELVAC® PRRS-HPE

Boehringer Ingelheim **Bacterin-Vaccine**

Porcine Reproductive and Respiratory Syndrome Vaccine, Respiratory Form-Erysipelothrix Rhusiopathiae-Haemophilus Parasuis Bacterin, Modified Live Virus

U.S. Vet. Lic. No.: 319

Contents: This product contains the antigens described above in lyophilized form (for the modified live virus) and in a bacterin diluent.

Contains amphotericin B, gentamicin, and neomycin as preservatives.

Indications: Recommended for the vaccination of healthy, susceptible swine 3 weeks of age or older as an aid in the reduction of disease associated with Porcine Reproductive and Respiratory Syndrome Virus, Respiratory Form and as an aid in the prevention and control of Glasser's disease caused by *Haemophilus parasuis*.

Recommended for use in healthy, susceptible pigs in PRRS virus positive herds only, per label directions.

Dosage and Administration: Read entire insert before use.

Read the product label before use.

Rehydrate the vaccine by adding the full contents of the accompanying bacterin diluent to the vaccine vial. Shake well and use immediately. Rehydrate only with the bacterin diluent provided; do not mix with other materials. Other diluents may be virucidal.

Using aseptic technique, administer a single 2 mL dose, intramuscularly to swine 3 weeks of age or older. Administer only to healthy pigs in PRRS virus positive herds, and only by intramuscular injection. Administer the complete 2 mL dose to each pig vaccinated. Efficacy and safety of the vaccine at other than the dose or route prescribed on the label is unknown, and therefore, not recommended and not USDA approved.

For *Haemophilus parasuis* protection revaccination of pigs in 2 to 4 weeks with a Boehringer Erysipelothrix Rhusiopathiae-Haemophilus Parasuis Bacterin is recommended. Repeat

vaccination of breeding swine every six months with a Boehringer Erysipelothrix Rhusiopathiae-Haemophilus Parasuis Bacterin is recommended.
Contraindication(s): Do not vaccinate pregnant sows or gilts, or boars of breeding age.
Precaution(s): Store out of direct sunlight in the outer carton. Store at a temperature between 35-45°F (2-7°C). Do not freeze. Use entire contents when first opened. Do not use bottles of damaged product. Do not store reconstituted vaccine.
Disposal: After use, burn containers and all unused contents by a procedure allowed by local, state, and federal regulations.
Caution(s): Anaphylactoid reactions may occur.
Expiration Date: Consult the outer carton for the last date this package of vaccine is acceptable for use.
Antidote(s): Administer epinephrine.
Warning(s): Vaccinated pigs are not to be harvested for human consumption before 21 days after vaccination.
For veterinary use only; for use only in pigs in PRRS virus positive herds as directed.
If human exposure occurs, administer first aid and consult physician immediately.
Discussion: Many factors must be considered in determining a sound PRRS vaccination program for a particular farm. To be most effective, the vaccine must be administered properly to healthy animals maintained in a proper environment under good management. Stressed or immunosuppressed pigs should not be vaccinated as the efficacy of the vaccine in these animals is unknown. The level of individual animal and herd immunity required will vary with management practices, the degree of exposure to PRRS virus, and the level of susceptibility of each animal. The benefits and risks from vaccination will vary in part with the levels of PRRS virus in the herd, and the need for the herd or individual animals to maintain a particular status for virus isolation, serological or other diagnostic tests. Therefore, the vaccination program must be carefully planned and implemented in collaboration with the herd veterinarian following label and insert indications and precautions.
Previous or Active PRRS Virus or Other Infection: The effect of concurrent or previous infections at or around the time of vaccination on the efficacy of this vaccine in reducing or modifying PRRS virus disease in pigs is not known.
Shedding and Transmission of Vaccine Virus by Vaccinates: Vaccine virus may be shed and transmitted to other populations of swine which are in contact with vaccinated swine. The duration of potential vaccine virus transmission may vary.
Research (Gorcyca et.al., unpublished) indicates that vaccine virus is found at varying times post vaccination at locations (tonsil, nasal mucosa, urine, feces) from which the potential for shedding exists. The chances of vaccine virus shedding may be increased when animals are treated with glucocorticoids, and possibly by disease or environmental conditions which stress pigs and elevate levels of endogenous glucocorticoids.
One field study (Torrison, 1996) indicated that non-vaccinated pigs in contact with INGELVAC® PRRS-HPE vaccinated pigs, may seroconvert to vaccine virus. Use of the vaccine on farms or transport of pigs from the farms where vaccine has been used to farms wanting to remain PRRS virus seronegative is contraindicated.
Breeding Animals: Do not vaccinate pregnant sows or gilts, or boars of breeding age.
Vaccination during the latter part of gestation of pregnant sows or gilts, either intramuscularly (Gorcyca et.al., 1995b) or oronasally (Mengeling et.al., 1995), which are PRRS virus naive and previously unvaccinated can result in piglets born vaccine viremic. The impact of vaccine viremia in the newborn pig is not known.
Vaccination of PRRS negative herds prior to breeding may result in a transient reduction of reproductive performance.
Vaccination of adult boars may result in the shedding of vaccine virus in the semen (Molitor et.al., 1995; Nielsen et.al., 1995; Christoper-Hennings et.al., 1995). Because the impact of shedding is not known, do not use in boars of breeding age.
This vaccine is not USDA licensed for use in pregnant swine or breeding boars.
References: Available upon request.
Presentation: Porcine Reproductive and Respiratory Syndrome Vaccine, Respiratory Form-Erysipelothrix Rhusiopathiae-Haemophilus Parasuis Bacterin, modified live virus is supplied in 10 dose and 50 dose cartons containing the lyophilized modified live virus in amber glass vials together with either 20 mL or 100 mL of bacterin diluent in plastic vials.
Compendium Code No.: 10280700

INGELVAC® PRRS MLV

Boehringer Ingelheim **Vaccine**

Porcine Reproductive and Respiratory Syndrome Vaccine, Reproductive & Respiratory Forms, Modified Live Virus
U.S. Vet. Lic. No.: 124
Contents: This product contains the antigens listed above.
Preservative: Neomycin.
Indications: Recommended for the vaccination of healthy, susceptible swine as an aid in the reduction of disease associated with Porcine Reproductive and Respiratory Syndrome virus reproductive and respiratory forms.
Recommended for use in healthy, susceptible swine in PRRS virus positive herds only, per label directions.
Dosage and Administration: Read entire insert before use.
Read the product label before use.
Rehydrate the vaccine by adding the full contents of the accompanying liquid diluent to the vaccine vial. Shake well and use immediately. Rehydrate only with the diluent provided; do not mix with other materials. Other diluents may be virucidal.
Sows and gilts: Using aseptic technique, inject a single 2 mL dose intramuscularly 3-4 weeks prior to breeding for the reproductive form of PRRS. The duration of immunity is at least 4 months or throughout gestation. Revaccinate prior to each subsequent breeding. Do not vaccinate pregnant sows or gilts.
Piglets: Using aseptic technique, inject a single 2 mL dose intramuscularly to swine 3 weeks of age or older for respiratory form of PRRS. The duration of immunity is at least 4 months or throughout the finishing period.
Administer only to healthy pigs, gilts, or sows in PRRS virus positive herds, and only by intramuscular injection. Administer the complete 2 mL dose to each pig, gilt, or sow vaccinated. Efficacy and safety of the vaccine at other than the dose or route prescribed on the label is unknown and, therefore, not recommended and not USDA approved.
Contraindication(s): Do not vaccinate pregnant sows or gilts or breeding age boars.
Precaution(s): Storage Before Use: Store out of direct sunlight in the outer carton. Store at a temperature between 35-45°F (2-7°C). Do not freeze. Use entire contents when first opened. Do not use bottles of damaged product. Do not store reconstituted vaccine.
Disposal: After use, burn containers and all unused contents by a procedure allowed by local, state, and Federal regulations.
Expiration Date: Consult the outer carton for the last date the package of vaccine is acceptable for use.
Caution(s): Breeding Animals: For use in non-pregnant females 3 to 4 weeks prior to breeding only in PRRS virus positive herds. Do not vaccinate pregnant sows, pregnant gilts, or breeding age boars.
Vaccination during the latter part of gestation of pregnant sows or gilts (Gorcyca, et. al., 1995b) which are PRRS virus naive and previously unvaccinated can result in piglets born viremic. The impact of vaccine viremia in the newborn pig is not known.
Vaccination of PRRS negative herds prior to breeding may result in a transient reduction of reproductive performance.
Vaccination of adult boars may result in the shedding of vaccine virus in the semen (Molitor et. al., 1995; Nielsen et. al., 1995; Christoper-Hennings et. al., 1995). Because the impact of shedding is not known, do not use in boars of breeding age.
This vaccine is not USDA licensed for use in pregnant swine or breeding boars.
For veterinary use only; for use only in swine as directed.
Anaphylactoid reactions may occur.
Antidote(s): Epinephrine.
Warning(s): Withdrawal Period: Vaccinated pigs, gilts, or sows are not to be harvested for human consumption before 21 days after vaccination.
If human exposure occurs, administer first aid and consult physician immediately.
Discussion: Many factors must be considered in determining a sound PRRS vaccination program for a particular farm. To be most effective, the vaccine must be administered properly to healthy animals maintained in a proper environment under good management. Stressed or immunosuppressed pigs should not be vaccinated as the efficacy of the vaccine in these animals is unknown. The level of individual animal and herd immunity required will vary with management practices, the degree of exposure to PRRS virus, and the level of susceptibility of each animal. The benefits and risks from vaccination will vary in part with the level of PRRS virus in the herd, and the need for the herd or individual animals to maintain a particular status for virus isolation, serological, or other diagnostic tests. Therefore, the vaccination program must be carefully planned and implemented in collaboration with the herd veterinarian following label and insert indications and precautions.
Previous or Active PRRS Virus or Other Infection: The effect of concurrent or previous infections at or around the time of vaccination on the efficacy of this vaccine in reducing or modifying PRRS virus disease in pigs, gilts, and sows is not known.
Shedding of vaccine virus by vaccinates: Vaccine virus may be shed and transmitted to other populations of swine which are in contact with vaccinated swine. The duration of potential vaccine virus transmission may vary.
Research (Gorcyca, et. al., unpublished) indicates that vaccine virus is found at varying times post vaccination at locations (tonsil, nasal mucosa, urine, feces) from which the potential for shedding exists. The chances of vaccine virus shedding may be increased when animals are treated with glucocorticoids and possibly by disease or environmental conditions which stress pigs and elevate levels of endogenous glucocorticoids.
One field study (Torrison, 1996) indicated that non-vaccinated pigs in contact with Ingelvac® PRRS MLV vaccinated pigs may seroconvert to vaccine virus. Use of the vaccine on farms or transport of pigs from the farms where vaccine has been used to farms wanting to remain PRRS virus seronegative is contraindicated.
References: Reference literature cited is available upon request.
Presentation: Porcine Reproductive and Respiratory Syndrome Vaccine, Reproductive and Respiratory Forms, Modified Live Virus is supplied in 10 dose and 50 dose amber glass vials together with either 20 mL or 100 mL of sterile diluent in plastic vials contained in an outer carton.
Compendium Code No.: 10280681 BI S124511-RP-1 10/00

INGELVAC® PRV-G1

Boehringer Ingelheim **Vaccine**

Pseudorabies Vaccine, Modified Live Virus
U.S. Vet. Lic. No.: 124
Contents: INGELVAC® PRV-G1 vaccine is prepared from a modified live INGELVAC® PRV-G1 Bartha strain (K-61) that is cytopathic in tissue culture.
It is a naturally attenuated gI negative vaccine. Antibody produced solely by vaccination with INGELVAC® PRV-G1 can be differentiated from antibody produced by infection, using the HerdChek® Anti-PRV gI assay.
The virus is stabilized, dispensed into amber, light-restricting bottles and freeze-dried to preserve the maximum concentration of viable vaccine virus at the time of use.
The vaccine contains neomycin as a preservative.
Indications: INGELVAC® PRV-G1 is recommended for the vaccination of healthy, susceptible swine of all ages against disease caused by pseudorabies virus.
Dosage and Administration: Using aseptic technique, administer 2 mL intramuscularly or 2 mL intranasally (1 mL per nostril) in healthy, susceptible swine. Piglets suckling immune sows should be revaccinated 30-90 days later when maternal antibody levels have declined. Gilts should be vaccinated prior to breeding and three (3) weeks before farrowing. Pregnant, susceptible swine may be safely vaccinated for protection against pseudorabies virus in an emergency situation where exposure is imminent. Boars may be vaccinated at any time.
Directions: Rehydrate the vaccine by adding the accompanying liquid diluent to the vaccine vial. Shake well and use immediately.
Precaution(s): Store out of direct sunlight at a temperature not over 45°F (7°C).
Caution(s): Use the entire contents when first opened.
Burn the containers and all the unused contents. Anaphylactic reactions may occur.
Antidote(s): Administer epinephrine.
Warning(s): Do not vaccinate within 21 days before slaughter.
Presentation: The package contains one 50 dose vial of vaccine and one 100 mL vial of sterile diluent.
* HerdChek is a registered trademark of Idexx Corporation.
Compendium Code No.: 10280710

INJECTROLYTE ℞

Vetus **Fluid Therapy**

Replacement Electrolytes (Sterile Solution-Nonpyrogenic)
Active Ingredient(s): Each 100 mL Contains:

Sodium Chloride	526 mg
Sodium Acetate	222 mg
Sodium Gluconate	502 mg
Potassium Chloride	37 mg
Magnesium Chloride Hexahydrate	30 mg
Water for Injection	q.s.

I

May contain hydrochloric acid or sodium hydroxide for pH adjustment.

Electrolytes per 1000 mL (not including ions for pH adjustment):

Sodium	140 mEq
Potassium	5 mEq
Magnesium	3 mEq
Chloride	98 mEq
Acetate	27 mEq
Gluconate	23 mEq

295 mOsm/Liter (Calc.)

pH 5.5-7.5 Isotonic

Indications: INJECTROLYTE is a sterile, nonpyrogenic solution of balanced electrolytes indicated for replacing acute losses of extracellular fluid and electrolytes, and for correcting moderate to severe acidosis.

Dosage and Administration: Contents or lesser amount as determined by veterinarian as a single dose; usually 3-10% of body weight. In shock, up to 10% of body weight in 1-2 hours. For intravenous or subcutaneous use. Solution should be warmed to body temperature and administered slowly.

Precaution(s): Store between 15°C and 30°C (59°F-86°F). Protect from freezing.

Do not use this product if seal is broken or solution is not clear. Contains no preservative. If entire contents are not used, discard unused portion. Additives may be incompatible. When introducing additives, use aseptic technique, mix thoroughly and do not store.

Caution(s): Federal law restricts this drug to use by or on the order of a licensed veterinarian.

For animal use only.

Warning(s): Not for human use. Keep out of reach of children.

Presentation: 1000 mL(NDC 47611-778-10)

Manufactured by: Phoenix Scientific, Inc.

Distributed by: Burns Veterinary Supply, Inc.

Compendium Code No.: 14440900 Rev. 11-00

INNOCUGEL™ EQUINE

Butler **Equine Dietary Supplement**

Active Ingredient(s): Each 15 grams contains:

Vitamin A	11,200 I.U.
Vitamin D_3	2,320 I.U.
Vitamin B_{12}	9.8 mcg
Calcium pantothenate	9.9 mg
Riboflavin	10.9 mg
Thiamine	15.0 mg

Total Colony Forming Units: 2 billion CFU

Ingredients: Dried *Lactobacillus acidophilus* fermentation product, dried *L. casei* fermentation product, dried *L. plantarum* fermentation product, dried *Streptococcus faecium* fermentation product, dried *L. fermentum* fermentation product, vegetable oil, sucrose, silicon dioxide, titanium dioxide, vitamins (A, D_3, and B_{12}), calcium pantothenate, riboflavin, thiamine, certified coloring, polysorbate 80, ethoxyquin preservative.

Indications: A microbial product for foals and horses.

Contains a source of live (viable). naturally occurring microorganisms.

Directions for Use: Administer orally on back of tongue.

Foals: 15 mL day of birth at 12 to 24 hours of age and day four. Adult Horses: Post Worming/Antibiotics - At conclusion of treatment, 15 mL on days 1, 3, and 7. Transportation: Before transportation, 15 mL on days 3 and 1 and on first day following transportation. Performance Training: For one week time period, administer 15 mL every other day, when horse is off feed due to training.

Precaution(s): Keep cool. Not a drug.

Presentation: 30 mL.

Compendium Code No.: 10820980

INSTAMAG BOLUS

Vedco **Antacid-Laxative**

Laxative and Carminative

Active Ingredient(s): Each bolus contains:

Magnesium Oxide .... 276 gr (17.9 g)

(Equiv. to magnesium hydroxide, 400 gr)

Flavored with ginger, capsicum, and methyl salicylate. Artificial color added.

Indications: For oral administration to ruminants as an aid in the treatment of digestive disturbances requiring an antacid and mild laxative.

Dosage and Administration: Give 2 to 4 boluses to ruminants, depending on size and condition of animal. Lubricate boluses and administer with a balling gun.

Precaution(s): Store at controlled room temperature between 15° and 30°C (59°-86°F).

Keep tightly closed when not in use.

Caution(s): Avoid frequent or continued use.

For animal use only. Keep out of reach of children.

Presentation: 50 boluses.

Compendium Code No.: 10941110

IN-SYNCH™ ℞

AgriLabs **Prostaglandin**

dinoprost tromethamine sterile solution

Active Ingredient(s): Description: This product contains the naturally occurring prostaglandin F2 alpha (dinoprost) as the tromethamine salt. Each mL contains dinoprost tromethamine equivalent to 5 mg dinoprost: also, benzyl alcohol, 9.45 mg added as preservative. When necessary, pH was adjusted with sodium hydroxide and/or hydrochloric acid. Dinoprost tromethamine is a white or slightly off-white crystalline powder that is readily soluble in water at room temperature in concentrations to at least 200 mg/mL.

Indications: For intramuscular use for estrus synchronization, treatment of unobserved (silent) estrus and pyometra (chronic endometritis) in cattle; for abortion of feedlot and other non-lactating cattle; for parturition induction in swine; and for controlling the timing of estrus in estrous cycling mares and clinically anestrous mares that have a corpus luteum.

Cattle: IN-SYNCH™ Sterile Solution is indicated as a luteolytic agent.

IN-SYNCH™ is effective only in those cattle having a corpus luteum, i.e., those which ovulated at least five days prior to treatment. Future reproductive performance of animals that are not cycling will be unaffected by injection of IN-SYNCH™.

Swine: For intramuscular use for parturition induction in swine. IN-SYNCH™ Sterile Solution is indicated for parturition induction in swine when injected within 3 days of normal predicted farrowing.

Mares: IN-SYNCH™ Sterile Solution is indicated for its luteolytic effect in mares. This luteolytic effect can be utilized to control the timing of estrus in estrous cycling and clinically anestrous mares that have a corpus luteum.

Pharmacology:

General Biologic Activity: Prostaglandins occur in nearly all mammalian tissues. Prostaglandins, especially PGE's and PGF's, have been shown, in certain species, to 1) increase at time of parturition in amniotic fluid, maternal placenta, myometrium, and blood, 2) stimulate myometrial activity, and 3) to induce either abortion or parturition. Prostaglandins, especially PGF2α, have been shown to 1) increase in the uterus and blood to levels similar to levels achieved by exogenous administration which elicited luteolysis, 2) be capable of crossing from the uterine vein to the ovarian artery (sheep), 3) be related to IUD induced luteal regression (sheep), and 4) be capable of regressing the corpus luteum of most mammalian species studied to date. Prostaglandins have been reported to result in release of pituitary tropic hormones. Data suggest prostaglandins, especially PGE's and PGF's, may be involved in the process of ovulation and gamete transport. Also PGF2α has been reported to cause increase in blood pressure, bronchoconstriction, and smooth muscle stimulation in certain species.

Metabolism: A number of metabolism studies have been done in laboratory animals. The metabolism of tritium labeled dinoprost (^{3}H PGF2 alpha) in the rat and in the monkey was similar. Although quantitative differences were observed, qualitatively similar metabolites were produced. A study demonstrated that equimolar doses of ^{3}H PGF2 alpha Tham and ^{3}H PGF2 alpha free acid administered intravenously to rats demonstrated no significant differences in blood concentration of dinoprost. An interesting observation in the above study was that the radioactive dose of ^{3}H PGF2 alpha rapidly distributed in tissues and dissipated in tissues with almost the same curve as it did in the serum. The half-life of dinoprost in bovine blood has been reported to be on the order of minutes. A complete study on the distribution of decline of ^{3}H PGF2 alpha Tham in the tissue of rats was well correlated with the work done in the cow. Cattle serum collected during 24 hours after doses of 0 to 250 mg dinoprost have been assayed by RIA for dinoprost and the 15-keto metabolites. These data support previous reports that dinoprost has a half-life of minutes.

Dinoprost is a natural prostaglandin. All systems associated with dinoprost metabolism exist in the body; therefore, no new metabolic, transport, excretory, binding or other systems need be established by the body to metabolize injected dinoprost.

Dosage and Administration:

Cattle: IN-SYNCH™ Sterile Solution is supplied at a concentration of 5 mg dinoprost per mL. IN-SYNCH™ is luteolytic in cattle at 25 mg (5 mL) administered intramuscularly. As with any multidose vial, practice aseptic techniques in withdrawing each dose. Adequately clean and disinfect the vial closure prior to entry with a sterile needle.

Instructions for Use:

1. For Intramuscular Use for Estrus Synchronization in Beef Cattle and Non-Lactating Dairy Heifers. IN-SYNCH™ is used to control the timing of estrus and ovulation in estrous cycling cattle that have a corpus luteum.
   Inject a dose of 5 mL IN-SYNCH™ (25 mg PGF2α) intramuscularly either once or twice at a 10 to 12 day interval.
   With the single injection, cattle should be bred at the usual time relative to estrus.
   With the two injections cattle can be bred after the second injection either at the usual time relative to detected estrus or at about 80 hours after the second injection of IN-SYNCH™.
   Estrus is expected to occur 1 to 5 days after injection if a corpus luteum was present. Cattle that do not become pregnant to breeding at estrus on days 1 to 5 after injection will be expected to return to estrus in about 18 to 24 days.
2. For Intramuscular Use for Unobserved (Silent) Estrus in Lactating Dairy Cows with a Corpus Luteum. Inject a dose of 5 mL IN-SYNCH™ (25 mg PGF2α) intramuscularly. Breed cows as they are detected in estrus. If estrus has not been observed by 80 hours after injection, breed at 80 hours. If the cow returns to estrus breed at the usual time relative to estrus.

Management Considerations: Many factors contribute to success and failure of reproduction management, and these factors are important also when time of breeding is to be regulated with IN-SYNCH™ Sterile Solution. Some of these factors are:

a. Cattle must be ready to breed—they must have a corpus luteum and be healthy;
b. Nutritional status must be adequate as this has a direct effect on conception and the initiation of estrus in heifers or return of estrous cycles in cows following calving;
c. Physical facilities must be adequate to allow cattle handling without being detrimental to the animal;
d. Estrus must be detected accurately if timed AI is not employed;
e. Semen of high fertility must be used;
f. Semen must be inseminated properly.

A successful breeding program can employ IN-SYNCH™ effectively, but a poorly managed breeding program will continue to be poor when IN-SYNCH™ is employed unless other management deficiencies are remedied first.

Cattle expressing estrus following IN-SYNCH™ are receptive to breeding by a bull. Using bulls to breed large numbers of cattle in heat following IN-SYNCH™ will require proper management of bulls and cattle.

3. For Intramuscular Use for Treatment of Pyometra (chronic endometritis) in Cattle. Inject a dose of 5 mL IN-SYNCH™ (25 mg PGF2α) intramuscularly. In studies conducted with IN-SYNCH™, pyometra was defined as presence of a corpus luteum in the ovary and uterine horns containing fluid but not a conceptus based on palpation *per rectum.* Return to normal was defined as evacuation of fluid and return of the uterine horn size to 40mm or less based on palpation *per rectum* at 14 and 28 days. Most cattle that recovered in response to IN-SYNCH™ recovered within 14 days after injection. After 14 days, recovery rate of treated cattle was no different than that of nontreated cattle.
4. For Intramuscular Use for Abortion of Feedlot and Other Non-Lactating Cattle. IN-SYNCH™ is indicated for its abortifacient effect in feedlot and other non-lactating cattle during the first 100 days of gestation. Inject a dose of 25 mg intramuscularly. Cattle that abort will abort within 35 days of injection.
   Commercial cattle were palpated *per rectum* for pregnancy in six feedlots. The percent of pregnant cattle in each feedlot less than 100 days of gestation ranged between 26 and 84; 80% or more of the pregnant cattle were less than 150 days of gestation. The abortion rates following injection of IN-SYNCH™ increased with increasing doses up to about 25 mg. As examples, the abortion rates, over 7 feedlots on the dose titration study, were 22%, 50%, 71%, 90% and 78% for cattle up to 100 days of gestation when injected IM with IN-SYNCH™ doses of 0, 1 (5 mg), 2 (10 mg), 4 (20 mg) and 8 (40 mg) mL, respectively. The statistical predicted relative abortion rate based on the dose titration data, was about 93% for the 5 mL (25 mg) IN-SYNCH™ dose for cattle injected up to 100 days of gestation.

Swine: IN-SYNCH™ Sterile Solution will induce parturition in swine at 10 mg (2 mL) when injected intramuscularly.

As with any multidose vial, practice aseptic techniques in withdrawing each dose. Adequately clean and disinfect the vial closure prior to entry with a sterile needle.

Instructions for Use: The response to treatment varies by individual animals with a mean interval from administration of 2 mL IN-SYNCH™ (10 mg dinoprost) to parturition of approximately 30 hours. This can be employed to control the time of farrowing in sows and gilts in late gestation.

Management Considerations: Several factors must be considered for the successful use of IN-SYNCH™ Sterile Solution for parturition induction in swine. The product must be administered at a relatively specific time (treatment earlier than 3 days prior to normal predicted farrowing may result in increased piglet mortality). It is important that adequate records be maintained on (1) the average length of gestation period for the animals on a specific location, and (2) the breeding and projected farrowing dates for each animal. This information is essential to determine the appropriate time for administration of IN-SYNCH™.

Mares:

Instructions for Use: IN-SYNCH™ Sterile Solution is indicated for its luteolytic effect in mares. This luteolytic effect can be utilized to control the timing of estrus in estrous cycling and clinically anestrous mares that have a corpus luteum in the following circumstances:

1. Controlling Time of Estrus of Estrous Cycling Mares: Mares treated with IN-SYNCH™ during diestrus (4 or more days after ovulation) will return to estrus within 2 to 4 days in most cases and ovulate 8 to 12 days after treatment. This procedure may be utilized as an aid to scheduling the use of stallions.
2. Difficult-to-Breed Mares: In extended diestrus there is failure to exhibit regular estrous cycles which is different from true anestrus. Many mares described as anestrus during the breeding season have serum progesterone levels consistent with the presence of a functional corpus luteum.

   A proportion of "barren", maiden, and lactating mares do not exhibit regular estrous cycles and may be in extended diestrus. Following abortion, early fetal death and resorption, or as a result of "pseudopregnancy", there may be serum progesterone levels consistent with a functional corpus luteum.

   Treatment of such mares with IN-SYNCH™ usually results in regression of the corpus luteum followed by estrus and/or ovulation. In one study with 122 Standardbred and Thoroughbred mares in clinical anestrus for an average of 58 days and treated during the breeding season, behavioral estrus was detected in 81 percent at an average time of 3.7 days after injection with 5 mg IN-SYNCH™; ovulation occurred an average of 7.0 days after treatment. Of those mares bred, 59% were pregnant following an average of 1.4 services during that estrus.

   Treatment of "anestrous" mares which abort subsequent to 36 days of pregnancy may not result in return to estrus due to presence of functional endometrial cups.

1. Evaluate the reproductive status of the mare.
2. Administer a single intramuscular injection of 1 mg per 100 lbs (45.5 kg) body weight which is usually 1 mL to 2 mL IN-SYNCH™ Sterile Solution.
3. Observe for signs of estrus by means of daily teasing with a stallion, and evaluate follicular changes on the ovary by palpation of the ovary *per rectum.*
4. Some clinically anestrous mares will not express estrus but will develop a follicle which will ovulate. These mares may become pregnant if inseminated at the appropriate time relative to rupture of the follicle.
5. Breed mares in estrus in a manner consistent with normal management.

Dinoprost tromethamine is administered once as a single intramuscular injection of 1 mg per 100 lbs (45.5 kg) body weight which is usually 1 mL to 2 mL of IN-SYNCH™ containing 5 mg dinoprost as the tromethamine salt per milliliter.

Precaution(s): Storage Conditions: Store at controlled room temperature 20° to 25°C (68° to 77°F) [see USP].

Caution(s): Federal (USA) law restricts this drug to use by or on the order of a licensed veterinarian.

Cattle: Do not administer to pregnant cattle unless abortion is desired.

Do not administer intravenously (I.V.), as this route might potentiate adverse reactions.

Cattle administered a progestogen would be expected to have a reduced response to IN-SYNCH™ Sterile Solution.

Aggressive antibiotic therapy should be employed at the first sign of infection at the injection site whether localized or diffuse. As with all parenteral products careful aseptic techniques should be employed to decrease the possibility of post injection bacterial infections.

Swine: Do not administer to sows and/or gilts prior to 3 days of normal predicted farrowing, as increased number of stillborn and postnatal mortality may result.

Mares: IN-SYNCH™ Sterile Solution is ineffective when administered prior to day-5 after ovulation.

Pregnancy status should be determined prior to treatment, since IN-SYNCH™ has been reported to induce abortion and parturition when sufficient doses were administered.

Mares should not be treated if they suffer from either acute or subacute disorders of the vascular system, gastrointestinal tract, respiratory system, or reproductive tract.

Do not administer by intravenous route.

Nonsteroidal anti-inflammatory drugs (i.e., indomethacin) may inhibit prostaglandin synthesis, therefore these drugs should not be administered concurrently.

Warning(s):

Cattle: No milk discard or preslaughter drug withdrawal period is required for labeled uses.

Swine: No preslaughter drug withdrawal period is required for labeled uses.

Mares: Not for use in horses intended for food.

Not for human use.

Women of child-bearing age, asthmatics, and persons with bronchial and other respiratory problems should exercise extreme caution when handling this product. In the early stages, women may be unaware of their pregnancies. Dinoprost tromethamine is readily absorbed through the skin and can cause abortion and/or bronchiospasms. Direct contact with the skin should, therefore, be avoided. Accidental spillage on the skin should be washed off immediately with soap and water.

Use of this product in excess of the approved dose may result in drug residues.

Toxicology: Safety and Toxicity:

Laboratory Animals: Dinoprost was non-teratogenic in rats when administered orally at 1.25, 3.2, 10.0 and 20.0 mg/kg/day from day 6th-15th of gestation or when administered subcutaneously at 0.5 and 1.0 mg/kg/day on gestation days 6, 7 and 8 or 9, 10 and 11 or 12, 13 and 14. Dinoprost was non-teratogenic in the rabbit when administered either subcutaneously at doses of 0.5 and 1.0 mg/kg/day on gestation days 6, 7 and 8 or 9, 10 and 11 or 12, 13 and 14 or 15, 16 and 17 or orally at doses of 0.01, 0.1 and 1.0 mg/kg/day on days 6-18 or 5.0 mg/kg/day on days 8-18 of gestation. A slight and marked embryo lethal effect was observed in dams given 1.0 and 5.0 mg/kg/day respectively. This was due to the expected luteolytic properties of the drug.

A 14-day continuous intravenous infusion study in rats at 20 mg PGF2α per kg body weight indicated prostaglandins of the F series could induce bone deposition. However, such bone changes were not observed in monkeys similarly administered IN-SYNCH™ Sterile Solution at 15 mg PGF2α per kg body weight for 14 days.

Cattle: In cattle, evaluation was made of clinical observations, clinical chemistry, hematology, urinalysis, organ weights, and gross plus microscopic measurements following treatment with various doses up to 250 mg dinoprost administered twice intramuscularly at a 10 day interval or doses of 25 mg administered daily for 10 days. There was no unequivocal effect of dinoprost on the hematology or clinical chemistry parameters measured. Clinically, a slight transitory increase in heart rate was detected. Rectal temperature was elevated about 1.5°F through the 6th hour after injection with 250 mg dinoprost, but had returned to baseline at 24 hours after injection. No dinoprost associated gross lesions were detected. There was no evidence of toxicological effects. Thus, dinoprost had a safety factor of at least 10X on injection (25 mg luteolytic dose vs. 250 mg safe dose), based on studies conducted with cattle. At luteolytic doses, dinoprost had no effect on progeny. If given to a pregnant cow, it may cause abortion; the dose required for abortion varies considerably with the stage of gestation.

Induction of abortion in feedlot cattle at stages of gestation up to 100 days of gestation did not result in dystocia, retained placenta or death of heifers in the field studies. The smallness of the fetus at this early stage of gestation should not lead to complications at abortion. However, induction of parturition or abortion with any exogenous compound may precipitate dystocia, fetal death, retained placenta and/or metritis, especially at latter stages of gestation.

Swine: In pigs, evaluation was made of clinical observations, food consumption, clinical pathologic determinations, body weight changes, urinalysis, organ weights, and gross and microscopic observations following treatment with single doses of 10, 30, 50 and 100 mg dinoprost administered intramuscularly. The results indicated no treatment related effects from dinoprost treatment that were deleterious to the health of the animals or to their offspring.

Mares: Dinoprost tromethamine was administered to adult mares (weighing 320 to 485 kg; 2 to 20 years old), at the rates of 0, 100, 200, 400, and 800 mg per mare per day for 8 days. Route of administration for each dose group was both intramuscularly (2 mares) and subcutaneously (2 mares). Changes were detected in all treated groups for clinical (reduced sensitivity to pain; locomotor incoordination; hypergastromotility; sweating; hyperthermia; labored respiration), blood chemistry (elevated cholesterol, total bilirubin, LDH, and glucose), and hematology (decreased eosinophils; increased hemoglobin, hematocrit, and erythrocytes) measurements. The effects in the 100 mg dose, and to a lesser extent, the 200 mg dose groups were transient in nature, lasting for a few minutes to several hours. Mares did not appear to sustain adverse effects following termination of the side effects.

Mares treated with either 400 mg or 800 mg exhibited more profound symptoms. The excessive hyperstimulation of the gastrointestinal tract caused a protracted diarrhea, slight electrolyte imbalance (decreased sodium and potassium), dehydration, gastrointestinal irritation, and slight liver malfunction (elevated SGOT, SGPT at 800 mg only). Heart rate was increased but pH of the urine was decreased. Other measurements evaluated in the study remained within normal limits. No mortality occurred in any of the groups. No apparent differences were observed between the intramuscular and subcutaneous routes of administration. Luteolytic doses of dinoprost tromethamine are on the order of 5 to 10 mg administered on one day, therefore, IN-SYNCH™ was demonstrated to have a wide margin of safety. Thus, the 100 mg dose gave a safety margin of 10 to 20X for a single injection or 80 to 160X for the 8 daily injections.

Additional studies investigated the effects in the mare of single intramuscular doses of 0, 0.25, 1.0, 2.5, 3.0, 5.0, and 10.0 mg dinoprost tromethamine. Heart rate, respiration rate, rectal temperature, and sweating were measured at 0, 0.25, 0.50, 0.75, 1.0, 1.5, 2.0, 3.0, 4.0, 5.0, and 6.0 hr. after injection. Neither heart rate nor respiration rates were significantly altered ($P > 0.05$) when compared to contemporary control values. Sweating was observed for 0 of 9, 2 of 9, 7 of 9, 9 of 9, and 8 of 9 mares injected with 0.25, 1.0, 2.5, 3.0, 5.0, or 10.0 mg dinoprost tromethamine, respectively. Sweating was temporary in all cases and was mild for doses of 3.0 mg or less but was extensive (beads of sweat over the entire body and dripping) for the 10 mg dose. Sweating after the 5.0 mg dose was intermediate between that seen for mares treated with 3.0 and 10.0 mg. Sweating began within 15 minutes after injection and ceased by 45 to 60 minutes after injection. Rectal temperature was decreased during the interval 0.5 until 1.0, 3 to 4, or 5 hours after injection for 0.25 and 1.0 mg, 2.5 and 3.0, or 5.0 and 10.0 mg dose groups, respectively. Average rectal temperature during the periods of decreased temperature was on the order of 97.5 to 99.6, with the greatest decreases observed in the 10 mg dose group.

Adverse Reactions:

Cattle:

1. The most frequently observed side effect is increased rectal temperature at a 5X or 10X overdose. However, rectal temperature change has been transient in all cases observed and has not been detrimental to the animal.
2. Limited salivation has been reported in some instances.
3. Intravenous administration might increase heart rate.
4. Localized post injection bacterial infections that may become generalized have been reported. In rare instances such infections have terminated fatally. See Cautions.

Swine: The most frequently observed side effects were erythema and pruritus, slight incoordination, nesting behavior, itching, urination, defecation, abdominal muscle spasms, tail movements, hyperpnea or dyspnea, increased vocalization, salivation, and at the 100 mg (10X) dose only, possible vomiting. These side effects are transitory, lasting from 10 minutes to 3 hours, and were not detrimental to the health of the animal.

Mares: The most frequently observed side effects are sweating and decreased rectal temperature. However, these have been transient in all cases observed and have not been detrimental to the animal. Other reactions seen have been increase in heart rate, increase in respiration rate, some abdominal discomfort, locomotor incoordination, and lying down. These effects are usually seen within 15 minutes of injection and disappear within one hour. Mares usually continue to eat during the period of expression of side effects. One anaphylactic reaction of several hundred mares treated with IN-SYNCH™ Sterile Solution was reported but was not confirmed.

Presentation: IN-SYNCH™ Sterile Solution is available in 30 mL vials, NDC 57561-019-17.

Compendium Code No.: 10581620 802 336 000

INTEGRATOR™ ℞

Butler **Equine Dietary Supplement**

Active Ingredient(s): Each 60 g contains:

DL-methionine	10 g
Zinc	300 mg
Thiamine hydrochloride (B_1)	100 mg
Biotin	15 mg

In a palatable soybean meal base.

Indications: For use as a supplemental source of the nutrients methionine, zinc, thiamine, and biotin in horses.

Dosage and Administration: Mix 60 g (2 oz.) with grain or sweet feed for 15 days, then give

30 g (1 oz.) a day for maintenance. A plastic measuring scoop is provided. One (1) full scoop contains 30 g (1 oz.) of INTEGRATOR™.

Precaution(s): Store at a controlled room temperature between 15° and 30°C (59°-86°F).

Caution(s): Federal law restricts this drug to use by or on the order of a licensed veterinarian.

For veterinary use only.

Keep out of the reach of children.

Presentation: 63.5 oz. (3.97 lbs., 1,800 g) containers (NDC 11695-096-11).

Compendium Code No.: 10820991

INTENSIVE CARE GRUEL™ (ICG)

TechMix **Weaning Formula**

Guaranteed Analysis:

Crude Protein, Minimum	23.50%
Lysine, Minimum,	1.85%
Crude Fat, Minimum	10.00%
Crude Fiber, Maximum	0.30%
Calcium (Ca), Minimum	0.80%
Calcium (Ca), Maximum	1.00%
Phosphorus (P), Minimum	0.80%
Salt (NaCl), Minimum	1.50%
Salt (NaCl), Maximum	2.50%
Selenium (Se), Minimum	.0.3 ppm
Zinc (Zn), Minimum	2,000 ppm
Vitamin A, Minimum	7,500 I. Units/lb
Vitamin D, Minimum	1,250 I. Units/lb
Vitamin E, Minimum	45 I. Units/lb

Ingredients: Dried Whey, Dried Milk. Dried Whey Soluble, Animal Plasma, Soy Protein Isolate, Whey Protein Concentrate, Fish Meal, Spray Dried Animal Blood Cells, Animal Far (preserved with BHA), Vegetable Fat, Dried Yeast, Sucrose, Dextrose, Calcium Carbonate, Monocalcium Phosphate, Dicalcium Phosphate, Salt, Potassium Sulfate, Magnesium Sulfate, 1-Lysine Monohydrochloride, dl-Methionine, Citric Acid, Irradiated Dried Yeast, Fructo-Oligosaccharides, Hydrated Sodium Calcium Aluminosilicate, Vitamin A Acetate, D-Activated Animal Sterol (source of Vitamin D_3), dl-Alpha Tocopheryl Acetate (source of Vitamin E Activity), Riboflavin Supplement, Niacin Supplement, d-Calcium Pantothenate, Choline Chloride, Vitamin B_{12} Supplement, Menadione Sodium Bisulfate Complex (source of Vitamin K Activity), d-Biotin, Folic Acid, 1-Ascorbyl-2-Polyphosphate, Pyridoxine Hydrochloride, Thiamine Mononitrate, Betaine, Manganese Amino Acid Complex, Manganese Sulfate, Manganous Oxide, Zinc Amino Acid Complex, Zinc Sulfate, Zinc Oxide, Iron Amino Acid Complex, Iron (ferrous) Sulfate, Copper Amino Acid Chelate, Copper Sulfate, Ethylenediamine Dihydriodide, Sodium Selenite, Cobalt Carbonate, Dried *Lactobacillus acidophilus* Fermentation Product, Dried *Lactobacillus lactis* Fermentation Product, Dried *Enterococcus diacetylactis* Fermentation Product, Dried *Enterococcus faecium* Fermentation Product. Dried *Bacillus subtilis* Fermentation Product, Yucca Schidigera Extract, Natural and Artificial Flavors added, Ethoxyquin (a preservative).

Indications: A highly water soluble and nutrient dense transition product specifically designed to be mixed with water and fed as a gruel to stimulate feed intake in small weaned, starved or orphan piglets. When ICG™ is mixed into a gruel it forms a tasty, aromatic and highly digestible product which lures pigs and helps entice high nutrient intake.

Directions for Use: ICG™ can be fed to small piglets dry or as a gruel to aid in transitioning weaned or orphan pigs to conventional starter pellets For feeding dry, use the steps below without the water added.

Step 1: Mix 8 ounces of ICG™ with 4-6 ounces of warm water and stir to form a gruel. Feed this amount of gruel for every 8-10 pigs or a small amount that the pigs will clean up within 30 minutes. Feed about 4-5 hours after weaning. Repeat feeding 4-5 hours after initial feeding.

Step 2: Mix 4 ounces of ICG™ with 4 ounces of conventional starter pellets with 4-6 ounces of warm water and stir to form a gruel and feed to 8-10 pigs.

Step 3: For subsequent feedings, gradually decrease the amount of water and ICG™ and increase the amount of starter pellet when mixing the gruel. Thus will reduce the problems associated with transitioning pigs to dry starter feed.

Offer ICG™ in a shallow J-bolt feeder or mat in small amounts and feed frequently to maintain freshness and encourage consumption. Expected consumption is 2 to 16 ounces.

Precaution(s): Store ICG™ in a clean, dry feed room to maintain freshness.

Caution(s): For very small or orphan pigs using baby Pig ReStart™ One-4 as part or all of the gruel protocol may be beneficial. Piglets too weak to start eating can be drenched with Baby Pig Restart One-4 (4 ounces of Baby Pig ReStart™ in 8 ounces of water).

Presentation: 25 lb. (11.34 kg).

Compendium Code No.: 11440150 991011

INTERCEPTOR® FLAVOR TABS® ℞

Novartis **Parasiticide-Oral**

(milbemycin oxime)

NADA No.: 140-915

Active Ingredient(s): Cats: Each tablet is formulated to provide a minimum of 0.9 mg/lb (2.0 mg/kg) body weight of milbemycin oxime.

Dogs: Each tablet is formulated to provide a minimum of 0.23 mg/lb (0.5 mg/kg) body weight of milbemycin oxime.

Package color	Milbemycin oxime tablet
Brown	2.3 mg
Green	5.75 mg
Yellow	11.5 mg
White	23.0 mg

Indications: Cats: INTERCEPTOR® Flavor Tabs® for Cats are indicated for use in the prevention of heartworm disease caused by *Dirofilaria immitis*, and the removal of adult *Ancytostoma tubaeforme* (hookworm) and *Toxocara cati* (roundworm) in cats and kittens six weeks of age or greater and 1.5 lbs body weight or greater.

Dogs: INTERCEPTOR® Flavor Tabs® are indicated for use in the prevention of heartworm disease caused by *Diroflaria immitis*, the control of adult *Ancylostoma caninum* (hookworm), and the removal and control of adult *Toxocara canis* and *Toxascaris leonina* (roundworms) and *Trichuris vulpis* (whipworm) infections in dogs and in puppies four weeks of age or greater and two pounds body weight or greater.

Pharmacology: Milbemycin oxime consists of the oxime derivatives of 5-didehydromilbemycins in the ratio of approximately 80% A_4 ($C_{32}H_{45}NO_7$, MW 555.71) and 20% A_3 ($C_{31}H_{43}NO_7$, MW 541.68).

Dosage and Administration: Dosage:

Cats: INTERCEPTOR® Flavor Tabs® for Cats are given orally, once a month, at the recommended minimum dosage rate of 0.9 mg milbemycin oxime per pound of body weight (2.0 mg/kg).

Recommended Dosage Schedule for Cats:

Body Weight	Flavor Tab®
1.5 to 6 lbs.	One tablet (5.75 mg)
6.1-12 lbs.	One tablet (11.5 mg)
12.1-25 lbs.	One tablet (23.0 mg)

Cats over 25 lbs. are provided the appropriate combination of tablets.

Dogs: INTERCEPTOR® Flavor Tabs® are given orally, once a month, at the recommended minimum dosage rate of 0.23 mg milbemycin oxime per pound of body weight (0.5 mg/kg).

Recommended Dosage Schedule for Dogs:

Body Weight	INTERCEPTOR®
2-10 lbs.	One tablet (2.3 mg)
11-25 lbs.	One tablet (5.75 mg)
26-50 lbs.	One tablet (11.5 mg)
51-100 lbs.	One tablet (23.0 mg)

Dogs over 100 lbs are provided the appropriate combination of tablets.

Administration:

Cats: INTERCEPTOR® Flavor Tabs® for Cats are palatable and may be offered by the owner as a treat. As an alternative, the tablet may be offered in food or administered as other tablet medications. The tablets can be broken for ease of administration. Watch the cat closely following dosing to be sure the entire dose has been consumed. If it is not entirely consumed, redose once with the full recommended dose as soon as possible.

INTERCEPTOR® Flavor Tabs® for Cats must be administered monthly, preferably on the same date each month. The first dose should be administered within one month of the cat's first exposure to mosquitoes and monthly thereafter until the end of the mosquito season. If a dose is missed and a 30-day interval between dosing is exceeded, administer INTERCEPTOR® Flavor Tabs® for Cats immediately and resume the monthly dosing schedule. It is recommended that cats be tested for existing heartworm infection prior to starting treatment with INTERCEPTOR® Flavor Tabs® for Cats (See Cautions).

Dogs: INTERCEPTOR® Flavor Tabs® are palatable and most dogs will consume the tablet willingly when offered by the owner. As an alternative, the dual-purpose tablet may be offered in food or administered as other tablet medications. Watch the dog closely following dosing to be sure the entire dose has been consumed. If it is not entirely consumed, redose once with the full recommended dose as soon as possible.

INTERCEPTOR® Flavor Tabs® must be administered monthly, preferably on the same date each month. The first dose should be administered within one month of the dog's first exposure to mosquitoes and monthly thereafter until the end of the mosquito season. If a dose is missed and a 30-day interval between dosing is exceeded, administer INTERCEPTOR® Flavor Tabs® immediately and resume the monthly dosing schedule.

If INTERCEPTOR® Flavor Tabs® replaces diethylcarbamazine (DEC) for heartworm prevention, the first dose must be given within 30 days after the last dose of DEC.

Precaution(s): Storage Conditions: INTERCEPTOR® Flavor Tabs® should be stored at room temperature, between 59° and 86°F (15-30°C).

Caution(s): U.S. Federal law restricts this drug to use by or on the order of a licensed veterinarian.

Cats: Do not use in kittens less than six weeks of age or less than 1.5 lbs. body weight. Safety in heartworm positive cats has not been established. Safety in breeding, pregnant, and lactating queens and breeding toms has not been established.

Dogs: Do not use in puppies less than four weeks of age and less than two pounds of body weight. Prior to the initiation of the INTERCEPTOR® Flavor Tabs® treatment program, dogs should be tested for existing heartworm infections. Infected dogs should be treated to remove adult heartworms and microfiliariae prior to initiating treatment with INTERCEPTOR® Flavor Tabs®. Mild, transient hypersensitivity reactions manifested as labored respiration, vomiting, salivation and lethargy, have been noted in some treated dogs carrying a high number of circulating microfilariae. These reactions are presumably caused by release of protein from dead or dying microfilariae.

Adverse Reactions: Dogs: The following adverse reactions have been reported following the use of INTERCEPTOR®: Depression/lethargy, vomiting, ataxia, anorexia, diarrhea, convulsions, weakness and hypersalivation.

Discussion: Efficacy:

Cats: INTERCEPTOR® Flavor Tabs® for Cats eliminate the tissue stage of heartworm larvae and hookworm *(Ancylostoma tubaeforme)* and roundworm *(Toxocara cati)* infections when administered orally according to the recommended dosage schedule. The anthelmintic activity of milbemycin oxime is believed to be a result of interference with invertebrate neurotransmission.

Dogs: INTERCEPTOR® Flavor Tabs® eliminate the tissue stage of heartworm larvae and the adult stage of hookworm *(Ancylostoma caninum)*, roundworms *(Toxocara canis, Toxascaris leonina)* and whipworm *(Trichuris vulpis)* infestations when administered orally according to the recommended dosage schedule. The anthelmintic activity of milbemycin oxime is believed to be a result of interference with invertebrate neurotransmission.

Trial Data: Palatability:

Cats: Palatability trials conducted in 72 cats demonstrated that INTERCEPTOR® Flavor Tabs® for Cats were successfully dosed by the owner when they either offered the tablet as a treat, placed the tablet in the cat's mouth or placed the tablet in the cat's food in 72% of cats. About 16% of the cats were manually dosed and 13% of the cats were not successfully dosed according to the protocol.

Dogs: Palatability trials conducted in 244 dogs from 10 different U.S. veterinary practices demonstrated that INTERCEPTOR® Flavor Tabs® were willingly accepted from the owner by over 95% of dogs. The trial was comprised of dogs representing 60 different breeds and both sexes, with weights ranging from 2.1 lbs to 143.3 lbs, and ages ranging from 8 weeks to 15 years.

Safety:

Cats: INTERCEPTOR® Flavor Tabs® for Cats has been tested safely in over 8 different breeds of cats. In well-controlled clinical field studies 141 cats completed treatment with milbemycin oxime. Milbemycin oxime was used safely in animals receiving frequently used veterinary products such as vaccines, anthelmintics, anesthetics, antibiotics, steroids, flea collars, shampoos and dips.

Safety studies were conducted in young cats and kittens and doses of 1X, 3X and 5X the minimum recommended dose of 2.0 mg/kg demonstrated no drug-related effects. Tolerability studies at exaggerated doses of 10X also demonstrated no drug-related adverse effects in kittens and young adult cats.

Dogs: INTERCEPTOR® has been tested safely in over 75 different breeds of dogs, including collies, pregnant females, breeding males and females, and puppies over two weeks of age. In well-controlled clinical field studies 786 dogs completed treatment with milbemycin oxime. Milbemycin oxime was used safely in animals receiving frequently used veterinary products such as vaccines, anthelmintics, antibiotics, steroids, flea collars, shampoos and dips.

Two studies in heartworm-infected dogs were conducted which demonstrated mild, transient hypersensitivity reactions in treated dogs with high microfilaremia counts (see Cautions for reactions observed).

Safety studies in pregnant dogs demonstrated that high doses (1.5 mg/kg = 3X) of milbemycin oxime given in an exaggerated dosing regimen (daily from mating through weaning), resulted in measurable concentrations of the drug in the milk. Puppies nursing these females which received exaggerated dosing regimens demonstrated milbemycin-related effects. These effects were directly attributable to the exaggerated experimental dosing regimen. The product is normally intended for once-a-month administration only. Subsequent studies included using 3X daily from mating to one week before weaning and demonstrated no effects on the pregnant females or their litters. A second study where pregnant females were dosed once at 3X the monthly use rate either before, on the day of or shortly after whelping resulted in no effects on the puppies.

Some nursing puppies, at 2, 4, and 6 weeks of age, given greatly exaggerated oral INTERCEPTOR® doses (9.6 mg/kg = 19X) exhibited signs typified by tremors, vocalization and ataxia. These effects were all transient and puppies returned to normal within 24 to 48 hours. No effects were observed in puppies given the recommended dose of INTERCEPTOR® (0.5 mg/kg). This product has not been tested in dogs less than 1 kg weight.

A rising-dose safety study conducted in roughcoated collies, manifested a clinical reaction consisting of ataxia, pyrexia and periodic recumbency, in one of fourteen dogs treated with milbemycin oxime at 12.5 mg/kg (25X monthly use rate). Prior to receiving the 12.5 mg/kg dose (25X monthly use rate) on day 56 of the study, all animals had undergone an exaggerated dosing regimen consisting of 2.5 mg/kg milbemycin oxime (5X monthly use rate) on day 0, following by 5.0 mg/kg (10X monthly use rate) on day 14 and 10.0 mg/kg (20X monthly use rate) on day 32. No adverse reactions were observed in any of the collies treated with this regimen up through the 10.0 mg/kg (20X monthly use rate) dose.

Presentation:

Cats: INTERCEPTOR® Flavor Tabs® for Cats are available in three tablet sizes (see Dosage section), formulated according to the weight of the cat. Each tablet size is available in color-coded packages of 6 tablets each, which are packaged 10 per display carton.

Dogs: INTERCEPTOR® Flavor Tabs® are available in four tablet sizes (see Dosage section), formulated according to the weight of the dog. Each tablet size is available in color-coded packages of 6 or 12 tablets each, which are packaged 10 per display carton.

U.S. Patent No. 4,547,520

Compendium Code No.: 11310014 NAH/INT-FT-12P/VI/1 05/01 / NAH/INT-FTCF-12P/VI/1 05/01

INTERSEPT™ ACTIVATOR

Westfalia•Surge **Teat Dip**

Activator for Sanitizing Barrier Teat Dip

Active Ingredient(s): Contents:

Lactic Acid 1.2%
Inactive Ingredients: 99.8%*

*Contains 3% Glycerin.

Indications: This topical liquid product, when properly mixed with InterSept™ Base and used undiluted as a post milking teat dip, effectively aids in reducing the spread of mastitis.

For farm, commercial and industrial use only.

Directions for Use: Use only when properly mixed with InterSept™ Base. Do not dilute.

Always prepare mixture in a ventilated area: add one volume of INTERSEPT™ Activator and one volume of InterSept™ Base to a clean container. Mix thoroughly. Prepare only enough product for one milking of the herd.

Pre Dipping: Before milking, dip each teat with a Westfalia•Surge sanitizing teat dip. After 15 to 30 seconds, dry each teat thoroughly with a single service towel. If the udder and teats are heavily soiled, wash with a sanitizing solution and dry before application of a Westfalia•Surge sanitizing teat dip.

Post Dipping: Immediately after milking, dip each teat with INTERSEPT™. Allow teats to air dry. Do not wipe.

If outside temperature is below freezing, allow to air dry on the teat before the cow leaves the parlor to prevent freezing.

At the end of lactation, apply this product daily for one week after the last milking. In addition, begin application of this product about one week prior to calving.

If a common teat dip cup is used for application, a fresh solution should always be used at each milking. The teat dip cup should be emptied, cleaned and rinsed with potable water after each milking session or when cup becomes contaminated during milking. Do not pour remaining solution from dip cup back into original container.

Precautionary Statements: Danger. Contains materials which may irritate or burn eyes and skin. May be harmful or fatal if swallowed. Protect eyes and skin when handling. Do not take internally. Avoid breathing vapors when mixing this product with InterSept™ Base. Do not mix with any other chemical products. Refer to Material Safety Data Sheet (MSDS).

First Aid:

If in Eyes: Flush with large volumes of water for at least 15 minutes. Call a physician immediately.

If Swallowed: Do not induce vomiting. Rinse mouth promptly then give small amount / glass of milk or water (4-6 oz. child / 10-12 oz. adult) (120-180 mL child / 300-360 mL adult). Avoid alcohol. Call a physician immediately. Do not give anything by mouth to an unconscious or convulsing person.

If on Skin: While removing contaminated clothing and shoes, flush with large volumes of water for at least 15 minutes. If irritation develops and persists, get medical attention.

Inhalation of Vapors: If breathing difficulty or irritation occurs, remove to fresh air. If symptoms persist, get medical attention.

For assistance with medical emergency, call 1-800-451-8346.

Storage: Store this product in a cool dry area away from direct sunlight and heat to avoid deterioration. Keep containers closed to prevent contamination of this product. Keep from freezing.

Warning(s): Keep out of reach of children.

Presentation: Contact the company for container sizes available.

INTERSEPT is a Trademark of Westfalia•Surge, Inc.

Compendium Code No.: 10020071 7751-0598-024 (Rev 03-00)

INTERSEPT™ BASE

Westfalia•Surge **Teat Dip**

Base for Sanitizing Barrier Teat Dip

Active Ingredient(s): Contents:

Sodium Chlorite 0.7%
Inactive Ingredients: 99.3%*

*Contains 2% Glycerin.

Indications: This topical liquid product, when properly mixed with InterSept™ Activator and used undiluted as a post milking teat dip, effectively aids in reducing the spread of mastitis.

For farm, commercial and industrial use only.

Directions for Use: Use only when properly mixed with InterSept™ Activator. Do not dilute.

Always prepare mixture in a ventilated area: add one volume of InterSept™ Activator and one volume of INTERSEPT™ Activator to a clean container. Mix thoroughly. Prepare only enough product for one milking of the herd.

Pre Dipping: Before milking, dip each teat with a Westfalia•Surge sanitizing teat dip. After 15 to 30 seconds, dry each teat thoroughly with a single service towel. If the udder and teats are heavily soiled, wash with a sanitizing solution and dry before application of a Westfalia•Surge sanitizing teat dip.

Post Dipping: Immediately after milking, dip each teat with INTERSEPT™. Allow teats to air dry. Do not wipe.

If outside temperature is below freezing, allow to air dry on the teat before the cow leaves the parlor to prevent freezing.

At the end of lactation, apply this product daily for one week after the last milking. In addition, begin application of this product about one week prior to calving.

If a common teat dip cup is used for application, a fresh solution should always be used at each milking. The teat dip cup should be emptied, cleaned and rinsed with potable water after each milking session or when cup becomes contaminated during milking. Do not pour remaining solution from dip cup back into original container.

Precautionary Statements: Danger. Contains materials which may irritate or burn eyes and skin. May be harmful or fatal if swallowed. Protect eyes and skin when handling. Do not take internally. Avoid breathing vapors when mixing this product with InterSept™ Activator. Do not mix with any other chemical products. Refer to Material Safety Data Sheet (MSDS).

First Aid:

If in Eyes: Flush with large volumes of water for at least 15 minutes. Call a physician immediately.

If Swallowed: Do not induce vomiting. Rinse mouth promptly then give small amount / glass of milk or water (4-6 oz. child / 10-12 oz. adult) (120-180 mL child / 300-360 mL adult). Avoid alcohol. Call a physician immediately. Do not give anything by mouth to an unconscious or convulsing person.

If on Skin: While removing contaminated clothing and shoes, flush with large volumes of water for at least 15 minutes. If irritation develops and persists, get medical attention.

Inhalation of Vapors: If breathing difficulty or irritation occurs, remove to fresh air. If symptoms persist, get medical attention.

For assistance with medical emergency, call 1-800-451-8346.

Storage: Store this product in a cool dry area away from direct sunlight and heat to avoid deterioration. Keep containers closed to prevent contamination of this product. Keep from freezing.

Warning(s): Keep out of reach of children.

Presentation: Contact the company for container sizes available.

INTERSEPT is a Trademark of Westfalia•Surge, Inc.

Compendium Code No.: 10020081 7751-0598-025 (Rev 03-00)

INTESTI-SORB BOLUS

AgriPharm **Adsorbent**

Active Ingredient(s): Each bolus contains: Activated attapulgite, carob, flour, pectin, and magnesium trisilicate, in a suitable base.

Indications: To aid in the supportive treatment of intestinal disturbances in cattle and horses.

Dosage and Administration:

Horses . . . . ½ to 1 bolus
Cattle. . . . . 1 to 1½ boluses

Repeat at 4-hour intervals, if indicated.

Precaution(s): Store at a controlled room temperature between 59°-86°F (15°-30°C).

Caution(s): For animal use only. Keep out of the reach of children.

Presentation: 50 bolus containers.

Compendium Code No.: 14570470

INTESTI-SORB CALF BOLUS

AgriPharm **Adsorbent**

Active Ingredient(s): Each bolus contains activated attapulgite, carob flour, pectin, and magnesium trisilicate, in a suitable base.

Indications: For use as an aid in relief of simple noninfectious diarrhea in colts and calves.

Dosage and Administration: Administer orally. Give two (2) boluses to calves and foals.

Repeat the treatment at 4- to 6-hour intervals as needed. Discontinue use of the product after three (3) days. If symptoms persist after using the preparation for three (3) days, consult a veterinarian.

Precaution(s): Store at a controlled room temperature between 59°-86°F (15°-30°C).

Caution(s): Keep out of the reach of children. For animal use only.

Presentation: 50 bolus containers.

Compendium Code No.: 14570480

INTRA-TRAC®-II

Schering-Plough **Bacterin-Vaccine**

Canine Parainfluenza-Bordetella bronchiseptica Vaccine, Modified Live Virus, Avirulent Live Culture

U.S. Vet. Lic. No.: 165A

Contents: Canine parainfluenza, modified live virus and *Bordetella bronchiseptica*, avirulent live culture.

This vaccine contains penicillin, streptomycin and nystatin as preservatives.

Indications: INTRA-TRAC®-II is recommended for use as an aid in the control and prevention of disease associated with canine parainfluenza and *Bordetella bronchiseptica* infection in healthy dogs 3 weeks of age or older. These agents have been implicated as playing a role in the etiology of the condition known as canine cough.

Dosage and Administration:
Preparation of the Vaccine:
1. Rehydrate the vaccine with the accompanying sterile diluent.
2. Draw the vaccine back into the syringe.
3. Remove needle from syringe.
4. Apply nasal applicator tip to syringe.

How to Vaccinate: Instill the rehydrated vaccine into one or both nostrils of dogs as illustrated below.
When to Vaccinate: Vaccinate dogs at 3 weeks of age or older. Revaccinate annually.

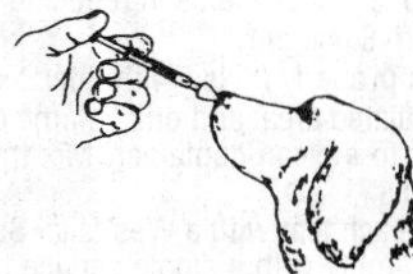

Precaution(s): Store at 2° to 7°C (35° to 45°F). Use entire contents when first opened. Burn containers and all unused contents.
Caution(s): This product is designed for intranasal use only with the enclosed applicators. Systemic reactions resulting from inadvertent intramuscular or subcutaneous injection have been reported. Symptoms may include vomiting, diarrhea, lethargy, inappetence, jaundice, and death associated with liver failure. Localized tissue necrosis at the injection site has also been reported. If inadvertent injection occurs, monitor the dog closely. Supportive therapy including IV fluids and treatment with gentamicin, tetracycline or trimethoprim/sulfa may be indicated.
Post vaccinal reactions consisting of mild canine cough syndrome may occur following use of this vaccine. If anaphylactoid reaction occurs, use epinephrine.
Warning(s): For intranasal use only. For veterinary use only.
Presentation: 25 x 1 mL single dose vials, 150 x 1 mL single dose vials, and 2 x 5 mL multiple dose vials, with sterile diluent and nasal applicators.
U.S. Pat. 4,225,583; 4,300,545; 4,381,773; Des. 270, 283
Compendium Code No.: 10471121

INTRA-TRAC®-II ADT*

Schering-Plough — **Bacterin-Vaccine**

Canine Parainfluenza-Bordetella bronchiseptica Vaccine, Modified Live Virus, Avirulent Live Culture
U.S. Vet. Lic. No.: 165A
Contents: Canine parainfluenza, modified live virus and *Bordetella bronchiseptica*, avirulent live culture.
This vaccine contains penicillin, streptomycin and nystatin as preservatives.
Indications: INTRA-TRAC® is recommended for use as an aid in the control and prevention of disease associated with canine parainfluenza and *Bordetella bronchiseptica* infections in healthy dogs 3 weeks of age or older. These agents have been implicated as playing a role in the etiology of the condition known as infectious canine cough.
Dosage and Administration:
When to Vaccinate: Vaccinate dogs at 3 weeks of age or older. Revaccinate annually.
Preparation of the Vaccine:
1. Hold the vaccine vial in an upright position. Flip the top up and pull to the left. The tear-off aluminum seal is connected to the flip top and will be easily removed. Remove, but do not discard the rubber stopper.
2. Hold the nasal applicator in an upright position and pull off the tip.
3. Carefully insert the tip of the nasal applicator into the upright vaccine vial.
4. Gently squeeze the diluent out of the nasal applicator into the vaccine vial. Do not discard the nasal applicator.
5. Replace the rubber stopper on the vaccine vial and shake gently until the vaccine is fully rehydrated.
6. Remove the rubber stopper from the vaccine vial and insert the tip of the nasal applicator into the upright vaccine vial.
7. Gently squeeze and release the nasal applicator so that the rehydrated vaccine is drawn back into the nasal applicator.
8. While holding the nasal applicator in an upright position, slide a nasal applicator tip over the top of the nasal applicator.
9. The vaccine is now ready for use.

How to Vaccinate: By gently squeezing the body of the nasal applicator, squirt the full 1 mL volume of rehydrated vaccine into one or both nostrils of the dog.
Precaution(s): Store at 2° to 7°C (35° to 45°F). Use entire contents when first opened. Burn all nasal applicators, vaccine vials and all unused contents.
Caution(s): This product is designed for intranasal use only with the enclosed diluent. Systemic reactions resulting from inadvertent intramuscular or subcutaneous injection have been reported. Symptoms may include vomiting, diarrhea, lethargy, inappetence, jaundice, and death associated with liver failure. Localized tissue necrosis at the injection site has also been reported. If inadvertent injection occurs, monitor the dog closely. Supportive therapy including IV fluids and treatment with gentamicin, tetracycline or trimethoprim/sulfa may be indicated.
Post vaccinal reactions consisting of mild canine cough syndrome may occur following use of this vaccine. If anaphylactoid reaction occurs, use epinephrine.
Warning(s): For intranasal use only. For veterinary use only.
Presentation: 25 x 1 mL and 150 x 1 mL dose vials, with ADT* diluents.
* Advanced Delivery Technology
U.S. Pat. 4,225,583; 4,381,773
Compendium Code No.: 10471131

INTRAUTERINE BOLUS

AgriLabs — **Uterine Bolus**

Active Ingredient(s): Each bolus contains:
Urea .... 13.4 g
Indications: For use as an antiseptic and proteolytic aid in beef and dairy cattle and sheep.
Dosage and Administration: For intra-uterine or topical use only. Insert boluses into uterus or dissolve in one (1) pint warm water to make a flush.
Cattle .... 2 to 4 boluses
Sheep .... ½ to 1 bolus
For a topical application, dissolve four (4) boluses in one (1) pint of warm water and thoroughly flush the wound.
Repeat treatment in 24 to 48 hours if necessary.
Precaution(s): Store in a cool, dry place. Keep the container tightly closed when not in use.
Caution(s): Do not administer orally.
Strict cleanliness must be observed to prevent introduction of further infections. Thoroughly cleanse hands and arms of operator and the external genital parts of the animal with soap and water before inserting boluses or flush.
Do not use in deep or puncture wounds or for serious burns. For animal use only.
Keep out of the reach of children.
Presentation: Jars of 50 boluses.
Compendium Code No.: 10580580

IODIDE POWDER

Neogen — **Iodine-Oral**

Dextrose Base-Iodide Feed Supplement
Active Ingredient(s): Each Pound (454 grams) Contains:
Ethylenediamine dihydroiodide .... 0.152 g
(Equivalent to 10 mg/30 g)
Dextrose .... q.s.
Indications: An iodide feed supplement for horses and cattle as an aid in correcting deficiencies where the use of iodide is indicated.
Dosage and Administration:
Horses and Cattle: Mix thoroughly one scoop (1 oz), that has been provided, with ration and feed per head per day. Each scoop provides 10 mg of ethylenediamine dihydroiodide, the recommended daily allowance.
Contraindication(s): Do not administer to animals showing symptoms of acute respiratory conditions.
Caution(s): Treat animals with caution until tolerance is determined as animals vary in susceptibility to iodides. For veterinary use only.
Warning(s): Livestock drug. Keep out of reach of children.
Presentation: 20 oz (567 g) (NDC: 59051-9162-5), 4 lbs (1.814 kg) (NDC: 59051-9163-6) and 20 lbs (9.072 kg) (NDC: 59051-9164-0).
Compendium Code No.: 14910311 — L424-0501 / L430-0501 / L435-0501

IODINE 7% TINCTURE

AgriLabs — **Topical Wound Dressing**

Active Ingredient(s): Contains:
Iodine .... 7.0% w/v
Potassium iodide .... 3.0% w/v
Isopropyl alcohol (99%) .... 82.0% v/v
Inert ingredients:
Water .... q.s.
Indications: For use as an antiseptic for topical use, and as a counter-irritant in chronic inflammatory conditions. May be used as a pre- and post-operative dressing.
Dosage and Administration: For superficial cuts, abrasions, insect bites or bruises, cleanse with soap and water. Apply lightly not more than once a day. If repeated, dilute with three (3) volumes of water. Do not bandage.
Contraindication(s): Not for use on burns, in deep wounds or in body cavities.
Precaution(s): Danger. Flammable. Keep tightly closed when not in use. Store in a cool place.
Caution(s): Poison. Keep out of the reach of children.
If redness, irritation, or swelling persists or increases, discontinue use. Avoid contact with the eyes and mucous membranes.
Antidote(s): Thin starch or flour water paste. To vomit, take mustard and warm water. Call a physician at once.
Presentation: 16 fl. oz. (473 mL) spray bottles and 1 gallon refills.
Compendium Code No.: 10580590

I.O. DINE COMPLEX™ BOLUS

PRN Pharmacal — **Topical Wound Dressing**

Active Ingredient(s): Each bolus contains: 250 mg available (active) iodine as polyvinylpyrrolidone iodine complex in a buffered urea base.
Indications: For flushing wounds or for topical disinfection.
Dosage and Administration: To prepare a solution of iodine for flushing wounds, or for topical disinfection: Dissolve one bolus in 50 to 100 mL water. Apply as a soak or cleanse area with solution on gauze.
Caution(s): For topical use only.
Warning(s): For external use only on non-food animals.
For veterinary use only. Keep out of reach of children.
Presentation: 50 boluses.
Compendium Code No.: 10900090

IODINE DISINFECTANT

Durvet — **Disinfectant**

EPA Reg. No.: 66171-10-12281
Active Ingredient(s):
Iodine* 1.75%
Inert Ingredients 98.25%
*from Nonylphenoxypoly (ethyleneoxy) ethanol-iodine complex
Indications: This product is for the disinfection of hospitals, veterinary clinics, other health care institutions, institutions, industry, schools, farm premises and poultry houses. It can also be used for sanitizing meat and food processing equipment and utensils, food grade egg shells, hands, poultry drinking water, and as a shoe bath sanitizer.
Directions for Use: It is a violation of Federal Law to use this product in a manner inconsistent with its labeling.
For disinfection remove gross filth or heavy soil. Apply IODINE DISINFECTANT with a cloth, mop or mechanical coarse spray device. When applied with a mechanical coarse spray device, surface must be sprayed until thoroughly wetted. Treated surfaces must remain wet for 10 minutes. Fresh solution should be prepared daily or more often if the solution becomes diluted or soiled.
IODINE DISINFECTANT is a proven "one-step" cleaner-disinfectant-sanitizer-deodorizer in the presence of moderate amounts of organic soil and 400 ppm hard water.
Disinfection - Hospitals, Veterinary Clinics, Other Health Care Institutions, Institutions, Industry, Schools, Farm Premises and Poultry Houses: Remove gross filth or heavy soil. Apply

½ oz. per gallon IODINE DISINFECTANT to walls, floors and other hard (inanimate) non-porous surfaces such as tables, chairs, countertops, tile, porcelain and bed frames. Allow surfaces to remain wet for at least 10 minutes. For heavily soiled areas, a preliminary cleaning is required.

For farms and poultry use, prior to disinfection, all poultry, other animals and their feeds must be removed from the premises. This includes emptying all troughs, racks and other feeding and water appliances. Removed all litter and droppings from floors, walls and other surfaces occupied or traversed by poultry or other animals.

After 10 minutes disinfection, ventilate buildings, coop and other closed spaces. Do not house poultry, or other animals or employ equipment until treatment has been absorbed, set or dried.

Sanitizing - Meat and food processing equipment and utensils: Remove heavy soils by flushing, scraping, or moping. Wash with 1 oz. per gallon of IODINE DISINFECTANT (or other good cleaner). Rinse with clean water and sanitize surfaces with 1 oz. IODINE DISINFECTANT per 5 gallons of water (25 ppm titratable iodine). Surface should remain in contact with solution for 1-2 minutes. Drain well and air dry. No potable water rinse is required.

Sanitizing Food Grade Egg Shells: To sanitize clean shell eggs intended for food or food products, spray with a solution of 1 ounce of product in 5 gallons of water (providing 25 ppm active). The solution must be equal to or warmer than the eggs, but not to exceed 130°F. Wet eggs thoroughly and allow to drain. Eggs that have been freshly washed may be sanitized with this compound only if the eggs are rinsed prior to application of the compound. A subsequent potable water rinse is not required. Eggs must be reasonably dry before casing or breaking. The solution must not be reused for sanitizing eggs.

Hand Sanitizing _ in food handling and meat cutting operations. Rinse and immerse hands in a 1 oz. IODINE DISINFECTANT per 5 gals of water solution (25 ppm titratable iodine).

Sanitizing Poultry Drinking Water - Add 1 ounce of IODINE DISINFECTANT per 10 gallons of drinking water (12.5 ppm titratable iodine).

Shoe Bath Sanitizer - To prevent tracking harmful organisms into animal areas, scrape shoes and place in a 3 oz. per gallon solution of IODINE DISINFECTANT for 30 seconds prior to entering area.

Precautionary Statements: Hazards to Humans and Domestic Animals:

Danger: Corrosive. Causes eye damage and skin irritation. Harmful if swallowed. Do not get in eyes, on skin or on clothes. Wear goggles or face shield and rubber gloves when handling. Wash thoroughly with soap and water after handling. Avoid contamination of food and foodstuffs. Avoid breathing spray mist. Remove contaminated clothing and wash before reuse.

Environmental Hazards: This product is toxic to fish. "Do not discharge effluent containing this product into lakes, streams, ponds, estuaries, oceans or other waters unless in accordance with the requirements of a National Pollutant Discharge Elimination System (NPDES) permit and the permitting authority has been notified in writing prior to discharge. Do not discharge effluent containing this product to sewer systems without previously notifying the local sewage treatment plant authority. For guidance contact your State Water Board or Regional Office of the EPA."

Physical and Chemical Hazards: Do not use, pour, spill or store near heat or open time.

Statement of Practical Treatment:

In case of contact, immediately flush eyes or skin with plenty of water for at least 15 minutes. For eyes, call a physician. Remove and wash contaminated clothing before reuse.

If swallowed, drink promptly large quantities of water. Avoid alcohol. Call a physician immediately.

Note to Physician: Probable mucosal damage may contraindicate the use of gastric lavage. Measures against circulatory shock, respiratory depression and convulsion may be needed.

Storage and Disposal:

1. Storage: Store only in tightly closed, original container in a secure area inaccessible to children. Do not contaminate water, food, or feed by storage or disposal.
2. Pesticide Disposal: Pesticide wastes are acutely hazardous. Improper disposal of excess pesticide, spray mixture, or rinsate is a violation of Federal Law. If these wastes cannot be disposed of by use according to label instructions, contact your State Pesticide or Environmental Control Agency, or the hazardous waste representative at the nearest EPA Regional Office for guidance.
3. Container Disposal: Do not reuse empty container. Triple rinse empty container with water. Return metal drums to reconditioner or puncture and dispose of in a sanitary landfill or by other procedures approved by state and local authorities. Plastic containers may be disposed of in a sanitary landfill, incinerated or, if allowed by local authorities, by burning. If burning stay out of smoke.
4. General: Consult Federal, State or local disposal authorities for approved alternative procedures.

Warning(s): Keep out of reach of children.
Presentation: 4 x 1 gallons.
Compendium Code No.: 10841780

IODINE SCRUB

A.A.H. **Surgical Scrub**

Povidone-Iodine Surgical Scrub

Active Ingredient(s): Povidone-Iodine Scrub is equivalent to 0.75% Titratable Iodine.

Indications: An antibacterial, non-irritating surgical scrub for pre-operative and post-operative scrubbing or washing by hospital personnel and for general use in the physician's office.

Directions for Use: Wet hands with water. Pour approximately 5 mL of IODINE SCRUB in palm of hand. Add enough water to make a lather. Lather thoroughly. Rinse thoroughly under running water.

For pre-operative use: Place approximately 5 mL of IODINE SCRUB into hands, rubbing with water. Scrub with brush around nails, under nails, and in nail and cuticle areas. Scrub entire hand and arm to elbow creases for five minutes. Rinse and repeat.

Precaution(s): Avoid storage in excessive heat.
Caution(s): For animal use only.
Warning(s): Keep out of reach of children.
Presentation: 4 x 3.78 L (128 fl oz) (1 gal) jugs per case.
Sold to veterinarians only.
Compendium Code No.: 11180230 1201

IODINE SHAMPOO

Evsco **Antidermatosis Shampoo**

Active Ingredient(s): IODINE SHAMPOO is a nonstaining, painless, medicated shampoo containing 0.2% titratable tamed iodine.

Contains povidone iodine 2.0% in an anionic shampoo base providing 0.2% titratable iodine.

Indications: For cleansing contaminated superficial wounds. Deep medicated cleaning action, good sudsing activity, easy rinsing, painless.

Dosage and Administration: Wet the animal with warm water. Apply IODINE SHAMPOO to the entire body. Work into a rich lather and rinse. Repeat the application and rinse again.

Caution(s): Keep out of the reach of children.

For external animal use only (not for use on cats or kittens).

Reasonable care should be taken to protect the eyes of the animal. May be harmful if swallowed. May discolor if stored in direct sunlight.

Presentation: 12 x 12 fl oz (355 mL) flip top bottles.
Compendium Code No.: 10050140

IODINE SHAMPOO

Tomlyn **Antidermatosis Shampoo**

Active Ingredient(s): Povidone iodine 2.0% in an anionic shampoo base providing 0.2% titratable iodine. Also contains aloe vera, as well as moisturizers and detanglers.

Indications: Tomlyn's IODINE SHAMPOO is a non-staining, painless, medicated shampoo containing 0.2% titratable tamed iodine. Excellent for cleansing contaminated superficial wounds. Deep medicated cleaning action, good for sudsing activity, easy rinsing, painless.

Directions: Wet animal with warm water. Apply IODINE SHAMPOO to the entire body. Work into a rich lather and rinse. Repeat application and rinse again.

Caution(s): Reasonable care should be taken to protect the eyes of the animal. May be harmful if swallowed. May discolor if stored in direct sunlight.

For external animal use only. (Not for use on cats or kittens.) Keep out of reach of children.

Presentation: 12 fl oz (355 mL) and 1 gallon (3.79 L).
Compendium Code No.: 11220071 616-1 6

IODINE SHAMPOO ℞

Vedco **Antidermatosis Shampoo**

Active Ingredient(s): Contains:

Nonylphenoxypoly (ethyleneoxy) ethanol-iodine complex 8.75%
(equivalent to 1.75% titratable iodine)
Inert ingredients 91.25%

Composed of: Linear alcohol ethoxylate sulfates, coco diethanolamides, ethoxylated linear alcohols, deionized water and buffering agents.

Indications: A mild and gentle form of complexed iodine incorporated into a sudsing shampoo base for the cleaning and grooming of dogs, cats, and horses. Iodine is a recognized antimicrobial showing broad-spectrum antiseptic action against gram-negative, and gram-positive bacteria, as well as fungi.

Dosage and Administration: Wet the hair with warm water. Apply the shampoo and work into a rich lather. Continue to massage the lather into the coat for a minimum of five minutes. Rewet the hair or coat and again massage into a rich lather. Rinse the animal with clean water to remove shampoo.

Precaution(s): Keep from freezing.

Caution(s): Federal law restricts this drug to use by or on the order of a licensed veterinarian.

For external use only.

Harmful if swallowed. Avoid contact with the eyes. In case of contact with eyes, flush with copious amounts of water. Contact a physician. Avoid contamination of feed and foodstuffs.

Warning(s): Keep out of reach of children.
Presentation: 1 gallon container.
Compendium Code No.: 10941121

IODINE TINCTURE 7%

AgriPharm **Topical Wound Dressing**

Active Ingredient(s):

Iodine .... 7.0% w/v
Potassium iodide .... 5.0% w/v
Isopropyl alcohol (99%) .... 82.0% v/v
Water .... q.s.

Indications: For topical application on the skin to disinfect superficial wounds, cuts, abrasions, insect bites and minor bruises.

Dosage and Administration: If necessary, clip hair from the area to be treated and cleanse with soap and water. Apply iodine with a swab.

Contraindication(s): Not for use in body cavities or in deep wounds. Do not use on burns.

Precaution(s): Flammable!

Keep away from heat and an open flame.
Keep the container closed when not in use.
Store at 36°-86°F (2°-30°C).
Protect from light.

Caution(s): Poison. May be fatal if swallowed.

For animal use only.
Keep out of the reach of children.

Do not apply under a bandage. Irritation may occur if used on tender skin areas. Avoid contact with the eyes and mucous membranes. In case of deep or puncture wounds or serious burns consult a veterinarian. If redness, irritation, or swelling persists or increases, discontinue use and consult a veterinarian.

Antidote(s): If swallowed give starch paste, milk, bread, egg white or activated charcoal. A 5% solution of sodium thiosulfate (photographic "hypo") may be administered orally at a rate of 10 mL per kilogram of body weight.

Presentation: 16 fl. oz (1 pt.) 1 gallon containers.
Compendium Code No.: 14570490

IODINE TINCTURE 7%

First Priority **Disinfectant**

Antiseptic/Disinfectant

Active Ingredient(s): Isopropyl Alcohol, Iodine, Potassium Iodide, Purified Water.

Indications: For topical application on the skin to disinfect superficial wounds, cuts, abrasions, insect bites and minor bruises.

Directions for Use: If necessary, clip hair from area to be treated and cleanse with soap and water. Apply iodine with a swab.

Precaution(s): Store at 2°-30°C (36°-86°F). Protect from light.

Flammable. Keep away from heat and open flame. Keep container closed when not in use.

Caution(s): Not for use in body cavities or deep wounds. Do not use on burns. Do not apply under bandage. Irritation may occur if used on tender skin areas. Avoid contact with eyes and mucous membranes. In case of deep or puncture wounds or serious burns consult a veterinarian. If redness, irritation, or swelling persists or increases, discontinue use and consult a veterinarian.

For animal use only.

Warning(s): Poison. May be fatal if swallowed.

Antidote: If swallowed give starch paste, milk, bread, egg-white or activated charcoal. A 5% solution of sodium thiosulfate (photographic "hypo") may be administered orally at a rate of 10 mL per kilogram of body weight.

Call a physician or poison control center.

Keep out of reach of children.

Presentation: 16 fl oz (473 mL) with trigger sprayer (NDC# 58829-230-16) and 1 gallon (3.785 L) (NDC# 58829-230-01).

Compendium Code No.: 11390413 Rev. 04-02 / Rev. 07-01

IODINE TINCTURE 7%

Phoenix Pharmaceutical **Topical Wound Dressing**

Active Ingredient(s): Contains:

Isopropyl Alcohol (by volume) 80%

Iodine .... 7% w/v

Indications: An antiseptic, disinfectant for application to superficial cuts, abrasions, insect bites or minor bruises.

Directions: Cleanse area with soap and water. Apply Iodine with swab.

Precaution(s): Flammable. Keep away from heat and open flame. Keep container closed when not in use. Store at 2° to 30°C (36°-86°F). Protect from light.

Caution(s): Do not apply under bandage. This product may irritate tender skin areas. In case of deep or puncture wounds or serious burns, consult veterinarian. If redness, irritation, or swelling persists or increases, discontinue use and consult veterinarian. Avoid contact with eyes and mucous membranes. Not for deep wounds or body cavities. Do not use on burns.

Poison. May be fatal if swallowed.

For animal use only.

Livestock drug.

Antidote(s): If swallowed, give starch paste, milk, bread, egg whites or activated charcoal. A 5% solution of sodium thiosulfate (photographic "hypo") may be administered orally at a rate of 10 mL per kilogram of body weight.

Call a physician or poison control center.

Warning(s): Keep out of reach of children.

Presentation: 1 gallon (3.785 L) containers (NDC 57319-394-09).

Compendium Code No.: 12560432

IODINE TINCTURE 7%

Vedco **Topical Wound Dressing**

Active Ingredient(s): Contains:

Iodine .... 7.0% W/V

Potassium iodide .... 3.0% W/V

Isopropyl alcohol .... 82.0% V/V

Inert ingredients:

Deionized water .... q.s.

Indications: For use as a topical antiseptic for chronic inflammatory conditions and the control of ringworm. An effective pre- and postoperative dressing.

Dosage and Administration: For superficial cuts, abrasions, insect bites or bruises. Cleanse the area with soap and water, apply once a day. If repeated, dilute with three (3) parts water. Do not bandage.

Note: When used on or near the teats or udder of dairy animals the teats and udder should be thoroughly washed before the next milking to prevent contamination of milk.

Contraindication(s): Not for burns, deep wounds or body cavities.

Precaution(s): Do not expose to heat or store at temperatures above 120°F. Store at 70°F or below.

Caution(s): Keep out of the reach of children. For external use only.

If redness, irritation or swelling persists or increases, discontinue use and consult a veterinarian.

Presentation: 16 fl oz (1 pt) and 128 fl oz (1 gallon) containers.

Compendium Code No.: 10941130

IODINE TOPICAL SOLUTION

A.A.H. **Topical Antibacterial**

Povidone Iodine Topical Solution, U.S.P.

Active Ingredient(s): Povidone IODINE TOPICAL SOLUTION, U.S.P. is equivalent to 1.0% Titratable Iodine.

Indications: For minor wounds and infections.

Directions for Use: For minor wounds and infections, apply directly to affected area. May be covered with gauze or adhesive bandage.

Precaution(s): Avoid storage in excessive heat.

Caution(s): Virtually non-irritating, film-forming, non-staining to skin, fur and natural fibers.

For animal use only.

Warning(s): Keep out of reach of children.

Presentation: 4 x 3.78 L (128 fl oz) (1 gal) jugs per case.

Compendium Code No.: 11180240 1201

IODINE WOUND SPRAY

AgriLabs **Topical Wound Dressing**

Active Ingredient(s): Contains:

Alpha (p-nonylphenyl) omega-hydroxypoly (oxyethylene) iodine complex .... 3.7% v/v (providing 1.00% minimum titratable iodine)

Isopropanol .... 30.0% v/v

Inert ingredients .... 66.3% v/v

Indications: A topical antiseptic for use on horses, cattle, swine and sheep prior to surgical procedures such as castrating and docking, for application to the navel of newborn animals; and as an aid in the treatment of minor cuts, bruises and abrasions.

Dosage and Administration: Hold the container approximately four (4) to six (6) inches from the area to be treated. Point the valve at the area to be sprayed. Pull the trigger of the valve and spray the area once lightly. May be repeated once a day, when necessary, until abraded area is healed.

Note: When sprayed on or near the teats or udders of dairy animals, the teats and udders should be thoroughly washed before the next milking to prevent contamination of milk.

Contraindication(s): Not for use on burns or in body cavities or in deep wounds.

Precaution(s): Store in a cool place. Flammable. Do not expose to heat or store at a temperature above 120°F. Do not use near an open flame.

Caution(s): If redness, irritation, or swelling persists or increases, discontinue use and consult a veterinarian.

Harmful if swallowed. Do not apply to the eyes, mucous membranes or large areas of abraded skin. Avoid inhalation of mist.

Livestock remedy. Not for human use. Keep out of the reach of children.

Presentation: 16 fl. oz. (473 mL) and 1 gallon (3.785 L) bottles.

Compendium Code No.: 10580600

IODINE WOUND SPRAY 1.0%

AgriPharm **Topical Wound Dressing**

Active Ingredient(s):

Alpha (p-nonylphenyl) omega-hydroxypoly (oxyethylene) iodine complex (providing 1.00% minimum titratable iodine) 3.7%

Isopropanol 30.0%

Inert ingredients 66.3%

Indications: A topical antiseptic for use prior to surgical procedures such as castrating and docking. For application to the navel of newborn animals, and for teat sores, minor cuts, bruises and abrasions.

Dosage and Administration: Remove the regular cap from the container and replace with the spray cap and tube. Hold the container approximately four (4) to six (6) inches from the area to be treated. Point the valve at the area to be sprayed. Pull the trigger of the valve and spray the area once lightly. May be repeated once a day, if necessary, until the area is healed.

Contraindication(s): Not for use on burns or in body cavities or deep wounds.

Precaution(s): Store in a cool place.

Flammable. Do not expose to heat or store at a temperature above 120°F. Do not use near an open flame.

Caution(s): Not for human use.

Keep out of the reach of children.

For external animal use only.

Harmful if swallowed. Do not apply to the eyes, mucous membranes or large areas of abraded skin. Avoid inhalation of mist.

If redness, irritation, or swelling persists or increases, discontinue use and consult a veterinarian.

Note: When used on or near the teats or udders of dairy animals, the teats and udders should be thoroughly washed before the next milking to prevent the contamination of milk.

Presentation: 16 fl. oz. (1 pt.) and 1 gallon containers.

Compendium Code No.: 14570500

IODINE WOUND SPRAY 2.44%

AgriPharm **Topical Wound Dressing**

Active Ingredient(s):

Alpha (p-nonylphenyl) omega-hydroxypoly (oxyethylene) iodine complex (providing 2.44% minimum titratable iodine) 8.7%

Isopropanol 52.8%

Inert ingredients 38.5%

Indications: A topical antiseptic for use prior to surgical procedures such as castrating and docking. For application to the navel of newborn animals, and for teat sores, minor cuts, bruises and abrasions.

Dosage and Administration: Remove the regular cap from the container and replace with the spray cap and tube. Hold the container approximately four (4) to six (6) inches from the area to be treated. Point the valve at the area to be sprayed. Pull the trigger of the valve and spray area once lightly. May be repeated once a day, if necessary, until the area is healed.

Contraindication(s): Not for use on burns or in body cavities or deep wounds.

Precaution(s): Store in a cool place.

Flammable. Do not expose to heat or store at a temperature above 120°F. Do not use near an open flame.

Caution(s): Not for human use.

Keep out of the reach of children.

For external animal use only.

Harmful if swallowed. Do not apply to the eyes, mucous membranes or large areas of abraded skin. Avoid inhalation of mist.

If redness, irritation, or swelling persists or increases, discontinue use and consult a veterinarian.

Note: When used on or near the teats or udders of dairy animals, the teats and udders should be thoroughly washed before the next milking to prevent the contamination of milk.

Presentation: 16 fl. oz. (1 pt.) and 1 gallon containers.

Compendium Code No.: 14570510

IODOJECT ℞

Vetus **Sodium Iodide**

Composition: Each 100 mL of sterile aqueous solution contains:

Sodium iodide .... 20 grams

Water for injection .... q.s.

Indications: For use as an aid in the treatment of actinomycosis (lumpy jaw) or actinobacillosis (wooden tongue), and necrotic stomatitis in cattle.

Dosage and Administration: Using aseptic procedures, administer slowly by intravenous injection. Inject carefully to avoid deposition outside of the vein. The usual dose is 30 mg per pound of body weight (15 mL/100 lb.). May be repeated at weekly intervals, if necessary.

Contraindication(s): The use of sodium iodide is contraindicated in pregnancy and in hyperthyroidism.

Precaution(s): Store between 15°C and 30°C (59°F-86°F).

Caution(s): Federal law restricts the drug to use by or on the order of a licensed veterinarian.

Animals vary in their susceptibility of iodides. Administer with caution until the animal's tolerance is determined. Discontinue treatment if adverse reactions occur.

Warning(s): Not for use in lactating dairy cows.

For animal only.

Keep out of reach of children.

Presentation: 250 mL multiple dose vials.

Compendium Code No.: 14440500

IOFEC®-20 DISINFECTANT

Loveland **Disinfectant**

EPA Reg. No.: 4959-15-134

Active Ingredient(s):

Titratable iodine* 1.75%
Inert ingredients. 98.25%
Total 100.00%

*From alpha-(p-nonylphenyl)-omega-hydroxypoly (oxyethylene)-iodine complex.

Indications: IOFEC®-20 Disinfectant is a concentrated, broad spectrum iodophor for use as a one-step cleaner, disinfectant and a no-rinse sanitizer in veterinary clinics, poultry and livestock drinking water, sanitizing commercial eggs, egg processing plants, dairy and poultry farms, meat and poultry plants, food processing plants, kennels, pet shops and zoos, hand sanitizing in food plants and animal handling facilities.

When used as directed IOFEC®-20 Disinfectant is effective against *Salmonella choleraesuis, Staphylococcus aureus, Pseudomonas aeruginosa, Mycobacterium tuberculosis* and pathogenic fungi.

Dosage and Administration: It is a violation of federal law to use the product in a manner inconsistent with its labeling.

The color of a IOFEC®-20 Disinfectant solution is proportional to the titratable iodine concentration. Prepare a fresh solution each day, or when there is a noticeable change in its rich amber color, or more often if the solution becomes diluted or soiled. Used as directed, IOFEC®-20 Disinfectant is effective in hard water (up to 400 ppm as $CaCO_3$) and in 5% organic serum load against *Salmonella choleraesuis, Staphylococcus aureus, Pseudomonas aeruginosa, Mycobacterium tuberculosis* and pathogenic fungi.

One-step cleaning and disinfecting:

Prior to use in veterinary clinics, animal handling facilities, farm premises, kennels, pet shops and zoos: Remove all animals and feed from premises, vehicles and enclosures. Remove all litter and manure from floors, walls and all surfaces to be treated. Empty all troughs, racks and other feeding and watering appliances. Then proceed as directed below.

To clean and disinfect: Before applying the disinfecting solution, food products and packaging materials must be removed from the room or carefully protected. Remove heavy soil deposits before applying the disinfecting solution. Using a solution of 3 oz. of IOFEC®-20 Disinfectant per five (5) gallons of warm water (68°F, 20°C or warmer), immerse the objects into the disinfecting solution, or apply the solution with a mop, sponge or brush. Where appropriate, use a mechanical sprayer. Allow a 10-minute contact time with the disinfecting solution. All food contact surfaces must be rinsed with potable water before reuse. Floors, walls and all other nonfood contact surfaces may be drained dry without rinsing.

Note: When mixing IOFEC®-20 Disinfectant with cold water (as low as 41°F, 6°C), increase the use to 6 oz. per five (5) gallons of water.

Before rehousing animals: Ventilate buildings, vehicles and other closed spaces. Do not house the animals or use equipment until the treatment is absorbed, set or dried. Thoroughly rinse all treated feed racks, mangers, troughs, automatic feeders, fountains and waterers with potable water before reuse.

Shoe bath: Routine use of shoe bath sanitizers reduces the spread of disease-causing organisms between poultry houses, farrowing houses, hog barns and other livestock buildings. Use 3 oz. of IOFEC®-20 Disinfectant per one (1) gallon of water. Place the sanitizing solution in shallow plastic or stainless steel pans inside all entrances to poultry and livestock buildings. Scrape the shoes outside the doorway and stand in the shoe bath for 30 seconds before entering the building. Replace the shoe bath once a day, or more often if the solution becomes soiled.

Sanitizing poultry and livestock drinking water: Add ½ oz. of IOFEC®-20 Disinfectant per 10 gallons of drinking water. Regular use in the drinking water reduces slime buildup and mineral deposits in watering equipment. Discontinue sanitizer use when treating the animals with other water medicants.

Sanitizing previously cleaned food contact surfaces: Sanitize previously cleaned and rinsed hard, nonporous surfaces such as glass, metal, plastic and porcelain with a solution containing 1 oz. of IOFEC®-20 Disinfectant per five (5) gallons of water. Spray or immerse the equipment with the sanitizing solution and allow one (1) minute of contact time. Drain the solution from the equipment, do not rinse. IOFEC®-20 Disinfectant used at 1 oz. per gallon of water contains 25 ppm titratable iodine and does not require a final rinse with potable water in accordance with Federal Food Additive Regulation 178.1010.

Sanitizing food-grade egg shells: Spray previously cleaned food-grade egg shells with a solution containing 1 oz. of IOFEC®-20 Disinfectant per five (5) gallons of water. The solution temperature should be warmer than the eggs, but not to exceed 130°F (53°C). Wet the eggs thoroughly for one (1) minute and allow to drain. A final potable water rinse is required only if the eggs are to be immediately broken for processing into the egg products. The eggs should be reasonably dry before casing or breaking. Do not reuse the solution to sanitize the eggs.

Hand sanitizing: Thoroughly wash and rinse the hands before sanitizing. Dip or rinse the hands in a solution containing 1 oz. of IOFEC®-20 Disinfectant per five (5) gallons of water. IOFEC®-20 Disinfectant may be injected directly into the wash or rinse water at a rate of 1 oz. per five (5) gallons of water. A final potable water rinse is not required.

Deodorizing: IOFEC®-20 Disinfectant destroys odors as it sanitizes and disinfects. For general deodorant applications (garbage pails, refuse containers, etc.), swab or spray the surface to be treated with a solution containing 1 oz. of IOFEC®-20 Disinfectant per gallon of water. Allow the treated surface to drain or air dry.

Use Dilution:

IOFEC®-20 Disinfectant/water = titratable iodine:

1 oz. to 10 gallons = 12.5 ppm
1 oz. to 5 gallons = 25 ppm
3 oz. to 5 gallons = 75 ppm
1 oz. to 1 gallon = 125 ppm
6 oz. to 5 gallons = 150 ppm

Precaution(s): Keep the container closed when not in use. Do not store below 25°F or above 100°F for extended periods of time.

Do not contaminate water, food or feed by storage or disposal. Open dumping is prohibited.

Pesticide Disposal: Pesticide wastes are acutely hazardous. Improper disposal of excess pesticide, spray mixture or rinsate is a violation of federal law. If these wastes cannot be disposed of according to label instructions, contact the state pesticide or environmental control agency, or the hazardous waste representative at the nearest EPA regional office for guidance.

Container Disposal: Triple rinse (or equivalent). Then offer for recycling or reconditioning, or puncture and dispose of in a sanitary landfill, or by incineration, or if allowed by state and local authorities, by burning. If burned, stay out of smoke.

Caution(s): Precautionary Statements:

Hazards to Humans and Domestic Animals: Keep out of the reach of children. Corrosive. Causes irreversible eye damage. Harmful if swallowed. Do not get in the eyes or on clothing. Avoid contact with the skin. Wear goggles or a face shield. Wash thoroughly with soap and water after handling. Remove contaminated clothing and wash before reuse.

Statement of Practical Treatment: In case of contact, immediately flush the eyes or the skin with plenty of water for at least 15 minutes. For eyes, call a physician. If swallowed, promptly drink a large quantity of water. Do not induce vomiting. Avoid alcohol. Get medical attention. Remove and wash all contaminated clothing before reuse.

Note to Physician: Probable mucosal damage may contraindicate the use of gastric lavage. Measures against circulatory shock, respiratory depression and convulsions may be needed.

Environmental Hazards: The product is toxic to fish. Keep out of lakes, ponds or streams. Do not contaminate water by the cleaning of equipment or the disposal of wastes. Do not discharge into lakes, streams, ponds or public waters unless in accordance with a NPDES permit. For guidance, contact the regional office of the EPA.

Presentation: 1 gallon (3.785 L) containers.

Compendium Code No.: 10860020

IOSAN®

WestAgro **Disinfectant**

EPA Reg. No.: 4959-23-AA

Active Ingredient(s):

Iodine* 1.75%
Phosphoric acid 15.95%
Inert ingredients:. 82.30%
Total 100.00%

*From nonylphenoxypoly (ethyleneoxy) ethanol-iodine complex and polypropoxypolyethoxy ethanol-iodine complex.

Indications: A concentrated manual detergent-germicide to be diluted with water. An IOSAN® solution can be used for sanitizing milking claws, milking utensils, bulk tanks and to wash and sanitize teats and udders prior to milking.

Dosage and Administration: It is a violation of federal law to use the product in a manner inconsistent with its labeling. The product is regulated by the U.S. Food and Drug Administration under the Food Additives Regulation for use on food-processing equipment and utensils up to 25 ppm titratable iodine without requiring a rinse with potable water.

IOSAN® detergent-germicide is its own indicator of germicidal activity. The amber or yellow color shows the presence of the active ingredient - iodine. When the color fades, prepare a fresh solution. IOSAN® detergent-germicide is not adversely affected by water hardness or cold water.

For use as an udder wash:

1. Prepare a water solution using 1 oz. of IOSAN® sanitizer to each 5 gallons of lukewarm water. The solution contains 25 ppm titratable iodine.
2. Dip a single service paper towel into the wash solution and wash the teats to the base of the udder.
3. Forestrip.
4. Dry the teat with an individual paper towel. Attach the milker unit.
5. Prepare a fresh solution if the wash solution fades noticeably or becomes diluted or soiled.

For sanitizing dairy equipment and utensils:

1. Wash the equipment to be sanitized using Super Kleenite™ Manual Cleaner, following label instructions. Rinse with potable water and drain.
2. Prepare a solution by mixing ½ oz. of IOSAN® sanitizer for each 5 gallons of water, or add ¼ oz. of sanitizer to a 10 qt. pail of water. This provides 12.5 ppm titratable iodine.
3. Immerse equipment (milking claws, liners, teat cups) into the solution making sure that all of the surfaces are in contact with the solution. A contact time of one (1) minute is required.
4. For equipment that cannot be immersed, spray a 25 ppm iodine solution onto all pre-cleaned surfaces.
5. Allow the solution to drain and air-dry.
6. Prepare a fresh solution at each milking or more frequently if the sanitizing solution fades noticeably or becomes diluted or soiled.

For milkstone removal:

1. Should a yellow color show on equipment after the first use of an IOSAN® solution, milkstone is indicated.
2. Remove it using an IOSAN® solution. Make a solution using equal parts IOSAN® detergent-germicide and lukewarm water. Spread over the surfaces to be cleaned.
3. Wait two (2) to three (3) minutes, then brush and rinse with potable water.

Precaution(s): Keep the container closed when not in use. Do not store below 20°F or above 100°F for extended periods. In case of a spill, flood areas with large quantities of water. Product or rinsates that cannot be used should be diluted with water before disposing in a sanitary sewer. Do not re-use the container, but place it in the trash collection. Do not contaminate food or feed by storage, disposal, or the cleaning of equipment.

Caution(s): Keep out of the reach of children.

Precautionary Statements:

Hazards to Humans and Domestic Animals: Danger. Corrosive. Causes eye and skin damage. Do not get in the eyes, on skin or on clothing. Wear goggles and rubber gloves when handling. Harmful or fatal if swallowed. Wash thoroughly with soap and water after handling.

Environmental Hazards: Keep out of lakes, ponds or streams. Do not contaminate water by the cleaning of equipment or the disposal of wastes.

Statement of Practical Treatment:

If swallowed: Promptly drink a large quantity of water. Do not induce vomiting. Avoid alcohol. Get medical attention.

If in eyes: Flush with plenty of water for 15 minutes. Get medical attention.

If on skin: Wash with plenty of soap and water. Get medical attention if irritation persists.

Note to Physician: Probable mucosal damage may contraindicate the use of gastric lavage.

Presentation: 1 gallon and 15 gallon drums.

Compendium Code No.: 10180010

IO-SHIELD® SANITIZING BARRIER TEAT DIP

Ecolab Food & Bev. Div. **Teat Dip**

Active Ingredient(s): .25% iodine (contains glycerine plus other emollients).

Indications: IO-SHIELD® is a unique germicidal 2500 ppm iodine teat dip that forms a protective barrier on the teat. Helps prevent common bacterial organisms known to cause mastitis from entering the teat canal and provides extended antimicrobial protection after dipping.

Benefits

Promotes Udder Health and Hygiene

NMC Protocol B study showed 79% reduction in new *Staph aureus* mastitis infections.

Contains .25% titratable iodine, providing both a germicide and a barrier film on the teat.

I

Equally effective against both infectious mastitis organisms and environmental types such as *E coli.*

Passes AOAC Germicidal and Detergent Sanitizer Test with a greater than 99.999% reduction of *Staph aureus* and *E coli* organisms.

Non-irritating formula aids teat conditioning; gentle on teats and hands.

Film former and wetting agent allows product to cling to the teat.

Versatile - Cost Effectiveness

Ready-to-use formula reduces wasteful, excessive consumption.

Easier to remove than latex barrier type dips - reduces prepping time.

Pharmacology: Properties:

Form	liquid
Color	dark brown
Odor	mild
Wetting Ability	excellent
Specific gravity	1.036
Pounds per gallon	8.6

Dosage and Administration: Important: Do not mix IO-SHIELD® with any other teat dip or other products. If transferred from the container to any other, make sure that other container is thoroughly pre-cleaned and bears the proper container labeling for IO-SHIELD®.

Use a post-milking teat dip on each teat as an aid in a complete cow-care program to help reduce the spread of organisms which may cause mastitis.

Immediately after milking, use IO-SHIELD® at full strength. Submerge entire teat in IO-SHIELD® solution. Allow to air dry. Do not wipe. Always use fresh, full strength IO-SHIELD®. If product in dip cup becomes visibly dirty, discard contents and replenish with undiluted product. Do not reuse or return unused product to the original container. Do not turn cows out in freezing weather until IO-SHIELD® is completely dry.

Wash teats thoroughly just prior to next milking with appropriate udder wash solution or pre-milking teat dip. Teats should then be dried with a single-service towel. Use proper procedures for udder washing or pre-dipping.

Precaution(s): Transport and store between 40°F (4°C) and 100°F (37.8°C). Do not freeze. Product damaged if frozen. Product that has been frozen and thawed may appear watery with clumps of material and will not produce a uniform film on the teat.

Caution(s): IO-SHIELD® is not intended to cure or help the healing of chapped or irritated teats. In case of teat irritation or chapping, have the condition examined and, if necessary, treated by a veterinarian.

Warning(s): For cautionary and first aid information, consult the Material Safety Data Sheet (MSDS).

Presentation: 4 x 1 gallon cases, 5 gallon pail, and 15 gallon drum.

Compendium Code No.: 14490040

IRON DEXTRAN-200

Durvet **Iron Injection**

(iron dextran injection) 200 mg/mL-Hematinic

ANADA No.: 200-256

Active Ingredient(s): Description: IRON DEXTRAN-200 (iron dextran injection) is a sterile solution containing ferric hydroxide in complex with a low molecular weight dextran fraction equivalent to 200 mg elemental iron per mL with 0.5% phenol as a preservative.

Indications: IRON DEXTRAN-200 (iron dextran injection) is intended for the prevention or treatment of anemia in baby pigs due to iron deficiency.

Dosage and Administration: For the prevention of anemia due to iron deficiency, administer an intramuscular injection of 200 milligrams of elemental iron (1 mL) at 1 to 3 days of age. For the treatment of anemia due to iron deficiency, administer an intramuscular injection of 200 milligrams of elemental iron (1 mL) at the first signs of anemia.

Directions for Use: Disinfect rubber stopper of vial as well as site of injection. Use small needle (20 gauge, ⅝ inch) that has been sterilized (boiled in water for 20 minutes). Injection should be intramuscular into the back of the ham. Place tension on the skin over the rear of the ham and inject to a depth of ½" or slightly more.

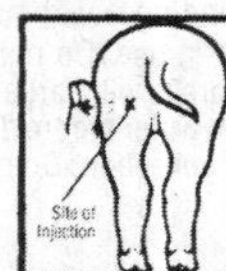

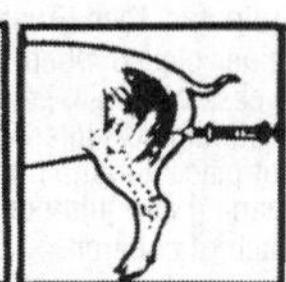

IRON DEXTRAN-200 (iron dextran injection) cannot be considered a substitute for sound animal husbandry. If disease is present in the litter, consult a veterinarian.

Precaution(s): Store at controlled room temperature 59°-86°F (15°-30°C).

Caution(s): For animal use only.

Warning(s): Keep out of reach of children.

Side Effects: Occasionally pigs may show a reaction to injectable iron, clinically characterized by prostration with muscular weakness. In extreme cases, death may result.

Notice: Organic iron preparation injected intramuscularly into pigs beyond 4 weeks of age may cause staining of the ham muscle.

Discussion: Actions: IRON DEXTRAN-200 (iron dextran injection) is easy and economical to use. Injection into the ham is rapid, safe, effective, quickly absorbed by the blood and goes to work immediately. With IRON DEXTRAN-200 (iron dextran injection), the right dosage can be given to every animal with assurance that it will be utilized. Iron deficiency anemia occurs commonly in the suckling pig, often within the first few days following birth. As body size and blood volume increase rapidly from the first few days following birth, hemoglobin levels in the blood fall due to diminishing iron reserves which cannot be replaced adequately from iron in the sow's milk. This natural deficiency lowers the resistance of the pig and scours, pneumonia or other infections may develop and lead to death of the animal. Pigs not hampered by iron deficiency anemia are more likely to experience normal growth and to maintain their normal level of resistance to disease. Adequate iron is necessary for normal, healthy, vigorous growth.

Presentation: IRON DEXTRAN-200 (iron dextran injection), 200 mg/mL is available in 100 mL multidose vials (NDC 30798-807-10).

Manufactured by: Phoenix Scientific, Inc., St. Joseph, MO 64503.

Compendium Code No.: 10841051 Iss. 12-98/Rev. 8-01

IRON DEXTRAN COMPLEX

Premier Farmtech **Iron Injection**

Iron Hydrogenated Dextran

NADA No.: 106-772

Active Ingredient(s): Each mL of IRON DEXTRAN contains 100 mg iron.

Indications: IRON DEXTRAN COMPLEX is for the prevention and treatment of baby pig anemia due to iron deficiency.

Dosage and Administration: For intramuscular injection.

Prevention: 1 mL at two (2) to four (4) days of age. Treatment: 1 mL repeated in 10 days.

Presentation: 100 mL bottles.

Compendium Code No.: 10320010

IRON DEXTRAN INJECTION

Durvet **Iron Injection**

Iron Hydrogenated Dextran

ANADA No.: 200-254

Active Ingredient(s): IRON DEXTRAN INJECTION is a sterile solution containing ferric hydroxide in complex with a low molecular weight dextran fraction equivalent to 100 mg elemental iron per mL with 0.5% phenol as a preservative.

Indications: IRON DEXTRAN INJECTION is intended for the prevention or treatment of iron deficiency anemia in baby pigs.

Dosage and Administration: Intramuscular Injection. Prevention: 1 mL (100 mg) at 2-4 days of age. Treatment: 1 mL (100 mg). May be repeated in approximately 10 days.

Directions for Use: Disinfect rubber stopper of vial as well as site of injection. Use small needle (20 gauge ⅝ inch) that has been sterilized (boiled in water for 20 minutes). Injection should be intramuscular into the back of the ham.

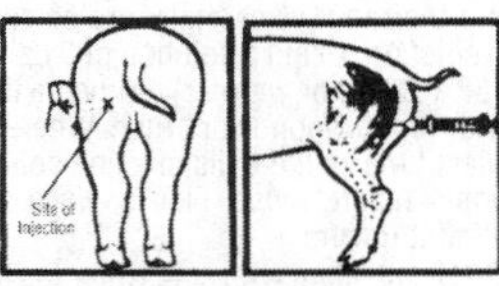

Notice: Organic iron preparation injected intramuscularly into pigs beyond 4 weeks of age may cause staining of muscle tissue.

Precaution(s): Store at controlled room temperature 59°-86°F (15°-30°C).

Caution(s): IRON DEXTRAN INJECTION cannot be considered a substitute for sound animal husbandry. If disease is present in the litter consult a veterinarian.

For intramuscular use only.

For animal use only. Keep out of reach of children.

Side Effects: Occasionally pigs may show a reaction to injectable iron, clinically characterized by prostration with muscular weakness. In extreme cases, death may result.

Discussion: IRON DEXTRAN INJECTION is easy and economical to use. Injection into the ham is rapid, safe, effective, quickly absorbed by the blood and goes to work immediately. With IRON DEXTRAN INJECTION the right dosage can be given to every animal with assurance that it will be utilized.

Treatment of baby pigs with IRON DEXTRAN INJECTION prevents anemia and reduces losses due to iron deficiency. Adequate iron is necessary for normal, healthy, vigorous growth.

Iron deficiency anemia occurs commonly in the suckling pig, often within the first few days following birth. As body size and blood volume increase rapidly from the first few days following birth, hemoglobin levels in the blood fall due to diminishing iron reserves which cannot be replaced adequately from iron in the sow's milk. This natural deficiency lowers the resistance of the pig and scours, pneumonia or other infections may develop and lead to death of the animal. Pigs not hampered by iron deficiency anemia are more likely to experience normal growth and to maintain their normal level of resistance to disease.

Presentation: IRON DEXTRAN INJECTION, 100 mg/mL is available in 100 mL multidose vials (NDC 30798-806-10).

Compendium Code No.: 10841041 Iss. 8-98

IRON DEXTRAN INJECTION

Phoenix Pharmaceutical **Iron Injection**

(Iron Hydrogenated Dextran)

ANADA No.: 200-254

Active Ingredient(s): IRON DEXTRAN INJECTION is a sterile solution containing ferric hydroxide in complex with a low molecular weight dextran fraction equivalent to 100 mg elemental iron per mL with 0.5% phenol as a preservative.

Indications: IRON DEXTRAN INJECTION is intended for the prevention or treatment of iron deficiency anemia in baby pigs. Iron deficiency anemia occurs commonly in the suckling pig, often within the first few days following birth. As body size and blood volume increase rapidly from the first few days following birth, hemoglobin levels in the blood fall due to diminishing iron reserves which cannot be replaced adequately from iron in the sow's milk. This natural deficiency lowers the resistance of the pig and scours, pneumonia or other infections may develop and lead to death of the animal. Pigs not hampered by iron deficiency anemia are more likely to experience normal growth and to maintain their normal level of resistance to disease.

Pharmacology: IRON DEXTRAN INJECTION is easy and economical to use. Injection into the ham is rapid, safe, effective, quickly absorbed by the blood and goes to work immediately. With IRON DEXTRAN INJECTION the right dosage can be given to every animal with assurance that it will be utilized.

Treatment of baby pigs with IRON DEXTRAN INJECTION prevents anemia and reduces losses due to iron deficiency. Adequate iron is necessary for normal, healthy, vigorous growth.

Dosage and Administration: Intramuscular Injection. Prevention: 1 mL (100 mg) at 2-4 days of age. Treatment 1 mL (100 mg). May be repeated in approximately 10 days.

Directions For Use: Disinfect rubber stopper of vial as well as site of injection. Use small needle (20 gauge ⅝ inch) that has been sterilized (boiled in water for 20 minutes). Injection should be intramuscular into the back of the ham.

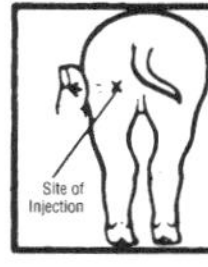

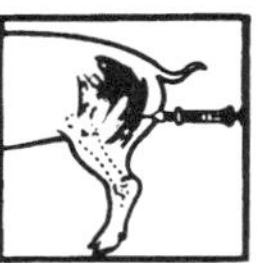

IRON DEXTRAN INJECTION cannot be considered a substitute for sound animal husbandry. If disease is present in the litter consult a veterinarian.

Precaution(s): Store at controlled room temperature 59°-86°F (15°-30°C).

Caution(s): For use in animals only.

For intramuscular use only.

Warning(s): Notice: Organic iron preparation injected intramuscularly into pigs beyond 4 weeks of age may cause staining of muscle tissue.

Keep out of reach of children.

Side Effects: Occasionally pigs may show a reaction to injectable iron, clinically characterized by prostration with muscular weakness. In extreme cases, death may result.

Presentation: IRON DEXTRAN INJECTION, 100 mg/mL is available in 100 mL multidose vials (NDC 57319-404-05).

Manufactured by: Phoenix Scientific, Inc., St. Joseph, MO 64503.

Compendium Code No.: 12560452 Rev. 5-00

IRON DEXTRAN INJECTION

Vedco **Iron Injection**

(Iron Hydrogenated Dextran)

ANADA No.: 200-254

Active Ingredient(s): IRON DEXTRAN INJECTION is a sterile solution containing ferric hydroxide in complex with a low molecular weight dextran fraction equivalent to 100 mg elemental iron per mL with 0.5% phenol as a preservative.

Indications: IRON DEXTRAN INJECTION is intended for the prevention or treatment of iron deficiency anemia in baby pigs.

Dosage and Administration: Intramuscular injection.

Prevention: 1 mL (100 mg) at 2-4 days of age.

Treatment: 1 mL (100 mg).

May be repeated in approximately 10 days.

Directions for Use: Disinfect rubber stopper of vial as well as site of injection. Use small needle (20 gauge, ⅝ inch) that has been sterilized (boiled in water for 20 minutes). Injection should be intramuscular into the back of the ham.

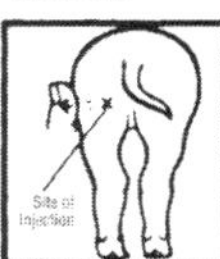

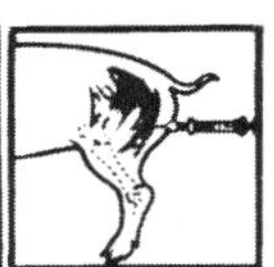

Notice: Organic iron preparation injected intramuscularly into pigs beyond 4 weeks of age may cause staining of muscle tissue.

Precaution(s): Store at controlled room temperature 59°-86°F (15°-30°C).

Caution(s): IRON DEXTRAN INJECTION cannot be considered a substitute for sound animal husbandry. If disease is present in the litter consult a veterinarian.

For intramuscular use only.

For use in animals only.

Warning(s): Keep out of reach of children.

Side Effects: Occasionally pigs may show a reaction to injectable iron, clinically characterized by prostration with muscular weakness. In extreme cases, death may result.

Discussion: IRON DEXTRAN INJECTION is easy and economical to use. Injection into the ham is rapid, safe, effective, quickly absorbed by the blood and goes to work immediately. With IRON DEXTRAN INJECTION the right dosage can be given to every animal with assurance that it will be utilized.

Iron deficiency anemia occurs commonly in the suckling pig, often within the first few days following birth. As body size and blood volume increase rapidly from the first few days following birth, hemoglobin levels in the blood fall due to diminishing iron reserves which cannot be replaced adequately from iron in the sow's milk. This natural deficiency lowers the resistance of the pig and scours, pneumonia or other infections may develop and lead to death of the animal. Pigs not hampered by iron deficiency anemia are more likely to experience normal growth and to maintain their normal level of resistance to disease.

Presentation: IRON DEXTRAN INJECTION is available in 100 mL multidose vials (NDC 50989-486-12).

Manufactured by: Phoenix Scientific, Inc., St. Joseph, MO 64503

Compendium Code No.: 10942470 Rev. 6-01

IRON DEXTRAN INJECTION-200

Aspen **Iron Injection**

Hematinic 200 mg/mL

ANADA No.: 200-256

Active Ingredient(s): IRON DEXTRAN INJECTION-200 in a sterile solution containing ferric hydroxide in complex with a low molecular weight dextran fraction equivalent to 200 mg elemental iron per mL with 0.5% phenol as a preservative.

Indications: For prevention or treatment of baby-pig anemia due to iron deficiency.

Dosage and Administration: For intramuscular injection only.

Prevention: 1 mL (200 mg iron) of 1-3 days of age.

Treatment: 1 mL (200 mg iron) at the first signs of iron deficiency.

Read package insert carefully before use.

Precaution(s): Store at controlled room temperature 59°-86°F (15°-30°C).

Caution(s): Use of this product after four (4) weeks of age may cause staining of the ham muscle.

Warning(s): For animal use only.

Keep out of reach of children.

Presentation: 100 mL.

Manufactured by: Phoenix Scientific, Inc.

Compendium Code No.: 14750460

IRON DEXTRAN INJECTION-200

Butler **Iron Injection**

200 mg/mL-Hematinic

ANADA No.: 200-256

Active Ingredient(s): Description: IRON DEXTRAN INJECTION-200 is a sterile solution containing ferric hydroxide in complex with a low molecular weight dextran fraction equivalent to 200 mg elemental iron per mL with 0.5% phenol as a preservative.

Indications: IRON DEXTRAN INJECTION-200 is intended for the prevention or treatment of anemia in baby pigs due to iron deficiency.

Pharmacology: Actions: IRON DEXTRAN INJECTION-200 is easy and economical to use. Injection into the ham is rapid, safe, effective, quickly absorbed by the blood and goes to work immediately. With IRON DEXTRAN INJECTION-200, the right dosage can be given to every animal with assurance that it will be utilized. Iron deficiency anemia occurs commonly in the suckling pig, often within the first few days following birth. As body size and blood volume increase rapidly from the first few days following birth, hemoglobin levels in the blood fall due to diminishing iron reserves which cannot be replaced adequately from iron in the sow's milk. This natural deficiency lowers the resistance of the pig and scours, pneumonia or other infections may develop and lead to death of the animal. Pigs not hampered by iron deficiency anemia are more likely to experience normal growth and to maintain their normal level of resistance to disease. Adequate iron is necessary for normal, healthy, vigorous growth.

Dosage and Administration: For the prevention of anemia due to iron deficiency, administer an intramuscular injection of 200 milligrams of elemental iron (1 mL) at 1 to 3 days of age. For the treatment of anemia due to iron deficiency, administer an intramuscular injection of 200 milligrams of elemental iron (1 mL) at the first signs of anemia.

Directions for Use: Disinfect rubber stopper of vial as well as site of injection. Use small needle (20 gauge, ⅝ inch) that has been sterilized (boiled in water for 20 minutes). Injection should be intramuscular into the back of the ham. Place tension on the skin over the rear of the ham and inject to a depth of ½" or slightly more.

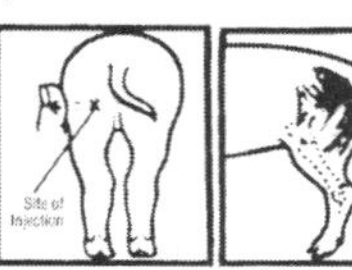

IRON DEXTRAN INJECTION-200 cannot be considered a substitute for sound animal husbandry. If disease is present in the litter, consult a veterinarian.

Precaution(s): Store between 15° and 30°C (59° and 86°F).

Caution(s): Notice: Organic iron preparation injected intramuscularly into pigs beyond 4 weeks of age may cause staining of ham muscle.

For animal use only.

Warning(s): Keep out of reach of children.

Side Effects: Occasionally pigs may show a reaction to injectable iron, clinically characterized by prostration with muscular weakness. In extreme cases, death may result.

Presentation: IRON DEXTRAN INJECTION-200, 200 mg/mL is available in 100 mL multidose vials (NDC 11695-3580-1).

Manufactured by: Phoenix Scientific, Inc., St. Joseph, MO 64503.

Compendium Code No.: 10821960 Iss. 09-01

IRON DEXTRAN INJECTION-200

Phoenix Pharmaceutical **Iron Injection**

200 mg/mL-Hematinic

ANADA No.: 200-256

Active Ingredient(s): Description: IRON DEXTRAN INJECTION-200 is a sterile solution containing ferric hydroxide in complex with a low molecular weight dextran fraction equivalent to 200 mg elemental iron per mL with 0.5% phenol as a preservative.

Indications: IRON DEXTRAN INJECTION-200 is intended for the prevention or treatment of anemia in baby pigs due to iron deficiency.

Pharmacology: Actions: IRON DEXTRAN INJECTION-200 is easy and economical to use. Injection into the ham is rapid, safe, effective, quickly absorbed by the blood and goes to work immediately. With IRON DEXTRAN INJECTION-200, the right dosage can be given to every animal with assurance that it will be utilized. Iron deficiency anemia occurs commonly in the suckling pig, often within the first few days following birth. As body size and blood volume increase rapidly from the first few days following birth, hemoglobin levels in the blood fall due to diminishing iron reserves which cannot be replaced adequately from iron in the sow's milk. This natural deficiency lowers the resistance of the pig and scours, pneumonia or other infections may develop and lead to death of the animal. Pigs not hampered by iron deficiency anemia are more likely to experience normal growth and to maintain their normal level of resistance to disease. Adequate iron is necessary for normal, healthy, vigorous growth.

Dosage and Administration: For the prevention of anemia due to iron deficiency, administer an intramuscular injection of 200 milligrams of elemental iron (1 mL) at 1 to 3 days of age. For the treatment of anemia due to iron deficiency, administer an intramuscular injection of 200 milligrams of elemental iron (1 mL) at the first signs of anemia.

Directions for Use: Disinfect rubber stopper of vial as well as site of injection. Use small needle (20 gauge, ⅝ inch) that has been sterilized (boiled in water for 20 minutes). Injection should be intramuscular into the back of the ham. Place tension on the skin over the rear of the ham and inject to a depth of ½" or slightly more.

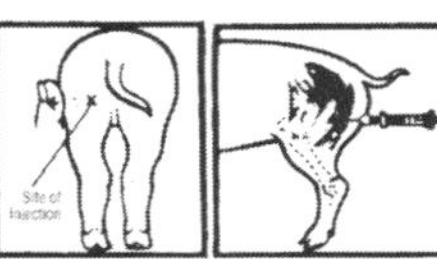

IRON DEXTRAN INJECTION-200 cannot be considered a substitute for sound animal husbandry. If disease is present in the litter, consult a veterinarian.

Precaution(s): Store at controlled room temperature 59°-86°F (15°-30°C).

Caution(s): For animal use only.

Warning(s): Keep out of reach of children.

Side Effects: Occasionally pigs may show a reaction to injectable iron, clinically characterized by prostration with muscular weakness. In extreme cases, death may result.

Notice: Organic iron preparation injected intramuscularly into pigs beyond 4 weeks of age may cause staining of ham muscle.

Presentation: IRON DEXTRAN INJECTION-200, 200 mg/mL is available in 100 mL multidose vials (NDC 57319-405-05).
Manufactured by: Phoenix Scientific, Inc., St. Joseph, MO 64503.
Compendium Code No.: 12560442 Rev. 8-01

IRON HYDROGENATED DEXTRAN INJECTION

Aspen **Iron Injection**

Active Ingredient(s): Each mL of sterile solution contains 100 mg of elemental iron stabilized with a low molecular weight hydrogenated dextran and 0.5% phenol as a preservative.
Indications: For the prevention or treatment of baby pig anemia due to iron deficiency.
Dosage and Administration: Administer by intramuscular injection only.
Prevention: 1 mL (100 mg) at two (2) to four (4) days of age.
Treatment: 1 mL (100 mg). May be repeated in approximately 10 days.
Precaution(s): Store at controlled temperature between 15°C and 30°C (59°F-86°F).
Protect from freezing.
Caution(s): Keep out of the reach of children.
Use of the product after four weeks of age may cause staining of the ham muscle.
Presentation: 100 mL vials.
Compendium Code No.: 14750470

IRON HYDROGENATED DEXTRAN INJECTION

V.L. **Iron Injection**

Hematinic
NADA No.: 138-255
Active Ingredient(s): IRON HYDROGENATED DEXTRAN INJECTION is a sterile solution containing 100 mg of elemental iron per mL, stabilized with a low molecular weight hydrogenated dextran and 0.5% phenol as a preservative.
Indications: For the prevention and treatment of anemia due to iron deficiency in baby pigs.
Dosage and Administration: For intramuscular injection only.

For the prevention of iron deficiency anemia, administer 1 mL (100 mg iron) at two (2) to four (4) days of age.

For the treatment of iron deficiency anemia, administer 1 mL (100 mg iron). The treatment may be repeated in 10 days.

Disinfect the rubber stopper of the vial and the injection site with a cotton ball moistened with rubbing alcohol or another suitable disinfectant. Use a small needle (20 gauge, ⅝ inch) and syringe that have been sterilized by boiling in water for 20 minutes. The injection should be made intramuscularly into the back of the ham. Apply tension to the skin at the injection site by pulling the skin and fat downward with pressure from the thumb or fingers. Inject into the muscle to a depth of approximately one-half (½) inch. Use a clean, sterile needle and syringe for each pig to avoid spreading infection.

The intramuscular injection of organic iron preparations into pigs beyond four (4) weeks of age may cause staining of muscle tissue.

Precaution(s): Store at a controlled room temperature between 15-30°C (59-86°F). Protect from freezing.
Caution(s): Keep out of the reach of children. For animal use only.
If disease or an abnormal condition is suspected, consult a veterinarian before administration.
Side Effects: Occasionally, pigs may exhibit a reaction to iron injection, clinically characterized by prostration and muscular weakness. In extreme cases, death may result.
Discussion: Iron deficiency anemia occurs commonly in the suckling pig, often within the first few days following birth. As body size and blood volume increase rapidly from the first few days following birth, hemoglobin levels in the blood fall due to diminishing iron reserves which cannot be adequately replaced from iron in the sow's milk. Thus, the need for a readily available outside source of iron is apparent. Without the additional iron many newborn pigs may develop anemia within the first few days of life. Anemia retards growth and lowers the body defenses against disease; scours, pneumonia, and other conditions may develop. Death from anemia or infections may occur, sometimes destroying entire litters.
Presentation: 100 mL multiple dose vials.
Compendium Code No.: 10510000

IRON-PLUS

Neogen **Iron-Oral**

Iron-Cobalt-Copper Preparation
Active Ingredient(s): Each Ounce Contains:

Ferric ammonium citrate	1200 mg
Copper gluconate	60 mg
Cobalt sulfate	15 mg

Sodium saccharin, imitation flavor, methylparaben, propylparaben as preservatives.
Indications: A high-potency iron supplement for nutritional anemia in animals.
Dosage and Administration: Dosage Orally:
Horses: 1 fluid ounce 2 to 3 times daily.
Dogs: 1 tablespoon 2 to 3 times daily.
Cattle: 2 fluid ounces 2 to 3 times daily.
Swine: ½ teaspoon 2 to 3 times daily.
Small Animals: Dose proportionately.
Caution(s): For veterinary use only.
Warning(s): Keep out of reach of children.
Presentation: 128 fl oz (1 gallon, 3.785 L) (NDC: 59051-9134-9).
Compendium Code No.: 14910322 L418-0501

I-SITE™

AgriLabs **Bacterin**

Moraxella bovis Bacterin
U.S. Vet. Lic. No.: 355
Active Ingredient(s): The vaccine contains formalin inactivated isolates of *Moraxella bovis.*
Indications: For use in healthy cattle to aid in the prevention and control of infectious bovine keratoconjunctivitis (pinkeye) caused by *Moraxella bovis.*
Dosage and Administration: Shake well before use. Administer a 2 mL dose subcutaneously to cattle five (5) months of age or older. Repeat the vaccination in 21 days.
Precaution(s): Store below 2°-7°C (35°-45°F).
Caution(s): For veterinary use only. Use the entire contents when first opened. If an anaphylactic reaction occurs, administer epinephrine or atropine.
Warning(s): Do not vaccinate within 21 days of slaughter.
Presentation: 20 mL (10 dose) and 100 mL (50 dose) vials.
Compendium Code No.: 10580570

ISOFLO® ℞

Abbott **Inhalation Anesthetic**

isoflurane, USP
Active Ingredient(s): Each mL contains 99.9% isoflurane.
Indications: ISOFLO® (isoflurane, USP) is used for induction and maintenance of general anesthesia in horses and dogs.
Pharmacology: Description: ISOFLO® (isoflurane, USP) is a nonflammable, nonexplosive general inhalation anesthetic agent. Its chemical name is 1-chloro-2,2,2-trifluoroethyl difluoromethyl ether, and its structural formula is:

```
    F   H       F
    |   |       |
F — C — C — O — C — H
    |   |       |
    F   Cl      F
```

Some physical constants are:

Molecular weight	184.5
Boiling point at 760 mm Hg	48.5°C
Refractive index n_D^{20}	1.2990-1.3005
Specific gravity 25°/25°C	1.496
Vapor pressure in mm Hg**:	
20°C	238
25°C	295
30°C	367
35°C	450

**Equation for vapor pressure calculation:

$$\log_{10}P_{vap} = A + \frac{B}{T}$$

where: A = 8.056 B = -1664.58 T = °C + 273.16

Partition coefficients at 37°C:	
Water/gas	0.61
Blood/gas	1.43
Oil/gas	90.8
Partition coefficients at 25°C - rubber and plastic:	
Conductive rubber/gas	62.0
Butyl rubber/gas	75.0
Polyvinyl chloride/gas	110.0
Polyethylene/gas	~2.0
Polyurethane/gas	~1.4
Polyolefin/gas	~1.1
Butyl acetate/gas	~2.5
Purity by gas chromatography	>99.9%
Lower limit of flammability in oxygen or nitrous oxide at 9 joules/sec. and 23°C	None
Lower limit of flammability in oxygen or nitrous oxide at 900 joules/sec. and 23°C	Greater than useful concentration in anesthesia

MAC (Minimum Alveolar Concentration) is 1.31% in horses[1] and 1.28% in dogs.[6]

Isoflurane is a clear, colorless, stable liquid containing no additives or chemical stabilizers. Isoflurane has a mildly pungent, musty, ethereal odor. Samples stored in indirect sunlight in clear, colorless glass for five years, as well as samples directly exposed for 30 hours to a 2 amp, 115 volt, 60 cycle long wave U.V. light were unchanged in composition as determined by gas chromatography. Isoflurane in one normal sodium methoxide-methanol solution, a strong base, for over six months consumed essentially no alkali, indicative of strong base stability. Isoflurane does not decompose in the presence of soda lime (at normal operating temperatures) and does not attack aluminum, tin, brass, iron or copper.

Clinical Pharmacology: ISOFLO® (isoflurane, USP) is an inhalation anesthetic. Induction and recovery from anesthesia with isoflurane are rapid.[2,5] The level of anesthesia may be changed rapidly with isoflurane. Isoflurane is a profound respiratory depressant. Respiration must be monitored closely in the horse and dog and supported when necessary. As anesthetic dose is increased, both tidal volume and respiratory rate decrease.[3,6] This depression is partially reversed by surgical stimulation, even at deeper levels of anesthesia.

Blood pressure decreases with induction of anesthesia but returns toward normal with surgical stimulation. Progressive increases in depth of anesthesia produce corresponding decreases in blood pressure; however, heart rhythm is stable and cardiac output is maintained with controlled ventilation and normal $PaCO_2$ despite the increasing depth of anesthesia. The hypercapnia which attends spontaneous ventilation during isoflurane anesthesia increases heart rate and raises cardiac output above levels observed with controlled ventilation.[3] Isoflurane does not sensitize the myocardium to exogenously administer epinephrine in the dog.

Muscle relaxation may be adequate for intra-abdominal operations at normal levels of anesthesia. However, if muscle relaxants are used to achieve greater relaxation, it should be noted that: all commonly used muscle relaxants are markedly potentiated with isoflurane, the effect being most profound with the nondepolarizing type. Neostigmine reverses the effect of nondepolarizing muscle relaxants in the presence of isoflurane but does not reverse the direct neuromuscular depression of isoflurane.

Dosage and Administration: Operating rooms should be provided with adequate ventilation to prevent the accumulation of anesthetic vapors.

Premedication: A premedication regimen, which may be employed depending upon the patient status, to avert excitement during induction, might include an anticholinergic, a tranquilizer, a muscle relaxant, and a short-acting barbiturate.

Inspired Concentration: The delivered concentration of ISOFLO® (isoflurane, USP) should be known. Isoflurane may be vaporized using a flow-through vaporizer specifically calibrated for isoflurane. Vaporizers delivering a saturated vapor which then is diluted (e.g. Verni-trol® vaporizer) also may be used. The delivered concentration from such a vaporizer may be calculated using the formula:

$$\%\ \text{isoflurane} = \frac{100\ P_V F_V}{F_T(P_A - P_V)}$$

Where: P_A = Pressure of atmosphere
P_V = Vapour pressure of isoflurane
F_V = Flow of gas through vaporizer (mL/min)
F_T = Total gas flow used (mL/min)

Isoflurane contains no stabilizer. Nothing in the drug product alters calibration or operation of these vaporizers.

Induction:

Horses: Inspired concentrations of 3.0 to 5.0% isoflurane alone with oxygen following a barbiturate anesthetic induction are usually employed to induce surgical anesthesia in the horse.

Dogs: Inspired concentrations of 2.0 to 2.5% isoflurane alone with oxygen following a barbiturate anesthetic induction are usually employed to induce surgical anesthesia in the dog.

These concentrations can be expected to produce surgical anesthesia in 5 to 10 minutes.

Maintenance: The concentration of vapor necessary to maintain anesthesia is much less than that required to induce it.

Horses: Surgical levels of anesthesia in the horse may be sustained with a 1.5 to 1.8% concentration of isoflurane in oxygen.

Dogs: Surgical levels of anesthesia in the dog may be sustained with a 1.5 to 1.8% concentration of isoflurane in oxygen.

The level of blood pressure during maintenance is an inverse function of isoflurane concentration in the absence of other complicating problems. Excessive decreases, unless related to hypovolemia, may be due to depth of anesthesia and in such instances may be corrected by lightening the level of anesthesia.

Recovery from isoflurane anesthesia is typically uneventful.[2]

Contraindication(s): ISOFLO® (isoflurane, USP) is contraindicated in horses and dogs with known sensitivity to isoflurane or to other halogenated agents.

Precaution(s): Store at room temperature 15°C-30°C (59°F-86°F).

Caution(s): Federal law restricts this drug to use by or on the order of a licensed veterinarian.

Increasing depth of anesthesia with ISOFLO® (isoflurane, USP) may increase hypotension and respiratory depression. The electroencephalographic pattern associated with deep anesthesia is characterized by burst suppression, spiking and isoelectric periods.[4]

Since levels of anesthesia may be altered easily and rapidly, only vaporizers producing predictable percentage concentrations of isoflurane should be used (see Dosage and Administration).

The action of nondepolarizing relaxants is augmented by isoflurane. Less than the usual amounts of these drugs should be used. If the usual amounts of nondepolarizing relaxants are given, the time for recovery from myoneural blockade will be longer in the presence of isoflurane than in the presence of other commonly used anesthetics.

ISOFLO® like some other inhalational anesthetics, can react with desiccated carbon dioxide (CO2) absorbents to produce carbon monoxide which may result in elevated carboxyhemoglobin levels in some patients. Case reports suggest that barium hydroxide lime and soda lime become desiccated when fresh gases are passed through the CO2 absorber canister at high flow rates over many hours or days. When a clinician suspects that CO2 absorbent may be desiccated, it should be replaced before the administration of ISOFLO®.

Warning(s): Not for use in horses intended for food.

Overdose: In the event of overdosage, or what may appear to be overdosage, the following action should be taken: Stop drug administration, establish that the airway is clear and initiate assisted or controlled ventilation with pure oxygen as circumstances dictate.

Adverse Reactions: Hypotension, respiratory depression and arrhythmias have been reported.

Trial Data: Usage in Pregnancy: Reproduction studies have been performed in mice and rats with no evidence of fetal malformation attributable to ISOFLO® (isoflurane, USP). Adequate data concerning the safe use of isoflurane in pregnant and breeding horses and dogs have not been obtained.

References: Available upon request.

Presentation: ISOFLO® (isoflurane, USP) is packaged in 100 mL and 250 mL amber-colored bottles.

ISOFLO® is a registered trademark of Abbott Laboratories.

Compendium Code No.: 10240040 — 5260-04-03 Revised November, 1996

ISOFLURANE, USP ℞

Halocarbon — **Inhalation Anesthetic**

Active Ingredient(s): Each mL contains 99.9% isoflurane.

Indications: ISOFLURANE, USP is used for induction and maintenance of general anesthesia in horses and dogs.

Pharmacology: Description: ISOFLURANE, USP is a nonflammable, nonexplosive general inhalation anesthetic agent. Its chemical name is 1-chloro-2,2,2-trifluoroethyl difluoromethyl ether, and its structural formula is:

```
     F   H       F
     |   |       |
 F — C — C — O — C — H
     |   |       |
     F   Cl      F
```

Some physical constants are:

Molecular weight	184.5
Boiling point at 760 mm Hg	48.5°C
Refractive index n_D^{20}	1.2990-1.3005
Specific gravity 25°/25°C	1.496
Vapor pressure in mm Hg**	
20°C	238
25°C	295
30°C	367
35°C	450

**Equation for vapor pressure calculation:

$$\log_{10}P_{vap} = A + \frac{B}{T}$$

where: A = 8.056 B = - 1664.58 T = °C + 273.16

Partition coefficients at 37°C:	
Water/gas	0.61
Blood/gas	1.43
Oil/gas	90.8

Partition coefficients at 25°C - rubber and plastic:	
Conductive rubber/gas	62.0
Butyl rubber/gas	75.0
Polyvinyl chloride/gas	110.0
Polyethylene/gas	~2.0
Polyurethane/gas	~1.4
Polyolefin/gas	~1.1
Butyl acetate/gas	~2.5

Purity by gas chromatography	>99.9%
Lower limit of flammability in oxygen or nitrous oxide at 9 joules/sec. and 23°C	None
Lower limit of flammability in oxygen or nitrous oxide at 900 joules/sec. and 23°C	Greater than useful concentration in anesthesia

MAC (Minimum Alveolar Concentration) is 1.31% in horses[1] and 1.28% in dogs.[6]

Isoflurane is a clear, colorless stable liquid containing no additives or chemical stabilizers. Isoflurane has a mildly pungent, musty, ethereal odor. Samples stored in indirect sunlight in clear, colorless glass for five years, as well as samples directly exposed for 30 hours to a 2 amp, 115 volt, 60 cycle long wave U.V. light were unchanged in composition as determined by gas chromatography. Isoflurane in one normal sodium methoxide-methanol solution, a strong base, for over six months consumed essentially no alkali, indicative of strong base stability. Isoflurane does not decompose in the presence of soda lime (at normal operating temperatures), and does not attack aluminum, tin, brass, iron or copper.

Clinical Pharmacology: ISOFLURANE, USP is an inhalation anesthetic. Induction and recovery from anesthesia with isoflurane are rapid.[2,5] The level of anesthesia may be changed rapidly with isoflurane. Isoflurane is a profound respiratory depressant. Respiration must be monitored closely in the horse and dog and supported when necessary. As anesthetic dose is increased, both tidal volume and respiratory rate decrease.[3,6] This depression is partially reversed by surgical stimulation, even at deeper levels of anesthesia.

Blood pressure decreases with induction of anesthesia but returns toward normal with surgical stimulation. Progressive increases in depth of anesthesia produce corresponding decreases in blood pressure; however, heart rhythm is stable and cardiac output is maintained with controlled ventilation and normal $PaCO_2$ despite increasing depth of anesthesia. The hypercapnia which attends spontaneous ventilation during isoflurane anesthesia increases heart rate and raises cardiac output above levels observed with controlled ventilation.[3] Isoflurane does not sensitize the myocardium to exogenously administered epinephrine in the dog.

Muscle relaxation may be adequate for intra-abdominal operations at normal levels of anesthesia. However, if muscle relaxants are used to achieve greater relaxation, it should be noted that: All commonly used muscle relaxants are markedly potentiated with isoflurane, the effect being most profound with the nondepolarizing type. Neostigmine reverses the effect of nondepolarizing muscle relaxants in the presence of isoflurane but does not reverse the direct neuromuscular depression of isoflurane.

Dosage and Administration: Caution: Operating rooms should be provided with adequate ventilation to prevent the accumulation of anesthetic vapors.

Premedication: A premedication regimen, which may be employed depending upon the patient status, to avert excitement during induction, might include an anticholinergic, a tranquilizer, a muscle relaxant, and a short-acting barbiturate.

Inspired Concentration: The delivered concentration of ISOFLURANE, USP should be known. Isoflurane may be vaporized using a flow-through vaporizer specifically calibrated for isoflurane. Vaporizers delivering a saturated vapor which then is diluted (e.g. Verni-trol® vaporizer) also may be used. The delivered concentration from such a vaporizer may be calculated using the formula:

$$\%\ \text{isoflurane} = \frac{100\ P_V F_V}{F_T(P_A - P_V)}$$

where: P_A = Pressure of atmosphere

P_V = Vapour pressure of isoflurane

F_V = Flow of gas through vaporizer (mL/min)

F_T = Total gas flow used (mL/min)

Isoflurane contains no stabilizer. Nothing in the drug product alters calibration or operation of these vaporizers.

Induction:

Horses: Inspired concentrations of 3.0 to 5.0% isoflurane alone with oxygen following a barbiturate anesthetic induction are usually employed to induce surgical anesthesia in the horse.

Dogs: Inspired concentrations of 2.0 to 2.5% isoflurane alone with oxygen following a barbiturate anesthetic induction are usually employed to induce surgical anesthesia in the dog.

These concentrations can be expected to produce surgical anesthesia in 5 to 10 minutes.

Maintenance: The concentration of vapor necessary to maintain anesthesia is much less than that required to induce it.

Horses: Surgical levels of anesthesia in the horse may be sustained with a 1.5 to 1.8% concentration of isoflurane in oxygen.

Dogs: Surgical levels of anesthesia in the dog may be sustained with a 1.5 to 1.8% concentration of isoflurane in oxygen.

The level of blood pressure during maintenance is an inverse function of isoflurane concentration in the absence of other complicating problems. Excessive decreases, unless related to hypovolemia, may be due to depth of anesthesia and in such instances may be corrected by lightening the level of anesthesia.

Recovery from isoflurane anesthesia is typically uneventful.[2]

Contraindication(s): ISOFLURANE, USP is contraindicated in horses and dogs with known sensitivity to isoflurane or to other halogenated agents.

Precaution(s): Storage: Store at room temperature 15°-30°C (59°-86°F).

Caution(s): Federal law restricts this drug to use by or on the order of a licensed veterinarian.

Increasing depth of anesthesia with ISOFLURANE, USP may increase hypotension and respiratory depression. The electroencephalographic pattern associated with deep anesthesia is characterized by burst suppression, spiking, and isoelectric periods.[4]

Since levels of anesthesia may be altered easily and rapidly, only vaporizers producing predictable percentage concentrations of isoflurane should be used (see Dosage and Administration).

The action of nondepolarizing relaxants is augmented by isoflurane. Less than the usual amounts of these drugs should be used. If the usual amounts of nondepolarizing relaxants are given, the time for recovery from myoneural blockade will be longer in the presence of isoflurane than in the presence of other commonly used anesthetics.

Isoflurane, like some other inhalational anesthetics, can react with desiccated carbon dioxide (CO_2) absorbents to produce carbon monoxide which may result in elevated carboxyhemoglobin levels in some patients. Case reports suggest that barium hydroxide lime and soda lime become desiccated when fresh gases are passed through the CO_2 abosorber cannister at high flow rates over many hours or days. When a clinician suspects that CO_2 absorbent may be desiccated, it should be replaced before the administration of isoflurane.

Warning(s): Not for use in horses intended for food.

Overdose: In the event of overdosage, or what may appear to be overdosage, the following action should be taken: Stop drug administration, establish that the airway is clear and initiate assisted or controlled ventilation with pure oxygen as circumstances dictate.

Adverse Reactions: Hypotension, respiratory depression and arrhythmias have been reported.

Trial Data: Usage in Pregnancy: Reproduction studies have been performed in mice and rats with no evidence of fetal malformation attributable to ISOFLURANE, USP. Adequate data concerning the safe use of isoflurane in pregnant and breeding horses and dogs have not been obtained.

References: Available upon request.

Presentation: ISOFLURANE, USP is packaged in 100 mL (NDC 12164-003-10) and 250 mL (NDC 12164-003-25) amber-colored bottles.

Compendium Code No.: 10700011 Revised 2-99

ISOFLURANE, USP ℞

Phoenix Pharmaceutical **Inhalation Anesthetic**

A nonflammable, nonexplosive anesthetic

Active Ingredient(s): Each mL contains 99.9% isoflurane.

Indications: ISOFLURANE, USP is used for induction and maintenance of general anesthesia in horses and dogs.

Pharmacology: Description: ISOFLURANE, USP, is a nonflammable, nonexplosive general inhalation anesthetic agent. Its chemical name is 1-chloro-2,2,2-trifluoroethyl difluoromethyl ether, and its structural formula is:

```
    F   H       F
    |   |       |
F — C — C — O — C — H
    |   |       |
    F   Cl      F
```

Some physical constants are:

Molecular weight 184.5
Boiling point at 760 mm Hg .... 48.5°C
Refractive index n_D^{20} 1.2990-1.3005
Specific gravity 25°/25°C 1.496
Vapor pressure in mm Hg**:
20°C 238
25°C 295
30°C 367
35°C 450

**Equation for vapor pressure calculation:

$$\log_{10}P_{vap} = A + \frac{B}{T}$$

where: A = 8.056 B = -1664.58 T = °C + 273.16

Partition coefficients at 37°C:
Water/gas 0.61
Blood/gas 1.43
Oil/gas 90.8

Partition coefficients at 25°C - rubber and plastic:
Conductive rubber/gas 62.0
Butyl rubber/gas 75.0
Polyvinyl chloride/gas 110.0
Polyethylene/gas .... ~2.0
Polyurethane/gas .... ~1.4
Polyolefin/gas .... ~1.1
Butyl acetate/gas .... ~2.5

Purity by gas chromatography .... >99.9%
Lower limit of flammability in oxygen or nitrous oxide at 9 joules/sec. and 23°C .... None
Lower limit of flammability in oxygen or nitrous oxide at 900 joules/sec. and 23°C .... Greater than useful concentration in anesthesia.

MAC (Minimum Alveolar Concentration) is 1.31% in horses[1] and 1.28% in dogs.[6]

Isoflurane is a clear, colorless stable liquid containing no additives or chemical stabilizers. Isoflurane has a mildly pungent, musty, ethereal odor. Samples stored in indirect sunlight in clear, colorless glass for five years, as well as samples directly exposed for 30 hours to a 2 amp, 115 volt, 60 cycle long wave U.V. light were unchanged in composition as determined by gas chromatography. Isoflurane in one normal sodium methoxide-methanol solution, a strong base, for over six months consumed essentially no alkali, indicative of strong base stability. Isoflurane does not decompose in the presence of soda lime (at normal operating temperatures), and does not attack aluminum, tin, brass, iron or copper.

Clinical Pharmacology: ISOFLURANE, USP is an inhalation anesthetic. Induction and recovery from anesthesia with isoflurane are rapid.[2,5] The level of anesthesia may be changed rapidly with isoflurane. Isoflurane is a profound respiratory depressant. Respiration must be monitored closely in the horse and dog and supported when necessary. As anesthetic dose is increased, both tidal volume and respiratory rate decrease.[3,6] This depression is partially reversed by surgical stimulation, even at deeper levels of anesthesia.

Blood pressure decreases with induction of anesthesia but returns toward normal with surgical stimulation. Progressive increases in depth of anesthesia produce corresponding decreases in blood pressure; however, heart rhythm is stable and cardiac output is maintained with controlled ventilation and normal $PaCO_2$ despite the increasing depth of anesthesia. The hypercapnia which attends spontaneous ventilation during isoflurane anesthesia increases heart rate and raises cardiac output above levels observed with controlled ventilation.[3] Isoflurane does not sensitize the myocardium to exogenously administer epinephrine in the dog.

Muscle relaxation may be adequate for intra-abdominal operations at normal levels of anesthesia. However, if muscle relaxants are used to achieve greater relaxation, it should be noted that: All commonly used muscle relaxants are markedly potentiated with isoflurane, the effect being most profound with the nondepolarizing type. Neostigmine reverses the effect of nondepolarizing muscle relaxants in the presence of isoflurane but does not reverse the direct neuromuscular depression of isoflurane.

Dosage and Administration:

Premedication: A premedication regimen, which may be employed depending upon the patient status, to avert excitement during induction, might include an anticholinergic, a tranquilizer, a muscle relaxant, and a short-acting barbiturate.

Inspired Concentration: The delivered concentration of ISOFLURANE, USP should be known. Isoflurane may be vaporized using a flow-through vaporizer specifically calibrated for isoflurane. Vaporizers delivering a saturated vapor which then is diluted (e.g. Vernitrol® vaporizer) also may be used. The delivered concentration from such a vaporizer may be calculated using the formula:

$$\%\ \text{isoflurane} = \frac{100\ P_V F_V}{F_T(P_A - P_V)}$$

where: P_A = Pressure of atmosphere
P_V = Vapour pressure of isoflurane
F_V = Flow of gas through vaporizer (mL/min)
F_T = Total gas flow used (mL/min)

Isoflurane contains no stabilizer. Nothing in the drug product alters calibration or operation of these vaporizers.

Induction:

Horses: Inspired concentrations of 3.0 to 5.0% isoflurane alone with oxygen following a barbiturate anesthetic induction are usually employed to induce surgical anesthesia in the horse.

Dogs: Inspired concentrations of 2.0 to 2.5% isoflurane alone with oxygen following a barbiturate anesthetic induction are usually employed to induce surgical anesthesia in the dog.

These concentrations can be expected to produce surgical anesthesia in 5 to 10 minutes.

Maintenance: The concentration of vapor necessary to maintain anesthesia is much less than that required to induce it.

Horses: Surgical levels of anesthesia in the horse may be sustained with a 1.5 to 1.8% concentration of isoflurane in oxygen.

Dogs: Surgical levels of anesthesia in the dog may be sustained with a 1.5 to 1.8% concentration of isoflurane in oxygen.

The level of blood pressure during maintenance is an inverse function of isoflurane concentration in the absence of other complicating problems. Excessive decreases, unless related to hypovolemia, may be due to depth of anesthesia and in such instances may be corrected by lightening the level of anesthesia.

Recovery from isoflurane anesthesia is typically uneventful.[2]

Contraindication(s): ISOFLURANE, USP is contraindicated in horses and dogs with known sensitivity to isoflurane or to other halogenated agents.

Precaution(s): Storage: Store at room temperature 15°-30°C (59°-86°F).

Caution(s): Federal law restricts this drug to use by or on the order of a licensed veterinarian.

Operating rooms should be provided with adequate ventilation to prevent the accumulation of anesthetic vapors.

Increasing depth of anesthesia with ISOFLURANE, USP may increase hypotension and respiratory depression. The electroencephalographic pattern associated with deep anesthesia is characterized by burst suppression, spiking and isoelectric periods.[4]

Since levels of anesthesia may be altered easily and rapidly, only vaporizers producing predictable percentage concentrations of isoflurane should be used (see Dosage and Administration).

The action of nondepolarizing relaxants is augmented by isoflurane. Less than the usual amounts of these drugs should be used. If the usual amounts of nondepolarizing relaxants are given, the time for recovery from myoneural blockade will be longer in the presence of isoflurane than in the presence of other commonly used anesthetics.

Isoflurane, like some other inhalational anesthetics, can react with desiccated carbon dioxide (CO_2) absorbents to produce carbon monoxide which may result in elevated carboxyhemoglobin levels in some patients. Case reports suggest that barium hydroxide lime and soda lime become desiccated when fresh gases are passed through the CO_2 absorber canister at high flow rates over many hours or days. When a clinician suspects that CO_2 absorbent may be desiccated, it should be replaced before the administration of isoflurane.

Warning(s): Not for use in horses intended for food.

Overdose: In the event of overdosage, or what may appear to be overdosage, the following action should be taken: Stop drug administration, establish that the airway is clear and initiate assisted or controlled ventilation with pure oxygen as circumstances dictate.

Adverse Reactions: Hypotension, respiratory depression and arrhythmias have been reported.

Trial Data: Usage in Pregnancy: Reproduction studies have been performed in mice and rats with no evidence of fetal malformation attributable to ISOFLURANE, USP. Adequate data concerning the safe use of isoflurane in pregnant and breeding horses and dogs have not been obtained.

References: Available upon request.

Presentation: ISOFLURANE, USP is packaged in 100 mL (NDC 57319-474-05) and 250 mL (NDC 57319-474-06) amber-colored bottles.

Manufactured by: Halocarbon Laboratories, P.O. Box 661, River Edge, NJ 07661.

Compendium Code No.: 12560461 Rev. 02-02

ISOPROPYL ALCOHOL 70%

AgriLabs **Counterirritant**

Active Ingredient(s): Contains:
Isopropyl alcohol .... 70% by volume

Indications: External solution for use as a topical antiseptic. May also be used for temporary relief of minor muscular aches or pain due to overexertion and fatigue.

Dosage and Administration: Scrub hands and arms with soap and water, rinse with water, then scrub with alcohol solution for disinfecting.

Apply full strength directly to affected area, wet thoroughly and massage briskly to stimulate circulation.

Precaution(s): Flammable. Keep away from fire or flame.

Store at controlled room temperature between 2°C and 30°C (36°F-86°F).

Caution(s): For external use only. If taken internally, serious gastric disturbances will result.

Avoid contact with eyes. In case of eye contact, flush thoroughly with water. Call a physician.

First Aid: Induce vomiting or use stomach pump.

For animal use only. For veterinary use only.

Warning(s): Keep out of reach of children.

Presentation: 1 gallon (3.785 L).

Compendium Code No.: 10580611 Rev. 0896

ISOPROPYL ALCOHOL 70%

AgriPharm **Counterirritant**

Active Ingredient(s):
Isopropyl alcohol .... 70% v/v
Water .... q.s.

Indications: For external use only as an antiseptic, disinfectant, and rubefacient.

Dosage and Administration: Use full strength as topical antiseptic or for disinfection of instruments.

May be used for temporary relief of minor muscular aches or pain due to overexertion and fatigue. Apply full strength to affected area and massage briskly to stimulate circulation.

Precaution(s): Store at controlled room temperature between 15°-30°C (59°-86°F).
Caution(s): In case of deep or puncture wounds or serious burns consult a veterinarian. If redness, irritation, or swelling persists or increases, discontinue use and consult a veterinarian. Do not apply to irritated skin or if excessive irritation develops.

If taken internally, serious gastric disturbance will result.

First Aid: Induce vomiting or use stomach pump. Call a physician immediately.

Avoid getting into eyes or on mucous membranes. In case of eye contact, flush thoroughly with water. Call a physician immediately.

Flammable. Keep away from heat and open flame. Keep container closed when not in use.
Presentation: 16 oz (1 pt) and 1 gallon containers.
Compendium Code No.: 14570520

ISOPROPYL ALCOHOL 70%

Aspen **Counterirritant**

Active Ingredient(s):
Isopropyl Alcohol . . . . . 70% v/v
water . . . . . 30% v/v
Indications: For external use only as an antiseptic, disinfectant and rubefacient in cattle, horses, sheep, swine, dogs and cats.
Dosage and Administration: Use full strength as a topical antiseptic or for disinfecting instruments. May also be used for the temporary relief of minor muscle aches or pain due to overexertion and fatigue; apply full strength to affected area and massage briskly to stimulate circulation.
Precaution(s): Store at controlled room temperature between 15°-30°C (59°-86°F).

Flammable: Do not store or use near heat or open flame.

Keep tightly closed when not in use.
Caution(s): In case of deep or puncture wounds or serious burns consult veterinarian. If redness, irritation or swelling persists or increases, discontinue use and consult veterinarian. Do not apply to irritated skin or if excessive irritation develops. Avoid getting into eyes or on mucous membranes.
Warning(s): For external use only. Not for internal use.

For animal use only. Keep out of reach of children.
Presentation: 1 gallon (3.785 L).
Compendium Code No.: 14750480

ISOPROPYL ALCOHOL 70%

Butler **Counterirritant**

Active Ingredient(s):
Isopropyl Alcohol . . . . . 70% w/v
Water . . . . . q.s.
Indications: For external use only as an antiseptic, disinfectant, and rubefacient.
Directions for Use: Use full strength as topical antiseptic or for disinfections of instruments.

May be used for temporary relief of minor muscle aches or pain due to overexertion and fatigue. Apply full strength to affected area and massage briskly to stimulate circulation.
Precaution(s): Store at controlled room temperature between 15°C-30°C (59°F-86°F).

Keep container closed when not in use.
Caution(s): In case of deep or puncture wounds or serious burns consult a veterinarian. If redness, irritation, or swelling persists or increases, discontinue use and consult a veterinarian. Do not apply to irritated skin or if excessive irritation develops.
Warning(s): If taken internally, serious gastric disturbance will result.

First Aid: Induce vomiting or use stomach pump. Call a physician immediately. Avoid getting into eyes or on mucous membranes. In case of eye contact, flush thoroughly with water. Call a physician immediately.

Flammable. Keep away from heat and open flame. For animal use only.

For external use only. Keep out of reach of children.
Presentation: 16 oz and 5 gallon containers.
Compendium Code No.: 10821000

ISOPROPYL ALCOHOL 70%

Centaur **Counterirritant**

Active Ingredient(s): Isopropyl alcohol 70%.
Indications: For use as an antiseptic and rubbing compound.

Pre-diluted solution for use by veterinarians and artificial inseminators as a bactericide and antiseptic.

May be used for temporary relief of minor muscular aches or pain due to over-exertion and fatigue.
Directions: Scrub hands and arms with soap and water, rinse with water, then scrub with alcohol solution.

May be used for temporary relief of minor muscular aches or pain due to over-exertion and fatigue. Apply directly to afflicted area, wet thoroughly and massage briskly to stimulate circulation.
Precaution(s): Flammable. Do not use near heat or open flame.

Store between 50°-85°F.
Caution(s): For external use only. If taken internally, serious gastric disturbances will result. Avoid contact with eyes. In case of eye contact, flush thoroughly with water. Call a physician.

First Aid: Induce vomiting or use stomach pump. For veterinary use only.
Warning(s): Keep out of reach of children.
Presentation: 1 pint (16 fl oz) 473 mL and 1 gallon (128 fl oz) 3.785 L.
Compendium Code No.: 14880190

ISOPROPYL ALCOHOL 70%

Durvet **Counterirritant**

Active Ingredient(s): Contents:
Isopropyl Alcohol . . . . . 70% v/v
Purified Water . . . . . 30% v/v
Indications: ISOPROPYL ALCOHOL 70% may be used for temporary relief of minor muscular aches or pain due to overexertion and fatigue.
Directions: Scrub hands and arms with soap and water, rinse with water, then scrub with alcohol solution.

Apply directly to affected area, wet thoroughly and massage briskly to stimulate circulation.
Precaution(s): Flammable. Do not use near heat or an open flame.
Caution(s): For external use only. If taken internally, serious gastric disturbance will result.

Avoid contact with eyes. In case of eye contact, flush thoroughly with water. Call a physician.

First Aid: Induce vomiting or use a stomach pump. Livestock drug. For animal use only.
Warning(s): Keep out of reach of children.
Presentation: 1 pint (16 oz) (NDC 30798-006-31) and 1 gallon.
Compendium Code No.: 10841061 6/01

ISOPROPYL ALCOHOL 70%

First Priority **Disinfectant**

Active Ingredient(s):
Isopropyl Alcohol . . . . . 70% w/v
Water . . . . . q.s.
Indications: For external use only as an antiseptic, disinfectant, and rubefacient.
Directions: Use full strength as topical antiseptic or for disinfection of instruments. May be used for temporary relief of minor muscular aches or pain due to overexertion and fatigue. Apply full strength to affected area and massage briskly to stimulate circulation.
Precaution(s): Storage: Store at controlled room temperature between 15°-30°C (59°-86°F). Keep container tightly closed when not in use.

Flammable. Keep away from heat and open flame.
Caution(s): In case of deep or puncture wounds or serious burns consult a veterinarian. If redness, irritation, or swelling persists or increases, discontinue use and consult a veterinarian. Do not apply to irritated skin or if excessive irritation develops.

For external use only.

For animal use only.
Warning(s): If taken internally, serious gastric disturbance will result.

First Aid: Induce vomiting or use stomach pump. Call a physician immediately. Avoid getting into eyes or on mucous membranes. In case of eye contact, flush thoroughly with water. Call a physician immediately. Keep out of reach of children.
Presentation: 16 fl oz (473 mL) (NDC# 58829-231-16), 32 fl oz (960 mL) (NDC# 58829-231-32), 1 gallon (3.785 L) (NDC# 58829-231-01) and 5 gallon (18.925 L) (NDC# 58829-231-31).
Compendium Code No.: 11390423 Rev. 9-99 / Rev. 08-01 / Rev. 07-01

ISOPROPYL ALCOHOL 70%

Phoenix Pharmaceutical **Counterirritant**

Active Ingredient(s):
Isopropyl Alcohol . . . . . 70% w/v
Water . . . . . q.s.
Indications: For external use only as an antiseptic, disinfectant and rubefacient.
Directions: Use full strength as topical antiseptic or for disinfection of instruments. May be used for temporary relief of minor muscular aches or pain due to overexertion and fatigue. Apply full strength to affected area and massage briskly to stimulate circulation.
Precaution(s): Store at a controlled room temperature between 15°-30°C (59°-86°F).

Keep container closed when not in use. Flammable! Keep away from heat and open flame.
Caution(s): In case of deep or puncture wounds or serious burns, consult a veterinarian.

If redness, irritation, or swelling persists or increases, discontinue use and consult a veterinarian. Do not apply to irritated skin or if excessive irritation develops.

For external use only. For animal use only.
Warning(s): If taken internally, serious gastric disturbance will result.

First Aid: Induce vomiting or use stomach pump. Call a physician immediately. Avoid getting into eyes or on mucous membranes. In case of eye contact, flush thoroughly with water. Call a physician immediately. Keep out of reach of children.
Presentation: 32 fl oz (NDC 57319-408-22) and 1 gallon (3.785 L) containers (NDC 57319-444-09).
Compendium Code No.: 12561061 Rev. 08-01

ISOPROPYL ALCOHOL 70%

Vedco **Counterirritant**

Active Ingredient(s): Contains:
Isopropyl alcohol 70%
Inert ingredient:
Water 30%
Indications: External solution for use as a topical antiseptic. May also be used for the temporary relief of minor muscular aches or pain due to overexertion and fatigue.
Dosage and Administration: Scrub hands and arms with soap and water, rinse with water, then scrub with the alcohol solution for disinfecting. For the temporary relief of minor muscular aches or pain due to overexertion and fatigue, apply full strength directly onto the afflicted area, wet thoroughly and massage briskly to stimulate circulation.
Precaution(s): Store at a controlled room temperature between 59-86°F (15-30°C). Flammable: Do not use near heat or an open flame.
Caution(s): For external use only.

If taken internally, serious gastric disturbance will result. Avoid contact with the eyes. In case of eye contact, flush thoroughly with water. Call a physician.

First Aid: Induce vomiting or use stomach pump.
Warning(s): Keep out of reach of children.
Presentation: 1 pint, 32 oz and 1 gallon containers.
Compendium Code No.: 10941141

ISOPROPYL ALCOHOL 99%

AgriLabs **Counterirritant**

Active Ingredient(s): Composition:
Isopropyl Alcohol . . . . . 99% v/v
Water . . . . . 1% v/v
Indications: For external use only as an antiseptic, disinfectant and rubefacient in cattle, horses, sheep, swine, dogs and cats.
Dosage and Administration: For use in making a standard solution (70%): Dilute by adding 1 part water to 2 parts of this 99% isopropyl alcohol.

Directions for use: Use standard strength (70%) as topical antiseptic or for disinfection of instruments. May also be used for temporary relief of minor muscular aches or pain due to overexertion and fatigue. Apply full strength to effected area and massage briskly to stimulate circulation.
Precaution(s): Flammable. Do not store or use near heat or open flame. Store at controlled room temperature between 15° and 30°C (59°-86°F).

Keep tightly closed when not in use.
Caution(s): In case of deep or puncture wounds or serious burns consult veterinarian. If redness,

I

irritation or swelling persists or increases, discontinue use and consult veterinarian. Do not apply to irritated skin or if excessive irritation develops. Avoid getting into eyes or in mucous membranes.

Not for internal use.

For animal use only.

Warning(s): Keep out of reach of children.

Presentation: 1 gallon (3.785 L) containers.

Compendium Code No.: 10580621 Iss. 2-95

ISOPROPYL ALCOHOL 99%

AgriPharm **Counterirritant**

Active Ingredient(s):

Isopropyl alcohol . . . . . 99% v/v

Water . . . . . q.s.

Indications: For external use only as an antiseptic, disinfectant and rubefacient.

Dosage and Administration: To make a standard solution (70%): Dilute by adding one (1) part water to two (2) parts of the 99% isopropyl alcohol.

Use full strength as topical antiseptic or for the disinfection of instruments.

May be used for the temporary relief of minor muscular aches or pain due to overexertion and fatigue. Apply full strength to the effected area and massage briskly to stimulate circulation.

Precaution(s): Flammable. Keep away from heat and anopen flame. Keep the container closed when not in use.

Store at a controlled room temperature between 59°-86°F (15°-30°C).

Caution(s): For animal use only.

Keep out of the reach of children.

If taken internally, serious gastric disturbance will result.

First aid: Induce vomiting or use a stomach pump. Call a physician immediately.

Avoid getting into the eyes or on mucous membranes. In case of eye contact, flush thoroughly with water. Call a physician immediately.

In case of deep or puncture wounds or serious burns, consult a veterinarian. If redness, irritation, or swelling persists or increases, discontinue use of the product and consult a veterinarian. Do not apply to irritated skin or if excessive irritation develops.

Presentation: 1 gallon containers.

Compendium Code No.: 14570530

ISOPROPYL ALCOHOL 99%

Aspen **Counterirritant**

Active Ingredient(s):

Isopropyl Alcohol 99%

Inert Ingredient:

Water 1%

Total 100%

Indications: External solution for use as a topical antiseptic. May also be used for temporary relief of minor muscular aches or pain due to overexertion and fatigue.

Dosage and Administration: As an antiseptic: Scrub hands and arms with soap and water, rinse with water, then scrub with alcohol solution for disinfecting.

For muscular aches: Apply full strength directly to affected area, wet thoroughly and massage briskly to stimulate circulation.

Precaution(s): Flammable. Do not expose to heat, sparks or open flame. Do not store above 120°F.

Warning(s): For external use only. If taken internally, serious gastric disturbance will result. Avoid contact with eyes. In case of eye contact, flush thoroughly with water. Call a physician.

First Aid: Induce vomiting or use stomach pump.

For animal use only.

Not for human use.

Keep out of reach of children.

Presentation: 1 gallon (3.785 L) containers.

Compendium Code No.: 14750490

ISOPROPYL ALCOHOL 99%

Centaur **Counterirritant**

Active Ingredient(s): Isopropyl Alcohol 99%.

Indications: Widely used by veterinarians and artificial inseminators as a bactericide and antiseptic. May also be used for temporary relief of minor muscular aches or pains due to overexertion or fatigue.

For use in manufacturing, processing or repackaging.

Directions: Dilute with water as desired. Scrub hands and arms with soap and water. Rinse with water and then scrub with alcohol. As a rub-down, apply full strength directly to affected area. Wet thoroughly and massage briskly to stimulate circulation.

Precaution(s): Flammable liquid. Store between 50°-85°F. Keep away from heat and open flame. Keep container closed.

Caution(s): Use only with adequate ventilation.

For external use only.

For animal use only.

Warning(s): Keep out of reach of children.

Presentation: 1 pint (16 fl oz) 473 mL and 1 gallon (128 fl oz) 3.785 L containers.

Manufactured by: Unavet, North Kansas City, MO 64116.

Compendium Code No.: 14880300

ISOPROPYL ALCOHOL 99%

First Priority **Disinfectant**

Active Ingredient(s):

Isopropyl Alcohol (min.) . . . . . 99% w/v

Indications: For external use only as an antiseptic, disinfectant, and rubefacient.

Directions for Use: Use full strength as topical antiseptic or for disinfections of instruments. May be used for temporary relief of minor muscular aches or pain due to overexertion and fatigue. Apply full strength to affected area and massage briskly to stimulate circulation.

To Make a Standard Solution (70%): Dilute by adding 1 part water to 2 parts of this 99% Isopropyl Alcohol.

Precaution(s): Storage: Store at controlled room temperature between 15°-30°C (59°-86°F). Keep container tightly closed when not in use.

Flammable. Keep away from heat and open flame.

Caution(s): In case of deep or puncture wounds or serious burns consult a veterinarian. If redness, irritation, or swelling persists or increases, discontinue use and consult a veterinarian. Do not apply to irritated skin or if excessive irritation develops.

For external use only.

For animal use only.

Warning(s): If taken internally, serious gastric disturbance will result.

First Aid: Induce vomiting or use stomach pump. Call a physician immediately. Avoid getting into eyes or on mucous membranes. In case of eye contact, flush thoroughly with water. Call a physician immediately.

Keep out of reach of children.

Presentation: 16 fl oz (473 mL) (NDC# 58829-232-16), 32 fl oz (960 mL) (NDC# 58829-232-32), 1 gallon (3.785 L) (NDC# 58829-232-01) and 5 gallon (18.925 L) (NDC# 58829-232-31).

Compendium Code No.: 11390433 Rev. 06-01 / Rev. 08-01 / Rev. 07-01

ISOPROPYL ALCOHOL 99%

Phoenix Pharmaceutical **Disinfectant**

Active Ingredient(s):

Isopropyl Alcohol . . . . . 99% w/v

Water . . . . . q.s.

Indications: For external use only as an antiseptic, disinfectant, and rubefacient.

Directions: To Make a Standard Solution (70%): Dilute by adding 1 part water to 2 parts of this 99% Isopropyl Alcohol.

Use full strength as topical antiseptic or for disinfections of instruments. May be used for temporary relief of minor muscular aches or pain due to overexertion and fatigue. Apply full strength to affected area and massage briskly to stimulate circulation.

Precaution(s): Store at controlled room temperature between 15°-30°C (59°-86°F).

Keep container closed when not in use.

Flammable! Keep away from heat and open flame.

Caution(s): In case of deep or puncture wounds or serious burns consult a veterinarian. If redness, irritation, or swelling persists or increases, discontinue use and consult a veterinarian. Do not apply to irritated skin or if excessive irritation develops.

For animal use only.

For external use only.

Warning(s): If taken internally, serious gastric disturbance will result.

First Aid: Induce vomiting or use stomach pump. Call a physician immediately. Avoid getting into eyes or on mucous membranes. In case of eye contact, flush thoroughly with water. Call a physician immediately.

Keep out of reach of children.

Presentation: 32 fl oz (NDC 57319-409-22) and 1 gallon (NDC 57319-409-09) containers.

Manufactured by: First Priority, Inc., Elgin, IL 60123-1146.

Compendium Code No.: 12561071 Rev. 03-02 / Rev. 7-00

ISOPROPYL ALCOHOL 99%

Vedco **Counterirritant**

Active Ingredient(s):

Isopropyl alcohol 99%

Inert Ingredient:

Water 1%

Total 100%

Indications: An external solution for use as a topical antiseptic.

Dosage and Administration: Scrub hands and arms with soap and water, rinse with water, then scrub with the alcohol solution for disinfecting.

May also be used for the temporary relief of minor muscular aches or pain due to overexertion and fatigue. Apply full strength to the affected area, wet thoroughly and massage briskly to stimulate circulation.

Precaution(s): Store at a controlled room temperature between 15° and 30°C (59°-86°F). Flammable: Do not use near heat or an open flame.

Caution(s): For external use only.

If taken internally, serious gastric disturbance will result. Avoid contact with the eyes. In case of eye contact, flush thoroughly with water. Call a physician.

First Aid: Induce vomiting or use a stomach pump.

For veterinary use only.

Warning(s): Keep out of reach of children.

Presentation: 32 oz and 1 gallon containers.

Compendium Code No.: 10941151

ISOPROPYL RUBBING ALCOHOL U.S.P.

Dominion **Counterirritant**

Active Ingredient(s):

Isopropyl Alcohol 70%

Indications: To relieve muscle stiffness or excessive perspiration.

Directions: Apply to animal and rub in well.

Precaution(s): Flammable: Keep away from open flames or sparks.

Caution(s): For external use only. May be poisonous if taken internally. Avoid inhalation of vapors. Keep out of reach of children.

Presentation: 500 mL bottle; 12 bottles/carton.

Compendium Code No.: 15080030

ISO-THESIA ℞

Vetus **Inhalation Anesthetic**

Isoflurane, U.S.P.

ANADA No.: 200-141

Active Ingredient(s): Each mL contains 99.9% isoflurane.

Indications: ISO-THESIA (isoflurane, U.S.P.) is used for the induction and maintenance of general anesthesia in horses and dogs.

Pharmacology: Description: Isoflurane is a nonflammable, nonexplosive general inhalation anesthetic agent. Its chemical name is 1-chloro-2,2,2-trifluoroethyl difluoromethyl ether.

Some physical constants are:

Molecular weight 184.5

Boiling point at 760 mm Hg . . . . . 48.5°C

Refractive index n^{20}_{D} 1.2990-1.3005

Specific gravity 25°/25°C 1.496

Vapor pressure in mm Hg**
20°C . . . 238
25°C . . . 295
30°C . . . 367
35°C . . . 450
**Equation for vapor pressure calculation:
$\log_{10}P_{vap} = A + B / T$
where: A = 8.056 B = -1664.58 T = °C + 273.16
Partition coefficients at 37°C:
Water/gas . . . 0.61
Blood/gas . . . 1.43
Oil/gas . . . 90.8
Partition coefficients at 25°C - rubber and plastic:
Conductive rubber/gas . . . 62.0
Butyl rubber/gas . . . 75.0
Polyvinyl chloride/gas . . . 110.0
Polyethylene/gas . . . ~2.0
Polyurethane/gas . . . ~1.4
Polyolefin/gas . . . ~1.1
Butyl acetate/gas . . . ~2.5
Purity by gas chromatography . . . >99.9%
Lower limit of flammability in oxygen or nitrous oxide at 9 joules/sec. and 23°C . . . None
Lower limit of flammability in oxygen or nitrous oxide at 900 joules/sec. and 23°C . . . Greater than useful concentration in anesthesia
MAC (Minimum Alveolar Concentration) is 1.31% in horses and 1.28% in dogs.

Isoflurane is a clear, colorless, stable liquid which does not contain additives or chemical stabilizers. Isoflurane has a mildly pungent, musty, ethereal odor. Samples stored in indirect sunlight in clear, colorless glass for five years, as well as samples directly exposed for 30 hours to a 2 amp, 115 volt, 60 cycle long wave U.V. light were unchanged in composition as determined by gas chromatography. Isoflurane in one normal sodium methoxide-methanol solution, a strong base, for over six months consumed essentially no alkali, indicative of strong base stability. Isoflurane does not decompose in the presence of soda lime, and does not attack aluminum, tin, brass, iron, or copper.

Clinical Pharmacology: ISO-THESIA (isoflurane, USP) is an inhalation anesthetic. Induction and recovery from anesthesia with isoflurane are rapid. The level of anesthesia may be changed rapidly with isoflurane. Isoflurane is a profound respiratory depressant. Respiration must be monitored closely in the horse and dog and supported when necessary. As anesthetic dose is increased, both tidal volume and respiratory rate decrease. This depression is partially reversed by surgical stimulation, even at deeper levels of anesthesia.

Blood pressure decreases with the induction of anesthesia but returns toward normal with surgical stimulation. Progressive increases in the depth of anesthesia produce corresponding decreases in blood pressure; however, heart rhythm is stable and cardiac output is maintained with controlled ventilation and normal $PaCO_2$ despite the increasing depth of anesthesia. The hypercapnia which attends spontaneous ventilation during isoflurane anesthesia increases the heart rate and raises cardiac output above levels observed with controlled ventilation. Isoflurane does not sensitize the myocardium to exogenously administered epinephrine in the dog.

Muscle relaxation may be adequate for intra-abdominal operations at normal levels of anesthesia. However, if muscle relaxants are used to achieve greater relaxation, it should be noted that all commonly used muscle relaxants are markedly potentiated with isoflurane, the effect being most profound with the nondepolarizing type. Neostigmine reverses the effect of nondepolarizing muscle relaxants in the presence of isoflurane but does not reverse the direct neuromuscular depression of isoflurane.

Dosage and Administration:

Premedication: A premedication regimen, which may be employed depending upon the patient status, to avert excitement during induction, might include an anticholinergic, a tranquilizer, a muscle relaxant, and a short-acting barbiturate.

Inspired Concentration: The delivered concentration of Isoflurane should be known. Isoflurane may be vaporized using a flow-through vaporizer specifically calibrated for isoflurane. Vaporizers delivering a saturated vapor which then is diluted (e.g., Vernitrol® vaporizer) also may be used. The delivered concentration from such a vaporizer may be calculated using the formula:

$$\%\ \text{isoflurane} = \frac{100\ P_V F_V}{F_T(P_A - P_V)}$$

where:
P_A = Pressure of atmosphere
P_V = Vapor pressure of isoflurane
F_V = Flow of gas through vaporizer (mL/min.)
F_T = Total gas flow used (mL/min.)

Isoflurane contains no a stabilizer. Nothing in the drug product alters calibration or the operation of these vaporizers.

Induction:

Horses: Inspired concentrations of 3.0 to 5.0% isoflurane alone with oxygen following a barbiturate anesthetic induction are usually employed to induce surgical anesthesia in the horse.

Dogs: Inspired concentrations of 2.0 to 2.5% isoflurane alone with oxygen following a barbiturate anesthetic induction are usually employed to induce surgical anesthesia in the dog.

These concentrations can be expected to produce surgical anesthesia in 5-10 minutes.

Maintenance: The concentration of vapor necessary to maintain anesthesia is much less than that required to induce it.

Horses and Dogs: Surgical levels of anesthesia in both horses and dogs may be sustained with a 1.5 to 1.8% concentration of isoflurane in oxygen.

The level of blood pressure during maintenance is an inverse function of isoflurane concentration in the absence of other complicating problems. Excessive decreases, unless related to hypovolemia, may be due to depth of anesthesia and in such instances may be corrected by lightening the level of anesthesia.

Recovery from isoflurane anesthesia is typically uneventful.

Contraindication(s): Contraindicated in horses and dogs with known sensitivity to isoflurane or to other halogenated agents.

Precaution(s): Store at controlled room temperature 15-30°C (59-85°F).

Caution(s): Federal law restricts this drug to use by or on the order of a licensed veterinarian.

Operating rooms should be provided with adequate ventilation to prevent the accumulation of anesthetic vapors.

Increasing depth of anesthesia with Isoflurane may increase hypotension and respiratory depression. The electro-encephalographic pattern associated with deep anesthesia is characterized by burst suppression, spiking, and isoelectric periods.

Since levels of anesthesia may be altered easily and rapidly, only vaporizers producing predictable percentage concentrations of isoflurane should be used (see Dosage and Administration).

The action of nondepolarizing relaxants is augmented by isoflurane. Less than the usual amounts of these drugs should be used. If the usual amounts of nondepolarizing relaxants are given, the time for recovery from myoneural blockade will be longer in the presence of isoflurane than in the presence of other commonly used anesthetics.

Warning(s): Not for use in horses intended for food.

For veterinary use in horses and dogs.

Overdose: In the event of overdosage, or what may appear to be overdosage, the following action should be taken:

Stop drug administration, establish that the airway is clear and initiate assisted or controlled ventilation with pure oxygen as circumstances dictate.

Adverse Reactions: Hypotension, respiratory depression and arrhythmias have been reported.

Trial Data: Usage in Pregnancy: Reproduction studies have been performed in mice and rats without evidence of fetal malformation attributable to ISO-THESIA (isoflurane, U.S.P.). Adequate data concerning the safe use of isoflurane in pregnant and breeding horses and dogs have not been obtained.

References: Available upon request.

Presentation: 100 mL and 250 mL amber-colored bottles.

Compendium Code No.: 14440511

ISOTONE-SA

Vet-A-Mix **Electrolytes-Oral**

Guaranteed Analysis:
Sodium chloride . . . 1.95 g
Potassium chloride . . . 0.95 g
Citric acid . . . 0.57 g
Sodium citrate . . . 0.03 g
Glycine . . . 1.50 g
Glucose . . . 11.00 g

Indications: An isotonic, buffered nutritional supplement for dogs and cats.

Dosage and Administration: Dosage: The recommended daily dose is one pint per 5-10 pounds body weight.

Do not exceed 3 packets per 10 pounds body weight in 24 hours.

Dissolve the contents of one packet (both compartments) in one pint of water. Allow free access to ISOTONE-SA in a plastic or stainless steel container or use as directed by your veterinarian.

Presentation: 16 grams.

Compendium Code No.: 10500120

I

IVERCIDE™ EQUINE PASTE 1.87%

Phoenix Pharmaceutical **Parasiticide-Oral**

(ivermectin) Anthelmintic and Boticide

ANADA No.: 200-286

Active Ingredient(s): Each syringe contains:
Ivermectin . . . 1.87%

Indications: Consult your veterinarian for assistance in the diagnosis, treatment, and control of parasitism. IVERCIDE™ (ivermectin) Equine Paste provides effective control of the following parasites in horses:

Large Strongyles (adults): *Strongylus vulgaris* (also early forms in blood vessels), *S. edentatus* (also tissue stages), *S. equinus, Triodontophorus* spp.

Small Strongyles including those resistant to some benzimidazole class compounds (adults and fourth-stage larvae): *Cyathostomum* spp., *Cylicocyclus* spp., *Cylicostephanus* spp., *Cylicodontophorus* spp.

Pinworms (adults and fourth-stage larvae): *Oxyuris equi.*

Ascarids (adults and third- and fourth-stage larvae): *Parascaris equorum.*

Hairworms (adults): *Trichostrongylus axei.*

Large-mouth Stomach Worms (adults): *Habronema muscae.*

Bots (oral and gastric stages): *Gasterophilus* spp..

Lungworms (adults and fourth-stage larvae): *Dictyocaulus arnfieldi.*

Intestinal Threadworms (adults): *Strongyloides westeri.*

Summer Sores caused by *Habronema* and *Draschia* spp. cutaneous third-stage larvae.

Dermatitis caused by neck threadworm microfilariae, *Onchocerca* sp.

Dosage and Administration: The syringe contains sufficient paste to treat one 1250 lb horse at the recommended dose rate of 91 mcg ivermectin per lb (200 mcg/kg) of body weight. Each weight marking on the syringe plunger delivers enough paste to treat 250 lb of body weight. (1) While holding plunger, turn the knurled ring on the plunger to the right so the side nearest the barrel is at the prescribed weight marking. (2) Make sure that horse's mouth contains no feed. (3) Remove the cover from the tip of the syringe. (4) Insert the syringe tip into the horse's mouth at the space between the teeth. (5) Depress the plunger as far as it will go, depositing paste on the back of the tongue. (6) Immediately raise the horse's head for a few seconds after dosing.

Parasite Control Program: All horses should be included in a regular parasite control program with particular attention being paid to mares, foals and yearlings. Foals should be treated initially at 6 to 8 weeks of age, and routine treatment repeated as appropriate.

Consult your veterinarian for a control program to meet your specific needs. IVERCIDE™ (ivermectin) Equine Paste effectively controls gastrointestinal nematodes and bots of horses. Regular treatment will reduce the chances of verminous arteritis caused by *S. vulgaris.*

Precaution(s): Store at controlled room temperature, 20° to 25°C (68° to 77°F).

Caution(s): IVERCIDE™ (ivermectin) Equine Paste has been formulated specifically for use in horses only. This product should not be used in other animal species as severe adverse reactions, including fatalities in dogs, may result. Ivermectin and excreted ivermectin residues may adversely affect aquatic organisms. Do not contaminate ground or surface water. Dispose of this syringe in approved landfill or by incineration.

Note to User: Swelling and itching reactions after treatment with IVERCIDE™ (ivermectin) Equine Paste have occurred in horses carrying heavy infections of neck threadworm *(Onchocera* sp.) microfilariae. These reactions were most likely the result of microfilariae dying in large numbers. Symptomatic treatment may be advisable. Consult your veterinarian should any such reactions occur. Healing of summer sores involving extensive tissue changes may require other appropriate therapy in conjunction with treatment with IVERCIDE™ (ivermectin) Equine Paste. Reinfection, and measures for its prevention should also be considered. Consult your veterinarian if the condition does not improve.

For oral use in horses only.

Warning(s): Residue Warning: Do not use in horses intended for food purposes.

Refrain from smoking and eating when handling. Wash hands after use. Avoid contact with eyes. Keep this and all drugs out of the reach of children.

Toxicology: Safety: IVERCIDE™ (ivermectin) Equine Paste may be used in horses of all ages including mares at any stage of pregnancy. Stallions may be treated without adversely affecting their fertility.

Presentation: 6.08 g (0.21 oz) syringe (NDC 57319-453-41).

Manufactured by: Phoenix Scientific, Inc., St. Joseph, MO 64503.

Compendium Code No.: 12561161

Rev. 08-01

IVERCIDE™ INJECTION FOR CATTLE AND SWINE

Phoenix Pharmaceutical **Parasiticide Injection**

(ivermectin) Injection 1% Sterile Solution

ANADA No.: 200-228

Active Ingredient(s): IVERCIDE™ Injection is a clear, ready-to-use, sterile solution containing 1% ivermectin, 40% glycerol formal, 1.5% benzyl alcohol (preservative), and propylene glycol, q.s. ad 100%. It is formulated to deliver the recommended dose level of 200 mcg ivermectin/kilogram of body weight in cattle when given subcutaneously at the rate of 1 mL/110 lb (50 kg).

In swine, IVERCIDE™ Injection is formulated to deliver the recommended dose level of 300 mcg ivermectin/kilogram body weight when given subcutaneously in the neck at the rate of 1 mL/75 lb (33 kg).

Indications: A parasiticide for the treatment and control of internal and external parasites of cattle and swine.

Cattle: IVERCIDE™ Injection is indicated for the effective treatment and control of the following harmful species of gastrointestinal roundworms, lungworms, grubs, sucking lice, and mange mites in cattle:

Gastrointestinal Roundworms (adults and fourth-stage larvae): *Ostertagia ostertagi* (including inhibited *O. ostertagi*), *O. lyrata, Haemonchus placei, Trichostrongylus axei, T. colubriformis, Cooperia oncophora, C. punctata, C. pectinata, Oesophagostomum radiatum, Bunostomum phlebotomum, Nematodirus helvetianus* (adults only), *N. spathiger* (adults only).

Lungworms (adults and fourth-stage larvae): *Dictyocaulus viviparus*.

Cattle Grubs (parasitic stages): *Hypoderma bovis, H. lineatum*.

Sucking Lice: *Linognathus vituli, Haematopinus eurysternus, Solenopotes capillatus*.

Mites (scabies): *Psoroptes ovis* (syn. *P. communis* var. *bovis*), *Sarcoptes scabiei* var. *bovis*.

Persistent Activity: IVERCIDE™ Injection has been proved to effectively control infections and to protect cattle from reinfection with *Dictyocaulus viviparus* for 21 days after treatment; *Ostertagia ostertagi* for 21 days after treatment; *Oesophagostomum radiatum, Haemonchus placei, Trichostrongylus axei, Cooperia punctata*, and *Cooperia oncophora* for 14 days after treatment.

Swine: IVERCIDE™ Injection is indicated for the effective treatment and control of the following harmful species of gastrointestinal roundworms, lungworms, lice, and mange mites in swine:

Gastrointestinal Roundworms (adults and fourth-stage larvae): Large roundworm: *Ascaris suum*.

Red stomach worm: *Hyostrongylus rubidus*.

Nodular worm: *Oesophagostomum* spp.

Threadworm: *Strongyloides ransomi* (adults only).

Somatic Roundworm Larvae:

Threadworm: *Strongyloides ransomi* (somatic larvae).

Sows must be treated at least seven days before farrowing to prevent infection in piglets.

Lungworms: *Metastrongylus* spp (adults).

Lice: *Haematopinus suis*.

Mange Mites: *Sarcoptes scabiei* var. *suis*.

Reindeer: For the treatment and control of warbles *(Oedemagena tarandi)* in reindeer (see Special Minor Use section under "Dosage and Administration").

American Bison: For the treatment and control of grubs *(Hypoderma bovis)* in American bison (see Special Minor Use section under "Dosage and Administration").

Pharmacology: Ivermectin is derived from the avermectins, a family of potent, broad-spectrum antiparasitic agents isolated from fermentation of *Streptomyces avermitilis*.

Mode of Action: Ivermectin is a member of the macrocyclic lactone class of endectocides which have a unique mode of action. Compounds of the class bind selectively and with high affinity to glutamate-gated chloride ion channels which occur in invertebrate nerve and muscle cells. This leads to an increase in the permeability of the cell membrane to chloride ions with hyperpolarization of the nerve or muscle cell, resulting in paralysis and death of the parasite. Compounds of this class may also interact with other ligand-gated chloride channels, such as those gated by the neurotransmitter gamma-aminobutyric acid (GABA).

The wide margin of safety is attributable to the fact that mammals do not have glutamate-gated chloride channels, the macrocyclic lactones have a low affinity for other mammalian ligand-gated chloride channels and they do not readily cross the blood-brain barrier.

Dosage and Administration: Dosage:

Cattle: IVERCIDE™ Injection should be given only by subcutaneous injection under the loose skin in front of or behind the shoulder at the recommended dose level of 200 mcg ivermectin per kilogram of body weight. Each mL of IVERCIDE™ contains 10 mg of ivermectin, sufficient to treat 110 lb (50 kg) of body weight (maximum 10 mL per injection site).

Body Weight (lb)	Dose (mL)
220	2
330	3
440	4
550	5
660	6
770	7
880	8
990	9
1100	10

Swine: IVERCIDE™ Injection should be given only by subcutaneous injection in the neck of swine at the recommended dose level of 300 mcg of ivermectin per kilogram (2.2 lb) of body weight. Each mL of IVERCIDE™ contains 10 mg of ivermectin, sufficient to treat 75 lb of body weight.

	Body Weight (lb)	Dose (mL)
Growing Pigs	19	1/4
	38	1/2
	75	1
	150	2
Breeding Animals (Sows, Gilts, and Boars)	225	3
	300	4
	375	5
	450	6

Administration:

Cattle: IVERCIDE™ Injection is to be given subcutaneously only, to reduce risk of potentially fatal clostridial infection of the injection site. Animals should be appropriately restrained to achieve the proper route of administration. Use of a 16-gauge ½ to ¾" needle is suggested. Inject under the loose skin in front of or behind the shoulder (see illustration).

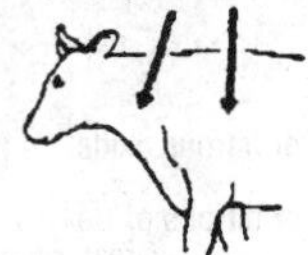

Any single-dose syringe or standard automatic syringe equipment may be used with the 50 mL package size. When using the 200 mL or 500 mL package size, use only automatic syringe equipment.

Use sterile equipment and sanitize the injection site by applying a suitable disinfectant. Clean, properly disinfected needles should be used to reduce the potential for injection site infection. No special handling or protective clothing is necessary.

Swine: IVERCIDE™ (ivermectin) Injection is to be given subcutaneously in the neck. Animals should be appropriately restrained to achieve the proper route of administration. Use of a 16- or 18-gauge needle is suggested for sows and boars, while an 18- or 20-gauge needle may be appropriate for young animals. Inject under the skin, immediately behind the ear (see illustration).

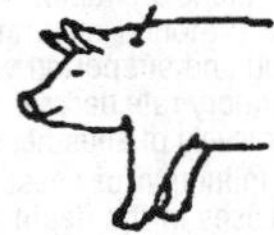

Any single-dose syringe or standard automatic syringe equipment may be used with the 50 mL package size. When using the 200 mL or 500 mL package size, use only automatic syringe equipment. As with any injection, sterile equipment should be used. The injection site should be cleaned and disinfected with alcohol before injection. The rubber stopper should also be disinfected with alcohol to prevent contamination of the contents. Mild and transient pain reactions may be seen in some swine following subcutaneous administration.

Recommended Treatment Program:

Swine: At the time of initiating any parasite control program, it is important to treat all breeding animals in the herd. After the initial treatment, use IVERCIDE™ (ivermectin) Injection regularly as follows:

Breeding Animals:

Sows: Treat prior to farrowing, preferably 7-14 days before, to minimize infection of piglets.

Gilts: Treat 7-14 days prior to breeding. Treat 7-14 days prior to farrowing.

Boars: Frequency and need for treatments are dependent upon exposure. Treat at least two times a year.

Feeder Pigs (Weaners/Growers/Finishers): All weaner/feeder pigs should be treated before placement in clean quarters.

Pigs exposed to contaminated soil or pasture may need retreatment if reinfection occurs.

Note:

1. IVERCIDE™ Injection has a persistent drug level sufficient to control mite infestations throughout the egg to adult life cycle. However, since the ivermectin effect is not immediate, care must be taken to prevent reinfestation from exposure to untreated animals or contaminated facilities. Generally, pigs should not be moved to clean quarters or exposed to uninfested pigs for approximately one week after treatment. Sows should be treated at least one week before farrowing to minimize transfer of mites to newborn baby pigs.
2. Louse eggs are unaffected by IVERCIDE™ Injection and may require up to three weeks to hatch. Louse infestations developing from hatching eggs may require retreatment.
3. Consult a veterinarian for aid in the diagnosis and control of internal and external parasites of swine.

Special Minor Use:

Reindeer: For the treatment and control of warbles *(Oedemagena tarandi)* in reindeer, inject 200 micrograms ivermectin per kilogram of body weight, subcutaneously. Follow use directions for cattle as described under Dosage and Administration.

American Bison: For the treatment and control of grubs *(Hypoderma bovis)* in American Bison, inject 200 micrograms ivermectin per kilogram of body weight, subcutaneously. Follow use directions for cattle as described under Dosage and Administration.

Consult your veterinarian for assistance in the diagnosis, treatment and control of parasitism.

Precaution(s): Store between 15°C-30°C (59°F-86°F).

Protect product from light.

Environmental Safety: Studies indicate that when ivermectin comes in contact with the soil, it readily and tightly binds to the soil and becomes inactive over time. Free ivermectin may adversely affect fish and certain water-borne organisms on which they feed. Do not permit water runoff from feedlots or production sites to enter lakes, streams, or ponds. Do not contaminate water by direct application or by the improper disposal of drug containers. Dispose of containers in an approved landfill or by incineration.

Caution(s): This product is not for intravenous or intramuscular use.

Use sterile equipment and sanitize the injection site by applying a suitable disinfectant. Clean, properly disinfected needles should be used to reduce the potential for injection site infections.

Transitory discomfort has been observed in some cattle following subcutaneous administration. A low incidence of soft tissue swelling at the injection site has been observed. These reactions have disappeared without treatment. For cattle, divide doses greater than 10 mL between two injection sites to reduce occasional discomfort or site reaction.

Observe cattle for injection site reactions. Reactions may be due to clostridial infection and should be aggressively treated with appropriate antibiotics. If injection site infections are suspected, consult your veterinarian.

IVERCIDE™ Injection for Cattle and Swine has been developed specifically for use in cattle, swine, reindeer and American bison only. This product should not be used in other animal species as severe adverse reactions, including fatalities in dogs, may result.

Warning(s): Residue Warning: Do not treat cattle within 35 days of slaughter. Because a withdrawal time in milk has not been established, do not use in female dairy cattle of breeding age.

Do not treat swine within 18 days of slaughter.

Do not treat reindeer or American bison within 8 weeks (56 days) of slaughter.

Keep this and all drugs out of the reach of children.

Not for use in humans.

Discussion: When to Treat Cattle with Grubs: IVERCIDE™ effectively controls all stages of cattle grubs. However, proper timing of treatment is important. For most effective results, cattle should be treated as soon as possible after the end of the heel fly (warble fly) season. Destruction of *Hypoderma* larvae (cattle grubs) at the period when these grubs are in vital areas may cause undesirable host-parasite reactions including the possibility of fatalities. Killing *Hypoderma lineatum* when it is in the tissue surrounding the esophagus (gullet) may cause salivation and bloat; killing *H. bovis* when it is in the vertebral canal may cause staggering or paralysis. These reactions are not specific to treatment with IVERCIDE™, but can occur with any successful treatment of grubs. Cattle should be treated either before or after these stages of grub development.

Consult your veterinarian concerning the proper time for treatment.

Cattle treated with IVERCIDE™ after the end of the heel fly season may be retreated with IVERCIDE™ during the winter for internal parasites, mange mites, or suckling lice without danger of grub-related reactions. A planned parasite control program is recommended.

Presentation: IVERCIDE™ Injection for Cattle and Swine is available in three ready-to-use sizes:

The 50 mL bottle (NDC 57319-459-04) contains sufficient solution to treat 10 head of 550 lb (250 kg) cattle or 100 head of 38 lb (17.3 kg) swine.

The 200 mL bottle (NDC 57319-459-42) contains sufficient solution to treat 40 head of 550 lb (250 kg) cattle or 400 head of 38 lb (17.3 kg) swine. Use automatic syringe equipment only.

The 500 mL bottle (NDC 57319-459-07) contains sufficient solution to treat 100 head of 550 lb (250 kg) cattle or 1000 head of 38 lb (17.3 kg) swine. Use automatic syringe equipment only.

Manufactured by: Phoenix Scientific, Inc., St. Joseph, MO 64503.

Compendium Code No.: 12561081 Rev. 7-01 / Rev. 12-01 / Iss. 01-01

IVERCIDE™ LIQUID FOR HORSES ℞

Phoenix Pharmaceutical **Parasiticide-Oral**

(ivermectin) 10 mg/mL

ANADA No.: 200-202

Active Ingredient(s): IVERCIDE™ (ivermectin) Liquid is a clear, ready-to-use solution with each mL containing 1% ivermectin (10 mg), 0.2 mL propylene glycol, 80 mg polysorbate 80, 9 mg sodium phosphate monobasic monohydrate, 1.3 mg sodium phosphate dibasic anhydrous, 1 mg butylated hydroxytoluene, 0.1 mg disodium edetate, 3% benzyl alcohol and water for injection q.s. ad 100%.

Indications: IVERCIDE™ (ivermectin) Liquid is indicated for the effective treatment and control of the following parasites or parasitic conditions in horses:

Large Strongyles: *Strongylus vulgaris* (adults and arterial larval stages), *S. edentatus* (adults and tissue stages), *S. equinus* (adults), *Triodontophorus* spp (adults).

Small Strongyles - including those resistant to some benzimidazole class compounds (adults and fourth-stage larvae): *Cyathostomum* spp, *Cylicocyclus* spp, *Cylicostephanus* spp, *Cylicodontophorus* spp.

Pinworms (adults and fourth-stage larvae): *Oxyuris equi.*

Ascarids (adults and third- and fourth-stage larvae): *Parascaris equorum.*

Hairworms (adults): *Trichostrongylus axei.*

Large-mouth Stomach Worms (adults): *Habronema muscae.*

Bots (oral and gastric stages): *Gasterophilus* spp.

Lungworms (adults and fourth-stage larvae): *Dictyocaulus arnfieldi.*

Intestinal Threadworms (adults): *Strongyloides westeri.*

Summer Sores caused by *Habronema* and *Draschia* spp cutaneous third-stage larvae.

Dermatitis caused by neck threadworm microfilariae, *Onchocerca* sp.

Pharmacology: Ivermectin is derived from the avermectins, a family of potent, broad-spectrum antiparasitic agents, which are isolated from fermentation of *Streptomyces avermitilis.*

Mode of Action: Ivermectin, one of the avermectins, kills certain parasitic roundworms and ectoparasites such as mites and lice. The avermectins are different in their action from other antiparasitic agents. This action involves a chemical that serves as a signal from one nerve cell to another, or from a nerve cell to a muscle cell. This chemical, a neurotransmitter, is called gamma-aminobutyric acid or GABA.

In roundworms, ivermectin stimulates the release of GABA from nerve endings and enhances binding of GABA to special receptors at nerve junctions, thus interrupting nerve impulses - thereby paralyzing and killing the parasite.

The enhancement of the GABA effect in arthropods such as mites and lice resembles that in roundworms except that nerve impulses are interrupted between the nerve ending and the muscle cell. Again, this leads to paralysis and death.

The principal peripheral neurotransmitter in mammals, acetylcholine, is unaffected by ivermectin. Ivermectin does not readily penetrate the central nervous system of mammals where GABA functions as a neurotransmitter.

Dosage and Administration: Dosage: IVERCIDE™ (ivermectin) Liquid for Horses is formulated for administration by stomach tube (nasogastric intubation) or as an oral drench. The recommended dose is 200 mcg of ivermectin per kilogram (91 mcg/lb) of body weight. Each mL contains sufficient ivermectin to treat 110 lb (50 kg) of body weight: 10 mL will treat an 1100 lb (500 kg) horse.

Administration: Use a calibrated dosing syringe inserted into the bottle to measure the appropriate dose, or pour the IVERCIDE™ (ivermectin) Liquid into a graduated cylinder for dose measurement. Use a clean syringe if accessing the bottle to avoid contaminating the remaining product.

Administration by stomach tube (gravity or positive flow): The recommended dose can be used undiluted or diluted up to 40 times with clean tepid water (see Notes to Veterinarian). Use tepid water to flush any drug remaining in the tube into the horse's stomach.

Administration by drench: For administration by this method, an undiluted dose is usually preferred. Clear the horse's mouth of any food material, elevate the horse's head, and using a syringe, deposit the appropriate dose in the back of the mouth. In order to avoid unnecessary coughing or the potential for material to enter the trachea and lungs, do not use excessive pressure (squirting), do not use a large (diluted) dose volume, and do not deposit the dose in the laryngeal area. Increased dose rejection may occur if the dose is deposited in the buccal space. Keep the horse's head elevated and observe the horse to insure the dose is retained.

Suggested Parasite Control Program: All horses should be included in a regular parasite control program with particular attention being paid to mares, foals and yearlings. Foals should be treated initially at 6 to 8 weeks of age, and routine treatment repeated as appropriate. IVERCIDE™ (ivermectin) effectively controls gastrointestinal nematodes and bots in horses. Regular treatment will reduce the chances of verminous arteritis and colic caused by *S. vulgaris.* With its broad spectrum, IVERCIDE™ (ivermectin) is well suited to be the major product in a parasite control program.

Contraindication(s): IVERCIDE™ (ivermectin) Liquid has been formulated specifically for use in horses only. This product should not be used in other animal species as severe adverse reactions, including fatalities in dogs, may result.

Precaution(s): Store in a tightly closed container at room temperature.

Protect IVERCIDE™ (ivermectin) Liquid (undiluted or diluted) from light.

Environmental Safety: Studies indicate that when ivermectin comes in contact with the soil, it readily and tightly binds to the soil and becomes inactive over time. Free ivermectin may adversely affect fish and certain water-borne organisms on which they feed. Do not contaminate lakes, streams, or ground water by direct application or by improper disposal of drug containers. Dispose of drug container in an approved landfill or by incineration.

Caution(s): Federal law restricts this drug to use by or on the order of a licensed veterinarian.

Notes to Veterinarian: Swelling and itching reactions after treatment with IVERCIDE™ (ivermectin) have occurred in horses carrying heavy infections of neck threadworm microfilariae, *Onchocerca* sp. These reactions were most likely the result of microfilariae dying in large numbers. Symptomatic treatment may be advisable.

Healing of summer sores involving extensive tissue changes may require other therapy in conjunction with IVERCIDE™ (ivermectin). Reinfection, and measures for its prevention, should also be considered.

Special consideration should be given to the effects or potential for injury from handling, restraint, and placement of the tube during administration by stomach tube. IVERCIDE™ (ivermectin) Liquid should be administered by drench if the risks associated with tubing are of concern. Due to the consequences of improper administration (also see Dosage and Administration), IVERCIDE™ (ivermectin) Liquid is intended for use by a veterinarian only and is not recommended for dispensing.

IVERCIDE™ (ivermectin) Liquid in 1 to 20 and 1 to 40 dilutions with tap water has been shown to be stable for 72 hours under the conditions recommended for this product (i.e., at room temperature, in a tightly closed container, protected from light). The diluted product does not promote the growth of common organisms. However, prolonged storage of the diluted product cannot be recommended, as the effects of possible contaminants and interactions with untested materials are unknown.

For veterinary use only.

Warning(s): Residue Warning: Do not use in horses intended for food purposes.

Refrain from smoking and eating when handling. Wash hands after use. Avoid contact with eyes. Keep this and all drugs out of the reach of children.

Trial Data: Safety: IVERCIDE™ (ivermectin) Liquid may be used in horses of all ages including mares at any stage of pregnancy. Stallions may be treated without adversely affecting their fertility. These horses have been treated with no adverse effects other than those noted under Notes to Veterinarian.

Discussion: IVERCIDE™ (ivermectin) Liquid for Horses has been formulated for professional administration by stomach tube or oral drench. One low-volume dose is effective against important internal parasites, including the arterial stages of *Strongylus vulgaris,* and bots.

Ivermectin is a potent antiparasitic agent whose chemical structure is different from those of other antiparasitic agents. Its convenience, broad-spectrum efficiency and safety margin make IVERCIDE™ (ivermectin) Liquid an ideal parasite control product for horses.

Presentation: IVERCIDE™ (ivermectin) Liquid for Horses is available in a 100 mL (NDC 57319-400-05) or 200 mL (NDC 57319-400-42) plastic bottle. The 100 mL bottle contains sufficient ivermectin to treat 10-500 kg (1100 lb) horses. The 200 mL bottle contains sufficient ivermectin to treat 20-500 kg (1100 lb) horses. Contents may be poured into a graduated cylinder for dose measurement. Alternatively, a clean syringe may be inserted directly into the bottle to draw off the appropriate dose.

Manufactured by: Phoenix Scientific, Inc., St. Joseph, MO 64503.

Compendium Code No.: 12560474 Rev. 6-00 / Rev. 3-02

IVERCIDE™ POUR-ON FOR CATTLE

Phoenix Pharmaceutical **Parasiticide-Topical**

(ivermectin) 5 mg per mL-Parasiticide

ANADA No.: 200-219

Active Ingredient(s): Contains 5 mg ivermectin/mL.

Indications: IVERCIDE™ Pour-On applied at the recommended dose level of 500 mcg/kg is indicated for the effective control of these parasites.

Gastrointestinal Roundworms: *Ostertagia ostertagi* (including inhibited stage) (adults and L_4), *Haemonchus placei* (adults and L_4), *Trichostrongylus axei* (adults and L_4), *T. colubriformis* (adults and L_4), *Cooperia* spp (adults and L_4), *Strongyloides papillosus* (adults), *Oesophagostomum radiatum* (adults and L_4), *Trichuris* spp (adults).

Lungworms: *Dictyocaulus viviparus* (adults and L_4).

Cattle Grubs (parasitic stages): *Hypoderma bovis, H. lineatum.*

Mites: *Sarcoptes scabiei* var. *bovis.*

Lice: *Linognathus vituli, Haematopinus eurysternus, Damalinia bovis, Solenopotes capillatus.*

Horn Flies: *Haematobia irritans.*

Pharmacology: Persistent Activity: IVERCIDE™ (ivermectin) Pour-On has been proved to effectively control infections and to protect cattle from reinfection with *Ostertagia ostertagi, Oesophagostomum radiatum, Haemonchus placei, Trichostrongylus axei, Cooperia punctata* and *Cooperia oncophora* for 14 days after treatment.

Mode of Action: Ivermectin as a member of the avermectin family kills certain parasitic roundworms and ectoparasites, such as mites, lice, horn flies and other insects. Its action is unique to the avermectin class of antiparasitic agents. This action involves a chemical that serves as a signal from one nerve cell to another, or from a nerve cell to a muscle cell. This chemical, a neurotransmitter, is called gamma-aminobutyric acid or GABA.

In roundworms, ivermectin stimulates the release of GABA from nerve endings and enhances binding of GABA to special receptors at nerve junctions, thus interrupting nerve impulses — thereby paralyzing and killing the parasite.

The enhancement of the GABA effect in arthropods such as mites, lice, and horn flies resembles that in roundworms except that nerve impulses are interrupted between the nerve ending and the muscle cell. Again, this leads to paralysis and death.

Ivermectin has no measurable effect against flukes or tapeworms, presumably because they do not have GABA as a nerve impulse transmitter.

The principal peripheral neurotransmitter in mammals, acetylcholine, is unaffected by ivermectin. Ivermectin does not readily penetrate the central nervous system of mammals where GABA functions as a neurotransmitter.

Dosage and Administration: Treatment for Cattle for Horn Flies: IVERCIDE™ Pour-On controls horn flies *(Haematobia irritans)* for up to 28 days after dosing. For best results, IVERCIDE™ Pour-On should be part of a parasite control program for both internal and external parasites based on the epidemiology of these parasites. Consult your veterinarian or an entomologist for the most effective timing of applications.

Dosage: The dose rate is 1 mL for each 22 lb of body weight. The formulation should be applied along the topline in a narrow strip extending from the withers to the tailhead.

Administration:

Dispensing Cap (1 L bottle): The enclosed dispensing cap is graduated in 5 mL increments. Each 5 mL will treat 110 lbs body weight. When body weight is between markings, use the next higher increment.

Attach the dispensing cap to the bottle.

Select the correct dose rate by rotating the adjuster top in either direction to position the dose indicator to the appropriate level.

Hold the bottle upright and gently squeeze it to deliver a slight excess of the required dose as indicated by the calibration lines.

By releasing the pressure, the dose automatically adjusts to the correct level. Tilt the bottle to deliver the dose. The off (stop) position will close the system between dosing.

Applicator Gun* (3.785 L bottle, 5 L backpack and 25 L carboy): Because of the solvents used in IVERCIDE™ Pour-On, only the IVERCIDE™ applicator gun from Simcro Tech Limited, or equivalent, is recommended. Other applicators may exhibit compatibility problems, resulting in locking, incorrect dosage or leakage.

Insert the brass end of the draw tube into the larger hole on the back side of the cap with the stem.

Slide one of the coil springs over one end of the draw-off tubing. Attach that end of the draw-off tubing to the stem on the applicator gun and slide the spring up to the connection. Slide the other coil spring over the other end of the draw-off tubing and connect that end to the cap that has the stem. Slide the spring to the connection. Replace the shipping cap with the cap having the draw-off tubing and draw tube attached. Tighten this draw-off cap to the bottle.

Directions For Use (IVERCIDE™ (ivermectin) Pour-On Applicator): This applicator has been designed for use with IVERCIDE™ Pour-On only, and is not recommended to be used with other products.

To Prime Applicator: Connect the delivery tube to the applicator and IVERCIDE™ Pour-On gallon bottle, squeeze the handle of the applicator several times until the pour-on is drawn through the tube filling the barrel. Point the applicator nozzle upwards and gently squeeze the handle several times until all air has been expelled from the applicator barrel.

To Set Dose: Turn the dose adjuster band clockwise to move the piston forward to the required dose setting marked on the barrel. Turning the dosage adjuster band clockwise decreases the dose while counter-clockwise increases the dose. The system is now ready for use.

Important - when adjusting the piston forward or back to a new dose setting, make sure the front face of the piston lines up with the printed mark on the barrel.

Follow the applicator gun manufacturer's directions for care of the applicator gun following use.

Weight	Dose
220 lb (100 kg)	10 mL
330 lb (150 kg)	15 mL
440 lb (200 kg)	20 mL
550 lb (250 kg)	25 mL
660 lb (300 kg)	30 mL
770 lb (350 kg)	35 mL
880 lb (400 kg)	40 mL
990 lb (450 kg)	45 mL
1100 lb (500 kg)	50 mL

*Additional Applicator Guns and Draw Tubes may be purchased from your Phoenix Pharmaceutical Distributor or through Phoenix Pharmaceutical, Inc.

When to Treat Cattle with Grubs: IVERCIDE™ Pour-On effectively controls all stages of cattle grubs. However, proper timing of treatment is important. For the most effective results, cattle should be treated as soon as possible after the end of the heel fly (warble fly) season. While this is not peculiar to ivermectin, destruction of *Hypoderma* larvae (cattle grubs) at the period when these grubs are in vital areas may cause undesirable host-parasite reactions. Killing *Hypoderma lineatum* when it is in the esophageal tissues may cause bloat; killing *H. bovis* when it is in the vertebral canal may cause staggering or paralysis. Cattle should be treated either before or after these stages of grub development.

Cattle treated with IVERCIDE™ Pour-On at the end of the fly season may be re-treated with IVERCIDE™ during the winter without danger of grub-related reactions. For further information and advice on a planned parasite control program, consult your veterinarian.

Consult your veterinarian for assistance in the diagnosis, treatment and control of parasitism.

Precaution(s): Flammable! Keep away from heat, sparks, open flame, and other sources of ignition.

Store between 15° and 30°C (59° and 86°F).

Store away from excessive heat (104°F/40°C) and protect from light.

Use only in well-ventilated areas or outdoors.

Close container tightly when not in use.

Cloudiness in the formulation may occur when IVERCIDE™ (ivermectin) Pour-On is stored at temperatures below 32°F. Allowing to warm at room temperature will restore the normal appearance without affecting efficacy.

Environmental Safety: Studies indicate that when ivermectin comes in contact with the soil, it readily and tightly binds to the soil and becomes inactive over time. Free ivermectin may adversely affect fish or certain water-borne organisms on which they feed. Do not permit cattle to enter lakes, streams or ponds for at least six hours after treatment. Do not contaminate water by direct application or by the improper disposal of drug containers. Dispose of containers in an approved landfill or by incineration.

Caution(s): Cattle should not be treated when hair or hide is wet since reduced efficacy may be experienced.

Do not use when rain is expected to wet cattle within six hours after treatment.

This product is for application to skin surface only. Do not give orally or parenterally.

Antiparasitic activity of ivermectin will be impaired if the formulation is applied to areas of the skin with mange scabs or lesions, or with dermatoses or adherent materials, e.g., caked mud or manure.

Ivermectin has been associated with adverse reaction in sensitive dogs; therefore, IVERCIDE™ Pour-On is not recommended for use in species other than cattle.

Warning(s): Residue Warning: Cattle must not be treated within 48 days of slaughter for human consumption. Because a withdrawal time in milk has not been established, do not use in female dairy cattle of breeding age.

Not for use in humans.

This product should not be applied to self or others because it may be irritating to human skin and eyes and absorbed through the skin. To minimize accidental skin contact, the user should wear a long-sleeved shirt and rubber gloves. If accidental skin contact occurs, wash immediately with soap and water. If accidental eye exposure occurs, flush eyes immediately with water and seek medical attention.

Keep this and all drugs out of the reach of children.

Discussion: IVERCIDE™ (ivermectin) Pour-On delivers internal and external parasite control in one convenient low-volume application. Ivermectin is a potent antiparasitic agent whose chemical structure is different from those of other antiparasitic agents.

Trial Data: Safety: Studies conducted in the U.S.A. have demonstrated the safety margin for ivermectin. Based on plasma levels, the topically applied formulation is expected to be at least as well tolerated by breeding animals as is the subcutaneous formulation which had no effect on breeding performance.

Presentation: IVERCIDE™ Pour-On is available in a 1 L (33.8 fl oz) (NDC 57319-406-08) bottle for use with the dispensing cap provided, or in a 3.785 L (1 gal) (NDC 57319-406-09) bottle, a 5 L (169 fl oz) (NDC 57319-406-40) backpack and a 25 L (6.6 gal) (NDC 57319-406-45) carboy for use with the appropriate automatic dosing applicator.

Manufactured by: Phoenix Scientific, Inc., St. Joseph, MO 64503.

Compendium Code No.: 12560482 Rev. 7-00 / Rev. 10-01 / Rev. 02-01 / Iss. 4-00

IVERHART™ PLUS FLAVORED CHEWABLES ℞

Virbac **Parasiticide-Oral**

(ivermectin/pyrantel)

ANADA No.: 200-302

Active Ingredient(s): Each chewable tablet contains:

Color Coding	Ivermectin Content	Pyrantel Content
Blue	68 mcg	57 mg
Green	136 mcg	114 mg
Brown	272 mcg	227 mg

Indications: For use in dogs to prevent canine heartworm disease by eliminating the tissue stage of heartworm larvae *(Dirofilaria immitis)* for a month (30 days) after infection and for the treatment and control of ascarids *(Toxocara canis, Toxascaris leonina)* and hookworms *(Ancylostoma caninum, Uncinaria stenocephala, Ancylostoma braziliense)*.

Dosage and Administration:

Dosage: IVERHART™ Plus (ivermectin/pyrantel) Flavored Chewables should be administered orally at monthly intervals at the recommended minimum dose level of 6 mcg of ivermectin per kilogram (2.72 mcg/lb) and 5 mg of pyrantel (as pamoate salt) per kg (2.27 mg/lb) of body weight. The recommended dosing schedule for prevention of canine heartworm disease and for the treatment and control of ascarids and hookworms is as follows:

Dog Weight	Flavored Chewable Per Month	Ivermectin Content	Pyrantel Content	Color Coding on Foil-Backing and Carton
Up to 25 lbs	1	68 mcg	57 mg	blue
26 to 50 lbs	1	136 mcg	114 mg	green
51 to 100 lbs	1	272 mcg	227 mg	brown

IVERHART™ Plus Flavored Chewables are recommended for dogs 6 weeks of age and older.

For dogs over 100 lbs use the appropriate combination of these flavored chewables.

Administration: Remove only one flavored chewable at a time from the foil-backed blister card. Because most dogs find IVERHART™ Plus Flavored Chewables palatable, the product can be offered to the dog by hand. Alternatively, it may be added intact to a small amount of dog food or placed in the back of the dog's mouth for forced swallowing. Care should be taken that the dog consumes the complete dose, and treated animals should be observed for a few minutes after administration to ensure that part of the dose is not lost or rejected. If it is suspected that any of the dose has been lost, redosing is recommended.

IVERHART™ Plus Flavored Chewables should be given at monthly intervals during the period of the year when mosquitoes (vectors), potentially carrying infective heartworm larvae, are active. The initial dose must be given within a month (30 days) after the dog's first exposure to mosquitoes. The final dose must be given within a month (30 days) after the dog's last exposure to mosquitoes.

When replacing another heartworm preventive product in a heartworm disease prevention program, the first dose of IVERHART™ Plus Flavored Chewables must be given within a month (30 days) of the last dose of the former medication.

If the interval between doses exceeds a month (30 days), the efficacy of ivermectin can be reduced. Therefore, for optimal performance, the chewable must be given once a month on or about the same day of the month. If treatment is delayed, whether by a few days or many, immediate treatment with IVERHART™ Plus Flavored Chewables and resumption of the recommended dosing regimen will minimize the opportunity for the development of adult heartworms.

Monthly treatment with IVERHART™ Plus Flavored Chewables also provides effective treatment and control of ascarids *(T. canis, T. leonina)* and hookworms *(A. caninum, U. stenocephala, A. braziliense)*. Clients should be advised of measures to be taken to prevent reinfection with intestinal parasites.

Efficacy: IVERHART™ Plus Flavored Chewables, given orally using the recommended dose and regimen, are effective against the tissue larval stage of *D. immitis* for a month (30 days) after infection and, as a result, prevent the development of the adult stage. IVERHART™ Plus Flavored Chewables are also effective against canine ascarids *(T. canis, T. leonina)* and hookworms *(A. caninum, U. stenocephala, A. braziliense)*.

Precaution(s): Store at controlled room temperature of 59°-86°F (15°-30°C).

Use product on or before expiration date. Discard or return unused tablets. Protect product from light.

Caution(s): Federal (U.S.A.) law restricts this drug to use by or on the order of a licensed veterinarian.

All dogs should be tested for existing heartworm infection before starting treatment with IVERHART™ Plus Flavored Chewables which are not effective against adult *D. immitis*. Infected dogs must be treated to remove adult heartworms and microfilariae before initiating a program with IVERHART™ Plus Flavored Chewables.

While some microfilariae may be killed by the ivermectin in IVERHART™ Plus Flavored Chewables at the recommended dose level, IVERHART™ Plus Flavored Chewables are not effective for microfilariae clearance. A mild hypersensitivity-type reaction, presumably due to dead or dying microfilariae and particularly involving a transient diarrhea, has been observed in clinical trials with ivermectin alone after treatment of some dogs that have circulating microfilariae.

Warning(s): Keep this and all drugs out of the reach of children.

In case of ingestion by humans, clients should be advised to contact a physician immediately. Physicians may contact a Poison Control Center for advice concerning cases of ingestion by humans.

Adverse Reactions: In clinical trials with ivermectin, vomiting or diarrhea within 24 hours of dosing was rarely observed (1.1% of administered doses). The following adverse reactions have been reported following the use of ivermectin: Depression/lethargy, vomiting, anorexia, diarrhea, mydriasis, ataxia, staggering, convulsions and hypersalivation.

For technical assistance or to report adverse drug reactions, please call 1-800-338-3659.

Trial Data: Acceptability: In a trial in client-owned dogs, IVERHART™ Plus Flavored Chewables were shown to be a palatable oral dosage form consumed at first offering by the majority of dogs.

Safety: Studies with ivermectin indicate that certain dogs of the Collie breed are more sensitive to the effects of ivermectin administered at elevated dose levels (more than 16 times the target use level of 6 mcg/kg) than dogs of other breeds. At elevated doses, sensitive dogs showed adverse reactions which included mydriasis, depression, ataxia, tremors, drooling, paresis, recumbency, excitability, stupor, coma and death. Ivermectin demonstrated no signs of toxicity at 10 times the recommended dose (60 mcg/kg) in sensitive Collies. Results of these trials and bioequivalency studies, support the safety of ivermectin products in dogs, including Collies, when used as recommended.

Ivermectin has shown a wide margin of safety at the recommended dose level in dogs, including pregnant or breeding bitches, stud dogs and puppies aged 6 or more weeks. In clinical trials, many commonly used flea collars, dips, shampoos, anthelmintics, antibiotics, vaccines and steroid preparations have been administered with ivermectin/pyrantel in a heartworm disease prevention program.

In one trial, where some pups had parvovirus, there was a marginal reduction in efficacy against intestinal nematodes, possibly due to a change in intestinal transit time.

Presentation: IVERHART™ Plus Flavored Chewables are available in three dosage strengths (see Dosage section) for dogs of different weights. Each strength comes in a box of 6 tablets, packed 10 boxes per display box and in a bulk dispenser carton containing 20 cards of 6 tablets per card.

Compendium Code No.: 10230691 0170DS, 0170DM, 0170DL, 0180TS, 0180TM, 0180TL

IVERMECTIN INJECTION FOR CATTLE AND SWINE

Aspen **Parasiticide Injection**

(ivermectin) Injection 1% Sterile Solution

ANADA No.: 200-228

Active Ingredient(s): IVERMECTIN INJECTION is a clear, ready-to-use, sterile solution containing 1% ivermectin, 40% glycerol formal, 1.5% benzyl alcohol (preservative), and propylene glycol, q.s. ad 100%. It is formulated to deliver the recommended dose level of 200 mcg ivermectin/kilogram of body weight in cattle when given subcutaneously at the rate of 1 mL/110 lb (50 kg).

In swine, IVERMECTIN INJECTION is formulated to deliver the recommended dose level of 300 mcg ivermectin/kilogram body weight when given subcutaneously in the neck at the rate of 1 mL/75 lb (33 kg).

Indications: A parasiticide for the treatment and control of internal and external parasites of cattle and swine.

Cattle: IVERMECTIN INJECTION is indicated for the effective treatment and control of the following harmful species of gastrointestinal roundworms, lungworms, grubs, sucking lice, and mange mites in cattle:

Gastrointestinal Roundworms (adults and fourth-stage larvae): *Ostertagia ostertagi* (including inhibited *O. ostertagi), O. lyrata, Haemonchus placei, Trichostrongylus axei, T. colubriformis, Cooperia oncophora, C. punctata, C. pectinata, Oesophagostomum radiatum, Bunostomum phlebotomum, Nematodirus helvetianus* (adults only), *N. spathiger* (adults only).

Lungworms (adults and fourth-stage larvae): *Dictyocaulus viviparus.*

Cattle Grubs (parasitic stages): *Hypoderma bovis, H. lineatum.*

Sucking Lice: *Linognathus vituli, Haematopinus eurysternus, Solenopotes capillatus.*

Mites (Scabies): *Psoroptes ovis* (syn. *P. communis* var. *bovis), Sarcoptes scabiei* var. *bovis.*

Persistent Activity: IVERMECTIN INJECTION has been proved to effectively control infections and to protect cattle from reinfection with *Dictyocaulus viviparus* for 21 days after treatment; *Ostertagia ostertagi* for 21 days after treatment; *Oesophagostomum radiatum, Haemonchus placei, Trichostrongylus axei, Cooperia punctata,* and *Cooperia oncophora* for 14 days after treatment.

Swine: IVERMECTIN INJECTION is indicated for the effective treatment and control of the following harmful species of gastrointestinal roundworms, lungworms, lice, and mange mites in swine:

Gastrointestinal Roundworms (adults and fourth-stage larvae): Large roundworm: *Ascaris suum.*

Red stomach worm: *Hyostrongylus rubidus.*

Nodular worm: *Oesophagostomum* spp.

Threadworm: *Strongyloides ransomi* (adults only).

Somatic Roundworm Larvae:

Threadworm: *Strongyloides ransomi* (somatic larvae).

Sows must be treated at least seven days before farrowing to prevent infection in piglets.

Lungworms: *Metastrongylus* spp (adults).

Lice: *Haematopinus suis.*

Mange Mites: *Sarcoptes scabiei* var. *suis.*

Reindeer: For the treatment and control of warbles *(Oedemagena tarandi)* in reindeer (see Special Minor Use section under "Dosage and Administration").

American Bison: For the treatment and control of grubs *(Hypoderma bovis)* in American bison (see Special Minor Use section under "Dosage and Administration").

Pharmacology: Product Description: Ivermectin is derived from the avermectins, a family of potent, broad-spectrum antiparasitic agents isolated from fermentation of *Streptomyces avermitilis.*

Mode of Action: Ivermectin is a member of the macrocyclic lactone class of endectocides which have a unique mode of action. Compounds of the class bind selectively and with high affinity to glutamate-gated chloride ion channels which occur in invertebrate nerve and muscle cells. This leads to an increase in the permeability of the cell membrane to chloride ions with hyperpolarization of the nerve or muscle cell, resulting in paralysis and death of the parasite. Compounds of this class may also interact with other ligand-gated chloride channels, such as those gated by the neurotransmitter gamma-aminobutyric acid (GABA).

The wide margin of safety is attributable to the fact that mammals do not have glutamate-gated chloride channels, the macrocyclic lactones have a low affinity for other mammalian ligand-gated chloride channels and they do not readily cross the blood-brain barrier.

Dosage and Administration: Dosage:

Cattle: IVERMECTIN should be given only by subcutaneous injection under the loose skin in front of or behind the shoulder at the recommended dose level of 200 mcg ivermectin per kilogram of body weight. Each mL of IVERMECTIN contains 10 mg of ivermectin, sufficient to treat 110 lb (50 kg) of body weight (maximum 10 mL per injection site).

Body Weight (lb)	Dose (mL)
220	2
330	3
440	4
550	5
660	6
770	7
880	8
990	9
1100	10

Swine: IVERMECTIN should be given only by subcutaneous injection in the neck of swine at the recommended dose level of 300 mcg of ivermectin per kilogram (2.2 lb) of body weight. Each mL of IVERMECTIN contains 10 mg of ivermectin, sufficient to treat 75 lb of body weight.

	Body Weight (lb)	Dose (mL)
Growing Pigs	19	¼
	38	½
	75	1
	150	2
Breeding Animals (Sows, Gilts, and Boars)	225	3
	300	4
	375	5
	450	6

Administration:

Cattle: IVERMECTIN INJECTION is to be given subcutaneously only, to reduce risk of potentially fatal clostridial infection of the injection site. Animals should be appropriately restrained to achieve the proper route of administration. Use of a 16-gauge ½ to ¾" needle is suggested. Inject under the loose skin in front of or behind the shoulder (see illustration).

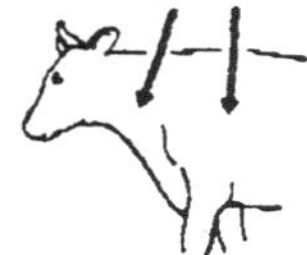

Any single-dose syringe or standard automatic syringe equipment may be used with the 50 mL package size. When using the 200 mL or 500 mL package size, use only automatic syringe equipment.

Use sterile equipment and sanitize the injection site by applying a suitable disinfectant. Clean, properly disinfected needles should be used to reduce the potential for injection site infections. No special handling or protective clothing is necessary.

Swine: IVERMECTIN INJECTION is to be given subcutaneously in the neck. Animals should be appropriately restrained to achieve the proper route of administration. Use of a 16- or 18-gauge needle is suggested for sows and boars, while an 18- or 20-gauge needle may be appropriate for young animals. Inject under the skin, immediately behind the ear (see illustration).

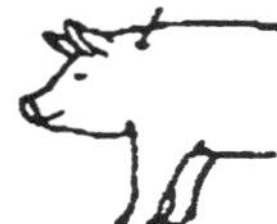

Any single-dose syringe or standard automatic syringe equipment may be used with the 50 mL package size. When using the 200 mL or 500 mL package size, use only automatic syringe equipment. As with any injection, sterile equipment should be used. The injection site should be cleaned and disinfected with alcohol before injection. The rubber stopper should also be disinfected with alcohol to prevent contamination of the contents. Mild and transient pain reactions may be seen in some swine following subcutaneous administration.

Recommended Treatment Program:

Swine: At the time of initiating any parasite control program, it is important to treat all breeding animals in the herd. After the initial treatment, use IVERMECTIN (ivermectin) INJECTION regularly as follows:

Breeding Animals:

Sows: Treat prior to farrowing, preferably 7-14 days before, to minimize infection of piglets.

Gilts: Treat 7-14 days prior to breeding. Treat 7-14 days prior to farrowing.

Boars: Frequency and need for treatments are dependent upon exposure. Treat at least two times a year.

Feeder Pigs (Weaners/Growers/Finishers): All weaner/feeder pigs should be treated before placement in clean quarters.

Pigs exposed to contaminated soil or pasture may need retreatment if reinfection occurs.

Note:

(1) IVERMECTIN INJECTION has a persistent drug level sufficient to control mite infestations throughout the egg to adult life cycle. However, since the ivermectin effect is not immediate,

care must be taken to prevent reinfestation from exposure to untreated animals or contaminated facilities. Generally, pigs should not be moved to clean quarters or exposed to uninfested pigs for approximately one week after treatment. Sows should be treated at least one week before farrowing to minimize transfer of mites to newborn baby pigs.

(2) Louse eggs are unaffected by IVERMECTIN INJECTION and may require up to three weeks to hatch. Louse infestations developing from hatching eggs may require retreatment.

(3) Consult a veterinarian for aid in the diagnosis and control of internal and external parasites of swine.

Special Minor Use:

Reindeer: For the treatment and control of warbles *(Oedemagena tarandi)* in reindeer, inject 200 micrograms ivermectin per kilogram of body weight, subcutaneously. Follow use directions for cattle as described under Dosage and Administration.

American Bison: For the treatment and control of grubs *(Hypoderma bovis)* in American Bison, inject 200 micrograms ivermectin per kilogram of body weight, subcutaneously. Follow use directions for cattle as described under Dosage and Administration.

Consult a veterinarian for assistance in the diagnosis, treatment and control of parasitism.

Contraindication(s): IVERMECTIN INJECTION FOR CATTLE AND SWINE has been developed specifically for use in cattle, swine, reindeer and American bison only. This product should not be used in other animal species as severe adverse reactions, including fatalities in dogs, may result.

Precaution(s): Protect product from light.

Store between 15°C-30°C (59°F-86°F).

Environmental Safety: Studies indicate that when ivermectin comes in contact with the soil, it readily and tightly binds to the soil and becomes inactive over time. Free ivermectin may adversely affect fish and certain water-borne organisms on which they feed. Do not permit water runoff from feedlots or production sites to enter lakes, streams, or ponds. Do not contaminate water by direct application or by the improper disposal of drug containers. Dispose of containers in an approved landfill or by incineration.

Caution(s): This product is not for intravenous or intramuscular use.

Use sterile equipment and sanitize the injection site by applying a suitable disinfectant. Clean, properly disinfected needles should be used to reduce the potential for injection site infections.

Transitory discomfort has been observed in some cattle following subcutaneous administration. A low incidence of soft-tissue swelling at the injection site has been observed. These reactions have disappeared without treatment. For cattle: divide doses greater than 10 mL between two injection sites to reduce occasional discomfort or site reaction.

Observe cattle for injection site reactions. Reactions may be due to clostridial infection and should be aggressively treated with appropriate antibiotics. If injection site infections are suspected, consult a veterinarian.

When to Treat Cattle with Grubs: IVERMECTIN effectively controls all stages of cattle grubs. However, proper timing of treatment is important. For most effective results, cattle should be treated as soon as possible after the end of the heel fly (warble fly) season.

Destruction of *Hypoderma* larvae (cattle grubs) at the period when these grubs are in vital areas may cause undesirable host-parasite reactions including the possibility of fatalities. Killing *Hypoderma lineatum* when it is in the tissue surrounding the esophagus (gullet) may cause salivation and bloat, killing *H. bovis* when it is in the vertebral canal may cause staggering or paralysis. These reactions are not specific to treatment with IVERMECTIN, but can occur with any successful treatment of grubs. Cattle should be treated either before or after these stages of grub development. Consult a veterinarian concerning the proper time for treatment.

Cattle treated with IVERMECTIN after the end of the heel fly season may be retreated with IVERMECTIN during the winter for internal parasites, mange mites, or sucking lice without danger of grub-related reactions. A planned parasite control program is recommended.

Keep this and all drugs out of the reach of children.

Not for use in humans.

Warning(s): Do not treat cattle within 35 days of slaughter. Because a withdrawal time in milk has not been established, do not use in female dairy cattle of breeding age.

Do not treat swine within 18 days of slaughter.

Do not treat reindeer or American bison within 8 weeks (56 days) of slaughter.

Presentation: IVERMECTIN INJECTION FOR CATTLE AND SWINE is available in three ready-to-use sizes:

The 50 mL bottle contains sufficient solution to treat 10 head of 550 lb (250 kg) cattle or 100 head of 38 lb (17.3 kg) swine.

The 200 mL bottle contains sufficient solution to treat 40 head of 550 lb (250 kg) cattle or 400 head of 38 lb (17.3 kg) swine. Use automatic syringe equipment only.

The 500 mL bottle contains sufficient solution to treat 100 head of 550 lb (250 kg) cattle or 1000 head of 38 lb (17.3 kg) swine. Use automatic syringe equipment only.

Manufactured by: Phoenix Scientific, Inc., St. Joseph, MO 64503.

Compendium Code No.: 14751030 Iss. 10-00

IVERMECTIN INJECTION FOR CATTLE AND SWINE

Durvet **Parasiticide Injection**

(ivermectin) Injection 1% Sterile Solution

ANADA No.: 200-228

Active Ingredient(s): IVERMECTIN INJECTION is a clear, ready-to-use, sterile solution containing 1% ivermectin, 40% glycerol formal, 1.5% benzyl alcohol (preservative), and propylene glycol, q.s. ad 100%. It is formulated to deliver the recommended dose level of 200 mcg ivermectin/kilogram of body weight in cattle when given subcutaneously at the rate of 1 mL/110 lb (50 kg).

In swine, IVERMECTIN INJECTION is formulated to deliver the recommended dose level of 300 mcg ivermectin/kilogram body weight when given subcutaneously in the neck at the rate of 1 mL/75 lb (33 kg).

Indications: A parasiticide for the treatment and control of internal and external parasites of cattle and swine.

Cattle: IVERMECTIN INJECTION is indicated for the effective treatment and control of the following harmful species of gastrointestinal roundworms, lungworms, grubs, sucking lice, and mange mites in cattle:

Gastrointestinal Roundworms (adults and fourth-stage larvae): *Ostertagia ostertagi* (including inhibited *O. ostertagi), O. lyrata, Haemonchus placei, Trichostrongylus axei, T. colubriformis, Cooperia oncophora, C. punctata, C. pectinata, Oesophagostomum radiatum, Bunostomum phlebotomum, Nematodirus helvetianus* (adults only), *N. spathiger* (adults only).

Lungworms (adults and fourth-stage larvae): *Dictyocaulus viviparus.*

Cattle Grubs (parasitic stages): *Hypoderma bovis, H. lineatum.*

Sucking Lice: *Linognathus vituli, Haematopinus eurysternus, Solenopotes capillatus.*

Mites (scabies): *Psoroptes ovis* (syn. *P. communis* var. *bovis), Sarcoptes scabiei* var. *bovis.*

Persistent activity: IVERMECTIN INJECTION has been proved to effectively control infections and to protect cattle from reinfection with *Dictyocaulus viviparus* for 21 days after treatment; *Ostertagia ostertagi* for 21 days after treatment; *Oesophagostomum radiatum, Haemonchus placei, Trichostrongylus axei, Cooperia punctata,* and *Cooperia oncophora* for 14 days after treatment.

Swine: IVERMECTIN INJECTION is indicated for the effective treatment and control of the following harmful species of gastrointestinal roundworms, lungworms, lice, and mange mites in swine:

Gastrointestinal Roundworms (adults and fourth-stage larvae): Large roundworm: *Ascaris suum.*

Red stomach worm: *Hyostrongylus rubidus.*

Nodular worm: *Oesophagostomum* spp.

Threadworm: *Strongyloides ransomi* (adults only).

Somatic Roundworm Larvae:

Threadworm: *Strongyloides ransomi* (somatic larvae).

Sows must be treated at least seven days before farrowing to prevent infection in piglets.

Lungworms: *Metastrongylus* spp (adults).

Lice: *Haematopinus suis.*

Mange Mites: *Sarcoptes scabiei* var. *suis.*

Reindeer: For the treatment and control of warbles *(Oedemagena tarandi)* in reindeer (see Special Minor Use section under "Dosage and Administration").

American Bison: For the treatment and control of grubs *(Hypoderma bovis)* in American bison (see Special Minor Use section under "Dosage and Administration").

Pharmacology: Product Description: Ivermectin is derived from the avermectins, a family of potent, broad-spectrum antiparasitic agents isolated from fermentation of *Streptomyces avermitilis.*

Mode of Action: Ivermectin is a member of the macrocyclic lactone class of endectocides which have a unique mode of action. Compounds of the class bind selectively and with high affinity to glutamate-gated chloride ion channels which occur in invertebrate nerve and muscle cells. This leads to an increase in the permeability of the cell membrane to chloride ions with hyperpolarization of the nerve or muscle cell, resulting in paralysis and death of the parasite. Compounds of this class may also interact with other ligand-gated chloride channels, such as those gated by the neurotransmitter gamma-aminobutyric acid (GABA).

The wide margin of safety is attributable to the fact that mammals do not have glutamate-gated chloride channels, the macrocyclic lactones have a low affinity for other mammalian ligand-gated chloride channels and they do not readily cross the blood-brain barrier.

Dosage and Administration: Dosage:

Cattle: IVERMECTIN should be given only by subcutaneous injection under the loose skin in front of or behind the shoulder at the recommended dose level of 200 mcg ivermectin per kilogram of body weight. Each mL of IVERMECTIN contains 10 mg of ivermectin, sufficient to treat 110 lb (50 kg) of body weight (maximum 10 mL per injection site).

Body Weight (lb)	Dose (mL)
220	2
330	3
440	4
550	5
660	6
770	7
880	8
990	9
1100	10

Swine: IVERMECTIN should be given only by subcutaneous injection in the neck of swine at the recommended dose level of 300 mcg of ivermectin per kilogram (2.2 lb) of body weight. Each mL of IVERMECTIN contains 10 mg of ivermectin, sufficient to treat 75 lb of body weight.

	Body Weight (lb)	Dose (mL)
Growing Pigs	19	¼
	38	½
	75	1
	150	2
Breeding Animals (Sows, Gilts, and Boars)	225	3
	300	4
	375	5
	450	6

Administration:

Cattle: IVERMECTIN INJECTION is to be given subcutaneously only, to reduce risk of potentially fatal clostridial infection of the injection site. Animals should be appropriately restrained to achieve the proper route of administration. Use of a 16-gauge ½ to ¾" needle is suggested. Inject under the loose skin in front of or behind the shoulder (see illustration).

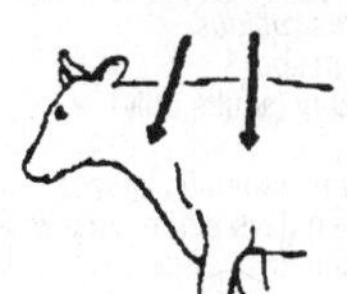

Any single-dose syringe or standard automatic syringe equipment may be used with the 50 mL package size. When using the 200 mL or 500 mL package size, use only automatic syringe equipment.

Use sterile equipment and sanitize the injection site by applying a suitable disinfectant. Clean, properly disinfected needles should be used to reduce the potential for injection site infections. No special handling or protective clothing is necessary.

Swine: IVERMECTIN (ivermectin) INJECTION is to be given subcutaneously in the neck. Animals should be appropriately restrained to achieve the proper route of administration. Use of a 16- or 18-gauge needle is suggested for sows and boars, while an 18- or 20-gauge needle may be appropriate for young animals. Inject under the skin, immediately behind the ear (see illustration).

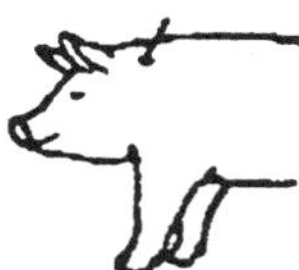

Any single-dose syringe or standard automatic syringe equipment may be used with the 50 mL package size. When using the 200 mL or 500 mL package size, use only automatic syringe equipment. As with any injection, sterile equipment should be used. The injection site should be cleaned and disinfected with alcohol before injection. The rubber stopper should also be disinfected with alcohol to prevent contamination of the contents. Mild and transient pain reactions may be seen in some swine following subcutaneous administration.

Recommended Treatment Program:

Swine: At the time of initiating any parasite control program, it is important to treat all breeding animals in the herd. After the initial treatment, use IVERMECTIN (ivermectin) INJECTION regularly as follows:

Breeding Animals:

Sows: Treat prior to farrowing, preferably 7-14 days before, to minimize infection of piglets.

Gilts: Treat 7-14 days prior to breeding. Treat 7-14 days prior to farrowing.

Boars: Frequency and need for treatments are dependent upon exposure. Treat at least two times a year.

Feeder Pigs (Weaners/Growers/Finishers): All weaner/feeder pigs should be treated before placement in clean quarters.

Pigs exposed to contaminated soil or pasture may need retreatment if reinfection occurs.

Note:

(1) IVERMECTIN INJECTION has a persistent drug level sufficient to control mite infestations throughout the egg to adult life cycle. However, since the ivermectin effect is not immediate, care must be taken to prevent reinfestation from exposure to untreated animals or contaminated facilities. Generally, pigs should not be moved to clean quarters or exposed to uninfested pigs for approximately one week after treatment. Sows should be treated at least one week before farrowing to minimize transfer of mites to newborn baby pigs.

(2) Louse eggs are unaffected by IVERMECTIN INJECTION and may require up to three weeks to hatch. Louse infestations developing from hatching eggs may require retreatment.

(3) Consult a veterinarian for aid in the diagnosis and control of internal and external parasites of swine.

Special Minor Use:

Reindeer: For the treatment and control of warbles *(Oedemagena tarandi)* in reindeer, inject 200 micrograms ivermectin per kilogram of body weight, subcutaneously. Follow use directions for cattle as described under Dosage and Administration.

American Bison: For the treatment and control of grubs *(Hypoderma bovis)* in American Bison, inject 200 micrograms ivermectin per kilogram of body weight, subcutaneously. Follow use directions for cattle as described under Dosage and Administration.

Consult your veterinarian for assistance in the diagnosis, treatment and control of parasitism.

Contraindication(s): IVERMECTIN INJECTION FOR CATTLE AND SWINE has been developed specifically for use in cattle, swine, reindeer and American bison only. This product should not be used in other animal species as severe adverse reactions, including fatalities in dogs, may result.

Precaution(s): Protect product from light.

Store between 15°C-30°C (59°F-86°F).

Environmental Safety: Studies indicate that when ivermectin comes in contact with the soil, it readily and tightly binds to the soil and becomes inactive over time. Free ivermectin may adversely affect fish and certain water-borne organisms on which they feed. Do not permit water runoff from feedlots or production sites to enter lakes, streams, or ponds. Do not contaminate water by direct application or by the improper disposal of drug containers. Dispose of containers in an approved landfill or by incineration.

Caution(s): The product is not for intravenous or intramuscular use.

Use sterile equipment and sanitize the injection site by applying a suitable disinfectant. Clean, properly disinfected needles should be used to reduce the potential for injection site infections.

Transitory discomfort has been observed in some cattle following subcutaneous administration. A low incidence of soft-tissue swelling at the injection site has been observed. These reactions have disappeared without treatment. For cattle, divide doses greater than 10 mL between two injection sites to reduce occasional discomfort or site reaction.

Observe cattle for injection site reactions. Reactions may be due to clostridial infection and should be aggressively treated with appropriate antibiotics. If injection site infections are suspected, consult your veterinarian.

When to Treat Cattle with Grubs: IVERMECTIN effectively controls all stages of cattle grubs. However, proper timing of treatment is important. For most effective results, cattle should be treated as soon as possible after the end of the heel fly (warble fly) season.

Destruction of *Hypoderma* larvae (cattle grubs) at the period when these grubs are in vital areas may cause undesirable host-parasite reactions including the possibility of fatalities. Killing *Hypoderma lineatum* when it is in the tissue surrounding the esophagus (gullet) may cause salivation and bloat, killing *H. bovis* when it is in the vertebral canal may cause staggering or paralysis. These reactions are not specific to treatment with IVERMECTIN, but can occur with any successful treatment of grubs. Cattle should be treated either before or after these stages of grub development. Consult your veterinarian concerning the proper time for treatment.

Cattle treated with IVERMECTIN after the end of the heel fly season may be retreated with IVERMECTIN during the winter for internal parasites, mange mites, or sucking lice without danger of grub-related reactions. A planned parasite control program is recommended.

Keep this and all drugs out of the reach of children.

Not for use in humans.

Warning(s): Do not treat cattle within 35 days of slaughter. Because a withdrawal time in milk has not been established, do not use in female dairy cattle of breeding age.

Do not treat swine within 18 days of slaughter.

Do not treat reindeer or American bison within 8 weeks (56 days) of slaughter.

Presentation: IVERMECTIN INJECTION FOR CATTLE AND SWINE is available in three ready-to-use sizes:

The 50 mL bottle contains sufficient solution to treat 10 head of 550 lb (250 kg) cattle or 100 head of 38 lb (17.3 kg) swine.

The 200 mL bottle contains sufficient solution to treat 40 head of 550 lb (250 kg) cattle or 400 head of 38 lb (17.3 kg) swine. Use automatic syringe equipment only.

The 500 mL bottle contains sufficient solution to treat 100 head of 550 lb (250 kg) cattle or 1000 head of 38 lb (17.3 kg) swine. Use automatic syringe equipment only.

Compendium Code No.: 10841791

Iss. 11-01

IVERMECTIN POUR-ON

Aspen **Parasiticide-Topical**

(ivermectin)

ANADA No.: 200-219

Active Ingredient(s): Contains 5 mg ivermectin/mL.

Indications: IVERMECTIN (ivermectin) POUR-ON applied at the recommended dose level of 500 mcg/kg is indicated for the effective control of these parasites.

Gastrointestinal Roundworms: *Ostertagia ostertagi* (including inhibited stage) (adults and L_4), *Haemonchus placei* (adults and L_4), *Trichostrongylus axei* (adults and L_4), *T. colubriformis* (adults and L_4), *Cooperia* spp (adults and L_4), *Strongyloides papillosus* (adults), *Oesophagostomum radiatum* (adults and L_4), *Trichuris* spp (adults).

Lungworms: *Dictyocaulus viviparus* (adults and L_4).

Cattle Grubs: *Hypoderma bovis, H. lineatum* (parasitic stages).

Mites: *Sarcoptes scabiei* var. *bovis.*

Lice: *Linognathus vituli, Haematopinus eurysternus, Damalinia bovis, Solenopotes capillatus.*

Horn Flies: *Haematobia irritans.*

Pharmacology: Persistent Activity: IVERMECTIN (ivermectin) Pour-On has been proved to effectively control infections and to protect cattle from re-infection with *Ostertagia ostertagi, Oesophagostomum radiatum, Haemonchus placei, Trichostrongylus axei, Cooperia punctata* and *Cooperia oncophora* for 14 days after treatment.

Mode of Action: Ivermectin as a member of the avermectin family kills certain parasitic roundworms and ectoparasites, such as mites, lice, horn flies and other insects. Its action is unique to the avermectin class of antiparasitic agents. This action involves a chemical that serves as a signal from one nerve cell to another, or from a nerve cell to a muscle cell. This chemical, a neurotransmitter, is called gamma-aminobutyric acid or GABA.

In roundworms, ivermectin stimulates the release of GABA from nerve endings and enhances binding of GABA to special receptors at nerve junctions, thus interrupting nerve impulses — thereby paralyzing and killing the parasite.

The enhancement of the GABA effect in arthropods such as mites, lice, and horn flies resembles that in roundworms except that nerve impulses are interrupted between the nerve ending and the muscle cell. Again, this leads to paralysis and death.

Ivermectin has no measurable effect against flukes or tapeworms, presumably because they do not have GABA as a nerve impulse transmitter.

The principal peripheral neurotransmitter in mammals, acetylcholine, is unaffected by ivermectin. Ivermectin does not readily penetrate the central nervous system of mammals where GABA functions as a neurotransmitter.

Dosage and Administration:

Treatment for Cattle for Horn Flies: IVERMECTIN (ivermectin) POUR-ON controls horn flies *(Haematobia irritans)* for up to 28 days after dosing. For best results IVERMECTIN (ivermectin) POUR-ON should be part of a parasite control program for both internal and external parasites based on the epidemiology of these parasites. Consult your veterinarian or an entomologist for the most effective timing of applications.

Dosage: The dose rate is 1 mL for each 22 lb of body weight. The formulation should be applied along the topline in a narrow strip extending from the withers to the tailhead.

Administration:

Measuring Cup (250 mL and 1 L bottles): The enclosed measuring cup is graduated in 5 mL increments. Each 5 mL will treat 110 lbs body weight. When body weight is between markings, use the next higher increment.

Applicator Gun* (3.785 L bottle, 5 L backpack and 25 L carboy): Because of the solvents used in IVERMECTIN (ivermectin) POUR-ON, only the Ivermectin (ivermectin) applicator gun from Simcro Tech Limited, or equivalent, is recommended. Other applicators may exhibit compatibility problems, resulting in locking, incorrect dosage or leakage.

Remove the draw-off cap and backpack strap from the indentation in the back of the bottle and refer to the diagram to fit the strap to the bottle.

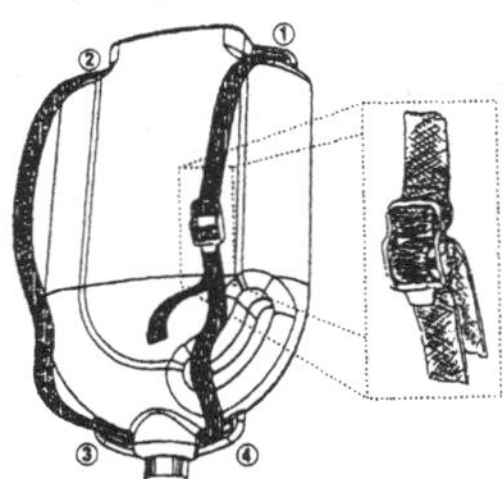

Thread the strap through the bottle eyelet number 1, then 2, 3, and 4, taking care to follow the diagram when connecting the strap to the buckle.

The strap is adjustable by lifting the tab on the buckle.

Slide one of the coil springs over one end of the draw-off tubing. Attach that end of the draw-off tubing to the stem on the applicator gun and slide the spring up to the connection. Slide the second coil spring over the other end of the draw-off tubing and connect that end to the cap that has the stem. Slide the spring to the connection. Replace the shipping cap with the cap having the draw-off tubing attached. Tighten this draw-off cap to the bottle. Invert the bottle and use as a backpack (for 5 L backpack).

Follow the applicator gun manufacturer's directions for priming the gun, adjusting the dose, and care of the applicator gun following use.

Weight	Dose
220 lb (100 kg)	10 mL
330 lb (150 kg)	15 mL
440 lb (200 kg)	20 mL
550 lb (250 kg)	25 mL
660 lb (300 kg)	30 mL
770 lb (350 kg)	35 mL
880 lb (400 kg)	40 mL
990 lb (450 kg)	45 mL
1100 lb (500 kg)	50 mL

*Additional Applicator Guns and Draw Tubes may be purchased from your local retail dealer or Aspen Veterinary Resources, Ltd.

When to Treat Cattle with Grubs: IVERMECTIN (ivermectin) POUR-ON effectively controls all stages of cattle grubs. However, proper timing of treatment is important. For the most effective results, cattle should be treated as soon as possible after the end of the heel fly (warble fly) season. While this is not peculiar to ivermectin, destruction of *Hypoderma* larvae (cattle grubs) at the period when these grubs are in vital areas may cause undesirable host-parasite reactions. Killing *Hypoderma lineatum* when it is in the esophageal tissues may cause bloat; killing *H. bovis* when it is in the vertebral canal may cause staggering or paralysis. Cattle should be treated either before or after these stages of grub development.

Cattle treated with IVERMECTIN (ivermectin) POUR-ON at the end of the fly season may be re-treated with IVERMECTIN (ivermectin) during the winter without danger of grub-related reactions. For further information and advice on a planned parasite control program, consult your veterinarian.

Consult your veterinarian for assistance in the diagnosis, treatment and control of parasitism.

Precaution(s): Flammable! Keep away from heat, sparks, open flame, and other sources of ignition.

Store between 15° and 30°C (59° and 86°F).

Store away from excessive heat (104°F/40°C) and protect from light.

Use only in well-ventilated areas or outdoors.

Close container tightly when not in use.

Cloudiness in the formulation may occur when IVERMECTIN (ivermectin) POUR-ON is stored at temperatures below 32°F. Allowing to warm at room temperature will restore the normal appearance without affecting efficacy.

Environmental Safety: Studies indicate that when ivermectin comes in contact with the soil, it readily and tightly binds to the soil and becomes inactive over time. Free ivermectin may adversely affect fish or certain water-borne organisms on which they feed. Do not permit cattle to enter lakes, streams or ponds for at least six hours after treatment. Do not contaminate water by direct application or by the improper disposal of drug containers. Dispose of containers in an approved landfill or by incineration.

Caution(s): Cattle should not be treated when hair or hide is wet since reduced efficacy may be experienced.

Do not use when rain is expected to wet cattle within six hours after treatment.

This product is for application to skin surface only. Do not give orally or parenterally.

Antiparasitic activity of ivermectin will be impaired if the formulation is applied to areas of the skin with mange scabs or lesions, or with dermatoses or adherent materials, e.g., caked mud or manure.

Ivermectin has been associated with adverse reactions in sensitive dogs; therefore, IVERMECTIN (ivermectin) POUR-ON is not recommended for use in species other than cattle.

Warning(s): Residue Warning: Cattle must not be treated within 48 days of slaughter for human consumption. Because a withdrawal time in milk has not been established, do not use in female dairy cattle of breeding age.

Not for use in humans.

This product should not be applied to self or others because it may be irritating to human skin and eyes and absorbed through the skin. To minimize accidental skin contact, the user should wear a long-sleeved shirt and rubber gloves. If accidental skin contact occurs, wash immediately with soap and water. If accidental eye exposure occurs, flush eyes immediately with water and seek medical attention.

Keep this and all drugs out of the reach of children.

Discussion: IVERMECTIN (ivermectin) Pour-On delivers internal and external parasite control in one convenient low-volume application. Ivermectin is a potent antiparasitic agent whose chemical structure is different from those of other antiparasitic agents.

Trial Data: Safety: Studies conducted in the U.S.A. have demonstrated the safety margin for ivermectin. Based on plasma levels, the topically applied formulation is expected to be at least as well tolerated by breeding animals as is the subcutaneous formulation which had no effect on breeding performance.

Presentation: IVERMECTIN (ivermectin) POUR-ON is available in a 250 mL (8.5 fl oz) bottle, a 1 L (33.8 fl oz) bottle for use with the dispensing cap provided, or a 3.785 L (1 gal) bottle, a 5 L (169 fl oz) backpack and a 25 L carboy for use with the appropriate automatic dosing applicator.

Manufactured by: Phoenix Scientific, Inc., St. Joseph, MO 64503

Compendium Code No.: 14750501

IVERMECTIN POUR-ON

Durvet **Parasiticide-Topical**

(ivermectin) Pour-On for Cattle

ANADA No.: 200-219

Active Ingredient(s): Contains 5 mg ivermectin/mL.

Indications: IVERMECTIN (ivermectin) POUR-ON applied at the recommended dose level of 500 mcg/kg is indicated for the effective control of these parasites.

Gastrointestinal Roundworms: *Ostertagia ostertagi* (including inhibited stage) (adults and L_4), *Haemonchus placei* (adults and L_4), *Trichostrongylus axei* (adults and L_4), *T. colubriformis* (adults and L_4), *Cooperia* spp (adults and L_4), *Strongyloides papillosus* (adults), *Oesophagostomum radiatum* (adults and L_4), *Trichuris* spp (adults).

Lungworms: *Dictyocaulus viviparus* (adults and L_4).

Cattle Grubs (parasitic stages): *Hypoderma bovis, H. lineatum.*

Mites: *Sarcoptes scabiei* var. *bovis.*

Lice: *Linognathus vituli, Haematopinus eurysternus, Damalinia bovis, Solenopotes capillatus.*

Horn Flies: *Haematobia irritans.*

Pharmacology: Persistent Activity: IVERMECTIN ivermectin) POUR-ON has been proved to effectively control infections and to protect cattle from re-infection with *Ostertagia ostertagi, Oesophagostomum radiatum, Haemonchus placei, Trichostrongylus axei, Cooperia punctata* and *Cooperia oncophora* for 14 days after treatment.

Mode of Action: Ivermectin as a member of the avermectin family kills certain parasitic roundworms and ectoparasites, such as mites, lice, horn flies and other insects. Its action is unique to the avermectin class of antiparasitic agents. This action involves a chemical that serves as a signal from one nerve cell to another, or from a nerve cell to a muscle cell. This chemical, a neurotransmitter, is called gamma-aminobutyric acid or GABA.

In roundworms, ivermectin stimulates the release of GABA from nerve endings and enhances binding of GABA to special receptors at nerve junctions, thus interrupting nerve impulses — thereby paralyzing and killing the parasite. The enhancement of the GABA effect in arthropods such as mites, lice, and horn flies resembles that in roundworms except that nerve impulses are interrupted between the nerve ending and the muscle cell. Again, this leads to paralysis and death.

Ivermectin has no measurable effect against flukes or tapeworms, presumably because they do not have GABA as a nerve impulse transmitter.

The principal peripheral neurotransmitter in mammals, acetylcholine, is unaffected by ivermectin. Ivermectin does not readily penetrate the central nervous system of mammals where GABA functions as a neurotransmitter.

Dosage and Administration: Treatment for Cattle for Horn Flies: IVERMECTIN (ivermectin) POUR-ON controls horn flies *(Haematobia irritans)* for up to 28 days after dosing. For best results, IVERMECTIN (ivermectin) POUR-ON should be part of a parasite control program for both internal and external parasites based on the epidemiology of these parasites. Consult a veterinarian or an entomologist for the most effective timing of applications.

Dosage: The dose rate is 1 mL for each 22 lb of body weight. The formulation should be applied along the topline in a narrow strip extending from the withers to the tailhead.

Administration:

Dispensing Cap (250 mL, 500 mL and 1 L bottles): The enclosed dispensing cap is graduated in 5 mL increments. Each 5 mL will treat 110 lbs body weight. When body weight is between markings, use the next higher increment.

Attach the dispensing cap to the bottle.

Select the correct dose rate by rotating the adjuster top in either direction to position the dose indicator to the appropriate level.

Hold the bottle upright and gently squeeze it to deliver a slight excess of the required dose as indicated by the calibration lines.

By releasing the pressure, the dose automatically adjusts to the correct level. Tilt the bottle to deliver the dose. The off (stop) position will close the system between dosing.

Applicator Gun* (3.785 L bottle, 5 L backpack and 25 L carboy): Because of the solvents used in IVERMECTIN (ivermectin) POUR-ON, only the Ivermectin (ivermectin) applicator gun from Simcro Tech Limited, or equivalent, is recommended. Other applicators may exhibit compatibility problems, resulting in locking, incorrect dosage or leakage.

Remove the draw-off cap and backpack strap from the indentation in the back of the bottle and refer to the diagram to fit the strap to the bottle.

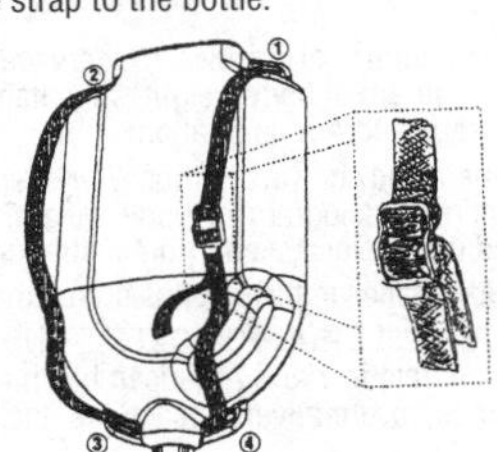

Thread the strap through the bottle eyelet number 1, then 2, 3, and 4, taking care to follow the diagram when connecting the strap to the buckle.

The strap is adjustable by lifting the tab on the buckle.

Slide one of the coil springs over one end of the draw-off tubing. Attach that end of the draw-off tubing to the stem on the applicator gun and slide the spring up to the connection. Slide the second coil spring over the other end of the draw-off tubing and connect that end to the cap that has the stem. Slide the spring to the connection. Replace the shipping cap with the cap having the draw-off tubing attached. Tighten this draw-off cap to the bottle. Invert the bottle and use as a backpack (for 5 L backpack).

Follow the applicator gun manufacturer's directions for priming the gun, adjusting the dose, and care of the applicator gun following use.

Weight	Dose
220 lb (100 kg)	10 mL
330 lb (150 kg)	15 mL
440 lb (200 kg)	20 mL
550 lb (250 kg)	25 mL
660 lb (300 kg)	30 mL
770 lb (350 kg)	35 mL
880 lb (400 kg)	40 mL
990 lb (450 kg)	45 mL
1100 lb (500 kg)	50 mL

*Additional Applicator Guns and Draw Tubes may be purchased from your Durvet Distributors, contact Durvet, Inc.

When to Treat Cattle with Grubs: IVERMECTIN (ivermectin) POUR-ON effectively controls all stages of cattle grubs. However, proper timing of treatment is important. For the most effective results, cattle should be treated as soon as possible after the end of the heel fly (warble fly) season. While this is not peculiar to ivermectin, destruction of *Hypoderma* larvae (cattle grubs) at the period when these grubs are in vital areas may cause undesirable host-parasite reactions. Killing *Hypoderma lineatum* when it is in the esophageal tissues may cause bloat; killing *H. bovis* when it is in the vertebral canal may cause staggering or paralysis. Cattle should be treated either before or after these stages of grub development.

Cattle treated with IVERMECTIN (ivermectin) POUR-ON at the end of the fly season may be re-treated with ivermectin during the winter without danger of grub-related reactions. For further information and advice on a planned parasite control program, consult a veterinarian. Consult a veterinarian for assistance in the diagnosis, treatment and control of parasitism.

Precaution(s): Flammable. Keep away from heat, sparks, open flame, and other sources of ignition.

Store between 15°-30°C (59°-86°F).

Store away from excessive heat (104°F/40°C) and protect from light.

Use only in well-ventilated areas or outdoors.

Close container tightly when not in use.

Cloudiness in the formulation may occur when IVERMECTIN (ivermectin) POUR-ON is stored at temperatures below 32°F. Allowing to warm at room temperature will restore the normal appearance without affecting efficacy.

Environmental Safety: Studies indicate that when ivermectin comes in contact with the soil, it readily and tightly binds to the soil and becomes inactive over time. Free ivermectin may adversely affect fish or certain water-borne organisms on which they feed. Do not permit cattle to enter lakes, streams or ponds for at least six hours after treatment. Do not contaminate water by direct application or by the improper disposal of drug containers. Dispose of containers in an approved landfill or by incineration.

Caution(s): Cattle should not be treated when hair or hide is wet since reduced efficacy may be experienced.

Do not use when rain is expected to wet cattle within six hours after treatment.

This product is for application to skin surface only. Do not give orally or parenterally.

Antiparasitic activity of ivermectin will be impaired if the formulation is applied to areas of the skin with mange scabs or lesions, or with dermatoses or adherent materials, e.g., caked mud or manure.

Ivermectin has been associated with adverse reactions in sensitive dogs; therefore, IVERMECTIN (ivermectin) POUR-ON is not recommended for use in species other than cattle.

Warning(s): Residue Warning: Cattle must not be treated within 48 days of slaughter for human consumption. Because a withdrawal time in milk has not been established, do not use on female dairy cattle of breeding age.

Not for use in humans.

This product should not be applied to self or others because it may be irritating to human skin and eyes and absorbed through the skin. To minimize accidental skin contact, the user should wear a long-sleeved shirt and rubber gloves. If accidental skin contact occurs, wash immediately with soap and water. If accidental eye exposure occurs, flush eyes immediately with water and seek medical attention.

Keep this and all drugs out of the reach of children.

Discussion: IVERMECTIN (ivermectin) POUR-ON delivers internal and external parasite control in one convenient low-volume application. Ivermectin is a potent antiparasitic agent whose chemical structure is different from those of other antiparasitic agents.

Trial Data: Safety: Studies conducted in the U.S.A. have demonstrated the safety margin for ivermectin. Based on plasma levels, the topically applied formulation is expected to be at least as well tolerated by breeding animals as is the subcutaneous formulation which had no effect on breeding performance.

Presentation: IVERMECTIN (ivermectin) POUR-ON is available in a 250 mL (8.5 fl oz) bottle, a 500 mL (16.9 fl oz) bottle, a 1 L (33.8 fl oz) bottle for use with the dispensing cap provided, or in a 3.785 L (1 gal) bottle, a 5 L (169 fl oz) backpack or a 25 L carboy for use with the appropriate automatic dosing applicator.

Compendium Code No.: 10841072 Rev. 10-01

IVER-ON™

Med-Pharmex **Parasiticide-Topical**

Ivermectin Pour-On-5 mg ivermectin/mL-Parasiticide

ANADA No.: 200-299

Active Ingredient(s): Contains 5 mg ivermectin/mL.

Indications: Ivermectin Pour-On applied at the recommended dose level of 500 mcg/kg is indicated for the effective control of these parasites.

Gastrointestinal Roundworms: *Ostertagia ostertagi* (adults and L4) (including inhibited stage), *Haemonchus placei* (adults and L4) *Trichostrongylus axei* (adults and L4), *T. colubriformis* (adults and L4), *Cooperia* spp. (adults and L4), *Strongyloides papillosus* (adults), *Oesophagostomum radiatum* (adults and L4), *Trichuris* spp. (adults).

Lungworms: *Dictyocaulus viviparus* (adults and L4).

Cattle Grubs (parasitic stages): *Hypoderma bovis, H. Lineatum.*

Mites: *Sarcoptes scabiei* var. *bovis.*

Lice: *Linognathus vituli, Haematopinus eurystemus, Damalinia bovis, Solenopotes capillatus.*

Horn Flies: *Haematobia irritans.*

Pharmacology: Persistent Activity: Ivermectin Pour-On has been proved to effectively control infections and to protect cattle from reinfection with *Ostertagia ostertagi, Oesophagostomum radiatum, Haemonchus placei, Trichostrongylus axei, Cooperia punctata* and *Cooperia oncophora* for 14 days after treatment.

Mode of Action: Ivermectin as a member of the avermectin family kills certain parasitic roundworms and ectoparasites, such as mites, lice, horn flies and other insects. Its action is unique to the avermectin class of antiparasitic agents. This action involves a chemical that serves as a signal from one nerve cell to another, or from a nerve cell to a muscle cell. This chemical, a neurotransmitter, is called gamma-amino-butyric add or GABA.

In roundworms, ivermectin stimulates the release of GABA from nerve endings and enhances binding of GABA to special receptors at nerve junctions, thus interrupting nerve impulses thereby paralyzing and killing the parasite.

The enhancement of the GABA effect in arthropods such as mites, lice and horn files resembles that in roundworms except that nerve impulses are interrupted between the nerve ending and the muscle cell. Again, this leads to paralysis and death.

Ivermectin has no measurable effect against flukes or tapeworms, presumably because they do not have GABA as a nerve impulse transmitter.

The principle peripheral neurotransmitter in mammals, acetylcholine, is unaffected by ivermectin. Ivermectin does not readily penetrate the central nervous system of mammals where GABA functions as a neurotransmitter.

Dosage and Administration:

Treatment of Cattle for Horn Flies: Ivermectin Pour-On controls horn flies *(Haematobia irritans)* for up to 28 days after dosing. For best results Ivermectin Pour-On should be part of a parasite control program for both internal and external parasites based on the epidemiology of these parasites. Consult your veterinarian or an entomologist for the most effective timing of applications.

Dosage: The dose rate is 1 mL for each 22 lb of body weight. The formulation should be applied along the topline in a narrow strip extending from the withers to the tailhead.

Administration:

Squeeze-Measure-Pour System (8.5 fl. oz./250 mL Bottle with 25 mL Measuring Cup): Measure the amount of solution to be used at the dose rate of 1 mL for each 22 lb of body weight into the measuring cup. When body weight is between markings use the higher setting.

Tilt the measuring cup to deliver the dose.

Squeeze-Measure-Pour System (33.8 fl. oz./1 L Bottle with 25 mL Measuring Cup): Measure the amount of solution to be used, at the dose rate of 1 mL for each 22 lbs of body weight, into the measuring cup. When body weight is between markings, use the higher setting.

Tilt the measuring cup to deliver the dose.

One Gallon Bottle and Collapsible Pack (84.5 fl. oz./2.5 L Pack and 169 fl. oz./5 L Pack):

Connect the applicator gun to the collapsible pack as follows: Attach the open end of the draw-off tubing to the dosing equipment. Replace the shipping cap with the draw-off cap and tighten down. Attach draw-off tubing to the draw-off cap.

Gently prime the applicator gun, checking for leaks.

Follow the manufacturer's directions for adjusting the dose.

When the interval between uses of the applicator gun is expected to exceed 12 hours, disconnect the gun and draw-off tubing from the product container and empty the product from the gun and tubing back into the product container. To prevent removal of special lubricants form the Protector Drench Gun, the gun and tubing must not be washed.

Consult your veterinarian for assistance in the diagnosis, treatment and control of parasitism.

Contraindication(s): Ivermectin has been associated with adverse reactions in sensitive dogs; therefore, Ivermectin Pour-On is not recommended for use in species other than cattle.

Precaution(s): Flammable. Keep away from heat, sparks, open flame and other sources of ignition.

Store away from excessive heat (104°F/40°C) and protect from light.

Use only in well-ventilated areas or outdoors.

Close container tightly when not in use.

Cloudiness in the formulation may occur when Ivermectin Pour-On is stored at temperatures below 32°F. Allowing to warn at room temperature will restore the normal appearance without affecting efficacy.

Environmental Safety: Studies indicate that when ivermectin comes in contact with the soil, it readily and tightly binds to the soil and becomes inactive over time. Free ivermectin may adversely affect fish or certain waterborne organisms on which they feed. Do not permit cattle to enter lakes, streams or ponds for at least six hours after treatment. Do not contaminate water by direct application or by the Improper disposal of drug containers. Dispose of containers in an approved landfill or by incineration.

Caution(s): Cattle should not be treated when hair or hide is wet since reduced efficacy may be experienced.

Do not use when rain is expected to wet cattle within six hours after treatment.

This product is for application to skin surface only. Do not give orally or parenterally.

Antiparasitic activity of ivermectin will be impaired if the formulation is applied to areas of the skin with mange scabs or lesions, or with dermatoses or adherent materials, e.g. caked mud or manure.

Warning(s): Cattle must not be treated within 48 days of slaughter for human consumption. Because a withdrawal time in milk has not been established, do not use in female dairy cattle of breeding age.

Not for use in humans.

This product should not be applied to self or others because it may be irritating to human skin and eyes and absorbed through the skin. To minimize accidental skin contact, the user should wear a long-sleeved shirt and rubber gloves. If accidental skin contact occurs, wash immediately with soap and water. If accidental eye exposure occurs, flush eyes immediately with water and seek medical attention.

Keep this and all drugs out of the reach of children.

Toxicology: Safety: Studies conducted in the USA have demonstrated the safety margin for ivermectin. Based on plasma levels, the topically applied formulation is expected to be at least as well tolerated by breeding animals as is the subcutaneous formulation which had no effect on breeding performance.

Discussion: Ivermectin Pour-On delivers internal and external parasite control in one convenient low-volume application. Discovered and developed by scientists from Merck Research Laboratories, Ivermectin Pour-On contains ivermectin, a unique chemical entity.

When to Treat Cattle with Grubs: Ivermectin Pour-On effectively controls all stages of cattle grubs. However, proper timing of treatment is important. For the most effective results, cattle should be treated as soon as possible after the end of the heel fly (warble fly) season. While this is not peculiar to ivermectin, destruction of *Hypoderma* larvae (cattle grubs) at the period when these grubs are in vital areas may cause undesirable hostparasite reactions. Killing *Hypoderma lineatum* when it is in esophageal tissues may cause bloat; killing *H. bovis* when it is in the vertebral canal may cause staggering or paralysis. Cattle should be treated either before or after these stages of grub development.

Cattle treated with Ivermectin Pour-On at the end of the fly season may be re-treated with ivermectin during the winter without danger of grub-related reactions. For further information and advice on a planned parasite control program, consult your veterinarian.

Presentation: Available in 8.5 fl. oz. (250 mL) and 33.8 fl. oz. (1 L) bottles, 84.5 fl. oz. (2.5 L) and 169 fl. oz. (5 L) collapsible packs.

Compendium Code No.: 10270150 November 2000

IVERSOL ℞

Med-Pharmex **Parasiticide-Oral**

(ivermectin) 10 mg/mL

ANADA No.: 200-292

Active Ingredient(s): IVERSOL (ivermectin) Liquid is a clear, ready-to-use solution with each mL containing 1% ivermectin (10 mg), 0.2 mL propylene glycol, 80 mg polysorbate 80, 9 mg sodium phosphate monobasic monohydrate, 1.3 mg sodium phosphate dibasic anhydrous, 1 mg butylated hydroxytoluene, 0.1 mg disodium edetate, 3% benzyl alcohol and purified water q.s. ad 100%.

Indications: IVERSOL (ivermectin) Liquid is indicated for the effective treatment and control of the following parasites or parasitic conditions in horses:

Large Strongyles: *Strongylus vulgaris* (adults and arterial larval stages), *S. edentatus* (adults and tissue stages), *S. equinus* (adults), *Triodontophorus* spp (adults).

Small Strongyles - including those resistant to some benzimidazole class compounds (adults and fourth-stage larvae): *Cyathostomum* spp, *Cylicocyclus* spp, *Cylicostephanus* spp, *Cylicodontophorus* spp.

Pinworms (adults and fourth-stage larvae): *Oxyuris equi.*

Ascarids (adults and third- and fourth-stage larvae): *Parascaris equorum.*

Hairworms (adults): *Trichostrongylus axei.*

Large-mouth Stomach Worms (adults): *Habronema muscae.*

Bots (oral and gastric stages): *Gastrophilus* spp.

Lungworms (adults and fourth-stage larvae): *Dictyocaulus arnfieldi*.
Intestinal Threadworms (adults): *Strongyloides westeri*.
Summer Sores caused by *Habronema* and *Draschia* spp cutaneous third-stage larvae.
Dermatitis caused by neck threadworm microfilariae, *Onchocerca* sp.

Pharmacology: Product Description: Ivermectin is derived from the avermectins, a family of potent, broad-spectrum antiparasitic agents, which are isolated from fermentation of *Streptomyces avermitilis*.

Mode of Action: Ivermectin, one of the avermectins, kills certain parasitic roundworms and ectoparasites such as mites and lice. The avermectins are different in their action from other antiparasitic agents. This action involves a chemical that serves as a signal from one nerve cell to another, or from a nerve cell to a muscle cell. This chemical, a neurotransmitter, is called gamma-aminobutyric acid or GABA.

In roundworms, ivermectin stimulates the release of GABA from nerve endings and enhances binding of GABA to special receptors at nerve junctions, thus interrupting nerve impulses-thereby paralyzing and killing the parasite.

The enhancement of the GABA effect in arthropods such as mites and lice resembles that in roundworms except that nerve impulses are interrupted between the nerve ending and the muscle cell. Again, this leads to paralysis and death.

The principal peripheral neurotransmitter in mammals, acetylcholine, is unaffected by ivermectin. Ivermectin does not readily penetrate the central nervous system of mammals where GABA functions as a neurotransmitter.

Dosage and Administration: Dosage: IVERSOL (ivermectin) Liquid for Horses is formulated for administration by stomach tube (nasogastric intubation) or as an oral drench. The recommended dose is 200 mcg of ivermectin per kilogram (91 mcg/lb) of body weight. Each mL contains sufficient ivermectin to treat 110 lb (50 kg) of body weight: 10 mL will treat an 1100 lb (500 kg) horse.

Administration: Use a calibrated dosing syringe inserted into the bottle to measure the appropriate dose, or pour the IVERSOL (ivermectin) Liquid into a graduated cylinder for dose measurement. Use a clean syringe if accessing the bottle to avoid contaminating the remaining product.

Administration by stomach tube (gravity or positive flow): The recommended dose can be used undiluted or diluted up to 40 times with clean tepid water (see Notes to Veterinarian). Use tepid water to flush any drug remaining in the tube into the horse's stomach.

I

Administration by drench: For administration by this method, an undiluted dose is usually preferred. Clear the horse's mouth of any food material, elevate the horse's head, and using a syringe, deposit the appropriate dose in the back of the mouth. In order to avoid unnecessary coughing or the potential for material to enter the trachea and lungs, do not use excessive pressure (squirting), do not use a large (diluted) dose volume, and do not deposit the dose in the laryngeal area. Increased dose rejection may occur if the dose is deposited in the buccal space. Keep the horse's head elevated and observe the horse to insure the dose is retained.

Suggested Parasite Control Program: All horses should be included in a regular parasite control program with particular attention being paid to mares, foals and yearlings. Foals should be treated initially at 6 to 8 weeks of age, and routine treatment repeated as appropriate. IVERSOL (ivermectin) Liquid effectively controls gastrointestinal nematodes and bots in horses. Regular treatment will reduce the chances of verminous arteritis and colic caused by *S. vulgaris*. With its broad spectrum, IVERSOL (ivermectin) Liquid is well suited to be the major product in a parasite control program.

Contraindication(s): IVERSOL (ivermectin) Liquid has been formulated specifically for use in horses only. This product should not be used in other animal species as severe adverse reactions, including fatalities in dogs, may result.

Precaution(s): Store in a tightly closed container at room temperature.

Do not store above 30°C (86°F).

Protect IVERSOL (ivermectin) Liquid (undiluted or diluted) from light.

Environmental Safety: Studies indicate that when ivermectin comes in contact with the soil, it readily and tightly binds to the soil and becomes inactive over time. Free ivermectin may adversely affect fish and certain water-borne organisms on which they feed. Do not contaminate lakes, streams, or ground water by direct application or by improper disposal of drug containers. Dispose of drug container in an approved landfill or by incineration.

Caution(s): Federal (U.S.A.) law restricts this drug to use by or on the order of a licensed veterinarian.

Refrain from smoking and eating when handling. Wash hands after use. Avoid contact with eyes.

For veterinary use only.

Warning(s): Do not use in horses intended for food purposes.

Keep this and all drugs out of the reach of children.

Toxicology: Safety: IVERSOL (ivermectin) Liquid may be used in horses of all ages including mares at any stage of pregnancy. Stallions may be treated without adversely affecting their fertility. These horses have been treated with no adverse effects other than those noted under Notes to Veterinarian.

Discussion: IVERSOL (ivermectin) Liquid for Horses has been formulated for professional administration by stomach tube or oral drench. One low-volume dose is effective against important internal parasites, including the arterial stages of *Strongylus vulgaris*, and bots.

Notes To Veterinarian: Swelling and itching reactions after treatment with IVERSOL (ivermectin) Liquid have occurred in horses carrying heavy infections of neck threadworm microfilariae, *Onchocerca* sp. These reactions were most likely the result of microfilariae dying in large numbers. Symptomatic treatment may be advisable.

Healing of summer sores involving extensive tissue changes may require other therapy in conjunction with IVERSOL (ivermectin) Liquid. Reinfection, and measures for its prevention, should also be considered.

Special consideration should be given to the effects or potential for injury from handling, restraint, and placement of the tube during administration by stomach tube. IVERSOL (ivermectin) Liquid should be administered by drench if the risks associated with tubing are of concern. Due to the consequences of improper administration (also see Dosage and Administration), IVERSOL (ivermectin) Liquid is intended for use by a veterinarian only and is not recommended for dispensing.

IVERSOL (ivermectin) Liquid in 1 to 20 and 1 to 40 dilutions with tap water has been shown to be stable for 72 hours under the conditions recommended for the product (i.e., at room temperature, in a tightly closed container, protected from light). The diluted product does not promote the growth of common organisms. However, prolonged storage of the diluted product cannot be recommended, as the effects of possible contaminants and interactions with untested materials are unknown.

Presentation: IVERSOL (ivermectin) Liquid for Horses is available in 50 mL, 100 mL and 250 mL plastic bottles.

Compendium Code No.: 10270160 Iss. 11-01

IVOMEC® 0.27% INJECTION FOR GROWER AND FEEDER PIGS

Merial **Parasiticide Injection**

(ivermectin) 0.27% Sterile Solution

NADA No.: 128-409

Active Ingredient(s): IVOMEC® Injection is a clear, ready-to-use, sterile solution containing 0.27% ivermectin, 40% glycerol formal, and propylene glycol, q.s. ad 100%.

Indications: A parasiticide for the treatment and control of internal and external parasites of grower and feeder pigs.

IVOMEC® Injection is indicated for the effective treatment and control of the following harmful species: gastrointestinal roundworms, lungworms, lice, and mange mites.

Gastrointestinal Roundworms:
Large roundworm, *Ascaris suum* (adults and fourth-stage larvae).
Red stomach worm, *Hyostrongylus rubidus* (adults and fourth-stage larvae).
Nodular worm, *Oesophagostomum* spp. (adults and fourth-stage larvae).
Threadworm, *Strongyloides ransomi* (adults).
Lungworms: *Metastrongylus* spp. (adults).
Lice: *Haematopinus suis*.
Mange Mites: *Sarcoptes scabiei* var. *suis*.

Ranch-Raised Foxes: For the treatment and control of ear mites *(Otodectes cynotis)* in ranch-raised fox (see Special Minor Use section under "Dosage and Administration").

Pharmacology: Product Description: Ivermectin is derived from the avermectins, a family of potent, broad-spectrum antiparasitic agents isolated from fermentation of *Streptomyces avermitilis*.

Mode of Action: Ivermectin is a member of the macrocyclic lactone class of endectocides which have a unique mode of action. Compounds of the class bind selectively and with high affinity to glutamate-gated chloride ion channels which occur in invertebrate nerve and muscle cells. This leads to an increase in the permeability of the cell membrane to chloride ions with hyperpolarization of the nerve or muscle cell, resulting in paralysis and death of the parasite. Compounds of this class may also interact with other ligand-gated chloride channels, such as those gated by the neurotransmitter gamma-aminobutyric acid (GABA).

The wide margin of safety is attributable to the fact that mammals do not have glutamate-gated chloride channels, the macrocyclic lactones have a low affinity for other mammalian ligand-gated chloride channels and they do not readily cross the blood-brain barrier.

Dosage and Administration: IVOMEC® Injection is formulated to deliver the recommended dose level of 300 mcg ivermectin/kilogram body weight when given subcutaneously in the neck at the rate of 1 mL per 20 lb (8.8 kg).

Dosage: IVOMEC® Injection should be given only by subcutaneous injection (under the skin), in the neck at the recommended dose level of 300 mcg ivermectin per kilogram (2.2 lb) of body weight. Each mL of IVOMEC® contains 2.7 mg of ivermectin, sufficient to treat 20 lb (8.8 kg) of body weight.

The table below indicates the dose volume of IVOMEC® Injection for growing pigs body weight:

Body Weight (lb)	Dose Volume (mL)	Doses per Pack
10	0.5	400
20	1.0	200
30	1.5	133
40	2.0	100
50	2.5	80
60	3.0	66
70	3.5	57

Administration: IVOMEC® (ivermectin) Injection is to be given subcutaneously (under the skin) immediately behind the ear (see illustration). Animals should be appropriately restrained to achieve the proper route of administration. An 18- or 20-gauge needle may be appropriate for young animals.

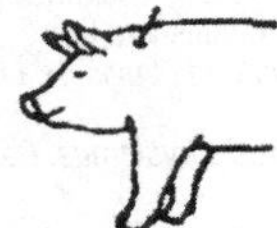

Use only automatic syringe equipment. As with any injection, sterile equipment should be used. The injection site should be cleaned and disinfected with alcohol before injection. The rubber stopper should also be disinfected with alcohol to prevent contamination of the contents. Mild and transient pain reactions may be seen in some swine following subcutaneous administration.

Recommended Treatment Program: All pigs should be treated before placement in clean quarters. Pigs exposed to contaminated premises, soil or pasture may need retreatment if reinfection occurs.

For pigs over 70 lbs body weight, use Ivomec® Injection for Swine 1% Sterile solution.

Note: (1) IVOMEC® Injection has a persistent drug level sufficient to control mite infestations throughout the egg to adult life cycle. However, since the ivermectin effect is not immediate, care must be taken to prevent reinfestation from exposure to untreated animals or contaminated facilities. Generally, pigs should not be moved to clean quarters or exposed to uninfested pigs for approximately one week after treatment.

(2) Louse eggs are unaffected by IVOMEC® Injection and may require up to three weeks to hatch. Louse infestations developing from hatching eggs may require retreatment.

(3) Consult a veterinarian for aid in the diagnosis and control of internal and external parasites of swine.

Special Minor Use:

Ranch-Raised Foxes: For the treatment and control of ear mites *(Otodectes cynotis)* in ranch-raised foxes. Inject 200 mcg ivermectin per kilogram (2.2 lb) of body weight, subcutaneously between the shoulder blades. Repeat treatment in 3 weeks.

Body Weight (lb)	Dose Volume (mL)
6.5	0.25
13	0.50
20	0.75

Consult your veterinarian for assistance in the diagnosis, treatment and control of parasitism.

Precaution(s): Protect product from light.

Environmental Safety: Studies indicate that when ivermectin comes in contact with the soil, it readily and tightly binds to the soil and becomes inactive over time. Free ivermectin may adversely affect fish and certain waterborne organisms on which they feed. Do not permit water runoff from feedlots or production sites to enter lakes, streams or ponds. Do not contaminate water by direct application or by the improper disposal of drug containers. Dispose of drug containers in an approved landfill or by incineration.

Caution(s): This product is for subcutaneous injection in the neck.

IVOMEC® Injection for Grower and Feeder Pigs has been developed specifically for use in swine and foxes only. This product should not be used in other animal species as severe adverse reactions, including fatalities in dogs, may result.

Warning(s): Residue Information: Do not treat swine within 18 days of slaughter.

Not for use in humans.

Keep this and all drugs out of the reach of children.

The Material Safety Data Sheet (MSDS) contains more detailed occupational safety information. To report adverse effects in users, to obtain an MSDS, or for assistance call 1-888-637-4251.

Discussion: IVOMEC® (ivermectin) Injection for Grower and Feeder Pigs is a dilute parasiticide for young pigs. A conveniently measured dose kills gastrointestinal roundworms, lungworms, lice, and mange mites that may impair the health of young pigs.

Discovered and developed by scientists from Merck Research Laboratories, ivermectin is a novel chemical entity. Its convenience, broad-spectrum efficacy and safety margin make IVOMEC® Injection a unique product for parasite control in young pigs.

Presentation: IVOMEC® Injection for Grower and Feeder Pigs is available in ready-to-use 200 mL soft, collapsible pack designed for use with automatic syringe equipment. Each pack contains sufficient solution to treat 100 head of 40 lb (18 kg) pigs.

IVOMEC is a registered trademark of Merial.

(Merial Limited: Registered in England and Wales [Reg. No. 3332571] with registered offices at 27 Knightsbridge, London SW1X 7QT, England and domesticated in Delaware, USA as Merial LLC).

U.S. Patent Nos. 4,199,569 and 4,853,372

Compendium Code No.: 11110301 8710508

IVOMEC® 1% INJECTION FOR CATTLE AND SWINE

Merial **Parasiticide Injection**

(ivermectin) 1% Sterile Solution

NADA No.: 128-409

Active Ingredient(s): IVOMEC® Injection is a clear, ready-to-use, sterile solution containing 1% ivermectin, 40% glycerol formal, and propylene glycol, q.s. ad 100%.

Indications: A parasiticide for the treatment and control of internal and external parasites in cattle and swine.

Cattle: IVOMEC® Injection is indicated for the effective treatment and control of the following harmful species of gastrointestinal roundworms, lungworms, grubs, sucking lice, and mange mites in cattle:

Gastrointestinal Roundworms (adults and fourth-stage larvae): *Ostertagia ostertagi* (including inhibited *O. ostertagi), O. lyrata, Haemonchus placei, Trichostrongylus axei, T. colubriformis, Cooperia oncophora, C. punctata, C. pectinata, Oesophagostomum radiatum, Bunostomum phlebotomum, Nematodirus helvetianus* (adults only), *N. spathiger* (adults only).

Lungworms (adults and fourth-stage larvae): *Dictyocaulus viviparus.*

Cattle Grubs (parasitic stages): *Hypoderma bovis, H. lineatum.*

Sucking Lice: *Linognathus vituli, Haematopinus eurysternus, Solenopotes capillatus.*

Mites (scabies): *Psoroptes ovis* (syn. *P. communis* var. *bovis), Sarcoptes scabiei* var. *bovis.*

Persistent Activity: IVOMEC® Injection has been proved to effectively control infections and to protect cattle from reinfection with *Dictyocaulus viviparus* for 28 days after treatment; *Ostertagia ostertagi* for 21 days after treatment; *Oesophagostomum radiatum, Haemonchus placei, Trichostrongylus axei, Cooperia punctata*, and *Cooperia oncophora* for 14 days after treatment.

Swine: IVOMEC® Injection is indicated for the effective treatment and control of the following harmful species of gastrointestinal roundworms, lungworms, lice, and mange mites in swine:

Gastrointestinal Roundworms:

Large roundworm: *Ascaris suum* (adults and fourth-stage larvae).

Red stomach worm: *Hyostrongylus rubidus* (adults and fourth-stage larvae).

Nodular worm: *Oesophagostomum* spp (adults and fourth-stage larvae).

Threadworm: *Strongyloides ransomi* (adults).

Somatic Roundworm Larvae:

Threadworm: *Strongyloides ransomi* (somatic larvae).

Sows must be treated at least seven days before farrowing to prevent infection in piglets.

Lungworms: *Metastrongylus* spp (adults).

Lice: *Haematopinus suis.*

Mange Mites: *Sarcoptes scabiei* var. *suis.*

Reindeer: For the treatment and control of warbles *(Oedemagena tarandi)* in reindeer (see Special Minor Use section under "Dosage and Administration").

American Bison: For the treatment and control of grubs *(Hypoderma bovis)* in American bison (see Special Minor Use section under "Dosage and Administration").

Pharmacology: Product Description: Ivermectin is derived from the avermectins, a family of potent, broad-spectrum antiparasitic agents isolated from fermentation of *Streptomyces avermitilis.*

Mode of Action: Ivermectin is a member of the macrocyclic lactone class of endectocides which have a unique mode of action. Compounds of the class bind selectively and with high affinity to glutamate-gated chloride ion channels which occur in invertebrate nerve and muscle cells. This leads to an increase in the permeability of the cell membrane to chloride ions with hyperpolarization of the nerve or muscle cell, resulting in paralysis and death of the parasite. Compounds of this class may also interact with other ligand-gated chloride channels, such as those gated by the neurotransmitter gamma-aminobutyric acid (GABA).

The wide margin of safety is attributable to the fact that mammals do not have glutamate-gated chloride channels, the macrocyclic lactones have a low affinity for other mammalian ligand-gated chloride channels and they do not readily cross the blood-brain barrier.

Dosage and Administration: IVOMEC® Injection is formulated to deliver the recommended dose level of 200 mcg ivermectin/kilogram of body weight in cattle when given subcutaneously at the rate of 1 mL/110 lb (50 kg). In swine, IVOMEC® Injection is formulated to deliver the recommended dose level of 300 mcg ivermectin/kilogram body weight when given subcutaneously in the neck at the rate of 1 mL per 75 lb (33 kg).

Dosage:

Cattle: IVOMEC® Injection should be given only by subcutaneous injection under the loose skin in front of or behind the shoulder at the recommended dose level of 200 mcg ivermectin per kilogram of body weight. Each mL of IVOMEC® contains 10 mg of ivermectin, sufficient to treat 110 lb (50 kg) of body weight (maximum 10 mL per injection site).

Body Weight (lb)	Dose Volume (mL)
220	2
330	3
440	4
550	5
660	6
770	7
990	9
1100	10

Swine: IVOMEC® Injection should be given only by subcutaneous injection in the neck of swine at the recommended dose level of 300 mcg of ivermectin per kilogram (2.2 lb) of body weight. Each mL of IVOMEC® contains 10 mg of ivermectin, sufficient to treat 75 lb of body weight.

	Body Weight (lb)	Dose Volume (mL)
Growing Pigs	19	1/4
	38	1/2
	75	1
	150	2
Breeding Animals (Sows, Gilts, and Boars)	225	3
	300	4
	375	5
	450	6

Administration:

Cattle: IVOMEC® Injection is to be given subcutaneously only, to reduce risk of potentially fatal clostridial infection of the injection site. Animals should be appropriately restrained to achieve the proper route of administration. Use of a 16-gauge ½" to ¾" needle is suggested. Inject under the loose skin in front of or behind the shoulder (see illustration).

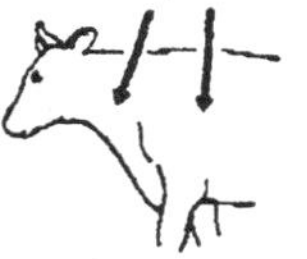

When using the 200, 500 or 1000 mL pack size, use only automatic syringe equipment.

Use sterile equipment and sanitize the injection site by applying a suitable disinfectant. Clean, properly disinfected needles should be used to reduce the potential for injection site infection.

No special handling or protective clothing is necessary.

Swine: IVOMEC® (ivermectin) Injection is to be given subcutaneously in the neck. Animals should be appropriately restrained to achieve the proper route of administration. Use of a 16- or 18-gauge needle is suggested for sows and boars, while an 18- or 20-gauge needle may be appropriate for young animals. Inject under the skin, immediately behind the ear (see illustration).

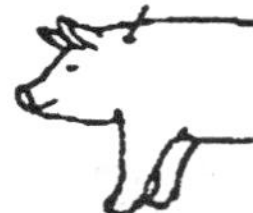

When using the 200 mL, 500 mL or 1000 mL pack size, use only automatic syringe equipment. As with any injection, sterile equipment should be used. The injection site should be cleaned and disinfected with alcohol before injection. The rubber stopper should also be disinfected with alcohol to prevent contamination of the contents. Mild and transient pain reactions may be seen in some swine following subcutaneous administration.

Recommended Treatment Program:

Swine: At the time of initiating any parasite control program, it is important to treat all breeding animals in the herd. After the initial treatment, use IVOMEC® Injection regularly as follows:

Breeding Animals:

Sows: Treat prior to farrowing, preferably 7-14 days before, to minimize infection of piglets.

Gilts: Treat 7-14 days prior to breeding. Treat 7-14 days prior to farrowing.

Boars: Frequency and need for treatments are dependent upon exposure.

Treat at least two times a year.

Feeder Pigs (Weaners/Growers/Finishers): All weaner/feeder pigs should be treated before placement in clean quarters.

Pigs exposed to contaminated soil or pasture may need retreatment if reinfection occurs.

Note: (1) IVOMEC® Injection has a persistent drug level sufficient to control mite infestations throughout the egg to adult life cycle. However, since the ivermectin effect is not immediate, care must be taken to prevent reinfestation from exposure to untreated animals or contaminated facilities. Generally, pigs should not be moved to clean quarters or exposed to uninfested pigs for approximately one week after treatment. Sows should be treated at least one week before farrowing to minimize transfer of mites to newborn baby pigs.

(2) Louse eggs are unaffected by IVOMEC® Injection and may require up to three weeks to hatch. Louse infestations developing from hatching eggs may require retreatment.

(3) Consult a veterinarian for aid in the diagnosis and control of internal and external parasites of swine.

Special Minor Use:

Reindeer: For the treatment and control of warbles *(Oedemagena tarandi)* in reindeer, inject 200 micrograms ivermectin per kilogram of body weight, subcutaneously. Follow use directions for cattle as described under Administration.

American Bison: For the treatment and control of grubs *(Hypoderma bovis)* in American bison, inject 200 micrograms ivermectin per kilogram of body weight, subcutaneously. Follow use directions for cattle as described under Administration.

When to Treat Cattle with Grubs: IVOMEC® effectively controls all stages of cattle grubs. However, proper timing of treatment is important. For most effective results, cattle should be treated as soon as possible after the end of the heel fly (warble fly) season. Destruction of *Hypoderma* larvae (cattle grubs) at the period when these grubs are in vital areas may cause undesirable host-parasite reactions including the possibility of fatalities. Killing *Hypoderma lineatum* when it is in the tissue surrounding the esophagus (gullet) may cause salivation and bloat, killing *H. bovis* when it is in the vertebral canal may cause staggering or paralysis. These reactions are not specific to treatment with IVOMEC®, but can occur with any successful treatment of grubs. Cattle should be treated either before or after these stages of grub development. Consult your veterinarian concerning the proper time for treatment.

Cattle treated with IVOMEC® after the end of the heel fly season may be retreated with IVOMEC® during the winter for internal parasites, mange mites, or sucking lice without danger of grub-related reactions. A planned parasite control program is recommended.

Consult your veterinarian for assistance in the diagnosis, treatment and control of parasitism.

Precaution(s): Protect product from light.

Environmental Safety: Studies indicate that when ivermectin comes in contact with the soil, it readily and tightly binds to the soil and becomes inactive over time. Free ivermectin may adversely affect fish and certain water-borne organisms on which they feed. Do not permit water runoff from feedlots or production sites to enter lakes, streams, or ponds. Do not contaminate water by direct application or by the improper disposal of drug containers. Dispose of containers in an approved landfill or by incineration.

Caution(s): This product is not for intravenous or intramuscular use.

Transitory discomfort has been observed in some cattle following subcutaneous administration. A low incidence of soft tissue swelling at the injection site has been observed. These reactions have disappeared without treatment. For cattle, divide doses greater than 10 mL between two injection sites to reduce occasional discomfort or site reaction.

Use sterile equipment and sanitize the injection site by applying a suitable disinfectant. Clean, properly disinfected needles should be used to reduce the potential for injection site infections.

Observe cattle for injection site reactions. Reactions may be due to clostridial infection and should be aggressively treated with appropriate antibiotics. If injection site infections are suspected, consult your veterinarian.

IVOMEC® Injection for Cattle and Swine has been developed specifically for use in cattle, swine, reindeer and American bison only. This product should not be used in other animal species as severe adverse reactions, including fatalities in dogs, may result.

Warning(s): Residue Information: Do not treat cattle within 35 days of slaughter. Because a withdrawal time in milk has not been established, do not use in female dairy cattle of breeding age. Do not treat swine within 18 days of slaughter.

Do not treat reindeer or American bison within 8 weeks (56 days) of slaughter.

Not for use in humans.

Keep this and all drugs out of the reach of children.

The Material Safety Data Sheet (MSDS) contains more detailed occupational safety information. To report adverse effects, obtain an MSDS or for assistance, contact Merial at 1-888-637-4251.

Discussion: IVOMEC® (ivermectin) is an injectable parasiticide for cattle and swine. One low-volume dose effectively treats and controls the following internal and external parasites that may impair the health of cattle and swine: gastrointestinal roundworms (including inhibited *Ostertagia ostertagi* in cattle), lungworms, grubs, sucking lice, and mange mites of cattle; and gastrointestinal roundworms, lungworms, lice, and mange mites of swine. Discovered and developed by scientists from Merck Research Laboratories, ivermectin is a novel chemical entity. Its convenience, broad-spectrum efficacy, and safety margin make IVOMEC® Injection a unique product for parasite control of cattle and swine.

Presentation: IVOMEC® Injection for Cattle and Swine is available in five ready-to-use pack sizes:

The 50 mL pack is a multiple dose, rubber-capped bottle. Each bottle contains sufficient solution to treat 10 head of 550 lb (250 kg) cattle or 100 head of 38 lb (17.3 kg) swine.

The 200 mL pack is a soft, collapsible pack designed for use with automatic syringe equipment. Each pack contains sufficient solution to treat 40 head of 550 lb (250 kg) cattle or 400 head of 38 lb (17.3 kg) swine.

The 500 mL pack is a soft, collapsible pack designed for use with automatic syringe equipment. Each pack contains sufficient solution to treat 100 head of 550 lb (250 kg) cattle or 1000 head of 38 lb (17.3 kg) swine.

The 2 x 500 mL includes two 500 mL packs with sufficient solution to treat 200 head of 550 lb (250 kg) cattle or 2000 head of 38 lb (17.3 kg) swine.

The 1000 mL pack is a soft, collapsible pack designed for use with automatic syringe equipment. Each pack contains sufficient solution to treat 200 head of 550 lb (250 kg) cattle or 2000 head of 38 lb (17.3 kg) swine.

IVOMEC is a registered trademark of Merial.

(Merial Limited: Registered in England and Wales [Reg. No. 3332751] with registered offices at 27 Knightsbridge, London, SW1X 7QT, England and domesticated in Delaware, USA as Merial LLC).

U.S. Patent Nos. 4,199,569 and 4,853,372

Compendium Code No.: 11110312 8913412

IVOMEC® 1% INJECTION FOR SWINE

Merial **Parasiticide Injection**

(ivermectin) 1% Sterile Solution

NADA No.: 128-409

Active Ingredient(s): IVOMEC® Injection is a clear, ready-to-use, sterile solution containing 1% ivermectin, 40% glycerol formal, and propylene glycol, q.s. ad 100%.

Indications: A parasiticide for the treatment and control of internal and external parasites of swine.

IVOMEC® Injection is indicated for the effective treatment and control of the following harmful species of gastrointestinal roundworms, lungworms, lice, and mange mites in swine.

Gastrointestinal Roundworms:

Large roundworm, *Ascaris suum* (adults and fourth-stage larvae).

Red stomach worm, *Hyostrongylus rubidus* (adults and fourth-stage larvae).

Nodular worm, *Oesophagostomum* spp (adults and fourth-stage larvae).

Threadworm, *Strongyloides ransomi* (adults).

Somatic Roundworm Larvae:

Threadworm, *Strongyloides ransomi* (somatic larvae).

Sows must be treated at least seven days before farrowing to prevent infection in piglets.

Lungworms: *Metastrongylus* spp (adults).

Lice: *Haematopinus suis.*

Mange Mites: *Sarcoptes scabiei* var. *suis.*

Pharmacology: Product Description: Ivermectin is derived from the avermectins, a family of potent, broad-spectrum antiparasitic agents isolated from fermentation of *Streptomyces avermitilis.*

Mode of Action: Ivermectin kills certain parasitic roundworms and ectoparasites, such as mites and lice. Its action is unique and not shared by other antiparasitic agents. This action involves a chemical that serves as a signal from one nerve cell to another, or from a nerve cell to a muscle cell. This chemical, a neurotransmitter, is called gamma-aminobutyric acid or GABA.

In roundworms, ivermectin stimulates the release of GABA from nerve endings and enhances binding of GABA to special receptors at nerve junctions, thus interrupting nerve impulses—thereby paralyzing and killing the parasite.

The enhancement of the GABA effect in arthropods such as mites and lice resembles that in roundworms except that nerve impulses are interrupted between the nerve ending and the muscle cell. Again, this leads to paralysis and death.

The principal peripheral neurotransmitter in mammals, acetylcholine, is unaffected by ivermectin. Ivermectin does not readily penetrate the central nervous system of mammals where GABA functions as a neurotransmitter.

Dosage and Administration: IVOMEC® Injection is formulated to deliver the recommended dose level of 300 mcg/kg given subcutaneously in the neck at the rate of 1 mL per 75 lb (33 kg).

Dosage: IVOMEC® Injection should be given only by subcutaneous injection in the neck of swine at the recommended dose level of 300 mcg ivermectin per kilogram (2.2 lb) of body weight. Each mL of IVOMEC® Injection contains 10 mg of ivermectin, sufficient to treat 75 lb (33 kg) of body weight.

The table below indicates the dose volume of IVOMEC® Injection for swine by animal body weight:

	Body Weight (lb)	Dose Volume (mL)
Growing Pigs	19	.25
	38	.5
	75	1
	150	2
Breeding Animals (Sows, Gilts, and Boars)	225	3
	300	4
	375	5
	450	6

Administration: IVOMEC® (ivermectin) Injection is to be given subcutaneously only in the neck. Animals should be appropriately restrained to achieve the proper route of administration. Use of a 16- or 18-gauge needle is suggested for sows and boars, while an 18- or 20-gauge needle may be appropriate for young animals. Inject under the skin, immediately behind the ear (see illustration).

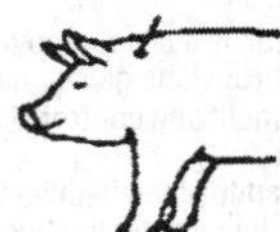

Any single-dose syringe or standard automatic syringe equipment may be used with the 50 mL pack size. Use only automatic syringe equipment when using the 200 mL or 500 mL pack size. As with any injection, sterile equipment should be used. The injection site should be cleaned and disinfected with alcohol before injection. The rubber stopper should also be disinfected with alcohol to prevent contamination of the contents. Mild and transient pain reactions may be seen in some swine following subcutaneous administration.

Recommended Treatment Program: At the time of initiating any parasite control program, it is important to treat all the animals in the herd. After the initial treatment, use IVOMEC® Injection regularly as follows:

Breeding Animals:

Sows: Treat prior to farrowing, preferably 7-14 days before, to minimize infection of piglets.

Gilts: Treat 7-14 days prior to breeding. Treat 7-14 days prior to farrowing.

Boars: Treat at least two times a year. Frequency of and need for treatments are dependent upon exposure.

Feeder Pigs (Weaners/Growers/Finishers): All weaner/feeder pigs should be treated before placement in clean quarters.

Pigs exposed to contaminated soil or pasture may need retreatment if reinfection occurs.

Note: (1) IVOMEC® Injection has a persistent drug level sufficient to control mite infestations throughout the egg to adult life cycle. However, since the ivermectin effect is not immediate, care must be taken to prevent reinfestation from exposure to untreated animals or contaminated facilities. Generally, pigs should not be moved to clean quarters or exposed to uninfested pigs for approximately one week after treatment. Sows should be treated at least one week before farrowing to minimize transfer of mites to newborn baby pigs.

(2) Louse eggs are unaffected by IVOMEC® Injection and may require up to three weeks to hatch. Louse infestations developing from hatching eggs may require retreatment.

(3) Consult a veterinarian for aid in the diagnosis and control of internal and external parasites of swine.

Consult your veterinarian for assistance in the diagnosis, treatment and control of parasitism.

Precaution(s): Protect product from light.

Environmental Safety: Studies indicate that when ivermectin comes in contact with the soil, it readily and tightly binds to the soil and becomes inactive over time. Free ivermectin may adversely affect fish and certain waterborne organisms on which they feed. Do not permit water runoff from feedlots or production sites to enter lakes, streams, or ponds. Do not contaminate water by direct application, or by the improper disposal of drug containers. Dispose of drug containers in an approved landfill or by incineration.

Caution(s): This product is for subcutaneous injection in the neck.

IVOMEC® Injection for Swine has been developed specifically for use in swine only. This product should not be used in other animal species as severe adverse reactions, including fatalities in dogs, may result.

Warning(s): Residue Information: Do not treat swine within 18 days of slaughter.

Not for human use.

Keep this and all drugs out of the reach of children.

The Material Safety Data Sheet (MSDS) contains more detailed occupational safety information. To report adverse effects in users, to obtain an MSDS, or for assistance, call 1-888-637-4251.

Discussion: IVOMEC® (ivermectin) is an injectable parasiticide for swine. A low volume dose effectively kills gastrointestinal roundworms, lungworms, lice, and mange mites that may impair the health of swine.

Discovered and developed by scientists from Merck Research Laboratories, ivermectin is a novel chemical entity. Its convenience, broad-spectrum efficacy and safety margin make IVOMEC® Injection a unique product for parasite control in swine.

Presentation: IVOMEC® Injection for Swine is available in three ready-to-use pack sizes:

50 mL pack is a multiple-dose, rubber capped bottle. Each bottle contains sufficient solution to treat 100 head of 38 lb (17.3 kg) swine.

The 200 mL pack is a soft, collapsible pack designed to use with automatic syringe equipment. Each pack contains sufficient solution to treat 400 head of 38 lb (17.3 kg) swine.

The 500 mL pack is a soft, collapsible pack designed to use with automatic syringe equipment. Each pack contains sufficient solution to treat 1000 head of 38 lb (17.3 kg) swine.

IVOMEC is a registered trademark of Merial.

(Merial Limited: Registered in England and Wales [Reg. No. 3332751] with registered offices at 27 Knightsbridge, London SW1X 7QT, England and domesticated in Delaware, USA as Merial LLC).

U.S. Patent Nos. 4,199,569 and 4,853,372

Compendium Code No.: 11110321 8662105

IVOMEC® EPRINEX® POUR-ON FOR BEEF AND DAIRY CATTLE

Merial **Parasiticide-Topical**

(eprinomectin) Parasiticide

NADA No.: 141-079

Active Ingredient(s): Contains 5 mg eprinomectin/mL.

Indications: For treatment and control of internal and external parasites.

IVOMEC® EPRINEX® Pour-On is indicated for the treatment and control of gastrointestinal roundworms (including inhibited *Ostertagia ostertagi),* lungworms, grubs, sucking and biting lice, chorioptic and sarcoptic mange mites, and horn flies in beef and dairy cattle of all ages, including lactating dairy cattle. Applied at the recommended dose volume of 1 mL/10 kg (22 lb) body weight, to achieve a dose level of 500 mcg eprinomectin/kg body weight, IVOMEC® EPRINEX® Pour-On is indicated for the effective treatment and control of the following parasites.

Gastrointestinal Roundworms: *Haemonchus placei* (adults and L4), *Ostertagia ostertagi* (including inhibited L4) (adults and L4), *Trichostrongylus axei* (adults and L4), *Trichostrongylus colubriformis* (adults and L4), *Trichostrongylus longispicularis* (adults only), *Cooperia oncophora* (adults and L4), *Cooperia punctata* (adults and L4), *Cooperia surnabada* (adults and L4), *Nematodirus helvetianus* (adults and L4), *Oesophagostomum radiatum* (adults and L4), *Bunostomum phlebotomum* (adults and L4), *Strongyloides papillosus* (adults only), *Trichuris* spp. (adults only).

Lungworms: *Dictyocaulus viviparus* (adults and L4).

Cattle Grubs (all parasitic stages): *Hypoderma lineatum, Hypoderma bovis.*

Lice: *Damalinia bovis, Linognathus vituli, Haematopinus eurysternus, Solenopotes capillatus.*

Mange Mites: *Chorioptes bovis, Sarcoptes scabiei.*

Horn Flies: *Haematobia irritans.*

Persistent Activity: IVOMEC® EPRINEX® (eprinomectin) Pour-On for Beef and Dairy Cattle has been proved to effectively control infections and to protect cattle from re-infection with *Dictyocaulus viviparus* for 21 days after treatment and *Haematobia irritans* for 7 days after treatment.

Pharmacology: Mode of Action: Eprinomectin is a member of the macrocyclic lactone class of endectocides which have a unique mode of action. Compounds of the class bind selectively and with high affinity to glutamate-gated chloride ion channels which occur in invertebrate nerve and muscle cells.

This leads to an increase in the permeability of the cell membrane to chloride ions with hyperpolarization of the nerve or muscle cell, resulting in paralysis and death of the parasite. Compounds of this class may also interact with other ligand-gated chloride channels, such as those gated by the neurotransmitter gamma-aminobutyric acid (GABA).

The margin of safety for compounds of this class is attributable to the fact that mammals do not have glutamate-gated chloride channels, the macrocyclic lactones have a low affinity for other mammalian ligand-gated chloride channels and they do not readily cross the blood-brain barrier.

Dosage and Administration: Dosage: The product is formulated only for external application to beef and dairy cattle. The dose rate is 1 mL/10 kg (22 lb) of body weight. The product should be applied topically along the backline in a narrow strip extending from the withers to the tailhead.

Administration:

Squeeze-Measure-Pour System (250 mL/8.5 fl oz Bottle with 25 mL Metering Cup):

Attach the metering cup to the bottle.

Set the dose by turning the top section of the cup to align the correct body weight with the pointer on the knurled cap. When body weight is between markings, use the higher setting.

Hold the bottle upright and squeeze it to deliver a slight excess of the required dose as indicated by the calibration lines.

By releasing the pressure, the dose automatically adjusts to the correct level. The off (Stop) position will close the system between dosing. Tilt the bottle to deliver the dose.

Squeeze-Measure-Pour System (1 Liter/33.8 fl oz Bottle with 50 mL Metering Cup):

Attach the metering cup to the bottle.

Set the dose by turning the top section of the cup to align the correct body weight with the pointer on the knurled cap. When body weight is between markings, use the higher setting.

Hold the bottle upright and squeeze it to deliver a slight excess of the required dose as indicated by the calibration lines.

By releasing the pressure, the dose automatically adjusts to the correct level. When a 220 lb (10 mL) or 330 lb (15 mL) dose is required, turn the pointer to "Stop" before delivering the dose. The off (Stop) position will close the system between dosing. Tilt the bottle to deliver the dose.

Collapsible Pack (2.5 L/84.5 fl oz and 5 L/169 fl oz Packs):

Connect the dosing applicator and draw-off tubing to the collapsible pack as follows:

Attach the open end of the draw-off tubing to an appropriate dosing applicator. Attach the draw-off tubing to the cap with the stem that is included in the pack. Replace the shipping cap with the cap having the draw-off tubing.

Gently prime the dosing applicator, checking for leaks. Follow the dosing applicator manufacturer's directions for adjusting the dose and proper use and maintenance of the dosing applicator and draw-off tubing.

Use Conditions: Varying weather conditions, including rainfall, do not affect the efficacy of IVOMEC® EPRINEX® Pour-On.

Management Considerations for Treatment of External Parasites: For best results IVOMEC® EPRINEX® Pour-On should be applied to all cattle in the herd. Cattle introduced to the herd later should be treated prior to introduction. Consult your veterinarian or an entomologist for the most effective timing of applications for the control of external parasites.

Chorioptic Mange: In clinical studies evaluating the efficacy of IVOMEC® EPRINEX® Pour-On against chorioptic mange mites, mites were not recovered from skin scrapings taken 8 weeks after treatment; however, chronic skin lesions were still present on some animals.

Horn flies: For optimal control of horn flies, as IVOMEC® EPRINEX® Pour-On provides 7 days of persistent activity against horn flies, the product should be used as part of an integrated control program utilizing other control methods to provide extended control.

When to Treat Cattle with Grubs: IVOMEC® EPRINEX® Pour-On is highly effective against all stages of cattle grubs. However, proper timing of treatment is important. For the most effective results, cattle should be treated as soon as possible after the end of the heel fly (warble fly) season. While this is not peculiar to eprinomectin, destruction of *Hypoderma* larvae (cattle grubs) at the period when these grubs are in vital areas may cause undesirable host-parasite reactions. Killing *Hypoderma lineatum* when it is in the esophageal tissues may cause bloat; killing *H. bovis* when it is in the vertebral canal may cause staggering or paralysis. Cattle should be treated either before or after these stages of grub development.

Cattle treated with IVOMEC® EPRINEX® Pour-On at the end of the fly season may be re-treated with IVOMEC® EPRINEX® Pour-On during the winter without danger of grub-related reactions. For further information and advice on a planned parasite control program, consult your veterinarian.

Consult your veterinarian for assistance in the diagnosis, treatment and control of parasitism.

Precaution(s): Storage Conditions: Store bottle or pack in the carton to protect from light and at temperatures up to 86°F (30°C). Storage at temperatures up to 104°F (40°C) is permitted for a short period of time, however, such exposure should be minimized.

Environmental Safety: Studies indicate that when eprinomectin comes in contact with the soil it readily and tightly binds to the soil and becomes inactive. Free eprinomectin may adversely affect fish and certain aquatic organisms. Do not contaminate water by direct application or by the improper disposal of drug containers. Dispose of containers in an approved landfill or by incineration.

Caution(s): This product is for topical application only. Do not administer orally or by injection.

Do not apply to areas of the backline covered with mud or manure.

IVOMEC® EPRINEX® Pour-On is not recommended for use in species other than cattle. Severe adverse reactions have been reported in other species treated with products containing compounds of this class.

Warning(s): Residue Information: When used according to label directions, neither a pre-slaughter drug withdrawal period nor a milk discard time is required, therefore, meat and milk from cattle treated with IVOMEC® EPRINEX® (eprinomectin) Pour-On may be used for human consumption at any time following treatment.

Keep this and all drugs out of the reach of children.

Not for use in humans.

As with any topical medication intended for treatment of animals, skin contact should be avoided. If accidental skin contact occurs, wash immediately with soap and water. If accidental eye exposure occurs, flush eyes immediately with water. The material safety data sheet (MSDS) contains more detailed occupational safety information. To report adverse effects, obtain an MSDS or for assistance, contact Merial at 1-888-637-4251.

Adverse Reactions: No adverse reactions were observed during clinical trials.

Discussion: IVOMEC® EPRINEX® Pour-On delivers highly effective internal and external parasite control in one application. Discovered and developed by scientists from Merck Research Laboratories, IVOMEC® EPRINEX® Pour-On contains eprinomectin, a unique avermectin. Its broad-spectrum efficacy in a weatherproof formulation, margin of safety, zero slaughter withdrawal and zero milk discard, make it a convenient product for parasite control in beef and dairy cattle, including lactating dairy cattle.

Trial Data: Animal Safety: Tolerance and toxicity studies have demonstrated the margin of safety for eprinomectin in cattle. In toxicity studies, application of 3 times the recommended dose had no adverse effects on neonatal calves, and application of up to 5 times the recommended dose 3 times at 7 day intervals had no adverse effects on 8 week old calves. In the tolerance study, one of 6 cattle treated once at 10 times the recommended dose showed clinical signs of mydriasis. Application of 3 times the recommended dose had no adverse effect on breeding performance of cows or bulls.

Presentation: IVOMEC® EPRINEX® Pour-On for Beef and Dairy Cattle is available in a 250 mL (8.5 fl oz) or 1 L (33.8 fl oz) bottle with a squeeze-measure-pour system, or in a 2.5 L (84.5 fl oz), 5 L (169 fl oz) or 20 L collapsible pack intended for use with appropriate automatic dosing equipment.

IVOMEC and EPRINEX are registered trademarks of Merial.

(Merial Limited: Registered in England and Wales [Reg. No. 3332751] with registered offices at 27 Knightsbridge, London, SW1X 7QT, England and domesticated in Delaware, USA as Merial LLC).

U.S. Patent Nos. 4,427,663 and 5,602,107

Compendium Code No.: 11110331 8931504 / 8931604 / 8931705 / 8931804

IVOMEC® PLUS INJECTION FOR CATTLE

Merial **Parasiticide Injection**

(1% w/v ivermectin and 10% clorsulon in a sterile solution)

NADA No.: 140-833

Active Ingredient(s): IVOMEC® Plus is a ready-to-use sterile solution containing 1% w/v ivermectin, 10% clorsulon, 40% glycerol formal, and propylene glycol, q.s. ad 100%.

Indications: For the treatment and control of internal parasites, including adult liver flukes, and external parasites.

IVOMEC® Plus Injection is indicated for the effective treatment and control of the following parasites of cattle:

Gastrointestinal Roundworms (adults and fourth-stage larvae): *Ostertagia ostertagi* (including inhibited *O. ostertagi), O. lyrata, Haemonchus placei, Trichostongylus axei, T. colubriformis, Cooperia oncophora, C. punctata, C. pectinata, Bunostomum phlebotomum, Nematodirus helvetianus* (adults only), *N. spathiger* (adults only), *Oesophagostomum radiatum.*

Lungworms (adults and fourth-stage larvae): *Dictyocaulus viviparus.*

Liver Flukes: *Fasciola hepatica* (adults only).

Cattle Grubs (parasitic stages): *Hypoderma bovis, H. lineatum.*

Sucking Lice: *Linognathus vituli, Haematopinus eurysternus, Solenopotes capillatus.*

Mange Mites (cattle scab*): *Psoroptes ovis* (syn. *P. communis* var. *bovis), Sarcoptes scabiei* var. *bovis.*

Persistent Activity: IVOMEC® Plus Injection has been proved to effectively control infections and to protect cattle from reinfection with *Dictyocaulus viviparus* for 28 days and *Ostertagia ostertagi* for 21 days after treatment; *Oesophagostomum radiatum, Haemonchus placei, Trichostrongylus axei, Cooperia punctata,* and *Cooperia oncophora* for 14 days after treatment.

*Ivermectin has been approved as a scabicide by USDA/APHIS. Federal regulations require that cattle infested with or exposed to scabies (i.e., infestations with *Psoroptes ovis)* be treated. Ivermectin when used according to label instructions meets this requirement. Treated cattle may be shipped interstate, but they must not be mixed with other cattle for 14 days following treatment. The federal regulations make no restriction on the movement of cattle not affected with or exposed to scabies. However, individual states have additional regulations to govern the interstate shipment of cattle and the regulatory veterinarian in the state of destination should be consulted for applicable regulations on the use of ivermectin in the control of scabies.

Pharmacology: Mode of Action: Ivermectin is a member of the macrocyclic lactone class of endectocides which have a unique mode of action. Compounds of the class bind selectively and with high affinity to glutamate-gated chloride ion channels which occur in invertebrate nerve and muscle cells. This leads to an increase in the permeability of the cell membrane to chloride ions with hyperpolarization of the nerve or muscle cell, resulting in paralysis and death of the parasite. Compounds of this class may also interact with other ligand-gated chloride channels, such as those gated by the neurotransmitter gamma-aminobutyric acid (GABA).

The wide margin of safety is attributable to the fact that mammals do not have glutamate-gated chloride channels, the macrocyclic lactones have a low affinity for other mammalian ligand-gated chloride channels and they do not readily cross the blood-brain barrier.

Clorsulon is rapidly absorbed into the circulating blood. Erythrocytes with bound drug as well as plasma are ingested by *Fasciola hepatica.* Adult *Fasciola hepatica* are killed by clorsulon because of inhibition of enzymes in the glycolytic pathway, which is their primary source of energy.

Dosage and Administration: It is formulated to deliver the recommended dose level of 200 mcg ivermectin/kg and 2 mg clorsulon/kg given subcutaneously behind the shoulder at the rate of 1 mL per 110 lb (50 kg) body weight.

Dosage: IVOMEC® Plus should be given only by subcutaneous injection at a dose volume of 1 mL per 110 lb (50 kg) body weight. This volume will deliver 10 mg ivermectin and 100 mg clorsulon. For example:

Body Weight (lb)	Dose (mL)
220	2
330	3
440	4
550	5
660	6
770	7
880	8
990	9
1100	10

The dosage level of clorsulon supplied by IVOMEC® Plus is effective only against adult liver flukes *(Fasciola hepatica).*

Administration: IVOMEC® Plus (ivermectin and chlorsulon) Injection is to be given subcutaneously only. Animals should be appropriately restrained to achieve the proper route of administration. Use of a 16-gauge, ½" to ¾" sterile needle is recommended. Inject the solution subcutaneously (under the skin) behind the shoulder (see illustration).

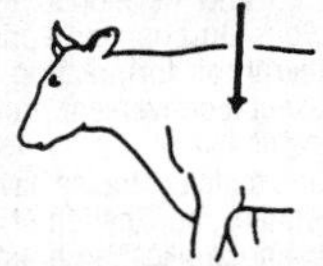

Any single-dose syringe or standard automatic syringe equipment may be used with the 50 mL pack size. When using the 200 mL or 500 mL pack size, use only automatic syringe equipment.

Use sterile equipment and sanitize the injection site by applying a suitable disinfectant. Clean, properly disinfected needles should be used to reduce the potential for injection site infections.

No special handling or protective clothing is necessary.

The viscosity of the product increases in cool temperatures. Administering IVOMEC® Plus at temperatures of 5°C (41°F) or below may be difficult. Users can make dosing easier by warming both the product and injection equipment to about 15°C (59°F).

When to Treat Cattle with Grubs: IVOMEC® Plus effectively controls all stages of cattle grubs. However, proper timing of treatment is important. For most effective results, cattle should be treated as soon as possible after the end of the heel fly (warble fly) season.

Destruction of *Hypoderma* larvae (cattle grubs) at the period when these grubs are in vital areas may cause undesirable host-parasite reactions including the possibility of fatalities. Killing *Hypoderma lineatum* when it is in the tissue surrounding the esophagus (gullet) may cause bloat; killing *H. bovis* when it is in the vertebral canal may cause staggering or paralysis. These reactions are not specific to treatment with IVOMEC® Plus, but can occur with any successful treatment of grubs. Cattle should be treated either before or after stages or grub development. Consult your veterinarian concerning the proper time for treatment.

Cattle treated with IVOMEC® Plus after the end of the heel fly season may be retreated with ivermectin during the winter for internal parasites, mange mites or sucking lice, without danger of grub-related reactions. A planned parasite control program is recommended.

Consult your veterinarian for assistance in the diagnosis, treatment and control of parasitism.

Precaution(s): Protect from light.

Environmental Safety: Studies indicate that when ivermectin comes in contact with the soil, it readily and tightly binds to the soil and becomes inactive over time. Free ivermectin may adversely affect fish and certain water-borne organisms on which they feed. Do not permit water runoff from feedlots to enter lakes, streams, or ponds. Do not contaminate water by direct application or by the improper disposal of drug containers. Dispose of containers in an approved landfill or by incineration.

Caution(s): Transitory discomfort has been observed in some cattle following subcutaneous administration. Soft-tissue swelling at the injection site has also been observed. These reactions have disappeared without treatment. Divide doses greater than 10 mL between two injection sites to reduce occasional discomfort or site reaction. Different injection sites should be used for other parenteral products.

IVOMEC® Plus Injection has been developed specifically for use in cattle only. This product should not be used in other animal species as severe adverse reactions, including fatalities in dogs, may result.

For subcutaneous injection in cattle only.

This product is not for intravenous or intramuscular use.

Warning(s): Residue Information: Do not treat cattle within 49 days of slaughter. Because a withdrawal time in milk has not been established, do not use in female dairy cattle of breeding age.

Not for use in humans.

Keep this and all drugs out of the reach of children.

The Material Safety Data Sheet (MSDS) contains more detailed occupational safety information. To report adverse effects, obtain an MSDS, or for assistance, contact Merial at 1-888-637-4251.

Discussion: The ability of Ivomec® (ivermectin) to deliver internal and external parasite control has been proven in cattle markets around the world. Now, Merck Research Laboratories combines ivermectin, the active ingredient of Ivomec®, with clorsulon, an effective adult flukicide.

A single injection of IVOMEC® Plus (ivermectin and clorsulon) offers all the benefits of Ivomec® plus control of adult *Fasciola hepatica.*

Trial Data: Animal Safety: In breeding animals (bulls and cows), ivermectin and clorsulon used at the recommended level had no effect on breeding performance.

Presentation: IVOMEC® Plus Injection is available in four ready-to-use pack sizes:

The 50 mL pack is a multiple-dose, rubber-capped bottle. Each bottle contains sufficient solution to treat 10 head of 550 lb (250 kg) cattle.

The 200 mL pack is a soft, collapsible pack designed for use with automatic syringe equipment. Each pack contains sufficient solution to treat 40 head of 550 lb (250 kg) cattle.

The 500 mL pack is a soft, collapsible pack designed for use with automatic syringe equipment. Each pack contains sufficient solution to treat 100 head of 550 lb (250 kg) cattle.

The 2 x 500 mL pack includes two 500 mL packs with sufficient solution to treat 200 head of 550 lb (250 kg) cattle.

The 1,000 mL pack is a soft, collapsible pack designed for use with automatic syringe equipment. Each pack contains sufficient solution to treat 200 head of 550 lb (250 kg) cattle.

IVOMEC is a registered trademark of Merial.

(Merial Limited: Registered in England and Wales [Reg. No. 3332751] with registered offices at 27 Knightsbridge, London, SW1X 7QT, England and domesticated in Delaware, USA as Merial LLC).

U.S. Patent Nos. 4,199,569 and 4,853,372

Compendium Code No.: 11110341

8862412

IVOMEC® POUR-ON FOR CATTLE

Merial **Parasiticide-Topical**

(ivermectin) Parasiticide

NADA No.: 140-841

Active Ingredient(s): Contains 5 mg ivermectin/mL.

Indications: IVOMEC® Pour-On applied at the recommended dose level of 500 mcg/kg is indicated for the effective control of these parasites.

Gastrointestinal Roundworms: *Ostertagia ostertagi* (including inhibited stage) (adults and L_4), *Haemonchus placei* (adults and L_4), *Trichostrongylus axei* (adults and L_4), *T. colubriformis* (adults and L_4), *Cooperia* spp. (adults and L_4), *Strongyloides papillosus* (adults), *Oesophagostomum radiatum* (adults and L_4), *Trichuris* spp. (adults).

Lungworms: *Dictyocaulus viviparus* (adults and L_4).

Cattle Grubs (parasitic stages): *Hypoderma bovis, H. lineatum.*

Mites: *Sarcoptes scabiei* var. *bovis.*

Lice: *Linognathus vituli, Haematopinus eurysternus, Damalinia bovis, Solenopotes capillatus.*

Horn Flies: *Haematobia irritans.*

Persistent Activity: IVOMEC® Pour-On has been proved to effectively control infections and to protect cattle from re-infection with *Ostertagia ostertagi, Oesophagostomum radiatum, Haemonchus placei, Trichostrongylus axei, Cooperia punctata* and *Cooperia oncophora* for 14 days after treatment.

Pharmacology: Mode of Action: Ivermectin as a member of the avermectin family kills certain parasitic roundworms and ectoparasites, such as mites, lice, horn flies and other insects. Its action is unique to the avermectin class of antiparasitic agents. This action involves a chemical that serves as a signal from one nerve cell to another, or from a nerve cell to a muscle cell. This chemical, a neurotransmitter, is called gamma-aminobutyric acid or GABA.

In roundworms, ivermectin stimulates the release of GABA from nerve endings and enhances binding of GABA to special receptors at nerve junctions, thus interrupting nerve impulses — thereby paralyzing and killing the parasite.

The enhancement of the GABA effect in arthropods such as mites, lice, and horn flies resembles that in roundworms except that nerve impulses are interrupted between the nerve ending and the muscle cell. Again, this leads to paralysis and death.

Ivermectin has no measurable effect against flukes or tapeworms, presumably because they do not have GABA as a nerve impulse transmitter.

The principal peripheral neurotransmitter in mammals, acetylcholine, is unaffected by ivermectin. Ivermectin does not readily penetrate the central nervous system of mammals where GABA functions as a neurotransmitter.

Dosage and Administration:

Treatment of Cattle for Horn Flies: IVOMEC® Pour-On controls horn flies *(Haematobia irritans)* for up to 28 days after dosing. For best results IVOMEC® Pour-On should be part of a parasite control program for both internal and external parasites based on the epidemiology of these parasites. Consult your veterinarian or an entomologist for the most effective timing of applications.

Dosage: The dose rate is 1 mL for each 22 lb of body weight. The formulation should be applied along the topline in a narrow strip from the withers to the tailhead.

Administration:

Squeeze-Measure-Pour System (8.5 fl oz/250 mL Bottle with 25 mL Metering Cup):

Attach the metering cup to the bottle.

Set the dose by turning the top section of the cup to align the correct body weight with the pointer on the knurled cap. When body weight is between markings, use the higher setting.

Hold the bottle upright and squeeze it to deliver a slight excess of the required dose as indicated by the calibration lines.

By releasing the pressure, the dose automatically adjusts to the correct level. The off (Stop) position will close the system between dosing.

Squeeze-Measure-Pour System (33.8 fl oz/1 Liter Bottle with 50 mL Metering Cup):

Attach the metering cup to the bottle.

Set the dose by turning the top section of the cup to align the correct body weight with the pointer on the knurled cap. When body weight is between markings, use the higher setting.

Hold the bottle upright and squeeze it to deliver a slight excess of the required dose as indicated by the calibration lines.

By releasing the pressure, the dose automatically adjusts to the correct level. Tilt the bottle to deliver the dose. When a 220 lb (10 mL) or 330 lb (15 mL) dose is required, turn the pointer to "Stop" before delivering the dose. The off (Stop) position will close the system between dosing.

Collapsible Pack (84.5 fl oz/2.5 L Pack and 169 fl oz/5 L Pack):

Connect the applicator gun to the collapsible pack as follows:

Attach the open end of the draw-off tubing to the dosing equipment. (Because of the solvents used in the formulation, only the Protector Drench Gun from Instrument Supplies Limited, or equivalent, is recommended. Other applicators may exhibit compatibility problems resulting in locking, incorrect dosage or leakage.)

Replace the shipping cap with the draw-off cap and tighten down. Attach draw-off tubing to the draw-off cap.

Gently prime the applicator gun, checking for leaks.

Follow the manufacturer's directions for adjusting the dose.

When the interval between uses of the applicator gun is expected to exceed 12 hours, disconnect the gun and draw-off tubing from the product container and empty the product from the gun and tubing back into the product container. To prevent removal of special lubricants from the Protector Drench Gun, the gun and tubing must not be washed.

Safety: Studies conducted in the U.S.A. have demonstrated the safety margin for ivermectin. Based on plasma levels, the topically applied formulation is expected to be at least as well tolerated by breeding animals as is the subcutaneous formulation which had no effect on breeding performance.

Consult your veterinarian for assistance in the diagnosis, treatment and control of parasitism.

Precaution(s): Flammable! Keep away from heat, sparks, open flame, and other sources of ignition.

Store away from excessive heat (104°F/40°C) and protect from light.

Use only in well-ventilated areas or outdoors.

Close container tightly when not in use.

Cloudiness in the formulation may occur when IVOMEC® (ivermectin) Pour-On is stored at temperatures below 32°F. Allowing to warm at room temperature will restore the normal appearance without affecting efficacy.

Environmental Safety: Studies indicate that when ivermectin comes in contact with the soil, it readily and tightly binds to the soil and becomes inactive over time. Free ivermectin may adversely affect fish or certain water-borne organisms on which they feed. Do not permit cattle to enter lakes, streams or ponds for at least six hours after treatment. Do not contaminate water by direct application or by the improper disposal of drug containers. Dispose of containers in an approved landfill or by incineration.

Caution(s): Cattle should not be treated when hair or hide is wet since reduced efficacy may be experienced.

Do not use when rain is expected to wet cattle within six hours after treatment.

This product is for application to skin surface only. Do not give orally or parenterally.

Antiparasitic activity of ivermectin will be impaired if the formulation is applied to areas of the skin with mange scabs or lesions, or with dermatoses or adherent materials, e.g., caked mud or manure.

Ivermectin has been associated with adverse reactions in sensitive dogs; therefore, IVOMEC® Pour-On is not recommended for use in species other than cattle.

Warning(s): Cattle must not be treated within 48 days of slaughter for human consumption. Because a withdrawal time in milk has not been established, do not use in female dairy cattle of breeding age.

Not for use in humans.

This product should not be applied to self or others because it may be irritating to human skin and eyes and absorbed through the skin. To minimize accidental skin contact, the user should wear a long-sleeved shirt and rubber gloves. If accidental skin contact occurs, wash immediately with soap and water. If accidental eye exposure occurs, flush eyes immediately with water and seek medical attention.

Keep this and all drugs out of the reach of children.

Discussion: When to Treat Cattle with Grubs: IVOMEC® Pour-On effectively controls all stages of cattle grubs. However, proper timing of treatment is important. For the most effective results, cattle should be treated as soon as possible after the end of the heel fly (warble fly) season. While this is not peculiar to ivermectin, destruction of *Hypoderma* larvae (cattle grubs) at the period when these grubs are in vital areas may cause undesirable host-parasite reactions. Killing *Hypoderma lineatum* when it is in the esophageal tissues may cause bloat; killing *H. bovis* when it is in the vertebral canal may cause staggering or paralysis. Cattle should be treated either before or after these stages of grub development.

Cattle treated with IVOMEC® Pour-On at the end of the fly season may be re-treated with IVOMEC® during the winter without danger of grub-related reactions. For further information and advice on a planned parasite control program, consult your veterinarian.

Presentation: IVOMEC® Pour-On is available in an 8.5 fl oz/250 mL bottle with a squeeze-measure-pour system, a 33.8 fl oz/1 L bottle with a squeeze-measure-pour system, or in a 84.5 fl oz/2.5 L collapsible pack, and a 169 oz/5 L collapsible pack intended for use with appropriate automatic dosing equipment.

® IVOMEC is a registered trademark of Merial.

U.S. Pat 4,199,569

Compendium Code No.: 11110350

IVOMEC® PREMIX FOR SWINE TYPE A MEDICATED ARTICLE

Merial **Feed Medication**

(ivermectin) Antiparasitic

Active Ingredient(s):

Ivermectin 0.6%

Ingredients: Ground corn cob.

Indications: For the treatment and control of gastrointestinal roundworms *(Ascaris suum*, adults and fourth-stage larvae; *Ascarops strongylina*, adults; *Hyostrongylus rubidus*, adults and fourth-stage larvae; *Oesophagostomum* spp., adults and fourth-stage larvae), kidneyworms *(Stephanurus dentatus*, adults and fourth-stage larvae), lungworms *(Metastrongylus* spp., adults), threadworms (*Strongyloides ransomi*, adults and somatic larvae, and prevention of transmission of infective larvae to piglets, via colostrum or milk, when fed during gestation), lice *(Haematopinus suis)* and mange mites *(Sarcoptes scabiei* var. *suis)* when incorporated into complete swine feeds at the level listed in the tables below. Follow mixing directions when preparing complete feeds.

Dosage and Administration: Important: Must be diluted in feed before use.

Mixing and Feeding Directions for Weaned/Growing/Finishing Pigs: Add IVOMEC® Premix (Type A Medicated Article) to starter, grower and finisher feeds at 300 g per ton to supply 1.8 g ivermectin per ton (2 ppm) of feed.

Use this Type C Medicated Feed as the only feed *ad libitum* for 7 consecutive days. This provides approximately 0.1 mg ivermectin per kg (2.2 lb) of body weight per day.

Mixing and Feeding Directions for Adult and Breeding Animals: The recommended dose level for breeding animals is 0.1 mg ivermectin/kg body weight daily for seven consecutive days. Add IVOMEC® Premix (Type A Medicated Article) to complete feed at 1.5 kg (3.3 lb) per ton to supply 9.1 g ivermectin per ton (10 ppm) of feed. Feed this Type C Medicated Feed at the rate of 1 lb (454 g) per 100 lb of body weight daily for seven consecutive days. On a daily basis, any additional non-medicated feed should not be given until the medicated feed is consumed. For heavy animals being fed less than 1% of their body weight per day, the ivermectin level in the Type C Medicated Feed can be up to 11.8 g per ton.

As sow feeding practices vary during the different phases of their reproductive cycle (i.e., limited feeding during gestation and *ad libitum* during lactation), the inclusion rate of ivermectin per ton of complete feed can be adjusted accordingly to obtain the 0.1 mg/kg treatment level.

As an example, the following inclusion rates for IVOMEC® Premix w/w (Type A Medicated Article) based on body weight and feed intake are determined by the formula.

$$\frac{\text{average body weight (lb)}}{\text{average daily intake (lb) per head X 30}} = \text{lb of IVOMEC® Premix (Type A Medicated Article) per ton of feed}$$

Average Body Weight (lb)	Daily Feed Intake (lb)	Premix (0.6%) per ton Type C Feed (lb)	Ivermectin Level in Type C Feed (g/ton)
400	4.0	3.33	9.1
	5.0	2.67	7.3
	6.0	2.22	6.1
500	4.0	4.17	11.3
	5.0	3.33	9.1
	6.0	2.78	7.6

IVOMEC® Premix (Type A Medicated Article) should be thoroughly and evenly mixed in the feed in accordance with good manufacturing practices for medicated feeds.

Dispersion of IVOMEC® Premix in the feed is enhanced by diluting 1 part of this 0.6% Type A Medicated Article with 14 parts of finely ground feed ingredients to provide an intermediate premix.

Recommended Treatment Program:

Weaned/Growing/Finish Pigs: All weaners/feeder pigs should be treated upon placement in clean quarters. Frequency of and need for additional treatments are dependent upon parasite exposure.

Adult and Breeding Animals: At the time of initiating any parasite control program, it is important to treat all animals in the herd. After the initial treatment, use IVOMEC® Premix regularly as follows:

Sows: Treat, preferably, 14-21 days prior to farrowing to minimize parasitism of piglets.

Gilts: Treat, preferably, 14-21 days prior to breeding.

Treat, preferably, 14-21 days prior to farrowing.

Boars: Treat at least 2 times per year.

Frequency of and need for additional treatments are dependent upon parasite exposure.

Note: (1) Since the effect of ivermectin on mange mites is not immediate, avoid contact between treated pigs and mange-free pigs for approximately one week after completion of treatment. Exposure of treated pigs to mange-infested pigs may result in reinfestation.

(2) Louse eggs are unaffected by ivermectin and may require up to three weeks to hatch. Louse infestations developing from hatching eggs may require retreatment.

Consult your veterinarian for assistance in the diagnosis, treatment and control of parasitism.

Precaution(s): Environmental Safety: Studies show that when ivermectin comes in contact with the soil, it readily and tightly binds to the soil and becomes inactive over time. Free ivermectin may adversely affect fish and certain water-borne organisms on which they feed. Do not permit water runoff from swine production sites to directly enter lakes, streams or ponds. Do not contaminate water by direct application or by the improper disposal of drug containers. Dispose of containers in an approved landfill or by incineration.

Caution(s): This product contains IVOMEC® brand ivermectin and has been formulated specifically for use in swine only. This product should not be used for other animal species.

Warning(s): Withdraw 5 days before slaughter.

Keep this and all drugs out of the reach of children.

Presentation: 50 lb (22.68 kg).

® IVOMEC is a registered trademark of Merial.

U.S. Pat. 4,199,569

Compendium Code No.: 11110360

IVOMEC® SHEEP DRENCH

Merial **Parasiticide-Oral**

Ivermectin 0.08% Solution

NADA No.: 131-392

Active Ingredient(s): IVOMEC® Sheep Drench is an 0.08% w/v pale amber colored solution of ivermectin.

Indications: IVOMEC® Sheep Drench is indicated for the effective treatment of gastro-intestinal roundworms (including *Haemonchus contortus)*, lungworms and nasal bots in sheep.

When used as recommended, it provides effective control of the parasites listed.

IVOMEC® Sheep Drench kills the following parasites:

Gastro-intestinal roundworms: *Haemonchus contortus* (adults and fourth-stage larvae), *Haemonchus placei* (adults), *Ostertagia circumcincta* (adults and fourth-stage larvae), *Trichostrongylus axei* (adults and fourth-stage larvae), *Trichostrongylus colubriformis* (adults and fourth-stage larvae), *Cooperia curticei* (adults and fourth-stage larvae), *Cooperia oncophora* (adults), *Oesophagostomum columbianum* (adults and fourth-stage larvae), *Oesophagostomum venulosum* (fourth-stage larvae), *Nematodirus battus* (adults and fourth-stage larvae), *Nematodirus spathiger* (adults and fourth-stage larvae), *Strongyloides papillosus* (adults), *Chabertia ovina* (adults), and *Trichuris ovis* (adults). Lungworms: *Dictyocaulus filaria* (adults and fourth-stage larvae). Nasal bots: *Oestrus ovis* (all larval stages).

Pharmacology: Ivermectin is derived from the avermectins, a family of highly active broad-spectrum, antiparasitic agents which are produced from the fermentation products of *Streptomyces avermitilis*.

The avermectin family of compounds of which ivermectin is a member, kills certain parasitic nematodes (roundworms) and arthropods. The action is unique and not shared by other antiparasitic agents and involves a chemical that serves as a signal from one nerve cell to another, or from a nerve cell to a muscle cell. This chemical, a neurotransmitter, is called gamma aminobutyric acid or GABA.

In roundworms, ivermectin stimulates the release of GABA from nerve endings and enhances binding of GABA to special receptors at nerve junctions, thus interrupting nerve impulses, thereby paralyzing and killing the parasite.

The enhancement of the GABA effect in arthropods resembles that in roundworms except that nerve impulses are interrupted between the nerve ending and the muscle cell. Again, this leads to paralysis and death in most species.

Ivermectin has no measurable effect against flukes or tapeworms, presumably because they do not have GABA as a nerve impulse transmitter.

Recommended doses of ivermectin have a wide safety margin in livestock. The principal peripheral neurotransmitter in mammals, acetylcholine, is unaffected by ivermectin. Ivermectin does not readily penetrate the central nervous system of mammals where GABA functions as a neurotransmitter.

Dosage and Administration: IVOMEC® Sheep Drench should be administered orally at the recommended dose level of 200 mcg ivermectin per kg of body weight. Three (3) mL of IVOMEC® Sheep Drench contains sufficient ivermectin to treat 26 pounds of body weight.

Sheep Body Weight Dosed	Volume
26 lbs.	3 mL
52 lbs.	6 mL
78 lbs.	9 mL
104 lbs.	12 mL
130 lbs.	15 mL
156 lbs.	18 mL
182 lbs.	21 mL
208 lbs.	24 mL
234 lbs.	27 mL
260 lbs.	30 mL

To avoid underdosing, it is important to get the dose according to the weight of the heaviest sheep in a group (ewes, lambs or rams), not the average weight. Several of the largest sheep should be weighed, judgment by the eye can be deceiving.

Any standard drenching equipment or any equipment which provides a consistent dose volume, can be used. Dose rates and equipment should be checked before drenching commences. Be sure the head is properly positioned for each sheep to receive the full dose. IVOMEC® Sheep Drench is readily accepted by sheep, but inconsequential coughing may be observed in some animals during and for several minutes after drenching. If slobbering occurs, the dose may be lost, and that sheep should be redosed.

Frequency of Dosing: Resistant parasites are a particular problem for sheep.

Please consult a veterinarian, county extension office or animal health supplier for the control program recommended in your area.

Safety: IVOMEC® Sheep Drench has been demonstrated to have a wide safety margin at the recommended dose level and may be used in sheep of all ages. Ewes may be treated at any stage of pregnancy.

Acceptability: Coughing may be observed in some animals during and for several minutes following drenching.

Precaution(s): IVOMEC® Sheep Drench is stable for 60 months when stored under normal conditions. Protect from light.

Environmental Safety: Studies indicate that when ivermectin comes in contact with the soil, it readily and tightly binds to the soil and becomes inactive over time. Free ivermectin may adversely affect fish and certain waterborn organisms on which they feed. Do not permit water run off from feedlots to enter lakes, streams, or ground water. Do not contaminate water by direct application or by the improper disposal of drug containers. Spills of IVOMEC® Sheep Drench should be contained and soaked up with absorbent towels or into loose soils. Gloves should be worn to prevent skin exposure. All the collected material (contaminated towels and soil), as well as all used drug containers, should be placed in an impervious film bag (plastic) and disposed of by incineration or in an approved landfill.

This product is not to be used parenterally. Protect from light.

Caution(s): IVOMEC® Sheep Drench has been formulated for use in sheep only. This product should not be used in other animal species as severe adverse reactions, including fatalities in dogs, may result.

Keep this and all drugs out of the reach of children.

Human Safety: When used as recommended in sheep, IVOMEC® Sheep Drench does not pose a hazard to human health. As a routine precaution, it is advisable to wash hands after use.

Contact with skin and eyes should be avoided, but protective clothing is not required.

Warning(s): Sheep must not be treated within 11 days of slaughter for human consumption.

Presentation: 960 mL (4 to a case) and 4,800 mL (4 to a case) containers.

® IVOMEC is a registered trademark of Merial Limited, Iselin, NJ.

Compendium Code No.: 11110390

IVOMEC® SR BOLUS

Merial **Parasiticide-Oral**

(ivermectin)

NADA No.: 140-988

Active Ingredient(s): Each bolus contains 1.72 g ivermectin.

Indications: The IVOMEC® (ivermectin) Sustained Release (SR) Bolus controls internal and external parasites in cattle throughout the grazing season.

Nematodes:

The IVOMEC® SR Bolus is indicated for the treatment of established infections and, throughout its approximately 130-day ivermectin delivery period, prevents the establishment of infection by newly ingested larvae of the following nematode species:

Gastrointestinal Roundworms: *Haemonchus placei, Ostertagia ostertagi, Trichostrongylus axei, Trichostrongylus colubriformis, Cooperia* spp, *Nematodirus helvetianus* (adults only), *Bunostomum phlebotomum, Oesophagostomum radiatum.*

Lungworms: *Dictyocaulus viviparus.*

IVOMEC® SR Bolus controls established infections of hypobiotic (inhibited) fourth-stage larvae of *Ostertagia ostertagi.*

Mange Mites:

The IVOMEC® SR Bolus provides control of established infestations of the following mange mites and prevents reinfestation for 135 days.

Psoroptes ovis, Sarcoptes scabiei var. *bovis*

Sucking Lice:

The IVOMEC® SR Bolus provides control of established infestations of the following sucking lice and prevents reinfestation for 135 days.

Linognathus vituli, Solenopotes capillatus

Cattle Grubs:

Initially, control is provided against migrating *Hypoderma* larvae (grubs) acquired prior to administration of the IVOMEC® SR Bolus; thereafter, prophylaxis is provided for approximately 135 days against newly acquired larvae.

Hypoderma spp

Ticks:

Control of the following tick will be provided by interfering with engorgement with blood and completion of the reproductive portion of the life cycle of newly acquired young adult females during the period of ivermectin delivery. However, larvae, nymphs and adult males, as well as young adult females already on the host at the time of treatment and actively in the engorgement process, may not be visibly affected.

Amblyomma americanum

Pharmacology: Mode of Action: Ivermectin is a member of the macrocyclic lactone class of endectocides which have a unique mode of action. Compounds of the class bind selectively and with high affinity to glutamate-gated chloride ion channels which occur in invertebrate nerve and muscle cells. This leads to an increase in the permeability of the cell membrane to chloride ions with hyperpolarization of the nerve or muscle cell, resulting in paralysis and death of the parasite. Compounds of this class may also interact with other ligand-gated chloride channels, such as those gated by the neurotransmitter gamma-aminobutyric acid (GABA).

The wide margin of safety is attributable to the fact that mammals do not have glutamate-gated chloride channels, the macrocyclic lactones have a low affinity for other mammalian ligand-gated chloride channels and they do not readily cross the blood-brain barrier.

Dosage and Administration: One IVOMEC® SR Bolus is given to cattle weighing at least 275 lb (125 kg) and not more than 660 lb (300 kg) body weight on the day of administration. Calves must be ruminating and greater than 12 weeks of age. Each bolus contains 1.72 g ivermectin.

Care should be exercised in handling and administering the IVOMEC® SR Bolus to ensure that the outer membrane is not damaged. Administer the bolus directly into the pharynx using an appropriate balling gun.

Remove the bolus from the container and insert into the retaining cup of the balling gun.

Place the instrument centrally into the animal's mouth just beyond the back of the tongue (i.e. pharynx) using gentle pressure and allowing the animal to swallow. Release the bolus by slowly depressing the plunger or trigger. If there is any resistance to release of the bolus, reposition the bolus cup.

Following release of the bolus, withdraw the balling gun. Once swallowed, the IVOMEC® SR Bolus has sufficient density to be retained in the rumen/reticulum for an extended duration. Some calves may not successfully complete the swallowing reflex upon initial administration; observe each animal briefly prior to release. Regurgitation of the bolus, although infrequent, has been observed during the first day after administration and throughout the delivery period.

Consult your veterinarian for assistance in the diagnosis, treatment and control of parasitism.

For Customer Service, contact: Merial Customer Service, 4545 Oleatha Avenue, St. Louis, MO 63116.

Contraindication(s): The IVOMEC® SR Bolus is specifically formulated for use in calves 275-660 lb (125-300 kg) body weight on the day of bolus administration. Calves must be ruminating and greater than 12 weeks of age. Do not administer in calves weighing less than 275 lbs (125 kg).

Administration to calves weighing less than 275 lb (125 kg) may result in esophageal injuries including obstruction or perforation with associated complications, including fatalities.

Precaution(s): Store below 86°F/30°C. Protect from excessive heat (104°F/40°C).

The IVOMEC® SR Bolus is stable for two years when stored below 86°F/30°C.

Studies indicate that when ivermectin comes in contact with the soil, it readily and tightly binds to the soil and becomes inactive over time. Free ivermectin may adversely affect fish and certain water-borne organisms on which they feed. Damaged boluses should be disposed of safely (e.g., by burying at an approved landfill or incinerating). Do not contaminate lakes, streams or ground water.

Caution(s): Remove each bolus from its container only immediately prior to use.

Do not administer a damaged bolus.

The IVOMEC® SR Bolus was specifically designed for use in cattle, and is not intended for use in other animal species.

Avoid using excessive force during administration.

Only a balling gun which has suitable dimensions and will deliver the IVOMEC® SR Bolus into the pharynx should be used for administration. Instruments intended for administration of other types of boluses may result in delivery into the oral cavity and the teeth may cause damage to the bolus.

Warning(s): Do not slaughter cattle within 180 days of treatment (day of administration). Because a milk withdrawal time has not been established, do not use in female dairy cattle of breeding age.

Not for human use. Keep out of reach of children. Wash hands after use. The material safety data sheet (MSDS) contains more detailed occupational safety information. To report adverse reactions in users, to obtain more information, or to obtain a MSDS call Merck's National Service Center.

Trial Data: Safety: In a study to investigate the effects of exaggerated doses of ivermectin administered via multiple boluses, groups of 6 calves weighing 142 to 200 kg were treated with ivermectin administered by SR bolus at (1X), (3X) or (5X) the therapeutic dose. Between one and 6 SR boluses were administered to each animal to deliver the assigned dose level of ivermectin. Mild digestive disturbances were observed in some calves given 3 or more boluses and calves in the groups treated at 3X and 5X gained less weight than untreated controls. These signs were attributed to effects from the physical mass of multiple devices in the rumen. Mild symmetrical mydriasis was observed in 4 of the 6 calves treated at 3X dose and in 2 of the 6 calves treated at 5X dose and one calf treated at 3X dose showed mild depression. No other clinical signs were observed during the study.

The effects of ivermectin sustained release bolus on reproductive performance in breeding bulls and cows have not been evaluated. However, the injectable ivermectin formulation (immediate release) had no effects on reproductive performance in studies in breeding bulls and cows.

Presentation: IVOMEC® SR Bolus is packaged 12 boluses per carton or 72 boluses per carton.

® IVOMEC is a registered trademark of Merial Limited, Iselin, NJ.

Compendium Code No.: 11110401

J

J-5 ESCHERICHIA COLI BACTERIN

Hygieia **Bacterin**

J-5 Escherichia coli Bacterin, in Freund's Incomplete Adjuvant

CA Vet. Biol. Lic. No.: 86

Contents: This product contains the antigen listed above.

Indications: J-5 *E. coli* bacterin is intended for use in conjunction with appropriate management practices to help prevent coliform mastitis in healthy bovine, caprine and porcine species.

Dosage and Administration: Recommended dose, route, and regimen are as follows:

Cows: 5.0 cc SQ in neck at 7 and 8 months gestation, and postparturient.

Does: 2.0 cc SQ in neck at 3 and 4 months gestation, and postparturient.

Sows: 2.0 cc IM under ear at breeding, 2 months gestation, and postparturient.

Precaution(s): Keep refrigerated at 35-45°F. Shake well before using.

Entire contents of this bottle should be used when first opened.

Caution(s): Do not use in septic, toxemic or mastitic animals. Administration should be under the supervision of a licensed veterinarian. Occasionally, anaphylactic or other adverse reactions may occur. If adverse reactions occur, appropriate therapy with epinephrine or other antianaphylactic drugs should be instituted immediately.

Any adverse reactions following vaccination should be immediately reported to the manufacturer.

Warning(s): Do not vaccinate within 42 days of slaughter.

This product contains oil adjuvant. In the event of accidental self injection, seek medical attention immediately.

Presentation: 20 dose (100 mL) and 50 dose (250 mL) bottles.

Compendium Code No.: 15060010

JENCINE® 4

Schering-Plough **Vaccine**

Bovine Rhinotracheitis-Virus Diarrhea-Parainfluenza$_3$-Respiratory Syncytial Virus Vaccine, Modified Live Virus

U.S. Vet. Lic. No.: 165A

Contents: This product contains the antigens listed above.

Contains gentamicin as a preservative.

Indications: JENCINE® 4 vaccine is for the vaccination of healthy cattle as an aid in the prevention of disease caused by infectious bovine rhinotracheitis (IBR), bovine virus diarrhea (BVD) type 1, bovine parainfluenza$_3$ (PI$_3$), bovine respiratory syncytial virus (BRSV) and BVD type 2. Vaccination of dams prior to breeding aids in the prevention of fetal infection by BVD type 1, a cause of persistent viremia in calves.

Dosage and Administration: For use in healthy cattle. Transfer entire contents of diluent vial to vaccine vial, using aseptic technique and sterile syringes and needles. Inject 2 mL intramuscularly or subcutaneously into each animal using aseptic technique. Annual revaccination with a single 2 ml dose is recommended. Calves vaccinated under 6 months of age should be revaccinated at 6 months of age or at weaning.

Precaution(s): Store at 35°-45°F (2°-7°C). Use entire contents when first opened. Do not use chemical disinfectants to sterilize syringes or needles. Burn container and all unused contents.

Caution(s): This product has been tested under laboratory conditions and shown to meet all Federal standards for safety and efficacy. This level of performance may be affected by conditions of use such as stress, weather, nutrition, disease, parasitism, other treatments, individual idiosyncrasies or impaired immunological competency. These factors should be considered by the user when evaluating product performance or freedom from reactions.

Anaphylactoid reactions may occur following use.

For veterinary use only.

Antidote(s): Epinephrine.

Warning(s): Do not vaccinate within 21 days of slaughter. Do not vaccinate calves under 2 weeks of age. Do not vaccinate pregnant cows or calves nursing pregnant cows.

Presentation: 10 doses with 20 mL diluent (NDC-0061-5257-01).

Compendium Code No.: 10472140 P19306-11

JORVET™ J-322 DIP QUICK STAIN

Jorgensen **Diagnostic Stain/Reagent**

Kit Contents: Fixative #1 component, Stain #2 component, Counter stain #3 component.

Indications: Used to stain blood smears for cell differential counts and evaluation. Can be used for general diagnostic cytology.

Directions for Use:

1. The slide is allowed to air dry.
2. After air drying the slide is repeatedly dipped directly into the wide mouth bottle marked #1 fixative for a total of 5 seconds. The slide is held up out of the bottle and excess fixative drained off.
3. The slide is repeatedly dipped directly in bottle with component #2 for a total of 5 seconds. It also is held up out of the bottle to drain off excess stain.
4. The slide is finally repeatedly dipped in component #3 bottle for 3-5 seconds.
5. Gently rinse with distilled water and gently blot dry with a paper towel.

Always close the lid tightly in the component bottles to avoid evaporation loss.

These polychromic stains will color acid groups blue (DNA/RNA), basic groups orange (protein eosinophil granules), and metachromic substances violet (mast cell and basophil granules).

Storage: Store at room temperature.

Caution(s): Danger! May be fatal or cause blindness if swallowed. Poison. Flammable. Vapor harmful. Causes eye irritation.

Do not breathe vapor. Do not get in eyes, on skin, on clothing. Keep container closed. Use with adequate ventilation. Keep away from heat, sparks and open flame. Wash thoroughly after handling.

Cannot be made nonpoisonous.

First Aid: If swallowed, call a physician immediately. In case of contact, immediately flush eyes with plenty of water for at least 15 minutes. Call a physician.

Presentation: Introductory kit is available, 1 each x 180 mL wide mouth bottle of each component.

J-322A: Bulk refill kit is available, 1 each x 500 mL of each component.

Compendium Code No.: 11520020

JORVET™ J-323 GRAM STAIN KIT

Jorgensen **Diagnostic Stain/Reagent**

Reagents:

Reagent #1 . . . . Crystal Violet: Crystal Violet 0.5% w/v in Denatured Alcohol.
Reagent #2 . . . . Iodine Solution: PVP Iodine 1.9% w/v; Potassium Iodide 13% w/v.
Reagent #3 . . . . Decolorizer: Specially Denatured Alcohol/Acetone
Reagent #4 . . . . Safranin Counterstain: Safranin 0.5% in denatured alcohol w/v.

Indications: To differentiate gram positive and gram negative bacteria. For *in vitro* diagnostic use.

Sample Collection: Organisms being stained by the Gram method are usually taken from a solid or liquid medium on (in) which they have been cultured from their original source (e.g. wounds, throat swabs, sputum, etc.). An aqueous suspension is made, in the case of the solid medium, by taking a small amount of the material and suspending it in a drop of distilled water on a microscope slide. Care should be taken not to make the smear too thick. In the case of a liquid medium, a drop is used directly from the culture container. However, due to the solids from the medium, this method is not always satisfactory.

Directions for Use: The suspension made by either method is air dried then "fixed" by passing rapidly through a Bunsen burner flame two or three times. Allow the smear to cool before staining. (See Sources of Error section.)

Step by Step Procedure:

1. Allow smears to air dry thoroughly (until moisture is no longer visible) then "fix" by passing rapidly through a Bunsen burner flame two or three times. (See Sources of Error section.)
2. Place the "fixed" smears on a staining rack and cover completely with Crystal Violet (Reagent #1) for 30-60 seconds.
3. Wash off the stain with distilled water.
4. Cover the slide with Iodine Solution (Reagent #2) for 30 seconds.
5. Wash off with distilled water.
6. Decolorize (Reagent #3 for 10-15 seconds).
7. Wash thoroughly with distilled water.
8. Replace the slide on the stain rack and cover completely with Safranin Counterstain (Reagent #4) for 30-60 seconds.
9. Wash with distilled water, air dry and examine under immersion oil. Label clearly. Gram positive organisms stain a dark purple; gram negative organisms stain red.

Gram positive organisms such as cocci appear dark blue or black, and gram negative organisms, such as the coliforms and pseudomonads, appear pink. The nuclei of leukocytes stain pink. All fungi are gram positive.

Stability of Final Reaction: Stained smears, after being properly mounted with mounting medium, have been observed to retain their staining characteristics for at least two months.

Sources of Error:

1. Overheating (burning) during fixation can be avoided by just touching the back of the slide to the back of the hand each time the smear has been passed through the flame.
2. Do not stain smears which have only been air dried. Smears must also be "fixed".
3. Smears should not be too thick. After air drying, examine under a microscope. If there are no areas of bacteria separation, more water should be added to dilute the smear. Repeat air drying and "fixing" as in step #1 of the Step by Step Procedure section.
4. After staining, it is essential that the back surface of slide is wiped clean.
5. If washing with distilled water is not done adequately, crystallization of stain may appear on the slide.
6. The manufacturer recommends that a known Gram positive and Gram negative control be stained at the same time as the test culture as an additional measure of quality control.
7. Staining times may vary to suit the individual.
8. In steps #3, #5 and #7 of the Step by Step Procedure section slides should be removed from the staining rack and held at an angle while washing.

Storage:

#1. Crystal Violet: Store at room temperature.

#2 Iodine Solution: Store at room temperature.

#3 Decolorizer: Stable indefinitely. Store at room temperature.

#4 Safranin Counterstain: Store at room temperature.

Caution(s):

#1. Crystal Violet: Poison: Do not take internally. Avoid contact with eyes. Vapor harmful. Flammable.

#2 Iodine Solution: Poison: Do not take internally. Avoid contact with eyes. Avoid breathing vapor.

#3 Decolorizer: Poison: Do not take internally. Avoid contact with eyes. Avoid breathing vapor.

#4 Safranin Counterstain: No special handling precautions.

Presentation: 4 X 250 mL bottles.

Compendium Code No.: 11520030

JORVET™ J-324 NEW METHYLENE BLUE STAIN

Jorgensen **Diagnostic Stain/Reagent**

Indications: Used for reticulocyte counts, determining blood parasites and evaluating vaginal smears. New methylene blue can be used in wet mount preparation or in the more conventional air dried mount.

Directions for Use: Reticulocyte count/Heartworm screen.

1.) Two drops of blood and an equal amount of stain are left mixed for 15 to 20 minutes in a small test tube. A slide is then prepared from the mixture in the usual manner. The reticulum will stain intensely blue and the erythrocytes are seen as ghost outlines. The reticulocyte count is expressed in percentage after counting 500 RBCS.

Dry unfixed blood or cytology.

2.) One drip of stain is applied evenly over the dried film. The slide is immediately ready to read. Also since the stain is contained in physiology saline, the film is not permanent and will only last a few hours.

Gently shake before use.

Storage: Keep covered. Store at room temperature.

Presentation: 250 mL bottle.

Compendium Code No.: 11520040

JORVET™ J-325F LUGOL'S IODINE (STAIN CONCENTRATE)

Jorgensen **Diagnostic Stain/Reagent**

Indications: Lugol's iodine identifies hard to find protozoan (i.e. giardia) and helminth intestinal parasites. Lugol's iodine makes nuclear structures of protozoan cysts more evident and heavily stains glycogen masses. The Lugol's iodine stain can be used on fresh fecal mounts i.e. for looking for giardan trophozoites, or on fecal flotation for giardia cysts. Other suggested uses are:

1. Toxoplasma 2. Coccidi
3. Cryptospordium 4. Helminth (i.e. ascarids or hookworms)

Directions for Use:

1. Add 3 drops of Lugol's stain to either the fresh mount or fecal floatation.
2. Stain will appear light-orange when absorbed up by the parasite.

Storage: Keep bottle covered. Store at room temperature.

Presentation: 500 mL bottle with 4 oz dropper bottle.

Compendium Code No.: 11520060

JORVET™ J-325 SUDAN III FECAL STAIN

Jorgensen **Diagnostic Stain/Reagent**

Contents: 1% Sudan in 70% alcohol.

Indications: For microscopic examination of feces in order to estimate the completeness of digestion and/or absorption. Examination is made for fat droplets (neutral lipid).

Directions for Use: A fecal specimen from a normal dog should be used as a control comparison. Pancreatic exocrine insufficiency yields large amounts of neutral undigested lipid in the feces. In malabsorption syndrome there is normal digestion but inadequate absorption.

1. Add a few drops of Sudan III to a thin film of fresh feces on a glass slide. Neutral fat will stain orange in large goblets.
2. In a case of suspected malabsorption, the sample is first acidified with two drops of vinegar (acetic acid), then gently heated with a cigarette lighter. Unabsorbed fat will now stain strongly orange with Sudan III. Malabsorption syndrome is suspected when the fecal sample is first negative for staining on fresh feces but positive staining after using acetic acid and heating of the fecal sample.

Storage: Keep bottle covered. Store at room temperature.

Presentation: 250 mL bottle.

Compendium Code No.: 11520050

JORVET™ J-326AS ACID FAST STAIN

Jorgensen **Diagnostic Stain/Reagent**

(for *Cryptosporidium* sp.)

Contents:

Component #1 .... Kinyoun Carbol Fuchsin
Component #2 .... 50% Ethanol
Component #3 .... 1% Sulfuric Acid
Component #4 .... Loeffler Methylene Blue

Indications: This stain is useful in identifying microorganisms that are strongly acid or alcohol fast in staining. Recently they have been found to be useful in selectively staining cryptosporidium oocysts and various spirochetes.

Directions for Use:

1. Pick a portion of material with an applicator stick, mix the material in a drop of saline, spread it on a glass slide (1 x 3 inch), and allow to dry.
2. Fix the dried film in methanol for 1 minute and air dry the slide, (component A).
3. Flood the slide with Kinyoun Carbol Fuchsin (component #1), and stain for 5 minutes.
4. Wash slide with 50% Ethanol (component #2), and immediately rinse slide with water.
5. Decolorize the smear with 1% Sulfuric Acid (component #3) for 2 minutes, or until no color runs from the slide.
6. Wash the slide with water.
7. Counterstain the smear with Loeffler Methylene Blue (component #4) for 1 minute.
8. Rinse the slide with water, dry it, and examine the smear with Immersion Oil. Cryptosporidium oocysts stain bright red and background materials stain blue or pale red.

Storage: Always close the lid tightly on the component bottles to avoid evaporation loss.

Presentation: 4 oz.

Compendium Code No.: 11520080

JORVET™ J-326B LACTOPHENOL COTTON BLUE STAIN

Jorgensen **Diagnostic Stain/Reagent**

(for fungi)

Contents:

Phenol 21.7%
Lactic acid 21.7%
Methyl blue 0.25%
Water 21.7%
Glycerin 34.8%

Indications: Aids in visualizing fungal organisms. Two different methods can be used:

1. With a solution of Potassium Hydroxide (KOH).
2. Without KOH (see Directions step #5).

Directions:

1. Mix the specimen whether a skin scraping, fluid exudate or tissue with two drops of the 10% KOH on a clean slide.
2. Then add 2 drops of the lactophenol cotton blue.
3. Gently press a cover slip to make a thin mount. Also gently warming will aid in clearing the mount.
4. Scan under low power with reduced lighting. Switch to high power to check for the presence of suspected fungal elements.
5. If KOH is not available, the stain can still be used but start with step #2.

Lactophenol Cotton Blue: Lactic acid acts as a preservative for fungi.
The phenol portion kills the fungi.
The cotton blue stains the fungal elements.

Interpretation of Results: Fungal elements are stained a deep blue; background is pale blue. Do not overstain.

Caution(s): For *in vitro* diagnostic use only.

Harmful if swallowed. Wash with water if exposed to skin.

Storage: Store at room temperature.

Presentation: 4 oz with flip-top cap.

Compendium Code No.: 11520090

JORVET™ J-326 POTASSIUM HYDROXIDE, KOH (10%)

Jorgensen **Diagnostic Stain/Reagent**

Indications: Aids in the detection of dematophyte infections. Allows visualization of fungal structures such as hyphae and con idida.

Directions for Use:

1. Material is collected as for a skin scraping, together with plucked hairs or nails, and deposited on a slide.
2. Several drops of KOH solution are applied to the slide and a coverslip is added.
3. Next, the slide is either gently heated for 20 seconds or allowed to stand for 30 minutes at room temperature.
4. Only a really thin layer of hair should be placed on a slide. Several layers of hair will make fungal parts even more difficult to see.

Storage: Keep bottle covered. Store at room temperature.

Presentation: 250 mL bottle.

Compendium Code No.: 11520070

JORVET™ J-326S LIVE-DEAD SEMEN STAIN

Jorgensen **Diagnostic Stain/Reagent**

Contents: One bottle of eosin, negrosin and sodium citrate together.

Indications: The JORVET™ Live-Dead Semen Stain is a diagnostic tool for all animal species in the evaluation of spermatazoa morphology.

The JORVET™ Live-Dead Semen Stain is an eosin-nigrosin based stain.

Test Principles: The proper examination of semen is an important veterinary procedure. A fertility evaluation of spermatazoa should consist of 3 separate criteria.

1) Sperm number: This should be evaluated with a hemocytometer.
2) Sperm motility: Extreme care with environmental insults such as cold shock can immobilize sperm. Small portable slide warmers are available for this purpose.
3) Sperm morphology: The appearance of an increased number of abnormal sperm in the ejaculate is a reflection of lesions of the testes and or of the excurrent duct system.

Test Procedure: Gently shake before use.

1) Semen smears can be prepared by placing a small drop of semen and an equal amount of stain placed next to each other.
2) A second slide is placed on edge at about 45°.
3) This slide is gently worked back and forth to mix thoroughly the semen and stain.
4) This second slide is then pulled across the primary slide leaving a thin smear as in doing a normal blood smear.
5) Examination is under a high powered light microscope but phase contrast should also be used. Certain sperm defects cannot be observed under a standard light microscope.
6) Abnormal sperm are categorized and percentages recorded while counting a total of 200 sperm cells.
7) If the presence of leukocytes or bacteria is suggested the semen should also be stained with a Wright Giemsa stain such as the JorVet™ Dip Quick Stain (#J-322).

Interpretation of Results: The presence of 15% major abnormalities or more than 30% total abnormalities especially coupled with palpated testicular lesions is sufficient reason to classify an animal as an unsatisfactory potential breeder.

A repeat test should be done in 30 days to reconfirm any negative results.

See figures 1 and 2 below.

Additional Note:

1) Many sperm abnormalities may be present in sexually immature animals.
2) The semen evaluated are part of about a 60 day cycle and transient insults such as heat stress should be considered.
3) Bacterial overgrowth can occur if contaminated or if not refrigerated.

Storage: Keep refrigerated.

Caution(s): Fatal if swallowed, for *in vitro* use only.

Discussion:

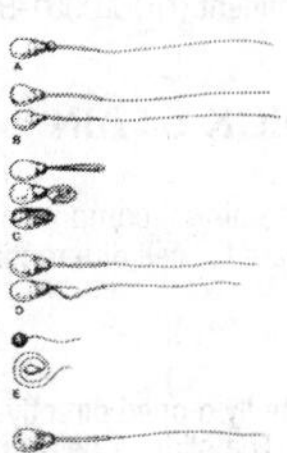

Figure 1. Major sperm abnormalities. A, Proximal cytoplasmic droplets. B, Pyriform heads. C, Strongly folded or coiled tails, tails coiled around the head. D, Middle piece defects. E, Maldeveloped. F, Craters.

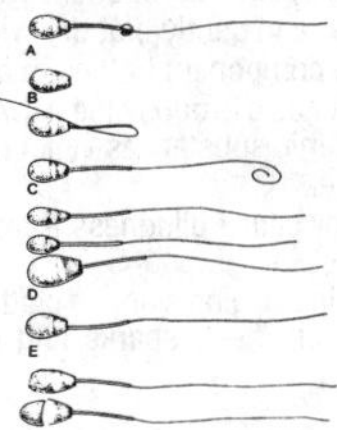

Figure 2. Minor sperm abnormalities. A, Distal cytoplasmic droplets. B, Tailless normal heads. C, Simple bend or terminally coiled tails. D. Narrow, small or giant heads. E, Abaxial implantation. F, Abnormal acrosomes (ruffled, detached).

Presentation: 2x7.5 mL bottles/kit.

Compendium Code No.: 11520100

JUST BORN® MILK REPLACER FOR KITTENS POWDERED FORMULA

Farnam **Milk Replacer**

Advanced Formula

Guaranteed Analysis: JUST BORN® Guaranteed Analysis (as a powder):

Crude Protein, min 33.5%
Crude Fat, min 18.0%
Crude Fiber, max 0.2%
Moisture, max 5.0%
Ash, max 8.0%

Ingredients: Non-fat dry milk, corn oil, soy protein isolate, sodium caseinate, corn syrup solids, maltodextrin, calcium carbonate, carrageenan, colostrum milk powder, magnesium phosphate, choline chloride, sodium ascorbate, potassium bicarbonate, dipotassium phosphate, natural and artificial flavors, ferrous sulfate, dl alpha tocopherol acetate (vitamin E), mono-diglycerides, niacinamide, zinc oxide, l-arginine, dl-methionine, cupric sulfate, calcium pantothenate, L-taurine, manganese sulfate, pyridoxine hydrochloride (vitamin B_6), thiamine hydrochloride, wheat starch, riboflavin, menadione, biotin, potassium iodide, folic acid, vitamin A palmitate, sodium selenite, cyanocobalamin (vitamin B_{12}), cholecalciferol (vitamin D_3), BHT and propyl gallate (preservatives).

Indications: JUST BORN® Milk Replacer for Kittens Powdered Formula is intended for intermittent or supplemental feeding only.

Directions for Use: Your veterinarian should be consulted for advice about the care and feeding of kittens.

Directions for Preparation and Use: Weigh the kitten. Prepare enough JUST BORN®, with the enclosed measuring scoop, for use within a 24 hour period. Kittens should be fed at least ½ ounce of liquid JUST BORN® for every 2 ounces of body weight, daily. Kittens should be allowed to consume as much formula as they want. The table below gives minimum feeding amounts for a 24 hour period. Mix 1 tablespoon powder into 1 tablespoon and 1 teaspoon water. Use tap or bottled water. Stir until smooth. Pour liquid into an appropriate sized, clean Just Born® nursing bottle. Heat liquid by placing bottle in a pan of tepid water. Test temperature on your wrist. It should feel lightly warm. Do not microwave. Store JUST BORN® powder in the refrigerator. Refrigerate unused reconstituted liquid for up to 24 hours.

1. Measure water.
2. Mix in JUST BORN®.
3. Stir until smooth.
4. Feed at temperature that feels slightly warm on your wrist.
5. Refrigerate unused portion.

After feeding, hold the kitten's head on your shoulder and rub his back gently until he burps. Make water available after kittens are 2 weeks old. Farnam small animal water bottles are recommended.

Weight of Animal	Minimum Amount of Liquid to Be Fed in 24 Hours (Ounces or Tablespoons)			Minimum Amount per Feeding if Fed Every... (Teaspoons)		
	Ounces		Tbs	8 hrs	6 hrs	4 hrs
2 Ounces	½ oz.	or	1 Tbs.	1 tsp.	¾ tsp.	½ tsp.
4 Ounces	1 oz.	or	2 Tbs.	2 tsp.	1½ tsp.	1 tsp.
8 Ounces	2 oz.	or	4 Tbs.	4 tsp.	3 tsp.	2 tsp.
16 Ounces	4 oz.	or	8 Tbs.	8 tsp.	6 tsp.	4 tsp.

Orphaned Kittens: If possible, kittens should nurse from their mother for the first 2 days of their lives to receive nutrient rich colostrum. Mother's colostrum provides temporary protection from numerous diseases and contains growth factors believed to stimulate protein synthesis, improve fat utilization, and promote cell growth. While mother's milk is always preferable, JUST BORN® contains nutrient rich colostrum milk powder harvested at USDA inspected facilities. It is extremely important to weigh kittens frequently (every day) to insure they are receiving adequate amounts of supplement. If a kitten loses weight after 48 hours, consult your veterinarian. Feed weak or small kittens every 4 hours, feed at 8 hour intervals if strong and active. Kittens' needs will vary and the time and amount may have to be increased or decreased, depending on the breed, growth rate and activity of the kitten. Orphan kittens must be kept warm for proper digestion to occur. Also, use a warm, moist washcloth and gently wipe the kitten's bottom until it wets and has a bowel movement, several times daily, to imitate a mother's care. This is required for young kitten survival.

Weaning Kittens: Healthy kittens may be weaned when they are about 25 days old or when they can lap formula from a bowl. At this age, blend a high quality dry kitten food with warm Just Born® Liquid Formula to make a paste. Feed the mixture 3-4 times a day for the first week. Each week, increase the amount of dry food in the mixture so that after 6-7 weeks the kitten is fully on dry food.

Pregnant and Lactating Queens: Mix 1 tablespoon of prepared JUST BORN® Milk Replacer per 5 pounds of body weight into the pregnant queen's daily ration. Continue until the kittens are weaned.

Supplementation: If a supplement is desired for a growing kitten, show cat, large litter, geriatric or convalescing cat, simply mix 1 tablespoon of prepared JUST BORN® Milk Replacer per 5 pounds of body weight into the cat's daily ration of food.

JUST BORN® Milk Replacer is also available in a ready-to-use liquid.

If you have questions or comments about JUST BORN® Milk Replacer, call Farnam's Technical Staff at 1-800-234-2269.

Precaution(s): Refrigerate after opening. Discard unused powder after three months.

Presentation: 170.1 g (6 oz) and 340.2 g (12 oz) fiber cans.

Compendium Code No.: 10000680 01-1506 / 01-1916

JUST BORN® MILK REPLACER FOR KITTENS READY-TO-USE LIQUID

Farnam **Milk Replacer**

Advanced Formula

Guaranteed Analysis: JUST BORN® Guaranteed Analysis (as a liquid):

Crude Protein, min 7.0%
Crude Fat, min 3.8%
Crude Fiber, max 0.2%
Moisture, max 83.0%
Ash, max 2.5%

Ingredients: Water, non-fat dry milk, corn oil, soy protein isolate, sodium caseinate, corn syrup solids, maltodextrin, calcium carbonate, carrageenan, colostrum milk powder, magnesium phosphate, choline chloride, sodium ascorbate, potassium bicarbonate, dipotassium phosphate, natural and artificial flavors, ferrous sulfate, dl alpha tocopherol acetate (vitamin E), mono-diglycerides, niacinamide, zinc oxide, l-arginine, dl-methionine, cupric sulfate, calcium pantothenate, L-taurine, manganese sulfate, pyridoxine hydrochloride (vitamin B_6), thiamine hydrochloride, wheat starch, riboflavin, menadione, biotin, potassium iodide, folic acid, vitamin A palmitate, sodium selenite, cyanocobalamin (vitamin B_{12}), cholecalciferol (vitamin D_3), BHT and propyl gallate (preservatives).

Indications: JUST BORN® Milk Replacer for Kittens Ready-To-Use Liquid is intended for intermittent or supplemental feeding only.

Directions for Use: Your veterinarian should be consulted for advice about the care and feeding of kittens.

Directions for Preparation and Use: Weigh the kitten. Feed at least ½ oz. of JUST BORN® for every 2 ounces of body weight, daily. Kittens should be allowed to consume as much formula as they want. Shake well before using. To open, unfold the corner and cut along the dotted line. Pour liquid into an appropriate sized, clean Just Born® nursing bottle. Reclose carton and refrigerate. Heat liquid by placing nursing bottle in a pan of tepid water. Test temperature on your wrist. It should feel slightly warm. Do not microwave. After feeding, hold the kitten's head on your shoulder and rub his back gently until he burps. Make water readily available after kittens are 2 weeks of age. Farnam water bottles are recommended.

Weight of Animal	Amount per Feeding if Fed Every ...		
	8 Hrs	6 Hrs	4 Hrs
2 oz.	1 tsp.	¾ tsp.	½ tsp.
4 oz.	2 tsp.	1½ tsp.	1 tsp.
8 oz.	4 tsp.	3 tsp.	2 tsp.
16 oz.	8 tsp.	6 tsp.	4 tsp.

Orphaned Kittens: If possible, kittens should nurse from their mother for the first 2 days of their lives to receive nutrient rich colostrum. Mother's colostrum provides temporary protection from numerous diseases and contains growth factors believed to stimulate protein synthesis, improve fat utilization, and promote cell growth. While mother's milk is always preferable, JUST BORN® contains nutrient rich colostrum milk powder harvested at USDA inspected facilities. It is extremely important to weigh kittens frequently (every day) to insure they are receiving adequate amounts of supplement. If a kitten loses weight after 48 hours, consult your veterinarian. Feed weak or small kittens every 4 hours, feed at 8 hour intervals if strong and active. Kittens' needs will vary and the time and amount may have to be increased or decreased, depending on the breed, growth rate and activity of the kitten. Orphan kittens must be kept warm for proper digestion to occur. Also, use a warm, moist washcloth and gently wipe the kitten's bottom until it wets and has a bowel movement, several times daily, to imitate a mother's care. This is required for young kitten survival.

Weaning Kittens: Healthy kittens may be weaned when they are about 25 days old or when they can lap formula from a bowl. At this age, blend a high quality dry kitten food with warm JUST BORN® Liquid Formula to make a paste. Feed the mixture 3-4 times a day for the first week. Each week, increase the amount of dry food in the mixture so that after 6-7 weeks the kitten is fully on dry food.

Pregnant and Lactating Queens: Mix 1 tablespoon of JUST BORN® Milk Replacer per 5 pounds of body weight into the pregnant queen's daily ration. Continue until the kittens are weaned.

Supplementation: If a supplement is desired for a growing kitten, show cat, large litter, geriatric or convalescing cat, simply mix 1 tablespoon per 5 pounds of body weight into the cat's daily ration of food.

JUST BORN® Milk Replacer is also available in a powder.

If you have questions or comments about JUST BORN® Milk Replacer, call Farnam's Technical Staff at 1-800-234-2269.

Precaution(s): Refrigerate after opening. Discard unused formula after 14 days.

Presentation: 236.6 mL (8 fl oz) Tetra Pak container.

Compendium Code No.: 10000690 01-1907

JUST BORN® MILK REPLACER FOR PUPPIES POWDERED FORMULA

Farnam **Milk Replacer**

Advanced Formula

Guaranteed Analysis: JUST BORN® Guaranteed Analysis (as a powder):

Crude Protein, min 29.0%
Crude Fat, min 28.0%
Crude Fiber, max. 0.2%
Moisture, max. 5.0%
Ash, max. 8.0%

Ingredients: Corn oil, non-fat dry milk, sodium caseinate, corn syrup solids, soy protein isolate, dicalcium phosphate, calcium carbonate, carregeenan, maltodextrin, dipotassium phosphate, colostrum milk powder, sodium ascorbate, potassium bicarbonate, natural and artificial flavors, choline chloride, zinc oxide, dl alphatocopherol acetate (vitamin E), magnesium sulfate, ferrous sulfate, mono-diglycerides, calcium pantothenate, l-arginine, dl-methionine, niacinamide, manganese sulfate, wheat starch, thiamine hydrochloride, cupric sulfate, vitamin A palmitate, pyridoxine hydrochloride, biotin, menadione, folic acid, cyanocobalamin (vitamin B_{12}), potassium iodide, sodium selenite, cholecalciferol (vitamin D_3), BHT and propyl gallate (preservatives).

Indications: JUST BORN® Milk Replacer for Puppies Powdered Formula is intended for intermittent or supplemental feeding only.

Directions for Use: Your veterinarian should be consulted for advice about the care and feeding of puppies.

Directions for Preparation and Use: Weigh the puppy. Prepare enough JUST BORN®, with the enclosed measuring scoop, for use within a 24 hour period. Puppies should be fed at least ½ ounce of liquid JUST BORN® for every 2 ounces of body weight, daily. Puppies should be allowed to consume as much formula as they want. The table at right gives minimum feeding amounts for a 24 hour period. For puppies 1-10 days old, mix 1 scoop powder into 2 scoops water. For puppies older than 10 days, mix 2 scoops powder into 3 scoops water. Use tap or bottled water. Stir until smooth. Pour liquid into an appropriate sized, clean Just Born® nursing bottle. Heat liquid by placing bottle in a pan of tepid water. Test temperature on your wrist. It should feel slightly warm. Do not microwave. Store JUST BORN® powder in the refrigerator. Refrigerate unused reconstituted liquid for up to 24 hours.

1. Measure water.
2. Mix in JUST BORN®.
3. Stir until smooth.
4. Feed at temperature that feels slightly warm on your wrist.
5. Refrigerate unused portion.

After feeding, hold the puppy's head on your shoulder and rub his back gently until he burps.

Make water available after puppies are 2 weeks old. Farnam puppy water bottles are recommended.

Weight of Animal	Minimum Amount of Liquid to Be Fed in 24 Hours (Ounces or Tablespoons)			Minimum Amount per Feeding if Fed Every... (Teaspoons)		
	Ounces		Tbs	8 Hrs	6 Hrs	4 Hrs
2 Ounces	½ oz.	or	1 Tbs.	1 tsp.	¾ tsp.	½ tsp.
4 Ounces	1 oz.	or	2 Tbs.	2 tsp.	1½ tsp.	1 tsp.
8 Ounces	2 oz.	or	4 Tbs.	4 tsp.	3 tsp.	2 tsp.
16 Ounces	4 oz.	or	8 Tbs.	8 tsp.	6 tsp.	4 tsp.

Orphaned Puppies: If possible, puppies should nurse from their mother for the first 2 days of their lives to receive nutrient rich colostrum. Mother's colostrum provides temporary protection from numerous diseases and contains growth factors believed to stimulate protein synthesis, improve fat utilization, and promote cell growth. While mother's milk is always preferable, JUST BORN® contains nutrient rich colostrum milk powder harvested at USDA inspected facilities. It is extremely important to weigh puppies frequently (every day) to insure they are receiving adequate amounts of supplement. If a puppy loses weight after 48 hours, consult your veterinarian. Feed weak or small puppies every 4 hours, feed at 8 hour intervals if strong and active. Puppies' needs will vary and the time and amount may have to be increased or decreased, depending on the breed, growth rate and activity of the puppy. Orphan puppies must be kept warm for proper digestion to occur. Also, use a warm, moist washcloth and gently wipe the puppy's bottom until it wets and has a bowel movement, several times daily, to imitate a mother's care. This is required for young puppy survival.

Weaning Puppies: Healthy puppies may be weaned when they are about 25 days old or when they can lap formula from a bowl. At this age, blend a high quality dry puppy food with warm Just Born® Liquid Formula to make a paste. Feed the mixture 3-4 times a day for the first week. Each week, increase the amount of dry food in the mixture so that after 6-7 weeks the puppy is fully on dry food.

Pregnant and Lactating Bitches: Mix 1 tablespoon of prepared JUST BORN® Milk Replacer per 5 pounds of body weight into the pregnant bitch's daily ration. Continue until the pups are weaned.

Supplementation: If a supplement is desired for a growing puppy, show dog, large litter, geriatric or convalescing dog, simply mix 1 tablespoon of prepared JUST BORN® Milk Replacer per 5 pounds of body weight into the dog's daily ration of food.

JUST BORN® Milk Replacer is also available in a ready-to-use liquid.

If you have questions or comments about JUST BORN® Milk Replacer, call Farnam's Technical Staff at 1-800-234-2269.

Precaution(s): Refrigerate after opening. Discard unused powder after three months.

Presentation: 340.2 g (12 oz) and 793.8 g (28 oz) fiber cans.

Compendium Code No.: 10000700 01-1917 / 01-1918

JUST BORN® MILK REPLACER FOR PUPPIES READY-TO-USE LIQUID

Farnam **Milk Replacer**

Advanced Formula

Guaranteed Analysis: JUST BORN® Guaranteed Analysis (as a liquid):

Crude Protein, min 6.5%
Crude Fat, min 6.5%
Crude Fiber, max 0.1%
Moisture, max 78.0%
Ash, max 2.5%

Ingredients: Water, corn oil, non-fat dry milk, sodium caseinate, corn syrup solids, soy protein isolate, dicalcium phosphate, calcium carbonate, carregeenan, maltodextrin, dipotassium phosphate, colostrum milk powder, sodium ascorbate, potassium bicarbonate, natural and artificial flavors, choline chloride, zinc oxide, dl alpha tocopherol acetate (vitamin E), magnesium sulfate, ferrous sulfate, mono-diglycerides, calcium pantothenate, l-arginine, dl-methionine, niacinamide, manganese sulfate, wheat starch, thiamine hydrochloride, cupric sulfate, vitamin A palmitate, pyridoxine hydrochloride, biotin, menadione, folic acid, cyanocobalamin (vitamin B_{12}), potassium iodide, sodium selenite, cholecalciferol (vitamin D_3), BHT and propyl gallate (preservatives).

Indications: JUST BORN® Milk Replacer for Puppies Ready-To-Use Liquid is intended for intermittent or supplemental feeding only.

Directions for Use: Your veterinarian should be consulted for advice about the care and feeding of puppies.

Directions for Preparation and Use: Weigh the puppy. Feed at least ½ oz. of JUST BORN® for every 2 ounces of body weight, daily. Puppies should be allowed to consume as much formula as they want. Shake well before using. To open, unfold the corner and cut along the dotted line. Pour liquid into an appropriate sized, clean Just Born® nursing bottle. Reclose carton and refrigerate. Heat liquid by placing nursing bottle in a pan of tepid water. Test temperature on your wrist. It should feel slightly warm. Do not microwave. After feeding, hold the puppy's head on your shoulder and rub his back gently until he burps. Make water readily available after puppies are 2 weeks of age. Farnam water bottles are recommended.

Weight of Animal	Amount Per Feeding if Fed Every ...		
	8 Hrs	6 Hrs	4 Hrs
2 oz.	1 tsp.	¾ tsp.	½ tsp.
4 oz.	2 tsp.	1½ tsp.	1 tsp.
8 oz.	4 tsp.	3 tsp.	2 tsp.
16 oz.	8 tsp.	6 tsp.	4 tsp.

Orphaned Puppies: If possible, puppies should nurse from their mother for the first 2 days of their lives to receive nutrient rich colostrum. Mother's colostrum provides temporary protection from numerous diseases and contains growth factors believed to stimulate protein synthesis, improve fat utilization, and promote cell growth. While mother's milk is always preferable, JUST BORN® contains nutrient rich colostrum milk powder harvested at USDA inspected facilities. It is extremely important to weigh puppies frequently (every day) to insure they are receiving adequate amounts of supplement. If a puppy loses weight after 48 hours, consult your veterinarian. Feed weak or small puppies every 4 hours, feed at 8 hour intervals if strong and active. Puppies' needs will vary and the time and amount may have to be increased or decreased, depending on the breed, growth rate and activity of the puppy. Orphan puppies must be kept warm for proper digestion to occur. Also, use a warm, moist washcloth and gently wipe the puppy's bottom until it wets and has a bowel movement, several times daily, to imitate a mother's care. This is required for young puppy survival.

Weaning Puppies: Healthy puppies may be weaned when they are about 25 days old or when they can lap formula from a bowl. At this age, blend a high quality dry puppy food with warm JUST BORN® Liquid Formula to make a paste. Feed the mixture 3-4 times a day for the first week. Each week, increase the amount of dry food in the mixture so that after 6-7 weeks the puppy is fully on dry food.

Pregnant and Lactating Bitches: Mix 1 tablespoon of JUST BORN® Milk Replacer per 5 pounds of body weight into the pregnant bitch's daily ration. Continue until the puppies are weaned.

Supplementation: If a supplement is desired for a growing puppy, show dog, large litter, geriatric or convalescing dog, simply mix 1 tablespoon per 5 pounds of body weight into the dog's daily ration of food.

JUST BORN® Milk Replacer is also available in a powder.

If you have questions or comments about JUST BORN® Milk Replacer, call Farnam's Technical Staff at 1-800-234-2269.

Precaution(s): Refrigerate after opening. Discard unused formula after 14 days.

Presentation: 236.6 mL (8 fl oz) Tetra Pak container.

Compendium Code No.: 10000710 01-1248

J-VAC®

Merial **Bacterin-Toxoid**

Escherichia Coli Bacterin-Toxoid

U.S. Vet. Lic. No.: 298

Contents: This product contains the antigen listed above.

Contains gentamicin and nystatin as preservatives.

Indications: For the vaccination of healthy cattle (cows, heifers) as an aid in prevention of mastitis due to *E. coli* and the effects of endotoxemia caused by *E. coli* and *Salmonella typhimurium*.

Dosage and Administration: Shake well before using.

As an aid in the prevention of mastitis, inject 2 mL (1 dose) intramuscularly or subcutaneously at 7 months of gestation or at dry off; revaccinate at 1 to 3 weeks before calving. Revaccinate annually as above.

As an aid in the prevention of the effects of endotoxemia, whole herd vaccination may be done at any time. Vaccinate with 2 mL (1 dose) followed by a second 2 mL dose 2 to 4 weeks later. Revaccinate annually as above.

Calves vaccinated under 6 months of age should be revaccinated after reaching 6 months of age.

Precaution(s): Store at 2-7°C (35-45°F). Do not freeze. Do not expose to heat or direct sunlight. Use entire contents when first opened. Do not use chemicals to sterilize syringes and needles.

Caution(s): In rare instances, administration of vaccines may cause lethargy, fever and inflammatory or hypersensitivity types of reactions. Treatment may include antihistamines, anti-inflammatories, and/or epinephrine.

For veterinary use only.

Warning(s): Do not vaccinate within 21 days prior to slaughter.

Presentation: 10 dose (20 mL) and 50 dose (100 mL) vials.

J-VAC is a registered trademark of Merial.

RM861R4 / RM865R4

Compendium Code No.: 11110412

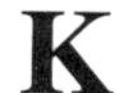

K

K9 ADVANTIX™

Bayer

Topical prevention and treatment of ticks, fleas and mosquitoes for monthly use on dogs and puppies 7 weeks of age and older.

Read The Entire Label Before Each Use

DO NOT USE ON CATS

For the Prevention and Treatment of Ticks, Fleas and Mosquitoes on Dogs

- Available only through licensed practicing veterinarians
- Repels and kills ticks including Deer ticks (vector of Lyme disease), American dog ticks (vector of Rocky Mountain spotted fever), Brown dog ticks (vector of ehrlichiosis), and Lone Star ticks for up to four weeks
- Kills 98-100% of the fleas on dogs within 12 hours and continues to prevent infestations for at least four weeks
- Kills fleas before they lay eggs
- Larval flea stages in the dog's surroundings are killed following contact with a K9 Advantix™ treated dog
- Repels and kills mosquitoes for up to four weeks
- Remains effective after bathing and swimming
- Convenient, easy to apply

Active Ingredients	% By Weight
Imidacloprid; 1-[(6-Chloro-3-pyridinyl) methyl]-N-nitro-2-imidazolidinimine	8.8%
Permethrin*	44.0%
Other Ingredients	47.2%
Total	100.0%

*cis/trans ratio: Max 55% (±) cis and min 45% (±) trans

KEEP OUT OF REACH OF CHILDREN

WARNING

See below for first aid and precautionary statements.

PRECAUTIONARY STATEMENTS

HAZARDS TO HUMANS

Causes eye irritation. Harmful if swallowed. Do not get in eyes or on clothing. Avoid contact with skin. Wash hands thoroughly with soap and warm water after handling.

HAZARDS TO DOMESTIC ANIMALS

For external use on dogs only.

Do not use on animals other than dogs.

Do not use on puppies under seven weeks of age. Do not get this product in dog's eyes or mouth. As with any product, consult your veterinarian before using this product on debilitated, aged, pregnant or nursing animals. Individual sensitivities, while rare, may occur after using ANY pesticide product for pets. If signs persist, or become more severe, consult a veterinarian immediately. If your animal is on medication, consult your veterinarian before using this or any other product.

DO NOT USE ON CATS

Due to their unique physiology and inability to metabolize certain compounds, this product must not be used on cats. If applied to a cat, or ingested by a cat which actively grooms a recently treated dog, this product may have serious harmful effects. If this occurs contact your veterinarian immediately.

For consumer questions call 1-800-255-6826.

For medical emergencies call 1-877-258-2280.

Environmental Hazards

This product is extremely toxic to fish. Do not add directly to water. Do not contaminate water when disposing of product or packaging.

First Aid

Have the product container or label with you when calling a poison control center or doctor, or going for treatment.

If in eyes: Hold eye open and rinse slowly and gently with water for 15-20 minutes. Remove contact lenses, if present, after the first 5 minutes, then continue rinsing eye. Call a poison control center or doctor for treatment advice.

If swallowed: Call poison control center or doctor immediately for treatment advice. Have person sip a glass of water if able to swallow. Do not induce vomiting unless told to do so by the poison control center or doctor. Do not give anything by mouth to an unconscious person.

If on skin or clothing: Take off contaminated clothing. Rinse skin immediately with plenty of water for 15-20 minutes. Call a poison control center or doctor for treatment advice.

To Physician: Treat the patient symptomatically.

Directions for Use

It is a violation of Federal Law to use this product in a manner inconsistent with its labeling. Do not contaminate feed or food.

How to Apply

1. Use only on dogs. DO NOT USE ON CATS or on other animals.
2. Remove applicator tube from the package.

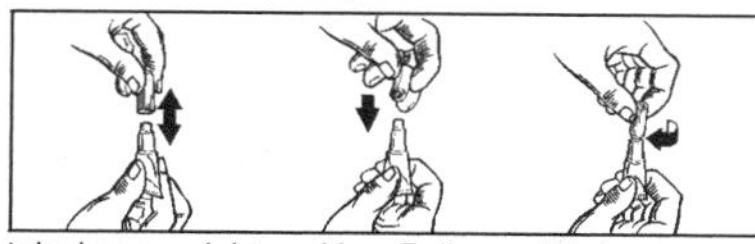

3. Hold applicator tube in an upright position. Pull cap off tube.
4. Turn the cap around and place other end of cap back on tube.
5. Twist cap to break seal, then remove cap from tube.
6. 10 lbs. and Under:

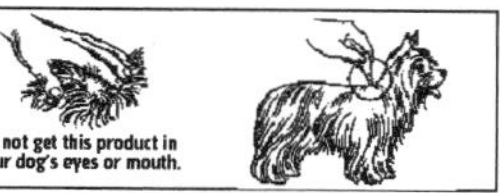

11-20 lbs.:

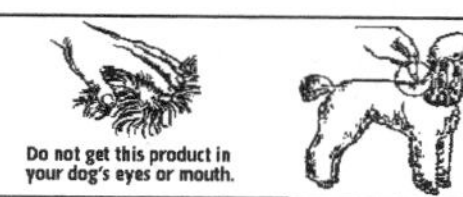

The dog should be standing for easy application. Part the hair on the dog's back, between the shoulder blades, until the skin is visible. Place the tip of the tube on the skin and squeeze the tube twice to expel the entire contents directly on the skin.

21-55 lbs.:

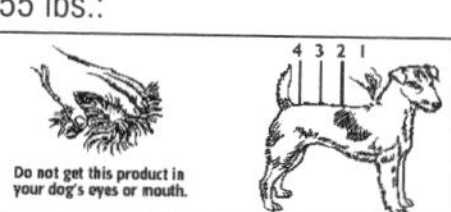

Over 55 lbs.:

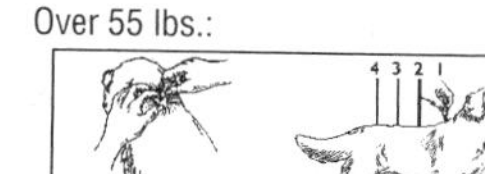

The dog should be standing for easy application. The entire contents of the K9 Advantix™ tube should be applied evenly to three or four spots on the top of the back from the shoulder to the base of the tail. At each spot, part the hair until the skin is visible. Place the tip of the tube on the skin and gently squeeze to expel a portion of the solution on the skin. Do not apply an excessive amount of solution at any one spot that could cause some of the solution to run off the side of the dog.

7. Discard empty tube as described in Storage and Disposal.

Kills fleas which may cause flea allergy dermatitis (FAD).

K9 Advantix™ kills 98-100% of the existing fleas on dogs within 12 hours. Reinfesting fleas are killed within 2 hours with protection against further flea infestation lasting at least four (4) weeks. Pre-existing pupae in the environment may continue to emerge for six (6) weeks or longer depending upon the climatic conditions.

Larval flea stages in the dog's surroundings are killed following contact with a K9 Advantix™ treated dog.

K9 Advantix™ remains efficacious following a shampoo treatment, swimming or after exposure to rain or sunlight.

Monthly treatments are required for optimal control and prevention of fleas and ticks.

Storage and Disposal

Do not contaminate water, food or feed by storage or disposal.

Storage: Store in a cool, dry place. Protect from freezing.

Pesticide Disposal:

If empty: Do not reuse this container. Place in trash or offer for recycling if available.

If partly filled: Call your local solid waste agency or 1-800-255-6826 for disposal instructions. Never place unused product down any indoor or outdoor drain.

Limited Warranty and Limitation of Damages

Bayer Corporation, Agriculture Division, Animal Health warrants that this material conforms to the chemical description on the label. BAYER CORPORATION MAKES NO OTHER EXPRESS OR IMPLIED WARRANTY, INCLUDING ANY OTHER EXPRESS OR IMPLIED WARRANTY OF FITNESS OR MERCHANTABILITY, and no agent of Bayer Corporation is authorized to do so except in writing with a specific reference to this warranty. Any damages arising from a breach of this warranty shall be limited to direct damages and shall not include consequential commercial damages such as loss of profits or values, etc.

Green/10 For Dogs and Puppies 7 Weeks and Older and 10 lbs. and Under
Code 02935094—Four 0.4 mL Tubes
Code 02935256—Six 0.4 mL Tubes
EPA Est. 11556-DEU-1 EPA Reg. No. 11556-132 02935094/02935256, R.0

Teal/20 For Dogs and Puppies 7 Weeks and Older and 11-20 lbs.
Code 02935132—Four 1.0 mL Tubes
Code 02935280—Six 1.0 mL Tubes
EPA Est. 11556-DEU-1 EPA Reg. No. 11556-133 02935132/02935280, R.0

Red/55 For Dogs and Puppies 7 Weeks and Older and 21-55 lbs.
Code 02935175—Four 2.5 mL Tubes
Code 02935310—Six 2.5 mL Tubes
EPA Est. 11556-DEU-1 EPA Reg. No. 11556-135 02935175/02935310, R.0

Blue/100 For Dogs and Puppies 7 Weeks and Older and Over 55 lbs.
Code 02935213—Four 4.0 mL Tubes
Code 02935353—Six 4.0 mL Tubes
EPA Est. 11556-DEU-1 EPA Reg. No. 11556-134 02935213/02935353, R.0

Made in Germany

Manufactured For Bayer Corporation, Agriculture Division, Animal Health, Shawnee Mission, Kansas 66201 USA

Compendium Code No.: 10400440

K-9 BLUELITE®

TechMix **Small Animal Dietary Supplement**

Active Ingredient(s): Guaranteed Analysis:

Crude fat, not less than	4.50% (9,072 mg/oz.)
Potassium (K), not less than	2.00% (7,938 mg/oz.)
Sodium (Na), not less than	1.75% (1,134 mg/oz.)
Calcium (Ca), not less than	0.25% (907 mg/oz.)
Phosphorus (P), not less than	0.20% (227 mg/oz.)
Zinc (Zn), not less than	0.07% (18 mg/oz.)
Magnesium (Mg), not less than	0.05% (3 mg/oz.)
Minimum vitamin content per pound:	
Vitamin A	50,000 I.U. (3,125 I.U./oz.)
Vitamin D_3	5,000 I.U. (312 I.U./oz.)
Vitamin E	100 I.U. (6.25 I.U./oz.)
Choline bitartrate	362 mg (22,600 mcg/oz.)
Niacin	30 mg (1,875 mcg/oz.)
d-Pantothenic acid	12.5 mg (780 mcg/oz.)
Riboflavin	7.5 mg (470 mcg/oz.)
Menadione (vitamin K activity)	3 mg (187.5 mcg/oz.)
Pyridoxine HCl	2 mg (125 mcg/oz.)
Thiamine HCl	2 mg (125 mcg/oz.)
Folic acid	0.5 mg (31.25 mcg/oz.)
d-Biotin	0.2 mg (12.5 mcg/oz.)
Vitamin B_{12}	0.025 mg (1.56 mcg/oz.)

Indications: Administer K-9 BLUELITE® in the water or on the dog food whenever dogs are dehydrated or are losing body condition as a result of debilitating stresses. K-9 BLUELITE® should be used to help prevent dehydration for dogs that are moved or shipped for competitive events such as shows, field trials, and long distance performance runs.

For use in minimizing the stress of dehydration as a result of extensive physical activity, diarrhea or conditions that may cause sudden losses of body fluid such as shipping, environmental changes and new surroundings.

For oral administration to dogs with gastritis and diarrhea.

K-9 BLUELITE® provides a digestive acidifying action in combination with multiple sources of energy. This acidifying action and the readily absorbed energy ingredients help provide optimum

K

digestive pH maximizing energy utilization and electrolyte absorption. This energizing-acidification action provides rehydration action in performance animals such as racing dogs and young puppies where prolonged dehydration and energy deficits may be a threat to normal health.

Dosage and Administration:

A. Drinking Water Administration: Mix one (1) pouch or one (1) heaping teaspoon to each one (1) to two (2) pints of drinking water depending upon the severity of dehydration. Keep K-9 BLUELITE® in all of the drinking water consumed by the dog for five (5) to seven (7) days or for as long as the signs of dehydration persist. It can be fed continuously as a vitamin-energy supplement in debilitated dogs.

B. Dog Food Applications: Mix K-9 BLUELITE® with the dog food or dissolve one (1) pouch or one (1) heaping teaspoon of K-9 BLUELITE® in about one-fourth (¼) cup of water and pour over the dog food. Feed one (1) pouch or one (1) heaping teaspoon per each 10-15 lbs. of body weight per day depending upon the condition of the dog.

C. K-9 BLUELITE® can be added to the drinking water at the recommended rate or diluted one (1) to four (4) (1 part K-9 BLUELITE® and 4 parts water) and used as an oral lavage in mature dogs or puppies suffering from dehydration.

Trial Data: K-9 BLUELITE® has been tested and evaluated in veterinary clinics, breeding kennels, sled dogs, greyhounds, lactating bitches and in nursing puppies. In these field trials, K-9 BLUELITE® helped restore and maintain normal body fluid balance in puppies that were afflicted with bacterial diarrhea and in mature dogs suffering from viral diarrhea. In an extensive trial in a breeding kennel, K-9 BLUELITE® helped maintain water intake in whelping-lactating bitches and increased water intake in dehydrated nursing puppies by 50%. K-9 BLUELITE®'s rehydration action is readily visible when administered in the water or in the dog food.

In some house pets and dogs with a selective taste and appetite, K-9 BLUELITE® should be added to the dog food, as any changes in water taste may delay water intake for a short duration.

Presentation: 14x2 lb. bags (28 lb. pail).

Compendium Code No.: 11440090

KANTRIM® ℞

Fort Dodge **Kanamycin**

Kanamycin Sulfate Injection

NADA No.: 041-836

Active Ingredient(s): Kanamycin is a water-soluble antibiotic produced through fermentation by *Streptomyces kanamyceticus*. KANTRIM® (kanamycin sulfate) Veterinary Injection is supplied as an aqueous solution of kanamycin sulfate, buffered with sodium citrate, preserved with methylparaben, propylparaben, sodium bisulfite, and sulfuric acid used to adjust pH.

Indications: This drug has been used successfully in the treatment of bacterial infections due to kanamycin susceptible organisms. Among these infections are:

Urinary-tract infections: Acute and chronic cystitis, nephritis, pyelonephritis and prostatitis.

Respiratory-tract infections: Sinusitis, tracheitis, lobar- and bronchopneumonia, lung abscesses, and tonsilitis.

Bacterial complication of canine distemper and feline pneumonitis.

Skin, soft-tissue and post-surgical infections: Abscesses, wound infections, cellulitis, pustular dermatitis.

Osteomyelitis, septic arthritis, periostitis, septicemia and bacteremia.

Gastrointestinal infections: Amebiasis, salmonellosis, gastroenteritis and staphylococcal enterocolitis.

Endometritis, mastitis, otitis media, pancreatitis.

While nearly all strains of *Staphylococcus aureus*, and the majority of strains of Proteus, *E. coli*, and *A. aerogenes* are highly susceptible to kanamycin, the invading organism should be cultured and its susceptibility demonstrated as a guide to therapy.

Pharmacology:

Description: Kanamycin is active against many gram-negative pathogens. These include coliforms, *Klebsiella pneumoniae, Enterobacter aerogenes*, Salmonella, strains of Proteus, Neisseria, *Pasteurella multocida* and Acinetobacter. Kanamycin's gram-positive spectrum includes Corynebacteria, *Bacillus anthracis, Staphylococcus albus*, and *Staphylococcus aureus* - including many strains resistant to other antibiotics. Bactericidal serum concentrations are obtained by average dosage. Bacterial resistance to kanamycin develops slowly among most susceptible organisms so far tested, particularly among the staphylococci.

Action: The drug is rapidly absorbed after subcutaneous or intramuscular injection. Peak serum levels are obtained approximately one hour after injection. Kanamycin diffuses readily into most body fluids (synovial fluid, bile, pleural and peritoneal fluids, bronchial secretions) but, under normal circumstances, poorly into spinal fluid. Kanamycin is poorly absorbed following oral administration. Systemic infections are preferably treated by subcutaneous injection; the drug may also be administered intramuscularly. Excretion of the drug is almost entirely by glomerular filtration. Virtually no tubular reabsorption of the drug occurs so that high concentrations are reached within the renal tubules. Renal excretion is rapid, approximately one-half of the injected dose clears the kidney within four hours in subjects with normal renal function, and excretion is complete in 24 to 48 hours. Subjects with impaired renal function excrete kanamycin much more slowly - roughly in proportion to the extent of renal damage, and such subjects must be well hydrated. Excessive accumulation of the drug greatly increases the risk of ototoxicity.

Dosage and Administration:

Dosage: The usual dose is 5 mg/lb body weight per day in equally divided doses at 12-hour intervals (see dosage table below). Kanamycin preferably should be administered by subcutaneous injection, but may also be given by the intramuscular route if desired. The remarks regarding excessive dosage under "Warning" should be noted. If definite clinical response does not occur within five days, therapy should be stopped and the antibiotic susceptibility pattern of the pathogenic organism rechecked. Failure of the infection to respond may be due to the presence of a resistant organism or septic foci requiring surgical drainage.

Dog and Cat Dosage Guide: Amount to be given every 12 hours.

Vial concentration 200 mg/mL:

Weight in lbs	Dosage every 12 hrs in mg	Dosage every 12 hrs in mL
20	50 mg	0.25 mL
40	100 mg	0.50 mL
60	150 mg	0.75 mL
80	200 mg	1.00 mL
100	250 mg	1.25 mL
120	300 mg	1.50 mL

Contraindication(s): Kanamycin should not be used following high doses or prolonged therapy with other antibiotics that may cause similar toxic reactions, e.g., streptomycin, neomycin. A history of allergic response to this drug is a contraindication. The use of concurrent drugs, other than analgesics, is not recommended. Do not administer to subjects undergoing general anesthesia.

Precaution(s): Unopened vials may occasionally darken during storage. This change of color does not affect potency.

Store at controlled room temperature 15° to 30°C (59° to 86°F).

Caution(s): Federal law restricts this drug to use by or on the order of a licensed veterinarian.

Warning(s): In subjects with normal renal function, when the recommended precautions and dosage are followed, the incidence of toxic reactions is negligible.

However, prolonged use of this antibiotic at doses in excess of those recommended may result in:

a) Ototoxicity from damage to both cochlear and vestibular portions of the auditory nerve. Such damage can be minimized by immediate withdrawal of the drug as soon as any evidence of eighth nerve injury (ataxia, incoordination) is noticed. In cats, weight loss often precedes ototoxicity.

b) Renal injury as evidenced by urinary sediments observed as pyuria, hematuria, proteinuria, and cylindruria, which frequently cease shortly after kanamycin therapy is stopped. Older patients and those with renal insufficiency show increased rates of kanamycin-related renal injury as is also the case with ototoxicity. Subjects should be thoroughly hydrated to reduce kanamycin levels in the nephron as much as possible.

When injected intramuscularly, kanamycin may cause moderately severe but transient pain.

For use in dogs and cats only.

Presentation: KANTRIM® (kanamycin sulfate) Veterinary Injection, 200 mg/mL.

10 grams in 50 mL vial (NDC 0856-2015-50).

Compendium Code No.: 10031001 4380F

KAOLIN PECTIN

Bimeda **Adsorbent**

Active Ingredient(s): Each fluid ounce contains:

Kaolin (colloidal) .... 90 gr.
Pectin .... 2 gr.

In a palatable vehicle.

Indications: For oral administration as an aid in the treatment of noninfectious diarrhea in horses, cattle, dogs and cats.

Dosage and Administration: Shake well before using.

For oral use.

Horses and Cattle: 6-10 ounces every two (2) to three (3) hours.

Colts and Calves: 3-4 ounces every two (2) to three (3) hours.

Dogs and Cats: 1-3 tablespoonfuls every one (1) to three (3) hours.

Precaution(s): Store at a controlled room temperature between 36°-86°F (2°-30°C).

Caution(s): If symptoms persist after using the product for two (2) or three (3) days, consult a veterinarian.

Warning(s): Not for human use.

Keep out of the reach of children.

Presentation: 1 gallon containers.

Compendium Code No.: 13990221

KAOLIN-PECTIN

Durvet **Adsorbent**

Anti-Diarrheal Liquid

Active Ingredient(s): Each fluid ounce contains:

Kaolin (colloidal) .... 90 gr.
Pectin (citrus) .... 2 gr.

In a palatable vehicle. Flavorings and color added.

Indications: A palatable, oral suspension for use in controlling simple diarrhea in horses, cattle, dogs and cats.

Dosage and Administration: Administer orally after first sign of diarrhea and after each loose bowel movement, or as needed.

Cattle and Horses: 6 to 10 fl oz

Calves and Foals: 3 to 4 fl oz

Dogs and Cats: 1 to 3 tablespoons

Precaution(s): Shake well before using. Protect from freezing.

Caution(s): If symptoms persist after using this product for 2 or 3 days, consult a veterinarian.

For animal use only.

Warning(s): Keep out of reach of children.

Presentation: 32 oz (NDC 30798-007-34) and 1 gallon (3.785 L) (NDC 30798-007-35).

Compendium Code No.: 10841081 Rev 2-02

KAOLIN-PECTIN PLUS

AgriPharm **Adsorbent**

Active Ingredient(s): Contains:

Kaolin .... 90 gr. (5.8 g)
Pectin .... 2 gr. (0.13 g)

In a palatable vehicle. Flavorings and color added.

Indications: For oral administration as an aid in the treatment of noninfectious diarrhea in horses and cattle.

Dosage and Administration: Shake well before using.

For oral use only.

Horses and cattle .... 6 to 10 fl. oz.
Colts and calves .... 3 to 4 fl. oz.

The dosage may be repeated after each loose bowel movement, or as needed.

Precaution(s): Store at a controlled room temperature between 59°-86°F (15°-30°C).

Protect from freezing.

Caution(s): For animal use only.

Keep out of the reach of children.

If symptoms persist after using the product for 2 or 3 days consult a veterinarian.

Presentation: 1 quart and 1 gallon containers.

Compendium Code No.: 14570540

KAOLIN PECTIN SUSPENSION

A.A.H. **Adsorbent**

Anti-Diarrheal Liquid

Active Ingredient(s): Composition: Each fluid ounce (2 tablespoonfuls) contains:

Kaolin.......... 90 gr (5.8 g)
Pectin.......... 4 gr (0.26 g)

In a palatable vehicle. Flavorings and color added.

Indications: For oral administration as an aid in the treatment of noninfectious diarrhea in horses, cattle, dogs and cats.

Dosage and Administration: Administer orally after first sign of diarrhea and after each loose bowel movement, or as needed.

Cattle and Horses: 6 to 10 fl oz
Calves and Foals: 3 to 4 fl oz
Dogs and Cats: 1 to 3 tablespoonfuls

Precaution(s): Store at controlled room temperature between 15° and 30°C (59°-86°F).

Protect from freezing. Shake well before using.

Caution(s): If symptoms persist after using this product for 2 or 3 days, consult your veterinarian.

For animal use only.

Warning(s): Keep out of reach of children.

Presentation: 4 x 3.78 L (128 fl oz) (1 gal) jugs per case.

Compendium Code No.: 11180250 1201

KAOLIN PECTIN SUSPENSION

First Priority **Adsorbent**

Anti-Diarrheal Liquid

Active Ingredient(s): Each fluid ounce (2 tablespoonfuls) contains:

Kaolin.......... 90 gr (5.8 g)
Pectin.......... 4 gr (0.268 g)

In a palatable vehicle. Flavorings and color added.

Indications: For oral administration as an aid in the treatment of noninfectious diarrhea in horses, cattle, dogs and cats.

Directions for Use: Administer orally after first sign of diarrhea and after each loose bowel movement, or as needed.

Cattle and Horses: 6 to 10 fl oz
Calves and Foals: 3 to 4 fl oz
Dogs and Cats: 1 to 3 tablespoonfuls

Precaution(s): Storage: Store at controlled room temperature between 15°-30°C (59°-86°F). Keep container tightly closed when not in use.

Protect from freezing. Shake well before using.

Caution(s): If symptoms persist after using this product for 2 to 3 days, consult your veterinarian.

For animal use only.

Warning(s): Keep out of reach of children.

Presentation: 32 fl oz (960 mL) (NDC# 58829-233-32) and 1 gallon (3.785 L) (NDC# 58829-233-01).

Compendium Code No.: 11390443 Rev. 03-02 / Rev. 08-01

KAOLIN PECTIN SUSPENSION

Vedco **Adsorbent**

Active Ingredient(s): Each fl. oz. contains:

Kaolin.......... 90 gr. (5.8 g)
Pectin.......... 2 gr. (0.13 g)

In a palatable vehicle. Flavorings and color added.

Indications: For use as an aid in the relief of uncomplicated diarrhea and gastro-enteritis.

Dosage and Administration: Shake well before using.

Administer orally after the first signs of diarrhea and after each loose bowel movement, or as needed.

Dogs and Cats: One (1) to three (3) tablespoonfuls. If symptoms persist after using the product for two (2) or three (3) days, the diagnosis and appropriate treatment should be reconsidered.

Precaution(s): Store at a controlled room temperature between 59-86°F (15-30°C). Protect from freezing.

Caution(s): Keep out of the reach of children. Not for human use.

Presentation: 1 gallon (3.785 L) containers.

Compendium Code No.: 10941160

KAO-PEC

AgriLabs **Adsorbent**

Active Ingredient(s): Each fl. oz. contains:

Kaolin (colloidal).......... 90 gr.
Pectin (citrus).......... 2 gr.

In a palatable vehicle.

Indications: For oral administration as an aid in the treatment of noninfectious diarrhea in horses, cattle, dogs and cats.

Dosage and Administration: Shake well before using.

Administer orally. May be repeated until condition improves.
Horses and Cattle: 6 to 10 oz. every two (2) to three (3) hours.
Colts and Calves: 3 to 4 oz. every two (2) to three (3) hours.
Dogs and Cats: One (1) to three (3) tablespoons every one (1) to three (3) hours.

Precaution(s): Keep from freezing.

Caution(s): Not for human use. Keep out of the reach of children.

If symptoms persist after using the product for two to three days consult a veterinarian.

Presentation: 1 gallon containers.

Compendium Code No.: 10580630

KAOPECTOLIN

Aspen **Adsorbent**

Active Ingredient(s): Each fluid ounce (2 tablespoonfuls) contains:

Kaolin.......... 90 gr (5.8 g)
Pectin.......... 2 gr (0.13 g)

In a colored and artificial flavored palatable vehicle.

Indications: For use as an aid in the relief of simple (uncomplicated) diarrhea.

Dosage and Administration: Administer orally after the first sign of diarrhea and after each loose bowel movement, or as needed.

Cattle and Horses: 8 to 10 fl oz.
Calves and Foals: 3 to 4 fl oz.
Dogs and Cats: 1 to 3 tablespoons.

If symptoms persist after using the product for 2 or 3 days, the diagnosis and appropriate treatment should be reconsidered.

Precaution(s): Protect from freezing.

Shake well before using.

Warning(s): For animal use only. Not for human use. Keep out of reach of children.

Presentation: 1 gallon (3.785 L) containers.

Compendium Code No.: 14750510

KAOPECTOLIN™

Butler **Adsorbent**

Active Ingredient(s): Each fluid ounce contains:

Kaolin (colloidal).......... 90 gr.
Pectin (citrus).......... 2 gr.

In a palatable vehicle.

Indications: For use as an aid in the control of noninfectious diarrhea by reducing hyperperistalsis and lessening the irritation to the gastro-intestinal mucosa by the absorbent action in counteracting toxins in the gastro-intestinal tract of cattle, horses, dogs and cats.

Dosage and Administration: Shake well before using. Administer orally. The dosage may be repeated until the condition improves.

Horses and Cattle: 6-10 ounces every two (2) to three (3) hours.
Foals and Calves: 3-4 ounces every two (2) to three (3) hours.
Dogs and Cats: 1-3 tablespoons every one (1) to three (3) hours.

Precaution(s): Store at a controlled room temperature between 15° and 30°C (59°-86°F).

Keep from freezing.

Caution(s): If symptoms persist after using the product for two to three days consult a veterinarian.

For veterinary use only.

Keep out of the reach of children.

Presentation: 1 gallon (3.79 L) containers.

Compendium Code No.: 10821010

KAO-PECT+

Phoenix Pharmaceutical **Adsorbent**

Anti-Diarrheal Liquid

Active Ingredient(s): Composition: Each fluid ounce (2 tablespoonfuls) contains:

Kaolin (colloidal).......... 90 gr.
Pectin (citrus).......... 2 gr.

In a palatable vehicle.
Flavorings and color added.

Indications: For use as an aid in the relief of simple (uncomplicated) diarrhea in horses, cattle, dogs and cats.

Dosage and Administration: Shake well before using.

Administer orally after the first signs of diarrhea and after each loose bowel movement.
Cattle: 6 to 10 fl oz.
Horses: 6 to 10 fl oz.
Foals: 3 to 4 fl oz.
Dogs and Cats: 1 to 3 tablespoons

Precaution(s): Store at a controlled room temperature between 15° and 30°C (59°-86°F). Protect from freezing.

Caution(s): If symptoms persist after using this product for 2-3 days, consult a veterinarian.

For animal use only.

Warning(s): Keep out of reach of children.

Presentation: 1 gallon (3.79 L) containers (NDC 57319-281-09).

Compendium Code No.: 12560492 Rev. 11/00

KAT-A-LAX* FELINE LAXATIVE

Veterinary Specialties **Laxative**

Feline Laxative

Active Ingredient(s): Contains: Cod liver oil, caramel, lecithin, malt syrup, white petrolatum, sodium benzoate 0.1% (as a preservative), vitamin E (dl-alpha-tocopheryl acetate), 0.036 IU/g (as an antioxidant), and purified water.

Indications: A palatable formula for the elimination and prevention of hair balls in cats.

Dosage and Administration: Many cats will accept KAT-A-LAX* Feline Laxative readily. For finicky animals, place a small amount on paw. The cat will lick its paw and become accustomed to the pleasant taste.

For Hairball Prevention: Administer two or three times per week.

For Hairball Removal: For average weight adult cats: administer once daily. Squeeze approximately one inch of KAT-A-LAX* from tube. For smaller cats, vary amount accordingly.

Your veterinarian may provide specific directions for treatment; in which case, follow his directions.

Warning(s): Keep out of reach of children. For veterinary use only.

Presentation: 56.70 gm (2 oz) tubes.

*Trademark, Veterinary Specialties, Inc.

Compendium Code No.: 10950000

K-CAPS ℞

Vetus **Vitamin K_1-Oral**

Contents: Each capsule contains 25 mg of Phytonadione.

Description: K-CAPS (Vitamin K_1 Capsules) contain phytonadione with excipients in an artificially colored soft gelatin shell.

Indications: K-CAPS (Vitamin K_1 Capsules) are indicated in dogs and cats to counter hypoprothrombinemia induced by ingestion of coumarin-based compounds, common ingredients of commercial rodenticides, and other drug induced hypoprothrombinemia where it is definitely shown that the result is due to interference with vitamin K metabolism, e.g. salicylates.

Dosage and Administration: Dogs and Cats: Hypoprothrombinemia (with hemorrhage) - Administer orally at the rate of 2.5-5 mg/kg body weight (1 capsule per each 22 pounds of body weight for lower dosage or 1 capsule per each 11 pounds body weight for higher dosage) daily as conditions require up to 3 weeks.

Frequency and amount of oral administration should be guided by regular determination of prothrombin time.

The smallest effective dose should be sought to minimize the risk of adverse reaction.

Contraindication(s): Hypersensitivity to any component of this medication.

Precaution(s): Protect from light at all times.

Caution(s): Federal law restricts this drug to use by or on the order of a licensed veterinarian.

Temporary resistance to prothrombin-depressing anticoagulants may result, especially when larger doses of phytonadione are used.

It is recommended that Vitamin K_1 oral capsules be used in follow-up therapy only after administration of Vitamin K_1 injection and hospitalization is no longer required. An immediate coagulant effect should not be expected after administration of phytonadione when administered orally.

Phytonadione will not counteract the anticoagulant action of heparin.

Repeated large doses of Vitamin K_1 are warranted in hepatic disease if the response to the initial therapy is unsatisfactory. Failure to respond to Vitamin K1 may indicate that the condition being treated is inherently unresponsive to Vitamin K_1.

Discussion: Actions: K-CAPS (Vitamin K_1 Capsules) for oral administration possesses the same type and degree of activity as does naturally occurring vitamin K. The primary function of Vitamin K is to stimulate the production via the liver of active prothrombin from a precursor protein. The mechanism by which vitamin K promotes formation of prothrombin at the molecular level has not been established.

Note: Regular determinations of prothrombin time response should be performed to guide in the initial and subsequent administration of Vitamin K_1 oral capsules. The dosage should be adjusted accordingly.

Presentation: Bottles of 50 capsules each.

Compendium Code No.: 14440520

KENNEL-JEC-2™

Durvet **Vaccine**

Canine Parainfluenza-Bordetella Bronchiseptica Vaccine, Modified Live Virus, Avirulent Live Culture

U.S. Vet. Lic. No.: 124

Contents: This product contains the antigens listed above.

Preservative: Neomycin.

Indications: For vaccination of healthy, susceptible dogs and puppies as an aid in the reduction of Canine Upper Respiratory Infection (Canine Cough) caused by canine parainfluenza and *Bordetella bronchiseptica*. Field studies support the safety of KENNEL-JEC-2™ when administered to puppies as young as 3 weeks of age.

Dosage and Administration: Rehydrate the vaccine with the accompanying sterile diluent. After dehydration, extract entire contents with the nasal pipette and administer entire dose intranasally. Do not vaccinate puppies under 3 weeks of age. Puppies vaccinated between 3-6 weeks of age should be revaccinated at 6 weeks. Annual revaccination is recommended.

Precaution(s): Store out of direct sunlight at 35-45°F (2-7°C). Burn containers and all unused contents.

Caution(s): For intranasal use in dogs only. Do not vaccinate dog parenterally. A very small percentage of dogs may show sneezing, coughing, or nasal discharge for 3-10 days following vaccination. While these are usually temporary symptoms, anti-bacterial therapy may be indicated. Anaphylactoid reactions may occur.

Antidote(s): Epinephrine.

Presentation: This package contains one 1 dose vial of vaccine, one 1 ml, vial of diluent, and one nasal pipette.

Manufactured by: Boehringer Ingelheim Vetmedica, Inc., St. Joseph, MO 64506 U.S.A.

Compendium Code No.: 10841800 10431-00

KENNELSOL™

Alpha Tech Pet **Detergent**

Germicidal Detergent & Deodorant

EPA Reg. No.: 47371-131-62472

Active Ingredient(s):

Didecyl dimethyl ammonium chloride 2.31%
n-Alkyl (C_{14} 50%, C_{12} 40%, C_{16} 10%) dimethyl benzyl ammonium chloride 1.54%
Inert Ingredients 96.15%

Indications: A multi-purpose germicidal detergent and deodorant effective in hard water up to 400 ppm hard water (calculated as $CaCO_3$) plus 5% organic serum. Disinfects, cleans, and deodorizes in one labor saving step.

Recommended for use in kennels, pet shops, tack shops, veterinary clinics, animal life science laboratories, breeding and grooming establishments, schools, colleges, equine farms, hospitals, nursing homes, airports, hotels and motels. For use in households.

Bactericidal at 1:64 dilution (2 ounces per gallon of water) against the following pathogenic bacteria according to the AOAC Use-Dilution Test method, current edition, modified in the presence of 400 ppm synthetic hard water (calculated as $CaCO_3$) plus 5% organic serum: *Pseudomonas aeruginosa, Proteus mirabilis, Staphylococcus aureus, Proteus vulgaris, Salmonella choleraesuis, Salmonella typhi, Bordetella bronchiseptica, Salmonella typhimurium, Chlamydia psittaci, Serratia marcescens, Escherichia coli* (antibiotic resistant), *Shigella flexneri, Escherichia coli, Shigella sonnei, Enterobacter aerogenes, Staphylococcus aureus* (antibiotic resistant), *Staphylococcus epidermidis* (antibiotic resistant), *Streptococcus faecalis* (antibiotic resistant), *Fusobacterium necrophorum, Enterobacter cloacae, Klebsiella pneumoniae, Klebsiella pneumoniae* (antibiotic resistant), *Pasteurella multocida, Streptococcus faecalis, Pseudomonas aeruginosa* (antibiotic resistant), *Streptococcus pyogenes*.

Fungicidal against *Trichophyton mentagrophytes* and *Candida albicans* according to the AOAC fungicidal test, modified in the presence of 400 ppm hard water (calculated as $CaCO_3$) plus 5% organic serum at 1:64 dilution.

Virucidal against canine parvovirus, canine distemper, feline leukemia, feline panleukopenia, feline picornavirus, *HIV-1 (AIDS virus), influenza A/Hong Kong, Herpes simplex type 1, Herpes simplex type 2, vaccinia, rubella, adenovirus type 4, rabies, porcine parvovirus, pseudorabies, infectious bovine rhinotracheitis, and infectious bronchitis (avian IBV) according to the virucidal qualification, modified in the presence of 400 ppm hard water plus 5% organic serum at a 1:64 dilution (2 ounces per gallon of water).

Directions for Use: It is a violation of Federal Law to use this product in a manner inconsistent with its labeling.

General Use Directions for Disinfecting: For use on hard, non-porous surfaces such as floors, walls, metal surfaces, stainless steel surfaces, porcelain, and plastic surfaces. Remove gross filth and heavy soil deposits then thoroughly wet surfaces. Use 2 ounces per gallon of water for a minimum contact time of 10 minutes in a single application. Can be applied with a cloth, mop, or sponge, as well as by spraying or soaking, or for use with steam or mechanical cleaning devices. The recommended use solution is prepared fresh for each use then discarded. Rinsing is not necessary unless floors are to be waxed or polished.

Mildewstatic Instructions: Will effectively control the growth of mold and mildew plus the odors caused by them when applied to hard, non-porous surfaces such as walls, floors, and table tops. Apply solution (2 ounces per gallon of water) with a cloth, mop, sponge or spray making sure to wet all surfaces completely. Let air dry. Repeat application weekly or when growth reappears.

*Kills HIV-1 (AIDS virus) on precleaned environmental surfaces/objects previously soiled with blood/body fluids in healthcare settings or other settings in which there is an expected likelihood of soiling of inanimate surfaces/objects with blood or body fluids, and in which the surface/object likely to be soiled with blood or body fluids can be associated with the potential for transmission of human immunodeficiency virus Type 1 (HIV-1) (associated with AIDS).

Special Instructions for Cleaning and Decontamination Against HIV-1 (AIDS Virus) of Surfaces/Objects Soiled with Blood/Body Fluids:

Personal Protection: Disposable latex or vinyl gloves, gowns, face masks, or eye coverings as appropriate, must be worn during all cleaning of body fluids, blood, and decontamination procedures.

Cleaning Procedures: Blood and body fluids must be thoroughly cleaned from surfaces and objects before application of disinfectant.

Contact Time: Effective against HIV-1 (AIDS virus) on hard, non-porous surfaces in the presence of a moderate amount of organic soil (5% blood serum) when used at a 1:64 dilution (providing 600 ppm of active quaternary) in 400 ppm $CaCO_3$ hard water for a contact time of 4 minutes at room temperature (20-25°C). Use a ten (10) minute contact time for disinfection against all other bacteria, fungi, and viruses claimed (listed on labeling).

Disposal of Infectious Materials: Blood and other body fluids should be autoclaved and disposed of according to federal, state, and local regulations for infectious waste disposal.

Precautionary Statements:

Hazards to Humans and Domestic Animals: Causes eye irritation. Avoid contact with eyes. Wash thoroughly after handling.

Statement of Practical Treatment: In case of contact, immediately flush eyes or skin with plenty of water for at least 15 minutes. For eyes call a physician.

Storage and Disposal:

Prohibitions: Do not contaminate water, food, or feed by storage or disposal. Open dumping is prohibited. Do not reuse empty container.

Pesticide Disposal: Wastes resulting from the use of this product may be disposed of on site or at an approved waste disposal facility.

Container Disposal:

Plastic Containers: Triple rinse (or equivalent). Then offer for recycling or reconditioning, or puncture and dispose of in a sanitary landfill, or incineration, or if allowed by state and local authorities, by burning. If burned, stay of out smoke.

For Household Use: Securely wrap original container in several layers of newspaper and discard in trash.

Fiber Drums with Liners: Completely empty liner by shaking and tapping sides and bottom to loose clinging particles. Empty residue into application equipment. Then dispose of liner in a sanitary landfill or by incineration if allowed by state and local authorities. If drum is contaminated and cannot be reused, dispose of in the same manner.

Metal Containers: Triple rinse (or equivalent). Then offer for recycling or reconditioning or puncture and dispose of in a sanitary landfill, or by other procedures approved by state and local authorities.

General: Consult federal, state, or local disposal authorities for approved alternative procedures such as limited open burning.

Warning(s): Keep out of reach of children.

Presentation: Available in pints (12 to a case), gallons (4 to a case), 5-gallon pail, 30-gallon drum, and 55-gallon drum.

Compendium Code No.: 10140040

KENNELSOL HC™

Alpha Tech Pet **Detergent**

One-Step Germicidal Detergent & Deodorant

EPA Reg. No.: 47371-129-62472

Active Ingredient(s):

Didecyl dimethyl ammonium chloride 9.70%
n-Alkyl (C_{14} 50%, C_{12} 40%, C_{16} 10%) dimethyl benzyl ammonium chloride 6.47%
Inert Ingredients 83.83%
Total 100.00%

Indications: Disinfectant, Bactericidal, Fungicidal, Mildewstatic, *Virucidal.

A multi-purpose, neutral pH, germicidal detergent and deodorant effective in hard water up to 400 ppm hard water (calculated as $CaCO_3$) in the presence of a moderate amount of soil (5% organic serum) according to the AOAC Use-dilution Test. Disinfects, cleans, and deodorizes in one labor-saving step.

Effective against the following pathogens: *Pseudomonas aeruginosa1*, *Adenovirus type 4, *Staphylococcus aureus1*, *Avian polyomavirus, *Salmonella choleraesuis*, *Canine distemper, *Acinetobacter calcoaceticus*, *Feline leukemia, *Bordetella bronchiseptica*, *Feline picornavirus, *Chlamydia psittaci*, *Herpes simplex type 1, *Enterobacter aerogenes*, *Herpes simplex type 2, *Enterobacter aerogenes*, *HIV-1 (AIDS virus), *Escherichia coli1*, *Infectious bovine rhinotracheitis, *Fusobacterium necrophorum*, *Infectious bronchitis (Avian IBV), *Klebsiella pneumoniae*, *Influenza A/Hong Kong, *Legionella pneumophila*, *Pseudorabies, *Listeria monocytogenes*, *Rabies, *Pasteurella multocida*, *Rubella (German Measles), *Proteus mirabilis*, *Transmissible gastroenteritis, *Proteus vulgaris*, *Vaccinia, *Salmonella enteritidis*, *Respiratory Syncytial virus (RSV), *Salmonella typhi, Salmonella typhimurium, Serratia marcescens, Shigella flexneri, Shigella sonnei, Staphylococcus aureus* (Methicillin resistant - MRSA), *Staphylococcus aureus* (Vancomycin Intermediate Resistant -VISA), *Staphylococcus epidermidis2*, *Streptococcus faecalis1*, *Aspergillus niger*, *Streptococcus pyogenes*, *Candida albicans*, *Enterococcus faecalis*, *Trichophyton mentagrophytes* (Vancomycin Resistant).

1 ATCC and antibiotic-resistant strain

2 antibiotic-resistant strain only

Directions for Use: It is a violation of Federal law to use this product in a manner inconsistent with its labeling.

This product is not to be used as a terminal sterilant / high level disinfectant on any surface or instrument that (1) is introduced directly into the human body, either into or in contact with the bloodstream or normally sterile areas of the body, or (2) contacts intact mucous membranes but which does not ordinarily penetrate the blood barrier or otherwise enter normally sterile areas of the body. This product may be used to preclean or decontaminate critical or semi-critical devices prior to sterilization or high-level disinfection.

Recommended for use in kennels, pet shops, veterinary clinics, animal life science laboratories, breeding establishments, grooming establishments, schools, colleges, federally inspected meat and poultry establishments, equine farms, tack shops, poultry farms, turkey farms, dairy farms, hog farms, and households. Disinfects, cleans, and deodorizes the following hard nonporous inanimate surfaces: floors, walls, metal surfaces, stainless steel surfaces, glazed porcelain, plastic surfaces (such as polypropylene, polystyrene, etc.).

Disinfection: Remove heavy soil deposits from surface. Then thoroughly wet surface with a solution ½ ounce of the concentrate per gallon of water. The solution can be applied with a cloth, mop, sponge, or coarse spray, or soaking. Let solution remain on surface for a minimum of 10 minutes. Rinse or allow to air dry. Rinsing of floors is not necessary unless they are to be waxed or polished. Food contact surfaces must be thoroughly rinsed with potable water. This product must not be used to clean the following food contact surfaces: utensils, glassware and dishes. Prepare a fresh solution daily or more often if the solution becomes visibly dirty or diluted.

USDA: For use in federally inspected meat and poultry plants as a disinfectant agent for use in all departments. Food products and packaging materials must be removed from the room or carefully protected. Use product in accordance with its label. All surfaces must be thoroughly rinsed with potable water.

Mildewstatic Instructions: Will effectively control the growth of mold and mildew plus the odors caused by them when applied to hard, nonporous surfaces such as walls, floors, and table tops. Apply solution (½ ounce per gallon of water) with a cloth, map, sponge, or coarse spray. Make sure to wet all surfaces completely. Let air dry. Repeat application weekly or when growth reappears.

Farm Premise, Livestock, Poultry and Turkey House Disinfectant:

Dilution: 1:256 (½ ounce per gallon of water).

1. Remove all animals and feeds from premises, trucks, coops, crates, and enclosures.
2. Remove all litter and manure from floors, walls, and surfaces of barns, pens, stalls, chutes, vehicles, and other facilities and fixtures occupied or traversed by animals.
3. Empty all troughs, racks, and other feeding and watering appliances.
4. Thoroughly clean all surfaces with soap or detergent, and rinse with water.
5. Saturate all surfaces with the recommended disinfecting solution for a period of 10 minutes.
6. Immerse all halters, ropes, and other types of equipment used in handling and restraining animals, as well as forks, shovels, and scrapers used for removing liter and manure.
7. Ventilate buildings, coops, cars, boats, and other closed spaces. Do not house animals or employ equipment until treatment has been absorbed, set, or dried.
8. After treatment with disinfectant, thoroughly scrub feed racks, troughs, automatic feeders, fountains, and waterers with soap or detergent, and rinse with potable water before reuse.

*Kills HIV-1 (AIDS virus) on precleaned, environmental surfaces/objects previously soiled with blood/body fluids in health care settings or other settings in which there is an expected likelihood of soiling of inanimate surfaces/objects with blood/body fluids, and in which the surfaces/objects likely to be soiled with blood/body fluids can be associated with the potential for transmission of Human Immunodeficiency Virus Type I (HIV-1) (associated with AIDS).

Special Instructions for Cleaning and Decontamination Against HIV-1 (AIDS Virus) of Surfaces/Objects Soiled with Blood/Body Fluids:

Personal Protection: Disposable latex or vinyl gloves, gowns, face masks, or eye coverings as appropriate, must be worn during all cleaning of blood/body fluids and during decontamination procedures.

Cleaning Procedures: Blood/body fluids must be thoroughly cleaned from surfaces/objects before application of disinfectant.

Contact Time: HIV-1 (AIDS virus) is inactivated after a contact time of 4 minutes at 25°C (room temperature). Uses 10-minute contact time for other viruses, fungi, and bacteria listed.

Disposal of Infectious Materials: Blood/body fluids should be autoclaved and disposed of according to federal, state, and local regulations for infectious waste disposal.

Precautionary Statements:

Hazards to Humans and Domestic Animals: Danger. Corrosive. Causes irreversible eye damage and skin burns. Harmful if swallowed. Do not get in eyes, on skin, or on clothing. When handling product, protect eyes by wearing goggles or face shield and protect skin by wearing rubber gloves. Wash thoroughly with soap and water after handling. Remove contaminated clothing and wash before reuse.

Statement of Practical Treatment: In case of contact, immediately flush eyes or skin with plenty of water for at least 15 minutes. For eyes or skin, call a physician. If swallowed, call a doctor or get medical attention. Do not induce vomiting or give anything by mouth to an unconscious person. Drink promptly a large quantity of milk, egg whites, gelatin solution, or if these are not available, drink large quantities of water. Avoid alcohol.

Note to Physician: Probable mucosal damage may contraindicate the use of gastric lavage. Measures against circulatory shock, respiratory depression and convulsion may be needed.

Environmental Hazards: Do not discharge effluent containing this product into lakes, streams, ponds, estuaries, oceans, or other waters unless in accordance with the requirements of a National Pollutant Discharge Elimination System (NPDES) permit and the permitting authority has been notified in writing prior to discharge. Do not discharge effluent containing this product to sewer systems without previously notifying the local sewage treatment plant authority. For guidance contact your State Water Board or Regional Office of the EPA.

Storage and Disposal:

(If container size is one gallon or less:) Keep product under locked storage, inaccessible to small children. Do not reuse empty container. Rinse thoroughly, securely wrap empty container in several layers of newspaper, and discard in trash.

(If container size is greater than one gallon:) Do not contaminate water, food, or feed by storage or disposal.

Pesticide Storage: Keep product under locked storage, inaccessible to children. Open dumping is prohibited. Do not reuse empty container.

Pesticide Disposal: Pesticide wastes are acutely hazardous. Improper disposal of excess pesticide, spray mixture, or rinsate is a violation of Federal law. If these wastes cannot be disposed of by use according to label instructions, contact your State Pesticide or Environmental Control Agency, or the Hazardous Waste representative at the nearest EPA Regional Office for guidance.

Container Disposal: (Plastic containers:) Triple rinse (or equivalent). Then offer for recycling or reconditioning, or puncture and dispose of in a sanitary landfill, or incinerate, or if allowed by state and local authorities, burn. If burned, stay of out smoke.

Warning(s): Keep out of reach of children.

Presentation: Available in gallons, 30-gallon drum, and 55-gallon drum.

Compendium Code No.: 10140020

KENNELSOL-NPV™

Alpha Tech Pet **Detergent**

Detergent & Deodorant

EPA Reg. No.: 1839-101-62472

Active Ingredient(s):

Alkyl (60% C_{14}, 30% C_{16}, 5% C_{12}, 5% C_{18}) dimethyl benzyl ammonium chlorides 0.80%
Alkyl (68% C_{12}, 32% C_{14}) dimethyl ethylbenzyl ammonium chlorides 0.80%
Inert Ingredients 98.40%
Total 100.00%

Indications: Cleaner, Detergent, Mildewstat (on hard inanimate surfaces), Canine Parvocidal, Disinfectant, Fungicide (against Pathogenic fungi), *Virucide.

Bactericidal Activity- When diluted at the rate of 4.5 ounces per gallon of water, this product exhibits disinfectant activity against the organisms: *Salmonella choleraesuis, Staphylococcus aureus* and *Escherichia coli.*

When diluted at the rate of 6 ounces per gallon of water, this product exhibits effective disinfectant activity against *Pseudomonas aeruginosa* in addition to the above microorganisms and meets all requirements for hospital use.

*Virucidal Activity - This product, when used on environmental inanimate hard nonporous surfaces at a dilution of 18 ounces per gallon of water exhibits effective virucidal activity against Canine Parvovirus.

Mildewstat - To control mold and mildew and the odors they cause on pre-cleaned, hard, non-porous surfaces add 4.5 ounces of this product per gallon of water. Apply solution with a cloth, mop or sponge making sure to wet all surfaces completely. Let air dry. Prepare a fresh solution for each use. Repeat application at weekly intervals or when mildew growth appears.

At the 4.5 ounces per gallon dilution KENNELSOL-NPV™ Detergent/Disinfectant is also fungicidal against the pathogenic fungi, *Trichophyton mentagrophytes.*

Efficacy tests have demonstrated that this product is an effective bactericide and fungicide in the presence of organic soil (5% blood serum).

Directions for Use: It is a violation of Federal Law to use this product in a manner inconsistent with its labeling.

KENNELSOL-NPV™ Detergent/Disinfectant has been designed to provide effective cleaning, deodorizing, and disinfection specifically for hospitals, nursing homes, households, schools, animal quarters, kennels, food processing plants, food service establishments and other institutions where housekeeping is of prime importance in controlling the hazard of cross contamination. This product, when used as directed, is formulated to disinfectant hard nonporous, inanimate environmental surfaces such as floors, walls, metal surfaces, stainless steel surfaces, porcelain, glazed ceramic tile, plastic surfaces, bathrooms, shower stalls, bathtubs, cabinets, tables, chairs, and telephones. For larger areas such as operating rooms, patient care facilities and restrooms, this product is designed to provide both heavy duty cleaning and disinfection. When used as directed, this product will remove most household dirt in a single application.

This product deodorizes those areas which generally are hard to keep fresh smelling, such as garbage storage areas, empty garbage bins and cans, toilet bowls and other areas which are prone to odors caused by microorganisms.

Disinfection - To disinfect hard inanimate surfaces apply solution with a mop, cloth, sponge or hand pump trigger sprayer so as to wet all surfaces thoroughly. Allow to remain wet for 10 minutes and then let air dry.

General Disinfection - Add 4.5 ounces of this product per gallon of water.

To disinfect toilet bowls, flush toilet, add 4.5 ounces of this product directly to the bowl water. Swab the bowl completely using a scrub brush or toilet mop, making sure to get under the rim. Let stand for 10 minutes and flush.

Hospital Disinfection - Add 6 ounces of this product per gallon of water.

For heavily soiled areas, a pre-cleaning step is required. Prepare a fresh solution for each use.

For Disinfection Against Canine Parvovirus - Add 18 ounces of this product per gallon of water.

Disinfection of Poultry Equipment, Animal Quarters and Kennels - For disinfection of pre-cleaned poultry equipment brooders, watering founts, feeding equipment), animal quarters and kennels, apply a solution of 6 ounces of this product per gallon of water. Remove all poultry, animals, and feed from premises, trucks, coops, and crates. Remove all litter and droppings from floors, walls and surfaces of facilities occupied or traversed by poultry or animals. Empty all troughs, racks, and other feeding and watering appliances. Thoroughly clean all surfaces with soap or detergent and rinse with water. Saturate the surfaces with the disinfecting solution for a period of 10 minutes. Ventilate building, coops, and other closed spaces. Do not house poultry or animals or employ equipment until treatment has been absorbed, set or dried. All treated equipment that will contact feed or drinking water must be rinsed with potable water before reuse.

Precautionary Statements: Hazards to Humans and Domestic Animals:

Danger: Keep out of reach of children. Corrosive.

Causes severe eye and skin damage. Do not get in eyes, on skin or on clothing. Wear goggles or face shield and rubber gloves when handling. Harmful or fatal if swallowed. Avoid contamination of food. Remove contaminated clothing and wash before reuse. Wash thoroughly with soap and water after handling.

Statement of Practical Treatment: In case of contact, immediately flush eyes or skin with plenty of water for at least 15 minutes. For eyes, call a physician. If swallowed, drink promptly large quantities of water. Do not induce vomiting. Avoid alcohol. Call physician immediately.

Note to Physician: Probable mucosal damage may contraindicate the use of gastric lavage.

Environmental Hazards: This pesticide is toxic to fish. Do not discharge effluent containing this product into lakes, streams, ponds, estuaries, oceans or other waters unless in accordance with the requirements of a National Pollutant Discharge Elimination System (NPDES) permit and the permitting authority has been notified in writing prior to discharge. Do not discharge effluent containing this product to sewer systems without previously notifying the local sewage treatment plant authority. For guidance contact your State Water Board or Regional Office of the EPA.

Storage and Disposal: Do not contaminate water, food, or feed by storage or disposal.

Storage - Store in a dry place no lower in temperature than 50°F or higher than 120°F.

Container Disposal - Do not reuse empty container. Triple rinse empty container with water. Return metal drum or offer for reconditioning or puncture and dispose of in a sanitary landfill, or by other procedures approved by State and local authorities. Plastic containers may be disposed of in a sanitary landfill, incinerated, or if allowed by local authorities, by burning. If burned stay out of smoke.

For Containers 1 Gallon or Less: Do not reuse empty container. Rinse thoroughly before discarding in trash.

Pesticide Disposal - Pesticide wastes are acutely hazardous. Improper disposal of excess pesticide, spray mixture, or rinsate is a violation of Federal Law. If these wastes cannot be disposed of by use according to label instructions contact your State Pesticide or Environmental Control Agency, or the Hazardous Waste representative at the nearest EPA Regional Office for guidance.

Presentation: Available in gallons, 5-gallon pail, 15-gallon drum, 30-gallon drum, and 55-gallon drum.

Compendium Code No.: 10140030

KERASOLV® GEL ℞

DVM **Grooming Product**

Keratolytic Humectant Gel for Hyperkeratotic Conditions

Active Ingredient(s): KERASOLV® is a topical gel containing salicylic acid 6.6%, sodium lactate and urea in a propylene glycol gel. Salicylic acid has been shown to produce desquamation of the horny layer of the skin while not affecting the qualitative or quantitative structure of the viable epidermis. Sodium lactate, urea and propylene glycol are humectants.

Indications: KERASOLV® is a topical aid in the removal of excessive keratin in hyperkeratotic skin disorders (calluses, thickened foot pads, planum nasale, etc.). Especially useful on geriatric animals.

Safe for use on dogs, cats and horses.

Dosage and Administration: Apply once daily, preferably after cleansing and hydration of the affected areas. Be sure to rub KERASOLV® in well so that no excess medication is visible on hair or surrounding area. Upon improvement, occasional use (2-3 times a week) will maintain remission. Hands should be rinsed thoroughly after application.

Caution(s): Federal law restricts this drug to use by, or on the order of, a licensed veterinarian.

For external use on dogs, cats and horses. Avoid contact with eyes and mucous membranes. Should erythema (swelling and redness) develop, decrease frequency of use or discontinue use and consult your veterinarian.

Presentation: 1 fl oz (30 mL) tubes (NDC 47203-375-01).

Compendium Code No.: 11420381 Rev 1197

KETAFLO™ ㊂

Abbott **General Anesthetic**

Ketamine Hydrochloride Injection, USP

ANADA No.: 200-279

Active Ingredient(s): It is chemically designated *dl* 2-(o-chlorophenyl)-2-(methylamino) cyclohexanone hydrochloride and is supplied as a slightly acid (pH 3.5 to 5.5) solution for intramuscular injection in a concentration containing the equivalent of 100 mg ketamine base per milliliter and contains 0.1 mg/mL benzethonium chloride as a preservative.

Indications: KETAFLO™ may be used in cats for restraint or as the sole anesthetic agent for diagnostic or minor, brief, surgical procedures that do not require skeletal muscle relaxation. It may be used in subhuman primates for restraint.

Pharmacology: Ketamine Hydrochloride Injection, USP is a rapid-acting, nonnarcotic, nonbarbiturate agent for anesthetic use in cats and for restraint in subhuman primates.

Action: Ketamine Hydrochloride Injection, USP is a rapid-acting agent whose pharmacological action is characterized by profound analgesia, normal pharyngeal-laryngeal reflexes, mild cardiac stimulation and respiratory depression. Skeletal muscle tone is variable and may be normal, enhanced or diminished. The anesthetic state produced does not fit into the conventional classification of stages of anesthesia, but instead Ketamine Hydrochloride Injection, USP produces a state of unconsciousness which has been termed "dissociative" anesthesia in that it appears to selectively interrupt association pathways to the brain before producing somesthetic sensory blockade.

In contrast to other anesthetics, protective reflexes, such as coughing and swallowing are maintained under Ketamine Hydrochloride Injection, USP anesthesia. The degree of muscle tone is dependent upon level of dose; therefore, variations in body temperature may occur. At low dosage levels there may be an increase in muscle tone and a concomitant slight increase in body temperature. However, at high dosage levels there is some diminution in muscle tone and a resultant decrease in body temperature, to the point where supplemental heat may be advisable.

In cats, there is usually some transient cardiovascular stimulation, increased cardiac output with slight increase in mean systolic pressure with little or no change in total peripheral resistance. At higher doses the respiratory rate is usually decreased.

The assurance of a patent airway is greatly enhanced by virtue of maintained pharyngeal-laryngeal reflexes. Although some salivation is occasionally noted, the persistence of the swallowing reflex aids in minimizing the hazards associated with ptyalism. Salivation may be effectively controlled with atropine sulfate in dosages of 0.04 mg/kg (0.02 mg/lb) in cats and 0.01 to 0.05 mg/kg (0.005 to 0.025 mg/lb) in subhuman primates.

Other reflexes, e.g., corneal, pedal, etc., are maintained during Ketamine Hydrochloride Injection, USP anesthesia, and should not be used as criteria for judging depth of anesthesia. The eyes normally remain open with the pupils dilated. It is suggested that a bland ophthalmic ointment be applied to the cornea if anesthesia is to be prolonged.

Following administration of recommended doses, cats become ataxic in about 5 minutes with anesthesia usually lasting from 30 to 45 minutes at higher doses. At the lower doses, complete recovery usually occurs in 4 to 5 hours but with higher doses recovery time is more prolonged and may be as long as 24 hours.

In studies involving 14 species of subhuman primates represented by at least 10 anesthetic episodes for each species, the median time to restraint ranged from 1.5 [*Aotus trivirgatus* (night monkey) and *Cebus capucinus* (white-throated capuchin)] to 5.3 minutes [*Macaca nemestrina* (pig-tailed macaque)]. The median duration of restraint ranged between 20 and 55 minutes in all but five of the species studied. Total time from injection to end of restraint ranged from 43 [*Saimiri sciureus* (squirrel monkey)] to 183 minutes [*Macaca nemestrina* (pig-tailed macaque)] after injection. Recovery is generally smooth and uneventful. The duration is dose related.

By single intramuscular injection, Ketamine Hydrochloride Injection, USP usually has a wide margin of safety in cats and subhuman primates. In cats, cases of prolonged recovery and death have been reported.

Dosage and Administration: Ketamine Hydrochloride Injection, USP is well tolerated by cats and subhuman primates when administered by intramuscular injection.

Fasting prior to induction of anesthesia or restraint with Ketamine Hydrochloride Injection, USP is not essential; however, when preparing for elective surgery, it is advisable to withhold food for at least six hours prior to administration of Ketamine Hydrochloride Injection, USP.

Anesthesia may be of shorter duration in immature cats. Restraint in subhuman primate neonates (less than 24 hours of age) is difficult to achieve.

As with other anesthetic agents, the individual response to Ketamine Hydrochloride Injection, USP is somewhat varied depending upon the dose, general condition and age of the subject so that dosage recommendations cannot be absolutely fixed.

Dosage —

Cats: A dose of 11 mg/kg (5 mg/lb) is recommended to produce restraint. Dosages from 22 to 33 mg/kg (10 to 15 mg/lb) produce anesthesia that is suitable for diagnostic or minor surgical procedures that do not require skeletal muscle relaxation.

Subhuman Primates: The recommended restraint dosages of Ketamine Hydrochloride Injection, USP for the following species are: *Cercocebus torquatus* (white-collared mangabey), *Papio cynocephalus* (yellow baboon), *Pan troglodytes verus* (chimpanzee), *Papio anubis* (olive baboon), *Pongo pygmaeus* (orangutan), *Macaca nemestrina* (pig-tailed macaque) 5 to 7.5 mg/kg; *Presbytis entellus* (entellus langur) 3 to 5 mg/kg; *Gorilla gorilla gorilla* (gorilla) 7 to 10 mg/kg; *Aotus trivirgatus* (night monkey) 10 to 12 mg/kg; *Macaca mulatta* (rhesus monkey) 5 to 10 mg/kg; *Cebus capucinus* (white-throated capuchin) 13 to 15 mg/kg; and *Macaca fascicularis* (crab-eating macaque), *Macaca radiata* (bonnet macaque) and *Saimiri sciureus* (squirrel monkey) 12 to 15 mg/kg.

A single intramuscular injection produces restraint suitable for TB testing; radiography, physical examination or blood collection.

Contraindication(s): Ketamine Hydrochloride Injection, USP is contraindicated in cats and subhuman primates suffering from renal or hepatic insufficiency.

Ketamine Hydrochloride Injection, USP is detoxified by the liver and excreted by the kidneys; therefore, any preexistent hepatic or renal pathology or impairment of function can be expected to result in prolonged anesthesia; related fatalities have been reported.

Precaution(s): Storage: Store at controlled room temperature 15°-30°C (59°-86°F). Protect from light.

Caution(s): Federal law restricts this drug to use by or on the order of a licensed veterinarian.

In cats, doses in excess of 50 mg/kg during any single procedure should not be used. The maximum recommended dose in subhuman primates is 40 mg/kg.

To reduce the incidence of emergence reactions, animals should not be stimulated by sound or handling during the recovery period. However, this does not preclude the monitoring of vital signs.

Apnea, respiratory arrest, cardiac arrest and death have occasionally been reported with ketamine used alone, and more frequently when used in conjunction with sedatives or other anesthetics. Close monitoring of patients is strongly advised during induction, maintenance and recovery from anesthesia.

Warning(s): For use in cats and subhuman primates only.

Adverse Reactions: Respiratory depression may occur following administration of high doses of Ketamine Hydrochloride Injection, USP. If at any time respiration becomes excessively depressed and the animal becomes cyanotic, resuscitative measures should be instituted promptly. Adequate pulmonary ventilation using either oxygen or room air is recommended as a resuscitative measure.

Adverse reactions reported have included emesis, salivation, vocalization, erratic recovery and prolonged recovery, spastic jerking movements, convulsions, muscular tremors, hypertonicity, opisthotonos, dyspnea and cardiac arrest. In the cat, myoclonic jerking and/or mild tonic convulsions can be controlled by ultrashort-acting barbiturates which should be given to effect. The barbiturates should be administered intravenously at a dose level of one-sixth to one-fourth the usual dose for the product being used. Acepromazine may also be used. However, some information indicates that some phenothiazine derivatives may potentiate the toxic effects of organic phosphate compounds such as found in flea collars and certain anthelmintics. A study has indicated that ketamine hydrochloride alone does not potentiate the toxic effects of organic phosphate compounds.

Trial Data: Clinical Studies: Ketamine Hydrochloride Injection, USP has been clinically studied in subhuman primates in addition to those species listed under Administration and Dosage. Dosages for restraint in these additional species, based on limited clinical data are: *Cercopithecus aethiops* (grivet), *Papio papio* (guinea baboon) 10 to 12 mg/kg; *Erythrocebus patas patas* (patas monkey) 3 to 5 mg/kg; *Hylobates lar* (white-handed gibbon) 5 to 10 mg/kg; *Lemur catta* (ringtailed lemur) 7.5 to 10 mg/kg; *Macaca fuscata* (Japanese macaque) 5 mg/kg; *Macaca speciosa* (stumptailed macaque) and *Miopithecus talapoin* (mangrove monkey) 5 to 7.5 mg/kg; and *Symphalangus syndactylus* (siamangs) 5 to 7 mg/kg.

Presentation: KETAFLO™ (ketamine hydrochloride injection, USP) is available in a 10 mL vial. Each vial contains the concentration equivalent to 100 mg ketamine base per milliliter, supplied as the hydrochloride.

Compendium Code No.: 10240050 58-6004 /R4 January, 2000

KETAJECT® ㊂

Phoenix Pharmaceutical **General Anesthetic**

Ketamine Hydrochloride Injection, USP

ANADA No.: 200-042

Active Ingredient(s): KETAJECT® (ketamine hydrochloride injection, USP) is chemically designated *dl* 2-(o-chlorophenyl)-2-(methylamino) cyclohexanone hydrochloride and is supplied as a slightly acid (pH 3.5 to 5.5) solution in a concentration containing the equivalent of 100 mg ketamine base per mL and contains not more than 0.1 mg/mL benzethonium chloride as a preservative.

Indications: KETAJECT® (ketamine hydrochloride injection, USP) is a rapid-acting, non-narcotic, non-barbiturate agent for anesthetic use in cats and for restraint in subhuman primates.

KETAJECT® may be used in cats for restraint or as the sole anesthetic agent for diagnostic or minor, brief, surgical procedures that do not require skeletal muscle relaxation. It may be used in subhuman primates for restraint.

Pharmacology: Action: KETAJECT® is a rapid acting agent whose pharmacological action is characterized by profound analgesia, normal pharyngeal-laryngeal reflexes, mild cardiac stimulation and respiratory depression. Skeletal muscle tone is variable and may be normal, enhanced or diminished. The anesthetic state produced does not fit into the conventional classification of stages of anesthesia, but instead KETAJECT® produces a state of unconsciousness which has been termed "dissociative" anesthesia in that it appears to selectively interrupt the association pathways to the brain before producing somesthetic sensory blockade.

In contrast to other anesthetics, protective reflexes, such as coughing and swallowing are maintained under KETAJECT® anesthesia. The degree of muscle tone is dependent upon the level of dose, therefore, variations in body temperature may occur. At low dosage levels there may be an increase in muscle tone and a concomitant slight increase in body temperature. However, at high dosage levels there is some diminution in muscle tone and a resultant decrease in body temperature to the point where supplemental heat may be advisable.

In cats, there is usually some transient cardiovascular stimulation, increased cardiac output with slight increase in mean systolic pressure with little or no change in total peripheral resistance. At higher doses, the respiratory rate is usually decreased.

The assurance of a patent airway is greatly enhanced by the virtue of maintained pharyngeal-laryngeal reflexes. Although some salivation is occasionally noted, the persistence of the swallowing reflex aids in minimizing the hazards associated with ptyalism. Salivation may be effectively controlled with atropine sulfate in dosages of 0.04 mg/kg (0.02 mg/lb) in cats and 0.01 to 0.05 mg/kg (0.005 to 0.025 mg/lb) in subhuman primates.

Other reflexes, e.g., corneal, pedal, etc., are maintained during KETAJECT® (ketamine hydrochloride injection, USP) anesthesia, and should not be used as criteria for judging the depth of anesthesia. The eyes normally remain open with the pupils dilated. It is suggested that a bland ophthalmic ointment be applied to the cornea if anesthesia is to be prolonged.

Following administration of recommended doses, cats become ataxic in about 5 minutes with anesthesia usually lasting from 30 to 45 minutes at higher doses. At the lower doses, complete recovery usually occurs in 4 to 5 hours but with higher doses recovery time is more prolonged and may be as long as 24 hours.

In studies involving 14 species of subhuman primates represented by at least ten anesthetic episodes for each species, the median time to restraint ranged from 1.5 [*Aotus trivirgatus* (night monkey) and *Cebus capucinus* (white throated capuchin)] to 5.3 minutes [*Macaca nemestrina* (pig tailed macaque)]. The median duration of restraint ranged between 20 and 55 minutes in all but five of the species studied. Total time from injection to end of restraint ranged from 43 [*Saimiri sciureus* (squirrel monkey)] to 183 minutes [*Macaca nemestrina* (pig tailed macaque)] after injection. Recovery is generally smooth and uneventful. The duration is dose related.

By single intramuscular injection, KETAJECT® usually has a wide margin of safety in cats and subhuman primates. In cats, cases of prolonged recovery and death have been reported.

Dosage and Administration: KETAJECT® is well tolerated by cats and subhuman primates when administered by intramuscular injection.

Fasting prior to the induction of anesthesia or restraint with KETAJECT® is not essential; however, when preparing for elective surgery, it is advisable to withhold food for at least six hours prior to the administration of KETAJECT®.

Anesthesia may be of shorter duration in immature cats. Restraint in subhuman primate neonates (less than 24 hours of age) is difficult to achieve.

As with other anesthetic agents, the individual response to KETAJECT® is somewhat varied depending upon the dose, general condition and age of the subject so that dosage recommendations cannot be absolutely fixed.

Dosage:

Cats: A dose of 11 mg/kg (5 mg/lb) is recommended to produce restraint. Dosages from 22 to 33 mg/kg (10 to 15 mg/lb) produce anesthesia that is suitable for diagnostic or minor surgical procedures that do not require skeletal muscle relaxation.

Subhuman Primates: The recommended restraint dosages of KETAJECT® (ketamine hydrochloride injection, USP) for the following species are: *Cercocebus torquatus* (white collared mangabey), *Papio cynocephalus* (yellow baboon), *Pan troglodytes verus* (chimpanzee), *Papio anubis* (olive baboon), *Pongo pygmaeus* (orangutan), *Macaca nemestrina* (pig tailed macaque) 5 to 7.5 mg/kg: *Presbytis entellus* (entellus langur) 3 to 5 mg/kg: *Gorilla gorilla gorilla* (gorilla) 7 to 10 mg/kg: *Aotus trivirgatus* (night monkey) 10 to 12 mg/kg: *Macaca mulatta* (rhesus monkey) 5 to 10 mg/kg: *Cebus capucinus* (white throated capuchin) 13 to 15 mg/kg: and *Macaca fascicularis* (crab eating macaque), *Macaca radiata* (bonnet macaque) and *Saimiri sciureus* (squirrel monkey) 12 to 15 mg/kg.

A single intramuscular injection produces restraint suitable for TB testing, radiography, physical examination or blood collection.

Clinical studies: Ketamine hydrochloride injection, USP has been clinically studied in subhuman primates in addition to those species listed above. Dosages for restraint in these additional species, based on limited clinical data, are: *Cercopithecus aethiops* (grivet), *Papio papio* (guinea baboon) 10 to 12 mg/kg; *Erythrocebus patas patas* (patas monkey) 3 to 5 mg/kg; *Hylobates lar* (white handed gibbon) 5 to 10 mg/kg; *Lemur catta* (ringtailed lemur) 7.5 to 10 mg/kg; Macaca fuscata (Japanese macaque) 5 mg/kg; *Maccaca speciosa* (stumptailed macaque) and *Miopithecus talapoin* (mangrove monkey) 5 to 7.5 mg/kg; and *Symphalangus syndactylus* (siamangs) 5 to 7 mg/kg.

Contraindication(s): KETAJECT® is contraindicated in cats and subhuman primates suffering from renal or hepatic insufficiency.

Precaution(s): Store between 15° and 30°C (59° and 86°F). Protect from light.

Color of solution may vary from colorless to very slightly yellowish and may darken upon prolonged exposure to light. This darkening does not affect potency. Do not use if a precipitate appears.

Caution(s): Federal law restricts this drug to use by or on the order of a licensed veterinarian.

For intramuscular use in cats and subhuman primates only.

KETAJECT® is detoxified by the liver and excreted by the kidneys, therefore, any pre-existent hepatic or renal pathology or impairment of function can be expected to result in prolonged anesthesia. Related fatalities have been reported.

In cats, doses in excess of 50 mg/kg during any single procedure should not be used. The maximum recommended dose in subhuman primates is 40 mg/kg.

To reduce the incidence of emergence reactions, animals should not be stimulated by sound or handling during the recovery period. However, it does not preclude the monitoring of vital signs.

Apnea, respiratory arrest, cardiac arrest and death have occasionally been reported with ketamine used alone, and more frequently when used in conjunction with sedatives or other anesthetics. Close monitoring of patients is strongly advised during induction, maintenance and recovery from anesthesia.

Adverse Reactions: Respiratory depression may occur following administration of high doses of KETAJECT® (ketamine hydrochloride injection, USP). If at any time respiration becomes excessively depressed and the animal becomes cyanotic, resuscitative measures should be instituted promptly. Adequate pulmonary ventilation using either oxygen or room air is recommended as a resuscitative measure.

Adverse reactions reported have included emesis, salivation, vocalization, erratic recovery and prolonged recovery, spastic jerking movements, convulsions, muscular tremors, hypertonicity, opisthotonos, dyspnea and cardiac arrest. In the cat, myoclonic jerking and/or mild tonic convulsions can be controlled by ultrashort-acting barbiturates which should be given to effect. The barbiturates should be administered intravenously at a dose level of one-sixth to one-fourth the usual dose for the product being used. Acepromazine may also be used. However, recent information indicates that some phenothiazine derivatives may potentiate the toxic effects of organic phosphate compounds such as those found in flea collars and certain anthelmintics. A study has indicated that ketamine hydrochloride alone does not potentiate the toxic effects of organic phosphate compounds.

Presentation: KETAJECT® is supplied in 10 mL vials (NDC 57319-291-02).

Manufactured by: Phoenix Scientific, Inc., St. Joseph, MO 64503.

Compendium Code No.: 12560502 Rev. 02-02

KETASET® Ⓒ III

Fort Dodge **General Anesthetic**

Ketamine Hydrochloride Injection, USP

NADA No.: 045-290

Active Ingredient(s): Supplied as a slightly acid (pH 3.5 to 5.5) solution for intramuscular injection in a concentration containing the equivalent of 100 mg ketamine base per milliliter and contains not more than 0.1 mg/mL of benzethonium chloride as a preservative.

Indications: KETASET® may be used in cats for restraint or as the sole anesthetic agent for diagnostic or minor, brief, surgical procedures that do not require skeletal muscle relaxation. It may be used in subhuman primates for restraint.

Pharmacology: KETASET® (ketamine hydrochloride injection, USP) is a rapid-acting, nonnarcotic, nonbarbiturate agent for anesthetic use in cats and for restraint in subhuman primates. It is chemically designated *dl* 2-(o-chlorophenyl)-2-(methylamino) cyclohexanone hydrochloride.

Action: KETASET® is a rapid-acting agent whose pharmacological action is characterized by profound analgesia, normal pharyngeal-laryngeal reflexes, mild cardiac stimulation and respiratory depression. Skeletal muscle tone is variable and may be normal, enhanced or diminished. The anesthetic state produced does not fit into the conventional classification of stages of anesthesia, but instead KETASET® produces a state of unconsciousness which has been termed "dissociative" anesthesia in that it appears to selectively interrupt association pathways to the brain before producing somesthetic sensory blockade.

In contrast to other anesthetics, protective reflexes, such as coughing and swallowing are maintained under KETASET® anesthesia. The degree of muscle tone is dependent upon level of dose; therefore, variations in body temperature may occur. At low dosage levels there may be an increase in muscle tone and a concomitant slight increase in body temperature. However, at high dosage levels there is some diminution in muscle tone and a resultant decrease in body temperature, to the point where supplemental heat may be advisable.

In cats, there is usually some transient cardiovascular stimulation, increased cardiac output with slight increase in mean systolic pressure with little or no change in total peripheral resistance. At higher doses respiratory rate is usually decreased.

The assurance of a patent airway is greatly enhanced by virtue of maintained pharyngeal-laryngeal reflexes. Although some salivation is occasionally noted, the persistence of the swallowing reflex aids in minimizing the hazards associated with ptyalism. Salivation may be effectively controlled with atropine sulfate in dosages of 0.04 mg/kg (0.02 mg/lb) in cats and 0.01 to 0.05 mg/kg (0.005 to 0.025 mg/lb) in subhuman primates.

Other reflexes, e.g., corneal, pedal, etc., are maintained during KETASET® anesthesia, and should not be used as criteria for judging depth of anesthesia. The eyes normally remain open with the pupils dilated. It is suggested that a bland ophthalmic ointment be applied to the cornea if anesthesia is to be prolonged.

Following administration of recommended doses, cats become ataxic in about 5 minutes with anesthesia usually lasting from 30 to 45 minutes at higher doses. At the lower doses, complete recovery usually occurs in 4 to 5 hours but with higher doses recovery time is more prolonged and may be as long as 24 hours.

In studies involving 14 species of subhuman primates represented by at least 10 anesthetic episodes for each species, the median time to restraint ranged from 1.5 [*Aotus trivirgatus* (night monkey) and *Cebus capucinus* (white-throated capuchin)] to 5.3 minutes [*Macaca nemestrina* (pig-tailed macaque)]. The median duration of restraint ranged between 20 and 55 minutes in all but five of the species studied. Total time from injection to end of restraint ranged from 43 [*Saimiri sciureus* (squirrel monkey] to 183 minutes [*Macaca nemestrina* (pig-tailed macaque)] after injection. Recovery is generally smooth and uneventful. The duration is dose related.

By single intramuscular injection, KETASET® usually has a wide margin of safety in cats and subhuman primates. In cats, cases of prolonged recovery and death have been reported.

Dosage and Administration: KETASET® is well tolerated by cats and subhuman primates when administered by intramuscular injection.

Fasting prior to induction of anesthesia or restraint with KETASET® is not essential; however, when preparing for elective surgery, it is advisable to withhold food for at least six hours prior to administration of KETASET®.

Anesthesia may be of shorter duration in immature cats. Restraint in subhuman primate neonates (less than 24 hours of age) is difficult to achieve.

As with other anesthetic agents, the individual response to KETASET® is somewhat varied depending upon the dose, general condition and age of the subject so that dosage recommendations cannot be absolutely fixed.

Dosage — Cats: A dose of 11 mg/kg (5 mg/lb) is recommended to produce restraint. Dosages from 22 to 33 mg/kg (10 to 15 mg/lb) produce anesthesia that is suitable for diagnostic or minor surgical procedures that do not require skeletal muscle relaxation.

Subhuman Primates: The recommended restraint dosages of KETASET® for the following species are: *Cercocebus torquatus* (white-collared mangabey), *Papio cynocephalus* (yellow baboon), *Pan troglodytes verus* (chimpanzee), *Papio anubis* (olive baboon), *Pongo pygmaeus* (orangutan), *Macaca nemestrina* (pig-tailed macaque) 5 to 7.5 mg/kg; *Presbytis entellus* (entellus langur) 3 to 5 mg/kg; *Gorilla gorilla gorilla* (gorilla) 7 to 10 mg/kg; *Aotus trivirgatus* (night monkey) 10 to 12 mg/kg; *Macaca mulatta* (rhesus monkey) 5 to 10 mg/kg; *Cebus capucinus* (white-throated capuchin) 13 to 15 mg/kg; and *Macaca fascicularis* (crab-eating macaque), *Macaca radiata* (bonnet macaque) and *Saimiri sciureus* (squirrel monkey) 12 to 15 mg/kg.

A single intramuscular injection produces restraint suitable for TB testing; radiography, physical examination or blood collection.

Contraindication(s): KETASET® is contraindicated in cats and subhuman primates suffering from renal or hepatic insufficiency.

KETASET® is detoxified by the liver and excreted by the kidneys; therefore, any preexistent hepatic or renal pathology or impairment of function can be expected to result in prolonged anesthesia; related fatalities have been reported.

Precaution(s): Color of solution may vary from colorless to very slightly yellowish and may darken upon prolonged exposure to light. This darkening does not affect potency. Do not use if precipitate appears.

Store at controlled room temperature 15° to 30°C (59° to 86°F). Protect from light.

Caution(s): Federal law restricts this drug to use by or on the order of a licensed veterinarian.

In cats, doses in excess of 50 mg/kg during any single procedure should not be used. The maximum recommended dose in subhuman primates is 40 mg/kg.

To reduce the incidence of emergence reactions, animals should not be stimulated by sound or handling during the recovery period. However, this does not preclude the monitoring of vital signs.

Apnea, respiratory arrest, cardiac arrest and death have occasionally been reported with ketamine used alone, and more frequently when used in conjunction with sedatives or other anesthetics. Close monitoring of patients is strongly advised during induction, maintenance and recovery from anesthesia.

Veterinary injection for intramuscular use in cats and subhuman primates only.

Adverse Reactions: Respiratory depression may occur following administration of high doses of KETASET® (ketamine hydrochloride injection, USP). If at any time respiration becomes excessively depressed and the animal becomes cyanotic, resuscitative measures should be instituted promptly. Adequate pulmonary ventilation using either oxygen or room air is recommended as a resuscitative measure.

Adverse reactions reported have included emesis, salivation, vocalization, erratic recovery and prolonged recovery, spastic jerking movements, convulsions, muscular tremors, hypertonicity, opisthotonos, dyspnea and cardiac arrest. In the cat, myoclonic jerking and/or mild tonic convulsions can be controlled by ultrashort-acting barbiturates which should be given to effect. The barbiturates should be administered intravenously at a dose level of one-sixth to one-fourth the usual dose for the product being used. Acepromazine may also be used. However, recent information indicates that some phenothiazine derivatives may potentiate the toxic effects of organic phosphate compounds such as found in flea collars and certain anthelmintics. A study has indicated that ketamine hydrochloride alone does not potentiate the toxic effects of organic phosphate compounds.

Trial Data: Clinical Studies: KETASET® has been clinically studied in subhuman primates in addition to those species listed under Administration and Dosage. Dosages for restraint in these additional species, based on limited clinical data, are: *Cercopithecus aethiops* (grivet), *Papio papio* (guinea baboon) 10 to 12 mg/kg; *Erythrocebus patas patas* (patas monkey) 3 to 5 mg/kg; *Hylobates lar* (white-handed gibbon) 5 to 10 mg/kg; *Lemur catta* (ringtailed lemur) 7.5 to 10 mg/kg; *Macaca fuscata* (Japanese macaque) 5 mg/kg; *Macaca speciosa* (stumptailed macaque) and *Miopithecus talapoin* (mangrove monkey) 5 to 7.5 mg/kg; and *Symphalangus syndactylus* (siamangs) 5 to 7 mg/kg.

References: Available upon request.

Presentation: KETASET® (ketamine hydrochloride injection, USP) is supplied as the hydrochloride in concentrations equivalent to ketamine base.

Each 10 mL vial contains 100 mg/mL (NDC 0856-2013-01).

Compendium Code No.: 10031011 4401G

KETA-STHETIC™ ℞

RXV **General Anesthetic**

Ketamine Hydrochloride Injection, USP

ANADA No.: 200-042

Active Ingredient(s): KETA-STHETIC™ (ketamine hydrochloride injection, USP) is chemically designated *dl* 2- (o-chlorophenyl) -2- (methylamino) cyclohexanone hydrochloride and is supplied as a slightly acid (pH 3.5 to 5.5) solution for intramuscular injection in a concentration containing the equivalent of 100 mg ketamine base per milliliter and contains 0.1 mg/mL benzethonium chloride as a preservative.

Indications: For intramuscular use in cats and subhuman primates only.

KETA-STHETIC™ may be used in cats for restraint or as the sole anesthetic agent for diagnostic or minor, brief, surgical procedures that do not require skeletal muscle relaxation. It may be used in subhuman primates for restraint.

K

Pharmacology: KETA-STHETIC™ is a rapid-acting agent whose pharmacological action is characterized by profound analgesia, normal pharyngeal-laryngeal reflexes, mild cardiac stimulation and respiratory depression. Skeletal muscle tone is variable and may be normal, enhanced or diminished. The anesthetic state produced does not fit into the conventional classification of stages of anesthesia, but instead KETA-STHETIC™ produces a state of unconsciousness which has been termed "dissociative" anesthesia in that it appears to selectively interrupt association pathways to the brain before producing somesthetic sensory blockade.

In contrast to other anesthetics, protective reflexes, such as coughing and swallowing are maintained under KETA-STHETIC™ anesthesia. The degree of muscle tone is dependent upon level of dose; therefore, variations in body temperature may occur. At low dosage levels there may be an increase in muscle tone and a concomitant slight increase in body temperature. However, at high dosage levels there is some diminution in muscle tone and a resultant decrease in body temperature, to the point where supplemental heat may be advisable.

In cats, there is usually some transient cardiovascular stimulation, increased cardiac output with slight increase in mean systolic pressure with little or no change in total peripheral resistance. At higher doses respiratory rate is usually decreased.

The assurance of a patent airway is greatly enhanced by virtue of maintained pharyngeal-laryngeal reflexes. Although some salivation is occasionally noted, the persistence of the swallowing reflex aids in minimizing the hazards associated with ptyalism. Salivation may be effectively controlled with atropine sulfate in dosages of 0.04 mg/kg (0.02 mg/lb) in cats and 0.01 to 0.05 mg/kg (0.005 to 0.025 mg/lb) in subhuman primates.

Other reflexes, e.g., corneal, pedal, etc., are maintained during KETA-STHETIC™ (ketamine hydrochloride injection, USP) anesthesia, and should not be used as criteria for judging depth of anesthesia. The eyes normally remain open with the pupils dilated. It is suggested that a bland ophthalmic ointment be applied to the cornea if anesthesia is to be prolonged.

Following administration of recommended doses, cats become ataxic in about 5 minutes with anesthesia usually lasting from 30 to 45 minutes at higher doses. At the lower doses, complete recovery usually occurs in 4 to 5 hours but with higher doses recovery time is more prolonged and may be as long as 24 hours.

In studies involving 14 species of subhuman primates represented by at least ten anesthetic episodes for each species, the median time to restraint ranged from 1.5 [*Aotus trivirgatus* (night monkey) and *Cebus capucinus* (white-throated capuchin)] to 5.3 minutes [*Macaca nemestrina* (pig-tailed macaque)]. The median duration of restraint ranged between 20 and 55 minutes in all but five of the species studied. Total time from injection to end of restraint ranged from 43 [*Saimiri sciureus* (squirrel monkey)] to 183 minutes [*Macaca nemestrina* (pig-tailed macaque)] after injection. Recovery is generally smooth and uneventful. The duration is dose related.

By single intramuscular injection, KETA-STHETIC™ usually has a wide margin of safety in cats and subhuman primates. In cats, cases of prolonged recovery and death have been reported.

Dosage and Administration: KETA-STHETIC™ is well tolerated by cats and subhuman primates when administered by intramuscular injection.

Fasting prior to induction of anesthesia or restraint with KETA-STHETIC™ is not essential; however, when preparing for elective surgery, it is advisable to withhold food for at least six hours prior to administration of KETA-STHETIC™.

Anesthesia may be of shorter duration in immature cats. Restraint in subhuman primate neonates (less than 24 hours of age) is difficult to achieve.

As with other anesthetic agents, the individual response to KETA-STHETIC™ is somewhat varied depending upon the dose, general condition and age of the subject so that dosage recommendations cannot be absolutely fixed.

Dosage:

Cats: A dose of 11 mg/kg (5 mg/lb) is recommended to produce restraint. Dosages from 22 to 33 mg/kg (10 to 15 mg/lb) produce anesthesia that is suitable for diagnostic or minor surgical procedures that do not require skeletal muscle relaxation.

Subhuman Primates: The recommended restraint dosages of KETA-STHETIC™ (ketamine hydrochloride injection, USP) for the following species are: *Cercocebus torquatus* (white-collared mangabey), *Papio cynocephalus* (yellow baboon), *Pan troglodytes verus* (chimpanzee), *Papio anubis* (olive baboon), *Pongo pygmaeus* (orangutan), *Macaca nemestrina* (pig-tailed macaque) 5 to 7.5 mg/kg; *Presbytis entellus* (entellus langur) 3 to 5 mg/kg; *Gorilla gorilla gorilla* (gorilla) 7 to 10 mg/kg; *Aotus trivirgatus* (night monkey) 10 to 12 mg/kg; *Macaca mulatto* (rhesus monkey) 5 to 10 mg/kg; *Cebus capucinus* (white-throated capuchin) 13 to 15 mg/kg; and *Macaca fascicularis* (crab-eating macaque), *Macaca radiata* (bonnet macaque) and *Saimiri sciureus* (squirrel monkey) 12 to 15 mg/kg.

A single intramuscular injection produces restraint suitable for TB testing; radiography, physical examination or blood collection.

Contraindication(s): KETA-STHETIC™ is contraindicated in cats and subhuman primates suffering from renal or hepatic insufficiency.

Precaution(s): Store at controlled room temperature between 15°-30°C (59°-86°F).

Protect from light.

Color of solution may vary from colorless to very slightly yellowish and may darken upon prolonged exposure to light. This darkening does not affect potency. Do not use if precipitate appears.

Not more than 0.1 mg/mL benzethonium chloride added as a preservative.

Caution(s): Federal law restricts this drug to use by or on the order of a licensed veterinarian.

KETA-STHETIC™ is detoxified by the liver and excreted by the kidneys; therefore, any pre-existent hepatic or renal pathology or impairment of function can be expected to result in prolonged anesthesia; related fatalities have been reported.

In cats, doses in excess of 50 mg/kg during any single procedure should not be used. The maximum recommended dose in subhuman primates is 40 mg/kg.

To reduce the incidence of emergence reactions, animals should not be stimulated by sound or handling during the recovery period. However, this does not preclude the monitoring of vital signs.

Apnea, respiratory arrest, cardiac arrest and death have occasionally been reported with ketamine used alone, and more frequently when used in conjunction with sedatives or other anesthetics. Close monitoring of patients is strongly advised during induction, maintenance and recovery from anesthesia.

Side Effects: Respiratory depression may occur following administration of high doses of KETA-STHETIC™ (ketamine hydrochloride injection, USP). If at any time respiration becomes excessively depressed and the animal becomes cyanotic, resuscitative measures should be instituted promptly. Adequate pulmonary ventilation using either oxygen or room air is recommended as a resuscitative measure.

Adverse reactions reported have included emesis, salivation, vocalization, erratic recovery and prolonged recovery, spastic jerking movements, convulsions, muscular tremors, hypertonicity, opisthotonos, dyspnea and cardiac arrest. In the cat, myoclonic jerking and/or mild tonic convulsions can be controlled by ultrashort-acting barbiturates which should be given to effect. The barbiturates should be administered intravenously at a dose level of one-sixth to one-fourth the usual dose for the product being used. Acepromazine may also be used. However, recent information indicates that some phenothiazine derivatives may potentiate the toxic effects of organic phosphate compounds such as found in flea collars and certain anthelmintics. A study has indicated that ketamine hydrochloride alone does not potentiate the toxic effects of organic phosphate compounds.

Trial Data: Clinical Studies: Ketamine hydrochloride injection, USP has been clinically studied in subhuman primates in addition to those species listed under Administration and Dosage. Dosages for restraint in these additional species, based on limited clinical data, are: *Cercopithecus aethiops* (grivet), *Papio papio* (guinea baboon) 10 to 12 mg/kg; *Erythrocebus patas patas* (patas monkey) 3 to 5 mg/kg; *Hylobates lar* (white-handed gibbon) 5 to 10 mg/kg; *Lemur catta* (ringtailed lemur) 7.5 to 10 mg/kg; *Macaca fuscata* (Japanese macaque) 5 mg/kg; *Macaca speciosa* (stumptailed macaque) and *Miopithecus talapoin* (mangrove monkey) 5 to 7.5 mg/kg; and *Symphalangus syndactylus* (siamangs) 5 to 7 mg/kg.

Presentation: 10 mL vial.

Compendium Code No.: 10910080

KETA-THESIA™ Ⓒⅲ

Vetus **General Anesthetic**

Ketamine Hydrochloride Injection, USP

ANADA No.: 200-279

Active Ingredient(s): It is chemically designated *dl* 2-(o-chlorophenyl)-2-(methylamino) cyclohexanone hydrochloride and is supplied as a slightly acid (pH 3.5 to 5.5) solution for intramuscular injection in a concentration containing the equivalent of 100 mg ketamine base per milliliter and contains 0.1 mg/mL benzethonium chloride as a preservative.

Indications: KETA-THESIA™ may be used in cats for restraint or as the sole anesthetic agent for diagnostic or minor, brief, surgical procedures that do not require skeletal muscle relaxation. It may be used in subhuman primates for restraint.

Pharmacology: Ketamine Hydrochloride Injection, USP is a rapid-acting, nonnarcotic, nonbarbiturate agent for anesthetic use in cats and for restraint in subhuman primates.

Action: Ketamine Hydrochloride Injection, USP is a rapid-acting agent whose pharmacological action is characterized by profound analgesia, normal pharyngeal-laryngeal reflexes, mild cardiac stimulation and respiratory depression. Skeletal muscle tone is variable and may be normal, enhanced or diminished. The anesthetic state produced does not fit into the conventional classification of stages of anesthesia, but instead Ketamine Hydrochloride Injection, USP produces a state of unconsciousness which has been termed "dissociative" anesthesia in that it appears to selectively interrupt association pathways to the brain before producing somesthetic sensory blockade.

In contrast to other anesthetics, protective reflexes, such as coughing and swallowing are maintained under Ketamine Hydrochloride Injection, USP anesthesia. The degree of muscle tone is dependent upon level of dose; therefore, variations in body temperature may occur. At low dosage levels there may be an increase in muscle tone and a concomitant slight increase in body temperature. However, at high dosage levels there is some diminution in muscle tone and a resultant decrease in body temperature, to the point where supplemental heat may be advisable.

In cats, there is usually some transient cardiovascular stimulation, increased cardiac output with slight increase in mean systolic pressure with little or no change in total peripheral resistance. At higher doses the respiratory rate is usually decreased.

The assurance of a patent airway is greatly enhanced by virtue of maintained pharyngeal-laryngeal reflexes. Although some salivation is occasionally noted, the persistence of the swallowing reflex aids in minimizing the hazards associated with ptyalism. Salivation may be effectively controlled with atropine sulfate in dosages of 0.04 mg/kg (0.02 mg/lb) in cats and 0.01 to 0.05 mg/kg (0.005 to 0.025 mg/lb) in subhuman primates.

Other reflexes, e.g., corneal, pedal, etc., are maintained during Ketamine Hydrochloride Injection, USP anesthesia, and should not be used as criteria for judging depth of anesthesia.

The eyes normally remain open with the pupils dilated. It is suggested that a bland ophthalmic ointment be applied to the cornea if anesthesia is to be prolonged.

Following administration of recommended doses, cats become ataxic in about 5 minutes with anesthesia usually lasting from 30 to 45 minutes at higher doses. At the lower doses, complete recovery usually occurs in 4 to 5 hours but with higher doses recovery time is more prolonged and may be as long as 24 hours.

In studies involving 14 species of subhuman primates represented by at least 10 anesthetic episodes for each species, the median time to restraint ranged from 1.5 [*Aotus trivirgatus* (night monkey) and *Cebus capucinus* (white-throated capuchin)] to 5.3 minutes [*Macaca nemestrina* (pig-tailed macaque)]. The median duration of restraint ranged between 20 and 55 minutes in all but five of the species studied. Total time from injection to end of restraint ranged from 43 [*Saimiri sciureus* (squirrel monkey)] to 183 minutes [*Macaca nemestrina* (pig-tailed macaque)] after injection. Recovery is generally smooth and uneventful. The duration is dose related.

By single intramuscular injection, Ketamine Hydrochloride Injection, USP usually has a wide margin of safety in cats and subhuman primates. In cats, cases of prolonged recovery and death have been reported.

Dosage and Administration: Ketamine Hydrochloride Injection, USP is well tolerated by cats and subhuman primates when administered by intramuscular injection.

Fasting prior to induction of anesthesia or restraint with Ketamine Hydrochloride Injection, USP is not essential; however, when preparing for elective surgery, it is advisable to withhold food for at least six hours prior to administration of Ketamine Hydrochloride Injection, USP.

Anesthesia may be of shorter duration in immature cats. Restraint in subhuman primate neonates (less than 24 hours of age) is difficult to achieve.

As with other anesthetic agents, the individual response to Ketamine Hydrochloride Injection, USP is somewhat varied depending upon the dose, general condition and age of the subject so that dosage recommendations cannot be absolutely fixed.

Dosage —

Cats: A dose of 11 mg/kg (5 mg/lb) is recommended to produce restraint. Dosages from 22 to 33 mg/kg (10 to 15 mg/lb) produce anesthesia that is suitable for diagnostic or minor surgical procedures that do not require skeletal muscle relaxation.

Subhuman Primates: The recommended restraint dosages of Ketamine Hydrochloride Injection, USP for the following species are: *Cercocebus torquatus* (white-collared mangabey), *Papio cynocephalus* (yellow baboon), *Pan troglodytes verus* (chimpanzee), *Papio anubis* (olive baboon), *Pongo pygmaeus* (orangutan), *Macaca nemestrina* (pig-tailed macaque) 5 to 7.5 mg/kg; *Presbytis entellus* (entellus langur) 3 to 5 mg/kg; *Gorilla gorilla gorilla* (gorilla) 7 to 10 mg/kg; *Aotus trivirgatus* (night monkey) 10 to 12 mg/kg; *Macaca mulatta* (rhesus monkey) 5 to 10 mg/kg; *Cebus capucinus* (white-throated capuchin) 13 to 15 mg/kg; and *Macaca fascicularis* (crab-eating macaque), *Macaca radiata* (bonnet macaque) and *Saimiri sciureus* (squirrel monkey) 12 to 15 mg/kg.

A single intramuscular injection produces restraint suitable for TB testing; radiography, physical examination or blood collection.

Contraindication(s): Ketamine Hydrochloride Injection, USP is contraindicated in cats and subhuman primates suffering from renal or hepatic insufficiency.

Ketamine Hydrochloride Injection, USP is detoxified by the liver and excreted by the kidneys; therefore, any preexistent hepatic or renal pathology or impairment of function can be expected to result in prolonged anesthesia; related fatalities have been reported.

Precaution(s): Storage: Store at controlled room temperature 15°-30°C (59°-86°F). Protect from light.

Caution(s): Federal law restricts this drug to use by or on the order of a licensed veterinarian.

Veterinary injection for intramuscular use in cats and subhuman primates only.

In cats, doses in excess of 50 mg/kg during any single procedure should not be used. The maximum recommended dose in subhuman primates is 40 mg/kg.

To reduce the incidence of emergence reactions, animals should not be stimulated by sound or handling during the recovery period. However, this does not preclude the monitoring of vital signs.

Apnea, respiratory arrest, cardiac arrest and death have occasionally been reported with ketamine used alone, and more frequently when used in conjunction with sedatives or other anesthetics. Close monitoring of patients is strongly advised during induction, maintenance and recovery from anesthesia.

For use in cats and subhuman primates only.

Adverse Reactions: Respiratory depression may occur following administration of high doses of Ketamine Hydrochloride Injection, USP. If at any time respiration becomes excessively depressed and the animal becomes cyanotic, resuscitative measures should be instituted promptly. Adequate pulmonary ventilation using either oxygen or room air is recommended as a resuscitative measure.

Adverse reactions reported have included emesis, salivation, vocalization, erratic recovery and prolonged recovery, spastic jerking movements, convulsions, muscular tremors, hypertonicity, opisthotonos, dyspnea and cardiac arrest. In the cat, myoclonic jerking and/or mild tonic convulsions can be controlled by ultrashort-acting barbiturates which should be given to effect. The barbiturates should be administered intravenously at a dose level of one-sixth to one-fourth the usual dose for the product being used. Acepromazine may also be used. However, some information indicates that some phenothiazine derivatives may potentiate the toxic effects of organic phosphate compounds such as found in flea collars and certain anthelmintics. A study has indicated that ketamine hydrochloride alone does not potentiate the toxic effects of organic phosphate compounds.

Trial Data: Clinical Studies: Ketamine Hydrochloride Injection, USP has been clinically studied in subhuman primates in addition to those species listed under Administration and Dosage. Dosages for restraint in these additional species, based on limited clinical data are: *Cercopithecus aethiops* (grivet), *Papio papio* (guinea baboon) 10 to 12 mg/kg; *Erythrocebus patas patas* (patas monkey) 3 to 5 mg/kg; *Hylobates lar* (white-handed gibbon) 5 to 10 mg/kg; *Lemur catta* (ringtailed lemur) 7.5 to 10 mg/kg; *Macaca fuscata* (Japanese macaque) 5 mg/kg; *Macaca speciosa* (stumptailed macaque) and *Miopithecus talapoin* (mangrove monkey) 5 to 7.5 mg/kg; and *Symphalangus syndactylus* (siamangs) 5 to 7 mg/kg.

References: Available upon request.

Presentation: KETA-THESIA™ (ketamine hydrochloride injection, USP) is available in a 10 mL vial. Each vial contains the concentration equivalent to 100 mg ketamine base per milliliter, supplied as the hydrochloride (NDC# 47611-486-70).

Manufactured by: Abbott Laboratories, North Chicago, IL 60064.

Distributed by: Burns Veterinary Supply, Inc., Westbury, NY 11590.

Compendium Code No.: 14441050 58-6511-R2-Rev. July, 2001

KETAVED™ ℞

Vedco **General Anesthetic**

Ketamine Hydrochloride Injection, USP

ANADA No.: 200-042

Active Ingredient(s): KETAVED™ (ketamine hydrochloride injection, USP) is chemically designated dl 2-(o-chlorophenyl)-2-(methylamino) cyclohexanone hydrochloride and is supplied as a slightly acid (pH 3.0 to 5.0) solution in a concentration containing the equivalent of 100 mg ketamine base per mL and contains not more than 0.1 mg/mL benzethonium chloride as a preservative.

Indications: KETAVED™ may be used in cats for restraint or as the sole anesthetic agent for diagnostic or minor, brief, surgical procedures that do not require skeletal muscle relaxation. It may be used in subhuman primates for restraint.

Pharmacology: KETAVED™ is a rapid acting agent with a pharmacological action that is characterized by profound analgesia, normal pharyngeal-laryngeal reflexes, mild cardiac stimulation and respiratory depression. Skeletal muscle tone is variable and may be normal, enhanced or diminished. The anesthetic state produced does not fit into the conventional classification of stages of anesthesia, but instead KETAVED™ produces a state of unconsciousness which has been termed "dissociative" anesthesia in that it appears to selectively interrupt the association pathways to the brain before producing somesthetic sensory blockade.

In contrast to other anesthetics, protective reflexes, such as coughing and swallowing are maintained under KETAVED™ anesthesia. The degree of muscle tone is dependent upon the level of dose, therefore, variations in body temperature may occur. At low dosage levels there may be an increase in muscle tone and a concomitant slight increase in body temperature. However, at high dosage levels there is some diminution in muscle tone and a resultant decrease in body temperature to the point where supplemental heat may be advisable.

In cats, there is usually some transient cardiovascular stimulation, increased cardiac output with slight increase in mean systolic pressure with little or no change in total peripheral resistance. At higher doses, the respiratory rate is usually decreased.

The assurance of a patent airway is greatly enhanced by the virtue of maintained pharyngeal-laryngeal reflexes. Although some salivation is occasionally noted, the persistence of the swallowing reflex aids in minimizing the hazards associated with ptyalism. Salivation may be effectively controlled with atropine sulfate in dosages of 0.04 mg/kg (0.02 mg/lb.) in cats and 0.01 to 0.05 mg/kg (0.005 to 0.025 mg/lb) in subhuman primates.

Other reflexes, e.g., corneal, pedal, etc., are maintained during KETAVED™ (ketamine hydrochloride injection, USP) anesthesia, and should not be used as criteria for judging the depth of anesthesia. The eyes normally remain open with the pupils dilated. It is suggested that a bland ophthalmic ointment be applied to the cornea if anesthesia is to be prolonged.

Following the administration of recommended doses, cats become ataxic in about 5 minutes with anesthesia usually lasting from 30 to 45 minutes at higher doses. At the lower doses, complete recovery usually occurs in 4 to 5 hours but with higher doses recovery time is more prolonged and may be as long as 24 hours.

In studies involving 14 species of subhuman primates represented by at least ten anesthetic episodes for each species, the median time to restraint ranged from 1.5 [*Aotus trivirgatus* (night monkey) and *Cebus capucinus* (white throated capuchin)] to 5.3 minutes [*Macaca nemestrina* (pig tailed macaque)]. The median duration of restraint ranged between 20 and 55 minutes in all but five of the species studied. Total time from injection to end of restraint ranged from 43 [*Saimiri sciureus* (squirrel monkey)] to 183 minutes [*Macaca nemestrina* (pig tailed macaque)] after injection. Recovery is generally smooth and uneventful. The duration is dose related.

By single intramuscular injection, KETAVED™ usually has a wide margin of safety in cats and subhuman primates. In cats, cases of prolonged recovery and death have been reported.

Dosage and Administration: KETAVED™ is well tolerated by cats and subhuman primates when administered by intramuscular injection.

Fasting prior to the induction of anesthesia or restraint with KETAVED™ is not essential. However, when preparing for elective surgery, it is advisable to withhold food for at least six hours prior to the administration of KETAVED™.

Anesthesia may be of shorter duration in immature cats. Restraint in subhuman primate neonates (less than 24 hours of age) is difficult to achieve.

As with other anesthetic agents, the individual response to KETAVED™ is somewhat varied depending upon the dose, general condition and age of the subject so that dosage recommendations cannot be absolutely fixed.

Cats: A dose of 11 mg/kg (5 mg/lb) is recommended to produce restraint. Dosages from 22 to 33 mg/kg (10 to 15 mg/lb) produce anesthesia that is suitable for diagnostic or minor surgical procedures that do not require skeletal muscle relaxation.

Subhuman primates: The recommended restraint dosages of KETAVED™ (ketamine hydrochloride injection, USP) for the following species are *Cercocebus torquatus* (white collared mangabey), *Papio cynocephalus* (yellow baboon), *Pan anubis* (olive baboon), *Pongo pygmaeus* (orangutan), *Macaca nemestrina* (pig tailed macaque) 5 to 7.5 mg/kg: *Presbytis entellus* (entellus langur) 3 to 5 mg/kg: *Gorilla gorilla gorilla* (gorilla) 7 to 10 mg/kg: *Aotus trivirgatus* (night monkey) 10 to 12 mg/kg: *Macaca mulatta* (rhesus monkey) 5 to 10 mg/kg: *Cebus capucinus* (white throated capuchin) 13 to 15 mg/kg: and *Macaca fascicularis* (crab eating macaque), *Macaca radiata* (bonnet macaque) and *Saimiri sciureus* (squirrel monkey) 12 to 15 mg/kg.

A single intramuscular injection produces restraint suitable for TB testing, radiography, physical examination or blood collection.

Clinical studies: Ketamine hydrochloride injection, USP has been clinically studied in subhuman primates in addition to those species listed above. Dosages for restraint in these additional species, based on limited clinical data, are: *Cercopithecus aethicps* (grivet), *Papio papio* (guinea baboon) 10 to 12 mg/kg: *Erythrocebus patas patas* (patas monkey) 3 to 5 mg/kg: *Hylobates lar* (white handed gibbon) 5 to 10 mg/kg: *Lemur catta* (ringtailed lemur) 7.5 to 10 mg/kg: Macaca fuscata (Japanese macaque) 5 mg/kg: *Maccaca speciosa* (stumptailed macaque) and *Miopithecus talapoin* (mangrove monkey) 5 to 7.5 mg/kg: and *Symphalangus syndactylus* (siamangs) 5 to 7 mg/kg.

Contraindication(s): KETAVED™ is contraindicated in cats and subhuman primates suffering from renal or hepatic insufficiency.

Precaution(s): Store at a controlled room temperature between 59°-86°F (15°-30°C). Protect from light.

Caution(s): Federal law restricts the drug to use by or on the order of a licensed veterinarian.

For use in cats and subhuman primates only.

KETAVED™ is detoxified by the liver and excreted by the kidneys, therefore, any pre-existent hepatic or renal pathology or impairment of function can be expected to result in prolonged anesthesia. Related fatalities have been reported.

In cats, doses in excess of 50 mg/kg during any single procedure should not be used.

The maximum recommended dose in subhuman primates is 40 mg/kg.

To reduce the incidence of emergence reactions, animals should not be stimulated by sound or handling during the recovery period. However, it does not preclude the monitoring of vital signs.

Apnea, respiratory arrest, cardiac arrest and death have occasionally been reported with ketimune use alone, and more frequently when used in conjunction with sedatives or other anesthetics. Close monitoring of patients is strongly advised during induction, maintenance and recovery from anesthesia.

Side Effects: Respiratory depression may occur following administration of high doses of KETAVED™ (ketamine hydrochloride injection, USP). If at any time respiration becomes excessively depressed and the animal becomes cyanotic, resuscitative measures should be instituted promptly. Adequate pulmonary ventilation using either oxygen or room air is recommended as a resuscitative measure.

Adverse reactions reported have included emesis, salivation, vocalization, erratic recovery, spastic jerking movements, convulsions, muscular tremors, hypertonicity, opisthotonos, dyspnea and cardiac arrest. In the cat, myoclonic jerking and/or mild tonic convulsions can be controlled by ultrashort acting barbiturates which should be given to effect. The barbiturates should be administered intravenously at a dose level of one-sixth to one-fourth the usual dose for the product being used. Acepromazine may also be used. However, recent information indicates that some phenothiazine derivatives may potentiate the toxic effects of organic phosphate compounds such as those found in flea collars and certain anthelmintics. A study has indicated that ketamine hydrochloride alone does not potentiate the toxic effects of organic phosphate compounds.

Presentation: KETAVED™ is supplied in 10 mL vials.

Compendium Code No.: 10941170

KETO AMINO FORTE™

Butler — **Electrolytes-Oral**

Active Ingredient(s): Each 1,000 mL of aseptically filled aqueous solution contains:

Dextrose • H_2O	300.0 g
Sodium chloride	5.4 g
Sodium acetate, anhydrous	3.0 g
Potassium acetate	1.0 g
Calcium chloride • $2H_2O$	330.0 mg
Magnesium chloride • $6H_2O$	260.0 mg
L-glutamic acid	560.0 mg
L-arginine hydrochloride	450.0 mg
L-proline	400.0 mg
L-lysine hydrochloride	240.0 mg
L-leucine	160.0 mg
L-phenylalanine	110.0 mg
L-valine	110.0 mg
L-threonine	100.0 mg
L-isoleucine	70.0 mg
L-histidine hydrochloride	40.0 mg
L-methionine	40.0 mg
L-tyrosine	24.0 mg
Methylparaben (preservative)	0.09%
Propylparaben (preservative)	0.01%

Indications: For use as a supplemental source of dextrose, electrolytes, and amino acids in cattle.

Dosage and Administration: Administer orally as a drench or by the use of a stomach tube. The usual recommended dose in adult cattle is 500 to 1,000 mL, depending upon the size and condition of the animal.

Precaution(s): Store at a controlled room temperature between 15° and 30°C (59°-86°F).

Caution(s): Not for human use.

Keep out of the reach of children.

Presentation: 1,000 mL vials.

Compendium Code No.: 10821021

KETOCHECK™

Great States — **Ketone Test**

Description: Ketone test powder for milk, urine or plasma.

Ingredients: Sodium carbonate, ammonium sulfate, nitroprusside.

Indications: KETOCHECK™ is a test material used to detect the presence of ketone bodies in milk, urine or plasma. Ketosis, or the presence of ketones (acetones) in lactating cows, occurs within a few days to six to eight weeks after calving. The disease is usually indicated by the cow going off feed, loss of weight, nervousness, and high excitability. There is also a loss of milk production.

Test Procedure:

1. Place small quantity (1-2 g) of KETOCHECK™ powder on a plain white surface.
2. Deposit one to two drops of milk, urine or plasma onto the powder.
3. Read results after two minutes, noting any change in color of the powder.

Test Interpretation: A purple color denotes a positive test. If the test shows positive, contact a veterinarian. Colostrum milk during the first 96 hours after calving may not provide a suitable test sample.

Storage: Keep tightly closed.

Warning(s): Keep out of reach of children

Presentation: Available in 20 g and 50 g sizes.

Compendium Code No.: 14110011

KETOCHLOR™ SHAMPOO ℞

Virbac — **Antidermatosis Shampoo**

Medicated Shampoo-Antimicrobial-Antifungal Antibacterial Cleansing

Active Ingredient(s):

Chlorhexidine gluconate	2%
Ketoconazole	1%

Indications: KETOCHLOR™ is an antifungal, antibacterial shampoo to be used in the management of fungal skin conditions and bacterial dermatitis (pyoderma) responsive to ketoconazole and chlorhexidine.

Uses: KETOCHLOR™ is an antifungal and antibacterial shampoo for use on dogs and cats of any age.

Directions: Shake well before use. Wet the coat with warm water and apply sufficient shampoo to create rich lather. Massage KETOCHLOR™ into wet coat, lather freely. Rinse and repeat. Allow to remain on hair for 5 to 10 minutes, then rinse thoroughly with clean water.

Frequency of use: Initially two to three times a week for four weeks, then reducing to once a week, or as directed by a veterinarian.

Precaution(s): Storage: Store at controlled room temperature of 59°-86°F.

Caution(s): Federal law (USA) restricts this drug to use by or on the order of a licensed veterinarian.

For external use only on dogs and cats. Avoid contact with eyes or mucous membranes. If undue skin irritation develops or increases, discontinue use and consult a veterinarian.

Available through licensed veterinarians only.

Warning(s): Keep out of reach of children. Wash hands after use.

Presentation: 8 fl oz (237 mL) bottle (NDC 56311-028-08).

Compendium Code No.: 10230700

KETOFEN® ℞

Fort Dodge — **Analgesic-Anti-inflammatory**

Ketoprofen Sterile Solution, 100 mg/mL

NADA No.: 140-269

Active Ingredient(s): Each mL of KETOFEN® (ketoprofen) contains 100 mg of ketoprofen in an aqueous formulation containing: L-Arginine, 70 mg; citric acid (to adjust pH); benzyl alcohol, 0.025 mg (as preservative).

Indications: KETOFEN® (ketoprofen) is recommended for the alleviation of inflammation and pain associated with musculoskeletal disorders in the horse.

Pharmacology: Ketoprofen is a non-steroidal anti-inflammatory agent of the propionic acid class that includes ibuprofen, naproxen and fenoprofen.

KETOFEN® is a non-narcotic, non-steroidal anti-inflammatory agent with analgesic and antipyretic properties.

In horses, intravenous doses of ketoprofen ranging from 0.5 to 1.5 mg/lb resulted in dosage dependent anti-inflammatory effects in the chronic adjuvant carpitis model as depicted in the following graph.

Maximum Flexion (intravenous ketoprofen, mean ± sem, n = 4)*

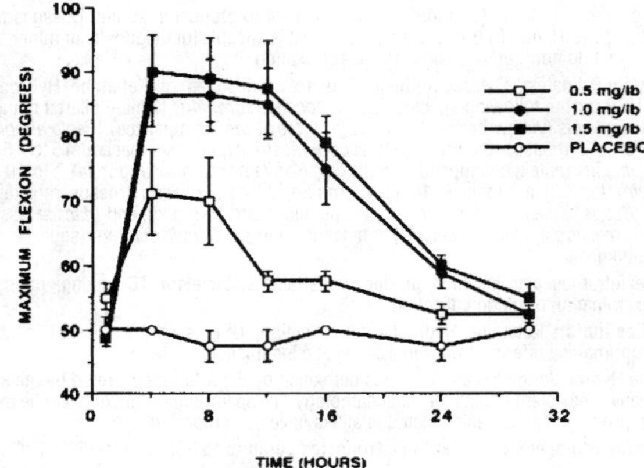

*sem = standard error of the mean

n = number of animals

Additional studies using the same model in horses have shown that the effects of ketoprofen are maximal by 12 hours and still measurable at 24 hours after each dosage as depicted in the following graph.

Maximum Flexion (mean ± sem, n = 6)*

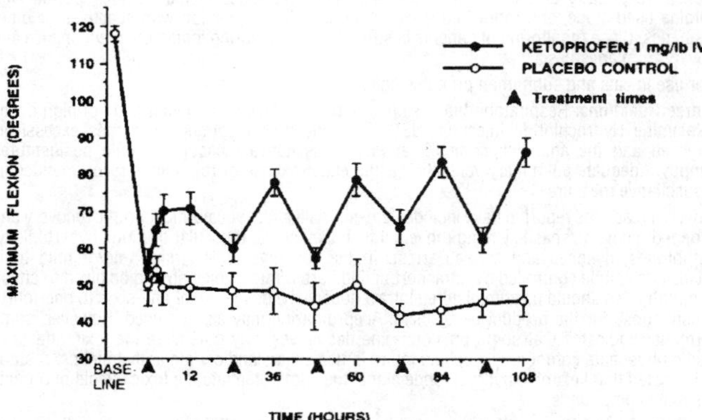

*sem = standard error of the mean

n = number of animals

Dosage and Administration: The recommended dosage is 1 mg/lb (1 mL/100 lbs) of body weight once daily. Treatment is administered by intravenous injection and may be repeated for up to five (5) days. Onset of activity is within two (2) hours with the peak response by 12 hours.

Contraindication(s): There are no known contraindications to this drug when used as directed. Intra-arterial injection should be avoided. Do not use in a horse if it has previously shown hypersensitivity to ketoprofen.

Precaution(s): Store at controlled room temperature 15° to 30°C (59° to 86°F).

Caution(s): Federal law restricts this drug to use by or on the order of a licensed veterinarian.

This product should not be used in breeding animals since the effects of KETOFEN® on fertility, pregnancy or fetal health in horses have not been determined.

Studies to determine activity of KETOFEN® when administered concomitantly with other drugs have not been conducted. Drug compatibility should be monitored closely in patients requiring adjunctive therapy.

For intravenous use in horses only.

Warning(s): Not for use in horses intended for food.

Toxicology: Toxicity: Horses were found to tolerate ketoprofen given intravenously at dosages of 0, 1, 3 and 5 mg/lb once daily for 15 consecutive days (up to five times the recommended dosage for three times the usual duration) with no evidence of toxic effects. In clinical studies, intravenous injection of 1 mg/lb/day for five days resulted in no injection site irritation or other side effects.

At 15-fold overdose (15 mg/lb/day) for five days one of two horses developed severe laminitis, but no gross lesions or histologic changes were observed. The toxic effects observed in the horses given a 25-fold overdose (25 mg/lb/day) for five days included inappetence, depression, icterus, abdominal swelling and postmortem findings of gastritis, nephritis and hepatitis.

Side Effects: During investigational studies, no significant side effects were reported.

Presentation: KETOFEN® (ketoprofen) Solution 100 mg/mL is available in 50 mL (NDC 0856-4396-01) and 100 mL (NDC 0856-4396-02) multidose bottles.

By arrangement with Rhone-Poulenc France

U.S. Patent No. 3,641,127

Compendium Code No.: 10031021 4390G

KETO-GEL™

Jorgensen **Acetonemia Preparation**

Guaranteed Analysis:

Propylene Glycol . . . . . 290 gm or 93.5%
Niacin . . . . . 6 gm or 1.9%
Choline . . . . . 6 gm or 1.9%
Methionine . . . . . 5 gm or 1.6%
Vitamin A . . . . . 40,000 IU/310 gm
Vitamin A . . . . . 10,000 IU/310 gm
Vitamin A . . . . . 100 IU/310 gm

Indications: KETO-GEL™ is a high energy gel, packed with vitamins, amino acids and trace minerals. It is used as an aid to help maintain normal blood glucose (sugar) levels during stress periods when ketosis (acetonemia) often develops.

Directions: One tube can be administered twice daily, or one tube can be administered after IV treatment of dextrose.

Administration: Load cartridge in standard dose gun and remove protective end cap. Place the nozzle near the back of the oral cavity and empty contents, allowing the cow to swallow.

Caution(s): Cow must have swallowing reflex. Nozzle should be placed near the back of the mouth. Extra care should be taken to not puncture the pharyngeal wall. If puncture occurs, you need to cease administration and contact your veterinarian.

Warning(s): For oral use only.

For veterinary use only.

Presentation: 447 gm tube, 12/case.

Compendium Code No.: 11520110

KETO-NIA-FRESH™

Vets Plus **Large Animal Dietary Supplement**

Oral High Energy Nutrient Supplement

Guaranteed Analysis: (min):

	Per Tube	Per lb.
Propylene Glycol	275 g	416 g
Vitamin A	210,000 IU	317,800 IU
Vitamin D	90,000 IU	136,200 IU
Vitamin E	75 IU	56 IU
Vitamin B_{12}	374 mcg	565 mcg
Vitamin B_6	18 mg	27 mg
Niacin	9 g	14 g
Riboflavin	37 mg	56 mg
d-Calcium Pantothenate	150 mg	227 mg
Folic Acid	10 mg	16 mg
Vitamin C	75 mg	113 mg

Ingredients: Propylene Glycol, Niacinamide, Vitamin A Acetate, d-Activated Animal Sterol (Vitamin D_3), Cyanocobalamin (Vitamin B_{12}), DL-alpha-Tocopheryl Acetate (Vitamin E), Riboflavin, d-Calcium Pantothenate, Folic Acid, Pyridoxine Hydrochloride (Vitamin B_6), Choline Bitartrate, Dextrose, Silica, Ascorbic Acid (Vitamin C), and Xanthan Gum.

Indications: Administer to every fresh cow or heifer before and after calving. KETO-NIA-FRESH™ provides propylene glycol, niacin, and other B complex vitamins to lower the incidence of ketosis, boost energy and stimulate appetite.

Dosage and Administration: Give one tube at the first sign of freshening and give another tube 6 to 12 hours post calving, repeat as needed. If the first dose is missed, a post calving dose is still beneficial.

Feeding Directions: Place the tube in a dosing gun and remove the cap. Hold the head of the cow in a slightly elevated position and place the nozzle on the back of the tongue. Administer the entire contents of the tube slowly, allowing the cow time to swallow. Do not give to cows that are unable to swallow.

Precaution(s): Keep in a cool dry place. Avoid freezing.

Caution(s): Keep out of the reach of children. Contact with eyes or wounds or prolonged contact with skin can cause irritation. Single dose unit. Properly dispose of unused portion.

Animal use only.

Presentation: 12x300 cc (300 gm) tubes per case.

Compendium Code No.: 10730090

KETO ORAL GEL

Phoenix Pharmaceutical **Acetonemia Preparation**

Nutritional Supplement

Guaranteed Analysis: Per Tube:

Propylene Glycol . . . . . 275 g
Niacin, Min . . . . . 9.6 g
Vitamin A, Min . . . . . 210,000 IU
Vitamin D_3, Min . . . . . 90,000 IU
Vitamin E, Min . . . . . 75 IU
Vitamin B_{12}, Min . . . . . 374.4 mcg
Ascorbic Acid, Min . . . . . 75 mg
Riboflavin, Min . . . . . 37.2 mg
d-Pantothenic Acid, Min . . . . . 150 mg
Folic Acid, Min . . . . . 10.8 mg
Pyridoxine Hydrochloride, Min . . . . . 18 mg
Choline, Min . . . . . 374.4 mg

Ingredients: Propylene Glycol, Niacin Supplement, Water, Vitamin A acetate (stability improved), D-activated animal sterol source of Vitamin E), Riboflavin Supplement, Calcium Pantothenic, Folic Acid, Pyridoxine Hydrochloride, Choline bitartrate, Ascorbic Acid, Starch and Xanthum Gum.

Indications: This preparation supplies these elements to ensure normal nutritional levels before, during and after calving.

A nutritional supplement for dairy cattle and calves.

Dosage and Administration: Place the tube in a dosing gun and remove the cap. Hold the head of the cow in a normal to slightly elevated position and carefully place the nozzle into the back of the mouth. Administer the entire contents of one tube per feeding to cows. Do not give to cows or calves that are unable to swallow.

Give one tube following calving. Give additional tubes as needed. As a supplement and energy source, for calves, give 15-20 mL per animal (approximately 15-20 doses per 300 mL tube) - 3-4 clicks of the delivery system.

Caution(s): Contact with eyes or wounds or prolonged contact with skin can cause irritation.

For animal use only.

Warning(s): Keep out of reach of children.

Presentation: 300 mL tube (NDC 57319-458-29).

Compendium Code No.: 12560511 Iss. 7-00

KETO PLUS GEL™

AgriLabs **Acetonemia Preparation**

Active Ingredient(s): Guaranteed analysis per tube:

Niacin, min. . . . . . 8 g
Propylene glycol . . . . . 235 mL
Vitamin A, min. . . . . . 175,000 I.U.
Vitamin D_3, min. . . . . . 75,000 I.U.
Vitamin E, min. . . . . . 62.5 mg
Vitamin B_{12}, min. . . . . . 312 mcg
Ascorbic acid, min. . . . . . 62.5 mg
Riboflavin, min. . . . . . 31 mg
d-Pantothenic acid, min. . . . . . 126 mg
Pyridoxine hydrochloride . . . . . 15 mg
Folic acid, min. . . . . . 9 mg
Choline, min. . . . . . 312 mg

Ingredients: Propylene glycol, niacin supplement, water, vitamin A acetate (stability improved), d-activated animal sterol (source of vitamin D_3), cyanocobalamin (source of vitamin B_{12}), d-alpha tocopheryl acetate (source of vitamin E), riboflavin supplement, d-pantothenic acid, folic acid, pyridoxine hydrochloride, choline bitartrate, starch and xanthan gum.

Indications: A nutritional supplement preparation that supplies the above elements to ensure normal levels in the blood before, during and after calving.

Dosage and Administration: Give one (1) tube following calving. Give additional tubes as needed.

Place the tube in a dosing gun and remove the cap. Hold the head of the cow in a normal to slightly elevated position and carefully place the nozzle into the back of the mouth. Administer the entire contents of one (1) tube per feeding. Do not give to cows that are unable to swallow.

Precaution(s): Store at 20°C.

Caution(s): Contact with the eyes or wounds, or prolonged contact with the skin can cause irritation.

Keep out of the reach of children.

A single dose unit, discard unused portion.

Presentation: 10.7 oz. (305 g) tubes.

Compendium Code No.: 10580640

KETO-PLUS GEL

AgriPharm **Acetonemia Preparation**

Active Ingredient(s): Minimum contents of 300 mL dose:

Cobalt . . . . . 0.150 g - 0.04%
Magnesium . . . . . 6 g - 1.6%
Propylene Glycol . . . . . 270 g
Propionic Acid . . . . . 10 g
Niacin . . . . . 15 g
Choline . . . . . 3 g
Vitamin A . . . . . 50,000 I.U.
Vitamin D_3 . . . . . 10,000 I.U.
Vitamin E . . . . . 100 I.U.
Vitamin B_{12} . . . . . 1000 mcg

Ingredients: Propylene glycol, silicon dioxide, niacin, vitamin A propionate, vitamin A palmitate, d-activated animal sterol (source of vitamin D_3), dl-alpha tocopherol acetate (source of vitamin E), vitamin B_{12} (cyanocobalamin), choline, cobalt sulfate, magnesium sulfate, polysorbate 80, preserved with propionic acid and ethoxyquin.

Indications: For use in cattle as an aid in prevention of ketosis.

Dosage and Administration: One tube can be administered daily to aid in prevention of ketosis or after IV treatment of dextrose.

1. Hold head of the cow in a slightly elevated position.
2. Place nozzle near rear of mouth. Use of hook nozzle recommended.
3. Discharge entire contents of the tube.
4. Hold up head of cow and allow animal time to swallow.

Precaution(s): Do not freeze. Keep cool.

Warning(s): For animal use only.

Keep out of reach of children.

Presentation: 300 mL.

Compendium Code No.: 14570550

KETO "PLUS" GEL

Durvet — **Acetonemia Preparation**

Active Ingredient(s): Minimum contents of 300 mL dose:

Propylene Glycol	270 gm
Propionic Acid	10 gm
Niacin	15 gm
Choline	3 gm
Vitamin A	50,000 I.U.
Vitamin D_3	10,000 I.U.
Vitamin E	100 I.U.
Vitamin B_{12}	1,000 I.U.

Ingredients: Propylene Glycol, Silicon Dioxide, Niacin, Vitamin A Propionate, Vitamin A Palmitate, D-activated animal sterol (source of vitamin D_3), dl-Alpha Tocopheryl Acetate (source of vitamin E), Vitamin B_{12} (Cyanocobalamin), Choline, Cobalt Sulfate, Magnesium Sulfate, Polysorbate 80, preserved with Propionic Acid and Ethoxyquin.

Indications: For use as an aid in the prevention of ketosis.

Directions for Use:

1. Hold head of the cow in a slightly elevated position.
2. Place nozzle near rear of mouth. Use of a hook nozzle is recommended.
3. Discharge entire contents of the tube.
4. Hold head up and allow animal time to swallow.

Give one tube prior to or after calving and a second tube 12 to 24 hours after calving.

Precaution(s): Do not freeze.

Caution(s): For animal use only. Not for human use.

Warning(s): Not a drug. No withdrawal time.

Keep out of reach of children.

Presentation: 300 mL tube (NDC: 30798-562-15).

Patent Pending

Compendium Code No.: 10841091 — 6/01

KETO PLUS ORAL GEL

Butler — **Acetonemia Preparation**

Active Ingredient(s): Minimum contents of 300 mL dose:

Cobalt	0.15 g (0.04%)
Magnesium	6 g (1.6%)
Propylene glycol	270 g
Propionic acid	10 g
Niacin	15 g
Choline	3 g
Vitamin A	50,000 I.U.
Vitamin D_3	10,000 I.U.
Vitamin E	100 I.U.
Vitamin B_{12}	1,000 mcg

Ingredients: Propylene glycol, silicon dioxide, niacin, vitamin A propionate, vitamin A palmitate, d-activated animal sterol (source of vitamin D_3), dl-alpha tocopheryl acetate (source of vitamin E), vitamin B_{12} (cyanocobalamin), choline, cobalt sulfate, magnesium sulfate, polysorbate 80, preserved with propionic acid and ethoxyquin.

Indications: For use as an aid in the prevention of ketosis.

Dosage and Administration:

1. Hold the head of the cow in a slightly elevated position.
2. Place the nozzle near the rear of the mouth. The use of a hook nozzle is recommended.
3. Discharge the entire contents of the tube.
4. Hold the head up and allow the animal time to swallow.

One (1) tube can be administered every day to aid in the prevention of ketosis or after I.V. administration of dextrose.

Precaution(s): Keep cool.

Presentation: 300 mL tube.

Compendium Code No.: 10821030

KETOPRO ORAL GEL

Vedco — **Acetonemia Preparation**

Ingredient(s): Polyethylene glycol, silicon dioxide, niacin, vitamin A propionate, vitamin A palmitate, vitamin D_3, dl-alpha tocopheryl acetate, cyanocobalamin, choline, cobalt sulfate, magnesium sulfate, polysorbate 80, preserved with propionic acid and ethoxyquin.

Minimum contents of 300 mL dose:

Cobalt	0.150 g - 0.04%
Magnesium	6 g - 1.6%
Propylene Glycol	270 g
Propionic Acid	10 g
Niacin	15 g
Choline	3 g
Vitamin A	50,000 I.U.
Vitamin D_3	10,000 I.U.
Vitamin E	100 I.U.
Vitamin B_{12}	1000 mcg

Indications: A high energy gel to be used as an aid in the prevention of ketosis.

Dosage and Administration: One tube can be administered daily to aid in prevention of ketosis or after IV treatment of dextrose.

1. Hold head of the cow in a slightly elevated position.
2. Place nozzle near rear of mouth.
3. Discharge entire contents of the tube.
4. Hold head up and allow animal time to swallow.

Precaution(s): Keep cool.

Presentation: One dose (300 mL).

Compendium Code No.: 10941180

KILTIX®

Topical Tick Control

Bayer

Pleasant Citrus Scent

Tick Control for Dogs and Puppies over 12 Weeks of Age

- Kills and Repels Ticks for up to 4 weeks.
- Kills and Repels Deer Ticks (vector of Lyme Disease) for up to 4 weeks.
- Kills and Repels Brown Dog Ticks *(Rhipicephalus sanguineus)* for up to 3 to 4 weeks.
- Kills and Repels American Dog Ticks *(Dermacentor variabilis)* for up to 3 to 4 weeks.
- Protects against Blood Feeding Mosquitoes (vector of Heartworm) for up to 4 weeks.
- Monthly Application.

Active Ingredients

*Permethrin	45%
Other Ingredients	55%
Total	100%

*cis/trans ratio: Max 55% (±) cis and min 45% (±) trans

KEEP OUT OF REACH OF CHILDREN

CAUTION

DO NOT USE ON CATS

READ ENTIRE LABEL BEFORE EACH USE

USE ONLY ON DOGS OVER 12 WEEKS OF AGE

PRECAUTIONARY STATEMENTS

HAZARDS TO HUMANS AND DOMESTIC ANIMALS

CAUTION

Hazards to Humans: Harmful if swallowed. Avoid contact with eyes or clothing. Causes moderate eye irritation. Wash thoroughly with soap and water after handling.

Hazards to Domestic Animals: FOR EXTERNAL USE ON DOGS ONLY. Do not use on puppies under 12 weeks of age. Consult a veterinarian before using this product on debilitated, aged, medicated, pregnant, or nursing dogs. Consult a veterinarian before using on dogs with known organ dysfunction. **DO NOT USE ON CATS** or animals other than dogs. Cats which actively groom or engage in close physical contact with recently treated dogs may be at risk of toxic exposure. Certain medications can interact with pesticides. It is advisable to consult a veterinarian before using this product with any other pesticide or drug.

FIRST AID

If Swallowed:

Call a poison control center or doctor immediately for treatment advice.

Have person sip a glass of water if able to swallow.

Do not induce vomiting unless told to do so by a poison control center or doctor.

Do not give anything by mouth to an unconscious person.

If in Eyes:

Hold eyes open and rinse slowly and gently with water for 15-20 minutes.

Remove contact lenses, if present, after the first five minutes, then continue rinsing eyes.

Call a poison control center or doctor for treatment advice.

HOT LINE NUMBER

Have a product container or label with you when calling a poison control center or doctor for treatment. You may also contact the product information center at 1-800-255-6826, or for emergency medical treatment information call 1-877-258-2280.

Adverse Reactions: Some animals may be sensitive to ingredients in this product. Reactions in dogs may include skin sensitivity. Dogs may show lethargy, increased pruritis (itchiness), erythema (redness), rash and hair discoloration or hair loss at the application site. Observe the dog following treatment. Sensitivity may occur after using ANY pesticide product on pets. If signs of sensitivity occur bathe your dog with a mild, non-insecticidal shampoo and rinse with large amounts of water. If signs continue, consult a veterinarian immediately.

PHYSICAL OR CHEMICAL HAZARDS

DO NOT USE OR STORE NEAR HEAT OR OPEN FLAMES

ENVIRONMENTAL HAZARDS

This product is extremely toxic to fish. Do not add directly to water. Do not contaminate water when disposing of product or packaging.

DIRECTIONS FOR USE

It is a violation of Federal Law to use this product in a manner inconsistent with its labeling.

DO NOT USE ON CATS or animals other than dogs. Do not get this product in your dog's eyes or mouth. Repeat applications may be made if necessary, but do not apply more often than once every 3 weeks, except to reapply after shampooing the dog.

For Dogs Weighing Less Than 33 Pounds: Apply one tube (1.5 mL) of KILTIX® Topical Tick Control as a spot between the shoulder blades or as a stripe to the dog's back.

For Dogs Weighing More Than 33 Pounds: Apply one tube (1.5 mL) of KILTIX® Topical Tick Control as a spot to the dog's shoulder blades or as a stripe to the dog's back and apply a second tube (1.5 mL) as a spot directly in the front of the base of the tail or as a stripe to the dog's back.

How To Apply:

1. Remove product tube from package.
2. Holding tube with notched end pointing up and away from face and body, snap off narrow end at notches.
3. Invert tube over dog and use open end to part dog's hair.
4. Squeeze tube firmly to apply all of the solution to the dog's skin.
5. Wrap tube and put in trash.

STORAGE AND DISPOSAL

Do not contaminate water, food or feed by storage or disposal.

Storage: Store in cool, dry place. Protect from freezing.

Pesticide Disposal: Securely wrap original container in several layers of newspaper and discard in trash.

Container Disposal: Do not reuse empty container. Wrap container and put in trash.

NOTICE OF WARRANTY

Seller makes no warranty of merchantability, fitness for any particular purpose, or otherwise, expressed or implied concerning this product or its uses which extend beyond the use of the product under normal conditions in accordance with the statements made on this label.

SUPPLIED:

Code 061799 — 1.5 mL Applicator

EPA Reg. No.: 270-279-11556

EPA Est. No.: 73634-NJ-001 — 79006170 R.2

EPA Est. No.: 73353-CAN-001 — MADE IN CANADA — 79006171 R.1

Manufactured For: Bayer Corporation, Agriculture Division, Animal Health, Shawnee Mission, Kansas 66201 U.S.A.

Compendium Code No.: 10400262

KITTEN FORMULA

Vet Solutions **Milk Replacer**

Guaranteed Analysis:

Crude Protein (min) 22%
Crude Protein from milk sources (min) 22%
Crude Fat (min) 23%
Crude Fiber (max) 0.25%
Moisture. 7%
Ash. 6.5%
Sodium 0.65%
Calcium 1.15%
Phosphorus 0.85%
Iron . . . . . 90 mg/kg
Manganese. . . . . 48 mg/kg
Zinc . . . . . 110 mg/kg
Selenium . . . . . 0.3 mg/kg
Vitamin A . . . . . 15,000 IU/kg
Vitamin D_3 . . . . . 2,000 IU/kg
Vitamin E . . . . . 100 IU/kg
Thiamine . . . . . 12 mg/kg
Riboflavin. . . . . 20 mg/kg
Niacin. . . . . 50 mg/kg
Vitamin B_{12}. . . . . 50 µg/kg
Biotin . . . . . 250 µg/kg
Ascorbic Acid . . . . . 100 mg/kg
Taurine. . . . . 1000 mg/kg

Additionally Contains:

Colostrum . . . . . 25 mg/kg
Eicosapentaenoic acid (EPA) . . . . . 68 mg/kg
Decosahexaenoic acid (DHA) . . . . . 268 mg/kg

Ingredients: Dried whey/whey product, homogenized and spray-dried animal/vegetable fat containing BHA and BHT, dried skimmed milk, corn syrup solids, dextroglucose, lecithin, L-lysine, DL-methionine, L-threonine, calcium formate, citric acid, phosphoric acid, dicalcium phosphate, taurine, Vitamin A, Vitamin D_3, Vitamin E, menadione sodium bisulphite, thiamin hydrochloride, riboflavin, niacinamide, pyridoxine hydrochloride, sodium ascorbate, choline chloride, folic acid, D-biotin, Vitamin B_{12}, iron sulphate, zinc sulphate, manganous sulphate, magnesium oxide, sodium chloride, copper sulphate, ethylene diamine dihydroiodide, cobalt sulphate, sodium selenite, silica dioxide, fish oil, flavor and aroma agents, dry colostrum.

Indications: Mother's milk replacer for kittens and food supplement for adult cats containing Colostrum and Docosahexaenoic acid (DHA).

Vet Solutions KITTEN FORMULA is a nutritionally complete milk replacer to be fed as a nutritional supplement when the supply of queen's milk is inadequate or as the sole ration for orphan kittens. When indicated, KITTEN FORMULA may be used to fortify the ration of queens to help meet the increased nutritional requirements in late gestation and early lactation. Whenever possible kittens should receive colostrum (queen's first milk) for the first 2 days, since this supplies antibodies essential to disease resistance in early life.

Dosage and Administration: Mixing Instructions: Prepare enough KITTEN FORMULA, with the enclosed measuring scoop, for use in a 24-hour period. Add 1 scoop (1 Tbsp.) per 2 scoops (1 ounce) of warm water. Stir or mix until smooth.

Feeding Instructions: Reconstituted KITTEN FORMULA solution should be fed at body temperature. Use of a nurser bottle is recommended. Feed kittens at least 2 tablespoons (30 mL) per 4 ounces (113 g) of body weight daily. Divide the daily feeding amount into equal portions for each feeding. For the first 4 days of feeding KITTEN FORMULA, the daily amount should be divided into 6 to 8 feedings. The number of feedings can then be gradually reduced to 4 per day (dividing the daily volumes into 4 equal parts). Kittens should be allowed to consume as much formula as they want during each feeding. Stool consistency provides a measure of the appropriate feeding level. If diarrhea develops, reduce the concentration of the solution (i.e. maintain water level but reduce the level of KITTEN FORMULA by 10-20% until stool consistency returns to normal). Should diarrhea persist, consult a veterinarian for advice. Cleanliness of feeding equipment (nursing bottle/bowl) is extremely important. Always wash with hot, soapy water, rinse and dry well after each use.

Weaning Kittens: When kittens are old enough to lap, begin offering reconstituted formula in a shallow bowl. Wean kittens between 4-6 weeks of age. Mix equal parts of KITTEN FORMULA and weaning cereal or kitten food and add enough water to make a soupy gruel. Gradually increase the proportion of kitten food until kitten is on solid food. Ensure a source of clean water is always available.

Pregnant and lactating queens: Feed 2 teaspoons (4 g) per 5 lbs. (2.2 kg) body weight until 2 weeks after queening.

Growing Kittens, Show Cats and convalescing Cats: Supplement regular ration with 1 teaspoons (2 g) of KITTEN FORMULA per 5 lbs. (2.2 kg) body weight daily.

Precaution(s): Storage: Moisture and high temperature will degrade KITTEN FORMULA. Store sealed container at controlled room temperature. May be stored indefinitely in the freezer. Do not mix more than will be consumed within 24 hours. Reconstituted KITTEN FORMULA should be refrigerated.

Presentation: 200 g (7.05 oz) and 8 oz.

Compendium Code No.: 10610190 010701

K-JECT ℞

Vetus **Vitamin K_1-Injection**

Active Ingredient(s): K-JECT is a yellow, sterile aqueous colloidal solution of vitamin K1 (phytonadione), available for injection by the intravenous, intramuscular and subcutaneous routes.

Each mL contains:

Phytonadione . . . . . 10 mg

Inactive Ingredients:

Polyoxyethylated fatty acid derivative. . . . . 70 mg
Dextrose Monohydrate. . . . . 37.4 mg
Water for Injection . . . . . q.s.

Added as a preservative:

Benzyl Alcohol . . . . . 0.9% w/v

Indications: For injection by the IV, IM, and SC routes. Indicated in cattle, calves, horses, swine, sheep, goats, dogs and cats to counter hypoprothrombinemia induced by ingestion of coumarin-based compounds, common ingredients in commercial rodenticides. K-JECT is also indicated to counter hypoprothrombinemia caused by consumption of bishydroxycoumarin found in spoiled and moldy sweet clover.

Dosage and Administration: Cattle, Calves, Horses, Swine, Sheep and Goats: Acute Hypoprothrombinemia (with Hemorrhage) - intravenously, 0.5-2.5 mg/kg body weight, at a rate not to exceed 10 mg/minute in mature animals and 5 mg/minute in newborn and very young animals.

Non-Acute Hypoprothrombinemia - Intramuscularly or subcutaneously, 0.5-2.5 mg/kg body weight.

Dogs and Cats: Acute Hypoprothrombinemia (with Hemorrhage) - Intravenously, 0.25-2.5 mg/kg body weight, at a rate not to exceed 5 mg/minute.

Non-Acute Hypoprothrombinemia - Intramuscularly or subcutaneously, 0.25-2.5 mg/kg body weight.

Whenever possible, K-JECT should be given by the intramuscular or subcutaneous routes. When intravenous injection is considered unavoidable, the drug should be given very slowly, at the rate indicated above. **Monitor prothrombin time and adjust dosage accordingly.**

Frequency and amount of subsequent doses should be guided by regular determination of prothrombin time response and clinical condition. If in 6 to 8 hours after parenteral administration the prothrombin time has not been shortened satisfactorily, the dose should be repeated.

In the event of shock or excessive blood loss, the use of whole blood or component therapy is indicated. The smallest effective dose sought to minimize the risk of adverse reaction.

Directions for Dilution: K-JECT may be diluted with 0.9% sodium chloride injection, 5% dextrose injection, or 5% dextrose w/sodium chloride injection. Other diluents should not be used. When dilutions are indicated, administration should be started immediately after mixture with the diluent, and unused portions of the dilution should be discarded.

Contraindication(s): Hypersensitivity to any component of this medication.

Precaution(s): Protect from light at all times.

Store at 15°C-30°C (59°F-86°F).

Caution(s): Federal law restricts this drug to use by or on the order of a licensed veterinarian.

Regular determinations of prothrombin time response should be performed to guide in the initial and subsequent administration of K-JECT. The dosage should be adjusted accordingly.

An immediate coagulant effect should not be expected after administration of phytonadione. A minimum of 1 to 2 hours is required for measurable improvement in the prothrombin time.

Whole blood or component therapy may be necessary if the bleeding is severe.

Phytonadione will not counteract the anticoagulant action of heparin.

Repeated large doses of vitamin K are not warranted in hepatic disease if the response to the initial therapy is unsatisfactory. Failure to respond to vitamin K may indicate that the condition being treated is inherently unresponsive to vitamin K.

Temporary resistance to prothrombin-depressing anticoagulants may result, especially when larger doses of phytonadione are used.

Side Effects: Adverse Reactions: Deaths have occurred following intravenous injection.

Intravenous Use: Severe reactions, including fatalities, have occurred during and immediately after intravenous injection of phytonadione, even when precautions have been taken to dilute the Vitamin K_1 and to avoid rapid infusion. Typically, these severe reactions have resembled hypersensitivity or anaphylaxis, including shock and cardiac and/or respiratory arrest. Some animals have exhibited these severe reactions on receiving K-JECT for the first time. Therefore, the intravenous route should be restricted to those situations where other routes are not feasible and the serious risk involved is considered justified.

Pain, swelling, and tenderness at the injection site may occur. The possibility of allergic sensitivity, including an anaphylactoid reaction, should be kept in mind.

Discussion: Actions: K-JECT, an aqueous colloidal solution of vitamin K1 for parenteral injection, possesses the same type and degree of activity as does naturally occurring vitamin K. The primary function of vitamin K is to stimulate the production via the liver of active prothrombin from a precursor protein. The mechanism by which vitamin K promotes formation of prothrombin at the molecular level has not been established.

The active of the aqueous colloidal solution, when administered intravenously, is generally detectable within an hour or two and hemorrhage is usually controlled within 3 to 6 hours. A normal prothrombin level may often be obtained in 12 to 14 hours.

Presentation: 100 mL vials.

Compendium Code No.: 14440531

KLEEN-ASEPTIC®

Metrex **Disinfectant**

EPA Reg. No.: 38526

Active Ingredient(s):

Diisobutylphenoxyethoxyethyl dimethyl benzyl ammonium chloride. 0.25%
Isopropanol. 14.85%
Inert ingredients 84.90%

Indications: A broad-spectrum surface disinfectant cleanser for use in hospital areas such as operating and emergency rooms, medical and dental offices, laboratories, neonatal nurseries and other critical areas where the control of disease causing micro-organisms is necessary. May be used on non-porous surfaces such as stainless steel, glass, painted surfaces, plexiglass, plastic, chrome, tile and vinyl. Ideal for use on infant incubators, anesthesia and respiratory equipment, bassinets, laboratory equipment and countertops. Safe for use in veterinary and animal care facilities.

KLEEN-ASEPTIC® is effective against: *Pseudomonus aeruginosa, Staphylococcus aureus, Salmonella choleraesuis, Mycobacterium tuberculosis var. bovis,* and *Trichophyton mentagrophytes.* It also inhibits the growth of mold and mildew.

Deodorizer: Suppresses malodor at its source.

Dosage and Administration: Shake well before using. Hold the dispenser 6" to 8" from the surface to be cleaned and sanitized. Spray thoroughly and wipe with a clean cloth or paper towel. To control mold and mildew, repeat the application once a week or when new growth appears.

Precaution(s): Disposal: Do not re-use the empty container. Wrap the container and put it in the trash collection.

Caution(s): Keep out of the reach of children.

Warning(s): Contents under pressure. Do not use near fire, sparks or flame. Do not puncture or incinerate container. Exposure to temperatures above 130°F may cause bursting.

Avoid spraying in the eyes or on food or foodstuffs.

May be harmful if swallowed.

In case of contact, immediately flush eyes with plenty of water. If irritation persists, get medical attention.

Presentation: 16 oz. spray.

Compendium Code No.: 13400011

KMR® 2ND STEP™ KITTEN WEANING FOOD

Pet-Ag **Weaning Formula**

Guaranteed Analysis:

Crude Protein, min. 34%
Crude Fat, min. 11%
Crude Fiber, max. 4%
Moisture, max 8%
Ash, max 8.5%

Ingredients: Rice flour, dried milk protein concentrate, dried skimmed milk, animal fat preserved with BHA and BHT, dried meat solubles, condensed whey product, dicalcium phosphate, vegetable oil, potassium chloride, dried whey protein concentrate, calcium carbonate, sodium chloride, zinc methionine, taurine, lecithin, artificial flavor, sodium silico aluminate, dl-methionine, silicon dioxide, iron choline citrate, vitamin E supplement, zinc choline citrate, manganese sulfate, calcium pantothenate, niacin supplement, copper choline citrate, vitamin A supplement, cobalt choline citrate, riboflavin supplement, calcium iodate, thiamine mononitrate, menadione sodium bisulfite complex, pyridoxine hydrochloride, folic acid, d-biotin supplement, vitamin D_3 supplement, vitamin B_{12} supplement.

Indications: Recommended as the transition diet to take kittens from nursing to solid food.

Directions for Use: 2ND STEP™ Kitten Weaning Food is a complete food for growing kittens. 2ND STEP™ Kitten Weaning Food may be mixed with water, however, for a more gradual change from queen's milk to a solid diet it is recommended that it be mixed with KMR®. 2ND STEP™ Kitten Weaning Food should be fed until kittens are 10 to 11 weeks old when they can be fed commercial kitten or cat food. All changes should be made gradually over a one week period.

Mix 2ND STEP™ Kitten Weaning Food using one of the methods in the table below.

Mixing Directions[1]:

2ND STEP™ Kitten Weaning Food	KMR® Powder	KMR® Liquid[2]	Water[2]
1/4 cup	2 tbls		3/4 cup
1/4 cup		3/4 cup	
1/4 cup			3/4 cup

[1]Amounts given are per pound bodyweight per day. Feed at least 3 times per day. Divide the amount per day by the number of feedings to give amount per feeding.

[2]Reduce to 1/2 cup after 5-6 days or when kittens are eating well.

Provide fresh clean water at all times.

Weaning from the Queen: Introduce 2ND STEP™ Kitten Weaning Food at about 4 weeks of age or as soon as the kittens begin to start eating the queen's food. Offer only a small quantity at first to reduce waste. Do not leave food with kittens for more than 2 hours. If desired kittens may be weaned entirely to 2ND STEP™ Kitten Weaning Food at 6 weeks of age.

Orphaned bottle-reared kittens: Kittens that are on their feet and are lapping their pre-mixed KMR® are ready for introduction to solid food.

Note: Weigh the kittens at least once a week to monitor weight gain and adequacy of feeding. A veterinarian should be consulted about sound kitten care practice. More or less food may be needed by individual kittens to satisfy their food requirements for optimum performance.

Presentation: 14 oz can, 12 per case.

Compendium Code No.: 10970182

KMR® LIQUID

Pet-Ag **Milk Replacer**

Guaranteed Analysis:

Crude protein, min. 7.5%
Crude fat, min. 4.5%
Crude fiber .... None
Moisture, max. 82.0%
Ash, max. 1.5%

Ingredients: Skimmed milk, water, soy oil, sodium caseinate, calcium caseinate, butter, egg yolk, lecithin, calcium carbonate precipitated, l-arginine, potassium chloride, potassium phosphate monobasic, choline chloride, magnesium sulfate, carrageenan, potassium phosphate dibasic, ascorbic acid, taurine, iron sulfate, zinc sulfate, vitamin E supplement, vitamin A supplement, copper sulfate, niacin supplement, calcium pantothenate, vitamin B_{12} supplement, manganese sulfate, thiamine hydrochloride, riboflavin, vitamin D_3 supplement, folic acid, potassium iodide, and pyridoxine hydrochloride.

Indications: Recommended as a food source for orphaned or rejected kittens or those nursing, but needing supplemental feeding. Also recommended for growing kittens or adult cats that are stressed and require a source of highly digestible nutrients.

Dosage and Administration:

Orphaned Kittens: All kittens should receive the queen's milk for at least two (2) days, if possible. The colostrum milk provides extra nutrition and temporary immunity against some diseases. Reconstituted KMR® Liquid may be fed at a daily rate of two (2) tablespoons per four (4) ounces (1/4 lb) of body weight. The daily feeding rate should be divided into equal portions for each feeding. Kittens' needs will vary and the amount fed will need to be increased or decreased, depending on the individual. Small and weak kittens should be fed every three (3) to four (4) hours, while larger kittens will do well when fed every eight (8) hours. Weigh the kittens three (3) times a week to assure adequate feeding. Kittens from large litters should be supplemented with KMR®. Feed at room temperature. Consult a veterinarian for advice.

Food Supplement: Feed KMR® Liquid as a food supplement for growing kittens, show cats, old or convalescing cats at a rate of one (1) tablespoon per 5 lbs (2.2 kg) of body weight.

Pregnant and Lactating Queens: Mix KMR® Liquid into the daily ration at the rate of two (2) tablespoons per 5 lbs (2.2 kg) of body weight until two (2) weeks after queening.

Precaution(s): Shake well before use. Refrigerate after opening. Discard after 72 hours. Do not freeze.

Presentation: 8 oz (24 per case) and 12.5 oz (12 per case) cans.

Compendium Code No.: 10970192

KMR® POWDER

Pet-Ag **Milk Replacer**

Guaranteed Analysis:

Crude Protein, min. 40.0%
Crude Fat, min. 27.0%
Crude Fiber. 0.0%
Moisture, max. 5.0%
Ash, max. 7.0%

Ingredients: Whey protein concentrate, casein, dried skimmed milk, vegetable oil, butter fat, corn syrup solids, egg yolk, monocalcium phosphate, lactose, L-arginine, lecithin, calcium carbonate, potassium chloride, choline chloride, potassium phosphate monobasic, dicalcium phosphate, magnesium carbonate, taurine, potassium phosphate dibasic, magnesium sulfate, ferrous sulfate, vitamin E supplement, zinc sulfate, dipotassium phosphate, silico aluminate, niacin supplement, ascorbic acid, copper sulfate, vitamin A supplement, vitamin B_{12} supplement, calcium pantothenate, manganese sulfate, vitamin D_3 supplement, ethylenediamine dihydroiodide, folic acid, riboflavin, thiamine hydrochloride, pyridoxine hydrochloride, biotin, and mono and diglycerides.

Indications: Recommended as a food source for orphaned or rejected kittens or those nursing, but needing supplemental feeding. Also recommended for growing kittens or adult cats that are stressed and require a source of highly digestible nutrients.

Directions for Use: For very young (less than 7 days old) or severely malnourished kittens, mix 1 measure KMR® with 2 measures of warm water. For older kittens (7 to 10 days old with eyes open) mix 2 measures KMR® with 3 measures of warm water.

All kittens should receive the mother's milk for at least 2 days, if possible. This colostrum milk gives extra nutrition and temporary immunity against some diseases.

Warm reconstituted KMR® to room or body temperature. Feed kittens 2 tablespoons per 4 ounces (115 g) of body weight daily. Small and/or weak kittens should be fed every 3 to 4 hours. Larger and/or older kittens can do well being fed every 8 hours. Divide the daily feeding amount into equal portions for each feeding. The amount required should be increased or decreased to meet the individual requirements for each kitten. Weigh the kitten daily to assure that they are receiving adequate KMR®.

Consult your veterinarian for advice.

The Pet-Ag 2 oz (60 mL) Esbilac® Small Animal Nurser is suited for feeding most kittens. When kittens are old enough to lap, begin offering reconstituted KMR® in a saucer. During the 3rd week, mix reconstituted KMR® with Pet-Ag Kitten Weaning Formula. Use of the KMR® and Weaning Formula will allow the kitten to be gradually switch to solid food.

Pregnant and lactating queens: Feed 2 teaspoons (4 g) KMR® Powder per 5 lbs (2.2 kg) body weight daily until 2 weeks after queening.

Growing kittens, show cats, and/or convalescing cats: Feed 1 teaspoon (2 g) KMR® Powder per 5 lbs (2.2 kg) body weight daily.

Precaution(s): Reconstituted KMR® Powder may be refrigerated up to 24 hours. Opened powder may be refrigerated 3 months.

Presentation: 6 oz cans (12 per case), 12 oz cans (12 per case), 28 oz cans (6 per case), and 3/4 oz pouch (48 per case).

KMR® Emergency Feeding Kit includes: 3/4 oz (21 g) KMR® Emergency powder pack, 2 oz nurser bottle and nipple, .035 oz (1 g) Bene-Bac™ "One Shot" and the Guide to Saving Little Lives (12 per case).

Compendium Code No.: 10970202

K.O. DYNE®

Westfalia•Surge **Udder Wash**

EPA Reg. No.: 1072-11

Active Ingredient(s):

Nonylphenoxypoly (ethyleneoxy) ethanol iodine complex
(provides 1.75% titratable iodine) 13.75%
Phosphoric acid 6.00%
Hydroxyacetic acid 7.00%
Inert ingredients 73.25%

Formula contains not more than 1.9% phosphorous or 0.12 g (3.8 L) per gallon average use concentration.

Indications: K.O. DYNE® is an iodine detergent sanitizer.

Directions for Use: It is a violation of federal law to use the product in a manner inconsistent with its labeling.

Sanitizing dairy equipment: After cleaning and before use sanitize all milk contact surfaces with a 25 ppm solution of K.O. DYNE® as required by state and local health authorities. Refer to table of proportions for proper dilution rate. Contact time should be at least two (2) minutes. Drain thoroughly.

Udder washing: Prepare a sanitizing solution in warm water (not over 100°F-43°C). Refer to table of proportions for proper dilution rate. Use a clean single service towel for each cow. Wash and massage teats and udder. Never dip used towel back into solution. Discard solution if visibly dirty. Prepare fresh solution for each milking. Dry teats and udder with clean single service towel prior to attachment of milking machine.

Do not use as a teat dip.

Note: Amber to brown color of use dilution is an indicator of solution strength. A fresh solution should be prepared if noticeable change occurs in the initial color of solution.

Table of Proportions:
25 ppm - 1 oz. (30 mL) in 5 gallons (18.9 L) water;
50 ppm - 1 oz. (30 mL) in 2.5 gallons (9.45 L) water.

Precautionary Statements: Hazards to Humans and Domestic Animals: Corrosive. Concentrate causes eye damage. Protect eyes when handling. Do not get in eyes or on clothing. Avoid skin contact. Harmful if swallowed. Avoid contamination of food.

First Aid: In case of contact with eyes, flush immediately with plenty of water for at least 15 minutes. Call a physician. For skin, wash promptly. Remove and wash contaminated clothing before use.

If swallowed, promptly drink large quantities of water. Avoid alcohol. Call a physician.

Environmental Hazards: This product is toxic to fish. Keep out of lakes, streams or ponds. Treated effluent may not be discharged into lakes, streams, ponds or public waters without a valid discharge permit. For guidance, contact the regional office of the Environmental Protection Agency.

State and Local Regulations: Consult a dealer, state or local health authorities for additional information.

Storage and Disposal: Store in cool, dry area away from direct sunlight. In case of spill, flood area with large quantities of water. Do not contaminate food or feed by storage, disposal or cleaning of equipment.

Pesticide Disposal: Pesticide wastes are acutely hazardous. Improper disposal of excess pesticide, spray mixture, or rinsate is a violation of federal law. If these wastes cannot be disposed of by use according to label instructions, contact a State Pesticide or Environmental Control Agency, or the hazardous waste representative at the nearest EPA Regional office for guidance.

Container Disposal: Triple rinse (or equivalent) and dispose in an incinerator or landfill approved for pesticide containers.

Keep from freezing. If frozen, separation may occur. Thaw completely and mix well prior to use.

Warning(s): Danger - Keep out of the reach of children.

Presentation: Contact the company for container sizes available.

Compendium Code No.: 10020091

K • O • E™, KENNEL ODOR ELIMINATOR

Thornell **Deodorant Product**

Description: Does not contain enzymes, bacteria, nor oxidizers. Nontoxic, nonirritating, biodegradable, nonflammable. Water soluble for easy cleanup.

Indications: To eliminate even old deeply impregnated animal odors from cages, runs, tables, floors, walls and other large areas.

Can be added to cleaner, rinse or spray. It is compatible with cleaners and germicides.

K • O • E™ works chemically through bonding, absorption and counteraction. It contains inhibitors to control odors caused by further biological (organic) decomposition (putrefaction), and residuals that re-activate after the initial application to combat and prevent odors.

Dosage and Administration: Add ¼ oz. to one (1) gallon of cleaning solution or rinse, whatever is done last. The same dilution in water may be applied to specific areas with plastic lawn/garden type pump up sprayer. For high pressure wash, add to detergent tank at the rate of ⅓ oz. to six (6) gallons (1 to 1,536). Ratios may be varied to achieve desired results.

Eight (8) ounce self measuring bottle makes 32 gallons.

Precaution(s): K • O • E™ has an indefinite shelf life.

Caution(s): The effectiveness dramatically decreases if used with chlorine solutions. Although safe, as with all chemicals, K • O • E™ should be kept out of the reach of children. For external use only.

Presentation: 8 oz. self measuring bottle and 1 gallon jugs.

Compendium Code No.: 11210050

KOPERTOX®

Fort Dodge **Topical Antifungal**

NADA No.: 012-991

Active Ingredient(s):

Copper naphthenate	37.5%
Inert ingredients	62.5%
Total	100.0%

Indications: Recommended as an aid in treating horses and ponies with thrush due to organisms susceptible to copper naphthenate.

Dosage and Administration:

General directions: Clean the hoof thoroughly removing debris and necrotic material prior to application of KOPERTOX®. Apply daily to affected hoofs with a narrow paint brush (about 1") until fully healed.

Note: KOPERTOX® is easily removed from hands, clothing and surfaces with light grade fuel oil or any type of lighter fluid.

Precaution(s): Store at controlled room temperature 15°C to 30°C (59° to 86°F).

Caution(s): Combustible mixture. Use in a well-ventilated place. Avoid fire, flame, sparks or heaters.

If swallowed, do not induce vomiting; call physician immediately. Avoid breathing vapor. Avoid contact with skin and eyes.

Do not allow runoff of excess KOPERTOX® onto hair since contact with KOPERTOX® may cause some hair loss. Do not contaminate feed.

Keep out of reach of children and pets.

For external use only.

Warning(s): Do not use on animals which are raised for food production.

Not for use on horses intended for food.

Presentation: ½ pint (8 oz., 236 mL) (NDC 0856-9910-01) and 1 pint (16 oz., 473 mL) (NDC 0856-9910-02), 12 in a case.

Compendium Code No.: 10031030 0755G

K-SOL

Alpharma **Vitamin K_3-Oral**

Ingredient(s): Sucrose, potassium chloride, sodium chloride, menadione dimethylpyrimidinol bisulfite.

Each 60 grain teaspoonful (3.9 g) contains 50 mg of menadione supplied by menadione dimethylpyrimidinol bisulfite.

Indications: Synthetic vitamin K soluble crystals for use in poultry drinking water.

Directions: Use 1 tsp of powder to each 5 gallons of poultry drinking water or 1 packet per 2 gallons* of stock solution for 5-7 days. Prior to management practices such as beak trimming or comb dubbing, K-SOL may be used at a rate up to 1 tsp of powder per gallon of poultry drinking water or 5 packets per 2 gallons* of stock solution for 1 day.

Mix fresh solutions daily.

*When used in proportioners set to deliver 1 oz per gallon of drinking water.

Precaution(s): Poultry drinking water containing synthetic vitamin K should be kept out of direct sunlight.

Store in cool, dry place.

Caution(s): Livestock remedy - Not for human use - Hazardous.

For oral animal use only.

Keep out of reach of children.

Presentation: 188 g (48 teaspoonsful) packages.

Compendium Code No.: 10220411 AHF-045 0007

KV WOUND POWDER

KenVet **Topical Antibacterial**

Nitrofurazone for Topical Application

NADA No.: 140-910

Active Ingredient(s):

Nitrofurazone 0.2%

In a water soluble base.

Indications: KV WOUND POWDER is a water soluble antibacterial powder for the prevention or treatment of surface bacterial infections of wounds, burns, skin ulcers and abscesses. For use only on dogs, cats and horses (not for food use).

Dosage and Administration: Shake or rotate to loosen powder.

Apply several times a day to the lesion or affected area directly from the plastic squeeze bottle.

Precaution(s): Avoid exposure to direct sunlight, strong fluorescent lighting, excessive heat and alkaline materials.

Caution(s): In case of deep or puncture wounds or serious burns, use only as recommended by a veterinarian. If redness, irritation or swelling persists or increases, discontinue use and consult a veterinarian.

Restricted drug - Use only as directed.

Keep out of the reach of children.

Warning(s): Do not use on horses intended for food.

Human Warnings: Carcinogenesis: Nitrofurazone has been shown to produce mammary tumors in rats and ovarian tumors in mice.

Some people may be hypersensitive to the product. Either wear gloves when applying, or wash hands afterwards.

Presentation: 45 g plastic squeeze bottle.

Compendium Code No.: 11340010

KWIK-STOP® STYPTIC POWDER

ARC **Hemostatic**

Active Ingredient(s): KWIK-STOP® contains: Ferric subsulfate, aluminum chloride, diatomite, bentonite, copper sulfate, ammonium chloride, and iodophor complex.

Indications: For use as an aid to stop bleeding caused by clipping nails, docking tails and trimming beaks and minor cuts. For external veterinary use only to control bleeding for dogs, cats and birds.

Dosage and Administration: Apply with moistened cotton tipped applicator to the cut nail or other superficial bleeding area using moderate constant pressure for 5-10 seconds. Do not use in deep wounds or body cavities or on burns.

Pressure bandaging should be used in conjunction with the product following tail docking.

Caution(s): Keep out of the reach of children.

Presentation: 14 g and 42 g jars.

Compendium Code No.: 10960040

K-ZYME® CAT GRANULES

BioZyme **Small Animal Dietary Supplement**

with the Amaferm® advantage

Active Ingredient(s): **Aspergillus oryzae* fermentation extract.

Guaranteed Analysis: Each teaspoon (2.3 grams) contains:

Calcium	39.0 mg
Min.	1.7%
Max.	2.7%
Phosphorus	30.0 mg
Min.	1.3%
Copper	0.2 mg Min.
Iodine	.1 mg Min.
Iron	4.0 mg Min.
Manganese	1.0 mg Min.
Potassium	20.0 mg Min.
Selenium	0.003 mg Min.
Zinc	5.0 mg Min.
Vitamin A	4,500.0 IU Min.
Vitamin D_3	250.0 IU Min.
Ascorbic Acid	1.0 mg Min.
Vitamin E	25.0 IU Min.
Thiamine	0.3 mg Min.
Riboflavin	0.2 mg Min.
Pyridoxine	0.2 mg Min.
Vitamin B_{12}	0.002 mg Min.
Biotin	0.01 mg Min.
Choline	100.0 mg Min.
Folic Acid	0.02 mg Min.
Niacin	1.0 mg Min.
Pantothenic Acid	0.3 mg Min.
dl-Methionine	1.0% - 23.0 mg Min.
Taurine	50.0 mg Min.
Linoleic Acid	114.0 mg Min.
Linolenic Acid	8.0 mg Min.
Arachidonic Acid	10.0 mg Min.
Eicosapentaenoic Acid	13.0 mg Min.
Docosahexaenoic Acid	8.0 mg Min.
Docosapentaenoic Acid	2.0 mg Min.
Total Fatty Acids	155.0 mg Min.

Ingredients: Desiccated liver meal, alfalfa powder, dried *Aspergillus oryzae* fermentation extract*, dried whey, brewers yeast, dextrose, dried egg, safflower oil, canola oil, steamed bone meal, calcium carbonate, dicalcium phosphate, fish oil, choline chloride, taurine, ferrous sulfate, magnesium oxide, potassium sulfate, manganese sulfate, vitamin A supplement, niacin supplement, dl-alpha-tocopherol acetate (a source of vitamin E), ascorbic acid, riboflavin supplement, d-activated animal sterol (a source of vitamin D_3), calcium pantothenate, thiamine mononitrate, potassium iodide, zinc oxide, copper sulfate, vitamin B_{12} supplement, sodium selenite.

Indications: A highly palatable (liver flavor) digestive enhancer fortified with vitamins and minerals. Supplement for cats.

Dosage and Administration:

For healthy kittens: ¼ teaspoon daily, top dress or mix in food.

For healthy cats: 1 teaspoon daily, top dress or mix in food.

For lactating queens: 1½ teaspoons daily, top dress or mix in food.

Presentation: 1 lb jar and 5 lb pail.

*Amaferm® is a product of a patented process, U.S. Patent #3043748

Compendium Code No.: 14960000

The Green pages list brands available for each non-proprietary name.

K

K-ZYME® CHEWABLE DOG TABLETS

BioZyme **Small Animal Dietary Supplement**

with the Amaferm® advantage

Active Ingredient(s): **Aspergillus oryzae* fermentation extract.

Guaranteed Analysis: Each chewable tablet weighs 2.5 grams and contains:

Calcium (min. 6.0%, max. 7.2%)	150.0 mg
Phosphorus (min. 4.9%)	123.0 mg
Copper	0.5 mg
Iodine	0.5 mg
Iron	4.0 mg
Magnesium	66.0 mg
Manganese	3.0 mg
Potassium	33.0 mg
Selenium	.003 mg
Zinc	5.0 mg
Vitamin A	2900.0 IU
Vitamin D_3	350.0 IU
Vitamin E	7.0 IU
Thiamine	0.5 mg
Riboflavin	0.5 mg
Pyridoxine	0.5 mg
Vitamin B_{12}	0.01 mg
Vitamin K	0.05 mg
Biotin	0.04 mg
Choline	35.0 mg
Folic Acid	0.06 mg
Niacin	5.0 mg
Pantothenic Acid	3.0 mg

Ingredients: Dicalcium phosphate, sucrose, liver powder, hydrolyzed vegetable protein, magnesium oxide, yeast culture, dried *Aspergillus oryzae* fermentation extract*, choline chloride, potassium sulfate, stearic acid, silicone dioxide, vitamin E supplement, iron oxide, manganese sulfate, zinc oxide, niacin supplement, vitamin A supplement, calcium pantothenate, copper sulfate, potassium iodide, d-activated animal sterol (a source of vitamin D_3), pyridoxine hydrochloride, thiamine mononitrate, riboflavin supplement, vitamin B_{12} supplement, menadione sodium bisulfite complex, folic acid, biotin, sodium selenite.

Indications: A highly palatable (roast beef and liver flavor) digestive enhancer fortified with vitamins and minerals. Supplement for dogs.

Dosage and Administration:

Dogs under 20 lbs: ½ tablet daily, top dress or mix in food.

Dogs over 20 lbs: 1 tablet daily, top dress or mix in food.

Presentation: Jar of 100 and 500 tablets and pail of 2,500 tablets.

*Amaferm® is a product of a patented process, U.S. Patent #3043748

Compendium Code No.: 14960010

K

Seeking additional information?
Consult the product manufacturer.
Their addresses appear in
the Manufacturer / Distributor Index.

K-ZYME® DOG GRANULES

BioZyme **Small Animal Dietary Supplement**

with the Amaferm® advantage

Active Ingredient(s): **Aspergillus oryzae* fermentation extract.

Guaranteed Analysis: Each teaspoon (2.8 grams) contains:

Calcium	160.0 mg
Min.	5.0%
Max.	7.2%
Phosphorus	123.0 mg
Min.	4.9%
Copper	0.5 mg Min.
Iodine	0.5 mg Min.
Iron	4.0 mg Min.
Magnesium	66.0 mg Min.
Manganese	3.0 mg Min.
Potassium	33.0 mg Min.
Selenium	0.003 mg Min.
Zinc	10.0 mg Min.
Vitamin A	3,000.0 IU Min.
Vitamin D_3	300.0 IU Min.
Ascorbic Acid	1.0 mg Min.
Vitamin E	25.0 IU Min.
Thiamine	0.9 mg Min.
Riboflavin	1.0 mg Min.
Pyridoxine	0.5 mg Min.
Vitamin B_{12}	0.01 mg Min.
Biotin	0.04 mg Min.
Choline	35.0 mg Min.
Folic Acid	0.06 mg Min.
Niacin	10.0 mg Min.
Pantothenic Acid	3.0 mg Min.
Linoleic Acid	114.0 mg Min.
Linolenic Acid	8.0 mg Min.
Arachidonic Acid	10.0 mg Min.
Eicosapentaenoic Acid	13.0 mg Min.
Docosahexaenoic Acid	8.0 mg Min.
Docosapentaenoic Acid	2.0 mg Min.
Total Fatty Acids	155.0 mg Min.

Ingredients: Desiccated liver meal, dicalcium phosphate, alfalfa powder, dried *Aspergillus oryzae* fermentation extract*, dried whey, brewers yeast, dextrose, safflower oil, canola oil, calcium carbonate, fish oil, ferrous sulfate, choline chloride, onion flavor, tocopherols (a preservative), magnesium oxide, potassium sulfate, manganese sulfate, vitamin A supplement, niacin supplement, dl-alpha-tocopherol acetate (a source of vitamin E), ascorbic acid, riboflavin supplement, d-activated animal sterol (a source of vitamin D_3), calcium pantothenate, thiamine mononitrate, potassium iodide, zinc oxide, copper sulfate, vitamin B_{12} supplement, sodium selenite.

Indications: A highly palatable (liver flavor) digestive enhancer fortified with vitamins and minerals. Supplement for dogs.

Dosage and Administration:

For healthy puppies: ¼ teaspoon daily, top dress or mix in food.

For healthy dogs: 1 teaspoon daily, top dress or mix in food.

For breeding and nursing dogs: 1½ teaspoons daily, top dress or mix in food.

For sporting dogs in training: 1½ teaspoons daily, top dress or mix in food.

Presentation: 1 lb jar, 5 lb, 20 lb and 40 lb pail.

*Amaferm® is a product of a patented process, U.S. Patent #3043748

Compendium Code No.: 14960020

L

LAB-EZ®/EIA

Synbiotics **EIA Test**

U.S. Vet. Lic. No.: 312

Description: Equine infectious anemia antibody test kit.

Components:

EIA Antigen (Bottle A) ... 1 vial
EIA Positive Control Serum (Bottle B) ... 3 vials
EIA Negative Control Serum (Bottle C) ... 1 vial

Package insert with instructions for conducting the test.

Indications: The agar gel immunodiffusion (AGID) test for the diagnosis of Equine Infectious Anemia (EIA) was described by Coggins and Norcross, *Cornell Veterinarian,* April 1970. The test has proven to reliably diagnose infection by detecting specific antibody against EIAV in the serum of infected horses.

Test Principles: The immunodiffusion test is based upon the concurrent movement of antigen and corresponding specific antibody toward each other in an agar gel, forming a visible precipitin line. Making use of this principle, the AGID test can reliably detect specific antibody that is formed after one to four weeks of infection with the EIA virus.

LAB-EZ®/EIA AGID uses a highly purified recombinant protein from the EIA virus which will form a specific line of identity with infected serum antibody. No precipitin lines will form if the serum is negative for EIAV.

Test Procedure: Use only horse serum for test specimens. Specimens may be stored at 2°-7°C for up to five days. If longer storage is desired, store at -20°C (-4°F). The presence of gross turbidity, hemolysis or bacterial growth may interfere with the performance and accuracy of the test.

A. Preparation of Agar Gel

1. Borate Buffer is prepared by mixing:
   2g Sodium Hydroxide (NaOH)
   9g Boric Acid (H_3BO_3)
   1 liter distilled water
   The resulting pH should be adjusted to 8.6 ± 0.2.
2. A one percent solution of Noble agar is prepared in the borate buffer and dissolved by either of two methods:
   a. Boil the suspension to dissolve the agar and autoclave for seven minutes.
   b. Microwave agar solution for a total of 3 minutes at 30 second intervals or until agar dissolves.
3. Add 15 mL of agar to a 100 mm diameter petri dish.
4. Plates are cooled for 1 hour at room temperature and then stored at 2°-7°C. If uncut, plates can be stored up to one week.

B. Cutting Wells in Agar

1. A seven-well pattern is used with one center well encircled by 6 wells. The wells are 2.4 mm apart and 5.3 mm in diameter. Cutting tools can be obtained from the National Veterinary Services Laboratory, P.O. Box 844, Ames, Iowa 50010
2. Wells are cut while the agar is cold and the same day as used. Remove the agar plugs and leave lids ajar for 30 minutes before adding reagents and serum samples. Any remaining moisture in the wells should be suctioned out or allowed to evaporate.

C. Filling Wells and Incubation of Agar Plates

Note: The negative control (Bottle C) should be run in at least one well for every group of plates. It should be pipetted into a test well in place of a test serum.

1. Fill each alternate outside well (see diagram 1) with one of the three test sera (or the kit negative control) but without overflowing onto the agar surface. Use a separate disposable pipette or pipette tip for each sample.
2. Fill the center well with purified EIA Antigen (Bottle A) in the same manner.
3. Fill the three remaining outside wells with EIA Positive Control Serum (Bottle B) in the same manner.
4. Incubate plates for 24-48 hours at room temperature in a moist chamber.

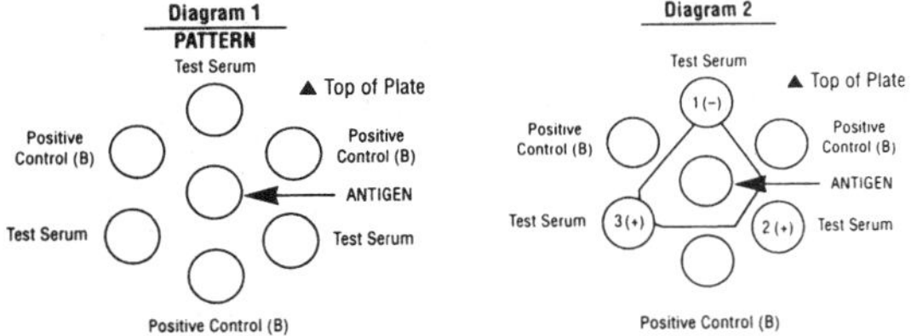

Test Interpretation: Interpretation of Results (See Diagram 2):

1. Negative - Reagent serum control lines continue into the test sample well without bending or with a slight bend back towards the reagent serum well.
2. Positive - Control lines join with and form a continuous line with the line between the test serum and antigen.
3. Weak positive - Control lines bend slightly towards the antigen well and away from the positive control serum well but do not form a complete line between antigen and test serum.
4. Very strong positive - Control lines turn towards the antigen well before they reach the well containing the test serum, and may continue on as a broad or hazy line which will be close to the antigen well. A more distinct line will usually form if the sample is diluted 1:2, 1:4 and 1:8 and retested.
5. Weak immunodiffusion reactions may be due to the following:
   a. Foals nursed by infected mares may produce positive results. The foal should be retested at 6 months of age to determine whether it is negative. If a mare is negative her positive foal should be considered infected.
   b. Weak positives have been observed during the incubation period of EIA. If a second sample is obtained 2 to 3 weeks later, the reaction should be stronger.
   c. Inapparent carriers that have no clinical signs of EIA for long periods of time may have weak reactions in the AGID. In these cases, retesting rarely results in a change in the strength of the reaction.
6. Any questionable sample should be sent to the National Veterinary Services Laboratory (NVSL) for verification.

Controls

Positive Control Serum (Bottle B) - If the positive reagent serum included in the kit does not react by forming a precipitin line with the EIA antigen (Bottle A), do not use the kit. Call Synbiotics' Technical Services at 800-228-4305

Negative Control Serum (Bottle C) - The negative control can be used as a comparison when testing weak reacting samples. If the negative control produces any pricipitin line with the EIA antigen reagent, do not use the kit. Call Synbiotics' Technical Services at 800-228-4305.

Storage: Store contents of kit at 2°-7°C (36°-45°F).

Caution(s): Sale and use restricted to laboratories approved by state and federal (U.S.D.A.) animal health officials.

For veterinary use only.

Antigen and accompanying antiserum have been standardized and should be used together. Do not allow reagents to stand at room temperature for excessive periods of time while performing tests. Handle all reagents and equipment as if capable of transmitting EIA. Burn all containers and all unused contents. Autoclave all disposable test components and test specimens after use. The negative control is to be used in place of a test serum. Do not substitute the negative control serum for a positive control serum well.

Presentation: 300 test kits.

Compendium Code No.: 11150131

LACTATED RINGERS ℞

Vet Tek **Fluid Therapy**

Sterile Solution

Active Ingredient(s): Each 100 mL contains:

Sodium Chloride ... 600 mg
Sodium Lactate ... 310 mg
Potassium Chloride ... 30 mg
Calcium Chloride Dihydrate ... 20 mg
Water for Injection ... q.s.

The Calcium, Potassium and Sodium contents are approximately 2.7, 4.0, and 130 mEq/liter, respectively.

Total Osmolar Concentration: 269 mOsm per liter (calculated).

This product contains no preservatives.

Indications: For the correction of electrolyte depletion, metabolic acidosis and dehydration of cattle, calves, horses, sheep and swine.

Dosage and Administration: May be injected intravenously, subcutaneously or intraperitoneally (except in horses) using strict aseptic technique.

Cattle and Horses: 2 to 5 mL per pound of body weight depending on size and condition of animal, repeated 1 to 3 times daily or as needed.

Swine and Sheep: 2 to 5 mL per pound of body weight depending on size and condition of animal, repeated 1 to 3 times daily or as needed.

If administered subcutaneously divide the dosage into several sites of injection and massage points of injection to aid in absorption and help prevent inflammation and/or sloughing.

Precaution(s): Store between 15°C and 30°C (59°F-86°F).

Solution should be warmed to body temperature prior to administration and administered at a slow rate. This is a single dose unit. Use entire contents when first opened.

Caution(s): Federal law restricts this drug to use by or on the order of a licensed veterinarian.

For animal use only.

Warning(s): Do not administer to horses by intraperitoneal injection. Do not administer to animals with inadequate renal function. Not for use in lactic acidosis.

Keep out of reach of children.

Presentation: 1000 mL (NDC 60270-030-20)

Manufactured by: Phoenix Scientific, Inc. St. Joseph, MO 64506.

Compendium Code No.: 14200111 Iss. 7-95

LACTATED RINGERS INJECTION ℞

Phoenix Pharmaceutical **Fluid Therapy**

Sterile Nonpyrogenic Solution

Active Ingredient(s): Each 100 mL contains:

Sodium Chloride ... 600 mg
Sodium Lactate ... 310 mg
Potassium Chloride ... 30 mg
Calcium Chloride Dihydrate ... 20 mg
Water for Injection ... q.s.

The Calcium, Potassium and Sodium contents are approximately 2.7, 4.0, and 130 mEq/liter, respectively.

Total Osmolar Concentration: 269 mOsm per liter (calculated).

This product contains no preservatives.

Indications: For the correction of electrolyte depletion, metabolic acidosis and dehydration of cattle, calves, horses, sheep and swine.

Dosage and Administration: May be injected intravenously, subcutaneously or intraperitoneally (except in horses) using strict aseptic technique.

Cattle and Horses: 2 to 5 mL per pound of body weight depending on size and condition of animal, repeated 1 to 3 times daily or as needed.

Swine and Sheep: 2 to 5 mL per pound of body weight depending on size and condition of animal, repeated 1 to 3 times daily or as needed.

If administered subcutaneously divide the dosage into several sites of injection and massage points of injection to aid in absorption and help prevent inflammation and/or sloughing.

Contraindication(s): Do not administer to horses by intraperitoneal injection. Do not administer to animals with inadequate renal function. Not for use in lactic acidosis.

Precaution(s): Store between 15° and 30°C (59°-86°F).

Use entire contents when first opened.

Caution(s): Federal law restricts this drug to use by or on the order of a licensed veterinarian.

Solution should be warmed to body temperature prior to administration and administered at a slow rate.

For animal use only.

Warning(s): Keep out of reach of children.

Presentation: 1000 mL single dose units (NDC 57319-084-08).

Manufactured by: Phoenix Scientific, Inc., St. Joseph, MO 64503.

Compendium Code No.: 12560522 Rev. 8-01

LACTATED RINGER'S INJECTION ℞

Vedco **Fluid Therapy**

Active Ingredient(s): Each 100 mL contains:

Sodium chloride	600 mg
Sodium lactate anhydrous	310 mg
Potassium chloride	30 mg
Calcium chloride	20 mg
Water for injection	q.s.

May contain hydrochloric acid or sodium hydroxide for pH adjustment.

Electrolytes per 100 mL (not including ions for adjusting pH):

Sodium	130 mEq
Potassium	4 mEq
Calcium	3 mEq
Chloride	109 mEq
Lactate	28 mEq
mOsm/L	273
Caloric value	9 per liter
Approximate pH	6.3
Isotonic	

Does not contain preservatives.

Indications: A sterile solution for the replacement of acute fluid and electrolyte losses and for correcting mild acidosis.

Dosage and Administration: Contents or a lesser amount as determined by a veterinarian as a single dose; usually 3-10% of body weight. For intravenous or subcutaneous use. The solution should be warmed to body temperature and administered slowly.

Caution(s): Federal law restricts this drug to use by or on the order of a licensed veterinarian.

Keep out of the reach of children.

Do not administer calcium containing solutions concurrently with stored blood.

Do not use the product if the seal is broken or the solution is not clear.

If the entire contents are not used, discard any unused portion.

Additives may be incompatible. When introducing additives, use aseptic technique, mix thoroughly and do not store.

Presentation: 1,000 mL containers.

Compendium Code No.: 10941190

LACTATED RINGERS INJECTION ℞

Vetus **Fluid Therapy**

Sterile Nonpyrogenic Solution

Active Ingredient(s): Each 100 mL contains:

Sodium Chloride	600 mg
Sodium Lactate	310 mg
Potassium Chloride	30 mg
Calcium Chloride Dihydrate	20 mg
Water for Injection	q.s.

The Calcium, Potassium and Sodium contents are approximately 2.7, 4.0, and 130 mEq/liter, respectively. Total Osomolar Concentration: 269 mOsm per liter (calculated).

Indications: For the correction of electrolyte depletion, metabolic acidosis and dehydration of cattle, calves, horses, sheep and swine.

Dosage and Administration: May be injected intravenously, subcutaneously or intraperitoneally (except in horses) using strict aseptic technique.

Cattle and Horses: 2 to 5 mL per pound of body weight depending on size and condition of animal, repeated 1 to 3 times daily or as needed.

Swine and Sheep: 2 to 5 mL per pound of body weight depending on size and condition of animal, repeated 1 to 3 times daily or as needed.

If administered subcutaneously divide the dosage into several sites of injection and massage points of injection to aid in absorption and help prevent inflammation and/or sloughing.

Precaution(s): Store between 15°C and 30°C (59°F-86°F).

This is a single dose unit. It contains no preservatives. Use entire contents when first opened.

Caution(s): Federal law restricts this drug to use by or on the order of a licensed veterinarian.

Solution should be warmed to body temperature prior to administration and administered at a slow rate.

Do not administer to horses by intraperitoneal injection. Do not administer to animals with inadequate renal function. Not for use in lactic acidosis.

For animal use only.

Warning(s): Keep out of reach of children.

Presentation: 1000 mL (NDC 47611-777-10).

Manufactured by: Phoenix Scientific, Inc.

Distributed by: Burns Veterinary Supply, Inc.

Compendium Code No.: 14440910 Rev. 01-01

LACTATED RINGERS INJECTION SC ℞

Butler **Fluid Therapy**

Sterile Nonpyrogenic Solution

Active Ingredient(s): Each 100 mL contains:

Sodium Chloride	600 mg
Sodium Lactate	310 mg
Potassium Chloride	30 mg
Calcium Chloride Dihydrate	20 mg
Water for Injection	q.s.

The Calcium, potassium and sodium contents are approximately 2.7, 4.0, and 130 meq/liter, respectively. Total Osomolar Concentration: 269 mOsm per liter (calculated).

Indications: For the correction of electrolyte depletion, metabolic acidosis and dehydration of cattle, calves, horses, sheep and swine.

Dosage and Administration: May be injected intravenously, subcutaneously or intraperitoneally (except in horses) using strict aseptic technique.

Cattle and Horses: 2 to 5 mL per pound of body weight depending on size and condition of animal, repeated 1 to 3 times daily or as needed.

Swine and Sheep: 2 to 5 mL per pound of body weight depending on size and condition of animal, repeated 1 to 3 times daily or as needed.

If administered subcutaneously divide the dosage into several sites of injection and massage points of injection to aid in absorption and help prevent inflammation and/or sloughing.

Contraindication(s): Do not administer to horses by intraperitoneal injection. Do not administer to animals with inadequate renal function. Not for use in lactic acidosis.

Precaution(s): Store between 15°C and 30°C (59°F-86°F).

Caution(s): Federal law restricts this drug to use by or on the order of a licensed veterinarian.

Solution should be warmed to body temperature prior to administration and administered at a slow rate. This is a single dose unit. It contains no preservatives. Use entire contents when first opened.

Warning(s): For animal use only. Keep out of reach of children.

Presentation: 1000 mL.

Manufactured by: Phoenix Scientific, Inc.

Compendium Code No.: 10821040

LACTATED RINGER'S INJECTION, USP ℞

AgriLabs **Fluid Therapy**

Active Ingredient(s): Contains no preservatives. Each 100 mL contains:

Sodium chloride	600 mg
Sodium lactate anhydrous	310 mg
Calcium chloride dihydrate	20 mg
Potassium chloride	30 mg
Water for injection	q.s.

May contain hydrochloric acid or sodium hydroxide for pH adjustment.

Electrolytes per 1,000 mL (not including ions for adjusting pH):

Sodium	130 mEq
Potassium	4 mEq
Calcium	2.7 mEq
Chloride	109 mEq
Lactate	28 mEq

273 mOsm/liter (calc).

pH 6.0-7.5 isotonic.

Indications: For the replacement of acute fluid and electrolyte losses and for correcting mild acidosis.

Dosage and Administration: Use the entire contents or a lesser amount as determined by a veterinarian as a single dose, usually 3-10% of body weight. For intravenous or subcutaneous use. The solution should be warmed to body temperature and administered slowly.

Precaution(s): Protect from freezing.

Caution(s): Federal law restricts this drug to use by or on the order of a licensed veterinarian. For animal use only. Not for human use. Keep out of the reach of children.

Do not administer calcium containing solutions concurrently with stored blood. Do not use the product if the seal is broken or if the solution is not clear. If the entire contents are not used, discard the unused portion. Additives may be incompatible. When introducing additives, use the aseptic technique, mix thoroughly and do not store.

Warning(s): Not for use in the treatment of lactic acidosis.

Presentation: 1,000 mL containers.

Compendium Code No.: 10581630 601608122-791

LACTATED RINGER'S INJECTION, USP ℞

Bimeda **Fluid Therapy**

Active Ingredient(s): Each 100 mL contains:

Sodium chloride	600 mg
Sodium lactate anhydrous	310 mg
Potassium chloride	30 mg
Calcium chloride dihydrate	20 mg
Water for injection	q.s.

May contain hydrochloric acid or sodium hydroxide for pH adjustment.

Electrolytes per 1,000 mL (not including ions for adjusting pH):

Sodium	130 mEq
Potassium	4 mEq
Calcium	2.7 mEq
Chloride	109 mEq
Lactate	28 mEq
mOsm/L (calc.)	273
pH (isotonic)	6.0-7.5

Contains no preservative.

Indications: For the replacement of acute fluid and electrolyte losses and for correcting mild acidosis.

Dosage and Administration: Contents or lesser amount as determined by a veterinarian as a single dose; usually 3-10% of body weight. For intravenous or subcutaneous use. The solution should be warmed to body temperature and administered slowly.

Precaution(s): Protect from freezing.

Caution(s): Federal law restricts this drug to use by or on the order of a licensed veterinarian.

Do not administer calcium containing solutions concurrently with stored blood. Do not use the product if the seal is broken or if the solution is not clear. If the entire contents are not used, discard the unused portion. Additives may be incompatible. When introducing additives, use aseptic technique, mix thoroughly and do not store.

For animal use only. Not for human use.

Keep out of the reach of children.

Warning(s): Not for use in the treatment of lactic acidosis.

Presentation: 1,000 mL vials.

Compendium Code No.: 13990230

LACTATED RINGER'S SOLUTION ℞

RXV **Fluid Therapy**

Active Ingredient(s): Each 100 mL of sterile aqueous solution contains:

Sodium Chloride	600 mg
Sodium Lactate	310 mg
Potassium Chloride	30 mg
Calcium Chloride • $2H_2O$	20 mg
Water for Injection	q.s.

Milliequivalents per liter:

Sodium	130 mEq/L
Potassium	4.0 mEq/L
Calcium	2.7 mEq/L
Total Osmolar Concentration	276 mOsm/L

Indications: For rehydration and the replacement of electrolytes in cattle, horses, sheep and swine.

Dosage and Administration: May be administered intravenously or intraperitoneally in cattle, sheep and swine. Administer to horses by intravenous injection only.

Warm solution to body temperature and administer 1 to 2 mL/lb of body weight, or as determined by condition of animal, at a rate of 10 to 30 mL per minute under strict asepsis. May be repeated as necessary.

Therapy requiring several vials of this product should be accompanied by laboratory analysis of serum electrolytes.

Precaution(s): Store at a temperature between 2°-30°C (36°-86°F).

This product contains no preservatives. Use entire contents when first opened. Discard any unused solution.

Caution(s): Federal law restricts this drug to use by or on the order of a licensed veterinarian.

Not for use in the treatment of lactic acidosis. Do not administer intraperitoneally to horses.

Not for human use.

Presentation: 1,000 mL vials.

Manufactured by: American Veterinary Products, Ft. Collins, CO 80524

Compendium Code No.: 10910320 Rev. 0793

LAMB & KID PASTE

Durvet **Large Animal Dietary Supplement**

Guaranteed Analysis: Total lactic acid producing bacteria: 5 x 10^7 CFU/g.

Lactobacillus acidophilus, Bifidobacterium thermophilum, Enterococcus faecium, Bifidobacterium longum, Bacillus subtillus, Lactase (A. oryzae) . . . . 200 µg lactose hydrolyzed/minute/g.

Ingredients: Vegetable Oil, Dried Egg Yolk, Hydrated Sodium Aluminosilicate, Sorbitan Monostearate, Dried Whey, Dried *Lactobacillus acidophilus* fermentation product, Dried *Bifidobacterium thermophilum* fermentation product, Dried *Enterococcus faecium* fermentation product, Dried *Bifidobacterium longum* fermentation product, Dried *Bacillus subtillus* fermentation product, Dried *Aspergillus oryzae* fermentation extract.

Indications: A source of live natural microorganisms used to minimize intestinal disorders and enhance the digestion of food.

Protects lambs and kids during the first critical 24 hours. Aids in the control of scours. Gives lambs and kids an immediate energy boost at birth. Use at first sign of health problems and to supplement colostrum. Protective coating allows bacteria to be used with antibiotics.

Directions: Dosage: Administer 3 to 5 grams on back of tongue of newborn lambs or kids. Administer 5 to 15 grams to older animals. Repeat dosage as needed.

Precaution(s): Store in cool, dry place.

Presentation: 15 g tubes.

Compendium Code No.: 10842060

LAND O LAKES® INSTANT AMPLIFIER® MAX

Land O'Lakes **Medicated Milk Replacer**

with Architect® Formulation System-Dairy Herd & Beef Calf Milk Replacer

Active Ingredient(s):

Oxytetracycline . . . . 125 grams per ton
Neomycin Base (from Neomycin Sulfate) . . . . 250 grams per ton

Guaranteed Analysis:

Crude Protein, not less than 22.0%
Crude Fat, not less than 20.0%
Crude Fiber, not more than 0.15%
Calcium (Ca), not less than 0.75%
Calcium (Ca), not more than 1.25%
Phosphorus (P), not less than 0.70%
Vitamin A, not less than . . . . 20,000 IU/lb
Vitamin D_3, not less than . . . . 5,000 IU/lb
Vitamin E, not less than . . . . 100 IU/lb

Ingredients: Dried whey, dried whey protein concentrate, dried whey product, dried skimmed milk, dried milk protein, animal fat (preserved with ethoxyquin), lecithin, polyethylene glycol (400) monooleate, dicalcium phosphate, calcium carbonate, vitamin A acetate, d-activated animal sterol (source of vitamin D_3), vitamin E supplement, thiamine mononitrate, pyridoxine hydrochloride, folic acid, vitamin B_{12} supplement, choline chloride, roughage products, sodium silico aluminate, manganese sulfate, zinc sulfate, ferrous sulfate, copper sulfate, cobalt sulfate, ethylenediamine dihydriodide and sodium selenite.

Indications: To aid in the prevention of bacterial diarrhea (scours) in calves.

Directions: Mixing Directions:

Accelerated Growth Program (Recommended):

Use the plastic cup provided to measure the milk replacer powder.

Add 1 full cup* of milk replacer powder to 2 quarts of 110-120°F water and mix thoroughly.

Large Batches: Mix 6¼ pounds (10 full cups) of milk replacer powder to 5 gallons of 110-120°F water.

Feed each calf according to the schedule listed below.

*One measuring cup holds approximately 10 ounces (weight) of dry milk replacer powder.

Conventional Program:

Use the plastic cup provided to measure the milk replacer powder.

Fill cup with milk replacer powder to 8 ounce mark and add to 2 quarts of 110-120°F water and mix thoroughly.

Large Batches: Mix 5 pounds (8 full cups) of milk replacer powder to 5 gallons of 110-120°F water. Feed each calf according to the schedule listed below.

Feeding Directions (4 days of age to weaning):

Large Breeds: Feed 2 quarts reconstituted liquid milk replacer twice a day.

Small Breeds: Feed 1½-2 quarts reconstituted liquid milk replacer twice a day.

In extremely cold weather it may be beneficial to feed another feeding of calf milk replacer in the middle of the day. Add ½ cup of milk replacer powder to 1 quart of 110-120°F water, mix and feed to 1 calf at midday.

A characteristic of this product is a slight layering that occurs approximately 7 minutes after mixing.

General Recommendations:

1. Newborn calves should receive 3 quarts of colostrum in the first feeding as soon after birth as possible (within 1 hour) and again 12 hours later.
2. For Days 2 and 3 of life, feed 2 quarts of colostrum twice daily to calves.
3. For best mixing, continuously stir with wire whip while adding powder to 110-120°F water (hot as you can tolerate on your hand). Use correct water temperature to avoid product separation. Feed milk replacer at 90-100°F.
4. Provide fresh, clean water and a high quality, palatable calf starter from 4 days after birth and continue on a free-choice basis.
5. Observe calves closely during the milk replacer feeding period. Avoid underfeeding which may result in starvation, or overconsumption which may increase incidence of scours.
6. Continue to feed milk replacer until the calf is consuming a minimum of 1½ pounds of calf starter per day, which usually occurs at 4-6 weeks of age.

Warning(s): Withdraw from calves 30 days before slaughter.

A withdrawal period has not been established for this product in pre-ruminating calves. Do not use in calves to be processed for veal.

Presentation: 25 lb (11.34 kg) and 50 lb (22.68 kg) bags.

® Registered Trademark of Land O'Lakes, Inc.

Compendium Code No.: 10380001

LAND O LAKES® INSTANT AMPLIFIER® SELECT

Land O'Lakes **Medicated Milk Replacer**

with Architect® Formulation System-Dairy Herd & Beef Calf Milk Replacer

Active Ingredient(s):

Oxytetracycline . . . . 125 grams per ton
Neomycin Base (from Neomycin Sulfate) . . . . 250 grams per ton

Guaranteed Analysis:

Crude Protein, not less than 18.0%
Crude Fat, not less than 20.0%
Crude Fiber, not more than 0.15%
Calcium (Ca), not less than 0.75%
Calcium (Ca), not more than 1.25%
Phosphorus (P), not less than 0.70%
Vitamin A, not less than . . . . 20,000 I.U./lb
Vitamin D_3, not less than . . . . 5,000 I.U./lb
Vitamin E, not less than . . . . 100 I.U./lb

Ingredients: Dried whey, dried whey protein concentrate, dried whey product, dried skimmed milk, dried milk protein, animal fat (preserved with ethoxyquin), lecithin, polyethylene glycol (400) monooleate, dicalcium phosphate, calcium carbonate, l-lysine, dl-methionine, vitamin A acetate, d-activated animal sterol (source of vitamin D_3), vitamin E supplement, thiamine mononitrate, pyridoxine hydrochloride, folic acid, vitamin B_{12} supplement, choline chloride, roughage products, sodium silico aluminate, manganese sulfate, zinc sulfate, ferrous sulfate, copper sulfate, cobalt sulfate, ethylenediamine dihydriodide and sodium selenite.

Indications: To aid in the prevention of bacterial diarrhea (scours) in calves.

Directions: Mixing Directions:

Accelerated Growth Program (Recommended):

Use the plastic cup provided to measure the milk replacer powder.

Add 1 full cup* of milk replacer powder to 2 quarts of 110-120°F water and mix thoroughly.

Large Batches: Mix 6¼ pounds (10 full cups) of milk replacer powder to 5 gallons of 110-120°F water.

Feed each calf according to the schedule listed below.

*One measuring cup holds approximately 10 ounces (weight) of dry milk replacer powder.

Conventional Program:

Use the plastic cup provided to measure the milk replacer powder.

Fill cup with milk replacer powder to 8 ounce mark and add to 2 quarts of 110-120°F water and mix thoroughly.

Large Batches: Mix 5 pounds (8 full cups) of milk replacer powder to 5 gallons of 110-120°F water. Feed each calf according to the schedule listed below.

Feeding Directions (4 days of age to weaning):

Large Breeds: Feed 2 quarts reconstituted liquid milk replacer twice a day.

Small Breeds: Feed 1½-2 quarts reconstituted liquid milk replacer twice a day.

In extremely cold weather it may be beneficial to feed another feeding of calf milk replacer in the middle of the day. Add ½ cup of milk replacer powder to 1 quart of 110-120°F water, mix and feed to 1 calf at midday.

A characteristic of this product is a slight layering that occurs approximately 7 minutes after mixing.

General Recommendations:

1. Newborn calves should receive 3 quarts of colostrum in the first feeding as soon after birth as possible (within 1 hour) and again 12 hours later.
2. For Days 2 and 3 of life, feed 2 quarts of colostrum twice daily to calves.
3. For best mixing, continuously stir with wire whip while adding powder to 110-120°F water (hot as you can tolerate on your hand). Use correct water temperature to avoid product separation. Feed milk replacer at 90-100°F.
4. Provide fresh, clean water and a high quality, palatable calf starter from 4 days after birth and continue on a free-choice basis.
5. Observe calves closely during the milk replacer feeding period. Avoid underfeeding, which may result in starvation, or overconsumption which may increase incidence of scours.
6. Continue to feed milk replacer until the calf is consuming a minimum of 1½ pounds of calf starter per day, which usually occurs at 4-6 weeks of age.

Warning(s): Withdraw from calves 30 days before slaughter.

A withdrawal period has not been established for this product in pre-ruminating calves. Do not use in calves to be processed for veal.

Presentation: 25 lb (11.34 kg) and 50 lb (22.68 kg) bags.

® Registered Trademark of Land O'Lakes, Inc.

Compendium Code No.: 10380011

LAND O LAKES® INSTANT AMPLIFIER® SELECT PLUS

Land O'Lakes **Medicated Milk Replacer**

Guaranteed Analysis:

Crude Protein, not less than 20.0%
Crude Fat, not less than 20.0%
Crude Fiber, not more than 0.15%
Calcium (Ca), not less than 0.75%
Calcium (Ca), not more than 1.25%
Phosphorus (P), not less than 0.70%
Vitamin A, not less than . . . . 20,000 IU/lb.
Vitamin D_3, not less than . . . . 5,000 IU/lb.
Vitamin E, not less than . . . . 100 IU/lb.

Ingredients: Dried Whey, Dried Whey Protein Concentrate, Dried Whey Product, Dried Skimmed Milk, Dried Milk Protein, Animal Fat (preserved with Ethoxyquin), Lecithin, Polyethylene

Glycol (400) Monooleate, DiCalcium Phosphate, Calcium Carbonate, Vitamin A Acetate, D-Activated Animal Sterol (Source of Vitamin D_3), Vitamin E Supplement, Thiamine Mononitrate, Pyridoxine Hydrochloride, Folic Acid, Vitamin B_{12} Supplement, Choline Chloride, Roughage Products, Sodium Silico Aluminate, Manganese Sulfate, Zinc Sulfate, Ferrous Sulfate, Copper Sulfate, Cobalt Sulfate, Ethylenediamine Dihydriodide and Sodium Selenite.

Indications: Dairy herd and beef calf milk replacer.

Directions: Mixing Directions:

Increased Growth Program (Recommended):

Use the plastic cup provided to measure the milk replacer powder.

Add 1 full cup* of milk replacer powder to 2 quarts of 110-120°F. water and mix thoroughly.

Large Batches: Mix 6¼ pounds (10 full cups) of milk replacer powder to 5 gallons of 110-120°F. water.

Feed each calf according to the schedule listed below.

*One measuring cup holds approximately 10 ounces (weight) of dry milk replacer powder.

Conventional Program:

Use the plastic cup provided to measure the milk replacer powder.

Fill cup with milk replacer powder to 8 ounce mark and add to 2 quarts of 110-120°F. water and mix thoroughly.

Large Batches: Mix 5 pounds (8 full cups) of milk replacer powder to 5 gallons of 110-120°F. water. Feed each calf according to the schedule listed below.

Feeding Directions (4 days of age to weaning):

Large Breeds: Feed 2 quarts reconstituted liquid milk replacer twice a day.

Small Breeds: Feed 1½-2 quarts reconstituted liquid milk replacer twice a day.

In extremely cold weather it may be beneficial to feed another feeding of calf milk replacer in the middle of the day. Add ½ cup of milk replacer powder to 1 quart of 110-120°F. water, mix and feed to 1 calf at midday.

A characteristic of this product is a slight layering that occurs approximately 7 minutes after mixing.

General Recommendations:

1. Newborn calves should receive 3 quarts of colostrum in the first feeding as soon after birth as possible (within 1 hour) and again 12 hours later.
2. For days 2 and 3 of life, feed 2 quarts of colostrum twice daily to calves.
3. For best mixing, continuously stir with wire whip while adding powder to 110-120°F. water (hot as you can tolerate on your hand). Use correct water temperature to avoid product separation. Feed milk replacer at 90-100°F.
4. Provide fresh, clean water and a high quality, palatable calf starter from 4 days after birth and continue on a free-choice basis.
5. Observe calves closely during the milk replacer feeding period. Avoid underfeeding, which may result in starvation, or overconsumption which may increase incidence of scours.
6. Continue to feed milk replacer until the calf is consuming a minimum of 1½ pounds of calf starter per day, which usually occurs at 4-6 weeks of age.

Presentation: 25 lb (11.34 kg) and 50 lb (22.68 kg) bags.

® Registered Trademark of Land O'Lakes, Inc.

Patent No. 5,571,542

Compendium Code No.: 10380100

LAND O LAKES® INSTANT COW'S MATCH™

Land O'Lakes **Medicated Milk Replacer**

Medicated Dairy Herd & Beef Calf Milk Replacer

Active Ingredient(s):

Oxytetracycline .... 100 g/ton
Neomycin Base (from Neomycin Sulfate) .... 200 g/ton

Guaranteed Analysis:

Crude Protein, not less than 28.0%
Crude Fat, not less than 20.0%
Crude Fiber, not more than 0.15%
Calcium (Ca), not less than 0.75%
Calcium (Ca), not more than 1.25%
Phosphorus (P), not less than 0.70%
Vitamin A, not less than .... 10,000 I.U./lb
Vitamin D_3, not less than .... 2,500 I.U./lb
Vitamin E, not less than .... 50 I.U./lb

Ingredients: Dried Whey, Dried Whey Protein Concentrate, Dried Whey Product, Dried Milk Protein, Animal Fat (preserved with Ethoxyquin), Lecithin, Polyethylene Glycol (400) Monooleate, DiCalcium Phosphate, Calcium Carbonate, Methionine Supplement, L-Lysine, Vitamin A Acetate, D-Activated Animal Sterol (Source of Vitamin D_3), Vitamin E Supplement, Thiamine Mononitrate, Riboflavin, Niacin Supplement, Calcium Pantothenate, Biotin, Ascorbic Acid, Pyridoxine Hydrochloride, Folic Acid, Vitamin B_{12} Supplement, Choline Chloride, Roughage Products, Sodium Silico Aluminate, Manganese Sulfate, Zinc Sulfate, Ferrous Sulfate, Copper Sulfate, Cobalt Sulfate, Ethylenediamine Dihydriodide and Sodium Selenite.

Indications: To aid in the prevention of bacterial diarrhea (scours) in calves.

Directions: Mixing Directions:

Small Batch: While stirring, pour 1.5 pounds (24 oz) of milk replacer powder into 3 quarts of 110-120°F water. Mix thoroughly and add 110-120°F water to bring to a total volume of 1 gallon of milk replacer solution.

Large Batch: While stirring, pour 7.5 pounds of milk replacer powder into 2 gallons of 110-120°F water. Mix thoroughly and add 110-120°F water to a total volume of 5 gallons of milk replacer solution.

Powder should be weighed for precision and best calf performance.

Feeding Directions (2 Days of Age to Weaning):

Large Breeds:

Week 1: Feed 2½ quarts of milk replacer solution twice daily.

Week 2 until 1 week prior to weaning: Feed 3½ quarts of milk replacer solution twice daily.

Last Weak on Milk: Feed 3½ quarts of milk replacer solution once per day.

(The above mixing and feeding rates are designed for optimal calf growth from COW'S MATCH™ calf milk replacer).

A characteristic of this product is a slight layering that occurs approximately 7 minutes after mixing. If layering occurs, re-mix before feeding.

General Recommendations:

1. Newborn calves should receive 3 quarts of colostrum in the first feeding as soon after birth as possible (within 1 hour) and again 12 hours later.
2. Begin feeding COW'S MATCH™ at two days of age at the recommended rate.
3. Provide fresh, clean water on day 2 and provide continuously on a free-choice basis.
4. Begin feeding a calf starter recommended for intensive feeding at two days of age and offer continuously on a free-choice basis.
5. The week of weaning, transition calves from twice per day feeding to once per day feeding of COW'S MATCH™. This will encourage the calf to eat more calf starter and assures an effective weaning.
6. Continue to feed appropriate intensive calf starter up to 12 weeks of age - no hay fed separately.
7. Begin feeding a calf grower recommended for intensive feeding at 12 weeks of age at the recommended rate.

Warning(s): Withdraw from calves 30 days before slaughter.

A withdrawal period has not been established for this product in pre-ruminating calves. Do not use in calves to be processed for veal.

Discussion: Intensified Calf Feeding and Management Program: Implementing an intensified calf feeding and management program will require specialized and detailed calf management. Calf to calf variations such as calf weight and health must be considered in implementing a program. Consult with your feed specialist for specific feeding and management recommendations to match with your calf performance goals and expectations. COW'S MATCH™ calf milk replacer is specifically designed to be fed as a calf milk replacer along with a specific calf starter designed for intensified feeding.

Presentation: 50 lb (22.68 kg) bag.

™ COW'S MATCH is a trademark of Land O'Lakes, Inc.

Patent No. 5,571,542

Compendium Code No.: 10380091 101

LAND O LAKES® INSTANT KID MILK REPLACER

Land O'Lakes **Milk Replacer**

Active Ingredient(s): Guaranteed Analysis:

Crude protein, not less than 26.00%
Crude fat, not less than 20.00%
Crude fiber, not more than 0.15%
Ash, not more than 11.00%
Added minerals, not more than 0.06%
Vitamin A, not less than .... 20,000 I.U./lb
Vitamin D_3, not less than .... 5,000 I.U./lb
Vitamin E, not less than .... 100 I.U./lb

Ingredients: Dried whey, dried whey protein concentrate, dried whey product, dried skimmed milk, dried milk protein, animal fat (preserved with ethoxyquin), lecithin, vitamin A acetate, d-activated animal sterol (source of vitamin D_3), vitamin E supplement, thiamine mononitrate, pyridoxine hydrochloride, folic acid, vitamin B_{12} supplement, choline chloride, sodium silico aluminate, manganese sulfate, zinc sulfate, ferrous sulfate, copper sulfate, cobalt sulfate, ethylenediamine dihydriodide and sodium selenite.

Indications: A milk replacer for kids from two days of age to weaning.

Dosage and Administration:

Mixing Directions: Use the plastic cup provided to measure the milk replacer powder. Each cup holds about ¼ lb. of powder. Mix one (1) level cup of LAND O LAKES® Instant Kid Milk Replacer in one and one-half (1½) pints (or pounds) of 110°-120°F water by slowly adding the powder to the water while stirring.

Hand Feeding Guidelines: Use the following schedule as a guideline for feeding reconstituted milk replacer:

Age of Kid (days)	No. feedings per day	Maximum pints per kid daily
1	4	Colostrum
2-3	4	1
4-5	3	1
6-10	2	1½
11-weaning	2	2-3

Free Choice Feeding - Use of a free choice device (ie. lamb bar) requires that the milk replacer solution be kept cold (about 40°F) to prevent overconsumption. Kids may need to be trained to suckle from nipples. However, they will adapt readily within one (1) or two (2) days.

Discussion: General Recommendations:

1. Keep all of the equipment used for mixing and feeding thoroughly cleaned.
2. Newborn kids should receive colostrum as soon after birth as possible (within 3-4 hours).
3. When hand-feeding by bottle or a shallow pan, the milk replacer should be about 90° to 100°F.
4. Provide fresh clean water and a high quality dry feed on a free choice basis after kids are seven days of age.
5. If scouring occurs due to bacterial infection, the kids may need treatment with an oral antibiotic. If scours persist, seek assistance from a veterinarian.

Presentation: 25 lb. bags.

Compendium Code No.: 10380020

LAND O LAKES® INSTANT MAXI CARE®

Land O'Lakes **Medicated Milk Replacer**

Dairy Herd & Beef Calf Milk Replacer

Active Ingredient(s):

Oxytetracycline .... 125 grams per ton
Neomycin Base (from Neomycin Sulfate) .... 250 grams per ton

Guaranteed Analysis:

Crude Protein, not less than 22.0%
Crude Fat, not less than 20.0%
Crude Fiber, not more than 0.5%
Calcium (Ca), not less than 0.75%
Calcium (Ca), not more than 1.25%
Phosphorus (P), not less than 0.70%
Vitamin A, not less than .... 20,000 I.U./lb
Vitamin D_3, not less than .... 5,000 I.U./lb
Vitamin E, not less than .... 100 I.U./lb

Ingredients: Dried whey, dried whey protein concentrate, dried whey product, dried skimmed milk, dried milk protein, protein modified soy flour, animal fat (preserved with ethoxyquin), lecithin, dicalcium phosphate, calcium carbonate, vitamin A acetate, d-activated animal sterol (source of vitamin D_3), vitamin E supplement, thiamine mononitrate, pyridoxine hydrochloride, folic acid, vitamin B_{12} supplement, choline chloride, sodium silico aluminate, manganese sulfate, zinc sulfate, ferrous sulfate, copper sulfate, cobalt sulfate, ethylenediamine dihydriodide and sodium selenite.

Indications: To aid in the prevention of bacterial diarrhea (scours) in calves.

Directions: Mixing Directions:

Accelerated Growth Program (Recommended):

Use the plastic cup provided to measure the milk replacer powder.

Add 1 full cup* of milk replacer powder to 2 quarts of 110-120°F water and mix thoroughly.

Large Batches: Mix 6¼ pounds (10 full cups) of milk replacer powder to 5 gallons of 110-120°F water.

Feed each calf according to the schedule listed below.

*One measuring cup holds approximately 10 ounces (weight) of dry milk replacer powder.

Conventional Program:

Use the plastic cup provided to measure the milk replacer powder.

Fill cup with milk replacer powder to 8 ounce mark and add to 2 quarts of 110-120°F water and mix thoroughly.

Large Batches: Mix 5 pounds (8 full cups) of milk replacer powder to 5 gallons of 110-120°F water. Feed each calf according to the schedule listed below.

Feeding Directions (4 days of age to weaning):

Large Breeds: Feed 2 quarts reconstituted liquid milk replacer twice a day.

Small Breeds: Feed 1½-2 quarts reconstituted liquid milk replacer twice a day.

In extremely cold weather it may be beneficial to feed another feeding of calf milk replacer in the middle of the day. Add ½ cup of milk replacer powder to 1 quart of 110-120°F water, mix and feed to 1 calf at midday.

General Recommendations:

1. Newborn calves should receive 3 quarts of colostrum in the first feeding as soon after birth as possible (within 1 hour) and again 12 hours later.
2. For Days 2 and 3 of life, feed 2 quarts of colostrum twice daily to calves.
3. For best mixing, continuously stir with wire whip while adding powder to 110-120°F water (hot as you can tolerate on your hand). Use correct water temperature to avoid product separation. Feed milk replacer at 90-100°F.
4. Provide fresh, clean water and a high quality, palatable calf starter from 4 days after birth and continue on a free-choice basis.
5. Observe calves closely during the milk replacer feeding period. Avoid underfeeding which may result in starvation, or overconsumption which may increase incidence of scours.
6. Continue to feed milk replacer until the calf is consuming a minimum of 1½ pounds of calf starter per day, which usually occurs at 4-6 weeks of age.

Warning(s): Withdraw from calves 30 days before slaughter.

A withdrawal period has not been established for this product in pre-ruminating calves. Do not use in calves to be processed for veal.

Presentation: 25 lb (11.34 kg) and 50 lb (22.68 kg) bags.

® Registered Trademark of Land O'Lakes, Inc.

Compendium Code No.: 10380031

LAND O LAKES® INSTANT NURSING FORMULA

Land O'Lakes **Milk Replacer**

Dairy Herd & Beef Calf Milk Replacer

Active Ingredient(s):

Oxytetracycline .... 125 grams per ton
Neomycin Base (from Neomycin Sulfate) .... 250 grams per ton

Guaranteed Analysis:

Crude Protein, not less than 22.0%
Crude Fat, not less than 20.0%
Crude Fiber, not more than 0.15%
Calcium (Ca), not less than 0.75%
Calcium (Ca), not more than 1.25%
Phosphorus (P), not less than 0.70%
Vitamin A, not less than .... 20,000 I.U./lb
Vitamin D_3, not less than .... 5,000 I.U./lb
Vitamin E, not less than .... 100 I.U./lb

Ingredients: Dried whey, dried whey protein concentrate, dried whey product, dried skimmed milk, dried milk protein, animal fat (preserved with ethoxyquin), lecithin, polyethylene glycol (400) monooleate, dicalcium phosphate, calcium carbonate, vitamin A acetate, d-activated animal sterol (source of vitamin D_3), vitamin E supplement, thiamine mononitrate, pyridoxine hydrochloride, folic acid, vitamin B_{12} supplement, choline chloride, sodium silico aluminate, manganese sulfate, zinc sulfate, ferrous sulfate, copper sulfate, cobalt sulfate, ethylenediamine dihydriodide and sodium selenite.

Indications: To aid in the prevention of bacterial diarrhea (scours) in calves.

Directions: Mixing Directions:

Accelerated Growth Program (Recommended):

Use the plastic cup provided to measure the milk replacer powder.

Add 1 full cup* of milk replacer powder to 2 quarts of 110-120°F water and mix thoroughly.

Large Batches: Mix 6¼ pounds (10 full cups) of milk replacer powder to 5 gallons of 110-120°F water.

Feed each calf according to the schedule listed below.

*One measuring cup holds approximately 10 ounces (weight) of dry milk replacer powder.

Conventional Program:

Use the plastic cup provided to measure the milk replacer powder.

Fill cup with milk replacer powder to 8 ounce mark and add to 2 quarts of 110-120°F water and mix thoroughly.

Large Batches: Mix 5 pounds (8 full cups) of milk replacer powder to 5 gallons of 110-120°F water. Feed each calf according to the schedule listed below.

Feeding Directions (4 days of age to weaning):

Large Breeds: Feed 2 quarts reconstituted liquid milk replacer twice a day.

Small Breeds: Feed 1½-2 quarts reconstituted liquid milk replacer twice a day.

In extremely cold weather it may be beneficial to feed another feeding of calf milk replacer in the middle of the day. Add ½ cup of milk replacer powder to 1 quart of 110-120°F water, mix and feed to 1 calf at midday.

General Recommendations:

1. Newborn calves should receive 3 quarts of colostrum in the first feeding as soon after birth as possible (within 1 hour) and again 12 hours later.
2. For Days 2 and 3 of life, feed 2 quarts of colostrum twice daily to calves.
3. For best mixing, continuously stir with wire whip while adding powder to 110-120°F water (hot as you can tolerate on your hand). Use correct water temperature to avoid product separation. Feed milk replacer at 90-100°F.
4. Provide fresh, clean water and a high quality, palatable calf starter from 4 days after birth and continue on a free-choice basis.
5. Observe calves closely during the milk replacer feeding period. Avoid underfeeding which may result in starvation, or overconsumption which may increase incidence of scours.
6. Continue to feed milk replacer until the calf is consuming a minimum of 1½ pounds of calf starter per day, which usually occurs at 4-6 weeks of age.

Warning(s): Withdraw from calves 30 days before slaughter.

A withdrawal period has not been established for this product in pre-ruminating calves. Do not use in calves to be processed for veal.

Presentation: 25 lb (11.34 kg) and 50 lb (22.68 kg) bags.

® Registered Trademark of Land O'Lakes, Inc.

Compendium Code No.: 10380041

LAND O LAKES® LITTERMILK®

Land O'Lakes **Medicated Milk Replacer**

Active Ingredient(s):

Oxytetracycline .... 140 g/ton
Neomycin base (from neomycin sulfate) .... 140 g/ton

Guaranteed Analysis:

Crude protein, not less than 28.0%
Crude fat, not less than 10.0%
Crude fiber, not more than 0.15%
Vitamin A, not less than .... 20,000 I.U./lb
Vitamin D_3, not less than .... 5,000 I.U./lb
Vitamin E, not less than .... 100 I.U./lb

Ingredients: Dried skimmed milk, dried whey, dried whey product, dried milk protein, animal fat (preserved with ethoxyquin), lecithin, vitamin A acetate, d-activated animal sterol (source of vitamin D_3), vitamin E supplement, thiamine mononitrate, riboflavin, niacin supplement, calcium pantothenate, biotin, ascorbic acid, pyridoxine hydrochloride, folic acid, vitamin B_{12} supplement, choline chloride, sodium silico aluminate, manganese sulfate, zinc sulfate, ferrous sulfate, copper sulfate, cobalt sulfate, ethylenediamine dihydriodide and sodium selenite.

Indications: For use as an aid in the treatment of bacterial enteritis (scours) in pigs.

Dosage and Administration: How to Mix and Feed LAND O LAKES® LITTERMILK®:

1. Mix three (3) level cups (15 oz.) of LAND O LAKES® LITTERMILK® powder (plastic cup provided) for each gallon of warm water (110°-120°F) required as determined by the number of pigs and amounts to feed on the feeding schedule below. (The plastic cup level full will hold about 0.31 lbs. of milk replacer powder).
2. Feed LAND O LAKES® LITTERMILK® at nursery room temperature for the entire milk feeding period.
3. Mix and feed LAND O LAKES® LITTERMILK® once each day using the LAND O LAKES® LITTERMILK® feeder.
   Important: Keep all equipment clean. Rinse the feeding equipment each day and thoroughly clean (use detergent and/or disinfectant).
4. Small or weak pigs may require assistance in receiving the milk replacer. A short rubber tube on a syringe (without needle) can be used effectively to force feed the milk replacer.
5. Daily Feeding Directions:

Pig Age (days)	Dry Powder Weight (oz.)	Fluid oz. of Water	Total Fluid oz./Pig[a]	Pints/Pig
1-3	3	27	30	1.90
4-5	5	45	50	3.10
6-7	6	54	60	3.75
8-12	8	72	80	5.00
*13-16	5	45	50	3.10
17-20	2	18	20	1.25
21	0	0	Wean	0.00

(a) To determine the total amount of LAND O LAKES® LITTERMILK® to be fed to each group, add up the daily amounts for each pig in that group.

*Begin at day 13 to provide a fresh, clean, high quality creep feed and provide fresh clean water at all times.

Warning(s): Withdraw the product from pigs 10 days before slaughter.

Discussion: Tips for Best Results

Equipment
- 4' x '4 raised nursery deck
- Maximum 8 pigs per pen
- Wire flooring or similar material
- Use LAND O LAKES® LITTERMILK® feeder

Environment
- Warm, dry, draft free
- Temperature 90°F; Use heat lamp
- Ventilation - no drafts
  - 1 cfm/pig, winter
  - 10 cfm/pig, spring-fall
  - 25 cfm/pg, summer

Management
- Select biggest pigs from litter to feed LITTERMILK®; leave small pigs on sow
- Disinfect navels at birth
- Use injectable iron at 3 and 10 days of age

Other Systems
- Empty farrowing crates - divide 8 pigs per side
- Milk supplement for pigs nursing thin gilts or sows.

General Recommendations
- Reseal bag between feedings.
- Do not underfeed - starvation may occur.
- Avoid overfeeding the pigs, as it may make weaning to dry feed more difficult.
- Insure pigs receive colostrum from sow as soon as possible after birth.
- Do not group small, weak pigs with big, healthy pigs.
- Do not group pigs of ages more than 7 days apart.
- Do not re-feed milk replacer that is left over more than 24 hours; clean out the old milk, if any.

Twice a day supervision required.
If scours occur:
First - Check environment for drafts and proper temperature.
Second - Evaluate sanitation.
Third - If scours persist, treat with suitable antibiotic doser.
Fourth - If scours continue, seek assistance from local veterinarian.

Presentation: 25 lb. packages.

Compendium Code No.: 10380050

LAND O LAKES® MARE'S MATCH®

Land O'Lakes **Milk Replacer**

Active Ingredient(s): Guaranteed Analysis:
Crude protein, not less than 24.0%
Crude fat, not less than 16.0%
Crude fiber, not more than 0.15%

Ingredients: Dried whey, dried whey protein concentrate, dried whey product, dried skimmed milk, dried milk protein, animal fat (preserved with ethoxyquin), lecithin, vitamin A acetate, d-activated animal sterol (source of vitamin D_3), vitamin E supplement, thiamine mononitrate, riboflavin, niacin supplement, calcium pantothenate, biotin, ascorbic acid, pyridoxine hydrochloride, folic acid, vitamin B_{12} supplement, choline chloride, sodium silico aluminate, calcium carbonate, manganese sulfate, zinc sulfate, ferrous sulfate, copper sulfate, cobalt sulfate, ethylenediamine dihydriodide and sodium selenite.

Indications: A foal milk replacer for orphan foals, foals with an inadequate milk supply, foals whose mare will not allow them to nurse or foals from sick mares.

Dosage and Administration: Use the plastic cup provided to measure the milk replacer powder. Each cup (½ pint) holds about ¼ lb of powder. Mix one (1) level cup of LAND O LAKES® MARE'S MATCH® in one (1) quart of 110-120°F water by slowly adding the powder to water while stirring. Feeding temperature should be 90-100°F.

Use the following schedule as a guideline for feeding reconstituted milk replacer:

Age of Foal	No. feedings per day	Feeding rates (quarts) per foal daily*
1 day	—	colostrum
2-7 days	4	4-8
2nd week**	4	6-12
3rd week and 4th week	3	8-15
5th week	3	6-12
6th week-8th week	2	4-8

*Higher feeding rates are designed for larger foals where a maximum growth rate is desired. Ponies should be fed at one-half (½) the lowest feeding rate for each age period.

**Begin feeding in small amounts a high quality foal creep ration and provide fresh clean water at all times. Gradually increase the feeding rate over time.

Discussion: General Recommendations:
1. Ensure that the foals receive colostrum from the mare as soon as possible after birth.
2. Completely sanitize the feeding equipment each day.
3. Buckets are an acceptable means of providing liquid MARE'S MATCH® to foals.
4. If persistent scours occur, consult a veterinarian.
5. Reseal the bag between feedings to maintain freshness.
6. Keep foals in a dry, draft-free environment.
7. Do not refeed milk replacer that is left over for more than two hours.

Presentation: 10 lb and 25 lb bags; 8 lb and 20 lb pails.

Compendium Code No.: 10380060

LAND O LAKES® MARE'S MATCH® FOAL PELLETS

Land O'Lakes **Equine Dietary Supplement**

Guaranteed Analysis:
Crude Protein, min. 26.0%
Crude Fat, min. 10.0%
Crude Fiber, max. 1.5%
Calcium, min. 1.40%
Calcium, max. 2.40%
Phosphorus, min. 0.90%
Copper, min. .... 30 ppm
Zinc, min. .... 120 ppm
Selenium, min. .... 0.30 ppm
Vitamin A, min. .... 20,000 I.U./lb
Vitamin D_3, min. .... 2,000 I.U./lb
Vitamin E, min. .... 100 I.U./lb

Ingredients: Dried whey, soy flour, dried whey protein concentrate, dried milk protein, dried skimmed milk, animal fat (preserved with ethoxyquin), calcium carbonate, dicalcium phosphate, vitamin A acetate, d-activated animal sterol (source of vitamin D_3), vitamin E supplement, thiamine mononitrate, riboflavin, niacin supplement, calcium pantothenate, biotin, ascorbic acid, pyridoxine hydrochloride, folic acid, vitamin B_{12} supplement, choline chloride, l-lysine, methionine supplement, manganese sulfate, zinc sulfate, zinc oxide, ferrous sulfate, copper sulfate, cobalt sulfate, ethylenediamine dihydriodide, sodium selenite and natural and artificial flavor.

Indications: A milk-base supplement designed for young foals and weanling horses.

Directions: Feeding Directions:

Orphaned/Early Weaned Foals:

Reconstituted MARE'S MATCH® Powder	MARE'S MATCH® Foal Pellets	Foal Feed
Feed according to directions on the MARE'S MATCH® Foal Milk Replacer package.	Can be fed free choice up to 2 pounds or 4 cups* per day.	Feed recommended foal feed according to directions.

Nursing Foals: MARE'S MATCH® Foal Pellets can be fed free-choice up to 1.5 pounds or 3 cups* per day.

Weanlings/Yearlings: Feed normal protein roughage/grain ration. If additional condition is desired feed 0.5 to 1.5 pounds (1-3 cups) of MARE'S MATCH® Foal Pellets.

Broodmares:

Gestation: Depending on the condition of the mare, supplement the mare's ration with 0.5 to 1.5 pounds (1-3 cups) of MARE'S MATCH® Foal Pellets daily. Do not allow the mare to become fat.

Lactation: If supplementation is needed feed 0.5 to 1.5 pounds (1-3 cups) daily depending upon condition of the mare.

Performance Horses: Supplement the ration with 0.5 to 1.5 pounds (1-3 cups) daily to maintain condition.

*Cup enclosed holds approximately 0.5 pound of Mare's Match Foal Pellets.

Presentation: 25 lb (11.34 kg).

® Registered Trademark of Land O'Lakes, Inc.

Compendium Code No.: 10380071

LAND O LAKES® ULTRA FRESH® LAMB MILK REPLACER

Land O'Lakes **Milk Replacer**

Active Ingredient(s): Guaranteed Analysis:
Crude protein, not less than 24.0%
Crude fat, not less than 35.0%
Crude fiber, not more than 0.15%
Vitamin A, not less than .... 20,000 I.U./lb
Vitamin D_3, not less than .... 5,000 I.U./lb
Vitamin E, not less than .... 100 I.U./lb

Ingredients: Dried whey, dried whey protein concentrate, dried skimmed milk, dried milk protein, animal fat (preserved with ethoxyquin), dried corn syrup, lecithin, vitamin A acetate, d-activated animal sterol (source of vitamin D_3), vitamin E supplement, thiamine mononitrate, pyridoxine hydrochloride, folic acid, vitamin B_{12} supplement, choline chloride, sodium silico aluminate, calcium propionate, malic acid, manganese sulfate, zinc sulfate, ferrous sulfate, copper sulfate, cobalt sulfate, ethylenediamine dihydriodide, sodium selenite and natural and artificial flavor.

Indications: Lamb milk replacer.

Dosage and Administration: Mixing and Feeding Directions:
1. Lambs should receive colostrum milk soon after birth. Remove lambs from ewes one (1) day after birth, if possible, and start the lambs on ULTRA FRESH® Lamb Milk Replacer.
2. Use the plastic cup provided in the bag to measure Lamb Milk Replacer powder. Mix one (1) level measure (about ¼ lb.) of ULTRA FRESH® Lamb Milk Replacer in one (1) pint of water, or for large batches mix 2 lbs. of ULTRA FRESH® Lamb Milk Replacer with one (1) gallon of water.
3. Mix with warm (110-120°F) water; stir while adding ULTRA FRESH® Lamb Milk Replacer.
4. Hand Feeding - When hand feeding by bottle, ULTRA FRESH® Lamb Milk Replacer should be fed at body temperature. The following feeding schedule is recommended:
   After colostrum feeding to three (3) days of age - Feed ⅓ cup of reconstituted ULTRA FRESH® Lamb Milk Replacer four (4) to six (6) times a day at 4-hour intervals.
   Four (4) days to two (2) weeks of age - Gradually decrease the number of feedings and increase the amount of ULTRA FRESH® Lamb Milk Replacer per feeding. At two (2) weeks of age, one (1) cup of reconstituted ULTRA FRESH® Lamb Milk Replacer three (3) times per day is sufficient.
   Two (2) weeks to weaning - Feed reconstituted ULTRA FRESH® Lamb Milk Replacer twice a day and in gradually increased quantities.
5. Free Choice Feeding - If using devices to give lambs free access to ULTRA FRESH® Lamb Milk Replacer, it should be fed cold at about 40°F. Cold milk is used to limit intake and prevent overeating. When starting lambs on nipples they will require assistance. However, they will adapt readily and nurse independently within one (1) or two (2) days.
6. Keep the milk replacer feeding equipment clean.
7. Provide a high quality creep feed at a few days of age and continue on a free choice basis. Fresh, clean water should be provided at all times.
8. Lambs should be weaned from milk at four (4) to six (6) weeks of age or at about 25 lbs. of weight. Abrupt weaning can be used. However, reduced milk replacer feeding a few days prior to weaning to encourage creep intake may be desirable.
9. If scours occur:
   a. Check the environment for drafts and proper temperature.
   b. Evaluate sanitation.
   c. If scours persist, treat with a suitable antibiotic as recommended by a veterinarian.

Presentation: 10 lb. and 25 lb. bags.

Compendium Code No.: 10380080

LANODINE™

Butler **Topical Wound Dressing**

NDC No.: 11695-2160-6

Active Ingredient(s): Povidone-iodine (1% titratable iodine).
Enriched with lanolin.

Indications: Antibacterial and antifungal ointment for wounds, cuts, and abrasions.

Water-resistant formula adheres to the wound to provide long-lasting protection even in harsh weather. Contains lanolin as an emollient and protectant.

Dosage and Administration: Apply to the wound after cleansing and drying. Apply as needed to maintain coverage. May bandage if necessary.

Caution(s): For veterinary use only. For deep or puncture wounds, use as directed by a veterinarian. Keep out of the reach of children.

Presentation: 1 lb. (16 oz.) containers.

Compendium Code No.: 10821060

LARVADEX® 1% PREMIX

Novartis **Feed Additive**

EPA Reg. No.: 70585-1

Active Ingredient(s):
Cyromazine: *N*-cyclopropyl-1,3,5-triazine-2,4,6-triamine 1.0%
Inert ingredients 99.0%
Total 100.0%

Indications: For fly control in and around:
1. Caged or slatted flooring layer chicken operations.
2. Breeder chicken operations.

LARVADEX® 1% Premix is a premix which, when blended into a poultry ration according to the "Directions for Use" given below, will control certain fly species which develop in poultry manure. LARVADEX® 1% Premix is intended for use only in poultry (chickens) layer and breeder operations.

Directions for Use:

Important: Read the entire "Directions for Use" and the "Conditions of Sale and Warranty" before using the product. If the terms are not acceptable, return the unopened product container at once.

It is a violation of federal law to use the product in a manner inconsistent with its labeling.

Failure to follow directions and precautions on the label may result in injury, poor fly control, and/or illegal residues.

Blending and Feeding LARVADEX® 1% Premix:

Housefly, soldier fly, lesser housefly: Mix 1 lb. of LARVADEX® 1% Premix per ton of feed. Feed the treated feed as a daily ration. Begin feeding when adult flies become active and continue the treatment as prescribed through the fly season.

LARVADEX® 1% Premix will provide a high degree of fly control and will give the best results when integrated with a well-managed fly control program which includes minimization of fly breeding sites, a determination of the degree of fly control desired, a monitoring of adult fly populations in and around the operation; and frequent examinations of manure for maggot activity.

When and How to Use LARVADEX® 1% Premix: First, monitor adult flies in and near the poultry house. When the population reaches a level to cause concern, use a registered adulticide spray or fog to reduce the breeding potential. Then, examine manure in the pits for maggot activity. If maggots are active, start LARVADEX® 1% Premix in the ration.

Feed LARVADEX® 1% Premix continuously as directed for four (4) to six (6) weeks. Usually, this is enough time for LARVADEX® 1% Premix to thoroughly cover the droppings and break the fly population cycle in the poultry house.

After a minimum of four (4) to six (6) weeks of LARVADEX® 1% Premix feeding, carefully examine the manure pits. If little or no activity is observed in the manure, discontinue LARVADEX® 1% Premix and continue the sanitary and management program. Continue monitoring the manure pits. If maggots become active again, repeat the procedure.

Use bait, sprays, or fogs as needed during and between LARVADEX® 1% Premix feeding periods to control any adult flies.

During the winter months or during periods of low fly pressure, discontinue LARVADEX® 1% Premix use for at least four (4) consecutive months per year.

Consult with local extension service poultry entomologists or the State Agricultural Experiment station for additional localized fly control suggestions.

Note: Do not feed LARVADEX® 1% Premix treated feed to broiler poultry. LARVADEX® 1% Premix use in poultry is limited to use as a feed-through in chicken layer and breeder operations only and may not be fed to any other poultry species.

Manure from chickens fed LARVADEX® 1% Premix may be used as a soil fertilizer supplement. Do not apply more than three (3) tons of manure per acre per year. Do not apply to small grain crops that will be harvested or grazed or illegal residues may result. Do not feed manure from chickens fed LARVADEX® 1% Premix to animals.

Precautionary Statements: Hazards to Humans and Domestic Animals: Harmful if inhaled or absorbed through the skin. Avoid breathing dust. Avoid contact with the skin or clothing. May cause skin sensitization reactions in certain individuals. Wash thoroughly with soap and water after handling.

Statement of Practical Treatment:

If on skin: Immediately wash with plenty of soap and water. Get medical attention if irritation develops or persists.

If inhaled: Remove victim to fresh air. If not breathing, give artifical respiration, preferably mouth-to-mouth, and get medical attention.

If in eyes: Flush with plenty of water. Get medical attention if irritation develops or persists.

Environmental Hazards: Keep out of lakes, ponds, or streams. Do not contaminate water by cleaning of equipment or disposal of wastes.

Storage and Disposal: Do not contaminate water, food, or feed by storage or disposal practices. Store in a dry place.

Pesticide: Wastes resulting from the use of the product may be disposed of on site or at an approved waste disposal facility.

Container: Completely empty the bag into a mixer. Dispose of the empty bags in a sanitary landfill, or by incineration, or by burning if allowed by state and local authorities. If burned, stay out of smoke.

In case of fire, accident, major spillage, or other emergency, contact Novartis at 1-800-888-8372, day or night.

Warning(s): To avoid illegal residues, LARVADEX® 1% Premix treated feed must be removed at least three (3) days (72 hours) before slaughter.

Important Note to Feed Mill Operators: LARVADEX® 1% Premix feed formulators (those mixing as a service to customers) must inform the feed user that treated feed must be removed from layers and breeders at least three (3) days before slaughter. The following label statement is suggested for use on treated feed containers: "This poultry feed is formulated with 5.0 ppm (0.01 lb./ton) cyromazine. Treated feed must not be fed to layers and breeders for a minimum of three (3) days (72 hours) before slaughter for food."

Keep out of the reach of children.

Disclaimer: Conditions of Sale and Warranty: The "Directions for Use" of the product reflect the opinion of experts based on field use and tests. The directions are believed to be reliable and should be followed carefully. However, it is impossible to eliminate all risks inherently associated with the use of the product. Injury, ineffectiveness, or other unintended consequences may result because of factors such as weather conditions, presence of other materials, or the manner of use or application all of which are beyond the control of Novartis or the seller. All such risks shall be assumed by the buyer.

Novartis warrants that the product conforms to the chemical description on the label and is reasonably fit for the purposes referred to in the "Directions for Use" subject to the inherent risks referred to above. Novartis makes no other express or implied warranty of fitness or merchantability or any other express or implied warranty. In no case shall Novartis or the seller be liable for consequential, special, or indirect damages resulting from the use or handling of the product. Novartis and the seller offer the product, and the buyer and user accept it, subject to the foregoing "Conditions of Sale and Warranty", which may be varied only by agreement in writing signed by a duly authorized representative of Novartis .

Discussion: Fly control in poultry operations should include appropriate sanitary and management practices to reduce the number and size of fly breeding sites. A successful sanitary and management program may allow less than constant use of insecticides. This, in turn, should prolong the effective life of such agents.

Eliminating Fly Breeding Sites: Certain conditions around poultry operations encourage flies and should be brought under control or eliminated as an aid to fly control. These include:

1. Removing broken eggs and dead birds.
2. Cleaning up of feed spills, manure spills, especially if wet.
3. Reducing feed spills in the manure pits.
4. Reducing moisture in manure in the pits.
5. Repairing water leaks that cause wet manure.
6. Cleaning out weed-choked water drainage ditches.
7. Minimizing sources from other fly-infested animal operations in close proximity to the poultry house.

Determining the Threshold of Fly Tolerance: Fly pressure can vary depending upon farm location, season of the year, and emphasis on sanitation. Newer, controlled environment poultry houses are known to be less susceptible to fly populations re-establishing, once brought under control. The frequency of manure removal and proximity of the farm to neighbors or residential areas will greatly influence the expected degree of fly control. Each farm must determine the level of fly control required and follow an appropriate control program.

Presentation: 25 pounds.

LARVADEX® trademark of Novartis

Compendium Code No.: 11310022 NAH/LDX1/1 10/97

LARVADEX® 2SL

Novartis **Premise Insecticide**

EPA Reg. No.: 70585-2

Active Ingredient(s):

Cyromazine: N-cyclopropyl-1,3,5-triazine-2,4,6-triamine 2%
Inert ingredients 98%
Total 100%

Contains 0.17 lb. cyromazine per gallon.

Indications: For fly control in and around chicken layer and breeder operations only.

LARVADEX® 2SL is a soluble concentrate, which, when diluted with water according to the "Directions for Use" given below, will act as a larvicide to control fly species which develop in poultry manure and refuse. LARVADEX® 2SL controls fly infestations by breaking the life cycle at the maggot stage.

Directions for Use:

Important: Read the entire "Directions for Use" and the "Conditions of Sale and Warranty" before using this product. If the terms are not acceptable, return the unopened product container at once.

It is a violation of federal law to use this product in a manner inconsistent with its labeling.

Failure to follow directions and precautions on the label may result in injury, poor fly control, and/or illegal residues.

Do not apply this product in such a manner as to directly or through spray drift expose workers or other persons.

When and How to Use LARVADEX® 2SL: First, monitor adult flies in and near the poultry house. When the population reaches a level to cause concern, use registered adulticide baits, sprays, or fog to reduce fly numbers and breeding potential. Then, examine manure and other fly breeding areas for maggot activity. If maggots are active, treat breeding sites with LARVADEX® 2SL.

Mixing Application: Dilute LARVADEX® 2SL with water to make 0.1% spray (see following Dilution Chart). Apply 1 gallon of finished spray per 100 sq. ft. of area over surface of manure, manure storage areas, spilled feed, and other sites where maggots are active. Do not apply LARVADEX® 2SL more frequently than once every 21 days.

Registered baits, sprays, or fogs should be used to reduce adult flies present at the onset of larvicide program and the best management practices should be followed. They should also be used to help control any influx of adult flies from other areas.

Notes:

Do not apply LARVADEX® 2SL directly to poultry or poultry feed as illegal residues may result.

Do not feed manure treated with LARVADEX® 2SL to animals.

Do not use LARVADEX® 2SL in conjunction with Larvadex® 1% Premix. If chickens have been fed LARVADEX®-treated feed, do not apply LARVADEX® 2SL to manure.

Manure treated with LARVADEX® 2SL may be used as a soil fertilizer supplement. Do not apply more than 4 tons of manure treated with LARVADEX® 2SL per acre per year.

Do not apply treated manure to small grain crops that will be harvested or grazed, or illegal residues may result.

LARVADEX® 2SL Dilution Chart:

Gallons of Finished Spray Needed	Amount of LARVADEX® 2SL to Use for 0.1% Finished Spray
1	6.5 fl. oz. (13 tablespoons)
5	32.00 fl. oz. (4 cups or 2 pints)
25	160.00 fl. oz. (20 cups or 10 pints)

Precautionary Statements: Hazards to Humans and Domestic Animals: Causes moderate eye irritation. Harmful if swallowed, absorbed through the skin or inhaled. Avoid contact with the eyes, skin, or clothing. Do not breathe vapors or spray mist. Wash thoroughly with soap and water after handling. Remove contaminated clothing and wash before reuse.

Statement of Practical Treatment:

If on skin: Wash with plenty of soap and water. If irritation develops or persists, get medical attention.

If in eyes: Flush with plenty of water. If irritation develops or persists, get medical attention.

If inhaled: Move to fresh air.

Environmental Hazards: Do not contaminate water by the cleaning of equipment or the disposal of wastes.

Physical or Chemical Hazards: Corrosive to tin.

Storage and Disposal: Do not contaminate water, food, or feed by storage or disposal, or the cleaning of equipment. Store at temperatures above 32°F. Crystals may form at lower temperatures. If this occurs, place the product in a warm room (72°F or above) and shake the container at frequent intervals until all of the crystals are dissolved. Since this formulation contains water, it can also freeze solid at temperatures below 32°F. However, when reconstituted and the crystals redissolved, the product performance is not affected.

Pesticide: Improper disposal of unused pesticide, spray mixture, or rinsate is a violation of federal law. Pesticide, spray mixture, or rinsate that cannot be used according to label instruction, must be disposed of according to federal, state, or local procedures. For guidance in proper disposal methods, contact a State Pesticide or Environmental Control Agency, or the Hazardous Waste representative at the nearest EPA regional office.

Container: Do not reuse the empty container. Triple rinse (or equivalent) and offer for recycling or reconditioning, or puncture and dispose of in a sanitary landfill, by incineration, or by open burning if allowed by state and local authorities. If burned, keep out of smoke.

For minor spills, leaks, etc., follow all precautions indicated on this label and clean up immediately. Take special care to avoid the contamination of equipment and facilities during cleanup procedures and disposal of wastes. In the event of a major spill, fire, or other emergency, call 1-800-637-0281, day or night.

Warning(s): To avoid illegal residues, allow 1 day (24 hours) between the last application and slaughter.

Keep out of the reach of children.

Conditions of Sale and Warranty: The "Directions for Use" of this product reflect the opinion of experts based on field use and tests. The directions are believed to be reliable and should be followed carefully. However, it is impossible to eliminate all risks inherently associated with the use of this product. Injury, ineffectiveness, or other unintended consequences may result because of factors such as weather conditions, presence of other materials, or the manner of use or application all of which are beyond the control of Novartis or the seller. All such risks shall be assumed by the buyer.

Novartis warrants that this product conforms to the chemical description on the label and is reasonably fit for the purposes referred to in the "Directions for Use" subject to the inherent risks referred to above. Novartis makes no other express or implied warranty of fitness or merchantability or any other express or implied warranty. In no case shall Novartis or the seller be liable for consequential, special, or indirect damages resulting from the use or handling of this product. Novartis and the seller offer this product, and the buyer and user accept it, subject to the foregoing "Conditions of Sale and Warranty", which may be varied only by agreement in writing signed by a duly authorized representative of Novartis.

Discussion: For housefly, lesser housefly, and soldier fly control in poultry operations, including layer and breeder chickens: Fly control in poultry operations should include appropriate sanitary and management practices to reduce the number and size of fly breeding sites. A successful sanitary and management program may allow less than constant use of insecticides. This, in turn, should prolong the effective life of such agents.

Eliminating Fly Breeding Sites: Certain conditions around poultry operations encourage flies and should be brought under control or eliminated as an aid to fly control. These include:

1. Removing broken eggs and dead birds.
2. Cleaning up of feed spills, manure spills, especially if wet.
3. Reducing feed spills in the manure pits.
4. Reducing moisture in manure in the pits.
5. Repairing water leaks that cause wet manure.
6. Cleaning out weed-choked water drainage ditches.
7. Minimizing sources from other fly-infested animal operations in close proximity to the poultry house.

Presentation: 1 gallon (U.S.).

LARVADEX® is a trademark of Novartis

Compendium Code No.: 11310031 NAH/LDX2SL/1 09/98

LARYNGO-VAC™

Fort Dodge **Vaccine**

Fowl Laryngotracheitis Vaccine, Modified Live Virus

U.S. Vet. Lic. No.: 112

Contents: This product contains the antigen listed above.

Contains gentamicin as a preservative.

Indications: LARYNGO-VAC™ is recommended for the intraocular, drinking-water, or coarse spray vaccination of healthy chickens as an aid in the prevention of infectious laryngotracheitis.

Directions: Read in full, follow directions carefully.

Vaccinate birds when they are 4 weeks old; or, if conditions dictate, birds may be vaccinated as early as 10 days of age.

Revaccinate replacement birds at 16 to 20 weeks of age.

Fowl Laryngotracheitis Vaccine is recommended for the immunization of healthy birds; should an outbreak of laryngotracheitis occur on the premises, immediately institute a program of vaccination of birds farthest from the infected and work towards the diseased birds.

For intraocular vaccination (1,000 dose bottles only)

1. To rehydrate 1 vial of vaccine with 1 vial of diluent, remove aluminum seal and rubber stopper from vaccine vial and diluent bottle. Avoid contamination of the stoppers and the contents.
2. Half-fill the vaccine vial with diluent.
3. Replace the stopper and shake the vial until vaccine material is dissolved.
4. Carefully pour the rehydrated-dissolved vaccine into the plastic diluent bottle. Replace the bottle stopper and shake once again to obtain a uniform mixture.
5. Remove diluent-bottle closure and fit drop dispenser into bottle. The vaccine is now ready for use.
6. To vaccinate intraocularly, hold bird and place 1 drop of vaccine into the eye. Allow the vaccine to spread over the eye before releasing the bird into a holding area for vaccinated birds.

For drinking-water vaccination (1,000 or 5,000 dose bottles): This vaccine is recommended for the vaccination of healthy chickens 10 days of age or older. Revaccinate replacement birds at 16 to 20 weeks of age.

1. Discontinue use of medications or sanitizing agents in the drinking water 24 hours before vaccinating. Do not resume use for 24 hours following vaccination.
2. Water used for the drinking-water administration of a live virus vaccine must be non-chlorinated.
3. Provide enough waterers, so two-thirds of the birds may drink at one time. Scrub waterers with fresh, clean, non-chlorinated water, and use no disinfectant. Let the waterers drain dry.
4. Turn off automatic waterers, so the only available water is the vaccine water. Do not give vaccine water through medication tanks.
5. Withhold water for 2 to 4 hours before vaccinating. Do not deprive the birds of water if the temperature is extremely high.
6. Remove seal from vaccine vial.
7. Remove stopper and half-fill with clean, cool, non-chlorinated water.
8. Replace stopper and shake until dissolved.
9. Use a clean container two-thirds filled with cool, clean, non-chlorinated water. Add dried milk at a rate of 31.25 ounces (887.5 grams) per 62.5 gallons (237.5 liters) of the final volume of vaccine solution. Stir the mixture until the dried milk is dissolved.
10. Add the rehydrated vaccine from the vial and again stir the contents thoroughly.
11. Next, add the mixture to the final volume of water, as follows:

Add this amount of vaccine	to this final volume of water	
	for chickens 2 to 8 weeks old	for chickens over 8 weeks old
5,000 doses	12.5 to 25 gallons (47 to 95 liters)	25 to 50 gallons (95 to 189 liters)

12. Give 1 dose of vaccine per bird.
13. Distribute the final volume of (vaccine) water evenly among the clean waterers. Do not place the waterers in direct sunlight. Resume regular water administration only after all the vaccine water has been consumed.

For spray vaccination (1,000 or 5,000 dose bottles): This vaccine may be used for the vaccination of healthy chickens 10 days of age or older by spraying the vaccine solution above the chickens. A sprayer that delivers a fine mist quickly and evenly is recommended. Revaccinate replacement birds at 16 to 20 weeks of age.

1. Remove seal from a vial of vaccine.
2. Remove the stopper and half-fill vial with cool, distilled water.
3. Replace stopper and shake until vaccine is in solution.
4. Pour rehydrated vaccine into a clean container and add 500 mL cool, distilled water per 5,000 doses vaccine. Shake thoroughly.
5. Apply at the rate of 100 mL rehydrated vaccine per 1,000 birds. For example, 5,000 birds will require 500 mL rehydrated vaccine. Place the vaccine solution in the sprayer canister, set the discharge control for a coarse spray (droplet size of 75 to 120 microns) and walk through the house. Direct the spray above the heads of the birds.
6. This spray method of vaccination should be employed in poultry houses where air movement can be reduced to a minimum. Before spraying the vaccine solution, close the house and shut off mechanical ventilation. Maintain these conditions both during spraying and for 20 minutes afterwards.
7. Wear goggles and a face mask while spraying.
8. Any sprayer used for application of a live virus vaccine should be used for no other purpose.

Records: Keep a record of vaccine serial number and expiration date; date of receipt and date of vaccination; where vaccination takes place; and any reactions observed.

Precaution(s): Store this vaccine at not above 45°F (7°C).

Use entire contents of vial when first opened.

Burn this container and all unused contents.

This vaccine is nonreturnable.

Caution(s): This product should be stored, transported, and administered in accordance with the directions.

The use of this vaccine is subject to state laws, wherever applicable.

1. Rehydrate the vaccine outside the pens. Rehydrate 1 vial at a time and use entire contents immediately after rehydration. Do not stretch the number of doses to a larger number of birds than recommended: 1 dose per bird.
2. Vaccinate all susceptible birds on the premises at the same time.
3. Vaccinate healthy birds only.
4. A mild conjunctival reaction may occur approximately 4 days following vaccination. This occurs more often in dry, dusty houses than in well-managed quarters. Such a reaction will disappear in about 3 days.
5. Take care not to spill or spatter the vaccine. As a precautionary measure, curb traffic for 10 to 14 days between premises where birds have been vaccinated and areas where there are nonvaccinated susceptible birds.

Warning(s): Do not vaccinate within 21 days before slaughter.

For veterinary use only.

Presentation: 10 x 1,000 dose and 10 x 5,000 dose vials.

Compendium Code No.: 10031041 10560B

LASOTA M41 CONN.™

L.A.H.I. (New Jersey) **Vaccine**

Newcastle-Bronchitis Vaccine, B_1 Type, LaSota Strain, Mass. and Conn. Types, Live Virus

U.S. Vet. Lic. No.: 196

Contents: This product contains Newcastle disease live virus, B_1 type, LaSota strain, and infectious bronchitis live viruses, Massachusetts and Connecticut types.

Contains neomycin as a preservative.

The product is manufactured from SPF (Specific Pathogen Free) eggs and is a combination live virus vaccine of chicken embryo origin for the prevention of Newcastle disease and Massachusetts and Connecticut types infectious bronchitis.

The strains of viruses in this product were carefully selected to protect against field challenges yet provide minimum reaction when used as directed.

This vaccine was carefully produced and passed all tests in accordance with the U.S. government requirements.

Indications: The product is recommended for initial vaccination and revaccination of chickens for the prevention of Newcastle disease and Massachusetts and Connecticut types infectious bronchitis. Initial vaccination is administered to birds at 5 weeks of age. This product is also used in replacement birds before 16 weeks of age that were previously vaccinated. For drinking water use.

This vaccine will stimulate protective antibodies in susceptible birds. However, the duration of immunity resulting from the use of this vaccine is not permanent, therefore, revaccinations are necessary.

Consult a poultry pathologist for recommendations on revaccination based on conditions existing in a designated area at any given time.

Dosage and Administration: Preparation of Vaccine: Remove the aluminum overseal and stopper and add clean, non-sanitized water. Replace the stopper and shake well. Pour the contents into a quart jar ¾ full of non-sanitized water. Shake well and dilute as outlined in the chart below.

Method of Vaccination: Withhold all medication and disinfectants from the drinking water 24 hours before and 24 hours after vaccinating. Rinse waterers with clean, non-sanitized water. Water starve the birds for at least two hours prior to vaccination. Provide adequate space so that at least two-thirds of the birds can drink at one time.

Add mixture to water as per the following chart:

1,000 Doses:

Age of birds	Heavy	Leghorn
5-8 weeks	8 gals. of water	5 gals. of water
9-15 weeks	10 gals. of water	8 gals. of water
16-20 weeks	13 gals. of water	10 gals. of water

10,000 Doses:

Age of birds	Heavy	Leghorn
5-8 weeks	80 gals. of water	50 gals. of water
9-15 weeks	100 gals. of water	80 gals. of water
16-20 weeks	130 gals. of water	100 gals. of water

Divide mixed vaccine into the waterers.

Provide no other drinking water until all vaccine has been consumed.

Contraindication(s): Vaccinate healthy chickens only that are free of PPLO and without previous history of a respiratory disease.

If there are susceptible laying birds on the premises there is the possibility that the virus might spread from the vaccinated to the susceptible birds and affect egg production.

Precaution(s): Keep vaccine in the dark between 2-7°C (35-45°F).

Use entire contents when first opened. Burn this container and all unused contents.

Caution(s): Federal regulations prohibit the repackaging or sale of the contents of the package in fractional units. Do not accept if seal is broken.

Warning(s): Do not vaccinate within 21 days before slaughter.

It is imperative that the user of this product comply with the indications for use, contraindications, and method of vaccination stated on the direction sheet. The vaccine must be prepared and administered as directed to obtain best results.

Care should be taken to avoid contaminating hands, eyes and clothing with the vaccine. Newcastle disease virus can cause a mild inflammation of the conjunctiva lasting for 3 to 5 days.

If chicks are to be vaccinated at a very young age, the vaccination must be done at the point of destination to avoid violation of the Postal Laws and regulations.

For veterinary use only.

Presentation: 1,000 and 10,000 doses.

Compendium Code No.: 10080243

LAXADE BOLUS

AgriPharm **Antacid-Laxative**

Active Ingredient(s): Each bolus contains:

Magnesium oxide. . . . . 0.276 gr. (17.9 g)

(equivalent to magnesium hydroxide, 400 gr.)

In a flavored base.

Indications: For oral administration as an aid in the treatment of digestive disturbances requiring an antacid or mild laxative in cattle.

Dosage and Administration: Give two (2) to four (4) boluses depending upon the size and condition of the animal. Lubricate the boluses and administer with a balling gun. Three (3) boluses are equivalent to one quart of milk of magnesia.

Precaution(s): Store at a controlled room temperature between 59°-86°F (15°-30°C).

Keep tightly closed when not in use.

Caution(s): For animal use only. Keep out of the reach of children.

Do not exceed the recommended dosage. Avoid frequent or continued use.

Warning(s): Milk that has been taken from animals during treatment and for 24 hours (2 milkings) after the last treatment with this drug must not be used for food.

Presentation: Jars of 50 boluses.

Compendium Code No.: 14570570

LAXADE POWDER

AgriPharm **Antacid-Laxative**

Active Ingredient(s): Each pound contains:

Magnesium hydroxide . . . . 10.35 oz.

In a flavored base.

One pound contains magnesium hydroxide equivalent to 1 gallon milk of magnesia.

Indications: A mild laxative and antacid for use in ruminant animals with simple indigestion.

Dosage and Administration: Mature bovine, stir one (1) pound of LAXADE POWDER into one (1) gallon of water and mix thoroughly. Administer as a drench or via a stomach tube. For sheep, goats and calves administer one (1) pint to one (1) quart depending upon the size of the animals. Frequent or continued use should be avoided.

Precaution(s): Do not store above 86°F (30°C).

Caution(s): For animal use only. Keep out of the reach of children.

Warning(s): Milk that has been taken from animals during treatment and for 12 hours (1 milking) after the last treatment with this drug must not be used for food.

Presentation: 16 oz. (1 lb.) containers.

Compendium Code No.: 14570580

LAX'AIRE®

Pfizer Animal Health **Laxative**

Active Ingredient(s): Contains: Liquid petrolatum, cod liver oil, soybean oil, peptonized iron in a palatable base.

Indications: A laxative and lubricant for cats and dogs.

Directions: LAX'AIRE® has been formulated with high taste appeal. Place a small amount on your pet's nose or on your cat's paw to stimulate initial taste interest.

Dosage:

Cats—½- to 1½-inch ribbon of ointment daily for 2-3 days, then ½-1 inch 2-3 times a week.

Dogs—½- to 2-inch ribbon of ointment 2-3 times a week.

Precaution(s): Store between 15°-30°C (59°-86°F).

Caution(s): Keep out of reach of children.

Presentation: 3 oz (85.1 g) tube.

Compendium Code No.: 36901160 10-8022-05

LAXA-STAT™

Tomlyn **Laxative**

Lubricant for Hair Ball Elimination and Prevention

Ingredient(s): White petroleum USP, light mineral oil NF, corn syrup, malt syrup, soybean oil (source of Linoleic and Linolenic Acid), cane molasses, water, gelatin by-products, Sodium Benzoate (preservative), Iron Proteinate, artificial flavor.

Indications: LAXA-STAT™ is a smooth, gentle lubricant for the prevention and elimination of hair balls in an easy-to-use "irrestible taste" gel form.

Directions: Place a small amount of LAXA-STAT™ on animal's nose to stimulate taste interest. For best results, feed between meals. Do not mix with food.

Dosage: Cats - For hair balls give ½-1 teaspoonful for 2-3 days, then ¼-½ teaspoonful 2-3 times a week.

Precaution(s): Store in a cool area.

Caution(s): For veterinary use only.

Keep out of reach of children.

Presentation: 4.25 oz (120.5 g) tube.

Compendium Code No.: 11220081 676-2 5

LAXATONE® & TUNA FLAVOR LAXATONE®

Evsco **Laxative**

Ingredients: White petrolatum and liquid petrolatum, linoleic acid and linolenic acid, and iron peptonized in a special palatable base.

Tuna Flavor: White petrolatum and liquid petrolatum in a palatable base. Also contains linoleic acid, linolenic acid, iron peptonized and tuna flavoring.

Indications: A laxative and lubricant for hair ball removal, with supplemental iron.

Dosage and Administration: Place a small amount of LAXATONE® on animal's nose to stimulate taste interest.

Cats:

For Hair Balls: ½-1 teaspoonful for 2-3 days then ¼-½ teaspoonful for 2-3 times a week.

Laxative: ¼-½ teaspoonful 2-3 times a week.

Dogs:

Laxative: ½-1 teaspoonful 2-3 times a week.

Precaution(s): Store in a cool place.

Warning(s): For veterinary use only.

Presentation: 12 x 2.5 oz (70.9 g) tubes, 2.5 oz (70.9 g) tubes (tuna flavor), and 4.25 oz. tubes (regular flavor).

Compendium Code No.: 10050151

LAXATONE® FOR CATS

Tomlyn **Laxative**

Ingredient(s): White Petrolatum USP, Light Mineral Oil NF, Corn Syrup, Malt Syrup, Soybean Oil, Cane Molasses, Water, Gelatin by-products, Sodium Benzoate (Preservative), Iron Proteinate, Artificial Flavor.

Indications: A lubricant for hair ball elimination and prevention in cats.

Directions: Place a small amount of LAXATONE® on animal's nose or directly into mouth to stimulate taste interest.

Dosage:

Cats: For Hair Balls - ½-1 teaspoonful for 2-3 days then ¼-½ teaspoonful 2-3 times a week.

Precaution(s): Store in a cool place.

Caution(s): For veterinary use only.

Warning(s): Keep out of reach of children.

Presentation: 2.5 oz (70.9 g) tubes.

Compendium Code No.: 11220280 6782 5

LAXATONE® FOR FERRETS & OTHER SMALL ANIMALS

Tomlyn **Laxative**

Ingredient(s): White Petrolatum USP, Light Mineral Oil NF, Corn Syrup, Malt Syrup, Soybean Oil, Cane Molasses, Water, Gelatin by-products, Sodium Benzoate (Preservative), Iron Proteinate, Artificial Flavor.

Indications: A lubricant for hair ball elimination and prevention in ferrets and other small animals.

Directions: Place a small amount of LAXATONE® on animal's nose or directly into mouth to stimulate taste interest.

Dosage: Ferrets and Other Small Animals for Hair Balls - ¼-½ teaspoonful for 2-3 days then ¼ teaspoonful 2-3 times a week.

Precaution(s): Store in a cool place.

Caution(s): For veterinary use only.

Warning(s): Keep out of reach of children.

Presentation: 2.5 oz (70.9 g) tubes.

Compendium Code No.: 11220290 726-4 2

LAYERMUNE® 2

Biomune **Vaccine**

Newcastle-Bronchitis Vaccine, Mass. Type, Killed Virus

U.S. Vet. Lic. No.: 368

Contents: LAYERMUNE® 2 contains Newcastle disease virus and infectious bronchitis virus of the Mass. serotype, Holland strain. The viruses are inactivated and suspended in an oil emulsion.

The vaccine has undergone rigid potency, safety and purity tests and meets Biomune and USDA requirements.

Indications: The vaccine is indicated for use in healthy chickens prior to the onset of egg production for the prevention of diseases caused by Newcastle disease virus and infectious bronchitis virus of the Mass. serotype. One dose of LAYERMUNE® 2 provides uniform and high serological titers throughout the lay cycle eliminating the need for use of live Newcastle-bronchitis vaccines during lay.

Dosage and Administration: Revaccination during molt is recommended.

A prime with live bronchitis vaccine of the Mass. type is recommended at least four (4) weeks in advance of administration of the inactivated vaccine.

Administration: Vaccinate chickens with 0.5 mL per bird. The vaccine is to be administered by the subcutaneous route in the back of the neck, midway between the head and the body, in a direction away from the head. Do not inject into muscle or vertebrae.

Refer to the product label for specific use directions and precautions.

Precaution(s): Store the vaccine at 35°-45°F (2°-7°C). Do not freeze.

Warning(s): Do not vaccinate with oil emulsion vaccine within 42 days before slaughter.

Avoid injection of the vaccine into a human. Should accidental injection of a human occur, seek medical attention immediately since a serious localized reaction may result.

Presentation: 1,000 dose (500 mL) bottle.

Compendium Code No.: 11290042

LAYERMUNE® 3

Biomune **Bacterin-Vaccine**

Newcastle-Bronchitis Vaccine, Mass. Type, Killed Virus-Salmonella enteritidis Bacterin

U.S. Vet. Lic. No.: 368

Contents: This product combines inactivated Newcastle disease virus and infectious bronchitis virus, Massachusetts type, with *Salmonella enteritidis.* The antigenic isolates are fully inactivated and suspended in an oil-emulsion adjuvant.

This vaccine is thoroughly tested before sale and meets the requirements of the U.S. Department of Agriculture.

Indications: LAYERMUNE® 3 is recommended for the vaccination of healthy chickens prior to the onset of egg production for the prevention of diseases caused by Newcastle disease virus and infectious bronchitis virus of the Mass. serotype. Also recommended to help reduce colonization of the internal organs, including the reproductive tract, by *Salmonella enteritidis* (SE) strains that have been proven to infect the ovary and consequently contaminate the egg. It will also help reduce colonization of the intestinal tract by SE, thereby reducing the risk of SE shed in the environment and egg shell contamination. The SE isolates used in this product have demonstrated proven efficacy against all phage types including the highly invasive phage type 4. Vaccination with Layermune® SE at least 4 weeks prior to vaccination with LAYERMUNE® 3 will provide maximum protection. Revaccination during molt is recommended.

Dosage and Administration: Vaccinate chickens with 0.5 mL (½ cc) per bird. The product is to be administered by the subcutaneous route in the back of the neck, midway between the head and the body, in a direction away from the head or subcutaneously in the shoulder of the bird. Do not inject into muscle or vertebrae.

Precaution(s): Store the vaccine at 35°-45°F (2°-7°C). Do not freeze.

Caution(s): Vaccination of breeder pullets should be in accordance with provisions established by NPIP. Priming with a live Newcastle disease vaccine and a live bronchitis vaccine of the Mass. type is recommended at least four weeks in advance of administration of the inactivated vaccine for best results.

Warning(s): Do not vaccinate with oil-emulsion vaccine within 42 days before slaughter.

Avoid injection of this vaccine into a human. Should accidental injection of a human occur, seek expert medical attention immediately since a serious localized reaction may result.

Presentation: 1,000 dose (500 mL) bottle.

Compendium Code No.: 11290091

LAYERMUNE® 5

Biomune **Vaccine**

Bursal Disease-Newcastle Disease-Bronchitis Vaccine, Standard and Variant, Mass. Type, Killed Virus

U.S. Vet. Lic. No.: 368

Contents: LAYERMUNE® 5 is an inactivated oil emulsion vaccine containing three bursal disease viruses (the standard type and two variants), Newcastle disease virus and infectious bronchitis virus of the Mass. serotype, Holland strain. All viruses in LAYERMUNE® 5 are of chicken embryo or bursal tissue origin.

The vaccine has undergone rigid potency, safety and purity tests and meets Biomune and USDA requirements.

Indications: The vaccine is indicated for use in healthy chickens prior to the onset of egg production against diseases caused by infectious bursal disease viruses (standard and variant types), Newcastle disease virus and infectious bronchitis virus of the Mass. serotype. One dose of LAYERMUNE® 5 provides uniform and high serological titers eliminating the need for use of live Newcastle-bronchitis vaccines during lay.

Breeder vaccination provides maternal antibody to the progeny of breeder hens for the prevention of early exposure to bursal disease.

Dosage and Administration: A prime with live infectious bursal disease vaccine and bronchitis vaccine of the Mass. type is recommended at least four (4) weeks in advance of administration of the inactivated vaccine.

Vaccinate chickens with 0.5 mL per bird. The vaccine is to be administered by the subcutaneous route in the back of the neck, midway between the head and the body, in a direction away from the head. Do not inject into muscle or vertebrae.

Revaccination during molt is recommended.

Refer to the product label for specific use directions and precautions.

Precaution(s): Store the vaccine at 35°-45°F (2°-7°C). Do not freeze.

Warning(s): Do not vaccinate with oil emusIsion vaccine within 42 days before slaughter.

Avoid injection of the vaccine into a human. Should accidental injection of a human occur, seek medical attention immediately since a serious localized reaction may result.

Presentation: 1,000 dose (500 mL) bottle.

Compendium Code No.: 11290052

LAYERMUNE® IB

Biomune **Vaccine**

Bronchitis Vaccine, Mass. Type, Killed Virus

U.S. Vet. Lic. No.: 368

Contents: LAYERMUNE® IB contains infectious bronchitis virus of the Mass. serotype, Holland strain. The vaccine is fully inactivated and suspended in an oil emulsion.

The vaccine has undergone rigid potency, safety and purity tests and meets Biomune and USDA requirements.

Indications: The vaccine is indicated for use in healthy chickens prior to the onset of egg production against disease caused by infectious bronchitis virus of the Mass. serotype. One dose of LAYERMUNE® IB provides uniform and high serological titers throughout the lay cycle eliminating the need for use of live bronchitis vaccine during lay.

Dosage and Administration: Vaccinate chickens with 0.5 mL per bird prior to the onset of egg production. The vaccine is to be administered by the subcutaneous route in the back of the neck, midway between the head and the body, in a direction away from the head. Do not inject into muscle or vertebrae.

Revaccination during molt is recommended.

A prime with live bronchitis vaccine of the Mass. type is recommended at least four (4) weeks in advance of administration of the inactivated vaccine.

Refer to the product label for specific use directions and precautions.

Precaution(s): Store the vaccine at 35°-45°F (2°-7°C). Do not freeze.

Warning(s): Do not vaccinate with oil emulsion vaccine within 42 days before slaughter.

Avoid injection of the vaccine into a human. Should accidental injection of a human occur, seek medical attention immediately since a serious localized reaction may result.

Presentation: 1,000 dose (500 mL) bottle.

Compendium Code No.: 11290062

LAYERMUNE® ND

Biomune **Vaccine**

Newcastle Disease Vaccine, Killed Virus

U.S. Vet. Lic. No.: 368

Contents: LAYERMUNE® ND contains inactivated Newcastle disease virus suspended in an oil emulsion.

The vaccine has undergone rigid potency, safety and purity tests and meets Biomune and USDA requirements.

Indications: The vaccine is indicated for use in chickens in the prevention of Newcastle disease. One dose of LAYERMUNE® ND prior to the onset of egg production provides uniform and high serological titers throughout the lay cycle eliminating the need for use of live Newcastle vaccine in the laying house.

Dosage and Administration: Vaccinate chickens with 0.5 mL per bird prior to the onset of egg production. The vaccine is to be administered by the subcutaneous route in the back of the neck, midway between the head and the body, in a direction away from the head. Do not inject into muscle or vertebrae.

Revaccination during molt is recommended.

Refer to the product label for specific use directions and precautions.

Precaution(s): Store the vaccine at 35°-45°F (2°-7°C). Do not freeze.

Warning(s): Do not vaccinate with an oil emulsion vaccine within 42 days before slaughter.

Avoid injection of the vaccine into a human. Should accidental injection of a human occur, seek medical attention immediately since a serious localized reaction may result.

Presentation: 1,000 dose (500 mL) bottle.

Compendium Code No.: 11290072

LAYERMUNE SE®

Biomune **Bacterin**

Salmonella enteritidis Bacterin

U.S. Vet. Lic. No.: 368

Contents: LAYERMUNE SE® bacterin is an inactivated bacterial vaccine emulsified in an oil adjuvant. The bacterin contains selected antigenic isolates of *Salmonella enteritidis* (SE) to aid in the protection against invasive field exposure. Since the *Salmonella* isolates in LAYERMUNE SE® are fully inactivated (killed), there is not risk of infection or spread of SE.

The product has been carefully produced and tested to comply with purity, safety, sterility, efficacy and potency requirements of Biomune and USDA regulations.

Indications: The product is indicated for use in pullets at least 12 weeks of age as an aid in the reduction of colonization by SE of the internal organs, including the reproductive tract, by strains of SE proven to infect the ovary with consequent contamination of the egg. The bacterin will also aid in the reduction of colonization of the intestinal tract by SE thereby reducing the risk of shed in the environment and egg shell contamination. Two injections at least four weeks apart will provide maximum protection. Revaccination during molt is recommended.

Dosage and Administration: The dose is 0.5 mL injected subcutaneously in the lower region of the back of the neck in a direction away from the head. Direct the needle just under the skin avoiding muscle and bone, toward the body and in line with the neck. Vaccinate only healthy chickens.

Refer to the product label for specific use directions and precautions.

Caution(s): Vaccination of breeder pullets should be in accordance with the provisions established by NPIP so as not to interfere with pullorum-typhoid testing.

Vaccination is additive to a salmonella control program and should be used in conjunction with biosecurity, cleaning and sanitation practices and rodent control.

Warning(s): Do not vaccinate within 42 days prior to slaughter with oil emulsion vaccine.

Ensure precautions against injection of humans with oil emulsion products. Should accidental human injection occur, seek immediate medical attention to avoid serious consequences.

Presentation: 1,000 dose (500 mL) bottle.

Compendium Code No.: 11290082

LD® 1 UDDER WASH BASE CONCENTRATE

Alcide **Udder Wash**

Active Ingredient(s):

Sodium Chlorite	3.03%
Inert Ingredients:	96.97%
Total:.	100.00%

Indications: Preparation for use as a sanitizing udder wash.

For use only with LD® Activator Concentrate.

Directions for Use: Do not mix Activator and Base directly. Follow Directions for Use.

It is a violation of Federal Law to use this product in a manner inconsistent with its labeling.

Preparation for use as a sanitizing udder wash: Base concentrate must be diluted with water prior to adding Activator Concentrate. Improper preparation can result in excessive generation of chlorine dioxide fumes. Use in a well ventilated area. Avoid breathing fumes.

1. Measure one part LD® Base Concentrate (Part 1) into a clean, empty, non-metallic container.
2. Add 16 parts cool tap water (at or below 77°F).
3. Add one part LD® Activator Concentrate (Part 2) and mix.
4. To apply, use a single service towel saturated in the udder wash solution or spray directly on the teat surfaces. Do not place used towel back into solution. Discard towel. Dry teats thoroughly with a clean towel to avoid contamination of milk. Apply milking unit. LD® Udder Wash is not a post milking teat dip.

Once mixed, the product has an effective shelf-life of 24 hours. Discard unused solution after 24 hours.

Mixed solution may be diluted with water and flushed safely down the drain.

Caution(s): This statement refers only to the unmixed Base Concentrate.

Hazards to Humans and Domestic Animals: Harmful if swallowed, inhaled, or absorbed through the skin. Causes eye irritation. Avoid contact with eyes, skin or clothing. Wash thoroughly with soap and water after handling.

First Aid:

If on Skin: Wash with plenty of soap and water. Get medical attention.

If in Eyes: Flush with plenty of water. Call a physician if irritation persists.

Storage and Disposal: Store unmixed concentrates in a cool, dark, dry place in the original containers. Always replace covers. Keep upright. Store mixed solution in a cool, dark place. Rinse mixing container after use. Wash empty concentrate containers thoroughly with water and offer for recycling or discard in trash. Do not reuse containers. Do not contaminate water, food or feed by storage or disposal. Wastes resulting from the use of this product may be disposed of on site or at an approved waste disposal facility.

Ventilation: Always use in a well-ventilated area. Avoid breathing fumes. When used in confined or large-volume area, the quantity of chlorine dioxide in the air may exceed OSHA Permissible Exposure Limits (PELs) and may require respiratory protection. Limits are defined as 0.1 ppm for an 8 hour time weighted average, and 0.3 ppm for a 15 minute short term exposure limit (29 CFR PART 1910.134 and Section 1910.1000, Air Contaminates, Table Z-1). Refer to MSDS for information on appropriate protective gear.

Warning(s): Keep out of reach of children.

Disclaimer: Distributor's and Alcide's liability on any claim, whether in negligence or any other tort or in contract or otherwise, with respect to products delivered hereunder, any use of such products or any technique recommended by Distributor or Alcide relating to such products or such use, shall not exceed the purchase price of the products sold or, if Distributor and Alcide shall so elect, buyer shall be entitled only to replacement of product. In no event shall Distributor

or Alcide be liable for buyer's incidental or consequential damages. Consult your veterinarian or milking equipment service personnel if cow's teats become irritated.
Presentation: Available in 1 and 5 gallon sizes.
Foreign Patents Issued and Pending
LD® is a registered trademark of Alcide Corporation.
Distributed by: IBA Inc., Animal Health Division, 27 Providence Road, Millbury, MA 01527.
Compendium Code No.: 14760042 L7710B Rev. 02 9-99

LD® 2 UDDER WASH ACTIVATOR CONCENTRATE

Alcide **Udder Wash**

Active Ingredient(s): 16.7% Organic Acid.
Indications: Preparation for use as a sanitizing udder wash.
For use only with LD® Base Concentrate.
Directions for Use: Do not mix Activator and Base directly. Follow Directions for Use.
It is a violation of Federal Law to use this product in a manner inconsistent with its labeling.
Preparation for use as a sanitizing udder wash: Base concentrate must be diluted with water prior to adding Activator Concentrate. Improper preparation can result in excessive generation of chlorine dioxide fumes. Use in a well ventilated area. Avoid breathing fumes.

1. Measure one part LD® Base Concentrate (Part 1) into a clean, empty, non-metallic container.
2. Add 16 parts cool tap water (at or below 77°F).
3. Add one part LD® Activator Concentrate (Part 2) and mix.
4. To apply, use a single service towel saturated in the udder wash solution or spray directly on the teat surfaces. Do not place used towel back into solution. Discard towel. Dry teats thoroughly with a clean towel to avoid contamination of milk. Apply milking unit. LD® Udder Wash is not a post milking teat dip.

Once mixed, the product has an effective shelf-life of 24 hours. Discard unused, mixed solution after 24 hours.
Mixed solution may be diluted with water and flushed safely down the drain.
Caution(s): This statement refers only to the unmixed Activator Concentrate.
Hazards to Humans and Domestic Animals: Harmful if swallowed, inhaled, or absorbed through the skin. Causes eye irritation. Avoid contact with eyes, skin or clothing. Wash thoroughly with soap and water after handling.
First Aid:
If on Skin: Wash with plenty of soap and water. Get medical attention.
If in Eyes: Flush with plenty of water. Call a physician if irritation persists.
Storage and Disposal: Store unmixed concentrates in a cool, dark, dry place in the original containers. Always replace covers. Keep upright. Store mixed solution in a cool, dark place. Rinse mixing container after use. Wash empty concentrate containers thoroughly with water and offer for recycling or discard in trash. Do not reuse containers. Do not contaminate water, food or feed by storage or disposal. Wastes resulting from the use of this product may be disposed of on site or at an approved waste disposal facility.
Ventilation: Always use in a well-ventilated area. Avoid breathing fumes. When used in confined or large-volume area, the quantity of chlorine dioxide in the air may exceed OSHA Permissible Exposure Limits (PELs) and may require respiratory protection. Limits are defined as 0.1 ppm for an 8 hour time weighted average, and 0.3 ppm for a 15 minute short term exposure limit (29 CFR PART 1910.134 and Section 1910.1000, Air Contaminates, Table Z-1). Refer to MSDS for information on appropriate protective gear.
Warning(s): Keep out of reach of children.
Disclaimer: Distributor's and Alcide's liability on any claim, whether in negligence or any other tort or in contract or otherwise, with respect to products delivered hereunder, any use of such products or any technique recommended by Distributor or Alcide relating to such products or such use, shall not exceed the purchase price of the products sold or, if Distributor and Alcide shall so elect, buyer shall be entitled only to replacement of product. In no event shall Distributor or Alcide be liable for buyer's incidental or consequential damages. Consult your veterinarian or milking equipment service personnel if cow's teats become irritated.
Presentation: Available in 1 and 5 gallon sizes.
Foreign Patents Issued and Pending
LD® is a registered trademark of Alcide Corporation.
Distributed by: IBA Inc., Animal Health Division, 27 Providence Road, Millbury, MA 01527.
Compendium Code No.: 14760052 L7710A Rev. 02 9-99

LDC-19™

Intercon **Disinfectant**

EPA Reg. No.: 48211-21
Active Ingredient(s):
Alkyl (C_{14}, 58%; C_{16}, 28%; C_{12}, 14%) dimethyl benzyl ammonium chloride 2.00%
Inert ingredients 98.00%
Total ingredients 100.00%
Indications: This disinfectant reduces the surface tension of water, improving its wettability. Microbes are capable of mass reproduction in sub-visible pores, scratches and cracks of surfaces. The wettability of this product improves the penetration of the use solution into areas that otherwise might not be reached. This disinfectant is effective against a wide variety of gram-positive and gram-negative bacteria. It is also a deodorant and is especially effective in controlling odors that are bacterial in origin. Has a pleasant lemon odor.
This disinfectant mixes with water to form clear, stable use solutions. Use solutions are noncorrosive and nonstaining to plastic, vinyl, synthetics, enamel, tile and most common metals.
This disinfectant is effective at 5 oz. per gallon against *Pseudomonas aeruginosa* PRD-10, *Salmonella choleraesuis* ATCC 10708, and *Staphylococcus aureus* ATCC 6538 when tested by the A.O.A.C. use dilution test method for precleaned, hard nonporous, inanimate environmental surfaces.
This disinfectant is also an effective virucide at 5 oz./gallon for influenza virus, type A, Brazil and herpes simplex type 2 on inanimate environmental surfaces.
Dosage and Administration: It is a violation of federal law to use the product in a manner inconsistent with its labeling.
Application Information: Select the proper dilution of this product for your use from the directions below. Apply the use solution with a clean mop, sponge, cloth, squeegee, mechanical scrubber or mechanical spraying device.
Prepare fresh use solutions daily. Do not re-use solutions. Discard solutions when they become visibly soiled. For disinfection, thoroughly wet the surfaces to be treated. Surfaces must remain moist for at least 10 minutes to assure proper germicidal action.
This product may be used for cleaning and disinfecting hard, nonporous, inanimate environmental surfaces (glass, metal, glazed porcelain, linoleum, tile, smooth leather, vinyl, enameled and finished wood surfaces) on walls, floors, appliances and furnishings.
Cleaning: To clean and deodorize or to preclean prior to disinfection. Depending on the soil level of the area to be cleaned, use 12-16 oz. of this product per gallon of water.
When applied as directed to precleaned hard, nonporous surfaces, this disinfectant also kills the following organisms at 5 oz. per gallon: *Candida albicans, Escherichia coli, Streptococcus pyogenes, Enterobacter aerogenes, Shigella sonnei.*
This product may be used for cleaning and deodorizing, one-step cleaning and disinfection, or disinfection of precleaned, nonporous, inanimate hard surfaces.
Hospitals, veterinary clinics, nursing homes: Use 10 oz. of this product per one and one-half (1½) gallons of water (1 part to 18 parts water) for one-step cleaning and disinfection of areas with light to medium soil loads. For heavily soiled areas, preclean as described above and then disinfect with this product at 5 oz. per gallon (1 part to 24 parts water).
Industrial areas, food and meat processing plants (nonfood processing areas), other nonmedical uses: Preclean surfaces. Then, disinfect with a solution of 4 oz. of this product in one and one-third (1⅓) gallons of water (1 part to 41 parts water). Alternatively, clean and disinfect in one operation using 10 oz. of this product per one and one-half (1½) gallons of water (1 part to 18 parts water).
For deodorizing garbage cans and garbage handling equipment. It is especially important to preclean for the product to perform properly. Then, apply a wetting concentration of 16 oz. of this product per gallon of water (1 part to 7 parts water).
For mildew control: Follow directions for hospital disinfection. Repeat treatment every seven (7) days, or when new growth appears.
This product may be used through automatic floor scrubbing equipment.
This product must not be used on food contact surfaces.
Precaution(s): Do not contaminate water, food or feed by storage or disposal.
Pesticide Disposal: Pesticide wastes are acutely hazardous. Improper disposal of excess pesticide, spray mixture, or rinsate is a violation of federal law. If these wastes cannot be disposed of by use according to label instructions, contact the nearest State Pesticide or Environmental Control Agency, or the Hazardous Waste representative at the nearest EPA Regional Office for guidance.
Container Disposal: Triple rinse (or equivalent). Then offer for recycling or reconditioning or puncture and dispose of in a sanitary landfill, or by incineration, or if allowed by state and local authorities by burning. If burned, stay out of smoke. Metal container: Triple rinse (or equivalent), then offer for recycling or reconditioning, or dispose of in a sanitary landfill, or by other procedures approved by state and local authorities
If container is one gallon size, use this container disposal statement: Do not re-use empty container. Wrap container and put in trash.
Caution(s): Keep out of the reach of children.
Avoid contamination of food. Avoid breathing spray mist.
Precautionary Statements: Hazard to Humans and Domestic Animals:
Statement of Practical Treatment: In case of contact, immediately flush eyes or skin with plenty of water for at least 15 minutes. For eyes, call a physician. Remove and wash contaminated clothing before re-use.
If swallowed, promptly drink a large quantity of milk, raw egg whites, gelatin solution or, if these are not readily available, drink a large quantity of water. Avoid alcohol. Call a physician immediately.
Environmental Hazards: This product is toxic to fish. Do not discharge into lakes, streams, ponds, or public water unless in accordance with an NPDES permit.
Do not contaminate water by cleaning of equipment or by disposing of wastes.
Presentation: 4x1 gallon and 5 gallon containers, and 55 gallon drums.
Compendium Code No.: 10130020

LEGACY® ℞

AgriLabs **Gentamicin**

Gentamicin Sulfate Solution-100 mg/mL
ANADA No.: 200-137
Active Ingredient(s): Description: Each mL of LEGACY® (Gentamicin Sulfate Solution) contains: Gentamicin sulfate equivalent to 100 mg gentamicin base; 3.2 mg sodium metabisulfite; 0.1 mg edetate disodium; 1.8 mg methylparaben and 0.2 mg propylparaben as preservatives; water for injection q.s.
Indications: LEGACY® (Gentamicin Sulfate Solution) is recommended for the control of bacterial infections of the uterus (metritis) in horses and as an aid in improving conception in mares with uterine infections caused by bacteria sensitive to gentamicin.
Bacteriologic studies should be conducted to identify the causative organism and to determine its sensitivity to gentamicin sulfate. Sensitivity discs of the drug are available for this purpose.
Pharmacology: Chemistry: Gentamicin is a mixture of aminoglycoside antibiotics derived from the fermentation of *Micromonospora purpurea*. Gentamicin sulfate is a mixture of sulfate salts of the antibiotics produced in this fermentation. The salts are weakly acidic, freely soluble in water, and stable in solution.
Antibacterial Activity: *In vitro* antibacterial activity has shown that gentamicin is active against most gram-negative and gram-positive bacteria isolated from domestic animals.[1] Gentamicin is active against *Pseudomonas aeruginosa*, indole-positive and -negative *Proteus* species, *Escherichia coli, Klebsiella* species, *Enterobacter* species, *Alcaligenes* species, *Staphylococcus* species, and *Streptococcus* species.
Studies in man indicate that recommended doses of gentamicin produce serum concentrations bactericidal for most bacteria sensitive to gentamicin within an hour after intramuscular injection; these concentrations last for 6 to 12 hours.[2] Some 30% of the administered dose of gentamicin is bound by serum proteins and released as the drug is excreted.
Gentamicin is excreted almost entirely by glomerular filtration. High concentrations of the active form are found in the urine. Fifty to 100% of the gentamicin injected can be recovered unchanged within 24 hours from the urine of patients with normal renal function. A small amount is excreted into the bile.
Dosage and Administration: The recommended dose is 20 to 25 mL (2.0-2.5 grams) gentamicin sulfate solution per day for 3 to 5 days during estrus. Each dose should be diluted with 200-500 mL of sterile physiological saline before aseptic uterine infusion.
Contraindication(s): There are no known contraindications to this drug when used as directed.
Precaution(s): Store between 2° and 30°C (36° and 86°F). Protect from freezing.
Caution(s): Federal law restricts this drug to use by or on the order of a licensed veterinarian.
If hypersensitivity to any of the components develops, or if an overgrowth of nonsusceptible bacteria, fungi, or yeasts occurs, treatment with LEGACY® (Gentamicin Sulfate Solution) should be discontinued and appropriate therapy instituted.
Although LEGACY®(Gentamicin Sulfate Solution) is not spermicidal, treatment should not be given the day of breeding.
For intra-uterine use in horses only.
For animal use only.

Not for human use.

Warning(s): Not for use in horses intended for food.

Keep out of reach of children.

Toxicology: Toxicity Studies: No toxic effects were observed in rats given gentamicin sulfate 20 mg/kg/day for 24 days; in cats given 10 mg/kg/day for 40 days. Gentamicin sulfate given to dogs at 6 mg/lb/day, 6 days weekly for 3 weeks, caused no detectable kidney damage. At higher doses, impairment of equilibrium and renal function were observed in these species.

Side Effects: There have been no reports of drug hypersensitivity or adverse side effects following the recommended intrauterine infusion of gentamicin sulfate solution combined with sterile physiological saline in mares.

References: Available upon request.

Presentation: LEGACY® (Gentamicin Sulfate Solution), 100 mg per mL for intrauterine use, is available in 100 mL and 250 mL multiple dose vials.

Compendium Code No.: 10581640 Iss. 10-99

LEGEND® ℞

(hyaluronate sodium) Injectable Solution

Bayer

For Intravenous Or Intra-Articular Use in Horses Only

CAUTION: Federal law restricts this drug to use by or on the order of a licensed veterinarian.

DESCRIPTION: Legend® (hyaluronate sodium) Injectable Solution is a clear, colorless solution of low viscosity. Legend Injectable Solution is pyrogen free, sterile and does not contain a preservative. It is administered by intravenous or intra-articular injection.

Hyaluronic acid, the conjugate acid of hyaluronate sodium, is extracted from the capsule of *Streptococcus* spp. and purified, resulting in a form which is essentially free of protein and nucleic acids.

Legend Injectable Solution is supplied in 2 mL (20 mg) and 4 mL (40 mg) vials. Each mL contains 10 mg hyaluronate sodium, 8.5 mg sodium chloride, 0.223 mg sodium phosphate dibasic and 0.04 mg sodium phosphate monobasic. The pH is adjusted to between 6.5 and 8.0 with sodium hydroxide or hydrochloric acid.

CHEMISTRY: Hyaluronic acid, a glycosaminoglycan, can exist in the following forms depending upon the chemical environment in which it is found: as the acid, hyaluronic acid; as the sodium salt, sodium hyaluronate (hyaluronate sodium); or as the hyaluronate anion. These terms may be used interchangeably but in all cases, reference is made to the glycosaminoglycan composed of repeating subunits of D-glucuronic acid and N-acetyl-D-glucosamine linked together by glycosidic bonds. Since this product originates from a microbial source, there is no potential for contamination with dermatan or chondroitin sulfate or any other glycosaminoglycan.

PHARMACOLOGY: Hyaluronic acid is a naturally occurring substance present in connective tissue, skin, vitreous humour and the umbilical cord in all mammals. High concentrations of hyaluronic acid are also found in the synovial fluid. It also constitutes the major component of the capsule of certain microorganisms. The hyaluronic acid produced by bacteria is of the same structure and configuration as that found in mammals.

The actual mechanism of action for hyaluronate sodium in the healing of degenerative joint disease is not completely understood. One major function appears to be the regulation of normal cellular constituents. This effect decreases the impact of exudation, enzyme release and subsequent degradation of joint integrity. Additionally, hyaluronate sodium exerts an anti-inflammatory action by inhibiting the movement of granulocytes and macrophages[1].

Hyaluronate molecules are long chains which form a filter network interspersed with normal cellular fluids. It is widely accepted that injection directly into the joint pouch enhances the healing of inflamed synovium by restoring lubrication of the joint fluid. This further supplements the visco-elastic properties of normal joint fluid.

CONTRAINDICATIONS: There are no known contraindications for the use of Legend® (hyaluronate sodium) Injectable Solution in horses.

TOXICOLOGY: Legend Injectable Solution was administered to normal horses at one, three and five times the recommended intra-articular dosage of 20 mg and the intravenous dosage of 40 mg. Treatments were given once weekly for nine consecutive weeks (three times the maximum duration). No systemic clinical signs were observed nor were there any adverse effects upon hematology or clinical chemistry parameters. A transient, slight to mild post-injection swelling of the joint capsule occurred in some of the animals treated intra-articularly with Legend Injectable Solution as it did in the saline treated control horses. No gross or histological lesions were observed in the soft tissues or the surface areas of the treated joint.

CLINICAL STUDIES: Forty-six horses with lameness in either the carpal or fetlock joints were treated intravenously or intra-articularly with Legend Injectable Solution in a well controlled clinical field trial conducted at four locations. One, two or three injections were given based on clinical improvement.

Overall clinical improvement was judged as excellent or good in 90% of the cases treated intravenously and 96% of those treated intra-articularly with Legend Injectable Solution.

SIDE EFFECTS OR ADVERSE REACTIONS: No local or systemic side effects were observed in the clinical field trials with either intravenous or intra-articular injections.

PRECAUTIONS: Radiographic evaluation should be carried out in cases of acute lameness to ensure that the joint is free from serious fractures. As with any intra-articular treatment, special precautions must be followed as to injection technique and sterility for the prevention of possible swelling or infection. Intra-articular injections should not be made through skin that has been recently fired or blistered, or that has excessive scurf and counterirritant on it.

WARNING: Not for use in horses intended for food.

Safety in breeding animals has not been determined with Legend Injectable Solution.

INDICATIONS: Legend® (hyaluronate sodium) Injectable Solution is indicated in the treatment of joint dysfunction of the carpus or fetlock in horses due to non-infectious synovitis associated with equine osteoarthritis.

DOSAGE AND ADMINISTRATION:

Intravenous-4 mL (40 mg). Intra-articular-2 mL (20 mg) in the carpus or fetlock. Treatment may be repeated at weekly intervals for a total of three treatments.

Strict aseptic technique should be observed when administering by intra-articular injection. As with any intra-articular procedure, proper injection site disinfection and animal restraint are important. Excess joint fluid should be aseptically removed prior to injection. Care should be taken to avoid scratching the cartilage surface with the tip of the injection needle. Diffuse swelling lasting 24 to 48 hours may result from movement of the needle while in the joint space.

For intravenous administration, use aseptic technique and inject slowly into the jugular vein.

Horses should be given stall rest after treatment before gradually resuming normal activity.

Discard any unused portion of the drug and the empty vial after opening.

HOW SUPPLIED:

Code 0175	Carton containing six 2 mL (20 mg) vials.	79001750, R.9 December, 2000
Code 0176	Carton containing six 4 mL (40 mg) vials.	79001760, R.5 December, 2000

REFERENCE:

[1]Swanstrom, O.G. 1978. Hyaluronate (hyaluronic acid) and its use. Proc. American Assoc. Equine Pract., 24th annual convention, pp. 345-348.

U.S. Patent Nos. 4,782,046 and 4,808,576

Bayer Corporation, Agriculture Division, Animal Health, Shawnee Mission, Kansas 66201 U.S.A.

Compendium Code No.: 10400281

LEPTO 5

AgriLabs **Bacterin**

Leptospira canicola-grippotyphosa-hardjo-icterohaemorrhagiae-pomona Bacterin

U.S. Vet. Lic. No.: 272

Active Ingredient(s): Contains chemically inactivated cultures of *Leptospira canicola, L. grippotyphosa, L. hardjo, L. icterohaemorrhagiae* and *L. pomona.*

Indications: For the immunization of healthy cattle and swine against leptospirosis caused by *Leptospira canicola, L. grippotyphosa, L. hardjo, L. icterohaemorrhagiae* and *L. pomona.*

Dosage and Administration: Shake thoroughly before use. Administer 2 mL intramuscularly or subcutaneously in healthy cattle or swine. In swine a second vaccination in two (2) to four (4) weeks is required. Annual revaccination with a single 2 mL dose is recommended.

Precaution(s): Store at 35-45°F (2-7°C).

Caution(s): Use the entire contents when first opened. In case of anaphylactic reactions use epinephrine.

Warning(s): Do not vaccinate within 21 days before slaughter.

Presentation: 20 mL (10 dose) and 100 mL (50 dose) vials.

Compendium Code No.: 10580650

LEPTO-5

Boehringer Ingelheim **Bacterin**

Leptospira Canicola-Grippotyphosa-Hardjo-Icterohaemorrhagiae-Pomona Bacterin

U.S. Vet. Lic. No.: 124

Composition: This product consists of chemically inactivated aluminum hydroxide adsorbed highly antigenic whole cultures of the organisms listed. Contains gentamicin and a fungistat as preservatives.

Indications: Recommended for the vaccination of healthy, susceptible cattle and swine against disease caused by *Leptospira canicola, L. grippotyphosa, L. hardjo, L. icterohaemorrhagiae* and *L. pomona.*

Dosage and Administration: Using aseptic technique, inject 2 mL intramuscularly. A second dose is recommended 3 to 6 weeks later. Cattle and swine vaccinated at an early age should be revaccinated after weaning. Repeat with a single 2 mL booster dose annually or prior to each breeding.

Precaution(s): Store out of direct sunlight at a temperature between 35-45°F (2-7°C). Avoid freezing. Shake well before using. Use entire contents when first opened.

Caution(s): Anaphylactoid reactions may occur.

Antidote(s): Epinephrine.

Warning(s): Do not vaccinate within 21 days before slaughter.

Animal inoculation only.

Presentation: 50 doses (100 mL).

Compendium Code No.: 10280740

LEPTO-5

Colorado Serum **Bacterin**

Leptospira Canicola-Grippotyphosa-Hardjo-Icterohaemorrhagiae-Pomona Bacterin

U.S. Vet. Lic. No.: 188

Contents: Inactivating whole cultures of *L. canicola, L. grippotyphosa, L. hardjo, L. icterohaemorrhagiae,* and *L. pomona,* aluminum hydroxide adsorbed.

Indications: For vaccination of healthy cattle and swine in areas where the serotypes named are known to be prevalent.

Dosage and Administration: Shake well. Aseptically inject 2.0 mL subcutaneously or intramuscularly. For swine, a second dose should be administered 2-4 weeks later. Annual re-vaccination is recommended for both species.

When to Vaccinate: Vaccination of both cattle and swine at least 3 weeks prior to breeding is recommended (1) on premises having a history of leptospirosis (2) when the disease exists in the area, and (3) when animals may be exposed to carriers of the micro-organisms.

Precaution(s): Store in dark at 2° to 7°C.

Use entire contents when bottle is first opened.

Caution(s): Anaphylactoid reaction sometimes follows administration of products of this nature. If noted, administer adrenalin or equivalent.

Warning(s): Do not vaccinate within 21 days before slaughter.

Discussion: Leptospirosis is one of the more serious diseases of cattle and swine. It is directly transmitted by contact with sick animals, through urine and mucous of the eyes, nose, and mouth; indirectly through water tanks and streams carrying live micro-organisms after being shed by infected animals. Clinical signs of the disease vary greatly from mild to severe and because of this it is difficult to list common symptoms. The following, however, have been reported as having been observed.

In calves, symptoms may include a rapid rise in temperature with depression and loss of appetite. The urine may become coffee-colored and sometimes streaked with blood. Animals may be anemic. Death losses can, in some instances, reach substantial proportions in calves under one year of age.

In older cattle the disease usually follows a milder course, with animals showing only a loss of appetite and depression for several days until death losses or abortions occur. *L. hardjo* infection, for instance, is clinically insignificant but is increasing in the number of isolations.

In dairy cattle the disease may result in a sharp reduction in milk production and this may be the first indication of infection. Udder secretions may be of a thick, yellowish nature. Frequently, the symptoms may he mistaken for common mastitis but the udder is not generally inflamed. In swine there are often no signs of infection until abortions occur. Sows generally abort two to four weeks before delivery date and the rate may be high. In some instances, sows may carry to full term but litters may contain dead and/or weak pigs.

When to Vaccinate: Vaccination of both cattle and swine at least 3 weeks prior to breeding is recommended (1) on premises having a history of leptospirosis (2) when the disease exists in the area, and (3) when animals may have been exposed to carriers of the micro-organisms.

Hogs being raised for market should also be vaccinated if contact with the disease is likely.

These animals should not thereafter be offered for slaughter until the full withdrawal time, as shown above, has been observed.

Best results are to be expected when the bacterin is administered prior to exposure of the animals. However, if infection has appeared in the herd, isolate the sick animals and vaccinate all those that are apparently unaffected. Some vaccinates may thereafter develop symptoms because immune response from administration of bacterin is not immediate. Vaccination of infected herds is suggested as Leptospira bacterins have been found to be of help in stopping spread of disease and bringing outbreaks under control.

Vaccination is recommended also for healthy herds suspected of having been exposed to leptospirosis and for herds into which replacement stock is periodically introduced. Such replacement stock should be vaccinated as well and hold separately until protective immunity is established. Isolation of new stock should be a rigid practice in herd management not only for aid in preventing leptospirosis but other diseases as well.

Revaccinate animals retained for breeding and those held beyond a normal marketing period, on an annual basis. In heavily contaminated areas semi-annual vaccination should be practiced. Occasionally, it may be necessary to vaccinate very young calves. If so, these should be revaccinated at 3-4 months of age.

Presentation: 10 dose (20 mL) and 50 dose (100 mL) vials.

Compendium Code No.: 11010252

LEPTO 5

Durvet **Bacterin**

Leptospira Canicola-Grippotyphosa-Hardjo-Icterohaemorrhagiae-Pomona Bacterin

U.S. Vet. Lic. No.: 303

Composition: This bacterin contains inactivated cultures of *Leptospira canicola, L. grippotyphosa, L. hardjo, L. icterohaemorrhagiae* and *L. pomona.*

Contains thimerosal as a preservative.

Indications: For use in healthy cattle and swine as an aid in the prevention and control of disease caused by *Leptospira canicola, L. grippotyphosa, L. hardjo, L. icterohaemorrhagiae* and *L. pomona.*

Dosage and Administration: Shake well before using. Administer 2 mL intramuscularly. For swine give a second dose in 3-4 weeks. Revaccination annually.

Precaution(s): Store at 35°F-45°F (2°C-7°C). Do not freeze. Use entire contents when first opened.

Caution(s): Anaphylactic reactions may occur following the use of this biological.

Symptomatic treatment: Epinephrine.

Warning(s): Do not vaccinate within 21 days prior to slaughter.

Presentation: 10 dose (20 mL) and 50 dose (100 mL).

Manufactured by: Advance Biologics, Inc. Freeman, SD 57209.

Compendium Code No.: 10841101 8/99

LEPTO 5

Premier Farmtech **Bacterin**

Leptospira canicola-grippotyphosa-hardjo-icterohaemorrhagiae-pomona Bacterin, Aluminum Hydroxide Adsorbed

U.S. Vet. Lic. No.: 272

Contents: Inactivated cultures of *Leptospira canicola, L grippotyphosa, L hardjo, L icterohaemorrhagiae* and *L pomona,* aluminum hydroxide adsorbed.

Indications: For the immunization of healthy cattle against infection by the organisms represented.

Dosage and Administration: Shake well. Administer 2 mL subcutaneously. Revaccinate once annually to maintain a high level of immunity.

Precaution(s): Store at 35°F - 45°F (2°C - 7°C). Use entire contents when first opened.

Caution(s): In case of anaphylactoid reactions, epinephrine should be administered immediately.

Antidote(s): Epinephrine.

Warning(s): Do not vaccinate within 21 days before slaughter.

For veterinary use only.

Presentation: 10 dose (20 mL) and 50 dose (100 mL) vials.

Compendium Code No.: 10320020

LEPTO 5 VACCINE

Aspen **Bacterin**

Leptospira canicola-grippotyphosa-hardjo-icterohaemorrhagiae-pomona Bacterin

U.S. Vet. Lic. No.: 272

Active Ingredient(s): Contains inactivated cultures of *Leptospira canicola, L grippotyphosa, L hardjo, L icterohaemorrhagiae* and *L pomona.*

Indications: For the immunization of healthy cattle and swine against infections caused by *Leptospira canicola, L grippotyphosa, L hardjo, L icterohaemorrhagiae* and *L pomona.*

Dosage and Administration: Shake well and inject 2 mL intramuscularly or subcutaneously.

Revaccinate once annually to maintain a high level of immunity. To ensure a high level of immunity in swine, a second vaccination in 2-4 weeks is necessary for the primary immunization.

Precaution(s): Store at 35°-45°F (2°-7°C). Do not freeze.

Caution(s): Use the entire contents when first opened.

If an allergic response occurs, epinephrine should be administered immediately.

Antidote(s): Epinephrine.

Warning(s): Do not vaccinate within 21 days before slaughter. For veterinary use only.

Presentation: 10 dose (20 mL) and 50 dose (100 mL) vials.

Compendium Code No.: 14750520

LEPTOFERM-5®

Pfizer Animal Health **Bacterin**

Leptospira Canicola-Grippotyphosa-Hardjo-Icterohaemorrhagiae-Pomona Bacterin

U.S. Vet. Lic. No.: 189

Description: LEPTOFERM-5® contains chemically inactivated whole cultures of the 5 *Leptospira* serovars listed above.

Indications: LEPTOFERM-5® is for vaccination of healthy swine and cattle as an aid in preventing leptospirosis caused by *Leptospira canicola, L. grippotyphosa, L. hardjo, L. icterohaemorrhagiae,* and *L. pomona.*

Directions:

1. General Directions: Vaccination of healthy swine and cattle is recommended. Shake well. Aseptically administer 2 mL intramuscularly. In accordance with Beef Quality Assurance guidelines, this product should be administered in the muscular region of the neck.
2. Primary Vaccination: Administer a single 2-mL dose to healthy cattle. Healthy swine should receive 2 doses administered 3-6 weeks apart.
3. Revaccination: Annual revaccination with a single dose is recommended for both species.
4. Good animal husbandry and herd health management practices should be employed.

Precaution(s): Store at 2°-7°C. Prolonged exposure to higher temperatures may adversely affect potency. Do not freeze.

Use entire contents when first opened.

Sterilized syringes and needles should be used to administer this vaccine.

Caution(s): As with many vaccines, anaphylaxis may occur after use. Initial antidote of epinephrine is recommended and should be followed with appropriate supportive therapy.

This product has been shown to be efficacious in healthy animals. A protective immune response may not be elicited if animals are incubating an infectious disease, are malnourished or parasitized, are stressed due to shipment or environmental conditions, are otherwise immunocompromised, or the vaccine is not administered in accordance with label directions.

Warning(s): Do not vaccinate within 21 days before slaughter.

For veterinary use only.

Discussion: Disease Description: Leptospirosis is a worldwide disease of animals and humans and causes serious economic loss to the livestock industry.[1] The disease is usually transmitted by direct or indirect contact with leptospire-infected urine.

Leptospirosis in swine is characterized by poor productivity, fever, anemia, kidney inflammation, and abortions; late-term abortions are the most important effect. In calves, clinical signs of leptospirosis may include fever, prostration, loss of appetite, shortness of breath, anemia, and blood in the urine. In adult cattle, the most common clinical sign is reproductive loss, including abortion and premature or full-term birth of weak calves. Decreased milk production may also occur.[2] *Leptospira* spp. are known zoonotic pathogens.

All the above *Leptospira* serovars produce identical clinical signs, yet immunity to leptospirosis is serovar-specific.[1] Vaccination against each serovar, therefore, is indicated for protection.

Trial Data: Safety and Efficacy: During developmental tests and in extensive field use of LEPTOFERM-5®, no significant postvaccination reactions were reported.

Although *L. hardjo* has been isolated from field cases of leptospirosis, attempts to experimentally induce clinical disease with that serovar had yielded unreliable results. Hence, no valid challenge-of-immunity tests on *L. hardjo* bacterin had been possible. Recent reports, however, have identified a method to induce clinical *L. hardjo* infection in cattle[2] and have also identified 2 distinct genotypes of *L. hardjo* in cattle.[3,4]

Accordingly, challenge-of-immunity tests were conducted to determine the efficacy of LEPTOFERM-5® against both *L. hardjo* genotypes.[5] Seventeen healthy heifers were divided into 2 groups of 6 vaccinates each and a group of 5 nonvaccinated controls. Vaccinates were administered the *L. hardjo* fraction of LEPTOFERM-5® in 1- or 2-dose regimens. Subsequently all cattle were challenged with disease-causing strains of both *L. hardjo* genotypes. After challenge, leptospires were recovered from the urine of all controls, which continued shedding leptospires in the urine until necropsy at 31-49 days after challenge. Three controls (60%) also experienced fever and developed leptospires in the blood. Conversely, leptospires were not recovered from the urine or kidneys of any vaccinates, and leptospires were recovered from the blood of only 1 vaccinate (8%) for 1 day.

Thus, efficacy of the *L. hardjo* fraction against both genotypes in cattle was confirmed. These results are similar to results of previously conducted challenge-of-immunity tests on the other 4 fractions of LEPTOFERM-5® in both cattle and swine. In those studies also, vaccinated animals remained healthy after challenge, while nonvaccinated animals developed clinical signs of leptospirosis.

References: Available upon request.

Presentation: 10 dose and 50 dose vials.

Compendium Code No.: 36900570 75-4475-02

LEPTO SHIELD™ 5

Novartis Animal Vaccines **Bacterin**

Leptospira canicola-grippotyphosa-hardjo-icterohaemorrhagiae-pomona Bacterin

U.S. Vet. Lic. No.: 303

Composition: *Leptospira canicola, L. grippotyphosa, L. hardjo, L. icterohaemorrhagiae,* and *L. pomona* bacterin.

Indications: For the prevention of *Leptospira canicola, grippotyphosa, hardjo, icterohaemorrhagiae,* and *pomona* infections in susceptible cattle and swine.

Dosage and Administration: Shake well before using. Inject 2 mL intramuscularly into cattle and swine using aseptic techniques. For swine, give a second dose in three (3) to four (4) weeks. Revaccinate during each pregnancy.

Precaution(s): Store in the dark at 35°-45°F (2°-7°C). Do not freeze. Use the entire contents when first opened.

Caution(s): Anaphylactic reactions may occur with this bacterin. Symptomatic treatment: Epinephrine.

Warning(s): Do not vaccinate within 21 days of slaughter.

Discussion: Leptospirosis is a contagious disease of both man and animals and has been estimated to cause losses in excess of 100 million dollars per year to the livestock industry, according to the USDA. This loss is due primarily to abortions and stillbirths in breeding stock, lowered milk production, and by sickness and death in young animals. Abortion rates can be 30% or higher in affected cattle herds before the disease can be stopped.

The causative organisms belong to a group of pathogens called *Leptospira interrogans,* with five major serovars incriminated: *L. grippotyphosa, L. hardjo, L. pomona, L. canicola,* and *L. icterohaemorrhagiae.*

This disease is spread to domestic livestock by the shedding of the organism in the urine, which contaminates feed or water. These organisms survive well in surface waters. The organism may be found in the udder and be secreted in the milk to suckling calves or piglets, thus infecting them.

Many wildlife species may be infected with these organisms, with some of the more common ones being rats, raccoons, skunks, foxes, and opossums. Dogs are also often infected.

The incubation period varies from one (1) to four (4) days and is followed by a leptospiremia (bacteria in the blood) which lasts for one (1) to five (5) days. With the appearance of antibody in the animal's blood, the leptospiremic phase is terminated. The organisms may remain in the kidney and multiply in this location, then are shed in the urine for months or years, infecting other farm animals.

Young animals that are acutely ill with leptospirosis may show a transient fever, loss of appetite, and difficulty in breathing, with death losses approaching 15% due to severe anemia. Lactating cows exhibit a loss of milk production with a milk secretion that is yellow, clotted, and often blood-tinged. Severely affected animals develop anemia, jaundice, hemoglobinuria and pneumonia.

In pregnant cows, the organism may infect the fetus, which dies and is aborted one (1) to four (4) weeks after the leptospiremic phase, usually in the last trimester of pregnancy.

Swine are infected similarly, with the most common serotypes being *L. pomona*, which is shed from pig to pig via the urine, and *L. icterohaemorrhagiae* which is spread to pigs from dogs and rats.

Symptoms in swine vary widely. Many of the infections are subclinical and are only recognized by seroconversion, by isolation of the organism from the kidneys and urine, or by cases of leptospirosis in other animals from the swine herd. The most common signs are abortions and stillbirths in pregnant animals, mainly late abortions. Common clinical signs include loss of appetite, intestinal problems and reduced weight gain. Acute or subacute infections are observed in young pigs, with fever and high death loss the primary signs.

As leptospirosis can be an occupational hazard for the dairy worker, the veterinarian should inform the dairy owner of the public health aspects of the disease whenever an outbreak occurs. Using antibiotic therapy and vaccination decreases the hazard by reducing the shedding of leptospires in the urine.

Presentation: Available in 50 dose (100 mL) bottles.

Compendium Code No.: 11140192

LEPTO SHIELD™ 5 HARDJO BOVIS

Novartis Animal Vaccines **Bacterin**

Leptospira Canicola-Grippotyphosa-Hardjo-Icterohaemorrhagiae-Pomona Bacterin

U.S. Vet. Lic. No.: 303

Composition: This bacterin contains inactivated cultures of *Leptospira canicola, grippotyphosa, hardjo-bovis, icterohaemorrhagiae,* and *pomona* adjuvanted with aluminum hydroxide. Contains thimerosal as a preservative.

Indications: For use in healthy cattle as an aid in the prevention and control of disease caused by *Leptospira canicola, grippotyphosa, hardjo, icterohaemorrhagiae,* and *pomona.*

Dosage and Administration: Shake well before using. Administer 2 mL intramuscularly. Revaccinate annually.

Precaution(s): Store in the dark at 35°-45°F (2°-7°C). Do not freeze. Use entire contents when first opened.

Caution(s): Anaphylactic reactions may occur following the use of this biological. Symptomatic treatment: Epinephrine.

For veterinary use only.

Warning(s): Do not vaccinate within 21 days prior to slaughter.

Presentation: 10 dose (20 mL) and 50 dose (100 mL) bottles.

Compendium Code No.: 11140740 F276 / F277

LEUKOCELL® 2

Pfizer Animal Health **Vaccine**

Feline Leukemia Vaccine, Killed Virus

U.S. Vet. Lic. No.: 189

Description: LEUKOCELL® 2 is prepared by propagating FeLV, subgroups A, B, and C, in FeLV-transformed lymphoid cells. Viral antigens are chemically inactivated, combined with a sterile adjuvant to enhance the immune response, and packaged in liquid form.

LEUKOCELL® 2 is prepared from an FeLV-transformed lymphoid cell line that releases FeLV viral particles which are soluble in a cell culture medium.[1] The practical benefit of this unique, patented feature is that production of immunosuppressive effects characteristic of fully assembled FeLV antigens, whether live or killed, is reduced.2-4 (See Safety and Efficacy).

Contains gentamicin as preservative.

Indications: LEUKOCELL® 2 is a multiple viral antigen vaccine for vaccination of healthy cats 9 weeks of age or older as an aid in preventing persistent viremia, lymphoid tumors caused by feline leukemia virus (FeLV), and diseases associated with FeLV infection.

Directions:

1. General Directions: Shake well. Aseptically administer 1 mL subcutaneously.
2. Primary Vaccination: Healthy cats 9 weeks of age or older should receive 2 doses administered 3-4 weeks apart.
3. Revaccination: Annual revaccination with a single dose is recommended.

Precaution(s): Store at 2°-7°C. Prolonged exposure to higher temperatures may adversely affect potency. Do not freeze.

Use entire contents when first opened.

Sterilized syringes and needles should be used to administer this vaccine.

Caution(s): Certain postvaccination reactions may occur. (See Safety and Efficacy)

As with many vaccines, anaphylaxis may occur after use. Initial antidote of epinephrine is recommended and should be followed with appropriate supportive therapy.

This product has been shown to be efficacious in healthy animals. A protective immune response may not be elicited if animals are incubating an infectious disease, are malnourished or parasitized, are stressed due to shipment or environmental conditions, are otherwise immunocompromised, or the vaccine is not administered in accordance with label directions.

Warning(s): For veterinary use only.

Discussion: LEUKOCELL® 2 is a second generation vaccine derived from and comparable to Leukocell, the first federally licensed FeLV vaccine. Licensed in the United States in November 1984, LEUKOCELL® originally was indicated for 3 intramuscular (IM) doses, a regimen demonstrated to be efficacious in preventing persistent viremia, lymphoid tumors, and FeLV-associated diseases. After basic development studies were performed to demonstrate suitability for licensing, additional data has been published attesting to the vaccine's safety and efficacy. Lymphocyte blastogenesis assays (LBA) showed that soluble vaccine proteins produced no significant effect on LBA of cat lymphocytes when compared with control samples,[5,6] an indication that the vaccine is not immunosuppressive. In a related test, cats were vaccinated with a 10-fold concentration of enhanced vaccine, and lymphocytes from these cats showed no change in LBA response, nor did their LBA values differ appreciably from those of nonvaccinated cats.[5,6] Other studies showed that LEUKOCELL® was an aid in protecting vaccinated cats from latent FeLV infection, even when repeated immunosuppressive treatment was administered.[5,7,8] Another series of tests showed that LEUKOCELL® consistently elicited marked levels of complement-dependent cytotoxic (CDC) antibodies, demonstrating that the vaccine's immunizing properties are not limited to its ability to stimulate anti-gp70 and anti-feline oncornavirus-associated membrane antigen (FOCMA) antibodies.[5,9,10] Clinical reports by independent practitioners have demonstrated that the vaccine protected cats in high-risk environments where frequent or continuous contact with known leukemic cats occurred.[11]

LEUKOCELL® 2 was licensed with a 2-dose subcutaneous (SC) indication. In multiple tests conducted to determine suitability for licensing, using minimal potency vaccine, LEUKOCELL® 2 was shown to be:

- Highly immunogenic, producing and priming for antibody responses to gp70, FOCMA, and virus neutralizing (VN) antigens.
- Highly efficacious, protecting more than 70% of artificially immunosuppressed vaccinates against persistent viremia after challenge.
- Safe, as no change in normal blood cell values of vaccinated cats was observed during the vaccination period.

Disease Description: FeLV is associated with a complex of feline diseases. These include 2 forms of cancer: (1) lymphosarcoma, characterized by presence of tumors, and (2) leukemia, characterized by presence of malignant cells in the bloodstream. In addition, FeLV is associated with a variety of non-neoplastic diseases, including aplastic anemia, reproduction failure, stomatitis, Fading Kitten Syndrome (thymic atrophy), and upper respiratory infections. The pathological process is enhanced by the virus's role as an immunosuppressive agent. Following chronic infection, immunosuppression persists until cancer or disease of microbial origin develops, usually after a period of months or years.

The causative agent of FeLV disease is a retrovirus, which was named "feline leukemia virus" after its discovery in 1964. The designation is somewhat inaccurate in view of the variety of clinical conditions that result from FeLV infection, only a minority of which are leukemic. Three FeLV subgroups, designated A, B, and C, have been identified, with subgroup A predominating. Structurally, the FeLV envelope consists of 2 proteins, gp70 and p15e. The gp70 protein is the more prominent. It is considered to be the primary immunogenic antigen inasmuch as gp70 antibodies will neutralize FeLV. A variety of other FeLV proteins have been identified (including p10, p12, p15, and p27) although their correlation with FeLV disease has not been established.

Lymphosarcoma is the most common form of cancer caused by FeLV. Lymphosarcomas resulting from FeLV infections express a nonviral antigen on the surface of the malignant cells. This tumor-specific antigen is designated feline oncornavirus-associated cell membrane antigen (FOCMA). Postexposure antibodies to FOCMA have been shown to confer immunity to FeLV-induced lymphosarcoma and are an important factor in successful resistance to tumor development.[12] Studies have shown that cats that develop FeLV malignancies do not have high FOCMA antibody titers,[12] and that inadequate anti-FOCMA response is a cause, rather than an effect, of ensuing FeLV lymphosarcoma.[13]

Trial Data: Safety and Efficacy: The vaccine's safety and lack of immunosuppression have been demonstrated by the lymphocyte blastogenesis assay (LBA), differential and complete blood counts (CBC). LEUKOCELL® 2 stimulates and primes for antibody responses to gp70 glycoprotein, the tumor-specific antigen FOCMA (see Disease Description), as well as VN antigens.

In an immunogenicity study, 25 specific pathogen free (SPF) cats were vaccinated with a 2-dose primary regimen (2 doses were given 3 weeks apart). After the second dose, significant levels of antibodies to gp70 and FOCMA were detected as well as VN antibodies.

After challenge with the Rickard strain of FeLV, which infected 100% of the control cats, more than 70% of the vaccinates were protected against establishment of persistent viremia. In contrast, 60% of nonvaccinated control cats developed persistent viremia.

In assessing these results, it should be noted that test cats were subjected to a far more rigorous challenge regimen than could be expected under normal exposure conditions (normal FeLV incidence after exposure is 30%[14,15]). All test cats (including vaccinates) were artificially immunosuppressed before challenge to enhance susceptibility to FeLV infection and tumor development. Challenge virus was administered intranasally to ensure uniform exposure that conforms to the natural route of infection, and assures optimum delivery of challenge virus.

Demonstrated safety is particularly critical in the case of an FeLV vaccine. Whole FeLV (live or killed) contains a specific envelope protein, designated p15e, that is responsible for host immunosuppression.[2-4,16,17] Rigorous safety tests of LEUKOCELL® 2 did not demonstrate any immunosuppressive effects. Kittens vaccinated with LEUKOCELL® 2 had normal postvaccination white blood cell (WBC) counts, did not become viremic, remained clinically normal, and developed gp70, FOCMA, and VN antibodies.

Postvaccination reactions have been observed in about 2% of vaccinated cats. These included stinging on injection, transient listlessness, depression, and brief temperature elevations. Hypersensitivity evidenced by myxedema and gastrointestinal distress (vomiting and bowel evacuation) occasionally has been reported.

Although a diagnostic test for FeLV antigen is not required prior to vaccination with LEUKOCELL® 2, such a test may be beneficial in evaluating candidates for vaccination. Vaccination is of no known therapeutic value in cats with existing FeLV infection, nor will it alter the natural course of disease.

References: Available upon request.

Presentation: Cartons of 50 x 1 dose vials.

U.S. Patent No. 4,332,793

Compendium Code No.: 36901170 75-4363-07

LEVAMISOLE INJECTABLE

AgriLabs **Parasiticide Injection**

(Levamisole Phosphate Injectable Solution 13.65%) Sterile Anthelmintic

ANADA No.: 200-271

Active Ingredient(s): Each mL of solution contains levamisole phosphate equivalent to 136.5 mg of levamisole hydrochloride.

Indications: Levamisole Phosphate is a broad-spectrum anthelmintic for subcutaneous injection in cattle and is effective against the following nematode infections in cattle:

Stomach Worms: *(Haemonchus, Ostertagia, Trichostrongylus).*

Intestinal Worms: *(Trichostrongylus, Cooperia, Nematodirus, Bunostomum, Oesophagostomum, Chabertia).*

Lungworms: *(Dictyocaulus).*

Dosage and Administration: Dosage: Inject subcutaneously in the mid-neck region at the rate of 2 mL per 100 lb body weight. It is recommended that no more than 10 mL be injected at one site.

Consult a veterinarian for assistance in the diagnosis, treatment, and control of parasitism.

The maturation of some helminth species may be arrested at a pre-adult stage when adult worm populations are heavy.

Cattle that are severely parasitized or maintained under conditions of constant helminth exposure may require retreatment with two to four weeks after the first treatment.

Administration: Thoroughly clean and disinfect syringes and needles by boiling in water for twenty minutes. Use 14 or 16 gauge ½ to 1 inch needles.

Do not remove rubber stopper from the bottle, but clean and disinfect it with 70% alcohol. With syringe attached to needle, insert needle through the rubber stopper and withdraw the required dose.

A clean sterile needle should be used for each animal to avoid the spread of infection.

Precaution(s): Storage Conditions: To assure maximum potency and efficacy, store at or below 70°F. Refrigeration advisable. Avoid freezing.

Caution(s): Careful cattle weight estimates are essential for proper performance of this product. It is recommended that Levamisole Phosphate be injected only in cattle in stocker or feeder condition. Cattle nearing slaughter weight and condition may show objectionable reactions at the site of injection. An occasional animal in stocker or feeder flesh may show swelling at injection site. The swelling will subside in 7 to 14 days and is no more severe than that observed from commonly used vaccines and bacterins.

The mid-neck region is the preferred injection site. Always use sterile needles and syringes. Non-sterile equipment may cause abscesses at the site of injection. Contents should be used as soon as possible after the seal has been broken. It is recommended that the cap be wiped with alcohol prior to withdrawing solution. Also, skin at the injection site should be swabbed with alcohol to avoid infection.

Muzzle foam may be observed; however, this reaction will disappear within a few hours. If this condition persists, a veterinarian should be consulted. Follow recommended dosages carefully.

Experience under field conditions indicates that stressful procedures such as vaccination, castration, dehorning, concurrent exposure to cholinesterase-inhibiting drugs, pesticides or chemicals, may increase the risk associated with the use of this product. Such concurrent stresses should be avoided when using this product.

Consult veterinarian before using in severely debilitated animals.

For subcutaneous injection in cattle.

Warning(s): Do not administer to cattle within 7 days of slaughter for food to avoid tissue residues. To prevent residues in milk, do not administer to dairy animals of breeding age.

Keep this and all drugs out of reach of children.

Presentation: Available in 500 mL vials.

Compendium Code No.: 10580661 Iss. 5-00

LEVAMISOLE PHOSPHATE

Durvet **Parasiticide Injection**

Injectable Solution, 13.65%-Sterile Anthelmintic

ANADA No.: 200-271

Active Ingredient(s): Each mL of solution contains levamisole phosphate equivalent to 136.5 mg of levamisole hydrochloride.

Indications: LEVAMISOLE PHOSPHATE is a sterile solution recommended for the treatment of cattle infected with the following parasites:

Stomach Worms: *Haemonchus, Ostertagia, Trichostrongylus.*

Intestinal Worms: *Trichostrongylus, Cooperia, Nematodirus, Bunostomum, Oesophagostomum, Chabertia.*

Lungworms: *Dictyocaulus.*

Dosage and Administration: Dosage: Inject subcutaneously in the mid-neck region at the rate of 2 mL per 100 lb body weight. It is recommended that no more than 10 mL be injected at one site.

Consult your veterinarian for assistance in the diagnosis, treatment, and control of parasitism.

The maturation of some helminth species may be arrested at pre-adult stage when adult worm populations are heavy.

Cattle that are severely parasitized or maintained under conditions of constant helminth exposure may require retreatment with two to four weeks after the first treatment.

Administration: Thoroughly clean and disinfect syringes and needles by boiling in water for twenty minutes. Use 14 or 16 gauge ½ to 1 inch needles.

Do not remove rubber stopper from the bottle, but clean and disinfect it with 70% alcohol. With syringe attached to needle, insert needle through the rubber stopper and withdraw the required dose.

The proper method of injection site preparation by swabbing with 70% alcohol or other suitable disinfectant, and the proper method of administration under a fold of skin in the mid-neck region are demonstrated below. A clean, sterile needle should be used for each animal to avoid spreading infection.

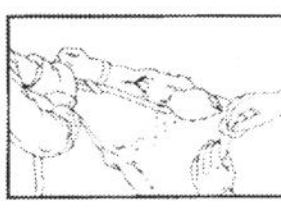

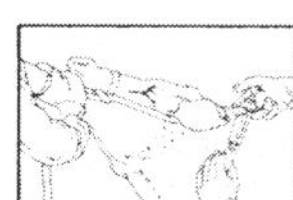

Precaution(s): Storage Conditions: To assure maximum potency and efficacy, store at or below 70°F. Refrigeration advisable. Avoid freezing.

Caution(s): Careful cattle weight estimates are essential for proper performance of this product. It is recommended that LEVAMISOLE PHOSPHATE be injected only in cattle in stocker or feeder condition. Cattle nearing slaughter weight and condition may show objectionable reactions at the site of injection. An occasional animal in stocker or feeder flesh may show swelling at the injection site. The swelling will subside in 7 to 14 days and is no more severe than that observed from commonly used vaccines and bacterins.

The mid-neck region is the preferred injection site. Always use sterile needles and syringes. Non-sterile equipment may cause abscesses at the site of injection. Contents should be used as soon as possible after the seal has been broken. It is recommended that the cap be wiped with alcohol prior to withdrawing solution. Also, skin at injection site should be swabbed with alcohol to avoid infection.

Muzzle foam may be observed; however, the reaction will disappear within a few hours. If this condition persists, a veterinarian should be consulted.

Follow recommended dosage carefully.

Experience under field conditions indicates that stressful procedures such as vaccination, castration, dehorning, concurrent exposure to cholinesterase-inhibiting drugs, pesticides, or chemicals, may increase the risk associated with the use of this product. Such concurrent stress should be avoided when using this product.

Consult veterinarian before using in severely debilitated animals.

Warning(s): Do not administer to cattle within 7 days of slaughter for food to avoid tissue residues. To prevent residues in milk, do not administer to dairy animals of breeding age.

Keep this and all drugs out of the reach of children.

Presentation: Available in 500 mL vials.

Compendium Code No.: 10842000 Iss. 11-00

LEVAMISOLE PHOSPHATE INJECTABLE SOLUTION, 13.65%

AgriPharm **Parasiticide Injection**

Sterile Anthelmintic

Active Ingredient(s): Each mL of solution contains levamisole phosphate equivalent to 136.5 mg of levamisole hydrochloride.

Indications: LEVAMISOLE PHOSPHATE INJECTABLE SOLUTION, 13.65% is a sterile solution recommended for the treatment of cattle infected with the following parasites:

Stomach Worms: *Haemonchus, Ostertagia, Trichostrongylus.*

Intestinal Worms: *Trichostrongylus, Cooperia, Nematodirus, Bunostomum, Oesophagostomum, Chabertia.*

Lungworms: *Dictyocaulus.*

Dosage and Administration: Inject subcutaneously in the mid-neck region at the rate of 2 mL per 100 lbs. of body weight. It is recommended that not more than 10 mL be injected at one site.

Consult a veterinarian for assistance in the diagnosis, treatment and control of parasitism.

The maturation of some helminth species may be arrested at a pre-adult stage when adult worm populations are heavy.

Cattle that are severely parasitized or maintained under conditions of constant helminth exposure may require retreatment with two (2) to four (4) weeks after the first treatment.

Thoroughly clean and disinfect syringes and needles by boiling in water for 20 minutes. Use 14 or 16 gauge one-half (½) to one (1) inch needles.

Do not remove the rubber stopper from the bottle, but clean and disinfect it with 70% alcohol. With the syringe attached to a needle, insert the needle through the rubber stopper and withdraw the required dose.

A clean sterile needle should be used for each animal to avoid the spread of infection.

Precaution(s): To ensure maximum potency and efficacy, store at or below 70°F. Refrigeration is advisable. Avoid freezing.

Caution(s): Careful cattle weight estimates are essential for the proper performance of the product. It is recommended that LEVAMISOLE PHOSPHATE INJECTABLE SOLUTION, 13.65% be injected in cattle in stocker or feeder condition only. Cattle nearing slaughter weight and condition may show objectionable reactions at the site of injection. An occasional animal in stocker or feeder flesh may show swelling at the injection site. The swelling will subside in 7-14 days and is not more severe than that observed from commonly used vaccines and bacterins.

The mid-neck region is the preferred injection site. Always use sterile needles and syringes. Non-sterile equipment may cause abscesses at the site of injection. Care should be used in maintaining the sterility of the solution. The contents should be used as soon as possible after the seal has been broken. It is recommended that the cap be wiped with alcohol prior to withdrawing any solution. Also, the skin at the injection site should be swabbed with alcohol to avoid infection.

Muzzle foam may be observed; however, the reaction will disappear within a few hours. If the condition persists, a veterinarian should be consulted.

Follow the recommended dosage carefully.

Experience under field conditions indicates that stressful procedures such as vaccination, castration, dehorning, concurrent exposure to cholinesterase-inhibiting drugs, pesticides, or chemicals, may increase the risk associated with the use of the product. Such concurrent stresses should be avoided when using the product.

Consult a veterinarian before using in severely debilitated animals.

Warning(s): Keep this and all drugs out of the reach of children.

Do not administer to cattle within seven (7) days of slaughter for food to avoid tissue residues. To prevent residues in milk, do not administer to dairy animals of breeding age.

Presentation: 500 mL vials.

Compendium Code No.: 14571210

LEVAMISOLE PHOSPHATE INJECTABLE SOLUTION, 13.65%

Aspen **Parasiticide Injection**

Sterile Anthelmintic

NADA No.: 102-437

Active Ingredient(s): Each mL of solution contains levamisole phosphate equivalent to 136.5 mg of levamisole hydrochloride.

Indications: LEVAMISOLE PHOSPHATE INJECTABLE SOLUTION, 13.65% is a sterile solution recommended for the treatment of cattle infected with the following parasites:

Stomach Worms: *Haemonchus, Ostertagia, Trichostrongylus.*

Intestinal Worms: *Trichostrongylus, Cooperia, Nematodirus, Bunostomum, Oesophagostomum, Chabertia.*

Lungworms: *Dictyocaulus.*

Dosage and Administration: Inject subcutaneously in the mid-neck region at the rate of 2 mL per 100 lbs of body weight. It is recommended that not more than 10 mL be injected at one site.

Consult a veterinarian for assistance in the diagnosis, treatment and control of parasitism.

The maturation of some helminth species may be arrested at a pre-adult stage when adult worm populations are heavy.

Cattle that are severely parasitized or maintained under conditions of constant helminth exposure may require retreatment with two (2) to four (4) weeks after the first treatment.

Thoroughly clean and disinfect syringes and needles by boiling in water for 20 minutes. Use 14 or 16 gauge one-half (½) to one (1) inch needles.

Do not remove the rubber stopper from the bottle, but clean and disinfect it with 70% alcohol. With the syringe attached to a needle, insert the needle through the rubber stopper and withdraw the required dose.

A clean sterile needle should be used for each animal to avoid the spread of infection.

Precaution(s): To ensure maximum potency and efficacy, store at or below 70°F. Refrigeration is advisable. Avoid freezing.

Caution(s): Careful cattle weight estimates are essential for the proper performance of the product. It is recommended that LEVAMISOLE PHOSPHATE INJECTABLE SOLUTION, 13.65% be injected in cattle in stocker or feeder condition only. Cattle nearing slaughter weight and condition may show objectionable reactions at the site of injection. An occasional animal in stocker or feeder flesh may show swelling at the injection site. The swelling will subside in 7-14 days and is not more severe than that observed from commonly used vaccines and bacterins.

The mid-neck region is the preferred injection site. Always use sterile needles and syringes. Non-sterile equipment may cause abscesses at the site of injection. Care should be used in maintaining the sterility of the solution. The contents should be used as soon as possible after the seal has been broken. It is recommended that the cap be wiped with alcohol prior to withdrawing any solution. Also, the skin at the injection site should be swabbed with alcohol to avoid infection.

Muzzle foam may be observed; however, the reaction will disappear within a few hours. If the condition persists, a veterinarian should be consulted. Follow the recommended dosage carefully.

Experience under field conditions indicates that stressful procedures such as vaccination, castration, dehorning, concurrent exposure to cholinesterase-inhibiting drugs, pesticides, or chemicals, may increase the risk associated with the use of the product. Such concurrent stresses should be avoided when using the product.

Consult a veterinarian before using in severely debilitated animals.

Warning(s): Keep this and all drugs out of the reach of children.

Do not administer to cattle within seven (7) days of slaughter for food to avoid tissue residues. To prevent residues in milk, do not administer to dairy animals of breeding age.

Presentation: 500 mL vials.

Compendium Code No.: 14750530

LEVAMISOLE SOLUBLE PIG WORMER

AgriLabs **Water Medication**

(Levamisole Hydrochloride) Anthelmintic

NADA No.: 112-049

Active Ingredient(s): This bottle contains 18.15 grams of levamisole hydrochloride.

Indications: Levamisole Hydrochloride is a broad-spectrum anthelmintic and is effective against the following nematode infections in swine:

Large Roundworms: *(Ascaris suum).*
Nodular Worms: *(Oesophagostomum* spp.)
Lungworms: *(Metastrongylus* spp.)
Intestinal Threadworms: *(Strongyloides ransomi.)*

Dosage and Administration: For use in drinking water.

This bottle contains 18.15 grams of levamisole hydrochloride activity which will treat the following:

200 - 25 lb. pigs or
100 - 50 lb. pigs or
50 - 100 lb. pigs or
25 - 200 lb. pigs

Directions for Preparing Soluble Pig Wormer Solution: When you are ready to worm your pigs, add water to the powder in this bottle up to the 500 mL mark. Agitate to mix thoroughly before using. If any solution is left over, it may be stored for up to 3 months in this tightly capped bottle; agitate well before using.

Directions for Use: Withholding water from pigs prior to treatment is not necessary for optimum anthelmintic efficacy and is not recommended during hot weather. Add 10 mL (2 teaspoons) of the solution from this bottle to 1 gallon of water; mix thoroughly. Allow one gallon of medicated water for each 100 pounds body weight of pigs to be treated. No other source of water should be offered. As soon as pigs have consumed all the medicated water, resume use of regular water.

Note: Careful estimates of pig weights are essential for proper performance of this product. Pigs maintained under conditions of constant worm exposure may require retreatment within 4-5 weeks after the first treatment due to reinfection.

Caution(s): Consult veterinarian before administering Levamisole Hydrochloride to sick swine. Consult your veterinarian for assistance in the diagnosis, treatment and control of parasitism. Salivation or muzzle foam may be observed. This reaction is occasionally seen and will disappear in a short time after medication.

If pigs are infected with mature lungworms, coughing and vomiting may be observed soon after medicated water is consumed. This reaction is due to the expulsion of worms from the lungs and will be over in several hours. Follow recommended dosage carefully to assure removal of worms and avoid an overdose of Levamisole Hydrochloride.

Warning(s): Do not administer within 72 hours of slaughter for food.

Keep out of reach of children.

Presentation: 0.71 oz. (20.17 g) bottle.

Compendium Code No.: 10580670

L

LEVASOLE® CATTLE WORMER BOLUSES

Schering-Plough **Parasiticide-Oral**

(levamisole hydrochloride) Anthelmintic

NADA No.: 091-826

Active Ingredient(s): Each bolus contains 2.19 g of levamisole hydrochloride activity.

Indications: LEVASOLE® (levamisole hydrochloride) is a broad-spectrum anthelmintic and is effective against the following nematode infections:

Stomach Worms: *Haemonchus, Trichostrongylus, Ostertagia.*
Intestinal Worms: *Trichostrongylus, Cooperia, Nematodirus, Bunostomum, Oesphagostomum.*
Lungworms: *Dictyocaulus.*

Dosage and Administration: Single Oral Dosage for Cattle:

Weight	No. Boluses
250 to 450 lb	½
450 to 750 lb	1
750 to 1050 lb	1½

Consult your veterinarian for a routine deworming program.

Caution(s): Muzzle foam may be observed. However, this reaction will disappear within a few hours. If this condition persists, a veterinarian should be consulted. Follow the recommended dosage carefully.

Cattle maintained under conditions of constant helminth exposure may require retreatment within 2 to 4 weeks after the first treatment.

Consult a veterinarian before using in severely debilitated animals.

Consult your veterinarian for assistance in the diagnosis, treatment and control of parasitism.

For oral use in cattle.

Warning(s): Do not administer within 48 hours of slaughter for food.

Do not administer to dairy animals of breeding age.

Keep out of reach of children.

Presentation: 1 box (50 boluses) (NDC 0061-5083-01).

Compendium Code No.: 10471162 Rev. 8/97

LEVASOLE® INJECTABLE SOLUTION, 13.65%

Schering-Plough **Parasiticide Injection**

(levamisole phosphate)-Sterile Anthelmintic

NADA No.: 102-437

Active Ingredient(s): Each mL of solution contains levamisole phosphate equivalent to 136.5 mg of levamisole hydrochloride.

Indications: LEVASOLE® (levamisole phosphate) is a broad-spectrum anthelmintic and is effective in the following nematode infections in cattle:

Stomach Worms: *Haemonchus, Ostertagia, Trichostrongylus.*
Intestinal Worms: *Trichostrongylus, Cooperia, Nematodirus, Bunostomum, Oesophagostomum, Chabertia.*
Lungworms: *Dictyocaulus.*
For subcutaneous injection in cattle.

Dosage and Administration: Dosage: Inject subcutaneously in the mid-neck region at the rate of 2 mL per 100 lb body weight. It is recommended that not more than 10 mL be injected at one site.

Consult your veterinarian for assistance in the diagnosis, treatment and control of parasitism.

The maturation of some helminth species may be arrested at a pre-adult stage when adult worm populations are heavy.

Cattle that are severely parasitized or maintained under conditions of constant helminth exposure may require retreatment with two to four weeks after the first treatment.

Administration: Thoroughly clean and disinfect syringes and needles by boiling in water for twenty minutes. Use 14 or 16 gauge ½ to 1 inch needles.

Do not remove rubber stopper from the bottle, but clean and disinfect it with 70% alcohol. With syringe attached to needle, insert needle through the rubber stopper and withdraw the required dose.

The proper method of injection site preparation, is swabbing with 70% alcohol or other suitable disinfectant, and the proper method of administration is under a fold of the skin in the mid-neck region as demonstrated. A clean sterile needle should be used for each animal to avoid spreading infection.

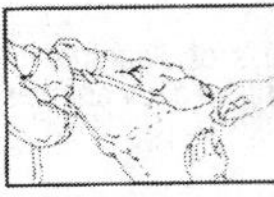

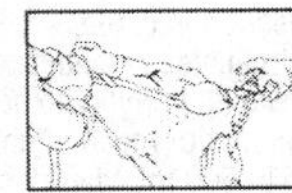

Precaution(s): Store at or below 70°F. Refrigeration is advisable. Avoid freezing.

Caution(s): Careful cattle weight estimates are essential for the proper performance of this product. It is recommended that LEVASOLE® Injectable Solution, 13.65% be injected only in cattle in stocker or feeder condition. Cattle nearing slaughter weight and condition may show objectionable reactions at the site of injection. An occasional animal in stocker or feeder flesh may show swelling at the injection site. The swelling will subside in 7 to 14 days and is no more severe than that observed from commonly used vaccines and bacterins.

The mid-neck region is the preferred injection site. Always use sterile needles and syringes. Non-sterile equipment may cause abscesses at the site of injection. Contents should be used as soon as possible after the seal has been broken. It is recommended that the cap be wiped with alcohol prior to withdrawing solution. Also, skin at the injection site should be swabbed with alcohol to avoid infection.

Muzzle foam may be observed; however, this reaction will disappear within a few hours. If this condition persists, a veterinarian should be consulted. Follow recommended dosage carefully.

Experience under field conditions indicates that stressful procedures such as vaccination, castration, dehorning, concurrent exposure to cholinesterase-inhibiting drugs, pesticides, or chemicals, may increase the risk associated with the use of this product. Such concurrent stresses should be avoided when using this product.

Consult a veterinarian before using in severely debilitated animals.

Warning(s): Do not administer to cattle within 7 days of slaughter for food to avoid tissue residues. To prevent residues in milk, do not administer to dairy animals of breeding age.

Keep this and all drugs out of reach of children.

Presentation: 100 mL (NDC 0061-5042-02) and 500 mL (NDC 0061-5042-01) vials.

Manufactured by: Boehringer Ingelheim Animal Health, Inc., St. Joseph, MO 64506.

Compendium Code No.: 10471173 Rev. 10/97

LEVASOLE® SHEEP WORMER BOLUSES

Schering-Plough **Parasiticide-Oral**

(levamisole hydrochloride) Anthelmintic

NADA No.: 112-052

Active Ingredient(s): Each bolus contains 0.184 g of levamisole hydrochloride activity.

Indications: LEVASOLE® (levamisole hydrochloride) is a broad-spectrum anthelmintic and is effective against the following nematode infections:

Stomach Worms: *Haemonchus, Trichostrongylus, Ostertagia.*
Intestinal Worms: *Trichostrongylus, Cooperia, Nematodirus, Bunostomum, Oesophagostomum, Chabertia.*
Lungworms: *Dictyocaulus.*

Dosage and Administration: Single Oral Dosage for Sheep:

Weight	No. Boluses
25 lb	½
50 lb	1
75 lb	1½
100 lb	2
150 lb	3

Sheep maintained under conditions of constant helminth exposure may require retreatment within 2 to 4 weeks after the first treatment. Consult your veterinarian for assistance in the diagnosis, treatment and control of parasitism.

Caution(s): Consult a veterinarian before using in severely debilitated animals. Follow the recommended dosage carefully.

Warning(s): Do not administer within 72 hours of slaughter for food.

Keep out of reach of children.

Presentation: Bottle of 100 boluses (NDC 0061-5082-01).

Compendium Code No.: 10471182 Rev. 8/97

LEVASOLE® SOLUBLE DRENCH POWDER

Schering-Plough **Parasiticide-Oral**

(levamisole hydrochloride) Anthelmintic

NADA No.: 112-051

Active Ingredient(s): Each packet contains 46.8 grams of levamisole hydrochloride activity.

The bottle contains 544.5 grams of levamisole hydrochloride activity.

Indications: LEVASOLE® (levamisole hydrochloride) is a broad-spectrum anthelmintic and is effect against the following nematode infections in cattle and sheep:

Stomach Worms: *Haemonchus, Trichostrongylus, Ostertagia.*
Intestinal Worms: *Trichostrongylus, Cooperia, Nematodirus, Bunostomum, Oesophagostomum [Chabertia*-Sheep only].
Lungworms: *Dictyocaulus.*

Dosage and Administration: Packet Administration:

Cattle-

Standard Drench Solution-Place the contents of the packet in a 1 quart (32 fl. oz.) container, fill with water; swirl until dissolved. Administer as a single drench dose according to the following table:

Weight	Drench Dosage	Packet Will Treat
200 lb	½ fl. oz.	64 head
400 lb	1 fl. oz.	32 head
600 lb	1½ fl. oz.	21 head
800 lb	2 fl. oz.	16 head

Concentrated Drench Solution-For use with 20 mL Automatic Syringe. Place the contents of the packet in a standard household measuring container and add water to the 8¾ fl. oz. level; or use the measuring container available from your supplier and add water to the mark. Swirl until dissolved. Give 2 mL (milliliter) per 100 lb body weight. Refer to the table above for the number of cattle each packet will treat.

Sheep-

Standard Drench Solution-Place the contents of the packet in a 1 gallon (128 fl. oz.) container, fill with water; swirl until dissolved. Administer as a single drench dose according to the following table:

Weight	Drench Dosage	Packet Will Treat
50 lb	½ fl. oz.	256 head
100 lb	1 fl. oz.	128 head
150 lb	1½ fl. oz.	84 head
200 lb	2 fl. oz.	64 head

Concentrated Drench Solution-For use with the 20 mL Automatic Syringe. Place the contents of the packet in a standard household measuring container and add water to the 17½ fl. oz. level. Swirl until dissolved. Give 2 mL per 50 lb body weight. Refer to the table above for the number of sheep each packet will treat.

Bottle Administration-

When you are ready to deworm your cattle or sheep, add water to the powder in the bottle up to the 3 liter mark. Swirl to mix thoroughly before using. If any solution left over it may be stored for up to 3 months in the tightly capped bottle. Shake well before using.

Administer as a single drench dose as follows:

Cattle — 2 mL per 100 lb body weight

Weight	Drench Dosage	Bottle Will Treat
100 lb	2 mL	1,500 head
300 lb	6 mL	500 head
500 lb	10 mL	300 head
700 lb	14 mL	214 head
1,000 lb	20 mL	150 head

Sheep — 1 mL per 50 lb body weight

Weight	Drench Dosage	Bottle Will Treat
50 lb	1 mL	3,000 head
100 lb	2 mL	1,500 head
150 lb	3 mL	1,000 head
200 lb	4 mL	750 head

Note: Careful weight estimates are essential for proper performance of this product. Prepare solutions as needed. However, excess solutions may be stored in clean closed containers for up to 90 days without loss of anthelmintic activity.

Cattle and Sheep maintained under conditions of constant helminth exposure may require retreatment within 2 to 4 weeks after the first treatment.

Consult your veterinarian for assistance in the diagnosis, treatment, and control of parasitism.

Caution(s): Muzzle foam may be observed. However, this reaction will disappear within a few hours. If this condition persists, a veterinarian should be consulted. Follow recommended dosage carefully. Consult veterinarian before using in severely debilitated animals.

Warning(s): Do not administer to cattle within 48 hours of slaughter for food. Do not administer to sheep within 72 hours of slaughter for food. To prevent residues in milk, do not administer to dairy animals of breeding age.

Keep out of the reach of children.

Presentation: 1.8 oz (52 g) packets (NDC 0061-5044-01) and 21.34 oz. (1.3 lb) (605 g) bottles (NDC 0061-5043-01).

Compendium Code No.: 10471193 Rev. 8/97

LEVASOLE® SOLUBLE DRENCH POWDER (Sheep)

Schering-Plough **Parasiticide-Oral**

(levamisole hydrochloride) Anthelmintic

NADA No.: 112-050

Active Ingredient(s): Each packet contains 11.7 g levamisole hydrochloride activity.

Indications: LEVASOLE® (levamisole hydrochloride) is a broad-spectrum anthelmintic and is effective against the following nematode infections in sheep:

Stomach Worms: *Haemonchus, Trichostrongylus, Ostertagia.*

Intestinal Worms: *Trichostrongylus, Cooperia, Nematodirus, Bunostomum, Oesophagostomum, Chabertia.*

Lungworms: *Dictyocaulus.*

Dosage and Administration: For oral use in sheep.

Administer as a standard drench with a standard drench syringe or administer as a concentrated drench solution with an automatic drenching syringe.

Preparation of Standard Drench Solution: For use with a standard drench syringe. Place the contents of 1 packet in a 1 quart (32 fl. oz.) container. Fill with water and swirl briefly until dissolved. Administer as a single drench dose according to the following table:

Weight	Standard Drench Dosage	One Packet Will Treat
50 lbs.	½ fl. oz.	64 head
100 lbs.	1 fl. oz.	32 head
150 lbs.	1½ fl. oz.	21 head
200 lbs.	2 fl. oz.	16 head

Preparation of Concentrated Drench Solution: For use with an automatic drenching syringe: Place the contents of 1 packet in a household measuring container and add water to the 10.9 fl. oz. level. Swirl briefly to dissolve and then administer at the rate of 1 mL per 10 lb body weight. Refer to the table above for the number of sheep each packet will treat.

Note: Careful sheep weight estimates are essential for the proper performance of this product. Prepare solutions as needed. However, excess solutions may be stored in clean closed containers for up to 90 days without loss of anthelmintic activity.

Sheep maintained under conditions of constant helminth exposure may require retreatment with 2 to 4 weeks after the first treatment.

Consult your veterinarian for assistance in the diagnosis, treatment and control of parasitism.

Caution(s): Consult a veterinarian before using in severely debilitated animals.

Follow the recommended dosage carefully.

Warning(s): Do not administer within 72 hours of slaughter for food.

Keep out of reach of children.

Presentation: 0.46 oz (13 g) packet (NDC 0061-5158-01).

Compendium Code No.: 10471202 Rev. 10/97

LEVASOLE® SOLUBLE PIG WORMER

Schering-Plough **Parasiticide-Oral**

(levamisole hydrochloride) Anthelmintic

NADA No.: 112-049

Active Ingredient(s): Each bottle contains 18.15 g of levamisole hydrochloride activity which will treat the following: 200-25 lb. pigs, or 100-50 lb. pigs, or 50-100 lb. pigs, or 25-200 lb. pigs.

Indications: LEVASOLE® (levamisole hydrochloride) is a broad-spectrum anthelmintic, and is effective against the following nematode infections in swine:

Large Roundworms: *Ascaris suum.*

Nodular Worms: *Oesophagostomum* spp.

Lungworms: *Metastrongylus* spp.

Intestinal Threadworms: *Strongyloides ransomi.*

Dosage and Administration: For use in drinking water.

Directions for Preparing Soluble Pig Wormer Solution: When ready to deworm pigs, add water to the powder in the bottle up to the 500 mL mark. Agitate to mix thoroughly before using. If any solution is left over, it may be stored for up to 3 months in the tightly capped bottle; shake well before using.

Directions for Use: Withholding water from pigs prior to treatment is not necessary for optimum anthelmintic efficacy and is not recommended during hot weather. Add 10 mL (2 teaspoonfuls) of the solution from the bottle to 1 gallon of water; mix thoroughly. Allow one gallon of medicated water for each 100 pounds of body weight of pigs to be treated. No other source of water should be offered. As soon as pigs have consumed all of the medicated water resume the use of regular water.

Note: Careful estimates of pig weights are essential for the proper performance of this product. Pigs maintained under conditions of constant worm exposure may require retreatment within 4-5 weeks after the first treatment due to reinfection.

Caution(s): Consult a veterinarian before administering levamisole to sick swine.

Consult your veterinarian for assistance in the diagnosis, treatment and control of parasitism.

Salivation or muzzle foam may be observed. The reaction is occasionally seen and will disappear in a short time after the medication.

If pigs are infected with mature lungworms, coughing and vomiting may be observed soon after medicated water is consumed. The reaction is due to the expulsion of worms from the lungs and will be over in several hours. Follow the recommended dosage carefully to ensure the removal of worms and avoid an overdose of levamisole.

Warning(s): Do not administer within 72 hours of slaughter for food.

Keep out of reach of children.

Presentation: 0.712 oz (20.17 g) bottle (NDC 0061-5023-01).

Compendium Code No.: 10471211 Rev. 9/01

LEVO-POWDER ℞

Vetus **Thyroid Therapy**

Active Ingredient(s): Each pound (453.6 g) contains: Levothyroxine Sodium, USP - 0.22% (1.0 g).

One level teaspoon contains approximately 12 mg of Levothyroxine; one level measure (1 tablespoon) contains approximately 36 mg of Levothyroxine.

Indications: For use in equine as a supplemental source of the thyroid hormone - T4 (Levothyroxine).

Dosage and Administration: The usual starting dose for an adult horse is 35 - 100 mg (1 - 3 measures or 1 - 3 tablespoons) daily. Each individual animal should be evaluated weekly until the proper maintenance dose is established.

Precaution(s): Store in a cool, dry place.

Caution(s): Federal law restricts this drug to use by or on the order of a licensed veterinarian.

Extreme caution should be used when giving to horses with heart disease, hypertension, or other conditions that would be adversely affected by an increased metabolism. The use of LEVO-POWDER in pregnant mares has not been evaluated.

Warning(s): Not for use in horses intended for food.

For equine use only.

For veterinary use only.

Keep out of the reach of children.

Presentation: 1 lb (16 oz) (453.6 g) and 10 lbs (4.536 kg).

Compendium Code No.: 14440550

LEVOTABS ℞

Vetus **Thyroid Therapy**

Active Ingredient(s): Each LEVOTAB provides synthetic crystalline levothyroxine sodium (L-thyroxine). LEVOTABS Tablets are available in the following strengths: 0.1 mg, 0.2 mg, 0.3 mg, 0.4 mg, 0.5 mg, 0.6 mg, 0.7 mg, and 0.8 mg.

Indications: Provides thyroid replacement therapy in all conditions of inadequate production of thyroid hormones in the dog.

Pharmacology: Levothyroxine sodium acts, as does endogenous thyroxine, to stimulate metabolism, growth, development and differentiation of tissue. It increases the rate of energy exchange and increases the maturation rate of the epiphyses. Levothyroxine sodium is absorbed rapidly from the gastrointestinal tract after oral administration. Following absorption, the compound becomes bound to the serum alpha globulin fraction. For purposes of comparison, 0.1 mg of levothyroxine sodium elicits a clinical response approximately equal to that produced by one grain (65 mg) of desiccated thyroid.

Dosage and Administration: The initial recommended daily dose is 0.1 mg per 10 lbs. (4.5 kg)

L

of body weight. The dose may then be adjusted according to the patient's response by monitoring T4 blood levels at time intervals of four (4) weeks.

Thyroxine tablets may be administered orally or placed in the food.

Contraindication(s): Levothyroxine sodium therapy is contraindicated in thyrotoxicosis, acute myocardial infraction and uncorrected adrenal insufficiency. Its use in pregnant bitches has not been evaluated.

Precaution(s): Do not store above 104°F (40°C). Protect from light.

Caution(s): Federal law restricts this drug to use by or on the order of a licensed veterinarian.

The effects of levothyroxine sodium therapy are slow in being manifested. An overdose of any thyroid drug may produce the signs and symptoms of thyrotoxicosis including, but not limited to, polydipsia, polyuria, polyphagia, reduced heat tolerance and hyperactivity or personality change. Administer with caution to animals with clinically significant heart disease, hypertension or other complications for which sharply increased metabolic rate might prove hazardous.

Side Effects: There are not any particular adverse reactions connected with L-thyroxine therapy at the recommended dose levels. Overdose will result in the signs of thyrotoxicosis listed above under Cautions.

Discussion: Hypothyroidism is the generalized metabolic disease resulting from deficiency of the thyroid hormones levothyroxine (T4) and liothyronine (T3). LEVOTABS will provide levothyroxine (T4) as a substrate for the physiologic deiodination to liothyronine (T3). Administration of levothyroxine sodium alone will result in complete physiologic thyroid replacement.

Canine hypothyroidism is primary, due to atrophy of the thyroid gland. In the majority of cases the atrophy is associated with lymphocytic thyroiditis and in the remainder it is non-inflammatory and of yet unknown etiology. Less than 10 percent of cases of hypothyroidism are secondary due to deficiency of the thyroid stimulating hormone (TSH). TSH deficiency may occur as a component of congenital hypopituitarism or as an acquired disorder in adult dogs, in which case it is invariably due to the growth of a pituitary tumor.

Hypothyroidism usually occurs in middle-aged and older dogs, although the condition will sometimes be seen in younger dogs of the larger breeds. Neutered animals of either sex are also frequently affected, regardless of age. The following are clinical signs of hypothyroidism in dogs: Lethargy, lack of endurance, increased sleeping; Reduced interest, alertness and excitability; Slow heart rate, weak apex beat and pulse, low voltage on ECG; Preference for warmth, low body temperature, cool skin; Increased body weight; Stiff and slow movements, dragging of the front feet; Head tilt, disturbed balance, unilateral facial paralysis; Atrophy of epidermis, thickening of dermis, surface and follicular hyperkeratosis, pigmentation; Puffy face, blepharoptosis, tragic expression, dry, coarse, sparse coat, slow regrowth after clipping; Retarded turnover of hair (carpet coat of boxers); Shortening or absence of estrus, lack of libido; Dry feces, occasional diarrhea; Hypercholesterolemia; Normochromic, normocytic anemia and Elevated serum creatinine phosphokinase.

Presentation: Available in bottles of 180 and 1,000 tablets.

Compendium Code No.: 14440561

LEVOXINE™ POWDER ℞

First Priority — **Thyroid Therapy**

Active Ingredient(s): Each pound (453.6 g) contains:

Levothyroxine Sodium USP .... 0.22% (1.0 g)

One level teaspoonful contains 12 mg of T_4; one level tablespoonful contains 36 mg of T_4.

Indications: For use in horses and ponies for correction of conditions associated with low circulating thyroid hormone (hypothyroidism).

Dosage and Administration: Dosage: Doses should be individualized and animals should be monitored daily for clinical signs of hyperthyroidism or hypersensitivity. Suggested initial doses are 1-10 mg levothyroxine sodium (T_4)/100 lb body weight (2-20 mg/100 kg) once per day or in divided doses. Response to the administration of LEVOXINE™ Powder should be evaluated clinically every week until an adequate maintenance dose is established. In most horses, this is usually in the range of 35 to 100 mg total daily dose of T_4 (1-3 level tablespoonfuls LEVOXINE™ Powder).

Administration: LEVOXINE™ Powder may be top dressed or mixed with the daily ration.

Precaution(s): Storage: Store at controlled room temperature between 15°-30°C (59°-86°F). Keep container tightly closed when not in use.

Caution(s): Federal law restricts this drug to use by or on the order of a licensed veterinarian.

Administer with caution to animals with clinically significant heart disease, hypertension or other complications for which a sharply increased metabolic rate might prove hazardous. Use in pregnant mares has not been evaluated.

Use only as directed.

For animal use only.

Warning(s): Keep out of reach of children.

Presentation: 1 lb (453.6 g) (NDC# 58829-278-16) and 10 lb (4.5 kg) (NDC# 58829-278-07).

Compendium Code No.: 11390453 Rev. 03-02 / Iss. 12-98

LIB

Neogen — **Iron-Oral**

Liver-Iron-B_{12}

Active Ingredient(s): Each Ounce Contains:

Ferrous Sulfate (Iron) .... 1500 mg

Dessicated liver, vitamin B_{12}, copper gluconate, cobalt sulfate, flavor, dextrose, sodium saccharin.

Indications: For use in animals as a hematinic to aid in the prevention and treatment of nutritional anemia or for convalescence.

Action: LIB provides therapeutic quantities of iron in combination with liver and the important factors of the vitamin B complex.

Dosage and Administration:

Horses: ½ to 1 ounce 1 or 2 times daily.

Cattle: ½ to 1 ounce 2 or 3 times daily.

Dogs: ½ teaspoon 1 or 2 times daily.

Swine: ½ ounce 2 times daily.

Precaution(s): Store in a dry place. Keep lid tightly closed.

Caution(s): For veterinary use only.

Warning(s): Keep out of reach of children.

Presentation: 4 lbs (1.814 kg) (NDC: 59051-9165-6) and 20 lbs (9.072 kg) (NDC: 59051-9166-0).

Compendium Code No.: 14910332 L423-0501 / L436-0501

LICKABLES™ CHARGE UP!™

A.A.H. — **Small Animal Dietary Supplement**

Senior Pet Health Formula-Nutritional Gel

Guaranteed Analysis: per teaspoon (6 grams):

Crude Protein (Min)	1.6%
Crude Fat (Min)	32.5%
Crude Fiber (Max)	3.2%
Moisture (Max)	13.5%
Calcium (Min)	(0.0026%) 0.16 mg
Calcium (Max)	(0.0033%) 0.20 mg
Phosphorus (Min)	(0.0006%) 0.03 mg
Potassium (Min)	(0.0027%) 0.16 mg
Magnesium (Min)	(0.0067%) 0.42 mg
Iron (Min)	(0.0088%) 0.53 mg
Manganese (Min)	(0.0176%) 1 mg
Iodine (Min)	(0.0088%) 0.53 mg
Vitamin A (Min)	1042 IU
Vitamin D (Min)	60 IU
Vitamin E (Min)	6 IU
Thiamine (Vit. B1) (Min)	1.8 mg
Riboflavin (Vit. B2) (Min)	0.2 mg
d-Pantothenic Acid (Min)	1 mg
Niacin (Min)	2 mg
Pyridoxine (Vit. B6) (Min)	0.8 mg
Folic Acid (Min)	0.2 mg
Vitamin B12 (Min)	2 mcg
Omega 3* (Min)	1041 mg
Omega 6* (Min)	135 mg
L-Carnitine (Min)	15000 ppm

*Not recognized as an essential nutrient by the AAFCO Dog or Cat Food Nutrient Profiles.

Ingredients: Malt Syrup, Corn Syrup, Soybean Oil, Methylcellulose, Cane Molasses, Water, L-Carnitine, Cod Liver Oil, Soy Protein Concentrate, dl-Alpha Tocopherol Acetate, Sorbic Acid (a preservative), Potassium Sorbate (a preservative), Manganese Sulfate, Iron Proteinate, Thiamine Hydrochloride, Niacinamide, Calcium Pantothenate, Magnesium Sulfate, Pyridoxine Hydrochloride, Vitamin A Supplement, Vitamin D3 Supplement, Potassium Iodide, Riboflavin-5'-Phosphate, Folic Acid, Vitamin A Palmitate and Vitamin B12 Supplement.

Indications: CHARGE UP!™ is formulated with Omega-6 and Omega-3 fatty acids, Soy Protein Concentrate and L-Carnitine. It is formulated in a concentrated form to provide supplemental caloric and nutritional intake for senior dogs and cats.

Directions: A few tasty licks provides additional calories and nutrition.

Feed a 2½" ribbon (1 teaspoon) per 10 pounds of body weight 3 times a day. Calorie content: 4420 kcal/kg (26.5 kcal/6 g).

CHARGE UP!™ tastes like a treat and is accepted by picky seniors. Feed CHARGE UP!™ right from your finger or mix with food from a dish.

Precaution(s): Store in a cool place.

Caution(s): For supplemental feeding only For animal use only.

Warning(s): Keep out of reach of children and pets.

Presentation: 5 oz (141.7 g) tube.

Compendium Code No.: 11180100

LICKABLES™ HAIRBALL RELIEF

A.A.H. — **Laxative**

Nutritional Gel

Guaranteed Analysis: per teaspoon (6 grams):

Crude Protein (Min)	0.5%
Crude Fat (Min)	18.5%
Crude Fiber (Max)	1.2%
Moisture (Max)	9.6%

Ingredients: Corn Syrup, Malt Syrup, Petrolatum, Cane Molasses, Soybean Oil, Mineral Oil, Water, Soy Protein Concentrate, Chamomile, Maple Flavor, Potassium Sorbate (a preservative), Sorbic Acid (a preservative), Vanilla Flavor.

Indications: Hairball Relief for cats and kittens eliminates swallowed hair and hairballs.

Directions: A few tasty licks from your finger or from a dish, will start your cat on a life free from hairballs.

Dosage: For cats - Start with a 1¼ to 2½ half inch ribbon (1 half or 1 full teaspoon) for the first 2-3 days. Lower dose to a ¾ inch ribbon (one third teaspoon) 2-3 times per week. For kittens over 4 weeks, use half doses.

Precaution(s): Store in a cool place.

Caution(s): For supplemental feeding only. For animal use only.

Warning(s): Keep out of reach of children and pets.

Presentation: 3 oz (85.0 g) tube.

Compendium Code No.: 11180070

LICKABLES™ HAIRBALL RELIEF CAVIAR FLAVORED

A.A.H. — **Laxative**

Nutritional Gel

Guaranteed Analysis: per teaspoon (6 grams):

Crude Protein (Min)	0.5%
Crude Fat (Min)	18.5%
Crude Fiber (Max)	1.2%
Moisture (Max)	9.6%

Ingredients: Corn Syrup, Malt Syrup, Petrolatum, Cane Molasses, Soybean Oil, Tuna Oil, Mineral Oil, Water, Caviar, Soy Protein Concentrate, Potassium Sorbate (a preservative), Sorbic Acid (a preservative), Chamomile.

Indications: Eliminates swallowed hair and hairballs. Caviar flavored for cats and kittens.

Directions: For the most discriminating felines. A few tasty licks from your finger (or from a silver or crystal dish), will start your cat on a life free from nasty hairballs.

Dosage: For cats - Start with a 1¼ to 2½ half inch ribbon (1 half or 1 full teaspoon) for the first 2-3 days.

Lower dose to a ¾ inch ribbon (one third teaspoon) 2-3 times per week.

For kittens over 4 weeks, use half doses.

Precaution(s): Store in a cool place.

Caution(s): For supplemental feeding only. For animal use only.

Warning(s): Keep out of reach of children and pets.

Presentation: 3 oz (85.0 g) tube.

Compendium Code No.: 11180080

LICKABLES™ HEARTY CAT™

A.A.H. **Small Animal Dietary Supplement**

Nutritional Gel

Guaranteed Analysis: per teaspoon (6 grams):

Crude Protein (Min)	1.2%
Crude Fat (Min)	17.4%
Crude Fiber (Max)	8.7%
Moisture (Max)	14.5%
Calcium (Min)	(0.9%) 55 mg
Calcium (Max)	(1.1%) 67 mg
Phosphorus (Min)	(0.7%) 42 mg
Potassium (Min)	(0.0015%) 0.09 mg
Salt (Min)	(0.045%) 2.7 mg
Salt (Max)	(0.055%) 3.3 mg
Magnesium (Min)	(0.0736%) 4.42 mg
Iron (Min)	(0.0125%) 0.75 mg
Copper (Min)	(0.0018%) 0.11 mg
Manganese (Min)	(0.0040%) 24 mg
Zinc (Min)	(0.0057%) 0.34 mg
Iodine (Min)	(0.0047%) 0.28 mg
Vitamin A (Min)	1480 IU
Vitamin D (Min)	148 IU
Vitamin E (Min)	6 IU
Menadione (Min)	0.77 mg
Thiamine (Vit. B1) (Min)	1.4 mg
Riboflavin (Vit. B2) (Min)	1.5 mg
d-Pantothenic Acid (Min)	2 mg
Niacin (Min)	7.4 mg
Pyridoxine (Vit. B6) (Min)	1.2 mg
Folic Acid (Min)	0.044 mg
Vitamin B12 (Min)	6 mcg
Choline (Min)	35 mg
Taurine (Min)	100 mg
Cobalt* (Min)	(0.0013%) 0.08 mg

*Not recognized as an essential nutrient by the AAFCO Cat Food Nutrient Profiles.

Ingredients: Corn Syrup, Malt Syrup, Soybean Oil, Calcium Phosphate, Cod Liver Oil, Cane Molasses, Methylcellulose, Poultry By-products, Fish By-products, Taurine, Water, Choline Bitartrate, Magnesium Sulfate, Niacinamide, dl-Alpha Tocopherol Acetate, Sorbic Acid (a preservative), Potassium Sorbate (a preservative), Iron Proteinate, Calcium Pantothenate, Riboflavin-5'-Phosphate, Salt, Thiamine Hydrochloride, Pyridoxine Hydrochloride, Vitamin A Supplement, Vitamin D3 Supplement, Zinc Sulfate, Menadione Sodium Bisulfite Complex, Manganese Sulfate, Potassium Iodide (source of Iodine and Potassium), Cobalt Sulfate, Copper Sulfate, Folic Acid, Tuna Oil, and Vitamin B12 Supplement.

Indications: Multi-vitamin with taurine. Antioxidant vitamins. Tuna flavor for cats and kittens.

Directions: Squeeze a ribbon of HEARTY CAT™ on your finger (or feed from a dish). Cats accept HEARTY CAT™ immediately, licking up their tasty daily dose without urging.

Adult Cats: A 2½ inch ribbon = one level teaspoon - approx. 6 grams.

Kittens: A 1¼ inch ribbon = one half level teaspoon - approx. 3 grams.

Precaution(s): Store in a cool place.

Caution(s): For supplemental feeding only.

For animal use only.

Warning(s): Keep out of reach of children and pets.

Presentation: 3 oz (85.0 g) tube.

Compendium Code No.: 11180090

LICKABLES ™ HEARTY DOG™

A.A.H. **Small Animal Dietary Supplement**

Nutritional Gel

Guaranteed Analysis: per teaspoon (6 grams):

Crude Protein (Min)	0.9%
Crude Fat (Min)	16.2%
Crude Fiber (Max)	1.5%
Moisture (Max)	13.5%
Calcium (Min)	(0.020%) 1.2 mg
Calcium (Max)	(0.026%) 1.6 mg
Phosphorus (Min)	(0.006%) 0.34 mg
Potassium (Min)	(0.004%) 0.23 mg
Magnesium (Min)	(0.004%) 0.25 mg
Iron (Min)	(0.009%) 0.53 mg
Manganese (Min)	(0.023%) 1.4 mg
Iodine (Min)	(0.012%) 0.72 mg
Vitamin A (Min)	21500 IU
Vitamin D (Min)	1051 IU
Vitamin E (Min)	72 IU
Thiamine (Vit. B1) (Min)	20 mg
Riboflavin (Vit. B2) (Min)	3.5 mg
d-Pantothenic Acid (Min)	7.4 mg
Niacin (Min)	22 mg
Pyridoxine (Vit. B6) (Min)	16 mg
Folic Acid (Min)	0.54 mg
Vitamin B12 (Min)	9 mcg

Ingredients: Corn Syrup, Malt Syrup, Soybean Oil, Cod Liver Oil, Cane Molasses, Water, Methylcellulose, dl-Alpha Tocopherol Acetate (Vit. E), Beef Flavor, Niacinamide, Thiamine, Pyridoxine Hydrochloride, Calcium Pantothenate (source of d-Pantothenic Acid), Vitamin A Supplement, Vitamin D3 Supplement, Vitamin A Palmitate, Potassium Sorbate (a preservative), Sorbic Acid (a preservative), Riboflavin-5'-Phosphate, Manganese Sulfate, Iron Proteinate, Magnesium Sulfate, Potassium Iodide (source of Iodine and Potassium), Folic Acid, and Vitamin B12 Supplement.

Indications: Heavily fortified with antioxidant vitamins. A few tasty licks supplies vitamins and minerals essential for good nutrition. For dogs and puppies. The gourmet taste of sirloin tips.

Directions: Squeeze a ¾ inch ribbon of HEARTY DOG™ onto your finger (or feed from a dish). Dogs, even those picky eaters, accept the gourmet flavor of HEARTY DOG™, licking up their tasty portion without urging.

Feed a ¾ inch ribbon per 10 lbs of body weight daily = a ¼ teaspoon = approximately 1.5 grams.

Precaution(s): Store in a cool place.

Caution(s): For supplemental feeding only.

For animal use only.

Warning(s): Keep out of reach of children and pets.

Presentation: 5 oz (141.7 g) tube.

Compendium Code No.: 11180110

LICKABLES™ SUPER CHARGER™

A.A.H. **Small Animal Dietary Supplement**

Nutritional Gel

Guaranteed Analysis: per teaspoon (6 grams):

Crude Protein (Min)	0.7%
Crude Fat (Min)	26.5%
Crude Fiber (Max)	3.0%
Moisture (Max)	13.5%
Calcium (Min)	(0.0026%) 0.16 mg
Calcium (Max)	(0.0033%) 0.20 mg
Phosphorus (Min)	(0.0006%) 0.03 mg
Potassium (Min)	(0.0027%) 0.16 mg
Magnesium (Min)	(0.0067%) 0.42 mg
Iron (Min)	(0.0088%) 0.53 mg
Manganese (Min)	(0.0176%) 1 mg
Iodine (Min)	(0.0088%) 0.53 mg
Vitamin A (Min)	1042 IU
Vitamin D (Min)	60 IU
Vitamin E (Min)	6 IU
Thiamine (Vit. B1) (Min)	1.8 mg
Riboflavin (Vit. B2) (Min)	0.2 mg
d-Pantothenic Acid (Min)	1 mg
Niacin (Min)	2 mg
Pyridoxine (Vit. B6) (Min)	0.8 mg
Folic Acid (Min)	0.2 mg
Vitamin B12 (Min)	2 mcg
Omega 3* (Min)	1041 mg
Omega 6* (Min)	135 mg

*Not recognized as an essential nutrient by the AAFCO Dog or Cat Food Nutrient Profiles.

Ingredients: Malt Syrup, Corn Syrup, Soybean Oil, Methylcellulose, Cane Molasses, Cod Liver Oil, Water, dl-Alpha Tocopherol Acetate, Sorbic Acid (a preservative), Potassium Sorbate (a preservative), Manganese Sulfate, Iron Proteinate, Thiamine Hydrochloride, Niacinamide, Calcium Pantothenate, Magnesium Sulfate, Pyridoxine Hydrochloride, Vitamin A Supplement, Vitamin D3 Supplement, Potassium Iodide, Riboflavin-5'-Phosphate, Folic Acid, Vitamin A Palmitate and Vitamin B12 Supplement.

Indications: For dogs and cats who won't eat. A few tasty licks supplies calories, protein, Omega 3 and 6 fatty acids, antioxidant vitamins and minerals.

SUPER CHARGER™ is formulated with Omega-6 and Omega-3 fatty acids, in a low volume form.

Directions: A few tasty licks provide supplemental caloric and nutritional intake. When the animal's caloric or nutritional intake is to be supplemented, give a 3¾ inch ribbon = 1½ teaspoons per 10 pounds of body weight daily. When animal is not consuming full feed ration, give a 7½ inch ribbon = 3 teaspoons (1 tablespoon) per 10 pounds of body weight daily. Calorie content; 4420 kcal/kg (26.5 kcal/6 g).

SUPER CHARGER™ tastes like a treat. A great way to bond with your pet is to feed SUPER CHARGER™ right from your finger. SUPER CHARGER™ may also be fed from a dish or mixed with food.

Precaution(s): Store in a cool place.

Caution(s): For supplemental feeding only.

For animal use only.

Warning(s): Keep out of reach of children and pets.

Presentation: 5 oz (141.7 g) tube.

Compendium Code No.: 11180120

LIDOCAINE 2% INJECTABLE ℞

Bimeda **Local Anesthetic**

20 mg/mL-Local Anesthetic

Active Ingredient(s): Composition: Each mL of sterile aqueous solution contains:

Lidocaine Hydrochloride	2.0%
Propylene Glycol	5.2%
Sodium Chloride	0.5%
Sodium Lactate	0.5%

With Methylparaben 0.15%, Sodium Metabisulfite 0.10%, Propylparaben 0.03% and Disodium Edetate 0.001% as preservatives.

Indications: LIDOCAINE is a potent local anesthetic for producing epidural, nerve conduction and infiltration anesthesia.

Dosage and Administration:

Epidural:

Cattle and Horses: 5 to 15 mL.

Dogs and Cats: 1 mL per 10 lbs of body weight.

Nerve block:

Cattle and Horses: 5 to 20 mL.

Infiltration: Dilute to 0.5% concentration (1 mL of 2% solution diluted with 3 mL of sterile water = 4 mL of a 0.5% solution).

Contraindication(s): LIDOCAINE is contraindicated in animals with a known hypersensitivity to the drug.

L

Precaution(s): Store at controlled room temperature between 15°C-30°C (59°F-86°F).
Caution(s): Federal law restricts this drug to use by or on the order of a licensed veterinarian.
LIDOCAINE is usually well tolerated. Nevertheless, as with all local anesthetics, untoward effects may occur due to hypersensitivity, faulty technique, overdosage and inadvertent intravascular or subarachnoid injection. In case of respiratory arrest, immediate resuscitation with oxygen is indicated.
For animal use only.
Warning(s): Keep out of reach of children.
Presentation: 100 mL (NDC # 61133-1298-8) and 250 mL (NDC # 61133-1298-7).
Manufactured by: Bimeda-MTC Animal Health, Inc., Cambridge, ON Canada N3C 2W4.
Compendium Code No.: 13990241

Iss. 1.01

LIDOCAINE 2% INJECTABLE ℞

Butler **Local Anesthetic**

Active Ingredient(s): Composition: Each mL of sterile aqueous solution contains:

Lidocaine Hydrochloride	2.0%
Propylene Glycol	5.2%
Sodium Chloride	0.5%
Sodium Lactate	0.5%

with Methylparaben 0.15%, Sodium Metabisulfite 0.10%, Propylparaben 0.03% and Disodium Edetate 0.001% as preservatives.
Indications: Lidocaine is a potent local anesthetic for producing epidural, nerve conduction and infiltration anesthesia.
Dosage and Administration:
Epidural:
Cattle and Horses—5 to 15 mL.
Dogs and Cats—1 mL per 10 pounds of body weight.
Nerve Block:
Cattle and Horses—5 to 20 mL.
Infiltration: Dilute to 0.5% concentration (1 mL of 2% solution diluted with 3 mL of sterile water = 4 mL of a 0.5% solution).
Contraindication(s): Lidocaine is contraindicated in animals with a known hypersensitivity to the drug.
Precaution(s): Store at controlled room temperature between 15° and 30°C (59°-86°F).
Caution(s): Federal law restricts this drug to use by or on the order of a licensed veterinarian.
Lidocaine is usually well tolerated. Nevertheless, as with all local anesthetics, untoward effects may occur due to hypersensitivity, faulty technique, overdosage and inadvertent intravascular or subarachnoid injection. In case of respiratory arrest, immediate resuscitation with oxygen is indicated.
Warning(s): For animal use only.
Keep out of reach of children.
Presentation: 100 mL (NDC 11695-3514-1) and 250 mL (NDC 11695-4135-5) vials.
Compendium Code No.: 10821070

L

LIDOCAINE HCl 2% ℞

RXV **Local Anesthetic**

Active Ingredient(s): Each mL contains:

Lidocaine HCl monohydrate	20 mg
Sodium chloride	2.2 mg
Methylparaben (as preservative)	1.0 mg
Potassium phosphate monobasic	2.0 mg
Potassium phosphate dibasic	2.4 mg
Water for injection	q.s.

pH adjusted with hydrochloric acid or sodium hydroxide.
Indications: For local anesthesia of cattle, dogs, and horses.
Dosage and Administration:
Epidural:
Cattle and Horses: 5 to 15 mL.
Dogs: 1 mL per 10 lbs. of body weight.
Nerve Block:
Cattle and Horses: 5 to 20 mL.
Infiltration: Dilute to 0.5% concentration (1 mL of 2% solution diluted with 3 mL of sterile water = 4 mL of a 0.5% solution).
Precaution(s): Store at a controlled room temperature between 59°-86°F (15°-30°C).
Caution(s): Federal law restricts this drug to use by or on the order of a licensed veterinarian.
For animal use only.
Keep out of the reach of children.
Presentation: 100 mL sterile multiple dose vials.
Compendium Code No.: 10910090

LIDOCAINE HCl INJECTABLE 2% ℞

Aspen **Local Anesthetic**

Active Ingredient(s): Each mL of sterile aqueous solution contains:

Lidocaine Hydrochloride	2.0%
Sodium Chloride	0.2%
Potassium Phosphate Monobasic	0.2%
Potassium Phosphate Dibasic	0.2%
Methylparaben (preservative)	0.1%
Water For Injection	q.s

Indications: Lidocaine is a potent local anesthetic for producing epidural and nerve conduction anesthesia.
Dosage and Administration:
Epidural:
Cattle and Horses - 5 to 15 mL.
Dogs and Cats - 1 mL per 10 pounds of body weight.
Nerve Block:
Cattle and Horses - 5 to 20 mL.
Contraindication(s): Lidocaine is contraindicated in animals with a known hypersensitivity to the drug.
Precaution(s): Store between 15°C and 30°C (59°F-86°F).
Caution(s): Federal law restricts this drug to use by or on the order of a licensed veterinarian.
Lidocaine is usually well tolerated. Nevertheless, as with all local anesthetics, untoward effects may occur due to hypersensitivity, faulty technique, overdosage and inadvertent intravascular or subarachnoid injection. In case of respiratory arrest, immediate resuscitation with oxygen is indicated.
Warning(s): For animal use only.
Keep out of reach of children.
Presentation: 100 mL.
Compendium Code No.: 14750540

LIDOCAINE HYDROCHLORIDE 2% ℞

Vet Tek **Local Anesthetic**

Sterile Solution
Active Ingredient(s): Composition: Each mL of sterile aqueous solution contains:

Lidocaine Hydrochloride	2.0%
Sodium Chloride	0.7%
Potassium Phosphate Monobasic	0.2%
Potassium Phosphate Dibasic	0.2%
Methylparaben (preservative)	0.1%
Water For Injection	q.s.

Indications: Lidocaine is a potent local anesthetic for producing epidural and nerve conduction anesthesia.
Dosage and Administration:
Epidural:
Cattle and Horses - 5 to 15 mL.
Dogs and Cats - 1 mL per 10 pounds of body weight.
Nerve Block:
Cattle and Horses - 5 to 20 mL.
Contraindication(s): Lidocaine is contraindicated in animals with a known hypersensitivity to the drug.
Precaution(s): Store between 15°C and 30°C (59°F-86°F).
Caution(s): Federal law restricts this drug to use by or on the order of a licensed veterinarian.
Lidocaine is usually well tolerated. Nevertheless, as with all local anesthetics, untoward effects may occur due to hypersensitivity, faulty technique, overdosage and inadvertent intravascular or subarachnoid injection. In case of respiratory arrest, immediate resuscitation with oxygen is indicated.
For animal use only.
Warning(s): Keep out of reach of children.
Presentation: 100 mL vials (NDC 60270-025-10).
Manufactured by: Phoenix Scientific, Inc., St. Joseph, MO 64506.
Compendium Code No.: 14200121

Iss. 7-95

LIDOCAINE HYDROCHLORIDE INJECTABLE-2% ℞

Phoenix Pharmaceutical **Local Anesthetic**

Active Ingredient(s): Composition: Each mL of sterile aqueous solution contains:

Lidocaine Hydrochloride	2.0%
Sodium Chloride	0.2%
Potassium Phosphate Monobasic	0.2%
Potassium Phosphate Dibasic	0.2%
Methylparaben	0.1%
Water for Injection	q.s.

Indications: Lidocaine is a potent local anesthetic for producing epidural and nerve conduction anesthesia.
Dosage and Administration:
Epidural:
Cattle and Horses: 5 to 15 mL.
Dogs and Cats: 1 mL per 10 pounds of body weight.
Nerve Block:
Cattle and Horses: 5 to 20 mL.
Contraindication(s): Lidocaine is contraindicated in animals with a known hypersensitivity to the drug.
Precaution(s): Store between 15°C and 30°C (59°F and 86°F).
Caution(s): Federal law restricts this drug to use by or on the order of a licensed veterinarian.
Lidocaine is usually well tolerated. Nevertheless, as with all local anesthetics, untoward effects may occur due to hypersensitivity, faulty technique, overdosage and inadvertent intravascular or subarachnoid injection. In case of respiratory arrest, immediate resuscitation with oxygen is indicated.
For animal use only.
Warning(s): Keep out of reach of children.
Presentation: 100 mL (NDC 57319-093-05) and 250 mL (NDC 57319-093-06) vials.
Manufactured by: Phoenix Scientific, Inc., St. Joseph, MO 64503.
Compendium Code No.: 12560532

Rev. 8-01 / Iss. 1-02

LIDOCAINE HYDROCHLORIDE INJECTION 2% ℞

AgriLabs **Local Anesthetic**

Active Ingredient(s): Each mL contains:

Lidocaine HCl	20 mg
Sodium bisulfite	0.5 mg
Methylparaben	1.0 mg
Potassium phosphate monobasic	2.0 mg
Potassium phosphate dibasic	2.4 mg
Sodium chloride	2.2 mg
Water for injection	q.s.

Indications: For all minor nerve blocking procedures in horses.
Dosage and Administration: Inject 3 to 5 mL over several areas. When larger volumes are required, only solutions with epinephrine should be used.
Caution(s): Federal law restricts this drug to use by or on the order of a licensed veterinarian.
For veterinary use only.
Presentation: 100 mL sterile multiple dose vials.
Compendium Code No.: 10581650

Iss. 8-89

LIDOCAINE INJECTABLE 2% ℞

Vedco **Local Anesthetic**

NADA No.: 045-578

Active Ingredient(s): Each mL contains:

Lidocaine hydrochloride	2.0%
Propylene glycol	5.2%
Sodium chloride	0.5%
Sodium lactate	0.5%
Preservatives:	
Methylparaben	0.15%
Sodium metabisulfite	0.10%
Propylparaben	0.03%
Disodium edetate	0.001%

Indications: LIDOCAINE is a potent local anesthetic for producing epidural, nerve conduction and infiltration anesthesia.

Dosage and Administration:

Epidural:

Cattle and Horses: 5 to 15 mL.

Dogs and Cats: 1 mL per 10 pounds of body weight.

Nerve block:

Cattle and Horses: 5 to 20 mL.

Infiltration: Dilute to 0.5% concentration (1 mL of 2% solution diluted with 3 mL of sterile water = 4 mL of a 0.5% solution).

Contraindication(s): LIDOCAINE is contraindicated in animals with a known hypersensitivity to the drug.

Precaution(s): Store at a controlled room temperature between 59-86°F (15-30°C).

Caution(s): Federal law restricts this drug to use by or on the order of a licensed veterinarian.

Keep out of the reach of children.

Lidocaine is usually well tolerated. Nevertheless, as with all local anesthetics, untoward effects may occur due to hypersensitivity, faulty technique, overdosage and inadvertent intravascular or subarachnoid injection. In case of respiratory arrest, immediate resuscitation with oxygen is indicated.

Presentation: 100 mL and 250 mL containers.

Compendium Code No.: 10941200

LIDOJECT ℞

Vetus **Local Anesthetic**

Composition: Each mL of sterile aqueous solution contains:

Lidocaine Hydrochloride	2.0%
Sodium Chloride	0.2%
Potassium Phosphate Monobasic	0.2%
Potassium Phosphate Dibasic	0.2%
Methylparben (preservative)	0.1%
Water For Injection	q.s.

Indications: Lidocaine is a potent local anesthetic for producing epidural and nerve conduction anesthesia in horses, cattle, dogs, and cats.

Dosage and Administration:

Epidural:

Cattle and Horses - 5 to 15 mL.

Dogs and Cats - 1 mL per 10 pounds of body weight.

Nerve Block:

Cattle and Horses - 5 to 20 mL.

Contraindication(s): Lidocaine is contraindicated in animals with a known hypersensitivity to the drug.

Precaution(s): Store between 15°C and 30°C (59°F-86°F).

Caution(s): Federal law restricts this drug to use by or on the order of a licensed veterinarian.

For animal use only.

Keep out of the reach of children.

Lidocaine is usually well tolerated. Nevertheless, as with all local anesthetics, untoward effects may occur due to hypersensitivity, faulty technique, overdosage and inadvertent intravascular or subarachnoid injection. In case of respiratory arrest, immediate resuscitation with oxygen is indicated.

Presentation: Available in 100 mL vials.

Compendium Code No.: 14440570

LIFEGARD® 256 PLUS

Rochester Midland **Disinfectant**

One-Step Germicidal Detergent and Deodorant

EPA Reg. No.: 47371-129-527

Active Ingredient(s):

Didecyl dimethyl ammonium chloride	9.22%
n-Alkyl (C_{14} 50%, C_{12} 40%, C_{18} 10%) dimethyl benzyl ammonium chloride	6.14%
Inert Ingredients	84.64%

Indications: A multi-purpose, neutral pH, germicidal detergent and deodorant effective in hard water up to 400 ppm (calculated as $CaCO_3$) in the presence of a moderate amount of soil (5% organic serum) according to the AOAC Use-dilution test. Disinfects, cleans and deodorizes in one labor saving step. Effective against the following pathogens: *Pseudomonas aeruginosa*[1], *Staphylococcus aureus*[1], *Salmonella chloeraesuis, Acinetobacter calcoaceticus, Bordetella bronchiseptica, Chlamydia psittaci, Enterobacter aerogenes, Enterobacter cloacae, Escherichia coli*[1], *Fuscobacterium necrophorum, Klebsiella pneumoniae, Listeria monocytogenes, Pasteurella multocida, Proteus mirabilis, Proteus vulgaris, Salmonella enteritidis, Salmonella typhi, Salmonella typhimurium, Serratia marcescens, Staphylococcus aureus* (methicillin resistant), *Staphylococcus epidermis*[2], *Streptococcus faecalis*[1], *Streptococcus pyogenes, Enterococcus faecalis* (Vancomycin resistant), *Shigella flexneri, Shigella sonnei,* *Adenovirus Type 4, *Canine distemper, *Feline leukemia, *Feline picornavirus, *Herpes simplex type 1, *Herpes simplex type 2, *HIV-1 (AIDS virus), *Infectious bovine rhinotracheitis, *Infectious bronchitis (Avian IBV), *Influenza A/Hong Kong, *Pseudorabies, *Rabies, *Respiratory syncytial virus (RSV), *Rubella (German measles), *Transmissible gastroenteritis virus (TGE), *Vaccinia, *Aspergillus niger, *Candida albicans, *Trichophyton mentagrophytes

[1]ATCC and antibiotic-resistant strain

[2]Antibiotic-resistant strain only

Directions for Use: It is a violation of federal law to use this product in a manner inconsistent with its labeling.

General Use Directions: Recommended for use in veterinary clinics, animal science laboratories, federally inspected meat and poultry establishments, equine farms, tack shops, pet shops, kennels, poultry farms, turkey farms, dairy farms, hog farms, breeding establishments, and grooming establishments. Disinfects, cleans and deodorizes floors, walls, metal surfaces, stainless steel surfaces, glazed porcelain, plastic surfaces (such as polypropylene, polystyrene, etc.), and other hard, non-porous surfaces.

Application: Remove heavy soil deposits from surface. Then thoroughly wet surface with a solution of ½ ounce of the concentrate per gallon of water. The solution can be applied with a cloth, mop, sponge, or coarse spray, or soaking. Let solution remain on surface for a minimum of 10 minutes. Rinse or allow to air dry. Rinsing of floors is not necessary unless they are to be waxed or polished. Prepare a fresh solution daily or more often if the solution becomes visibly dirty or diluted.

USDA: For use in federally inspected meat and poultry plants as a disinfectant agent for use in all departments. Food products and packaging materials must be removed from the room or carefully protected. Use product in accordance with its label. All surfaces must be thoroughly rinsed with potable water.

Farm Premise, Livestock, Poultry and Turkey House Disinfectant

1. Remove all animals from premises, trucks, coops, crates, and enclosures.
2. Remove all litter and manure from floors, walls, and surfaces of barns, pens, stalls, chutes, vehicles, and other facilities and fixtures occupied or traversed by animals.
3. Empty all troughs, racks, and other feeding and watering appliances.
4. Thoroughly clean all surfaces with soap or detergent, and rinse with water.
5. Saturate all surfaces with the recommended disinfecting solution for a period of 10 minutes.
6. Immerse all halters, ropes, and other types of equipment using in handling and restraining animals, as well as forks, shovels, and scrapers used for removing litter and manure.
7. Ventilate buildings, coops, cars, boats, and other closed spaces. Do not house animals or employ equipment until treatment has been absorbed, set, or dried.
8. After treatment with disinfectant, thoroughly scrub feed racks, troughs, automatic feeders, fountains, and waterers with soap or detergent, and rinse with potable water before reuse.

Mildewstatic Instructions: Will effectively control the growth of mold and mildew plus the odors caused by them when applied to hard, non-porous surfaces such as walls, floors and table tops. Apply solution (½ ounce per gallon of water) with a cloth, mop, sponge, or coarse spray. Make sure to wet all surfaces completely. Repeat application weekly or when growth reappears.

*Kills HIV-1 (AIDS virus) on precleaned, environmental surfaces/objects previously soiled with blood/body fluids in health care settings or other settings in which there is an expected likelihood of soiling of inanimate surfaces/objects with blood/body fluids, and in which the surfaces/objects likely to be soiled with bloody/body fluids can be associated with the potential for transmission of Human immunodeficiency virus Type 1 (HIV-1)(Associated with AIDS).

Special Instructions for Cleaning and Decontamination Against HIV-1 (AIDS Virus) of Surfaces/Objects Soiled with Blood/Body Fluids:

Personal Protection: Disposable latex or vinyl gloves, gowns, face masks, or eye coverings as appropriate must be worn during all cleaning of blood/body fluids decontamination procedures.

Cleaning procedures: Blood/body fluids must be thoroughly cleaning from surfaces/objects before application of disinfectant.

Contact Time: HIV-1 (AIDS Virus) is inactivated after a contact time of 4 minutes at 25°C (room temperature). Use a 10 minute contact time for other viruses, fungi, and bacteria listed.

Disposal of Infectious Materials: Blood/body fluids should be autoclaved and disposed of according to federal, state, and local regulations for infectious waste disposal.

L

Precautionary Statements: Hazards to Humans and Domestic Animals:

Danger: Corrosive. Causes eye damage and severe skin irritation. Harmful if swallowed. Do not get in eyes, on skin, or on clothing. When handling product, protect eyes by wearing goggles or face shield and protect skin by wearing rubber gloves. Wash thoroughly with soap and water after handling. Remove contaminated clothing and wash before reuse.

Statement of Practical Treatment:

In case of contact, immediately flush eyes or skin with plenty of water for at least 15 minutes. For eyes, call a physician. If swallowed, immediately drink a large quantity of water. Avoid alcohol. Get medical attention.

Note to Physician: Probable mucosal damage may contraindicate the use of gastric lavage. Measures against circulatory shock, respiratory depression, and convulsion may be needed.

Environmental Hazard: Do not discharge effluent containing this product into lakes, streams, ponds, estuaries, oceans or other waters unless in accordance with the requirements of a National Pollutant Discharge Elimination System (NPDES) permit and the permitting authority has been notified in writing prior to its discharge. Do not discharge effluent containing this product to sewer systems without previously notifying the local sewage treatment plant authority. For guidance contact your State Water Board or Regional Office of the EPA.

Storage and Disposal: Keep product under locked storage, inaccessible to children. Do not contaminate water, food, or feed by storage or disposal. Open dumping is prohibited. Do not reuse empty container.

Pesticide Disposal: Pesticide wastes are acutely hazardous. Improper disposal of excess pesticide, spray mixture, or rinsate is a violation of Federal law. If these wastes cannot be disposed of by use according to label instructions, contact your State Pesticide or Environmental Control Agency, or the Hazardous Waste representative at the nearest EPA Regional Office for guidance.

Container Disposal: Triple rinse (or equivalent). Then offer for recycling or reconditioning, or puncture and dispose of in a sanitary landfill, or incinerate, or if allowed by state and local authorities, burn, if burned, stay out of smoke.

Warning(s): Keep out of reach of children.

Presentation: 1 U.S. gallon (3.8 liters), 4x1 U.S. gallon (3.8 liters) per case, 5 gallon (18.9 liters) pail, and 55 gallons (208.2 liters).

Compendium Code No.: 13690011

REV. 8/28/96

LIFEGARD® 800

Rochester Midland **Cleaning Product**

Ingredient(s): Polymeric dispersant (No CAS #), Potassium hydroxide (1310-58-3), Sodium metasilicate (6834-92-0), Water (7732-18-5).

Indications: LIFEGARD® 800 is an aluminum safe cleaner designed for use primarily in rack and tunnel washers in pharmaceutical and cosmetic manufacturing, animal laboratory, medical research and other life science facilities.

Claims: No carcinogenic ingredients.

Directions for Use: LIFEGARD® 800 removes starch, protein, fats and oils. It is effective in both hard and soft, cold or hot water.

Aluminum safe, when diluted 1:10 or greater.

Automatic Washers/Central Pressure Wash Systems/Portable Pressure Washers: Dilute ¼ to 4 ounces per gallon of hot water.

Automatic Floor Scrubbers: Dilute ½ to 2 ounces per gallon depending upon soil conditions.

Manual Applications: Apply LIFEGARD® 800, diluted 1 to 4 ounces per gallon of water with sponge, brush or mop.

Rinse all cleaned surfaces with potable water.

Mix only with water.

Caution(s): May cause burns to eyes, skin and mucous membranes. Burns may not be immediately painful or visible. May cause respiratory irritation or be harmful if inhaled. Harmful if swallowed. Do not get in eyes, on skin or clothing, or breathe mist, dust or vapors. Wear goggles, rubber gloves, rubber shoes or boots, and other appropriate protective clothing when handling. Liquid may penetrate leather shoes and cause delayed burns. If ventilation is inadequate, a suitable respirator may be needed. Keep container closed when not in use. Refer to the product Material Safety Data Sheet for other safety information.

Warning(s): If in eyes: Immediately flush with plenty of water for at least 15 minutes while holding eyelids open. Get immediate medical attention. If on skin: Immediately wash with water for at least 15 minutes while removing all contaminated clothing and shoes. Get medical attention. If inhaled: Remove to fresh air. If not breathing, give artificial respiration. If breathing is difficult, give oxygen. Get medical attention. If swallowed: Do Not Induce Vomiting. Give a glass of water or milk to dilute. Get immediate medical attention. Never give anything by mouth to an unconscious person.

Keep out of reach of children.

Presentation: 5 gallon (18.9 liters) pail, 30 gallons (113.6 liters), and 55 gallons (208.2 liters).

Compendium Code No.: 13690061

LIFEGARD® 855 PLUS

Rochester Midland **Cleaning Product**

Liquid Chlorinated Alkaline Low Foam Cleaner

Ingredient(s): Detergent mixture (No CAS #), Potassium hydroxide (1310-58-3), Sodium hypochlorite (7681-52-9), Sodium silicate (1344-09-8), Water (7732-18-5), Sodium metasilicate (6834-92-0).

Indications: A low foam cleaner recommended for use in veterinary clinics, animal science laboratories, pet shops, kennels, poultry farms, hatchery sanitation programs, dairy farms, hog farms, and breeding establishments. Suggested for cleaning laboratory animal cages constructed of aluminum, galvanized and mild steel, and laboratory glassware. It is also used for cleaning trays, racks, plastic boxes, and plastic egg flats.

Aluminum safe when used according to directions.

Authorized by USDA for use in federally inspected meat and poultry plants.

Directions for Use: LIFEGARD® 855 Plus is especially effective in removing starch, protein, fats and oils. It is effective in both hard and soft, cold and hot water.

Warning: Contents may be under pressure. Open the cap slightly to vent any pressure in the container. Continue to open the cap after all pressure has been relieved.

Aluminum Safe: LIFEGARD® 855 Plus when diluted 12 ounces per gallon or less.

Automatic Washers/Central Pressure Wash Systems/Portable Pressure Washers: Use LIFEGARD® 855 Plus at ¼ to 4 ounces per gallon of hot water (150°F).

Automatic Floor Scrubbers: Use LIFEGARD® 855 Plus at 1 to 4 ounces per gallon depending upon soil conditions.

Manual Applications: Apply LIFEGARD® 855 Plus, 1 to 4 ounces per gallon of water with sponge, brush or mop.

Rinse all cleaned food contact surfaces with potable water. Do not mix with other cleaners. Keep from freezing. Keep container closed when not in use.

Cooling and Retort Water Treatment: Add ½ to 1 fl. oz. of LIFEGARD® 855 Plus per gallon to the retort water, washing spray, or cooling water for canned products.

Note: Do not mix with acids, ammonia, or any other cleaning chemicals as dangerous fumes may result.

Mix only with water.

Caution(s): Danger: Causes severe burns to eyes, skin and mucous membranes. Burns may not be immediately painful or visible. Harmful or fatal if swallowed or inhaled. Do not get in eyes, on skin or clothing, or breathe mist, dust or vapors. Wear goggles, face shield, rubber gloves, rubber shoes or boots, and other appropriate protective clothing when handling. Liquid may penetrate leather shoes and cause delayed burns. If working in mist, dust or vapors, use an appropriate respirator. Keep container closed when not in use. Refer to the product Material Safety Data Sheet for other safety information.

Contact with acid releases chlorine gas.

Warning(s): If in eyes: Immediately flush with plenty of water for at least 15 minutes while holding eyelids open. Get immediate medical attention. If on skin: Immediately wash with water for at least 15 minutes while removing all contaminated clothing and shoes. Get medical attention. If inhaled: Remove to fresh air. If not breathing, give artificial respiration. If breathing is difficult, give oxygen. Get medical attention. If swallowed: Do not induce vomiting. Give a glass of water or milk to dilute. Get immediate medical attention. Never give anything by mouth to an unconscious person.

Keep out of reach of children.

Presentation: 55 gallon (208.0 liter) drums.

Compendium Code No.: 13690081 REV. 12/22/98

LIFEGARD™ 900

Rochester Midland **Cleaning Product**

Liquid Alkaline Cleaner

Active Ingredient(s): Detergent mixture (No CAS #), Tetrasodium EDTA (64-02-8), Water (7732-18-5).

Indications: LIFEGARD™ 900 is a liquid alkaline cleaner effective in removing organic soils including starch and proteinaceous soils, and body oils from cages, racks and accessories. LIFEGARD™ 900 is a highly chelated, non-caustic product especially formulated with polymers, a wetting agent, and a dispersant. LIFEGARD™ 900 is safe to use on glass, plastics, polycarbonate cages, aluminum, galvanized steel, and stainless steel surfaces. It is designed to be used in CIP systems, pressure washers, soak tanks, automatic rack and tunnel washing equipment, cart and cage washers, bottle washers, and by bucket and brush application.

LIFEGARD™ 900 is hard water tolerant and free rinsing, leaving no residue on equipment surfaces. Recommended for use in pharmaceutical and cosmetic manufacturing, animal laboratories, poultry farms, hatchery sanitation programs, medical research, and other life science facilities. Used cleaning solutions containing LIFEGARD™ 900 have outstanding oil/water separation for appropriate waste water management.

Pharmacology: Physical Properties:

Biodegradable: Yes
Foam Generation: Nil to very low
Emulsification/Solubility: Rapid
Specific Gravity @ 75°F: 1.1 - 1.2
Appearance and Odor: Clear, light blue liquid; odorless
Rinsing: Excellent
Hard Water Tolerance: Moderate
pH 1.0% dilution: 9.9 ± 0.2
Pounds/Gallon: 9.2

Directions for Use: LIFEGARD™ 900 is highly effective in wash solutions with temperatures from 120°F (35°C) up to 190°F (74°C). It produces very low foam when water temperature is 120°F (35°C) or higher.

CIP Systems/Automatic Washers/Pressure Washers: Dilute LIFEGARD™ 900 ¼-½ ounce per gallon of water (512:1 - 256:1).

Manual Applications: Apply LIFEGARD™ 900 diluted 1 - 2 ounces per gallon of water (128:1 64:1).

Use Test Kit RF-3000-7.

Caution(s): May cause eye or respiratory irritation. Do not get in eyes. Avoid breathing mist, dust or vapors. Wash thoroughly after handling.

If in eyes: Rinse immediately with plenty of water for 15 minutes while holding eyelids open.
If on skin: Wash with water.
If inhaled: Remove to fresh air. Aid breathing as needed.
If swallowed, or if irritation persists: Get medical attention.
Medical Emergency Telephone: 1-800-535-5053 (U.S.). Outside the U.S. 1-352-323-3500.

Warning(s): Keep out of reach of children.

Disclaimer: All data statements and information presented herein are believed to be accurate and reliable but are not to be taken as a guarantee, express warranty or implied warranty or merchantability or fitness for a particular purpose, or representation, express or implied, for which seller assumes legal responsibility, and they are offered solely for your consideration, investigation and verification. Statements or suggestions concerning possible use of this product are made without representation or warranty that any such use is free of patent infringement and are not recommendations to infringe on any patent.

Presentation: 55 gallon (208.2 L) drum.

Compendium Code No.: 13690120 Form 1210-BLK/Form 1030C

LIFEGARD® 7000

Rochester Midland **Detergent**

Phosphoric Acid Cleaner and Brightener

Ingredient(s): Detergent mixture (No CAS #), Phosphoric acid (7664-38-2), Water (7732-18-5).

No carcinogenic ingredients.

Indications: LIFEGARD® 7000 is a specially formulated, controlled foam acid cleaner for pharmaceutical and cosmetic manufacturing and medical research, laboratory animal, and other life science facilities.

LIFEGARD® 7000 removes uric salts, rust, scale, mold, mildew, starch and protein. It is designed for use in tunnel and rack washers, CIP systems, and manually.

Directions for Use: LIFEGARD® 7000 dilution will vary depending upon type and quantity of soil.

For use in rack and tunnel washers and CIP systems, start with 2-3 oz per gallon of water.

For manual use, start with a dilution of 20 oz/gal. in warm water.

LIFEGARD® 7000 cleaning solutions are most effective at 140° to 150°F.

Rinse with potable water.

Do not mix with chlorine containing products or bleach — releases chlorine gas.

Mix only with water.

Do not use on aluminum, tin or zinc-plated surfaces. Pitting or surface deterioration may result.

Caution(s): Danger: Causes severe burns to eyes, skin and mucous membranes. Burns may not be immediately painful or visible. Harmful or fatal if swallowed or inhaled. Do not get in eyes, on skin or clothing, or breathe mist, dust or vapors. Wear goggles, rubber gloves, rubber shoes or boots, and other appropriate protective clothing when handling. Liquid may penetrate leather shoes and cause delayed burns. A face shield may be needed if splashes are likely. If ventilation is inadequate, a suitable respirator may be needed. Keep container closed when not in use. Refer to the product Material Safety Data Sheet for other safety information.

Warning(s): If in eyes: Immediately flush with plenty of water for at least 15 minutes while holding eyelids open. Get immediate medical attention. If on skin: Immediately wash with water for at least 15 minutes while removing all contaminated clothing and shoes. Get medical attention. If inhaled: Remove to fresh air. If not breathing, give artificial respiration. If breathing is difficult, give oxygen. Get medical attention. If swallowed: Do Not Induce Vomiting. Give a glass of water or milk to dilute. Get immediate medical attention. Never give anything by mouth to an unconscious person. Medical Emergency Telephone 1-800-535-5053 (U.S.). Outside the U.S. 1-352-323-3500.

Keep out of reach of children.

Presentation: 1 gallon container, 30 gallon (113.6 liter) and 55 gallon (208.2 liter) drums.

Compendium Code No.: 13690022 REV. 10/2/00

LIFEGARD® 7500F

Rochester Midland **Detergent**

Liquid Phosphoric Acid Foam Cleaner

Ingredient(s): Detergent mixture (No CAS #), Phosphoric acid (7664-38-2), Water (7732-18-5).

Indications: LIFEGARD® 7500F is a concentrated acid cleaner designed for foam, spray and manual cleaning of stainless steel equipment in pharmaceutical and cosmetic plants, and laboratory animal, medical research and other life science facilities.

Claims: No carcinogenic ingredients.

Directions for Use: LIFEGARD® 7500F removes scale, rust, lime deposits, uric salts, mold, mildew, starch and protein.

LIFEGARD® 7500F dilution ratios will vary depending on soil conditions. Dilute 1 part to 5 parts water for rust and heavy scale accumulations. Adjust dilution as necessary. Agitate and rinse with potable water.

Foam Application: Dilute 12 ounces per gallon or less and apply through foam generating equipment. Agitate with stiff brush or abrasive pad if necessary, and rinse with potable water.

Recommended use temperature is 140°-150°F.

Mix only with water.

Do not use on aluminum, tin or zinc-plated surfaces. Pitting or surface deterioration may result.

Do not mix with chlorine containing products or bleach - releases chlorine gas.

Caution(s): Danger: Causes severe burns to eyes, skin and mucous membranes. Burns may not be immediately painful or visible. Harmful or fatal if swallowed or inhaled. Do not get in eyes, on skin or clothing, or breathe mist, dust or vapors. Wear goggles, rubber gloves, face shield, rubber shoes or boots, and other appropriate protective clothing when handling. Liquid may penetrate leather shoes and cause delayed burns. If ventilation is inadequate, a suitable respirator may be needed. Keep container closed when not in use. Refer to the product Material Safety Data Sheet for other safety information.

Warning(s): If in eyes: Immediately flush with plenty of water for at least 15 minutes while holding eyelids open. Get immediate medical attention. If on skin: Immediately wash with water for at least 15 minutes while removing all contaminated clothing and shoes. Get medical attention. If inhaled: Remove to fresh air. If not breathing, give artificial respiration. If breathing is difficult, give oxygen. Get medical attention. If swallowed: Do Not Induce Vomiting. Give a glass of water or milk to dilute. Get immediate medical attention. Never give anything by mouth to an unconscious person. Medical Emergency Telephone 1-800-535-5053 (U.S.). Outside the U.S. 1-352-323-3500.

Keep out of reach of children.

Presentation: 30 gallon (113.6 liter) and 55 gallon (208.2 liter) drums.

Compendium Code No.: 13690042

LIFEGARD® 7700

Rochester Midland **Detergent**

Ingredient(s): Detergent mixture (No CAS #), Phosphoric acid (7664-38-2), Water (7732-18-5).

Indications: LIFEGARD® 7700 is a specially formulated, controlled foam, concentrated acid cleaner for pharmaceutical, cosmetic, manufacturing, and medical research, laboratory animal and other life science facilities. LIFEGARD® 7700 removes uric salts, rust, scale, mold, mildew, starch and protein. It is designed for use in tunnel and rack washers, CIP systems and manually.

Claims: No carcinogenic ingredients.

Dosage and Administration: LIFEGARD® 7700 dilution ratios will vary depending on soil conditions. Adjust to a higher or lower dilution as necessary.

For use in rack and tunnel washers or CIP systems, begin with 1-2 oz per gallon of water.

For manual use, start with a dilution of 10 oz/gal. in warm water.

LIFEGARD® 7700 cleaning solutions are most effective at 140° to 150°F.

Rinse with potable water.

Mix only with water.

Do not use on aluminum, tin or zinc-plated surfaces. Pitting or surface deterioration may result.

Do not mix with chlorine containing products or bleach - releases chlorine gas.

Caution(s): Danger: Causes severe burns to eyes, skin and mucous membranes. Burns may not be immediately painful or visible. Harmful or fatal if swallowed or inhaled. Do not get in eyes, on skin or clothing, or breathe mist, dust or vapors. Wear goggles, rubber gloves, rubber shoes or boots, and other appropriate protective clothing when handling. Liquid may penetrate leather shoes and cause delayed burns. A face shield may be needed if splashes are likely. If ventilation is inadequate, a suitable respirator may be needed. Keep container closed when not in use. Refer to the product Material Safety Data Sheet for other safety information.

Warning(s): If in eyes: Immediately flush with plenty of water for at least 15 minutes while holding eyelids open. Get immediate medical attention. If on skin: Immediately wash with water for at least 15 minutes while removing all contaminated clothing and shoes. Get medical attention. If inhaled: Remove to fresh air. If not breathing, give artificial respiration. If breathing is difficult, give oxygen. Get medical attention. If swallowed: Do Not Induce Vomiting. Give a glass of water or milk to dilute. Get immediate medical attention. Never give anything by mouth to an unconscious person.

Keep out of reach of children.

Presentation: 30 gallons (113.6 liters) and 55 gallons (208.2 liters).

Compendium Code No.: 13690051

LIFEGARD® 7700ND

Rochester Midland **Detergent**

Ingredient(s): Detergent mixture (No CAS #), Phosphoric acid (7664-38-2), Water (7732-18-5).

Indications: LIFEGARD® 7700ND is a specially formulated, controlled foam, concentrated acid cleaner for pharmaceutical, cosmetic, manufacturing, and medical research, laboratory animal and other life science facilities. LIFEGARD® 7700ND removes uric salts, rust, scale, mold, mildew, starch and protein. It is designed for use in tunnel and rack washers, CIP systems and manually.

Claims: No carcinogenic ingredients.

Directions for Use: LIFEGARD® 7700ND dilution ratios will vary depending on soil conditions. Adjust to a higher or lower dilution as necessary.

For use in rack and tunnel washers or CIP systems, begin with 1-2 oz per gallon of water.

For manual use, start with a dilution of 10 oz/gal. in warm water.

LIFEGARD® 7700ND cleaning solutions are most effective at 140° to 150°F.

Rinse with potable water.

Mix only with water.

Do not use on aluminum, tin or zinc-plated surfaces. Pitting or surface deterioration may result.

Do not mix with chlorine containing products or bleach - releases chlorine gas.

Caution(s): Danger: Causes severe burns to eyes, skin and mucous membranes. Burns may not be immediately painful or visible. Harmful or fatal if swallowed or inhaled. Do not get in eyes, on skin or clothing, or breathe mist, dust or vapors. Wear goggles, rubber gloves, rubber shoes or boots, and other appropriate protective clothing when handling. Liquid may penetrate leather shoes and cause delayed burns. A face shield may be needed if splashes are likely. If ventilation is inadequate, a suitable respirator may be needed. Keep container closed when not in use. Refer to the product Material Safety Data Sheet for other safety information.

Warning(s): If in eyes: Immediately flush with plenty of water for at least 15 minutes while holding eyelids open. Get immediate medical attention. If on skin: Immediately wash with water for at least 15 minutes while removing all contaminated clothing and shoes. Get medical attention. If inhaled: Remove to fresh air. If not breathing, give artificial respiration. If breathing is difficult, give oxygen. Get medical attention. If swallowed: Do Not Induce Vomiting. Give a glass of water or milk to dilute. Get immediate medical attention. Never give anything by mouth to an unconscious person.

Keep out of reach of children.

Presentation: 30 gallons (113.6 liters) and 55 gallons (208.2 liters).

Compendium Code No.: 13690130

LINCOCIN® ℞

Pharmacia & Upjohn **Lincomycin**

Lincomycin hydrochloride products

NADA No.: 033-887 (Tablets) / 040-587 (Aquadrops) / 034-025 (Sterile Solution)

Active Ingredient(s):

Tablets:

100 mg: Each scored tablet contains lincomycin hydrochloride equivalent to lincomycin, 100 mg.

200 mg: Each scored tablet contains lincomycin hydrochloride equivalent to lincomycin, 200 mg.

500 mg: Each scored tablet contains lincomycin hydrochloride equivalent to lincomycin, 500 mg.

AQUADROPS®: Each mL containing lincomycin hydrochloride equivalent to lincomycin, 50 mg; preserved with methylparaben 0.075%, propylparaben 0.025%, and sorbic acid 0.1%.

Sterile Solution: Each mL containing lincomycin hydrochloride equivalent to lincomycin, 100 mg; also Benzyl Alcohol, 9.45 mg added as preservative.

Indications: LINCOCIN® products are indicated in infections caused by gram-positive organisms which are sensitive to its action, particularly streptococci and staphylococci. The drug has proven effective in eradicating causative organisms in most of the common upper respiratory tract infections, in septicemia, and in infections of the skin and adjoining tissues.

Systemic therapy with LINCOCIN® has been shown to be of benefit in many animals with pustular dermatitis. As with all antibiotics, *in vitro* sensitivity studies should be performed before LINCOCIN® is utilized as sole antibiotic therapy.

LINCOCIN® has been demonstrated to be effective in the treatment of staphylococcal infections resistant to other antibiotics and sensitive to lincomycin. The drug may be administered in combination therapy with other antimicrobial agents when indicated.

No serious hypersensitivity reactions have been reported and many animals have received LINCOCIN® repeatedly without developing evidence of hypersensitivity.

In dogs, LINCOCIN® has demonstrated excellent efficacy in the treatment of upper respiratory infections and of skin diseases, particularly those caused by staphylococcus and streptococcus organisms. LINCOCIN® has demonstrated efficacy even in some chronic conditions of long standing and in infections which have resisted treatment with other antibacterial agents.

Infections successfully treated with LINCOCIN® include pustular dermatitis, abscesses, infected wounds (including bite and fight wounds), tonsillitis, laryngitis, metritis, and secondary bacterial infections associated with the canine distemper-hepatitis complex.

In cats, LINCOCIN® has demonstrated efficacy in the treatment of localized infections, such as abscesses following fight wounds, pneumonitis, and feline rhinotracheitis.

Success in the treatment of viral diseases must be attributed to the control of susceptible secondary bacterial invaders rather than to any effect of LINCOCIN® on the virus.

Pharmacology: LINCOCIN® products contain lincomycin hydrochloride, an antibiotic produced by *Streptomyces lincolnensis var. lincolnensis*, which is chemically distinct from all other clinically available antibiotics and is isolated as a white crystalline solid. It is stable in the dry state and in aqueous solution for at least 24 months. Lincomycin hydrochloride is readily soluble in water at room temperature in concentrations up to 500 mg/mL. Physical stability of aqueous solutions can be maintained at drug concentrations up to 345 mg/mL at temperatures as low as 4° C. The solubility in 95 percent ethanol is 80 mg/mL.

LINCOCIN® products have been shown to be effective against most of the common gram-positive pathogens. Depending on the sensitivity of the organism and concentration of the antibiotic, it may be either bactericidal or bacteriostatic. It has not shown cross resistance with other available antibiotics. Microorganisms have not developed resistance to LINCOCIN® rapidly when tested by *in vitro* or *in vivo* methods.

Actions:

Biological Studies—*In vitro* studies indicate that the spectrum of activity includes *Staphylococcus aureus, Staphylococcus albus, β-hemolytic Streptococcus, Streptococcus viridans, Clostridium tetani, Erysipelothrix insidiosa, Mycoplasma* spp., and *Clostridium perfringens*. The drug is not active against gram-negative organisms or yeasts.

In vivo experimental animal studies demonstrated the effectiveness of LINCOCIN® in protecting animals infected with *Streptococcus viridans, β-hemolytic Streptococcus, Staphylococcus aureus, Erysipelothrix insidiosa, Mycoplasma* spp., and *Leptospira pomona*. It was ineffective in *Klebsiella, Pasteurella, Pseudomonas,* and *Salmonella* infections.

Cross resistance has not been demonstrated with penicillin, erythromycin, triacetyloleandomycin, chloramphenicol, novobiocin, streptomycin, or the tetracyclines. Staphylococci develop resistance to LINCOCIN® in a slow, stepwise manner based on *in vitro*, serial subculture experiments. This pattern of resistance development is unlike that shown for streptomycin.

Clinical Absorption and Excretion—Administered intramuscularly, LINCOCIN® Sterile Solution is very rapidly absorbed. In studies with dogs, peak serum levels were reached in from ten minutes to two hours with detectable levels for 16 to 24 hours. The concentration of LINCOCIN® in the blood serum varies with the dose administered and with the individual animal. Levels are maintained above the *in vitro* minimum inhibitory concentration for most gram-positive organisms for six to eight hours following a therapeutic dose. Intravenous administration also provides very rapid absorption, but should be administered with normal saline or 5% glucose as an intravenous drip infusion.

Administered orally to dogs, LINCOCIN® was also rapidly absorbed with serum levels present within one-half hour; peak values were reached at two to four hours; and detectable levels persisted for 16 to 24 hours.

Tissue level studies indicate that bile is an important route of excretion. Significant levels of LINCOCIN® have been demonstrated in the majority of body tissues. After a single oral administration of LINCOCIN® to a dog, fecal excretion amounted to 77 percent of the dose; urinary excretion to 14 percent. After a single intramuscular injection, fecal excretion equaled 38 percent of the dose; and urinary excretion, 49 percent. Urinary excretion was essentially complete in less than 24 hours and fecal excretion by 48 hours after either route of administration. LINCOCIN® has also been shown to be excreted in the milk of lactating cows, goats, rats, and women.

Dosage and Administration:

Oral: 10 mg per pound of body weight every 12 hours or 7 mg per pound every 8 hours.

Intramuscular: 10 mg per pound of body weight once a day or 5 mg per pound every 12 hours.

Intravenous: 5 to 10 mg per pound of body weight one or two times per day diluted with 5 percent glucose in water or normal saline and given as a drip infusion.

Treatment with LINCOCIN® products may be continued for periods as long as 12 days if clinical judgment indicates.

As with any multi-dose vial, practice aseptic techniques in withdrawing each dose. Adequately clean and disinfect the vial closure prior to entry with a sterile needle and syringe.

Contraindication(s): As with all drugs, the use of LINCOCIN® products is contraindicated in animals previously found to be hypersensitive to the drug.

LINCOCIN® should not be given to animals with known preexisting monilial infections.

The following species are sensitive to the gastrointestinal effects of lincomycin: rabbits, hamsters, guinea pigs and horses. Therefore, the administration of LINCOCIN® should be avoided in these species.

Precaution(s): Store at controlled room temperature 20° to 25°C (68° to 77°F) [see USP].

Caution(s): Federal (USA) law restricts this drug to use by or on the order of a licensed veterinarian.

The use of antibiotics occasionally results in overgrowth of nonsusceptible organisms—particularly yeasts. Should superinfections occur, appropriate measures should be taken.

For use in animals only.

Warning(s): Not for human use.

Toxicology:

Animal Toxicology—The acute LD_{50} intraperitoneally in mice is 1000 mg/kg and orally in rats is 15,645 mg/kg. LINCOCIN® was well tolerated orally in rats and dogs at doses up to 300 mg/kg/day for periods up to one year. Parenteral dosages of up to 60 mg/kg/day for 30 days subcutaneously in the rat and intramuscularly in the dog produced no significant systemic effects or pathological findings at necropsy.

LINCOCIN® at a daily dose level of 75 mg/kg subcutaneously was injected into mature male and female rats during a prebreeding period of 60 days and throughout two mating cycles (84 days). No evidence was obtained that LINCOCIN® exerted any effects on breeding performance and no drug-induced anomalies were discovered in the young. Similarly no evidence was obtained that LINCOCIN®, when given in sustained parenteral dosage of 50 mg/kg daily to pregnant bitches, produced a teratogenic effect on the canine embryo.

The subcutaneous LD_{50} value in the newborn rat was determined to be 783 mg/kg. Newborn rats and canine pups have tolerated multiple doses of 30-90 mg/kg/day of the drug without evidence of ill effects.

Adverse Reactions: Loose stools occasionally have been observed in dogs and cats on oral doses. Vomiting in cats has occasionally been reported following oral administration.

Intramuscularly and intravenously, LINCOCIN® products have demonstrated excellent local tolerance with no reports of pain or inflammation following injection.

Presentation: LINCOCIN® products for veterinary use are available in the following dosage forms and strengths:

Tablets:

100 mg: Supplied in bottles of 500 (NDC 0009-0595-05).
200 mg: Supplied in bottles of 250 (NDC 0009-0596-02).
500 mg: Supplied in bottles of 100 (NDC 0009-0475-01).

AQUADROPS®: Supplied in 20 mL bottles with graduated dropper (NDC 0009-0570-01).
Sterile Solution: Supplied in 20 mL vials (NDC 0009-0617-01).
LINCOCIN® Tablets manufactured by Global Pharm Inc., Canada

Compendium Code No.: 10490221 810 411 716

LINCOCIN® INJECTABLE

AgriLabs **Lincomycin**

brand of lincomycin injection, USP

NADA No.: 034-025

Active Ingredient(s):

25 mg/mL: Special baby pig concentration: Each mL contains lincomycin hydrochloride equivalent to lincomycin, 25 mg; also benzyl alcohol, 9.45 mg added as preservative.

300 mg/mL: For use in swine weighing 300 pounds and more. Each mL contains lincomycin hydrochloride equivalent to lincomycin, 300 mg; also Benzyl Alcohol, 9.45 mg added as preservative.

Indications: Swine: LINCOCIN® Injectable is indicated for the treatment of infectious forms of arthritis caused by organisms sensitive to its activity. This includes most of the organisms responsible for the various infectious arthritides in swine, such as staphylococci, streptococci, *Erysipelothrix* and *Mycoplasma* spp.

It is also indicated for the treatment of mycoplasma pneumonia.

Pharmacology: LINCOCIN® Injectable contains lincomycin hydrochloride, an antibiotic produced by *Streptomyces lincolnensis var. lincolnensis,* which is chemically distinct from all other clinically available antibiotics and is isolated as a white crystalline solid.

Dosage and Administration: For arthritis or mycoplasma pneumonia—5 mg per pound of body weight intramuscularly once daily for three to seven days as needed. When using LINCOCIN® Injectable containing 25 mg/mL, 1 mL/5 lb body weight will provide 5 mg/lb. When using LINCOCIN® Injectable containing 300 mg/mL, 1 mL/60 lb body weight will provide 5 mg/lb.

For optimal results, initiate treatment as soon as possible.

As with any multi-dose vial, practice aseptic techniques in withdrawing each dose. Adequately clean and disinfect the vial closure prior to entry with a sterile needle and syringe. No vial closure should be entered more than 20 times.

Contraindication(s): As with all drugs, the use of LINCOCIN® Injectable is contraindicated in animals previously found to be hypersensitive to the drug.

Precaution(s): Store at controlled room temperature 20° to 25°C (68° to 77°F) [see USP].

Caution(s): If no improvement is noted within 48 hours, consult a veterinarian.

For intramuscular use in swine only.

Restricted Drug—Use only as directed (California). For use in animals only.

Warning(s): Swine intended for human consumption should not be slaughtered within 48 hours of latest treatment. Not for human use.

Adverse Reactions: The intramuscular administration to swine may cause a transient diarrhea or loose stools. Although this effect has rarely been reported, one must be alert to the possibility that it may occur.

Should this occur, it is important that the necessary steps be taken to prevent the effects of dehydration.

Presentation: LINCOCIN® Injectable is available in two concentrations: 25 mg/mL and 300 mg/mL.

25 mg/mL: Supplied in 100 mL (3.3 fl oz) vials.
300 mg/mL: Supplied in 100 mL (3.3 fl oz) vials.

Manufactured by: Pharmacia & Upjohn Co., Kalamazoo, MI 49001
*LINCOCIN is a registered trademark of Pharmacia & Upjohn Company.

Compendium Code No.: 10581300 818 298 000 / 818 306 000

LINCOCIN® STERILE SOLUTION*

Durvet **Lincomycin**

brand of lincomycin injection, USP

NADA No.: 034-025

Active Ingredient(s):

25 mg/mL: Special baby pig concentration. Each mL contains lincomycin hydrochloride equivalent to lincomycin, 25 mg; also Benzyl Alcohol, 9.45 mg added as preservative.

100 mg/mL: Each mL contains lincomycin hydrochloride equivalent to lincomycin, 100 mg; also Benzyl Alcohol, 9.45 mg added as preservative.

300 mg/mL: For use in swine weighing 300 pounds and more. Each mL contains lincomycin hydrochloride equivalent to lincomycin, 300 mg; also Benzyl Alcohol, 9.45 mg added as preservative.

Indications: Swine: LINCOCIN® Sterile Solution is indicated for the treatment of infectious forms of arthritis caused by organisms sensitive to its activity. This includes most of the organisms responsible for the various infectious arthritides in swine, such as staphylococci, streptococci, *Erysipelothrix* and *Mycoplasma* spp.

It is also indicated for the treatment of mycoplasma pneumonia.

Pharmacology: LINCOCIN® Sterile Solution contains lincomycin hydrochloride, an antibiotic produced by *Streptomyces lincolnensis var. lincolnensis,* which is chemically distinct from all other clinically available antibiotics and is isolated as a white crystalline solid.

Dosage and Administration: For arthritis or mycoplasma pneumonia — 5 mg per pound of body weight intramuscularly once daily for three to seven days as needed. When using LINCOCIN® Sterile Solution containing 25 mg/mL, 1 mL/5 lb body weight will provide 5 mg/lb. When using LINCOCIN® Sterile Solution containing 300 mg/mL, 1 mL/60 lb body weight will provide 5 mg/lb.

For optimal results, initiate treatment as soon as possible.

As with any multi-dose vial, practice aseptic techniques in withdrawing each dose. Adequately clean and disinfect the vial closure prior to entry with a sterile needle and syringe. No vial closure should be entered more than 20 times.

Contraindication(s): As with all drugs, the use of LINCOCIN® Sterile Solution is contraindicated in animals previously found to be hypersensitive to the drug.

Precaution(s): Store at controlled room temperature 20° to 25°C (68° to 77°F) [see USP].

Caution(s): If no improvement is noted within 48 hours, consult a veterinarian.

For intramuscular use in swine only.

Restricted Drug-Use only as directed (California). For use in animals only.

Warning(s): Swine intended for human consumption should not be slaughtered within 48 hours of latest treatment. Not for human use.

Adverse Reactions: The intramuscular administration to swine may cause a transient diarrhea or loose stools. Although this effect has rarely been reported, one must be alert to the possibility that it may occur.

Should this occur, it is important that the necessary steps be taken to prevent the effects of dehydration.

Presentation: LINCOCIN® Sterile Solution is available in three concentrations: 25 mg/mL, 100 mg/mL, and 300 mg/mL.

25 mg/mL: Supplied in 100 mL (3.3 fl oz) vials (NDC 30798-674-10).
100 mg/mL: Supplied in 100 mL (3.3 fl oz) vials (NDC 30798-675-10).
300 mg/mL: Supplied in 100 mL (3.3 fl oz) vials (NDC 30798-676-10).

Manufactured by: Pharmacia & Upjohn Co., Kalamazoo, MI 49001.
*LINCOCIN is a registered trademark of Pharmacia & Upjohn Company.

Compendium Code No.: 10841812 2/01

LINCOCIN® STERILE SOLUTION (Swine)

Pharmacia & Upjohn **Lincomycin**

lincomycin injection, USP

NADA No.: 034-025

Active Ingredient(s): Each mL contains lincomycin hydrochloride equivalent to lincomycin, 100 mg; also benzyl alcohol, 9.45 mg added as preservative.

Indications: Swine: LINCOCIN® is indicated for the treatment of infectious forms of arthritis caused by organisms sensitive to its activity. This includes most of the organisms responsible for the various infectious arthritides in swine, such as staphylococci, streptococci, *Erysipelothrix* and *Mycoplasma* spp.

It is also indicated for the treatment of Mycoplasma pneumonia.

Pharmacology: LINCOCIN® Sterile Solution contains lincomycin hydrochloride, an antibiotic produced by *Streptomyces lincolnensis var. lincolnensis*, which is chemically distinct from all other clinically available antibiotics and is isolated as a white crystalline solid. It is stable in the dry state and in aqueous solution for at least 24 months. Lincomycin hydrochloride is readily soluble in water at room temperature in concentrations up to 500 mg/mL. Physical stability of aqueous solutions can be maintained at drug concentrations up to 345 mg/mL at temperatures as low as 4° C. The solubility in 95 percent ethanol is 80 mg/mL.

Lincomycin hydrochloride has been shown to be effective against most of the common gram-positive pathogens. Depending on the sensitivity of the organism and concentration of the antibiotic, it may be either bactericidal or bacteriostatic. It has not shown cross resistance with other available antibiotics. Microorganisms have not developed resistance to lincomycin hydrochloride rapidly when tested by *in vitro* or *in vivo* methods.

Biological Studies—*In vitro* studies indicate that the spectrum of activity includes *Staphylococcus aureus, Staphylococcus albus,* β-hemolytic *Streptococcus, Streptococcus viridans, Clostridium tetani, Erysipelothrix insidiosa, Mycoplasma* spp., and *Clostridium perfringens.* The drug is not active against gram-negative organisms or yeasts.

In vivo experimental animal studies demonstrated lincomycin hydrochloride is effective in protecting animals infected with *Streptococcus viridans,* β-hemolytic Streptococcus, *Staphylococcus aureus, Erysipelothrix insidiosa, Mycoplasma* spp., and *Leptospira pomona.* It was ineffective in *Klebsiella, Pasteurella, Pseudomonas,* and *Salmonella* infections.

Cross resistance has not been demonstrated with penicillin, erythromycin, triacetyloleandomycin, chloramphenicol, novobiocin, streptomycin, or the tetracyclines. Staphylococci develop resistance to lincomycin hydrochloride in a slow, stepwise manner based on *in vitro,* serial subculture experiments. This pattern of resistance development is unlike that shown for streptomycin.

When lincomycin hydrochloride was administered intramuscularly in swine at various dose levels, high levels were found in peritoneal fluid, pericardial fluid and bile at five to six hours. At 24 hours, detectable levels were still present in these fluids. At 48 hours, all tissues were free of drug.

Tissue level studies indicate that bile is an important route of excretion. Significant levels of lincomycin hydrochloride have been demonstrated in the majority of body tissues. After a single oral administration of lincomycin hydrochloride to a dog, fecal excretion amounted to 77 percent of the dose; urinary excretion to 14 percent. After a single intramuscular injection, fecal excretion equaled 38 percent of the dose; and urinary excretion, 49 percent. Urinary excretion was essentially complete in less than 24 hours and fecal excretion by 48 hours after either route of administration. Lincomycin hydrochloride has also been shown to be excreted in the milk of lactating cows, goats, rats and women.

Dosage and Administration: For arthritis or mycoplasma pneumonia—5 mg per pound of body weight intramuscularly once daily for three to seven days as needed. When using LINCOCIN® containing 100 mg/mL, 1 mL/20 lb body weight will provide 5 mg/lb.

For optimal results in infectious forms of arthritis, initiate treatment as soon as possible.

As with any multi-dose vial, practice aseptic techniques in withdrawing each dose. Adequately clean and disinfect the vial closure prior to entry with a sterile needle and syringe.

Contraindication(s): As with all drugs, the use of LINCOCIN® is contraindicated in animals previously found to be hypersensitive to the drug.

LINCOCIN® should not be given to animals with known preexisting monilial infections.

The following species are sensitive to the gastrointestinal effects of lincomycin: rabbits, hamsters, guinea pigs and horses. Therefore, the administration of LINCOCIN® should be avoided in these species.

Precaution(s): Store at controlled room temperature 20° to 25°C (68° to 77°F) [see USP].
Caution(s): For intramuscular use in swine.

For use in animals only.

If no improvement is noted within 48 hours, consult a veterinarian.

Warning(s): Not for human use.

Swine intended for human consumption should not be slaughtered within 48 hours of latest treatment.

Toxicology: Animal Toxicology—The acute LD_{50} intraperitoneally in mice is 1000 mg/kg and orally in rats is 15,645 mg/kg. Lincomycin hydrochloride was well tolerated orally in rats and dogs at doses up to 300 mg/kg/day for periods up to one year. Parenteral dosages of up to 60 mg/kg/day for 30 days subcutaneously in the rat and intramuscularly in the dog produced no significant systemic effects or pathological findings at necropsy.

Swine receiving lincomycin hydrochloride intramuscularly at 10, 25, and 50 mg/lb (two, five, and ten times overdose) for 14 days tolerated all injections well, gained weight normally, and showed normal hematology, urinalysis, and blood chemistry values. Diarrhea was noted in the 50 mg/lb group with a lessening gradation of soft stools seen in the 25 mg/lb and 10 mg/lb groups. These changes in stool consistency did not adversely affect performance or blood electrolyte values. By the tenth day of the trial period, all stools were again normal.

Lincomycin hydrochloride at a daily dose level of 75 mg/kg subcutaneously was injected into mature male and female rats during a prebreeding period of 60 days and throughout two mating cycles (84 days). No evidence was obtained that lincomycin hydrochloride exerted any effects on breeding performance and no drug-induced anomalies were discovered in the young. Similarly no evidence was obtained that lincomycin hydrochloride, when given in sustained parenteral dosage of 50 mg/kg daily to pregnant bitches, produced a teratogenic effect on the canine embryo.

The subcutaneous LD_{50} value in the newborn rat was determined to be 783 mg/kg. Newborn rats and canine pups have tolerated multiple doses of 30-90 mg/kg/day of the drug without evidence of ill effects.

Adverse Reactions: The intramuscular administration to swine may cause a transient diarrhea or loose stools. Although this effect has rarely been reported, one must be alert to the possibility that it may occur.

Should this occur, it is important that the necessary steps be taken to prevent the effects of dehydration.

Presentation: LINCOCIN® Sterile Solution lincomycin injection, USP 100 mg/mL, is available in 100 mL vials (NDC 0009-0617-09).

Compendium Code No.: 10490241 810 595 108

LINCOMIX® 20 FEED MEDICATION

Pharmacia & Upjohn **Feed Additive**

(Type A Medicated Article) 20 grams/lb

NADA No.: 097-505

Active Ingredient(s): Each pound contains:

Lincomycin (as lincomycin hydrochloride agricultural grade) .... 20 grams

Inactive Ingredients: Soybean hulls, #20 grind; mineral oil, USP.

Indications:

Broilers: For increase in rate of weight gain, for improved feed efficiency, and for the control of necrotic enteritis caused or complicated by *Clostridium* spp. or other organisms susceptible to lincomycin in broilers.

Swine: For the treatment and control of swine dysentery, and the control of porcine proliferative enteropathies (ileitis) caused by *Lawsonia intracellularis.* For reduction in the severity of swine mycoplasmal pneumonia caused by *Mycoplasma hyopneumoniae.* For increase in rate of weight gain in growing-finishing swine.

Directions for Use: Important: Must be thoroughly mixed in feeds before use.

Broilers:

For increase in rate of weight gain and improved feed efficiency: LINCOMIX® 20, 20 grams/lb, should be mixed into the complete feed supplied to broiler chickens so that the final feed contains 2 to 4 grams of lincomycin per ton of feed.

For the control of necrotic enteritis: LINCOMIX® 20, 20 grams/lb, should be mixed into the complete feed supplied to broiler chickens so that the final feed contains 2 grams of lincomycin per ton of feed.

Mixing Directions:

Intermediate Premix Amount of LINCOMIX® 20 per 1000 lb (454 kg) of Feed Ingredients	Complete Feed Amount of Intermediate Premix to use to Provide Desired Grams of lincomycin per ton of Type C Medicated Feed		
	lincomycin per ton of feed		
	2 grams	3 grams	4 grams
50 lbs	2 lbs	3 lbs	4 lbs
10 lbs	10 lbs	15 lbs	20 lbs
5 lbs	20 lbs	30 lbs	40 lbs

Swine:

For the treatment of swine dysentery, and the control of porcine proliferative enteropathies (ileitis) caused by *Lawsonia intracellularis:* Feed 100 grams of lincomycin per ton of complete feed as the sole ration for three weeks, or until signs of disease (watery, mucoid, or bloody stools) disappear.

For the treatment and control of swine dysentery, and the control of porcine proliferative enteropathies (ileitis) caused by *Lawsonia intracellularis:* Feed 100 grams of lincomycin per ton of complete feed as the sole ration for three weeks, or until signs of disease (watery, mucoid, or bloody stools) disappear, followed by 40 grams of lincomycin per ton.

For the control of swine dysentery and porcine proliferative enteropathies (ileitis) caused by *Lawsonia intracellularis:* Feed 40 grams of lincomycin per ton of complete feed as the sole ration. For use in animals or on premises with a history of swine dysentery, but where symptoms have not yet occurred.

For reduction in the severity of swine mycoplasmal pneumonia: Feed 200 grams of lincomycin per ton of complete feed as the sole ration for 21 days.

For increase in rate of weight gain in growing-finishing swine: Feed 20 grams of lincomycin per ton of complete feed as the sole ration from weaning to market weight.

Mixing Directions:

Type C Medicated Feeds:

For treatment of swine dysentery and the control of porcine proliferative enteropathies (ileitis) caused by *Lawsonia intracellularis:* To make complete feed containing 100 grams of lincomycin, add 5 lbs of LINCOMIX® 20 per ton.

For control of swine dysentery and porcine proliferative enteropathies (ileitis) caused by *Lawsonia intracellularis:* To make complete feed containing 40 grams of lincomycin, add 2 lbs of LINCOMIX® 20 per ton.

For reduction in the severity of mycoplasmal pneumonia: To make complete feed containing 200 grams of lincomycin, add 10 lbs of LINCOMIX® 20 per ton.

For increase in rate of weight gain in growing-finishing swine: To make complete feed containing 20 grams of lincomycin, add 1 lb of LINCOMIX® 20 per ton.

Precaution(s): Store opened bag in dry place to prevent caking.

Store at room temperature.

Caution(s): Not for use in layers, breeders, or turkeys.

Occasionally, swine fed lincomycin may within the first two days after the onset of treatment develop diarrhea and/or swelling of the anus. On rare occasions, some pigs may show reddening of the skin and irritable behavior. These conditions have been self-correcting within five to eight days without discontinuing the lincomycin treatment. Not to be fed to swine that weigh more than 250 pounds.

Do not allow rabbits, hamsters, guinea pigs, horses, or ruminants access to feeds containing lincomycin. Ingestion by these species may result in severe gastrointestinal effects.

Good Manufacturing Practices should be observed in preparing feeds containing LINCOMIX® 20. This includes appropriate clean-out procedures to avoid cross-contamination.

Restricted Drug—Use only as directed (California).

Warning(s): When using LINCOMIX® 20 in approved combinations with other drugs, follow the required withdrawal times for those drugs. No drug withdrawal period is required before slaughter of birds fed LINCOMIX® 20 at approved concentrations (2 to 4 grams lincomycin per ton of feed).

When using LINCOMIX® in approved combinations with other drugs, follow the required withdrawal times for those drugs. No drug withdrawal period is required before slaughter of swine fed LINCOMIX® at approved concentrations (20, 40, 100 or 200 grams lincomycin per ton of feed).

Not for human use.

Presentation: 50 lb (22.6 kg) (NDC 0009-0494-17).

Made by Pharmacia Animal Health, Orangeville, Ontario, Canada L9W 3T3

Compendium Code No.: 10490262 814 511 310

LINCOMIX® 50 FEED MEDICATION

Pharmacia & Upjohn **Feed Additive**

(Type A Medicated Article) 50 grams/lb

NADA No.: 097-505

Active Ingredient(s): Each pound contains:

Lincomycin (as lincomycin hydrochloride agricultural grade) .... 50 grams

Inactive Ingredients: Soybean hulls, #20 grind; Mineral Oil, USP.

Indications:

Broilers: For increase in rate of weight gain, for improved feed efficiency, and for the control of necrotic enteritis caused or complicated by *Clostridium* spp. or other organisms susceptible to lincomycin in broilers.

Swine: For the treatment and control of swine dysentery, and the control of porcine proliferative enteropathies (ileitis) caused by *Lawsonia intracellularis.* For reduction in the severity of swine mycoplasmal pneumonia caused by *Mycoplasma hyopneumoniae.* For increase in rate of weight gain in growing-finishing swine.

Directions for Use: Important: Must be thoroughly mixed in feeds before use.

Broilers:

For increase in rate of weight gain and improved feed efficiency: LINCOMIX® 50, 50 grams/lb, should be mixed into the complete feed supplied to broiler chickens so that the final feed contains 2 to 4 grams of lincomycin per ton of feed.

For the control of necrotic enteritis: LINCOMIX® 50, 50 grams/lb, should be mixed into the complete feed supplied to broiler chickens so that the final feed contains 2 grams of lincomycin per ton of feed.

Mixing Directions:

Intermediate Premix Amount of LINCOMIX® 50 per 1000 lb (454 kg) of Feed Ingredients	Complete Feed Amount of Intermediate Premix to use to Provide Desired Grams of lincomycin per ton of Type C Medicated Feed		
	lincomycin per ton of feed		
	2 grams	3 grams	4 grams
20 lbs	2 lbs	3 lbs	4 lbs
4 lbs	10 lbs	15 lbs	20 lbs
2 lbs	20 lbs	30 lbs	40 lbs

Swine:

For the treatment of swine dysentery, and the control of porcine proliferative enteropathies (ileitis) caused by *Lawsonia intracellularis:* Feed 100 grams of lincomycin per ton of complete feed as the sole ration for three weeks, or until signs of disease (watery, mucoid, or bloody stools) disappear.

For the treatment and control of swine dysentery, and the control of porcine proliferative enteropathies (ileitis) caused by *Lawsonia intracellularis:* Feed 100 grams of lincomycin per ton of complete feed as the sole ration for three weeks, or until signs of disease (watery, mucoid, or bloody stools) disappear, followed by 40 grams of lincomycin per ton.

For the control of swine dysentery and porcine proliferative enteropathies (ileitis) caused by *Lawsonia intracellularis:* Feed 40 grams of lincomycin per ton of complete feed as the sole ration. For use in animals or on premises with a history of swine dysentery, but where symptoms have not yet occurred.

For reduction in the severity of swine mycoplasmal pneumonia: Feed 200 grams of lincomycin per ton of complete feed as the sole ration for 21 days.

For increase in rate of weight gain in growing-finishing swine: Feed 20 grams of lincomycin per ton of complete feed as the sole ration from weaning to market weight.

Mixing Directions:

Type C Medicated Feeds:

For treatment of swine dysentery, and the control of porcine proliferative enteropathies (ileitis) caused by *Lawsonia intracellularis:* To make complete feed containing 100 grams of lincomycin, add 2 lbs of LINCOMIX® 50 per ton.

For control of swine dysentery and porcine proliferative enteropathies (ileitis) caused by *Lawsonia intracellularis:* To make complete feed containing 40 grams of lincomycin, add 0.8 lbs of LINCOMIX® 50 per ton.

For reduction in the severity of mycoplasmal pneumonia: To make complete feed containing 200 grams of lincomycin, add 4 lbs of LINCOMIX® 50 per ton.

For increase in rate of weight gain in growing-finishing swine: To make complete feed containing 20 grams of lincomycin, add 0.4 lbs of LINCOMIX® 50 per ton.

L

Additional mixing directions to make complete feed containing 20 or 40 grams of lincomycin per ton are provided below:

Intermediate Premix Amount of LINCOMIX® 50 per 1000 lb (454 g) of Feed Ingredients	Complete Feed Amount of Intermediate Premix to use to Provide Desired Grams of lincomycin per ton of Type C Medicated Feed	
	lincomycin per ton of feed	
	20 grams	40 grams
50 lbs	8 lbs	16 lbs
40 lbs	10 lbs	20 lbs
20 lbs	20 lbs	40 lbs

Precaution(s): Store opened bag in dry place to prevent caking.

Store at room temperature.

Caution(s): Not for use in layers, breeders, or turkeys.

Occasionally, swine fed lincomycin may within the first two days after the onset of treatment develop diarrhea and/or swelling of the anus. On rare occasions, some pigs may show reddening of the skin and irritable behavior. These conditions have been self-correcting within five to eight days without discontinuing the lincomycin treatment. Not to be fed to swine that weigh more than 250 pounds.

Do not allow rabbits, hamsters, guinea pigs, horses, or ruminants access to feeds containing lincomycin. Ingestion by these species may result in severe gastrointestinal effects.

Good Manufacturing Practices should be observed in preparing feeds containing LINCOMIX® 50. This includes appropriate clean-out procedures to avoid cross contamination.

Restricted Drug—Use only as directed (California).

Warning(s): When using LINCOMIX® 50 in approved combinations with other drugs, follow the required withdrawal times for those drugs. No drug withdrawal period is required before slaughter of birds fed LINCOMIX® 50 at approved concentrations (2 to 4 grams lincomycin per ton of feed).

When using LINCOMIX® 50 in approved combinations with other drugs, follow the required withdrawal times for those drugs. No drug withdrawal period is required before slaughter of swine fed LINCOMIX® 50 at approved concentrations (20, 40, 100 or 200 grams lincomycin per ton of feed).

Not for human use.

Presentation: 50 lb (22.6 kg) (NDC 0009-0487-05).

Made by Pharmacia Animal Health, Orangeville, Ontario, Canada L9W 3T3

Compendium Code No.: 10490272 810 731 718

LINCOMIX® INJECTABLE

Pharmacia & Upjohn **Lincomycin**

brand of lincomycin hydrochloride, USP

NADA No.: 034-025

Active Ingredient(s): LINCOMIX® Injectable contains lincomycin hydrochloride, an antibiotic produced by *Streptomyces lincolnensis var. lincolnensis*, which is chemically distinct from all other clinically available antibiotics and is isolated as a white crystalline solid.

L

LINCOMIX® Injectable is available in three concentrations: 300 mg/mL, 100 mg/mL, and 25 mg/mL.

300 mg/mL: For use in swine weighing 300 pounds or more. Each mL contains lincomycin hydrochloride equivalent to lincomycin, 300 mg; also benzyl alcohol, 9.45 mg added as preservative.

100 mg/mL: Each mL contains lincomycin hydrochloride equivalent to lincomycin, 100 mg; also benzyl alcohol, 9.45 mg added as preservative.

25 mg/mL: Special baby pig concentration. Each mL contains lincomycin hydrochloride equivalent to lincomycin, 25 mg; also benzyl alcohol, 9.45 mg added as preservative.

Indications: LINCOMIX® Injectable is indicated for the treatment of infectious forms of arthritis caused by organisms sensitive to its activity. This includes most of the organisms responsible for the various infectious arthritides in swine, such as the staphylococci, streptococci, *Erysipelothrix* and *Mycoplasma* spp.

It is also indicated for the treatment of mycoplasma pneumonia.

Dosage and Administration: For arthritis or mycoplasma pneumonia - 5 mg per pound of body weight intramuscularly once daily for three to seven days as needed. When using LINCOMIX® Injectable containing 25 mg/mL, 1 mL/5 lb body weight will provide 5 mg/lb. When using LINCOMIX® Injectable containing 100 mg/mL, 1 mL/20 lb body weight will provide 5 mg/lb. When using LINCOMIX® Injectable containing 300 mg/mL, 1 mL/60 lb body weight will provide 5 mg/lb.

For optimal results, initiate treatment as soon as possible.

As with any multi-dose vial, practice aseptic techniques in withdrawing each dose. Adequately clean and disinfect the vial closure prior to entry with a sterile needle and syringe. No vial closure should be entered more than 20 times.

Contraindication(s): As with all drugs, the use of LINCOMIX® Injectable is contraindicated in animals previously found to be hypersensitive to the drug.

Precaution(s): Store at controlled room temperature 20° to 25°C (68° to 77°F) [see USP].

Caution(s): If no improvement is noted within 48 hours, consult a veterinarian.

Not for human use.

For intramuscular use in swine only.

Warning(s): Swine intended for human consumption should not be slaughtered within 48 hours of latest treatment.

Adverse Reactions: The intramuscular administration to swine may cause a transient diarrhea or loose stools. Although this effect has rarely been reported, one must be alert to the possibility that it may occur.

Should this occur, it is important that the necessary steps be taken to prevent the effects of dehydration.

Presentation: Supplied in 100 mL vials (NDC 0009-0617-13, 0009-3072-06, 0009-3256-01).

Compendium Code No.: 10490280 810 601 211

LINCOMIX® SOLUBLE POWDER

Pharmacia & Upjohn **Water Medication**

Lincomycin hydrochloride (agricultural grade) soluble powder-Antibacterial

NADA No.: 111-636

Active Ingredient(s): Each 40 g packet contains as active ingredient:

Lincomycin hydrochloride, equivalent to lincomycin .... 16 grams

Each 80 g packet contains as active ingredient:

Lincomycin hydrochloride, equivalent to lincomycin .... 32 grams

Indications:

Swine: LINCOMIX® Soluble Powder is indicated for the treatment of swine dysentery (bloody scours).

Broiler Chickens: LINCOMIX® Soluble Powder is indicated for the control of necrotic enteritis caused by *Clostridium perfringens* susceptible to lincomycin.

Dosage and Administration:

Swine:

Dosage: Administer at a dose rate of 250 mg of lincomycin per gallon of drinking water. In clinical studies, this dose rate provided an average of 3.8 mg of lincomycin per pound of body weight per day.

Treatment Period: The drug should be administered for a minimum of 5 consecutive days beyond the disappearance of symptoms (bloody stools) up to a maximum of 10 consecutive days. If water treatment is discontinued prior to this time, a lincomycin treatment program may be continued with lincomycin premix at 100 grams lincomycin per ton of complete feed as the sole ration according to label directions.

Administration: Each 40 g packet will medicate 64 gallons of drinking water providing 250 mg/gallon and each 80 g packet will mediation 128 gallons of drinking water providing 250 mg/gallon. A dose of 3.8 mg lincomycin per pound of body weight may be maintained by medicating the drinking water at a concentration of 250 mg per gallon of drinking water when pigs are consuming 1.5 gallons per 100 lbs of body weight per day. Under these circumstances the concentration of lincomycin required in medicated water may be adjusted to compensate for variations in age and weight of animals, the nature and severity of disease symptoms, environmental temperature and humidity, each of which affects water consumption.

For use in automatic water proportioners, prepare the stock solution by dissolving two packets in one gallon of water: then adjust the proportioner to deliver 1 ounce of stock solution per gallon of drinking water.

Note: After a treatment program is discontinued, a control program for swine dysentery may be followed by feeding lincomycin premix at 40 grams lincomycin per ton of complete feed as the sole ration.

Broiler Chickens:

Dosage: Administer at a dose rate of 64 mg of lincomycin per gallon of drinking water.

Treatment Period: Start medication as soon as the diagnosis of necrotic enteritis is determined. If improvement is not noted within 24 to 48 hours, consult a licensed veterinarian or veterinary diagnostic laboratory to determine diagnosis. The drug should be administered for 7 consecutive days.

Administration: Each 40 g packet will medicate 250 gallons of drinking water providing 64 mg/gallon and each 80 g packet will medicate 500 gallons of drinking water providing 64 mg/gallon.

Note: After water medication is discontinued, a control program for necrotic enteritis may be followed by feeding lincomycin premix at 2 grams lincomycin per ton of complete feed.

Precaution(s): Store at controlled room temperature 20° to 25°C (68° to 77°F) [see USP].

Caution(s): For oral use in swine and broiler chickens only.

Restricted Drug—Use only as directed (California).

1. Discard medicated drinking water if not used within 2 days. Fresh stock solution should be prepared daily. 2. If clinical signs of bloody scours (watery, mucoid or bloody stools) have not improved during the first 6 days of medication, discontinue treatment and redetermine the diagnosis. 3. Occasionally, swine fed lincomycin may within the first two days after the onset of treatment develop diarrhea and/or swelling of the anus. On rare occasions, some pigs may show reddening of the skin and irritable behavior. These conditions have been self-correcting within five to eight days without discontinuing the lincomycin treatment. 4. Not for use in swine weighing more than 250 pounds. 5. Do not allow rabbits, hamsters, guinea pigs, horses, or ruminants access to water containing lincomycin. Ingestion by these species may result in severe gastrointestinal effects. 6. Do not use the water treatment and the feed treatment simultaneously. 7. Not for use in layer and breeder chickens.

Warning(s):

1. No drug withdrawal period is required before slaughter of swine receiving LINCOMIX® Soluble Powder at the approved level of 250 mg per gallon of drinking water, nor before slaughter of birds receiving LINCOMIX® Soluble Powder at the approved level of 64 mg per gallon of drinking water.
2. Not for human use.

Presentation: 48-40 g (1.4 oz) (NDC 0009-0962-13) and 24-80 g (2.8 oz) (NDC 0009-0962-18) packets per pail.

Compendium Code No.: 10490291 815 935 103 / 814 632 207

LINCOMYCIN HYDROCHLORIDE SOLUBLE POWDER

Durvet **Water Medication**

Antibacterial

NADA No.: 111-636

Active Ingredient(s): The 80 g packet contains as active ingredient:

Lincomycin hydrochloride (agricultural grade), equivalent to lincomycin .... 32 grams

Indications:

Swine: LINCOMYCIN HYDROCHLORIDE SOLUBLE POWDER is indicated for the treatment of swine dysentery (bloody scours).

Broiler Chickens: LINCOMYCIN HYDROCHLORIDE SOLUBLE POWDER is indicated for the control of necrotic enteritis caused by *Clostridium perfringens* susceptible to lincomycin.

Directions for Use:

Swine:

Dosage: Administer at a dose rate of 250 mg of lincomycin per gallon of drinking water. In clinical studies, this dose rate provided an average of 3.8 mg of lincomycin per pound of body weight per day.

Treatment Period: The drug should be administered for a minimum of 5 consecutive days beyond the disappearance of symptoms (bloody stools) up to a maximum of 10 consecutive days. If water treatment is discontinued prior to this time, a lincomycin treatment program may be continued with lincomycin premix at 100 grams lincomycin per ton of complete feed as the sole ration according to label directions.

Administration: This packet will medicate 128 gallons of drinking water providing 250 mg/gallon. A dose of 3.8 mg lincomycin per pound of body weight may be maintained by medicating the drinking water at a concentration of 250 mg per gallon of drinking water when pigs are consuming 1.5 gallons per 100 lbs of body weight per day. Under these circumstances, the concentration of lincomycin required in medicated water may be adjusted to compensate for variations in age and weight of animals, the nature and severity of disease symptoms, environmental temperature and humidity, each of which affects water consumption.

For use in automatic water proportioners, prepare the stock solution by dissolving one packet in one gallon of water: then adjust the proportioner to deliver 1 ounce of stock solution per gallon of drinking water.

Note: After a treatment program is discontinued, a control program for swine dysentery may be followed by feeding lincomycin premix at 40 grams lincomycin per ton of complete feed as the sole ration.

Broiler Chickens:

Dosage: Administer at a dose rate of 64 mg of lincomycin per gallon of drinking water.

Treatment Period: Start medication as soon as the diagnosis of necrotic enteritis is determined. If improvement is not noted within 24 to 48 hours, consult a licensed veterinarian or veterinary diagnostic laboratory to determine diagnosis. The drug should be administered for 7 consecutive days.

Administration: This packet will medicate 500 gallons of drinking water providing 64 mg/gallon.

Note: After water medication is discontinued. a control program for necrotic enteritis may be followed by feeding lincomycin premix at 2 grams lincomycin per ton of complete feed.

Precaution(s): Store at controlled room temperature 20° to 25°C (68° to 77°F) [see USP].

Caution(s): Restricted Drug—Use only as directed (California).

1. Discard medicated drinking water if not used within 2 days. Fresh stock solution should be prepared daily.
2. If clinical signs of bloody scours (watery, mucoid or bloody stools) have not improved during the first 6 days of medication, discontinue treatment and redetermine the diagnosis.
3. Occasionally, swine fed lincomycin may within the first two days after the onset of treatment develop diarrhea and/or swelling of the anus. On rare occasions, some pigs may show reddening of the skin and irritable behavior. These conditions have been self-correcting within five to eight days without discontinuing the lincomycin treatment.
4. Not for use in swine weighing more than 250 pounds.
5. Do not allow rabbits, hamsters, guinea pigs, horses, or ruminants access to water containing lincomycin. Ingestion by these species may result in severe gastrointestinal effects.
6. Do not use the water treatment and the feed treatment simultaneously.
7. Not for use in layer and breeder chickens.

Warning(s): For oral use in swine and broiler chickens only.

1. No drug withdrawal period is required before slaughter of swine receiving LINCOMYCIN HYDROCHLORIDE SOLUBLE POWDER at the approved level of 250 mg per gallon of drinking water, nor before slaughter of birds receiving LINCOMYCIN HYDROCHLORIDE SOLUBLE POWDER at the approved level of 64 mg per gallon of drinking water.
2. Not for human use.

Presentation: 1.41 oz (40 grams) and 2.82 oz (80 grams).

Compendium Code No.: 10841110 817 893 000

LINCOMYCIN SOLUBLE

Alpharma **Water Medication**

Lincomycin Hydrochloride-Antibacterial

ANADA No.: 200-189

Active Ingredient(s): Each 40 g packet contains:

Lincomycin HCl equivalent to lincomycin .... 16 g

Each 80 g packet contains:

Lincomycin HCl equivalent to lincomycin .... 32 g

Indications:

Broiler Chickens: LINCOMYCIN SOLUBLE is indicated for the control of necrotic enteritis caused by *Clostridium perfringens* susceptible to lincomycin.

Swine: LINCOMYCIN SOLUBLE is indicated for the treatment of swine dysentery (bloody scours).

Directions for Use:

Broiler Chickens:

Dosage: Administer at a dose rate of 64 mg of lincomycin per gallon of drinking water.

Treatment Period: Start medication as soon as the diagnosis of necrotic enteritis is determined. If improvement is not noted within 24 to 48 hours, consult a licensed veterinarian or veterinary diagnostic laboratory to determine diagnosis. The drug should be administered for 7 consecutive days.

Administration: The 40 g packet will medicate 250 gallons of drinking water providing 64 mg/gallon.

The 80 g packet will medicate 500 gallons of drinking water providing 64 mg/gallon.

Note: After water medication is discontinued, a recommended control program for necrotic enteritis consists of feeding lincomycin premix at 2 g lincomycin per ton of complete feed.

Swine:

Dosage: Administer at a dose rate of 250 mg of lincomycin per gallon of drinking water. In clinical studies, this dose rate provided an average of 3.8 mg of lincomycin per lb of body weight per day.

Treatment Period: The drug should be administered for a minimum of 5 consecutive days beyond the disappearance of symptoms (bloody stools) up to a maximum of 10 consecutive days. If water treatment is discontinued prior to this time, a lincomycin treatment program may be continued with lincomycin premix at 100 grams lincomycin per ton of complete feed as the sole ration according to label directions.

Administration: The 40 g packet will medicate 64 gallons of drinking water providing 250 mg/gallon.

The 80 g packet will medicate 128 gallons of drinking water providing 250 mg/gallon.

A dose of 3.8 mg lincomycin per lb of body weight may be maintained by medicating the drinking water at a concentration of 250 mg per gallon of drinking water when pigs are consuming 1.5 gallons per 100 lbs of body weight per day. Under these circumstances the concentration of lincomycin required in medicated water may be adjusted to compensate for variations in age and weight of animals, the nature and severity of disease symptoms, environmental temperature and humidity, each of which affects water consumption. For use in automatic water proportioners, prepare the stock solution by dissolving two 40 g packets or one 80 g packet in one gallon of water; then adjust the proportioner to deliver 1 oz of stock solution per gallon of drinking water.

Note: After a treatment program is discontinued, a control program for swine dysentery may be followed by feeding lincomycin premix at 40 g lincomycin per ton of complete feed as the sole ration.

Precaution(s): Store below 86°F (30°C).

Caution(s):

1. Discard medicated drinking water if not used within 2 days. Fresh stock solution should be prepared daily.
2. If clinical signs of bloody scours (water, mucoid or bloody stools) have not improved during the first 6 days of medication, discontinue treatment and redetermine the diagnosis.
3. Occasionally, swine fed lincomycin may within the first 2 days after the onset of treatment develop diarrhea and/or swelling of the anus. On rare occasions, some pigs may show reddening of the skin and irritable behavior. These conditions have been self-correcting within 5 to 8 days without discontinuing the lincomycin treatment.
4. Not for use in swine weighing more than 250 pounds.
5. Do not allow rabbits, hamsters, guinea pigs, horses, or ruminants access to water containing lincomycin. Ingestion by these species may result in severe gastrointestinal effects.
6. Do not use the water treatment and the feed treatment simultaneously.

For oral use in swine and broiler chickens only.

Restricted Drug - Use only as directed (CA).

Warning(s):

1. Do not slaughter swine for human consumption for 6 days following last treatment.
2. No drug withdrawal period is required before slaughter of birds receiving LINCOMYCIN SOLUBLE at the approved level of 64 mg per gallon of drinking water.
3. Not for human use.

Not for use in layer and breeder chickens.

Keep out of reach of children.

Presentation: 1.41 oz (40 gram) and 2.82 oz (80 gram) packets.

Compendium Code No.: 10220422 AHF-023 0107 / AHF-055 0107

LINCOMYCIN SOLUBLE POWDER

AgriLabs **Water Medication**

lincomycin hydrochloride soluble powder-Antibacterial

NADA No.: 111-636

Active Ingredient(s): Each 40 g packet contains as active ingredient:

Lincomycin hydrochloride, equivalent to lincomycin (agricultural grade) .... 16 g

Each 80 g packet contains as active ingredient:

Lincomycin hydrochloride, equivalent to lincomycin (agricultural grade) .... 32 g

Indications:

Swine: Lincomycin hydrochloride soluble powder is indicated for the treatment of swine dysentery (bloody scours).

Broiler Chickens: Lincomycin hydrochloride soluble powder is indicated for the control of necrotic enteritis caused by *Clostridium perfringens* susceptible to lincomycin.

Directions for Use:

Swine:

Dosage: Administer at a dose rate of 250 mg of lincomycin per gallon of drinking water. In clinical studies, this dose rate provided an average of 3.8 mg of lincomycin per pound of body weight per day.

Treatment Period: The drug should be administered for a minimum of 5 consecutive days beyond the disappearance of symptoms (bloody stools) up to a maximum of 10 consecutive days. If water treatment is discontinued prior to this time, a lincomycin treatment program may be continued with lincomycin premix at 100 grams lincomycin per ton of complete feed as the sole ration according to label directions.

Administration: Each 40 g packet will medicate 64 gallons of drinking water providing 250 mg/gallon and each 80 g packet will mediation 128 gallons of drinking water providing 250 mg/gallon. A dose of 3.8 mg lincomycin per pound of body weight may be maintained by medicating the drinking water at a concentration of 250 mg per gallon of drinking water when pigs are consuming 1.5 gallons per 100 lbs of body weight per day. Under these circumstances the concentration of lincomycin required in medicated water may be adjusted to compensate for variations in age and weight of animals, the nature and severity of disease symptoms, environmental temperature and humidity, each of which affects water consumption.

For use in automatic water proportioners, prepare the stock solution by dissolving two packets in one gallon of water: then adjust the proportioner to deliver 1 ounce of stock solution per gallon of drinking water.

Note: After a treatment program is discontinued, a control program for swine dysentery may be followed by feeding lincomycin premix at 40 grams lincomycin per ton of complete feed as the sole ration.

Broiler Chickens:

Dosage: Administer at a dose rate of 64 mg of lincomycin per gallon of drinking water.

Treatment Period: Start medication as soon as the diagnosis of necrotic enteritis is determined. If improvement is not noted within 24 to 48 hours, consult a licensed veterinarian or veterinary diagnostic laboratory to determine diagnosis. The drug should be administered for 7 consecutive days.

Administration: Each 40 g packet will medicate 250 gallons of drinking water providing 64 mg/gallon and each 80 g packet will medicate 500 gallons of drinking water providing 64 mg/gallon.

Note: After water medication is discontinued, a control program for necrotic enteritis may be followed by feeding lincomycin premix at 2 grams lincomycin per ton of complete feed.

Precaution(s): Store at controlled room temperature 20° to 25°C (68° to 77°F) [see USP].

Caution(s): 1. Discard medicated drinking water if not used within 2 days. Fresh stock solution should be prepared daily. 2. If clinical signs of bloody scours (watery, mucoid or bloody stools) have not improved during the first 6 days of medication, discontinue treatment and redetermine the diagnosis. 3. Occasionally, swine fed lincomycin may within the first two days after the onset of treatment develop diarrhea and/or swelling of the anus. On rare occasions, some pigs may show reddening of the skin and irritable behavior. These conditions have been self-correcting within five to eight days without discontinuing the lincomycin treatment. 4. Not for use in swine weighing more than 250 pounds. 5. Do not allow rabbits, hamsters, guinea pigs, horses, or ruminants access to water containing lincomycin. Ingestion by these species may result in severe gastrointestinal effects. 6. Do not use the water treatment and the feed treatment simultaneously. 7. Not for use in layer and breeder chickens.

For oral use in swine and broiler chickens only.

Restricted Drug—Use only as directed (California).

Warning(s):

1. No drug withdrawal period is required before slaughter of swine receiving lincomycin hydrochloride soluble powder at the approved level of 250 mg per gallon of drinking water, nor before slaughter of birds receiving lincomycin hydrochloride soluble powder at the approved level of 64 mg per gallon of drinking water.
2. Not for human use.

Presentation: 1.41 oz (40 g) and 2.82 oz (80 g) packets.

Compendium Code No.: 10581310 817 858 000

LINCOSOL SOLUBLE POWDER

Med-Pharmex **Water Medication**

Brand of lincomycin hydrochloride soluble powder

ANADA No.: 200-241

Active Ingredient(s): Each gram of powder contains:

Lincomycin hydrochloride equivalent to lincomycin .... 400 mg

The 40 g packet contains as active ingredient:

Lincomycin hydrochloride equivalent to lincomycin .... 16.0 g

The 80 g packet contains as active ingredient:

Lincomycin hydrochloride equivalent to lincomycin .... 32.0 g

Indications:

Swine: LINCOSOL SOLUBLE POWDER is indicated for the treatment of swine dysentery (bloody scours).

Broiler Chickens: LINCOSOL SOLUBLE POWDER is indicated for the control of necrotic enteritis caused by *Clostridium perfringens* susceptible to lincomycin.

Directions for Use: Swine:

Dosage: Administer at a dose rate of 250 mg of lincomycin per gallon of drinking water. In clinical studies, this dose rate provided an average of 3.8 mg of lincomycin per pound of body weight per day.

Treatment Period: The drug should be administered for a minimum of 5 consecutive days beyond the disappearance of symptoms (bloody stools) up to a maximum of 10 consecutive days. If water treatment is discontinued prior to this time, a lincomycin treatment program may be continued with lincomycin premix at 100 grams lincomycin per ton of complete feed as the sole ration according to label directions.

Administration: One scoop (provided) of this powder will medicate 64 gallons of drinking water providing 250 mg/gallon. The 1.41 oz (40 g) packet will medicate 64 gallons of drinking water providing 250 mg/gallon. The 2.82 oz (80 g) packet will medicate 128 gallons of drinking water providing 250 mg/gallon. A dose of 3.8 mg lincomycin per pound of body weight may be maintained by medicating the drinking water at a concentration of 250 mg per gallon of drinking water when pigs are consuming 1.5 gallons per 100 lbs of body weight per day. Under these circumstances the concentration of lincomycin required in medicated water may be adjusted to compensate for variations in age and weight of animals, the nature and severity of disease symptoms, environmental temperature and humidity, each of which affects water consumption.

For use in automatic water proportioners, prepare the stock solution by dissolving two scoops, two 1.41 oz (40 g) packets, or one 2.82 oz (80 g) packet in one gallon of water: then adjust the proportioner to deliver 1 ounce of stock solution per gallon of drinking water.

Note: After a treatment program is discontinued, a control program for swine dysentery may be followed by feeding lincomycin premix at 40 grams lincomycin per ton of complete feed as the sole ration.

Broiler Chickens:

Dosage: Administer at a dose rate of 64 mg of lincomycin per gallon of drinking water.

Treatment Period: Start medication as soon as the diagnosis of necrotic enteritis is determined. If improvement is not noted within 24 to 48 hours, consult a licensed veterinarian or veterinary diagnostic laboratory to determine diagnosis. The drug should be administered for 7 consecutive days.

L

Administration: One scoop (provided) of this powder will medicate 250 gallons of drinking water providing 64 mg/gallon.

The 1.41 oz (40 g) packet will medicate 250 gallons of drinking water providing 64 mg/gallon.

The 2.82 oz (80 g) packet will medicate 500 gallons of drinking water providing 64 mg/gallon.

Note: After water medication is discontinued, a control program for necrotic enteritis may be followed by feeding lincomycin premix at 2 grams lincomycin per ton of complete feed.

Precaution(s): Store at controlled room temperature 15° to 30°C (59° to 86°F).

Caution(s):

1. Discard medicated drinking water if not used within 2 days. Fresh stock solution should be prepared daily.
2. If clinical signs of bloody scours (water, mucoid or bloody stools) have not improved during the first 6 days of medication, discontinue treatment and redetermine the diagnosis.
3. Occasionally, swine fed lincomycin may within the first two days after the onset of treatment develop diarrhea and/or swelling of the anus. On rare occasions, some pigs may show reddening of the skin and irritable behavior. These conditions have been self-correcting within five to eight days without discontinuing the lincomycin treatment.
4. Not for use in swine weighing more than 250 pounds.
5. Do not allow rabbits, hamsters, guinea pigs, horses, or ruminants access to water containing lincomycin. Ingestion by these species may result in severe gastrointestinal effects.
6. Do not use the water treatment and the feed treatment simultaneously.

Warning(s): Do not slaughter swine for human consumption for 6 days following last treatment.

No drug withdrawal period is required before slaughter of birds receiving LINCOSOL SOLUBLE POWDER at the approved level of 64 mg per gallon of drinking water.

Not for use in layer and breeder chickens.

Not for human use.

For oral use in swine and broiler chickens only.

Restricted drug - Use only as directed (California).

Presentation: 1.41 oz (40 g) and 2.82 oz (80 g) packets, and 32 oz (0.907 kg).

Compendium Code No.: 10270050

LINCO-SPECTIN® STERILE SOLUTION

Pharmacia & Upjohn **Lincomycin-Spectinomycin**

Active Ingredient(s): Each mL contains:

Lincomycin hydrochloride, equivalent to lincomycin .... 50 mg

Spectinomycin sulfate tetrahydrate equivalent to spectinomycin .... 100 mg

Also contains:

Benzyl alcohol added as preservative .... 9.45 mg

When necessary, pH was adjusted with sodium hydroxide and/or hydrochloric acid.

Indications: For use in semen extenders.

Precaution(s): Store at room temperature.

Caution(s): For use in semen extenders only.

Not for drug use.

Presentation: 20 mL vials (NDC 0009-0618-01).

Compendium Code No.: 10490211 811 334 504/811 334 604

LINIMENT GEL

First Priority **Liniment**

Ingredient(s): Contains: Camphor, Menthol, Thymol, Witch Hazel, Isopropyl Alcohol in a specially prepared base.

Indications: A topical liniment gel for horses to be used for temporary relief of minor muscle stiffness and soreness due to overexertion.

Directions for Use: LINIMENT GEL may be used concentrated or diluted depending on the condition. It will not burn or blister.

For horses in training: Use before and after workouts, under bandages, either wet or dry.

In shipping horses: Apply on legs and use a cotton bandage.

Method of Use: Be certain skin and hair are clean. It is advised that the area to be treated be washed first. Apply by rubbing deeply into hair in the first application, assuring contact with the skin. Following first application, apply a generous amount for the second application. Use as often as indicated.

For using as a diluted application the indications are: Use after strenuous exercise for any type of performance animal.

Use as a therapeutic bodywash when a coolant is indicated.

Directions for Using: Mix 2 tablespoons of LINIMENT GEL to a quart of warm water. Apply with a sponge, covering the horse's entire body. Use a brisk rubbing motion when applying. Guard against creating heat or irritation by overrubbing.

Precaution(s): It is important to keep the cap on tight, thereby avoiding evaporation.

Store in a cool, dry area. Do not store near heat.

Caution(s): Do not apply any other type of external medicants to the same area where LINIMENT GEL has been administered.

Avoid contact with eyes and mucous membranes. If the condition for which this preparation is used persists, or if a rash develops, discontinue use and consult your veterinarian.

Warning(s): Not for use on food producing animals.

Keep out of reach of children.

Presentation: 1 lb (453.6 g) (NDC# 58829-170-16).

Compendium Code No.: 11390461 Rev. 04-02

LINIMENT GEL WITH BENZOCAINE

First Priority **Liniment**

Ingredient(s): Benzocaine, Camphor, Menthol, Thymol, Witch Hazel, Isopropyl Alcohol in a specially prepared base.

Indications: A topical anesthetic, LINIMENT GEL WITH BENZOCAINE is to be used for temporary relief of minor muscle stiffness and soreness due to overexertion.

Directions for Use: LINIMENT GEL WITH BENZOCAINE may be used concentrated or diluted depending on the condition. It will not burn or blister.

Be certain skin and hair are clean. It is advised that the area to be treated be washed first. Apply by rubbing deeply into hair in the first application, assuring contact with the skin. Following first application, apply a generous amount for the second application. Use as often as indicated.

Dilution: Use after strenuous exercise for any type of performance animal. Use as a therapeutic bodywash when a coolant is indicated. Mix 2 tablespoons of LINIMENT GEL WITH BENZOCAINE to a quart of warm water. Apply with a sponge, covering the horse's entire body. Use a brisk rubbing motion when applying. Guard against creating heat or irritation by over-rubbing.

For horses in training: Use before and after workouts, under bandages, either wet or dry.

In shipping horses: Apply on legs and use a cotton bandage. LINIMENT GEL WITH BENZOCAINE will not burn or blister under bandages.

Contraindication(s): Racetracks: When saliva and urine tests are to be conducted, do not administer before or after racing as horses may pick up components by licking and the ingredients may show up in testing.

Precaution(s): Storage: Store at controlled room temperature between 15°-30°C (59°-86°F). Keep container tightly closed when not in use. It is important to keep the cap on tight, thereby avoiding evaporation. Store in a cool, dry area. Do not store near heat.

Caution(s): Do not apply any other type of external medicants to the same area where LINIMENT GEL WITH BENZOCAINE has been administered.

Avoid contact with eyes and mucous membranes. If the condition for which this preparation is used persists, or if a rash develops, discontinue use and consult your veterinarian.

For animal use only.

Warning(s): Not for use on food producing animals.

Keep out of reach of children.

Presentation: 4 oz (113.3 g) (NDC# 58829-171-04) and 1 lb (453.6 g) (NDC# 58829-171-16).

Compendium Code No.: 11390472 Rev. 06-99 / Rev. 08-01

LIN-O-GEL®

Hawthorne **Liniment**

Active Ingredient(s): Each 16 U.S. oz contains:

Alcohol .... 60.0 g

Camphor .... 4.8 g

Menthol .... 3.7 g

Iodine .... 3.7 g

and essential oils.

Indications: For aid in the temporary relief of minor stiffness and soreness caused by over-exertion.

Dosage and Administration: Apply freely to leg. Rub against and with hair. Next apply with hair only. Wrap with paper towel and bandage. Leave on leg 48 to 72 hours. Repeat if necessary. Leave LIN-O-GEL® on leg while working or walking. Remove with warm water.

Precaution(s): Keep in a cool, dry place.

Caution(s): Keep away from children. Consult veterinarian if condition persists.

Warning(s): Do not use on food animals.

Presentation: 16 U.S. oz.

Compendium Code No.: 10670070

LIPOCAPS

Vetus **Small Animal Dietary Supplement**

NDC No.: 47611-600-10

Active Ingredient(s): Each capsule provides:

Choline bitartrate ... 240 mg
Racemethionine ... 110 mg
Inositol ... 83 mg
Vitamin B_1 (thiamine mononitrate) ... 3 mg
Vitamin B_2 (riboflavin) ... 3 mg
Vitamin B_6 (pyridoxine HCl) ... 2 mg
Vitamin B_{12} (cobalamin concentrate) ... 2 mcg
Niacinamide ... 10 mg
Dexpanthenol ... 2 mg
Desiccated liver concentrate ... 86 mg

Indications: For use in dogs and cats to support the metabolism of fat in the liver, as a nutritional support in the detoxification of metabolic wastes, and to increase the solubility and emulsification of fats so that they may be carried in the blood.

Dosage and Administration: Give one (1) capsule per 20 lbs. of body weight per day to dogs and cats, or as directed by a veterinarian.

The capsules may be opened to disperse the contents onto the food if desired.

Precaution(s): To preserve the quality and freshness, keep the bottle tightly closed. Store in a cool, dry place between 59°F-86°F (15°C-30°C).

Caution(s): For veterinary use only. Keep out of the reach of children.

Presentation: Bottles of 1,000 capsules.

Compendium Code No.: 14440580

LIPO-FORM

Vet-A-Mix **Small Animal Dietary Supplement**

Tasty chewable lipotropic and vitamin supplement for dogs

Guaranteed Analysis: per Tablet:

(All Values are minimum quantities unless otherwise stated).

Vitamins and Others:

Choline chloride ... 125 mg
DL-Methionine ... 100 mg
Niacin ... 10 mg
Vitamin E ... 10 IU
D-Pantothenic acid ... 0.25 mg
Riboflavin ... 0.22 mg
Pyridoxine hydrochloride ... 0.11 mg
Thiamine mononitrate ... 0.1 mg
Folic acid ... 22. mcg
Vitamin B_{12} ... 3.5 mcg

Ingredients: Brewer's dried yeast, Extracted glandular meal (pork), Choline chloride, Lactose, DL-methionine, Glycerin, Starch, Soybean flour, Animal liver meal (pork), Silicon dioxide, Gelatin, Inositol, Cod liver oil, DL-alpha tocopheryl acetate, Niacin, Vitamin B_{12} supplement, Thiamine mononitrate, Pantothenic acid, Riboflavin, Pyridoxine hydrochloride, Folic acid.

Indications: Use as a supplementary dietary source of the lipotropic factors: choline and methionine in the canine.

Dosage and Administration: Feed free choice, from the hand or crumble and mix into the food. The usual daily dose is 1 to 2 tablets per 10 kilograms (22 pounds) of body weight.

Precaution(s): Store at room temperature. Protect from light. Avoid excessive heat (40°C or 104°F).

Caution(s): Avoid prolonged excessive dosage administration. In rare cases animals may experience gastrointestinal irritation. In the event of stomach upset, administer tablets during or after feeding.

Warning(s): Keep out of reach of children.

Presentation: Bottles of 50 and 500 tablets.

Compendium Code No.: 10500131 0499

LIPOGEN FORTE™

Novartis (Aqua Health) **Bacterin**

Aeromonas salmonicida-Vibrio anguillarum-ordalii-salmonicida Bacterin

U.S. Vet. Lic. No.: 335

Contents: Contains formalin inactivated cultures of *Aeromonas salmonicida, Vibrio anguillarum* Types 1 and 2, *Vibrio ordalii* and *Vibrio salmonicida* 1 and 2 in liquid emulsion with an oil-based adjuvant.

Indications: Uses: As an aid in the prevention of furunculosis, vibriosis and cold water vibriosis by injection of healthy salmonids.

Dosage and Administration: Vaccination Program: This bacterin has been shown to be safe and effective when administered by manual intraperitoneal injection to salmonids 10 g or larger. Vaccination should precede exposure of vaccinates to the disease agent by 400 degree-days (number of days multiplied by the mean water temperature (°C) during period).

Fish are anesthetized to immobilize and given a 0.1 mL injection intraperitoneally one fin length ahead of the pelvic fins along the midline. Warming of the vaccine by leaving at room temperature overnight (15-20°C) may facilitate injection.

Precaution(s): Shake well before using. Store between 2-7°C (35-45°F). Do not freeze. Use entire contents when first opened.

Caution(s): Vaccinate healthy fish only. If accidental injection of the operator occurs, the operator should discontinue activity and seek medical advice immediately. For veterinary use only.

Warning(s): Do not vaccinate within 60 days of slaughter.

Presentation: 750 mL and 1000 mL bags.

Distributed by: Mr. J. Zinn, Buhl, Idaho 83316

Compendium Code No.: 14970062 L-029-1 / L-029-1.1

LIPOGEN TRIPLE

Novartis (Aqua Health) **Bacterin**

Aeromonas Salmonicida-Vibrio Anguillarum-Ordalii-Salmonicida Bacterin

U.S. Vet. Lic. No.: 335

Contents: Contains only formalin inactivated cultures of *Aeromonas salmonicida, Vibrio anguillarum, Vibrio ordalii* and *Vibrio salmonicida* in liquid emulsion with an oil-based adjuvant.

Indications: As an aid to the prevention of Furunculosis, Vibriosis and Cold Water Vibriosis by injection of healthy salmonids.

Dosage and Administration: Shake well before using.

Vaccination Program: This bacterin has been shown to be safe and effective when administered by manual intraperitoneal injection to Atlantic salmon 10 g or larger. Vaccination should precede exposure of vaccinates to the disease agent by 400 degree-days (number of days multiplied by the mean water temperature (°C) during period).

Fish are anesthetized to immobilize and given a 0.2 mL injection intraperitoneally. Warming of the vaccine to 15-20°C may facilitate injection.

Precaution(s): Store between 2-7°C (35-45°F). Do not freeze.

Caution(s): Use entire contents when first opened.

Vaccinate healthy fish only.

Warning(s): Do not vaccinate within 60 days of slaughter.

If accidental injection of the operator occurs, the operator should discontinue activity and seek medical advice immediately.

For veterinary use only.

Presentation: 1000 mL bags.

Distributed by: Mr. J. Zinn, Buhl, Idaho 83316

Compendium Code No.: 14970071

LIPOTINIC

Vet-A-Mix **Large Animal Dietary Supplement**

Active Ingredient(s): Each bolus contains:

Niacin ... 6,000 mg
Thiamine mononitrate ... 250 mg
Riboflavin ... 250 mg
Pyridoxine hydrochloride ... 100 mg
Vitamin B_{12} ... 100 mcg

Ingredients: Nicotinic acid, thiamine mononitrate, riboflavin, pyridoxine hydrochloride, vitamin B_{12} supplement, dextrin, starch, lactose, modified cellulose, magnesium stearate, artificial coloring.

Indications: For use as a niacin and B vitamin supplement in lactating dairy cattle.

Dosage and Administration: Administer one (1) bolus in the morning and one (1) bolus in the evening for 10 consecutive days to high producing dairy cows when supplementation of nicotinic acid (niacin) is required.

It is recommended that all high producing dairy cows receive two (2) boluses per day for 10 days starting the day before freshening.

LIPOTINIC boluses may be given with a balling gun or broken and mixed into the feed.

Presentation: Bottles of 20 boluses.

Compendium Code No.: 10500140

LIQUAMYCIN® LA-200®

Pfizer Animal Health **Oxytetracycline Injection**

(oxytetracycline injection) Antibiotic

NADA No.: 113-232

Active Ingredient(s): Each mL contains 200 mg of oxytetracycline base as oxytetracycline dihydrate.

Indications: LIQUAMYCIN® LA-200® is intended for use in the treatment of the following diseases in beef cattle; dairy cattle; calves, including preruminating (veal) calves; and swine when due to oxytetracycline-susceptible organisms:

Cattle: LIQUAMYCIN® LA-200® is indicated in the treatment of pneumonia and shipping fever complex associated with *Pasteurella* spp. and *Hemophilus* spp.; infectious bovine keratoconjunctivitis (pinkeye) caused by *Moraxella bovis;* foot rot and diphtheria caused by *Fusobacterium necrophorum;* bacterial enteritis (scours) caused by *Escherichia coli;* wooden tongue caused by *Actinobacillus lignieresii;* leptospirosis caused by *Leptospira pomona;* and wound infections and acute metritis caused by strains of staphylococci and streptococci organisms sensitive to oxytetracycline.

Swine: LIQUAMYCIN® LA-200® is indicated in the treatment of bacterial enteritis (scours, colibacillosis) caused by *Escherichia coli;* pneumonia caused by *Pasteurella multocida;* and leptospirosis caused by *Leptospira pomona.*

In sows, LIQUAMYCIN® LA-200® is indicated as an aid in the control of infectious enteritis (baby pig scours, colibacillosis) in suckling pigs caused by *Escherichia coli.*

Dosage and Administration: Read entire package insert carefully before using this product.

Dosage:

Cattle: LIQUAMYCIN® LA-200® is to be administered by subcutaneous (SC, under the skin), or intravenous injection according to Beef Quality Assurance Guidelines.

A single dosage of 9 mg of LIQUAMYCIN® LA-200® per lb of body weight administered subcutaneously is recommended in the treatment of the following conditions: 1) bacterial pneumonia caused by *Pasteurella* spp. (shipping fever) in calves and yearlings, where retreatment is impractical due to husbandry conditions, such as cattle on range, or where their repeated restraint is inadvisable; 2) infectious bovine keratoconjunctivitis (pinkeye) caused by *Moraxella bovis.*

LIQUAMYCIN® LA-200® can also be administered by subcutaneous or intravenous injection at a level of 3-5 mg of oxytetracycline per lb of body weight per day. In the treatment of severe foot rot and advanced cases of other indicated diseases, a dosage level of 5 mg/lb of body weight per day is recommended. Treatment should be continued 24-48 hours following remission of disease signs; however, not to exceed a total of 4 consecutive days. Consult your veterinarian if improvement is not noted within 24-48 hours of the beginning of treatment.

Swine: A single dose of 9 mg of LIQUAMYCIN® LA-200® per lb of body weight administered intramuscularly in the neck region is recommended in the treatment of bacterial pneumonia caused by *Pasteurella multocida* in swine, where retreatment is impractical due to husbandry conditions or where repeated restraint is inadvisable.

LIQUAMYCIN® LA-200® can also be administered by intramuscular injection at a level of 3-5 mg of oxytetracycline per lb of body weight per day. Treatment should be continued 24-48 hours following remission of disease signs; however, not to exceed a total of 4 consecutive days. Consult your veterinarian if improvement is not noted within 24-48 hours of the beginning of treatment.

For sows, administer once intramuscularly in the neck region 3 mg of oxytetracycline per lb of body weight approximately 8 hours before farrowing or immediately after completion of farrowing.

For swine weighing 25 lb of body weight and under, LIQUAMYCIN® LA-200® should be administered undiluted for treatment at 9 mg/lb but should be administered diluted for treatment at 3 or 5 mg/lb.

Body Weight	9 mg/lb Dosage Volume of Undiluted LIQUAMYCIN® LA-200®	3 or 5 mg/lb Dosage Volume of Diluted LIQUAMYCIN® LA-200®		
	9 mg/lb	3 mg/lb	Dilution*	5 mg/lb
5 lb	0.2 mL	0.6 mL	1:7	1.0 mL
10 lb	0.5 mL	0.9 mL	1:5	1.5 mL
25 lb	1.1 mL	1.5 mL	1:3	2.5 mL

* To prepare dilutions, add 1 one part LIQUAMYCIN® LA-200® to 3, 5, or 7 parts of sterile water, or 5% dextrose solution as indicated; the diluted product should be used immediately.

Directions for Use: LIQUAMYCIN® LA-200® is intended for use in the treatment of disease due to oxytetracycline-susceptible organisms in beef cattle; dairy cattle; calves, including preruminating (veal) calves; and swine. A thoroughly cleaned, sterile needle and syringe should be used for each injection (needles and syringes may be sterilized by boiling in water for 15 minutes). In cold weather, LIQUAMYCIN® LA-200® should be warmed to room temperature before administration to animals. Before withdrawing the solution from the bottle, disinfect the rubber cap on the bottle with suitable disinfectant, such as 70% alcohol. The injection site should be similarly cleaned with the disinfectant. Needles of 16-18 gauge and 1-1½ inches long are adequate for intramuscular and subcutaneous injections. Needles 2-3 inches are recommended for intravenous use.

Intramuscular Administration: Intramuscular injections in swine should be made by directing the needle of suitable gauge and length into the fleshy part of a thick muscle in the neck region; avoid blood vessels and major nerves. Before injecting the solution, pull back gently on the plunger. If blood appears in the syringe, a blood vessel has been entered; withdraw the needle and select a different site. No more than 5 mL should be injected at any one site in adult swine; rotate injection sites for each succeeding treatment.

Subcutaneous Administration: Subcutaneous injections in beef cattle, dairy cattle, and calves, including preruminating (veal) calves, should be made by directing the needle of suitable gauge and length through the loose folds of the neck skin in front of the shoulder. Care should be taken to ensure that the tip of the needle has penetrated the skin but is not lodged in muscle. Before injecting the solution, pull back gently on the plunger. If blood appears in the syringe, a blood vessel has been entered; withdraw the needle and select a different site. The solution should be injected slowly into the area between the skin and muscles. No more than 10 mL should be injected subcutaneously at any one site in adult beef cattle and dairy cattle; rotate injection sites for each succeeding treatment. The volume administered per injection site should be reduced according to age and body size so that 1-2 mL per site is injected in small calves.

Intravenous Administration: LIQUAMYCIN® LA-200® may be administered intravenously to beef and dairy cattle. As with all highly concentrated materials, LIQUAMYCIN® LA-200® should be administered slowly by the intravenous route.

Preparation of the Animal for Injection:

1. Approximate location of vein. The jugular vein runs in the jugular groove on each side of the neck from the angle of the jaw to just above the brisket and slightly above and to the side of the windpipe (see Fig. I).
2. Restraint. A stanchion or chute is ideal for restraining the animal. With a halter, rope, or cattle leader (nose tongs), pull the animal's head around the side of the stanchion, cattle chute, or post in such a manner to form a bow in the neck (see Fig. II), then snub the head securely to prevent movement. By forming the bow in the neck, the outside curvature of the bow tends to expose the jugular vein and make it easily accessible. Caution: Avoid restraining the animal with a tight rope or halter around the throat or upper neck which might impede blood flow. Animals that are down present no problem so far as restraint is concerned.
3. Clip hair in area where injection is to be made (over the vein in the upper third of the neck). Clean and disinfect the skin with alcohol or other suitable antiseptic.

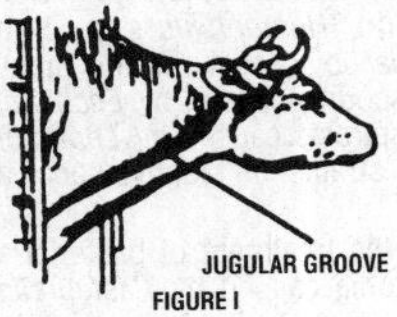

FIGURE I

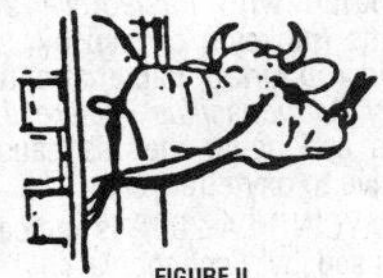
FIGURE II

Entering the Vein and Making the Injection:

1. Raise the vein. This is accomplished by tying the choke rope tightly around the neck close to the shoulder. The rope should be tied in such a way that it will not come loose and so that it can be untied quickly by pulling the loose end (see Fig. II). In thick-necked animals, a block of wood placed in the jugular groove between the rope and the hide will help considerably in applying the desired pressure at the right point. The vein is a soft flexible tube through which blood flows back to the heart. Under ordinary conditions it cannot be seen or felt with the fingers. When the flow of blood is blocked at the base of the neck by the choke rope, the vein becomes enlarged and rigid because of the back pressure. If the choke rope is sufficiently tight, the vein stands out and can be easily seen and felt in thin-necked animals. As a further check in identifying the vein, tap it with the fingers in front of the choke rope. Pulsations that can be seen or felt with the fingers in front of the point being tapped will confirm the fact that the vein is properly distended. It is impossible to put the needle into the vein unless it is distended. Experienced operators are able to raise the vein simply by hand pressure, but the use of a choke rope is more certain.
2. Inserting the needle. This involves 3 distinct steps. First, insert the needle through the hide. Second, insert the needle into the vein. This may require 2 or 3 attempts before the vein is entered. The vein has a tendency to roll away from the point of the needle, especially if the needle is not sharp. The vein can be steadied with the thumb and finger of one hand. With the other hand, the needle point is placed directly over the vein, slanting it so that its direction is along the length of the vein, either toward the head or toward the heart. Properly positioned this way, a quick thrust of the needle will be followed by a spurt of blood through the needle, which indicates that the vein has been entered. Third, once in the vein, the needle should be inserted along the length of the vein all the way to the hub, exercising caution to see that the needle does not penetrate the opposite side of the vein. Continuous steady flow of blood through the needle indicates that the needle is still in the vein. If blood does not flow continuously, the needle is out of the vein (or clogged) and another attempt must be made. If difficulty is encountered, it may be advisable to use the vein on the other side of the neck.
3. While the needle is being placed in proper position in the vein, an assistant should get the medication ready so that the injection can be started without delay after the vein has been entered.
4. Making the injection. With the needle in position as indicated by continuous flow of blood, release the choke rope by a quick pull on the free end. This is essential — the medication cannot flow into the vein while it is blocked. Immediately connect the syringe containing LIQUAMYCIN® LA-200® to the needle and slowly depress the plunger. If there is resistance to depression of the plunger, this indicates that the needle has slipped out of the vein (or is clogged) and the procedure will have to be repeated. Watch for any swelling under the skin near the needle, which would indicate that the medication is not going into the vein. Should this occur, it is best to try the vein on the opposite side of the neck.
5. Removing the needle. When injection is complete, remove needle with straight pull. Then apply pressure over the area of injection momentarily to control any bleeding through needle puncture, using cotton soaked in alcohol or other suitable antiseptic.

Precaution(s): Exceeding the highest recommended level of drug per lb of body weight per day, administering more than the recommended number of treatments, and/or exceeding 10 mL subcutaneously per injection site in adult beef cattle and dairy cattle, and 5 mL intramuscularly per injection site in adult swine, may result in antibiotic residues beyond the withdrawal period.

Consult with your veterinarian prior to administering this product in order to determine the proper treatment required in the event of an adverse reaction. At the first sign of any adverse reaction, discontinue use of the product and seek the advice of your veterinarian. Some of the reactions may be attributed either to anaphylaxis (an allergic reaction) or to cardiovascular collapse of unknown cause.

Shortly after injection, treated animals may have transient hemoglobinuria resulting in darkened urine.

As with all antibiotic preparations, use of this drug may result in overgrowth of nonsusceptible organisms, including fungi. A lack of response by the treated animal, or the development of new signs, may suggest that an overgrowth of nonsusceptible organisms has occurred. If any of these conditions occur, consult your veterinarian.

Since bacteriostatic drugs may interfere with the bactericidal action of penicillin, it is advisable to avoid giving LIQUAMYCIN® LA-200® in conjunction with penicillin.

Storage: Store at room temperature 15°-30°C (59°-86°F). Keep from freezing.

LIQUAMYCIN® LA-200® does not require refrigeration; however, it is recommended that it be stored at room temperature, 15°-30°C (59°-86°F).

Caution(s): When administered to cattle, muscle discoloration may necessitate trimming of the injection site(s) and surrounding tissues during the dressing procedure.

For animal use only.

Restricted Drug (California)—Use only as directed.

Not for human use.

Warning(s): Discontinue treatment at least 28 days prior to slaughter of cattle and swine. Milk taken from animals during treatment and for 96 hours after the last treatment must not be used for food. Rapid intravenous administration may result in animal collapse. Oxytetracycline should be administered intravenously slowly over a period of at least 5 minutes.

Adverse Reactions: Reports of adverse reactions associated with oxytetracycline administration include injection site swelling, restlessness, ataxia, trembling, swelling of eyelids, ears, muzzle, anus and vulva (or scrotum and sheath in males), respiratory abnormalities (labored breathing), frothing at the mouth, collapse and possibly death. Some of these reactions may be attributed to anaphylaxis (an allergic reaction) or to cardiovascular collapse of unknown cause.

Discussion: LIQUAMYCIN® LA-200® (oxytetracycline injection) is a sterile, ready-to-use solution for the administration of the broad-spectrum antibiotic oxytetracycline (Terramycin®) by injection. Terramycin, discovered by Pfizer scientists, is an antimicrobial agent that is effective in the treatment of a wide range of diseases caused by susceptible gram-positive and gram-negative bacteria.

LIQUAMYCIN® LA-200® administered to cattle or swine for the treatment of bacterial pneumonia at a dosage of 9 mg of oxytetracycline per lb of body weight has been demonstrated in clinical trials to be as effective as 2 or 3 repeated, daily treatments of Terramycin® Injectable at 3-5 mg/lb of body weight.

The antibiotic activity of oxytetracycline is not appreciably diminished in the presence of body fluids, serum, or exudates.

Care of Sick Animals: The use of antibiotics in the management of diseases is based on an accurate diagnosis and an adequate course of treatment. When properly used in the treatment of diseases caused by oxytetracycline-susceptible organisms, most animals that have been treated with LIQUAMYCIN® LA-200® show a noticeable improvement within 24-48 hours. It is recommended that the diagnosis and treatment of animal diseases be carried out by a veterinarian. Since many diseases look alike but require different types of treatment, the use of professional veterinary and laboratory services can reduce treatment time, costs, and needless losses. Good housing, sanitation, and nutrition are important in the maintenance of healthy animals, and are essential in the treatment of diseased animals.

Presentation: 100 mL, 250 mL and 500 mL vials.

U.S. Patent No. 4,018,889

Compendium Code No.: 36900822

79-4984-00-2 May 2001

LIQUATONE™

Westfalia•Surge **Udder Wash**

EPA Reg. No.: 1072-16

Active Ingredient(s):

n-Alkyl (C_{14} 60%, C_{16} 30%, C_{12} 5%, C_{18} 5%)
dimethyl benzyl ammonium chlorides 10%
n-Alkyl (C_{12} 68%, C_{14} 32%) dimethyl ethylbenzyl ammonium chlorides 10%
Inert ingredients 80%
Total 100%

Indications: A sanitizer used for sanitizing dairy equipment and for udder washing.

Directions for Use: It is a violation of federal law to use the product in a manner inconsistent with its labeling.

Sanitizing dairy equipment: After cleaning and before use, sanitize all milk contact surfaces with a 200 ppm solution of LIQUATONE™ as required by state and local health authorities. The contact time should be at least two (2) minutes. Drain thoroughly and air dry.

Udder washing: Prepare a sanitizing solution by mixing ⅛ oz. (3.7 mL) of LIQUATONE™ in one (1) gallon (3.8 L) of warm [110°F (43°C)] water. Use a clean single service towel for each cow. Wash and massage the teats and udder. Never dip the used towel back into the solution.

Discard the solution if it is visibly dirty. Prepare a fresh solution for each milking. Dry teats and udder with a clean single service towel prior to the attachment of the milking machine.

Do not use as a teat dip.

Precautionary Statements: Hazards to Humans and Domestic Animals: Concentrate causes eye and skin damage. Protect the eyes when handling. Do not get in the eyes or on clothing. Avoid skin contact. Harmful if swallowed. Avoid contamination of food.

First Aid: In case of contact with the eyes, flush immediately with plenty of water for at least 15 minutes. Call a physician. For skin, wash promptly. Remove and wash contaminated clothing before reuse.

Environmental Hazards: The product is toxic to fish. Keep out of lakes, streams, or ponds. Treated effluent may not be discharged into lakes, streams, ponds or public waters without a valid discharge permit. For guidance, contact the regional office of the Environmental Protection Agency.

State and Local Regulations: Consult a dealer, state or local health authorities for additional information.

Storage and Disposal: Store in a cool, dry area away from direct sunlight. Keep from freezing. If frozen, separation may occur. Thaw completely and mix well. In case of a spill, flood the area with large quantities of water. Do not contaminate food or feed by storage, disposal or the cleaning of equipment.

Pesticide Disposal: Pesticide wastes are acutely hazardous. Improper disposal of excess pesticide, spray mixture, or rinsate is a violation of federal law. If these wastes cannot be disposed of by use according to label instructions, contact a State Pesticide or Environmental Control Agency, or the Hazardous Waste representative at the nearest EPA regional office for guidance.

Container Disposal: Triple rinse (or equivalent) and dispose in an incinerator or landfill approved for pesticide containers.

Warning(s): Danger. Keep out of the reach of children.

Presentation: Contact the company for container sizes available.

Compendium Code No.: 10020101

LIQUICAL™

Butler — **Small Animal Dietary Supplement**

Caloric Supplement in Concentrated Form

Active Ingredient(s): Ingredients: Each 100 grams contains Vitamin A 7500 I.U., Vitamin D 1500 I.U., Vitamin E 100 I.U., Thiamine HCl (B_1) 35 mg., Riboflavin (B_2) 3.5 mg., Pyridoxine (B_6) 17 mg., Cyanocobalamin (B_{12}) 35 mcg., Nicotinamide 35 mg., Calcium Panthothenate 35 mg., Folic Acid 3.5 mg., Dextrose, Maltose, Maltotriose, Higher Saccharides, Palmitic, Stearic, Oleic, Linoleic, Linolenic acids, Polysorbate 60, Xanthan gum, Potassium Sorbate, Potassium Benzoate, FDC approved flavor and color.

Indications: LIQUICAL™ is a high calorie liquid dietary supplement containing 335 calories per 100 grams. It has been formulated to be highly palatable and easily digested without straining the animal's digestive system. Useful for stressed animals, pregnancy/lactation and undernourished neonates.

Dosage and Administration: Dosage: 1 mL per 2 lbs. of body weight, given from 1 to 3 times daily, or as indicated.

Precaution(s): Shake well. Refrigerate after opening. Store in a cool, dry place.

Caution(s): For veterinary use only.

Warning(s): Keep out of reach of children.

Presentation: 2 oz and 8 oz.

Compendium Code No.: 10821970

LIQUI-CHAR®-VET

King Animal Health — **Adsorbent**

Aqueous Suspension-Activated Charcoal, USP

Active Ingredient(s): 50 g of activated charcoal in a unit dose tube.

Indications: Recommended as an emergency treatment for ingestion of acute toxins.

Dosage and Administration: The recommended dosage for LIQUI-CHAR®-VET is 5 mL or 5 cc per 1 pound (454 grams) animal body weight. One 240 mL tube provides sufficient LIQUI-CHAR®-VET suspension to treat a 50 lb (22.7 kg) animal.

Usage Instructions: LIQUI-CHAR®-VET should be kneaded and vigorously shaken prior to administration. Administration with a stomach or rumen tube is recommended; the tip of the LIQUI-CHAR®-VET tube should be snipped with scissors and the contents of the LIQUI-CHAR®-VET tube squeezed directly into the stomach tube. For ease of administration two fittings are provided to adapt LIQUI-CHAR®-VET tip to the desired opening. After administration, rinse the stomach tube with water and then remove.

Animals should be closely observed after treatment; specific and/or systemic treatment may need to be repeated. Repeated administration of LIQUI-CHAR®-VET is usually indicated only if the animal's condition worsens or remains unchanged within a 2 hour period from initial LIQUI-CHAR®-VET treatment.

Precaution(s): Do not reuse container.

Discard all unused portions of LIQUI-CHAR®-VET suspension. Store unopened tubes of LIQUI-CHAR®-VET at controlled room temperature of 15°-30° Celsius (59°-86° Fahrenheit).

Caution(s): The use of LIQUI-CHAR®-VET is not recommended as an antidote for heavy metal poisoning.

LIQUI-CHAR®-VET is ineffective for mineral acids, alkalies, and substances insoluble in aqueous acidic solutions.

For veterinary use only.

Discussion: LIQUI-CHAR®-VET should be administered at a level to inactivate at least 80% of the ingested toxin. A combination of normal body detoxification and specific and/or symptomatic antidotal therapy may be used to augment the effectiveness of LIQUI-CHAR®-VET aqueous suspension.

For best prognosis, LIQUI-CHAR®-VET suspension should be administered as soon as ingestion of toxin is suspected, or upon onset of symptomatic toxicity.

LIQUI-CHAR®-VET may also be administered daily or it may be mixed in feed in subacute or chronic toxicoses, or to aid in excretion of the body-burden of a toxicant. When LIQUI-CHAR®-VET is administered repeatedly on a daily basis, it may suppress adsorption of vitamins, as well as suppressing the adsorption of antibacterial drugs, such as sulfonamides and antibiotics.

LIQUI-CHAR®-VET may be used to treat toxic enteritis and toxic overload in ruminants. LIQUI-CHAR®-VET may be effective in the adsorption of bacterial exotoxins.

Presentation: 240 mL tubes.

Compendium Code No.: 11320011

LIQUI-CHAR®-VET WITH SORBITOL

King Animal Health — **Adsorbent**

Activated Charcoal, USP in a Sorbitol Base

Active Ingredient(s): Each 8 fl oz (240 mL) contains 50 grams activated charcoal, USP and 25 grams sorbitol, USP (base).

Indications: An adsorbent for use in poisoning and overdosages.

Dosage and Administration: The recommended dosage of LIQUI-CHAR®-VET is 5 mL per 1 lb. One 8 oz tube (240 mL) will treat a 50 lb animal. Observe patient carefully and if no improvement is seen in 2 hours post treatment, repeat initial dosage.

Knead and shake vigorously before using.

Precaution(s): Discard any unused portion.

Store at room temperature 15°-30° C (59°-86° F).

Do not refrigerate.

Presentation: 8 fl oz (240 mL) tubes.

Compendium Code No.: 11320021

LIQUID ASP-RIN™

AgriLabs — **Water Medication**

Antipyretic and Analgesic-Liquid Concentrate for Drinking Water Solutions

Active Ingredient(s): Each quart (32 fl oz) contains:

Sodium Salicylate (14,375 mg per oz) .... 460 gm

Excipients: Acetic Acid, Disodium Salt of 6-Hydroxy-5-[(2-Methoxy-5-Methyl-4-Sulfophenyl)Azo]-2-Naphthalenesulfonic Acid, Ethyl Heptonate, Ethyl Lactate, Propylene Glycol, Strawberry Aldehyde, Water.

Indications: For use in the drinking water of poultry and swine as an aid in reducing fever and as a mild analgesic.

Directions for Use: Mix 0.3 oz of LIQUID ASP-RIN™ for each 1000 lbs body weight to be treated in a sufficient amount of drinking water to be consumed in each 8-12 hour period. This can ordinarily be accomplished in poultry and swine by mixing 8 oz into each gallon of stock solution, and metering at 1 oz stock per gallon of drinking water. Prepare fresh solutions daily. Repeat as necessary.

Contraindication(s): Not for use in cats or dogs.

Precaution(s): Storage: Keep container tightly closed. Store at room temperature. Protect from temperature extremes.

Caution(s): For animal use only.

Not for human use.

Warning(s): Keep out of reach of children.

Presentation: 32 fl oz.

Compendium Code No.: 10581320

Iss. 11-00

LIQUID B COMPLEX

Alpharma — **Vitamin B-Complex**

Active Ingredient(s): Each 100 mL contains:

Thiamine Hydrochloride	877 mg
Riboflavin	17.54 mg
Dexpanthenol	87 mg
Niacinamide	877 mg
Pyridoxine Hydrochloride	17.54 mg
Vitamin B_{12}	17.54 µg
Sodium Chloride	274 mg
Sodium Acetate	141 mg
Potassium Chloride	13.70 mg
Magnesium Chloride Hexahydrate	10 mg
Calcium Chloride Dihydrate	8.20 mg
Dextrose	1,177 mg
Propylparaben	30 mg
Methylparaben	180 mg
Propylene Glycol	1.60 mL
Sorbitol Solution (70%)	1.67 mL
Menadione Sodium Bisulfite (Vitamin K)	4.60 mg

Contains: Sorbitol, dextrose, vitamin K_3 and electrolytes in proper proportions.

Ingredients: Deionized water, sorbitol solution, propylene glycol, thiamine HCl, dextrose, niacinamide, sodium chloride, methylparaben, sodium acetate, dexpanthenol, propylparaben, riboflavin-5'-phosphate, pyridoxine HCl, potassium chloride, magnesium chloride, calcium chloride, menadione sodium bisulfite, cyanocobalamin.

Preserved with methylparaben and propylparaben.

Indications: A supplementary nutrition in healthy, sick or convalescing poults.

Dosage and Administration: 2 teaspoons per gallon of drinking water (0.2 mL per poult). For proportioners, use product undiluted.

Precaution(s): Recommended storage conditions: Store below 77°F) (25°C).

Warning(s): Keep out of reach of children. Not for human use.

Presentation: 1520 mL.

Compendium Code No.: 10220431

AHL-460 0109

LIQUID VITAMIN PREMIX

Alpharma — **Dietary Supplement**

Active Ingredient(s): The product contains water, dl-alpha-tocopheryl acetate, niacinamide, menadione sodium bisulfite complex, thiamine HCl, pyridoxine HCl, inositol, dexpanthenol, vitamin A propionate, riboflavin 5 phosphate, d-activated animal sterol, folic acid, biotin and cyanocobalamin.

Guaranteed analysis per fluid ounce:

Vitamin A	125,000 I.U.
Vitamin D_3	58,750 I.U.
Vitamin E	465 I.U.
Vitamin B_{12}	250 mcg
Riboflavin	26 mg
Niacinamide	305 mg
d-Pantothenic acid	60 mg
Menadione SBC	135 mg
Folic acid	1,725 mcg
Thiamine HCl	130 mg
Pyridoxine HCl	130 mg
Inositol	115 mg
Biotin	1,560 mcg

Indications: LIQUID VITAMIN PREMIX is a nutritional supplement for use in poultry drinking water.

Dosage and Administration: Mix 6 fl. oz. in 128 gallons of drinking water.

Caution(s): For oral animal use only.

Keep out of the reach of children.

Presentation: 30 oz.

Compendium Code No.: 10220440

L

LIQUI-LUBE

Vetus **Lubricant**

NDC No.: 47611-205-90

Active Ingredient(s): LIQUI-LUBE contains USP purified water, propylene glycol and sodium carboxymethylcellulose. Methylparaben and propylparaben are added as preservatives.

Indications: A nonspermicidal, bacteriostatic, nonirritating, nontoxic, greaseless lubricating jelly which minimizes irritation to the skin of the operator and the mucous membranes of the animal during examination. LIQUI-LUBE is water soluble.

Dosage and Administration: For coating the hands, the arms, the instruments, and the subject area in performing gynecological procedures and for rectal examinations, apply liberally immediately before use.

Precaution(s): Avoid storing at excessive heat.

Caution(s): Keep out of the reach of children. For veterinary use only.

Presentation: 1 gallon containers.

Compendium Code No.: 14440590

LIQUI-PRIN™

AgriPharm **Water Medication**

Antipyretic and Analgesic

Active Ingredient(s): Each quart (32 fl. oz.) contains:

Sodium Salicylate (14,375 mg per oz.) .... 460 gm

Excipients: Acetic Acid, Disodium Salt of 6-Hydroxy-5-[(2-Methoxy-5-Methyl-4-Sulfo-phenyl)Azo]-2-Naphthalenesulfonic Acid, Ethyl Heptonate, Ethyl Lactate, Propylene Glycol, Strawberry Aldehyde, Water.

Indications: For use in the drinking water of poultry and swine as an aid in reducing fever and as a mild analgesic.

Directions for Use: Mix 0.3 oz. of LIQUI-PRIN™ for each 1000 lbs body weight to be treated in a sufficient amount of drinking water to be consumed in each 8-12 hour period. This can ordinarily be accomplished in poultry and swine by mixing 8 oz. into each gallon of stock solution, and metering at 1 oz. stock per gallon of drinking water. Prepare fresh solutions daily. Repeat as necessary.

Precaution(s): Storage: Keep container tightly closed. Store at room temperature. Protect from temperature extremes.

Caution(s): Not for use in cats or dogs.

Not for human use. For animal use only.

Warning(s): Keep out of reach of children.

Presentation: 32 fl. oz. and 12x32 fl. oz.

Compendium Code No.: 14571220 Iss. 4-01

LIQUI-PRIN™

First Priority **Water Medication**

Antipyretic and Analgesic

Active Ingredient(s): Each quart (32 fl. oz.) contains:

Sodium Salicylate (14,375 mg per oz.) .... 460 gm

Excipients: Acetic Acid, Disodium Salt of 6-Hydroxy-5-[(2-Methoxy-5-Methyl-4-Sulfo-phenyl)Azo]-2-Naphthalenesulfonic Acid, Ethyl Heptonate, Ethyl Lactate, Propylene Glycol, Strawberry Aldehyde, Water.

Indications: For use in the drinking water of poultry and swine as an aid in reducing fever and as a mild analgesic.

Directions for Use: Mix 0.3 oz. of LIQUI-PRIN™ for each 1000 lbs body weight to be treated in a sufficient amount of drinking water to be consumed in each 8-12 hour period. This can ordinarily be accomplished in poultry and swine by mixing 8 oz. into each gallon of stock solution, and metering at 1 oz. stock per gallon of drinking water. Prepare fresh solutions daily. Repeat as necessary.

Precaution(s): Storage: Keep container tightly closed. Store at room temperature. Protect from temperature extremes.

Caution(s): Not for use in cats or dogs.

Not for human use. For animal use only.

Warning(s): Keep out of reach of children.

Presentation: 32 fl. oz. (960 mL) (NDC# 58829-306-32).

Compendium Code No.: 11390790 Iss. 5-01

LITTERGUARD®

Pfizer Animal Health **Bacterin**

Escherichia Coli Bacterin

U.S. Vet. Lic. No.: 189

Description: The bacterin is prepared from chemically inactivated strains of *E. coli.* A sterile adjuvant is used to enhance the immune response.

Indications: LITTERGUARD® is for vaccination of healthy pregnant sows and gilts for passive transfer of protective maternal antibodies to their pigs against neonatal diarrhea caused by enterotoxigenic strains of *Escherichia coli* having the K99, K88, 987P, or F41 adherence factors. The addition of F41 now offers broader protection than previously available.

Directions:

1. General Directions: Shake well. Aseptically administer 2 mL intramuscularly or subcutaneously.
2. Primary Vaccination: Healthy pregnant swine should receive 2 doses administered 3 weeks apart during the last half of pregnancy. The second dose should be given at least 2 weeks before farrowing.
3. Revaccination: Pregnant swine should be revaccinated with a single dose at least 2 weeks before each subsequent farrowing.
4. Good animal husbandry and herd health management practices should be employed.

Precaution(s): Store at 2°-7°C. Prolonged exposure to higher temperatures may adversely affect potency. Do not freeze.

Use entire contents when first opened.

Sterilized syringes and needles should be used to administer this vaccine.

Caution(s): As with many vaccines, anaphylaxis may occur after use. Initial antidote of epinephrine is recommended and should be followed with appropriate supportive therapy.

This product has been shown to be efficacious in healthy animals. A protective immune response may not be elicited if animals are incubating an infectious disease, are malnourished or parasitized, are stressed due to shipment or environmental conditions, are otherwise immunocompromised, or the vaccine is not administered in accordance with label directions.

For veterinary use only.

Warning(s): Do not vaccinate within 21 days before slaughter.

Discussion: Disease Description: Enterotoxigenic strains of *E. coli* are among the most important etiologic agents of porcine neonatal diarrhea. Studies have shown that enterotoxigenic *E. coli* isolated from diarrheic pigs have 2 characteristics in common: (1) they have pili, surface antigenic structures which attach the bacteria to cells of the intestinal epithelium; and (2) they express enterotoxins, causing the intestinal cells to secrete body fluids and electrolytes into the gut lumen. The results are diarrhea, dehydration, and in severe cases, death. The 4 major pili types associated with neonatal enteric colibacillosis in swine are K99, K88, 987P,[1] and F41.[2]

Trial Data: Safety and Efficacy: No adverse reactions to LITTERGUARD® were reported in experimental tests, or in clinical trials conducted by independent veterinarians. Anaphylaxis occasionally has been observed in field use (see Cautions). Susceptible pigs are protected by receiving colostral antibodies from vaccinated dams. Thus, adequate and timely consumption of colostrum by the neonatal pig is essential for protection. Controlled challenge-of-immunity tests were conducted involving 110 gilts and sows and their litters. Fractions of LITTERGUARD® were tested for effectiveness separately and in combination. Results showed that vaccination of pregnant swine with 2 doses of LITTERGUARD® significantly reduced the incidence and severity of neonatal diarrhea in their litters.

References: Available upon request.

Presentation: 50 dose vials.

K88 component under Pfizer contract with Cetus Corporation.

Compendium Code No.: 36900561 75-4400-04

LITTERGUARD® LT

Pfizer Animal Health **Bacterin-Toxoid**

Escherichia Coli Bacterin-Toxoid

U.S. Vet. Lic. No.: 189

Description: The bacterin-toxoid is prepared from chemically inactivated strains of *E. coli.* A sterile adjuvant is used to enhance the immune response.

Indications: LITTERGUARD® LT is for vaccination of healthy, pregnant sows and gilts for passive transfer of protective maternal antibodies to their pigs as an aid in preventing neonatal diarrhea caused by enterotoxigenic strains of *Escherichia coli* producing heat-labile toxin or having the K99, K88, 987P, or F41 adherence factors. The addition of F41 now offers broader protection than previously available.

Directions:

1. General Directions: Shake well. Aseptically administer 2 mL intramuscularly or subcutaneously.
2. Primary Vaccination: Healthy, pregnant swine should receive 2 doses administered 3 weeks apart during the last half of pregnancy. The second dose should be given at least 2 weeks before farrowing.
3. Revaccination: Pregnant swine should be revaccinated with a single dose at least 2 weeks before each subsequent farrowing.
4. Good animal husbandry and herd health management practices should be employed.

Precaution(s): Store at 2°-7°C. Prolonged exposure to higher temperatures may adversely affect potency. Do not freeze.

Use entire contents when first opened.

Sterilized syringes and needles should be used to administer this vaccine.

Caution(s): As with many vaccines, anaphylaxis may occur after use. Initial antidote of epinephrine is recommended and should be followed with appropriate supportive therapy.

This product has been shown to be efficacious in healthy animals. A protective immune response may not be elicited if animals are incubating an infectious disease, are malnourished or parasitized, are stressed due to shipment or environmental conditions, are otherwise immunocompromised, or the vaccine is not administered in accordance with label directions.

For veterinary use only.

Warning(s): Do not vaccinate within 21 days before slaughter.

Discussion: Disease Description: Enterotoxigenic strains of *E. coli* are among the most important etiologic agents of porcine neonatal diarrhea. Studies have shown that enterotoxigenic *E. coli* isolated from diarrheic pigs have 2 characteristics in common: (1) they have pili, surface antigenic structures which attach the bacteria to cells of the intestinal epithelium; and (2) they express enterotoxins, causing the intestinal cells to secrete body fluids and electrolytes into the gut lumen. The results are diarrhea, dehydration, and in severe cases, death. The 4 major pili types associated with neonatal enteric colibacillosis in swine are K99, K88, 987P,[1] and F41.[2]

Trial Data: Safety and Efficacy: No adverse reactions to LITTERGUARD® LT were reported in experimental tests, or in clinical trials conducted by independent veterinarians. Anaphylaxis occasionally has been observed in field use (see Cautions). Susceptible pigs are protected by receiving colostral antibodies from vaccinated dams. Thus, adequate and timely consumption of colostrum by the neonatal pig is essential for protection. Controlled challenge-of-immunity tests were conducted involving 110 gilts and sows and their litters. Fractions of LITTERGUARD® LT were tested for effectiveness separately and in combination. Results showed that vaccination of pregnant swine with 2 doses of LITTERGUARD® LT significantly reduced the incidence and severity of neonatal diarrhea in their litters.

References: Available upon request.

Presentation: 10 dose and 50 dose vials.

K88 component under Pfizer contract with Cetus Corporation.

Compendium Code No.: 36900841 75-4426-06

LITTERGUARD® LT-C

Pfizer Animal Health **Bacterin-Toxoid**

Clostridium Perfringens Type C-Escherichia Coli Bacterin-Toxoid

U.S. Vet. Lic. No.: 189

Description: The bacterin-toxoid is prepared from chemically inactivated strains of *E. coli* and *Cl. perfringens* type C beta toxoid. A sterile adjuvant is used to enhance the immune response.

Indications: LITTERGUARD® LT-C is for vaccination of healthy pregnant sows and gilts for passive transfer of protective maternal antibodies to their pigs against neonatal diarrhea caused by beta toxin produced by *Clostridium perfringens* type C and enterotoxigenic strains of *Escherichia coli* producing heat-labile toxin or having the K99, K88, 987P, or F41 adherence factors.

Directions:

1. General Directions: Shake well. Aseptically administer 2 mL intramuscularly or subcutaneously.
2. Primary Vaccination: Healthy, pregnant swine should receive 2 doses administered 3 weeks apart during the last half of pregnancy. The second dose should be given at least 2 weeks before farrowing.
3. Revaccination: Pregnant swine should be revaccinated with a single dose at least 2 weeks before each subsequent farrowing.

4. Good animal husbandry and herd health management practices should be employed.

Precaution(s): Store at 2°-7°C. Prolonged exposure to higher temperatures may adversely affect potency. Do not freeze.

Use entire contents when first opened.

Sterilized syringes and needles should be used to administer this vaccine.

Caution(s): As with many vaccines, anaphylaxis may occur after use. Initial antidote of epinephrine is recommended and should be followed with appropriate supportive therapy.

This product has been shown to be efficacious in healthy animals. A protective immune response may not be elicited if animals are incubating an infectious disease, are malnourished or parasitized, are stressed due to shipment or environmental conditions, are otherwise immunocompromised, or the vaccine is not administered in accordance with label directions.

For veterinary use only.

Warning(s): Do not vaccinate within 21 days before slaughter.

Discussion: Disease Description: Enterotoxigenic strains of *E. coli* are among the most important etiologic agents of porcine neonatal diarrhea. Studies have shown that enterotoxigenic *E. coli* isolated from diarrheic pigs have 2 characteristics in common: (1) they have pili, surface antigenic structures which attach the bacteria to cells of the intestinal epithelium; and (2) they express enterotoxins, causing the intestinal cells to secrete body fluids and electrolytes into the gut lumen. The results are diarrhea, dehydration, and in severe cases, death. The 4 major pili types associated with neonatal enteric colibacillosis in swine are K99, K88, 987P,[1] and F41.[2]

Cl. perfringens type C produces a highly fatal enteritis, usually in pigs less than 1 week old. It is characterized clinically by dehydration, weakness, and diarrhea, which is hemorrhagic in peracute and acute cases. Although morbidity rates vary greatly between herds and even between litters in the same herd, mortality is consistently high in pigs clinically affected. Death may be caused by one or more of the consequences of enterotoxemia. In some cases secondary bacteremia occurs, usually involving *E. coli* or other *Cl. perfringens* types.[3]

Trial Data: Safety and Efficacy: No adverse reactions to LITTERGUARD® LT-C were reported in experimental tests, or in clinical trials conducted by independent veterinarians. Efficacy of LITTERGUARD® LT-C was demonstrated in challenge-of-immunity tests involving pregnant sows and gilts and their litters. Newborn pigs from vaccinated dams experienced significantly lower incidence and severity of neonatal diarrhea than newborn pigs from nonvaccinated dams. No immunologic interference was demonstrated among the various fractions of LITTERGUARD® LT-C.

LITTERGUARD® LT-C protects pigs by means of maternally derived antibodies present in colostrum and milk of vaccinated dams. Newborn pigs' adequate and timely consumption of the colostrum and milk is therefore essential for protection.

References: Available upon request.

Presentation: 10 dose and 50 dose vials.

K88 component under Pfizer contract with Cetus Corporation.

Compendium Code No.: 36900551 75-4408-06

LIVER 7 INJECTION ℞

Neogen **Vitamin B-Complex**

Active Ingredient(s): Each mL contains:

Crude Liver Extract	10 mg
Cyanocobalamin	100 mcg
Thiamine HCL	10 mg
Riboflavin 5 Sodium Phosphate, U.S.P.	2 mg
Pyridoxine HCL	10 mg
Niacinamide	10 mg
d-Panthenol	10 mg
Benzyl Alcohol	2%
Water for Injection	qs

Indications: For treatment and prevention of deficiencies of B vitamins in horses, cattle, sheep, swine, dogs and cats.

Dosage and Administration:

Horses, cattle, sheep and swine - 1 mL to 2 mL per 100 lbs body weight by intravenous or intramuscular injection.

Dogs and cats - 0.1 mL to 0.2 mL per 10 lbs body weight by intravenous or intramuscular injection.

Precaution(s): Store at refrigerated temperature between 2°-8°C (36°-46°F).

Caution(s): Federal Law restricts this drug to use by or on the order of a licensed veterinarian.

Anaphylactogenesis to parenteral thiamine has occurred. Administer with caution in doses over 50 mg.

For animal use only.

Warning(s): Keep out of reach of children.

Presentation: 100 mL sterile-multiple dose vials (NDC: 59051-8884-5).

Manufactured by: Omega Laboratories, Montreal, QC.

Compendium Code No.: 14910341 L335-0501

LIXOTINIC®

Pfizer Animal Health **Dietary Supplement**

Vitamin-Iron Supplement

Guaranteed Analysis: per fl oz (30 mL): (All values are minimum quantities unless otherwise stated.)

Minerals:	
Calcium	
Minimum	0.0%
Maximum	0.5%
Phosphorus	0.0%
Salt	
Minimum	0.0%
Maximum	0.5%
Iron	75 mg
Copper	1.2 mg
Vitamins and Others:	
Thiamine	12.0 mg
Riboflavin	6.0 mg
Niacin	60.0 mg
Pyridoxine	6.0 mg
Vitamin B_{12}	12.5 mcg

Ingredients: Corn syrup, water, sucrose, glycerin, liver paste, iron proteinate, sodium citrate, carmel color, citric acid, niacinamide, potassium sorbate, cyanocobalamin, thiamine hydrochloride, pyridoxine hydrochloride, riboflavin, cupric sulfate, anise flavor, sodium hydroxide.

Indications: LIXOTINIC® is a premium quality vitamin and mineral supplement providing nutrients in a highly available and palatable form. Useful as a nutritional aid for: Adult and yearling horses, foals and weanling horses more than 1 week old, cats and dogs.

Dosage and Administration: Recommended Daily Use:

Horses	1-2 oz
Foals more than 1 week of age	½-1 oz
Cats and Dogs	⅙ oz (1 tsp) (per 25 lb of body wt)

Administer orally or pour over feed.

Precaution(s): Store in amber bottle at controlled room temperature 15°-30°C (59°-86°F).

Keep bottle tightly closed to preserve freshness.

Caution(s): Do not feed to cattle or other ruminants.

Presentation: 1 gal (128 fl oz) (3.78 L).

Compendium Code No.: 36901181 85-8047-07

LONGLIFE® 90 DAY™ BRAND COLLAR FOR CATS

Hartz Mountain **Parasiticide Collar**

EPA Reg. No.: 2596-49

Active Ingredient(s): By Weight (Nom.):

Tetrachlorvinphos (CAS# 22248-79-9)	14.55%
Other Ingredients:	85.45%
Total	100.00%

Indications: For use only on cats. Kills fleas and ticks, including the Deer Tick, which may carry Lyme Disease, for 60 days and continue to aid in their control an additional 30 days.

Directions for Use: It is a violation of Federal Law to use this product in a manner inconsistent with its labeling.

Read entire label before each use.

Remove collar from package, unroll and stretch to activate insecticide generator.

Do not use on kittens under 12 weeks of age. Do not unroll collar until ready to use. Place the LONGLIFE® 90 DAY™ Brand Collar around the cat's neck, adjust for proper fit, and buckle in place. The collar must be worn loosely to allow for growth of the cat and to permit the collar to move about the neck. Generally, a properly fitted collar is one that when fastened will snugly slide over the cat's head. Leave 2 or 3 inches on the collar for extra adjustment and cut off and dispose of the extra length. Consult a veterinarian before using this product on debilitated aged, medicated, pregnant or nursing animals. Sensitivities may occur after using any pesticide product for pets. Some animals may become irritated by any collar if it is applied too tightly. If this occurs, loosen the collar. If irritation continues, remove the collar from the animal. If signs of sensitivity occur, remove the collar and bathe your pet with mild soap and rinse with large amounts of water. If signs continue, consult a veterinarian immediately. Do not use this product on animals simultaneously or within 30 days before or after treatment with or exposure to cholinesterase inhibiting drugs, pesticides, or chemicals. However, flea & tick collars may be immediately replaced. This collar is intended for use as an insecticide generator.

For continuous flea protection under normal conditions, replace the collar every 3 months. Under conditions where cats are exposed to severe flea infestation, it may be necessary to replace the collar every 2 months. Ticks may be an occasional problem for cats. The collar will kill ticks, including the Deer Tick, which may carry Lyme Disease, for 60 days and continue to aid in their control an additional 30 days. The cat should be examined from time to time and the collar replaced when mature tick or flea populations begin to appear. Wetting will not impair the collar's effectiveness or pet's protection. If the cat is out in the rain, it is not necessary to remove the collar. LONGLIFE® 90 DAY™ Brand Collar may be worn with a regular collar.

Disposal: Do not use empty pouch. Dispose in trash collection.

Warning(s): Do not let children play with this collar.

Presentation: 1 Collar, 0.4 oz (11 g).

Compendium Code No.: 10360580 RM138993 554475

LONGLIFE® 90 DAY™ BRAND COLLAR FOR DOGS

Hartz Mountain **Parasiticide Collar**

EPA Reg. No.: 2596-50

Active Ingredient(s): By Weight (Nom.):

Tetrachlorvinphos (CAS# 22248-79-9)	14.55%
Other Ingredients:	85.45%
Total	100.00%

Indications: For use only on dogs. Kills fleas and ticks, including the Rocky Mountain Wood Tick, carrier of Rocky Mountain Spotted Fever, and the Deer Tick, which may carry Lyme Disease, for 60 days and continue to aid in their control an additional 30 days.

Directions for Use: It is a violation of Federal Law to use this product in a manner inconsistent with its labeling.

Read entire label before each use.

Remove collar from package, unroll and stretch to activate insecticide generator.

Do not use on puppies less than 6 weeks of age. Do not unroll collar until ready to use. Place the LONGLIFE® 90 DAY™ Brand Collar around the dog's neck, adjust for proper fit, and buckle in place. The collar must be worn loosely to allow for growth of the dog and to permit the collar to move about the neck. Generally, a properly fitted collar is one that when fastened will snugly slide over the dog's head. Leave 2 or 3 inches on the collar for extra adjustment and cut off and dispose of the extra length. Consult a veterinarian before using this product on debilitated aged, medicated, pregnant or nursing animals. Sensitivities may occur after using any pesticide product for pets. Some animals may become irritated by any collar if it is applied too tightly. If this occurs, loosen the collar. If irritation continues, remove the collar from the animal. If signs of sensitivity occur, remove the collar and bathe your pet with mild soap and rinse with large amounts of water. If signs continue, consult a veterinarian immediately. Do not use this product on animals simultaneously or within 30 days before or after treatment with or exposure to cholinesterase inhibiting drugs, pesticides, or chemicals. However, flea & tick collars may be immediately replaced. This collar is intended for use as an insecticide generator.

For continuous flea protection under normal conditions, replace the collar every 3 months. Under conditions where dogs are exposed to severe flea infestation, it may be necessary to replace the collar every 2 months. Ticks may be an occasional problem for dogs. The collar will kill ticks, including the Rocky Mountain Wood Tick, carrier of Rocky Mountain Spotted Fever, and the Deer Tick, which may carry Lyme Disease, for 60 days and continue to aid in their control an additional 30 days. The dog should be examined from time to time and the collar replaced when mature tick or flea populations begin to appear. Wetting will not impair the collar's effectiveness or pet's protection. If the dog goes swimming or is out in the rain, it is not necessary to remove the collar. The LONGLIFE® 90 DAY™ Brand Collar may be worn with a regular collar.

Disposal: Do not use empty pouch. Dispose in trash collection.

Warning(s): Do not let children play with this collar.

Presentation: 1 Collar, 0.67 oz (19 g). For dogs with necks to 21".

Compendium Code No.: 10360591 RM138994 554474

LOUSE POWDER WITH RABON®

LeGear **Topical Insecticide**

EPA Reg. No.: 34704-307-1910

Active Ingredient(s):

Tetrachlorvinphos: 2-chloro-1-(2,4,5-trichlorophenyl) vinyl dimethyl phosphate...... 3.00%
Inert ingredients.......... 97.00%
Total.......... 100.00%

Indications: A ready-to-use insecticide dust to control horn flies, lice and to aid in the control of face flies on horses, beef, and dairy cattle. Helps to control lice on swine and northern fowl mites, chicken mites and lice on or around poultry.

Dosage and Administration: It is a violation of federal law to use the product in a manner inconsistent with its labeling.

Applications: The product is a ready to use insecticide dust which can be applied by hand. There is no withholding period from last application to slaughter. Wear long sleeved shirt and pants, chemical resistant gloves, shoes and socks.

Beef cattle: For the control of horn flies apply approximately 2 oz. of dust by shaker can, rotary duster or by spoon to the upper portions of the back, neck and poll and to the face as an aid in the control of face flies. Rub in lightly to carry the dust beneath the hair. Repeat as necessary.

Dairy cattle: For the control of face flies and lice apply approximately 2 oz. of dust by shaker can, rotary duster or by spoon to the upper portions of the back, neck and poll and to the face as an aid in the control of face flies. Rub in lightly to carry the dust beneath the hair. Repeat as necessary.

Swine: For the control of lice apply 3-4 oz. of dust by conventional hand or power duster to each animal with special attention given to the neck and around the ears. Repeat as necessary but not more often than once every 14 days. In severe infestations, both individual animals and bedding may be treated. One lb. of 3% dust should be applied per 150 sq. ft. of bedding.

Poultry:

Wire Cages: Apply 1 lb./300 birds using a plunger, rotary type duster or shaker can duster. For individual treatment direct dust to vent and fluff area. Group treatment may be preferred. Dust should reach the skin. Do not repeat more often than every 14 days. Wire rungs and corners should also be treated.

Note: For northern fowl mites on roosters, thorough individual application of the dust will assure long lasting control and reduce reinfestation of breeding flocks.

Litter floor management: Apply 1 lb./100 sq. ft. using a plunger or rotary type duster. Treat evenly and thoroughly. Also treat roosts, cracks and crevices where pests may hide.

Dust box floor management: Apply 2 lb./100 birds. Use a box about 2 ft. by 1 ft. deep.

Roost paint floor management: Apply 1 lb./100 ft. - make thick slury by mixing 1 lb. of dust with one (1) pint of water while continually stirring. Treat roosts thoroughly, particularly the cracks and crevices.

Precaution(s): Storage and Disposal:

Prohibitions: Do not contaminate water, food or feed by storage or disposal.

Storage: Store in a cool, dry place in the original container.

Pesticide Disposal: Wastes resulting from the use of the product may be disposed of on site or at an approved waste disposal facility.

Container Disposal: Completely empty the container into the application equipment. Then dispose of the empty container in a sanitary landfill or by incineration, or, if allowed by state and local authorities, by burning. If burned, stay out of smoke.

Caution(s): Keep out of the reach of children.

Precautionary Statements:

Hazards to Humans and Domestic Animals: May be fatal if swallowed, inhaled or absorbed through skin. Avoid breathing dust. Do not get in eyes, on skin, or on clothing. If the material gets into the eyes, wash with plenty of water. If irritation persists, see a physician. Wash thoroughly with soap and water after handling and before eating or smoking. Avoid contamination of feed and foodstuffs. Do not apply in dwellings.

Environmental Hazards: The product is toxic to fish. Drift and runoff may be hazardous to aquatic organisms in adjacent areas. Do not apply directly to water or wetlands (swamps, bogs, marshes and potholes). Do not contaminate water when disposing of equipment washwater.

The product is highly toxic to bees exposed to direct treatment on blooming crops or weeds. Do not apply the product or allow it to drift to blooming crops or weeds if bees are visiting the area.

Warning(s): Notice of Warranty: Seller makes no warranty of merchantability, fitness for any purpose, or otherwise express or implied, concerning the product or its use which extend beyond the statements of the label.

Presentation: Available in 2 lb. canisters.

Compendium Code No.: 11530000

L-S 50 WATER SOLUBLE® POWDER

Pharmacia & Upjohn **Water Medication**

lincomycin-spectinomycin-Antibacterial and Antimycoplasmal

NADA No.: 046-109

Active Ingredient(s): The packet contains:

Lincomycin hydrochloride, equivalent to lincomycin.......... 16.7 grams
Spectinomycin sulfate tetrahydrate, equivalent to spectinomycin.......... 33.3 grams
Total Antibiotic Activity 50.0 grams

Indications: For use in chickens up to 7 days of age as an aid in the control of:

Airsacculitis caused by either *Mycoplasma synoviae* or *Mycoplasma gallisepticum* susceptible to lincomycin-spectinomycin.

Complicated Chronic Respiratory Disease (Air Sac Infection) caused by *Escherichia coli* and *M. gallisepticum* susceptible to lincomycin-spectinomycin.

Dosage and Administration: Dosage: Provide 2 grams (g) antibiotic activity per gallon of drinking water. Administer as the sole source of water for the first 5 to 7 days of life.

Administration:

Amount of L-S 50	Amount of Drinking Water
1 packet	25 gallons
For proportioners delivering 1 ounce of solution per gallon of drinking water, dissolve contents of 5 packets in each gallon of proportioner solution.	

Important: Chickens should consume water at the following approximate rate to insure intake of the required dose of lincomycin-spectinomycin indicated:

Broiler and Layer Replacements (Light and Heavy):

Age (Weeks)	Daily Water Intake Gallons/1000	Dosage Mg Antibiotic/Lb
1	5	50-65

Precaution(s): Store at room temperature.

Caution(s): Discard medicated drinking water daily and replace with fresh medicated drinking water.

Restricted Drug—Use Only as Directed (California).

For use in chickens only.

Warning(s): Not for human use.

Presentation: 2.65 oz (75.0 gram) packets (NDC 0009-0108-06).

Compendium Code No.: 10490201 813 526 004

LT BLEN®

Merial Select **Vaccine**

Fowl Laryngotracheitis Vaccine, Modified Live Virus

U.S. Vet. Lic. No.: 279

Contents: This vaccine contains a modified live fowl laryngotracheitis virus for the initial vaccination or revaccination of healthy chickens four weeks of age or older by eyedrop or by drinking water as an aid in the prevention of fowl laryngotracheitis.

Notice: Merial Select's vaccines have met the requirements of the USDA in regard to safety, purity, potency, and the capability to protect susceptible chickens. This vaccine has been tested by the Master Seed immunogenicity test for efficacy.

Contains Gentamicin as a bacteriostatic agent.

Indications: This vaccine is recommended for the protection of healthy chickens. It is essential that the chickens be maintained under good environmental conditions and that exposure to disease viruses be reduced as much as possible.

Dosage and Administration:

Intraocular Vaccination: The vaccine used for intraocular vaccination is accompanied by diluent and is recommended for the vaccination of healthy chickens four weeks of age or older using only the 1,000 dose or 2,000 dose vial.

1. Reconstitute each 1,000 doses of vaccine with 30 mL of diluent.
   a. Remove aluminum seal and rubber stopper from vaccine vial and diluent vial. Avoid contamination of stoppers and contents.
   b. Add diluent to half-fill the vaccine vial. Replace stopper in vial and shake it so that all contents are dissolved.
   c. Pour the reconstituted vaccine into the diluent container. Replace stopper in diluent container and shake.
   d. Remove stopper and fit drop-dispenser tip into diluent container.
2. Holding the diluent container with the dropper tip down, gently press the sides, dropping one drop of vaccine on the bird's eye. Be sure the vaccine spreads over the eye before releasing the bird.

Drinking Water Vaccination Using Pouring Application: Drinking water vaccination is recommended for healthy chickens at least four weeks of age.

1. Remove all medications, sanitizers and disinfectants from the drinking water 72 hours (three days) prior to vaccination.
2. Provide sufficient waterers so that all the chickens can drink at one time. Shut off water supply and allow chickens to consume all the water in the lines.
3. Raise water lines above the chickens' heads. Clean and rinse the waterers thoroughly.
4. Withhold all water from the chickens for a minimum of two hours in warm weather to four hours in cool weather prior to vaccination to stimulate thirst. Withdrawal time should be reduced if half-house brooding is in process.
5. Do not open or mix vaccine until ready to vaccinate.
6. Drinking water for vaccine delivery should contain one ounce (29 gram) of non-fat dry milk per gallon (3.8 liters) of non-chlorinated water, or should contain milk product based stabilizer prepared according to the manufacturer's instructions.
7. Reconstitute the vaccine in 3 gallons (11 liters) of milk-water during cool weather or 4 gallons (15 liters) of milk-water during warm weather for each 1,000 doses.
8. Distribute vaccine solution among waterers. Avoid direct sunlight.
9. Lower waterers and allow the chickens to drink freely. Add the remaining vaccine solution to the water lines as the chickens drink.
10. Do not provide additional drinking water until all the vaccine is consumed.

Drinking Water Vaccination Using Proportioner Application: Drinking water vaccination is recommended for healthy chickens at least four weeks of age. Several types of medicator/proportioners are commercially available. Set proportioner to deliver one ounce (30 mL) of vaccine concentrate per one gallon (3.8 liters) of water.

1. Remove all medications, sanitizers and disinfectants from the drinking water 72 hours (three days) prior to vaccination.
2. Clean all containers, hoses and waterers prior to vaccination.
3. Withhold all water from the chickens for a minimum of two hours in warm weather to four hours in cool weather prior to vaccination to stimulate thirst. Withdrawal time should be reduced if half-house brooding is in process.
4. Do not open or mix vaccine until ready to vaccinate.
5. Calculate to supply vaccine solution at a rate of 3 gallons (11 liters) per 1,000 chickens in cool weather and 4 gallons (15 liters) per 1,000 chickens in warm weather. The age of the chickens should be considered when calculating water supply. Always use non-chlorinated water when vaccinating chickens.

Example

1,000 chickens in cool weather x 3 gallons (11 liters) = 3 gallons (11 liters).
1,000 chickens in warm weather x 4 gallons (15 liters) = 4 gallons (15 liters).

6. Prepare vaccine stock solution as follows:
   a. Determine the quantity of vaccine concentrate required by multiplying one ounce (30 mL) x gallons of water needed for vaccine/drinking water.

Example

For 1,000 chickens: 3 gallons x 1 ounce (30 mL) = 3 ounces (90 mL).

b. Add 3 ounces (85 gm) of non-fat dry milk per 16 ounces (480 mL) of cool water, or use a commercial milk product based stabilizer according to the manufacturer's instructions. For 1,000 chickens add 0.5 ounces (16 gm) non-fat dry milk to the 3 ounces (90 mL) of water.
c. Reconstitute the dried vaccine with the milk solution. Rinse the vaccine vial to remove all the vaccine.
7. Insert proportioner hose into the vaccine stock solution and start water flow. Continue until all solution has been consumed before changing water supply to direct flow.
8. Do not medicate or use disinfectants for 24 hours after vaccination.

Precaution(s): Store vaccine at 35-45°F (2-7°C). Do not freeze. Use entire vial contents within four hours of opening. Burn this container and all unused contents.

This vaccine is non-returnable.

Caution(s): The capability of this vaccine to produce satisfactory results depends upon many factors, including — but not limited to — conditions of storage and handling by the user, administration of the vaccine, health and responsiveness of individual chickens, and degree of field exposure. Therefore, directions for use should be followed carefully. The use of this vaccine is subject to applicable state and federal laws and regulations.

When the vaccine is administered by eyedrop, a mild conjunctivitis often associated with slight lacrimation appearing at about the fourth or fifth day post-vaccination and disappearing about the seventh or eighth day post-vaccination is frequently seen in some birds. The conjunctivitis may be accentuated in dry and dusty houses because of the additional irritation of dust particles.

Vaccinate all chickens on the premises at one time.

For eyedrop vaccination, mix the vaccine and diluent one vial at a time, and use within four hours of opening.

Do not attempt to save any unused portion of vaccine and do not stretch the dosage.

Do not spill or splatter the vaccine and avoid contaminating your hands, eyes and clothing with the vaccine.

The vaccine is prepared for the vaccination of healthy birds. Improper handling or administration may result in variable responses.

Avoid stress conditions during and following vaccination.

Do not vaccinate diseased chickens.

Do not place chickens in contaminated facilities.

Exposure to disease must be minimized as much as possible.

Warning(s): Do not vaccinate within 21 days of slaughter.

For veterinary use only.

Presentation: 30 mL (25 x 1,000 dose), 60 mL (25 x 2,000 dose) and 150 mL (25 x 5,000 dose) vials. A bottle of liquid (dilution) is provided with each package of the vaccine (except 5,000 dose vial) for mixing with the dried virus material.

Compendium Code No.: 11050221 PA-1M/PB-2M/PC-5M 1199

LT-IVAX®

Schering-Plough **Vaccine**

Fowl Laryngotracheitis Vaccine, Modified Live Virus

U.S. Vet. Lic. No.: 165A

Active Ingredient(s): LT-IVAX® is a live virus vaccine containing a carefully selected fowl laryngotracheitis virus strain modified by passage in tissue culture. Because of the highly modified character of this vaccine, it does not offer the same degree of protection usually obtained from more virulent products. The vaccine contains a very mild attenuated virus and there is no danger of seeding down the premises with laryngotracheitis virus which can spread and cause the disease. The vaccine contains gentamicin as a preservative.

Indications: For use in chickens four weeks of age or older, as an aid in preventing fowl laryngotracheitis through immunization by the eye drop method.

Dosage and Administration:

When to Vaccinate:

Initial Vaccination: Four (4) weeks of age.

Revaccination: 10 weeks of age or older.

Vaccination Program: The development of a durable, strong protection depends upon the use of an effective vaccination program as well as many other circumstances such as administration techniques, environment and flock health at the time of vaccination. Also, the immune response to one (1) vaccination under field conditions is seldom complete for all animals within a given flock. Even when vaccination is successful, the protection stimulated in individual animals against different diseases may not be life-long.

If necessary, the vaccine may be used to aid in limiting the spread of an outbreak; however, only birds not yet infected with the virulent outbreak virus can be protected.

Examination of birds for vaccination takes is unnecessary and so-called takes are not to be expected. As with all live virus vaccines, a mild transitory reaction may occur in a small portion of the flock, and with LT-IVAX® this is generally limited to a mild, localized eye reaction of short duration.

Preparation of the Vaccine:

1. Do not open and rehydrate the vaccine until ready for use.
2. Mix only one (1) vial at a time and use the entire contents within two (2) hours.
3. Remove the tear-off aluminum seal and stopper from the vial containing the dried vaccine.
4. Remove the tear-off aluminum seal and stopper from the bottle containing the diluent.
5. Hold the diluent bottle firmly in an upright position and insert the vaccine vial on the adapter of the diluent bottle. The neck of the vaccine vial should snap into position and should be seated securely on the adapter on the diluent bottle.
6. Invert the two (2) containers so that the vaccine vial is on the bottom and allow the diluent to flow into the vaccine vial. If the diluent does not flow freely, squeeze the bottle gently and the diluent will flow into the vaccine vial. The vaccine vial should be completely filled with diluent to prevent excess foaming.
7. Hold the joined containers by the ends and shake vigorously until the vaccine plug is completely dissolved.
8. Return the joined containers to their original position (diluent bottle on the bottom). Allow the vaccine to flow into the diluent bottle. If the rehydrated vaccine does not flow into the diluent bottle, tap or squeeze the diluent bottle gently and release to draw the vaccine into the diluent bottle. Be sure that all of the vaccine is removed from the vaccine vial.
9. Remove the vaccine vial and adapter from the neck of the diluent bottle and insert the dropper applicator into the plastic diluent bottle.
10. The vaccine is now ready for eye drop use.

How to Vaccinate: Vaccination for laryngotracheitis by the eye drop method is conducted by allowing one (1) full drop of rehydrated vaccine to fall into the open eye of the bird and holding until the bird swallows. Hold the dropper bottle in a vertical position throughout the vaccination to avoid wasting the vaccine.

Records: Keep a record of the vaccine type, quantity, serial number, expiration date, and place of purchase; the date and time of vaccination; the number, age, and location of the birds; the names of operators performing the vaccination and any observed reactions.

Contraindication(s): The application of Newcastle or bronchitis vaccine, either singly or in combination should be avoided for a three-day period prior to and for three days after the application of LT-IVAX®.

Precaution(s): Store at 35° to 45°F (2° to 7°C).

Caution(s): For veterinary use only.

1. Vaccinate healthy birds only. Although disease may not be evident, coccidiosis, chronic respiratory disease, mycoplasma infection, lymphoid leukosis, infectious bursal disease, Marek's disease, or other disease conditions may cause serious complications or reduce protection.
2. An eye reaction may be noticed if the birds are incubating coryza or other infectious organisms, or if there is an excess amount of ammonia or dust in the air of the housing facilities.
3. In outbreak situations, vaccinate healthy birds first, progressing toward outbreak areas in order to vaccinate diseased birds last.
4. Do not spill or spatter the vaccine. Use the entire contents of the vial when first opened. Burn the empty bottles, caps and all unused vaccine and accessories.
5. Wash hands thoroughly after using the vaccine.
6. Do not dilute the vaccine or otherwise stretch the dosage.

Warning(s): Do not vaccinate within 21 days before slaughter.

Presentation: Supplied in 10 x 1,000 dose units with diluent.

Compendium Code No.: 10471230

LUBISEPTOL

AgriPharm **Lubricant**

Non-Spermicidal Lubricant

Active Ingredient(s): Contains: Propylene glycol, sodium carboxy methyl cellulose, methyl and propyl paraben in an inert base.

Indications: For use as a lubricant on hands, arms and instruments when performing obstetrical, vaginal and rectal examinations.

Dosage and Administration: Apply LUBISEPTOL to gloves, sleeves or instruments when performing vaginal and rectal examinations. After use, rinse thoroughly with water to remove excess lubricant from exposed areas of patient.

Precaution(s): Store at controlled room temperature between 15°-30°C (59°-86°F).

Caution(s): Failure to rinse after use may result in local irritation in some cases.

Not for human use.

Keep out of reach of children.

Presentation: 1 gallon containers.

Compendium Code No.: 14570600

LUBRI-NERT™

Life Science **Lubricant**

Ingredients: LUBRI-NERT™ (O.B. lubricant) is an unmedicated, non-irritating aqueous base lubricant.

Methyl and propyl parabens are added as preservatives.

Indications: For lubrication of the arm or glove for rectal and obstetrical procedures in large or small animals; for the lubrication of devices such as stomach tubes, enema nozzles, catheters and obstetrical instruments before insertion into body cavities; and as an aid in delivery at dry birth.

Dosage and Administration: Formulated for use either diluted or as a concentrate.

Distribute a small amount of LUBRI-NERT™ evenly to a wet or dry glove, arm or instruments.

To prepare a bulk lubricant to aid in dry birth, add LUBRI-NERT™ to two (2) quarts of water until the desired viscosity is reached.

Caution(s): For animal use only.

Not for human use.

Keep out of the reach of children.

Presentation: 1 gallon (3.785 L) container.

Compendium Code No.: 10870090

LUBRIVET™

Butler **Lubricant**

Active Ingredient(s): A solution of sodium carboxymethylcellulose in propylene glycol. Propyl and methyl parahydroxybenzoate included as preservatives.

Indications: For coating hands, arms, instruments and subject area in performing gynecological procedures and rectal examinations. The bland lubricating qualities minimize irritation to the skin of the operator and the delicate mucous membranes of the animal.

Dosage and Administration: Apply liberally immediately before use.

Caution(s): Keep out of the reach of children. For veterinary use only.

Presentation: 8 oz. flask, 1 gallon and 2.5 gallon containers.

Compendium Code No.: 10821080

LUGOL'S SOLUTION

Butler **Iodine**

Active Ingredient(s): Contains: 5% free iodine and 10% potassium iodide in an aqueous solution.

Indications: For use where iodine therapy is indicated, such as exophthalmic goiter, chronic vaginitis and chronic metritis.

Dosage and Administration: May be given internally as prescribed by the attending veterinarian. As a douche, dilution with sterile water or glycerine may be used or as prescribed by the attending veterinarian.

Precaution(s): Store at 2° to 30°C (36°-86°F).

Caution(s): Prolonged use may cause iodism.

Poison.

Antidote(s): If swallowed, give starch paste, milk, bread, egg white or activated charcoal. A 5% solution of sodium thiosulfate (photographic "hypo") may be administered orally at a rate of 10 mL per kilogram of body weight.

Call a physician or poison control center.

Warning(s): Keep out of the reach of children.

Presentation: 1 gallon (3.785 L) container.

Compendium Code No.: 10821092

LUSTRE GROOM MIST™

Butler **Grooming Product**

Active Ingredient(s): LUSTRE GROOM MIST™ is an alcohol-free spray which contains a mixture of mink oil, jojoba oil, dl-panthenol (vitamin B_5), keratin proteins and a blend of nonoily detanglers.

The ingredients in the product are biodegradable.

Indications: The conditioners in LUSTRE GROOM MIST™ will produce a high sheen without drying out the coat. LUSTRE GROOM MIST™ has been designed to be used on all types of canine and feline coats and is absorbed into the hair to provide for a healthy, nonoily, full body coat. Because LUSTRE GROOM MIST™ is antistatic, it will not attract dirt.

Dosage and Administration:

Detangler: Saturate mats and tangles. Comb out tangles and proceed with grooming.

Conditioning: After shampooing, apply LUSTRE GROOM MIST™ to the coat using a light mist from the head to the tail. Allow to dry and lightly brush to a high sheen.

Presentation: 236 mL containers.

Compendium Code No.: 10821100

LUTALYSE® STERILE SOLUTION ℞

Pharmacia & Upjohn **Prostaglandin**

Dinoprost tromethamine

NADA No.: 108-901

Active Ingredient(s): This product contains the naturally occurring prostaglandin F2 alpha (dinoprost) as the tromethamine salt. Each mL contains dinoprost tromethamine equivalent to 5 mg dinoprost: also, benzyl alcohol, 9.45 mg added as preservative. When necessary, pH was adjusted with sodium hydroxide and/or hydrochloric acid. Dinoprost tromethamine is a white or slightly off-white crystalline powder that is readily soluble in water at room temperature in concentrations to at least 200 mg/mL.

Indications: For intramuscular use for estrus synchronization, treatment of unobserved (silent) estrus and pyometra (chronic endometritis) in cattle; for abortion of feedlot and other non-lactating cattle; for parturition induction in swine; and for controlling the timing of estrus in estrous cycling mares and clinically anestrous mares that have a corpus luteum.

Cattle: LUTALYSE® Sterile Solution is indicated as a luteolytic agent.

LUTALYSE® is effective only in those cattle having a corpus luteum, i.e., those which ovulated at least five days prior to treatment. Future reproductive performance of animals that are not cycling will be unaffected by injection of LUTALYSE®.

Swine: For intramuscular use for parturition induction in swine. LUTALYSE® Sterile Solution is indicated for parturition induction in swine when injected within 3 days of normal predicted farrowing.

Mares: LUTALYSE® Sterile Solution is indicated for its luteolytic effect in mares. This luteolytic effect can be utilized to control the timing of estrus in estrous cycling and clinically anestrous mares that have a corpus luteum.

Pharmacology:

General Biologic Activity: Prostaglandins occur in nearly all mammalian tissues. Prostaglandins, especially PGE's and PGF's, have been shown, in certain species, to 1) increase at time of parturition in amniotic fluid, maternal placenta, myometrium, and blood, 2) stimulate myometrial activity, and 3) to induce either abortion or parturition. Prostaglandins, especially PGF2α, have been shown to 1) increase in the uterus and blood to levels similar to levels achieved by exogenous administration which elicited luteolysis, 2) be capable of crossing from the uterine vein to the ovarian artery (sheep), 3) be related to IUD induced luteal regression (sheep), and 4) be capable of regressing the corpus luteum of most mammalian species studied to date. Prostaglandins have been reported to result in release of pituitary tropic hormones. Data suggest prostaglandins, especially PGE's and PGF's, may be involved in the process of ovulation and gamete transport. Also PGF2α has been reported to cause increase in blood pressure, bronchoconstriction, and smooth muscle stimulation in certain species.

Metabolism: A number of metabolism studies have been done in laboratory animals. The metabolism of tritium labeled dinoprost (^{3}H PGF2 alpha) in the rat and in the monkey was similar. Although quantitative differences were observed, qualitatively similar metabolites were produced. A study demonstrated that equimolar doses of ^{3}H PGF2 alpha Tham and ^{3}H PGF2 alpha free acid administered intravenously to rats demonstrated no significant differences in blood concentration of dinoprost. An interesting observation in the above study was that the radioactive dose of ^{3}H PGF2 alpha rapidly distributed in tissues and dissipated in tissues with almost the same curve as it did in the serum. The half-life of dinoprost in bovine blood has been reported to be on the order of minutes. A complete study on the distribution of decline of ^{3}H PGF2 alpha Tham in the tissue of rats was well correlated with the work done in the cow. Cattle serum collected during 24 hours after doses of 0 to 250 mg dinoprost have been assayed by RIA for dinoprost and the 15-keto metabolites. These data support previous reports that dinoprost has a half-life of minutes.

Dinoprost is a natural prostaglandin. All systems associated with dinoprost metabolism exist in the body; therefore, no new metabolic, transport, excretory, binding or other systems need be established by the body to metabolize injected dinoprost.

Dosage and Administration:

Cattle: LUTALYSE® Sterile Solution is supplied at a concentration of 5 mg dinoprost per mL. LUTALYSE® is luteolytic in cattle at 25 mg (5 mL) administered intramuscularly. As with any multidose vial, practice aseptic techniques in withdrawing each dose. Adequately clean and disinfect the vial closure prior to entry with a sterile needle.

Instructions for Use:

1. For Intramuscular Use for Estrus Synchronization in Beef Cattle and Non-Lactating Dairy Heifers. LUTALYSE® is used to control the timing of estrus and ovulation in estrous cycling cattle that have a corpus luteum.

   Inject a dose of 5 mL LUTALYSE® (25 mg PGF2α) intramuscularly either once or twice at a 10 to 12 day interval.

   With the single injection, cattle should be bred at the usual time relative to estrus.

   With the two injections cattle can be bred after the second injection either at the usual time relative to detected estrus or at about 80 hours after the second injection of LUTALYSE®.

   Estrus is expected to occur 1 to 5 days after injection if a corpus luteum was present. Cattle that do not become pregnant to breeding at estrus on days 1 to 5 after injection will be expected to return to estrus in about 18 to 24 days.

2. For Intramuscular Use for Unobserved (Silent) Estrus in Lactating Dairy Cows with a Corpus Luteum. Inject a dose of 5 mL LUTALYSE® (25 mg PGF2α) intramuscularly. Breed cows as they are detected in estrus. If estrus has not been observed by 80 hours after injection, breed at 80 hours. If the cow returns to estrus breed at the usual time relative to estrus.

Management Considerations: Many factors contribute to success and failure of reproduction management, and these factors are important also when time of breeding is to be regulated with LUTALYSE® Sterile Solution. Some of these factors are:

a. Cattle must be ready to breed—they must have a corpus luteum and be healthy;
b. Nutritional status must be adequate as this has a direct effect on conception and the initiation of estrus in heifers or return of estrous cycles in cows following calving;
c. Physical facilities must be adequate to allow cattle handling without being detrimental to the animal;
d. Estrus must be detected accurately if timed AI is not employed;
e. Semen of high fertility must be used;
f. Semen must be inseminated properly.

A successful breeding program can employ LUTALYSE® effectively, but a poorly managed breeding program will continue to be poor when LUTALYSE® is employed unless other management deficiencies are remedied first.

Cattle expressing estrus following LUTALYSE® are receptive to breeding by a bull. Using bulls to breed large numbers of cattle in heat following LUTALYSE® will require proper management of bulls and cattle.

3. For Intramuscular Use for Treatment of Pyometra (chronic endometritis) in Cattle. Inject a dose of 5 mL LUTALYSE® (25 mg PGF2α) intramuscularly. In studies conducted with LUTALYSE®, pyometra was defined as presence of a corpus luteum in the ovary and uterine horns containing fluid but not a conceptus based on palpation *per rectum.* Return to normal was defined as evacuation of fluid and return of the uterine horn size to 40mm or less based on palpation *per rectum* at 14 and 28 days. Most cattle that recovered in response to LUTALYSE® recovered within 14 days after injection. After 14 days, recovery rate of treated cattle was no different than that of nontreated cattle.
4. For Intramuscular Use for Abortion of Feedlot and Other Non-Lactating Cattle. LUTALYSE® is indicated for its abortifacient effect in feedlot and other non-lactating cattle during the first 100 days of gestation. Inject a dose of 25 mg intramuscularly. Cattle that abort will abort within 35 days of injection.

   Commercial cattle were palpated *per rectum* for pregnancy in six feedlots. The percent of pregnant cattle in each feedlot less than 100 days of gestation ranged between 26 and 84; 80% or more of the pregnant cattle were less than 150 days of gestation. The abortion rates following injection of LUTALYSE® increased with increasing doses up to about 25 mg. As examples, the abortion rates, over 7 feedlots on the dose titration study, were 22%, 50%, 71%, 90% and 78% for cattle up to 100 days of gestation when injected IM with LUTALYSE® doses of 0, 1 (5 mg), 2 (10 mg), 4 (20 mg) and 8 (40 mg) mL, respectively. The statistical predicted relative abortion rate based on the dose titration data, was about 93% for the 5 mL (25 mg) LUTALYSE® dose for cattle injected up to 100 days of gestation.

Swine: LUTALYSE® Sterile Solution will induce parturition in swine at 10 mg (2 mL) when injected intramuscularly.

As with any multidose vial, practice aseptic techniques in withdrawing each dose. Adequately clean and disinfect the vial closure prior to entry with a sterile needle.

Instructions for Use: The response to treatment varies by individual animals with a mean interval from administration of 2 mL LUTALYSE® (10 mg dinoprost) to parturition of approximately 30 hours. This can be employed to control the time of farrowing in sows and gilts in late gestation.

Management Considerations: Several factors must be considered for the successful use of LUTALYSE® Sterile Solution for parturition induction in swine. The product must be administered at a relatively specific time (treatment earlier than 3 days prior to normal predicted farrowing may result in increased piglet mortality). It is important that adequate records be maintained on (1) the average length of gestation period for the animals on a specific location, and (2) the breeding and projected farrowing dates for each animal. This information is essential to determine the appropriate time for administration of LUTALYSE®.

Mares:

Instructions for Use: LUTALYSE® Sterile Solution is indicated for its luteolytic effect in mares. This luteolytic effect can be utilized to control the timing of estrus in estrous cycling and clinically anestrous mares that have a corpus luteum in the following circumstances:

1. Controlling Time of Estrus of Estrous Cycling Mares: Mares treated with LUTALYSE® during diestrus (4 or more days after ovulation) will return to estrus within 2 to 4 days in most cases and ovulate 8 to 12 days after treatment. This procedure may be utilized as an aid to scheduling the use of stallions.
2. Difficult-to-Breed Mares: In extended diestrus there is failure to exhibit regular estrous cycles which is different from true anestrus. Many mares described as anestrus during the breeding season have serum progesterone levels consistent with the presence of a functional corpus luteum.

   A proportion of "barren", maiden, and lactating mares do not exhibit regular estrous cycles and may be in extended diestrus. Following abortion, early fetal death and resorption, or as a result of "pseudopregnancy", there may be serum progesterone levels consistent with a functional corpus luteum.

   Treatment of such mares with LUTALYSE® usually results in regression of the corpus luteum followed by estrus and/or ovulation. In one study with 122 Standardbred and Thoroughbred mares in clinical anestrus for an average of 58 days and treated during the breeding season, behavioral estrus was detected in 81 percent at an average time of 3.7 days after injection with 5 mg LUTALYSE®; ovulation occurred an average of 7.0 days after treatment. Of those mares bred, 59% were pregnant following an average of 1.4 services during that estrus.

   Treatment of "anestrous" mares which abort subsequent to 36 days of pregnancy may not result in return to estrus due to presence of functional endometrial cups.

a. Evaluate the reproductive status of the mare.
b. Administer a single intramuscular injection of 1 mg per 100 lbs (45.5 kg) body weight which is usually 1 mL to 2 mL LUTALYSE® Sterile Solution.
c. Observe for signs of estrus by means of daily teasing with a stallion, and evaluate follicular changes on the ovary by palpation of the ovary *per rectum.*
d. Some clinically anestrous mares will not express estrus but will develop a follicle which will ovulate. These mares may become pregnant if inseminated at the appropriate time relative to rupture of the follicle.
e. Breed mares in estrus in a manner consistent with normal management.

Dinoprost tromethamine is administered once as a single intramuscular injection of 1 mg per 100 lbs (45.5 kg) body weight which is usually 1 mL to 2 mL of LUTALYSE® containing 5 mg dinoprost as the tromethamine salt per milliliter.

Precaution(s): Store at controlled room temperature 20° to 25°C (68° to 77°F) [see USP].

Caution(s): Federal (USA) law restricts this drug to use by or on the order of a licensed veterinarian.

Cattle: Do not administer to pregnant cattle unless abortion is desired.

Do not administer intravenously (I.V.), as this route might potentiate adverse reactions.

Cattle administered a progestogen would be expected to have a reduced response to LUTALYSE® Sterile Solution.

Aggressive antibiotic therapy should be employed at the first sign of infection at the injection site whether localized or diffuse. As with all parenteral products careful aseptic techniques should be employed to decrease the possibility of post injection bacterial infections.

Swine: Do not administer to sows and/or gilts prior to 3 days of normal predicted farrowing, as increased number of stillborn and postnatal mortality may result.

Mares: LUTALYSE® Sterile Solution is ineffective when administered prior to day-5 after ovulation.

Pregnancy status should be determined prior to treatment, since LUTALYSE® has been reported to induce abortion and parturition when sufficient doses were administered.

Mares should not be treated if they suffer from either acute or subacute disorders of the vascular system, gastrointestinal tract, respiratory system, or reproductive tract.

Do not administer by intravenous route.

Nonsteroidal anti-inflammatory drugs (i.e., indomethacin) may inhibit prostaglandin synthesis, therefore these drugs should not be administered concurrently.

Warning(s):

Cattle: No milk discard or preslaughter drug withdrawal period is required for labeled uses.

Swine: No preslaughter drug withdrawal period is required for labeled uses.

Mares: Not for use in horses intended for food.

Not for human use.

Women of child-bearing age, asthmatics, and persons with bronchial and other respiratory problems should exercise extreme caution when handling this product. In the early stages, women may be unaware of their pregnancies. Dinoprost tromethamine is readily absorbed through the skin and can cause abortion and/or bronchiospasms. Direct contact with the skin should, therefore, be avoided. Accidental spillage on the skin should be washed off immediately with soap and water.

Use of this product in excess of the approved dose may result in drug residues.

Toxicology: Safety and Toxicity:

Laboratory Animals: Dinoprost was non-teratogenic in rats when administered orally at 1.25, 3.2, 10.0 and 20.0 mg/kg/day from day 6th-15th of gestation or when administered subcutaneously at 0.5 and 1.0 mg/kg/day on gestation days 6, 7 and 8 or 9, 10 and 11 or 12, 13 and 14. Dinoprost was non-teratogenic in the rabbit when administered either subcutaneously at doses of 0.5 and 1.0 mg/kg/day on gestation days 6, 7 and 8 or 9, 10 and 11 or 12, 13 and 14 or 15, 16 and 17 or orally at doses of 0.01, 0.1 and 1.0 mg/kg/day on days 6-18 or 5.0 mg/kg/day on days 8-18 of gestation. A slight and marked embryo lethal effect was observed in dams given 1.0 and 5.0 mg/kg/day respectively. This was due to the expected luteolytic properties of the drug.

A 14-day continuous intravenous infusion study in rats at 20 mg PGF2α per kg body weight indicated prostaglandins of the F series could induce bone deposition. However, such bone changes were not observed in monkeys similarly administered LUTALYSE® Sterile Solution at 15 mg PGF2α per kg body weight for 14 days.

Cattle: In cattle, evaluation was made of clinical observations, clinical chemistry, hematology, urinalysis, organ weights, and gross plus microscopic measurements following treatment with various doses up to 250 mg dinoprost administered twice intramuscularly at a 10 day interval or doses of 25 mg administered daily for 10 days. There was no unequivocal effect of dinoprost on the hematology or clinical chemistry parameters measured. Clinically, a slight transitory increase in heart rate was detected. Rectal temperature was elevated about 1.5° F through the 6th hour after injection with 250 mg dinoprost, but had returned to baseline at 24 hours after injection. No dinoprost associated gross lesions were detected. There was no evidence of toxicological effects. Thus, dinoprost had a safety factor of at least 10X on injection (25 mg luteolytic dose vs. 250 mg safe dose), based on studies conducted with cattle. At luteolytic doses, dinoprost had no effect on progeny. If given to a pregnant cow, it may cause abortion; the dose required for abortion varies considerably with the stage of gestation.

Induction of abortion in feedlot cattle at stages of gestation up to 100 days of gestation did not result in dystocia, retained placenta or death of heifers in the field studies. The smallness of the fetus at this early stage of gestation should not lead to complications at abortion. However, induction of parturition or abortion with any exogenous compound may precipitate dystocia, fetal death, retained placenta and/or metritis, especially at latter stages of gestation.

Swine: In pigs, evaluation was made of clinical observations, food consumption, clinical pathologic determinations, body weight changes, urinalysis, organ weights, and gross and microscopic observations following treatment with single doses of 10, 30, 50 and 100 mg dinoprost administered intramuscularly. The results indicated no treatment related effects from dinoprost treatment that were deleterious to the health of the animals or to their offspring.

Mares: Dinoprost tromethamine was administered to adult mares (weighing 320 to 485 kg; 2 to 20 years old), at the rates of 0, 100, 200, 400, and 800 mg per mare per day for 8 days. Route of administration for each dose group was both intramuscularly (2 mares) and subcutaneously (2 mares). Changes were detected in all treated groups for clinical (reduced sensitivity to pain; locomotor incoordination; hypergastromotility; sweating; hyperthermia; labored respiration), blood chemistry (elevated cholesterol, total bilirubin, LDH, and glucose), and hematology (decreased eosinophils; increased hemoglobin, hematocrit, and erythrocytes) measurements. The effects in the 100 mg dose, and to a lesser extent, the 200 mg dose groups were transient in nature, lasting for a few minutes to several hours. Mares did not appear to sustain adverse effects following termination of the side effects.

Mares treated with either 400 mg or 800 mg exhibited more profound symptoms. The excessive hyperstimulation of the gastrointestinal tract caused a protracted diarrhea, slight electrolyte imbalance (decreased sodium and potassium), dehydration, gastrointestinal irritation, and slight liver malfunction (elevated SGOT, SGPT at 800 mg only). Heart rate was increased but pH of the urine was decreased. Other measurements evaluated in the study remained within normal limits. No mortality occurred in any of the groups. No apparent differences were observed between the intramuscular and subcutaneous routes of administration. Luteolytic doses of dinoprost tromethamine are on the order of 5 to 10 mg administered on one day, therefore, LUTALYSE® was demonstrated to have a wide margin of safety. Thus, the 100 mg dose gave a safety margin of 10 to 20X for a single injection or 80 to 160X for the 8 daily injections.

Additional studies investigated the effects in the mare of single intramuscular doses of 0, 0.25, 1.0, 2.5, 3.0, 5.0, and 10.0 mg dinoprost tromethamine. Heart rate, respiration rate, rectal temperature, and sweating were measured at 0, 0.25, 0.50, 0.75, 1.0, 1.5, 2.0, 3.0, 4.0, 5.0, and 6.0 hr. after injection. Neither heart rate nor respiration rates were significantly altered ($P > 0.05$) when compared to contemporary control values. Sweating was observed for 0 of 9, 2 of 9, 7 of 9, 9 of 9, and 8 of 9 mares injected with 0.25, 1.0, 2.5, 3.0, 5.0, or 10.0 mg dinoprost tromethamine, respectively. Sweating was temporary in all cases and was mild for doses of 3.0 mg or less but was extensive (beads of sweat over the entire body and dripping) for the 10 mg dose. Sweating after the 5.0 mg dose was intermediate between that seen for mares treated with 3.0 and 10.0 mg. Sweating began within 15 minutes after injection and ceased by 45 to 60 minutes after injection. Rectal temperature was decreased during the interval 0.5 until 1.0, 3 to 4, or 5 hours after injection for 0.25 and 1.0 mg, 2.5 and 3.0, or 5.0 and 10.0 mg dose groups, respectively. Average rectal temperature during the periods of decreased temperature was on the order of 97.5 to 99.6, with the greatest decreases observed in the 10 mg dose group.

Adverse Reactions:

Cattle:

1. The most frequently observed side effect is increased rectal temperature at a 5X or 10X overdose. However, rectal temperature change has been transient in all cases observed and has not been detrimental to the animal.
2. Limited salivation has been reported in some instances.
3. Intravenous administration might increase heart rate.
4. Localized post injection bacterial infections that may become generalized have been reported. In rare instances such infections have terminated fatally. See Cautions.

Swine: The most frequently observed side effects were erythema and pruritus, slight incoordination, nesting behavior, itching, urination, defecation, abdominal muscle spasms, tail movements, hyperpnea or dyspnea, increased vocalization, salivation, and at the 100 mg (10X) dose only, vomiting. These side effects are transitory, lasting from 10 minutes to 3 hours, and were not detrimental to the health of the animal.

Mares: The most frequently observed side effects are sweating and decreased rectal temperature. However, these have been transient in all cases observed and have not been detrimental to the animal. Other reactions seen have been increase in heart rate, increase in respiration rate, some abdominal discomfort, locomotor incoordination, and lying down. These effects are usually seen within 15 minutes of injection and disappear within one hour. Mares usually continue to eat during the period of expression of side effects. One anaphylactic reaction of several hundred mares treated with LUTALYSE® Sterile Solution was reported but was not confirmed.

Presentation: LUTALYSE® Sterile Solution is available in 10 and 30 mL vials.

Compendium Code No.: 10490300

LYMDYP™

DVM **Antidermatosis Rinse**

Pet Dip-Scented Lime Sulfur Concentrate

Active Ingredient(s):

Sulfurated Lime Solution	97.8%
Inert Ingredients	2.2%
Total	100.0%

Indications: For treatment of non-specific dermatoses and parasites responsive to the active ingredient. For dogs, cats, puppies and kittens.

LYMDYP™ is a scented sulfur concentrate which provides antimicrobial and antiparasitic activity.

Directions for Use: Shake well before use. Dilute 4 ounces in one gallon of water. Apply as a rinse or dip at 5 to 7 day intervals. Do not rinse. For more chronic and resistant cases, may be used at 8 ounces per gallon.

Precaution(s): Store at room temperature.

Caution(s): May stain light colored dogs/cats and porous (e.g. cement) surfaces. Will change color of jewelry.

For topical use on dogs and cats. May cause skin irritation. If irritation develops, decrease the frequency of use or discontinue use. Avoid contact with eyes. If contact occurs, rinse thoroughly with water. Note: If a precipitate or crust forms, immerse the sealed container in warm water for 15 minutes and shake well. Then use according to the directions.

Warning(s): Keep out of reach of children.

Presentation: 16 fl oz (473 mL) and 1 gallon (3.78 L).

Compendium Code No.: 11420391

Rev 1197

LymeCHEK®

Synbiotics **Lyme Disease Test**

U.S. Vet. Lic. No.: 312

Contents:

B. burgdorferi antigen coated wells	8 x 12 wells
Bottle A positive antibody control (red cap)	1 vial (3.0 mL)
Bottle B negative antibody control (grey cap)	11 vial (3.0 mL)
Bottle C HRP-*B. burgdorferi* conjugate (blue cap)	1 vial (7.0 mL)
Bottle D chromogen (green cap)	1 vial (7.0 mL)
Bottle E substrate buffer (white cap)	1 vial (7.0 mL)

Additional material provided: Holder for microtiter wells, and transfer pipets.

Material required, but not provided:

1. Timer/stopwatch.
2. Marking pen.
3. Deionized water (for plasma or sera).
4. Normal saline (for whole blood).

Indications: For use in the detection of canine antibodies to *Borrelia burgdorferi*.

Test Principle: The plastic wells are coated with inactivated *B. burgdorferi* antigens. These same antigens in a separate reagent are labelled with the enzyme horseradish peroxidase (HRP) and are used to detect the presence of *B. burgdorferi* antibodies. The specimen, either canine whole blood, plasma or serum, is incubated with the enzyme-linked antigen simultaneously in the antigen coated plastic wells. Anti-*Borrelia burgdorferi* antibody, if present in the sample, will attach to the solid phase and the conjugate. Excess conjugate and irrelevant sample proteins are washed away. After a brief incubation with the chromogenic reagent, a positive or negative result is determined visually.

LymeCHEK® is highly specific, sensitive and simple to perform. The test results can be obtained in 10 minutes. The diagnostic test kit contains a positive control and a negative control which should be included each time the assay is performed. Visual comparison of the color of the sample well with the positive and negative control wells allows accurate detection of the presence of antibodies to *B. burgdorferi*.

Test Procedure: 50 microliters (0.05 mL) of either whole blood (anticoagulated with EDTA, heparin, etc.), plasma or serum are required. Specimens may be stored at 2-7°C for up to seven (7) days. If longer storage is desired, store the serum or plasma at -20°C. Hemolysis does not significantly interfere with the test if adequate washing is performed.

Results: For the test to be valid, the fluid in the positive control well must be distinctly blue, while that in the negative control well must show little or no color change from initial substrate color.

A color change in the test sample of greater intensity than the negative control indicates the presence of *B. burgdorferi* antibodies. Because serum antibody levels in animals can remain elevated for several months following infection, a positive result is not necessarily indicative of an active infection. Since antibody development occurs over a three (3) to six (6) week period following infection, an early infection may show negative results due to low or absent antibody levels. Weak positive results obtained in the test may be indicative of an early infection, these animals should be retested in three (3) to four (4) weeks. Confirmatory diagnosis of the presence of an active *B. burgdorferi* infection should not be made solely on the results of the test, but rather on the basis of patient history, clinical symptoms, and response to antibiotic therapy in addition to the LymeCHEK® serology results.

Set up and conjugate:

1. Place one (1) well in the holder for the positive control, one (1) well for the negative control and one (1) well for each specimen. Leave the wells attached to each other.
2. Place one (1) drop of positive control (bottle A - red cap) into the first well and one (1) drop of negative control (bottle B - grey cap) into the second well. Place 50 mcg (one (1) drop using the pipet provided) of the sample into subsequent wells (wells 3, 4, etc.).
   If several samples are run simultaneously, only one (1) set of controls is needed.
   If a device is not available to accurately pipet 50 mcg of the sample, four (4) drops from a 20 gauge needle or six (6) drops from a 22 gauge needle may be used.
3. Place one (1) drop of HRP *B. burgdorferi* conjugate (bottle C - blue cap) into each well. Mix gently by tapping the holder several times (10-15 seconds). Incubate for five (5) minutes at room temperature (70°-78°F, 21°-25°C).

Blot and wash:

4. Discard the fluid from the wells by inverting and blotting onto a paper towel.

Develop:

5. Wash by vigorously filling the wells to overflowing with normal (isotonic) saline when using whole blood, or with distilled or deionized water when using serum or plasma. Discard the fluid from the wells and blot after each wash. Repeat washing five (5) times and blot dry on a paper towel after the final wash. Cross-contamination positives cannot occur from overflow during washing. The wells cannot be overwashed.
6. Place one (1) drop of chromogen (bottle D - green cap) into each well, followed by one (1) drop of substrate buffer (bottle E - white cap). Mix by gently tapping the holder several times. Incubate for five (5) minutes. After incubating, gently tap the holder for five (5) seconds, then read the results.

Note:

1. Leave the required number of wells attached to each other.
2. Whole blood must be anticoagulated with EDTA or heparin.
3. Washing is the most important step.
4. When washing, completely fill and empty all the wells each time, blotting between each wash. Spillage between the wells during washing will not affect the results. It is impossible to wash too much.
5. Always compare the results to the positive and negative control.

Precaution(s):

1. Store the test kit at 2-7°C. Do not store below 2°C as a precaution against freezing.
2. Allow the components to come to room temperature (70-78°F, 21-25°C) prior to use. The color intensity will vary with temperature.
3. Use a separate pipet for each specimen.
4. Include positive and negative controls provided each time the test is performed.
5. Follow the instructions exactly. Improper washing or contamination of the reagents may produce nonspecific color development. Immediate intense color development of negative control and samples usually indicates inadequate washing.
6. Handle all the samples and reagents as if capable of transmitting *B. burgdorferi* spirochetes. Burn or properly dispose of all unused biological components.
7. If properly stored, reagents should be stable until the expiration date.

Caution(s): Do not mix reagents from different kit lots.

For veterinary use only.

Discussion: Lyme disease is caused by the spirochete *Borrelia burgdorferi*, which is transmitted by ticks. Lyme disease is known to affect a variety of mammals, including dogs, cats, horses and humans. The diagnosis of Lyme disease is based upon clinical symptomology and elevated serum antibody titers to *B. burgdorferi*. In dogs, the most common symptoms are anorexia, lethargy, lameness and painful joint abnormalities. Depression and swollen lymph nodes can also occur.[1] Exposure to the spirochete results in the production of serum antibodies to *B. burgdorferi* over a period of three to six weeks. Following infection, these antibody levels remain elevated for a period of several months.[2] Exposure to the spirochete can be determined by serological evaluation for the presence of these antibodies to *B. burgdorferi* in canine blood. LymeCHEK® is an immunoenzymetric assay which specifically recognizes antibodies to *B. burgdorferi* in canine blood, plasma or serum. The assay provides for the rapid and accurate identification of dogs exposed to *B. burgdorferi*.

References: Available upon request.

Presentation: 8-22 tests.

Compendium Code No.: 11150140

LYMEVAX®

Fort Dodge **Bacterin**

Borrelia Burgdorferi Bacterin

U.S. Vet. Lic. No.: 112

Contents: This product contains the antigen listed above.

Thimerosal added as a preservative.

Indications: For vaccination of healthy dogs 9 weeks of age or older as an aid in the prevention of the disease caused by *Borrelia burgdorferi*.

Dosage and Administration: Dogs, inject one 1 mL dose subcutaneously using aseptic technique. A second dose should be administered 2 to 3 weeks later. Annual revaccination with one dose is recommended.

InfoVax-ID® System: The InfoVax-ID® System provides a simple and effective method of recording pertinent information on the vaccines administered to animals in a veterinary practice.

For vaccines requiring reconstitution, remove label from both vials and affix both labels to the animal's medical chart.

Using the InfoVax-ID® System:

1. Grasp the lower right hand corner of the tab at the arrow marked "Peel Here" between your thumb and forefinger.
2. Pull steadily at a slight upward angle until the top portion of the label is separated from the vial.
3. Place the label on the animal's medical chart. Press down on the label to ensure adhesion.

Precaution(s): Store in dark at 2° to 7°C (35° to 45°F). Avoid freezing. Shake well.

Caution(s): In the absence of a veterinarian-client-patient relationship, Federal law prohibits the relabeling, repackaging, resale, or redistribution of the individual contents of this package. (9 CFR 112.6)

In case of anaphylactoid reaction, administer epinephrine.

For use in dogs only. For veterinary use only.

Presentation: 10 dose (10 mL vial of vaccine) and 50 dose (50 x 1 mL vials of vaccine), featuring the InfoVax-ID® System.

U.S. Patents Pending and U.S. Patent No. 4,721,617

U.S. Pat. No. 5,704,648 (InfoVax-ID® System)

Made under license from MGI Pharma, Inc.

Compendium Code No.: 10031051 1404M

LYSIGIN®

Boehringer Ingelheim **Bacterin**

Staphylococcus Aureus Bacterin

U.S. Vet. Lic. No.: 124

Composition: A lysed culture of highly antigenic polyvalent somatic antigen containing phage types I, II, III, IV and miscellaneous groups of *Staphylococcus aureus*.

Indications: Recommended for the vaccination of healthy, susceptible cattle as an aid in the prevention of mastitis caused by *Staphylococcus aureus*.

Dosage and Administration: Using aseptic technique, inject 5 mL intramuscularly. Repeat in 14 days. Follow with a single 5 mL booster dose each 5 to 6 months. Start vaccinating all heifers at 6 months of age.

Precaution(s): Store out of direct sunlight at a temperature between 35-45°F (2-7°C). Avoid freezing. Shake well before using. Use entire contents when first opened.

Caution(s): Anaphylactoid reactions may occur.

Antidote(s): Epinephrine.

Warning(s): Do not vaccinate within 21 days before slaughter.

Presentation: 10 doses (50 mL) and 50 doses (250 mL).

Compendium Code No.: 10280752 BI 1041-8R-1 12/01

LYSING SOLUTION

Centaur **Heartworm Test**

Indications: Diagnostic reagent for *in vitro* use only for the detection of microfilariae in dogs.

Precaution(s): Store at room temperature. Keep out of direct sunlight.

Presentation: 0.5 gallon (1.89 L).

Compendium Code No.: 14880200

LYSING SOLUTION

Vedco **Heartworm Test**

Description: Lysing solution (diagnostic reagent).

Ingredient(s): Formaldehyde. Also contains Versene and green and yellow dye.

Indications: To be used in test protocols designed for the detection of microfilariae in blood. Sold to veterinarians only.

Storage: Store at room temperature.

Warning(s): For *in vitro* use only.

Presentation: 64 oz container.

Compendium Code No.: 10941210

LYSOL® I.C.™ BRAND QUATERNARY DISINFECTANT CLEANER

Reckitt Benckiser **Disinfectant**

Pseudomonacidal-Salmonellacidal-Fungicidal-Mildewstatic-Staphylocidal-Bactericidal-Virucidal*-Disinfectant

EPA Reg. No.: 47371-129-675

Active Ingredient(s):

Didecyl dimethyl ammonium chloride 9.70%
n-Alykl (C_{14} 50%, C_{12} 40%, C_{16} 10%) dimethyl benzyl ammonium chloride 6.47%
Inert Ingredients: 83.83%
Total: 100.00%

Indications: A multi-purpose, neutral pH germicidal detergent, deodorant effective in hard water up to 400 ppm (calculated as $CaCO_3$) in the presence of a moderate amount of soil (5% organic serum) according to the AOAC Use-dilution Test. Disinfects, cleans and deodorizes in one labor-saving step.

Effective against the following pathogens:

Bacteria: *Pseudomonas aeruginosa*[1], *Salmonella choleraesuis, Staphylococcus aureus* (Methicillin Resistant), *Staphylococcus aureus*[1], *Acinetobacter calcoaceticus, Bordetella bronchiseptica, Chlamydia psittaci, Enterobacter aerogenes, Enterobacter cloacae, Escherichia coli*[1], *Fusobacterium necrophorum, Klebsiella pneumoniae*[1], *Listeria monocytogenes, Pasteurella multocida, Proteus mirabilis, Proteus vulgaris, Salmonella enteritidis, Legionella pneumophila, Salmonella typhi, Salmonella typhimurium, Serratia marsescens, Shigella flexneri, Shigella sonnei, Staphylococcus epidermidis*[2], *Streptococcus faecalis*[1], *Streptococcus pyogenes, Enterococcus faecalis* (Vancomycin Resistant).

[1] ATTC and antibiotic-resistant strain

[2] Antibiotic-resistant strain only

Fungi: *Aspergillus niger, Candida albicans, Trichophyton mentagrophytes.*

Viruses: HIV-1 (AIDS Virus), Herpes Simplex Type 1, Herpes Simplex Type 2, Respiratory Syncytial Virus (RSV), Rubella (German Measles), Adenovirus Type 4, Vaccinia, Influenza A/Hong Kong.

Animal Viruses: Canine Distemper, Feline Leukemia, Pseudorabies, Feline Picornavirus, Transmissable Gastroenteritis Virus (TGE), Rabies, Infectious Bronchitis (Avian IBV), Infectious Bovine Rhinotracheitis.

Disinfects, cleans and deodorizes the following hard nonporous inanimate surfaces: floors, walls, (non-medical) metal surfaces, (non-medical) stainless steel surfaces, glazed porcelain, plastic surfaces (such as polypropylene, polystyrene, etc.).

Recommended for use in Hospitals, Nursing Homes, Schools, Colleges, Industrial Institutions, Office Buildings, Veterinary Clinics, Animal Life Science Laboratories, Equine Farms, Tack Shops, Pet Shops, Airports, Kennels, Hotels, Poultry Farms, Dairy Farms, Breeding Establishments, Grooming Establishments and Households.

Directions for Use: It is a violation of Federal law to use this product in a manner inconsistent with its labeling.

Disinfection/Cleaning/Deodorizing Directions: Remove heavy soil deposits from surface, then thoroughly wet surface with a solution of ½ ounce of the concentrate per gallon of water. The solution can be applied with a cloth, mop, sponge, or coarse spray or soaking. Let solution remain on surface for a minimum of 10 minutes. Rinse or allow to air dry. Rinsing of floors is not necessary unless they are to be waxed or polished. Food contact surfaces must be thoroughly rinsed with potable water. This product must not be used to clean the following food contact surfaces: utensils, glassware and dishes. Prepare a fresh solution daily or more often if the solution becomes visibly dirty or diluted.

Dilution Chart:

Correct Solution Strength: 0.39% (1:256, ½ oz. per gallon)

Product	Water
½ oz.	1 gallon
2½ oz.	5 gallons

Fungicidal Directions: For use in areas such as locker rooms, dressing rooms, shower and bath areas and exercise facilities follow disinfection directions.

Mildewstatic Directions: Will effectively control the growth of mold and mildew plus the odors caused by them when applied to hard nonporous surfaces such as walls, floors, and table tops. Apply solution (½ oz. per gallon of water) with a cloth, mop, sponge, or coarse spray. Make sure to wet all surfaces completely. Let air dry. Repeat application weekly or when growth reappears.

Farm Premise, Livestock, Poultry and Turkey House Disinfectant:

1. Remove all animals and feeds from premises, trucks, coops, crates and enclosures.
2. Remove all litter and manure from floors, walls, and surfaces of barns, pens, stalls, chutes, vehicles, and other facilities and fixtures occupied or traversed by animals.
3. Empty all troughs, racks, and other feeding and watering appliances.
4. Thoroughly clean all surfaces with soap or detergent, and rinse with water.
5. Saturate all surfaces with a ½ oz. per gallon of water disinfecting solution for a period of 10 minutes.
6. Immerse all halters, ropes, and other types of equipment used in handling and restraining animals, as well as forks, shovels, and scrapers used for removing litter and manure.
7. Ventilate buildings, coops, cars, trucks, boats, and other closed spaces. Do not house animals or employ equipment until treatment has been absorbed, set, or dried.
8. After treatment with disinfectant, thoroughly scrub feed racks, troughs, automatic feeders, fountains, and waterers with soap or detergent, and rinse with potable water before reuse.

Veterinary Practice/Animal Care/Animal Laboratory/Zoos/Pet Shop/Kennels/Disinfection Directions:

For cleaning and disinfecting the following hard nonporous surfaces: equipment not used for animal food or water, utensils, instruments, cages, kennels, stables, catteries, etc. Remove all animals and feeds from premises, animal transportation vehicles, crates, etc. Remove all litter, droppings and manure from floors, walls and surfaces of facilities occupied or traversed by animals. Thoroughly clean all surfaces with soap or detergent and rinse with water. Saturate surfaces with a use-solution of ½ oz. of LYSOL® Brand I.C.™ Quaternary Disinfectant Cleaner per gallon of water (or equivalent dilution) for a period of 10 minutes. Ventilate buildings and other closed spaces. Do not house animals or employ equipment until treatment has been absorbed, set or dried.

Precautionary Statements: Hazards to Humans and Domestic Animals: Danger: Corrosive. Causes irreversible eye damage and skin burns. Harmful if swallowed. Do not get in eyes, on skin or on clothing. When handling product, protect eyes by wearing goggles or face shield and protect skin by wearing rubber gloves. Wash thoroughly with soap and water after handling. Remove contaminated clothing and wash before reuse.

First Aid: In case of contact, immediately flush eyes or skin with plenty of water for at least 15 minutes. For eyes or skin, call a physician. If swallowed, call a doctor or get medical attention. Do not induce vomiting or give anything by mouth to an unconscious person. Drink promptly a large quantity of milk, egg whites, gelatin solution, or if these are not available, drink large quantities of water. Avoid alcohol.

Note to Physician: Probable mucosal damage may contraindicate the use of gastric lavage. Measures against circulatory shock, respiratory depression and convulsion may be needed.

Storage and Disposal: Keep product under locked storage, inaccessible to small children. Do not reuse empty container. Rinse thoroughly, securely wrap empty container in several layers of newspaper, then discard in trash.

Warning(s): Keep out of reach of children.

Presentation: 1 gallon (3.79 liters).

Compendium Code No.: 10011050 368992

Looking for a particular vaccine?
Check the Blue pages.

LYSOL® BRAND II I.C.™ DISINFECTANT SPRAY

Reckitt Benckiser **Disinfectant**

Surface Disinfectant-Tuberculocidal-Ready To Use

EPA Reg. No.: 777-72-675

Active Ingredient(s):

Alkyl (50% C_{14}, 40% C_{12}, 10% C_{16}) Dimethyl Benzyl Ammonium Saccharinate 0.1%
Ethanol 79.0%
Inert Ingredients: 20.9%
Total 100.0%

Indications: LYSOL® Brand II I.C.™ Disinfectant Spray meets AOAC Germicidal Spray Product Test standards for hospital aerosol disinfectants: Germicidal, Fungicidal, Tuberculocidal, Virucidal.*

On environmental surfaces, LYSOL® Brand II I.C.™ Disinfectant Spray kills the following bacteria and fungi:

Bacteria: *Mycobacterium tuberculosis* var bovis, *Staphylococcus aureus, Salmonella choleraesuis, Pseudomonas aeruginosa, Campylobacter jejuni, Enterobacter aerogenes, Corynebacterium diphtheriae, Enterococcus faecalis, Escherichia coli, Klebsiella pneumoniae, Listeria monocytogenes, Proteus vulgaris, Serratia marcescens, Neisseria elongata, Shigella dysenteriae, Staphylococcus aureus* (Methicillin and Gentamicin resistant), *Streptococcus pyogenes.*

Fungi: *Aspergillus niger, Candida albicans, Trichophyton mentagrophytes.*

It also kills hydrophilic and lipophilic viruses*: Human Immunodeficiency Virus Type 1 (HIV-1) (AIDS Virus), Adenovirus Type 2, Cytomegalovirus, Echovirus Type 12, Hepatitis A Virus, Herpes Simplex Type 1, Herpes Simplex Type 2, Influenza A_2 (Japan), Influenza Type B (Hong Kong), Poliovirus Type 1, Respiratory Synctial Virus, Rhinovirus Type 39, Rotavirus WA, Vaccinia.

For Use In: Hospitals, Ambulances, Nursing Homes, Kennels, Clinics, Veterinary Offices, Dental Offices, Day Care Centers, Physician Offices, Health Clubs.

Directions for Use: It is a violation of Federal law to use this product in a manner inconsistent with its labeling.

Hold can upright 6" to 8" from surface.

To Disinfect: Spray precleaned surface 2 to 3 seconds until covered with mist. Allow to stand 10 minutes to air dry.

Sanitizes: Kills 99.9% of *Staphylococcus aureus* and *Klebsiella pneumoniae* on hard, nonporous surfaces in 30 seconds

To Deodorize: Spray on surfaces as needed.

Eliminates Odors: LYSOL® Brand II I.C.™ Disinfectant Spray deodorizes by killing many germs that cause odor. It eliminates odors at their source. To eliminate odors retained in fabrics, spray on draperies curtains and upholstered furniture.

Precautionary Statements: Hazards to Humans and Domestic Animals: Causes eye irritation. Do not spray in eyes on skin or on clothing.

First Aid: In case of eye contact, immediately flush eyes thoroughly with water, remove any contact lenses, and continue to flush eyes with plenty of water for at least 15 minutes. Get medial attention if irritation persists.

Physical Hazards:

Flammable: Contents under pressure. Keep away from heat, sparks and open flame. Do not puncture or incinerate container. Exposure to temperatures above 130°F may cause bursting. Do not use on polished wood, rayon fabrics, leather, or acrylic plastics.

Storage and Disposal: Store in original container in areas inaccessible to small children. Replace cap and discard in trash. Do not puncture or incinerate. Do not reuse empty container.

Warning(s): Keep out of reach of children.

Presentation: 12 x 19 oz (1 lb 3 oz) 538.65 g cans.

Compendium Code No.: 10011040 368994

LYTAR® SHAMPOO

DVM **Antidermatosis Shampoo**

Full Strength Antiseborrheic Antipruritic Conditioning Formulation

Active Ingredient(s): Coal tar 3%, sulfur 2% and salicylic acid 2%.

Indications: For the relief of oiliness, scaling, itching and inflammation associated with seborrheic dermatitis.

LYTAR® is a full strength, degreasing, antiseborrheic, antipruritic, soap-free formulation complemented with protein and coat conditioners.

Directions for Use: Shake well before use. Wet coat thoroughly. Apply and lather shampoo over entire body, allowing for 5-10 minutes of contact time. Rinse completely. Repeat procedure if necessary. Use once or twice weekly or as directed by veterinarian.

Precaution(s): Store at room temperature.

Caution(s): For topical use on dogs. Avoid contact with eyes. If contact occurs, rinse thoroughly with water. If irritation develops, discontinue and consult your veterinarian.

Warning(s): Keep out of reach of children.

Presentation: 8 fl oz (237 mL) (NDC 47203-300-08), 12 fl oz (355 mL) (NDC 47203-300-12) and 1 gallon (3.78 L) (NDC 47203-300-28).

Compendium Code No.: 11420401 Rev 0199

L

Disclaimer

Every effort has been made to ensure the accuracy of the information published. However, it remains the responsibility of the readers to familiarize themselves with the product information contained on the product label or package insert.

Inclusion or omission of products does not imply endorsement or criticism by the Publisher or anyone involved in the publication. Inclusion does not imply product availability and/or product registration. The Publisher, Editorial Team and all people involved in the production of this book cannot be held responsible for publication errors or any consequence that could result from the use of published information.

M

MAGESTIC™ 7 WITH SPUR®*

Intervet — **Bacterin-Vaccine**

Parvovirus Vaccine, Killed Virus-Erysipelothrix Rhusiopathiae-Leptospira Canicola-Grippotyphosa-Hardjo-Icterohaemorrhagiae-Pomona Bacterin

U.S. Vet. Lic. No.: 286

Contents: This product contains the antigens listed above.

Contains gentamicin as a preservative.

Indications: For use as an aid in the prevention of disease caused by porcine parvovirus, *Erysipelothrix rhusiopathiae,* and *Leptospira* serovars *canicola, grippotyphosa, hardjo, icterohaemorrhagiae* and *pomona* in healthy, breeding age swine.

Dosage and Administration: Shake well before using. Administer 2 mL intramuscularly to breeding animals. One dose six (6) weeks before breeding followed by a second dose in 14 to 28 days. Revaccination with a single dose is recommended prior to each breeding (semi-annually). Boars should be vaccinated semi-annually).

Precaution(s): Store at 35° to 45°F (2° to 7°C). Use entire contents when first opened. Burn the container and all unused contents.

Caution(s): Allergic reactions may follow the use of products of this nature.

For use in animals only.

Antidote(s): Epinephrine.

Warning(s): Do not vaccinate within 21 days of slaughter.

Presentation: 50 doses (100 mL).

*Adjuvant—Intervet's Proprietary Technology

Compendium Code No.: 11060840

MAGNALAX BOLUS

Phoenix Pharmaceutical — **Antacid-Laxative**

Antacid-Laxative-480 Grains

Active Ingredient(s): Composition: Each bolus contains:

Magnesium Oxide (equiv. to Magnesium Hydroxide 400 gr) .... 276 gr (17.9 g)

Flavored with Ginger, Capsicum, and Methyl Salicylate. Artificial color added.

Indications: For oral administration to ruminants as an aid in the treatment of digestive disturbances requiring an antacid and mild laxative.

Dosage and Administration: Give 2 to 4 boluses to ruminants, depending on size and condition of animal. Lubricate boluses and administer with a balling gun.

One and one-half MAGNALAX BOLUSES are equivalent to one pint of milk of magnesia.

Precaution(s): Store in a cool, dry place. Keep tightly closed when not in use.

Caution(s): For animal use only. Avoid frequent or continued use.

Warning(s): Keep out of reach of children.

Presentation: 50 boluses (NDC 57319-047-12).

Compendium Code No.: 12560541 — Rev. 06-00

MAGNALAX BOLUSES

Aspen — **Antacid-Laxative**

Active Ingredient(s): Each bolus contains:

Magnesium oxide (equivalent to magnesium hydroxide, 400 gr).................. 276 gr

Flavored with ginger, capsicum, and methyl salicylate. Artificial color added.

Indications: For oral administration to ruminants as an aid in the treatment of digestive disturbances requiring an antacid and mild laxative.

Dosage and Administration: Give two (2) to four (4) boluses to ruminants, depending upon the size and the condition of the animal. Lubricate the boluses and administer with a balling gun.

One and one-half (1½) MAGNALAX BOLUSES are equivalent to one (1) pint of milk of magnesia.

Precaution(s): Store at controlled room temperature between 15° and 30°F (59°-86°F). Keep tightly closed when not in use.

Caution(s): Keep out of the reach of children. Avoid frequent or continued use.

Presentation: 50 boluses.

Compendium Code No.: 14750550

MAGNALAX BOLUSES

Bimeda — **Antacid-Laxative**

Active Ingredient(s): Each bolus contains:

Magnesium hydroxide .... 27 g (416 gr.)

Other ingredients: Capsicum, ginger, methyl salicylate and other inert ingredients.

Indications: For oral administration as an aid in the treatment of digestive disturbances requiring an antacid and mild laxative in cattle.

Dosage and Administration: Give two (2) to four (4) boluses depending upon the size and the condition of the animal.

Three (3) boluses are equivalent to one (1) quart of milk of magnesia.

Lubricate the boluses with mineral oil or other nonirritating lubricants before administering.

Precaution(s): Keep in a cool, dry place.

Caution(s): For animal use only. Not for human use.

Keep out of the reach of children.

Warning(s): Milk that has been taken from animals during treatment and for 24 hours (2 milkings) after the last treatment with this drug must not be used for food.

Presentation: 50 boluses.

Compendium Code No.: 13990250

MAGNALAX BOLUSES

First Priority — **Antacid-Laxative**

Magnesium oxide

Active Ingredient(s): Each bolus contains:

Magnesium Oxide .... 276 gr (17.9 g)

Flavored with ginger, capsicum, and methyl salicylate. Artificial color added.

Indications: For oral administration to ruminants as an aid in the treatment of digestive disturbances requiring an antacid and mild laxative.

Dosage and Administration: Give 2 to 4 boluses to ruminants, depending on the size and condition of animal. Lubricate boluses and administer with a balling gun.

One and one-half MAGNALAX BOLUSES are equivalent to one pint of milk of magnesia.

Precaution(s): Store at controlled room temperature between 15° and 30°F (59°-86°F).

Keep tightly closed when not in use.

Caution(s): Avoid frequent or continued use.

Warning(s): For animal use only. Keep out of the reach of children.

Presentation: 50 boluses.

Compendium Code No.: 11390500

MAGNALAX POWDER

Bimeda — **Antacid-Laxative**

Active Ingredient(s): Each pound contains:

Magnesium hydroxide.. 10.35 oz.

In a flavored base.

One pound contains magnesium hydroxide equivalent to one gallon milk of magnesia.

Indications: A mild laxative, antacid for use in ruminant animals with simple indigestion.

Dosage and Administration: Mature bovine, stir 1 lb. of MAGNALAX POWDER into one (1) gallon of water and mix thoroughly. Administer as a drench or via a stomach tube. For sheep, goats and calves, administer one (1) pint to one (1) quart depending upon the size of the animal.

Frequent or continued use should be avoided.

Precaution(s): Do not store above 86°F (30°C).

Caution(s): For animal use only. Not for human use. Keep out of the reach of children.

Warning(s): Milk that has been taken from animals during treatment and for 24 hours (2 milkings) after the last treatment must not be used for food.

Presentation: 1 lb. and 25 lb. jars.

Compendium Code No.: 13990260

MAGNALAX POWDER

Phoenix Pharmaceutical — **Antacid-Laxative**

Antacid-Laxative-Adsorbent

Active Ingredient(s): Each pound contains:

Magnesium Hydroxide .... 10.35 oz

In a flavored base.

Indications: A mild laxative, antacid for use in ruminant animals with simple ingestion.

Directions: Mature bovine, stir one pound of MAGNALAX POWDER into one gallon of water and mix thoroughly. Administer as a drench or via a stomach tube. For sheep, goats and calves, administer one pint to one quart depending on size of animals. Frequent or continued use should be avoided.

One pound of MAGNALAX POWDER contains magnesium hydroxide equivalent to 1 gallon of milk of magnesia.

Precaution(s): Do not store above 30°C (86°F). Store in a cool, dry place. Keep lid tightly closed when not in use.

Caution(s): For animal use only. Keep out of reach of children.

Warning(s): Milk that has been taken from animals during treatment and for 12 hours (1 milking) after the latest treatment must not be used for food.

Presentation: 16 oz (1 lb) jars (NDC 57319-114-27).

Compendium Code No.: 12560551 — Rev. 06-00

MAGNALAX POWDER

Vedco — **Antacid-Laxative**

Active Ingredient(s): Each bolus contains:

Magnesium oxide .... 10.35 oz.

With kaolin and flavoring agents (capsicum, ginger and methyl salicylate).

One pound contains magnesium hydroxide equivalent to one gallon milk of magnesia.

Indications: A mild laxative, anti-acid and detoxicant for simple indigestions of ruminants.

Dosage and Administration:

For mature bovine: Mix one (1) pound thoroughly with one (1) gallon of water and administer as a drench or with a stomach tube. Dose smaller animals according to size and weight.

Sheep or Goats: Two (2) ounces mixed with water. Shake well before administering.

Precaution(s): Do not store above 86°F (30°C).

Caution(s): Keep out of the reach of children. Frequent or continued use should be avoided.

Warning(s): Milk that has been taken from animals during treatment and for 24 hours (2 milkings) after the latest treatment must not be used for food.

Presentation: 1 lb. and 25 lb. containers.

Compendium Code No.: 10941220

MAGNA-LYTE

First Priority — **Electrolytes-Oral**

Guaranteed Analysis:

Calcium (Ca) not less than 0.15%
Calcium (Ca) not more than 0.50%
Salt (Nacl) not less than 9.25%
Salt (Nacl) not more than 11.00%
Sodium (Na) not less than 3.50%
Potassium (K) not less than 0.60%
Magnesium (Mg) not less than 0.05%
Glucose (not more than)........................ 78.00%

Ingredients: Dextrose, salt, potassium chloride, calcium lactate, magnesium sulfate, sodium citrate, silicon dioxide.

Indications: MAGNA-LYTE is a concentrated electrolyte powder for use in cattle, swine, sheep and horses. MAGNA-LYTE provides a balanced electrolyte solution with dextrose.

Dosage and Administration:

For use in drinking water: Dissolve contents of one full bag - 16 oz (454 grams) in approximately 40 gallons of drinking water.

For drenching: Dissolve 4 oz (113.5 grams) of powder per 6 gallons of drinking water. Use proper drenching procedures to provide 1 quart per 100 lbs (45 kg) of body weight for sheep and swine. Give 2 quarts per 100 lbs (45 kg) of body weight for cattle and horses.

Warning(s): For oral use only. For use in animals only.

Keep out of reach of children.

Presentation: 1 lb (453.6 g).

Compendium Code No.: 11390481

MAGNAPASTE™

Butler **Poultice**

Decongestant Poultice

Active Ingredient(s): Composition:

Magnesium Sulphate (epsom salt) 60%
Methyl Salicylate .... q.s.

In a water soluble base.

Indications: A poultice paste for use on horses and cattle. For strains, sprains, and bruises. An osmotic agent for external application.

Directions: Apply locally as a poultice (without rubbing) to acute swellings, sprains, contusions, acute mastitis, swollen glands. May be repeated within 24 hours, as indicated.

Precaution(s): Keep container tightly closed. Store in a cool, dry place.

Caution(s): Avoid contact with eyes and mucous membranes.

For animal use only.

Keep out of reach of children.

Presentation: 20 oz (NDC 11695-2185-2).

Compendium Code No.: 10821112 Iss. 6-00

MAGNA-POULTICE™

First Priority **Poultice**

Active Ingredient(s):

Magnesium Sulphate (epsom salt) 60%
Methyl Salicylate .... q.s.

In a water soluble base.

Indications: A decongestant poultice paste for strains, sprains and bruises for use on horses and cattle.

An osmotic agent for external application.

Directions for Use: Apply locally as a poultice (without rubbing) to acute swellings, sprains, contusions, acute mastitis, swollen glands. May be repeated within 24 hours, as indicated.

Precaution(s): Storage: Store at controlled room temperature between 15°-30°C (59°-86°F). Keep container tightly closed when not in use.

Caution(s): Avoid contact with eyes and mucous membranes.

For animal use only.

Warning(s): Keep out of reach of children.

Presentation: 1.25 lb (567 g) (NDC# 58829-273-20).

Compendium Code No.: 11390492 Rev. 11-01

MAGSALT™

SSI Corp. **Hoof Product**

Active Ingredient(s):

Magnesium (Mg) 4.27%
Sulfur (S) 7.06%
Inert 88.67%

Indications: Aids in the prevention of footwarts (Papillomatous Digital Dermatitis) in dairy cattle.

Directions: MAGSALT™ can be applied in two ways:

Spraying for Prevention (Preferred Method): Use as a direct topical spray by mixing one (1) part MAGSALT™ to three (3) parts water. Clean affected area beforehand as well as possible. Spray all animals, all feet, or at least the back feet, four to five milkings straight. MAGSALT™ can be used in your rotation program every fourth to fifth week.

Foot Baths (Optional Method): Mix one (1) quart MAGSALT™ to fifty (50) gallons of water. Change every 150 head. Foot bath may need to be cleaned and recharged more often than every 150 head depending on environment and hygiene conditions. When using foot baths a product rotation is best. Footbaths require careful management. If not properly managed results are reduced significantly.

Precaution(s): Keep from freezing.

Caution(s): Eye irritant. In case of eye contact, flush for 15 minutes. If irritation persists, call a physician.

Warning(s): Keep out of the reach of children.

Discussion: MAGSALT™ is specifically formulated to be used in a rotational program of products for the prevention of footwarts (papillomatous digital dermatitis). MAGSALT™ can be used in your prevention program with SSI's Hoofpro+® and Rotational Zinc™ as well as E-Z Copper™. A regularly scheduled preventative maintenance program for all animals should be implemented as risk of reoccurrence of footwarts is very likely.

Presentation: 2.5, 5 and 30 gallon drums.

Compendium Code No.: 14930031

MAKE YOUR OWN CHLORHEXIDINE SHAMPOO

Davis **Antidermatosis Shampoo**

Directions for Use: To make a 1% chlorhexidine shampoo, dilute 6 oz of Davis 20% CHLORHEXIDINE GLUCONATE in one gallon of non-medicated shampoo and mix thoroughly. Wet animal's coat completely with warm water. Do not get shampoo into eyes. Apply shampoo on head and ears, then lather. Repeat procedure with neck, chest, middle and hind quarter, finishing legs last. Allow pet to stand for 5 to 10 minutes. Rinse pet thoroughly. For best results, repeat procedure.

After bathing, a chlorhexidine rinse may result in greater residual activity. To make a .50% solution, dilute 3 oz of Davis 20% CHLORHEXIDINE GLUCONATE in one gallon of water. Mix thoroughly.

To make a 2% chlorhexidine solution, dilute 12 oz of Davis 20% CHLORHEXIDINE GLUCONATE to one gallon of water.

Use under the direction of a licensed veterinarian.

To reconstitute MAKE YOUR OWN CHLORHEXIDINE SHAMPOO follow these four steps:

1) Pour 1 gallon Davis Gold Shampoo into 5 gallon bucket.
2) Pour 32 ounces Davis 20% Chlorhexidine Gluconate into the 5 gallon bucket and stir.
3) Pour 3 ounces Fresh & Clean Fragrance into bucket and stir.
4) Fill the rest of the bucket with water and stir well before using.

Precautionary Statements: Product may be harmful if swallowed and irritating to eyes, respiratory system and skin.

First Aid:

If Swallowed: Contact a physician immediately. Drink two glasses of water and induce vomiting. Never give anything by mouth to an unconscious person.

If In Eyes or On Skin: Flush affected areas immediately with plenty of water. If irritation persists, consult a physician. Remove contaminated clothing and shoes.

If Inhaled: Remove to fresh air. Give artificial respiration and/or oxygen if breathing is difficult.

Storage: Avoid exposure to heat and/or direct sunlight.

Warning(s): For external use only. Keep out of reach of children.

Presentation: Reconstituted to 5 gallons.

Compendium Code No.: 11410230

MAKE YOUR OWN FLEA & TICK SHAMPOO

Davis **Parasiticide Shampoo**

EPA Reg. No.: 50591-2 (Davis Pyrethrins®)

Active Ingredient(s):

In Davis Pyrethrins®:

Pyrethrins 7.5%
Piperonyl butoxide, technical* 75.0%
Inert ingredients 17.5%
Total 100.0%

Davis Pyrethrins® is a concentrate to be added to shampoo for use on cats and dogs to kill fleas and ticks.

To reconstitute MAKE YOUR OWN FLEA & TICK SHAMPOO follow these four steps:

1) Pour 1 gallon Davis Gold Shampoo into 5 gallon bucket.
2) Pour 5 ounces Davis Pyrethrins into 5 gallon bucket and stir.
3) Pour 3 ounces Fresh & Clean Fragrance into bucket and stir.
4) Fill the rest of the bucket with water and stir.

Indications: For dogs, cats, puppies and kittens.

Dosage and Administration: It is a violation of federal law to use the product in a manner inconsistent with its labeling.

To shampoo and kill fleas and ticks, follow these steps:

1. Wet the animal thoroughly.
2. Apply a generous amount of the shampoo mixture to the coat, massaging the lather well into the coat and skin.
3. Allow the lather to remain on the animal for five (5) minutes to permit the pyrethrins to take their full effect.
4. Rinse the animal thoroughly.

Precaution(s): Do not re-use the empty container. Wrap it in newspaper and discard it with the trash. Do not use or store near heat or an open flame.

Environmental Hazards: The product is toxic to fish. Do not dispose of in lakes, streams or open ponds.

Caution(s): Keep out of the reach of children. To be applied only by or under the supervision of a licensed veterinarian or pet groomer.

Precautionary Statements: Hazards to Humans: Harmful if swallowed. Do not get in the eyes. Wash hands thoroughly after each use and before eating or smoking.

Hazards to Domestic Animals: Do not apply directly to or on the eyes, mouth or genitals of pets. Do not treat or cause exposure to kittens or puppies of less than four weeks of age.

Warning(s): Statement of Practical Treatment:

If swallowed: Contact a physician or poison control center immediately. Do not induce vomiting. The product contains petroleum distillate. Vomiting may cause aspiration pneumonia.

If in eyes or on skin: Flush the affected areas with plenty of water. Contact a physician if irritation persists.

Buyer assumes all risks of use, storage or handling of the material not in strict accordance with directions given on the label.

Presentation: Reconstituted to 5 gallons.

Compendium Code No.: 11410240

MALASEB™ FLUSH

DVM **Antifungal**

Active Ingredient(s): Miconazole base 0.174% w/v (equivalent to Miconazole Nitrate 0.2% w/v), Chlorhexidine Gluconate 0.2% w/v.

Indications: For conditions associated with infections responsive to Miconazole and Chlorhexidine Gluconate.

Product Description: MALASEB™ Flush combines a unique formulation of antibacterial and antifungal agents enhances with phospholipids for optimal therapeutic effectiveness.

A medicated formulation for dogs and cats.

Directions: Apply MALASEB™ Flush liberally to affected area. Use cotton or absorbent material to clean excess solution. Apply twice daily or as directed by your veterinarian.

Precaution(s): Store at room temperature.

Caution(s): For external use on animals only. Do not instill in eyes or on sensitive membranes that are damages or compromised.

Warning(s): Keep out of reach of children.

Presentation: 4 fl oz (118 mL) (NDC 47203-595-04) and 12 fl oz (355 mL) (NDC 47203-595-12).

Compendium Code No.: 11420630 Rev. 1100

MALASEB™ PLEDGETS

DVM **Antifungal**

Active Ingredient(s): Each MALASEB™ PLEDGET applicator (2.25 inch in diameter, 70% Rayon, 30% Polyester) contains approximately 17.4 mg of Miconazole (equivalent to 20 mg Miconazole Nitrate), 20 mg of Chlorhexidine Gluconate.

Also contains SDA 3C Ethyl Alcohol 30% v/v.

Indications: For dermatological conditions associated with infections responsive to Miconazole and Chlorhexidine Gluconate. A localized treatment to be used between generalized therapy.

Medicated pads for dogs, cats, and horses.

Directions for Use: Treat affected area(s) 2-3 times daily, or as directed by veterinarian. Use pledgets to wipe affected area thoroughly. Distract animal for several minutes following treatment to prevent licking. Each pledget should be used once and discarded.

Precaution(s): Flammable: Keep away from extreme heat or flame. Store at room temperature.

Caution(s): For topical use on dogs, cats and horses. Avoid contact with eyes. Wash hands thoroughly after use. If irritation develops, discontinue and consult your veterinarian. Keep out of reach of children.

Presentation: 60 pledgets (NDC 47203-590-60).

U.S. Patent No. 5536742

Compendium Code No.: 11420590 REV 0900

MALASEB™ SHAMPOO

DVM **Antifungal Shampoo**

Medicated Shampoo Formulation

Active Ingredient(s): Miconazole nitrate 2%, chlorhexidine gluconate 2%.

Indications: For dermatological conditions associated with infections responsive to miconazole nitrate and chlorhexidine gluconate for dogs, cats and horses.

Product Description: MALASEB™'s unique formulation provides antibacterial and antifungal agents for optimal therapeutic effectiveness.

Directions for Use: Wet coat thoroughly with water. Apply and lather shampoo over the entire body, allowing 10 minutes of contact time. Rinse completely with water. Repeat twice weekly until symptoms subside, then weekly, or as directed by veterinarian.

Precaution(s): Store at room temperature.

Caution(s): For topical use only on dogs, cats, and horses. Avoid contact with eyes. If irritation develops, discontinue and consult your veterinarian.

Warning(s): Keep out of reach of children.

Presentation: 8 fl oz (237 mL), 12 fl oz (355 mL) (NDC 47203-585-12) and 1 gallon (3.78 L) (NDC 47203-585-28).

Compendium Code No.: 11420602 Rev 0200

MALASEB™ SPRAY

DVM **Antifungal**

Active Ingredient(s): Miconazole 1.74% w/v (equivalent to 2.0% w/v miconazole nitrate), Chlorhexidine Gluconate 2% w/v.

Also contains SDA 3C Ethyl Alcohol 30% v/v.

Indications: For dermatological conditions associated with infections responsive to Miconazole and Chlorhexidine Gluconate. A localized treatment to be used between generalized therapy.

Medicated spray formulation for dogs, cats and horses.

Directions for Use: Spray directly onto the affected area(s) 2-3 times daily, or as directed by veterinarian. Distract animal for several minutes following treatment to prevent licking.

Precaution(s): Flammable: Keep away from extreme heat or flame. Store at room temperature.

Caution(s): For topical use on dogs, cats and horses. Avoid contact with eyes. If irritation develops, discontinue and consult your veterinarian. Keep out of reach of children.

Presentation: 8 fl. oz. (237 mL) (NDC 47203-590-08).

U.S. Patent No. 5536742

Compendium Code No.: 11420610 REV 0800

MALOTIC® OINTMENT ℞

Vedco **Otic Antimicrobial-Corticosteroid**

(Gentamicin Sulfate, Betamethasone Valerate, USP and Clotrimazole, USP Ointment)

Active Ingredient(s): Each gram of MALOTIC® Ointment contains gentamicin sulfate USP equivalent to 3 mg gentamicin base; betamethasone valerate, USP equivalent to 1 mg betamethasone; and 10 mg clotrimazole, USP in a mineral oil-based system containing a plasticized hydrocarbon gel.

Indications: MALOTIC® Ointment is indicated for the treatment of canine acute and chronic otitis externa associated with yeast *(Malassezia pachydermatis (Pityrosporum canis))* and/or bacteria susceptible to gentamicin.

Pharmacology: Gentamicin sulfate is an aminoglycoside antibiotic active against a wide variety of pathogenic gram-negative and gram-positive bacteria. *In vitro* tests have determined that gentamicin is bactericidal and acts by inhibiting normal protein synthesis in susceptible microorganisms. Specifically, gentamicin is active against the following organisms commonly isolated from canine ears: *Staphylococcus aureus*, other *Staphylococcus* spp., *Pseudomonas aeruginosa*, *Proteus* spp., and *Escherichia coli*.

Betamethasone valerate is a synthetic adrenocorticoid for dermatologic use. Betamethasone, an analog of prednisolone, has a high degree of corticosteroid activity and a slight degree of mineral corticosteroid activity. Betamethasone valerate, the 17-valerate ester of betamethasone, has been shown to provide anti-inflammatory and anti-pruritic activity in the topical management of corticosteroid-responsive otitis externa. Topical corticosteroids can be absorbed from normal, intact skin. Inflammation can increase percutaneous absorption. Once absorbed through the skin, topical corticosteroids are handled through pharmacokinetic pathways similar to systemically administered corticosteroids.

Clotrimazole is a broad-spectrum antifungal agent that is used for the treatment of dermal infections caused by various species of pathogenic dermatophytes and yeasts. The primary action of clotrimazole is against dividing and growing organisms. *In vitro*, clotrimazole exhibits fungistatic and fungicidal activity against isolates of *Trichophyton rubrum, Trichophyton mentagrophytes, Epidermophyton floccosum, Microsporum canis, Candida* spp., and *Malassezia pachydermatis (Pityrosporum canis)*. Resistance to clotrimazole is very rare among the fungi that cause superficial mycoses. In an induced otitis externa infected with *Malassezia pachydermatis*, 1% clotrimazole in the MALOTIC® Ointment vehicle was effective both microbiologically and clinically in terms of reduction of exudate odor and swelling.

In studies of the mechanism of action, the minimum fungicidal concentration of clotrimazole caused leakage of intracellular phosphorus compounds into the ambient medium with concomitant breakdown of cellular nucleic acids and accelerated potassium efflux. These events began rapidly and extensively after addition of the drug. Clotrimazole is very poorly absorbed following dermal application.

MALOTIC® Ointment: By virtue of its three active ingredients, gentamicin, betamethasone and clotrimazole has anti-bacterial, anti-inflammatory, and anti-fungal activity. In component efficacy studies, the compatibility and additive effect of each of the components were demonstrated. In clinical field trials MALOTIC® was effective in the treatment of otitis externa associated with bacteria and *Malassezia pachydermatis*.

MALOTIC® Ointment reduced discomfort, redness, swelling, exudate, and odor, and exerted a strong antimicrobial effect.

Dosage and Administration: The external ear should be thoroughly cleaned and dried before treatment. Remove foreign material, debris, crusted exudates, etc., with suitable non-irritating solutions. Excessive hair should be clipped from the treatment area. After verifying that the eardrum is intact, instill 4 drops (2 drops from the 215 g bottle) of MALOTIC® Ointment twice daily into the ear canal of dogs weighing less than 30 lbs. Instill 8 drops (4 drops from the 215 g bottle) twice daily into the ear canal of dogs weighing 30 lbs. or more. Therapy should continue for 7 consecutive days.

Contraindication(s): If hypersensitivity to any of the components occurs, treatment should be discontinued and appropriate therapy instituted. Concomitant use of drugs known to induce ototoxicity should be avoided. Do not use in dogs with known perforation of eardrums.

Precaution(s): Store between 2° and 25°C (36° and 77°F).

Shake well before use when using the 215 gram bottle.

Caution(s): Federal law restricts this drug to use by or on the order of a licensed veterinarian.

The use of MALOTIC® Ointment has been associated with deafness or partial hearing loss in a small number of sensitive dogs (eg, geriatric). The hearing deficit is usually temporary. If hearing or vestibular dysfunction is noted during the course of treatment, discontinue use of MALOTIC® Ointment immediately and flush the ear canal thoroughly with a non-ototoxic solution. Corticosteroids administered to dogs, rabbits, and rodents during pregnancy have resulted in cleft palate in offspring. Other congenital anomalies including deformed forelegs, phocomelia, and anasarca have been reported in offspring of dogs which received corticosteroids during pregnancy. Clinical and experimental data have demonstrated that corticosteroids administered orally or parenterally to animals may induce the first stage of parturition if used during the last trimester of pregnancy and may precipitate premature parturition followed by dystocia, fetal death, retained placenta, and metritis.

Identification of infecting organisms should be made either by microscopic roll smear evaluation or by culture as appropriate. Antibiotic susceptibility of the pathogenic organism(s) should be determined prior to use of this preparation. If overgrowth of non-susceptible bacteria, fungi, or yeasts occur, or if hypersensitivity develops, treatment should be discontinued and appropriate therapy instituted. Administration of recommended doses of MALOTIC® Ointment beyond 7 days may result in delayed wound-healing. Avoid ingestion. Adverse systemic reactions have been observed following the oral ingestion of some topical corticosteroid preparations. Patients should be closely observed for the usual signs of adrenocorticoid overdosage which include sodium retention, potassium loss, fluid retention, weight gain, polydipsia, and/or polyuria. Prolonged use or overdosage may produce adverse immunosuppressive effects. Use of corticosteroids, depending on dose, duration, and specific steroid, may result in endogenous steroid production inhibition following drug withdrawal. In patients presently receiving or recently withdrawn from corticosteroid treatments, therapy with a rapidly acting corticosteroid should be considered in especially stressful situations.

Before instilling any medication into the ear, examine the external ear canal thoroughly to be certain the tympanic membrane is not ruptured in order to avoid the possibility of transmitting infection to the middle ear as well as damaging the cochlea or vestibular apparatus from prolonged contact.

Warning(s): Keep out of reach of children.

Toxicology: Clinical and safety studies with MALOTIC® Ointment have shown a wide safety margin at the recommended dose level in dogs (see Cautions/Side Effects).

Side Effects:

Gentamicin: While aminoglycosides are absorbed poorly from skin, intoxication may occur when aminoglycosides are applied topically for prolonged periods of time to large wounds, burns, or any denuded skin, particularly if there is renal insufficiency. All aminoglycosides have the potential to produce reversible and irreversible vestibular, cochlear, and renal toxicity.

Betamethasone: Side effects such as SAP and SGPT enzyme elevations, weight loss, anorexia, polydipsia, and polyuria have occurred following the use of parenteral or systemic synthetic corticosteroids in dogs. Vomiting and diarrhea (occasionally bloody) have been observed in dogs and cats. Cushing's syndrome in dogs has been reported in association with prolonged or repeated steroid therapy.

Clotrimazole: The following have been reported occasionally in humans in connection with the use of clotrimazole: erythema, stinging, blistering, peeling, edema, pruritus, urticaria, and general irritation of the skin not present before therapy.

Presentation: MALOTIC® Ointment is available in 7.5 g and 15 g tubes as well as in a 215 g plastic bottle.

Compendium Code No.: 10942240

MANGE TREATMENT™

LeGear **Parasiticide-Topical**

EPA Reg. No.: 1910-1

Active Ingredient(s):

Benzyl benzoate	36% w/w
Total inert ingredients	64% w/w
Total	100% w/w

Indications: For the control of sarcoptes mites which cause mange in dogs.

Dosage and Administration: Apply MANGE TREATMENT™ with a swab and rub in thoroughly. Apply once a week until the condition clears up. If improvement is not noted within 10 days, consult a veterinarian.

Provide clean disinfectant sleeping quarters by using a disinfectant according to label directions.

Do not apply to areas equivalent to more than one-third (⅓) of the body at one time. Treat such areas on alternate days.

Precaution(s): Avoid freezing.

Storage: Replace the cap immediately after use. Do not expose to elevated temperatures.

Disposal: Securely wrap the original container in several layers of newspaper and discard it in the trash.

Caution(s): Do not use on cats or rabbits.

Precautionary Statements:

Hazards to Humans and Domestic Animals: Avoid contamination of food and foodstuffs. Do not allow to get into the eyes of animals. Use only as directed. May be absorbed through the skin. Wash hands thoroughly after using on a dog. Harmful if swallowed. Avoid contact with the skin. Do not apply to nursing bitches or puppies under three months of age. Do not use on sick or convalescing animals.

Physical or Chemical Hazards: Flammable. Keep away from heat and open flame.

Presentation: Available in 6 oz. glass bottles.

Compendium Code No.: 11530010

MANNIJECT ℞

Vetus **Diuretic**

NDC No.: 47611-963-82

Active Ingredient(s): Each mL contains:

Mannitol . . . 180 mg

Water for injection . . . q.s.

Total osmolar concentration is 989 mOsm per liter.

Indications: A sterile solution for use as an aid in diuresis and in the removal of extracellular fluids.

Dosage and Administration: For diuresis, administer by intravenous infusion only.

9.2-12.2 mL (1.65-2.2 g) per kilogram of body weight.

Note: The solution may form crystals on chilling. The crystals may be dissolved with adequate warming and agitation.

Caution(s): Federal law restricts the drug to use by or on the order of a licensed veterinarian.

For veterinary use only. Keep out of the reach of children.

Presentation: 100 mL sterile single dose vials.

Compendium Code No.: 14440600

MANNITOL ℞

Butler **Diuretic**

Active Ingredient(s): Each mL contains:

Mannitol . . . 180 mg

Water for injection . . . q.s.

Total osmolar concentration is 989 mOsm per liter.

Indications: A sterile solution for use as an aid in diuresis and in the removal of extracellular fluids.

Dosage and Administration: For diuresis, administer by intravenous infusion only.

Dosage: 1.65-2.2 g (9.2-12.2 mL) per kilogram of body weight.

Note: The solution may form crystals on chilling. Crystals may be dissolved with adequate warming and agitation.

Caution(s): Federal law restricts this drug to use by or on the order of a licensed veterinarian.

For veterinary use only.

Keep out of the reach of children.

Presentation: 100 mL single dose vials.

Compendium Code No.: 10821130

MANNITOL INJECTION ℞

Vedco **Diuretic**

Active Ingredient(s): Each mL contains:

Mannitol . . . 180 mg

Water for injection . . . q.s.

Total osmolar concentration is 989 mOsm per liter.

Indications: A sterile solution for use as an aid in diuresis and in the removal of extracellular fluids.

Dosage and Administration: For diuresis administer by intravenous infusion only.

Dosage: 1.65-2.2 g (9.2-12.2 mL) per kilogram of body weight.

Note: The solution may form crystals on chilling. Crystals may be dissolved with adequate warming and agitation.

Caution(s): Federal law restricts this drug to use by or on the order of a licensed veterinarian.

Keep out of the reach of children.

Presentation: 100 mL sterile single dose vials.

Compendium Code No.: 10941230

MANNITOL INJECTION 20% ℞

Neogen **Diuretic**

Sterile Solution

Active Ingredient(s): Each 100 mL contains:

Mannitol USP . . . 20 g

Water for injection . . . q.s.

This solution contains 1098 mOsmols/Liter.

This is a single dose vial that contains no preservatives.

Indications: MANNITOL INJECTION 20% is indicated for use as an osmotic diuretic in canine species. Mannitol is essentially inert metabolically. When given parenterally, it is freely filtered at the glomerulus which produces osmotic diuresis as more than 90% of the mannitol injected escapes reabsorption.

Dosage and Administration: The usual canine dosage administered intravenously is 1.5-2.0 g per kg body weight given over a 30 minute period. This is approximately 3.4-4.5 mL/lb of body weight.

Precaution(s): Store at controlled room temperature between 15°-30°C (59°-86°F).

Use entire contents when first opened or resterilize by autoclaving.

Caution(s): Federal law (U.S.A.) restricts this drug to use by or on the order of a licensed veterinarian.

For animal use only.

Note: Crystals of mannitol may form in a 20% saturated solution of mannitol. Dissolve the crystals by warming in hot water or autoclaving for 15 minutes. Cool to body temperature before administering.

Warning(s): Keep out of reach of children.

Presentation: 12 x 100 mL glass single-dose vials per carton (NDC: 59051-9061-5).

Manufactured by: Omega Laboratories, Montreal, Quebec H3M 3E4.

Compendium Code No.: 14910062 L566-0201

MANNITOL INJECTION 20% ℞

Phoenix Pharmaceutical **Diuretic**

Sterile Solution

Active Ingredient(s): Each 100 mL contains:

Mannitol USP . . . 20 g

Water for Injection . . . q.s.

This solution contains 1098 mOsmols/Liter.

This is a single dose vial that contains no preservatives.

Indications: MANNITOL INJECTION 20% is indicated for use as an osmotic diuretic in canine species. Mannitol is essentially inert metabolically. When given parenterally, it is freely filtered at the glomerulus which produces osmotic diuresis as more than 90% of the mannitol injected escapes reabsorption.

Dosage and Administration: The usual canine dosage administered intravenously is 1.5-2.0 g per kg body weight given over a 30 minute period. This is approximately 3.4-4.5 mL/lb of body weight.

Precaution(s): Store between 15° and 30°C (59° and 86°F).

Use entire contents when first opened or resterilize by autoclaving.

Caution(s): Federal law restricts this drug to use by or on the order of a licensed veterinarian.

For animal use only.

Note: Crystals of mannitol may form in a 20% saturated solution of mannitol. Dissolve the crystals by warming in hot water or autoclaving for 15 minutes. Cool to body temperature before administering.

Warning(s): Keep out of reach of children.

Presentation: 100 mL single-dose vials (NDC 57319-472-05).

Manufactured by: Phoenix Scientific, Inc., St. Joseph, MO 64503

Compendium Code No.: 12561190 Iss. 1-02

MAN O'WAR™ SHAMPOO

Equicare **Grooming Shampoo**

Ingredient(s): Di-water, sodium lauryl ether sulfate, sodium lauryl sulfate, coconut diethanolamide, sodium chloride, lanolin, FD&C yellow #5.

Indications: Shampoo for horses.

Directions for Use: Wet animal with water and apply a sufficient amount of shampoo to work into a rich lather. Rinse thoroughly. Remove excess water and dry animal as desired.

Presentation: 32 oz and 3.785 L (1 gallon).

Compendium Code No.: 14470101

MANPRO 80

Zinpro **Feed Additive**

Manganese Methionine

Typical Analysis:

Manganese . . . 8.0%

Methionine . . . 18.0%

Protein . . . 17.0%

Fat . . . 0.0%

Fiber . . . 22.0%

Ash . . . 19.5%

Salt . . . 1.3%

Indications: Recommended as a nutritional feed additive for livestock and poultry. When used as a commercial feed ingredient it must be declared as manganese methionine.

Physical Description: A light brown, granular powder. MANPRO 80 weighs approximately 30 lbs/cu ft.

Feeding Instructions:

Swine: Add 1 lb (454 grams) per ton of complete ration.

Laying Hens, Broilers and Turkeys: Add 1 lb (454 grams) per ton of complete ration.

Dairy Cattle: Feed 2.5 grains per head daily, or 1 ounce per 12 head daily.

Beef Cattle: Feed 2.5 grams per head daily, or 1 ounce per 12 head daily.

Sheep: Feed 0.50 grams per head daily, or 1 ounce per 60 head daily.

Horses: Feed 2.5 grams per head daily.

Toxicology: When correctly used, there is no toxicity hazard in the use of MANPRO 80.

Presentation: MANPRO 80 is packaged in 50 lb multiwall bags.

Compendium Code No.: 11300150

MANPRO 160

Zinpro **Feed Additive**

Manganese Methionine

Typical Analysis:

Manganese . . . 16.0%

Methionine . . . 36.0%

Protein . . . 21.2%

Fat . . . 0.0%

Fiber . . . 0.0%

Ash . . . 45.0%

Salt . . . 0.1%

Indications: Recommended as a nutritional feed additive for livestock and poultry. When used as a commercial feed ingredient it must be declared as manganese methionine.

Physical Description: An off-white fine powder. MANPRO 160 weighs approximately 25 lbs/cu ft.

Feeding Instructions:

Swine: Add ½ lb (225 grams) per ton of complete ration.

Laying Hens, Broilers and Turkeys: Add ½ lb (225 grams) per ton of complete ration.

Dairy Cattle: Feed 1.25 grains per head daily, or 1 ounce per 24 head daily.

Beef Cattle: Feed 1.25 grams per head daily, or 1 ounce per 24 head daily.

Sheep: Feed 0.25 gram per head daily, or 1 ounce per 120 head daily.

Horses: Feed 1.25 grams per head daily.

Contraindication(s): This product is not recommended for water use.

Toxicology: When correctly used, there is no toxicity hazard in the use of MANPRO 160.

Presentation: MANPRO 160 is packaged in 50 lb multiwall bags with 2 mil inserted polyethylene liners.

Compendium Code No.: 11300140

MAP®-5

Bioniche Animal Health (formerly Vetrepharm) **Embryo Transfer**

Description: Hyaluronic acid is a natural, highly charged, polyanionic molecule composed of alternating units of D-glucuronic and 2-acetamido-2-deoxy-D-glucose. These unbranched, coiled, elongated polysaccharide chains maintain a large negative electrostatic charge that attracts water molecules and allow the deformation of the molecular coil as ice crystallization occurs during freezing and thawing. Hyaluronic acid coats and protects cells and tissues by attaching to the CD44 (hyaluronan) receptor sites on cells. The purity, defined molecular weight, and molecular chain length of the sodium hyaluronic acid in MAP®-5 ensure that cells are completely coated and protected during all phases of handling and storage.

Indications: Sterile solution for embryo transfer, *in vitro*, cellular handling and cryopreservation.

MAP®-5 is a patented salt of hyaluronic acid in normal saline for use in the collection, handling, culture and cryopreservation of embryo, ova, sperm and other cells. Sterile MAP®-5 acts as a replacement for serum and serum products in cell handling and freezing solution, and thereby reduces the risk of contaminating microorganisms that may contaminate serum product.

Directions for Use: MAP®-5 should be added to collection, handling, culture and freezing solutions to replace serum and serum products normally used in these media. MAP®-5 is compatible with all common cell supporting media, cell surfactants and cryopreservative solutions used in embryo transfer and *in vitro* fertilization procedures. The inclusion concentration depends on the procedure and the prior results and experiences of individual veterinarians and cell biologists. Studies have demonstrated that a 0.1% w/v MAP®-5 replaces 20% v/v of serum in holding and cryopreservative solutions. The common final concentration of MAP®-5 used in freezing solutions is 1 mg/mL (0.1% w/v). Flushing and collection solutions commonly employ 0.1 to 0.5 mg/mL of MAP®-5.

Use strict aseptic techniques to add the required amount of MAP®-5 to the appropriate handling or freezing solution.

Precaution(s): Store at 60-85°F (15-30°C). MAP®-5 contains no preservatives. Discard unused portions of the vials.

Warning(s): For use in embryo transfer procedures, *in vitro* cellular handling and the cryopreservation of embryo, ova, sperm and other cells and tissues. Not for use as a therapeutic in animals or humans.

Presentation: MAP®-5 is supplied in two formats to reduce wastage and facilitate its addition to the required solutions.

MAP®-5 (10 mg/mL) 2 mL vial - one vial/20 mL cryopreservative solution.

MAP®-5/50 (5 mg/mL) 10 mL vial - one vial/100-500 mL flushing solution.

US Patent No. 5,102,783

Compendium Code No.: 11070041

MARCICIDE II

M.A.R.C. **Disinfectant**

EPA No.: 12204-18

Active Ingredient(s):

Pine oil. 3.95%
Alkyl (C_{14}, 58%; C_{16}, 28%; C_{12}, 14%) dimethyl benzyl ammonium chloride 1.97%
Inert ingredients. 94.08%
Total ingredients 100.00%

Indications: MARCICIDE II is effective against a wide variety of gram-positive and gram-negative bacteria. It is also a deodorant and is effective in controlling odors that are bacterial in origin.

MARCICIDE II mixes with water to form clear, stable use solutions. Use solutions are noncorrosive and nonstaining to plastic, vinyl, synthetics, enamel, tile and most common metals.

The disinfectant is effective at 6 oz./gallon against *Pseudomonas aeruginosa* PRD-10, *Salmonella choleraesuis* ATCC 10708, and *Staphylococcus aureus* ATCC 6538 when tested by the A.O.A.C. Use Dilution Test Method for precleaned, hard, nonporous surfaces.

The disinfectant is also an effective virucide at 6 oz./gallon for Influenza virus, type A, Brazil on inanimate, environmental surfaces.

The product may be used for cleaning and deodorizing, one-step cleaning and disinfection, or disinfection of precleaned, nonporous, inanimate, hard surfaces.

When applied as directed to precleaned hard, nonporous surfaces, this disinfectant also kills the following organisms at 6 oz. per gallon: *Candida albicans, Escherichia coli, Streptococcus pyogenes, Enterobacter aerogenes, Shigella sonnei.*

Dosage and Administration: It is a violation of federal law to use the product in a manner inconsistent with its labeling.

Select the proper dilution of MARCICIDE II for use from the directions that follow. Apply the use solution with a clean mop, sponge, cloth, squeegee, or mechanical scrubber.

Prepare fresh use solutions daily. Do not re-use solutions. Discard solutions when they become visibly soiled. For disinfection, thoroughly wet the surfaces to be treated. Surfaces must remain moist for at least 10 minutes to assure proper germicidal action.

The product may be used for cleaning and disinfecting hard, nonporous, inanimate, environmental surfaces (glass, metal, glazed porcelain, linoleum, tile, smooth leather, vinyl, enameled and finished wood surfaces) on walls, floors, appliances and furnishings.

Cleaning: To clean and deodorize or to preclean prior to disinfection, use 3 to 12 oz. of MARCICIDE II per gallon of water depending upon the soil level of the area to be cleaned.

Disinfecting:

Hospitals and veterinary clinics: Use 7½ oz. of MARCICIDE II per gallon of water (1 part to 16 parts water) for one-step cleaning and disinfection of areas with light to medium soil loads. For heavily soiled areas, preclean as described earlier and then disinfect with MARCICIDE II at 6 oz. per gallon of water (1 part to 20 parts water).

Industrial areas, restrooms, food and meat processing plants (nonfood processing areas), other nonmedical uses: Preclean surfaces. Then, disinfect with a solution of 4 oz. of MARCICIDE II in a gallon of water (1 part to 31 parts water). Alternatively, clean and disinfect in one operation using 7½ oz. of MARCICIDE II per gallon of water.

For deodorizing garbage cans, garbage trucks, industrial waste receptacles, and garbage handling equipment. It is important to preclean for the product to perform properly. Then, apply a wetting concentration of 16 oz. of MARCICIDE II per gallon of water.

For mildew control: Follow the directions for hospital disinfection. Repeat the treatment every seven (7) days or when new growth appears.

MARCICIDE II may be used through automatic floor scrubbing equipment.

MARCICIDE II must not be used on food contact surfaces.

Precaution(s): Store only in a tightly closed, original container in a secure area inaccessible to children. Do not contaminate water, food, or feed by storage or disposal.

Pesticide wastes are acutely hazardous. Improper disposal of excess pesticide, spray mixture, or rinsate is a violation of federal law. If the wastes cannot be disposed of according to label instructions, contact a State Pesticide or Environmental Control Agency, or the hazardous waste representative at the nearest EPA Regional Office for guidance.

Do not re-use the empty container. Triple rinse the empty container with water. Return the metal drums to a reconditioner or puncture and dispose of them in a sanitary landfill or by other procedures approved by state and local authorities. Plastic containers may be disposed of in a sanitary landfill, incinerated or, if allowed by local authorities, by burning. If burned, stay out of smoke.

Caution(s): Danger - Keep out of the reach of children.

Precautionary Statements:

Hazards to Humans and Domestic Animals: Causes severe eye and skin damage. Do not get into the eyes, on skin, or on clothing. Harmful if swallowed. Avoid the contamination of food. Wear goggles or a face mask and rubber gloves when handling.

Environmental Hazards: The product is toxic to fish. Do not discharge into lakes, streams, ponds, or public water unless in accordance with an NPDES Permit.

Physical or Chemical Hazards: Do not use or store near heat or open flame.

Practical Treatment (First Aid): In case of contact, immediately flush the eyes or skin with plenty of water for at least 15 minutes. For eyes, call a physician.

Remove and wash contaminated clothing before re-use.

If swallowed, promptly drink a large quantity of milk, raw egg whites, gelatin solution, or if these are not readily available, drink a large quantity of water. Avoid alcohol. Call a physician immediately.

Presentation: 1 gallon jug, 5 gallon pail, 20 gallon, 35 gallon and 55 gallon drums.

Compendium Code No.: 10110000

MAREK'S DISEASE VACCINE (Chicken and Turkey)

Merial Select **Vaccine**

Marek's Disease Vaccine, Live Chicken and Turkey Herpesvirus

U.S. Vet. Lic. No.: 279

Active Ingredient(s): The vaccine contains the FC-126 strain of turkey herpesvirus and the SB-I strain of chicken herpesvirus.

Penicillin and streptomycin sulfate are added as bacteriostatic agents.

Contains fungizone as a fungistatic agent.

Notice: The vaccine has met the requirements of the USDA in regards to safety, purity, potency and the capability to immunize normally susceptible chickens. The vaccine has been tested by the master seed immunogenicity test for efficacy.

Indications: The vaccine is recommended for use in healthy one day old chickens as an aid in the prevention of Marek's disease.

Chickens to be vaccinated must be healthy and free of all diseases. It is essential that the chickens be maintained under good environmental conditions, and that exposure to disease viruses be reduced as much as possible in the field.

Dosage and Administration: Frozen Vaccine:

Preparation of the Vaccine for Use:

Important: Sterilize the vaccinating equipment by autoclaving for a minimum of 15 minutes at 250°F (121°C) or by boiling in water for at least 20 minutes. Never allow chemical disinfectants to come into contact with the vaccinating equipment.

1. Use 200 mL of sterile diluent for each 1,000 doses of vaccine indicated on the ampule.
2. Remove only one (1) ampule of vaccine at a time from the liquid nitrogen container. Thaw and use immediately. Do not hold the ampule toward the face when removing it from a liquid nitrogen container. Never refreeze a vaccine ampule after thawing.
3. The contents of the ampule are thawed rapidly by immersing in water at room temperature (15-25°C). Gently swirl the ampule to disperse the contents. Break the ampule at its neck and quickly proceed as described below.
4. Remove the cover from the diluent container. Draw the contents of the ampule into a sterile 10 mL syringe fitted with an 18 to 20 gauge needle. Slowly add the contents of the vaccine ampule to the appropriate volume of diluent. Withdraw a small amount of the diluent, rinse the ampule once and add this to the vaccine-diluent mixture. Mix the contents of the diluent container thoroughly by swirling and inverting the container. Do not shake vigorously.
5. Use the vaccine-diluent mixture immediately as described below.

Method of Vaccination:

1. Give subcutaneously only.
2. Use a sterile automatic syringe with a 20-22 gauge, ⅜"-½" needle which is set to accurately deliver 0.2 mL per dose. Check the accuracy of delivery several times during the vaccination procedure.
3. Dilute the vaccine only as directed, observing all precautions and warnings for handling.
4. Keep the bottle of diluted vaccine in an ice bath and agitate continuously.
5. Inject chickens under the loose skin at the back of the neck (subcutaneously), holding the chickens by the back of the neck just below the head. The loose skin in this area is raised by gently pinching with the thumb and forefinger. Insert the needle beneath the skin in a direction away from the head. Inject 0.2 mL per chicken. Avoid hitting the muscles and bones in the neck.
6. Use the entire contents of the vaccine container within one (1) hour after mixing the vaccine with the diluent.

Precaution(s):

Ampules: Store in a liquid nitrogen container.

Liquid nitrogen container: Carefully observe all liquid nitrogen precautions, including wearing eye protection and gloves. Store in a cool, well-ventilated area. Check the liquid nitrogen level once a day. Keep the container away from incubator intakes and chicken boxes.

Liquid Nitrogen Precautions: The liquid nitrogen containers and vaccines should be handled by properly trained personnel only. These persons should be familiar with the Union Carbide publication "Precautions and Safe Practices - Liquid Atmospheric Gases", form #9888. Liquid nitrogen is extremely cold. Accidental contact with the skin or eyes can cause serious frostbite. Protect the eyes with goggles or a face shield. Wear gloves and long sleeves when removing and handling frozen ampules or when adding liquid nitrogen to the container. Storage and handling of liquid nitrogen containers should be in a well-ventilated area. Excessive amounts of nitrogen reduces the concentration of oxygen in the air of an unventilated space and can cause asphyxiation. If drowsiness occurs, get fresh air quickly and ventilate the entire area. If a person becomes groggy or loses consciousness while working with liquid nitrogen, get the person to a well-ventilated area immediately. If breathing has stopped, begin artificial respiration. Call a physician immediately.

Caution(s): Do not vaccinate diseased birds.

Vaccinate all of the birds on the premises at one time.

Administer a minimum of one dose for each bird.

Avoid stress conditions during and following vaccination.

Do not place chickens in contaminated facilities.

Exposure to disease must be minimized as much as possible.

For veterinary use only.

Administer only as recommended.

Use entire contents when first opened.

Burn the container and all unused contents.

The capability of the vaccine to produce satisfactory results depends upon many factors, including, but not limited to, conditions of storage and handling by the user, administration of the vaccine, health and the responsiveness of individual animals and the degree of field exposure. Directions for use should be followed carefully.

The use of the vaccine is subject to applicable local and federal laws and regulations.

Warning(s): Do not vaccinate within 21 days before slaughter.

Presentation: 5 x 1,000 dose and 5 x 2,000 dose ampules of virus, with 200 mL of diluent for each ampule.

Compendium Code No.: 11050231

MAREK'S DISEASE VACCINE (FC-126 Strain)

Merial Select **Vaccine**

Marek's Disease Vaccine, Live Turkey Herpesvirus

U.S. Vet. Lic. No.: 279

Active Ingredient(s): The vaccine contains the FC-126 strain of the live turkey herpesvirus.

Penicillin and streptomycin sulfate are added as bacteriostatic agents.

Contains fungizone as a fungistatic agent.

Notice: The vaccine has met the requirements of the USDA in regards to safety, purity, potency and the capability to immunize normally susceptible chickens. The vaccine has been tested by the master seed immunogenicity test for efficacy.

Indications: The vaccine is recommended for use in healthy one day old chickens for the prevention of Marek's disease.

Chickens to be vaccinated must be healthy and free of all diseases. It is essential that the chickens be maintained under good environmental conditions, and that exposure to disease viruses be reduced as much as possible in the field.

Dosage and Administration: Frozen Vaccine:

Preparation of the Vaccine for Use:

Important: Sterilize the vaccinating equipment by autoclaving for a minimum of 15 minutes at 250°F (121°C) or by boiling in water for at least 20 minutes. Never allow chemical disinfectants to come into contact with the vaccinating equipment.

1. Use 200 mL of sterile diluent for each 1,000 doses of vaccine indicated on the ampule.
2. Remove only one (1) ampule of vaccine at a time from the liquid nitrogen container. Thaw and use immediately. Do not hold the ampule toward the face when removing it from a liquid nitrogen container. Never refreeze a vaccine ampule after thawing.
3. The contents of the ampule are thawed rapidly by immersing it in water at room temperature (15-25°C). Gently swirl the ampule to disperse the contents. Break the ampule at its neck and quickly proceed as described below.
4. Remove the cover from the diluent container. Draw contents of the ampule into a sterile 10 mL syringe fitted with an 18 to 20 gauge needle. Slowly add the contents of the vaccine ampule to the appropriate volume of diluent. Withdraw a small amount of the diluent, rinse the ampule once and add this to the vaccine-diluent mixture. Mix the contents of the diluent container thoroughly by swirling and inverting the container. Do not shake vigorously.
5. Use the vaccine-diluent mixture immediately as described below.

Method of Vaccination:

1. Give subcutaneously only.
2. Use a sterile automatic syringe with a 20-22 gauge, 3/8"-1/2" needle which is set to accurately deliver 0.2 mL per dose. Check the accuracy of delivery several times during the vaccination procedure.
3. Dilute the vaccine only as directed, observing all precautions and warnings for handling.
4. Keep the bottle of diluted vaccine in an ice bath and agitate continuously.
5. Inject chickens under the loose skin at the back of the neck (subcutaneously), holding the chickens by the back of the neck just below the head. The loose skin in this area is raised by gently pinching with the thumb and forefinger. Insert the needle beneath the skin in a direction away from the head. Inject 0.2 mL per chicken. Avoid hitting the muscles and bones in the neck.
6. Use the entire contents of the vaccine container within one (1) hour after mixing the vaccine with the diluent.

Precaution(s):

Ampules: Store in a liquid nitrogen container.

Liquid nitrogen container: Carefully observe all liquid nitrogen precautions, including wearing eye protection and gloves. Store in a cool, well-ventilated area. Check the liquid nitrogen level once a day. Keep the container away from incubator intakes and chicken boxes.

Liquid Nitrogen Precautions: The liquid nitrogen containers and vaccines should be handled by properly trained personnel only. These persons should be familiar with the Union Carbide publication "Precautions and Safe Practices - Liquid Atmospheric Gases", form #9888. Liquid nitrogen is extremely cold. Accidental contact with the skin or eyes can cause serious frostbite. Protect the eyes with goggles or a face shield. Wear gloves and long sleeves when removing and handling frozen ampules or when adding liquid nitrogen to the container. Storage and handling of liquid nitrogen containers should be in a well-ventilated area. Excessive amounts of nitrogen reduces the concentration of oxygen in the air of an unventilated space and can cause asphyxiation. If drowsiness occurs, get fresh air quickly and ventilate the entire area. If a person becomes groggy or loses consciousness while working with liquid nitrogen, get the person to a well-ventilated area immediately. If breathing has stopped, begin artificial respiration. Call a physician immediately.

Caution(s): Do not vaccinate diseased birds.

Vaccinate all of the birds on the premises at one time.

Administer a minimum of one dose for each bird.

Avoid stress conditions during and following vaccination.

Do not place chickens in contaminated facilities.

Exposure to disease must be minimized as much as possible.

For veterinary use only.

Administer only as recommended.

Use the entire contents when first opened.

Burn the container and all unused contents.

The capability of the vaccine to produce satisfactory results depends upon many factors, including, but not limited to, conditions of storage and handling by the user, administration of the vaccine, health and the responsiveness of individual animals and the degree of field exposure. Directions for use should be followed carefully.

The use of the vaccine is subject to applicable local and federal laws and regulations.

Warning(s): Do not vaccinate within 21 days before slaughter.

Presentation: 5 x 1,000 doses and 5 x 2,000 doses.

Compendium Code No.: 11050241

MAREK'S DISEASE VACCINE (Rispens CVI 988 Strain)

Merial Select **Vaccine**

Marek's Disease Vaccine, Live Chicken Herpesvirus

U.S. Vet. Lic. No.: 279

Contents: This vaccine contains the Rispens CVI 988 strain of chicken herpesvirus, live virus. This product is used as an aid in the prevention of very virulent Marek's disease in chickens.

Penicillin and streptomycin sulfate are added as bacteriostatic agents.

Contains amphotericin B as a fungistatic agent.

Indications: This Marek's disease vaccine is recommended for use in healthy one day-old chickens. It is essential that the chickens be maintained under good environmental conditions and that exposure to disease viruses be reduced as much as possible.

Dosage and Administration: Preparation of Vaccine for Use:

Important: Sterilize vaccinating equipment by autoclaving a minimum of 15 minutes at 250°F (121°C) or boiling in water for at least 20 minutes. Never allow chemical disinfectants to come in contact with vaccinating equipment.

1. Use 200 mL of sterile diluent for each 1,000 doses of vaccine indicated on the ampule.
2. Remove only one ampule of vaccine at a time from the liquid nitrogen container. Thaw and use immediately. Caution: Do not hold ampule toward face when removing from a liquid nitrogen container. Never refreeze a vaccine ampule after thawing.
3. The contents of the ampule are thawed rapidly by immersing in water at room temperature (15-25°C). Gently swirl the ampule to disperse contents. Break ampule at its neck and quickly proceed as described below.
4. Remove the cover from the diluent container. Draw contents of the ampule into a sterile 10 mL syringe fitted with an 18 to 20 gauge needle. Slowly add the contents of the vaccine ampule to the appropriate volume of diluent. Withdraw a small amount of the diluent, rinse the ampule once and add this to the vaccine-diluent mixture. Mix the contents of the diluent container thoroughly by swirling and inverting the container. Do not shake vigorously.
5. Use the vaccine-diluent mixture immediately as described below.

Method Of Vaccination:

1. Give subcutaneously only.
2. Use a sterile automatic syringe with a 20-22 gauge 3/8"-1/2" needle that is set to accurately deliver 0.2 mL per dose. Check the accuracy of delivery several times during the vaccination procedure.
3. Dilute the vaccine only as directed, observing all precautions and warnings for handling.
4. Keep the bottle of diluted vaccine in an ice bath and agitate continuously.
5. Inject chickens under the loose skin at the back of the neck (subcutaneous), holding the chicken by the back of the neck just below the head. The loose skin in this area is raised by gently pinching with the thumb and forefinger. Insert the needle beneath the skin in a direction away from the head. Inject 0.2 mL per chicken. Avoid hitting the muscles and bones in the neck.
6. Use the entire contents of vaccine container within one hour after mixing the vaccine with the diluent.

Precaution(s): Storage Conditions:

Ampules: Store in liquid nitrogen container.

Diluent: Store at room temperature.

Liquid Nitrogen Container: Carefully observe all liquid nitrogen precautions, including wearing eye protection and gloves. Store in a cool, well-ventilated area. Check liquid nitrogen level daily. Keep container away from incubator intakes and chicken boxes.

Use entire contents when first opened.

Burn this container and all unused contents.

Caution(s): Do not vaccinate diseased birds.

Vaccinate all birds on the premises at one time.

Administer a full dose to each bird.

Avoid stress conditions during and following vaccination.

Do not place chickens in contaminated facilities.

Exposure to disease must be minimized as much as possible.

Give subcutaneously only.

Administer only as recommended.

The capability of this vaccine to produce satisfactory results depends upon many factors, including — but not limited to — conditions of storage and handling by the user, administration of the vaccine, health and responsiveness of individual chickens and degree of field exposure. Therefore, directions for use should be followed carefully. The use of this vaccine is subject to applicable local and federal laws and regulations.

Warning(s): Do not vaccinate within 21 days before slaughter.

For veterinary use only.

Liquid Nitrogen Precautions: The liquid nitrogen containers and vaccines should be handled only by properly trained personnel. These persons should be familiar with the Union Carbide publication "Precautions and Safe Practices — Liquid Atmospheric Gases," form #9888. Liquid nitrogen is extremely cold. Accidental contact with skin or eyes can cause severe frostbite. Protect eyes with goggles or face shield. Wear gloves and long sleeves when removing and handling frozen ampules or when adding liquid nitrogen to the container. Storage and handling of liquid nitrogen containers should be in a well ventilated area. Excessive amounts of nitrogen reduce the concentration of oxygen in the air of an unventilated space and can cause asphyxiation. If drowsiness occurs, get fresh air quickly and ventilate the entire area. If a person becomes groggy or loses consciousness while working with liquid nitrogen, get the person to a well-ventilated area immediately. If breathing has stopped, begin artificial respiration. Call a physician immediately.

Trial Data: Merial Select's vaccines have met the requirements of the USDA in regard to safety, purity, potency and the capability to protect susceptible chickens. This vaccine has been tested by the Master Seed immunogenicity test for efficacy.

Presentation: 5 x 1,000 doses and 5 x 2,000 doses.

Compendium Code No.: 11050261

MAREK'S DISEASE VACCINE (Rispens CVI 988 Strain + FC-126 Strain)

Merial Select **Vaccine**

Marek's Disease Vaccine, Live Chicken and Turkey Herpesvirus

U.S. Vet. Lic. No.: 279

Contents: This vaccine contains the Rispens CVI 988 strain of chicken herpesvirus and the FC-126 strain of turkey herpesvirus, live virus. This product is used as an aid in the prevention of very virulent Marek's disease in chickens. The product consists of one ampule of vaccine and a container of diluent.

Penicillin and streptomycin sulfate are added as bacteriostatic agents.

Contains amphotericin B as a fungistatic agent.

Indications: This Marek's disease vaccine is recommended for use in healthy one day-old chickens. It is essential that the chickens be maintained under good environmental conditions and that exposure to disease viruses be reduced as much as possible.

Dosage and Administration:

Preparation of Vaccine for Use: Read full instructions which must be followed exactly for best results. Guard against exposure to Marek's disease for at least two weeks.

Important: Sterilize vaccinating equipment by autoclaving a minimum of 15 minutes at 250°F

(121°C) or boiling in water for at least 20 minutes. Never allow chemical disinfectants to come in contact with vaccinating equipment.

1. Know and follow all precautions and safety practices for handling liquid nitrogen.
2. Before withdrawing vaccine from liquid nitrogen, protect hands with gloves, wear long sleeves and protect face with a plastic face shield or wear protective goggles.
3. Remove from the liquid nitrogen only the ampules that are going to be used immediately. Match the dosage size of the vaccine ampules and diluent bottle using 200 mL of sterile diluent for each 1,000 doses of vaccine indicated on the ampule. Move quickly, but carefully.
4. Place the ampule(s) in a large, clean container of lukewarm water (75° to 85°F) to thaw ampule quickly. Gentle agitation promotes rapid thawing and evenly distributes the vaccine in the ampule. Thaw the entire contents.
5. Mix vaccine with room temperature diluent immediately after thawing. Remove closure from top of diluent bottle. Draw vaccine from the ampule into a sterile 10 mL mixing syringe fitted with an 18 to 20 gauge needle.
6. Slowly expel contents into the diluent bottle. Rinse the ampule once with the diluted vaccine.
7. Place the diluted vaccine into an ice bath. Agitate as needed to ensure a uniform suspension of the cells.
8. Use the vaccine/diluent mixture immediately as described below.

Method Of Vaccination:

1. Give subcutaneously only.
2. Use a sterile automatic syringe with a 20-22 gauge 3/8"-1/2" needle that is set to accurately deliver 0.2 mL per dose. Check the accuracy of delivery several times during the vaccination procedure.
3. Dilute the vaccine only as directed, observing all precautions and warnings for handling.
4. Keep the bottle of diluted vaccine in an ice bath and agitate continuously.
5. Inject chickens under the loose skin at the back of the neck (subcutaneously), holding the chicken by the back of the neck just below the head. The loose skin in this area is raised by gently pinching with the thumb and forefinger. Insert the needle beneath the skin in a direction away from the head. Inject 0.2 mL per chicken. Avoid hitting the muscles and bones in the neck.
6. Use the entire contents of vaccine container within one hour after mixing the vaccine with the diluent.
7. Burn all discarded containers and unused contents. Do not vaccinate within 21 days before slaughter.

Precaution(s): Storage Conditions:

Ampules: Store in liquid nitrogen container.

Diluent: Store at room temperature.

Liquid Nitrogen Container: Carefully observe all liquid nitrogen precautions including wearing eye protection and gloves. Store in a cool, well-ventilated area. Check liquid nitrogen level daily. Keep container away from incubator intakes and chicken boxes.

Use entire contents when first opened.

Burn this container and all unused contents.

Caution(s): Do not vaccinate diseased birds.

Vaccinate all birds on the premises at one time.

Administer a full dose to each bird.

Avoid stress conditions during and following vaccination.

Do not place chickens in contaminated facilities.

Exposure to disease must be minimized as much as possible.

Give subcutaneously only.

Administer only as recommended.

The capability of this vaccine to produce satisfactory results depends upon many factors, including — but not limited to — conditions of storage and handling by the user, administration of the vaccine, health and responsiveness of individual chickens and degree of field exposure. Therefore, directions for use should be followed carefully. The use of this vaccine is subject to applicable local and federal laws and regulations.

Warning(s): Do not vaccinate within 21 days before slaughter.

For veterinary use only.

Liquid Nitrogen Precautions: The liquid nitrogen containers and vaccines should be handled only by properly trained personnel. These persons should be familiar with the Union Carbide publication "Precautions and Safe Practices — Liquid Atmospheric Gases," form #9888. Liquid nitrogen is extremely cold. Accidental contact with skin or eyes can cause severe frostbite. Protect eyes with goggles or face shield. Wear gloves and long sleeves when removing and handling frozen ampules or when adding liquid nitrogen to the container. Storage and handling of liquid nitrogen containers should be in a well ventilated area. Excessive amounts of nitrogen reduce the concentration of oxygen in the air of an unventilated space and can cause asphyxiation. If drowsiness occurs, get fresh air quickly and ventilate the entire area. If a person becomes groggy or loses consciousness while working with liquid nitrogen, get the person to a well-ventilated area immediately. If breathing has stopped, begin artificial respiration. Call a physician immediately.

Trial Data: Merial Select's vaccines have met the requirements of the USDA in regard to safety, purity, potency and the capability to protect susceptible chickens. This vaccine has been tested by the Master Seed immunogenicity test for efficacy.

Presentation: 5 x 1,000 doses and 5 x 2,000 doses.

Compendium Code No.: 11050251

MAREK'S DISEASE VACCINE (SB-1 Strain)

Merial Select **Vaccine**

Marek's Disease Vaccine, Live Chicken Herpesvirus

U.S. Vet. Lic. No.: 279

Active Ingredient(s): The vaccine contains the SB-1 strain of the chicken herpesvirus.

Penicillin and streptomycin sulfate are added as bacteriostatic agents.

Contains fungizone as a fungistatic agent.

Notice: The vaccine has met the requirements of the USDA in regards to safety, purity, potency and the capability to immunize normally susceptible chickens. The vaccine has been tested by the master seed immunogenicity test for efficacy.

Indications: The vaccine is recommended for use in healthy one day old chickens to aid in the prevention of Marek's disease.

Chickens to be vaccinated must be healthy and free of all diseases. It is essential that the chickens be maintained under good environmental conditions, and that exposure to disease viruses be reduced as much as possible in the field.

Dosage and Administration: Frozen Vaccine:

Preparation of the Vaccine for Use:

Important: Sterilize the vaccinating equipment by autoclaving for a minimum of 15 minutes at 250°F (121°C) or by boiling in water for at least 20 minutes. Never allow chemical disinfectants to come into contact with vaccinating equipment.

1. Use 200 mL of sterile diluent for each 1,000 doses of vaccine indicated on the ampule.
2. Remove only one (1) ampule of vaccine at a time from the liquid nitrogen container. Thaw and use immediately. Do not hold the ampule toward the face when removing it from a liquid nitrogen container. Never refreeze a vaccine ampule after thawing.
3. The contents of the ampule are thawed rapidly by immersing in water at room temperature (15-25°C). Gently swirl the ampule to disperse the contents. Break the ampule at its neck and quickly proceed as described below.
4. Remove the cover from the diluent container. Draw the contents of the ampule into a sterile 10 mL syringe fitted with an 18 to 20 gauge needle. Slowly add the contents of the vaccine ampule to the appropriate volume of diluent. Withdraw a small amount of the diluent, rinse the ampule once and add this to the vaccine-diluent mixture. Mix the contents of the diluent container thoroughly by swirling and inverting the container. Do not shake vigorously.
5. Use the vaccine-diluent mixture immediately as described below.

Method of Vaccination:

1. Give subcutaneously only.
2. Use a sterile automatic syringe with a 20-22 gauge, 3/8"-1/2" needle which is set to accurately deliver 0.2 mL per dose. Check the accuracy of delivery several times during the vaccination procedure.
3. Dilute the vaccine only as directed, observing all precautions and warnings for handling.
4. Keep the bottle of diluted vaccine in an ice bath and agitate continuously.
5. Inject chickens under the loose skin at the back of the neck (subcutaneously), holding the chickens by the back of the neck just below the head. The loose skin in this area is raised by gently pinching with the thumb and forefinger. Insert the needle beneath the skin in a direction away from the head. Inject 0.2 mL per chicken. Avoid hitting the muscles and bones in the neck.
6. Use the entire contents of the vaccine container within one (1) hour after mixing the vaccine with the diluent.

Precaution(s):

Ampules: Store in a liquid nitrogen container.

Liquid nitrogen container: Carefully observe all liquid nitrogen precautions, including wearing eye protection and gloves. Store in a cool, well-ventilated area. Check the liquid nitrogen level once a day. Keep the container away from incubator intakes and chicken boxes.

Liquid Nitrogen Precautions: The liquid nitrogen containers and vaccines should be handled by properly trained personnel only. These persons should be familiar with the Union Carbide publication "Precautions and Safe Practices - Liquid Atmospheric Gases", form #9888. Liquid nitrogen is extremely cold. Accidental contact with the skin or eyes can cause serious frostbite. Protect the eyes with goggles or a face shield. Wear gloves and long sleeves when removing and handling frozen ampules or when adding liquid nitrogen to the container. Storage and handling of liquid nitrogen containers should be in a well-ventilated area. Excessive amounts of nitrogen reduces the concentration of oxygen in the air of an unventilated space and can cause asphyxiation. If drowsiness occurs, get fresh air quickly and ventilate the entire area. If a person becomes groggy or loses consciousness while working with liquid nitrogen, get the person to a well-ventilated area immediately. If breathing has stopped, begin artificial respiration. Call a physician immediately.

Caution(s): Do not vaccinate diseased birds.

Vaccinate all of the birds on the premises at one time.

Administer a minimum of one dose for each bird.

Avoid stress conditions during and following vaccination.

Do not place chickens in contaminated facilities.

Exposure to disease must be minimized as much as possible.

For veterinary use only.

Administer only as recommended.

Use the entire contents when first opened.

Burn the container and all unused contents.

The capability of the vaccine to produce satisfactory results depends upon many factors, including, but not limited to, conditions of storage and handling by the user, administration of the vaccine, health and the responsiveness of individual animals and the degree of field exposure. Directions for use should be followed carefully.

The use of the vaccine is subject to applicable local and federal laws and regulations.

Warning(s): Do not vaccinate within 21 days before slaughter.

Presentation: 5 x 1,000 doses and 5 x 2,000 doses.

Compendium Code No.: 11050271

MARE-PLUS®

Farnam **Large Animal Dietary Supplement**

Guaranteed Analysis: Each pound contains not less than:

Calcium (minimum)	5.800%
Calcium (maximum)	6.800%
Phosphorus (minimum)	5.000%
Salt (minimum)	1.000%
Salt (maximum)	1.500%
Potassium (minimum)	1.880%
Magnesium (minimum)	0.395%
Cobalt (minimum)	300 ppm
Copper (minimum)	250 ppm
Iodine (minimum)	40 ppm
Iron (minimum)	3,960 ppm
Manganese (minimum)	4,400 ppm
Selenium (minimum)	4 ppm
Zinc (minimum)	2,000 ppm
Vitamin A	800,000 I.U.
Vitamin D	80,000 I.U.
Vitamin E	960 I.U.
Vitamin B_{12}	3,240 mg
Riboflavin	800 mg
d-Pantothenic Acid	1,000 mg
Thiamine	800 mg
Niacin	2,000 mg
Vitamin B_6	200 mg
Folic Acid	144 mg
Choline	7,200 mg
P-Amino Benzoic Acid	800 mg

M

Ingredients: Wheat Middlings, Dehydrated Alfalfa Meal, Pulverized Corn, Dicalcium Phosphate, Calcium Carbonate, Vitamin A Acetate, Cholecalciferol (source of Vitamin D_3), dl-Alpha Tocopherol Acetate (source of Vitamin E), Choline Chloride, Thiamine Mononitrate, Riboflavin Supplement, Niacinamide, Pyridoxine Hydrochloride (source of Vitamin B_6), Calcium Pantothenate, Cyanocobalamin (source of Vitamin B_{12}), Folic Acid, Para-Aminobenzoic Acid, Cobalt Sulfate, Copper Sulfate, Zinc Sulfate, Manganous Oxide, Magnesium Sulfate, Potassium Chloride, Salt, Sodium Selenite, Beta Carotene and Cane Molasses.

Indications: Supplement for mares.

A vitamin-mineral supplement to bring the mare's system into a properly balanced condition, optimal for conception, parturition and lactation.

Dosage and Administration: Feed one ounce of MARE-PLUS® twice daily with the feed - once in the morning and again in the evening. Mix right with regular ration. A handy measuring cup is packed inside. One level cupful hold exactly one ounce.

Caution(s): Follow label directions. The addition to feed of higher levels of this premix containing selenium is not permitted.

Presentation: 3 lb, 7 lb (3.18 kg), 20 lb and 100 lb containers.

Compendium Code No.: 10000281

MAREXINE®

Intervet **Vaccine**

Marek's Disease Vaccine, Live Turkey Herpesvirus, Cell Associated

U.S. Vet. Lic. No.: 286

Active Ingredient(s): MAREXINE® is of chicken tissue culture origin using SPF (Specific Pathogen Free) eggs. The product contains the FC-126 strain of turkey herpesvirus. It is packaged in two separate units. One is an ample containing 1,000 doses of frozen live cell associated herpesvirus and the other is a bottle of sterile diluent. The ampules are inserted in metal canes and shipped in a liquid nitrogen (LN) container. The diluent is packaged in separate cartons in bottles of 200 mL, 1,200 mL or 1,600 mL. The vaccine may contain either neomycin or gentamicin in an individual ampule as a preservative.

Indications: The vaccine is recommended for use in healthy one-day-old chickens. The product is used for the prevention of Marek's disease in chickens. The virus will infect chickens even though they may be carrying maternal antibodies to Marek's disease herpesvirus (MDHV).

Dosage and Administration: Preparation of Vaccine:

Caution: Read the safety precaution advice on handling the vaccine ampule. Sterilize vaccinating equipment by boiling it in water for 30 minutes or by autoclaving (20 minutes at 121°C). Do not use chemical disinfectants.

1. Use the contents of one (1) ampule with 200 mL of sterile diluent per 1,000 chickens.
2. Before withdrawing the vaccine from the liquid nitrogen canister, protect the hands with gloves, wear long sleeves and use a face mask or goggles. It is possible that an accident could occur with either the liquid nitrogen or the ampules of vaccine. When removing an ampule from the cane, hold the palm of the gloved hand away from the body and the face.
3. When withdrawing a cane of ampules from the canister in the liquid nitrogen refrigerator, expose only the ampule to be used immediately. We recommend handling only one (1) ampule at a time. After removing the ampule from the cane, the remaining ampules should be replaced immediately in the canister of the liquid nitrogen refrigerator.
4. The contents of the ampule are thawed rapidly by immersing in water at room temperature. Shake the ampule to disperse the contents. Then break the ampule at its neck and immediately proceed. One (1) ampule of MAREXINE® is added to the 200 mL bottle of diluent, six (6) to the 1,200 mL bottle and eight (8) to the 1,600 mL bottle. Caution: Ampules have been known to explode on sudden temperature changes. Do not thaw in hot or ice cold water.
5. Draw the contents of the ampule into a sterile 5 or 10 mL syringe, mounted with an 18-gauge needle.
6. Dilute immediately by filling the syringe slowly with a portion of the diluent. Important: The diluent should be at room temperature (15°-25°C) at the time of mixing.
7. The contents of the filled syringe are then added to the remaining diluent. It is important that this be done slowly. Slowly empty the syringe, allowing the vaccine to run down the side of the bottle. Gently shake the bottle as the vaccine is being mixed. Withdraw a portion of the diluent with the syringe to flush the ampule. Inject the washing back into the diluent bottle. Remove the syringe.
8. Fill the previously sterilized automatic syringe according to the manufacturer's recommendations and set the dose for 0.20 mL.
9. The vaccine is now ready for use.

Method of Vaccination: Subcutaneous administration:

1. Hold the chicken by the back of the neck just below the head. The loose skin in the area is raised by gently pinching with the thumb and forefinger. Insert the needle beneath the skin in a downward direction away from the head. Inject 0.20 mL per chicken. The bottle of vaccine should be kept in an ice bath and swirled frequently.
2. Avoid hitting the muscles and bones in the neck.
3. The entire contents of the bottle must be used within one (1) hour after mixing or discarded.

Records: Keep a record of vaccine, quantity, serial number, expiration date, and place of purchase; the date and time of vaccination; the number, age, breed, and locations of chickens; names of operators performing the vaccination and any observed reactions.

Precaution(s):

Ampules: Store in a liquid nitrogen container.

Diluent: Store at room temperature.

Container: Store the liquid nitrogen container securely in an upright position in a dry, well ventilated area and away from incubator intakes and chicken boxes.

Safety Precautions: The liquid nitrogen container and the vaccine should be handled only by properly trained personnel who are thoroughly conversant with the Union Carbide publication and instruction booklet regarding the use of, precautions and safe practices for liquified atmospheric gases (particularly nitrogen).

When removing the ampule cane, handling the frozen ampules, or adding the liquid nitrogen, wear long sleeves, a plastic face shield and gloves to protect the skin from contact with the liquid nitrogen. All storage and handling of the liquid nitrogen container must be in a dry, ventilated area. Do not inhale liquid nitrogen vapors. If drowsiness occurs, get fresh air quickly, then ventilate the entire area. If breathing difficulty occurs, apply artificial respiration. If any of these difficulties persist or there is a loss of consciousness, summon a physician immediately. Care should be exercised to prevent contamination of the hands, the eyes and the clothing with the vaccine.

Use only as directed. Store vaccines in liquid nitrogen. The product is not returnable.

Caution(s): Good management practices are recommended to reduce exposure to MDHV for at least three weeks following vaccination. Therefore, the directions should be followed carefully.

1. Do not mix any substance, other than SB-1 type Marek's vaccine, with this vaccine.
2. Gloves and a visor should be worn when handling liquid nitrogen.
3. Do not dilute or otherwise stretch the dosage of the vaccine.
4. Read the directions carefully.
5. Only healthy chickens should be vaccinated.
6. Store the vaccine in liquid nitrogen at a temperature below -150°C.
7. Once diluted the vaccine should be used within one hour and the unused vaccine discarded into disinfectant or burned.
8. Once thawed, the product should not be refrozen.

Warning(s): Do not vaccinate within 21 days before slaughter.

Discussion: The vaccine has undergone rigid potency, safety and purity tests, and meets Intervet America Inc. and USDA requirements. It is designed to stimulate effective immunity when used as directed, but the user must be advised that the response to the product depends upon many factors, including, but not limited to, conditions of storage and handling by the user, administration of the vaccine, health and responsiveness of the individual chickens, and the degree of field exposure.

The use of the vaccine is subject to applicable federal and local laws and regulations.

Presentation: 1 x 1,000 dose ampule with 1 x 200 mL bottle of diluent.

Compendium Code No.: 11060891

MAREXINE-89/03®

Intervet **Vaccine**

Bursal Disease-Marek's Disease Vaccine, Variant, Serotype 3, Live Virus

U.S. Vet. Lic. No.: 286

Description: MAREXINE-89/03® is a frozen vaccine which contains the FC-126 strain of turkey herpesvirus and the 89/03 strain of infectious bursal disease virus. 89/03 virus is a Delaware type IBD virus which protects against IBD standard and variant strains.

This vaccine contains Gentamicin as a preservative.

Quality tested for purity, potency, and safety.

Indications: MAREXINE-89/03® is recommended for vaccination of healthy one-day-old chickens against Marek's Disease and Infectious Bursal Disease (Standard, Delaware and GLS Variants) by subcutaneous injection.

Dosage and Administration: Preparation of Vaccine:

Caution: Read "Safety Precautions" advice on handling vaccine ampule. Sterilize vaccinating equipment by boiling in water for 30 minutes or by autoclaving (20 minutes at 121°C). Do not use chemical disinfectants.

1. Use 1,000 doses of vaccine with 200 mL sterile diluent per 1,000 chickens.
2. Before withdrawing vaccine from liquid nitrogen canister, protect hands with gloves, wear long sleeves and use a face mask or goggles. It is possible an accident could occur with either the liquid nitrogen or the ampules of vaccine. When removing an ampule from the cane, hold palm of gloved hand away from body and face.
3. When withdrawing a cane of ampules from canister in liquid nitrogen refrigerator, expose only the ampule to be used immediately. The manufacturer recommends handling only one ampule at a time. After removing the ampule from the cane, the remaining ampules should be replaced immediately in the canister of the liquid nitrogen refrigerator.
4. The contents of the ampule are thawed rapidly by immersing in water at room temperature. Shake ampule to disperse contents. Then break ampule at its neck and immediately proceed as below. 1,000 doses of MAREXINE 89/03® is added for each 200 mL of diluent. Caution: Ampules have been known to explode on sudden temperature changes. Do not thaw in hot or ice cold water.
5. Draw contents of ampule into a sterile 5 or 10 mL syringe, mounted with an 18-guage needle.
6. Dilute immediately by filling the syringe slowly with a portion of the diluent. Important: The diluent should be at room temperature (60°-80°F) at time of mixing.
7. The contents of the filled syringe are then added to the remaining diluent. It is important that this be done slowly. Slowly empty the syringe, allowing the vaccine to run down the side of the diluent container. Gently swirl the container as the vaccine is being mixed. Withdraw a portion of the diluent with the syringe to flush ampule. Inject the washing back into the diluent bottle. Remove the syringe.
8. Fill the previously sterilized automatic syringe according to the manufacturer's recommendations and set the dose for 0.2 mL.
9. The vaccine is now ready for use.

Method of Vaccination:

Subcutaneous Administration:

1. Hold the chicken by the back of the neck just below the head. The loose skin in the area is raised by gently pinching with the thumb and forefinger. Insert the needle beneath the skin in a downward direction away from the head. Inject 0.2 mL per chicken.
2. Avoid hitting the muscles and bones in the neck.
3. Entire contents of bottle must be used within 1 hour after mixing or discarded.
4. After reconstitution the vaccine should be kept cool and swirled frequently - every 5 minutes.

Records: Keep a record of vaccine, quantity, serial number, expiration date and place of purchase; the date and time of vaccination; the number, age, breed and locations of chickens; names of operators performing the vaccination and any observed reactions.

Precaution(s): Important: Storage Conditions:

Ampules - Store in liquid nitrogen container.

Diluent - Store at room temperature.

Container - Store liquid nitrogen container securely in an upright position in a dry, well-ventilated area and away from incubator intakes and chicken boxes.

Safety Precautions: Liquid nitrogen container and vaccine should be handled only by properly trained personnel who are thoroughly conversant with the Union Carbide publication and instruction booklet regarding the use of precautions and safe practice for liquified atmospheric gases (particularly liquid nitrogen).

When removing ampule cane, handling frozen ampules, or adding liquid nitrogen, wear long sleeves, a plastic face shield and gloves to protect the skin from contact with the liquid nitrogen. All storage and handling of the liquid nitrogen container must be in a dry, ventilated area. Do not inhale liquid nitrogen vapors. If drowsiness occurs, get fresh air quickly; then ventilate entire area. If breathing difficulty occurs, apply artificial respiration. If any of these difficulties persist or there is a loss of consciousness, summon a physician immediately. Care should be exercised to prevent contaminating your hands, eyes and clothing with the vaccine.

Do not mix any substance not approved by Intervet, Inc. with this vaccine.

Store vaccine in liquid nitrogen at a temperature below -150°C.

Gloves and visor should be worn when handling liquid nitrogen.

Once thawed, the product should not be refrozen.

Once mixed with diluent, the vaccine should be swirled frequently, every 5 minutes.

Once mixed with diluent, the vaccine should be used within 1 hour.

Burn the container and all unused contents.

This product is non-returnable.

Caution(s): Use only in localities where permitted and on premises with a history of Infectious Bursal Disease.

Good management practices are recommended to reduce exposure to Marek's Disease and Infectious Bursal Disease viruses for at least three weeks following vaccination. Therefore, directions should be followed carefully.

Do not dilute or otherwise stretch the dosage of this vaccine.

Only healthy chickens should be vaccinated.

For veterinary use only.

Read the directions carefully.

Notice: This vaccine has undergone rigid potency, safety and purity tests, and meets Intervet Inc. and USDA requirements. It is designed to stimulate effective immunity when used as directed, but the user must be advised that the response to the product depends upon many factors, including, but not limited to, conditions of storage and handling by the user, administration of the vaccine, health and responsiveness of the individual chickens, and the degree of field exposure.

This product is not hazardous when used according to directions supplied. A material safety data sheet (MSDS) is available upon request. This and any other consumer information can be obtained by calling Intervet Customer Service at 1-800-441-8272 or 1-302-934-8051.

The use of this vaccine is subject to applicable local and federal laws and regulations.

Use only as directed.

Warning(s): Do not vaccinate within 21 days before slaughter.

Presentation: 1 x 1,000 dose ampule and 1 x 2,000 dose ampule with 200 mL diluent per 1,000 doses.

MAREXINE-89/03® is packaged in two separate units. One is an ampule containing either 1,000 or 2,000 doses of frozen live cell associated herpesvirus and infectious bursal disease virus, and the other is a bottle or bag of sterile diluent. The ampules are inserted into metal canes and shipped in a liquid nitrogen (LN) container. The diluent is packaged in separate containers at the rate of 200 mL diluent per 1,000 doses of vaccine.

U.S. Patent No. 5,919,461

Compendium Code No.: 11060851

MAREXINE-SB-89/03®

Intervet **Vaccine**

Bursal Disease-Marek's Disease Vaccine, Variant Strain, Serotypes 2 & 3, Live Virus

U.S. Vet. Lic. No.: 286

Description: MAREXINE-SB-89/03® is a frozen vaccine that contains the FC-126 strain of turkey herpesvirus, the SB-1 strain of chicken herpesvirus and the 89/03 strain of Infectious Bursal Disease virus (IBDV). 89/03 is a Delaware type IBDV that protects against IBDV standard and variant strains.

This vaccine contains gentamicin as a preservative.

Quality tested for purity, potency, and safety.

Indications: MAREXINE-SB-89/03® is recommended for vaccination of healthy one-day-old chickens by subcutaneous (SC) injection to aid in the prevention of very virulent Marek's disease and Infectious Bursal Disease (Standard, Delaware and GLS variants).

Dosage and Administration: Preparation of Vaccine:

Caution: Read "Safety Precautions" advice on handling vaccine ampule. Sterilize vaccinating equipment by boiling in water for 30 minutes or by autoclaving (20 minutes at 121°C). Do not use chemical disinfectants.

1. Use 1,000 doses of vaccine with 200 mL sterile diluent per 1,000 chickens.
2. Before withdrawing vaccine from liquid nitrogen canister, protect hands with gloves, wear long sleeves and use a face mask or goggles. It is possible an accident could occur with either liquid nitrogen or the ampules of vaccine. When removing an ampule from the cane, hold palm of gloved hand away from body and face.
3. When withdrawing a cane of ampules from canister in liquid nitrogen refrigerator, expose only the ampule to be used immediately. The manufacturer recommends handling only one ampule at a time. After removing the ampule from the cane, the remaining ampules should be replaced immediately in the canister of the liquid nitrogen refrigerator.
4. The contents of the ampule are thawed rapidly by immersing in water at room temperature. Shake ampule to disperse contents. Then break the ampule at its neck and immediately proceed as below. 1,000 doses of MAREXINE-SB-89/03® is added for each 200 mL of diluent. Caution: Ampules have been known to explode on sudden temperature changes. Do not thaw in hot or ice cold water.
5. Draw contents of ampule into a sterile 10 mL syringe, mounted with an 18-gauge needle.
6. Dilute immediately by filling the syringe slowly with a portion of the diluent. Important: The diluent should be at room temperature (60°-80°F) at time of mixing.
7. The contents of the filled syringe are then added to the remaining diluent. It is important that this be done slowly. Slowly empty the syringe, allowing the vaccine to run down the side of the diluent container. Gently swirl the container as the vaccine is being mixed. Withdraw a portion of the diluent with the syringe to flush ampule. Inject the washing back into the diluent bottle. Remove the syringe.
8. Fill the previously sterilized automatic syringe according to the manufacturer's recommendations and set the dose at 0.2 mL.
9. The vaccine is now ready for use.

Method of Vaccination:

Subcutaneous Administration:

1. Hold the chicken by the back of the neck just below the head. The loose skin in the area is raised by gently pinching with the thumb and forefinger. Insert the needle beneath the skin in a downward direction away from the head. Inject 0.2 mL per chicken.
2. Avoid hitting the muscles and bones in the neck.
3. Entire contents of container must be used within 1 hour after mixing or be discarded according to Precaution(s).
4. After reconstitution the vaccine should be kept cool and swirled frequently - every 5 minutes.

Records: Keep a record of vaccine, quantity, serial number, expiration date and place of purchase; the date and time of vaccination; the number, age, breed and locations of chickens; names of operators performing the vaccination and any observed reactions.

Precaution(s): Important: Storage Conditions:

Ampules - Store in liquid nitrogen container.

Diluent - Store at room temperature.

Container - Store liquid nitrogen container securely in upright position in a dry, well-ventilated area away from incubator intakes and chicken boxes.

Safety Precautions: Liquid nitrogen container and vaccine should be handled only by properly trained personnel who are thoroughly conversant with the Union Carbide publication and instruction booklet regarding the use of, precautions and safe practices for liquified atmospheric gases (particularly liquid nitrogen).

When removing ampule cane, handling frozen ampules, or adding liquid nitrogen, wear long sleeves, a plastic face shield and gloves to protect the skin from contact with the liquid nitrogen. All storage and handling of the liquid nitrogen container must be in a dry, ventilated area. Do not inhale liquid nitrogen vapors. If drowsiness occurs, get fresh air quickly; then ventilate entire area. If breathing difficulty occurs, apply artificial respiration. If any of these difficulties persist or there is a loss of consciousness, summon a physician immediately.

Care should be exercised to prevent contaminating your hands, eyes and clothing with the vaccine.

Do not mix any substance not approved by Intervet with this vaccine.

Store vaccine in liquid nitrogen at a temperature below -150°C.

Gloves and visor should be worn when handling liquid nitrogen.

Once thawed, the product should not be refrozen.

Once mixed with diluent, the vaccine should be swirled frequently, every 5 minutes.

Once mixed with diluent, the vaccine should be used within 1 hour.

Burn the container and all unused contents.

This product is non-returnable.

Caution(s): Use only in localities where permitted and on premises with a history of Infectious Bursal Disease.

Good management practices are recommended to reduce exposure to Marek's disease and IBDV for at least three weeks following vaccination. Therefore, directions should be followed carefully.

Do not dilute or otherwise stretch the dosage of this vaccine.

Only healthy chickens should be vaccinated.

Cell associated serotype 2 Marek's disease vaccines have been shown to augment development of lymphoid leukosis in susceptible chickens.

For veterinary use only.

Read the directions carefully.

Notice: This vaccine has undergone rigid potency, safety and purity tests, and meets Intervet Inc. and USDA requirements. It is designed to stimulate effective immunity when used as directed, but the user must be advised that the response to the product depends upon many factors, including, but not limited to, conditions of storage and handling by the user, administration of the vaccine, health and responsiveness of the individual chickens, and the degree of field exposure.

This product is not hazardous when used according to directions supplied. A material safety data sheet (MSDS) is available upon request. This and any other consumer information can be obtained by calling Intervet Inc. Customer Service at 1-800-441-8272 or 1-302-934-8051.

The use of this vaccine is subject to applicable local and federal laws and regulations.

Use only as directed.

Warning(s): Do not vaccinate within 21 days before slaughter.

Presentation: 1 x 1,000 dose ampule with 200 mL sterile diluent per 1,000 does.

MAREXINE-SB-89/03® is packaged in two separate units. One is an ampule containing 1,000 doses of frozen, live, cell-associated, turkey and chicken herpesviruses, and frozen, live, 89/03. The second is a container of sterile diluent. The ampules are inserted in metal canes and shipped in a liquid nitrogen container. The diluent is packaged in separate containers at the rate of 200 mL of diluent per 1,000 doses of vaccine.

U.S. Patent No. 5,919,461

Compendium Code No.: 11060871 27403 AL166

MAREXINE® SB-VAC®

Intervet **Vaccine**

Marek's Disease Vaccine, Serotypes 2 & 3, Live Virus-Combination Package

U.S. Vet. Lic. No.: 286

Description: The combination package of Marexine® and SB-Vac® is a frozen vaccine that contains the FC-126 strain of turkey herpesvirus and the SB-1 strain of chicken herpesvirus.

This vaccine contains Gentamicin as a preservative.

Quality tested for purity, potency, and safety.

Indications: This vaccine is recommended for vaccination of healthy one-day-old chickens by subcutaneous injection to aid in the prevention of very virulent Marek's disease. The viruses will infect chickens even though they may possess maternal antibodies to Marek's disease virus (MDV).

Dosage and Administration: Preparation of Vaccine:

Caution: Read "Safety Precautions" advice on handling vaccine ampule. Sterilize vaccinating equipment by boiling it in water for 30 minutes or by autoclaving (20 minutes at 121°C). Do not use chemical disinfectants.

1. Use 1,000 doses of Marexine® and 1,000 doses of SB-Vac® with 200 mL sterile diluent per 1,000 chickens.
2. Before withdrawing vaccine from liquid nitrogen canister, protect hands with gloves, wear long sleeves and use a face mask or goggles. It is possible an accident could occur with either the liquid nitrogen or the ampules of vaccine. When removing an ampule from the cane, hold palm of gloved hand away from body and face.
3. When withdrawing a cane of ampules from the canister in liquid nitrogen refrigerator, expose only the ampule to be used immediately. The manufacturer recommends handling only one ampule at a time. After removing the ampule from the cane, the remaining ampules should be replaced immediately in the canister of the liquid nitrogen refrigerator.
4. The contents of the ampule are thawed rapidly by immersing in water at room temperature. Shake ampule to disperse contents. Then break ampule at its neck and immediately proceed as below. 1,000 doses of Marexine® and 1,000 doses of SB-Vac® are added for each 200 mL of diluent. Caution: Ampules have been known to explode on sudden temperature changes. Do not thaw in hot or ice cold water.

5. Draw contents of ampule into a sterile 10 mL syringe, mounted with an 18-gauge needle.
6. Dilute immediately by filling the syringe slowly with a portion of the diluent. Important: The diluent should be at room temperature (60°-80°F) at time of mixing.
7. The contents of the filled syringe are then added to remaining diluent. It is important that this be done slowly. Slowly empty the syringe, allowing the vaccine to run down the side of the diluent container. Gently swirl the container as the vaccine is being mixed. Withdraw a portion of the diluent with the syringe to flush the ampule. Inject the washing back into the diluent bottle. Remove the syringe.
8. Fill the previously sterilized automatic syringe according to the manufacturer's recommendations and set the dose at 0.2 mL.
9. The vaccine is now ready for use.

Method of Vaccination:

Subcutaneous Administration:

1. Hold the chicken by the back of the neck just below the head. The loose skin in the area is raised by gently pinching with the thumb and forefinger. Insert the needle beneath the skin in a downward direction away from the head. Inject 0.2 mL per chicken.
2. Avoid hitting the muscles and bones in the neck.
3. Entire contents of container must be used within 1 hour after mixing or be discarded according to Precaution(s).
4. After reconstitution, the vaccine should be kept cool and swirled frequently - every 5 minutes.

Records: Keep a record of vaccine, quantity, serial number, expiration date, and place of purchase; the date and time of vaccination; the number, age, breed, and locations of chickens; names of operators performing the vaccination and any observed reactions.

Precaution(s): Important: Storage Conditions:

Ampules - Store in liquid nitrogen container.

Diluent - Store at room temperature.

Container - Store liquid nitrogen container securely in upright position in a dry, well-ventilated area and away from incubator intakes and chicken boxes.

Safety Precautions: Liquid nitrogen container and vaccine should be handled only by properly trained personnel who are thoroughly conversant with the Union Carbide publication and instruction booklet regarding the use of, precautions and safe practices for liquified atmospheric gases (particularly nitrogen).

When removing ampule cane, handling frozen ampules, or adding liquid nitrogen, wear long sleeves, a plastic face shield and gloves to protect the skin from contact with the liquid nitrogen. All storage and handling of the liquid nitrogen container must be in a dry, ventilated area. Do not inhale liquid nitrogen vapors. If drowsiness occurs, get fresh air quickly; then ventilate the entire area. If breathing difficulty occurs, apply artificial respiration. If any of these difficulties persist or there is a loss of consciousness, summon a physician immediately.

Care should be exercised to prevent contaminating your hands, eyes and clothing with the vaccine.

Do not mix any substances not approved by Intervet Inc. with this vaccine.

Store vaccine in liquid nitrogen at a temperature below -150°C.

Gloves and visor should be worn when handling liquid nitrogen.

Once thawed, the product should not be refrozen.

Once mixed with diluent, the vaccine should be swirled frequently, every 5 minutes.

Once mixed with diluent, the vaccine should be used within 1 hour.

Burn the container and all unused contents.

This product is non-returnable.

Caution(s): Good management practices are recommended to reduce exposure to Marek's disease for at least three weeks following vaccination. Directions should be followed carefully.

Do not dilute or otherwise stretch the dosage of this vaccine.

Only healthy chickens should be vaccinated.

Cell-associated serotype 2 Marek's disease vaccines have been shown to augment development of lymphoid leukosis in susceptible chickens.

For veterinary use only.

Read the directions carefully.

Notice: This vaccine has undergone rigid potency, safety and purity tests, and meets Intervet Inc. and USDA requirements. It is designed to stimulate effective immunity when used as directed, but the user must be advised that the response to the product depends upon many factors, including, but not limited to, conditions of storage and handling by the user, administration of the vaccine, health and responsiveness of the individual chickens, and the degree of field exposure.

This product is not hazardous when used according to directions supplied. A material safety data sheet (MSDS) is available upon request. This and any other consumer information can be obtained by calling Intervet Inc. Customer Service at 1-800-441-8272 or 1-302-934-8051.

The use of this vaccine is subject to applicable local and federal laws and regulations.

Use only as directed.

Warning(s): Do not vaccinate within 21 days before slaughter.

Presentation: Two 1,000 dose ampules with 200 mL sterile diluent per 1,000 doses.

The vaccine is packaged in three separate units. One is an ampule containing 1,000 doses of frozen, live, cell-associated turkey herpesvirus. The second is an ampule containing 1,000 doses of frozen, live, cell-associated chicken herpesvirus. The third is a container of sterile diluent. The ampules are inserted in metal canes and shipped in a liquid nitrogen container. The diluent is packaged in separate containers and is used at the rate of 200 mL of diluent per 1,000 doses of vaccine.

Compendium Code No.: 11060881 Rev. 01801901 AL168

M

MARQUIS™ ℞

(15% w/w ponazuril) Antiprotozoal Oral Paste

Bayer

Caution: Federal (U.S.A.) Law restricts this drug to use by or on the order of a licensed veterinarian.

For The Treatment Of Equine Protozoal Myeloencephalitis (EPM) In Horses

For Oral Use Only

DESCRIPTION: Marquis (15% w/w ponazuril) Antiprotozoal Oral Paste is supplied in ready-to-use syringes containing 127 grams of paste. Each gram of paste contains 150 mg of ponazuril (15% w/w). Marquis (ponazuril) is designed to be delivered as an orally administered paste.

Each syringe barrel of Marquis (ponazuril) contains enough paste to treat one (1) 1,200 lb (544 kg) horse for seven (7) days, at a dose rate of 5 mg/kg (2.27 mg/lb) body weight. The plunger contains a dosage ring calibrated for a dose rate of 5 mg/kg (2.27 mg/lb) body weight and marked for horse weight from 600 to 1,200 lbs (272 to 544 kg). The syringe barrels are packaged in units of four with one reusable plunger. This package provides sufficient paste to treat one 1,200 lb (544 kg) horse for 28 days at a dose rate of 5 mg/kg (2.27 mg/lb) body weight.

Ponazuril is an anticoccidial (antiprotozoal) compound with activity against several genera of the phylum Apicomplexa.

CHEMICAL NOMENCLATURE AND STRUCTURE: Ponazuril

1,3,5-Triazine-2,4,6(1H, 3H, 5H)-trione,1-methyl-3-[3-methyl-4-[4-[(trifluoromethyl)sulfonyl] phenoxy]phenyl]-(9Cl)

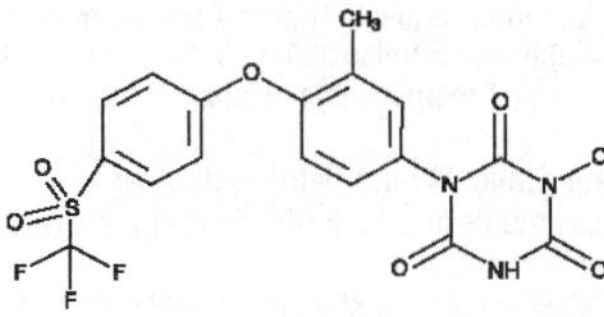

CLINICAL PHARMACOLOGY: The activity of ponazuril has been demonstrated in several Apicomplexans[1-6]. Lindsay, Dubey and Kennedy[7] showed that the concentration of ponazuril necessary to kill *Sarcocystis neurona in vitro* was 0.1 to 1.0 µg/mL. Furr and Kennedy[8] evaluated the pharmacokinetics of ponazuril in serum and CSF in normal horses treated daily at 5 mg/kg for 28 days. The time to peak serum concentration (T_{max}) was 18.20 (±5.9) days and the maximum serum concentration (C_{max}) was 5.59 (±0.92) µg/mL. The terminal elimination half-life for serum (calculated using Day 28 to 42 data) was 4.50 (±0.57) days. In CSF, T_{max} was 15.40 (±7.9) days and C_{max} was 0.21 (±0.072) µg/mL.

INDICATIONS: Marquis (ponazuril) is indicated for the treatment of equine protozoal myeloencephalitis (EPM) caused by *Sarcocystis neurona*.

EFFECTIVENESS SUMMARY: A field study was conducted at six sites with seven investigators across the United States.[9] The study was conducted using historical controls. In this study, each animal's response to treatment was compared to its pre-treatment values. The following standardized neurologic scale was used to grade the horses:

0 - Normal, no deficit detected

1 - Deficit just detected at normal gait

2 - Deficit easily detected and is exaggerated by backing, turning, swaying, loin pressure or neck extension

3 - Deficit very prominent on walking, turning, loin pressure or neck extension

4 - Stumbling, tripping and falling down spontaneously

5 - Recumbent, unable to rise

Improvement was defined as a decrease of at least one grade.

Naturally-occurring clinical cases of EPM, characterized by signalment and laboratory diagnosis, were randomly allotted to one of two treatment doses (5 or 10 mg/kg/day for a period of 28 days), then evaluated for clinical changes through 118 days. Acceptance into the study was based on the results from a standardized neurological examination including radiography, serum *S. neurona* IgG level determination by Western Blot (WB), and a positive cerebrospinal fluid (CSF) for *S. neurona* IgG level by WB.

Response to treatment was determined by the investigator to be acceptable when a clinical improvement of at least one grade occurred by no later than 3 months after treatment, regardless of whether the CSF by WB was positive or negative.

Changes in clinical condition were evaluated first by the subjective scoring of the investigator, then by masked assessment of videotapes of the neurological examination. At 5 mg/kg for 28 days, 28 of 47 horses (60%) improved at least one grade by Day 118. Seventy-five percent (75%) of those improved, that had also been videotaped, were corroborated successes by videotape assessment. At 10 mg/kg, 32 of 55 animals (58%) improved at least one grade by Day 118 and 56% of those improved, that had also been videotaped, were corroborated successes using videotape assessment. With respect to the clinical investigators' scores there was no statistical difference between 5 mg/kg and 10 mg/kg treatment group results (p = 0.8867).

WARNING: For use in animals only. Not for use in horses intended for food. Not for human use. Keep out of the reach of children.

PRECAUTIONS: Prior to treatment, EPM should be distinguished from other diseases that may cause ataxia in horses. Injuries or lameness may also complicate the evaluation of an animal with EPM. In most instances, ataxia due to EPM is asymmetrical and affects the hind limbs.

Clinicians should recognize that clearance of the parasite by ponazuril may not completely resolve the clinical signs attributed to the natural progression of the disease. The prognosis for animals treated for EPM may be dependent upon the severity of disease and the duration of the infection prior to treatment.

The safe use of Marquis (ponazuril) in horses used for breeding purposes, during pregnancy, or in lactating mares, has not been evaluated. The safety of Marquis (ponazuril) with concomitant therapies in horses has not been evaluated.

ADVERSE REACTIONS: In the field study, eight animals were noted to have unusual daily observations. Two horses exhibited blisters on the nose and mouth at some point in the field study, three animals showed a skin rash or hives for up to 18 days, one animal had loose stools throughout the treatment period, one had a mild colic on one day and one animal had a seizure while on medication. The association of these reactions to treatment was not established.

ANIMAL SAFETY SUMMARY: Marquis (ponazuril) was administered to 24 adult horses (12 males and 12 females) in a target animal safety study. Three groups of 8 horses each received 0, 10, or 30 mg/kg (water as control, 2X and 6X for a 5 mg/kg [2.27 mg/lb] dose). Horses were dosed after feeding. One half of each group was treated for 28 days and the other half for 56 days followed by necropsy upon termination of treatment. There were several instances of loose feces in all animals in the study irrespective of treatment, sporadic inappetence and one horse at 10 mg/kg (2X) lost weight while on test. Loose feces were treatment related. Histopathological findings included moderate edema in the uterine epithelium of three of the four females in the 6X group (two treated for 28 days and one for 56 days).

For a copy of the Material Safety Data Sheet (MSDS) or to report Adverse Reactions, call Bayer Customer Service at (800) 633-3796.

DOSAGE: Marquis (ponazuril) is to be used at a dose of 5 mg/kg (2.27 mg/lb) body weight once daily for a period of 28 days.

ADMINISTRATION:

Paste syringe assembly:

Before administration, the syringe barrel and plunger require assembly. Ensure plunger is clean and dry.

Step 1. End cap **must** be on syringe barrel when inserting plunger.

Step 2. Carefully insert reusable plunger into base of syringe barrel until it snaps into place, then remove end cap and gently apply pressure to the plunger until paste is seen at the tip of the syringe barrel.

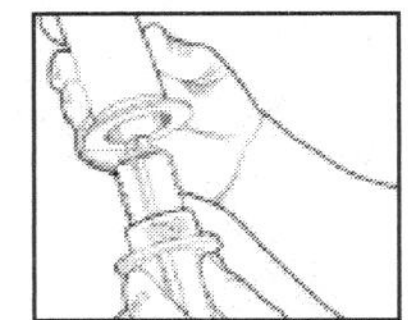

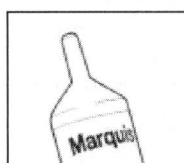

Step 3. Return end cap to tip of paste syringe.

Administering Marquis (ponazuril) to the horse:

NOTE: The paste syringe is a multi-dose package. Ensure that the correct dose is administered with each use.

Step 1. Remove end cap and gently apply pressure to the plunger until paste is seen at the tip of the syringe barrel. Return end cap to tip of paste syringe.

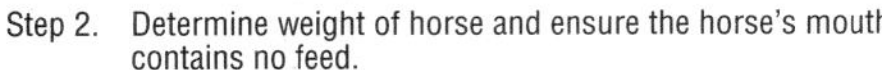

Step 2. Determine weight of horse and ensure the horse's mouth contains no feed.

Step 3. To measure dose, dosage ring collar and barrel collar should be flush. Hold plunger and rotate dosage ring with the other hand to the weight of the horse.

Step 4. Remove end cap from tip of syringe barrel.

Step 5. The selected dose of paste should be deposited onto the back and top of the horse's tongue. Introduce tip of paste syringe into the side of the horse's mouth at the space between the front (incisor) and back (molar) teeth. Deposit paste on the horse's tongue by depressing the plunger of the syringe as far as the dose ring permits. Remove tip of syringe from horse's mouth.

Step 6. To aid swallowing of paste, immediately raise horse's head for a few seconds after dosing.

Step 7. Clean the tip of the syringe with a clean disposable towel and return end cap to tip of syringe barrel.

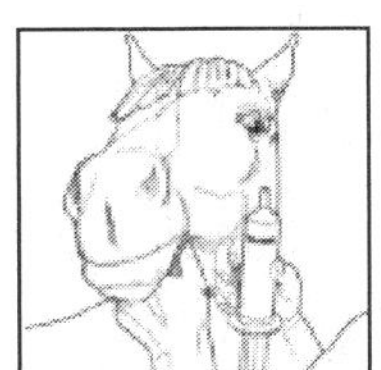

Step 8. For the next daily dose, repeat steps 1-7.

NOTE: *When the paste syringe barrel is empty,* ***remove plunger for re-use and assembly with a new syringe barrel.*** *When removed, the plunger may retain a seal from the empty paste syringe barrel. If this occurs, remove the seal before plunger is inserted into the base of the new paste syringe barrel. At the end of the prescribed treatment period, partially used syringes should be discarded.*

STORAGE: Store at Controlled Room Temperature 15-30° C (59-86° F).

HOW SUPPLIED:

Code: 045799 Carton contains four (4) x 127 gram syringe applicators and one (1) reusable syringe plunger

REFERENCES:

1. Mehlhorn, H., Ortmann-Falkenstein, G., Haberkorn, A.: (1984) The effects of the sym. Trianzinons on developmental stages of *Eimeria tenella, E. maxima* and *E. acervulina:* a light and electron microscopical study. Zeitschr Parsitenk 70: 173-182.
2. Bohrmann, R.: (1991) Treatment with toltrazuril in a natural outbreak of coccidiosis in calves. Dtsch. Tierarzl. Wschr. 98: 343-345.
3. Stafford, K.J., West, D.M., Vermunt, J.J., Pomroy, W., Adlington, B.A., Calder, S.M.: (1994) The effect of repeated doses of toltrazuril on coccidial oocyst output and weight gain in infected lambs. NZ Vet J 42(3): 117-119.
4. Haberkorn, A.G., Stoltefuss, D.I.J.: (1987) Studies on the activity spectrum of toltrazuril, a new anticoccidial compound. Vet. Med. Review 1: 22-32.
5. Koudela, B., Vodstricilova, M., Klimes, B., Vladik, P., Vitovec, J.: (1991) Application of the anticoccidiosis drug Toltrazuril in the coccidiosis of neonatal pigs. Veterinami medicina (Praha) 36: 657-663.
6. Benoit, E., Buronfosse, T., Delatour, P.: (1994) Effect of Cytochrome P-450 1A induction on enantioselective metabolism and pharmacokinetics of an aryltrifluoromethyl sulfide in the rat. Chirality 6(5): 372-377.
7. Lindsay, D.S., Dubey, J.P., Kennedy, T.J.: (2000) Determination of the activity of ponazuril against *Sarcocystis neurona* in cell cultures. Vet Parasit 92: 165-169.
8. Furr, M., Kennedy, T.: Pharmacokinetics of ponazuril in horses. Study 150-717 Bayer Corporation.
9. Furr, M., Andrews, F., MacKay, R., Reed, S., Bernard, W., Bain, F., Byars, D., Kennedy, T.: Treatment of equine protozoal myeloencephalitis (EPM) with various doses of ponazuril. Study Report 150-664 Bayer Corporation.

U.S. Patent No. 5,833,095

79004570, R.1
July, 2001

Manufactured by Bayer Corporation, Agriculture Division, Animal Health, Shawnee Mission, Kansas 66201 U.S.A.

NADA #141-188, Approved by FDA

Compendium Code No.: 10400390

MASTER GUARD™ 10

AgriLabs **Bacterin-Vaccine**

Bovine Rhinotracheitis-Virus Diarrhea-Parainfluenza$_3$-Respiratory Syncytial Virus Vaccine, Modified Live and Killed Virus-Leptospira Canicola-Grippotyphosa-Hardjo-Icterohaemorrhagiae-Pomona Bacterin

U.S. Vet. Lic. No.: 213

Contents: This product contains the antigens listed above.

Indications: For the vaccination of healthy dairy and beef cattle 5 months of age or older, including pregnant cows, as an aid in the prevention of disease caused by infectious bovine rhinotracheitis virus (IBR), bovine virus diarrhea virus, Type I and Type II (BVD), parainfluenza$_3$ (PI$_3$), bovine respiratory syncytial virus (BRSV) and as an aid in the prevention of disease caused by Leptospira canicola-grippotyphosa-hardjo-icterohaemorrhagiae-pomona.

Dosage and Administration: Rehydrate the desiccated vial of Titanium™ 2 with the accompanying vial of Master Guard™ 8 and shake well. Inject 5 mL subcutaneously or intramuscularly using aseptic technique. Repeat the dose in 14 to 28 days. Annual revaccination is recommended.

Precaution(s): Store at 35° to 45°F (2° to 7°C). Do not freeze. Use entire contents when first opened. Burn container and all unused contents.

Caution(s): Allergic reactions may follow the use of vaccines.

Antidote(s): Epinephrine.

Warning(s): Do not vaccinate within 21 days before slaughter.

Presentation: 10 dose (50 mL) and 20 dose (100 mL).

Manufactured by: Diamond Animal Health, Inc., Des Moines, Iowa 50317 U.S.A.

Compendium Code No.: 10580692

MASTER GUARD® 10

Intervet **Bacterin-Vaccine**

Bovine Rhinotracheitis-Virus Diarrhea-Parainfluenza$_3$-Respiratory Syncytial Virus Vaccine, Modified Live and Killed Virus-Leptospira Canicola-Grippotyphosa-Hardjo-Icterohaemorrhagiae-Pomona Bacterin

U.S. Vet. Lic. No.: 213

Contents: This product contains the antigens listed above.
Contains gentamicin as a preservative.

Indications: For the vaccination of healthy dairy and beef cattle 5 months of age or older, including pregnant cows, as an aid in the prevention of disease caused by infectious bovine rhinotracheitis virus (IBR), bovine virus diarrhea virus, Type I and Type II (BVD), bovine parainfluenza$_3$ virus (PI$_3$), bovine respiratory syncytial virus (BRSV) and as an aid in the prevention of disease caused by *Leptospira canicola, L. grippotyphosa, L. hardjo, L. icterohaemorrhagiae, L. pomona.*

Dosage and Administration: Rehydrate the desiccated vial of Titanium® 2 with the accompanying vial of Master Guard® 8 and shake well. Inject 5 mL subcutaneously or intramuscularly using aseptic technique. Repeat the dose in 14 to 28 days. Annual revaccination is recommended.

Precaution(s): Store at 35° to 45°F (2° to 7°C). Do not freeze. Use entire contents when first opened. Burn container and all unused contents.

Caution(s): Allergic reactions may follow the use of vaccines. For use in animals only.

Antidote(s): Epinephrine.

Warning(s): Do not vaccinate within 21 days before slaughter.

Presentation: 10 doses (50 mL) and 20 doses (100 mL).

MASTER GUARD® is a registered trademark of Agri Laboratories, Ltd.

Manufactured by: Diamond Animal Health, Inc., Des Moines, IA 50327.

Compendium Code No.: 11062621 03279-2 / 03280-2

MASTER GUARD® 10 + VIBRIO

AgriLabs **Bacterin-Vaccine**

Bovine Rhinotracheitis-Virus Diarrhea-Parainfluenza$_3$-Respiratory Syncytial Virus Vaccine, Modified Live and Killed Virus-Campylobacter Fetus-Leptospira Canicola-Grippotyphosa-Hardjo-Icterohaemorrhagiae-Pomona Bacterin

U.S. Vet. Lic. No.: 213

Contents: This product contains the antigens listed above.

Indications: For the vaccination of healthy dairy and beef cattle, including pregnant cows and heifers, as an aid in the prevention of disease caused by infectious bovine rhinotracheitis virus (IBR), bovine virus diarrhea virus, Type I and Type II (BVD), parainfluenza$_3$ (PI$_3$), bovine respiratory syncytial virus (BRSV) and as an aid in the prevention of disease caused by *Campylobacter fetus* and *Leptospira canicola-grippotyphosa-hardjo-icterohaemorrhagiae-pomona.*

Dosage and Administration: Rehydrate the desiccated vial of Titanium® 2 with the accompanying vial of Master Guard® 8 + Vibrio and shake well. Inject 5 mL subcutaneously or intramuscularly using aseptic technique. Repeat the dose in 14 to 28 days. Annual revaccination is recommended.

Precaution(s): Store at 35° to 45°F (2° to 7°C). Do not freeze. Use entire contents when first opened. Burn container and all unused contents.

Caution(s): Allergic reactions may follow the use of vaccines.

Antidote(s): Epinephrine.

Warning(s): Do not vaccinate within 21 days before slaughter.

Presentation: 10 dose (50 mL) and 20 dose (100 mL) vials.

Manufactured by: Diamond Animal Health, Inc., Des Moines, IA 50327

Compendium Code No.: 10581360 03323

MASTER GUARD® J5

AgriLabs **Bacterin**

Escherichia Coli Bacterin

U.S. Vet. Lic. No.: 303

Contents: Contains chemically inactivated culture of J5 Mutant *Escherichia coli* and Suprimm® adjuvant.

Indications: As an aid in the prevention of endotoxemia caused by *E. coli* in healthy cattle six months of age or older.

Dosage and Administration: Directions and Dosage: Three 2 mL doses at three week intervals administered intramuscularly or subcutaneously. Annual booster doses are recommended at dry-off and two to three weeks prior to calving.

Precaution(s): Store at 2-7°C. Shake thoroughly before use. Use entire contents when first opened.

Caution(s): In case of anaphylactoid reactions administer epinephrine. Transient, local swelling may occur at the injection site. For animal use only.

Warning(s): Do not vaccinate within 60 days of slaughter. Keep out of reach of children.

Presentation: 10 doses (20 mL) and 50 doses (100 mL).

Manufactured by: ImmTech Biologics, LLC, Bucyrus, KS 66013.

Compendium Code No.: 10581331

MASTER GUARD™ PREG 5

AgriLabs **Vaccine**

Bovine Rhinotracheitis-Virus Diarrhea-Parainfluenza$_3$-Respiratory Syncytial Virus Vaccine, Modified Live and Killed Virus

U.S. Vet. Lic. No.: 213

Contents: This product contains the antigens listed above.

Indications: For the vaccination of healthy dairy and beef cattle 5 months of age or older, including pregnant cows, as an aid in the prevention of disease caused by infectious bovine rhinotracheitis virus (IBR), bovine virus diarrhea virus, Type I and Type II (BVD), parainfluenza$_3$ (PI$_3$), bovine respiratory syncytial virus (BRSV).

Dosage and Administration: Rehydrate the desiccated vial of Titanium™ 2 with the accompanying vial of Master Guard™ 3 and shake well. Inject 5 mL subcutaneously or intramuscularly using aseptic technique. Repeat the dose in 14 to 28 days. Annual revaccination is recommended.

Precaution(s): Store at 35° to 45°F (2° to 7°C). Do not freeze. Use entire contents when first opened. Burn container and all unused contents.

Caution(s): Allergic reactions may follow the use of vaccines.

Antidote(s): Epinephrine.

Warning(s): Do not vaccinate within 21 days before slaughter.

Presentation: 10 dose (50 mL) and 20 dose (100 mL).

Manufactured by: Diamond Animal Health, Inc., Des Moines, Iowa 50317 U.S.A.

Compendium Code No.: 10580700

MASTER GUARD® PREG 5

Intervet **Vaccine**

Bovine Rhinotracheitis-Virus Diarrhea-Parainfluenza$_3$-Respiratory Syncytial Virus Vaccine, Modified Live and Killed Virus

U.S. Vet. Lic. No.: 213

Contents: This product contains the antigens listed above.

Contains gentamicin as a preservative.

Indications: For the vaccination of healthy dairy and beef cattle 5 months of age or older, including pregnant cows, as an aid in the prevention of disease caused by infectious bovine rhinotracheitis virus (IBR), bovine virus diarrhea virus, Type I and Type II (BVD), bovine parainfluenza$_3$ virus (PI$_3$), bovine respiratory syncytial virus (BRSV).

Dosage and Administration: Rehydrate the desiccated vial of Titanium® 2 with the accompanying vial of Master Guard® 3 and shake well. Inject 5 mL subcutaneously or intramuscularly using aseptic technique. Repeat the dose in 14 to 28 days. Annual revaccination is recommended.

Precaution(s): Store at 35° to 45°F (2° to 7°C). Do not freeze. Use entire contents when first opened. Burn container and all unused contents.

Caution(s): Allergic reactions may follow the use of vaccines. For use in animals only.

Antidote(s): Epinephrine.

Warning(s): Do not vaccinate within 21 days before slaughter.

Presentation: 10 doses (50 mL) and 20 doses (100 mL).

MASTER GUARD® is a registered trademark of Agri Laboratories, Ltd.

Manufactured by: Diamond Animal Health, Inc., Des Moines, IA 50327.

Compendium Code No.: 11062631 03277-3 / 03276-2

MASTI-CLEAR™

G.C. Hanford **Mastitis Therapy**

Penicillin G Procaine in Sesame Oil-Lactating Cow Mastitis Treatment

Active Ingredient(s): Each 10 mL single dose syringe contains:

Penicillin G procaine.......... 100,000 units

Indications: This product is intended for the treatment of bovine mastitis in dry cows. This product is effective against udder infection caused by the following susceptible microorganisms: *Streptococcus agalactiae, Streptococcus dysgalactiae* and *Streptococcus uberis.* For the best results, it should be used promptly at the first signs of mastitis.

Signs of mastitis include:

1. Inflammation of the udder or teat. Inflammation may be recognized by redness, swelling, elevated temperature, or pain in the affected part.
2. Abnormal milk. Presence of flakes or clots, in the milk, or milk of a watery character is usually indicative of a mastitis infection.
3. High white-cell counts. The routine use of the California Mastitis Test is encouraged. A high incidence of scores in excess of CMT 2 or a high CMT score on bulk milk samples may indicate a potential mastitis problem. In these situations a veterinarian should be consulted for a definitive diagnosis and recommendations.

Dosage and Administration: The dose is 10 mL of this product per infected quarter administered by intramammary infusion. Treatment may be repeated at intervals of 12 hours. Do not administer more than three consecutive doses. If abnormal milk, redness, or swelling persists or increases, discontinue use and consult your veterinarian.

Milk out udder completely. Wash udder and teats thoroughly with warm water containing a suitable dairy disinfectant. Dry thoroughly. Saturate a small piece of cotton with a suitable antiseptic such as 70 percent alcohol and wipe off teat, using a separate piece of cotton for each teat. The hands of the operator should be washed and dried before the administration of each treatment. Appropriate sanitation and management procedures to prevent and/or control bovine mastitis should be instituted.

When using this product remove plastic cover from tip of syringe and, while holding teat firmly, insert tip into streak canal; then push plunger and inject entire contents. After injection, grasp the end of the teat firmly, then gently massage the medication up the teat canal into the milk cistern.

Treated quarters should not be milked for at least six hours after treatment but should be milked at regular intervals thereafter. Treatment may be repeated at 12 hour intervals, up to a total of three doses, as indicated by the clinical response.

Note: Mastitis cannot be considered cured until bacteriologic examination of milk samples taken approximately three weeks after treatment demonstrates the absence of causative microorganisms.

Precaution(s): Discard empty container; do not reuse.

Store at room temperature: 59°-86°F (15°-30°C).

This product was manufactured by a non-sterilizing process.

Warning(s): For udder instillation in lactating cattle only.

1. Milk that has been taken from animals during treatment and for 60 hours (5 milkings) after the latest treatment must not be used for food.
2. Animals shall not be slaughtered for food during treatment or within three (3) days after the latest treatment.
3. Administration of more than three consecutive doses may result in drug residues in the milk and meat beyond the discard periods.

Restricted drug (California) - Use only as directed. Keep out of reach of children.

Presentation: 12x10 mL single dose syringe with 12 alcohol pads.

Compendium Code No.: 10340011

MASTIK™

ImmuCell **Mastitis Test**

Mastitis Antibiotic Susceptibility Testing Kit

Test Description: MASTiK™ is a rapid antibiotic susceptibility test for mastitis. The results may be obtained in 12 hours in most cases, with a range of 6 to 24 hours. The MASTiK™ test principally consists of reagent vials containing milk media with pH indicator dye and 96 well polystyrene plates with various antimicrobials in different concentrations, packaged separately. The box containing MASTiK™ Reagent should be removed from the kit on arrival and stored at refrigeration temperature 2°-8°C or 36°-46°F) until used. The other kit components may be stored at room temperature. Three different samples can be tested per plate against 3 or 4 concentrations of 8 different antimicrobials as shown below.

Antimicrobial	Range (ug/ml)
Negative Control	Growth inhibitor
Positive Control	None
Erythromycin	0.5-4.0
*Oxacillin + 2% NaCL	0.5-4.0
**Ampicillin	0.25-4.0
Penicillin	0.12-2.0
***Cephalothin	0.5-16.0
Pirlimycin	0.25-4.0
Oxytetracycline	2.0-16.0
Sulfadimethoxine	0.125-2.0

* Oxacillin is the parent compound for Cloxacillin.

** Ampicillin is the parent compound for Amoxicillin and Hetacillin.

*** Cephalothin is the parent compound for Cephapirin and Ceftiofur.

Note: If the bacteria are sensitive to the parent compound it means that they will also be susceptible to the daughter compounds. For example, if test results indicate that oxacillin is effective, then it follows that Coxacillin (its daughter compound) is also effective. The reverse may or may not be true.

These concentrations of antimicrobials are obtained when 0.05 ml (50 microliters) of culture is added to the well. The lowest concentration well is at a level usually lower than that which is achieved in milk when the cow is treated with commonly used doses. The highest concentration well is at a level that may be difficult to maintain throughout the therapeutic period when commonly used dosages are chosen.

The distribution of the controls and the concentrations of the antimicrobials in ug/ml after reconstitution with the treated sample are detailed in the MASTiK™ record card.

Contents: Materials

	3 Test Kit	15 Test Kit	30 Test Kit
1. 96 well antimicrobial plates (3 tests per plate)	1	5	10
2. Adhesive seals	2	5	10
3. Pad of record cards	1	1	1
4. Sterile transfer pipettes	4	18	36
5. Flip-top collections tubes, sterile inside	3	15	30
6. Package insert	1	1	1
7. MASTiK™ Reagent - vials contain 3 ml milk media with indicator dye	4	18	36

Materials needed but not included with MASTiK™:

1. Alcohol swabs
2. Incubator (34°-39°C or 93°-102°F).

Indications: Use of the Test: MASTiK™ is a rapid *in-vitro* antibiotic susceptibility test for clinical mastitis in the bovine due to the following major mastitis-causing bacteria: *Staphylococcus aureus, Streptococcus agalactiae, Streptococcus uberis, Streptococcus dysgalactiae, E. coli, Klebsiella* species, and *Actinomyces pyogenes.* Results are usually obtained in 12 hours or less, but range from 6 to 24 hours. Organisms which can cause mastitis much less frequently (and are usually unsuccessfully treated with antibiotics) such as *Pseudomonas* species, *Prototheca, Mycoplasma* species, and yeast will not show evidence of growth in this test. A test result of no growth in the positive control well usually means antibiotic therapy is not indicated.

MASTiK™ is not intended for use on specimens other than mastitic milk.

Samples to be tested must be aseptically drawn from quarters with mastitis. Affected cows may or may not be sick, but they must not have been recently treated with antibiotics by any route. Always take a sample from a cow before you treat her and refrigerate it in case you wish to run a test later. Chronic or subclinical cases can usually be successfully tested, although they will require a longer incubation time with the reagent before transferring to the test plate.

Test Principles: A milk sample is drawn under sterile conditions from the affected quarter and mixed with a MASTiK™ reagent (sterile milk and the purple dye BCP, a pH color indicator) and incubated from 0 to 8 hours, usually 1-3 hours at 35°-37°C (65°-98.6°F) to allow bacterial multiplication. A small quantity of this mixture (0.05 ml) is then added to each of 32 wells (1/3) of the MASTiK™ plate containing 8 antibiotics at 3 or 4 concentrations each. The plate is covered with a clear adhesive seal and incubated at 35°-37°C until results are obtained. Since the major mastitis-causing bacteria ferment lactose, producing lactic acid, their growth will lower the pH of the milk media gradually changing the color from purple to yellow. If the growth of the bacteria is inhibited by the antibiotic, there will be little or no lactic acid produced and thus little or no change in color from the original purple.

In MASTiK™ the antibiotic susceptibility of the organisms is tested in approximately the same concentration of organisms as the environment (milk media) present in the udder to be treated. Thus the result is expected to produce a more realistic correlation between the *in-vitro* sensitivity test and the response to treatment. The uncommon microorganisms of mastitis which do not ferment lactose will not cause any change in color of the media.

Test Procedure: The MASTiK™ Panel (Three tests per plate)

	1	2	3	4	5	6	7	8	9	10	11	12
A	CTRL POS	ERY .5	ERY 1	ERY 4	CTRL POS	ERY .5	ERY 1	ERY 4	CTRL POS	ERY .5	ERY 1	ERY 4
B	CTRL NEG	OXA .5	OXA 1	OXA 4	CTRL NEG	OXA .5	OXA 1	OXA 4	CTRL NEG	OXA .5	OXA 1	OXA 4
C	AMP .25	AMP .5	AMP 1	AMP 4	AMP .25	AMP .5	AMP 1	AMP 4	AMP .25	AMP .5	AMP 1	AMP 4
D	PEN .125	PEN .25	PEN .5	PEN 2	PEN .125	PEN .25	PEN .5	PEN 2	PEN .125	PEN .25	PEN .5	PEN 2
E	CEP .5	CEP 2	CEP 4	CEP 16	CEP .5	CEP 2	CEP 4	CEP 16	CEP .5	CEP 2	CEP 4	CEP 16
F	PIR .25	PIR .5	PIR 1	PIR 4	PIR .25	PIR .5	PIR 1	PIR 4	PIR .25	PIR .5	PIR 1	PIR 4
G	OXY 2	OXY 4	OXY 8	OXY 16	OXY 2	OXY 4	OXY 8	OXY 16	OXY 2	OXY 4	OXY 8	OXY 16
H	SDM .125	SDM .25	SDM .5	SDM 2	SDM .125	SDM .25	SDM .5	SDM 2	SDM .125	SDM .25	SDM .5	SDM 2

Note: Three sample can be tested with each antimicrobial plate. The milk samples must be collected and handled under aseptic conditions at all time.

Collection of Samples: (Important Note: If the sample is not collected under sterile conditions as outlined in steps 1-4, contamination will make these test results meaningless).

1. After washing hands thoroughly wash the teat with udder wash and water and dry with paper towels.
2. Discard first stripping of milk.
3. Vigorously swab teat end with alcohol swab and let air dry.
4. Flip up cap from collection tube. While holding both tube and teat at a 45° angle, squirt at least 2 ml (one stripping) of milk into the tube and cap the tube. Refrigerate the sample if a delay of more than 6 hours is anticipated before testing the sample. Freeze if the anticipated delay is more that 4 days.

Testing of Samples (See below for quick steps)

5. Open the cap of a MASTiK™ Reagent vial and pour approximately 1 ml of the mastitis sample into the reagent vial by filling the reagent vial up to the 4 ml line on the label. Do not use the pipettes provided in the kit to add the milk to the reagent vial. Recap the reagent vial, invert to mix and label it appropriately. If the sample is from a highly acute case and the cow is very sick, skip step 6 and proceed to step 7.
6. Incubate the reagent vial at 35-37°C (95-99°F) for 1-3 hours. The sample-reagent mixture should retain its blue-purple color. If the sample-reagent mixture begins to change color (from purple to blue-green or yellow), pour approximately 1 ml of the sample-reagent mixture into a fresh reagent vial and proceed to the next step. Note: If the sample is from a case of subclinical or chronic mastitis instead of clinical or acute mastitis, then prolong the initial incubation time to 6-8 hours.
7. Remove the plate from the foil package. Three samples can be run concurrently on this plate. For running one sample, begin with Section A1-H4. At a later time, a 2nd sample can be run in the middle four columns and a 3rd sample in the last four columns. Label the sections of the plate as required (see The MASTiK™ Panel).
8. Mix by inverting the incubated sample-reagent vial containing the milk sample several times. Using a separate sterile disposable transfer pipette for each sample, add 2 drops of sample-reagent mixture to each of the 32 wells of the appropriate section. Do not touch wells with the pipette. Solids, flakes, or clots should be avoided. Place leftover pre-incubated vial in refrigerator.
9. Remove the clear plastic adhesive sheet from its paper backing and cover the plate and all wells. The adhesive seal should remain on the plate to protect any unused wells. When testing subsequent samples pull the adhesive seal back to expose unused wells.
10. Incubate the plate at 35-37°C or 95-99°F.
11. When handling the plate, be sure not to turn it upside down. Examine the plate for color change after 4 to 8 hours of incubation and thereafter every 4 to 8 hours until the color of the positive control well has changed from purple to yellow.
    Do not incubate the plate more than 24 hours in total. The bottom of the plate should be checked for color changes by holding the plate level over your head. Most plates will be ready to read in 8 to 12 hours. In general, the more acute the case, the faster the results.

Reading the Test Results

12. Do not turn the plate over. Hold it level over your head and examine the bottoms of the wells for color changes. Note the positions of the letters (A-H) and numbers (1-12) on the top of the plate - make sure you match the positions on the plate with the record sheet when recording the results. The test results are ready to read if growth has occurred in the positive control well causing it to change color from purple to yellow. Wells A1, A5, and A9 are positive control wells and contain no antibiotics. Yellow in these wells is recorded on the results sheet as Positive. No color change in the positive control well indicates the probable presence of non-lactose fermenting organisms or the absence of living bacteria.
13. Wells B1, B5, B9 are negative control wells and should always inhibit growth. Therefore, the negative control well should always be purple or the original color of the sample. Purple in these wells should be recorded on the results sheet as Negative. Purple color in all wells, including both controls, indicates the probable presence of non-lactose fermenting organisms or the absence of living bacteria.
14. Record the result of the test wells as S, R, or I on the record card provided.
    Purple = No Growth = S (Susceptible)
    Yellow = Growth = R (Resistant)
    Intermediate color = I (partial growth)
    Any test well that has not changed color and is similar in color to the negative control well is recorded on the results sheet as S (Susceptible). Any well that has changed color toward yellow and is similar in color to the positive control well is indicative of growth and recorded as R (Resistant). A well intermediate in color between the positive and negative control wells is recorded as I (Intermediate).
    Note: If color changes are not dramatic, continue incubation another 4 to 8 hours but not more than 24 hours total and re-read results.
    Read each section of the plate independent of the other sections based upon the appropriate changes in the control wells as described above.

Quick-Step Chart

1. Pour approximately 1 ml of mastitis sample into MASTiK™ reagent tube (fill to 4 ml line on label). Recap, invert to mix and label tube. If case is acute and highly severe, skip step 2 and proceed to step 3.
2. Incubate sample-reagent mixture for 1-3 hours (6-8 hours if mastitis is chronic or subclinical) at 95-99°F (35-37°C).
3. Remove plate from foil pouch. Using supplied pipette, add 2 drops of mixture to each of the 32 test wells (4 columns of 8 wells per sample).
4. Remove clear plastic adhesive sheet from paper backing and cover all 96 wells.
5. Incubate plate at 95-99°F (35-37°C).
6. Examine plate for color changes every 4-8 hours until positive control well has changed from purple to yellow.
7. Hold plate overhead and record colors on MASTiK™ record sheet, making sure you match the positions of the wells with the sheet. The negative control well should have retained its original purple color. For other wells, record yellow as resistant and purple as susceptible.

Interpretation of Results: MASTiK™ is an *in-vitro* susceptibility test and the test results should be used as an aid only, in selecting the drug of choice for treatment. The concentration of the antimicrobials in the lowest concentration well is at a level lower than what is usually achieved in milk when the cow is treated with the commonly used dosages; the highest concentration well is at a level that is sometimes higher than the concentration achieved by usual therapeutic dosages.

Thus, in general, when choosing an antimicrobial for therapy, the best choice is one in which all of its wells displayed no growth (retained the original purple color). The second best choice would be the drug in which only the lowest concentration well showed growth (changed in color from purple to yellow).

When all wells, including the positive and negative controls, remain purple, infection with non-lactose fermenting organisms such as *Mycoplasma bovis, Pseudomonas aeruginosa,* yeast or *Prototheca* should be suspected.

Use in Dry Treatment Selection: If you are depending on dry treatment to cure subclinical mastitis, it makes sense, especially in high producing cows, to use an antibiotic to which the bacteria are susceptible. If you are using the same dry treatment on all quarters of all cows, chances are it will work no better than using the same antibiotic all the time to treat all cases of clinical mastitis.

If a cow is near drying off and you know she has subclinical mastitis from culture results or somatic cell counting, identify the problem quarter(s) by culture or CMT* test. You may then run MASTiK™ with a simple modification; increase the incubation time of the sample-reagent mixture outlined in step 6 to 6-8 hours.

* Contact ImmuCell to obtain CMT.

Limitations: MASTiK™ susceptibility test is effective only with lactose fermenting bacteria. It does not reveal the sensitivity of non-lactose fermenting organisms. Good correlations between the test results and treatment response is expected but can not be assumed in all cases.

Troubleshooting

Problem: No Color Changes After Recommended Incubation Time

1. No bacteria in sample (case is not bacterial mastitis).
   Solution: Do standard culture and identification.
2. Bacteria in sample are totally engulfed by leukocytes in milk.
   Solution: Re-sample cow and repeat test.
   Note that most commonly used antibiotics cannot enter these cells are not indicated in these cases.
3. Organism in sample is not *Staphylococcus, Streptococcus, Actinomyces,* or coliform.
   Solution: Culture and identify organism.
4. Not enough bacteria in sample. Occurs most often when testing subclinical or chronic cases.
   Solution: Continue incubating and check test every 4 hours. Problem often avoided if preincubation (step 6) period is extended to 6-8 hours.
   Laboratory Note: MASTiK™ may be run from colonies isolated on agar by standardizing the inoculum.
5. Slow growing bacteria.
   Solution: Continue incubation of plate and check for color changes every 4 hours.
6. Cow was treated with an antibiotic before sample was taken.
   Solution: Sample only cases not treated within past 48 hours. Always aseptically sample the cow before initiating treatment.

Problem: Overgrowth - All Wells Change Color

1. Occurs in cases with unusually high numbers of bacteria, especially if plate is not checked every 4 hours.
   Solution: Re-run the test with the remainder of the original sample that has been refrigerated. Skip step 6 (2 hour pre-incubation) and immediately fill plate. If the quantity left is insufficient to fill the plate (less than 1½ ml) add a small amount of MASTiK™ Reagent, incubate for 30 minutes, and then fill plate.
2. Can occur with contaminated sample.
   Solution: Must use proper sampling technique.
   Must handle sample and fill plate using aseptic technique.

Problem: Color Changes Not Dramatic
   Solution: Continue incubation.

Problem: Skips - Growth occurs in high concentration well, but not in low concentration well of the same drug.

1. Uneven distribution of bacterial numbers when filling plate.
   Solution: One skip on a plate occasionally is acceptable and can be ignored.
2. Flakes (coated with high numbers of bacteria) were pipetted into wells.
   Solution: Avoid pipetting clumps and flakes from sample.

M

Problem: Sample began to change color in sample vial after preincubation (step 6) and before filling plate.

Solution: Add approximately one ml of the mixture to a fresh vial of MASTiK™ Reagent. Immediately fill the plate and incubate it. Check the plate every 2 hours for color changes.

Treatment Failure: Although MASTiK™ is highly accurate, some cases may not respond to the recommended antibiotic. Some causes for this phenomenon include:

1. Sample was contaminated.
2. Pathogenic bacteria were intracellular, not in milk.
3. Case is due to a pathogen often unresponsive to antibiotics such as *Pseudomonas, Actinomyces,* yeasts, *Prototheca,* or *Mycoplasma.*
4. The quarter is infected with two or more pathogens growing at different rates.
5. Course of treatment was too short or infrequent.
6. Case was due to chronic infection with Staphylococcus aureus.
7. Test was misread.
8. Antibiotic administered by the intramammary route did not disperse and distribute evenly throughout gland due to low volume of dose, improper vehicle, antibiotic kinetics, or inflammatory by-products.
9. Drug was administered improperly.
10. Administered drug (intramammary) was contaminated.
11. Sample did not contain a major mastitis pathogen.
12. Cow was too clinically ill.

Some of the above pitfalls can be avoided if the sample is simultaneously cultured and identified while running the MASTiK™ test.

Examples of Mastitis Preparation Trade Names

Antibiotic	Trade Name	Maker
A. Erythromycin (ERY)	Erythro-36™	Sanofi
	Erythro-Dry™	Sanofi
	Gallimycin-36™	AgriLabs
	Gallimycin Dry Cow™	AgriLabs
	Uddermate™	Anchor
B. Oxacillin (OXA) (daughter compound: cloxacillin	Dariclox™	Pfizer
	Orbenin-DC™	Pfizer
	Dry-Clox™	Fort Dodge
C. Ampicillin (AMP) (daughter compounds: amoxicillin, hetacillin)	Amoxi-Mast™	Pfizer
	Hetacin-K™	Fort Dodge
D. Penicillin (PEN) or penicillin combination products	Go-Dry™	G.C. Hanford
	Albacillin™	Pharmacia & Upjohn
	Albadry-Plus™	Pharmacia & Upjohn
	Quartermaster™	Pharmacia & Upjohn
E. Cephalothin (CEP) (daughter compounds: cephapirin, ceftiofur)	Cefa-Lak™	Fort Dodge
	Cefa-Dri™	Fort Dodge
	Today™	Fort Dodge
	Tomorrow™	Fort Dodge
F. Pirlimycin (PIR)	Pirsue™	Pharmacia & Upjohn

M

Storage: Storage and Shelf Life: The plates should be stored at room temperature (15-25°C or 59-77°F) away from direct sunlight or heat. Use the plate prior to the expiration date printed on the label. If the package has been damaged in any manner, the plate in the package should be discarded. A silica gel desiccant is included in each foil package. The desiccant should be blue upon opening the package. Do not use the plate if the desiccant did not retain its blue color or if the foil pouch is not intact.

MASTiK™ Reagent must be stored at refrigerated temperature (2-8°C or 36-46°F). Use the MASTiK™ Reagent prior to the expiration date printed on the label. If the reagent has not retained its blue-purple color (i.e. it appears yellow or green) it may be contaminated and should not be used.

Caution(s):

1. Strict aseptic measures should be followed in collection of samples and running the test.
2. The test is for diagnostic use only.
3. Since microorganisms present in the samples tested with this product can be infectious, proper handling and disposal methods should be established.
4. Only personnel adequately trained in such methods should perform this type of diagnostic procedure.

The used plates, reagent vials and the samples should be disposed of properly, according to state and local regulations.

Discussion: General Information: Despite great improvements in recent years in mastitis prevention, both clinical and subclinical mastitis remains a most common and costly disease of dairy cows. Most cases are due to the bacteria *Staphylococcus aureus, Streptococcus agalactiae, Streptococcus dysgalactiae, Streptococcus uberis, Klebsiella* and *E. coli.* Early diagnosis and treatment of clinical mastitis with an effective antibiotic is usually a cost-effective approach. Losses due to clinical mastitis include not only unsalable milk during the treatment and drug withdrawal period and medicine, but the biggest loss to the dairyman is decreased milk production over the remainder of the lactation. Clinical mastitis that is not totally cured but becomes subclinical will also result in lowered milk production.

Because traditional antibiotic susceptibility tests are usually slow (often taking several days) and often inaccurate (they are human not bovine tests) veterinarians and dairy farmers most commonly treat cows with clinical mastitis by guessing which antibiotic will work. These guesses are usually based on what has been working lately or simply intuition. Because of the emergence of so many antibiotic resistant strains of mastitis-causing bacteria and the ever-shrinking profit margin in dairying, there is a need for a rapid, cost-effective, and accurate antibiotic susceptibility test for mastitis. MASTiK™ is such a test which is run in milk rather than laboratory media using bacteria that exists in the cow's udder rather than a standardized concentration. The results should be used as an aid in choosing an approved antibiotic at an approved dosage for mastitis therapy.

Important Information: Please Read Carefully Before Proceeding:

MASTiK™ is a laboratory diagnostic test kit to be used only as an aid in selecting FDA approved antibiotics for mastitis therapy. Examples of approved over-the-counter antibiotics are penicillin, cephapirin and erythromycin. Examples of approved antibiotics which may be used with a veterinarian's prescription include hetacillin, pirlimycin, amoxicillin, and cloxacillin. The antibiotics listed above are available under a variety of trade name and must be used according to label directions. The dosage or frequency of treatment of these antibiotics cannot be increased without a veterinarian's prescription.

Oxytetracycline and sulfadimethoxine are examples of antibiotics which cannot be used to treat mastitis unless prescribed by a veterinarian in an extra-label fashion. These drugs are included in the MASTiK™ panel solely for the veterinarian's information.

Presentation: 3, 15, or 30 tests per kit.

Compendium Code No.: 11200060

MAXI-B 1000

Durvet **Vitamin B-Complex**

Injection

Active Ingredient(s): Each mL of sterile aqueous solution contains:

Thiamine Hydrochloride (B_1) . . . . . 12.5 mg
Niacinamide . . . . . 12.5 mg
Pyridoxine Hydrochloride (B_6) . . . . . 5.0 mg
d-Panthenol . . . . . 5.0 mg
Riboflavin (B_2) (as Riboflavin 5' phosphate sodium) . . . . . 2.0 mg
Cyanocobalamin (B_{12}) . . . . . 1000 mcg

with benzyl alcohol 1.5% v/v as preservative, ammonium sulfate 0.1%.

Indications: For use as a supplemental source of B complex vitamins in cattle, swine and sheep.

Dosage and Administration: Subcutaneous or intramuscular injection is recommended. May be administered intravenously at the discretion of a veterinarian. The following are suggested dosages, depending on the condition of the animal and the desired response.

Adult Cattle: 1 to 2 mL per 500 pounds of body weight.

Calves, Swine and Sheep: 1 to 2 mL. May be repeated once or twice weekly.

Precaution(s): Store at controlled room temperature between 15° to 30°C (59°-86°F).

Protect from light.

Caution(s): Hypersensitivity reactions to the parenteral administration of products containing thiamine have been reported. Administer with caution and keep treated animals under close observation.

Warning(s): For animal use only. Livestock drug.

Keep out of reach of children.

Presentation: 100 mL and 250 mL vials.

Compendium Code No.: 10841130

MAXIBAN® 72

Elanco **Feed Medication**

Narasin and Nicarbazin-Type A Medicated Article

NADA No.: 138-952

Active Ingredient(s):

Narasin . . . . . 36 g per lb
Nicarbazin . . . . . 36 g per lb
Contains: Verxite (non-nutritive) 1-2%

Indications: For the prevention of coccidiosis in broiler chickens caused by *Eimeria necatrix, E. tenella, E. acervulina, E. brunetti, E. mivati,* and *E. maxima.*

Directions: Important: Must be thoroughly mixed into feeds before use.

Mixing Directions: (Broiler Chickens): Thoroughly mix the following amounts of MAXIBAN® 72 in one ton of complete feed to provide from 27 to 45 g per ton each of narasin and nicarbazin. The dosage should be adjusted to meet the severity of the coccidial challenge, which varies with environmental and management conditions.

It is recommended that a preblend of the MAXIBAN® 72 in 15-20 lbs of feed be made before incorporating into the total amount of the finished feed.

Narasin and Nicarbazin (Grams Per Ton)	MAXIBAN® 72 (Lbs Per Ton of Type C Feed)
54	0.75
72	1.00
90	1.25

Feeding Directions: Feed continuously as the sole ration.

Do not feed undiluted.

Precaution(s): Store in a cool, dry place.

Not to be used after the date printed on top of bag.

When mixing and handling MAXIBAN® 72, use protective clothing, impervious gloves, and a dust mask. Operators should wash thoroughly with soap and water after handling. If accidental eye contact occurs, immediately rinse thoroughly with water.

Caution(s): Nicarbazin medicated broilers may show reduced heat tolerance if exposed to high temperature and high humidity. Provide adequate drinking water and ventilation during these periods. Do not allow adult turkeys, horses, or other equines access to formulations containing narasin. Ingestion of narasin by these species has been fatal. Do not feed to laying hens.

For use in broiler chicken feeds only.

Warning(s): Feeds containing MAXIBAN® must be withdrawn 5 days prior to slaughter.

Presentation: 50 lb (22.68 kg) bags.

Compendium Code No.: 10310041

BG 1510 AMB

MAXI/GUARD® NASAL VAC

Addison **Bacterin**

Bordetella Bronchiseptica Vaccine, Avirulent Live Culture

U.S. Vet. Lic. No.: 355

Contents: This product contains the antigen listed above.

Indications: For use as an aid in the prevention of respiratory disease associated with virulent *Bordetella bronchiseptica* in swine.

Dosage and Administration: Shake well. Administer 1 mL intranasally (½ mL into each nostril) into piglets at one (1) to three (3) days of age.

Precaution(s): Store at not over 45°F or 7°C.

Caution(s): Use the entire contents when first opened. Burn the container and all unused contents.

Warning(s): Do not vaccinate within 21 days before slaughter.

Presentation: 30 mL (30 dose) vial.

Compendium Code No.: 11270000

MAXI/GUARD® ORAL CLEANSING GEL

Addison **Dental Preparation**

Active Ingredient(s): Deionized water, zinc gluconate, ascorbic acid (vitamin C), methylcellulose, taurine, methylparaben, propylparaben, F.D.&C. blue no. 1. May also contain zinc sulfate.

Indications: An oral cleansing gel that cleanses and freshens with or without brushing.

Directions: Remove cap and applicator tip. Pour attached vial contents into gel. Snap applicator tip into place and replace cap. After ascorbic acid has dropped to bottom of gel, shake until dissolved. Holding your pet's head steady with one hand, place the applicator tip inside the corner of the mouth. Gently squeeze a small amount of gel onto the outside of the back upper molar teeth and gums. A natural cleansing action will distribute gel to remote areas. Use daily for best results.

Precaution(s): Storage: The mixed product should be refrigerated or stored in a a cool dark cabinet. Keep out of direct sunlight. A blue or green color denotes freshness.

Caution(s): Keep out of reach of children.

Presentation: 4 fl. oz. (112 mL) bottles.

Compendium Code No.: 11270010

MAXI/GUARD® PINKEYE BACTERIN

Addison **Bacterin**

Moraxella Bovis Bacterin

U.S. Vet. Lic. No.: 355

Composition: This vaccine contains formalin inactivated isolates of *Moraxella bovis.*

Indications: For use in prevention and control of pinkeye (infectious bovine keratoconjunctivitis) in healthy cattle caused by *Moraxella bovis.*

Dosage and Administration: Shake well. Administer a 2 mL dose subcutaneously to cattle 2 months of age or older. Repeat vaccination in 21 days.

Precaution(s): Store at not over 45°F or 7°C. Do not freeze. Shake well before and during use. Use entire contents when first opened.

Antidote(s): In case of anaphylactic reaction; administer epinephrine or atropine.

Warning(s): Do not vaccinate within 21 days before slaughter.

For veterinary use only.

Presentation: 10 doses (20 mL) and 50 doses (100 mL).

Compendium Code No.: 11270020 Cat. No. 0100-1, R298

MAXI/GUARD® Zn7™ DERM

Addison **Topical Wound Dressing**

Antipruritic-Astringent

Ingredient(s): Deionized water, glycerin, carboxymethylcellulose, zinc gluconate, L-lysine, taurine, methylparaben, propylparaben.

Indications: A protective astringent and counterirritant topical to aid in the management of superficial wounds, abrasions or raw skin of dogs or cats. Zn7™ Derm is a natural (patented) neutralized zinc topical that provides relief from itching and drying of raw skin conditions.

Directions for Use: Thoroughly cleanse and dry the skin to be treated. Saturate affected areas by applying directly twice daily. Affected areas may be bandaged or exposed. Please consult your veterinarian.

Caution(s): If no improvement is observed within 7 days of treatment, consult your veterinarian.

Keep out of reach of children.

Presentation: 2 fl oz (60 mL).

Compendium Code No.: 11270030

MAXI/GUARD® Zn7™ DERM SPRAY

Addison **Topical Product**

Antipruritic/Fosters Healing-Skin Care Spray

Ingredient(s): Patented Ingredients: Deionized water, glycerin, zinc gluconate, L-lysine, taurine, carboxymethylcellulose, methylparaben, propylparaben.

Patented neutralized zinc (pH 6.8-7.0).

Indications: A protective counterirritant topical to aid in the management of superficial wounds, abrasions or raw skin of dogs or cats. Zn7™ Derm is a natural (patented) neutralized zinc topical that provides relief from itching and drying of raw skin conditions. Can be used as an adjunct to standard antibiotic or steroid therapy.

Directions: Thoroughly clean and dry affected skin, then spray site. Apply once or twice daily. Affected areas may be bandaged or exposed. Please consult your veterinarian for additional advice or clinical evaluation.

Caution(s): If no improvement is observed within 7 days of treatment, consult your veterinarian.

For veterinary use only.

Warning(s): Keep out of reach of children.

Presentation: 1 fl oz (30 mL) spray.

Compendium Code No.: 11270050

MAXI/GUARD® Zn7™ EQUINE WOUND CARE FORMULA

Addison **Topical Product**

Equine Skin Conditioner-Antipruritic/Astrigent

Ingredient(s): Deionized water, Glycerin, Zinc gluconate, Carboxymethylcellulose, L-lysine, Taurine, Methylparaben, Propylparaben.

Natural Ingredients: Patented Neutralized Zinc (pH 6.8-7.0).

Indications: A protective topical aid in management of superficial wounds, abrasions of skin, or pruritic skin conditions (saddle or bridle sores, burns, dermatoses). Can be used as an adjunct to standard antibiotic or steroid therapy.

Also safe for dogs, cats and small animals.

Directions: Thoroughly clean and dry affected skin, then spray site. Apply once or twice daily. Affected areas may be bandaged or exposed. Please consult your veterinarian for additional advice or clinical evaluations.

Caution(s): If no improvement is observed within 7 days of treatment, consult your veterinarian.

For veterinary use only.

Presentation: 4 fl oz (120 mL) spray.

Compendium Code No.: 11270040

MAXIM-200®

Phoenix Pharmaceutical **Oxytetracycline Injection**

(Oxytetracycline Injection) Antibiotic

ANADA No.: 200-123

Active Ingredient(s): MAXIM-200® (oxytetracycline injection) is a sterile preconstituted solution of the broad spectrum antibiotic oxytetracycline. Each mL contains 200 mg of oxytetracycline base as amphoteric oxytetracycline and, on a w/v basis, 40.0% 2-pyrrolidone, 5.0% povidone, 1.8% magnesium oxide, 0.2% sodium formaldehyde sulfoxylate (as a preservative), monoethanolamine and/or hydrochloric acid as required to adjust pH.

Indications: MAXIM-200® (oxytetracycline injection) is intended for use in the treatment of the following diseases in beef cattle, non-lactating dairy cattle; calves, including preruminating (veal) calves; and swine when due to oxytetracycline-susceptible organisms:

Cattle: In cattle, MAXIM-200® (oxytetracycline injection) is indicated in the treatment of pneumonia and shipping fever complex associated with *Pasteurella* spp. and *Hemophilus* spp; infectious bovine keratoconjunctivitis (pinkeye) caused by *Moraxella bovis;* foot-rot and diphtheria caused by *Fuscobacterium necrophorum;* bacterial enteritis (scours) caused by *Escherichia coli;* wooden tongue caused by *Actinobacillus ligniersii;* leptospirosis caused by *Leptospira pomona;* and wound infections and acute metritis caused by strains of staphylococci and streptococci organisms sensitive to oxytetracycline.

Swine: In swine, MAXIM-200® (oxytetracycline injection) is indicated in the treatment of bacterial enteritis (scours, colibacillosis) caused by *Escherichia coli;* pneumonia caused by *Pasteurella multocida;* and leptospirosis caused by *Leptospira pomona.*

In sows, MAXIM-200® (oxytetracycline injection) is indicated as an aid in the control of infectious enteritis (baby pig scours, colibacillosis) in suckling pigs caused by *Escherichia coli.*

Dosage and Administration: Dosage:

Cattle: MAXIM-200® (oxytetracycline injection) is to be administered by intramuscular, subcutaneous or intravenous injection to beef cattle and non-lactating dairy cattle and calves, including preruminating (veal) calves.

A single dosage of 9 milligrams of MAXIM-200® (oxytetracycline injection) per pound of body weight administered intramuscularly or subcutaneously is recommended in the treatment of the following conditions: 1) bacterial pneumonia caused by *Pasteurella* spp. (shipping fever) in calves and yearlings, where re-treatment is impractical due to husbandry conditions, such as cattle on range, or where their repeated restraint is inadvisable; 2) infectious bovine keratoconjunctivitis (pinkeye) caused by *Moraxella bovis.*

MAXIM-200® (oxytetracycline injection) can also be administered by intravenous, subcutaneous or intramuscular injection at a level of 3 to 5 milligrams of oxytetracycline per pound of body weight per day. In the treatment of severe foot-rot and advanced cases of other indicated diseases, dosage level of 5 milligrams per pound of body weight per day is recommended. Treatment should be continued 24 to 48 hours following remission of disease signs; however, not to exceed a total of four consecutive days. Consult your veterinarian if improvement is not noted within 24 to 48 hours of the beginning of treatment.

Swine: In swine a single dosage of 9 milligrams of MAXIM-200® (oxytetracycline injection) per pound of body weight administered intramuscularly is recommended in the treatment of bacterial pneumonia caused by *Pasteurella multocida* in swine, where re-treatment is impractical due to husbandry conditions or where repeated restraint is inadvisable.

MAXIM-200® (oxytetracycline injection) can also be administered by intramuscular injection at a level of 3 to 5 milligrams of oxytetracycline per pound of body weight per day. Treatment should be continued 24 to 48 hours following remission of the disease signs; however, not to exceed a total of four consecutive days. Consult your veterinarian if improvement is not noted within 24 to 48 hours of the beginning of treatment.

For sows, administer once intramuscularly 3 milligrams of oxytetracycline per pound of body weight approximately 8 hours before farrowing or immediately after completion of farrowing.

For swine weighing 25 lb of body weight and under, MAXIM-200® (oxytetracycline injection) should be administered undiluted for treatment at 9 mg/lb but should be administered diluted for treatment at 3 to 5 mg/lb body weight.

	9 mg/lb Dosage Volume of Undiluted MAXIM-200® (oxytetracycline injection)	3 or 5 mg/lb Dosage Volume of Diluted MAXIM-200® (oxytetracycline injection)		
Body Weight	9 mg/lb	3 mg/lb	Dilution*	5 mg/lb
5 lb	0.2 mL	0.6 mL	1:7	1.0 mL
10 lb	0.5 mL	0.9 mL	1:5	1.5 mL
25 lb	1.1 mL	1.5 mL	1:3	2.5 mL

*To prepare dilutions, add one part MAXIM-200® (oxytetracycline injection) to three, five or seven parts of sterile water, or 5 percent dextrose solution as indicated; the diluted product should be used immediately.

Directions for Use: MAXIM-200® (oxytetracycline injection) is intended for use in the treatment of disease due to oxytetracycline-susceptible organisms in beef cattle, non-lactating dairy cattle, calves, including preruminating (veal) calves and swine. A thoroughly cleaned, sterile needle and syringe should be used for each injection (needles and syringes may be sterilized by boiling in water for 15 minutes). In cold weather, MAXIM-200® (oxytetracycline injection) should be warmed to room temperature before administration to animals. Before withdrawing the solution from the bottle, disinfect the rubber cap on the bottle with suitable disinfectant, such as 70 percent alcohol. The injection site should be similarly cleaned with the disinfectant. Needles of 16 to 18 gauge and 1 to 1½ inches long are adequate for intramuscular injections. Needles 2 to 3 inches are recommended for intravenous use.

Intramuscular Administration: Intramuscular injections should be made by directing the needle of suitable gauge length into the fleshy part of a thick muscle such as in the rump, hip, or thigh regions; avoid blood vessels and major nerves. Before injecting the solution, pull back gently on the plunger. If blood appears in the syringe, a blood vessel has been entered; withdraw the needle and select a different site. No more than 10 mL should be injected intramuscularly at any one site in adult beef cattle and non-lactating dairy cattle, and not more than 5 mL per site in adult swine; rotate injection sites for each succeeding treatment. The volume administered per injection site should be reduced according to age and body size so that 1 to 2 mL per site is injected in small calves.

Subcutaneous Administration: Subcutaneous injections in beef cattle, non-lactating dairy cattle and calves, including preruminating (veal) calves, should be made by directing the needle of suitable gauge and length through the loose folds of the neck skin in front of the shoulder. Care should be taken to ensure that the tip of the needle has penetrated the skin but is not lodged in muscle. Before injecting the solution, pull back gently on the plunger. If blood appears in the syringe, a blood vessel has been entered; withdraw the needle and select a different site. The solution should be injected slowly into the area between the skin and muscles. No more than 10 mL should be injected subcutaneously at any one site in adult beef cattle and non-lactating dairy cattle; rotate injection sites for each succeeding treatment. The volume administered per injection site should be reduced according to age and body size so that 1-2 mL per site is injected in small calves.

Intravenous Administration: MAXIM-200® (oxytetracycline injection) may be administered intravenously to beef cattle and non-lactating dairy cattle. As with all highly concentrated materials, MAXIM-200® (oxytetracycline injection) should be administered slowly by the intravenous route.

Preparation of the Animal for Injection:

1. Approximate location of vein. The jugular vein runs in the jugular groove on each side of the neck from the angle of the jaw to just above the brisket and slightly above and to the side of the windpipe. (See Fig. I)
2. Restraint. A stanchion or chute is ideal for restraining the animal. With a halter, rope, or cattle leader (nose tongs), pull the animal's head around the side of the stanchion, cattle chute, or post in such a manner to form a bow in the neck (See Fig. II), then snub the head securely to prevent movement. By forming the bow in the neck, the outside curvature of the bow tends to expose the jugular vein and make it easily accessible. Caution: Avoid restraining the animal with a tight rope or halter around the throat or upper neck which might impede blood flow. Animals that are down present no problem so far as restraint is concerned.
3. Clip hair in area where injection is to be made (over the vein in the upper third of the neck). Clean and disinfect the skin with alcohol or other suitable antiseptic.

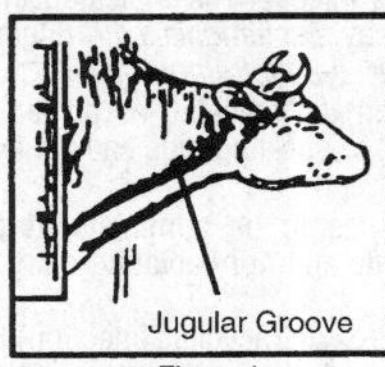

Figure I

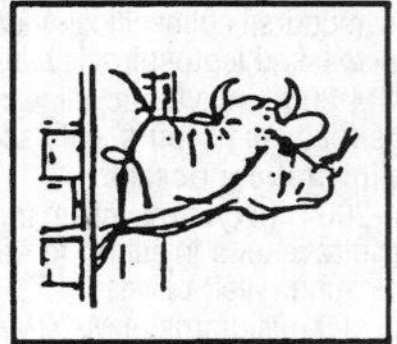
Figure II

Entering the Vein and Making the Injection:

1. Raise the vein. This is accomplished by tying the choke rope tightly around the neck close to the shoulder. The rope should be tied in such a way that it will not come loose and so that it can be untied quickly by pulling the loose end (See Fig. II). In thick-necked animals, a block of wood placed in the jugular groove between the rope and hide will help considerably in applying the desired pressure at the right point. The vein is a soft flexible tube through which blood flows back to the heart. Under ordinary conditions it cannot be seen or felt with the fingers. When the flow of blood is blocked at the base of the neck by the choke rope, the vein becomes enlarged and rigid because of the back pressure. If the choke rope is sufficiently tight, the vein stands out and can be easily seen and felt in thin-necked animals. As a further check in identifying the vein, tap it with the fingers in front of the choke rope. Pulsations that can be seen or felt with the fingers in front of the point being tapped will confirm the fact that the vein is properly distended. It is impossible to put the needle into the vein unless it is distended. Experienced operators are able to raise the vein simply by hand pressure, but the use of a choke rope is more certain.
2. Inserting the needle. This involves three distinct steps. First, insert the needle through the hide. Second, insert the needle into the vein. This may require two or three attempts before the vein is entered. The vein has a tendency to roll away from the point of the needle, especially if the needle is not sharp. The vein can be steadied with the thumb and finger of one hand. With the other hand, the needle point is placed directly over the vein, slanting it so that its direction is along the length of the vein, either toward the head or toward the heart. Properly positioned this way, a quick thrust of the needle will be followed by a spurt of blood through the needle, which indicates that the vein has been entered. Third, once in the vein, the needle should be inserted along the length of the vein all the way to the hub exercising caution to see that the needle does not penetrate the opposite side of the vein. Continuous steady flow of blood through the needle indicates that the needle is still in the vein. If blood does not flow continuously, the needle is out of the vein (or clogged) and another attempt must be made. If difficulty is encountered, it may be advisable to use the vein on the other side of the neck.
3. While the needle is being placed in proper position in the vein, an assistant should get the medication ready so that the injection can be started without delay after the vein has been entered.
4. Making the injection. With the needle in position as indicated by continuous flow of blood, release the choke rope by a quick pull on the free end. This is essential - the medication cannot flow into the vein while it is blocked. Immediately connect the syringe containing MAXIM-200® (oxytetracycline injection) to the needle and slowly depress the plunger. If there is resistance to depression of the plunger, this indicates that the needle has slipped out of the vein (or is clogged) and the procedure will have to be repeated. Watch for any swelling under the skin near the needle which would indicate that the medication is not going into the vein. Should this occur, it is best to try the vein on the opposite side of the neck.
5. Removing the needle. When injection is complete, remove needle with straight pull. Then apply pressure over the area of injection momentarily to control any bleeding through needle puncture, using cotton soaked in alcohol or other suitable antiseptic.

Precaution(s): Storage: MAXIM-200® (oxytetracycline injection) does not require refrigeration; however, it is recommended that it be stored at room temperature, 15°-30°C (59°-86°F). The antibiotic activity of oxytetracycline is not appreciably diminished in the presence of body fluids, serum, or exudates. Keep from freezing.

Caution(s): Rapid intravenous administration may result in animal collapse. Oxytetracycline should be administered slowly over a period of at least 5 minutes.

Exceeding the highest recommended dosage level of drug per pound of body weight per day, administering more than the recommended number of treatments, and/or exceeding 10 mL intramuscularly or subcutaneously per injection site in adult beef cattle and non-lactating dairy cattle, and 5 mL intramuscularly per injection site in adult swine, may result in antibiotic residues beyond the withdrawal period.

Consult with your veterinarian prior to administering this product in order to determine the proper treatment required in the event of an adverse reaction. At the first sight of any adverse reaction, discontinue use of product and seek the advice of your veterinarian. Some of the reactions may be attributed either to anaphylaxis (an allergic reaction) or to cardiovascular collapse of unknown cause.

Shock may be observed following intravenous administration, especially where highly concentrated materials are involved. To minimize this occurrence, it is recommended that MAXIM-200® (oxytetracycline injection) be administered slowly by this route. Shortly after injection, treated animals may have transient hemoglobinuria resulting in darkened urine.

As with all antibiotic preparations, use of the drug may result in overgrowth of nonsusceptible organisms, including fungi. A lack of response by the treated animal, or the development of new signs, may suggest that an overgrowth of nonsusceptible organisms has occurred. If any of these conditions occur, consult your veterinarian.

Since bacteriostatic drugs may interfere with the bactericidal action of penicillin, it is advisable to avoid giving MAXIM-200® (oxytetracycline injection) in conjunction with penicillin.

Restricted Drug (California), use only as directed.

For animal use only.

Warning(s): Discontinue treatment at least 28 days prior to slaughter of cattle and swine. Not for use in lactating dairy animals.

Livestock drug, not for human use. Keep out of reach of children.

Adverse Reactions: Reports of adverse reactions associated with oxytetracycline administration include injection site swelling, restlessness, ataxia, trembling, swelling of eyelids, ears, muzzle, anus and vulva (or scrotum and sheath in males), respiratory abnormalities (labored breathing), frothing at the mouth, collapse and possibly death. Some of these reactions may be attributed either to anaphylaxis (an allergic reaction) or to cardiovascular collapse of unknown cause.

Discussion: Care of Sick Animals: The use of antibiotics in the management of diseases is based on an accurate diagnosis and an adequate course of treatment. When properly used in the treatment of diseases caused by oxytetracycline-susceptible organisms, most animals that have been treated with oxytetracycline injection show a noticeable improvement within 24 to 48 hours. It is recommended that the diagnosis and treatment of animal diseases be carried out by a veterinarian. Since many diseases look alike but require different types of treatment, the use of professional veterinary and laboratory services can reduce treatment time, costs and needless losses. Good housing, sanitation and nutrition are important in the maintenance of healthy animals, and are essential in the treatment of diseased animals.

Presentation: 100 mL (NDC 57319-311-05), 250 mL (NDC 57319-311-06) and 500 mL (NDC 57319-311-07).

Compendium Code No.: 12560562 Rev. 9-01

MAXIMUNE® 4

Biomune **Vaccine**

Bursal Disease-Newcastle Vaccine, Standard and Variants, Killed Virus

U.S. Vet. Lic. No.: 368

Contents: MAXIMUNE® 4 is an inactivated oil emulsion vaccine containing Newcastle disease virus and three infectious bursal disease viruses, the standard type and two variants. All viruses in MAXIMUNE® 4 are noncloned isolates produced in chicken embryos or bursal tissue. The origin of the bursal disease virus fraction is greater than 90% bursal derived.

The vaccine has undergone rigid potency, safety and purity tests and meets Biomune and USDA requirements.

Indications: The vaccine is indicated for use in healthy chickens against Newcastle disease and infectious bursal disease caused by standard and variant viruses. Breeder vaccination provides maternal antibody to progeny of breeder hens for the prevention of early exposure to bursal disease.

Dosage and Administration: A prime with live infectious bursal disease vaccine is recommended at least four (4) weeks in advance of administration of the inactivated vaccine.

Vaccinate chickens with 0.5 mL per bird. The vaccine is to be administered by the subcutaneous route in the back of the neck, midway between the head and the body, in a direction away from the head. Do not inject into muscle or vertebrae.

Refer to the product label for specific use directions and precautions.

Precaution(s): Store the vaccine at 35°-45°F (2°-7°C). Do not freeze.

Warning(s): Do not vaccinate with oil emulsion vaccine within 42 days before slaughter.

Avoid injection of the vaccine into a human. Should accidental injection of a human occur, seek medical attention immediately since a serious localized reaction may result.

Presentation: 1,000 dose (500 mL) bottle.

Compendium Code No.: 11290102

MAXIMUNE® 6

Biomune **Vaccine**

Bursal Disease-Reovirus Vaccine, Standard and Variants, Killed Virus

U.S. Vet. Lic. No.: 368

Contents: MAXIMUNE® 6 is an inactivated oil emulsion vaccine containing three infectious bursal disease viruses, the standard type and two variant strains, and three reoviruses including strain S1133 (a tenosynovitis pathotype), strain 2408 (a malabsorption pathotype) and strain SS412 (a distinct serotype from the S1133 type reoviruses and a causative agent of proventriculitis and malabsorption in broilers).

All viruses in MAXIMUNE® 6 are noncloned isolates produced in chicken embryos or bursal tissue. The origin of the bursal disease virus fraction is greater than 90% bursal derived.

The vaccine has undergone rigid potency, safety and purity tests and meets Biomune and USDA requirements.

Indications: The vaccine is indicated for use in healthy breeder replacement chickens and breeder hens against diseases caused by infectious bursal disease viruses (standard and variant types) and reoviruses (standard and SS412 types). Breeder vaccination provides maternal antibody to the progeny of breeder hens for the prevention of early exposure to bursal disease, tenosynovitis (viral arthritis) and malabsorption syndrome which includes feed passage and proventriculitis.

Dosage and Administration: Optimum results with MAXIMUNE® 6 require that chickens are adequately primed with live infectious bursal disease vaccine and a tenosynovitis vaccine at least four (4) weeks in advance of administration of the inactivated vaccine.

Vaccinate chickens with 0.5 mL per bird. The vaccine is to be administered by the subcutaneous route in the back of the neck, midway between the head and the body, in a direction away from the head. Do not inject into muscle or vertebrae.

Refer to the product label for specific use directions and precautions.

Precaution(s): Store the vaccine at 35°-45°F (2°-7°C). Do not freeze.

Warning(s): Do not vaccinate with an oil emulsion vaccine within 42 days before slaughter.

Avoid injection of the vaccine into a human. Should accidental injection of a human occur, seek medical attention immediately since a serious localized reaction may result.

Presentation: 1,000 dose (500 mL) bottle.

Compendium Code No.: 11290112

MAXIMUNE® 7

Biomune **Vaccine**

Bursal Disease-Newcastle Disease-Reovirus Vaccine, Standard and Variants, Killed Virus

U.S. Vet. Lic. No.: 368

Contents: MAXIMUNE® 7 is an inactivated oil emulsion vaccine containing three infectious bursal disease viruses, the standard type and two variant strains, Newcastle disease virus, and three reoviruses including strain S1133 (a tenosynovitis pathotype), strain 2408 (a malabsorption pathotype) and strain SS412 (a distinct serotype from the S1133 type reoviruses and a causative agent of proventriculitis and malabsorption in broilers).

All of the viruses in MAXIMUNE® 7 are noncloned isolates produced in chicken embryos or bursal tissue. The origin of the bursal disease virus fraction is greater than 90% bursal derived.

The vaccine has undergone rigid potency, safety and purity tests and meets Biomune and USDA requirements.

Indications: The vaccine is indicated for use in healthy breeder replacement chickens and breeder hens against diseases caused by infectious bursal disease viruses (standard and variant types), Newcastle disease virus and reoviruses (standard and SS412 types). Breeder vaccination provides maternal antibody to the progeny of breeder hens for the prevention of early exposure to bursal disease, tenosynovitis (viral arthritis) and malabsorption syndrome which includes feed passage and proventriculitis.

Dosage and Administration: Optimum results with MAXIMUNE® 7 require that chickens are adequately primed with live infectious bursal disease vaccine and tenosynovitis vaccine at least four (4) weeks in advance of administration of the inactivated vaccine.

Vaccinate chickens with 0.5 mL per bird. The vaccine is to be administered by the subcutaneous route in the back of the neck, midway between the head and the body, in a direction away from the head. Do not inject into muscle or vertebrae.

Refer to the product label for specific use directions and precautions.

Precaution(s): Store the vaccine at 35°-45°F (2°-7°C). Do not freeze.

Warning(s): Do not vaccinate with oil emulsion vaccine within 42 days before slaughter.

Avoid injection of the vaccine into a human. Should accidental injection of a human occur, seek medical attention immediately since a serious localized reaction may result.

Presentation: 1,000 dose (500 mL) bottle.

Compendium Code No.: 11290122

MAXIMUNE® 8

Biomune **Vaccine**

Bursal Disease-Newcastle Disease-Bronchitis-Reovirus Vaccine, Standard and Variants, Mass. Type, Killed Virus

U.S. Vet. Lic. No.: 368

Contents: MAXIMUNE® 8 is an inactivated oil emulsion vaccine containing three infectious bursal disease viruses (the standard type and two variant strains) and three reoviruses including strain S1133 (a tenosynovitis pathotype), strain 2408 (a malabsorption pathotype) and strain SS412 (a distinct serotype from the S1133 type reoviruses and a causative agent of proventriculitis and malabsorption in broilers). MAXIMUNE® 8 also contains Newcastle disease virus and infectious bronchitis virus of the Mass. serotype.

All viruses in MAXIMUNE® 8 are noncloned isolates produced in chicken embryos or bursal tissue. The origin of the bursal disease virus fraction is greater than 90% bursal derived.

The vaccine has undergone rigid potency, safety and purity tests and meets Biomune and USDA requirements.

Indications: The vaccine is indicated for use in healthy breeder replacement chickens and breeder hens against diseases caused by infectious bursal disease viruses (standard and variant types), Newcastle disease virus, infectious bronchitis virus (Mass. type) and reoviruses (standard and SS412 types). Breeder vaccination provides maternal antibody to progeny of breeder hens for the prevention of early exposure to bursal disease, tenosynovitis (viral arthritis) and malabsorption syndrome which includes feed passage and proventriculitis.

Dosage and Administration: Optimum results with MAXIMUNE® 8 require that chickens are adequately primed with live infectious bursal disease vaccine, tenosynovitis vaccine and bronchitis vaccine of the Mass. type at least four (4) weeks in advance of administration of the inactivated vaccine.

Vaccinate chickens with 0.5 mL per bird. The vaccine is to be administered by the subcutaneous route in the back of the neck, midway between the head and the body, in a direction away from the head. Do not inject into muscle or vertebrae.

Refer to the product label for specific use directions and precautions.

Precaution(s): Store the vaccine at 35°-45°F (2°-7°C). Do not freeze.

Warning(s): Do not vaccinate with oil emulsion vaccine within 42 days before slaughter.

Avoid injection of the vaccine into a human. Should accidental injection of a human occur, seek medical attention immediately since a serious localized reaction may result.

Presentation: 1,000 dose (500 mL) bottle.

Compendium Code No.: 11290132

MAXIMUNE® IBD

Biomune **Vaccine**

Bursal Disease Vaccine, Standard and Variants, Killed Virus

U.S. Vet. Lic. No.: 368

Contents: MAXIMUNE® IBD is an inactivated oil emulsion vaccine containing three infectious bursal disease viruses, the standard type and two variants. The viruses in MAXIMUNE® IBD are noncloned isolates produced in chicken embryos or bursal tissue. The origin of the bursal disease virus fraction is greater than 90% bursal derived.

Indications: The vaccine is intended for use in healthy replacement chickens and breeder hens against disease caused by infectious bursal disease virus of the standard and variant types. Breeder vaccination provides maternal antibody to the progeny of breeder hens for the prevention of early exposure to bursal disease.

Dosage and Administration: A prime with live infectious bursal disease vaccine is recommended at least four (4) weeks in advance of administration of the inactivated vaccine.

Vaccinate chickens with 0.5 mL per bird. The vaccine is to be administered by the subcutaneous route in the back of the neck, midway between the head and the body, in a direction away from the head. Do not inject into muscle or vertebrae.

Refer to the product label for specific use directions and precautions.

Precaution(s): Store the vaccine at 35°-45°F (2°-7°C). Do not freeze.

Warning(s): Do not vaccinate with oil emulsion vaccine within 42 days before slaughter.

Avoid injection of the vaccine into a human. Should accidental injection of a human occur, seek medical attention immediately since a serious localized reaction may result.

Presentation: 1,000 dose (500 mL) bottle.

Compendium Code No.: 11290142

MAXI-SORB BOLUS

Durvet **Adsorbent**

NDC No.: 30798-016-69

Active Ingredient(s): Each bolus contains activated attapulgite, carob flour, pectin and magnesium trisilicate, in a palatable base.

Indications: For use as an aid in the relief of non-infectious diarrhea in horses and cattle.

Dosage and Administration: Administer orally.

Give two (2) boluses to adult cattle and horses.

Give one (1) bolus to calves and foals.

Repeat the treatment at four (4) to six (6) hour intervals, as needed.

Discontinue use of the product after three (3) days.

Precaution(s): Store at a controlled room temperature between 59°-86°F (15°C and 30°C).

Caution(s): If symptoms persist after using the preparation for three days, consult a veterinarian.

Keep out of the reach of children.

For animal use only.

Presentation: 50 boluses.

Compendium Code No.: 10841140

MAXI SORB CALF BOLUS

Durvet **Antidiarrheal-Adsorbent**

Antidiarrheal-Demulcent

Active Ingredient(s): Each bolus contains: Activated attapulgite, carob flour, pectin, and magnesium trisilicate, in a suitable base.

Indications: For use as an aid in relief of simple non-infectious diarrhea in colts and calves.

Dosage and Administration: Administer orally. Give two (2) boluses to calves and foals.

Repeat treatment at 4 to 6 hour intervals as needed. Discontinue use of product after 3 days. If symptoms persist after using this preparation for 3 days, consult a veterinarian.

Precaution(s): Store at controlled room temperature between 15° and 30°C (59°-86°F).

Warning(s): For animal use only.

Keep out of reach of children.

Presentation: 50 boluses.

Compendium Code No.: 10841120

MAXIVAC® EXCELL™

SyntroVet **Vaccine**

Swine Influenza Vaccine, H1N1 and H3N2, Killed Virus

U.S. Vet. Lic. No.: 165A

Contents: MAXIVAC® EXCELL™ Swine influenza vaccine is an inactivated vaccine containing swine influenza virus type A, subtypes H1N1 and H3N2, in a proprietary dual-acting adjuvant (Emunade®).

Preservatives: Gentamicin and thimerosal.

Indications: The product is indicated for use in healthy pigs 4 weeks of age or older as an aid in the prevention of disease associated with swine influenza virus subtypes H1N1 and H3N2. The vaccine has been demonstrated to reduce clinical signs, pneumonia and virus shedding following challenge.

Dosage and Administration: Shake well. Using aseptic technique, inject 2 mL intramuscularly (IM) into healthy pigs at 4 weeks of age or older. Revaccinate with 2 mL 2-3 weeks after initial vaccination. Pigs nursing non-immune dams can be safely and effectively vaccinated at weaning. Pigs from immune dams should be vaccinated when maternal antibody levels will allow active immunization. Duration of immunity to H3N2 has been demonstrated by challenge to be at least two months following vaccination. Challenge studies to confirm longer duration of immunity are in progress.

Precaution(s): Store at 2°-7°C (35°-45°F). Do not freeze. Use entire contents when first opened.

Caution(s): If allergic response occurs, administer epinephrine.

For veterinary use only.

Warning(s): Do not vaccinate within 21 days of slaughter.

Extreme caution should be used when injecting an oil emulsion vaccine to avoid injecting your own finger or hand. Accidental injection can cause serious local reaction. Contact a physician immediately if accidental injection occurs.

Presentation: 50 dose (100 mL), 125 dose (250 mL) and 250 dose (500 mL) (NDC-0061-5263-03) vials.

Compendium Code No.: 11170050 P19018-10

MAXIVAC®-FLU

SyntroVet **Vaccine**

Swine Influenza Vaccine, Killed Virus

U.S. Vet. Lic. No.: 165A

Contents: The vaccine contains a type A subtype H1N1 field isolate and is adjuvanted to enhance immunity. Field and laboratory data indicate that the vaccine is safe and effective in weaning age pigs, is safe for use in pregnant females at any stage of gestation, and provides immunity for at least three months following vaccination. Contains gentamicin and thimerosal as preservatives.

Indications: For the vaccination of healthy swine against swine influenza due to Type A H1N1 subtype.

Dosage and Administration: For use in swine only. Shake well and administer 2 mL intramuscularly. Pigs nursing non-immune dams can be safely and effectively vaccinated at weaning. Pigs from immune dams should be vaccinated when maternal antibody levels will allow active immunization. For primary vaccination, administer a second dose in 3 to 4 weeks.

Precaution(s): Store at 35°-45°F (2°-7°C). Use entire contents when first opened.

Caution(s): Anaphylactoid reactions may occur.

Antidote(s): Epinephrine.

Warning(s): Do not vaccinate within 21 days of slaughter.

Presentation: 10 dose (20 mL), 50 dose (100 mL) (NDC-0061-5145-02) and 100 dose (200 mL) (NDC-0061-5145-03) vials.

Compendium Code No.: 11170002 P19003-10 / P19005-10

M

MAXIVAC®-M+

SyntroVet **Bacterin-Vaccine**

Swine Influenza Vaccine, Killed Virus, Mycoplasma Hyopneumoniae Bacterin

U.S. Vet. Lic. No.: 165A

Contents: MAXIVAC®-M+ inactivated vaccine contains a swine influenza type A virus, subtype H1 N1 Field Isolate, in combination with *Mycoplasma hyopneumoniae* in a proprietary dual acting adjuvant (Emunade®).

Preservatives: Ampicillin, Gentamicin, and Thimerosal.

Indications: For use is healthy pigs 3-4 weeks of age or older as an aid in the prevention of pneumonia caused by swine influenza virus, type A, subtype H1N1, and *Mycoplasma hyopneumoniae,* and as an aid in the reduction of clinical signs and virus shedding caused by swine influenza virus, type A, subtype H1N1.

Dosage and Administration: Shake well. Using aseptic technique, inject 2 mL intramuscularly (IM) to healthy pigs at 3-4 weeks of age or older. Revaccinate with 2 mL 2-3 weeks after initial vaccination. Pigs nursing nonimmune dams can be safely and effectively vaccinated at weaning. Pigs from immune dams should be vaccinated when maternal antibody levels will allow active immunization. Revaccinate with a single 2 mL dose annually.

Precaution(s): Store at 2°-7°C (35°-45°F). Do not freeze. Use entire contents when first opened.

Caution(s): Transient local reaction may occur at the injection site. If allergic response occurs, administer epinephrine.

Warning(s): Do not vaccinate within 60 days of slaughter. For veterinary use only.

Extreme caution should be used when injecting an oil emulsion vaccine to avoid injecting your own finger or hand. Accidental injection can cause serious local reaction. Contact a physician immediately if accidental injection occurs.

Presentation: 50 dose (100 mL) and 100 dose (200 mL) vials.

Compendium Code No.: 11170010 P17919-10

MAXUM® CRUMBLES

Horse Health **Equine Dietary Supplement**

Guaranteed Analysis: per pound:

Crude Protein, min.	13%
Lysine, min.	0.7275%
Methionine, min.	0.1929%
Crude Fat, min.	2.0%
Crude Fiber, max.	11%
Calcium, min.	3.0000%
Calcium, max.	4.0000%
Phosphorous, min.	2.7500%
Salt, min.	0.8000%
Salt, max.	1.3000%
Potassium, min.	1.3000%
Magnesium, min.	0.4000%
Iron, min.	1.0580%
Copper, min.	1,060 mg
Cobalt, min.	35 mg
Zinc, min.	4,400 mg
Manganese, min.	2,820 mg
Iodine, min.	35 mg
Selenium, min.	35 mg
Vitamin A, min.	256,000 I.U.
Vitamin D_3, min.	25,600 I.U.
Vitamin E, min.	1,200 I.U.
Vitamin B_{12}.	0.64 mg
Riboflavin, min.	448 mg
d-Pantothenic Acid, min.	200 mg
Thiamine, min.	226 mg
Niacinamide, min.	1,000 mg
Vitamin B_6	160 mg
Folic Acid, min.	24 mg
Choline, min.	2,000 mg
Biotin, min.	0.25 mg

Ingredients: Wheat Middlings, Dehydrated Alfalfa Meal, Monocalcium Phosphate, Ferrous Sulfate, Soybean Meal, Ground Corn, Lignin Sulfonate, Salt, Choline Chloride, Potassium Chloride, Magnesium Oxide, L-Lysine, Sodium Selenite, Yucca Schidegera Extract (a natural flavoring agent), *Lactobacillus acidophilus* Fermentation Product Dehydrated, Dried Seaweed Meal, Calcium Carbonate, Vitamin A Supplement, Vitamin D_3 Supplement, Vitamin E Supplement, Vitamin B_{12} Supplement, Riboflavin, Niacinamide, d-Calcium Pantothenate, Menadione Sodium Bisulfite Complex, Folic Acid, Pyridoxine Hydrochloride, Thiamine mononitrate, Biotin, Manganous Oxide, Zinc Oxide, Copper Oxide, Ethylenediamine Dihydriodide, Cobalt Carbonate, and Propionic and Acetic Acid (as preservatives).

Indications: MAXUM® is a concentrated supplement for horses, formulated to provide supplemental vitamins, minerals and amino acids that may be lacking or in insufficient quantities in the horse's regular feed ration.

Directions: Feeding Directions: MAXUM® can be mixed into a complete feed at the rate of 12½ lbs. per ton.

Individual Supplementation: Feed 1 to 2 ounces of MAXUM® daily.

Precaution(s): Close container after each use. Store in cool, dry place. Store in area inaccessible to children and animals.

Caution(s): Follow label directions. The addition to feed of higher levels of this premix containing selenium is not permitted. Excessive amounts of selenium may be toxic.

For animal use only.

Warning(s): Keep out of reach of children.

Presentation: 2.5 lb, 15 lb (6.8 kg) and 25 lb.

Compendium Code No.: 15000031

McKILLIP'S DUSTING POWDER

Butler **Hemostatic**

Active Ingredient(s):

Sodium alum	10.0% w/w
Chloroxylenol	1.0% w/w

In a free-flowing absorbent base. Not sterilized.

Indications: For use as an antiseptic and astringent dressing powder for superficial wounds, cuts and abrasions on horses.

Dosage and Administration: Dust the powder freely onto wounds, cuts, or abrasions. Repeat as necessary to keep the wounds dry. May be applied under a gauze bandage if desired.

Precaution(s): Store at a controlled room temperature between 15° and 30°C (59°-86°F).

Keep the container tightly closed when not in use.

Caution(s): In case of deep or puncture wounds or serious burns consult a veterinarian. If redness, irritation, or swelling persists or increases, discontinue use and consult a veterinarian. Avoid contact with the eyes and mucous membranes. Do not apply to large areas of broken skin.

Not for human use. Keep out of the reach of children.

Presentation: 5 oz. (142 g) containers.

Compendium Code No.: 10821140

McKILLIP'S DUSTING POWDER

First Priority **Hemostatic**

Topical Antiseptic-Astringent

Active Ingredient(s):

Ammonium Alum	10.0%
Chloroxylenol	1.0%

In a free-flowing starch base. Not sterilized.

Indications: For use as an antiseptic and astringent dressing powder for superficial wounds, cuts and abrasions on horses.

Directions for Use: Dust powder freely onto wounds, cuts, or abrasions. Repeat as necessary to keep wounds dry. May be applied under a gauze bandage if desired.

Precaution(s): Storage: Store at controlled room temperature between 15°-30°C (59°-86°F). Keep container tightly closed when not in use.

Caution(s): In case of deep or puncture wounds or serious burns, consult veterinarian. If redness, irritation, or swelling persists or increases, discontinue use and consult veterinarian. Avoid contact with the eyes and mucous membranes. Do not apply to large areas of broken skin.

For animal use only. For external use only. For veterinary use only.

Warning(s): Keep out of reach of children.

Presentation: 5 oz (142 g) (NDC# 58829-180-05).

Compendium Code No.: 11390512 Rev. 06-01

MD-VAC® CAF FROZEN

Fort Dodge **Vaccine**

Marek's Disease Vaccine, Serotype 3, Live Virus

U.S. Vet. Lic. No.: 112

Contents: This product contains the antigen listed above.

Contains gentamicin as a preservative.

Indications: This product is recommended for the subcutaneous vaccination of healthy one-day-old chicks or the *in ovo* vaccination of 18 to 19 day old embryonated chicken eggs, to aid in the prevention of the signs and lesions of Marek's disease. Use only the Fort Dodge Animal Health sterile diluent included.

Dosage and Administration: Read in full, follow directions carefully.

Directions for Subcutaneous Administration:

1. Vaccinate healthy one-day-old chicks only.
2. Avoid early exposure of chicks to Marek's disease, to allow for development of protection.
3. The exact amount of diluent is provided for each shipment of vaccine. Use Fort Dodge Animal Health diluent only. Store diluent at not over 80°F (27°C).
4. Wear protective clothing when withdrawing vaccine from liquid-nitrogen refrigerator; protect hands with gloves, wear long sleeves, and use a face mask or goggles.
5. Before opening liquid-nitrogen refrigerator, prepare a clean, wide-mouthed container with a capacity of 1 to 5 gallons (3.8-19 liters). Half-fill this container with water 80°F (27°C).
6. When withdrawing a cane of vials from the liquid-nitrogen refrigerator, expose only the vial to be used immediately. When removing a vial from the cane, hold palm of gloved hand away from face and body. Dilute only 1 vial at a time. Immediately replace cane with remaining vials into the canister in the liquid-nitrogen refrigerator.
7. Place the vial into prepared container half-filled with water 80°F (27°C). The frozen material thaws rapidly. When thawed, towel-dry vial.
8. The vials are pre-scored below the gold band. Before snapping off the top portion, wrap vial with a cloth, holding the top part away from face and body.
9. For subcutaneous route of vaccination, use 400 mLs of diluent per 2,000 doses of vaccine. For example: 2,000 doses of vaccine-400 mLs diluent; 6,000 doses of vaccine-1,200 mLs of diluent.
10. Using a sterile mixing syringe with a 1½-inch (3.8 cm) 18-gauge needle, draw up a small amount of diluent. Then draw the contents from the vaccine vial into the syringe and swirl gently. Insert needle into diluent bottle and slowly expel contents of syringe. Mix well by gently swirling the bottle. Withdraw a small amount of the reconstituted vaccine and use to rinse each vial injecting the rinses back into reconstituted vaccine. The vaccine is ready for use.
11. While vaccinating, maintain the diluted vaccine (in the diluent bottle) at 70° to 80°F (21° to 27°C). If the temperature cannot be held as low as 80°F (27°C), place the diluent bottle containing the diluted vaccine in an ice bath.
12. For vaccination, an automatic syringe with 22- to 20-gauge needles, ⅜- to ½-inch (0.95 to 1.27 cm) long, is recommended. Make certain that all equipment is sterilized and change needles frequently.
13. Inject each chick subcutaneously with 0.2 mL of the vaccine.
14. After diluting, use the vaccine within 2 hours. Do not save any vaccine that has been diluted. Burn vaccine containers and all unused contents.

Directions for use with Embrex Inovoject® Egg Injection System:

1. Vaccinate using the *in ovo* route of vaccination in 18 to 19 day old healthy embryonated chicken eggs only.
2. The exact amount of diluent is provided for each shipment of vaccine. Use Fort Dodge Animal Health diluent only. Store diluent at not over 80°F (27°C).
3. Sanitize the Inovoject® Egg Injection System in accordance with the procedures described in the Inovoject® operator's manual.
4. Wear protective clothing when withdrawing vaccine from liquid-nitrogen refrigerator; protect hands with gloves, wear long sleeves, and use a face mask or goggles.
5. Before opening liquid-nitrogen refrigerator, prepare a clean, wide-mouthed container with a capacity of 1 to 5 gallons (3.8-19 liters). Half-fill this container with water at 80°F (27°C).
6. When withdrawing a cane of vials from the liquid-nitrogen refrigerator, expose only the vials to be used immediately. When removing a vial from the cane, hold palm of gloved hand away from face and body. Dilute only 4 vials at a time. Immediately replace the cane with remaining vials into the canister in the liquid-nitrogen refrigerator.

7. Place the vials into a prepared container half-filled with water 80°F (27°C). The frozen material thaws rapidly. When thawed, towel-dry vial.
8. The vials are pre-scored below the gold band. Before snapping off the top portion, wrap the vial with a cloth, holding the top part away from face and body.
9. For *in ovo* route of vaccination, use 100 mLs diluent per 2,000 doses of vaccine.
10. Using 4 sterile mixing syringes with a 1½-inch (3.8 cm) 18-gauge needle, draw up a small amount of diluent into each syringe. Then draw the contents from one vaccine vial into the syringe and swirl gently. Repeat this step with the other 3 syringes. Insert needle into diluent container and slowly expel contents of syringe. Repeat this step with the other 3 syringes. Mix well by gently swirling the container. Withdraw a small amount of the reconstituted vaccine and use to rinse each vial injecting the rinses back into reconstituted vaccine. The vaccine is ready for use.
11. While vaccinating, maintain the diluted vaccine (in the diluent container at 70° to 80°F (21° to 27°C). If the temperature cannot be held as low as 80°F (27°C), place the diluent container containing the diluted vaccine in an ice bath.
12. Carefully read and follow the Inovoject® operator's manual before initiating vaccination. Failure to follow instructions for Inovoject® operation may result in personal injury and/or embryonic morbidity and mortality.
13. The Inovoject® Egg Injection machine is equipped with an automatic injection system which utilizes a 20-gauge needle and deposits the vaccine about 1-inch deep into the egg.
14. Inject each egg *in ovo* with 0.05 mL of the vaccine solution.
15. After diluting, use the vaccine solution within 2 hours. Do not save any vaccine that has been diluted. Burn all unused material.

Records: Keep a record of vaccine serial number and expiration date; date of receipt and date of vaccination; where vaccination takes place; and any reactions observed.

Precaution(s): Store in liquid nitrogen. Dilute before using. Use entire contents of vial when first opened. Burn vaccine container and all unused contents.

This product is nonreturnable.

Caution(s): This product should be stored, transported, and administered in accordance with the instructions and directions.

The use of this vaccine is subject to state laws, wherever applicable.

Combining this product with other biological products is not recommended.

Warning(s): Do not vaccinate within 21 days before slaughter.

Take all precautionary measures, including the use of gloves and face shield or goggles, to avoid potential hazards of handling liquid nitrogen and the possibility of explosion of glass vials as they are taken from the liquid-nitrogen refrigerator or canister or holding cane, or as they are placed in the thawing container. When removing the vial from the cane, hold palm of the gloved hand away from face and body.

Only vaccines, diluents etc., that have been approved by Embrex and are labeled appropriately for *in ovo* use can be used in the Inovoject® Egg Injection System.

Before using this vaccine, be certain to read directions.

For veterinary use only.

Disclaimer: Having cautioned the user concerning the handling of liquid nitrogen and the possibility of explosion of glass ampules as they are removed from the nitrogen or holding cane, or when placed in the thawing container, and having no control over the safety measures taken other than cautioning against possible dangers, Fort Dodge Animal Health shall not be responsible for personal injury and/or property damage resulting from said handling and/or the possibility of explosion.

Presentation: 5 x 2,000 doses.

Inovoject is a registered trademark of Embrex, Inc.

U.S. Patent No. 3,642,574 (MD-Vac)

Compendium Code No.: 10031060 15994A

MD-VAC® CFL

Fort Dodge **Vaccine**

Marek's Disease Vaccine, Serotype 3, Live Virus

U.S. Vet. Lic. No.: 112

Contents: This product contain the antigens listed above.

Contains gentamicin as a preservative.

Indications: MD-VAC® CFL with and without ACM™ 1 (acemannan) is recommended for the vaccination of healthy one-day-old chicks only, to aid in the prevention of the signs and lesions of Marek's disease. Use only the Fort Dodge Animal Health, Inc., sterile diluent included.

Directions: Read in full, follow directions carefully.

No. 2874: Directions for MD-VAC® CFL:

1. Vaccinate healthy one day old chicks only.
2. Avoid early exposure of chicks to Marek's virus challenge.
3. Use Fort Dodge Animal Health, Inc. diluent only. The exact amount of diluent is provided for each shipment of vaccine. Store diluent at not over 80°F (27°C).
4. 1,000 Doses: Rehydrate only 1 vial (1,000 doses) with 200 mL of Fort Dodge Animal Health diluent.
   2,000 Doses: Rehydrate only 1 vial (2,000 doses) with 400 mL of Fort Dodge Animal Health diluent.
5. Remove the central tab of the aluminum seal of the vaccine vial, leaving the outer ring intact. Sanitize the rubber stopper with alcohol. Also, sanitize with alcohol the rubber stopper of the bottle of diluent.
6. Using a sterile syringe and needle, withdraw 3 mL (3 cc) diluent. Then, insert needle through stopper of vaccine vial and discharge syringe contents.
7. Remove syringe and needle. Mix gently until vaccine is dissolved. Pull back on syringe plunger to admit 2 or 3 mL of air. This is very important.
8. Reinsert needle into vaccine vial. Barely penetrate the stopper. Expel the air into the vial (to break vacuum).
9. With syringe and needle still in place, invert the vial and pull back plunger so that all the contents (the rehydrated vaccine) are drawn from vial into syringe.
10. Now, insert the needle into diluent and expel syringe contents into the diluent. Gently swirl until the mixture is uniform. The vaccine is ready for use.
11. During vaccination, maintain the rehydrated vaccine (in the diluent bottle) at 70° to 80°F (21° to 27°C). If the temperature cannot be held as low as 80°F (27°C), place the diluent bottle containing the rehydrated vaccine in an ice bath.
12. For vaccination, an automatic syringe with 22- to 20-gauge needles, ⅜-inch to ½-inch in length, is recommended. Make certain that all equipment is sterilized and change needles frequently.
13. Inject each chick subcutaneously with 0.2 mL (two-tenths of a milliliter) of the vaccine.
14. Use all the vaccine from 1 vial within 1 hour after rehydrating. Do not save any vaccine that has been rehydrated. Burn vaccine containers and all unused contents.

No. 06860: Directions for MD-VAC® CFL and ACM™ 1:

1. Vaccinate healthy one day old chicks only.
2. Avoid early exposure of chicks to Marek's virus challenge.
3. Use Fort Dodge Animal Health, Inc. diluent only. The exact amount of diluent and ACM™ 1 is provided for each shipment of vaccine. Store diluent at not over 80°F (27°C).
4. Using a sterile mixing syringe with a 1½ inch (3.8 cm) 16-gauge needle, reconstitute 1,000 doses ACM™ 1 using 15 mL of the diluent provided. Gently mix. Wait 5 minutes for the product to become well suspended. Add the contents of a 1,000 dose bottle to 200 mL diluent or contents of a 2,000 dose bottle to 400 mL diluent. Withdraw 15 mL of diluent containing ACM™ 1 and use to rinse each bottle. Inject the rinses back into the diluent. After ACM™ 1 is added to the diluent, wait at least 30 minutes before adding the vaccine. The diluent should be used within 8 hours after adding ACM™ 1 and within 1 hour after adding the Marek's vaccine (see #14).
5. Remove the central tab of the aluminum seal of the vaccine vial, leaving the outer ring intact. Sanitize the rubber stopper with alcohol. Also, sanitize with alcohol the rubber stopper of the bottle of diluent.
6. Using a sterile syringe and needle, withdraw 3 mL (3 cc) diluent containing ACM™ 1. Then, insert needle through the stopper of vaccine vial and discharge syringe contents.
7. Remove syringe and needle. Mix gently until vaccine is dissolved. Pull back on syringe plunger to admit 2 or 3 mL of air. This is very important.
8. Reinsert needle into vaccine vial. Barely penetrate the stopper. Expel the air into the vial (to break vacuum).
9. With syringe and needle still in place, invert the vial and pull back plunger so that all the contents (the rehydrated vaccine) are drawn from vial into syringe.
10. Now, insert the needle into diluent containing ACM™ 1 and expel syringe contents into the diluent. Gently swirl until the mixture is uniform. The vaccine is ready for use.
11. During vaccination, maintain the rehydrated vaccine (in the diluent bottle) at 70° to 80°F (21° to 27°C). If the temperature cannot be held as low as 80°F (27°C), place the diluent bottle containing the rehydrated vaccine in an ice bath.
12. For vaccination, an automatic syringe with 22- to 20-gauge needles, ⅜-inch to ½-inch in length, is recommended. Make certain that all equipment is sterilized and change needles frequently.
13. Inject each chick subcutaneously with 0.2 mL (two-tenths of a milliliter) of the vaccine.
14. Use all the vaccine from 1 vial within 1 hour after rehydrating. Do not save any vaccine that has been rehydrated. Burn vaccine containers and all unused contents.

Records: Keep a record of vaccine serial number and expiration date; date of receipt and date of vaccination; where vaccination took place; and any reactions observed.

Precaution(s): Store at not over 45°F (7°C).

Use entire contents of vial when first opened.

Dispose of all materials in a proper manner.

Burn vaccine containers and all unused contents.

This vaccine is nonreturnable.

Caution(s): This product should be stored, transported, and administered in accordance with the directions.

The use of this vaccine is subject to state laws, wherever applicable.

Warning(s): Do not vaccinate within 21 days before slaughter.

Give subcutaneously only.

For veterinary use only.

Presentation: 10 x 1,000 doses
10 x 2,000 doses

Compendium Code No.: 10031070 10800C

MECADOX® 10

Phibro **Feed Medication**

Carbadox-Type A Medicated Article

NADA No.: 041-061

Active Ingredient(s):

Carbadox. . . . . 2.2% (10 g/lb)

Indications: Control of swine dysentery (vibrionic dysentery, bloody scours or hemorrhagic dysentery); control of bacterial swine enteritis (salmonellosis or necrotic enteritis caused by *Salmonella choleraesuis);* increased rate of weight gain and improved feed efficiency in swine.

Directions: Mixing and Use Directions:

Complete Swine Feed:

Indications for Use	Amount of Drug	lb of MECADOX® 10/ton of Complete Feed
Increased rate of weight gain and improved feed efficiency.	0.0011-0.00275% (10-25 g/ton)	1.0-2.5 lb
Control of swine dysentery (vibrionic dysentery, bloody scours or hemorrhagic dysentery); control of bacterial swine enteritis (salmonellosis or necrotic enteritis caused by *Salmonella choleraesuis);* increased rate of weight gain and improved feed efficiency.	0.0055% (50 g/ton)	5.0 lb

Protein Supplement:

Amount of Supplement per Ton of Complete Feed (lb)	lb of MECADOX® 10 per Ton of Protein Supplement		
	Desired Level of MECADOX® in Complete Feed		
	0.0055% (50 g/ton)	0.00275% (25 g/ton)	0.0011% (10 g/ton)
1000	10	5	2
667	15	7	3
500	20	10	4
250	40	20	8
100	100	50	20
75	133	67	27
50	200	100	40
40	250	125	50
20	500	250	100

Precaution(s): Store in a dry, cool place.

Caution(s): For use in the manufacture of complete swine feeds and/or swine protein supplement feeds only.

Not for use in pregnant swine or swine intended for breeding purposes. Do not mix in feeds containing bentonite.

Warning(s): Do not feed to swine within 42 days of slaughter.

Certain components of animal feeds, including medicated premixes, possess properties that may be a potential health hazard or a source of personal discomfort to certain individuals who are exposed to them. Human exposure should, therefore, be minimized by observing the general industry standards for occupational health and safety.

Precautions such as the following should be considered: dust masks or respirators and protective clothing should be worn; dust-arresting equipment and adequate ventilation should be utilized; personal hygiene should be observed; wash before eating or leaving a work site; be alert for signs of allergic reactions—seek prompt medical treatment if such reactions are suspected.

Presentation: 40 lb (18.2 kg) bags.

MECADOX is a registered trademark of Phibro Animal Health, for carbadox.

U.S. Patent Nos. 3,371,080 and 3,433,871

Compendium Code No.: 36930061

MEDALONE CREAM ℞

Med-Pharmex **Topical Corticosteroid**

Triamcinolone Acetonide Cream USP

ANADA No.: 200-275

Active Ingredient(s): Description: Triamcinolone Acetonide Cream USP provides 1 mg triamcinolone acetonide per gram (0.1%) in a vanishing cream base containing propylene glycol, cetostearyl alcohol (and) ceteareth-20, white petrolatum, sorbitol solution, glyceryl monostearate, polyethylene glycol monostearate, simethicone, sorbic acid and purified water.

Indications: Triamcinolone Acetonide Cream USP is indicated for topical treatment of allergic dermatitis and summer eczema in dogs.

Pharmacology: Actions: Triamcinolone Acetonide Cream USP is a corticosteroid that provides prompt relief of itching, burning, inflamed skin lesions by virtue of its anti-inflammatory, antipruritic and anti-allergic effects.

Dosage and Administration: Apply Triamcinolone Acetonide Cream USP by rubbing into the affected areas two to four times daily for 4 to 10 days.

Contraindication(s): Triamcinolone Acetonide Cream USP should not be used ophthalmically.

Precaution(s): Store at room temperature; avoid freezing. Do not store above 30°C (86°F).

Caution(s): Federal law restricts this drug to use by or on the order of a licensed veterinarian.

If local infection exists, suitable concomitant antimicrobial therapy should be administered. If favorable response does not occur promptly, application of Triamcinolone Acetonide Cream USP should be discontinued until the infection is adequately controlled by appropriate measures. Avoid ingestion. Oral or parenteral use of corticosteroids, depending on dose, duration and specific steroid, may result in inhibition of endogenous steroid production following drug withdrawal.

Warning(s): Triamcinolone Acetonide Cream USP is indicated for use on dogs only. Do not use Triamcinolone Acetonide Cream USP on animals which are raised for food production.

Absorption of triamcinolone acetonide through topical application on the skin and by licking does occur. Therefore, dogs receiving Triamcinolone Acetonide Cream USP therapy should be observed closely for signs of polydipsia, polyuria and increased weight gain, particularly when used over large areas or for extended periods of time.

M

Clinical and experimental data have demonstrated that corticosteroids administered orally or by injection to animals may induce the first stage of parturition if used during the last trimester of pregnancy and may precipitate premature parturition followed by dystocia, fetal death, retained placenta and metritis.

Additionally, corticosteroids administered to dogs, rabbits and rodents during pregnancy have resulted in cleft palate in offspring. Corticosteroids administered to dogs during pregnancy have also resulted in other congenital anomalies including deformed forelegs, phocomelia and anasarca.

For topical use on dogs only.

Side Effects: SAP and SGPT (ALT) enzyme elevations, polydipsia and polyuria have occurred following parenteral or systemic use of synthetic corticosteroids in dogs. Vomiting and diarrhea (occasionally bloody) have been observed in dogs.

Cushing's Syndrome in dogs has been reported in association with prolonged or repeated steroid therapy.

Presentation: Triamcinolone Acetonide Cream USP is supplied in 7.5 gram and 15 gram tubes.

Compendium Code No.: 10270061

MEDICATED UDDER BALM

First Priority **Udder Product**

Ingredient(s): Purified water, mineral oil, stearic acid, glycerol stearate, petrolatum, glycerine, cetyl alcohol, propylene glycol, lanolin, triethanolamine, fragrance, methylparaben, parachlorometaxylenol, vitamin A, vitamin E, aloe vera, propylparaben, para aminobenzoic acid, vitamin D, FD&C Blue #1.

Indications: MEDICATED UDDER BALM is used as an aid in the treatment of dry, cracked, and/or chapped udders in cattle. Contains humectants which assist in maintaining the moisture balance of skin. MEDICATED UDDER BALM is recommended for use on teats, udders, and other skin areas that are exposed to sun, weather changes, and frequent washing. This non-sticky formula is quickly absorbed, discouraging dirt and manure from sticking to the skin or udders.

Directions for Use: Apply daily or as often as needed after milking to help reduce dryness and aid in soothing and softening of the skin. Thoroughly wash treated areas, using individual towels, before each milking to avoid contamination of milk. After each milking, bathe with plenty of warm water, strip milk out, dry skin, and apply MEDICATED UDDER BALM.

Precaution(s): Storage: Store at controlled room temperature between 15°-30°C (59°-86°F). Keep container tightly closed when not in use.

Caution(s): If animal shows signs of uncontrolled generalized skin infections, consult your veterinarian. Wash teats and udder thoroughly before milking.

For animal use only.

Warning(s): Keep out of reach of children.

Presentation: 4 oz (113.3 g) jar, 1 lb (453.6 g) and 4 lb (1.8 kg).

Compendium Code No.: 11390522 Rev. 03-02 / Rev. 07-01

MEDICATED WOUND CREAM

First Priority **Topical Wound Dressing**

Active Ingredient(s): Zinc bacitracin, lanolin, aloe vera and vitamins A, D, and E.

Indications: MEDICATED WOUND CREAM provides soothing relief, helps prevent bacterial infection, promotes rapid healing and helps to minimize scarring. Safe and effective in treating minor cuts and abrasions, skin irritations, dry or chapped skin, and cracked heels. Safe for use in all racing, shows, and events.

Directions for Use: Thoroughly cleanse the affected area. Rinse with warm water and pat dry. Apply generous amounts of MEDICATED WOUND CREAM to the affected area. If needed, cover with light gauze or clean wrap. Change the wrap daily, cleaning wound thoroughly and re-applying MEDICATED WOUND CREAM. Continue treatment until wound is completely healed.

Precaution(s): Storage: Store at a controlled room temperature between 32°F and 90°F.

Caution(s): Not for use on deep or puncture wounds. If redness, irritation, or swelling persists or increases, discontinue use and consult a veterinarian.

For animal use only.

Warning(s): Do not use on animals intended for food.

Keep out of reach of children.

Presentation: 4 oz (113.3 g) and 1 lb (453.6 g) (NDC# 58829-280-16).

Compendium Code No.: 11390532 Rev. 05-01

MEDICATED WOUND POWDER

First Priority **Topical Wound Dressing**

Anti-Bacterial, Anti-Fungal

Active Ingredient(s): Zinc bacitracin and zinc undecylenate in a specially prepared base.

Indications: Helps prevent bacterial infection while promoting rapid healing. MEDICATED WOUND POWDER is specially formulated with anti-bacterial and anti-fungal agents to help prevent infections and act as an effective drying agent to help most wounds heal quickly. A safe and effective aid in the treatment of minor cuts and abrasions, scratches, and skin irritations. Safe for use in all racing, shows and events.

Directions for Use: Thoroughly cleanse the affected area. Rinse with warm water and pat dry. Dust wound or skin irritation with generous amounts of MEDICATED WOUND POWDER. For treatment of scratches, dust generously and apply bandage or wrap. Change bandage or wrap daily. Continue treatment until wound is completely healed.

Precaution(s): Storage: Store at controlled room temperature between 15°-30°C (59°-86°F). Keep container tightly closed when not in use.

Caution(s): Do not use in deep or puncture wounds or serious burns. If redness, irritation or swelling persists or increases, discontinue use and consult a veterinarian.

For animal use only.

Warning(s): Do not use on animals intended for food.

Keep out of reach of children.

Presentation: 6 oz (170 g) (NDC# 58829-285-06).

Compendium Code No.: 11390542 Iss. 06-01

MEDROL® ℞

Pharmacia & Upjohn **Corticosteroid-Oral**

brand of methylprednisolone tablets

NADA No.: 011-403

Active Ingredient(s): Each 4 mg tablet contains 4 mg methylprednisolone.

Indications: The indications for MEDROL® Tablets are the same as those for other anti-inflammatory steroids and comprise the various collagen, dermal, allergic, ocular, otic, and musculoskeletal conditions known to be responsive to the anti-inflammatory corticosteroids. Representative of the conditions in which the use of steroid therapy and the benefits to be derived therefrom have had repeated confirmation in the veterinary literature are: (1) dermal conditions, such as non-specific eczema, summer dermatitis, and burns; (2) allergic manifestations, such as acute urticaria, allergic dermatitis, drug and serum reactions, bronchial asthma, and pollen sensitivities; (3) ocular conditions, such as iritis, iridocyclitis, secondary glaucoma, uveitis, and chorioretinitis; (4) otic conditions, such as otitis externa; (5) musculoskeletal conditions, such as myositis, rheumatoid arthritis, osteoarthritis, and bursitis; (6) various chronic or recurrent diseases of unknown etiology such as ulcerative colitis and nephrosis.

In acute adrenal insufficiency, MEDROL® may be effective because of its ability to correct the defect in carbohydrate metabolism and relieve the impaired diuretic response to water characteristic of primary or secondary adrenal insufficiency. However, because this agent lacks significant mineralocorticoid activity, the parent hormones, Solu-Cortef® containing hydrocortisone sodium succinate, Cortef® containing hydrocortisone, or cortisone should be used when salt retention is indicated.

Pharmacology: Methylprednisolone, a potent anti-inflammatory steroid synthesized and developed in the Research Laboratories of The Upjohn Company is the 6-methyl derivative of prednisolone. It has a greater anti-inflammatory potency than prednisolone and even less tendency than prednisolone to induce sodium and water retention. Its advantage over the older corticoids lies in its ability to achieve equal anti-inflammatory effect with lower dose, while at the same time enhancing the split between anti-inflammatory and mineralocorticoid activities.

Dosage and Administration: For oral use in dogs and cats.

Dosage: Average total daily oral doses for dogs and cats are as follows:

5 to 15 lb body wt.	2 mg
15 to 40 lb body wt.	2 to 4 mg
40 to 80 lb body wt.	4 to 8 mg

The total daily dose should be given in divided doses, 6 to 10 hours apart.

Administration: The keystone of satisfactory therapeutic management with MEDROL® Tablets, as with its steroid predecessors, is individualization of dosage in reference to the severity of the disease, the anticipated duration of steroid therapy, and the animal patient's threshold or tolerance for steroid excess. The prime objective of steroid therapy should be to achieve a satisfactory degree of control with a minimum effective daily dose.

The dosage recommendations are suggested average total daily doses and are intended as guides. As with other orally administered corticosteroids, the total daily dose of MEDROL® should be given in equally divided doses. The initial suppressive dose level is continued until a satisfactory clinical response is obtained, a period usually of 2 to 7 days in the case of musculoskeletal diseases, allergic conditions affecting the skin or respiratory tract, and ocular inflammatory diseases. If a satisfactory response is not obtained in 7 days, reevaluation of the case to confirm the original diagnosis should be made. As soon as a satisfactory clinical response is obtained, the daily dose should be reduced gradually, either to termination of treatment in the case of acute conditions (eg, seasonal asthma, dermatitis, acute ocular inflammations) or to the minimal effective maintenance dose level in the case of chronic conditions (eg, rheumatoid arthritis). In chronic conditions, and in rheumatoid arthritis especially, it is important that the reduction in dosage from initial to maintenance dose levels be accomplished slowly. The maintenance dose level should be adjusted from time to time as required by fluctuation in the activity of the disease and the animal's general status. Accumulated experience has shown that the long-term benefits to be gained from continued steroid maintenance are probably greater the lower the maintenance dose level. In rheumatoid arthritis in particular, maintenance steroid therapy should be at the lowest possible level.

Important: In the therapeutic management of animal patients with chronic diseases such as rheumatoid arthritis, methylprednisolone should be regarded as a highly valuable adjunct, to be used in conjunction with but not as replacement for standard therapeutic measures.

Contraindication(s): MEDROL® Tablets like prednisolone, are contraindicated in animals with arrested tuberculosis, peptic ulcer, acute psychoses, and Cushingoid syndrome. The presence of diabetes, osteoporosis, chronic psychotic reactions, predisposition to thrombophlebitis, hypertension, congestive heart failure, renal insufficiency, and active tuberculosis necessitates carefully controlled use. Some of the above conditions occur only rarely in dogs and cats but should be kept in mind.

Precaution(s): Store at controlled room temperature 20° to 25° C (68° to 77° F) [see USP].

Caution(s): Federal (USA) law restricts this drug to use by or on the order of a licensed veterinarian.

Because of its inhibitory effect on fibroplasia, methylprednisolone may mask the signs of infection and enhance dissemination of the infecting organism. Hence, all animal patients receiving methylprednisolone should be watched for evidence of intercurrent infection. Should infection occur, it must be brought under control by use of appropriate antibacterial measures, or administration of methylprednisolone should be discontinued.

MEDROL® Tablets, like prednisolone and other adrenocortical steroids is a potent therapeutic agent influencing the biochemical behavior of most, if not all, tissues of the body. Because this anti-inflammatory steroid manifests little sodium-retaining activity, the usual early sign of cortisone or hydrocortisone overdosage (ie, increase in body weight due to fluid retention) is not a reliable index of overdosage. Hence, recommended dose levels should not be exceeded, and all animal patients receiving MEDROL® should be under close medical supervision. All cautions pertinent to the use of prednisolone apply to methylprednisolone. Moreover, the veterinarian should endeavor to keep informed of current studies with MEDROL® as they are reported in the veterinary literature.

Warning(s): Not for human use. Clinical and experimental data have demonstrated that corticosteroids administered orally or parenterally to animals may induce the first stage of parturition when administered during the last trimester of pregnancy and may precipitate premature parturition followed by dystocia, fetal death, retained placenta, and metritis.

Additionally, corticosteroids administered to dogs, rabbits and rodents during pregnancy have resulted in cleft palate in offspring. Corticosteroids administered to dogs during pregnancy have also resulted in other congenital anomalies including deformed forelegs, phocomelia, and anasarca.

Adverse Reactions: With therapeutically equivalent doses, the likelihood of occurrence of troublesome side effects is less with methylprednisolone than with prednisolone; moreover, side effects actually have been conspicuously absent during clinical trials with MEDROL® Tablets in dogs and cats. However, methylprednisolone is similar to prednisolone in regard to kinds of side effects and metabolic alterations to be anticipated when treatment is intensive or prolonged. In animal patients with diabetes mellitus, use of methylprednisolone may be associated with an increase in the insulin requirement. Negative nitrogen balance may occur, particularly in animals that require protracted maintenance therapy; measures to counteract persistent nitrogen loss include a high protein intake and the administration when indicated, of a suitable anabolic agent. Excessive loss of potassium, like excessive retention of sodium, is not likely to be induced by effective maintenance doses of MEDROL®. However, these effects should be kept in mind and the usual regulatory measures employed as indicated. Ecchymotic manifestations, while not noted during the clinical evaluation in dogs and cats, may occur. If such reactions do occur and are serious, reduction in dosage or discontinuance of methylprednisolone therapy may be indicated. Concurrent use of daily oral supplements of ascorbic acid may be of value in helping to control ecchymotic tendencies.

Since methylprednisolone, like prednisolone, suppresses endogenous adrenocortical activity, it is highly important that the animal patient receiving MEDROL® be under careful observation, not only during the course of treatment but for some time after treatment is terminated. Adequate adrenocortical supportive therapy with cortisone or hydrocortisone, and including ACTH, must be employed promptly if the animal is subjected to any unusual stress such as surgery, trauma, or severe infection.

Presentation: Veterinary MEDROL® Tablets are compressed cross-scored tablets available in bottles of 500 (NDC 0009-3547-01).

Compendium Code No.: 10490310

812 602 308

MEGA CMPK BOLUS

AgriPharm **Calcium-Oral**

Calcium, Magnesium, Phosphorus, Potassium and Vitamin Bolus

Guaranteed Analysis:

	Per Bolus	Per Pound
Calcium (Ca), min.	4.4 gm	12.2%
Calcium (Ca), max.	5.3 gm	14.7%
Phosphorus (P), min.	3.7 gm	10.2%
Potassium (K), min.	1.5 gm	4.1%
Magnesium (Mg), min.	1.4 gm	3.8%
Vitamin D_3, min.	50,000 IU	630,000 IU

Ingredients: Dicalcium phosphate, calcium carbonate, potassium chloride, microcrystalline cellulose, magnesium oxide, magnesium stearate, vitamin D_3 supplement, sodium carboxymethylcellulose, dried whey, lactose, dextrose, starch, beet pulp, distillers dried grain with solubles, brewers dried yeast, natural and artificial flavors.

Indications: MEGA CMPK BOLUS is a nutritional supplement that provides additional nutritional support of the minerals calcium, phosphorus, potassium and magnesium for cattle, horses, sheep and swine.

Dosage and Administration: Administer orally with a balling gun in accordance to the following as described below or consult a veterinarian.

	For Daily Supplementation	For Increased Nutrient Intake
Cattle and Horses	1 to 2 boluses per day, 3 to 5 days preceding shipment or parturition.	2 to 3 boluses per day, 3 to 5 days following parenteral therapy.
Sheep and Swine	½ to 1 bolus per day, 3 to 5 days preceding shipment or parturition.	1 to 2 boluses per day, 3 to 5 days following parenteral therapy.

Boluses may be administered by crushing and sprinkled on the daily feed ration or suspended in milk or water and given as a drench. A balanced ration and access to ample water supply should be provided.

Precaution(s): Keep container tightly closed when not in use. Store in a cool, dry place.

Caution(s): For animal use only. Keep out of reach of children.

Presentation: 50 boluses (36 g per bolus).

Compendium Code No.: 14570610

MEGAN® VAC 1

Megan **Vaccine**

Salmonella Typhimurium Vaccine, Live Bacteria, Gene Modified

U.S. Vet. Lic. No.: 240

Contents: This product contains the antigen listed above.

Indications: This vaccine is recommended as an aid in the reduction of *Salmonella typhimurium, Salmonella enteritidis* and *Salmonella heidelberg* colonization of the internal organs of young growing chickens and as an aid in the reduction of colonization of the digestive tract excluding the ceca. The ovaries and oviducts were not evaluated and therefore this vaccine is not indicated for use in older chickens.

This vaccine is recommended for use at 1 day of age by spray. A second dose should be given at 14 days of age in the drinking water.

Dosage and Administration:

Spray Method: Rehydrate the vaccine with cool, sterile, non-chlorinated water, which contains no antimicrobials, in an amount sufficient to vaccinate the required number of chickens according to the directions of the spray cabinet or sprayer manufacturer. This is usually about 500 mL per 5000 chicks. Use 5000 doses of vaccine to vaccinate 5000 chickens. Do not dilute.

Wear a mask and gloves while handling the vaccine. Avoid breathing the aerosolized vaccine.

Drinking Water Method: Remove disinfectant, sanitizers and antimicrobials from the drinking water 24 hours prior to and after vaccination. Mix vaccine in clean water which contains no sanitizing agents or antimicrobials. Use 50 liters of water for each 5000 birds. Provide ample space for all birds to drink easily. Water containing vaccine should be consumed in 2 hours or less. To assure all birds drink, withhold water for one hour prior to vaccination.

Precaution(s): Store at not over 45°F (7°C). Use entire contents when vial opened.

Burn all vials and unused contents. Follow vaccine storage directions.

Caution(s): Vaccinate only healthy birds.

Keep permanent vaccination records including vaccine serial number.

This vaccine has been carefully manufactured and has passed all tests for purity and potency according to the requirements of the Company and of the United States Department of Agriculture. For veterinary use only.

Warning(s): Do not vaccinate within 21 days of slaughter.

Presentation: 10 x 5,000 dose and 10 x 10,000 dose vials.

Manufactured by: Lohmann Animal Health.

Exclusively distributed by: Lohmann Animal Health.

U.S. Patent Reg. No. 5,389,368

Compendium Code No.: 15040002

MELALEUCA MIST

Davis **Grooming Spray**

Active Ingredient(s): MELALEUCA MIST is formulated using a synergistic combination of natural oils, penetrants and emollients, with Melaleuca alternifolia oil.

Indications: MELALEUCA MIST is an all-natural spray for use on dogs, cats, puppies and kittens to help most problem areas without irritating the skin.

Dosage and Administration: To use on pets with skin problems, mist the pet starting with the head, neck and ears, then repeat the procedure with the chest, middle and hindquarter, finishing with the legs. Use enough of the mist to penetrate the skin.

Presentation: 16 oz.

Compendium Code No.: 11410251

MELALEUCA SHAMPOO

Davis **Grooming Shampoo**

Active Ingredient(s): Contains: *Melaleuca alternifolia* oil, hydrolyzed keratin panthenol, vitamin E, wheat germ oil, rosemary, coconut oil in a mild shampoo base.

Indications: For dogs, cats, puppies and kittens.

For conditions caused by seborrheic dermatitis, skin bacteria and fungus.

Directions for Use: To use Davis MELALEUCA SHAMPOO on pets with skin problems, dilute 3 parts water to 1 part shampoo (3:1). For pets with severe skin conditions, dilute 1 part water to 1 part shampoo (1:1). To use as a general grooming and cleansing shampoo, dilute 5 parts water to 1 part shampoo (5:1).

Wet pet's coat thoroughly with warm water. Do not get shampoo into eyes. Apply shampoo on head and ears, then lather. Repeat procedure with neck, chest, middle and hind quarter, finishing legs last. Let the pet stand for 5 to 10 minutes. (This is an important part of the grooming procedure). Rinse pet thoroughly. For best results, repeat procedure.

Caution(s): Do not use on puppies and kittens under 4 weeks of age. For external use only. Do not use if human or pet is allergic to this product.

Warning(s): Keep out of reach of children.

Discussion: Davis MELALEUCA SHAMPOO is formulated with a synergistic combination of natural oils, penetrants and emollients featuring the natural soothing action of oil of melaleuca alternifolia. Melaleuca oil has been used as a natural healer for over 60 years in Australia where it is obtained by steam distillation of the foliage and branches of one of the Australian Tea Trees, *Melaleuca alternifolia.*

Davis MELALEUCA SHAMPOO helps soothe the skin conditions caused by dry skin, flea and tick problems, itching, scaling and will not irritate the skin. A healthy skin grows a healthy coat.

Presentation: 12 oz (355 mL) and 1 gallon (3.785 L) containers.

Compendium Code No.: 11410262

METHAPLEX INJECTION ℞

PRN Pharmacal **Vitamin B-Complex**

B-Complex Injection 150 High Potency

Active Ingredient(s): Each mL contains:

Thiamine Hydrochloride . . . 150 mg
Riboflavin 5' Sodium Phosphate USP . . . 2 mg
Niacinamide . . . 150 mg
d-Panthenol . . . 10 mg
Pyridoxine HCL . . . 10 mg
Inositol . . . 20 mg

Choline Chloride.......... 20 mg
Benzyl Alcohol (as preservative).......... 2% v/v
Water for injection.......... q.s.
Indications: As a source of B complex vitamins for use in the treatment of deficiencies of these vitamins in cattle, sheep, and horses.
Dosage and Administration: Administer by intramuscular, subcutaneous or slow intravenous injection. Dosage may be repeated once or twice weekly as needed.
1 to 5 mL per 100 lbs of body weight.
Precaution(s): Store at refrigerated temperature between 2°-8°C (36°-46°F).
Caution(s): Federal law restricts this drug to use by or on the order of a licensed veterinarian.
Parenteral administration of thiamine has resulted in anaphylactic shock. Administer slowly and with caution in doses over ⅓ mL (50 mg thiamine).
Warning(s): For animal use only.
Keep out of reach of children.
Presentation: 100 mL.
Compendium Code No.: 10900100

METHIGEL®

Evsco **Urinary Acidifier**

Active Ingredient(s): Guaranteed analysis per teaspoon (5 g):
dl-methionine.......... 400 mg (8%)
Ingredients: Corn syrup, malt syrup, white petrolatum, dl-methionine, soybean oil, cane molasses, mineral oil, cod liver oil, water, methylcellulose, peptones, and sodium benzoate (preservative).
Indications: For use as a supplemental source of methionine, aids in maintaining an acidic urine.
Dosage and Administration: METHIGEL® is palatable. To stimulate taste interest place a small amount of METHIGEL® on the animal's nose or directly into the mouth.
Cats: One-half (½) to one (1) teaspoonful twice a day.
Dogs: One (1) teaspoonful twice a day.
Precaution(s): Store at room temperature.
Caution(s): For veterinary use only.
Warning(s): METHIGEL® should not be administered to animals with severe liver or kidney disease. METHIGEL® should not be administered to animals on an empty stomach. Large doses may cause gastro-intestinal upset. Control of urinary tract infection is essential.
Presentation: 12 x 4¼ oz. (120.5 g) tubes.
Compendium Code No.: 10050170

METHIO-FORM® CHEWABLE TABLETS ℞

Vet-A-Mix **Urinary Acidifier**

DL-Methionine
Active Ingredient(s): Each tablet contains:
DL-Methionine.......... 500 mg (6.7 mEq)
In a palatable protein base.
Indications: For use as an aid in acidifying the urine of dogs and cats. METHIO-FORM® is also an aid in controlling the odor from feline and canine urine residues.
METHIO-FORM® Chewable Tablets may be used as a source of the essential amino acid, DL-Methionine.
Dosage and Administration: Administration: METHIO-FORM® Chewable Tablets may be fed free choice, from the hand or maybe crumbled and mixed into the food. Dosing one time each day is appropriate, but daily doses may be administered in 2 or 3 divided doses if more convenient or in rare cases where animals may vomit a single daily dose.
Dosage: Daily dosages vary with diet and the amount of acidification needed. After dosages have been determined, they may be used continuously.
Cats: The usual daily dose is 2.5 to 5.0 mEq (188-375 mg)/kg body weight or ½ to 1 tablet per 1 to 1.5 kg (2.5 to 3 lb) of body weight. Average size adult cats normally should receive 1½ to 3 tablets (10-20 mEq) daily.
Dogs: The usual daily dose is 2 to 4 mEq (150-300 mg)/kg body weight. Small breeds - 7 kg (15 lb) or under, ½ to 4 tablets. Medium breeds - 7 to 15 kg (15 to 33 lb), 2 to 7 tablets. Large breeds - 15-30 kg (33-66 lb), 4 to 13 tablets.
Note: METHIO-FORM® tablets can be crumbled and sprinkled on the animal's food. A level teaspoonful of a crumbled tablet contains 746 mg (10.0 mEq) of DL-methionine.
Contraindication(s): Do not administer to animals with severe liver, kidney or pancreatic disease, or which are acidotic.
Precaution(s): Storage: Store at room temperature and protect from light. Avoid excessive heat (104°F).
Caution(s): Federal law restricts this drug to use by or on the order of a licensed veterinarian.
In rare cases, animals may experience gastrointestinal disturbance. In those cases, administer during feeding or in two to three divided doses.
Warning(s): Over-consumption may result if access to open bottles occurs. The effect may be severe and could result in life-threatening metabolic acidosis if veterinary treatment is not initiated.
Keep out of reach of children.
Presentation: Bottles of 50, 150, and 500 tablets.
Patent Pending
Compendium Code No.: 10500151 0197/Rev. 0799

METHIO-TABS® ℞

Vet-A-Mix **Urinary Acidifier**

Active Ingredient(s): Each scored tablet contains either:
Dl-methionine.......... 200 mg (2.68 mEq)
Dl-methionine.......... 500 mg (6.70 mEq)
Indications: For use as an aid in acidifying the urine of dogs and cats.
Dosage and Administration: Daily dosages vary with diet and the amount of acidification needed. After dosages have been determined, they may be used continuously.
Cats: The usual daily dose is 2.5-5.0 mEq/kg of body weight.
200 mg tablets: 1-2 tablets per 1 to 1.5 kg (2.5 to 3 lbs.) of body weight. Average size adult cats normally should receive 4-8 tablets (10-20 mEq) daily.
500 mg tablets: ½-1 tablet per 1 to 1.5 kg (2.5 to 3 lbs.) of body weight. Average size adult cats normally should receive 1½-3 tablets (10-20 mEq) daily.
Dogs: The usually daily dose is 2-4 mEq/kg of body weight.
200 mg tablets: Small breeds - 7 kg (15 lbs.) or under, 1-10 tablets. Medium breeds - 7-15 kg (15-33 lbs.), 5-18 tablets. Large breeds - 15-30 kg (33-66 lbs.), 10-32 tablets.
500 mg tablets: Small breeds - 7 kg (15 lbs.) or under, ½-4 tablets. Medium breeds - 7-15 kg (15-33 lbs.), 2-7 tablets. Large breeds - 15-30 kg (33-66 lbs.), 4-13 tablets.
Contraindication(s): Do not administer to animals with severe liver, kidney or pancreatic disease, or which are acidotic.
Precaution(s): Store at room temperature and protect from light. Avoid excessive heat (104°F).
Caution(s): U.S. federal law restricts this drug to use by or on the order of a licensed veterinarian.
Keep out of the reach of children.
In rare cases, animals may experience gastro-intestinal disturbance. In those cases, administer tablets during or after feeding or in two to three divided doses.
Presentation: Bottles of 1,000 tablets.
Compendium Code No.: 10500160

METH-IRON 65

Zinpro **Feed Additive**

Iron Methionine
Typical Analysis:
Iron.......... 14.5%
Methionine.......... 33.0%
Protein.......... 21.0%
Fat.......... 0.0%
Fiber.......... 0.0%
Ash.......... 34.7%
Salt.......... 0.6%
Indications: Recommended as a nutritional feed additive for livestock and poultry. When used as a commercial feed ingredient it must be declared as iron methionine.
Physical Description: A light brown water soluble powder with characteristic methionine-like odor. METH-IRON 65 weighs approximately 25 lbs/cu ft.
Feeding Instructions:
Swine:
Sows--Add 2 lbs (908 grams) per ton of gestation-farrowing-lactation ration.
Pig Starters--Add 2 lbs (908 grams) per ton of complete ration.
Growing and Finishing Swine--Add 1 lb (454 grams) per ton of complete ration.
Dairy Cattle: Feed 4.5 grams per head daily, or 1 lb per 100 head daily.
Beef Cattle: Feed 4.5 grams per head daily, or 1 lb per 100 head daily.
Calves: Feed 1 lb (454 grams) per 500 head daily.
Sheep: Feed 1 lb (454 (grams) per 500 head daily.
Chickens and Turkeys: Add 2 lbs (908 grams) per ton of complete ration.
Horses: Feed 4.5 grams per head daily.
Toxicology: When correctly used, there is no toxicity hazard in the use of METH-IRON 65.
Presentation: METH-IRON 65 is packaged in 50 lb multiwall bags with 2 mil inserted polyethylene liners.
Compendium Code No.: 11300160

METHOCOL™ CAPSULES

Life Science **Small Animal Dietary Supplement**

Dietary Supplement with Lipotropics
Active Ingredient(s): Each Capsule Contains:
Choline Bitartrate.......... 240 mg
dl-Methionine.......... 110 mg
Inositol.......... 83 mg
Vitamin B_{12} (Cyanocobalamin).......... 2 mcg
Thiamine Mononitrate.......... 3 mg
Riboflavin.......... 3 mg
Pyridoxine HCl.......... 2 mg
Niacinamide.......... 10 mg
d-Calcium Pantothenate.......... 2 mg
Desiccated Liver.......... 86 mg
Indications: Use: As a dietary supplement for small animals.
Dosage and Administration: Give one capsule per 20 lbs body weight or as directed by a veterinarian.
Precaution(s): Keep in a cool, dry place.
Caution(s): For animal use only.
Warning(s): Keep out of reach of children.
Presentation: Bottles of 1,000 capsules.
Compendium Code No.: 10870101 Rev. 0-7196

METHYLENE BLUE

Centaur **Diagnostic Stain/Reagent**

Active Ingredient(s):
Methylene Blue.......... 1% (w/v) solution (in water).
Indications: Suitable for use as a dye, laboratory indicator and reagent.
Precaution(s): Protect from freezing.
Caution(s): For animal use only.
Warning(s): Keep out of reach of children.
Presentation: 1 pint (16 fl oz) 473 mL and 1 gallon (128 fl oz) 3.785 L).
Compendium Code No.: 14880210

METHYLPREDNISOLONE TABLETS ℞

Boehringer Ingelheim **Corticosteroid-Oral**

NADA No.: 135-771
Active Ingredient(s): Each tablet contains 2 mg methylprednisolone.
Indications: The indications are the same as those for other anti-inflammatory steroids and comprise the various collagen, dermal, allergic, ocular, otic and musculoskeletal conditions known to be responsive to the anti-inflammatory corticosteroids. Representative of the conditions in which the use of steroid therapy and the benefits to be derived therefrom have had repeated confirmation in the veterinary literature are:
Dermal conditions, such as non-specific eczema and summer dermatitis.[1,2,4]
Allergic manifestations, such as acute urticaria, allergic dermatitis, drug and serum reactions, non-specific pruritus, bronchial asthma and pollen sensitivities.[1,2,3,4,5]
Ocular conditions such as iritis, iridocyclitis, secondary glaucoma, uveitis and chorioretinitis.[1,3,4,5]
Otic conditions, such as otitis externa.[4]

Musculoskeletal conditions, such as myositis, rheumatoid arthritis, osteoarthritis and bursitis.[1,2,3,4,5]

Various chronic or recurrent diseases of unknown etiology such as ulcerative colitis and nephrosis.[1,2,3,5]

In acute adrenal insufficiency, methylprednisolone may be effective because of its ability to correct the defect in carbohydrate metabolism and relieve the impaired diuretic response to water, characteristic of primary or secondary adrenal insufficiency. However, because this agent lacks significant mineralocorticoid activity, hydrocortisone sodium succinate or cortisone should be used when salt retention is indicated.[6]

Pharmacology: Methylprednisolone, a potent glucocorticoid and anti-inflammatory agent, is a synthetic 6-methyl derivative of prednisolone. It has a greater anti-inflammatory potency than prednisolone and is less likely to induce sodium and water retention. Its advantage over the older corticoids lies in its ability to achieve an equal anti-inflammatory effect with a lower dose, while at the same time enhancing the split between anti-inflammatory and mineralocorticoid activities.[1,2,3]

Glucocorticoids exert a regulatory influence on lymphocytes, erythrocytes and eosinophils of the blood and on the structure and function of lymphoid tissues.[1,4,5] A primary feature of the glucocorticoids is their anti-inflammatory activity with minimum sodium and water retention which is often associated with the mineralocorticoids.[1,2,3,4,5,6] Glucocorticoids not only inhibit early phases of the inflammatory process (edema, fibrin deposition, capillary dilatation, migration of leukocytes into the inflamed area and phagocytic activity) but also the later manifestations (capillary proliferation, fibroblast proliferation and the deposition of collagen).[3,4,6] The exact mechanism is not known, but the glucocorticoids obviously suppress normal tissue response to injury and alleviate symptoms from many conditions.[2]

Dosage and Administration: The keystone of satisfactory therapeutic management with methylprednisolone, as with its steroid predecessors, is the individualization of dosage in reference to the severity of the disease, the anticipated duration of steroid therapy and the animal's threshold or tolerance for steroid excess. The prime objective of steroid therapy should be to achieve a satisfactory degree of control with a minimum effective daily dose.

The dosage recommendations are suggested average total daily doses and are intended as guides. As with other orally administered corticosteroids, the total daily dose of methylprednisolone tablets should be given in equally divided doses. The initial suppressive dose level is continued until a satisfactory clinical response is obtained, a period usually of two (2) to seven (7) days in the case of musculoskeletal diseases, allergic conditions affecting the skin or respiratory tract and ocular inflammatory diseases. If a satisfactory response is not obtained in seven (7) days, a re-evaluation of the case to confirm the original diagnosis should be made. As soon as a satisfactory clinical response is obtained, the daily dose should be reduced gradually, either to the termination of treatment in the case of acute conditions (e.g. seasonal asthma, dermatitis, acute ocular inflammations) or to the minimal effective maintenance dose level in the case of chronic conditions (e.g. rheumatoid arthritis). In chronic conditions, and in rheumatoid arthritis especially, it is important that the reduction in dosage from initial to maintenance dose levels be accomplished slowly. The maintenance dose level should be adjusted from time to time as required by the fluctuation in the activity of the disease and the animal's general status. Accumulated experience has shown that the long-term benefits to be gained from continued steroid maintenance are probably greater the lower the maintenance dose level. In rheumatoid arthritis in particular, maintenance steroid therapy should be at the lowest possible level.

Important: In the therapeutic management of animals with chronic diseases, such as rheumatoid arthritis, methylprednisolone should be regarded as a highly valuable adjunct, to be used in conjunction with but not as a replacement for standard therapeutic measures.

Recommended Dosage Schedule: Average total daily doses for dogs and cats are as follows:

5 to 15 lb. of body wt. .... 2 mg
15 to 40 lb. of body wt. .... 2 to 4 mg
40 to 80 lb. of body wt. .... 4 to 8 mg

The total daily dose should be given in divided doses, 6-10 hours apart.

Contraindication(s): Do not use in viral infections. Methylprednisolone, like prednisolone, is contraindicated in animals with arrested tuberculosis, peptic ulcer, acute psychoses, corneal ulcer and Cushingoid syndrome. The presence of diabetes, osteoporosis, chronic psychotic reactions, predisposition to thrombophlebitis, hypertension, congestive heart failure, renal insufficiency and active tuberculosis necessitates carefully controlled use. Some of the above conditions occur rarely in dogs and cats but should be kept in mind.

Precaution(s): Methylprednisolone, like prednisolone and other adrenocortical steroids, is a potent therapeutic agent influencing the biochemical behavior of most, if not all, tissues of the body. Because this anti-inflammatory steroid manifests little sodium-retaining activity, the usual early sign of cortisone or hydrocortisone overdosage (i.e., increase in body weight due to fluid retention) is not a reliable index of overdosage. Hence, the recommended dosage levels should not be exceeded, and all animals receiving methylprednisolone should be under close medical supervision. All precautions pertinent to the use of prednisolone apply to methylprednisolone. Moreover, the veterinarian should endeavor to keep informed of current studies with methylprednisolone as they are reported in the veterinary literature.

The use of corticosteroids, depending upon dose, duration and specific steroid may result in the inhibition of endogenous steroid production following drug withdrawal. In patients presently receiving or recently withdrawn from systemic corticosteroid treatments, therapy with a rapid acting corticosteroid should be considered only in unusually stressful situations.

Caution(s): Federal law restricts this drug to use by or on the order of a licensed veterinarian.

Keep out of the reach of children.

Warning(s): Because of its inhibitory effect on fibroplasia, methylprednisolone may mask the signs of infection and enhance the dissemination of the infecting organism. Hence, all animals receiving methylprednisolone should be watched for any evidence of intercurrent infection. Should infection occur, it must be brought under control by the use of appropriate antibacterial measures and the administration of methylprednisolone should be discontinued.

Not for human use. Clinical and experimental data have demonstrated that corticosteroids administered orally or parenterally to animals may induce the first stage of parturition when administered during the last trimester of pregnancy and may precipitate premature parturition followed by dystocia, fetal death, retained placenta and metritis.

Additionally, corticosteroids administered to dogs, rabbits and rodents during pregnancy have produced cleft palate. Other congenital anomalies including deformed forelegs, phocomelia and anasarca have been reported in offspring of dogs which received corticosteroids during pregnancy.

Side Effects: Methylprednisolone is similar to prednisolone in regard to the kinds of side effects and metabolic alterations to be anticipated when treatment is intensive or prolonged. In animals with diabetes mellitus, the use of methylprednisolone may be associated with an increase in the insulin requirement. Negative nitrogen balance may occur, particularly in animals that require protracted maintenance therapy; measures to counteract persistent nitrogen loss include a high protein intake and the administration, when indicated, of a suitable anabolic agent. Excessive loss of potassium, like excessive retention of sodium, is not likely to be induced by effective maintenance doses of methylprednisolone. However, these effects should be kept in mind and the usual regulatory measures employed as indicated. Ecchymotic manifestations, while not noted during the clinical evaluation in dogs and cats, may occur. If such reactions do occur and are serious, a reduction in the dosage or the discontinuance of methylprednisolone therapy may be indicated. Concurrent use of daily oral supplements of ascorbic acid may be of value in helping to control ecchymotic tendencies.

Side effects, such as SAP and SGPT enzyme elevations, weight loss, anorexia, polydipsia and polyuria have occurred following the use of synthetic corticosteroids in dogs. Vomiting and diarrhea (occasionally bloody) have been observed in dogs and cats. Cushing's syndrome in dogs has been reported in association with prolonged or repeated steroid therapy.

References: Available upon request.

Presentation: Bottles of 1,000 tablets.

Compendium Code No.: 10280770

METHYLPREDNISOLONE TABLETS ℞

Butler **Corticosteroid-Oral**

NADA No.: 135-771

Active Ingredient(s): Each tablet contains 2 mg methylprednisolone.

Indications: The indications are the same as those for other anti-inflammatory steroids and comprise the various collagen, dermal, allergic, ocular, otic and musculoskeletal conditions known to be responsive to the anti-inflammatory corticosteroids. Representative of the conditions in which the use of steroid therapy and the benefits to be derived therefrom have had repeated confirmation in the veterinary literature are:

Dermal conditions, such as non-specific eczema and summer dermatitis.[1,2,4]

Allergic manifestations, such as acute urticaria, allergic dermatitis, drug and serum reactions, non-specific pruritus, bronchial asthma and pollen sensitivities.[1,2,3,4,5]

Ocular conditions such as iritis, iridocyclitis, secondary glaucoma, uveitis and chorioretinitis.[1,3,4,5]

Otic conditions, such as otitis externa.[4]

Musculoskeletal conditions, such as myositis, rheumatoid arthritis, osteoarthritis and bursitis.[1,2,3,4,5]

Various chronic or recurrent diseases of unknown etiology such as ulcerative colitis and nephrosis.[1,2,3,5]

In acute adrenal insufficiency, methylprednisolone may be effective because of its ability to correct the defect in carbohydrate metabolism and relieve the impaired diuretic response to water, characteristic of primary or secondary adrenal insufficiency. However, because this agent lacks significant mineralocorticoid activity, hydrocortisone sodium succinate or cortisone should be used when salt retention is indicated.[6]

Pharmacology: Description: Methylprednisolone, a potent glucocorticoid and anti-inflammatory agent, is a synthetic 6-methyl derivative of prednisolone. It has a greater anti-inflammatory potency than prednisolone and is less likely to induce sodium and water retention. Its advantage over the older corticoids lies in its ability to achieve an equal anti-inflammatory effect with a lower dose, while at the same time enhancing the split between anti-inflammatory and mineralocorticoid activities.[1,2,3]

Actions: Glucocorticoids exert a regulatory influence on lymphocytes, erythrocytes and eosinophils of the blood and on the structure and function of lymphoid tissues.[1,4,5] A primary feature of the glucocorticoids is their anti-inflammatory activity with minimum sodium and water retention which is often associated with the mineralocorticoids.[1,2,3,4,5,6] Glucocorticoids not only inhibit the early phases of the inflammatory process (edema, fibrin deposition, capillary dilatation, migration of leukocytes into the inflamed area and phagocytic activity) but also the later manifestations (capillary proliferation, fibroblast proliferation and the deposition of collagen).[3,4,6] The exact mechanism is not known, but the glucocorticoids obviously suppress normal tissue response to injury and alleviate symptoms from many conditions.[2]

Dosage and Administration: The keystone of satisfactory therapeutic management with methylprednisolone, as with its steroid predecessors, is the individualization of dosage in reference to the severity of the disease, the anticipated duration of steroid therapy and the animal's threshold or tolerance for steroid excess. The prime objective of steroid therapy should be to achieve a satisfactory degree of control with a minimum effective daily dose.

The dosage recommendations are suggested average total daily doses and are intended as guides. As with other orally administered corticosteroids, the total daily dose of methylprednisolone tablets should be given in equally divided doses. The initial suppressive dose level is continued until a satisfactory clinical response is obtained, a period usually of 2 to 7 days in the case of musculoskeletal diseases, allergic conditions affecting the skin or respiratory tract and ocular inflammatory diseases. If a satisfactory response is not obtained in 7 days, a re-evaluation of the case to confirm the original diagnosis should be reduced gradually, either to the termination of treatment in the case of acute conditions (e.g. seasonal asthma, dermatitis, acute ocular inflammations) or to the minimal effective maintenance dose level in the case of chronic conditions (e.g. rheumatoid arthritis). In chronic conditions, and in rheumatoid arthritis especially, it is important that the reduction in dosage from initial to maintenance dose levels be accomplished slowly. The maintenance dose level should be adjusted from time to time as required by the fluctuation in the activity of the disease and the animal's general status. Accumulated experience has shown that the long-term benefits to be gained from continued steroid maintenance are probably greater the lower the maintenance dose level. In rheumatoid arthritis in particular, maintenance steroid therapy should be at the lowest possible level.

Important: In the therapeutic management of animals with chronic diseases, such as rheumatoid arthritis, methylprednisolone should be regarded as a highly valuable adjunct, to be used in conjunction with but not as a replacement for standard therapeutic measures.

Recommended Dosage Schedule:

Average total daily doses for dogs and cats are as follows:

5 to 15 lb body wt. .... 2 mg
15 to 40 lb body wt. .... 2 to 4 mg
40 to 80 lb body wt. .... 4 to 8 mg

The total daily dose should be given in divided doses, 6 to 10 hours apart.

Contraindication(s): Do not use in viral infections. Methylprednisolone, like prednisolone, is contraindicated in animals with arrested tuberculosis, peptic ulcer, acute psychoses, corneal ulcer and Cushingoid syndrome. The presence of diabetes, osteoporosis, chronic psychotic reactions, predisposition to thrombophlebitis, hypertension, congestive heart failure, renal insufficiency and active tuberculosis necessitates carefully controlled use. Some of the above conditions occur rarely in dogs and cats but should be kept in mind.

Caution(s): Federal law restricts this drug to use by or on the order of a licensed veterinarian.

Because of its inhibitory effect on fibroplasia, methylprednisolone may mask the signs of infection and enhance the dissemination of the infecting organism. Hence, all animals receiving methylprednisolone should be watched for any evidence of intercurrent infection. Should infection occur, it must be brought under control by the use of appropriate antibacterial measures and the administration of methylprednisolone should be discontinued.

Not for human use. Clinical and experimental data have demonstrated that corticosteroids administered orally or parenterally to animals may induce the first stage of parturition when administered during the last trimester of pregnancy and may precipitate premature parturition followed by dystocia, fetal death, retained placenta and metritis.

Additionally, corticosteroids administered to dogs, rabbits and rodents during pregnancy have produced cleft palate. Other congenital anomalies including deformed forelegs, phocomelia and anasarca have been reported in offspring of dogs which received corticosteroids during pregnancy.

Methylprednisolone, like prednisolone and other adrenocortical steroids, is a potent therapeutic agent influencing the biochemical behavior of most, if not all, tissues of the body. Because this anti-inflammatory steroid manifests little sodium-retaining activity, the usual early sign of cortisone or hydrocortisone overdosage (i.e., increase in body weight due to fluid retention) is not a reliable index of overdosage. Hence, the recommended dosage levels should not be exceeded, and all animals receiving methylprednisolone should be under close medical supervision. All precautions pertinent to the use of prednisolone apply to methylprednisolone. Moreover, the veterinarian should endeavor to keep informed of current studies with methylprednisolone as they are reported in the veterinary literature.

The use of corticosteroids, depending on dose, duration and specific steroid may result in the inhibition of endogenous steroid production following drug withdrawal. In patients presently receiving or recently withdrawn from systemic corticosteroid treatments, therapy with a rapid acting corticosteroid should be considered only in unusually stressful situations.

For oral use in dogs and cats only.

Warning(s): Keep out of reach of children.

Adverse Reactions: Methylprednisolone is similar to prednisolone in regard to the kinds of side effects and metabolic alterations to be anticipated when treatment is intensive or prolonged. In animals with diabetes mellitus, the use of methylprednisolone may be associated with an increase in the insulin requirement. Negative nitrogen balance may occur, particularly in animals that require protracted maintenance therapy; measures to counteract persistent nitrogen loss include a high protein intake and the administration, when indicated, of a suitable anabolic agent. Excessive loss of potassium, like excessive retention of sodium, is not likely to be induced by effective maintenance doses of methylprednisolone. However, these effects should be kept in mind and the usual regulatory measures employed as indicated. Ecchymotic manifestations, while not noted during the clinical evaluation in dogs and cats, may occur. If such reactions do occur and are serious, a reduction in the dosage or the discontinuance of methylprednisolone therapy may be indicated. Concurrent use of daily oral supplements of ascorbic acid may be of value in helping to control ecchymotic tendencies.

Side effects, such as SAP and SGPT enzyme elevations, weight loss, anorexia, polydipsia and polyuria have occurred following the use of synthetic corticosteroids in dogs. Vomiting and diarrhea (occasionally bloody) have been observed in dogs and cats. Cushing's syndrome in dogs has been reported in association with prolonged or repeated steroid therapy.

References: Available upon request.

Presentation: Bottles of 1000 tablets.

Compendium Code No.: 10821980

METHYLPREDNISOLONE TABLETS ℞

Vedco **Corticosteroid-Oral**

NADA No.: 135-771

Active Ingredient(s): Each tablet contains 2 mg of methylprednisolone.

Indications: The indications are the same as those for other anti-inflammatory steroids and comprise the various collagen, dermal, allergic, ocular, otic and musculoskeletal conditions known to be responsive to the anti-inflammatory corticosteroids. Representative of the conditions in which the use of steroid therapy and the benefits to be derived therefrom have had repeated confirmation in the veterinary literature are:

M

Dermal Conditions, such as non-specific eczema and summer dermatitis.[1,2,4]

Allergic Manifestations, such as acute urticaria, allergic dermatitis, drug and serum reactions, non-specific pruritus, bronchial asthma and pollen sensitivities.[1,2,3,4,5]

Ocular Conditions, such as iritis, iridocyclitis, secondary glaucoma, uveitis and chorioretinitis.[1,3,4,5]

Otic Conditions, such as otitis externa.[4]

Musculoskeletal Conditions, such as myositis, rheumatoid arthritis, osteoarthritis and bursitis.[1,2,3,4,5]

Various chronic or recurrent diseases of unknown etiology such as ulcerative colitis and nephrosis.[1,2,3,5]

In acute adrenal insufficiency, methylprednisolone may be effective because of its ability to correct the defect in carbohydrate metabolism and relieve the impaired diuretic response to water, characteristic of primary or secondary adrenal insufficiency. However, because this agent lacks significant mineralocorticoid activity, hydrocortisone sodium succinate or cortisone should be used when salt retention is indicated.[6]

Pharmacology: Methylprednisolone, a potent glucocorticoid and anti-inflammatory agent, is a synthetic 6-methyl derivative of prednisolone. It has a greater anti-inflammatory potency than prednisolone and is less likely to induce sodium and water retention. Its advantage over the older corticoids lies in its ability to achieve equal anti-inflammatory effect with a lower dose, while at the same time enhancing the split between anti-inflammatory and mineralocorticoid activities.[1,2,3]

Glucocorticoids exert a regulatory influence on lymphocytes, erythrocytes and eosinophils of the blood and on the structure and function of lymphoid tissues.[1,4,5] A primary feature of the glucocorticoids is their anti-inflammatory activity with minimum sodium and water retention which is often associated with the mineralocorticoids.[1,2,3,4,5,6] Glucocorticoids not only inhibit early phases of the inflammatory process (edema, fibrin deposition, capillary dilatation, migration of leukocytes into the inflamed area and phagocytic activity) but also the later manifestations (capillary proliferation, fibroblast proliferation and deposition of collagen).[3,4,6] The exact mechanism is not known, but the glucocorticoids obviously suppress normal tissue response to injury and alleviate symptoms from many conditions.[2]

Dosage and Administration: The keystone of satisfactory therapeutic management with methylprednisolone, as with its steroid predecessors, is individualization of dosage in reference to the severity of the disease, the anticipated duration of steroid therapy and the animal's threshold or tolerance for steroid excess. The prime objective of steroid therapy should be to achieve a satisfactory degree of control with a minimum effective daily dose.

The dosage recommendations are suggested average total daily doses and are intended as guides. As with other orally administered corticosteroids, the total daily dose of methylprednisolone tablets should be given in equally divided doses. The initial suppressive dose level is continued until a satisfactory clinical response is obtained, a period usually of 2 to 7 days in the case of musculoskeletal diseases, allergic conditions affecting the skin or respiratory tract and ocular inflammatory diseases. If a satisfactory response is not obtained in 7 days, re-evaluation of the case to confirm the original diagnosis should be made. As soon as a satisfactory clinical response is obtained, the daily dose should be reduced gradually, either to termination of treatment in the case of acute conditions (e.g., seasonal asthma, dermatitis, acute ocular inflammations) or to the minimal effective maintenance dose level in the case of chronic conditions (e.g., rheumatoid arthritis). In chronic conditions, and in rheumatoid arthritis especially, it is important that the reduction in dosage from initial to maintenance dose levels be accomplished slowly. The maintenance dose level should be adjusted from time to time as required by fluctuation in the activity of the disease and the animal's general status. Accumulated experience has shown that the long-term benefits to be gained from continued steroid maintenance are probably greater the lower the maintenance dose level. In rheumatoid arthritis in particular, maintenance steroid therapy should be at the lowest possible level.

Important: In the therapeutic management of animals with chronic diseases, such as rheumatoid arthritis, methylprednisolone should be regarded as a highly valuable adjunct, to be used in conjunction with but not as a replacement for standard therapeutic measures.

Recommended Dosage Schedule: Average total daily doses for dogs and cats are as follows:

5 to 15 lb body wt.	2 mg
15 to 40 lb body wt.	2 to 4 mg
40 to 80 lb body wt.	4 to 8 mg

The total daily dose should be given in divided doses, 6 to 10 hours apart.

Contraindication(s): Do not use in viral infections. Methylprednisolone, like prednisolone, is contraindicated in animals with arrested tuberculosis, peptic ulcer, acute psychoses, corneal ulcer and Cushingoid syndrome. The presence of diabetes, osteoporosis, chronic psychotic reactions, predisposition to thrombophlebitis, hypertension, congestive heart failure, renal insufficiency and active tuberculosis necessitates carefully controlled use. Some of the above conditions occur only rarely in dogs and cats but should be kept in mind.

Precaution(s): Methylprednisolone, like prednisolone and other adrenocortical steroids, is a potent therapeutic agent influencing the biochemical behavior of most, if not all, tissues of the body. Because this anti-inflammatory steroid manifests little sodium-retaining activity, the usual early sign of cortisone or hydrocortisone overdosage (i.e., increase in body weight due to fluid retention) is not a reliable index of overdosage. Hence, recommended dosage levels should not be exceeded, and all animals receiving methylprednisolone should be under close medical supervision. All precautions pertinent to the use of prednisolone apply to methylprednisolone. Moreover, the veterinarian should endeavor to keep informed of current studies with methylprednisolone as they are reported in the veterinary literature.

Use of corticosteroids, depending on dose, duration and specific steroid, may result in inhibition of endogenous steroid production following drug withdrawal. In patients presently receiving or recently withdrawn from systemic corticosteroid treatments, therapy with a rapid acting corticosteroid should be considered in unusually stressful situations.

Caution(s): Federal law restricts this drug to use by or on the order of a licensed veterinarian.

For oral use in dogs and cats only.

Keep out of reach of children.

Warning(s): Because of its inhibitory effect on fibroplasia, methylprednisolone may mask the signs of infection and enhance dissemination of the infecting organism. Hence, all animals receiving methylprednisolone should be watched for evidence of intercurrent infection. Should infection occur, it must be brought under control by use of appropriate antibacterial measures and administration of methylprednisolone should be discontinued.

Not for human use. Clinical and experimental data have demonstrated that corticosteroids administered orally or parenterally to animals may induce the first stage of parturition when administered during the last trimester of pregnancy and may precipitate premature parturition followed by dystocia, fetal death, retained placenta and metritis.

Additionally, corticosteroids administered to dogs, rabbits and rodents during pregnancy have produced cleft palate. Other congenital anomalies including deformed forelegs, phocomelia and anasarca have been reported in offspring of dogs which received corticosteroids during pregnancy.

Side Effects: Methylprednisolone is similar to prednisolone in regard to kinds of side effects and metabolic alterations to be anticipated when treatment is intensive or prolonged. In animals with diabetes mellitus, use of methylprednisolone may be associated with an increase in the insulin requirement. Negative nitrogen balance may occur, particularly in animals that require protracted maintenance therapy; measures to counteract persistent nitrogen loss include a high protein intake and the administration, when indicated, of a suitable anabolic agent. Excessive loss of potassium, like excessive retention of sodium, is not likely to be induced by effective maintenance doses of methylprednisolone. However, these effects should be kept in mind and the usual regulatory measures employed as indicated. Ecchymotic manifestations, while not noted during the clinical evaluation in dogs and cats, may occur. If such reactions do occur and are serious, reduction in dosage or discontinuance of methylprednisolone therapy may be indicated. Concurrent use of daily oral supplements of ascorbic acid may be of value in helping to control ecchymotic tendencies.

Side effects, such as SAP and SGPT enzyme elevations, weight loss, anorexia, polydipsia and polyuria have occurred following the use of synthetic corticosteroids in dogs. Vomiting and diarrhea (occasionally bloody) have been observed in dogs and cats. Cushing's syndrome in dogs has been reported in association with prolonged or repeated steroid therapy.

References: Available upon request.

Presentation: Bottles of 1000 tablets.

Compendium Code No.: 10941240

METRICIDE®

Metrex **Disinfectant**

(Glutaraldehyde 2.6%) 14-Day Sterilizing & Disinfecting Solution

Active Ingredient(s):

Glutaraldehyde	2.6%
Inert ingredients:	97.4%
Total	100.0%

Indications:

1. Germicide Level of Activity: METRICIDE® Activated Dialdehyde Solution is a liquid chemical sterilant and high-level disinfectant, when used according to the "Directions for Use".

   Sterilant: METRICIDE® solution is a sterilant when used or reused, according to "Directions for Use", at full strength for a maximum of 14 days at 25°C with an immersion time of at least 10 hours.

   High-Level Disinfectant: METRICIDE® solution is a high-level disinfectant when used or reused, according to "Directions for Use", at full strength for a maximum of 14 days at 25°C with an immersion time of at least 45 minutes.

2. Reuse Period: METRICIDE® solution has also demonstrated efficacy in the presence of 2% organic soil contamination and a simulated amount of microbiological burden during reuse. METRICIDE® solution can be reused for a period not to exceed 14 days provided the required conditions of glutaraldehyde concentration, pH, and temperature exist based upon monitoring described in "Directions for Use". Do not rely solely on days in use. Efficacy of this product during its use-life must be verified by a 1.5% glutaraldehyde concentration

indicator to determine that at least the minimum effective concentration (MEC) of 1.5% glutaraldehyde is present.

3. General Information on Selection and Use of Germicides for Medical Device Reprocessing: Choose a germicide with the level of microbicidal activity that is appropriate for the reusable medical device or equipment surface. Follow the reusable device labeling and standard institutional practices. In the absence of complete instructions, use the following process: First, for patient-contacting devices, determine whether the reusable device to be reprocessed is a critical or semi-critical device.
- A critical device presents a high risk of infection if not sterile. Critical devices routinely penetrate the skin or mucous membranes during use, or are otherwise used in normally sterile tissue of the body.
- A semi-critical device makes contact with mucous membranes, but does not ordinarily penetrate normally sterile areas of the body.
Second, determine the level of germicidal activity that is needed for the reusable device.
Critical Device: Sterilization required (e.g.: products that enter sterile tissue or the vascular system, such as laparoscopes and microsurgical instruments).
Semi-critical Device: Sterilization recommended when practical, otherwise, High-Level Disinfection is acceptable (e.g.: GI endoscopes, anesthesia equipment for the airway, diaphragm-fitting rings, etc.).
Third, select a germicide that is labeled for the appropriate germicidal level and is compatible with the reusable device. Follow directions for the germicide.

4. Microbicidal Activity: The following indicates the spectrum of activity as demonstrated by testing of METRICIDE®* solution:
Bacteria:
Spores: *Bacillus subtilis, Clostridium sporogenes.*
Vegetative Organisms: *Staphylococcus aureus, Salmonella choleraesuis, Pseudomonas aeruginosa, Mycobacterium tuberculosis.*
Fungi: Trichophyton mentagrophytes.
Viruses:
Non-Enveloped: Poliovirus Types 1 and 2, Rhinovirus Type 14, Adenovirus Type 2, Vaccinia.
Enveloped: Cytomegalovirus, Influenza virus Type A_2HK, HIV-1 (AIDS Virus), Herpes simplex Types 1 and 2.
*Testing was done after 14 days of simulated reuse using prescribed testing methods.

5. Material Compatibility: METRICIDE® is compatible with the following reusable devices and materials: Rigid and flexible endoscopes, respiratory therapy equipment, anesthesia equipment, rubber, most stainless steel instruments, plastic, most dental instruments (not including dental handpieces), many types of metals, such as stainless steel, carbon steel, and aluminum, and plated metals such as nickel plating or chrome plating.
For a listing of specific device manufacturers that have reported device compatibility with METRICIDE®, see Table 1 below.
Table 1. Manufacturers Reporting Device Compatibility with METRICIDE®:

Company	Instrumentation
Acoustic Imaging	Transducers
Acuson Computed Sonography	Biplane Tranesophageal and External Transducers
Bard Interventional Products	Automatic Endoscope Washers (Models 000187, 000387, and 000487)
Circon - ACMI	Cystoscopes
Hewlett Packard	Omniplane TEE Probe
Instrumentation Industries	Plastics used in Respiratory Therapy
Medivators, Inc.	Automatic Endoscope Washers
Olympus Corporation	Olympus Flexible Endoscopes
Pentax Precision Instrument Corporation	Upper GI Fiberscopes
Pilling Surgical Instruments	Rubber Bougies
Karl Storz	Rigid Cystoscopes
Welch Allyn	Flexible Sigmoidoscopes

Please refer to labeling of the reusable device for additional instructions, or call the reusable device manufacturer directly.

Please Note: METRICIDE® is incompatible with the following reusable devices and materials: Type IV dental stone impression material and Heidbrink Expiratory Valve.

6. Precleaning Agent Compatibility: METRICIDE® solution is compatible with enzymatic detergents which are mild in pH, low foaming, and easily rinsed from equipment. Detergents that are either highly acidic or alkaline are contraindicated as precleaning agents since improper rinsing could affect the efficacy of the METRICIDE® solution by altering their pH.

Directions for Use: It is a violation of Federal Law to use this product in a manner inconsistent with its labeling.

Note: Contents of the attached vial must be added to solution before this product is effective.

1. Activation: Activate the METRICIDE® solution by adding the entire contents of the Activator 14 activator vial which is attached to the METRICIDE® solution container. Shake well. Activated solution immediately changes color to green, thereby indicating solution is ready to use. METRICIDE® solution is intended for use in manual (bucket and tray) systems made from polypropylene, ABS, polyethylene, glass-filled polypropylene or specially molded polycarbonate plastics. Record the date of activation (mixing date) and expiration date on the METRICIDE® solution container label in the space provided, in a log book, or on a label affixed to any secondary container used for the activated solution.
2. Cleaning/Decontamination: Blood and other body fluids must be thoroughly cleaned from surfaces, lumens, and objects before application of the disinfectant or sterilant. Blood and other body fluids should be autoclaved and disposed of according to all applicable federal, state and local regulations for infectious waste disposal.
For complete disinfection or sterilization of medical instruments and equipment, thoroughly clean, rinse and rough dry objects before immersing in METRICIDE® solution. Cleanse and rinse the lumens of hollow instruments before filling with METRICIDE® solution. Refer to the reusable device manufacturer's labeling far additional instructions on disassembly, decontamination, cleaning and leak testing of their equipment.
3. Usage: It is a violation of Federal Law to use this product in a manner inconsistent with its labeling.
   a. Sterilization (Bucket/Tray Manual System): Immerse medical equipment/device completely in METRICIDE® solution for a minimum of 10 hours at 25°C to eliminate all microorganisms including *Clostridium sporogenes* and *Bacillus subtilis* spores. Remove equipment from the solution using sterile technique and rinse thoroughly with sterile water following the rinsing instructions below.
   b. High-Level Disinfection (Bucket/Tray Manual System): Immerse medical equipment/device completely in METRICIDE® solution for a minimum of 45 minutes at 25°C to destroy all pathogenic microorganisms, except for large numbers of bacterial endospores, but including *Mycobacterium tuberculosis* (Quantitative TB Method). Remove devices and equipment from the solution and rinse thoroughly following the rinsing instructions below.
   c. Rinsing Instructions: Following immersion in METRICIDE® solution, thoroughly rinse the equipment or medical device by immersing it completely in three separate copious volumes of water. Each rinse should be a minimum of one minute in duration unless otherwise noted by the device or equipment manufacturer. Use fresh portions of water for each rinse. Discard the water following each rinse. Do not reuse the water for rinsing or any other purpose, as it will be contaminated with glutaraldehyde.
   Refer to the reusable device/equipment manufacturer's labeling for additional rinsing instructions.
   Sterile Water Rinse: The following devices should be rinsed with sterile water, using sterile technique when rinsing and handling.
   1. Devices intended for use in normally sterile areas of the body;
   2. Devices intended for use in known immunocompromised patients, or potentially immunocompromised patients based on institutional procedures (e.g.: high risk population served) and;
   3. When practicable, bronchoscopes, due to a risk of atypical *Mycobacteria* contamination from potable water supply.
   Potable Water Rinse: For all other devices a sterile water rinse is recommended when practicable, otherwise a high-quality potable tap water rinse is acceptable. A high-quality potable water is one that meets Federal Clean Water Standards at the point of use. When using potable water for rinsing, the user should be aware of the increased risk of recontaminating the device or medical equipment with *Pseudomonas* and atypical (fast growing) *Mycobacteria* often present in potable water supplies. A device (e.g.: colonoscope) that is not completely dried provides an ideal situation for rapid colonization of bacteria. Additionally, *Mycobacteria* are highly resistant to drying; therefore, rapid drying will avoid possible colonization but may not result in a device free from atypical *Mycobacteria*. Although these bacteria are not normally pathogenic in patients with healthy immune systems. AIDS patients or other immunocompromised individuals may be placed at high risk of infection by these opportunistic microorganisms. A final rinse using a 70% isopropyl alcohol solution is useful to speed the drying process and reduce the numbers of any organism present as a result of rinsing with potable water.
   d. Reusage: METRICIDE® solution has also demonstrated efficacy in the presence of 2% organic soil contamination and a simulated amount of microbiological burden during reuse. This solution may be used and reused within the limitations indicated above for up to 14 days after activation. Do not use activated solution beyond 14 days. Efficacy of this product during its use-life must be verified by a 1.5% glutaraldehyde concentration indicator to determine that the minimum effective concentration (MEC) of 1.5% is present.
4. Monitoring of Germicide to Ensure Specifications are Met: During the usage of METRICIDE® solution, as a high-level disinfectant and/or sterilant, it is recommended that a thermometer and timer be utilized to ensure that the optimum usage conditions are met. In addition, it is recommended that the METRICIDE® solution be tested with a 1.5% glutaraldehyde concentration indicator prior to each usage. This is to ensure that the appropriate concentration of glutaraldehyde is present and to guard against a dilution which may lower the effectiveness of the solution below its MEC. The pH of the activated solution may also be periodically checked to verify that the pH of the solution is between 7.5 and 8.5.
5. Post-Processing Handling and Storage of Reusable Devices: Sterilized or disinfected reusable devices are either to be immediately used or stored in a manner to minimize recontamination. Note that only terminal sterilization (sterilization in a suitable wrap) provides maximum assurance against recontamination. Refer to the reusable device-equipment manufacturer's labeling for additional storage and/or handling instructions.

User Proficiency: It is a violation of Federal Law to use this product in a manner inconsistent with its labeling. The user should be adequately trained in the decontamination and disinfection or sterilization of medical devices and the handling of toxic substances such as liquid chemical germicides.

Contraindication(s):

1. Sterilant Usage: Routine biological monitoring is not feasible with METRICIDE® solution, and therefore, this solution should not be used to sterilize reusable medical devices that are compatible with other available methods of sterilization that can be biologically monitored, e.g.: heat, ethylene oxide, or peroxide gas plasma. METRICIDE® solution should not be used for sterilization of critical devices intended for single use (e.g.: catheters).
2. High-Level Disinfectant Usage: METRICIDE® solution should not be used to high-level disinfect a semi-critical device when sterilization is practical.
3. Endoscope Usage: METRICIDE® solution is not the method of choice for sterilization of rigid endoscopes which the device manufacturer indicates is compatible with steam sterilization. In general, glutaraldehyde solutions that do not contain surfactants (e.g.: METRICIDE® solution) are more appropriate for flexible endoscopes, because glutaraldehyde solutions containing surfactants (e.g.: MetriCide® 28 and MetriCide Plus 30® solutions) are more difficult to rinse from the devices. However, these surfactant containing disinfectants may be used for reprocessing of flexible endoscopes if a validated protocol for rinsing and leak testing is employed.

Storage and Disposal: Storage Conditions and Expiration Date:

1. Prior to activation, METRICIDE® solution should be stored in its original sealed container at room temperature. Once the METRICIDE® solution has been activated, it should be stored in the original container until transferred to the containers in which the immersion for disinfection or sterilization is to take place. Containers should be stored in a well-ventilated, low traffic area at room temperature.
2. The expiration date of the unactivated METRICIDE® solution will be found on the immediate container.
3. The use period for activated METRICIDE® solution is for no longer than 14 days following activation or as indicated by a 1.5% glutaraldehyde concentration indicator. Once activated, the solution requires no further dilution prior to its usage.

Disposal Information:

Germicide Disposal: Discard residual solution in drain. Flush thoroughly with water.

Container Disposal:

One Quart (946 mL) and One Gallon (3.8 L) Size Containers: Do not reuse empty container. Wrap container and put in trash.

Caution(s):

1. Protective gloves (butyl rubber, nitrile rubber, polyethylene or double-gloved latex), eye protection, face masks, and liquid-proof gowns should be warn when cleaning and sterilizing/disinfecting soiled devices and equipment.

2. Contaminatedc reusable devices must be thoroughly cleaned prior to disinfection or sterilization, because residual contamination will decrease effectiveness of the germicide.
3. The user must adhere to the "Directions for Use", because any modification will affect the safety and effectiveness of the germicide.
4. The reusable device manufacturer should provide the user with a validated reprocessing procedure for that device using METRICIDE® solution.
5. The use of METRICIDE® solution in automated endoscope washers must be part of a validated reprocessing procedure provided by the washer manufacturer. Contact the manufacturer of the endoscope washer for instructions on the maximum number of reprocessing cycles which may be used before refilling with fresh METRICIDE® solution. Use a 1.5% glutaraldehyde concentration indicator to monitor glutaraldehyde concentration before each cycle to detect unexpected dilution.

Warning(s): METRICIDE® Activated Dialdehyde Solution is hazardous to humans and domestic animals.

Danger: Keep out of reach of children. Contains glutaraldehyde.

1. Direct contact is corrosive to exposed tissue, causing eye damage and skin irritation/damage. Do not get into eyes, on skin, or on clothing.
2. Avoid contamination of food.
3. Use in well-ventilated area in closed containers.

In case of contact, immediately flush eyes or skin with plenty of water for at least 15 minutes. For eyes, get medical attention.
Harmful if swallowed. Drink large quantities of water and call a physician immediately. Probable mucosal damage from oral exposure may contraindicate the use of gastric lavage.
Emergency, safety, or technical information about METRICIDE® solution can be obtained from Metrex Research Corporation Customer Care Department at 1-800-841-1428, or by contacting your local Metrex Research Corporation sales representative.

References: Available upon request.

Presentation: 16 x 1 qt (946 mL) bottles per case and 4 x 1 gallon (128 fl oz) (3.8 L) bottles per case.

Compendium Code No.: 13400071 1001-13

METRICIDE® 28

Metrex **Disinfectant**

(Glutaraldehyde 2.5%) 28-Day Sterilizing & Disinfecting Solution

Active Ingredient(s):

Glutaraldehyde 2.5%
Inert ingredients: 97.5%
Total 100.0%

Contains sodium nitrite as a corrosion inhibitor.

Indications:

1. Germicide Level of Activity: METRICIDE® 28 Long-Life Activated Dialdehyde Solution is a liquid chemical sterilant and high-level disinfectant, when used according to the "Directions for Use".

Sterilant: METRICIDE® 28 solution is a sterilant when used or reused, according to "Directions for Use", at full strength for a maximum of 28 days at 25°C with an immersion time of at least 10 hours.

High-Level Disinfectant: METRICIDE® 28 solution is a high-level disinfectant when used or reused, according to "Directions for Use", at full strength for a maximum of 28 days at 25°C with an immersion time of at least 90 minutes.

M

2. Reuse Period: METRICIDE® 28 solution has also demonstrated efficacy in the presence of 2% organic soil contamination and a simulated amount of microbiological burden during reuse. METRICIDE® 28 solution can be reused for a period not to exceed 28 days provided the required conditions of glutaraldehyde concentration, pH, and temperature exist based upon monitoring described in "Directions for Use". Do not rely solely on days in use. Efficacy of this product during its use-life must be verified by a 1.8% glutaraldehyde concentration indicator to determine that at least the minimum effective concentration (MEC) of 1.8% glutaraldehyde is present.
3. General Information on Selection and Use of Germicides for Medical Device Reprocessing: Choose a germicide with the level of microbicidal activity that is appropriate for the reusable medical device or equipment surface. Follow the reusable device labeling and standard institutional practices. In the absence of complete instructions, use the following process:
First, for patient-contacting devices, determine whether the reusable device to be reprocessed is a critical or semi-critical device.
- A critical device presents a high risk of infection if not sterile. Critical devices routinely penetrate the skin or mucous membranes during use, or are otherwise used in normally sterile tissue of the body.
- A semi-critical device makes contact with mucous membranes, but does not ordinarily penetrate normally sterile areas of the body.
Second, determine the level of germicidal activity that is needed for the reusable device.
Critical Device: Sterilization required (e.g.: products that enter sterile tissue or the vascular system, such as laparoscopes and microsurgical instruments).
Semi-critical Device: Sterilization recommended when practical, otherwise, High-Level Disinfection is acceptable (e.g.: GI endoscopes, anesthesia equipment for the airway. diaphragm-fitting rings, etc.).
Third, select a germicide that is labeled for the appropriate germicidal level and is compatible with the reusable device. Follow directions for the germicide.
4. Microbicidal Activity: The following indicates the spectrum of activity as demonstrated by testing of METRICIDE® 28* solution:
Bacteria:
Spores: *Bacillus subtilis, Clostridium sporogenes.*
Vegetative Organisms: *Staphylococcus aureus, Salmonella choleraesuis, Pseudomonas aeruginosa, Mycobacterium tuberculosis.*
Fungi: Trichophyton mentagrophytes.
Viruses:
Non-Enveloped: Poliovirus Types 1 and 2, Rhinovirus Type 14, Adenovirus Type 2, Vaccinia, Coxsackievirus B5a.
Enveloped: Cytomegalovirus, Influenza virus Type A_2HK, HIV-1 (AIDS Virus), Herpes simplex Types 1 and 2.

*Testing was done after 28 days of simulated reuse using prescribed testing methods.

5. Material Compatibility: METRICIDE® 28 is compatible with the following reusable devices and materials: Respiratory therapy equipment, anesthesia equipment, rubber, most stainless steel instruments, plastic, most dental instruments (not including dental handpieces), many types of metals, such as stainless steel, carbon steel, and aluminum, and plated metals such as nickel plating or chrome plating.

For a listing of specific device manufacturers that have reported device compatibility with METRICIDE® 28, see Table 1 below.

Table 1. Manufacturers Reporting Device Compatibility with METRICIDE® 28:

Company	Instrumentation
Acoustic Imaging	Transducers
Advanced Technology Lab	Ultrasound Scanheads
Hewlett Packard	Omniplane TEE Probe
Instrumentation Industries	Respiratory Therapy Equipment

Please refer to labeling of the reusable device for additional instructions, or call the reusable device manufacturer directly.

Please Note: METRICIDE® 28 is incompatible with the following specific reusable devices: Acuson V510B transesophageal transducers, high-frequency cables, coagulating forceps, resectoscope instruments, and devices that have the potential for electrosurgical malfunctioning.

6. Precleaning Agent Compatibility: METRICIDE® 28 solution is compatible with enzymatic detergents which are mild in pH, low foaming, and easily rinsed from equipment. Detergents that are either highly acidic or alkaline are contraindicated as precleaning agents since improper rinsing could affect the efficacy of the METRICIDE® 28 solution by altering its pH.

Directions for Use: It is a violation of Federal Law to use this product in a manner inconsistent with its labeling.

Note: Contents of the attached vial must be added to solution before this product is effective.

1. Activation: Activate the METRICIDE® 28 solution by adding the entire contents of the Activator Plus activator vial which is attached to the METRICIDE® 28 solution container. Shake well. Activated solution immediately changes color to bluish-green, thereby indicating solution is ready to use. METRICIDE® 28 solution is intended for use in manual (bucket and tray) systems made from polypropylene, ABS, polyethylene, glass-filled polypropylene or specially molded polycarbonate plastics. Record the date of activation (mixing date) and expiration date on the solution container label in the space provided, in a log book, or on a label affixed to any secondary container used for the activated solution.
2. Cleaning/Decontamination: Blood and other body fluids must be thoroughly cleaned from surfaces, lumens, and objects before application of the disinfectant or sterilant. Blood and other body fluids should be autoclaved and disposed of according to all applicable federal, state and local regulations for infectious waste disposal.
For complete disinfection or sterilization of medical instruments and equipment, thoroughly clean, rinse and rough dry objects before immersing in METRICIDE® 28 solution. Cleanse and rinse the lumens of hollow instruments before filling with METRICIDE® 28 solution. Refer to the reusable device manufacturer's labeling for additional instructions on disassembly, decontamination, cleaning and leak testing of their equipment.
3. Usage: It is a violation of Federal Law to use this product in a manner inconsistent with its labeling.
   a. Sterilization (Bucket/Tray Manual System): Immerse medical equipment/device completely in METRICIDE® 28 solution for a minimum of 10 hours at 25°C to eliminate all microorganisms including *Clostridium sporogenes* and *Bacillus subtilis* spores. Remove equipment from the solution using sterile technique and rinse thoroughly with sterile water following the rinsing instructions below.
   b. High-Level Disinfection (Bucket/Tray Manual System): Immerse medical equipment/device completely in METRICIDE® 28 solution for a minimum of 90 minutes at 25°C to destroy all pathogenic microorganisms, except for large numbers of bacterial endospores, but including *Mycobacterium tuberculosis* (Quantitative TB Method). Remove devices and equipment from the solution and rinse thoroughly following the rinsing instructions below.
   c. Rinsing Instructions: Following immersion in METRICIDE® 28 solution, thoroughly rinse the equipment or medical device by immersing it completely in three separate copious volumes of water. Each rinse should be a minimum of one minute in duration unless otherwise noted by the device or equipment manufacturer. Use fresh portions of water for each rinse. Discard the water following each rinse. Do not reuse the water for rinsing or any other purpose, as it will be contaminated with glutaraldehyde.
   Refer to the reusable device/equipment manufacturer's labeling for additional rinsing instructions.
   Sterile Water Rinse: The following devices should be rinsed with sterile water, using sterile technique when rinsing and handling.
   1. Devices intended for use in normally sterile areas of the body;
   2. Devices intended for use in known immunocompromised patients, or potentially immunocompromised patients based on institutional procedures (e.g.: high risk population served) and;
   3. When practicable, bronchoscopes, due to a risk of atypical *Mycobacteria* contamination from potable water supply.
   Potable Water Rinse: For all other devices a sterile water rinse is recommended when practicable, otherwise a high-quality potable tap water rinse is acceptable. A high-quality potable water is one that meets Federal Clean Water Standards at the point of use. When using potable water for rinsing, the user should be aware of the increased risk of recontaminating the device or medical equipment with *Pseudomonas* and atypical (fast growing) *Mycobacteria* often present in potable water supplies. A device (e.g.: colonoscope) that is not completely dried provides an ideal situation for rapid colonization of bacteria. Additionally, *Mycobacteria* are highly resistant to drying; therefore, rapid drying will avoid possible colonization but may not result in a device free from atypical *Mycobacteria.* Although these bacteria are not normally pathogenic in patients with healthy immune systems, AIDS patients or other immunocompromised individuals may be placed at high risk of infection by these opportunistic microorganisms. A final rinse using a 70% isopropyl alcohol solution is useful to speed the drying process and reduce the numbers of any organism present as a result of rinsing with potable water.
   d. Reusage: METRICIDE® 28 solution has also demonstrated efficacy in the presence of 2% organic soil contamination and a simulated amount of microbiological burden during reuse. These solutions may be used and reused within the limitations indicated above for up to 28 days after activation. Do not use activated solution beyond 28 days. Efficacy of this product during its use-life must be verified by a 1.8% glutaraldehyde concentration indicator to determine that the minimum effective concentration (MEC) of 1.8% is present.
4. Monitoring of Germicide to Ensure Specifications are Met: During the usage of METRICIDE® 28 solution, as a high-level disinfectant and/or sterilant, it is recommended that a thermometer and timer be utilized to ensure that the optimum usage conditions are met. In addition, it is recommended that the METRICIDE® 28 solution be tested with a 1.8%

glutaraldehyde concentration indicator prior to each usage. This is to ensure that the appropriate concentration of glutaraldehyde is present and to guard against a dilution which may lower the effectiveness of the solution below its MEC. The pH of the activated solution may also be periodically checked to verify that the pH of the solution is between 7.5 and 8.5.

5. Post-Processing Handling and Storage of Reusable Devices: Sterilized or disinfected reusable devices are either to be immediately used or stored in a manner to minimize recontamination. Note that only terminal sterilization (sterilization in a suitable wrap) provides maximum assurance against recontamination. Refer to the reusable device-equipment manufacturer's labeling for additional storage and/or handling instructions.

User Proficiency: It is a violation of Federal Law to use this product in a manner inconsistent with its labeling. The user should be adequately trained in the decontamination and disinfection or sterilization of medical devices and the handling of toxic substances such as liquid chemical germicides.

Contraindication(s):

1. Sterilant Usage: Routine biological monitoring is not feasible with METRICIDE® 28 solution, and therefore, this solution should not be used to sterilize reusable medical devices that are compatible with other available methods of sterilization that can be biologically monitored. e.g.: heat, ethylene oxide, or peroxide gas plasma. METRICIDE® 28 solution should not be used for sterilization of critical devices intended for single use (e.g.: catheters).
2. High-Level Disinfectant Usage: METRICIDE® 28 solution should not be used to high-level disinfect a semi-critical device when sterilization is practical.
3. Endoscope Usage: METRICIDE® 28 solution is not the method of choice for sterilization of rigid endoscopes which the device manufacturer indicates is compatible with steam sterilization. In general, glutaraldehyde solutions that do not contain surfactants (e.g.: MetriCide® solution) are more appropriate for flexible endoscopes, because glutaraldehyde solutions containing surfactants (e.g.: METRICIDE® 28 and MetriCide Plus 30® solutions) are more difficult to rinse from the devices. However, these surfactant-containing disinfectants may be used for reprocessing of flexible endoscopes if a validated protocol for rinsing and leak testing is employed.

Storage and Disposal: Storage Conditions and Expiration Date:

1. Prior to activation, METRICIDE® 28 solution should be stored in its original sealed container at room temperature. Once the METRICIDE® 28 solution has been activated, it should be stored in the original container until transferred to the containers in which the immersion for disinfection or sterilization is to take place. Containers should be stored in a well-ventilated, low traffic area at room temperature.
2. The expiration date of the unactivated METRICIDE® 28 solution will be found on the immediate container.
3. The use period for activated METRICIDE® 28 solution is for no longer than 28 days following activation or as indicated by a 1.8% glutaraldehyde concentration indicator. Once activated, the solution requires no further dilution prior to its usage.

Disposal Information:

Germicide Disposal: Discard residual solution in drain. Flush thoroughly with water.

Container Disposal:

One Quart (946 mL) and One Gallon (3.8 L) Size Containers: Do not reuse empty container. Wrap container and put in trash.

Caution(s):

1. Protective gloves (butyl rubber, nitrile rubber, polyethylene or double-gloved latex), eye protection, face masks, and liquid-proof gowns should be worn when cleaning and sterilizing/disinfecting soiled devices and equipment.
2. Contaminated, reusable devices must be thoroughly cleaned prior to disinfection or sterilization, because residual contamination will decrease effectiveness of the germicide.
3. The user must adhere to the "Directions for Use", because any modification will affect the safety and effectiveness of the germicide.
4. The reusable device manufacturer should provide the user with a validated reprocessing procedure for that device using METRICIDE® 28 solution.
5. The use of METRICIDE® 28 solution in automated endoscope washers must be part of a validated reprocessing procedure provided by the washer manufacturer. Contact the manufacturer of the endoscope washer for instructions on the maximum number of reprocessing cycles which may be used before refilling with fresh METRICIDE® 28 solution. Use a 1.8% glutaraldehyde concentration indicator to monitor glutaraldehyde concentration before each cycle to detect unexpected dilution.

Warning(s): METRICIDE® 28 Activated Dialdehyde Solution is hazardous to humans and domestic animals.

Danger: Keep out of reach of children. Contains glutaraldehyde.

1. Direct contact is corrosive to exposed tissue, causing eye damage and skin irritation/damage. Do not get into eyes, on skin, or on clothing.
2. Avoid contamination of food.
3. Use in well-ventilated area in closed containers.

In case of contact, immediately flush eyes or skin with plenty of water for at least 15 minutes. For eyes, get medical attention.

Harmful if swallowed. Drink large quantities of water and call a physician immediately. Probable mucosal damage from oral exposure may contraindicate the use of gastric lavage. Emergency, safety, or technical information about METRICIDE® 28 solution can be obtained from Metrex Research Corporation Customer Care Department at 1-800-841-1428, or by contacting your local Metrex Research Corporation sales representative.

References: Available upon request.

Presentation: 16 x 1 qt (946 mL) bottles per case and 4 x 1 gallon (128 fl oz) (3.8 L) bottles per case.

Compendium Code No.: 13400080 2000-14

METRICIDE PLUS 30®

Metrex **Disinfectant**

(Glutaraldehyde 3.4%) 28-Day Sterilizing & Disinfecting Solution

Active Ingredient(s):

Glutaraldehyde 3.4%
Inert ingredients: 96.6%
Total 100.0%

Contains sodium nitrite as a corrosion inhibitor.

Indications:

1. Germicide Level of Activity: METRICIDE PLUS 30® Long-Life Activated Dialdehyde Solution is a liquid chemical sterilant and high-level disinfectant, when used according to the "Directions for Use".

Sterilant: METRICIDE PLUS 30® solution is a sterilant when used or reused, according to "Directions for Use", at full strength for a maximum of 28 days at 25°C with an immersion time of at least 10 hours.

High-Level Disinfectant: METRICIDE PLUS 30® solution is a high-level disinfectant when used or reused, according to "Directions for Use", at full strength for a maximum of 28 days at 25°C with an immersion time of at least 90 minutes.

2. Reuse Period: METRICIDE PLUS 30® solution has also demonstrated efficacy in the presence of 2% organic soil contamination and a simulated amount of microbiological burden during reuse. METRICIDE PLUS 30® solution can be reused for a period not to exceed 28 days provided the required conditions of glutaraldehyde concentration, pH, and temperature exist based upon monitoring described in "Directions for Use". Do not rely solely on days in use. Efficacy of this product during its use-life must be verified by a 1.8% glutaraldehyde concentration indicator to determine that at least the minimum effective concentration (MEC) of 1.8% glutaraldehyde is present.
3. General Information on Selection and Use of Germicides for Medical Device Reprocessing: Choose a germicide with the level of microbicidal activity that is appropriate for the reusable medical device or equipment surface. Follow the reusable device labeling and standard institutional practices. In the absence of complete instructions, use the following process: First, for patient-contacting devices, determine whether the reusable device to be reprocessed is a critical or semi-critical device.

   - A critical device presents a high risk of infection if not sterile. Critical devices routinely penetrate the skin or mucous membranes during use, or are otherwise used in normally sterile tissue of the body.
   - A semi-critical device makes contact with mucous membranes, but does not ordinarily penetrate normally sterile areas of the body.

   Second, determine the level of germicidal activity that is needed for the reusable device.
   Critical Device: Sterilization required (e.g.: products that enter sterile tissue or the vascular system, such as laparoscopes and microsurgical instruments).
   Semi-critical Device: Sterilization recommended when practical, otherwise, High-Level Disinfection is acceptable (e.g.: GI endoscopes, anesthesia equipment for the airway, diaphragm-fitting rings, etc.).
   Third, select a germicide that is labeled for the appropriate germicidal level and is compatible with the reusable device. Follow directions for the germicide.
4. Microbicidal Activity: The following indicates the spectrum of activity as demonstrated by testing of METRICIDE PLUS 30®* solution:
   Bacteria:
   Spores: *Bacillus subtilis, Clostridium sporogenes.*
   Vegetative Organisms: *Staphylococcus aureus, Salmonella choleraesuis, Pseudomonas aeruginosa, Mycobacterium tuberculosis.*
   Fungi: Trichophyton mentagrophytes.
   Viruses:
   Non-Enveloped: Poliovirus Types 1 and 2, Rhinovirus Type 14, Adenovirus Type 2, Vaccinia, Coxsackievirus B5a.
   Enveloped: Cytomegalovirus, Influenza virus Type A_2HK, HIV-1 (AIDS Virus), Herpes simplex Types 1 and 2.

*Testing was done after 28 days of simulated reuse using prescribed testing methods.

5. Material Compatibility: METRICIDE PLUS 30® is compatible with the following reusable devices and materials: Respiratory therapy equipment, anesthesia equipment, rubber, most stainless steel instruments, plastic, most dental instruments (not including dental handpieces), many types of metals, such as stainless steel, carbon steel, and aluminum, and plated metals such as nickel plating or chrome plating.

For a listing of specific device manufacturers that have reported device compatibility with METRICIDE PLUS 30®, see Table 1 below.

Table 1. Manufacturers Reporting Device Compatibility with METRICIDE PLUS 30®:

Company	Instrumentation
Acoustic Imaging	Transducers
Advanced Technology Lab	Ultrasound Scanheads
Hewlett Packard	Omniplane TEE Probe
Instrumentation Industries	Respiratory Therapy Equipment

Please refer to labeling of the reusable device for additional instructions, or call the reusable device manufacturer directly.

Please Note: METRICIDE PLUS 30® is incompatible with the following specific reusable devices: Acuson V510B transesophageal transducers, high-frequency cables, coagulating forceps, resectoscope instruments, and devices that have the potential for electrosurgical malfunctioning.

6. Precleaning Agent Compatibility: METRICIDE PLUS 30® solution is compatible with enzymatic detergents which are mild in pH, low foaming, and easily rinsed from equipment. Detergents that are either highly acidic or alkaline are contraindicated as precleaning agents since improper rinsing could affect the efficacy of the METRICIDE PLUS 30® solution by altering its pH.

Directions for Use: It is a violation of Federal Law to use this product in a manner inconsistent with its labeling.

Note: Contents of the attached vial must be added to solution before this product is effective.

1. Activation: Activate the METRICIDE PLUS 30® solution by adding the entire contents of the Activator Plus activator vial which is attached to the METRICIDE PLUS 30® solution container. Shake well. Activated solution immediately changes color to bluish-green, thereby indicating solution is ready to use. METRICIDE PLUS 30® solution is intended for use in manual (bucket and tray) systems made from polypropylene, ABS, polyethylene, glass-filled polypropylene or specially molded polycarbonate plastics. Record the date of activation (mixing date) and expiration date on the solution container label in the space provided, in a log book, or on a label affixed to any secondary container used for the activated solution.
2. Cleaning/Decontamination: Blood and other body fluids must be thoroughly cleaned from surfaces, lumens, and objects before application of the disinfectant or sterilant. Blood and other body fluids should be autoclaved and disposed of according to all applicable federal, state and local regulations for infectious waste disposal.
   For complete disinfection or sterilization of medical instruments and equipment, thoroughly clean, rinse and rough dry objects before immersing in METRICIDE PLUS 30® solution. Cleanse and rinse the lumens of hollow instruments before filling with METRICIDE PLUS 30® solution. Refer to the reusable device manufacturer's labeling for additional instructions on disassembly, decontamination, cleaning and leak testing of their equipment.
3. Usage: It is a violation of Federal Law to use this product in a manner inconsistent with its labeling.
   a. Sterilization (Bucket/Tray Manual System): Immerse medical equipment/device completely in METRICIDE PLUS 30® solution for a minimum of 10 hours at 25°C to

M

eliminate all microorganisms including *Clostridium sporogenes* and *Bacillus subtilis* spores. Remove equipment from the solution using sterile technique and rinse thoroughly with sterile water following the rinsing instructions below.

b. High-Level Disinfection (Bucket/Tray Manual System): Immerse medical equipment/device completely in METRICIDE PLUS 30® solution for a minimum of 90 minutes at 25°C to destroy all pathogenic microorganisms, except for large numbers of bacterial endospores, but including *Mycobacterium tuberculosis* (Quantitative TB Method). Remove devices and equipment from the solution and rinse thoroughly following the rinsing instructions below.

c. Rinsing Instructions: Following immersion in METRICIDE PLUS 30® solution, thoroughly rinse the equipment or medical device by immersing it completely in three separate copious volumes of water. Each rinse should be a minimum of one minute in duration unless otherwise noted by the device or equipment manufacturer. Use fresh portions of water for each rinse. Discard the water following each rinse. Do not reuse the water for rinsing or any other purpose, as it will be contaminated with glutaraldehyde. Refer to the reusable device/equipment manufacturer's labeling for additional rinsing instructions.

Sterile Water Rinse: The following devices should be rinsed with sterile water, using sterile technique when rinsing and handling.

1. Devices intended for use in normally sterile areas of the body;
2. Devices intended for use in known immunocompromised patients, or potentially immunocompromised patients based on institutional procedures (e.g.: high risk population served) and;
3. When practicable, bronchoscopes, due to a risk of atypical *Mycobacteria* contamination from potable water supply.

Potable Water Rinse: For all other devices a sterile water rinse is recommended when practicable, otherwise a high-quality potable tap water rinse is acceptable. A high-quality potable water is one that meets Federal Clean Water Standards at the point of use. When using potable water for rinsing, the user should be aware of the increased risk of recontaminating the device or medical equipment with *Pseudomonas* and atypical (fast growing) *Mycobacteria* often present in potable water supplies. A device (e.g.: colonoscope) that is not completely dried provides an ideal situation for rapid colonization of bacteria. Additionally, *Mycobacteria* are highly resistant to drying; therefore, rapid drying will avoid possible colonization but may not result in a device free from atypical *Mycobacteria*. Although these bacteria are not normally pathogenic in patients with healthy immune systems, AIDS patients or other immunocompromised individuals may be placed at high risk of infection by these opportunistic microorganisms. A final rinse using a 70% isopropyl alcohol solution is useful to speed the drying process and reduce the numbers of any organism present as a result of rinsing with potable water.

d. Reusage: METRICIDE PLUS 30® solution has also demonstrated efficacy in the presence of 2% organic soil contamination and a simulated amount of microbiological burden during reuse. These solutions may be used and reused within the limitations indicated above for up to 28 days after activation. Do not use activated solution beyond 28 days. Efficacy of this product during its use-life must be verified by a 1.8% glutaraldehyde concentration indicator to determine that the minimum effective concentration (MEC) of 1.8% is present.

4. Monitoring of Germicide to Ensure Specifications are Met: During the usage of METRICIDE PLUS 30® solution, as a high-level disinfectant and/or sterilant, it is recommended that a thermometer and timer be utilized to ensure that the optimum usage conditions are met. In addition, it is recommended that the METRICIDE PLUS 30® solution be tested with a 1.8% glutaraldehyde concentration indicator prior to each usage. This is to ensure that the appropriate concentration of glutaraldehyde is present and to guard against a dilution which may lower the effectiveness of the solution below its MEC. The pH of the activated solution may also be periodically checked to verify that the pH of the solution is between 7.5 and 8.5.
5. Post-Processing Handling and Storage of Reusable Devices: Sterilized or disinfected reusable devices are either to be immediately used or stored in a manner to minimize recontamination. Note that only terminal sterilization (sterilization in a suitable wrap) provides maximum assurance against recontamination. Refer to the reusable device-equipment manufacturer's labeling for additional storage and/or handling instructions.

User Proficiency: It is a violation of Federal Law to use this product in a manner inconsistent with its labeling. The user should be adequately trained in the decontamination and disinfection or sterilization of medical devices and the handling of toxic substances such as liquid chemical germicides.

Contraindication(s):

1. Sterilant Usage: Routine biological monitoring is not feasible with METRICIDE PLUS 30® solution, and therefore, this solution should not be used to sterilize reusable medical devices that are compatible with other available methods of sterilization that can be biologically monitored. e.g.: heat, ethylene oxide, or peroxide gas plasma. METRICIDE PLUS 30® solution should not be used for sterilization of critical devices intended for single use (e.g.: catheters).
2. High-Level Disinfectant Usage: METRICIDE PLUS 30® solution should not be used to high-level disinfect a semi-critical device when sterilization is practical.
3. Endoscope Usage: METRICIDE PLUS 30® solution is not the method of choice for sterilization of rigid endoscopes which the device manufacturer indicates is compatible with steam sterilization. In general, glutaraldehyde solutions that do not contain surfactants (e.g.: MetriCide® solution) are more appropriate for flexible endoscopes, because glutaraldehyde solutions containing surfactants (e.g.: MetriCide® 28 and METRICIDE PLUS 30® solutions) are more difficult to rinse from the devices. However, these surfactant-containing disinfectants may be used for reprocessing of flexible endoscopes if a validated protocol for rinsing and leak testing is employed.

Storage and Disposal: Storage Conditions and Expiration Date:

1. Prior to activation, METRICIDE PLUS 30® solution should be stored in its original sealed container at room temperature. Once the METRICIDE PLUS 30® solution has been activated, it should be stored in the original container until transferred to the containers in which the immersion for disinfection or sterilization is to take place. Containers should be stored in a well-ventilated, low traffic area at room temperature.
2. The expiration date of the unactivated METRICIDE PLUS 30® solution will be found on the immediate container.
3. The use period for activated METRICIDE PLUS 30® solution is for no longer than 28 days following activation or as indicated by a 1.8% glutaraldehyde concentration indicator. Once activated, the solution requires no further dilution prior to its usage.

Disposal Information:

Germicide Disposal: Discard residual solution in drain. Flush thoroughly with water.

Container Disposal:

One Quart (946 mL) and One Gallon (3.8 L) Size Containers: Do not reuse empty container. Wrap container and put in trash.

Caution(s):

1. Protective gloves (butyl rubber, nitrile rubber, polyethylene or double-gloved latex), eye protection, face masks, and liquid-proof gowns should be worn when cleaning and sterilizing/disinfecting soiled devices and equipment.
2. Contaminated, reusable devices must be thoroughly cleaned prior to disinfection or sterilization, because residual contamination will decrease effectiveness of the germicide.
3. The user must adhere to the "Directions for Use", because any modification will affect the safety and effectiveness of the germicide.
4. The reusable device manufacturer should provide the user with a validated reprocessing procedure for that device using METRICIDE PLUS 30® solution.
5. The use of METRICIDE PLUS 30® solution in automated endoscope washers must be part of a validated reprocessing procedure provided by the washer manufacturer. Contact the manufacturer of the endoscope washer for instructions on the maximum number of reprocessing cycles which may be used before refilling with fresh METRICIDE PLUS 30® solution. Use a 1.8% glutaraldehyde concentration indicator to monitor glutaraldehyde concentration before each cycle to detect unexpected dilution.

Warning(s): METRICIDE PLUS 30® Activated Dialdehyde Solution is hazardous to humans and domestic animals.

Danger: Keep out of reach of children. Contains glutaraldehyde.

1. Direct contact is corrosive to exposed tissue, causing eye damage and skin irritation/damage. Do not get into eyes, on skin, or on clothing.
2. Avoid contamination of food.
3. Use in well-ventilated area in closed containers.

In case of contact, immediately flush eyes or skin with plenty of water for at least 15 minutes. For eyes, get medical attention.

Harmful if swallowed. Drink large quantities of water and call a physician immediately. Probable mucosal damage from oral exposure may contraindicate the use of gastric lavage. Emergency, safety, or technical information about METRICIDE PLUS 30® solution can be obtained from Metrex Research Corporation Customer Care Department at 1-800-841-1428, or by contacting your local Metrex Research Corporation sales representative.

References: Available upon request.

Presentation: 16 x 1 qt (946 mL) bottles per case and 4 x 1 gallon (128 fl oz) (3.8 L) bottles per case.

Compendium Code No.: 13400090 5130-11

METRICLEAN2®

Metrex **Detergent**

Low Foaming-Multi-Purpose Instrument Cleaner & Polisher

Contents: METRICLEAN2® contains powerful detergents, wetting agents, rust and stain inhibitors and chelating agents (to remove mineral deposits). METRICLEAN2® is biodegradable.

Indications: METRICLEAN2® is a low-foaming, concentrated instrument cleaner and polisher for use in ultrasonic cleaners, washer/sterilizers or decontaminators, automatic cart washers, and certain specialized instrument cleaning equipment. METRICLEAN2® is specially formulated to clean and condition stainless steel instruments.

Chemically Engineered to Replace: Manual Cleaning Detergents, Ultrasonic Detergents, Cart Washer Detergents, Washer/Sterilizer Detergents, Rust, Stain and Scale Removers.

Directions for Use: Ultrasonic Cleaners:

Room Temperature: One ounce of METRICLEAN2® to one gallon of water.

Hot Water: One half ounce per one gallon of water. Process instruments according to manufacturer's directions.

Washer-Sterilizer/Decontaminator: Attach concentrate container to the machine's automatic dispensing unit. Add one to three ounces of METRICLEAN2® per wash load (5 to 10 gallons). Actual quantity depends on water characteristics and dilution factors of specific machines.

Manual Cleaning: One ounce of METRICLEAN2® to one gallon of water. Soak instruments as needed in warm water. A minimum of 5 minutes is recommended, but not longer than 1 hour. Following soak period, visually inspect for cleanliness. Use soft brush or cloth to remove any remaining debris. A power spray unit will assist in thoroughly rinsing any remaining residue.

Automatic Cart Washers: One ounce of METRICLEAN2® to ten gallons of water.

Note: Under normal conditions, the hotter the water, the less METRICLEAN2® is required. METRICLEAN2® is not recommended for use on lensed equipment or prolonged contact with soft metals.

Storage and Disposal: Keep in a cool place.

Solution Disposal: Dispose of in accordance with all Federal, State and Local regulations.

Container Disposal: Rinse empty container thoroughly with water and discard clean, empty container as general trash.

Warning(s): Contains alkalies which can cause burns to eyes and nose. Prolonged exposure to concentrate solution may cause burns to skin. If concentrate solution gets in eyes or on skin, flush with water for 15 minutes and call a physician. Use with recommended attire where exposure to blood and body fluids is expected. This includes protective eye gear, impervious gloves and clothing.

Do not take internally.

Keep out of reach of children.

Presentation: 4 x 1 gallon (128 fl oz) (3.8 L) bottles, 5 gallon bottles, 15 gallon, 30 gallon and 55 gallon drums.

Compendium Code No.: 13400100 2910-5

METRIGUARD®

Metrex **Disinfectant**

Surface Disinfectant Decontaminant Cleaner-Bactericidal-Fungicidal-Virucidal*-Tuberculocidal**

EPA Reg. No.: 46781-6

Active Ingredient(s):

Diisobutylphenoxyethoxyethyl dimethyl benzyl ammonium chloride 0.28%
Isopropanol 17.20%
Inert Ingredients: 82.52%
Total: 100.00%

Indications: Effective Against: *Staphylococcus aureus, Pseudomonas aeruginosa, Salmonella choleraesuis, Mycobacterium tuberculosis* var. *bovis* (BCG)**, Methicillin Resistant *Staphylococcus aureus* (MRSA), Vancomycin Resistant *Enterococcus faecalis* (VRE), Trichophyton mentagrophytes, Herpes simplex virus types 1 and 2*, Human Immunodeficiency Virus (HIV-1)*, and Canine parvovirus**.

M

*On inanimate surfaces.
**In 10 minutes at room temperature 20°C.

Directions for Use: It is a violation of U.S. Federal law to use this product in a manner inconsistent with its labeling.

Description: METRIGUARD® is a multi-purpose, broad spectrum, ready-to-use, highly effective cleaner and disinfectant for use on the surfaces of inanimate objects. It is especially useful in hospital operating rooms, isolation areas, animal care facilities, and other areas where the control of cross contamination is important. METRIGUARD® will effectively clean and disinfect, when used as directed, such items as: infant incubators and bassinets, anesthesia machines and respiratory therapy equipment surfaces, operating room tables and lights, and other inanimate surfaces, including those made of plastics (such as: polycarbonate, polyvinylchloride, polypropylene and polystyrene non-porous vinyl and upholstery, stainless steel, painted surfaces, Plexiglas®, glass, and other hard non-porous surfaces.

Applications:

Surfaces: (Where appropriate, follow Universal Precautions.)

For disinfecting non-critical devices/medical equipment and surfaces: Apply METRIGUARD® to precleaned surface, thoroughly wetting area to be disinfected. Allow to remain wet for 3 minutes at room temperature (69°F/20°C). (**For Tuberculocidal Activity - Allow 10 minutes.) Follow by wiping surface using a clean paper or cloth towel or rinse and either allow surface to air dry or wipe rinsed surface dry using a clean paper or cloth towel. Discard towel.

For precleaning medical equipment and other surfaces prior to disinfection: Apply directly to surface. Allow to remain wet for 30 seconds. Wipe surface clean using paper or cloth towel or rinse surface and either wipe dry or allow to air dry. Discard dirty towel.

Instruments: (Where appropriate, follow Universal Precautions.)

For use as an instrument preclean decontamination spray: Place instruments into a suitable container. Thoroughly spray METRIGUARD® solution onto instruments so as to thoroughly drench all surfaces. Cover instruments and transport to appropriate cleaning area. Rinse instruments, follow with appropriate cleaning and disinfection process. (Critical and semi-critical devices must be followed by appropriate terminal sterilization/high-level preclean disinfection process.)

METRIGUARD® effectively kills HIV on precleaned environmental surfaces previously soiled with blood/body fluids in healthcare settings or other settings in which there is an expected likelihood of soiling of inanimate surfaces/objects with blood/body fluids, and in which the surfaces/objects can be associated with the potential for transmission of Human Immunodeficiency Virus Type 1 (HIV-1).

Special Instructions for Cleaning and Decontamination Against HIV-1 (Human Immunodeficiency Virus) of Surface/Objects Soiled with Blood/Body Fluid:

Personal Protection: Wear appropriate barrier protection such as latex gloves, gowns, masks or eye coverings.

Cleaning Procedure: Blood and other bodily fluids must be thoroughly cleaned from surfaces and objects before disinfection with METRIGUARD®.

Contact Time: While the HIV-1 virus is inactivated in 2 minutes, use the recommended contact time for the disinfection of other organisms listed under "Indications".

Infectious Materials Disposal: Cleaning materials used that may contain, blood or other bodily fluids should be autoclaved and/or disposed of in accordance with local regulations for infectious materials disposal.

**This product is not to be used as a terminal sterilant/high-level disinfectant on any surface or instrument that (1) is introduced directly into the human body, either into or in contact with the bloodstream or normally sterile areas of the body, or (2) contacts intact mucous membranes but which does not ordinarily penetrate the blood barrier or otherwise enter normally sterile areas of the body. This product, may be used to preclean or decontaminate critical or semi-critical medical devices prior to sterilization/high-level disinfection.

Precautionary Statements: Hazards to Humans and Domestic Animals. Causes moderate eye irritation. Avoid contact with eyes or clothing. Wash hands thoroughly with soap and water after handling. In case of direct eye contact, immediately flush eyes with plenty of water for at least 15 minutes. If irritation persists, seek medical attention.

Storage and Disposal: Store in a cool place.

Pesticide Disposal: Dilute with water. Dispose of in ordinary sanitary sewer.

Container Disposal: Triple rinse. Then offer for recycling, or puncture and dispose of in sanitary landfill, or incineration, or, if allowed by state/local authorities, by burning. If burned, keep out of smoke.

Warning(s): Keep out of reach of children.

Presentation: 12 x 32 fl oz (946 mL) spray bottles.

Compendium Code No.: 13400110 7006-5

METRILUBE®

Metrex **Instrument Lubricant**

Instrument Lubricant Concentrate

Indications: For the care of surgical instruments. Lubricates all moving parts. Helps prevent spotting, staining and rusting. Safe for use in automated washers. Anticorrosive. Silicone free. Nongreasy.

Directions: Shake well before use.

Manual Cleaning: Mix 1 part METRILUBE® with up to 15 parts of deionized or distilled water. (The dilution may be as low as 6 parts of water.)

Immerse cleaned instruments in bath for 30-45 seconds. Remove instruments and let drain, then autoclave. Rinsing and wiping are unnecessary.

Automated Washer/Disinfectors: Mechanically feed in the Lubrication/Final Rinse cycle of automated washer/disinfectors. Dispense at equipment manufacturer's recommendations. METRILUBE® can be used in the dilution range of ¼ oz to 2 oz per gallon.

For best results, use in conjunction with MetriWash™ Instrument Detergent.

Storage and Disposal: Keep in a cool place.

Solution must be disposed of weekly or more frequently as necessary depending on number of instruments processed.

Used solution should be disposed of according to federal, state and local regulations.

Rinse empty container thoroughly with water and discard clean, empty container as general trash.

Caution(s): METRILUBE® is not a detergent or sterilant. Instruments must be autoclaved after treatment. The lubricant bath should be replaced at least weekly or more frequently as necessary depending on number of instruments processed.

Warning(s): Keep out of reach of children.

Presentation: 12 x 24 oz spray bottles, 4 x 1 gallon (128 fl oz) (3.8 L) and 5 gallon bottles, 15 gallon and 30 gallon drums.

Compendium Code No.: 13400121 3900-3

METRIMIST®

Metrex **Deodorant Product**

Natural Aromatic Deodorizer

Indications: Eliminates offensive odors by cleaning the air, not masking the smell.

Effectively neutralizes airborne odors.

For use in all clinical settings to eliminate offensive odors where needed.

Inert. Biodegradable.

Directions for Use: Use sparingly — a little goes a long way. Spray METRIMIST® in air or directly on surfaces emanating odors. METRIMIST® is safe to use on surfaces.

METRIMIST® is an environmentally friendly, more effective alternative to aerosol air fresheners. It is non-toxic, non-poisonous and non-flammable.

METRIMIST® is suggested for use anywhere offensive odors need to be eliminated.

Warning(s): Important: If METRIMIST® is accidentally splashed in the eyes or on the skin, immediately flush with water. If accidentally ingested, drink large amounts of water.

Keep out of reach of children.

Presentation: 100 x 1 fl oz (30 mL) and 12 x 8 fl oz (239 mL) spray bottles.

Compendium Code No.: 13400150 1158-3

METRISPONGE®

Metrex **Detergent**

Ingredient(s): Proteolytic enzymes, propylene glycol, non-ionic surfactants, water and inerts.

Saturated with MetriZyme® Dual Enzymatic Detergent.

Indications: Easy-to-use pre-moistened sponge.

Dual proteolytic enzymes help ensure thorough pre-cleaning.

Directions for Use: Gloves, eye gear and impervious gown must be worn.

- Remove METRISPONGE® from bag and squeeze to the point of foam. Immerse in water and thoroughly scrub surfaces. Allow a minimum of 2-5 minutes contact time. Visually inspect for cleanliness.
- For more thorough cleaning, even in hard-to-reach places, use MetriZyme® Dual Enzymatic Detergent solution, per manufacturer's label directions.
- Rinse all surfaces thoroughly with warm water.

If chemically disinfecting or sterilizing, rough dry, then immerse in a Disinfecting/Sterilizing Solution according to manufacturer's label directions.

Note: MetriZyme® is not a sterilant/disinfectant.

Precaution(s): Storage: Keep in a cool place.

Caution(s): For professional use only.

For one-time use only - do not reuse.

Warning(s): Use with protective eye gear, gloves and clothing, especially where exposure to blood and body fluids is expected. If accidental eye contact occurs, flush immediately with water for 15 minutes and seek medical attention. Temporary redness of the eye may occur.

Risk Phrase(s):

- May cause eye and skin irritation.
- May cause throat, mouth, and stomach irritation if ingested.
- Repeated inhalation may result in sensitization and allergic reaction in hypersensitive individuals.

Precautionary Measures:

- Avoid contact with strong oxidizing agents (bleach).
- Long exposure of product to heat and/or humidity may reduce product's activity.
- Keep in a cool place.

Personal Protective Equipment: Protective gloves, eye gear, and impervious gown must be worn.

First Aid Measures:

Eyes: Flush immediately with water for 15 minutes. Seek medical attention.

Skin: Wash with soap and water.

Inhalation: Seek fresh air. Consult physician if allergic response exhibited.

Ingestion: Do not induce vomiting. Consult physician.

For Further Information Refer To: Metrex Research METRISPONGE® Material Safety Data Sheet.

Presentation: 25 pre-moistened sponges per box, 4 boxes per case.

Compendium Code No.: 13400160 4026-7/8310-2

METRIWASH™

Metrex **Detergent**

Instrument Detergent Concentrate

Indications: For manual and ultrasonic cleaning of surgical instruments.

No phosphates, chlorides or hydroxides. Biodegradable.

Rinses freely. Non-corrosive.

Directions:

1. Dilute METRIWASH™ ¼ oz to 2 oz per gallon of tap water.
2. May be used manually or in ultrasonic/automated cleaning systems.
3. Rinse thoroughly.

(Do not use for cleaning spinal syringes or needles.)

For best results use in conjunction with MetriLube® Instrument Lubricant.

Storage and Disposal: Keep in a cool place.

Solution must be disposed of daily or more frequently if visibly soiled.

Used solution should be disposed of according to federal, state and local regulations.

Rinse empty container thoroughly with water and discard clean, empty container as general trash.

Caution(s): METRIWASH™ Instrument Detergent, as with all detergents, should not be used for cleaning spinal syringes or needles.

Warning(s): Eye Irritant - contains nonionic detergents. In case of eye contact, rinse eye thoroughly with copious amounts of water and consult physician.

Accidental ingestion may be hazardous and require medical attention.

Keep out of reach of children.

Presentation: 4 x 1 gallon (128 fl oz) (3.8 L) and 5 gallon bottles, 15 gallon and 30 gallon drums.

Compendium Code No.: 13400130 3910-3

M

METRIWIPES®

Metrex **Disinfectant**

Germicidal Disposable Cloth

EPA Reg. No.: 9480-5-46781

Active Ingredient(s):

n-Alkyl (68% C_{12}, 32% C_{14}) dimethyl ethylbenzyl ammonium chlorides 0.14%
n-Alkyl (60% C_{14}, 30% C_{16}, 5% C_{12}, 5% C_{18}) dimethyl benzyl ammonium chlorides ... 0.14%
Isopropyl alcohol 8.00%
Inert Ingredients........ 91.72%
Total 100%

Indications: A dual chain quaternary/alcohol solution impregnated in a wiping cloth.

Disinfects environmental surfaces.

Effective against *Staphylococcus aureus, Salmonella choleraesuis, Pseudomonas aeruginosa, Klebsiella pneumoniae* in 5 minutes.

Kills viruses such as Influenza A2/HK and Herpes Simplex Type II in 30 seconds.

Kills *Mycobacterium bovis* BCG (Tuberculosis) in 10 minutes at 20°C.

Kills HIV on pre-cleaned environmental surfaces or objects previously soiled with blood or body fluids in 30 seconds at room temperature (20-25°C) in healthcare settings or other settings in which there is an expected likelihood of soiling of inanimate surfaces/objects with blood or body fluids, and in which the surfaces/objects likely to be soiled with blood or body fluids can be associated with the potential for transmission of Human Immunodeficiency Virus Type 1 (HIV 1).

A non-woven disposable cloth for use in hospitals and other critical care areas where control of the hazards of cross-contamination is required. Use on surfaces and equipment such as stainless steel, Formica, glass tables, carts, baskets, counters, cabinets, telephones and other hard non-porous surfaces.

Some Areas of Use: Hard surfaces in: surgery, recovery, anesthesia, x-ray, CAT lab, emergency room, new-born nursery, respiratory therapy, radiology and central supply.

This product is not used as a terminal sterilant/high level disinfectant on any surface or instrument that (1) is introduced directly into the human body, either into or in contact with the bloodstream or normally sterile areas of the body, or (2) contacts intact mucous membranes but which does not ordinarily penetrate the blood barrier or otherwise enter normally sterile areas of the body. This product may be used to preclean or decontaminate critical or semi-critical medical devices prior to sterilization or high level disinfection.

Directions for Use: It is a violation of Federal law to use this product in a manner inconsistent with its labeling.

Dispenser Directions: To start feed, remove large cover. From center of towelette roll, pull up a towelette corner, twist it into a point and thread it through the hole in the container cover. Pull through about one inch. Replace cover. Pull out first towelette and snap off at a 90° angle. Remaining towelettes feed automatically ready for next use. When through using, keep small center cap closed to prevent moisture loss. Open, unfold, wipe to remove gross filth. Use second towel to thoroughly wet surface. Allow to remain wet 5 minutes where required. Let air dry.

Special Instructions for Cleaning and Decontamination Against HIV-1 for Surfaces or Objects Soiled with Blood or Body Fluids:

Personal Protection: When using the germicidal cloth, wear disposable protective gloves, protective gowns, face masks, or eye coverings as appropriate when handling HIV-1 infected blood or body fluids.

Cleaning Procedures: All blood and other body fluids must be thoroughly cleaned from surface and objects before disinfection by the germicidal cloth. Open, unfold first germicidal cloth to remove gross filth.

Contact Time: Use second germicidal cloth to thoroughly wet surface. Allow to remain wet for 30 seconds. Let air dry. Although efficacy at a 30 second contact time has been shown to be adequate against HIV-1 (AIDS Virus), this time would not be sufficient for other organisms. Use listed disinfection times against all of the organisms claimed.

Disposal of Infectious Materials: Dispose of used towelette in accordance with local regulations for infectious waste disposal.

Precautionary Statements: Hazards to Humans and Domestic Animals:

Caution: Avoid contact with eyes. In case of eye contact, flush with plenty of water for at least 15 minutes. If irritation persists, call a physician.

Storage and Disposal: Towelette: Do not reuse towel. Dispose of used towel in trash.

Dispenser: Do not reuse empty container. Wrap container and put in trash collection.

Do not store near heat or open flame.

Warning(s): Keep out of reach of children.

Presentation: 12 x 160 (6 x 6.75") premoistened cloths per unit.

Compendium Code No.: 13400141 1070-5

METRIZYME®

Metrex **Detergent**

Active Ingredient(s): A proprietary formulation of non-animal enzymes with a light lemon fragrance.

Indications: METRIZYME® is a low-foaming, quick cleaning, enzyme detergent specifically designed for use in all areas where instruments and/or cloth materials may become soiled with organic or inorganic debris. METRIZYME® does not contain animal enzymes. METRIZYME® effectively reaches those hard-to-reach places such as lumens, channels and instrument box locks. METRIZYME® safely disintegrates blood and protein from delicate instruments, equipment, linens, clothing and surgical scrubs and it's one-step cleaning process decreases the need and hazards associated with the manual handling of contaminated items.

When used as directed, METRIZYME®'s pH neutral formula is safe for use on rubber, plastic and stainless steel instruments and equipment as well as linens, clothing, surgical scrubs, etc. METRIZYME® is compatible with all medical and surgical equipment, including endoscopes and other lensed instruments. METRIZYME® is non-flammable, non-toxic, non-caustic and 100% biodegradable. METRIZYME® may be used in temperatures up to 180°F.

When used according to label instructions, METRIZYME® may be used:

1. As a manual cleaner.
2. As a presoak for blood contaminated linens, clothing and surgical scrubs.
3. In endoscope reprocessors.
4. In ultrasonic units.
5. In washer sterilizer/decontaminators.

Dosage and Administration: Add 1 oz. METRIZYME® to each gallon of hot water. Immerse instruments and allow to soak for two (2) to five (5) minutes. Thoroughly rinse. Follow with an appropriate disinfection or sterilization process before patient use.

Precaution(s): Store at room temperature.

Presentation: 8 oz, 1 quart, ½ gallon, and 1 gallon.

Compendium Code No.: 13400021

METZ IODINE DETERGENT

Metz **Disinfectant**

EPA Reg. No.: 8781-4

Active Ingredient(s): Contains biodegradable detergents.

Nonylphenoxypoly (ethyleneoxy) ethanol-iodine complex........ 18.6%
(Providing 1.75% titratable iodine.)
Phosphoric acid 6.5%
Inert ingredients 74.9%

Indications: An iodine detergent germicide.

Dosage and Administration:

Milking machines: After each use, flush with warm water. Prepare a cleaning solution by adding one (1) ounce of METZ IODINE DETERGENT for each five (5) gallons of water (provides 25 ppm available iodine). Disassemble the machine. Immerse and brush in the cleaning solution. Rinse in a separate solution containing one-half (½) ounce of METZ IODINE DETERGENT for each five (5) gallons of water to prevent recontamination from the rinse water (provides 12.5 ppm available iodine). Immediately before re-use, sanitize by flushing with one-quarter (¼) ounce of METZ IODINE DETERGENT in 10 quarts of water.

Bulk tanks: Immediately after milk is removed rinse with warm water. Place sufficient warm water in the tank to wash effectively and add one (1) ounce of METZ IODINE DETERGENT for each five (5) gallons of water (provides 25 ppm available iodine). Brush thoroughly, drain and rinse for two (2) minutes. Valves should be removed and washed in a similar solution and rinsed. Where the code permits, sanitize by brushing with a solution containing one-quarter (¼) ounce of METZ IODINE DETERGENT in 10 quarts of water immediately before re-use.

Udder washing: Prepare a solution containing one-half (½) ounce of METZ IODINE DETERGENT in 10 quarts of warm water (provides 25 ppm available iodine). Just before milking wipe udders and teats with a clean cloth or paper towel saturated with the solution. Use a clean towel for each cow. Do not return used towels to the solution.

Precaution(s): Keep capped in a cool place. Keep from freezing.

Caution(s): Keep out of the reach of children.

METZ IODINE DETERGENT is a disinfectant containing phosphoric acid and iodine. Do not take internally. Harmful if swallowed. Avoid the contamination of food. Avoid getting the concentrate in the eyes or on skin. In case of contact, immediately flush with plenty of water for at least 15 minutes. If relief is not obtained, get medical attention.

Presentation: 1, 5, 15, 30 and 55 gallon containers.

Compendium Code No.: 10190020

METZ IODINE TEAT DIP (0.25%)

Metz **Teat Dip**

NDC No.: 050748-020

Active Ingredient(s): Contains glycerine, minimum pH 4.0, a-(p-nonylphenyl)-omega-hydroxypoly (oxyethylene) iodine complex, (provides 0.25% minimum titratable iodine). Equivalent to 2,500 parts per million titratable iodine.

Indications: For use as an aid in controlling the spread of bacteria that may cause mastitis.

Dosage and Administration: Do not dilute the product. Use at full strength. Discard the dip solution when it becomes visibly dirty or if sediment is present. If teats are chapped or sore, consult a veterinarian before beginning or continuing to use the product.

As a pre-dip: Remove all visible dirt by washing the teats and the base of the udder, using a minimal amount of an approved udder wash solution and a clean single service towel. Dry the teats and the udder completely with a clean single service towel. Dip or spray the teats with METZ IODINE TEAT DIP (0.25%). Allow a 30 second contact time. Before attaching the milker, remove the teat dip by drying thoroughly with a clean single service paper towel.

As a post-dip: Immediately after the milker is removed, dip or spray the teats with undiluted METZ IODINE TEAT DIP. If the cow will be returned to a below freezing temperature environment, allow the teat dip to air dry before discharging her from the milking area.

Caution(s): Keep out of the reach of children.

Avoid contact with food.

Presentation: 1 gallon, 5 gallon, 15 gallon, 30 gallon, and 55 gallon containers.

Compendium Code No.: 10190030

METZ IODINE TEAT DIP (0.5%)

Metz **Teat Dip**

NDC No.: 050748-018

Active Ingredient(s): Contains glycerine, minimum pH 4.0, a-(p-nonylphenyl)-omega-hydroxypoly (oxyethylene) iodine complex, (provides 0.5% minimum titratable iodine). Equivalent to 5,000 parts per million titratable iodine.

Indications: For use as an aid in controlling the spread of bacteria that may cause mastitis.

Dosage and Administration: Immediately after each cow is milked, dip the teats in undiluted METZ IODINE TEAT DIP. Ideally a fresh teat dip solution should be provided for each cow and in no case should the same cup of solution be used for more than three (3) or four (4) cows before discarding and providing a fresh solution. Just prior to the next milking thoroughly wash the treated udder and teats in potable water. Use a fresh towel for each cow and never dip used towels back into the solution. When a cow is being dried off, dip the teats for three (3) or four (4) days after the last milking. Do not use for cleaning and/or sanitizing milk equipment.

Caution(s): Keep out of the reach of children. Avoid contact with food.

Presentation: 1 gallon, 5 gallon, 15 gallon, 30 gallon, and 55 gallon containers.

Compendium Code No.: 10190040

METZ IODINE TEAT DIP (1.0%)

Metz **Teat Dip**

NDC No.: 050748-017

Active Ingredient(s): Contains 10% glycerine, minimum pH 4.0, a-(p-nonylphenyl)-omega-hydroxypoly (oxyethylene) iodine complex, (provides 1.0% minimum titratable iodine). Equivalent to 10,000 parts per million titratable iodine.

Indications: For use as an aid in controlling the spread of bacteria that may cause mastitis.

Dosage and Administration: Immediately after each cow is milked, dip the teats in undiluted METZ IODINE TEAT DIP. Ideally a fresh teat dip solution should be provided for each cow and in no case should the same cup of solution be used for more than three (3) or four (4) cows before discarding and providing a fresh solution. Just prior to the next milking thoroughly wash the treated udder and teats in potable water. Use a fresh towel for each cow and never dip used

towels back into the solution. When a cow is being dried off, dip the teats for three (3) or four (4) days after the last milking. Do not use for cleaning and/or sanitizing milk equipment.
Caution(s): Keep out of the reach of children. Avoid contact with food.
Presentation: 1 gallon, 5 gallon, 15 gallon, 30 gallon, and 55 gallon containers.
Compendium Code No.: 10190050

METZ SOFT-KOTE TEAT DIP

Metz **Teat Dip**

NDC No.: 050748-019
Active Ingredient(s): Contains glycerine and chlorhexidine gluconate 0.5% w/w.
Indications: A teat dip containing chlorhexidine in a glycerine emollient base to aid in controlling the spread of bacteria that may cause mastitis.
Dosage and Administration: Immediately after each cow is milked, dip the teats in undiluted METZ SOFT-KOTE TEAT DIP. Ideally a fresh teat dip solution should be provided for each cow and in no case should the same cup of solution be used for more than three (3) or four (4) cows before discarding and providing a fresh solution. Just prior to the next milking thoroughly wash the treated udder and teats in potable water. Use a fresh towel for each cow and never dip used towels back into the solution. When a cow is being dried off, dip the teats for three (3) or four (4) days after the last milking. Do not use for cleaning and/or sanitizing milk equipment.
Precaution(s): Store in a cool, dark place. Keep from freezing. If frozen, thaw completely and agitate well by shaking or rolling the container before use.
Caution(s): May be harmful if swallowed. Keep out of the reach of children.
Avoid contact with food.
If swallowed, drink large quantities of milk or water and induce vomiting. Call a physician immediately. May irritate the eyes and mucous membranes. Flush gently with large amounts of water and see a physician.
Presentation: 1 gallon, 5 gallon, 15 gallon, 30 gallon, and 55 gallon containers.
Compendium Code No.: 10190060

METZ SOFT-KOTE TEAT SPRAY

Metz **Teat Dip**

NDC No.: 050748-021
Active Ingredient(s): Contains glycerine and chlorhexidine gluconate 0.5% w/w.
Indications: A teat dip containing chlorhexidine in a glycerine emollient base to aid in controlling the spread of bacteria that may cause mastitis.
Dosage and Administration: Immediately after each cow is milked, spray or dip the teats in undiluted METZ SOFT-KOTE TEAT SPRAY. If cows are sprayed be sure to cover the entire teat. If cows are dipped, ideally a fresh teat dip solution should be provided for each cow and in no case should the same cup of solution be used for more than three (3) or four (4) cows before discarding and providing a fresh solution. Just prior to the next milking thoroughly wash the treated udder and teats in potable water. Use a fresh towel for each cow and never dip used towels back into the solution. When a cow is being dried off, dip the teats for three (3) or four (4) days after the last milking. Do not use for cleaning and/or sanitizing milk equipment.
Precaution(s): Store in a cool, dark place. Keep from freezing. If frozen, thaw completely and agitate well by shaking or rolling the container before use.
Caution(s): May be harmful if swallowed. Keep out of the reach of children.
Avoid contact with food.
If swallowed, drink large quantities of milk or water and induce vomiting. Call a physician immediately. May irritate the eyes and mucous membranes. Flush gently with large amounts of water and see a physician.
Presentation: 5 gallon, 15 gallon, 30 gallon, and 55 gallon containers.
Compendium Code No.: 10190070

M.F.O. SOLUTION

AgriLabs **Large Animal Dietary Supplement**

Active Ingredient(s): Each 500 mL of aqueous solution contains:
Calcium (as calcium borogluconate) .... 10.0 g
Phosphorus (as sodium hypophosphite • H_2O) .... 6.0 g
Magnesium (as magnesium chloride • H_2O) .... 2.8 g
Potassium (as potassium chloride) .... 0.5 g
Dextrose • H_2O .... 75.0 g
Preservatives:
Methylparaben 0.18%
Propylparaben 0.02%
Ethylparaben 0.01%
Indications: For use as a supplemental source of calcium, phosphorus, magnesium, potassium and dextrose in cattle.
Dosage and Administration: Administer orally as a drench. The usual dose for adult cattle is 500 mL.
Precaution(s): Store at a controlled temperature between 15-30°C (59-86°F).
Caution(s): Not for human use. Keep out of the reach of children.
Presentation: 500 mL bottles.
Compendium Code No.: 10580680

MGA® 200 PREMIX

Pharmacia & Upjohn **Feed Additive**
(Type A Medicated Article)

NADA No.: 034-254
Active Ingredient(s): Each pound contains:
Melengestrol Acetate .... 200 mg
Inactive Ingredients:
Soybean hulls, #20 grind 96.0%
Starch 2.98%
Mineral Oil 1.0%
Indications:
Heifers Fed in Confinement for Slaughter: For increased rate of weight gain, improved feed efficiency and suppression of estrus (heat).
Heifers Intended for Breeding: For suppression of estrus (heat).
Dosage and Administration:
Heifers Fed in Confinement for Slaughter: MGA® 200 Premix (Type A Medicated Article) should be thoroughly mixed in the supplement of feedlot heifers to provide 0.25 to 0.50 mg of melengestrol acetate per head per day. Average daily intakes approximating the middle of this range provide the most optimal and economical improvements in rate of gain and feed utilization. Constant daily intakes of 0.35 to 0.50 mg per head per day give a high degree of estrus suppression. Levels of 0.25 to 0.35 mg provide a lower but still effective degree of estrus suppression.
Heifers Intended for Breeding: MGA® 200 Premix (Type A Medicated Article) should be thoroughly mixed in the supplement to provide 0.5 mg of melengestrol acetate per head per day.
Mixing Directions: Thoroughly mix 1.25 to 10 pounds of MGA® 200 Premix (Type A Medicated Article) per ton of non-medicated feed to prepare a Type C medicated feed containing 0.25 to 2.0 grams of melengestrol acetate per ton. The following table may be used as a guide in determining the amount of MGA® 200 Premix (Type A Medicated Article) to be added to prepare a ton of Type C medicated feed.

Amount of Supplement Fed (lb/head/day)	Melengestrol Acetate (mg/head/day)	Pounds MGA® 200 per Ton of Supplement
0.5	0.25	5.00
0.5	0.30	6.00
0.5	0.35	7.00
0.5	0.40	8.00
0.5	0.45	9.00
0.5	0.50	10.00
1.0	0.25	2.50
1.0	0.30	3.00
1.0	0.35	3.50
1.0	0.40	4.00
1.0	0.45	4.50
1.0	0.50	5.00
1.5	0.25	1.67
1.5	0.30	2.00
1.5	0.35	2.33
1.5	0.40	2.67
1.5	0.45	3.00
1.5	0.50	3.33
2.0	0.25	1.25
2.0	0.30	1.50
2.0	0.35	1.75
2.0	0.40	2.00
2.0	0.45	2.25
2.0	0.50	2.50

Type B medicated feeds containing 4 to 10 grams melengestrol acetate per ton may be manufactured by thoroughly mixing 20 to 50 lbs of MGA® 200 Premix with 1980 to 1950 lbs of non-medicated feed. Labeling for such Type B feeds shall contain directions for manufacturing Type C medicated feeds containing 0.25 to 2.0 grams melengestrol acetate per ton (0.125-1.0 mg/lb). The Type C medicated feed, containing melengestrol acetate, must be top dressed on grain or roughage or mixed with a complete ration at the rate of 0.5 to 2.0 pounds per head per day.
Precaution(s): Store in a dry place to prevent caking.
Store at room temperature.
Caution(s): Heifers Fed in Confinement for Slaughter: Withdrawal periods of three to five days or more should be avoided to prevent the possibility that the heifers may come into estrus (heat) at loading time.
Heifers Intended for Breeding: Do not exceed 24 days of feeding of melengestrol acetate to heifers intended for breeding. A reduced conception rate can be expected if heifers are bred at estruses observed within 1 to 12 days after withdrawal of melengestrol acetate, whereas heifers bred at subsequent observed estruses are expected to have normal conception rates.
Use only as directed. Excessive contact with skin should be avoided. Destroy empty container. Do not reuse.
For manufacturing, processing or repacking. To be mixed with feed prior to animal use.
Not for human use.
Restricted Drug — Use only as directed (California).
Not effective in steers and spayed heifers.
Good manufacturing procedures should be observed in preparing supplements containing MGA® 200.
Presentation: 50 lb (22.6 kg).
Compendium Code No.: 10490320

M

MGA® 500 LIQUID PREMIX

Pharmacia & Upjohn **Feed Efficiency Enhancer**
(Type A Medicated Article)

NADA No.: 039-402
Active Ingredient(s): Each Pound Contains:
Melengestrol Acetate (as melengestrol acetate and its propylene glycol ketal) .... 500 mg
Inactive Ingredient:
Propylene Glycol, U.S.P. 99.89%
Indications: Heifers Fed in Confinement for Slaughter: For increased rate of weight gain, improved feed efficiency and suppression of estrus (heat).
Heifers Intended for Breeding: For suppression of estrus (heat).
Directions for Use: Heifers Fed in Confinement for Slaughter: MGA® 500 Liquid Premix (Type A Medicated Article) should be thoroughly mixed in liquid Type C medicated feed which must be fed at 0.5 to 2.0 pounds per head daily to provide 0.25 to 0.5 mg of melengestrol acetate per head per day. Average daily intakes approximating the middle of this range provide the most optimal and economical improvements in rate of gain and feed utilization. Constant daily intakes of 0.35 to 0.50 mg per head per day give a high degree of estrus suppression. Levels of 0.25 to 0.35 mg provide a lower but still effective degree of estrus suppression.
Heifers Intended for Breeding: MGA® 500 Liquid Premix (Type A Medicated Article) should be thoroughly mixed in the supplement to provide 0.5 mg of melengestrol acetate per head per day.
Mixing Directions: Liquid Type B and C medicated feeds containing melengestrol acetate must have a pH of 4.0 to 8.0 and their labels must bear appropriate mixing directions. Mixing directions for liquid Type B or C feeds stored in recirculation tank systems are: "Recirculate immediately prior to use for no less than 10 minutes, moving not less than 1 percent of the tank contents from the bottom of the tank to the top. Recirculate daily, as directed in this paragraph even when the Type B (or C) feed is not used." Mixing directions for liquid Type B and C feeds stored in

mechanical, air or other agitation-type tank systems are: "Agitate immediately prior to use for not less than 10 minutes, creating a turbulence at the bottom of the tank that is visible at the top. Agitate daily, as directed in this paragraph, even when the Type B (or C) feed is not used."

Intermediate premixes should not be made from MGA® 500 Liquid Premix (Type A Medicated Article) except as a part of a continuous mixing operation to make a complete liquid Type B or Type C medicated feed.

Thoroughly mix 0.5 to 4 pounds of MGA® 500 Liquid Premix (Type A Medicated Article) per ton of a non-medicated feed to prepare a Type C medicated feed containing 0.25 to 2.0 grams of melengestrol acetate per ton.

The following Table may be used as a guide in determining the amount of MGA® 500 Liquid Premix (Type A Medicated Article) to be added to prepare a ton of Type C medicated feed.

Amount of Supplement Fed (lb/head/day)	Melengestrol acetate (mg/head/day)	MGA® 500 Liquid Premix Per Ton of Liquid Supplement	
		When Added by Weight (lb)	When Added by Volume (mL)
0.5	0.25	2.00	876
0.5	0.30	2.40	1051
0.5	0.35	2.80	1226
0.5	0.40	3.20	1402
0.5	0.45	3.60	1577
0.5	0.50	4.00	1752
1.0	0.25	1.00	438
1.0	0.30	1.20	526
1.0	0.35	1.40	613
1.0	0.40	1.60	701
1.0	0.45	1.80	788
1.0	0.50	2.00	876
1.5	0.25	0.66	289
1.5	0.30	0.80	350
1.5	0.35	0.93	407
1.5	0.40	1.07	469
1.5	0.45	1.20	526
1.5	0.50	1.33	582
2.0	0.25	0.50	219
2.0	0.30	0.60	263
2.0	0.35	0.70	307
2.0	0.40	0.80	350
2.0	0.45	0.90	394
2.0	0.50	1.00	438

Type B medicated feed containing 4 to 10 grams melengestrol acetate per ton may be manufactured by thoroughly mixing 8 to 20 lbs of MGA® 500 Liquid Premix with 1992 to 1980 lbs of non-medicated feed. Labeling for such Type B feed shall contain directions for manufacturing Type C medicated feeds containing 0.25 to 2.0 grams melengestrol acetate per ton (0.125 to 1.0 mg/lb). The Type C medicated feed, containing melengestrol acetate, must be top dressed on grain or roughage or mixed with a complete ration at the rate of 0.5 to 2.0 pounds per head per day.

M

Good manufacturing practice regulations must be adhered to in manufacturing feeds containing MGA® 500.

Precaution(s): Store at room temperature

Caution(s): For manufacturing, processing, or repacking. To be mixed with feed prior to animal use. Use only as directed. Excessive contact with skin should be avoided. Destroy empty container. Do not reuse.

Restricted Drug—Use Only As Directed (California).

Not effective in steers and spayed heifers.

Warning(s): Not for human use.

Heifers Fed in Confinement for Slaughter: Withdrawal periods of three to five days or more should be avoided to prevent the possibility that the heifers may come into estrus (heat) at loading time.

Heifers Intended for Breeding: Do not exceed 24 days of feeding of melengestrol acetate to heifers intended for breeding. A reduced conception rate can be expected if heifers are bred at estruses observed within 1 to 12 days after withdrawal of melengestrol acetate, whereas heifers bred at subsequent observed estruses are expected to have normal conception rates.

Presentation: 40 lbs (18 kg) (4.627 gal [17.5 L]) (NDC 0009-0547-01).

Compendium Code No.: 10490331 813 925 107

MG-BAC®

Fort Dodge **Bacterin**

Mycoplasma Gallisepticum Bacterin

U.S. Vet. Lic. No.: 112

Contents: This product contains the antigen listed above.

Penicillin added as a preservative.

Indications: For the subcutaneous or intramuscular vaccination of chickens and turkeys as an aid in the prevention of clinical signs associated with *Mycoplasma gallisepticum* infection.

Dosage and Administration: Inject 0.5 mL (0.5 cc) subcutaneously (in the lower neck region) for birds 1 to 10 weeks of age using aseptic technique. For birds 10 weeks of age or older, may vaccinate intramuscularly or subcutaneously. Vaccinate only healthy birds prior to field exposure. The vaccination program should be completed prior to the point of lay. For optimum results, vaccinate twice, allowing at least 4 weeks between vaccinations. Revaccinate birds during molt before the second laying period.

Precaution(s): Store in the dark at 36° to 45°F (2° to 7°C). Do not freeze. Warm to 72°F (22°C) and shake well before using. Use entire contents when first opened.

Caution(s): Do not vaccinate broilers or meat turkeys by the intramuscular route of administration. If birds are vaccinated during lay, a drop in egg production may occur.

Warning(s): Do not vaccinate within 42 days before slaughter.

In case of accidental human injection seek immediate medical attention, stating the vaccine is an oil emulsion type.

For veterinary use only.

Presentation: 1,000 dose (500 mL) vials.

Compendium Code No.: 10031081 10221B

M.G. BACTERIN

L.A.H.I. (New Jersey) **Bacterin**

Mycoplasma gallisepticum Bacterin

U.S. Vet. Lic. No.: 196

Active Ingredient(s): This product is a formalin inactivated oil base suspension of highly immunogenic strains of *Mycoplasma gallisepticum.* The bacterin is used for the prevention of clinical signs associated with *Mycoplasma gallisepticum* infection in chickens.

The bacterin is manufactured in accordance with a detailed production outline which has been filed with the Veterinary Services of the USDA. The production seeds are derived from a master seed culture which have been fully tested for purity, safety and immunogenicity. The organisms are grown under special growth conditions. After the organisms are inactivated by formalin, their concentration is adjusted and oil adjuvant with emulsifiers is mycoplasma added to the suspensions. After homogenization, 600 mL plastic bottles are filled with 500 mL of the emulsion and stoppers and aluminum overseals are applied.

Quality Control: The cultures used to manufacture this product have been tested for purity and serological type. The product is fully tested for purity and safety according to the standard requirements for inactivated bacterial products published as part 113, in particular, 113.85 of title 9 of the federal regulations by the Animal and Plant Health Inspection Service of the USDA.

Each serial is tested for: Live bacteria and fungi; safety tests. Efficacy is demonstrated by a challenge protection test.

Samples and complete test reports on each serial are submitted to the Veterinary Services Laboratory of the USDA and no vaccine is released for sale or shipment until this governmental agency has provided its authorization to release.

Indications: The product is used for vaccination of chickens at one to ten weeks of age or older for the prevention of clinical signs associated with *Mycoplasma gallisepticum* infection.

Dosage and Administration: The vaccine should be administered subcutaneously in the mid-portion of the neck. Chickens should be vaccinated with a 0.5 mL dose.

Birds should be vaccinated twice allowing at least four (4) weeks between vaccinations. If birds are to be kept for a second year of production, they should be revaccinated during molt.

Precaution(s): The bacterin should be stored in the dark, at a temperature between 35 to 45°F (2 to 7°C). The product must not be frozen. Expiration date: 24 months.

Caution(s): It is imperative that the user of this product comply with the indications for use, contraindications, and method of vaccination stated on the direction sheet. The product must be prepared and administered as directed to obtain best results. For veterinary use only.

Warning(s): Do not market birds for at least six (6) weeks after vaccinating so that there is no swelling at the site of vaccine administration.

Presentation: 1,000 doses.

Compendium Code No.: 10080252

MICAVED® LOTION 1% ℞

Vedco **Topical Antifungal**

(Miconazole Nitrate)

ANADA No.: 200-196

Active Ingredient(s): MICAVED® (miconazole nitrate) Lotion is a synthetic antifungal agent for use in dogs and cats. It contains: 1.15% miconazole nitrate (equivalent to 1% miconazole base by weight), polyethylene glycol 400 and ethyl alcohol 55%.

Indications: MICAVED® (miconazole nitrate) Lotion is indicated for the treatment of fungal infections in dogs and cats caused by *Microsporum canis, Microsporum gypseum* and *Trichophyton mentagraphytes.*

Dosage and Administration: Accurate diagnosis of the infecting organism is essential. Identification should be made either by direct microscopic examination of a mounting of infected tissue in a solution of potassium hydroxide, or by culture on an appropriate medium.

Apply a light covering of MICAVED® (miconazole nitrate) Lotion to affected areas, once daily, for 2 to 4 weeks. Application is best accomplished using a gauze pad or cotton swab. Medication must be continued until the infecting organism is completely eradicated as indicated by appropriate clinical or laboratory examination. If no improvement is noticed within 2 weeks, diagnosis should be re-evaluated. Difficult cases may require treatment for 6 weeks.

General measures in regard to hygiene should be observed to control sources of infection or reinfection. Clipping of hair around and over the sites of infection should be done at the start of treatment and again as necessary.

Caution(s): Federal law restricts this drug to use by or on the order of a licensed veterinarian.

In the event of sensitization or irritation due to MICAVED® Lotion, treatment should be discontinued. Avoid contact with eyes, since irritation may result. Wash hands thoroughly after administration to avoid spread of fungal infection.

Presentation: MICAVED® (miconazole nitrate) Lotion in 60 mL containers.

Compendium Code No.: 10941250

MICAVED® SPRAY 1% ℞

Vedco **Topical Antifungal**

(Miconazole Nitrate)

ANADA No.: 200-196

Active Ingredient(s): MICAVED® (miconazole nitrate) Spray is a synthetic antifungal agent for use in dogs and cats. It contains: 1.15% miconazole nitrate (equivalent to 1% miconazole base by weight), polyethylene glycol 400 and ethyl alcohol 55%.

Indications: MICAVED® (miconazole nitrate) Spray is indicated for the treatment of fungal infections in dogs and cats caused by *Microsporum canis, Microsporum gypseum* and *Trichophyton mentagraphytes.*

Dosage and Administration: Accurate diagnosis of the infecting organism is essential. Identification should be made either by direct microscopic examination of a mounting of infected tissue in a solution of potassium hydroxide, or by culture on an appropriate medium.

Spray affected areas from a distance of 2 to 4 inches to apply a light covering, once daily for 2 to 4 weeks. Medication must be continued until the infecting organism is completely eradicated as indicated by appropriate clinical or laboratory examination. If no improvement is noticed within 2 weeks, diagnosis should be re-evaluated. Difficult cases may require treatment for 6 weeks.

General measures in regard to hygiene should be observed to control sources of infection or reinfection. Clipping of hair around and over the sites of infection should be done at the start of treatment and again as necessary.

Caution(s): Federal law restricts this drug to use by or on the order of a licensed veterinarian.

In the event of sensitization or irritation due to MICAVED® Spray, treatment should be discontinued. Avoid contact with eyes, since irritation may result. Wash hands thoroughly after administration to avoid spread of fungal infection.

Presentation: MICAVED® (miconazole nitrate) Spray in 120 mL and 240 mL containers.

Compendium Code No.: 10941260

MICAZOLE LOTION 1% ℞

Vetus **Topical Antifungal**

(Miconazole Nitrate)

ANADA No.: 200-196

Active Ingredient(s): MICAZOLE (miconazole nitrate) Lotion is a synthetic antifungal agent for use in dogs and cats. It contains: 1.15% miconazole nitrate (equivalent to 1% miconazole base by weight), polyethylene glycol 400 and ethyl alcohol 55%.

Indications: MICAZOLE (miconazole nitrate) Lotion is indicated for the treatment of fungal infections in dogs and cats caused by *Microsporum canis, Microsporum gypseum* and *Trichophyton mentagraphytes.*

Dosage and Administration: Accurate diagnosis of the infecting organism is essential. Identification should be made by either direct microscopic examination of a mounting of infected tissue in a solution of potassium hydroxide, or by culture on an appropriate medium.

Apply a light covering of MICAZOLE (miconazole nitrate) Lotion to affected areas, once daily, for 2 to 4 weeks. Application is best accomplished using a gauze pad or cotton swab. Medication must be continued until the infecting organism is completely eradicated as indicated by appropriate clinical or laboratory examination. If no improvement is noticed within 2 weeks, diagnosis should be re-evaluated. Difficult cases may require treatment for 6 weeks.

General measures in regard to hygiene should be observed to control sources of infection or reinfection. Clipping of hair around and over the sites of infection should be done at the start of treatment and again as necessary.

Caution(s): Federal law restricts this drug to use by or on the order of a licensed veterinarian.

In the event of sensitization or irritation due to MICAZOLE Lotion, treatment should be discontinued. Avoid contact with eyes, since irritation may result. Wash hands thoroughly after administration to avoid spread of fungal infection.

Presentation: MICAZOLE (miconazole nitrate) Lotion in 60 mL containers.

Compendium Code No.: 14440610

MICAZOLE SPRAY 1% ℞

Vetus **Topical Antifungal**

(Miconazole Nitrate)

ANADA No.: 200-196

Active Ingredient(s): MICAZOLE (miconazole nitrate) Spray is a synthetic antifungal agent for use in dogs and cats. It contains: 1.15% miconazole nitrate (equivalent to 1% miconazole base by weight), polyethylene glycol 400 and ethyl alcohol 55%.

Indications: MICAZOLE (miconazole nitrate) Spray is indicated for the treatment of fungal infections in dogs and cats caused by *Microsporum canis, Microsporum gypseum* and *Trichophyton mentagraphytes.*

Dosage and Administration: Accurate diagnosis of the infecting organism is essential. Identification should be made by either direct microscopic examination of a mounting of infected tissue in a solution of potassium hydroxide, or by culture on an appropriate medium.

Spray affected areas from a distance of 2 to 4 inches to apply a light covering, once daily, for 2 to 4 weeks. Medication must be continued until the infecting organism is completely eradicated as indicated by appropriate clinical or laboratory examination. If no improvement is noticed within 2 weeks, diagnosis should be re-evaluated. Difficult cases may require treatment for 6 weeks.

General measures in regard to hygiene should be observed to control sources of infection or reinfection. Clipping of hair around and over the sites of infection should be done at the start of treatment and again as necessary.

Caution(s): Federal law restricts this drug to use by or on the order of a licensed veterinarian.

In the event of sensitization or irritation due to MICAZOLE Spray, treatment should be discontinued. Avoid contact with eyes, since irritation may result. Wash hands thoroughly after administration to avoid spread of fungal infection.

Presentation: MICAZOLE (miconazole nitrate) Spray in 120 mL and 240 mL containers.

Compendium Code No.: 14440620

MICONAZOLE NITRATE LOTION 1% ℞

Butler **Topical Antifungal**

(Miconazole Nitrate) Topical antifungal agent

ANADA No.: 200-196

Active Ingredient(s): MICONAZOLE NITRATE LOTION is a synthetic antifungal agent for use in dogs and cats. It contains: 1.15% miconazole nitrate (equivalent to 1% miconazole base by weight), polyethylene glycol 400 and ethyl alcohol 55%.

Indications: MICONAZOLE NITRATE LOTION is indicated for the treatment of fungal infections in dogs and cats caused by *Microsporum canis, Microsporum gypseum* and *Trichophyton mentagrophytes.*

Dosage and Administration: Accurate diagnosis of the infecting organism is essential. Identification should be made either by direct microscopic examination of a mounting of infected tissue in a solution of potassium hydroxide, or by culture on an appropriate medium.

Apply a light covering of MICONAZOLE NITRATE LOTION to affected areas, once daily, for 2 to 4 weeks. Application is best accomplished using a gauze pad or cotton swab. Medication must be continued until the infecting organism is completely eradicated as indicated by appropriate clinical or laboratory examination. If no improvement is noticed within 2 weeks, diagnosis should be re-evaluated. Difficult cases may require treatment for 6 weeks.

General measures in regard to hygiene should be observed to control sources of infection or reinfection. Clipping of hair around and over the sites of infection should be done at the start of treatment and again as necessary.

Caution(s): Federal law restricts this drug to use by or on the order of a licensed veterinarian.

In the event of sensitization or irritation due to MICONAZOLE NITRATE LOTION, treatment should be discontinued. Avoid contact with eyes, since irritation may result. Wash hands thoroughly after administration to avoid spread of fungal infection.

Presentation: MICONAZOLE NITRATE LOTION in 60 mL containers.

Manufactured by: Med-Pharmex, Inc.

Compendium Code No.: 10821150

MICONAZOLE NITRATE SPRAY 1% ℞

Butler **Topical Antifungal**

(Miconazole Nitrate) Topical antifungal agent

ANADA No.: 200-196

Active Ingredient(s): MICONAZOLE NITRATE SPRAY is a synthetic antifungal agent for use in dogs and cats. It contains: 1.15% miconazole nitrate (equivalent to 1% miconazole base by weight), polyethylene glycol 400 and ethyl alcohol 55%.

Indications: MICONAZOLE NITRATE SPRAY is indicated for the treatment of fungal infections in dogs and cats caused by *Microsporum canis, Microsporum gypseum* and *Trichophyton mentagrophytes.*

Dosage and Administration: Accurate diagnosis of the infecting organism is essential. Identification should be made either by direct microscopic examination of a mounting of infected tissue in a solution of potassium hydroxide, or by culture on an appropriate medium.

Spray affected areas from a distance of 2 to 4 inches to apply a light covering, once daily for 2 to 4 weeks. Medication must be continued until the infecting organism is completely eradicated as indicated by appropriate clinical or laboratory examination. If no improvement is noticed within 2 weeks, diagnosis should be re-evaluated. Difficult cases may require treatment for 6 weeks.

General measures in regard to hygiene should be observed to control sources of infection or reinfection. Clipping of hair around and over the sites of infection should be done at the start of treatment and again as necessary.

Caution(s): Federal law restricts this drug to use by or on the order of a licensed veterinarian.

In the event of sensitization or irritation due to MICONAZOLE NITRATE SPRAY, treatment should be discontinued. Avoid contact with eyes, since irritation may result. Wash hands thoroughly after administration to avoid spread of fungal infection.

Presentation: MICONAZOLE NITRATE SPRAY in 120 mL and 240 mL containers.

Manufactured by: Med-Pharmex, Inc.

Compendium Code No.: 10821160

MICONOSOL LOTION 1% ℞

Med-Pharmex **Topical Antifungal**

(Miconazole Nitrate) Topical antifungal agent

ANADA No.: 200-196

Active Ingredient(s): MICONOSOL (miconazole nitrate) LOTION is a synthetic antifungal agent for use in dogs and cats. It contains: 1.15% miconazole nitrate (equivalent to 1% miconazole base by weight), polyethylene glycol 400 and ethyl alcohol 55%.

Indications: MICONOSOL (miconazole nitrate) LOTION is indicated for the treatment of fungal infections in dogs and cats caused by *Microsporum canis, Microsporum gypseum* and *Trichophyton mentagrophytes.*

Dosage and Administration: Accurate diagnosis of the infecting organism is essential. Identification should be made either by direct microscopic examination of a mounting of infected tissue in a solution of potassium hydroxide, or by culture on an appropriate medium.

Apply a light covering of MICONOSOL (miconazole nitrate) LOTION to affected areas, once daily, for 2 to 4 weeks. Application is best accomplished using a gauze pad or cotton swab. Medication must be continued until the infecting organism is completely eradicated as indicated by appropriate clinical or laboratory examination. If no improvement is noticed within 2 weeks, diagnosis should be re-evaluated. Difficult cases may require treatment for 6 weeks.

General measures in regard to hygiene should be observed to control sources of infection or reinfection. Clipping of hair around and over the sites of infection should be done at the start of treatment and again as necessary.

Caution(s): Federal law restricts this drug to use by or on the order of a licensed veterinarian.

In the event of sensitization or irritation due to MICONOSOL LOTION, treatment should be discontinued. Avoid contact with eyes, since irritation may result. Wash hands thoroughly after administration to avoid spread of fungal infection.

Presentation: MICONOSOL (miconazole nitrate) LOTION in 60 mL containers.

Compendium Code No.: 10270070

MICONOSOL SPRAY 1% ℞

Med-Pharmex **Topical Antifungal**

(Miconazole Nitrate) Topical antifungal agent

ANADA No.: 200-196

Active Ingredient(s): MICONOSOL (miconazole nitrate) SPRAY is a synthetic antifungal agent for use in dogs and cats. It contains: 1.15% miconazole nitrate (equivalent to 1% miconazole base by weight), polyethylene glycol 400 and ethyl alcohol 55%.

Indications: MICONOSOL (miconazole nitrate) SPRAY is indicated for the treatment of fungal infections in dogs and cats caused by *Microsporum canis, Microsporum gypseum* and *Trichophyton mentagrophytes.*

Dosage and Administration: Accurate diagnosis of the infecting organism is essential. Identification should be made either by direct microscopic examination of a mounting of infected tissue in a solution of potassium hydroxide, or by culture on an appropriate medium.

Spray affected areas from a distance of 2 to 4 inches to apply a light covering, once daily for 2 to 4 weeks. Medication must be continued until the infecting organism is completely eradicated as indicated by appropriate clinical or laboratory examination. If no improvement is noticed within 2 weeks, diagnosis should be re-evaluated. Difficult cases may require treatment for 6 weeks.

General measures in regard to hygiene should be observed to control sources of infection or reinfection. Clipping of hair around and over the sites of infection should be done at the start of treatment and again as necessary.

Caution(s): Federal law restricts this drug to use by or on the order of a licensed veterinarian.

In the event of sensitization or irritation due to MICONOSOL SPRAY, treatment should be discontinued. Avoid contact with eyes, since irritation may result. Wash hands thoroughly after administration to avoid spread of fungal infection.

Presentation: MICONOSOL (miconazole nitrate) SPRAY in 120 mL and 240 mL containers.

Compendium Code No.: 10270080

MICOTIL® 300 INJECTION ℞

Elanco **Tilmicosin**

Tilmicosin Injection, USP

NADA No.: 140-929

Active Ingredient(s): MICOTIL® is a solution of the antibiotic tilmicosin. Each mL contains 300 mg of tilmicosin base as tilmicosin phosphate in 25% propylene glycol, phosphoric acid as needed to adjust pH and water for injection, q.s. Tilmicosin, USP is produced semi-synthetically and is in the macrolide class of antibiotics.

Indications: MICOTIL® is indicated for the treatment of bovine respiratory disease (BRD) associated with *Pasteurella haemolytica.* For the control of respiratory disease in cattle at high risk of developing BRD associated with *Pasteurella haemolytica.*

Pharmacology: Actions: Activity—Tilmicosin has an *in vitro** antibacterial spectrum that is predominantly gram-positive with activity against certain gram-negative microorganisms. Activity against several mycoplasma species has also been detected.

Ninety-five percent of the *Pasteurella haemolytica* isolates were inhibited by 3.12 μg/mL or less.

M

Microorganism	MIC (µg/mL)
Pasteurella haemolytica	3.12
Pasteurella multocida	6.25
Haemophilus somnus	6.25
Mycoplasma dispar	0.097
M. bovirhinis	0.024
M. bovoculi	0.048

*The clinical significance of this *in vitro* data in cattle has not been demonstrated.

A single subcutaneous injection of MICOTIL® at 10 mg/kg of body weight dose in cattle resulted in peak tilmicosin levels within one hour and detectable levels (0.07 µg/mL) in serum beyond 3 days. However, lung concentrations of tilmicosin remained above the tilmicosin MIC 95% of 3.12 µg/mL for *P. haemolytica* for at least three days following the single injection. Serum tilmicosin levels are a poor indicator of total body tilmicosin. The lung/serum tilmicosin ratio in favor of lung tissue appeared to equilibrate by three days post injection at approximately 60. In a study with radioactive tilmicosin, 24% and 68% of the dose was recovered from urine and feces respectively over 21 days.

Directions: Inject subcutaneously in cattle only. Administer a single subcutaneous dose of 10 mg/kg of body weight (1 mL/30 kg or 1.5 mL per 100 lbs). Do not inject more than 15 mL per injection site.

If no improvement is noted within 48 hours, the diagnosis should be reevaluated.

Injection under the skin behind the shoulders and over the ribs is suggested.

Note—Swelling at the subcutaneous site of injection may be observed but is transient and usually mild.

Contraindication(s): Do not use in automatically powered syringes. Do not administer intravenously to cattle. Intravenous injection in cattle will be fatal. Do not administer to animals other than cattle. Injection of this antibiotic has been shown to be fatal in swine and non-human primates, and it may be fatal in horses.

Precaution(s): Storage: Store at room temperature, 86°F (30°C) or below. Protect from direct sunlight.

Caution(s): Federal (USA) law restricts this drug to use by or on the order of a licensed veterinarian.

Do not administer to swine. Injection in swine has been shown to be fatal.

The safety of tilmicosin has not been established in pregnant cattle and in animals used for breeding purposes. Intramuscular injection will cause a local reaction which may result in trim loss.

Warning(s): Animals intended for human consumption must not be slaughtered within 28 days of last treatment. Do not use in female dairy cattle 20 months of age or older. Use of tilmicosin in this class of cattle may cause milk residues.

Human Warnings: Not for human use. Injection of this drug in humans may be fatal. Keep out of reach of children. Do not use in automatically powered syringes. Exercise extreme caution to avoid accidental self injection. In case of human injection, consult a physician immediately. Emergency medical telephone numbers are 1-800-722-0987 or 1-317-276-2000. Avoid contact with eyes.

Note to Physician: The cardiovascular system appears to be the target of toxicity. This antibiotic persists in tissues for several days. The cardiovascular system should be monitored closely and supportive treatment provided. Dobutamine partially offset the negative inotropic effects induced by MICOTIL® in dogs. β-adrenergic antagonists, such as propranolol, exacerbated the negative inotropy of MICOTIL®-induced tachycardia in dogs. Epinephrine potentiated lethality of MICOTIL® in pigs.

M

Toxicology: The heart is the target of toxicity in laboratory and domestic animals given MICOTIL® 300 by oral or parenteral routes. The primary cardiac effects are increased heart rate (tachycardia) and decreased contractility (negative inotropy).

Upon injection subcutaneously, the acute median initial dose of tilmicosin in mice is 97 mg per kg, and in rats is 185 mg/kg of body weight. Given orally, the median lethal dose is 800 mg/kg and 2250 mg/kg in fasted and non-fasted rats, respectively. No compound-related lesions were found at necropsy.

In monkeys, a single intramuscular dose of 10 mg/kg caused no signs of toxicity. A single dose of 20 mg/kg caused vomiting and 30 mg/kg caused the death of the only monkey tested.

In swine, intramuscular injection of 10 mg/kg caused increased respiration, emesis, and a convulsion, 20 mg/kg resulted in mortality in 3 of 4 pigs, and 30 mg/kg caused the death of all 4 pigs tested.

Results of genetic toxicology studies were all negative. Results of teratology and reproduction studies in rats were negative. The no effect level in dogs after daily oral doses for up to one year is 4 mg/kg of body weight.

In cattle, subcutaneous doses of 10, 30, and 50 mg/kg of body weight, each injected three times at 72 hour intervals did not cause any deaths. As expected edema at the site of injection was noted. The only lesion observed at necropsy was minimal myocardial necrosis in some animals in the 50 mg/kg group. Subcutaneous doses of 150 mg/kg injected at 72-hour intervals resulted in deaths. Edema was marked at the site of injection. Minimal myocardial necrosis was the only lesion observed at necropsy. Deaths of cattle have been observed with a single intravenous dose of 5 mg/kg of body weight.

Presentation: MICOTIL® is supplied in 50 mL, 100 mL and 250 mL multidose bottles sold by individual bottles or in cases of 6 or 12.

MICOTIL® is a trademark of Eli Lilly and Company.

Compendium Code No.: 10310052 PI 3795 AMP

MICROBAN® X-580 INSTITUTIONAL SPRAY PLUS

Microban **Premise Insecticide-Disinfectant**

EPA Reg. No.: 70263-3

Active Ingredient(s):

o-Phenylphenol	0.22%
Diisobutylphenoxyethoxy ethyl dimethyl benzyl ammonium chloride monohydrate	0.70%
N-octyl bicycloheptene dicarboximide	0.33%
Piperonyl butoxide technical	0.20%
Pyrethrins	0.10%
Inert Ingredients	98.45%
Total	100%

[equivalent to (butylcarbityl) (6-propyl piperonyl) ether: 0.16% and related compounds: 0.04%]

Indications: A mildewcide, bactericide, fungicide, disinfectant, antimicrobial, insecticide and deodorant for institutional, household, farm premise uses and animal quarters.

MICROBAN® Formula X-580 Institutional Spray Plus is a broad spectrum disinfectant against most bacteria and is also effective in controlling insects, fungus and bacterial or organic odors.

Directions for Use: Shake well before and during use.

Test fabric or surface in an inconspicuous area for color fastness or adversive reaction.

It is a violation of Federal Law to use this product in a manner inconsistent with its labeling.

MICROBAN® Formula X-580 Institutional Spray Plus should be applied with hand or power operated sprayers, foggers, automated metering systems or gravity drip dispensers as an insecticide, bactericide, mold and mildewcide, fungicide and deodorizing agent, to previously cleaned surfaces. Spray areas until thoroughly moist, giving special attention to cracks and crevices. Allow ten to twenty minutes for drying. It is not necessary to wipe the sprayed surface. MICROBAN® Formula X-580 Institutional Spray Plus should not stain those materials not stained by water.

Direct and repeat spraying of ants, roaches, bedbugs, silverfish and other harmful insects and in the cracks, crevices and hidden surfaces where they hide are necessary for control. Apply every 28 days or as often as needed.

To Kill Fleas and Ticks: Remove and destroy old animal bedding. Spray sleeping quarters of animals, floor areas, around baseboards, window and door frames, cracks, crevices and wherever the presence of these insects are suspected. Repeat as necessary. Thoroughly vacuum rugs and carpets prior to application. Do not spray animals. Put fresh bedding in animal quarters after spray has dried. Treat animals with a registered flea and tick control product before allowing them to enter treated area.

To Kill Sowbugs, Centipedes, Firebrats and Mites: Contact as many insects as possible with the spray. Also thoroughly spray all parts of the room suspected of harboring these pests. Special attention should be paid to cracks, crevices, hidden surfaces under sinks, basement and utility rooms, floors, doorjams, behind and under stoves and refrigerators.

To Kill Flies, Mosquitoes, Gnats and Wasps: Close all doors and windows and spray upward into center of room with a slow sweeping motion. Spray 5-10 seconds for average room. Keep room closed for 15 minutes after spraying. Ventilate room thoroughly before re-entry. Sweep up and destroy fallen insects. Before spraying cover exposed food and utensils.

To Kill Carpet Beetles, Lice and Moths: Clean all articles prior to application. Thoroughly spray top and undersides of rugs and carpets. Thoroughly spray the interiors of lockers, trunks, closets, cupboards and other storage areas. Spray directly on restroom fixtures. When treating upholstered furniture and mattresses thoroughly spray exterior, paying particular attention to seams and folds. Interior should be treated to eliminate hidden infestations.

General Method of Application: Surfaces and objects must be cleaned of gross filth with suitable detergent before treatment. Spray surfaces and articles until thoroughly wet, use enough so that treated surfaces and objects remain wet for at least 10 minutes. May be applied with a sponge to pre-cleaned, hard non-porous surfaces, allowing to dry for 10 minutes. For fogging and other large volume applications use appropriate spraying equipment, protective clothing, gloves and respirator. Heavily treated spaces should be adequately ventilated and not re-entered for at least one hour after treatment.

As a Mildewcide, Fungicide and Broad-Spectrum Disinfectant: (Kills most gram negative and gram positive bacteria and influenza virus.) In hospitals, operating rooms, emergency rooms, lobbies, hallways, patient rooms, wards, washrooms, scrub stations, mop rooms, morgues, pathology labs, nurse's stations, laboratories, veterinary clinics and other health care facilities; in schools, hotels, motels, restaurants, offices, homes and industrial buildings.

For use on pre-cleaned hard non-porous surfaces such as glazed tiled porcelain, waste receptacles, compactors, on, in and around rest room fixtures, toilet seats, locker rooms, telephones, door knobs, hospital apparatus and equipment, furniture and empty containerized storage units. For athletes foot fungus on floors, shower stalls and rest rooms. Follow method of application specified above.

As a Bacteriostat, Fungistat and Deodorizing Agent: Apply MICROBAN® Formula X-580 Institutional Spray Plus as directed to floors, walls, ceilings that have been damaged by smoke, fire, floods and sewage backups. For cleanup operations in areas such as attics, wall voids, basements, areas above suspended ceilings and similar inaccessible spaces in buildings. Spray avian, rodent and other animal and human wastes and carcasses as directed above, prior to removal and disposal. Treat spaces and surfaces as specified in method of application. For use as a bacteriostat, fungistat and deodorizing agent on carpeting found in schools, hotels, motels, homes, shelters, commercial, industrial and public buildings. After flood or water damage, vacuum or extract as much water as possible before application. Apply full strength with sprayer until moist to carpet nap and rake or brush in. To treat the backing and padding a fogger is recommended. Allow to remain dry. For best results, carpets should be cleaned before application.

This product is not to be used as a terminal sterilant/high level disinfectant on any surface or instrument that (1) is introduced directly into the human body, either into or in contact with the bloodstream or normally sterile areas of the body, or (2) contacts intact mucous membranes but which does not ordinarily penetrate the blood barrier or otherwise enter normally sterile areas of the body. This product may be used to preclean or decontaminate critical or semi-critical medical devices prior to sterilization or high level disinfection.

To Disinfect Farm Premises, Poultry Houses, Animal Pens and Vehicles: Remove all animals and feed from premises, vehicles and enclosures. Remove all litter and manure from floors, walls and surfaces of barns, pens, stalls, chutes and other facilities and fixtures occupied or traversed by animals. Empty all troughs, racks and other feeding and watering appliances. Thoroughly clean all surfaces with soap or detergent and rinse with water. Saturate all surfaces with the recommended disinfecting solution for a period of 10 minutes. Immerse all halters, ropes and other types of equipment used in handling and restraining animals, as well as forks, shovels and scrapers used for removing litter and manure. Ventilate buildings, cars, boats and other closed spaces. Do not house livestock or employ equipment until treatment has been absorbed, set or dried. Thoroughly scrub all treated feed racks, mangers, troughs, automatic feeders, fountains and waterers, with soap or detergent and rinse with potable water before reuse. Apply MICROBAN® Formula X-580 Institutional Plus full strength as directed in general method of application until thoroughly wet. Allow all surfaces to dry thoroughly, ventilate enclosed spaces adequately. Do not house animals in treated areas until thoroughly dry and free from odors.

Precautionary Statements: Hazards to Humans and Domestic Animals:

Warning: May be harmful if swallowed (inhaled or absorbed through the skin). Do not breathe vapors (dust or spray mist). Causes eye (and skin) irritation. Do not get in eyes, on skin or on clothing.

Statements of Practical Treatment:

First Aid: In case of contact flush eyes and skin with plenty of water for at least fifteen minutes.

For eyes get medical attention. If swallowed drink promptly large quantities of water. Do not induce vomiting. Remove and wash contaminated clothing before reuse.

Physical and Chemical Hazards: Flammable. Keep away from heat and open frame.

Storage and Disposal: Storage: Keep from freezing. Store in ventilated areas. Do not contaminate water, food or feed by storage and disposal. Dispose left overs in landfill approved for pesticides. Pesticide Disposal: Wastes resulting from the use of this product may be disposed of on site or at an approved waste disposal facility. Container Disposal: Large containers (55 gallon drums and 5 gallon pails): Triple rinse (or equivalent) all containers and offer for recycling or reconditioning or puncture and dispose of in a sanitary landfill or by procedures approved by the state and local authorities. Small container (1 gallon or less): Rinse thoroughly and discard with trash.

Warning(s): Keep out of reach of children.

Presentation: 1 quart, 1 gallon, 5 gallons and 55 gallons.

Compendium Code No.: 10090002 Revised 2000 MSI

MICROCILLIN

Anthony **Penicillin Injection**

Penicillin G Procaine Aqueous Suspension

NADA No.: 065-505

Active Ingredient(s): Each mL contains:

Penicillin G procaine	300,000 units
Methylparaben	1.3 mg
Propylparaben	0.2 mg
Sodium citrate	10 mg
Sodium carboxymethylcellulose	1 mg
Povidone	5 mg
Lecithin	6 mg
Sodium formaldehyde sulfoxylate	0.2 mg
Procaine hydrochloride	20 mg
In water for injection	q.s.

Indications: Penicillin G is an effective bactericide in the treatment of infections caused primarily by penicillin-sensitive organisms, such as *Streptococcus equi* and *Erysipelothrix insidiosa*, as well as the gram-negative organism *Pasteurella multocida*.

MICROCILLIN is indicated for the treatment of:

1. Cattle and Sheep: Bacterial pneumonia (shipping fever) caused by *Pasteurella multocida*.
2. Swine: Erysipelas caused by *Erysipelothrix insidiosa*.
3. Horses: Strangles caused by *Streptococcus equi*.

Dosage and Administration: The suspension should be administered by deep intramuscular injection within the fleshy muscles of the hip, rump, round or thigh, or into the neck, changing the site for each injection. Do not inject subcutaneously, into a blood vessel, or near a major nerve.

Use a 16- or 18-gauge needle, 1.5 inches long. The needle and syringe should be washed thoroughly before use. The needle and syringe should then be sterilized by placing them in boiling water for 15 to 20 minutes.

The injection site should be washed with soap and water and painted with a germicide such as tincture of iodine or 70% alcohol. The product should then be administered by using the following procedure:

1. Warm the vial to room temperature and shake thoroughly to ensure uniform suspension.
2. Wipe the rubber stopper on the top of the vial with a piece of absorbent cotton soaked in 70% alcohol.
3. Inject air into the vial for easier withdrawal.
4. After filling the syringe, make sure that the needle is empty by pulling back the plunger until a small air bubble appears. Then detach the needle from the syringe.
5. Insert the needle deeply into the muscle, attach the syringe and withdraw the plunger slightly. If blood appears, withdraw the needle and insert it in a different location.
6. Inject the dose slowly. Do not massage the site of injection.
7. Not more than 10 mL should be injected in one location.

Daily treatment should be continued for at least 48 hours after the temperature has returned to normal and other signs of infection have subsided. Animals treated with MICROCILLIN should show noticeable improvement within 36 to 48 hours.

The dosage for cattle, sheep, swine, and horses is 3,000 units per pound of body weight, or 1.0 mL for each 100 pounds of body weight once a day. Treatment should not exceed 7 days in non-lactating dairy and beef cattle, sheep, and swine, or 5 days in lactating dairy cattle. If no improvement is observed within 48 hours, consult your veterinarian.

Precaution(s): MICROCILLIN should be stored in a cold room at a temperature between 2° and 8°C (36°-46°F). Avoid freezing the product.

Caution(s): Restricted drug (under California law). Use only as directed.

Sensitivity reactions to penicillin and procaine, such as hives or respiratory distress, may occur in some animals. If such signs of sensitivity occur, stop medication and call a veterinarian. In some instances, particularly if respiratory distress is severe, immediate injection of epinephrine or antihistamine may be necessary.

As with any antibiotic preparation, prolonged use may result in the overgrowth of non-susceptible organisms, including fungi. If this condition is suspected, stop medication and consult a veterinarian.

For animal use only.

Warning(s):

1. Not for use in horses intended for food.
2. Milk that has been taken from animals during treatment and for 48 hours (4 milkings) after the last treatment must not be used for food. The daily treatment schedule should not exceed 7 days of treatment in non-lactating dairy and beef cattle, sheep and swine, or 5 days in lactating dairy cattle.
3. The drug should be discontinued for the following time periods before treated animals are slaughtered for food:

Cattle	4 days
Sheep	8 days
Swine	6 days
Non-ruminating calves	7 days

Presentation: MICROCILLIN is supplied in 100 mL, 250 mL and 500 mL multiple-dose vials.

Compendium Code No.: 10250021 Rev. 6/00

MICRO-D® 500

Alpharma **Feed Additive**

Guaranteed Analysis: Vitamin D_3 500,000 International Chick Units per gram (226,800,000 ICU per pound).

Ingredients: Activated 7-dehydrocholesterol, butylated hydroxytoluene (preservative), vegetable oil, modified edible starch, certified food color.

Indications: Source of cholecalciferol, vitamin D_3.

Dosage and Administration: Use as needed.

Precaution(s): Store in a cool dry location. Keep container closed. Do not accept if container has been opened.

Caution(s): For manufacturing feedstuffs only.

Presentation: 55.1 lb (25 kg).

Compendium Code No.: 10220460

MICRO-D® 1000

Alpharma **Feed Additive**

Guaranteed Analysis: Vitamin D_3 1,000,000 International Chick Units per gram (453,590,000 ICU per pound).

Ingredients: Activated 7-dehydrocholesterol, butylated hydroxytoluene (preservative), vegetable oil, modified edible starch, certified food color.

Indications: Source of cholecalciferol, vitamin D_3.

Dosage and Administration: Use as needed.

Precaution(s): Store in a cool dry location. Keep container closed. Do not accept if container has been opened.

Caution(s): For manufacturing feedstuffs only.

Presentation: 55.1 lb (25 kg).

Compendium Code No.: 10220450

MICROMASTER® ALERT™ CALF BOLUS

Loveland **Large Animal Dietary Supplement**

Guaranteed Analysis:

Lactobacillus acidophilus	3×10^7 cfu/gm
Bifidobacterium thermophilum	3×10^7 cfu/gm
Bifidobacterium longum	3×10^7 cfu/gm
Streptococcus faecium	3×10^7 cfu/gm
Saccharomyces cerevisiae	1×10^7 cfu/gm

Ingredients: Dried egg, dried *Lactobacillus acidophilus* fermentation product, dried *Bifidobacterium thermophilum* fermentation product, dried *Streptococcus faecium* fermentation product, *Saccharomyces cerevisiae*, powdered cellulose, hydrated sodium calcium aluminosilicate, lactose, magnesium stearate, artificial color.

Indications: A source of live (viable) naturally occurring microorganisms for young or weak calves.

Dosage and Administration: Administer one (1) bolus within the first 12 hours to newborn calves. Repeat or increase dosage as needed.

Precaution(s): Keep in a cool, dry place. Protect from direct sunlight.

Notice: Loveland Industries, Inc. warrants that this product conforms to the chemical description on the label thereof and is reasonably fit for the purposes stated on such label only when used in accordance with the directions under normal use conditions. It is impossible to eliminate all risks inherently associated with the use of this product. Crop injury, equipment damage or other unintended consequences may result because of such factors as weather conditions, presence of other materials or the manner of application or use all of which are beyond the control of Loveland Industries, Inc. In no case shall Loveland Industries, Inc. be liable for consequential, special or indirect damages resulting from the use or handling of this product. All such risks shall be assumed by the buyer. Loveland Industries, Inc. makes no warranties of merchantability or fitness for a particular purpose nor any other express or implied warranty except as stated above.

Presentation: 12 boluses, 0.30 oz (8.5 grams) per bolus.

Compendium Code No.: 10860030

MICROMASTER® AVIAN PAC™ HT

Loveland **Poultry Dietary Supplement**

Guaranteed Analysis:

Microencapsulated *Lactobacillus acidophilus* . . . 3×10^7 (30 million) CFU's/g

LI Avian specific strain #12

LI Avian specific strain #18

Rhizopus Species Fermentation Extract

Activity	Units / gram
Amylase	2,200
Protease	300
Lipase	90
Cellulase	115
Pectinase	57.5

Ingredients: Calcium carbonate, grain by-products, dried egg, vegetable oil.

Indications: A source of live (viable) naturally occurring microorganisms.

Dosage and Administration: For use in pelleted or mash feeds, mix 500 to 1,000 grams per metric ton.

Precaution(s): Store in cool, dry place. Keep out of direct sunlight.

Notice: Loveland Industries, Inc. warrants that the product conforms to the chemical description on the label thereof and is reasonably fit for the purposes stated on such label only when used in accordance with the directions under normal use conditions. It is impossible to eliminate all risks inherently associated with the use of this product. In no case shall Loveland Industries, Inc. be liable for consequential, special or indirect damages resulting from use or handling of this product. All such risks shall be assumed by the buyer. Loveland Industries, Inc. makes no warranties of merchantability or fitness for a particular purpose nor any other express or implied warranty except as stated above.

Presentation: 1 kg.

Compendium Code No.: 10860040

MICROMASTER® AVIAN PAC™ ROUTINE

Loveland **Poultry Dietary Supplement**

Guaranteed Analysis:

Microencapsulated *Lactobacillus acidophilus*. . . . . 3 x 10^7 (30 million) CFU's/g

LI Avian specific strain #12

LI Avian specific strain #18

Saccharomyces cerevisiae . . . . 5.5 x 10^9 (5.5 billion) CFU's/g

Ingredients: Calcium carbonate, grain by-products, vegetable oil.

Indications: A source of live (viable) naturally occurring microorganisms for use in broilers, breeders and layers.

Dosage and Administration: 500 to 1,000 grams per metric ton. 1 to 2 pounds per short ton.

Precaution(s): Store in cool, dry place. Keep out of direct sunlight.

Notice: Loveland Industries, Inc. warrants that the product conforms to the chemical description on the label thereof and is reasonably fit for the purposes stated on such label only when used in accordance with the directions under normal use conditions. It is impossible to eliminate all risks inherently associated with the use of this product. In no case shall Loveland Industries, Inc. be liable for consequential, special or indirect damages resulting from use or handling of this product. All such risks shall be assumed by the buyer. Loveland Industries, Inc. makes no warranties of merchantability or fitness for a particular purpose nor any other express or implied warranty except as stated above.

Presentation: 1 kg.

Compendium Code No.: 10860050

MICROMASTER® AVIAN PAC™ SOLUBLE

Loveland **Poultry Dietary Supplement**

Guaranteed Analysis:

Lactobacillus acidophilus. . . . . 1.5 x 10^8 (150 million) CFU's/g

LI Avian specific strain #12

LI Avian specific strain #18

Streptococcus faecium. . . . . 1.5 x 10^8 (150 million) CFU's/g

LI Avian specific strain #7

Ingredients: Citric acid.

Indications: A source of live (viable) naturally occurring microorganisms for use in avian water supplies.

Dosage and Administration: Dissolve one 50 gram packet into 120 gallons of drinking water for every 10,000 birds. Change every 24 hours. For metering systems: Add one 50 gram packet to one gallon of water. Set proportioner to meter one ounce per gallon of water.

Precaution(s): Store in cool, dry place. Keep out of direct sunlight.

Notice: Loveland Industries, Inc. warrants that the product conforms to the chemical description on the label thereof and is reasonably fit for the purposes stated on such label only when used in accordance with the directions under normal use conditions. It is impossible to eliminate all risks inherently associated with the use of this product. In no case shall Loveland Industries, Inc. be liable for consequential, special or indirect damages resulting from use or handling of this product. All such risks shall be assumed by the buyer. Loveland Industries, Inc. makes no warranties of merchantability or fitness for a particular purpose nor any other express or implied warranty except as stated above.

Presentation: 50 g packet.

Compendium Code No.: 10860060

M

MICROMASTER® AVIAN PAC™ SOLUBLE PLUS

Loveland **Poultry Dietary Supplement**

Guaranteed Analysis:

Lactobacillus acidophilus. . . . . 1.0 x 10^8 (100 million) CFU's/g

LI Avian specific strain #12

LI Avian specific strain #18

Streptococcus faecium. . . . . 1.0 x 10^8 (100 million) CFU's/g

LI Avian specific strain #7

Ingredients: Citric acid, dried egg.

Indications: A source of live (viable) naturally occurring microorganisms for use in avian water supplies.

Dosage and Administration: Dissolve 150 grams of AVIAN PAC™ Soluble Plus 120 gallons of drinking water for every 10,000 birds. Repeat dosage for 2-3 days.

Precaution(s): Store in cool, dry place. Keep out of direct sunlight.

Notice: Loveland Industries, Inc. warrants that the product conforms to the chemical description on the label thereof and is reasonably fit for the purposes stated on such label only when used in accordance with the directions under normal use conditions. It is impossible to eliminate all risks inherently associated with the use of this product. In no case shall Loveland Industries, Inc. be liable for consequential, special or indirect damages resulting from use or handling of this product. All such risks shall be assumed by the buyer. Loveland Industries, Inc. makes no warranties of merchantability or fitness for a particular purpose nor any other express or implied warranty except as stated above.

Presentation: 150 g.

Compendium Code No.: 10860070

MICROMASTER® AVIAN PULSE PAC™

Loveland **Poultry Dietary Supplement**

Guaranteed Analysis:

Microencapsulated *Lactobacillus acidophilus*. . . . . 3 x 10^7 (30 million) CFU's/g

LI Avian specific strain #20

LI Avian specific strain #26

Ingredients: Calcium carbonate, grain by-products, dried egg, vegetable oil.

Indications: A source of live (viable) naturally occurring microorganisms for layers and breeders.

Dosage and Administration: 1 kg per metric ton; 1 week on, 2 weeks off.

1 to 2 pounds per short ton.

Precaution(s): Store in cool, dry place. Keep out of direct sunlight.

Notice: Loveland Industries, Inc. warrants that the product conforms to the chemical description on the label thereof and is reasonably fit for the purposes stated on such label only when used in accordance with the directions under normal use conditions. It is impossible to eliminate all risks inherently associated with the use of this product. In no case shall Loveland Industries, Inc. be liable for consequential, special or indirect damages resulting from use or handling of this product. All such risks shall be assumed by the buyer. Loveland Industries, Inc. makes no warranties of merchantability or fitness for a particular purpose nor any other express or implied warranty except as stated above.

Presentation: 1 kg.

Compendium Code No.: 10860080

MICROMASTER® BOVINE PASTE

Loveland **Large Animal Dietary Supplement**

Guaranteed Analysis: As colony-forming units per gram

Lactobacillus acidophilus (LI 1B) . . . . 1 x 10^8 Cfu/gm

Lactobacillus lactis (LI 12B) . . . . 1 x 10^8 Cfu/gm

Bifidobacterium longum (LI 16B) . . . . 1 x 10^8 Cfu/gm

Bifidobacterium thermophilus (LI 3B). . . . . 3 x 10^8 Cfu/gm

Streptococcus faecium (LI 80B) . . . . 1 x 10^8 Cfu/gm

Saccharomyces cerevisiae (LI 11). 2 x 10^9 Cfu/gm

Ingredients: Corn oil, silicon dioxide, dextrose, whey, dried egg, sorbitan monostearate, potassium sorbate.

Indications: A source of live (viable) naturally occurring microorganisms in beef cattle, dairy cattle and calves.

Dosage and Administration: 6 to 8 grams of paste for each animal per day.

Precaution(s): Store product at 50°-65°F.

Notice: Loveland Industries, Inc. warrants that the product conforms to the chemical description on the label thereof and is reasonably fit for the purposes stated on such label only when used in accordance with the directions under normal use conditions. It is impossible to eliminate all risks inherently associated with the use of this product. In no case shall Loveland Industries, Inc. be liable for consequential, special or indirect damages resulting from the use or handling of this product. All such risks shall be assumed by the buyer. Loveland Industries, Inc. makes no warranties of merchantability or fitness for a particular purpose nor any other express or implied warranty except as stated above.

Presentation: 300 grams.

Compendium Code No.: 10860090

MICROMASTER® CALF PAC™ SOLUBLE

Loveland **Large Animal Dietary Supplement**

Guaranteed Analysis:

Lactobacillus acidophilus . . . . 1.4 x 10^6 (1.4 million) CFU's/g

Bifidobacterium longum . . . . 3.5 x 10^6 (3.5 million) CFU's/g

Bifidobacterium thermophilus . . . . 3.5 x 10^6 (3.5 million) CFU's/g

Streptococcus faecium . . . . 1.4 x 10^6 (1.4 million) CFU's/g

Saccharomyces cerevisiae . . . . 1.5 x 10^9 (1.5 million) CFU's/g

Ingredients: Whey, dextrose, dried egg.

Indications: A source of live (viable) naturally occurring microorganisms for cattle and sheep.

Dosage and Administration: Add to milk replacer or dry feed.

Cattle: Feed 10 grams per head per day; For 14 to 21 days as needed.

Sheep: Feed 10 grams per 5 head per day; For 14 to 21 days as needed.

Precaution(s): Store in cool, dry place. Keep out of direct sunlight.

Notice: Loveland Industries, Inc. warrants that the product conforms to the chemical description on the label thereof and is reasonably fit for the purposes stated on such label only when used in accordance with the directions under normal use conditions. It is impossible to eliminate all risks inherently associated with the use of this product. In no case shall Loveland Industries, Inc. be liable for consequential, special or indirect damages resulting from the use or handling of this product. All such risks shall be assumed by the buyer. Loveland Industries, Inc. makes no warranties of merchantability or fitness for a particular purpose nor any other express or implied warranty except as stated above.

Presentation: 5 kg.

Compendium Code No.: 10860100

MICROMASTER® DAIRY PAC™

Loveland **Large Animal Dietary Supplement**

Guaranteed Analysis:

Saccharomyces cerevisiae . . . . 2.3 x 10^9 (2.3 million) CFU's/g

Lactobacillus acidophilus . . . . 2.0 x 10^7 (20 million) CFU's/g

Streptococcus faecium . . . . 2.0 x 10^7 (20 million) CFU's/g

Aspergillus oryzae fermentation extract

Activity Units / gram

Carbohydrase 12,000

Ingredients: Extruded wheat middlings.

Indications: A source of live (viable) naturally occurring microorganisms for dairy cattle.

Dosage and Administration: 10 grams per head per day. Top dressed or mixed in ration.

Precaution(s): Store in cool, dry place. Keep out of direct sunlight.

Notice: Loveland Industries, Inc. warrants that the product conforms to the chemical description on the label thereof and is reasonably fit for the purposes stated on such label only when used in accordance with the directions under normal use conditions. It is impossible to eliminate all risks inherently associated with the use of this product. In no case shall Loveland Industries, Inc. be liable for consequential, special or indirect damages resulting from use or handling of this product. All such risks shall be assumed by the buyer. Loveland Industries, Inc. makes no warranties of merchantability or fitness for a particular purpose nor any other express or implied warranty except as stated above.

Presentation: 10 kg.

Compendium Code No.: 10860110

MICROMASTER® EQUINE GEL

Loveland — **Equine Dietary Supplement**

Guaranteed Analysis:

Streptococcus faecium, Lactobacillus acidophilus	5 billion CFU's total
Saccharomyces cerevisiae	30 billion CFU's total
Vitamin A	12,000 IU
Vitamin E	10 IU
Thiamine	15 mg
Riboflavin	12 mg
Niacin	15 mg
Pyridoxine	1.5 mg
Pantothenic acid	10 mg
Folic acid	1.5 mg
Vitamin B_{12}	15 mcg
Vitamin D_3	1,200 IU

Ingredients: Vegetable oil, corn starch, silicon dioxide, anhydrous dextrose, apple flavor.

Indications: A source of lactic bacteria for gastrointestinal supplementation in horses.

Dosage and Administration: Administer Equine Gel orally on back of tongue.

Foals: Administer 5 cc at birth. Repeat 3-5 days later and at weaning. Adult horses: Administer 10 cc prior to changing feed, water, environment, or training conditions, or prior to transporting.

Precaution(s): Store product at 50°-65°F.

Notice: Loveland Industries, Inc. warrants that the product conforms to the chemical description on the label thereof and is reasonably fit for the purposes stated on such label only when used in accordance with the directions under normal use conditions. It is impossible to eliminate all risks inherently associated with the use of this product. In no case shall Loveland Industries, Inc. be liable for consequential, special or indirect damages resulting from the use or handling of this product. All such risks shall be assumed by the buyer. Loveland Industries, Inc. makes no warranties of merchantability or fitness for a particular purpose nor any other express or implied warranty except as stated above.

Presentation: 60 cc.

Compendium Code No.: 10860120

MICROMASTER® PET GEL

Loveland — **Small Animal Dietary Supplement**

Guaranteed Analysis:

Enterococcus faecium, Lactobacillus acidophilus	4 billion CFU's total
Saccharomyces cerevisiae	500 million CFU's total
Vitamin A	2,000 IU
Vitamin E	20 IU
Vitamin D_3	200 IU

Ingredients: Vegetable oil, silicon dioxide, dextrose, active dry yeast *(Saccharomyces cerevisiae)*, dried *Enterococcus faecium* fermentation product, dried *Lactobacillus acidophilus* fermentation product, vitamin A acetate, D-activated animal sterol (source of D_3), Dl-Alpha tocopherol acetate (source of vitamin E).

Indications: A live probiotic culture for dogs and cats. Contains a source of live (viable) naturally occurring microorganisms.

Dosage and Administration: Administer Pet Gel between lower teeth and cheek, or top dress on feed.

Cats: 1 cc

Dogs less than 25 lbs: 1 cc

Dogs greater than 25 lbs: 2 cc

Precaution(s): Store product at 50°-65°F.

Notice: Loveland Industries, Inc. warrants that the product conforms to the chemical description on the label thereof and is reasonably fit for the purposes stated on such label only when used in accordance with the directions under normal use conditions. It is impossible to eliminate all risks inherently associated with the use of this product. In no case shall Loveland Industries, Inc. be liable for consequential, special or indirect damages resulting from the use or handling of this product. All such risks shall be assumed by the buyer. Loveland Industries, Inc. makes no warranties of merchantability or fitness for a particular purpose nor any other express or implied warranty except as stated above.

Presentation: 15 cc.

Compendium Code No.: 10860130

MICROMASTER® PORCINE PAC™ HT

Loveland — **Large Animal Dietary Supplement**

Guaranteed Analysis:

Microencapsulated *Lactobacillus acidophilus*	1.0 x 10^7 (10 million) CFU's/g
Microencapsulated *Lactobacillus lactis*	1.0 x 10^7 (10 million) CFU's/g
Microencapsulated *Streptococcus faecium*	1.0 x 10^7 (10 million) CFU's/g

Rhizopus Species Fermentation Extract

Activity	Units / gram
Amylase	2,200
Protease	300
Lipase	90
Cellulase	115
Pectinase	57.5

Ingredients: Wheat flour, calcium carbonate.

Indications: A source of live (viable) naturally occurring microorganisms for swine.

Dosage and Administration: Administer on pelleted or mash feeds.

500 to 1,000 grams per metric ton for grower-finisher.

300 grams per metric ton for dry sows.

500 grams per metric ton for pre-farrow (3 weeks) and lactating sows.

Precaution(s): Store in cool, dry place. Keep out of direct sunlight.

Notice: Loveland Industries, Inc. warrants that the product conforms to the chemical description on the label thereof and is reasonably fit for the purposes stated on such label only when used in accordance with the directions under normal use conditions. It is impossible to eliminate all risks inherently associated with the use of this product. In no case shall Loveland Industries, Inc. be liable for consequential, special or indirect damages resulting from use or handling of this product. All such risks shall be assumed by the buyer. Loveland Industries, Inc. makes no warranties of merchantability or fitness for a particular purpose nor any other express or implied warranty except as stated above.

Presentation: 1 kg.

Compendium Code No.: 10860140

MICROMASTER® PORCINE PASTE

Loveland — **Large Animal Dietary Supplement**

Guaranteed Analysis: As colony-forming units per gram

Lactobacillus acidophilus (LI 7P)	1 x 10^8 Cfu/gm
Lactobacillus lactis (LI 12P)	1 x 10^8 Cfu/gm
Bifidobacterium longum (LI 44P)	1 x 10^8 Cfu/gm
Bifidobacterium thermophilus (LI 16P)	1 x 10^8 Cfu/gm
Streptococcus faecium (LI 14P)	1 x 10^8 Cfu/gm
Saccharomyces cerevisiae (LI 11)	1 x 10^9 Cfu/gm

Ingredients: Corn oil, silicon dioxide, dextrose, whey, dried egg, sorbitan monostearate, potassium sorbate.

Indications: A source of live (viable) naturally occurring microorganisms for gastrointestinal supplementation in swine.

Dosage and Administration: 3 to 4 grams of paste for each animal per day.

Precaution(s): Store product at 50°-65°F.

Notice: Loveland Industries, Inc. warrants that the product conforms to the chemical description on the label thereof and is reasonably fit for the purposes stated on such label only when used in accordance with the directions under normal use conditions. It is impossible to eliminate all risks inherently associated with the use of this product. In no case shall Loveland Industries, Inc. be liable for consequential, special or indirect damages resulting from the use or handling of this product. All such risks shall be assumed by the buyer. Loveland Industries, Inc. makes no warranties of merchantability or fitness for a particular purpose nor any other express or implied warranty except as stated above.

Presentation: 300 grams.

Compendium Code No.: 10860150

MICROMASTER® PORCINE STARTER PAC™

Loveland — **Large Animal Dietary Supplement**

Guaranteed Analysis:

Microencapsulated *Lactobacillus acidophilus*	1.0 x 10^7 (10 million) CFU's/g
Microencapsulated *Lactobacillus lactis*	1.0 x 10^7 (10 million) CFU's/g
Microencapsulated *Streptococcus faecium*	1.0 x 10^7 (10 million) CFU's/g

Ingredients: Wheat flour, dried egg, vegetable oil.

Indications: A source of live (viable) naturally occurring microorganisms for pre-starter and starter pigs.

Dosage and Administration: Use in pelleted or mash feeds at a rate of 500 to 1,000 grams per metric ton.

Precaution(s): Store in cool, dry place. Keep out of direct sunlight.

Notice: Loveland Industries, Inc. warrants that the product conforms to the chemical description on the label thereof and is reasonably fit for the purposes stated on such label only when used in accordance with the directions under normal use conditions. It is impossible to eliminate all risks inherently associated with the use of this product. In no case shall Loveland Industries, Inc. be liable for consequential, special or indirect damages resulting from use or handling of this product. All such risks shall be assumed by the buyer. Loveland Industries, Inc. makes no warranties of merchantability or fitness for a particular purpose nor any other express or implied warranty except as stated above.

Presentation: 1 kg.

Compendium Code No.: 10860160

MICROMASTER® PORCINE STARTER PAC™ SOLUBLE

Loveland — **Large Animal Dietary Supplement**

Guaranteed Analysis:

Microencapsulated *Lactobacillus acidophilus*	1.0 x 10^8 (100 million) CFU's/g
Microencapsulated *Lactobacillus lactis*	1.0 x 10^8 (100 million) CFU's/g
Microencapsulated *Streptococcus faecium*	1.0 x 10^8 (100 million) CFU's/g

Ingredients: Whey, dextrose, dried egg, vegetable oil.

Indications: A source of live (viable) naturally occurring microorganisms for use in porcine water supplies.

Dosage and Administration:

Routine Use: Add 50 grams to water for 800 pigs.

Short Term Pulse Inoculation Use: Add 50 grams to water for 100 pigs.

Precaution(s): Store in cool, dry place. Keep out of direct sunlight.

Notice: Loveland Industries, Inc. warrants that the product conforms to the chemical description on the label thereof and is reasonably fit for the purposes stated on such label only when used in accordance with the directions under normal use conditions. It is impossible to eliminate all risks inherently associated with the use of this product. In no case shall Loveland Industries, Inc. be liable for consequential, special or indirect damages resulting from use or handling of this product. All such risks shall be assumed by the buyer. Loveland Industries, Inc. makes no warranties of merchantability or fitness for a particular purpose nor any other express or implied warranty except as stated above.

Presentation: 10 kg.

Compendium Code No.: 10860171

MICRO PEARLS ADVANTAGE™ BENZOYL-PLUS™ ℞

Evsco — **Antidermatosis Shampoo**

Active Ingredient(s): Contains 2.5% benzoyl peroxide in a mild shampoo base containing water, decyl polyglucose, glycerin, carbomer, tocopheryl acetate, glyceryl stearate, sodium hydroxide, dimethicone, cholesterol, C12-15 alkyl benzoate, potassium cocoate, potassium oleate, propylene glycol, nonoxynol-20, octoxynol-5, methylchloroisothiazolinone, methylisothiazolinone, tetrasodium EDTA.

Indications: Safe for use on dogs and cats.

Indicated for topical therapy of pyoderma, folliculitis and seborrhea complex. May be used as a moisturizing, antiseptic shampoo for routine use as directed by your veterinarian. For pretreatment cleansing, Micro Pearls Advantage™ Hydra-Pearls™ Shampoo may be used prior to the application of BENZOYL-PLUS™.

Dosage and Administration: Shake well. Wet coat thoroughly before applying shampoo. Work shampoo into coat until a mild lather is produced. Allow to stand for 5-10 minutes and then rinse thoroughly. Repeat if necessary. BENZOYL-PLUS™ Shampoo may be used daily or weekly as directed by your veterinarian.

Precaution(s): Store at controlled room temperature. May bleach colored fabrics.

Caution(s): Federal law (USA) restricts this drug to use by or on the order of a licensed veterinarian.

For topical use only on dogs and cats. Avoid contact with eyes and mucous membranes.

Discontinue use if skin becomes irritated or inflamed. Systemic antibiotic treatment may be indicated if condition does not improve.
Warning(s): Keep out of reach of children. For animal use only.
Discussion: BENZOYL-PLUS™ contains microtargeted Novasome® microvesicles and the recognized bacteria fighting ingredient benzoyl peroxide. The Novasome® microvesicles are designed to deliver long lasting moisture to the hair shafts and epidermal layers. These microvesicles counteract the drying effects of an oxidizing benzoyl peroxide shampoo.
Presentation: 12 fl. oz (355 mL) bottle and gallon containers.
® Novasome is a registered trademark of Micro Pak, Inc.
Compendium Code No.: 10050180

MICRO PEARLS ADVANTAGE™ DERMAL-SOOTHE™ ANTI-ITCH CREAM RINSE

Evsco **Antidermatosis Rinse**

Active Ingredient(s): Contains 1% Pramoxine HCl in a concentrated cream rinse with Novasome® microvesicles, Colloidal Oatmeal and Skin Respiratory Factor.
Indications: Anti-itch cream rinse for dogs, cats and horses.
Dosage and Administration: Apply a liberal amount after shampooing. Work into coat and let stand 5-10 minutes and then rinse thoroughly. As with any medicated product, gloves should be worn when applying this product.
Caution(s): For topical use only on dogs, cats and horses. Avoid contact with eyes and mucous membranes. Discontinue use if skin becomes irritated or inflamed.
Warning(s): Keep out of reach of children. For animal use only.
Discussion: An itch relieving, moisturizing cream rinse for application after shampooing. May be used on normal, dry or sensitive skin to provide itch relief, lasting moisture and coat luster. May be used with other medicated shampoos as directed by your veterinarian.

DERMAL-SOOTHE™ Anti-Itch Cream Rinse contains itch relieving Pramoxine HCl and Novasome® microvesicles designed to deliver long lasting moisture factors to the hair and epidermal layers in a rich cream rinse base that relieves itching dry skin and leaves the hair coat soft, supple and lustrous.
Presentation: 12 fl. oz. (355 mL) bottle and gallon containers.
® Novasome is a trademark of Micro Pak, Inc.
Compendium Code No.: 10050190

MICRO PEARLS ADVANTAGE™ DERMAL-SOOTHE™ ANTI-ITCH SHAMPOO

Evsco **Antidermatosis Shampoo**

Active Ingredient(s): 1% Pramoxine HCl in a concentrated shampoo base with Novasome® microvesicles, Colloidal Oatmeal and Skin Respiratory Factor.
Indications: Anti-itch shampoo for dogs, cats and horses.
Dosage and Administration: Wet coat thoroughly before applying shampoo. Work into coat until a lather is produced. Allow to stand for 5-10 minutes and rinse thoroughly. As with any medicated shampoo, gloves should be worn when applying this product.
Caution(s): For topical use only on dogs, cats and horses. Avoid contact with eyes and mucous membranes. Discontinue use if skin becomes irritated or inflamed.
Warning(s): Keep out of reach of children. For animal use only.
Discussion: A conditioning shampoo for relieving itching and dry skin. Excellent for use on animals with normal, dry or sensitive skin.

DERMAL-SOOTHE™ Anti-Itch Shampoo contains itch relieving Pramoxine HCl and Novasome® microvesicles designed to deliver long lasting moisture factors to the hair and epidermal layers in a shampoo. The result is an itch relieving shampoo that leaves your pet a coat that is soft, supple and lustrous.
Presentation: 12 fl. oz. (355 mL) bottle and gallon containers.
® Novasome is a trademark of Micro Pak, Inc.
Compendium Code No.: 10050200

MICRO PEARLS ADVANTAGE™ DERMAL-SOOTHE™ ANTI-ITCH SPRAY

Evsco **Antidermatosis Spray**

Active Ingredient(s): Pramoxine HCl 1%, in base containing Lactamide MEA (a Lactic Acid derivative emollient) and Novasome® microvesicles.
Indications: Anti-itch spray for dogs, cats and horses.

A soothing, anti-itch, moisturizing spray for application after shampooing or between shampoos as needed. Aids in the relief of itching and flaking due to dry skin. May be used with other medicated shampoos as directed by your veterinarian.
Dosage and Administration: Shake well. Spray liberally onto damp or dry coat, allowing spray to reach the skin. Repeat as necessary.
Caution(s): For topical use only on dogs, cats and horses. Avoid contact with eyes and mucous membranes. Discontinue use if skin becomes irritated or inflamed.
Warning(s): Keep out of reach of children. For animal use only.
Discussion: DERMAL-SOOTHE™ Anti-Itch Spray contains itch relieving Pramoxine HCl and Novasome® microvesicles designed to deliver long lasting moisture factors to the hair and epidermal layers in a humidifying spray containing Lactamide MEA. The result is an itch relieving shampoo that leaves your pet a coat that is soft, supple and lustrous.
Presentation: 12 fl. oz. (355 mL) container.
® Novasome is a trademark of Micro Pak, Inc.
Compendium Code No.: 10050210

MICRO PEARLS ADVANTAGE™ EVSCO-TAR™ SHAMPOO

Evsco **Antidermatosis Shampoo**

Active Ingredient(s): Contains 5% coal tar topical solution U.S.P. (equivalent to 1% coal tar) with Novasome® encapsulated moisturizers in a concentrated shampoo base.
Indications: For dogs.

A keratolytic, keratoplastic, antipruritic shampoo for the treatment of seborrhea and pruritic dermatoses. Controls crusting, scaling, and odor related to seborrhea complex. May be used in conjunction with Micro Pearls Advantage™ Seba-Moist Shampoo, as directed by your veterinarian. For pretreatment cleansing, Micro Pearls Advantage™ Hydra-Pearls™ Shampoo may be used prior to application of EVSCO-TAR™ Shampoo.
Dosage and Administration: Shake well. Wet the coat thoroughly before applying the shampoo. Work into the coat until a mild lather is produced. Allow to stand for 5-10 minutes and then rinse thoroughly. Repeat if necessary, depending upon the severity of the condition. MICRO PEARLS ADVANTAGE™ may be used 2-3 times weekly as an initial therapy, and then at required intervals.
Caution(s): For topical use on dogs only. Avoid contact with the eyes and mucus membranes. Discontinue use if skin becomes irritated or inflamed.
Warning(s): Keep out of the reach of children. For animal use only.
Discussion: EVSCO-TAR™ Shampoo contains microtargeted Novasome® microvesicles, designed to deliver long-lasting moisture factors to the hair shafts and epidermal layers. This is combined with a non-steroidal pH balanced medicated shampoo containing an antiseborrheic and antipruritic agent. EVSCO-TAR™ Shampoo gently medicates as soothing moisture is released from the Novasome® microvesicles to inhibit drying of the skin and haircoat. Safe for use on dogs.
Presentation: 12 fl oz (355 mL) bottle and gallon containers.
® Novasome is a registered trademark of Micro Pak, Inc.
Compendium Code No.: 10050220

MICRO PEARLS ADVANTAGE™ HYDRA-PEARLS™ CREAM RINSE

Evsco **Grooming Rinse**

Active Ingredient(s): Contains Novasome® encapsulated moisturizers in a pH balanced concentrated cream rinse.
Indications: For dogs, cats and horses.

A soothing, moisturizing cream rinse for application after shampooing. May be used on normal, dry or sensitive skin. Counteracts the drying effects of the environment, as well as the drying effects of flea control products and medicated shampoos. May be used after the application of Micro Pearls Advantage™ medicated shampoos as directed by your veterinarian.
Dosage and Administration: Apply a liberal amount after shampooing. Work into coat and then rinse thoroughly.
Caution(s): For topical use only on dogs, cats and horses. Avoid contact with eyes and mucous membranes. Discontinue use if skin becomes irritated or inflamed.
Warning(s): Keep out of reach of children. For animal use only.
Discussion: HYDRA-PEARLS™ contains microtargeted Novasome® microvesicles designed to deliver long lasting moisture factors to the hairshafts and epidermal layers. HYDRA-PEARLS™ leaves even dry, flaking skin soft and supple and the haircoat silky and lustrous. Safe for use on dogs and cats.
Presentation: 12 fl. oz. (355 mL) bottle and gallon containers.
® Novasome is a registered trademark of Micro Pak, Inc.
Compendium Code No.: 10050230

MICRO PEARLS ADVANTAGE™ HYDRA-PEARLS™ REHYDRATING SPRAY

Evsco **Grooming Spray**

Active Ingredient(s): Contains Lactamide MEA, a lactic acid derivative emollient with Novasome® encapsulated moisturizers in an oil-free base.
Indications: For dogs, cats and horses.

A soothing non-oily moisturizing spray for application after shampooing or between shampoos as needed. Aids in the relief of flaking and scaling skin. Counteracts the drying effects of the environment, as well as the drying effects of flea control products and medicated shampoos. May be used after the application of Micro Pearls Advantage™ shampoos as directed by your veterinarian.
Dosage and Administration: Shake well. Apply spray liberally to damp or dry coat. Allow to dry and then brush as necessary.
Caution(s): For topical use only on dogs, cats and horses. Avoid contact with eyes and mucous membranes. Discontinue use if skin becomes irritated or inflamed.
Warning(s): Keep out of reach of children. For animal use only.
Discussion: HYDRA-PEARLS™ Spray combines microtargeted Novasome® microvesicles designed to deliver long-lasting moisture factors to the hair shafts and epidermal layers, with a humidifying spray containing lactamide MEA. The result is a coat that is soft, supple and lustrous. Safe for use on dogs and cats.
Presentation: 12 fl. oz. (355 mL) bottle.
® Novasome is a registered trademark of Micro Pak, Inc.
Compendium Code No.: 10050240

MICRO PEARLS ADVANTAGE™ HYDRA-PEARLS™ SHAMPOO

Evsco **Grooming Shampoo**

Active Ingredient(s): Contains Novasome® encapsulated moisturizers in a pH balanced concentrated shampoo base.
Indications: For dogs, cats and horses.

A pH balanced, conditioning shampoo for routine cleansing and moisturizing of normal, dry, or sensitive skin. Counteracts the drying effects of the environment, as well as the drying effects of flea control products and medicated shampoos. May be used prior to the application of Micro Pearls Advantage™ medicated shampoos as directed by your veterinarian.
Dosage and Administration: Wet coat thoroughly before applying shampoo. Work shampoo into coat until a mild lather is produced. Rinse thoroughly. Repeat if necessary.
Caution(s): For topical use only on dogs, cats and horses. Avoid contact with eyes and mucous membranes. Discontinue use if skin becomes irritated or inflamed.
Warning(s): Keep out of reach of children. For animal use only.
Discussion: HYDRA-PEARLS™ Shampoo contains microtargeted Novasome® microvesicles designed to deliver long lasting moisture factors to the hairshafts and epidermal layers. The result is a healthy, lustrous coat that is cleaned and moisturized. Safe for use on dogs and cats.
Presentation: 12 fl. oz. (355 mL) bottle and gallon containers.
® Novasome is a registered trademark of Micro Pak, Inc.
Compendium Code No.: 10050250

MICRO PEARLS ADVANTAGE™ MICONAZOLE™ SHAMPOO ℞

Evsco **Antidermatosis Shampoo**

Anti-fungal Shampoo
Active Ingredient(s): Miconazole nitrate 2%.

Other Ingredients: Water, sodium C14-16 olefin sulfonate, lauramidopropyl betaine, glycerin, cocamide DEA, polyquaternium-7, glycol stearate, DMDM hydantoin, glyceryl stearate, chlorhexidine gluconate, dimethicone, cholesterol, C12-15 alkyl benzoate, potassium cocoate, potassium oleate, propylene glycol, nonoxynol-20, octoxynol-5, methylchloroisothiazolinone, methylisothiazolinone, tetrasodium EDTA.
Indications: For the treatment of fungal infections such as ringworm, and superficial skin infections caused by yeast *(Candida albicans)*. Safe for use on dogs, cats and horses.

Dosage and Administration: Wet coat thoroughly before applying shampoo. Work into coat until a lather is produced. Allow to stand at least 10 minutes, then rinse thoroughly. As with any medicated shampoo, gloves should be worn when applying this product. May be used 2-3 times weekly as an initial therapy, then at required intervals as directed by your veterinarian. If irritation occurs or if there is no improvement within four weeks, discontinue use and consult your veterinarian.

Caution(s): Federal law (USA) restricts this drug to use by or on the order of a licensed veterinarian.

Discontinue use if skin becomes irritated or inflamed.

Warning(s): For topical use only on dogs, cats and horses. Not for use on animals intended for food. Avoid contact with eyes and mucous membranes.

Keep out of reach of children. For animal use only.

Discussion: MICONAZOLE™ Shampoo contains the anti-fungal agent miconazole nitrate and Novasome® microvesicles designed to deliver long lasting moisture factors to the hair and epidermal layers.

Presentation: 12 fl oz (355 mL) bottles.

Novasome® is a registered trademark of Micro Pak, Inc.

Compendium Code No.: 10050260

MICRO PEARLS ADVANTAGE™ MICONAZOLE™ SPRAY ℞

Evsco **Antidermatosis Spray**

Anti-fungal Spray

Active Ingredient(s): Miconazole nitrate 2%.

Other Ingredients: PEG-4, SD alcohol 40B, Polysorbate 20, BHT.

Indications: For the treatment of fungal infections such as ringworm, and superficial skin infections caused by yeast *(Candida albicans)*. Safe for use on dogs, cats and horses.

Dosage and Administration: Clean and dry affected area thoroughly before applying. Apply a thin layer twice daily or as directed by your veterinarian. If irritation occurs or if there is no improvement within four weeks, discontinue use and consult your veterinarian.

Caution(s): Federal law (USA) restricts this drug to use by or on the order of a licensed veterinarian.

Discontinue use if skin becomes irritated or inflamed.

Warning(s): For topical use only on dogs, cats and horses. Not for use on animals intended for food. Avoid contact with eyes and mucous membranes.

Keep out of reach of children. For animal use only.

Presentation: 4 fl oz (118 mL) bottles.

Compendium Code No.: 10050270

MICRO PEARLS ADVANTAGE™ SEBA-HEX™ SHAMPOO ℞

Evsco **Antidermatosis Shampoo**

2% Chlorhexidine Gluconate

Active Ingredient(s): Chlorhexidine gluconate 2%.

Other Ingredients: Contains water, sodium C14-16 olefin sulfonate, cocamide DEA, glycol stearate, hydrolyzed keratin, salicylic acid, sulfur, glyceryl stearate, cetyl alcohol, fragrance, dimethicone, cholesterol, methylparaben, C12-15 alkyl benzoate, potassium cocoate, potassium oleate, propylene glycol, propylparaben, nonoxynol-20, octoxynol-5, methylchloroisothiazolinone, methylisothiazolinone, tetrasodium EDTA.

Indications: Indicated for topical therapy of pyoderma, folliculitis and seborrhea complex. Safe for use on dogs, cats and horses.

Dosage and Administration: Wet coat thoroughly before applying shampoo. Work into coat until a lather is produced. Allow to stand at least 10-15 minutes, then rinse thoroughly. As with any medicated shampoo, gloves should be worn when applying product. May be used 2-3 times a week or as directed by your veterinarian.

Caution(s): Federal law (USA) restricts this drug to use by or on the order of a licensed veterinarian.

Discontinue use if skin becomes irritated or inflamed.

Warning(s): For topical use only on dogs, cats and horses. Not for use on animals intended for food. Avoid contact with eyes and mucous membranes.

Keep out of reach of children.

For animal use only.

Discussion: SEBA-HEX™ Shampoo has a keratolytic and keratoplastic shampoo base with Novasome® microvesicles designed to deliver long lasting moisture factors to the hair and epidermal layers.

Presentation: 12 fl oz (355 mL) and 1 gallon (128 fl oz - 3.79 L) containers.

Novasome® is a registered trademark of Micro Pak, Inc.

Compendium Code No.: 10050280

MICRO PEARLS ADVANTAGE™ SEBA-MOIST™ SHAMPOO

Evsco **Antidermatosis Shampoo**

Active Ingredient(s): Contains 2% sulfur and 2% salicylic acid with Novasome® encapsulated moisturizers in a concentrated shampoo base.

Indications: For dogs.

A keratolytic, keratoplastic, antipruritic shampoo for the treatment of seborrhea and pruritic dermatoses. Effectively decreases scaling and flaking. May be used in conjunction with Micro Pearls Advantage™ Evsco-Tar™ Shampoo, as directed by your veterinarian. For pre-treatment cleansing, Micro Pearls Advantage™ Hydra-Pearls™ Shampoo may be used prior to application of SEBA-MOIST™ Shampoo.

Dosage and Administration: Shake well. Wet the coat thoroughly before applying the shampoo. Work the shampoo into the coat until a mild lather is produced. Allow to stand for 5-10 minutes and then rinse thoroughly. Repeat if necessary. MICRO PEARLS ADVANTAGE™ SEBA-MOIST™ Shampoo may be used 2-3 times weekly as an initial therapy, and then at required intervals.

Caution(s): For topical use on dogs only. Avoid contact with the eyes and mucous membranes. Discontinue use if skin becomes irritated or inflamed.

Warning(s): Keep out of the reach of children.

For animal use only.

Discussion: SEBA-MOIST™ Shampoo combines microtargeted Novasome® microvesicles designed to deliver long-lasting moisture factors to the hair shafts and epidermal layers with the synergistic antiseborrheic properties of sulfur and salicylic acid. The result is a shampoo that gently medicates, normalizing keratin production to decrease scaling and flaking. Safe for use on dogs.

Presentation: 12 fl oz (355 mL) bottle and gallon containers.

® Novasome is a registered trademark of Micro Pak, Inc.

Compendium Code No.: 10050290

MICRO-VET™ EQUINE TRADITIONAL BLEND

Boehringer Ingelheim **Large Animal Dietary Supplement**

Vitamin-Mineral Supplement

Guaranteed Analysis: Per Pound:

Crude Protein not less than	14.5%
Crude Fat not less than	2.0%
Crude Fiber not more than	24.0%
Calcium (minimum)	0.75%
Calcium (maximum)	1.25%
Phosphorus (minimum)	1.0%
Zinc (minimum)	1,500 ppm
Iron (minimum)	750 ppm
Manganese (minimum)	100 ppm
Copper (minimum)	50 ppm
Iodine (minimum)	30 ppm
Selenium (minimum)	20 ppm
Vitamin A (minimum)	600,000 IU
Vitamin D_3 (minimum)	60,000 IU
Vitamin E (minimum)	400 IU
Thiamine (minimum)	200 mg
Riboflavin (minimum)	400 mg
d-Pantothenic acid (minimum)	65 mg
Niacin (minimum)	1,000 mg
Vitamin B_{12} (minimum)	1,450 mcg
Total CFU (Colony Forming Units), minimum	6.2 Billion

Ingredients: Dehydrated alfalfa meal, yeast culture, soybean meal, wheat middlings, cane molasses, monosodium phosphate, potassium chloride, potassium sulfate, zinc methionine, copper proteinate, manganese proteinate, iron proteinate, cobalt proteinate, potassium iodide, sodium selenite, vitamin A supplement, D-activated animal sterol (source of vitamin D_3), vitamin E supplement, menadione sodium metabisulfite complex (source of vitamin K), vitamin B_{12} supplement, thiamine mononitrate, riboflavin supplement, niacin, d-calcium pantothenate, biotin, choline chloride, folic acid, pyridoxine hydrochloride (vitamin B_6), beta carotene, ascorbic acid, magnesium sulfate, sodium bentonite, zinc oxide, ferrous sulfate, copper oxide, manganous oxide, DL-methionine, L-lysine monohydrochloride, dried *Enterococcus faecium* fermentation product, dried *Bacillus subtilis* fermentation product, dried *Bacillus licheniformis* fermentation product, dried *Lactobacillus acidophilus* fermentation product, dried *Lactobacillus plantarum* fermentation product, dried *Aspergillus oryzae* fermentation extract, dried *Bacillus subtilis* fermentation extract, natural and artificial flavors.

Indications: MICRO-VET™ Equine is a vitamin and mineral supplement for horses containing electrolytes, chelated trace minerals and live (viable) naturally occurring microorganisms.

Dosage and Administration: Feed as a top-dressing.

Horses in training: 2 scoops per day.
Lactating mares: 2 scoops per day.
Brood mares, last ⅓ of pregnancy: 1½ scoops per day.
Brood mares, open or first ⅓ of pregnancy: 1 scoop per day.
Stallions, in service: 2 scoops per day.
Stallions, not in service: 1½ scoops per day.
Working horses: 2 scoops per day.
Pleasure horses: 1 scoop per day.
Weaned horses, yearlings and ponies: 1 scoop per day.
Suckling foals on dry feed: ½ scoop per day.
There are approximately 12 scoops per lb, or 1⅓ oz (38 gm) per scoop.

For maximum effect of MICRO-VET™ Equine feed a palatable and nutritious ration.

Precaution(s): Keep tightly closed when not in use. Store in cool, dry place. Protect from direct sunlight.

Warning(s): No withdrawal period required. Not for human use. For oral use in livestock only. Keep out of reach of children.

Presentation: 6 lb and 20 lb containers.

Compendium Code No.: 10280780

MICROZYME BOLUS FOR CATTLE

Vedco **Large Animal Dietary Supplement**

Active Ingredient(s): Guaranteed Analysis:

Ash	16% max.
Zinc	0.41% min.
Iron	0.32% min.
Cobalt	0.159% min.
Selenium	0.0032% min.
Vitamin A	2,185,000 I.U./lb.
Vitamin D	832,000 I.U./lb.
Vitamin E	2,590 I.U./lb.
Choline	1,050 mg/lb.
Niacin	32,500 mg/lb.
d-Pantothenic acid	78 mg/lb.
Riboflavin	52 mg/lb.
Thiamine	11 mg/lb.
Vitamin B_{12}	130 mcg/lb.

Ingredients: Dextrose, potassium sulfate, dried *Aspergillus oryzae* fermentation extract*, yeast culture, active dry yeast, dried whey, calcium phosphate dibasic, cellulose, vitamin A supplement, d-activated animal sterol (source of vitamin D_3), dl-alpha-tocopheryl (source of vitamin E), choline chloride, niacin supplement, calcium pantothenate, riboflavin supplement, thiamine hydrochloride, vitamin B_{12} supplement, zinc sulfate, ferrous sulfate, copper sulfate, manganese sulfate, cobalt sulfate, and sodium selenite.

Indications: A source of soluble vitamins, minerals, dried *Aspergillus oryzae* fermentation extract* and yeast that dissolves quickly.

Dosage and Administration: Recommended Use:

Cattle over 350 lbs.: One (1) 28 g bolus each day.

Precaution(s): Store in a cool, dry place. Protect from direct sunlight.

Caution(s): Administer with proper procedure noting the animal's ability to accommodate bolus size. Not for human use. For oral use in livestock only. Keep out of the reach of children.

Presentation: 50 x 28 g boluses.

* Amaferm® is a product of a patented process. U.S. patent # 3043748.

Compendium Code No.: 10941280

MILBEMITE™ OTIC SOLUTION ℞

Novartis **Otic Parasiticide**

(0.1% milbemycin oxime)

NADA No.: 141-163

Active Ingredient(s): Each plastic tube contains 0.25 mL of MILBEMITE™ Otic Solution as a 0.1% solution of milbemycin oxime.

Indications: MILBEMITE™ Otic Solution is indicated for treatment of ear mite *(Otodectes cynotis)* infestations in cats and kittens four weeks of age and older. Effectiveness is maintained throughout the life cycle of the ear mite.

Pharmacology: Milbemycin oxime consists of the oxime derivatives of 5-didehydromilbemycins in the ratio of approximately 80% A_4 ($C_{32}H_{45}NO_7$, MW 555.71) and 20% A_3 ($C_{31}H_{43}NO_7$, MW 541.68).

Dosage and Administration: Dosage: MILBEMITE™ Otic Solution should be administered topically into the external ear canal as the entire contents of a single dose tube per ear. The volume delivered will be approximately 0.2 mL, with 0.05 mL residual volume remaining in dispensing tube.

Repeat the treatment one time if necessary, based upon the ear mite life cycle and the response to treatment.

Administration: MILBEMITE™ Otic Solution should be administered as one tube per ear as a single treatment. Each foil pouch contains two tubes of solution, one for each ear. Open the tube by snapping off the cap. Squeeze the tube to administer the contents of one tube into each external ear canal. Massage the base of the ear for optimal distribution. In clinical field trials, ears were not cleaned and many animals still had debris in their ears at the end of the study. Cleaning of the external ear canal prior to treatment may be performed, but is not necessary to provide effectiveness.

Precaution(s): Storage Conditions: MILBEMITE™ Otic Solution should be stored at room temperature, between 59° and 77°F (15°-25°C).

Caution(s): U.S. Federal law restricts this drug to use by, or on the order of a licensed veterinarian.

The safe use of MILBEMITE™ Otic Solution in cats used for breeding purposes, during pregnancy, or in lactating queens, has not been evaluated.

Warning(s): Human Warnings: Not for human use. Keep this and all drugs out of the reach of children.

Adverse Reactions: No adverse reactions caused by MILBEMITE™ Otic Solution have been reported in controlled effectiveness studies in adult cats and kittens (4 weeks of age).

Trial Data: Effectiveness: The clinical effectiveness of milbemycin oxime 0.1% solution was evaluated in a placebo-controlled clinical field trial of client-owned cats. *Otodectes cynotis* infestation was diagnosed by direct microscopic visualization of ear swab debris. Test or placebo treatment was administered to both ears of the cat following the pre-treatment examination. Cats' ears were examined by ear swab microscopy at multiple intervals throughout the life cycle of the mite (up to day 30). Ninety-nine percent (99%) of the milbemycin oxime treated group were ear mite negative at the microscopic exams.

Safety: A study was conducted using otic doses of 0.1, 0.3 or 0.5% milbemycin oxime solutions administered once weekly for six applications in kittens that were 4 weeks of age at the initiation of the study. Otic doses of 0.1 and 0.3% did not produce adverse systemic or local effects. One kitten treated with 0.5% was lethargic 8 hours after the second treatment. The kitten was offered milk replacer and by 10 hours post-treatment it appeared normal. In this kitten, lethargy was not observed after subsequent treatments. A study was conducted to evaluate the safety of a 0.1% milbemycin oxime solution in adult cats. Topical doses at 1X, 3X or 5X the recommended dose applied in one ear did not produce adverse effects.

Presentation: MILBEMITE™ Otic Solution is supplied in individual white polypropylene tubes, paired in a foil overlay pouch. The product is packaged in a box of 10 pouches of 2 tubes of 0.25 mL each.

U.S. Patent No. 4,547,520

Compendium Code No.: 11310111 NAH/MIL-LE/VI/3 0202

"MILD" IODINE WOUND SPRAY

Centaur **Topical Wound Dressing**

Topical Antiseptic

Active Ingredient(s):

Alpha (p-nonylphenyl) omega-hydroxypoly (oxyethylene) iodine complex (providing 1.00% minimum titratable iodine) 9.4%

Inert Ingredients 90.6%

Indications: A topical antiseptic for use on large and small animals prior to surgical procedures such as castrating and docking. For application to the navel of newborn animals, and for aid in treatment of minor cuts, bruises and abrasions.

Directions: Apply freely to infected area. When spraying hold container approximately 4 to 6 inches from the area to be treated. Point valve at the area to be sprayed. Pull trigger of valve and spray area once lightly. May be repeated daily, when necessary, until abraded area is healed.

Contraindication(s): Not for use on burns or in body cavities or deep wounds.

Precaution(s): Store in a cool place. Do not expose to heat or store at a temperature above 120°F. Do not use near an open flame.

Caution(s): If redness, irritation, or swelling persists or increases, discontinue use and consult a veterinarian.

Harmful if swallowed. Do not apply to the eyes, mucous membranes or large areas of abraded skin. Avoid inhalation of mist.

Note: When used on or near the teats or udders of dairy animals, the teats and udders should be thoroughly washed before the next milking to prevent contamination of milk.

For animal use only. Hazardous. Livestock remedy.

Warning(s): Keep out of reach of children. Not for human use.

Presentation: 1 pint (16 fl oz) 473 mL and 1 gallon (128 fl oz) 3.785 L.

Manufactured by: Unavet, North Kansas City, MO 64116.

Compendium Code No.: 14880220 Rev. 4-97

MILDVAC-ARK®

Intervet **Vaccine**

Bronchitis Vaccine, Arkansas Type, Live Virus

U.S. Vet. Lic. No.: 286

Description: MILDVAC-ARK®, a live virus vaccine, is prepared from a mild Arkansas strain of Arkansas type bronchitis. The mild Arkansas infectious bronchitis strain was developed by Intervet research and selected for its low reactivity and high immunogenicity. The virus has been propagated using SPF (Specific Pathogen Free) substrates. The immunizing capability has also been proven by the Master Seed Immunogenicity Test.

This vaccine contains gentamicin as a preservative. Quality tested for purity, potency, and safety.

Indications: Beak-O-Vac or Coarse Spray - Vaccination of healthy chickens one day of age or older (spray) for protection against Arkansas type bronchitis.

Dosage and Administration: Vaccination Programs: Many factors must be considered in determining a sound vaccination program for a particular farm or poultry complex. To be fully effective, the vaccine must be administered properly to healthy, receptive animals maintained in a proper environment under good management. In addition, the response may be influenced by the age of the animals and their immune status. Seldom does one live virus vaccination under field conditions produce lifetime protection for all individuals in a given flock. The level of immunity required will vary with operational practices and the degree of exposure. Therefore, a program of periodic revaccinations may be necessary.

Preparation of Vaccine:

Beak-O-Vac Use: Do not open and mix the vaccine until ready to begin vaccination. Use vaccine immediately after mixing.

1. Remove the tear-off seal and stopper from vial containing the dried vaccine.
2. Remove the seal and stopper from the bottle of diluent.
3. Pour a small amount of diluent into vial of vaccine.
4. Insert the rubber stopper and shake.
5. Pour the rehydrated vaccine back into the bottle containing the rest of the diluent. Replace the stopper and shake.
6. Place the vaccine in an appropriate container.

The vaccine is now ready for use by the following methods. For best results, be sure to follow the directions carefully!

Beak-O-Vac Administration - For Chickens One Day of Age:

1. Attach the container holding the vaccine to the Beak-O-Vac machine and adjust the delivery of 33-35 doses per mL.
2. Hold the chicken in such a manner that the chicken's beak is opened in the direction of the nozzle so the vaccine is deposited on the roof of the mouth as the beak is burned.

Preparation of Vaccine:

For Coarse Spray Use: Do not open and mix the vaccine until ready to begin vaccination. Use vaccine immediately after mixing.

1. Remove the tear-off seal and stopper from vial containing the dried vaccine.
2. Carefully pour clean, cool non-chlorinated tap water into the vaccine vial until the vial is approximately two-thirds full.
3. Insert the rubber stopper and shake vigorously until all material is dissolved.
4. The vaccine is now ready for coarse spray use in accordance with directions below. For best results, be sure to follow directions carefully!

Coarse Spray Vaccination - For Chickens One Day of Age:

1. Use rehydrated vaccine as indicated for specific coarse spray vaccination machine. For example, a machine which dispenses 20 mL in 3 seconds to a box of 100 chickens; - total volume for 1,000 doses is 200 mL, and 10,000 doses is 2,000 mL of deionized water. Mix thoroughly.
2. Add the prepared vaccine solution to reservoir on the machine.
3. Prime and adjust machine as instructed in manual accompanying the specific machine.
4. Place boxes holding 100 chickens each on the conveyor belt or in machine. Activate spray head.

Coarse Spray Administration - For Chickens Two Days of Age or Older:

1. Do not use any disinfectants or skim milk in sprayer.
2. Use sprayer only for administration of vaccine.
3. Shut off all fans while spray vaccinating. Turn on fan immediately after spraying.
4. Be careful in hot weather.
5. Spray chickens by walking slowly through the house.
6. Follow the manufacturer's directions regarding water volume.
7. Use only clean, cool, deionized water.
8. Individual(s) spraying chickens should wear face mask and goggles.

Records: Keep a record of vaccine, quantity, serial number, expiration date, and place of purchase; the date and time of vaccination; the number, age, breed and locations of chickens; name of operators performing the vaccination and any observed reactions.

Precaution(s): Store vaccine between 2 and 7°C (35 and 45°F).

Do not spill or splash the vaccine. Use entire contents when first opened.

Burn containers and all unused contents. This product is non-returnable.

Caution(s): Vaccinate only healthy chickens. Although disease may not be evident, coccidiosis, Mycoplasma infection, infectious bursal disease, Marek's disease, and other disease conditions may cause complications or reduce immunity.

All susceptible chickens on the same premises should be vaccinated at the same time.

The revaccination of laying hens against bronchitis may be detrimental to the flock and cannot be generally recommended. In some areas where infectious bronchitis is a severe continuing problem the local poultry pathologists are recommending revaccination of the laying hens for bronchitis at specified intervals. If used, such recommendations should be strictly followed. A delay in revaccination may result in some layers becoming susceptible to bronchitis. If these hens are exposed to the virus they can experience a disturbance in egg production.

Efforts should be taken to reduce stress conditions at the time of vaccination and during the reaction period.

Do not dilute the vaccine or otherwise stretch the dosage. For veterinary use only.

Notice: This vaccine has undergone rigid potency, safety and purity tests, and meets Intervet Inc. and USDA requirements. It is designed to stimulate effective immunity when used as directed, but the user must be advised that the response to the product depends upon many factors, including, but not limited to, conditions of storage and handling by the user, administration of the vaccine, health and responsiveness of individual chickens, and the degree of field exposure. Therefore, directions should be followed carefully!

This product is not hazardous when used according to directions supplied. A material safety data sheet (MSDS) is available upon request. This and any other consumer information can be obtained by calling Intervet Customer Service at 1-800-441-8272 or 1-302-934-8051.

The use of this vaccine is subject to applicable federal and local laws and regulations.

Use only as directed.

Warning(s): Do not vaccinate within 21 days before slaughter.

Presentation: 10 x 10,000 doses for coarse spray use, 10 x 10,000 doses with diluent for Beak-O-Vac use and 10 x 25,000 doses for coarse spray use.

Compendium Code No.: 11060912 16106 AL 144

MILDVAC-Ma5®

Intervet **Vaccine**

Bronchitis Vaccine, Massachusetts Type, Live Virus

U.S. Vet. Lic. No.: 286

Active Ingredient(s): MILDVAC-Ma5®, a live virus vaccine, is prepared from the cloned Ma5 strain of Massachusetts type bronchitis. The Ma5 infectious bronchitis strain was developed by Intervet research and selected for its low reactivity and high immunogenicity. The Ma5 strain is unique from other infectious bronchitis viruses in its ability to spontaneously hemagglutinate chicken red blood cells. The viruses have been propagated using SPF substrates. The immunizing capability has also been proven by the Master Seed Immunogenicity Test. The vaccine contains gentamicin as a preservative.

Indications:

Drinking water: Vaccination of healthy chickens at two weeks of age or older for protection against Mass. type bronchitis.

Beak-O-Vac or coarse spray: Vaccination of healthy chickens at one day of age for protection against Mass. type bronchitis.

Dosage and Administration: Many factors must be considered in determining a sound vaccination program for a particular farm or poultry complex. To be fully effective, the vaccine must be administered properly to healthy, receptive birds maintained in a proper environment under good management. In addition, the response may be influenced by the age of the birds and their immune status. Seldom does one live virus vaccination under field conditions produce lifetime protection for all individuals in a given flock. The level of immunity required will vary with operational practices and the degree of exposure. Therefore, a program of periodic revaccinations may be necessary.

Preparation of Vaccine: For Beak-O-Vac use:

Do not open and mix the vaccine until ready to begin vaccination. Use the vaccine immediately after mixing.

1. Remove the tear-off seal and stopper from the vial containing the dried vaccine.
2. Remove the seal and stopper from the bottle of diluent.
3. Pour a small amount of the diluent into the vial of dried vaccine.
4. Insert the rubber stopper and shake.
5. Pour the rehydrated vaccine into the bottle containing the rest of the diluent. Replace the stopper and shake.
6. Place the vaccine into an appropriate container.

The vaccine is now ready for use by the following methods. For the best results, be sure to follow the directions carefully.

Beak-O-Vac Administration: For chickens one (1) day of age.

1. Attach the container holding the vaccine to the Beak-O-Vac machine and adjust for a delivery of 33-35 doses per mL.
2. Hold the chicken in such a manner that the chicken's beak is opened in the direction of the nozzle so that the vaccine is deposited on the roof of the mouth as the beak is turned.

Preparation of Vaccine: For drinking water or coarse spray use:

Do not open and mix the vaccine until ready to begin vaccination. Use the vaccine immediately after mixing.

1. Remove the tear-off seal and stopper from the vial containing the dried vaccine.
2. Carefully pour clean, cool non-chlorinated tap water into the vaccine vial until the vial is approximately two-thirds (⅔) full.
3. Insert the rubber stopper and shake vigorously until all of the material is dissolved.
4. The vaccine is now ready for drinking water or coarse spray use. For the best results, be sure to follow the directions carefully.

Drinking Water Administration: For chickens two (2) weeks of age or older:

1. Do not use any disinfectants in the drinking water for 48 hours before vaccinating and for 24 hours after vaccination.
2. Withhold drinking water from the chickens until they are thirsty. Withholding periods will vary from two (2) to eight (8) hours according to the age of the chickens and the climatic conditions.
3. Scrub the waterers and rinse thoroughly with fresh, clean water. Do not use disinfectants for cleaning the waterers.
4. Rehydrate the vaccine.
5. Mix the rehydrated vaccine with clean, cool, non-chlorinated tap water.

Age of chickens	Water per 1,000 doses vaccine
2-4 weeks	6 gallons (23 L)
4-8 weeks	10 gallons (38 L)
8 weeks or older	16 gallons (60 L)

As an aid in preserving the virus, 3.2 oz. (100 g) of non-fat powdered milk may be added with each 10 gallons (38 L) of water used for mixing vaccine. Add the dried milk first and mix until dissolved. Then add the rehydrated vaccine from the vial and again mix thoroughly.

6. Distribute the vaccine solution among the waterers provided for the chickens. Avoid placing the waterers in direct sunlight.
7. Do not provide any other drinking water until all of the vaccine-water solution has been consumed.

Coarse Spray Administration: For chickens one (1) day of age:

1. Use the rehydrated vaccine as indicated for a specific coarse spray vaccination machine. For example, a machine which dispenses 20 mL in three (3) seconds to a box of 100 chickens; - total volume for 2,000 doses is 400 mL, and 10,000 doses is 2,000 mL of deionized water. Mix thoroughly.
2. Add the prepared vaccine solution to the reservoir on the machine.
3. Prime and adjust the machine as instructed in the manual accompanying the specific machine.
4. Place the boxes holding 100 chickens each on the conveyor belt or in the machine. Activate the spray head.

Coarse Spray Administration: For chickens two (2) days of age or older:

1. Do not use any disinfectants or skim milk in the sprayer.
2. Use the sprayer for administration of the vaccines only.
3. Shut off all fans while spray vaccinating. Turn on the fan immediately after spraying.
4. Be careful in hot weather.
5. Spray the chickens by walking slowly through the house.
6. Follow the manufacturer's directions regarding water volume.
7. Use only clean, cool, deionized water.
8. Individual(s) spraying chickens should wear a face mask and goggles.

Records: Keep a record of vaccine, quantity, serial number, expiration date, and place of purchase; the date and time of vaccination; the number, age, breed, and locations of chickens; names of operators performing the vaccination and any observed reactions.

Precaution(s): Use only as directed. Store the vaccine between 2-7°C (35-45°F). The product is not returnable.

Caution(s):

1. Vaccinate healthy chickens only. Although disease may not be evident, coccidiosis, mycoplasma infection, infectious bursal disease, Marek's disease, and other disease conditions may cause complications or reduce immunity.
2. All susceptible chickens on the same premises should be vaccinated at the same time.
3. The revaccination of laying hens with live bronchitis may be detrimental to the flock and cannot be generally recommended. Consult an Intervet representative for more information.
4. Efforts should be taken to reduce stress conditions at the time of vaccination and during the reaction period.
5. Do not spill or splash the vaccine.
6. Do not dilute the vaccine or otherwise stretch the dosage.
7. Use the entire contents when first opened.
8. Burn the containers and all unused contents.

Warning(s): Do not vaccinate within 21 days before slaughter.

Discussion: The vaccine has undergone rigid potency, safety and purity tests, and meets Intervet America Inc. and USDA requirements. It is designed to stimulate effective immunity when used as directed, but the user must be advised that the response to the product depends upon many factors, including, but not limited to, conditions of storage and handling by the user, administration of the vaccine, health and responsiveness of individual chickens, and the degree of field exposure. Therefore, directions should be followed carefully.

The use of the vaccine is subject to applicable federal and local laws and regulations.

Presentation: 10 x 10,000 doses for drinking water or coarse spray use.
With diluent for Beak-O-Vac use.

* U.S. Patent No. 4,751,079.

Compendium Code No.: 11060920

MILKIN MIX

Skylabs **Large Animal Dietary Supplement**

Active Ingredient(s):

Vitamin A (avg.)	348,143 I.U./kg
Vitamin D_3 (avg.)	58,024 I.U./kg
Vitamin E (avg.)	870 I.U./kg
Vitamin B_{12} (avg.)	1,335 mcg/kg
Vitamin K (act.)	335 mg/kg
Calcium pantothenate (act.)	928 mg/kg
Niacin (act.)	1,740 mg/kg
Riboflavin (act.)	232 mg/kg
Pyridoxine (act.)	116 mg/kg
Folic acid (act.)	11.6 mg/kg
Thiamine (act.)	116 mg/kg
Biotin (avg.)	2,901 mcg/kg
Iron (act.)	3,746 mg/kg
Iodine (act.)	25.4 mg/kg
Manganese (act.)	435 mg/kg
Copper (act.)	250 mg/kg
Zinc (act.)	2,100 mg/kg
Cobalt (act.)	3.09 mg/kg

Ingredients: Vitamin A acetate, d-activated animal sterol, dl-alpha tocopherol acetate, biotin, vitamin B_{12} supplement, menadione sodium bisulfite, calcium pantothenate, niacin, riboflavin supplement, folic acid, pyridoxine hydrochloride, thiamine hydrochloride, zinc sulfate, manganous oxide, ethylenediamine dihydroiodide, copper sulfate, cobalt carbonate, ferrous sulfate.

Indications: MILKIN MIX may assist in preventing constipation in sows during gestation and farrowing when most milking problems are experienced.

Dosage and Administration: To be used as a source of vitamin and trace mineral supplementation two (2) weeks prior to farrowing and through lactation. During this period, add one (1) bag (5 kg) of MILKIN MIX per ton of complete feed. After farrowing, be sure that the sows receive and consume at least 5 kg to 6 kg of complete lactation feed per day per sow.

Presentation: 11 lb.

Compendium Code No.: 10920001

MILK OF MAGNESIA

Neogen **Antacid-Laxative**

Active Ingredient(s): Each teaspoonful contains magnesium hydroxide 400 mg.

Indications: For the relief of heartburn, sour stomach and/or acid indigestion, and mild constipation in dogs and horses.

Directions: Shake well before use.

Dosage:

Horses: Consult veterinarian.

Dogs: ½ to 1 teaspoonful as an antacid.

½ to 1 tablespoonful as a laxative.

Precaution(s): Keep from freezing.

Caution(s): For veterinary use only.

Warning(s): Keep out of reach of children.

Presentation: 128 fl oz (1 gallon) 3.785 L (NDC: 59051-9135-9).

Compendium Code No.: 14910351 L420-0501

MINERAL OIL

AgriLabs **Laxative**

Active Ingredient(s): Contains mineral oil.

Indications: For relief of obstruction or impaction of the intestinal tract of cattle, sheep, goats, swine and horses.

Dosage and Administration:

Cattle	2 to 4 quarts
Horses	2 to 4 quarts

M

Sheep . . . . . . 1 to 2 pints
Swine . . . . . . 1 to 2 pints
Goats . . . . . . 1 to 2 pints
Dogs . . . . . . 1 to 4 tbsp. daily
Caution(s): Keep out of the reach of children.
If there is no response to the use of this product, consult a veterinarian.
If no response to dosage, consult a veterinarian.
Presentation: 1 gallon (3.785 L) containers.
Compendium Code No.: 10580710

MINERAL OIL
AgriPharm
Laxative
Active Ingredient(s): Mineral oil.
Indications: A mild laxative for the lubrication of the intestinal tract.
Dosage and Administration: Dose Chart:
Horses . . . . . . 1 qt.
Cattle . . . . . . 1 qt.
Sheep . . . . . . 5 oz.
Hogs . . . . . . 1 pt.
Dogs:
Toy breeds and Pups . . . . . . 1 oz.
Adult dogs . . . . . . 2 oz.
According to size.
Caution(s): Not for human use.
Keep out of the reach of children.
Exercise care in administering to avoid aspiration into the lungs and possible foreign body pneumonia. Prolonged use or frequently repeated use may interfere with the normal absorption of nutrients from the digestive tract.
Not recommended for frequently repeated or extended repeated administration. If the condition persists, consult a veterinarian.
Presentation: 32 fl. oz. (1 qt.) and 1 gallon containers.
Compendium Code No.: 14570620

MINERAL OIL
Aspen
Laxative
Active Ingredient(s): Mineral oil.
Indications: For use as a mild laxative. Softens and lubricates stools to help relieve simple constipation.
Dosage and Administration: Suggested dosage for oral administration, according to the size of the animal:
Adult Cattle and Horses . . . . . . 1 pt to 2 qt
Calves and Colts . . . . . . 2-4 fl oz
Pigs, Sheep and Goats . . . . . . 1-10 fl oz
Dogs . . . . . . 1 tsp-4 tbsp
Cats . . . . . . ½-2 tsp
Precaution(s): Store at controlled room temperature between 15°-30°C (59°-86°F).
Caution(s): Keep out of the reach of children. Not recommended for frequent or extended use. Continuous or too frequent use may interfere with the absorption of fat, soluble vitamins and other nutrients.
Use care to avoid getting into the respiratory tract (windpipe and lungs). Accidental introduction into the respiratory tract can result in serious complications, including foreign body pneumonia.
If constipation is not relieved after one or two doses, consult a veterinarian.
Presentation: 1 gallon (3.785 L) containers.
Compendium Code No.: 14750560

MINERAL OIL
Dominion
Laxative
Active Ingredient(s):
Mineral Oil 100%
Indications: MINERAL OIL is recommended as an intestinal lubricant to relieve constipation, a dry skin softener, and as a coat dressing.
Dosage and Administration: As a Laxative:
Cattle and Horses: 240 to 960 mL depending on body weight and severity of condition.
Sheep, Goats and Swine: 60 to 240 mL.
Dogs and Cats: 5 to 120 mL.
Repeat dosage daily until condition is corrected. Habitual constipation may be relieved by administering 1 to 2 times weekly.
As a Coat Dressing: Mix 1 L alcohol, 1 L water, and 2 L mineral oil; shake vigorously to make an emulsion. Massage into the coat and skin. Follow with a good brushing.
For use as a spray, dissolve 30 grams of soap in 450 mL of hot water. Let cool, then add 450 mL of oil. Then use 30 mL of this mixture to 180 mL of water for spraying.
Caution(s): Keep out of reach of children.
Presentation: 4 liter jug; 4 jugs/carton.
Compendium Code No.: 15080040

MINERAL OIL
Durvet
Laxative
Active Ingredient(s): Mineral oil.
Indications: Uses: A mild laxative for the lubrication of the intestinal tract.
Dosage and Administration: Dose Chart:
Horses . . . . . . 1 qt.
Cattle . . . . . . 1 qt.
Sheep . . . . . . 5 oz.
Hogs . . . . . . 1 pt.
Dogs - toy breeds, pups . . . . . . 1 oz.
Adult dogs . . . . . . 2 oz.
According to size.
Precaution(s): Store at a controlled room temperature between 15° and 30°C (59°F-86°F). Keep tightly closed and protect from light.
Caution(s): Exercise care in administering to avoid aspiration into the lungs and possible foreign body pneumonia. Prolonged use or frequent repeated usage may interfere with normal absorption of nutrients from the digestive tract.
Not recommended for frequent repeat or extended repeated administration. If condition persists consult veterinarian.
For animal use only.
Warning(s): Keep out of reach of children.
Presentation: 1 gallon (3.785 L) (NDC: 30798-784-35).
Compendium Code No.: 10841151
Rev. 7-98

MINERAL OIL
Vedco
Laxative
Active Ingredient(s): Contains mineral oil.
Indications: A mild laxative for the lubrication of the intestinal tract.
Dosage and Administration:
Horse . . . . . . 1 qt.
Cattle . . . . . . 1 qt.
Sheep . . . . . . 5 oz.
Hogs . . . . . . 1 pt.
Dogs (toy breeds, pups) . . . . . . 1 oz.
Adult dogs . . . . . . 2 oz. (according to size)
Precaution(s): Store at a controlled room temperature between 59-86°F (15-30°C).
Caution(s): Exercise care in administering to avoid aspiration into the lungs and possible foreign body pneumonia. Prolonged use or frequently repeated use may interfere with the normal absorption of nutrients from the digestive tract.
Warning(s): Keep out of reach of children.
Presentation: 1 gallon and 5 gallon containers.
Compendium Code No.: 10941291

MINERAL OIL 95 V
Butler
Laxative
NDC No.: 11695-2172-1
Active Ingredient(s): Mineral oil.
Indications: A mild laxative for the lubrication of the intestinal tract.
Dosage and Administration:
Horse . . . . . . 1 pt
Cattle . . . . . . 1 pt
Sheep . . . . . . 5 oz
Hogs . . . . . . 1 pt
Dogs-toy breeds/pups . . . . . . 1 oz
Adult dogs . . . . . . 2 oz
According to size.
Precaution(s): Store at controlled room temperature between 15° and 30°C (59°F-86°F).
Keep tightly closed, protect from light.
Caution(s): Exercise care in administering to avoid aspiration into the lungs and possible foreign body pneumonia. Prolonged use or frequent repeat use may interfere with normal absorption of nutrients from the digestive tract. Keep out of reach of children.
Not recommended for frequent repeat or extended repeated administration. If condition persists consult veterinarian.
Warning(s): Livestock drug. For animal use only.
Keep out of reach of children.
Presentation: 1 gallon (3.785 L).
Compendium Code No.: 10821170

MINERAL OIL 95 VISCOSITY
First Priority
Laxative
Active Ingredient(s): Mineral oil.
Indications: A mild laxative for the lubrication of the intestinal tract.
Dosage and Administration:
Horse . . . . . . 1 pt
Cattle . . . . . . 1 pt
Sheep . . . . . . 5 oz
Hogs . . . . . . 1 pt
Dogs-toy breeds and pups . . . . . . 1 oz
Adult dogs . . . . . . 2 oz
According to size.
Precaution(s): Storage: Store at controlled room temperature between 15° and 30°C (59°-86°F).
Keep container tightly closed, protect from light.
Caution(s): Not recommended for frequent repeated or extended repeated administration. If condition persists consult veterinarian.
Exercise care in administering to avoid aspiration into the lungs and possible foreign body pneumonia. Prolonged use or frequent repeat use may interfere with normal absorption of nutrients from the digestive tract.
For animal use only.
Warning(s): Keep out of reach of children.
Presentation: 1 gallon (3.785 L) (NDC# 58829-234-01).
Compendium Code No.: 11390552
Rev. 06-01

MINERAL OIL 150 VISCOSITY
First Priority
Laxative
Active Ingredient(s): Mineral oil.
Indications: A mild laxative for the lubrication of the intestinal tract.
Dosage and Administration: Dose Chart:
Horses . . . . . . 1 pt
Cattle . . . . . . 1 pt
Sheep . . . . . . 5 oz
Hogs . . . . . . 1 pt
Dogs-toy breeds/pups . . . . . . 1 oz
Adult dogs . . . . . . 2 oz
According to size.
Precaution(s): Storage: Store at controlled room temperature between 15°-30°C (59°-86°F). Keep container tightly closed when not in use.
Caution(s): Exercise care in administering to avoid aspiration into the lungs and possible foreign body pneumonia. Prolonged use or frequent repeated use may interfere with normal absorption of nutrients from the digestive tract.

Not recommended for frequent repeated or extended repeated administration. If condition persists consult veterinarian.

For animal use only.

Warning(s): Keep out of reach of children.

Presentation: 1 gallon (3.785 L) (NDC# 58829-287-01) and 2.5 gallons (9.46 L) (NDC# 58829-287-25).

Compendium Code No.: 11390563 Rev. 07-01 / Iss. 12-01

MINERAL OIL LIGHT

Centaur **Laxative**

Active Ingredient(s): Mineral oil.

Indications: For use as a mild laxative for lubrication of intestinal tract.

For relief of obstruction or impaction of the intestinal tract in livestock and pets. Also used as an excellent general purpose veterinary lubricant and coat conditioner. Indicated for use on horses, cattle, sheep, swine, goats and dogs.

Dosage and Administration: As a laxative and gut protectant use following dosage chart:

Cattle: 2 to 4 quarts
Horses: 2 to 4 quarts.
Sheep: 1 to 2 pints
Swine: 1 to 2 pints
Goats: 1 to 2 pints
Dogs:
Toy Breeds and Pups 1 ounce
Adult Dogs 2 ounces

As a conditioner-lubricant, apply a small amount to coat and work in with fingers or brush.

Precaution(s): Store between 50°-85°F.

Caution(s): If no response to dosage, consult a veterinarian.

For animal use only.

Warning(s): Keep out of reach of children.

Presentation: 1 gallon (128 fl oz) 3.785 L containers.

Manufactured by: Unavet, North Kansas City, MO 64116.

Compendium Code No.: 14880230

MINERAL OIL LIGHT

Phoenix Pharmaceutical **Laxative**

Mild Laxative

Active Ingredient(s): Mineral oil.

Indications: For use as a mild laxative. Softens and lubricates stools to help relieve simple constipation.

Dosage and Administration: Suggested dosage for oral administration, according to the size of the animal:

Adult Cattle and Horses: 1 pint to 2 quarts.
Calves and Colts: 2 to 4 fl. oz.
Pigs, Sheep and Goats: 1 to 10 fl. oz.
Dogs: 1 tsp.-4 tbsp.
Cats: ½-2 tsp.

Caution(s): Not recommended for frequent or extended use. Continuous or too frequent use may interfere with absorption of fat-soluble vitamins and other nutrients.

Use great care to avoid getting into the respiratory tract (wind-pipe and lungs). Accidental introduction into the respiratory tract can result in serious complications, including foreign body pneumonia.

If constipation is not relieved after one or two doses, consult a veterinarian.

For animal use only.

For external use only.

Warning(s): Keep out of reach of children.

Presentation: 1 gallon (3.785 L) containers (NDC 57319-429-09).

Compendium Code No.: 12561090 Rev. 11-00

MINERAL VET 5

Neogen **Equine Dietary Supplement**

Mineral Supplement

Guaranteed Analysis:

Calcium
not more than 11.4%
not less than 9.5%
Phosphorus
not less than 0.3%
Salt
not more than 2.5%
not less than 2.0%
Iodine, not less than 0.001%
Magnesium, not less than 2.0%
Iron, not less than 1.2%
Zinc, not less than 2100 ppm
Copper, not less than 510 ppm
Cobalt, not less than 40 ppm

Ingredients: Calcium Carbonate, Calcium Oxide, Tricalcium Phosphate, Bentonite, Salt, Potassium Iodide, Magnesium Oxide, Zinc Sulphate, Copper Oxide, Cobalt Carbonate.

Indications: A mineral supplement for all grain fed horses.

Dosage and Administration: Feeding Instructions:

Ponies: 1 ounce daily.
Stallions: 2 ounces daily.
Working Horses: 3 ounces daily.

Precaution(s): Keep lid tightly closed.

Caution(s): For veterinary use only.

Warning(s): Keep out of reach of children.

Presentation: 6 lbs (2.721 kg) (NDC: 59051-9167-0) and 16 lbs (7.27 kg) (NDC: 59051-9168-0).

Compendium Code No.: 14910361 L438-0501 / L439-0501

MINT DISINFECTANT

Air-Tite **Disinfectant/Detergent**

Germicidal Detergent and Deodorant

Pseudomonacidal, Staphylocidal, Salmonellacidal, Fungicidal, *Virucidal

EPA Reg. No.: 47371-130-9854

Active Ingredient(s):

Didecyl dimethyl ammonium chloride 4.61%
n-Alkyl (C_{14} 50%, C_{12} 40%, C_{18} 10%) dimethyl benzyl ammonium chloride 3.07%
Inert Ingredients 92.32%

Indications: Recommended for use in hospitals, nursing homes, schools, colleges, veterinary clinics, animal life science laboratories, equine farms, tack shops, pet shops, airports, kennels, hotels and motels, poultry and turkey farms, dairy farms and hog farms, breeding and grooming establishments.

Bactericidal at 1:128 dilution (1 ounce per gallon of water) against *Pseudomonas aeruginosa, Staphylococcus aureus,* and *Salmonella choleraesuis* according to the current AOAC Use-Dilution Test method, modified in the presence of 400 ppm synthetic hard water (calculated as $CaCO_3$) plus 5% organic serum.

Fungicidal against *Trichophyton interdigitale* and *Candida albicans* according to the AOAC fungicidal test, modified in the presence of 400 ppm hard water (calculated as a $CaCO_3$) plus 5% organic serum at a 1:128 dilution.

Virucidal against *HIV-1 (AIDS virus), influenza A/Hong Kong, Herpes simplex type I, herpes simplex type II, vaccinia, rubella, adenovirus type IV, canine parvovirus, canine distemper, feline panleukopenia, feline picornavirus, feline leukemia, rabies, porcine parvovirus, pseudorabies, infectious bovine rhinotracheitis and infectious bronchitis (avian IBV) according to the virucidal qualification, modified in the presence of 400 ppm hard water plus 5% organic serum at 1:128 dilution (1 ounce per gallon of water).

Directions for Use: It is a violation of Federal Law to use this product in a manner inconsistent with its labeling.

General Use Directions for Disinfecting: For use on hard non-porous surfaces such as floors, walls, metal surfaces, stainless steel surfaces, porcelain, and plastic surfaces. Remove gross filth and heavy soil deposits then thoroughly wet surfaces. Use 1 ounce per gallon of water for a minimum contact time of 10 minutes in a single application. Can be applied with a mop, sponge, or cloth as well as spraying or soaking. The recommended use solution is prepared fresh for each use then discarded. Rinsing is not necessary unless floors are to be waxed or polished.

Mildewstatic Instructions: Will effectively control the growth of mold and mildew plus the odors caused by them when applied to hard, nonporous surfaces such as walls, floors, and table tops. Apply solution (1 ounce per gallon of water) with cloth, mop, sponge, or spray making sure to wet all surfaces completely. Let air dry. Repeat application weekly or when growth reappears.

*Kills HIV-1 (AIDS virus) on precleaned, environmental surfaces/objects previously soiled with blood/body fluids in healthcare settings or other settings in which there is an expected likelihood of soiling of inanimate surfaces/objects with blood or body fluids, and in which the surfaces/objects likely to be soiled with blood or body fluids can be associated with the potential for transmission of human immunodeficiency virus Type 1 (HIV-1) (associated with AIDS).

Special Instructions for Cleaning and Decontamination Against HIV-1 (AIDS Virus) of Surfaces/Objects Soiled with Blood/Body Fluids:

Personal Protection: Disposable latex or vinyl gloves, gowns, face masks, or eye coverings as appropriate, must be worn during all cleaning of body fluids, blood, and decontamination procedures.

Cleaning Procedures: Blood and body fluids must be thoroughly cleaned from surfaces and objects before application of disinfectant.

Contact Time: Effective against HIV-1 (AIDS virus) on hard nonporous surfaces in the presence of a moderate amount of organic soil (5% blood serum) when used at a 1:128 dilution (providing 600 ppm of active quaternary) in 400 ppm $CaCO_3$ hard water for a contact time of 4 minutes at room temperature (20-25°C). Use a ten (10) minute contact time for disinfection against all other bacteria, fungi, viruses claimed (listed on labeling).

Disposal of Infectious Materials: Blood and other body fluids should be autoclaved and disposed of according to federal, state, and local regulations for infectious waste disposal.

Precautionary Statements: Hazards to Humans and Domestic Animal:

Corrosive: Causes eye damage and severe skin irritation. Do not get in eyes, on skin, or on clothing. To protect eyes wear goggles or face shield and to protect skin, wear rubber gloves when handling. Wash thoroughly with soap and water after handling. Remove contaminated clothing and wash before reuse. Harmful if swallowed.

Statement of Practical Treatment: In case of contact, immediately flush eyes or skin with plenty of water for at least 15 minutes. For eyes call a physician. If swallowed, drink promptly a large quantity of milk, egg whites, gelatin solution or, if these are not available, drink large quantities of water. Avoid alcohol. Get medical attention.

Note to Physician: Probable mucosal damage may contraindicate the use of gastric lavage. Measures against circulatory shock, respiratory depression and convulsion may be needed.

Storage and Disposal:

Prohibitions: Do not contaminate water, food or feed by storage or disposal. Open dumping is prohibited. Do not reuse empty container.

Pesticide Disposal: Pesticide wastes are acutely hazardous. Improper disposal of excess pesticide, spray mixture, or rinsate is a violation of Federal Law. If these wastes cannot be disposed of by use according to label instructions, contact your State Pesticide or Environmental Control Agency, or the Hazardous Waste representative at the nearest EPA Regional Office for guidance.

Container Disposal Plastic Containers: Triple rinse (or equivalent). Then offer for recycling or reconditioning, or puncture and dispose of in a sanitary landfill, or incineration, or if allowed by state and local authorities, by burning. If burned, stay out of smoke.

General: Consult federal, state or local disposal authorities for approved alternative procedures such as limited open burning.

Warning(s): Keep out of reach of children.

Discussion: A concentrated, multi-purpose germicidal detergent and deodorant effective in hard water up to 400 ppm hard water (calculated as $CaCO_3$) plus 5% organic serum. Disinfects, cleans, and deodorizes in one step. Effective against the following pathogenic bacteria according to the AOAC Use-Dilution, current edition, modified in the presence of 400 ppm synthetic hard water (calculated as $CaCO_3$) plus 5% organic serum: *Pseudomonas aeruginosa, Staphylococcus aureus, Salmonella choleraesuis, Bordetella bronchiseptica, Chlamydia psittaci, E coli, E coli* (antibiotic resistant), *Enterobacter aerogenes, Enterobacter cloacae, Fusobacterium necrophorum, Klebsiella pneumoniae, Klebsiella pneumoniae* (antibiotic resistant), *Pasteurella multocida, Pseudonomas aeruginosa* (antibiotic resistant), *Proteus mirabilis, Proteus vulgaris, Salmonella typhi, Salmonella typhimurium, Serratia marcescens, Shigella flexneri, Shigella sonnei, Staphylococcus aureus* (antibiotic resistant), *Staphylococcus epidermidis* (antibiotic resistant), *Streptococcus faecalis* (antibiotic resistant), *Streptococcus faecalis, Streptococcus pyogenes.*

Presentation: 1 gallon.

Compendium Code No.: 11510000

MIRRA-COAT® (EQUINE SYSTEM)

Pet-Ag **Large Animal Dietary Supplement**

Guaranteed Analysis: (minimums)

Linoleic Acid (as glycerides) 12.5%
Zinc 0.10%
Vitamin A .... 36,000 I.U./lb.
Vitamin E .... 240 I.U./lb.
Vitamin B_6 .... 30 mg/lb.
Biotin .... 1 mg/lb.

Ingredients: Soy flour with soybean oil added, vegetable oil, dextrose, silicon dioxide, zinc methionine, vitamin E supplement, natural and artificial flavors added, preserved with tertiary butyl hydroquinolone and citric acid, vitamin A supplement, pyridoxine hydrochloride, biotin.

Indications: MIRRA-COAT® Nutritional Supplement for Skin and Coat is a balanced blend of essential fatty acids, biotin, and zinc, formulated specifically to develop and a healthy skin and haircoat. MIRRA-COAT® contains nutrients essential for the maintenance of normal skin cells. The results are a pliable, moisturized skin that reduces dandruff and develops a glossy "show" coat. And horses love the taste of MIRRA-COAT®. They lick their feed buckets clean when MIRRA-COAT® is added to their feed.

Directions: Feeding Directions:

Horses: For the first two weeks, mix 2 scoops (enclosed) of MIRRA-COAT® into the horse's daily ration. After two weeks, reduce to 1 scoop daily.

Dogs: Mix into the dog's regular ration daily. Feed ¼ scoop per 20 lbs. bodyweight.

If a poor skin and coat condition persists, other than dietary factors may be involved and your veterinarian should be consulted.

Presentation: Equine System: 5 lb. (2.27 kg) (4 per case) and 25 lb. pails, and 40 lb. bags. Formula V™: 5 lb. buckets and 25 lb. pails.

Compendium Code No.: 10970210 304F, ENG304B

MIRRA-COAT® FOR CATS

Pet-Ag **Small Animal Dietary Supplement**

Guaranteed Analysis:

Arachadonic acid, min. 2.2%
Linoleic acid, min. 33.0%
Linolenic acid, min. 3.3%
Vitamin A, min. .... 110,000 I.U./lb.
Vitamin E, min. .... 900 I.U./lb.
Vitamin B_6, min. .... 40 mg/lb.
Biotin, min. .... 0.54 mg/lb.
Zinc, min. .... 100 mg/lb.

Ingredients: Vegetable oil, fish oil, water, vitamin E supplement, lecithin, zinc chloride, pyridoxine hydrochloride, natural and artificial flavors added, vitamin A supplement, biotin, preserved with propionic acid, BHA, propyl gallate and citric acid.

Indications: Recommended for use as a supplement for cats that need special attention to help control shedding, scratching, dull coat and dry, flaky skin. Use to aid in restoring the skin and coat condition after treatment for non-nutritional problems such as parasites, trauma and allergies. Improvements are seen within two weeks of use.

Dosage and Administration: Add one-half (½) teaspoon (2.5 mL or 4 pumps) to the cat's food each day for each 6 lbs. (2.7 kg) of body weight.

Consult a veterinarian if conditions persist.

Precaution(s): Store under cool, dry conditions.

Caution(s): For animal use only.

Discussion:

Essential fatty acids (EFA): Arachadonic acid: Cell membrane formation, improves skin barrier function.

Vitamin A: Prevents plugged hair follicles.

Vitamin E: Prevents cellular EFA oxidation, balances vitamin A concentration, activates EFA metabolism.

Vitamin B_6: Prevents dermatitis and hair loss, activates EFA and protein metabolism.

Biotin: Prevents scaly dermatitis and hair loss, improves hair color and luster, activates EFA and protein metabolism.

Zinc: Prevents scaly dermatitis and hair loss, activates EFA and protein enzyme systems.

Does not contain Vitamin D: Excess vitamin D causes bone dysfunction and soft tissue calcification.

Presentation: 4 oz. (12 per case) and 8 oz. (12 per case) bottles.

Compendium Code No.: 10970221

MIRRA-COAT® POWDER AND LIQUID

Pet-Ag **Small Animal Dietary Supplement**

Active Ingredient(s): Guaranteed Analysis:

	Powder	Liquid
Linoleic acid, min.	12.50%	52.75%
Linolenic acid, min.	1.30%	4.40%
Vitamin A, min.	36,100 I.U./lb.	66,000 I.U./lb.
Vitamin E, min.	240 I.U./lb.	660 I.U./lb.
Vitamin B_6, min.	30.300 mg/lb.	50.000 mg/lb.
Biotin, min.	0.475 mg/lb.	0.800 mg/lb.
Zinc, min.	238.000 mg/lb.	400.000 mg/lb.

Ingredients:

Powder: Soy flour with soybean oil added, vegetable oil, sugar, silicon dioxide, zinc methionine, vitamin E supplement, natural and artificial flavors added, preserved with tertiary butyl hydroquinone and citric acid, vitamin A supplement, pyridoxine hydrochloride, and biotin.

Liquid: Vegetable oil, water, zinc chloride, lecithin, vitamin E supplement, natural and artificial flavors added, vitamin A supplement, pyridoxine hydrochloride, biotin, preserved with tertiary butyl hydroquinone and citric acid.

Indications: Recommended for use as a concentrated supplement for dogs and other animals that need special attention to help control shedding, scratching, dull coat and dry, flaky skin. Use to aid in restoring the skin and coat condition after treatment for non-nutritional problems such as parasites, trauma and allergies. Improvements are seen within two weeks of use.

Dosage and Administration:

Powder: Add one (1) tablespoon a day to the dog's food for each 20 lbs. of body weight.

Liquid: Add one (1) teaspoon (5 mL or 7 pumps) to the dog's food for each 20 lbs. of body weight.

May be used in wirehaired breeds at one-half (½) the recommended levels. Higher levels will result in a soft coat.

Consult a veterinarian if conditions persist.

Precaution(s): Store in cool, dry conditions.

Caution(s): For animal use only.

Discussion:

Essential fatty acids (EFA): Cell membrane formation, improves skin barrier function.

Vitamin A: Prevents plugged hair follicles.

Vitamin E: Prevents cellular EFA oxidation, balances vitamin A concentration, activates EFA metabolism.

Vitamin B_6: Prevents dermatitis and hair loss, activates EFA and protein metabolism.

Biotin: Prevents scaly dermatitis and hair loss, improves hair color and luster, activates EFA and protein metabolism.

Zinc: Prevents scaly dermatitis and hair loss, activates EFA and protein enzyme systems.

Does not contains Vitamin D: Excess vitamin D causes bone dysfunction and soft tissue calcification.

Presentation:

Form	Size	Units
Powder	1 lb. can	12 per case
	2½ lb. can	6 per case
	20 lb. drum	1
Liquid	8 oz. bottle	12 per case
	16 oz. bottle	12 per case
	64 oz. bottle	6 per case

Compendium Code No.: 10970230

MITABAN® ℞

Pharmacia & Upjohn **Parasiticide-Topical**

Amitraz liquid concentrate

NADA No.: 120-299

Active Ingredient(s): MITABAN® Liquid Concentrate (amitraz) contains 19.9% N'-(2,4-dimethylphenyl)-N-[[2,4-dimethylphenyl) imino] methyl]-N-methyl-methanimidamide (w/w), and also xylol, propylene oxide, and a blend of alkyl benzene sulfonates and exthoxylated polyethers.

Indications: MITABAN® (amitraz) is indicated for treatment of generalized demodicosis *(Demodex canis)* in dogs. Current data do not support use for treatment of localized demodicosis or scabies.

Pharmacology: Amitraz, a diamide, is pale yellow, has a melting point of 86° to 87° C, is not hygroscopic, is stable to heating, soluble in most organic solvents, and sparingly soluble in water.

Amitraz is hydrolyzed to 2,4-dimethyl-formanilide and N-(2,4-dimethylphenyl)-N'-methylformamidine; these metabolites are further metabolized to 2,4-dimethylaniline and ultimately to 4-amino-3-methylbenzoic acid, which was the principle metabolite in the urine and liver.

Radiolabeled amitraz was administered to beagles as a single oral treatment at a level of 4 mg/kg. Peak blood levels were reached between 1.5 and 6 hours posttreatment; the half-life was approximately 12 hours during the initial 48 hours. Radioactivity was extremely low in whole blood and plasma at 72 (0.05-0.06 ppm) and 96 (0.03-0.06 ppm) hours. The organs having residues at levels greater than plasma concentrations at 96 hours included: liver, skin, eyes, bile, kidney, medulla, cerebrum, lungs, gonads, fat, thyroid, spleen, and large intestine. The main metabolite isolated from these tissues was identified as 4-amino-3-methylbenzoic acid, which is nontoxic for the dog.

Studies have not been conducted to quantitatively determine absorption by the dog following topical or dermal treatment with amitraz. The technical drug (amitraz) and formulated material (MITABAN® Liquid Concentrate) have been extensively evaluated in laboratory and domesticated animals in a series of acute, subchronic and chronic studies.

The mechanism of action for amitraz is unknown, however data currently available suggest the drug may act on the central nervous system. *In vitro* housefly tests indicated amitraz does not have significant cholinesterase inhibitory activity.

Dosage and Administration: Long and medium-haired dogs should be clipped closely before treating. Prior to the initial treatment, all dogs should be bathed with a mild soap and water and towel dried. The entire animal should then be topically treated with MITABAN® (amitraz) at a rate of 10.6 milliliters (contents of one bottle) per 2 gallons of warm water (250 ppm active drug). Two bottles (21.2 milliliters) per four gallons of water may be necessary to treat large dogs. The entire dog should be thoroughly and completely wetted with the mixture, and then allowed to air dry. Do not rinse or towel dry the dog after treatment with MITABAN®. A fresh MITABAN®-water mixture should be prepared for each patient; using the same mixture for more than one patient can spread other dermal infections and also the concentration of MITABAN® could be reduced to a level which would be less effective than the recommended concentration.

Three to six topical treatments (14 days apart) are recommended for treatment of generalized demodicosis. It is important to continue the treatment until no viable (alive) mites are found in the skin scrapings at two successive treatments, or until six treatments have been applied. Severe (chronic) cases and dogs which are reinfested may require a second and third series of treatments, and again the treatment should be applied at 14 day intervals. Discontinue treatment of dogs which do not respond clinically.

When employing MITABAN® for treatment of demodicosis, other dogs in the home also should be examined for lesions to ascertain whether treatment of these animals is warranted.

Contraindication(s): Fertility impairment studies have not been conducted in the canine with MITABAN® (amitraz). It is not known whether MITABAN® may cause impairment of fertility in dogs.

Reproduction studies during pregnancy have not been conducted with MITABAN®. It is not known whether MITABAN® may harm the embryo or fetus.

The safety of MITABAN® has not been established for dogs less than four months of age.

Precaution(s): Store at controlled room temperature 20° to 25°C (68° to 77°F) [see USP].

Caution: Federal (USA) law restricts this drug to use by or on the order of a licensed veterinarian.

Though eye or dermal irritation was not reported during controlled experiments, such effects have been infrequently reported from clinical use. Consistent with good veterinary practice, it is recommended that a protectant be used in the eyes of patients prior to facial treatment with any topical therapy.

Well-controlled experiments with MITABAN® (amitraz) have not been conducted to determine the compatibility range with other products.

For topical use on dogs.

For use in animals only.

Warning(s): Toxicology studies conducted in the dog and other species suggest amitraz may alter the animal's ability to maintain homeostasis. Animals treated with MITABAN® (amitraz) should not be subjected to stress for a period of at least 24 hours posttreatment. Adverse reactions including three fatalities were reported during the clinical studies. In excess of 1100 patients with generalized demodicosis were topically treated with MITABAN®.

Information for Clients: Clients should be informed that animals treated with MITABAN® (amitraz) should not be subjected to additional stress for a period of at least 24 hours posttreatment. Refer to additional warnings below.

Not for human use. Keep out of reach of children.

MITABAN® (amitraz) may be harmful if swallowed by humans. If swallowed, do not induce vomiting (contains xylol) and immediately call a physician. Avoid inhalation of vapors (xylol) and contamination of feed and food stuffs.

MITABAN® is flammable; when diluted with water, the mixture is not flammable.

MITABAN® (concentrate or diluted) may cause eye or skin irritation in sensitive persons. Do not get in eyes, on skin or on clothing. If in eyes, wash with water for 15 minutes and call a physician immediately.

Protect exposed skin (e.g. with rubber gloves, etc.) when mixing MITABAN® with water and treating animals. Wash hands and arms with soap and water after treatment of the pet(s). Dispose of unused MITABAN®-water solution by flushing down the drain. Rinse the MITABAN® container with water and do not reuse.

Avoid handling pets immediately after treatment. Contact may cause skin irritation in sensitive individuals during the first few days after treatment.

Amitraz, the active ingredient in MITABAN®, has been shown to cause liver tumors in female mice.

Ingestion or inhalation may cause central nervous system depression.

Toxicology:

Dermal Studies—Dog: Acute and subchronic dermal toxicity studies were conducted with nondiseased beagles using the recommended concentration (250 ppm active drug) and exaggerated concentrations of MITABAN® (amitraz). A single treatment with 250 ppm, 1250 ppm or 2500 ppm was topically applied to healthy dogs. Transient sedation was observed within 8 hours posttreatment in 1 of 6 dogs at 250 ppm, and all of the animals at 1250 ppm and 2500 ppm; all of the animals were normal at 24 hours posttreatment. There was a significant depression of rectal temperatures at 4 hours posttreatment in the 1250 ppm and 2500 ppm groups. Blood glucose values were elevated at 4 hours posttreatment in the 250 ppm female group, and in both sexes at the 1250 ppm and 2500 ppm concentrations. Rectal temperatures and glucose values returned to normal within 24 hours posttreatment. In another study, groups of healthy beagles were topically treated with either 250 ppm, 750 ppm or 1250 ppm of active drug at 14 day intervals and for 12 weeks. Blood glucose values were elevated at the 750 ppm concentration at 4 hours posttreatment after 3 of 6 treatments, and after 5 of 6 treatments at the 1250 ppm level. In the 750 ppm group, serum glucose values returned to normal at 24 hours posttreatment, however for the 1250 ppm group, at 24 hours and after 3 of 6 treatments the levels remained significantly elevated.

Dermal or ocular responses were not observed when MITABAN® was applied at recommended or exaggerated concentrations to the skin and incidentally to the eyes of dogs (in controlled experiments simulating recommended use). However, such responses have been infrequently reported from clinical use. (See Cautions).

Oral Studies—Dog: An acute oral toxicity study was conducted with amitraz utilizing nondiseased beagles. Death occurred in one of two dogs given a single oral dose of 100 mg/kg. Clinical signs included CNS depression, ataxia, hypothermia, bradycardia, muscular weakness, vomition, uncontrolled vocal spasm and micturition. Clinical laboratory data indicated a hemoconcentration, and transient elevations in blood glucose, blood urea nitrogen, serum potassium and alkaline phosphatase values. Dogs given 20 mg/kg (single oral dose) showed similar, though less pronounced, clinical signs and were clinically normal at three days posttreatment. Hemoconcentration and increased blood urea nitrogen were noted in both dogs; increased and transient blood glucose and serum alkaline phosphatase values were observed in one dog. Dogs given 4 mg/kg (single oral dose) had decreased rectal temperatures within three hours and were normal at 24 hours posttreatment.

Amitraz was orally administered to nondiseased beagles at levels of 0, 0.25, 1 and 4 mg/kg once daily for 90 days. There were no deaths in any of the groups. At 3 hours posttreatment and for only the initial three days of the 90 day experiment, dogs treated with 4 mg/kg exhibited CNS depression and ataxia; the effects remained for 3 to 6 hours and the dogs were normal within 24 hours posttreatment. Vomition occurred in two dogs on only the initial two days of the study. Thereafter (days 4 through 90) the dogs appeared to be subdued for approximately 6 hours after dosing, and ataxia was nearly impossible to detect. In the initial 48 to 72 hours, dogs treated with 1 mg/kg/day exhibited signs of depression (without ataxia) for 4-6 hours; subsequently the depression became less marked and of shorter duration. At 3 hours after dosing, dogs treated with 1 or 4 mg/kg consistently had subnormal rectal temperatures and pulse rates; both parameters returned to normal within 24 hours posttreatment. At 0.25 mg/kg/day, the dogs appeared normal throughout the experiment. Hyperglycemia consistently occurred in dogs treated with 1 and 4 mg/kg/day and rarely occurred in dogs at the 0.25 mg/kg level; this response was maximal within 6 hours posttreatment and serum glucose values returned to normal within 24 hours after treatment. Grossly there was a significant increase in liver weights for dogs treated at the 4 mg/kg level, however microscopically the findings were minimal and consisted of a slight enlargement of the central and midzonal hepatocytes; the degree of enlargement was not dose related. However, at the two higher doses the area affected appeared more prominent as reflected by an increase of the periportal hepatocytes. In the adrenal gland, several dogs treated with the two higher levels had thinning of the zonae fasiculata and reticularis, which may be associated with slight hyperplasia of the zona glomerulosa.

Side Effects: Ingestion of MITABAN® may increase the risk of adverse effects. Therefore, appropriate care should be exercised both during and immediately after MITABAN® application to minimize the opportunity for exposure by the oral route.

The most frequently observed adverse reaction in the clinical studies was transient sedation, which occurred in approximately 8% of the generalized demodicosis patients. This effect was observed within 2 to 6 hours posttreatment, and usually dissipated within 24 to 72 hours. In approximately 40% of the affected generalized demodicosis patients, the effect dissipated in less than 24 hours. Sedation often was less apparent when additional MITABAN® (amitraz) treatments were applied, however in approximately 35% of the generalized demodicosis patients sleepiness was observed after each treatment. Transient pruritus, which clinical investigators considered to be an indirect effect due to an inflammatory reaction associated with dead mites, occurred in less than 3% of the generalized demodicosis patients. This effect usually occurred and dissipated within 24-48 hours posttreatment. Other observations noted by the clinical investigators and/or clients were a low incidence (less than 1%) of convulsions, ataxia, hyperexcitability, personality change, hypothermia, appetite stimulation, bloat, polyuria, vomition, diarrhea, anorexia, edema, erythema and other varying degrees of skin irritation. Three fatalities were recorded.

Trial Data: Canine Efficacy:

Controlled Studies: The efficacy of MITABAN® (amitraz) was extensively evaluated on dogs experimentally or naturally parasitized with *Demodex canis*. Three to six MITABAN® treatments (250 ppm active drug), at 14 day intervals, were highly efficacious for treatment of naturally acquired demodicosis. MITABAN® treatment was continued until all *Demodex* in the skin scrapings were dead or the dogs no longer harbored mites at two successive treatments, or the animal received six treatments. Ninety-six percent of the dogs were cleared of mites.

Clinical Studies: Investigators at university veterinary clinics, small animal practitioners, and dermatology specialists clinically evaluated MITABAN®. A total of 1107 generalized demodicosis patients were included in these investigations. A variety of breeds, ages, hair conditions and lengths, and weights of dogs were included in these field investigations. The pre- and posttreatment demodicosis indices were used to quantify the degree and extent of involvement. Of the generalized cases, greater than 95% clinically improved (posttreatment clinical condition better than pre-treatment condition), and the average clinical response [(mean pretreatment index - mean posttreatment index) X 100 ÷ mean pretreatment index] was greater than 90%; these patients received an average of 5 treatments. Seventy-five percent of the generalized demodicosis patients were negative for viable mites prior to administration of the final MITABAN® treatment.

Eighty percent of the generalized demodicosis patients were returned to clinical normalcy and did not require additional therapy after receiving one treatment series. Twenty percent of all patients with generalized demodicosis required a second treatment series. When retreated, the 14 day treatment interval was again followed, and these patients received an average of 5 treatments. Greater than 90% of the dogs clinically improved, and the average clinical response of these patients was approximately 80%. Greater than 96% of all generalized demodicosis patients returned to normalcy after receiving one or two treatment series and did not require further therapy. Between 3 and 4% of all generalized demodicosis patients were returned to the investigators and required therapy beyond the second treatment series; these patients received a third or fourth series of MITABAN® treatments. Greater than 99% of all generalized demodicosis patients returned to normalcy after receiving one, two, or three treatment series, and did not require further therapy; less than 1% of the patients required additional therapy.

Presentation: MITABAN® Liquid Concentrate (amitraz) is available in cartons of 12—10.6 mL bottles.

Manufactured by: Pharmacia & Upjohn Animal Health, Canada.

Compendium Code No.: 10490340

MITA-CLEAR™

Pfizer Animal Health **Otic Parasiticide**

EPA Reg. No.: 37425-14-1007

Active Ingredient(s):

Pyrethrins	0.15%
Piperonyl butoxide, technical*	1.50%
N-octyl bicycloheptene dicarboximide	0.50%
Di-n-propyl isocinchomeronate	1.00%
Inert ingredients	96.85%
Total	100.00%

*Equivalent to 1.20% of butylcarbityl (6-propyl-piperonyl) ether and 0.30% of related compounds.

Indications: Kills ear mites in dogs, puppies, cats, and kittens.

Directions: It is a violation of Federal law to use this product in a manner inconsistent with its labeling.

To Kill Ear Mites:

Clean ear with an otic solution. Place a sufficient amount of MITA-CLEAR™ into each ear to thoroughly coat the surface of the ear canal. Gently massage the base of the ear. Leave lotion in ear for a few minutes and carefully wipe the excess lotion from the ear with cotton. Lotion to be applied twice at 7-day intervals.

Precautionary Statements: Hazards to Humans and Domestic Animals: Caution:

Human: Harmful if swallowed. Avoid breathing vapors. Avoid contact with eyes. In case of contact, immediately flush eyes with plenty of water. Obtain medical attention if irritation persists. If swallowed, do not induce vomiting. Wash hands with soap and water after using.

Animal: Avoid contact with eyes. If in eyes, flush with water. Do not use on puppies or kittens under 12 weeks of age. Consult a veterinarian before using this product on debilitated, aged, medicated, pregnant, or nursing animals.

Sensitivities may occur after using any pesticide product for pets. If signs of sensitivity occur, consult a veterinarian immediately.

Environmental Hazards: This product is toxic to fish. Do not add directly to water.

First Aid:

If swallowed: Call physician or poison control center. Do not induce vomiting. Do not give anything by mouth to an unconscious person.

If in eyes: Flush eyes with plenty of water. Call a physician if irritation persists.

If on skin: Wash with plenty of soap and water. See physician if irritation persists.

Storage and Disposal:

Storage: Store in a cool, dry area away from heat and open flame. Do not contaminate water, food or feed by storage or disposal. Do not transfer contents to other containers.

Disposal: Do not reuse empty container. Rinse thoroughly and wrap container in several layers of newspaper and discard in trash.

Warning(s): Keep out of reach of children.

Read entire label before use.

Use only on dogs or cats.

Presentation: 22 mL.

Compendium Code No.: 36901190 79-9654-65-0, 05-9655-65-0

MITAPLEX-P™

Tomlyn **Otic Parasiticide**

EPA Reg. No.: 45087-21-50414

Active Ingredient(s):

Pyrethrins	0.05%
Piperonyl butoxide, technical	0.50%
Inert Ingredients	99.45%

*Equivalent to 0.4% (butycarbityl) (6-propylpiperonyl) ether and 0.1% related compounds.

Indications: Kills ear mites. For dogs and cats.

Directions for Use: It is a violation of Federal Law to use this product in a manner inconsistent with its labeling.

Read entire label before each use.

Use only on dogs and cats.

Remove excess dirt and wax. Do not injure the delicate tissue of the ear. Place recommended dose in each ear. Reapply every day for 7 to 10 days.

Body Weight Dose	
Weight of Pet	Amount of MITAPLEX-P™
1-15 lbs	3-5 drops
15-30 lbs	5-10 drops
30 lbs and over	10-15 drops

Precautionary Statements: Hazards to Humans and Animals:

Caution: Not for human use. Harmful if swallowed or absorbed through skin. Avoid breathing vapors. If ingested, vomiting should not be induced. Consult physician. In case of contact, flush eyes or skin with plenty of water. See physician if irritation persists.

For animals, discontinue use and consult veterinarian if irritation develops. Do not use on puppies or kittens under 12 weeks of age. Consult a veterinarian before using this product on debilitated, aged, pregnant or nursing animals or animals on medication.

Sensitivity may occur after using any pesticide product for pets. If signs of sensitivity occur, bathe your pet with mild soap and rinse with large amounts of water. If signs continue, consult a veterinarian immediately.

Physical Hazard: Do not use or store near heat or open flame.

Storage and Disposal: Storage: Store in original container in locked storage area.

Disposal: Securely wrap original container in several layers of newspaper and discard in trash. Do not reuse container. Rinse thoroughly before discarding in trash.

Warning(s): Keep out of reach of children.

Discussion: Ear mites normally cause a dry, dark brown waxy exudate with crusts in the ears of dogs and cats. Mites are easily observed by placing some ear wax on a dark surface and watching closely for moving white specks. Inflamed, watery or blocked ear canals indicate a more serious condition which requires services of a veterinarian.

Presentation: 4 fl oz (118 mL) containers.

Compendium Code No.: 11220380

M-NINEVAX®

Schering-Plough **Vaccine**

Pasteurella Multocida Vaccine, Avirulent Live Culture, Avian Isolate

U.S. Vet. Lic. No.: 165A

Contents: M-NINEVAX® vaccine is a live bacterial vaccine containing the mild avirulent M-9 strain of *Pasteurella multocida*, Heddleston Type 3-4 cross, in a freeze-dried preparation sealed under vacuum. This vaccine strain has been shown to offer protection against fowl cholera in turkeys. The seed culture used to make this vaccine has been laboratory tested for protection against challenge with the P1059 (Type 3) strain of *P. multocida*.

Indications: For use in healthy turkeys 6 weeks of age or older as an aid in preventing pasteurellosis (fowl cholera) due to *Pasteurella multocida* Type 3, through vaccination by the drinking water method.

Dosage and Administration: When to Vaccinate: Best results are obtained when vaccine is administered initially to turkeys 6 to 8 weeks of age, followed by a booster dose three weeks later, and repeated every 4 to 6 weeks thereafter as necessary according to exposure conditions.

Your Vaccination Program: The development of a durable, strong protection to this disease depends upon the use of an effective vaccination program as well as many other circumstances such as administration techniques, environment and flock health at the time of vaccination. Also, the immune response to one vaccination under field conditions is seldom complete for all animals within a given flock. Even when vaccination is successful, the protection stimulated in individual animals against different diseases may not be life long. Therefore, a program of periodic revaccination may be necessary.

Preparation of the Vaccine:

1. Assemble the vaccine and equipment needed to vaccinate the entire flock at one time.
2. Do not open and rehydrate the vaccine until ready for use.
3. Remove the tear-off aluminum seal from the vaccine vial without disturbing the rubber stopper.
4. Use cool, clean, non-chlorinated tap water to which powdered milk has been added as directed under How to Vaccinate.
5. Remove the rubber stopper from the vaccine vial and rehydrate the vaccine by filling the vial about half-full with tap water (milk added).
6. Reseat the stopper and shake to thoroughly dissolve the vaccine.

How to Vaccinate: Do not mix the vaccine into the drinking water until ready for use. Drinking water for vaccination should be mixed with powdered milk to prevent inactivation from chlorine or other water additives and also to stabilize the vaccine bacteria. The powdered milk should be added to the water at the rate of 3 grams per 11 liters (one heaped teaspoon per 3 U.S. gallons or 2.5 Imp. gallons); or 87 grams per 190 liters (one heaped cupful per 50 U.S. gallons or 41 Imp. gallons).

Use only clean waterers and equipment free of disinfectants or sanitizers. All water must be withheld for at least 2 hours prior to vaccination to assure that all turkeys drink. Mix the rehydrated vaccine in the quantity of drinking water (milk added) which will be consumed by thirsty turkeys in approximately 2 hours.

The following schedule is a general guideline for the amount of water to use with the vaccine. These amounts will vary depending upon the individual management conditions, climate, age and sex of the birds.

Age	Sex	Climate	Amount of Water for Each 1,000 Doses		
			L	U.S. gal.	Imp. gal.
6-8 weeks	Toms	Hot	95	25	21
6-8 weeks	Hens	Hot	76	20	17
6-8 weeks	Toms	Cold	49	13	11
6-8 weeks	Hens	Cold	38	10	8
10-14 weeks	Toms	Hot	133	35	29
10-14 weeks	Hens	Hot	103	27	22,
10-14 weeks	Toms	Cold	68	18	15
10-14 weeks	Hens	Cold	53	14	12

Another helpful guideline for daily water consumption is 3.8 liters (one U.S. gallon or 0.8 Imp. gallon) of water per week of age per 100 poults; figure 40% of this amount. This 40% is about a three hour supply for the flock.

Distribute 500 doses of vaccine in water as used by 500 turkeys, 1,000 doses of vaccine in water as used by 1,000 turkeys or 2,000 doses of vaccine in water as used by 2,000 turkeys. Provide ample water space so that all turkeys can drink easily. Do not administer through water lines with a proportioner or medication tank.

Records: Keep a record of vaccine type, quantity, serial number, expiration date, and place of purchase; the date and time of vaccination; the number, age, breed, and location of the birds; names of operators performing the vaccination and any observed reactions.

Contraindication(s): Turkeys must be healthy and free of environmental or physical stress at the time of vaccination. Initial vaccination with this vaccine should not be conducted in turkeys older than 12 weeks of age. Do not use this vaccine within 2 weeks before or 2 weeks after vaccinating turkeys with live Newcastle virus vaccine.

Precaution(s): Store at 2° to 7°C (35° to 45°F).

Do not spill or spatter the vaccine. Burn empty bottles, caps and all unused vaccine and accessories. Use entire contents of vial when first opened.

Caution(s):

1. For veterinary use only.
2. To avoid interference with the development of protection, turkeys to be vaccinated should not be given any antibiotic and/or sulfonamide medication used in the prevention or treatment of fowl cholera for 3 days before and 5 days after vaccination.
3. Vaccinate only healthy birds. Coccidiosis, respiratory disease, mycoplasma infection, or other disease conditions may cause serious complications or reduce protection. Vaccinated flocks should be watched closely and medicated as necessary to control more severe reactions. Avoid exposing birds other than turkeys to the vaccine.
4. All birds within a flock should be vaccinated on the same day. Isolate other susceptible birds on the premises from the birds being vaccinated.
5. In outbreak situations, vaccinate healthy birds first progressing toward outbreak areas in order to vaccinate diseased birds last. Vaccination in the face of an acute outbreak is not recommended. Under these conditions, use an effective fowl cholera treatment, wait at least 3 days or until the outbreak subsides and then vaccinate.
6. Wash hands thoroughly after using the vaccine.
7. Do not dilute the vaccine or otherwise stretch the dosage.

Warning(s): Do not vaccinate within 21 days of slaughter.

Avoid contact of open wounds with the vaccine since this might cause a bacterial infection. If this occurs, consult a physician immediately to obtain proper treatment.

Presentation: Supplied in 10 x 1,000 doses (NDC 0138-0852-01) and 10 x 2,000 doses (NDC 0138-0852-03).

Compendium Code No.: 10471261

M-NINEVAX®-C

Schering-Plough **Vaccine**

Pasteurella multocida Vaccine, Avirulent Live Culture, Avian Isolate

U.S. Vet. Lic. No.: 165A

Active Ingredient(s): M-NINEVAX®-C is a live bacterial vaccine containing the mild avirulent M-9 strain of *Pasteurella multocida*, Heddleston type 3-4 cross, in a freeze-dried preparation sealed under vacuum.

The seed culture used to make the vaccine has been laboratory tested for protection against challenge with the X-73 (type 1) strain of *P. multocida*.

Indications: For the vaccination of healthy breeder and layer chickens as an aid in the prevention of fowl cholera due to *P. multocida*.

Dosage and Administration:

When to Vaccinate: The vaccine is administered initially to chickens 10 to 12 weeks of age and must be repeated once at 18 to 20 weeks of age. There should be at least six (6) weeks and no more than 10 weeks between vaccinations.

Vaccination Program: The development of a durable, strong protection to this disease depends upon the use of an effective vaccination program as well as many other circumstances such as administration techniques, environment and flock health at the time of vaccination. Also, the immune response to one (1) vaccination under field conditions is seldom complete for all animals within a given flock. Even when vaccination is successful, the protection stimulated in individual animals against different diseases may not be life-long. Therefore, a program of revaccination may be necessary.

Preparation of the Vaccine:

1. Do not open and mix the vaccine until ready for use.
2. Mix only one (1) vial at a time and use the entire contents within two (2) hours.
3. Remove the tear-off aluminum seal and stopper from the vial containing the dried vaccine.
4. Remove the tear-off aluminum seal and stopper from the bottle containing the diluent.
5. Hold the diluent bottle firmly in an upright position and insert the shorter end of the transfer tube. Still holding the diluent bottle in an upright position, insert the neck of the vaccine vial over the longer end of the transfer tube. The vaccine vial should snap into position, connecting the two (2) vials securely.
6. Invert the two (2) containers so that the vaccine vial is on the bottom and allow the diluent to flow into the vaccine vial. If the diluent does not flow freely, squeeze the diluent bottle gently and the diluent will flow into the vaccine vial. The vaccine vial should be completely filled with diluent to prevent excess foaming.
7. Hold the joined containers by the ends and shake vigorously until the vaccine plug is completely dissolved.
8. Hold the joined containers so that the vaccine vial is on the bottom and the diluent bottle is on the top. Allow the rehydrated vaccine to flow into the vaccine vial. If the rehydrated vaccine does not flow into the vaccine vial, squeeze the diluent bottle gently and release to force the rehydrated vaccine into the vaccine vial. Be sure that all of the vaccine is removed from the diluent bottle.
9. Remove the diluent bottle and transfer tube from the neck of the vaccine vial.
10. The vaccine is now ready for use.

How to Vaccinate: Vaccination is accomplished by dipping the needle applicator into the mixed vaccine and piercing the webbed portion of the underside of the wing. Avoid piercing through feathers which may wipe off the vaccine, and avoid hitting the wing muscle or bone to minimize reaction. The applicator is designed to pick up the proper amount of vaccine on the needle, which is deposited in the tissues when the wing is pierced. Redip the applicator in the vaccine before each application. Excess vaccine adhering to the applicator should be removed by touching the applicator to the inside of the vial.

Reactions: Examination for Takes: Normally, no overall clinical reaction is observed. At 5-10 days following vaccination, a swelling of the skin (subcutaneous granuloma) will develop in the wing-web at the point of inoculation. The absence of this local reaction may mean that the birds were immune before vaccination or that improper vaccination methods were used. Examination for these takes may be used to ensure that the proper vaccination has been conducted. Protection will normally develop within 14 days after vaccination.

Records: Keep a record of the vaccine type, quantity, serial number, expiration date, and place

M

of purchase; the date and time of vaccination; the number, age, breed, and location of the birds; the names of operators performing the vaccination, and any observed reactions.

Contraindication(s): Initial vaccination in chickens over 12 weeks of age may be undesirable because larger granulomas may develop at the site of inoculation and this may result in the downgrading of carcasses at slaughter.

Precaution(s): Store at 35° to 45°F (2° to 7°C).

Caution(s): For veterinary use only.

1. Vaccinate healthy birds only. Although disease may not be evident, coccidiosis, chronic respiratory disease, mycoplasma infection, lymphoid leukosis, infectious bursal disease, Marek's disease, or other disease conditions may cause serious complications or reduce protection.
2. To avoid interference with the development of protection, the chickens to be vaccinated should not be given any antibiotic and/or sulfonamide medication used in the prevention or treatment of fowl cholera for three days before and five days after vaccination.
3. All birds within a flock should be vaccinated on the same day. Isolate other susceptible birds on the premises from the birds being vaccinated.
4. In outbreak situations, vaccinate healthy birds first, progressing toward outbreak areas in order to vaccinate diseased birds last.
5. Do not spill or spatter the vaccine. Use the entire contents of the vial when first opened. Burn the empty bottles, caps and all unused vaccine and accessories.
6. Avoid contact of open wounds or inoculation of vaccinating personnel with the vaccine since this might cause a bacterial infection. If this occurs, consult a physician immediately to obtain proper treatment. The vaccine organism, as with any *P. multocida* stain, may accidently act as a human pathogen and precautions should be taken to avoid exposure.
7. Wash hands thoroughly after using the vaccine.
8. Do not dilute the vaccine or otherwise stretch the dosage.

Warning(s): Do not vaccinate within 21 days before slaughter.

Presentation: Supplied in 10 x 1,000 dose units with diluent and wing-web stabbers.

Compendium Code No.: 10471250

MOMETAMAX™ OTIC SUSPENSION ℞

Schering-Plough **Otic Antibiotic-Anti-Inflammatory-Antifungal (Gentamicin Sulfate, USP; Mometasone Furoate Monohydrate; and Clotrimazole, USP, Otic Suspension)-Veterinary**

NADA No.: 141-177

Active Ingredient(s): Description: Each gram of MOMETAMAX™ Otic Suspension contains gentamicin sulfate, USP equivalent to 3 mg gentamicin base; mometasone furoate monohydrate equivalent to 1 mg mometasone; and 10 mg clotrimazole, USP in a mineral oil-based system containing a plasticized hydrocarbon gel.

Indications: MOMETAMAX™ Otic Suspension is indicated for the treatment of canine otitis externa associated with yeast *(Malassezia pachydermatis)* and/or bacteria susceptible to gentamicin in dogs.

Pharmacology:

Gentamicin: Gentamicin sulfate is an aminoglycoside antibiotic active against a wide variety of gram-negative and gram-positive bacteria. *In vitro* tests have determined that gentamicin is bactericidal and acts by inhibiting normal protein synthesis in susceptible microorganisms. In clinical trials, gentamicin was shown to have a range of activity against the following organisms commonly isolated from infected canine ears: *Staphylococcus intermedius, Staphylococcus aureus,* other *Staphylococcus* spp., *Pseudomonas aeruginosa, Proteus* spp., and *Escherichia coli.*

Mometasone: Mometasone furoate monohydrate is a synthetic adrenocorticoid characterized by a novel (2') furoate 17-ester having chlorine at the 9 and 21 positions, which have shown to possess high topical potency.

Systemic absorption of mometasone furoate ointment was found to be minimal (2%) over 1 week when applied topically to dogs with intact skin. In a 6-month dermal toxicity study using 0.1% mometasone ointment on healthy intact skin in dogs, systemic effects typical of corticosteroid therapy were noted.

The extent of percutaneous absorption of topical corticosteroids is determined by many factors including the integrity of the epidermal barrier. Topical corticosteroids can be absorbed from normal, intact skin. Inflammation can increase percutaneous absorption. Once absorbed through the skin, topical corticosteroids are handled through pharmacokinetic pathways similar to systemically administered corticosteroids.

Clotrimazole: Clotrimazole is a broad-spectrum antifungal agent that is used for the treatment of dermal infections caused by various species of dermatophytes and yeast. The primary action of clotrimazole is against dividing and growing organisms.

In vitro, clotrimazole exhibits fungistatic and fungicidal activity against isolates of *Trichophyton rubrum, Trichophyton mentagrophytes, Epidermophyton floccosum, Microsporum canis, Candida* spp., and *Malassezia pachydermatis.* Resistance to clotrimazole is very rare among the fungi that cause superficial mycoses. In an induced otitis externa study using dogs infected with *Malassezia pachydermatis,* 1% clotrimazole in the vehicle formulation was effective both microbiologically and clinically in terms of reduction of exudate, odor, and swelling.

In studies of the mechanism of action, the minimum fungicidal concentration of clotrimazole caused leakage of intracellular phosphorus compounds into the ambient medium with concomitant breakdown of cellular nucleic acids and accelerated potassium efflux. These events began rapidly and extensively after addition of the drug. Clotrimazole is very poorly absorbed following dermal application.

Gentamicin-Mometasone-Clotrimazole: By virtue of its three active ingredients, MOMETAMAX™ Otic Suspension has antibacterial, anti-inflammatory, and antifungal activity. In a clinical field trial, MOMETAMAX™ Otic Suspension was effective in the treatment of otitis externa associated with bacteria and *Malassezia pachydermatis.* MOMETAMAX™ Otic Suspension reduced discomfort, redness, swelling, exudate, and odor.

Dosage and Administration: The external ear canal should be thoroughly cleaned and dried before treatment. Verify that the eardrum is intact. For dogs weighing less than 30 lbs, instill 4 drops from the 15 g and 30 g bottles (2 drops from the 215 g bottle) of MOMETAMAX™ Otic Suspension twice daily into the ear canal. For dogs weighing 30 lbs or more, instill 8 drops from the 15 g and 30 g bottles (4 drops from the 215 g bottle) twice daily into the ear canal. Therapy should continue for 7 consecutive days.

Contraindication(s): If hypersensitivity to any of the components occurs, treatment should be discontinued and appropriate therapy instituted. Concomitant use of drugs known to induce ototoxicity should be avoided. Do not use in dogs with known perforation of eardrums.

Precaution(s): Store between 2° and 25°C (36° and 77°F). Shake well before use.

Caution(s): Federal law restricts this drug to use by or on the order of a licensed veterinarian.

Keep this and all drugs out of the reach of children.

Before instilling any medication into the ear, examine the external ear canal thoroughly to be certain the tympanic membrane is not ruptured in order to avoid the possibility of transmitting infection to the middle ear as well as damaging the cochlea or vestibular apparatus from prolonged contact.

Administration of recommended doses of MOMETAMAX™ Otic Suspension beyond 7 days may result in delayed wound healing.

If overgrowth of nonsusceptible bacteria or fungi occurs, treatment should be discontinued and appropriate therapy instituted.

Avoid ingestion. Adverse systemic reactions have been observed following the oral ingestion of some topical corticosteroid preparations. Patients should be closely observed for the usual signs of adrenocorticoid overdosage which include sodium retention, potassium loss, fluid retention, weight gain, polydipsia, and/or polyuria. Prolonged use or overdosage may produce adverse immunosuppressive effects.

Use of corticosteroids, depending on dose, duration, and specific steroid, may result in endogenous steroid production inhibition following drug withdrawal. In patients presently receiving or recently withdrawn from corticosteroid treatments, therapy with a rapidly acting corticosteroid should be considered in especially stressful situations.

For otic use in dogs only.

Warning(s): The use of these components has been associated with deafness or partial hearing loss in a small number of sensitive dogs (e.g. geriatric). The hearing deficit is usually temporary. If hearing or vestibular dysfunction is noted during the course of treatment, discontinue use of MOMETAMAX™ Otic Suspension immediately and flush the ear canal thoroughly with a non-ototoxic solution.

Corticosteroids administered to dogs, rabbits, and rodents during pregnancy have resulted in cleft palate in offspring. Other congenital anomalies including deformed forelegs, phocomelia, and anasarca have been reported in offspring of dogs that received corticosteroids during pregnancy.

Clinical and experimental data have demonstrated that corticosteroids administered orally or parenterally to animals may induce the first stage of parturition if used during the last trimester of pregnancy and may precipitate premature parturition followed by dystocia, fetal death, retained placenta, and metritis.

Toxicology: Clinical and safety studies with MOMETAMAX™ Otic Suspension have shown a wide safety margin at the recommended dose level in dogs (see Cautions/Adverse Reactions).

Adverse Reactions:

Gentamicin: While aminoglycosides are absorbed poorly from skin, intoxication may occur when aminoglycosides are applied topically for prolonged periods of time to large wounds, burns, or any denuded skin, particularly if there is renal insufficiency. All aminoglycosides have the potential to produce reversible and irreversible vestibular, cochlear, and renal toxicity.

Mometasone: ALP (SAP) and ALT (SGPT) enzyme elevations, weight loss, anorexia, polydipsia, polyuria, neutrophilia, and lymphopenia have occurred following the use of parenteral, high-dose and/or prolonged or systemic synthetic corticosteroids in dogs. Cushing's syndrome in dogs has been reported in association with prolonged or repeated steroid therapy.

Clotrimazole: The following have been reported occasionally in humans in connection with the use of clotrimazole: erythema, stinging, blistering, peeling, edema, pruritus, urticaria, and general irritation of the skin not present before therapy.

MOMETAMAX™ Otic Suspension: In a clinical field trial following treatment with MOMETAMAX™ Otic Suspension, inflammation of the pinna and diarrhea were observed in less than 1% of 141 dogs.

Presentation: MOMETAMAX™ Otic Suspension is available in 12 x 15 g (NDC 0061-1246-04), 6 x 30 g (NDC 0061-1246-01), and 1 x 215 g (NDC 0061-1246-02) plastic bottles.

Compendium Code No.: 10472121 23873605

MO' MILK® FEED MIX AND TOP DRESS

TechMix **Laxative**

Active Ingredient(s): Guaranteed Analysis:

Calcium (Ca), not more than	2.000%
Calcium (Ca), not less than	1.000%
Phosphorus (P), not less than	0.800%
Salt (NaCl)	None added
Iodine (I), not less than	0.025%
Iron (Fe), not less than	1.500%
Vitamin A, not less than	100,000 I.U./lb.
Vitamin D_3, not less than	50,000 I.U./lb.
Vitamin E, not less than	100 I.U./lb.

Ingredients: Blood albumin, ground psyllium seed and husks, potassium chloride, dried whey, condensed fish solubles, glycine, sodium bicarbonate, potassium sulfate, magnesium sulfate, dicalcium phosphate, monocalcium phosphate, monosodium phosphate, calcium carbonate, sodium sulfate, dried streptomyces fermentation product, corn distiller's dried grains with solubles, yeast culture, brewer's dried yeast, l-Lysine monohydrochloride, sodium silico aluminate (anti-caking agent), iron oxide, zinc oxide, manganese sulfate, magnesium oxide, copper sulfate, copper oxide, ethylene diamine dihydriodide, cobalt carbonate, d-methionine, iron (ferrous), sulfate monohydrate, zinc methionine, ferric methionine, vitamin A acetate (stability improved), d-activated animal sterol (source of vitamin D_3), dl-alpha tocopheryl acetate (source of vitamin E activity), choline chloride, niacin, d-calcium pantothenate, riboflavin supplement, vitamin B_{12} supplement, thiamine mononitrate, folic acid, menadione sodium bisulfite complex (source of vitamin K activity), pyridoxine hydrochloride, ascorbic acid (vitamin C), d-biotin, artificial flavor added, and ethoxyquin (a preservative).

Indications: MO' MILK® Feed Mix and MO' MILK® Top Dress are designed for use at farrowing time to help alleviate problems of constipation with specific ingredients that provide a safe laxative action. These ingredients produce a soothing, mucilaginous, stool-softening action that helps facilitate normal elimination and bowel movements.

Dosage and Administration:

MO' MILK® Feed Mix Feeding Directions: Start feeding MO' MILK® at about 14-21 days prior to farrowing until pigs are 7-10 days of age, or whenever signs of constipation appear in the pregnant sow or gilt. Mix one (1) bag of MO' MILK® Feed Mix (8 lbs. or 3.63 kg) to each ton of complete ration, or one (1) pound of MO' MILK® Feed Mix to each 250 lbs. of complete ration. Maintain MO' MILK® in the gestating-farrowing-lactation ration until pigs are weaned.

MO' MILK® Top Dress Feeding Directions: Feed MO' MILK® Top Dress as follows:

1. Feed MO' MILK® Top Dress to all gilts and sows on the first feeding when gilts and sows are moved into the farrowing crates, pens, or stalls.
2. For sows-gilts showing signs of constipation, top dress one (1) scoopful (approximately 4 oz.) on top of the gestation-farrowing ration. Continue feeding MO' MILK® Top Dress at this rate on each feeding until stools return to the desired consistency.
3. To help stimulate feed intake in sows or gilts that are constipated, off feed, or eating less than the normal amount expected, mix MO' MILK® Top Dress with one (1) quart of warm water or milk. Shake or stir well and pour the suspension of MO' MILK® Top Dress over the

M

feed in a trough or bowl and continue feeding MO' MILK® Top Dress for an additional three (3) to four (4) days.

Discussion: One of the primary causes of agalactia and lactation failure is intestinal stasis or constipation. Many sows and gilts encounter this problem in the farrowing crate due to lack of exercise, poor appetite, and changes of environment-management. Sows or gilts that are constipated for a significant period of time have poorer digestion and feed utilization. Lactating animals in this condition frequently develop hypoglycemia (reduced blood sugar) and depressed milk flow. Inadequate levels of blood sugar impede and disrupt normal milk production thereby causing nursing piglets to suffer from inadequate nutrition. Sows or gilts in this condition frequently develop excess udder edema (caking).

The active ingredients in MO' MILK® Feed Mix and MO' MILK® Top Dress provide mucilaginous lubricating action in the digestive tract that facilitates normal bowel movement without dehydrating the sow or gilt. This lubricating action can be demonstrated by mixing two tablespoons of MO' MILK® Top Dress with several ounces of water in a small glass. Within minutes, the MO' MILK® Top Dress will form an oily-slippery, lubricating film on the walls of the glass just as it does on the lining of the digestive tract when it comes in contact with liquid ingesta. This action helps produce a soft, oil stool in the sow or gilt to help facilitate normal elimination without creating a severe, watery stool than can lead to dehydration. MO' MILK® Feed Mix, in addition to its natural laxative action, also provides electrolyte, vitamin and trace mineral fortification to help assure adequate intake of essential nutrients at farrowing.

Presentation: MO' MILK® Feed Mix: 6x8 lb. (3.63 kg) (48 lb. case) and 40 lb. (18.18 kg) bags.
MO' MILK® Top Dress: 12x2 lb. (0.90 kg) bags (24 lb. pail) and 25 lb. (11.30 kg) pails.

Compendium Code No.: 11440100

MONARCH® MON-O-DINE

Ecolab Food & Bev. Div. **Udder Wash**

Active Ingredient(s):
Alpha (para-nonylphenyl) omega-hydroxpoly (oxyethylene) iodine complex 18.75%
(Providing 1.75% titratable iodine.)
Phosphoric acid 8.0%
Inert ingredients 73.25%

Indications: A detergent sanitizer for use in the dairy food industry.

Dosage and Administration: Mon-O-Dine is a concentrated product. Must be diluted before using.

Sanitizing with Mon-O-Dine: To sanitize previously cleaned equipment and utensils, dip, brush, or spray the equipment with a solution of Mon-O-Dine at 1 oz. of Mon-O-Dine to four (4) gallons of water. Provides 25 ppm titratable iodine. Allow at least a two (2) minute contact time. Allow the equipment to drain well but do not rinse. When used at levels not exceeding 25 ppm titratable iodine, Mon-O-Dine does not require a potable water rinse.

Udder washing with Mon-O-Dine: Approximately one (1) minute before applying the milking unit, wash and massage the teats with a clean paper towel wetted with a solution of Mon-O-Dine at ½ oz. to two (2) gallons of water at 110°F. Provides 25 ppm titratable iodine. Never reuse towels or dip a used towel back into the solution. Always use freshly prepared solutions and non-corrodible utensils.

For general cleaning and disinfecting in one (1) operation, use 3 oz. Mon-O-Dine to four (4) gallons of water. For porous or extremely dirty surfaces, use 6 oz. to four (4) gallons of water. Food contact surfaces should be rinsed with potable water whenever the use rate exceeds 1 oz. to four (4) gallons water.

Precaution(s): Keep from freezing.

Caution(s): Danger. Corrosive - Causes eye damage and skin irritation. Keep out of the reach of children.

M

First Aid: Do not get in eyes, on skin or on clothing. Protect the eyes and skin when handling. Harmful if swallowed. Avoid the contamination of food.

In case of contact, immediately flush the eyes or skin with plenty of water for at least 15 minutes. For eyes, call a physician. Remove and wash contaminated clothing before reuse.

If swallowed, promptly drink a large quantity of milk, egg whites, gelatin solution or if these are not available, drink large quantities of water. Call a physician immediately.

Note to physician: Probable mucosal damage may contraindicate the use of gastric lavage. Measures against circulatory shock, respiratory depression and convulsion may be needed. Rinse the empty container thoroughly with water and discard it.

Warning(s): The manufacturer's only obligation shall be to replace or pay for any material proved defective. Beyond the purchase price of materials supplied by the manufacturer we assume no liability for damages of any kind and the user accepts the products "as is" and without warranties, express or implied. The suitability of the product for an intended use shall be solely up to the user.

Presentation: 4 x 1 gallon case, 5 gallon pail, and 15 gallon drum.

Compendium Code No.: 14490071

MONARCH® PREP UDDER WASH

Ecolab Food & Bev. Div. **Udder Wash**

Active Ingredient(s):
Chlorhexidine acetate 1.20%
Inert ingredients 98.80%
Total 100.00%

Indications: Udder wash.

Dosage and Administration: PREP UDDER WASH is a concentrated product and must be diluted before using.

1. Prepare the udder wash solution in a plastic pail using 1 oz. of PREP UDDER WASH in each two and one-half (2½) imp. gallons of 110°-115°F warm water, or ½ oz. to each one and one-quarter (1¼) imp. gallons. PREP UDDER WASH may also be applied as a spray by using an in-line proportioner to meter the proper amount of udder wash into the spray.
2. Approximately one (1) minute before applying the milking unit, wash and massage the teats with a clean paper towel wet with the udder wash solution.
3. Discard the used towel. Do not reuse towels or dip the used towels back into the udder wash solution.

Precaution(s): Keep from freezing. If frozen, thaw completely and shake well before using.

Caution(s): For veterinary use only.
Causes eye damage and skin irritation. Keep out of the reach of children.
May be harmful if swallowed.
Contains chlorhexidine acetate.
Avoid contact with the eyes. In case of eye contact flush eyes immediately with water.
Contact a physician. If swallowed, drink milk or water and get medical attention.
Do not use for cleaning and/or sanitizing milk equipment.

Presentation: 4 x 1 gallon and 5 gallon.

Compendium Code No.: 14490081

MONARCH® PROTEK® SPRAY

Ecolab Food & Bev. Div. **Teat Dip**

Active Ingredient(s):
Chlorhexidine acetate 0.5%

Indications: The product is formulated to be used full strength as a post-milking teat dip to aid in the prevention of the spread of mastitis causing organisms.

Dosage and Administration: Immediately after each cow is milked, dip the teats in undiluted MONARCH® PROTEK® Spray. When the cow is being dried off, the teats should be dipped once a day for several days after last milking. With freshening cows, begin dipping teats twice a day for about 10 days before calving.

Precaution(s): Keep from freezing. If frozen, thaw completely and shake well before using.

Caution(s): If swallowed, may cause slight irritation.
Do not induce vomiting, contact a physician.
Avoid contact with the eyes. If accidental contact should occur, flush with water.
Contact a physician.
Consult the Material Safety Data Sheet for additional information.
Keep out of the reach of children. Do not use for cleaning and/or sanitizing milk equipment.

Presentation: 4 x 1 gallon, 5 gallon, 15 gallon, and 55 gallon.

Compendium Code No.: 14490091

MONARCH® PROTEK® TEAT DIP

Ecolab Food & Bev. Div. **Teat Dip**

Active Ingredient(s): Chlorhexidine acetate 0.5% with polyvinylpyrridone and glycerin 3.0% in an aqueous base.

Indications: The product is formulated to be used full strength as a post-milking teat dip to aid in the prevention of the spread of mastitis causing organisms.

Dosage and Administration: Immediately after each cow is milked, dip the teat in undiluted MONARCH® PROTEK® Teat Dip. Replace the solution if it becomes visibly dirty. When the cow is being dried off, the teats should be dipped once a day for several days after the last milking. With freshening cows, begin dipping teats twice a day for about 10 days before calving. Using an approved udder wash and a single service clean towel, thoroughly wash udder and teats of treated cows before milking to avoid the contamination of milk.

Precaution(s): Keep from freezing.

Caution(s): Do not use for cleaning and/or sanitizing milk equipment.
For veterinary use only. Keep out of the reach of children.
Eye irritant, may be harmful if swallowed. Contains chlorhexidine acetate.
Avoid contact with the eyes. In case of eye contact flush eyes immediately with water.
Contact a physician. If swallowed, drink milk or water and get medical attention.

Presentation: 4 x 1 gallon case, 5 gallon pail, 15 gallon drum, and 55 gallon drum.

Compendium Code No.: 14490101

MONARCH® SUPER KABON®

Ecolab Food & Bev. Div. **Udder Wash**

EPA Reg. No.: 4524-24

Active Ingredient(s):
N-Alkyl (50% C_{14}, 40% C_{12}, 10% C_{16}) dimethylbenzyl ammonium chloride 10.0%
Ethanol 2.5%
Inert ingredients:
Water 87.5%
Total 100.0%

Indications:
In the milk house: For milking machines, inflations, pipeline milkers, cream separators, farm bulk tanks, dipping teat cups, etc.
In the dairy barn: As an udder wash.
In farrowing houses, etc.: To wash floors, walls, etc.

Dosage and Administration:
For the dairy farm: Sanitizing with SUPER KABON®:
In the milk house: For milking machines, inflations, pipeline milkers, cream separators, farm bulk tanks, dipping teat cups, etc.
1. Flush all traces of detergent from equipment.
2. Sanitize by immersion or recirculation with SUPER KABON® solution containing 1 oz. SUPER KABON® to 13 qts. of water (provides over 200 ppm quaternary).
3. Drain, allow to dry.
4. Store according to the recommendations of the local health authorities.

In the dairy barn: For use as an udder wash.
1. Add 1 oz. SUPER KABON® to 13 qts. of 130°F water.
2. One (1) minute before milking wash the udders and flanks with a towel which has been dipped into the above solution.
3. Use an individual cloth, or paper towel for each cow.

In farrowing houses, etc. - Wash floors, walls, etc. with solution containing 1 oz. SUPER KABON® per 4 qts. of hot water. SUPER KABON® may be added to lye solutions to improve their germicidal properties.

Directions for Dilution:
Stir 1 oz. SUPER KABON® 10% into 13 qts. water = 200 ppm solution (1:5,000).

Caution(s): SUPER KABON® is a potent germicide and should be diluted before using as directed. SUPER KABON® solution must not come in contact with foods. SUPER KABON® solutions should not be used with soap or anionic detergents.
Note: Have all surfaces cleaned and rinsed before using germicide.
Keep out of the reach of children.

Presentation: 4 x 1 gallon.

Compendium Code No.: 14490111

MONTEBAN® 45

Elanco **Feed Medication**

Narasin-Type A Medicated Article

NADA No.: 118-980

Active Ingredient(s):
Narasin .... 45 g/lb.
Verxite (non-nutritive) 1-2%

Indications: For the prevention of coccidiosis caused by *Eimeria necatrix, E. tenella, E. acervulina, E. brunetti, E. mivati,* and *E. maxima.*

Directions: Important: Must be thoroughly mixed into feeds before use.

Mixing Directions—Thoroughly mix the following amounts of MONTEBAN® to provide 54 through 72 g of narasin in one ton of feed. The dosage should be adjusted to meet the severity of the coccidial challenge, which varies with environmental and management conditions.

It is recommended that a preblend of MONTEBAN® in 15-20 lbs of feed be made before incorporating into the total amount of the finished feed.

Narasin (Grams/Ton)	MONTEBAN® 45 (Lbs/Ton of Type C Feed)
	Lbs
54	1.20
59	1.31
63	1.40
68	1.51
72	1.60

Feeding Directions—Feed continuously as the only ration.

Do not feed undiluted.

Precaution(s): Store in a cool, dry place.

Not to be used after the date printed on top of bag.

When mixing and handling MONTEBAN®, use protective clothing, impervious gloves, and a dust mask. Operators should wash thoroughly with soap and water after handling. If accidental eye contact occurs, immediately rinse thoroughly with water.

Caution(s): Do not allow adult turkeys, horses, or other equines access to formulations containing MONTEBAN®. Ingestion of MONTEBAN® by these species has been fatal.

For use in broiler chicken feeds only.

Presentation: 50 lb (22.68 kg) bags.

Compendium Code No.: 10310061 BG 1500 AMB

MOORMAN'S® BEEF CATTLE BOOST® BT

ADM **Feed Medication**

Type B Medicated Feed

Active Ingredient(s):

Lasalocid . . . . 400 grams per ton (200 milligrams per pound)

Guaranteed Analysis:

Crude Protein, not less than 40.0%

(This includes not more than 4.0% equivalent crude protein from non-protein nitrogen.)

Crude Fat, not less than 0.5%

Crude Fiber, not more than 9.5%

Calcium (Ca), not less than 1.7%

Calcium (Ca), not more than 2.2%

Phosphorus (P), not less than 1.0%

Salt (NaCl), not less than 1.3%

Salt (NaCl), not more than 1.8%

Potassium (K), not less than 1.3%

Vitamin A, not less than . . . . 120,000 IU/lb

Ingredients: Dehulled Soybean Meal, Soybean Feed, Wheat Middlings, Cottonseed Meal, Calcium Carbonate, Monocalcium Phosphate, Dicalcium Phosphate, Salt, Urea, Animal Fat, BHT (A Preservative), Corn Gluten Feed, Calcium Sulfate, Cane Molasses, Vitamin E Supplement, Manganous Oxide, Zinc Oxide, Copper Sulfate, Vitamin A Acetate, Magnesium Oxide, Defluorinated Phosphate, Linseed Meal, Ferrous Sulfate, Mineral Oil, Potassium Sulfate, Potassium Iodide, Sodium Selenite, Cobalt Carbonate, D-Activated Animal Sterol (Source of Vitamin D_3).

Indications: For improved feed efficiency in beef cattle fed in confinement for slaughter.

Directions: Instructions for Mixing and Feeding: Start cattle on MOORMAN'S® BEEF CATTLE BOOST® BT by feeding 1 lb per head per day of this product thoroughly mixed with grain or grain-roughage mixtures before feeding. When starting cattle on grain, roughage must be fed either free-choice or mixed in the ration. Feed 1 lb of this product with not less than 5 lb of grain and a minimum of 8 lb roughage per head per day for the first 4 to 7 days to provide no more than 30 gram lasalocid per ton of final ration. After cattle are eating well, gradually increase the amount of grain mixed with 1 lb/hd/day of this product until the desired level of grain intake is reached. Adjust roughage to the desired level. The amount of grain-roughage mixture fed must equal a minimum of 13 lb per head per day. Feed continuously. This product is designed to be fed at the rate of 1 lb per head per day. Do not feed more than 1 lb of this product per head per day. Provide sufficient bunk space so all cattle can eat at one time.

Drug Level: When fed at the rate of 1 lb per head per day, this product provides 200 mg lasalocid. The complete ration should contain from 10 to 30 grams per ton of lasalocid.

Caution(s): Consumption of this product by sheep and goats may result in copper toxicity. The safety of lasalocid in unapproved species has not been established. Do not allow horses or other equines access to formulations containing lasalocid as ingestion may be fatal. Feeding undiluted or mixing errors resulting in excessive concentrations of lasalocid could be fatal to cattle.

Warning(s): This feed should be used only in accordance with instructions furnished on the label. A withdrawal period has not been established for this product in pre-ruminating cattle. Do not use in calves to be processed for veal.

Do not feed to lactating dairy cows.

Presentation: Available in bulk and 50 lb bags.

Compendium Code No.: 10410181

MOORMAN'S® BMD® 30

ADM **Feed Medication**

Type A Medicated Article

NADA No.: 046-592

Active Ingredient(s):

Bacitracin methylene disalicylate . . . . 30 g bacitracin per lb. (master standard)

A dried precipitated fermentation product obtained by culturing *B. licheniformis* Tracy on media adapted for microbiological production of bacitracin; calcium carbonate.

Indications: For use in medicating swine, broiler chickens, growing turkeys, pheasants, quail and feedlot beef cattle rations.

Swine: For increased weight gain and improved feed efficiency. For control of swine dysentery associated with *Treponema hyodysenteriae.*

Broiler chickens: For increased weight gain and improved feed efficiency. For use as an aid in the prevention of necrotic enteritis caused or complicated by *Clostridium spp.* or organisms susceptible to bacitracin. For use as an aid in the control of necrotic enteritis caused or complicated by *Clostridium spp.* or organisms susceptible to bacitracin.

Growing Turkeys: For increased rate of weight gain and improved feed efficiency. For use as an aid in the control of transmissible enteritis in growing turkeys complicated by organisms susceptible to bacitracin methylene disalicylate.

Pheasants: For increased rate of weight gain and improved feed efficiency.

Quail: For increased rate of weight gain and improved feed efficiency in birds up to five weeks of age. For the prevention of ulcerative enteritis in growing quail due to *Clostridium colinum* susceptible to bacitracin methylene disalicylate.

Feedlot beef cattle: For the reduction in the number of liver condemnations due to abscesses.

Dosage and Administration: Thoroughly mix sufficient MOORMAN'S® BMD® 30 with nonmedicated feed to supply the desired level of antibiotic. Make a preblend by mixing the proper amount of MOORMAN'S® BMD® 30 with part of the feed ingredients. Mix the preblend with the remaining ingredients to give the desired level of medication per ton. BMD™ 30 contains 30 g (30,000 mg) bacitracin per lb. The amount of product needed varies with the desired purpose according to the following:

For medicating complete feed:

The following information gives the purpose, required amount of bacitracin and the amount of MOORMAN'S® BMD® 30 needed to medicate one (1) ton of complete feed.

Swine:

For increased weight gain and improved feed efficiency: Add 0.33 to 1.0 lbs. BMD® 30 to one (1) ton of complete feed. This will give 10 to 30 g per ton of bacitracin.

For the control of swine dysentery associated with *Treponema hyodysenteriae*: Feed 250 g per ton of complete feed on premises with a history of swine dysentery but where signs of the disease have not yet occurred or following an approved treatment of the disease condition.

Feed containing an approved level of bacitracin methylene disalicylate should be fed as the sole ration. The 250 g/ton level will provide 5 to 7 mg/lb. in swine weighing 40 to 250 lbs. Add 8.33 lbs. BMD® 30 to one (1) ton of complete feed. This will give 250 g per ton of bacitracin.

Broiler chickens:

For increased weight gain and improved feed efficiency: Add 0.13 to 1.67 BMD® 30 to one (1) ton of complete feed. This will give 4 to 50 g per ton of bacitracin.

For use as an aid in the prevention of necrotic enteritis caused or complicated by *Clostridium* spp., or organisms susceptible to bacitracin: Add 1.67 lbs. BMD® 30 to one (1) ton of complete feed. This will give 50 g per ton of bacitracin.

For use as an aid in the control of necrotic enteritis caused or complicated by *Clostridium* spp., or organisms susceptible to bacitracin: Add 3.33 to 6.67 lbs. BMD® 30 to one (1) ton of complete feed. This will give 100 to 200 g per ton of bacitracin.

To control a necrotic enteritis outbreak, start medication at the first clinical signs of disease. The dosage range permitted provides for different levels based on the severity of the infection. Consult a poultry diagnostic laboratory or pathologist to determine the diagnosis and advice regarding the optimal level of drug. Administer continuously for five (5) to seven (7) days or as long as clinical signs persist, and then reduce the medication to the prevention level (50 g/ton).

Growing turkeys:

For increased rate of weight gain and improved feed efficiency: Add 0.13 to 1.67 lbs. BMD® 30 to one (1) ton complete feed. This will give 4 to 50 g per ton of bacitracin.

For use as an aid in control of transmissible enteritis in growing turkeys complicated by organisms susceptible to bacitracin methylene disalicylate: Add 6.67 lbs. BMD® 30 to one (1) ton of complete feed. This will give 200 g per ton of bacitracin.

Pheasants:

For increased rate of weight gain and improved feed efficiency: Add 0.13 to 1.67 lbs. BMD® 30 to one (1) ton of complete feed. This will give 4 to 50 g per ton bacitracin.

Quail:

For increased rate of weight gain and improved feed efficiency in birds up to five (5) weeks of age: Add 0.167 to 0.67 lbs. BMD® 30 to one (1) ton of complete feed. This will give 5 to 20 g per ton bacitracin.

For the prevention of ulcerative enteritis in growing quail due to *Clostridium colinum* susceptible to bacitracin methylene disalicylate: Add 6.67 lbs. BMD® 30 to one (1) ton of complete feed. This will give 200 g per ton of bacitracin.

For medicating animals on per head per day basis:

The following information gives the purpose, daily dose of bacitracin and the amount of MOORMAN'S® BMD® 30 needed per ton, for one (1) pound per head per day medicated mix.

Feedlot beef cattle:

For a reduction in the number of liver condemnations due to abscesses: Add 4.67 lbs. BMD® 30 to one (1) ton of complete feed. This will give 70 mg bacitracin to feed per head per day on a continuous feed; or add 16.67 lbs. BMD® 30 to one (1) ton of complete feed. This will give 250 mg bacitracin per head daily for five (5) days. Then do not feed BMD® 30 for 25 subsequent days. Repeat the pattern during the feeding period.

Caution(s): Swine: The diagnosis should be confirmed by a veterinarian when results are not satisfactory. Not for use in swine weighing more than 250 lbs.

Presentation: 50 lb bags.

* BMD is a registered trademark of Alpharma Inc.

Compendium Code No.: 10410012

MOORMAN'S® CBX

ADM **Feed Medication**

Type B Medicated Feed

NADA No.: 041-061

Active Ingredient(s):

Carbadox (Mecadox®). . . . . 0.55% (2.5 g per lb.)

Ingredients: Rice hulls, ground corn, calcium carbonate, mineral oil, sodium propionate (a preservative).

Indications: For the control of swine dysentery (vibrionic dysentery, bloody scours or hemorrhagic dysentery), control of bacterial swine enteritis (salmonellosis or necrotic enteritis caused by *Salmonella choleraesuis,* increase rate of weight gain and improved feed efficiency.

Dosage and Administration: Thoroughly mix 20 lbs. of MOORMAN'S® CBX with 1,980 lbs. of an approved ration recommended for the age of the pigs being fed to make one (1) ton of complete swine feed containing 50 g carbadox.

The resultant complete feed is to be fed continuously as the sole ration and may be fed up to 75 lbs. of body weight. Then switch to an approved swine ration for pigs of this weight.

Caution(s): Do not mix in feeds containing bentonite.

Warning(s): Do not feed to swine weighing more than 75 lbs. of body weight. Do not feed to swine within 10 weeks of slaughter. Do not mix in complete feeds containing less than 15% crude protein.

Presentation: 50 lb bags.

* Mecadox is Phibro Animal Health's trademark for carbadox.

Compendium Code No.: 10410051

MOORMAN'S® DUST WITH CO-RAL®* INSECTICIDE

ADM **Topical Insecticide**

EPA Reg. No.: 11556-14-1157

Active Ingredient(s):

0,0 diethyl 0-(3-chloro-4-methyl-2-oxo-(2H)-1-benzopyran-7-yl) phosphorothioate 1.0%
Inert ingredients 99.0%
Total 100.0%

Indications: For the control of horn flies and lice on beef and dairy cattle, and for the reduction of face flies on beef and dairy cattle.

Directions for Use: It is a violation of federal law to use the product in a manner inconsistent with its labeling.

DUST WITH CO-RAL®* Insecticide is to be used to fill cattle dust bags. When used as recommended, DUST WITH CO-RAL®* Insecticide controls horn flies and lice and reduces face flies on beef and dairy cattle.

Recommended Application: Control of horn flies and lice on beef and dairy cattle, reduction of face flies on beef and dairy cattle.

Dust bag: Place the contents of the package in any commercially available dust bag. Suspend bags in areas frequented by cattle or in gateways or lanes through which the animals pass daily for water, feed or minerals. The bags may also be suspended in loafing sheds or in front of protected mineral feeders. For lactating dairy cows, the bags may be suspended in the exit through which cows leave the milking barn. In all cases, the bags should be adjusted so that the bottom of the bag will hang four (4) to six (6) inches below the topline of the cattle. For the reduction of face flies, the bags must be located so that the animals will be forced to use them daily and hung at a height to ensure that the faces of the cattle will be dusted.

No interval is required between treatment and slaughter or between treatment and use of milk for food.

Use Restrictions: For external insecticidal use only on the above-specified animals. Do not contaminate feed, troughs, water, or water utensils. Provide thorough ventilation while dusting. Do not apply to sick, stressed or convalescent animals.

Precautionary Statements: Hazards to Humans and Domestic Animals: Harmful if swallowed, inhaled, or absorbed through the skin. Avoid inhaling dust. Avoid contact with the eyes, skin and clothing.

Practical Treatments:

If swallowed, call a physician or poison control center immediately. Drink one or two glasses of water and induce vomiting by touching the back of the throat with a finger. Repeat until the vomit fluid is clear. Do not induce vomiting or give anything by mouth to an unconscious person.

If inhaled, remove victim to fresh air. Apply artificial respiration if indicated. Get medical attention if the victim displays signs of poisoning.

If on skin, remove contaminated clothing and wash the affected areas with soap and water.

If in eyes, flush eyes with plenty of water. Call a physician immediately.

Note to Physician: Prolonged exposure will result in cholinesterase depression. Atropine sulfate is antidotal. 2-PAM is also antidotal and may be administered in conjunction with atropine.

Environmental Hazards: The product is toxic to fish, birds and other wildlife. Keep out of lakes, streams and ponds. Do not contaminate water by the cleaning of equipment or the disposal of wastes. Apply the product only as specified on the label.

Storage and Disposal: Do not contaminate water, food or feed by storage or disposal.

Storage: Store in a cool, dry place.

Pesticide Disposal: Wastes resulting from the use of the product may be disposed of on site or at an approved waste disposal facility.

M

Container Disposal: Completely empty the bag into the application equipment. Then dispose of the empty bag in a sanitary landfill or by incineration, or, if allowed by state and local authorities, by burning. If burned, stay out of smoke.

Warning(s): Keep out of the reach of children.

Disclaimer: Warranty and Limitation of Damages: Use only as directed.

Moorman Manufacturing Company warrants that this material conforms to the chemical description on the label and is reasonably fit for the purposes referred to in the Directions for Use and Restrictions, subject to the risks referred to therein. Moorman Manufacturing Company makes no other express or implied warranty, including any other express or implied warranty of fitness or of merchantability. Any damages arising from a breach of the warranty shall be limited to direct damages, and shall not include consequential commercial damages such as loss of profits or values, etc.

Presentation: 6¼ lb containers.

* CO-RAL is a registered trademark of the parent company of Farbenfabriken Bayer GmbH, Leverkusen.

Compendium Code No.: 10410061

MOORMAN'S® FLY SPRAY

ADM **Premise and Topical Insecticide**

EPA Reg. No.: 606-103-1157

Active Ingredient(s):

Pyrethrins 0.10%
Piperonyl butoxide technical* 1.00%
Refined petroleum distillates 98.90%
Total 100.00%

*Equivalent to 0.80% of (butylcarbityl) (6-propylpiperonyl) ether and 0.20% of related compounds.

Indications: For use on dairy cows, in dairy barns and on beef cattle and horses for the control of face flies, horn flies, stable flies, house flies, horse flies, mosquitoes and gnats.

Directions for Use: MOORMAN'S® Fly Spray is to be used full strength and should be applied to livestock as a mist spray only. Only efficient hand type spray guns or insecticide foggers should be used. A fine mist with considerable force is desirable. A coarse spray is wasteful and inefficient. Make sure that the sprayer is in perfect working condition.

On dairy cows and calves: Use the spray before milking or feeding. Do not contaminate milk or feed with the spray. For the greatest efficiency spray cows inside the barn with windows and doors closed during, and for 10 minutes after, spraying. Outside spraying and spraying open barns takes more spray to control flies.

Using a spray gun: Spray the cows from the rear holding the spray gun 15 to 20 inches away from the surface to be sprayed. At each spraying use 1-1.5 ounces for the average size cow (1 pint for each 12 to 16 head). Use proportionally less for calves and younger animals. In addition to covering the back and sides of the cows and calves, the spray mist goes into the air above the animals thus helping to kill the flies in the building. Spray the legs and under parts lightly. The hair should be dampened, not soaked. Allow the spray to settle before milking.

Using an insecticide fogger: Make sure that the fogger is located properly and operating satisfactorily. Follow the manufacturer's instructions as to the area the fogger will adequately handle. Locate the fogger high enough so that some cows are not overexposed and that their feed is not contaminated. Locate the fogger so the rear of the cows are exposed to the mist and the eyes are protected from direct spraying. Do not expose the cows to excessive fog which may produce bronchial troubles.

Close the windows and doors for the best fogging results. Usually five (5) minutes of fogging is sufficient.

Spray building liberally for better control: To obtain the most complete control of face flies, stable flies, house flies, horse flies, mosquitoes and gnats, MOORMAN'S® Fly Spray should be used on the animals and also in the barns or nearby sheds where insects may congregate. After closing the doors and windows, spray or fog liberally directing the spray toward the ceiling. Keep closed for 10 minutes after spraying.

Spraying beef cattle and horses: MOORMAN'S® Fly Spray may be used in the same way on beef cattle and horses and in other buildings for killing flies, mosquitoes and gnats.

Precautionary Statements: Keep out of the reach of children. Do not spray near or toward an open flame. Avoid the contamination of milk, milk utensils and feed. Harmful if swallowed.

Prevention Important: Effective control of flies requires the frequent removal of all manure, litter and other breeding places of flies.

Not for household use. To make the effect of MOORMAN'S® Fly Spray more lasting, an oil base is used. It is not recommended for household use.

Storage and Disposal: Do not contaminate water, food or feed by storage or disposal.

Storage: Do not store near heat or open flame. Store the container in the upright position. Store in the original container. Keep the container closed.

Pesticide Disposal: Wastes resulting from the use of the product may be disposed of on site or at an approved waste disposal facility.

Container Disposal: Triple rinse (or equivalent). Then offer for recycling or reconditioning, or puncture and dispose of in a sanitary landfill, or incineration, or, if allowed by state and local authorities, by burning. If burned, stay out of smoke.

Presentation: 2½ gallon containers.

Compendium Code No.: 10410072

MOORMAN'S® HI-MAG IGR MINERALS®

ADM **Feed Additive**

EPA Reg. No.: 1157-44

Active Ingredient(s):

S-methoprene (CAS Number 65733-16-6)* 0.02%
Other Ingredients: 99.98%
Total 100.00%

Guaranteed Analysis:

Calcium (Ca), not less than 9.2%
Calcium (Ca), not more than 11.0%
Phosphorus (P), not less than 6.0%
Salt (NaCl), not less than 13.4%
Salt (NaCl), not more than 16.0%
Magnesium (Mg), not less than 14.0%
Potassium (K), not less than 0.2%
Copper (Cu), not less than .... 1100 ppm
Selenium (Se), not less than .... 39 ppm
Zinc (Zn), not less than .... 3800 ppm
Vitamin A, not less than .... 200,000 IU/lb

Feed Ingredients: Magnesium Oxide, Monocalcium Phosphate, Dicalcium Phosphate, Salt, Defluorinated Phosphate, Soybean Meal, Calcium Carbonate, Petrolatum, Cane Molasses, Magnesium-Mica, Manganous Oxide, Calcium Sulfate, Iron Oxide, Brewer's Condensed Solubles, Zinc Oxide, Potassium Sulfate, Copper Sulfate, Dried Corn Syrup, Ferrous Sulfate, Vitamin A Acetate, Ethylenediamine Dihydriodide, Potassium Iodide, Sodium Selenite, Cobalt Carbonate, Mineral Oil, Cholecalciferol (Source of Vitamin D_3).

Indications: To prevent the breeding of horn flies in the manure of treated cattle only.

A pesticidally active mineral feed for beef and dairy cattle containing methoprene* insect growth regulator for continuous feeding during the fly season.

Directions for Use: It is a violation of Federal law to use this product in a manner inconsistent with its labeling.

This product only prevents emergence of adult horn flies from the manure of treated cattle. Begin use in the spring before horn flies appear on cattle and continue feeding until cold weather restricts horn fly activity. Introduction of the product when significant numbers of adult horn flies are present may require the use of adulticide sprays or dusts.

Free-Choice Feeding (self-feeding): Make sure cattle are not starved for minerals or salt by providing them before feeding MOORMAN'S® HI-MAG IGR MINERALS®. Then remove salt or mineral supplement and start continuous feeding of MOORMAN'S® HI-MAG IGR MINERALS®.

The recommended consumption of MOORMAN'S® HI-MAG IGR MINERALS® is 0.25 lb (¼ lb) to 0.5 lb (½ lb) per 100 lb of body weight per month. Place MOORMAN'S® HI-MAG IGR MINERALS® near watering or loafing areas and provide one feeder for each 15 to 20 head. Put out only a 5-7 day supply of MOORMAN'S® HI-MAG IGR MINERALS® at one time and protect it from rain.

If consumption of MOORMAN'S® HI-MAG IGR MINERALS® is above 0.5 lb (½ lb) per 100 lb of body weight per month, reduce the number of feeding stations or relocate feeders in areas frequented less by cattle.

If consumption of MOORMAN'S® HI-MAG IGR MINERALS® is below 0.25 lb (¼ lb) per 100 lb of body weight per month, increase the number of feeding stations or relocate feeders in areas more frequented by cattle.

Mixed Ration Feeding (hand-feeding): When cattle are on supplemental feeds or if mineral consumption is not as recommended, mix MOORMAN'S® HI-MAG IGR MINERALS® with other non-medicated feeds and feed daily to provide 0.25 lb (¼ lb) to 0.5 lb (½ lb) of MOORMAN'S® HI-MAG IGR MINERALS® per 100 lb of body weight per month.

Storage and Disposal: Do not contaminate water or food by storage or disposal.

Storage: Store in a dry area. Do not contaminate with pesticides or fertilizer.

Pesticide Disposal: Wastes resulting from the use of this product may be disposed of on site or at an approved waste disposal facility.

Container Disposal: Completely empty bag into application equipment. Then dispose of empty bag in a sanitary landfill or by incineration, or, if allowed by State and local authorities, by burning. If burned, stay out of smoke.

Warning(s): Keep out of reach of children.

Presentation: 50 lb (22.67 kg) bag.

*As the insect growth regulator Altosid® CP-10, a registered trademark of Wellmark International.

Compendium Code No.: 10410200

MOORMAN'S® IGR CATTLE CONCENTRATE

ADM **Feed Additive**

EPA Reg. No.: 1157-46

Active Ingredient(s):

Methoprene [isopropyl (E,E)-1,1-methoxy-3,7,11-trimethyl-2,4-dodecadienoate]* 0.40%
Inert ingredients 99.60%
Total 100.00%

Guaranteed Analysis:
Crude protein, not less than 35%
Crude fat, not less than 5%
Crude fiber, not more than 6%

Feed Ingredients: Soybean meal, dehulled soybean meal, corn distillers dried grains with solubles, corn gluten feed, mineral oil, cane molasses.

Indications: To prevent the breeding of horn flies in the manure of treated cattle.

A pesticidally active feed concentrate for cattle containing methoprene* insect growth regulator for continuous feeding during the fly season.

Directions for Use: It is a violation of federal law to use the product in a manner inconsistent with its labeling.

The product prevents emergence of adult horn flies from the manure of the treated cattle. Begin use in the spring before horn flies appear on cattle and continue feeding until the cold weather restricts horn fly activity. Introduction of the product when significant numbers of adult flies are present requires the use of adulticide sprays or dusts.

The dosage of MOORMAN'S® IGR Cattle Concentrate is proportional to body weight. The recommended consumption of the product is 0.0125 lbs. to 0.025 lbs. per 100 lbs. of body weight per month (30 days). Feed by either of the following methods.

Mixed with a free-choice-fed MoorMan® Cattle Minerals: Mix MOORMAN'S® IGR Cattle Concentrate with a free-choice-fed MoorMan® mineral to produce an IGR Cattle Concentrate and mineral mixture containing 0.02% active ingredient (methoprene) as shown in the following table:

IGR Cattle Concentrate .... 5 lbs. (5%)
Free-choice MoorMan® minerals .... 95 lbs. (95%)
Total .... 100 lbs. (100%)

Place the mixture of IGR Cattle Concentrate and minerals near watering or loafing areas and provide one (1) feeder for each 15 to 20 head. Put out only a five (5) to seven (7) day supply of the mixture at one time and protect it from the rain.

When the recommended mixture of IGR Cattle Concentrate and minerals is consumed at the rate of 0.25 lbs. to 0.5 lbs. per 100 lbs. of body weight per month, the mixture provides 0.0125 lbs. to 0.025 lbs. of IGR Cattle Concentrate per 100 lbs. of body weight per month.

Mixed-ration feeding: Thoroughly mix IGR Cattle Concentrate with grain or supplement to provide 0.0125 lbs. to 0.025 lbs. of IGR Cattle Concentrate per 100 lbs. of body weight per month.

Use the following table as a guide for determining the proper mixing rate:

	Daily Grain or Supplement Consumption (Lbs. of IGR Cattle Concentrate needed/ton of grain or suppl. feed)	
Body Weight (lbs.)	2-4	5-10
500	2.1	—
600	2.5	1.0
700	2.9	1.2
800	3.3	1.3
900	3.8	1.5
1,000	4.1	1.7
1,100	4.6	1.8
1,200	5.0	2.0
1,300	5.4	2.2
1,400	5.8	2.3
1,500	6.3	2.5
1,600	6.7	2.7

Storage and Disposal: Do not contaminate water or feed by storage or disposal.

Storage: Store in a dry area. Do not contaminate with pesticides or fertilizer.

Pesticide Disposal: Wastes resulting from the use of this product may be disposed of on site or at an approved waste disposal facility.

Container Disposal: Completely empty the bag by shaking it and tapping the sides and bottom to loosen clinging particles. Empty the residue into the application equipment. Then dispose of the empty bag in a sanitary landfill or by incineration, or, if allowed by state and local authorities, by burning. If burned, stay out of smoke.

Warning(s): Keep out of the reach of children.

Presentation: 25 lb bags.

* As the insect growth regulator Altosid®, a trademark of Wellmark International (U.S. Patents 3,904,662 and 3,912,815).

Compendium Code No.: 10410081

MOORMAN'S® IGR CATTLE MIX

ADM **Feed Additive**

EPA Reg. No.: 1157-45

Active Ingredient(s):

Methoprene [isopropyl (E,E)-1,1-methoxy-3,7,11-trimethyl-2,4-dodecadienoate]* 0.02%
Inert ingredients 99.98%
Total 100.00%

Guaranteed Analysis:
Crude protein, not less than 40.0%
Crude fat, not less than 1.5%
Crude fiber, not more than 8.0%

Feed Ingredients: Soybean meal, corn distillers dried grains with solubles, corn gluten feed, mineral oil, cane molasses.

Indications: To prevent the breeding of horn flies in the manure of treated cattle only.

A pesticidally active feed for cattle containing methoprene* insect growth regulator for continuous feeding during the fly season.

Directions for Use: It is a violation of federal law to use the product in a manner inconsistent with its labeling.

The product only prevents emergence of adult horn flies from the manure of the treated cattle. Begin use in the spring before horn flies appear on cattle and continue feeding until the cold weather restricts horn fly activity. Introduction of the product when significant numbers of adult flies are present requires the use of adulticide sprays or dusts.

The dosage of MOORMAN'S® IGR Cattle Mix is proportional to body weight. The recommended consumption of the product is 0.25 lbs. to 0.5 lbs. per 100 lbs. of body weight per month (30 days). Feed by either of the following methods:

Top-dress and hand-mix feeding: Top-dress or hand-mix with supplemental feeds to provide 0.25 lbs. to 0.5 lbs. of IGR Cattle Mix per 100 lbs. of body weight per month. When top-dress feeding IGR Cattle Mix, have sufficient bunk space to allow all of the animals to eat at the same time.

Use the following table as a guide for determining the daily feeding rate of IGR Cattle Mix:

	Amount of IGR Cattle Mix required/head/day	
Body Weight (lbs.)	By Weight	By Volume
500-699	1.2 oz. (0.075 lbs.)	¼ cup*
700-999	1.6 oz. (0.100 lbs.)	⅓ cup*
1,000-1,600	2.4 oz. (0.150 lbs.)	½ cup*

*Standard household measuring cup.

Mixed-ration feeding: Thoroughly mix IGR Cattle Mix with the daily grain or supplement to provide 0.25 lbs. to 0.5 lbs. of IGR Cattle Mix per 100 lbs. of body weight per month.

Use the following table as a guide for determining the proper mixing rate:

	Daily Grain or Supplemental Feed Consumption (Lbs. of IGR Cattle Mix needed/ton of grain or suppl. feed)			
Body Weight (lbs.)	2-4	5-10	11-22	23-46
500	41.6	16.6	—	—
600	50.0	20.0	—	—
700	58.3	23.3	—	—
800	66.6	26.6	—	—
900	75.0	30.0	13.6	—
1,000	83.3	33.3	15.2	—
1,100	91.6	36.6	16.6	7.9
1,200	100.0	40.0	18.2	8.7
1,300	108.3	43.3	19.7	9.4
1,400	116.6	46.6	21.2	10.1
1,500	125.0	50.0	22.7	10.9
1,600	133.3	53.3	24.2	11.6

Storage and Disposal: Do not contaminate water or food by storage or disposal.

Storage: Store in a dry area. Do not contaminate with pesticides or fertilizer.

Pesticide Disposal: Wastes resulting from the use of the product may be disposed of on site or at an approved waste disposal facility.

Container Disposal: Completely empty the bag by shaking it and tapping the sides and bottom to loosen clinging particles. Empty the residue into the application equipment. Then dispose of the empty bag in a sanitary landfill or by incineration, or, if allowed by state and local authorities, by burning. If burned, stay out of smoke.

Warning(s): Keep out of the reach of children.

Presentation: 50 lb bags.

* As the insect growth regulator, Altosid®, a trademark of Wellmark International (U.S. Patents 3,904,662 and 3,912,815).

Compendium Code No.: 10410091

M

MOORMAN'S® IGR MINERALS®

ADM **Feed Additive**

EPA Reg. No.: 1157-41

Active Ingredient(s):

S-methoprene (CAS Number 65733-16-6)* 0.02%
Other Ingredients 99.98%
Total 100.00%

Guaranteed Analysis:
Calcium (Ca), not less than 16.0%
Calcium (Ca), not more than 19.2%
Phosphorus (P), not less than 8.0%
Salt (NaCl), not less than 13.5%
Salt (NaCl), not more than 16.2%
Magnesium (Mg), not less than 2.5%
Potassium (K), not less than 0.2%
Copper (Cu), not less than .... 1100 ppm
Selenium (Se), not less than .... 39 ppm
Zinc (Zn), not less than .... 3800 ppm
Vitamin A, not less than .... 200,000 IU/lb

Feed Ingredients: Monocalcium Phosphate, Dicalcium Phosphate, Calcium Carbonate, Salt, Defluorinated Phosphate, Magnesium Oxide, Petrolatum, Soybean Meal, Cane Molasses, Calcium Sulfate, Magnesium-Mica, Iron Oxide, Manganous Oxide, Brewers Condensed Solubles, Zinc Oxide, Potassium Sulfate, Copper Sulfate, Dried Corn Syrup, Ferrous Sulfate, Vitamin A Acetate, Ethylenediamine Dihydriodide, Potassium Iodide, Sodium Selenite, Cobalt Carbonate, Mineral Oil, Cholecalciferol (Source of Vitamin D_3).

Indications: To prevent the breeding of horn flies in the manure of treated cattle only.

A pesticidally active mineral feed for beef and dairy cattle containing methoprene* insect growth regulator for continuous feeding during the fly season.

Directions for Use: It is a violation of Federal law to use this product in a manner inconsistent with its labeling.

Free-Choice Feeding (self-feeding): Make sure cattle are not starved for minerals or salt by providing them before feeding MOORMAN'S® IGR MINERALS®. Then remove salt or mineral supplement and start continuous feeding of MOORMAN'S® IGR MINERALS® in the spring before horn flies appear on cattle and continue feeding until cold weather restricts horn fly activity.

The recommended consumption of MOORMAN'S® IGR MINERALS® is 0.25 lb (¼ lb) to 0.5 lb (½ lb) per 100 lb of body weight per month. Place MOORMAN'S® IGR MINERALS® near watering or loafing areas and provide one feeder for each 15 to 20 head. Put out only a 5-7 day supply of MOORMAN'S® IGR MINERALS® at one time and protect it from rain.

If consumption of MOORMAN'S® IGR MINERALS® is above 0.5 lb (½ lb) per 100 lb of body weight per month, reduce the number of feeding stations or relocate feeders to areas frequented less by cattle.

If consumption of MOORMAN'S® IGR MINERALS® is below 0.25 lb (¼ lb) per 100 lb of body weight per month, increase the number of feeding stations or relocate to areas more frequented by cattle.

Mixed Ration Feeding (hand-feeding): When cattle are on supplemental feeds or if mineral consumption is not as recommended, mix MOORMAN'S® IGR MINERALS® with other non-medicated feeds and feed daily to provide 0.25 lb (¼ lb) to 0.5 lb (½ lb) of MOORMAN'S® IGR MINERALS® per 100 lb of body weight per month. Start continuous feeding in the spring before horn flies appear on cattle and continue feeding until the cold weather restricts horn fly activity.

Storage and Disposal: Do not contaminate water or food by storage or disposal.

Storage: Store in a dry area. Do not contaminate with pesticides or fertilizer.

Pesticide Disposal: Wastes resulting from the use of the product may be disposed of on site or at an approved waste disposal facility.

Container Disposal: Completely empty bag into application equipment. Then dispose of empty bag in a sanitary landfill or by incineration, or, if allowed by State and local authorities, by burning. If burned, stay out of smoke.

Warning(s): Keep out of reach of children.

Presentation: 50 lb (22.67 kg) bags.

* As the insect growth regulator, Altosid® CP-10, a registered trademark of Wellmark International.

Compendium Code No.: 10410101

MOORMAN'S® LN 10

ADM **Feed Medication**

NADA No.: 132-659

Active Ingredient(s):

Lincomycin (lincomycin hydrochloride) . . . . 10 g per lb.

Ingredients: Rice hulls, ground corn, calcium carbonate, mineral oil, sodium propionate (as preservative).

Indications: For the treatment and control of swine dysentery. For a reduction in the severity of swine mycoplasmal pneumonia caused by *Mycoplasma hyopneumoniae.*

For increased rate of weight gain in growing-finishing swine. For increased rate of weight gain and improved feed efficiency in broiler chickens.

Dosage and Administration:

Swine:

For the treatment of swine dysentery: Thoroughly mix 10 lbs. of MOORMAN'S® LN 10 with 1,990 lbs. of an approved ration recommended for the age of the pigs being fed to make one (1) ton of complete feed containing 100 g lincomycin per ton. The resultant complete feed is to be fed as the sole ration for three (3) weeks or until signs of the disease (watery, mucoid, or bloody stools) disappear.

For the treatment and control of swine dysentery: Thoroughly mix 10 lbs. of MOORMAN'S® LN 10 with 1,990 lbs. of an approved ration recommended for the age of the pigs being fed to make one (1) ton of complete feed containing 100 g lincomycin per ton. The resultant complete feed is to be fed continuously as the sole ration for three (3) weeks or until signs of the disease (watery, mucoid, or bloody stools) disappear. Following treatment with 100 g lincomycin per ton, thoroughly mix 4 lbs. of MOORMAN'S® LN 10 with 1,996 lbs. of an approved ration recommended for the age of the pigs being fed to make one (1) ton of complete feed containing 40 g lincomycin per ton. The resultant complete feed is to be fed continuously as the sole ration.

For the control of swine dysentery: For use in animals or on premises with a history of swine dysentery but where symptoms have not yet occurred. Thoroughly mix 4 lbs. of MOORMAN'S® LN 10 with 1,996 lbs. of an approved ration recommended for the age of the pigs being fed to make one (1) ton of complete feed containing 40 g lincomycin per ton. The resultant complete feed is to be fed continuously as the sole ration.

For the reduction in the severity of swine mycoplasmal pneumonia: Thoroughly mix 20 lbs. of MOORMAN'S® LN 10 with 1,980 lbs. of an approved ration recommended for the age of the pigs being fed to make one (1) ton of complete feed containing 200 g lincomycin per ton. The resultant complete feed is to be fed continuously as the sole ration for three (3) weeks.

For increased rate of weight gain in growing-finishing swine: Thoroughly mix 2 lbs. of MOORMAN'S® LN 10 with 1,998 lbs. of an approved ration recommended for the body weight of the pigs being fed to make one (1) ton of complete feed containing 20 g lincomycin per ton. Feed the resultant complete ration continuously as the sole ration.

Broiler chickens:

Thoroughly mix 0.2 to 0.4 lbs. of LN 10 with part of a ton of complete broiler feed to make a preblend. Thoroughly mix the preblend with the remainder of the ton of complete broiler feed to make a complete feed containing 2 to 4 g of lincomycin per ton. Feed the resultant complete feed continuously as the sole ration.

Precaution(s): Must be thoroughly mixed in feeds before use. Store the opened bag in a dry place to prevent caking. Store at room temperature.

Caution(s): Occasionally, swine fed lincomycin may, within the first two days after the onset of treatment, develop diarrhea and/or swelling of the anus. On rare occasions, some pigs may show reddening of the skin and irritable behavior. These conditions have been self-correcting within five to eight days without discontinuing the lincomycin treatment.

Not to be fed to swine that weigh more than 250 lbs.

Do not allow rabbits, hamsters, guinea pigs, horses, or ruminants access to feeds containing lincomycin. Ingestion by these species may result in severe gastrointestinal effects.

Warning(s): Do not slaughter swine for human consumption for six (6) days following last treatment.

Not for human use.

Presentation: 50 lb bags.

Compendium Code No.: 10410111

MOORMAN'S® MOORGUARD® SWINE DEWORMER

ADM **Feed Medication**

NADA No.: 131-675

Active Ingredient(s):

Fenbendazole . . . . 0.45% (2.04 g per lb.)

Ingredients: Rice hulls, calcium carbonate, ground corn, mineral oil.

Indications: For the removal of: Adult large roundworm *(Ascaris suum)**, adult whipworm *(Trichuris suis)**, nodular worm *(Oesophagostomum dentatum, O. quadrispinulatum)*, small stomach worm *(Hyostrongylus rubidus)*, kidneyworm (mature and immature *Stephanurus dentatus)*, lungworm *(Metastrongylus apri* and *Metastrongylus pudendoctectus)* in swine.

Dosage and Administration: Administer a total of 9 mg/kg of body weight over a period of 4-12 days.

*When a total of 9 mg/kg is administered over a 3-day period, fenbendazole is also effective for removal and control of immature (L_3, L_4 stages - liver, lung, intestinal forms) large roundworms *(A. suum)*, and immature ($L_{2,3,4}$ stages - intestinal mucosal forms) whipworms *(T. suis)*.

Thoroughly mix the recommended amount of MOORGUARD® into a 3- to 12-day supply of complete feed. When the recommended dose is split over a 3-day treatment period the dewormer is more effective against the immature stages of large roundworm and whipworms than when the MOORGUARD® dose is split over a treatment period of more than three (3) days. When used as directed, the medicated complete ration should provide a total intake of 4.08 mg of fenbendazole per pound of body weight (9 mg/kg).

One (1) pound of MOORGUARD® (⅕ of package) will provide sufficient fenbendazole to deworm 500 lbs. of pork or ten 50 lb. pigs.]

The following table can be used to determine the amount of MOORGUARD® Swine Dewormer for a 3-day deworming treatment and a 4- to 12-day deworming treatment.

Pig Weight (lb.)	Total pounds of MOORGUARD® needed	Approximate number of pigs dewormed per 5 lb. package
30	0.06	83
40	0.08	62
50	0.10	50
75	0.15	33
100	0.20	25
Gilts, sows, boars:		
300	0.60	8
400	0.80	6
500	1.00	5

Consult a veterinarian for assistance in the diagnosis, treatment and control of parasitism. Swine maintained under conditions of constant worm exposure may require retreatment within four (4) weeks after the first treatment due to re-infection.

Presentation: 5 lb bags.

Compendium Code No.: 10410141

MOORMAN'S® NT 10/10

ADM **Feed Medication**

NADA No.: 143-919

Active Ingredient(s):

Neomycin base . . . . 7 g per lb.

(equivalent to 10 g per lb. of neomycin sulfate)

Oxytetracycline . . . . 10 g per lb.

(from oxytetracycline quaternary salt, equivalent to oxytetracycline hydrochloride)

Ingredients: Rice hulls, ground corn, calcium carbonate, mineral oil, sodium propionate (as preservative).

Indications:

Swine, baby pigs, growing-finishing pigs and sows: Bacterial enteritis (scours), baby pig diarrhea (in baby pigs only), vibrionic dysentery, bloody and salmonellosis (necro or necrotic enteritis).

Sows to be fed during gestation and lactation: For use as an aid in the maintenance of weight gains and feed consumption in the presence of atrophic rhinitis.For use as an aid in the treatment of bacterial enteritis.

Calves: For use as an aid in the prevention and treatment of bacterial enteritis (scours).

Chickens: For use as an aid in the prevention of disease from oxytetracycline-susceptible organisms during periods of stress. Aid in the prevention of bacterial enteritis and in the control of neomycin-sensitive organisms associated with bluecomb (mud fever or nonspecific enteritis).

Extended period of high egg production, to improve feed efficiency, to improve fertility, to improve egg production and feed efficiency in the presence of disease and at times of stress, to improve egg shell quality.

Prevention of complicated chronic respiratory disease (air-sac infection) and the control of complicated CRD by lowering mortality and severity during outbreaks.

Dosage and Administration: Thoroughly mix the specified amount of MOORMAN'S® NT 10/10 with an approved ration recommended for the age of the species to be fed. NT 10/10 contains 7 g neomycin base per lb. and 10 g oxytetracycline per lb. The amount of NT 10/10 needed per ton of complete feed varies with the desired purpose as given below.

For medicating complete feed:

The following information gives the purpose, required amounts of neomycin base and oxytetracycline, and the amount of NT 10/10 needed to medicate one (1) ton of complete feed.

Swine, baby pigs, growing-finishing pigs and sows:

For the prevention of bacterial enteritis, (scours) vibrionic dysentery, bloody dysentery and salmonellosis (necro or necrotic enteritis): Add 5 lbs. NT 10/10 to one (1) ton of complete feed. This will give 50 g per ton oxytetracycline and 35 g per ton neomycin base.

For the treatment of bacterial enteritis (scours), vibrionic dysentery, bloody dysentery and salmonellosis (necro or necrotic enteritis): Add 10 lbs. NT 10/10 to one (1) ton of complete feed. This will give 100 g per ton of oxytetracycline and 70 g per ton of neomycin base.

Sows to be fed during gestation and lactation: For use as an aid in the maintenance of weight gains and feed consumption in the presence of atrophic rhinitis. For use as an aid in the treatment of bacterial enteritis: Add 10 to 15 lbs. NT 10/10 to one (1) ton of complete feed. This will give 100 to 150 g per ton of oxytetracycline and 70 to 105 g per ton of neomycin base.

Calves:

For the prevention of bacterial enteritis (scours): Add 5 lbs. NT 10/10 to one (1) ton of complete feed. This will give 50 g per ton oxytetracycline and 35 g per ton neomycin base.

For the treatment of bacterial enteritis (scours): Add 10 lbs. NT 10/10 to one (1) ton of complete feed. This will give 100 g per ton oxytetracycline and 70 g per ton neomycin base.

Chickens:

For use as an aid in the prevention of disease from oxytetracycline-susceptible organisms, prevention of bacterial enteritis and in the control of neomycin-sensitive organisms associated with bluecomb (mud fever or nonspecific enteritis): Add 5 lbs. NT 10/10 to one (1) ton of complete feed. This will give 50 g per ton oxytetracycline and 35 g per ton neomycin base.

For extended period of high egg production, to improve feed efficiency, to improve fertility, to improve egg production and feed efficiency in presence of disease and at times of stress, to improve egg shell quality: Add 5 to 10 lbs. NT 10/10 to one (1) ton of complete feed. This will give 50 to 100 g per ton oxytetracycline and 35 to 70 g per ton neomycin base.

For the prevention of complicated chronic respiratory disease (air-sac infection) and the control of complicated CRD by lowering mortality and severity during outbreaks: Add 10 to 20 lbs. NT 10/10 to one (1) ton of complete feed. This will give 100 to 200 g per ton oxytetracycline and 70 to 140 g per ton neomycin base.

Warning(s): The combination, when fed at the level of 1.4 g of neomycin base plus 2 g oxytetracycline head each day, requires withdrawal from feed seven (7) days before slaughter of calves. Withdrawal is not required at lower levels.

Withdraw NT 10/10 from swine feed five (5) days before slaughter.

Withdraw NT 10/10 from feed five (5) days before slaughter of broilers and 14 days before slaughter of laying hens.

Presentation: 50 lb bags.

Compendium Code No.: 10410151

MOORMAN'S® SPECIAL MIX CATTLE BOOST® BT

ADM **Feed Medication**

Type B Medicated Feed

Active Ingredient(s):

Lasalocid . . . . . 400 grams per ton (200 milligrams per pound)

Guaranteed Analysis:

Crude Protein, not less than 40.0%
(This includes not more than 8.0% equivalent crude protein from non-protein nitrogen.)
Crude Fat, not less than 0.5%
Crude Fiber, not more than 9.5%
Calcium (Ca), not less than 3.7%
Calcium (Ca), not more than 4.7%
Phosphorus (P), not less than 1.0%
Salt (NaCl), not less than 1.3%
Salt (NaCl), not more than 1.8%
Potassium (K), not less than 1.0%
Vitamin A, not less than . . . . . 120,000 IU/lb

Ingredients: Dehulled Soybean Meal, Soybean Feed, Wheat Middlings, Calcium Carbonate, Cottonseed Meal, Urea, Monocalcium Phosphate, Dicalcium Phosphate, Salt, Animal Fat, BHT (A Preservative), Calcium Sulfate, Corn Gluten Feed, Cane Molasses, Manganous Oxide, Vitamin E Supplement, Zinc Oxide, Copper Sulfate, Vitamin A Acetate, Magnesium Oxide, Defluorinated Phosphate, Linseed Meal, Ferrous Sulfate, Mineral Oil, Potassium Sulfate, Potassium Iodide, Cobalt Carbonate, Sodium Selenite, D-Activated Animal Sterol (Source of Vitamin D_3).

Indications: For improved feed efficiency in beef cattle fed in confinement for slaughter.

Directions: Instructions for Mixing and Feeding: Start cattle on MOORMAN'S® SPECIAL MIX CATTLE BOOST® BT by feeding 1 lb per head per day of this product thoroughly mixed with grain or grain-roughage mixtures before feeding. When starting cattle on grain, roughage must be fed either free-choice or mixed in the ration. Feed 1 lb of this product with not less than 5 lb of grain and a minimum of 8 lb roughage per head per day for the first 4 to 7 days to provide no more than 30 gram lasalocid per ton of final ration. After cattle are eating well, gradually increase the amount of grain mixed with 1 lb/hd/day of this product until the desired level of grain intake is reached. Adjust roughage to the desired level. The amount of grain-roughage mixture fed must equal a minimum of 13 lb per head per day. Feed continuously. This product is designed to be fed at the rate of 1 lb per head per day. Do not feed more than 1 lb of this product per head per day. Provide sufficient bunk space so all cattle can eat at one time.

Drug Level: When fed at the rate of 1 lb per head per day, this product provides 200 mg lasalocid. The complete ration should contain from 10 to 30 grams per ton of lasalocid.

Caution(s): Consumption of this product by sheep and goats may result in copper toxicity. The safety of lasalocid in unapproved species has not been established. Do not allow horses or other equines access to formulations containing lasalocid as ingestion may be fatal. Feeding undiluted or mixing errors resulting in excessive concentrations of lasalocid could be fatal to cattle.

Warning(s): This feed should be used only in accordance with instructions furnished on the label. A withdrawal period has not been established for this product in pre-ruminating cattle. Do not use in calves to be processed for veal. Do not feed to lactating dairy cows.

Presentation: Available in bulk and 50 lb bags.

Compendium Code No.: 10410191

MOORMAN'S® TYS 5/5

ADM **Feed Medication**

Type B Medicated Feed

Active Ingredient(s):

Tylosin (as tylosin phosphate) . . . . . 5 grams per pound
Sulfamethazine . . . . . 1.1% (5 grams per pound)

Ingredients: Rice hulls, ground corn, calcium carbonate, mineral oil, sodium propionate (a preservative).

Indications: For maintaining weight gains and feed efficiency in the presence of atrophic rhinitis; lowering incidence and severity of *Bordetella bronchiseptica* rhinitis; prevention of swine dysentery (vibrionic); control of swine pneumonias caused by bacterial pathogens *(Pasteurella multocida* and/or *Actinomyces pyogenes)* when fed according to directions.

Dosage and Administration: Thoroughly mix 20 pounds of MOORMAN'S® TYS 5/5 with 1980 pounds of a MoorMan approved ration recommended for the age of the pigs being fed to make one ton of complete feed containing 100 grams tylosin and 100 grams sulfamethazine per ton. The resultant complete feed is to be fed continuously as the sole ration.

Caution(s): Must be thoroughly mixed in feeds before use. Do not use in any finished feed (supplement, concentrate or complete feed) containing in excess of 2% bentonite.

Warning(s): Withdraw feeds containing TYS 5/5 15 days before slaughter.

Presentation: 50 lb (22.67) bags.

Compendium Code No.: 10410161

MOORMAN'S® WDC

ADM **Feed Medication**

NADA No.: 092-955

Active Ingredient(s):

Carbadox (Mecadox®) . . . . . 0.55% (2.5 g per lb.)
Pyrantel tartrate (Banminth®). . . . . 1.06% (4.8 g per lb.)

Ingredients: Rice hulls, ground corn, calcium carbonate, mineral oil, sodium propionate (as preservative).

Indications: For the control of swine dysentery (vibrionic dysentery, bloody scours or hemorrhagic dysentery), control of bacterial swine enteritis (salmonellosis or necrotic enteritis caused by *Salmonella choleraesuis),* and aids in the prevention of migration and establishment of large roundworm *(Ascaris suum)* infections, aid in the prevention of establishment of nodular worm (oesophagostomum) infections in swine.

Dosage and Administration: Thoroughly mix 20 lbs. of MOORMAN'S® WDC with 1,980 lbs. of an approved ration recommended for the age of the pigs being fed to make one (1) ton of complete swine feed containing 50 g carbadox and 96 g pyrantel tartrate.

The resultant complete feed is to be fed continuously as the sole ration and may be fed up to 75 lbs. of body weight. Then switch to an approved swine ration for pigs of that weight.

Caution(s): Consult a veterinarian before using in severely debilitated animals. Consult a veterinarian for assistance in the diagnosis, treatment, and control of parasitism. Do not mix in feeds containing bentonite.

Warning(s): Do not feed to swine weighing more than 75 lbs. of body weight. Do not feed to swine within 10 weeks of slaughter. Do not mix in complete feeds containing less than 15% crude protein.

Presentation: 50 lb bags.

* Mecadox is Phibro Animal Health's trademark for carbadox.
Banminth is Phibro Animal Health's trademark for pyrantel tartrate.

Compendium Code No.: 10410171

M+PAC®

Schering-Plough **Bacterin**

Mycoplasma Hyopneumoniae Bacterin

U.S. Vet. Lic. No.: 165A

Contents: This product contains the antigen listed above. M+PAC® bacterin contains the proprietary dual adjuvant Emunade®.

Preservatives: Ampicillin, gentamicin and thimerosal.

Indications: Recommended for use as an aid in the prevention of pneumonia caused by *Mycoplasma hyopneumoniae* infection in swine.

Dosage and Administration: For vaccination of healthy swine. Using aseptic technique. Vaccinate pigs subcutaneously or intramuscularly at 7-10 days of age or older with a 1 mL dose followed by a second 1 mL dose 14 days later. For herds that use a single dose program, vaccinate pigs intramuscularly at 6 weeks of age or older with a single 2 mL dose. Intramuscular vaccination with a single 2 mL dose of M+PAC® at 6 weeks of age has been demonstrated to provide at least 4 months duration of immunity.

Precaution(s): Store at 2°-7°C (35°-45°F). Do not freeze. Use entire contents when first opened.

Caution(s): For veterinary use only. Transient local reaction may occur at the injection site. Anaphylactoid reactions may occur after use.

Antidote(s): Epinephrine.

Warning(s): Do not vaccinate within 21 days of slaughter.

Extreme caution should be used when injecting any oil emulsion vaccine to avoid injecting your own finger or hand. Accidental injection can cause serious local reaction. Contact a physician immediately if accidental injection occurs.

Presentation: 50 mL (25 doses/50 doses), 100 mL (50 doses/100 doses), 250 mL (125 doses/250 doses) and 500 mL (250 doses/500 doses).

Compendium Code No.: 10471283 P17946-10/P17947-10/P17948-10/P17949-10

M+PARAPAC™

Schering-Plough **Bacterin**

Haemophilus Parasuis-Mycoplasma Hyopneumoniae Bacterin

U.S. Vet. Lic. No.: 165A

Contents: This product contains the antigens listed above.

Preservatives: Ampicillin, Gentamicin, and Thimerosal. This product contains the adjuvant Emunade™.

Indications: Recommended for use in healthy swine as an aid in the prevention of Glasser's disease caused by *Haemophilus parasuis* and pneumonia caused by *Mycoplasma hyopneumoniae.*

Dosage and Administration: Using aseptic technique, inject 2 mL intramuscularly at 7-10 days of age or older. Revaccinate with 2 mL 2 to 3 weeks after initial vaccination. Revaccinate with a single 2 mL dose annually.

Precaution(s): Store at 2°-7°C (35°-45°F). Do not freeze. Use entire contents when first opened.

Caution(s): Transient local reaction may occur at the injection site. If allergic response occurs, administer epinephrine.

Warning(s): Do not vaccinate within 60 days before slaughter.

Extreme caution should be used when injecting any oil emulsion vaccine to avoid injecting your own finger or hand. Accidental injection can cause serious local reaction. Contact a physician immediately if accidental injection occurs. For veterinary use only.

Presentation: 100 dose (200 mL) vials.

Compendium Code No.: 10471240

MRS. ALLEN'S SHED-STOP® GRANULES FOR CATS

Farnam **Small Animal Dietary Supplement**

Microencapsulated Omega Fatty Acid

Guaranteed Analysis: Per 15-gram scoop:

Vegetable Oils
(Safflower, Sunflower, Soybean, Flax Seed, Borage, and Evening Primrose Oils) . . 2500 mg
Marine Lipid Concentrates . . . . . 500 mg
Vitamin A . . . . . 1,000 IU
Vitamin D3 . . . . . 100 IU
Vitamin E . . . . . 10 IU
Vitamin B1 (Thiamine) . . . . . 1,000 mcg
Vitamin B2 (Riboflavin) . . . . . 1,000 mcg
Vitamin B3 (Niacin) . . . . . 10 mg
Vitamin B6 (Pyridoxine) . . . . . 1,000 mcg
Vitamin B12 (Cyanocobalamin) . . . . . 10 mcg
Choline . . . . . 20 mg
Inositol . . . . . 10 mg
Copper (as Copper Sulfate) . . . . . 10 mg
Manganese (as Manganese Sulfate) . . . . . 10 mg
Zinc (as Zinc Sulfate) . . . . . 10 mg
Selenium . . . . . 10 mcg

Indications: Formulated with high levels of Omega 6 and Omega 3 fatty acids, plus a complete listing of essential vitamins and minerals to optimize the health of an animal's coat providing for glossy thick coats on cats.

M

Dosage and Administration: 1 scoop daily.

In extreme cases, double the dose for the first ten days, then return to the regular dose. Initial results should be seen in four to six weeks.

Warning(s): Keep out of reach of children.

Presentation: 450 g.

SHED-STOP® is a registered trademark of Stabar Enterprises, Inc.

Compendium Code No.: 10000870 0B1

MRS. ALLEN'S SHED-STOP® GRANULES FOR DOGS

Farnam **Small Animal Dietary Supplement**

Microencapsulated Omega Fatty Acids

Guaranteed Analysis: Per 7.5-gram scoop:

Vegetable Oils	
(Safflower, Sunflower, Soybean, Flax Seed, Borage, and Evening Primrose)	1400 mg
Marine Lipid Concentrates	100 mg
Copper, min.	5 mg
Manganese, min.	5 mg
Zinc, min.	5 mg
Selenium	5 mcg
Vitamin A	500 IU
Vitamin D3	50 IU
Vitamin E	5 IU
Vitamin B1 (Thiamine)	500 mcg
Vitamin B2 (Riboflavin)	500 mcg
Vitamin B3 (Niacin)	5 mg
Vitamin B6 (Pyridoxine)	500 mcg
Vitamin B12 (Cyanocobalamin)	5 mcg
Choline	10 mg
Inositol	5 mg

Composition: Crude Protein (min.) 1.0%, Crude Fat (min.) 20.0%, Fiber (max.) 30.0%, Moisture (max.) 15.0%.

Ingredients: Natural flavors (roast beef, liver and fish), vegetable oils (safflower, sunflower, soybean, flax seed, borage and evening primrose oils), marine lipid concentrates, taurine, Vitamin A, Vitamin D3, Vitamin E, Vitamin B1, Vitamin B2, Vitamin B3, Vitamin B6, Vitamin B12, Choline Chloride, Inositol, Copper Sulfate, Manganese Sulfate, Zinc Sulfate, and Selenium.

Indications: SHED-STOP® for Dogs: Formulated with an ideal ratio of Omega 6 and Omega 3 fatty acids of 6:1. Includes essential vitamins and minerals to assist in minimizing non-seasonal shedding and to enhance overall skin and coat quality.

Dosage and Administration: Mix with dog food or administer as a treat. For the first week, to ensure acceptance of this product, gradually mix into the pet's diet.

Up to 25 lbs.: 1 scoop daily   26 to 60 lbs.: 2 scoops daily   Over 60 lbs.: 3 scoops daily

In extreme cases, double the dose for several weeks, then return to the regular dose. Initial results should be seen in four to six weeks.

When introducing any new items into your pet's diet, it is advisable to consult with your veterinarian.

Warning(s): Keep out of reach of children.

Presentation: 450 g.

SHED-STOP® is a registered trademark of Stabar Enterprises, Inc.

Compendium Code No.: 10000880 0D1

M

MRS. ALLEN'S VITA CARE® VITAMINS FOR CATS

Farnam **Small Animal Dietary Supplement**

Guaranteed Analysis: per tablet:

Fatty Acid:	
Linoleic Acid, min.	22 mg
Minerals:	
Calcium, min.	3.6% (40 mg)
Phosphorus, min.	1.4% (31 mg)
Potassium, min.	31 mcg
Magnesium, min.	30 mg
Iron, min.	5 mg
Copper, min.	200 mcg
Manganese, min.	200 mcg
Zinc, min.	300 mcg
Iodine, min.	100 mcg
Cobalt, min.	100 mcg
Vitamins:	
Vitamin A, min.	1500 I.U.
Vitamin D, min.	150 I.U.
Vitamin E, min.	4 I.U.
Thiamin (B1), min.	810 mcg
Riboflavin, min.	1 mg
d-Pantothenic Acid, min.	1 mg
Niacin, min.	4 mg
Pyridoxine, min.	410 mcg
Choline, min.	50 mg
Taurine, min.	50 mg
Inositol, min.	10 mg

Ingredients: Whey, dried corn syrup, artificial flavoring, beef livers meal, stearic acid, sucrose, choline bitartrate, taurine, dried brewers yeast, calcium phosphate, magnesium stearate, fish protein concentrate, linoleic acid, soybean flour, malted milk, safflower oil, soy protein isolate, inositol, vitamin E supplement, ferrous fumerate, silicon dioxide, niacin supplement, vitamin A acetate, vitamin D3 supplement, d-calcium pantothenate, riboflavin supplement, thiamine mononitrate, pyridoxine hydrochloride, zinc gluconate, copper gluconate, manganese sulfate, cobalt sulfate, and potassium iodide.

Indications: Vitamin tablets for cats. Contains antioxidants and taurine.

Dosage and Administration: For Dietary Supplement:

Mature cats: 1 tablet daily.   Kittens: 1/4 to 1 tablet daily.

For sick, convalescing, pregnant or nursing cats: 2 tablets daily.

Administer liver-flavored VITA CARE® cat vitamins by hand prior to feeding or crumble and mix with food.

Warning(s): Keep out of reach of children.

Presentation: Bottles of 60 tablets.

Compendium Code No.: 10000890 0B1

MRS. ALLEN'S VITA CARE® VITAMINS FOR DOGS

Farnam **Small Animal Dietary Supplement**

Guaranteed Analysis: per tablet:

Fatty Acid:	
Linoleic Acid, min.	30 mg
Minerals:	
Calcium, min.	4.23% (151 mg)
Phosphorus, min.	3.30% (116.2 mg)
Potassium, min.	16 mcg
Magnesium, min.	230 mcg
Iron, min.	1 mg
Copper, min.	50 mcg
Manganese, min.	60 mcg
Zinc, min.	1.5 mg
Iodine, min.	52 mcg
Cobalt, min.	14 mcg
Vitamins:	
Vitamin A, min.	1000 I.U.
Vitamin D, min.	100 I.U.
Vitamin E, min.	2.1 I.U.
Thiamin (B1), min.	810 mcg
Riboflavin, min.	1 mg
Niacin, min.	10 mg
Pyridoxine, min.	82 mcg
Vitamin B12, min.	0.2 mcg

Ingredients: Wheat germ meal, dried corn syrup, kaolin, beef livers meal, calcium phosphate, stearic acid, animal digest, sucrose, lactose, safflower oil, gelatin, linoleic acid, whey, silicon dioxide, corn starch, niacin supplement, vitamin E supplement, vitamin A acetate, zinc oxide, iron proteinate, riboflavin supplement, magnesium stearate, vitamin D3 supplement, pyridoxine hydrochloride, manganese sulfate, potassium iodide, copper sulfate monohydrate, cobalt sulfate, and vitamin B12 supplement.

Indications: Vitamin tablets for dogs. Contains antioxidants.

Dosage and Administration: For Dietary Supplement:

Dogs under 10 lbs.: 1/2 tablet daily.

Dogs over 10 lbs.: 1 tablet daily.

Liver-flavored VITA CARE® dog vitamins with antioxidants provide a special taste appeal.

Administer by hand prior to feeding or crumble and mix with food.

Warning(s): Keep out of reach of children.

Presentation: Bottles of 60 tablets.

Compendium Code No.: 10000900 0B1

MS-BAC™

Fort Dodge **Bacterin**

Mycoplasma Synoviae Bacterin

U.S. Vet. Lic. No.: 112

Contents: This product contains the antigen listed above.

Penicillin added as a preservative.

Indications: For the vaccination of chickens and turkeys as an aid in the prevention of clinical signs associated with *Mycoplasma synoviae.*

Dosage and Administration: Inject 0.5 mL (0.5 cc) subcutaneously (in the lower neck region) for birds 1 to 10 weeks of age using aseptic technique. If 10 weeks of age or older, may vaccinate intramuscularly or subcutaneously. Vaccinate only healthy birds prior to field exposure. For optimum results, vaccinate twice, allowing at least 4 weeks between vaccinations. Revaccinate birds during molt before the second laying period.

Precaution(s): Store in the dark at 36° to 45°F (2° to 7°C). Do not freeze. Warm to 72°F (22°C) and shake well before using. Use entire contents when first opened.

Warning(s): Do not vaccinate within 42 days before slaughter.

In case of accidental human injection seek immediate medical attention.

For veterinary use only.

Presentation: 1,000 dose (500 mL) vials.

Compendium Code No.: 10031091 10261B

MULTI-ELECTROLYTES

Neogen **Electrolytes-Oral**

Guaranteed Analysis: per lb:

Sodium	22.6%
Potassium	11.7%
Chloride	45.0%
Vitamin A	100,000 1 unit
Vitamin D_3	5,000 1 unit
Vitamin E	500 1 unit

Ingredients: Sodium chloride, Potassium chloride, Starch, Calcium lactate, Citric acid, Vitamin A acetate, D-activated animal sterol (source of Vitamin D_3), dL-alpha tocopheryl acetate, Ferrous sulfate, Zinc sulfate, Manganese sulfate, Copper sulfate, Cobalt sulfate, Dextrose, Artificial flavor added.

Indications: For use as a nutritional supplement in the horse where a deficiency exists.

Directions: Add at the rate of 2 ozs per 10 gallons of water or into feed at the same rate of 2 ozs per 10 lbs of grain ration.

Caution(s): Sold to licensed veterinarians only.

For the horse only.

For animal use only.

Warning(s): Keep out of reach of children.

Presentation: 5 lbs.

Compendium Code No.: 14910272 L107-0997 Rev 11/01

MULTIMAX™

SureNutrition **Equine Dietary Supplement**

Comprehensive Vitamin & Mineral Equine Supplement-Amino Acids (Free Form)-Probiotic Enzyme (Lactobacillus Acidophilus)

Guaranteed Analysis: per lb.:

Amino Acids:

Lysine, min. .... 0.77% (3500 mg)
Methionine, min. .... 0.55% (2500 mg)

Minerals/Vitamins:

Calcium, min. 4.0%
Calcium, max. 4.8%
Phosphorous, min. 3.0%
Magnesium, min. 2.21%
Potassium, min. 0.70%
Sulfur, min. 0.33%
Copper, min. .... 440 ppm
Zinc, min. .... 1,300 ppm
Iron, min. .... 3,800 ppm
Manganese, min. .... 1,100 ppm
Cobalt, min. .... 20 ppm
Iodine, min. .... 20 ppm
Selenium, min. .... 8.8 ppm
Vitamin A, min. .... 100,000 IU
Vitamin D, min. .... 20,000 IU
Vitamin E, min. .... 4,000 IU
Vitamin B_{12}, min. .... 22 mg
Menadione, min. .... 4 mg
Riboflavin, min. .... 1,000 mg
Pantothenic Acid, min. .... 200 mg
Thiamine, min. .... 224 mg
Niacin, min. .... 500 mg
Vitamin B_6, min. .... 243 mg
Folic Acid, min. .... 80 mg
Choline, min. .... 3,333 mg
Biotin, min. .... 8 mg
Inositol, min. .... 6 mg
PABA, min. .... 175 mg
Ascorbic Acid, min. .... 500 mg
Beta Carotene, min. .... 8 mg
Lactobacillus Acidophilus .... 1×10^7 CFU
Lactobacillus Lactis .... 2×10^6 CFU
Lactobacillus Plantarum .... 2×10^6 CFU
Enterococcus Cremoris .... 2×10^6 CFU
Enterococcus Diacetylactis .... 2×10^6 CFU
Bacillus Subtilis .... 1×10^6 CFU
Aspergillus Oryzae .... 1×10^6 CFU

Ingredients: Dehydrated Alfalfa Meal, Dicalcium Phosphate, Sugar, Mineral Oil, Magnesium Oxide, Ferrous Fumarate, Ferrous Sulfate, Monosodium Phosphate, Calcium Carbonate, Wheat Middlings, Artificial Flavoring, Potassium Chloride, Sulfur, Artificial Sweetener, Yeast Culture, Dried Whey, Vitamin A Supplement, D-Activated Animal Sterol (source of Vitamin D_3), Vitamin E Supplement, Riboflavin Supplement, Niacin Supplement, Choline Chloride, Calcium Pantothenate, Menadione Sodium Bisulfite Complex, L-Lysine Hydrochloride, DL Methionine, Vitamin B_{12} Supplement, Folic Acid, Pyridoxine Hydrochloride, D-Biotin, Para Amino Benzoic Acid, Thiamine Mononitrate, Ascorbic Acid, Manganese Proteinate, Zinc Proteinate, Copper Proteinate, Cobalt Proteinate, Ethylene Dihydriodide, Sodium Selenite, Dried *Lactobacillus Acidophilus* Fermentation Product, Dried *Lactobacillus Lactis* Fermentation Product, Dried *Lactobacillus Plantarum* Fermentation Product, Dried *B-Subtillus* Fermentation Product, Dried *Aspergillus Oryzae* Fermentation Product, and Dried Brewers Yeast.

Indications: A comprehensive vitamin and mineral equine supplement.

Dosage and Administration: Feeding Directions: Feed at the rate of 1-2 ounces per head per day.

The enclosed scoop holds 1½ ounces when rounded full.

Presentation: 5 lb (2.2 kg), 10 lb (4.4 kg) and 20 lb (8.8 kg) pails.

Compendium Code No.: 12060020 0BB1 / 0A1

MULTI-MILK™

Pet-Ag **Milk Replacer**

Active Ingredient(s): Guaranteed Analysis:

Crude protein, min. 30.00000%
Crude fat, min. 55.00000%
Crude fiber, max. 0.25000%
Ash, max. 8.00000%
Moisture, max. 5.00000%
Calcium, min. 1.00000%
Calcium, max. 1.50000%
Phosphorus, min. 0.85000%
Sodium 0.45000%
Potassium 0.70000%
Magnesium 0.07000%
Chloride 0.70000%
Iron 0.00500%
Copper 0.00100%
Zinc 0.00500%
Manganese 0.00090%
Iodine 0.00080%
Selenium, added 0.00002%

Minimum per Pound

Vitamin A .... 40,000 I.U.
Vitamin D_3 .... 4,000 I.U.
Vitamin E .... 90 I.U.
Vitamin B_{12} .... 30.0 mcg
Menadione .... 0.60 mg
Riboflavin .... 3.00 mg
d-Pantothenic acid .... 25.00 mg
Thiamine .... 1.90 mg
Niacin .... 24.00 mg
Vitamin B_6 .... 1.50 mg
Folic acid .... 0.30 mg
Choline .... 1,450.00 mg
Biotin .... 0.10 mg

Ingredients: Animal fat (preserved with BHA, and citric acid), casein, dicalcium phosphate, calcium carbonate, lecithin, potassium chloride, choline chloride, magnesium sulfate, vitamin E supplement, vitamin A supplement, zinc methionine, ferrous sulfate, calcium pantothenate, vitamin B_{12} supplement, niacin supplement, manganese sulfate, copper sulfate, vitamin D_3 supplement, riboflavin supplement, thiamine mononitrate, pyridoxine hydrochloride, menadione sodium bisulfite complex, folic acid, calcium iodate, biotin, sodium selenite, mono and di-glycerides.

Indications: MULTI-MILK™ is a high fat milk protein powder containing traces of lactose and fortified with vitamins and minerals.

MULTI-MILK™ has been developed as a milk replacer for animals with lactose intolerance, and as a base to blend with Esbilac®, KMR®, or Foal-Lac® milk replacers to yield a variety of milks.

It is also useful as a supplement to provide highly digestible sources of protein, fat, vitamins and minerals for added nutrition.

MULTI-MILK™ can be mixed into food as a powder or mixed with water for tubular feeding.

Dosage and Administration:

Mixing Directions: There are some variations in the weight per unit volume of milk replacer powders. Therefore, the most accurate measurements are made by actually weighing the powder and water. For example, 25 g of MULTI-MILK™ plus 75 g of water will 100 g of a reconstituted milk replacer containing 25% solids.

If weighing is not possible, the following volume measurements can be used to reconstitute MULTI-MILK™ to the indicated approximate concentrations:

MULTI-MILK™	Water	% Solids	% Protein	% Fat	% Lactose
1 part	1 part	25.0	7.5	13.8	nil
3 parts	4 parts	20.0	6.0	11.0	nil
1 part	2 parts	14.3	4.3	7.9	nil
2 parts	5 parts	11.8	3.5	6.5	nil

One (1) part is a volume measurement such as a tablespoon or cup. The volume relationships shown above were calculated from the following weight-volume measurements. All weights were made on level measurements.

	Weight in grams	
Utensil	MULTI-MILK™	Water
Tablespoon (enclosed)	4.6	14.0
Standard measuring tablespoon	5.5	15.0
¼ Standard measuring cup	20.0	60.0
⅓ Standard measuring cup	26.0	80.0

Precaution(s): Store in a cool, dry place.

If MULTI-MILK™ is blended with Esbilac® Powder or KMR® Powder, the blended powder should be refrigerated until used. Any milk replacer reconstituted with water should be refrigerated until used preferably within 24 hours.

Presentation: 1½ lb. can, 4 lb. pail, and 15 lb. drum.

Compendium Code No.: 10970240

M

MULTIMIN™ ℞

Multimin **Mineral Injection**

An injectable supplemental source of zinc, manganese, selenium, and copper

Guaranteed Analysis:

Zinc, not less than .... 20 mg/mL
Manganese, not less than .... 20 mg/mL
Selenium, not less than .... 5 mg/mL
Copper, not less than .... 10 mg/mL

Ingredients: Manganese sulfate, zinc oxide, soda ash, copper carbonate, sodium selenite, disodium EDTA, sodium hydroxide.

Directions: Use only in cattle by subcutaneous injection only.

Bulls: 7 mL 3 times per year
Cows: 5 mL + 3 weeks before calving
5 mL + 6 weeks after calving
5 mL + 5 months into lactation
Calves: 3 mL at weaning (+ 3 months)
Heifers: 5 mL every 3 months until breeding
NB: 5 mL + 3 weeks before first insemination
Additional: 5 mL every 2 months in wet conditions
Administration: Use standard sterile procedures during administration of injections.

Precaution(s): Store in a cool dry place.

Caution(s): Federal law restricts this drug to use by or on the order of a licensed veterinarian.

Slight local reaction may occur for about 30 sec. after injection. A slight swelling may be observed at injection site for a few days after administration.

Warning(s): Use only in cattle.

Keep out of reach of children.

Presentation: 100 mL.

Manufactured by: Animalia CC, Republic of South Africa

Compendium Code No.: 12680000

MULTIMUNE® CU

Biomune **Vaccine**

Pasteurella multocida Vaccine, Avirulent Live Culture, Avian Isolate

U.S. Vet. Lic. No.: 368

Active Ingredient(s): MULTIMUNE® CU is a live bacterial vaccine containing the Clemson University (CU) strain of *Pasteurella multocida* type 3 X 4 in a freeze-dried preparation. The CU vaccine strain has been shown to offer protection against naturally occurring field strains of *P. multocida* in most important turkey areas. The seed culture used to make the vaccine has been laboratory tested as required by USDA for protection against challenge with *P. multocida* strains P-1059 (type 3) and P-1662 (type 4).

Indications: MULTIMUNE® CU is recommended for use in healthy turkeys six weeks of age or older as an aid in preventing fowl cholera due to *Pasteurella multocida* types 3 and 4.

Dosage and Administration: Administer a 1,000 dose vial of vaccine in the water to be consumed by 1,000 turkeys. The best results are obtained when the vaccine is administered initially to turkeys 6 to 8 weeks of age and repeated 4 to 6 weeks later. Older market turkeys and breeders may require additional revaccination at 4 to 6 week intervals. Initial vaccination should not be conducted in turkeys older than 12 weeks of age.

Do not mix the vaccine until ready for use. Drinking water for vaccination should be mixed with powdered milk to prevent possible vaccine inactivation from chlorine or other water additives and also to stabilize the vaccine. The powdered milk should be added to the water at the rate of one (1) heaped teaspoonful per three (3) gallons, or one (1) heaped cupful per 50 gallons. Rehydrate the vaccine by filling the vaccine vial approximately half (½) full with tap water to which milk has been added and mix until completely dissolved. Use only clean waterers and equipment free of disinfectants or sanitizers. All water must be withheld for at least two (2) hours prior to vaccination to ensure that all of the turkeys drink. Mix the rehydrated vaccine in the quantity of drinking water (milk added) which will be consumed by thirsty turkeys in approximately two (2) hours. The following schedule is a general guideline for the amount of water to use with the vaccine. These amounts will vary depending upon the individual management conditions, climate, age and sex of the turkeys.

Age	Sex	Climate	Amount of water for each 1,000 doses
6-8 wks.	Toms	Hot	25 gallons
6-8 wks.	Hens	Hot	20 gallons
6-8 wks.	Toms	Cold	13 gallons
6-8 wks.	Hens	Cold	10 gallons
10-14 wks.	Toms	Hot	35 gallons
10-14 wks.	Hens	Hot	27 gallons
10-14 wks.	Toms	Cold	18 gallons
10-14 wks.	Hens	Cold	14 gallons

Distribute 1,000 doses of vaccine in water to be consumed by 1,000 turkeys. Provide ample water space so that all of the turkeys can easily drink. Do not administer through water lines with a proportioner or medication tank.

Precaution(s): Keep MULTIMUNE® CU refrigerated until use. Store between 35°-45°F (2°-7°C).

Caution(s): Avoid the use of live Newcastle vaccine two weeks prior to two weeks following vaccination with MULTIMUNE® CU. Turkeys to be vaccinated should not be given any antibiotic and/or sulfonamide medication for three days before and five days after vaccination to avoid interference with vaccine immunity.

The capacity of the vaccine to produce satisfactory immunity is dependent upon many factors, including but not limited to, the conditions of storage and handling by the user, and technique of administration as measured by the user's care in following directions and good management. It has been noted by others that the use of the product may cause an increase in flock mortality, usually due to some turkeys being subclinically ill at the time of administration. Vaccinated flocks should be watched closely and medicated as necessary to control more severe reactions. Avoid exposing birds other than turkeys to the vaccine.

Since MULTIMUNE® CU is a live bacterial culture, caution should be used to avoid contact with open wounds or the accidental inoculation of personnel. If accidental inoculation of personnel occurs, consult a physician immediately as the vaccine may act as a human pathogen. Vaccinating crew personnel must wash their hands after using the vaccine.

Use the entire contents of the vial when first opened. Burn all of the containers and unused contents.

Warning(s): Do not vaccinate within 21 days before slaughter.

Presentation: 10 x 1,000 dose vials of vaccine.

Compendium Code No.: 11290151

M

MULTIMUNE® K

Biomune **Bacterin**

Pasteurella Multocida Bacterin, Avian Isolates Types 1, 3 and 4, Oil Emulsion

U.S. Vet. Lic. No.: 368

Contents: This product contains the antigens listed above.

Contains gentamicin as a preservative.

Indications: This bacterin is recommended for use in healthy chickens and turkeys as an aid in the prevention of fowl cholera caused by *Pasteurella multocida* type 1 in chickens and types 3 and 4 in turkeys.

Dosage and Administration: Give 0.5 mL subcutaneously in the lower neck region in a direction away from the head and parallel with the neck. In turkeys, the injection site is in the feathered area of the neck. Do not inject into muscle tissue or neck vertebrae. Turkeys should be initially vaccinated at 6 weeks of age or older and chickens should be initially vaccinated at 12 weeks of age of older. Birds should be revaccinated 3 to 4 weeks later.

Precaution(s): The bacterin should be stored, transported and administered in accordance with the instructions and directions.

Do not freeze. Store in the dark at 35°-45°F (2°-7°C).

Warm to room temperature and shake well before using and during use.

Use entire contents when first opened.

Caution(s): This product contains an oil based adjuvant and accidental injection of this bacterin into a human may cause a serious localized reaction. Seek expert medical attention immediately.

This product is non-returnable.

For veterinary use only.

Warning(s): Do not vaccinate within 42 days before slaughter.

Presentation: 1000 dose (500 mL) bottles.

Compendium Code No.: 11290161 214

MULTIMUNE® K5

Biomune **Bacterin**

Pasteurella Multocida Bacterin, Avian Isolates Types 1, 3, 4 and 3 x 4, Oil Emulsion

U.S. Vet. Lic. No.: 368

Contents: This bacterin contains five strains consisting of four serotypes of *Pasteurella multocida*, including two strains of serotype 3 x 4. The bacterin is emulsified in an oil adjuvant.

Indications: This bacterin is recommended for use in healthy chickens and turkeys as an aid in the prevention of fowl cholera caused by *Pasteurella multocida* type 1 in chickens and types 3, 4 and 3 x 4 in turkeys.

Dosage and Administration: Give 0.5 mL subcutaneously in the lower neck region in a direction away from the head and parallel with the neck. In turkeys, the injection site is in the feathered area of the neck. Do not inject into muscle tissue or neck vertebrae. Turkeys should be initially vaccinated at 18 weeks of age or older and chickens should be initially vaccinated at 12 weeks of age or older. Birds should be revaccinated 3 to 4 weeks later.

Precaution(s): The bacterin should be stored, transported and administered in accordance with the instructions and directions.

Do not freeze. Store in the dark at 35°-45°F (2°-7°C).

Warm to room temperature and shake well before and during use.

Use entire contents when first opened.

Caution(s): This product contains an oil based adjuvant and accidental injection of this bacterin into a human may cause a serious localized reaction. Seek expert medical attention immediately.

This product is non-returnable. For veterinary use only.

Warning(s): Do not vaccinate within 42 days before slaughter.

Presentation: 1000 doses (500 mL).

Compendium Code No.: 11290380 243

MULTIMUNE® M

Biomune **Vaccine**

Pasteurella Multocida Vaccine, Avirulent Live Culture, Avian Isolate

U.S. Vet. Lic. No.: 368

Active Ingredient(s): MULTIMUNE® M is a live bacterial vaccine containing the avirulent M-9 strain of *Pasteurella multocida* in a freeze-dried preparation. The M-9 strain has been shown to offer protection against naturally occurring field strains of *P. multocida*. The seed culture used to make the vaccine has been laboratory tested as required by the USDA for protection against challenge with *P. multocida* strains P-1059 (type 3) and P-1662 (type 4).

Indications: MULTIMUNE® M is recommended for use in healthy turkeys six weeks of age or older as an aid in preventing pasteurellosis (fowl cholera) due to *Pasteurella multocida* types 3 and 4.

Dosage and Administration: The contents of one vial of vaccine is administered to 1,000 turkeys by wing web stab (0.01 mL). The best results are obtained when the vaccine is administered initially to turkeys 6 to 12 weeks of age and repeated as needed according to current flock conditions. High disease challenge situations may require revaccination every 4 to 6 weeks.

Vaccinate healthy turkeys only. The initial vaccination should not be conducted in turkeys older than 12 weeks of age, as it may result in larger granulomas at the site of inoculation which may cause possible carcass downgrading at slaughter.

Rehydrate the vaccine vial with the entire contents of one (1) 10 mL vial of diluent (packaged separately) and mix well. Use the entire contents of one (1) 1,000 dose vial of vaccine within two (2) hours. Vaccinate by dipping the applicator needle into the rehydrated vaccine and piercing the webbed portion under the wing. Do not let the needle contact the feathers as they will absorb the vaccine preventing the turkey from receiving an adequate dose. Avoid piercing the wing muscle, bone or large blood vessels. Refill the needle between each vaccination by dipping the needle into the vial.

Usually there is not a clinical reaction to the vaccine. Vaccination sites should be examined five (5) to 10 days after vaccination for the presence of a reaction which is a small granuloma referred to as a vaccine "take". If a reaction is not seen, the birds may have already been immune or the vaccination may not have been properly conducted.

Precaution(s): Keep MULTIMUNE® M vaccine refrigerated until use. Store the vaccine between 35°-45°F (2°-7°C).

Caution(s): Turkeys to be vaccinated should not be given any antibiotic and/or sulfonamide medication for three days before and five days after vaccination to avoid interference with vaccine immunity. Avoid vaccination with live Newcastle vaccine two weeks before and two weeks after vaccination with MULTIMUNE® M.

Since MULTIMUNE® M is a live bacterial culture, caution should be used to avoid contact with open wounds or accidental inoculation of personnel. If accidental inoculation occurs, consult a physician immediately as the vaccine may act as a human pathogen. Vaccinating crew personnel must wash their hands after using the vaccine.

Use the entire contents of the vial when first opened. Burn all unused contents.

Warning(s): Do not vaccinate within 21 days before slaughter.

Presentation: 10 x 1,000 dose vials of vaccine/box and 10 x 10 mL vials of diluent with vaccine applicators/box.

Compendium Code No.: 11290181

MULTI-PAK/256

Alpharma **Large Animal Dietary Supplement**

Ingredient(s): Niacinamide, sodium bicarbonate, vitamin E supplement, ascorbic acid, potassium chloride, d-calcium pantothenic acid, vitamin A supplement, biotin supplement, citric acid, menadione sodium bisulfite complex, magnesium sulfate, B_{12} supplement, vitamin D_3 supplement, thiamine HCl, riboflavin, pyridoxine HCl, folic acid.

Guaranteed analysis per pound:

Vitamin A	16,000,000 IU
Vitamin D_3	5,000,000 IU
Vitamin E	25,000 IU
Vitamin B_{12}	50 mg
Riboflavin	7,200 mg
Niacinamide	80,809 mg
Pantothenic acid	35,000 mg
Menadione SBC	18,182 mg
Folic acid	2,000 mcg
Biotin	240 mg
Thiamine HCl	9,000 mg
Pyridoxine HCl	7,300 mg
Ascorbic acid	48,000 mg
Magnesium	0.573%
Potassium	4.40%

This product also contains citric acid and sodium bicarbonate.

Indications: MULTI-PAK/256 is for use in commercial layers, heavy breeders, turkeys and swine to ensure adequate intake of vitamins.

Dosage and Administration: To assure adequate intake of vitamins in commercial layers, heavy breeders, turkeys and swine: Use one 4 oz packet in 256 gallons (968 L) water, or one 4 oz packet in 2 gallons of stock solution. Do not mix in closed container.

Precaution(s): Store in cool, dry place.

Caution(s): For oral animal use only.

Not for human use. Keep out of reach of children.

Presentation: 4 oz (113.4 g) packages.

Compendium Code No.: 10220471 AHF-042 0005

MULTI-PURPOSE DISINFECTANT

LeGear **Disinfectant**

EPA Reg. No.: 2155-117-1910

Active Ingredient(s): Didecyl dimethyl ammonium chloride, N-alkyl (C_{14} 50%, C_{12} 40%, C_{16} 10%), dimethyl benzyl ammonium chloride.

Indications: A one-step disinfectant, germicide, deodorizer for barns, hog houses, equine and dairy quarters, poultry farms, pet shops, kennels, veterinary clinics, meat and poultry establishments.

Dosage and Administration: Mix 1 oz. per gallon of water for use on floors, walls, porcelain, metal and plastic surfaces.

Presentation: Available in 1 quart bottles and 1 gallon containers.

Compendium Code No.: 11530020

MULTI-QUAT 128

Intercon **Disinfectant**

One Step Germicidal Detergent and Deodorant-Disinfectant-Bactericidal-Pseudomonacidal-Staphylocidal-Salmonellacidal-Fungicidal-*Virucidal

EPA Reg. No.: 47371-130-48211

Active Ingredient(s):

Didecyl dimethyl ammonium chloride	4.61%
n-Alkyl (C_{14}, 50%; C_{12}, 40%; C_{16}, 10%) dimethyl benzyl ammonium chloride	3.07%
Inert Ingredients	92.32%

Indications: A multi-purpose, neutral pH, germicidal detergent and deodorant effective in hard water up to 400 ppm (calculated as $CaCO_3$) in the presence of a moderate amount of soil (5% organic serum) according to the AOAC Use Dilution Test.

Disinfects, cleans, and deodorizes in one labor saving step. Effective against the following pathogens: *Pseudomonas aeruginosa*[1], *Staphylococcus aureus*[1], *Salmonella choleraesuis, Acinetobacter calcoaceticus, Bordetella bronchiseptica, Chlamydia psittaci, Enterobacter aerogenes, Enterobacter cloacae, Escherichia coli*[1], *Fusobacterium necrophorum, Klebsellia pneumonae*[1], *Legionella pneumophile, Listeria monocytogenes, Pasteurella multocida, Proteus miribilis, Proteus vulgaris, Salmonella enteritidis, Salmonella typhi, Salmonella typhimurium, Serratia marcescens, Shigella flexneri, Shigella sonnei, Staphylococcus aureus* (methicillin resistant), *Staphylococcus epidermidae*[2], *Streptococcus faecalis*[1], *Streptococcus pyogenes, Enterococcus faecalis* (Vancomycin Resistant), *Adenovirus type 4, *Avian polyomavirus, *Canine distemper, *Feline leukemia, *Feline picornavirus, *Herpes simplex Type 1, *Herpes simplex Type 2, *HIV-1 (AIDS virus), *Infectious bovine rhinotracheitis, *Infectious bronchitis (Avian IBV), *Influenza A/Hong Kong, *Pseudorabies, *Rabies, *Respiratory syncytial virus (RSV), *Rubella (German Measles), *Transmissible gastroenteritis virus (TGE), *Vaccinia, *Aspergillus niger, Candida albicans, Trichophyton metagrophytes.*

[1]ATCC and antibiotic-resistant strain

[2]antibiotic-resistant strain only

Recommended for use in hospitals, nursing homes, schools and colleges, commercial and industrial institutions, office buildings, veterinary clinics and animal life science laboratories, federally inspected meat and poultry establishments, equine farms, tack shops, pet shops, airports, kennels, hotels and motels, poultry and turkey farms, dairy farms and hog farms, breeding and grooming establishments. Disinfects, cleans, and deodorizes floors, walls, metal surfaces, stainless steel surfaces, glazed porcelain, plastic surfaces (such as polypropylene, polystyrene, etc.) and other hard, non-porous surfaces.

Directions for Use: Dilution: 1:128 (600 ppm quat) 1 ounce per gallon of water.

It is a violation of Federal Law to use this product in a manner inconsistent with its labeling.

This product is not to be used as a terminal sterilant/high level disinfectant on any surface or instrument that (1) is introduced directly into the human body, either into or in contact with the bloodstream or normally sterile areas of the body, or (2) contacts intact mucous membranes but which does not ordinarily penetrate the blood barrier or otherwise enter normally sterile areas of the body. This product may be used to preclean or decontaminate critical or semi-critical devices prior to sterilization or high-level disinfection.

Application: Remove heavy soil deposits from surface. Then thoroughly wet surfaces with a solution of 1 ounce of the concentrate per gallon of water. The solution can be applied with a cloth, mop, sponge, or coarse spray, or soaking. Let solution remain on surface for a minimum of 10 minutes. Rinse or allow to air dry. Rinsing of floors is not necessary unless they are to be waxed or polished. Prepare a fresh solution daily or more often if the solution becomes visibly dirty or diluted.

Mildewstatic Instructions: Will effectively control the growth of mold and mildew plus odors caused by them when applied to hard, non-porous surfaces such as walls, floors, and table tops. Apply solution (1 ounce per gallon of water) with a cloth, mop, sponge, or coarse spray. Make sure to wet all surfaces completely. Let air dry. Repeat application weekly or when growth reappears.

*Kills HIV on precleaned, environmental surfaces/objects previously soiled with blood/body fluids in health care settings or other settings in which there is an expected likelihood of soiling of inanimate surfaces/objects with blood/body fluids, and which the surfaces/objects likely to be soiled with blood/body fluids can be associated with the potential for transmission of Human Immunodeficiency virus Type 1 (HIV-1) (associated with AIDS).

"Special Instructions for Cleaning and Decontamination Against HIV-1 (AIDS Virus) of Surfaces/Objects Soiled with Blood/Body Fluids."

Personal Protection: Disposable latex or vinyl gloves, gowns, face masks, or eye coverings as appropriate must be worn during all cleaning of blood/body fluids and during decontamination procedures.

Cleaning Procedure: Blood/body fluids must be thoroughly cleaned from surface/objects before application of disinfectant.

Contact Time: HIV-1 (AIDS virus) is inactivated after a contact time of 4 minutes at 25°C (room temperature). Use a 10-minute contact time for other viruses, fungi, and bacteria listed.

Disposal of Infectious Materials: Blood/body fluids should be autoclaved and disposed of according to federal, state, and local regulations for infectious waste disposal.

Precautionary Statements: Hazards to Humans and Domestic Animals:

Danger. Corrosive: Causes eye damage and severe skin irritation. Harmful if swallowed. Do not get in eyes, on skin, or on clothing. When handling product, protect eyes by wearing goggles or face shield and protect skin by wearing rubber gloves. Wash thoroughly with soap and water after handling. Remove contaminated clothing and wash before reuse.

Statement of Practical Treatment: In case of contact, immediately flush eyes or skin with plenty of water for at least 15 minutes. For eyes, call a physician. If swallowed, immediately drink a large quantity of water. Avoid alcohol. Get medical attention.

Note to Physician: Probable mucosal damage may contraindicate the use of gastric lavage. Measures against circulatory shock, respiratory depression and convulsion may be needed.

Storage and Disposal: Keep product under locked storage, inaccessible to children. Do not contaminate water, food, or feed by storage or disposal. Open dumping is prohibited. Do not reuse empty container.

Pesticide Disposal: Pesticide wastes are acutely hazardous. Improper disposal of excess pesticide, spray mixture, or rinsate is a violation of Federal Law. If these wastes cannot be disposed of by use according to label instructions, contact your State Pesticide or Environmental Control Agency, or the Hazardous Waste Representative at the nearest EPA Regional Office for guidance.

Container Disposal: Do not reuse empty container. Rinse thoroughly, securely wrap in several layers of newspaper, and discard empty container in trash.

Warning(s): Keep out of reach of children.

Presentation: 4x1 gallon (3.78 L), 5 gallon pails and 55 gallon drums.

Compendium Code No.: 10130040

MULTI QUAT TB™

Intercon **Disinfectant**

Tuberculocidal, Disinfectant, *Virucide, Fungicide (against pathogenic fungi), Mildewstat (on hard, inanimate surfaces), Cleaner, Deodorizer

EPA Reg. No.: 1839-83-48211

Active Ingredient(s):

n-Alkyl (60% C_{14}; 30% C_{16}; 5% C_{12}, 5% C_{18}) dimethyl benzyl ammonium chlorides	0.105%
n-Alkyl (68% C_{12}; 32% C_{14}) dimethyl ethylbenzyl ammonium chlorides	0.105%
Inert Ingredients	99.790%
Total	100.000%

Indications: This product is designed specifically as a general non-acid cleaner and disinfectant for use in hospitals, nursing homes, schools, hotels and restaurants. It is formulated to disinfect hard, non-porous, inanimate environmental surfaces such as floors, walls, metal surfaces, stainless steel surfaces, porcelain, glazed ceramic tile, plastic surfaces, bathrooms, shower stalls, bathtubs, and cabinets. May be used in the kitchen on counters, sinks, appliances and stove tops. A rinse with potable water is required for surfaces in direct contact with food. In addition, this product deodorizes those areas which generally are hard to keep fresh smelling, such as garbage storage areas, empty garbage bins and cans, basements, restrooms and other areas which are prone to odors caused by microorganisms.

Tuberculocidal Activity - This product exhibits disinfectant efficacy against *Mycobacterium tuberculosis* (BCG) in 10 minutes at 20 degrees Centigrade when used as directed on previously cleaned hard non-porous inanimate surfaces.

Bactericidal Activity - When used as directed, this product exhibits effective disinfectant activity against the organisms: *Staphylococcus aureus, Salmonella choleraesuis, Pseudomonas aeruginosa, Escherichia coli* 0157:H7, and meets the requirements for hospital use.

*Virucidal Activity - This product, when used on environmental, inanimate, non-porous surfaces, exhibits effective virucidal activity against HIV-1 (associated with AIDS) and Canine Parvovirus.

Fungicidal Activity - This product is fungicidal against the pathogenic fungi, *Trichophyton mentagrophytes* (Athletes Foot Fungus) when used as directed on hard surfaces found in bathrooms, shower stalls, locker rooms, or other clean, non-porous, hard surfaces commonly contacted by bare feet.

Efficacy tests have demonstrated that this product is an effective bactericide, fungicide, and virucide in the presence of organic soil (5% blood serum).

Directions for Use: It is a violation of Federal Law to use this product in a manner inconsistent with its labeling.

Disinfection, Deodorizing and Cleaning - Remove gross filth or heavy soil prior to application of the product. Hold container six to eight inches from surface to be treated. Spray area until it is covered with the solution. Allow product to penetrate and remain wet for 10 minutes. No scrubbing is necessary. Wipe off with a clean cloth, mop or sponge. The product will not leave grit or soap scum.

Kills HIV on pre-cleaned environmental surfaces/objects previously soiled with blood/body fluids in health care settings (hospitals, nursing homes) or other settings in which there is an expected likelihood of soiling of inanimate surfaces/objects with blood or body fluids, and in which the surfaces/objects likely to be soiled with blood or body fluids can be associated with the potential for transmission of Human Immunodeficiency Virus Type 1 (HIV-1) (associated with AIDS).

Special Instructions for Cleaning and Decontamination Against HIV-1 of Surfaces/Objects Soiled with Blood/Body Fluids.

Personal Protection: When handling items soiled with blood or body fluids use disposable latex gloves, gowns, masks, or eye coverings.

Cleaning Procedures: Blood and other body fluids must be thoroughly cleaned from surfaces and objects before application of this product.

Contact Time: Allow surface to remain wet for 10 minutes.

Disposal of Infectious Materials: Blood and other body fluids should be autoclaved and disposed of according to local regulations for infectious waste disposal.

Mildewstat - To control mold and mildew on pre-cleaned, hard, non-porous surfaces spray surface to be treated making sure to wet completely. Let air dry. Repeat application at weekly intervals or when mildew growth appears.

Precautionary Statements:

Hazards to Humans and Domestic Animals: Causes eye and skin irritation. Do not get in eyes, on skin or on clothing. Harmful if swallowed. Avoid contamination of food. Remove contaminated clothing and wash before reuse. Wash thoroughly with soap and water after handling.

Statement of Practical Treatment:

In case of contact, immediately flush eyes or skin with plenty of water for at least 15 minutes. For eyes, call a physician.

If swallowed, drink egg whites or gelatin solution, or if these are not available, drink large quantities of water. Call a physician immediately.

Note to Physician: Probable mucosal damage may contraindicate the use of gastric lavage.

Storage and Disposal: Do not contaminate water, food or feed by storage or disposal.

Container Disposal - Do not reuse container (bottle, can or jar). Rinse thoroughly before discarding in trash.

Storage - Store in a dry place no lower in temperature than 50°F or higher than 120°F.

Warning(s): Keep out of reach of children.

Presentation: 4x1 gallon (3.78 L) containers and 12 qt. cases.

Compendium Code No.: 10130030

M

MULTI SERUM

Durvet **Antibodies**

Actinomyces Pyogenes-Escherichia Coli-Pasturella Haemolytica-Multocida-Salmonella Typhimurium Antibody, Bovine Origin

U.S. Vet. Lic. No.: 303

Composition: This product is prepared from the blood of cattle hyperimmunized with *Actinomyces pyogenes, Escherichia coli, Pasteurella haemolytica, Pasteurella multocida,* and *Salmonella typhimurium.* Contains phenol and thimerosal as preservatives.

Indications: For use as an aid in the prevention and treatment of enteric and respiratory conditions in cattle and sheep caused by *Actinomyces pyogenes, Escherichia coli, Pasteurella haemolytica, Pasteurella multocida,* and *Salmonella typhimurium.*

Dosage and Administration: Shake well before using. Administer the following dosage intramuscularly or subcutaneously.

	Prevention	Treatment
Calves (as soon after birth as possible)	20-40 mL	40-100 mL
Cattle	50-75 mL	75-150 mL
Sheep	10-15 mL	20-40 mL

The recommended dose for treatment is to be administered at 12-24 hour intervals until improvement is noted.

Precaution(s): Store in the dark at 35°- 45°F (2°-7°C). Do not freeze. Use entire contents when first opened.

Caution(s): Anaphylactic reactions may occur following the use of this biological. Symptomatic treatment: Epinephrine.

Warning(s): Do not administer within 21 days prior to slaughter.

Presentation: 250 mL.

Manufactured by: Advance Biologics, Inc., Freeman, SD 57029

Compendium Code No.: 10841860 DV 214

MU-SE® ℞

Schering-Plough **Vitamin E-Selenium**

(Selenium, Vitamin E) Injection-Veterinary

NADA No.: 030-314

Active Ingredient(s): MU-SE® (selenium, vitamin E) is an emulsion of selenium-tocopherol. Each mL contains: 10.95 mg sodium selenite (equivalent to 5 mg selenium), 50 mg (68 USP units) vitamin E (as d-alpha tocopheryl acetate), 250 mg polysorbate 80, 2% benzyl alcohol (preservative), water for injection q.s. Sodium hydroxide and/or hydrochloric acid may be added to adjust pH.

Indications: MU-SE® (selenium, vitamin E) is recommended for the prevention and treatment of STD syndrome in weanling calves and breeding beef cows. Clinical signs are: Stiffness and lameness, chronic persistent diarrhea, unthriftiness, abortions and/or weak premature calves.

Pharmacology: Actions: It has been demonstrated that selenium and tocopherol exert physiological effects and that these effects are intertwined with sulfur metabolism. Additionally, tocopherol appears to have a significant role in the oxidation process, thus suggesting an interrelationship between selenium and tocopherol in overcoming sulfur-induced depletion and restoring normal metabolism. Although oral ingestion of adequate amounts of selenium and tocopherol would seemingly restore normal metabolism, it is apparent that the presence of sulfur and, perhaps other factors interfere during the digestive process with the proper utilization of selenium and tocopherol. When selenium and tocopherol are injected, they bypass the digestive process and exert their full metabolic effects promptly on cell metabolism. Anti-inflammatory action has been demonstrated by selenium-tocopherol in the Selye Pouch Technique and experimentally induced polyarthritis study in rats.

Dosage and Administration: Inject subcutaneously or intramuscularly.

Weanling Calves: 1 mL per 200 pounds of body weight.

Breeding Beef Cows: 1 mL per 200 pounds of body weight during the middle third of pregnancy, and 30 days before calving.

Contraindication(s): Do not use in adult dairy cattle. Premature births and abortions have been reported in dairy cattle injected with this product during the third trimester of pregnancy.

Precaution(s): Storage: Store between 2° and 30°C (36° and 86°F). Protect from freezing.

Caution(s): Federal law restricts this drug to use by or on the order of a licensed veterinarian.

Selenium-Tocopherol Deficiency (STD) syndrome produces a variety and complexity of symptoms often interfering with a proper diagnosis. Even in selenium deficient areas there are other disease conditions which produce similar clinical signs. It is imperative that all these conditions be carefully considered prior to the treatment of STD syndrome. Selenium levels, elevated SGOT, and creatine serum levels may serve as aids in arriving at a diagnosis of STD, when associated with other indices.

Important: Use only the selenium-tocopherol product recommended for each species. Each formulation is designed for the species indicated to produce the maximum efficacy and safety.

Selenium is toxic if administered in excess. A fixed dose schedule is therefore important (read package insert for each selenium-tocopherol product carefully before using).

Anaphylactoid reactions, some of which have been fatal, have been reported in cattle administered the MU-SE® product. Signs include excitement, sweating, trembling, ataxia, respiratory distress, and cardiac dysfunction.

For veterinary use only.

Warning(s): Use only as directed in weanling calves and breeding beef cows. Discontinue use 30 days before the treated cattle are slaughtered for human consumption.

Presentation: 100 mL sterile, multiple dose vial (NDC 0061-0950-04).

Compendium Code No.: 10471311 Rev. 10/98

MVT™ BOLUS WET GRANULATION FORMULA

Butler **Antacid-Laxative**

NDC No.: 11695-4131-3

Active Ingredient(s): Each bolus contains:

Magnesium Oxide .... 276 gr (17.9 g)

(Equiv. to Magnesium Hydroxide, 400 gr).

Flavored with ginger, capsicum and methyl salicylate, artificial color added.

One and one-half MVT™ boluss are equivalent to one pint of milk of magnesia.

Indications: For oral administration to ruminants as an aid in the treatment of digestive disturbances requiring an antacid and mild laxative.

Dosage and Administration: Give 2 to 4 boluses to ruminants, depending on size and condition of animal. Lubricate boluses and administer with a balling gun.

Precaution(s): Store at controlled temperature between 15° and 30°C (59°-86°F).

Keep tightly closed when not in use.

Caution(s): Avoid frequent or continued use.

Warning(s): For animal use only.

Keep out of the reach of children.

Presentation: 50 boluses.

Compendium Code No.: 10821190

MVT POWDER™

Butler **Antacid-Laxative**

Active Ingredient(s): Each pound contains:

Magnesium hydroxide............ 10.4 oz.

Kaolin .... 5.5 oz.

Flavored with capiscum, ginger and methyl salicylate. Artificial color added.

One pound of MVT POWDER™ contains magnesium hydroxide equivalent to one gallon of milk of magnesia.

Indications: For oral administration to ruminants as an aid in the treatment of digestive disturbances requiring an antacid, mild laxative and adsorbent.

Dosage and Administration: Mix one (1) pound of MVT POWDER™ into one (1) gallon of water and stir thoroughly. Shake well before using. Administer with a stomach tube or as a drench.

Cattle: One (1) gallon of mixture.

Sheep and Calves: One (1) pint to one (1) quart of mixture, depending upon the size of the animal.

Precaution(s): Avoid frequent or continued use.

Store in a cool, dry place.

Keep the lid tightly closed when not in use.

Caution(s): Not for human use.

Keep out of the reach of children.

Warning(s): Milk that has been taken from animals during treatment and for 24 hours (2 milkings) after the last treatment with this drug must not be used for food.

Presentation: 1 lb. and 25 lb. containers.

Compendium Code No.: 10821180

MYCASEPTIC®

Neogen **Disinfectant**

Active Ingredient(s): Limonene, B-Ionone.

Indications: For use as a disinfectant.

Directions for Use: Use in conjunction with debridement for hoof disinfection in cattle (including dairy cattle), horses and sheep. Spray area until saturated. Disinfection may continue daily until no longer needed. Shake well before using.

Precaution(s): Store at room temperature. Product is flammable.

Caution(s): Avoid eye and skin contact. Use only with sprayer attached.

For veterinary use only.

Warning(s): For external use. Wash hands after handling. Keep out of reach of children.

Presentation: 460 mL (NDC: 59051-8895-0).

Compendium Code No.: 14910372 696-0401

MYCASEPTIC® E

Neogen **Disinfectant**

Ingredient(s): Limonene, B-Ionone.

Indications: For use as a disinfectant. MYCASEPTIC® E is a natural hoof disinfectant spray.

Directions for Use: Shake well before use. Use in conjunction with debridement for hoof disinfection in horses, sheep, and cattle (including dairy cattle). Spray hoof daily or based upon severity of condition. Spray hoof until saturated. Turn sprayer to off position when not in use.

Precaution(s): Store at room temperature. Product is flammable.

Caution(s): Do not spray above coronet band. Avoid eye and skin contact. May irritate skin. Use only with sprayer attached.

For veterinary use only.

For external use only.

Warning(s): Wash hands after handling. Keep out of reach of children.

Presentation: 460 mL (15.3 oz).

Compendium Code No.: 14910510 L416-0501

MYCITRACIN® STERILE OINTMENT ℞

Pharmacia & Upjohn **Ophthalmic Antibiotic**

brand of bacitracin, polymyxin B sulfate and neomycin sulfate-sterile ointment

Active Ingredient(s): Description: Each gram contains Bacitracin Zinc 400 units, Neomycin Sulfate 5 mg (equivalent to 3.5 mg of Neomycin Base), Polymyxin B Sulfate 10,000 units, in a base of White Petrolatum and Mineral Oil.

Indications: In the treatment of superficial bacterial infections of the eyelid and conjunctiva in dogs and cats when due to organisms susceptible to the antibiotics contained in the ointment. Laboratory tests should be conducted including *in vitro* culturing and susceptibility tests on samples collected prior to treatment.

Pharmacology: Actions: The three antibiotics present in MYCITRACIN® Sterile Ointment provide a broad spectrum of activity against the gram-positive and gram-negative bacteria commonly involved in superficial infections of the eyelid and conjunctiva. Bacitracin is effective against gram-positive bacteria including hemolytic and non-hemolytic Streptococci and Staphylococci. Resistant strains rarely develop. Neomycin is effective against both gram-positive and gram-negative bacteria including *Staphylococci, Escherichia coli,* and *Haemophilus influenzae* and many strains of Proteus and Pseudomonas. Polymyxin B is bactericidal to gram-negative bacteria especially Pseudomonas. No resistant strains have been found to develop *in vivo.*

Dosage and Administration: Apply a thin film over the cornea three or four times daily in dogs and cats. The area should be properly cleansed prior to the use of MYCITRACIN® Sterile Ointment. Foreign bodies, crusted exudates and debris should be carefully removed.

Precaution(s): Store at room temperature.

Caution(s): Federal (USA) law restricts this drug to use by or on the order of a licensed veterinarian.

Sensitivity to MYCITRACIN® Sterile Ointment is rare; however, if a reaction occurs, discontinue use of the preparation. As with any antibiotic preparation, prolonged use may result in the overgrowth of nonsusceptible organisms including fungi. Appropriate measures should be taken if this occurs. If infection does not respond to treatment in two or three days, the diagnosis and therapy should be reevaluated.

Care should be taken not to contaminate the applicator tip of the tube during application of the preparation. Do not allow the applicator tip to come in contact with any tissue.

Do not use this product as a pre-surgical ocular lubricant.

Adverse reactions of ocular irritation and corneal ulceration have been reported in association with such use.

Adverse Reactions: Itching, burning or inflammation may occur in animals sensitive to the product. Discontinue use in such cases.

Presentation: MYCITRACIN® Sterile Ointment is available in 3.5 gram tubes (NDC 0009-3354-02).

Manufactured by: Altana Inc., Melville, NY 11747.

Compendium Code No.: 10490351 812 553 303

MYCOBACTIN J

Allied Monitor **Mycobacterium Growth Factor**

Active Ingredient(s): MYCOBACTIN J is an iron chelated cell extract.

Indications: MYCOBACTIN J is for use in media as a growth promoter for the isolation of *Mycobacterium* sp. Incorporation of MYCOBACTIN J into culture medium reduces the period of cultivation of approximately six to eight weeks for *Mycobacterium paratuberculosis*, and enhances the growth of strains of fastidious mycobacteria which otherwise could not be isolated.

Dosage and Administration:

MYCOBACTIN J[1] Reconstitution and Use: MYCOBACTIN J is shipped in dry form. It is highly soluble in 95% ethyl alcohol (ETOH). The dry product is shipped in heavy-walled containers in 2 mg, 100 mg, 200 mg, and 1,000 mg sizes. The weight of mycobactin contained in each vial is clearly indicated on the label. MYCOBACTIN J in dry form remains effective for an indefinite period.

Bottling MYCOBACTIN J is not a sterile process. Airborne contaminants are killed by the alcohol and heat treatment of the medium to which the mycobactin is added.

MYCOBACTIN J is equivalent to MYCOBACTIN J, lot MB-2 (control obtained from Dr. R.S. Merkel of the National Animal Disease Center, Ames Iowa USA) as a supplement for laboratory culture media for the growth of *Mycobacterium paratuberculosis* isolated in primary culture from feces from a paratuberculous bovine. Tested at a concentration of 2.0 mg per liter of Herrold's egg yolk culture medium, incubated at 37°C.

To reconstitute dry mycobactin, add ETOH to the vial (e.g. 4 mL to mg of product) and allow to dissolve 2 mg is sufficient for supplementing 1 L of Herrold's egg yolk culture medium[2] for isolation of *Mycobacterium paratuberculosis*.[3]

1. Flush down the inner sidewalls when ETOH is added.
2. Pour the mycobactin solution directly into the medium being prepared, not down the inner glass wall.
3. Identify slants containing MYCOBACTIN J, the mycobactin does not impart any color or other quality to distinguish it from mycobactin-free medium.
4. 2 mg is sufficient for supplementing 1 L of culture medium[2] for the isolation of *M. paratuberculosis*.[3]
5. Avoid pH levels above 8.

References: Available upon request.

Presentation: 2 mg, 100 mg, 200 mg, and 1,000 mg containers.

Compendium Code No.: 10800031

MYCODEX® ALL-IN-ONE™ SPRAY

V.P.L. **Flea Control & Topical Parasiticide**

EPA Reg. No.: 37425-44

Active Ingredient(s):

Pyrethrins	0.15%
Nylar® 2-[1-Methyl-2-(4-phenoxyphenoxy) ethoxy] pyridine	0.15%
Piperonyl butoxide, technical*	1.50%
N-Octyl bicycloheptene dicarboximide	0.50%
Inert ingredients**	97.70%
Total	100.00%

*Equivalent to 1.20% butylcarbityl (6-propylpiperonyl) ether and .30% related compounds.

**Inert ingredients include grooming additives to ease combing and brushing of the coat to remove dead fleas and ticks.

Indications: Insecticide, insect growth regulator, waterproofing agent and repellent for use on dogs, cats, nursing puppies and kittens.

Directions for Use: It is a violation of Federal law to use this product in a manner inconsistent with its labeling.

Use only in a well ventilated area.

Dogs and Cats: To prevent harm to you or your pet, read entire label before use. Consult your veterinarian before using this product on pregnant or lactating females, old, sick, or debilitated animals, or on animals undergoing drug or other pesticide treatment. Cover animal's eyes with hand and with a firm, fast stroke to get a proper spray mist, spray head, ears and chest until damp. With fingertips, rub into face around mouth, nose and eyes. Then spray neck, middle and hindquarters, finishing legs last. For best penetration of spray to the skin, direct spray against the natural lay of the hair. On long-haired dogs, rub your hand against the lay of the hair, spraying the ruffled hair directly behind the hand. Make sure spray thoroughly wets ticks. Repeat treatment as needed.

Nursing Puppies and Kittens: Avoid treatment of pets under 12 weeks of age. If treatment is necessary, spray only along pet's back or on your fingertips and massage into fur.

Precautionary Statements: Warning: Hazards to Humans and Domestic Animals:

Human: Causes substantial but temporary eye injury. Harmful if swallowed or absorbed through skin. Do not get in eyes or on clothing. Avoid contact with skin. Wash thoroughly with soap and water after handling. Remove contaminated clothing and wash before reuse.

Animal: Avoid treatment of nursing puppies and kittens. If treatment is necessary, consult your veterinarian. Do not oversaturate, especially on cats. Avoid spraying of genital areas. Use of this product is contraindicated in animals with known liver disease. Some animals may be sensitive to ingredients in this product. Following treatment observe your pet for possible signs of sensitivity or adverse reactions to the product, such as non-formed feces, tremors, hyperactivity, excessive salivation, gastrointestinal disorders, decreased or no food consumption, body weight loss, or reduced body weight gain.

Statement of Practical Treatment:

If in Eyes: Call physician. Flush eyes with gentle stream of water for 15 minutes.

If Swallowed: Call physician or Poison Control Center. Drink promptly a large quantity of milk, egg white, or gelatin mixture, or if these are unavailable a large quantity of water.

If on Skin: Wash with plenty of soap and water. Get medical attention.

If animal has adverse effects after the use of this product, discontinue use and immediately seek veterinary advice.

Environmental Hazards: This product is toxic to fish. Do not add directly to water. Do not apply where runoff is likely to occur.

Physical or Chemical Hazards: Flammable. Keep away from heat and open flame. Contains alcohol. Do not apply to painted or finished wood surfaces.

Storage and Disposal: Storage: Store in a cool, dry area away from heat and open flame.

Disposal: Do not reuse container. Rinse thoroughly and wrap container in several layers of newspaper and discard in trash.

Warning(s): Keep out of reach of children.

Presentation: 16 oz plastic bottle with trigger sprayer.

Nylar is a registered trademark of McLaughlin, Gormley, King Co.

Compendium Code No.: 11430171

MYCODEX® ENVIRONMENTAL CONTROL™ AEROSOL HOUSEHOLD SPRAY

V.P.L. **Premise Insecticide**

EPA Reg. No.: 37425-38

Active Ingredient(s):

2-[1-Methyl-2-(4-phenoxyphenoxy) ethoxy] pyridine	0.015%
Tetramethrin [(1-Cyclohexene-1,2-dicarboximido) methyl 2,2-dimethyl-3-(2 methylpropenyl) cyclopropanecarboxylate]	0.400%
3-Phenoxybenzyl-(1RS, 3RS: 1RS, 3SR)-2,2-dimethyl-3-(2-methylprop-1-enyl) cyclopropanecarboxylate	0.300%
Inert Ingredients	99.285%
Total	100.000%

Indications: A ready-for-use, water-based aerosol household spray that contains adulticides for quick kill and rapid knockdown of adult fleas and an IGR to kill immature fleas for 120 days.

Directions for Use: It is a violation of Federal law to use this product in a manner inconsistent with its labelling.

For indoor use only.

Fleas and Ticks: Shake Well. Hold can 2 or 3 feet from surfaces to be treated. Be sure to apply uniformly using a sweeping motion to carpets, rugs, drapes and all surfaces of upholstered furniture. Be sure to treat pet bedding as this is a primary hiding place for fleas. No need to remove pet bedding after treatment. Do not treat pets. Use a registered Mycodex® product for flea and tick control on your pets in conjunction with this treatment. Retreat as necessary. Avoid wetting furniture and carpeting. A fine mist or spray applied uniformly is all that is necessary to kill fleas and ticks.

Precautionary Statements: Hazards to Humans and Domestic Animals:

Caution: Harmful if swallowed or absorbed through skin. Contains petroleum distillate. Do not induce vomiting because of aspiration pneumonia hazard. Do not breathe vapors or spray mist. Avoid contact with skin or eyes. In case of contact, flush with water. Wash with soap and water after use. Obtain medical attention if irritation persists. Avoid contamination of food.

Do not use in commercial food processing, preparation, food storage or serving areas. In the home, all food processing surfaces and utensils should be covered during treatment, or thoroughly washed before use. Exposed food should be covered or removed. Remove pets, birds, and cover fish aquariums before spraying.

Physical or Chemical Hazards: Contents under pressure. Keep away from heat, sparks and open flame. Do not puncture or incinerate container. Exposure to temperatures above 130°F may cause bursting.

Statement Of Practical Treatment:

If swallowed: Call a physician or Poison Control Center immediately. Do not induce vomiting because of aspiration pneumonia hazard.

If in eyes: Flush with water. Get medical attention if irritation persists.

If on skin or clothing: Remove contaminated clothing and wash before reuse. Wash skin with soap and warm water. Get medical attention if irritation persists.

If inhaled: Remove victim to fresh air. Apply artificial respiration if indicated.

Storage and Disposal:

Storage: Store in cool, dry place. Keep container closed.

Disposal: Do not reuse container. Wrap container in several layers of newspaper and discard in trash.

Warning(s): Keep out of the reach of children. For external use only.

This product is restricted for sale exclusively through veterinary clinics, practices and hospitals.

Presentation: Available in 16 oz, hand-held can.

Compendium Code No.: 11430180

MYCODEX® ENVIRONMENTAL CONTROL™ AEROSOL ROOM FOGGER

V.P.L. **Premise Insecticide**

EPA Reg. No.: 37425-37

Active Ingredient(s):

2-[1-Methyl-2-(4-phenoxyphenoxy) ethoxy] pyridine	0.100%
Pyrethrins	0.050%
*N-Octyl bicycloheptenedicarboximide	0.400%
Permethrin [**(3-Phenoxyphenyl) methyl ± cis, trans-3-(2,2-dichloroethenyl) 2,2-dimethylcyclopropanecarboxylate]	0.400%
Related compounds	0.035%
Inert Ingredients	99.015%
Total	100.000%

*MGK® 264, Insecticide Synergist

**cis-trans isomer ratio: Min. 25% ± cis Max 65% ± trans

Indications: A ready-for-use, water-based automatic room fogger that contains adulticides to kill adult and preadult fleas, and an IGR to kill larval fleas and flea eggs for 210 days.

Directions for Use: It is a violation of Federal law to use this product in a manner inconsistent with its labelling.

Shake well before use.

Keep container upright.

This product will kill ants, cockroaches, crickets, fleas, houseflies, mosquitos, rice weevils, saw-toothed grain beetles, small flying moths, and ticks. It will also prevent preadult fleas from developing into the adult biting stage up to 210 days. Cover exposed food, dishes and food-handling equipment. Open cabinets and doors of area to be treated. Shut off fans and air conditioners. Put out all flames and pilot lights. Close doors and windows. Point valve opening away from face and eyes when releasing. Use one unit for each 6,000 cubic feet of unobstructed area. Use additional units for remote rooms or where free flow of mist is not assured. Do not remain in the area during treatment and ventilate thoroughly before re-entry.

M

To Operate Valve: To lock valve in open position for automatic discharge, press the valve button all the way down, hooking the catch. Then place fogger on stand or table in the center of the room with valve locked open, placing several layers of newspaper or pad under fogger. Leave building at once and keep building closed for two hours before airing out. Open all doors and windows and allow to air for 30 minutes. Repeat spraying in two weeks or when necessary.

Precautionary Statements: Hazards to Humans and Domestic Animals:

Caution: Harmful if swallowed or absorbed through skin. Do not breathe vapors or spray mist. Avoid contact with skin or eyes. In case of contact, flush with water. Wash with soap and water after use. Obtain medical attention if irritation persists. Avoid contamination of food.

Statement of Practical Treatment:

If Swallowed: Call a physician or Poison Control Center immediately.

If in Eyes: Flush with water. Get medical attention if irritation persists.

If on Skin or Clothing: Remove contaminated clothing and wash before reuse. Wash skin with soap and warm water. Get medical attention if irritation persists.

If Inhaled: Remove victim to fresh air if effects occur and call a physician.

Environmental Hazards: Do not contaminate water when disposing of equipment washwaters.

Physical or Chemical Hazards: Contents under pressure. Keep away from heat, sparks and open flame. Do not puncture or incinerate container. Exposure to temperatures above 130°F may cause bursting. Extremely flammable.

Storage and Disposal:

Storage: Store in cool, dry area away from heat or open flame.

Disposal: Replace cap and discard container in trash. Do not incinerate or puncture.

Warning(s): Keep out of the reach of children. For external use only.

This product is restricted for sale exclusively through veterinary clinics, practices and hospitals.

Presentation: Available in 6 oz one-time use can.

Compendium Code No.: 11430190

MYCODEX® ODOR NEUTRALIZER

V.P.L. **Deodorant Product**

Indications: Removes unwanted odors associated with cats, dogs and other household pets.

Will not harm clothes, fabrics, upholstery or furniture.

MYCODEX® Odor Neutralizer doesn't just cover pet odor. It eliminates odors in pet bedding, carpets, rugs, upholstered furniture and other areas frequented by pets - even the toughest odors such as urine, feces, vomit and anal glands. If you normally avoid using fragrant products around your birds, carefully test this product prior to use.

Water-based. Leaves a fresh, clean scent.

Directions for Use: Turn sprayer nozzle to the "On" position and spray evenly until slightly damp. For anal gland use, spray a towel until slightly damp. Apply over animal's anal area. For fabrics and upholstery, test spray first in an inconspicuous spot as some fibers may be adversely affected by any liquid product. Strong odors may require additional applications. Repeat as necessary. Do not spray directly toward face. Always use in a well ventilated area.

Caution(s): MYCODEX® Odor Neutralizer will not damage clothes, fabrics, upholstery or furniture. However, it is not recommended for silk or suede. Always test fabrics for colorfastness or watermarking.

Warning(s): Keep out of reach of children. For eye contact, flush with clear running water for 15 minutes. If irritation persists, consult with a physician. Seek fresh air if needed.

Presentation: 24 oz spray.

Compendium Code No.: 11430470 01-1631

M

MYCODEX® PEARLESCENT GROOMING SHAMPOO

V.P.L. **Grooming Shampoo**

Ingredients:

Ingredient	
Polymer JR-400 (polyquaternium-10)	0.25%
Sodium Lauryl Sulfate Solution*	29.00%
Ethylene Glycol Monostearate	1.00%
Polyoxyethylene Lanolins	0.50%
Lauric-Linoleic Diethanolamide	6.00%
Color, fragrance, other trace elements	—
Water	q.s.

*8.4% Sodium Lauryl Sulfate

Indications: A routine cleansing and grooming shampoo to restore natural luster and body to the hair-coats of dogs and cats. Deodorizes.

Directions for Use: Thoroughly wet the entire hair-coat of the cat or dog with warm water, then apply enough shampoo to make a lather and work well into coat. Rinse thoroughly.

Repeat as often as needed. As a precaution, a bland ophthalmic ointment should be placed in the eyes prior to bathing to prevent irritation.

Caution(s): Harmful if swallowed. Avoid contact with eyes. In case of eye contact, flush eyes immediately with water.

Warning(s): Keep out of reach of children.

For external use only.

Presentation: Available in 8 oz and 1 gallon plastic bottles.

Compendium Code No.: 11430200

MYCODEX® PET SHAMPOO WITH 3X PYRETHRINS

V.P.L. **Parasiticide Shampoo**

EPA Reg. No.: 2097-17

Active Ingredient(s):

Ingredient	
Pyrethrins	0.15%
*Piperonyl Butoxide, technical	1.50%
Inert Ingredients	98.35%
Total	100.00%

*Equivalent to 1.2% of butylcarbityl (6-propylpiperonyl) ether and to 0.3% of related compounds.

Indications: Kills fleas and ticks on dogs and fleas on cats.

Directions for Use: It is a violation of Federal law to use this product in a manner inconsistent with its labeling.

As a precaution, a bland ophthalmic ointment should be placed in the eyes prior to bathing to prevent possible irritation.

Thoroughly wet entire hair-coat with warm water and then apply enough shampoo to make a lather and work into the coat and skin. For best results allow lather to remain in contact with skin for 5 minutes before rinsing. Rinse thoroughly. Product contains emollient and may be repeated semiweekly or weekly as required.

Precautionary Statements: Hazards to Humans and Domestic Animal:

Human: May be harmful if swallowed or absorbed through skin. Avoid skin contact. May cause eye irritation. Avoid contact with eyes. Wash thoroughly after handling.

Animals: Avoid treatment of nursing puppies and kittens under 12 weeks of age unless prescribed by a veterinarian. Do not use on lactating animals.

Environment Hazards: This product is extremely toxic to aquatic invertebrates. Do not contaminate water by cleaning of equipment or disposal of wastes.

Practical Treatment: If in eyes flush with water. Get medical attention if irritation persists. If on skin wash thoroughly with soap and water, remove contaminated clothing. If irritation persists, consult physician.

Storage and Disposal:

Storage: Store in a cool, dry area.

Disposal: Do not reuse container. Rinse thoroughly and wrap container in several layers of newspaper and discard in trash.

Warning(s): Keep out of reach of children.

For external use only.

Presentation: Available in 6 oz, 12 oz and 1 gallon plastic bottles.

Compendium Code No.: 11430210

MYCODEX® PET SHAMPOO WITH CARBARYL

V.P.L. **Parasiticide Shampoo**

EPA Reg. No.: 2097-8

Active Ingredient(s):

Ingredient	
Carbaryl (1-Naphthyl N-Methylcarbamate)	0.50%
Inert Ingredients	99.50%
Total	100.00%

Indications: A routine cleansing shampoo to restore natural luster to the hair-coat of dogs and cats. Kills fleas, lice and ticks.

Directions for Use: It is a violation of Federal law to use this product in a manner inconsistent with its labeling.

As a precaution, a bland ophthalmic ointment should be placed in the eyes prior to bathing to prevent possible irritation.

Thoroughly soak animal with warm water taking 2-3 minutes to wet hair. Apply MYCODEX® Pet Shampoo with Carbaryl on head and ears and lather, then repeat procedure with neck, chest, middle, and hindquarters, finishing legs last. For best effects, allow lather to remain in contact with skin for 5 minutes before rinsing. Rinse thoroughly. Use no more than once weekly. Do not allow to get into eyes or on scrotum.

Precautionary Statements: Hazards to Humans and Domestic Animals: Caution:

Human: Avoid contact with eyes, skin, or clothing. In case of contact immediately flush eyes or skin with water. Obtain medical attention if irritation persists. Harmful if swallowed.

Animals: Do not treat puppies or kittens under 12 weeks of age. Do not use on pregnant animals.

Environmental Hazards: This product is extremely toxic to aquatic invertebrates. Do not contaminate water by cleaning of equipment or disposal of wastes.

Storage and Disposal:

Storage: Store in a cool, dry area.

Disposal: Do not reuse container. Rinse thoroughly and wrap container in several layers of newspaper and discard in trash.

Warning(s): Keep out of reach of children.

For external use only.

Presentation: Available in 6 oz, 12 oz and 1 gallon plastic bottles.

Compendium Code No.: 11430220

MYCODEX® SENSICARE™ FLEA & TICK SHAMPOO

V.P.L. **Parasiticide Shampoo**

EPA Reg. No.: 2097-11

Active Ingredient(s):

Ingredient	
d-trans Allethrin	0.12%
Piperonyl Butoxide, technical*	0.50%
Inert Ingredients	99.38%
Total	100.00%

*Equivalent to 0.4% of butylcarbityl (6-propylpiperonyl) ether and 0.1% related compounds.

Indications: A routine cleansing and deodorizing shampoo to restore natural luster to the hair-coat of dogs and cats, and to kill fleas.

Directions for Use: It is a violation of Federal law to use this product in a manner inconsistent with its labeling.

As a precaution, a bland ophthalmic ointment should be placed in the eyes prior to bathing to prevent possible irritation.

Thoroughly soak animal with warm water taking 2-3 minutes to wet hair. Apply MYCODEX® SENSICARE™ Flea & Tick Shampoo on head and ears and lather, then repeat procedure with neck, chest, middle, and hindquarters, finishing legs last. For best effects, allow lather to remain in contact with skin for 5 minutes before rinsing. Rinse thoroughly. For a complete flea and tick control program consult your veterinarian.

Precautionary Statements: Hazards to Humans and Domestic Animals:

Caution: Avoid contact with eyes. In case of contact, immediately flush eyes with water. Obtain medical attention if irritation persists. Harmful if swallowed.

Storage and Disposal: Storage: Store in a cool, dry area at room temperature. Container not for household use.

Disposal: Do not reuse container. Rinse thoroughly and wrap container in several layers of newspaper and discard in trash.

Warning(s): Keep out of reach of children.

For external use only.

Presentation: Available in 12 oz (355 mL) and 1 gallon plastic bottles.

Compendium Code No.: 11430231

MYCODEX® SENSICARE™ FLEA & TICK SPRAY

V.P.L. **Parasiticide Spray**

EPA Reg. No.: 2097-15

Active Ingredient(s):

Ingredient	
Pyrethrins	0.20%
*Piperonyl Butoxide, technical	2.00%
Inert Ingredients	97.80%
Total	100.00%

*Equivalent to 1.6% of butylcarbityl (6-propylpiperonyl) ether and 0.3% related compounds.

Indications: A water-based flea and tick spray for puppies, kittens, dogs and cats.
Directions for Use: It is a violation of Federal law to use this product in a manner inconsistent with its labeling.

Cover animal's eyes with hand and with a firm, fast stroke to get a proper spray mist, spray head, ears and chest until damp. With fingertips, rub into face and around mouth, nose and eyes. Then spray neck, middle and hindquarters, finishing legs last. For best penetration of spray to the skin, direct spray against the natural lay of the hair. On long-haired dogs, rub your hand against the lay of the hair, spraying the ruffled hair directly behind the hand. Make sure spray thoroughly wets ticks. Repeat treatment as needed.
Precautionary Statements: Hazards to Humans and Domestic Animals: Caution:

Human: Harmful if swallowed or inhaled. Avoid breathing mist. Avoid contamination of food. Wash hands with soap and water after using.

Animal: Avoid treatment of nursing puppies and kittens. If treatment is necessary, spray on tips of fingers and rub into coat.

Environmental Hazards: This product is toxic to fish. Do not add directly to water. Do not apply where runoff is likely to occur.
Storage and Disposal:

Storage: Store in a cool, dry area.

Disposal: Do not reuse empty container. Rinse thoroughly and wrap container in several layers of newspaper and discard in trash.
Warning(s): Keep out of reach of children.

For external use only.
Presentation: Available in 16 oz (473 mL) plastic bottle with trigger sprayer.
Compendium Code No.: 11430240

MYCOPLASMA BOVIS BACTERIN

Biomune **Bacterin**

Mycoplasma Bovis Bacterin
U.S. Vet. Lic. No.: 368
Contents: This product contains the antigen listed above.
Indications: This bacterin is recommended as an aid in the prevention of mastitis caused by *Mycoplasma bovis*.
Dosage and Administration: Shake well before use. Using aseptic technique, a 2 mL dose is subcutaneously administered in the neck. It is recommended that animals are vaccinated 3 times at 2-4 week intervals prior to calving. The third dose should be administered at least 2 to 3 weeks prior to calving. A booster dose should be administered whenever field conditions warrant. It is recommended to vaccinate a few animals and observe for any unexpected reactions prior to vaccinating the entire herd. Administer epinephrine in the event of anaphylactic reaction.
Precaution(s): Do not freeze. Store at 35-45°F (2-7°C). Use entire contents when first opened.
Caution(s): Notice: This product is conditionally licensed. Potency and efficacy studies are in progress.

Non-returnable product.

For veterinary use only.
Warning(s): Do not vaccinate within 21 days before slaughter.

Product contains an adjuvant, and accidental injection into a human may cause a serious localized reaction. Seek medical attention immediately.
Presentation: 10 doses (20 mL) and 50 doses (100 mL).
Patent pending
Compendium Code No.: 11290391 700

MYCOPLASMA GALLISEPTICUM NOBILIS® ANTIGEN TEST KIT

Intervet **Plate Agglutination Test**

S-6 Serotype, Plate Stained Antigen for Plate Agglutination Test
U.S. Vet. Lic. No.: 286
Description: This antigen is a suspension of killed, stained S-6 Adler Strain *Mycoplasma gallisepticum* (MG) antigen for serum plate testing of chicken and turkey serum. The reactivity has been standardized against a reference serum.

Contains neomycin as a preservative.

Quality tested for purity and effectiveness.
Indications: The antigen is used for the detection of MG antibody in chickens and turkeys. It is possible that not all birds in an infected flock will show a positive reaction, thus it is strongly recommended to use the serum plate agglutination (SPA) test for flock diagnosis and not for the individual identification of infected birds.

MG infection can be subtly present in a flock. It is therefore recommended only to consider a flock as negative when the test has been repeated several times and has given a negative result each time. Before officially designating a flock as being infected or not infected, consult your poultry pathologist. Plate testing is a screening method only. Do not destroy a flock based on results of testing with this antigen.
Test Procedure: The testing sequence for a flock should be as follows:

1. Conduct SPA test using Intervet NOBILIS® Antigen.
2. Test positive SPA serum samples with HI antigen.
3. Utilize HI results, additional tests (i.e., culture, etc.) and your local poultry pathologist before determining *Mycoplasma* status of a flock. Always refer to the NPIP manual as mentioned under "References".

The serum plate test for MG is conducted by contacting and mixing 0.05 mL of test serum with 0.05 mL of serum plate antigen on a glass plate at room temperature. The standard procedure is:

1. Do not dilute this antigen.
2. Allow antigen and test serums to warm up to room temperature before use. Do not allow serum to be frozen prior to plate testing.
3. Dispense test serums in 0.05 mL amounts with a pipette (rinsed between samples) to 1½" squares on a ruled glass plate. Limit the number of samples (no more than 25) to be set up at one time according to the speed of the operator. Serum should not dry out before being mixed with antigen.
4. Shake antigen prior to use. Dispense 0.05 mL of antigen beside the test serum on each square. Hold antigen dispensing dropper vertically.
5. Mix the serum and antigen, using a multimixing device if large numbers are to be run at one time.
6. Rotate the plate for 5 seconds. At the end of the first minute, rotate the plate again for 5 seconds and read 55 seconds later.
7. A positive reaction is characterized by the formation of definite clumps, usually starting at the periphery of the mixture. Most samples that are positive will react within the two-minute test period. Whenever samples are run, the antigen should be tested against known positive and negative control serums.

The serum plate MG test should be considered a basic screening test for antibodies. Under normal circumstances, the rate of nonspecific reactions is low. However, nonspecific reactions may occasionally be high for a variety of reasons.
Test Interpretation: The hemagglutination inhibition (HI) test is too cumbersome for routine screening use. Positive HI reactions are generally accurate, however, and are useful in evaluating serum samples that react with the plate antigen. The test should be conducted with four HA units. Titers of 1:80 or greater for both chicken and turkey sera are considered positive, while a 1:40 titer would be suspicious and additional tests are required. Titers of 1:20 or less are considered negative.
Storage: The antigen should be stored in a dark area at 2-7°C (35-45°F).
Caution(s): This product is not hazardous when used according to directions supplied. A material safety data sheet (MSDS) is available upon request. This and any other consumer information can be obtained by calling Intervet Customer Service at 1-800-441-8272 or 1-302-934-8051.

For veterinary use only.
References: For additional information on *Mycoplasma* test procedures, refer to the following references: Proc. 77th Annual Meeting, U.S. Animal Health Association, 1973; Isolation and Identification of Avian Pathogens, 2nd edition; Methods for Examining Poultry Biologics and for Identifying and Quantifying Avian Pathogens, 1971; and the National Poultry Improvement Plan and Auxiliary Provisions Manual, USDA-APHIS, June 1985.
Presentation: 200 tests (10 mL). Ten mL of antigen is packaged in a glass bottle with a separate dropper top. This top is calibrated to deliver 0.05 mL of antigen per test.
Compendium Code No.: 11060961 65005 AL113

MYCOPLASMA GALLISEPTICUM VACCINE

Merial Select **Vaccine**

Mycoplasma gallisepticum, Live Culture, MG TS-11
U.S. Vet. Lic. No.: 279
Active Ingredient(s): The vaccine contains the TS-11 strain of *Mycoplasma gallisepticum* (MG), live culture.

Contains amoxicillin as a preservative.

Notice: The vaccine has met the requirements of the USDA in regards to safety, purity, potency, and the capability to protect susceptible chickens. The vaccine has been tested by the master seed immunogenicity test for efficacy.
Indications: The vaccine is for the vaccination of healthy chickens nine weeks of age or older as an aid in the prevention of clinical signs of MG infection.

The vaccine is recommended for use in healthy chickens only. It is essential that the chickens be maintained under good environmental conditions and that exposure to disease viruses be reduced as much as possible in the field. Do not use in breeder chickens where negative MG serology is desired or required.
Dosage and Administration: Read the full directions carefully.

Eyedrop Vaccination:

1. Bottles should be rapidly thawed in warm water (Caution: No warmer than 30°C or 86°F). Shake well before removing the cap.
2. Remove the cap and stopper and insert the dropper tip.
3. Hold each bird with its head tilted to one side.
4. Place one (1) drop on the eye allowing the drop to spread over the eye before releasing the bird.
5. Use the entire contents when first thawed.

Precaution(s): MYCOPLASMA GALLISEPTICUM VACCINE is a frozen vaccine; store at -40°F (-40°C) or lower until ready for use.
Caution(s): Do not vaccinate MG positive or diseased birds.

Vaccinate all of the birds on the premises at one time.

Administer a minimum of one dose for each bird.

Vaccination should be carried out at least three weeks before expected exposure to the field type MG.

Avoid stress conditions during and following vaccination.

Do not place chickens in contaminated facilities.

For veterinary use only.

Do not medicate chickens with antibacterial drugs 14 days before or seven days after vaccination.

The capability of the vaccine to produce satisfactory results depends upon many factors including, but not limited to, conditions of storage and handling by the user, administration of the vaccine, health and responsiveness of individual animals and the degree of field exposure. Directions for use should be followed carefully. The use of the vaccine is subject to applicable local and federal laws and regulations.

Use the entire contents when first opened. Burn the container and all unused contents.

Use only in localities where permitted.

Do not use in breeders.
Warning(s): Do not vaccinate within 21 days before slaughter.
Presentation: 10 x 1,000 doses.
Compendium Code No.: 11050280

MYCOPLASMA MELEAGRIDIS NOBILIS® ANTIGEN TEST KIT

Intervet **Plate Agglutination Test**

H-Serotype, Plate Stained Antigen for Plate Agglutination Test
U.S. Vet. Lic. No.: 286
Description: This antigen is a suspension of killed, stained Yamamoto 529 Strain *Mycoplasma meleagridis* (MM) antigen for serum plate testing of turkey serum. The reactivity has been standardized against a reference serum.

Contains neomycin as a preservative.

Quality tested for purity and effectiveness.
Indications: The antigen is used for the detection of MM antibody in turkeys. It is possible that not all birds in an infected flock will show a positive reaction, thus it is strongly recommended to use the serum plate agglutination (SPA) test for flock diagnosis and not for the individual identification of infected birds.

MM infection can be subtly present in a flock. It is therefore recommended only to consider a flock as negative when the test has been repeated several times and has given a negative result each time. Before officially designating a flock as being infected or not infected, consult your poultry pathologist. Plate testing is a screening method only. Do not destroy a flock based upon results of testing with this antigen.

Test Procedure: The testing sequence for a flock should be as follows:

1. Conduct SPA test using Intervet Antigen.
2. Test positive SPA serum samples with HI antigen.
3. Utilize HI results, additional tests (i.e., culture, etc.) and your local poultry pathologist before determining *Mycoplasma* status of a flock. Always refer to the NPIP manual as mentioned under "References".

The serum plate test for MM is conducted by contacting and mixing 0.05 mL of test serum with 0.05 mL of serum plate antigen on a glass plate at room temperature. The standard procedure is:

1. Do not dilute this antigen.
2. Allow antigen and test serums to warm up to room temperature before use. Do not allow serum to be frozen prior to plate testing.
3. Dispense test sera in 0.05 mL amounts with a pipette (rinsed between samples) to 1½" squares on a ruled glass plate. Limit the number of samples (no more than 25) to be set up at one time according to the speed of the operator. Serum should not dry out before being mixed with antigen.
4. Do not dilute serum.
5. Shake antigen prior to use. Dispense 0.05 mL of antigen beside the test serum on each square. Hold antigen dispensing dropper vertically.
6. Mix the serum and antigen, using a multimixing device if large numbers are to be run at one time.
7. Rotate the plate for 5 seconds. At the end of the first minute, rotate the plate again for 5 seconds and read 55 seconds later.
8. A positive reaction is characterized by the formation of definite clumps, usually starting at the periphery of the mixture. Most samples that are positive will react within the two minute test period. Whenever samples are run, the antigen should be tested against known positive and negative control serums.

This serum plate MM test should be considered a basic screening test for antibodies. Under normal circumstances, the rate of nonspecific false positive reactions is low. However, nonspecific reactions may occasionally be high for a variety of reasons.

Test Interpretation: The hemagglutination inhibition (HI) test is too cumbersome for routine screening use. Positive HI reactions are generally accurate, however, and are useful in evaluating serum samples that react with the plate antigen. The test should be conducted with four HA units. Titers of 1:80 or greater for turkey sera are considered positive, while a 1:40 titer would be suspicious, and additional tests are required. Titers of 1:20 or less are considered negative.

Storage: The antigen should be stored in a dark area at 2-7°C (35-45°F).

Caution(s): This product is not hazardous when used according to directions supplied. A material safety data sheet (MSDS) is available upon request. This and any other consumer information can be obtained by calling Intervet Customer Service at 1-800-441-8272 or 1-302-934-8051.

For veterinary use only.

References: For additional information on *Mycoplasma* test procedures, refer to the following references: Proc. 77th Annual Meeting, U.S. Animal Health Association, 1973; Isolation and Identification of Avian Pathogens, 2nd Edition; Methods for Examining Poultry Biologics and for Identifying and Quantifying Avian Pathogens, 1971; and the National Poultry Improvement Plan and Auxiliary Provisions Manual, USDA-APHIS, June 1985.

Presentation: 200 tests (10 mL). Ten mL of antigen is packaged in a glass bottle with a dropper top. This top is calibrated to deliver 0.05 mL of antigen per test.

Compendium Code No.: 11060971 65206 AL 136

M

MYCOPLASMA SYNOVIAE NOBILIS® ANTIGEN TEST KIT

Intervet **Plate Agglutination Test**

S-Serotype, Plate Stained Antigen for Plate Agglutination Test

U.S. Import Permit No.: 286A

Description: This antigen is a suspension of killed, stained WVU-1853 strain *Mycoplasma synoviae* (MS) antigen for serum plate testing of chicken and turkey serum. The reactivity has been standardized against a reference serum.

Contains neomycin as a preservative.

Quality tested for purity and effectiveness.

Indications: The antigen is used for the detection of MS antibody in chickens and turkeys. It is possible that not all birds in an infected flock will show a positive reaction, thus it is strongly recommended to use the serum plate agglutination for flock diagnosis and not for the individual identification of infected birds.

MS infection can be subtly present in a flock. It is therefore recommended only to consider a flock as negative when the test has been repeated several times and has given a negative result each time. Current technical information indicates that turkey flocks may become infected with MS and not react with the serum plate test antigen. Under these conditions consult your poultry pathologist.

Before officially designating a flock as being infected, consult your poultry pathologist. Plate testing is a screening method only. Do not destroy a flock based upon results of testing with this antigen.

Test Procedure: The testing sequence for a flock should be as follows:

1. Conduct SPA test using Intervet NOBILIS® Antigen.
2. Test positive SPA serum samples with HI antigen.
3. Utilize HI results, additional tests (i.e., culture, etc.) and your local poultry pathologist before determining *Mycoplasma* status of a flock. Always refer to the NPIP manual as mentioned under "References".

The serum plate test for MS is conducted by contacting and mixing 0.05 mL of test serum with 0.05 mL of serum plate antigen on a glass plate at room temperature. The standard procedure is:

1. Do not dilute this antigen.
2. Allow antigen and test serums to warm up to room temperature before use. Do not allow serum to be frozen prior to plate testing.
3. Dispense test serums in 0.05 mL amounts with a pipette (rinsed between samples) to 1½" squares on a ruled glass plate. Limit the number of samples (no more than 25) to be set up at one time according to the speed of the operator. Serum should not dry out before being mixed with antigen.
4. Shake antigen prior to use. Dispense 0.05 mL of antigen beside the test serum on each square. Hold antigen dispensing dropper vertically.
5. Mix the serum and antigen, using a multimixing device if large numbers are to be run at one time.
6. Rotate the plate for 5 seconds. At the end of the first minute, rotate the plate again for 5 seconds and read 55 seconds later.
7. A positive reaction is characterized by the formation of definite clumps, usually starting at the periphery of the mixture. Most samples that are positive will react within the two-minute test period. Whenever samples are run, the antigen should be tested against known positive and negative control serums.

The serum plate MS test should be considered a basic screening test for antibodies. Under normal circumstances, the rate of nonspecific reactions is low. However, nonspecific reactions may occasionally be high for a variety of reasons.

Test Interpretation: The hemagglutination inhibition (HI) test is too cumbersome for routine screening use. Positive HI reactions are generally accurate, however, and are useful in evaluating serum samples that react with the plate antigen. The test should be conducted with four HA units. Titers of 1:80 or greater for both chicken and turkey sera are considered positive, while a 1:40 titer would be suspicious, and additional tests are required. Titers at 1:20 or less are considered negative.

Storage: The antigen should be stored in a dark area at 2-7°C (35-45°F).

Caution(s): This product is not hazardous when used according to directions supplied. A material safety data sheet (MSDS) is available upon request. This and any other consumer information can be obtained by calling Intervet Customer Service at 1-800-441-8272 or 1-302-934-8051.

For veterinary use only.

References: For additional information on *Mycoplasma* test procedures, refer to the following references: Proc. 77th Annual Meeting, U.S. Animal Health Association, 1973; Isolation and Identification of Avian Pathogens, 2nd Edition; Methods for Examining Poultry Biologics and for Identifying and Quantifying Avian Pathogens, 1971; and the National Poultry Improvement Plan and Auxiliary Provisions Manual, USDA-APHIS, June 1985.

Presentation: 200 tests (10 mL). Ten mL of antigen is packaged in a glass bottle with a separate dropper top. This top is calibrated to deliver 0.05 mL of antigen per test.

Manufactured by: Intervet International B.V., Boxmeer, Holland.

Compendium Code No.: 11060981 651061 AL133

MYCO SHIELD™

Novartis Animal Vaccines **Bacterin**

Mycoplasma hyopneumoniae Bacterin

Composition: This bacterin contains inactivated cultures of *Mycoplasma hyopneumoniae*. Contains penicillin and thimerosal as preservatives.

Indications: For use in healthy swine as an aid in the prevention and control of pneumonia caused by *Mycoplasma hyopneumoniae*.

Dosage and Administration: Shake well before using.

Administer 1 mL intramuscularly at 2 weeks of age or older. Revaccinate in 2 weeks.

Precaution(s): Store in the dark at 35°-45°F (2°-7°C). Do not freeze. Use entire contents when opened.

Caution(s): Anaphylactic reactions may occur following the use of this biological. Symptomatic treatment: Epinephrine.

For veterinary use only.

Warning(s): Do not vaccinate within 21 days prior to slaughter.

Discussion: Enzootic pneumonia of swine, caused by *Mycoplasma hyopneumoniae*, is an extremely common disease with a worldwide incidence. Slaughter checks have revealed evidence of the disease in 30-80% of the slaughter-weight swine in the United States.

Mycoplasma is most common in co-mingled groups of pigs. Spread within a herd often occurs from sows to their piglets, and then from piglet to piglet once litters are mixed together. Transmission requires direct contact with respiratory secretions from infected pigs which contain high levels of organisms. There is also some evidence that airborne transmissions may occur between groups that are housed within one mile of each other.

Symptoms are most common in pigs over 6 weeks of age, and often don't show up until pigs are 3-6 months of age. The disease has a slow onset with a long incubation. It spreads slowly throughout the herd. Uncomplicated *Mycoplasma hyopneumoniae* infections show a high morbidity but low to no mortality. Often the only clinical sign will be a chronic, non-productive cough in pigs with an "unthrifty" appearance. The main effect is economic, since affected pigs will show decreased rates of gain and a decreased feed conversion ratio.

Unfortunately for swine producers, almost all *M. hyopneumoniae* infections are complicated by secondary pneumonias, which can result in high death losses and severe economic hardship. *Mycoplasma* infection predisposes pigs to *Pasteurella* and *Actinobacillus pleuropneumoniae*, both of which can be devastating. *Mycoplasma* infections can also occur concurrently with other bacteria, viruses, mycoplasmas and migrating parasites. Often changes in weather or other stresses will precipitate severe pneumonias from these mixed infections. Severe disease is often due to a complex interaction between *Mycoplasma*, bacteria, a poor environment and sub-optimal management levels.

On post-mortem, lungs of pigs with *M. hyopneumoniae* infections will show purple to gray areas of "meaty" consolidation, almost always in the cranio-ventral portions of the lungs. Lesions are usually clearly demarcated from surrounding areas of the normal lung. Pigs suffering from severe, mixed infections will have lungs with appearances typical of the secondary infections.

Diagnosis is based on a combination of clinical signs, post-mortem lesions, histopathology, serology and tests such as fluorescent antibody staining of affected lung tissue. Diagnosis by culturing the organism is unreliable, since *Mycoplasma* is extremely difficult to culture even from known infected lungs. Differential diagnosis must include swine influenza, bacterial pneumonias, and parasites such as ascarids and lungworms.

Various antibiotics have been used to treat *Mycoplasma* infections, with mixed results. Prevention of the disease involves maintaining an optimum environment and a strict all-in / all-out program to minimize pig-to-pig spread of the disease. Management systems such as the SPF program and various medicated early weaning (MEW) programs are also helpful.

The final step to preventing *Mycoplasma* problems involves incorporating a vaccination program into the management system. Vaccination has been shown to greatly reduce both the severity of disease and the economic losses associated with *M. hyopneumoniae* infections. MYCO SHIELD™ is a convenient 1 mL dose vaccine that can be given to any pig 2 weeks of age or older. Revaccination with a booster dose in 2 weeks produces elevated and extended immunity to help prevent the potentially devastating effects of *Mycoplasma hyopneumoniae* infections.

Trial Data:

Weight Gain:

	Avg. wt. 5 days	Avg. wt. 83 days	Avg. wt. 155 days
MYCO SHIELD™ Vaccinates	5.78 lbs	66 lbs	195.3 lbs
Controls	5.94 lbs	62 lbs	179.7 lbs
Wt. gain advantage of vaccinates	-.16 lbs	+4 lbs	+15.6 lbs

Piglets from 20 litters were divided evenly between vaccinate and control groups. Vaccinates were inoculated with two doses of MYCO SHIELD™ and weights were taken at 5 days of age, 83 days of age, and 155 days of age. Vaccinates, even though they were lighter at 5 days of age, showed significant weight gain advantages at both 83 days of age and 155 days of age.

Vaccination and Challenge:
Trial #1:

	Nr.	Avg. % Lung Consolidation
Vaccinates	20	1.85%
Controls	10	10.9%

All pigs were challenged with *M. hyopneumoniae* on four different occasions beginning 3 weeks after the second dose of MYCO SHIELD™. Pigs were necropsied 9 weeks post-challenge, at which time lung consolidation scores were measured. Pigs from the vaccinated group showed statistically significant reductions in the degree of lung lesions present.
Trial #2

	Nr.	Avg. % Lung Consolidation
Vaccinates	10	1.2%
Controls	10	10.4%

(P=0.0001)
Pigs in each group were challenged and lung lesion scores were subsequently measured. In addition, attempts were made to isolate *M. hyopneumoniae* from both vaccinates and controls. Isolation was successful in only one of the vaccinates (10%) versus five of the controls (50%), indicating the effectiveness of vaccinating with MYCO SHIELD™.
References: Available upon request.
Presentation: Available in 100 dose (100 mL) and 250 dose (250 mL) bottles.
Compendium Code No.: 11140203

MYCO SILENCER® BPM

Intervet **Bacterin-Toxoid**
Bordetella Bronchiseptica-Mycoplasma Hyopneumoniae-Pasteurella Multocida Bacterin-Toxoid
U.S. Vet. Lic. No.: 286
Contents: An inactivated, adjuvanted culture of *Bordetella bronchiseptica, Mycoplasma hyopneumoniae* and *Pasteurella multocida* non-toxigenic type A and toxigenic type D.
Contains gentamicin and thimerosal as preservatives.
Indications: For use in healthy swine as an aid in the prevention of atrophic rhinitis and pneumonia caused by *B. bronchiseptica* and *P. multocida* non-toxigenic type A and toxigenic types A and D, and pneumonia caused by *M. hyopneumoniae.*
Dosage and Administration: Shake well, inject intramuscularly or subcutaneously.
Sows and Gilts: One 2 mL dose at 5 weeks and 2 weeks prefarrowing; one 2 mL dose at 1-2 weeks before subsequent farrowings.
Baby Pigs: One 1 mL dose at 5-7 days of age; one 1 mL dose at 23-28 days of age.
Feeder Pig Vaccination: One 1 mL dose at weaning (3 weeks of age); one 1 mL dose 3 weeks later.
Boars: One 2 mL dose annually.
Precaution(s): Store in the dark at not over 45°F (7°C). Do not freeze. Use entire contents when first opened; do not save partial contents.
Caution(s): Use only in healthy swine.
If allergic reaction occurs, treat with epinephrine. Transient local swelling may occur at site of injection. Not to be used as a diluent for viral products. For veterinary use only.
Warning(s): Do not vaccinate within 21 days of slaughter.
Presentation: 50 sow/100 piglet dose (100 mL) and 250 sow/500 piglet dose (500 mL) vials.
U.S. Patent No. 5,968,525
Compendium Code No.: 11061561 7155001

MYCO SILENCER® BPME*

Intervet **Bacterin-Toxoid**
Bordetella Bronchiseptica-Erysipelothrix Rhusiopathiae-Mycoplasma Hyopneumoniae-Pasteurella Multocida Bacterin-Toxoid
U.S. Vet. Lic. No.: 286
Contents: An inactivated, adjuvanted bacterin-toxoid product containing *Bordetella bronchiseptica, Erysipelothrix rhusiopathiae, Mycoplasma hyopneumoniae, and Pasteurella multocida* non-toxigenic type A and toxigenic type D.
Contains gentamicin, thimerosal, and polymyxin B.
Indications: For use in healthy swine as an aid in the prevention of atrophic rhinitis and pneumonia caused by *B. bronchiseptica, P. multocida* (toxigenic types A and D, non-toxigenic type A), pneumonia caused by *M. hyopneumoniae,* and erysipelas caused by *E. rhusiopathiae.*
Dosage and Administration: Shake well, inject intramuscularly (IM) or subcutaneously (SC).
Sows and Gilts: Administer a 2 mL dose at 5 weeks and again at 2 weeks before farrowing. For subsequent farrowings, administer one 2 mL dose at 1-2 weeks before farrowing.
Baby Pigs from Vaccinated Sows: Administer one 1 mL dose at 5-7 days and again at 23-28 days of age.
Feeder Pig Vaccination: Administer one 1 mL dose at weaning (3 weeks of age); one 1 mL dose 3 weeks later.
Boars: Administer two 2 mL doses three weeks apart prior to breeding herd introduction. Annual revaccination with one 2 mL dose is recommended.
Precaution(s): Store in the dark at not over 45°F (7°C). Do not freeze. Use entire contents when first opened.
Caution(s): If allergic reaction occurs, treat with epinephrine. Not to be used as a diluent for viral products. For veterinary use only.
Warning(s): Do not vaccinate within 21 days of slaughter.
Presentation: 50 sow/100 piglet dose (100 mL) and 250 sow/500 piglet dose (500 mL) vials.
*U.S. Patent No. 5,968,525
Compendium Code No.: 11062600 71625001

MYCO SILENCER® M

Intervet **Bacterin**
Mycoplasma Hyopneumoniae Bacterin
U.S. Vet. Lic. No.: 286
Contents: An inactivated, adjuvanted culture of *Mycoplasma hyopneumoniae.*
Contains gentamicin and thimerosal as preservatives.
Indications: For use in healthy swine as an aid in the prevention of pneumonia caused by *Mycoplasma hyopneumoniae.*
Dosage and Administration: Shake well, inject intramuscularly or subcutaneously.
Sows and Gilts: One 2 mL dose at 5 weeks and 2 weeks prefarrowing; one 2 mL dose at 1-2 weeks before subsequent farrowings.
Baby Pigs: One 1 mL dose at 5-7 days of age; one 1 mL dose at 23-28 days of age.
Feeder Pig Vaccination: One 1 mL dose at weaning (3 weeks of age); one 1 mL dose 3 weeks later.
Boars: One 2 mL dose annually.
Precaution(s): Store in the dark at not over 45°F (7°C). Do not freeze. Use entire contents when first opened; do not save partial contents.
Caution(s): Use only in healthy swine.
If allergic reaction occurs, treat with epinephrine. Transient local swelling may occur at site of injection. Not to be used as a diluent for viral products.
For veterinary use only.
Warning(s): Do not vaccinate within 21 days of slaughter.
Presentation: 50 sow/100 piglet dose (100 mL) and 250 sow/500 piglet dose (500 mL) vials.
Compendium Code No.: 11061581 71425001

MYCO SILENCER® MEH

Intervet **Bacterin**
Erysipelothrix Rhusiopathiae-Haemophilus Parasuis-Mycoplasma Hyopneumoniae Bacterin
U.S. Vet. Lic. No.: 286
Contents: This product contains inactivated cultures of *Mycoplasma hyopneumoniae, Erysipelothrix rhusiopathiae* and two strains of *Haemophilus parasuis* in Diluvac Forte® adjuvant.
Contains thimerosal, gentamicin and polymyxin B as preservatives.
Indications: For use in healthy swine as an aid in the prevention of pneumonia caused by *Mycoplasma hyopneumoniae,* erysipelas caused by *Erysipelothrix rhusiopathiae* and polyserositis (Glasser's Disease) caused by *Haemophilus parasuis.*
Dosage and Administration: Shake well, aseptically inject intramuscularly (IM). Administer a 2.0 mL dose at 3 weeks of age or older, followed by one 2.0 mL dose 3 weeks later.
Precaution(s): Store in the dark at not over 45°F (7°C). Do not freeze. Do not save partial contents. Burn the container and all unused product.
Caution(s): Use only in healthy swine. If allergic reaction occurs, treat with epinephrine.
For veterinary use only.
Warning(s): Do not vaccinate within 21 days of slaughter.
Presentation: 50 doses (100 mL).
*U.S. Patent Nos. 5,650,155, 5,667,784 and 5,968,525.
Compendium Code No.: 11062640 7655002

MYCO SILENCER® ONCE

Intervet **Bacterin**
Mycoplasma Hyopneumoniae Bacterin
U.S. Vet. Lic. No.: 286
Contents: This product contains the antigen listed above.
This product contains an inactivated culture in Microsol Diluvac Forte®.
Contains gentamicin and thimerosal as preservatives.
Indications: For use in healthy swine as an aid in the prevention of pneumonia caused by *Mycoplasma hyopneumoniae* for up to 6 months.
Dosage and Administration: Shake well, aseptically inject intramuscularly (IM). Administer a single 2 mL dose at 3 weeks of age or older.
Precaution(s): Store in the dark at not over 45°F (7°C). Do not freeze. Do not save partial contents. Burn the container and all unused product.
Caution(s): Use in healthy swine. If allergic reaction occurs, treat with epinephrine.
For veterinary use only.
Warning(s): Do not vaccinate within 21 days of slaughter.
Presentation: 50 dose (100 mL) and 250 dose (500 mL) bottles.
Compendium Code No.: 11062540 78825001

MYCOVAC-L®

Intervet **Vaccine**
Mycoplasma Gallisepticum Vaccine, Live Culture
U.S. Vet. Lic. No.: 286
Description: MYCOVAC-L® is a live vaccine, prepared from the Intervet 6/85 strain of *Mycoplasma gallisepticum* in a freeze-dried preparation sealed under vacuum. The 6/85 strain is unique in that it is highly immunogenic for chickens and non-pathogenic for turkeys, does not readily spread to adjacent houses of chicken and is biologically stable.
MYCOVAC-L® has been propagated under exacting standards. The immunizing capability of this vaccine has been proven by various procedures including the Master Seed Immunogenicity Test.
This vaccine contains no preservative.
Quality tested for purity, potency, and safety.
Indications: Fine Spray — Vaccination of healthy chickens six weeks of age or older for protection against clinical signs of MG.
Dosage and Administration: Vaccination Programs: Many factors must be considered in determining a sound vaccination program for a particular farm or poultry complex. To be fully effective, the vaccine must be administered properly to healthy, receptive animals maintained in a proper environment under good management. In addition, the response may be influenced by the age of the animals and their immune status. The level of immunity required will vary with operational practices and the degree of exposure. Therefore, a program of periodic revaccination may be necessary.
Preparation of Vaccine:
For Fine Spray Use: Do not open and mix the vaccine until ready to begin vaccination. Use vaccine immediately after mixing.
1. Remove the tear-off seal and stopper from vial containing the vaccine.
2. Carefully pour clean, cool, non-chlorinated water, preferably distilled, into the vaccine vial until the vial is approximately two-thirds full.
3. Insert the rubber stopper and shake moderately until all material is dissolved.
4. The vaccine is now ready for fine spray application in accordance with the directions below. For best results, be sure to follow directions carefully.

Fine Spray Administration:
For Chickens Six Weeks of Age or Older:
1. Spray vaccination should be of fine spray of less than 20 microns.
2. Do not use any disinfectants or skim milk in sprayer.
3. Use sprayer only for administration of vaccines. Clean thoroughly after each use.

4. Shut off all fans while spray vaccinating. Turn on fans immediately after spraying. Be careful in hot weather.
5. Spray chickens by walking slowly through the house.
6. Follow the recommendation of the manufacturer of the sprayer regarding water volume.
7. Use only clean, cool, non-chlorinated water, preferably distilled.
8. Individual(s) spraying chickens should wear face mask and goggles.

Records: Keep a record of vaccine, quantity, serial number, expiration date, and place of purchase; the date and time of vaccination; the number, age, breed, and locations of chickens; name of operators performing the vaccination and any observed reactions.

Precaution(s): Store in the dark in a refrigerator between 2-7°C (35-45°F). Do not freeze.

Do not spill, splash or mix this vaccine with any substance.

Use entire contents when first opened.

Burn containers and all unused contents.

This product is non-returnable.

Caution(s): Vaccinate only healthy chickens. Although disease may not be evident, coccidiosis, respiratory virus infection, infectious bursal disease, avian reovirus disease, Marek's disease, and other disease conditions may cause complications or reduce immunity.

All susceptible chickens on the same premises should be vaccinated at the same time.

The 6/85 strain of MG is not pathogenic for turkeys, but care should be taken in the application of the vaccine and handling of the chickens so as to maintain tight disease security.

Efforts should be taken to reduce stress conditions at the time of vaccination and during the reaction period.

Do not dilute the vaccine or otherwise stretch the dosage.

For veterinary use only.

This vaccine is to be used only in states where its usage is permitted and is to be used in compliance with applicable state and federal regulations.

Notice: This vaccine has undergone rigid potency, safety and purity tests, and meets Intervet Inc. and USDA requirements. It is designed to stimulate effective immunity when used as directed, but the user must be advised that the response to the product depends upon many factors, including, but not limited to, conditions of storage and handling by the user, administration of the vaccine, health and responsiveness of the individual chickens, and the degree of field exposure. Therefore, directions should be followed carefully.

This product is not hazardous when used according to directions supplied. A material safety data sheet (MSDS) is available upon request. This and any other consumer information can be obtained by calling Intervet Customer Service at 1-800-441-8272 or 1-302-934-8051.

The use of this vaccine is subject to applicable local and federal laws and regulations. This vaccine is to be used only in states where its usage is permitted.

Use only as directed.

Warning(s): Do not vaccinate within 21 days before slaughter.

Do not medicate chickens with antibacterial drugs - especially chlortetracycline, oxytetracycline or sulfonamide - five days prior to or after vaccination.

This vaccine should not be administered within two weeks of any live Newcastle, bronchitis or laryngotracheitis vaccination.

Do not administer this vaccine within four weeks of onset of egg production or after egg production has begun.

Presentation: 10 x 1,000 doses for fine spray use.

U.S. Patent No. 5,064,647

Compendium Code No.: 11060991

Rev. 24005 AL145

M

MYOSAN™ CREAM

Life Science — **Topical Antifungal**

Active Ingredient(s): Carbamide, benzalkonium chloride, and allantoin in an ointment base.

Indications: Ringworm control and antiseptic for horses, dogs and cats.

Dosage and Administration: Gently apply MYOSAN™ Cream directly onto the lesion and rub gently until the cream disappears into the skin. Apply each day until new hair growth occurs. Leave the treated area uncovered.

Fresh ringworm lesions normally show visible clinical results within 7-10 days, if not, consult a veterinarian.

Note: Efficacy is neutralized by soap or detergent residues.

Caution(s): For external animal use only.

Keep out of the reach of children.

In case of contact with eyes or mucous membranes, flush immediately with water. Obtain medical attention for eye irritation.

Warning(s): Not for use on animals intended for food.

Presentation: 4 oz (113 g) container.

Compendium Code No.: 10870110

MYOSAN™ SOLUTION

Life Science — **Topical Antifungal**

Active Ingredient(s): Carbamide, benzalkonium chloride, and allantoin in an aqueous base.

Indications: For use on horses, dogs and cats as an aid in the control of summer itch, girth itch, ringworm and other fungal problems.

Dosage and Administration: Soak the affected area liberally with MYOSAN™ Solution. Apply each day until the hair begins to grow. Leave the treated area uncovered. Rinse the treated areas with clear water before re-applying. If improvement is not noted within seven (7) days, consult a veterinarian.

Note: Efficiency is neutralized by soap or detergent residues.

Caution(s): For external veterinary use only.

Not for human use.

Keep out of the reach of children.

In case of contact with eyes or mucous membranes, flush immediately with water. Obtain medical attention for eye irritation.

Warning(s): Not for use on animals intended for food.

Presentation: 8 fl oz (237 mL) and 32 fl oz (946 mL) containers.

Compendium Code No.: 10870121

MYSTIQUE®

Intervet — **Bacterin**

Ehrlichia Risticii Bacterin

U.S. Vet. Lic. No.: 286

Contents: The bacterin contains inactivated, purified, concentrated, adjuvanted, tissue culture origin *Ehrlichia Risticii.*

Contains gentamicin as a preservative.

Indications: For vaccination of healthy horses 3 months of age or older as an aid in the prevention of Potomac Horse Fever (equine monocytic ehrlichiosis) caused by *E. risticii.*

Dosage and Administration: For primary immunization aseptically inject 1 mL intramuscularly. Repeat the dose in 3 to 4 weeks. A 1 mL booster dose should be administered annually and at any time epidemic conditions exist or are reported and exposure is imminent.

Precaution(s): Store at 35° to 45°F (2° to 7°C). Do not freeze. Shake well before using. Use entire contents when first opened.

Caution(s): Local reactions may occur if this product is given subcutaneously. Inject deep in the muscle only. Anaphylactoid reactions may occur.

For use in animals only.

Antidote(s): Epinephrine.

Warning(s): Do not vaccinate within 21 days before slaughter.

Presentation: 10 dose (10 x 1 mL) syringes with separate sterile needle and 10 dose (10 mL) vial.

Compendium Code No.: 11061001

MYSTIQUE® II

Intervet — **Bacterin-Vaccine**

Rabies Vaccine, Killed Virus-Ehrlichia Risticii Bacterin

U.S. Vet. Lic. No.: 286

Contents: MYSTIQUE® II is a liquid suspension of inactivated rabies virus propagated in a stable cell line, combined with an inactivated suspension of *Ehrlichia risticii.*

Contains gentamicin as a preservative.

Indications: For vaccination of healthy horses 3 months of age or older against disease caused by rabies virus and as an aid in the prevention of Potomac Horse Fever (equine monocytic ehrlichiosis) caused by *E. risticii.*

Dosage and Administration: For primary immunization aseptically inject 1 mL intramuscularly. For *E. risticii*, repeat the dose in 3 to 4 weeks using this product or Mystique®. Repeat the dose annually or at any time epidemic conditions exist or are reported and exposure is imminent.

Precaution(s): Store at 35°-45°F (2°-7°C). Do not freeze. Shake well before using. Use entire contents when first opened.

Caution(s): Vaccinating animals whose immune response is compromised by stress, disease, etc. may not produce the desired results. Anaphylactic reactions may occur.

Antidote(s): Epinephrine.

Warning(s): Do not vaccinate within 21 days of slaughter.

Trial Data: The efficacy of this combination vaccine has been demonstrated in controlled vaccination challenge tests and the safety in thorough field evaluations.

Presentation: 10 dose (10 mL) vial.

Sold to veterinarians only.

Compendium Code No.: 11061011

N

NAQUASONE® BOLUS ℞

Schering-Plough **Diuretic-Anti-inflammatory**

(Trichlormethiazide and dexamethasone) Bolus

NADA No.: 030-136

Active Ingredient(s): NAQUASONE® Bolus contains 200 mg trichlormethiazide and 5 mg dexamethasone.

Indications: NAQUASONE® is recommended for the treatment of physiological parturient udder edema of the mammary gland and associated structures in cattle.

Pharmacology: NAQUASONE® Bolus combines the effective diuretic activity of trichlormethiazide with the specific anti-inflammatory activity of dexamethasone. This combination of activities is complementary in the reduction of physiological parturient edema of the mammary gland and associated structures in cattle. Because the two drugs are complementary in action, effects are achieved with minimum dosage of trichlormethiazide.

The mechanism of action by which Naqua® (trichlormethiazide) effects diuresis in edematous conditions is by an inhibitory effect on the re-absorption of sodium and chloride in the renal tubules, thereby enhancing excretion of sodium chloride and water, while apparently having a considerably lessened and more temporary effect on the excretion of potassium and bicarbonate.

The corticosteroid Azium® (dexamethasone) possesses remarkable anti-inflammatory and antistress activity. Clinical experience shows that udder edema is greatly reduced in many cases following parenteral treatment with 10 to 20 mg dexamethasone alone. In the majority of these cases, udder congestion is greatly reduced in 48 hours. Effective doses apparently do not cause sodium and fluid retention or potassium loss when used for a short treatment period as recommended, but rather enhance the action of the diuretic in NAQUASONE® by the specific anti-inflammatory effect exerted by corticosteroids.

Trichlormethiazide is an orally administered, highly effective diuretic agent of the benzothiadiazine series. Studies in man and experimental animals show that trichlormethiazide presents a favorable pattern of less potassium excretion than chlorothiazide or hydrochlorothiazide. The clinically determined saluretic potency of trichlormethiazide is estimated to be 10 to 20 times that of hydrochlorothiazide and, correspondingly, 100 to 200 times that of chlorothiazide. Furthermore, trichlormethiazide more closely approaches the ideal saluretic agent in that sodium and chloride excretions tend to be equivalent. The possible occurrence of hypochloremic alkalosis, therefore, is lessened compared to hydrochlorothiazide with which chloride excretion in relation to sodium output may be excessive. In addition to an enhanced saluretic potency, trichlormethiazide exhibits a higher sodium to potassium ratio than either hydrochlorothiazide or chlorothiazide. The lesser potassium diuresis may be significant in decreasing the incidence of hypokalemic manifestations.

Experimental animal studies show that dexamethasone is a highly effective corticosteroid possessing remarkable anti-inflammatory activity in the bovine and other species. Veterinary clinical evidence shows dexamethasone to have anti-inflammatory activity approximately twenty times that of prednisolone in the bovine. In laboratory studies for mineralocorticoid activity (i.e., the capacity to induce retention of sodium and water in the adrenalectomized rat preparation), dexamethasone did not cause sodium or water retention.

Dosage and Administration: One (1) or two (2) boluses initially followed by one-half (½) to one (1) bolus daily depending on the size and response of the animal and the severity of the edema. Total duration of treatment should not exceed three (3) days.

The usual case of edema seen under field conditions will generally begin to respond within 24-48 hours after NAQUASONE® therapy is initiated. Most cases will subside in three (3) to four (4) days. If results are not evident in three (3) days, it is recommended the animal be re-examined.

Precaution(s): Store between 2-30°C (36-86°F).

Caution(s): Federal law restricts this drug to use by or on the order of a licensed veterinarian.

For all the beneficial effects of the corticosteroids one should be aware of the possible untoward reactions resulting from their use. Dexamethasone, like cortisone and all other corticoid derivatives, is capable of causing side effects, especially during long continued and/or high dosage. Some side effects produced by injudicious use of corticosteroids are: suppression of inflammation, reduction of fever, increased protein degradation and its conversion to carbohydrate leading to a negative nitrogen balance, sodium retention and potassium diuresis, retardation of wound healing, lowering of resistance to many infectious agents such as bacteria and fungi, reduction in numbers of circulating lymphocytes.

NAQUASONE® may be administered to animals with acute or chronic bacterial infections providing the infections are controlled with appropriate antibiotic or chemotherapeutic agents.

It is recommended that the veterinarian determine by all practical means whether or not associated infections are present with the edema. When infections are believed to be present, one must choose the logical antimicrobial treatment and determine whether the infection should be treated first or concurrently with NAQUASONE® Boluses.

It should be kept in mind that dexamethasone, like all corticosteroids, through its anti-inflammatory action may mask the signs of infection and by this action, could give a false impression of the progress of the antimicrobial treatment.

Dexamethasone is an extremely potent drug with profound physiologic effects. All of the precautions and contraindications for adrenocortical hormones must be followed. Animals receiving the drug should be under close observation.

Unless studies should prove otherwise, the possible action of dexamethasone in delaying wound healing should be kept in mind.

Trichlormethiazide is an extremely potent nonmercurial diuretic agent required in low milligram doses for saluretic effectiveness and should be used accordingly. Electrolyte depletion effects may be seen with over vigorous therapy and maximum doses should not be used over an extended period of time. Potassium supplements have not generally been necessary with trichlormethiazide and their administration routinely should not be required. Hypochloremia is less likely with trichlormethiazide than with hydrochlorothiazide at equivalent saluretic levels. Animals with severe renal function impairments should be checked for hyperkalemia and acidosis, since therapy with benzothiadiazine diuretics like trichlormethiazide may be contraindicated in these patients.

The use of corticosteroids, depending upon dose, duration, and specific steroid, may result in the inhibition of endogenous steroid production following drug withdrawal. In patients presently receiving or recently withdrawn from systemic corticosteroid treatments, therapy with a rapidly acting corticosteroid should be considered in unusually stressful situations.

Warning(s): Milk taken from dairy animals during treatment and for 72 hours after the latest treatment must not be used for food.

Clinical and experimental data have demonstrated that corticosteroids administered orally or parenterally to animals may induce the first stage of parturition when administered during the last trimester of pregnancy and may precipitate premature parturition followed by dystocia, fetal death, retained placenta, and metritis.

Additionally, corticosteroids administered to dogs, rabbits, and rodents during pregnancy have produced cleft palate. Other congenital anomalies including deformed forelegs, phocomelia, and anasarca have been reported in offspring of dogs which received corticosteroids during pregnancy.

Side Effects: Side effects such as SAP and SGPT enzyme elevations, weight loss, anorexia, polydipsia, and polyuria have occurred following the use of synthetic corticosteroids in dogs. Vomiting and diarrhea (occasionally bloody) have been observed in dogs and cats.

Cushing's syndrome in dogs has been reported in association with prolonged or repeated steroid therapy.

Presentation: Boxes of 30 and 100 boluses.

Compendium Code No.: 10471320

NARAMUNE-2™

Boehringer Ingelheim **Vaccine**

Canine Parainfluenza-Bordetella Bronchiseptica Vaccine, Modified Live Virus, Avirulent Live Culture

U.S. Vet. Lic. No.: 124

Contents: This product contains the antigens listed above.

Preservative: Neomycin.

Indications: For vaccination of healthy susceptible dogs and puppies against Canine Upper Respiratory Infection (Canine Cough) caused by canine parainfluenza and *Bordetella bronchiseptica*. Field studies support the safety of NARAMUNE-2™ when administered to puppies as young as 3 weeks of age.

Dosage and Administration: Rehydration: Rehydrate to desired dose volume with accompanying sterile diluent. For five 0.5 mL doses, reconstitute with 2.5 mL of diluent. For five 1 mL doses, reconstitute with 5 mL of diluent. Shake well and use immediately.

Using aseptic technique, administer entire dose intranasally. Use enclosed applicator tip on hub of syringe in place of syringe needle. Apply new nasal applicator tip for each dog vaccinated. Do not vaccinate puppies under 3 weeks of age. Puppies vaccinated between 3 and 6 weeks of age should be revaccinated at 6 weeks of age. Annual revaccination is recommended.

Precaution(s): Store out of direct sunlight at a temperature between 35-45°F (2-7°C). Use entire contents when first opened. Burn containers and all unused contents.

Caution(s): For intranasal use in dogs only; do not vaccinate dogs parenterally. Anaphylactoid reactions may occur.

Antidote(s): Epinephrine.

Discussion: Description and General Information: NARAMUNE-2™ Canine Parainfluenza Vaccine, Modified Live Virus, Bordetella Bronchiseptica Vaccine, Avirulent Live Culture is designed to be administered intranasally for convenient, rapid prevention of Canine Upper Respiratory Infection (Canine Cough). Both of these organisms are widespread, common etiologic agents of this syndrome which appears as a mild, self-limiting disease involving the trachea and bronchi of dogs of any age. It spreads rapidly among dogs that are closely confined as in hospitals, kennels and pet stores. The disease is highly contagious and is transmitted via the airborne route.

Both of the organisms in NARAMUNE-2™ are avirulent so that they can be safely administered intranasally with little or no symptoms of disease. By instilling these organisms into the nasal passages, it becomes possible for these agents to infect target cells of the nasal-pharyngeal region, mimicking the pathogenesis of natural field infection. A very small percentage of dogs may show sneezing, coughing or nasal discharge for 3-10 days following vaccination. While these are usually temporary symptoms, antibacterial therapy may be indicated.

Presentation: 20 x 1 dose (1 mL) and 5 dose (5 mL) vials.

Compendium Code No.: 10280791 10423-01 / 10421-01/10422-01

NASALGEN® IP VACCINE

Schering-Plough **Vaccine**

Bovine Rhinotracheitis-Parainfluenza$_3$ Vaccine, Modified Live Virus

U.S. Vet. Lic. No.: 314

Contents: This lyophilized vaccine contains the antigens listed above. Contains gentamicin as a preservative.

Indications: For the vaccination of healthy cattle as an aid in the prevention of disease caused by infectious bovine rhinotracheitis and parainfluenza$_3$ virus.

Dosage and Administration: For intranasal use only: For use in healthy cattle 6 months of age or older. Slowly transfer entire contents of diluent vial to vaccine vial, using aseptic technique and sterile syringes and needles. The 2 mL dose may be administered into one nostril or 1 mL into each nostril. Use a separate disposable cannula for each animal. Calves vaccinated under 6 months of age should be revaccinated at 6 months of age or weaning.

Precaution(s): Store at 35°-45°F (2°-7°C). Use entire contents when first opened. Do not use chemical disinfectants to sterilize syringes, needles or cannulas. Burn container and all unused contents.

Caution(s): Anaphylactoid reactions may occur following use.

Antidote(s): Epinephrine.

Warning(s): Do not vaccinate within 21 days before slaughter.

For veterinary use only.

Presentation: 10 x 1 dose (2 mL), 10 dose (20 mL), and 50 dose (100 mL) vials with diluent.

Compendium Code No.: 10471330

NASAL-VAX™

AgriPharm **Vaccine**

Bovine Rhinotracheitis-Parainfluenza$_3$ Vaccine, Modified Live Virus

U.S. Vet. Lic. No.: 165A

Contents: This lyophilized vaccine contains the antigens listed above.

Contains gentamicin as a preservative.

Indications: For the vaccination of healthy cattle as an aid in the prevention of disease caused by infectious bovine rhinotracheitis and parainfluenza$_3$ virus.

Dosage and Administration: For intranasal use only. For use in healthy cattle 6 months of age or older. Slowly transfer entire contents of diluent vial to vaccine vial, using aseptic technique and sterile syringes and needles. The 2 mL dose may be administered into one nostril or 1 mL into each nostril. Use a separate disposable cannula for each animal. Calves vaccinated under 6 months of age should be revaccinated at 6 months of age or weaning.

Precaution(s): Store at 35°-45°F (2°-7°C). Use entire contents when first opened. Do not use chemical disinfectants to sterilize syringes, needles or cannulas. Burn container and all unused contents.

Caution(s): Anaphylactoid reactions may occur following use.

For veterinary use only.

Antidote(s): Epinephrine.

Warning(s): Do not vaccinate within 21 days before slaughter.

Presentation: 10 x 1 dose (2 mL), 10 dose (20 mL), and 50 dose (100 mL) vials with diluent.

Compendium Code No.: 14571300

NATURAL MINT LINIMENT™

Horses Prefer **Liniment**

Ingredient(s): D.I. Water, Mineral Oil, Peppermint Oil, Glycerin, Polysorbate, Propylene Glycol, Triethanolamine, Carbomer, Vitamin E, DMDM Hydantoin, Methyl Paraben, Propyl Paraben.

No artificial fragrance added.

Indications: NATURAL MINT LINIMENT™ contains Peppermint, Oil, Aloe Vera, and other emollients. The special combination of these ingredients aids in soothing and moisturizing the tired, aching muscles and ligaments.

Directions: Apply liberally to the tired, overused, aching muscles and joints 2-3 times daily or as needed.

Discontinue use if excessive irritation occurs.

If condition persists, contact a veterinarian.

Caution(s): Avoid contact with eyes and nose. In the event of contact, rinse with water.

For animal use.

For external use only.

Warning(s): Keep out of reach of children.

Presentation: 8 oz.

Compendium Code No.: 36950031

NATURAL SOLVENT™

Butler **Topical Product**

Ingredient(s): NATURAL SOLVENT™ is an organically based solvent cleaner derived from citrus fruits.

Indications: NATURAL SOLVENT™ is designed to quickly dissolve tar, adhesive gum and oil from the fur of household pets. It can also be added to cleaning solutions for floors, walls, exam rooms, kennels, and other areas throughout the clinic.

Directions for Use: Apply solvent to the area of the animal that requires treatment. Avoid contact with the eyes, nose and mouth. Allow to sit for 30-60 seconds, then wipe area clean. Repeat as needed. After area has been cleaned, rinse with clean water or use a clean damp cloth to remove any remaining residue.

To use as a general cleaner, add 6-10 oz. per gallon of water or cleaning solution to enhance cleaning effectiveness and leave the area smelling fresh.

Caution(s): For veterinary use only.

Warning(s): Keep out of reach of children.

Combustible.

Presentation: 32 fl oz and 128 fl oz containers.

Compendium Code No.: 10821201

NAXCEL® ℞

Pharmacia & Upjohn **Cephalosporin(s)**

brand of ceftiofur sodium sterile powder

NADA No.: 140-338

Active Ingredient(s): Each mL of the reconstituted drug contains ceftiofur sodium equivalent to 50 mg ceftiofur. The pH was adjusted with sodium hydroxide and monobasic potassium phosphate.

Indications: For intramuscular and subcutaneous injection in cattle only. For intramuscular injection in swine, sheep, goats and horses. For subcutaneous injection in dogs, day-old chickens and day-old turkey poults. This product may be used in lactating dairy cattle, sheep and goats.

Cattle: NAXCEL® Sterile Powder is indicated for treatment of bovine respiratory disease (shipping fever, pneumonia) associated with *Pasteurella haemolytica, Pasteurella multocida* and *Haemophilus somnus.* NAXCEL® Sterile Powder is also indicated for treatment of acute bovine interdigital necrobacillosis (foot rot, pododermatitis) associated with *Fusobacterium necrophorum* and *Bacteroides melaninogenicus.*

Swine: NAXCEL® Sterile Powder is indicated for treatment/control of swine bacterial respiratory disease (swine bacterial pneumonia) associated with *Actinobacillus (Haemophilus) pleuropneumoniae, Pasteurella multocida, Salmonella choleraesuis* and *Streptococcus suis* type 2.

Sheep: NAXCEL® Sterile Powder is indicated for treatment of sheep respiratory disease (sheep pneumonia) associated with *Pasteurella haemolytica* and *Pasteurella multocida.*

Goats: NAXCEL® Sterile Powder is indicated for treatment of caprine respiratory disease (goat pneumonia) associated with *Pasteurella haemolytica* and *Pasteurella multocida.*

Horses: NAXCEL® Sterile Powder is indicated for treatment of respiratory infections in horses associated with *Streptococcus zooepidemicus.*

Dogs: NAXCEL® Sterile Powder is indicated for the treatment of canine urinary tract infections associated with *Escherichia coli* and *Proteus mirabilis.*

Day-Old Chickens: NAXCEL® Sterile Powder is indicated for the control of early mortality, associated with *E. coli* organisms susceptible to ceftiofur, in day-old chicks.

Day-Old Turkey Poults: NAXCEL® Sterile Powder is indicated for the control of early mortality, associated with *E. coli* organisms susceptible to ceftiofur, in day-old turkey poults.

Pharmacology: NAXCEL® Sterile Powder contains the sodium salt of ceftiofur which is a broad spectrum cephalosporin antibiotic active against gram-positive and gram-negative bacteria including β-lactamase-producing strains. Like other cephalosporins, ceftiofur is bactericidal *in vitro*, resulting from inhibition of cell wall synthesis.

Chemical Structure of Ceftiofur Sodium:

Chemical Name of Ceftiofur Sodium: 5-Thia-1-azabicyclo[4.2.0]oct-2-ene-2-carboxylic acid, 7-[[(2-amino-4-thiazolyl)(methoxyimino)-acetyl]amino]-3-[[(2-furanyl-carbonyl)thio] methyl]-8-oxo-, monosodium salt, [6R-[6α,7β(Z)]]-

Clinical Microbiology:

Animal	Organism	n	MIC Range (mcg/mL)	MIC_{90} (mcg/mL)	Date tested
Bovine *	*Pasteurella haemolytica (Mannheimia* spp.)	461	≤0.03-0.13	0.06	1988-1992
	Pasteurella multocida	318	≤0.03-0.25	0.06	1988-1992
	Haemophilus somnus	109	≤0.03-0.13	0.06	1988-1992
	Fusobacterium necrophorum	17	≤0.06	≤0.06	1994
**	*Salmonella* spp.	28	0.06-2.0	1.0	1994
	Bacteroides fragilis group	29	≤0.06->16.0	16.0	1994
	Bacteroides spp., non-fragilis group	12	0.13->16.0	16.0	1994
	Peptostreptococcus anaerobius	12	0.13-2.0	2.0	1994
	Moraxella bovis	100	0.03-0.5	0.25	1998
Swine **	*Actinobacillus pleuropn.*	83	≤0.03-0.06	≤0.03	1993
	Pasteurella multocida	74	≤0.03-0.06	≤0.03	1993
	Streptococcus suis	94	≤0.03-1.0	0.25	1993
	Salmonella choleraesuis	50	1.0-2.0	1.0	1993
	Escherichia coli	84	0.25-4.0	1.0	1993
	Salmonella typhimurim	98	1.0-2.0	2.0	1993
	Staphylococcus hyicus	100	0.13-1.0	1.0	1992
	beta-hemolytic *Streptococcus* spp.	24	≤0.03-0.06	≤0.03	1993
	Actinobacillus suis	77	0.0019-0.0078	0.0078	1998
	Haemophilus parasuis	76	0.0039-0.25	0.06	1998
Sheep *	*Pasteurella haemolytica*	39	≤0.03-0.13	0.13	1992
	Pasteurella multocida	23	≤0.03	≤0.03	1992
Horses **	*Streptococcus equi* subsp. *equi*	12	≤0.0019	≤0.0019	1994
	Streptococcus zooepidemicus	48	≤0.0019	≤0.0019	1994
	Rhodococcus equi	67	≤0.03-2.0	8.0	1998
	Bacteroides fragilis group	32	0.13->16.0	>16.0	1995
	Bacteroides spp. non-fragilis group	12	0.25-4.0	4.0	1995
	Fusobacterium necrophorum	16	≤0.06	≤0.06	1995
Canine *	*Escherichia coli*	44	0.06-64.0	4.0	1992
	Escherichia coli	18	0.013-0.5	0.25	1990
	Proteus mirabilis	17	≤0.06-0.5	≤0.06	1990
	Proteus mirabilis	23	≤0.06-4.0	1.0	1992
Turkey Poults *	*Escherichia coli*	1204	0.13->32.0	1.0	1995
**	*Citrobacter* spp.	37	0.5->32.0	1.0	1995
	Enterobacter spp.	51	0.13->32.0	0.5	1995
	Klebsiella spp.	100	0.13-2.0	0.5	1995
	Proteus spp.	19	0.06-32.0	0.13	1995
	Pseudomonas spp.	31	0.06->32.0	32.0	1995
	Salmonella spp.	24	0.5-1.0	1.0	1995
	Staphylococcus spp. (coagulase positive)	17	1.0-2.0	1.0	1995
	Staphylococcus spp. (coagulase negative)	26	0.13->32.0	2.0	1995
	Streptococcus spp. and *Enterococcus* spp.	55	≤0.03->32.0	>32.0	1995

* Clinical isolates supported by clinical data and indications for use.

** Clinical isolates not supported by clinical data, the clinical significance of these data is not known.

MIC_{90} Minimum inhibitory concentration for 90% of the isolates.

MIC_{50} Minimum inhibitory concentration for 50% of the isolates.

n Number of isolates.

Dosage and Administration:

Cattle: Administer to cattle at the dosage of 0.5 to 1.0 mg ceftiofur per pound of body weight (1-2 mL reconstituted sterile solution per 100 lb body weight). Treatment should be repeated at 24-hour intervals for a total of three consecutive days. Additional treatments may be given on days four and five for animals which do not show a satisfactory response (not recovered) after the initial three treatments. Selection of dosage (0.5 to 1.0 mg/lb) should be based on the practitioner's judgment of severity of disease (i.e., for respiratory disease, extent of elevated body temperature, depressed physical appearance, increased respiratory rate, coughing and/or loss of appetite; and for foot rot, extent of swelling, lesion and severity of lameness).

Swine: Administer to swine at a dosage of 1.36 to 2.27 mg ceftiofur/lb (3.0 to 5.0 mg/kg) of body weight (1 mL of reconstituted sterile solution 22 to 37 pounds of body weight). Treatment should be repeated at 24-hour intervals for a total of three consecutive days.

Sheep: Administer to sheep at the dosage of 0.5 to 1.0 mg ceftiofur per pound of body weight (1-2 mL reconstituted sterile solution per 100 lbs body weight). Treatment should be repeated at 24-hour intervals for a total of three consecutive days. Additional treatments may be given on days four and five for animals which do not show a satisfactory response (not recovered) after the initial three treatments. Selection of dosage (0.5 to 1.0 mg/lb) should be based on the practitioner's judgment of severity of disease (i.e., extent of elevated body temperature, depressed physical appearance, increased respiratory rate, coughing and/or loss of appetite).

Goats: Administer to goats at the dosage of 0.5 to 1.0 mg ceftiofur per pound of body weight (1-2 mL reconstituted sterile solution per 100 lbs body weight). Treatment should be repeated at 24-hour intervals for a total of three consecutive days. Additional treatment may be given on days four and five for animals which do not show a satisfactory response (not recovered) after the initial three treatments. Selection of dosage (0.5 to 1.0 mg/lb) should be based on the practitioner's judgment of severity of disease (i.e., extent of elevated body temperature, depressed physical appearance, increased respiratory rate, coughing and/or loss of appetite). Pharmacokinetic data indicate that elimination of the drug is more rapid in lactating does. For lactating does, the high end of the dose range is recommended.

Horses: Administer to horses at a dosage of 1.0 to 2.0 mg ceftiofur per pound of body weight (2-4 mL reconstituted sterile solution per 100 lb body weight). A maximum of 10 mL may be administered per injection site. Treatment should be repeated at 24-hour intervals, continued for 48 hours after clinical signs have disappeared and should not exceed 10 days.

Dogs: Administer to dogs by subcutaneous injection at a dosage of 1.0 mg ceftiofur per pound of body weight (0.1 mL reconstituted sterile solution per 5 lbs of body weight). Treatment should be repeated at 24-hour intervals for 5-14 days.

Day-Old Chickens: Administer by subcutaneous injection in the neck region of day-old chicks at a dosage of 0.08 to 0.20 mg ceftiofur/chick. One mL of the 50 mg/mL reconstituted solution will treat approximately 250 to 625 day-old chicks.

Day-Old Turkey Poults: Administer by subcutaneous injection in the neck region of day-old turkey poults at a dosage of 0.17 to 0.5 mg ceftiofur/poult. One mL of the 50 mg/mL reconstituted solution will treat approximately 100 to 294 day-old turkey poults.

Administration:

Cattle: Reconstituted NAXCEL® Sterile Powder is to be administered by intramuscular or subcutaneous injection only.

Swine, Sheep, Goats and Horses: Reconstituted NAXCEL® Sterile Powder is to be administered by intramuscular injection only.

Dogs: Reconstituted NAXCEL® Sterile Powder is to be administered to dogs by subcutaneous injection. No vial closure should be entered more than 20 times. Therefore, only the 1 gram vial is approved for use in dogs.

Day-Old Chickens: Reconstituted NAXCEL® Sterile Powder is to be administered by subcutaneous injection only. A sterile 26 gauge needle and syringe or properly cleaned automatic injection machine should be used.

Day-Old Turkey Poults: Reconstituted NAXCEL® Sterile Powder is to be administered by subcutaneous injection only.

Reconstitution of the Sterile Powder: NAXCEL® Sterile Powder should be reconstituted as follows:

1 gram vial—Reconstitute with 20 mL Sterile Water for Injection. Each mL of the resulting solution contains ceftiofur sodium equivalent to 50 mg ceftiofur.

4 gram vial—Reconstitute with 80 mL Sterile Water for Injection. Each mL of the resulting solution contains ceftiofur sodium equivalent to 50 mg ceftiofur.

Contraindication(s): As with all drugs, the use of NAXCEL® Sterile Powder is contraindicated in animals previously found to be hypersensitive to the drug.

Precaution(s): Storage Conditions: Store unreconstituted product at controlled room temperature 20° to 25°C (68° to 77°F) [see USP].

Store reconstituted product either in a refrigerator 2° to 8°C (36° to 46°F) for up to 7 days or at controlled room temperature 20° to 25°C (68° to 77°F) [see USP] for up to 12 hours.

Reconstituted NAXCEL® Sterile Powder can be frozen for up to 8 weeks without loss in potency or other chemical properties. Carefully thaw the frozen material under warm to hot running water, gently swirling the container to accelerate thawing. The frozen material may also be thawed at room temperature.

Protect from light. Color of the cake may vary from off-white to a tan color. Color does not affect potency.

Caution(s): Federal (USA) law restricts this drug to use by or on the order of a licensed veterinarian.

Following subcutaneous administration of ceftiofur sodium in the neck of cattle, small areas of discoloration at the site may persist beyond five days, potentially resulting in trim loss of edible tissues at slaughter.

As with any parenteral injection, localized post-injection bacterial infections may result in abscess formation. Attention to hygienic procedures can minimize their occurrence.

The safety of ceftiofur has not been determined for swine, horses, or dogs intended for breeding, or pregnant dogs.

The administration of antimicrobials to horses under conditions of stress may be associated with acute diarrhea that could be fatal. If acute diarrhea is observed, discontinue use of this antimicrobial and initiate appropriate therapy.

Warning(s): Residue Warnings: Neither a pre-slaughter drug withdrawal interval nor a milk discard time is required when this product is used according to label indications, dosage, and route of administration. Use of dosages in excess of those indicated or by unapproved routes of administration, such as intramammary, may result in illegal residues in edible tissues and/or in milk. Not for use in horses intended for human consumption.

Not for human use. Keep out of reach of children.

Penicillins and cephalosporins can cause allergic reactions in sensitized individuals. Topical exposure to such antimicrobials, including ceftiofur, may elicit mild to severe allergic reactions in some individuals. Repeated or prolonged exposure may lead to sensitization. Avoid direct contact of the product with the skin, eyes, mouth, and clothing.

Persons with a known hypersensitivity to penicillin or cephalosporins should avoid exposure to this product.

In case of accidental eye exposure, flush with water for 15 minutes. In case of accidental skin exposure, wash with soap and water. Remove contaminated clothing. If allergic reaction occurs (e.g., skin rash, hives, difficult breathing), seek medical attention.

The material safety data sheet contains more detailed occupational safety information. To report adverse effects in users, to obtain more information or obtain a material safety data sheet, call 1-800-253-8600.

Toxicology: Animal Safety:

Cattle: Results from a five-day tolerance study in normal feeder calves indicated that formulated ceftiofur was well tolerated at 25 times (25 mg/lb/day) the highest recommended dose of 1.0 mg/lb/day for five consecutive days. Ceftiofur administered intramuscularly had no adverse systemic effects.

In a 15-day safety/toxicity study, five steer and five heifer calves per group were intramuscularly administered formulated ceftiofur at 0 (vehicle control), 1, 3, 5 and 10 times the highest recommended dose of 1.0 mg/lb/day to determine the safety factor. There were no adverse systemic effects indicating that the formulated ceftiofur has a wide margin of safety when injected intramuscularly into the feeder calves at 10 times (10 mg/lb/day) the recommended dose for three times (15 days) the recommended three to five days of therapy. The formulation was shown to be a slight muscle irritant based on results of histopathological evaluation of the injection sites at 1 and 3 times the highest recommended dose of 1.0 mg/lb/day. The histopathological evaluations were conducted at post-treatment days 1, 3, 7 and 14.

The injection of NAXCEL® Sterile Powder at the recommended dose administered SC in the neck of cattle was well tolerated. However, a several square centimeter area of yellow-red discoloration resulting from a single SC injection persisted in many of the cattle beyond 4.5 days post injection. Also, one of the animals developed an abscess at the injection site.

Swine: Results from a five-day tolerance study in normal feeder pigs indicated that formulated ceftiofur was well tolerated when administered at 57 mg/lb (more than 25 times the highest recommended daily dosage of 2.27 mg/lb of body weight) for five consecutive days. Ceftiofur administered intramuscularly to pigs produced no overt adverse signs of toxicity.

To determine the safety factor and to measure the muscle irritancy potential in swine, a safety/toxicity study was conducted. Five barrows and five gilts per group were intramuscularly administered formulated ceftiofur at 0, 2.27, 6.81 and 11.36 mg/lb of body weight for 15 days which is 0, 1, 3 and 5 times the highest recommended dose of 2.27 mg/lb of body weight/day and 5 times the recommended treatment length of 3 days. There were no adverse systemic effects indicating that formulated ceftiofur has a wide margin of safety when injected intramuscularly into feeder pigs at the highest recommended dose of 2.27 mg/lb/day for 3 days or at levels up to 5 times the highest recommended dose for 5 times the recommended length of treatment. The formulation was shown to be a slight muscle irritant based on results of histopathological evaluation of the injection sites at post-treatment days 1, 2, 3 and 4. By day 10 post injection the muscle reaction was subsiding and at day 15 post injection there was little evidence of muscle damage in any of the pigs in any of the treatment groups.

Sheep: In a 15-day safety/toxicity study in sheep, three wether and three ewe lambs per group were given formulated ceftiofur sodium by the intramuscular route 0 (sterile water vehicle), 1, 3 or 5 times the recommended dose of 1.0 mg/lb/day for 3 times the recommended maximum duration of 5 days of treatment. There were no adverse systemic effects indicating that formulated ceftiofur is well tolerated and has a wide margin of safety in sheep. Based on examination of injection sites from study days 9, 11, 13 and 15, a low incidence of visual changes and histopathologic findings of mild, reversible inflammation from all groups including the controls indicated that the formulation is a slight muscle irritant.

Goats: In a 15-day safety-toxicity study, 5 lactating does, 5 dry does, and 5 wethers were given formulated ceftiofur by the intramuscular route with 11 mg/kg/day for 15 days. This constitutes 5 times the recommended dose for 3 times the recommended maximum duration of 5 days of treatment. There were no adverse systemic effects indicating that formulated ceftiofur is well tolerated and has a wide margin of safety in goats.

Horses: In a safety study, horses received a daily intramuscular injection of either 0 mg/lb/day (saline control), 1.0 mg/lb/day (50 mg/mL), 3.0 mg/lb/day (100 mg/mL), or 5.0 mg/lb/day (200 mg/mL) of an aqueous solution of ceftiofur sodium for 30 or 31 days. Ceftiofur sodium was well tolerated when administered intramuscularly to male and female horses at doses up to 5.0 mg/lb/day for 30 or 31 days. No clinical evidence of irritation was noted at any dose. The drug-related changes detected in this study were limited to a transient decrease in food consumption in horses receiving 3.0 or 5.0 mg/lb/day ceftiofur, and general mild skeletal muscle irritation at the injection sites which resolved by regeneration of muscle fibers.

In a tolerance study, horses received a single daily intravenous infusion of either 0 (saline), 10.0 or 25.0 mg/lb/day of an aqueous solution (50 mg/mL) of ceftiofur for 10 days. The results indicated that ceftiofur administered intravenously at a dose of 10.0 or 25.0 mg/lb/day apparently can change the bacterial flora of the large intestine thereby leading to inflammation of the large intestine with subsequent diarrhea and other clinical signs (loose feces, eating bedding straw, dehydration, rolling or colic and a dull, inactive demeanor). Decreased food consumption, a loss of body weight, hematologic changes related to acute inflammation and stress, and serum chemistry changes related to decreased food consumption and diarrhea were also associated with treatment at these doses. The adverse effects were most severe a few days after dosing was initiated and tended to become less severe toward the end of the 10-day dosing period.

Dogs: Ceftiofur sodium was well tolerated at the therapeutic dose and is safe for the treatment of urinary tract infections in dogs. In the acute safety study, ceftiofur was well tolerated by dogs at the recommended level (1.0 mg/lb) for 5-14 days. When administered subcutaneously for 42 consecutive days, one of four females developed thrombocytopenia (15 days) and anemia (36 days). Thrombocytopenia and anemia also occurred at the 3X and 5X dose levels. In the reversibility phase of the study (5X dose), the thrombocytopenia reversed within 8 days, and of the two anemic animals the male recovered within 6 weeks and the female was sacrificed due to the severity of the anemia.

In the 15-day tolerance study in dogs, high subcutaneous doses (25 and 125 times the recommended therapeutic dose) produced a progressive and dose-related thrombocytopenia, with some dogs also exhibiting anemia and bone marrow changes. The hematopoietic changes noted in dogs treated with ceftiofur were similar to those associated with long-term cephalosporin administration in dogs and also man. The hematopoietic effects are not expected to occur as a result of recommended therapy.

Day-Old Chickens: In an acute toxicity study of ceftiofur in day-old chicks, a total of 60 male and 60 female chicks were each given single subcutaneous injections of 10, 100 or 1,000 mg/kg of body weight. Treatment on day 1 was followed by 6 days of observation; body weight was determined on days 1, 4 and 7; and selected hematology parameters were evaluated on day 4. No meaningful differences were noted among the treated and control groups of chicks for the parameters evaluated. Histopathologic evaluation of all deaths and chicks surviving to termination did not reveal a target organ or tissue of potential toxicity of ceftiofur when administered at up to 20 times (100 mg/kg) the intended highest use dosage.

Day-Old Turkey Poults: In an acute toxicity study of ceftiofur in day-old turkey poults, a total of 30 male and 30 female poults were each administered single subcutaneous injections of 100, 400 or 800 mg/kg body weight. Injection on day 1 was followed by 6 days of observation; body weight on days 1, 4, and 7; and selected hematology parameters on day 4. No meaningful differences were noted between the treated groups at 100 or 400 mg ceftiofur/kg and a negative control group for the parameters evaluated. Histopathologic evaluation of deaths and poults surviving to termination did not reveal a target organ or tissue of potential toxicity of ceftiofur when administered at up to 50 times (400 mg/kg) the highest use dosage. A dose of 800 mg/kg (100 times the intended highest use dosage) was toxic, resulting in clinical signs and deaths accompanied by gross and microscopic morphologic tissue alterations.

Adverse Reactions: The use of ceftiofur may result in some signs of immediate and transient local pain to the animal.

Presentation: NAXCEL® Sterile Powder is available in the following package sizes:
1 gram vial (NDC 0009-3362-03)
4 gram vial (NDC 0009-3362-04)

Manufactured by: GlaxoSmithKline, Research Triangle Park, NC 27709.

U.S. Patent No. 4,464,367

Compendium Code No.: 10490363 814 055 419

NB BLEN® PLUS

Merial Select **Vaccine**

Newcastle-Bronchitis Vaccine, B_1 Type, LaSota Strain Mass. and Conn. Types, Live Virus

Contents: This product contains the antigens listed above.

This vaccine is composed of live viruses in a lyophilized preparation sealed under vacuum.

Contains gentamicin as a bacteriostatic agent.

Notice: Merial Select's vaccines have met the requirements of the USDA in regard to safety, purity, potency, and the capability to protect susceptible chickens. This vaccine has been tested by the Master Seed immunogenicity test for efficacy.

Indications: This vaccine is recommended for vaccination of healthy chickens at least four days of age by eyedrop and 21 days of age by drinking water as an aid in the prevention of Newcastle disease and Massachusetts and Connecticut types bronchitis. Revaccination approximately four weeks after the initial vaccination is recommended.

This vaccine is recommended for the protection of healthy chickens. It is essential that the chickens be maintained under good environmental conditions and that exposure to disease viruses be reduced as much as possible.

Dosage and Administration:

Intraocular Vaccination: The vaccine used for intraocular vaccination is accompanied by diluent and is recommended for the vaccination of healthy chickens four days of age or older using the 2,000 dose vial.

1. Reconstitute each 1,000 doses of vaccine with 30 mL of diluent.
   a. Remove aluminum seal and rubber stopper from vaccine vial and diluent vial. Avoid contamination of stoppers and contents.
   b. Add diluent to half-fill the vaccine vial. Replace stopper in vial and shake it so that all contents are dissolved.
   c. Pour the reconstituted vaccine into the diluent container. Replace stopper in diluent container and shake.
   d. Remove stopper and fit drop-dispenser tip into diluent container.
2. Holding the diluent container with the dropper tip down, gently press the sides, dropping one drop of vaccine on the bird's eye. Be sure the vaccine spreads over the eye before releasing the bird.

Drinking Water Vaccination Using Pouring Application: Drinking water vaccination is recommended for healthy chickens at least 21 days of age.

1. Remove all medications, sanitizers and disinfectants from the drinking water 72 hours (three days) prior to vaccination.
2. Provide sufficient waterers so that all the chickens can drink at one time. Shut off water supply and allow chickens to consume all the water in the lines.
3. Raise water lines above the chickens' heads. Clean and rinse the waterers thoroughly.
4. Withhold all water from the chickens for a minimum of two hours in warm weather to four hours in cool weather prior to vaccination to stimulate thirst. Withdrawal time should be reduced if half-house brooding is in process.
5. Do not open or mix vaccine until ready to vaccinate.
6. Drinking water for vaccine delivery should contain one ounce (29 gm) of non-fat dry milk per gallon (3.8 liters) of non-chlorinated water, or should contain milk product based stabilizer prepared according to the manufacturer's instructions.
7. Reconstitute the vaccine in 3 gallons (11 liters) of milk-water during cool weather or 4 gallons (15 liters) of milk-water during warm weather for each 1,000 doses.
8. Distribute vaccine solution among waterers. Avoid direct sunlight.
9. Lower waterers and allow the chickens to drink freely. Add the remaining vaccine solution to the water lines as the chickens drink.
10. Do not provide additional drinking water until all the vaccine is consumed.

N

Drinking Water Vaccination Using Proportioner Application: Drinking water vaccination is recommended for healthy chickens at least 21 days of age. Several types of medicator/proportioners are commercially available. Set proportioner to deliver one ounce (30 mL) of vaccine concentrate per one gallon (3.8 liters) of water.

1. Remove all medications, sanitizers and disinfectants from the drinking water 72 hours (three days) prior to vaccination.
2. Clean all containers, hoses and waterers prior to vaccination.
3. Withhold all water from the chickens for a minimum of two hours in warm weather to four hours in cool weather prior to vaccination to stimulate thirst. Withdrawal time should be reduced if half-house brooding is in process.
4. Do not open or mix vaccine until ready to vaccinate.
5. Calculate to supply vaccine solution at a rate of 3 gallons (11 liters) per 1,000 chickens in cool weather and 4 gallons (15 liters) per 1,000 chickens in warm weather. The age of the chickens should be considered when calculating water supply. Always use non-chlorinated water when vaccinating chickens.
   Example:
   1,000 chickens in cool weather x 3 gallons (11 liters) = 3 gallons (11 liters).
   1,000 chickens in warm weather x 4 gallons (15 liters) = 4 gallons (15 liters).
6. Prepare vaccine stock solution as follows:
   a. Determine the quantity of vaccine concentrate required by multiplying one ounce (30 mL) x gallons of water needed for vaccine/drinking water.
   Example:
   For 1,000 chickens: 3 gallons x 1 ounce (30 mL) = 3 ounces (90 mL).
   b. Add 3 ounces (85 gm) of non-fat dry milk per 16 ounces (480 mL) of cool water, or use a commercial milk product based stabilizer according to the manufacturer's instructions. For 1,000 chickens add 0.5 ounces (16 gm) non-fat dry milk to the 3 ounces (90 mL) of water.
   c. Reconstitute the dried vaccine with the milk solution. Rinse the vaccine vial to remove all the vaccine.
7. Insert proportioner hose into the vaccine stock solution and start water flow. Continue until all solution has been consumed before changing water supply to direct flow.
8. Do not medicate or use disinfectants for 24 hours after vaccination.

Precaution(s): Store at 35-45°F (2-7°C). Do not freeze. Use entire contents within eight hours of opening. Burn the container and all unused contents.

Mix only the amount of vaccine to be used immediately and use promptly. Use all at one time and do not stretch the dosage.

Improper storage or handling of the vaccine may result in loss of potency.

Caution(s): Newcastle disease can cause inflammation of the eyelids of humans. Eye protection must be worn when rehydrating and administering this vaccine. Avoid contaminating hands and clothing with the vaccine. Hand washing is recommended after exposure to the product.

Birds should be vaccinated before they reach maturity since bronchitis virus may cause permanent damage to the reproductive tract of mature birds, resulting in eggs with poor interior quality and shell texture.

Infectious bronchitis is highly contagious when non-vaccinated birds are kept in close contact with vaccinated birds during the period of respiratory signs. The vaccine should be used with caution around non-vaccinated laying birds.

Do not vaccinate diseased chickens.

Vaccinate all chickens on the premises at one time.

Administer a minimum of one dose per chicken.

Avoid stress conditions during and following vaccination.

Do not place chickens in contaminated facilities.

Exposure to disease must be minimized as much as possible.

The capability of this vaccine to produce satisfactory results depends upon many factors, including, but not limited to, conditions of storage and handling by the user, administration of the vaccine, health and responsiveness of individual chickens, and degree of field exposure. Therefore, directions for use should be followed carefully. The use of this vaccine is subject to applicable state and federal laws and regulations.

For veterinary use only.

Warning(s): Do not vaccinate within 21 days of slaughter.

Presentation: 25 x 2,000 doses (eyedrop and water).

Compendium Code No.: 11050291 0699

NEIGH-LOX®

K.P.P. **Antacid**

Equine Antacid

Guaranteed Analysis:

Crude Protein (min)	8.0%
Calcium (min)	0.9%
Calcium (max)	1.1%
Phosphorus (min)	3.0%

Ingredients: Ground wheat, ground oat groats, dried whey, dihydroxy-aluminum sodium carbonate, aluminum phosphate, soybean oil, dicalcium carbonate, preserved with ethyoxyquin and propionic acid.

Indications: An aid in the reduction of excess gastric acid in horses and foals caused by high grain intakes.

Directions: Feeding Directions:

Young Growing Horses (6-12 months of age): Add 2 oz (1 scoop) to each grain meal. Do not exceed a total daily intake of 8 oz.

Yearlings (12-24 months of age): Add 4 oz (2 scoops) to each grain meal. Do not exceed a total daily intake of 16 oz.

Horses in Training: Add 4 oz (2 scoops) to each grain meal. Do not exceed a total daily intake of 16 oz.

Precaution(s): Store in a cool, dry place.

Presentation: 3.5 lbs (1.59 kg) and 25 lbs (11.36 kg).

U.S. Patent No. 6,284,265

Compendium Code No.: 10790001 02-205

NEMEX™ TABS

Pfizer Animal Health **Parasiticide-Oral**

(pyrantel pamoate) Canine Anthelmintic Tablets

NADA No.: 101-331

Active Ingredient(s): For small dogs and puppies, each tablet contains 22.7 mg pyrantel base as pyrantel pamoate.

For large dogs, each tablet contains 113.5 mg pyrantel base as pyrantel pamoate.

Indications: For removal of ascarids *(Toxocara canis, Toxascaris leonina)* and hookworms *(Anclyostoma caninum, Uncinaria stenocephala)* in dogs and puppies.

To prevent reinfection of *T. canis* in puppies and adult dogs and in lactating bitches after whelping.

Directions:

For Small Dogs and Puppies: For the removal of large roundworms (ascarids) and hookworms, give 1 tablet for each 10 lb of body weight (Dosage is designed to provide at least 2.27 mg per lb of body weight for dogs weighing over 5 lb and at least 4.54 mg per lb of body weight for dogs weighing less than 5 lb). For dogs weighing more than 10 lb, tablets may be broken in half to provide ½ tablet for each additional 5 lb of body weight.

For Large Dogs: For the removal of large roundworms (ascarids) and hookworms, give 1 tablet for each 50 lb of body weight. Tablets may be broken in half to provide ½ tablet for 25 lb of body weight.

Place tablet directly into back of mouth or conceal tablet in a small amount of food. A follow-up fecal examination should be conducted 2-4 weeks after first treatment to determine the need for retreatment.

Because anthelmintics cannot be relied upon to prevent reinfection or to remove larvae not present in the intestinal tract at the time of initial treatment, for maximum control, it is recommended that puppies be treated at 2, 3, 4, 6, 8 and 10 weeks of age. Lactating bitches should be treated 2-3 weeks after whelping. Adult dogs should be routinely treated at monthly intervals to protect against environmental *T. canis* reinfection. Retreatment of adult dogs may be necessary at monthly intervals as determined by laboratory fecal examinations or in animals kept in known contaminated quarters. Consult your veterinarian for assistance in the diagnosis, treatment, and control of parasitism.

The presence of these parasites should be confirmed by laboratory fecal examination. Do not withhold food from dog prior to or after treatment.

Caution(s): If dog looks or acts sick, do not treat with this product.

For use only as directed on label.

Restricted Drug (California)—Use only as directed.

For veterinary use only.

Warning(s): Not for human use. Keep out of reach of children.

Presentation: For Small Dogs and Puppies: Bottles of 100 tablets.
For Large Dogs: Bottles of 50 tablets.

Compendium Code No.: 36901201 01-4167-35-3 / 01-4166-35-3

NEMEX™-2 SUSPENSION

Pfizer Animal Health **Parasiticide-Oral**

(pyrantel pamoate) Canine Anthelmintic Suspension

NADA No.: 100-237

Active Ingredient(s): NEMEX™-2 is a suspension of pyrantel pamoate in a palatable caramel-flavored vehicle. Each mL contains 4.54 mg of pyrantel base as pyrantel pamoate.

Indications: NEMEX™-2 Suspension is a highly palatable formulation intended as a single treatment for the removal of large roundworms *(Toxocara canis* and *Toxascaris leonina)* and hookworms *(Anclyostoma caninum* and *Uncinaria stenocephala)* in dogs and puppies. The presence of these parasites should be confirmed by laboratory fecal examination. Consult your veterinarian for assistance in the diagnosis, treatment, and control of parasitism.

NEMEX™-2 Suspension may also be used to prevent reinfestation of *T. canis* in puppies and adult dogs and in lactating bitches after whelping.

Pharmacology: Pyrantel pamoate is a compound belonging to a family classified chemically as tetrahydropyrimidines. It is a yellow, water-insoluble crystalline salt of the tetrahydropyrimidine base and pamoic acid containing 34.7% base activity. The chemical structure and name are given below:

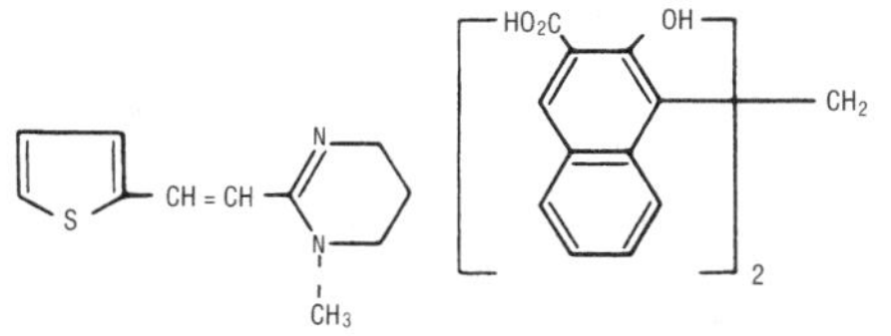

HO_2C OH CH_2 CH = CH S N N CH_3 2

(E)-1,4,5,6-Tetrahydro-1-methyl-2-[2-(2-thienyl) vinyl] pyrimidine 4,4' methylenebis [3-hydroxy-2-naphtoate] (1:1)

Directions for Use: Administer 1 teaspoon (5 mL) for each 10 lb of body weight. It is not necessary to withhold food prior to or after treatment. Dogs usually find this dewormer very palatable and will lick the dose from the bowl willingly. If there is reluctance to accept the dose, mix in a small quantity of dog food to encourage consumption. It is recommended that dogs maintained under conditions of constant exposure to worm infestation should have a follow-up fecal exam within 2-4 weeks after treatment.

For maximum control and prevention of reinfestation, it is recommended that puppies be treated at 2, 3, 4, 6, 8, and 10 weeks of age. Lactating bitches should be treated 2-3 weeks after whelping. Adult dogs kept in heavily contaminated quarters may be treated at monthly intervals to prevent *T. canis* reinfestation.

Precaution(s): This product is a suspension and as such will separate. To ensure uniform resuspension and to achieve proper dosage, it is extremely important that the product be shaken thoroughly before every use.

Store below 30°C (86°F).

Caution(s): Keep out of reach of children.

For animal use only.

Toxicology: One of the most significant features of NEMEX™-2 is its wide margin of therapeutic safety in dogs. The acute oral LD_{50} of pyrantel pamoate administered in gelatin capsules to female and male dogs is greater than 314 mg base per lb of body weight, which indicates a therapeutic index in excess of 138 times the recommended dosage. In subacute and chronic studies, no significant morphological abnormalities could be attributed to NEMEX™-2 when administered to dogs at daily dose rates of up to 94 mg base per lb of body weight (40x) for periods of 19, 30, and 90 days. Clinical studies conducted in a wide variety of geographic locations using more than 40 different breeds of dogs showed no drug-induced toxic effects. Included in these studies were nursing pups, weaned pups, adults, pregnant bitches, and males at stud. Additional data have demonstrated the safe use of NEMEX™-2 in dogs having heartworm infestations and/or receiving medication for heartworms, dogs exposed to organophosphate flea collars or flea/tick dip treatments, and dogs undergoing concurrent treatment or medication at the time of worming such as immunization and antibacterial treatment.

Trial Data: Critical (worm count) studies in dogs demonstrated that NEMEX™-2 at the recommended dosage is highly efficacious against *T. leonina* (99%), *T. canis* (85%), *A. caninum* (97%), and *U. stenocephala* (94%).

Presentation: Available in 2 fl oz (60 mL) and 15 fl oz (473 mL) bottles.

Compendium Code No.: 36901210 75-7991-00

NEO-325 SOLUBLE POWDER

Bimeda **Water Medication**

Neomycin Sulfate (commercial grade)-Antibacterial

ANADA No.: 200-050

Active Ingredient(s): Each 100 g Packet Contains: 71.4 g neomycin sulfate (commercial grade) equivalent to 50 g neomycin.

Each 200 g Packet Contains: 142.8 g neomycin sulfate (commercial grade) equivalent to 100 g neomycin.

Each Pound Contains: 325 g neomycin sulfate (commercial grade) equivalent to 277.5 g neomycin.

Indications: For the treatment and control of colibacillosis (bacterial enteritis) caused by *Escherichia coli* susceptible to neomycin sulfate in cattle (excluding veal calves), swine, sheep and goats. For the control of mortality associated with *Escherichia coli* organisms susceptible to neomycin sulfate in growing turkeys.

Dosage and Administration: Add to drinking water — Not for use in liquid supplements.

Administer to cattle (excluding veal calves), swine, sheep and goats at a dose of 10 mg neomycin sulfate per pound of body weight per day in divided doses for a maximum of 14 days. Administer to turkeys at a dose of 10 mg neomycin sulfate per pound of body weight per day for 5 days.

Herd/Flock Treatment: Each 100 g packet will treat 7,150 pounds body weight. Each 200 g packet will treat 14,300 pounds body weight. Therefore, estimate the total number of pounds of body weight of the animals to be treated and administer one (1) 100 g packet (or portion thereof) for each 7,150 pounds, or one (1) 200 g packet (or portion thereof) for each 14,300 pounds. The product should be added to the amount of drinking water estimated to be consumed in 12-24 hours. Provide medicated water as the sole source of water each day until consumed, followed by non-medicated water as required. Fresh medicated water should be prepared each day.

Individual Animal Treatment: To provide 10 mg neomycin sulfate per pound of body weight, mix one (1) level teaspoon in water or milk for each 160 pounds body weight. Administer daily either as a drench in divided doses or in the drinking water to be consumed in 12-24 hours.

Drinking Water: Swine — Use the number of packets indicated below in 256 gallons of water, or in two gallons of stock solution used in proportioner set to meter one once per gallon.

	No. of 100 g Packets	No. of 200 g Packets
Pigs Weighing 25 to 50 Pounds	2	1
Pigs Weighing 50 to 100 Pounds	3	1.5
Pigs Weighing Over 100 Pounds	4	2

Using measuring spoons, the recommended dosage can be determined as follows.

Daily Schedule for Drinking Water:

Swine:

One tablespoonful* of NEO-325 added to water consumed in one day will treat	Weight of each pig
50 pigs	10 pounds
20 pigs	25 pounds
10 pigs	50 pounds

Cattle:

One tablespoonful* of NEO-325 added to water or milk consumed in one day will treat	Weight of each calf
10 calves	50 pounds
7 calves	75 pounds
4 calves	125 pounds

Turkeys:

One tablespoonful* of NEO-325 added to water or milk consumed in one day will treat	Weight of each bird
1000 birds	0.5 pounds
500 birds	1 pound
100 birds	5 pounds
50 birds	10 pounds

*Level Tablespoonful = US Standard Measure

The product should be added to the amount of drinking water estimated to be consumed in 12-24 hours. Provide medicated water as the sole source of water each day until consumed, followed by non-medicated water as required. Fresh medicated water should be prepared each day. For a stock solution, add six level tablespoonfuls to one gallon of water. Each pint of this stock solution will medicate 5 gallons of drinking water.

For use in automatic proportioners delivering 2 ounces of stock solution per gallon of drinking water, dissolve 9 level tablespoonfuls in a gallon of water to make the stock solution.

Precaution(s): Fold opened packet tightly to keep out moisture.

When storing partially used containers, securely close bags and keep container tightly closed to prevent contents from caking.

Store at controlled room temperature.

Caution(s): To administer the stated dosage, the concentration of neomycin required in medicated water must be adjusted to compensate for variation in age and weight of animal, the nature and severity of disease signs, and environmental temperature and humidity, each of which affects water consumption.

If symptoms persist after using this preparation for 2 or 3 days, consult a veterinarian. If symptoms such as fever, depression, or going off feed develop, oral neomycin is not indicated as the sole treatment since systemic levels of neomycin are not obtained due to low absorption from the gastrointestinal tract.

Important: Treatment should continue 24 to 48 hours beyond remission of disease symptoms, but not to exceed a total of 14 consecutive days for cattle, swine, sheep and goats and 5 days for turkeys. Animals not drinking or eating should be treated individually by drench.

For animal use only.

Not for human use.

Restricted Drug — Use only as directed (California).

Warning(s): Discontinue treatment prior to slaughter by at least the number of days listed below for appropriate species:

Cattle. . . . . 1 day
Swine and goats . . . . 3 days
Sheep . . . . 2 days
Turkeys. . . . . 0 days

A withdrawal period has not been established for this product in pre-ruminating calves. Do not use in calves to be processed for veal.

A milk discard has not been established for this product in lactating dairy cattle.

Do not use in female dairy cattle 20 months of age or older.

Keep out of reach of children.

Presentation: 100 g (3.5 oz) packet, 200 g (7 oz) packet, and 50 lb (22.7 kg) bag.

Compendium Code No.: 13990271 8NEO008-602 / 8NEO008-802 / 8NEO003-1201

NEOBACIMYX® ℞

Schering-Plough **Ophthalmic-Antibiotic**

(Bacitracin-Neomycin-Polymyxin) Ophthalmic Ointment-Sterile, Veterinary Antibacterial

NADA No.: 065-016

Active Ingredient(s): Description: Each gram contains: 400 units bacitracin zinc, 5 mg neomycin sulfate (equivalent to 3.5 mg neomycin base), 10,000 units polymyxin B sulfate, in a base of white petrolatum and mineral oil.

Indications: In the treatment of superficial bacterial infections of the eyelid and conjunctiva in dogs and cats when due to organisms susceptible to the antibiotics contained in the ointment. Laboratory tests should be conducted including *in vitro* culturing and susceptibility tests on samples collected prior to treatment.

Pharmacology: Actions: The three antibiotics present in NEOBACIMYX® Ophthalmic Ointment provide a broad spectrum of activity against the gram-positive and gram-negative bacteria commonly involved in superficial infections of the eyelid and conjunctiva. Bacitracin is effective against gram-positive bacteria including hemolytic and non-hemolytic Streptococci and Staphylococci. Resistant strains rarely develop. Neomycin is effective against both gram-positive and gram-negative bacteria including Staphylococci, *Escherichia coli, Haemophilus* influenzae and many strains of Proteus and Pseudomonas. Polymyxin B is bactericidal to gram-negative bacteria especially Pseudomonas. No resistant strains have been found to develop *in vivo.*

Dosage and Administration: Apply a thin film over the cornea three or four times daily in dogs

N

and cats. The area should be properly cleansed prior to the use of NEOBACIMYX® Ophthalmic Ointment. Foreign bodies, crusted exudates and debris should be carefully removed.

Contraindication(s): Do not use this product as a pre-surgical ocular lubricant. Adverse reactions of ocular irritation and corneal ulceration have been reported in association with such use.

Precaution(s): Store at room temperature.

Caution(s): Federal law restricts this drug to use by or on the order of a licensed veterinarian.

Sensitivity to NEOBACIMYX® Ophthalmic Ointment is rare, however, if a reaction occurs, discontinue use of the preparation. As with any antibiotic preparation, prolonged use may result in the overgrowth of non-susceptible organisms including fungi. Appropriate measures should be taken if this occurs. If infection does not respond to treatment in 2 or 3 days, the diagnosis and therapy should be re-evaluated.

Care should be taken not to contaminate the applicator tip of the tube during application of the preparation. Do not allow the applicator tip to come in contact with any tissue.

Adverse Reactions: Itching, burning, or inflammation may occur in animals sensitive to the product. Discontinue use in such cases.

Presentation: Cartons of 12 x 3.5 g sterile, tamper-proof tubes (NDC 0061-0039-01).

Manufactured by: Altana, Inc., Melville, NY 11747.

Compendium Code No.: 10471341 Rev. 2/98

NEOBACIMYX®-H ℞

Schering-Plough **Ophthalmic Antimicrobial-Corticosteroid**

(Bacitracin-Neomycin-Polymyxin-Hydrocortisone Acetate 1%) Sterile, Veterinary Ophthalmic Ointment

NADA No.: 065-015

Active Ingredient(s): Description: Each gram contains: 400 units bacitracin zinc, 0.5% neomycin sulfate (equivalent to 3.5 mg neomycin base), 10,000 units polymyxin B sulfate, 1% hydrocortisone acetate, in a base of white petrolatum and mineral oil.

Indications: It may be used in acute or chronic conjunctivitis, when caused by organisms susceptible to the antibiotics contained in this ointment. Laboratory tests should be conducted including *in vitro* culturing and susceptibility tests on samples collected prior to treatment.

Pharmacology: Actions: The overlapping spectra of these three antibiotics provide effective bactericidal action against most commonly occurring gram-positive and gram-negative bacteria associated with infections of the eyes. The range of bactericidal activity encompasses many bacteria which are, or have become, resistant to other antibiotics, notably Pseudomonas and Staphylococcus. In susceptible organisms, resistance rarely develops, even on repeated or prolonged usage. Hydrocortisone acetate exerts a marked anti-inflammatory action at the tissue level and effectively suppresses inflammation in many disorders of the anterior segment of the eye. Local application to the eye often gives rapid relief of pain and photophobia, particularly in lesions of the cornea.

The combined anti-inflammatory and antimicrobial activity of NEOBACIMYX®-H Ophthalmic Ointment permits effective management of many disorders of the anterior segment of the eye in which combined activity is needed.

Dosage and Administration: Apply a thin film over the cornea three or four times daily. The area to be treated should be properly cleansed prior to use. Foreign bodies, crusted exudates and debris should be carefully removed. Insert the tip of the tube beneath the lower lid and express a small quantity of the ointment into the conjunctival sac in dogs and cats.

Contraindication(s): Ophthalmic preparations containing corticosteroids are contraindicated in the treatment of those deep, ulcerative lesions of the cornea where the inner layer (endothelium) is involved, in fungal infections and in the presence of viral infections.

Precaution(s): Store at room temperature.

Caution(s): Federal law restricts this drug to use by or on the order of a licensed veterinarian.

Sensitivity to this ophthalmic ointment is rare, however, if reactions occur, discontinue use of the preparation.

N

The prolonged use of antibiotic containing preparations may result in overgrowth of non-susceptible organisms including fungi. Appropriate measures should be taken if this occurs. If infection does not respond to treatment in 2 or 3 days, the diagnosis and therapy should be re-evaluated. Animals under treatment with this product should be observed for usual signs of corticosteroid overdose which include polydipsia and occasionally an increase in weight.

Use of corticosteroids, depending on dose, duration, and specific steroid, may result in inhibition of endogenous steroid production following drug withdrawal. In patients presently receiving or recently withdrawn from systemic corticosteroid treatments, therapy with a rapidly action corticosteroid should be considered in unusually stressful situations. Care should be taken not to contaminate the applicator tip during administration of the preparation.

All topical ophthalmic preparations containing corticosteroids with or without an antimicrobial agent, are contraindicated in the initial treatment of corneal ulcers. They should not be used until the infection is under control and corneal regeneration is well under way.

Clinical and experimental data have demonstrated that corticosteroids administered orally or by injection to animals may induce the first stage of parturition if used during the last trimester of pregnancy and may precipitate premature parturition followed by dystocia, fetal death, retained placenta, and metritis.

Additionally, corticosteroids administered to dogs, rabbits, and rodents during pregnancy have resulted in cleft palate in offspring. Corticosteroids administered to dogs during pregnancy have also resulted in other congenital anomalies including deformed forelegs, phocomelia, and anasarca.

Adverse Reactions: Itching, burning, or inflammation may occur in animals sensitive to the product. Discontinue use in such cases.

SAP and SGPT (ALT) enzyme elevations, polydipsia, and polyuria have occurred following parenteral or systemic use of synthetic corticosteroids in dogs. Vomiting and diarrhea (occasionally bloody) have been observed in dogs.

Cushing's syndrome in dogs has been reported in association with prolonged or repeated steroid therapy.

Presentation: Cartons of 12 x 3.5 g sterile, tamper-proof tubes.

Manufactured by: Altana, Inc., Melville, NY 11747.

Compendium Code No.: 10471351 Rev. 1/99

NEOGUARD™

Intervet **Vaccine**

Neospora Caninum Vaccine, Killed Protozoa

U.S. Vet. Lic. No.: 286

Contents: This product contains the antigen listed above.

Contains neomycin as a preservative.

Indications: NEOGUARD™ with Spur®* is for use in healthy pregnant cattle as an aid in the reduction of abortions caused by *Neospora caninum.*

Dosage and Administration: During the first trimester inject 5 mL subcutaneously, followed by a second 5 mL dose 3-4 weeks later. Revaccination with two doses is recommended for subsequent pregnancies.

Precaution(s): Store at 35-45°F (2-7°C). Shake well before using. Use entire contents when first opened.

Caution(s): Anaphylactoid reactions may occur.

For veterinary use only.

Antidote(s): Epinephrine.

Warning(s): Do not vaccinate within 21 days before slaughter.

Presentation: 50 dose (250 mL) vial.

*Adjuvant-Intervet's proprietary technology.

Neospora Caninum Vaccine - U.S. Patent No. 5,707,617

Compendium Code No.: 11061021 9805002

NEOMIX® 325 SOLUBLE POWDER

Pharmacia & Upjohn **Water Medication**

neomycin sulfate (commercial grade)-Antibacterial

NADA No.: 011-315

Active Ingredient(s): Each 3.5 oz (100 g) packet contains: 71.5 gm neomycin sulfate (commercial grade) equivalent to 50 gm neomycin.

Each pound contains: 325 gm neomycin sulfate equivalent to 227.5 gm neomycin.

Indications: For the treatment and control of colibacillosis (bacterial enteritis) caused by *Escherichia coli* susceptible to neomycin sulfate in cattle, swine, sheep and goats.

For the control of mortality associated with *Escherichia coli* organisms susceptible to neomycin sulfate in growing turkeys.

Dosage and Administration: Administer to turkeys at a dose of 10 mg neomycin sulfate per pound of body weight per day for 5 days. Administer to cattle, swine, sheep and goats at a dose of 10 mg neomycin sulfate per pound of body weight per day in divided doses for a maximum of 14 days.

How to Mix 3.5 oz Packet:

Herd/Flock Treatment: Each packet will treat 7150 pounds body weight. Therefore, estimate the total number of pounds of body weight of the animals to be treated and administer one (1) packet (or portion thereof) for each 7150 pounds. The product should be added to the amount of drinking water estimated to be consumed in 12-24 hours. Provide medicated water as the sole source of water each day until consumed, followed by non-medicated water as required. Fresh medicated water should be prepared each day.

Drinking Water: Use the number of packets indicated below in 256 gallons of water, or in two gallons of stock solution used in proportioners set to meter one ounce per gallon.

Swine:

Pigs Weighing 25 to 50 Pounds . . . . 2 Packets
Pigs Weighing 50 to 100 Pounds . . . . 3 Packets
Pigs Weighing Over 100 Pounds . . . . 4 Packets

How to Mix Using Measuring Spoons: Daily Schedule for Drinking Water

Swine		Cattle		Turkey	
One tablespoonful* of NEOMIX® 325 added to water consumed in one day will treat	Weight of each pig	One tablespoonful* of NEOMIX® 325 added to water or milk consumed in one day will treat	Weight of each calf	One tablespoonful* of NEOMIX® 325 added to water consumed in one day will treat	Weight of each bird
50 pigs	10 pounds	10 calves	50 pounds	1000 birds	.5 pound
20 pigs	25 pounds	7 calves	75 pounds	500 birds	1 pound
10 pigs	50 pounds	4 calves	125 pounds	100 birds	5 pounds
				50 birds	10 pounds

*Level Tablespoonful=US Standard Measure

The product should be added to the amount of drinking water estimated to be consumed in 12-24 hours. Provide medicated water as the sole source of water each day until consumed, followed by non-medicated water as required. Fresh medicated water should be prepared each day. For a Stock Solution, add six level tablespoonfuls to one gallon of water. Each pint of this stock solution will medicate 5 gallons of drinking water.

For use in Automatic Proportioners delivering 2 ounces of stock solution per gallon of drinking water, dissolve 9 level tablespoonfuls in a gallon of water to make the stock solution.

Individual Animal Treatment: To provide 10 mg neomycin sulfate per pound of body weight, mix one (1) level teaspoon in water or milk for each 160 pounds body weight. Administer daily either as a drench in divided doses or in the drinking water to be consumed in 12-24 hours.

Precaution(s): Store at room temperature.

Fold opened packet tightly to keep out moisture.

Keep container tightly closed.

Important: Store in a dry place. When storing partially used containers, securely close bags to prevent contents from caking.

Caution(s): To administer the stated dosage, the concentration of neomycin required in medicated water must be adjusted to compensate for variation in age and weight of animal, the nature and severity of disease signs, and environmental temperature and humidity, each of which affects water consumption.

If symptoms persist after using this preparation for 2 or 3 days, consult a veterinarian. If symptoms such as fever, depression, or going off feed develop, oral neomycin is not indicated as the sole treatment since systemic levels of neomycin are not obtained due to low absorption from the gastrointestinal tract.

Important: Treatment should continue 24 to 48 hours beyond remission of disease symptoms, but not to exceed a total of 14 consecutive days for cattle, swine, sheep, goats and 5 days for turkeys. Animals not drinking or eating should be treated individually by drench.

Restricted Drug—Use only as directed (California).

For use in animals only.

Add to drinking water—Not for use in liquid supplements.

Warning(s): Not for human use. Keep out of reach of children.

Discontinue treatment prior to slaughter by at least the number of days listed below for the appropriate species:

Turkeys . . . . 0 days
Cattle . . . . 1 day
Sheep . . . . 2 days
Swine and goats . . . . 3 days

A withdrawal period has not been established for this product in pre-ruminating calves. Do not use in calves to be processed for veal. A milk discard period has not been established for this product in lactating dairy cattle. Do not use in female dairy cattle 20 months of age or older.

Presentation: 3.5 oz (100 gram) packets (NDC 0009-0553-40) and 50 lb (22.6 kg) bags (NDC 0009-0553-05).

Compendium Code No.: 10490391 813 860 006 / 813 288 208

NEOMIX® AG 325 MEDICATED PREMIX

Pharmacia & Upjohn **Feed Medication**

neomycin sulfate (agricultural grade)-Type A Medicated Article-Antibacterial

NADA No.: 140-976

Active Ingredient(s): Neomycin sulfate, 325 gm/lb.

Inert Ingredient: Sucrose.

Indications: For use in the manufacture of medicated feeds including medicated milk replacers.

For the treatment and control of colibacillosis (bacterial enteritis) caused by *Escherichia coli* susceptible to neomycin sulfate in cattle, swine, sheep, goats and their offspring.

For use as a Type A medicated article in the preparation of Type B or Type C medicated feeds. Type C medicated feeds may be either medicated solid feeds or medicated milk replacers.

Dosage and Administration: Administer 10 mg neomycin sulfate per pound of body weight per day for a maximum of 14 days.

It is recommended that NEOMIX® AG 325 be diluted to prepare an intermediate or working premix prior to addition to final feed. Working premixes typically contain one part NEOMIX® AG 325 to 4 to 19 parts feed.

Type B Feeds: Type B medicated feeds may contain 1.61 to 160.7 grams of NEOMIX® AG 325 per pound of medicated feed (to provide 1.13 to 112.5 grams of neomycin sulfate) per pound of Type B feed.

Type C Medicated Solid Feeds:

Animal	Use Level
Cattle, swine, sheep or goats	Will vary depending on animal consumption and weight. Medicated feeds may contain 250 to 2250 g/ton of neomycin sulfate in complete feed.

Type C Medicated Milk Replacers:

Mixing Directions:

1000 grams per ton	1600 grams per ton
Mix 3.08 lb NEOMIX® AG 325 in 1 ton of milk replacer	Mix 4.92 lb NEOMIX® AG 325 in 1 ton of milk replacer

Example Feeding Directions for Milk Replacers: Note that the examples are based on the following assumptions: Young animals will consume milk replacer at 10% of their body weight per day. Calf and kid milk replacers will contain 12.5% solids after reconstitution. Lamb and piglet milk replacers will contain 20% solids after reconstitution.

Animal	Use level of neomycin sulfate	lb of NEOMIX® AG 325/ton
Calf	10 mg/lb body weight daily	4.92[1]
Kid	10 mg/lb body weight daily	4.92[2]
Lamb	10 mg/lb body weight daily	3.08[3]
Piglet	10 mg/lb body weight daily	3.08[4]

1. Calf weighing 100 lb consuming 1.25 lb dry milk replacer mixed with 1.1 gallon (140 fluid ounces) of water.
2. Kid weighing 20 lb consuming 0.25 lb dry milk replacer mixed with 1.75 pints (28 fluid ounces) of water.
3. Lamb weighing 20 lb consuming 0.4 lb dry milk replacer mixed with 1.6 pints (26 fluid ounces) of water.
4. Piglet weighing 10 lb consuming 0.2 lb dry milk replacer mixed with 0.8 pints (13 fluid ounces) of water.

Precaution(s): Important: Store in a dry place. When storing partially used containers, securely close bags to prevent contents from caking.

Store at room temperature.

Keep container tightly closed.

Caution(s): To administer the stated dosage, the concentration of neomycin required in medicated feed or in medicated milk replacer must be adjusted to compensate for variation in age and weight of animal, the nature and severity of disease signs, and environmental temperature and humidity, each of which affects feed consumption. If symptoms persist after using this preparation for 2 or 3 days, consult a veterinarian. If symptoms such as fever, depression or going off feed develop, oral neomycin is not indicated as the sole treatment since systemic levels of neomycin sulfate are not obtained due to low absorption from the gastrointestinal tract.

Important: Treatment should continue for 24 to 48 hours beyond remission of disease symptoms, but not to exceed a total of 14 consecutive days for cattle, swine, sheep, goats and their offspring.

For use in dry feeds only — not for use in liquid feed supplements.

Restricted Drug—Use only as directed (California). For use in animals only.

Warning(s): Not for human use. Keep out of reach of children.

Discontinue treatment prior to slaughter by at least the number of days listed below for the appropriate species:

Cattle/Ruminating Calves . . . . 1 day
Swine/Piglets . . . . 3 days
Sheep/Lambs . . . . 2 days
Goats/Kids . . . . 3 days

A withdrawal period has not been established for this product in pre-ruminating calves. Do not use in calves to be processed for veal.

A milk discard time has not been established for this product in lactating dairy cattle or lactating dairy goats. Do not use in female dairy cattle 20 months of age or older or female dairy goats 12 months of age or older.

Presentation: 50 lb (22.7 kg) (NDC 0009-0799-12).

Compendium Code No.: 10490402 818 036 201

NEOMIX® AG 325 SOLUBLE POWDER

Pharmacia & Upjohn **Water Medication**

neomycin sulfate (agricultural grade)-Antibacterial

NADA No.: 011-315

Active Ingredient(s): Contains per pound: 325 gm neomycin sulfate equivalent to 227.5 gm neomycin.

Indications: For the treatment and control of colibacillosis (bacterial enteritis) caused by *Escherichia coli* susceptible to neomycin sulfate in cattle, swine, sheep, and goats. For the control of mortality associated with *Escherichia coli* organisms susceptible to neomycin sulfate in growing turkeys.

Dosage and Administration: Administer to turkeys at a dose of 10 mg neomycin sulfate per pound of body weight per day for 5 days. Administer to cattle, swine, sheep and goats at a dose of 10 mg neomycin sulfate per pound of body weight per day in divided doses for a maximum of 14 days. Using measuring spoons, the recommended dosage can be determined as follows:

Daily Schedule for Drinking Water

Swine

One tablespoonful* of NEOMIX® AG 325 added to water consumed in one day will treat	Weight of each pig
50 pigs	10 pounds
20 pigs	25 pounds
10 pigs	50 pounds

Cattle

One tablespoonful* of NEOMIX® AG 325 added to water or milk consumed in one day will treat	Weight of each calf
10 calves	50 pounds
7 calves	75 pounds
4 calves	125 pounds

Turkey

One tablespoonful* of NEOMIX® AG 325 added to water consumed in one day will treat	Weight of each bird
1000 birds	.5 pound
500 birds	1 pound
100 birds	5 pounds
50 birds	10 pounds

*Level Tablespoonful = US Standard Measure

The product should be added to the amount of drinking water estimated to be consumed in 12-24 hours. Provide medicated water as the sole source of water each day until consumed, followed by non-medicated water as required. Fresh medicated water should be prepared each day. For a Stock Solution, add six level tablespoonfuls to one gallon of water. Each pint of this stock solution will medicate 5 gallons of drinking water.

For use in Automatic Proportioners delivering 2 ounces of stock solution per gallon of drinking water, dissolve 9 level tablespoonfuls in a gallon of water to make the stock solution.

Individual Animal Treatment–To provide 10 mg neomycin sulfate per pound of body weight, mix one (1) level teaspoon in water or milk for each 160 pounds of body weight. Administer daily either as a drench in divided doses or in the drinking water to be consumed in 12-24 hours.

Precaution(s): Important: Store in a dry place. When storing partially used containers, securely close bags to prevent contents from caking.

Keep container tightly closed.

Store at room temperature.

Caution(s): To administer the stated dosage, the concentration of neomycin required in medicated water must be adjusted to compensate for variation in age and weight of animal, the nature and severity of disease signs, and environmental temperature and humidity, each of which affects water consumption. If symptoms persist after using this preparation for 2 or 3 days, consult a veterinarian. If symptoms such as fever, depression or going off feed develop, oral neomycin is not indicated as the sole treatment since systemic levels of neomycin are not obtained due to low absorption from the gastrointestinal tract.

Important: Treatment should continue 24 to 48 hours beyond the remission of disease symptoms, but not to exceed a total of 14 consecutive days for cattle, swine, sheep, goats, and 5 days for turkeys. Animals not drinking or eating should be treated individually by drench.

Restricted Drug—Use only as directed (California).

For oral use in animals only.

Add to drinking water—Not for use in liquid supplements.

Not for human use. Keep out of reach of children.

Warning(s): Discontinue treatment prior to slaughter by at least the number of days listed below for appropriate species:

Turkeys . . . . 0 days
Cattle . . . . 1 days
Sheep . . . . 2 days
Swine and goats . . . . 3 days

A withdrawal period has not been established for this product in pre-ruminating calves. Do not use in calves to be processed for veal. A milk discard period has not been established for this product in lactating dairy cattle. Do not use in female dairy cattle 20 months of age or older.

Presentation: 50 lb (22.6 kg) drums (NDC 0009-0799-04).

Compendium Code No.: 10490410 813 275 209

NEOMYCIN 200

Aspen **Water Medication**

Neomycin Oral Solution

ANADA No.: 200-118

Active Ingredient(s): Each mL contains:

Neomycin Sulfate . . . . 200 mg
(equivalent to 140 mg neomycin base)

Indications: For the treatment and control of colibacillosis (bacterial enteritis) caused by *Escherichia coli* susceptible to neomycin sulfate in cattle (excluding veal calves), swine, sheep and goats. Antibacterial for oral use only.

Dosage and Administration: Administer to cattle (excluding veal calves), swine, sheep and goats at a dose of 10 mg neomycin sulfate per pound of body weight in divided doses for a maximum of 14 days.

Dosage Schedule for Treatment of Colibacillosis:

Pounds of Body Weight	Amount of Neomycin Oral Solution per Day in Divided Doses
25 lb	1.2 mL (¼ tsp*)
50 lb	2.5 mL (½ tsp*)
100 lb	5 mL (1 tsp*)
300 lb	15 mL (1 tbsp*)
591.5 lb	29.5 mL (1 fl oz)

Neomycin Oral Solution may be given undiluted or diluted with water.

Herd Treatment: Each 3.785 L (1 gal) will treat 75700 pounds of body weight. Therefore, estimate the total number of pounds of body weight of the animals to be treated and administer 29.5 mL (1 fl oz) for 591.5 pounds. The product should be added to the amount of drinking water estimated to be consumed in 12-24 hours. Provide medicated water as the sole source of water each day until consumed, followed by non-medicated water as required. Fresh medicated water should be prepared each day.

Individual Animal Treatment: To provide 10 mg neomycin sulfate per pound of body weight, mix 5 mL (1 tsp*) in water or milk for each 100 pounds of body weight. Administer daily either as a drench in divided dosages or in the drinking water to be consumed in 12-24 hours.

*Teaspoon (tsp) / Tablespoon (tbsp) is equal to U.S. Standard Measure.

Precaution(s): Store at controlled room temperature between 15° and 30°C (59°-86°F).

Caution(s): To administer the stated dosage, the concentration of neomycin required in medicated water must be adjusted to compensate for variation in age and weight of animal, the nature and severity of disease signs, and environmental temperature and humidity, each of which affects water consumption.

If symptoms persist after using this preparation for 2 or 3 days, consult a veterinarian. If symptoms such as fever, depression, or going off feed develop, oral neomycin is not indicated as the sole treatment since systemic levels of neomycin are not obtained due to poor absorption from the gastrointestinal tract.

Important: Treatment should continue 24 to 48 hours beyond remission of disease symptoms, but not to exceed a total of 14 consecutive days.

Animals not drinking or eating should be treated individually by drench.

Warning(s): Discontinue treatment prior to slaughter by at least the number of days listed below for appropriate species:

Cattle .... 1 day
(not to be used in veal calves)
Sheep .... 2 days
Swine and Goats .... 3 days

A withdrawal period has not been established for this product in pre-ruminating calves. Do not use in calves to be processed for veal.

A milk discard period has not been established for this product in lactating dairy cattle. Do not use in female dairy cattle 20 months of age or older.

Restricted Drug - Use only as directed (California).

For animal use only. Keep out of reach of children.

Presentation: 1 gallon (3.785 L) containers.

Compendium Code No.: 14750570

NEOMYCIN 325

AgriLabs **Water Medication**

Soluble Powder Neomycin Sulfate (Commercial Grade)

ANADA No.: 200-050

Active Ingredient(s): Each Packet Contains: 71.4 g neomycin sulfate (commercial grade) equivalent to 50 g neomycin.

Indications: For the treatment and control of colibacillosis (bacterial enteritis) caused by *Escherichia coli* susceptible to neomycin sulfate in cattle (excluding veal calves), swine, sheep and goats.

Dosage and Administration: Administer to cattle (excluding veal calves), swine, sheep and goats at a dose of 10 mg neomycin sulfate per pound of body weight per day in divided dosed for a maximum of 14 days.

Herd Treatment: Each packet will treat 7150 pounds body weight. Therefore, estimate the total number of pounds of body weight of the animals to be treated and administer one (1) packet (or portion thereof) for each 7150 pounds. The product should be added to the amount of drinking water estimated to be consumed in 12-24 hours. Provide medicated water at the sole source of water each day until consumed, followed by non-medicated water as required. Fresh medicated water should be prepared each day.

Individual Animal Treatment: To provide 10 mg neomycin sulfate per pound of body weight, mix one (1) level teaspoon in water or milk for each 160 pounds body weight. Administer daily either as a drench in divided doses or in the drinking water to be consumed in 12-24 hours.

Drinking Water: Swine — Use the number of packets indicated below in 256 gallons of water, or in two gallons of stock solution used in proportioner set to meter one once per gallon.

Pigs Weighing 25 to 50 Pounds .... 2 Packets
Pigs Weighing 50 to 100 Pounds .... 3 Packets
Pigs Weighing Over 100 Pounds .... 4 Packets

Treatment should continue 24 to 48 hours beyond remission of disease symptoms, but not to exceed a total of 14 consecutive days. Animals not drinking or eating should be treated individually by drench.

Precaution(s): Store at room temperature. Fold opened packet tightly to keep out moisture.

Caution(s): To administer the stated dosage, the concentration of neomycin required in medicated water must be adjusted to compensate for variation in age and weight of animal, the nature and severity of disease signs, and environmental temperature and humidity, each of which affects water consumption.

If symptoms persist after using this preparation for 2 or 3 days, consult a veterinarian. If symptoms such as fever, depression, or going off feed develop, oral neomycin is not indicated as the sole treatment since systemic levels of neomycin are not obtained due to low absorption from the gastrointestinal tract.

Add to drinking water — Not for use in liquid supplements.

Warning(s): Discontinue treatment prior to slaughter by at least the number of days listed below for appropriate species:

Cattle and goats (Not to be used in veal calves) .... 30 days
Swine and sheep .... 20 days

For Animal Use Only. Not For Human Use. Keep Out of Reach of Children.

Restricted Drug — Use Only As Directed (California).

Presentation: 100 Grams (3.5 Oz).

Compendium Code No.: 10580720

NEOMYCIN 325

Durvet **Water Medication**

Soluble Powder-neomycin sulfate (commercial grade)-Antibacterial

ANADA No.: 200-050

Active Ingredients: Each Packet Contains 71.4 g neomycin sulfate (commercial grade) equivalent to 50 g neomycin.

Indications: For the treatment and control of colibacillosis, (bacterial enteritis) caused by *Escherichia coli* susceptible to neomycin sulfate in cattle (excluding veal calves), swine, sheep and goats.

Dosage and Administration: Add to drinking water — Not for use in liquid supplements.

Administer to cattle (excluding veal calves), swine, sheep and goats at a dose of 10 mg neomycin sulfate per pound of body weight per day in divided doses for a maximum of 14 days.

Herd Treatment: Each packet will treat 7150 pounds body weight. Therefore, estimate the total number of pounds of body weight of the animals to be treated and administer one (1) packet (or portion thereof) for each 7150 pounds. The product should be added to the amount of drinking water estimated to be consumed in 12-24 hours. Provide medicated water as the sole source of water each day until consumed, followed by non-medicated water as required. Fresh medicated water should be prepared each day.

Individual Animal Treatment: To provide 10 mg neomycin sulfate per pound of body weight, mix one (1) level teaspoon in water or milk for each 160 pounds of body weight. Administer daily either as a drench in divided doses or in the drinking water to be consumed in 12-24 hours.

Drinking Water: Swine—Use the number of packets indicated below in 256 gallons of water, or in two gallons of stock solution used in proportioner set to meter one ounce per gallon.

Pigs Weighing 25 to 50 Pounds .... 2 Packets
Pigs Weighing 50 to 100 Pounds .... 3 Packets
Pigs Weighing Over 100 Pounds .... 4 Packets

Precaution(s): Store at room temperature.

Fold opened packet tightly to keep out moisture.

Cautions: To administer the stated dosage, the concentration of neomycin required in medicated water must be adjusted to compensate for variation in age and weight of animal, the nature and severity of disease signs, and environmental temperature and humidity, each of which affects water consumption.

If symptoms persist after using this preparation for 2 or 3 days, consult a veterinarian. If symptoms such as fever, depression, or going off feed develop, oral neomycin is not indicated as the sole treatment since systemic levels of neomycin are not obtained due to low absorption from the gastrointestinal tract.

Important: Treatment should continue 24 to 48 hours beyond remission of disease symptoms, but not to exceed a total of 14 consecutive days. Animals not drinking or eating should be treated individually by drench.

For animal use only.

Not for human use.

Restricted Drug - Use only as directed (California).

Warning(s): Discontinue treatment prior to slaughter by at least the number of days listed below for appropriate species:

Cattle .... 1 day
Swine and goats .... 3 days
Sheep .... 2 days

A withdrawal period has not been established for this product in pre-ruminating calves. Do not use in calves to be processed for veal.

A milk discard period has not been established for this product in lactating dairy cattle. Do not use in female dairy cattle 20 months of age or older.

Keep out of reach of children.

Presentation: 100 g (3.5 oz.) packet.

Compendium Code No.: 10841161 598

NEOMYCIN ORAL SOLUTION

AgriLabs **Water Medication**

Antibacterial

ANADA No.: 200-118

Active Ingredients: Composition: Each mL contains:

Neomycin Sulfate .... 200 mg
(equivalent to 140 mg neomycin base)

Indications: For the treatment and control of colibacillosis (bacterial enteritis) caused by *Escherichia coli* susceptible to neomycin sulfate in cattle (excluding veal calves), swine, sheep and goats.

Dosage and Administration: Administer to cattle (excluding veal calves), swine, sheep and goats at a dose of 10 mg neomycin sulfate per pound of body weight in divided doses for a maximum of 14 days.

Dosage Schedule for Treatment of Colibacillosis:

Pounds of Body Weight	Amount of NEOMYCIN ORAL SOLUTION per Day in Divided Doses
25 Lb	1.2 mL (¼ tsp*)
50 Lb	2.5 mL (½ tsp*)
100 Lb	5 mL (1 tsp*)
300 Lb	15 mL (1 tbsp*)
591.5 Lb	29.5 mL (1 Fl Oz)

NEOMYCIN ORAL SOLUTION may be given undiluted or diluted with water.

Herd Treatment: Each 473.1 mL (1 Pt) will treat 9464 pounds of body weight. Therefore, estimate the total number of pounds of body weight of the animals to be treated and administer 29.5 mL (1 Fl Oz) for 591.5 pounds. The product should be added to the amount of drinking water estimated to be consumed in 12-24 hours. Provide medicated water as the sole source of water each day until consumed, followed by non-medicated water as required. Fresh medicated water should be prepared each day.

Individual Animal Treatment: To provide 10 mg neomycin sulfate per pound of body weight, mix 5 mL (1 tsp*) in water or milk for each 100 pounds of body weight. Administer daily either as a drench in divided dosages or in the drinking water to be consumed in 12-24 hours.

* Teaspoon (tsp) / Tablespoon (tbsp) is equal to U.S. Standard Measure.

Precaution(s): Store at controlled room temperature between 15° and 30°C (59°-86°F).

Cautions: To administer the stated dosage, the concentration of neomycin required in medicated water must be adjusted to compensate for variation in age and weight of animal, the nature and severity of disease signs, and environmental temperature and humidity, each of which affects water consumption.

If symptoms persist after using this preparation for 2 or 3 days, consult a veterinarian. If symptoms such as fever, depression, or going off feed develop, oral neomycin is not indicated as the sole treatment since systemic levels of neomycin are not obtained due to poor absorption from the gastrointestinal tract.

Important: Treatment should continue 24 to 48 hours beyond remission of disease symptoms, but not to exceed a total of 14 consecutive days. Animals not drinking or eating should be treated individually by drench.

Restricted drug — Use only as directed (California).

Warning(s): Discontinue treatment prior to slaughter by at least the number of days listed below for appropriate species:

Cattle .... 1 day
(not to be used in veal calves)
Sheep........ 2 days
Swine and Goats .... 3 days

A withdrawal period has not been established for this product in pre-ruminating calves. Do not use in calves to be processed for veal.

A milk discard period has not been established for this product in lactating dairy cattle. Do not use in female dairy cattle 20 months of age or older.

For oral use only. For animal use only. Keep out of reach of children.

Presentation: 473.1 mL (1 pint) and 3.785 L (1 gallon).

Compendium Code No.: 10580730 Rev. 10-98

NEOMYCIN ORAL SOLUTION

Durvet **Water Medication**

Antibacterial

ANADA No.: 200-118

Active Ingredients: Each mL contains:

Neomycin Sulfate........ 200 mg
(equivalent to 140 mg neomycin base)

Indications: For the treatment and control of colibacillosis (bacterial enteritis) caused by *Escherichia coli* susceptible to neomycin sulfate in cattle (excluding veal calves), swine, sheep and goats.

Dosage and Administration: Administer to cattle (excluding veal calves), swine, sheep and goats at a dose of 10 mg neomycin sulfate per pound of body weight in divided doses for a maximum of 14 days.

Dosage Schedule for Treatment of Colibacillosis:

Pounds of Body Weight	Amount of NEOMYCIN ORAL SOLUTION per Day in Divided Doses
25 Lb	1.2 mL (¼ tsp*)
50 Lb	2.5 mL (½ tsp*)
100 Lb	5 mL (1 tsp*)
300 Lb	15 mL (1 tbsp*)
591.5 Lb	29.5 mL (1 Fl Oz)

NEOMYCIN ORAL SOLUTION may be given undiluted or diluted with water.

Herd Treatment: Each 473.1 mL (1 Pt) will treat 9464 pounds of body weight. Each 3.785 L (1 Gal) will treat 75700 pounds of body weight. Therefore, estimate the total number of pounds of body weight of the animals to be treated and administer 29.5 mL (1 Fl Oz) for 591.5 pounds. The product should be added to the amount of drinking water estimated to be consumed in 12-24 hours. Provide medicated water as the sole source of water each day until consumed, followed by non-medicated water as required. Fresh medicated water should be prepared each day.

Individual Animal Treatment: To provide 10 mg neomycin sulfate per pound of body weight, mix 5 mL (1 tsp*) in water or milk for each 100 pounds of body weight. Administer daily either as a drench in divided dosages or in the drinking water to be consumed in 12-24 hours.

* Teaspoon (tsp) / Tablespoon (tbsp) is equal to U.S. Standard Measure.

Precaution(s): Store at controlled room temperature between 15° and 30°C (59°-86°F).

Cautions: To administer the stated dosage, the concentration of neomycin required in medicated water must be adjusted to compensate for variation in age and weight of animal, the nature and severity of disease signs, and environmental temperature and humidity, each of which affects water consumption.

If symptoms persist after using this preparation for 2 or 3 days, consult a veterinarian. If symptoms such as fever, depression, or going off feed develop, oral neomycin is not indicated as the sole treatment since systemic levels of neomycin are not obtained due to poor absorption from the gastrointestinal tract.

Important: Treatment should continue 24 to 48 hours beyond remission of disease symptoms, but not to exceed a total of 14 consecutive days. Animals not drinking or eating should be treated individually by drench.

Restricted drug — Use only as directed (California).

Warning(s): Discontinue treatment prior to slaughter by at least the number of days listed below for appropriate species:

Cattle .... 1 day
(not to be used in veal calves)
Sheep........ 2 days
Swine and Goats .... 3 days

A withdrawal period has not been established for this product in pre-ruminating calves. Do not use in calves to be processed for veal.

A milk discard period has not been established for this product in lactating dairy cattle. Do not use in female dairy cattle 20 months of age or older.

For oral use only. For animal use only. Keep out of reach of children.

Presentation: 473.1 mL (1 pint) and 3.785 L (1 gallon).

Compendium Code No.: 10841170

NEOMYCIN ORAL SOLUTION

Phoenix Pharmaceutical **Water Medication**

Antibacterial

ANADA No.: 200-118

Active Ingredient(s): Composition: Each mL contains:

Neomycin Sulfate........ 200 mg
(equivalent to 140 mg neomycin base)

Indications: For the treatment and control of colibacillosis (bacterial enteritis) caused by *Escherichia coli* susceptible to neomycin sulfate in cattle (excluding veal calves), swine, sheep and goats.

Dosage and Administration: Administer to cattle (excluding veal calves), swine, sheep and goats at a dose of 10 mg neomycin sulfate per pound of body weight in divided doses for a maximum of 14 days.

Dosage Schedule for Treatment of Colibacillosis:

Pounds of Body Weight	Amount of NEOMYCIN ORAL SOLUTION per Day in Divided Doses
25 Lb	1.2 mL (¼ tsp*)
50 Lb	2.5 mL (½ tsp*)
100 Lb	5 mL (1 tsp*)
300 Lb	15 mL (1 tbsp*)
591.5 Lb	29.5 mL (1 fl oz)

*Teaspoon (tsp)/Tablespoon (tbsp) is equal to U.S. Standard Measure.

NEOMYCIN ORAL SOLUTION may be given undiluted or diluted with water.

Herd Treatment: Each 3.785 L (1 Gal) will treat 75700 pounds of body weight. Therefore, estimate the total number of pounds of body weight of the animals to be treated and administer 29.5 mL (1 fl oz) for 591.5 pounds. The product should be added to the amount of drinking water estimated to be consumed in 12-24 hours. Provide medicated water as the sole source of drinking water each day until consumed, followed by non-medicated water as required. Fresh medicated water should be prepared each day.

Individual Animal Treatment: To provide 10 mg neomycin sulfate per pound of body weight, mix 5 mL (1 tsp*) in water or milk for each 100 pounds of body weight. Administer daily either as a drench in divided dosages or in the drinking water to be consumed in 12-24 hours.

Precaution(s): Store at controlled room temperature between 15° and 30°C (59°-86°F).

Caution(s): To administer the stated dosage, the concentration of neomycin required in medicated water must be adjusted to compensate for variation in age and weight of animal, the nature and severity of disease signs, and environmental temperature and humidity, each of which affects water consumption.

If symptoms persist after using this preparation for 2 or 3 days, consult a veterinarian. If symptoms such as fever, depression, or going off feed develop, oral neomycin is not indicated as the sole treatment since systemic levels of neomycin are not obtained due to poor absorption from the gastrointestinal tract.

Important: Treatment should continue 24 to 48 hours beyond remission of disease symptoms, but not to exceed a total of 14 consecutive days. Animals not drinking or eating should be treated individually by drench.

For animal use only.

For oral use only.

Warning(s): Discontinue treatment prior to slaughter by at least the number of days listed below for appropriate species:

Cattle........ 1 day
(not to be used in veal calves)
Sheep .... 2 days
Swine and Goats........ 3 days

A withdrawal period has not been established for this product in pre-ruminating calves Do not use in calves to be processed for veal.

A milk discard period has not been established for this product in lactating dairy cattle. Do not use in female dairy cattle 20 months of age or older.

Restricted Drug - Use only as directed (California).

Keep out of reach of children.

Presentation: 473.1 mL (1 pint) (NDC 57319-309-21) and 3.785 L (1 gal) (NDC 57319-308-09).

Manufactured by: Phoenix Scientific, Inc.

Compendium Code No.: 12560571 Rev. 9-00 / Rev. 1-99

NEO-OXY 10/5 MEAL

PennField **Feed Medication**

(Type B Medicated Feed)

NADA No.: 138-939

Active Ingredient(s): Oxytetracycline (quaternary salt) equivalent to 5 grams oxytetracycline HCl, neomycin sulfate 10 g (equivalent to 7 g neomycin base)/lb.

Ingredients: Roughage products, neomycin sulfate, calcium carbonate, oxytetracycline and mineral oil.

Guaranteed Analysis:

Crude Protein, Not Less Than 1.5%
Crude Fat, Not Less Than 0.3%
Crude Fiber, Not More Than 0.20%

Indications: An antimicrobial premix for use in the prevention, control and treatment of diseases caused by microorganisms sensitive to the drugs included in the formula. For use in the feed of chickens, turkeys, swine and calves.

Directions for Use:

Chickens:

Prevention of diseases from oxytetracycline-susceptible organisms during periods of stress. As an aid in the prevention of bacterial enteritis and in the control of neomycin-sensitive organisms associated with bluecomb (mud fever or nonspecific enteritis).

Drug Ingredient	Use Levels	lbs. of NEO-OXY 10/5 per ton
Oxytetracycline Neomycin Base	50 g/ton 70 g/ton	10.0

Chickens (first 2 weeks).

Prevention of early chick mortality due to oxytetracycline-susceptible organisms. As an aid in the prevention of bacterial enteritis and in the control of neomycin-sensitive organisms associated with bluecomb (mud fever or nonspecific enteritis).

Drug Ingredient	Use Levels	lbs. of NEO-OXY 10/5 per ton
Oxytetracycline Neomycin Base	50-100 g/ton 70-140 g/ton	10.0-20.0

Chickens:

To extend period of high egg production, to improve feed efficiency, to improve egg production and feed efficiency in presence of disease and at time of stress. As an aid in maintaining and improving hatchability where birds are suffering stress from moving, vaccinations, culling, extreme temperature changes, and worming; to improve livability of progeny when losses are due to oxytetracycline-susceptible organisms, to improve egg shell quality, prevention of bluecomb (mud fever or nonspecific enteritis). As an aid in the prevention of bacterial enteritis and in the control of neomycin-sensitive organisms associated with bluecomb (mud fever or nonspecific enteritis).

Drug Ingredient	Use Levels	lbs. of NEO-OXY 10/5 per ton
Oxytetracycline Neomycin Base	50-100 g/ton 70-140 g/ton	10.0-20.0

Chickens:

Prevention of complicated chronic respiratory disease (air-sac infection) and control of complicated chronic respiratory disease by lowering mortality and severity during outbreaks. As an aid in the prevention of bacterial enteritis and in the control of neomycin-sensitive organisms associated with bluecomb (mud fever or nonspecific enteritis).

Drug Ingredient	Use Levels	lbs. of NEO-OXY 10/5 per ton
Oxytetracycline Neomycin Base	100 g/ton 140 g/ton	20.0

Turkeys (first 4 weeks):

As an aid in the prevention of early poult mortality due to oxytetracycline-sensitive organisms. As an aid in the prevention of bacterial enteritis and in the control of neomycin-sensitive organisms associated with bluecomb (mud fever or nonspecific enteritis).

Drug Ingredient	Use Levels	lbs. of NEO-OXY 10/5 per ton
Oxytetracycline Neomycin Base	50-100 g/ton 70-140 g/ton	10.0-20.0

Turkeys:

As an aid in prevention of diseases from oxytetracycline-susceptible organisms during periods of stress. As an aid in the prevention of bacterial enteritis and in the control of neomycin-sensitive organisms associated with bluecomb (mud fever or nonspecific enteritis).

Drug Ingredient	Use Levels	lbs. of NEO-OXY 10/5 per ton
Oxytetracycline Neomycin Base	50 g/ton 70 g/ton	10.0

To extend period of high egg production, to improve egg production, to improve fertility, to improve egg production and feed efficiency in the presence of disease and at time of stress; as an aid in maintaining and improving hatchability where birds are suffering from stress exposure, moving, vaccination, culling, extreme losses due to oxytetracycline-susceptible organisms and to improve egg shell quality, prevention of hexamitiasis. As an aid in the prevention of bacterial enteritis and in the control of neomycin-sensitive organisms associated with bluecomb (mud fever or nonspecific enteritis).

Drug Ingredient	Use Levels	lbs. of NEO-OXY 10/5 per ton
Oxytetracycline Neomycin Base	50-100 g/ton 70-140 g/ton	10.0-20.0

Control of bluecomb (mud fever or nonspecific enteritis), infectious sinusitis and hexamitiasis, prevention of infectious synovitis. As an aid in the prevention of bacterial enteritis and in the control of neomycin-sensitive organisms associated with bluecomb (mud fever or nonspecific enteritis).

Drug Ingredient	Use Levels	lbs. of NEO-OXY 10/5 per ton
Oxytetracycline Neomycin Base	100 g/ton 140 g/ton	20.0

Swine:

As an aid in the prevention of bacterial enteritis (scours), baby pig diarrhea (in baby pigs only), vibrionic dysentery, bloody dysentery and salmonellosis (necro or necrotic enteritis).

Drug Ingredient	Use Levels	lbs. of NEO-OXY 10/5 per ton
Oxytetracycline Neomycin Base	50 g/ton 70 g/ton	10.0

As an aid in the maintenance of weight gain and feed consumption in the presence of atrophic rhinitis. As an aid in the treatment of bacterial enteritis.

Drug Ingredient	Use Levels	lbs. of NEO-OXY 10/5 per ton
Oxytetracycline Neomycin Base	50-100 g/ton 70-140 g/ton	10.0-20.0

Calves, Beef and Nonlactating Dairy Cattle:

As an aid in the prevention of bacterial enteritis (scours).

Drug Ingredient	Use Levels	lbs. of NEO-OXY 10/5 per ton
Oxytetracycline Neomycin Base	50 g/ton 70 g/ton	10.0

As an aid in the treatment of bacterial enteritis (scours). (See Warnings)

Drug Ingredient	Use Levels	lbs. of NEO-OXY 10/5 per ton
Oxytetracycline Neomycin Base	100 g/ton 140 g/ton	20.0

Calves:

As an aid in the prevention of bacterial diarrhea (scours).

Drug Ingredient	Use Levels	lbs. of NEO-OXY 10/5 per ton
Oxytetracycline Neomycin Base	8-100 mg/gal reconstituted milk replacer 100-200 mg/gal reconstituted milk replacer	

As an aid in the treatment of bacterial diarrhea (scours).

Drug Ingredient	Use Levels	lbs. of NEO-OXY 10/5 per ton
Oxytetracycline Neomycin Base	40-200 mg/gal reconstituted milk replacer 200-400 mg/gal reconstituted milk replacer	

Warning(s):

Chickens: Withdraw from feed 5 days before slaughter of broilers and 14 days before slaughter of laying hens.

Turkeys: Withdraw from feed 14 days before slaughter.

Swine: Withdraw from feed 5 days before slaughter.

Calves, Beef and Nonlactating Dairy Cattle:

When fed at the level of 1.4 g neomycin base plus 2 g oxytetracycline per head daily, requires withdrawal from feed 7 days before slaughter. No withdrawal is required at lower levels. A withdrawal period has not been established for this product in pre-ruminating calves. Do not use in calves to be processed for veal.

All use levels in milk replacers for calves require a 30 day withdrawal period before slaughter.

For use in the manufacture of medicated feeds.

For use in dry feeds only - Not for use in liquid feed supplements.

Restricted drug (California) - Use only as directed.

Presentation: 50 lb (22.7 kg).

Compendium Code No.: 10450011

REV. 1-93

NEO-OXY 10/10 MEAL

PennField **Feed Medication**

(Type B Medicated Feed)

NADA No.: 138-939

Active Ingredient(s): Oxytetracycline (quaternary salt) equivalent to 10 grams oxytetracycline HCl, neomycin sulfate 10 g (equivalent to 7 g neomycin base)/lb.

Ingredients: Dried oxytetracycline fermentation meal, neomycin sulfate,* magnesium-mica, calcium carbonate, roughage products and mineral oil.

*Neomycin sulfate manufactured by The Upjohn Company.

Guaranteed Analysis:

Crude Protein, not less than 1.5%
Crude Fat, not less than 0.1%
Crude Fiber, not more than 23.0%
Calcium (Ca), not less than 4.0%
Calcium (Ca), not more than 5.0%
Ash, not more than 60.0%

Indications: An antimicrobial premix for use in the prevention, control and treatment of diseases caused by microorganisms sensitive to the drugs included in the formula. For use in the feed of chickens, turkeys, swine and calves.

Directions for Use: (Use levels are as neomycin base* and oxytetracycline HCl.) Mix quantity of NEO-OXY 10/10 per ton of feed.

Chickens:

Prevention of diseases from oxytetracycline-susceptible organisms during periods of stress. As an aid in the prevention of bacterial enteritis and in the control of neomycin-sensitive organisms associated with bluecomb (mud fever or nonspecific enteritis).

Drug Ingredient	Use Levels	lbs of NEO-OXY 10/10 per ton
Oxytetracycline Neomycin Base	50 g/ton 35 g/ton	5.0

Chickens (first 2 weeks).

Prevention of early chick mortality due to oxytetracycline-susceptible organisms. As an aid in the prevention of bacterial enteritis and in the control of neomycin-sensitive organisms associated with bluecomb (mud fever or nonspecific enteritis).

Drug Ingredient	Use Levels	lbs of NEO-OXY 10/10 per ton
Oxytetracycline Neomycin Base	50-100 g/ton 35-70 g/ton	5.0-10.0

Chickens:

To extend period of high egg production, to improve feed efficiency, to improve egg production and feed efficiency in presence of disease and at time of stress. As an aid in maintaining and improving hatchability where birds are suffering stress from moving, vaccinations, culling, extreme temperature changes, and worming; to improve livability of progeny when losses are due to oxytetracycline-susceptible organisms, to improve egg shell quality, prevention of bluecomb (mud fever or nonspecific enteritis). As an aid in the prevention of bacterial enteritis and in the control of neomycin-sensitive organisms associated with bluecomb (mud fever or nonspecific enteritis).

Drug Ingredient	Use Levels	lbs of NEO-OXY 10/10 per ton
Oxytetracycline Neomycin Base	50-100 g/ton 35-70 g/ton	5.0-10.0

Chickens:

Prevention of complicated chronic respiratory disease (air-sac infection) and control of complicated chronic respiratory disease by lowering mortality and severity during outbreaks. As an aid in the prevention of bacterial enteritis and in the control of neomycin-sensitive organisms associated with bluecomb (mud fever or nonspecific enteritis).

Drug Ingredient	Use Levels	lbs of NEO-OXY 10/10 per ton
Oxytetracycline Neomycin Base	100-200 g/ton 70-140 g/ton	10.0-20.0

Turkeys (first 4 weeks):

As an aid in the prevention of early poult mortality due to oxytetracycline-sensitive organisms. As an aid in the prevention of bacterial enteritis and in the control of neomycin-sensitive organisms associated with bluecomb (mud fever or nonspecific enteritis).

Drug Ingredient	Use Levels	lbs of NEO-OXY 10/10 per ton
Oxytetracycline Neomycin Base	50-100 g/ton 35-70 g/ton	5.0-10.0

As an aid in reducing mortality in birds which have suffered an attack of air-saculitis (it is recommended, wherever possible, to feed from time of attack to marketing).

Drug Ingredient	Use Levels	lbs of NEO-OXY 10/10 per ton
Oxytetracycline Neomycin Base	100-150 g/ton 70-105 g/ton	10.0-15.0

Turkeys:

As an aid in the prevention of diseases from oxytetracycline-susceptible organisms during periods of stress. As an aid in the prevention of bacterial enteritis and in the control of neomycin-sensitive organisms associated with bluecomb (mud fever or nonspecific enteritis).

Drug Ingredient	Use Levels	lbs of NEO-OXY 10/10 per ton
Oxytetracycline Neomycin Base	50 g/ton 35 g/ton	5.0

To extend period of high egg production, to improve egg production, to improve feed efficiency, to improve fertility, to improve egg production, and feed efficiency in the presence of disease and at time of stress; as an aid in maintaining and improving hatchability where birds are suffering stress from exposure, moving, vaccination, culling, extreme losses due to oxytetracycline-susceptible organisms, and to improve egg shell quality, prevention of hexamitiasis. As an aid in the prevention of bacterial enteritis and in the control of neomycin-sensitive organisms associated with bluecomb (mud fever or nonspecific enteritis).

Drug Ingredient	Use Levels	lbs of NEO-OXY 10/10 per ton
Oxytetracycline Neomycin Base	50-100 g/ton 35-70 g/ton	5.0-10.0

As an aid in reducing mortality in birds which have suffered an attack of air-saculitis (it is recommended, wherever possible, to feed from time of attack to marketing). As an aid in the prevention of bacterial enteritis and in the control of neomycin-sensitive organisms associated with bluecomb (mud fever or nonspecific enteritis).

Drug Ingredient	Use Levels	lbs of NEO-OXY 10/10 per ton
Oxytetracycline Neomycin Base	100-150 g/ton 70-105 g/ton	10.0-15.0

Control of bluecomb (mud fever or nonspecific enteritis), infectious sinusitis and hexamitiasis, prevention of infectious synovitis. As an aid in the prevention of bacterial enteritis and in the control of neomycin-sensitive organisms associated with bluecomb (mud fever or nonspecific enteritis).

Drug Ingredient	Use Levels	lbs of NEO-OXY 10/10 per ton
Oxytetracycline Neomycin Base	100-200 g/ton 70-140 g/ton	10.0-20.0

Control of infectious synovitis. For the treatment of bacterial enteritis and bluecomb (mud fever or nonspecific enteritis).

Drug Ingredient	Use Levels	lbs of NEO-OXY 10/10 per ton
Oxytetracycline Neomycin Base	200 g/ton 140 g/ton	20.0

Swine (baby pigs, growing-finishing pigs and sows):

As an aid in the prevention of bacterial enteritis (scours), baby pig diarrhea (in baby pigs only), vibrionic dysentery, bloody dysentery and salmonellosis (necro or necrotic enteritis).

Drug Ingredient	Use Levels	lbs of NEO-OXY 10/10 per ton
Oxytetracycline Neomycin Base	50 g/ton 35 g/ton	5.0

As an aid in the treatment of bacterial enteritis (scours), baby pig diarrhea (in baby pigs only), vibrionic dysentery, bloody dysentery and salmonellosis (necro or necrotic enteritis).

Drug Ingredient	Use Levels	lbs of NEO-OXY 10/10 per ton
Oxytetracycline Neomycin Base	100 g/ton 70 g/ton	10.0

As an aid in the maintenance of weight gains and feed consumption in the presence of atrophic rhinitis. As an aid in the treatment of bacterial enteritis. (When used in sows: to be fed during the gestation and lactation periods.)

Drug Ingredient	Use Levels	lbs of NEO-OXY 10/10 per ton
Oxytetracycline Neomycin Base	100-150 g/ton 70-105 g/ton	10.0-15.0

Calves:

As an aid in the prevention of bacterial enteritis (scours).

Drug Ingredient	Use Levels	lbs of NEO-OXY 10/10 per ton
Oxytetracycline Neomycin Base	50 g/ton 35 g/ton	5.0

As an aid in the treatment of bacterial enteritis (scours). (See Warnings)

Drug Ingredient	Use Levels	lbs of NEO-OXY 10/10 per ton
Oxytetracycline Neomycin Base	100 g/ton 70 g/ton	10.0

As an aid in the prevention of bacterial enteritis (scours).

Drug Ingredient	Use Levels	lbs of NEO-OXY 10/10 per ton
Oxytetracycline Neomycin Base	8-100 mg/gal reconstituted milk replacer 100-200 mg/gal reconstituted milk replacer	

As an aid in the treatment of bacterial enteritis (scours).

Drug Ingredient	Use Levels	lbs of NEO-OXY 10/10 per ton
Oxytetracycline Neomycin Base	40-200 mg/gal reconstituted milk replacer 200-400 mg/gal reconstituted milk replacer	

Warning(s):

Chickens: Withdraw from feed 5 days before slaughter of broilers and 14 days before slaughter of laying hens.

Turkeys: Withdraw from feed 14 days before slaughter.

Swine: Withdraw from feed 5 days before slaughter.

Calves:

A withdrawal period has not been established for this product in preruminating calves. Do not use in calves to be processed for veal.

This product, when fed to calves at a level of 1.4 g neomycin base plus 2 grams oxytetracycline per head daily, requires withdrawal from feed 7 days before slaughter. No withdrawal is required at lower levels.

All use levels in milk replacers for calves require a 30 day withdrawal period before slaughter.

For use in the manufacture of medicated animal feeds.

For use in dry feeds only - Not for use in liquid feed supplements.

Restricted drug (California) - Use only as directed.

Presentation: 50 lb (22.7 kg).

Compendium Code No.: 10450001

NEO-OXY 50/50 MEAL

PennField **Feed Medication**

(Type A Medicated Feed)

NADA No.: 138-939

Active Ingredient(s): Oxytetracycline (quaternary salt) equivalent to 50 grams oxytetracycline HCl, neomycin sulfate 50 g (equivalent to 35 g neomycin base)/lb.

Ingredients: Dried oxytetracycline fermentation meal, neomycin sulfate,* magnesium-mica, calcium carbonate, roughage products and mineral oil.

*Neomycin sulfate manufactured by The Upjohn Company.

Indications: An antimicrobial premix for use in the prevention, control and treatment of diseases caused by microorganisms sensitive to the drugs included in the formula. For use in the feed of chickens, turkeys, swine and calves.

Directions for Use: (Use levels are as neomycin base* and oxytetracycline HCl.) Mix quantity of NEO-OXY 50/50 per ton of feed.

Chickens:

Prevention of diseases from oxytetracycline-susceptible organisms during periods of stress. As an aid in the prevention of bacterial enteritis and in the control of neomycin-sensitive organisms associated with bluecomb (mud fever or nonspecific enteritis).

Drug Ingredient	Use Levels	lbs of NEO-OXY 50/50 per ton
Oxytetracycline Neomycin Base	50 g/ton 35 g/ton	1.0

Chickens (first 2 weeks).

Prevention of early chick mortality due to oxytetracycline-susceptible organisms. As an aid in the prevention of bacterial enteritis and in the control of neomycin-sensitive organisms associated with bluecomb (mud fever or nonspecific enteritis).

Drug Ingredient	Use Levels	lbs of NEO-OXY 50/50 per ton
Oxytetracycline Neomycin Base	50-100 g/ton 35-70 g/ton	1.0-2.0

Chickens:

To extend period of high egg production, to improve feed efficiency, to improve egg production and feed efficiency in presence of disease and at time of stress. As an aid in maintaining and improving hatchability where birds are suffering stress from moving, vaccinations, culling, extreme temperature changes, and worming; to improve livability of progeny when losses are due to oxytetracycline-susceptible organisms, to improve egg shell quality, prevention of bluecomb (mud fever or nonspecific enteritis). As an aid in the prevention of bacterial enteritis and in the control of neomycin-sensitive organisms associated with bluecomb (mud fever or nonspecific enteritis).

Drug Ingredient	Use Levels	lbs of NEO-OXY 50/50 per ton
Oxytetracycline Neomycin Base	50-100 g/ton 35-70 g/ton	1.0-2.0

Chickens:

Prevention of complicated chronic respiratory disease (air-sac infection) and control of complicated chronic respiratory disease by lowering mortality and severity during outbreaks. As an aid in the prevention of bacterial enteritis and in the control of neomycin-sensitive organisms associated with bluecomb (mud fever or nonspecific enteritis).

Drug Ingredient	Use Levels	lbs of NEO-OXY 50/50 per ton
Oxytetracycline Neomycin Base	100-200 g/ton 70-140 g/ton	2.0-4.0

Turkeys (first 4 weeks):

As an aid in the prevention of early poult mortality due to oxytetracycline-sensitive organisms. As an aid in the prevention of bacterial enteritis and in the control of neomycin-sensitive organisms associated with bluecomb (mud fever or nonspecific enteritis).

Drug Ingredient	Use Levels	lbs of NEO-OXY 50/50 per ton
Oxytetracycline Neomycin Base	50-100 g/ton 35-70 g/ton	1.0-2.0

As an aid in reducing mortality in birds which have suffered an attack of air-saculitis (it is recommended, wherever possible, to feed from time of attack to marketing).

Drug Ingredient	Use Levels	lbs of NEO-OXY 50/50 per ton
Oxytetracycline Neomycin Base	100-150 g/ton 70-105 g/ton	2.0-3.0

Turkeys:

As an aid in the prevention of diseases from oxytetracycline-susceptible organisms during periods of stress. As an aid in the prevention of bacterial enteritis and in the control of neomycin-sensitive organisms associated with bluecomb (mud fever or nonspecific enteritis).

Drug Ingredient	Use Levels	lbs of NEO-OXY 50/50 per ton
Oxytetracycline Neomycin Base	50 g/ton 35 g/ton	1.0

To extend period of high egg production, to improve egg production, to improve feed efficiency, to improve fertility, to improve egg production, and feed efficiency in the presence of disease and at time of stress; as an aid in maintaining and improving hatchability where birds are suffering stress from exposure, moving, vaccination, culling, extreme losses due to oxytetracycline-susceptible organisms, and to improve egg shell quality, prevention of hexamitiasis. As an aid in the prevention of bacterial enteritis and in the control of neomycin-sensitive organisms associated with bluecomb (mud fever or nonspecific enteritis).

Drug Ingredient	Use Levels	lbs of NEO-OXY 50/50 per ton
Oxytetracycline Neomycin Base	50-100 g/ton 35-70 g/ton	1.0-2.0

As an aid in reducing mortality in birds which have suffered an attack of air-saculitis (it is recommended, wherever possible, to feed from time of attack to marketing). As an aid in the prevention of bacterial enteritis and in the control of neomycin-sensitive organisms associated with bluecomb (mud fever or nonspecific enteritis).

Drug Ingredient	Use Levels	lbs of NEO-OXY 50/50 per ton
Oxytetracycline Neomycin Base	100-150 g/ton 70-105 g/ton	2.0-3.0

Control of bluecomb (mud fever or nonspecific enteritis), infectious sinusitis and hexamitiasis, prevention of infectious synovitis. As an aid in the prevention of bacterial enteritis and in the control of neomycin-sensitive organisms associated with bluecomb (mud fever or nonspecific enteritis).

Drug Ingredient	Use Levels	lbs of NEO-OXY 50/50 per ton
Oxytetracycline Neomycin Base	100-200 g/ton 70-140 g/ton	2.0-4.0

Control of infectious synovitis. For the treatment of bacterial enteritis and bluecomb (mud fever or nonspecific enteritis).

Drug Ingredient	Use Levels	lbs of NEO-OXY 50/50 per ton
Oxytetracycline Neomycin Base	200 g/ton 140 g/ton	4.0

Swine (baby pigs, growing-finishing pigs and sows):

As an aid in the prevention of bacterial enteritis (scours), baby pig diarrhea (in baby pigs only), vibrionic dysentery, bloody dysentery and salmonellosis (necro or necrotic enteritis).

Drug Ingredient	Use Levels	lbs of NEO-OXY 50/50 per ton
Oxytetracycline Neomycin Base	50 g/ton 35 g/ton	1.0

As an aid in the treatment of bacterial enteritis (scours), baby pig diarrhea (in baby pigs only), vibrionic dysentery, bloody dysentery and salmonellosis (necro or necrotic enteritis).

Drug Ingredient	Use Levels	lbs of NEO-OXY 50/50 per ton
Oxytetracycline Neomycin Base	100 g/ton 70 g/ton	2.0

As an aid in the maintenance of weight gains and feed consumption in the presence of atrophic rhinitis. As an aid in the treatment of bacterial enteritis. (When used in sows: to be fed during the gestation and lactation periods.)

Drug Ingredient	Use Levels	lbs of NEO-OXY 50/50 per ton
Oxytetracycline Neomycin Base	100-150 g/ton 70-105 g/ton	2.0-3.0

Calves:

As an aid in the prevention of bacterial enteritis (scours).

Drug Ingredient	Use Levels	lbs of NEO-OXY 50/50 per ton
Oxytetracycline Neomycin Base	50 g/ton 35 g/ton	1.0

As an aid in the treatment of bacterial enteritis (scours). (See Warnings)

Drug Ingredient	Use Levels	lbs of NEO-OXY 50/50 per ton
Oxytetracycline Neomycin Base	100 g/ton 70 g/ton	2.0

As an aid in the prevention of bacterial enteritis (scours).

Drug Ingredient	Use Levels	lbs of NEO-OXY 50/50 per ton
Oxytetracycline Neomycin Base	8-100 mg/gal reconstituted milk replacer 100-200 mg/gal reconstituted milk replacer	

As an aid in the treatment of bacterial enteritis (scours).

Drug Ingredient	Use Levels	lbs of NEO-OXY 50/50 per ton
Oxytetracycline Neomycin Base	40-200 mg/gal reconstituted milk replacer 200-400 mg/gal reconstituted milk replacer	

Warning(s):

Chickens: Withdraw from feed 5 days before slaughter of broilers and 14 days before slaughter of laying hens.

Turkeys: Withdraw from feed 14 days before slaughter.

Swine: Withdraw from feed 5 days before slaughter.

Calves:

A withdrawal period has not been established for this product in preruminating calves. Do not use in calves to be processed for veal.

This product, when fed to calves at a level of 1.4 g neomycin base plus 2 grams oxytetracycline per head daily, requires withdrawal from feed 7 days before slaughter. No withdrawal is required at lower levels.

All use levels in milk replacers for calves require a 30 day withdrawal period before slaughter.

For use in the manufacture of medicated animal feeds.

For use in dry feeds only - Not for use in liquid feed supplements.

Restricted drug (California) - Use only as directed.

Presentation: 50 lb (22.7 kg).

Compendium Code No.: 10450041

NEO-OXY 100/50 MEAL

PennField **Feed Medication**

(Type A Medicated Feed)

NADA No.: 138-939

Active Ingredient(s): Oxytetracycline (quaternary salt) equivalent to 50 grams oxytetracycline HCl, neomycin sulfate 100 g (equivalent to 70 g neomycin base)/lb.

Ingredients: Dried oxytetracycline fermentation meal, neomycin sulfate,* magnesium-mica, calcium carbonate, roughage products and mineral oil.

*Neomycin sulfate manufactured by The Upjohn Company.

Indications: An antimicrobial premix for use in the prevention, control and treatment of diseases caused by microorganisms sensitive to the drugs included in the formula. For use in the feed of chickens, turkeys, swine and calves.

Directions for Use: (Use levels are as neomycin base* and oxytetracycline HCl.) Mix quantity of NEO-OXY 100/50 per ton of feed.

Chickens:

Prevention of diseases from oxytetracycline-susceptible organisms during periods of stress. As an aid in the prevention of bacterial enteritis and in the control of neomycin-sensitive organisms associated with bluecomb (mud fever or nonspecific enteritis).

Drug Ingredient	Use Levels	lbs of NEO-OXY 100/50 per ton
Oxytetracycline Neomycin Base	50 g/ton 70 g/ton	1.0

Chickens (first 2 weeks).

Prevention of early chick mortality due to oxytetracycline-susceptible organisms. As an aid in the prevention of bacterial enteritis and in the control of neomycin-sensitive organisms associated with bluecomb (mud fever or nonspecific enteritis).

Drug Ingredient	Use Levels	lbs of NEO-OXY 100/50 per ton
Oxytetracycline Neomycin Base	50-100 g/ton 70-140 g/ton	1.0-2.0

Chickens:

To extend period of high egg production, to improve feed efficiency, to improve egg production and feed efficiency in presence of disease and at time of stress. As an aid in maintaining and improving hatchability where birds are suffering stress from moving, vaccinations, culling, extreme temperature changes, and worming; to improve livability of progeny when losses are due to oxytetracycline-susceptible organisms, to improve egg shell quality, prevention of bluecomb (mud fever or nonspecific enteritis). As an aid in the prevention of bacterial enteritis and in the control of neomycin-sensitive organisms associated with bluecomb (mud fever or nonspecific enteritis).

Drug Ingredient	Use Levels	lbs of NEO-OXY 100/50 per ton
Oxytetracycline Neomycin Base	50-100 g/ton 70-140 g/ton	1.0-2.0

Chickens:

Prevention of complicated chronic respiratory disease (air-sac infection) and control of complicated chronic respiratory disease by lowering mortality and severity during outbreaks. As an aid in the prevention of bacterial enteritis and in the control of neomycin-sensitive organisms associated with bluecomb (mud fever or nonspecific enteritis).

Drug Ingredient	Use Levels	lbs of NEO-OXY 100/50 per ton
Oxytetracycline Neomycin Base	100-200 g/ton 140-280 g/ton	2.0-4.0

Turkeys (first 4 weeks):

As an aid in the prevention of early poult mortality due to oxytetracycline-sensitive organisms. As an aid in the prevention of bacterial enteritis and in the control of neomycin-sensitive organisms associated with bluecomb (mud fever or nonspecific enteritis).

Drug Ingredient	Use Levels	lbs of NEO-OXY 100/50 per ton
Oxytetracycline Neomycin Base	50-100 g/ton 70-140 g/ton	1.0-2.0

As an aid in reducing mortality in birds which have suffered an attack of air-saculitis (it is recommended, wherever possible, to feed from time of attack to marketing).

Drug Ingredient	Use Levels	lbs of NEO-OXY 100/50 per ton
Oxytetracycline Neomycin Base	100-150 g/ton 140-210 g/ton	2.0-3.0

Turkeys:

As an aid in the prevention of diseases from oxytetracycline-susceptible organisms during periods of stress. As an aid in the prevention of bacterial enteritis and in the control of neomycin-sensitive organisms associated with bluecomb (mud fever or nonspecific enteritis).

Drug Ingredient	Use Levels	lbs of NEO-OXY 100/50 per ton
Oxytetracycline Neomycin Base	50 g/ton 70 g/ton	1.0

To extend period of high egg production, to improve egg production, to improve feed efficiency, to improve fertility, to improve egg production, and feed efficiency in the presence of disease and at time of stress; as an aid in maintaining and improving hatchability where birds are suffering stress from exposure, moving, vaccination, culling, extreme losses due to oxytetracycline-susceptible organisms, and to improve egg shell quality, prevention of hexamitiasis. As an aid in the prevention of bacterial enteritis and in the control of neomycin-sensitive organisms associated with bluecomb (mud fever or nonspecific enteritis).

Drug Ingredient	Use Levels	lbs of NEO-OXY 100/50 per ton
Oxytetracycline Neomycin Base	50-100 g/ton 70-140 g/ton	1.0-2.0

As an aid in reducing mortality in birds which have suffered an attack of air-saculitis (it is recommended, wherever possible, to feed from time of attack to marketing). As an aid in the prevention of bacterial enteritis and in the control of neomycin-sensitive organisms associated with bluecomb (mud fever or nonspecific enteritis).

Drug Ingredient	Use Levels	lbs of NEO-OXY 100/50 per ton
Oxytetracycline Neomycin Base	100-150 g/ton 140-210 g/ton	2.0-3.0

Control of bluecomb (mud fever or nonspecific enteritis), infectious sinusitis and hexamitiasis, prevention of infectious synovitis. As an aid in the prevention of bacterial enteritis and in the control of neomycin-sensitive organisms associated with bluecomb (mud fever or nonspecific enteritis).

Drug Ingredient	Use Levels	lbs of NEO-OXY 100/50 per ton
Oxytetracycline Neomycin Base	100-200 g/ton 140-280 g/ton	2.0-4.0

Control of infectious synovitis. For the treatment of bacterial enteritis and bluecomb (mud fever or nonspecific enteritis).

Drug Ingredient	Use Levels	lbs of NEO-OXY 100/50 per ton
Oxytetracycline Neomycin Base	200 g/ton 280 g/ton	4.0

Swine (baby pigs, growing-finishing pigs and sows):

As an aid in the prevention of bacterial enteritis (scours), baby pig diarrhea (in baby pigs only), vibrionic dysentery, bloody dysentery and salmonellosis (necro or necrotic enteritis).

Drug Ingredient	Use Levels	lbs of NEO-OXY 100/50 per ton
Oxytetracycline Neomycin Base	50 g/ton 70 g/ton	1.0

As an aid in the treatment of bacterial enteritis (scours), baby pig diarrhea (in baby pigs only), vibrionic dysentery, bloody dysentery and salmonellosis (necro or necrotic enteritis).

Drug Ingredient	Use Levels	lbs of NEO-OXY 100/50 per ton
Oxytetracycline Neomycin Base	100 g/ton 140 g/ton	2.0

As an aid in the maintenance of weight gains and feed consumption in the presence of atrophic rhinitis. As an aid in the treatment of bacterial enteritis. (When used in sows: to be fed during the gestation and lactation periods.)

Drug Ingredient	Use Levels	lbs of NEO-OXY 100/50 per ton
Oxytetracycline Neomycin Base	100-150 g/ton 140-210 g/ton	2.0-3.0

Calves:

As an aid in the prevention of bacterial enteritis (scours).

Drug Ingredient	Use Levels	lbs of NEO-OXY 100/50 per ton
Oxytetracycline Neomycin Base	50 g/ton 70 g/ton	1.0

As an aid in the treatment of bacterial enteritis (scours). (See Warnings)

Drug Ingredient	Use Levels	lbs of NEO-OXY 100/50 per ton
Oxytetracycline Neomycin Base	100 g/ton 140 g/ton	2.0

As an aid in the prevention of bacterial enteritis (scours).

Drug Ingredient	Use Levels	lbs of NEO-OXY 100/50 per ton
Oxytetracycline Neomycin Base	8-100 mg/gal reconstituted milk replacer 100-200 mg/gal reconstituted milk replacer	

As an aid in the treatment of bacterial enteritis (scours).

Drug Ingredient	Use Levels	lbs of NEO-OXY 100/50 per ton
Oxytetracycline Neomycin Base	40-200 mg/gal reconstituted milk replacer 200-400 mg/gal reconstituted milk replacer	

Warning(s):

Chickens: Withdraw from feed 5 days before slaughter of broilers and 14 days before slaughter of laying hens.

Turkeys: Withdraw from feed 14 days before slaughter.

Swine: Withdraw from feed 5 days before slaughter.

Calves:

A withdrawal period has not been established for this product in preruminating calves. Do not use in calves to be processed for veal.

This product, when fed to calves at a level of 1.4 g neomycin base plus 2 grams oxytetracycline per head daily, requires withdrawal from feed 7 days before slaughter. No withdrawal is required at lower levels.

All use levels in milk replacers for calves require a 30 day withdrawal period before slaughter.

For use in the manufacture of medicated animal feeds.

For use in dry feeds only - Not for use in liquid feed supplements.

Restricted drug (California) - Use only as directed.

Presentation: 50 lb (22.7 kg).

Compendium Code No.: 10450021

NEO-OXY 100/50 MR

PennField **Feed Medication**

(Type A Medicated Article)

NADA No.: 138-939

Active Ingredient(s):

Oxytetracycline (As Quaternary Salt) equivalent to Oxytetracycline Hydrochloride .... 50 g/lb.

Neomycin base from neomycin sulfate .... 100 g/lb.

Indications:

Calves (Milk Replacer): Aid in the prevention and treatment of bacterial enteritis (scours).

Baby Pigs (Milk Replacer): Aid in the prevention and treatment of bacterial enteritis (scours).

Directions for Use: Mixing and Use Directions: Mix NEO-OXY 100/50 MR with nonmedicated milk replacer to provide the following dosages:

Indications for use	Oxytetracycline(1)	Neomycin(1) base	lb of NEO-OXY 100/50 MR/ton(2)
Calves (Milk Replacer)			
Aid in the prevention of bacterial enteritis (scours)	50-100 mg/gal	100-200 mg/gal	2-4
Aid in the treatment of bacterial enteritis (scours)	100-200 mg/gal	200-400 mg/gal	4-8
Baby Pigs (Milk Replacer)			
Aid in the prevention of bacterial enteritis (scours)	50 g/ton	100 g/ton	1
Aid in the treatment of bacterial enteritis (scours)	50-70 g/ton	100-140 g/ton	1-1.4

(1) The dosage in calves is expressed in mg/gallon of reconstituted milk replacer whereas in baby pigs the dosage is expressed in g/ton of dry milk replacer.

(2) Mixing directions for calves are for example only and are based on mixing 1 lb of dry milk replacer with 1 gallon of water.

Warning(s): In calves withdraw from feed 30 days prior to slaughter. In pigs withdraw from feed 10 days before slaughter when neomycin base level is 140 g/ton and 5 days withdrawal when the neomycin base level is below 140 g/ton. A withdrawal period has not been established for this product in preruminating calves. Do not use in calves to be processed for veal.

For use in the manufacture of medicated feeds.

For use in dry feeds only. Not for use in liquid feed supplements.

Restricted drug (California) - Use only as directed.

Presentation: 100 lb (48.6 kg) drum.

Compendium Code No.: 10450030

Revised 1/2000 Label AH12

NEO-OXY 100/100 MEAL

PennField **Feed Medication**

(Type A Medicated Article)

NADA No.: 138-939

Active Ingredient(s): Oxytetracycline (Quaternary Salt) equivalent to 100 grams Oxytetracycline HCl, Neomycin Sulfate 100 g (equivalent to 70 g Neomycin Base)/lb.

Ingredients: Calcium Carbonate, Roughage Products, Neomycin Sulfate and Mineral Oil.

Indications: For use in the manufacture of medicated animal feeds.

An antimicrobial premix for use in the prevention, control and treatment of diseases caused by microorganisms sensitive to the drugs included in the formula. For use in the feed of chickens, turkeys, swine and calves.

Directions for Use: (Use levels are as Neomycin Base and Oxytetracycline HCl. Mix quantity of NEO-OXY 100/100 per ton of feed).

Chickens:

Prevention of diseases from oxytetracycline-susceptible organisms during periods of stress. As an aid in the prevention of bacterial enteritis and in the control of neomycin-sensitive organisms associated with bluecomb (mud fever or nonspecific enteritis).

Drug Ingredient	Use Levels	lbs of NEO-OXY 100/100 per ton
Oxytetracycline Neomycin Base	50 g/ton 35 g/ton	0.5

Chickens (first 2 weeks):

Prevention of early chick mortality due to oxytetracycline-susceptible organisms. As an aid in the prevention of bacterial enteritis and in the control of neomycin-sensitive organisms associated with bluecomb (mud fever or nonspecific enteritis).

Drug Ingredient	Use Levels	lbs of NEO-OXY 100/100 per ton
Oxytetracycline Neomycin Base	50-100 g/ton 35-70 g/ton	0.5-1.0

Chickens:

To extend period of high egg production, to improve feed efficiency, to improve egg production and feed efficiency in presence of disease and at time of stress. As an aid in maintaining and improving hatchability where birds are suffering stress from moving, vaccinations, culling, extreme temperature changes, and worming; to improve livability of progeny when losses are due to oxytetracycline-susceptible organisms, to improve egg shell quality, prevention of bluecomb (mud fever or nonspecific enteritis). As an aid in the prevention of bacterial enteritis and in the control of neomycin-sensitive organisms associated with bluecomb (mud fever or nonspecific enteritis).

Drug Ingredient	Use Levels	lbs of NEO-OXY 100/100 per ton
Oxytetracycline Neomycin Base	50-100 g/ton 35-70 g/ton	0.5-1.0

Chickens:

Prevention of complicated chronic respiratory disease (air-sac infection) and control of complicated chronic respiratory disease by lowering mortality and severity during outbreaks. As an aid in the prevention of bacterial enteritis and in the control of neomycin-sensitive organisms associated with bluecomb (mud fever or nonspecific enteritis).

Drug Ingredient	Use Levels	lbs of NEO-OXY 100/100 per ton
Oxytetracycline Neomycin Base	100-200 g/ton 70-140 g/ton	1.0-2.0

Turkeys (first 4 weeks):

As an aid in the prevention of early poult mortality due to oxytetracycline-sensitive organisms. As an aid in the prevention of bacterial enteritis and in the control of neomycin-sensitive organisms associated with bluecomb (mud fever or nonspecific enteritis).

Drug Ingredient	Use Levels	lbs of NEO-OXY 100/100 per ton
Oxytetracycline Neomycin Base	50-100 g/ton 35-70 g/ton	0.5-1.0

Turkeys:

As an aid in the prevention of disease from oxytetracycline-susceptible organisms during periods of stress. As an aid in the prevention of bacterial enteritis and in the control of neomycin-sensitive organisms associated with bluecomb (mud fever or nonspecific enteritis).

Drug Ingredient	Use Levels	lbs of NEO-OXY 100/100 per ton
Oxytetracycline Neomycin Base	50 g/ton 35 g/ton	0.5

Turkeys:

To extend period of high egg production, to improve egg production, to improve fertility, to improve egg production, and feed efficiency in the presence of disease and at time of stress; as an aid in maintaining and improving hatchability where birds are suffering stress from exposure, moving, vaccination, culling, extreme losses due to oxytetracycline-susceptible organisms, and to improve egg shell quality, prevention of hexamitiasis. As an aid in the prevention of bacterial enteritis and in the control of neomycin-sensitive organisms associated with bluecomb (mud fever or nonspecific enteritis).

Drug Ingredient	Use Levels	lbs of NEO-OXY 100/100 per ton
Oxytetracycline Neomycin Base	50-100 g/ton 35-70 g/ton	0.5-1.0

As an aid in reducing mortality in birds which have suffered an attack of air-saculitis (it is recommended, wherever possible, to feed from time of attack to marketing). As an aid in the prevention of bacterial enteritis and in the control of neomycin-sensitive organisms associated with bluecomb (mud fever or nonspecific enteritis).

Drug Ingredient	Use Levels	lbs of NEO-OXY 100/100 per ton
Oxytetracycline Neomycin Base	100-150 g/ton 70-105 g/ton	1.0-1.5

Control of bluecomb (mud fever or nonspecific enteritis), infectious sinusitis and hexamitiasis, prevention of infectious synovitis. As an aid in the prevention of bacterial enteritis and in the control of neomycin-sensitive organisms associated with bluecomb (mud fever or nonspecific enteritis).

Drug Ingredient	Use Levels	lbs of NEO-OXY 100/100 per ton
Oxytetracycline Neomycin Base	100-200 g/ton 70-140 g/ton	1.0-2.0

Control of infectious synovitis. For the treatment of bacterial enteritis and bluecomb (mud fever or nonspecific enteritis).

Drug Ingredient	Use Levels	lbs of NEO-OXY 100/100 per ton
Oxytetracycline Neomycin Base	200 g/ton 140 g/ton	2.0

Swine:

As an aid in the prevention of bacterial enteritis (scours), baby pig diarrhea (in baby pigs only), vibrionic dysentery, bloody dysentery and salmonellosis (necro or necrotic enteritis).

Drug Ingredient	Use Levels	lbs of NEO-OXY 100/100 per ton
Oxytetracycline Neomycin Base	50 g/ton 35 g/ton	0.5

As an aid in the maintenance of weight gain and feed consumption in the presence of atrophic rhinitis. As an aid in the treatment of bacterial enteritis.

Drug Ingredient	Use Levels	lbs of NEO-OXY 100/100 per ton
Oxytetracycline Neomycin Base	100-150 g/ton 70-105 g/ton	1.0-1.5

Calves:

As an aid in the prevention of bacterial enteritis (scours).

Drug Ingredient	Use Levels	lbs of NEO-OXY 100/100 per ton
Oxytetracycline Neomycin Base	50 g/ton 35 g/ton	0.5

As an aid in the treatment of bacterial enteritis (scours). (See Warnings)

Drug Ingredient	Use Levels	lbs of NEO-OXY 100/100 per ton
Oxytetracycline Neomycin Base	100 g/ton 70 g/ton	1.0

As an aid in the prevention of bacterial enteritis (scours).

Drug Ingredient	Use Levels	lbs of NEO-OXY 100/100 per ton
Oxytetracycline Neomycin Base	8-100 mg/gal reconstituted milk replacer 100-200 mg/gal reconstituted milk replacer	

As an aid in the treatment of bacterial enteritis (scours).

Drug Ingredient	Use Levels	lbs of NEO-OXY 100/100 per ton
Oxytetracycline Neomycin Base	40-200 mg/gal reconstituted milk replacer 200-400 mg/gal reconstituted milk replacer	

Caution(s): For use in dry feeds only - not for use in liquid feed supplements.

Restricted Drug (California - Use only as directed.

Warning(s):

Chickens: Withdraw from feed 5 days before slaughter of broilers and 14 days before slaughter of laying hens.

Turkeys: Withdraw from feed 14 days before slaughter.

Swine: Withdraw from feed 5 days before slaughter.

Calves: When fed at the level of 1.4 g Neomycin base plus 2 g Oxytetracycline per head daily, requires withdrawal from feed 7 days before slaughter. No withdrawal is required at lower levels. A withdrawal period has not been established for this product in pre-ruminating calves. Do not use in calves to be processed for veal.

All use levels in milk replacers for calves require a 30 day withdrawal period before slaughter.

Presentation: 50 lb (22.7 kg) bag.

Compendium Code No.: 10450200 Rev. 2/01 Bag N1

NEOPAR®

NeoTech **Vaccine**

Canine Parvovirus Vaccine, Modified Live Virus

U.S. Vet. Lic. No.: 472

Description: NEOPAR® is a modified live virus vaccine containing a high antigenic mass per dose of a highly immunogenic strain of canine parvovirus.

Gentamicin and Amphotericin B are used as preservatives.

Indications: NEOPAR® is for the vaccination of healthy dogs against disease due to canine parvovirus. NEOPAR® is designed to be used primarily where the severe threat of canine parvovirus infections exists in the resident dog population.

This vaccine gives reliable protection against infections by other known strains of canine parvovirus.

NEOPAR® overrides moderate to high antibody levels such as those found in puppies having maternal antibodies or in dogs from pre-existing vaccination. It can be used successfully as a booster for a pre-existing vaccination.

Puppies vaccinated with NEOPAR® generated high levels of the IgM and IgG classes of antibodies. Secretory immunity was engendered in the gut. Reversion to virulence does not occur. Field studies indicate that this vaccine is safe in puppies 3 weeks of age or older.

Dosage and Administration: Aseptically inject 1 mL subcutaneously or intramuscularly into healthy dogs. Administer the initial dose at or about 42 days of age. Because there is potential for maternal antibody to interfere with the immune response to the original vaccination, revaccinate every 14 to 21 days until the dog is 18 weeks of age. Dogs over 18 weeks should receive a single dose (1 mL). Revaccinate annually with one dose.

Precaution(s): Store between 2° and 7°C (35° and 45°F). Do not freeze. Shake well before using. Use entire contents when first opened. Burn this container and all unused contents.

Caution(s): Do not vaccinate pregnant bitches or obviously sick or debilitated dogs. The use of this vaccine may produce anaphylaxis and/or other inflammatory reactions.

For use in dogs only.

For veterinary use only.

Antidote(s): Epinephrine, corticosteroids, and antihistamines may all be indicated depending on the nature and severity of the reaction.

Presentation: 10 dose (10 mL) and 1 dose (1 mL) vials.

Compendium Code No.: 12670000

NEO-PREDEF® WITH TETRACAINE POWDER ℞

Pharmacia & Upjohn **Topical Antimicrobial-Corticosteroid**

brand of neomycin sulfate, isoflupredone acetate, tetracaine hydrochloride topical powder

NADA No.: 015-433

Active Ingredient(s): NEO-PREDEF® with Tetracaine Powder contains in each gram neomycin sulfate, 5 mg (equivalent to 3.5 mg neomycin); isoflupredone acetate, 1 mg; tetracaine hydrochloride, 5 mg; myristyl-gamma-picolinium chloride, 0.2 mg; also lactose hydrous. Because of the prompt, potent, and specific actions of the individual components, this combination is well suited for the treatment of certain ear and skin conditions occurring in dogs, cats and horses.

Indications: NEO-PREDEF® with Tetracaine Powder is indicated in the treatment or adjunctive therapy of certain ear and skin conditions in dogs, cats and horses caused by or associated with neomycin-susceptible organisms and/or allergy. In addition, it is indicated as superficial dressing applied to minor cuts, wounds, lacerations, abrasions, and for post-surgical application where reduction of pain and inflammatory response is deemed desirable. NEO-PREDEF® with Tetracaine Powder may be used as a dusting powder following amputation of tails, claws, and dew-claws; following ear trimming and castrating; and following such surgical procedure as ovariohysterectomies.

Applied superficially, it has been used successfully in the treatment of acute otitis externa in dogs, acute moist dermatitis and interdigital dermatitis in the dog, and as a dusting powder to various minor cuts, lacerations, and abrasions in the horse, cat and dog.

Pharmacology:

Isoflupredone Acetate: Isoflupredone acetate markedly inhibits inflammatory reaction through its controlling influence on connective tissue and vascular components. Topically applied isoflupredone acetate is usually rapidly effective. In otitis externa, wounds of the concha, ulcerations of the ear flaps, and irritated lesions of the skin, the inflammatory response may also be effectively inhibited by isoflupredone acetate. Chronic conditions respond more slowly and relapses are more frequent.

Neomycin: Neomycin is an antibiotic substance derived from cultures of the soil organism *Streptomyces fradiae*. Its antimicrobial range includes both gram-positive and gram-negative organisms commonly responsible for or associated with otic infections, such as staphylococci, streptococci, *Escherichia coli, Aerobacter aerogenes*, and many strains of Proteus and Pseudomonas organisms. It is not active against fungi. Neomycin is unusually nontoxic for epithelial cells in tissue culture and is nonirritating in therapeutic concentrations. The presence of neomycin in NEO-PREDEF® with Tetracaine Powder affords control of neomycin-sensitive organisms.

Tetracaine: Tetracaine hydrochloride is a topical anesthetic agent that is more potent than either procaine or cocaine in comparable concentration. The duration of anesthetic action of tetracaine exceeds that produced by either butacaine or phenacaine.

Many investigators have demonstrated that local anesthesia plays a significant part in the promotion of healing, especially where pain is a prominent factor. It is believed that trauma stimulates local pain receptors, which results in reflex vasodilation, edema, tenderness, and muscular spasm.

If the reflex is abolished through use of a local anesthetic such as tetracaine, amelioration of these tissue changes that interfere with healing is favored. The local anesthetic action of tetracaine has proved to be of great value in alleviating the pain reflex in painful skin and ear conditions.

Myristyl-Gamma-Picolinium Chloride: Myristyl-gamma-picolinium Chloride is highly germicidal, nonirritating and relatively nontoxic. In solution it reduces surface tension (a surfactant), possesses detergent and emulsifying actions, and exhibits properties which favor the penetration and wetting of tissue surfaces. The drug is effective against a wide range of organisms, its active ingredient killing in ten minutes *Staphylococcus aureus* in dilutions up to 1:85,000 at 37 degrees Centigrade; E. typhosa in dilutions up to 1:140,000; *Esch. coli* in dilutions up to 1:40,000, and *S. dysenteriae* in dilutions up to 1:80,000.

Myristyl-gamma-picolinium Chloride has been used, per se, for preoperative disinfection of the skin, for application to superficial injuries, for irrigating deep wounds, and for application to infections and wounds of mucous membranes.

Dosage and Administration: For topical ear and skin use in dogs, cats and horses.

Application: After cleansing the affected area, NEO-PREDEF® with Tetracaine Powder is applied by compressing the sides of the container with short, sharp squeezes. In most instances a single daily application will be sufficient; however, it may be applied one to three times daily, as required.

Precaution(s): Storage: Store in a dry place at controlled room temperature 20° to 25°C (68° to 77°F) [see USP].

Because of the hygroscopic properties of neomycin sulfate, the bottle should be stored in a dry place. The cap should be replaced when the bottle is not in use. The puffer bottle has been designed to permit dusting when held in any position. Protecting the outlet from moisture will aid in assuring proper function; therefore, the tip should not be allowed to come in contact with moist membranes or weeping surfaces.

Caution(s): Federal (USA) law restricts this drug to use by or on the order of a licensed veterinarian.

Incomplete response or exacerbation of corticosteroid-response lesions may be due to the presence of nonsusceptible organisms or to prolonged use of antibiotic-containing preparations resulting in overgrowth of nonsusceptible organisms, particularly Monilia. Thus, if improvement is not noted within two or three days, or if redness, irritation, or swelling persists or increases, the diagnosis should be redetermined and appropriate therapeutic measures initiated.

Before instilling any medication into the ear, examine the external ear canal thoroughly to be certain the tympanic membrane is not ruptured in order to avoid the possibility of transmitting infection to the middle ear as well as damaging the cochlea or vestibular apparatus from prolonged contact. If hearing or vestibular dysfunction is noted during the course of treatment discontinue use of NEO-PREDEF® with Tetracaine Powder.

For use in animals only.

Presentation: NEO-PREDEF® with Tetracaine Powder is available in 15 gram plastic insufflator bottles (NDC 0009-0584-01).

Compendium Code No.: 10490381 812 605 205

NEO-SOL® 50

Alpharma **Water Medication**

Neomycin Sulfate-Antibacterial

ANADA No.: 200-130

Active Ingredient(s): Each packet contains: 71.5 gm neomycin sulfate equivalent to 50 gm neomycin.

Indications: For the treatment and control of colibacillosis (bacterial enteritis) caused by *Escherichia coli* susceptible to neomycin sulfate in cattle (excluding veal calves), swine, sheep and goats.

Dosage and Administration: Administer to cattle (excluding veal calves), swine, sheep and goats at a dose of 10 mg neomycin sulfate per pound of body weight per day in divided doses for a maximum of 14 days.

Herd Treatment: Each packet will treat 7150 pounds body weight. Therefore, estimate the total number of pounds of body weight of the animals to be treated and administer one (1) packet (or portion thereof) for each 7150 pounds. The product should be added to the amount of drinking water estimated to be consumed in 12-18 hours. Provide medicated water as the sole source of water each day until consumed, followed by non-medicated water as required.

Fresh medicated water should be prepared every 18 hours.

Individual Animal Treatment: To provide 10 mg neomycin sulfate per pound of body weight, mix one (1) level teaspoon in water or milk for each 160 pounds body weight. Administer daily either as a drench in divided doses or in the drinking water to be consumed in 12-18 hours.

Drinking Water: Swine - Use the number of packets indicated below in 256 gallons of water, or in two gallons of stock solution used in proportioner set to meter one ounce per gallon.

Pigs Weighing 25 to 50 pounds . . . . . 2 Packets
Pigs Weighing 50 to 100 pounds . . . . . 3 Packets
Pigs Weighing Over 100 pounds . . . . . 4 Packets

Note: To maintain drug potency, use only non-rustable pre-dosing mixing containers such as stainless steel or plastic buckets.

Precaution(s): Store at room temperature.

Caution(s): To administer the stated dosage, the concentration of neomycin required in medicated water must be adjusted to compensate for variation in age and weight of animal, the nature and severity of disease signs, and environmental temperature and humidity, each of which affects water consumption.

If symptoms persist after using this preparation for 2 or 3 days, consult a veterinarian. If symptoms such as fever, depression, or going off feed develop, oral neomycin is not indicated as the sole treatment since systemic levels of neomycin are not obtained due to low absorption from the gastrointestinal tract.

Important: Treatment should continue 24 to 48 hours beyond remission of disease symptoms, but not to exceed a total of 14 consecutive days. Animals not drinking or eating should be treated individually by drench.

For use in animals only.

Restricted drug. Use only as directed (CA).

Add to drinking water - Not for use in liquid supplements.

Warning(s): Not for human use. Keep out of reach of children. Discontinue treatment prior to slaughter by at least the number of days listed below for the appropriate species:

Cattle . . . . . 1 day
Sheep . . . . . 2 days
Swine and Goats . . . . . 3 days

A withdrawal period has not been established for this product in pre-ruminating calves. Do not use in calves to be processed for veal.

A milk discard period has not been established for this product in lactating dairy cattle. Do not use in female dairy cattle 20 months of age or older.

Presentation: 3.5 oz (100 g) packets.

Compendium Code No.: 10220481 AHF-009A 0008

NEOSOL-ORAL

Med-Pharmex **Water Medication**

(Neomycin Oral Solution) Antibacterial

ANADA No.: 200-289

Active Ingredient(s): Composition: Each mL contains:

Neomycin Sulfate (equivalent to 140 mg of neomycin base) . . . . . 200 mg.

Indications: For the treatment and control of colibacillosis (bacterial enteritis) caused by *Escherichia coli* susceptible to neomycin sulfate in cattle (excluding veal calves), swine, sheep and goats.

Dosage and Administration: Administer to cattle (excluding veal calves), swine, sheep and goats at a dose of 10 mg neomycin sulfate per pound of body weight in divided doses for a maximum of 14 days.

Dosage schedule for treatment of colibacillosis.

Pounds of Body Weight	Amount of Neomycin Oral Solution Per Day in Divided Doses
25 lbs.	1.2 mL (1/4 teaspoonful)
50 lbs.	2.5 mL (1/2 teaspoonful)
100 lbs.	5.0 mL (1 teaspoonful)
300 lbs.	15 mL (1 tablespoonful)
591.5 lbs.	29.5 mL (1 fluid ounce)

Teaspoon = U.S. Standard Measure

Neomycin Oral Solution may be given undiluted or diluted with water.

Herd Treatment: Each 473 mL (1 pt) will treat 9464 pounds of body weight. Therefore estimate the total number of pounds of body weight of animals to be treated and administer 29.5 mL (1 fl. oz.) for each 591.5 lbs. The product should be added to the amount of drinking water estimated to be consumed in 12-24 hours. Provide medicated water as the sole source of water each day until consumed, followed by non-medicated water as required. Fresh medicated water should be prepared each day.

Individual Animal Treatment: To provide 10 mg neomycin sulfate per pound of body weight, mix 5 mL (1 tsp) in water or milk for each 100 lbs. of body weight. Administer daily either as a drench in divided dosages or in the drinking water to be consumed in 12-24 hours.

Precaution(s): Store at controlled room temperature 15°C to 30°C (59°-86°F).

Caution(s): To administer the stated dosage, the concentration of neomycin required in medicated water must be adjusted to compensate for variation in age and weight of animal, the nature and severity of disease signs, and environmental temperature and humidity, each of which affects water consumption.

If symptoms persist after using this preparation for 2 or 3 days, consult a veterinarian. If symptoms such as fever, depression or going off feed develop, oral neomycin is not indicated as the sole treatment since systemic levels of neomycin are not obtained due to poor absorption from the gastrointestinal tract.

Important: Treatment should continue 24 to 48 hours beyond remission of disease symptoms, but not to exceed a total of 14 consecutive days. Animals not drinking or eating should be treated individually by drench.

Restricted Drug - Use Only as Directed (California).

For oral use only.

For animal use only.

Warning(s): Discontinue treatment prior to slaughter as follows:

Cattle - 1 day

Sheep - 2 days

Swine and Goats - 3 days

Keep out of reach of children.

Presentation: 1 pint (473 mL) and 1 gallon (3.785 L).

Compendium Code No.: 10270170

NEOSOL SOLUBLE POWDER

Med-Pharmex **Water Medication**

Neomycin Sulfate

ANADA No.: 200-235

Active Ingredient(s): Each packet contains: Neomycin sulfate equivalent to 50 gm neomycin.

Contains per pound: Neomycin sulfate equivalent to 227.5 gm neomycin.

Indications: For the treatment and control of colibacillosis (bacterial enteritis) caused by *Escherichia coli* susceptible to neomycin sulfate in cattle (excluding veal calves), swine, sheep and goats.

Dosage and Administration: Add to drinking water - Not for use in liquid supplements.

3.5 oz (100 gram) Packets:

Administer to cattle (excluding veal calves), swine, sheep and goats at a dose of 10 mg neomycin sulfate per pound of body weight per day in divided doses for a maximum of 14 days.

Herd Treatment: Each packet will treat 7150 pounds body weight. Therefore, estimate the total number of pounds of body weight of the animals to be treated and administer one (1) packet (or portion thereof) for each 7150 pounds. The product should be added to the amount of drinking water estimated to be consumed in 12-24 hours. Provide medicated water as the sole source of water each day until consumed, followed by non-medicated water as required. Fresh medicated water should be prepared each day.

Individual Animal Treatment: To provide 10 mg neomycin sulfate per pound of body weight, mix one (1) level teaspoon in water or milk for each 160 pounds body weight. Administer daily either as a drench in divided doses or in the drinking water to be consumed in 12-24 hours.

Drinking Water: Swine - Use the number of packets indicated below in 256 gallons of water, or in two gallons of stock solution used in proportioner set to meter one ounce per gallon.

Pigs Weighing 25 to 50 Pounds . . . . . 2 Packets
Pigs Weighing 50 to 100 Pounds . . . . . 3 Packets
Pigs Weighing Over 100 Pounds . . . . . 4 Packets

50 lb (22.6 kg) Drum:

Administer 10 mg neomycin sulfate per pound of body weight per day in divided doses for a maximum of 14 days. Using measuring spoons, the recommended dosage can be determined as follows:

Daily Schedule for Drinking Water:

Swine	
One tablespoonful* of NEOSOL SOLUBLE POWDER added to water consumed in one day will treat	Weight of each pig
50 pigs	10 pounds
20 pigs	25 pounds
10 pigs	50 pounds

Cattle	
One tablespoonful* of NEOSOL SOLUBLE POWDER added to water or milk consumed in one day will treat	Weight of each calf
10 calves	50 pounds
7 calves	75 pounds
4 calves	125 pounds

*Level Tablespoonful - US Standard Measure

The product should be added to the amount of drinking water estimated to be consumed in 12-24 hours. Provide medicated water as the sole source of water each day until consumed, followed by non-medicated water as required. Fresh medicated water should be prepared each day. For a stock solution, add six level tablespoonfuls to one gallon of water. Each pint of this stock solution will medicate 5 gallons of drinking water. For use in Automatic Proportioners delivering 2 ounces of stock solution per gallon of drinking water, dissolve 9 level tablespoonfuls in a gallon of water to make the stock solution.

Individual Animal Treatment - To provide 10 mg neomycin sulfate per pound of body weight, mix one (1) level teaspoon in water or milk for each 160 pounds of body weight. Administer daily either as a drench in divided doses or in the drinking water to be consumed in 12-24 hours.

Important: Treatment should continue 24 to 48 hours beyond remission of disease symptoms, but not to exceed a total of 14 consecutive days. Animals not drinking or eating should be treated individually by drench.

Precaution(s): Store in a dry place. When storing partially used containers, securely close bags to prevent contents from caking.

Keep container tightly closed.

Store at room temperature.

Caution(s): To administer the stated dosage, the concentration of neomycin required in medicated water must be adjusted to compensate for variation in age and weight of animal, the nature and severity of disease signs, and environmental temperature and humidity, each of which affects water consumption. If symptoms persist after using this preparation for 2 or 3 days, consult a veterinarian. If symptoms such as fever, depression, or going off feed develop, oral neomycin is not indicated as the sole treatment since systemic levels of neomycin are not obtained due to low absorption from the gastrointestinal tract.

Warning(s): Discontinue treatment prior to slaughter by at least the number of days listed below for appropriate species.

Cattle and goats . . . . . 30 days
(Not to be used in veal calves)
Swine and sheep . . . . . 20 days

Restricted drug - Use only as directed (California).

For oral use in animals only. Not for human use. Keep out of reach of children.

Presentation: 3.5 oz (100 gram) packets and 50 lb (22.6 kg) drums.

Compendium Code No.: 10270090

NEO-TERRAMYCIN® 50/50

Phibro **Feed Medication**

NADA No.: 094-975

Active Ingredient(s):

Terramycin®* . . . . . 50 g/lb.
Neomycin sulfate (providing 35 g neomycin base per lb.) . . . . . 50 g/lb.

*Oxytetracycline (from oxytetracycline quaternary salt) equivalent to oxytetracycline hydrochloride.

Ingredients: Rice hulls, calcium carbonate, mineral oil and sodium aluminosilicate.

Moisture: Not more than 10.0%.

Screen analysis: Not more than 10% on 20 U.S. Standard sieve mesh. Not more than 25% through 100 U.S. Standard sieve mesh.

N

Bulk density: Loose, 32 to 36 lbs./cu. ft. packed, 38 to 42 lbs./cu. ft.

Indications:

Chickens: As an aid in the prevention of diseases from oxytetracycline susceptible organisms during periods of stress.

As an aid in the prevention of bacterial enteritis and in the control of neomycin-sensitive organisms associated with bluecomb (mud fever or transmissible enteritis).

Prevention of early chick mortality due to oxytetracycline susceptible organisms.

To extend period of high egg production, to improve feed efficiency, to improve fertility, to improve egg production and feed efficiency in presence of disease and at times of stress; as an aid in maintaining and improving hatchability where birds are suffering stress from moving, vaccinations, culling, extreme temperature changes and worming; to improve livability of progeny when losses are due to oxytetracycline susceptible organisms, to improve egg shell quality, prevention of bluecomb (mud fever or transmissible enteritis).

Prevention of complicated chronic respiratory disease (air-sac infection) and control of complicated CRD by lowering mortality and severity during outbreaks.

Turkeys: As an aid in the prevention of diseases from oxytetracycline susceptible organisms during periods of stress.

As an aid in the prevention of bacterial enteritis and in the control of neomycin-sensitive organisms associated with bluecomb (mud fever or transmissible enteritis).

To extend period of high egg production, to improve feed efficiency, to improve fertility, to improve egg production and feed efficiency in presence of disease and at times of stress; as an aid in maintaining and improving hatchability where birds are suffering stress from exposure, moving, vaccinations, culling, extreme losses due to oxytetracycline susceptible organisms, and to improve egg shell quality, prevention of hexamitiasis.

As an aid in the prevention of early poult mortality due to oxytetracycline susceptible organisms.

As an aid in reducing mortality in birds which have suffered an attack of airsaculitis. (It is recommended, whenever possible, to feed from time of attack to marketing.)

Control of bluecomb (mud fever or transmissible enteritis), infectious sinusitis and hexamitiasis; prevention of infectious synovitis.

Control of infectious synovitis.

For the treatment of bacterial enteritis and bluecomb (mud fever or transmissible enteritis).

Swine (baby pigs, growing-finishing pigs and sows): As an aid in the prevention of bacterial enteritis (scours), baby pig diarrhea (in baby pigs only), vibrionic dysentery, bloody dysentery and salmonellosis (necrotic enteritis).

As an aid in the treatment of bacterial enteritis (scours), baby pig diarrhea (in baby pigs only), vibrionic dysentery, bloody dysentery and salmonellosis (necrotic enteritis).

When used in sows to be fed during the gestation and lactation periods: As an aid in the maintenance of weight gains and feed consumption in the presence of atrophic rhinitis.

As an aid in the treatment of bacterial enteritis.

Calves (starter feeds): Aid in the prevention of bacterial enteritis (scours).

Aid in the treatment of bacterial enteritis (scours).

Mink: Aid in the prevention of bacterial enteritis (scours).

Aid in the treatment of bacterial enteritis (scours).

Dosage and Administration:

Chickens:

1. As an aid in the prevention of diseases from oxytetracycline susceptible organisms during periods of stress.
2. As an aid in the prevention of bacterial enteritis and in the control of neomycin-sensitive organisms associated with bluecomb (mud fever or transmissible enteritis).

Grams of Antibiotic/ton NEO-TERRAMYCIN®:

Terramycin®	Neomycin (base)	lbs. of Terramycin® 50/50/ton
50	35-140	1

N

3. Prevention of early chick mortality due to oxytetracycline susceptible organisms (first 2 weeks).
4. As an aid in the prevention of bacterial enteritis and in the control of neomycin-sensitive organisms associated with bluecomb (mud fever or transmissible enteritis).

Grams of Antibiotic/ton NEO-TERRAMYCIN®:

Terramycin®	Neomycin (base)	lbs. of Terramycin® 50/50/ton
50-100	35-70	1-2

5. To extend period of high egg production, to improve feed efficiency, to improve fertility, to improve egg production and feed efficiency in presence of disease and at times of stress; as an aid in maintaining and improving hatchability where birds are suffering stress from moving, vaccinations, culling, extreme temperature changes and worming; to improve livability of progeny when losses are due to oxytetracycline susceptible organisms, to improve egg shell quality, prevention of bluecomb (mud fever or transmissible enteritis).
6. As an aid in the prevention of bacterial enteritis and in the control of neomycin-sensitive organisms associated with bluecomb (mud fever or transmissible enteritis).

Grams of Antibiotic/ton NEO-TERRAMYCIN®:

Terramycin®	Neomycin (base)	lbs. of Terramycin® 50/50/ton
50-100	35-70	1-2

7. Prevention of complicated chronic respiratory disease (air-sac infection) and control of complicated CRD by lowering mortality and severity during outbreaks.
8. As an aid in the prevention of bacterial enteritis and in the control of neomycin-sensitive organisms associated with bluecomb (mud fever or transmissible enteritis).

Grams of Antibiotic/ton NEO-TERRAMYCIN®:

Terramycin®	Neomycin (base)	lbs. of Terramycin® 50/50/ton
100-200	70-140	2-4

Special Considerations: Oxytetracycline in low calcium feeds (0.18-0.55% dietary calcium) should not be fed for more than five (5) days and should not be fed to laying hens.

Turkeys:

1. As an aid in the prevention of diseases from oxytetracycline susceptible organisms during periods of stress.
2. As an aid in the prevention of bacterial enteritis and in the control of neomycin-sensitive organisms associated with bluecomb (mud fever or transmissible enteritis).

Grams of Antibiotic/ton NEO-TERRAMYCIN®:

Terramycin®	Neomycin (base)	lbs. of Terramycin® 50/50/ton
50	35	1

3. To extend period of high egg production, to improve feed efficiency, to improve fertility, to improve egg production and feed efficiency in presence of disease and at times of stress; as an aid in maintaining and improving hatchability where birds are suffering stress from exposure, moving, vaccinations, culling, extreme losses due to oxytetracycline susceptible organisms, and to improve egg shell quality, prevention of hexamitiasis.
4. As an aid in the prevention of bacterial enteritis and in the control of neomycin-sensitive organisms associated with bluecomb (mud fever or transmissible enteritis).

Grams of Antibiotic/ton NEO-TERRAMYCIN®:

Terramycin®	Neomycin (base)	lbs. of Terramycin® 50/50/ton
50-100	35-70	1-2

5. As an aid in the prevention of early poult mortality due to oxytetracycline susceptible organisms (first 4 weeks).

Grams of Antibiotic/ton NEO-TERRAMYCIN®:

Terramycin®	Neomycin (base)	lbs. of Terramycin® 50/50/ton
50-100	35-70	1-2

6. As an aid in reducing mortality in birds which have suffered an attack of airsaculitis. (It is recommended, whenever possible, to feed from time of attack to marketing.)
7. As an aid in the prevention of bacterial enteritis and in the control of neomycin-sensitive organisms associated with bluecomb (mud fever or transmissible enteritis).

Grams of Antibiotic/ton NEO-TERRAMYCIN®:

Terramycin®	Neomycin (base)	lbs. of Terramycin® 50/50/ton
100-150	70-105	2-3

8. Control of bluecomb (mud fever or transmissible enteritis), infectious sinusitis and hexamitiasis; prevention of infectious synovitis.
9. As an aid in the prevention of bacterial enteritis and in the control of neomycin-sensitive organisms associated with bluecomb (mud fever or transmissible enteritis).

Grams of Antibiotic/ton NEO-TERRAMYCIN®:

Terramycin®	Neomycin (base)	lbs. of Terramycin® 50/50/ton
100-200	70-140	2-4

10. Control of infectious synovitis.
11. For the treatment of bacterial enteritis and bluecomb (mud fever or transmissible enteritis).

Grams of Antibiotic/ton NEO-TERRAMYCIN®:

Terramycin®	Neomycin (base)	lbs. of Terramycin® 50/50/ton
200	140	4

Swine (baby pigs, growing-finishing pigs and sows):

1. As an aid in the prevention of bacterial enteritis (scours), baby pig diarrhea (in baby pigs only), vibrionic dysentery, bloody dysentery and salmonellosis (necrotic enteritis).

Grams of Antibiotic/ton NEO-TERRAMYCIN®:

Terramycin®	Neomycin (base)	lbs. of Terramycin® 50/50/ton
50	35	1

2. As an aid in the treatment of bacterial enteritis (scours), baby pig diarrhea (in baby pigs only), vibrionic dysentery, bloody dysentery and salmonellosis (necrotic enteritis).

Grams of Antibiotic/ton NEO-TERRAMYCIN®:

Terramycin®	Neomycin (base)	lbs. of Terramycin® 50/50/ton
100	70	2

When used in sows to be fed during the gestation and lactation periods.

1. As an aid in the maintenance of weight gains and feed consumption in the presence of atrophic rhinitis.
2. As an aid in the treatment of bacterial enteritis.

Grams of Antibiotic/ton NEO-TERRAMYCIN®:

Terramycin®	Neomycin (base)	lbs. of Terramycin® 50/50/ton
50-150	70-105	2-3

Calves (starter feeds):

1. As an aid in the prevention of bacterial enteritis (scours).

Grams of Antibiotic/ton NEO-TERRAMYCIN®:

Terramycin®	Neomycin (base)	lbs. of Terramycin® 50/50/ton
50	35	1

2. As an aid in the treatment of bacterial enteritis (scours).

Grams of Antibiotic/ton NEO-TERRAMYCIN®:

Terramycin®	Neomycin (base)	lbs. of Terramycin® 50/50/ton
100	70	2

Mink:

1. As an aid in the prevention of bacterial enteritis (scours).

Grams of Antibiotic/ton NEO-TERRAMYCIN®:

Terramycin®	Neomycin (base)	lbs. of Terramycin® 50/50/ton
50	70	1A

2. As an aid in the treatment of bacterial enteritis (scours).

Grams of Antibiotic/ton NEO-TERRAMYCIN®:

Terramycin®	Neomycin (base)	lbs. of Terramycin® 50/50/ton
100	140	2B

A. To achieve the approved level, the addition of 35 g of neomycin base per ton of feed is required. This may be added as Phibro's neomycin sulfate 325.

B. To achieve the approved level, the addition of 70 g of neomycin base per ton of feed is required. This may be added as Phibro's neomycin sulfate 325.

*Neomycin use levels are expressed as grams of neomycin base per ton (70% neomycin sulfate level). For example, 140 g neomycin base is equivalent to 200 g neomycin sulfate.

Caution(s): For use in dry feeds only.

Not for use in liquid feed supplements.

Warning(s):

Chickens: This combination requires withdrawal from feed five (5) days before slaughter of broilers and 14 days before slaughter of laying hens.

Turkeys: This combination requires withdrawal from feed 14 days before slaughter.

Swine: This combination requires withdrawal from feed five (5) days before slaughter when used at the above levels.

Calves: This combination, when fed at the level of 1.4 g of neomycin base plus 2 g oxytetracycline head daily, requires withdrawal from feed seven (7) days before slaughter. No withdrawal is required at lower levels.

Discussion: Terramycin® broad-spectrum antibiotic used in animal health, has proved effective against a wide variety of infectious diseases caused by susceptible gram-positive and gram-negative bacteria. Terramycin® is effective in the control of disease complexes, such as shipping fever in cattle and CRD in chickens.

NEO-TERRAMYCIN® is a combination of two antibiotics: terramycin and neomycin. Neomycin has a proven record of effectiveness against scours. This antibiotic is primarily effective against gram-negative bacteria, including *E. coli* and Salmonella, and it is also effective against certain gram-positive bacteria. Terramycin® combats disease-producing organisms in both the blood and gastro-intestinal tract, while neomycin concentrates its anti-infective action in the gastro-intestinal tract.

Presentation: 50 lb. multiwall paper bags.

Terramycin is a registered trademark of Pfizer Inc., licensed to Phibro Animal Health, for oxytetracycline.

Compendium Code No.: 36930071

NEO-TERRAMYCIN® 50/50D

Phibro **Feed Medication**

NADA No.: 094-975

Active Ingredient(s):

Terramycin®*. . . . . 50 g/lb.
Neomycin base from neomycin sulfate† . . . . 50 g/lb.

*Oxytetracycline (from oxytetracycline quaternary salt) equivalent to oxytetracycline hydrochloride.

†Equivalent to approximately 70 g/lb of neomycin sulfate.

Ingredients: Sucrose, sodium aluminosilicate, and mineral oil.

Moisture: Not more than 5%.

Screen analysis: No retention on 20 U.S. Standard sieve mesh; 55% average passage through 100 U.S. Standard sieve mesh.

Indications:

Calves (milk replacer): For use as an aid in the prevention of bacterial enteritis (scours).

For use as an aid in the treatment of bacterial enteritis (scours).

Baby pigs (milk replacer): For use as an aid in the prevention of bacterial enteritis (scours).

For use as an aid in the treatment of bacterial enteritis (scours).

Dosage and Administration: Mix NEO-TERRAMYCIN® 50/50D with non-medicated milk replacer to provide the following dosages:

Calves (milk replacer):

1. For use as an aid in the prevention of bacterial enteritis (scours).

Oxytetracycline*	Neomycin** (base)	lbs. of Neo-Terramycin® 50/50D/ton
100 mg/gallon	100 mg/gallon	1

2. For use as an aid in the treatment of bacterial enteritis (scours).

Oxytetracycline*	Neomycin** (base)	lbs. of Neo-Terramycin® 50/50D/ton
200 mg/gallon	200 mg/gallon	1

Baby pigs (milk replacer):

1. For use as an aid in the prevention of bacterial enteritis (scours).

Oxytetracycline*	Neomycin** (base)	lbs. of Neo-Terramycin® 50/50D/ton
50 g/ton	50 g/ton	1

2. For use as an aid in the treatment of bacterial enteritis (scours).

Oxytetracycline*	Neomycin** (base)	lbs. of Neo-Terramycin® 50/50D/ton
70-140 g/ton	70-140 g/ton	1.4-2.8

* The dosage in calves is expressed in mg/gallon of reconstituted milk replacer whereas in baby pigs the dosage is expressed in g/ton of dry milk replacer.

** Mixing directions for calves are for example only and are based on mixing 1 lb. of dry milk replacer with one (1) gallon of water.

Precaution(s): Store in a dry, cool place.

Caution(s): For use in dry feeds only.

Not for use in liquid feed supplements.

For use in manufacturing medicated animal feeds only.

Certain components of animal feeds, including medicated premixes, possess properties that may be a potential health hazard or a source of personal discomfort to certain individuals who are exposed to them. Human exposure should, therefore, be minimized by observing the general industry standards for occupational health and safety.

Precautions such as the following should be considered: dust masks or respirators and protective clothing should be worn, dust arresting equipment and adequate ventilation should be utilized, personal hygiene should be observed, wash before eating or leaving a work site, be alert for signs of allergic reactions. Seek prompt medical treatment if such reactions are suspected.

Warning(s): In calves, withdraw from feed 30 days prior to slaughter. In pigs, withdraw from feed 10 days prior to slaughter when neomycin base level is 140 g/ton and five (5) days withdrawal when the neomycin base level is below 140 g/ton.

Discussion: NEO-TERRAMYCIN® is a combination of two antibiotics: terramycin® and neomycin. NEO-TERRAMYCIN® 50/50D is a dispersible formulation designed specifically for use in milk replacers.

Terramycin, a broad-spectrum antibiotic, has proved effective against a wide variety of infectious diseases caused by susceptible gram-positive and gram-negative bacteria. Terramycin is effective in the control of disease complexes, such as shipping fever.

Neomycin has a reliable record of effectiveness against scours. This antibiotic is primarily effective against gram-negative bacteria, including *E. coli* and Salmonella, and it is also effective against certain gram-positive bacteria. Terramycin combats disease-producing organisms in both the blood and gastro-intestinal tract, while neomycin concentrates its anti-infective action in the gastro-intestinal tract.

Presentation: 50 lb. multiwall paper bags.

Terramycin is a registered trademark of Pfizer Inc., licensed to Phibro Animal Health, for oxytetracycline.

Compendium Code No.: 36930081

NEO-TERRAMYCIN® 100/50

Phibro **Feed Medication**

NADA No.: 094-975

Active Ingredient(s):

Terramycin®* . . . . 50 g/lb.
Neomycin sulfate (providing 70 g neomycin base per lb.) . . . . 100 g/lb.

*Oxytetracycline (from oxytetracycline quaternary salt) equivalent to oxytetracycline hydrochloride.

Ingredients: Roughage products, mineral oil, and sodium aluminosilicate.

Moisture: Not more than 8%.

Screen analysis: Less than 1% average retention on 20 U.S. Standard sieve mesh; 50% average passage through 100 U.S. Standard sieve mesh.

Indications:

Chickens: Prevention of diseases from oxytetracycline-susceptible organisms during periods of stress.

For use as an aid in the prevention of bacterial enteritis and in the control of neomycin-sensitive organisms associated with bluecomb (mud fever or transmissible enteritis).

Prevention of early chick mortality due to oxytetracycline-susceptible organisms.

To extend the period of high egg production, to improve feed efficiency, to improve fertility, to improve egg production and feed efficiency in the presence of disease and at times of stress; as an aid in maintaining and improving hatchability where birds are suffering stress from moving, vaccinations, culling, extreme temperature changes and worming; to improve livability of progeny when losses are due to oxytetracycline-susceptible organisms, to improve egg shell quality, and for the prevention of bluecomb (mud fever or transmissible enteritis).

Prevention of complicated chronic respiratory disease (air-sac infection) and control of complicated CRD by lowering mortality and severity during outbreaks.

Turkeys: For use as an aid in the prevention of diseases from oxytetracycline-susceptible organisms during periods of stress.

For use as an aid in the prevention of bacterial enteritis and in the control of neomycin-sensitive organisms associated with bluecomb (mud fever or transmissible enteritis).

To extend the period of high egg production, to improve feed efficiency, to improve fertility, to improve egg production and feed efficiency in the presence of disease and at times of stress; as an aid in maintaining and improving hatchability where birds are suffering stress from exposure, moving, vaccinations, culling, extreme losses due to oxytetracycline-susceptible organisms, and to improve egg shell quality, and for the prevention of hexamitiasis.

For use as an aid in the prevention of early poult mortality due to oxytetracycline-susceptible organisms.

Control of bluecomb (mud fever or transmissible enteritis), infectious sinusitis and hexamitiasis; prevention of infectious synovitis.

Swine (baby pigs, growing-finishing pigs and sows): For use as an aid in the prevention of bacterial enteritis (scours), baby pig diarrhea (in baby pigs only), vibrionic dysentery, bloody dysentery and salmonellosis (necrotic enteritis).

For use as an aid in the treatment of bacterial enteritis (scours), baby pig diarrhea (in baby pigs only), vibrionic dysentery, bloody dysentery and salmonellosis (necrotic enteritis).

When used in sows to be fed during the gestation and lactation periods: For use as an aid in the maintenance of weight gains and feed consumption in the presence of atrophic rhinitis.

For use as an aid in the treatment of bacterial enteritis.

Calves (starter feeds): For use as an aid in the prevention of bacterial enteritis (scours).

For use as an aid in the treatment of bacterial enteritis (scours).

Mink: For use as an aid in the prevention of bacterial enteritis (scours).

For use as an aid in the treatment of bacterial enteritis (scours).

Dosage and Administration: Thoroughly mix the amount of the premix according to the table in the Directions for Use with non-medicated feed.

Chickens:

1. Prevention of diseases from oxytetracycline-susceptible organisms during periods of stress.
2. For use as an aid in the prevention of bacterial enteritis and in the control of neomycin-sensitive organisms associated with bluecomb (mud fever or transmissible enteritis).

g/ton Terramycin®	g/ton Neomycin (base)	lbs. of Neo-Terramycin® 100/50/ton
50	700	1

3. Prevention of early chick mortality due to oxytetracycline-susceptible organisms (first 2 weeks).
4. For use as an aid in the prevention of bacterial enteritis and in the control of neomycin-sensitive organisms associated with bluecomb (mud fever or transmissible enteritis).

g/ton Terramycin®	g/ton Neomycin (base)	lbs. of Neo-Terramycin® 100/50/ton
50-100	70-140	1-2

5. To extend the period of high egg production, to improve feed efficiency, to improve fertility, to improve egg production and feed efficiency in the presence of disease and at times of stress; as an aid in maintaining and improving hatchability where birds are suffering stress from moving, vaccinations, culling, extreme temperature changes and worming; to improve livability of progeny when losses are due to oxytetracycline-susceptible organisms, to improve egg shell quality, and for the prevention of bluecomb (mud fever or transmissible enteritis).
6. For use as an aid in the prevention of bacterial enteritis and in the control of neomycin-sensitive organisms associated with bluecomb (mud fever or transmissible enteritis).

g/ton Terramycin®	g/ton Neomycin (base)	lbs. of Neo-Terramycin® 100/50/ton
50-100	70-140	1-2

7. Prevention of complicated chronic respiratory disease (air-sac infection) and control of complicated CRD by lowering mortality and severity during outbreaks.
8. For use as an aid in the prevention of bacterial enteritis and in the control of neomycin-sensitive organisms associated with bluecomb (mud fever or transmissible enteritis).

g/ton Terramycin®	g/ton Neomycin (base)	lbs. of Neo-Terramycin® 100/50/ton
100	140	2

Special Considerations: Oxytetracycline in low calcium feeds (0.18-0.55% dietary calcium) should not be fed for more than five (5) days and should not be fed to laying hens.

Turkeys:

1. For use as an aid in the prevention of diseases from oxytetracycline-susceptible organisms during periods of stress.
2. For use as an aid in the prevention of bacterial enteritis and in the control of neomycin-sensitive organisms associated with bluecomb (mud fever or transmissible enteritis).

g/ton Terramycin®	g/ton Neomycin (base)	lbs. of Neo-Terramycin® 100/50/ton
50	70	1

3. To extend the period of high egg production, to improve feed efficiency, to improve fertility, to improve egg production and feed efficiency in the presence of disease and at times of stress; as an aid in maintaining and improving hatchability where birds are suffering stress from exposure, moving, vaccinations, culling, extreme losses due to oxytetracycline-susceptible organisms, and to improve egg shell quality, and for the prevention of hexamitiasis.
4. For use as an aid in the prevention of bacterial enteritis and in the control of neomycin-sensitive organisms associated with bluecomb (mud fever or transmissible enteritis).

g/ton Terramycin®	g/ton Neomycin (base)	lbs. of Neo-Terramycin® 100/50/ton
50-100	70-140	1-2

5. For use as an aid in the prevention of early poult mortality due to oxytetracycline-susceptible organisms (first 4 weeks).
6. For use as an aid in the prevention of bacterial enteritis and in the control of neomycin-sensitive organisms associated with bluecomb (mud fever or transmissible enteritis).

g/ton Terramycin®	g/ton Neomycin (base)	lbs. of Neo-Terramycin® 100/50/ton
50-100	70-140	1-2

7. Control of bluecomb (mud fever or transmissible enteritis), infectious sinusitis and hexamitiasis; prevention of infectious synovitis.
8. For use as an aid in the prevention of bacterial enteritis and in the control of neomycin-sensitive organisms associated with bluecomb (mud fever or transmissible enteritis).

g/ton Terramycin®	g/ton Neomycin (base)	lbs. of Neo-Terramycin® 100/50/ton
100	140	2

Swine (baby pigs, growing-finishing pigs and sows):

1. For use as an aid in the prevention of bacterial enteritis (scours), baby pig diarrhea (in baby pigs only), vibrionic dysentery, bloody dysentery and salmonellosis (necrotic enteritis).

g/ton Terramycin®	g/ton Neomycin (base)	lbs. of Neo-Terramycin® 100/50/ton
50	70	1

2. For use as an aid in the treatment of bacterial enteritis (scours), baby pig diarrhea (in baby pigs only), vibrionic dysentery, bloody dysentery and salmonellosis (necrotic enteritis).

g/ton Terramycin®	g/ton Neomycin (base)	lbs. of Neo-Terramycin® 100/50/ton
50-100	70-140	1-2

When used in sows to be fed during the gestation and lactation periods.

g/ton Terramycin®	g/ton Neomycin (base)	lbs. of Neo-Terramycin® 100/50/ton
50-100	70-140	1-2

3. For use as an aid in the maintenance of weight gains and feed consumption in the presence of atrophic rhinitis.
4. For use as an aid in the treatment of bacterial enteritis.

g/ton Terramycin®	g/ton Neomycin (base)	lbs. of Neo-Terramycin® 100/50/ton
50-100	70-140	1-2

Calves (starter feeds):

1. For use as an aid in the prevention of bacterial enteritis (scours).

g/ton Terramycin®	g/ton Neomycin (base)	lbs. of Neo-Terramycin® 100/50/ton
50	70	1

2. For use as an aid in the treatment of bacterial enteritis (scours).

g/ton Terramycin®	g/ton Neomycin (base)	lbs. of Neo-Terramycin® 100/50/ton
100	140	2

Mink:

1. For use as an aid in the prevention of bacterial enteritis (scours).

g/ton Terramycin®	g/ton Neomycin (base)	lbs. of Neo-Terramycin® 100/50/ton
50	70	1

2. For use as an aid in the treatment of bacterial enteritis (scours).

g/ton Terramycin®	g/ton Neomycin (base)	lbs. of Neo-Terramycin® 100/50/ton
100	140	2

Precaution(s): Store in a dry, cool place.

Caution(s): For use in dry feeds only.

Not for use in liquid feed supplements.

For use in manufacturing medicated animal feeds only.

Certain components of animal feeds, including medicated premixes, possess properties that may be a potential health hazard or a source of personal discomfort to certain individuals who are exposed to them. Human exposure should, therefore, be minimized by observing the general industry standards for occupational health and safety.

Precautions such as the following should be considered: dust masks or respirators and protective clothing should be worn, dust arresting equipment and adequate ventilation should be utilized, personal hygiene should be observed, wash before eating or leaving a work site, be alert for signs of allergic reactions. Seek prompt medical treatment if such reactions are suspected.

Warning(s):

Chickens: This combination requires withdrawal from feed five (5) days before slaughter of broilers and 14 days before slaughter of laying hens.

Turkeys: This combination requires withdrawal from feed 14 days before slaughter.

Swine: This combination requires withdrawal from feed five (5) days before slaughter when used at the above levels.

Calves: This combination, when fed at the level of 1.4 g of neomycin base plus 2 g oxytetracycline per head daily, requires withdrawal from feed seven (7) days before slaughter. No withdrawal is required at lower levels.

Discussion: NEO-TERRAMYCIN® is a combination of two antibiotics: terramycin® and neomycin.

Terramycin, a broad-spectrum antibiotic, has proved effective against a wide variety of infectious diseases caused by susceptible gram-positive and gram-negative bacteria. Terramycin is effective in the control of disease complexes, such as shipping fever.

Neomycin has a reliable record of effectiveness against scours. This antibiotic is primarily effective against gram-negative bacteria, including *E. coli* and Salmonella, and it is also effective against certain gram-positive bacteria. Terramycin combats disease-producing organisms in both the blood and gastro-intestinal tract, while neomycin concentrates its anti-infective action in the gastro-intestinal tract.

Presentation: 50 lb. multiwall paper bags.

Terramycin is a registered trademark of Pfizer Inc., licensed to Phibro Animal Health, for oxytetracycline.

Compendium Code No.: 36930091

NEO-TERRAMYCIN® 100/50D

Phibro **Feed Medication**

NADA No.: 094-975

Active Ingredient(s):

Terramycin®* . . . . 50 g/lb.
Neomycin base from neomycin sulfate† . . . . 100 g/lb.

*Oxytetracycline (from oxytetracycline quaternary salt) equivalent to oxytetracycline hydrochloride.

†Equivalent to approximately 140 g/lb of neomycin sulfate.

Ingredients: Sucrose, sodium aluminosilicate, and mineral oil.

Moisture: Not more than 8%.

Screen analysis: Less than 1% average retention on 20 U.S. Standard sieve mesh; 71% average passage through 100 U.S. Standard sieve mesh.

Indications:

Calves (milk replacer): For use as an aid in the prevention of bacterial enteritis (scours).
For use as an aid in the treatment of bacterial enteritis (scours).
Baby pigs (milk replacer): For use as an aid in the prevention of bacterial enteritis (scours).
For use as an aid in the treatment of bacterial enteritis (scours).
Mink (milk replacer): For use as an aid in the prevention of bacterial enteritis (scours).
For use as an aid in the treatment of bacterial enteritis (scours).

Dosage and Administration: Mix NEO-TERRAMYCIN® 100/50D with non-medicated milk replacer to provide the following dosages:

Calves (milk replacer):

1. For use as an aid in the prevention of bacterial enteritis (scours).

Oxytetracycline*	Neomycin** (base)	lbs. of Neo-Terramycin® 100/50D/ton
50-100 mg/gallon	100-200 mg/gallon	2-4

2. For use as an aid in the treatment of bacterial enteritis (scours).

Oxytetracycline*	Neomycin** (base)	lbs. of Neo-Terramycin® 100/50D/ton
100-200 mg/gallon	200-400 mg/gallon	4-8

Baby pigs (milk replacer):

1. For use as an aid in the prevention of bacterial enteritis (scours).

Oxytetracycline*	Neomycin** (base)	lbs. of Neo-Terramycin® 100/50D/ton
50 g/ton	100 g/ton	1

2. For use as an aid in the treatment of bacterial enteritis (scours).

Oxytetracycline*	Neomycin** (base)	lbs. of Neo-Terramycin® 100/50D/ton
50-70 g/ton	100-140 g/ton	1-1.4

Mink (milk replacer):

1. For use as an aid in the prevention of bacterial enteritis (scours).

Oxytetracycline*	Neomycin** (base)	lbs. of Neo-Terramycin® 100/50D/ton
50 g/ton	100 g/ton	1

2. For use as an aid in the treatment of bacterial enteritis (scours).

Oxytetracycline*	Neomycin** (base)	lbs. of Neo-Terramycin® 100/50D/ton
100 g/ton	200 g/ton	2

* The dosage in calves is expressed in mg/gallon of reconstituted milk replacer whereas in baby pigs and mink the dosage is expressed in g/ton of dry milk replacer.

** Mixing directions for calves are for example only and are based on mixing 1 lb. of dry milk replacer with one (1) gallon of water.

Precaution(s): Store in a dry, cool place.

Caution(s): For use in dry feeds only.

Not for use in liquid feed supplements.

For use in manufacturing medicated animal feeds only.

Certain components of animal feeds, including medicated premixes, possess properties that may be a potential health hazard or a source of personal discomfort to certain individuals who are exposed to them. Human exposure should, therefore, be minimized by observing the general industry standards for occupational health and safety.

Precautions such as the following should be considered: dust masks or respirators and protective clothing should be worn, dust arresting equipment and adequate ventilation should be utilized, personal hygiene should be observed, wash before eating or leaving a work site, be alert for signs of allergic reactions. Seek prompt medical treatment if such reactions are suspected.

Warning(s): In calves, withdraw from feed 30 days prior to slaughter. In pigs, withdraw from feed 10 days prior to slaughter when neomycin base level is 140 g/ton and five (5) days withdrawal when the neomycin base level is below 140 g/ton.

Discussion: NEO-TERRAMYCIN® is a combination of two antibiotics: terramycin® and neomycin. NEO-TERRAMYCIN® 100/50D is a dispersible formulation designed specifically for use in milk replacers.

Terramycin, a broad-spectrum antibiotic, has proved effective against a wide variety of infectious diseases caused by susceptible gram-positive and gram-negative bacteria. Terramycin is effective in the control of disease complexes, such as shipping fever.

Neomycin has a reliable record of effectiveness against scours. This antibiotic is primarily effective against gram-negative bacteria, including *E. coli* and Salmonella, and it is also effective against certain gram-positive bacteria. Terramycin combats disease-producing organisms in both the blood and gastro-intestinal tract, while neomycin concentrates its anti-infective action in the gastro-intestinal tract.

Presentation: 50 lb. multiwall paper bags.

Terramycin is a registered trademark of Pfizer Inc., licensed to Phibro Animal Health, for oxytetracycline.

Compendium Code No.: 36930101

NEOVED 200

Vedco **Water Medication**

Neomycin Oral Solution

ANADA No.: 200-118

Active Ingredient(s): Each mL contains:

Neomycin Sulfate . . . . . 200 mg
(equivalent to 140 mg neomycin base)

Indications: For the treatment and control of colibacillosis (bacterial enteritis) caused by *Escherichia coli* susceptible to neomycin sulfate in cattle (excluding veal calves), swine, sheep and goats.

Dosage and Administration: Administer to cattle (excluding veal calves), swine, sheep and goats at a dose of 10 mg neomycin sulfate per pound of body weight in divided doses for a maximum of 14 days.

Dosage Schedule for Treatment of Colibacillosis:

Pounds of Body Weight	Amount of Neomycin Oral Solution per Day in Divided Doses
25 Lb	1.2 mL (¼ tsp*)
50 Lb	2.5 mL (½ tsp*)
100 Lb	5 mL (1 tsp*)
300 Lb	15 mL (1 tbsp*)
591.5 Lb	29.5 mL (1 fl oz)

* Teaspoon (tsp) / Tablespoon (tbsp) is equal to U.S. Standard Measure.

Neomycin Oral Solution may be given undiluted or diluted with water.

Herd Treatment: Each 3.785 L (1 Gal) will treat 75,700 pounds of body weight. Therefore, estimate the total number of pounds of body weight of the animals to be treated and administer 28.5 mL (1 fl oz) for 591.5 pounds. The product should be added to the amount of drinking water estimated to be consumed in 12-24 hours. Provide medicated water as the sole source of drinking water each day until consumed, followed by non-medicated water as required. Fresh medicated water should be prepared each day.

Individual Animal Treatment: To provide 10 mg neomycin sulfate per pound of body weight, mix 5 mL (1 tsp*) in water or milk for each 100 pounds of body weight. Administer daily either as a drench in divided dosages or in the drinking water to be consumed in 12-24 hours.

Precaution(s): Store at controlled room temperature between 15° and 30°C (59°-86°F).

Caution(s): To administer the stated dosage, the concentration of neomycin required in medicated water must be adjusted to compensate for variation in age and weight of animal, the nature and severity of disease signs, and environmental temperature and humidity, each of which affects water consumption.

If symptoms persist after using this preparation for 2 or 3 days, consult a veterinarian. If symptoms such as fever, depression, or going off feed develop, oral neomycin is not indicated as the sole treatment since systemic levels of neomycin are not obtained due to poor absorption from the gastrointestinal tract.

Important: Treatment should continue 24 to 48 hours beyond remission of disease symptoms, but not to exceed a total of 14 consecutive days. Animals not drinking or eating should be treated individually by drench.

For oral use only.

Restricted drug - Use only as directed (California).

For animal use only.

Keep out of reach of children.

Warning(s): Discontinue treatment prior to slaughter by at least the number of days listed below for appropriate species:

Cattle and goats . . . . . 30 days
(not to be used in veal calves)

Swine and sheep . . . . . 20 days

Presentation: 473.1 mL (1 pt) and 3.785 L (1 Gal).

Compendium Code No.: 10941300

NEOVET 325/100

AgriPharm **Water Medication**

Soluble Powder

neomycin sulfate (commercial grade)

ANADA No.: 200-130

Active Ingredient(s): Each packet contains 71.5 g neomycin sulfate (commercial grade) equivalent to 50 gm neomycin.

Indications: For the treatment and control of colibacillosis (bacterial enteritis) caused by *Escherichia coli* susceptible to neomycin sulfate in cattle (excluding veal calves), swine, sheep and goats.

Dosage and Administration: Administer to cattle (excluding veal calves), swine, sheep and goats at a dose of 10 mg neomycin sulfate per pound of body weight per day in divided doses for a maximum of 14 days.

Herd Treatment: Each packet will treat 7150 pounds body weight. Therefore, estimate the total number of pounds of body weight of the animals to be treated and administer one (1) packet (or portion thereof) for each 7150 pounds. The product should be added to the amount of drinking water estimated to be consumed in 12-18 hours. Provide medicated water as the sole source of water each day until consumed, followed by non-medicated water as required. Fresh medicated water should be prepared every 18 hours.

Individual Animal Treatment: To provide 10 mg neomycin sulfate per pound of body weight, mix one (1) level teaspoon in water or milk for each 160 pounds body weight. Administer daily either as a drench in divided doses or in the drinking water to be consumed in 12-18 hours.

Drinking Water: Swine - Use the number of packets indicated below in 256 gallons of water, or in two gallons of stock solution used in proportioner set to meter one ounce per gallon.

Pigs weighing 25 to 50 pounds. . . . . 2 packets
Pigs weighing 50 to 100 pounds. . . . . 3 packets
Pigs weighing over 100 pounds . . . . . 4 packets

Note: To maintain drug potency, use only non-rustable pre-dosing mixing containers such as stainless steel or plastic buckets.

Precaution(s): Store at room temperature.

Caution(s): Restricted Drug - Use only as directed (California).

For use in animals only.

Add to drinking water - Not for use in liquid supplements.

To administer the stated dosage, the concentration of neomycin required in medicated water must be adjusted to compensate for variation in age and weight of animal, the nature and severity of disease signs, and environmental temperature and humidity, each of which affects water consumption.

If symptoms persist after using this preparation for 2 or 3 days, consult a veterinarian. If symptoms such as fever, depression, or going off feed develop, oral neomycin is not indicated as the sole treatment since systemic levels of neomycin are not obtained due to low absorption from the gastrointestinal tract.

Important: Treatment should continue 24 to 48 hours beyond remission of disease symptoms, but not to exceed a total of 14 consecutive days. Animals not drinking or eating should be treated individually by drench.

Warning(s): Not for human use. Keep out of reach of children. Discontinue treatment prior to slaughter by at least the number of days listed below for the appropriate species:

Cattle. . . . . 1 day
Swine and Goats. . . . . 3 days
Sheep . . . . . 2 days

A withdrawal period has not been established for this product in pre-ruminating calves. Do not use in calves to be processed for veal.

A milk discard period has not been established for this product in lactating dairy cattle. Do not use in female dairy cattle 20 months of age or older.

Presentation: 3.5 oz (100 gram) packets.

Compendium Code No.: 14570640

NEOVET® NEOMYCIN ORAL SOLUTION

AgriPharm **Water Medication**

Antibacterial

ANADA No.: 200-118

Active Ingredient(s): Each mL contains:

Neomycin sulfate . . . . . 200 mg
(equivalent to 140 mg neomycin base)

Indications: For the treatment and control of colibacillosis (bacterial enteritis) caused by *Escherichia coli* susceptible to neomycin sulfate in cattle (excluding veal calves), swine, sheep and goats.

Dosage and Administration: Administer to cattle (excluding veal calves), swine, sheep and goats at a dose of 10 mg neomycin sulfate per pound of body weight in divided doses for a maximum of 14 days.

Dosage Schedule for Treatment of Colibacillosis:

Pounds of Body Weight	Amount of Neomycin Oral Solution per Day in Divided Doses
25 lb.	1.2 mL (¼ tsp*)
50 lb.	2.5 mL (½ tsp*)
100 lb.	5 mL (1 tsp*)
300 lb.	15 mL (1 tbsp*)
591.5 lb.	29.5 mL (1 fl. oz.)

Neomycin Oral Solution may be given undiluted or diluted with water.

Herd Treatment: Each 473.1 mL (1 pt.) will treat 9,464 pounds of body weight. Each 3.785 L (1 gal.) will treat 75,700 pounds of body weight. Therefore, estimate the total number of pounds of body weight of the animals to be treated and administer 29.5 mL (1 fl. oz.) for 591.5 pounds. The product should be added to the amount of drinking water estimated to be consumed in 12-24 hours. Provide medicated water as the sole source of water each day until consumed, followed by non-medicated water as required. Fresh medicated water should be prepared each day.

Individual Animal Treatment: To provide 10 mg neomycin sulfate per pound of body weight, mix 5 mL (1 tsp*) in water or milk for each 100 pounds of body weight. Administer daily either as a drench in divided dosages or in the drinking water to be consumed in 12-24 hours.

* Teaspoon (tsp) / Tablespoon (tbsp) is equal to U.S. standard measure.

Precaution(s): Store at controlled room temperature between 15° and 30°C (59°-86°F).

Caution(s): To administer the stated dosage, the concentration of neomycin required in medicated water must be adjusted to compensate for variation in age and weight of animal, the nature and severity of disease signs, and environmental temperature and humidity, each of which affects water consumption.

If symptoms persist after using this preparation for 2 or 3 days, consult a veterinarian. If symptoms such as fever, depression, or going off feed develop, oral neomycin is not indicated as the sole treatment since systemic levels of neomycin are not obtained due to poor absorption from the gastrointestinal tract.

Important: Treatment should continue 24 to 48 hours beyond remission of disease symptoms, but not to exceed a total of 14 consecutive days.

Animals not drinking or eating should be treated individually by drench.

Restricted drug - Use only as directed (California).

For oral use only.

For animal use only.

Keep out of reach of children.

Warning(s): Discontinue treatment prior to slaughter by at least the number of days listed below for appropriate species:

Cattle and goats . . . . . 30 days
(not to be use in veal calves)

Swine and sheep. . . . . 20 days

Presentation: 473.1 mL (1 pt.), 12 per case and 3.785 L (1 gal.), 4 per case.

Compendium Code No.: 14570650

NEUROSYN™ TABLETS ℞

Boehringer Ingelheim **Anticonvulsant**

(Primidone)

NADA No.: 117-689

Active Ingredient(s): Each tablet contains 250 mg of primidone.

Indications: Use only in dogs to treat:

Idiopathic epilepsy: Archibald[6] has reported on the use of primidone in the treatment of idiopathic epilepsy in dogs previously treated with other anticonvulsants without success. In this experience, primidone was found to be an effective agent completely controlling the convulsions in most of the cases studied and reducing the number and severity of seizures in the remaining small percentage.

Epileptiform convulsions: Clinically these convulsions are similar to those of true epilepsy. Primidone may be useful as symptomatic treatment of these convulsions of unknown etiology.

Virus encephalitis, distemper, hardpad disease which occurs as a clinically recognizable lesion in certain entities in dogs: Primidone provides an effective means of controlling convulsions associated with infectious neuropathies such as virus encephalitis, distemper, or hardpad disease. Supplementation of therapy with primidone is recommended as soon as a diagnosis is made. Oliver and Hoerlin (1965), reported that primidone has been the most effective agent in the dog for the control of seizures associated with post distemper convulsions. Clinical experience has revealed that once the seizure of a dog cannot be controlled with primidone, none of the other anticonvulsants are likely to do any better.[7] However, it must be borne in mind that primidone does not correct the primary causes of these disorders, but is a valuable adjunct to therapy, making possible control of seizures without hypnosis or interference with proper nutrition.

Primidone has not proved useful in the treatment of chorea.

Pharmacology: Primidone, 5-ethyldihydro-5-phenyl-4,6(1H,-5H)- pyrimidinedione is a white crystalline substance, and a pyrimidine derivative. Studies of chronic administration of primidone indicate it can metabolize into two active metabolites, phenobarbital and phenylethylmalonamide (PEMA).[1,2,3]

Although primidone is less potent than phenobarbital as a general CNS depressant, primidone is more potent than phenobarbital in the protection of animals against maximal seizures induced by both electroshock and pentylenetetrazole.[4,5,10] As indicated above, primidone may undergo a somewhat complex metabolism involving the production of phenobarbital and the practitioner should take this into consideration if administering other drugs such as other antiepileptics concurrently.

Primidone acts upon the central nervous system to raise the seizure threshold, hence its value as an anticonvulsant, whether the seizure is induced electrically or is a symptom of a primary disease process.

Dosage and Administration: The initial dose of primidone is gradually increased until the optimum control of convulsions is achieved, and the dosage level necessary to establish this effect is usually maintained.

Usual daily dosage: 25 mg/lb. of body weight (55 mg/kg of body weight). Tablets may be administered whole or crushed and mixed with food. When convulsions are frequent, the daily dosage should be divided and administered at intervals. When convulsions occur only every few days, or less often, the daily dosage should be given at one time.[10] A reduction in dosage should be made gradually and should never be discontinued abruptly.

Precaution(s): Do not use in cats. Primidone appears to have specific neurotoxicity in cats. In long-term therapy using primidone there is the possibility of Serum Alkaline Phosphatase (SAP) elevation to slightly above normal. When primidone therapy is discontinued, SAP should return to normal unless the elevation was caused by other abnormal conditions, such as bone disease, healing fractures or pregnancy.

Caution(s): Federal law restricts this drug to use by or on the order of a licensed veterinarian.

Keep out of reach of children.

N

Side Effects: Primidone is well tolerated at effective therapeutic levels. Side effects such as staggering and drowsiness occur infrequently and usually disappear with an adjustment in dosage.

Several investigators have successfully treated megaloblastic anemia associated with long-term primidone with folic acid, vitamin B_{12} and iron.[8,9]

References: Available upon request.

Presentation: Bottles of 100 and 1,000 tablets.

Compendium Code No.: 10280820

NEW BRONZ®

Fort Dodge **Vaccine**

Newcastle-Bronchitis Vaccine, Mass. Type, Killed Virus

U.S. Vet. Lic. No.: 112

Contents: This product contains the antigens listed above.

Gentamicin added as a preservative.

Indications: For the revaccination of healthy chickens 3 weeks of age or older as an aid in the prevention of Newcastle disease and infectious bronchitis, Massachusetts type.

Dosage and Administration: Inject 0.5 mL (0.5 cc) intramuscularly or subcutaneously (in the lower neck region) using aseptic technique. Vaccinate only healthy birds.

Precaution(s): Store in the dark at 36° to 45°F (2° to 7°C). Do not freeze. Warm to 72°F (22°C) and shake well before using. Use entire contents when first opened.

Warning(s): Do not vaccinate within 42 days before slaughter.

In case of accidental human injection seek immediate medical attention.

For veterinary use only.

Presentation: 1,000 dose (500 mL) vials.

Compendium Code No.: 10031101

10321C

NEW BRONZ® MG

Fort Dodge **Bacterin-Vaccine**

Newcastle-Bronchitis Vaccine, Mass. Type, Killed Virus-Mycoplasma Gallisepticum Bacterin

U.S. Vet. Lic. No.: 112

Contents: This product contains the antigens listed above.

Penicillin and streptomycin added as preservatives.

Indications: For the vaccination of healthy chickens 3 weeks of age or older as an aid in the prevention of Newcastle disease, infectious bronchitis, Massachusetts type, and the clinical signs associated with *Mycoplasma gallisepticum* infection.

It is essential for best protection to prime the birds at least once with live virus Newcastle and bronchitis vaccine.

Dosage and Administration: Inject 0.5 mL (0.5 cc) intramuscularly or subcutaneously (in the lower neck region) using aseptic technique. Vaccinate only healthy birds.

Precaution(s): Store in the dark at 36° to 45°F (2° to 7°C). Do not freeze. Warm to 72°F (22°C) and shake well before using. Use entire contents when first opened.

Warning(s): Do not vaccinate within 42 days before slaughter.

In case of accidental human injection seek immediate medical attention.

For veterinary use only.

Presentation: 1,000 dose (500 mL) vials.

Compendium Code No.: 10031110

10241C

NEWCASTLE B₁+BRONCHITIS CONN

Fort Dodge **Vaccine**

Newcastle-Bronchitis Vaccine, B1 Type, B1 Strain, Connecticut Type, Live Virus

U.S. Vet. Lic. No.: 112

Contents: This product contains the antigens listed above.

Contains gentamicin as a preservative.

Indications: This vaccine is recommended for administration to healthy chickens, as an aid in the prevention of Newcastle disease and infectious bronchitis, Connecticut serotype.

Directions: Read in full. Follow directions carefully.

For Intranasal or Intraocular Vaccination: This Newcastle-Bronchitis Vaccine accompanied by diluent is recommended for the vaccination of healthy chickens one day of age or older.

1. Rehydrate 1 vial of vaccine with 1 vial of diluent.
2. Remove seal and stopper from vaccine and diluent vials. Avoid contamination of stoppers and contents.
3. Add diluent to half-fill the vaccine vial. Replace stopper and shake until contents are dissolved.
4. Pour the rehydrated vaccine into the diluent container. Replace stopper and shake.
5. Remove stopper and fit drop-dispenser tip into diluent container.
6. To vaccinate intranasally, place finger over one of the bird's nostrils and place 1 drop of vaccine in the other nostril. Do not release bird until vaccine has been inhaled.
7. To vaccinate intraocularly, place 1 drop of vaccine in the eye.

For Drinking-Water Vaccination: This Newcastle-Bronchitis Vaccine is recommended for the vaccination of healthy chickens 2 weeks of age or older. If birds are vaccinated by this route before 2 weeks of age, they should be revaccinated.

1. Discontinue use of medications or sanitizing agents in the drinking water 24 hours before vaccinating. Do not resume use for 24 hours following vaccination.
2. Water used for the drinking-water administration of a live virus vaccine must be non-chlorinated.
3. Provide enough waterers so two-thirds of the birds may drink at one time. Scrub waterers with fresh, clean, non-chlorinated water, and use no disinfectant. Let the waterers drain dry.
4. Turn off automatic waterers, so the only available water is the vaccine water. Do not give vaccine water through medication tanks.
5. Withhold water for 2 hours before vaccinating. Do not deprive the birds of water if the temperature is extremely high.
6. Remove seal from vaccine vial.
7. Remove stopper and half-fill with clean, cool, non-chlorinated water.
8. Replace stopper and shake until dissolved.
9. Use a clean container two-thirds filled with cool, clean, non-chlorinated water. Add dried milk. Use 1 ounce (28.4 grams) dried milk if final volume of water per 1,000 doses of vaccine is to be 2½ gallons (9.5 liters); 2 ounces (56.8 grams) dried milk if final volume of water is to be 5 gallons (19.0 liters); and 4 ounces (113.6 grams) dried milk for a final volume of 10 gallons (38.0 liters). Stir the mixture until the dried milk is dissolved.
10. Add the rehydrated vaccine from the vial and again stir the contents thoroughly.
11. Next, add the mixture to the final volume of water, as follows:

Add this amount of vaccine	to this final volume of water	
	for chickens 2 to 8 weeks old	for chickens over 8 weeks old
1,000 doses	2½ to 5 gallons (9.5 to 19.0 liters)	5 to 10 gallons (19.0 to 38.0 liters)

12. Give 1 dose of vaccine per bird.
13. Distribute the final volume of vaccine water evenly among the clean waterers. Do not place the waterers in direct sunlight. Resume regular water administration only after all the vaccine water has been consumed.

For Spray Vaccination: This vaccine may be used for the revaccination of healthy chickens 4 weeks of age or older by spraying the vaccine solution above the chickens. A sprayer that delivers a fine mist quickly and evenly is recommended.

1. Remove seal from a vial of vaccine.
2. Remove the stopper and half-fill vial with cool, distilled water.
3. Replace stopper and shake until vaccine is in solution.
4. Pour rehydrated vaccine into a clean container and add 100 mL cool, distilled water per 1,000 doses vaccine. Shake thoroughly.
5. Apply at the rate of 100 mL rehydrated vaccine per 1,000 birds. For example, 20,000 birds will require 2,000 mL (approx. 2 quarts) rehydrated vaccine. Place the vaccine solution in the sprayer canister, set the discharge control at "low" and walk through the house, spraying at the rate of 1,000 birds per minute. Direct the spray above the heads of the birds.
6. Whatever volume of vaccine solution is used in the sprayer, take care to administer 1,000 doses vaccine per 1,000 birds.
7. This spray method of vaccination should be employed in poultry houses where air movement can be reduced to a minimum. Before spraying the vaccine solution, close the house and shut off mechanical ventilation. Maintain these conditions both during spraying and for 20 minutes afterwards.
8. Wear goggles and a face mask while spraying.
9. Any sprayer used for application of a live virus vaccine should be used for no other purpose.

Records: Keep a record of vaccine serial number and expiration date; date of receipt and date of vaccination; where vaccination takes place; and any reactions observed.

Precaution(s): Store this vaccine at not over 45°F (7°C). Use entire contents when vial is first opened. Burn vaccine container and all unused contents.

This vaccine is nonreturnable.

Caution(s): If possible, vaccinate all susceptible birds on the premises at the same time. For 10 to 14 days after vaccinating, avoid carrying vaccine particles on shoes, clothing, etc., into areas where there are unvaccinated birds.

Newcastle Disease Vaccine virus is capable of causing a mild, irritating eye infection in humans, lasting about 3 days. Do not allow vaccine to contact the eyes.

This product should be stored, transported, and administered in accordance with the instructions and directions.

The use of this vaccine is subject to state laws, wherever applicable.

Warning(s): Do not vaccinate within 21 days before slaughter.

For veterinary use only.

Presentation: 10 x 1,000 doses.

Compendium Code No.: 10031121

10870A

NEWCASTLE B$_1$+BRONCHITIS CONN MASS (1,000 DOSE)

Fort Dodge **Vaccine**

Newcastle-Bronchitis Vaccine, B1 Type, B1 Strain, Massachusetts and Connecticut Types, Live Virus

U.S. Vet. Lic. No.: 112

Contents: This product contains the antigens listed above.

Contains gentamicin as a preservative.

Indications: This vaccine is recommended for administration to healthy chickens, as an aid in the prevention of Newcastle disease and infectious bronchitis, Massachusetts and Connecticut serotypes.

Directions: Read in full. Follow directions carefully.

For Intranasal or Intraocular Vaccination: This Newcastle-Bronchitis Vaccine accompanied by diluent is recommended for the vaccination of healthy chickens one day of age or older.

1. Rehydrate 1 vial of vaccine with 1 vial of diluent.
2. Remove seal and stopper from vaccine and diluent vials. Avoid contamination of stoppers and contents.
3. Add diluent to half-fill the vaccine vial. Replace stopper and shake until contents are dissolved.
4. Pour the rehydrated vaccine into the diluent container. Replace stopper and shake.
5. Remove stopper and fit drop-dispenser tip into diluent container.
6. To vaccinate intranasally, place finger over one of the bird's nostrils and place 1 drop of vaccine in the other nostril. Do not release bird until vaccine has been inhaled.
7. To vaccinate intraocularly, place 1 drop of vaccine in the eye.

For Drinking-Water Vaccination: This Newcastle-Bronchitis Vaccine is recommended for the vaccination of healthy chickens 2 weeks of age or older. If birds are vaccinated by this route before 2 weeks of age, they should be revaccinated.

1. Discontinue use of medications or sanitizing agents in the drinking water 24 hours before vaccinating. Do not resume use for 24 hours following vaccination.
2. Water used for the drinking-water administration of a live virus vaccine must be non-chlorinated.
3. Provide enough waterers so two-thirds of the birds may drink at one time. Scrub waterers with fresh, clean, non-chlorinated water, and use no disinfectant. Let the waterers drain dry.
4. Turn off automatic waterers, so the only available water is the vaccine water. Do not give vaccine water through medication tanks.
5. Withhold water for 2 hours before vaccinating. Do not deprive the birds of water if the temperature is extremely high.
6. Remove seal from vaccine vial.
7. Remove stopper and half-fill with clean, cool, non-chlorinated water.
8. Replace stopper and shake until dissolved.
9. Use a clean container two-thirds filled with cool, clean, non-chlorinated water. Add dried milk. Use 1 ounce (28.4 grams) dried milk if final volume of water per 1,000 doses of vaccine is to be 2½ gallons (9.5 liters); 2 ounces (56.8 grams) dried milk if final volume of water is to be 5 gallons (19.0 liters); and 4 ounces (113.6 grams) dried milk for a final volume of 10 gallons (38.0 liters). Stir the mixture until the dried milk is dissolved.
10. Add the rehydrated vaccine from the vial and again stir the contents thoroughly.
11. Next, add the mixture to the final volume of water, as follows:

Add this amount of vaccine	to this final volume of water	
	for chickens 2 to 8 weeks old	for chickens over 8 weeks old
1,000 doses	2½ to 5 gallons (9.5 to 19.0 liters)	5 to 10 gallons (19.0 to 38.0 liters)

12. Give 1 dose of vaccine per bird.
13. Distribute the final volume of vaccine water evenly among the clean waterers. Do not place the waterers in direct sunlight. Resume regular water administration only after all the vaccine water has been consumed.

For Spray Vaccination: This vaccine may be used for the revaccination of healthy chickens 4 weeks of age or older by spraying the vaccine solution above the chickens. A sprayer that delivers a fine mist quickly and evenly is recommended.

1. Remove seal from a vial of vaccine.
2. Remove the stopper and half-fill vial with cool, distilled water.
3. Replace stopper and shake until vaccine is in solution.
4. Pour rehydrated vaccine into a clean container and add 100 mL cool, distilled water per 1,000 doses vaccine. Shake thoroughly.
5. Apply at the rate of 100 mL rehydrated vaccine per 1,000 birds. For example, 20,000 birds will require 2,000 mL (approx. 2 quarts) rehydrated vaccine. Place the vaccine solution in the sprayer canister, set the discharge control at "low" and walk through the house, spraying at the rate of 1,000 birds per minute. Direct the spray above the heads of the birds.
6. Whatever volume of vaccine solution is used in the sprayer, take care to administer 1,000 doses vaccine per 1,000 birds.
7. This spray method of vaccination should be employed in poultry houses where air movement can be reduced to a minimum. Before spraying the vaccine solution, close the house and shut off mechanical ventilation. Maintain these conditions both during spraying and for 20 minutes afterwards.
8. Wear goggles and a face mask while spraying.
9. Any sprayer used for application of a live virus vaccine should be used for no other purpose.

Records: Keep a record of vaccine serial number and expiration date; date of receipt and date of vaccination; where vaccination takes place; and any reactions observed.

Precaution(s): Store this vaccine at not over 45°F (7°C). Use entire contents when vial is first opened. Burn vaccine container and all unused contents.

This vaccine is nonreturnable.

Caution(s): If possible, vaccinate all susceptible birds on the premises at the same time. For 10 to 14 days after vaccinating, avoid carrying vaccine particles on shoes, clothing, etc., into areas where there are unvaccinated birds.

Newcastle Disease Vaccine virus is capable of causing a mild, irritating eye infection in humans, lasting about 3 days. Do not allow vaccine to contact the eyes.

This product should be stored, transported, and administered in accordance with the instructions and directions.

The use of this vaccine is subject to state laws, wherever applicable.

Warning(s): Do not vaccinate within 21 days before slaughter.

For veterinary use only.

Presentation: 10 x 1,000 doses.

Compendium Code No.: 10031131

10870A

NEWCASTLE B$_1$+BRONCHITIS CONN MASS (5,000 AND 10,000 DOSE)

Fort Dodge **Vaccine**

Newcastle-Bronchitis Vaccine, B1 Type, B1 Strain, Mass. and Conn. Types, Live Virus

U.S. Vet. Lic. No.: 112

Contents: This product contains the antigens listed above.

Indications: This vaccine is recommended for mass administration to healthy chickens, as an aid in the prevention of Newcastle disease and of infectious bronchitis, Massachusetts and Connecticut serotypes.

Dosage and Administration: Read in full, follow directions carefully.

Directions:

For drinking-water vaccination: This product is recommended for the vaccination of healthy chickens 2 weeks of age or older. If birds are vaccinated by this route before 2 weeks of age, they should be revaccinated.

1. Discontinue use of medications or sanitizing agents in the drinking water 24 hours before vaccinating. Do not resume use for 24 hours following vaccination.
2. Water used for the drinking-water administration of a live virus vaccine must be non-chlorinated.
3. Provide enough waterers, so two-thirds of the birds may drink at one time. Scrub waterers with fresh, clean, non-chlorinated water, and use no disinfectant. Let the waterers drain dry.
4. Turn off automatic waterers, so the only available water is the vaccine water. Do not give vaccine water through medication tanks.
5. Withhold water for 2 to 4 hours before vaccinating. Do not deprive the birds of water if the temperature is extremely high.
6. Remove seal from vaccine vial.
7. Remove stopper and half-fill vial with clean, cool, non-chlorinated water.
8. Replace stopper and shake until dissolved.
9. Use a clean container two-thirds filled with cool, clean, non-chlorinated water. Add dried milk at a rate of 12.5 ounces (355 grams) per 25 gallons (95 liters) of the final volume of vaccine solution. Stir the mixture until the dried milk is dissolved.
10. Add the rehydrated vaccine from the vial and again stir the contents thoroughly.
11. Next, add the mixture to the final volume of water, as follows:

Add this amount of vaccine	to this final volume of water	
	for chickens 2 to 8 weeks old	for chickens over 8 weeks old
5,000 doses	12.5 to 25 gallons (47.5 to 95 liters)	25 to 50 gallons (95 to 190 liters)
10,000 doses	25 to 50 gallons (95 to 190 liters)	50 to 100 gallons (190 to 380 liters)

12. Give 1 dose of vaccine per bird.
13. Distribute the final volume of (vaccine) water evenly among the clean waterers. Do not place the waterers in direct sunlight. Resume regular water administration only after all the vaccine water has been consumed.

For spray vaccination: This vaccine may be used for the revaccination of healthy chickens 4 weeks of age or older by spraying the vaccine solution above the chickens. A sprayer that delivers a fine mist quickly and evenly is recommended.

1. Remove seal from a vial of vaccine.
2. Remove the stopper and half-fill vial with cool, distilled water.
3. Replace stopper and shake until vaccine is in solution.
4. Pour rehydrated vaccine into a clean container and add approximately 500 mL cool, distilled water per 5,000 doses vaccine or 1,000 mL cool, distilled water per 10,000 doses vaccine.
5. Apply at the rate of 100 mL rehydrated vaccine per 1,000 birds. For example, 10,000 birds will require 1,000 mL (approx. 1 quart) rehydrated vaccine. Place the vaccine solution in the sprayer canister, set the discharge control at "low" and walk through the house, spraying at the rate of 1,000 birds per minute. Direct the spray above the heads of the birds.
6. Whatever volume of vaccine solution is used in the sprayer, take care to administer 1,000 doses vaccine per 1,000 birds.
7. This spray method of vaccination should be employed in poultry houses where air movement can be reduced to a minimum. Before spraying the vaccine solution, close the house and shut off mechanical ventilation. Maintain these conditions both during spraying and for 20 minutes afterwards.
8. Wear goggles and a face mask while spraying.
9. Any sprayer used for application of a live virus vaccine should be used for no other purpose.

Records: Keep a record of vaccine serial number and expiration date; date of receipt and date of vaccination; where vaccination takes place; and any reactions observed.

Precaution(s): Store this vaccine at not over 45°F (7°C).

Use entire contents when vial is first opened.

Burn vaccine container and all unused contents.

This product is nonreturnable.

Caution(s): This product should be stored, transported, and administered in accordance with the instructions and directions.

The use of this vaccine is subject to state laws, wherever applicable.

If possible, vaccinate all susceptible birds on the premises at the same time. For 10 to 14 days after vaccinating, avoid carrying vaccine particles on shoes, clothing, etc., into areas where there are unvaccinated birds.

Newcastle Disease Vaccine virus is capable of causing a mild, irritating eye infection in humans, lasting about 3 days. Do not allow vaccine to contact the eyes.

Warning(s): Do not vaccinate within 21 days before slaughter.

For veterinary use only.

Presentation: 10 x 5,000 doses and 10 x 10,000 doses.

Compendium Code No.: 10031141

10880A

NEWCASTLE B_1+BRONCHITIS MASS

Fort Dodge **Vaccine**

Newcastle-Bronchitis Vaccine, B1 Type, B1 Strain, Massachusetts Type, Live Virus

U.S. Vet. Lic. No.: 112

Contents: This product contains the antigens listed above.

Contains gentamicin as a preservative.

Indications: This vaccine is recommended for administration to healthy chickens, as an aid in the prevention of Newcastle disease and infectious bronchitis, Massachusetts serotype.

Directions: Read in full. Follow directions carefully.

For Intranasal or Intraocular Vaccination: This Newcastle-Bronchitis Vaccine accompanied by diluent is recommended for the vaccination of healthy chickens one day of age or older.

1. Rehydrate 1 vial of vaccine with 1 vial of diluent.
2. Remove seal and stopper from vaccine and diluent vials. Avoid contamination of stoppers and contents.
3. Add diluent to half-fill the vaccine vial. Replace stopper and shake until contents are dissolved.
4. Pour the rehydrated vaccine into the diluent container. Replace stopper and shake.
5. Remove stopper and fit drop-dispenser tip into diluent container.
6. To vaccinate intranasally, place finger over one of the bird's nostrils and place 1 drop of vaccine in the other nostril. Do not release bird until vaccine has been inhaled.
7. To vaccinate intraocularly, place 1 drop of vaccine in the eye.

For Drinking-Water Vaccination: This Newcastle-Bronchitis Vaccine is recommended for the vaccination of healthy chickens 2 weeks of age or older. If birds are vaccinated by this route before 2 weeks of age, they should be revaccinated.

1. Discontinue use of medications or sanitizing agents in the drinking water 24 hours before vaccinating. Do not resume use for 24 hours following vaccination.
2. Water used for the drinking-water administration of a live virus vaccine must be non-chlorinated.
3. Provide enough waterers so two-thirds of the birds may drink at one time. Scrub waterers with fresh, clean, non-chlorinated water, and use no disinfectant. Let the waterers drain dry.
4. Turn off automatic waterers, so the only available water is the vaccine water. Do not give vaccine water through medication tanks.
5. Withhold water for 2 hours before vaccinating. Do not deprive the birds of water if the temperature is extremely high.
6. Remove seal from vaccine vial.
7. Remove stopper and half-fill with clean, cool, non-chlorinated water.
8. Replace stopper and shake until dissolved.
9. Use a clean container two-thirds filled with cool, clean, non-chlorinated water. Add dried milk. Use 1 ounce (28.4 grams) dried milk if final volume of water per 1,000 doses of vaccine is to be 2½ gallons (9.5 liters); 2 ounces (56.8 grams) dried milk if final volume of water is to be 5 gallons (19.0 liters); and 4 ounces (113.6 grams) dried milk for a final volume of 10 gallons (38.0 liters). Stir the mixture until the dried milk is dissolved.
10. Add the rehydrated vaccine from the vial and again stir the contents thoroughly.
11. Next, add the mixture to the final volume of water, as follows:

Add this amount of vaccine	to this final volume of water	
	for chickens 2 to 8 weeks old	for chickens over 8 weeks old
1,000 doses	2½ to 5 gallons (9.5 to 19.0 liters)	5 to 10 gallons (19.0 to 38.0 liters)

12. Give 1 dose of vaccine per bird.
13. Distribute the final volume of vaccine water evenly among the clean waterers. Do not place the waterers in direct sunlight. Resume regular water administration only after all the vaccine water has been consumed.

N

For Spray Vaccination: This vaccine may be used for the revaccination of healthy chickens 4 weeks of age or older by spraying the vaccine solution above the chickens. A sprayer that delivers a fine mist quickly and evenly is recommended.

1. Remove seal from a vial of vaccine.
2. Remove the stopper and half-fill vial with cool, distilled water.
3. Replace stopper and shake until vaccine is in solution.
4. Pour rehydrated vaccine into a clean container and add 100 mL cool, distilled water per 1,000 doses vaccine. Shake thoroughly.
5. Apply at the rate of 100 mL rehydrated vaccine per 1,000 birds. For example, 20,000 birds will require 2,000 mL (approx. 2 quarts) rehydrated vaccine. Place the vaccine solution in the sprayer canister, set the discharge control at "low" and walk through the house, spraying at the rate of 1,000 birds per minute. Direct the spray above the heads of the birds.
6. Whatever volume of vaccine solution is used in the sprayer, take care to administer 1,000 doses vaccine per 1,000 birds.
7. This spray method of vaccination should be employed in poultry houses where air movement can be reduced to a minimum. Before spraying the vaccine solution, close the house and shut off mechanical ventilation. Maintain these conditions both during spraying and for 20 minutes afterwards.
8. Wear goggles and a face mask while spraying.
9. Any sprayer used for application of a live virus vaccine should be used for no other purpose.

Records: Keep a record of vaccine serial number and expiration date; date of receipt and date of vaccination; where vaccination takes place; and any reactions observed.

Precaution(s): Store this vaccine at not over 45°F (7°C). Use entire contents when vial is first opened. Burn vaccine container and all unused contents.

This vaccine is nonreturnable.

Caution(s): If possible, vaccinate all susceptible birds on the premises at the same time. For 10 to 14 days after vaccinating, avoid carrying vaccine particles on shoes, clothing, etc., into areas where there are unvaccinated birds.

Newcastle Disease Vaccine virus is capable of causing a mild, irritating eye infection in humans, lasting about 3 days. Do not allow vaccine to contact the eyes.

This product should be stored, transported, and administered in accordance with the instructions and directions.

The use of this vaccine is subject to state laws, wherever applicable.

Warning(s): Do not vaccinate within 21 days before slaughter.

For veterinary use only.

Presentation: 10 x 1,000 doses.

Compendium Code No.: 10031151 10870A

NEWCASTLE B_1+BRONCHITIS MASS+ARK

Fort Dodge **Vaccine**

Newcastle-Bronchitis Vaccine, B1 Type, B1 Strain, Mass. and Ark. Types, Live Virus

U.S. Vet. Lic. No.: 112

Contents: This product contains the antigens listed above.

Contains gentamicin as a preservative.

Indications: Newcastle-Bronchitis Vaccine, B1 Type, B1 Strain, Massachusetts and Arkansas Types Live Virus, is recommended for mass administration to healthy chickens, as an aid in the prevention of Newcastle disease and of infectious bronchitis, Massachusetts and Arkansas serotypes.

Directions: Read in full, follow directions carefully.

For Drinking-Water Administration: Use this product to vaccinate healthy chickens through the drinking water when they are 2 weeks of age or older. If the product is used prior to 2 weeks of age, less than optimum results may be encountered.

1. If medications or sanitizing agents are being given or used in the drinking water, discontinue their use at least 24 hours before vaccinating and do not resume their use for 24 hours following consumption of the vaccine water.
2. Water used for the drinking-water administration of a live-virus vaccine must be non-chlorinated.
3. Provide enough waterers so that at least two-thirds of the birds may drink at one time. Scrub waterers with fresh, clean, non-chlorinated water, and use no disinfectant. Then, let the waterers drain dry.
4. Turn off automatic waterers, so that the only available water is the vaccine water (from ordinary waterers). Do not give vaccine water through medication tanks.
5. To stimulate thirst, withhold water for 2 hours before vaccinating.
6. Remove aluminum seal from vial.
7. Remove rubber stopper and half-fill vial with clean, cool, non-chlorinated water.
8. Replace stopper in vial and shake it until vaccine is in solution.
9. Use a clean container two-thirds filled with cool, clean, non-chlorinated water. To this add dried milk. Use 10 oz. (284 grams) dried milk if final volume of water per 10,000 doses of vaccine is to be 25 gallons (95 liters); 20 oz. (568 grams) dried milk if final volume of water is to be 50 gal. (190 liters); 40 oz. (1136 grams) dried milk for a final volume of 100 gal. (380 liters); etc. Shake or stir until the dried milk is in solution.
10. Add the rehydrated vaccine from the vial to the water containing dried milk and shake or stir thoroughly.
11. Next, add this solution containing the 10,000 doses to water to make the final volume as follows:

For chickens 2 to 8 weeks old - 25 to 50 gallons (95 to 190 liters)

For chickens over 8 weeks old - 50 to 100 gallons (190 to 380 liters)

12. Never provide less than 1 dose of vaccine per bird.
13. Distribute the final volume of vaccine water evenly among the clean waterers. Do not place the waterers in direct sunlight. Resume regular water administration only after all the vaccine water has been consumed.

Records: Keep a record of vaccine serial number and expiration date; date of receipt and date of vaccination; where vaccination takes place; and any reactions observed.

Precaution(s): Store at not over 45°F (7°C).

Use entire contents of vial when first opened.

Burn vaccine container and all unused contents.

This vaccine is nonreturnable.

Caution(s): Use of this product is restricted to states in which officials have permitted it.

This product should be stored, transported, and administered in accordance with the instructions and directions. The use of this vaccine is subject to state laws, wherever applicable.

If possible, vaccinate all susceptible birds on the premises at the same time. For 10 to 14 days after vaccinating, exercise particular care to avoid carrying particles on shoes, clothing, etc., into areas where there are unvaccinated birds. Newcastle Disease Vaccine virus is capable of causing a mild but irritating eye infection in humans, lasting perhaps 3 days. Do not allow vaccine to contact the eyes.

Warning(s): Do not vaccinate within 21 days before slaughter.

For veterinary use only.

Presentation: 10 x 10,000 doses.

Compendium Code No.: 10031161 10890A

NEWCASTLE-BRONCHITIS VACCINE

L.A.H.I. (New Jersey) **Vaccine**

Newcastle-Bronchitis Vaccine, Killed Virus

U.S. Vet. Lic. No.: 196

Active Ingredient(s): This product is an inactivated viral vaccine used as an aid in the prevention of Newcastle disease and Massachusetts type infectious bronchitis. The vaccine is presented as an oil emulsion.

The vaccine is manufactured in accordance with a detailed production outline, which has been filed with the Veterinary Services of the USDA. Only specific pathogen free (SPF) eggs are used for production purposes. Seed virus is derived from a master seed virus lot which has been fully tested for purity, safety and immunogenicity. The fill volume for these products is 500 mL in a 625 mL plastic bottle. The bottles are sealed with a rubber stopper and an aluminum overseal.

Quality Control: The flocks producing SPF eggs are under constant observation by experienced personnel and routinely sampled and tested serologically to confirm absence of exposure to a large variety of avian pathogens. Shipments from the supplier are accompanied by regular reports on test results for each flock from which eggs were obtained.

These products are fully tested for purity, safety and potency according to the standard requirements for Newcastle disease and infectious bronchitis vaccines published as part 113, in particular, sections 113.125 of title 9 of the federal regulations by the Animal and Plant Health Inspection Service of the USDA, and according to the production outline submitted to the U.S. Department of Agriculture.

Each serial is tested for: Bacteria, fungi, and salmonella.

Potency is tested according to the outline approved by the USDA.

Indications: This product is packaged for subcutaneous vaccination in chickens three weeks of age or older. The recommended age for vaccination is 18 to 20 weeks of age. At least three weeks prior to the administration of the killed vaccine, a live Newcastle and Mass. type bronchitis vaccine should be used in any of the recommended methods of application for priming. Prevaccination with live vaccine is an absolute necessity for the effective use of the killed vaccine. If birds are to be kept for a second year of production, they should be revaccinated during molt.

Dosage and Administration: Immediately prior to use, shake the vaccine vigorously for 30 seconds to one (1) minute. Remove the aluminum overseal and the vaccine is ready to use.

Method of Vaccination: The inoculation should be given subcutaneously in the mid-portion of the neck. Each bird should receive 0.5 mL of vaccine in this manner.

Precaution(s): The vaccine shall be stored in the dark in a refrigerator between 2-7°C (35-45°F). Expiration date: 24 months.

Caution(s): It is imperative that the user of this product comply with the indications for use, contraindications, cautions and method of vaccination stated on the directions sheet packed with the product. The vaccine must be prepared and administered as directed to obtain the best results. For veterinary use only.

Warning(s): Do not market birds for at least six (6) weeks after vaccinating so that there is no swelling at the site of vaccine administration.

Presentation: 1,000 and 10,000 doses.

Compendium Code No.: 10080312

NEWCASTLE-BRONCHITIS VACCINE (B_1 Strain, Mass. Type)

Merial Select **Vaccine**

Newcastle-Bronchitis Vaccine, B1 Type, B1 Strain, Massachusetts Type, Live Virus

U.S. Vet. Lic. No.: 279

Active Ingredient(s): These vaccines contain the live virus B_1 strain of the Newcastle disease virus and a selected strain of infectious bronchitis virus of the Massachusetts type. The virus has been propagated in fertile eggs from specific pathogen free flocks. The immunizing capability of each vaccine has been proven by a master seed immunogenicity test. These vaccines offer proven immunity with mild reactions.

Penicillin and streptomycin sulfate are added as bacteriostatic agents.

Contains fungizone as a fungistatic agent.

These vaccines have met the requirements of the USDA in regards to safety, purity, potency and the capability to immunize normally susceptible chickens. These vaccines have been tested by the master seed immunogenicity test for efficacy.

Indications: These vaccines are recommended for use in healthy chickens as an aid in the prevention of Newcastle disease and bronchitis diseases, Massachusetts serotype.

The frozen vaccine is recommended for use in healthy one day old chickens.

The 5,000 and 25,000 dose size of the freeze-dried vaccine is recommended for healthy one day old chickens using the coarse spray method or for the revaccination of 14-28 day old broiler type chickens using drinking water or aerosol spray application. The use of an aerosol spray is recommended for revaccination only. The 15,000 dose size is for the vaccination of healthy chickens 14 days of age or older.

Chickens to be vaccinated must be healthy and free of all diseases. It is essential that the chickens be maintained under good environmental conditions, and that exposure to disease viruses be reduced as much as possible in the field.

Dosage and Administration:

A. Frozen Vaccine: For healthy one (1) day old chickens.

Preparation of the Vaccine for Use:

Important: Sterilize the vaccinating equipment by autoclaving for a minimum of 15 minutes at 250°F (121°C) or by boiling in water for at least 20 minutes. Never allow chemical disinfectants to come into contact with the vaccinating equipment.

1. Remove only one (1) ampule of vaccine at a time from the liquid nitrogen container. Thaw and use immediately. Do not hold the ampule towards the face when removing it from a liquid nitrogen container. Never refreeze a vaccine ampule after thawing.
2. The contents of the ampule are thawed rapidly by immersing it in water at room temperature (15-25°C). Gently swirl the ampule to disperse the contents. Break the ampule at its neck and quickly proceed as described below.
3. Transfer the contents of the ampule into a sterile 2 mL or 5 mL syringe fitted with an 18 to 20 gauge needle to cool, distilled, de-ionized water (10,000 doses to 700 mL of water).
4. Use the vaccine mixture immediately as described below.

Method of Vaccination:

1. Use the coarse spray application method.
2. Attach the spray head to the container and set the nozzle at a coarse spray setting.
3. To each box of 100 chickens, administer the vaccine by spraying 18-24 inches above the box.
4. Each box of 100 chickens should receive approximately 7 mL of vaccine. The exact amount can be determined by spraying into a calibrated tube or container to arrive at the number of applications needed to deliver 7 mL of vaccine.
5. Whatever the volume of vaccine used, take care to administer 1,000 doses to 1,000 chickens.

B. Freeze-dried Vaccine (5,000 doses): The vaccines are recommended for the vaccination of healthy chickens at one (1) day of age using the coarse spray method or for the vaccination of healthy chickens 14 days of age or older administered either in the drinking water or by aerosol spray. The use of an aerosol spray is recommended for revaccination only.

Directions for Coarse Spray Vaccination:

1. Be certain that all of the vaccinating equipment is clean before use. Never allow chemical disinfectants to come into contact with the vaccinating equipment.
2. Do not open and mix the vaccine until ready to use.
3. Remove the aluminum seal and rubber stopper from the vial.
4. Aseptically transfer 3-5 mL of cool, distilled water into the vaccine vial and mix gently.
5. Transfer the dissolved vaccine into cool, distilled water; 350 mL for 5,000 doses. Mix thoroughly.
6. Attach the spray head to the container and adjust the nozzle for coarse spray.
7. Administer the vaccine by spraying 18-24 inches above each tray of chicks.
8. Each tray of 100 chickens should receive approximately 7 mL of vaccine. The exact amount can be determined by spraying into a calibrated tube to arrive at the number of applications necessary to deliver 7 mL of vaccine.
9. Whatever volume of vaccine is used in the spray, take care to administer 5,000 doses to 5,000 birds.
10. Since coarse spray application is of a large droplet size, aerosol-like mist of the vaccine is reduced. However, always wear goggles and a face mask while spraying a live virus vaccine.
11. Any equipment used for the application of a live virus vaccine should not be used for any other purpose.

Directions for Drinking Water Vaccination: Do not use the drinking water method for vaccination of chickens younger than two (2) weeks of age or less than satisfactory results may be obtained.

1. Do not open or mix the vaccine until ready to use.
2. Remove all medications, sanitizers and disinfectants from the drinking water 72 hours prior to vaccination. Clean and rinse the waterers thoroughly.
3. Provide sufficient waterers so that all of the birds can drink at one time.
4. Withhold all water from the birds for two (2) to four (4) hours prior to vaccination to stimulate thirst.
5. Add nonfat dry milk to the water at the rate of 1 oz. per gallon before mixing the vaccine.
6. Remove the aluminum seal and rubber stopper from the vial.
7. Fill the vaccine vial with 3-5 mL of clean, cool water and mix gently.
8. Mix the dissolved vaccine with water as shown below:

Age of birds	Water per 5,000 doses vaccine
2-4 weeks	12.5 gallons (49.5 L)
4-8 weeks	25 gallons (94.5 L)
8 weeks or older	50 gallons (189.5 L)

9. Distribute the vaccine solution among waterers. Avoid direct sunlight.
10. Do not provide any other drinking water until all of the vaccine solution has been consumed.

Directions for Aerosol Spray Vaccination: Do not use for initial vaccination. Use only for revaccination of healthy chickens two (2) weeks of age or older.

Use a sprayer delivering an aerosol mist to disperse the rehydrated vaccine quickly and evenly throughout the chicken house.

1. Prior to spraying, reduce the air flow to a minimum. Keep the air flow reduced for 20 minutes following spray vaccination.
2. Remove the aluminum seal from a vial of the vaccine.
3. Remove the rubber stopper and fill the vial with 3-5 mL of cool, distilled water.
4. Pour the rehydrated vaccine into a clean container and add 500 mL of cool, distilled water per 5,000 doses of vaccine. Mix thoroughly.
5. For aerosol spray vaccination, apply at the rate of 500 mL per 5,000 chickens.
6. Place the vaccine solution in the sprayer canister, set the discharge control and walk through the house spraying at the rate of 1,000 chickens per minute. Direct the spray above the heads of the birds.
7. Whatever volume of vaccine solution is used, take care to administer 5,000 doses of vaccine per 5,000 birds.
8. Avoid direct contact with the vaccine solution. Wear goggles and a face mask while spraying a live virus vaccine.
9. Any equipment used for the application of a live virus vaccine should not be used for any other purpose.

C. Freeze-dried Vaccine (15,000 doses): For the vaccination of healthy chickens 14 days of age or older.

Drinking Water Vaccination - Pouring Application: For use in houses containing between 10,000 and 15,000 chickens.

1. Do not open or mix the vaccine until ready to vaccinate.
2. Remove all medications, sanitizers and disinfectants from the drinking water 72 hours (3 days) prior to vaccination.
3. Provide sufficient waterers so that all of the chickens can drink at one time. Shut off the water supply and allow the chickens to drink the troughs dry.
4. Raise the water troughs above the chickens' heads. Clean and rinse the waterers thoroughly.
5. Withhold all water from the chickens for a minimum of two (2) hours in warm weather to four (4) hours in cool weather prior to vaccination to stimulate thirst. The water withdrawal time should be reduced if half-house brooding is in process.
6. Calculate to supply the vaccine solution at a rate of three (3) gallons (11 L) per 1,000 chickens in cool weather and four (4) gallons (15 L) per 1,000 chickens in warm weather. The age of the chickens should be considered when calculating the water supply. Always use nonchlorinated water when vaccinating chickens.
   Example:
   10,000 chickens in cool weather x 3 gallons (11 L) = 30 gallons (114 L).
   14,500 chickens in warm weather x 4 gallons (15 L) = 58 gallons (220 L).
7. Add one of the following to pouring water for vaccine distribution:
   a. One (1) ounce (30 mL) of nonfat, dry milk per gallon (4 L) of water, or
   b. Four (4) ounces (118 mL) of fresh skim milk per gallon (4 L) of water.
8. Prepare the vaccine concentrate as follows:
   a. Prepare a container of milk/water figuring one (1) ounce (30 mL) of concentrate for one (1) gallon (4 L) of water to be used.
   b. Add cool milk/water to the vial until the dried vaccine is dissolved. Add the vaccine to the container of milk/water to make the vaccine concentrate. Rinse the vaccine vial to remove all of the vaccine.
9. To make the vaccine solution, add one (1) ounce (30 mL) of concentrate for each gallon (4 L) of water needed.
10. Distribute the vaccine solution among the waterers. Avoid direct sunlight.
11. Lower the water troughs and allow the birds to drink freely. Add the remaining vaccine solution to the troughs as the birds drink.
12. Do not provide any additional drinking water until all of the vaccine solution is consumed.

Drinking Water Vaccination - Proportioner Application: Several types of medicator/proportioners are commercially available. Set the proportioner to deliver one (1) ounce (30 mL) of vaccine concentrate per one (1) gallon (4 L) of water.

1. Do not open or mix the vaccine until ready to vaccinate.
2. Remove all medications, sanitizers and disinfectants from the proportioner 72 hours (3 days) prior to vaccination.
3. Clean all containers, hoses, and waterers prior to vaccination.
4. Withhold all water from the chickens for a minimum of two (2) hours in warm weather to four (4) hours in cool weather prior to vaccination to stimulate thirst.
5. Calculate to supply the vaccine solution at a rate of three (3) gallons (11 L) per 1,000 chickens in cool weather and four (4) gallons (15 L) per 1,000 chickens in warm weather. The age of the chickens should be considered when calculating the water supply. Always use nonchlorinated water when vaccinating chickens.
   Example:
   10,000 chickens in cool weather x 3 gallons (11 L) = 30 gallons (114 L).
   14,500 chickens in warm weather x 4 gallons (15 L) = 58 gallons (220 L).
6. Prepare the vaccine concentrate as follows:
   a. Add three (3) ounces (90 mL) of nonfat, dry milk per 16 ounces (473 mL) of cool water, or
   b. Use undiluted, cool, fresh skim milk.
7. To make the vaccine solution, add one (1) ounce (30 mL) of concentrate for each gallon (4 L) of water needed.
8. Add the milk solution to the vial until the dried vaccine is dissolved. Rinse the vaccine vial to remove all of the vaccine.
9. Insert the proportioner hose into the vaccine concentrate and start the water flow. Continue until all of the concentrate has been consumed before changing the water supply to direct flow.

10. Do not medicate or use disinfectants for 24 hours after vaccination.

Coarse Spray Application: For use in houses containing between 10,000 and 15,000 chickens. Spray application is recommended for revaccination only and not as a primary vaccination. Use a sprayer delivering a coarse spray pattern to dispense the rehydrated vaccine quickly and evenly throughout a house of chickens.

1. Prior to spraying, reduce the air flow by raising curtains or stopping fans. Air movement should be limited for 15 minutes following vaccination.
2. Fill the vaccine container with cool, distilled, de-ionized water.
3. Pour the reconstituted vaccine into a clean container and add five (5) ounces (150 mL) of cool water for each 1,000 chickens to be vaccinated.
4. Place the vaccine solution into a spray canister and walk through the house spraying at the rate of 1,000 chickens per minute. Direct spray directly above the heads of the chickens.
5. Avoid direct contact with the vaccine solution. Wear goggles and a face mask while spraying.
6. Do not use vaccinating equipment for any other purpose.

D. Freeze-dried Vaccine (25,000 doses): For vaccination or revaccination of 14-28 day old broiler type chickens.

Directions for Drinking Water Vaccination: For use in houses containing between 15,000 and 25,000 chickens. Do not use the drinking water vaccination method for chickens under 14 days of age.

Drinking Water - Pouring Application:

1. Do not open or mix the vaccine until ready to pour the vaccine solution into water troughs.
2. Stop use of medication, sanitizers and disinfectants such as iodine in the drinking water 72 hours (3 days) prior to vaccination.
3. Shut off the water supply and allow the chickens to drink the troughs dry. Water should be withheld from chickens for a minimum of two (2) hours in warm weather to four (4) hours in cold weather. The water withdrawal times should be reduced if half-house brooding is in process.
4. Raise the water troughs above the chickens heads. Clean and rinse the waterers thoroughly.
5. Calculate to supply the vaccine solution at a rate of three (3) gallons per 1,000 chickens in cold weather and four (4) gallons per 1,000 chickens in warm weather.
   Example:
   17,000 chickens in cool weather x 3 gallons = 51 gallons.
   22,500 chickens in warm weather x 4 gallons = 90 gallons.
6. Add one of the following to pouring water for vaccine distribution:
   a. One (1) ounce of nonfat dry milk per gallon of water, or
   b. Four (4) ounces of fresh skim milk per gallon of water.
   Milk or milk solids are added to neutralize low levels of virucidal chemicals which may be present in farm water.
7. Prepare the vaccine concentrate as follows:
   a. Prepare a container of milk/water figuring one (1) ounce of concentrate for one (1) gallon of water to be used.
   b. Open the vaccine container by removing the aluminum seal and stopper.
   c. Add cool milk/water to the vial until the dried vaccine is dissolved. Add the vaccine to the container of milk/water to make the vaccine concentrate. Rinse the vaccine bottle to remove all of the vaccine.
8. To make the vaccine solution, add one (1) ounce of concentrate for each gallon of pouring water needed. Mix well.
9. Fill all of the water troughs full with the vaccine solution. Avoid direct sunlight.
10. Lower the water troughs and allow the birds to drink freely. Add the remaining vaccine solution to the troughs as the birds drink.
11. Do not provide any additional drinking water until all of the vaccine solution has been consumed.

N

Drinking Water - Proportioner Application: Several types of medicator/proportioners are commercially available, such as the dosmatic liquid dispenser. Set the proportioner to deliver one (1) ounce of vaccine concentrate per one (1) gallon of water.

1. Stop use of medication, sanitizers and disinfectants such as iodine in the dispenser 72 hours (3 days) prior to vaccination. Clean all containers and hoses prior to vaccination. Do not use medicator containers for vaccine use.
2. Shut off the water supply for four (4) hours in cool weather and two (2) hours in warm weather before vaccination to stimulate thirst.
3. Calculate three (3) gallons of vaccine solution per 1,000 birds in cool weather and four (4) gallons in warm weather.
4. Calculate one (1) ounce of vaccine concentrate per gallon of water to make vaccine solution for bird consumption.
5. Vaccine concentrate preparation:
   a. Add three (3) ounces of dried nonfat milk per 16 ounces of cool water, or
   b. Use undiluted, cool, fresh skim milk.
6. Open the vaccine container by removing the aluminum seal and stopper.
7. Add the milk solution to the bottle, mix well, and add to the vaccine concentrate container. Rinse the vaccine bottle to remove all of the vaccine. Mix well.
8. Insert the dosmatic hose into the vaccine concentrate and start the water flow. Continue until all of the concentrate has been consumed before changing the water supply to direct flow.
9. Do not medicate or use disinfectants for 24 hours after vaccination.

Spray Application: For use in houses containing between 15,000 and 25,000 chickens. Spray application is recommended only for revaccination and not as a primary vaccination.

Coarse Aerosol Application: Use a sprayer delivering a coarse aerosol mist to dispense the rehydrated vaccine quickly and evenly throughout a house of chickens.

Directions:

1. Prior to spraying, reduce the air flow by raising curtains or stopping fans. Air movement should be limited for 15 minutes following vaccination.
2. Remove the aluminum seal and rubber stopper. Fill the vaccine container with cool water.
3. Pour the reconstituted vaccine into a clean container and add 150 mL (5 oz.) of cool water for each 1,000 chickens to be vaccinated.
4. Place the vaccine solution into a spray canister and walk through the house spraying at the rate of 1,000 birds per minute. Direct spray directly above the heads of the chickens.
5. Use all of the vaccine solution for each house containing 15,000 to 25,000 birds.
6. Avoid direct contact with the vaccine solution. Wear goggles and a face mask while spraying.
7. Do not use vaccinating equipment for any other purpose.

Precaution(s):

A. Storage Conditions for Frozen Vaccine:

Ampules: Store in a liquid nitrogen container.

Liquid nitrogen container: Carefully observe all liquid nitrogen precautions, including wearing eye protection and gloves. Store in a cool, well-ventilated area. Check the liquid nitrogen level once a day. Keep the container away from incubator intakes and chicken boxes.

Liquid Nitrogen Precautions: The liquid nitrogen containers and vaccines should be handled by properly trained personnel only. These persons should be familiar with the Union Carbide publication "Precautions and Safe Practices - Liquid Atmospheric Gases", form #9888. Liquid nitrogen is extremely cold. Accidental contact with the skin or eyes can cause serious frostbite. Protect the eyes with goggles or a face shield. Wear gloves and long sleeves when removing and handling frozen ampules or when adding liquid nitrogen to the container. Storage and handling of liquid nitrogen containers should be in a well-ventilated area. Excessive amounts of nitrogen reduces the concentration of oxygen in the air of an unventilated space and can cause asphyxiation. If drowsiness occurs, get fresh air quickly and ventilate the entire area. If a person becomes groggy or loses consciousness while working with liquid nitrogen, get the person to a well-ventilated area immediately. If breathing has stopped, begin artificial respiration. Call a physician immediately.

B. Storage Conditions for Freeze-dried Vaccine:

Store the vaccine at 35-45°F (2-7°C). Do not freeze.

Caution(s):

A. Frozen Vaccine:

Do not vaccinate diseased birds.
Vaccinate all of the birds on the premises at one time.
Administer a minimum of one dose for each bird.
Avoid stress conditions during and following vaccination.
Do not place chickens in contaminated facilities.
Exposure to disease must be minimized as much as possible.
For veterinary use only.

The capability of the vaccine to produce satisfactory results depends upon many factors, including, but not limited to, conditions of storage and handling by the user, administration of the vaccine, health and the responsiveness of individual animals and the degree of field exposure. Therefore, directions for use should be followed carefully.

The use of the vaccine is subject to applicable state and federal laws and regulations.
Use only in localities where permitted.

Newcastle disease virus can cause inflammation of the eyelids of humans. Care should be taken to avoid contamination of the eyes, hands and clothing with the vaccine.

Administer only as recommended.
Use the entire contents when first opened.
Burn the container and all unused contents.

B. Freeze-dried Vaccine:

Do not vaccinate diseased birds.
Birds should be free of respiratory disease and parasite infestations.
Vaccinate all of the birds on the premises at one time.
Administer a minimum of one dose for each bird (ie. 5,000 doses to 5,000 chickens).
Avoid stress conditions during and following vaccination.
Do not place chickens in contaminated facilities.
Exposure to disease must be minimized as much as possible.
Do not start the vaccination program for replacement pullets after birds are 16 weeks old.
For veterinary use only.

The capability of the vaccine to produce satisfactory results depends upon many factors, including, but not limited to, conditions of storage and handling by the user, administration of the vaccine, health and the responsiveness of individual animals and the degree of field exposure. Therefore, directions for use should be followed carefully.

The use of the vaccine is subject to applicable state and federal laws and regulations.
Use only in states where permitted.
Use the entire vial contents when first opened.
Burn the container and all unused contents.

Newcastle disease virus can cause inflammation of the eyelids of humans. Care should be taken to avoid contamination of the eyes, hands and clothing with the vaccine.

Warning(s): Do not vaccinate within 21 days before slaughter.

Presentation: Frozen vaccine: 5 x 10,000 dose vials.
Freeze-dried vaccine: 25 x 5,000 and 15 x 25,000 dose vials.

Compendium Code No.: 11050341

NEWCASTLE-BRONCHITIS VACCINE (B1 Type, LaSota Strain and Mass. Type, Holland Strain)

Merial Select **Vaccine**

Newcastle-Bronchitis Vaccine, B1 Type, LaSota Strain, Mass. Type, Live Virus, Holland Strain

U.S. Vet. Lic. No.: 279

Contents: This live virus vaccine contains the B1 type, LaSota strain of Newcastle disease virus and infectious bronchitis virus of the Massachusetts type, Holland strain.

Indications: This vaccine is recommended for vaccination of healthy chickens at 14 days of age or older using the drinking water or coarse aerosol spray application methods.

This vaccine is recommended for the protection of healthy chickens. It is essential that the chickens be maintained under good environmental conditions and that exposure to disease viruses be reduced as much as possible.

Dosage and Administration:

Drinking Water Vaccination:

Pouring Application: Drinking water vaccination is recommended for healthy chickens 14 days of age or older.

1. Do not open or mix vaccine until ready to vaccinate.
2. Remove all medications, sanitizers and disinfectants from the drinking water 72 hours (three days) prior to vaccination.
3. Provide sufficient waterers so that all the chickens can drink at one time. Shut off water supply and allow chickens to drink troughs dry.
4. Raise water troughs above chickens' heads. Clean and rinse the waterers thoroughly.
5. Withhold all water from the chickens for a minimum of two hours in warm weather to four hours in cool weather prior to vaccination to stimulate thirst. Withdrawal time should be reduced if half-house brooding is in process.
6. Calculate to supply vaccine solution at a rate of 3 gallons (11 liters) per 1,000 chickens in cool weather and 4 gallons (15 liters) per 1,000 chickens in warm weather. The age of the chickens should be considered when calculating water supply. Always use non-chlorinated water when vaccinating chickens.
   Example:
   10,000 chickens in cool weather x 3 gallons (11 liters) = 30 gallons (114 liters).

10,000 chickens in warm weather x 4 gallons (15 liters) = 40 gallons (152 liters).

7. Add to pouring water for vaccine distribution one of the following:
   a. One ounce (30 mL) of non-fat dry milk per gallon (3.8 liters) of water, or
   b. Four ounces (118 mL) of fresh skim milk per gallon (3.8 liters) of water.
8. Prepare vaccine concentrate as follows:
   a. Prepare a container of milk/water figuring one ounce (30 mL) of concentrate for one gallon (3.8 liters) of water to be used.
   b. Add cool milk/water to vial until dried vaccine is dissolved. Add vaccine to container of milk/water to make vaccine concentrate. Rinse vaccine vial to remove all vaccine.
9. To make vaccine solution, add one ounce (30 mL) of concentrate for each gallon (3.8 liters) of water needed.
10. Distribute vaccine solution among waterers. Avoid direct sunlight.
11. Lower troughs and allow the chickens to drink freely. Add remaining vaccine solution to troughs as chickens drink.
12. Do not provide additional drinking water until all vaccine is consumed.

Drinking Water Vaccination:

Proportioner Application: Drinking water vaccination is recommended for healthy chickens 14 days of age or older. Several types of medicator/proportioners are commercially available. Set proportioner to deliver one ounce (30 mL) of vaccine concentrate per one gallon (3.8 liters) of water.

1. Do not open or mix vaccine until ready to vaccinate.
2. Remove all medications, sanitizers and disinfectants from the drinking water 72 hours (3 days) prior to vaccination.
3. Clean all containers, hoses and waterers prior to vaccination.
4. Withhold all water from the chickens for a minimum of two hours in warm weather to four hours in cool weather prior to vaccination to stimulate thirst. Withdrawal time should be reduced if half-house brooding is in process.
5. Calculate to supply vaccine solution at a rate of 3 gallons (11 liters) per 1,000 chickens in cool weather and 4 gallons (15 liters) per 1,000 chickens in warm weather. The age of the chickens should be considered when calculating water supply. Always use non-chlorinated water when vaccinating chickens.
   Example:
   10,000 chickens in cool weather x 3 gallons (11 liters) = 30 gallons (114 liters).
   10,000 chickens in warm weather x 4 gallons (15 liters) = 40 gallons (152 liters).
6. Prepare vaccine concentrate as follows:
   a. Add 3 ounces (90 mL) of non-fat dry milk per 16 ounces (480 mL) of cool water, or
   b. Use undiluted cool, fresh skim milk.
7. To make vaccine solution, add one ounce (30 mL) of concentrate for each gallon (3.8 liters) of water needed.
8. Add milk solution to vial until dried vaccine is dissolved. Rinse vaccine vial to remove all vaccine.
9. Insert proportioner hose into vaccine concentrate and start water flow. Continue until all concentrate has been consumed before changing water supply to direct flow.
10. Do not medicate or use disinfectants for 24 hours after vaccination.

Coarse Aerosol Spray Application: Coarse aerosol spray application is recommended only for revaccination of healthy chickens 14 days of age or older and not as a primary vaccination. Use a sprayer delivering a coarse aerosol spray pattern to dispense rehydrated vaccine quickly and evenly throughout a house of chickens.

1. Prior to spraying, reduce air flow by raising curtains or stopping fans. Air movement should be limited for 20 minutes following vaccination.
2. Fill vaccine container with cool, distilled water.
3. Pour reconstituted vaccine into a clean container and add 5 ounces (150 mL) of cool water for each 1,000 chickens to be vaccinated.
4. Place the vaccine solution into spray canister and walk through the house spraying at the rate of 1,000 chickens per minute. Aim spray directly above the heads of the chickens.
5. Avoid direct contact with the vaccine solution. Wear goggles and mask while spraying.
6. Do not use vaccinating equipment for any other purpose.

Caution(s): Do not vaccinate diseased chickens.

Vaccinate all chickens on the premises at one time.

Administer a minimum of one dose for each bird. Avoid stress conditions during and following vaccination.

Do not place chickens in contaminated facilities.

Exposure to disease must be minimized as much as possible.

The capability of this vaccine to produce satisfactory results depends upon many factors, including — but not limited to — conditions of storage and handling by the user, administration of the vaccine, health and responsiveness of individual chickens, and degree of field exposure. Therefore, directions for use should be followed carefully. The use of this vaccine is subject to applicable state and federal laws and regulations.

Warning(s): Newcastle disease virus can cause inflammation of the eyelids of humans. Care should be taken to avoid contamination of eyes, hands and clothing with this vaccine.

For veterinary use only.

Trial Data: Merial Select's vaccines have met the requirements of the USDA in regard to safety, purity, potency and the capability to protect susceptible chickens. This vaccine has been tested by the Master Seed immunogenicity test for efficacy.

Presentation: 25 x 5,000 doses.

Compendium Code No.: 11050351

NEWCASTLE-BRONCHITIS VACCINE (Conn. Type)

Merial Select **Vaccine**

Newcastle-Bronchitis Vaccine, B1 Type, B1 Strain, Conn. Type, Live Virus

U.S. Vet. Lic. No.: 279

Active Ingredient(s): These vaccines contain the freeze-dried B_1 strain of Newcastle disease virus and selected strains of infectious bronchitis virus of the Connecticut serotype. The virus has been propagated in fertile eggs from specific pathogen free flocks. The immunizing capability of these vaccines have been proven by a master seed immunogenicity test. The vaccine offers proven immunity with mild reactions.

Contains streptomycin and penicillin as bacteriostatic agents.

Contains fungizone as a fungistatic agent.

Notice: These vaccines have met the requirements of the USDA in regards to safety, purity, potency and the ability to immunize normal, susceptible chickens.

Indications: These vaccines are recommended for the vaccination of healthy chickens as an aid in the prevention of Newcastle disease and infectious bronchitis, Connecticut serotype.

The frozen vaccine is recommended for use in healthy one day old chickens.

The freeze-dried vaccine is recommended for the vaccination of healthy one day old chickens using the coarse spray method or for the vaccination of healthy chickens 14 days of age or older administered either in the drinking water or by aerosol spray. The use of an aerosol spray is recommended for revaccination only.

Chickens to be vaccinated must be healthy and free of all diseases. It is essential that the chickens be maintained under good environmental conditions, and that exposure to disease viruses be reduced as much as possible in the field.

Dosage and Administration:

A. Frozen Vaccine: For one (1) day old chickens.

Preparation of the Vaccine for Use:

Important: Sterilize the vaccinating equipment by autoclaving for a minimum of 15 minutes at 250°F (121°C) or by boiling in water for at least 20 minutes. Never allow chemical disinfectants to come into contact with the vaccinating equipment.

1. Remove only one (1) ampule of vaccine at a time from the liquid nitrogen container. Thaw and use immediately. Do not hold the ampule towards the face when removing it from a liquid nitrogen container. Never refreeze a vaccine ampule after thawing.
2. The contents of the ampule are thawed rapidly by immersing it in water at room temperature (15-25°C). Gently swirl the ampule to disperse the contents. Break the ampule at its neck and quickly proceed as described below.
3. Transfer the contents of the ampule into a sterile 2 mL or 5 mL syringe fitted with an 18 to 20 gauge needle to cool, distilled, de-ionized water (10,000 doses to 700 mL of water).
4. Use the vaccine mixture immediately as described below.

Method of Vaccination:

1. Use the coarse spray application method.
2. Attach the spray head to the container and set the nozzle at a coarse spray setting.
3. To each box of 100 chickens, administer the vaccine by spraying 18-24 inches above the box.
4. Each box of 100 chickens should receive approximately 7 mL of vaccine. The exact amount can be determined by spraying into a calibrated tube or container to arrive at the number of applications needed to deliver 7 mL of vaccine.
5. Whatever the volume of vaccine used, take care to administer 1,000 doses to 1,000 chickens.

B. Freeze-dried Vaccine: For one (1) day old chickens.

Directions for Coarse Spray Vaccination:

1. Be certain all vaccinating equipment is clean before use. Never allow chemical disinfectants to come into contact with the vaccinating equipment.
2. Do not open and mix the vaccine until ready to use.
3. Remove the aluminum seal and rubber stopper from vial.
4. Aseptically transfer 3-5 mL of cool, distilled water into vaccine vial and mix gently.
5. Transfer the dissolved vaccine into cool, distilled water; 350 mL for 5,000 doses. Mix thoroughly.
6. Attach the spray head to the container and adjust the nozzle for coarse spray.
7. Administer the vaccine by spraying 18-24 inches above each tray of chicks.
8. Each tray of 100 chickens should receive approximately 7 mL of vaccine. The exact amount can be determined by spraying into a calibrated tube to arrive at the number of applications necessary to deliver 7 mL of vaccine.
9. Whatever volume of vaccine is used in the spray, take care to administer 5,000 doses to 5,000 birds.
10. Since coarse spray application is of a large droplet size, aerosol-like mist of the vaccine is reduced. However, always wear goggles and a face mask while spraying a live virus vaccine.
11. Any equipment used for the application of a live virus vaccine should not be used for any other purpose.

Directions for Drinking Water Vaccination: Do not use the drinking water method for vaccination of chickens younger than two (2) weeks of age or less than satisfactory results may be obtained.

N

1. Do not open or mix the vaccine until ready to use.
2. Remove all medications, sanitizers and disinfectants from the drinking water 72 hours prior to vaccination. Clean and rinse waterers thoroughly.
3. Provide sufficient waterers so that all of the birds can drink at one time.
4. Withhold all water from the birds for two (2) to four (4) hours prior to vaccination to stimulate thirst.
5. Add nonfat dry milk to the water at the rate of 1 oz. per gallon before mixing the vaccine.
6. Remove the aluminum seal and rubber stopper from the vial.
7. Fill the vaccine vial with 3-5 mL of clean, cool water and mix gently.
8. Mix the dissolved vaccine with water as shown below:

Age of birds	Water per 5,000 doses vaccine
2-4 weeks	12.5 gallons (49.5 L)
4-8 weeks	25 gallons (94.5 L)
8 weeks or older	50 gallons (189.5 L)

9. Distribute the vaccine solution among the waterers. Avoid direct sunlight.
10. Do not provide any other drinking water until all of the vaccine solution has been consumed.

Directions for Aerosol Spray Vaccination: Do not use for initial vaccination. Use only for revaccination of healthy chickens two (2) weeks of age or older.

Use a sprayer delivering an aerosol mist to disperse the rehydrated vaccine quickly and evenly throughout the chicken house.

1. Prior to spraying, reduce the air flow to a minimum. Keep the air flow reduced for 20 minutes following spray vaccination.
2. Remove the aluminum seal from a vial of the vaccine.
3. Remove the rubber stopper and fill the vial with 3-5 mL of cool, distilled water.
4. Pour the rehydrated vaccine into a clean container and add 500 mL of cool, distilled water per 5,000 doses of vaccine. Mix thoroughly.
5. For aerosol spray vaccination, apply at the rate of 500 mL per 5,000 chickens.
6. Place the vaccine solution in the sprayer canister, set the discharge control and walk through the house spraying at the rate of 1,000 chickens per minute. Direct the spray above the heads of the birds.
7. Whatever volume of vaccine solution is used, take care to administer 5,000 doses of vaccine to 5,000 birds.
8. Avoid direct contact with the vaccine solution. Wear goggles and a face mask while spraying a live virus vaccine.
9. Any equipment used for the application of a live virus vaccine should not be used for any other purpose.

Precaution(s):

A. Storage Conditions for Frozen Vaccine:

Ampules: Store in a liquid nitrogen container.

Liquid nitrogen container: Carefully observe all liquid nitrogen precautions, including wearing eye protection and gloves. Store in a cool, well-ventilated area. Check the liquid nitrogen level once a day. Keep the container away from incubator intakes and chicken boxes.

Liquid Nitrogen Precautions: The liquid nitrogen containers and vaccines should be handled by properly trained personnel only. These persons should be familiar with the Union Carbide publication "Precautions and Safe Practices - Liquid Atmospheric Gases", form #9888. Liquid nitrogen is extremely cold. Accidental contact with the skin or eyes can cause serious frostbite. Protect the eyes with goggles or a face shield. Wear gloves and long sleeves when removing and handling frozen ampules or when adding liquid nitrogen to the container. Storage and handling of liquid nitrogen containers should be in a well-ventilated area. Excessive amounts of nitrogen reduces the concentration of oxygen in the air of an unventilated space and can cause asphyxiation. If drowsiness occurs, get fresh air quickly and ventilate the entire area. If a person becomes groggy or loses consciousness while working with liquid nitrogen, get the person to a well-ventilated area immediately. If breathing has stopped, begin artificial respiration. Call a physician immediately.

B. Storage Conditions for Freeze-dried Vaccine:

Store the freeze-dried vaccine at 35-45°F (2-7°C). Do not freeze.

Caution(s):

A. Frozen Vaccine:

Do not vaccinate diseased birds.

Vaccinate all of the birds on the premises at one time.

Administer a minimum of one dose for each bird.

Avoid stress conditions during and following the vaccination.

Do not place chickens on contaminated premises.

Exposure to disease must be minimized as much as possible.

For veterinary use only.

The capability of these vaccines to produce satisfactory results depends upon many factors, including, but not limited to, conditions of storage and handling by the user, administration of the vaccine, health and the responsiveness of individual animals and the degree of field exposure. Therefore, directions for use should be followed carefully.

The use of these vaccines is subject to applicable local and federal laws and regulations.

Use only in localities where permitted.

Newcastle disease virus can cause inflammation to the eyelids of humans. Care should be taken to avoid contamination of the eyes, hands and clothing with the vaccine.

Administer only as recommended.

Use the entire contents when first opened.

Burn the container and all unused contents.

B. Freeze-dried Vaccine:

Do not vaccinate diseased chickens.

Birds should be free of respiratory disease and parasite infestations.

Vaccinate all of the birds on the same premises at the same time.

Administer 5,000 doses to 5,000 chickens.

Avoid stress conditions during and following the vaccination.

Do not place chickens on contaminated premises.

Exposure to disease must be minimized as much as possible.

Do not start the vaccination program for replacement pullets after birds are 16 weeks old.

The vaccine is designed to stimulate effective immunity when used as directed, but the user must be advised that the response to the product depends upon many factors, including, but not limited to, conditions of storage and handling by the user, administration of the vaccine, health and the responsiveness of individual birds, and the degree of field exposure. Therefore, directions for use should be followed carefully.

The product must be stored, transported, and administered in accordance with instructions and directions.

N

The use of the vaccine is subject to state laws wherever applicable.

Use only in states where permitted.

Use the entire contents when first opened.

Burn the container and all unused contents.

Since Newcastle disease virus can cause inflammation to the eyelids of humans, care should be taken to avoid contamination of the eyes, hands and clothing with the vaccine.

Warning(s): Do not vaccinate within 21 days before slaughter.

Presentation: Frozen vaccine: 5 x 10,000 dose vials.
Freeze-dried vaccine: 25 x 5,000 dose vials.

Compendium Code No.: 11050361

NEWCASTLE-BRONCHITIS VACCINE (LaSota Strain, Mass. Type)

Merial Select **Vaccine**

Newcastle-Bronchitis Vaccine, B_1 Type, LaSota Strain, Mass. Type, Live Virus

U.S. Vet. Lic. No.: 279

Contents: This vaccine contains the B_1 type, LaSota strain of Newcastle disease virus and Massachusetts type bronchitis virus.

Contains streptomycin sulfate and penicillin as bacteriostatic agents and amphotericin B as a fungistatic agent.

Notice: Merial Select's vaccines have met the requirements of the USDA in regard to safety, purity, potency, and the capability to protect susceptible chickens. This vaccine has been tested by the Master Seed immunogenicity test for efficacy.

Indications: It is recommended for the vaccination of healthy chickens 14 days of age or older using the eyedrop or drinking water method, or for the revaccination at 14 days of age or older using coarse aerosol spray as an aid in the prevention of Newcastle disease and Massachusetts type bronchitis.

This vaccine is recommended for the protection of healthy chickens. It is essential that the chickens be maintained under good environmental conditions and that exposure to disease viruses be reduced as much as possible.

Dosage and Administration:

Intraocular Vaccination: The vaccine used for intraocular vaccination is accompanied by diluent and is recommended for the vaccination of healthy chickens 14 days of age or older using the 1,000 dose vial only.

1. Reconstitute each 1,000 doses of vaccine with 30 mL of diluent.
   a. Remove aluminum seal and rubber stopper from vaccine vial and diluent vial. Avoid contamination of stoppers and contents.
   b. Add diluent to half-fill the vaccine vial. Replace stopper in vial and shake it so that all contents are dissolved.
   c. Pour the reconstituted vaccine into the diluent container. Replace stopper in diluent container and shake.
   d. Remove stopper and fit drop-dispenser tip into diluent container.
2. Holding the diluent container with the dropper tip down, gently press the sides, dropping one drop of vaccine on the bird's eye. Be sure the vaccine spreads over the eye before releasing the bird.

Drinking Water Vaccination Using Pouring Application: Drinking water vaccination is recommended for healthy chickens 14 days of age or older.

1. Remove all medications, sanitizers and disinfectants from the drinking water 72 hours (three days) prior to vaccination.
2. Provide sufficient waterers so that all the chickens can drink at one time. Shut off water supply and allow chickens to consume all the water in the lines.
3. Raise water lines above the chickens' heads. Clean and rinse the waterers thoroughly.
4. Withhold all water from the chickens for a minimum of two hours in warm weather to four hours in cool weather prior to vaccination to stimulate thirst. Withdrawal time should be reduced if half-house brooding is in process.
5. Do not open or mix vaccine until ready to vaccinate.
6. Drinking water for vaccine delivery should contain one ounce (29 gm) of non-fat dry milk per gallon (3.8 liters) of non-chlorinated water, or should contain milk product based stabilizer prepared according to the manufacturer's instructions.
7. Reconstitute the vaccine in 3 gallons (11 liters) of milk-water during cool weather or 4 gallons (15 liters) of milk-water during warm weather for each 1,000 doses.
8. Distribute vaccine solution among waterers. Avoid direct sunlight.
9. Lower waterers and allow the chickens to drink freely. Add the remaining vaccine solution to the water lines as the chickens drink.
10. Do not provide additional drinking water until all the vaccine is consumed.

Drinking Water Vaccination Using Proportioner Application: Drinking water vaccination is recommended for healthy chickens 14 days of age or older. Several types of medicator/proportioners are commercially available. Set proportioner to deliver one ounce (30 mL) of vaccine concentrate per one gallon (3.8 liters) of water.

1. Remove all medications, sanitizers and disinfectants from the drinking water 72 hours (three days) prior to vaccination.
2. Clean all containers, hoses and waterers prior to vaccination.
3. Withhold all water from the chickens for a minimum of two hours in warm weather to four hours in cool weather prior to vaccination to stimulate thirst. Withdrawal time should be reduced if half-house brooding is in process.
4. Do not open or mix vaccine until ready to vaccinate.
5. Calculate to supply vaccine solution at a rate of 3 gallons (11 liters) per 1,000 chickens in cool weather and 4 gallons (15 liters) per 1,000 chickens in warm weather. The age of the chickens should be considered when calculating water supply. Always use non-chlorinated water when vaccinating chickens.
   Example:
   1,000 chickens in cool weather x 3 gallons (11 liters) = 3 gallons (11 liters).
   1,000 chickens in warm weather x 4 gallons (15 liters) = 4 gallons (15 liters).
6. Prepare vaccine stock solution as follows:
   a. Determine the quantity of vaccine concentrate required by multiplying one ounce (30 mL) x gallons of water needed for vaccine/drinking water.
   Example:
   For 1,000 chickens: 3 gallons x 1 ounce (30 mL) = 3 ounces (90 mL).
   b. Add 3 ounces (85 gm) of non-fat dry milk per 16 ounces (480 mL) of cool water, or use a commercial milk product based stabilizer according to the manufacturer's instructions. For 1,000 chickens add 0.5 ounces (16 gm) non-fat dry milk to the 3 ounces (90 mL) of water.
   c. Reconstitute the dried vaccine with the milk solution. Rinse the vaccine vial to remove all the vaccine.
7. Insert proportioner hose into the vaccine stock solution and start water flow. Continue until all solution has been consumed before changing water supply to direct flow.
8. Do not medicate or use disinfectants for 24 hours after vaccination.

Coarse Aerosol Spray Application: Coarse aerosol spray application is recommended for revaccination of healthy chickens 14 days of age or older. Use a sprayer delivering a coarse aerosol spray pattern to dispense rehydrated vaccine quickly and evenly throughout a house of chickens. Do not use vaccinating equipment for any other purpose.

1. Prior to spraying, reduce air flow by raising curtains or stopping fans. Air movement should be limited for 20 minutes following vaccination.
2. Do not open or mix vaccine until ready to vaccinate.
3. Fill vaccine container with cool, distilled water.
4. Pour reconstituted vaccine into a clean container and add 5 ounces (150 mL) of cool water for each 1,000 chickens to be vaccinated.
5. Place the vaccine solution into spray canister and walk through the house spraying at the rate of 1,000 chickens per minute. Aim spray directly above the heads of the chickens.
6. Avoid direct contact with the vaccine solution. Wear goggles and mask while spraying.

Precaution(s): Store at 35-45°F (2-7°C). Do not freeze. Use entire contents when first opened. Burn the container and all unused contents.

Caution(s): Newcastle disease can cause inflammation of the eyelids of humans. Eye protection must be worn when rehydrating and administering this vaccine. Avoid contaminating hands and clothing with the vaccine. Hand washing is recommended after exposure to the product.

Do not vaccinate diseased chickens.

Vaccinate all chickens on the premises at one time.

Administer a minimum of one dose per chicken.

Avoid stress conditions during and following vaccination.

Do not place chickens in contaminated facilities.

Exposure to disease must be minimized as much as possible.

The capability of this vaccine to produce satisfactory results depends upon many factors, including, but not limited to, conditions of storage and handling by the user, administration of the vaccine, health and responsiveness of individual chickens, and degree of field exposure. Therefore, directions for use should be followed carefully. The use of this vaccine is subject to applicable state and federal laws and regulations.

For veterinary use only.

Warning(s): Do not vaccinate within 21 days of slaughter.

Presentation: 50 x 2,000 dose, 25 x 5,000 dose and 10 x 15,000 dose vials.

Compendium Code No.: 11050301 1199

NEWCASTLE-BRONCHITIS VACCINE LS MASS II™

Fort Dodge **Vaccine**

Newcastle-Bronchitis Vaccine, B1 Type, LaSota Strain, Massachusetts Type, Live Virus

U.S. Vet. Lic. No.: 112

Contents: LS MASS II™ is a combination live-virus vaccine. The Newcastle fraction is the B1 type, LaSota strain, and the bronchitis fraction is prepared from a modified strain of infectious-bronchitis virus, Massachusetts type.

Contains gentamicin as a preservative.

Indications: This vaccine is recommended as an aid in the prevention of Newcastle disease and of infectious bronchitis, Massachusetts serotype.

Directions: Read in full, follow directions carefully.

For intranasal, intraocular or drinking-water administration.

For intranasal or intraocular vaccination: This vaccine accompanied by diluent is recommended for the vaccination of healthy chickens one day of age or older.

1. Rehydrate 1 vial of vaccine with 1 vial of diluent.
2. Remove seal and stopper from vaccine and diluent vials. Avoid contamination of stoppers and contents.
3. Add diluent to half-fill the vaccine vial. Replace stopper and shake until contents are dissolved.
4. Pour the rehydrated vaccine into the diluent container. Replace stopper and shake.
5. Remove stopper and fit drop-dispenser tip into diluent container.
6. To vaccinate intranasally, place finger over one of the bird's nostrils and place 1 drop of vaccine in the other nostril. Do not release bird until vaccine has been inhaled.
7. To vaccinate intraocularly, place 1 drop of vaccine in the eye.

For drinking-water vaccination: This vaccine is recommended for the vaccination of healthy chickens 2 weeks of age or older. If chickens are vaccinated by this route before 2 weeks of age, they should be revaccinated.

1. Discontinue use of medications or sanitizing agents in the drinking water for 24 hours before vaccinating. Do not resume their use for 24 hours following vaccination.
2. Water used for the drinking-water administration of a live virus vaccine must be non-chlorinated.
3. Provide enough waterers so two-thirds of the birds may drink at one time. Scrub waterers with fresh, clean, non-chlorinated water, and use no disinfectant. Let the waterers drain dry.
4. Turn off automatic waterers, so the only available water is the vaccine water. Do not give vaccine water through medication tanks.
5. Withhold water for 2 to 4 hours before vaccinating. Do not deprive the birds of water if the temperature is extremely high.
6. Remove seal from vaccine vial.
7. Remove stopper and half-fill vial with clean, cool, non-chlorinated water.
8. Replace stopper and shake until dissolved.
9. Use a clean container two-thirds filled with cool, clean, non-chlorinated water. Add dried milk at a rate of 1 ounce (28.4 grams) dried milk if final volume of water per 1,000 doses of vaccine is to be 2½ gallons (9.5 liters); 2 ounces (56.8 grams) dried milk if final volume of water is to be 5 gallons (19.0 liters); and 4 ounces (113.6 grams) dried milk for a final volume of 10 gallons (38.0 liters). Stir the mixture until the dried milk is dissolved.
10. Add the rehydrated vaccine from the vial and again stir the contents thoroughly.
11. Next, add the mixture to the final volume of water, as follows:

Add this amount of vaccine	to this final volume of water	
	for chickens 2 to 8 weeks old	for chickens over 8 weeks old
1,000 doses	2½ to 5 gallons (9.5 to 19.0 liters)	5 to 10 gallons (19.0 to 38.0 liters)

12. Give 1 dose of vaccine per bird.
13. Distribute the final volume of (vaccine) water evenly among the clean waterers. Do not place the waterers in direct sunlight. Resume regular water administration only after all the vaccine water has been consumed.

Revaccination: For growing chickens intended for replacement flocks or breeder flocks, it is advisable to revaccinate in advance of the onset of egg production.

Records: Keep a record of vaccine serial number and expiration date; date of receipt and date of vaccination; where vaccination takes place; and any reactions observed.

Precaution(s): Store this vaccine at not over 45°F (7°C).

Use entire contents when vial is first opened.

Burn vaccine container and all unused contents.

This product is nonreturnable.

Caution(s): This product should be stored, transported, and administered in accordance with the instructions and directions.

The use of this vaccine is subject to state laws, wherever applicable.

If possible, vaccinate all susceptible birds on the premises at the same time. For 10 to 14 days after vaccinating, avoid carrying vaccine particles on shoes, clothing, etc., into areas where there are unvaccinated birds.

Newcastle Disease Vaccine virus is capable of causing a mild, irritating eye infection in humans, lasting about 3 days. Do not allow vaccine to contact the eyes.

Warning(s): Do not vaccinate within 21 days before slaughter.

For veterinary use only.

Presentation: 10 x 1,000 doses.

Compendium Code No.: 10031211 10930A

NEWCASTLE-BRONCHITIS VACCINE (Mass. & Ark. Types)

Merial Select **Vaccine**

Newcastle-Bronchitis Vaccine, B1 Type, B1 Strain, Mass. & Ark. Types, Live Virus

U.S. Vet. Lic. No.: 279

Active Ingredient(s): These vaccines contain the B_1 strain of Newcastle disease virus and selected strains of infectious bronchitis viruses of the Massachusetts and Arkansas serotypes. The virus has been propagated in fertile eggs from specific pathogen free flocks. The immunizing capability of these vaccines have been proven by a master seed immunogenicity test for efficacy. These vaccines offer proven immunity with mild reactions.

Contains streptomycin and penicillin as bacteriostatic agents.

Contains fungizone as a fungistatic agent.

Notice: These vaccines have met the requirements of the USDA in regard to safety, purity, potency and the capacity to immunize normal, susceptible chickens.

Indications: These vaccines are recommended for the vaccination of healthy chickens as an aid in the prevention of Newcastle disease and infectious bronchitis, Massachusetts and Arkansas serotypes.

The frozen vaccine is recommended for use in healthy one day old chickens.

The 5,000 and 25,000 dose size of the freeze-dried vaccine is recommended for the vaccination of healthy chickens at one day of age using the coarse spray method or for the vaccination of healthy chickens 14 days of age or older administered either in the drinking water or by aerosol spray. The use of an aerosol spray is recommended for revaccination only.

Dosage and Administration:

A. Frozen Vaccine: For healthy one (1) day old chickens.

Preparation of the Vaccine for Use:

Important: Sterilize the vaccinating equipment by autoclaving for a minimum of 15 minutes at 250°F (121°C) or by boiling in water for at least 20 minutes. Never allow chemical disinfectants to come into contact with the vaccinating equipment.

1. Remove only one (1) ampule of vaccine at a time from the liquid nitrogen container. Thaw and use immediately. Do not hold the ampule towards the face when removing it from a liquid nitrogen container. Never refreeze a vaccine ampule after thawing.
2. The contents of the ampule are thawed rapidly by immersing it in water at room temperature (15-25°C). Gently swirl the ampule to disperse the contents. Break the ampule at its neck and quickly proceed as described below.
3. Transfer the contents of the ampule into a sterile 2 mL or 5 mL syringe fitted with an 18 to 20 gauge needle to cool, distilled, de-ionized water (10,000 doses to 700 mL of water).
4. Use the vaccine mixture immediately as described below.

Method of Vaccination:

1. Use the coarse spray application method.
2. Attach the spray head to the container and set the nozzle at a coarse spray setting.
3. To each box of 100 chickens, administer the vaccine by spraying 18-24 inches above the box.
4. Each box of 100 chickens should receive approximately 7 mL of vaccine. The exact amount can be determined by spraying into a calibrated tube or container to arrive at the number of applications needed to deliver 7 mL of vaccine.
5. Whatever the volume of vaccine used, take care to administer 1,000 doses to 1,000 chickens.

B. Freeze-dried Vaccine (5,000 doses): The vaccines are recommended for the vaccination of healthy chickens at one (1) day of age using the coarse spray method or for the vaccination of healthy chickens 14 days of age or older administered either in the drinking water or by aerosol spray. The use of an aerosol spray is recommended for revaccination only.

Directions for Coarse Spray Vaccination:

1. Be certain that all vaccinating equipment is clean before use. Never allow chemical disinfectants to come into contact with the vaccinating equipment.
2. Do not open and mix the vaccine until ready to use.
3. Remove the aluminum seal and rubber stopper from the vial.
4. Aseptically transfer 3-5 mL of cool, distilled water into the vaccine vial and mix gently.
5. Transfer the dissolved vaccine into cool, distilled water; 350 mL for 5,000 doses. Mix thoroughly.
6. Attach the spray head to the container and adjust the nozzle for coarse spray.
7. Administer the vaccine by spraying 18-24 inches above each tray of chicks.
8. Each tray of 100 chickens should receive approximately 7 mL of vaccine. The exact amount can be determined by spraying into a calibrated tube to arrive at the number of applications necessary to deliver 7 mL of vaccine.
9. Whatever volume of vaccine is used in the spray, take care to administer 5,000 doses to 5,000 birds.
10. Since coarse spray application is of a large droplet size, aerosol-like mist of the vaccine is reduced. However, always wear goggles and a face mask while spraying a live virus vaccine.
11. Any equipment used for the application of a live virus vaccine should not be used for any other purpose.

Directions for Drinking Water Vaccination: Do not use the drinking water method for the vaccination of chickens younger than two (2) weeks of age or less than satisfactory results may be obtained.

1. Do not open or mix the vaccine until ready to use.
2. Remove all medications, sanitizers and disinfectants from the drinking water 72 hours prior to vaccination. Clean and rinse waterers thoroughly.
3. Provide sufficient waterers so that all of the birds can drink at one time.
4. Withhold all water from the birds for two (2) to four (4) hours prior to vaccination to stimulate thirst.
5. Add nonfat, dry milk to the water at the rate of 1 oz. per gallon before mixing the vaccine.
6. Remove the aluminum seal and rubber stopper from the vial.
7. Fill the vaccine vial with 3-5 mL of clean, cool water and mix gently.
8. Mix the dissolved vaccine with water as shown below:

Age of birds	Water per 5,000 doses vaccine
2-4 weeks	12.5 gallons (49.5 L)
4-8 weeks	25 gallons (94.5 L)
8 weeks or older	50 gallons (189.5 L)

9. Distribute the vaccine solution among the waterers. Avoid direct sunlight.
10. Do not provide any other drinking water until all of the vaccine solution has been consumed.

Directions for Aerosol Spray Vaccination: Do not use for initial vaccination. Use only for revaccination of healthy chickens two (2) weeks of age or older.

Use a sprayer delivering an aerosol mist to disperse the rehydrated vaccine quickly and evenly throughout the chicken house.

1. Prior to spraying, reduce the air flow to a minimum. Keep the air flow reduced for 20 minutes following spray vaccination.
2. Remove the aluminum seal from a vial of the vaccine.
3. Remove the rubber stopper and fill the vial with 3-5 mL of cool, distilled water.
4. Pour the rehydrated vaccine into a clean container and add 500 mL of cool, distilled water per 5,000 doses of vaccine. Mix thoroughly.
5. For aerosol spray vaccination, apply at the rate of 500 mL per 5,000 chickens.
6. Place the vaccine solution in the sprayer canister, set the discharge control and walk through the house spraying at the rate of 1,000 chickens per minute. Direct the spray above the heads of the birds.
7. Whatever volume of vaccine solution is used, take care to administer 5,000 doses of vaccine per 5,000 birds.
8. Avoid direct contact with the vaccine solution. Wear goggles and a face mask while spraying a live virus vaccine.
9. Any equipment used for the application of a live virus vaccine should not be used for any other purpose.

C. Freeze-dried Vaccine (25,000 doses): For 14-28 day old broiler type chickens.

Directions for Drinking Water Vaccination: For use in houses containing between 15,000 and

25,000 chickens. Do not use the drinking water vaccination method for chickens under 14 days of age.

Drinking Water - Pouring Application:

1. Do not open or mix the vaccine until ready to pour the vaccine solution into the water troughs.
2. Stop use of medication, sanitizers and disinfectants such as iodine in the drinking water 72 hours (3 days) prior to vaccination.
3. Shut off the water supply and allow the chickens to drink the troughs dry. Water should be withheld from chickens for a minimum of two (2) hours in warm weather to four (4) hours in cold weather. The water withdrawal time should be shortened if half-house brooding is in process.
4. Raise the water troughs above the chickens heads. Clean and rinse waters thoroughly.
5. Calculate to supply the vaccine solution at a rate of three (3) gallons per 1,000 chickens in cold weather and four (4) gallons per 1,000 chickens in warm weather.
   Example:
   17,000 chickens in cool weather x 3 gallons = 51 gallons.
   22,500 chickens in warm weather x 4 gallons = 90 gallons.
6. Add one of the following to pouring water for vaccine distribution:
   a. One (1) ounce of nonfat dry milk per gallon of water, or
   b. Four (4) ounces of fresh skim milk per gallon of water.
   Milk or milk solids are added to neutralize low levels of virucidal chemicals which may be present in farm water.
7. Prepare the vaccine concentrate as follows:
   a. Prepare a container of milk/water figuring one (1) ounce of concentrate for one (1) gallon of water to be used.
   b. Open the vaccine container by removing the aluminum seal and stopper.
   c. Add cool milk/water to the vial until the dried vaccine is dissolved. Add the vaccine to the container of milk/water to make the vaccine concentrate. Rinse the vaccine bottle to remove all of the vaccine.
8. To make the vaccine solution, add one (1) ounce of concentrate for each gallon of pouring water needed. Mix well.
9. Fill all of the water troughs full with the vaccine solution. Avoid direct sunlight.
10. Lower the water troughs and allow the birds to drink freely. Add the remaining vaccine solutions to the troughs as the birds drink.
11. Do not provide any additional drinking water until all of the vaccine solution has been consumed.

Drinking Water - Proportioner Application: Several types of medicator/proportioners are commercially available. Set the proportioner to deliver one (1) ounce of vaccine concentrate per one (1) gallon of water.

1. Stop use of medication, sanitizers and disinfectants such as iodine from dispenser 72 hours (3 days) prior to vaccination. Clean all containers and hoses prior to vaccination. Do not use medicator containers for vaccine use.
2. Shut off the water supply for four (4) hours in cool weather and two (2) hours in warm weather before vaccination to stimulate thirst. The water withdrawal time should be reduced if half-house brooding is in process.
3. Calculate three (3) gallons of the vaccine solution per 1,000 birds in cool weather and four (4) gallons in warm weather.
4. Calculate one (1) ounce of the vaccine concentrate per gallon of water to make the vaccine solution for bird consumption.
5. Vaccine concentrate preparation:
   a. Add three (3) ounces of dried nonfat milk per 16 ounces of cool water, or
   b. Use undiluted, cool, fresh skim milk.
6. Open the vaccine container by removing the aluminum seal and stopper.
7. Add the milk solution to the bottle, mix well and add to the vaccine concentrate container. Rinse the vaccine bottle to remove all of the vaccine. Mix well.
8. Insert the dosmatic hose into the vaccine concentrate and start the water flow. Continue until all of the concentrate has been consumed before changing the water supply to direct flow.
9. Do not medicate or use disinfectants for 24 hours after vaccination.

Spray Application: For use in houses containing between 15,000 and 25,000 chickens. Spray application is recommended for revaccination only and not as a primary vaccination.

Coarse Aerosol Application: Use a sprayer delivering a coarse aerosol mist to dispense the rehydrated vaccine quickly and evenly throughout a house of chickens.

Directions:

1. Prior to spraying, reduce the air flow by raising curtains or stopping fans. Air movement should be limited for 15 minutes following vaccination.
2. Remove the aluminum seal and rubber stopper. Fill the vaccine container with cool water.
3. Pour the reconstituted vaccine into a clean container and add 150 mL (5 oz.) of cool water for each 1,000 chickens to be vaccinated.
4. Place the vaccine solution into a spray canister and walk through the house spraying at the rate of 1,000 birds per minute. Direct the spray directly above the heads of the chickens.
5. Use all of the vaccine solution for each house containing 15,000 to 25,000 birds.
6. Avoid direct contact with the vaccine solution. Wear goggles and a face mask while spraying.
7. Do not use vaccinating equipment for any other purposes.

Precaution(s):

A. Storage Conditions for Frozen Vaccine:

Ampules: Store in a liquid nitrogen container.

Liquid nitrogen container: Carefully observe all liquid nitrogen precautions, including wearing eye protection and gloves. Store in a cool, well-ventilated area. Check the liquid nitrogen level once a day. Keep the container away from incubator intakes and chicken boxes.

Liquid Nitrogen Precautions: The liquid nitrogen containers and vaccines should be handled by properly trained personnel only. These persons should be familiar with the Union Carbide publication "Precautions and Safe Practices - Liquid Atmospheric Gasses", form #9888. Liquid nitrogen is extremely cold. Accidental contact with the skin or eyes can cause serious frostbite. Protect the eyes with goggles or a face shield. Wear gloves and long sleeves when removing and handling frozen ampules or when adding liquid nitrogen to the container. Storage and handling of liquid nitrogen containers should be in a well-ventilated area. Excessive amounts of nitrogen reduces the concentration of oxygen in the air of an unventilated space and can cause asphyxiation. If drowsiness occurs, get fresh air quickly and ventilate the entire area. If a person becomes groggy or loses consciousness while working with liquid nitrogen, get the person to a well-ventilated area immediately. If breathing has stopped, begin artificial respiration. Call a physician immediately.

B. Storage Conditions for Freeze-dried Vaccine:

Store the freeze-dried vaccine at 35-45°F (2-7°C). Do not freeze.

Caution(s):

A. Frozen Vaccine:

Do not vaccinate diseased birds.

Vaccinate all of the birds on the premises at one time.

Administer a minimum of one dose for each bird.

Avoid stress conditions during and following vaccination.

Do not place chickens in contaminated facilities.

Exposure to disease must be minimized as much as possible.

For veterinary use only.

The capability of the vaccine to produce satisfactory results depends upon many factors, including, but not limited to, conditions of storage and handling by the user, administration of the vaccine, health and the responsiveness of individual animals and the degree of field exposure. Therefore, directions for use should be followed carefully.

The use of the vaccine is subject to applicable state and federal laws and regulations.

Use only in localities where permitted.

Newcastle disease virus can cause inflammation of the eyelids of humans. Care should be taken to avoid contamination of the eyes, hands and clothing with this vaccine.

Administer only as recommended.

Use the entire contents when first opened.

Burn the container and all unused contents.

B. Freeze-dried Vaccine:

Do not vaccinate diseased birds or birds exhibiting respiratory distress.

Birds should be free of respiratory disease and parasite infestations.

Vaccinate all of the birds on the premises at one time.

Administer a minimum of one dose for each bird (ie. 5,000 doses to 5,000 chickens).

Avoid stress conditions during and following vaccination.

Do not place chickens in contaminated facilities.

Exposure to disease must be minimized as much as possible.

Do not start vaccination program for replacement pullets after birds are 16 weeks old.

For veterinary use only.

The capability of the vaccine to produce satisfactory results depends upon many factors, including, but not limited to, conditions of storage and handling by the user, administration of the vaccine, health and the responsiveness of individual animals and the degree of field exposure. Therefore, directions for use should be followed carefully.

The use of the vaccine is subject to applicable state and federal laws and regulations.

Use only in states where permitted.

Use the entire vial contents when first opened.

Burn the container and all unused contents.

Newcastle disease virus can cause inflammation of the eyelids of humans lasting up to three days. Care should be taken to avoid contamination of the eyes, hands and clothing with this vaccine.

Warning(s): Do not vaccinate within 21 days before slaughter.

Presentation: Frozen vaccine: 5 x 10,000 dose vials.

Freeze-dried vaccine: 25 x 5,000, 10 x 15,000 and 15 x 25,000 dose vials.

Compendium Code No.: 11050371

NEWCASTLE-BRONCHITIS VACCINE (Mass. & Conn. Types)

Merial Select **Vaccine**

Newcastle-Bronchitis Vaccine, B1 Type, B1 Strain, Mass. & Conn. Types, Live Virus

U.S. Vet. Lic. No.: 279

Active Ingredient(s): These vaccines contain the B_1 strain of the Newcastle disease virus and selected strains of infectious bronchitis virus of the Massachusetts and Connecticut types. The virus has been propagated in fertile eggs from specific pathogen free flocks. The immunizing capability of each vaccine has been proven by a master seed immunogenicity test. These vaccines offer proven immunity with mild reactions.

Penicillin and streptomycin sulfate are added as bacteriostatic agents.

Contains fungizone as a fungistatic agent.

Notice: These vaccines have met the requirements of the USDA in regards to safety, purity, potency and the capability to immunize normally susceptible chickens. These vaccines have been tested by the master seed immunogenicity test for efficacy.

Indications: These vaccines are recommended for administration to healthy chickens as an aid in the prevention of Newcastle disease and infectious bronchitis, Massachusetts and Connecticut serotypes.

The frozen vaccine is recommended for use in healthy one day old chickens.

The freeze-dried vaccine is recommended for the vaccination of healthy chickens at one day of age using the coarse spray method or for the vaccination of healthy chickens 14 days of age or older administered either in the drinking water or by aerosol spray. The use of an aerosol spray is recommended for revaccination only.

Dosage and Administration:

A. Frozen Vaccine: For healthy one (1) day old chickens.

Preparation of the Vaccine for Use:

Important: Sterilize the vaccinating equipment by autoclaving for a minimum of 15 minutes at 250°F (121°C) or by boiling in water for at least 20 minutes. Never allow chemical disinfectants to come into contact with the vaccinating equipment.

1. Remove only one (1) ampule of vaccine at a time from the liquid nitrogen container. Thaw and use immediately. Do not hold the ampule towards the face when removing it from a liquid nitrogen container. Never refreeze a vaccine ampule after thawing.
2. The contents of the ampule are thawed rapidly by immersing it in water at room temperature (15-25°C). Gently swirl the ampule to disperse the contents. Break the ampule at its neck and quickly proceed as described below.
3. Transfer the contents of the ampule into a sterile 2 mL or 5 mL syringe fitted with an 18 to 20 gauge needle to cool, distilled, de-ionized water (10,000 doses to 700 mL of water).
4. Use the vaccine mixture immediately as described below.

Method of Vaccination:

1. Use the coarse spray application method.
2. Attach the spray head to the container and set the nozzle at a coarse spray setting.
3. To each box of 100 chickens, administer the vaccine by spraying 18-24 inches above the box.
4. Each box of 100 chickens should receive approximately 7 mL of vaccine. The exact amount can be determined by spraying into a calibrated tube or container to arrive at the number of applications needed to deliver 7 mL of vaccine.
5. Whatever the volume of vaccine used, take care to administer 1,000 doses to 1,000 chickens.

B. Freeze-dried Vaccine (5,000 doses): The vaccines are recommended for the vaccination of healthy chickens at one (1) day of age using the coarse spray method or for the vaccination of healthy chickens 14 days of age or older administered either in the drinking water or by aerosol spray. The use of an aerosol spray is recommended for revaccination only.

Directions for Coarse Spray Vaccination:

1. Be certain that all of the vaccinating equipment is clean before use. Never allow chemical disinfectants to come into contact with the vaccinating equipment.
2. Do not open and mix the vaccine until ready to use.
3. Remove the aluminum seal and rubber stopper from the vial.
4. Aseptically transfer 3-5 mL of cool, distilled water into the vaccine vial and mix gently.
5. Transfer the dissolved vaccine into cool, distilled water; 350 mL for 5,000 doses. Mix thoroughly.
6. Attach the spray head to the container and adjust the nozzle for coarse spray.
7. Administer the vaccine by spraying 18-24 inches above each tray of chicks.
8. Each tray of 100 chickens should receive approximately 7 mL of vaccine. The exact amount can be determined by spraying into a calibrated tube to arrive at the number of applications necessary to deliver 7 mL of vaccine.
9. Whatever volume of vaccine is used in the spray, take care to administer 5,000 doses to 5,000 birds.
10. Since coarse spray application is of a large droplet size, aerosol-like mist of the vaccine is reduced. However, always wear goggles and a face mask while spraying a live virus vaccine.
11. Any equipment used for the application of a live virus vaccine should not be used for any other purpose.

Directions for Drinking Water Vaccination: Do not use the drinking water method for vaccination of chickens younger than two (2) weeks of age or less than satisfactory results may be obtained.

1. Do not open or mix the vaccine until ready to use.
2. Remove all medications, sanitizers and disinfectants from the drinking water 72 hours prior to vaccination. Clean and rinse the waterers thoroughly.
3. Provide sufficient waterers so that all of the birds can drink at one time.
4. Withhold all water from the birds for two (2) to four (4) hours prior to vaccination to stimulate thirst.
5. Add nonfat, dry milk to the water at the rate of 1 oz. per gallon before mixing the vaccine.
6. Remove the aluminum seal and rubber stopper from the vial.
7. Fill the vaccine vial with 3-5 mL of clean, cool water and mix gently.
8. Mix the dissolved vaccine with water as shown below:

Age of birds	Water per 5,000 doses vaccine
2-4 weeks	12.5 gallons (49.5 L)
4-8 weeks	25 gallons (94.5 L)
8 weeks or older	50 gallons (189.5 L)

9. Distribute the vaccine solution among the waterers. Avoid direct sunlight.
10. Do not provide any other drinking water until all of the vaccine solution has been consumed.

Directions for Aerosol Spray Vaccination: Do not use for initial vaccination. Use only for revaccination of healthy chickens two (2) weeks of age or older.

Use a sprayer delivering an aerosol mist to disperse the rehydrated vaccine quickly and evenly throughout the chicken house.

1. Prior to spraying, reduce the air flow to a minimum. Keep the air flow reduced for 20 minutes following spray vaccination.
2. Remove the aluminum seal from a vial of the vaccine.
3. Remove the rubber stopper and fill the vial with 3-5 mL of cool, distilled water.
4. Pour the rehydrated vaccine into a clean container and add 500 mL of cool, distilled water per 5,000 doses of vaccine. Mix thoroughly.
5. For aerosol spray vaccination, apply at the rate of 500 mL per 5,000 chickens.
6. Place the vaccine solution in the sprayer canister, set the discharge control and walk through the house spraying at the rate of 1,000 chickens per minute. Direct the spray above the heads of the birds.
7. Whatever volume of vaccine solution is used, take care to administer 5,000 doses of vaccine per 5,000 birds.
8. Avoid direct contact with the vaccine solution. Wear goggles and a face mask while spraying a live virus vaccine.
9. Any equipment used for the application of a live virus vaccine should not be used for any other purpose.

C. Freeze-dried Vaccine (15,000 doses): For healthy chickens 14 days of age or older.

Drinking Water - Pouring Application: For use in houses containing between 10,000 and 15,000 chickens.

1. Do not open or mix the vaccine until ready to vaccinate.
2. Remove all medications, sanitizers and disinfectants from the drinking water 72 hours (3 days) prior to vaccination.
3. Provide sufficient waterers so that all of the chickens can drink at one time. Shut off the water supply and allow the chickens to drink the troughs dry.
4. Raise the water troughs above the chicken's heads. Clean and rinse the waters thoroughly.
5. Withhold all of the water from the chickens for a minimum of two (2) hours in warm weather to four (4) hours in cool weather prior to vaccination to stimulate thirst. The water withdrawal times should be reduced if half-house brooding is in process.
6. Calculate to supply the vaccine solution at a rate of three (3) gallons (11 L) per 1,000 chickens in cool weather and four (4) gallons (15 L) per 1,000 chickens in warm weather. The age of the chickens should be considered when calculating the water supply. Always use nonchlorinated water when vaccinating chickens.
   Example:
   10,000 chickens in cool weather x 3 gallons (11 L) = 30 gallons (114 L).
   14,500 chickens in warm weather x 4 gallons (15 L) = 58 gallons (220 L).
7. Add one of the following to pouring water for vaccine distribution:
   a. One (1) ounce (30 mL) of nonfat, dry milk per gallon (4 L) of water, or
   b. Four (4) ounces (118 mL) of fresh skim milk per gallon (4 L) of water.
8. Prepare the vaccine concentrate as follows:
   a. Prepare a container of milk/water figuring one (1) ounce (30 mL) of concentrate for one (1) gallon (4 L) of water to be used.
   b. Add cool milk/water to the vial until the dried vaccine is dissolved. Add the vaccine to the container of milk/water to make the vaccine concentrate. Rinse the vaccine vial to remove all of the vaccine.
9. To make the vaccine solution, add one (1) ounce (30 mL) of concentrate for each gallon (4 L) of water needed.
10. Distribute the vaccine solution among the waterers. Avoid direct sunlight.
11. Lower the water troughs and allow the birds to drink freely. Add the remaining vaccine solution to the troughs as the birds drink.
12. Do not provide any additional drinking water until all of the vaccine solution is consumed.

Drinking Water Vaccination - Proportioner Application: Several types of medicator/proportioners are commercially available. Set the proportioner to deliver one (1) ounce (30 mL) of vaccine concentrate per one (1) gallon (4 L) of water.

1. Do not open or mix the vaccine until ready to vaccinate.
2. Remove all medications, sanitizers and disinfectants from the proportioner 72 hours (3 days) prior to vaccination.
3. Clean all containers, hoses, and waterers prior to vaccination.
4. Withhold all water from the chickens for a minimum of two (2) hours in warm weather to four (4) hours in cool weather prior to vaccination to stimulate thirst.
5. Calculate to supply the vaccine solution at a rate of three (3) gallons (11 L) per 1,000 chickens in cool weather and four (4) gallons (15 L) per 1,000 chickens in warm weather. The age of the chickens should be considered when calculating the water supply. Always use nonchlorinated water when vaccinating chickens.
   Example:
   10,000 chickens in cool weather x 3 gallons (11 L) = 30 gallons (114 L).
   14,500 chickens in warm weather x 4 gallons (15 L) = 58 gallons (220 L).
6. Prepare the vaccine concentrate as follows:
   a. Add three (3) ounces (90 mL) of nonfat, dry milk per 16 ounces (473 mL) of cool water, or
   b. Use undiluted, cool, fresh skim milk.
7. To make the vaccine solution, add one (1) ounce (30 mL) of concentrate for each gallon (4 L) of water needed.
8. Add the milk solution to the vial until the dried vaccine is dissolved. Rinse the vaccine vial to remove all of the vaccine.
9. Insert the proportioner hose into the vaccine concentrate and start the water flow. Continue until all of the concentrate has been consumed before changing the water supply to direct flow.
10. Do not medicate or use disinfectants for 24 hours after vaccination.

Coarse Spray Application: For use in houses containing between 10,000 and 15,000 chickens. Use a sprayer delivering a coarse spray pattern to disperse the rehydrated vaccine quickly and evenly throughout a house of chickens.

1. Prior to spraying, reduce the air flow by raising curtains or stopping fans. Air movement should be limited for 15 minutes following vaccination.
2. Fill the vaccine container with cool, distilled, de-ionized water.
3. Pour the reconstituted vaccine into a clean container and add five (5) ounces (150 mL) of cool water for each 1,000 chickens to be vaccinated.
4. Place the vaccine solution into a spray canister and walk through the house spraying at the rate of 1,000 chickens per minute. Direct spray directly above the heads of the chickens.
5. Avoid direct contact with the vaccine solution. Wear goggles and a face mask while spraying.
6. Do not use vaccinating equipment for any other purposes.

D. Freeze-dried Vaccine (25,000 doses): For healthy chickens 14 days of age or older.

Drinking Water - Pouring Application: For use in houses containing between 15,000 and 25,000 chickens.

1. Do not open or mix the vaccine until ready to vaccinate.
2. Remove all medications, sanitizers and disinfectants from the drinking water 72 hours (3 days) prior to vaccination.
3. Provide sufficient waterers so that all of the chickens can drink at one time. Shut off the water supply and allow the chickens to drink the troughs dry.
4. Raise the water troughs above the chicken's heads. Clean and rinse all of the containers, hoses, and waters thoroughly prior to vaccination.
5. Withhold all water from the chickens for a minimum of two (2) hours in warm weather to four (4) hours in cool weather prior to vaccination to stimulate thirst. The water withdrawal times should be reduced if half-house brooding is in process.
6. Calculate to supply the vaccine solution at a rate of three (3) gallons (11 L) per 1,000 chickens in cool weather and four (4) gallons (15 L) per 1,000 chickens in warm weather. The age of the chickens should be considered when calculating the water supply. Always use nonchlorinated water when vaccinating chickens.
   Example:
   17,000 chickens in cool weather x 3 gallons (11 L) = 51 gallons (193 L).
   22,500 chickens in warm weather x 4 gallons (15 L) = 90 gallons (340 L).
7. Add one of the following to pouring water for vaccine distribution:
   a. One (1) ounce (30 mL) of nonfat, dry skim milk per gallon (4 L) of water, or
   b. Four (4) ounces (118 mL) of fresh skim milk per gallon (4 L) of water.
8. Prepare the vaccine concentrate as follows:
   a. Prepare a container of milk/water figuring one (1) ounce (30 mL) of concentrate for one (1) gallon (4 L) of water to be used.
   b. Add cool milk/water to the vial until the dried vaccine is dissolved. Add the vaccine to the container of milk/water to make the vaccine concentrate. Rinse the vaccine vial to remove all of the vaccine.
9. To make the vaccine solution, add one (1) ounce (30 mL) of concentrate for each gallon (4 L) of water needed.
10. Distribute the vaccine solution among the waterers. Avoid direct sunlight.
11. Lower the water troughs and allow the birds to drink freely. Add the remaining vaccine solution to the troughs as the birds drink.
12. Do not provide any additional drinking water until all of the vaccine solution is consumed.

Drinking Water Vaccination - Proportioner Application: Several types of medicator/proportioners are commercially available. Set the proportioner to deliver one (1) ounce (30 mL) of vaccine concentrate per one (1) gallon (4 L) of water.

1. Do not open or mix the vaccine until ready to vaccinate.
2. Remove all medications, sanitizers and disinfectants from the proportioner 72 hours (3 days) prior to vaccination.
3. Provide sufficient waterers so that all of the chickens can drink at one time. Shut off the water supply and allow the chickens to drink the troughs dry.
4. Raise the water troughs above the chicken's heads. Clean and rinse all of the containers, hoses, and waterers thoroughly prior to vaccination.
5. Withhold all water from the chickens for a minimum of two (2) hours in warm weather to four (4) hours in cool weather prior to vaccination to stimulate thirst. The water withdrawal times should be reduced if half-house brooding is in process.
6. Calculate to supply the vaccine solution at a rate of three (3) gallons (11 L) per 1,000 chickens in cool weather and four (4) gallons (15 L) per 1,000 chickens in warm weather. The age of

the chickens should be considered when calculating the water supply. Always use nonchlorinated water when vaccinating chickens.

Example:

17,000 chickens in cool weather x 3 gallons (11 L) = 51 gallons (193 L).

22,500 chickens in warm weather x 4 gallons (15 L) = 90 gallons (340 L).

7. Prepare the vaccine concentrate as follows:
   a. Add three (3) ounces (90 mL) of dried, nonfat skim milk per 16 ounces (473 mL) of cool water, or
   b. Use undiluted, cool, fresh skim milk.
8. To make the vaccine solution, add one (1) ounce (30 mL) of concentrate for each gallon (4 L) of water needed.
9. Add the milk solution to the vial until the dried vaccine is dissolved. Rinse the vaccine vial to remove all of the vaccine.
10. Insert the proportioner hose into the vaccine concentrate and start the water flow. Continue until all of the concentrate has been consumed before changing the water supply to direct flow.
11. Do not medicate or use disinfectants for 24 hours after vaccination.

Coarse Spray Application: For use in houses containing between 15,000 and 25,000 chickens. Spray application is recommended for revaccination only and not as a primary vaccination. Use a sprayer delivering a coarse spray pattern to disperse the rehydrated vaccine quickly and evenly throughout a house of chickens.

1. Prior to spraying, reduce the air flow by raising curtains or stopping fans. Air movement should be limited for 15 minutes following vaccination.
2. Fill the vaccine container with cool, distilled, de-ionized water.
3. Pour the reconstituted vaccine into a clean container and add five (5) ounces (150 mL) of cool, distilled, de-ionized water for each 1,000 chickens to be vaccinated.
4. Place the vaccine solution into a spray canister and walk through the house spraying at the rate of 1,000 chickens per minute. Direct the spray directly above the heads of the chickens.
5. Avoid direct contact with the vaccine solution. Wear goggles and a face mask while spraying.
6. Do not use vaccinating equipment for any other purposes.

Precaution(s):

A. Storage Conditions for Frozen Vaccine:

Ampules: Store in a liquid nitrogen container.

Liquid nitrogen container: Carefully observe all liquid nitrogen precautions, including wearing eye protection and gloves. Store in a cool, well-ventilated area. Check the liquid nitrogen level once a day. Keep the container away from incubator intakes and chicken boxes.

Liquid Nitrogen Precautions: The liquid nitrogen containers and vaccines should be handled by properly trained personnel only. These persons should be familiar with the Union Carbide publication "Precautions and Safe Practices - Liquid Atmospheric Gases", form #9888. Liquid nitrogen is extremely cold. Accidental contact with the skin or eyes can cause serious frostbite. Protect the eyes with goggles or a face shield. Wear gloves and long sleeves when removing and handling frozen ampules or when adding liquid nitrogen to the container. Storage and handling of liquid nitrogen containers should be in a well-ventilated area. Excessive amounts of nitrogen reduces the concentration of oxygen in the air of an unventilated space and can cause asphyxiation. If drowsiness occurs, get fresh air quickly and ventilate the entire area. If a person becomes groggy or loses consciousness while working with liquid nitrogen, get the person to a well-ventilated area immediately. If breathing has stopped, begin artificial respiration. Call a physician immediately.

B. Storage Conditions for Freeze-dried Vaccine:

Store the freeze-dried vaccine at 35-45°F (2-7°C). Do not freeze.

Caution(s):

A. Frozen Vaccine:

Do not vaccinate diseased birds.

Vaccinate all of the birds on the premises at one time.

Administer a minimum of one dose for each bird.

Avoid stress conditions during and following vaccination.

Do not place chickens in contaminated facilities.

Exposure to disease must be minimized as much as possible.

For veterinary use only.

The capability of the vaccine to produce satisfactory results depends upon many factors, including, but not limited to, conditions of storage and handling by the user, administration of the vaccine, health and the responsiveness of individual animals and the degree of field exposure. Therefore, directions for use should be followed carefully.

The use of the vaccine is subject to applicable state and federal laws and regulations.

Use only in localities where permitted.

Newcastle disease virus can cause inflammation of the eyelids of humans. Care should be taken to avoid contamination of the eyes, hands and clothing with the vaccine.

Administer only as recommended.

Use the entire contents when first opened.

Burn the container and all unused contents.

B. Freeze-dried Vaccine:

Do not vaccinate diseased birds.

Birds should be free of respiratory disease and parasite infestations.

Vaccinate all of the birds on the premises at one time.

Administer a minimum of one dose for each bird (ie. 5,000 doses to 5,000 chickens).

Avoid stress conditions during and following vaccination.

Do not place chickens in contaminated facilities.

Exposure to disease must be minimized as much as possible.

Do not start the vaccination program for replacement pullets after birds are 16 weeks old.

For veterinary use only.

The capability of the vaccine to produce satisfactory results depends upon many factors, including, but not limited to, conditions of storage and handling by the user, administration of the vaccine, health and the responsiveness of individual animals and the degree of field exposure. Therefore, directions for use should be followed carefully.

The use of the vaccine is subject to applicable state and federal laws and regulations.

Use only in states where permitted.

Use the entire vial contents when first opened.

Burn the container and all unused contents.

Newcastle disease virus can cause inflammation of the eyelids of humans. Care should be taken to avoid contamination of the eyes, hands and clothing with the vaccine.

Warning(s): Do not vaccinate within 21 days before slaughter.

Presentation: Frozen vaccine: 5 x 10,000 dose vials.

Freeze-dried vaccine: 50 x 2,000, 25 x 5,000, 10 x 15,000, and 25 x 25,000 dose vials.

Compendium Code No.: 11050381

NEWCASTLE DISEASE-FOWL POX VACCINE (Recombinant)

Merial Select **Vaccine**

Newcastle Disease-Fowl Pox Vaccine, Fowl Pox Vector

U.S. Vet. Lic. No.: 279

Contents: This vaccine contains a live strain of fowlpox vectored virus that has been shown to aid in the prevention of Newcastle disease and fowlpox. It is recommended for subcutaneous injection of one day-old chickens.

Penicillin and streptomycin sulfate are added as bacteriostatic agents.

Contains amphotericin B as a fungistatic agent.

Indications: This vaccine is recommended for use in healthy one-day-old chickens for the prevention of Newcastle disease and fowlpox. It is essential that the chickens be maintained under good environmental conditions, and that exposure to disease viruses be reduced as much as possible. The chickens should be revaccinated at 10 to 21 days of age with a vaccine containing a conventional Newcastle disease virus.

Dosage and Administration: Preparation of Vaccine for Use:

Important: Sterilize vaccinating equipment by autoclaving a minimum of 15 minutes at 121°C or boiling in water for at least 20 minutes. Never allow chemical disinfectants to come in contact with vaccinating equipment.

1. Use 200 mL of sterile diluent for each 1,000 doses of vaccine indicated on the ampule.
2. Remove only one ampule of vaccine at a time from the liquid nitrogen container. Thaw and use immediately. Caution: Do not hold ampule toward face when removing from a liquid nitrogen container. Never refreeze a vaccine ampule after thawing.
3. The contents of the ampule are thawed rapidly by immersing in room temperature (15-25°C) water. Gently swirl the ampule to disperse contents. Break ampule at its neck and quickly proceed as described below.
4. Remove the cover from the diluent container. Draw contents of the ampule into a sterile 10 mL syringe fitted with an 18 to 20 gauge needle. Slowly add the contents of the vaccine ampule to the appropriate volume of diluent. Withdraw a small amount of the diluent, rinse the ampule once and add this to the vaccine-diluent mixture. Mix the contents of the diluent container thoroughly by swirling and inverting the container. Do not shake vigorously.
5. Use the vaccine-diluent mixture immediately as described below.

Method of Vaccination:

1. Give subcutaneously only.
2. Use a sterile automatic syringe with a 20-22 gauge 3/8"-1/2" needle which is set to accurately deliver 0.2 mL per dose. Check the accuracy of delivery several times during the vaccination procedure.
3. Dilute the vaccine only as directed observing all precautions and warnings for handling.
4. Keep the container of diluted vaccine in an ice bath and agitate continuously.
5. Inject each chicken under the loose skin at the back of the neck (subcutaneously), holding the chicken by the back of the neck just below the head. The loose skin in this area is raised by gently pinching with the thumb and forefinger. Insert the needle beneath the skin in a direction away from the head. Inject 0.2 mL per chicken. Avoid hitting the muscles and bones in the neck.
6. Use the entire contents of the vaccine container within one hour after mixing the vaccine with the diluent.

Precaution(s): Storage Conditions:

Ampules: Store in liquid nitrogen container.

Diluent: Store at room temperature.

Liquid Nitrogen Container: Carefully observe all liquid nitrogen precautions including wearing eye protection and gloves. Store in a cool, well-ventilated area. Check liquid nitrogen level daily. Keep container away from incubator intakes and chicken boxes.

Use entire contents when first opened.

Burn this container and all unused contents.

Caution(s): Do not vaccinate diseased birds.

Vaccinate all birds on the premises at one time.

Administer a full dose to each bird.

Avoid stress conditions during and following vaccination.

Do not place chickens in contaminated facilities.

Exposure to disease must be minimized as much as possible.

Administer subcutaneously only.

The capability of this vaccine to produce satisfactory results depends upon many factors, including, but not limited to, conditions of storage and handling by the user, administration of the vaccine, health and responsiveness of individual chickens and degree of field exposure. Therefore, directions for use should be followed carefully. The use of this vaccine is subject to applicable local and federal laws and regulations.

Warning(s): Do not vaccinate within 21 days before slaughter.

For veterinary use only.

Liquid Nitrogen Precautions: The liquid nitrogen containers and vaccines should be handled only by properly trained personnel. These persons should be familiar with the Union Carbide publication "Precautions and Safe Practices — Liquid Atmospheric Gases," form #9888.

Liquid nitrogen is extremely cold. Accidental contact with skin or eyes can cause severe frostbite. Protect eyes with goggles or face shield. Wear gloves and long sleeves when removing and handling frozen ampules or when adding liquid nitrogen to the container. Storage and handling of liquid nitrogen containers should be in a well-ventilated area.

Excessive amounts of nitrogen reduce the concentration of oxygen in the air of an unventilated space and can cause asphyxiation. If drowsiness occurs, get fresh air quickly and ventilate the entire area. If a person becomes groggy or loses consciousness while working with liquid nitrogen, get the person to a well-ventilated area immediately. If breathing has stopped, begin artificial respiration. Call a physician immediately.

Trial Data: Merial Select's vaccines have met the requirements of the USDA in regard to safety, purity, potency and the capability to protect susceptible chickens. This vaccine has been tested by the Master Seed immunogenicity test for efficacy.

Presentation: 5 x 1,000 doses.

Compendium Code No.: 11050331

NEWCASTLE DISEASE VACCINE

L.A.H.I. (New Jersey) **Vaccine**

Newcastle Disease Vaccine, Killed Virus

U.S. Vet. Lic. No.: 196

Active Ingredient(s): This product is an inactivated viral vaccine used as an aid in the prevention of Newcastle disease in chickens and turkeys.

The vaccine is manufactured in accordance with a detailed production outline, which has been filed with the Veterinary Services of the USDA. Only specific pathogen free (SPF) eggs are used for production purposes. Seed virus is derived from a master seed virus lot which has been fully tested for purity, safety and immunogenicity. The fill volume for these products is 500 mL in a 625 mL plastic bottle. The bottles are sealed with a rubber stopper and an aluminum overseal.

Quality Control: The flocks producing SPF eggs are under constant observation by experienced personnel and routinely sampled and tested serologically to confirm absence of exposure to a large variety of avian pathogens. Shipments from the supplier are accompanied by regular reports on test results for each flock from which eggs were obtained.

These products are fully tested for purity, safety and potency according to the standard requirements for Newcastle disease and infectious bronchitis vaccines published as part 113, in particular, section 113.125 of title 9 of the federal regulations by the Animal and Plant Health Inspection Service of the USDA, and according to the production outline submitted to the U.S. Department of Agriculture.

Each serial is tested for: Bacteria, fungi, and salmonella.

Potency is tested according to the outline approved by the USDA.

Indications: This product is packaged for subcutaneous or intramuscular vaccination for the prevention of Newcastle disease in chickens or turkeys.

Dosage and Administration:

Chickens:

1st vaccination: Three (3) weeks of age or older.

2nd vaccination: 20 to 22 weeks of age.

Turkeys:

1st vaccination: Three (3) to six (6) weeks of age.

2nd vaccination: 20 to 22 weeks of age.

If birds are to be kept for a second year of production, they should be revaccinated during molt.

Preparation of Vaccine: Immediately prior to use, shake the vaccine vigorously for 30 seconds to one (1) minute. Remove the aluminum overseal and the vaccine is ready to use.

Method of Vaccination: The vaccine should be administered subcutaneously in the neck or intramuscularly in the leg. No other route is suggested or implied. Subcutaneous inoculation should be given in the mid-portion of the neck. Each bird should receive 0.5 mL of vaccine in this manner. Intramuscular injection in a dose of 0.5 mL should be given in the back of the leg into the thigh muscle.

Precaution(s): The vaccine shall be stored in the dark in a refrigerator between 2-7°C (35-45°F).

Expiration date: 26 months.

Caution(s): Vaccinate healthy birds only.

It is imperative that the user of this product comply with the indications for use, contraindications, cautions and method of vaccination stated on the directions sheet packed with the product. The vaccine must be prepared and administered as directed to obtain the best results. For veterinary use only.

Warning(s): Do not market birds for at least six (6) weeks after vaccinating so that there is no swelling at the site of vaccine administration.

Presentation: 1,000, 2,500 and 10,000 doses.

Compendium Code No.: 10080262

NEWCASTLE DISEASE VACCINE (B_1 Strain)

Merial Select **Vaccine**

Newcastle Disease Vaccine, B1 Type, B1 Strain, Live Virus

U.S. Vet. Lic. No.: 279

Active Ingredient(s): These vaccines contain the B_1 strain of Newcastle disease virus. The virus has been propagated in fertile eggs from specific pathogen free flocks. The immunizing capability of these vaccines have been proven by the master seed immunogenicity test. These vaccines offer proven immunity with mild reactions.

Contains streptomycin and penicillin as bacteriostatic agents.

Contains fungizone as a fungistatic agent.

Notice: These vaccines have met the requirements of the USDA in regard to safety, purity, potency and the capacity to immunize normal, susceptible chickens. These vaccines have been tested by the master seed immunogenicity test for efficacy.

Indications: These vaccines are recommended for the initial vaccination and revaccination of healthy chickens as an aid in the prevention of Newcastle disease.

The frozen vaccine is recommended for use in healthy one day old chickens.

The 5,000 dose size of the freeze-dried vaccine is recommended for the initial vaccination of healthy one day old chickens using the coarse spray application method, or for vaccination of healthy chickens 14 days of age or older using the drinking water application method or aerosol spray. Spray vaccination is recommended for revaccination only. Revaccination is recommended at four weeks and 16 weeks of age.

The 15,000 and 25,000 dose sizes of the freeze-dried vaccine are recommended for the primary vaccination or revaccination of 14-28 day old broiler type chickens using the drinking water or aerosol spray application. The 15,000 dose size is for the vaccination of healthy chickens 14 days of age or older.

These vaccines are recommended for the protection of healthy chickens which are free of all diseases. It is essential that the chickens be maintained under good environmental conditions and that exposure to disease viruses be reduced as much as possible in the field.

Dosage and Administration:

A. Frozen Vaccine: For healthy one (1) day old chickens.

Preparation of the Vaccine for Use:

Important: Sterilize the vaccinating equipment by autoclaving for a minimum of 15 minutes at 250°F (121°C) or by boiling in water for at least 20 minutes. Never allow chemical disinfectants to come into contact with the vaccinating equipment.

1. Remove only one (1) ampule of vaccine at a time from the liquid nitrogen container. Thaw and use immediately. Do not hold the ampule towards the face when removing it from a liquid nitrogen container. Never refreeze a vaccine ampule after thawing.
2. The contents of the ampule are thawed rapidly by immersing it in water at room temperature (15-25°C). Gently swirl the ampule to disperse the contents. Break the ampule at its neck and quickly proceed as described below.
3. Transfer the contents of the ampule into a sterile 2 mL or 5 mL syringe fitted with an 18 to 20 gauge needle to cool, distilled, de-ionized water (10,000 doses to 700 mL of water).
4. Use the vaccine mixture immediately as described below.

Method of Vaccination:

1. Use the coarse spray application method.
2. Attach the spray head to the container and set the nozzle at a coarse spray setting.
3. To each box of 100 chickens, administer the vaccine by spraying 18-24 inches above the box.
4. Each box of 100 chickens should receive approximately 7 mL of vaccine. The exact amount can be determined by spraying into a calibrated tube or container to arrive at the number of applications needed to deliver 7 mL of vaccine.
5. Whatever the volume of vaccine used, take care to administer 1,000 doses to 1,000 chickens.

B. Freeze-dried Vaccine (5,000 doses): For healthy chickens 14 days of age or older.

Directions for Coarse Spray Vaccination:

1. Be certain that all of the vaccinating equipment is clean before use. Never allow chemical disinfectants to come into contact with the vaccinating equipment.
2. Do not open and mix the vaccine until ready to vaccinate.
3. Remove the aluminum seal and rubber stopper from the vaccine vial.
4. Aseptically transfer a small amount (3-5 mL) of cool distilled water into the vaccine vial and gently mix.
5. Transfer the dissolved vaccine into cool, distilled water (5,000 doses in 350 mL) and gently mix.
6. Attach the spray head to the container and set the nozzle at a coarse spray setting.
7. To each tray of 100 birds, administer the vaccine by spraying 18-24 inches above tray.
8. Each tray of 100 birds should receive approximately 7 mL of vaccine. The exact amount can be determined by spraying into a calibrated tube to arrive at the number of applications needed to deliver 7 mL of vaccine.
9. Whatever volume of vaccine is used in the spray, take care to administer 5,000 doses to 5,000 birds.
10. Since coarse spray application is of a large droplet size, aerosol-like mist of the vaccine is reduced; however, always wear eye goggles and a face mask while spraying a live virus vaccine.
11. Any equipment used for the application of a live virus vaccine should not be used for any other purpose.

Directions for Drinking Water Vaccination:

1. Do not open or mix the vaccine until ready to vaccinate.
2. Remove all medication, sanitizers and disinfectants such as iodine from the drinking water 72 hours prior to vaccination.
3. Provide sufficient waterers so that all of the birds can drink at one time. Clean and rinse the waterers thoroughly.
4. Withhold all water from the birds for two (2) to four (4) hours prior to vaccination to stimulate thirst.
5. Add nonfat dry milk to the water at the rate of one (1) ounce per gallon before mixing the vaccine.
6. Remove the aluminum seal and rubber stopper from a vaccine vial.
7. Fill the vaccine vial two-thirds (2/3) full with clean, cool water and mix gently.
8. Mix the dissolved vaccine with water as shown below.

Age of birds	Water per 5,000 doses vaccine
2-4 weeks	12.5 gallons (45.5 L)
4-8 weeks	25 gallons (96 L)
8 weeks or older	50 gallons (189.5 L)

9. Distribute the vaccine solution among the waterers. Avoid direct sunlight.
10. Do not provide any other drinking water until all of the vaccine mixture has been consumed.

Spray Aerosol Vaccination: Use only for revaccination of healthy chickens two (2) weeks of age or older. Do not use for initial vaccination.

Use a sprayer delivering an aerosol-like mist to disperse the rehydrated vaccine quickly and evenly throughout a house of chickens.

1. Remove the aluminum seal and rubber stopper from the vaccine vial.
2. Fill the vaccine vial full with cool, distilled water. Pour the dissolved vaccine into a container and add approximately 500 mL of cool, distilled water per 5,000 doses of vaccine. Mix thoroughly.
3. For spray aerosol vaccination of a house of chickens, apply at the rate of 500 mL per 5,000 chickens.
4. Example: 20,000 birds will require 2,000 mL (approximately 2 quarts) of rehydrated vaccine.
5. Place the vaccine solution into the sprayer canister, set the discharge control to the coarsest setting and walk through the house spraying at the rate of 1,000 birds per minute. Direct the spray above the heads of the birds.
6. Whatever volume of vaccine solution is used, take care to administer 5,000 doses of vaccine to 5,000 birds.
7. Prior to spraying, reduce air flow to a minimum. Keep the air flow reduced for 20 minutes following spray vaccination.
8. Avoid direct contact with the vaccine solution. Wear goggles and a mask while spraying a live virus vaccine.
9. Any equipment used for the application of a live virus vaccine should not be used for any other purpose.

C. Freeze-dried Vaccine (15,000 doses): For healthy chickens 14 days of age or older.

Drinking Water Vaccination - Pouring Application:

1. Do not open or mix the vaccine until ready to vaccinate.
2. Remove all medications, sanitizers and disinfectants from the drinking water 72 hours (3 days) prior to vaccination.
3. Provide sufficient waterers so that all of the chickens can drink at one time. Shut off the water supply and allow the chickens to drink the troughs dry.
4. Raise the water troughs above the chickens' heads. Clean and rinse the waterers thoroughly.
5. Withhold all water from the chickens for a minimum of two (2) hours in warm weather to four (4) hours in cool weather prior to vaccination to stimulate thirst. The water withdrawal time should be reduced if half-house brooding is in process.
6. Calculate to supply the vaccine solution at a rate of three (3) gallons (11 L) per 1,000 chickens in cool weather and four (4) gallons (15 L) per 1,000 chickens in warm weather. The age of the chickens should be considered when calculating the water supply. Always use nonchlorinated water when vaccinating chickens.

   Example:

   10,000 chickens in cool weather x 3 gallons (11 L) = 30 gallons (114 L).

   14,500 chickens in warm weather x 4 gallons (15 L) = 58 gallons (220 L).

7. Add one of the following to pouring water for vaccine distribution:
   a. One (1) ounce (30 mL) of nonfat, dry milk per gallon (4 L) of water, or
   b. Four (4) ounces (118 mL) of fresh skim milk per gallon (4 L) of water.
8. Prepare the vaccine concentrate as follows:
   a. Prepare a container of milk/water figuring one (1) ounce (30 mL) of concentrate for one (1) gallon (4 L) of water to be used.
   b. Add cool milk/water to the vial until the dried vaccine is dissolved. Add the vaccine to the container of milk/water to make the vaccine concentrate. Rinse the vaccine vial to remove all of the vaccine.
9. To make the vaccine solution, add one (1) ounce (30 mL) of concentrate for each gallon (4 L) of water needed.
10. Distribute the vaccine solution among the waterers. Avoid direct sunlight.
11. Lower the water troughs and allow the birds to drink freely. Add the remaining vaccine solution to the troughs as the birds drink.
12. Do not provide any additional drinking water until all of the vaccine solution is consumed.

Drinking Water Vaccination - Proportioner Application: Several types of medicator/proportioners are commercially available. Set the proportioner to deliver one (1) ounce (30 mL) of vaccine concentrate per one (1) gallon (4 L) of water.

1. Do not open or mix the vaccine until ready to vaccinate.
2. Remove all medications, sanitizers and disinfectants from the proportioner 72 hours (3 days) prior to vaccination.
3. Clean all containers, hoses, and waterers prior to vaccination.
4. Withhold all water from the chickens for a minimum of two (2) hours in warm weather to four (4) hours in cool weather prior to vaccination to stimulate thirst.
5. Calculate to supply the vaccine solution at a rate of three (3) gallons (11 L) per 1,000 chickens in cool weather and four (4) gallons (15 L) per 1,000 chickens in warm weather. The age of the chickens should be considered when calculating the water supply. Always use nonchlorinated water when vaccinating chickens.
   Example:
   10,000 chickens in cool weather x 3 gallons (11 L) = 30 gallons (114 L).
   14,500 chickens in warm weather x 4 gallons (15 L) = 58 gallons (220 L).
6. Prepare the vaccine concentrate as follows:
   a. Add three (3) ounces (90 mL) of nonfat, dry milk per 16 ounces (473 mL) of cool water, or
   b. Use undiluted, cool, fresh skim milk.
7. To make the vaccine solution, add one (1) ounce (30 mL) of concentrate for each gallon (4 L) of water needed.
8. Add the milk solution to the vial until the dried vaccine is dissolved. Rinse the vaccine vial to remove all of the vaccine.
9. Insert the proportioner hose into the vaccine concentrate and start the water flow. Continue until all of the concentrate has been consumed before changing the water supply to direct flow.
10. Do not medicate or use disinfectants for 24 hours after vaccination.

Coarse Spray Application: For use in houses containing between 10,000 and 15,000 chickens. Coarse spray application is recommended for revaccination only and not as a primary vaccination. Use a sprayer delivering a coarse spray pattern to dispense the rehydrated vaccine quickly and evenly throughout a house of chickens.

1. Prior to spraying, reduce the air flow by raising curtains or stopping fans. Air movement should be limited for 15 minutes following vaccination.
2. Fill the vaccine container with cool, distilled, de-ionized water.
3. Pour the reconstituted vaccine into a clean container and add five (5) ounces (150 mL) of cool water for each 1,000 chickens to be vaccinated.
4. Place the vaccine solution into the spray canister and walk through the house spraying at the rate of 1,000 chickens per minute. Direct the spray directly above the heads of the chickens.
5. Avoid direct contact with the vaccine solution. Wear goggles and a mask while spraying.
6. Do not use vaccinating equipment for any other purposes.

D. Freeze-dried Vaccine (25,000 doses): For 14-28 day old broiler type chickens.

Directions of Drinking Water Vaccination: For use in houses containing between 15,000 and 25,000 chickens. Do not use the drinking water vaccination method for chickens under 14 days of age.

Drinking Water - Pouring Application:

1. Do not open or mix the vaccine until ready to pour the vaccine solution into the water troughs.
2. Stop use of medication, sanitizers and disinfectants such as iodine from the drinking water 72 hours (3 days) prior to vaccination.
3. Shut off the water supply and allow the chickens to drink the troughs dry. Water should be withheld from chickens for a minimum of two (2) hours in warm weather to four (4) hours in cold weather. The water withdrawal times should be reduced if half-house brooding is in process.
4. Rinse the water troughs above the chickens heads. Clean and rinse the waterers thoroughly.
5. Calculate to supply the vaccine solution at a rate of three (3) gallons per 1,000 chickens in cold weather and four (4) gallons per 1,000 chickens in warm weather.
   Example:
   17,000 chickens in cool weather x 3 gallons = 51 gallons.
   22,500 chickens in warm weather x 4 gallons = 90 gallons.
6. Add one of the following to pouring water for vaccine distribution:
   a. One (1) ounce of nonfat dry milk per gallon of water, or
   b. Four (4) ounces of fresh skim milk per gallon of water.
   Milk or milk solids are added to neutralize low levels of virucidal chemicals which may be present in farm water.
7. Prepare the vaccine concentrate as follows:
   a. Prepare a container of milk/water figuring one (1) ounce of concentrate for one (1) gallon of water to be used.
   b. Open the vaccine container by removing the aluminum seal and stopper.
   c. Add cool milk/water to the vial until the dried vaccine is dissolved. Add the vaccine to the container of milk/water to make the vaccine concentrate. Rinse the vaccine bottle to remove all of the vaccine.
8. To make the vaccine solution, add one (1) ounce of concentrate for each gallon of pouring water needed. Mix well.
9. Fill all of the water troughs full with the vaccine solution. Avoid direct sunlight.
10. Lower the water troughs and allow the birds to drink freely. Add the remaining vaccine solution to the troughs as the birds drink.
11. Do not provide any additional drinking water until all of the vaccine solution has been consumed.

Drinking Water - Proportioner Application: Several types of medicator/proportioners are commercially available such as the dosmatic liquid dispenser. Set the proportioner to deliver one (1) ounce of vaccine concentrate per one (1) gallon of water.

1. Stop use of medication, sanitizers and disinfectants such as iodine from dispenser 72 hours (3 days) prior to vaccination. Clean all containers and hoses prior to vaccination. Do not use medicator containers for vaccine use.
2. Shut off the water supply for four (4) hours in cool weather and two (2) hours in warm weather before vaccination to stimulate thirst.
3. Calculate three (3) gallons of vaccine solution per 1,000 birds in cool weather and four (4) gallons in warm weather.
4. Calculate one (1) ounce of vaccine concentrate per gallon of water to make vaccine solution for bird consumption.
5. Vaccine concentrate preparation:
   a. Add three (3) ounces of dried nonfat milk per 16 ounces of cool water, or
   b. Use undiluted, cool, fresh skim milk.
6. Open the vaccine container by removing the aluminum seal and stopper.
7. Add the milk solution to the bottle, mix well, and add to the vaccine concentrate container. Rinse the vaccine bottle to remove all of the vaccine. Mix well.
8. Insert the dosmatic hose into the vaccine concentrate and start the water flow. Continue until all of the concentrate has been consumed before changing the water supply to direct flow.
9. Do not medicate or use disinfectants for 24 hours after vaccination.

Spray Application: For use in houses containing between 15,000 and 25,000 chickens. Spray application is recommended only for revaccination and not as a primary vaccination.

Coarse Aerosol Application: Use a sprayer delivering a coarse aerosol mist to dispense the rehydrated vaccine quickly and evenly throughout a house of chickens.

Directions:

1. Prior to spraying, reduce the air flow by raising curtains or stopping fans. Air movement should be limited for 15 minutes following vaccination.
2. Remove the aluminum seal and rubber stopper. Fill the vaccine container with cool water.
3. Pour the reconstituted vaccine into a clean container and add 150 mL (5 oz.) of cool water for each 1,000 chickens to be vaccinated.
4. Place the vaccine solution into the spray canister and walk through the house spraying at the rate of 1,000 birds per minute. Direct the spray directly above the heads of the chickens.
5. Use all of the vaccine solution for each house containing 15,000 to 25,000 birds.
6. Avoid direct contact with the vaccine solution. Wear goggles and a mask while spraying.
7. Do not use vaccinating equipment for other purposes.

Precaution(s):

A. Storage Conditions for Frozen Vaccine:

Ampules: Store in liquid nitrogen container.

Liquid nitrogen container: Carefully observe all liquid nitrogen precautions, including wearing eye protection and gloves. Store in a cool, well-ventilated area. Check the liquid nitrogen level daily. Keep the container away from incubator intakes and chicken boxes.

Liquid Nitrogen Precautions: The liquid nitrogen containers and vaccines should be handled only by properly trained personnel. These persons should be familiar with the Union Carbide publication "Precautions and Safe Practices - Liquid Atmospheric Gases", form #9888. Liquid nitrogen is extremely cold. Accidental contact with skin or eyes can cause serious frostbite. Protect eyes with goggles or a face shield. Wear gloves and long sleeves when removing and handling frozen ampules or when adding liquid nitrogen to the container. Storage and handling of liquid nitrogen containers should be in a well-ventilated area. Excessive amounts of nitrogen reduces the concentration of oxygen in the air of an unventilated space and can cause asphyxiation. If drowsiness occurs, get fresh air quickly and ventilate the entire area. If a person becomes groggy or loses consciousness while working with liquid nitrogen, get the person to a well-ventilated area immediately. If breathing has stopped, begin artificial respiration. Call a physician immediately.

B. Storage Conditions for Freeze-dried Vaccine:

Store freeze-dried vaccine at 35-45°F (2-7°C). Do not freeze.

Caution(s):

A. Frozen Vaccine:

Do not vaccinate diseased birds.

Vaccinate all of the birds on the premises at one time.

Administer a minimum of one dose for each bird.

Avoid stress conditions during and following vaccination.

Do not place chickens in contaminated facilities.

Exposure to disease must be minimized as much as possible.

For veterinary use only.

The capability of this vaccine to produce satisfactory results depends upon many factors, including, but not limited to, conditions of storage and handling by the user, administration of the vaccine, health and responsiveness of individual animals and degree of field exposure. Therefore, directions for use should be followed carefully.

The use of this vaccine is subject to applicable state and federal laws and regulations.

Use only in localities where permitted.

Newcastle disease virus can cause inflammation of the eyelids of humans. Care should be taken to avoid contamination of eyes, hands and clothing with this vaccine.

Administer only as recommended.

Use the entire contents when first opened.

Burn the container and all unused contents.

B. Freeze-dried Vaccine:

Do not vaccinate diseased birds or birds exhibiting respiratory distress and parasite infestations.

Vaccinate all birds on the same premises at the same time.

Administer a minimum of one dose for each bird.

Avoid stress conditions during and following vaccination.

Do not place chickens in contaminated premises.

Exposure to disease must be minimized as much as possible.

For veterinary use only.

Do not start vaccination program for replacement pullets after birds are 16 weeks old.

Use the entire contents when first opened.

Burn this container and all unused contents.

Since Newcastle disease virus can cause inflammation of the eyelids of humans lasting up to

N

three days, care should be taken to avoid contamination of eyes, hands and clothing with this vaccine.

The capability of these vaccines to produce satisfactory results depends upon many factors, including, but not limited to, conditions of storage and handling by the user, administration of the vaccine, health and responsiveness of individual animals and degree of field exposure. Therefore, directions for use should be followed carefully.

The use of these vaccines is subject to applicable state and federal laws and regulations.

Warning(s): Do not vaccinate within 21 days before slaughter.

Presentation: Frozen vaccine: 5 x 10,000 dose vials.
Freeze-dried vaccine: 25 x 5,000 dose and 15 x 25,000 dose vials.

Compendium Code No.: 11050311

NEWCASTLE DISEASE VACCINE (B1 TYPE, B1 STRAIN, LIVE VIRUS)

Fort Dodge Vaccine

Newcastle Disease Vaccine, B1 Type, B1 Strain, Live Virus

U.S. Vet. Lic. No.: 112

Contents: This product contains the antigens listed above.

Contains gentamicin as a preservative.

Indications: This vaccine is recommended for administration to healthy chickens, as an aid in the prevention of Newcastle disease.

Directions: Read in full, follow directions carefully.

For intranasal, intraocular, drinking-water or spray administration.

For intranasal or intraocular vaccination: This Newcastle Disease Vaccine accompanied by diluent is recommended for the vaccination of healthy chickens one day of age or older.

1. Rehydrate 1 vial of vaccine with 1 vial of diluent.
2. Remove seal and stopper from vaccine and diluent vials. Avoid contamination of stoppers and contents.
3. Add diluent to half-fill the vaccine vial. Replace stopper and shake until contents are dissolved.
4. Pour the rehydrated vaccine into the diluent container. Replace stopper and shake.
5. Remove stopper and fit drop-dispenser tip into diluent container.
6. To vaccinate intranasally, place finger over one of the bird's nostrils and place 1 drop of vaccine in the other nostril. Do not release bird until vaccine has been inhaled.
7. To vaccinate intraocularly, place 1 drop of vaccine in the eye.

For Drinking-Water Vaccination: This Newcastle Disease Vaccine is recommended for the vaccination of healthy chickens 2 weeks of age or older.

1. Discontinue use of medications or sanitizing agents in the drinking water 24 hours before vaccinating. Do not resume use for 24 hours following vaccination.
2. Water used for the drinking-water administration of a live virus vaccine must be non-chlorinated.
3. Provide enough waterers so two-thirds of the birds may drink at one time. Scrub waterers, with fresh, clean, non-chlorinated water, and use no disinfectant. Let the waterers drain dry.
4. Turn off automatic waterers, so the only available water is the vaccine water. Do not give vaccine water through medication tanks.
5. Withhold water for 2 hours before vaccinating. Do not deprive the birds of water if the temperature is extremely high.
6. Remove seal from vaccine vial.
7. Remove stopper and half-fill with clean, cool, non-chlorinated water.
8. Replace stopper and shake until dissolved.
9. Use a clean container two-thirds filled with cool, clean, non-chlorinated water. Add dried milk. Use 1 ounce (28.4 grams) dried milk if final volume of water per 1,000 doses of vaccine is to be 2½ gallons (9.5 liters); 2 ounces (56.8 grams) dried milk if final volume of water is to be 5 gallons (19.0 liters); and 4 ounces (113.6 grams) dried milk for a final volume of 10 gallons (38.0 liters). Stir the mixture until the dried milk is dissolved.
10. Add the rehydrated vaccine from the vial and again stir the contents thoroughly.
11. Next, add the mixture to the final volume of water, as follows:

Add this amount of vaccine	to this final volume of water	
	for chickens 2 to 8 weeks old	for chickens over 8 weeks old
1,000 doses	2½ to 5 gallons (9.5 to 19.0 liters)	5 to 10 gallons (19.0 to 38.0 liters)

12. Give 1 dose of vaccine per bird.
13. Distribute the final volume of vaccine water evenly among the clean waterers. Do not place the waterers in direct sunlight. Resume regular water administration only after all the vaccine water has been consumed.

For Spray Vaccination: This Newcastle Disease Vaccine may be used for the revaccination of healthy chickens 4 weeks of age or older by spraying the vaccine solution above the chickens. A sprayer that delivers a fine mist quickly and evenly is recommended.

1. Remove seal from a vial of vaccine.
2. Remove the stopper and half-fill vial with cool, distilled water.
3. Replace stopper and shake until vaccine is in solution.
4. Pour rehydrated vaccine into a clean container and add 100 mL cool, distilled water per 1,000 doses vaccine. Shake thoroughly.
5. Apply at the rate of 100 mL rehydrated vaccine per 1,000 birds. For example, 20,000 birds will require 2,000 mL (approx. 2 quarts) rehydrated vaccine. Place the vaccine solution in the sprayer canister, set the discharge control at "low" and walk through the house, spraying at the rate of 1,000 birds per minute. Direct the spray above the heads of the birds.
6. Whatever volume of vaccine solution is used in the sprayer, take care to administer 1,000 doses vaccine per 1,000 birds.
7. This spray method of vaccination should be employed in poultry houses where air movement can be reduced to a minimum. Before spraying the vaccine solution, close the house and shut off mechanical ventilation. Maintain these conditions both during spraying and for 20 minutes afterwards.
8. Wear goggles and a face mask while spraying.
9. Any sprayer used for application of a live virus vaccine should be used for no other purpose.

Records: Keep a record of vaccine serial number and expiration date; date of receipt and date of vaccination; where vaccination takes place; and any reactions observed.

Precaution(s): Store this vaccine at not over 45°F (7°C).

Use entire contents of vial when first opened.

Burn vaccine container and all unused contents.

This vaccine is nonreturnable.

Caution(s): If possible, vaccinate all susceptible birds on the premises at the same time. For 10 to 14 days after vaccinating, avoid carrying vaccine particles on shoes, clothing, etc., into areas where there are unvaccinated birds.

Newcastle Disease Vaccine virus is capable of causing a mild, irritating eye infection in humans, lasting about 3 days. Do not allow vaccine to contact the eyes.

This product should be stored, transported, and administered in accordance with the instructions and directions.

The use of this vaccine is subject to state laws, wherever applicable.

Warning(s): Do not vaccinate within 21 days before slaughter.

For veterinary use only.

Presentation: 10 x 1,000 doses.

Compendium Code No.: 10031171 10840B

NEWCASTLE DISEASE VACCINE (B_1 Type, B_1 Strain, Live Virus)

L.A.H.I. (New Jersey) Vaccine

Newcastle Disease Vaccine, B_1 Type, B_1 Strain, Live Virus

U.S. Vet. Lic. No.: 196

Active Ingredient(s): This product contains Newcastle disease live virus, B_1 type, B_1 strain.

This product is manufactured with SPF (Specific Pathogen Free) eggs and is a live virus vaccine of chicken embryo origin for the prevention of Newcastle disease in chickens.

The strain of virus in this product was carefully selected to protect against field challenges yet provide minimum reaction when used as directed.

This vaccine was carefully produced and passed all tests in accordance with the U.S. Government requirements.

Contains neomycin as a preservative.

Indications: This product is used for initial vaccination and revaccination of chickens for the prevention of Newcastle disease. Initial vaccination is administered at 2 weeks of age by the intranasal, intraocular or drinking water routes, and at 5 weeks of age by the aerosol spray route. If birds are vaccinated under the recommended age limit, revaccination is required. This product is also used in replacement birds before 16 weeks of age that were previously vaccinated.

This vaccine will stimulate protective antibodies in susceptible birds. However, the duration of immunity resulting from the use of this vaccine is not permanent, therefore, revaccinations are necessary.

Consult your poultry pathologist for recommendations on revaccination based on conditions existing in your area at any given time.

Dosage and Administration: 1,000 Dose: Preparation of Vaccine for Intranasal and Intraocular Use: Remove aluminum overseal and rubber stopper from the vaccine bottle and pour part of the diluent into the bottle. Shake well and pour the vaccine back into the remaining diluent and place the dropper tip on the diluent bottle. The vaccine is now ready for intranasal or intraocular use.

Method of Vaccination: The vaccine may be administered by way of the nostril (intranasally) or the eye (intraocularly). When the vaccine is administered by way of the nostril, the chick's beak is held shut, a finger is placed over one nostril and a drop of vaccine, from the special applicator, is dropped into the other nostril.

When used intraocularly, birds are held on their side and one drop of the mixed vaccine allowed to fall into the open eye. Bird should be held until the drop of vaccine disappears. Care must be taken to prevent injury to the cornea of the eye with the dropper tip.

Preparation of Vaccine for Aerosol Use: Remove the aluminum overseal and stopper from the vaccine bottle and pour part of the diluent into the bottle. Shake well and pour the vaccine back into the remaining diluent. Pour the entire contents into the reservoir of a sprayer containing 70 mL of deionized water or 5 mL of glycerine and 65 mL of deionized water. Before the vaccination the sprayer should be calibrated so that 100 mL will be delivered in 3 minutes.

Method of Vaccination: Confine the birds to a corner of the house with fences and direct the stream from the sprayer over the heads of the birds. Extreme caution should be taken to prevent birds from smothering during this operation.

1,000 and 2,500 Doses: Preparation of Vaccine for Drinking Water Use: Remove the aluminum overseal and stopper and add clean non-sanitized water. Replace the stopper and shake well. Pour the contents into a quart jar ¾ full of non-sanitized water. Shake well and dilute the vaccine for 1,000 doses or 2,500 doses as the case may be as outlined in the chart below. A dried skim milk powder should be used as a vaccine stabilizer at the rate of 8.0 grams per gallon of water. The powdered milk is added prior to the reconstitution of the vaccine.

Method of Vaccination: Withhold all medication and disinfectants from the drinking water 24 hours before and 24 hours after vaccinating. Rinse waterers with clean non-sanitized water and remove all water from chicks for at least two hours prior to vaccination. Provide adequate space so that at least two-thirds of the birds can drink at one time.

Add mixture to water as per following charts:

1,000 Doses:

Age of Birds	Heavy per 1,000 birds	Leghorn per 1,000 birds
2 Weeks-3 Weeks	3 Gals. of Water	3 Gals. of Water
4 Weeks-8 Weeks	8 Gals. of Water	5 Gals. of Water
9 Weeks-15 Weeks	10 Gals. of Water	8 Gals. of Water
16 Weeks-20 Weeks	13 Gals. of Water	10 Gals. of Water

2,500 Doses:

Age of Birds	Heavy per 2,500 birds	Leghorn per 2,500 birds
2 Weeks-3 Weeks	7 Gals. of Water	7 Gals. of Water
4 Weeks-8 Weeks	20 Gals. of Water	12 Gals. of Water
9 Weeks-15 Weeks	25 Gals. of Water	20 Gals. of Water
16 Weeks-20 Weeks	30 Gals. of Water	25 Gals. of Water

Divide the mixed vaccine into the waterers.

Provide no other drinking water until all vaccine has been consumed.

Contraindication(s): Vaccinate healthy chickens only that are free of PPLO and without previous history of a respiratory disease.

If there are susceptible laying birds on the premises there is the possibility that the virus might spread from the vaccinated to the susceptible birds and affect egg production.

Precaution(s): Keep vaccine in the dark between 2-7°C (35-45°F).

Use entire contents when first opened. Burn this container and all unused contents.

Caution(s): It is imperative that the user of this product comply with the indications for use, contraindication, and method of vaccination stated on the direction sheet. The vaccine must be prepared and administered as directed to obtain best results.

If chicks are to be vaccinated at a very young age, the vaccination must be done at the point of destination to avoid violation of the Postal Laws and Regulations.

Warning(s): Do not vaccinate within 21 days before slaughter.

Care should be taken to avoid contaminating hands, eyes and clothing with the vaccine since the Newcastle disease virus can cause a mild inflammation of the conjunctiva lasting for 3-5 days.

For veterinary use only.

Presentation: 1,000 and 2,500 doses.

Compendium Code No.: 10080273

NEWCASTLE DISEASE VACCINE (B_1 Type, B_1 Strain, Live Virus) (Drinking Water Use)

L.A.H.I. (New Jersey) **Vaccine**

Newcastle Disease Vaccine, B_1 Type, B_1 Strain, Live Virus

U.S. Vet. Lic. No.: 196

Description: This product is manufactured from SPF (Specific Pathogen Free) eggs and is a live virus vaccine of chicken embryo origin for the prevention of Newcastle Disease in chickens.

The strain of virus in this product was carefully selected to protect against field challenges yet provide minimum reaction when used as directed.

This vaccine was carefully produced and passed all tests in accordance with the U.S. Government requirements.

Contains neomycin as a preservative.

Indications: This product is used for initial vaccination and revaccination of chickens for the prevention of Newcastle Disease. Initial vaccination is administered to birds at 2 weeks of age. If birds are vaccinated under 2 weeks of age, revaccination is required. This product is also used in replacement birds before 16 weeks of age that were previously vaccinated.

This vaccine will stimulate protective antibodies in susceptible birds. However, the duration of immunity resulting from the use of this vaccine is not permanent, therefore, revaccinations are necessary.

Consult your poultry pathologist for recommendations on revaccination based conditions existing in your area at any given time.

For drinking water use.

Dosage and Administration: Read instructions before use.

10,000 Doses:

Preparation of Vaccine: Remove the aluminum overseal and stopper and add clean non-sanitized water. Replace the stopper and shake well. Pour the contents into a quart jar ¾ full of non-sanitized water. Shake well and dilute as outlined in the chart below.

Method of Vaccination: Withhold all medication and disinfectants from the drinking water 24 hours before and 24 hours after vaccination. Rinse waterers with clean non-sanitized water and remove all water from chicks for at least two hours prior to vaccination. Provide adequate space so that at least two-thirds of the birds can drink at one time.

Add mixture to water as per following chart:

Age of Birds	Heavy	Leghorn
2-3 Weeks	30 Gals. of Water	30 Gals. of Water
4-8 Weeks	80 Gals. of Water	50 Gals. of Water
9-15 Weeks	100 Gals. of Water	80 Gals. of Water
16-20 Weeks	130 Gals. of Water	100 Gals. of Water

Divide mixed vaccine into the waterers.

Provide no other drinking water until all vaccine has been consumed.

N

Contraindication(s): Vaccinate healthy chickens only that are free of PPLO and without previous history of a respiratory disease.

If there are susceptible laying birds on the premises there is the possibility that the virus might spread from the vaccinated to the susceptible birds and affect egg production.

Precaution(s): Keep vaccine in the dark between 2-7°C (35-45°F).

Use entire contents when first opened. Burn this container and all unused contents.

Caution(s): It is imperative that the user of this product comply with the "Indications", "Contraindications", and "Method of Vaccination" stated on the direction sheet. The vaccine must be prepared and administered as directed to obtain best results.

If chicks are to be vaccinated at a very young age, the vaccination must be done at the point of destination to avoid violation of the Postal Laws and Regulations.

Warning(s): Do not vaccinate within 21 days before slaughter.

Care should be taken to avoid contaminating hands, eyes and clothing with the vaccine since the Newcastle Disease virus can cause a mild inflammation of the conjunctiva lasting for 3 to 5 days.

For veterinary use only.

Presentation: 10,000 dose vial.

Compendium Code No.: 10080661 R582150

NEWCASTLE DISEASE VACCINE (B1 TYPE, LASOTA STRAIN, LIVE VIRUS)

Fort Dodge **Vaccine**

Newcastle Disease Vaccine, B1 Type, LaSota Strain, Live Virus

U.S. Vet. Lic. No.: 112

Contents: This product contains the antigens listed above.

Contains gentamicin as a preservative.

Indications: This vaccine is recommended for administration to healthy chickens, as an aid in the prevention of Newcastle disease.

Directions: Read in full, follow directions carefully.

For intranasal, intraocular, drinking-water or spray administration.

For intranasal or intraocular vaccination: This Newcastle Disease Vaccine accompanied by diluent is recommended for the vaccination of healthy chickens one day of age or older.

1. Rehydrate 1 vial of vaccine with 1 vial of diluent.
2. Remove seal and stopper from vaccine and diluent vials. Avoid contamination of stoppers and contents.
3. Add diluent to half-fill the vaccine vial. Replace stopper and shake until contents are dissolved.
4. Pour the rehydrated vaccine into the diluent container. Replace stopper and shake.
5. Remove stopper and fit drop-dispenser tip into diluent container.
6. To vaccinate intranasally, place finger over one of the bird's nostrils and place 1 drop of vaccine in the other nostril. Do not release bird until vaccine has been inhaled.
7. To vaccinate intraocularly, place 1 drop of vaccine in the eye.

For Drinking-Water Vaccination: This Newcastle Disease Vaccine is recommended for the vaccination of healthy chickens 2 weeks of age or older.

1. Discontinue use of medications or sanitizing agents in the drinking water 24 hours before vaccinating. Do not resume use for 24 hours following vaccination.
2. Water used for the drinking-water administration of a live virus vaccine must be non-chlorinated.
3. Provide enough waterers so two-thirds of the birds may drink at one time. Scrub waterers, with fresh, clean, non-chlorinated water, and use no disinfectant. Let the waterers drain dry.
4. Turn off automatic waterers, so the only available water is the vaccine water. Do not give vaccine water through medication tanks.
5. Withhold water for 2 hours before vaccinating. Do not deprive the birds of water if the temperature is extremely high.
6. Remove seal from vaccine vial.
7. Remove stopper and half-fill with clean, cool, non-chlorinated water.
8. Replace stopper and shake until dissolved.
9. Use a clean container two-thirds filled with cool, clean, non-chlorinated water. Add dried milk. Use 1 ounce (28.4 grams) dried milk if final volume of water per 1,000 doses of vaccine is to be 2½ gallons (9.5 liters); 2 ounces (56.8 grams) dried milk if final volume of water is to be 5 gallons (19.0 liters); and 4 ounces (113.6 grams) dried milk for a final volume of 10 gallons (38.0 liters). Stir the mixture until the dried milk is dissolved.
10. Add the rehydrated vaccine from the vial and again stir the contents thoroughly.
11. Next, add the mixture to the final volume of water, as follows:

Add this amount of vaccine	to this final volume of water	
	for chickens 2 to 8 weeks old	for chickens over 8 weeks old
1,000 doses	2½ to 5 gallons (9.5 to 19.0 liters)	5 to 10 gallons (19.0 to 38.0 liters)

12. Give 1 dose of vaccine per bird.
13. Distribute the final volume of vaccine water evenly among the clean waterers. Do not place the waterers in direct sunlight. Resume regular water administration only after all the vaccine water has been consumed.

For Spray Vaccination: This Newcastle Disease Vaccine may be used for the revaccination of healthy chickens 4 weeks of age or older by spraying the vaccine solution above the chickens. A sprayer that delivers a fine mist quickly and evenly is recommended.

1. Remove seal from a vial of vaccine.
2. Remove the stopper and half-fill vial with cool, distilled water.
3. Replace stopper and shake until vaccine is in solution.
4. Pour rehydrated vaccine into a clean container and add 100 mL cool, distilled water per 1,000 doses vaccine. Shake thoroughly.
5. Apply at the rate of 100 mL rehydrated vaccine per 1,000 birds. For example, 20,000 birds will require 2,000 mL (approx. 2 quarts) rehydrated vaccine. Place the vaccine solution in the sprayer canister, set the discharge control at "low" and walk through the house, spraying at the rate of 1,000 birds per minute. Direct the spray above the heads of the birds.
6. Whatever volume of vaccine solution is used in the sprayer, take care to administer 1,000 doses vaccine per 1,000 birds.
7. This spray method of vaccination should be employed in poultry houses where air movement can be reduced to a minimum. Before spraying the vaccine solution, close the house and shut off mechanical ventilation. Maintain these conditions both during spraying and for 20 minutes afterwards.
8. Wear goggles and a face mask while spraying.
9. Any sprayer used for application of a live virus vaccine should be used for no other purpose.

Records: Keep a record of vaccine serial number and expiration date; date of receipt and date of vaccination; where vaccination takes place; and any reactions observed.

Precaution(s): Store this vaccine at not over 45°F (7°C).

Use entire contents of vial when first opened.

Burn vaccine container and all unused contents.

This vaccine is nonreturnable.

Caution(s): If possible, vaccinate all susceptible birds on the premises at the same time. For 10 to 14 days after vaccinating, avoid carrying vaccine particles on shoes, clothing, etc., into areas where there are unvaccinated birds.

Newcastle Disease Vaccine virus is capable of causing a mild, irritating eye infection in humans, lasting about 3 days. Do not allow vaccine to contact the eyes.

This product should be stored, transported, and administered in accordance with the instructions and directions.

The use of this vaccine is subject to state laws, wherever applicable.

Warning(s): Do not vaccinate within 21 days before slaughter.

For veterinary use only.

Presentation: 10 x 1,000 doses.

Compendium Code No.: 10031181 10840B

NEWCASTLE DISEASE VACCINE (B_1 Type, Lasota Strain, Live Virus)

L.A.H.I. (New Jersey) **Vaccine**

Newcastle Disease Vaccine, B_1 Type, LaSota Strain, Live Virus

U.S. Vet. Lic. No.: 196

Active Ingredient(s): This product contains Newcastle disease live virus, B_1 type, LaSota strain. Contains neomycin as a preservative.

It is manufactured from SPF (Specific Pathogen Free) eggs and is a live virus vaccine of chicken embryo origin for the prevention of Newcastle disease in chickens.

The strain of virus in this product was carefully selected to protect against field challenges yet provide minimum reaction when used as directed.

This vaccine was carefully produced and passes all tests in accordance with the U.S. Government requirements.

Indications: This product is used for initial vaccination and revaccination of chickens for the prevention of Newcastle disease. Initial vaccination is administered at 2 weeks of age by the intranasal or intraocular or intramuscular routes, and at 5 weeks of age by aerosol spray. If birds are vaccinated under the recommended age limit, revaccination is required. This product is also used in replacement birds before 16 weeks of age that were previously vaccinated.

This vaccine will stimulate protective antibodies in susceptible birds. However, the duration of immunity resulting from the use of this vaccine is not permanent, therefore, revaccinations are necessary.

Consult your poultry pathologist for recommendations on revaccination based on conditions existing in your area at any given time.

Dosage and Administration: Preparation of Vaccine for Intranasal and Intraocular Use: Remove aluminum overseal and stopper from the vaccine bottle and pour part of the diluent into the bottle. Shake well and pour the vaccine back into the remaining diluent and place the dropper tip on the diluent bottle. The vaccine is now ready for intranasal or intraocular use.

Method of Vaccination: The vaccine may be administered by way of the nostril (intranasally) or the eye (intraocularly). When the vaccine is administered by way of the nostril, the chick's beak is held shut, a finger is placed over one nostril and a drop of vaccine, from the special applicator, is dropped into the other nostril.

When used intraocularly, birds are held on their side and one drop of the mixed vaccine allowed to fall into the open eye. Bird should be held until the drop of vaccine disappears. Care must be taken to prevent injury to the cornea of the eye with the dropper tip.

Preparation of Vaccine for Aerosol Use: Remove the aluminum overseal and stopper from the vaccine bottle and pour part of the diluent into the bottle. Shake well and pour the vaccine back into the remaining diluent. Pour the entire contents into the reservoir of a sprayer containing 70 mL of deionized water or 5 mL of glycerine and 65 mL of deionized water. Before the vaccination the sprayer should be calibrated so that 100 mL will be delivered in 3 minutes.

Method of Vaccination: Confine the birds to a corner of the house with fences and direct the stream from the sprayer over the heads of the birds. Extreme caution should be taken to prevent birds from smothering during this operation.

1,000 Doses and 2,500 Doses: Preparation of Vaccine for Drinking Water Use: Remove the aluminum overseal and stopper and add clean non-sanitized water. Replace the stopper and shake well. Pour the contents into a quart jar ¾ full of non-sanitized water. Shake well and dilute the vaccine for 1,000 doses or 2,500 doses as the case may be as outlined in the chart below. A dried skim milk powder should be used as a vaccine stabilizer at the rate of 8.0 grams per gallon of water. The powdered milk is added prior to the reconstitution of the vaccine.

Method of Vaccination: Withhold all medication and disinfectants from the drinking water 24 hours before and 24 hours after vaccinating. Rinse waterers with clean non-sanitized water and remove all water from chicks for at least two hours prior to vaccination. Provide adequate space so that at least two-thirds of the birds can drink at one time.

Add mixture to water as per following charts:

1,000 Doses:

Age of Birds	Heavy per 1,000 birds	Leghorn per 1,000 birds
2 Weeks-3 Weeks	3 Gals. of Water	3 Gals. of Water
4 Weeks-8 Weeks	8 Gals. of Water	5 Gals. of Water
9 Weeks-15 Weeks	10 Gals. of Water	8 Gals. of Water
16 Weeks-20 Weeks	13 Gals. of Water	10 Gals. of Water

2,500 Doses:

Age of Birds	Heavy per 2,500 birds	Leghorn per 2,500 birds
2 Weeks-3 Weeks	7 Gals. of Water	7 Gals. of Water
4 Weeks-8 Weeks	20 Gals. of Water	12 Gals. of Water
9 Weeks-15 Weeks	25 Gals. of Water	20 Gals. of Water
16 Weeks-20 Weeks	30 Gals. of Water	25 Gals. of Water

Divide the mixed vaccine into the waterers.

Provide no other drinking water until all vaccine has been consumed.

Contraindication(s): Vaccinate healthy chickens only.

If there are susceptible laying birds on the premises there is a possibility that the virus might spread from the vaccinated to the susceptible birds and affect egg production.

Precaution(s): Keep vaccine in the dark between 2-7°C (35-45°F).

Use entire contents when first opened. Burn this container and all unused contents.

Caution(s): It is imperative that the user of this product comply with the indications for use, contraindications, and method of vaccination stated on the direction sheet. The vaccine must be prepared and administered as directed to obtain best results.

If chicks are to be vaccinated at a very young age, the vaccination must be done at the point of destination to avoid violation of the Postal Laws and regulations.

Warning(s): Do not vaccinate within 21 days before slaughter.

Care should be taken to avoid contaminating your hands, eyes and clothing with the vaccine since the Newcastle disease virus can cause a mild inflammation of the conjunctiva lasting for 3 to 5 days.

For veterinary use only.

Presentation: 1,000 and 2,500 doses.

Compendium Code No.: 10080282

NEWCASTLE DISEASE VACCINE (Killed Virus)

L.A.H.I. (New Jersey) **Vaccine**

Newcastle Disease Vaccine, Killed Virus

U.S. Vet. Lic. No.: 196

Active Ingredient(s): The product is manufactured from SPF (Specific Pathogen Free) eggs and consists of one inactivated virus strain of Newcastle disease. The virus used in this product is an antigen strain and is presented with Novasome™ adjuvant.

The vaccine was carefully produced and passed all tests in accordance with the U.S. government requirements.

Indications: The vaccine is used for protection against Newcastle disease in chickens.

Dosage and Administration: Shake the vaccine for two (2) minutes before use.

Inject each bird with a 0.5 mL dose subcutaneously in the mid portion of the neck or intramuscularly in the breast or thigh muscle.

The first vaccination should be done when the birds are three (3) weeks of age or older. The second vaccination should be done at 18 to 20 weeks. If birds are to be kept for a second year of production, they should be vaccinated during molt.

Preparation of Vaccine: Remove the aluminum overseal and the vaccine is ready to use. Should greater than four (4) hours elapse between the first and last use of the vaccine from any one container, it is recommended that the vaccine be shaken again before continuing with the vaccinations.

Precaution(s): Keep the vaccine in the dark between 35-45°F (2-7°C). Do not freeze.

Caution(s): For veterinary use only.

Use aseptic precautions. Sterilize needles, syringes and stopper.

Vaccinate healthy birds only. Consult a poultry pathologist before vaccinating.

Burn the vaccine containers and all unused contents.

Use the entire contents when first opened.

It is imperative that the user of this product comply with the instructions stated in the direction sheet packed with each product. The vaccine must be prepared and administered as directed to obtain the best results.

The use of nonsterile needles under field vaccination may result in abscess formation and condemnation of the birds.

Warning(s): Do not market birds for at least six (6) weeks after vaccinating. Make sure that the birds marketed do not have swellings at the site of vaccine administration since this may result in condemnations of the birds.

Presentation: 1,000 dose (500 mL) bottles.

Compendium Code No.: 10080292

NEWCASTLE DISEASE VACCINE (LaSota Strain)

Merial Select **Vaccine**

Newcastle Disease Vaccine, B1 Type, LaSota Strain, Live Virus

U.S. Vet. Lic. No.: 279

Active Ingredient(s): The vaccine contains the LaSota strain of Newcastle disease virus. The virus has been propagated in fertile eggs from specific pathogen free flocks. The immunizing capability of the vaccine has been proven by the master seed immunogenicity test. The vaccine offers proven immunity with mild reactions.

Contains streptomycin and penicillin as bacteriostatic agents.

Contains fungizone as a fungistatic agent.

Notice: The vaccine has undergone rigid potency, safety, and purity tests and meets Merial Select, Inc., and USDA requirements.

Indications: The vaccine is recommended for administration to healthy chickens as an aid in the prevention of Newcastle disease.

The vaccine is recommended for the vaccination of healthy chickens 14 days of age or older by drinking water administration or by aerosol spray. Spray vaccination is recommended for revaccination only. Revaccination is recommended at four weeks and 16 weeks of age.

Dosage and Administration: Freeze-dried Vaccine:

Directions for Drinking Water Vaccination:

1. Do not open and mix the vaccine until ready to vaccinate.
2. Remove all medication, sanitizers and disinfectants from the drinking water 72 hours prior to vaccination.
3. Provide sufficient waterers so that all of the birds can drink at one time. Clean and rinse the waterers thoroughly.
4. Withhold all water from the birds for two (2) to four (4) hours prior to vaccination to stimulate thirst.
5. Add nonfat dry milk to the water at the rate of one (1) ounce per gallon before mixing the vaccine.
6. Remove the aluminum seal and rubber stopper from a vaccine vial.
7. Fill the vaccine vial two-thirds (⅔) full with clean, cool water and mix gently.
8. Mix the dissolved vaccine with water as shown below:

Age of birds	Water per 1,000 doses vaccine
2-4 weeks	2.5 gallons (9.9 L)
4-8 weeks	5 gallons (18.9 L)
8 weeks or older	10 gallons (37.9 L)

9. Distribute the vaccine solution among the waterers. Avoid direct sunlight.
10. Do not provide any other drinking water until all of the vaccine mixture has been consumed.

Spray Aerosol Vaccination: Use only for revaccination of healthy chickens two (2) weeks of age or older. Do not use for initial vaccination.

Use a sprayer delivering an aerosol-like mist to disperse the rehydrated vaccine quickly and evenly throughout a house of chickens.

Directions:

1. Remove the aluminum seal and rubber stopper from the vaccine vial.
2. Fill the vaccine vial full with cool, distilled water. Pour the dissolved vaccine into a container and add approximately 500 mL of cool, distilled water per 5,000 doses of vaccine. Mix thoroughly.
3. For spray aerosol vaccination of a house of chickens, apply at the rate of 500 mL per 5,000 chickens.
4. Example: 20,000 birds will require 2,000 mL (approximately 2 quarts) of rehydrated vaccine.
5. Place the vaccine solution into the sprayer canister, set the discharge control and walk through the house spraying at the rate of 1,000 birds per minute. Direct the spray above the heads of the birds.
6. Whatever volume of vaccine solution is used, take care to administer 5,000 doses of vaccine to 5,000 birds.
7. Prior to spraying, reduce the air flow to a minimum. Keep air flow reduced for 20 minutes following spray vaccination.
8. Avoid direct contact with the vaccine solution. Wear goggles and a mask while spraying a live virus vaccine.
9. Any equipment used for the application of a live virus vaccine should not be used for any other purpose.

Precaution(s): Store at 35-45°F (2-7°C). Do not freeze.

Caution(s): Do not vaccinate diseased birds.

Birds should be free of respiratory diseases and parasite infestations.

Vaccinate all of the birds on the same premises at the same time.

Administer 5,000 doses to 5,000 birds.

Avoid stress conditions during and following vaccination.

Do not place chickens on contaminated premises.

Exposure to disease must be minimized as much as possible.

For veterinary use only.

Do not start vaccination program for replacement pullets after birds are 16 weeks old.

Use the entire contents when first opened.

Burn the container and all unused contents.

Since Newcastle disease virus can cause inflammation of the eyelids of humans lasting up to three days, care should be taken to avoid contamination of the eyes, hands and clothing with the vaccine.

The capability of these vaccines to produce satisfactory results depends upon many factors, including, but not limited to, conditions of storage and handling by the user, administration of the vaccine, health and the responsiveness of individual animals and the degree of field exposure. Therefore, directions for use should be followed carefully.

The use of these vaccines is subject to applicable state and federal laws and regulations.

Warning(s): Do not vaccinate within 21 days before slaughter.

Presentation: 25 x 5,000 dose vials.

Compendium Code No.: 11050321

NEWCASTLE-K

Fort Dodge **Vaccine**

Newcastle Disease Vaccine, Killed Virus

U.S. Vet. Lic. No.: 112

Contents: This product contains the antigen listed above.

Gentamicin added as a preservative.

Indications: For the vaccination of healthy chickens 3 weeks of age or older as an aid in the prevention of Newcastle disease.

Dosage and Administration: Inject 0.5 mL (0.5 cc) intramuscularly or subcutaneously (in the lower neck region) using aseptic technique. Vaccinate only healthy birds. For primed birds, a single dose between 16 and 22 weeks (approximately 4 weeks prior to lay) is indicated.

Precaution(s): Store in the dark at 36° to 45°F (2° to 7°C). Do not freeze. Warm to 72°F (22°C) and shake well before using. Use entire contents when first opened.

Warning(s): Do not vaccinate within 42 days before slaughter.

In case of accidental human injection seek immediate medical attention.

For veterinary use only.

Presentation: 1,000 dose (500 mL) vials.

Compendium Code No.: 10031221 10271C

NEWCASTLE LASOTA+BRONCHITIS MASS

Fort Dodge **Vaccine**

Newcastle-Bronchitis Vaccine, B1 Type, LaSota Strain, Massachusetts Type, Live Virus

U.S. Vet. Lic. No.: 112

Contents: This product contains the antigens listed above.

Contains gentamicin as a preservative.

Indications: This vaccine is recommended for administration to healthy chickens, as an aid in the prevention of Newcastle disease and infectious bronchitis, Massachusetts serotype.

Directions: Read in full. Follow directions carefully.

For Intranasal or Intraocular Vaccination: This Newcastle-Bronchitis Vaccine accompanied by diluent is recommended for the vaccination of healthy chickens one day of age or older.

1. Rehydrate 1 vial of vaccine with 1 vial of diluent.
2. Remove seal and stopper from vaccine and diluent vials. Avoid contamination of stoppers and contents.
3. Add diluent to half-fill the vaccine vial. Replace stopper and shake until contents are dissolved.
4. Pour the rehydrated vaccine into the diluent container. Replace stopper and shake.
5. Remove stopper and fit drop-dispenser tip into diluent container.
6. To vaccinate intranasally, place finger over one of the bird's nostrils and place 1 drop of vaccine in the other nostril. Do not release bird until vaccine has been inhaled.
7. To vaccinate intraocularly, place 1 drop of vaccine in the eye.

For Drinking-Water Vaccination: This Newcastle-Bronchitis Vaccine is recommended for the vaccination of healthy chickens 2 weeks of age or older. If birds are vaccinated by this route before 2 weeks of age, they should be revaccinated.

1. Discontinue use of medications or sanitizing agents in the drinking water 24 hours before vaccinating. Do not resume use for 24 hours following vaccination.
2. Water used for the drinking-water administration of a live virus vaccine must be non-chlorinated.
3. Provide enough waterers so two-thirds of the birds may drink at one time. Scrub waterers with fresh, clean, non-chlorinated water, and use no disinfectant. Let the waterers drain dry.
4. Turn off automatic waterers, so the only available water is the vaccine water. Do not give vaccine water through medication tanks.
5. Withhold water for 2 hours before vaccinating. Do not deprive the birds of water if the temperature is extremely high.
6. Remove seal from vaccine vial.
7. Remove stopper and half-fill with clean, cool, non-chlorinated water.
8. Replace stopper and shake until dissolved.
9. Use a clean container two-thirds filled with cool, clean, non-chlorinated water. Add dried milk. Use 1 ounce (28.4 grams) dried milk if final volume of water per 1,000 doses of vaccine is to be 2½ gallons (9.5 liters); 2 ounces (56.8 grams) dried milk if final volume of water is to be 5 gallons (19.0 liters); and 4 ounces (113.6 grams) dried milk for a final volume of 10 gallons (38.0 liters). Stir the mixture until the dried milk is dissolved.
10. Add the rehydrated vaccine from the vial and again stir the contents thoroughly.
11. Next, add the mixture to the final volume of water, as follows:

Add this amount of vaccine	to this final volume of water	
	for chickens 2 to 8 weeks old	for chickens over 8 weeks old
1,000 doses	2½ to 5 gallons (9.5 to 19.0 liters)	5 to 10 gallons (19.0 to 38.0 liters)

12. Give 1 dose of vaccine per bird.
13. Distribute the final volume of vaccine water evenly among the clean waterers. Do not place the waterers in direct sunlight. Resume regular water administration only after all the vaccine water has been consumed.

For Spray Vaccination: This vaccine may be used for the revaccination of healthy chickens 4 weeks of age or older by spraying the vaccine solution above the chickens. A sprayer that delivers a fine mist quickly and evenly is recommended.

1. Remove seal from a vial of vaccine.
2. Remove the stopper and half-fill vial with cool, distilled water.
3. Replace stopper and shake until vaccine is in solution.
4. Pour rehydrated vaccine into a clean container and add 100 mL cool, distilled water per 1,000 doses vaccine. Shake thoroughly.
5. Apply at the rate of 100 mL rehydrated vaccine per 1,000 birds. For example, 20,000 birds will require 2,000 mL (approx. 2 quarts) rehydrated vaccine. Place the vaccine solution in the sprayer canister, set the discharge control at "low" and walk through the house, spraying at the rate of 1,000 birds per minute. Direct the spray above the heads of the birds.
6. Whatever volume of vaccine solution is used in the sprayer, take care to administer 1,000 doses vaccine per 1,000 birds.
7. This spray method of vaccination should be employed in poultry houses where air movement can be reduced to a minimum. Before spraying the vaccine solution, close the house and shut off mechanical ventilation. Maintain these conditions both during spraying and for 20 minutes afterwards.
8. Wear goggles and a face mask while spraying.
9. Any sprayer used for application of a live virus vaccine should be used for no other purpose.

Records: Keep a record of vaccine serial number and expiration date; date of receipt and date of vaccination; where vaccination takes place; and any reactions observed.

Precaution(s): Store this vaccine at not over 45°F (7°C). Use entire contents when vial is first opened. Burn vaccine container and all unused contents.

This vaccine is nonreturnable.

Caution(s): If possible, vaccinate all susceptible birds on the premises at the same time. For 10 to 14 days after vaccinating, avoid carrying vaccine particles on shoes, clothing, etc., into areas where there are unvaccinated birds.

Newcastle Disease Vaccine virus is capable of causing a mild, irritating eye infection in humans, lasting about 3 days. Do not allow vaccine to contact the eyes.

This product should be stored, transported, and administered in accordance with the instructions and directions. The use of this vaccine is subject to state laws, wherever applicable.

Warning(s): Do not vaccinate within 21 days before slaughter. For veterinary use only.

Presentation: 10 x 1,000 doses.

Compendium Code No.: 10031191 10870A

NEWHATCH-C2-M™

Intervet **Vaccine**

Newcastle-Bronchitis Vaccine, B_1 Type, C2 Strain, Mass. Type, Live Virus

U.S. Vet. Lic. No.: 286

Description: NEWHATCH-C2-M™, a live virus vaccine, is prepared from a B_1 Type, C2 Strain of Newcastle disease virus and a mild Massachusetts strain of Infectious Bronchitis virus. The viruses have been propagated using SPF substrates.

This vaccine contains gentamicin as a preservative.

Quality tested for purity, potency, and safety.

Indications: The vaccine is recommended for vaccination of healthy chickens, one day of age or older for protection against Newcastle disease and Infectious Bronchitis disease (Massachusetts strain) by coarse spray administration.

Dosage and Administration: Vaccination Program: Many factors must be considered in determining a sound vaccination program for a particular farm or poultry complex. To be fully effective, the vaccine must be administered properly to healthy, receptive chickens maintained in a proper environment under good management. In addition, the response may be influenced by the age of the chickens and their immune status. Seldom does one live virus vaccination under field conditions produce lifetime protection for all individuals in a given flock. The level of immunity required will vary with operational practices and the degree of exposure. Therefore, a program of periodic revaccinations may be necessary.

Preparation of Vaccine:

For Coarse Spray: Do not open and mix the vaccine until ready to begin vaccination. Use vaccine immediately after mixing.

1. Remove the tear-off seal and stopper from the vial containing the dried vaccine.
2. Carefully pour clean, cool, deionized water into the vaccine vial until the vial is approximately two-thirds full.
3. Insert the rubber stopper and shake vigorously until all material is dissolved.
4. The vaccine is now ready for coarse spray use in accordance with the following directions. For best results, be sure to follow directions carefully!

Coarse Spray Administration - For Chickens One Day of Age:

1. Use rehydrated vaccine as indicated for specific coarse spray vaccination machine. For example, a machine which dispenses 20 mL to a box of 100 chickens - total volume for 10,000 doses is 2,000 mL of deionized water. Mix thoroughly.
2. Add the prepared vaccine solution to reservoir on the machine.
3. Prime and adjust machine as instructed in manual accompanying the specific machine.
4. Place boxes holding 100 chickens each on the conveyor belt or in machine. Activate spray head.

Records: Keep a record of vaccine, quantity, serial number, expiration date and place of purchase; the date and time of vaccination; the number, age, breed and locations of chickens; names of operators performing the vaccination and any observed reactions.

Precaution(s): Store vaccine in refrigerator between 2 and 7°C (35 and 45°F).

Do not spill or splash the vaccine.

Use entire contents when first opened.

Burn containers and all unused contents.

Avoid exposure of this vaccine to sunlight.

This product is nonreturnable.

Caution(s): Vaccinate only healthy chickens. Although disease may not be evident, Coccidiosis, Mycoplasma infection, Infectious Bursal disease, Chicken Infectious Anemia, Reovirus infection, Marek's disease and other disease conditions may cause complications or reduce immunity.

All susceptible chickens on the same premises should be vaccinated at the same time.

The revaccination of laying hens with live Newcastle/Bronchitis vaccine may be detrimental to the flock and cannot be generally recommended. This caution applies to all live Newcastle/Bronchitis vaccines currently available. Consult your Intervet representative for more information.

Efforts should be taken to reduce stress conditions at the time of vaccination and during the reaction period.

Do not dilute the vaccine or otherwise stretch the dosage.

Do not use less than 1 dose per bird.

For veterinary use only.

Notice: This vaccine has undergone rigid potency, safety and purity tests and meets Intervet Inc. and USDA requirements. It is designed to stimulate effective immunity when used as directed, but the user must be advised that the response to the product depends upon many factors, including, but not limited to, conditions of storage and handling by the user, administration of the vaccine, health and responsiveness of individual chickens and the degree of field exposure. Therefore, directions should be followed carefully.

This product is not hazardous when used according to directions supplied. A material safety data sheet (MSDS) is available upon request. This and any other consumer information can be obtained by calling Intervet Customer Service at 1-800-441-8272 or 1-302-934-8051.

The use of this vaccine is subject to applicable federal and local laws and regulations.

Use only as directed.

Warning(s): Do not vaccinate within 21 days before slaughter.

Newcastle virus occasionally causes conjunctivitis in humans. Avoid any contact of vaccine with eyes.

Presentation: 10 x 10,000 doses.

U.S. Patent No. 5,750,111

Compendium Code No.: 11062830 20803 AL176

NEWHATCH-C2-MC™

Intervet **Vaccine**

Newcastle-Bronchitis Vaccine, B_1 Type, C2 Strain, Mass. and Conn. Types, Live Virus

U.S. Vet. Lic. No.: 286

Description: NEWHATCH-C2-MC™, a live virus vaccine, is prepared from a B_1 Type, C2 Strain of Newcastle disease virus and the mild Massachusetts and Connecticut types of Infectious Bronchitis virus. The viruses have been propagated using SPF substrates.

This vaccine contains gentamicin as a preservative.

Quality tested for purity, potency, and safety.

Indications: The vaccine is recommended for vaccination of healthy chickens, one day of age or older for protection against Newcastle disease and Infectious Bronchitis disease (Massachusetts and Connecticut strains) by coarse spray administration.

Dosage and Administration: Vaccination Program: Many factors must be considered in determining a sound vaccination program for a particular farm or poultry complex. To be fully effective, the vaccine must be administered properly to healthy, receptive chickens maintained in a proper environment under good management. In addition, the response may be influenced by the age of the chickens and their immune status. Seldom does one live virus vaccination under field conditions produce lifetime protection for all individuals in a given flock. The level of immunity required will vary with operational practices and the degree of exposure. Therefore, a program of periodic revaccinations may be necessary.

Preparation of Vaccine:

For Coarse Spray: Do not open and mix the vaccine until ready to begin vaccination. Use vaccine immediately after mixing.

1. Remove the tear-off seal and stopper from the vial containing the dried vaccine.
2. Carefully pour clean, cool, deionized water into the vaccine vial until the vial is approximately two-thirds full.
3. Insert the rubber stopper and shake vigorously until all material is dissolved.
4. The vaccine is now ready for coarse spray use in accordance with the following directions. For best results, be sure to follow directions carefully!

Coarse Spray Administration - For Chickens One Day of Age:

1. Use rehydrated vaccine as indicated for specific coarse spray vaccination machine. For example, a machine which dispenses 20 mL to a box of 100 chickens - total volume for 10,000 doses is 2,000 mL of deionized water. Mix thoroughly.
2. Add the prepared vaccine solution to reservoir on the machine.
3. Prime and adjust machine as instructed in manual accompanying the specific machine.
4. Place boxes holding 100 chickens each on the conveyor belt or in machine. Activate spray head.

Records: Keep a record of vaccine, quantity, serial number, expiration date and place of purchase; the date and time of vaccination; the number, age, breed and locations of chickens; names of operators performing the vaccination and any observed reactions.

Precaution(s): Store vaccine in refrigerator between 2 and 7°C (35 and 45°F).

Do not spill or splash the vaccine.

Use entire contents when first opened.

Burn containers and all unused contents.

Avoid exposure of this vaccine to sunlight.

This product is nonreturnable.

Caution(s): Vaccinate only healthy chickens. Although disease may not be evident, Coccidiosis, Mycoplasma infection, Infectious Bursal disease, Chicken Infectious Anemia, Reovirus infection, Marek's disease and other disease conditions may cause complications or reduce immunity.

All susceptible chickens on the same premises should be vaccinated at the same time.

The revaccination of laying hens with live Newcastle/Bronchitis vaccine may be detrimental to the flock and cannot be generally recommended. This caution applies to all live Newcastle/Bronchitis vaccines currently available. Consult your Intervet representative for more information.

Efforts should be taken to reduce stress conditions at the time of vaccination and during the reaction period.

Do not dilute the vaccine or otherwise stretch the dosage.

Do not use less than 1 dose per bird.

For veterinary use only.

Notice: This vaccine has undergone rigid potency, safety and purity tests and meets Intervet Inc. and USDA requirements. It is designed to stimulate effective immunity when used as directed, but the user must be advised that the response to the product depends upon many factors, including, but not limited to, conditions of storage and handling by the user, administration of the vaccine, health and responsiveness of individual chickens and the degree of field exposure. Therefore, directions should be followed carefully.

This product is not hazardous when used according to directions supplied. A material safety data sheet (MSDS) is available upon request. This and any other consumer information can be obtained by calling Intervet Customer Service at 1-800-441-8272 or 1-302-934-8051.

The use of this vaccine is subject to applicable federal and local laws and regulations.

Use only as directed.

Warning(s): Do not vaccinate within 21 days before slaughter.

Newcastle virus occasionally causes conjunctivitis in humans. Avoid any contact of vaccine with eyes.

Presentation: 10 x 10,000 doses.

U.S. Patent No. 5,750,111

Compendium Code No.: 11062840 20703 AL175

NEW-HOOF™ CONCENTRATE

Vets Plus **Hoof Product**

Ingredient(s):

Ionized Copper (Cu) 0.67%
Nonionized Surfactants 7.00%
Inert Ingredients.......... 92.33%

Indications: For use in footbaths to lower the occurrence of hairy heel wart, foot rot or other foot conditions. NEW-HOOF™ Concentrate contains ionized copper to kill bacteria that can cause foot problems.

Directions for Use: For maximum results, treatment and prevention programs must both be in place.

Treatment: Use the New-Hoof Topical™ ready-to-use spray, or for larger operations, prepare a mixture using one part NEW-HOOF™ Concentrate and two parts water. Clean the hoof as thoroughly as possible as exposure to the NEW-HOOF™ solution is important. Spray the affected area to the saturation point to achieve maximum exposure to the NEW-HOOF™ solution. Continue to spray the affected area prior to every milking until the lesions dry up or drop off. To promote healing, the wound can then be treated with an antiseptic salve and wrapped for protection from the elements.

Prevention: Use NEW-HOOF™ Concentrate in the foot bath as part of your hoof health program. Prepare the foot bath solution using one quart of NEW-HOOF™ Concentrate per 50 gallons of water (1:200 dilution). Change the foot bath every other day or every 500 head. It is recommended that NEW-HOOF™ be used in rotation with other prevention protocols.

Precaution(s): Keep in a cool, dry place. Avoid freezing. Environmentally safe.

Disposal: NEW-HOOF™ is environmentally friendly. After use, NEW-HOOF™ may be disposed of in the manure lagoon without detrimental effects on the natural digestion process. As with any product, follow local guidelines for soil or foliar application.

Caution(s): Keep out of the reach of children. Can cause eye irritation. In case of eye contact, flush for 15 minutes with cool water. If irritation persists call your physician.

For animal use only.

Discussion: Management Information: NEW-HOOF™ Concentrate/New-Hoof Topical™ is only part of the solution for proper hoof care. Healthy hooves are dependent on proper nutrition, clean environment, good management and proper health care. Any one element alone will not prevent or control hoof problems.

Presentation: 4 x 1 gallon (3.8 L) containers per case, 5 gallon pail, 15 and 55 gallon drums by special order.

Compendium Code No.: 10730111

NEW-HOOF TOPICAL™

Vets Plus **Hoof Product**

Ingredient(s):

Ionized copper (Cu) 0.268%
Non-ionized surfactants 2.800%
Inert ingredients 96.932%

Indications: For topical use on hooves to treat hairy heel wart, foot rot or other foot conditions. NEW-HOOF TOPICAL™ provides ionized copper to kill bacteria that can cause foot problems.

Directions for Use: For maximum results, treatment and prevention programs must both be in place.

Treatment: NEW HOOF TOPICAL™ is a convenient ready-to-use solution designed for direct application to the hoof. Clean the hoof as thoroughly as possible as exposure to the New-Hoof™ solution is important. Spray the affected area to the saturation point to achieve maximum exposure to the New-Hoof™ solution. Continue to spray the affected area during each milking until the lesions dry up or drop off. To promote healing, the wound can then be treated with an antiseptic salve and wrapped for protection from the elements.

Prevention: Use New-Hoof™ Concentrate in the foot bath as part of your hoof health program. Prepare the foot bath solution using one quart of New-Hoof™ Concentrate per 50 gallons of water (1:200 dilution). Change the foot bath every other day or every 500 head. It is recommended that New-Hoof™ be used in rotation with other prevention protocols.

Precaution(s): Keep in a cool, dry place. Avoid freezing. Environmentally safe.

Caution(s): Can cause eye irritation. In case of eye contact, flush for 15 minutes with cool water. If irritation persist, call your physician.

Keep out of the reach of children. For animal use only.

Discussion: Management Information: New-Hoof™/NEW-HOOF TOPICAL™ is only part of the solution for proper hoof care. Healthy hooves are dependent on proper nutrition, clean environment, good management and proper health care. Any one element alone will not prevent or control hoof problems. New-Hoof™/NEW-HOOF TOPICAL™ is only one part of the total program, where management is the key. Any one element alone will not prevent or control hoof infections.

Presentation: 1 quart (0.95 Liter).

Compendium Code No.: 10730100

NEWVAX®

Schering-Plough **Vaccine**

Newcastle Disease Vaccine, B_1 Type, B_1 Strain Live Virus

U.S. Vet. Lic. No.: 165A

Active Ingredient(s): NEWVAX® is a live virus vaccine of chicken embryo origin containing the mild B_1 Newcastle strain. This virus has the ability to stimulate protection against a wide variety of Newcastle field strains while causing only a minimum of respiratory distress in healthy birds. The vaccine contains gentamicin as a preservative.

Indications: For the vaccination of healthy chickens as an aid in preventing Newcastle disease through vaccination by the water route at four days of age or older (initial vaccination) or the spray route (revaccination).

Dosage and Administration:

When to Vaccinate:

Initial Vaccination (Water): Four (4) days to 16 weeks of age.

Birds vaccinated initially before four (4) weeks of age should be revaccinated as below.

Revaccination (Spray): Four (4) weeks of age or older.

Vaccination Program: The development of a durable, strong protection to both diseases depends upon the use of an effective vaccination program as well as many circumstances such as administration techniques, environment and flock health at the time of vaccination. Also, the immune response to one (1) vaccination under field conditions is seldom complete for all animals within a given flock. Even when vaccination is successful, the protection stimulated in individual animals against different diseases may not be life-long. Therefore, a program of periodic revaccination may be necessary.

Preparation of the Vaccine:

1. Assemble the equipment needed to vaccinate the entire flock at one time.
2. Do not open and mix the vaccine until ready for use.
3. Remove the tear-off aluminum seal from the vaccine vial without disturbing the rubber stopper.
4. Use cool, clean, nonchlorinated tap water to which powdered milk has been added as directed under How to Vaccinate.
5. Hold the vial submerged in a pail of water or under a running stream of water. Lift the lip of the rubber stopper so that the water (milk added) is sucked into the vial.
6. Reseat the stopper and shake to thoroughly dissolve the vaccine.

How to Vaccinate:

1. Drinking Water Method: Do not mix the vaccine into the drinking water until ready for use. Drinking water for vaccination should be mixed with powdered milk to prevent inactivation from chlorine or other water additives and also to stabilize the vaccine virus. The powdered milk should be added to the water at the rate of one (1) heaped teaspoon per three (3) U.S. gallons or 2.5 imperial gallons (3 g per 11 L); or one (1) heaped cupful per 80 U.S. gallons or 66 imperial gallons (90 g per 300 L).
   Withhold water from the birds for several hours before vaccinating so that the birds are thirsty. Thoroughly clean and rinse all watering containers so that no residual disinfectants remain. Dilute the vaccine immediately before use with cool, clean, nonchlorinated water (milk added). Pour the dissolved vaccine material into the following amounts of water and mix thoroughly.

Each 5,000 Birds	U.S. Gallons	Imperial Gallons	Metric Liters
4 days to 4 weeks	12.5	10	50
4 weeks to 8 weeks	25.0	20	100
Over 8 weeks	50.0	40	200

   Distribute the diluted vaccine so that all of the birds are able to drink within a 1-hour period and do not add any more water until the vaccine is consumed. Avoid placing water in direct sunlight.
2. Spray Method: Use this method for revaccination only. Proper spray application of the vaccine is only accomplished through the use of a clean sprayer emitting a very a fine aerosol (mist) which floats and disseminates easily through the air. Only use the spray method in houses that can be closed during vaccination and for at least 15 minutes thereafter. Cross winds, drafts, or operating ventilation fans prevent effective application.
   Rehydrate the vaccine according to the above instructions. Further dilute each 5,000 doses of vaccine to 500 mL using distilled water. Place the vaccine in the sprayer and set at the lowest output. Spray droplets of 17 to 20 microns average size and the application of about 700 doses of vaccine per minute are desirable.
   Apply the vaccine over all of the birds at the rate of one (1) dose per square foot, or one (1) dose per bird, whichever is greater.
   Use protective goggles during vaccination to avoid eye contact with Newcastle vaccine.

Records: Keep a record of the vaccine type, quantity, serial number, expiration date, and place of purchase; the date and time of vaccination; the number, age, breed, and location of the birds; the names of operators performing the vaccination; and any observed reactions.

Precaution(s): Store at 35° to 45° F (2° to 7°C).

Caution(s): For veterinary use only.

1. Vaccinate healthy birds only. Although disease may not be evident, coccidiosis, chronic respiratory disease, mycoplasma infection, lymphoid leukosis, infectious bursal disease, Marek's disease, or other disease conditions may cause serious complications or reduce protection.
2. All birds within a house should be vaccinated on the same day. Isolate other susceptible birds on the premises from the birds being vaccinated.
3. In outbreak situations, vaccinate healthy birds first, progressing toward outbreak areas in order to vaccinate diseased birds last.
4. Do not spill or spatter the vaccine. Use the entire contents of the vial when first opened. Burn the empty bottles, caps, and all unused vaccine and accessories.
5. Wash hands thoroughly after using the vaccine.
6. Do not dilute the vaccine or otherwise stretch the dosage.
7. Newcastle virus occasionally causes inflammation of the eyelids in humans, lasting two or three days. Avoid contact of the eyes with the vaccine.

Warning(s): Do not vaccinate within 21 days before slaughter.

Presentation: Supplied in 10 x 5,000 dose units.

Compendium Code No.: 10471360

N

NEW Z® DIAZINON INSECTICIDE CATTLE EAR TAGS

Farnam **Insecticide Ear Tags**

EPA Reg. No.: 270-260

Active Ingredient(s):

Diazinon [0,0-Diethyl 0-(2-isopropyl-6-methyl-4-pyrimidinyl) phosphorothioate] 18.0%
Piperonyl Butoxide Technical* 2.0%
Other Ingredients 80.0%

*Equivalent to 1.6% (butylcarbityl)(6-propylpiperonyl) ether and 0.4% related compounds.

Indications: For use on beef and non-lactating dairy cattle to control horn flies (including pyrethroid resistant populations), and as an aid in control of face flies, house flies, stable flies, gulf coast ticks and spinose ear ticks.

Directions for Use: It is a violation of Federal Law to use this product in a manner inconsistent with its labeling. This labeling must be in the possession of the user at the time of pesticide application.

For optimum pest control and to minimize development of insect resistance, apply two tags per animal (one in each ear) in May to June or when flies first become a problem in the spring. Replace as necessary. NEW Z® Diazinon Insecticide Cattle Ear Tags have been proven effective against pyrethroid resistant Horn Flies for a minimum of 4 months. Remove tags in the fall. Calves less than 3 months of age should not be tagged as ear damage may result. Tags are easily applied and designed for use with the unique New Z® Applicator.

Tagging Instructions: Refer to illustrations below.

1. Put pin in tag loading position.

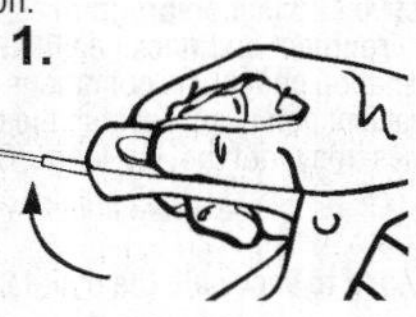

2. Insert pin in tag.

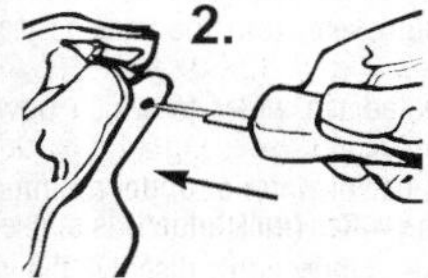

3. Straighten self-piercing tip and push down onto pin. Seat the tag fully on the pin.

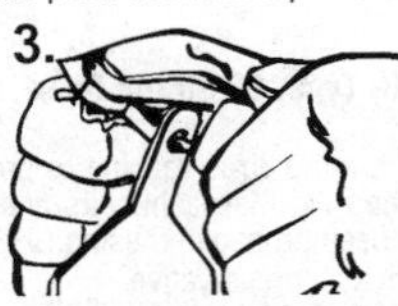

4. Rotate tag to the side. Flip loaded pin down into tagging position.

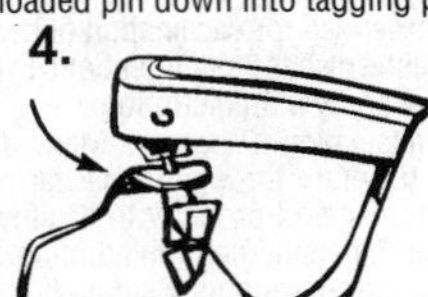

5. To insert tag in ear, squeeze handles firmly together.
   Suggested tagging position. Try not to use existing ear tag holes.

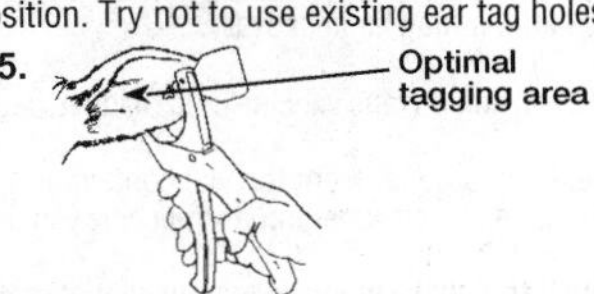

6. To remove tagger pull away from animal's ear - Tagger pin automatically flips up to ensure no ripped ears during tagging.
   Do not release handles!

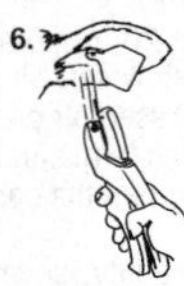

Precautionary Statements: Hazards to Humans:

Caution: Harmful if absorbed through the skin or if swallowed. Avoid contact with skin and eyes. Wash thoroughly with soap and water after handling and before eating or smoking. Avoid contamination of feed and foodstuffs. If rubbed in eyes, flush with plenty of water. If swallowed or if eye irritation persists, call a physician. Wear clean gloves daily when applying tags.

Note to Physician: This product is a cholinesterase inhibitor. If symptoms of cholinesterase inhibition are present, atropine sulfate by injection is antidotal. 2-PAM is also antidotal and may be administered, but only in conjunction with atropine.

Environmental Hazards: This pesticide is toxic to fish. Do not apply directly to water. Do not contaminate water by disposal of used tags.

Storage and Disposal: Do not contaminate water, food or feed by storage or disposal.

Storage: Store in cool location away from direct sunlight. Opened pouches containing ear tags should be resealed for storage.

Pesticide Disposal: Remove tags before slaughter. Securely wrap used tags in several layers of newspaper and discard in trash.

Container Disposal: Do not reuse bag. Discard bag in trash.

Warning(s): Remove tags before slaughter.

Keep out of reach of children.

Disclaimer: Notice of Warranty: Farnam Companies, Inc. makes no warranty of merchantability, fitness for any particular purpose, or otherwise expressed or implied concerning this product or its uses which extend beyond the use of the product under normal conditions in accordance with the statements made on the label.

Presentation: 20 x 12 g tags.

Compendium Code No.: 10000720 0BO

NEW Z® PERMETHRIN INSECTICIDE CATTLE EAR TAGS

Farnam **Insecticide Ear Tags**

EPA Reg. No.: 52637-1-270

Active Ingredient(s):

Permethrin (3-phenoxphenyl) methyl (±) Cis, trans-3-(2,2-dichloroethenyl)-2,2-dimethylopropane carboxylate* 10.0%
Inert Ingredients 90.0%

*cis/trans ratio: min. 20% (±) Cis and max. 80% (±) trans.

Indications: Controls horn flies, face flies, Gulf Coast ticks and spinose ear ticks on dairy and beef cattle and calves.

Directions for Use: It is a violation of Federal Law to use this product in a manner inconsistent with its labeling.

Attach one tag to each ear when flies or ticks first appear in the spring. Tags may remain effective for up to 4 or 5 months.

Replace as necessary.

Tags are easily applied and designed for use with the unique New Z® Applicator.

Tagging Instructions: Refer to illustrations below.

1. Put pin in tag loading position.

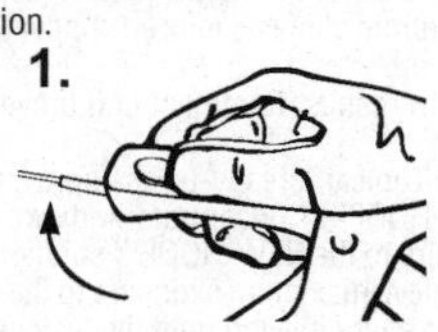

2. Insert pin in tag.

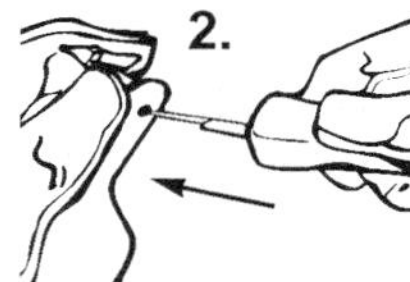

3. Straighten self-piercing tip and push down onto pin. Seat the tag fully on the pin.

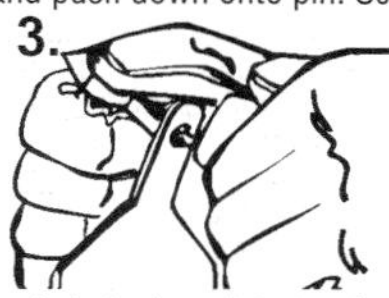

4. Rotate tag to the side. Flip loaded pin down into tagging position.

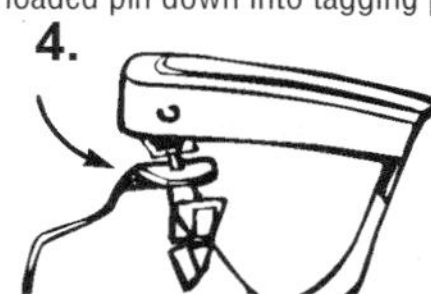

5. To insert tag in ear, squeeze handles firmly together.
   Suggested tagging position. Try not to use existing ear tag holes.

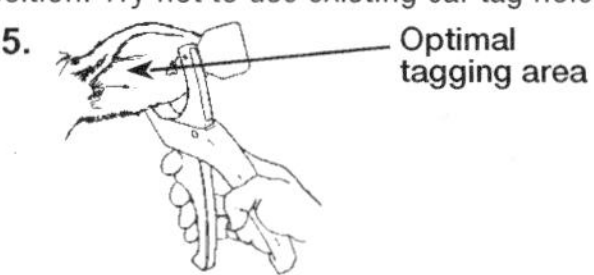

6. To remove tagger pull away from animal's ear - Tagger pin automatically flips up to ensure no ripped ears during tagging.
   Do not release handles!

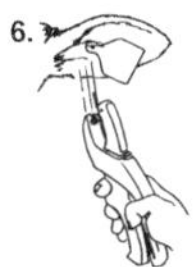

Precautionary Statements: Hazards to Humans and Domestic Animals:

Caution: Wash thoroughly with soap and water after handling and before eating or smoking. Avoid contamination of feed and foodstuffs.

Environmental Hazards: This pesticide is toxic to fish. Do not add directly to water. Do not contaminate water by disposal of used tags.

Storage and Disposal: Store in cool place. Do not contaminate water, food or feed by storage or disposal. Remove tags before slaughter. Do not reuse bag. Discard bag in trash along with used tags.

Warning(s): Remove tags before slaughter.

Keep out of reach of children.

Disclaimer: Notice of Warranty: Farnam Companies, Inc. makes no warranty of merchantability, fitness for any particular purpose, or otherwise expressed or implied concerning this product or its uses which extend beyond the use of the product under normal conditions in accordance with the statements made on the label.

Presentation: 20 x 10 g tags.

Compendium Code No.: 10000730 9EE9

NEXABAND® LIQUID

Abbott **Surgical Glue**

Description: NEXABAND® Liquid topical tissue adhesive (2-octyl cyanoacrylate) contains a purified cyanoacrylate monomer and stabilizers. NEXABAND® Liquid topical tissue adhesive is a colorless formulation that has been demonstrated to be useful for closing surgical incisions in cat declaw procedures.

Indications: NEXABAND® Liquid topical tissue adhesive is indicated for veterinary use only. NEXABAND® Liquid topical tissue adhesive is indicated for closing surgical incisions in cat declaw procedures.

Pharmacology: Action: NEXABAND® Liquid topical tissue adhesive is a monomeric formulation which, upon contact with an alkaline pH environment, polymerizes to form a thin, flexible bandage. NEXABAND® Liquid topical tissue adhesive polymerizes within seconds after contact with moist wound surfaces. Polymerization is slower on a dry field.

Tissue regeneration and wound healing occur under the applied NEXABAND® Liquid topical tissue adhesive layer. The NEXABAND® Liquid topical tissue adhesive bandage is sloughed naturally as healing occurs.

Dosage and Administration:

1. The successful application of NEXABAND® Liquid topical tissue adhesive requires proper preparation of the wound site. If antiseptic treatment is desired for the wound site, wash the area with a povidone or chlorhexidine gluconate (4%) solution. Do not use other topical ointments or salves as they may interfere with the formation of the NEXABAND® Liquid topical tissue adhesive bandage.
2. After preparing the wound site, pat the wound with dry, sterile gauze to remove excess fluid and assure direct tissue contact for adherence of NEXABAND® Liquid topical tissue adhesive to the skin by removing any accumulating blood or moisture from the wound. Do not apply NEXABAND® Liquid topical tissue adhesive over a pool of blood or fluid. Moisture accelerates the polymerization and may affect wound closure results by causing premature sloughing of the bandage.
3. Do not bury this product. It metabolizes very slowly, which could lead to the development of a foreign body reaction.
4. Insert the extension tube into the tip of the NEXABAND® Liquid topical tissue adhesive bottle. The extension tube can be bent, improving the control over the size and placement of the drops.

   Note: The extension tube can be left in place over an extended period of time. If replacing the cap, always remember to wipe clean the tip on the NEXABAND® Liquid topical tissue adhesive bottle before replacing the cap to prevent sealing the cap onto the bottle.
5. Approximate wound edges with gloved fingers or sterile forceps. Hold the tip of the bottle, fitted with the extension tube, slightly above the wound. Slowly apply NEXABAND® Liquid topical tissue adhesive drops until the wound is completely covered. The product coverage should extend slightly beyond the wound, onto healthy tissue.

For declaw procedures: Apply 1-2 drops per socket.

Note: Do not over apply NEXABAND® Liquid topical tissue adhesive. A thin, light coat is better than a thick, heavy coat.

Contraindication(s): NEXABAND® Liquid topical tissue adhesive is contraindicated in the management of infected and deep puncture wounds. NEXABAND® Liquid topical tissue adhesive is not intended to be used as a replacement for suture material that would normally be buried (i.e. absorbable sutures).

Precaution(s): Storage Conditions: Store NEXABAND® Liquid topical tissue adhesive at room temperature. Protect from freezing and extreme heat.

Avoid contact with surgical instruments and apparatus (such as gloves). Avoid contact with clothing since the stain will be permanent.

The product should not be used beyond the indicated expiration date.

Caution(s): Avoid unintended placement on skin and eyes.

Removal of NEXABAND® Liquid Topical Tissue Adhesive: NEXABAND® Liquid topical tissue adhesive can be removed from skin or other surfaces with acetone.

Presentation: NEXABAND® Liquid topical tissue adhesive (2-octyl cyanoacrylate) is supplied in individual packages, list number 5295, with each package containing: One dropper bottle containing 1.5 mL (approximately 150 drops), extension tubes and a package insert.

Manufactured by: Closure Medical Corporation, Raleigh, NC 27616.

Compendium Code No.: 10240140 04-3629/R2

NEXABAND® S/C

Abbott **Surgical Glue**

Description: NEXABAND® S/C topical tissue adhesive (2-octyl cyanoacrylate) contains a purified cyanoacrylate monomer, thickener and stabilizers. NEXABAND® S/C topical tissue adhesive is a colorless formulation that has been demonstrated to be useful for skin closure in spays, neuters and other soft tissue surgeries.

Indications: NEXABAND® S/C topical tissue adhesive is indicated for veterinary use only. NEXABAND® S/C topical tissue adhesive is indicated as a tissue bridge, providing subcutaneous suture is used (when appropriate), in the following procedures: Spays, Lacerations, Neuters, Laparotomies, Tumor removals, Incisions.

Pharmacology: Action: NEXABAND® S/C topical tissue adhesive is a monomeric 2-octyl cyanoacrylate formulation, which, upon contact with most bodily fluids or with an alkaline pH environment, polymerizes to form a thin, flexible, waterproof bridge/bandage. When NEXABAND® S/C topical tissue adhesive is used along an approximated surgical incision, the initial contact of the product will rapidly polymerize at the tissue junction. The remaining material that forms the tissue bridge will polymerize at a slower rate. The formation of the tissue bridge holds the approximated wound edges together.

NEXABAND® S/C topical tissue adhesive has been formulated as a colorless fluid to maximize visibility of approximated wound edges during application. Tissue regeneration and wound healing occurs under the NEXABAND® S/C topical tissue adhesive layer and is sloughed naturally as the incision heals.

Dosage and Administration:

1. The successful application of NEXABAND® S/C topical tissue adhesive requires proper preparation of the wound site. If antiseptic treatment is desired for the wound site, wash the area with a povidone or chlorhexidine gluconate (4%) solution. Do not use other topical ointments or salves as they may interfere with the formation of the NEXABAND® S/C topical tissue adhesive bandage.
2. The normal surgical procedure should be followed with the exception of the skin-closing step. Subcutaneous tissue should be closed with absorbable suture, resulting in a tension-free wound.
3. Suture the subcutaneous tissue to approximate the skin edges as closely as possible minimizing exposed subcutaneous tissue between skin edges. If gaps in the primary tissue closure are apparent, press the skin edges together with gloved fingers or sterile forceps while slowly applying the NEXABAND® S/C topical tissue adhesive.
4. Insert the pipette into the bottle. Apply pressure then release to draw the NEXABAND® S/C topical tissue adhesive into the pipette.
5. Hold the pipette tip slightly above the incision line and squeeze the pipette to release the NEXABAND® S/C topical tissue adhesive in a thin line to the surface of the approximated skin edges. Do not over apply.
6. The wound edges need to be manually apposed for approximately 1 minute or until adequate wound strength is achieved. Full polymerization is expected when the top NEXABAND® S/C topical tissue adhesive layer is no longer tacky.
7. Do not bury this product. It metabolizes very slowly, which could lead to the development of a foreign body reaction.
8. Do not apply NEXABAND® S/C topical tissue adhesive over a pool of blood or fluid. This will cause improper polymerization and adherence to the skin, resulting in the premature sloughing of the NEXABAND® S/C topical tissue adhesive.

Contraindication(s): NEXABAND® S/C topical tissue adhesive is contraindicated in the management of infected or deep puncture wounds. NEXABAND® S/C topical tissue adhesive is not intended to be used as a replacement for suture material that would normally be buried (i.e. absorbable sutures).

Precaution(s): Storage Conditions: Store NEXABAND® S/C topical tissue adhesive at room temperature. Protect from freezing and extreme heat.

Avoid contact with surgical instruments and apparatus (such as gloves). Before replacing the screw-top cap, wipe excess solution from the lip of the bottle with an absorbent lint-free wipe so as not to seal the top to the container. The product should not be used beyond the indicated expiration date.

Caution(s): Avoid unintended placement on skin and eyes.

Removal of NEXABAND® S/C Topical Tissue Adhesive: NEXABAND® S/C topical tissue adhesive can be removed from skin or other surfaces with acetone.

Presentation: NEXABAND® S/C topical tissue adhesive (2-octyl cyanoacrylate) is supplied in individual packages, list number 5297, with each package containing: One 1.5 mL bottle, disposable pipettes and a package insert.

Manufactured by: Closure Medical Corporation, Raleigh, NC 27616.

Compendium Code No.: 10240150 04-3630/R2

NFZ® PUFFER

AgriLabs **Topical Antibacterial**

NADA No.: 011-154

Active Ingredient(s): Contains 0.2% nitrofurazone in a water soluble base.

Indications: For pinkeye in cattle, sheep and goats, eye and ear infections in dogs and cats, and surface wounds, cuts and abrasions on all livestock.

Dosage and Administration: Shake or rotate to loosen powder.

For pinkeye in cattle, sheep and goats and eye infections in dogs and cats: Remove the cap and squeeze the container to force a stream of powder directly into the eye. Repeat the treatment once a day. Animals with pinkeye are sensitive to sunlight. Confine in darkened quarters if possible. If there is not improvement after four (4) days, a new diagnosis should be made or a veterinarian consulted.

For ear infections in dogs and cats: Clean out the inside of the ear and the ear canal with a cotton pledget. Prepared cotton swabs are best for cleaning out the ear canal. Insert the nozzle of the container into the ear canal and squeeze twice. Repeat once a day until an improvement is noted.

For surface wounds, cuts and abrasions on all livestock: Apply once a day until danger from infection is eliminated, or until healing takes place.

Precaution(s): Protect from heat.

Caution(s): Keep out of the reach of children. Restricted drug (California) - Use only as directed.

Human Warnings: Carcinogenesis: Nitrofurazone has been shown to produce mammary tumors in rats and ovarian tumors in mice.

Some people may be hypersensitive to the product. Either wear gloves when applying, or wash hands afterwards.

Warning(s): A withdrawal period has not been established in preruminating calves. Do not use on veal calves.

Presentation: 1.59 oz. puffer bottles.

Compendium Code No.: 10580741

NFZ® PUFFER

AgriPharm **Topical Antibacterial**

NADA No.: 011-154

Active Ingredient(s): Contains 0.2% nitrofurazone in a water soluble base.

Indications: For pink eye in cattle, sheep and goats, eye and ear infections in dogs and cats, and surface wounds, cuts and abrasions on all livestock.

Dosage and Administration: For Pink Eye in Cattle, Sheep and Goats and eye infections in Dogs and Cats — remove cap and squeeze container to force a stream of powder directly into the eye. Repeat treatment daily. If there is no improvement after 4 days, a new diagnosis should be made or a veterinarian consulted.

(Animals with pink eye are sensitive to sunlight. Confine in darkened quarters if possible.)

For Ear Infections in Dogs and Cats — clean out inside of ear and ear canal with cotton pledget. Prepared cotton swabs which may be obtained at any drug store are best for cleaning out the ear canal. Insert nozzle of container into ear canal and squeeze twice. Repeat daily until improvement is noted.

For Surface Wounds, Cuts and Abrasions on all livestock — apply daily until danger from infection is eliminated or until healing takes place.

Precaution(s): Protect from heat.

Warning(s): A withdrawal period has not been established for this product in preruminating calves. Do not use in calves to be processed for veal.

Human Warnings: Carcinogenesis: Nitrofurazone has been shown to produce mammary tumors in rats and ovarian tumors in mice.

Some people may be hypersensitive to this product. Either wear gloves when applying or wash the hands afterwards. Restricted drug (California). Keep out of reach of children.

Presentation: 1.59 oz (45 g).

® nfz is a registered trademark of Hess & Clark, Inc.

Compendium Code No.: 14570661

NFZ® PUFFER

Aspen **Topical Antibacterial**

NADA No.: 011-154

Active Ingredient(s): Contains 0.2% Nitrofurazone in a water soluble base.

Indications: For eye and ear infections in dogs and cats. For surface wounds, cuts and abrasions.

Directions: Shake or rotate to loosen powder.

For Eye Infections in Dogs and Cats — remove cap and squeeze container to force a stream of powder directly into the eye. Repeat treatment daily. If there is no improvement after 4 days, a new diagnosis should be made or a veterinarian consulted.

For Ear Infections in Dogs and Cats — clean out inside of ear and ear canal with cotton pledget. Prepared cotton swabs which may be obtained at any drug store are best for cleaning out the ear canal. Insert nozzle of container into ear canal and squeeze twice. Repeat daily until improvement is noted.

For Surface Wounds, Cuts and Abrasions — apply daily until danger from infection is eliminated or until healing takes place.

Precaution(s): Protect from heat.

Caution(s): Federal Law prohibits the use of this product in food-producing animals.

Restricted Drug—(California). Use only as directed.

Warning(s): Human Warnings: Carcinogenesis: Nitrofurazone has been shown to product mammary tumors in rats and ovarian tumors in mice.

Some people may be hypersensitive to this product. Either wear gloves when applying, or wash hands afterwards.

Keep out of reach of children.

Presentation: 1.59 oz (45 gm) container.

NFZ is a registered trademark of Hess & Clark, Inc.

Compendium Code No.: 14750582 AUT-23

NFZ® PUFFER

Durvet **Topical Antibacterial**

NADA No.: 011-154

Active Ingredient(s): Contains 0.2% Nitrofurazone in a water soluble base.

Indications: For eye and ear infections in dogs and cats, and surface wounds, cuts and abrasions.

Directions: Shake or rotate to loosen powder.

For Eye Infections in Dogs and Cats: Remove cap and squeeze container to force a stream of powder directly into the eye. Repeat treatment daily. If there is no improvement after 4 days a new diagnosis should be made or a veterinarian consulted.

For Ear Infections in Dogs and Cats: Clean out inside of ear and ear canal with a cotton pledget. Prepared cotton swabs are best for cleaning out the ear canal. Insert nozzle of container into ear canal and squeeze twice. Repeat daily until improvement is noted.

For Surface Wounds, Cuts and Abrasions: Apply daily until danger from infection is eliminated, or until healing takes place.

Precaution(s): Protect from heat.

Caution(s): Federal law prohibits the use of this product in food producing animals.

Restricted drug - (California). Use only as directed.

Warning(s): Human Warnings: Carcinogenesis: Nitrofurazone has been shown to produce mammary tumors in rats and ovarian tumors in mice.

Some people may be hypersensitive to this product. Either wear gloves when applying, or wash hands afterwards. Keep out of reach of children.

Presentation: 1.59 oz. (45 g) puffer bottles.

® NFZ is a registered trademark of Hess and Clark, Inc.

Compendium Code No.: 10841182 5/99

NFZ® PUFFER

Loveland **Topical Antibacterial**

NADA No.: 011-154

Active Ingredient(s): Contains 0.2% nitrofurazone in a water soluble base.

Indications: For pink eye in cattle, sheep and goats, eye and ear infections in dogs and cats, and surface wounds, cuts and abrasions on all livestock.

Dosage and Administration: Shake or rotate to loosen powder.

For pink eye in cattle, sheep and goats and eye infections in dogs and cats: Remove the cap and squeeze the container to force a stream of powder directly into the eye. Repeat the treatment once a day. If there is not improvement after four (4) days, a new diagnosis should be made or a veterinarian consulted.

(Animals with pink eye are sensitive to sunlight. Confine in darkened quarters if possible.)

For ear infections in dogs and cats: Clean out the inside of the ear and the ear canal with a cotton pledget. Prepared cotton swabs are best for cleaning out the ear canal. Insert the nozzle of the container into the ear canal and squeeze twice. Repeat once a day until an improvement is noted.

For surface wounds, cuts and abrasions on all livestock: Apply once a day until danger from infection is eliminated, or until healing takes place.

Precaution(s): Protect from heat.

Caution(s): Keep out of the reach of children. Restricted drug (California). Use only as directed.

Human Warnings: Carcinogenesis: Nitrofurazone has been shown to produce mammary tumors in rats and ovarian tumors in mice.

Some people may be hypersensitive to the product. Wear gloves when applying, or wash the hands after use.

Warning(s): A withdrawal period has not been established in preruminating calves.

Do not use on veal calves.

Presentation: 1.59 oz. puffer bottles.

Compendium Code No.: 10860181

NFZ® WOUND DRESSING

Loveland **Topical Antibacterial**

Nitrofurazone Preparation

NADA No.: 140-851

Active Ingredient(s):

Nitrofurazone 0.2%

In a water soluble base.

Indications: NFZ® Wound Dressing is a water soluble antibacterial ointment for the prevention or treatment of surface bacterial infections of wounds, burns and cutaneous ulcers. For use on dogs, cats and horses (not for food use).

Dosage and Administration: Apply directly onto the lesion with a spatula, or first place on a piece of gauze. The application of a bandage is optional.

The preparation should be in contact with the lesion for at least 24 hours. The dressing may be changed several times a day or left on the lesion for a longer period.

Precaution(s): Avoid exposure to direct sunlight, strong fluorescent lighting, excessive heat and alkaline materials.

Caution(s): Keep out of the reach of children.

In case of deep or puncture wounds or serious burns, use only as recommended by a veterinarian. If redness, irritation, or swelling persists or increases, discontinue use and consult a veterinarian.

Avoid exposure to alkaline material and fluorescent lighting.

Human Warnings: Carcinogenesis: Nitrofurazone has been shown to produce mammary tumors in rats and ovarian tumors in mice.

Some people may be hypersensitive to the product. Wear gloves when applying, or wash hands after use.

Warning(s): Do not use on horses intended for food purposes.

Presentation: 16 oz. (453.6 g) containers.

Compendium Code No.: 10860190

NIA-BOL™

Great States **Niacin**

Niacin Bolus Nutritional Supplement

Guaranteed Analysis: Each 15 g bolus contains:

Niacin (Nicotinic Acid). . . . . 6 g

Ingredients: Niacin, dicalcium phosphate, microcrystalline cellulose and magnesium stearate.

Indications: For use as a supplemental nutritional source of niacin when supplementation is indicated in high-producing dairy cows during calving time and the start of lactation.

Directions for Use: During calving time administer bolus orally beginning 1 or 2 days prior to calving and 8-10 days following calving for a total of 10 days. Administer one bolus both in the morning and in the evening. Bolus may be administered either with balling gun or crushed and mixed with feed.

Precaution(s): Store in controlled room temperature between 15-30°C (59-86°F). Keep lid tightly closed when not in use.

Caution(s): For animal use only.

Warning(s): Keep out of reach of children.

Presentation: Jars of 20 boluses.

Compendium Code No.: 14110021

NIACIN BOLUS

Vets Plus **Niacin**

Guaranteed Analysis: Per bolus (min):

Nicotinic Acid .... 6.0 g

Ingredients: Dextrose, nicotinic acid, lactose, and magnesium stearate.

Indications: NIACIN BOLUS is a nutritional supplement providing nicotinic acid for high producing dairy cows.

Dosage and Administration: Administer 2 boluses per day (1 in morning and 1 in evening) for additional nutritional support of nicotinic acid.

Precaution(s): Keep lid tightly closed. Store in a cool, dry place.

Caution(s): Keep out of reach of children. For animal use only.

Presentation: 20 boluses, 15 g each.

Compendium Code No.: 10730120

NIACIN-ENERGY DRENCH PLUS VITAMINS

AgriLabs **Acetonemia Preparation**

Oral Nutritional Supplement For Ketotic Cattle

Guaranteed Analysis: (per 200 mL feeding)

Niacin, Min. .... 11,500 mg
Vitamin B_6 .... 60 mg
Vitamin B_{12} .... 600 mcg
Propylene Glycol .... 90 gm

Indications: Use on every fresh heifer and on ketotic cows NIACIN-ENERGY DRENCH provides niacin to counteract ketosis, propylene glycol for the energy deficient heifer and B vitamins to stimulate the appetite.

Dosage and Administration: Provide one 200 mL feeding immediately following calving. Give additional feedings as needed. Administer using a drench gun. The drench should be administered slowly between the cheek and the teeth. Do not administer to a cow without a swallowing reflex.

Presentation: 1 gallon.

Compendium Code No.: 10580750

NIACIN-ENERGY DRENCH PLUS VITAMINS

Durvet **Acetonemia Preparation**

Guaranteed Analysis: (per 200 mL feeding)

Niacin, Min. .... 11,500 Mg
Vitamin B_6, Min. .... 60 Mg
Vitamin B_{12}, Min. .... 600 Mcg

Ingredients: Propylene glycol, niacin, vitamin A acetate, D-activated animal sterol, cyanocobalamin, D-alpha tocopheryl acetate, riboflavin supplement, calcium pantothenate, folic acid, pyridoxine hydrochloride, choline bitartrate and ascorbic acid.

Indications: Use on every fresh heifer and on ketotic cows. NIACIN-ENERGY DRENCH provides niacin to counteract ketosis, propylene glycol for the energy deficient fresh heifer and B vitamins to stimulate the appetite.

Dosage and Administration: Shake well before use. Provide on 200 mL feeding immediately following calving. Give additional feedings as needed. Administer using a drench gun. The drench should be administered slowly between the cheek and the teeth. Do not administer to a cow without a swallowing reflex.

Warning(s): For animal use only. Not for human use. Keep out of reach of children.

Presentation: 3.785 L (1 gallon).

Compendium Code No.: 10841190

NICARB® 25%

Phibro **Feed Medication**

(nicarbazin) Type A Medicated Article with Microtracer®

NADA No.: 009-476

Active Ingredient(s):

Nicarbazin 25%

Ingredients: Wheat Middlings, Soybean Oil and Microtracer®.

Indications: As an aid in preventing outbreaks of cecal *(Eimeria tenella)* and intestinal *(E. acervulina, E. maxima, E. necatrix, and E. brunetti)* coccidiosis in chickens.

Directions: Mixing Directions: NICARB® (nicarbazin) 25% should be thoroughly and evenly mixed in the feed in accordance with current good manufacturing practice for feed. Type C medicated feeds should contain 0.0125% nicarbazin. Uniformly mix 1 pound of NICARB® 25% with 1,999 pounds of feed ingredients to produce a finished feed containing 0.0125% nicarbazin.

Suggested Directions for Feed Tags:

Use Directions: Use nicarbazin Type C medicated feed as the only ration from the time chicks are placed on litter until past the time when coccidiosis is ordinarily a hazard.

Contraindication(s): Do not use as a treatment for outbreaks of coccidiosis. Do not use in flushing mashes.

Caution(s): To be used only in the manufacture of registered feeds.

If losses exceed 0.5 percent in a 2-day period, obtain an accurate diagnosis and follow the instructions of your veterinarian or poultry pathologist.

Broilers fed feed medicated with NICARB® 25% may show reduced heat tolerance when exposed to high temperature and high humidity to which they have not been accustomed and under severe conditions, fatalities may result. An ample supply of drinking water and adequate ventilation will improve the birds' tolerance of heat.

Warning(s): Discontinue medication 4 days before marketing the birds for human consumption to allow for elimination of the drug from the edible tissue.

Do not feed to laying hens in production. Keep this and all drugs out of the reach of children.

Presentation: 50 lb (22.68 kg).

NICARB Reg. TM Koffolk, Inc.
Microtracer Reg. TM Micro-Tracers, Inc., San Francisco, CA.

Compendium Code No.: 36930370 101-9018-01

NIK STOP® STYPTIC POWDER

Tomlyn **Hemostatic**

Ingredient(s): Benzocaine 0.2%, ferric subsulfate, bentonite, diatomaceous earth, aluminum chloride, ammonium chloride, copper sulfate, iodoform.

Indications: An aid to stop minor external bleeding and to temporarily relieve pain caused by clipping nails or dew claws and minor cuts.

Dosage and Administration: Apply directly to bleeding area. Pressure bandage is sometimes required if nails are cut too short. If bleeding persists, or in the case of a deep puncture wounds, consult your veterinarian immediately.

Caution(s): For external animal use only. Keep out of reach of children and pets.

Presentation: 1 oz (28.4 g).

Compendium Code No.: 11220100

NITRO-CHOL®

Arko **Vaccine**

Pasteurella multocida vaccine, Avirulent Live Culture, Avian Isolate

U.S. Vet. Lic. No.: 337

Active Ingredient(s): NITRO-CHOL® is a live bacterial vaccine, preserved as a frozen preparation. Freezing maximizes the numbers of organisms preserved and viability at the time of administration.

Indications: *Pasteurella multocida* vaccine (NITRO-CHOL®) is recommended for use in healthy turkeys to reduce losses due to naturally occurring field strains of *P. multocida* (fowl cholera).

The vaccine is recommended for oral immunization of healthy turkeys beginning at six to eight weeks of age. Booster doses should be given every three to five weeks depending on field exposure. Turkeys must be healthy and free from any outside stresses at the time of vaccination. NITRO-CHOL® will provide a successful vaccination, but the immune response in the birds also depends on administration techniques, previous exposure to immunosuppressing agents and the environment. Prevaccination exposure to field coryza, Newcastle, hemorrhagic enteritis and other disease agents can influence the birds ability to respond to vaccination. Do not use NITRO-CHOL® within 14 days of vaccinating for Newcastle disease.

This vaccine will produce effective immunity. It has passed potency, safety and purity tests meeting all the requirements set forth by Arko Laboratories Ltd. and the USDA. The response to the product, the stimulation of antibodies within the turkey and the resultant level of immunity may be affected by other factors: Management conditions, concurrent infections and stress levels at vaccination.

Dosage and Administration: The first dose of vaccine should be administered in the drinking water at six (6) to eight (8) weeks of age. Repeat vaccinations should be given every three (3) to five (5) weeks.

1. Medications and disinfecting products in the drinking water are not compatible with NITRO-CHOL® vaccine. Discontinue their use at least three (3) days before vaccinating and do not resume their use for three (3) days after vaccination.
2. Do not use chlorinated water for vaccination. Scrub and clean all waterers before vaccination with nonchlorinated water.
3. Flush the water lines with one (1) pound of powdered milk per 100 gallons of water prior to vaccinating to protect the vaccine and prevent possible inactivation by chlorine.
4. Thaw the vaccine at room temperature just prior to vaccinating. Shake each vial of vaccine before removing the aluminum seal.
5. The vaccine is to be used at a rate of one (1) vial of vaccine for every 1,000 birds. Generally water may be withheld for up to two (2) hours prior to vaccinating to assure that all the turkeys will drink. The vaccine should be administered in an amount of drinking water (milk added) that would be consumed by thirsty turkeys in approximately two (2) hours. Provide ample water space so that all turkeys can drink easily.
6. Daily water consumption for each flock needs to be determined just prior to vaccination. Water consumption is affected by weather, management conditions and the age of the birds. The following table will serve as a general guideline to determine the amount of water to be used with the vaccine if more specific information is not available.

Water consumption per 1,000 doses:

Age in weeks	Gallons of water consumed by 1,000 turkeys per day (average temperatures)
4	40
5	50
6	60
7	75
8	95
9	115
10	125
12	150
15	165

Vaccinate only healthy birds. Do not vaccinate in the face of a challenge due to cholera or any other disease. Vaccination during a challenge can cause complications and reduce immunity. Do not use this vaccine within two (2) weeks on either side of a vaccination with live Newcastle virus vaccine. Discontinue all medications and antibiotics for three (3) days prior to vaccination. Resume medications three (3) days post vaccination if needed.

Precaution(s): Store this vaccine frozen. Protect from sunlight.

It is advised to record the vaccine serial number, the expiration date, the date of vaccination and any reactions observed. This product should be stored, transported, and administered in accordance with the instructions and directions.

Caution(s): Use only proper hygiene when handling the vaccine. Clean any spills with disinfectants. Keep the vaccine away from open wounds. Wear gloves if necessary. Consult a physician if contamination occurs. Wash hands thoroughly after using the vaccine.

Use the entire contents when first opened. Burn the vaccine container and all unused contents.

Warning(s): Do not vaccinate within 21 days before slaughter.

Discussion: Fowl cholera is a contagious, widely distributed disease in turkeys occurring as a

septicemia with a sudden onset. Pneumonia is particularly common in turkeys resulting in high morbidity and mortality.
Trial Data: Challenge: NITRO-CHOL® protected isolated turkeys in controlled laboratory experimentation against challenge with the P1059 (type 3) strain of *Pasteurella multocida*.
Presentation: 1,000 dose vials.
Compendium Code No.: 11230050

NITROFURAZONE

Aspen **Topical Antibacterial**
Active Ingredient(s): 0.2% nitrofurazone in a water soluble base of polyethylene glycols.
Indications: For the prevention or treatment of surface bacterial infections of wounds, burns and cutaneous ulcers on dogs, cats and horses.
Dosage and Administration: Apply directly onto the lesion with a spatula, or first place on a piece of gauze. Use of a bandage is optional. The preparation should remain on the lesion for at least 24 hours. The dressing may be changed several times a day or left on the lesion for a longer period.
Precaution(s): Keep away from excessive heat or direct sunlight.
Caution(s): Keep out of the reach of children.
In case of deep or puncture wounds or serious burns, consult a veterinarian. If redness, irritation, or swelling persists or increases, discontinue use and consult a veterinarian.
Avoid exposure to alkaline material and fluorescent lighting.
Warning(s): Not for use on animals intended for food.
Carcinogenesis: Nitrofurazone, the active ingredient, has been shown to produce mammary tumors in rats and ovarian tumors in mice. Additionally, some people may be hypersensitive to this product.
Either wear gloves when applying, or wash hands afterwards.
Presentation: 1 lb containers.
Compendium Code No.: 14750590

NITROFURAZONE DRESSING

Durvet **Topical Antibacterial**
Antibacterial Preparation
Active Ingredient(s): Contents: 0.2% nitrofurazone in a water-soluble base of polyethylene glycols.
Indications: For the prevention or treatment of surface bacterial infections of wounds, burns and cutaneous ulcers For use only on dogs, cats and horses (not for food use).
Dosage and Administration: Apply directly on the lesion with a spatula, or first place on a piece of gauze. Application of a bandage is optional.
This preparation should be in contact with the lesion for at least 24 hours. The dressing may be changed several times daily or left on the lesion for a longer period.
Precaution(s): Avoid exposure to excessive heat or direct sunlight and strong fluorescent lighting.
Caution(s): In case of deep or puncture wounds or serious burns, consult veterinarian. If redness, irritation or swelling persists or increases, discontinue use and veterinarian.
Warning(s): Do not use on horses intended for food.
Not to be used on animals intended for food purposes.
Human Warnings:
Carcinogenesis: Nitrofurazone, the active ingredient of NITROFURAZONE DRESSING, has been shown to produce mammary tumors in rats and ovarian tumors in mice.
Additionally, some people may be hypersensitive to this product.
Either wear gloves when applying or wash hands afterwards.
Presentation: 1 lb. (NDC 30798-219-41).
Compendium Code No.: 10841910 Rev. 8/92

NITROFURAZONE DRESSING 0.2%

AgriLabs **Topical Antibacterial**
An Antibacterial Preparation for Topical Application
NADA No.: 125-797
Active Ingredient(s): 0.2% nitrofurazone in a water soluble base of polyethylene glycols.
Indications: For the prevention or treatment of surface bacterial infections of wounds, burns and cutaneous ulcers. For use only on dogs, cats and horses.
Dosage and Administration: Apply directly on the lesion with a spatula, or first place on a piece of gauze. Application of a bandage is optional.
This preparation should be in contact with the lesion for at least 24 hours. The dressing may be changed several times a day or left on the lesion for a longer period of time.
Precaution(s): Avoid exposure to excessive heat or direct sunlight and strong fluorescent lighting.
Caution(s): In case of deep or puncture wounds or serious burns, consult a veterinarian. If redness, irritation, or swelling persists or increases, discontinue use and consult a veterinarian.
Warning(s): Not to be used on animals intended for food purposes.
Do not use on horses intended for food.
Presentation: 16 oz. (1 lb.) containers.
Compendium Code No.: 10580760

NITROFURAZONE DRESSING 0.2%

AgriPharm **Topical Antibacterial**
Active Ingredient(s): 0.2% nitrofurazone in a water soluble base of polyethylene glycols.
Indications: For the prevention and treatment of surface bacterial infections of wounds, burns and cutaneous ulcers. For use only on dogs, cats and horses.
Dosage and Administration: Apply directly on the lesion with a spatula, or first place on a piece of gauze. Application of a bandage is optional.
The preparation should be in contact with the lesion for at least 24 hours. The dressing may be changed several times a day or left on the lesion for a longer period of time.
Precaution(s): Avoid exposure to excessive heat or direct sunlight and strong fluorescent lighting.
Caution(s): Keep out of the reach of children.
In case of deep or puncture wounds or serious burns, consult a veterinarian. If redness, irritation, or swelling persists or increases, discontinue use and consult a veterinarian.
Warning(s): Not to be used on animals intended for food purposes.
Do not use on horses intended for food.
Presentation: 16 oz. (1 lb. - 454 g) containers.
Compendium Code No.: 14570670

NITROFURAZONE OINTMENT

Phoenix Pharmaceutical **Topical Antibacterial**
NADA No.: 132-427
Active Ingredient(s): Contents: 0.2% Nitrofurazone in a water-soluble base of polyethylene glycols.
Indications: An antibacterial preparation for topical application. For the prevention or treatment of surface bacterial infections of wounds, burns, cutaneous ulcers. For use in horses only.
Dosage and Administration: Apply directly on the lesion with a spatula or first place on a piece of gauze. Application of a bandage is optional.
The preparation should be in contact with the lesion for at least 24 hours. The dressing may be changed several times a day or left on the lesion for a longer period.
Precaution(s): Avoid exposure to alkaline material and fluorescent lighting.
Keep away from excessive heat or direct sunlight.
Caution(s): In case of deep or puncture wounds or serious burns, use only as recommended by a veterinarian. If redness, irritation, or swelling persists or increases, discontinue use, reconsult a veterinarian.
Warning(s): Federal law prohibits the use of this product in food producing animals.
Not to be used on horses intended for food.
Human Warning: Carcinogenesis:
Nitrofurazone, the active ingredient of NITROFURAZONE OINTMENT, has been shown to produce mammary tumors in rats and ovarian tumors in mice.
Some people may be hypersensitive to this product. Either wear gloves when applying, or wash hands afterwards. Keep out of reach of children.
Presentation: 1 lb (454 g) jars (NDC 57319-425-27).
Compendium Code No.: 12560581 Rev. 9/99

NITROFURAZONE SOLUBLE DRESSING

Butler **Topical Antibacterial**
An Antibacterial Preparation for Topical Application
NADA No.: 140-881
Active Ingredient(s): 0.2% nitrofurazone in a water soluble base of polyethylene glycols.
Indications: For the prevention or treatment of surface bacterial infections of wounds, burns, and cutaneous ulcers. For use on dogs, cats and horses only.
Dosage and Administration: Apply directly onto the lesion with a spatula or first place on a piece of gauze. The application of a bandage is optional.
The preparation should be in contact with the lesion for at least 24 hours. The dressing may be changed several times a day or left on the lesion for a longer period of time.
Caution(s): In case of deep or puncture wounds or serious burns, consult a veterinarian. If redness, irritation, or swelling persists or increases, discontinue use of the product and consult a veterinarian. Avoid exposure to excessive heat or direct sunlight and strong fluorescent lighting.
Warning(s): Do not use on horses intended for food.
Presentation: 1 lb. containers.
Compendium Code No.: 10821210

NITROFURAZONE SOLUBLE DRESSING

Med-Pharmex **Topical Antibacterial**
NADA No.: 140-881
Active Ingredient(s): 0.2% Nitrofurazone in a water soluble base.
Indications: For the prevention or treatment of surface bacterial infections of wounds, burns and cutaneous ulcers of dogs, cats and horses (not for food use).
Dosage and Administration: Apply directly on the lesion with a spatula or first place on a piece of gauze. Use of a bandage is optional. The preparation should remain on the lesion for at least 24 hours. The dressing may be changed several times daily or left on the lesion for a longer period.
Precaution(s): Keep away from excessive heat or direct sunlight.
Caution(s): In case of deep or puncture wounds or serious burns, consult veterinarian. If redness, irritation or swelling persists or increases, discontinue use and veterinarian.
Avoid exposure to alkaline material and strong fluorescent lighting.
Warning(s): Not for use in horses intended for food.
Carcinogenesis: Nitrofurazone has been shown to produce mammary tumors in rats and ovarian tumors in mice.
Some people may be hypersensitive to this product. Either wear gloves when applying or wash hands afterwards.
Presentation: 16 oz (454 g).
Compendium Code No.: 10270100

NITRO-SAL

Arko **Vaccine**
Salmonella choleraesuis Vaccine
U.S. Vet. Lic. No.: 337
Active Ingredient(s): NITRO-SAL is an avirulent live culture offering protection to swine against naturally occurring field strains of *Salmonella choleraesuis*. NITRO-SAL is preserved as a frozen preparation.
Indications: Recommended for the subcutaneous vaccination of healthy, susceptible swine five weeks of age or older against disease caused by *Salmonella choleraesuis*. Pigs must be free from any outside stresses at the time of the vaccination.
Dosage and Administration: Thaw the vaccine at room temperature just prior to the vaccination. Shake well before using. Inject ½ mL subcutaneously at five (5) weeks of age or older.
NITRO-SAL will provide a successful vaccination, but the immune response in the pigs also depends upon the administration techniques, previous exposure to immunosuppressing agents and the environment.
Precaution(s): Store the frozen vaccine at a temperature of 14°F (-10°C). Freezing maximizes the number of organisms preserved and viability at the time of administration.
Trial Data: Twenty randomly selected four to five week old pigs were vaccinated subcutaneously with a dose of *Salmonella choleraesuis* vaccine (NITRO-SAL). Twenty more randomly selected pigs were held as controls. All of the pigs were challenged with a laboratory Salmonella culture from the National Veterinary Services Laboratory.

Results: All of the control pigs experienced clinical disease. Fourteen pigs died. Six pigs survived for two weeks exhibiting typical signs and lesions of salmonellosis. The vaccine provided protection to the vaccinated pigs. Clinical problems were not detected in the vaccinated pigs.

The field evaluation of NITRO-SAL in *Salmonella choleraesuis* infected herds resulted in reduced mortality, improved feed conversion and increased rate of gain. One shot protection provides a means of controlling a significant swine disease.

Presentation: 20 dose, 50 dose and 100 dose.

Compendium Code No.: 11230060

NITRO-SAL F.D.

Arko **Vaccine**

Salmonella Choleraesuis Vaccine, Avirulent Live Culture

U.S. Vet. Lic. No.: 337

Contents: NITRO-SAL F.D. is an avirulent live culture offering protection to swine against naturally occurring field strains of *Salmonella choleraesuis.*

Indications: Recommended for the vaccination of healthy, susceptible swine five weeks of age or older against salmonellosis associated with *Salmonella choleraesuis.* Pigs must be healthy and free from any outside stresses at the time of vaccination.

Dosage and Administration: Reconstitute the vaccine with the accompanying diluent. Shake well before using. Administer to pigs 5 weeks of age or older either via the drinking water or by the subcutaneous injection of ½ mL per pig. Administer orally in an amount of vaccine-laden drinking water that the herd will consume in 4 hours.

Oral Administration:

1) Medications and disinfecting products in the drinking water are not compatible with oral administration of Salmonella Choleraesuis Vaccine.
2) Do not use chlorinated water for vaccination.
3) Flush the water lines with ⅓ pound (2 cups) of human grade non-fat dry skim milk per 100 gallons of drinking water prior to vaccinating to protect the vaccine and prevent possible inactivation from chlorine residue.
4) Milk diluent should be used as stock solution for the vaccination. Milk diluent can be made by adding 2 cups of human grade non-fat dry skim milk to one gallon of cool, clean non-chlorinated water.
5) Rehydrate the vaccine with the diluent provided. Mix the rehydrated vaccine into the milk stock solution. The vaccine is to be used at a rate of 1 vial of vaccine for every 100 pigs. Generally water may be withheld up to 2 hours prior to vaccinating to assure all pigs will drink. The vaccine should be administered orally in an amount of drinking water (milk added) that would be consumed by thirsty pigs in approximately 4 hours. Provide ample water space so that all the pigs can drink easily.
6) Daily water consumption for each vaccination needs to be determined just prior to use. Water consumption is affected by weather, management conditions and the age of the pigs. When specific water consumption information is not available please refer to a reference table. The following table will serve as a general guideline to determine the amount of water to be used with the vaccine if more specific information is not available.

Size of Animals	Gallons of Drinking Water per 100 head in a 4 Hour Consumption Period
15 to 40 lbs	12.5 to 25 gallons
40 to 110 lbs	25 to 37.5 gallons
110 to 240 lbs	37.5 to 50 gallons

No. of Animals	Vials of Vaccine	4 Hour consumption	
		Drinking Water Gallons	Stock Solution Ounces
15 lb Pigs			
100	1	12.5	12.5
200	2	25	25
300	3	37.5	37.5
400	4	50	50
500	5	62.5	62.5
40 lb Pigs			
100	1	25	25
200	2	50	50
300	3	75	75
400	4	100	100
500	5	125	125
110 lb Pigs			
100	1	37.5	37.5
200	2	75	75
300	3	112.5	112.5
400	4	150	150
500	5	187.5	187.5
240 lb Pigs			
100	1	50	50
200	2	100	100
300	3	150	150
400	4	200	200
500	5	250	250

All figures based on 1 ounce stock solution to 1 gallon drinking water.

NITRO-SAL will provide a successful vaccination but the immune response in the pigs also depends on administration techniques, previous exposure to immunosuppressing agents and environment.

Precaution(s): Store at a temperature of 35-45°F (2-7°C). Do not freeze.

Caution(s): Needles and syringes should be sterilized by boiling. Do not use chemical sterilization as traces of chemicals may inactivate the vaccine. Use only proper hygiene when handling the vaccine. Clean any spills with disinfectants. Keep the vaccine away from open wounds. Wear gloves if necessary. Consult a physician if contamination occurs. Wash hands thoroughly after using the vaccine. Use entire contents when first opened. Burn this container and all unused contents. Anaphylactoid reactions may occur.

It is advised to record the vaccine serial number, the expiration date, the date of vaccination and any reactions observed. This product should be stored, transported and administered in accordance with the instructions and directions.

Antidote(s): Administer epinephrine.

Warning(s): Do not vaccinate within 21 days before slaughter.

Presentation: 100 dose (50 mL) vial.

Compendium Code No.: 11230070

NITROZONE™ OINTMENT

Bimeda **Topical Antibacterial**

Topical Antibacterial Ointment

NADA No.: 126-504

Active Ingredient(s): Contains:

Nitrofurazone 0.2%

In a water soluble base of polyethylene glycol.

Indications: For the prevention or treatment of surface infections of wounds, burns, and cutaneous ulcers, caused by organisms sensitive to nitrofurazone. For use on dogs and cats, and only on horses not intended for food use.

Dosage and Administration: Apply directly onto the lesion with a spatula or on a piece of gauze. The application of a bandage is optional. The preparation should be in contact with the lesion for at least 24 hours. The dressing may be changed several times a day or left on the lesion for a longer period of time.

Precaution(s): Keep away from excessive heat or direct sunlight.

Do not freeze.

Caution(s): In case of deep puncture wounds or serious burns, consult a veterinarian. If redness, irritation, or swelling persists or increases, discontinue use and consult a veterinarian.

Avoid exposure to alkaline material and fluorescent lighting.

For animal use only. Not for human use.

Keep out of the reach of children.

Warning(s): Not for use on horses intended to be used for food.

Human Warnings:

Carcinogenesis: Nitrofurazone, the active ingredient of NITROZONE™, has been shown to produce mammary tumors in rats and ovarian tumors in mice. Additionally, some people may be hypersensitive to the product. Either wear gloves when applying, or wash hands afterwards.

Presentation: 1 lb. (453.6 g) containers.

Compendium Code No.: 13990280

NO CHEW SPRAY

Vetus **Topical Product**

Active Ingredient(s): Water, Propylene Glycol, Bitrex®, Fragrance.

Indications: Bitter Spray contains Bitrex® (Denatonium Benzoate NF) a substance that tastes so bad, it discourages licking, biting and chewing by animals.

Directions: Shake well before use. apply to bandages, casts, hair or household furniture twice daily or as directed by a veterinarian.

Caution(s): Avoid contact with broken skin, eyes or mucous membranes. If in contact, wash with copious amounts of cool water. Before applying to extensive areas of furniture, test the effect of this product on small inconspicuous areas.

For veterinary use only.

Warning(s): Keep out of reach of children.

Presentation: 4 fl oz (120 mL) bottle (NDC: 47611-363-97).

Distributed by: Burns Veterinary Supply, Inc.

Compendium Code No.: 14440990

N

NOLVA-CLEANSE™

Fort Dodge **Otic Cleanser**

Ear Cleaning Solution

Active Ingredient(s): A unique combination of nonirritating surfactants to enhance cleansing.

Indications: NOLVA-CLEANSE™ is a topical cleaner for the routine cleaning of ears of dogs and cats to aid in the removal of wax, dirt, and/or debris.

The external ear canal of dogs and cats must be cleaned to remove accumulations of wax, dirt, and other debris, in preparation for the use of treatment drugs, in infected ears. Healthy ears, which have accumulations of wax and debris, should be cleaned routinely.

Directions for Use: NOLVA-CLEANSE™ should be used as directed by a veterinarian. Apply liberally into the ear canal. Gently massage the base of the ear, allowing the solution to come in contact with wax, dirt and/or debris. Use cotton or other suitable material, such as gauze or facial tissue, to remove wax, dirt and/or debris. It may be necessary to repeat the procedure two to three times daily in dogs having excessively dirty ears. Use of NOLVA-CLEANSE™ in cats should be limited to once weekly. In animals that are prone to recurring ear problems, NOLVA-CLEANSE™ should be used weekly to keep the ears clean.

Precaution(s): Do not store above 104°F (40°C).

Caution(s): Not for use in the eye. Do not use if there is suspected damage to the ear drum. NOLVA-CLEANSE™ should be used as directed by a veterinarian.

In case of irritation or inflammation of ears, discontinue use and consult your veterinarian. Propylene glycol may cause temporary flushing (reddening) of the treated area, especially in white-haired dogs and cats.

Warning(s): For veterinary use only.

For external use only.

Keep out of reach of children.

Presentation: Available in 4 fl oz and 8 fl oz (236 mL) dispensing bottles.

Compendium Code No.: 10031231 12852A

NOLVADENT®

Fort Dodge **Dental Preparation**

Oral Cleansing Solution

Active Ingredient(s): 0.1% Chlorhexidine acetate formulated with special surfactant, peppermint flavored base, FD&C Red 40 & Red 33; 6% ethyl alcohol by volume.

Indications: To assist in the daily maintenance of a healthy and pleasant smelling mouth in dogs and cats through the removal of food particles and other debris from the teeth and gum line.

Dosage and Administration: Instructions: Apply NOLVADENT® either as an oral rinse or with a toothbrush.

Oral Rinse: Holding the animal's head steady with one hand, gently insert the applicator inside the corner of the mouth and apply a small amount of NOLVADENT® between the teeth and side of the mouth. Massage the mouth over the teeth to work NOLVADENT® over the surface of the teeth. Repeat on the opposite side of the mouth so that the gum surfaces are thoroughly wet on both sides of the mouth.

Tooth Brushing: Place a small amount of NOLVADENT® in a clean dish or cup. Holding the animal's head steady with one hand, dip the toothbrush into the solution and carefully brush the teeth with a gentle motion. Re-wet the brush with NOLVADENT® as needed.

Special Note: Use of NOLVADENT® should not be considered a substitute for sound veterinary dental treatment. This product should be used under the direction of a veterinarian who can advise on a complete oral health program.

Precaution(s): Store at controlled room temperature 15° to 30°C (59° to 86°F). Protect from freezing.

Caution(s): For external use only as oral rinse. Not for use in eyes. Keep out of reach of children.

Side Effects: Published literature has reported some staining of teeth surfaces after prolonged usage of rinses containing chlorhexidine. Build up of stain can be prevented by applying the solution with a toothbrush.

Presentation: 4 fl oz bottle with sprayer (NDC 0856-0281-01) and 8 fl oz bottles (NDC 0856-0281-02).

Compendium Code No.: 10031250 0283F

NOLVALUBE®

Fort Dodge **Lubricant**

Active Ingredient(s): A lubricant containing Nolvasan® (0.1% chlorhexidine acetate).

Indications: A ready to use, antiseptic lubricant for topical or intrauterine application. Non-greasy; free from irritating effects; will not injure rubber appliances or surgical instruments.

Dosage and Administration: Suggested Usage:

Topical: Remove sufficient amount to cover hand and arm or instruments as required. If desired, a small amount of water can be used.

Intrauterine: Add approximately four (4) ounces of NOLVALUBE® per gallon of warm water and mix well.

Precaution(s): Keep container tightly closed.

Store at controlled room temperature 15° to 30°C (59° to 86°F).

Caution(s): Keep out of reach of children.

For animal use only.

Presentation: 8 fl oz (236 mL) (NDC 0856-3602-01) and 8 lb (NDC 0856-3602-02) containers.

Compendium Code No.: 10031260 3603I

NOLVASAN® 5% TEAT DIP CONCENTRATE

Fort Dodge **Teat Dip**

Chlorhexidine Acetate

Active Ingredient(s):

Chlorhexidine acetate .... 5% (94.6 g)
Inert Ingredients .... q.s.
(Including 60% glycerin)

Indications: For use as an aid in controlling bacteria that cause bovine mastitis.

Directions:

To Prepare 0.5% Teat Dip Solution: This ½ gallon of NOLVASAN® 5% Teat Dip Concentrate should be reconstituted to 5 gallons of 0.5% teat dip solution. Place entire contents in a clean 5 gallon container and add clean, potable water to yield 5 gallons of teat dip solution. (Use of "hard water" may result in some precipitation. If the 0.5% solution is to be held longer than 1 week, it is advisable to use distilled or deionized water.)

To prepare smaller quantity of final 0.5% solution, use one part of this NOLVASAN® 5% Teat Dip Concentrate and add nine parts clean potable water.

N

Use of 0.5% Teat Dip Solution: Teat dipping should start 1 week before the cow freshens. During lactation, dip each teat into 0.5% solution immediately after the cow is milked. When the cow is dried off, the teats should continue to be dipped in the solution once a day for 3 to 4 days. Dip each teat so that the lower 1 inch of the teat has been covered with the solution.

Udder and teats of the cow should be thoroughly washed before milking.

If minor irritation or chapping of the teats should occur during lactation, it is helpful to dilute the 0.5% solution half and half with clean water for a couple of days and then gradually return to use of the 0.5% solution.

Precaution(s): Store at controlled room temperature 15° to 30°C (59° to 86°F). Avoid freezing or exposure to excessive heat.

Caution(s): May be irritating to eyes or mucous membranes. May be harmful if swallowed. Avoid contamination of feed or feedstuffs. If in contact, flush thoroughly with water. Rinse empty container with water and discard.

Warning(s): Do not use this solution undiluted. Dip teats only in a properly prepared 0.5% solution as directed. Do not use this solution for cleaning milking equipment.

Keep out of reach of children.

For veterinary us only.

Presentation: 64 fl oz (1.8 L) containers (NDC 0856-0656-01).

Compendium Code No.: 10031280 0656G

NOLVASAN® ANTISEPTIC OINTMENT

Fort Dodge **Topical Wound Dressing**

NADA No.: 009-782

Active Ingredient(s): 1% chlorhexidine acetate in a hydrophilic ointment base which contains 10% stearyl alcohol.

Indications:

Dogs, Cats and Horses - For use as a topical antiseptic ointment for surface wounds.

Dosage and Administration:

Suggested usage:

Dogs, Cats and Horses - Carefully cleanse the wound area and apply daily.

Precaution(s): Store at controlled room temperature 15° to 30°C (59° to 86°F). Protect from freezing.

Caution(s): In case of deep or puncture wounds or serious burns consult veterinarian. If redness, irritation or swelling persists or increases, discontinue use and consult veterinarian.

Keep out of reach of children.

Warning(s): Not to be used on horses intended for use as food.

Presentation: 1 oz. tubes (NDC 0856-7371-01), 7 oz. jar (NDC 0856-7371-02), and 16 oz.jar (NDC 0856-7371-03).

Compendium Code No.: 10031290 3715G

NOLVASAN® CAP-TABS®

Fort Dodge **Intrauterine Antiseptic**

Chlorhexidine

NADA No.: 009-809

Active Ingredient(s): Each CAP-TAB® contains 1 g chlorhexidine hydrochloride incorporated in an effervescent base.

Indications: For prevention or treatment of metritis and vaginitis in mares when caused by pathogens sensitive to chlorhexidine hydrochloride.

Dosage and Administration: Unattached placental membranes and any excess uterine fluid or debris should be removed from the uterus. The external genitalia should be carefully cleaned and 1 or 2 CAP-TABS® placed deep into each uterine horn. The operator should wear a clean obstetrical sleeve while inserting the CAP-TABS® into the uterus so that no contamination is introduced.

In a uterus which contains little or no uterine fluid, the effervescent CAP-TAB® may cause some localized irritation. For treatment of such a uterus, or where the cervix is tightly constricted, the CAP-TAB® should be dissolved in an appropriate amount of clean, boiled water and the solution infused into the uterus using a clean, sterile catheter. Treatment may be repeated in 48 to 72 hours.

Precaution(s): Store at controlled room temperature 15° to 30°C (59° to 86°F).

Caution(s): Keep bottle tightly closed to avoid deterioration by moisture or heat.

For use in horses only.

Keep out of reach of children.

Warning(s): Not for use in horses intended for food.

Presentation: Bottle of 50 CAP-TABS® (NDC 0856-1551-01).

Compendium Code No.: 10031300 5514J

NOLVASAN® OTIC

Fort Dodge **Otic Cleanser**

Cleansing Solution

Active Ingredient(s): Contains special solvent and surfactant.

Indications: For general cleaning of ears of dogs and cats to aid in removal of debris.

Dosage and Administration:

For Use in Cleaning Ears: Apply liberally into the ear canal. Gently massage the base of the ear. Carefully clean excess fluid from accessible portion of external ear with cotton. Repeat one to three times daily, if necessary, depending on condition of ear and amount of debris to be removed.

Precaution(s): Store at controlled room temperature 15° to 30°C (59° to 86°F).

Caution(s): For external use only. Not for use in the eye. Do not apply if there is suspected damage to the ear drum. It is advised to use under the direction of a veterinarian.

Keep out of reach of children.

Presentation: 4 fl oz (118 mL) and 16 fl oz (473 mL) containers.

Compendium Code No.: 10031310 0225F

NOLVASAN® S

Fort Dodge **Disinfectant**

Chlorhexidine diacetate-Scented Disinfectant-Bactericide-Virucide†

EPA Reg. No.: 1117-48

Active Ingredient(s):

1,1'-Hexamethylenebis [5-(p-chlorophenyl) biguanide] diacetate 2%
Other Ingredients 98%
100%

Indications: For cleaning, disinfection, deodorizing.

†For disinfection of inanimate objects to aid in control of canine distemper virus, equine influenza virus, transmissible gastroenteritis virus, hog cholera virus, parainfluenza-3 virus, bovine rhinotracheitis virus, bovine virus diarrhea virus, infectious bronchitis virus, Newcastle virus, Venezuelan equine encephalitis virus, equine rhinopneumonitis virus, feline rhinotracheitis virus, pseudorabies virus, equine arteritis virus and canine coronavirus.

For disinfection of veterinary or farm premises.

Directions for Use: It is a violation of federal law to use this product in a manner inconsistent with its labeling.

When applying by wiping, mopping, or spraying: Applicators or other handlers must wear long-sleeve shirt and long pants, socks plus shoes, and rubber gloves.

Do not apply this product in a way that will contact workers or other persons, either directly or through drift. Only protected handlers may be in the area during application.

Entry Restrictions: Thoroughly ventilate buildings, vehicles, and closed spaces following application. Do not enter, allow other persons to enter, house livestock, or use equipment in the treated area until ventilation is complete and the liquid chlorhexidine diacetate has been absorbed, set or dried.

User Safety: Follow manufacturer's instructions for cleaning/maintaining personal protective equipment. If there are no such instructions for washables, use detergent and hot water. Keep and wash personal protective equipment separately from other laundry.

Users should wash hands before eating, drinking, chewing gum, using tobacco, or using the toilet. Users should remove clothing immediately if pesticide gets on or inside it, then wash both skin and clothing thoroughly and put on clean clothes. Users should remove personal protective equipment immediately after handling this product. Wash the outside of gloves before removing. As soon as possible, wash skin and clothing thoroughly and change into clean clothes.

NOLVASAN® Solution final use dilutions may be applied by wiping, mopping, or spraying on the inanimate surface.

Veterinary or Farm Premises:

1. Remove all animals and feed from premises, vehicles and other equipment.
2. Remove all litter and manure from floors, walls and surfaces of barns, pens, stalls, chutes and other facilities and fixtures occupied or traversed by animals.
3. Empty all troughs, racks and other feeding and watering appliances.
4. Thoroughly clean all surfaces with soap or detergent and rinse with water.
5. Saturate all surfaces with the recommended disinfecting solution for a period of 10 minutes.
6. Immerse all halters, ropes and other types of equipment used in handling and restraining animals, as well as forks, shovels and scrapers used for removing litter and manure.
7. Thoroughly scrub all treated feed racks, mangers, troughs, automatic feeders, fountains and waterers with soap or detergent, and rinse with potable water before reuse.

Recommended Concentration For Use:

†For disinfection of inanimate objects to aid in control of canine distemper virus, equine influenza virus, transmissible gastroenteritis virus, hog cholera virus, parainfluenza-3 virus, bovine rhinotracheitis virus, bovine virus diarrhea virus, infectious bronchitis virus, Newcastle virus, Venezuelan equine encephalitis virus, equine rhinopneumonitis virus, feline rhinotracheitis virus, pseudorabies virus, equine arteritis virus and canine coronavirus — 3 ounces (6 tablespoonfuls) per gallon of clean water. NOLVASAN® S has been shown to be virucidal *in vitro* against rabies virus (CVS strain) in laboratory tests when used as directed above.

For disinfection of veterinary or farm premises — 1 ounce (2 tablespoonfuls) per gallon of clean water.

Not effective against *Pseudomonas aeruginosa* or gram-positive cocci on inanimate surfaces.*

*According to A.O.A.C. Use Dilution Test Method.

Precautionary Statements: Hazards to Humans (and Domestic Animals): Danger.

Corrosive: Causes irreversible eye damage. Wear protective eyewear (Goggles, face shield or safety glasses). Harmful if swallowed or absorbed through skin or inhaled. May be fatal if inhaled. Avoid breathing spray mist.

Avoid contact with skin or clothing and do not swallow. Wear rubber gloves when handling or applying.

Statement of Practical Treatment:

If in eyes: Hold eyelids open and flush with a steady, gentle stream of water for 15 minutes. Get medical attention.

If inhaled: Remove victim to fresh air. If not breathing, give artificial respiration, preferably mouth-to-mouth. Get medical attention.

If swallowed: Call a physician or Poison Control Center. Drink 1 or 2 glasses of water and induce vomiting by touching back of throat with finger. If person is unconscious, do not give anything by mouth and do not induce vomiting.

If on skin: Wash with plenty of soap and water. Get medical attention if irritation observed.

Note to Physician: Probable mucosal damage may contraindicate the use of gastric lavage.

Environmental Hazards: Do not discharge effluent containing this product into lakes, streams, ponds, estuaries, oceans, or other waters unless in accordance with the requirements of a National Pollutant Discharge Elimination System (NPDES) permit and the permitting authority has been notified in writing prior to discharge. Do not discharge effluent containing this product to sewer systems without previously notifying the local sewage treatment plant authority. For guidance contact your State Water Board or Regional Office of the EPA. Do not contaminate water by cleaning of equipment or disposal of waste.

Storage and Disposal:

Prohibition: Do not contaminate water, food or feed by storage or disposal. Open dumping is prohibited. Do not reuse empty container. Protect from freezing. Do not use or store near heat or open flame.

Pesticide Disposal: Wastes resulting from use of this product may be disposed of on site or at an approved waste disposal facility.

Container Disposal: Do not reuse containers. Rinse thoroughly with water and discard in trash.

General: Consult federal, state or local disposal authorities for approved alternative procedures such as limited open burning.

Warning(s): Keep out of reach of children.

For animal premises use only.

Presentation: 1 pint and 1 gallon (3.7 L) containers.

For further information contact Fort Dodge Animal Health at 1-800-477-1365

Compendium Code No.: 10031321 04060

NOLVASAN® SHAMPOO

Fort Dodge **Grooming Shampoo**

Antiseptic with Conditioner

Active Ingredient(s): Contains 0.5% chlorhexidine acetate.

Indications: NOLVASAN® Shampoo cleans and restores luster to the hair coat of dogs, cats and horses. NOLVASAN® Shampoo has excellent cleansing and deodorizing properties.

Directions: Wet animal thoroughly with warm water. Apply enough shampoo to make a lather, adding more water if necessary. Massage into the hair coat for 2 to 5 minutes. Rinse hair and skin thoroughly with clean water. A second application of shampoo may be applied if necessary. Dry thoroughly.

Precaution(s): Store at controlled room temperature 15° to 30°C (59° to 86°F). Protect from freezing.

Caution(s): Avoid contact with eyes. Keep out of reach of children.

Warning(s): Not to be used on horses intended for food.

Presentation: 8 oz bottles, package of 12 (NDC 0856-0722-01) and 1 gallon (3.7 L) containers (NDC 0856-0722-02).

Compendium Code No.: 10031330 0726L

NOLVASAN® SKIN AND WOUND CLEANSER

Fort Dodge **Topical Wound Dressing**

Active Ingredient(s): Contains 2% (w/v) chlorhexidine acetate in a stable detergent base.

Indications: For external use only as a skin and wound cleanser. NOLVASAN® Skin and Wound Cleanser possesses a wide range of antimicrobial activity and provides a rapid and residual antimicrobial effect.

Directions for Use:

General Skin Cleansing: Thoroughly rinse area to be cleansed with water. Apply sufficient NOLVASAN® Skin and Wound Cleanser and wash gently. Rinse again thoroughly.

Wound Cleansing: Rinse the area to be cleansed with clean water. A moistened gauze pad may be used to apply a small amount of NOLVASAN® Skin and Wound Cleanser to the affected area. Gently cleanse for 2-4 minutes. Additional water may be needed to obtain adequate sudsing. Repeat cleaning if necessary. Wipe away excess foam with a clean gauze pad. After cleansing, an antiseptic ointment or suitable dressing may be applied.

Precaution(s): Store at controlled room temperature 15° to 30°C (59° to 86°F).

Caution(s): In case of deep or puncture wounds or serious burns contact a veterinarian. If redness, irritation, or swelling persists or increases, consult a veterinarian.

Avoid contact with the eyes and mucous membranes. If contact is made, flush promptly and thoroughly with clean water. Hypersensitivity to NOLVASAN® is rare; however, if reactions should occur, discontinue use.

Keep out of reach of children.

For animal use only.

Presentation: 4 fl oz (NDC 0856-0253-01) and 8 fl oz (236 mL) bottles (NDC 0856-0253-02), packages of 12.

Compendium Code No.: 10031340 0252G

NOLVASAN® SOLUTION

Fort Dodge **Disinfectant**

Chlorhexidine diacetate-Disinfectant-Bactericide-Virucide†

EPA Reg. No.: 1117-30

Active Ingredient(s):

Chlorhexidine (1,1'-Hexamethylenebis [5-(p-chlorophenyl) biguanide]) diacetate 2%
Other Ingredients 98%
100%

The product contains the active ingredient at 0.168 pounds per gallon.

Indications: †For disinfection of inanimate objects to aid in control of canine distemper virus, equine influenza virus, transmissible gastroenteritis virus, hog cholera virus, parainfluenza-3 virus, bovine rhinotracheitis virus, bovine virus diarrhea virus, infectious bronchitis virus, Newcastle virus, Venezuelan equine encephalitis virus, equine rhinopneumonitis virus, feline rhinotracheitis virus, pseudorabies virus, equine arteritis virus and canine coronavirus.

For disinfection of veterinary or farm premises.

For use in federally inspected meat, poultry, rabbit and egg establishments.

For dipping teats as an aid in controlling bacteria that causes mastitis.

Directions for Use: It is a violation of federal law to use this product in a manner inconsistent with its labeling.

NOLVASAN® Solution final use dilutions may be applied by wiping, mopping, or spraying on the inanimate surface. It may also be used in fogging (wet misting) operations as an adjunct either preceding or following regular cleaning and disinfecting procedures. Fog (wet mist) until the area is moist using automatic foggers according to manufacturer's directions.

When applying by wiping, mopping, or spraying: Applicators or other handlers must wear long-sleeve shirt and long pants, socks plus shoes, and rubber gloves.

When applying by wet-mist fogging: Applicators and other handlers exposed to the fog during wet-mist fogging applications and until the fog has dissipated and the enclosed area has been thoroughly ventilated must wear: Long-sleeve shirt and long pants, rubber gloves, socks plus shoes, and a full face respirator with a canister approved for pesticides (MSHA/NIOSH approval number prefix TC-14-G).

Do not apply this product in a way that will contact workers or other persons, either directly or through drift. Only protected handlers may be in the area during application.

Entry Restrictions: Thoroughly ventilate buildings, vehicles, and closed spaces following application. Do not enter, allow other persons to enter, house livestock, or use equipment in the treated area until ventilation is complete and the liquid chlorhexidine diacetate has been absorbed, set or dried.

For entry into fogged areas before ventilation is complete and the fog has completely dissipated, absorbed, set, or dried, all persons must wear: Long-sleeve shirt and long pants, rubber gloves, socks plus shoes and a full face respirator with a canister approved for pesticides (MSHA/NIOSH approval number prefix TC-14-G).

User Safety: Follow manufacturer's instructions for cleaning/maintaining personal protective equipment. If there are no such instructions for washables, use detergent and hot water. Keep and wash personal protective equipment separately from other laundry.

Users should wash hands before eating, drinking, chewing gum, using tobacco, or using the toilet. Users should remove clothing immediately if pesticide gets on or inside it, then wash both skin and clothing thoroughly and put on clean clothes. Users should remove personal protective equipment immediately after handling this product. Wash the outside of gloves before removing. As soon as possible, wash skin and clothing thoroughly and change into clean clothes.

Veterinary or Farm Premises:

1. Remove all animals and feed from premises, vehicles and other equipment.
2. Remove all litter and manure from floors, walls and surfaces of barns, pens, stalls, chutes and other facilities and fixtures occupied or traversed by animals.
3. Empty all troughs, racks and other feeding and watering appliances.
4. Thoroughly clean all surfaces with soap or detergent and rinse with water.
5. Saturate all surfaces with the recommended disinfecting solution for a period of 10 minutes.
6. Immerse all halters, ropes and other types of equipment used in handling and restraining animals, as well as forks, shovels and scrapers used for removing litter and manure.
7. Thoroughly scrub all treated feed racks, mangers, troughs, automatic feeders, fountains and waterers with soap or detergent, and rinse with potable water before reuse.

For use in federally inspected meat, poultry, rabbit and egg establishments:

1. All food products and packaging material must be removed from the room or carefully covered and protected.
2. Remove any loose dirt, litter, etc., that might be lying on floor or attached to the equipment.
3. Thoroughly clean all surfaces with soap or detergent and rinse with water.
4. Saturate all surfaces with the recommended disinfecting solution for a period of 10 minutes.
5. Expose or soak all equipment and/or utensils with the recommended disinfecting solution for a period of 10 minutes.
6. After disinfection all equipment and/or utensils must be thoroughly rinsed with potable water before operations are resumed.

For dipping teats as an aid in controlling bacteria that causes mastitis: Immediately after the cow is milked dip each teat into the dipping solution. Teat dipping should start one week before the cow freshens. When drying off a cow the teats should continue to be dipped once a day for 3 to 4 days. Udder and teats of the cow must be thoroughly washed before milking.

Recommended Concentration for Use:

1. †For disinfection of inanimate objects to aid in control of canine distemper virus, equine influenza virus, transmissible gastroenteritis virus, hog cholera virus, parainfluenza-3 virus, bovine rhinotracheitis virus, bovine virus diarrhea virus, infectious bronchitis virus, Newcastle virus, Venezuelan equine encephalitis virus, equine rhinopneumonitis virus, feline rhinotracheitis virus, pseudorabies virus, equine arteritis virus and canine coronavirus — 3 ounces (6 tablespoonfuls) per gallon of clean water. NOLVASAN® Solution has been shown to be virucidal *in vitro* against rabies virus (CVS strain) in laboratory tests when used as directed above.
2. For disinfection of veterinary or farm premises — 1 ounce (2 tablespoonfuls) per gallon of clean water.
3. For use in federally inspected meat, poultry, rabbit and egg establishments — 1 ounce (2 tablespoonfuls) of NOLVASAN® Solution to each gallon clean water.
4. For dipping teats as an aid in controlling bacteria that causes mastitis. Make up a final dipping solution by putting 32 ounces (one quart) of NOLVASAN® Solution in a clean gallon container, adding 6 ounces of glycerin and then adding clean potable water until you have a total volume of one gallon.

Not effective against *Pseudomonas aeruginosa* or gram-positive cocci on inanimate surfaces*.

*According to A.O.A.C. Use Dilution Test Method.

Precautionary Statements: Hazards to Humans (and Domestic Animals): Danger.

Corrosive: Causes irreversible eye damage. Wear protective eyewear (Goggles, face shield or safety glasses). Harmful if swallowed or absorbed through skin or inhaled. May be fatal if inhaled. Avoid breathing spray mist.

Avoid contact with skin or clothing and do not swallow. Wear rubber gloves when handling or applying.

Statement of Practical Treatment:

If in eyes: Hold eyelids open and flush with a steady, gentle stream of water for 15 minutes. Get medical attention.

If inhaled: Remove victim to fresh air. If not breathing, give artificial respiration, preferably mouth-to-mouth. Get medical attention.

If swallowed: Call a physician or Poison Control Center. Drink 1 or 2 glasses of water and induce vomiting by touching back of throat with finger. If person is unconscious, do not give anything by mouth and do not induce vomiting.

If on skin: Wash with plenty of soap and water. Get medical attention if irritation observed.

Note to Physician: Probable mucosal damage may contraindicate the use of gastric lavage.

Environmental Hazards: Do not discharge effluent containing this product into lakes, streams, ponds, estuaries, oceans, or other waters unless in accordance with the requirements of a National Pollutant Discharge Elimination System (NPDES) permit and the permitting authority has been notified in writing prior to discharge. Do not discharge effluent containing this product to sewer systems without previously notifying the local sewage treatment plant authority. For guidance contact your State Water Board or Regional Office of the EPA. Do not contaminate water by cleaning of equipment or disposal of waste.

Storage and Disposal: Do not contaminate water, food or feed by storage or disposal. Open dumping is prohibited. Do not reuse empty container. Protect from freezing.

Pesticide Storage: Store the product in a dry and cool place, where it is not reachable by children.

Pesticide Disposal: Wastes resulting from use of this product may be disposed of on site or at an approved waste disposal facility.

Container Disposal: Do not reuse containers. Rinse thoroughly with water and discard in trash.

General: Consult federal, state or local disposal authorities for approved alternative procedures such as limited open burning.

Warning(s): Keep out of reach of children. For animal premises use only.

Presentation: 1 gallon (3.7 L) containers.

For further information contact Fort Dodge Animal Health at 1-800-477-1365

Compendium Code No.: 10031351 0626O

NOLVASAN® SURGICAL SCRUB

Fort Dodge **Surgical Scrub**

(Chlorhexidine) Antimicrobial skin and wound cleanser

Active Ingredient(s): Contains 2% (w/v) chlorhexidine acetate in a stable detergent base.

Indications: NOLVASAN® Surgical Scrub possesses a wide range of antimicrobial activity and provides a rapid and residual antimicrobial effect.

Directions for Use: Rinse the area to be cleansed with clean water. Apply 1 to 5 mL of NOLVASAN® Surgical Scrub to the area and wash with a sponge or brush for 2 to 4 minutes. It may be necessary to apply additional water to obtain adequate sudsing. Wipe away excess foam with sterile sponge.

Precaution(s): Store at controlled room temperature 15° to 30°C (59° to 86°F).

Caution(s): For external use only. Avoid contact with the eyes and mucous membranes. If contact is made, flush promptly and thoroughly with clean water. Hypersensitivity to NOLVASAN® is rare; however, if reactions should occur, discontinue use.

Keep out of reach of children.

For veterinary use only.

Presentation: 2 oz (NDC 0856-1041-01), 16 fl oz (473 mL) (NDC 0856-1041-02) and 1 gallon (NDC 0856-1041-03) containers.

Compendium Code No.: 10031361 0253I

NOLVASAN® SUSPENSION

Fort Dodge **Intrauterine Antiseptic**

(Chlorhexidine)

NADA No.: 010-434

Active Ingredient(s): Each 28 mL syringe contains 1 g chlorhexidine hydrochloride in a special base.

Indications: For prevention and treatment of metritis and vaginitis in mares caused by pathogens sensitive to chlorhexidine hydrochloride.

Dosage and Administration: Unattached placental membranes and any excess uterine fluid or debris should be removed from the uterus. The external genitalia should be carefully cleaned and a clean, sterile inseminating pipette should be passed through the cervix and the NOLVASAN® Suspension infused into the uterus.

Treatment may be repeated in 48 to 72 hours.

Precaution(s): Store at controlled room temperature 15° to 30°C (59° to 86°F).

Caution(s): Keep out of reach of children. For use in horses only.

Warning(s): Not for use in horses intended for food.

Presentation: 0.95 fl. oz. (28 mL) syringe (NDC 0856-1050-01).

Compendium Code No.: 10031371 0501M

NOLVASAN® TEAT DIP CONCENTRATE

Fort Dodge **Teat Dip**

Chlorhexidine Acetate

Active Ingredient(s):

Chlorhexidine acetate . . . . . 4% (18.9 g)
Inert Ingredients . . . . . q.s.
(Including 39% glycerin)

Indications: For use as an aid in controlling bacteria that cause bovine mastitis.

Directions:

To Prepare 0.5% Teat Dip Solution: This 1 pint of NOLVASAN® Teat Dip Concentrate should be reconstituted to 1 gallon of 0.5% teat dip solution. Place entire contents in a clean 1 gallon container and add clean, potable water to yield 1 gallon of teat dip solution. (Use of "hard water" may result in some precipitation. If the 0.5% solution is to be held longer than 1 week, it is advisable to use distilled or deionized water.)

Use of 0.5% Teat Dip Solution: Teat dipping should start 1 week before the cow freshens. During lactation, dip each teat into the 0.5% solution immediately after the cow is milked. When the cow is dried off, the teats should continue to be dipped in the solution once a day for 3 to 4 days. Dip each teat so that the lower 1 inch of the teat has been covered with the solution.

Udder and teats of the cow should be thoroughly washed before milking.

If minor irritation or chapping of the teats should occur during lactation, it is often helpful to dilute the 0.5% solution half and half with clean water for a couple of days and then gradually return to use of the 0.5% solution.

Precaution(s): Store at controlled room temperature 15° to 30°C (59° to 86°F).

Caution(s): May be irritating to eyes or mucous membranes. May be harmful if swallowed. Avoid contamination of feed or feedstuffs. If in contact, flush thoroughly with water. Rinse empty container with water and discard.

Warning(s): Do not use this solution undiluted. Dip teats only in a properly prepared 0.5% solution as directed. Do not use this solution for cleaning milking equipment.

Keep out of reach of children.

For veterinary use only.

Presentation: 16 fl oz (473 mL) containers (NDC 0856-1075-01).

Compendium Code No.: 10031380 0632F

NOLVASAN® UDDER WASH CONCENTRATE

Fort Dodge **Udder Wash**

Chlorhexidine Acetate

Active Ingredient(s):

Chlorhexidine acetate 4%
Inert Ingredients . . . . . q.s.

Indications: A special formula of surfactant and the antimicrobial agent, chlorhexidine acetate, to be used in washing the udder and teats prior to milking. As an aid in sanitizing; and reducing bacteria from the surface of the udder and teats.

Directions: To prepare the final udder wash product add 1 fluid ounce (2 tablespoonfuls) of NOLVASAN® Udder Wash Concentrate to four (4) gallons of clean, potable water. Prepare fresh wash for each milking.

To wash the udder and teats use a separate clean paper towel for each cow; soak the paper towel in the prepared udder wash; and thoroughly wash the entire udder and teats of the cow within 2 minutes of applying the milk machine. Discard the paper towel after use. When washing be careful to remove all dirt and debris from the surface of the udder. (If udder or teats are excessively dirty, a second paper towel should be soaked and the udder/teats washed the second time).

After the udder/teats are washed with the udder wash another paper towel should be used to thoroughly wipe dry the surface of the udder and teats before the milk machine cups are placed on the cow.

Washing of udder/teats should be conducted before each milking. It is also advised to use the Nolvasan® Teat Dip to dip all teats after milking. This will aid in control of bacteria that cause bovine mastitis.

Precaution(s): Store at controlled room temperature 15° to 30°C (59° to 86°F). Avoid freezing or exposure to excessive heat.

Caution(s): Concentrate may be irritating to eyes or mucous membranes. May be harmful if swallowed. Avoid contamination of feed or feedstuffs. If in contact, flush thoroughly with water. Rinse empty container with water and discard.

Warning(s): Do not use this solution undiluted. Wash udder and teats only with properly diluted udder wash and then wipe off udder and teats with clean towel as directed. Do not use this solution for washing of milking equipment.

Keep out of reach of children.

For veterinary use only.

Presentation: 16 fl oz (473 mL) (NDC 0856-0554-01) and 1 gallon (NDC 0856-0554-02) containers.

Compendium Code No.: 10031391 0554H

NON-SPERMICIDAL - STERILE LUBRICATING JELLY

First Priority **Lubricant**

NDC No.: 58829-200-05

Active Ingredient(s): Contains: Propylene glycol, HP methylcellulose, carbomer, purified water and sodium hydroxide to adjust pH.

Indications: NON-SPERMICIDAL - STERILE LUBRICATING JELLY is a sterile non-spermicidal water soluble lubricating jelly for all types of medical procedures.

Dosage and Administration: Apply liberally as needed.

Caution(s): Sterility is not guaranteed after the tube is opened or if damaged.

Presentation: 5 fl oz (150 mL) tube.

Compendium Code No.: 11390571

NORCALCIPHOS™ ℞

Pfizer Animal Health **Calcium-Combination Therapy**

Parenteral Solution

Active Ingredient(s): Contains: Calcium borogluconate, dextrose, magnesium borogluconate, calcium hypophosphite and base.

Total calcium chemically equivalent to calcium borogluconate 26.0%
Dextrose 15.0%
Magnesium borogluconate 6.0%
Total phosphorus in amounts chemically equivalent to elemental phosphorus 0.5%

Indications: For intravenous use in milk fever, and in calcium, phosphorus, magnesium and glucose deficiency in animals.

Dosage and Administration: Dosage: Cattle, 500 mL. For milk fever prophylaxis, give 200-500 mL at time of calving. Horses, 250-500 mL; Sheep 50-125 mL. Repeat in 2 to 6 hours if needed. This product contains no preservative. Unused portion remaining in bottle must be discarded.

Note: Intravenous administration is always preferable. If used subcutaneously, always distribute dose in several places and massage to facilitate absorption.

Precaution(s): Store at controlled room temperature 15°-30°C (59°-86°F). Protect from freezing.

Caution(s): Federal law restricts this drug to use by or on the order of a licensed veterinarian.

Large doses administered intravenously may have toxic action on heart if the blood level of calcium is raised excessively. Doses should be carefully regulated according to severity of hypocalcemia and injected slowly so that administration may be stopped if toxic action becomes evident.

Presentation: Cartons of 12 x 500 mL nonbreakable plastic bottles.

Manufactured by: Phoenix Scientific, Inc., St. Joseph, MO 64506, USA

Compendium Code No.: 36900710 85-7150-09

NORMAL EQUINE SERUM

Colorado Serum **Equine Serum**

Normal Serum, Equine Origin

U.S. Vet. Lic. No.: 188

Active Ingredient(s): The serum is prepared from the blood of normal, healthy horses. Antigenic substances are not administered to production animals for the purpose of stimulating antibody response. Thus, the final product is referred to as normal serum.

Contains phenol and thimerosal as preservatives.

Indications: Indicated as an aid in the nonspecific treatment of equine infections and disease conditions.

Dosage and Administration: Inject subcutaneously, intramuscularly, or intravenously, 50 mL to 250 mL, depending upon the weight of the animal and the judgement of the veterinarian administering. Repeat doses may be given.

When to Vaccinate: NORMAL EQUINE SERUM is recommended for the nonspecific treatment of horses with anemia, haemorrhage, shock that may occur following injury, and for physically debilitating conditions for which blood enrichment is considered desirable.

Precaution(s): Store in the dark at 2-7°C.

Sterilize syringes and needles by boiling in clean water. Use the entire contents when first opened.

Caution(s): Anaphylactic reactions sometimes follow administration of products of this nature. If noted, administer adrenaline or an equivalent drug.

A condition referred to as serum hepatitis infrequently occurs in horses. The literature associates this with the injection of biologics containing equine serum or tissue. The connection is based, at the present time, upon supposition and not upon scientific evidence as efforts to experimentally reproduce such a condition in horses have not been successful. It seems prudent, however, in view of the published implications, to make horse owners aware of it.

For veterinary use only.

Warning(s): Do not vaccinate within 21 days before slaughter.

Presentation: 100 mL and 250 mL vials.

Compendium Code No.: 11010260

NORMAL SERUM-EQUINE

Professional Biological **Equine Serum**

Normal Serum, Equine Origin

U.S. Vet. Lic. No.: 188

Active Ingredient(s): Preserved serum prepared from the blood of normal, healthy horses.

Contains phenol and thimerosal as preservatives.

Indications: Indicated as an aid in the nonspecific treatment of equine infections and disease conditions.

Dosage and Administration: Inject subcutaneously, intramuscularly, or intravenously, 50 mL to 250 mL, depending upon the weight of the animal and the judgement of the veterinarian administering. Repeat doses may be given.

Precaution(s): Store in dark at 2° to 7°C.

Caution(s): Anaphylactic reactions sometime follow administration of products of this nature. If noted, administer adrenaline or equivalent. Use the entire contents when first opened.

A condition referred to as "serum hepatitis" infrequently occurs in horses. The literature associates this partially with the injection of biologics containing equine serum or tissue. This connection is based, at the present time, upon supposition and not upon scientific evidence as efforts to experimentally reproduce such a condition in horses have not been successful. It seems prudent, however, in view of the published implications, to make horse owners aware of it.

For veterinary use only.

Warning(s): Do not vaccinate within 21 days before slaughter.

Presentation: 100 mL and 250 mL vials.

Compendium Code No.: 14250021

NORMOSOL®-R ℞

Abbott **Fluid Therapy**

Replacement Electrolytes and Water

Active Ingredient(s): Description: NORMOSOL®-R is a sterile, nonpyrogenic isotonic solution of balanced electrolytes in water for injection. The solution is administered by intravenous infusion for parenteral replacement of acute losses of extracellular fluid.

Each 100 mL of NORMOSOL®-R contains sodium chloride, 526 mg; sodium acetate, 222 mg; sodium gluconate, 502 mg; potassium chloride, 37 mg; magnesium chloride hexahydrate, 30 mg. May contain HCl and/or NaOH for pH adjustment. (pH 6.6 (5.5 - 8.0): 294 mOsmol/liter (calc.).)

Electrolytes per 1000 mL (not including pH adjustment): Sodium 140 mEq; potassium 5 mEq; magnesium 3 mEq; chloride 98 mEq; acetate 27 mEq; gluconate 23 mEq.

The solution contains no bacteriostat, antimicrobial agent or added buffer (except for pH adjustment) and is intended only for use as a single-dose injection. When smaller doses are required the unused portion should be discarded.

Contains no preservative.

Indications: NORMOSOL®-R is indicated for replacement of acute extracellular fluid volume losses in surgery, trauma, burns or shock. NORMOSOL®-R also can be used as an adjunct to restore a decrease in circulatory volume in patients with moderate blood loss. NORMOSOL®-R is not intended to supplant transfusion of whole blood or packed red cells in the presence of uncontrolled hemorrhage or severe reductions of red cell volume.

Pharmacology: NORMOSOL®-R is a parenteral fluid and electrolyte replenisher.

Sodium Chloride, USP is chemically designated NaCl, a white crystalline powder freely soluble in water.

Potassium Chloride, USP is chemically designated KCl, a white granular powder freely soluble in water.

Magnesium Chloride, USP is chemically designated magnesium chloride hexahydrate ($MgCl_2 \cdot 6H_2O$) deliquescent crystals very soluble in water.

Sodium Acetate, USP, is chemically designated sodium acetate anhydrous ($C_2H_3NaO_2$), a hygroscopic powder soluble in water. It has the following structural formula:

```
    H   O
    |   ‖
H — C — C — ONa
    |
    H
```

Sodium gluconate is chemically designated $C_6H_{11}NaO_7$, the normal sodium salt of gluconic acid soluble in water. It has the following structural formula:

```
         H    H    OH   H
         |    |    |    |
HOCH₂— C  — C  — C  — C — COONa
         |    |    |    |
         OH   OH   H    OH
```

Water for Injection, USP is chemically designated H2O.

The flexible plastic container is fabricated from a specially formulated polyvinylchloride. Water can permeate from inside the container into the overwrap but not in amounts sufficient to affect the solution significantly. Solutions inside the plastic container also can leach out certain of its chemical components in very small amounts before the expiration period is attained. However, the safety of the plastic has been confirmed by tests in animals according to USP biological standards for plastic containers.

Clinical Pharmacology: When administered intravenously, NORMOSOL®-R provides water and electrolytes for replacement of acute extracellular fluid losses without disturbing normal electrolyte relationships. The electrolyte composition approaches that of the principal ions of normal plasma (extracellular fluid). The electrolyte concentration is approximately isotonic in relation to the extracellular fluid (approx. 280 mOsmol/liter) and provides a physiologic sodium to chloride ratio, normal plasma concentrations of potassium and magnesium and two bicarbonate alternates, acetate and gluconate.

Sodium chloride in water dissociates to provide sodium (Na+) and chloride (Cl^-) ions. Sodium (Na^+) is the principal cation of the extracellular fluid and plays a large part in the therapy of fluid and electrolyte disturbances. Chloride (Cl^-) has an integral role in buffering action when oxygen and carbon dioxide exchange occurs in the red blood cells. The distribution and excretion of sodium (Na^+) and chloride (Cl^-) are largely under the control of the kidney which maintains a balance between intake and output.

Potassium chloride in water dissociates to provide potassium (K^+) and chloride (Cl^-) ions. Potassium is the chief cation of body cells (160 mEq/liter of intracellular water). It is found in low concentration in plasma and extracellular fluids (3.5 to 5.0 mEq/liter in a healthy adult). Potassium plays an important role in electrolyte balance.

Normally about 80 to 90% of the potassium intake is excreted in the urine; the remainder in the stools and to a small extent, in the perspiration. The kidney does not conserve potassium well so that during fasting or in patients on a potassium-free diet, potassium loss from the body continues resulting in potassium depletion.

Magnesium chloride in water dissociates to provide magnesium (Mg^{++}) and chloride (Cl^-) ions. Magnesium is the second most plentiful cation of the intracellular fluids. It is an important cofactor for enzymatic reactions and plays an important role in neurochemical transmission and muscular excitability. Normal plasma concentration ranges from 1.5 to 2.5 or 3.0 mEq/liter. Magnesium is excreted solely by the kidney at a rate proportional to the plasma concentration and glomerular filtration.

Sodium acetate provides sodium (Na^+) and acetate (CH_3COO^-) ions, the latter anion (a source of hydrogen ion acceptors) serving as an alternate source of bicarbonate (HCO_3^-) by metabolic conversion. This has been shown to proceed readily even in the presence of severe liver disease. Thus, acetate anion exerts a mild systemic antiacidotic action that may be advantageous during fluid and electrolyte replacement therapy.

Sodium gluconate provides sodium (Na^+) and gluconate ($C_6H_{11}O_7^-$)ions. Gluconate is a theoretical alternate metabolic source of bicarbonate (HCO_3^-) anion.

Water is an essential constituent of all body tissues and accounts for approximately 70% of total body weight. Average normal adult daily requirement ranges from two to three liters (1.0 to 1.5 liters each for insensible water loss by perspiration and urine production).

Water balance is maintained by various regulatory mechanisms. Water distribution depends primarily on the concentration of electrolytes in the body compartments and sodium (Na^+) plays a major role in maintaining physiologic equilibrium.

Dosage and Administration: NORMOSOL®-R is administered by intravenous infusion. It may also be administered subcutaneously. The amount to be infused is based on replacement of losses of extracellular fluid volume in the individual patient. Up to 3 times the volume of estimated blood loss during and after surgery can be given to correct circulatory volume when there is only a moderate loss of blood.

Drug Interactions: Additives may be incompatible. Consult with Additive Manufacturer. When introducing additives, use aseptic technique, mix thoroughly and do not store.

Parenteral drug products should be inspected visually for particulate matter or discoloration prior to administration, whenever solution and container permit. See Cautions.

NORMOSOL®-R does not contain calcium to avoid precipitation of calcium salts that may occur when certain drugs are added. Solutions which contain calcium in amounts exceeding the normal plasma concentration may enhance clotting on contact with citrated blood. Hence, NORMOSOLL®-R can be used for starting blood transfusion.

Instructions For Use:

To Open: Tear outer wrap at notch and remove solution container. If supplemental medication is desired, follow directions below before preparing for administration. Some opacity of the plastic due to moisture absorption during the sterilization process may be observed. This is normal and does not affect the solution quality or safety. The opacity will diminish gradually.

To Add Medication:

1. Prepare additive port.
2. Using aseptic technique and an additive delivery needle of appropriate length, puncture resealable additive port at target area, inner diaphragm and inject. Withdraw needle after injecting medication.
3. The additive port may be protected by covering with an additive cap.
4. Mix container contents thoroughly.

Preparation for Administration (Use aseptic technique):

1. Close flow control clamp of administration set.
2. Remove cover from outlet port at bottom of container.
3. Insert piercing pin of administration set into port with a twisting motion until the set is firmly seated. Note: See full directions on administration set carton.
4. Suspend container from hanger.
5. Squeeze and release drip chamber to establish proper fluid level in chamber.
6. Open flow control clamp and clear air from set. Close clamp.

7. Attach set to venipuncture device. If device is not indwelling, prime and make venipuncture.
8. Regulate rate of administration with flow control clamp.

Contraindication(s): None known.
Precaution(s): Exposure of pharmaceutical products to heat should be minimized. Avoid excessive heat. Protect from freezing. It is recommended that the product be stored at room temperature (25°C); however, brief exposure up to 40°C does not adversely affect the product.
Caution(s): Federal (USA) law restricts this drug to use by or on the order of a licensed veterinarian.

NORMOSOL®-R should be used with caution in severe renal impairment because of the danger of hyperkalemia. As with all intravenous solutions, care should be taken to avoid circulatory overload, especially in patients with cardiac or pulmonary disorders. NORMOSOL®-R is not intended to correct acidosis or large deficits of individual electrolytes, nor to replace blood or plasma expanders when these are indicated.

Clinical evaluation and periodic laboratory determinations are necessary to monitor changes in fluid balance, electrolyte concentrations and acid-base balance during prolonged parenteral therapy or whenever the condition of the patient warrants such evaluation.

Caution must be exercised in the administration of parenteral fluids, especially those containing sodium ions, to patients receiving corticosteroids or corticotropin.

Solutions containing acetate or gluconate ions should be used with caution, as excess administration may result in metabolic alkalosis.

Do not administer unless solution is clear and container is undamaged. Discard unused portion.

For animal use only.

Warning(s): Solutions containing sodium ions should be used with great care, if at all, in patients with congestive heart failure, severe renal insufficiency and in clinical states in which there exists edema with sodium retention.

Solutions which contain potassium should be used with great care, if at all, in patients with hyperkalemia, severe renal failure and in conditions in which potassium retention is present.

In patents with diminished renal function, administration of solutions containing sodium or potassium ions may result in sodium or potassium retention.

Solutions containing acetate or gluconate ions should be used with great care in patients with metabolic or respiratory alkalosis. Acetate or gluconate should be administered with great care in those conditions in which there is an increased level or an impaired utilization of these ions, such as severe hepatic insufficiency.

The intravenous administration of this solution can cause fluid and/or solute overloading resulting in dilution of serum electrolyte concentrations, overhydration, congested states or pulmonary edema.

The risk of dilutional states is inversely proportional to the electrolyte concentrations of administered parenteral solutions. The risk of solute overload causing congested states with peripheral and pulmonary edema is directly proportional to the electrolyte concentrations of such solutions.

Overdose: In the event of overhydration or solute overload, re-evaluate the patient and institute appropriate corrective measures. See warnings, Cautions and adverse reactions.
Adverse Reactions: Reactions which may occur because of the solution or the technique of administration include febrile response, infection at the site of injection, venous thrombosis or phlebitis extending from the site of injection, extravasation and hypervolemia.

If an adverse reaction does occur, discontinue the infusion, evaluate the patient, institute appropriate therapeutic countermeasures and save the remainder of the fluid for examination if deemed necessary.

Presentation: NORMOSOL®-R is supplied in a 3000 mL single-dose flexible plastic container (List No. 210701).
NORMOSOL®-R is a registered trademark of Abbott Laboratories.
Compendium Code No.: 10240060 06-9416/RI

N

NOVA PEARLS™ 5 TO 1 CONCENTRATE SHAMPOO

Tomlyn **Grooming Shampoo**

Active Ingredient(s): Contains Novasome® encapsulated moisturizers in a pH balanced concentrated shampoo base.
Indications: A concentrated, moisturizing grooming shampoo for use on dogs and cats.
Directions: Shake well and dilute one part shampoo to four parts water. Wet coat thoroughly before applying shampoo. Work shampoo into coat until a mild lather is produced. Rinse and repeat as necessary.
Precaution(s): Store at room temperature.
Caution(s): For topical use only on dogs and cats. Avoid contact with eyes and mucous membranes. Discontinue use if skin becomes irritated or inflamed.

Keep out of reach of children.

Presentation: 4 x 1 gallon (128 fl oz - 3.79 L) -- One gallon makes 5 gallons.
Novasome® is a registered trademark of Micro Pak, Inc.
Compendium Code No.: 11220110 679-1

NOVA PEARLS™ ANTISEBORRHEIC SHAMPOO

Tomlyn **Antidermatosis Shampoo**

Active Ingredient(s):
Sulfur 2%
Salicylic acid 2%

Also contains Novasome™ encapsulated moisturizers in a concentrated shampoo base.

Indications: NOVA PEARLS™ antiseborrheic formulation shampoo contains micro-targeted Novasome™ microvesicles designed to deliver long lasting moisture factors to the hair shafts and skin along with antiseborrheic medications. The result is a shampoo that aids in decreasing the drying and scaling of seborrhea.

Formulated for dry, flaking, itchy skin for medicated cleansing and conditioning in dogs.

Dosage and Administration: Shake well. Wet the coat thoroughly before applying the shampoo. Work the shampoo into the coat until a mild lather is produced. Allow to stand for 5-10 minutes and then rinse thoroughly. Repeat as necessary. NOVA PEARLS™ antiseborrheic formulation shampoo may be used two (2) to three (3) times a week initially, and then at required intervals as directed by a veterinarian.
Caution(s): For veterinary use only.

For topical use only on dogs. Avoid contact with the eyes and mucous membranes. Discontinue use if the skin becomes irritated or inflamed.

Keep out of the reach of children.

Presentation: 355 mL and 3.79 L.
* Novasome is a trademark of Micro Pak, Inc. Produced under licensing agreement with Micro Vesicular Systems, Inc.
Compendium Code No.: 11220120

NOVA PEARLS™ COAL TAR SPRAY

Tomlyn **Antidermatosis Spray**

Medical Coal Tar Spray

Active Ingredient(s):
Coal tar topical solution U.S.P. 3.5%
(Equivalent to 0.7% coal tar.)

Also contains Novasome® encapsulated moisturizers in an oil free base.

Indications: NOVA PEARLS™ Coal Tar Spray medicates as Power Moisturizers™ are slow-released to keep the skin moisture-rich for days after.

Formulated to help stop the itching of seborrhea, minor skin irritations, inflammations and rashes as it soothes and moisturizes.

Directions: Shake well. Apply spray to damp or dry coat after shampooing or between shampoo treatments. Use as necessary to control scaling, flaking and itching. Allow spray to dry, then brush as needed.
Caution(s): For topical use only on dogs. Avoid contact with eyes and mucous membranes. Discontinue use if skin becomes irritated or inflamed.

Keep out of reach of children.

For animals use only.

Warning(s): This product contains coal tar, a chemical known to the State of California to cause cancer.
Presentation: 12 fl oz (355 mL).
Novasome is a registered trademark of Micro Pak, Inc.
Compendium Code No.: 11220131 026-2 5

NOVA PEARLS™ DRY SKIN BATH FOR DOGS

Tomlyn **Grooming Shampoo**

Active Ingredient(s):
Sulfur 2%
Salicylic Acid 2%

Also contains Novasome® encapsulated moisturizers in a concentrated shampoo base.

Indications: A moisturizing grooming shampoo formulated to relieve excessive dryness, flaking and itching due of seborrhea.
Directions: Shake well. Wet coat thoroughly before applying shampoo. Work shampoo into coat until a mild lather is produced. Allow to stand for 5-10 minutes and then rinse thoroughly. Repeat as necessary. NOVA PEARLS™ Dry Skin Bath with sulfur & salicylic acid may be used 2-3 times weekly Initially, and then at required intervals as directed by a veterinarian. As with all medicated shampoos, the applicator should wear gloves when applying this product.
Precaution(s): Store in a cool place.
Caution(s): For topical use only on dogs. Avoid contact with eyes and mucous membranes. Discontinue use if skin becomes irritated or inflamed.

Keep out of reach of children.

For animal use only.

Presentation: 12 x 12 fl oz (355 mL) and 4 x 1 gallon (128 fl oz - 3.79 L).
Novasome® is a registered trademark of Micro Pak, Inc.
Compendium Code No.: 11220140 029-2, 030-2

NOVA PEARLS™ FRESH SCENT DEODORANT SPRAY FOR DOGS AND CATS

Tomlyn **Grooming Spray**

Ingredient(s): Contains Lactamide MEA a lactic acid derivative emollient with Novasome® encapsulated moisturizers in an oil-free base.
Indications: Moisturizing deodorizing spray for dogs and cats.

Formulated to provide instant deodorizing and moisture surge to aid in the elimination of pet odor, the revitalization of dry dull coat and the relief of flaking and scaling due to dry skin.

Directions: Shake well. Apply NOVA PEARLS™ Power Moisturizing Deodorizing Spray liberally to damp or dry coat. Use as necessary to control odor, scaling and flaking due to excessive dryness. Allow spray to dry, then brush as needed.
Caution(s): For topical use only on dogs and cats.

Avoid contact with eyes and mucous membranes.

Discontinue use if skin becomes irritated or inflamed.

For animal use only.

Warning(s): Keep out of reach of children.
Discussion: Tomlyn NOVA PEARLS™ products are the only dry skin treatments with Power Moisturizers™ encapsulated in Novasome® microcarriers.

Power Moisturizers™ are coupled with conditioners in a humidifying spray with Lactamide MEA for a soft, supple, lustrous coat.

Power Moisturizers™ are, slow-released for long-lasting moisturization to keep the skin and coat moisture-rich and fresh for days after. Safe for use on dogs and cats.

Presentation: 12 fl oz (355 mL).
Novasome is a registered trademark of Micro Pak, Inc.
Compendium Code No.: 11220310 0321 1

NOVA PEARLS™ FRESH SCENT DEODORANT SPRAY FOR FERRETS

Tomlyn **Deodorant Product**

Active Ingredient(s): Contains Lactamide MEA, a lactic acid derivative emollient with Novasome® encapsulated moisturizers in an oil-free base.
Indications: A conditioning and deodorant spray for use on ferrets. It may also be used on other small animals.
Directions: Shake well. Apply NOVA PEARLS™ power moisturizing deodorizing spray for ferrets liberally to damp or dry coat. Use as necessary to control odor, scaling and flaking due to excessive dryness. Allow spray to dry, then brush as needed.
Precaution(s): Store in a cool place.
Caution(s): For topical use only on ferrets and other small animals. Avoid contact with eyes and mucous membranes. Discontinue use if skin becomes irritated or inflamed.

Keep out of reach of children.

For animal use only.

Presentation: 12 x 6 fl oz (177 mL).
Novasome® is a registered trademark of Micro Pak, Inc.
Compendium Code No.: 11220150 726-0

NOVA PEARLS™ POWER MOISTURIZING SPRAY MIST

Tomlyn

Active Ingredient(s): Contains lactic acid derivative emolient with Novasome® encapsulated moisturizers in an oil-free base.
Indications: A conditioning spray for use on dogs and cats.
Directions: Shake well. Apply NOVA PEARLS® Power Moisturizing Spray Mist liberally to damp or dry coat. Use as necessary to control scaling and flaking. Allow spray to dry, then brush as needed.
Precaution(s): Store in a cool place.
Caution(s): For topical use only on dogs and cats. Avoid contact with eyes and mucous membranes. Discontinue use if skin becomes irritated or inflamed.
Keep out of reach of children.
Presentation: 12 x 12 fl oz (355 mL).
Novasome® is a registered trademark of Micro Pak, Inc.
Compendium Code No.: 11220160 031-2

NOVA PEARLS™ SENSITIVE SKIN SHAMPOO

Tomlyn **Grooming Shampoo**

Active Ingredient(s): Contains Novasome® encapsulated moisturizers in a pH balanced concerntrated shampoo base.
Indications: A moisturizing grooming shampoo for dogs and cats.
Directions: Shake well. Wet coat thoroughly before applying shampoo. Work shampoo into coat until a mild lather is produced. Rinse and repeat as necessary.
Precaution(s): Store at room temperature.
Caution(s): For topical use only on dogs and cats. Avoid contact with eyes and mucous membranes. Discontinue use if it skin becomes irritated or inflamed.
Keep out of reach of children.
For animal use only.
Presentation: 12 x 12 fl oz (355 mL) and 4 x 1 gallon (128 fl oz - 3.79 L).
Novasome® is a registered trademark of Micro Pak, Inc.
Compendium Code No.: 11220170 027-2, 028-2

NOVA PEARLS™ SPRAY ON MOISTURIZER FOR CAT DANDER

Tomlyn **Allergy Relief Spray**

Active Ingredient(s): Contains Lactamide MEA, a lactic acid derivative emollient with Novasome® encapsulated moisturizers in an oil-free base.
Indications: Recommended to help reduce the amount of dander shed by cats. Dander causes undesirable reactions in allergic people.
Directions: Shake well. Apply NOVA PEARLS™ Spray On Moisturizer to damp or dry coat before and after brushing to keep dander in check. Spray with and against the lay of the hair to insure penetration to the skin. Use to prevent and control scaling and flaking due to dry skin every time you groom your pet.
Precaution(s): Store in a cool place.
Caution(s): For topical use on cats. Avoid contact with eyes and mucous membranes. Discontinue use if skin becomes irritated or inflamed.
Keep out of reach of children.
For animal use only.
Presentation: 12 x 12 fl oz (355 mL).
Novasome® is a registered trademark of Micro Pak, Inc.
Compendium Code No.: 11220180 033-1

NOVA PEARLS™ THERAPEUTIC COAL TAR SHAMPOO

Tomlyn **Antidermatosis Shampoo**

Active Ingredient(s): Coal Tar Topical Solution USP 5% (Equivalent to 1% Coal Tar).
Also contains Novasome® encapsulated moisturizers in a pH balanced concentrated shampoo base.
Indications: Controls seborrheic dermatitis in dogs.
Formulated to help stop the itching of seborrhea, minor skin irritations, inflammations and rashes as it cleanses and moisturizes.
Directions: Shake well. Wet coat thoroughly before applying shampoo. Work into coat until a mild lather is produced. Allow to stand for 5-10 minutes and then rinse thoroughly. Repeat as necessary, depending on severity of the condition. NOVA PEARLS™ Coal Tar Shampoo may be used 2-3 times weekly initially, and then at required intervals as directed by a veterinarian. As with all medicated shampoos, the applicator should wear gloves when applying this product.
Caution(s): For topical use only on dogs. Avoid contact with eyes and mucous membranes. Discontinue use if skin becomes irritated or inflamed.
For animal use only.
Warning(s): Keep out of reach of children.
This product contains coal tar, a chemical known to the State of California to cause cancer.
Discussion: Tomlyn's NOVA PEARLS™ products are the only dry skin treatments with Power Moisturizers™ encapsulated in Novasome® microcarriers. Power Moisturizers™ are coupled with a non-steroidal pH balanced medicated shampoo containing 5% coal tar topical solution, an antiseborrheic and anti-itch agent. NOVA PEARLS™ Coal Tar Shampoo medicates as Power Moisturizers™ are slow-released to keep the skin moisture-rich for days after Safe for use on dogs only.
Presentation: 1 gallon (128 fl oz - 3.79 L).
Novasome is a registered Trademark of Micro Pak, Inc.
Compendium Code No.: 11220320 025-2 5

NRG-PLUS™

Bimeda **Large Animal Dietary Supplement**

Guaranteed Analysis:
Crude Protein, not less than 9.0%
Crude Fat, not less than 0.25%
Crude Fiber, not more than 1.0%
Crude Ash, not more than 4.0%

Ingredients: Nutrients: Dextrose, dried skimmed milk, dried whey, enzymatic hydrolysates of yeast, sodium caseinate, soy protein, dl-methionine and corn starch.
Vitamins: Vitamin A (as acetate and palmitate), vitamin D_3, vitamin E, riboflavin (vitamin B_2), d-pantothenic acid (vitamin B_5), niacin (vitamin B_3), choline bitartrate, menadione sodium bisulphite complex (source of vitamin K), folic acid, thiamine mononitrate (vitamin B_1), ascorbic acid (vitamin C), pyridoxine hydrochloride (vitamin B_6), cyanocobalamin (vitamin B_{12}).
Electrolytes: Sodium chloride, potassium chloride, sodium bicarbonate and potassium phosphate.
Trace Minerals: Polysaccharide complexes of zinc, cobalt, manganese, iron and copper.
Indications: NRG-PLUS™ is a source of amino acids, energy, vitamins and electrolytes. It is designed for oral use in calves.
Dosage and Administration: Give 1 pound per 500-1000 pounds body weight. Suspend product in at least 2 quarts of lukewarm water and administer through a stomach tube or as a drench. Repeat as indicated. Consult your veterinarian concerning correct drenching procedure. Prepare fresh solution daily.
Warning(s): For animal use only. Not for human use.
Keep out of reach of children.
Presentation: 1 pound (454 gram) pouch and 20 lb pail.
Compendium Code No.: 13990290

NUFLOR® INJECTABLE SOLUTION 300 MG/ML ℞

Schering-Plough **Florfenicol**

NADA No.: 141-063
Active Ingredient(s): Description: NUFLOR® Injectable is a solution of the synthetic antibiotic florfenicol. Each millimeter of sterile NUFLOR® Injectable Solution contains 300 mg of florfenicol, 250 mg n-methyl-2-pyrrolidone, 150 mg propylene glycol, and polyethylene glycol q.s.
Indications: NUFLOR® Injectable Solution is indicated for treatment of bovine respiratory disease (BRD), associated with *Pasteurella haemolytica, Pasteurella multocida*, and *Haemophilus somnus*, and for the treatment of bovine interdigital phlegmon (foot rot, acute interdigital necrobacillosis, infectious pododermatitis) associated with *Fusobacterium necrophorum* and *Bacteroides melaninogenicus*. Also, it is indicated for the control of respiratory disease in cattle at high risk of developing BRD associated with *Pasteurella haemolytica, Pasteurella multocida*, and *Haemophilus somnus*.
Pharmacology: Clinical Pharmacology: The pharmacokinetic disposition of NUFLOR® Injectable Solution was evaluated in feeder calves following single intramuscular administration at the recommended dose of 20 mg/kg. NUFLOR® Injectable Solution was also administered intravenously to the same cattle in order to calculate the volume of distribution, clearance, and percent bioavailability[1] (Table 1).
Table 1: Pharmakokinetic Parameter Values for Florfenicol following IM Administration of 20 mg/kg Body Weight to Feeder Calves (n=10).

Parameter	Median	Range
C_{MAX} (μg/mL)	3.07*	1.43 - 5.60
T_{MAX} (hr)	3.33	0.75 - 8.00
T½, (hr)	18.3**	8.30 - 44.0
AUC (μg•min/mL)	4242	3200 - 6250
Bioavailability (%)	78.5	59.3 - 106
Vd_{ss} (L/kg)***	0.77	0.68 - 0.85
Cl_t (mL/min/kg)***	3.75	3.17 - 4.31

* harmonic mean
** mean value
*** following I.V. administration
C_{MAX} Maximum serum concentration
T_{MAX} Time at which C_{MAX} is observed
T½ Biological half-life
AUC Area under the curve
Vd_{ss} Volume of distribution at steady state
Cl_t Total body clearance

N

Florfenicol was detectable in the serum of most animals through 60 hours after intramuscular administration with a mean concentration of 0.19 μg/mL. The protein binding of florfenicol was 12.7%, 13.2%, and 18.3% at serum concentrations of 0.5, 3.0, and 16.0 μg/mL, respectively.
Microbiology: Florfenicol is a synthetic, broad-spectrum antibiotic active against many gram-negative and gram-positive bacteria isolated from domestic animals. It is primarily bacteriostatic and acts by binding to the 50S ribosomal subunit and inhibiting bacterial protein synthesis. *In vitro* and *in vivo* activity has been demonstrated against commonly isolated bacterial pathogens involved in bovine respiratory disease (BRD), including *Pasteurella haemolytica, Pasteurella multocida*, and *Haemophilus somnus*, as well as against commonly isolated bacterial pathogens involved in bovine interdigital phlegmon including *Fusobacterium necrophorum* and *Bacteroides melaninogenicus*.
The minimum inhibitory concentrations (MICs) of florfenicol for BRD organisms were determined using isolates obtained from natural infections from 1990 to 1993. The MICs for interdigital phlegmon organisms were determined using isolates obtained from natural infections from 1973 to 1997 (Table 2).
Table 2: MIC Values* of Florfenicol Against Bacterial Isolates From Natural Infection of Cattle

Organism	Isolate Numbers	MIC_{50}** (μg/mL)	MIC_{90}** (μg/mL)
Pasteurella haemolytica	398	0.50	1.00
Pasteurella multocida	350	0.50	0.50
Haemophilus somnus	66	0.25	0.50
Fusobacterium necrophorum	33	0.25	0.25
Bacteroides melaninogenicus	20	0.25	0.25

*The correlation between the *in vitro* susceptibility data (MIC values) and clinical response has not been confirmed.
**The minimum inhibitory concentration for 50% and 90% of the isolates.
Dosage and Administration: For treatment of bovine respiratory disease (BRD) and bovine interdigital phlegmon (foot rot): NUFLOR® Injectable Solution should be administered by intramuscular injection to cattle at a dose rate of 20 mg/kg body weight (3 mL/100 lbs). A second dose should be administered 48 hours later. Alternatively, NUFLOR® Injectable Solution can be administered by a single subcutaneous injection to cattle at a dose rate of 40 mg/kg body weight (6 mL/100 lbs). Do not administer more than 10 mL at each site. The injection should be given only in the neck.
Note: Intramuscular injection may result in local tissue reaction which persists beyond 28 days. This may result in trim loss of edible tissue at slaughter. Tissue reaction at injection sites other than the neck are likely to be more severe.
For control of respiratory disease in cattle at high-risk of developing BRD: NUFLOR® Injectable Solution should be administered by a single subcutaneous injection to cattle at a dose rate of

40 mg/kg body weight (6 mL/100 lbs). Do not administer more than 10 mL at each site. The injection should be given only in the neck.

Animal Weight (lbs)	NUFLOR® Dosage Guide IM NUFLOR® Dosage 3.0 mL/100 lb Body Weight (mL)	SC NUFLOR® Dosage 6.0 mL/100 lb Body Weight (mL)
100	3.0	6.0
200	6.0	12.0
300	9.0	18.0
400	12.0	24.0
500	15.0	30.0
600	18.0	36.0
700	21.0	42.0
800	24.0	48.0
900	27.0	54.0
1000	30.0	60.0

Do not inject more than 10 mL per injection site.

Recommended Injection Location:

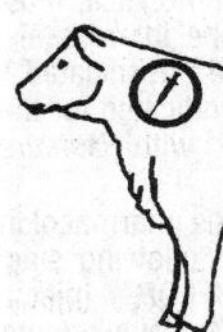

Clinical improvement should be evident in most treated subjects within 24 hours of initiation of treatment. If a positive response is not noted within 72 hours of initiation of treatment, the diagnosis should be re-evaluated.

Precaution(s): Storage Conditions: Store between 2°-30°C (36°-86°F). Refrigeration is not required. The solution is light yellow to straw colored. Color does not affect potency.

Caution(s): Federal law restricts this drug to use by or on the order of a licensed veterinarian.

Not for use in cattle of breeding age. The effects of florfenicol on bovine reproductive performance, pregnancy, and lactation have not been determined. Intramuscular injection may result in local tissue reaction which persists beyond 28 days. This may result in trim loss of edible tissue at slaughter. Tissue reaction at injection sites other than the neck are likely to be more severe.

For intramuscular and subcutaneous use in cattle only.

Warning(s): Residue Warnings: Animals intended for human consumption must not be slaughtered within 28 days of the last intramuscular treatment. Animals intended for human consumption must not be slaughtered within 38 days of subcutaneous treatment. Do not use in female dairy cattle 20 months of age or older. Use of florfenicol in this class of cattle may cause milk residues. A withdrawal period has not been established in pre-ruminating calves. Do not use in calves to be processed for veal.

Not for human use. Keep out of reach of children. This product contains materials that can be irritating to skin and eyes. Avoid direct contact with skin, eyes, and clothing. In case of accidental skin exposure, wash with soap and water. Remove contaminated clothing. Consult a physician if irritation persists. Accidental injection of this product may cause local irritation. Consult a physician immediately. The Material Safety Data Sheet (MSDS) contains more detailed occupational safety information.

N

For customer service, adverse effects reporting, and/or a copy of the MSDS, call 1-800-211-3573.

Toxicology: A 10X safety study was conducted in feeder calves. Two intramuscular injections of 200 mg/kg were administered at a 48-hour interval. The calves were monitored for 14 days after the second dose. Marked anorexia, decreased water consumption, decreased body weight, and increased serum enzymes were observed following dose administration. These effects resolved by the end of the study.

A 1X, 3X, and 5X (20, 60, and 100 mg/kg) safety study was conducted in feeder calves for 3X the duration of treatment (6 injections at 48-hour intervals. Slight decrease in feed and water consumption was observed in the 1X dose group. Decreased feed and water consumption, body weight, urine pH, and increased serum enzymes, were observed in the 3X and 5X dose groups. Depression, soft stool consistency, and dehydration were also observed in some animals (most frequently at the 3X and 5X dose levels), primarily near the end of dosing.

A 43-day controlled study was conducted in healthy cattle to evaluate effects of NUFLOR® Injectable Solution administered at the recommended dose on feed consumption. Although a transient decrease in feed consumption was observed, NUFLOR® Injectable Solution administration had no long-term effect on body weight, rate of gain, or feed consumption.

Adverse Reactions: Inappetence, decreased water consumption, or diarrhea may occur transiently following treatment.

References: Available upon request.

Presentation: NUFLOR® Injectable Solution is packaged in 100 mL (NDC 0061-1116-04), 250 mL (NDC 0061-1116-05), and 500 mL (NDC 0061-1116-06) glass sterile multiple-dose vials.

Compendium Code No.: 10471372 Rev. 12/01 / Rev. 1/99 / Rev. 6/99

NU-KETO™ BOLUS

Butler **Niacin**

Active Ingredient(s): Each 15 g bolus contains:

Niacin (nicotinic acid) . . . . 6 g

Indications: For use as a supplementary source of niacin when such supplementation is indicated in high-producing dairy cows.

Dosage and Administration: Give one (1) bolus in the morning and one (1) bolus in the evening. Administer orally with a balling gun or crush the bolus and feed with the high energy ration.

Precaution(s): Store at a controlled room temperature between 15° and 30°C (59°-86°F).

Caution(s): For veterinary use only.

Keep out of the reach of children.

Presentation: Boxes of 20 boluses.

Compendium Code No.: 10821220

NURTURALL®-C FOR KITTENS

V.P.L. **Milk Replacer**

Balanced Milk Replacer

Guaranteed Analysis: (as a powder):

Crude Protein, min 33.5%
Crude Fat, min 18.0%
Crude Fiber, max. 0.2%
Moisture, max. 5.0%
Ash, max. 8.0%

Ingredients: Nonfat Dry Milk, Corn Oil, Soy Protein Isolate, Sodium Caseinate, Corn Syrup Solids, Maltodextrin, Calcium Carbonate, Carrageenan, Colostrum Milk Powder, Magnesium Phosphate, Choline Chloride, Sodium Ascorbate, Potassium Bicarbonate, Dipotassium Phosphate, Natural and Artificial Flavors, Ferrous Sulfate, Vitamin E Acetate, Mono-Diglycerides, Niacinamide, Zinc Oxide, L-Arginine, DL-Methionine, Cupric Sulfate, Calcium Pantothenate, L-Taurine, Manganese Sulfate, Pyridoxine Hydrochloride (Vitamin B_6), Thiamine Hydrochloride, Wheat Starch, Riboflavin, Menadione, Biotin, Potassium Iodide, Folic Acid, Vitamin A Palmitate, Sodium Selenite, Cyanocobalamin (Vitamin B_{12}), Cholecalciferol (Vitamin D_3), BHT and Propyl Gallate (preservatives).

Powder Form: Fortified with colostrum.

Indications: Mother's milk replacer for kittens and food supplement for adult cats.

This product is intended for intermittent or supplemental feeding only.

Directions: Directions for Preparation and Use: Weigh the kitten. Prepare enough NURTURALL®-C, with the enclosed measuring scoop, for use within a 24-hour period. Kittens should be fed at least ½ ounce of liquid NURTURALL®-C for every two ounces of body weight, daily. Kittens should be allowed to consume as much formula as they want. The table below gives minimum feeding amounts for a 24-hour period. Mix one scoop powder into one scoop of water. Use tap or bottled water. Stir until smooth. Pour liquid into a clean Nurturall® nurser. Heat liquid by placing bottle in a pan of tepid water. Test temperature on your wrist. It should feel slightly warm. Do not microwave. Store NURTURALL®-C powder in the refrigerator. Refrigerate any unused reconstituted liquid for up to 24 hours.

After feeding, hold the kitten's head on your shoulder and rub his back gently until he burps. Make water available after kittens are two weeks old. Small animal water bottles are recommended.

1. Measure water.
2. Mix in NURTURALL®-C.
3. Stir until smooth.
4. Feed at temperature that feels slightly warm on your wrist.
5. Refrigerate unused portion.

Weight of Animal	Minimum Amount of Liquid to be Fed in 24 Hours (Ounces or Tablespoons)			Minimum Amount per Feeding if Fed Every... (Teaspoons)		
	oz		Tbs	8 hrs	6 hrs	4 hrs
2 ounces	½ oz	or	1 Tbs	1 tsp	¾ tsp	½ tsp
4 ounces	1 oz	or	2 Tbs	2 tsp	1½ tsp	1 tsp
8 ounces	2 oz	or	4 Tbs	4 tsp	3 tsp	2 tsp
16 ounces	4 oz	or	8 Tbs	8 tsp	6 tsp	4 tsp

Orphaned kittens: If possible, kittens should nurse from their mother for the first two days of their lives to receive nutrient rich colostrum. Mother's colostrum provides temporary protection from numerous diseases and contains growth factors believed to stimulate protein synthesis, improve fat utilization, and promote cell growth. While mother's milk is always preferable, NURTURALL®-C contains nutrient rich colostrum milk powder harvested at USDA inspected facilities. It is extremely important to weigh kittens frequently (everyday) to insure they are receiving adequate amounts of supplement. If a kitten loses weight after 48 hours, consult your veterinarian. Feed weak or small kittens every four hours; feed at eight-hour intervals if the kitten is strong and active. Kittens' needs will vary and the time and amount may have to be increased or decreased, depending on the breed, growth rate and activity of the kittens. Orphan kittens must be kept warm for proper digestion to occur. Also, use a warm, moist washcloth and gently wipe the kitten's bottom until it wets and has a bowel movement, several times daily, to imitate a mother's care. This is required for young kitten survival.

Weaning kittens: Kittens may be weaned when they are about 25 days old. As soon as they are able to lap up formula, mix equal parts of prepared NURTURALL®-C Milk Replacer with a weaning cereal until a soupy mixture is produced. Place mixture in a shallow bowl. As the kitten grows, gradually increase the portion of cereal while decreasing the formula.

Pregnant and lactating queens: Mix one tablespoon of liquid NURTURALL®-C Milk Replacer per five pounds of body weight into the pregnant queen's daily ration. Continue until the kittens are weaned.

Supplementation: If a supplement is desired for a growing kitten, show cat, nursing mother, geriatric or convalescing cat, simply mix one tablespoon of the liquid per five pounds of body weight into the cat's daily ration of food.

NURTURALL®-C Milk Replacer is also available in a ready to use liquid.

Product is filled by weight not volume.

Your veterinarian should be consulted for advice about the care and feeding of kittens.

Precaution(s): Refrigerate after opening. Discard unused powder after three months.

Presentation: Powder: 170.1 g (6 oz) and 340.2 g (12 oz) containers.
Liquid (without colostrum): 236.6 mL (8 fl oz) container.

Compendium Code No.: 11430490 01-1089

NURTURALL®-C FOR PUPPIES

V.P.L. **Milk Replacer**

Balanced Milk Replacer

Guaranteed Analysis: (as a powder):

Crude Protein, min 29.0%
Crude Fat, min 28.0%
Crude Fiber, max. 0.2%
Moisture, max. 5.0%
Ash, max. 8.0%

Ingredients: Corn Oil, Nonfat Dry Milk, Sodium Caseinate, Corn Syrup Solids, Soy Protein Isolate, Dicalcium Phosphate, Calcium Carbonate, Carrageenan, Maltodextrin, Dipotassium Phosphate, Colostrum Milk Powder, Sodium Ascorbate, Potassium Bicarbonate, Natural and Artificial Flavors, Choline Chloride, Zinc Oxide, DL-Alpha-Tocopherol Acetate (Vitamin E), Magnesium Sulfate, Ferrous Sulfate, Mono-Diglycerides, Calcium Pantothenate, L-Arginine, DL-Methionine, Niacinamide, Manganese Sulfate, Wheat Starch, Thiamine Hydrochloride, Cupric

Sulfate, Vitamin A Palmitate, Pyridoxine Hydrochloride, Biotin, Menadione, Folic Acid, Cyanocobalamin (Vitamin B_{12}), Potassium Iodide, Sodium Selenite, Cholecalciferol (Vitamin D_3), BHT and Propyl Gallate (preservatives).

Powder Form: Fortified with colostrum.

Indications: Mother's milk replacer for puppies and food supplement for adult dogs.

This product is intended for intermittent or supplemental feeding only.

Directions: Directions for Preparation and Use: Weigh the puppy. Prepare enough NURTURALL®-C, with the enclosed measuring scoop, for use within a 24-hour period. Puppies should be fed at least ½ ounce of liquid NURTURALL®-C for every two ounces of body weight, daily. Puppies should be allowed to consume as much formula as they want. The table below gives minimum feeding amounts for a 24-hour period. For puppies 1-10 days old, mix one scoop powder into two scoops water. For puppies older than 10 days, mix two scoops powder into three scoops water. Use tap or bottled water. Stir until smooth. Pour liquid into a clean Nurturall® nurser. Heat liquid by placing bottle in a pan of tepid water. Test temperature on your wrist. It should feel slightly warm. Do not microwave. Store NURTURALL®-C powder in the refrigerator. Refrigerate any unused reconstituted liquid for up to 24 hours.

After feeding, hold the puppy's head on your shoulder and rub his back gently until he burps. Make water available after puppies are two weeks old. Small animal water bottles are recommended.

1. Measure water.
2. Mix in NURTURALL®-C.
3. Stir until smooth.
4. Feed at temperature that feels slightly warm on your wrist.
5. Refrigerate unused portion.

Weight of Animal	Minimum Amount of Liquid to be Fed in 24 Hours (Ounces or Tablespoons)			Minimum Amount per Feeding if Fed Every... (Teaspoons)		
	Ounces		Tbs	8 hrs	6 hrs	4 hrs
2 ounces	½ oz	or	1 Tbs	1 tsp	¾ tsp	½ tsp
4 ounces	1 oz	or	2 Tbs	2 tsp	1½ tsp	1 tsp
8 ounces	2 oz	or	4 Tbs	4 tsp	3 tsp	2 tsp
16 ounces	4 oz	or	8 Tbs	8 tsp	6 tsp	4 tsp

Orphaned puppies: If possible, puppies should nurse from their mother for the first two days of their lives to receive nutrient rich colostrum. Mother's colostrum provides temporary protection from numerous diseases and contains growth factors believed to stimulate protein synthesis, improve fat utilization, and promote cell growth. While mother's milk is always preferable, NURTURALL®-C contains nutrient rich colostrum milk powder harvested at USDA inspected facilities. It is extremely important to weigh puppies frequently (everyday) to insure they are receiving adequate amounts of supplement. If a puppy loses weight after 48 hours, consult your veterinarian. Feed weak or small puppies every four hours; feed at eight-hour intervals if the puppy is strong and active. Puppies' needs will vary and the time and amount may have to be increased or decreased, depending on the breed, growth rate and activity of the puppies. Orphan puppies must be kept warm for proper digestion to occur. Also, use a warm, moist washcloth and gently wipe the puppy's bottom until it wets and has a bowel movement, several times daily, to imitate a mother's care. This is required for young puppy survival.

Weaning puppies: Puppies may be weaned when they are about 25 days old. As soon as they are able to lap up formula, mix equal parts of prepared NURTURALL®-C Milk Replacer with a weaning cereal until a soupy mixture is produced. Place mixture in a shallow bowl. As the puppy grows, gradually increase the portion of cereal while decreasing the formula.

Pregnant and lactating bitches: Mix one tablespoon of liquid NURTURALL®-C Milk Replacer per five pounds of body weight into the pregnant bitch's daily ration. Continue until the puppies are weaned.

Supplementation: If a supplement is desired for a growing puppy, show dog, large litter, geriatric or convalescing dog, simply mix one tablespoon of the liquid per five pounds of body weight into the dog's daily ration of food.

NURTURALL®-C Milk Replacer is also available in a ready to use liquid.

Product is filled by weight not volume.

Your veterinarian should be consulted for advice about the care and feeding of puppies.

Precaution(s): Refrigerate after opening. Discard unused powder after three months.

Presentation: Powder: 340.2 g (12 oz) and 793.8 g (28 oz) containers.
Liquid (without colostrum): 236.6 mL (8 fl oz) container.

Compendium Code No.: 11430500 01-1090

NUSAL-T® SHAMPOO

DVM **Antidermatosis Shampoo**

Antiseborrheic Antipruritic Conditioning Formulation

Active Ingredient(s): Salicylic acid 3%, coal tar 2%, menthol 1%.

Indications: An antiseborrheic, antiseptic, keratolytic, antipruritic, that relieves irritation, itching and skin flaking associated with seborrheic, atopic and non-specific dermatoses.

NUSAL-T® is an antiseborrheic, mentholated, fragranced soap-free shampoo consisting of a unique combination of surfactants and coat conditioners.

Directions for Use: Shake well before use. Wet coat thoroughly with water. Apply and lather shampoo over the entire body, allowing for 5-10 minutes of contact time. Rinse completely. Repeat procedure if necessary. Use once or twice weekly, or as directed by veterinarian.

Precaution(s): Store at room temperature.

Caution(s): For topical use on dogs. Avoid contact with eyes. If contact occurs, rinse thoroughly with water. If irritation develops, discontinue and consult your veterinarian.

Warning(s): Keep out of reach of children.

Presentation: 8 fl oz (237 mL) (NDC 47203-340-08), 12 fl oz (355 mL) (NDC 47203-340-12), and 1 gallon (3.78 L) (NDC 47203-340-28).

Compendium Code No.: 11420411 Rev 0597

NUTRA-SURE™ CAT VITAMINS

Farnam **Small Animal Dietary Supplement**

Guaranteed Analysis: per tablet:

Fatty Acid:
Linoleic Acid, min. .... 22 mg
Minerals:
Calcium, min. .... 3.6% (40 mg)
Phosphorus, min.. .... 1.4% (31 mg)
Potassium, min. .... 31 mcg
Magnesium, min. .... 30 mg
Iron, min. .... 5 mg
Copper, min. .... 200 mcg
Manganese, min. .... 200 mcg
Zinc, min. .... 300 mcg
Iodine, min.. .... 100 mcg
Cobalt, min. .... 100 mcg
Vitamins:
Vitamin A, min. .... 1500 I.U.
Vitamin D, min. .... 150 I.U.
Vitamin E, min. .... 4 I.U.
Thiamine (B1), min. .... 810 mcg
Riboflavin, min. .... 1 mg
d-Pantothenic Acid, min.. .... 1 mg
Niacin, min.. .... 4 mg
Pyridoxine, min. .... 410 mcg
Choline, min.. .... 50 mg
Taurine, min.. .... 50 mg
Inositol, min.. .... 10 mg

Ingredients: Wheat germ meal, dextran, dicalcium phosphate, microcrystalline cellulose, hydrolyzed fish meal, animal liver meal, safflower oil, sorbitol, potassium chloride, magnesium oxide, ferrous sulfate, copper sulfate, manganese sulfate, zinc oxide, calcium iodate, cobalt sulfate, taurine, choline chloride, inositol, niacin, d-calcium pantothenate, riboflavin, thiamine hydrochloride, pyridoxine hydrochloride, vitamin A supplement, vitamin D supplement, vitamin E supplement, corn starch, silicon dioxide, stearic acid, and magnesium stearate.

Indications: Essential vitamins and minerals with linoleic acid for healthy skin and coat. Chewable liver-flavored tablets for cats.

Dosage and Administration: For Dietary Supplement:
Mature cats: 1 tablet daily.
Kittens: ¼ to 1 tablet daily.
For sick, convalescing, pregnant or nursing cats: 2 tablets daily.

Administer liver-flavored NUTRA-SURE™ cat vitamins by hand prior to feeding or crumble and mix with food.

Warning(s): Keep out of reach of children.

Presentation: Bottles of 60 tablets.

Compendium Code No.: 10000910 01-1286

NUTRI-CAL®

Evsco **Small Animal Dietary Supplement**

Active Ingredient(s): Guaranteed analysis per teaspoon (6 g):

Crude protein (min.) 1.5%
Crude fat (min.). 34.5%
Crude fiber (max.). 3.7%
Moisture (max.) 14%
Calories (calculated) 30
Calcium (min.) .... 0.16 mg (0.0026%)
Calcium (max.) .... 0.20 mg (0.0033%)
Phosphorus .... 0.03 mg (0.0006%)
Iron. .... 0.53 mg (0.0088%)
Iodine .... 0.53 mg (0.0088%)
Magnesium. .... 0.42 mg (0.0067%)
Manganese .... 1 mg (0.0176%)
Potassium. .... 0.16 mg (0.0027%)
Vitamin A .... 1,045 I.U.
Vitamin D_3. .... 60 I.U.
Vitamin E .... 6 I.U.
Vitamin B_1 (thiamine HCl) .... 2 mg
Vitamin B_2 (riboflavin). .... 0.2 mg
Vitamin B_6 (pyridoxine HCl) .... 1 mg
Vitamin B_{12} .... 2 mcg
Folic acid. .... 0.2 mg
Nicotinamide. .... 2 mg
Pantothenic acid .... 2 mg

Ingredients: Corn syrup, soybean oil, malt syrup, cod liver oil, cane molasses, methylcellulose, water, peptones, dl-alpha tocopheryl acetate (vit. E), sodium benzoate (preservative), manganese sulfate, iron peptonate, thiamine HCl, nicotinamide, calcium pantothenate (source of calcium and pantothenic acid), magnesium sulfate, pyridoxine HCl, vitamin A palmitate, potassium iodide (source of iodine and potassium), riboflavin 5' phosphate sodium (source of vit. B_2 and phosphorus), vitamin A palmitate and D_3 concentrate, folic acid and cyanocobalamin (vit. B_{12}).

Indications: A high calorie dietary supplement in a low volume form, to provide supplemental caloric and nutritional intake to dogs and cats.

Dosage and Administration: Provides an added source of energy for hunting and working dogs. When the animal's caloric or nutritional intake is to be supplemented, give 1½ teaspoons per 10 lbs. of body weight once a day. When the animal is not consuming a full feed ration, give three (3) teaspoons (1 tablespoon) per 10 lbs. of body weight once a day.

Each teaspoon (6 g) provides 30 calories.

NUTRI-CAL® is palatable. To acquaint the animal with the flavor, place a small amount of NUTRI-CAL® in the animal's mouth.

Precaution(s): Store in a cool area.

Presentation: 4¼ oz. (120.5 g) tubes.

Compendium Code No.: 10050301

NUTRI-CAL® FOR DOGS AND CATS

Tomlyn **Small Animal Dietary Supplement**

High Calorie Palatable Dietary Supplement

Active Ingredient(s): Minimum guaranteed analysis per teaspoon (6 grams):

Crude Protein 0.7%
Crude Fat 34.5%
Calcium. .... 0.16 mg (0.0026%)
Phosphorus .... 0.02 mg (0.0003%)
Iron. .... 0.47 mg (0.0078%)
Iodine .... 0.50 mg (0.0083%)
Magnesium. .... 0.38 mg (0.0063%)
Manganese .... 0.90 mg (0.0167%)
Potassium. .... 0.15 mg (0.0025%)
Vitamin A .... 940 IU

N

Vitamin D_3	54 IU
Vitamin E	5 IU
Vitamin B_1 (Thiamine)	1.7 mg
Vitamin B_2 (Riboflavin)	0.2 mg
Vitamin B_6 (Pyridoxine)	0.8 mg
Vitamin B_{12}	1.9 mcg
Folic Acid	0.2 mg
Niacin	1.9 mg
d-Pantothenic Acid	0.9 mg

Also a source of: Linoleic, Linolenic, Eicosapentanoic Acid, Docosahexanoic Acid and Omega-6 and Omega-3 Fatty Acids.

Ingredients: Corn Syrup, Soybean Oil, Malt Syrup, Cod Liver Oil, Cane Molasses, Methylcellulose, Water, Gelatin By-products, dl-Alpha Tocopheryl Acetate (Vit. E), Sodium Benzoate (Preservative), Manganese Sulfate, Iron Proteinate, Thiamine HCl, Niacin, Calcium Pantothenate (Source of Calcium and Pantothenic Acid), Magnesium Sulfate, Pyridoxine HCl, Potassium Iodide (Source of Iodine and Potassium), Riboflavin 5'-Phosphate Sodium (Source of Vit. B_2 and Phosphorus), Vitamin A Palmitate and D_3 supplement, Folic Acid and Cyanocobalamin (Vit. B_{12}).

Indications: Uses: To provide supplemental caloric and nutritional intake in dogs and cats. Provides an added source of energy for hunting and working dogs.

Directions: When the animal's caloric or nutritional intake is to be supplemented, give 1½ teaspoons per 10 pounds of body weight daily. When animal is not consuming full feed ration, give 3 teaspoons (1 tablespoon) per 10 pounds of body weight daily. Calorie content: 4420 kcal/kg (26.5 kcal/6 g).

NUTRI-CAL® is extremely palatable. To acquaint the animal with the flavor, place a small amount of NUTRI-CAL® in the animal's mouth.

Precaution(s): Store in a cool area.

Caution(s): For veterinary use only.

Warning(s): Keep out of reach of children.

Presentation: 4.25 oz (120.5 g) tubes.

Compendium Code No.: 11220330 6786 4

NUTRI-CAL® FOR FERRETS

Tomlyn **Dietary Supplement**

High Calorie Palatable Dietary Supplement

Active Ingredient(s): Minimum guaranteed analysis per teaspoon (6 grams):

Crude Protein	0.7%
Crude Fat	34.5%
Calcium	0.16 mg (0.0026%)
Phosphorus	0.02 mg (0.0003%)
Iron	0.47 mg (0.0078%)
Iodine	0.50 mg (0.0083%)
Magnesium	0.38 mg (0.0063%)
Manganese	0.90 mg (0.0167%)
Potassium	0.15 mg (0.0025%)
Vitamin A	940 IU
Vitamin D_3	54 IU
Vitamin E	5 IU
Vitamin B_1 (Thiamine)	1.7 mg
Vitamin B_2 (Riboflavin)	0.7 mg
Vitamin B_6 (Pyridoxine)	0.8 mg
Vitamin B_{12}	1.9 mcg
Folic Acid	0.2 mg
Niacin	1.9 mg
d-Pantothenic Acid	0.9 mg

Also a source of: Linoleic, Linolenic, Eicosapentanoic Acid, Docosahexanoic Acid and Omega-6 and Omega-3 Fatty-Acids.

Ingredients: Corn Syrup, Soybean Oil, Malt Syrup, Cod Liver Oil, Cane Molasses, Methylcellulose, Water, Gelatin By-Products, dl-Alpha Tocopheryl Acetate (Vit. E), Sodium Benzoate (Preservative), Manganese Sulfate, Iron Proteinate, Thiamine HCl, Niacin, Calcium Pantothenate (Source of Calcium and Pantothenic Acid), Magnesium Sulfate, Pyridoxine HCl, Vitamin A Palmitate, Potassium Iodide (Source of Iodine and Potassium). Riboflavin 5'-Phosphate Sodium (Source of Vit. B_2 and Phosphorus), Vitamin D_3 supplement, Folic Acid and Cyancobalamin (Vit. B_{12}).

Indications: Uses: To provide supplemental caloric and nutritional intake in ferrets.

Directions: When the animal's caloric or nutritional intake is to be supplemented, give ⅛ teaspoon per pound of body weight daily.

When animal is not consuming full feed ration, give ¼ teaspoon per pound of body weight daily.

Calorie content: 4420 kcal/kg (26.5 kcal/6 g).

NUTRI-CAL® is extremely palatable. To acquaint the animal with the flavor, place a small amount of NUTRI-CAL® in the animal's mouth.

Precaution(s): Store in a cool area.

Caution(s): For veterinary use only.

Warning(s): Keep out of reach of children.

Presentation: 4.25 oz (120.5 g) tubes.

Compendium Code No.: 11220340 726-3 2

NUTRI-CAL® FOR FERRETS & OTHER SMALL ANIMALS

Tomlyn **Dietary Supplement**

High Calorie Palatable Dietary Supplement in a Low Volume Form

Active Ingredient(s): Guaranteed Analysis per Teaspoon (6 grams):

Crude Protein (Min)	0.7%
Crude Fat (Min)	34.5%
Crude Fiber (Max)	3.8%
Moisture (Max)	14%
Calcium (Min)	0.16 mg (0.0026%)
Calcium (Max)	0.20 mg (0.0033%)
Phosphorus (Min)	0.03 mg (0.0006%)
Iron (Min)	0.53 mg (0.0088%)
Iodine (Min)	0.53 mg (0.0088%)
Magnesium (Min)	0.42 mg (0.0067%)
Manganese (Min)	1 mg (0.0176%)
Potassium (Min)	0.16 mg (0.0027%)
Vitamin A (Min)	1045 IU
Vitamin D_3 (Min)	60 IU
Vitamin E (Min)	6 IU
Vitamin B_1 (Thiamine)(Min)	1.8 mg
Vitamin B_2 (Riboflavin)(Min)	0.2 mg
Vitamin B_6 (Pyridoxine)(Min)	0.8 mg
Vitamin B_{12} (Min)	2 mcg
Folic Acid (Min)	0.2 mg
Niacinamide (Min)	2 mg
d-Pantothenic Acid (Min)	1 mg

Ingredients: Corn Syrup, Soybean Oil, Malt Syrup, Cod Liver Oil, Cane Molasses, Methylcellulose, Water, Gelatin By-products, dl-Alpha Tocopheryl Acetate (Vit. E), Sodium Benzoate (Preservative), Manganese Sulfate, Iron Proteinate, Thiamine HCl, Niacinamide, Calcium Pantothenate (Source of Calcium and Pantothenic Acid), Magnesium Sulfate, Pyridoxine HCl, Vitamin A Palmitate, Potassium Iodide (Source of Iodine and Potassium), Riboflavin 5'-Phosphate Sodium (Source of Vit. B_2 and Phosphorus), Folic Acid, Vitamin D_3 Supplement and Cyanocobalamin (Vit. B_{12}).

Indications: Uses: To provide supplemental caloric and nutritional intake in ferrets and other small animals.

Directions: When the animal's caloric or nutritional intake is to be supplemented, give ⅛ teaspoon per pound of body weight daily. When animal is not consuming full feed ration, give ¼ teaspoon per pound of body weight daily. Calorie content: 4420 kcal/kg (26.5 kcal/6 g).

NUTRI-CAL® is extremely palatable. To acquaint the animal with the flavor, place a small amount of NUTRI-CAL® in the animal's mouth.

Precaution(s): Store in a cool area.

Caution(s): For veterinary use only.

Warning(s): Keep out of reach of children.

Presentation: 4.25 oz (120.5 g) tubes.

Compendium Code No.: 11220350 726-3 2

NUTRI-STAT™

Tomlyn **Small Animal Dietary Supplement**

High Calorie Food Supplement with Omega Acids

Active Ingredient(s): Minimum guaranteed analysis per teaspoon (6 grams):

Crude Protein	0.7%
Crude Fat	34.5%
Calcium	0.16 mg (0.0026%)
Phosphorus	0.02 mg (0.0003%)
Iron	0.47 mg (0.0078%)
Iodine	0.50 mg (0.0083%)
Magnesium	0.38 mg (0.0063%)
Manganese	0.90 mg (0.0167%)
Potassium	0.15 mg (0.0025%)
Vitamin A	940 IU
Vitamin D_3	64 IU
Vitamin E	5 IU
Vitamin B_1 (Thiamin)	1.7 mg
Vitamin B_2 (Riboflavin)	0.2 mg
Vitamin B_6 (Pyridoxine)	0.8 mg
Vitamin B_{12}	1.9 mcg
Folic Acid	0.2 mg
Niacin	1.9 mg
d-Pantothenic Acid	0.9 mg

Also a source of: Linoleic, Linolenic, Eicosapemanoic Acid, Docosahexanoic Acid and Omega-6 and Omega-3 Acids.

Ingredients: Corn Syrup, Soybean Oil (source of LA and ALA), Malt Syrup, Cod Liver Oil (source of EPA and DHA), Cane Molasses, Methylcellulose, Water, Gelatin By-products, dl-Alpha Tocopheryl Acetate (Vit. E), Sodium Benzoate (Preservative), Manganese Sulfate, Icon Proteinate, Thiamine HCl, Niacin, Calcium Pantothenate (Source of Calcium and Pantothenic Acid), Magnesium Sulfate, Pyridoxine HCl, Vitamin A Palmitate and D_3 supplement, Potassium Iodide (Source of Iodine and Potassium). Riboflavin 5'- Phosphate Sodium (Source of Vit. B_2 and Phosphorus), Folic Acid and Cyancobalamin (Vit. B_{12}).

Indications: NUTRI-STAT™ is formulated with Omega-6 (LA) and Omega-3 (ALA, EPA, DHA) fatty acids, in a low volume form to provide supplemental caloric and nutritional intake when an added source of energy is required.

Directions: When the animal's caloric or nutritional intake is to be supplemented, give 1½ teaspoons per 10 pounds of body weight daily. When animal is not consuming full feed ration, give 3 teaspoons (1 tablespoon) per 10 pounds of body weight daily. Calorie content: 4420 kcal/kg (26.5 kcal/6 g).

NUTRI-STAT™ has "irresistible taste". To acquaint the animal with the flavor, place a small amount of NUTRI-STAT™ in the animal's mouth.

Precaution(s): Store in a cool area.

Caution(s): For veterinary use only.

Warning(s): Keep out of reach of children.

Presentation: 4.25 oz (120.5 g) tubes.

Compendium Code No.: 11220360 677-2 5

NUTRIVED™ B-COMPLEX PLUS IRON LIQUID

Vedco **Small Animal Dietary Supplement**

Active Ingredient(s): Each teaspoonful (5 mL) contains:

Liver fraction 1	250 mg
Minerals:	
Copper (from copper sulfate)	250 mcg
Iron (from iron peptonized)	25 mg
Vitamins:	
Vitamin B_1 (thiamine)	7.5 mcg
Vitamin B_2 (riboflavin)	1.5 mg
Vitamin B_6 (pyridoxine)	1.5 mg
Vitamin B_{12} (cyanocobalamin)	2.5 mcg
Choline	7.5 mg
Folic acid	10.0 mcg
Inositol	20.0 mg
Niacin	20.0 mg
Pantothenic acid	7.5 mg

Indications: For supplementation of the diet to aid in the prophylaxis and treatment of iron, copper, amino acid, and vitamin B-complex deficiencies in young or orphaned dogs and cats and convalescent or debilitated dogs and cats.

Dosage and Administration:

Dogs and Cats: Approximately ½ teaspoonful (2.5 mL) per 25 lbs. of body weight twice a day. Administer directly into the pet's mouth, or mix with food.

Precaution(s): NUTRIVED™ B-Complex Plus Iron Liquid does not require refrigeration.

Presentation: 4 oz. containers.

Compendium Code No.: 10941320

NUTRIVED™ CALCIUM PLUS CHEWABLE TABLETS

Vedco **Small Animal Dietary Supplement**

Active Ingredient(s): Each chewable tablet contains:

Minerals:

Calcium (from calcium phosphate) ... 600 mg
Phosphorus (from calcium phosphate) ... 470 mg

Vitamins:

Vitamin A ... 750 I.U.
Vitamin C ... 10 mg
Vitamin D_3 ... 400 I.U.

Proteins:

Includes the following amino acids: Alanine, arginine, aspartic acid, cysteine, cystine, glutamic acid, glycine, histidine, hydroxyproline, isoleucine, leucine, lysine, methionine, phenylalanine, proline, serine, threonine, tyrosine, tryptophan, and valine.

Indications: Intended as a dietary supplement, particularly for fast growing large breeds of puppies, pregnant and lactating bitches, or whenever aid is required in the control of calcium, vitamin A, vitamin C, and vitamin D_3 deficiencies.

Dosage and Administration: For diet supplementation:

Dogs under 10 lbs. ... ½ tablet a day
Dogs 10 lbs. and over ... 1 to 2 tablets a day

Administer free choice just prior to feeding, or crumble and mix with food.

Presentation: Bottles of 60 tablets.

Compendium Code No.: 10941330

NUTRIVED™ CHEWABLE VITAMINS FOR ACTIVE DOGS

Vedco **Small Animal Dietary Supplement**

Active Ingredient(s): Each chewable tablet contains:

Minerals:

Calcium (from calcium phosphate) ... 160 mg
Chloride (from sodium chloride) ... 3 mg
Chromium (from chromium chloride) ... 1 mcg
Cobalt (from cobalt sulfate) ... 500 mcg
Copper (from copper gluconate) ... 500 mcg
Fluoride (from sodium fluoride) ... 10 mcg
Iodine (from potassium iodide) ... 600 mcg
Iron (from ferrous fumarate) ... 10 mg
Magnesium (from magnesium sulfate) ... 3 mg
Manganese (from manganese sulfate) ... 500 mcg
Molybdenum (from molybdenum trioxide) ... 1 mcg
Nickel (from nickel chloride) ... 1 mcg
Phosphorus (from calcium phosphate) ... 123 mg
Potassium (from potassium iodide) ... 185 mcg
Selenium (from selenium powder) ... 4 mcg
Silicon (from silicon dioxide) ... 1 mcg
Sodium (from sodium chloride) ... 2 mg
Tin (from tin powder) ... 1 mcg
Vanadium (from vanadium oxide) ... 1 mcg
Zinc (from zinc oxide) ... 2.5 mg

Vitamins:

Vitamin A ... 5,000 I.U.
Vitamin B_1 (thiamine) ... 3 mg
Vitamin B_2 (riboflavin) ... 5 mg
Vitamin B_6 (pyridoxine) ... 3 mg
Vitamin B_{12} (cyanocobalamin) ... 50 mcg
Vitamin C ... 20 mg
Vitamin D_3 ... 200 I.U.
Vitamin E ... 25 I.U.
Vitamin K ... 300 mcg
Biotin ... 30 mcg
Choline ... 60 mg
Folic acid ... 200 mcg
Inositol ... 15 mg
Niacin ... 25 mg
Pantothenic acid ... 2 mg

Essential Fatty Acids:

Linoleic acid ... 30 mg

Linolenic acid, arachidonic acid, eicosapentaenoic acid, docosahexaenoic acid, docosapentaenoic acid.

Proteins:

Includes the following amino acids: Alanine, arginine, aspartic acid, cysteine, cystine, glutamic acid, glycine, histidine, hydroxyproline, isoleucine, leucine, lysine, methionine, phenylalanine, proline, serine, threonine, tyrosine, tryptophan, and valine.

Indications: For supplementation of the diet for dogs with special nutritional needs due to sickness, debilitation, convalescence, pregnancy, nursing, stress, or high activity requirements.

Dosage and Administration: For diet supplementation:

Dogs under 10 lbs. ... ½ tablet a day
Dogs 10 lbs. and over ... 1 to 2 tablets a day

Administer free choice just prior to feeding, or crumble and mix with food.

Presentation: Bottles of 60 tablets.

Compendium Code No.: 10941340

NUTRIVED™ CHEWABLE VITAMINS FOR CATS

Vedco **Small Animal Dietary Supplement**

Active Ingredient(s): Each chewable tablet contains:

Taurine ... 100 mg

Minerals:

Calcium (from calcium phosphate) ... 50 mg
Chloride (from sodium chloride) ... 4 mg
Chromium (from chromium chloride) ... 1 mcg
Cobalt (from cobalt sulfate) ... 100 mcg
Copper (from copper gluconate) ... 200 mcg
Fluoride (from sodium fluoride) ... 6 mcg
Iodine (from potassium iodide) ... 200 mcg
Iron (from ferrous fumarate) ... 5 mg
Manganese (from manganese sulfate) ... 200 mcg
Molybdenum (from molybdenum trioxide) ... 1 mcg
Nickel (from nickel chloride) ... 1 mcg
Phosphorus (from calcium phosphate) ... 39 mg
Potassium (from potassium iodide) ... 62 mcg
Selenium (from selenium powder) ... 4 mcg
Silicon (from silicon dioxide) ... 1 mcg
Sodium (from sodium chloride) ... 2 mg
Tin (from tin powder) ... 1 mcg
Vanadium (from vanadium oxide) ... 1 mcg
Zinc (from zinc oxide) ... 300 mcg

Vitamins:

Vitamin A ... 1,500 I.U.
Vitamin B_1 (thiamine) ... 810 mcg
Vitamin B_2 (riboflavin) ... 1 mg
Vitamin B_6 (pyridoxine) ... 410 mcg
Vitamin B_{12} (cyanocobalamin) ... 4 mcg
Vitamin C ... 4 mg
Vitamin D_3 ... 150 I.U.
Vitamin E ... 4 I.U.
Biotin ... 10 mcg
Choline ... 50 mg
Folic acid ... 20 mcg
Inositol ... 20 mg
Niacin ... 4 mg
Pantothenic acid ... 1 mg

Essential Fatty Acids:

Linoleic acid ... 30 mg

Linolenic acid, arachidonic acid, eicosapentaenoic acid, docosahexaenoic acid, docosapentaenoic acid.

Proteins:

Includes the following amino acids: Alanine, arginine, aspartic acid, cysteine, cystine, glutamic acid, glycine, histidine, hydroxyproline, isoleucine, leucine, lysine, methionine, phenylalanine, proline, serine, threonine, tyrosine, tryptophan, and valine.

Indications: For supplementation of the diet for cats to aid in the prophylaxis and treatment of multiple vitamin and mineral deficiencies.

Dosage and Administration: For diet supplementation:

Cats ... 1 tablet a day

For sick, convalescing, pregnant, or nursing cats:

Cats ... 2 tablets a day

Administer free choice just prior to feeding, or crumble and mix with food.

Presentation: Bottles of 60 tablets.

Compendium Code No.: 10941350

NUTRIVED™ CHEWABLE VITAMINS FOR DOGS

Vedco **Small Animal Dietary Supplement**

Ingredient(s): Each chewable tablet contains:

Essential Fatty Acids:

Linoleic acid ... 30 mg

Linolenic acid, arachidonic acid, eicosapentaenoic acid, docosahexaenoic acid, docosapentaenoic acid.

Proteins:

Includes the following amino acids: Alanine, arginine, aspartic acid, cysteine, cystine, glutamic acid, glycine, histidine, hydroxyproline, isoleucine, leucine, lysine, methionine, phenylalanine, proline, serine, threonine, tyrosine, tryptophan, and valine.

Minerals:

Calcium (from calcium phosphate) ... 160 mg
Chloride (from sodium chloride) ... 3 mg
Chromium (from chromium chloride) ... 1 mcg
Cobalt (from cobalt sulfate) ... 14 mcg
Copper (from copper gluconate) ... 500 mcg
Fluoride (from sodium fluoride) ... 10 mcg
Iodine (from potassium iodide) ... 52 mg
Iron (from ferrous fumarate) ... 10 mg
Magnesium (from magnesium sulfate) ... 1 mg
Manganese (from manganese sulfate) ... 60 mcg
Molybdenum (from molybdenum trioxide) ... 1 mcg
Nickel (from nickel chloride) ... 1 mcg
Phosphorus (from calcium phosphate) ... 123 mg
Potassium (from potassium iodide) ... 16 mcg
Selenium (from selenium powder) ... 4 mcg
Silicon (from silicon dioxide) ... 1 mcg
Sodium (from sodium chloride) ... 2 mg
Tin (from tin powder) ... 1 mcg
Vanadium (from vanadium oxide) ... 1 mcg
Zinc (from zinc oxide) ... 2.5 mg

Vitamins:

Vitamin A ... 1300 I.U.
Vitamin B_1 (thiamine) ... 810 mcg
Vitamin B_2 (riboflavin) ... 1 mg
Vitamin B_6 (pyridoxine) ... 820 mcg

Vitamin B_{12} (cyanocobalamin) .... 10 mcg
Vitamin C .... 5 mg
Vitamin D_3 .... 150 I.U.
Vitamin E .... 3 I.U.
Biotin .... 10 mcg
Choline .... 20 mg
Folic acid .... 40 mcg
Inositol .... 5 mg
Niacin .... 10 mg
Pantothenic acid .... 2 mg

Indications: For supplementation of the diet for dogs to aid in prophylaxis and treatment of multiple vitamin and mineral deficiencies in dogs.

Dosage and Administration: For diet supplementation:

Dogs under 10 pounds .... ½ tablet daily
Dogs 10 pounds and over .... 1 to 2 tablets daily

For sick, convalescing, pregnant, or nursing dogs:

Dogs under 10 pounds .... 1 tablet daily
Dogs 10 pounds and over .... 2 tablets daily

NUTRIVED™ Vitamins are made with a special taste appeal for dogs (roast beef and liver flavor). Administer free choice just prior to feeding, or crumble and mix with food.

Presentation: Bottles of 60 and 180 tablets.

Compendium Code No.: 10941360

NUTRIVED™ CHEWABLE VITAMINS FOR KITTENS

Vedco **Small Animal Dietary Supplement**

Active Ingredient(s): Each chewable tablet contains:

Taurine .... 50 mg

Minerals:

Calcium (from calcium phosphate) .... 25 mg
Chloride (from sodium chloride) .... 2 mg
Chromium (from chromium chloride) .... 0.5 mcg
Cobalt (from cobalt sulfate) .... 50 mcg
Copper (from copper gluconate) .... 100 mcg
Fluoride (from sodium fluoride) .... 3 mcg
Iodine (from potassium iodide) .... 100 mcg
Iron (from ferrous fumarate) .... 2.5 mg
Manganese (from manganese sulfate) .... 100 mcg
Molybdenum (from molybdenum trioxide) .... 0.5 mcg
Nickel (from nickel chloride) .... 0.5 mcg
Phosphorus (from calcium phosphate) .... 19.5 mg
Potassium (from potassium iodide) .... 31 mcg
Selenium (from selenium powder) .... 2 mcg
Silicon (from silicon dioxide) .... 0.5 mcg
Sodium (from sodium chloride) .... 1 mg
Tin (from tin powder) .... 0.5 mcg
Vanadium (from vanadium oxide) .... 0.5 mcg
Zinc (from zinc oxide) .... 150 mcg

Vitamins:

Vitamin A .... 750 I.U.
Vitamin B_1 (thiamine) .... 405 mcg
Vitamin B_2 (riboflavin) .... 500 mcg
Vitamin B_6 (pyridoxine) .... 205 mcg
Vitamin B_{12} (cyanocobalamin) .... 2 mcg
Vitamin C .... 2 mg
Vitamin D_3 .... 75 I.U.
Vitamin E .... 2 I.U.
Biotin .... 5 mcg
Choline .... 25 mg
Folic acid .... 10 mcg
Inositol .... 10 mg
Niacin .... 2 mg
Pantothenic acid .... 500 mcg

Essential Fatty Acids:

Linoleic acid (from vegetable oil) .... 15 mg

Linolenic acid, arachidonic acid, eicosapentaenoic acid, docosahexaenoic acid, docosapentaenoic acid.

Proteins:

Includes the following amino acids: Alanine, arginine, aspartic acid, cysteine, cystine, glutamic acid, glycine, histidine, hydroxyproline, isoleucine, leucine, lysine, methionine, phenylalanine, proline, serine, threonine, tyrosine, tryptophan, and valine.

Indications: For supplementation of the diet for kittens to aid in the prophylaxis and treatment of multiple vitamin and mineral deficiencies.

Dosage and Administration: For diet supplementation:

Growing kittens .... 1 tablet a day
For sick, convalescing kittens .... 2 tablets a day
Cats .... 4 tablets a day

Administer free choice just prior to feeding, or crumble and mix with food.

Presentation: Bottles of 50 tablets.

Compendium Code No.: 10941370

NUTRIVED™ CHEWABLE VITAMINS FOR PUPPIES

Vedco **Small Animal Dietary Supplement**

Active Ingredient(s): Each chewable tablet contains:

Minerals:

Calcium (from calcium phosphate) .... 100 mg
Chloride (from sodium chloride) .... 3 mg
Chromium (from chromium chloride) .... 1 mcg
Cobalt (from cobalt sulfate) .... 10 mcg
Copper (from copper gluconate) .... 300 mcg
Fluoride (from sodium fluoride) .... 10 mcg
Iodine (from potassium iodide) .... 26 mcg
Iron (from ferrous fumarate) .... 3 mg
Magnesium (from magnesium sulfate) .... 700 mcg
Manganese (from manganese sulfate) .... 40 mcg
Molybdenum (from molybdenum trioxide) .... 1 mcg
Nickel (from nickel chloride) .... 1 mcg
Phosphorus (from calcium phosphate) .... 77 mg
Potassium (from potassium iodide) .... 8 mcg
Selenium (from selenium powder) .... 4 mcg
Silicon (from silicon dioxide) .... 1 mcg
Sodium (from sodium chloride) .... 2 mg
Tin (from tin powder) .... 1 mcg
Vanadium (from vanadium oxide) .... 1 mcg
Zinc (from zinc oxide) .... 1.5 mg

Vitamins:

Vitamin A .... 1,000 I.U.
Vitamin B_1 (thiamine) .... 405 mcg
Vitamin B_2 (riboflavin) .... 1 mg
Vitamin B_6 (pyridoxine) .... 410 mcg
Vitamin B_{12} (cyanocobalamin) .... 5 mcg
Vitamin C .... 3 mg
Vitamin D_3 .... 100 I.U.
Vitamin E .... 2 I.U.
Biotin .... 5 mcg
Choline .... 10 mg
Folic acid .... 20 mcg
Inositol .... 3 mg
Niacin .... 5 mg
Pantothenic acid .... 1 mg

Essential Fatty Acids:

Linoleic acid .... 20 mg

Linolenic acid, arachidonic acid, eicosapentaenoic acid, docosahexaenoic acid, docosapentaenoic acid.

Proteins:

Includes the following amino acids: Alanine, arginine, aspartic acid, cysteine, cystine, glutamic acid, glycine, histidine, hydroxyproline, isoleucine, leucine, lysine, methionine, phenylalanine, proline, serine, threonine, tyrosine, tryptophan, and valine.

Indications: For supplementation of the diet for puppies to aid in the prophylaxis and treatment of multiple vitamin and mineral deficiencies.

Dosage and Administration: For diet supplementation:

Growing puppies .... 2 tablets a day
For sick, convalescing puppies .... 4 tablets a day

Administer free choice just prior to feeding, or crumble and mix with food.

Presentation: Bottles of 50 tablets.

Compendium Code No.: 10941380

NUTRIVED™ CHEWABLE ZINPRO® TABLETS

Vedco **Small Animal Dietary Supplement**

Active Ingredient(s): Guaranteed Analysis:

	Per Tablet	Per Kilogram
Zinc	15 mg	6 g
Methionine	30 mg	12 g

Ingredients: Zinc methionine, liver meal, roast beef flavor, dried whey, calcium carbonate, and artificial color.

Indications: A chewable dietary supplement of soluble zinc methionine for dogs.

Dosage and Administration: Administer one (1) chewable tablet each day to provide 15 mg of zinc per day for each 20 lbs. of body weight.

Caution(s): The product is intended for intermittent or supplemental feeding only.

For animal use only.

Presentation: Bottles of 100 tablets.

* ZINPRO® is a registered trademark of Zinpro Corporation.

Compendium Code No.: 10941390

NUTRIVED™ ENERGEL FORTE

Vedco **Large Animal Dietary Supplement**

Guaranteed Analysis:

Vitamin E, minimum .... 122 I.U./lb.
Sodium (Na), maximum 5.50%
Sodium (Na), minimum 6.00%
Potassium (K), minimum 1.40%
Magnesium (Mg), minimum 0.15%
Lactic acid bacteria, minimum
(L. acidophilus, L. casei, L. fermentum, L. plantarum, S. faecium) .... 907,200,000 CFU/lb.

Ingredients: Glucose, guar gum, sodium chloride, sodium bicarbonate, potassium chloride, lecithin, citric acid, magnesium sulfate, glycine, dried *Lactobacillus acidophilus* fermentation product, dried *Lactobacillus casei* fermentation product, dried *Lactobacillus fermentum* fermentation product, dried *Lactobacillus plantarum* fermentation product, dried *Streptococcus faecium* fermentation product, sodium sulfate, sodium silico aluminate, monocalcium phosphate, corn syrup solids, active yeast (Saccharomyces cerevisiae), vitamin A acetate, d-activated animal sterol (source of vitamin D_3), vitamin E supplement, vitamin B_{12} supplement, riboflavin supplement, niacin supplement, calcium pantothenate, menadione dimethylpyrimidinol bisulphite, folic acid, pyridoxine hydrochloride, thiamine hydrochloride, d-biotin, fumaric acid, dried citrus pulp, ascorbic acid, zinc proteinate, cobalt proteinate, ferrous proteinate, copper proteinate, buttermilk, cellulose gum and manganese proteinate.

Indications: A blend of ingredients as a source of electrolytes, nutrients and sugars for energy in young calves, veal, foals and lambs. Contains a source of live (viable) naturally occurring micro-organisms.

Dosage and Administration: Mix two-thirds (⅔) cup (100 g) into two (2) quarts of warm water or milk replacer and shake or mix thoroughly.

Calves, Veal and Foals: Feed the mixture per calf twice a day for two (2) days. Receiving calves should be given two (2) feedings prior to the regular milk program.

Lambs: Feed the above mixture at the rate of four (4) fluid ounces per five (5) pounds of body weight, three (3) times a day for two (2) days.

Presentation: 32 x 100 g packets/pail and 10 lb (4.536 kg) pail.

Compendium Code No.: 10941421

NUTRIVED™ FLATUEX CHEWABLE TABLETS

Vedco **Antiflatulent**

Active Ingredient(s): Each tablet contains:

Simethicone .... 80 mg

Includes the following amino acids: Alanine, arginine, aspartic acid, cysteine, cystine, glutamic acid, glycine, histidine, hydroxyproline, isoleucine, leucine, lysine, methionine, phenylalanine, proline, serine, threonine, tyrosine, tryptophan, and valine.

Indications: For use as an aid in prophylaxis and treatment of canine gas/flatulence.

Dosage and Administration:

Dogs under 20 pounds: 1 tablet after each feeding and at bedtime daily.

Dogs 20 pounds and over: 2 to 4 tablets after each feeding and at bedtime daily.

Administer free choice after feeding and at bedtime, or crumble and mix with food.

Presentation: 60 tablets.

Compendium Code No.: 10941430

NUTRIVED™ HYPO ALLERGENIC CHEWABLE TABLETS

Vedco **Small Animal Dietary Supplement**

Ingredient(s): Each chewable tablet contains:

Essential Fatty Acids (Linoleic Acid, Arachidonic Acid) .... 30 mg

Proteins: Includes the following amino acids: Alanine, arginine, aspartic acid, cysteine, cystine, glutamic acid, glycine, histidine, hydroxyproline, isoleucine, leucine, lysine, methionine, phenylalanine, proline, serine, threonine, tyrosine, tryptophan, and valine.

Minerals: Calcium 160 mg; molybdenum 1 mcg; chloride 3 mg; nickel 1 mcg; chromium 1 mcg; phosphorus 123 mg; cobalt 14 mcg; potassium 16 mcg; copper 500 mcg; selenium 4 mcg; fluoride 10 mcg; silicon 1 mcg; iodine 52 mcg; sodium 2 mg; iron 10 mg; tin 1 mcg; magnesium 1 mg; vanadium 1 mcg; manganese 60 mcg; zinc 2.5 mg.

Vitamins: Vitamin A 1300 I.U.; vitamin B_1 810 mcg; vitamin B_2 1 mg; vitamin B_6 820 mcg; vitamin B_{12} 10 mcg; vitamin C 5 mg; vitamin D_3 150 I.U.; biotin 10 mcg; choline 10 mcg; folic acid 40 mcg; inositol 5 mg; niacin 10 mg; pantothenic acid 2 mg; vitamin E 3 I.U.

Indications: For supplementation of the diet to aid in prophylaxis and treatment of multiple vitamin and mineral deficiencies for dogs which may have food sensitivities to: beef, pork, fish, corn or wheat.

Dosage and Administration: For diet supplementation:

Dogs under 10 pounds .... ½ tablet daily
Dogs 10 pounds and over .... 1 to 2 tablets daily

For sick, convalescing, pregnant or nursing dogs:

Dogs under 10 pounds .... 1 tablet daily
Dogs 10 pounds and over .... 2 tablet daily

Administer free choice just prior to feeding or crumble with food.

Presentation: 60 tablet container.

Compendium Code No.: 10941440

NUTRIVED™ HYPO-K GRANULES

Vedco **Small Animal Dietary Supplement**

Potassium Gluconate

Active Ingredient(s): Each 650 mg scoop dose contains 78.2 mg Potassium (2 mEq Potassium) contained in 468 mg Potassium Gluconate, along with 50 mg essential fatty acids and amino acids.

Each bottle will yield 185 level scoop doses. Roast beef and liver flavor added.

Indications: Indicated for use as a supplement in potassium deficient states in cats and dogs.

Dosage and Administration: In Cats: 650 mg or one level scoop twice daily with moist food. In Dogs: 650 mg or one level scoop per 10 lbs body weight, not to exceed 3,900 mg (6 scoops), twice daily with moist food.

Presentation: Bottles containing 120 grams.

Compendium Code No.: 10941460

NUTRIVED™ O.F.A. CHEWABLE TABLETS FOR CATS

Vedco **Small Animal Dietary Supplement**

Active Ingredient(s): Each chewable tablet contains:

Marine lipid concentrates .... 135 mg
Vegetable oils .... 28.5 mg
Total fatty acids .... 163.5 mg

Vitamins:

Vitamin A .... 750 I.U.
Vitamin D_3 .... 150 I.U.
Vitamin E .... 12.5 I.U.
Choline .... 775 mcg
Inositol .... 550 mcg

Minerals:

Zinc .... 1 mg

Proteins:

Includes the following amino acids: Alanine, arginine, aspartic acid, cysteine, cystine, glutamic acid, glycine, histidine, hydroxyproline, isoleucine, leucine, lysine, methionine, phenylalanine, proline, serine, threonine, tyrosine, tryptophan, and valine.

Indications: NUTRIVED™ O.F.A. Chewable Tablets for Cats are a supplemental source of omega fatty acids, vitamins A, D_3, and E, and zinc, which are beneficial to cats for the maintenance of healthy skin and coats.

Dosage and Administration: For diet supplementation:

Cats under 10 lbs. .... ½ to 1 tablet a day
Cats 10 lbs. and over .... 1 to 2 tablets a day

Administer free choice just prior to feeding, or crumble and mix with food.

Presentation: Bottles of 60 tablets.

Compendium Code No.: 10941470

NUTRIVED™ O.F.A. CHEWABLE TABLETS FOR LARGE DOGS

Vedco **Small Animal Dietary Supplement**

Active Ingredient(s): Each chewable tablet contains:

Essential fatty acids micro-encapsulated omega 3 fatty acids .... 200 mg

Eicosapentaenoic acid, docosahexaenoic acid, docosapentaenoic acid, gamma linolenic and linolenic acid.

Polyunsaturated fatty acids other than omega 3 acids .... 60 mg

Linoleic acid and oleic acid.

Vitamins:

Vitamin A .... 3,000 I.U.
Vitamin D_3 .... 600 I.U.
Vitamin E .... 50 I.U.
Choline .... 3,100 mcg
Inositol .... 2, 200 mcg

Minerals:

Zinc .... 4 mg

Proteins:

Includes the following amino acids: Alanine, arginine, aspartic acid, cysteine, cystine, glutamic acid, glycine, histidine, hydroxyproline, isoleucine, leucine, lysine, methionine, phenylalanine, proline, serine, threonine, tyrosine, tryptophan, and valine.

Indications: For supplementation of the diet to aid in the prophylaxis and treatment of fatty acids, zinc, and vitamins A, D_3, and E deficiencies. As such, NUTRIVED™ O.F.A. Chewable Tablets for Large Dogs should prove beneficial in the improvement and maintenance of healthy skin and coats on dogs.

Dosage and Administration: For diet supplementation:

Dogs 20 to 50 lbs. .... 1 tablet a day
Dogs over 50 lbs. .... 1 to 2 tablets a day

Administer free choice just prior to feeding, or crumble and mix with food.

Presentation: Bottles of 60 tablets.

Compendium Code No.: 10941480

NUTRIVED™ O.F.A. CHEWABLE TABLETS FOR SMALL AND MEDIUM DOGS

Vedco **Small Animal Dietary Supplement**

Active Ingredient(s): Each chewable tablet contains:

Marine lipid concentrates .... 270 mg
Vegetable oils .... 57 mg
Total fatty acids .... 327 mg

Vitamins:

Vitamin A .... 1,500 I.U.
Vitamin D_3 .... 300 I.U.
Vitamin E .... 25 I.U.
Choline .... 1,550 mcg
Inositol .... 1,100 mcg

Minerals:

Zinc .... 2 mg

Proteins:

Includes the following amino acids: Alanine, arginine, aspartic acid, cysteine, cystine, glutamic acid, glycine, histidine, hydroxyproline, isoleucine, leucine, lysine, methionine, phenylalanine, proline, serine, threonine, tyrosine, tryptophan, and valine.

Indications: NUTRIVED™ O.F.A. Chewable Tablets for small and medium dogs are a supplemental source of omega fatty acids, vitamins A, D_3, and E, and zinc, which are beneficial in dogs for the maintenance of healthy skin and coats.

Dosage and Administration: For diet supplementation:

Dogs under 10 lbs. .... ½ to 1 tablet a day
Dogs 10 lbs. and over .... 1 to 2 tablets a day

Administer free choice just prior to feeding, or crumble and mix with food.

Presentation: Bottles of 60 tablets.

Compendium Code No.: 10941490

NUTRIVED™ O.F.A. GEL CAPS FOR LARGE DOGS

Vedco **Small Animal Dietary Supplement**

Active Ingredient(s): Eicosapentanoic acid, gamma linolenic acid, decahexanoic acid, linolenic acid, safflower oil (containing linoleic acid and oleic acid), natural glycerin, d-alpha tocopherol (vitamin E), and gelatin.

Nutritional information:

Calories per capsule .... less than 10
Protein .... less than 1 g
Carbohydrates .... less than 1 g
Fat .... 1 g

Indications: A concentrated omega fatty acid dietary supplement for the skin of large dogs.

Dosage and Administration: One (1) capsule per 50-70 lbs. of body weight per day.

Note: The capsule may be punctured and the liquid contents squeezed onto the food if desired.

Precaution(s): Store the container in a cool, dry place.

Caution(s): For veterinary use only.

Keep out of the reach of children.

Presentation: Bottles of 60 capsules.

Compendium Code No.: 10941500

NUTRIVED™ O.F.A. GEL CAPS FOR SMALL AND MEDIUM DOGS

Vedco **Small Animal Dietary Supplement**

Active Ingredient(s): Eicosapentanoic acid, gamma linolenic acid, decahexanoic acid, linolenic acid, safflower oil (containing linoleic acid and oleic acid), natural glycerin, d-alpha tocopherol (vitamin E), and gelatin.

Nutritional information:

Calories per capsule .... less than 5
Protein .... less than 1 g
Carbohydrates .... less than 1 g
Fat .... 1 g

Indications: A concentrated omega fatty acid dietary supplement for the skin of small and medium size dogs.
Dosage and Administration: One (1) capsule per 20 lbs. of body weight per day.
Note: The capsule may be punctured and the liquid contents squeezed onto the food if desired.
Precaution(s): Store the container in a cool, dry place.
Caution(s): For veterinary use only.
Keep out of the reach of children.
Presentation: Bottles of 60 capsules.
Compendium Code No.: 10941510

NUTRIVED™ O.F.A. GRANULES FOR CATS

Vedco — **Small Animal Dietary Supplement**

Active Ingredient(s): Each 10 g (approximately 1 scoop) contains:

Taurine	100 mg
Essential Fatty Acids:	
Linoleic acid	458 mg
Linolenic acid	34 mg
Arachidonic acid	81 mg
Eicosapentaenoic acid	55 mg
Docosahexaenoic acid	32 mg
Docosapentaenoic acid	8 mg
Total fatty acids (as glycerides)	845 mg
Minerals:	
Calcium (from calcium phosphate)	50 mg
Chloride (from sodium chloride)	4 mg
Chromium (from chromium chloride)	1 mcg
Cobalt (from cobalt sulfate)	100 mcg
Copper (from copper gluconate)	200 mcg
Fluoride (from sodium fluoride)	6 mcg
Iodine (from potassium iodide)	200 mcg
Iron (from ferrous fumarate)	5 mg
Manganese (from manganese sulfate)	200 mcg
Molybdenum (from molybdenum trioxide)	1 mcg
Nickel (from nickel chloride)	1 mcg
Phosphorus (from calcium phosphate)	39 mg
Potassium (from potassium iodide)	62 mcg
Selenium (from selenium powder)	4 mcg
Silicon (from silicon dioxide)	1 mcg
Sodium (from sodium chloride)	2 mg
Tin (from tin powder)	1 mcg
Vanadium (from vanadium oxide)	1 mcg
Zinc (from zinc oxide)	300 mcg
Vitamins:	
Vitamin A	1,500 I.U.
Vitamin B_1 (thiamine)	810 mcg
Vitamin B_2 (riboflavin)	1 mg
Vitamin B_6 (pyridoxine)	410 mcg
Vitamin B_{12} (cyanocobalamin)	4 mcg
Vitamin C	4 mg
Vitamin D_3	150 I.U.
Vitamin E	4 I.U.
Biotin	10 mcg
Choline	50 mg
Folic acid	20 mcg
Inositol	20 mg
Niacin	4 mg
Pantothenic acid	1 mg

Proteins:
Includes the following amino acids: Alanine, arginine, aspartic acid, cysteine, cystine, glutamic acid, glycine, histidine, hydroxyproline, isoleucine, leucine, lysine, methionine, phenylalanine, proline, serine, threonine, tyrosine, tryptophan, and valine.
Indications: For supplementation of the diet to aid in the prophylaxis and treatment of fatty acid, multiple vitamin and mineral deficiencies. As such NUTRIVED™ O.F.A. Granules should prove beneficial in the improvement and maintenance of healthy skin and coats on cats.
Dosage and Administration: For diet supplementation:

Cats	1 scoop a day
For sick, convalescing, pregnant, or nursing cats:	
Cats	2 scoops a day

Administer by mixing with, or sprinkling on food.
Presentation: 650 g container.
Compendium Code No.: 10941520

NUTRIVED™ O.F.A. GRANULES FOR DOGS

Vedco — **Small Animal Dietary Supplement**

Active Ingredient(s): Each 10 g (approximately 1 scoop) contains:

Essential Fatty Acids:	
Linoleic acid	458 mg
Linolenic acid	34 mg
Arachidonic acid	81 mg
Eicosapentaenoic acid	55 mg
Docosahexaenoic acid	32 mg
Docosapentaenoic acid	8 mg
Total fatty acids (as glycerides)	845 mg
Minerals:	
Calcium (from calcium phosphate)	160 mg
Chloride (from sodium chloride)	3 mg
Chromium (from chromium chloride)	1 mcg
Cobalt (from cobalt sulfate)	14 mcg
Copper (from copper gluconate)	500 mcg
Fluoride (from sodium fluoride)	10 mcg
Iodine (from potassium iodide)	52 mcg
Iron (from ferrous fumarate)	10 mg
Magnesium (from magnesium sulfate)	1 mg
Manganese (from manganese sulfate)	60 mcg
Molybdenum (from molybdenum trioxide)	1 mcg
Nickel (from nickel chloride)	1 mcg
Phosphorus (from calcium phosphate)	123 mg
Potassium (from potassium iodide)	16 mcg
Selenium (from selenium powder)	4 mcg
Silicon (from silicon dioxide)	1 mcg
Sodium (from sodium chloride)	2 mg
Tin (from tin powder)	1 mcg
Vanadium (from vanadium oxide)	1 mcg
Zinc (from zinc oxide)	2.5 mg
Vitamins:	
Vitamin A	1,300 I.U.
Vitamin B_1 (thiamine)	810 mcg
Vitamin B_2 (riboflavin)	1 mg
Vitamin B_6 (pyridoxine)	820 mcg
Vitamin B_{12} (cyanocobalamin)	10 mcg
Vitamin C	5 mg
Vitamin D_3	150 I.U.
Vitamin E	3 I.U.
Biotin	10 mcg
Choline	20 mg
Folic acid	40 mcg
Inositol	5 mg
Niacin	10 mg
Pantothenic acid	2 mg

Proteins:
Includes the following amino acids: Alanine, arginine, aspartic acid, cysteine, cystine, glutamic acid, glycine, histidine, hydroxyproline, isoleucine, leucine, lysine, methionine, phenylalanine, proline, serine, threonine, tyrosine, tryptophan, and valine.
Indications: For supplementation of the diet to aid in the prophylaxis and treatment of fatty acid, multiple vitamin and mineral deficiencies. As such, NUTRIVED™ O.F.A. Granules should prove beneficial in the improvement and maintenance of healthy skin and coats on dogs.
Dosage and Administration: For diet supplementation:

Dogs under 10 lbs.	½ scoop a day
Dogs 10 lbs. and over	1 to 2 scoops a day
For sick, convalescing, pregnant, or nursing dogs:	
Dogs under 10 lbs.	1 scoop a day
Dogs 10 lbs. and over	2 scoops a day

Administer by mixing with, or sprinkling on food.
Presentation: 650 g container.
Compendium Code No.: 10941530

NUTRIVED™ O.F.A. LIQUID

Vedco — **Small Animal Dietary Supplement**

Active Ingredient(s): Each mL contains:

Vitamins:	
Vitamin A	300 I.U.
Vitamin D_3	60 I.U.
Vitamin E	5 I.U.
Choline	310 mcg
Inositol	220 mcg
Essential Fatty Acids:	
Linoleic acid	426 mg
Linolenic acid	61 mg
Arachidonic acid	15 mg
Eicosapentaenoic acid	10 mg
Docosahexaenoic acid	6 mg
Docosapentaenoic acid	1 mg
Total fatty acids (as glycerides)	739 mg
Proteins	10 mg

Indications: For supplementation of the diet to aid in the prophylaxis and treatment of fatty acid and vitamin A, D_3, and E deficiencies. As such, NUTRIVED™ O.F.A. Liquid should prove beneficial in the improvement and maintenance of healthy skin and coats on dogs and cats.
Dosage and Administration: Administer once a day according to the following schedule:

Body Weight	Dose
Under 15 lbs.	2 mL
15 to 30 lbs.	4 mL
31 to 50 lbs.	6 mL
51 lbs. and over	8 mL

Administer by mixing with food.
Precaution(s): NUTRIVED™ O.F.A. Liquid does not require refrigeration.
Presentation: 8 oz. container.
Compendium Code No.: 10941540

NUTRIVED™ POTASSIUM CITRATE GRANULES FOR CATS AND DOGS

Vedco — **Small Animal Dietary Supplement**

Active Ingredient(s): Each 5 grams (approximately 1 scoop) contains:

Special Nutrient:	
Potassium Citrate (coated):*	300 mg
Essential Fatty Acids:	
Total Fatty Acids (as glycerides)	423 mg

Proteins: Includes the following amino acids: Alanine, arginine, aspartic acid, cysteine, cystine, glutamic acid, glycine, histidine, hydroxyproline, isoleucine, leucine, lysine, methionine, phenylalanine, proline, serine, threonine, tyrosine, and valine.
Ingredients: Wheat, liver powder, whey, sugar, dicalcium phosphate, vegetable oil, potassium citrate (coated), stearic acid, hydrolyzed vegetable protein, fish oil, choline chloride, silicone dioxide.
Indications: For supplementation of the diet to aid in prophylaxis of urinary stone formation in cats and dogs. Vedco Microencapsulated Potassium Citrate Granules help decrease the possibility of calcium oxalate stone formation.

Dosage and Administration: Cats: 1 scoop per day for prophylaxis. Dogs: 1 scoop per day for every 10 pounds of body weight for prophylaxis.

Vedco Coated Potassium Citrate Granules are made with a special microencapsulated potassium citrate in a liver and roast beef flavor base. Administer by mixing with or sprinkling on food. Your veterinarian may give you specific directions increasing or decreasing these dosages - Follow your veterinarian's advice closely.

Presentation: Bulk container containing 300 grams which equals 60 doses.

Compendium Code No.: 10941550

NUTRIVED™ T-4 CHEWABLE TABLETS ℞

Vedco **Thyroid Therapy**

Active Ingredient(s): Tablets are available in several concentrations. Each scored, round, chewable tablet contains 0.2 mg, 0.3, 0.5, or 0.8 Levothyroxine sodium, USP in a proprietary roast beef and liver flavor base.

Indications: For use in the canine for correction of conditions associated with low circulating thyroid hormone (hypothyroidism).

Dosage and Administration: The initial daily dose is 0.05 to 0.1 mg/10 lb (4.5 kg) body weight. Response should be evaluated every four weeks until an adequate maintenance dose is established. In most dogs, with the exception of the toy breeds, this is usually in the range of 0.2 mg (200 mcg) to 0.8 mg (800 mcg) total daily dose. NUTRIVED™ T-4 Chewable Tablets may be fed free choice, from the hand, or crumbled and placed on the food.

Precaution(s): Store at controlled room temperature 15° to 30°C and protect from light.

Caution(s): Federal law restricts this drug to use by or on the order of a licensed veterinarian.

Administer with caution to animals with clinically significant heart disease, hypertension, or other complications for which a sharply increased metabolic rate might prove hazardous. Use in pregnant bitches has not been evaluated.

Warning(s): Keep out of the reach of children.

Presentation: 0.2 mg: Bottles of 120 and 1000 tablets.
0.3 mg: Bottles of 120 and 1000 tablets.
0.5 mg: Bottles of 120 and 1000 tablets.
0.8 mg: Bottles of 120 and 1000 tablets.

Compendium Code No.: 10941561

N

N

Disclaimer
Every effort has been made to ensure the accuracy of the information published. However, it remains the responsibility of the readers to familiarize themselves with the product information contained on the product label or package insert.
Inclusion or omission of products does not imply endorsement or criticism by the Publisher or anyone involved in the publication. Inclusion does not imply product availability and/or product registration. The Publisher, Editorial Team and all people involved in the production of this book cannot be held responsible for publication errors or any consequence that could result from the use of published information.

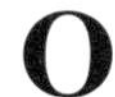

O

OATMEAL & ALOE SHAMPOO

Davis **Grooming Shampoo**

Active Ingredient(s): 2% Colloidal oatmeal and aloe in a mild hypoallergenic base.
Indications: For dogs, cats, puppies and kittens.
Hypoallergenic formula helps soothe dry, sensitive and irritated skin with superior moisturizers.
Claims: Recommended and used by veterinarians.
Dosage and Administration: To use Davis OATMEAL & ALOE SHAMPOO as a general grooming and cleansing shampoo, dilute 12 parts water to 1 part shampoo (12:1). For sensitive pets, dilute 3 parts water to 1 part shampoo (3:1).
Wet pet's coat thoroughly with warm water. Do not get shampoo into eyes. Apply shampoo to head and ears, then lather. Repeat procedure with neck, chest, middle and hind quarter, finishing legs last. Add more shampoo if necessary. Rinse thoroughly. May be used daily.
Warning(s): For external use only.
Keep out of reach of children.
Discussion: Davis OATMEAL & ALOE SHAMPOO contains colloidal oatmeal, known for centuries to benefit skin that has been damaged, abraded or distressed due to a wide variety of reasons. Colloidal oatmeal is consistently recommended for use in baths and lotions for its highly moisturizing and anti-itch properties. Sensitive skin will respond to this mild shampoo as it soothes with Aloe Vera and cleanses dry, itchy, and scaly skin.
Helpful in relieving irritation and redness caused by exposure to harsh soaps.
Excellent emollient attributes. Helpful in treating skin itching.
Soothing effect for pets with sensitive skin.
Assists in relieving itching due to seborrheic dermatitis. Excellent anti-pruritic agent.
Non irritating to skin. Acts as soap free cleanser.
Presentation: 12 oz (355 mL) and 1 gallon (3.785 L).
Compendium Code No.: 11410291

O B LUBE

AgriLabs **Lubricant**

Active Ingredient(s): Contains propylene glycol, sodium carboxymethylcellulose, methylparaben and propylparaben in an inert base.
Indications: Can be used as a lubricant for operator's hands and arms in obstetrical work, vaginal examinations and rectal examinations. May be used as a lubricant for catheters and stomach tubes.
Dosage and Administration: Apply O B LUBE to gloves or sleeves when performing gynecological procedures and rectal examinations. After use, rinse thoroughly with water to remove excess from the exposed surfaces of the animal. May be used with or without water. Use on large or small animals.
Caution(s): If skin irritation should develop when using the product, discontinue use.
Warning(s): Keep out of reach of children.
Presentation: 1 gallon container.
Compendium Code No.: 10580771

O B LUBE

Centaur **Lubricant**

Ingredient(s): Propylene glycol, sodium carboxy methyl cellulose, methyl and propyl paraben in an inert base.
Indications: Can be used as a lubricant for operator's hands and arms in obstetrical work, vaginal examinations and rectal examinations. May be used as a lubricant for catheters and stomach tubes.
Directions: Apply O B LUBE to gloves or sleeves when performing gynecological procedures and rectal examinations. After use, rinse thoroughly with water to remove excess from exposed surfaces of animal.
May be used with or without water.
Use on large or small animals.
Caution(s): In case skin irritation should develop when using this product, discontinue use.
For animal use only.
Warning(s): Keep out of reach of children.
Presentation: 8 fl oz (236.5 mL) and 1 gallon (128 fl oz) 3.785 L containers.
Manufactured by: Unavet, North Kansas City, MO 64116.
Compendium Code No.: 14880240

OCU-GUARD® MB

Boehringer Ingelheim **Bacterin**

Moraxella Bovis Bacterin
U.S. Vet. Lic. No.: 124
Composition: This vaccine contains inactivated isolates of *Moraxella bovis*.
Indications: For use as an aid in the prevention and control of pinkeye (infectious bovine keratoconjunctivitis) in healthy cattle caused by *Moraxella bovis*.
Dosage and Administration: Shake well. Administer a 2 mL dose subcutaneously to cattle 2 months of age or older. Repeat vaccination in 21 days.
Precaution(s): Store out of direct sunlight at a temperature between 35-45°F (2-7°C). Do not freeze. Shake well before and during use. Use entire contents when first opened.
Caution(s): Anaphylactoid reactions may occur.
Antidote(s): Epinephrine.
Warning(s): Do not vaccinate within 21 days before slaughter.
Presentation: 10 dose (20 mL) and 50 dose (100 mL) vials.
Compendium Code No.: 10280831 BI 1052-1 6/01

OCUVAX®

Schering-Plough **Vaccine**

Fowl Laryngotracheitis Vaccine, Live Virus
U.S. Vet. Lic. No.: 165A
Active Ingredient(s): OCUVAX®* is a live virus vaccine containing a carefully selected fowl laryngotracheitis virus strain adapted to passage in chicken embryos. The vaccine contains gentamicin as a preservative.
Indications: For the vaccination of healthy chickens 10 weeks of age or older, as an aid in preventing fowl laryngotracheitis.
Dosage and Administration:
When to Vaccinate: Vaccinate at 10 weeks of age.
Vaccination Program: The development of a durable, strong protection depends upon the use of an effective vaccination program as well as many circumstances such as administration techniques, environment and flock health at the time of vaccination. Also, the immune response to one (1) vaccination under field conditions is seldom complete for all animals within a given flock. Even when vaccination is successful, the protection stimulated in individual animals against different diseases may not be life-long.
If necessary, the vaccine may be used to aid in limiting the spread of an outbreak; however, only birds not yet infected with the virulent outbreak virus can be protected.
Examination of birds for vaccination takes is unnecessary and so-called takes are not to be expected. As with all live virus vaccines, a mild transitory reaction may occur. This is generally limited to a mild, localized eye reaction of short duration.
Preparation of the Vaccine:

1. Do not open and mix the vaccine until ready for use.
2. Mix only one (1) vial at a time and use the entire contents within two (2) hours.
3. Remove the tear-off aluminum seal and stopper from the vial containing the dried vaccine.
4. Remove the tear-off aluminum seal and stopper from the bottle containing the diluent.
5. Hold the diluent bottle firmly in an upright position and insert the vaccine vial on the adapter of the diluent bottle. The neck of the vaccine vial should snap into position and should be seated securely on the adapter on the diluent bottle.
6. Invert the two (2) containers so that the vaccine vial is on the bottom and allow the diluent to flow into the vaccine vial. If the diluent does not flow freely, squeeze the bottle gently and the diluent will flow into the vaccine vial. The vaccine vial should be completely filled with diluent to prevent excess foaming.
7. Hold the joined containers by the ends and shake vigorously until the vaccine plug is completely dissolved.
8. Return the joined containers to their original position (diluent bottle on the bottom). Allow the vaccine to flow into the diluent bottle. If the rehydrated vaccine does not flow into the diluent bottle, tap or squeeze the diluent bottle gently and release to draw the vaccine into the diluent bottle. Be sure that all of the product is removed from the vaccine vial.
9. Remove the vaccine vial and adapter from the neck of the diluent bottle and insert the dropper applicator into the plastic diluent bottle.
10. The vaccine is now ready for use.

How to Vaccinate: Vaccination for laryngotracheitis by the eyedrop method is conducted by allowing one (1) full drop of vaccine to fall into the open eye of the bird and holding until the bird swallows. Hold the dropper bottle in a vertical position throughout the vaccination to avoid wasting the vaccine.
Records: Keep a record of the vaccine type, quantity, serial number, expiration date, and place of purchase; the date and time of vaccination; the number, age, breed, and location of the birds; the names of operators performing the vaccination; and any observed reactions.
Precaution(s): Store at 35° to 45° F (2° to 7°C).
Caution(s): For veterinary use only.

1. Vaccinate healthy birds only. Although disease may not be evident, coccidiosis, chronic respiratory disease, mycoplasma infection, lymphoid leukosis, infectious bursal disease, Marek's disease, or other disease conditions may cause serious complications or reduce protection.
2. Increased eye reactions may be noticed if birds are incubating coryza or other infectious organisms, or if there is an excess amount of ammonia or dust in the air of the housing facilities.
3. All birds within a house should be vaccinated on the same day. Isolate other susceptible birds on the premises from the birds being vaccinated.
4. In outbreak situations, vaccinate healthy birds first, progressing toward outbreak areas in order to vaccinate diseased birds last.
5. Do not spill or spatter the vaccine. Use the entire contents of the vial when first opened. Burn the empty bottles, caps, and all unused vaccine and accessories.
6. Wash hands thoroughly after using the vaccine.
7. Do not dilute the vaccine or otherwise stretch the dosage.

Warning(s): Do not vaccinate within 21 days before slaughter.
Presentation: Supplied in 10 x 1,000 dose units with diluent.
* Restricted to sales in California only.
Compendium Code No.: 10471380

ODOR DESTROYER

Davis **Deodorant Product**

Active Ingredient(s): 1-(3-chloroallyl)-3,5,7-Triaza-1-Azoniaadamantane Chloride.
Indications: For the elimination of malodors caused by: urine, feces, vomit, decaying organic matter.
Dosage and Administration: For the treatment of offensive malodors or decaying matter, spray Davis ODOR DESTROYER full strength, directly on malodor. (Do not use on any surface you are unsure of. If in doubt, test a small inconspicuous area before applying product.)
When using as a washdown, or as an additive to mopwater, dilute two (2) ounces of Davis ODOR DESTROYER with one (1) gallon of water. Continue normal procedure for use.
Davis ODOR DESTROYER must contact the malodor to be effective. Upon contact, Davis ODOR DESTROYER interacts with the molecular structure of the malodor in a unique and selective manner to capture and control odors, limited to certain molecular configurations, eg. Mercaptans, amines, sulphides etc. ... (Pleasing odors remain unaffected).
Caution(s): Do not take internally. Avoid contact with eyes, open wounds, skin and clothing. Wash thoroughly after handling. Avoid breathing mist. May irritate eyes or respiratory system. This product not tested for use on animals.
Warning(s): Keep out of reach of children.
Discussion: Davis ODOR DESTROYER is a Exothermic Reaction Synthesis creating a proprietary, one of a kind blend.

1. Captures malodor molecules and holds them hostage.
2. Breaks down the molecular structure of malodors.
3. Contains a fragrance to freshen the air.

Will not affect pleasing odors.
Davis ODOR DESTROYER begins to destroy malodors almost immediately upon contact...then continues to effectively capture and destroy malodors until the offending odor is completely broken down and destroyed.
Presentation: 32 oz and one gallon (3.785 L).
Compendium Code No.: 11410300

OMEGA-3 FATTY ACID CAPSULES FOR LARGE & GIANT BREEDS

Vet Solutions **Small Animal Dietary Supplement**

A Dietary Supplement for Large and Giant Breeds

Active Ingredient(s): Each capsule contains: Eicosapentaenoic acid (EPA), 360 mg; docosahexaenoic acid (DHA), 240 mg; vitamin A, 400 IU; vitamin D, 100 IU; and vitamin E, 4 IU.

Ingredients: Fish oil (source of omega-3 fatty acids), gelatin, glycerin, water, dl-alpha tocopheryl, (source of vitamin E), vitamin A palmitate, vitamin D3.

Description: Vet Solutions OMEGA-3 FATTY ACID CAPSULES contain a concentrated source of omega-3 fatty acids supplemented with vitamins A, D and E.

Indications: A supplementary source of Omega-3 Fatty Acids where dietary intake is inadequate or when the skin and coat condition indicate that supplementation would be of benefit to the animal.

For pets over 27.3 kg (60 lbs.).

Directions for Use: Administer orally 1 capsule daily for animals 27.3-36.4 kg (60-80 lbs.) or 2 capsules for animals over 36.4 kg (80 lbs.) body weight. Capsules may be punctured and liquid content squeezed onto food if desired.

Precaution(s): Storage: Store at controlled room temperature.

Caution(s): Sold exclusively through veterinarians.

Presentation: 60 and 250 capsules (600 mg).

Compendium Code No.: 10610130 000102

OMEGA-3 FATTY ACID CAPSULES FOR MEDIUM BREEDS

Vet Solutions **Small Animal Dietary Supplement**

A Dietary Supplement for Medium Breeds

Active Ingredient(s): Each capsule contains: Eicosapentaenoic acid (EPA), 180 mg; docosahexaenoic acid (DHA), 120 mg; vitamin A, 400 IU; vitamin D, 100 IU; and vitamin E, 4 IU.

Ingredients: Fish oil (source of omega-3 fatty acids), gelatin, glycerin, water, dl-alpha tocopheryl, (source of vitamin E), vitamin A palmitate, vitamin D3.

Description: Vet Solutions OMEGA-3 FATTY ACID CAPSULES contain a concentrated source of omega-3 fatty acids supplemented with vitamins A, D and E.

Indications: A supplementary source of Omega-3 Fatty Acids where dietary intake is inadequate or when the skin and coat condition indicate that supplementation would be of benefit to the animal.

For pets over 13.6-27.3 kg (30-60 lbs.).

Directions for Use: Administer orally 1 capsule daily for animals 13.6-27.3 kg (30-60 lbs.) body weight. Capsules may be punctured and liquid content squeezed onto food if desired.

Precaution(s): Storage: Store at controlled room temperature.

Caution(s): Sold exclusively through veterinarians.

Presentation: 60 and 250 capsules (300 mg).

Compendium Code No.: 10610140 000102

OMEGA-3 FATTY ACID CAPSULES FOR SMALL BREEDS

Vet Solutions **Small Animal Dietary Supplement**

A Dietary Supplement for Small Breeds

Active Ingredient(s): Each capsule contains: Eicosapentaenoic acid (EPA), 110 mg; docosahexaenoic acid (DHA), 73 mg; vitamin A, 200 IU; vitamin D, 50 IU; and vitamin E, 2 IU.

Ingredients: Fish oil (source of omega-3 fatty acids), gelatin, glycerin, water, dl-alpha tocopheryl, (source of vitamin E), vitamin A palmitate, vitamin D3.

Description: Vet Solutions OMEGA-3 FATTY ACID CAPSULES contain a concentrated source of omega-3 fatty acids supplemented with vitamins A, D and E.

Indications: A supplementary source of Omega-3 Fatty Acids where dietary intake is inadequate or when the skin and coat condition indicate that supplementation would be of benefit to the animal.

For pets over 4.5-13.6 kg (10-30 lbs.).

Directions for Use: Administer orally 1 capsule daily for animals 4.5-13.6 kg (10-30 lbs.) body weight. Capsules may be punctured and liquid content squeezed onto food if desired.

Precaution(s): Storage: Store at controlled room temperature.

Caution(s): Sold exclusively through veterinarians.

Presentation: 60 and 250 capsules (183 mg).

Compendium Code No.: 10610150 000102

OMEGA-3 FATTY ACID LIQUID

Vet Solutions **Small Animal Dietary Supplement**

Economy Size-A Dietary Supplement for Companion Animals

Active Ingredient(s): Each mL contains:

Eicosapentaenoic acid (EPA) .... 166.5 mg
Docosahexaenoic acid (DHA) .... 111 mg
Vitamin A .... 200 IU
Vitamin D .... 50 IU
Vitamin E .... 4 IU

Ingredients: Fish oils, (source of omega-3 fatty acids), dl-alpha tocopheryl acetate, (source of vitamin E), vitamin A palmitate, vitamin D3.

Description: Vet Solutions OMEGA-3 FATTY ACID LIQUID is an economical, concentrated source of omega-3 fatty acids supplemented with vitamins A, D and E.

Indications: A supplementary source of Omega-3 Fatty Acids where dietary intake is inadequate or when the skin and coat condition indicate that supplementation would be of benefit to the animal.

Directions for Use: Administer supplement to pet's food once per day.

Animal Weight	Recommended Daily Dose
3.6-8.65 kg (8-19 lbs.)	½ pump
9-17.7 kg (20-39 lbs.)	1 pump
18-26.8 kg (40-59 lbs.)	2 pumps
27-36 kg (60-79 lbs.)	3 pumps
36.4-45 kg (80-100 lbs.)	4 pumps
Each pump contains:	1 mL

Precaution(s): Storage: Store at controlled room temperature.

Caution(s): Sold exclusively through veterinarians.

Presentation: 237 mL (8 fl. oz.) and 1 gallon.

Compendium Code No.: 10610160 000103

OMEGA EFA™ CAPSULES

Butler **Small Animal Dietary Supplement**

Active Ingredient(s): Eicosapentanoic acid, gamma linolenic acid, decahexanoic acid, safflower oil, natural glycerin, d-alpha tocopherols (vitamin E), and gelatin.

Nutritional information:

Calories .... less than 5
Protein .... less than 1 g
Carbohydrates .... less than 1 g
Fat .... 1 g

Indications: A concentrated fatty acid dietary supplement for the skin of small and medium breeds of dogs and cats.

Dosage and Administration: One (1) capsule per 20 lbs. of body weight per day.

Note: The capsule may be punctured and the liquid contents squeezed onto the food if desired.

Precaution(s): Store the container in a cool, dry place.

Caution(s): For veterinary use only. Keep out of the reach of children.

Presentation: Bottles of 90 capsules.

Compendium Code No.: 10821230

OMEGA EFA™ CAPSULES XS

Butler **Small Animal Dietary Supplement**

Active Ingredient(s): Eicosapentanoic acid, gamma linolenic acid, decahexanoic acid, safflower oil, natural glycerin, d-alpha tocopherols (vitamin E), and gelatin.

Nutritional information:

Calories .... less than 10
Protein .... less than 1 g
Carbohydrates .... less than 1 g
Fat .... 1 g

Indications: A concentrated fatty acid dietary supplement for the skin of medium and large breeds of dogs.

Dosage and Administration: One (1) capsule per 50-70 lbs. of body weight per day.

Note: The capsule may be punctured and the liquid contents squeezed onto the food if desired.

Precaution(s): Store the container in a cool, dry place.

Caution(s): For veterinary use only. Keep out of the reach of children.

Presentation: Bottles of 90 capsules.

Compendium Code No.: 10821240

OMEGA EFA™ LIQUID

Butler **Small Animal Dietary Supplement**

Active Ingredient(s): Eicosapentanoic acid, gamma linolenic acid, decahexanoic acid, safflower oil, natural glycerin, and d-alpha tocopherols (vitamin E).

Nutritional information (at 1.0 mL):

Calories .... less than 5
Protein .... less than 1 g
Carbohydrates .... less than 1 g
Fat .... 1 g

Indications: A concentrated fatty acid dietary supplement for the skin of small and medium breeds of dogs and cats.

Dosage and Administration:

Animal Weight — Recommended Daily Dosage
10 lbs. .... 0.5 mL
20 lbs. .... 1.0 mL
30 lbs. .... 1.5 mL

Caution(s): For professional veterinary use only.

Presentation: 2 oz. (60 mL) bottles.

Compendium Code No.: 10821250

OMEGA EFA™ LIQUID XS

Butler **Small Animal Dietary Supplement**

Active Ingredient(s): Eicosapentanoic acid, gamma linolenic acid, decahexanoic acid, safflower oil, natural glycerin, and d-alpha tocopherols (vitamin E).

Nutritional information (at 1.0 mL):

Calories .... less than 10
Protein .... less than 1 g
Carbohydrates .... less than 1 g
Fat .... 1 g

Indications: A concentrated fatty acid dietary supplement for the skin of medium and large breeds of dogs and cats.

Dosage and Administration:

Animal Weight — Recommended Daily Dosage
30 lbs. .... 0.5 mL
60 lbs. .... 1.0 mL
90 lbs. .... 1.5 mL

Caution(s): For professional veterinary use only.

Presentation: 2 oz. (60 mL) bottles.

Compendium Code No.: 10821260

OMEGA-GLO E SHAMPOO

Vedco **Grooming Shampoo**

Ingredient(s): Vitamin E, all natural vegetable oil (containing the omega fatty acids of linoleic and liolenic acid), sodium lactate and glycerin as natural emollients and deionized water in a low allergen, cleansing system.

Indications: To be used for bathing and as an aid in grooming and restoring the natural luster to the haircoat.

Recommended for normal, dry and sensitive skin.

Dosage and Administration: Wet coat, apply shampoo and lather. Rinse thoroughly. Repeat if necessary. Before use, the shampoo may be diluted 4:1 in water. It may be used as often as desired.

Precaution(s): Store in a cool place.

Warning(s): For external use only. Avoid contact to eyes. Keep out of reach of children.

Presentation: Sold to graduate veterinarians only in 8 fl oz and 1 gallon.

Compendium Code No.: 10941570

OMNITROL IGR 1.3% EMULSIFIABLE CONCENTRATE

Vedco **Flea Control**

EPA Reg. No.: 28293-216-44084

Active Ingredient(s):

2-[1-Methyl-2-(4-phenoxyphenoxy) ethoxyl] pyridine	1.30%
Inert Ingredients:	98.70%
	100.00%

Indications: Prevents adult flea emergence indoors for 7 months (210 days).

Directions for Use: It is a violation of Federal Law to use this product in a manner inconsistent with its labeling.

Read all directions completely before use.

For best results, follow directions for specific use areas. Do not use this product in or on electrical equipment due to possibility of shock hazard. Avoid excessive wetting of carpet, draperies and furniture. Always test in an inconspicuous (hidden) area prior to use as some natural and synthetic fibers may be adversely affected by any liquid product.

For Flea Control: The active ingredient in this concentrate is Nylar®, an insect growth regulator. It is similar to insect growth hormones that occurs naturally in insects and acts on the immature life stages of the flea, preventing the adult flea from developing. Flea eggs deposited on treated areas will not develop into adult fleas. Flea larvae crawling onto treated surfaces will also not develop into adult fleas. The unique properties of Nylar® eliminates the flea population, when used as directed. It causes a gradual reduction and ultimate elimination of the flea population by breaking the reproduction cycle. It stops the flea life cycle and inhibits the development of the immature stages of the flea for 7 months preventing them from reaching the biting adult stage. Existing adult fleas and flea pupae are not affected.

If a high population of adult fleas are present, the use of an adulticide may be necessary for immediate relief. This concentrate may also be combined with a flea adulticide. This product compliments the rapid activity of the adulticide by providing long term control of preadult fleas before they grow up to be biting adults.

Flea control on pets is important in the prevention of the introduction of adult fleas. Pets, their bedding and the areas they frequent should also be treated with EPA registered flea and tick control products, as part of a complete flea control program in conjunction with this application to minimize the introduction of adult fleas.

This Concentrate can be used prior to the flea season. Application of this product in areas where pets and other animals are known to frequent and where previous infestations have been known to occur, will prevent the emergence of adult fleas and also control stages of fleas that don't resemble fleas. This early usage could reduce the need for conventional insecticides when used alone as directed. Pretreatment of these areas before the fleas become biting and reproductive adults will aid in reducing developing populations.

Indoors: Prior to treatment, carpets, draperies and upholstered furniture should be vacuumed thoroughly and the vacuum cleaner bag disposed of in an outdoor trash receptacle.

Instructions for Use: This Concentrate is intended to be mixed with water and applied with spray equipment such as any low pressure sprayer (tank type sprayer) (trigger sprayer) typically used for indoor application.

Spray Preparation: Prepare a diluted spray solution by adding 1 ounce per gallon of water. Partially fill the mixing container with water, add Concentrate, agitate and fill to final volume. Do not allow spray mixture to stand overnight. Mix before each use.

In Conjunction with an Adulticide Insecticide: This Concentrate may be combined with an insecticide registered for adult control of fleas. The combination would provide immediate relief of adult fleas and inhibit the development of the immature stages of the flea for 7 months. This application should conform to accepted use precautions and directions for both products. Use this Concentrate at application rates specified above.

General Surface Application: Apply diluted spray at the rate of 1 gallon per 1,500 square feet of surface area. Treat all areas which may harbor fleas, including carpets, furniture, pet sleeping areas and throw rugs. Treat under cushions of upholstered furniture. Do not allow children or pets to contact treated surfaces until spray has dried. Repeat as necessary.

In Kennels and Doghouses: Treatment of these areas will control the development of preadult fleas from becoming biting and reproductive adult flea. Using an adjustable hose-end sprayer, tank type sprayer or sprinkling can, prepare a diluted spray solution by adding 1 ounce per gallon water. Partially fill the sprayer with water, add required amount of concentrate in sprayer, agitate and fill to final volume. Agitate before each spray. Do not allow the spray mixture to stand overnight.

Apply at a rate of 1 gallon diluted solution per 1,500 square feet of surface area. Apply to building, resting areas, walls, floor, animal bedding and run areas. Remove animals before spraying and do not return animals to treated areas until spray has dried completely. Pets and their bedding should also be treated with EPA registered flea and tick control products, in conjunction with this application as part of a complete flea control program to prevent the introduction of adult fleas. Repeat as necessary.

For German, Asian, and Brown Banded Cockroach Control: The active ingredient in the Concentrate is Nylar®, an insect growth regulator. It is similar to insect growth hormones that occur naturally in insects and acts on the immature life stages of the cockroach preventing nymphal cockroaches from developing into adults. Shortly after application of this Concentrate, cockroaches with twisted wings will begin to appear indicating that it has taken effect - those cockroaches with twisted wings are unable to reproduce. The unique properties of this Concentrate eliminates the cockroach population, when used as directed. One treatment works for 6 months against hatching cockroaches.

If a high population of adult cockroaches are present, the use of an adulticide may be necessary for immediate relief. Nylar® causes a gradual reduction in the cockroach population by interrupting the life cycle of the cockroach and preventing the cockroaches from breeding. This Concentrate may also be combined with a cockroach adulticide. This Concentrate compliments the rapid activity of the adulticide by providing long term control of cockroach nymphs before they become breeding adults.

Indoors:

Instructions for Use: This Concentrate is intended to be mixed with water and applied with spray equipment such as any low pressure sprayer (tank type sprayer) (trigger sprayer) typically used for indoor applications.

Spray Preparation: Prepare a diluted spray solution by added 2 ounces per gallon of water. Partially fill the mixing container with water, add Concentrate, agitate and fill to the final volume. Agitate before each spray. Do not allow spray mixture to stand overnight.

In Conjunction with an Adulticide Insecticide: This Concentrate may be combined with an insecticide registered for adult control of cockroaches. The combination would provide immediate relief of adult cockroaches and inhibit the development of the immature stages of the cockroach for 6 months. This application should conform to accepted use precautions and directions for both products. Use this Concentrate at application rates specified above.

General Surface Application:

Cockroaches - Brown Banded Cockroach, Asian Cockroach, German Cockroach and Cricket: Apply diluted spray at the rate of 1 gallon per 1,000 square feet of surface area as a spot treatment, surface application and crack and crevice spray. Contact as many insects as possible with this spray in addition to thorough spraying of all parts of the room suspected of harboring these pests. Special attention should be paid to hiding places such as beneath sinks, behind and beneath stoves and refrigerators, cracks and crevices, around garbage cans, cabinets, along the outside of baseboards, door and window sills, door and window frames and floors, around and on drains, pipes, plumbing, behind bookcases, storage and other utility installation areas, infested furniture and the inside of cabinets and closets hitting insects with spray whenever possible. Repeat as necessary.

Note: Not labeled for use in food areas of food handling establishments.

Spot and Crack and Crevice Applications: Apply diluted spray solution using a pressurized spray system capable of delivering a pin-point or variable spray pattern.

Crack and Crevice applications may be made directly to areas such as but not limited to crevices, baseboards, floors, ceilings, walls, expansion joints, molding, areas around water and sewer pipes, voids where pests can hide and similar areas. Spot treatments may also be made to areas including but not limited to storage area, closets, around water pipes, doors and windows, behind and under refrigerators, cabinets, sinks, stoves and other equipment shelves, drawers and similar areas.

Precautionary Statements:

Hazards to Humans and Domestic Animals:

Caution: Harmful if swallowed or absorbed through skin. Do not breathe vapors or spray mist. Avoid contact with skin or eyes. In case of contact flush with plenty of water. Wash with soap and water after use. Obtain medical attention if irritation persists. Avoid contamination of food or feedstuffs.

Physical or Chemical Hazards: Do not use or store near heat or open flame.

Statement of Practical Treatment:

If in Eyes: Flush with plenty of water. Get medical attention if irritation persists.

If Swallowed: Call a physician or Poison Control Center immediately. Do not induce vomiting.

If on Skin or Clothing: Remove contaminated clothing and wash before reuse. Wash skin with soap and warm water. Get medical attention if irritation persists.

Storage and Disposal:

Storage: Store in a cool, dry place. Keep container closed.

Disposal: Do not reuse empty container. Wrap container in several layers of newspaper and discard in trash.

Warning(s): Keep out of reach of children.

Presentation: 1 oz. 1 fl oz treats 1,500 sq. ft.

Nylar®-Registered trademark of McLaughlin Gormley King Co.

Compendium Code No.: 10941580

OMNITROL IGR FOGGER

Vedco **Househole Insecticide**

EPA Reg. No.: 28293-214-44084

Active Ingredient(s):

2-[1-Methyl-2-(4-phenoxyphenoxy) ethoxy] pyridine	0.100%
Pyrethrins	0.050%
*N-octyl bicycloheptene dicarboximide	0.400%
Permethrin [**(3-phenoxyphenyl) methyl (±) cis-trans-3-(2,2-dichloroethenyl) 2,2-dimethylcyclopropanecarboxylate)	0.400%
Related compounds	0.035%
Inert ingredients:	99.015%

*MGK® 264, insecticide synergist

**cis-trans isomers ratio: Max. 35% (±) cis and Min. 65% (±) trans

Indications: Kills adult and preadult fleas, ticks, cockroaches, spiders and ants. Prevents reinfestation for 7 months (210 Days).

Stops the flea from developing into egg laying adults. Keeps working in areas exposed to the sun. Prevents fleas from developing into biting adult stage. Stops preadult fleas from developing into biting adults. Flea eggs deposited on treated areas will not develop into adult fleas. Larvae crawling onto treated areas will not develop into adult fleas.

Kills deer ticks and other ixodid species that may carry and transmit lyme disease.

For use in: Apartments, attics, basements, closed porches, garages, homes, kennels, pet sleeping areas, and storage areas.

Directions for Use: It is a violation of Federal law to use this product in a manner inconsistent with its labeling.

Read all directions completely before use.

For use only when building has been vacated by human beings and pets. Ventilate area for 30 minutes before re-entry.

For best results, treat all infested areas (sites). Use one (12 oz) fogger for each 12,000 cubic feet (approximately 54 ft. x 54 ft. x 16 ft. ceiling) of unobstructed area. Use additional units for remote rooms or where the free flow of fog is not assured.

Note: Do not use more than one unit per average size room. Do not use this unit in a cabinet or under a counter or table. Do not use 12 oz fogger in an area less than 200 cubic feet. Preparation: Remove or cover exposed food, dishes, utensils, surfaces and food-handling equipment. Shut off fans and air conditioners. Put out all flames and pilot lights. Close outside doors and windows. Remove pets and birds but leave pets bedding as this is a primary hiding place for fleas and must be treated for best results. No need to discard pet bedding after treatment. Cover or remove fish tanks and bowls. Leave rugs, draperies and upholstered furniture in place. This product will not harm furniture when used as directed. Open interior closet doors and cabinets or areas to be treated. Cover waxed furniture and waxed wood floors in the immediate area surrounding the fogger. Newspapers may be used.

For more effective control of storage pests open all cupboard doors, kitchen, bathrooms, pantry, and drawers for better penetration of fog. Remove all infested foodstuffs and dispose of in outdoor trash.

For flea and tick control, thoroughly vacuum all carpeting, upholstered furniture, along baseboards, under furniture and in closets. Put vacuum bag into a sack and dispose of in outside trash. Mop all hard floor surfaces.

Read all directions and cautions before using. To Start Fogging: Shake Fogger Well Before Using: Hold can at arm's length with top of can pointing away from face and eyes. Push down on finger pad until it locks. This will start fogging action. Set canister in an upright position on a table, stand, etc. (up to 30" inches in height in the center of the area) and place several thicknesses of newspaper under the canister to prevent marring of the surface. Treat the whole dwelling using multiple units in homes with more than one level and numerous rooms. Leave the building at once. Do Not Re-Enter Building For Two Hours: After two hours, open all outside doors and windows, turn on air conditioner and/or fans and let treated area air for 30 minutes before reoccupying. If additional units are used for remote rooms or where free flow of fog is not assured, increase airing-out time accordingly.

Precautionary Statements:

Hazards to Humans and Domestic Animals: Harmful if swallowed. Avoid breathing vapors or spray mist. Avoid contact with skin or eyes. In case of contact, flush with plenty of water. Wash with soap and warm water after use. Obtain medical attention if irritation persists. Avoid contamination of food or feedstuffs. In the home, all food processing surfaces and utensils should be covered during treatment or thoroughly washed before use. Remove pets, birds, and cover fish aquariums before spraying.

Statement of Practical Treatment:

If Swallowed: Call a physician or poison control center immediately. If In Eyes: Flush with plenty of water. Get medical attention if irritation persists. If on Skin or Clothing: Remove contaminated clothing and wash before reuse. Wash skin with soap and warm water. Get medical attention if irritation persists. If Inhaled: Remove victim to fresh air if effects occur, and call a physician.

Physical or chemical hazards: Contents under pressure. Keep away from heat, sparks, and open flame. Do not puncture or incinerate container. Exposure to temperatures above 130°F may cause bursting.

Storage and Disposal:

Storage: Store in a cool, dry area away from heat or open flame.

Disposal: Replace cap and discard container in trash. Do not incinerate or puncture.

Warning(s): Keep out of reach of children.

Discussion: Nylar®, an insect growth regulator, is similar to growth hormones that occur naturally in insects. It inhibits development of the immature stages of flea for 7 months, preventing them from reaching the biting stage. This product contains a combination of three insecticides that stops the flea life cycle in three ways and controls other listed insects. The first insecticide is Nylar®, an insect growth regulator, that will not allow the flea to reproduce thereby providing long term control. The second insecticide is the botanical Pyrethrum, (an extract of Chrysanthemum flower), which provides effective, quick-kill of insects upon direct contact and an added benefit of flushing the insects from their hiding place to aid in a more complete control. Permethrin, the third active insecticide, provides activity until Nylar® takes effect. This product contains a combination of ingredients that kills both adult fleas and preadult fleas. Kills preadult fleas before they grow up to bite. The insect growth regulator in this product continues to kill hatching fleas for 7 months by preventing their development into adults. The product reaches fleas and other listed insects hidden in carpets, rugs, drapes upholstery, pet bedding, floor cracks and open cabinets. Occasionally adult fleas may be present in treated areas when reintroduced form infested animals. To protect your pet against and to minimize reintroduction of adult fleas from outdoors, use EPA registered flea and tick products, in conjunction with this application and prior to re-entry. As part of complete flea control program use an EPA registered outdoor spray. Kills insects on contact such as: Cockroaches (adults and nymphs), waterbugs (adults and nymphs), palmetto bugs (adults and nymphs), carpet beetles, fire ants, pharaoh ants, carpenter ants, sowbugs, millipedes, beetles, boxelder bugs, earwigs, lice, pillbugs, clover mites, centipedes, rice weevil, flies, gnats, mosquito, silverfish, flying moths (small), hornets, carpenter bees, wasps, yellowjackets, fleas (adults, larvae, eggs), ticks that may carry Lyme disease, brown dog ticks, lone star ticks, deer tick, other ixodid species, American dog tick, gulf coast tick.

Presentation: 12 oz fogger.

Nylar® - Registered trademark of McLaughlin Gormley King Co.

Compendium Code No.: 10941591

ONCE PMH®

Intervet — **Vaccine**

Pasteurella Haemolytica-Multocida Vaccine, Avirulent Live Culture

U.S. Vet. Lic. No.: 286

Contents: This product contains the antigens listed above.

This product contains streptomycin as a preservative.

Indications: For use in the vaccination of healthy cattle against respiratory disease caused by *Pasteurella haemolytica* and *Pasteurella multocida*.

Directions: Aseptically rehydrate vial of desiccated product with accompanying vial of diluent. Shake well. Administer 2 mL I.M. Annual revaccination with a single 2 mL dose is recommended.

Precaution(s): Store in the dark, 35°F-45°F (2°C-7°C). Do not freeze. Use entire contents when first rehydrated. Care should be taken to avoid chemical or microbial contamination of the product. Burn the containers and all unused contents.

Caution(s): In case of anaphylactoid reactions, epinephrine should be administered immediately.

For veterinary use only.

Warning(s): Do not vaccinate within 21 days before slaughter.

Presentation: 10 doses (20 mL), 25 doses (50 mL) and 50 doses (100 mL) with sterile diluent.

Compendium Code No.: 11061032

ONE DAY RESPONSE™

Farnam, Livestock Div. — **Large Animal Dietary Supplement**

Nutritional Supplement

Guaranteed Analysis:

Salt (NaCl), minimum	4.5%
Salt (NaCl), maximum	5.5%
Sodium, minimum	4%
Potassium, minimum	1%
Magnesium, minimum	0.2%

Ingredients: Psyllium seed husk, sucrose, salt (sodium chloride), sodium citrate, sodium bicarbonate, medium chain triglycerides, potassium chloride, glycine, silicon dioxide, magnesium hydroxide.

Contains no artificial colors or flavorings.

Indications: ONE DAY RESPONSE™ is an oral rehydrant for young calves. When mixed with water and administered, ONE DAY RESPONSE™ provides fluids, fiber and synergistic nutrients essential for maintaining normal activity.

Dosage and Administration: Feeding Instructions (includes 1.25 oz scoop):

1) Mix 2 scoops or 1 packet (2.5 oz) with 2 quarts of warm water.
2) Administer the mixture orally to the calf every 12 hours for 4 feedings.
3) Resume regular diet within 48 hours (or less if calf responds favorably after one or two feedings).

Note:

Feed immediately after mixing. Do not pre-mix - the solution will become too thick to feed.

Many calves are ready to resume regular diets after only one or two feedings.

1 quart of milk may be substituted for 1 quart of water in the 4th feeding. In that case, mix 1 scoop with 1 quart warm water and 1 scoop with 1 quart milk and combine for the final feeding.

Bucket feeding: mix with a whisk for best results.

Bottle feeding: to eliminate clumping, pour 2.5 oz of powdered into bottle, and 1 pint water and shake well until powder is thoroughly mixed. Then add 3 more pints of water to bottle and shake well before feeding.

1st Feeding (0 Hours): 2 scoops or 1 packet ONE DAY RESPONSE™ + 2 quarts warm water

2nd Feeding (12 Hours): 2 scoops or 1 packet ONE DAY RESPONSE™ + 2 quarts warm water

3rd Feeding (24 Hours): 2 scoops or 1 packet ONE DAY RESPONSE™ + 2 quarts warm water

4th Feeding (36 Hours): 1 scoop or ½ packet ONE DAY RESPONSE™ + 1 quart warm water combined with 1 scoop or ½ packet ONE DAY RESPONSE™ + 1 quart milk

Resume Regular Feeding (48 Hours) or sooner if calf responds well after 1st or 2nd feeding

Precaution(s): Store packets and pails in a cool, dry place.

Warning(s): Specifically formulated for calves. Do not feed to other animals or humans.

Presentation: 2.5 oz pouch, 3.15 lbs and 6.3 lbs pails.

Compendium Code No.: 14990000

ONE SHOT®

Pfizer Animal Health — **Bacterin-Toxoid**

Pasteurella Haemolytica Bacterin-Toxoid

U.S. Vet. Lic. No.: 189

Description: ONE SHOT® is an inactivated freeze-dried product prepared from whole cultures propagated to increase the production of leukotoxin and capsular and cell-associated antigens. A sterile diluent containing adjuvant to enhance the immune response is used to rehydrate the freeze-dried bacterin-toxoid.

Indications: ONE SHOT® is a bacterin-toxoid for vaccination of healthy cattle as an aid in preventing bovine pneumonic pasteurellosis caused by Pasteurella haemolytica type A1.

Directions:

1. General Directions: Vaccination of healthy cattle is recommended. Aseptically rehydrate the freeze-dried bacterin-toxoid with the accompanying adjuvant-containing sterile diluent, shake well, and administer 2 mL subcutaneously. In accordance with Beef Quality Assurance guidelines, this product should be administered subcutaneously (SC) under the skin. Healthy cattle should be vaccinated a minimum of 14 days prior to weaning, shipping, or exposure to stress or infectious conditions.
2. Primary Vaccination: Administer a single dose to healthy cattle. Only a single dose is necessary to confer active immunity. Good management practices support revaccination whenever subsequent stress or exposure is likely.
3. Good animal husbandry and herd health management practices should be employed.

Precaution(s): Store at 2°-7°C. Prolonged exposure to higher temperatures may adversely affect potency. Do not freeze.

Use entire contents when first opened.

Sterilized syringes and needles should be used to administer this vaccine.

Caution(s): As with many vaccines, anaphylaxis may occur after use. Initial antidote of epinephrine is recommended and should be followed with appropriate supportive therapy.

This product has been shown to be efficacious in healthy animals. A protective immune response may not be elicited if animals are incubating an infectious disease, are malnourished or parasitized, are stressed due to shipment or environmental conditions, are otherwise immunocompromised, or the vaccine is not administered in accordance with label directions.

Warning(s): Do not vaccinate within 21 days before slaughter.

For veterinary use only.

Discussion: Disease Description: Pneumonic pasteurellosis caused by *Pasteurella haemolytica* type A1 has resulted in substantial economic losses in the cattle industry.[1] The disease condition, known as shipping fever, often prevents optimal weight gain in infected cattle and may result in death. Clinical signs may include difficult breathing, nasal discharge, reduced feed intake, fever, and increased pulse rate.

Pasteurella haemolytica type A1, a normal constituent of the bovine nasopharynx, increases greatly in number when an animal undergoes stress (transport, change in climate, viral infections). This rapid increase in bacterial population adds to the deposition of organisms in the lungs. In the lung, *P. haemolytica* type A1 may grow rapidly and produce a leukotoxin which incapacitates leukocytes (alveolar macrophages and polymorphonuclear neutrophils).[2] When the bacterium is engulfed by a weakened leukocyte, the leukocyte is unable to destroy the bacterium, allowing the bacterium to produce leukotoxin, which kills the leukocyte. As the leukocyte dies, it releases enzymes that add to the fibrinopurulent consolidation and local areas of necrosis characteristic of pneumonic pasteurellosis (shipping fever).

Trial Data: Safety and Efficacy: ONE SHOT® is considered safe in cattle of all ages. Following vaccination, animals remained alert, and they exhibited no signs of pain or soreness.

The product was observed to cause moderate swelling at the injection site in some animals, primarily in dairy calves. Resolution occurred in most cases within 14-28 days; while in a few animals, small swelling was noticeable 60 days postvaccination.

Efficacy of ONE SHOT® was demonstrated in challenge-of-immunity studies. Cattle (400-550 lb) vaccinated with 1 dose of ONE SHOT® were subjected to severe experimental challenge at 2 weeks postvaccination with a heterologous strain of *P. haemolytica* type A1. Six days postchallenge, animals were necropsied and individual lungs were evaluated for lung damage and lesions characteristic of *P. haemolytica* type A1 infection. Subcutaneous vaccinates demonstrated statistically significant reduction in lung damage compared to placebo controls.

References: Available upon request.

Presentation: 5, 10 and 50 dose vials.

Compendium Code No.: 36900390 — 75-4991-06

ONE SHOT ULTRA™ 7

Pfizer Animal Health — **Bacterin-Toxoid**

Clostridium Chauvoei-Septicum-Novyi-Sordellii-Perfringens Types C & D-Pasteurella Haemolytica Bacterin-Toxoid

U.S. Vet. Lic. No.: 189

Description: The freeze-dried component is a preparation of inactivated whole cultures of *P. haemolytica* propagated to increase the production of leukotoxin and capsular and cell-associated antigens. The liquid component consists of killed, standardized cultures of *Cl. chauvoei, Cl. septicum, Cl. novyi, Cl. sordellii,* and *Cl. perfringens* types C and D, with a special, water-soluble adjuvant (Stimugen™) to enhance the immune response.

Contains formalin as a preservative.

Indications: ONE SHOT ULTRA™ 7 is for vaccination of healthy cattle as an aid in preventing blackleg caused by *Clostridium chauvoei*, malignant edema caused by *Cl. septicum*, black disease caused by *Cl. novyi*, gas-gangrene caused by *Cl. sordellii*, enterotoxemia and enteritis caused by *Cl. perfringens* types B, C, and D, and bovine pneumonic pasteurellosis caused by *Pasteurella haemolytica* type A1. Although *Cl. perfringens* type B is not a significant problem in North America, immunity is provided by the beta toxoid of type C and the epsilon toxoid of type D.

Directions:

1. General Directions: Vaccination of healthy cattle is recommended. Aseptically rehydrate the freeze-dried bacterin-toxoid (ONE SHOT ULTRA™ 7) with the accompanying vial of diluent (UltraChoice™ 7), shake well, and administer 2 mL subcutaneously. In accordance with Beef Quality Assurance guidelines, this product should be administered subcutaneously (SC) under the skin.
2. Primary Vaccination: Administer a single 2-mL dose to healthy cattle, followed by a second 2-mL dose of UltraChoice™ 7, 4-6 weeks later.
3. Revaccination: Annual revaccination with a single dose of UltraChoice™ 7 is recommended. Good management practices support revaccination with One Shot® whenever subsequent stress or exposure is likely.
4. Good animal husbandry and herd health management practices should be employed.

Precaution(s): Store at 2°-7°C. Prolonged exposure to higher temperatures may adversely affect potency. Do not freeze.

Use entire contents when first opened.

Sterilized syringes and needles should be used to administer this vaccine.

Caution(s): Not for use in sheep.

Temporary local swelling at injection site may occur after administration.

As with many vaccines, anaphylaxis may occur after use. Initial antidote of epinephrine is recommended and should be followed with appropriate supportive therapy.

This product has been shown to be efficacious in healthy animals. A protective immune response may not be elicited if animals are incubating an infectious disease, are malnourished or parasitized, are stressed due to shipment or environmental conditions, are otherwise immunocompromised, or the vaccine is not administered in accordance with label directions.

Warning(s): Do not vaccinate within 21 days before slaughter.

For veterinary use only.

Discussion: Disease Description: Pneumonic pasteurellosis caused by *P. haemolytica* type A1 has resulted in substantial economic losses in the cattle industry.[1] The disease condition, known as shipping fever, often prevents optimal weight gain in infected cattle and may result in death. Clinical signs may include difficult breathing, nasal discharge, reduced feed intake, fever, and increased pulse rate.

P. haemolytica type A1, a normal constituent of the bovine nasopharynx, increases greatly in number when an animal undergoes stress (transport, change in climate, viral infections). This rapid increase in bacterial population adds to the deposition of organisms in the lungs. In the lung, *P. haemolytica* type A1 may grow rapidly and produce a leukotoxin which incapacitates leukocytes (alveolar macrophages and polymorphonuclear neutrophils).[2] When the bacterium is engulfed by a weakened leukocyte, the leukocyte is unable to destroy the bacterium, allowing the bacterium to produce leukotoxin, which kills the leukocyte. As the leukocyte dies, it releases enzymes that add to the fibrinopurulent consolidation and local areas of necrosis characteristic of pneumonic pasteurellosis (shipping fever).

Trial Data: Safety and Efficacy: In safety studies involving 595 animals, no untoward reactions were noted following vaccination. Vaccination did result in small, temporary injection site swellings.

Efficacy of the *P. haemolytica* fraction in ONE SHOT ULTRA™ 7 was demonstrated in a challenge-of-immunity study. Cattle (300-550 lb) vaccinated with 1 dose of One Shot Ultra™ 8 were subjected to severe experimental challenge at 2 weeks postvaccination with a heterologous strain of *P. haemolytica* type A1. Four days postchallenge, animals were necropsied and individual lungs were evaluated for lung damage and lesions characteristic of *P. haemolytica* type A1 infection. Vaccinates demonstrated a statistically significant reduction (82.6%) in lung damage compared to animals receiving a placebo. Immunogenicity of the clostridial fractions was confirmed by serologic studies.

References: Available upon request.

Presentation: 10 doses and 50 doses.

Compendium Code No.: 36900730

75-5074-00

ONE SHOT ULTRA™ 8

Pfizer Animal Health **Bacterin-Toxoid**

Clostridium Chauvoei-Septicum-Haemolyticum-Novyi-Sordellii-Perfringens Types C & D-Pasteurella Haemolytica Bacterin-Toxoid

U.S. Vet. Lic. No.: 189

Description: The freeze-dried component is a preparation of inactivated whole cultures of P. haemolytica propagated to increase the production of leukotoxin and capsular and cell-associated antigens. The liquid component consists of killed, standardized cultures of *Cl. chauvoei, Cl. septicum, Cl. haemolyticum, Cl. novyi, Cl. sordellii,* and *Cl. perfringens* types C and D, with a special, water-soluble adjuvant (Stimugen™) to enhance the immune response.

Contains formalin as a preservative.

Indications: ONE SHOT ULTRA™ 8 is for vaccination of healthy cattle as an aid in preventing blackleg caused by *Clostridium chauvoei;* malignant edema caused by *Cl. septicum;* bacillary hemoglobinuria caused by *Cl. haemolyticum;* black disease caused by *Cl. novyi;* gas-gangrene caused by *Cl. sordellii;* enterotoxemia and enteritis caused by *Cl. perfringens* types B, C, and D; and bovine pneumonic pasteurellosis caused by *Pasteurella haemolytica* type A1. Although *Cl. perfringens* type B is not a significant problem in North America, immunity is provided by the beta toxoid of type C and the epsilon toxoid of type D.

Directions:

1. General Directions: Vaccination of healthy cattle is recommended. Aseptically rehydrate the freeze-dried bacterin-toxoid (ONE SHOT ULTRA™ 8) with the accompanying vial of diluent (UltraChoice™ 8), shake well, and administer 2 mL subcutaneously. In accordance with Beef Quality Assurance guidelines, this product should be administered subcutaneously (SC) under the skin.
2. Primary Vaccination: Administer a single 2-mL dose to healthy cattle, followed by a second 2-mL dose of UltraChoice™ 8, 4-6 weeks later. For *Cl. haemolyticum* repeat the dose every 6 months in animals subject to reexposure.
3. Revaccination: Annual revaccination with a single dose of UltraChoice™ 8 is recommended. Good management practices support revaccination with One Shot® whenever subsequent stress or exposure is likely.
4. Good animal husbandry and herd health management practices should be employed.

Precaution(s): Store at 2°-7°C. Prolonged exposure to higher temperatures may adversely affect potency. Do not freeze.

Use entire contents when first opened.

Sterilized syringes and needles should be used to administer this vaccine.

Not for use in sheep.

7. Temporary local swelling at injection site may occur after administration.

8. As with many vaccines, anaphylaxis may occur after use. Initial antidote of epinephrine is recommended and should be followed with appropriate supportive therapy.

9. This product has been shown to be efficacious in healthy animals. A protective immune response may not be elicited if animals are incubating an infectious disease, are malnourished or parasitized, are stressed due to shipment or environmental conditions, are otherwise immunocompromised, or the vaccine is not administered in accordance with label directions.

Warning(s): Do not vaccinate within 21 days before slaughter.

For veterinary use only.

Discussion: Disease Description: Pneumonic pasteurellosis caused by *P. haemolytica* type A1 has resulted in substantial economic losses in the cattle industry.[1] The disease condition, known as shipping fever, often prevents optimal weight gain in infected cattle and may result in death. Clinical signs may include difficult breathing, nasal discharge, reduced feed intake, fever, and increased pulse rate.

P. haemolytica type A1, a normal constituent of the bovine nasopharynx, increases greatly in number when an animal undergoes stress (transport, change in climate, viral infections). This rapid increase in bacterial population adds to the deposition of organisms in the lungs. In the lung, *P. haemolytica* type A1 may grow rapidly and produce a leukotoxin which incapacitates leukocytes (alveolar macrophages and polymorphonuclear neutrophils).[2] When the bacterium is engulfed by a weakened leukocyte, the leukocyte is unable to destroy the bacterium, allowing the bacterium to produce leukotoxin, which kills the leukocyte. As the leukocyte dies, it releases enzymes that add to the fibrinopurulent consolidation and local areas of necrosis characteristic of pneumonic pasteurellosis (shipping fever).

Trial Data: Safety and Efficacy: In safety studies involving 595 animals, no untoward reactions were noted following vaccination. Vaccination did result in small, temporary injection site swellings.

Efficacy of ONE SHOT ULTRA™ 8 against *P. haemolytica* was demonstrated in a challenge-of-immunity study. Cattle (300-550 lb) vaccinated with 1 dose of ONE SHOT ULTRA™ 8 were subjected to severe experimental challenge at 2 weeks postvaccination with a heterologous strain of *P. haemolytica* type A1. Four days postchallenge, animals were necropsied and individual lungs were evaluated for lung damage and lesions characteristic of *P. haemolytica* type A1 infection. Vaccinates demonstrated a statistically significant reduction (82.6%) in lung damage compared to animals receiving a placebo. Immunogenicity of the clostridial fractions was confirmed by serologic studies.

References: Available upon request.

Presentation: 10 doses and 50 doses.

Compendium Code No.: 36900740

75-5076-00

ONE STEP

Vedco **Disinfectant**

EPA Reg. No.: 4959-15-44084

Active Ingredient(s):

Iodine* 1.75%

Inert Ingredients 98.25%

*From alpha-(p-nonylphenyl)-omega-hydroxypoly (oxyethylene)-iodine complex.

Indications: Concentrated broad spectrum iodophor for use as a one step cleaner-disinfectant and no-rinse sanitizer.

Used as directed ONE STEP is effective in hard water (up to 400 ppm as CaCO3) and in 5% organic serum load against the following viruses, bacteria and pathogenic fungi: Polio1*, Vaccinia*, Herpes Simplex Type 1*, Influenza A2/Japan 305*, and Canine Parvovirus*, bactericidal against *Salmonella cholerasuis, Staphylococcus aureus, Pseudomonas aeruginosa,* and *E coli;* is fungicidal against *Trichophyton mentagrophytes* (the athlete's foot fungus).

For veterinary hospital use only.

Dosage and Administration: It is a violation of Federal Law to use this product in a manner inconsistent with its labeling.

Use Dilution Table: ONE STEP/Water Titratable Iodine

1 oz to 10 gal 12.5 ppm

1 oz to 5 gal 25 ppm

3 oz to 5 gal 75 ppm

1 oz to 1 gal 125 ppm

6 oz to 5 gal 150 ppm

Not for residential use.

The color of ONE STEP solution is proportional to the titratable iodine concentration. Prepare a fresh solution daily, or when there is a noticeable change in its rich color, or more often if the solution becomes diluted or soiled. Used as directed, ONE STEP is effective in hard water (up to 400 ppm CaCO3) and in 5% organic serum load against listed bacteria and pathogenic fungi.

ONE STEP Cleaning and Disinfecting: Prior to use in veterinary clinics, animal holding facilities, farm premises, kennels, pet shops and zoos: Remove all animals and feeds from premises, vehicles and enclosures. Remove all litter and manure from floors, walls, and all surfaces to be treated. Empty all troughs, racks and other feeding and watering appliances. Then proceed as directed below.

To Clean and Disinfect: Before applying disinfecting solution, food products and packaging materials must be removed from the room or carefully protected. Remove heavy soil deposits before applying the disinfecting solution. Using a solution of 3 ounces ONE STEP per 5 gallons of warm water (68°F, 20°C or warmer), immerse objects in disinfecting solution, or apply solution with a mop, sponge or brush. When appropriate, use a mechanical sprayer to produce coarse spray. Allow a 10 minute contact time with disinfecting solution. For efficacy against Canine Parvovirus, allow a 120 minute contact time; surface must remain wet. All food contact surfaces must be rinsed with potable water before reuse. Floors, walls and all other non-food contact surfaces may drain dry without rinsing.

Note: When mixing ONE STEP with cold water (as low as 41°F, 5°C), increase use to 6 oz per 5 gallons of water.

Before Rehousing Animals: Ventilate buildings, vehicles and other closed spaces. Do not house animals or use equipment until treatment absorbs, sets or dries. Thoroughly rinse all treated feed racks, mangers, troughs, automatic feeders, fountains and waterers with potable water before reuse.

Shoe Bath: Routine use of shoe bath sanitizers helps reduce the spread of disease causing organisms between poultry houses, farrowing houses, hog barns and other livestock buildings. Use 3 ounces of ONE STEP per 1 gallon of water. Place sanitizing solution in shallow plastic or stainless steel pans inside all entrances to poultry and livestock buildings. Scrape shoes outside doorway and stand in shoe bath for 30 seconds before entering building. Replace shoe bath daily or more often if solution becomes soiled.

Cleaning Milking Equipment and Bulk Tanks: Immediately after milking, flush milking equipment and utensils with lukewarm (100°F, 38°C) water to wash out all milk. Take apart milking machines and immerse air hoses, inflations, metal parts (except pulsator) and utensils in a solution containing 1 ounce of ONE STEP per 5 gallons of water. Brush all parts thoroughly. Drain completely, rinse with water and allow to air dry. After emptying bulk tanks, flush tanks thoroughly with 100°F (38°C) water to wash out all milk. Brush tanks thoroughly with a solution containing 1 ounce ONE STEP per 5 gallons of water. Allow wash solution to drain, rinse with water and air dry.

Sanitizing Milking Machines and Bulk Tanks: Before each milking, flush assembled milking machines and empty bulk tanks with a solution containing 1 ounce ONE STEP per 5 gallons of water. Allow a 1 minute contact time. Drain thoroughly and air dry before use.

Sanitizing Previously Cleaned Food Contact Surfaces: Sanitize previously cleaned and rinsed hard, non-porous surfaces such as glass, metal, plastic and porcelain with a solution containing 1 ounce of ONE STEP per 5 gallons of water. Spray or immerse equipment with sanitizing solution and allow 1 minute of contact time. Drain solution from equipment; do not rinse. ONE STEP used at 1 ounce per 5 gallons of water contains 25 ppm titratable iodine and does not require a final rinse with potable water in accordance with Federal Food Additive Regulation 178.1010.

Sanitizing Food-Grade Egg Shells: Coarse spray previously cleaned food-grade egg shells with a solution containing 1 ounce of ONE STEP Disinfectant per 5 gallons of water. Solution temperature should be warmer than the eggs, but not to exceed 130°F (53°C). Wet eggs thoroughly for 1 minute and allow to drain. A final potable water rinse is not required. Eggs should be reasonably dry before casing or breaking. Do not reuse solution to sanitize eggs.

Precaution(s): Storage: Keep container closed when not in use. Do not store below 25°F or above 100°F for extended periods.

Prohibitions: Do not contaminate water, food or feed by storage or disposal. Open dumping is prohibited.

Pesticide Disposal: Pesticide wastes are acutely hazardous. Improper disposal of excess pesticide, spray mixture or rinsate is a violation of Federal Law. If these wastes cannot be disposed of by use according to label instructions, contact your State Pesticide or Environmental Control Agency, or the Hazardous Waste representative at the nearest EPA Regional Office for guidance.

Container Disposal: Triple rinse (or equivalent). Then offer for recycling or reconditioning, or puncture and dispose of in a sanitary landfill, or incinerate, or, if allowed by State and local authorities, burn container. If burned, stay out of smoke.

Environmental Hazards: This product is toxic to fish. Keep out of lakes, ponds or streams. Do not contaminate water by cleaning of equipment or disposal of wastes. Do not discharge effluent containing this product into lakes, streams, ponds, estuaries, oceans or other water unless in accordance with the requirements of a National Pollutant Discharge Elimination System (NPDES) permit and the permitting authority has been notified in writing prior to discharge. Do not discharge effluent containing this product to sewer systems without previously notifying the local sewage treatment plant authority. For guidance, contact your State Water Board or Regional Office of the EPA.

Caution(s): Precautionary Statements:

Hazards to Humans and Domestic Animals: Danger: Corrosive: Causes irreversible eye damage. Harmful if swallowed. Do not get in eyes or on clothing. Avoid contact with skin. Wear goggles or face shield. Wash thoroughly with soap and water after handling. Remove contaminated clothing and wash before reuse. Sold to veterinarians only.

Warning(s): Statement of Practical Treatment:

In case of contact, immediately flush the eyes or skin with plenty of water for at least 15 minutes. For eyes, call a physician. If swallowed, drink promptly a large quantity of water. Call a physician immediately. Do not induce vomiting. Avoid alcohol. Get medical attention. Remove and wash all contaminated clothing before reuse.

Note to Physician: Probable mucosal damage may contraindicate the use of gastric lavage. Measures against circulatory shock, respiratory depression and convulsions may be needed.

Keep out of reach of children.

Presentation: 1 gallon.

Compendium Code No.: 10941600

ONO™

PRN Pharmacal **Odor Product-Oral**

Active Ingredient(s): Chlorine Dioxide (Orex™).

Indications: For use in the dry or canned food of cats, dogs and small mammals in order to eliminate odors associated with urine, feces, cat spray and other animal by-products.

Directions: Spray over the entire surface of the animal's food at every feeding.

For best results, mix thoroughly.

Average size feline: 3 to 4 full sprays.

Small Canine: 2 to 4 full sprays.

Medium Canine: 5 to 6 full sprays.

Large Canine: 7 to 10 full sprays.

For other mammals, follow instructions as with other above named species.

Contraindication(s): Do not give to pregnant or nursing animals.

Precaution(s): Keep out of direct sunlight and store at room temperature.

Caution(s): For animal use only. Keep out of children's reach.

Available through veterinarians only.

Presentation: Available in 16 fl oz containers.

A trademark of: PRN Pharmacal, Inc.

Compendium Code No.: 10900110

OPTICLEAR™ EYE WASH SOLUTION

Tomlyn **Ophthalmic Solution**

Active Ingredient(s):

Sodium chloride 0.44%
Sodium phosphate, monobasic 0.14%
Sodium phosphate, dibasic 0.84%

Other Ingredients: Purified water, preserved with benzalkonium chloride (0.01%) and disodium edetate (0.05%).

Indications: Tomlyn's OPTICLEAR™ Eye Wash is a sterile buffered isotonic solution that has the same salt concentration as normal tear fluid.

OPTICLEAR™ is used to wash away dried mucous secretions and discharges from the eyes of cats and dogs. It is useful for the removal of hair from the eye after grooming or clipping.

Dosage and Administration: Wipe away excess matter that may have collected in the corner of the eye. Flush the eye gently with a fine stream, controlling the rate of flow of solution by pressure on the bottle. Repeat as necessary.

Caution(s): To avoid contamination, do not touch the tip of the container to any surface. Replace the cap after using. Consult a veterinarian for excessive or persistent redness or irritation of the eye. If the solution changes color or becomes cloudy, do not use.

Keep out of the reach of children. For external animal use only. For veterinary use only.

Presentation: 118 mL.

Compendium Code No.: 11220190

OPTIMMUNE® ℞

Schering-Plough **Ophthalmic Preparation**

0.2% Cyclosporine, USP Ophthalmic Ointment

NADA No.: 141-052

Active Ingredient(s): Each gram of OPTIMMUNE® Ophthalmic Ointment contains 2 mg of cyclosporine, USP; petrolatum, USP; corn oil, NF; and Amerchol® CAB base. Cyclosporine (cyclosporin A), the active ingredient of OPTIMMUNE® Ophthalmic Ointment, is a cyclic undecapeptide metabolite of the fungus *Tolypocladium inflatum gams.*

Indications: OPTIMMUNE® Ophthalmic Ointment is indicated for management of chronic keratoconjunctivitis sicca (KCS) and chronic superficial keratitis (CSK) in dogs.

Mode of Action: When applied ophthalmically, cyclosporine is believed to act as a local immunomodulator of diseases suspected to be immune-mediated such as keratoconjunctivitis sicca (KCS) and chronic superficial keratitis (CSK). In the management of KCS, the mechanism by which cyclosporine causes an increase in lacrimation is poorly understood. Clinical improvement in cases in aqueous tear production (as measured by the Schirmer Tear Test [STT]). See Efficacy.

Dosage and Administration: Remove debris with suitable nonirritating solutions. Apply a ¼ inch strip of ointment to the affected eye(s) every 12 hours. The ointment may be placed directly on the cornea or into the conjunctival sac.

It is recommended that dogs exhibiting chronic recurring conjunctivitis be tested for adequate tear production to determine if they are suffering from early stages of chronic KCS.

For best results in treating KCS, cyclosporine ophthalmic ointment should be administered early in the course of the disease before irreversible damage to the lacrimal tissue, or dense corneal scarring or pigmentation occurs.

Dogs afflicted with KCS or CSK will most likely require lifelong consistent therapy (see Efficacy section). For CSK, because environmental factors such as ultraviolet (UV) radiation are implicated in the pathogenesis, clinical signs may subside in the winter months when light intensity is reduced or if the dog is moved to a lower altitude, or indoors, and thus exposed to less UV radiation.[1]

In cases refractory to cyclosporine, the diagnosis should be re-evaluated and a different course of therapy considered. Periodic reassessment of the need for OPTIMMUNE® Ophthalmic Ointment therapy is recommended.

Precaution(s): Store between 2° and 30°C (36° and 86°F).

Caution(s): US Federal law restricts this drug to use by or on the order of a licensed veterinarian.

The clinical effects of OPTIMMUNE® Ophthalmic Ointment have not been determined in dogs with KCS due to the following conditions: congenital alacrima, sulfonamide usage, canine distemper virus, metabolic disease, surgical removal of the third eyelid gland, and facial nerve paralysis with loss of the palpebral reflex. Some of the underlying conditions which may lead to KCS can be either transient (eg, facial nerve trauma) or correctable with appropriate treatment. Consequently, recovery from clinical signs attributed to KCS may be observed and treatment options may need reconsideration.

When switching to cyclosporine from another therapeutic agent (eg, frequent application of an artificial tear preparation) for KCS or CSK, it should be kept in mind that clinical efficacy is not necessarily apparent immediately after initiation of OPTIMMUNE® Ophthalmic Ointment therapy. Several days to a few weeks may be required before the clinical effects are of OPTIMMUNE® Ophthalmic Ointment are of sufficient magnitude such that a previously initiated therapy can be safely withdrawn. Abrupt cessation of a therapeutic agent immediately upon initiation of OPTIMMUNE® Ophthalmic Ointment therapy can result in rapid clinical relapse which may be erroneously interpreted as an adverse reaction to the OPTIMMUNE® Ophthalmic Ointment.

The safety of OPTIMMUNE® Ophthalmic Ointment has not been determined in cases of preexisting viral or fungal ocular infections. It is recommended that in such cases, OPTIMMUNE® Ophthalmic Ointment therapy be delayed until the fungal/viral ocular infection has been successfully treated.

The safety of OPTIMMUNE® Ophthalmic Ointment in puppies, pregnant bitches, or dogs used for breeding has not been determined.

Warning(s): Keep this and all drugs out of the reach of children.

For ophthalmic use in dogs only.

Safety: A target animal safety study and clinical field studies with OPTIMMUNE® Ophthalmic Ointment showed a wide safety margin in adult dogs. In the 6-month target animal safety study, dogs were subjected twice daily to up to 10 times the approved concentration of OPTIMMUNE® Ophthalmic Ointment. No apparent toxicity or adverse reactions were observed. Dogs in this study were vaccinated with commercially available vaccines. No effect on antibody titer response was noted. Epiphora was noted in all groups, including the placebo group, and was not associated with any inflammatory change, nor was there any correlation to gross and histopathological changes.

Adverse Reactions: In the KCS clinical field trial, there were 20 adverse reactions reported out of 132 cases enrolled. This corresponds to an adverse reaction rate of 12.9% (13 of 101 cases) for OPTIMMUNE® Ophthalmic Ointment treated dogs and 22.6% (7 of 31) for placebo treated dogs. The reactions described were primarily ocular and periocular inflammatory reactions. These were likely a function of therapy being unable to fully control the keratoconjunctivitis, rather than a true "adverse reaction." Similarly, in the CSK trial, of 36 cases evaluated for safety, adverse reactions were noted in 2 animals (5.6%). One involved transient hyperemia, epiphora, and mild discomfort of the eye. The other involved periocular/palpebral inflammation and mild alopecia.

On rare occasion, instillation of OPTIMMUNE® Ophthalmic Ointment may be associated with local irritation as manifested by periocular redness, lid spasm, and excessive rubbing. As the eyes of dogs with KCS often demonstrate considerable inflammation, it will be difficult to determine whether this local irritation constitutes a hypersensitivity to OPTIMMUNE® Ophthalmic Ointment. If this ocular irritation persists beyond 7 days, hypersensitivity to a component of OPTIMMUNE® Ophthalmic Ointment should be suspected and therapeutic options reassessed.

Efficacy: 1. KCS A well-controlled clinical field trial was conducted by veterinary ophthalmologists in 9 states and included 132 dogs afflicted with KCS of which 124 were evaluated for efficacy. Dogs were randomly assigned to BID treatment with either 0.2% (OPTIMMUNE® Ophthalmic Ointment) or 0% (placebo vehicle) cyclosporine ophthalmic ointment for 12 weeks. Treatment with OPTIMMUNE® Ophthalmic Ointment resulted in an average 8 to 9 mm increase in STT by the end of the study period (vs 3 to 4 mm for the placebo vehicle). Most of the increase in STT, approximately 6 mm, occurred in the first week of therapy. Some dogs improved clinically (ie, exhibited a decrease in conjunctival and/or corneal pathology) without an increase in STT values. This is thought to occur through suppression of inflammation by cyclosporine on the ocular surface. In this clinical field trial, OPTIMMUNE® Ophthalmic Ointment therapy was also associated with an improvement in clinical signs in comparison to the placebo. Blepharitis, blepharospasm, and "other signs of ocular discomfort" (eg, pawing at eyes), were markedly reduced. Improvement in conjunctival health as manifested by reduced conjunctival hypertrophy, reduced hyperemia, reduced conjunctival discharge volume, and improved character of discharge was evident. Improvement in corneal health as manifested by improved corneal surface contour, reduced corneal edema and corneal neovascularization was also noted. Overall improvement was noted in 81% of eyes treated with OPTIMMUNE® Ophthalmic Ointment.

Withdrawal of OPTIMMUNE® Ophthalmic Ointment therapy resulted in rapid clinical regression in all but one test eye indicating the need for long-term continual therapy for almost all cases of chronic KCS.

2. CSK The efficacy of OPTIMMUNE® Ophthalmic Ointment was determined in a historically controlled clinical field trial conducted by veterinary ophthalmologists in four countries and included 36 dogs afflicted with CSK. Dogs, primarily German shepherds, a breed disposed to CSK (German shepherd pannus), were treated twice daily with OPTIMMUNE® Ophthalmic Ointment for 6 weeks. Clinical improvement was noted by the investigators in 90.3% of eyes treated with OPTIMMUNE® Ophthalmic Ointment when compared to baseline.

References: Available upon request.

Presentation: OPTIMMUNE® Ophthalmic Ointment is available in a 3.5 g tube, carton of 6.

U.S. Pats. 4,839,342 & 5,411,952

Compendium Code No.: 10471390

OPTIMUNE® 4

Biomune **Vaccine**

Bursal Disease-Newcastle Disease Vaccine, Standard and Variants, Killed Virus

U.S. Vet. Lic. No.: 368

Contents: OPTIMUNE® 4 is an inactivated oil emulsion vaccine containing Newcastle disease virus and three infectious bursal disease viruses, the standard type and two variants. All viruses in OPTIMUNE® 4 are noncloned isolates produced in chicken embryos or bursal tissue.

The vaccine has undergone rigid potency, safety and purity tests and meets Biomune and USDA requirements.

Indications: The vaccine is indicated for use in healthy chickens against Newcastle disease and infectious bursal disease caused by standard and variant viruses. Breeder vaccination provides maternal antibody to the progeny of breeder hens for the prevention of early exposure to bursal disease.

Dosage and Administration: A prime with live infectious bursal disease vaccine is recommended at least four (4) weeks in advance of administration of the inactivated vaccine.

Vaccinate chickens with 0.5 mL per bird. The vaccine is to be administered by the subcutaneous route in the back of the neck, midway between the head and the body, in a direction away from the head. Do not inject into muscle or vertebrae.

Refer to the product label for specific use directions and precautions.

Precaution(s): Store the vaccine at 35°-45°F (2°-7°C). Do not freeze.

Warning(s): Do not vaccinate with oil emulsion vaccine within 42 days before slaughter.

Avoid injection of the vaccine into a human. Should accidental injection of a human occur, seek medical attention immediately since a serious localized reaction may result.

Presentation: 1,000 dose (500 mL) bottle.

Compendium Code No.: 11290192

OPTIMUNE® 6

Biomune **Vaccine**

Bursal Disease-Reovirus Vaccine, Standard and Variants, Killed Virus

U.S. Vet. Lic. No.: 368

Contents: OPTIMUNE® 6 is an inactivated oil emulsion vaccine containing three infectious bursal disease viruses, the standard type and two variant strains, and three reoviruses including strain S1133 (a tenosynovitis pathotype), strain 2408 (a malabsorption pathotype) and strain SS412 (a distinct serotype from the S1133 type reoviruses and a causative agent of proventriculitis and malabsorption in broilers).

All viruses in OPTIMUNE® 6 are noncloned isolates produced in chicken embryos or bursal tissue.

The vaccine has undergone rigid potency, safety and purity tests and meets Biomune and USDA requirements.

Indications: The vaccine is indicated for use in healthy breeder replacement chickens and breeder hens against diseases caused by infectious bursal disease viruses (standard and variant types) and reoviruses (standard and SS412 types). Breeder vaccination provides maternal antibody to the progeny of breeder hens for the prevention of early exposure to bursal disease, tenosynovitis (viral arthritis) and malabsorption syndrome which includes feed passage and proventriculitis.

Dosage and Administration: Optimum results with OPTIMUNE® 6 require that chickens are adequately primed with live infectious bursal disease vaccine and tenosynovitis vaccine at least four (4) weeks in advance of administration of the inactivated vaccine.

Vaccinate chickens with 0.5 mL per bird. The vaccine is to be administered by the subcutaneous route in the back of the neck, midway between the head and the body, in a direction away from the head. Do not inject into muscle or vertebrae.

Refer to the product label for specific use directions and precautions.

Precaution(s): Store the vaccine at 35°-45°F (2°-7°C). Do not freeze.

Warning(s): Do not vaccinate with oil emulsion vaccine within 42 days before slaughter.

Avoid injection of the vaccine into a human. Should accidental injection of a human occur, seek medical attention immediately since a serious localized reaction may result.

Presentation: 1,000 dose (500 mL) bottle.

Compendium Code No.: 11290202

OPTIMUNE® 7

Biomune **Vaccine**

Bursal Disease-Newcastle Disease-Reovirus Vaccine, Standard and Variants, Killed Virus

U.S. Vet. Lic. No.: 368

Contents: OPTIMUNE® 7 is an inactivated oil emulsion vaccine containing three infectious bursal disease viruses, the standard type and two variant strains, Newcastle disease virus, and three reoviruses including strain S1133 (a tenosynovitis pathotype), strain 2408 (a malabsorption pathotype) and strain SS412 (a distinct serotype from the S1133 type reoviruses and a causative agent of proventriculitis and malabsorption in broilers).

All viruses in OPTIMUNE® 7 are noncloned isolates produced in chicken embryos or bursal tissue.

The vaccine has undergone rigid potency, safety and purity tests and meets Biomune and USDA requirements.

Indications: The vaccine is indicated for use in healthy breeder replacement chickens and breeder hens against diseases caused by infectious bursal disease viruses (standard and variant types), Newcastle disease virus and reoviruses (standard and SS412 types). Breeder vaccination provides maternal antibody to the progeny of breeder hens for the prevention of early exposure to bursal disease, tenosynovitis (viral arthritis) and malabsorption syndrome which includes feed passage and proventriculitis.

Dosage and Administration: Optimum results with OPTIMUNE® 7 require that chickens are adequately primed with live infectious bursal disease vaccine and tenosynovitis vaccine at least four (4) weeks in advance of administration of the inactivated vaccine.

Vaccinate chickens with 0.5 mL per bird. The vaccine is to be administered by the subcutaneous route in the back of the neck, midway between the head and the body, in a direction away from the head. Do not inject into muscle or vertebrae.

Refer to the product label for specific use directions and precautions.

Precaution(s): Store the vaccine at 35°-45°F (2°-7°C). Do not freeze.

Warning(s): Do not vaccinate with oil emulsion vaccine within 42 days before slaughter.

Avoid injection of the vaccine into a human. Should accidental injection of a human occur, seek medical attention immediately since a serious localized reaction may result.

Presentation: 1,000 dose (500 mL) bottle.

Compendium Code No.: 11290212

OPTIMUNE® 8

Biomune **Vaccine**

Bursal Disease-Newcastle-Bronchitis-Reovirus Vaccine, Standard and Variants, Mass. Type, Killed Virus

U.S. Vet. Lic. No.: 368

Contents: OPTIMUNE® 8 is an inactivated oil emulsion vaccine containing three infectious bursal disease viruses, the standard type and two variant strains, and three reoviruses including strain S1133 (a tenosynovitis pathotype), strain 2408 (a malabsorption pathotype) and strain SS412 (a distinct serotype from the S1133 type reoviruses and a causative agent of proventriculitis and malabsorption in broilers). OPTIMUNE® 8 also contains Newcastle disease virus and infectious bronchitis virus of the Mass. serotype.

All viruses in OPTIMUNE® 8 are noncloned isolates produced in chicken embryos or bursal tissue.

The vaccine has undergone rigid potency, safety and purity tests and meets Biomune and USDA requirements.

Indications: The vaccine is indicated for use in healthy breeder replacement chickens and breeder hens against diseases caused by infectious bursal disease viruses (standard and variant types), Newcastle disease virus, infectious bronchitis virus (Mass. type) and reoviruses (standard and SS412 types). Breeder vaccination provides maternal antibody to the progeny of breeder hens for the prevention of early exposure to bursal disease, tenosynovitis (viral arthritis) and malabsorption syndrome which includes feed passage and proventriculitis.

Dosage and Administration: Optimum results with OPTIMUNE® 8 require that chickens are adequately primed with live infectious bursal disease vaccine, tenosynovitis vaccine and bronchitis vaccine of the Mass. type at least four (4) weeks in advance of administration of the inactivated vaccine.

Vaccinate chickens with 0.5 mL per bird. The vaccine is to be administered by the subcutaneous route in the back of the neck, midway between the head and the body, in a direction away from the head. Do not inject into muscle or vertebrae.

Refer to the product label for specific use directions and precautions.

Precaution(s): Store the vaccine at 35°-45°F (2°-7°C). Do not freeze.

Warning(s): Do not vaccinate with oil emulsion vaccine within 42 days before slaughter.

Avoid injection of the vaccine into a human. Should accidental injection of a human occur, seek medical attention immediately since a serious localized reaction may result.

Presentation: 1,000 dose (500 mL) bottle.

Compendium Code No.: 11290222

OPTIMUNE® IBD

Biomune **Vaccine**

Bursal Disease Vaccine, Standard and Variants, Killed Virus

U.S. Vet. Lic. No.: 368

Contents: OPTIMUNE® IBD is an inactivated oil emulsion vaccine containing three infectious bursal disease viruses, the standard type and two variants. The viruses in OPTIMUNE® IBD are noncloned isolates produced in chicken embryos or bursal tissue.

The vaccine has undergone rigid potency, safety and purity tests and meets Biomune and USDA requirements.

Indications: The vaccine is intended for use in healthy breeder replacement chickens and breeder hens against disease caused by infectious bursal disease viruses or the standard and variant types. Breeder vaccination provides maternal antibody to the progeny of breeder hens for the prevention of early exposure to bursal disease.

Dosage and Administration: A prime with live infectious bursal disease vaccine is recommended at least four (4) weeks in advance of administration of the inactivated vaccine.

Vaccinate chickens with 0.5 mL per bird. The vaccine is to be administered by the subcutaneous route in the back of the neck, midway between the head and the body, in a direction away from the head. Do not inject into muscle or vertebrae.

Refer to the product label for specific use directions and precautions.

Precaution(s): Store the vaccine at 35°-45°F (2°-7°C). Do not freeze.

Warning(s): Do not vaccinate with oil emulsion vaccine within 42 days before slaughter.

Avoid injection of the vaccine into a human. Should accidental injection of a human occur, seek medical attention immediately since a serious localized reaction may result.

Presentation: 1,000 dose (500 mL) bottle.

Compendium Code No.: 11290232

ORACHOL®

Schering-Plough **Vaccine**

Pasteurella multocida Vaccine, Avirulent Live Culture, Avian Isolate

U.S. Vet. Lic. No.: 165A

Active Ingredient(s): ORACHOL® is a live bacterial vaccine containing the known avirulent isolate of *Pasteurella multocida* type 3/4, Clemson University strain, in a freeze-dried preparation sealed under vacuum

The seed culture used to make the vaccine has been laboratory tested for protection against challenge with *P. multocida* strains P-1059 (type 3) and P-1662 (type 4).

Indications: For the vaccination of healthy turkeys six weeks of age or older as an aid in preventing pasteurellosis (fowl cholera) due to *P. multocida* types 3 and 4.

Dosage and Administration:

When to Vaccinate: The best results are obtained when the vaccine is administered initially to turkeys six (6) to eight (8) weeks of age and repeated every four (4) to six (6) weeks thereafter as necessary according to exposure conditions.

Vaccination Program: The development of a durable, strong protection to this disease depends upon the use of an effective vaccination program as well as many other circumstances such as

O

administration techniques, environment and flock health at the time of vaccination. Also, the immune response to one (1) vaccination under field conditions is seldom complete for all animals within a given flock. Even when vaccination is successful, the protection stimulated in individual animals against different diseases may not be life-long. Therefore, a program of periodic revaccination may be necessary.

Preparation of the Vaccine:

1. Assemble the vaccine and equipment needed to vaccinate the entire flock at one time.
2. Do not open and rehydrate the vaccine until ready for use.
3. Remove the tear-off aluminum seal from the vaccine vial without disturbing the rubber stopper.
4. Use cool, clean, nonchlorinated tap water to which powdered milk has been added as directed under How to Vaccinate.
5. Remove the rubber stopper from the vaccine vial and rehydrate the vaccine by filling the vial about half-full with tap water (milk added).
6. Reseat the stopper and shake to thoroughly dissolve the vaccine.

How to Vaccinate: Do not mix the vaccine into the drinking water until ready for use. Drinking water for vaccination should be mixed with powdered milk to prevent possible inactivation from chlorine or other water additives and also to stabilize the vaccine bacteria. The powdered milk should be added to the water at the rate of one (1) heaped teaspoon per 3 U.S. gallons or 2.5 imperial gallons (3 g per 11 L); or one (1) heaped cupful per 50 U.S. gallons or 41 imperial gallons (87 g per 190 L).

Use only clean waterers and equipment free of disinfectants or sanitizers. All water must be withheld from the birds for at least two (2) hours prior to vaccination to ensure that all turkeys drink. Mix the rehydrated vaccine in the quantity of drinking water (milk added) which will be consumed by thirsty turkeys in approximately two (2) hours.

The following schedule is a general guideline for the amount of water to use with the vaccine. These amounts will vary depending upon the individual management conditions, climate, age and sex of the birds.

Age	Sex	Climate	Amount of water for each 1,000 doses		
			U.S. Gallons	Imperial Gallons	Liters
6-8 weeks	Toms	Hot	25	21	95
6-8 weeks	Hens	Hot	20	17	76
6-8 weeks	Toms	Cold	13	11	49
6-8 weeks	Hens	Cold	10	8	38
10-14 weeks	Toms	Hot	35	29	133
10-14 weeks	Hens	Hot	27	22	103
10-14 weeks	Toms	Cold	18	15	68
10-14 weeks	Hens	Cold	14	12	53

Another helpful guideline for daily water consumption is one (1) U.S. gallon or 0.8 imperial gallon (3.8 L) of water per week of age per 100 poults; figure 40% of this amount. This 40% is about a 3-hour supply for the flock.

Distribute 1,000 doses of vaccine in water as used by 1,000 turkeys. Provide ample watering space so that all of the turkeys can drink easily. Do not administer through water lines with a proportioner or medication tank.

Records: Keep a record of the vaccine type, quantity, serial number, expiration date, and place of purchase; the date and time of vaccination; the number, age, breed, and location of the birds; the names of operators performing the vaccination and any observed reactions.

Contraindication(s): Turkeys must be healthy and free of environmental or physical stress at the time of vaccination. Initial vaccination with this vaccine should not be conducted in turkeys older than 12 weeks of age. Do not use this vaccine within two weeks before or two weeks after vaccinating turkeys with a live virus Newcastle vaccine.

Precaution(s): Store at 35° to 45°F (2° to 7°C).

Caution(s): For veterinary use only.

1. To avoid interference with the development of protection, turkeys to be vaccinated should not be given any antibiotic and/or sulfonamide medication used in the prevention or treatment of fowl cholera for three days before and five days after vaccination.
2. Vaccinate healthy birds only. Coccidiosis, respiratory disease, mycoplasma infection, or other disease conditions may cause serious complications or reduce protection. Vaccinated flocks should be watched closely and medicated as necessary to control more severe reactions. Avoid exposing birds other than turkeys to the vaccine.
3. All birds within a flock should be vaccinated on the same day. Isolate other susceptible birds on the premises from the birds being vaccinated.
4. In outbreak situations, vaccinate healthy birds first, progressing toward outbreak areas in order to vaccinate diseased birds last. Vaccination in the face of an acute outbreak is not recommended. Under these conditions, use an effective fowl cholera treatment, wait at least three days or until the outbreak subsides and then vaccinate.
5. Do not spill or spatter the vaccine. Burn the empty bottles, caps and all unused vaccine and accessories. Use the entire contents of the vial when first opened.
6. Wash hands thoroughly after using the vaccine.
7. Do not dilute the vaccine or otherwise stretch the dosage.

Warning(s): Do not vaccinate within 21 days before slaughter.

Presentation: Supplied in 10 x 1,000 dose units.

Compendium Code No.: 10471400

ORAL CALCIUM DRENCH

DVM Formula **Calcium-Oral**

Guaranteed Analysis: Per 200 mL Feeding:

Calcium, Min. .... 25 gm
Calcium, Max. .... 31 gm

Ingredients: Water, calcium chloride, magnesium chloride, propylene glycol, potassium chloride, riboflavin, cyanocobalamin (vitamin B_{12}), thiamine hydrochloride, pyridoxine hydrochloride (vitamin B_6), and d-calcium pantothenate.

Indications: Use on every fresh cow or heifer before and after calving. ORAL CALCIUM DRENCH is a liquid oral supplement designed to provide calcium, vitamin B complex, and propylene glycol in a readily absorbable formula. ORAL CALCIUM DRENCH rapidly elevates serum calcium levels and helps reduce the incidence of milk fever, displaced abomassum, and retained placenta. ORAL CALCIUM DRENCH can also be used as a follow up to intravenous treatment.

Dosage and Administration: Administer a 200 mL dose at the first sign of freshening and another 200 mL 6 to 12 hours after calving, repeat as needed. If the first dose is missed, a post calving dose is still beneficial. Shake well before using.

Feeding Directions: Administer orally using a drench gun. Hold the head of the animal in a slightly elevated position and place the nozzle between the cheek and teeth. Administer the recommended dose slowly, allowing the animal time to swallow. Do not give to animals without a swallowing reflex.

Use only with an approved drench gun.

Presentation: 1 gallon jug and 15 gallon drum.

Compendium Code No.: 15030030

ORAL CALCIUM GEL

DVM Formula **Calcium-Oral**

Guaranteed Analysis:

	Per Pound	Per Tube
Calcium, Min.	65 gm	54 gm
Calcium, Max.	70 gm	58 gm
Vitamin B_{12}, Min.	121 mcg	100 mcg
Vitamin C, Min.	6 mg	5 mg
Vitamin E, Min.	60 IU	50 IU
Niacinamide, Min.	121 mg	100 mg
Thiamine Hydrochloride, Min.	12 mg	100 mg
d-Calcium Pantothenate	12 mg	10 mg
Riboflavin, Min.	6 mg	5 mg

Ingredients: Calcium chloride, tri-calcium phosphate, DL-alpha-tocopherol acetate (vitamin E), thiamine hydrochloride, riboflavin, niacinamide, d-calcium pantothenate, pyridoxine hydrochloride (vitamin B_6), cyanocobalamin (vitamin B_{12}), ascorbic acid (vitamin C), and xanthan gum.

Indications: Use ORAL CALCIUM GEL on every fresh cow or heifer before and after calving. ORAL CALCIUM GEL provides calcium to lower the incidence of milk fever and vitamins to stimulate appetite. ORAL CALCIUM GEL can be used as a follow up to intravenous treatment.

Dosage and Administration: Give one tube at the first sign of freshening and give another tube 6 to 12 hours after calving, repeat every 12 hours as needed. If the first dose is missed, a post calving dose is still beneficial.

Feeding Directions: Place the tube in a dosing gun and remove the cap. Hold the head of the animal in a slightly elevated position and place the nozzle on the back of the tongue. Administer the entire contents of the tube slowly, allowing the animal time to swallow. Do not give to animals without a swallowing reflex.

Presentation: 300 cc tube.

Compendium Code No.: 15030040

ORAL CAL MPK

Durvet **Calcium-Oral**

Calcium-Phosphorus-Magnesium-Potassium-Dextrose Oral Solution

Active Ingredient(s): Composition: Each 500 mL of aqueous solution contains:

Calcium (as calcium borogluconate) .... 10.0 g
Phosphorus (as sodium hypophosphate • H_2O) .... 6.0 g
Magnesium (as magnesium chloride • $6H_2O$) .... 2.8 g
Potassium (as potassium chloride) .... 8.0 g
Dextrose • H_2O .... 75.0 g

With methylparaben 0.18%, propylparaben 0.02%, and ethylparaben 0.01% added as preservatives.

Indications: For use as a supplemental nutritive source of calcium, phosphorus, magnesium, potassium and dextrose in cattle.

Dosage and Administration: Administer orally as a drench. The usual dose for adult cattle is 500 mL.

Precaution(s): Store at a controlled room temperature between 15°C - 30°C (59°F - 86°F).

Caution(s): For animal use only.

Warning(s): Keep out of reach of children.

Presentation: 500 mL (NDC 30798-032-17).

Compendium Code No.: 10841211

ORAL CMPK GEL

DVM Formula **Calcium-Oral**

Guaranteed Analysis:

	Per Pound	Per Tube
Calcium, Min.	61 mg	54 gm
Calcium, Max.	68 mg	58 gm
Phosphorus, Min.	11 mg	10 mg
Magnesium, Min.	3 gm	3 gm
Potassium, Min.	2 gm	2 gm

Ingredients: Calcium chloride, tri-calcium phosphate, magnesium chloride, potassium chloride, and xanthan gum.

Indications: Use on every fresh cow or heifer before and after calving to lower the incidence of milk fever. ORAL CMPK GEL can also be used as a follow up to intravenous treatment.

Dosage and Administration: Give one tube at the first signs of freshening and give another tube within 6 to 12 hours after calving, repeat every 12 hours as needed. If the first dose is missed, a post calving dose is still beneficial.

Feeding Directions: Place the tube in a dosing gun and remove the cap. Hold the head of the animal in a slightly elevated position and place the nozzle on the back of the tongue. Administer the entire contents of the tube slowly, allowing the animal time to swallow. Do not give to animals without a swallowing reflex.

Presentation: 300 cc tube.

Compendium Code No.: 15030050

ORAL CPMK GEL

First Priority **Calcium-Oral**

Guaranteed Analysis: Per Tube:

Calcium (Ca), Min. 11.5% .... 47.3 g
Calcium (Ca), Max. 16.5% .... 67.6 g
Phosphorus (P), Min. 1.5% .... 6.2 g
Magnesium (Mg), Min. 0.7% .... 2.9 g
Potassium (K), Min. 0.2% .... 1.0 g

Ingredients: Calcium Chloride, Purified Water, Phosphoric Acid, Tri-Sodium Phosphate, Magnesium Hydroxide, Glucose, Potassium Chloride, Silicon Dioxide, Sodium Citrate, Artificial Flavorings.

Indications: A nutritional supplement for dairy cattle during calving. This preparation supplies the necessary elements to ensure normal nutritional levels before, during and after calving.

Directions for Use: Place the tube in a dosing gun and remove the cap. Hold the head of the cow in a normal to slightly elevated position and carefully place the nozzle into the back of the mouth. Administer the entire contents of one tube per feeding. Do not give to cows or calves that are unable to swallow.

Give one tube within 6 to 12 hours prior to calving. Give another tube within 6 to 12 hours after calving.

Precaution(s): Storage: Store at controlled room temperature between 15°-30°C (59°-86°F).

Single dose unit. Discard unused portion.

Caution(s): Contact with eyes or wounds or prolonged contact with skin can cause irritation.

For animal use only.

Warning(s): Keep out of reach of children.

Presentation: 300 mL tube (NDC# 58829-275-40).

Compendium Code No.: 11390583 Rev. 04-02

ORALDENT

Phoenix Pharmaceutical **Dental Preparation**

Cleansing Solution

Active Ingredient(s): 0.1% Chlorhexidine formulated with special surfactant, peppermint flavor base, FD & C Red 40 and Red 33, and 6% Ethyl Alcohol by volume.

Indications: To assist in the daily maintenance of a healthy and pleasant smelling mouth in dogs and cats through the removal of food particles and other debris from the teeth and gum line.

Directions: Instructions: Apply ORALDENT either as an oral rinse or with a toothbrush.

Oral Rinse: Holding the animal's head steady with one hand, spray inside the corner of the mouth, gently inserting the sprayer a short distance from the cheek. Spray a small amount of ORALDENT between the teeth and the side of the mouth. Massage the mouth over the teeth to work ORALDENT over the surface of the teeth. Repeat on the opposite side of the mouth so that the gum surfaces are thoroughly wet on both sides of the mouth.

Tooth Brushing: Place a small amount of ORALDENT in a clean dish or cup. Holding the animal's head steady with one hand, dip the toothbrush into the solution and carefully brush the teeth with a gentle motion. Rewet the brush with ORALDENT as needed.

Precaution(s): Store at room temperature. Avoid exposure to temperatures over 120°F.

Caution(s): Special Note: The use of ORALDENT should not be considered a substitute for sound veterinary dental treatment. The product should be used under the direction of a veterinarian who can advise on a complete oral breath program. Published literature has reported some staining of the teeth surfaces after the prolonged use of rinses containing chlorhexidine. Build-up of stain can be prevented by applying the solution with a toothbrush.

For external use only as an oral rinse.

Not for use in eyes.

Warning(s): Keep out of reach of children.

Presentation: 8 fl oz containers (NDC 57319-055-20).

Compendium Code No.: 12560592 Rev. 11-01

ORAL KETO ENERGEL

First Priority **Large Animal Dietary Supplement**

Guaranteed Analysis: Per Tube:

Cobalt .... 0.150 g (0.04%)
Magnesium .... 6.0 g (1.6%)
Propylene Glycol .... 250 g
Propionic Acid .... 10 g
Niacin .... 15 g
Choline .... 3.0 g
Vitamin A .... 50,000 IU
Vitamin D_3 .... 10,000 IU
Vitamin E .... 100 IU
Vitamin B_{12} .... 1,000 mcg

Ingredients: Propylene Glycol, Magnesium Sulfate Heptahydrate, Choline Bitartrate, Niacin, Cobalt Sulfate, Propionic Acid, Ethoxyquin, Polysorbate 80, Cab-O-Sil, Vitamin A Palmitate, Vitamin D_3, Vitamin E, Cyanocobalamin (B_{12}).

Indications: A nutritional supplement for dairy cattle and calves. This preparation supplies the necessary elements to ensure normal nutritional levels before, during and after calving.

Directions for Use: Place the tube in a dosing gun and remove the cap. Hold the head of the cow in a normal to slightly elevated position and carefully place the nozzle into the back of the mouth. Administer the entire contents of one tube per feeding to cows. Do not give to cows or calves that are unable to swallow.

Give one tube following calving. Give additional tubes as needed. As a supplement and energy source, for calves, give 15-20 mL per animal (approximately 15-20 doses per 300 mL tube) - 3-4 clicks of the delivery system.

Precaution(s): Storage: Store at controlled room temperature between 15°-30°C (59°-86°F). Keep container tightly closed when not in use.

Caution(s): Contact with eyes or wounds or prolonged contact with skin can cause irritation.

For animal use only.

Warning(s): Keep out of reach of children.

Presentation: 300 mL tube (NDC# 58829-277-30).

Compendium Code No.: 11390592 Rev. 04-02

ORAL KETO-ENERGY DRENCH

DVM Formula **Acetonemia Preparation**

Guaranteed Analysis: Per 200 mL Feeding:

Niacin, Min. .... 11,500 mg
Vitamin B_6, Min. .... 60 mg
Vitamin B_{12}, Min. .... 600 mcg

Ingredients: Propylene glycol, niacinamide, vitamin A acetate, d-activated animal sterol (vitamin D_3), cyanocobalamin (vitamin B_{12}), DL-alpha-tocopheryl acetate (vitamin E), riboflavin, pantothenate, folic acid, pyridoxine hydrochloride (vitamin B_6), choline bitartrate, ascorbic acid, and xanthan gum.

Indications: Use on every fresh cow or heifer before and after calving. ORAL KETO-ENERGY DRENCH provides niacin, propylene glycol, and vitamins to lower the incidence of ketosis, boost energy, and stimulate appetite.

Dosage and Administration: Administer a 200 mL dose at the first sign of freshening and another 200 mL 6 to 12 hours after calving, repeat as needed. If the first dose is missed, a post calving dose is still beneficial. Shake well before using.

Feeding Directions: Administer orally using a drench gun. Hold the head of the animal in a slightly elevated position and place the nozzle between the teeth and cheek. Administer the recommended dose slowly, allowing the animal time to swallow. Do not give to animals without a swallowing reflex.

Use only with an approved an drench gun.

Presentation: 1 gallon jug and 15 gallon drum.

Compendium Code No.: 15030060

ORAL KETO-ENERGY GEL

DVM Formula **Acetonemia Preparation**

Guaranteed Analysis: Per Tube:

Propylene Glycol .... 275.0 gm
Niacin, Min. .... 9.6 gm
Vitamin A, Min. .... 210,000 IU
Vitamin B_6 (Pyridoxine) .... 18.0 mg
Vitamin B_{12}, Min. .... 374.4 mcg
Vitamin C, Min. .... 75.0 mg
Vitamin D_3, Min. .... 90,000 IU
Vitamin E, Min. .... 75 IU
Riboflavin, Min. .... 37.2 mg
d-Pantothenic Acid, Min. .... 150.0 mg
Folic Acid, Min. .... 10.8 mg

Ingredients: Propylene glycol, niacin, vitamin a acetate, d-activated animal sterol (vitamin D_3), cyanocobalamin (vitamin B_{12}), DL-alpha-tocopheryl acetate (vitamin E), riboflavin, d-calcium pantothenate, folic acid, pyridoxine hydrochloride (vitamin B_6), choline bitartrate, ascorbic acid (vitamin C), and xanthan gum.

Indications: Use on every fresh cow or heifer before and after calving. ORAL KETO-ENERGY GEL provides niacin, vitamins, and propylene glycol to lower the incidence of ketosis, boost energy and stimulate appetite.

Dosage and Administration: Give one tube at the first signs of freshening and give another tube 6 to 12 hours post calving, repeat as needed. If the first dose is missed, a post calving dose is still beneficial.

Feeding Directions: Place the tube in a dosing gun and remove the cap. Hold the head of the animal in a slightly elevated position and place the nozzle on the back of the tongue. Administer the entire contents of the tube slowly, allowing the animal time to swallow. Do not give to animals without a swallowing reflex.

Presentation: 300 cc tube.

Compendium Code No.: 15030070

ORAL PROBIOTIC CALF PAK

AgriPharm **Large Animal Dietary Supplement**

Active Ingredient(s): Dried colostrum whey, dried *Lactobacillus acidophilus* fermentation product, dried *Lactobacillus lactis* fermentation product, dried *Streptococcus faecium* fermentation product, dried milk protein, feed fat (preserved with BHA), dried whey product, lecithin, vitamin A acetate, D-activated animal sterol (source of vitamin D), D-alpha tocopharol acetate (source of vitamin E), vitamin B_{12} supplement, choline chloride, riboflavin supplement, niacin supplement, folic acid, calcium pantothenate, thiamine mononitrate, calcium carbonate, silicon dioxide, citric acid, magnesium oxide, manganese sulfate, ferrous sulfate, zinc sulfate, copper sulfate, ethylenediamine dihydroiodide, sodium selenite and polyoxethylen glycol (400) mono and dioleates.

Guaranteed analysis:

Crude protein .... min. 18%/wt.
Crude fat .... min. 14%/wt.
Crude Fibre .... max. 0.15%/wt.
Ash .... max. 12%/wt.
Added minerals .... max. 2%/wt.
Vitamin A .... 85,000 I.U./lb.
Vitamin D .... 54,000 I.U./lb.
Vitamin E .... 1,000 I.U./lb.

Total dried viable cultures of *Lactobacillus acidophilis*, 4 billion CFU/lb.

Total dried viable cultures of *Lactobacillus lactis*, 4 billion CFU/lb.

Total dried viable cultures of *Streptococcus faecium*, 1.8 billion CFU/lb.

Indications: A dietary supplement for calves.

Dosage and Administration: All incoming calves, when colostrum intake is unknown: Mix 1.76 oz. (1 packet) in one (1) pint (0.47 L) of warm nonmedicated milk, milk replacer, or water and feed upon arrival. Repeat the dosage on the second day for weak calves, or those that do not appear thrifty.

Calves/cattle following stresses from clinical/drug therapy, shipping, ration change, and severe weather change: Mix 1.76 oz. (1 packet) in one (1) pint (0.47 L) of warm nonmedicated milk, milk replacer, or water and feed upon arrival. Repeat the dosage on the second day for weak calves, or those that do not appear thrifty.

For cattle over 400 lbs.: Mix two (2) paks in one (1) pint (0.47 L) of warm nonmedicated milk, milk replacer or water. Repeat the dosage on the second day for weak calves, or those that do not appear thrifty.

Caution(s): For animal use only.

Keep out of the reach of children.

Presentation: 1.76 oz. (50 g) packets.

Compendium Code No.: 14570680

ORALVAX-HE™

Schering-Plough **Vaccine**

Hemorrhagic Enteritis Vaccine, Live Virus

U.S. Vet. Lic. No.: 165A

Active Ingredient(s): ORALVAX-HE™ is a live virus vaccine containing a turkey avirulent type II avian adenovirus of pheasant origin. The virus is grown in the RP-19 cell line and freeze-dried (lyophilized) and sealed under vacuum. The vaccine contains gentamicin and amphotericin B as preservatives.

Indications: It is a high titer vaccine recommended for use in healthy turkeys six weeks of age or older as an aid in the control and prevention of hemorrhagic enteritis through immunization by the drinking water method.

Dosage and Administration:

When to Vaccinate: Vaccinate at six (6) weeks of age or older.

Preparation of the Vaccine:

1. Assemble the vaccine and the equipment needed to vaccinate the entire flock at one time.
2. Do not open and rehydrate the vaccine until ready for use.
3. Remove the tear-off seal from the vaccine vial without disturbing the rubber stopper.
4. Use cool, clean, nonchlorinated tap water to which powdered milk has been added as directed under How to Vaccinate.
5. Remove the rubber stopper from the vaccine vial and rehydrate the vaccine by filling the vial about half-full with tap water (milk added).
6. Reseat the stopper and shake to thoroughly dissolve the vaccine.

How to Vaccinate: Do not mix the vaccine into the drinking water until ready for use. Drinking water for vaccination should be mixed with powdered milk to prevent possible inactivation from chlorine or other water additives and also to stabilize the vaccine virus. The powdered milk should be added to the water at the rate of one (1) heaped teaspoon per 3 U.S. gallons or 2.5 imperial gallons (3 g per 11 L); or one (1) heaped cupful per 50 U.S. gallons or 41 imperial gallons (87 g per 190 L).

Use only clean waterers and equipment free of disinfectants or sanitizers. All water must be withheld from the birds for at least two (2) hours prior to vaccination to ensure that all turkeys drink. Mix the rehydrated vaccine in the quantity of drinking water (milk added) which will be consumed by the thirsty turkeys in approximately two (2) hours.

The following schedule is a general guideline for the amount of water to use with the vaccine. These amounts will vary depending upon the individual management conditions, climate, age and sex of the birds.

Each 5,000 birds:

Age	U.S. Gallons	Imperial Gallons	Liters
6 weeks	460	120	100
7 weeks	530	140	115
8 weeks	610	160	135
9 weeks	680	180	150
10 weeks	760	200	170

Distribute 5,000 doses of the vaccine in water as used by 5,000 turkeys. Provide ample watering space so that all of the turkeys can drink easily. Do not administer through water lines with a proportioner or medication tank.

Records: Keep a record of the vaccine type, quantity, serial number, expiration date and place of purchase; the date and time of the vaccination; the number, age, breed, and location of the birds; the names of operators performing the vaccination; and any observed reactions.

Precaution(s): Store at 35° to 45°F (2° to 7°C).

Caution(s): For veterinary use only.

1. Vaccinate healthy birds only.
2. Avoid exposing birds other than turkeys to the vaccine.
3. Do not use to vaccinate pheasants.
4. All birds within a flock should be vaccinated on the same day.
5. In outbreak situations, vaccinate healthy flocks first, progressing toward outbreak areas in order to vaccinate the affected birds last.
6. Do not spill or spatter the vaccine. Burn the empty bottles, caps and all the unused vaccine and accessories. Use the entire contents of the vial when first opened.
7. Wash hands thoroughly after using the vaccine.
8. Do not dilute the vaccine or otherwise stretch the dosage.

Warning(s): Do not vaccinate within 21 days before slaughter.

Presentation: Supplied in 5 x 2,000 and 5 x 5,000 dose units.

Compendium Code No.: 10471410

ORA-LYTE™ POWDER

Butler **Electrolytes-Oral**

Guaranteed Analysis: Analysis, (not less than):

Calcium (Ca)	.04%
Salt	.25%
Potassium (K)	.50%
Magnesium (Mg)	.02%
Iron (Fe)	400 ppm
Zinc (Zn)	500 ppm
Thiamine	130 mg per lb
Niacin	220 mg per lb
Ascorbic Acid	220 mg per lb

Ingredients: Dextrose, salt, potassium chloride, calcium gluconate, magnesium sulfate, sodium citrate, niacin, thiamine hydrochloride, ascorbic acid, zinc sulfate, ferrous sulfate, melojel.

Indications: ORA-LYTE™ Powder is a water soluble oral nutritional supplement intended for use in horses.

ORA-LYTE™ Powder is formulated to provide supplemental nutrients during training, racing, shipping, and periods of high activity.

Directions for Use: Mix one or two ounces of ORA-LYTE™ Powder per one to two gallons of water. Allow the horse to drink small amounts of mixture at short intervals.

Prepare fresh solutions daily.

Precaution(s): Store in a cool, dry place.

Caution(s): For use in animals only. For veterinary use only.

Warning(s): Keep out of the reach of children.

Presentation: 5 lbs and 25 lbs.

Compendium Code No.: 10821271

ORBAX™ TABLETS ℞

Schering-Plough **Orbifloxacin**

NADA No.: 141-081

Active Ingredient(s): ORBAX™ Tablets contain orbifloxacin in concentrations of 5.7 mg, 22.7 mg and 68 mg.

Indications: ORBAX™ (orbifloxacin) Tablets are indicated for the management of diseases in dogs and cats associated with bacteria susceptible to orbifloxacin.

Efficacy Confirmation: Clinical efficacy was established in skin and soft tissue infections (wounds and abscesses) in the dog and cat, and urinary tract infections (cystitis) in the dog, associated with bacteria susceptible to orbifloxacin. Specific bacterial pathogens isolated in clinical field trials are listed in the Microbiology section.

Pharmacology: Orbifloxacin is a synthetic broad-spectrum antibacterial agent from the class of fluoroquinolone carboxylic acid derivatives. Orbifloxacin is the international nonproprietary name for 1-cyclopropyl-5,6,8-trifluoro-1,4-dihydro-7-(*cis*-3,5-dimethyl-1-piperazinyl)-4-oxoquinoline-3-carboxylic acid. The chemical formula for orbifloxacin is $C_{19}H_{20}F_3N_3O_3$ and its molecular weight is 395.38.

The compound is slightly soluble in water; however, solubility increases in both acidic and alkaline conditions. The compound has two dissociation constants (pKa's): 5.95 and 9.01.

Figure 1. Chemical structure of orbifloxacin.

Clinical Pharmacology: Pharmacokinetics in healthy adult beagle dogs and healthy adult cats: In fasted animals, orbifloxacin is rapidly and almost completely absorbed from the gastrointestinal tract following oral administration. Absorption of orally administered orbifloxacin increases proportionately with dose (exhibits linear pharmacokinetics) up to 37.5 mg/kg when given daily for 30 days. The absolute bioavailability (F) of an oral dose is approximately 100%. Peak plasma concentrations are usually attained within 1 hour of administration. The effects of concomitant feeding on the absorption of orbifloxacin has not been studied. Divalent cations are generally known to diminish the absorption of fluoroquinolones. (See Drug Interactions.)

The relatively large volume of distribution at steady state (V_{SS}) is indicative of a widespread distribution and penetration into body tissues. Within 24 hours of administration, approximately 40% of an oral dose was excreted into the urine unchanged in dogs with normal renal function. This supports the efficacy of orbifloxacin in the treatment of urinary tract infections. Based on the plasma elimination half-life and the dosing interval, negligible drug accumulation is expected with multiple dosing.

Pharmacokinetic parameters estimated in a randomized two-period, two-sequence crossover study using single intravenous and oral doses are summarized in Tables 2 and 3 and Figures 2 and 3.

Table 2: Mean Pharmcokinetic Parameters Estimated in 12 Adult Beagle Dogs and 12 Adult Cats After a Single IV Bolus of Orbifloxacin at 2.5 mg/kg:

Pharmacokinetic Parameter	Dog Estimate (SD)	Cat Estimate (SD)
Total body clearance, mL/min/kg	2.9 ± 0.2	4.09 ± 0.7
Volume of distribution at steady state, V_{SS} (L/kg)	1.2 ± 0.2	1.3 ± 0.13
$AUC_{0-\infty}$ (μg•h/mL)	14.3 ± 0.9	10.6 ± 2.4
Terminal plasma elimination half-life, $t_{1/2}$ (hrs)	5.4 ± 1.1	4.5 ± 1.8

Table 3: Mean Pharmacokinetic Parameters Estimated in 12 Adult Beagle Dogs and 12 Adult Cats After a Single Oral Dose of Orbifloxacin at 2.5 mg/kg:

Pharmacokinetic Parameter	Dog Estimate (SD)	Cat Estimate (SD)
Total body clearance/F, mL/min/kg	3.0 ± 0.2	3.98 ± 0.8
Maximum concentration, C_{max} (μg/mL)	2.3 ± 0.3	2.06 ± 0.6
Time of maximum concentration, T_{max} (minutes)	46 ± 27	60 ± 27
$AUC_{0-\infty}$ (μg•h/mL)	14.3 ± 1.4	10.82 ± 2.6
Terminal plasma elimination half-life, $t_{1/2}$ (hrs)	5.6 ± 1.1	5.52 ± 2.66

Plasma Concentration of Orbifloxacin vs. Time in Dogs

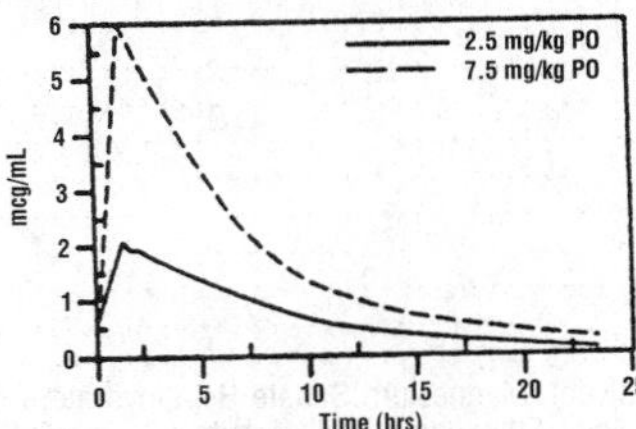

Figure 2. Mean plasma concentration of orbifloxacin vs. time in dogs (2.5 mg/kg = observed values, 7.5 mg/kg = extrapolated values).

Plasma Concentration of Orbifloxacin vs. Time in Cats

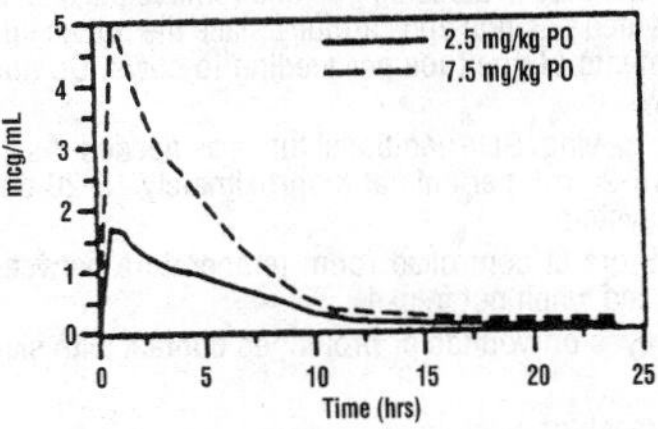

Figure 3. Mean plasma concentration of orbifloxacin vs. time in cats (2.5 mg/kg = normalized from an actual mean dose of 3.32 mg/kg; 7.5 mg/kg = extrapolated values).

Microbiology: Orbifloxacin is bactericidal against a wide range of gram-negative and gram-positive organisms and exerts its antibacterial effect through interference with the bacterial enzyme DNA gyrase which is needed for the maintenance and synthesis of bacterial DNA. The minimum inhibitory concentrations (MICs) of pathogens isolated in multicentered clinical field trials performed in the United States was determined using National Committee for Clinical Laboratory Standards (NCCLS), and is shown in Tables 4, 5, and 6.

Table 4: MIC Values* (μg/mL) of Orbifloxacin Against Urinary Pathogens Isolated Between 1994 and 1996 From Clinical Infections in Dogs:

Bacteria Name	Number of Isolates	MIC_{50}	MIC_{90}	MIC Range
Staphylococcus intermedius	5	**	**	0.0975 - 0.39
Proteus mirabilis	19	0.78	1.56	0.048 - 1.56
Escherichia coli	35	0.0975	0.39	0.024 - ≥25
Enterococcus faecalis	5	**	**	0.003 - 3.12

*The correlation between the *in vitro* susceptibility data (MIC Values) and clinical response has not been determined.

**There were an insufficient number of isolates to calculate the MIC_{50} or MIC_{90}.

Table 5: MIC Values* (μg/mL) of Orbifloxacin Against Dermal Pathogens Isolated Between 1994 and 1996 From Clinical Infections of Dogs:

Bacteria Name	Number of Isolates	MIC_{50}	MIC_{90}	MIC Range
Staphylococcus intermedius	51	0.195	0.39	0.003 - 1.56
Staphylococcus aureus	8	**	**	0.195 - ≥25
Coagulase +ve staphylococci	59	0.195	0.39	0.003 - ≥25
Pasteurella multocida	5	**	0	0.003 - 0.78
Proteus mirabilis	7	**	**	0.39 - 1.56
Pseudomonas aeruginosa	14	3.125	12.5	0.39 - ≥25
Pseudomonas spp	18	3.125	12.5	0.02 - ≥25
Klebsiella pneumoniae	9	**	**	0.0975 - 0.195
Escherichia coli	28	0.0975	0.39	0.012 - 6.25
Enterobacter spp	24	0.0975	0.39	0.012 - 6.25
Citrobacter spp	4	**	**	0.024 - 0.0975
Enterococcus faecalis	11	**	**	0.3 - ≥25
Streptococcus β-hemolytic (Grp G)	22	0.39	1.56	0.006 - 3.12
Streptococcus equisimilis	10	**	**	0.003 - 0.78

*The correlation between the *in vitro* susceptibility data (MIC Values) and clinical response has not been determined.

**There were an insufficient number of isolates to calculate the MIC_{50} or MIC_{90}.

Table 6: MIC Values* (μg/mL) of Orbifloxacin Against Dermal Pathogens Isolated Between 1994 and 1996 From Clinical Infections of Cats:

Bacteria Name	Number of Isolates	MIC_{50}	MIC_{90}	MIC Range
Staphylococcus intermedius	25	0.39	0.39	0.024 - 3.125
Staphylococcus aureus	7	**	**	0.195 - 0.39
Coagulase +ve staphylococci	32	0.39	0.39	0.024 - 3.125
Pasteurella multocida	47	0.012	0.048	0.003 - 0.195
Proteus mirabilis	7	**	**	0.39 - 1.56
Pseudomonas aeruginosa	3	**	**	0.39 - 3.125
Pseudomonas spp	10	**	**	0.195 - 6.25
Escherichia coli	17	0.048	0.195	0.024 - 25
Enterobacter spp	12	**	**	0.024 - 0.78
Enterococcus faecalis	10	**	**	1.56 - 3.125
Streptococcus β-hemolytic (Grp G)	14	**	**	0.006 - 1.56

*The correlation between the *in vitro* susceptibility data (MIC Values) and clinical response has not been determined.

**There were an insufficient number of isolates to calculate the MIC_{50} or MIC_{90}.

Dosage and Administration: For routine outpatient treatment of infection caused by a susceptible organism, in an otherwise healthy dog or cat, the dose of ORBAX™ (orbifloxacin) Tablets is 2.5 to 7.5 mg/kg of body weight administered once daily. (See Drug Interactions and Target Animal Safety section.) The determination of dosage for any particular patient must take into consideration such factors as the severity and nature of the infection, the susceptibility of the causative organism, and the integrity of the patient's host-defense mechanisms. Antibiotic susceptibility of the pathogenic organism(s) should be determined prior to use of this preparation. Therapy with ORBAX™ (orbifloxacin) Tablets may be initiated before results of these tests are known. Once results become available, continue with appropriate therapy.

For the treatment of skin and associated soft tissue infections, ORBAX™ Tablets should be given for two (2) to three (3) days beyond the cessation of clinical signs to a maximum of 30 days. For the treatment of urinary tract infections, ORBAX™ Tablets should be administered for at least 10 consecutive days. If no improvement is seen within five (5) days, the diagnosis should be re-evaluated and a different course of therapy considered.

To administer a total daily dose of 2.5 mg/kg, ORBAX™ Tablets may be dispensed as indicated in Table 1.

Table 1: Dose Table for ORBAX™ Tablets (2.5 mg/kg total daily dose).

	Weight of Dog/Cat (lbs)								
	5	10	20	30	40	50	60	90	120
No of 5.7 mg tablets	1	2							
No. of 22.7 mg tablets		½	1	1½	2	2½			
No. of 68 mg tablets				½			1	1½	2

Drug Interactions: Compounds (eg, sucralfate, antacids, and multivitamins) containing divalent and trivalent cations (eg, iron, aluminum, calcium, magnesium, and zinc) may substantially interfere with the absorption of quinolones resulting in a decrease in product bioavailability. Therefore, the concomitant oral administration of quinolones with foods, supplements, or other preparations containing these compounds should be avoided.

Contraindication(s): Orbifloxacin and other quinolones have been shown to cause arthropathy in immature animals of most species tested, the dog being particularly sensitive to this side effect. Orbifloxacin is contraindicated in immature dogs during the rapid growth phase (between 2 and 8 months of age in small and medium-sized breeds, and up to 18 months of age in large and giant breeds).

Orbifloxacin is contraindicated in dogs and cats known to be hypersensitive to quinolones.

Precaution(s): Store between 2° and 30°C (36° and 86°F). Protect from excessive moisture.

Caution(s): Federal (USA) law restricts this drug to use by or on the order of a licensed veterinarian.

Quinolones should be used with caution in animals with known or suspected central nervous system (CNS) disorders. In such animals, quinolones have, in rare instances, been associated with CNS stimulation which may lead to convulsive seizures. Quinolones have been shown to produce erosions of cartilage of weight-bearing joints and other signs of arthropathy in immature animals of various species.

Safety in breeding or pregnant dogs and cats has not been established.

Warning(s): Federal law prohibits the use of this drug in food or food producing animals.

Human Warnings: For use in animals only. Keep out of the reach of children.

Avoid contact with eyes. In case of contact, immediately flush eyes with copious amounts of water for 15 minutes. In case of dermal contact, wash skin with soap and water. Consult a physician if irritation persists following ocular or dermal exposure. Individuals with a history of hypersensitivity to quinolones should avoid this product. In humans, there is a risk of user photosensitization within a few hours after excessive exposure to quinolones. If excessive accidental exposure occurs, avoid direct sunlight.

For oral use in dogs and cats only.

Target Animal Safety: Orbifloxacin administered to young, clinically healthy, adult dogs and cats at doses of 7.5 mg/kg, 22.5 mg/kg, and 37.5 mg/kg for 30 consecutive days was well tolerated. At the exaggerated doses of 22.5 and 37.5 mg/kg/day, orbifloxacin caused mild gastrointestinal effects (soft feces) in both male and female cats. Emesis (males only), diarrhea (males only), reduced food consumption with subsequent reduced bodyweight were evident in cats administered ORBAX™ at 75 mg/kg/day for 10 days. Orbifloxacin and other quinolones have been shown to cause arthropathy in immature animals of most species tested, the dog being particularly sensitive to this side effect. In 8- to 10-week-old beagle puppies dosed daily with orbifloxacin for 30 days, microscopic lesions consistent with fluoroquinolone-induced arthropathy of the articular cartilage was seen in only one of eight dogs dosed at 12.5 mg/kg, and in all eight dogs dosed at 25 mg/kg (see Contraindications). No arthropathy was noted in 12-week-old kittens administered orbifloxacin at doses as high as 25 mg/kg for 1 month.

Adverse Reactions: In clinical trials, when the drug was administered at 2.5 mg/kg/day, no drug-related adverse reactions were reported.

Presentation: ORBAX™ (orbifloxacin) Tablets are available in the following presentations:

5.7 mg: Bottles of 250 yellow tablets.

22.7 mg: Bottles of 250 green, E-Z Break, single-scored tablets.

68 mg: Bottles of 100 blue, E-Z Break, single-scored tablets.

Compendium Code No.: 10471420

ORBENIN®-DC ℞

Pfizer Animal Health **Mastitis Therapy**

(benzathine cloxacillin) Dry Cow Intramammary Infusion

NADA No.: 055-069

Active Ingredient(s): Description: ORBENIN®-DC (benzathine cloxacillin) is a stable, nonirritating suspension of benzathine cloxacillin containing the equivalent of 500 mg of cloxacillin per disposable syringe. ORBENIN®-DC is manufactured by a nonsterilizing process.

Indications: ORBENIN®-DC is indicated in the treatment and prophylaxis of bovine mastitis in nonlactating cows due to *Staphylococcus aureus* and *Streptococcus agalactiae*.

Pharmacology: Benzathine cloxacillin is a semisynthetic penicillin derived from the penicillin nucleus, 6-amino-penicillanic acid. Benzathine cloxacillin is the benzathine salt of 6-[3-(2-chlorophenyl)-5-methylisoxazolyl-4-carboxamido] penicillanic acid.

The low solubility of ORBENIN®-DC results in an extended period of activity. Therefore, directions for use should be followed explicitly.

Action: Benzathine cloxacillin is bactericidal in action against susceptible organisms during the stage of active multiplication. It acts through the inhibition of biosynthesis of cell wall mucopeptide. It is active against gram-positive organisms associated with mastitis such as *Staphylococcus aureus* and *Streptococcus agalactiae* and, because of its resistance to penicillinase, penicillin G-resistant staphylococci which may be the cause of mastitis.

Appropriate laboratory tests should be conducted, including *in vitro* culturing and susceptibility tests on pretreatment milk samples collected aseptically.

Susceptibility Test: The Kirby-Bauer* procedure, utilizing antibiotic susceptibility disks, is a quantitative method that may be adapted to determining the sensitivity of bacteria in milk to ORBENIN®-DC.

For testing the effectiveness of ORBENIN®-DC in milk, follow the Kirby-Bauer procedure using the 1 mcg oxacillin susceptibility disk. Zone diameters for interpreting susceptibility are:

Resistant	Intermediate	Susceptible
≤ 10 mm	11-12 mm	≥ 13 mm

* Bauer AW, Kirby WMM, Sherris JC, et al: Antibiotic testing by a standardized single disk method, Am J Clin Path 45:493, 1966. Standardized Disk Susceptibility Test, Federal Register 37:20527-29, 1972.

Dosage and Administration: At the last milking of lactation, milk the cow out normally. Clean and disinfect the teats with alcohol swabs provided in the carton, and infuse 1 syringe of ORBENIN®-DC, which has been warmed to room temperature, into each quarter. Do not milk out. The cow may be milked as usual when she calves.

The extent of subclinical and latent mastitis in a herd is frequently greater than suspected. In untreated herds a significant buildup of subclinical mastitis may occur during the dry period, which results in clinical severity after a few lactations. The adverse influence of subclinical mastitis on milk yield, the risk of cross-infection, and the chance of clinical mastitis flare-up make it necessary to treat the matter as a herd problem. Clinical studies have proven the value of treating all the cows in heavily infected herds as they are dried off. When the herd infection has been reduced, it may be desirable to be more selective in treating infected quarters.

Each carton contains 12 alcohol swabs to facilitate proper cleaning and disinfecting of the teat orifice.

Contraindication(s): Because benzathine cloxacillin is relatively insoluble, ORBENIN®-DC's activity will be prolonged. Therefore, ORBENIN®-DC should not be used for the occasional cow which may have a dry period of less than 4 weeks. This precaution will avoid residues in the milk following removal of the colostrum.

Precaution(s): Do not store above 24°C (75°F).

Caution(s): Federal law restricts this drug to use by or on the order of a licensed veterinarian.

Because it is a derivative of 6-amino-penicillanic acid, ORBENIN®-DC has the potential for producing allergic reactions. Such reactions are rare; however, should they occur, the subject should be treated with the usual agents (antihistamines, pressor amines).

Warning(s): For use in dry cows only. Do not use within 4 weeks (28 days) of calving. Treated animals must not be slaughtered for food purposes within 4 weeks (28 days) of treatment.

Presentation: ORBENIN®-DC is supplied in cartons of 12 single-dose syringes with 12 alcohol swabs. Each disposable syringe contains 500 mg of cloxacillin as the benzathine salt in 7.5 g of suitable base.

ORBENIN® is a trademark owned by and used under license from SmithKline Beecham.

Manufactured by: G.C. Hanford Mfg. Co., Syracuse, NY 13201

Compendium Code No.: 36900161 75-8163-00

ORGANIC IODIDE

Butler **Iodine-Oral**

Active Ingredient(s): Ethylenediamine dihydriodide 320 grs. (equivalent to 20 grs. per ounce) and dextrose/salt, q.s.

ORGANIC IODIDE is available in either a sugar base or a salt base.

Indications: An iodine feed supplement for use as an aid in correcting nutritional deficiencies where the use of iodine is indicated.

Dosage and Administration: Cattle: Feed 50 mg per head per day in feed or salt continuously.

Caution(s): For veterinary use only. Keep out of the reach of children.

Feed the product to animals with caution until their tolerance is determined because of the variation in susceptibility to iodine.

Warning(s): Not to be fed to dairy cattle in production.

Presentation: 1 lb. and 25 lb. containers.

Compendium Code No.: 10821290

ORGANIC IODIDE 20

Durvet **Iodine-Oral**

Organic Iodide Nutritional Supplement

Active Ingredient(s): Minimum Guaranteed Analysis:

Iodine (equivalent to 20,825 mg EDDI/lb) 3.65%

In salt base.

Artificial color added for identification.

Indications: For routine supplementation of iodine in the diet of beef and dairy cattle.

Directions for Use: Add this product to the ration (protein mix, grain mix, or salt) in proportions that will provide EDDI at the rate of 10 mg per head per day.

Mix thoroughly to obtain uniform distribution in ration.

Protein Mix: Add ½ lb of this product to each ton of protein mix. Feed at the rate of not more than 2 lbs per head per day.

Grain Mix: Add 1 oz of this product to each ton of grain mix. Feed at the rate of not more than 15 lbs per head per day.

Salt: Add 1 lb of this product to 130 lbs of feeding salt. Then feed 1 oz of salt mixture per head per day.

Precaution(s): Store in a cool, dry place. Keep tightly closed when not in use.

Caution(s): For animal use only.

Warning(s): Keep out of reach of children.

Presentation: 453.6 g (1 lb) and 11.34 kg (25 lb).

Compendium Code No.: 10841222 Rev. 1001

ORGANIC IODIDE 40

Durvet **Iodine-Oral**

Organic Iodide Nutritional Supplement

Active Ingredient(s): Minimum Guaranteed Analysis:

Iodine (equivalent to 41,650 mg EDDI/lb) 7.30%

In salt base.

Artificial color added for identification.

Indications: For routine supplementation of iodine in the diet of beef and dairy cattle.

Directions for Use: Add this product to the ration (protein mix, grain mix, or salt) in proportions that will provide EDDI at the rate of 10 mg per head per day. Mix thoroughly to obtain uniform distribution in ration.

Protein Mix: Add ¼ lb. of this product to each ton of protein mix. Feed at the rate of not more than 2 lbs. per head per day.

Grain Mix: Add ½ oz. of this product to each ton of grain mix. Feed at the rate of not more than 15 lbs. per head per day.

Salt: Add 1 lb. of this product to 260 lbs. of feeding salt. Then feed 1 oz. of salt mixture per head per day.

Precaution(s): Store in a cool, dry place. Keep tightly closed when not in use.

Caution(s): For animal use only.

Warning(s): Keep out of reach of children.

Presentation: 453.6 g (1 lb) and 25 lb.

Compendium Code No.: 10841231 Rev. 10-01 / Rev. 7-93

ORGANIC IODIDE POWDER

Neogen **Iodine-Oral**

Active Ingredient(s): Each lb (454 g) contains:

Ethylenediamine Dihydriodide .... 20.0 g

(Equivalent to 1.3 g per oz)

Sucrose .... q.s.

Indications: An iodine feed supplement as an aid in correcting nutritional deficiencies where the use of iodine is indicated.

Dosage and Administration: As per veterinarian's instructions.

Caution(s): Do not administer to animals showing symptoms of acute respiratory conditions. Treat animals with caution until tolerance is determined as animals vary in susceptibility to iodides.

Sold to licensed veterinarians only.

For animal use only.

Warning(s): Do not administer to dairy cattle in production.

Keep out of reach of children.

Presentation: 1 lb.

Compendium Code No.: 14910381 L104-0299 Rev 11/01

ORGANIC IODINE

AgriLabs **Iodine-Oral**

Active Ingredient(s): Guaranteed analysis:

ORGANIC IODINE 20:

Ethylenediamine dihydriodide (equiv. to 20 grains/oz.; 21,000 mg/lb.; 46 mg/g) 4.6%

ORGANIC IODINE 40:

Ethylenediamine dihydriodide (equiv. to 40 grains/oz.; 42,000 mg/lb.; 92 mg/g) 9.2%

Ingredients: Ethylenediamine dihydriodide (EDDI), sodium chloride/sugar*, mineral oil, and iron oxide.

Indications: For routine iodine supplementation in feeds for cattle, swine, sheep, horses, goats and poultry.

Dosage and Administration:

ORGANIC IODINE 20:

Protein feeds: Mix ½ lb. ORGANIC IODINE 20 per ton of feed. Do not feed more than 2 lbs. of this mixture per head per day.

Mix 1 oz. of ORGANIC IODINE 20 thoroughly into the feed of 130 feedings for cattle, swine, sheep, horses or goats to provide the level of 10 mg EDDI per head per day.

Mix 1 lb. of ORGANIC IODINE 20 per ton of complete poultry feed. Feed for only five (5) to seven (7) days.

Mix 2 lbs. of ORGANIC IODINE 20 to each 100 lbs. of feeding salt or mineral and feed 4 oz. per head per day to provide 10 mg EDDI.

ORGANIC IODINE 40:

Protein feeds: Mix ¼ lb. ORGANIC IODINE 40 per ton of feed. Do not feed more than 1 lb. of this mixture per head per day.

Mix ½ oz. of ORGANIC IODINE 40 thoroughly into the feed of 130 feedings for cattle, swine, sheep, horses or goats to provide the level of 10 mg EDDI per head per day.

Mix ½ lb. of ORGANIC IODINE 40 per ton of complete poultry feed. Feed for only five (5) to seven (7) days.

Mix 1 lb. of ORGANIC IODINE 40 to each 100 lbs. of feeding salt or mineral and feed 4 oz. per head per day to provide 10 mg EDDI.

Caution(s): Keep out of the reach of children. Do not feed more than 10 mg per head per day of EDDI.

Warning(s): Not for use in lactating dairy cows.

Presentation: Available in 1 lb. (16 oz.) and 25 lb. containers.

Compendium Code No.: 10580780

ORGANIC IODINE

AgriPharm **Iodine-Oral**

Active Ingredient(s): Each pound (454 g) contains either:

Ethylenediamine dihydroiodide (EDDI) .... 20.8 g

(equivalent to 20 grains EDDI/oz.)

Ethylenediamine dihydroiodide (EDDI) .... 41.4 g

(equivalent to 40 grains EDDI/oz)

In a salt base. Artificial color added for identification.

Indications: For the routine supplementation of iodine in the diet of beef cattle.

Dosage and Administration: Cattle: 10 mg/head/day.

To be added to the feed ration in proportions that will obtain the suggested dosage.

Directions: Add the product to the feed ration (protein mix, grain mix, or salt) in proportions that will provide EDDI at the rate of 10 mg per head per day. Mix thoroughly to obtain a uniform distribution.

ORGANIC IODINE 20:

Protein mix: Add ½ lb. of organic iodine to each ton of grain mix and feed at the rate of not more that 15 lbs. per head per day.

Salt: Add 2 lbs. of organic iodine to each 100 lbs. of feeding salt.

ORGANIC IODINE 40:

Protein mix: Add ¼ lb. of ORGANIC IODINE 40 to each ton of protein mix and feed at the rate of not more than 2 lbs. per head per day.

Grain mix: Add ½ oz. of ORGANIC IODINE 40 to each ton of grain mix and feed at the rate of not more than 15 lbs. per head per day.

Salt: Add 1 lb. of ORGANIC IODINE 40 to each 100 lbs. of feeding salt.

Precaution(s): Store in a cool, dry place, not above 86°F (30°C).

Keep tightly closed when not in use.

Caution(s): For animal use only. Keep out of the reach of children.

Presentation: 1 lb. and 25 lb. containers.

Compendium Code No.: 14570690

OSTEO-FORM POWDER

Vet-A-Mix **Large Animal Dietary Supplement**

Calcium-phosphorous and vitamin powder supplement for horses

Guaranteed Analysis:	Per Pound
Calcium, maximum	32.0%
Calcium, minimum	27.0%
Phosphorus, minimum	16.5%
Vitamin A, minimum	153,000 IU
Vitamin D_3, minimum	15,300 IU

Ingredients: Dicalcium phosphate, Bone ash, Calcium carbonate, Soybean flour, Bone meal steamed, Polysorbate 80, Citric acid, Ascorbic acid, Vitamin A acetate and Cholecalciferol.

Indications: For use as an aid in the prevention of dietary deficiencies of calcium, phosphorus and vitamins A and D.

Dosage and Administration: Dosage: To aid in the prevention of dietary deficiencies, give 1 to 3 slightly rounded tablespoonfuls to foals and 3 to 5 tablespoonfuls to yearlings and adults each day for as long as indicated.

Administration: OSTEO-FORM may be added to the daily ration or mixed with milk or water. To facilitate proper adhesion of OSTEO-FORM to the ration, slightly moisten the grain with water or liquid supplement.

Each slightly rounded tablespoonful of OSTEO-FORM contains approximately 12 g. A tablespoon measure is enclosed.

When using OSTEO-FORM as a maintenance dietary supplement, calcium and phosphorus from other food sources should be considered.

Contraindication(s): Do not feed to cattle or other ruminants.

Warning(s): Keep out of reach of children.

Presentation: 1 lb. (453.6 g) bottles and 25 lb. pails.

Compendium Code No.: 10500191 0299

OSTEO-FORM SA

Vet-A-Mix **Small Animal Dietary Supplement**

Content(s): Contents per 350 grams:
Calcium, not more than 32.4%
Calcium, not less than 27.0%
Phosphorus, not less than 16.5%
Vitamin A .... 115,000 IU
Vitamin D_3 .... 11,500 IU

Ingredients: Bone ash, vitamin A acetate, cholecalciferol (source of vitamin D_3), calcium carbonate, calcium phosphate dibasic, soy flour, ascorbic acid, bone meal, and stabilizers.
Indications: For use as an aid in the prevention of dietary deficiencies of calcium, phosphorous and vitamins A and D in dogs, cats, birds and reptiles.
Dosage and Administration: Dogs and Cats - To aid in the prevention of dietary deficiencies give 1 to 2 slightly rounded teaspoonfuls for each 20 pounds body weight per day as long as indicated.

Many reptile and avian diets are low in calcium and high in phosphorus. Evaluation of the entire diet is necessary before recommending the exact dose of OSTEO-FORM SA, which may be added to the daily ration or mixed with milk or water. To facilitate proper adhesion of OSTEO-FORM SA to dry food, slightly moisten food with water.

Each slightly rounded teaspoonful of OSTEO-FORM SA contains approximately 4 grams. A teaspoon measure is enclosed. When using OSTEO-FORM SA as a maintenance dietary supplement, calcium and phosphorus from other food sources should be considered.
Warning(s): Keep out of reach of children.
Presentation: 350 grams.
Compendium Code No.: 10500200

OSTEO-FORM TABLETS

Vet-A-Mix **Small Animal Dietary Supplement**

Ingredient(s): Each tablet contains: Minerals: Calcium min. 18.5% - max. 22.2% (600 mg) and phosphorus min. 10.0% (335 mg). Vitamins: Vitamins A 750 IU and vitamin D_3 75 IU.

Ingredients: Dicalcium phosphate, calcium carbonate, torula dried yeast, extracted glandular meal, bone ash, lactose, starch, propylene glycol, animal liver meal, bone meal steamed, magnesium stearate, ascorbic acid, vitamin A palmitate, ethoxyquin, cholecalciferol, BHT.
Indications: Use as an aid in the prevention of dietary deficiencies of calcium, phosphorus and vitamins A and D in dogs and cats.
Dosage and Administration: Feed free choice, from the hand or crumble and mix into the food.

As an aid in the prevention of dietary deficiencies give 1 to 2 tablets per 5 kilograms (11 pounds) of body weight per day.

Note: Two OSTEO-FORM Chewable Tablets are equivalent to one slightly rounded teaspoonful of Osteo-Form SA powder.
Caution(s): When using OSTEO-FORM Chewable Tablets as a maintenance dietary supplement, calcium and phosphorus from other food sources should be considered.
Warning(s): Keep out of reach of children.
Presentation: Bottles of 50, 150, and 500 tablets.
Compendium Code No.: 10500210

OT 200

Vetus **Oxytetracycline Injection**

(Oxytetracycline)
ANADA No.: 200-123
Active Ingredient(s): OT 200 (oxytetracycline injection) is a sterile preconstituted solution of the broad spectrum antibiotic oxytetracycline. Each mL contains 200 mg of oxytetracycline base as amphoteric oxytetracycline and, on a w/v basis, 40.0% 2-pyrrolidone, 5.0% povidone, 1.8% magnesium oxide, 0.2% sodium formaldehyde sulfoxylate (as a preservative), monoethanolamine and/or hydrochloric acid as required to adjust pH.
Indications: For use in beef cattle, nonlactating dairy cattle and swine. For use in the treatment of the following diseases in beef cattle, nonlactating dairy cattle and swine when due to oxytetracycline-susceptible organisms:

Cattle: Indicated in the treatment of pneumonia and shipping fever complex associated with *Pasteurella* spp. and *Hemophilus* spp; infectious bovine keratoconjunctivitis (pinkeye) caused by *Moraxella bovis;* foot-rot and diphtheria caused by *Fuscobacterium necrophorum;* bacterial enteritis (scours) caused by *Escherichia coli;* wooden tongue caused by *Actinobacillus lignieresii;* leptospirosis caused by *Leptospira pomona;* and wound infections and acute metritis caused by strains of staphylococci and streptococci organisms sensitive to oxytetracycline.

Swine: Indicated in the treatment of bacterial enteritis (scours, colibacillosis) caused by *Escherichia coli;* pneumonia caused by *Pasteurella multocida;* and leptospirosis caused by *Leptospira pomona.*

In sows, OT 200 is indicated as an aid in the control of infectious enteritis (baby pig scours, colibacillosis) in suckling pigs caused by *Escherichia coli.*
Dosage and Administration: Read entire package insert carefully before using this product.

Cattle: To be administered by intramuscular or intravenous injection to beef cattle and nonlactating dairy cattle.

A single dosage of 9 milligrams per pound of body weight administered intramuscularly is recommended in the treatment of the following conditions: 1) bacterial pneumonia caused by *Pasteurella* spp. (shipping fever) in calves and yearlings, where re-treatment is impractical due to husbandry conditions, such as cattle on range, or where their repeated restraint is inadvisable; 2) infectious bovine keratoconjunctivitis (pinkeye) caused by *Moraxella bovis.*

OT 200 can also be administered by intravenous or intramuscular injection at a level of 3 to 5 milligrams of oxytetracycline per pound of body weight per day. In the treatment of severe foot-rot and advanced cases of other indicated diseases, dosage level of 5 milligrams per pound of body weight per day is recommended. Treatment should be continued 24 to 48 hours following remission of disease signs; however, not to exceed a total of four consecutive days. Consult your veterinarian if improvement is not noted within 24 to 48 hours of the beginning of treatment.

Swine: In swine a single dosage of 9 milligrams of OT 200 per pound of body weight administered intramuscularly is recommended in the treatment of bacterial pneumonia caused by *Pasteurella multocida* in swine, where re-treatment is impractical due to husbandry conditions or where repeated restraint is inadvisable.

OT 200 can also be administered by intramuscular injection at a level of 3 to 5 milligrams of oxytetracycline per pound of body weight per day. Treatment should be continued 24 to 48 hours following remission of the disease signs; however, not to exceed a total of four consecutive days. Consult your veterinarian if improvement is not noted within 24 to 48 hours of the beginning of treatment.

For sows, administer once intramuscularly 3 milligrams of oxytetracycline per pound of body weight approximately 8 hours before farrowing or immediately after completion of farrowing.

For swine weighing 25 lb of body weight and under, OT 200 should be administered undiluted for treatment at 9 mg/lb but should be administered diluted for treatment at 3 to 5 mg/lb body weight.

9 mg/lb Dosage Volume of Undiluted OT 200		3 or 5 mg/lb Dosage Volume of Diluted OT 200		
Body Weight	9 mg/lb	3 mg/lb	Dilution*	5 mg/lb
5 lb	0.2 mL	0.6 mL	1:7	1.0 mL
10 lb	0.5 mL	0.9 mL	1:5	1.5 mL
25 lb	1.1 mL	1.5 mL	1:3	2.5 mL

*To prepare dilutions, add one part OT 200 to three, five or seven parts of sterile water, or 5 percent dextrose solution as indicated; the diluted product should be used immediately.

A thoroughly cleaned, sterile needle and syringe should be used for each injection (needles and syringes may be sterilized by boiling in water for 15 minutes). In cold weather, OT 200 should be warmed to room temperature before administration to animals. Before withdrawing the solution from the bottle, disinfect the rubber cap on the bottle with suitable disinfectant, such as 70 percent alcohol. The injection site should be similarly cleaned with the disinfectant. Needles of 16 to 18 gauge and 1 to 1½ inches long are adequate for intramuscular injections. Needles 2 to 3 inches are recommended for intravenous use.
Precaution(s): Store at room temperature, 15°-30°C (59°-86°F). Keep from freezing.
Caution(s): Exceeding the highest recommended dosage level of drug per pound of body weight per day, administering more than the recommended number of treatments, and/or exceeding 10 mL intramuscularly per injection site in adult beef cattle and nonlactating dairy cattle, and 5 mL intramuscularly per injection site in adult swine, may result in antibiotic residues beyond the withdrawal period.

Reactions of an allergic or anaphylactic nature, sometimes fatal, have been known to occur in hypersensitive animals following the injection of oxytetracycline. Such adverse reactions can be characterized by signs such as restlessness, erection of hair, muscle trembling; swelling of eyelids, ears, muzzle, anus and vulva (or scrotum and sheath in males); labored breathing, defecation and urination, glassy-eyed appearance, eruption of skin plaques, frothing from the mouth, and prostration. Pregnant animals that recover may subsequently abort. At the first sign of any adverse reaction, discontinue use of this product and administer epinephrine at the recommended dosage levels. Call a veterinarian immediately.

Shock may be observed following intravenous administration, especially where highly concentrated materials are involved. To minimize this occurrence, it is recommended that OT 200 be administered slowly by this route.

Shortly after injection, treated animals may have transient hemoglobinuria resulting in darkened urine.

As with all antibiotic preparations, use of the drug may result in overgrowth of nonsusceptible organisms, including fungi. A lack of response by the treated animal, or the development of new signs, may suggest that an overgrowth of nonsusceptible organisms has occurred. If any of these conditions occur, consult your veterinarian.

Since bacteriostatic drugs may interfere with the bactericidal action of penicillin, it is advisable to avoid giving OT 200 in conjunction with penicillin.
Warning(s): Discontinue treatment at least 28 days prior to slaughter of cattle and swine. Not for use in lactating dairy animals.

Livestock drug, not for human use. For animal use only. Restricted drug (California), use only as directed. Keep out of reach of children.
Discussion: OT 200 (oxytetracycline injection) is a sterile, ready-to-use solution for the administration of the broad-spectrum antibiotic oxytetracycline by injection. Oxytetracycline is an antimicrobial agent that is effective in the treatment of a wide range of diseases caused by susceptible gram-positive and gram-negative bacteria. The antibiotic activity of oxytetracycline is not appreciably diminished in the presence of body fluids, serum, or exudates.

Care of Sick Animals: The use of antibiotics in the management of diseases is based on an accurate diagnosis and an adequate course of treatment. When properly used in the treatment of diseases caused by oxytetracycline susceptible organisms, most animals that have been treated with oxytetracycline injection show a noticeable improvement within 24 to 48 hours. It is recommended that the diagnosis and treatment of animal diseases be carried out by a veterinarian. Since many diseases look alike but require different types of treatment, the use of professional veterinary and laboratory services can reduce treatment time, costs and needless losses. Good housing, sanitation and nutrition are important in the maintenance of healthy animals, and are essential in the treatment of diseased animals.
Presentation: 500 mL vials.
Compendium Code No.: 14440670

OTC 50

Durvet **Feed Medication**

Oxytetracycline (Type A Medicated Article)
Active Ingredient(s): Oxytetracycline (from oxytetracycline quaternary salt) equivalent to 50 grams oxytetracycline hydrochloride/lb.

Ingredients: Oxytetracycline, calcium carbonate, roughage products and mineral oil.
Indications: An antimicrobial premix for use in the feed of chickens, turkeys, sheep, swine, calves, beef cattle, and non-lactating dairy cattle. It can also be administered to honey bees.

Recommended for the prevention and control of diseases caused by microorganisms sensitive to oxytetracycline, and also for other production uses.
Directions for Use:

Indications for Use	Use Levels of Oxytetracycline	lbs of OTC 50 per ton
Chickens:		
For Broiler/Fryer Chickens: For an increased rate of weight gain and improved feed efficiency. (Use continuously.)	10-50 g/ton	0.2-1.0
For Chickens: Control of infectious synovitis caused by *Mycoplasma synoviae;* control of fowl cholera caused by *Pasteurella multocida* sensitive to oxytetracycline. (Feed continuously for 7-14 days.)	100-200 g/ton	2.0-4.0
For Chickens: Control of chronic respiratory disease (CRD) and air sac infection caused by *Mycoplasma gallisepticum* and *Escherichia coli* susceptible to oxytetracycline. (Feed continuously for 7-14 days.)	400 g/ton	8.0
Broiler Chickens: Reduction of mortality due to air succulitis (air-sac infection) caused by *Escherichia coli* susceptible to oxytetracycline. (Feed for 5 days.)	500 g/ton	10.0

Turkeys:		
For Turkeys: Growing Turkeys: For an increased rate of weight gain and improved feed efficiency. (Use continuously.)	10-50 g/ton	0.2-1.0
For Turkeys: Control of infectious synovitis caused by *Mycoplasma synoviae* susceptible to oxytetracycline. (Feed continuously for 7-14 days.)	200 g/ton	4.0
For Turkeys: Control of hexamitiasis caused by *Hexamita meleagrides* susceptible to oxytetracycline. (Feed continuously 7-14 days.)	100 g/ton	2.0
For Turkeys: Control of complicating bacterial organisms associated with bluecomb (transmissible enteritis, coronaviral enteritis) susceptible to oxytetracycline. (Feed continuously for 7-14 days.)	25 mg/lb body weight/day	

Sheep:		
For Sheep: For an increased rate of weight gain and improved feed efficiency. (Use continuously.)	10-20 g/ton	0.20-0.4
For Sheep: Treatment of bacterial enteritis caused by *Escherichia coli* and bacterial pneumonia caused by *Pasteurella multocida* susceptible to oxytetracycline. (Feed continuously 7-14 days.)	10 mg/lb	

Swine:		
For Swine: For an increased rate of weight gain and improved feed efficiency. (Use continuously.)	10-50 g/ton	0.20-1.0
For Swine: Treatment of bacterial enteritis caused by *Escherichia coli* and *Salmonella choleraesuis* susceptible to oxytetracycline and treatment of bacterial pneumonia caused by *Pasteurella multocida* susceptible to oxytetracycline. (Feed continuously 7-14 days.)	10.0 mg/lb	
For Breeding Swine: Prevention and treatment of Leptospirosis (reducing the instances of abortions and shedding of leptospirae) caused by *Leptospira pomona* susceptible to oxytetracycline. (Feed continuously for 14 days.)	10 mg/lb	

Calves, Beef Cattle, and Non-Lactating Dairy Cattle:	
For Calves (up to 250 lbs): For an increased weight gain and improved feed efficiency. (Use continuously.)	0.05-0.1 mg/lb
For Calves (250-400 lbs): For an increased weight gain and improved feed efficiency. (Use continuously.)	25 mg/head/day
For Growing Cattle (over 400 lbs): For an increased weight gain, improved feed efficiency and reduction of liver condemnation due to liver abscesses. (Use continuously.)	75 mg/head/day
For the prevention and treatment of the early stages of the shipping fever complex. (Feed 3-5 days before and after arrival in feedlots.)	0.5-2.0 g/head/day
For Calves and Beef Cattle: Treatment of bacterial enteritis caused by *Escherichia coli* and bacterial pneumonia (shipping fever complex) caused by *Pasteurella multocida* susceptible to oxytetracycline. (Feed continuously for 7-14 days.) Note: When used in milk replacers, the treatment claim (10 mg/lb) is limited to bacterial enteritis caused by *Escherichia coli* only.	10 mg/lb

Honey Bees:	
For Honey Bees: For control of American Foulbrood caused by *Bacillus larvae*, and European Foulbrood caused by *Streptococcus pluton* susceptible to oxytetracycline. (Use directions available upon request.)	200 mg/colony

Caution(s): For use in the manufacture of medicated feeds.

For use in dry feeds only - Not for use in liquid feed supplements.

Restricted Drug (California) — Use only as directed.

Warning(s):

Chickens:

When used at levels of 400 g/ton and above: Do not administer to chickens producing eggs for human consumption. In low calcium feeds withdraw 3 days before slaughter.

When used at levels of 400 g/ton: Zero-day withdrawal period. In low calcium feeds withdraw 3 days before slaughter.

When used at levels of 500 g/ton: 24 hours withdrawal period. In low calcium feeds withdraw 3 days before slaughter.

Turkeys:

When used at levels of 200 g/ton or higher: Withdraw 5 days before slaughter.

When used at levels below 200 g/ton: Zero-day withdrawal period.

For all levels of use: Do not administer to turkeys producing eggs for human consumption.

Sheep:

When used at levels of 10 mg/lb: Withdraw 5 days before slaughter.

Swine:

When used at levels of 10 mg/lb: Withdraw 5 days before slaughter.

Cattle:

When used at levels of 10 mg/lb: Withdraw 5 days before slaughter.

Honey Bees: Remove at least 6 weeks prior to main honey flow.

Presentation: 50 lb (22.7 kg) (NDC: 30798-375-56).

Compendium Code No.: 10841241 7/97

OTC™ JUG

SureNutrition **Electrolytes-Oral**

Electrolytes & Vitamins

Guaranteed Analysis: 1 Full Tube Contains:

Amino Acids:

Arginine, min.	0.31%
Histidine, min.	0.22%
Isoleucine, min.	0.31%
Leucine, min.	0.68%
Lysine, min.	0.62%
Cystine, min.	0.22%
Methionine, min.	0.12%
Tyrosine, min.	0.48%
Phenylalanine, min.	0.39%
Threonine, min.	0.29%
Tryptophan, min.	0.15%
Aspartic Acid, min.	1.61%
Alanine, min.	0.61%
Valine, min.	0.50%
Glutamic Acid, min.	2.90%
Proline, min.	0.69%
Glycine, min.	0.63%
Serine, min.	0.32%

Minerals/Vitamins/lb:

Calcium, min.	0.50%
Calcium, max.	0.70%
Sodium, min.	5.00%
Sodium, max.	6.00%
Magnesium, min.	0.50%
Potassium, min.	1.40%
Phosphorus, min.	1.00%
Copper, min.	350 ppm
Iron, min.	3500 ppm
Manganese, min.	350 ppm
Cobalt, min.	2 ppm
Zinc, min.	1000 ppm
Vitamin B12, min.	1013 mcg
Menadione, min.	500 mg
Riboflavin, min.	81 mg
Pantothenic Acid, min.	46 mg
Thiamine, min.	992 mg
Niacin, min.	465 mg
Vitamin B6, min.	37 mg
Inositol, min.	183 mg
Ascorbic Acid, min.	2000 mg

Ingredients: Water, Dextrose, Potassium Amino Acid Complex, Sodium Chloride, Ascorbic Acid, Magnesium Amino Acid Chelate, Calcium Amino Acid Chelate, Phosphorus, Amino Acid Complex, Menadione Sodium Bisulfate, Liver Fraction, Iron Amino Acid Chelate, Thiamine Hydrochloride, Niacinamide, Zinc Amino Acid Chelate, Inositol, Riboflavin, Pyridoxine Hydrochloride, Copper Amino Acid Chelate, Manganese Amino Acid Chelate, D-Calcium Pantothenate, Folic Acid, Cobalt, Amino Acid Complex, Cyanocobalimin, Xanthan Gum, Corn Oil, Sorbic Acid.

Indications: Use before or after an event to replace vitamins, minerals and amino acids lost during excessive exercise or heat. Keep ample drinking water supplied.

Electrolytes and vitamins for all classes of horses.

Directions: 1 full tube onto back of tongue equals Vet. Electrolyte Jug. A ½ tube before or after light workout during hot weather to prevent dehydration.

Contraindication(s): Do not feed to cattle or other ruminants.

Caution(s): This product intended for livestock only.

Presentation: 1 x 60 cc (68 g) and 6 x 60 cc (68 g) tubes.

Compendium Code No.: 12060030 0AA1

OTIBIOTIC OINTMENT ℞

Vetus **Otic Antimicrobial-Corticosteroid**

Gentamicin Sulfate USP, Betamethasone Valerate, USP and Clotrimazole, USP Ointment

ANADA No.: 200-229

Active Ingredient(s): Each gram of OTIBIOTIC OINTMENT (gentamicin-betamethasone-clotrimazole ointment) contains gentamicin sulfate USP equivalent to 3 mg gentamicin base; betamethasone valerate, USP equivalent to 1 mg betamethasone; and 10 mg clotrimazole, USP in a mineral oil-based system containing a plasticized hydrocarbon gel.

Indications: OTIBIOTIC OINTMENT (gentamicin-betamethasone-clotrimazole ointment) is indicated for the treatment of canine acute and chronic otitis externa associated with yeast *(Malassezia pachydermatis*, formerly *Pityrosporum canis)* and/or bacteria susceptible to gentamicin.

Pharmacology:

Gentamicin: Gentamicin sulfate is an aminoglycoside antibiotic active against a wide variety of pathogenic gram-negative and gram-positive bacteria. *In vitro* tests have determined that gentamicin is bactericidal and acts by inhibiting normal protein synthesis in susceptible microorganisms. Specifically, gentamicin is active against the following organisms commonly isolated from canine ears: *Staphylococcus aureus*, other *Staphylococcus* spp., *Pseudomonas aeruginosa*, *Proteus* spp., and *Escherichia coli*.

Betamethasone: Betamethasone valerate is a synthetic adrenocorticoid for dermatologic use. Betamethasone, an analog of prednisolone, has a high degree of corticosteroid activity and a slight degree of mineralocorticosteroid activity. Betamethasone valerate, the 17-valerate ester of betamethasone, has been shown to provide anti-inflammatory and anti-pruritic activity in the topical management of corticosteroid-responsive otitis externa. Topical corticosteroids can be absorbed from normal, intact skin. Inflammation can increase percutaneous absorption. Once absorbed through the skin, topical corticosteroids are handled through pharmacokinetic pathways similar to systemically administered corticosteroids.

Clotrimazole: Clotrimazole is a broad-spectrum antifungal agent that is used for the treatment of dermal infections caused by various species of pathogenic dermatophytes and yeasts. The primary action of clotrimazole is against dividing and growing organisms.

In vitro, clotrimazole exhibits fungistatic and fungicidal activity against isolates of *Trichophyton rubrum, Trichophyton mentagrophytes, Epidermophyton floccosum, Microsporum canis, Candida* spp. and *Malassezia pachydermatis (Pityrosporum canis)*. Resistance to clotrimazole is very rare among the fungi that cause superficial mycoses. In an induced otitis externa infected with *Malassezia pachydermatis*, 1% clotrimazole in the gentamicin-betamethasone-clotrimazole ointment vehicle was effective both microbiologically and clinically in terms of reduction of exudate odor and swelling.

In studies of the mechanism of action, the minimum fungicidal concentration of clotrimazole caused leakage of intracellular phosphorus compounds into the ambient medium with concomitant breakdown of cellular nucleic acids and accelerated potassium efflux. These events began rapidly and extensively after addition of the drug. Clotrimazole is very poorly absorbed following dermal application.

Gentamicin-Betamethasone-Clotrimazole: By virtue of its three active ingredients, OTIBIOTIC OINTMENT (gentamicin-betamethasone-clotrimazole) has antibacterial, anti-inflammatory, and antifungal activity. In component efficacy studies, the compatibility and additive effect of each of the components were demonstrated. In clinical field trials, gentamicin-betamethasone-clotrimazole was effective in the treatment of otitis externa associated with bacteria and *Malassezia pachydermatis*. OTIBIOTIC OINTMENT (gentamicin sulfate USP, betamethasone valerate, USP and clotrimazole, USP ointment) reduced discomfort, redness, swelling, exudate, and odor, and exerted a strong antimicrobial effect.

Dosage and Administration: The external ear should be thoroughly cleaned and dried before treatment. Remove foreign material, debris, crusted exudates, etc., with suitable non-irritating solutions. Excessive hair should be clipped from the treatment area. After verifying that the eardrum is intact, instill 4 drops (2 drops from the 215 g bottle) of OTIBIOTIC OINTMENT (gentamicin-betamethasone-clotrimazole ointment) twice daily into the ear canal of dogs weighing less than 30 lbs. Instill 8 drops (4 drops from the 215 g bottle) twice daily into the ear canal of dogs weighing 30 lbs or more. Therapy should continue for 7 consecutive days.

Contraindication(s): If hypersensitivity to any of the components occurs, treatment should be discontinued and appropriate therapy instituted. Concomitant use of drugs known to induce ototoxicity should be avoided. Do not use in dogs with known perforation of eardrums.

Precaution(s): Store between 2° and 25°C (36° and 77°F). Shake well before use when using the 215 gram bottle.

Caution(s): Federal law restricts this drug to use by or on the order of a licensed veterinarian.

The use of OTIBIOTIC OINTMENT (gentamicin-betamethasone-clotrimazole ointment) has been associated with deafness or partial hearing loss in a small number of sensitive dogs (eg. geriatric). The hearing deficit is usually temporary. If hearing or vestibular dysfunction is noted during the course of treatment, discontinue use of OTIBIOTIC OINTMENT (gentamicin-betamethasone-clotrimazole ointment) immediately and flush the ear canal thoroughly with a non-ototoxic solution. Corticosteroids administered to dogs, rabbits, and rodents during pregnancy have resulted in cleft palate in offspring. Other congenital anomalies including deformed forelegs, phocomelia, and anasarca have been reported in offspring of dogs which received corticosteroids during pregnancy.

Clinical and experimental data have demonstrated that corticosteroids administered orally or parenterally to animals may induce the first stage of parturition if used during the last trimester of pregnancy and may precipitate premature parturition followed by dystocia, fetal death, retained placenta and metritis.

Identification of infecting organisms should be made either by microscopic roll smear evaluation or by culture as appropriate. Antibiotic susceptibility of the pathogenic organism(s) should be determined prior to use of this preparation.

If overgrowth of nonsusceptible bacteria, fungi, or yeasts occur, or if hypersensitivity develops, treatment should be discontinued and appropriate therapy instituted.

Administration of recommended doses of OTIBIOTIC OINTMENT (gentamicin-betamethasone-clotrimazole ointment) beyond 7 days may result in delayed wound healing.

Avoid ingestion. Adverse systemic reactions have been observed following the oral ingestion of some topical corticosteroid preparations. Patients should be closely observed for the usual signs of adrenocorticoid overdosage which include sodium retention, potassium loss, fluid retention, weight gain, polydipsia and/or polyuria. Prolonged use or overdosage may produce adverse immunosuppressive effects.

Use of corticosteroids, depending on dose, duration, and specific steroid, may result in endogenous steroid production inhibition following drug withdrawal. In patients presently receiving or recently withdrawn from corticosteroid treatments, therapy with a rapidly acting corticosteroid should be considered in especially stressful situations.

Before instilling any medication into the ear, examine the external ear canal thoroughly to be certain the tympanic membrane is not ruptured in order to avoid the possibility of transmitting infection to the middle ear as well as damaging the cochlea or vestibular apparatus from prolonged contact.

Warning(s): For otic use in dogs only.

Keep this and all drugs out of the reach of children.

Toxicology: Clinical and safety studies with OTIBIOTIC OINTMENT (gentamicin sulfate USP, betamethasone valerate, USP and clotrimazole, USP ointment) have shown a wide safety margin at the recommended dose level in dogs (see Cautions/Side Effects).

Side Effects:

Gentamicin: While aminoglycosides are absorbed poorly from skin, intoxication may occur when aminoglycosides are applied topically for prolonged periods of time to large wounds, burns, or any denuded skin, particularly if there is renal insufficiency. All aminoglycosides have the potential to produce reversible and irreversible vestibular, cochlear, and renal toxicity.

Betamethasone: Side effects such as SAP and SGPT enzyme elevations, weight loss, anorexia, polydipsia, and polyuria have occurred following the use of parenteral or systemic synthetic corticosteroids in dogs. Vomiting and diarrhea (occasionally bloody) have been observed in dogs and cats.

Cushing's syndrome in dogs has been reported in association with prolonged or repeated steroid therapy.

Clotrimazole: The following have been reported occasionally in humans in connection with the use of clotrimazole: erythema, stinging, blistering, peeling, edema, pruritus, urticaria, and general irritation of the skin not present before therapy.

Presentation: OTIBIOTIC OINTMENT (gentamicin-betamethasone-clotrimazole ointment) is available in 7.5 gram, 10 gram, 15 gram and 25 gram tubes as well as in a 215 gram plastic bottle.

Compendium Code No.: 14440681

OTICALM™ CLEANSING SOLUTION

DVM — **Otic Cleanser**

Cleansing Solution for Ears

Ingredient(s): Water, propylene glycol, poloxamer 407, salicylic acid, benzoic acid, malic acid and eucalyptus oil.

Indications: For general cleansing of waxy, dirty, or exudative ears.

OTICALM™ is an astringent, general cleansing formulation for use in the ears of dogs and cats.

Directions:

For Routine Ear Cleansing: Apply OTICALM™ liberally into ear canal. Gently massage base of ear to help break up any accumulated internal wax and crust. Use cotton or absorbent material to clean any excess solution and debris from open area of ear. Apply once or twice weekly, or as directed by your veterinarian.

For Otitis Externa: Follow the above directions and apply 1-2 times daily for as many days as directed by your veterinarian.

Precaution(s): Store this product at room temperature.

Caution(s): For external use on animals only.

Warning(s): Keep out of reach of children.

Presentation: 4 fl oz (118 mL) and 12 fl oz (355 mL).

Compendium Code No.: 11420421

Rev 0201 / Rev 0497

OTI-CARE®-B DRYING EAR CREME

ARC — **Otic Dryer**

Ingredients: Contains: 70% isopropyl alcohol, silicon dioxide, salicylic acid, boric acid, fragrance, polysorbate 60, zinc oxide, talc, PEG 75 lanolin oil, sucrose octyl acetate, acetic acid, propylene glycol, FD&C blue no. 1.

Indications: OTICARE®-B Drying Ear Creme is safe and recommended for long term, continuous use in dogs and cats which have recurring problems with moist, odorous ears. This is common in spaniels, poodles, cockapoos and any dogs which swim or hunt. OTICARE®-B dries to a powder which helps keep the ear canal dry. It does not contain cortisone or antibiotics.

Directions: Before using, clean ears with OtiClean®-A Ear Lotion. Shake well. Apply OTICARE®-B Drying Ear Creme to the opening of the ear canal. Massage base of ear to allow contact with entire ear surface. Remove excess creme with facial tissue. Repeat 3 to 5 times weekly or as otherwise directed by your veterinarian. Before each use, clean ears with OtiClean®-A Ear Lotion. Use before and after bathing or swimming.

Precaution(s): Flammable - Keep away from open flame or heat.

Caution(s): Keep out of reach of children. Avoid contact with eyes and mucous membranes. If eyes contacted, wash with water immediately. Harmful if swallowed. First Aid - Call a physician or poison control center. For external veterinary use only.

Available only from veterinarians.

Presentation: 2 fl. oz. (59 mL) and 8 fl. oz. (237 mL).

Compendium Code No.: 10960051

OTICARE®-P EAR POWDER

ARC — **Otic Dryer**

Active Ingredient(s): Rosin.

Indications: For use to help keep the ears dry and reduce ear odors in dogs and cats.

Also used to help remove hair from the ear canal of dogs.

Dosage and Administration: First clean the ears with a suitable ear cleaning lotion. Next puff OTICARE®-P Ear Powder into the ear canal.

To help remove hair from the ear canal of dogs: With electric clippers or scissors remove the excess hair that surrounds the opening of the ear canal. Puff OTICARE®-P Ear Powder into the ear. With forceps or tweezers, remove any hair growing in the ear canal.

Presentation: 6 g container.

Compendium Code No.: 10960071

OTIC CLEAR

Butler — **Otic Cleanser**

Active Ingredient(s): Deionized water, isopropyl alcohol, propylene glycol, glycerine, fragrance, salicylic acid, PEG 75 lanolin oil, lidocaine hydrochloride, boric acid, acetic acid, FD&C blue #1.

Indications: OTIC CLEAR is used on dogs and cats for the routine cleaning and odor control of the ear canal.

Dosage and Administration: Fill the ear canal with OTIC CLEAR and gently massage. Ear debris and excess solution should be wiped from the inner ear surface. For dirty ears, repeat the process. To keep ears clean and fresh-smelling, use upon the direction of a veterinarian. May be used before and after bathing or swimming.

Precaution(s): Flammable: Keep away from heat or open flame.

Caution(s): Harmful if swallowed. If swallowed, call a physician or poison control center. Avoid contact with the eyes and mucous membranes. If in eyes, wash with copious amounts of cool water.

For external veterinary use only.

Keep out of the reach of children.

Sold only through veterinarians.

Presentation: 4 oz., 8 oz. and 1 gallon containers.

Compendium Code No.: 10821300

OTICLEAN®-A EAR CLEANING AND DEODORANT PADS

ARC — **Otic Cleaner**

Ingredients: Absorbent pads with 35% isopropyl alcohol, salicylic acid, fragrance, P E G 75 lanolin oil, acetic acid, propylene glycol, glycerin, FD & C blue no. 1; pH adjusted to 3.

Indications: Ear cleaning and deodorant pads for dogs and cats.

Dosage and Administration: As you clean the ear allow some lotion to reach the lower ear canal. Massage the ear canal, which can be felt under the skin.

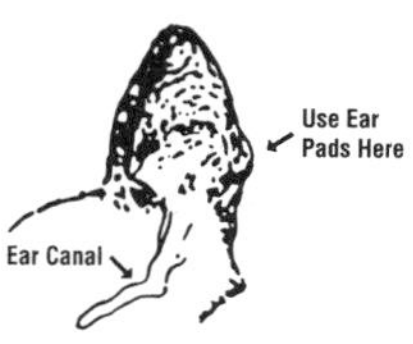

Repeat procedure for very dirty ears. Use twice weekly or as otherwise directed by your veterinarian to clean and help reduce ear odors. Use before and after bathing or swimming. In hounds and Spaniels, dogs that swim or hunt or any dogs which have recurring problems with moist, odorous ears, use OtiCare®-B Drying Ear Cream after the ears have been cleaned with OTICLEAN®-A Ear Cleaning Lotion or Pads.

For Ear Mites and Ear Ticks: First clean the ears with OTICLEAN®-A Ear Cleaning Lotion or Pads, and then apply OtiCare®-M Ear Mite Treatment.

Precaution(s): Flammable - Keep away from open flame or heat.

Warning(s): Avoid contact with eyes and mucous membranes. If eyes contacted, wash with water immediately. Harmful if swallowed. First Aid - Call a physician or poison control center. For external veterinary use only. Keep out of reach of children.
Discussion: The ears of dogs and cats are especially susceptible to problems. After a medical problem has been treated by your veterinarian, it is important to continue taking care of the ears on a regular basis. Proper aftercare will reduce the likelihood of recurring ear problems.
The canal is deep, curved structure. The deep ear canal does not drain well and tends to accumulate dirt, wax, and moisture. This can lead to bacterial growth and odors if the ears are not cleaned at regular intervals.
Presentation: 35 pads/jar (Net Wt. 200 g).
Compendium Code No.: 10960081

OTICLEAN®-A EAR CLEANING LOTION

ARC **Otic Cleanser**

Active Ingredient(s): Contains: 35% isopropyl alcohol, salicylic acid, fragrance, PEG 75, lanolin oil, acetic acid, propylene glycol, glycerine, FD&C blue no. 1.
OTICLEAN®-A Ear Cleaning Lotion pH is 3.0.
Indications: For cleaning and odor control of the ear canal in dogs and cats.
Hospital Use: To flush the ear canal.
Home Use: For routine cleansing and odor control. Use before or after bathing, swimming or hunting.
Directions: Fill the ear canal with lotion. Gently rub and massage the deep ear canal. Use facial tissue to remove excess lotion, dirt and debris. Repeat procedure for very dirty ears. Use twice weekly or as otherwise directed by your veterinarian to clean and help reduce ear odors. Use before and after bathing or swimming.
Precaution(s): Flammable - Keep away from open flame or heat.
Caution(s): Keep out of reach of children. Avoid contact with the eyes and mucous membranes. If eyes contacted, wash with water immediately. Harmful if swallowed. First Aid - Call a physician or poison control center. For external veterinary use only.
Available only from veterinarians.
Presentation: 2 fl. oz., 4 fl. oz., 16 fl. oz. and 1 gallon containers.
OTICLEAN®-A Cleaning and Deodorant Pads - 10 and 35 pads per jar.
Compendium Code No.: 10960090

OTI-CLENS®

Pfizer Animal Health **Otic Cleanser**

Active Ingredient(s): Contains: Propylene glycol, malic acid, benzoic acid, salicylic acid.
Indications: OTI-CLENS® is a nontoxic, ear-cleaning agent for use in dogs and cats. Routine use helps maintain good ear hygiene.
Dosage and Administration: General Directions: Apply liberally to the ear. Massage the base of the ear. Clean the accessible portion of the ear with a cotton ball. Repeat if necessary. Use once or twice weekly on a routine basis. OTI-CLENS® may be used up to 3 times daily over extended periods. Use as directed by your veterinarian.
Precaution(s): Store at controlled room temperature 15°-30°C (59°-86°F).
Caution(s): For external use only. Irritating to the eye.
Keep out of reach of children.
Warning(s): For veterinary use only.
Presentation: 4 fl oz (120 mL).
Compendium Code No.: 36901220 50-8055-04

OTIFOAM™ EAR CLEANSER

DVM **Otic Cleanser**

Foaming Action Ear Cleanser
Active Ingredient(s): OTIFOAM™ contains surface acting agents which loosen and dislodge excessive wax formation. Ingredients: Water, cocamidopropyl betaine, PEG-60 almond glycerides, mackalene 426, salicylic acid and oil of eucalyptus.
Indications: To breakdown and dislodge excessive wax and debris within the ear canal prior to flushing ears with OtiRinse™ Cleansing/Drying Ear Solution.
Directions: Apply OTIFOAM™ liberally into ear canal. Gently massage base of ear to help break up accumulated internal wax and crust. Remain in ear 1-2 minutes for foaming action. Use DVM's OtiRinse™ to flush excess wax and dry ear canal. Repeat process once or twice weekly or as directed by your veterinarian.
Precaution(s): Store this product at room temperature.
Caution(s): For external use on animals only.
Warning(s): Keep out of reach of children.
Presentation: 8 fl oz (237 mL) and 1 gallon (3.78 L).
Compendium Code No.: 11420431 Rev 0599 / Rev 0999

OTIPAN® CLEANSING SOLUTION

Harlmen **Otic Cleanser**

Active Ingredient(s): Propylene glycol, hydroxypropyl cellulose, octoxynol and a phosphate buffer system (phosphoric acid and potassium hydroxide). The pH is adjusted to 2.5 or less.
Indications: For veterinary use only on cats and dogs. OTIPAN® cleansing solution is a patented formula designed to cleanse wax, necrotic tissue debris and exudate from the external ear canal.
The solution is colorless, odorless and has a viscosity which promotes adherence to tissue. The solution will not irritate delicate mucous membranes.
Dosage and Administration: Instill 1 to 2 mL into the ear canal each day for 14 days, or as directed by a veterinarian. Use a liberal amount of solution and rub any excess into the chapped or pigmented skin around the external auditory meatus.
Caution(s): For topical use only. Keep out of the reach of children.
Presentation: 2 oz. (12's) and 16 oz. (for clinic use) bottles. Each size is furnished with a bottle of Otipan® Blue Stain.
Compendium Code No.: 14500030

OTIRINSE™ CLEANSING/DRYING EAR SOLUTION

DVM **Otic Preparation**

Antiseptic Ear Solution
Ingredient(s): Water, propylene glycol, SD alcohol 40, dioctyl sodium sulfosuccinate (DSS), glycerin, nonoxynol-12, salicylic acid, lactic acid, benzoic acid, benzyl alcohol, fragrance and aloe vera.
Indications: For cleaning of wax and debris within the ear canal.
OTIRINSE™ is formulated to clean and dry ear canals in dogs and cats.
Directions: Apply OTIRINSE™ liberally into ear canal. Gently massage base of ear to help break up accumulated internal wax and crust. Use cotton or absorbent material to clean excess solution and debris from open area of ear. Apply once or twice weekly or as directed by your veterinarian.
Precaution(s): Store this product at room temperature.
Caution(s): For external use on animals only. Keep out of reach of children.
Presentation: 8 fl oz (237 mL) and 1 gallon (3.78 L).
Compendium Code No.: 11420441 Rev 0599 / Rev 0999

OTISOL™

Wysong **Otic Cleanser**

Active Ingredient(s): Copper chelate of chlorophyll, essential oils of eucalyptus, peppermint, cajeput, juniper, wintergreen, clove, jojoba oil, aloe vera extract, benzocaine, carbolic acid and natural oleoresins, menthol in a coconut soap, sodium metasilicate, isopropanol base. Stabilized with rosemary extract and vitamin E.
Indications: Designed for use in animals without serious ear disorders. OTISOL™ is effective in preventing the buildup of dirt and residue which provide a medium for pathogenic growth. To be used where exudate and waxes have accumulated in the ear, or where cleaning, anti-inflammatory or antimicrobial actions, or tissue healing are needed.
Dosage and Administration: Shake well before using. Instill several drops into the ear two (2) to three (3) times a day. Massage into the ear canal well and remove any excess with a cotton or tissue. Repeat the procedure if the ears are excessively dirty. Use before and after bathing if the ears are particularly sensitive. For routine ear cleansing, use once a week.
Caution(s): Keep out of the reach of children. Chlorophyll pigments may stain. Do not use in excess and be sure to remove overflow.
Presentation: 1.25 oz. (36.96 mL) and 16 oz. (480 mL) containers.
Compendium Code No.: 14070001

OTISOL-O™

Wysong **Otic Cleanser**

Active Ingredient(s): Copper chelate of chlorophyll, jojoba oil, aloe vera, arnica, and essential oils of eucalyptus, peppermint, cajeput, juniper, wintergreen, clove, and menthol in a base of extra virgin olive oil stabilized with Wysong oxherphol (tocopherol epimers of vitamin E, botanical oleoresins, ascorbate oxidase and glutathione peroxidase).
Indications: Designed for use in animals without serious ear disorders. OTISOL-O™ is effective in preventing the buildup of dirt and residue which provide a medium for pathogenic growth. To be used where exudate and waxes have accumulated in the ear, or where cleaning, anti-inflammatory or antimicrobial actions, or tissue healing are needed.
Dosage and Administration: Instill several drops into the ear two (2) to three (3) times a day. Work well into the ear canal by massaging and compressing the ear canal as it can be felt lying under the skin. Remove any excess at the ear opening with a cotton or tissue. Do not probe into the ear canal with instruments. Repeat the procedure if the ears are excessively soiled. Use before and after bathing if the ears are particularly sensitive. For routine ear cleansing, use once a week.
Caution(s): Keep out of the reach of children.
Presentation: 1.25 oz. (36.96 mL) and 16 oz. (480 mL) containers.
Compendium Code No.: 14070011

OTOCETIC SOLUTION

Vedco **Otic Cleanser**

Active Ingredient(s): 2% Boric acid and 2% acetic acid with surfactants.
Indications: OTOCETIC SOLUTION is specifically designed for the routine cleaning and drying of moist ears. The product does not contain ingredients that are ototoxic. It acidifies, controls yeast and swimmers ear.
It is also useful for the removal of ceruminolytic material and in controlling odor problems associated with the ear.
Dosage and Administration: For the routine cleansing of ears, apply in the outer ear while massaging the base of the ear. Excess material can be easily removed with a cotton ball. Repeat as necessary. In the rare cases where the ear has become ulcerated, it is recommended to dilute OTOCETIC SOLUTION 1:1 with water.
For the treatment of otitis externa, follow the directions as indicated above and repeat 2-3 times daily, or as directed by your veterinarian.
Precaution(s): Store in a cool place.
Warning(s): For external use only. Avoid contact to eyes.
Keep out of reach of children.
Presentation: 4 fl oz and 16 fl oz.
Sold to graduate veterinarians only.
US patent pending.
Compendium Code No.: 10941610

OTO HC-B

RXV **Topical Corticosteroid**

Hydrocortisone and Burow's Solution
Active Ingredient(s):

Hydrocortisone	10 mg
Burow's Solution	20 mg

In a water miscible base containing Propylene Glycol.
Indications: Topical treatment for the relief of discomfort caused by inflammatory pruritis in dogs.
Hydrocortisone is an anti-inflammatory and anti-pruritic agent.
Burow's Solution is used as an astringent for drying of moist dermatitis. It provides cooling relief for discomfort.
Dosage and Administration: Apply 3 to 4 times daily.
Contraindication(s): As with any topical hydrocortisone product OTO HC-B should not be used in the presence of tuberculosis of the skin.
Caution(s): For topical use only. Not intended for deep-seated infections. Not for use in the eyes. For animal use only.
Warning(s): Keep out of reach of children.
Presentation: 1 oz (NDC# 14049-160-10) and 16 oz (NDC# 14049-160-16).
Compendium Code No.: 10910360 Iss. 06-01

OTOMAX® ℞

Schering-Plough **Otic Antimicrobial-Corticosteroid**

(Gentamicin Sulfate Veterinary, Betamethasone Valerate, USP and Clotrimazole, USP Ointment)

NADA No.: 140-896

Active Ingredient(s): Each gram of OTOMAX® contains gentamicin sulfate veterinary equivalent to 3 mg gentamicin base; betamethasone valerate, USP equivalent to 1 mg betamethasone; and 10 mg clotrimazole, USP in a mineral oil-based system containing a plasticized hydrocarbon gel.

Indications: OTOMAX® is indicated for the treatment of canine acute and chronic otitis externa associated with yeast *(Malassezia pachydermatis*, formerly *Pityrosporum canis)* and/or bacteria susceptible to gentamicin.

Pharmacology:

Gentamicin: Gentamicin sulfate is an aminoglycoside antibiotic active against a wide variety of pathogenic gram-negative and gram-positive bacteria. *In vitro* tests have determined that gentamicin is bactericidal and acts by inhibiting normal protein synthesis in susceptible microorganisms. Specifically, gentamicin is active against the following organisms commonly isolated from canine ears: *Staphylococcus aureus*, other *Staphylococcus* spp., *Pseudomonas aeruginosa*, *Proteus* spp., and *Escherichia coli*.

Betamethasone: Betamethasone valerate is a synthetic adrenocorticoid for dermatologic use. Betamethasone, an analog of prednisolone, has a high degree of corticosteroid activity and a slight degree of mineralocorticosteroid activity. Betamethasone valerate, the 17-valerate ester of betamethasone, has been shown to provide anti-inflammatory and anti-pruritic activity in the topical management of corticosteroid-responsive otitis externa.

Topical corticosteroids can be absorbed from normal, intact skin. Inflammation can increase percutaneous absorption. Once absorbed through the skin, topical corticosteroids are handled through pharmacokinetic pathways similar to systemically administered corticosteroids.

Clotrimazole: Clotrimazole is a broad-spectrum antifungal agent that is used for the treatment of dermal infections caused by various species of pathogenic dermatophytes and yeasts. The primary action of clotrimazole is against dividing and growing organisms.

In vitro, clotrimazole exhibits fungistatic and fungicidal activity against isolates of *Trichophyton rubrum, Trichophyton mentagrophytes, Epidermophyton floccosum, Microsporum canis, Candida* spp., and *Malassezia pachydermatis (Pityrosporum canis)*. Resistance to clotrimazole is very rare among the fungi that cause superficial mycoses.

In an induced otitis externa infected with *Malassezia pachydermatis*, 1% clotrimazole in the OTOMAX® vehicle was effective both microbiologically and clinically in terms of reduction of exudate odor and swelling.

In studies of the mechanism of action, the minimum fungicidal concentration of clotrimazole caused leakage of intracellular phosphorus compounds into the ambient medium with concomitant breakdown of cellular nucleic acids and accelerated potassium efflux. These events began rapidly and extensively after addition of the drug.

Clotrimazole is very poorly absorbed following dermal application.

Gentamicin-Betamethasone-Clotrimazole: By virtue of its three active ingredients, OTOMAX® has antibacterial, anti-inflammatory, and antifungal activity.

In component efficacy studies, the compatibility and additive effect of each of the components were demonstrated.

In clinical field trials, OTOMAX® was effective in the treatment of otitis externa associated with bacteria and *Malassezia pachydermatis*. OTOMAX® reduced discomfort, redness, swelling, exudate, and odor, and exerted a strong antimicrobial effect.

Dosage and Administration: The external ear should be thoroughly cleaned and dried before treatment. Remove foreign material, debris, crusted exudates, etc., with suitable non-irritating solutions. Excessive hair should be clipped from the treatment area. After verifying that the eardrum is intact, instill 4 drops (2 drops from the 215 g bottle) of OTOMAX® twice daily into the ear canal of dogs weighing less than 30 lbs. Instill 8 drops (4 drops from the 215 g bottle) twice daily into the ear canal of dogs weighing 30 lbs. or more. Therapy should continue for 7 consecutive days.

Contraindication(s): If hypersensitivity to any of the components occurs, treatment should be discontinued and appropriate therapy instituted. Concomitant use of drugs known to induce ototoxicity should be avoided. Do not use in dogs with known perforation of eardrums.

Precaution(s): Store between 2° and 25°C (36° and 77°F).

Shake well before use when using the 215 gram bottle.

Caution(s): Federal law restricts this drug to use by or on the order of a licensed veterinarian.

The use of OTOMAX® has been associated with deafness or partial hearing loss in a small number of sensitive dogs (eg, geriatric). The hearing deficit is usually temporary. If hearing or vestibular dysfunction is noted during the course of treatment, discontinue use of OTOMAX® immediately and flush the ear canal thoroughly with a non-ototoxic solution.

Identification of infecting organisms should be made either by microscopic roll smear evaluation or by culture as appropriate. Antibiotic susceptibility of the pathogenic organism(s) should be determined prior to use of this preparation.

If overgrowth of nonsusceptible bacteria, fungi, or yeasts occur, or if hypersensitivity develops, treatment should be discontinued and appropriate therapy instituted.

Administration of recommended doses of OTOMAX® beyond 7 days may result in delayed wound healing.

Avoid ingestion. Adverse systemic reactions have been observed following the oral ingestion of some topical corticosteroid preparations. Patients should be closely observed for the usual signs of adrenocorticoid overdosage which include sodium retention, potassium loss, fluid retention, weight gain, polydipsia, and/or polyuria. Prolonged use or overdosage may produce adverse immunosuppressive effects.

Use of corticosteroids, depending on dose, duration, and specific steroid, may result in endogenous steroid production inhibition following drug withdrawal. In patients presently receiving or recently withdrawn from corticosteroid treatments, therapy with a rapidly acting corticosteroid should be considered in especially stressful situations.

Before instilling any medication into the ear, examine the external ear canal thoroughly to be certain the tympanic membrane is not ruptured in order to avoid the possibility of transmitting infection to the middle ear as well as damaging the cochlea or vestibular apparatus from prolonged contact. If hearing or vestibular dysfunction is noted during the course of treatment, discontinue use of OTOMAX®.

Warning(s): Corticosteroids administered to dogs, rabbits, and rodents during pregnancy have resulted in cleft palate in offspring. Other congenital anomalies including deformed forelegs, phocomelia, and anasarca have been reported in offspring of dogs which received corticosteroids during pregnancy.

Clinical and experimental data have demonstrated that corticosteroids administered orally or parenterally to animals may induce the first stage of parturition if used during the last trimester of pregnancy and may precipitate premature parturition followed by dystocia, fetal death, retained placenta, and metritis.

Keep this and all drugs out of the reach of children.

Toxicology: Clinical and safety studies with OTOMAX® have shown a wide safety margin at the recommended dose level in dogs (see Cautions/Side Effects).

Side Effects:

Gentamicin: While aminoglycosides are absorbed poorly from skin, intoxication may occur when aminoglycosides are applied topically for prolonged periods of time to large wounds, burns, or any denuded skin, particularly if there is renal insufficiency. All aminoglycosides have the potential to produce reversible and irreversible vestibular, cochlear, and renal toxicity.

Betamethasone: Side effects such as SAP and SGPT enzyme elevations, weight loss, anorexia, polydipsia, and polyuria have occurred following the use of parenteral or systemic synthetic corticosteroids in dogs. Vomiting and diarrhea (occasionally bloody) have been observed in dogs and cats.

Cushing's syndrome in dogs has been reported in association with prolonged or repeated steroid therapy.

Clotrimazole: The following have been reported occasionally in humans in connection with the use of clotrimazole: erythema, stinging, blistering, peeling, edema, pruritus, urticaria, and general irritation of the skin not present before therapy.

Presentation: OTOMAX® is available in 12 x 7.5 gram and 12 x 15 gram tubes, as well as in 12 x 12.5 gram, 1 x 215 gram, and 6 x 30 gram plastic bottles.

Compendium Code No.: 10471431

OTOMITE® PLUS

Virbac **Otic Parasiticide**

Ear Mite Treatment

EPA Reg. No.: 2382-116

Active Ingredient(s):

Pyrethrins	0.15%
Technical piperonyl butoxide*	1.50%
N-octyl bicycloheptene dicarboximide	0.5%
Di-n-propyl isocinchomeronate	1.0%
Inert ingredients	96.85%

*Equivalent to 0.4% (butylcarbityl)(6-propyl-piperonyl) ether and 0.1% related components.

Indications: Ear mite treatment for dogs, cats, puppies and kittens.

Directions for Use: It is a violation of federal law to use this product in a manner inconsistent with its labeling.

Directions: Cleanse ear thoroughly with a low pH ear cleanser. Place sufficient OTOMITE® Plus in each ear to wet external ear canal and massage base of ear. Retreat in 7 days. If it is necessary to again clean the ears sooner, retreat with OTOMITE® Plus.

Precautionary Statements:

Hazards to Humans and Domestic Animals: Harmful if swallowed. Avoid contact with eyes. Wash hands after using.

Statement of Practical Treatment:

If in Eyes: Flush eyes with plenty of water. Get medical attention if irritation persists.

Storage and Disposal:

Storage: Do not use or store near heat or open flame.

Disposal: Do not reuse empty container. Wrap container and put in trash.

Warning(s): For veterinary use only.

Keep out of reach of children.

Presentation: 0.5 fl oz (15 mL).

Compendium Code No.: 10230380

OTO SOOTHE® OINTMENT ℞

RXV **Otic Antimicrobial-Corticosteroid**

Gentamicin Sulfate USP, Betamethasone Valerate, USP and Clotrimazole, USP Ointment

ANADA No.: 200-229

Active Ingredient(s): Description: Each gram of gentamicin-betamethasone-clotrimazole ointment contains gentamicin sulfate USP equivalent to 3 mg gentamicin base; betamethasone valerate, USP equivalent to 1 mg betamethasone; and 10 mg clotrimazole, USP in a mineral oil-based system containing a plasticized hydrocarbon gel.

Indications: Gentamicin-betamethasone-clotrimazole ointment is indicated for the treatment of canine acute and chronic otitis externa associated with yeast *(Malassezia pachydermatis*, formerly *Pityrosporum canis)* and/or bacteria susceptible to gentamicin.

Pharmacology:

Gentamicin: Gentamicin sulfate is an aminoglycoside antibiotic active against a wide variety of pathogenic gram-negative and gram-positive bacteria. *In vitro* tests have determined that gentamicin is bactericidal and acts by inhibiting normal protein synthesis in susceptible microorganisms. Specifically, gentamicin is active against the following organisms commonly isolated from canine ears: *Staphylococcus aureus*, other *Staphylococcus* spp., *Pseudomonas aeruginosa*, *Proteus* spp., and *Escherichia coli*.

Betamethasone: Betamethasone valerate is a synthetic adrenocorticoid for dermatologic use. Betamethasone, an analog of prednisolone, has a high degree of corticosteroid activity and a slight degree of mineralocorticosteroid activity. Betamethasone valerate, the 17-valerate ester of betamethasone, has been shown to provide anti-inflammatory and anti-pruritic activity in the topical management of corticosteroid-responsive otitis externa. Topical corticosteroids can be absorbed from normal, intact skin. Inflammation can increase percutaneous absorption. Once absorbed through the skin, topical corticosteroids are handled through pharmacokinetic pathways similar to systemically administered corticosteroids.

Clotrimazole: Clotrimazole is a broad-spectrum antifungal agent that is used for the treatment of dermal infections caused by various species of pathogenic dermatophytes and yeasts. The primary action of clotrimazole is against dividing and growing organisms.

In vitro, clotrimazole exhibits fungistatic and fungicidal activity against isolates of *Trichophyton rubrum, Trichophyton mentagrophytes, Epidermophyton floccosum, Microsporum canis, Candida* spp. and *Malassezia pachydermatis (Pityrosporum canis)*. Resistance to clotrimazole is very rare among the fungi that cause superficial mycoses.

In an induced otitis externa infected with *Malassezia pachydermatis*, 1% clotrimazole in the gentamicin-betamethasone-clotrimazole ointment vehicle was effective both microbiologically and clinically in terms of reduction of exudate odor and swelling.

In studies of the mechanism of action, the minimum fungicidal concentration of clotrimazole caused leakage of intracellular phosphorus compounds into the ambient medium with concomitant breakdown of cellular nucleic acids and accelerated potassium efflux. These events began rapidly and extensively after addition of the drug. Clotrimazole is very poorly absorbed following dermal application.

Gentamicin-Betamethasone-Clotrimazole: By virtue of its three active ingredients,

O

gentamicin-betamethasone-clotrimazole ointment has antibacterial, anti-inflammatory, and antifungal activity.

In component efficacy studies, the compatibility and additive effect of each of the components were demonstrated. In clinical field trials, gentamicin-betamethasone-clotrimazole was effective in the treatment of otitis externa associated with bacteria and *Malassezia pachydermatis*. Gentamicin sulfate USP, betamethasone valerate, USP and clotrimazole, USP ointment reduced discomfort, redness, swelling, exudate, and odor, and exerted a strong antimicrobial effect.

Dosage and Administration: The external ear should be thoroughly cleaned and dried before treatment. Remove foreign material, debris, crusted exudates, etc., with suitable non-irritating solutions. Excessive hair should be clipped from the treatment area. After verifying that the eardrum is intact, instill 4 drops (2 drops from the 215 g bottle) of gentamicin-betamethasone-clotrimazole ointment twice daily into the ear canal of dogs weighing less than 30 lbs. Instill 8 drops (4 drops from the 215 g bottle) twice daily into the ear canal of dogs weighing 30 lbs or more. Therapy should continue for 7 consecutive days.

Contraindication(s): If hypersensitivity to any of the components occurs, treatment should be discontinued and appropriate therapy instituted. Concomitant use of drugs known to induce ototoxicity should be avoided. Do not use in dogs with known perforation of eardrums.

Precaution(s): Store between 2° and 25°C (36° and 77°F).

Shake well before use when using the 215 gram bottle.

Caution(s): Federal law restricts this drug to use by or on the order of a licensed veterinarian.

The use of gentamicin-betamethasone-clotrimazole ointment has been associated with deafness or partial hearing loss in a small number of sensitive dogs (eg. geriatric). The hearing deficit is usually temporary. If hearing or vestibular dysfunction is noted during the course of treatment, discontinue use of gentamicin-betamethasone-clotrimazole ointment immediately and flush the ear canal thoroughly with a non-ototoxic solution. Corticosteroids administered to dogs, rabbits, and rodents during pregnancy have resulted in cleft palate in offspring. Other congenital anomalies including deformed forelegs, phocomelia, and anasarca have been reported in offspring of dogs which received corticosteroids during pregnancy.

Clinical and experimental data have demonstrated that corticosteroids administered orally or parenterally to animals may induce the first stage of parturition if used during the last trimester of pregnancy and may precipitate premature parturition followed by dystocia, fetal death, retained placenta and metritis.

Identification of infecting organisms should be made either by microscopic roll smear evaluation or by culture as appropriate. Antibiotic susceptibility of the pathogenic organism(s) should be determined prior to use of this preparation.

If overgrowth of nonsusceptible bacteria, fungi or yeasts occur, or if hypersensitivity develops, treatment should be discontinued and appropriate therapy instituted.

Administration of recommended doses of gentamicin-betamethasone-clotrimazole ointment beyond 7 days may result in delayed wound healing.

Avoid ingestion. Adverse systemic reactions have been observed following the oral ingestion of some topical corticosteroid preparations. Patients should be closely observed for the usual signs of adrenocorticoid overdosage which include sodium retention, potassium loss, fluid retention, weight gain, polydipsia and/or polyuria. Prolonged use or overdosage may produce adverse immunosuppressive effects.

Use of corticosteroids, depending on dose, duration, and specific steroid, may result in endogenous steroid production inhibition following drug withdrawal. In patients presently receiving or recently withdrawn from corticosteroid treatments, therapy with a rapidly acting corticosteroid should be considered in especially stressful situations.

Before instilling any medication into the ear, examine the external ear canal thoroughly to be certain the tympanic membrane is not ruptured in order to avoid the possibility of transmitting infection to the middle ear as well as damaging the cochlea or vestibular apparatus from prolonged contact.

Warning(s): For otic use in dogs only.

Keep this and all drugs out of the reach of children.

Toxicology: Clinical and safety studies with gentamicin sulfate USP, betamethasone valerate, USP and clotrimazole, USP ointment have shown a wide safety margin at the recommended dose level in dogs (see Cautions/Side Effects).

Side Effects:

Gentamicin: While aminoglycosides are absorbed poorly from skin, intoxication may occur when aminoglycosides are applied topically for prolonged periods of time to large wounds, burns, or any denuded skin, particularly if there is renal insufficiency. All aminoglycosides have the potential to produce reversible and irreversible vestibular, cochlear and renal toxicity.

Betamethasone: Side effects such as SAP and SGPT enzyme elevations, weight loss, anorexia, polydipsia, and polyuria have occurred following the use of parenteral or systemic synthetic corticosteroids in dogs. Vomiting and diarrhea (occasionally bloody) have been observed in dogs and cats.

Cushing's syndrome in dogs has been reported in association with prolonged or repeated steroid therapy.

Clotrimazole: The following have been reported occasionally in humans in connection with the use of clotrimazole: erythema, stinging, blistering, peeling, edema, pruritus, urticaria, and general irritation of the skin not present before therapy.

Presentation: Gentamicin-betamethasone-clotrimazole ointment is available in 7.5 gram and 15 gram tubes as well as in 215 gram plastic bottles.

Compendium Code No.: 10910390 January 2001

OVABAN® TABLETS ℞

Schering-Plough **Progestogen**

(Megestrol Acetate) Veterinary

NADA No.: 091-603

Active Ingredient(s): Description: Each tablet contains megestrol acetate in a dried yeast base. Two strengths are available: 5 mg and 20 mg tablets.

Indications: OVABAN® (Megestrol Acetate) is recommended for the postponement of estrus and the alleviation of false pregnancy in the dog.

Pharmacology: Megestrol acetate is a tasteless, odorless, crystalline powder with a melting point of about 217°C and a molecular weight of 384.5. It is a potent oral progestogen with marked anti-estrogenic properties and more active in the Clauberg assay than progesterone given subcutaneously.[1]

Megestrol acetate is rapidly metabolized. In dogs given the recommended oral dose for 8 days, the drug (as metabolites) was recovered from feces and urine. An average of 50% of the total dose was excreted by the last treatment day and 90% within an additional 15 days.[2]

Dosage and Administration: OVABAN® Tablets are palatable and may be given intact or crushed and mixed in the food. It is recommended that the full dosage regimen be completed to produce the desired effect. In addition, OVABAN® Tablets should not be administered for more than two consecutive treatments.

Postponement of estrus: Treatment regimens for the postponement of estrus depend on the stage of the estrus cycle when therapy is initiated.

Proestrus treatment: Administer 1 mg per pound of body weight per day for 8 days. An 8-day course of OVABAN® is recommended for dogs in proestrus. Vaginal bleeding and vulvar swelling will usually disappear in 3 to 8 days. The time until the next estrus occurs is dependent on the timing of the dose and will vary with individual dogs. In clinical studies, return to estrus ranged from 2 to 9 months with the majority recurring in 4 to 6 months.

Treatment should be initiated during the first 3 days of proestrus for best results. Examination of vaginal smears is strongly recommended prior to OVABAN® therapy to confirm detection of proestrus.

Once therapy is started, the dog should be confined for 3 to 8 days or until cessation of bleeding, since dogs in proestrus may accept a male. Once bleeding stops, male dogs should not be attracted.

Anestrus treatment: Administer 0.25 mg per pound of body weight per day for 32 days. A 32-day course of OVABAN® therapy is recommended for dogs in anestrus. The dog will remain anestrus as long as therapy is continued.

The next estrus may occur any time after cessation of treatment. In clinical studies, there was a range of 2 to 9 months, though most dogs returned to estrus in 4 to 6 months.

Alleviation of false pregnancy: Administer 1 mg per pound of body weight per day for 8 days. OVABAN® can be administered to alleviate the physical and nervous symptoms of false pregnancy. Remission of symptoms will usually occur in 3 to 8 days. For best results, treatment should be initiated at the first signs of false pregnancy.

Contraindication(s): OVABAN® Tablets must not be used in dogs when there is evidence of uterine disease, or in the presence of disease in any of the reproductive organs.

OVABAN® Tablets should not be used in dogs prior to or during their first estrus cycle.

OVABAN® Tablets must not be used in pregnant dogs. It should be established that there was no exposure to a male dog during the previous heat period.

OVABAN® Tablets must not be used in dogs with mammary tumors. Growth of some mammary tumors may be stimulated by exogenous progestogens.

Should estrus occur within 30 days after cessation of treatment with OVABAN® Tablets, mating should be prevented.

Precaution(s): Store between 2° and 30°C (36° and 86°F).

Caution(s): Federal law restricts this drug to use by or on the order of a licensed veterinarian.

Clinical studies indicate the full dosage regimen must be completed to produce the desired effect.

OVABAN® Tablets should not be administered for more than two consecutive treatments.

For use in dogs only.

Toxicology: Toxicity Studies: Megestrol acetate at 0.1 to 0.25 mg/kg/day orally in dogs for 36 months did not produce any gross abnormalities. Histologically, cystic endometrial hyperplasia was observed at 36 months. These uterine changes were reversed when dosing ceased and the dogs were observed for an additional 15 months.

In another study, megestrol acetate was administered orally at the rate of 0.5 mg/kg/day for 5 months. At this observation period, no abnormalities were noted except signs of mild uterine hyperplasia which regressed at the final observation period which was 4 months from cessation of treatment.

Additionally, dogs were treated with 2 mg/kg/day for 64 days. Uterine biopsies were taken at day 32 and day 64. Uteri were found to be normal at day 32. At day 64, signs of early cystic endometritis were evident. No other abnormalities were observed.

Cox[3] compared several progestogens in dogs and determined megestrol acetate did not produce cystic endometrial hyperplasia at the recommended doses.

Burke[4] reported studies in dogs that show no effects on conception, litter size, mortality, or sex ratios following megestrol acetate at recommended dosage for 32 days.

Megestrol acetate at 0.25 mg/lb. for 32 days did not affect the dam or litter when administered during the first half of pregnancy, however, reduced litter size and livability resulted when the dose was given during the last half of pregnancy.

Side Effects: Oral doses of megestrol acetate are well tolerated. Occasionally, the following transient progestational side effects were noted in clinical studies; mammary enlargement, lactation, listlessness, increased appetite, and temperament change. In clinical studies, confirmed cases of pyometra occurred in 0.6% of the cases.

References: Available upon request.

Presentation: OVABAN® Tablets, 5 mg (NDC 0061-0867) and 20 mg (NDC 0061-0509), are available in bottles of 100 tablets.

Compendium Code No.: 10471442 Rev. 1/00

OVA FLOAT ZN 118™

Butler **Fecal Flotation**

Active Ingredient(s): Zinc sulfate.

Indications: OVA FLOAT Zn 118™ is a premeasured amount of zinc sulfate to be reconstituted and used for flotation techniques of fecal analysis.

Dosage and Administration: Fill the container with warm water to the brim, secure the cap and shake well. Repeat shaking - do not add additional water. This will produce a specific gravity of 1.18.

Warning(s): Keep out of the reach of children.

Presentation: 1 gallon container.

Compendium Code No.: 10821311

OVASOL ℞

Vedco **Fecal Flotation**

Description: Fecal flotation medium.

Ingredient(s): Zinc sulfate.

Indications: OVASOL is a premeasured amount of zinc sulfate heptahydrate to be reconstituted and used for flotation techniques of fecal analysis.

Procedure: Fill container with warm water up to the brim, secure cap and shake well. Repeat shaking - Do not add additional water. This will produce a specific gravity of 1.18.

Caution(s): Federal law restricts this drug to use by or on the order of a licensed veterinarian.

Warning(s): For veterinary use only.

Keep out of reach of children.

Presentation: 2.9 lbs (1.32 kg).

Compendium Code No.: 10941620

OVASSAY® PLUS

Synbiotics **Fecal Flotation**

U.S. Vet. Lic. No.: 312

Components: Fecal floatation analysis kit and collection devices.

Indications: For the examination of fecal samples for ova.

Test Principle: Salts and sugars have been used to produce high specific gravity media to aid in the separation of common parasite ova from the debris in fecal matter. The fecal flotation method has been adapted for use in the kit. When a fecal specimen is homogenized in a solution with specific gravity of approximately 1.2, the common ova float at the top of the liquid while most of the fecal debris settles to the bottom. The top portion of the liquid is then collected on a coverslip and examined microscopically.

Test Procedure: Materials required, but not provided:

1. Microscope slides and coverslips (22 mm^2).
2. Microscope capable of low and 100X magnification.

Specimen information:

1. Approximately 2 g of feces are required.
2. Prompt processing of the specimen will aid in the accurate diagnosis of parasitic infection.

Time required for the test:
Total time: 10-15 minutes.
Working time: Approximately five (5) minutes.
Set up time: 30-45 seconds.
Reading time: Three (3) to four (4) minutes.

Examine the specimen for any visible adult parasites or tapeworm segments.

Prepare the zinc sulfate solution according to the directions on the bottle of OVASSAY® plus zinc sulfate crystals.

How to collect a stool sample:

1. Remove insert. A little cup-like area forms the bottom of the insert.
2. Fill small end by pressing it into stool. Loose stools may need to be scooped into the small end of insert.
3. Place loaded insert back into the device.

Analyzing the Fecal Sample

1. With the filled insert in place, add OVASSAY® Plus Zinc Sulfate Solution until fluid level reaches about half way up the device.
2. Mix thoroughly by rotating the insert. This separates eggs and cysts from fecal sample.
3. With the bottom edge of the cap, apply pressure on the insert until it is firmly seated in the device.
4. Carefully fill the device to the brim with flotation solution to form a meniscus.
5. Place a 22 mm^2 cover slip on the meniscus for 5 minutes.
6. Then transfer slip to slide for microscopic examination. Examine under low power and 100x for ova.

Close the cap tightly for easy disposal.

Examination of the slide: Moving the slide systematically, scan the entire preparation. Identify all parasite eggs and grade the quantity of eggs to relate to light, medium or heavy infections. Do not confuse epithelial cells, air bubbles, etc. with the ova.

Limitation of procedure: Generally, the ova of common nematode parasites are readily detected by the technique. Tapeworm eggs would be detected if gravid proglotids are found in the samples or if they burst and disseminate eggs into the feces.

Discussion: The OVASSAY® Plus fecal diagnostic system has been found to compare favorably with standard flotation techniques for identifying parasitic infections. It requires a minimum of manipulative procedures, and the materials and remaining debris are disposable in a manner that minimizes chances of contamination of the technician's hands or laboratory area.

Presentation: 50 tests per kit.

Compendium Code No.: 11150150

OVINE ECOLIZER®

Novartis Animal Vaccines **Antiserum**

Escherichia coli Antiserum

U.S. Vet. Lic. No.: 303

Composition: OVINE ECOLIZER® is prepared from the blood of horses hyperimmunized with four whole cell cultures of *Escherichia coli*, each containing K99 pilus antigen. The antiserum contains phenol, thimerosal, and oxytetracycline as preservatives.

Indications: For the use in the prevention and treatment of colibacillosis caused by *Escherichia coli* in newborn lambs.

Dosage and Administration: Administer 5 mL orally to each lamb within 12 hours after birth. Slowly syringe the contents into the back of the lamb's mouth. Colostrum should be fed to each lamb.

Precaution(s): Store in the dark at 35-45°F (2-7°C). Do not freeze. Use the entire contents when first opened.

Caution(s): Anaphylactic reactions may occur following the use of this biological. Symptomatic treatment: Epinephrine.

Warning(s): Do not administer within 21 days of slaughter.

Discussion: OVINE ECOLIZER® consists of antibodies to the K99 antigen that is present on four different whole cell cultures of *E. coli*. This is a natural method of antibody production using hyperimmunized horses.

The K99 antigen is one of the main attributes of virulence found on the enterotoxigenic strains of *E. coli* (ETEC) isolated from calves, sheep and pigs. This pilus has been shown to be one of the main attachment mechanisms which allow the ETEC to colonize in the small intestine. Since colonization is an essential step in the pathogenesis of diarrhea, interference of attachment will prevent this disease. Controlled challenge studies have shown that the K99 pilus antibody will prevent the attachment of the *E. coli* bacteria, thus preventing fatal enterotoxigenic diarrhea. The absorption of the K99 antibodies from the lamb's intestine and entrance into the general circulatory system will have a significant effect on the lamb also, helping to prevent the septicemic form of the disease.

Colibacillosis is an acute contagious infection in young lambs characterized by enteritis and septicemia caused by *E. coli*.

The disease is very common in young lambs that are being raised in closely confined operations where the presence of *E. coli* bacteria is such that oral ingestion cannot be prevented.

The disease causes diarrhea and dehydration and may result in death despite heroic treatment that includes antibiotics, electrolytes, and other antishock procedures. Death could occur before diarrhea appears due to the severe septicemia that can occur.

Trial Data: OVINE ECOLIZER® Challenge Study:

Group	Cumulative Average Clinical Score	% of Protection Against Death
Controls	20.1	50%
OVINE ECOLIZER®	7.8	83%

Study over seven days. Data on file at Novartis Animal Vaccines, Inc.

Presentation: Available in 2 dose (10 mL) disposable syringes (12 disposable syringes per box).

Compendium Code No.: 11140213

OVINE ECTHYMA VACCINE

Colorado Serum **Vaccine**

Ovine Ecthyma Vaccine, Live Virus

U.S. Vet. Lic. No.: 188

Active Ingredient(s): Contains dried ovine ecthyma vaccine and a bottle of sterile rehydrating fluid labeled as sterile diluent.

Penicillin and streptomycin are added as preservatives.

Indications: Recommended for vaccinating both sheep and goats against disease caused by ovine ecthyma virus or against sore mouth infection.

Dosage and Administration: It is advisable to vaccinate each new lamb and kid crop because dried scabs retain the infective virus which is resistant to heat and cold and can be expected to survive from year to year. Exposure to infection can occur during shipping. Range lambs moving into feedlots should be vaccinated at least 10 days before shipment to prevent the spread of the disease after arrival.

Normally only healthy animals should be vaccinated but experience has shown that in outbreaks of sore mouth, vaccination of the infected sheep and lambs tends to shorten the course of disease.

OVINE ECTHYMA VACCINE is a live virus vaccine. Do not use within 24 hours of dipping or spraying.

Rehydrating: Rehydrate the vaccine just prior to use. Contents of the diluent vial may be withdrawn with a sterile syringe and needle, without removing the stoppers, and transferred to the bottle of dried vaccine. If a syringe is not convenient the aluminum seals may be pried off the bottles with a pocket knife and the diluent poured into the vaccine bottle.

Shake the vaccine bottle until the dried virus substance is completely restored to liquid form. Live virus products contain a stabilizer that may slow rehydration slightly but complete liquefaction will take place within a few moments. The vaccine is then ready to use. When rehydrating the vaccine use only the diluent that is supplied with the product.

The bottle of vaccine contains 100 doses. Select a wool free area of skin, such as the inside of the flank and scarify the outer layer by scratching with the notched handle of the applicator furnished as a part of the package. Scratching need not be deep enough to cause bleeding but should be sufficient to adequately roughen the skin. An area of at least one (1) square inch should be scarified. The vaccine can be applied by dipping the brush into the vaccine bottle or by placing a drop of vaccine on the scarified area and brushing vigorously.

Reddening and a slight swelling of the site of administration should be observed a few days after vaccination. This will develop into raised areas that will rupture and scab over representing a take that indicates successful vaccination. Scabs will dry and fall of in about three (3) weeks.

Precaution(s): Store in the dark at 2-7°C. Do not use chemical disinfectants with the vaccine.

Use the entire contents when the bottle is first opened. Burn the container and all unused contents.

Caution(s): Humans have been accidently infected with ovine ecthyma virus. Lesions that have been described in man are most often on the hands and arms. Usually such infections are not serious but all individuals handling the vaccine should take precautions against infecting themselves with the virus.

Brushes and scarifiers should be used only in a single flock of sheep. If there is a need to use the instrument a second time, it should be sterilized by boiling in water for several minutes.

For veterinary use only.

Warning(s): Do not vaccinate within 21 days before slaughter.

Discussion: Ovine ecthyma (sore mouth) is a contagious disease of sheep and goats caused by a virus. Most commonly this is characterized by vesicular and pustular lesions that progress to the formation of thick scabs on the lips or the skin. The disease exists wherever sheep and goats are raised.

Infected suckling young may transmit the infection to the udder of susceptible ewes. Sores on the mouths of the young and on the udders of the ewes greatly limits feeding and there is a severe economic impact from loss of weight and condition. Uncomplicated cases heal spontaneously in four to five weeks, usually without treatment. If secondary bacterial infections and maggot infestation develop, such invaders can cause fatalities ranging from 10 to 50 percent of the animals.

Treatment is difficult. In small flocks scabs can be removed and the lesions cleansed of maggots. A penetrating antiseptic may be of limited value with respect to bacterial infections. The use of a fly spray will help to restrict maggot re-infestation.

Presentation: 100 dose vials.

Compendium Code No.: 11010270

OVINE POSITIVE REAGENT

Allied Monitor **Mycobacterium Test Reagent**

Active Ingredient(s): Serum obtained from adult sheep, confirmed paratuberculous by culture and necropsy. It is sterile-filtered and lyophilized.

Indications: For use as a positive control in ELISA and AGID against PPA antigen.

Presentation: 1 mL.

Compendium Code No.: 10800041

OVINE TETANUS SHIELD™

Novartis Animal Vaccines **Toxoid**

Tetanus Toxoid

U.S. Vet. Lic. No.: 303

Composition: This product is a highly antigenic toxoid prepared from cultures of *Clostridium tetani* adjuvanted with aluminum hydroxide. Contains penicillin and streptomycin as preservatives.

Indications: For use in healthy sheep as an aid in the prevention and control of disease caused by *Clostridium tetani*.

Dosage and Administration: Shake well before using. Administer 2 mL intramuscularly or subcutaneously. Revaccinate in 2-4 weeks and once annually.

Precaution(s): Store in the dark at 35°-45°F (2°-7°C). Do not freeze. Use entire contents when first opened.

Caution(s): Anaphylactic reactions may occur following the use of this biological. Symptomatic treatment: Epinephrine.

For veterinary use only.

Warning(s): Do not vaccinate within 21 days prior to slaughter.

Discussion: Tetanus is a sporadic disease that affects a wide variety of domestic animals as well as man. The causative agent, *Clostridium tetani,* is an obligate anaerobe, which means that it only grows where there is no oxygen present. The bacteria are present in manure and soil as spores, which are highly resistant to destruction. When these spores are carried into a wound such as a puncture, castration or tail docking wound, tissue damage can produce an area devoid of oxygen, which allows the spores to begin growing. These growing bacteria produce a potent neurotoxin, which travels along nerve tissue to the central nervous system (CNS), where it produces the visible symptoms of tetanus. If large amounts of toxin are produced at the wound site, this toxin can also diffuse in the lymph system and blood and be carried to the CNS in this manner. There is also some evidence that preformed toxin can be absorbed through wounds in the mouth when the toxin is consumed in spoiled feeds.

Tetanus usually affects animals less than six months of age, in large part because this is the time when procedures such as tail docking and castration are normally performed. Symptoms usually appear after a 4-10 day incubation period. The first symptoms noticed are erect ears, a stiff tail, and prolapsed third eyelids. These progress to generalized muscle spasms and a tightly clenched jaw (hence the name "lockjaw"). All four limbs will be rigid and extended, causing the animal to assume a "sawhorse" stance. The animal is overly sensitive to touch and sound, either of which can precipitate severe spasms. Death is caused by respiratory failure and usually occurs within 3-10 days after symptoms appear. The mortality rate approaches 100% of affected animals.

In the early stages of the disease, tetanus may be confused with strychnine poisoning, hypomagnesemia or acute laminitis. Treatment of tetanus is usually futile, although large doses of penicillin and antitoxin may be helpful. Prevention includes removal of any sharp objects that may cause puncture wounds, and using clean techniques when performing surgeries such as castration. The best prevention is the use of OVINE TETANUS SHIELD™ to build up active immunity in the animals prior to time of exposure to the disease. Sheep are given a 2 mL dose either subcutaneously or intramuscularly, with revaccination in 2-4 weeks, followed by an annual booster to maintain solid immunity.

Trial Data:

Geometric Mean Tetanus ELISA Titers[1]			
Treatment	Initial Titers	14 Days Post 1st Vac. Titer	14 Days Post 2nd Vac. Titer
IM Vaccinates	3.1	6.2	34.9
SQ Vaccinates	2.8	13.4	22.6
Controls - No Vaccine	2.6	3.1	3.7

IM = Intramuscular SQ = Subcutaneous

Animals were vaccinated with two doses of product administered two weeks apart. Both the IM and SQ vaccinates showed strong increases in ELISA titers, indicating an excellent response to the vaccine regardless of route of administration.

Antitoxin Titers[1]			
Treatment	Initial Titers	14 Days Post 1st Vac. Titer	14 Days Post 2nd Vac. Titer
IM Vaccinates	<0.1 AU	>0.1 AU	>0.1 AU
SQ Vaccinates	<0.1 AU	>0.1 AU	>0.1 AU
Controls - No Vaccine	<0.1 AU	<0.1 AU	<0.1 AU

IM = Intramuscular SQ = Subcutaneous AU = Antitoxin Units

Both the IM and SQ vaccine groups showed responses above the 0.1 American Tetanus Antitoxin Units per milliliter required to demonstrate adequate protection.

[1]Data on file at Novartis Animal Vaccines, Inc. and with USDA.

O

References: Available upon request.

Presentation: Available in 50 dose (100 mL) bottles (F207).

Compendium Code No.: 11140222

OVUM FLOTATION DRY

Centaur **Fecal Flotation**

Fecal Flotation Medium

Active Ingredient(s): OVUM FLOTATION DRY is a pre-measured amount of zinc sulfate to be reconstituted.

Indications: Used for flotation techniques of fecal analysis.

Directions: Shake well before using.

Fill container with warm water to brim, secure cap and shake well. Repeat shaking - do not add additional water. This will product a specific gravity of 1.18.

Precaution(s): Protect from freezing. Keep tightly closed when not in use.

Caution(s): For animal use only.

Presentation: 1.32 kg (2.9 lbs).

Manufactured by: Unavet, North Kansas City, MO 64116.

Compendium Code No.: 14880250 Iss. 11-94

OVUM FLOTATION DRY

Phoenix Pharmaceutical **Fecal Flotation**

Active Ingredient(s): OVUM FLOTATION DRY is a pre-measured amount of zinc sulfate to be reconstituted.

Indications: Used for flotation techniques of fecal analysis.

Directions: Shake well before using.

Fill the container with warm water to brim, secure cap and shake well. Repeat shaking - do not add additional water. This will product a specific gravity of 1.18.

Precaution(s): Protect from freezing. Keep tightly closed when not in use.

Caution(s): For animal use only.

Warning(s): Keep out of reach of children.

Presentation: 1 gallon (1.32 kg, 2.9 lbs) (NDC 57319-360-09).

Manufactured by: Ameri-Pac Inc., St. Joseph, MO 64502

Compendium Code No.: 12560601 Rev. 6-01

OVUPLANT™ ℞

Fort Dodge **Deslorelin**

Deslorelin-Implantable Sustained Release Gonadotropin Releasing Hormone (GnRH) Analog (Deslorelin) for Ovulation Induction in Mares

NADA No.: 141-044

Active Ingredient(s): Implant Description: Each implant contains 2.1 mg deslorelin (as deslorelin acetate) in an inert matrix. The implant is white, cylindrical and approximately 2.3 mm in diameter and 3.6 mm in length.

Indications: OVUPLANT™ is indicated for inducing ovulation within 48 hours in estrous mares with an ovarian follicle greater than 30 mm in diameter. Follicular size should be determined by rectal palpation and/or ultrasonography prior to treatment.

Pharmacology: Description: OVUPLANT™ (deslorelin) is a synthetic GnRH analog in a biocompatible sustained release subcutaneous implant with the indication to induce ovulation in the estrous mare within 48 hours. OVUPLANT™ is formulated as a cylindrical implant in a preloaded syringe with an attached needle (implanter).

Chemical Structure:

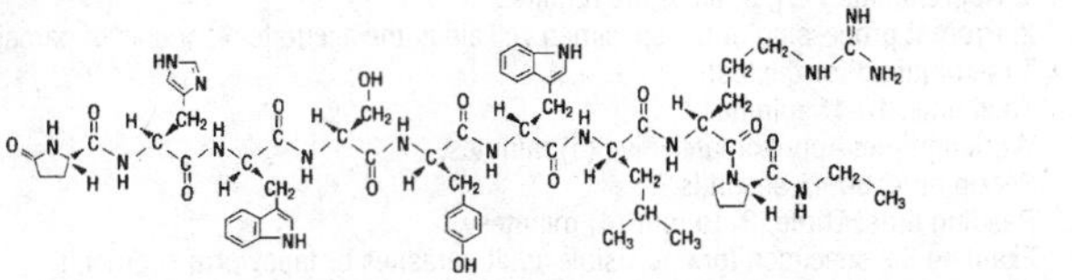

[(6-D-tryptophan-9-(N-ethyl-L-prolinamide)-10-deglycinamide)] GnRH

Clinical Pharmacology: The long duration of estrus in mares and the varying time from the onset of estrus to ovulation typically results in the need for multiple breedings, or inseminations, in order to achieve conception. OVUPLANT™ has been shown to induce ovulation within 48 hours after treatment in more than 86% of mares with a developing follicle greater than 30 mm in diameter. Deslorelin induces ovulation by increasing the levels of endogenous LH. Induction of ovulation decreases the duration of estrus and reduces the number of breedings or inseminations required.

This product is intended to optimize breeding management through shortening the estrous period. By reducing the number of breedings to achieve conception, stallions may be more efficiently managed. When used to induce ovulation in mares being bred by artificial insemination of fresh cooled or frozen semen, the number of inseminations can be reduced. Abnormalities in neonatal viability and foal behavior related to the use of deslorelin have not been observed in foals born to treated mares.

Dosage and Administration: Breeding or insemination prior to ovulation has been shown to produce higher conception rates than post-ovulation breedings or inseminations. To manage a breeding properly, a mare in estrus with an ovarian follicle greater than 30 mm should be implanted with OVUPLANT™. The mare should then be bred or inseminated prior to ovulation within the next 48 hours. The mare should be monitored to ensure ovulation did occur and further breedings are not required. If ovulation does not occur within the 48 hour period, continue breeding according to routine reproductive management procedures.

One implant should be placed subcutaneously in the neck of an estrous mare that has been determined by rectal palpation and/or ultrasonography to have an ovarian follicle greater than 30 mm in diameter. Effectiveness is contingent upon accurate diagnosis of estrus and detection of a developing follicle greater than 30 mm in diameter. Only one (1) implant should be administered per mare during a given estrus.

Select the implant site by locating an area midway between the head and shoulder over the muscle mass of the neck and away from subcutaneous nerves and vessels. Prepare the implantation site by thoroughly cleaning the skin with an appropriate disinfectant.

Insert the entire length of the needle subcutaneously and fully depress the implanter plunger. Slowly withdraw the needle while pressing the skin at the insertion site. Examine the implanter to verify the implant has not remained in the syringe or needle. It may be possible to palpate the implant *in situ.* This biocompatible implant is absorbed and does not require removal.

Do not attempt to reuse the implanter. Dispose of the implanter appropriately.

Precaution(s): Store at refrigerator temperature 2° to 8°C (36° to 46°F).

Caution(s): Federal law (USA) restricts this drug to use by or on the order of a licensed veterinarian.

Warning(s): Not for use in horses intended for food. Keep out of reach of children. Not for human use. Exercise caution to avoid accidental injection. In case of human injection, consult a physician immediately. Do not use if the foil pouch is broken.

Adverse Reactions: Systemic adverse reactions have not been observed with the use of OVUPLANT™ (deslorelin) at the recommended dosage in more than 550 mares.

Trial Data: Safety: Minor local swellings, sensitivity to touch, and elevated skin temperature at the implantation site have been observed. These signs resolved uneventfully without treatment in 1-5 days.

In a tolerance study, administration of ten times the recommended dose of OVUPLANT™ to reproductively sound mares caused neuroendocrine downregulation resulting in inactive ovaries. No other adverse effects were observed.

In a combined target animal safety and reproductive safety study, mares receiving 1x, 3x or 5x the recommended dose of OVUPLANT™ for 3 consecutive cycles did not show any clinical adverse effects. During the second and third estrus, the 3x and 5x treatment groups showed a dose related increase in the interestrous interval, the duration of estrus, and slower growth of the lead follicle. These short-term signs of interference with neuroendocrine regulation did not prevent cyclicity, appearance of estrus or ovulations and did not impair fertility.

Presentation: NDC 0856-5200-01 — Five (5) implants per carton.

OVUPLANT™ (deslorelin) is formulated as a cylindrical implant in a preloaded syringe with an attached needle (implanter). Each preloaded implanter is individually packaged in a foil pouch.

Manufactured by: Wildlife Pharmaceuticals, Inc.

Developed by: Peptech Animal Health Pty Limited, North Ryde NSW 2113 Australia.

Compendium Code No.: 10031400 5200C

OXOJECT ℞

Vetus **Oxytocin**

(Oxytocin Injection)

NADA No.: 099-169

Active Ingredient(s): Each mL contains: Oxytocin activity equivalent to 20 USP posterior pituitary units with sodium hydroxide/acetic acid for pH adjustment.

Chlorobutanol (as preservative) . . . . 2.4 mg

Water for Injection . . . . q.s.

Indications: Oxytocin may be used as a uterine contractor to precipitate and accelerate normal parturition and the postpartum evacuation of uterine debris. In surgery, it may be used postoperatively following caesarean section to facilitate involution and resistance to the large inflow of blood. It will contract smooth muscle cells of the mammary gland for milk letdown if the udder is in the proper physiological state.
Dosage and Administration: (Intravenous, Intramuscular or Subcutaneous)

	U.S.P Units
For obstetrical use:	
Horses and Cows	100 (5 mL)
Sows and Ewes	30-50 (1½ to 2½ mL)
For milk letdown:	
Cows	10-20 (½ to 1 mL)
Sows	5-20 (¼ to 1 mL)

Contraindication(s): Do not use in dystocia due to the abnormal presentation of the fetus until a correction is accomplished.
Precaution(s): Store at controlled room temperature between 15°C and 30°C (59°F-86°F). Do not freeze.
As this is a multi-dose container, this preparation should be handled under aseptic conditions.
Caution(s): Federal law restricts this drug to use by or on the order of a licensed veterinarian.
For animal use only.
Keep out of reach of children.
For prepartum use, full relaxation of the cervix should be accomplished, either naturally or by the administration of estrogen prior to oxytocin therapy.
Hazardous - Not for human use (California).
Presentation: 100 mL sterile, multiple dose vial.
Compendium Code No.: 14440690

OXY 500 CALF BOLUS

Boehringer Ingelheim **Oxytetracycline-Oral**
Oxytetracycline HCl-Broad Spectrum Antibiotic
NADA No.: 141-002
Active Ingredient(s): Each bolus contains 500 mg oxytetracycline hydrochloride.
Indications: OXY 500 CALF BOLUS is recommended for oral administration for the control and treatment of the following diseases of beef and dairy calves caused by organisms sensitive to oxytetracycline: bacterial enteritis caused by *Salmonella typhimurium* and *Escherichia coli* (colibacillosis); bacterial pneumonia (shipping fever complex, pasteurellosis) caused by *Pasteurella multocida.*
Pharmacology: OXY 500 CALF BOLUS is an oral formulation containing oxytetracycline, a broad-spectrum antibiotic that possesses a high order of stability and potent antimicrobial activity, for use in beef and dairy calves.
Dosage and Administration: Read the entire leaflet carefully before using this product.
Dosage Levels: For the control of bacterial enteritis and bacterial pneumonia in beef and dairy calves: administer orally half a bolus (250 mg oxytetracycline hydrochloride) per 100 lb of body weight every 12 hours (5 mg/lb body weight in divided doses) for up to four consecutive days.
For the treatment of bacterial enteritis and bacterial pneumonia in beef and dairy calves: administer orally one bolus (500 mg oxytetracycline hydrochloride) per 100 lb of body weight every 12 hours (10 mg/lb body weight in divided doses) for up to four consecutive days.
Dosage should continue until the animal returns to normal and for 24 to 48 hours after symptoms have subsided. Treatment should not exceed four consecutive days.
Precaution(s): Recommended Storage: Store at room temperatures 15°-30°C (59°-86°F).
Caution(s): Exceeding the recommended dosage level of one bolus (500 mg oxytetracycline hydrochloride) per 100 lb body weight every 12 hours, or administration at the recommended level for more than four consecutive days, may result in antibiotic residues beyond the withdrawal time.
Organisms may vary in their degree of susceptibility to any chemotherapy. If no improvement is observed after recommended treatment, diagnosis and susceptibility should be reexamined.
Rarely do side reactions or allergic manifestations occur in calves treated with OXY 500 CALF BOLUS. If any unusual reactions are noted, discontinue use of the drug immediately and call a veterinarian.
Since bacteriostatic drugs may interfere with the bactericidal action of penicillin, it is advisable to avoid giving OXY 500 CALF BOLUS in conjunction with penicillin.
Restricted drug (California) - Use only as directed.
For use in animals only.
Warning(s): There is no pre-slaughter withdrawal period when used at the recommended dosage level. Not for use in lactating dairy cattle. A withdrawal period has not been established for this product in pre-ruminating calves. Do not use in calves to be processed for veal.
Discussion: Care of Sick Animals: The use of antibiotics in the management of disease is based on an accurate diagnosis and an adequate course of treatment. When properly used in the treatment of disease caused by oxytetracycline susceptible organisms, most animals treated with OXY 500 CALF BOLUS show a noticeable improvement within 24 to 48 hours. It is recommended that the diagnosis and treatment of animal diseases be carried out by a veterinarian. Since many diseases look alike but require different types of treatment, the use of professional veterinary and laboratory services can reduce treatment time, costs and needless losses. Good housing, sanitation and nutrition are important in the maintenance of healthy animals and are essential in the treatment of disease.
Presentation: 25 bolus and 100 bolus containers.
Compendium Code No.: 10281210 BI 6834-1 1/01

OXY 1000 CALF BOLUS

Boehringer Ingelheim **Oxytetracycline-Oral**
Oxytetracycline HCl-Broad-Spectrum Antibiotic
NADA No.: 141-002
Active Ingredient(s): Each bolus contains 1000 mg oxytetracycline hydrochloride.
Indications: OXY 1000 CALF BOLUS is recommended for oral administration for the control and treatment of the following diseases of beef and dairy calves caused by organisms sensitive to oxytetracycline: bacterial enteritis caused by *Salmonella typhimurium* and *Escherichia coli* (colibacillosis); bacterial pneumonia (shipping fever complex, pasteurellosis) caused by *Pasteurella multocida.*
Pharmacology: OXY 1000 CALF BOLUS is an oral formulation containing oxytetracycline, a broad-spectrum antibiotic that possesses a high order of stability and potent antimicrobial activity, for use in beef and dairy calves.
Dosage and Administration: Read entire leaflet carefully before using this product.
Dosage Levels: For the control of bacterial enteritis and bacterial pneumonia in beef and dairy calves: administer orally half a bolus (500 mg oxytetracycline hydrochloride) per 200 lb of body weight every 12 hours (5 mg/lb body weight in divided doses) for up to four consecutive days.
For the treatment of bacterial enteritis and bacterial pneumonia in beef and dairy calves: administer orally one bolus (1000 mg oxytetracycline hydrochloride) per 200 lb of bodyweight every 12 hours (10 mg/lb body weight in divided doses) for up to four consecutive days.
Dosage should continue until the animal returns to normal and for 24 to 48 hours after symptoms have subsided. Treatment should not exceed four consecutive days.
Precaution(s): Recommended Storage: Store at room temperature 15°-30°C (59°-86°F).
Caution(s): Exceeding the recommended dosage level of one bolus (1000 mg oxytetracycline hydrochloride) per 200 lb body weight every 12 hours, or administration at the recommended level for more than four consecutive days, may result in antibiotic residues beyond the withdrawal time.
Organisms may vary in their degree of susceptibility to any chemotherapy. If no improvement is observed after recommended treatment, diagnosis and susceptibility should be re-examined.
Rarely do side reactions or allergic manifestations occur in calves treated with OXY 1000 CALF BOLUS. If any unusual reactions are noted, discontinue use of the drug immediately and call a veterinarian.
Since bacteriostatic drugs may interfere with the bactericidal action of penicillin, it is advisable to avoid giving OXY 1000 CALF BOLUS in conjunction with penicillin.
Restricted drug (California) - Use only as directed.
Use only as directed.
For use in animals only.
Warning(s): There is no pre-slaughter withdrawal period when used at the recommended dosage level. Not for use in lactating dairy cattle. A withdrawal period has not been established for this product in pre-ruminating calves. Do not use in calves to be processed for veal.
Discussion: Care of Sick Animals: The use of antibiotics in the management of disease is based on an accurate diagnosis and an adequate course of treatment. When properly used in the treatment of disease caused by oxytetracycline susceptible organisms, most animals treated with OXY 1000 CALF BOLUS show a noticeable improvement within 24 to 48 hours. It is recommended that the diagnosis and treatment of animal diseases be carried out by a veterinarian. Since many diseases look alike but require different types of treatment, the use of professional veterinary and laboratory services can reduce treatment time, costs and needless losses. Good housing, sanitation and nutrition are important in the maintenance of healthy animals and are essential in the treatment of disease.
Presentation: 25 bolus and 100 bolus containers.
Compendium Code No.: 10281221 BI 6836-1 1/01

OXYBIOTIC™-100

Butler **Oxytetracycline Injection**
(Oxytetracycline Hydrochloride Injection) 100 mg/mL
NADA No.: 108-963
Active Ingredient(s): Each mL contains:
Oxytetracycline hydrochloride .... 100 mg
Magnesium chloride hexahydrate .... 5.75% w/v
Water for injection .... 17.0% w/v
Sodium formaldehyde sulfoxylate (as preservative) .... 1.3% w/v
Propylene glycol .... q.s.
Also contains 2-aminoethanol to adjust pH.
Indications: Oxytetracycline hydrochloride injection is for the treatment of diseases caused by pathogens susceptible to oxytetracycline hydrochloride in beef cattle and nonlactating dairy cattle only.
Dosage and Administration: Inject 3-5 mg per pound of body weight intravenously once a day for a maximum of four (4) consecutive days.
Precaution(s): Do not store at temperatures above 77°F (25°C).
Caution(s): Keep out of the reach of children. For intravenous use only.
Warning(s): Discontinue treatment at least 19 days prior to slaughter. Not for use in lactating dairy cattle.
Presentation: 500 mL sterile multiple-dose vials.
Compendium Code No.: 10821320

OXYBIOTIC™-200

Butler **Oxytetracycline Injection**
(Oxytetracycline injection)
ANADA No.: 200-123
Active Ingredient(s): OXYBIOTIC™-200 (Oxytetracycline Injection) is a sterile preconstituted solution of the broad spectrum antibiotic oxytetracycline. Each mL contains 200 mg of oxytetracycline and, on a w/v basis, 40.0% 2-pyrrolidone, 5.0% povidone, 1.8% magnesium oxide, 0.2% sodium formaldehyde sulfoxylate (as a preservative), monoethanolamine and/or hydrochloric acid is required to adjust pH.
Indications: OXYBIOTIC™-200 is intended for use in the treatment of the following diseases in beef cattle, nonlactating dairy cattle and swine when due to oxytetracycline-susceptible organisms:
Cattle: In cattle, OXYBIOTIC™-200 is indicated in the treatment of pneumonia and shipping fever complex associated with *Pasteurella* spp. and *Hemophilus* spp; infectious bovine keratoconjunctivitis (pinkeye) caused by *Moraxella bovis;* foot-rot and diphtheria caused by *Fusobacterium necrophorum;* bacterial enteritis (scours) caused by *Escherichia coli;* wooden tongue caused by *Actinobacillus ligniersii;* leptospirosis caused by *Leptospira pomona;* and wound infections and acute metritis caused by strains of staphylococci and streptococci organisms sensitive to oxytetracycline.
Swine: In swine, OXYBIOTIC™-200 (oxytetracycline injection) is indicated in the treatment of bacterial enteritis (scours, colibacillosis) caused by *Escherichia coli;* pneumonia caused by *Pasteurella multocida;* and leptospirosis caused by *Leptospira pomona.*
In sows, OXYBIOTIC™-200 is indicated as an aid in the control of infectious enteritis (baby pig scours, colibacillosis) in suckling pigs caused by *Escherichia coli.*
Dosage and Administration: Dosage:
Cattle: OXYBIOTIC™-200 is to be administered by intramuscular or intravenous injection to beef cattle and nonlactating dairy cattle.
A single dosage of 9 milligrams of OXYBIOTIC™-200 per pound of body weight administered intramuscularly is recommended in the treatment of the following conditions: 1) bacterial pneumonia caused by *Pasteurella* spp. (shipping fever) in calves and yearlings, where

O

re-treatment is impractical due to husbandry conditions, such as cattle on range, or where their repeated restraint is inadvisable; 2) infectious bovine keratoconjunctivitis (pinkeye) caused by *Moraxella bovis.*

OXYBIOTIC™-200 can also be administered by intravenous or intramuscular injection at a level of 3 to 5 milligrams of oxytetracycline per pound of body weight per day. In the treatment of severe foot-rot and advanced cases of other indicated diseases, dosage level of 5 milligrams per pound of body weight per day is recommended. Treatment should be continued 24 to 48 hours following remission of disease signs; however, not to exceed a total of four consecutive days. Consult your veterinarian if improvement is not noted within 24 to 48 hours of the beginning of treatment.

Swine: In swine a single dosage of 9 milligrams of OXYBIOTIC™-200 per pound of body weight administered intramuscularly is recommended in the treatment of bacterial pneumonia caused by *Pasteurella multocida* in swine, where re-treatment is impractical due to husbandry conditions or where repeated restraint is inadvisable.

OXYBIOTIC™-200 can also be administered by intramuscular injection at a level of 3 to 5 milligrams of oxytetracycline per pound of body weight per day. Treatment should be continued 24 to 48 hours following remission of the disease signs; however, not to exceed a total of four consecutive days. Consult your veterinarian if improvement is not noted within 24 to 48 hours of the beginning of treatment.

For sows, administer once intramuscularly 3 milligrams of oxytetracycline per pound of body weight approximately 8 hours before farrowing or immediately after completion of farrowing.

For swine weighing 25 lb of body weight and under, OXYBIOTIC™-200 should be administered undiluted for treatment at 9 mg/lb but should be administered diluted for treatment at 3 to 5 mg/lb body weight.

	9 mg/lb Dosage Volume of Undiluted OXYBIOTIC™-200	3 or 5 mg/lb Dosage Volume of Diluted OXYBIOTIC™-200		
Body Weight	9 mg/lb	3 mg/lb	Dilution*	5 mg/lb
5 lb	0.2 mL	0.6 mL	1:7	1.0 mL
10 lb	0.5 mL	0.9 mL	1:5	1.5 mL
25 lb	1.1 mL	1.5 mL	1:3	2.5 mL

*To prepare dilutions, add one part OXYBIOTIC™-200 to three, five or seven parts of sterile water, or 5 percent dextrose solution as indicated; the diluted product should be used immediately.

Directions for Use: OXYBIOTIC™-200 is intended for use in the treatment of disease due to oxytetracycline-susceptible organisms in beef cattle, nonlactating dairy cattle and swine. A thoroughly cleaned, sterile needle and syringe should be used for each injection (needles and syringes may be sterilized by boiling in water for 15 minutes). In cold weather, OXYBIOTIC™-200 should be warmed to room temperature before administration to animals. Before withdrawing the solution from the bottle, disinfect the rubber cap on the bottle with suitable disinfectant, such as 70 percent alcohol. The injection site should be similarly cleaned with the disinfectant. Needles of 16 to 18 gauge and 1 to 1½ inches long are adequate for intramuscular injections. Needles 2 to 3 inches are recommended for intravenous use.

Intramuscular Administration: Intramuscular injections should be made by directing the needle of suitable gauge length into the fleshy part of a thick muscle such as in the rump, hip, or thigh regions; avoid blood vessels and major nerves. Before injecting the solution, pull back gently on the plunger. If blood appears in the syringe, a blood vessel has been entered; withdraw the needle and select a different site. No more than 10 mL should be injected intramuscularly at any one site in adult beef cattle and nonlactating dairy cattle, and not more than 5 mL per site in adult sine; rotate injection sites for each succeeding treatment. The volume administered per injection site should be reduced according to age and body size so that 1 to 2 mL per site is injected in small calves.

Intravenous Administration: OXYBIOTIC™-200 (oxytetracycline injection) may be administered intravenously to beef cattle and nonlactating dairy cattle. As with all highly concentrated materials, OXYBIOTIC™-200 should be administered slowly by the intravenous route.

O

Preparation of the Animal for Injection:

1. Approximate location of vein. The jugular vein runs in the jugular groove on each side of the neck from the angle of the jaw to just above the brisket and slightly above and to the side of the windpipe. (See Fig. I)
2. Restraint. A stanchion or chute is ideal for restraining the animal. With a halter, rope, or cattle leader (nose tongs), pull the animal's head around the side of the stanchion, cattle chute, or post in such a manner to form a bow in the neck (See Fig. II), then snub the head securely to prevent movement. By forming the bow in the neck, the outside curvature of the bow tends to expose the jugular vein and make it easily accessible. Caution: Avoid restraining the animal with a tight rope or halter around the throat or upper neck which might impede blood flow. Animals that are down present no problem so far as restraint is concerned.
3. Clip hair in area where injection is to be made (over the vein in the upper third of the neck). Clean and disinfect the skin with alcohol or other suitable antiseptic.

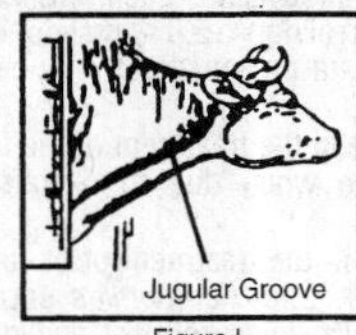

Figure I

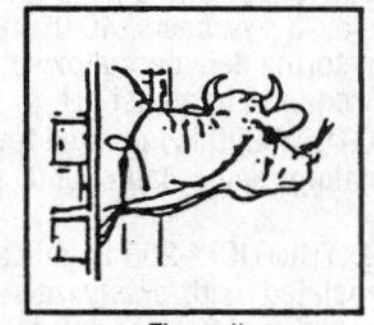
Figure II

Entering the Vein and Making the Injection:

1. Raise the vein. This is accomplished by tying the choke rope tightly around the neck close to the shoulder. The rope should be tied in such a way that it will not come loose and so that it can be untied quickly by pulling the loose end (See Fig. II). In thick-necked animals, a block of wood placed in the jugular groove between the rope and hide will help considerably in applying the desired pressure at the right point. The vein is a soft flexible tube through which blood flows back to the heart. Under ordinary conditions it cannot be seen or felt with the fingers. When the flow of blood is blocked at the base of the neck by the choke rope, the vein becomes enlarged and rigid because of the back pressure. If the choke rope is sufficiently tight, the vein stands out and can be easily seen and felt in thin-necked animals. As a further check in identifying the vein, tap it with the fingers in front of the choke rope. Pulsations that can be seen or felt with the fingers in front of the point being tapped will confirm the fact that the vein is properly distended. It is impossible to put the needle into the vein unless it is distended. Experienced operators are able to raise the vein simply by hand pressure, but the use of a choke rope is more certain.
2. Inserting the needle. This involves three distinct steps. First, insert the needle through the hide. Second, insert the needle into the vein. This may require two or three attempts before the vein is entered. The vein has a tendency to roll away from the point of the needle, especially if the needle is not sharp. The vein can be steadied with the thumb and finger of one hand. With the other hand, the needle point is placed directly over the vein, slanting it so that its direction is along the length of the vein, either toward the head or toward the heart. Properly positioned this way, a quick thrust of the needle will be followed by a spurt of blood through the needle, which indicates that the vein has been entered. Third, once in the vein, the needle should be inserted along the length of the vein all the way to the hub exercising caution to see that the needle does not penetrate the opposite side of the vein. Continuous steady flow of blood through the needle indicates that the needle is still in the vein. If blood does not flow continuously, the needle is out of the vein (or clogged) and another attempt must be made. If difficulty is encountered, it may be advisable to use the vein on the other side of the neck.
3. While the needle is being placed in proper position in the vein, an assistant should get the medication ready so that the injection can be started without delay after the vein has been entered.
4. Making the injection. With the needle in position as indicated by continuous flow of blood, release the choke rope by a quick pull on the free end. This is essential - the medication cannot flow into the vein while it is blocked. Immediately connect the syringe containing OXYBIOTIC™-200 (oxytetracycline injection) to the needle and slowly depress the plunger. If there is resistance to depression of the plunger, this indicates that the needle has slipped out of the vein (or is clogged) and the procedure will have to be repeated. Watch for any swelling under the skin near the needle which would indicate that the medication is not going into the vein. Should this occur, it is best to try the vein on the opposite side of the neck.
5. Removing the needle. When injection is complete, remove needle with straight pull. Then apply pressure over the area of injection momentarily to control any bleeding through needle puncture, using cotton soaked in alcohol or other suitable antiseptic.

Precaution(s): OXYBIOTIC™-200 does not require refrigeration; however, it is recommended that it be stored at room temperature. 15°-30°C (59°-86°F). The antibiotic activity of oxytetracycline is not appreciably diminished in the presence of body fluids, serum, or exudates. Keep from freezing.

Caution(s): Exceeding the highest recommended dosage level of drug per pound of body weight per day, administering more than the recommended number of treatments, and/or exceeding 10 mL intramuscularly per injection site in adult beef cattle and nonlactating dairy cattle, and 5 mL intramuscularly per injection site in adult swine, may result in antibiotic residues beyond the withdrawal period.

Reactions of an allergic or anaphylactic nature, sometimes fatal, have been known to occur in hypersensitive animals following the injection of oxytetracycline. Such adverse reactions can be characterized by signs such as restlessness, erection of hair, muscle trembling; swelling of eyelids, ears, muzzle, anus and vulva (or scrotum and sheath in males); labored breathing, defecation and urination, glassy-eyes appearance, eruption of skin plaques, frothing from the mouth, and prostration. Pregnant animals that recover may subsequently abort. At the first sign of any adverse reaction, discontinue use of this product and administer epinephrine at the recommended dosage levels. Call a veterinarian immediately.

Shock may be observed following intravenous administration, especially where highly concentrated materials are involved. To minimize this occurrence, it is recommended that OXYBIOTIC™-200 be administered slowly by this route.

Shortly after injection, treated animals may have transient hemoglobinuria resulting in darkened urine.

As with all antibiotic preparations, use of the drug may result in overgrowth of nonsusceptible organisms, including fungi. A lack of response by the treated animal, or the development of new signs, may suggest that an overgrowth of nonsusceptible organisms has occurred. If any of these conditions occur, consult your veterinarian.

Since bacteriostatic drugs may interfere with the bactericidal action of penicillin, it is advisable to avoid giving OXYBIOTIC™-200 in conjunction with penicillin.

Warning(s): Discontinue treatment at least 28 days prior to slaughter of cattle and swine. Not for use in lactating dairy animals.

Livestock drug, not for human use.

Restricted drug (California), use only as directed.

Discussion: Care of Sick Animals: The use of antibiotics in the management of diseases is based on an accurate diagnosis and an adequate course of treatment. When properly used in the treatment of diseases caused by oxytetracycline susceptible organisms, most animals that have been treated with oxytetracycline injection show a noticeable improvement within 24 to 48 hours. It is recommended that the diagnosis and treatment of animal diseases be carried out by a veterinarian. Since many diseases look alike but require different types of treatment, the use of professional veterinary and laboratory services can reduce treatment time, costs and needless losses. Good housing, sanitation and nutrition are important in the maintenance of healthy animals, and are essential in the treatment of diseased animals.

Presentation: 100, 250 and 500 mL vials.

Compendium Code No.: 10821331

OXYCURE™-100

Vedco **Oxytetracycline Injection**

(Oxytetracycline Hydrochloride Injection) Antibiotic 100 mg/mL

ANADA No.: 200-068

Active Ingredient(s): Each mL contains:

Oxytetracycline base (as HCl) . . . . . 100 mg
Magnesium Chloride • $6H_2O$ . . . . . 5.76% w/v
Water For Injection . . . . . 17% v/v
Propylene Glycol . . . . . q.s.

with sodium formaldehyde sulfoxylate, 1.3% w/v as a preservative and monoethanolamine for pH adjustment.

Indications: General Indications for Use: A great many of the pathogens involved in cattle diseases are known to be susceptible to oxytetracycline hydrochloride therapy. Many strains of organisms, however, have shown resistance to oxytetracycline. In the case of certain coliforms, streptococci and staphylococci, it may be advisable to conduct culture and sensitivity testing to determine susceptibility of the infecting organism to oxytetracycline. In this manner, the likelihood of successful treatment with OXYCURE™-100 (Oxytetracycline Hydrochloride Injection) solution can be determined in advance.

Diseases for Which OXYCURE™-100 (Oxytetracycline Hydrochloride Injection) is Indicated: The use of OXYCURE™-100 (Oxytetracycline Hydrochloride Injection) is indicated in beef cattle, beef calves, non-lactating dairy cattle and dairy calves for treatment of the following disease conditions caused by one or more of the oxytetracycline sensitive pathogens listed as follows:

Disease	Causative Organism(s) Which Show Sensitivity to OXYCURE™-100 (Oxytetracycline HCl Injection)
Bacterial pneumonia and shipping fever complex associated with *Pasteurella* spp.	*Pasteurella* spp.
Bacterial enteritis (scours)	*Escherichia coli*
Necrotic pododermatitis (foot rot)	*Fusobacterium necrophorum*
Calf diphtheria	*Fusobacterium necrophorum*
Wooden tongue	*Actinobacillus lignieresii*
Wound infections; acute metritis; traumatic injury	Caused by oxytetracycline-susceptible strains of streptococcal and staphylococcal organisms.

Pharmacology: Description: OXYCURE™-100 (Oxytetracycline Hydrochloride Injection) is a sterile ready-to-use preparation containing 100 mg/mL oxytetracycline HCl, for administration of the broad spectrum antibiotic, oxytetracycline, by injection.

Antibiotic Action of Oxytetracycline: Oxytetracycline is effective against a wide range of gram-negative and gram-positive organisms that are pathogenic for cattle. The antibiotic is primarily bacteriostatic in effect, and is believed to exert its antimicrobial action by the inhibition of microbial protein synthesis. The antibiotic activity of oxytetracycline is not appreciably diminished in the presence of body fluids, serum or exudates. Since the drugs in the tetracycline class have similar antimicrobial spectra, organisms can develop cross resistance among them. Oxytetracycline is concentrated by the liver in the bile and excreted in the urine and feces at high concentrations and in a biologically active form.

Dosage and Administration: Treat at the first clinical signs of disease.

The intravenous injection of 3 to 5 mg of oxytetracycline hydrochloride per pound of body weight per day (3 to 5 mL per 100 lbs body weight) is the recommended dosage.

Severe foot-rot and the severe forms of the indicated diseases should be treated with 5 mg per pound of body weight. Surgical procedures may be indicated in some forms of foot-rot or other conditions.

In disease treatment, the daily dose of OXYCURE™-100 (Oxytetracycline Hydrochloride Injection) should be continued to 24 to 48 hours following remission of disease symptoms; however, not to exceed a total of 4 consecutive days.

Dosage for Injection:

Refer to the table below for proper dosage according to body weight of the animal.

Weight of Animals, Lbs (Beef Cattle, Beef Calves, Non-Lactating Dairy Cattle, Dairy Calves)	Milligrams of Oxytetracycline Hydrochloride per 100 lbs of Body Weight Per Day	Daily Dosage of OXYCURE™-100 Injection (Oxytetracycline Hydrochloride Injection) (mL)
50 lbs	300-500 mg	1.5-2.5 mL
100 lbs	300-500 mg	3-5 mL
200 lbs	300-500 mg	6-10 mL
300 lbs	300-500 mg	9-15 mL
400 lbs	300-500 mg	12-20 mL
500 lbs	300-500 mg	15-25 mL
600 lbs	300-500 mg	18-30 mL
800 lbs	300-500 mg	24-40 mL
1000 lbs	300-500 mg	30-50 mL
1200 lbs	300-500 mg	36-60 mL
1400 lbs	300-500 mg	42-70 mL

Precaution(s): Store at 59°-86°F.

Note: Solution may darken on storage but potency remains unaffected.

Caution(s): If no improvement occurs within 24 to 48 hours, consult a veterinarian. Do not use the drug for more than 4 consecutive days. Use beyond 4 days or doses higher than maximum recommended dose may result in antibiotic tissue residues beyond the withdrawal period.

The improper or accidental injection of the drug outside of the vein will cause local tissue irritation manifested by temporary swelling and discoloration at the injection site.

Shortly after injection, treated animals may have a transient hemoglobinuria (darkened urine).

Reactions of an allergic or anaphylactic nature, sometimes fatal, have been known to occur in hypersensitive animals following the injection of oxytetracycline solutions, but such reactions are rare.

At the first sign of any adverse reaction or anaphylactic shock (noted by glassy eyes, increased salivation, grinding of the teeth, rapid breathing, muscular tremors, staggering, swelling of the eyelids or collapse), the product should be discontinued. Epinephrine solution at the recommended dosage levels should be administered and a veterinarian should be called immediately.

Because bacteriostatic drugs interfere with the bactericidal action of penicillin, do not give oxytetracycline hydrochloride in conjunction with penicillin.

As with other antibiotics, use of this drug may result in over-growth of non-susceptible organisms. If any unusual symptoms occur or in the absence of a favorable response following treatment, discontinue use immediately and call a veterinarian.

Warning(s): Discontinue treatment with OXYCURE™-100 (Oxytetracycline Hydrochloride Injection) at least 22 days prior to slaughter of the animal. Not for use in lactating dairy animals.

A withdrawal period has not been established for this product in pre-ruminating calves. Do not use in calves to be processed for veal.

For use in animals only.

Restricted Drug (California). Use only as directed.

Keep out of reach of children.

Discussion: Instructions for Care of Sick Animals: The use of antibiotics, as with most medications used in the management of diseases, is based on accurate diagnosis and adequate treatment. When properly used in the treatment of diseases caused by oxytetracycline-susceptible organisms, animals usually show a noticeable improvement within 24 to 48 hours. If improvement does not occur within this period of time, the diagnosis and treatment of animal diseases should be carried out by a veterinarian. The use of professional veterinary and laboratory services can reduce treatment costs, time and needless losses. Good management, housing, sanitation and nutrition are essential in the care of animals and in the successful treatment of disease.

Presentation: OXYCURE™-100 (Oxytetracycline Hydrochloride Injection) is available in 500 mL multidose vials.

Compendium Code No.: 10941640

OXYCURE™ 200

Vedco

Oxytetracycline Injection

(Oxytetracycline)

ANADA No.: 200-123

Active Ingredient(s): OXYCURE™ 200 (oxytetracycline injection) is a sterile preconstituted solution of the broad-spectrum antibiotic oxytetracycline. Each mL contains 200 mg of oxytetracycline base as amphoteric oxytetracycline and, on a w/v basis, 40.0% 2-pyrrolidone, 5.0% povidone, 1.8% magnesium oxide, 0.2% sodium formaldehyde sulfoxylate (as a preservative), monoethanolamine and/or hydrochloric acid as required to adjust pH.

Indications: OXYCURE™ 200 is intended for use in the treatment of the following diseases in beef cattle, nonlactating dairy cattle and swine when due to oxytetracycline-susceptible organisms:

Cattle: In cattle, OXYCURE™ 200 is indicated in the treatment of pneumonia and shipping fever complex associated with *Pasteurella* spp. and *Hemophilus* spp; infectious bovine keratoconjunctivitis (pinkeye) caused by *Moraxella bovis;* foot-rot and diphtheria caused by *Fusobacterium necrophorum;* bacterial enteritis (scours) caused by *Escherichia coli;* wooden tongue caused by *Actinobacillus lignieresii;* leptospirosis caused by *Leptospira pomona;* and wound infections and acute metritis caused by strains of staphylococci and streptococci organisms sensitive to oxytetracycline.

Swine: In swine, OXYCURE™ 200 (oxytetracycline injection) is indicated in the treatment of bacterial enteritis (scours, colibacillosis) caused by *Escherichia coli;* pneumonia caused by *Pasteurella multocida;* and leptospirosis caused by *Leptospira pomona.*

In sows, OXYCURE™ 200 is indicated as an aid in the control of infectious enteritis (baby pig scours, colibacillosis) in suckling pigs caused by *Escherichia coli.*

Dosage and Administration:

Cattle: OXYCURE™ 200 is to be administered by intramuscular or intravenous injection to beef cattle and nonlactating dairy cattle.

A single dosage of 9 milligrams of OXYCURE™ 200 per pound of body weight administered intramuscularly is recommended in the treatment of the following conditions: 1) bacterial pneumonia caused by *Pasteurella* spp. (shipping fever) in calves and yearlings, where re-treatment is impractical due to husbandry conditions, such as cattle on range, or where their repeated restraint is inadvisable; 2) infectious bovine keratoconjunctivitis (pinkeye) caused by *Moraxella bovis.*

OXYCURE™ 200 can also be administered by intravenous or intramuscular injection at a level of 3 to 5 milligrams of oxytetracycline per pound of body weight per day. In the treatment of severe foot-rot and advanced cases of other indicated diseases, dosage level of 5 milligrams per pound of body weight per day is recommended. Treatment should be continued 24 to 48 hours following remission of disease signs; however, not to exceed a total of four consecutive days. Consult your veterinarian if improvement is not noted within 24 to 48 hours of the beginning of treatment.

Swine: In swine a single dosage of 9 milligrams of OXYCURE™ 200 per pound of body weight administered intramuscularly is recommended in the treatment of bacterial pneumonia caused by *Pasteurella multocida* in swine, where re-treatment is impractical due to husbandry conditions or where repeated restraint is inadvisable.

OXYCURE™ 200 can also be administered by intramuscular injection at a level of 3 to 5 milligrams of oxytetracycline per pound of body weight per day. Treatment should be continued 24 to 48 hours following remission of disease signs; however, not to exceed a total of four consecutive days. Consult your veterinarian if improvement is not noted within 24 to 48 hours of the beginning of treatment.

For sows, administer once intramuscularly 3 milligrams of oxytetracycline per pound of body weight approximately 8 hours before farrowing or immediately after completion of farrowing.

For swine weighing 25 lb of body weight and under, OXYCURE™ 200 should be administered undiluted for treatment at 9 mg/lb but should be administered diluted for treatment at 3 to 5 mg/lb body weight.

9 mg/lb Dosage Volume of Undiluted OXYCURE™ 200		3 or 5 mg/lb Dosage Volume of Diluted OXYCURE™ 200		
Body Weight	9 mg/lb	3 mg/lb	Dilution*	5 mg/lb
5 lb	0.2 mL	0.6 mL	1:7	1.0 mL
10 lb	0.5 mL	0.9 mL	1:5	1.5 mL
25 lb	1.1 mL	1.5 mL	1:3	2.5 mL

*To prepare dilutions, add one part OXYCURE™ 200 to three, five or seven parts of sterile water, or 5 percent dextrose solution as indicated; the diluted product should be used immediately.

OXYCURE™ 200 is intended for use in the treatment of disease due to oxytetracycline-susceptible organisms in beef cattle, nonlactating dairy cattle and swine. A thoroughly cleaned, sterile needle and syringe should be used for each injection (needles and syringes may be sterilized by boiling in water for 15 minutes). In cold weather, OXYCURE™ 200 should be warmed to room temperature before administration to animals. Before withdrawing the solution from the bottle, disinfect the rubber cap on the bottle with suitable disinfectant, such as 70 percent alcohol. The injection site should be similarly cleaned with the disinfectant. Needles of 16 to 18 gauge and 1 to 1½ inches long are adequate for intramuscular injections. Needles 2 to 3 inches are recommended for intravenous use.

Intramuscular Administration: Intramuscular injections should be made by directing the needle of suitable gauge and length into the fleshy part of a thick muscle such as in the rump, hip, or thigh regions; avoid blood vessels and major nerves. Before injecting the solution, pull back gently on the plunger. If blood appears in the syringe, a blood vessel has been entered; withdraw the needle and select a different site. No more than 10 mL should be injected intramuscularly at any one site in adult beef cattle and nonlactating dairy cattle, and not more than 5 mL per site in adult swine; rotate injection sites for each succeeding treatment. The volume administered per injection site should be reduced according to age and body size so that 1 to 2 mL per site is injected in small calves.

Intravenous Administration: OXYCURE™ 200 (oxytetracycline injection) may be administered intravenously to beef cattle and nonlactating dairy cattle. As with all highly concentrated materials, OXYCURE™ 200 should be administered *slowly* by the intravenous route.

Precaution(s): Store at room temperature, 15°-30°C (59°-86°F). Keep from freezing.

Caution(s): Exceeding the highest recommended dosage level of drug per pound of body weight per day, administering more than the recommended number of treatments, and/or exceeding 10 mL intramuscularly per injection site in adult beef cattle and nonlactating dairy cattle, and 5 mL intramuscularly per injection site in adult swine, may result in antibiotic residues beyond the withdrawal period.

Reactions of an allergic or anaphylactic nature, sometimes fatal, have been known to occur in hypersensitive animals following the injection of oxytetracycline. Such adverse reactions can be characterized by signs such as restlessness, erection of hair, muscle trembling; swelling of eyelids, ears, muzzle, anus and vulva (or scrotum and sheath in males); labored breathing, defecation and urination, glassy-eyed appearance, eruption of skin plaques, frothing from the mouth, and prostration. Pregnant animals that recover may subsequently abort. At the first sign of any adverse reaction, discontinue use of this product and administer epinephrine at the recommended dosage levels. Call a veterinarian immediately.

Shock may be observed following intravenous administration, especially where highly concentrated materials are involved. To minimize this occurrence, it is recommended that OXYCURE™ 200 be administered slowly by this route.

Shortly after injection, treated animals may have transient hemoglobinuria resulting in darkened urine.

As with all antibiotic preparations, use of the drug may result in overgrowth of nonsusceptible organisms, including fungi. A lack of response by the treated animal, or the development of new signs, may suggest that an overgrowth of nonsusceptible organisms has occurred. If any of these conditions occur, consult your veterinarian.

Since bacteriostatic drugs may interfere with the bactericidal action of penicillin, it is advisable to avoid giving OXYCURE™ 200 in conjunction with penicillin.

Warning(s): Discontinue treatment at least 28 days prior to slaughter of cattle and swine. Not for use in lactating dairy animals.

Livestock drug, not for human use.

Restricted drug (California), use only as directed.

For animal use only.

Keep out of reach of children.

Discussion: OXYCURE™ 200 (oxytetracycline injection) is a sterile, ready-to-use solution for the administration of the broad-spectrum antibiotic oxytetracycline by injection. Oxytetracycline is an antimicrobial agent that is effective in the treatment of a wide range of diseases caused by susceptible gram-positive and gram-negative bacteria.

The antibiotic activity of oxytetracycline is not appreciably diminished in the presence of body fluids, serum, or exudates.

Care of Sick Animals: The use of antibiotics in the management of diseases is based on an accurate diagnosis and an adequate course of treatment. When properly used in the treatment of diseases caused by oxytetracycline-susceptible organisms, most animals that have been treated with oxytetracycline injection show a noticeable improvement within 24 to 48 hours. It is recommended that the diagnosis and treatment of animal diseases be carried out by a veterinarian. Since many diseases look alike but require different types of treatment, the use of professional veterinary and laboratory services can reduce treatment time, costs and needless losses. Good housing, sanitation and nutrition are important in the maintenance of healthy animals, and are essential in the treatment of diseased animals.

Presentation: 100 mL, 250 mL and 500 mL bottles.

Compendium Code No.: 10941631

OXYDEX® GEL ℞

DVM **Antidermatosis Shampoo**

Topical Antibacterial Therapy

Active Ingredient(s): Benzoyl peroxide (5%).

Indications: For the relief of signs associated with superficial and deep pyodermas, folliculitis, seborrhea complex, etc. — and of conditions where an antibacterial, antimicrobial, keratolytic formulation is of benefit. For external use only on dogs and cats.

Directions for Use: Apply once or twice daily to affected areas. Cleanse areas prior to treatment to enhance effect. Use only sufficient medicine as to impart a thin invisible film over the entire lesion. Rub in well so that no excess medication is visible on the hair or surrounding areas. Prevent pet from licking treated areas until gel has dried (1-2 minutes).

Contraindication(s): Contact sensitivity, although not reported in dogs, has been observed in humans (1-2%).

Precaution(s): Store at room temperature.

Caution(s): Federal law restricts this drug to use by, or on the order of, a licensed veterinarian.

Avoid contact with eyes.

May bleach colored fabrics. Rub in well so that no residue remains.

Warning(s): Keep out of reach of children.

Presentation: 1 fl oz (30 g) plastic tubes (NDC 47203-210-01).

U.S. Pat. No. 4,075,353

Compendium Code No.: 11420451 Rev 0199

OXYDEX® SHAMPOO

DVM **Antidermatosis Shampoo**

Antimicrobial Degreasing Cleansing Moisturizing Formulation

Active Ingredient(s): Benzoyl peroxide 2.5%.

Indications: For relief of signs associated with superficial and deep pyodermas, seborrhea complex, etc. and of conditions where an antimicrobial, follicular flushing is of benefit in dogs and cats.

OXYDEX® Shampoo is a potent, antimicrobial, cleansing and degreasing formulation in an elegant, fragranced, soap-free, lathering shampoo base.

Directions for Use: Shake well before use.

Wet coat thoroughly. Begin by applying to affected areas, and then proceed to apply product over entire body. When the entire coat is treated, allow to stand 5-10 minutes. Rinse thoroughly with water. OXYDEX® Shampoo may be used as often as necessary or as directed by veterinarian.

Precaution(s): Store at room temperature.

Caution(s): Avoid contact with eyes. If contact occurs, rinse thoroughly with water. If irritation develops, discontinue and consult your veterinarian.

May bleach colored fabrics.

Warning(s): Keep out of reach of children.

Presentation: 8 fl oz (237 mL) (NDC 47203-200-08), 12 fl oz (355 mL) (NDC 47203-200-12), and 1 gallon (3.78 L) (NDC 47203-200-28).

Compendium Code No.: 11420461 Rev 0199

Seeking additional information?
Consult the product manufacturer.
Their addresses appear in
the Manufacturer / Distributor Index.

OXY-GARD™ ACTIVATED PEROXIDE SANITIZING TEAT DIP

Ecolab Food & Bev. Div. **Teat Dip & Spray**

Active Ingredient(s): Active ingredients include hydrogen peroxide 0.5%, lactic acid 1.7%, and sodium linear alkylate sulfonate, 0.5%.

Indications: A peroxide-based teat dip that provides broad spectrum germicidal activity both before and after milking.

Dosage and Administration: To Use: Directions For Teat Dipping

Pre-Milking: Fill teat cup with OXY-GARD™. Do not dilute. Before each cow is milked, dip the teats as far as possible into the teat dip cup containing OXY-GARD™. Wipe teats dry after dipping, using single-service towels to avoid contamination of milk.

Udder and teats which are heavily soiled should be washed before using a pre-milking teat dip. Teats should then be dried with a single service towel and dipped in OXY-GARD™, wiping the teats dry before milking.

Post-Milking: Immediately after milking, use OXY-GARD™ at full strength. Submerge entire teat in OXY-GARD™ solution. Allow to air dry. Do not wipe. Always use fresh, full strength OXY-GARD™. If product in dip cup becomes visibly dirty, discard contents and replenish with undiluted product. Do not reuse or return used product to the original container Do not turn cows out in freezing weather until OXY-GARD™ is completely dry.

Use proper procedures for udder washing or pre-milking teat dipping just prior to next milking to avoid contamination of milk.

Important: Do not mix OXY-GARD™ with any other teat spray, dip or other products. If transferred from this container to any other, make sure that other container is thoroughly pre-cleaned and bears the proper container labeling for OXY-GARD™.

Directions For Teat Spraying: Use a post-milking spray on each teat as an aid in a complete cow-care program to help reduce the spread of organisms which may cause mastitis. Immediately after milking, use OXY-GARD™ at full strength. Spray entire teat with OXY-GARD™ solution. Allow to air dry. Do not wipe. Always use fresh, full strength OXY-GARD™. Do not turn cows out in freezing weather until OXY-GARD™ is completely dry.

Wash entire udder and teats thoroughly just prior to next milking with appropriate udder wash product solution to avoid contamination of milk. Use proper procedures for udder washing.

Precaution(s): Protect from freezing. If frozen, mix well by shaking or rolling container.

Caution(s): OXY-GARD™ is not intended to cure or help the healing of chapped or irritated teats. In case of teat irritation or chapping, have the condition examined and, if necessary, treated by a veterinarian.

Warning(s): For cautionary and first aid information, consult the Material Safety Data Sheet (MSDS).

Presentation: Available in 4/1 gallon (4/3.78 L) case, 5 gallon (18.9 L) pail, and 15 gallon (56.8 L) and 55 gallon (208.2 L) drums.

Compendium Code No.: 14490121

OXYGLOBIN® SOLUTION ℞

Biopure **Oxygen Carrying Fluid**

hemoglobin glutamer-200 (bovine)

NADA No.: 141-067

Active Ingredient(s): Description: OXYGLOBIN® contains 13 g/dL polymerized hemoglobin of bovine origin in a modified Lactated Ringer's Solution containing Water for Injection USP 100 g/dL, NaCl USP 113 mmol/L, KCl USP 4 mmol/L, $CaCl\text{-}2H_2O$ USP 1.4 mmol/L, NaOH NF 10 mmol/L, Sodium Lactate USP 27 mmol/L, N-acetyl-L-cysteine USP 200 mg/dL. It has an osmolality of 300 mOsm/kg. It is a sterile, clear dark purple solution with a pH of 7.8. It is a distribution of hemoglobin polymers with less than 5% of the hemoglobin as unstabilized tetramers, approximately 50% has a molecular weight between 65 and 130 kD, and no more than 10% has a molecular weight >500 kD. It contains less than the detectable level of 3.5 μg/mL free-glutaraldehyde and 0.05 EU/mL endotoxin.

Indications: OXYGLOBIN® is indicated for the treatment of anemia in dogs by increasing systemic oxygen content (plasma hemoglobin concentration) and improving the clinical signs associated with anemia, regardless of the cause of anemia (hemolysis, blood loss, or ineffective erythropoiesis) (See Effectiveness).

Pharmacology: OXYGLOBIN® is a hemoglobin-based oxygen carrying fluid which increases plasma and total hemoglobin concentration and thus increases arterial oxygen content. The terminal elimination half-life of the drug is estimated to range between 18 and 43 hours for dosages of 10-30 mL/kg (Table A) in dogs. The increase in half-life with dose suggests a saturable elimination process. Depending on the dose, greater than 95% of the administered dose is expected to be eliminated from the body at 4 to 9 days after infusion. A laboratory study in dogs established that an increase in total hemoglobin by as little as 0.7 mg/dL with a hemoglobin-based oxygen carrying fluid restored normal tissue oxygenation.[1]

Table A provides data from a laboratory study on the post-infusion duration (hours) for which plasma OXYGLOBIN® levels remained above this therapeutically critical level (1 g/dL).

Table A: Pharmacokinetic parameters at multiple dose levels after a single infusion of OXYGLOBIN®

Dose (mL/kg)	Immediate post infusion concentration (g/dL)	Duration (hours): OXYGLOBIN® levels over 1 g/dL	Terminal half-Life* (hours)	Cleared from plasma (days)***
10	1.5-2.0	11-23	18-26	4-5
15	2.0-2.5	23-39	19-30	4-6
21	3.4-4.3	66-70	25-34	5-7
30	3.6-4.8	74-82	22-43**	5-9**

* range based on mean ± SD

** range based on estimated mean value with bounds of a 95% prediction interval

*** range based on 5 terminal half-lives

Metabolism and Excretion: In a toxicokinetic study involving 24 healthy young adult male Beagle dogs, transient hemoglobinuria was noted for less than 4 hours after completion of the OXYGLOBIN® infusion. The duration of hemoglobinuria in diseased dogs has not been determined.

Dosage and Administration: The recommended dosage of OXYGLOBIN® is a one time dose of 10-30 mL/kg of body weight administered intravenously at a rate of up to 10 mL/kg/hr (See Cautions). The choice of dose within the recommended range will vary with the patient and the clinical situation. Pharmacokinetic data show that there is an increase in the duration of action with increasing dose. (See Pharmacology).

For recommendations on patient monitoring during and immediately following OXYGLOBIN® administration and discussion of conditions which may warrant adjustment in the administration rate see Cautions section. If desired, OXYGLOBIN® may be warmed to 37°C prior to administration.

Remove overwrap prior to use and use within 24 hours. OXYGLOBIN® should be administered using aseptic technique via a standard intravenous infusion set and catheter through a central or peripheral vein at a rate of 10 mL/kg/hr. Do not administer with other fluids or drugs via the same infusion set. Do not add medications or other solutions to the bag. Do not combine the contents of more than one bag.

Use of OXYGLOBIN® does not require cross-matching with recipient blood. A blood transfusion is not contraindicated in dogs which receive OXYGLOBIN® nor is OXYGLOBIN® contraindicated in dogs which have previously received a blood transfusion. OXYGLOBIN® is intended for single dose use. Any unused OXYGLOBIN® should be disposed of in accordance with local requirements for handling veterinary medical waste.

Contraindication(s): Plasma volume expanders, such as OXYGLOBIN®, are contraindicated in dogs with a pre-disposition to volume overload such as those with advanced cardiac disease (i.e., congestive heart failure) or otherwise severely impaired cardiac function or oliguria or anuria. The safety of OXYGLOBIN® was not assessed in dogs with these conditions.

Precaution(s): Storage Conditions: Store at room temperature or refrigerated (2-30°C). Do not freeze. OXYGLOBIN® remains stable for up to 36 months; the expiry date is printed on the bag.

Caution(s): Federal (USA) law restricts this drug to use by or on the order of a licensed veterinarian.

The safety and efficacy of repeat administration of OXYGLOBIN® have not been demonstrated in dogs. The safety of OXYGLOBIN® for use in breeding dogs and pregnant or lactating bitches has not been determined. Teratogenic effects were observed in preliminary reproductive toxicity studies in rats using a related polymerized bovine hemoglobin product. The safety and efficacy of OXYGLOBIN® have not been evaluated in dogs with disseminated intravascular coagulopathy, thrombocytopenia with active bleeding, hemoglobinemia and hemoglobinuria, or autoagglutination.

If an immediate hypersensitivity reaction occurs, infusion of OXYGLOBIN® should be immediately discontinued and appropriate treatment administered. If a delayed type of hypersensitivity reaction occurs, immunosuppressant therapy is recommended.

Concomitant treatment of the cause of anemia should be instituted.

Treatment with OXYGLOBIN® at a dosage of 30 mL/kg results in a mild decrease in PCV immediately post infusion. Due to the dilutional effects of OXYGLOBIN® at that dose, PCV and RBC count are not accurate measures of the degree of anemia for 24 hours following administration. Dilutional effects are not seen at a dosage of 15 mL/kg.

The animal should be adequately hydrated (but not overhydrated) prior to administration. Due to the plasma expanding properties of OXYGLOBIN®, the possibility of circulatory overload should be considered especially when administering adjunctive intravenous fluids, particularly colloidal solutions. If concurrent fluid therapy is administered, it should be temporarily discontinued during infusion of OXYGLOBIN®. Close monitoring of central venous pressure (CVP) during and immediately following administration of OXYGLOBIN® is recommended. If CVP measurement is not feasible, the patient should be carefully monitored for signs of circulatory overload. If CVP increases to a clinically unacceptable level and/or if signs of circulatory overload are observed, the infusion of OXYGLOBIN® should be temporarily discontinued and reinstituted at a slower rate when signs abate and/or CVP decreases. Use of a diuretic may be indicated.

For intravenous use in dogs only.

Warning(s): Overdosage or an excessively rapid administration rate (i.e., > 10 mL/kg/hr) may result in circulatory overload.

Not for human use.

Toxicology: Safety: The safety of OXYGLOBIN® was assessed in 40 healthy Beagle dogs with induced acute, severe normovolemic anemia (total hemoglobin concentration ≈ 5 g/dL). OXYGLOBIN® was administered at 0, 30, 60, and 90 mL/kg twice at a 72 hour interval (equivalent to 0, 1X, 2X, 3X the recommended dose given twice, respectively). 13% Human Serum Albumin (HSA) in Saline was a control (90 mL/kg twice at 72 hour interval) used to determine the effects of a protein load compared with OXYGLOBIN®. There was 100% survival in all groups.

The clinical and pathological effects associated with OXYGLOBIN® were: Transient clinical signs: yellow-orange discoloration of the skin, ear canals, pinnae, mucous membranes (gums), and sclera, red-dark-green discoloration of feces, brown-black discoloration of urine, red spotting of skin and/or lips (less common finding) and decreased appetite and thirst. Vomiting, diarrhea, and decreased skin elasticity occurred within 48 hours of dosing. The frequency and/or intensity of these clinical signs were dose dependent. Clinical pathology: transient, dose dependent red discoloration of plasma, increases in serum enzyme activity with no corresponding microscopic lesions in the liver: 8-fold mean increase in aspartate aminotransferase (AST) activity (peak activity 200 and 677 U/L at 1X and 2X doses given twice, respectively) and 5-fold mean increase in alanine aminotransferase (ALT) activity at 3X dose given twice only (peak activity 372 U/L), increase in serum total protein (peak concentration 9.9 and 14.6 g/dL at 1X and 3X doses given twice, respectively), and hemoglobinuria.

Gross pathology: Dark yellow-orange-brown discoloration (whole body) and dark areas on gall bladder serosa. Histopathology: Hemosiderin in the renal cortex, arteriolitis (limited duration) and activation of tissue macrophages in multiple organs occurred in all OXYGLOBIN® treated groups. Microscopic hemorrhage in the gall bladder and evidence of hepatic macrophage activation occurred in only the 2X and 3X dose groups given twice. Reversible, slight to mild renal tubular damage with limited distribution was seen in both the OXYGLOBIN® treated and HSA in Saline treated control dogs. All findings were dose dependent except for renal tubular protein droplets and casts (indicating saturation of tubular protein reabsorption) and a slight proliferative glomerulopathy (limited duration and distribution) seen in all OXYGLOBIN® treated groups.

Immunohistopathology: Immunofluorescent antibody staining was performed on kidneys of OXYGLOBIN® treated dogs in which a glomerulopathy was identified (5/24) to detect deposition of immune complexes. Only one dog with a glomerulopathy (graded slight) had a focal non-specific IgG deposit in a single area in the outer cortex of one kidney in an estimated amount of 30%. Deposits of <25% is considered normal in dogs.

Immunology: Low levels of canine immunoglobin-G class antibodies to bovine hemoglobin (anti-BvHb) were produced in 11/12 OXYGLOBIN® treated dogs. Due to the limited nature of the study, no relationship between anti-BvHb antibody titer and dose of OXYGLOBIN® administered could be demonstrated. Observed levels of IgG anti-BvHb are not expected to have any toxicological significance in dogs.

Overdose: Accidental overdosage or an excessive rate of administration (i.e., >10 mL/kg/hr) could result in immediate cardiopulmonary effects, in which case infusion of OXYGLOBIN® should be discontinued immediately until signs abate. Signs of circulatory overload such as pulmonary edema, pleural effusion, increased central venous pressure, dyspnea, or coughing may occur. Treatment of circulatory overload may be necessary.

Adverse Reactions: The clinical field trial included dogs with anemia (PCV 6-23%) due to hemolysis (immune mediated, naphthalene toxicity), blood loss (gastrointestinal, traumatic, surgical, rodenticide intoxication), and ineffective erythropoiesis (idiopathic, red cell aplasia, ehrlichiosis, chronic renal failure). Adverse reactions were tabulated by frequency in treated dogs (n=52). The following adverse reactions may be related to OXYGLOBIN® and/or the underlying disease.

Table C: Frequency of Adverse Reactions in OXYGLOBIN® Treated Dogs

Adverse Reaction	% of Treated Dogs with Adverse Reaction (n=52)
Discoloration	
Mucous Membranes[a]	69
Sclera (yellow, red, brown)	56
Urine (orange, red, brown)	52
Skin (yellow)	12
Cardiovascular	
Increased CVP[b]	33
Ventricular Arrhythmia[c]	15
Ecchymoses/Petechiae	8
Bradycardia	6
Gastrointestinal	
Vomiting	35
Diarrhea	15
Anorexia	8
Respiratory	
Tachypnea	15
Dyspnea	14
Pulmonary Edema	12
Harsh Lung Sounds/Crackles	8
Pleural Effusion	6
Miscellaneous	
Fever	17
Death/Euthanasia	15
Peripheral Edema	8
Hemoglobinuria[d]	6
Dehydration	6

[a] yellow, red, purple, brown

[b] measured in 17 dogs only

[c] AV block, tachycardia, ventricular premature contractions

[d] measured in 3 dogs only

Adverse reactions occurring in 4% of the dogs treated with OXYGLOBIN® included: coughing, disseminated intravascular coagulopathy, melena, nasal discharge/crusts (red), peritoneal effusion, respiratory arrest, and weight loss (5-7% body weight). Adverse reactions occurring in less than 2% of the dogs treated with OXYGLOBIN® included: abdominal discomfort on palpation, acidosis, cardiac arrest, cardiovascular volume overload (by echocardiography), collapse, cystitis, dark stool, discolored soft stool (red-brown) and tongue (purple), focal hyperemic areas on gums, forelimb cellulitis/lameness, hematemesis or hemoptysis (unable to differentiate), hypernatremia, hypotension, hypoxemia, lack of neurologic responses, left forebrain signs, nystagmus, pancreatitis, pendulous abdomen, polyuria, pulmonary thromboembolism, ptosis, reddened pinnae with papules/head shaking, reduction in heart rate, thrombocytopenia (worsening), and venous thrombosis.

Trial Data: Clinical Pathology:

Chemistry: The presence of OXYGLOBIN® in serum may result in artifactual increases or decreases in the results of serum chemistry tests, depending on the type of analyzer and reagents used.

Table B: Valid Analytes by Instrumentation

Idexx VetLab	Hitachi All Models	Johnson & Johnson Ektachem/Vitros	Dupont Dimension	Beckman CX7/CX3
sodium	sodium	sodium	sodium	sodium
potassium	potassium	potassium	potassium	potassium
chloride	chloride	chloride	chloride	chloride
BUN	BUN	BUN	BUN	BUN
CK	CK	CK	LDH	calcium
creatinine	glucose	AST	calcium	glucose
	ALT	calcium		
	AST	magnesium		
	calcium	lipase		
		glucose		

Hematology: No interference. Confirm that hemoglobin is measured, not calculated from red blood cell number.

Coagulation: Prothrombin time (PT) and activated partial thromboplastin time (aPTT) can be accurately determined using methods that are mechanical, magnetic, and light scattering. Optical methods are not reliable for coagulation assays in the presence of OXYGLOBIN®. Fibrin degradation products can be measured using the Thrombo-Wellcotest kit (Murex® Kent, England).

Urinalysis: Sediment examination is accurate. Dipstick measurements (i.e., pH, glucose, ketones, protein) are inaccurate while gross discoloration of the urine is present.

Effectiveness:

Dose Response Study: A controlled laboratory study was conducted in 30 healthy dogs with induced acute, severe normovolemic anemia (total hemoglobin concentration ≈ 3 g/dL). OXYGLOBIN®, administered once at a dose of 30 mL/kg, resulted in significantly ($p \leq 0.01$) increased arterial oxygen content at 60 minutes and 24 hours following dosing compared with control dogs. A positive correlation was established between arterial oxygen content (laboratory measured) and plasma hemoglobin concentration (clinically measured).

Clinical Field Study: A well controlled clinical field trial involving 64 client-owned dogs (2 months to 15 years old) weighing 2.1 to 71.8 kg with moderate-severe anemia (total hemoglobin concentration 1.7-6.9 g/dL and PCV 6-23%) was conducted at six clinical sites. Dogs were either treated with OXYGLOBIN® (30 mL/kg) or untreated (with an option to receive OXYGLOBIN® if condition worsened). Relative to pretreatment, plasma hemoglobin concentration significantly increased ($p \leq 0.001$) and clinical signs associated with anemia (lethargy/depression, exercise intolerance, and increased heart rate) significantly improved ($p \leq = 0.001$) in the OXYGLOBIN® treated group for at least 24 hours. Treatment success, defined as the lack of need for additional oxygen carrying support (i.e., a blood transfusion) for 24 hours, was 95% in the OXYGLOBIN® treated group compared with 32% in the control group.

The effectiveness of the lower end of the dose range is supported by controlled laboratory studies (See Pharmacology).

References: Available upon request.

Presentation: OXYGLOBIN® is available as follows: 125 mL single dose bags (NDC 63075-301-01).

OXYGLOBIN® Solution and its method of preparation are covered by one or more of the following United States Patents: No. 5,084,558; No. 5,618,919; No. 5,691,452 and No. 5,296,465.

OXYGLOBIN is a registered trademark of Biopure Corporation.

Compendium Code No.: 10530003 Revision Jan 02

OXY-MYCIN® 100

AgriPharm **Oxytetracycline Injection**

Oxytetracycline HCl

NADA No.: 140-582

Active Ingredient(s): Each mL contains:

Oxytetracycline hydrochloride .... 100 mg
Magnesium chloride hexahydrate.......... 5.7% w/v
Sodium formaldehyde sulfoxylate (as preservative).......... 1.3% w/v
2-aminoethanol .... to adjust pH
Water for injection .... 17.0% w/v
Propylene glycol.......... q.s.

Indications: Oxytetracycline hydrochloride injection is only for the treatment of diseases in beef cattle and nonlactating dairy cattle caused by pathogens susceptible to oxytetracycline HCl.

Dosage and Administration: For intravenous use only.

3-5 mg/lb. of body weight per day for a maximum of four (4) consecutive days.

Precaution(s): Do not store above 77°F (25°C).

Caution(s): Restricted drug (California). Use only as directed.

Keep out of the reach of children.

Warning(s): Discontinue treatment at least 19 days prior to slaughter. Not for use in lactating dairy cattle.

Do not use in calves to be processed for veal.

A withdrawal period has not been established for the product in preruminating calves.

Presentation: 500 mL vials.

Compendium Code No.: 14570790

OXY-MYCIN® 200

AgriPharm **Oxytetracycline Injection**

(Oxytetracycline Injection) Antibiotic

ANADA No.: 200-123

Active Ingredient(s): OXY-MYCIN® 200 (oxytetracycline injection) is a sterile preconstituted solution of the broad-spectrum antibiotic oxytetracycline. Each mL contains 200 mg of oxytetracycline base as amphoteric oxytetracycline and, on a w/v basis, 40.0% 2-pyrrolidone, 5.0% povidone, 1.8% magnesium oxide, 0.2% sodium formaldehyde sulfoxylate (as a preservative), monoethanolamine and/or hydrochloric acid as required to adjust pH.

Indications: For the treatment of disease in beef cattle, nonlactating dairy cattle and swine.

Dosage and Administration:

Cattle: A single dosage of 9 milligrams of oxytetracycline per pound of body weight (4.5 mL/100 lb) administered intramuscularly is recommended in the treatment of the following conditions: 1) bacterial pneumonia caused by *Pasteurella* spp (shipping fever) in calves and yearlings, where re-treatment is impractical due to husbandry conditions, such as cattle on range, or where repeated restraint is inadvisable; 2) infectious bovine keratoconjunctivitis (pinkeye) caused by *Moraxella bovis.*

Swine: A single dosage of 9 milligrams of oxytetracycline per pound of body weight (4.5 mL/100 lb) administered intramuscularly is recommended in the treatment of bacterial pneumonia caused by *Pasteurella multocida* in swine, where re-treatment is impractical due to husbandry conditions or where repeated restraint is inadvisable.

Precaution(s): Store at room temperature 15°C-30°C.

Keep from freezing.

Warning(s): Discontinue treatment at least 28 days prior to slaughter of cattle and swine. Not for use in lactating dairy animals.

Exceeding the highest recommended level of drug per pound of body weight per day, administering more than the recommended number of treatments, and/or exceeding 10 mL intramuscularly per injection site in adult beef cattle and nonlactating dairy cattle, and 5 mL intramuscularly per injection site in adult swine may result in antibiotic residues beyond the withdrawal period.

For animal use only.

Keep out of reach of children.

Presentation: 100 mL, 250 mL and 500 mL vials.

Compendium Code No.: 14570800

OXYTETRACYCLINE-343

Durvet **Water Medication**

Oxytetracycline Hydrochloride Soluble Powder

ANADA No.: 200-066

Active Ingredient(s): Each packet contains 102.4 grams of oxytetracycline HCl and will make:

512 gallons (1398 L) containing 200 mg oxytetracycline HCl per gallon.
256 gallons (969 L) containing 400 mg oxytetracycline HCl per gallon.
128 gallons (484 L) containing 800 mg oxytetracycline HCl per gallon.
Each packet will treat 10,240 pounds of swine.

Indications: Antibiotic for control of specific diseases in poultry and swine.

Directions for Use:

Mix fresh solutions daily - Use as sole source of drinking water - Do not mix this product directly with milk or milk replacers. Administer one hour or two hours after feeding milk or milk replacers.

Consult a poultry diagnostic laboratory or poultry pathologist for diagnosis and advice on dosage for chickens and turkeys. As a generalization, 200 chickens will drink one gallon of water per day for each week of age. Turkeys will consume twice that amount. Administer up to 5 days to swine and 7 to 14 days for chickens and turkeys.

Note: The concentration of drug required in medicated water must be adequate to compensate for variation in the age of the animals, feed consumption rate, and the environmental temperature and humidity, each of which affects water consumption.

Mixing Instructions for Water Medication (Chickens — Turkeys — Swine): For use in water proportioners—Add the following amount to one gallon of stock solution when proportioner is set to meter at the rate of one ounce per gallon.

Disease	Treatment Level	Packs/Gal. Stock Sol.
Chickens		
Control of infectious synovitis caused by *Mycoplasma synoviae*, susceptible to oxytetracycline.	200-400 mg	¼-½ (34-68 g)
Control of chronic respiratory disease (CRD) and air sac infections caused by *Mycoplasma gallisepticum* and *Escherichia coli*, susceptible to oxytetracycline.	400-800 mg	½-1 (68-135.5 g)
Control of fowl cholera caused by *Pasteurella multocida*, susceptible to oxytetracycline.	400-800 mg	½-1 (68-135.5 g)
Turkeys		
Control of hexamitiasis caused by *Hexamita meleagridis* susceptible to oxytetracycline.	200-400 mg	¼-½ (34-68 g)
Control of infectious synovitis caused by *Mycoplasma synoviae* susceptible to oxytetracycline.	400 mg	½ (68 g)
Growing Turkeys — Control of complicating bacterial organisms associated with bluecomb (transmissible enteritis, coronaviral enteritis) susceptible to oxytetracycline.	25 mg/lb body weight	Varies with age and water consumption
Swine		
For the Control and Treatment of the Following Diseases in Swine: Bacterial enteritis caused by *Escherichia coli* and *Salmonella choleraesuis*, susceptible to oxytetracycline. Bacterial pneumonia caused by *Pasteurella multocida*, susceptible to oxytetracycline. For Breeding Swine: Leptospirosis (reducing the incidence of abortions and shedding of leptospira) caused by *Leptospira pomona*, susceptible to oxytetracycline.	10 mg/lb body weight	Varies with age and water consumption

Precaution(s): Recommended Storage: Store below 77°F (25°C).

Caution(s): Use as sole source of oxytetracycline—Not to be used for more than 5 consecutive days in swine and 14 consecutive days in chickens and turkeys.

For use in drinking water only—Not for use in liquid feed supplements.

For use in animals only.

Warning(s): Do not feed to birds producing eggs for human consumption. Discontinue treatment of swine 13 days and turkeys 5 days prior to slaughter.

Keep out of reach of children.

Presentation: 50 x 4.78 oz (135.5 g) packets (NDC 30798-646-75).

Compendium Code No.: 10841251 0696

OXYTET SOLUBLE

Alpharma **Water Medication**

Oxytetracycline HCl-Antibiotic

NADA No.: 130-435

Active Ingredient(s): Each 70 g packet contains 25.6 g of oxytetracycline HCl.

Each 280 g packet contains 102.4 g of oxytetracycline HCl.

Each 1,400 g packet contains 512 g of oxytetracycline HCl.

Indications:

Chickens: Control of infectious synovitis caused by *Mycoplasma synoviae,* chronic respiratory disease (CRD) and air sac infections caused by *Mycoplasma gallisepticum* and *Escherichia coli,* and fowl cholera caused by *Pasteurella multocida,* susceptible to oxytetracycline.

Turkeys: Control of hexamitiasis caused by *Hexamita meleagridis,* infectious synovitis caused by *Mycoplasma synoviae,* susceptible to oxytetracycline.

Growing Turkeys - Control of complicating bacterial organisms associated with bluecomb (transmissible enteritis, coronaviral enteritis), susceptible to oxytetracycline.

Swine: For the control and treatment of the following diseases in swine - Bacterial enteritis caused by *Escherichia coli* and *Salmonella choleraesuis,* bacterial pneumonia caused by *Pasteurella multocida* susceptible to oxytetracycline.

For Breeding Swine: Leptospirosis (reducing the incidence of abortions and shedding of leptospira) caused by *Leptospira pomona,* susceptible to oxytetracycline.

Directions for Use: Mix fresh solutions daily. Use as sole source of drinking water. Do not mix this product directly with milk or milk replacers. Administer 1 hour before or 2 hours after feeding milk or milk replacers. Consult a poultry diagnostic laboratory or poultry pathologist for diagnosis and advice on dosage for chickens and turkeys. As a generalization, 200 chickens will drink 1 gallon of water per day for each week of age. Turkeys will consume twice that amount. Administer up to 5 days to swine and 7 to 14 days for chickens and turkeys.

Note: The concentration of drug required in medicated water must be adequate to compensate for variation in the age of the animal, feed consumption rate, and the environmental temperatures and humidity, each of which affects water consumption.

Mixing Directions for Water Medication: Chickens - Turkeys - Swine:

Water Proportioners: Add the following amount to 1 gallon of stock solution when proportioner is set to meter at the rate of 1 oz per gallon.

Disease	Treatment Level	Packs/Gallon Stock		Gallons/Pack Stock
		70 g packet	280 g packet	1,400 g packet
Chickens				
Control of infectious synovitis caused by *Mycoplasma synoviae*, susceptible to oxytetracycline	200-400 mg	1-2 (70-140 g)	¼-½ (70-140 g)	20-10
Control of chronic respiratory disease (CRD) and air sac infections caused by *Mycoplasma gallisepticum* and *Escherichia coli*, and fowl cholera caused by *Pasteurella multocida*, susceptible to oxytetracycline	400-800 mg	2-4 (140-280 g)	½-1 (140-280 g)	10-5
Turkeys				
Control of hexamitiasis caused by *Hexamita meleagridis*, susceptible to oxytetracycline	200-400 mg	1-2 (70-140 g)	¼-½ (70-140 g)	20-10
Control of infectious synovitis caused by *Mycoplasma synoviae*, susceptible to oxytetracycline	400 mg	2 (140 g)	½ (140 g)	10
Growing Turkeys — Control of complicating bacterial organisms associated with bluecomb (transmissible enteritis, coronaviral enteritis), susceptible to oxytetracycline	25 mg/lb body weight	Varies with age & water consumption	Varies with age & water consumption	Varies with age & water consumption
Swine				
For the control and treatment of the following diseases in swine - Bacterial enteritis caused by *Escherichia coli* and *Salmonella choleraesuis*, bacterial pneumonia caused by *Pasteurella multocida*, and leptospirosis in breeding swine (reducing the incidence of abortions and shedding of leptospira) caused by *Leptospira pomona*, susceptible to oxytetracycline	10 mg/lb body weight	Varies with age & water consumption	Varies with age & water consumption	Varies with age & water consumption

The 70 g packet contains 25.6 g of oxytetracycline HCl and will make:
128 gallons (484 L) containing 200 mg oxytetracycline HCl per gallon.
64 gallons (242 L) containing 400 mg oxytetracycline HCl per gallon.
32 gallons (121 L) containing 800 mg oxytetracycline HCl per gallon.
The 70 g packet will treat 2,560 lbs of swine.

The 280 g packet contains 102.4 g of oxytetracycline HCl and will make:
512 gallons (1936 L) containing 200 mg oxytetracycline HCl per gallon.
128 gallons (484 L) containing 800 mg oxytetracycline HCl per gallon.
The 280 g packet will treat 10,240 lbs of swine.

The 1,400 g packet contains 512 g of oxytetracycline HCl and will make:
2,560 gallons (9,690 L) containing 200 mg oxytetracycline HCl per gallon.
1,280 gallons (4,845 L) containing 400 mg oxytetracycline HCl per gallon.
640 gallons (2,422 L) containing 800 mg oxytetracycline HCl per gallon.
The 1,400 g packet will treat 51,200 lbs of swine.

Precaution(s): Recommended Packet Storage Conditions: Store below 77°F (25°C).

Caution(s): Use as sole source of oxytetracycline. Not to be used for more than five consecutive days in swine or 14 consecutive days in chickens and turkeys.

For use in drinking water only. Not for use in liquid Type B medicated feeds.

Restricted drug, use only as directed (CA).

Livestock remedy. Not for human use. Hazardous remedy.

Warning(s): Do not feed to birds producing eggs for human consumption.

Discontinue treatment of swine 13 days and turkeys 5 days prior to slaughter.

Keep out of reach of children.

Presentation: 2.46 oz (70 g), 9.87 oz (280 g), and 3.09 lb (1,400 g) packets.

Compendium Code No.: 10220492 AHF-049 0012 / AHF-031 0012 / AHF-039 0101

OXYTOCIN INJECTION ℞

AgriLabs **Oxytocin**

20 U.S.P. Units per mL

Active Ingredient(s): Each mL contains:
Oxytocin . . . . 20 U.S.P. units
Chlorobutanol (as a preservative) . . . . 5 mg
Acetic acid 0.25%
In water for injection.

Indications: For obstetrical use in horses and cows, and milk letdown in cows.

Dosage and Administration: For intravenous, intramuscular or subcutaneous use.
For obstetrical use:
Horses and Cows . . . . 100 U.S.P. units (5 mL)
For milk letdown:
Cows . . . . 10 to 20 U.S.P. units (0.5 to 1.0 mL)

Contraindication(s): Do not use in dystocia due to the abnormal presentation of the fetus until correction is accomplished.

Precaution(s): Avoid excessive exposure to heat. Store in a refrigerator between 36°-46°F (2°-8°C). Do not freeze.

Caution(s): Federal law restricts this drug to use by or on the order of a licensed veterinarian.

Keep this and all medications out of the reach of children. For veterinary use only.

Presentation: 100 mL sterile multiple dose vials.

Compendium Code No.: 10581660

OXYTOCIN INJECTION ℞

Aspen **Oxytocin**

NADA No.: 099-169

Active Ingredient(s): Each mL contains: Oxytocin activity equivalent to 20 USP posterior pituitary units with sodium hydroxide/acetic acid for pH adjustment.
Chlorobutanol (as preservative) . . . . 2.4 mg
Water For Injection . . . . q.s.

Indications: Oxytocin may be used as a uterine contractor to precipitate and accelerate parturition and postpartum evacuation of uterine debris. In surgery it may be used post-operatively following cesarean section to facilitate involution and resistance to the large inflow of blood. It will contract smooth muscle cells of the mammary gland for milk letdown if the udder is in proper physiological state.

Dosage and Administration: (Intravenous, Intramuscular or Subcutaneous)

For obstetrical use:	U.S.P. Units	
Horses and Cows	100	(5 mL)
Sows and Ewes	30-50	(1½ to 2½ mL)
Dogs	5-30	(¼ to 1½ mL)
Cats	5-10	(¼ to ½ mL)

For milk letdown:	U.S.P. Units	
Cows	10-20	(½ to 1 mL)
Sows	5-20	(¼ to 1 mL)

Contraindication(s): Do not use in dystocia due to abnormal presentation of fetus until correction is accomplished.

Precaution(s): Store at controlled room temperature between 15°C and 30°C (59°F-86°F).

Note: As this is a multi-dose container, this preparation should be handled under aseptic conditions. Do not freeze.

Caution(s): Federal law restricts this drug to use by or on the order of a licensed veterinarian.

For prepartum usage, full relaxation of the cervix should be accomplished either naturally or by the administration of estrogen prior to oxytocin therapy.

Warning(s): Hazardous - Not for human use (California).

For animal use only. Keep out of the reach of children.

Presentation: 100 mL vials.

Compendium Code No.: 14750600

OXYTOCIN INJECTION ℞

Bimeda **Oxytocin**

NADA No.: 130-136

Active Ingredient(s): Each mL contains:
Oxytocin . . . . 20 U.S.P. units
Chlorobutanol (as a preservative) . . . . 5 mg
Acetic acid 0.25%
In water for injection.

Indications: For obstetrical use in horses and cows, and milk letdown in cows.

Dosage and Administration: For intravenous, intramuscular or subcutaneous use.
For obstetrical use:
Horses and Cows . . . . 100 U.S.P. units (5 mL)
For milk letdown:
Cows . . . . 10-20 U.S.P. units (0.5-1.0 mL)

Contraindication(s): Do not use in dystocia due to the abnormal presentation of the fetus until a correction is accomplished.

Precaution(s): Avoid excessive exposure to heat. Store in a refrigerator at 36°-46°F (2°-8°C). Do not freeze.

Caution(s): Federal law restricts this drug to use by or on the order of a licensed veterinarian.

Keep this and all medication out of the reach of children.

Presentation: 100 mL sterile multiple dose vials.

Compendium Code No.: 13990310

OXYTOCIN INJECTION ℞

Butler **Oxytocin**

NADA No.: 130-136

Active Ingredient(s): Each mL contains:
Oxytocin . . . . 20 U.S.P. units
Chlorobutanol . . . . 5 mg
Acetic acid 0.25%
Water for injection . . . . q.s.

Indications: For obstetrical use in mares and cows, and for use as an aid in milk letdown in cows.

Dosage and Administration: For intravenous, intramuscular or subcutaneous use.
For obstetrical use:
Horses and Cows . . . . 100 U.S.P. units (5 mL)
For milk letdown:
Cows . . . . 10-20 U.S.P. units (0.5-1.0 mL)

Contraindication(s): Do not use in cases of dystocia due to the abnormal presentation of the fetus until the correction is accomplished.

Precaution(s): Avoid excessive exposure to heat. Store in a refrigerator at temperatures between 2°-8°C (36°-46°F). Do not freeze.
Caution(s): Federal law restricts this drug to use by or on the order of a licensed veterinarian.
For veterinary use only.
Keep this and all other medications out of the reach of children.
Presentation: 100 mL sterile multiple dose vials.
Compendium Code No.: 10821340

OXYTOCIN INJECTION ℞

Phoenix Pharmaceutical **Oxytocin**

NADA No.: 099-169
Active Ingredient(s): Each mL contains:
Oxytocic Activity Equivalent to 20 USP Posterior Pituitary units with Sodium Hydroxide/Acetic Acid for pH adjustment.
Chlorobutanol (as preservative) .... 2.4 mg
Water for Injection .... q.s.
Indications: Oxytocin may be used as a uterine contractor to precipitate and accelerate normal parturition and postpartum evacuation of uterine debris. In surgery it may be used post-operatively following caesarean section to facilitate involution and resistance to the large inflow of blood. It will contract smooth muscle cells of the mammary gland for milk letdown if the udder is in proper physiological state.
Dosage and Administration: (Intravenous, Intramuscular or Subcutaneous)
For obstetrical use:
Horses and Cows .... 100 U.S.P. units (5 mL)
Sows and Ewes .... 30-50 U.S.P. units (1½ to 2½ mL)
For milk letdown:
Cows .... 10-20 U.S.P. units (½ to 1 mL)
Sows .... 5-20 U.S.P. units (¼ to 1 mL)
Contraindication(s): Do not use in dystocia due to abnormal presentation of fetus, until correction is accomplished.
Precaution(s): Store between 15°C and 30°C (59°F-86°F). Do not freeze.
As this is a multi-dose container, this preparation should be handled under aseptic conditions.
Caution(s): Federal law restricts this drug to use by or on the order of a licensed veterinarian.
For prepartum usage, full relaxation of the cervix should be accomplished either naturally or by the administration of estrogen prior to oxytocin therapy.
For animal use only.
Warning(s): Hazardous — Not for human use (California).
Keep out of reach of children.
Presentation: 100 mL (NDC 57319-306-05).
Manufactured by: Phoenix Scientific, Inc., St. Joseph, MO 64503.
Compendium Code No.: 12560612 Rev. 5-01

OXYTOCIN INJECTION ℞

RXV **Oxytocin**

Purified Oxytocic Principle (20 U.S.P. Units per mL)
NADA No.: 130-136
Active Ingredient(s): OXYTOCIN INJECTION contains 20 U.S.P. units of oxytocin and less than 0.4 units of presser activity per mL. Each mL of the sterile solution also contains 0.9% w/v sodium chloride, 0.5% w/v chlorobutanol (as a preservative), with water for injection, q.s., and pH adjusted to approximately 3.3 with glacial acetic acid.
Indications: Because of the specific action of oxytocin upon the uterine musculature, it is recommended as an aid in the management of the following conditions:
1) To precipitate labor.
2) To accelerate normal parturition.
3) Postpartum evacuation of uterine debris.
4) Postoperative contraction of the uterus following cesarean section and control of uterine hemorrhage.

Oxytocin will contract the smooth muscle cells of the mammary gland to induce milk let-down if the udder is in a proper physiological state.
Pharmacology: OXYTOCIN INJECTION is a sterile aqueous solution of highly purified oxytocic principle derived by synthesis or obtained from the posterior lobe of the pituitary gland of healthy domestic animals used for food by humans.
Oxytocin acts directly on the smooth musculature of the uterus in all species to induce rhythmic contractions, although in some species the uterine cervix does not respond to oxytocin. The responsiveness of the uterine musculature to oxytocin varies greatly with the stage of the reproductive cycle. During the early phases of pregnancy the uterus is relatively insensitive to the effects of oxytocin, while in the late phases the sensitivity is markedly increased. Most authorities attribute this varying response to the varying levels of estrogen and progesterone during the course of pregnancy.
Oxytocin also has been shown to exert a milk-ejecting effect, occasionally referred to as the galactogogic effect. The actual mechanism by which oxytocin stimulates the release of milk from the mammary glands is not known with certainty, but oxytocin is presumed to act on certain smooth muscle elements in the gland.
Dosage and Administration: Inject aseptically by the intravenous, intramuscular, or subcutaneous route as follows:
Obstetrical Use:
Ewes and Sows .... 1.5 to 2.5 mL (30 to 50 U.S.P. units)
Cows and Horses .... 5.0 mL (100 U.S.P. units)
The dosages are recommended, and may be repeated as necessary.
Milk Let-down:
Sows .... 0.25 to 1.0 mL (5 to 20 U.S.P. units)
Cows .... 0.5 to 1.0 mL (10 to 20 U.S.P. units)
These dosages are recommended, and may be repeated as necessary.
Note: Oxytocin will not induce milk let-down unless the udder is in the proper physiological state.
Contraindication(s): Do not use in dystocia due to abnormal presentation of the fetus until correction is accomplished.
Precaution(s): Keep refrigerated at 2.2°-7.8°C (36°-46°F). Do not freeze.
Caution(s): Federal law restricts this drug to use by or on the order of a licensed veterinarian.
Oxytocin is a potent preparation, accordingly, it should be administered with due caution. For prepartum use, full dilation of the cervix should be accomplished either naturally or through the administration of estrogen prior to oxytocin therapy.
Warning(s): For animal use only. Keep out of reach of children.
Restricted drug (California). Use only as directed.
Presentation: OXYTOCIN INJECTION is available in 100 mL multiple dose vials.
Compendium Code No.: 10910100

OXYTOCIN INJECTION ℞

Vedco **Oxytocin**

NADA No.: 099-169
Active Ingredient(s): Each mL contains: Oxytocic activity equivalent to 20 USP posterior pituitary units with sodium hydroxide/acetic acid for pH adjustment.
Chlorobutanol (as preservative) .... 2.4 mg
Water for injection .... q.s.
Indications: Oxytocin may be used as a uterine contractor to precipitate and accelerate normal parturition and postpartum evacuation of uterine debris. In surgery it may be used postoperatively following cesarian section to facilitate involution and resistance to the large inflow of blood. It will contract smooth muscle cells of the mammary gland for milk letdown if the udder is in proper physiological state.
Dosage and Administration: (Intravenous, intramuscular or subcutaneous):
For obstetrical use:
Horses and Cows .... 100 U.S.P. units (5 mL)
Sows and Ewes .... 30-50 U.S.P. units (1½ to 2½ mL)
For milk letdown:
Cows .... 10-20 U.S.P. units (½-1 mL)
Sows .... 5-20 U.S.P. units (¼ to 1 mL)
Contraindication(s): Do not use in dystocia due to the abnormal presentation of the fetus until correction is accomplished.
Precaution(s): Store at controlled room temperature between 15°C and 30°C (59°-86°F).
Note: As the vial is a multi-dose container, this preparation should be handled under aseptic conditions.
Caution(s): Federal law restricts this drug to use by or on the order of a licensed veterinarian.
For prepartum usage, full relaxation of the cervix should be accomplished either naturally or by the administration of estrogen prior to oxytocin therapy.
For animal use only.
Warning(s): Hazardous - Not for human use (California).
Keep out of reach of children.
Presentation: 100 mL sterile, multiple dose vials (NDC 50989-420-12).
Manufactured by: Phoenix Scientific, Inc., St. Joseph, MO 64503.
Compendium Code No.: 10941661 Rev. 7-00

OXYTOCIN INJECTION ℞

Vet Tek **Oxytocin**

NADA No.: 099-169
Active Ingredient(s): Each mL Contains: Oxytocin Activity Equivalent to 20 USP Posterior Pituitary units with Sodium Hydroxide/Acetic Acid for pH adjustment.
Chlorobutanol (as preservative) .... 2.4 mg
Water For Injection .... q.s.
Indications: Oxytocin may be used as a uterine contractor to precipitate and accelerate normal parturity and postpartum evacuation of uterine debris. In surgery it may be used postoperatively following cesarean section to facilitate involution and resistance to the large inflow of blood. It will contact smooth muscle cells of the mammary gland for milk letdown if the udder is in proper physiological state.
Dosage and Administration: (Intravenous, Intramuscular or Subcutaneous).
For obstetrical use:
Horses and Cows .... 100 U.S.P. units (5 mL)
Sows and Ewes .... 30-50 U.S.P. units (1½ to 2½ mL)
For milk letdown:
Cows .... 10-20 U.S.P. units (½ to 1 mL)
Sows .... 5 to 20 U.S.P. units (¼ to 1 mL)
Contraindication(s): Do not use in dystocia due to abnormal presentation of fetus until correction is accomplished.
Precaution(s): Store at controlled room temperature between 15°C and 30°C (59°F-86°F). Do not freeze.
Note: As this is a multi-dose container, this preparation should be handled under aseptic conditions.
Caution(s): Federal law restricts this drug to use by or on the order of a licensed veterinarian.
For prepartum usage, full relaxation of the cervix should be accomplished either naturally or by the administration of estrogen prior to oxytocin therapy.
For animal use only.
Warning(s): Keep out of the reach of children.
Hazardous-Not for human use (California).
Presentation: 100 mL (NDC 60270-032-10).
Manufactured by: Phoenix Scientific, Inc., St. Joseph, MO 64506.
Compendium Code No.: 14200131 Rev. 10-95

P

P-128

First Priority **Detergent**

One-Step, Germicidal Detergent & Deodorant-Disinfectant-Pseudomonacidal-Staphylocidal-Salmonellacidal-Bactericidal-Fungicidal-Mildewstatic-*Virucidal

EPA Reg. No.: 47371-130-68077

Active Ingredient(s):

Didecyl dimethyl ammonium chloride 4.85%
n-Alkyl (C_{14} 50%, C_{12} 40%, C_{16} 10%) dimethyl benzyl ammonium chloride 3.23%
Inert Ingredients.......... 91.92%
Total 100.00%

Indications: A multi-purpose, neutral pH, germicidal detergent and deodorant effective in hard water up to 400 ppm (calculated as $CaCO_3$) in the presence of a moderate amount of soil (5% organic serum) according to the AOAC Use-dilution Test. Disinfects, cleans, and deodorizes in one step.

Effective against the following pathogens: *Pseudomonas aeruginosa*[1], *Staphylococcus aureus*[1], *Salmonella choleraesuis, Acinetobacter calcoaceticus, Bordetella bronchiseptica, Chlamydia psittaci, Enterobacter aerogenes, Enterobacter cloacae, Enterococcus faecalis*-Vancomycin Resistant (VRE), *Escherichia coli*[1], *Fusobacterium necrophorum, Klebsiella pneumoniae*[1], *Legionella pneumophila, Listeria monocytogenes, Pasteurella multocida, Proteus mirabilis, Proteus vulgaris, Salmonella enteritidis, Salmonella typhi, Salmonella typhimurium, Serratia marcescens, Shigella flexneri, Shigella sonnei, Staphylococcus aureus*-Methicillin resistant (MRSA), *Staphylococcus aureus*-Vancomycin intermediate resistant (VISA), *Staphylococcus epidermidis*[2], *Streptococcus faecalis*[1], *Streptococcus pyogenes,* Adenovirus type 4*, Avian polyomavirus*, Canine distemper*, Feline leukemia*, Feline picornavirus*, Herpes simplex type 1*, Herpes simplex type 2*, HIV-1 (AIDS virus)*, Infectious Bovine rhinotracheitis*, Infectious bronchitis (Avian IBV)*, Influenza A/Hong Kong*, Pseudorabies*, Rabies*, Respiratory syncytial virus (RSV)*, Rubella (German measles)*, Transmissible gastroenteritis virus (TGE)*, Vaccinia*, *Aspergillus niger, Candida albicans, Trichophyton mentagrophytes.*

[1] ATCC and Antibiotic - resistant strain

[2] Antibiotic - resistant strain only

*Kills HIV-1 (AIDS Virus) on precleaned, environmental surfaces/objects previously soiled with blood/body fluids in health care settings or other settings in which there is an expected likelihood of soiling of inanimate surfaces/objects with blood/body fluids, and in which the surfaces/objects likely to be soiled with blood/body fluids can be associated with the potential for transmission of Human Immunodeficiency Virus Type 1 (HIV-1) (associated with AIDS).

Directions for Use: It is a violation of Federal law to use this product in a manner inconsistent with its labeling.

Dilution: 1:128 (600 ppm quat) - 1 ounce per gallon of water.

This product is not to be used as a terminal sterilant/high level disinfectant on any surface or instrument that (1) is introduced directly into the human body, either into or in contact with the bloodstream or normally sterile areas of the body, or (2) contacts intact mucous membranes but which does not ordinarily penetrate the blood barrier or otherwise enter normally sterile areas of the body. This product may be used to preclean or decontaminate critical or semi-critical devices prior to sterilization or high-level disinfection.

Recommended for use in hospitals, nursing homes, schools, colleges, commercial and industrial institutions, office buildings, veterinary clinics, animal life science laboratories, federally inspected meat and poultry establishments, equine farms, tack shops, pet shops, airports, kennels, hotels, motels, poultry farms, turkey farms, dairy farms, hog farms, breeding establishments, grooming establishments and households. Disinfects, cleans, and deodorizes floors, walls, metal surfaces, stainless steel surfaces, glazed porcelain, plastic surfaces (such as polypropylene, polystyrene, etc.).

Disinfection: Remove heavy soil deposits from surface. Then thoroughly wet surface with a solution of 1 ounce of the concentrate per gallon of water. The solution can be applied with a cloth, mop, sponge, or coarse spray, or soaking. Let solution remain on surface for a minimum of 10 minutes. Rinse or allow to air dry. Rinsing of floors is not necessary unless they are to be waxed or polished. Food contact surfaces must be thoroughly rinsed with potable water. This product must not be used to clean the following food contact surfaces: utensils, glassware and dishes. Prepare a fresh solution daily or more often if the solution becomes visibly dirty or diluted.

USDA: For use in federally inspected meat and poultry plants as a disinfectant agent for use in all departments. Food products and packaging materials must be removed from the room or carefully protected. Use product in accordance with its label. All surfaces must be thoroughly rinsed with potable water.

Toilet Bowls: Swab bowl with brush to remove heavy soil prior to cleaning or disinfecting. Clean by applying diluted solution around the bowl and up under the rim. Stubborn stains may require brushing. To disinfect, first remove or expel over the inner trap the residual bowl water. Pour in three ounces of the diluted solution. Swab the bowl completely using a scrub brush or mop, making sure to get under rim. Let stand for ten minutes or overnight, then flush.

Mildewstatic Instructions: Will effectively control the growth of mold and mildew plus the odors caused by them when applied to hard, non-porous surfaces such as walls, floors, and table tops. Apply solution (1 ounce per gallon of water) with a cloth, mop, sponge, or coarse spray. Make sure to wet all surfaces completely. Let air dry. Repeat application weekly or when growth reappears.

Farm Premise, Livestock, Poultry and Turkey House Disinfectant - Directions for Use:

Dilution: 1:128 - 1 ounce per gallon of water.

1. Remove all animals and feeds from premises, trucks, coops, crates, and enclosures.
2. Remove all litter and manure from floors, walls and surfaces of barns, pens, stalls, chutes, vehicles, and other facilities and fixtures occupied or traversed by animals.
3. Empty all troughs, racks, and other feeding and watering appliances.
4. Thoroughly clean all surfaces with soap or detergent, and rinse with water.
5. Saturate all surfaces with the recommended disinfecting solution for a period of 10 minutes.
6. Immerse all halters, ropes, and other types of equipment used in handling and restraining animals, as well as forks, shovels, and scrapers used for removing litter and manure.
7. Ventilate buildings, coops, cars, boats, and other closed spaces. Do not house animals or employ equipment until treatment has been absorbed, set, or dried.
8. After treatment with disinfectant, thoroughly scrub feed racks, troughs, automatic feeders, fountains, and waterers with soap or detergent, and rinse with potable water before reuse.

Special Instructions for Cleaning and Decontamination Against HIV-1 (AIDS Virus) of Surfaces/Objects Soiled with Blood/Body Fluids:

Personal Protection: Disposable latex or vinyl gloves, gowns, face masks, or eye coverings as appropriate must be worn during all cleaning of blood/body fluids and during decontamination procedures.

Cleaning Procedures: Blood/body fluids must be thoroughly cleaned from surfaces/objects before application of disinfectant.

Contact Time: HIV-1 (AIDS virus) is inactivated after a contact time of 4 minutes at 25°C (room temperature). Use a 10-minute contact time for other viruses, fungi, and bacteria listed.

Disposal of Infectious Materials: Blood/body fluids should be autoclaved and disposed of according to federal, state, and local regulations for infectious waste disposal.

Precautionary Statements: Hazards to Humans and Domestic Animals: Danger.

Corrosive: Causes irreversible eye damage and skin burns. Harmful if swallowed. Do not get in eyes, on skin or on gloves. When handling product, protect eyes by wearing goggles or face shield and protect skin by wearing rubber gloves. Wash thoroughly with soap and water after handling. Remove contaminated clothing and wash before reuse.

Statement of Practical Treatment: In case of contact, immediately flush eyes or skin with plenty of water for at least 15 minutes. For eyes or skin, call a physician. If swallowed, call a doctor or get medical attention. Do not induce vomiting or give anything by mouth to an unconscious person. Drink promptly a large quantity of milk, egg whites, gelatin solution, or if these are not available, drink large quantities of water. Avoid alcohol.

Note to Physician: Probable mucosal damage may contraindicate the use of gastric lavage. Measures against circulatory shock, respiratory depression, and convulsion may be needed.

Storage and Disposal: Keep product under locked storage, inaccessible to children. Do not reuse empty container. Rinse thoroughly, securely wrap empty container in several layers of newspaper, and discard in trash.

Warning(s): Keep out of reach of children.

Presentation: 1 gallon (3.785 L).

Compendium Code No.: 11390601 Rev. 07-01

PABAC®

Fort Dodge **Bacterin**

Pasteurella Multocida Bacterin, Avian Isolates, Types 1, 3 & 4

U.S. Vet. Lic. No.: 112

Contents: This product contains the antigens listed above.

Gentamicin added as a preservative.

Indications: For the vaccination of healthy chickens and turkeys as an aid in the prevention of fowl cholera, types 1, 3 and 4.

Dosage and Administration: Inject 0.5 mL (0.5 cc) subcutaneously (in back of the neck) using aseptic technique. Vaccinate only healthy birds.

Turkeys: Vaccinate at 8 to 10 weeks of age or when birds go on range. Repeat 4 to 5 weeks later. If necessary, vaccinations may be repeated at 2 to 3 month intervals.

Chickens: Vaccinate at 12 weeks of age and repeat 4 to 5 weeks later.

Precaution(s): Store in the dark at 36° to 45°F (2° to 7°C). Do not freeze. Warm to 65° to 85°F (18° to 29°C) and shake well before using. Use entire contents when first opened.

Warning(s): Do not vaccinate within 42 days before slaughter.

In case of accidental human injection seek immediate medical attention.

For veterinary use only.

Presentation: 1,000 dose (500 mL) vials.

Compendium Code No.: 10031411 10342B

PAD-TOUGH™

Life Science **Topical Product**

Contents: Isopropyl alcohol, purified water, comfrey extract, ethyl alcohol, propylene glycol, benzoin, storax, tolu balsam and aloe vera.

Indications: Protective covering and toughening agent for dogs' pads.

Directions: Coat pads liberally with PAD-TOUGH™ prior to field trials, shows, hunting or other rigorous exercise. PAD-TOUGH™ should be used routinely prior to any extensive outdoor activity.

Precaution(s): Flammable.

Caution(s): For animal use only. For external use only.

Warning(s): Harmful if swallowed. Avoid contact with eyes. Keep out of reach of children.

Presentation: 4 fl oz (118 mL).

Compendium Code No.: 10870131

PALABIS™

PharmX **Adsorbent**

Palatable Bismuth Subsalicylate

Active Ingredient(s): Each tablet contains the equivalent of one tablespoonful of pink, regular strength bismuth subsalicylate preparations for humans (262 milligrams of bismuth subsalicylate).

Indications: For use in relieving distress from upset stomach and in some acute and chronic diarrheal syndromes.

Dosage and Administration: The total recommended daily dosage of PALABIS™ (bismuth subsalicylate is 17.5-52.5 milligrams per kilogram per day to be given t.i.d. or q.i.d.

5 kg (11 lb) dog	1⁄3 - 1 tablet per day
10 kg (22 lb) dog	2⁄3 - 2 tablets per day
20 kg (44 lb) dog	1 1⁄3 - 4 tablets per day
30 kg (66 lb) dog	2 - 6 tablets per day
40 kg (88 lb) dog	2 2⁄3 - 8 tablets per day

Contraindication(s): PALABIS™ should not be administered to dogs who are actively vomiting. Do not administer with aspirin. If symptoms persist for more than three days, discontinue use and consult your veterinarian. Do not administer to animals with known salicylate allergies or when salicylates are contraindicated.

Caution(s): Administer PALABIS™ in divided dosages. Bismuth subsalicylate may cause black stools.

Water must be available to prevent dehydration which may accompany diarrhea.

PALABIS™ may be administered alone or by mixing with food.

Warning(s): Keep out of reach of children and animals. In case of accidental overdose, contact a health professional immediately. For use in dogs only.

Presentation: 100 tablets.

Compendium Code No.: 10460000

PALAMEGA™ COMPLEX CHEWABLE TABLETS (Liver Flavor)

Schering-Plough **Small Animal Dietary Supplement**

Microencapsulated Omega Fatty Acids with Vitamins and Zinc

Guaranteed Analysis: Each chewable tablet contains:

Crude Protein . . . . . . 12% Min.
Crude Fat . . . . . . 12% Min.
Crude Fiber. . . . . . 15% Max.
Moisture. . . . . . 8% Max.
Linoleic acid . . . . . . 1.1% Min.
Zinc . . . . . . 2 mg Min.
Vitamin A . . . . . . 1350 I.U. Min.
Vitamin D_3 . . . . . . 270 I.U. Min.
Vitamin E . . . . . . 22.5 I.U. Min.

Ingredients: Includes the following: Calcium phosphate, powdered cellulose, fish oil, liver powder, hydrolyzed vegetable protein (roast beef flavor), sucrose, vitamin E acetate, vegetable oil, stearic acid, vitamin A acetate, choline chloride, zinc oxide, inositol, vitamin D_3 supplement, TBHQ (preservative).

Indications: A supplemental source of omega fatty acids, zinc, and vitamins A, D_3, and E. As such, PALAMEGA™ Complex Chewable Tablets for Cats and Dogs are beneficial for the maintenance of healthy skin and coats.

Dosage and Administration: For diet supplementation:

Cats . . . . . . ½ to 1 tablet daily
Dogs under 10 pounds . . . . . . ½ to 1 tablet daily
Dogs 10 - 50 pounds. . . . . . 1 to 2 tablets daily
Dogs over 50 pounds. . . . . . 2 to 4 tablets daily

Administer free choice just prior to feeding, or crumble and mix with food.

This product intended for intermittent or supplemental feeding only.

Presentation: 100 tablets.

Compendium Code No.: 10472190 Rev. 1/01

PALAPECTATE™

PharmX **Antidiarrheal-Adsorbent**

Palatable Attapulgite

Active Ingredient(s): Each PALAPECTATE™ tablet contains 750 milligrams of beef-flavored attapulgite.

Indications: PALAPECTATE™ contains attapulgite for relief of common canine diarrhea.

Dosage and Administration: Each tablet contains 750 mg attapulgite, the equivalent of one tablespoonful of the human anti-diarrheal product.

The recommended dose is 25 to 50 mg per kg every two to six hours, or after each loose stool.

For smaller dogs (less than 15 lbs) ¼ to ½ tablet every two to six hours.

For medium dogs (15-30 lbs) ½ to 1 tablet every two to six hours.

For large dogs (30-60 lbs) 1-2 tablets every two to six hours.

Precaution(s): Keep container tightly closed and dry.

Store at room temperature. Avoid excessive heat.

Caution(s): Do not exceed six tablets per day.

If diarrhea persists for more than three days, consult your veterinarian.

For diarrhea accompanied by high fever, or by bloody stools, contact your veterinarian.

Warning(s): Keep out of reach of children and animals. In case of accidental overdose, contact a health professional immediately. For use in dogs only.

Presentation: 100 tablets.

Compendium Code No.: 10460010

PALAPRIN® 65 ℞

PharmX **Non-Steroidal Anti-Inflammatory**

Palatable Buffered Aspirin

Active Ingredient(s): Each tablet contains 65 mg aspirin (1 grain).

Indications: For use in relieving pain, fever or inflammation.

Dosage and Administration: Give 1 tablet per 10 lbs every 12 hours.

Contraindication(s): PALAPRIN® tablets should not be administered to dogs having gastritis, enteritis, or other gastrointestinal conditions, except as directed by a veterinarian. If symptoms persist for more than three days, discontinue use and contact your veterinarian.

Precaution(s): Keep container tightly closed and dry.

Store at room temperature. Avoid excessive heat.

Caution(s): Federal law restricts this drug to use by or on the order of a licensed veterinarian.

PALAPRIN® may be administered alone or by mixing with food. Timing the administration to coincide with feeding reduces the chances of gastrointestinal irritation.

Warning(s): Keep out of reach of children and animals. In case of accidental overdose, contact a health professional immediately. For use in dogs only.

Presentation: 30 and 100 tablets.

Compendium Code No.: 10460031

PALAPRIN® 325 ℞

PharmX **Non-Steroidal Anti-Inflammatory**

Palatable Buffered Aspirin

Active Ingredient(s): Each tablet contains 325 mg aspirin (5 grains).

Indications: For use in relieving pain, fever or inflammation.

Dosage and Administration: Give ½ tablet per 25 lbs every 12 hours.

Contraindication(s): PALAPRIN® tablets should not be administered to dogs having gastritis, enteritis, or other gastrointestinal conditions, except as directed by a veterinarian. If symptoms persist for more than three days, discontinue use and contact your veterinarian.

Precaution(s): Keep container tightly closed and dry.

Store at room temperature. Avoid excessive heat.

Caution(s): Federal law restricts this drug to use by or on the order of a licensed veterinarian.

PALAPRIN® may be administered alone or by mixing with food. Timing the administration to coincide with feeding reduces the chances of gastrointestinal irritation.

Warning(s): Keep out of reach of children and animals. In case of accidental overdose, contact a health professional immediately. For use in dogs only.

Presentation: 30 and 100 tablets.

Compendium Code No.: 10460021

PANACUR® BEEF AND DAIRY CATTLE DEWORMER ℞

Intervet **Parasiticide-Oral**

(fenbendazole) Suspension 10%-100 mg/mL

NADA No.: 128-620

Active Ingredient(s): Each mL contains 100 mg of fenbendazole.

Indications:

Beef and Dairy Cattle: For the removal and control of:

Lungworm: *(Dictyocaulus viviparus)*.

Stomach worm (adults): *Ostertagia ostertagi* (Brown stomach worm).

Stomach worm (adults and 4th stage larvae): *Haemonchus contortus/placei* (barberpole worm), *Trichostrongylus axei* (small stomach worm).

Intestinal worm (adults and 4th stage larvae): *Bunostomum phlebotomum* (hookworm), *Nematodirus helvetianus* (thread-necked intestinal worm), *Cooperia punctata* and *C. oncophora* (small intestinal worm), *Trichostrongylus colubriformis* (bankrupt worm), *Oesophagostomum radiatum* (nodular worm).

Beef Cattle Only: For the removal and control of:

Stomach worm (4th stage inhibited larvae): *Ostertagia ostertagi* (Type II Ostertagiasis).

Tapeworm: *Moniezia benedeni.*

Dosage and Administration:

Beef and Dairy Cattle: 5 mg/kg (2.3 mg/lb.) for the removal and control of:

Lungworm: *(Dictyocaulus viviparus)*.

Stomach worm (adults): *Ostertagia ostertagi* (Brown stomach worm).

Stomach worm (adults and 4th stage larvae): *Haemonchus contortus/placei* (barberpole worm), *Trichostrongylus axei* (small stomach worm).

Intestinal worm (adults and 4th stage larvae): *Bunostomum phlebotomum* (hookworm), *Nematodirus helvetianus* (thread-necked intestinal worm), *Cooperia punctata* and *C. oncophora* (small intestinal worm), *Trichostrongylus colubriformis* (bankrupt worm), *Oesophagostomum radiatum* (nodular worm).

Beef Cattle Only: 10 mg/kg (4.6 mg/lb.) for the removal and control of:

Stomach worm (4th stage inhibited larvae): *Ostertagia ostertagi* (Type II Ostertagiasis).

Tapeworm: *Moniezia benedeni.*

Do not use in dairy cattle at 10 mg/kg.

Directions: Determine the proper dose according to estimated body weight. Administer orally. In beef and dairy cattle, the recommended dose of 5 mg/kg is achieved when 2.3 mL of the drug is given for each 100 lb. of body weight. In beef cattle only, the recommended dosage of 10 mg/kg for treatment of Ostertagiasis Type II (inhibited 4th stage larvae) or tapeworm is achieved when 4.6 mL of the drug is given for each 100 lb. of body weight.

Examples:

Dose (5 mg/kg)	Dose (10 mg/kg)	Cattle Weight
2.3 mL	4.6 mL	100 lb.
4.6 mL	9.2 mL	200 lb.
6.9 mL	13.8 mL	300 lb.
9.2 mL	18.4 mL	400 lb.
11.5 mL	23.0 mL	500 lb.
23.0 mL	46.0 mL	1000 lb.
34.5 mL	69.0 mL	1500 lb.

Under conditions of continued exposure to parasites, retreatment may be needed after 4 to 6 weeks.

Contraindication(s): There are no known contraindications to the use of the drug in cattle.

Precaution(s): Store at or below 25°C (77°F). Protect from freezing. Shake well before use.

Caution(s): Federal law restricts this drug to use by or on the order of a licensed veterinarian.

Warning(s): Residue Warnings: Cattle must not be slaughtered for human consumption within 8 days following treatment.

Do not use at 10 mg/kg in dairy cattle. Dose rate of 10 mg/kg is for beef cattle only. Dose rate of 10 mg/kg in dairy cattle could result in violative residues in milk.

For dairy cattle there is no milk withdrawal period at 5 mg/kg.

Keep this and all medication out of the reach of children.

Presentation: 1 gallon (3785 mL) bottles.

Manufactured by: DPT Laboratories, San Antonio, TX 78215.

Compendium Code No.: 11061121 697810-A/697815-A

PANACUR® GRANULES 22.2% ℞

Intervet **Parasiticide-Oral**

(fenbendazole) (222 mg/g) Dewormer

NADA No.: 121-473

Active Ingredient(s): PANACUR® Granules 22.2% contains 222 mg/g of fenbendazole.

Indications: For dogs and for only the carnivorous/omnivorous animals listed.

For the following carnivorous/omnivorous animals: Lions *(Panthera leo)*, Tigers *(Panthera tigris)*, Cheetahs *(Acinonyx jubatus)*, Pumas *(Felis concolor)*, Jaguars *(Panthera onca)*, Leopards *(Panthera pardus)*, Panthers *(Panthera* spp.), Grizzly Bears *(Ursus horribilis)*, Polar Bears *(Ursus maritimus)*, Black Bears *(Ursus americanus)*.

PANACUR® Granules 22.2% is used for control of the following internal parasites of the families *Felidae* and *Ursidae*.

Felidae: Lions *(Panthera leo)*. For control of ascarids *(Toxocara cati, Toxascaris leonina)*, hookworms *(Ancylostoma spp.)*.

Tigers *(Panthera tigris)*. For control of ascarids *(Toxocara cati, Toxascaris leonina)*, hookworms *(Ancylostoma spp.)*.

Cheetahs *(Acinonyx jubatus)*. For control of ascarids *(Toxocara cati, Toxascaris leonina)*.

Pumas *(Felis concolor)*, Panthers *(Panthera* spp.), Leopards *(Panthera pardus)*, Jaguars *(Panthera onca)*. For control of ascarids *(Toxocara cati, Toxascaris leonina)*, hookworms *(Ancylostoma spp.)*, tapeworms *(Taenia hydatigena, T. krabbei, T. taeniaeformis)*.

Ursidae: Black Bears *(Ursus americanus)*. For control of ascarids *(Baylisascaris transfuga, Toxacaris leonina)*, hookworms *(Ancylostoma caninum)*, tapeworms *(Taenia hydatigena, T. krabbei)*.

Polar Bears *(Ursus maritimus)* and Grizzly Bears *(Ursus horribilis)*. For control of ascarids *(Baylisascaris transfuga, Toxacaris leonina)*.

For dogs: For the removal of ascarids *(Toxocara canis, Toxascaris leonina)*, hookworms *(Anclyostoma caninum, Uncinaria stenocephaia)*, whipworms *(Trichuris vulpis)*, and tapeworms *(Taenia pisiformis)*.

Pharmacology: PANACUR® (fenbendazole) Granules 22.2% contains the active anthelmintic, fenbendazole. The chemical name of fenbendazole is methyl 5-(phenylthio)-2-benzimidazolecarbamate.

The CAS Registry Number is 43210-67-9.

The chemical structure is:

Actions: The antiparasitic action of PANACUR® Granules 22.2% is believed to be due to the inhibition of energy metabolism in the parasite.

Dosage and Administration: The dose of *Felidae* and *Ursidae* is 10 mg/kg bw daily for 3 consecutive days. Please see Indications for details as to claims for animal and parasite.

Directions: The daily dose of 10 mg/kg (4.54 mg/lb) can be achieved as follows:

Using a gram scale, weigh out 1 gram of PANACUR® Granules 22.2% for each 22 kg or 50 lbs body weight.

For Dogs: 50 mg/kg (22.7 mg/lb) daily for 3 consecutive days for the removal of ascarids *(Toxocara canis, Toxascaris leonina)*, hookworms *(Anclyostoma caninum, Uncinaria stenocephaia)*, whipworms *(Trichuris vulpis)*, and tapeworms *(Taenia pisiformis)*.

Directions: The daily dosage of 50 mg/kg (22.7 mg/lb) can be achieved as follows:

Using a gram scale, weight out 1 gram of PANACUR® (fenbendazole) Granules 22.2% for each 4.44 kg or 10 lbs body weight.

Daily dosages must be repeated for 3 consecutive days. Mix the appropriate amount of drug with a small amount of the usual food; dry dog food may require slight moistening to facilitate mixing with the drug.

Compatibilities: Drug Reactions: There are currently no data available to support the use of PANACUR® Granules 22.2% in conjunction with other nutritional and drug substances in *Felidae* and *Ursidae*. However, experience with the drug under actual conditions of use has not revealed any incompatibilities with PANACUR®.

PANACUR® Granules 22.2% has been administered to dogs in clinical trials along with a wide variety of other drugs including antibiotics, steroids, anesthetics, tranquilizers, vitamins, and minerals. No incompatibilities with other drugs are known at this time.

Contraindication(s): None known.

Precaution(s): Store at controlled room temperature 59 to 86°F (15 to 30°C).

Caution(s): Federal law restricts this drug to use by or on the order of a licensed veterinarian.

Medicated food must be fully consumed for PANACUR® to be effective. Dispensing containers must be labeled with drug identification and directions for use.

Warning(s): Do not use 14 days before or during the hunting season.

Keep this and all medication out of the reach of children.

Toxicology: PANACUR® has been fed to pregnant and non-pregnant females and to male animals including *Felidae* and *Ursidae* at ten times the recommended dose for twice the recommended treatment period without effect on reproduction. In one puma and one jaguar, ten times the recommended dose given for twice the recommended duration showed evidence of inappetence when administered the PANACUR® Granules.

PANACUR® Granules 22.2% did not cause toxicity when administered to weaned pups at doses equal to 5 times the recommended daily dose and for 2 times the duration of treatment.

Side Effects: In studies conducted in a variety of captive animals, loose stools have been reported in pumas, black bears, and ruminants. In one puma and one jaguar, periods of inappetence followed the initial consumption of fenbendazole at ten times the recommended treatment level.

Another benzimidazole has been reported to cause hepatotoxicity clinically in canines. However, this effect has not been reported during the clinical use of fenbendazole. In US clinical studies, 3 of 240 dogs vomited which may have been drug related.

Discussion: Efficacy is dependent on the correct dose level based on body weight over the appropriate treatment period. When possible, animals should be weighed to determine body weight accurately, otherwise weights can be estimated.

It is important that the appropriate dose of PANACUR® be ingested. This may be accomplished by applying the granules as a top dressing or mixing with a small portion of the food prior to offering the main meal.

Refer to the Dosage and Administration portion of the labeling for determining the appropriate dose for each species of animal.

Presentation: PANACUR® Granules 22.2% is supplied in 1 lb (454 g) jars.

Manufactured by: Global Pharm, Inc., Don Mills, Ontario, Canada.

Compendium Code No.: 11061052

PANACUR® GRANULES 22.2% (Dogs only) ℞

Intervet **Parasiticide-Oral**

(fenbendazole) (222 mg/g)

NADA No.: 121-473

Active Ingredient(s):

Fenbendazole .... 222 mg/g (22.2%)

Indications: For the control and removal of ascarids *(Toxocara canis, Toxascaris leonina)*, hookworms *(Ancylostoma caninum, Uncinaria stenocephala)*, whipworms *(Trichuris vulpis)*, and tapeworms *(Taenia pisiformis)* in dogs.

Dosage and Administration: The daily dose of 50 mg/kg (22.7 mg/lb) body weight can be achieved as follows:

Packet Size	Dog Weight
1 g	10 lbs
2 g	20 lbs
4 g	40 lbs

Daily dosage, must be repeated for 3 consecutive days. Retreatment schedules should be applied according to parasite contamination and life cycles.

Mix the appropriate amount of drug with a small amount of the usual food; dry dog food may require slight moistening to facilitate mixing with the drug.

Compatibilities: Drug Reactions: PANACUR® (fenbendazole) Granules 22.2% has been administered to dogs in clinical trials along with a variety of other drugs including antibiotics, steroids, anesthetics, tranquilizers, vitamins and minerals. No incompatibilities with other drugs are known at this time.

Contraindication(s): None known.

Precaution(s): Store at controlled room temperature (59 to 86°F).

Caution(s): Federal law restricts this drug to use by or on the order of a licensed veterinarian.

Medicated food must be fully consumed to be effective.

For dogs only.

Warning(s): Keep this and all medication out of the reach of children.

Toxicology: PANACUR® (fenbendazole) Granules 22.2% did not cause toxicity when administered to weaned pups at doses equal to 5 times the recommended daily dose and for 2 times the duration of treatment.

Adverse Reactions: Another benzimidazole has been reported to cause hepatotoxicity clinically in canines. However, this effect has not been reported during the clinical use of fenbendazole. In US clinical studies 3 of 240 dogs vomited which may have been drug related.

Presentation: 81 packets x 1 g each (10 lb), 60 packets x 2 g each (20 lb) and 42 packets x 4 g each (40 lb).

Manufactured by: Global Pharm, Inc., Don Mills, Ontario, Canada.

Compendium Code No.: 11061061

PANACUR® GRANULES 22.2% (Horse)

Intervet **Parasiticide-Oral**

(Fenbendazole) 22.2%

NADA No.: 111-278

Active Ingredient(s): Each gram contains 222 mg of fenbendazole.

Indications: For oral use in all horses, foals and ponies.

For the control of large strongyles *(Strongylus edentatus, S. equinus, S. vulgaris)*, small strongyles, pinworms *(Oxyuris equi)*, and ascarids *(Parascaris equorum)* in horses.

Dosage and Administration: The contents of one packet will deworm a horse weighing approximately 500 lbs. Each packet contains 1.15 g fenbendazole. Fenbendazole fed at the rate of 2.3 mg/lb controls the listed parasites. *Sprinkle the appropriate amount of drug on a small amount of the usual grain ration. Prepare for each horse individually. No need to withhold feed or water.

*Ascarid infections are most common in young animals. The dose of foals and weanlings (less than 18 months of age) is two packets for each 500 lbs body weight.

Regular deworming at intervals of six to eight weeks may be required. Consult your veterinarian for assistance in the diagnosis, treatment and control of parasitism.

Precaution(s): Store at controlled room temperature (59-86°F).

Caution(s): Keep this and all medication out of the reach of children.

Warning(s): Do not use in horses intended for food.

For veterinary use only.

Presentation: 20 x 0.18 oz (5.2 g) packets.

PANACUR Reg TM Hoechst AG

Compendium Code No.: 11061070

PANACUR® HORSE AND CATTLE DEWORMER ℞

Intervet **Parasiticide-Oral**

(fenbendazole) Suspension 10%-100 mg/mL

NADA No.: 104-494 (Horse)/128-620 (Cattle)

Active Ingredient(s): Each mL contains 100 mg of fenbendazole.

Indications: Horses: For the control of large strongyles *(Strongylus edentatus, S. equinus, S. vulgaris, Triodontophorus* spp.), small strongyles *(Cyathostomum* spp., *Cylicocyclus* spp., *Cylicostephanus* spp., *Cylicodontophorus* spp.), pinworms *(Oxyuris equi)*, and ascarids *(Parascaris equorum)*.

Beef and Dairy Cattle: For the removal and control of:

Lungworm: *(Dictyocaulus viviparus)*.

Stomach worm (adults): *Ostertagia ostertagi* (brown stomach worms).

Stomach worm (adults and 4th stage larvae): *Haemonchus contortus/placei* (barberpole worm), *Trichostrongylus axei* (small stomach worm).

Intestinal worms (adults and 4th stage larvae): *Bunostomum phlebotomum* (hookworm), *Nematodirus helvetianus* (thread-necked intestinal worm), *Cooperia punctata* and *C. oncophora* (small intestinal worm), *Trichostrongylus colubriformis* (bankrupt worm), *Oesophagostomum radiatum* (nodular worm).

Beef Cattle Only: For the removal and control of:

Stomach worm (4th stage inhibited larvae): *Ostertagia ostertagi* (Type II Ostertagiasis).

Tapeworm: *Moniezia benedeni*.

Dosage and Administration: Horses: 5 mg/kg (2.3 mg/lb.) for the control of large strongyles *(Strongylus edentatus, S. equinus, S. vulgaris, Triodontophorus* spp.), small strongyles *(Cyathostomum* spp., *Cylicocyclus* spp., *Cylicostephanus* spp., *Cylicodontophorus* spp.) and pinworms *(Oxyuris equi)*. Example: 2.3 mL/100 lb.; 23 mL/1000 lb.

10 mg/kg (4.6 mg/lb.) for the control of ascarids *(Parascaris equorum)*. Example: (10 mg/kg); 2.3 mL/50 lb.; 23 mL/500 lb.

Beef and Dairy Cattle: 5 mg/kg (2.3 mg/lb.) for the removal and control of:

Lungworm: *(Dictyocaulus viviparus)*.

Stomach worm (adults): *Ostertagia ostertagi* (brown stomach worms).

Stomach worm (adults and 4th stage larvae): *Haemonchus contortus/placei* (barberpole worm), *Trichostrongylus axei* (small stomach worm).

Intestinal worms (adults and 4th stage larvae): *Bunostomum phlebotomum* (hookworm), *Nematodirus helvetianus* (thread-necked intestinal worm), *Cooperia punctata* and *C. oncophora* (small intestinal worm), *Trichostrongylus colubriformis* (bankrupt worm), *Oesophagostomum radiatum* (nodular worm).

Beef Cattle Only: 10 mg/kg (4.6 mg/lb.) for the removal and control of:

Stomach worm (4th stage inhibited larvae): *Ostertagia ostertagi* (Type II Ostertagiasis).

Tapeworm: *Moniezia benedeni*.

Do not use in dairy cattle at 10 mg/kg.

In beef and dairy cattle, the recommended dose of 5 mg/kg is achieved when 2.3 mL of the drug are given for each 100 lb. of body weight. In beef cattle only, the recommended dosage of 10 mg/kg for the treatment of Ostertagiasis Type II (inhibited 4th stage larvae) or tapeworm is achieved when 4.6 mL of the drug is given for each 100 lb. of body weight.

Examples: (Horses and Cattle)

Dose (5 mg/kg)	Dose (10 mg/kg)	Animal Weight
2.3 mL	4.6 mL	100 lb.
4.6 mL	9.2 mL	200 lb.
6.9 mL	13.8 mL	300 lb.
9.2 mL	18.4 mL	400 lb.
11.5 mL	23.0 mL	500 lb.
23.0 mL	46.0 mL	1000 lb.
34.5 mL	69.0 mL	1500 lb.

Directions:

Beef and Dairy Cattle and Horses: Determine the proper dose according to estimated body weight. Administer orally by suitable dosing syringe. Insert nozzle of syringe through the interdental space and deposit the drug on the back of the tongue by depressing the plunger. The drug may also be administered by stomach tube.

PANACUR® (fenbendazole) Suspension 10% is approved for use concomitantly with an approved form of trichlorfon. Trichlorfon is approved for the treatment of stomach bots *(Gasterophilus* spp.) in horses. Refer to the manufacturer's label for directions for use and cautions for trichlorfon.

Regular deworming at intervals of six to eight weeks may be required for horses.

Under conditions of continued exposure to parasites, retreatment may be needed after 4-6 weeks.

Contraindication(s): There are no known contraindications to the use of the drug in cattle or horses.

Caution(s): Federal law restricts this drug to use by or on the order of a licensed veterinarian.

Warning(s): Residue Warnings: Do not use in horses intended for food.

Cattle must not be slaughtered for human consumption within 8 days following treatment.

Do not use at 10 mg/kg in dairy cattle. Dose rate of 10 mg/kg is for beef cattle only. Dose rate of 10 mg/kg in dairy cattle could result in violative residues in milk.

For dairy cattle, there is no milk withdrawal period at 5 mg/kg.

Keep this and all medication out of the reach of children.

Presentation: 1000 mL (33.8 fl oz) bottles.

Manufactured by: DPT Laboratories, San Antonio, TX 78215.

Compendium Code No.: 11061111 697700-A/697705-A

PANACUR® HORSE AND CATTLE DEWORMER (92 g)

Intervet **Parasiticide-Oral**

(fenbendazole) Paste 10% (100 mg/g)

NADA No.: 120-648 (horse)/132-872 (cattle)

Active Ingredient(s): Each gram of PANACUR® Paste 10% contains 100 mg of fenbendazole and is flavored with artificial apple-cinnamon liquid.

Indications: Horse: PANACUR® Paste 10% is indicated for the control of large strongyles *(Strongylus edentatus, S. equinus, S. vulgaris)*, encysted early 3rd stage (hypobiotic), late 3rd stage and 4th stage cysthostome larvae, small strongyles, pinworms *(Oxyuris equi)*, ascarids *(Parascaris equorum)*, and arteritis caused by 4th stage larvae of *Strongylus vulgaris* in horses.

PANACUR® Paste 10% is approved for use concomitantly with an approved form of trichlorfon. Trichlorfon is approved for the treatment of stomach bots *(Gasterophilus* spp) in horses. Refer to the manufacturer's label for directions for use and cautions for trichlorfon.

Beef and Dairy Cattle: PANACUR® Paste 10% is indicated for the removal and control of: Lungworm *(Dictyocaulus viviparus);* Stomach worms: *(Haemonchus contortus, Ostertagia ostertagi, Trichostrongylus axei);* Intestinal worms: *(Bunostomum phlebotomum, Nematodirus helvetianus, Cooperia punctata* and *C. oncophora, Trichostrongylus colubriformis, Oesophagostomum radiatum).*

Pharmacology: PANACUR® (fenbendazole) Paste 10% contains the active anthelmintic, fenbendazole. The chemical name of fenbendazole is methyl 5-(phenyl-thio)-2- benzimidazole carbamate.

The CAS Registry Number is 43210-67-9.

The chemical structure is:

H N NHCOOCH₃ S N

Actions: The antiparasitic action of PANACUR® Paste 10% is believed to be due to the inhibition of energy metabolism in the parasite.

Dosage and Administration: Treats 8 animals of 500 lbs each.

Horse: PANACUR® Paste 10% is administered orally at a rate of 2.3 mg/lb (5 mg/kg) for the control of large strongyles, small strongyles, and pinworms. Each mark on the plunger rod corresponds to a dose of 5 mg/kg (2.3 mg/lb) for 250 lbs body weight.

For foals and weanlings (less than 18 months of age) where ascarids are a common problem, the recommended dose is 4.6 mg/lb (10 mg/kg) or two marks will deworm a 250 lb horse.

For control of encysted early 3rd stage (hypobiotic), late 3rd stage and 4th stage cysthostome larvae and 4th stage larvae of *Strongylus vulgaris,* the recommended dose is 4.6 mg/lb (10 mg/kg) daily for 5 consecutive days; administer two marks for each 250 lbs body weight per day.

Retreatment Recommendations for Horses:

Internal Parasites: Regular deworming at intervals of six to eight weeks may be required due to the possibility of reinfection.

Migrating Tissue Parasites: In the case of 4th stage larvae of *Strongylus vulgaris,* treatment and retreatment should be based on the life cycle and the epidemiology. Treatment should be initiated in the spring and repeated in the fall after a six-month interval.

Optimum Deworming Program for Control of *S. vulgaris:* Optimum reduction of *S. vulgaris* infections is achieved by reducing the infectivity of the pastures. When horses are running on pasture, in temperate North America, maximum pasture infectivity occurs in October-December. If horses are removed from those pastures in January, pasture infectivity will decline to zero by July 1. Egg production of *S. vulgaris* is minimal from January through April, peaking in August and declining to minimal values in December.

Recommended Deworming Program: *December 1, February 1, April 1, June 1, August 1, October 1.

The April 1 and October 1 treatments are the recommended periods when the 5-day treatment regimen for the control of the migrating larvae of *S. vulgaris* should be performed.

*For other areas in the world, retreatment periods for the migrating larvae of *S. vulgaris* may be different; consult with your veterinarian.

Beef and Dairy Cattle: PANACUR® Paste 10% is administered orally at a rate of 2.3 mg/lb (5 mg/kg) or 11.5 g PANACUR® (fenbendazole) Paste for 500 lb body weight (227 kg). Under conditions of continuous exposure to parasites, retreatment may be needed after 4-6 weeks.

Directions for Use:

1. Determine the weight of the animal.
2. Remove the syringe tip.
3. Turn the dial ring until the edge of the ring nearest the tip lines up with zero.
4. Fully depress plunger and discard expelled paste. Syringe is ready for dosing.
5. Each mark on the plunger rod corresponds to a dose of 5 mg/kg (2.3 mg/lb) for 250 lbs body weight. Dial the ring edge nearest the tip back by one mark for each 250 lbs body weight (do not underdose).
   Examples:
   250 lbs: 1 mark
   500 lbs: 2 marks
   750 lbs: 3 marks
   1000 lbs: 4 marks
   1500 lbs: 6 marks
6. Animal's mouth should be free of food. Insert nozzle of syringe through the interdental space and deposit the paste on the back of the tongue by depressing the plunger.
7. Repeat steps 1, 5 and 6 for each additional animal.

Contraindication(s): There are no known contraindications for the use of PANACUR® Paste 10% in horses or cattle.

Precaution(s): Store at or below 25°C (77°F).

Caution(s): When using PANACUR® (fenbendazole) Paste 10% concomitantly with trichlorfon, refer to the manufacturer's labels for use and cautions for trichlorfon.

Consult your veterinarian for assistance in the diagnosis, treatment and control of parasitism.

Warning(s): Do not use in horses intended for food.

Cattle must not be slaughtered within 8 days following last treatment.

In dairy cattle, there is no milk withdrawal period.

Keep this and all medications out of the reach of children.

Side Effects: Horse: Side effects associated with PANACUR® Paste 10% could not be established in well-controlled safety studies in horses with single doses as high as 454 mg/lb (1,000 mg/kg) and 15 consecutive daily doses of 22.7 mg/lb (50 mg/kg). At higher dose levels, the lethal action of fenbendazole may cause the release of antigens by the dying parasites. This phenomenon may result in either a local or systemic hypersensitive reaction varying in severity from itching or a rash to increased respiration and collapse. A veterinarian should be consulted if this type of reaction is suspected.

PANACUR® Paste 10% has been evaluated for safety in pregnant mares during all stages of gestation with doses as high as 11.4 mg/lb (25 mg/kg) and in stallions with doses as high as 11.4 mg/lb (25 mg/kg). No adverse effects on reproductivity were detected. The recommended dose for control of 4th stage larvae of *Strongylus vulgaris,* 4.6 mg/lb (10 mg/kg) daily for 5 consecutive days, has not been evaluated for safety in stallions or pregnant mares.

Presentation: PANACUR® Paste 10% Horse and Cattle Dewormer is supplied in 92 gram (3.2 oz) syringes, 12 syringes per carton.

Manufactured by: DPT Laboratories, San Antonio, TX 78215.

Compendium Code No.: 11061091 798001-A

PANACUR® HORSE DEWORMER (25 g)

Intervet **Parasiticide-Oral**

(fenbendazole) Paste 10% (100 mg/g)

NADA No.: 120-648

Active Ingredient(s): Each gram of PANACUR® (fenbendazole) Paste 10% contains 100 mg of fenbendazole and is flavored with artificial apple-cinnamon liquid.

Indications: PANACUR® (fenbendazole) Paste 10% is indicated for the control of large strongyles *(Strongylus edentatus, S. equinus, S. vulgaris)*, encysted early third stage (hypobiotic), late third stage and fourth stage cyathostome larvae, small strongyles, pinworms *(Oxyuris equi)*, ascarids *(Parascaris equorum)*, and arteritis caused by 4th stage larvae of *Strongylus vulgaris* in horses.

PANACUR® (fenbendazole) Paste 10% is approved for use concomitantly with an approved form of trichlorfon. Trichlorfon is approved for the treatment of stomach bots *(Gasterophilus* spp.) in horses. Refer to the manufacturer's label for directions for use and cautions for trichlorfon.

Pharmacology: PANACUR® (fenbendazole) Paste 10% contains the active anthelmintic, fenbendazole. The chemical name of fenbendazole is methyl 5-(phenylthio)-2- benzimidazol-carbamate.

The chemical structure is:

H N NHCOOCH₃ S N

Actions: The antiparasitic action of PANACUR® (fenbendazole) Paste 10% is believed to be due to the inhibition of energy metabolism in the parasite.

Dosage and Administration: Horse: PANACUR® (fenbendazole) Paste 10% is administered orally at a rate of 2.3 mg/lb (5 mg/kg) for the control of large strongylus, small strongyles, and pinworms. One syringe will deworm a 1,100 lb horse. For foals and weanlings (less than 18 months of age) where ascarids are a common problem, the recommended dose is 4.6 mg/lb (10 mg/kg); one syringe will deworm a 550 lb horse. For control of encysted early third stage (hypobiotic), late third stage and fourth stage cyathostome larvae, and fourth stage larvae of *Strongylus vulgaris*, the recommended dose is 4.6 mg/lb (10 mg/kg) daily for 5 consecutive days; administer one syringe for each 550 lbs of body weight per day.

Directions for Use:

1. Determine the weight of the horse.
2. Remove syringe tip.
3. Turn the dial ring until the edge of the ring nearest the tip lines up with zero.
4. Depress plunger to advance paste to tip.
5. Now set the dial ring at the graduation nearest the weight of the horse (do not underdose).
6. Horse's mouth should be free of food.

7. Insert nozzle of syringe through the interdental space and deposit the paste on the back of the tongue by depressing the plunger.

Retreatment Recommendations:

Internal Parasites: Regular deworming at intervals of six to eight weeks may be required due to the possibility of reinfection.

Migrating Tissue Parasites: In the case of 4th stage larvae of *Strongylus vulgaris*, treatment and retreatment should be based on the life cycle and the epidemiology. Treatment should be initiated in the spring and repeated in the fall after a six-month interval.

Optimum Deworming Program for Control of *S. vulgaris*: Optimum reduction of *S. vulgaris* infections is achieved by reducing the infectivity of the pastures. When horses are running on pasture, in temperate North America, maximum pasture infectivity occurs in October-December. If horses are removed from those pastures in January, pasture infectivity will decline to zero by July 1. Egg production of *S. vulgaris* is minimal from January through April, peaking in August and declining to minimal values in December.

Recommended Deworming Program: *December 1, February 1, April 1, June 1, August 1, October 1.

The April 1st and October 1st treatments are the recommended periods when the 5 day treatment regimen for the control of the migrating larvae of *S. vulgaris* should be performed.

*For other areas in the world, retreatment periods for the migrating larvae of *S. vulgaris* may be different; consult with your veterinarian.

Contraindication(s): There are no known contraindications for the use of PANACUR® (fenbendazole) Paste 10% in horses.

Precaution(s): Store at or below 25°C (75°F).

Caution(s): When using PANACUR® (fenbendazole) Paste 10% concomitantly with trichlorfon, refer to the manufacturer's labels for use and cautions for trichlorfon.

Consult your veterinarian for assistance in the diagnosis, treatment and control of parasitism.

For use in animals only.

Warning(s): Do not use in horses intended for food.

Keep this and all medications out of the reach of children.

Side Effects: Side effects associated with PANACUR® (fenbendazole) Paste 10% could not be established in well-controlled safety studies in horses with single doses as high as 454 mg/lb (1,000 mg/kg) and 15 consecutive daily doses of 22.7 mg/lb (50 mg/kg). Particularly with higher doses, the lethal action of fenbendazole may cause the release of antigens by the dying parasites. This phenomenon may result in either a local or systemic hypersensitive reaction. As with any drug, these reactions should be treated symptomatically.

PANACUR® (fenbendazole) Paste 10% has been evaluated for safety in pregnant mares during all stages of gestation with doses as high as 11.4 mg/lb (25 mg/kg) and in stallions with doses as high as 11.4 mg/lb (25 mg/kg). No adverse effects on reproductivity were detected. The recommended dose for control of 4th stage larvae of *Strongylus vulgaris*, 4.6 mg/lb (10 mg/kg) daily for 5 consecutive days, has not been evaluated for safety in stallions or pregnant mares.

Presentation: PANACUR® (fenbendazole) Paste 10% Horse Wormer is supplied in 25 gram (0.88 oz) syringes, 12 per carton.

Manufactured by: DPT Laboratories, San Antonio, TX 78215.

Compendium Code No.: 11061081

PANACUR® HORSE DEWORMER (57 g)

Intervet **Parasiticide-Oral**

(fenbendazole) Paste 10% (100 mg/g)

NADA No.: 120-648

Active Ingredient(s): Each gram of PANACUR® (fenbendazole) Paste 10% contains 100 mg of fenbendazole and is flavored with artificial apple-cinnamon liquid.

Indications: PANACUR® (fenbendazole) Paste 10% is indicated for the control of large strongyles *(Strongylus edentatus, S. equinus, S. vulgaris)*, encysted early third stage (hypobiotic), late third stage and fourth stage cyathostome larvae, small strongyles, pinworms *(Oxyuris equi)*, ascarids *(Parascaris equorum)*, and arteritis caused by 4th stage larvae of *Strongylus vulgaris* in horses.

PANACUR® (fenbendazole) Paste 10% is approved for use concomitantly with an approved form of trichlorfon. Trichlorfon is approved for the treatment of stomach bots *(Gasterophilus* spp.) in horses. Refer to the manufacturer's label for directions for use and cautions and trichlorfon.

Pharmacology: PANACUR® (fenbendazole) Paste 10% contains the active anthelmintic, fenbendazole. The chemical name of fenbendazole is methyl 5-(phenylthio)-2- benzimidazol-carbamate.

The CAS Registry Number is 43210-67-9.

The chemical structure is:

Actions: The antiparasitic action of PANACUR® (fenbendazole) Paste 10% is believed to be due to the inhibition of energy metabolism in the parasite.

Dosage and Administration: Horse: PANACUR® (fenbendazole) Paste 10% is administered orally at a rate of 2.3 mg/lb (5 mg/kg) for the control of large strongylus, small strongyles, and pinworms. One syringe will deworm a 2,500 lb horse. For foals and weanlings (less than 18 months of age) where ascarids are a common problem, the recommended dose is 4.6 mg/lb (10 mg/kg); one syringe will deworm a 1,250 lb horse. For control of encysted early third stage (hypobiotic), late third stage and fourth stage cyathostome larvae, and fourth stage larvae of *Strongylus vulgaris* the recommended dose is 4.6 mg/lb (10 mg/kg) daily for 5 consecutive days; administer one syringe for each 1,250 lbs of body weight per day.

Directions for Use:

1. Determine the weight of the horse.
2. Remove syringe tip.
3. Turn the dial ring until the edge of the ring nearest the tip lines up with zero.
4. Depress plunger to advance paste to tip.
5. Now set the dial ring at the graduation nearest the weight of the horse (do not underdose).
6. Horse's mouth should be free of food.
7. Insert nozzle of syringe through the interdental space and deposit the paste on the back of the tongue by depressing the plunger.

Retreatment Recommendations:

Internal Parasites: Regular deworming at intervals of six to eight weeks may be required due to the possibility of reinfection.

Migrating Tissue Parasites: In the case of 4th stage larvae of *Strongylus vulgaris*, treatment and retreatment should be based on the life cycle and the epidemiology. Treatment should be initiated in the spring and repeated in the fall after a six-month interval.

Optimum Deworming Program for Control of *S. vulgaris*: Optimum reduction of *S. vulgaris* infections is achieved by reducing the infectivity of the pastures. When horses are running on pasture, in temperate North America, maximum pasture infectivity occurs in October-December. If horses are removed from those pastures in January, pasture infectivity will decline to zero by July 1. Egg production of *S. vulgaris* is minimal from January through April, peaking in August and declining to minimal values in December.

Recommended Deworming Program: *December 1, February 1, April 1, June 1, August 1, October 1.

The April 1st and October 1st treatments are the recommended periods when the 5-day treatment regimen for the control of the migrating larvae of *S. vulgaris* should be performed.

*For other areas in the world, retreatment periods for the migrating larvae of *S. vulgaris* may be different; consult with your veterinarian.

Contraindication(s): There are no known contraindications for the use of PANACUR® (fenbendazole) Paste 10% in horses.

Precaution(s): Store at or below 25°C (77°F).

Caution(s): When using PANACUR® (fenbendazole) Paste 10% concomitantly with trichlorfon, refer to the manufacturer's labels for use and cautions for trichlorfon.

Consult your veterinarian for assistance in the diagnosis, treatment and control of parasitism.

For use in animals only.

Warning(s): Do not use in horses intended for food.

Keep this and all medications out of the reach of children.

Side Effects: Side effects associated with PANACUR® (fenbendazole) Paste 10% could not be established in well-controlled safety studies in horses with single doses as high as 454 mg/lb (1000 mg/kg) and 15 consecutive daily doses of 22.7 mg/lb (50 mg/kg). Particularly with higher doses, the lethal actions of fenbendazole may cause the release of antigens by the dying parasites. This phenomenon may result in either a local or systemic hypersensitive reaction. As with any drug, these reactions should be treated symptomatically.

PANACUR® (fenbendazole) Paste 10% has been evaluated for safety in pregnant mares during all stages of gestation with doses as high as 11.4 mg/lb (25 mg/kg) and in stallions with doses as high as 11.4 mg/lb (25 mg/kg). No adverse effects on reproductivity were detected. The recommended dose for control of 4th stage larvae of *Strongylus vulgaris*, 4.6 mg/lb (10 mg/kg) daily for 5 consecutive days, has not been evaluated for safety in stallions or pregnant mares.

Presentation: PANACUR® (fenbendazole) Paste 10% Horse Wormer is supplied in 57 gram (2.01 oz) syringes, 5 per carton, in the Panacur® Powerpac and 57 gram (2.01 oz) syringes, 12 per carton.

Manufactured by: DPT Laboratories, San Antonio, TX 78215.

Compendium Code No.: 11061101

PANAKARE™ PLUS POWDER ℞

Neogen **Enzyme Preparation**

Pancreatic Enzyme Concentrate Plus Fat Soluble Vitamins

Active Ingredient(s): Each 2.8 g (1 teaspoonful) contains:

Lipase	71,400 USP units
Protease	388,000 USP units
Amylase	460,000 USP units
Vitamin A	1,000 IUs
Vitamin D_3	100 IUs
Vitamin E	10 IUs

Indications: PANAKARE™ Plus is used as a digestive aid in replacement therapy where digestion of protein, carbohydrate and fat is inadequate due to exocrine pancreatic insufficiency.

Description: PANAKARE™ Plus is a pancreatic enzyme supplement of porcine origin fortified with the fat soluble vitamins A, D and E.

Directions for Use: PANAKARE™ Plus is administered before each meal and is estimated according to condition and weight of the animal. PANAKARE™ Plus is added to moistened dog food (canned or dry). Thorough mixing is necessary to bring the enzymes into close contact with the food particles. After mixing, incubate at room temperature for 15-20 minutes.

Average amount/meal:

Dogs: ¾-1 teaspoonful (2.8 g/teaspoonful).

Cats: ¼-¾ teaspoonful.

Precaution(s): Store tightly closed container in a dry place at a temperature not exceeding 25°C (77°F).

Caution(s): Federal law restricts this drug to use by or on the order of a licensed veterinarian.

Discontinue use in animals with symptoms of sensitivity.

For animal use only.

Warning(s): Keep out of reach of children.

Presentation: Bottles containing 4 oz (113 g) (NDC: 59051-9064-1), 8 oz (227 g) (NDC: 59051-9065-2) and 12 oz (340.2 g) (NDC: 59051-9066-3).

Manufactured by: Tabs Limited, St. Joseph, MO.

Compendium Code No.: 14910073 0201

PANAKARE™ PLUS TABLETS ℞

Neogen **Enzyme Preparation**

Pancreatic Enzyme Concentrate Plus Fat Soluble Vitamins

Active Ingredient(s): Each tablet contains:

Lipase	9,000 USP units
Protease	57,000 USP units
Amylase	64,000 USP units
Vitamin A	1,000 IUs
Vitamin D_3	100 IUs
Vitamin E	10 IUs

Indications: PANAKARE™ Plus is used as a digestive aid in replacement therapy where digestion of protein, carbohydrate and fat is inadequate due to exocrine pancreatic insufficiency.

Description: PANAKARE™ Plus is a pancreatic enzyme concentrate of porcine origin fortified with the fat soluble Vitamins A, D and E.

Directions for Use: PANAKARE™ Plus is administered before each meal and is estimated according, to the severity of the condition and weight of the animal.

Average amount/meal:

Dogs: 2-3 tablets.

Cats: ½-1 tablet.

Precaution(s): Store tightly closed container in a dry place at a temperature not exceeding 25°C (77°F).

P

Caution(s): Federal law restricts this drug to use by or on the order of a licensed veterinarian.
Discontinue use in animals with symptoms of sensitivity.
For animal use only.
Warning(s): Keep out of reach of children.
Presentation: Bottles of 100 (NDC: 59051-9067-5) and 500 (NDC: 59051-9068-7) tablets.
Manufactured by: Tabs Limited, St. Joseph, MO.
Compendium Code No.: 14910083 0201

PANCREATIC PLUS POWDER

Butler **Enzyme Preparation**

Active Ingredient(s): Each 2.8 g (1 teaspoonful) contains:

Lipase	71,400 USP units
Protease	388,000 USP units
Amylase	460,000 USP units
Vitamin A	1,000 IUs
Vitamin D_3	100 IUs
Vitamin E	10 IUs

Pancreatic enzymes are of porcine origin.
Indications: As a digestive aid in replacement therapy for dogs and cats where digestion of protein, carbohydrate and fat is inadequate due to exocrine pancreatic insufficiency.
Dosage and Administration: Dose is administered before each meal and is estimated according to the severity of the condition and weight of the animal. PANCREATIC PLUS is added to moistened dog food (canned or dry). Thorough mixing is necessary to bring the enzymes into close contact with the food particles. After mixing, incubate at room temperature for 15-20 minutes.
Average dose/meal:
Dogs: ¾-1 teaspoon (2.8 g/teaspoon).
Cats: ¼-¾ teaspoon. Fortified with-soluble vitamins A, D, and E where metabolism of these essential vitamins is insufficient.
Precaution(s): Store tightly closed container in a dry place at a temperature not exceeding 25°C (77°F).
Caution(s): Discontinue use in animals with symptoms of sensitivity.
Presentation: 4 oz., 8 oz., and 12 oz. containers.
Compendium Code No.: 10821350

PANCREATIC PLUS TABLETS

Butler **Enzyme Preparation**

Active Ingredient(s): Each 2.8 g (1 teaspoonful) contains:

Lipase	9,000 USP units
Protease	57,000 USP units
Amylase	64,000 USP units
Vitamin A	1,000 IUs
Vitamin D_3	100 IUs
Vitamin E	10 IUs

Pancreatic enzymes are of porcine origin.
Indications: As a digestive aid in replacement therapy for dogs and cats where digestion of protein, carbohydrate and fat is inadequate due to exocrine pancreatic insufficiency. Fortified with-soluble vitamins A, D, and E where metabolism of these essential vitamins is insufficient.
Dosage and Administration: Dose is administered before each meal and is estimated according to the severity of the condition and weight of the animal. PANCREATIC PLUS is added to moistened dog food (canned or dry). Thorough mixing is necessary to bring the enzymes into close contact with the food particles. After mixing, incubate at room temperature for 15-20 minutes.
Average dose/meal:
Dogs: 2-3 tablets.
Cats: ½-1 tablet.
Precaution(s): Store in a tightly closed container in a dry place at a temperature not exceeding 25°C (77°F).
Caution(s): Discontinue use in animals with symptoms of sensitivity.
Presentation: Bottles of 100 and 500 tablets.
Compendium Code No.: 10821360

P

PANCREVED POWDER ℞

Vedco **Enzyme Preparation**

Pancreatic Enzyme Concentrate Plus Fat Soluble Vitamins
Active Ingredient(s): Each 2.8 g (1 teaspoonful) contains:

Lipase	71,400 USP units
Protease	388,000 USP units
Amylase	460,000 USP units
Vitamin A	1,000 IUs
Vitamin D_3	100 IUs
Vitamin E	10 IUs

Description: PANCREVED is a pancreatic enzyme concentrate of porcine origin fortified with fat-soluble vitamins A, D and E.
Indications: As a digestive aid in replacement therapy where digestion of protein, carbohydrate and fat is inadequate due to exocrine pancreatic insufficiency.
Dosage and Administration: Dosage: Dose is administered before each meal and is estimated according to the severity of the condition and weight of the animal. PANCREVED is added to moistened dog food (canned or dry). Thorough mixing is necessary to bring the enzymes into close contact with the food particles. After mixing, incubate at room temperature for 15-20 minutes.
Average dose/meal:
Dogs: ¾-1 teaspoon (2.8 g/teaspoon).
Cats: ¼-¾ teaspoon.
Precaution(s): Store tightly closed container in a dry place at a temperature not exceeding 25°C (77°F).
Caution(s): Federal law restricts this drug to use by or on the order of a licensed veterinarian.
Discontinue use in animals with symptoms of sensitivity.
For animal use only.
Warning(s): Keep out of reach of children.
Presentation: 4 oz (113 g) (NDC 50989-313-21), 8 oz (227 g) (NDC 50989-313-24), and 12 oz (340.5 g) (NDC 50989-313-25) containers.
Compendium Code No.: 10942250 0998 / 0998 / 0498

PANCREVED TABLETS ℞

Vedco **Enzyme Preparation**

Pancreatic Enzyme Concentrate Plus Fat Soluble Vitamins
Active Ingredient(s): Each 425 mg tablet contains:

Lipase	9,000 USP units
Protease	57,000 USP units
Amylase	64,000 USP units
Vitamin A	1,000 IUs
Vitamin D_3	100 IUs
Vitamin E	10 IUs

Description: PANCREVED is a pancreatic enzyme concentrate of porcine origin fortified with the fat-soluble vitamins A, D, and E.
Indications: As a digestive aid in replacement therapy where digestion of protein, carbohydrate and fat is inadequate due to exocrine pancreatic insufficiency.
Dosage and Administration: Dosage: Dose is administered before each meal and is estimated according to the severity of the condition and weight of the animal. Average dose/meal:
Dogs: 2-3 tablets.
Cats: ½-1 tablet.
Precaution(s): Store tightly closed container in a dry place at a temperature not exceeding 25°C (77°F).
Caution(s): Federal law restricts this drug to use by or on the order of a licensed veterinarian.
Discontinue use in animals with symptoms of sensitivity.
For animal use only.
Warning(s): Keep out of reach of children.
Presentation: Bottles of 100 (NDC 50989-313-51) and 500 (NDC 50989-313-25) tablets.
Compendium Code No.: 10942260 0998

PANCREZYME® ℞

King Animal Health **Enzyme Preparation**

Active Ingredient(s):
Each 425 mg tablet contains:

Lipase	9,000 U.S.P. units
Protease	57,000 U.S.P. units
Amylase	64,000 U.S.P. units

Each teaspoonful (2.8 g) contains:

Lipase	71,400 U.S.P. units
Protease	388,000 U.S.P. units
Amylase	460,000 U.S.P. units

PANCREZYME® is an enzymatic concentrate derived from porcine pancreas containing standardized lipase, protease and amylase plus esterases, peptidases, nucleases and elastase.
Indications: For use in animals with deficient exocrine pancreatic secretions, as a digestive aid in enzyme replacement therapy where digestion of carbohydrate, protein and fat is inadequate.
Dosage and Administration: The dose should be adjusted according to the severity of the condition and the weight of the animal.
Tablets:
Adult dogs: The average dose is 2-3 tablets with each meal.
Adult cats: ½-1 tablet with each meal.
Powder:
Adult dogs: ¾-1 teaspoonful with each meal.
Adult cats: ¼-¾ teaspoonful with each meal.
Mix well with moistened food (canned or dry) and let stand at room temperature for 15-20 minutes before feeding. Frequent feeding, at least three (3) times a day is important.
Precaution(s): Discontinue use in animals with symptoms of sensitivity.
Caution(s): Federal law restricts this drug to use by or on the order of a licensed veterinarian.
Presentation: PANCREZYME® Tablets 425 mg - Bottles of 100 and 500 tablets.
PANCREZYME® Powder - Bottles of 4 oz., 8 oz. and 12 oz.
Compendium Code No.: 11320042

PANMYCIN AQUADROPS® ℞

Pharmacia & Upjohn **Tetracycline-Oral**

brand of tetracycline liquid
NADA No.: 065-060
Active Ingredient(s): PANMYCIN AQUADROPS® Liquid contains tetracycline which is a broad spectrum antibiotic that can be conveniently administered to dogs and cats in a palatable liquid preparation. PANMYCIN AQUADROPS® contains in each mL tetracycline base equivalent to 100 mg of tetracycline hydrochloride, suspended in a chocolate-mint flavored aqueous vehicle. Methylparaben, 0.075%; propylparaben, 0.025%; and sodium metabisulfite, 0.5%; are present as preservatives. PANMYCIN AQUADROPS® is stable at room temperature.
Indications: PANMYCIN AQUADROPS® is indicated for oral administration to dogs and cats in the treatment of infections caused by organisms sensitive to tetracycline hydrochloride such as:
1. Bacterial gastroenteritis due to *E. coli*.
2. Urinary tract infections due to *Staphylococcus* spp. and *E. coli*.

Appropriate laboratory tests should be conducted including *in vitro* culturing and susceptibility tests on samples collected prior to treatment.
Pharmacology: Tetracycline is a bright yellow, crystalline, broad spectrum antibiotic produced by a species of Streptomyces. Although its chemical and physical properties as well as its antibacterial spectrum resemble those of oxytetracycline and chlortetracycline, tetracycline hydrochloride offers the advantage of greater stability in plasma and, on oral administration, fewer gastrointestinal side effects.

Action: Tetracycline has a wide range of antibacterial activity against gram-positive and gram-negative bacteria. These include *Streptococcus* spp., *Staphylococcus* spp., *Aerobacter aerogenes*, *E.coli*, *Klebsiella* spp., *Salmonella* spp., *(Haemophilus) and Pasteurella* spp. The antimicrobial activity of tetracycline also includes rickettsia and agents belonging to the psittacosislymphogranuloma group.

Administered by mouth, tetracycline is absorbed from the gastrointestinal tract and readily diffuses into various body fluids including blood serum, spinal fluid, pleural fluid, and peritoneal fluid, cord serum, and saliva. Maximum blood levels of the antibiotic are reached at about two hours after administration and are maintained at high levels for 6 to 8 hours. The blood levels were observed to be somewhat higher than those obtained with similar doses of oxytetracycline or chlortetracycline. Spinal fluid concentrations were found to be notably higher than those produced by the other tetracyclines, indicating the greater ease of tetracycline to pass the bloodbrain barrier. The urinary excretion of tetracycline is rapid, the rate being approximately equal to that of the other tetracyclines. A significant portion of the dose is not absorbed and appears in the feces.

Dosage and Administration: The dosage of PANMYCIN AQUADROPS®, as with other tetracycline drugs, will vary in different animal patients according to the severity of the infection, response to treatment, and susceptibility of the causative bacteria. The following average dosage is suggested:

Dogs and Cats: 25 mg tetracycline (5 drops PANMYCIN AQUADROPS®) per pound of body weight, per day, in divided doses every 6 hours.

Treatment should be continued until the temperature has been normal for 48 hours or characteristic symptoms of the disease have subsided. In dogs and cats tetracycline is usually well tolerated, but, if necessary, the drug may be given with a light diet.

To assure even distribution of the tetracycline the bottle should be shaken thoroughly before each dose.

Precaution(s): Storage Conditions: Store at controlled room temperature 20° to 25°C (68° to 77°F) [see USP].

Caution(s): Federal (USA) law restricts this drug to use by or on the order of a licensed veterinarian.

Use of tetracycline hydrochloride during tooth development (late prenatal, neonatal and early postnatal periods) may cause discoloration of the teeth (yellow-grey-brownish). This effect occurs mostly during long-term use of the drug. But it has also been observed following short treatment courses.

With the use of any broad spectrum antibiotic, prolonged use may result in overgrowth of nonsusceptible organisms, including *Candida (monilia) albicans*. Constant observation is essential. Should superinfection occur, the antibiotic should be discontinued and/or other appropriate measures taken.

For oral use in dogs and cats only.

For animal use only.

Warning(s): Not for use in animals which are raised for food production.

Not for human use.

Adverse Reactions: Tetracycline hydrochloride is generally well tolerated; however, in some instances a change in consistency of the stool may occur due to the wide antibacterial effects of tetracycline on the intestinal flora.

If allergic reactions occur or if individual idiosyncrasy appears, discontinue medication.

Presentation: PANMYCIN AQUADROPS® Liquid is supplied in 15 mL (NDC 0009-0571-06) and 30 mL (NDC 0009-0571-02) bottles with direction labels and calibrated droppers.

Compendium Code No.: 10490422 812 308 206

PANOLOG® CREAM ℞

Fort Dodge **Topical Antimicrobial-Corticosteroid**

Nystatin-Neomycin Sulfate-Thiostrepton-Triamcinolone Acetonide Cream USP

NADA No.: 096-676

Active Ingredient(s): PANOLOG® Cream (nystatin-neomycin sulfate-thiostrepton-triamcinolone acetonide cream USP) combines nystatin, neomycin sulfate, thiostrepton and triamcinolone acetonide.

Each gram contains 100,000 units nystatin, neomycin sulfate equivalent to 2.5 mg of neomycin base, 2,500 units thiostrepton, and 1.0 mg triamcinolone acetonide in an aqueous, nonirritating vanishing cream base with cetearyl alcohol (and) ceteareth-20, ethylenediamine hydrochloride, methylparaben, propylparaben, propylene glycol, sorbitol solution, titanium dioxide, sodium citrate, citric acid, white petrolatum, simethicone emulsion and purified water.

Indications: PANOLOG® Cream is indicated in the management of dermatologic disorders in dogs and cats, characterized by inflammation and dry or exudative dermatitis, particularly those caused, complicated or threatened by bacterial or candidal *(Candida albicans)* infections. It is also of value in eczematous dermatitis, contact dermatitis and seborrheic dermatitis; and as an adjunct in the treatment of dermatitis due to parasitic infestation.

Pharmacology: Actions: By virtue of its four active ingredients, PANOLOG® Cream provides four basic therapeutic effects: anti-inflammatory, antipruritic, antifungal and antibacterial. Triamcinolone acetonide is a potent synthetic corticosteroid providing rapid and prolonged symptomatic relief on topical administration. Inflammation, edema and pruritus promptly subside, and lesions are permitted to heal. Nystatin is the first well-tolerated antifungal antibiotic of dependable efficacy for the treatment of cutaneous infections caused by *Candida albicans* (Monilia). Nystatin is fungistatic *in vitro* against a variety of yeast and yeastlike fungi including many fungi pathogenic to animals. No appreciable activity is exhibited against bacteria. Thiostrepton has a high order of activity against gram-positive organisms, including many which are resistant to other antibiotics; neomycin exerts antimicrobial action against a wide range of gram-positive and gram-negative bacteria. Together they provide comprehensive therapy against those organisms responsible for most superficial bacterial infections.

Dosage and Administration: Frequency of administration is dependent on the severity of the condition. For mild inflammations, application may range from once daily to once a week; for severe conditions PANOLOG® Cream may be applied as often as 2 to 3 times daily, if necessary. Frequency of treatment may be decreased as improvement occurs.

Clean affected areas, removing any encrusted discharge or exudate. Apply PANOLOG® Cream sparingly in a thin film.

Contraindication(s): PANOLOG® Cream (nystatin-neomycin sulfate-thiostrepton-triamcinolone acetonide cream USP) should not be used ophthalmically.

Precaution(s): Do not store above 86°F (30°C).

Caution(s): Federal law restricts this drug to use by or on the order of a licensed veterinarian.

PANOLOG® Cream is not intended for the treatment of deep abscesses or deep-seated infections such as inflammation of the lymphatic vessels. Parenteral antibiotic therapy is indicated in these infections.

PANOLOG® Cream has been extremely well tolerated. The occurrence of systemic reactions is rarely a problem with topical administration. Sensitivity to neomycin may occur. If redness, irritation or swelling persists or increases, discontinue use. Do not use if pus is present since the drug may allow the infection to spread.

Avoid ingestion. Oral or parenteral use of corticosteroids, depending on dose, duration and specific steroid may result in inhibition of endogenous steroid production following drug withdrawal.

Absorption of triamcinolone acetonide through topical application and by licking may occur. Therefore animals should be observed closely for signs of polydipsia, polyuria and increased weight gain particularly when the preparation is used over large areas or for extended periods of time.

Clinical and experimental data have demonstrated that corticosteroids administered orally or by injection to animals may induce the first stage of parturition if used during the last trimester of pregnancy and may precipitate premature parturition followed by dystocia, fetal death, retained placenta, and metritis.

Additionally, corticosteroids administered to dogs, rabbits and rodents during pregnancy have resulted in cleft palate in offspring. Corticosteroids administered to dogs during pregnancy have also resulted in other congenital anomalies including deformed forelegs, phocomelia and anasarca.

Warning(s): PANOLOG® Cream is indicated for topical use in dogs and cats only. Not for use in animals which are raised for food.

Side Effects: SAP and SGPT (ALT) enzyme elevations, polydipsia and polyuria have occurred following parenteral or systemic use of synthetic corticosteroids in dogs. Vomiting and diarrhea (occasionally bloody) have been observed in dogs.

Cushing's syndrome in dogs has been reported in association with prolonged or repeated steroid therapy.

Presentation: PANOLOG® Cream is supplied in 7.5 gram and 15 gram tubes.

NDC 53501-583-01 — 7.5 gram tube.
NDC 53501-583-02 — 15 gram tube.
NDC 53501-583-03 — 72 x 15 gram tubes.

Compendium Code No.: 10031421 12830B

PANOLOG® OINTMENT ℞

Fort Dodge **Topical Antimicrobial-Corticosteroid**

Nystatin-Neomycin Sulfate-Thiostrepton-Triamcinolone Acetonide Ointment USP

NADA No.: 012-258

Active Ingredient(s): PANOLOG® Ointment (nystatin-neomycin sulfate-thiostrepton-triamcinolone acetonide ointment USP) combines nystatin, neomycin sulfate, thiostrepton and triamcinolone acetonide in a non-irritating, protective vehicle, Plastibase® (plasticized hydrocarbon gel), a polyethylene and mineral oil gel base.

Each mL contains 100,000 units nystatin, neomycin sulfate equivalent to 2.5 mg of neomycin base, 2,500 units thiostrepton, and 1.0 mg triamcinolone acetonide.

Indications: The preparation is intended for local therapy in a variety of cutaneous disorders of cats and dogs; it is especially useful in disorders caused, complicated or threatened by bacterial and/or candidal (monilial) infection.

PANOLOG® Ointment is particularly useful in the treatment of acute and chronic otitis of varied etiologies, in interdigital cysts in cats and dogs and in anal gland infections in dogs.

The preparation is also indicated in the management of dermatologic disorders characterized by inflammation and dry or exudative dermatitis, particularly those caused, complicated or threatened by bacterial or candidal *(Candida albicans)* infections. It is also of value in eczematous dermatitis, contact dermatitis and seborrheic dermatitis; and as an adjunct in the treatment of dermatitis due to parasitic infestation.

Pharmacology: Actions: By virtue of its four active ingredients, PANOLOG® Ointment provides four basic therapeutic effects; anti-inflammatory, antipruritic, antifungal and antibacterial. Triamcinolone acetonide is a potent synthetic corticosteroid providing rapid and prolonged symptomatic relief on topical administration. Inflammation, edema and pruritus promptly subside, and lesions are permitted to heal. Nystatin is the first well-tolerated antifungal antibiotic of dependable efficacy for the treatment of cutaneous infections caused by *Candida albicans* (Monilia). Nystatin is fungistatic *in vitro* against a variety of yeast and yeast-like fungi including many fungi pathogenic to animals. No appreciable activity is exhibited against bacteria. Thiostrepton has a high order of activity against gram-positive organisms, including many which are resistant to other antibiotics: neomycin exerts antimicrobial action against a wide range of gram-positive and gram-negative bacteria. Together they provide comprehensive therapy against those organisms responsible for most superficial bacterial infections.

Dosage and Administration: Frequency of administration is dependent on the severity of the condition. For mild inflammations, application may range from once daily to once a week; for severe conditions PANOLOG® Ointment may be applied as often as two to three times daily, if necessary. Frequency of treatment may be decreased as improvement occurs.

Otitis: Clean ear canal of impacted cerumen. Inspect canal and remove any foreign bodies such as grass awns, ticks, etc. Instill three to five drops of PANOLOG® Ointment.

Preliminary use of a local anesthetic such as Ophthaine® Solution Veterinary (proparacaine hydrochloride ophthalmic solution USP) may be advisable. The suggested dosage for Ophthaine is two drops instilled into the ear every five minutes for three doses just prior to cleaning - see package insert accompanying that product for complete information.

Infected anal glands, cystic areas, etc.: Drain gland or cyst and then fill with PANOLOG® Ointment.

Other dermatologic disorders: Clean affected areas, removing any encrusted discharge or exudate. Apply PANOLOG® Ointment sparingly in a thin film.

Precaution(s): Do not store above 86°F (30°C).

Caution(s): Federal law restricts this drug to use by or on the order of a licensed veterinarian.

Before instilling any medication into the ear, examine the external ear canal thoroughly to be certain the tympanic membrane is not ruptured in order to avoid the possibility of transmitting infection to the middle ear as well as damaging the cochlea or vestibular apparatus from prolonged contact. If hearing or vestibular dysfunction is noted during the course of treatment, discontinue use of PANOLOG® Ointment.

PANOLOG® Ointment (nystatin-neomycin sulfate-thiostrepton-triamcinolone acetonide ointment USP) is not intended for the treatment of deep abscesses or deep-seated infections such as inflammation of the lymphatic vessels. Parenteral antibiotic therapy is indicated in these infections.

PANOLOG® Ointment has been extremely well tolerated. Cutaneous reactions attributable to its use have been extremely rare. The occurrence of systemic reactions is rarely a problem with topical administration. There is some evidence that corticosteroids can be absorbed after topical application and cause systemic effects. Therefore, an animal receiving PANOLOG® Ointment therapy should be observed closely for signs such as polydipsia, polyuria and increased weight gain.

PANOLOG® Ointment is not generally recommended for the treatment of deep or puncture wounds or serious burns.

Sensitivity to neomycin may occur. If redness, irritation, or swelling persists or increases, discontinue use. Do not use if pus is present since the drug may allow the infection to spread.

Avoid ingestion. Oral or parenteral use of corticosteroids, depending on dose, duration and specific steroid, may result in inhibition of endogenous steroid production following drug withdrawal.

Clinical and experimental data have demonstrated that corticosteroids administered orally or by injection to animals may induce the first stage of parturition if used during the last trimester of pregnancy and may precipitate premature parturition followed by dystocia, fetal death, retained placenta and metritis.

Additionally, corticosteroids administered to dogs, rabbits and rodents during pregnancy have resulted in cleft palate in offspring. Corticosteroids administered to dogs during pregnancy have also resulted in other congenital anomalies including deformed forelegs, phocomelia and anasarca.

Warning(s): Keep this and all medications out of the reach of children.

For use in dogs and cats only.

Side Effects: SAP and SGPT (ALT) enzyme elevations, polydipsia and polyuria have occurred following parenteral or systemic use of synthetic corticosteroids in dogs. Vomiting and diarrhea (occasionally bloody) have been observed in dogs.

Cushing's Syndrome in dogs has been reported in association with prolonged or repeated steroid therapy. Temporary hearing loss has been reported in conjunction with treatment of otitis. However, regression usually occurred following withdrawal of the drug. If hearing dysfunction is noted during the course of treatment, discontinue use of PANOLOG® Ointment.

Presentation: PANOLOG® Ointment is supplied in tubes of ¼ fl. oz. (7.5 mL), ½ fl. oz. (15 mL), and 1 fl. oz. (30 mL), each with an elongated tip for easy application, and in dispensing packages of 8 fl. oz. (240 mL).

NDC 53501-581-19 — 7.5 mL tube.

NDC 53501-581-78 — 144 x 7.5 mL tube.

NDC 53501-581-17 — 15 mL tubes.

NDC 53501-581-28 — 30 mL tubes.

NDC 53501-581-82 — 240 mL tubes.

Plastibase® and Ophthaine® are E.R. Squibb & Sons, Inc. trademarks.

Compendium Code No.: 10031430 4212840B

PANTEK® CLEANSER

Loveland **Detergent**

Indications: PANTEK® Cleanser is a combination of cresols (50%) and soap which, when diluted with water, is used for cleaning poultry houses, hog barns and other livestock buildings. PANTEK® Cleanser can also be used to clean livestock trucks, stockyard pens, chutes and equipment.

Dosage and Administration: For all uses, mix one (1) part PANTEK® Cleanser with 200 parts water.

Before using, remove all livestock, equipment and feed from the house. Remove as much litter and other debris from the building as possible. Spray or wash the building with PANTEK® solution using between 20 to 40 gallons per 1,000 sq. ft. of floor space. For the best results, ensure that the spray gets into all cracks and crevices. Ventilate closed areas before re-entry or use.

To clean equipment requiring a smaller amount of the solution, mix approximately 2 oz. of PANTEK® Cleanser with three (3) gallons of water (1:200) and scrub all surfaces. Let stand for at least 10 minutes. Rinse thoroughly with clean water before using.

Precaution(s): Store in the original container and keep closed when not in use.

Caution(s): Keep out of the reach of children.

The product may be fatal if swallowed or absorbed through the skin. May produce severe burns to the skin, the eyes and mucous membranes. If taken internally, call a physician immediately. Do not induce vomiting. Vapors may be harmful in confined spaces. Do not get into the eyes, on the skin or on clothing. Wear eye protection while mixing or using the product. If the product comes into contact with the skin or the eyes, flush with water for 15 minutes and call a physician. Wash thoroughly after handling.

Presentation: 1 gallon containers.

Compendium Code No.: 10860201

PAPILLOMUNE™

Biomune **Vaccine**

Bovine Wart Vaccine, Killed Virus

U.S. Vet. Lic. No.: 368

Contents: PAPILLOMUNE™ contains a standardized, inactivated concentration of virus-laden tissue extract derived from bovine papillomas. The antigenic concentration contained in PAPILLOMUNE™ exceeds the minimum volume set by USDA and is labeled for a uniform 10 mL dose. PAPILLOMUNE™ is a uniformly clear, homogenous suspension that is easily syringeable.

Indications: PAPILLOMUNE™ is indicated for use as an aid in the prevention of viral warts in cattle. Vaccinate only healthy animals.

Dosage and Administration: Shake well before using. Administer 10 mL subcutaneously in two sites on the animal (5 mL each) using aseptic technique. Repeat dose in 3-5 weeks. Because the papilloma virus is so environmentally stable, many experienced bovine practitioners suggest continuation of the vaccination regime for at least one year after the last warts have been observed in a herd.

Precaution(s): Use entire contents when first opened. Store in the dark at 35°-45°F (2°-7°C).

Caution(s): Vaccinate only healthy animals. This vaccine is a tissue derived extract. In case of anaphylactic reaction use epinephrine or equivalent.

This vaccine has been carefully produced and has undergone purity and safety tests to meet Biomune's requirements and USDA regulations.

Warning(s): Do not vaccinate within 21 days of slaughter. @P1 = **Discussion:** Field testing of several hundred animals demonstrated PAPILLOMUNE™ to be safe, with no adverse reactions. Injection site swelling was minimal and of short duration.

In animals destined for the show-ring, and in seedstock cattle, warts (papillomas) can seriously impair the aesthetic, and ultimately the economic value of the animal. Benign, self limiting tumors, warts in cattle are caused by bovine papilloma virus. The virus replicates within the wart tissue with a great deal of the infective virus residing near the surface. When affected animals rub against fences, stanchions or other objects, they may transfer infective virus to the object leaving others in the herd vulnerable to infection should they receive skin abrasions from these objects.

Surgical instruments, needles, tattoo pliers and other instruments have also been suspected sources of virus spread between animals. While usually appearing on the head, neck and shoulders, warts can occur anywhere on the animal's body, including mucous membranes of the reproductive tract. Surgical removal or chemical treatment are often unacceptable to owners and may stimulate regrowth and spread of warts.

References: Available upon request.

Presentation: 1 dose (10 mL) and 5 dose (50 mL) vials.

Compendium Code No.: 11290240

PARACHEK™

Biocor **Mycobacterium Test**

Mycobacterium paratuberculosis Antibody Test Kit-Johne's Absorbed EIA

U.S. Vet. Lic. No.: 462A

Components: Kit Components:

1. Microtitre plates coated with *M. paratuberculosis*	2 x plates* with lids	30 x plates† with lids	Ready for use.
2. Positive Control Contains 0.01% w/v thimerosal	1 x 0.75 mL	1 x 2.0 mL	Ready for use.
3. Negative Control Contains 0.01% w/v thimerosal	1 x 0.75 mL	1 x 2.0 mL	Ready for use.
4. Green Diluent - serum diluent buffer Contains 0.01% w/v thimerosal	1 x 100 mL	3 x 501 mL	Ready for use.
5. Wash buffer - 20X conc. Contains 0.01% w/v thimerosal	1 x 100 mL	2 x 500 mL	Dilute with deionized or distilled water.
6. Conjugate - 100X conc. Horseradish peroxidase labelled anti-bovine Ig Contains 0.01% w/v thimerosal	1 x 0.5 mL	2 x 2 mL	Dilute with Blue Diluent.
7. Blue Diluent - conjugate diluent buffer Contains 0.01% w/v thimerosal	1 x 30mL	2 x 200 mL	Ready for use.
8. Enzyme substrate buffer solution Contains H_2O_2	1 x 30mL	2 x 200 mL	Ready for use.
9. Chromogen solution - 100X conc. Contains TMB in DMSO	1 x 0.5 mL	2 x 2 mL	Dilute with enzyme substrate buffer solution.
10. Enzyme stopping solution (0.5M H_2SO_4)	1 x 15 mL	1 x 200 mL	Ready for use.

*CSL Cat. No. 03010201 †CSL Cat. No. 03012501

Equipment Required: Accurate, replaceable-tip variable-volume pipettes (to deliver 475 µL, 25 µL and 10 to 120 µL), Graduated 1, 5 and 10 mL pipettes, Measuring cylinders - 100 mL, 1 L and 2 L, Suitable microtitre plate washer/dispenser, Multichannel pipetter (to deliver 50 and 100 µL), Suitable microtitre plate reader. This reader must be fitted with filters to read at 450 nm and 620-650 nm., Tubes, 1 mL plastic racked in 96 well format. Suitable tubes and racks are available from Bio-Rad.

Indications: *In vitro* diagnostic for the detection of bovine antibodies to *Mycobacterium paratuberculosis.*

Test Principles: The test involves four separate stages:

Stage 1: Serum samples are diluted and incubated in diluent buffer containing *M. phlei* to remove cross-reacting antibodies.

Stage 2: Diluted serum samples are reacted with *M. paratuberculosis* antigens bound to a solid support. Unreacted proteins are removed by washing after a suitable incubation time.

Stage 3: Conjugate (horseradish peroxidase labelled anti-bovine Ig) reacts with immunoglobulins bound to the solid-phase antigen. Unreacted conjugate is removed by washing after a suitable time.

Stage 4: Enzyme substrate is added. The rate of conversion of substrate is proportional to the amount of bound immunoglobulin. Reaction is terminated after a suitable time and the amount of colour development estimated spectrophotometrically.

Test Procedure: Preparation of Reagents:

1. Plates: Allow plates to equilibrate to room temperature for at least 30 minutes before unsealing plastic pouch. Strips not required should be removed from frame and resealed in the plastic pouch along with desiccant. Frames and lids are reusable.
2. Positive and negative controls: Bring to room temperature and mix each thoroughly.
3. Green Diluent: Serum diluent buffer. Bring to room temperature and mix thoroughly. Use undiluted.

   Note: Up to 2 hours may be required to ensure a full bottle of Green Diluent has reached room temperature. If a shorter equilibration time is desired, an ambient temperature water bath must be used.
4. Blue Diluent: Conjugate diluent buffer. Bring to room temperature and mix thoroughly. Use undiluted.
5. Conjugate 100X Concentrate: Conjugate 100X Concentrate must be stored at 2° to 7°C at all times.
6. Preparation of Conjugate: Bring Blue Diluent (conjugate diluent buffer) to room temperature then mix thoroughly with Conjugate 100X Concentrate to make Conjugate Reagent ready for use. Suitable volumes are presented in the Conjugate and Substrate Preparation Table. The working strength Conjugate Reagent should be used within 30 minutes of preparation and unused reagent immediately discarded. Return any unused Conjugate 100X Concentrate to 2° to 7°C immediately after use.
7. Wash Buffer: Prepare working strength wash buffer by thoroughly mixing one part 20X concentrate with 19 parts deionized or distilled water. Working strength wash buffer may be stored at room temperature for up to 2 weeks.
8. Enzyme substrate solution: Bring enzyme substrate reagents to room temperature for at least 30 minutes prior to mixing. Prepare enzyme substrate solution just prior to use by diluting the chromogen solution concentrate in enzyme substrate buffer as shown in the Conjugate and Substrate Preparation Table. Enzyme substrate solution should be colourless. Discard if blue coloration occurs.

   Use within 10 minutes of preparation.

   Note: If possible use plastic polypropylene disposable containers sterilized by irradiation to prepare the enzyme substrate solution.

   Do not use polystyrene containers or pipettes.

   Any glassware used with the enzyme substrate reagents should be rinsed thoroughly with 1N H_2SO_4 or HCl followed by at least three washes of deionized or distilled water, ensuring no acid residue remains on the glassware.

Conjugate and Substrate Preparation Table:

Number of Strips	Volume of Concentrate	Volume of Diluent
1	10 µL	1 mL
2	20 µL	2 mL
3	30 µL	3 mL
4	40 µL	4 mL
5	50 µL	5 mL

Number of Strips	Volume of Concentrate	Volume of Diluent
6	60 µL	6 mL
7	70 µL	7 mL
8	80 µL	8 mL
9	90 µL	9 mL
10	100 µL	10 mL
11	110 µL	11 mL
12	120 µL	12 mL

Procedural Notes:

1. Allow all reagents except the Conjugate 100X Concentrate to equilibrate to room temperature (22°C ± 5°C) for at least 30 minutes before use.
   Note: Refer to special requirements for Green Diluent (see Preparation of Reagents).
2. All kit components are to be stored at 2° to 7°C. Return to 2° to 7°C immediately after use. Working strength wash buffer may be stored at room temperature for up to 2 weeks.
3. The Conjugate 100X Concentrate must be left at 2° to 7°C at all times.
4. Once the assay has been started it should be completed without interruption.
5. Use a separate disposable tip for each sample to prevent cross contamination.
6. Test sera may be assayed in duplicate in adjacent wells.
7. Positive and negative controls must be assayed in duplicate. For convenience, controls may be located at the beginning of each plate (eg. negative controls in well A1 and B1, positive controls in wells C1 and D1).

Test Procedures:

Steps:

1. Equilibrate all reagents except the Conjugate 100X Concentrate.
2. Add 25 µL of test and control samples to their appropriate tubes. Allow 1 tube per sample and 1 tube for each of the controls.
3. Add 475 µL of Green Diluent to each of the tubes being very careful not to cross contaminate the tubes. If splashing or cross contamination does occur, discard the tubes and start again. Mix thoroughly either by pipetting up and down 3 to 5 times or by vortexing tubes several times.
4. Cover tubes and incubate at room temperature (22°C ± 5°C) for a minimum of 30 minutes. A longer period (up to 60 minutes) is not detrimental to the test.
5. Add 100 µL of test and control samples to appropriate wells.
   Add control samples after the test samples have been added. Shake plate. Controls may be positioned anywhere on the plate (see Procedural Notes).
6. Cover each plate with a lid and incubate at room temperature (22°C ± 5°C) for 30 minutes. Conjugate 100X Concentrate should be diluted ready for use at the end of this incubation.
7. Shake out diluted serum samples and wash trays 6 times at room temperature as follows. Fill wells with wash buffer taking care not to cross contaminate adjacent wells. Shake out wash fluid and repeat operation a further 5 times. After the sixth wash, tap trays face down several times on absorbent paper to remove as much remaining wash buffer as possible (refer to Technical Information for further instructions).
8. Add 100 µL of freshly prepared conjugate reagent to each well. Shake plate.
9. Cover each plate with a lid and incubate at room temperature for 30 minutes.
10. Wash plates as in Step 7.
    Note: The enzyme substrate solution is best prepared after this wash step.
11. Add 100 µL of freshly prepared enzyme substrate solution to each well.
12. Cover each plate with a lid, shake and incubate at room temperature. Optimal time of incubation is dependent on a number of variables. Time is best judged by reading the absorbance of the positive controls during colour development. A 620-650 nm filter must be used. Proceed to step 13 when the absorbance is between 0.35 and 0.40*.
    Note: Gently mix the contents of plates by tapping to evenly distribute colour in positive control wells before estimating intensity as above. Protect from direct sunlight.
13. Add 50 µL of enzyme stopping solution to each well, being careful not to transfer chromogen from well to well, then mix by gentle agitation.
    Note: The stopping solution should be added to wells in the same order and at the same speed as the enzyme substrate solution.
14. Read the absorbance of each well using a 450 nm filter between 2 and 20 minutes after terminating the reaction. The absorbance values will then be used to calculate results.

*If available, read plates using the monitored end point option (blank on air) of software, with the plate shaking option set to operate between each reading.

Caution(s): General Precautions:

1. Laboratory Safety: Correct laboratory procedures should be applied at all times.
2. Chromogen Solution: Caution. Avoid contact with skin. Handle chromogen solution with care since dimethyl sulphoxide (DMSO) is readily absorbed through the skin.
3. Stopping Solution: The enzyme stopping solution is a strong acid.
   Wipe up spills immediately.
   Flush the area of the spill with water.
   If the stopping solution contacts the skin or eyes, flush with copious quantities of water and seek medical attention.

For veterinary use only.

Approved diagnostic test for use in Australia's National Johne's Disease Market Assurance Program.

Discussion: Johne's disease is a chronic, debilitating enteritis of ruminants caused by infection with *Mycobacterium paratuberculosis*. During the active stage of infection and prior to onset of clinical disease, cattle generally develop antibodies to *M. paratuberculosis* antigens. Uninfected cattle lack specific antibodies to *M. paratuberculosis*, but may have cross-reacting antibodies to other mycobacteria. These cross-reacting antibodies can be removed by absorption of serum with *M. phlei* prior to commencement of the EIA.[1] This test is a solid phase, indirect enzyme immunoassay (EIA) to detect antibodies to *M. paratuberculosis* in bovine serum and may be used as a specific test for Johne's disease in cattle. In this test, cross-reacting antibodies are removed in a rapid absorption step where *M. phlei* antigens form part of the serum diluent buffer (Green Diluent). The test has been evaluated in cattle herds from Johne's disease-endemic and Johne's disease-free regions of Australia[2] and the United States.[3] The test specificities were 99% or greater. Calculations of sensitivity were affected by the history of the herd under test. However, the EIA detected up to 80% of animals before onset of clinical disease and 60-65% of faecal shedders were EIA positive on or before first detection of *M. paratuberculosis* in their faeces. The test should permit epidemiological studies and be a useful tool in the management and control of Johne's disease.

Technical Information: Follow the PARACHEK™ (Johne's Absorbed EIA) kit instructions as closely as possible, as any deviation may reduce the performance of the test and lead to erroneous results.

1. The kit instructions stipulate that 25 µL of serum is to be diluted with 475 µL of Green Diluent. Any variation to this instruction may reduce the performance of the kit by introducing excess dilution errors.
2. Vortex mixing of conjugate in the Blue Diluent may reduce kit performance if it is done too vigorously. Vortex mixing should be done at a moderate speed, "stop-starting" 3-4 times, in order to prevent or minimize frothing of the diluent. This approach should be used whenever vortex mixing any biological reagent.
   However, not mixing enough may also lead to problems. Remember, it is impossible to over mix, as long as it is done gently. For accurate and reproducible results always ensure the conjugate is evenly mixed throughout the diluent.
3. Incubating plates (with or without a lid) directly on the bench is not recommended. The cold solid surface may act as a heat sink and lead to the phenomenon commonly known as "edge effects". Plates should be incubated with a lid on, with the plate supported on an upturned, non-metal, test-tube rack so that air is free to circulate around the plate.
4. The kit instructions specify that when reagents are added to the plate, the plate should then be mixed by shaking. Deviation from this instruction may lower the reproducibility of the assay and lead to invalid results. After each reagent is added to the plate, the plate is to be placed on a plate shaker and shaken for one minute. The plate should also be similarly mixed before any optical reading is performed.
5. The use of a squeeze bottle to apply wash buffer to wash plates, instead of an EIA washer, may leave too much wash buffer in the plate wells after washing and may cause a significant number of bubbles. Excessive residual wash buffer may affect the performance of the substrate buffer. This may result in a significant reduction in the amount of colour developed by the EIA, manifested as an increased stop time. Because the amount of residual wash buffer varies well-to-well and plate-to-plate, the stop time will vary accordingly. The more wash buffer left in wells, the longer the stop time will be.
   The following methodology is recommended: Wash plates as detailed under Test Procedures. After the last wash, tip out or aspirate the contents of the wells. Wipe the bottom of the plate dry with tissue paper, cover with lid and place upright on the bench. Excess wash buffer will drain to the bottom of the wells. Now, but not before, make up the appropriate volume of conjugate or substrate, whichever is applicable. Do not cause the conjugate to froth when mixing. It is critical the conjugate is mixed thoroughly, but this must be done gently. If using a vortex mixer, use a relatively slow speed and "stop-start" 3-4 times to ensure mixing is complete.
   Now flick out the contents of the plate firmly, several times, until all the remaining wash buffer that has drained down into the bottom of the plate wells is removed. There should be virtually no wash buffer or bubbles visible in the wells. Gently wipe the top of the plate dry and proceed to add the conjugate or substrate. Place the plate on a shaker for about one minute to mix the well contents. Cover the plate with a lid and incubate, elevated off the bench surface, for the prescribed time. This is conveniently done by placing the plate on the grill base of an upturned plastic test-tube rack. This effectively maximizes air circulation around the plate and minimizes the so-called "edge effects" phenomenon.
6. Absorbent paper, such as paper hand towel material, is not ideal for pat drying plates. Paper lint is readily liberated and can stick onto the wet inner surfaces of wells which may cause the substrate to change colour. Use lint-free absorbent paper, or similar material, to dry plates.
7. Blanking of EIA readers can be problematic. It appears that different readers blanked differently result in vastly different absorbance readings for the negative control. All readers should be blanked using a new unused plate or strip.
8. For a plate to be valid, the mean positive control absorbance reading at 450 nm should always be between 0.9 - 1.2. If this is not routinely observed, the level of the "blue" reading at 620 nm, nominally up to 0.4, should be adjusted to a value that leads to the validation criteria being subsequently achieved. Prior to any absorbance reading, the contents of plate wells should be mixed to homogeneity (point 4 above). If available, select the reader option to do this step automatically before each reading.

Test Interpretation:

Validation of Test Performance: The control results must be examined before the sample results can be interpreted.

Determine the mean absorbance of negative and positive controls.

Acceptable range of means:

Negative control < 0.150

Note: The duplicates must not vary by more than 0.040

Positive control between 0.900 and 1.200

Note: The positive control values must not deviate by more than 30% from its mean absorbance.

The run is invalid if either of these criteria is not met and must be repeated.

Interpretation of Results: The cut-off value for a valid assay is the mean of the negative controls plus 0.100, e.g. if the two negative controls were 0.055 and 0.085, the cut-off would be 0.070 + 0.100 = 0.170.

A positive result is a sample absorbance value greater than the cut-off value.

A positive result indicates that the animal is likely to be infected with *M. paratuberculosis* and that there are potentially other infected animals within the herd.

A negative result on a single animal can only be interpreted when the paratuberculosis history and test results of the entire herd are known. Even though animals are generally infected as neonates, an immune response does not develop immediately. Current information suggests that seroconversion generally occurs before any clinical signs are apparent.

As with any biological test, this test may occasionally give a false positive or false negative result due to local conditions. A test should be interpreted in the context of all available clinical, historical and epidemiological information relevant to the animal(s) under test. Further confirmatory testing may be required in certain circumstances.

Responsibility for test interpretation and consequent animal husbandry decisions rests solely with the user, and any consulting veterinarian and appropriate animal health advisers or authorities. CSL accepts no responsibility for any loss or damage, howsoever caused, arising from the interpretation of test results.

References: Available upon request.

Presentation: 192 well and 2880 well test kits.

Manufactured by: CSL Limited, Victoria, Australia.

Compendium Code No.: 13940260 03010000M

P

PARACIDE-F

Argent **Parasiticide-Aquaculture**

Parasiticide for trout, salmon, catfish, largemouth bass & bluegill and fungicide for trout, salmon & esocid eggs

NADA No.: 140-831

Active Ingredient(s): Formalin (aqueous solution of formaldehyde).

Guaranteed Analysis:
Formaldehyde (CH_2O) 37%
Methanol 6-13%
Water and inert ingredients 50-57%

Indications: PARACIDE-F is effective for the control of external protozoan parasites on trout, salmon, catfish, largemouth bass and bluegill. Organisms controlled include the protozoa: *Ichthyophthirius* spp. ("Ich"), *Chilodonella* spp., *Costia* spp., *Epistylis* spp., *Scyphydia* spp., and *Trichodina* spp.; monogenic trematodes: *Cleidodiscus* spp., *Gyrodactylus* spp., and *Dactylogyrus* spp.

PARACIDE-F is effective for the control of fungi (Saprolegniaceae family) on eggs of salmonids and esocids.

Pharmacology: PARACIDE-F is the aqueous solution of formaldehyde gas and contains not less than 37% (by weight) of formaldehyde gas per weight of water and 6 to 13% (12%) methanol. In solution, formaldehyde is present chiefly as HO (CH_2O)H. Its molecular weight is 30.93. PARACIDE-F is readily miscible with water, methanol and ethanol and is slightly soluble in ether. It is a clear, colorless liquid (Heyden Newport Chemical Corporation, 1961).

Dosage and Administration:

For Trout, Salmon, Catfish, Largemouth Bass and Bluegill: Concentrations used for treatments are expressed as microliters (µL) of PARACIDE-F (37% formaldehyde) per liter of water and are equivalent to part per million (ppm).

Table 1: Concentrations required for control of parasites on the following fish.

Fish	Concentration of PARACIDE-F (µL/L)* in	
	Tanks and raceways (for up to 1 hour)	Earthen ponds (indefinitely)
Salmon and Trout		
above 50°F	up to 170	15-25
below 50°F	up to 250	15-25
Catfish, Largemouth Bass and Bluegill	up to 250	15-25[a]

[a]Use the lower concentrations when pond is heavily loaded with fish or phytoplankton.
*µL/L = microliters per liter.

Table 2: Amounts of PARACIDE-F needed to supply effective concentrations in selected volumes of water.

Volume of Water	Amount of PARACIDE-F needed to give the following concentration of µL/L			
	15	25	170	250
10 gallons	0.60 mL	0.95 mL	6.4 mL	9.5 mL
100 liters	1.50 mL	2.50 mL	17.0 mL	25.0 mL
1 acre foot	4.86 gal	8.10 gal		

Methods of Application:

Applications to tanks and raceways: Turn off water supply, provide aeration, apply appropriate amount of PARACIDE-F and thoroughly dilute and mix to assure equal distribution of PARACIDE-F. Treat for up to 1 hour, then drain the solution and refill the tank with fresh, well-aerated water. While tank is under treatment, adequate oxygen must be present to maintain the fish. If needed, aeration should be provided to prevent oxygen depletion. Treatments may be repeated daily until parasite control is achieved.

Application to ponds: Apply greatly diluted PARACIDE-F to the pond evenly using a pump, sprayer, boat bailer, or other suitable device to assure even distribution. Allow PARACIDE-F to dissipate naturally. Single treatments usually control most parasites but may be repeated in 5 to 10 days if needed. Treatments of *Ichthyophthirius* should be made at 2-day intervals until control is achieved.

For trout, salmon and esocid eggs: Apply concentration of 1,000 to 2,000 µL/L (3.8 to 7.6 mL/gallon of water). The most widely used concentration is about 1,670 µL/L.

Method of application: Apply as constant flow to water supply of incubating facilities for 15 minutes. Repeat treatment as often as necessary to control growth of fungi.

Precaution(s): The recommended storage temperature is 59°F (15°C). Do not expose to direct sunlight. Avoid prolonged storage at temperatures below 40°F (4.4°C).

Caution(s):

For trout, salmon, catfish, largemouth bass and bluegill: Do not use when the water temperature in ponds is above 27°C (80°F). Do not discharge contents of fish treatment tanks into natural waters without a 10x dilution.

For fish eggs of salmon, trout and esocids:

1. Do not use PARACIDE-F which has been subjected to temperatures lower than 40°F or allowed to freeze. Cold or freezing causes the formation of paraformaldehyde, a substance which is toxic to fish. Paraformaldehyde can be recognized as a white precipitate at the bottom or on the walls of the container.
2. Do not use on striped bass *(Morone saxatillis).* Tolerances to PARACIDE-F may vary with strains and species of fish. While the indicated concentrations are considered safe for the indicated fishes, a small number of each lot to be treated should be used to check for any unusual sensitivity to PARACIDE-F before processing. Striped bass *(Morone saxatilis)* are known to be highly sensitive to PARACIDE-F so pond treatments are not appropriate for this species.
3. Under some conditions, fish may be stressed by normal treatment concentrations. Heavily parasitized or diseased fish often have a greatly reduced tolerance to PARACIDE-F. Such fish do not tolerate the normal tank treatment regimen the first day they are treated. Therefore the time or dosage or both may need to be reduced if the fish show evidence of distress (by piping at the surface). The solution should be removed and replaced with fresh, well-aerated water. Careful observations should always be made throughout the treatment period whenever tank or raceway treatments are made. Treatments in tanks should never exceed 1 hour even if the fish show no signs of stress.
4. Do not apply PARACIDE-F to ponds with water warmer than 27°C (80°F) when a heavy bloom of phytoplankton is present or when the concentration of dissolved oxygen is less than 5 mg/L (5 ppm). PARACIDE-F may kill phytoplankton and can cause depletion of dissolved oxygen. If an oxygen depletion occurs, add fresh, well-aerated water to dilute the solution and to provide oxygen.
5. Do not discharge the contents of fish treatment tanks into natural streams or ponds without thorough dilution (greater than or equal to 10%). Do not discharge the contents of egg treatment tanks without a 75% dilution. This will avoid damage to PARACIDE-F sensitive phytoplankton, zooplankton, and fish populations and avoid depletion of dissolved oxygen.
6. Do not use PARACIDE-F in a tank or pond in which methylene blue or other dyes have been recently used.

Warning(s): Keep out of reach of children.

Harmful if inhaled or absorbed through the skin. Do not get in eyes or on skin. If PARACIDE-F is inhaled, remove the patient to fresh air. Irritation may be alleviated by inhalation of spirits of ammonia. If eyes or skin are exposed to PARACIDE-F, wash with water. Eyes should be flushed freely with water for at least 15 minutes and then treated by a physician.

Harmful if swallowed. PARACIDE-F should be diluted and removed from the stomach as rapidly as possible. Irritation may then be alleviated with demulcents.

Toxicology: The toxicity of PARACIDE-F was measured by standard methods in laboratory bioassays with rainbow trout, Atlantic salmon, lake trout, black bullhead, channel catfish, green sunfish, bluegill, smallmouth bass and largemouth bass. The 3, 6, 24 and 96-hour LC_{50} (lethal concentration for 50% of the animals) values for trout range from 1,230 to 100 µL/L; for catfish, from 495 to 65.8 µL/L; for bluegill, from 2,290 to 100 µL/L; and for largemouth bass, the values to 6 to 96 hours range from 1,030 to 143 µL/L (Bill *et al.*, 1977).

Presentation: 4 x 1 gallon (U.S.) cases, 5 gallon container and 55 gallon drum.

Compendium Code No.: 10260011

PARAGUARD™ SHAMPOO

First Priority **Antidermatosis Shampoo**

Anti-Ringworm, Anti-Fungal, Anti-Bacterial Therapeutic Shampoo

Active Ingredient(s):
Captan .... 2% w/w
Sulfur .... 1% w/w

Indications: A therapeutic shampoo for use as an aid in the control of fungal and bacterial infections of the skin often associated with parasitic infections in dogs, cats and horses.

Directions for Use: Shake well before using. Apply liberally and work vigorously into the animal's coat and rinse thoroughly. Repeat procedure adding ample water to create a sudsy lather. Work into skin areas with lesions allowing the shampoo to set for 5-10 minutes. Rinse completely and then dry.

Quantity Usage:
Dogs .... 1-2 fluid oz per 25 lbs
Cats .... 1 fluid oz
Horses .... Amount determined by surface area to be covered

Precaution(s): Storage: Store at controlled room temperature between 15°-30°C (59°-86°F). Keep container tightly closed when not in use.

Caution(s): If redness, irritation or swelling persists or increases, discontinue use and consult a veterinarian.

For animal use only.

Warning(s): Do not use on animals intended for food.

Keep out of reach of children.

Presentation: 16 fl oz (473 mL) (NDC# 58829-286-16), 32 fl oz (960 mL) (NDC# 58829-286-32), and 1 gallon (3.785 L) (NDC# 58829-286-01).

Compendium Code No.: 11390613 Rev. 06-01 / Iss. 12-98 / Rev. 07-01

PARAMUNE™-5

Biocor **Bacterin-Vaccine**

Canine Distemper-Hepatitis-Parainfluenza Vaccine, Modified Live Virus-Leptospira Bacterin

U.S. Vet. Lic. No.: 462

Contents: This product contains the antigens listed above.

This product contains gentamicin, amphotericin B and thimerosal as preservatives.

The live viruses contained have been attenuated to assure safety upon administration.

Indications: PARAMUNE™-5 is a multivalent vaccine recommended for use in the vaccination of healthy dogs against disease caused by the viral and bacterial fractions of canine distemper, canine hepatitis, canine parainfluenza and leptospirosis caused by *Leptospira canicola* and *Leptospira icterohaemorrhagiae.*

Directions: Aseptically rehydrate vial of desiccated virus with the accompanying vial of bacterin. Shake well. Administer entire contents (1 mL) IM or SC.

Persistence of maternal origin antibody in puppies should receive consideration in determining vaccination programs. Ideally puppies should be vaccinated at 9 weeks of age with revaccination every 2-4 weeks until at least 18 weeks of age. Dogs over 18 weeks of age should receive a 1 mL dose followed by a second dose approximately 2-4 weeks later. Annual revaccination with a single 1 mL dose is recommended.

Precaution(s): Store at 35°-45°F (2°-7°C). Do not freeze.

Use entire contents when first rehydrated.

Burn these containers and all unused contents.

Caution(s): Do not vaccinate pregnant bitches.

In case of anaphylactoid reactions, epinephrine should be administered immediately.

For use in dogs only.

For veterinary use only.

Presentation: Code 66211B - 25 x 1 dose (1 mL) vials with diluent.

Compendium Code No.: 13940121 BAH2225-1098

PARAPAC™

Schering-Plough **Bacterin**

Haemophilus parasuis Bacterin

U.S. Vet. Lic. No.: 165A

Active Ingredient(s): Contains chemically-inactivated cultures of *Haemophilus parasuis.*

Preservatives: Gentamicin and amphotericin B.

Indications: For use in healthy swine for prevention of Glasser's disease caused by *Haemophilus parasuis.*

Dosage and Administration: Shake well. Using aseptic technique, inject sows/gilts with 1 mL subcutaneously 6 to 7 weeks and 2 to 3 weeks prior to first farrowing, and 2 to 3 weeks prior to each subsequent farrowing. Inject piglets from vaccinated dams with 1 mL subcutaneously at 7 days of age and between 17 and 28 days of age.

Precaution(s): Store at 2° to 7°C (35° to 45°F). Do not freeze. Use entire contents when first opened.

Caution(s): Transient local reaction may occur at the injection site. If anaphylaxis occurs administer epinephrine.
Antidote(s): Epinephrine.
Warning(s): Do not vaccinate within 21 days prior to slaughter.
For veterinary use only.
Presentation: 50 dose (50 mL) and 100 dose (100 mL) vials.
Compendium Code No.: 10471460

PARAPLEURO SHIELD® P

Novartis Animal Vaccines **Bacterin**

Haemophilus parasuis-pleuropneumoniae-Pasteurella multocida Bacterin

U.S. Vet. Lic. No.: 303

Composition: The bacterin contains inactivated cultures of *Haemophilus parasuis, Haemophilus pleuropneumoniae* serotypes 1, 5, and 7 and *Pasteurella multocida* adjuvanted with aluminum hydroxide. Contains penicillin and streptomycin as preservatives.

Indications: For use in healthy swine as an aid in the prevention and control of diseases caused by *Haemophilus parasuis, Haemophilus pleuropneumoniae* and *Pasteurella multocida.*

Dosage and Administration: Shake well before and during use. Administer 1 mL intramuscularly to pigs under 30 lbs. and 2 mL to pigs over 30 lbs. Revaccinate two (2) to three (3) weeks later. Sows and gilts should receive two (2) doses prior to farrowing. The first dose should be given approximately five (5) weeks before farrowing and a second dose should be given two (2) to three (3) weeks later.

Precaution(s): Store at 35°-45°F (2°-7°C). Do not freeze. Use the entire contents when first opened.

Caution(s): Anaphylactic reactions can occur following the use of the product. Symptomatic treatment: Epinephrine.

Warning(s): Do not vaccinate within 21 days of slaughter.

Discussion: *Haemophilus parasuis* causes Glasser's disease in swine, which is an infection of the serous membranes throughout the body (polyserositis). The disease is found throughout the world. Pigs under four months of age are most commonly affected, with the majority of cases occurring in the month immediately after weaning. Older animals may be infected, with specific pathogen free (SPF) pigs especially susceptible due to their lack of natural exposure to disease organisms. The morbidity rate is variable, and the mortality rate may reach 50% of the infected animals.

More research must be done into how the disease spreads, but it is known that the organism is common on many farms, and that healthy carrier pigs play a role. Stress conditions such as weaning, inclement weather, and transporting are the usual triggering factors for a disease outbreak.

Infected pigs may show various clinical signs, depending upon which area of the body is most severely affected. Affected animals show fevers of 105° to 108°F. They may show purplish discolorations of the skin and edema around the eyelids, indicating a failure of the peripheral circulation. They may show signs of difficult breathing. One or more joints may be swollen and painful. Many animals show tremors, incoordination and inability to rise, indicating that there is central nervous system involvement. At least two reports suggest that *H. parasuis* may serve as an initiator or potentiator of pneumonia or atrophic rhinitis in pigs.[1,2]

At necropsy, the main lesions are fibrinous inflammations of the various serous membranes. The most commonly occurring abnormalities are in the brain (meningitis), the joints (arthritis), the chest and abdominal cavity (pleuritis and peritonitis), and the tissue surrounding the heart (pericarditis).

It is important to confirm a diagnosis of Glasser's disease by bacterial culture, since several other diseases show similar symptoms. These include Streptococcus infections, erysipelas, Mycoplasma infections, edema disease *(Escherichia coli)*, and pseudorabies.

Treatment must be started as soon as symptoms are noticed, and all pigs in the group should be treated. Penicillin, ampicillin and tetracycline are normally effective, but must be given in high doses in order to reach therapeutic levels in the brain and joints.

Haemophilus pleuropneumoniae is a major cause of pleuropneumonia in hogs. It is distributed throughout the world, but different serovars of the bacteria are more prevalent in certain areas. In the United States, serovars 1 and 5 are most common, with serovar 7 causing problems in some areas. Animals of all ages are susceptible, but the majority of cases occur during the growing and finishing stages of production. In acute outbreaks, the morbidity rate is usually high and may approach 100%. The mortality rate in untreated animals may also approach 100%.

Pleuropneumonia is spread by aerosol and through direct pig to pig contact. Animals may carry the organism without showing symptoms, and movement of these carrier animals spreads the disease to other herds. There is not evidence to indicate that other animals, such as rodents and birds, play any role in transmission. There is a slight possibility that the disease could spread by clothing and equipment moved from a herd experiencing an acute outbreak to a clean herd, since the bacteria can survive for a few days in the environment.

H. pleuropneumoniae is a very virulent organism, with as few as 100 organisms needed to cause disease in experimental animals. The disease can also progress very rapidly. Animals experimentally infected with high doses of the bacteria often die within six hours. Much of this can be attributed to the actions of a potent toxin produced by the bacteria as they grow.[3]

In natural infections, producers may find a dead pig as their first clue that something is wrong. On closer inspection, they may notice pigs that seem lethargic, and fevers of 107°F are not uncommon. Pigs rapidly progress to show very labored breathing, and there may be a bloody discharge from the mouth and nose. The disease rapidly progresses through the herd. Animals that recover often become chronic poor-doers.

At necropsy, lesions are confined mainly to the lungs and chest cavity. The lining of the chest cavity is inflamed, and the lungs are often tightly attached to it by adhesions. The lungs themselves show evidence of severe pneumonia.

Definite diagnosis can often be made on the basis of these characteristic signs and lesions. If there is doubt, culturing can be done to detect the organism responsible, since other bacterial infections may mimic *H. pleuropneumoniae.*

Response to treatment is variable. If the disease is detected early and is aggressively treated, animals can fully recover. Other animals may become permanently stunted. Penicillin or ampicillin are often the first drugs of choice, since many strains are sensitive to them. However, it is a good idea to test each strain for its antibiotic resistance pattern, since there are many exceptions to this rule.

Pasteurella multocida is another important cause of pneumonia in swine. It is found worldwide, and it is a common inhabitant of the respiratory tract of healthy animals. It can affect animals of any age.

P. multocida alone causes either no disease or a mild pneumonia. Its importance is as a secondary invader. When lungs are damaged due to some other cause, such as poor air quality, larval ascarid migrations, or other bacterial or mycoplasmal infections, Pasteurella will begin to invade and cause further lung damage, culminating in a severe pneumonia.

Animals infected by *P. multocida* show the typical signs associated with pneumonia - coughing, shortness of breath, "thumping", and high fevers (up to 107°F). If pigs are not treated, the disease tends to linger on, and many of the animals become chronic cases. Death loss is typically fairly low, but can be high in individual cases.

At necropsy, lung lesions are typical of a bronchopneumonia, and the lungs may adhere to the chest cavity. Lung cultures should be done to determine the exact causes, since most are mixed infections.

Treatment can be effective if the proper antibiotic is used. Antibacterial sensitivity of different strains of *P. multocida* varies greatly, which is another important reason culturing should be done. Sulfas, penicillin, tetracycline, and tylosin are commonly used drugs, and all are effective if used properly against sensitive strains.

References: Available upon request.
Presentation: Available in 50 dose (100 mL) bottles.
Compendium Code No.: 11140243

PARAPLEURO SHIELD® P+BE

Novartis Animal Vaccines **Bacterin**

Bordetella bronchiseptica-Erysipelothrix rhusiopathiae-Haemophilus parasuis-pleuropneumoniae-Pasteurella multocida Bacterin

U.S. Vet. Lic. No.: 303

Composition: The bacterin is prepared from highly antigenic inactivated cultures of *Bordetella bronchiseptica, Erysipelothrix rhusiopathiae, Haemophilus parasuis, Haemophilus pleuropneumoniae* serotypes 1, 5 and 7 and two strains of *Pasteurella multocida.* Contains penicillin and streptomycin as preservatives.

Indications: For use in healthy swine as an aid in the prevention and control of diseases caused by *Bordetella bronchiseptica, Erysipelothrix rhusiopathiae, Haemophilus parasuis, Haemophilus pleuropneumoniae* and *Pasteurella multocida.*

Dosage and Administration: Shake well before using. The product is designed for use in feeder pigs from sows previously vaccinated against *Bordetella bronchiseptica.* Vaccinate feeder pigs weighing 45 to 50 lbs. or more intramuscularly with a 5 mL dose. Repeat in 2-3 weeks.

Precaution(s): Store at 35°-45°F (2°-7°C). Do not freeze. Use the entire contents when first opened.

Caution(s): Anaphylactic reactions may occur following the use of the product. Symptomatic treatment: Epinephrine.

Warning(s): Do not vaccinate within 21 days prior to slaughter.

Discussion: *Haemophilus parasuis* causes Glasser's disease in swine, which is an infection of the serous membranes throughout the body (polyserositis). The disease is found throughout the world. Pigs under four months of age are most commonly affected, with the majority of cases occurring in the month immediately after weaning. Older animals may be infected, with specific pathogen free (SPF) pigs especially susceptible due to their lack of natural exposure to disease organisms. The morbidity rate is variable, and the mortality rate may reach 50% of the infected animals.

More research must be done into how the disease spreads, but it is known that the organism is common on many farms, and that healthy carrier pigs play a role. Stress conditions such as weaning, inclement weather, and transporting are the usual triggering factors for a disease outbreak.

Infected pigs may show various clinical signs, depending upon which area of the body is most severely affected. Affected animals show fevers of 105° to 108°F. They may show purplish discolorations of the skin and edema around the eyelids, indicating a failure of the peripheral circulation. The lungs may be affected. One or more joints may be swollen and painful. Many animals show tremors, incoordination and inability to rise, indicating that there is central nervous system involvement. At least two reports suggest that *H. parasuis* may serve as an initiator or potentiator of pneumonia or atrophic rhinitis in pigs.[1,2]

At necropsy, the main lesions are fibrinous inflammations of the various serous membranes. The most commonly occurring abnormalities are in the brain (meningitis), the joints (arthritis), the chest and abdominal cavity (pleuritis and peritonitis), and the tissue surrounding the heart (pericarditis).

It is important to confirm a diagnosis of Glasser's disease by bacterial culture, since several other diseases show similar symptoms. These include Streptococcus infections, erysipelas, Mycoplasma infections, edema disease *(Escherichia coli)*, and pseudorabies.

Haemophilus pleuropneumoniae (Actinobacillus pleuropneumoniae) is a major cause of pleuropneumonia in hogs. It is distributed throughout the world, but different serovars of the bacteria are more prevalent in certain areas. In the United States, serovars 1 and 5 are most common, with serovar 7 causing problems in some areas. Animals of all ages are susceptible, but the majority of cases occur during the growing and finishing stages of production. In acute outbreaks, the morbidity rate is usually high and may approach 100%. The mortality rate in untreated animals may also approach 100%.

Pleuropneumonia is spread by aerosol and through direct pig to pig contact. Animals may carry the organism without showing symptoms, and movement of these carrier animals spreads the disease to other herds. There is not evidence to indicate that other animals, such as rodents and birds, play any role in transmission. There is a slight possibility that the disease could spread by clothing and equipment moved from a herd experiencing an acute outbreak to a clean herd, since the bacteria can survive for a few days in the environment.

H. pleuropneumoniae is a very virulent organism, with as few as 100 organisms needed to cause disease in experimental animals. The disease can also progress very rapidly. Animals experimentally infected with high doses of the bacteria often die within six hours. Much of this can be attributed to the actions of a potent toxin produced by the bacteria as they grow.[3]

In natural infections, producers may find a dead pig as their first clue that something is wrong. On closer inspection, they may notice pigs that seem lethargic, and fevers of 107°F are not uncommon. Pigs rapidly progress and show very labored breathing, and there may be a bloody discharge from the mouth and nose. The disease rapidly progresses through the herd. Animals that recover often become chronic poor-doers.

At necropsy, lesions are confined mainly to the lungs and chest cavity. The lining of the chest cavity is inflamed, and the lungs are often tightly attached to it by adhesions. The lungs themselves show evidence of severe pneumonia.

Definite diagnosis can often be made on the basis of these characteristic signs and lesions. If there is doubt, culturing can be done to detect the organism responsible, since other bacterial infections may mimic *H. pleuropneumoniae.*

Pasteurella multocida is another important cause of pneumonia and atrophic rhinitis in swine. It is found worldwide, and it is a common inhabitant of the respiratory tract of healthy animals. It can affect animals of any age.

P. multocida is divided into two types, A and D. Type A is a common cause of pneumonia. Its importance is as a secondary invader. Lungs damaged by other causes such as poor air quality, ascarid (roundworm) migrations, or other infectious agents, can be invaded by Pasteurella, which causes further lung damage and culminates in a severe pneumonia. These animals will show typical pneumonia symptoms - coughing, shortness of breath, labored breathing ("thumping"),

P

and fevers up to 107°F. If not treated in the early stages, many animals become chronic cases. Death losses, while typically low, may be high in some cases.

Toxin-producing strains of *P. multocida* type D are an important cause of atrophic rhinitis. The bacteria colonize the nasal turbinates, then release a toxin which causes damage to the tissues and results in the typical signs of atrophic rhinitis (AR) - sneezing, sniffling, teary eyes and crooked snouts. An important feature with type D is that it can infect older pigs and cause severe AR, whereas piglets normally have to be infected with *B. bronchiseptica* within a few days after birth in order to develop AR.

Nasal turbinates damaged by AR are not able to do an effective job of filtering the air the pig breathes, allowing more bacteria access to the lungs. This, in turn, makes it more likely that the pig will develop severe pneumonia.

Bordetella bronchiseptica has long been established as a primary cause of AR and pneumonia. In the case of AR, *B. bronchiseptica* may act as a primary invader and, depending on the virulence of the strain, may act alone or may compromise the nasal epithelium so that secondary Pasteurella organisms can invade and cause more extensive damage.

The most common clinical signs of AR are sneezing, snuffling, rubbing the nose, black tear streaks from the eye and excessive nasal discharge.

A more severe clinical situation associated with *B. bronchiseptica* is bronchopneumonia. This can occur in piglets as young as three to five days of age and is considered a primary infection. The clinical signs of *B. bronchiseptica* bronchopneumonia are coughing and labored breathing. Morbidity and mortality can be high.

Erysipelothrix rhusiopathiae is the cause of swine erysipelas (SE) or diamond skin disease. The disease is worldwide in distribution and many apparently normal animals can carry and shed the organism. SE is generally divided into three general classifications - peracute, subacute, and chronic. The peracute septicemic form may be seen as sudden death, fever, lameness, and depression. Skin changes may occur as purplish-red discoloration of the ears and abdomen. There may in some cases be the characteristic diamond-shaped skin lesions. The subacute form is a milder manifestation of the acute form. The chronic form will usually follow recovery of acute or subacute cases, or appear in animals where immunity is not completely protective. The chronic form will most often appear as lameness and bacterial growths in the heart. The diagnosis of SE should be made by bacterial isolation from tissues.

Trial Data: *Haemophilus parasuis* Challenge Study: Two 2 mL doses of Para Shield®.

	No. of Pigs	Live After Challenge	% Protected
Para Shield®	11	9/11	82%
Controls	11	2/11	18%

*Vaccinated pigs demonstrated 74% less fibrin and fluid accumulation than the nonvaccinated controls.

* *H. parasuis* was re-isolated from none (0%) of the 11 vaccinated pigs as compared to six of the 11 (55%) nonvaccinated controls.

References: Available upon request.

Presentation: Available in 20 dose (100 mL), and 50 dose (250 mL) bottles.

Compendium Code No.: 11140253

PARA SHIELD®

Novartis Animal Vaccines **Bacterin**

Haemophilus parasuis Bacterin

U.S. Vet. Lic. No.: 303

Composition: The bacterin contains an inactivated culture of *Haemophilus parasuis* adjuvanted with aluminum hydroxide. Contains penicillin and streptomycin as preservatives.

Indications: For use in healthy swine as an aid in the prevention and control of diseases caused by *Haemophilus parasuis.*

Dosage and Administration: Shake well before and during use. Administer 2 mL of bacterin intramuscularly. Vaccinate piglets at three (3) to four (4) weeks of age or older with revaccination two (2) to three (3) weeks later.

Precaution(s): Store at 35°-45°F (2°-7°C). Do not freeze.

Caution(s): Anaphylactic reactions can occur following the use of the product. Symptomatic treatment: Epinephrine.

Warning(s): Do not vaccinate within 21 days of slaughter.

Discussion: *Haemophilus parasuis* causes Glasser's disease in swine, which is an infection of the serous membranes throughout the body (polyserositis). The disease is found throughout the world. Pigs under four months of age are most commonly affected, with the majority of cases occurring in the month immediately after weaning. Older animals may be infected, with specific pathogen free (SPF) pigs especially susceptible due to their lack of natural exposure to disease organisms. The morbidity rate is variable, and the mortality rate may reach 50% of the infected animals.

More research must be done into how the disease spreads, but it is known that the organism is common on many farms, and that healthy carrier pigs play a role. Stress conditions such as weaning, inclement weather, and transporting are the usual triggering factors for a disease outbreak. Miniats *et al.*[1] reported that Glasser's disease is one of the most immediate and frequent problems associated with mixing pigs of different health status and that field observations indicate that the true incidence of disease is at least 10-fold greater than recorded by diagnostic laboratories.

Infected pigs may show various clinical signs, depending upon which area of the body is most severely affected. Affected animals show fevers of 105° to 108°F. They may show purplish discolorations of the skin and edema around the eyelids, indicating a failure of the peripheral circulation. They may show signs of difficult breathing. One or more joints may be swollen and painful. Many animals show tremors, incoordination and inability to rise, indicating that there is central nervous system involvement. At least two reports suggest that *H. parasuis* may serve as an initiator or potentiator of pneumonia or atrophic rhinitis in pigs.[2,3]

At necropsy, the main lesions are fibrinous inflammations of the various serous membranes. The most commonly occurring abnormalities are in the brain (meningitis), the joints (arthritis), the chest and abdominal cavity (pleuritis and peritonitis), and the tissue surrounding the heart (pericarditis).

It is important to confirm a diagnosis of Glasser's disease by bacterial culture, since several other diseases show similar symptoms. These include Streptococcus infections, erysipelas, Mycoplasma infections, edema disease *(Escherichia coli),* and pseudorabies.

Treatment must be started as soon as the symptoms are noticed, and all pigs in the group should be treated. Penicillin, ampicillin and tetracycline are normally effective, but must be given in high doses in order to reach therapeutic levels in the brain and joints.

References: Available upon request.

Presentation: Available in 50 dose (100 mL) bottles.

Compendium Code No.: 11140233

PARASITE-S

Western Chemical **Parasiticide-Aquaculture**

Formalin (Aqueous formaldehyde solution)

NADA No.: 140-989

Active Ingredient(s): Formalin (Aqueous formaldehyde solution) that contains:

Formaldehyde (CH_2O) . . . . . . 37% w/w
Methanol 6-14%
Water and inert ingredients 49-57%
Total 100%

Indications: For control of external protozoa and monogenetic trematodes on salmonid fish and for control of fungi on the eggs of salmonid fish.

Formalin has been used since 1909 in the United States in the production of sport, commercial, and experimental fishes (Schnick 1973). It is used as a therapeutant and prophylactic for the control of external parasites on salmon, trout, catfish, largemouth bass, and bluegill, and for the control of fungi on salmon, trout, and esocid eggs. PARASITE-S has been used since the early 1970's to control external protozoans on penaeid shrimp (Johnson et al. 1973).

Chemistry: This product is the aqueous solution of formaldehyde gas. U.S.P. grade PARASITE-S contains not less than 37% (by weight) of formaldehyde gas per weight of water and 6 to 14% methanol. In solution, formaldehyde is present chiefly as $HO(CH_2O)H$. Its molecular weight is 30.93. This product is readily miscible with water, methanol, and ethanol and is slightly soluble in ether. It is a clear, colorless liquid (Heyden Newport Chemical Corporation, 1961).

Dosage and Administration: Directions for Use on Salmonid Fish:

PARASITE-S is effective for the control of external parasites on salmonid fish. Organisms controlled include the protozoa: *Ichthyophthirius* spp. ("Ich"), *Chilodonella* spp., *Costia* spp., *Scyphidia* spp., *Epistylis* spp., and *Trichodina* spp., and for the monogenetic trematodes: *Cleidodiscus* spp., *Gyrodactylus* spp., and *Dactylogyrus* spp.

Directions for Use on Fish:

Concentration: Concentrations used for treatment are expressed as microliter (μL) of formalin (37% formaldehyde) per liter of water and are equivalent to parts per million (ppm).

Table 1. Concentrations required for control of parasites on fish.

Fish	Concentration of Formalin (μL/L*) in	
	Tanks and raceway (for up to 1 hour)	Earthen ponds (indefinitely)
Salmonid Fish above 50°F below 50°F	up to 170 (62.9)	 15-25 (5.55-9.25) 15-25 (5.55-9.25)

Use the lower concentrations when the pond is heavily loaded with fish, shrimp or phytoplankton.

*μL/L = microliters per liter (ppm)

The figure in parentheses denotes the concentration of formaldehyde expressed as parts per million (ppm) by weight.

A single treatment usually controls most parasites but it may be repeated in 5-10 days, if needed.

Table 2. Amounts of PARASITE-S needed to supply effective concentrations in selected volumes of water.

Volume of water	Amount of PARASITE-S needed to give the following concentration of μL/L			
	15	25	170	250
100 L	1.50 mL	2.50 mL	17.0 mL	25.0 mL

Methods of Application:

Application to Tanks and Raceways: Turn off water supply, provide aeration, apply the appropriate amount of PARASITE-S and thoroughly dilute and mix to assure equal distribution of PARASITE-S. Treat for up to one (1) hour for fish, then drain the solution and refill the tank with fresh, well-aerated water. While the tank is under treatment, adequate oxygen must be present to maintain the fish or shrimp. If needed, aeration should be provided to prevent oxygen depletion. Treatments may be repeated once a day until parasite control is achieved.

Application to Ponds: Apply greatly diluted PARASITE-S to the pond evenly using a pump, sprayer, boat bailer, or another suitable device to assure even distribution. Allow PARASITE-S to dissipate naturally. Single treatments usually control most parasites but they may be repeated in 5-10 days if needed. Treatments for Ichthyophthirius should be made at 2-day intervals until control is achieved.

Use Directions for Salmonid Eggs:

PARASITE-S is also effective for the control of fungi (Saprolegniaceae) on eggs of salmonid fish.

Concentrations: Apply at a concentration of 1,000 to 2,000 μL/L. The most widely used concentration is about 1,670 μL/L (618 ppm formaldehyde).

Method of Application: Apply as constant flow to water supply of incubating facilities for 15 minutes. Repeat the treatment as often as is necessary to prevent growth of fungi.

Precaution(s): Recommended storage temperature is 59°F (15°C). Do not expose to direct sunlight. Store indoors away from direct sunlight, heat, sparks, and open flames, and ventilate storage area. Do not subject to temperatures below 40°F (4.4°C).

Caution(s): Poison.

EPA identified as a toxic pollutant and hazardous substance.

EPS/NPDES permits required at all facilities using the product.

PARASITE-S subjected to temperatures below 40°F causes the formation of paraformaldehyde, a substance which is toxic to fish. Paraformaldehyde can be recognized as a white precipitate at the bottom or on the walls of the container.

Tolerance to formalin may vary with strain and species of fish. While the indicated concentrations are considered safe for the indicated fishes, a small number of each lot to be treated should be used to check for any unusual sensitivity to formalin before proceeding.

Under some conditions, fish may be stressed by normal treatment concentrations. Heavily parasitized or diseased fish often have a greatly reduced tolerance to PARASITE-S. Such animals do not tolerate the normal tank treatment regimen the first time they are treated. Therefore, the time and dosage may need to be reduced. If they show evidence of distress (by piping at the surface), the solution should be removed and replaced with fresh, well aerated water. Careful observations should always be made throughout the treatment period whenever tank or raceway treatments are made. Treatment in tanks should never exceed one hour for fish even if the fish show no sign of distress.

Do not apply formalin to ponds with water warmer than 27°C (80°F), when a heavy bloom of phytoplankton is present, or when the concentration of dissolved oxygen is less than 5 mg/L (5 ppm). PARASITE-S may kill phytoplankton and can cause depletion of dissolved oxygen. If an oxygen depletion occurs, add fresh, well-aerated water to dilute the solution and to provide oxygen.

Do not discharge the contents of fish treatment tanks into natural streams or ponds without thorough dilution (greater than or equal to 10X). Do not discharge the contents of egg treatment tanks without a 75X dilution. This will avoid damage to PARASITE-S sensitive phytoplankton, zooplankton, and fish or invertebrate populations and avoid depletion of dissolved oxygen.

Do not use in a tank or pond in which methylene blue, or other dyes, which are absorbed, have been recently used.

Warning(s): Hazardous Ingredients: The ingredients listed below have been associated with one or more of the listed immediate and/or delayed(*) health hazards. Risk of damage and effects depends upon duration and level of exposure. Before using or handling, read and understand the MSDS.

50-00-0 *Formaldehyde

67-56-1 *Methanol

Attention: Potential cancer hazard, allergic skin reaction, respiratory sensitization, reproductive disorders, lung damage, liver damage, kidney damage, brain and nervous system damage.

Read entire instructions and MSDS before using the product.

Immediate Health Hazards:

Skin Absorption: May be harmful if absorbed through the skin.

Ingestion: May be harmful if swallowed.

If accidently swallowed, burns or irritation to mucous membranes, esophagus or gastro-intestinal tract can result. Can cause central nervous system depression.

Inhalation: May be harmful if inhaled. Liquid or vapor may cause irritation of nose, throat and lungs. Can cause central nervous system depression.

Skin: Causes irritation.

Eyes: Causes chemical burns.

Handling Precautions:

Skin Absorption: Avoid contact with the eyes, skin or clothing.

Inhalation: Avoid inhaling vapor. Use with adequate ventilation.

Skin: Avoid contact with the skin.

Eyes: Do not get in the eyes.

Wash thoroughly after handling.

First Aid:

Skin Absorption: In case of contact, immediately flush eyes or skin with plenty of water for at least 15 minutes while removing contaminated clothing and shoes. Wash clothing and shoes before reuse.

Ingestion: If accidently swallowed, dilute by drinking large quantities of water. Immediately contact a poison control center or hospital emergency room for any other additional treatment directions.

Inhalation: If inhaled, remove to fresh air. If not breathing, give artificial respiration, preferably mouth-to-mouth. Call a physician.

Skin Contact: Flush skin with plenty of water. Remove contaminated clothing. Call a physician if irritation persists.

Eye Contact: Immediately flush eyes with plenty of water for at least 15 minutes. Eyelids should be held apart during irrigation to ensure water contact with entire surface of eyes and lids. Call a physician.

Keep out of the reach of children.

Toxicology: Fish Toxicity Studies: The toxicity of PARASITE-S was measured by standard methods in laboratory bio-assays with rainbow trout, Atlantic salmon, and lake trout. The 3, 6, 24 and 96-hour LC_{50} (lethal concentration for 50% of the animals) values for trout range from 1,230 to 100 µL/L (455 to 37 ppm formaldehyde).

Presentation: 55 gallon drum.

Compendium Code No.: 10210001

PARATUBERCULOSIS PROTOPLASMIC ANTIGEN (PPA)

Allied Monitor **Mycobacterium Test Antigen**

Active Ingredient(s): The culture is grown from Mycobacterium strain 18. The cells are ruptured, then centrifuged to remove whole cells and cell walls. The supernatant protoplasm is dialized centrifuged and lyophilized. The resultant protoplasmic extract is checked for sterility.

Indications: To be used as an antigen in ELISA and AGID testing.

Presentation: 10 mg, 20 mg and 40 mg.

Compendium Code No.: 10800051

PARR QUAT

Butler **Disinfectant/Detergent**

Germicidal Detergent and Deodorant

EPA Reg. No.: 47371-131-6480

Active Ingredient(s):

Didecyl dimethyl ammonium chloride	2.43%
n-Alkyl (C_{14} 50%, C_{12} 40%, C_{16} 10%) dimethyl benzyl ammonium chloride	1.62%
Inert Ingredients	95.95%
Total	100.00%

Indications: Disinfectant, Pseudomonacidal, Staphylocidal, Salmonellacidal, Bactericidal, *Virucidal, Fungicidal, Mildewstatic.

Recommended for use in hospitals, nursing homes, schools, colleges, commercial and industrial institutions, office buildings, veterinary clinics, animal life science laboratories, tack shops, pet shops, airports, kennels, hotels, motels, dairy farms, hog farms, breeding establishments, grooming establishments, and households. Disinfects, cleans and deodorizes the following hard nonporous inanimate surfaces: floors, walls, metal surfaces, stainless steel surfaces, glazed porcelain, plastic surfaces (such as polypropylene, polystyrene, etc.).

A multi-purpose, neutral pH, germicidal detergent and deodorant effective in hard water up to 400 ppm (calculated as $CaCO_3$) in the presence of a moderate amount of soil (5% organic-serum) according to the AOAC Use-dilution Test. Disinfects, cleans, and deodorizes in one labor-saving step. Effective against the following pathogens:

Pseudomonas aeruginosa[1], *Staphylococcus aureus*[1], *Salmonella cholerasuis, Acinetobacter calcoaceticus, Bordetella bronchiseptica, Chlamydia psittaci, Enterobacter aerogenes, Enterobacter cloacae, Escherichia coli*[1], *Fusobacterium necrophorum, Klebsiella pneumoniae*[1], *Legionella pneumophila, Listeria monocytogenes, Pasteurella multocida, Proteus mirabilis, Proteus vulgaris, Salmonella enteritidis, Salmonella typhi, Salmonella typhimurium, Serratia marcascens, Shigella flexneri, Shigella sonnei, Staphylococcus aureus* - Methicillin Resistant (MRSA), *Staphylococcus epidermis*[2], *Adenovirus type 4, Avian polyomavirus, Canine distemper, Feline leukemia, Feline picomavirus , Herpes simplex type 1, Herpes simplex type 2, Infectious bovine rhinotracheitis, Infectious bronchitis (Avian IBV), Influenza A/Hong Kong, Pseudorabies, Rabies, Respiratory syncytial virus (RSV), Rubella (German Measles), Transmissible gastroenteritis virus (TGE), Vaccinia, *Aspergillus niger, Candida albicans, Trichophyton mentagrophytes, Streptococcus faecalis*[1], *Streptococcus pyogenes, Enterococcus faecalis* (Vancomycin Resistant).

[1] ATCC and antibiotic-resistant

[2] antibiotic-resistant strain only

Directions for Use: 2 ounces per gallon of water. Dilution 1:64 (630 ppm quat).

It is a violation of Federal Law to use this product in a manner inconsistent with its labeling.

This product is not to be used as a sterilant/high level disinfectant on any surface or instrument that (1) is introduced directly into the human body, either into or in contact with the blood stream or normally sterile areas of the body, (2) contacts intact mucous membranes but which does not ordinarily penetrate the blood barrier or otherwise enter normally sterile areas of the body. This product may be used to preclean or decontaminate critical or semi-critical devices prior to sterilization or high-level disinfection.

Disinfection: Remove heavy soil from surface. Then thoroughly wet surface with a solution of 2 ounces of the concentrate per gallon of water. The solution can be applied with a cloth, mop, sponge, or coarse spray, or soaking. Let solution remain on surface for a minimum of 10 minutes. Rinse or allow to air dry. Rinsing of floors is not necessary unless they are to be waxed or polished. Food contact surfaces must be thoroughly rinsed with potable water. This product must not be used to clean the following food contact surfaces: utensils, glassware and dishes. Prepare a fresh solution daily or more often if the solution becomes visibly dirty or diluted.

Mildewstatic Instructions: Will effectively control the growth of mold and mildew plus the odors caused by them when applied to hard, non-porous surfaces such as walls, floors, and table tops. Apply solution (2 ounce per gallon of water) with a cloth, mop, sponge, or coarse spray. Make sure to wet all surfaces completely. Let air dry. Repeat application weekly or when growth reappears.

Precautionary Statements: Hazards to Humans and Domestic Animals:

Caution: Causes moderate eye irritation. Harmful if absorbed through skin. Avoid contact with eyes, skin and clothing. Harmful if inhaled. Avoid breathing spray mist. Wash thoroughly with soap and water after handling. Remove contaminated clothing and wash before reuse.

Statement of Practical Treatment:

If In Eyes: Flush with plenty of water. Call a physician if irritation persists.

If On Skin: Wash with plenty of soap and water. Get medical attention.

If Inhaled: Remove victim to fresh air. If not breathing, give artificial respiration, preferably mouth to mouth. Get medical attention.

Storage and Disposal: Keep product under locked storage, inaccessible to small children. Do not reuse container. Rinse thoroughly, securely wrap empty container in several layers of newspaper and discard in the trash.

Container Disposal: Triple rinse (or equivalent). Then offer for recycling or reconditioning, or puncture and dispose of in a sanitary landfill, or incinerate, or if allowed by state and local authorities, burn. If burned, stay out of smoke.

Warning(s): Keep out of reach of children.

Presentation: 1 gallon.

Compendium Code No.: 10821370

PARR QUAT 4X

Butler **Disinfectant/Detergent**

Germicidal Detergent and Deodorant

EPA Reg. No.: 47371-129-6480

Active Ingredient(s):

Didecyl dimethyl ammonium chloride	9.70%
n-Alkyl (C_{14} 50%, C_{12} 40%, C_{16} 10%) dimethyl benzyl ammonium chloride	6.47%
Inert Ingredients	83.83%
	100.0%

Indications: Disinfectant, Pseudomonacidal, Staphylocidal, Salmonellacidal, Bactericidal, *Virucidal, Fungicidal, Mildewstatic.

Recommended for use in hospitals, nursing homes, schools, colleges, commercial and industrial institutions, office buildings, veterinary clinics, animal life science laboratories, tack shops, pet shops, airports, kennels, hotels, motels, dairy farms, hog farms, breeding establishments, grooming establishments, and households. Disinfects, cleans, and deodorizes the following hard nonporous inanimate surfaces: floors, walls, metal surfaces, stainless steel surface, glazed porcelain, plastic surfaces (such as polypropylene, polystyrene, etc.).

A multi-purpose, neutral pH, germicidal detergent and deodorant effective in hard water up to 400 ppm (calculated as $CaCO_3$) in the presence of a moderate amount of soil (5% organic-serum) according to the AOAC Use-dilution Test. Disinfects, cleans, and deodorizes in one labor-saving step. Effective against the following pathogens:

Pseudomonas aeruginosa[1], *Staphylococcus aureus*[1], *Salmonella cholerasuis, Acinetobacter calcoaceticus, Bordetella bronchiseptica, Chlamydia psittaci, Enterobacter aerogenes, Enterobacter cloacae, Escherichia coli*[1], *Fusobacterium necrophorum, Klebsiella pneumoniae*[1], *Legionella pneumophila, Listeria monocytogenes, Pasteurella multocida, Proteus mirabilis, Proteus vulgaris, Salmonella enteritidis, Salmonella typhi, Salmonella typhimurium, Serratia marcascens, Shigella flexneri, Shigella sonnei, Staphylococcus aureus* - Methicillin Resistant (MRSA), *Staphylococcus epidermis*[2], *Adenovirus type 4, Avian polyomavirus, Canine distemper, Feline leukemia, Feline picomavirus , Herpes simplex type 1, Herpes simplex type 2, Infectious bovine rhinotracheitis, Infectious bronchitis (Avian IBV), Influenza A/Hong Kong, Pseudorabies, Rabies, Respiratory syncytial virus (RSV), Rubella (German Measles), Transmissible gastroenteritis virus (TGE), Vaccinia, *Aspergillus niger, Candida albicans, Trichophyton mentagrophytes, Streptococcus faecalis*[1], *Streptococcus pyogenes, Enterococcus faecalis* (Vancomycin Resistant).

[1] ATCC and antibiotic-resistant

[2] antibiotic-resistant strain only

Directions for Use: 2 ounces per gallon of water. Dilution 1:256 (630 ppm quat).

It is a violation of Federal Law to use this product in a manner inconsistent with its labeling.

This product is not to be used as a sterilant/high level disinfectant on any surface or instrument that (1) is introduced directly into the human body, either into or in contact with the blood stream or normally sterile areas of the body, (2) contacts intact mucous membranes but which does not ordinarily penetrate the blood barrier or otherwise enter normally sterile areas of the body. This product may be used to preclean or decontaminate critical or semi-critical devices prior to sterilization or high-level disinfection.

Disinfection: Remove heavy soil from surface. Then thoroughly wet surface with a solution of ½ ounce of the concentrate per gallon of water. The solution can be applied with a cloth, mop, sponge, or coarse spray, or soaking. Let solution remain on surface for a minimum of 10 minutes. Rinse or allow to air dry. Rinsing of floors is not necessary unless they are to be waxed or polished. Food contact surfaces must be thoroughly rinsed with potable water. This product must not be used to clean the following food contact surfaces: utensils, glassware and dishes. Prepare a fresh solution daily or more often if the solution becomes visibly dirty or diluted.

Mildewstatic Instructions: Will effectively control the growth of mold and mildew plus the odors caused by them when applied to hard, non-porous surfaces such as walls, floors, and table tops. Apply solution (½ ounce per gallon of water) with a cloth, mop, sponge, or coarse spray. Make sure to wet all surfaces completely. Let air dry. Repeat application weekly or when growth reappears.

Precautionary Statements: Hazards to Humans and Domestic Animals:

Danger. Corrosive. Causes irreversible eye damage and skin burns. Harmful if swallowed. Do not get in eyes, on skin, or on clothing. When handling product, protect eyes by wearing goggles or face shield and protect skin by wearing rubber gloves. Wash thoroughly with soap and water after handling. Remove contaminated clothing and wash before reuse.

Statement of Practical Treatment: In case of contact, immediately flush eyes or skin with plenty of water for at least 15 minutes. For eyes or skin, call a physician. If swallowed, call a doctor or get medical attention. Do not induce vomiting or give anything by mouth to an unconscious person. Drink promptly a large quantity of milk, egg whites, gellatin solution, or if these are not available, drink large quantities of water. Avoid alcohol.

Note to Physician: Probable mucosal damage may contraindicate the use of gastric lavage. Measures against circulatory shock, respiratory depression, and convulsion may be needed.

Storage and Disposal: Keep product under locked storage, inaccessible to small children. Do not reuse container. Rinse thoroughly, securely wrap empty container in several layers of newspaper, and discard in the trash.

Warning(s): Keep out of reach of children.

Presentation: 1 gallon and 5 gallon.

Compendium Code No.: 10821380

PARVOCINE®

Biocor **Vaccine**

Parvovirus Vaccine, Killed Virus

U.S. Vet. Lic. No.: 462

Contents: This product contains the antigen listed above.

The Parvovirus is inactivated to assure safety.

This product contains gentamicin, amphotericin B and thimerosal as preservatives.

Indications: PARVOCINE® is a stable vaccine recommended for use in the vaccination of healthy dogs against disease caused by Canine Parvovirus.

Directions: Shake well. Administer 1 mL intramuscularly or subcutaneously at 9 weeks of age. For initial vaccination, a second dose is required 2-4 weeks later. Young animals vaccinated under 18 weeks of age should be revaccinated every 2-4 weeks until at least 18 weeks of age. Annual revaccination with a single 1 mL dose is recommended.

May be safely used in pregnant bitches. Persistence of maternal origin antibody in puppies should receive consideration in determining vaccination programs. Puppies from susceptible bitches and orphan puppies should begin vaccination at a very early age.

Precaution(s): Store at 35°-45°F (2°-7°C). Do not freeze. Use entire contents when first opened. Do not use chemically sterilized syringes or needles.

Caution(s): In case of anaphylactoid reactions, epinephrine should be administered immediately.

For use in dogs only. For veterinary use only.

Presentation: Code 66411B - 25 x 1 dose (1 mL) vials.
Code 66454B - 10 dose (10 mL) vials.

Compendium Code No.: 13940132 BAH9925-1098 / BAH998-1098

PARVO GUARD™

First Priority **Disinfectant**

Disinfectant-Cleaner-Sanitizer-Tuberculocide, Virucide*, Bactericide, Fungicide, Deodorizer

EPA Reg. No.: 4959-15-68077

Active Ingredient(s):

Iodine** 1.75%
Inert Ingredients 98.25%
Total 100.00%

**From alpha-(p-nonylphenyl)-omega-hydroxypoly (oxyethylene)-iodine complex

Indications: Concentrated broad spectrum iodophor for use as a one-step cleaner-disinfectant and no-rinse sanitizer in veterinary clinics, poultry drinking water, sanitizing commercial eggs, egg processing plants, dairy and poultry farms, meat and poultry plants, food processing plants, kennels, pet shops and zoos, hand sanitizing in food plants and animal handling facilities.

Used as directed PARVO GUARD™ is effective in hard water (up to 400 ppm as $CaCO_3$) and in 5% organic serum load against the following viruses, bacteria and pathogenic fungi: Polio 1*, Vaccinia*, Herpes Simplex Type 1*, Influenza A2/Japan 305*, and Canine Parvovirus*, bactericidal against *Salmonella cholerasuis, Staphylococcus aureus, Pseudomonas aeruginosa,* and *E coli;* is fungicidal against *Trichophyton mentagrophytes* (the athlete's foot fungus); on pre-cleaned food contact surfaces PARVO GUARD™ is effective against *Salmonella choleraesuis, Listeria monocytogens* and *Escherichia coli,* 0157:H7, Hemorrhagic.

Directions for Use: It is a violation of Federal law to use this product in a manner inconsistent with its labeling.

Use Dilution Table:

PARVO GUARD™/Water	Titratable Iodine
1 oz to 10 gal	12.5 ppm
1 oz to 5 gal	25 ppm
3 oz to 5 gal	75 ppm
1 oz to 1 gal	125 ppm
6 oz to 5 gal	150 ppm

Not for residential use.

The color of PARVO GUARD™ solution is proportional to the titratable iodine concentration. Prepare a fresh solution daily, or when there is a noticeable change in its rich amber color, or more often if the solution becomes diluted or soiled. Used as directed, PARVO GUARD™ is tuberculocidal when used in hard water (up to 400 ppm $CaCO_3$) on pre-cleaned surfaces at 20°C for a contact time of 10 minutes. Prepare a solution of 3 ounces PARVO GUARD™ to 5 gallons water (provides 75 ppm titratable iodine).

One-Step Cleaning and Disinfecting: Prior to use in veterinary clinics, animal handling facilities, farm premises, kennels, pet shops and zoos: Remove all animals and feeds from premises, vehicles and enclosures. Remove all litter and manure from floors, walls and all surfaces to be treated. Empty all troughs, racks and other feeding and watering appliances. Then proceed as directed below.

To Clean and Disinfect: Before applying disinfecting solution, food products and packaging materials must be removed from the room or carefully protected. Remove heavy soil deposits before applying the disinfecting solution. Using a solution of 3 ounces PARVO GUARD™ per 5 gallons of warm water (68°F, 20°C or warmer), immerse objects in disinfecting solution, or apply solution with a mop, sponge or brush. When appropriate, use a mechanical sprayer to produce coarse spray. Allow a 10 minute contact time with disinfecting solution. For efficacy against Canine Parvovirus, allow a 120 minute contact time; surface must remain wet. All food contact surfaces must be rinsed with potable water before reuse. Floors, walls and all other non-food contact surfaces may drain dry without rinsing.

Note: When mixing PARVO GUARD™ with cold water (as low as 41°F, 5°C), increase use to 6 oz per 5 gallons water.

Before Rehousing Animals: Ventilate buildings, vehicles and other closed spaces. Do not house animals or use equipment until treatment absorbs, sets or dries. Thoroughly rinse all treated feed racks, mangers, troughs, automatic feeders, fountains and waterers with potable water before reuse.

Shoe Bath: Routine use of shoe bath sanitizers helps reduce the spread of disease causing organisms between poultry houses, farrowing houses, hog barns and other livestock buildings. Use 3 ounces of PARVO GUARD™ per 1 gallon of water. Place sanitizing solution in shallow plastic or stainless steel pans inside all entrances to poultry and livestock buildings. Scrape shoes outside doorway and stand in shoe bath for 30 seconds before entering building. Replace shoe bath daily or more often if solution becomes soiled.

Cleaning Milking Equipment and Bulk Tanks: Immediately after milking, flush milking equipment and utensils with lukewarm (100°F, 38°C) water to wash out all milk. Take apart milking machines and immerse air hoses, inflations, metal parts (except pulsator) and utensils in a solution containing 1 ounce of PARVO GUARD™ per 5 gallons of water. Brush all parts thoroughly. Drain completely, rinse with water and allow to air dry. After emptying bulk tanks, flush tanks thoroughly with 100°F (38°C) water to wash out all milk. Brush tanks thoroughly with a solution containing 1 ounce PARVO GUARD™ per 5 gallons of water. Allow wash solution to drain, rinse with water and air dry.

Sanitizing Milking Machines and Bulk Tanks: Before each milking, flush assembled milking machines and empty bulk tanks with a solution containing 1 ounce PARVO GUARD™ per 5 gallons of water. Allow a 1 minute contact time. Drain thoroughly and air dry before use.

Removal of Milkstone and Hard Water Deposits: Yellow color may appear on equipment after the first use of PARVO GUARD™. This may indicate the presence of milkstone or hard water deposits. Remove these deposits by applying a solution containing equal parts of PARVO GUARD™ and lukewarm water. Wait 2-3 minutes, brush and then rinse with potable water. Daily use of PARVO GUARD™ will help prevent the formation of milkstone and hard water deposits.

Sanitizing Poultry Drinking Water: Add 1 ounce of PARVO GUARD™ per 10 gallons of drinking water. Regular use of this product in drinking water reduces the buildup of slime and mineral deposits in watering equipment. Do not use this product together with other water treatments such as medications.

Sanitizing Previously Cleaned Food Contact Surfaces: Sanitize previously cleaned and rinsed hard, non-porous surfaces such as glass, metal, plastic and porcelain with a solution containing 1 ounce of PARVO GUARD™ per 5 gallons of water. Spray or immerse equipment with sanitizing solution and allow 1 minute of contact time. Drain solution from equipment; do not rinse. PARVO GUARD™ used at 1 ounce per 5 gallons of water contains 25 ppm titratable iodine and does not require a final rinse with potable water in accordance with Federal Food Additive Regulation 178.1010.

Sanitizing Food-Grade Egg Shells: Coarse spray previously cleaned food-grade egg shells with a solution containing 1 ounce of PARVO GUARD™ per 5 gallons of water. Solution temperature should be warmer than the eggs, but not to exceed 130°F (53°C). Wet eggs thoroughly for 1 minute and allow to drain. A final potable water rinse is not required. Eggs should be reasonably dry before casing or breaking. Do not reuse solution to sanitize eggs.

Hand Sanitizing: Thoroughly wash and rinse hands before sanitizing. Dip or rinse hands in a solution containing 1 ounce of PARVO GUARD™ per 5 gallons of water. PARVO GUARD™ may be injected directly into wash or rinse water at a rate of 1 ounce per 5 gallons of water. A final potable water rinse is not required.

Precautionary Statements: Hazards to Humans and Domestic Animals:

Danger: Corrosive: Causes irreversible eye damage. Harmful if swallowed. Do not get in eyes or on clothing. Avoid contact with skin. Wear goggles or face shield. Wash thoroughly with soap and water after handling. Remove contaminated clothing and wash before reuse.

Environmental Hazards: This product is toxic to fish and aquatic organisms. Do not contaminate water by cleaning of equipment or disposal of wastes. Do not discharge effluent containing this product into lakes, streams, ponds, estuaries, oceans or other water unless in accordance with the requirements of a National Pollutant Discharge Elimination System (NPDES) permit and the permitting authority has been notified in writing prior to discharge. Do not discharge effluent containing this product to sewer systems without previously notifying the local sewage treatment plant authority. For guidance, contact your State Water Board or Regional Office of the EPA.

First Aid:

If in Eyes: Hold eye open and rinse slowly and gently with water for 15-20 minutes. Remove contact lenses, if present. after first 5 minutes. Then continue rinsing. Call a poison control center or doctor for treatment advice.

If on Skin: Take off contaminated clothing. Rinse skin immediately with plenty of water for 15-20 minutes. Call a poison control center or doctor for treatment advice.

If Swallowed: Call a poison control center or doctor for treatment advice. Have the person sip a glass of water if able to swallow. Do not induce vomiting unless told to do so by the poison control center or doctor. Do not give anything by mouth to an unconscious person.

If Inhaled: Move person to fresh air. If person is not breathing call 911 or an ambulance, then give artificial respiration, preferably mouth-to-mouth, if possible. Call a poison control center or doctor for treatment advice.

Note to Physician: Probable mucosal damage may contraindicate the use of gastric lavage. Measures against circulatory shock, respiratory depression and convulsions may be needed.

Storage and Disposal: Keep container closed when not in use. Do not store below 25°F or above 100°F for extended periods.

Prohibition: Do not contaminate water, food or feed by storage or disposal. Open dumping is prohibited.

Pesticide Disposal: Pesticide wastes are acutely hazardous. Improper disposal of excess pesticide, spray mixture or rinsate is a violation of Federal law. If these wastes cannot be disposed of by use according to label instructions, contact your State Pesticide or Environmental Control Agency, or the Hazardous Waste representative at the nearest EPA Regional Office for guidance.

Container Disposal: Triple rinse (or equivalent). Then offer for recycling or reconditioning, or puncture and dispose of in a sanitary landfill, or incinerate, or, if allowed by State and local authorities, burn container. If burned, stay out of smoke.

Warning(s): Keep out of reach of children.

Presentation: 1 gallon (3.785 L).

Compendium Code No.: 11390622 Rev. 08-01

PARVOSAN™

KenVet **Disinfectant**

Broad Spectrum Hospital Disinfectant

EPA Reg. No.: 134-65-36208

Active Ingredient(s):

2-(Hydroxymethyl)-2-Nitro-1, 3-Propanediol 19.20%
Alkyl (C12-67%, C14-25%, C16-7%, C8, C10, C18-1%)
dimethyl benzyl ammonium chloride 3.08%
Formaldehyde 2.28%
Inert Ingredients.......... 75.44%
Total.......... 100.00%

Indications: For control of canine parvovirus in veterinary clinics and kennels

Bactericidal, Fungicidal, Virucidal*.

General: PARVOSAN™ Disinfectant is a vapor phase broad-spectrum surface disinfectant effective against gram positive and gram negative microorganisms. PARVOSAN™ Disinfectant is a nonflammable and noncorrosive formulation. PARVOSAN™ Disinfectant can be used in the following areas: Swine Operations, Dairy Farms, Cattle Farms, Veal Farms, Equine Farms, Zoos, Veterinary Clinics, Kennels, Animal Life Sciences Laboratories and in farm foot baths. PARVOSAN™ Disinfectant can be used to disinfect pens, hutches, feeders, waterers and cages. PARVOSAN™ has proven effective as a disinfectant by the A.O.A.C. use dilution test modified for spray products against the following organisms. All dilutions 1:128 tested at 400 ppm water hardness (as calcium carbonate) and 5% calf serum.

Staphylococcus aureus, Escherichia coli, Salmonella choleraesuis, Klebsiella pneumoniae, Salmonella enteritidis, Mycoplasma pneumonia, Pseudomonas aeruginosa, Salmonella typhimurium, Pasteurella multocida, Proteus vulgaris, Clostridium perfringens, Streptococcus pyogenes, Campylobacter jejuni, Bordetella bronchiseptica, Enterobacter aerogenes, Actinobacillus suis.

*PARVOSAN™ has proven virucidal efficacy for use on hard, nonporous, inanimate environmental surfaces. All dilutions 1:128 tested with 400 ppm water hardness (as calcium carbonate) and 5% bovine serum.

Pseudorabies, Avian influenza, Transmissible gastroenteritis, Infectious Bronchitis virus, Avian laryngotracheitis, Swine influenza virus, Canine Parvovirus, Feline Panleukopenia, Newcastle disease, Porcine Respiratory and Reproductive Syndrome (PRRS).

PARVOSAN™ has proven effective fungicidal activity by the A.O.A.C. use dilution test modified for spray products. All dilutions 1:128 tested with tap water and 5% calf serum.

Candida albicans, Trichophyton mentagrophytes.

Directions for Use: It is a violation of Federal Law to use this product in a manner inconsistent with its labeling.

To be used in the disinfection of farm buildings and equipment which are used for livestock production and for other non-livestock buildings. Especially suited for equipment, which may harbor or spread many germs or microorganisms within the farm operation or to other farms. Apply PARVOSAN™ Disinfectant with a mechanical spray device. Spray all surfaces to be disinfected until thoroughly wet. Dilute PARVOSAN™ Disinfectant one ounce per gallon of water. Use as follows:

Livestock Buildings: Evacuate all animals from buildings. Remove all litter and manure from floors, walls and surfaces of barns, pens, stalls, chutes and other facilities and fixtures occupied or traversed by animals. Empty all troughs, racks and other feeding and watering appliances. Thoroughly clean all surfaces with soap or detergent and rinse with water. Spray all surfaces and allow PARVOSAN™ Disinfectant to saturate all surfaces for 10 minutes. Equipment inside the building should be first cleaned with soap or detergent, rinsed with water and then saturated as above with this product.

Ventilate buildings and other closed spaces. Do not house livestock or employ equipment until treatment has been absorbed, set or dried. Thoroughly scrub all treated feed racks, troughs, automatic feeders, fountains and waterers with soap or detergent and rinse with potable water before reuse.

Equipment: Empty all troughs, racks and other feeding and watering appliances. Thoroughly clean all surfaces with soap or detergent and rinse with water. Then thoroughly spray or soak all exposed parts of the cleaned equipment used in the livestock or veterinary operation.

All treated feed racks, food bowls, mangers, troughs, automatic feeders, fountains and waterers must be thoroughly scrubbed with detergents and rinsed with potable water prior to reuse.

Immerse cleaned halters, ropes and other types of equipment used in handling and restraining animals, forks, and all shovels and scrapers used for removing litter and manure or feces and allow PARVOSAN™ Disinfectant to saturate all surfaces for 10 minutes. Do not spray onto feed to be consumed by animals.

*For Canine Parvovirus and Feline Panleukopenia: PARVOSAN™ Disinfectant is effective against Canine Parvovirus when used at a three ounces per gallon dilution. To control Canine Parvovirus thoroughly clean all surfaces and mix three (3) ounces of PARVOSAN™ Disinfectant in one gallon of water. Apply as a spray. Allow to air dry or area may be rinsed after 45 minutes.

All Other Non-livestock Buildings and Facilities: Thoroughly clean all surfaces with soap or detergent and rinse with water. Spray all surfaces to be disinfected and allow to saturate all surfaces for 10 minutes. Ventilate buildings and other closed spaces.

Precautionary Statements: Precautionary Statements Hazards to Humans and Domestic Animals:

Danger: Causes severe eye irritation. Wear goggles or a face shield. Causes skin irritation. Harmful if inhaled or absorbed through skin. Do not get in eyes, on skin, or on clothing. Handlers must wear long-sleeved shirt and long pants, chemical resistant rubber gloves, shoes and socks. Wash thoroughly with soap and water after handling. Remove contaminated clothing and wash before reuse. Prolonged or frequently repeated skin contact may cause allergic reactions in some individuals. Do not use on animals.

Statement of Practical Treatment:

If in eyes- Hold eyelids open and flush with a steady, gentle stream of water for 15 minutes. Get medical attention.

If on skin- Wash with plenty of soap and water. Get medical attention.

If Inhaled- Remove victim to fresh air. If not breathing, give artificial respiration, preferably mouth-to-mouth. Get medical attention.

Storage and Disposal: Do not contaminate water, food or feed by storage or disposal.

Storage - Keep upright while moving and in storage. Container equipped with a pressure relief closure. Keep from freezing. Store in original container only, in safe manner. Do not store under conditions which might adversely affect the container or its ability to function properly. Reduce stacking height where local conditions can affect package strength. Open container in a well-ventilated area, avoid breathing vapor. Keep container tightly closed when not in use.

Spill Control- Soak up spill in a dry absorbent such as clay. Sweep it up, put into disposal containers and dispose as directed below. Wear protective clothing and equipment consistent with good pesticide handling procedures while exposed to spilled material.

Pesticide Disposal- "Pesticide wastes are toxic. Improper disposal of excess pesticide, spray mixture, or rinsate is a violation of Federal Law. If these wastes cannot be disposed of by use according to label instructions, contact your State Pesticide or Environmental Control Agency, or the Hazardous Waste representatives at the nearest EPA Regional Office for guidance."

Container Disposal - Triple rinse (or equivalent). Then offer for recycling or reconditioning, or puncture and dispose of in a sanitary landfill, or incineration, or, if allowed by State and Local authorities, by burning. If burned, stay out of smoke.

Warning(s): Keep out of reach of children.

Presentation: 1 gallon, 5 gallon and 55 gallon drum.

Compendium Code No.: 11340020 LIA198

PARVO SHIELD®

Novartis Animal Vaccines **Vaccine**

Parvovirus Vaccine, Killed Virus

U.S. Vet. Lic. No.: 303

Composition: The vaccine contains inactivated antigenic cultures of porcine parvovirus adjuvanted with aluminum hydroxide.

Contains amphotericin B, penicillin, streptomycin, and thimerosal as preservatives.

Indications: For use in healthy swine as an aid in the prevention and control of diseases caused by porcine parvovirus.

Dosage and Administration: Shake well before using. Administer 2 mL intramuscularly or subcutaneously three (3) to four (4) weeks prior to breeding. Revaccinate prior to each subsequent breeding. Vaccinate boars annually.

Precaution(s): Store in the dark at 35°-45°F (2°-7°C). Do not freeze. Use the entire contents when first opened.

Caution(s): Anaphylactic reactions may occur following the use of the product. Symptomatic treatment: Epinephrine. For veterinary use only.

Warning(s): Do not vaccinate within 21 days of slaughter.

Presentation: Available in 50 dose (100 mL) bottles.

Compendium Code No.: 11140262

PARVO SHIELD® L5

Novartis Animal Vaccines **Bacterin-Vaccine**

Parvovirus Vaccine-Leptospira canicola-grippotyphosa-hardjo-icterohaemorrhagiae-pomona Bacterin, Killed Virus

U.S. Vet. Lic. No.: 303

Composition: The bacterin contains inactivated antigenic cultures of porcine parvovirus, *Leptospira canicola, L. grippotyphosa, L. hardjo, L. icterohaemorrhagiae,* and *L. pomona* which are adjuvanted with aluminum hydroxide. Contains penicillin, streptomycin, and amphotericin B as preservatives.

Indications: For use in healthy swine as an aid in the prevention and control of diseases caused by porcine parvovirus, *Leptospira canicola, L. grippotyphosa, L. hardjo, L. icterohaemorrhagiae,* and *L. pomona.*

Dosage and Administration: Shake well before using. Inject 2 mL subcutaneously or intramuscularly to sows and gilts four (4) to six (6) weeks prior to breeding and again in three (3) to four (4) weeks. Revaccinate with a single dose four (4) to six (6) weeks prior to each subsequent breeding. Vaccinate boars semi-annually.

Precaution(s): Store at 35°-45°F (2°-7°C). Do not freeze. Use the entire contents when first opened.

Caution(s): Anaphylactic reactions may occur following the use of the product. Symptomatic treatment: Epinephrine.

Warning(s): Do not vaccinate within 21 days of slaughter.

Discussion: Leptospirosis has been recognized in the United States since 1950 and has established itself as a disease of great economic importance. Entrance of the disease into a susceptible herd results in losses due to aborted, stillborn or weak piglets.

All pathogenic strains of Lepto are serovars of *Leptospira interrogans.* The common serovars found in swine are *L. canicola, L. pomona, L. hardjo, L. grippotyphosa,* and *L. icterohaemorrhagiae.*

Leptospirosis is easily transmitted from the urine of infected animals into breaks in the skin, through the mucous membranes, or by way of the conjunctiva of the eye. It only takes a small number of the organisms to cause disease. Following exposure, an incubation period of one to two weeks occurs. The organism localizes in the kidneys and may be shed into the urine for a few weeks up to two years. Intra-uterine infections can occur in the last half of gestation, with abortions, stillbirths, and neonatal diseases being a common occurrence. Both acute and chronic forms of the disease can occur, with reproductive problems more likely to occur in animals with subclinical infections.

The control of leptospirosis is important both because of the economic losses associated with fetal death and because swine are an important reservoir of infection for other species of farm animals and humans. Since the disease can occur unnoticed in a herd, prevention is very important.

Porcine parvovirus is found in swine throughout the world. In major swine producing areas, such as the Midwest, infection is present in most herds. Gilts and sows that have not developed a natural immunity to the disease run a very high risk of infection with reproductive disease occurring. The most common routes of infection are oronasal in sows and gilts and transplacental to the unborn piglets.

Porcine parvovirus is a contagious disease of swine characterized by reproductive failure. Symptoms seen depend upon the stage of gestation when the infection occurs. Infection during the first half of gestation results in reproductive failure. Fetal death occurs, followed by re-absorption or mummification. Sows may return to estrus, fail to farrow even though they show signs of pregnancy, farrow small litters, or farrow a large proportion of mummified fetuses. Sometimes the only outward sign is a decrease in maternal abdominal size when the fetuses die and their associated fluids are re-absorbed. If infection occurs after mid-gestation, the fetuses are able to develop antibodies against the infection and will be unaffected.

Presentation: Available in 10 dose (20 mL) and 50 dose (100 mL) bottles.

Compendium Code No.: 11140272

PARVO SHIELD® L5E

Novartis Animal Vaccines **Bacterin-Vaccine**

Parvovirus Vaccine-Erysipelothrix rhusiopathiae-Leptospira canicola-grippotyphosa-hardjo-icterohaemorrhagiae-pomona Bacterin, Killed Virus

U.S. Vet. Lic. No.: 303

Composition: The product contains inactivated antigenic cultures of porcine parvovirus, *Erysipelothrix rhusiopathiae, Leptospira canicola, L. grippotyphosa, L. hardjo, L.*

icterohaemorrhagiae, and *L. pomona* which are adjuvanted with aluminum hydroxide. Contains penicillin, streptomycin, and amphotericin B as preservatives.

Indications: For use in healthy swine as an aid in the prevention and control of diseases caused by porcine parvovirus, *Erysipelothrix rhusiopathiae, Leptospira canicola, L. grippotyphosa, L. hardjo, L. icterohaemorrhagiae,* and *L. pomona.*

Dosage and Administration: Shake well before using. Inject 5 mL subcutaneously or intramuscularly to sows and gilts four (4) to six (6) weeks prior to breeding and again in three (3) to four (4) weeks. Revaccinate with a single dose four (4) to six (6) weeks prior to each subsequent breeding. Vaccinate boars semi-annually.

Precaution(s): Store at 35°-45°F (2°-7°C). Do not freeze. Use the entire contents when first opened.

Caution(s): Anaphylactic reactions may occur following the use of this biological. Symptomatic treatment: Epinephrine.

Warning(s): Do not vaccinate within 21 days of slaughter.

Discussion: Leptospirosis has been recognized in the United States since 1950 and has established itself as a disease of great economic importance. Entrance of the disease into a susceptible herd results in losses due to aborted, stillborn or weak piglets.

All pathogenic strains of Lepto are serovars of *Leptospira interrogans.* The common serovars found in swine are *L. canicola, L. pomona, L. hardjo, L. grippotyphosa,* and *L. icterohaemorrhagiae.*

Leptospirosis is easily transmitted from the urine of infected animals into breaks in the skin, through the mucous membranes, or by way of the conjunctiva of the eye. It only takes a small number of the organisms to cause disease. Following exposure, an incubation period of one to two weeks occurs. The organism localizes in the kidneys and may be shed into the urine for a few weeks up to two years. Intra-uterine infections can occur in the last half of gestation, with abortions, stillbirths, and neonatal diseases being a common occurrence. Both acute and chronic forms of the disease can occur, with reproductive problems more likely to occur in animals with subclinical infections.

The control of leptospirosis is important both because of the economic losses associated with fetal death and because swine are an important reservoir of infection for other species of farm animals and humans. Since the disease can occur unnoticed in a herd, prevention is very important.

Porcine parvovirus is found in swine throughout the world. In major swine producing areas, such as the Midwest, infection is present in most herds. Gilts and sows that have not developed a natural immunity to the disease run a very high risk of infection with reproductive disease occurring. The most common routes of infection are oronasal in the sows and transplacental to the unborn piglets.

Porcine parvovirus is a contagious disease of swine characterized by reproductive failure. Symptoms seen depend upon the stage of gestation when the infection occurs. Infection during the first half of gestation results in reproductive failure. Fetal death occurs, followed by re-absorption or mummification. Sows may return to estrus, fail to farrow even though they show signs of pregnancy, farrow small litters, or farrow a large proportion of mummified fetuses. Sometimes the only outward sign is a decrease in maternal abdominal size when the fetuses die and their associated fluids are re-absorbed. If infection occurs after mid-gestation, the fetuses are able to develop antibodies against the infection and will be unaffected.

Erysipelas in swine is caused by a bacteria, *Erysipelothrix rhusiopathiae.* Pigs become infected most commonly from ingesting the organism, although it may also enter the body through skin wounds. The source of the infection is usually other carrier pigs or wild animals such as rodents and birds.

Clinical signs of erysipelas in swine can be acute, subacute or chronic. In the acute form, animals show signs of systemic disease. They lie around and are reluctant to rise. If forced to rise, they will stand with their legs tucked under their bodies. Affected pigs are off feed and have fevers of 104°-108°F. Pregnant sows may abort. Raised red skin lesions ("diamond skin" lesions) often appear within two to three days, and animals that develop severe skin lesions usually die.

Subacute erysipelas includes many of the same symptoms, but they are less severe, sometimes to the point of being unnoticed.

Chronic erysipelas may follow cases of acute or subacute erysipelas, or it may show up in pigs that have not had previous signs of illness. Pigs with chronic erysipelas usually show signs of arthritis due to degenerative changes in the joints. The valves of the heart may also be affected, in which case the animals will show signs of heart disease such as shortness of breath.

Presentation: Available in 10 dose (50 mL), 20 dose (100 mL) and 50 dose (250 mL) bottles.

Compendium Code No.: 11140283

P

PARVOSOL® II RTU

KenVet **Disinfectant**

EPA Reg. No.: 1839-83-36208

Active Ingredient(s):

n-Alkyl (60% C_{14}, 30% C_{16}, 5% C_{12}, 5% C_{18}) dimethyl benzyl ammonium chlorides . . 0.105%
n-Alkyl (68% C_{12}, 32% C_{14}) dimethyl ethylbenzyl ammonium chlorides 0.105%
Inert Ingredients. 99.790%
Total 100.000%

Indications: A cleaner and disinfectant for use in home and hospitals. This product exhibits virucidal activity against canine parvovirus.

Directions for Use: It is a violation of Federal law to use this product in a manner inconsistent with its labeling. PARVOSOL® II RTU is designed specifically as a general non-acid cleaner and disinfectant for use in homes and hospitals: authorized by USDA for use in federally inspected meat and poultry processing plants. It is formulated to disinfect hard, non-porous, inanimate environmental surfaces such as floors, walls, metal surfaces, stainless steel surfaces, porcelain, glazed ceramic tile, plastic surfaces, and cabinets. A rinse with potable water is required for surfaces in direct contact with food. In addition, this product deodorizes those areas which generally are hard to keep fresh smelling, such as garbage storage areas, empty garbage bins and cans, basements, and other areas which are prone to odors caused by microorganisms.

Disinfection, Deodorizing and Cleaning - Remove gross filth or heavy soil prior to application of the product. Hold container six to eight inches from surface to be treated. Spray area until it is covered with the solution. Allow product to penetrate and remain wet for 10 minutes. No scrubbing is necessary. Wipe off with a clean cloth, mop or sponge. The product will not leave grit or soap scum.

Virucidal Activity - This product, when used on environmental, inanimate, non-porous surfaces, exhibits effective virucidal activity against Canine Parvovirus.

Tuberculocidal Activity - This product exhibits disinfectant efficacy against *Mycobacterium tuberculosis* (BCG) in 10 minutes at 20 degrees Centigrade when used as directed on previously cleaned hard non-porous inanimate surfaces.

Bactericidal Activity - When used as directed, this product exhibits effective disinfectant activity against the organisms: *Staphylococcus aureus, Salmonella choleraesuis, Pseudomonas aeruginosa, Escherichia coli* 0157:H7, and meets the requirements for hospital use.

Contact Time: Allow surface to remain wet for 10 minutes.

Mildewstat - To control mold and mildew on pre-cleaned, hard, non-porous surfaces, spray surface to be treated making sure to wet completely. Let air dry. Repeat application at weekly intervals or when mildew growth appears.

Fungicidal Activity - This product is fungicidal against the pathogenic fungi, *Trichophyton mentagrophytes* (Athlete's Foot Fungus) when used as directed on clean, non-porous, hard surfaces commonly contacted by bare feet.

Efficacy tests have demonstrated that this product is an effective bactericide, fungicide, and virucide in the presence of organic soil (5% blood serum).

Precautionary Statements: Hazards to Humans and Domestic Animals:

Warning: Keep out of reach of children.

Causes eye and skin irritation. Do not get in eyes, on skin or on clothing. Harmful if swallowed. Avoid contamination of food. Remove contaminated clothing and wash before reuse. Wash thoroughly with soap and water after handling.

Statement of Practical Treatment: In case of contact, immediately flush eyes or skin with plenty of water for at least 15 minutes. For eyes, call a physician.

Note to Physician: Probable mucosal damage may contraindicate the use of gastric lavage.

Storage and Disposal: Do not contaminate water, food, or feed by storage or disposal.

Container Disposal - Do not reuse container (bottle, can, or jar). Rinse thoroughly before discarding in trash.

Storage - Store in a dry place no lower in temperature than 50 degrees or higher than 120 degrees.

Disclaimer: Except as expressly provided herein, neither Loveland nor seller makes any warranties, guarantees, or representations of any kind, either by usage of trade, statutory or otherwise, with regard to the product sold, including, but not limited to merchantability, fitness for a particular purpose, use or eligibility of the product for any particular trade usage. Unintended consequences may result because of, but not limited to, such factors as presence of other materials, or the manner of use or application, all of which are beyond the control of Loveland Industries, Inc. or seller. In no case shall seller be liable for consequential, special, or indirect damages resulting from the use or handling of this product. All such risks shall be assumed by the buyer or user.

Applicator's or grower's exclusive remedy against Loveland Industries, Inc. or seller for any cause of action relating to the product is a claim for damages, and in no event shall damages or any other recovery exceed the purchase price of the product in respect of which such claim is made.

Presentation: 1 gallon.

Compendium Code No.: 11340031

PARVO-VAC®/LEPTOFERM-5®

Pfizer Animal Health **Bacterin-Vaccine**

Parvovirus Vaccine, Killed Virus-Leptospira Canicola-Grippotyphosa-Hardjo-Icterohaemorrhagiae-Pomona Bacterin

U.S. Vet. Lic. No.: 189

Description: The parvovirus fraction is a chemically inactivated, adjuvanted PPV strain grown on an established porcine cell line. The *Leptospira* fraction is prepared from whole cultures of *L. canicola, L. grippotyphosa, L. hardjo, L. icterohaemorrhagiae,* and *L. pomona.*

Contains gentamicin as preservative.

Indications: PARVO-VAC®/LEPTOFERM-5® is for vaccination of healthy swine as an aid in preventing reproductive failure caused by porcine parvovirus (PPV) and leptospirosis caused by *Leptospira canicola, L. grippotyphosa, L. hardjo, L. icterohaemorrhagiae,* and *L. pomona.*

Directions:

1. General Directions: Shake well. Aseptically administer 5 mL intramuscularly.
2. Primary Vaccination: Administer a single 5-mL dose to healthy sows 14-60 days before breeding. Healthy gilts, however, should receive a single 5-mL dose as near as possible to 14 days before breeding; if gilts are vaccinated sooner, persisting maternal antibodies may interfere with active immunization. For protection against leptospirosis, a second dose is recommended 3-6 weeks after the initial dose.
3. Revaccination: Semiannual revaccination with a single dose before breeding is recommended.

Precaution(s): Store at 2°-7°C. Prolonged exposure to higher temperatures may adversely affect potency. Do not freeze.

Use entire contents when first opened.

Sterilized syringes and needles should be used to administer this vaccine.

Caution(s): As with many vaccines, anaphylaxis may occur after use. Initial antidote of epinephrine is recommended and should be followed with appropriate supportive therapy.

This product has been shown to be efficacious in healthy animals. A protective immune response may not be elicited if animals are incubating an infectious disease, are malnourished or parasitized, are stressed due to shipment or environmental conditions, are otherwise immunocompromised, or the vaccine is not administered in accordance with label directions.

Warning(s): Do not vaccinate within 21 days before slaughter.

For use in swine only.

For veterinary use only.

Discussion: Disease Description: PPV is a major cause of swine reproductive failure. Infection in susceptible swine is generally subclinical. However, infection of pregnant females may involve the developing fetus. Stillbirths, mummified fetuses, embryonic death, and infertility (SMEDI) are the chief manifestations of the disease. The PPV agent is enzootic in the United States[1] and has a worldwide distribution. Thus, a large proportion of adult swine carry antibodies or disseminate the virus.[2] When maternally acquired antibodies decline below protective levels, stock is at risk.

Swine leptospirosis is characterized by poor production, anemia, and nephritis. Late-term abortions are the most important effect of the disease.

Trial Data: Safety and Efficacy: Postvaccination reactions were not observed in experimental pigs vaccinated with the PPV fraction or in swine vaccinated under field conditions in extensive safety trials. In efficacy studies, vaccination of seronegative gilts before breeding protected 95.7% of developing fetuses from infection and death after challenge with virulent PPV. In contrast, 46.3% of the fetuses from nonvaccinated control gilts became infected and died after the same challenge. Immunogenicity of the *Leptospira* fraction was confirmed by challenge-of-immunity or serologic tests.

References: Available upon request.

Presentation: 50 dose vials.

Compendium Code No.: 36900670 75-4581-07

PASTEURELLA HAEMOLYTICA MULTOCIDA BACTERIN

Colorado Serum **Bacterin**

Pasteurella haemolytica-multocida Bacterin, Bovine Isolates

U.S. Vet. Lic. No.: 188

Active Ingredient(s): Chemically killed, aluminum hydroxide adsorbed, cultures of *Pasteurella haemolytica*, and *Pasteurella multocida*, bovine isolates.

Contains thimerosal as a preservative.

Indications: For the vaccination of healthy cattle, sheep and goats against pasteurellosis, caused by the micro-organsims named.

Dosage and Administration: Inject 2.0 mL subcutaneously. A second dose should be administered at two (2) to four (4) weeks. Animals vaccinated when less than three (3) months old should be revaccinated at weaning or at four (4) to six (6) months of age.

Precaution(s): Shake well, each dose must have a proportionate share of the precipitate for a proper response. Store in the dark at 2-7°C. Do not freeze. Use the entire contents when first opened.

Caution(s): Anaphylactic reactions sometimes follow administration of products of this nature. If noted, administer adrenaline or an equivalent drug.

For veterinary use only.

Warning(s): Do not vaccinate within 21 days before slaughter.

Presentation: 10 dose (20 mL) and 50 dose (100 mL) vials.

Compendium Code No.: 11010280

PASTEURELLA MULTOCIDA BACTERIN (Types 1, 3, & 4)

L.A.H.I. (New Jersey) **Bacterin**

Pasteurella multocida Bacterin, Avian Isolates Types 1, 3 & 4, Emulsified

U.S. Vet. Lic. No.: 196

Active Ingredient(s): This product is a formalin inactivated oil base emulsion consisting of three strains (types 1, 3 and 4) of *Pasteurella multocida* with merthiolate added as a preservative.

The bacterin is manufactured in accordance with a detailed production outline which has been filed with the Veterinary Services of the USDA. The fill volume for this product is 500 mL in a 625 mL plastic bottle. The bottles are sealed with a rubber stopper and an aluminum overseal.

Quality Control: The bacterin is fully tested for purity, safety and potency according to the standard requirements for *Pasteurella multocida* bacterins, avian isolates, section 113.101, 113.102 and 113.103 of title 9 of the federal regulations by the Animal and Plant Health Inspection Service of the USDA.

Each serial is tested for: Bacteria and fungi; formaldehyde content; safety and potency tests in chickens and turkeys according to 9 CFR 113.102 and 113.103.

Samples and complete test reports on each serial are submitted to the Veterinary Services of the USDA and no merchandise is released for shipment until this government agency has given its release agreement.

Indications: This product is used for the prevention of fowl cholera in chickens and turkeys.

Dosage and Administration: Dosage: 0.5 mL per bird.

Vaccinating instrument: Glass or disposable syringe; needles, one-half (½) inch long, 18-20 gauge.

Site: Inject 0.5 mL subcutaneously (under the skin) in the mid-portion of the neck.

Age of birds to be vaccinated: Six (6) weeks of age or older.

Schedule of vaccination: Repeat vaccination three (3) to six (6) weeks after first vaccination. Revaccinate layers or breeders at 3-month intervals.

If a natural outbreak of the disease occurs on a farm, vaccinate the remaining birds, including birds in production. Immunity can be demonstrated in vaccinated birds 21 days after administration of the product.

Preparation of Bacterin: To prevent shock, allow bacterin to reach room temperature (70° to 95°F) before injecting under the skin of the birds. Sterilize syringes and needles by boiling or submerging in alcohol or other suitable antiseptic prior to use.

Apply an antiseptic solution to the rubber stopper of the bottle of bacterin before inserting needle through the stopper. Use all of the bacterin immediately once the stopper surface has been broken or the stopper removed.

Contraindication(s): The administration of this product to birds in egg production may result in a drop in production by the hens. This can be attributed to handling and administration of the bacterin. Before vaccinating birds in production, test its effect on a small group of birds to determine the effect on egg production.

Precaution(s): The bacterin shall be stored in the dark in a refrigerator between 35-45°F (2-7°C).

Expiration dating: 24 months.

Caution(s): It is imperative that the user of this product comply with the indications for use, contraindications, cautions and directions for use stated on the directions sheet packed with product. The bacterin must be prepared and administered as directed to obtain the best results. For veterinary use only.

Warning(s): Do not market birds for at least six (6) weeks after vaccinating so that there is no swelling at the site of vaccine administration.

Side Effects: Some birds may develop local tissue reactions and swellings at the site of vaccination. Injection should be made in the mid-portion of the neck under the skin, not into the musculature. Needles must be sharp. Injection equipment and needles must be free of contamination.

Presentation: 1,000 dose bottles.

Compendium Code No.: 10080332

PASTEURELLA MULTOCIDA BACTERIN (Types 1, 3, 4 & 3 x 4)

L.A.H.I. (New Jersey) **Bacterin**

Pasteurella multocida Bacterin, Emulsified, Avian Isolates Types 1, 3, 4 & 3 x 4

U.S. Vet. Lic. No.: 196

Active Ingredient(s): The product is a formalin inactivated oil base emulsion consisting of four strains (types 1, 3 and 4 and type 3 x 4) of *Pasteurella multocida.*

The vaccine is carefully produced and passes all tests in accordance with the U.S. government requirements. •

Indications: The product is used for the prevention of *P. multocida* type 1 infection in chickens and turkeys.

Dosage and Administration: Shake the vaccine for two (2) minutes before use.

Chickens should be 12 weeks of age or older and turkeys should be six (6) weeks of age or older at the time of first vaccination. Revaccination should be done three (3) to six (6) weeks after the first vaccination. Layers or breeders should be revaccinated at 3-month intervals. In the event of a natural outbreak, vaccinate the unaffected birds, .

Preparation of Vaccine: Remove the aluminum overseal and the vaccine is ready to use. Should greater than four (4) hours elapse between the first and last use of the product from any one container, it is recommended that the vaccine be shaken again before continuing with the vaccinations.

Inject each bird with a 0.5 mL dose subcutaneously in the mid portion of the neck.

Precaution(s): Keep the vaccine in the dark between 35°-45°F (2°-7°C). Do not freeze.

Caution(s): Use aseptic precautions. Sterilize needles, syringes, and stopper.

Vaccinate healthy birds only. Consult a poultry pathologist before vaccinating.

Burn the vaccine containers and all unused contents.

Use the entire contents when first opened.

It is imperative that the user of this product comply with the instructions. The vaccine must be prepared and administered as directed to obtain the best results. Use of nonsterile needles to administer the vaccine may result in abscess formation and condemnation of birds. Avoid self-injection with the vaccine. Consult a physician immediately if self-injection with the vaccine occurs.

For veterinary use only.

Warning(s): Do not market birds for at least six (6) weeks after vaccinating. Make sure that the birds marketed do not have swellings at the site of vaccine administration since this may result in condemnation of the birds.

Presentation: 1,000 dose (500 mL) bottles.

Compendium Code No.: 10080342

PATRIOT™ INSECTICIDE CATTLE EAR TAGS

Boehringer Ingelheim **Insecticide Ear Tags**

EPA Reg. No.: 4691-148

Active Ingredient(s):

Diazinon (CAS #333-41-5)	40.0%
Inert Ingredients:	60.0%
Total	100.0%

Indications: For use on beef and non-lactating dairy cattle to control horn flies (including pyrethroid resistant populations), gulf coast ticks, spinose ear ticks, and as an aid to control face flies, lice, stable flies and house flies.

Directions for Use: It is a violation of Federal law to use this product in a manner inconsistent with its labeling.

For adequate control of horn flies, attach one tag per animal. For optimum control of horn flies, control of ear ticks, and as an aid in the control of face flies, lice, stable flies and house flies, attach one tag to each ear (two per animal). Replace as necessary. PATRIOT™ tags have been proven to be effective against pyrethroid resistant horn flies for up to five months. Apply as indicated.

1. Disinfect pliers prior to use. Place female tag under clip by depressing lever. Collar on tag must be pointing down.
2. Slide male button on pin. Align tip of male button with female portion of tag. Tag and button are now ready for application.
3. Position tag on the inner flat surface in center of ear. Do not allow shaft of the male rivet to penetrate any cartilage rib or blood vessel or ear damage may result. Boehringer Ingelheim Vetmedica, Inc. recommends that tag be rotated at a 90° angle for ease of application. Tag may also be extended outward from the plier in a straight manner.
4. When properly positioned, the tag should hang as shown.

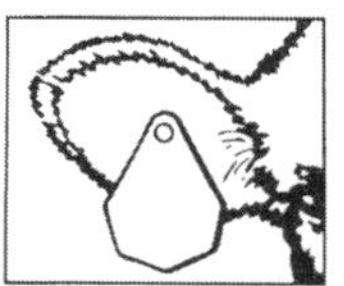

Precautionary Statements:

Hazards to Humans: Harmful if absorbed through the skin or if swallowed. Avoid contact with skin and eyes. Wash thoroughly with soap and water after handling and before eating or smoking. Wear non-permeable protective gloves when applying tags.

Environmental Hazards: This pesticide is toxic to fish. Do not apply directly to water. Do not contaminate water by disposal of used tags.

Statement of Practical Treatment:

If on Skin — Remove contaminated clothing and wash affected areas with soap and water.

If in Eyes — Flush eyes with plenty of water. Call a physician if irritation persists.

If Swallowed — Call a physician or Poison Control Center immediately. Drink one or two glasses of water and induce vomiting by touching the back of throat with finger. Do not induce vomiting or give anything by mouth to an unconscious or convulsing person.

Note to physician — This product is a cholinesterase inhibitor. If symptoms of cholinesterase inhibition are present, atropine sulfate by injection is antidotal. 2-PAM is also antidotal and may be administered, but only in conjunction with atropine.

Storage and Disposal: Store in a cool place in original container.

Opened pouches containing the ear tags should be resealed for storage. Do not contaminate water, food, or feed by storage or disposal.

Pesticide Disposal — Waste (spent tags) resulting from the use of this product may be disposed of on site or at an approved waste disposal facility.

Container Disposal — Dispose of empty container in a sanitary landfill or by incineration, or, if allowed by State and local authorities, by burning. If burned, stay out of smoke.

Warning(s): Calves less than 3 months of age should not be tagged as ear damage may result.

Remove tag prior to slaughter.

Keep out of reach of children.

Presentation: 20's and 120's.

Compendium Code No.: 10280841

PAYLEAN® 9

Elanco **Feed Medication**

Ractopamine Hydrochloride-Type A Medicated Article

NADA No.: 140-863

Active Ingredient(s): Ractopamine hydrochloride - 9 g per lb (20 g per kg).

Inert Ingredients: Ground corncobs.

Indications: For increased rate of weight gain, improved feed efficiency, and increased carcass leanness in finishing swine fed a complete ration containing at least 16% crude protein from 150 lb (68 kg) to 240 lb (109 kg) body weight.

Directions for Use: Do not feed undiluted.

Important: Must be thoroughly mixed into feeds before use. Follow label directions.

P

Indications	Appropriate Concentration of Ractopamine in Type C Medicated Feed
Increased Rate of Weight Gain, Improved Feed Efficiency, and Increased Carcass Leanness	4.5 grams/ton (5 ppm)
Improved Feed Efficiency and Increased Carcass Leanness	4.5 to 18 grams/ton (5 ppm to 20 ppm)

Carcass Measurements	Effect of Ractopamine	
	4.5 grams/ton (5 ppm)	9 - 18 grams/ton (10 - 20 ppm)
Carcass Fat	NC	↓
10th Rib Backfat (3/4 location)	NC	↓
Last Rib Backfat (midline)	NC	NC
Loineye Area (10th rib)	NC	↑
Rate of Lean Gain	NC	↑
Efficiency of Lean Gain	NC	↑
Dressing Percentage	NC	↑

NC = No Change, ↑ = increased, ↓ = decreased

Mixing Directions: Thoroughly mix PAYLEAN® 9 Type A Medicated Article into one ton of appropriate feed ingredients or diluents according to the table below to obtain the proper concentration in the Type B Medicated Feed (maximum 3600 g/ton).

The following table gives examples of how some Type B Medicated Feed concentrations can be prepared:

Pounds of PAYLEAN® 9 To Add Per Ton To Make a Type B Medicated Feed	Resulting Ractopamine Concentration in Type B Medicated Feed	
	grams/ton	grams/pound
100	900	0.45
200	1,800	0.90
300	2,700	1.35
400	3,600	1.80

Thoroughly mix PAYLEAN® 9 Type A Medicated Article into one ton of complete swine feed according to the table below to obtain the proper concentration in the Type C Medicated Feed. Prepare an intermediate pre-blend of the premix prior to mixing in a complete feed. Thoroughly mix the required amount in a convenient quantity of feed ingredients then add to the remaining feed ingredients to make a ton of complete feed.

Pounds PAYLEAN® 9 To Add Per Ton of Type C Medicated Feed	Resulting Ractopamine Concentration in Type C Medicated Feed
0.5	4.5 grams/ton (5 ppm)
1.0	9 grams/ton (10 ppm)
1.5	13.5 grams/ton (15 ppm)
2.0	18 grams/ton (20 ppm)

Feeding Directions: Feed continuously to finishing swine as the sole ration from 150 lb (68 kg) to 240 lb (109 kg) body weight.

Precaution(s): Store at room temperature.

Expiration Date and Lot Number are printed on the bag. Not to be used after the expiry date.

Caution(s): Pigs fed PAYLEAN® are at an increased risk for exhibiting the downer pig syndrome (also referred to as "slows," "subs," or "suspects"). Pig handling methods to reduce the incidence of downer pigs should be thoroughly evaluated prior to initiating use of PAYLEAN®. Not for use in breeding swine.

Warning(s): The active ingredient in PAYLEAN®, ractopamine hydrochloride, is a beta-adrenergic agonist. Individuals with cardiovascular disease should exercise special caution to avoid exposure. Not for use in humans. Keep out of the reach of children. The PAYLEAN® 9 formulation (Type A Medicated Article) poses a low dust potential under usual conditions of handling and mixing. When mixing and handling PAYLEAN®, use protective clothing, impervious gloves, protective eye wear, and a NIOSH-approved dust mask. Operators should wash thoroughly with soap and water after handling. If accidental eye contact occurs, immediately rinse eyes thoroughly with water. If irritation persists, seek medical attention. The material safety data sheet contains more detailed occupational safety information. To report adverse effects, access medical information, or obtain additional product information, call 1-800-428-4441.

For use in finishing swine feeds only.

Presentation: 25 lbs (11.34 kg) bag.

PAYLEAN® is a trademark of Eli Lilly and Company.

Compendium Code No.: 10310072 BG5001DEAML (Jun 01) - BGG090

PEARLYT™ SHAMPOO

DVM **Grooming Shampoo**

Soap-Free Conditioning Formulation with Oatmeal & Brightening Agents

Ingredient(s): Water, ammonium lauryl sulfate, ammonium laureth sulfate, glycol distearate, ammonium xylenesulfonate, oatmeal, propylene glycol, iodopropynyl butylcarbamate, carbomer, triethanolamine, methylparaben, butylparaben, fragrance, FD&C Blue #1, D&C Violet #2.

Indications: For general cleansing, grooming and conditioning of haircoat on dogs and cats. Soothes mild irritation and itching.

Product Description: A soap-free formulation combining the benefits of oatmeal, coat conditioners and brightening agents. PEARLYT™ soothes and moisturizes skin while enhancing luster and sheen of haircoat.

Directions for Use: Wet coat thoroughly. Apply sufficient PEARLYT™ Shampoo to lather well into haircoat. Rinse thoroughly. May be used as often as necessary.

Precaution(s): Store at room temperature.

Caution(s): For topical use on animals only. Avoid contact with eyes.

Warning(s): Keep out of reach of children.

Presentation: 12 fl oz (355 mL) and 1 gallon (3.78 L).

Compendium Code No.: 11420471 Rev 0598

PELLITOL® OINTMENT

Veterinary Specialties **Antiseptic**

Antiseptic-Protective

Active Ingredient(s): Contains: Resorcinol, 5%; bismuth subgallate, 1%; bismuth subnitrate, 9%; zinc oxide, 17%; calamine, 10%; juniper tar, 1%.

Indications: For use on domestic animals as an aid in the treatment of minor wounds, abrasions, and inflammation of the external ear canal. PELLITOL® Ointment forms a protective coating and helps reduce pain, irritation and itching.

Directions for Use: Apply a layer of PELLITOL® Ointment, approximately one-eighth inch thick, over the affected area once or twice daily. Cover with a bandage, if possible.

Ears should be checked for the presence of foreign bodies and/or parasites and treated as necessary before application of PELLITOL® Ointment. Attach applicator to tube and gently insert into the ear canal. Continually apply pressure to the tube as applicator is withdrawn from the ear canal. Apply a layer of PELLITOL® Ointment over any existing lesions on the outer surface of the ear. Repeat the application once or twice daily.

Warning(s): Do not use in eyes. Keep out of reach of children.

Presentation: One dozen tubes with each tube containing 1 ounce (28.35 g) of medication. Each tube will be packaged in an individual carton.

Compendium Code No.: 10950011

PEN-AQUEOUS

AgriPharm **Penicillin Injection**

(Sterile Penicillin G Procaine)

NADA No.: 065-505

Active Ingredient(s): Each mL contains:

Penicillin G procaine . . . . . 300,000 units
Sodium citrate. . . . . 10 mg
Povidone. . . . . 5 mg
Lecithin. . . . . 6 mg
Sodium carboxymethylcellulose . . . . . 1 mg
Methylparaben . . . . . 1.3 mg
Propylparaben. . . . . 0.2 mg
Sodium formaldehyde sulfoxylate. . . . . 0.2 mg
Procaine hydrochloride. . . . . 20 mg
Water for injection . . . . . q.s.

Indications: For the treatment of cattle and sheep for bacterial pneumonia (shipping fever) caused by *Pasteurella multocida*; swine for erysipelas caused by *Erysipelothrix rhusiopathiae (insidiosa)*; and horses for strangles caused by *Streptococcus equi*.

Dosage and Administration: Shake well before using.

The dosage for cattle, sheep, swine and horses is 3,000 units per pound of body weight or 1 mL for each 100 lbs. of body weight once a day.

Continue the treatment for at least one (1) day after symptoms disappear (usually 2 or 3 days).

Treatment should not exceed four (4) consecutive days. If improvement is not observed, consult a veterinarian.

PEN-AQUEOUS should be injected deep within the fleshy muscles of the hip, rump, round or thigh. Do not inject subcutaneously, into a blood vessel or near a major nerve. The site of each injection should be changed. Use a 16 or 18 gauge needle, one and one-half (1½) inches long. The needle and syringe should be washed thoroughly before use and sterilized in boiling water for 15 to 20 minutes before use. The injection site should be washed with soap and water and painted with a disinfectant, such as 70% alcohol.

Warm the product to room temperature and shake well. Wipe the rubber stopper in the vial with 70% alcohol. Withdraw the suspension from the vial and inject deep into the muscle. Do not inject more than 10 mL into one site.

Precaution(s): Store between 36°-46°F (2°-8°C). Avoid freezing.

Caution(s): Restricted drug (California). Keep out of reach of children. For animal use only.

Exceeding the highest recommended daily dosage of 3,000 units per pound of body weight, administering at recommended levels for more than 4 consecutive days, and/or exceeding 10 mL intramuscularly per injection site may result in antibiotic residues beyond the withdrawal time.

Warning(s): Not for use in horses intended for food.

Milk taken from animals during treatment and for 48 hours (4 milkings) after the last treatment with this drug must not be used for food. Treatment should not exceed five (5) consecutive days in lactating cattle. Discontinue use of the drug for the following time periods before treated animals are slaughtered for food:

Cattle. . . . . 4 days
Sheep . . . . . 8 days
Swine . . . . . 6 days
Nonruminating calves . . . . . 7 days

Presentation: 100 mL, 250 mL and 500 mL multiple dose vials.

Compendium Code No.: 14570810

PEN-AQUEOUS

Durvet **Penicillin Injection**

Penicillin G Procaine Injectable Suspension U.S.P-Antibiotic

NADA No.: 065-010

Active Ingredient(s): PEN-AQUEOUS is a suspension of penicillin G procaine. Each mL is designed to provide 300,000 units penicillin G as procaine in a stable suspension.

Penicillin G Potassium* . . . . . 300,000 units
Procaine Hydrochloride* . . . . . 139.0 mg
Procaine Hydrochloride. 2.0%
Potassium Phosphate, Monobasic . . . . . 3.0 mg
Potassium Phosphate, Dibasic . . . . . 6.0 mg
Sodium Formaldehyde Sulfoxylate 0.4%
Polysorbate 80 . . . . . 0.4 mg
Sorbitan Monolaurate (Span 20). 0.2%
Polyoxyethelene Sorbitan (Tween 20). . . . . 0.1 mg
Methyl Paraben 0.1%
Propyl Paraben. 0.01%
Sodium Carboxymethylcellulose 0.15%
Water for Injection . . . . . q.s.

*Penicillin G Potassium and Procaine Hydrochloride react to form penicillin G procaine.

Indications: Penicillin G Procaine is a potent antibacterial agent which is effective against a variety of pathogenic organisms, chiefly in the gram-positive category. PEN-AQUEOUS is recommended for treatment of bacterial pneumonia (shipping fever) caused by *Pasteurella multocida* in cattle

P

and sheep, erysipelas caused by *Erysipelothrix insidiosa* in swine, and strangles caused by *Streptococcus equi* in horses. For use in cattle, sheep, swine and horses.

Directions for Use: Read entire brochure carefully before using this product.

Shake well before using.

A thoroughly cleaned, sterile needle and syringe should be used for each injection (needles and syringes may be sterilized in boiling water for 15 minutes). Before withdrawing the solution from the bottle, disinfect the rubber cap top with 70% alcohol. The injection site should be similarly disinfected with alcohol. Needles of 16 to 18 gauge and 1 to 1.5 inches long are adequate for intramuscular injections.

In livestock intramuscular injections should be made by directing the needle of suitable gauge and length into the fleshy part of a thick muscle, such as rump, hip, or thigh region; avoid blood vessels and major nerves. Before injecting the solution, pull back gently on the plunger. If blood appears in the syringe, a blood vessel has been entered; withdraw the needle and select a different site.

Dosage: PEN-AQUEOUS should be administered by the intramuscular route. The product is ready for injection after warming the vial to room temperature and shaking to ensure a uniform suspension.

The recommended daily dosage of penicillin is 3,000 units per pound of body weight (one mL per 100 lbs body weight). Continue daily treatment until recovery is apparent and for at least one day after symptoms disappear, usually in two to three days. Treatment should not exceed four consecutive days. No more than 10 mL should be injected at any one site in adult livestock; rotate injection sites for each succeeding treatment.

Precaution(s): PEN-AQUEOUS should be stored between 2°-8°C (36°-46°F).

Caution(s): Penicillin G Procaine is a substance of low toxicity. However, side effects, or so-called allergic or anaphylactic reactions - sometimes fatal, have been known to occur in animals hypersensitive to penicillin and procaine. Such reactions can occur unpredictably with varying intensity. Animals administered Penicillin G Procaine should be kept under close observation for at least one half hour. Should allergic or anaphylactic reactions occur, discontinue use of the product and call a veterinarian. If respiratory distress is severe, immediate injection of epinephrine or antihistamine following manufacturer's recommendations may be necessary. As with all antibiotic preparations, use of this drug may result in overgrowth of nonsusceptible organisms, including fungi. A lack of response by the treated animal, or the development of new signs or symptoms suggest that an overgrowth of nonsusceptible organisms has occurred. In such instances, consult a veterinarian. Since bacterial drugs may interfere with the bacteriostatic action of tetracyclines, it is advisable to avoid giving penicillin in conjunction with tetracyclines.

Restricted Drug (California) - Use only as directed.

For animal use only. For intramuscular injection only.

Warning(s): Exceeding the recommended daily dosage of 3,000 units per pound of body weight, administering at the recommended level for more than four consecutive days and/or exceeding 10 mL intramuscularly per injection site, may result in antibiotic residues beyond the withdrawal time. Milk taken from treated dairy animals within 48 hours after the latest treatment must not be used for food. Discontinue use of this drug for the following time period before treated animals are slaughtered for food.

Cattle - 10 days, Sheep - 9 days, Swine - 7 days.

Not for use in horses intended for food.

A withdrawal period has not been established for this product in pre-ruminating calves. Do not use in calves to be processed for veal.

Keep out of reach of children.

Discussion: Care of Sick animals: The use of antibiotics in the management of diseases is based on an accurate diagnosis and an adequate course of treatment. When properly used in the treatment of diseases caused by penicillin-susceptible organisms, most animals treated with Pen-Aqueous show a noticeable improvement within 24 to 48 hours. If improvement does not occur within this period of time, the diagnosis and course of treatment should be re-evaluated. It is recommended that the diagnosis and treatment of animal diseases be carried out by a veterinarian.

Since many diseases look alike but require different types of treatment, the use of professional veterinary and laboratory services can reduce treatment time, costs and needless losses. Good housing, sanitation and nutrition are important in the maintenance of healthy animals and are essential in the treatment of disease.

Presentation: Available in 100 mL, 250 mL and 500 mL multiple dose vials.

Manufactured in the UK.

Compendium Code No.: 10841261 I01

PENE-MITE™

Farnam **Otic Parasiticide**

EPA Reg. No.: 270-168

Active Ingredient(s):

Pyrethrins 0.05%
Technical Piperonyl Butoxide* 0.50%
Inert Ingredients.......... 99.45%

*Equivalent to 0.4% (butylcarbityl) (6 propyl-piperonyl) ether and 0.1% related compounds.

Indications: For the treatment of ear mites *(Otodectes cynotis)* in rabbits, dogs and cats.

Directions for Use: It is a violation of Federal law to use this product in a manner inconsistent with its labeling.

Hold pet securely. Cleanse ear thoroughly. Fill outer ear canal half full with PENE-MITE™. Massage base of the ear to distribute solution into ear wax. Repeat every other day until condition is relieved. Symptoms should improve in 4 to 6 days. Continue treatment for 12 days. Since ear mites occasionally are found on other parts of the body, reinfestation may occur unless a suitable dip or other full-body treatment is used.

Precautionary Statements: Hazards to Humans and Domestic Animals:

Caution: Harmful if swallowed. Avoid contact with eyes. In case of eye contact, flush with plenty of water. Consult a physician if irritation persists (humans). Avoid contamination of foodstuffs or utensils. For animals, discontinue use if irritation develops.

Storage and Disposal: Do not contaminate water, food or feed by storage or disposal.

Storage: Keep away from heat.

Disposal: Do not reuse empty container. Wrap and put in trash collection.

Warning(s): Keep out of reach of children. For veterinary use only.

Discussion: Ear mites normally cause a dry, dark brown, waxy exudate with crusts in the ears of rabbits, dogs and cats. Mites are easily observed by placing some of the ear wax on a dark surface and watching closely for moving white specks. Do not injure the delicate tissue of the ear. Inflamed, watery or blocked ear canals indicate a more serious condition which requires special treatment.

Presentation: 0.5 fl oz (14.8 mL) plastic bottle with dropper cap.

Compendium Code No.: 10000740 9BB3

PENICILLIN 100

Alpharma **Feed Medication**

Penicillin G Procaine-Type A Medicated Article-Antibacterial

NADA No.: 046-666

Active Ingredient(s): 60 grams penicillin G (from penicillin G procaine) per pound.

Ingredients: Roughage products, Calcium carbonate, and Mineral oil.

Indications: For increased rate of weight gain and improved feed efficiency in swine, chickens, turkeys, pheasants and quail.

Dosage and Administration:

Species	Penicillin g/ton	Lb of PENICILLIN 100 Premix per ton of feed
Swine	10-50	0.167-0.834
Chickens	2.4-50	0.04-0.834
Turkeys	2.4-50	0.04-0.834
Pheasants	2.4-50	0.04-0.834
Quail	5-20	0.0834-0.333
Limitation: Not for use in quail over 5 weeks of age.		

Precautions: Keep container tightly closed to prevent contamination or moisture pick up.

Store at 50°-80°F (10°-27°C).

Precautions such as the following should be considered: dusk masks or respirators and protective clothing should be worn; dust-arresting equipment and adequate ventilation should be utilized; personal hygiene should be observed; wash before eating or leaving a work site; be alert for signs of allergic reactions - seek prompt medical treatment if such reactions are suspected.

Cautions: For use in manufacturing medicated animal feeds only.

Certain components of animal feeds, including medicated premixes, possess properties that may be a potential health hazard or a source of personal discomfort to certain individuals who are exposed to them. Human exposure should, therefore, be minimized by observing the general industry standards for occupational health and safety.

Restricted drug: For use in animals only.

Presentation: 50 lb (22.67 kg) bag.

Compendium Code No.: 10220501 AHM-057A 9907

PENICILLIN G POTASSIUM

AgriLabs **Water Medication**

Antibiotic for Drinking Water

ANADA No.: 200-103

Active Ingredient(s): 0.500 billion units penicillin G potassium.

Nonsterile.

Indications: For treatment of erysipelas in turkeys caused by *Erysipelothrix rhusiopathiae*.

Dosage and Administration: Administer orally at a dosage of 1,500,000 units of penicillin per gallon (3.8 liters) of drinking water for 5 consecutive days.

Add enough water (approx. 2 pints - 946 mL) to fill bottle two-thirds (⅔) full. Shake to dissolve. Allow the concentrated solution to stand until foam disappears. The concentrated solution should be used up or discarded within one hour of preparation.

Automatic Watering Systems: Pour the concentrated solution into a glass or plastic container then add enough water to make 2.6 gallons (9.9 liters) of stock solution. [This amount of solution will medicate 333 gallons (1260 liters) of drinking water.] The automatic waterer should be adjusted to deliver 1 ounce (30 mL) of stock solution per gallon (3.8 liters) of drinking water. Prepare fresh stock solutions and medicated drinking water solutions every 12 hours. All solutions in contact with galvanized metal should be changed every three (3) hours.

Gravity Flow Watering Systems: Pour the concentrated solution into enough water to make 333 gallons (1260 liters) of drinking water. In gravity flow watering systems, prepare fresh solution every 12 hours. All solutions in contact with galvanized metal should be changed every three (3) hours.

Drinking water prepared as directed above will contain 1,500,000 units of penicillin G potassium per gallon (3.8 liters).

Precaution(s): Store at or below 25°C (77°F). Protect from excessive heat, 40°C (104°F), and moisture.

Caution(s): For best results, the treatment should be started at the first sign of infection. If improvement is not noted after 3 to 4 days of treatment, consult a poultry pathologist or veterinarian. Keep this and all medication out of reach of children. Restricted drug (under California law). Use only as directed. Recommendations for conditions of storage and replacement of stock and medicated water solutions stated in the labeling must be followed to assure the performance of this drug product.

For oral use in turkeys only.

For animal use only.

Not for human use.

Keep out of reach of children.

Warning(s): Treated turkeys must not be slaughtered for food during treatment and for one day after last treatment.

Do not use in turkeys producing eggs for human consumption.

Presentation: 12 x 0.500 billion I.U.

Compendium Code No.: 10580800

PENICILLIN G POTASSIUM, USP

AgriPharm **Water Medication**

Antibiotic for Drinking Water

ANADA No.: 200-103

Active Ingredient(s): 0.500 billion units penicillin G potassium.

Nonsterile.

Indications: For treatment of erysipelas in turkeys caused by *Erysipelothrix rhusiopathiae*.

Dosage and Administration: Administer orally at a dosage of 1,500,000 units of penicillin per gallon (3.8 liters) of drinking water for five (5) consecutive days.

Add enough water (approx. 2 pints - 946 mL) to fill bottle two-thirds (⅔) full. Shake to dissolve. Allow the concentrated solution to stand until foam disappears. The concentrated solution should be used up or discarded within one (1) hour of preparation.

Automatic Watering Systems: Pour the concentrated solution into a glass or plastic container then add enough water to make 2.6 gallons (9.9 liters) of stock solution. [This amount of solution will medicate 333 gallons (1,260 liters) of drinking water.] The automatic waterer should be adjusted to deliver one (1) ounce (30 mL) of stock solution per gallon (3.8 liters) of drinking water. Prepare fresh stock solutions and medicated drinking water solutions every 12 hours. All solutions in contact with galvanized metal should be changed every three (3) hours.

Gravity Flow Watering Systems: Pour the concentrated solution into enough water to make 333 gallons (1,260 liters) of drinking water. In gravity flow watering systems, prepare fresh solution every 12 hours. All solutions in contact with galvanized metal should be changed every three (3) hours.

Drinking water prepared as directed above will contain 1,500,000 units of penicillin G potassium per gallon (3.8 liters).

Precaution(s): Store at or below 25°C (77°F).

Caution(s): For best results, the treatment should be started at the first sign of infection. If improvement is not noted after 3 to 4 days of treatment, consult a poultry pathologist or veterinarian. Keep this and all medication out of reach of children. Restricted drug (under California law). Use only as directed. Recommendations for conditions of storage and replacement of stock and medicated water solutions stated in the labeling must be followed to assure the performance of this drug product.

For oral use in turkeys only.

For animal use only.

Not for human use.

Keep out of reach of children.

Warning(s): Treated turkeys must not be slaughtered for food during treatment and for one (1) day after last treatment.

Do not use in turkeys producing eggs for human consumption.

Presentation: 12 - 0.500 billion units bottles per case.

Compendium Code No.: 14570820

PENICILLIN G POTASSIUM, USP

Bimeda **Water Medication**

Antibiotic for us in Drinking Water

ANADA No.: 200-103

Active Ingredient(s): Each 11.4 oz pack contains:

Penicillin G Potassium, USP. . . . . 0.500 billion I.U.

Indications: For the oral treatment of erysipelas in turkeys caused by *Erysipelothrix rhusiopathiae*.

Dosage and Administration: Administer orally at a dosage of 1,500,000 units of penicillin per gallon (3.8 liters) of drinking water for 5 consecutive days.

Add enough water (approx. 2 pints - 946 mL) to fill bottle two-thirds full. Shake to dissolve. Allow the concentrated solution to stand until foam disappears. The concentrated solution should be used up or discarded within one hour of preparation.

Automatic Watering Systems: Pour the concentrated solution into a glass or plastic container, then add enough water to make 2.6 gallons (9.9 liters) of stock solution. [This amount of solution will medicate 333 gallons (1,260 liters) of drinking water.] The automatic waterer should be adjusted to deliver 1 ounce (30 mL) of stock solution per gallon (3.8 liters) of drinking water. Prepare fresh stock solutions and medicated drinking water solutions every twelve (12) hours. All solutions in contact with galvanized metal should be changed every three (3) hours.

Gravity Flow Watering Systems: Pour the concentrated solution into enough water to make 333 gallons (1,260 liters) of drinking water. In gravity flow watering systems, prepare fresh solution every 12 hours. All solutions in contact with galvanized metal should be changed every three (3) hours.

Drinking water prepared as directed above will contain 1,500,000 units of penicillin G potassium per gallon (3.8 liters).

Precaution(s): Store at or below 25°C (77°F).

Protect from excessive heat 40°C (104°F), and moisture.

Recommendations for conditions of storage and replacement of stock and medicated water solutions stated in the labeling must be followed to assure the performance of this drug product.

Caution(s): For best results, the treatment should be started at the first sign of infection. If improvement is not noted within 3 to 4 days of treatment, consult a poultry pathologist or veterinarian.

Warning(s): Treated turkeys must not be slaughtered for food during treatment and for one day after last treatment.

Do not use in turkeys producing eggs for human consumption.

Restricted drug (California). Use only as directed.

For oral use in turkeys only.

For animal use only.

Not for human use.

Keep out of reach of children.

Presentation: 11.4 oz/0.500 billion I.U. (12 in a case).

Compendium Code No.: 13990320

PENICILLIN G POTASSIUM, USP

Durvet **Water Medication**

Antibiotic for Drinking Water-Nonsterile

ANADA No.: 200-103

Active Ingredient(s): 0.500 billion units penicillin G potassium.

Indications: For treatment of erysipelas in turkeys caused by *Erysipelothrix rhusiopathiae*.

Dosage and Administration: Administer orally at a dosage of 1,500,000 units of penicillin per gallon (3.8 liters) of drinking water for 5 consecutive days.

Directions: Add enough water (approx. 2 pints - 946 mL) to fill bottle two-thirds full. Shake to dissolve. Allow the concentrated solution to stand until foam disappears. The concentrated solution should be used up or discarded within one hour of preparation.

Automatic Watering Systems: Pour the concentrated solution into a glass or plastic container then add enough water to make 2.6 gallons (9.9 liters) of stock solution. [This amount of solution will medicate 333 gallons (1260 liters) of drinking water]. The automatic waterer should be adjusted to deliver 1 ounce (30 mL) of stock solution per gallon (3.8 liters) of drinking water. Prepare fresh stock solutions and medicated drinking water solutions every twelve (12) hours. All solutions in contact with galvanized metal should be changed every three (3) hours.

Gravity Flow Watering Systems: Pour the concentrated solution into enough water to make 333 gallons (1260 liters) of drinking water. In gravity flow watering systems, prepare fresh solution every 12 hours. All solutions in contact with galvanized metal should be changed every three (3) hours.

Drinking water prepared as directed above will contain 1,500,000 units of penicillin G per gallon (3.8 liters).

Precaution(s): Store at or below 25°C (77°F). Protect from excessive heat 40°C (104°F), and moisture. Label recommendations for conditions of storage and replacement of stock and medicated water solutions stated in the labeling must be followed to assure the performance of this drug product.

Caution(s): For best results, the treatment should be started at the first sign of infection. If improvement is not noted after 3 to 4 days of treatment, consult a poultry pathologist or veterinarian. Restricted drug (under California law). Use only as directed.

For oral use in turkeys only.

For animal use only.

Not for human use.

Warning(s): Treated turkeys must not be slaughtered for food during treatment and for one day after last treatment.

Do not use in turkeys producing eggs for human consumption.

Keep this and all medication out of reach of children.

Presentation: 0.500 billion units (NDC 30798-310-60).

Compendium Code No.: 10841271 598

PENICILLIN G POTASSIUM USP

Fort Dodge **Water Medication**

Antibiotic for drinking water

NADA No.: 055-060

Active Ingredient(s): 0.500 billion units penicillin G potassium. Nonsterile.

Indications: For the treatment of erysipelas in turkeys (caused by *Erysipelothrix rhusiopathiae*).

Dosage and Administration: Administer orally at a dosage of 1,500,000 units of penicillin per gallon (3.8 liters) of drinking water for 5 consecutive days.

Directions: Combine contents and approximately 1½ pints (710 mL) of water in a glass or plastic container. Stir to dissolve. Allow concentrated solution to stand until the foam disappears. The concentrated solution should be used up or discarded within one hour after preparation.

Automatic Watering Systems — Pour the concentrated solution into a glass or plastic container then add enough water to make 2.6 gallons (9.9 liters) of stock solution. [This amount of solution will medicate 333 gallons (1260 liters) of drinking water]. The automatic waterer should be adjusted to deliver 1 ounce (30 mL) of stock solution per gallon (3.8 liters) of drinking water. In automatic watering systems, prepare fresh solutions daily.

Gravity Flow Watering Systems — Pour the concentrated solution into enough water to make 333 gallons (1260 liters) of drinking water. In gravity flow watering systems, prepare fresh solutions every 12 hours.

Drinking water prepared as directed above will contain 1,500,000 units of penicillin G per gallon (3.8 liters).

Precaution(s): Store at room temperature; avoid excessive heat (104°F or 40°C).

Caution(s): For best results, the treatment should be started at the first sign of infection. If improvement is not noted after 3 to 4 days of treatment, consult a poultry pathologist or veterinarian.

Keep out of the reach of children.

Restricted drug (under California law) — Use only as directed.

For oral use in turkeys only.

For veterinary use only.

Warning(s): Treated turkeys must not be slaughtered for food during treatment and for one day after last treatment.

Do not use in turkeys producing eggs for human consumption.

Presentation: 313 grams (11 ounces) (NDC 53501-059-02).

Manufactured by: G.C. Hanford Manufacturing Co., Syracuse, NY 13201

Compendium Code No.: 10031440 12431B

PENICILLIN G PROCAINE

G.C. Hanford **Penicillin Injection**

Penicillin G Procaine Aqueous Suspension

NADA No.: 065-493

Active Ingredient(s): Each mL contains:

Penicillin G procaine	300,000 units
Sodium citrate	10 mg
Povidone	5 mg
Lecithin	6 mg
Sodium carboxymethylcellulose	1 mg
Methylparaben	1.3 mg
Propylparaben	0.2 mg
Sodium formaldehyde sulfoxylate	0.2 mg
Procaine hydrochloride	20 mg
Water for injection	q.s.

Indications: For the treatment of cattle and sheep for bacterial pneumonia (shipping fever) caused by *Pasteurella multocida;* swine for erysipelas caused by *Erysipelothrix rhusiopathiae (insidiosa);* and horses for strangles caused by *Streptococcus equi.*

Dosage and Administration: PENICILLIN G PROCAINE Suspension should be injected deep within the fleshy muscles of the hip, rump, round or thigh. Do not inject subcutaneously, into a blood vessel or near a major nerve. The site of each injection should be changed. Use a 16 or 18 gauge needle, one and one-half (1½) inches long. The needle and syringe should be washed thoroughly before use and sterilized in boiling water for 15 to 20 minutes before use. The injection site should be washed with soap and water and painted with a disinfectant, such as 70% alcohol.

Warm the product to room temperature and shake well. Wipe the rubber stopper in the vial with 70% alcohol. Withdraw the suspension from the vial and inject deep into the muscle. Do not inject more than 10 mL into one site.

The dosage for cattle, sheep, swine and horses is 3,000 units per lb. of body weight or 1 mL for each 100 lbs. of body weight, once a day.

Continue the treatment for at least one (1) day after the symptoms disappear (usually 2 or 3 days).

Precaution(s): PENICILLIN G PROCAINE Suspension should be stored in a refrigerator (36°-46°F, 2°-8°C). Protect from freezing.

Caution(s): Treatment should not exceed four consecutive days. If improvement is not observed, consult a veterinarian.

Sensitivity reactions to penicillin or procaine such as hives or respiratory distress, sometimes fatal, have been known to occur in some animals. If signs of sensitivity do occur, stop using the medication and call a veterinarian. If respiratory distress is severe, the immediate injection of epinephrine may be helpful.

As with any antibiotic preparation, prolonged use may result in the overgrowth of nonsusceptible organisms, including fungi. If this condition is suspected, stop using the medication and consult a veterinarian.

Warning(s): Not for use in horses intended for food.

Milk that has been taken from animals during treatment and for 48 hours (4 milkings) after the last treatment with this drug must not be used for food.

Discontinue the use of this drug before treated animals are slaughtered for food for 10 days in cattle, nine (9) days in sheep and seven (7) days in swine.

Milk withholding time for the product is based on human safety standards. The milk plant may advise additional testing to ensure compliance with industry requirements. It is strongly recommended that the processor be consulted to avoid possible penalties.

Presentation: 12x100 mL and 12x250 mL multiple dose vials. A 12x500 mL vial is available for use with automated injection equipment.

Compendium Code No.: 10340021

PENICILLIN G PROCAINE 50

Alpharma **Feed Medication**

Type A medicated article (antibacterial premix)

NADA No.: 046-666

Active Ingredient(s): Each gram provides 0.5 gram penicillin G procaine (equivalent to 0.3 gram penicillin G Master standard).

Inactive Ingredients: Calcium carbonate and calcium stearate.

Indications: For use in the manufacture of feeds for increased rate of weight gain and improved feed efficiency for chickens, turkeys, pheasants, quail, and swine.

Dosage and Administration: Mixing Directions: Mix with grain or non-medicated feed prior to use. A premix is recommended before the final mixing to obtain a uniform blend in the feed.

Species	Approved Label Claim	Penicillin g/ton	Grams of PENICILLIN G PROCAINE 50 Premix per ton of feed
Swine	For increased rate of weight gain and improved feed efficiency.	10-50	16.7-83.5
Chickens, Turkeys, Pheasants	For increased rate of weight gain and improved feed efficiency.	2.4-50	4-83.4
Quail	For increased rate of weight gain and improved feed efficiency. Limitation: Not for use in quail over 5 weeks of age.	5-20	8.4-33.6

Precautions: Store at 50°-80°F (10°-27°C). Keep container tightly closed to prevent contamination or moisture pick up.

Cautions: For feed manufacturing use only.

Restricted Drug: For use in animals only.

Presentation: 110 lb (50 kg) bags.

Compendium Code No.: 10220510

PENNCHLOR 50•G®

PennField **Feed Medication**

(Type A Medicated Feed)

NADA No.: 138-935

Active Ingredient(s): Chlortetracycline as chlortetracycline calcium complex equivalent to 50 grams chlortetracycline hydrochloride/lb.

Ingredients: Chlortetracycline, calcium carbonate, roughage products and mineral oil.

Indications: An antimicrobial premix for use in the feed of chickens, turkeys, sheep, swine, calves, beef cattle, and non-lactating dairy cattle.

Recommended for the prevention and control of diseases caused by microorganisms sensitive to chlortetracycline, and also for other production uses.

Directions for Use:

Indications for Use	Use Levels of Chlortetracycline	lbs of PENNCHLOR 50•G® per ton
Chickens		
For Broiler/fryer chickens: For an increased rate of weight gain and improved feed efficiency.	10-50 g/ton	0.2-1.0
For Chickens: Control of infectious synovitis caused by *Mycoplasma synoviae;* susceptible to chlortetracycline. (Feed continuously for 7-14 days.)	100-200 g/ton	2.0-4.0
For Chickens: Control of chronic respiratory disease (CRD) and air sac infection caused by *Mycoplasma gallisepticum* and *Escherichia coli* susceptible to chlortetracycline. (Feed continuously for 7-14 days.)	200-400 g/ton	4.0-8.0
For Chickens: Reduction of mortality due to *Escherichia coli* infections susceptible to chlortetracycline. (Feed for 5 days.)	500 g/ton	10.0
Turkeys		
For Turkeys: Growing Turkeys: For an increased rate of weight gain and improved feed efficiency.	10-50 g/ton	0.2-1.0
For Turkeys: Control of infectious synovitis caused by *Mycoplasma synoviae* susceptible to chlortetracycline. (Feed continuously for 7-14 days.)	200 g/ton	4.0
For Turkeys: Control of hexamitiasis caused by *Hexamita meleagrides* susceptible to chlortetracycline. (Feed continuously 7-14 days.)	400 g/ton	8.0
For Turkeys: Turkey poults not over 4 weeks of age: Reduction of mortality due to paratyphoid caused by *Salmonella typhimurium* susceptible to chlortetracycline.	400 g/ton	8.0
For Turkeys: Control of complicating bacterial organisms associated with bluecomb (transmissible enteritis, coronaviral enteritis) susceptible to chlortetracycline. (Feed continuously for 7-14 days.)	25 mg/lb body weight/day	
Sheep		
For Growing Sheep: For an increased rate of weight gain and improved feed efficiency.	20-50 g/ton	0.4-1.0
For Breeding Sheep: Reducing the incidence of (vibrionic) abortion caused by *Campylobacter fetus* infection susceptible to chlortetracycline.	80 mg/head/day	
Swine		
For Growing Swine: For an increased rate of weight gain and improved feed efficiency.	10-50 g/ton	0.20-1.0
For Swine: Reducing the incidence of cervical lymphadenitis (jowl abscesses) caused by *Group E Streptococci* susceptible to chlortetracycline.	50-100 g/ton	1.0-2.0
For Breeding Swine: Control of leptospirosis (reducing the instances of abortions and shedding of leptospirae) caused by *Leptospira pomona* susceptible to chlortetracycline. (Feed continuously for 14 days.)	400 g/ton	8.0
For Swine: Treatment of bacterial enteritis caused by *Escherichia coli* and *Salmonella choleraesuis* and bacterial pneumonia caused by *Pasteurella multocida* susceptible to chlortetracycline. (Feed for not more than 14 days.)	10 mg/lb body weight/day	
Calves, Beef Cattle, and Nonlactating Dairy Cattle		
For Calves (up to 250 lbs): For an increased weight gain and improved feed efficiency.	0.1 mg/lb body weight/day	
For Calves (250-400 lbs): For an increased weight gain and improved feed efficiency.	25-70 mg/head/day	
For Growing Cattle (over 400 lbs): For an increased weight gain, improved feed efficiency and reduction of liver condemnation due to liver abscesses.	70 mg/head/day	
For Cattle: For the control of bacterial pneumonia associated with shipping fever complex susceptible to chlortetracycline.	350 mg/head/day	
For Beef Cattle (under 700 lbs): Control of active infection of anaplasmosis caused by *Anaplasma marginale* susceptible to chlortetracycline.	350 mg/head/day	
For Beef Cattle (over 700 lbs): Control of active infection of anaplasmosis caused by *Anaplasma marginale* susceptible to chlortetracycline.	0.5 mg/lb body weight/day	
For Calves, Beef, and Nonlactating Dairy Cattle: For treatment of bacterial enteritis caused by *Escherichia coli* and bacterial pneumonia caused by *Pasteurella multocida* susceptible to chlortetracycline. (Treat for not more than 5 days.)	10 mg/lb body weight/day	

Caution(s): For use in the manufacture of medicated feeds.

For use in dry feeds only — Not for use in liquid feed supplements.

Restricted drug (California) - Use only as directed.

Warning(s):

Chickens:

When used at levels above 200 g/ton: Do not feed to chickens producing eggs for human consumption.

When used at levels up to 400 g/ton: Zero-day withdrawal period.

When used at levels of 500 g/ton: Withdraw 24 hours prior to slaughter.

Turkeys: When used at levels of 25 mg/lb body weight/day: Do not feed to turkeys producing eggs for human consumption. Zero-day withdrawal period.

Sheep: Zero-day withdrawal period.

Swine: Zero-day withdrawal period.

Cattle:

A withdrawal period has not been established for this product in pre-ruminating calves. Do not use in calves to be processed for veal.

When used in growing cattle at a level of 70 mg/head/day or less: Zero-day withdrawal period.

When used in beef cattle at a level of 0.5 mg/lb body weight/day and at 350 mg/head/day: Withdraw 1 day prior to slaughter.

When used in calves, beef cattle and non-lactating dairy cattle at levels of 10 mg/lb body weight/day: Withdraw 1 day prior to slaughter.

Presentation: 50 lb (22.7 kg) bag.

Patents Pending

Compendium Code No.: 10450060 REV. 5/99

PENNCHLOR™ 50 MEAL

PennField **Feed Medication**

Chlortetracycline (Type A Medicated Feed)

NADA No.: 138-935

Active Ingredient(s): Chlortetracycline as chlortetracycline calcium complex equivalent to 50 grams chlortetracycline hydrochloride/lb.

Ingredients: Chlortetracycline, calcium carbonate, roughage products and mineral oil.

Indications: An antimicrobial premix for use in the feed of chickens, turkeys, sheep, swine, calves, beef cattle, and nonlactating dairy cattle.

Recommended for the prevention and control of diseases caused by microorganisms sensitive to chlortetracycline, and also for other production uses.

P

Directions for Use:

Indications for Use	Use Levels of Chlortetracycline	lbs. of PENNCHLOR™ 50 per ton
Chickens		
For Broiler/fryer chickens: For an increased rate of weight gain and improved feed efficiency.	10-50 g/ton	0.2-1.0
For Chickens: Control of infectious synovitis caused by *Mycoplasma synoviae;* susceptible to chlortetracycline. (Feed continuously for 7-14 days.)	100-200 g/ton	2.0-4.0
For Chickens: Control of chronic respiratory disease (CRD) and air sac infection caused by *Mycoplasma gallisepticum* and *Escherichia coli* susceptible to chlortetracycline. (Feed continuously for 7-14 days.)	200-400 g/ton	4.0-8.0
For Chickens: Reduction of mortality due to *Escherichia coli* infections susceptible to chlortetracycline. (Feed for 5 days.)	500 g/ton	10.0
Turkeys		
For Turkeys: Growing Turkeys: For an increased rate of weight gain and improved feed efficiency.	10-50 g/ton	0.2-1.0
For Turkeys: Control of infectious synovitis caused by *Mycoplasma synoviae* susceptible to chlortetracycline. (Feed continuously for 7-14 days.)	200 g/ton	4.0
For Turkeys: Control of hexamitiasis caused by *Hexamita meleagrides* susceptible to chlortetracycline. (Feed continuously 7-14 days.)	400 g/ton	8.0
For Turkeys: Turkey poults not over 4 weeks of age: Reduction of mortality due to paratyphoid caused by *Salmonella typhimurium* susceptible to chlortetracycline.	400 g/ton	8.0
For Turkeys: Control of complicating bacterial organisms associated with bluecomb (transmissible enteritis, coronaviral enteritis) susceptible to chlortetracycline. (Feed continuously for 7-14 days.)	25 mg/lb body weight/day	
Sheep		
For Growing Sheep: For an increased rate of weight gain and improved feed efficiency.	20-50 g/ton	0.4-1.0
For Breeding Sheep: Reducing the incidence of (vibrionic) abortion caused by *Campylobacter fetus* infection susceptible to chlortetracycline.	80 mg/head/day	
Swine		
For Growing Swine: For an increased rate of weight gain and improved feed efficiency.	10-50 g/ton	0.20-1.0
For Swine: Reducing the incidence of cervical lymphadenitis (jowl abscesses) caused by *Group E Streptococci* susceptible to chlortetracycline.	50-100 g/ton	1.0-2.0
For Breeding Swine: Control of leptospirosis (reducing the instances of abortions and shedding of leptospirae) caused by *Leptospira pomona* susceptible to chlortetracycline. (Feed continuously for 14 days.)	400 g/ton	8.0
For Swine: Treatment of bacterial enteritis caused by *Escherichia coli* and *Salmonella choleraesuis* and bacterial pneumonia caused by *Pasteurella multocida* susceptible to chlortetracycline. (Feed for not more than 14 days.)	10 mg/lb body weight/day	
Calves, Beef Cattle, and Nonlactating Dairy Cattle		
For Calves (up to 250 lbs.): For an increased weight gain and improved feed efficiency.	0.1 mg/lb body weight/day	
For Calves (250-400 lbs.): For an increased weight gain and improved feed efficiency.	25-70 mg/head/day	
For Growing Cattle (over 400 lbs.): For an increased weight gain, improved feed efficiency and reduction of liver condemnation due to liver abscesses.	70 mg/head/day	
For Cattle: For the control of bacterial pneumonia associated with shipping fever complex susceptible to chlortetracycline.	350 mg/head/day	
For Beef Cattle (under 700 lbs.): Control of active infection of anaplasmosis caused by *Anaplasma marginale* susceptible to chlortetracycline.	350 mg/head/day	
For Beef Cattle (over 700 lbs.): Control of active infection of anaplasmosis caused by *Anaplasma marginale* susceptible to chlortetracycline.	0.5 mg/lb body weight/day	
For Calves, Beef, and Nonlactating Dairy Cattle: For treatment of bacterial enteritis caused by *Escherichia coli* and bacterial pneumonia caused by *Pasteurella multocida* susceptible to chlortetracycline. (Treat for not more than 5 days.)	10 mg/lb body weight/day	

Warning(s):

Chickens:

Do not feed to chickens producing eggs for human consumption.

When used at levels up to 400 g/ton: Zero-day withdrawal period.

When used at levels of 500 g/ton: Withdraw 24 hours prior to slaughter.

Turkeys: Do not feed to turkeys producing eggs for human consumption. Zero-day withdrawal period.

Sheep: Zero-day withdrawal period.

Swine: Zero-day withdrawal period.

Cattle:

A withdrawal period has not been established for this product in pre-ruminating calves. Do not use in calves to be processed for veal.

When used in growing cattle at a level of 70 mg/head/day or less: Zero-day withdrawal period.

When used in beef cattle at a level of 0.5 mg/lb body weight/day: Withdraw 1 day prior to slaughter.

When used in calves, beef cattle and nonlactating dairy cattle at levels of 10 mg/lb body weight/day: Withdraw 1 day prior to slaughter.

For use in the manufacture of medicated feeds.

For use in dry feeds only - Not for use in liquid feed supplements.

Restricted drug (California) - Use only as directed.

Presentation: 50 lb (22.7 kg) bag.

Compendium Code No.: 10450110

Rev. 8/99

PENNCHLOR™ 64 SOLUBLE POWDER

PennField **Water Medication**

Chlortetracycline HCl Soluble Powder Concentrate-Antibiotic

ANADA No.: 200-295

Active Ingredient(s): Each packet contains 102.4 g (64 g/lb) chlortetracycline HCl and will make:

1,024 gallons (3,876 L) containing 100 mg Pennchlor™ chlortetracycline HCl per gallon.

512 gallons (1,938 L) containing 200 mg Pennchlor™ chlortetracycline HCl per gallon.

256 gallons (969 L) containing 400 mg Pennchlor™ chlortetracycline HCl per gallon.

102.4 gallons (387 L) containing 1,000 mg Pennchlor™ chlortetracycline HCl per gallon.

Indications: A broad-spectrum, antibiotic powder intended for use in the drinking water of chickens, turkeys, calves and swine.

Dosage and Administration: Dosages in terms of packets per 512 gallons are based on stated dosages per unit of body weight and average water consumption of the species. Weather conditions, ambient temperature, humidity, age, class of livestock and other factors may affect consumption and, except where calves are drenched, the unit dosage should be used as a guide to effective use in drinking water. Animals must actually consume enough medicated water to provide the desired therapeutic dose under the conditions that prevail.

For the control or treatment of the following diseases caused by organisms susceptible to chlortetracycline, administer according to the table below:

Swine	Dose-10 mg/lb body wt/day
Bacterial Enteritis (Scours) *(Escherichia coli)*	5 packets per 512 gallons. (This will treat 51,200 lb of pigs for one day; that is five hundred twelve 100-lb pigs, providing 10 mg/lb body weight).
Bacterial Pneumonia *(Pasteurella* spp, *Actinobacillus pleuropneumoniae (Hemophilus* spp,) *Klebsiella* spp)	Administer at this rate in the total water consumed over a full, 24-hour period. Do not administer for more than 5 days.

Calves	Dose-10 mg/lb body wt/day
Bacterial Pneumonia *(Pasteurella* spp, *Actinobacillus pleuropneumoniae (Hemophilus* spp,) *Klebsiella* spp)	One standard teaspoonful of powder contains 500 mg. Administer four such teaspoonsful in solution to a 200-lb calf in divided doses.
Bacterial Enteritis *(Escherichia coli)*	Administer at this rate in the total water consumed over a full 24-hour period, or as a drench in divided doses. Do not administer for more than 5 days.

Chickens	Dose
	Administer at the indicated rates in the total water consumed over a full, 24-hour period.
Chronic Respiratory Disease (CRD) and Air-Sac Infection *(Mycoplasma gallisepticum, Escherichia coli)*	2-4 packets per 512 gallons (400-800 mg/gallon).
Infectious Synovitis *(Mycoplasma synoviae)*	1-2 packets per 512 gallons (200-400 mg/gallon).
For the control of mortality due to fowl cholera *(Pasteurella multocida)* in growing chickens	5 packets per 512 gallons (1000 mg/gallon).

Turkeys	Dose
Control of complicating bacterial organisms associated with Bluecomb (transmissible enteritis or Corona virus enteritis) susceptible to chlortetracycline	25 mg/lb body wt/day. Administer 1 packet for every 4,096 lb of turkeys in the total water consumed over a full, 24-hour period.
Infectious Synovitis *(Mycoplasma synoviae)*	2 packets per 512 gallons (400 mg/gallon). Administer at this rate in the total water consumed over a full, 24-hour period.

Medicate chickens and turkeys continuously at the first clinical signs of disease and continue for 7 to 14 consecutive days. The dosage ranges permitted provide for different levels based on the severity of the infection. If improvement is not noted in 24-48 hours, consult a veterinarian or a diagnostic laboratory to determine diagnoses and for advice regarding the optimal level of the drug where ranges are permitted.

Caution(s): When used in plastic or stainless steel waterers, or automatic waterers, prepare fresh solutions every 24 hours. When used in galvanized waterers, prepare fresh solutions every 12 hours. When feeding milk or milk replacers, administration one hour before or two hours after feeding is recommended.

For animal use in drinking water.

Warning(s): Use as the sole source of chlortetracycline. Not to be used for more than 14 consecutive days in chickens and turkeys, 5 days in calves, or 5 days in swine. Do not use in laying chickens. For growing turkeys only. Do not administer to calves within 1 day of slaughter. Do not administer to chickens at 1,000 mg/gallon of water (one packet per 102.4 gallons) within 24 hours of slaughter. Zero day withdrawal in swine.

Presentation: PENNCHLOR™ 64 is available in 25.6 oz (725.7 g) packets, packed 24 packets per pack.

Compendium Code No.: 10450121

Rev 8/00 F64-1

PENNCHLOR™ 70 MEAL

PennField **Feed Medication**

Chlortetracycline (Type A Medicated Feed)

NADA No.: 138-935

Active Ingredient(s): Chlortetracycline as chlortetracycline calcium complex equivalent to 70 grams chlortetracycline hydrochloride/lb.

Ingredients: Chlortetracycline, calcium carbonate, roughage products and mineral oil.

Indications: An antimicrobial premix for use in the feed of chickens, turkeys, sheep, swine, calves, beef cattle, and non-lactating dairy cattle.

Recommended for the prevention and control of diseases caused by microorganisms sensitive to chlortetracycline, and also for other production uses.

Directions for Use:

Indications for Use	Use Levels of Chlortetracycline	lbs of PENNCHLOR™ 70 per ton
Chickens		
For Broiler/fryer chickens: For an increased rate of weight gain and improved feed efficiency.	10-50 g/ton	0.143-0.714
For Chickens: Control of infectious synovitis caused by *Mycoplasma synoviae;* susceptible to chlortetracycline. (Feed continuously for 7-14 days.)	100-200 g/ton	1.43-2.86
For Chickens: Control of chronic respiratory disease (CRD) and air sac infection caused by *Mycoplasma gallisepticum* and *Escherichia coli* susceptible to chlortetracycline. (Feed continuously for 7-14 days.)	200-400 g/ton	2.86-5.72
For Chickens: Reduction of mortality due to *Escherichia coli* infections susceptible to chlortetracycline. (Feed for 5 days.)	500 g/ton	7.14
Turkeys		
For Turkeys: Growing Turkeys: For an increased rate of weight gain and improved feed efficiency.	10-50 g/ton	0.143-0.714
For Turkeys: Control of infectious synovitis caused by *Mycoplasma synoviae* susceptible to chlortetracycline. (Feed continuously for 7-14 days.)	200 g/ton	2.86
For Turkeys: Control of hexamitiasis caused by *Hexamita meleagrides* susceptible to chlortetracycline. (Feed continuously 7-14 days.)	400 g/ton	5.72
For Turkeys: Turkey poults not over 4 weeks of age: Reduction of mortality due to paratyphoid caused by *Salmonella typhimurium* susceptible to chlortetracycline.	400 g/ton	5.72
For Turkeys: Control of complicating bacterial organisms associated with bluecomb (transmissible enteritis, coronaviral enteritis) susceptible to chlortetracycline. (Feed continuously for 7-14 days.)	25 mg/lb body weight/day	
Sheep		
For Growing Sheep: For an increased rate of weight gain and improved feed efficiency.	20-50 g/ton	0.286-0.714
For Breeding Sheep: Reducing the incidence of (vibrionic) abortion caused by *Campylobacter fetus* infection susceptible to chlortetracycline.	80 mg/head/day	
Swine		
For Growing Swine: For an increased rate of weight gain and improved feed efficiency.	10-50 g/ton	0.143-0.714
For Swine: Reducing the incidence of cervical lymphadenitis (jowl abscesses) caused by *Group E Streptococci* susceptible to chlortetracycline.	50-100 g/ton	0.714-1.43
For Breeding Swine: Control of leptospirosis (reducing the instances of abortions and shedding of leptospirae) caused by *Leptospira pomona* susceptible to chlortetracycline. (Feed continuously for 14 days.)	400 g/ton	5.72
For Swine: Treatment of bacterial enteritis caused by *Escherichia coli* and *Salmonella choleraesuis* and bacterial pneumonia caused by *Pasteurella multocida* susceptible to chlortetracycline. (Feed for not more than 14 days.)	10 mg/lb body weight/day	
Calves, Beef Cattle, and Nonlactating Dairy Cattle		
For Calves (up to 250 lbs): For an increased weight gain and improved feed efficiency.	0.1 mg/lb body weight/day	
For Calves (250-400 lbs): For an increased weight gain and improved feed efficiency.	25-70 mg/head/day	
For Growing Cattle (over 400 lbs): For an increased weight gain, improved feed efficiency and reduction of liver condemnation due to liver abscesses.	70 mg/head/day	
For Cattle: For the control of bacterial pneumonia associated with shipping fever complex susceptible to chlortetracycline.	350 mg/head/day	
For Beef Cattle: Control of active infection of anaplasmosis caused by *Anaplasma marginale* susceptible to chlortetracycline.	350 mg/head/day	
For Beef Cattle (over 700 lbs): Control of active infection of anaplasmosis caused by *Anaplasma marginale* susceptible to chlortetracycline.	0.5 mg/lb body weight/day	
For Calves, Beef, and Nonlactating Dairy Cattle: For treatment of bacterial enteritis caused by *Escherichia coli* and bacterial pneumonia caused by *Pasteurella multocida* susceptible to chlortetracycline. (Treat for not more than 5 days.)	10 mg/lb body weight/day	

Caution(s): For use in the manufacture of medicated feeds.

For use in dry feeds only - Not for use in liquid feed supplements.

Restricted drug (California) - Use only as directed.

Warning(s):

Chickens:

When used at levels above 200 g/ton: Do not feed to chickens producing eggs for human consumption.

When used at levels up to 400 g/ton: Zero-day withdrawal period.

When used at levels of 500 g/ton: Withdraw 24 hours prior to slaughter.

Turkeys: When used at levels of 25 mg/lb body weight/day: Do not feed to turkeys producing eggs for human consumption. Zero-day withdrawal period.

Sheep: Zero-day withdrawal period.

Swine: Zero-day withdrawal period.

Cattle:

A withdrawal period has not been established for this product in pre-ruminating calves. Do not use in calves to be processed for veal.

When used in growing cattle at a level of 70 mg/head/day or less: Zero-day withdrawal period.

When used in beef cattle at a level of 0.5 mg/lb body weight/day and at 350 mg/head/day: Withdraw 1 day prior to slaughter.

When used in calves, beef cattle and non-lactating dairy cattle at levels of 10 mg/lb body weight/day: Withdraw 1 day prior to slaughter.

Presentation: 50 lb (22.7 kg) bag.

Compendium Code No.: 10450130

REV. 8/99

PENNCHLOR 90•G®

PennField **Feed Medication**

Chlortetracycline (Type A Medicated Article)

NADA No.: 138-935

Active Ingredient(s): Chlortetracycline as chlortetracycline calcium complex equivalent to 90 grams chlortetracycline hydrochloride/lb.

Ingredients: Chlortetracycline, calcium carbonate, roughage products and mineral oil.

Indications: Chlortetracycline is a broad spectrum antibiotic cleared for use in livestock and poultry feeds. Chlortetracycline is used in livestock and poultry to treat disease, and as an aid to increase weight, and improve feed/gain ratio. Chlortetracycline is effective against strains of both gram-positive and gram-negative organisms. Chlortetracycline is indicated to increase the rate of weight gain and improve feed efficiency in cattle, swine, chickens, turkeys and sheep.

Directions for Use: (Use level based on Chlortetracycline as HCl Salt. Mix quantity designated per ton of feed.)

Indications for Use	Use Levels of Chlortetracycline	lbs of PENNCHLOR 90•G® per ton
Chickens		
For Broiler/fryer chickens: For an increased rate of weight gain and improved feed efficiency.	10-50 g/ton	0.111-0.555
For Chickens: Control of infectious synovitis caused by *Mycoplasma synoviae;* susceptible to chlortetracycline. (Feed continuously for 7-14 days.)	100-200 g/ton	1.11-2.22
For Chickens: Control of chronic respiratory disease (CRD) and air sac infection caused by *Mycoplasma gallisepticum* and *Escherichia coli* susceptible to chlortetracycline. (Feed continuously for 7-14 days.)	200-400 g/ton	2.22-4.44
For Chickens: Reduction of mortality due to *Escherichia coli* infections susceptible to chlortetracycline. (Feed for 5 days.)	500 g/ton	5.55
Turkeys		
For Turkeys: Growing Turkeys: For an increased rate of weight gain and improved feed efficiency.	10-50 g/ton	0.111-0.555
For Turkeys: Control of infectious synovitis caused by *Mycoplasma synoviae* susceptible to chlortetracycline. (Feed continuously for 7-14 days.)	200 g/ton	2.22
For Turkeys: Control of hexamitiasis caused by *Hexamita meleagrides* susceptible to chlortetracycline. (Feed continuously 7-14 days.)	400 g/ton	4.44
For Turkeys: Turkey poults not over 4 weeks of age: Reduction of mortality due to paratyphoid caused by *Salmonella typhimurium* susceptible to chlortetracycline.	400 g/ton	4.44
For Turkeys: Control of complicating bacterial organisms associated with bluecomb (transmissible enteritis, coronaviral enteritis) susceptible to chlortetracycline. (Feed continuously for 7-14 days.)	25 mg/lb body weight/day	
Sheep		
For Growing Sheep: For an increased rate of weight gain and improved feed efficiency.	20-50 g/ton	0.222-0.555
For Breeding Sheep: Reducing the incidence of (vibrionic) abortion caused by *Campylobacter fetus* infection susceptible to chlortetracycline.	80 mg/head/day	
Swine		
For Growing Swine: For an increased rate of weight gain and improved feed efficiency.	10-50 g/ton	0.111-0.555
For Swine: Reducing the incidence of cervical lymphadenitis (jowl abscesses) caused by *Group E Streptococci* susceptible to chlortetracycline.	50-100 g/ton	0.555-1.11
For Breeding Swine: Control of leptospirosis (reducing the instances of abortions and shedding of leptospirae) caused by *Leptospira pomona* susceptible to chlortetracycline. (Feed continuously for 14 days.)	400 g/ton	4.44
For Swine: Treatment of bacterial enteritis caused by *Escherichia coli* and *Salmonella choleraesuis* and bacterial pneumonia caused by *Pasteurella multocida* susceptible to chlortetracycline. (Feed for not more than 14 days.)	10 mg/lb body weight/day	
Calves, Beef Cattle, and Nonlactating Dairy Cattle		
For Calves (up to 250 lbs): For an increased weight gain and improved feed efficiency.	0.1 mg/lb body weight/day	

P

Indications for Use	Use Levels of Chlortetracycline	lbs of PENNCHLOR 90•G® per ton
For Calves (250-400 lbs): For an increased weight gain and improved feed efficiency.	25-70 mg/head/day	
For Growing Cattle (over 400 lbs): For an increased weight gain, improved feed efficiency and reduction of liver condemnation due to liver abscesses.	70 mg/head/day	
For Cattle: For the control of bacterial pneumonia associated with shipping fever complex susceptible to chlortetracycline.	350 mg/head/day	
For Beef Cattle (under 700 lbs): Control of active infection of anaplasmosis caused by *Anaplasma marginale* susceptible to chlortetracycline.	350 mg/head/day	
For Beef Cattle (over 700 lbs): Control of active infection of anaplasmosis caused by *Anaplasma marginale* susceptible to chlortetracycline.	0.5 mg/lb body weight/day	
For Calves, Beef, and Nonlactating Dairy Cattle: For treatment of bacterial enteritis caused by *Escherichia coli* and bacterial pneumonia caused by *Pasteurella multocida* susceptible to chlortetracycline. (Treat for not more than 5 days.)	10 mg/lb body weight/day	

Warning(s):

Chickens:

When used at levels above 200 g/ton: Do not feed to chickens producing eggs for human consumption. Zero-day withdrawal period.

When used at levels of 500 g/ton: Do not feed to chickens producing eggs for human consumption. Withdraw 24 hours prior to slaughter.

Turkeys: When used at levels of 25 mg/lb body weight/day: Do not feed to turkeys producing eggs for human consumption. Zero-day withdrawal period.

Sheep: Zero-day withdrawal period.

Swine: Zero-day withdrawal period.

Cattle:

A withdrawal period has not been established for this product in pre-ruminating calves. Do not use in calves to be processed for veal.

When used in growing cattle at a level of 70 mg/head/day: Zero-day withdrawal period.

When used in beef cattle at a level of 0.5 mg/lb body weight/day: Withdraw 1 day prior to slaughter.

When used in calves, beef cattle, and non-lactating dairy cattle at levels of 10 mg/lb body weight/day: Withdraw 1 day prior to slaughter.

For use in the manufacture of medicated feeds.

For use in dry feeds only - Not for use in liquid feed supplements.

Restricted drug (California) - Use only as directed.

Presentation: PENNCHLOR 90•G® is available in 50 lb (22.7 kg) bags. Bags are light purple color-coded in gusset area.

Patents Pending

Compendium Code No.: 10450070

PENNCHLOR 100 HI-FLO™ MEAL

PennField **Feed Medication**

Chlortetracycline (Type A Medicated Feed)

NADA No.: 138-935

Active Ingredient(s): Chlortetracycline as chlortetracycline calcium complex equivalent to 100 grams chlortetracycline hydrochloride/lb.

Ingredients: Chlortetracycline, calcium carbonate, roughage products and mineral oil.

Indications: An antimicrobial premix for use in the feed of chickens, turkeys, sheep, swine, calves, beef cattle, and non-lactating dairy cattle. Recommended for the prevention and control of diseases caused by microorganisms sensitive to chlortetracycline, and also for other production uses.

Directions for Use:

Indications for Use	Use Levels of Chlortetracycline	lbs of PENNCHLOR 100 per ton
Chickens		
For Broiler/fryer chickens: For an increased rate of weight gain and improved feed efficiency.	10-50 g/ton	0.1-0.5
For Chickens: Control of infectious synovitis caused by *Mycoplasma synoviae;* susceptible to chlortetracycline. (Feed continuously for 7-14 days.)	100-200 g/ton	1.0-2.0
For Chickens: Control of chronic respiratory disease (CRD) and air sac infection caused by *Mycoplasma gallisepticum* and *Escherichia coli* susceptible to chlortetracycline. (Feed continuously for 7-14 days.)	200-400 g/ton	2.0-4.0
For Chickens: Reduction of mortality due to *Escherichia coli* infections susceptible to chlortetracycline. (Feed for 5 days.)	500 g/ton	5.0
Turkeys		
For Turkeys: Growing Turkeys: For an increased rate of weight gain and improved feed efficiency.	10-50 g/ton	0.1-0.5
For Turkeys: Control of infectious synovitis caused by *Mycoplasma synoviae* susceptible to chlortetracycline. (Feed continuously for 7-14 days.)	200 g/ton	2.0
For Turkeys: Control of hexamitiasis caused by *Hexamita meleagrides* susceptible to chlortetracycline. (Feed continuously 7-14 days.)	400 g/ton	4.0
For Turkeys: Turkey poults not over 4 weeks of age: Reduction of mortality due to paratyphoid caused by *Salmonella typhimurium* susceptible to chlortetracycline.	400 g/ton	4.0
For Turkeys: Control of complicating bacterial organisms associated with bluecomb (transmissible enteritis, coronaviral enteritis) susceptible to chlortetracycline. (Feed continuously for 7-14 days.)	25 mg/lb body weight/day	
Sheep		
For Growing Sheep: For an increased rate of weight gain and improved feed efficiency.	20-50 g/ton	0.2-0.5
For Breeding Sheep: Reducing the incidence of (vibrionic) abortion caused by *Campylobacter fetus* infection susceptible to chlortetracycline.	80 mg/head/day	
Swine		
For Growing Swine: For an increased rate of weight gain and improved feed efficiency.	10-50 g/ton	0.10-0.5
For Swine: Reducing the incidence of cervical lymphadenitis (jowl abscesses) caused by *Group E Streptococci* susceptible to chlortetracycline.	50-100 g/ton	0.5-1.0
For Breeding Swine: Control of leptospirosis (reducing the instances of abortion and shedding of leptospirae) caused by *Leptospira pomona* susceptible to chlortetracycline. (Feed continuously for 14 days.)	400 g/ton	4.0
For Swine: Treatment of bacterial enteritis caused by *Escherichia coli* and *Salmonella choleraesuis* and bacterial pneumonia caused by *Pasteurella multocida* susceptible to chlortetracycline. (Feed for not more than 14 days.)	10 mg/lb body weight/day	
Calves, Beef Cattle, and Nonlactating Dairy Cattle		
For Calves (up to 250 lbs): For an increased weight gain and improved feed efficiency.	0.1 mg/lb body weight/day	
For Calves (250-400 lbs): For an increased weight gain and improved feed efficiency.	25-70 mg/head/day	
For Growing Cattle (over 400 lbs): For an increased weight gain, improved feed efficiency and reduction of liver condemnation due to liver abscesses.	70 mg/head/day	
For Cattle: For the control of bacterial pneumonia associated with shipping fever complex susceptible to chlortetracycline.	350 mg/head/day	
For Beef Cattle (under 700 lbs): Control of active infection of anaplasmosis caused by *Anaplasma marginale* susceptible to chlortetracycline.	350 mg/head/day	
For Beef Cattle (over 700 lbs): Control of active infection of anaplasmosis caused by *Anaplasma marginale* susceptible to chlortetracycline.	0.5 mg/lb body weight/day	
For Calves, Beef, and Nonlactating Dairy Cattle: For treatment of bacterial enteritis caused by *Escherichia coli* and bacterial pneumonia caused by *Pasteurella multocida* susceptible to chlortetracycline. (Treat for not more than 5 days.)	10 mg/lb weight/day	

Warning(s):

Chickens:

When used at levels of 10-400 g/ton: Do not feed to chickens producing eggs for human consumption. Zero-day withdrawal period.

When used at levels of 500 g/ton: Do not feed to chickens producing eggs for human consumption. Withdraw 24 hours prior to slaughter.

Turkeys: Do not feed to turkeys producing eggs for human consumption. Zero-day withdrawal period.

Breeding Sheep: Zero-day withdrawal period.

Swine: Zero-day withdrawal period.

Calves, Beef Cattle, and Nonlactating Dairy Cattle: A withdrawal period has not been established for this product in pre-ruminating calves. Do not use in calves to be processed for veal.

Growing Cattle (over 400 lbs): When used at levels of 70 mg/head/day: Zero-day withdrawal period.

For Cattle and Beef Cattle (over 700 lbs): When used at levels of 350 mg/head/day or 0.5 mg/lb body weight/day: Withdraw 1 day prior to slaughter.

Calves, Beef Cattle, and Nonlactating Dairy Cattle: When used at levels of 10 mg/lb body weight/day: Withdraw 1 day prior to slaughter.

For use in the manufacture of medicated feeds.

For use in dry feeds only - Not for use in liquid feed supplements.

Restricted Drug: (California) - Use only as directed.

Presentation: 50 lb (22.7 kg).

Compendium Code No.: 10450050

PENNCHLOR™ 100-MR

PennField **Feed Medication**

Chlortetracycline (Type A Medicated Article)

NADA No.: 138-935

Active Ingredient(s):

Chlortetracycline equivalent to Chlortetracycline Hydrochloride .... 100 grams/lb.

Ingredient: Sucrose.

Indications: Chlortetracycline Antibacterial Premix for use in calf milk replacers or starter feeds for improved feed efficiency and treatment of bacterial enteritis.

Directions for Use: For An Increased Rate of Weight Gain and Improved Feed Efficiency in Replacement Calves Up To 250 Pounds:

Dose: 0.1 mg Chlortetracycline per pound body weight per day.

Mixing Directions: Mix 0.2 lb. PENNCHLOR™ 100-MR in 1 ton of milk replacer or starter feed.

For Treatment of Bacterial Enteritis Caused by *Escherichia coli* Organisms Susceptible to Chlortetracycline:

Dose: 10 mg Chlortetracycline per pound body weight per day. Feed for not more than 5 days.

Mixing Directions: Mix 20 lb. PENNCHLOR™ 100-MR in 1 ton of milk replacer or starter feed.

Feeding Directions for Milk Replacers or Starter Feeds				
Body Weight of Calf	75 lbs.	100 lbs.	150 lbs.	250 lbs.
Amount of Milk Replacer or Starter Feed for Calf Per Day	0.75 lbs.	1.0 lbs.	1.5 lbs.	2.5 lbs.

Warning(s): A withdrawal period is not required when fed at 0.1 mg/lb/day.

Withdraw 10 days before slaughter when fed at 10 mg/lb/day.

A withdrawal period has not been established for this product in pre-ruminating calves. Do not use in calves to be processed for veal.

For use in the manufacture of medicated feeds.

For animal use only.

Restricted drug (California) - Use only as directed.

Presentation: 25 lb pail and 100 lb (45.4 kg) drum.

Compendium Code No.: 10450100

Revised 10/97 Label AH7

PENNCHLOR SP 250®

PennField **Feed Medication**

Chlortetracycline, sulfamethazine, penicillin (Type B Medicated Article)

NADA No.: 138-935

Active Ingredient(s):

Chlortetracycline Calcium Complex equivalent to Chlortetracycline HCl .... 10 g per lb
Sulfamethazine.. 2.2% (10 g/lb)
Penicillin (from procaine penicillin) .... 5 g per lb

Guaranteed Analysis:

Calcium (Ca) not less than 1.5%
Calcium (Ca) not more than 2.0%
Magnesium (Mg) not less than 1.5%
Magnesium (Mg) not more than 2.0%
Crude Protein, not less than... 8.0%
Crude Fat, not less than 0.1%
Crude Fiber, not more than 60%

Ingredients: Roughage products, magnesium-mica, chlortetracycline, calcium carbonate, mineral oil, sulfamethazine, penicillin (from procaine penicillin).

Indications: For reduction of the incidence of cervical abscesses, treatment of bacterial swine enteritis (salmonellosis or necrotic enteritis caused by *Salmonella choleraesuis* and vibrionic dysentery); prevention of these diseases during times of stress; maintenance of weight gains in the presence of atrophic rhinitis; growth promotion and increased feed efficiency in swine weighing up to 75 pounds.

Directions: Mix at the rate of 10 pounds (4.54 kg) per ton (907.2 kg) with part of the feed ingredients to make a preblend. Add the remainder of the ingredients to give a final concentration of 100 g chlortetracycline, 100 g sulfamethazine and 50 g penicillin per ton of Type C feed and mix thoroughly.

Warning(s): Withdraw 15 days prior to slaughter.

For use in the manufacture of swine feeds.

Restricted drug: (California) - Use only as directed.

Presentation: 50 lb (22.7 kg).

Compendium Code No.: 10450081

REV. 8/98

PENNCHLOR SP 500®

PennField **Feed Medication**

Chlortetracycline, sulfamethazine, penicillin (Type A Medicated Article)

NADA No.: 138-935

Active Ingredient(s):

Chlortetracycline Calcium Complex equivalent to Chlortetracycline HCl .... 40 g per lb
Sulfamethazine.. 8.8% (40 g/lb)
Penicillin (from procaine penicillin) .... 20 g per lb

Inactive Ingredients: Roughage products, calcium carbonate and mineral oil.

Indications: For reduction of the incidence of cervical abscesses; treatment of bacterial swine enteritis (salmonellosis or necrotic enteritis caused by *Salmonella choleraesuis* and vibrionic dysentery); prevention of these diseases during times of stress; maintenance of weight gains in the presence of atrophic rhinitis; growth promotion and increased feed efficiency in swine weighing up to 75 pounds.

Directions: Mix 2.5 lbs. of Article with part of the feed ingredients to make a preblend. Add the remainder of the ingredients to give a final concentration of 100 g chlortetracycline, 100 g sulfamethazine and 50 g penicillin per ton of Type C feed and mix thoroughly.

Warning(s): Withdraw 15 days prior to slaughter.

For use in the manufacture of swine feeds.

Restricted drug: (California) - Use only as directed.

Presentation: PENNCHLOR SP 500® is available in 50 lb (22.7 kg) bags. Bags are fuchsia color-coded in gusset area.

Compendium Code No.: 10450091

PENNOX™ 50 MEAL

PennField **Feed Medication**

Oxytetracycline (Type A Medicated Feed)

NADA No.: 138-938

Active Ingredient(s): Oxytetracycline (as quaternary salt) equivalent to 50 grams oxytetracycline hydrochloride/lb.

Ingredients: Oxytetracycline, calcium carbonate, roughage products and mineral oil.

Indications: An antimicrobial premix for use in the feed of chickens, turkeys, sheep, swine, calves, beef cattle, and non-lactating dairy cattle. It can also be administered to honey bees.

Recommended for the prevention and control of diseases caused by microorganisms sensitive to oxytetracycline, and also for other production uses.

Directions for Use:

Indications for Use	Use Levels of Oxytetracycline	lbs of PENNOX™ 50 per ton
Chickens		
For Broiler/fryer chickens: For an increased rate of weight gain and improved feed efficiency. (Use continuously.)	10-50 g/ton	0.2-1.0
For Chickens: Control of infectious synovitis caused by *Mycoplasma synoviae;* control of fowl cholera caused by *Pasteurella multocida* sensitive to oxytetracycline. (Feed continuously for 7-14 days.)	100-200 g/ton	2.0-4.0
For Chickens: Control of chronic respiratory disease (CRD) and air sac infection caused by *Mycoplasma gallisepticum* and *Escherichia coli* susceptible to oxytetracycline. (Feed continuously for 7-14 days.)	400 g/ton	8.0
Broiler Chickens: Reduction of mortality due to air succulitis (air-sac infection) caused by *Escherichia coli* susceptible to oxytetracycline. (Feed for 5 days.)	500 g/ton	10.0
Turkeys		
For Turkeys: Growing Turkeys: For an increased rate of weight gain and improved feed efficiency. (Use continuously.)	10-50 g/ton	0.2-1.0
For Turkeys: Control of infectious synovitis caused by *Mycoplasma synoviae* susceptible to oxytetracycline. (Feed continuously for 7-14 days.)	200 g/ton	4.0
For Turkeys: Control of hexamitiasis caused by *Hexamita meleagrides* susceptible to oxytetracycline. (Feed continuously 7-14 days.)	100 g/ton	2.0
For Turkeys: Control of complicating bacterial organisms associated with bluecomb (transmissible enteritis, coronaviral enteritis) susceptible to oxytetracycline. (Feed continuously for 7-14 days.)	25 mg/lb body weight/day	
Sheep		
For Sheep: For an increased rate of weight gain and improved feed efficiency. (Use continuously.)	10-20 g/ton	0.20-0.4
For Sheep: Treatment of bacterial enteritis caused by *Escherichia coli* and bacterial pneumonia caused by *Pasteurella multocida* susceptible to oxytetracycline. (Feed continuously 7-14 days.)	10 mg/lb	
Swine		
For Swine: For an increased rate of weight gain and improved feed efficiency. (Use continuously.)	10-50 g/ton	0.20-1.0
For Swine: Treatment of bacterial enteritis caused by *Escherichia coli* and *Salmonella choleraesuis* susceptible to oxytetracycline and treatment of bacterial pneumonia caused by *Pasteurella multocida* susceptible to oxytetracycline. (Feed continuously 7-14 days.)	10.0 mg/lb	
For Breeding Swine: Prevention and treatment of Leptospirosis (reducing the instances of abortions and shedding of leptospirae) caused by *Leptospira pomona* susceptible to oxytetracycline. (Feed continuously for 14 days.)	10 mg/lb	
Calves, Beef Cattle, and Nonlactating Dairy Cattle		
For Calves (up to 250 lbs): For an increased weight gain and improved feed efficiency. (Use continuously.)	0.05-0.1 mg/lb	
For Calves (250-400 lbs): For an increased weight gain and improved feed efficiency. (Use continuously.)	25 mg/head/day	
For Growing Cattle (over 400 lbs): For an increased weight gain, improved feed efficiency and reduction of liver condemnation due to liver abscesses. (Use continuously.)	75 mg/head/day	
For the prevention and treatment of the early stages of the shipping fever complex. (Feed 3-5 days before and after arrival in feedlots.)	0.5-2.0 g/head/day	
For Calves and Beef Cattle: Treatment of bacterial enteritis caused by *Escherichia coli* and bacterial pneumonia (shipping fever complex) caused by *Pasteurella multocida* susceptible to oxytetracycline. (Feed continuously for 7-14 days.) Note: When used in milk replacers, the treatment claim (10 mg/lb) is limited to bacterial enteritis caused by *Escherichia coli* only.	10 mg/lb	
Honey Bees		
For Honey Bees: For control of American Foulbrood caused by *Bacillus larvae*, and European Foulbrood caused by *Streptococcus pluton* susceptible to oxytetracycline.	200 mg/colony	

Warning(s):

Chickens:

When used at levels of 400 g/ton and above: Do not administer to chickens producing eggs for human consumption. In low calcium feeds withdraw 3 days before slaughter.

When used at levels of 400 g/ton: Zero-day withdrawal period. In low calcium feeds withdraw 3 days before slaughter.

When used at levels of 500 g/ton: 24 hours withdrawal period. In low calcium feeds withdraw 3 days before slaughter.

Turkeys:

When used at levels of 200 g/ton or higher: Withdraw 5 days before slaughter.

When used at levels below 200 g/ton or higher: Zero-day withdrawal period.

For all levels of use: Do not administer to turkeys producing eggs for human consumption.

Sheep: When used at levels of 10 mg/lb body weight/day: Withdraw 5 days before slaughter.

Swine: When used at levels of 10 mg/lb body weight/day: Withdraw 5 days before slaughter.

Cattle: When used at levels of 10 mg/lb body weight/day: Withdraw 5 days before slaughter.

Honey Bees: Remove at least 6 weeks prior to main honey flow.

For use in the manufacture of medicated feeds.

For use in dry feeds only - Not for use in liquid feed supplements.

Restricted drug (California) - Use only as directed.

Presentation: 50 lb (22.7 kg).

Compendium Code No.: 10450190

PENNOX 100 HI-FLO™ MEAL

PennField **Feed Medication**

Oxytetracycline (Type A Medicated Feed)

NADA No.: 138-938

Active Ingredient(s): Oxytetracycline (as quaternary salt) equivalent to 100 grams oxytetracycline hydrochloride/lb.

Ingredients: Oxytetracycline, calcium carbonate, roughage products and mineral oil.

Indications: An antimicrobial premix for use in the feed of chickens, turkeys, sheep, swine, calves, beef cattle, and non-lactating dairy cattle. It can also be administered to honey bees.

Recommended for the prevention and control of diseases caused by microorganisms sensitive to oxytetracycline, and also for other production uses.

Directions for Use:

Indications for Use	Use Levels of Oxytetracycline	lbs of PENNOX 100 per ton
Chickens		
For Broiler/fryer chickens: For an increased rate of weight gain and improved feed efficiency. (Use continuously.)	10-50 g/ton	0.1-0.5
For Chickens: Control of infectious synovitis caused by *Mycoplasma synoviae;* control of fowl cholera caused by *Pasteurella multocida* sensitive to oxytetracycline. (Feed continuously for 7-14 days.)	100-200 g/ton	1.0-2.0
For Chickens: Control of chronic respiratory disease (CRD) and air sac infection caused by *Mycoplasma gallisepticum* and *Escherichia coli* susceptible to oxytetracycline. (Feed continuously for 7-14 days.)	400 g/ton	4.0
Broiler Chickens: Reduction of mortality due to air succulitis (air-sac infection) caused by *Escherichia coli* susceptible to oxytetracycline. (Feed for 5 days.)	500 g/ton	5.0
Turkeys		
For Turkeys: Growing Turkeys: For an increased rate of weight gain and improved feed efficiency. (Use continuously.)	10-50 g/ton	0.1-0.5
For Turkeys: Control of infectious synovitis caused by *Mycoplasma synoviae* susceptible to oxytetracycline. (Feed continuously for 7-14 days.)	200 g/ton	2.0
For Turkeys: Control of hexamitiasis caused by *Hexamita meleagrides* susceptible to oxytetracycline. (Feed continuously 7-14 days.)	100 g/ton	1.0
For Turkeys: Control of complicating bacterial organisms associated with bluecomb (transmissible enteritis, coronaviral enteritis) susceptible to oxytetracycline. (Feed continuously for 7-14 days.)	25 mg/lb body weight/day	
Sheep		
For Sheep: For an increased rate of weight gain and improved feed efficiency. (Use continuously.)	10-20 g/ton	0.10-0.20
For Sheep: Treatment of bacterial enteritis caused by *Escherichia coli* and bacterial pneumonia caused by *Pasteurella multocida* susceptible to oxytetracycline. (Feed continuously 7-14 days.)	10 mg/lb	
Swine		
For Swine: For an increased rate of weight gain and improved feed efficiency. (Use continuously.)	10-50 g/ton	0.10-0.5
For Swine: Treatment of bacterial enteritis caused by *Escherichia coli* and *Salmonella choleraesuis* susceptible to oxytetracycline and treatment of bacterial pneumonia caused by *Pasteurella multocida* susceptible to oxytetracycline. (Feed continuously 7-14 days.)	10.0 mg/lb	
For Breeding Swine: Prevention and treatment of Leptospirosis (reducing the instances of abortions and shedding of leptospirae) caused by *Leptospira pomona* susceptible to oxytetracycline. (Feed continuously for 14 days.)	10 mg/lb	
Calves, Beef Cattle, and Nonlactating Dairy Cattle		
For Calves (up to 250 lbs): For an increased weight gain and improved feed efficiency. (Use continuously.)	0.05-0.1 mg/lb	
For Calves (250-400 lbs): For an increased weight gain and improved feed efficiency. (Use continuously.)	25 mg/head/day	
For Growing Cattle (over 400 lbs): For an increased weight gain, improved feed efficiency and reduction of liver condemnation due to liver abscesses. (Use continuously.)	75 mg/head/day	
For the prevention and treatment of the early stages of the shipping fever complex. (Feed 3-5 days before and after arrival in feedlots.)	0.5-2.0 g/head/day	
For Calves and Beef Cattle: Treatment of bacterial enteritis caused by *Escherichia coli* and bacterial pneumonia (shipping fever complex) caused by *Pasteurella multocida* susceptible to oxytetracycline. (Feed continuously for 7-14 days.) Note: When used in milk replacers, the treatment claim (10 mg/lb) is limited to bacterial enteritis caused by *Escherichia coli* only.	10 mg/lb	
Honey Bees		
For Honey Bees: For control of American Foulbrood caused by *Bacillus larvae,* and European Foulbrood caused by *Streptococcus pluton* susceptible to oxytetracycline.	200 mg/colony	

Warning(s):

Chickens:

When used at levels of 400 g/ton and above: Do not administer to chickens producing eggs for human consumption. In low calcium feeds withdraw 3 days before slaughter.

When used at levels of 400 g/ton: Zero-day withdrawal period. In low calcium feeds withdraw 3 days before slaughter.

When used at levels of 500 g/ton: 24 hours withdrawal period. In low calcium feeds withdraw 3 days before slaughter.

Turkeys:

When used at levels of 200 g/ton or higher: Withdraw 5 days before slaughter.

When used at levels below 200 g/ton or higher: Zero-day withdrawal period.

For all levels of use: Do not administer to turkeys producing eggs for human consumption.

Sheep: When used at levels of 10 mg/lb body weight/day: Withdraw 5 days before slaughter.

Swine: When used at levels of 10 mg/lb body weight/day: Withdraw 5 days before slaughter.

Cattle: When used at levels of 10 mg/lb body weight/day: Withdraw 5 days before slaughter.

Honey Bees: Remove at least 6 weeks prior to main honey flow.

For use in the manufacture of medicated feeds.

For use in dry feeds only - Not for use in liquid feed supplements.

Restricted drug (California) - Use only as directed.

Presentation: 50 lb (22.7 kg).

Compendium Code No.: 10450140

PENNOX™ 100-MR

PennField **Feed Medication**

Oxytetracycline (Type A Medicated Feed)

NADA No.: 138-938

Active Ingredient(s): Oxytetracycline equivalent to 100 grams oxytetracycline hydrochloride/lb.

Ingredients: Oxytetracycline hydrochloride, sucrose.

Indications: Oxytetracycline Antibacterial Premix for use in calf milk replacers or starter feeds for improved feed efficiency and treatment of bacterial enteritis.

Directions for Use:

For an increased rate of weight gain and improved feed efficiency in replacement calves up to 250 pounds:

Dose: 0.1 mg oxytetracycline per pound body weight per day.

Mixing Directions: Mix 0.2 lb PENNOX™ 100-MR in 1 ton of milk replacer or starter feed.

For treatment of bacterial enteritis caused by *Escherichia coli* organisms susceptible to oxytetracycline:

Dose: 10 mg oxytetracycline per pound body weight per day. Feed for 7-14 days.

Mixing Directions: Mix 20 lb PENNOX™ 100-MR in 1 ton of milk replacer or starter feed.

Feeding Directions for Milk Replacers or Starter Feeds:

Body Weight of Calf	75 lbs	100 lbs	150 lbs	250 lbs
Amount of Milk Replacer or Starter Feed for Calf Per Day	0.75 lbs	1.0 lbs	1.5 lbs	2.5 lbs

Warning(s): When dosed at 0.1 mg/lb body weight/day: Zero-day withdrawal period.

When dosed at 10 mg/lb body weight/day: Withdraw 5 days before slaughter.

For use in the manufacture of medicated feeds.

For animal use only.

Restricted drug (California) - Use only as directed.

Presentation: 25 lb pail and 100 lb (45.4 kg) drum.

Compendium Code No.: 10450160

PENNOX 200 HI-FLO™ MEAL

PennField **Feed Medication**

Oxytetracycline (Type A Medicated Feed)

NADA No.: 138-938

Active Ingredient(s): Oxytetracycline (as quaternary salt) equivalent to 200 grams oxytetracycline hydrochloride/lb.

Ingredients: Oxytetracycline, calcium carbonate, roughage products and mineral oil.

Indications: An antimicrobial premix for use in the feed of chickens, turkeys, sheep, swine, calves, beef cattle, and non-lactating dairy cattle. It can also be administered to honey bees.

Recommended for the prevention and control of diseases caused by microorganisms sensitive to oxytetracycline, and also for other production uses.

Directions for Use:

Indications for Use	Use Levels of Oxytetracycline	lbs of PENNOX 200 per ton
Chickens		
For Broiler/fryer chickens: For an increased rate of weight gain and improved feed efficiency. (Use continuously.)	10-50 g/ton	0.05-0.25
For Chickens: Control of infectious synovitis caused by *Mycoplasma synoviae;* control of fowl cholera caused by *Pasteurella multocida* sensitive to oxytetracycline. (Feed continuously for 7-14 days.)	100-200 g/ton	0.5-1.0
For Chickens: Control of chronic respiratory disease (CRD) and air sac infection caused by *Mycoplasma gallisepticum* and *Escherichia coli* susceptible to oxytetracycline. (Feed continuously for 7-14 days.)	400 g/ton	2.0
Broiler Chickens: Reduction of mortality due to air succulitis (air-sac infection) caused by *Escherichia coli* susceptible to oxytetracycline. (Feed for 5 days.)	500 g/ton	2.5
Turkeys		
For Turkeys: Growing Turkeys: For an increased rate of weight gain and improved feed efficiency. (Use continuously.)	10-50 g/ton	0.05-0.25
For Turkeys: Control of infectious synovitis caused by *Mycoplasma synoviae* susceptible to oxytetracycline. (Feed continuously for 7-14 days.)	200 g/ton	1.0
For Turkeys: Control of hexamitiasis caused by *Hexamita meleagrides* susceptible to oxytetracycline. (Feed continuously 7-14 days.)	100 g/ton	0.5
For Turkeys: Control of complicating bacterial organisms associated with bluecomb (transmissible enteritis, coronaviral enteritis) susceptible to oxytetracycline. (Feed continuously for 7-14 days.)	25 mg/lb body weight/day	

Indications for Use	Use Levels of Oxytetracycline	lbs of PENNOX 200 per ton
Sheep		
For Sheep: For an increased rate of weight gain and improved feed efficiency. (Use continuously.)	10-20 g/ton	0.05-0.10
For Sheep: Treatment of bacterial enteritis caused by *Escherichia coli* and bacterial pneumonia caused by *Pasteurella multocida* susceptible to oxytetracycline. (Feed continuously 7-14 days.)	10 mg/lb body weight/day	
Swine		
For Swine: For an increased rate of weight gain and improved feed efficiency. (Use continuously.)	10-50 g/ton	0.05-0.25
For Swine: Treatment of bacterial enteritis caused by *Escherichia coli* and *Salmonella choleraesuis* susceptible to oxytetracycline and treatment of bacterial pneumonia caused by *Pasteurella multocida* susceptible to oxytetracycline. (Feed continuously 7-14 days.)	10.0 mg/lb body weight/day	
For Breeding Swine: Prevention and treatment of Leptospirosis (reducing the instances of abortions and shedding of leptospirae) caused by *Leptospira pomona* susceptible to oxytetracycline. (Feed continuously for 14 days.)	10 mg/lb body weight/day	
Calves, Beef Cattle, and Nonlactating Dairy Cattle		
For Calves (up to 250 lbs): For an increased weight gain and improved feed efficiency. (Use continuously.)	0.05-0.1 mg/lb body weight/day	
For Calves (250-400 lbs): For an increased weight gain and improved feed efficiency. (Use continuously.)	25 mg/head/day	
For Growing Cattle (over 400 lbs): For an increased weight gain, improved feed efficiency and reduction of liver condemnation due to liver abscesses. (Use continuously.)	75 mg/head/day	
For the prevention and treatment of the early stages of the shipping fever complex. (Feed 3-5 days before and after arrival in feedlots.)	0.5-2.0 g/head/day	
For Calves and Beef Cattle: Treatment of bacterial enteritis caused by *Escherichia coli* and bacterial pneumonia (shipping fever complex) caused by *Pasteurella multocida* susceptible to oxytetracycline. (Feed continuously for 7-14 days.) Note: When used in milk replacers, the treatment claim (10 mg/lb) is limited to bacterial enteritis caused by *Escherichia coli* only.	10 mg/lb body weight/day	
Honey Bees		
For Honey Bees: For control of American Foulbrood caused by *Bacillus larvae*, and European Foulbrood caused by *Streptococcus pluton* susceptible to oxytetracycline.	200 mg/colony	

Warning(s):

Chickens:

When used at levels of 400 g/ton: Zero-day withdrawal period. In low calcium feeds withdraw 3 days before slaughter. Do not administer to chickens producing eggs for human consumption.

When used at levels of 500 g/ton: 24 hours withdrawal period. In low calcium feeds withdraw 3 days before slaughter. Do not administer to chickens producing eggs for human consumption.

Turkeys: At 200 g/ton use level or higher, withdraw 5 days before slaughter. Zero-day withdrawal period for lower use levels.

Do not administer to turkeys producing eggs for human consumption.

Sheep: 5 days withdrawal at 10 mg/lb body weight/day dosage.

Swine and Breeding Swine: 5 days withdrawal at 10 mg/lb body weight/day dosage.

Calves, Beef Cattle and Nonlactating Dairy Cattle: 5 days withdrawal at 10 mg/lb body weight/day dosage.

Honey Bees: Remove at least 6 weeks prior to main honey flow.

For use in the manufacture of medicated feeds.

For use in dry feeds only - Not for use in liquid feed supplements.

Restricted drug (California) - Use only as directed.

Presentation: 50 lb (22.7 kg).

Compendium Code No.: 10450150

PENNOX™ 200 INJECTABLE

PennField **Oxytetracycline Injection**

Antibiotic

ANADA No.: 200-154

Active Ingredient(s): PENNOX™ 200 (oxytetracycline injection) is a sterile, preconstituted solution of the broad-spectrum antibiotic, oxytetracycline. Each mL contains 200 mg of oxytetracycline base as amphoteric oxytetracycline and on a w/v basis: 40.0% 2-pyrrolidone, 5.0% povidone, 1.8% magnesium oxide, 0.2% sodium formaldehyde sulfoxylate (as a preservative), monoethanolamine and/or hydrochloric acid as required to adjust pH.

Indications: PENNOX™ 200 (oxytetracycline injection) is a sterile, ready-to-use solution for the administration of the broad-spectrum antibiotic oxytetracycline by injection. Oxytetracycline is an antimicrobial agent that is effective in the treatment of a wide range of diseases caused by susceptible gram-positive and gram-negative bacteria.

PENNOX™ 200 is intended for the use in the treatment of the following diseases in beef cattle, non-lactating dairy cattle and swine when due to oxytetracycline-susceptible organisms.

Beef Cattle, Non-Lactating Dairy Cattle and Calves, Including Pre-Ruminating (Veal) Calves: In cattle, PENNOX™ 200 is indicated in the treatment of pneumonia and shipping fever complex associated with *Pasteurella* spp and *Hemophilus* spp; infectious bovine keratoconjunctivitis (pinkeye) caused by *Moraxella bovis;* foot-rot and diphtheria caused by *Fusobacterium necrophorum;* bacterial enteritis (scours) caused by *Escherichia coli;* wooden tongue caused by *Actinobacillus lignieresii;* leptospirosis caused by *Leptospira pomona;* and wound infections and acute metritis caused by strains of staphylococci and streptococci organisms susceptible to oxytetracycline.

Swine: In swine, PENNOX™ 200 is indicated in the treatment of bacterial enteritis (scours, colibacillosis) caused by *Escherichia coli;* pneumonia caused by *Pasteurella multocida;* and leptospirosis caused by *Leptospira pomona.*

In sows, PENNOX™ 200 is indicated as an aid in the control of infectious enteritis (baby pig scours, colibacillosis) in suckling pigs caused by *Escherichia coli.*

Dosage and Administration:

Beef Cattle, Non-Lactating Dairy Cattle and Calves, Including Pre-Ruminating (Veal) Calves: PENNOX™ 200 is to be administered by intramuscular or intravenous injection to beef cattle and non-lactating dairy cattle.

A single dosage of 9 milligrams of PENNOX™ 200 per pound of body weight administered intramuscularly or subcutaneously is recommended in the treatment of the following conditions: (1) bacterial pneumonia caused by *Pasteurella* spp (shipping fever) in calves and yearlings, where re-treatment is impractical due to husbandry conditions, such as cattle on the range, or where repeated restraint is inadvisable; and (2) infectious bovine keratoconjunctivitis (pinkeye) caused by *Moraxella bovis.*

PENNOX™ 200 can also be administered by intravenous or intramuscular injection at a level of 3 to 5 milligrams of oxytetracycline per pound of body weight per day. In the treatment of severe foot-rot and advanced cases of other indicated diseases, a dosage level of 5 milligrams per pound of body weight per day is recommended. Treatment should be continued for 24 to 48 hours following remission of disease signs; however, not to exceed a total of four consecutive days. Consult your veterinarian if improvement is not noted within 24 to 48 hours of the beginning of treatment.

Swine: In swine, a single dosage of 9 milligrams of PENNOX™ 200 per pound of body weight administered intramuscularly is recommended in the treatment of bacterial pneumonia caused by *Pasteurella multocida* in swine, where re-treatment is impractical due to husbandry conditions, or where repeated restraint is inadvisable. PENNOX™ 200 can also be administered by intramuscular injection at a level of 3 to 5 milligrams of oxytetracycline per pound of body weight per day. Treatment should be continued 24 to 48 hours following remission of disease signs; however, not to exceed a total of four consecutive days. Consult your veterinarian if improvement is not noted within 24 to 48 hours of the beginning of treatment.

For sows, administer once intramuscularly 3 milligrams of oxytetracycline per pound of body weight approximately 8 hours before farrowing or immediately after completion of farrowing.

For swine weighing 25 lb of body weight and under, PENNOX™ 200 should be administered undiluted for treatment at 9 mg/lb, but should be administered diluted for treatment at 3 or 5 mg/lb.

Body Weight	9 mg/lb Dosage Volume of Undiluted PENNOX™ 200	3 or 5 mg/lb Dosage Volume of Diluted PENNOX™ 200		
	9 mg/lb	3 mg/lb	Dilution*	5 mg/lb
5 lb	0.2 mL	0.6 mL	1:7	1.0 mL
10 lb	0.5 mL	0.9 mL	1:5	1.5 mL
25 lb	1.1 mL	1.5 mL	1:3	2.5 mL

*To prepare dilutions, add one part PENNOX™ 200 to three, five, or seven parts of sterile water, or 5 percent dextrose solution as indicated; the diluted product should be used immediately.

Directions for Use: A thoroughly cleaned, sterile needle and syringe should be used for each injection (needles and syringes may he sterilized by boiling in water for 15 minutes). In cold weather, PENNOX™ 200 should be warmed to room temperature before administration to animals. Before withdrawing the solution from the bottle, disinfect the rubber cap on the bottle with a suitable disinfectant, such as 70 percent alcohol. The injection site should be similarly cleaned with the disinfectant. Needles of 16 to 18 gauge and 1 to 1 ½ inches long are adequate for intramuscular injections. Needles 2 to 3 inches are recommended for intravenous use.

Subcutaneous Administration: Subcutaneous injections in beef cattle, non-lactating dairy cattle and calves, including pre-ruminating (veal) calves, should be made by directing the needle of suitable gauge and length through the loose folds of the neck skin in front of the shoulder. Care should be taken to ensure that the tip of the needle has penetrated the skin, but is not lodged in muscle. Before injecting the solution, pull back gently on the plunger. If blood appears in the syringe, a blood vessel has been entered; withdraw the needle and select a different site. The solution should be injected slowly into the area between the skin and muscles. No more than 10 mL should be injected subcutaneously at any one site in adult beef cattle and non-lactating dairy cattle; rotate injection sites for each succeeding treatment. The volume administered per injection site should be reduced according to age and body size so that 1 to 2 mL per site is injected in small calves.

Intramuscular Administration: Intramuscular injections should be made by directing the needle of suitable gauge and length into the fleshy part of a thick muscle such as in the rump, hip, or thigh regions, avoid blood vessels and major nerves. Before injecting the solution, pull back gently on the plunger. If blood appears in the syringe, a blood vessel has been entered; withdraw the needle and select a different site. No more than 10 mL should be injected intramuscularly at any one site in adult beef cattle and non-lactating dairy cattle, and not more than 5 mL per site in adult swine, rotate injection sites for each succeeding treatment. The volume administered per injection site should be reduced according to age and body size so that 1 to 2 mL per site is injected in small calves.

Intravenous Administration: PENNOX™ 200 (oxytetracycline injection) may be administered intravenously to beef cattle and non-lactating dairy cattle. As with all highly concentrated materials, PENNOX™ 200 should be administered slowly by the intravenous route.

Preparation of the Animal for Injection:

1. Approximate the location of a vein. The jugular vein runs in the jugular groove on each side of the neck from the angle of the jaw to just above the brisket and slightly above and to the side of the windpipe. (See Fig. 1)
2. Restraint. A stanchion or chute is ideal for restraining the animal. With a halter, rope, or cattle leader (nose tongs), pull the animal's head around the side of the stanchion, cattle chute or post in such a manner to form a bow in the neck (See Fig. 2); then snub the head securely to prevent movement. By forming the bow in the neck, the outside curvature of the bow tends to expose the jugular vein and make it easily accessible. Caution: avoid restraining the animal with a tight rope or halter around the throat or upper neck which might impede blood flow. Animals that are down present no problem so far as restraint is concerned.
3. Clip hair in the area where the injection is to be made (over the vein in the upper part of the neck). Clean and disinfect the skin with alcohol or other suitable antiseptic.

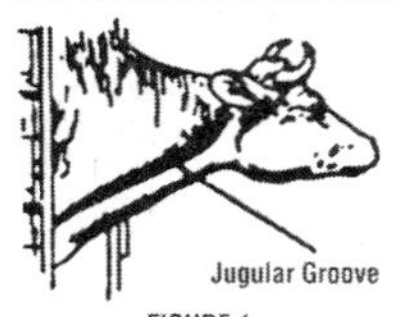

FIGURE 1

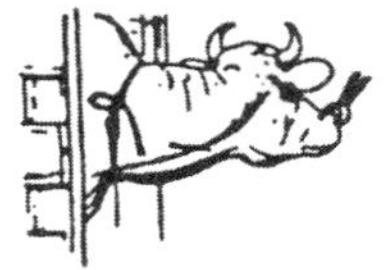
FIGURE 2

P

Entering the Vein and Making the Injection:

1. Raise the vein. This is accomplished by tying the choke rope tightly around the neck close to the shoulder. The rope should be tied in such a way that it will not come loose and so that it can be untied quickly by pulling the loose end (See Fig. 2). In thick-necked animals, a block of wood placed in the jugular groove between the rope and the hide will help considerably in applying the desired pressure at the right point. The vein is a soft flexible tube through which blood flows back to the heart. Under ordinary conditions, it cannot be seen or felt with the fingers. When the flow of blood is blocked at the base of the neck by the choke rope, the vein becomes enlarged and rigid because of back pressure. If the choke rope is sufficiently tight, the vein stands out and can easily be seen and felt in thin-necked animals. As a further check in identifying the vein, tap it with the fingers in front of the point being tapped will confirm the fact that the vein is properly distended. It is impossible to put the needle in to the vein unless it is distended. Experienced operators are able to raise the vein simply by hand pressure, but the use of a choke rope is more certain.
2. Inserting the needle. This involves three distinct steps. First, insert the needle through the hide. Second, insert the needle into the vein. This may require two or three attempts before the vein is entered. The vein has a tendency to roll away from the point of the needle, especially if the needle is not sharp. The vein can be steadied by the finger and thumb of one hand. With the other hand, the needle point is placed directly over the vein, slanting it so its direction is along the length of the vein, either toward the head or heart. Properly positioned this way, a quick thrust of the needle will be followed by a spurt of blood through the needle, which indicates the vein has been entered. Third, once in the vein, the needle should be inserted along the length of the vein all the way to the hub, exercising caution to see that the needle does not penetrate the opposite side of the vein. Continuously steady flow of blood through the needle indicates that the needle is still in the vein. If blood does not flow continuously, the needle is out of the vein (or clogged) and another attempt must be made. If difficulty is encountered, it may be advisable to use the vein on the other side of the neck.
3. While the needle is being placed in proper position in the vein, an assistant should get the medication ready so that injection can be started without delay after the vein has been entered.
4. Making the injection. With the needle in position as indicated by the continuous flow of blood, release the choke rope by a quick pull on the free end. This is essential. The medication cannot flow into the vein while it is blocked. Immediately connect the syringe containing PENNOX™ 200 (oxytetracycline injection) to the needle and slowly depress the plunger. If there is resistance to depression of the plunger, this indicates the needle has slipped out of the vein (or is clogged) and the procedure will have to be repeated. Watch for any swelling under the skin near the needle, which would indicate that the medication is not going into the vein. Should this occur, it is best to try the vein on the opposite side of the neck.
5. Removing the needle. When injection is complete, remove needle with a straight pull. Then apply pressure over the area of the injection momentarily to control any bleeding through needle puncture, using cotton soaked in alcohol or other suitable antiseptic.

Precaution(s): Storage: PENNOX™ 200 does not require refrigeration, however it is recommended that it be stored at controlled room temperature. 15°-30°C (59°-86°F). Keep from freezing.

Caution(s): Exceeding the highest recommended dosage level of drug per pound of body weight per day, administering more than the recommended number of treatments, and/or exceeding 10 mL intramuscularly or subcutaneously per injection site in adult beef cattle and non-lactating dairy cattle, and 5 mL intramuscularly per injection site in adult swine, may result in antibiotic residues beyond the withdrawal period.

Consult with your veterinarian prior to administering this product in order to determine the proper treatment required in the event of an adverse reaction. At the first sign of any adverse reaction, discontinue use of product and seek the advice of your veterinarian. Some of the reactions may be attributed either to anaphylaxis (an allergic reaction) or to cardiovascular collapse of unknown cause.

Shock may be observed following intravenous administration, especially where highly concentrated materials are involved. To minimize this occurrence, it is recommended that PENNOX™ 200 be administered slowly by this route.

Shortly after injection, treated animals may have transient hemoglobinuria resulting in darkened urine.

As with all antibiotic preparations, use of this drug may result in overgrowth of nonsusceptible organisms, including fungi. A lack of response by the treated animal, or the development of new signs, may suggest that an overgrowth of nonsusceptible organisms has occurred. If any of these conditions occur, consult your veterinarian.

Since bacteriostatic drugs may interfere with the bactericidal action of penicillin, it is advisable to avoid giving PENNOX™ 200 in conjunction with penicillin.

Rapid intravenous administration may result in animal collapse.

Oxytetracycline should be administered intravenously slowly over a period of at least 5 minutes.

Warning(s): Discontinue treatment at least 28 days prior to slaughter of cattle and swine.

Not for use in lactating dairy animals.

Livestock drug, not for human use.

Restricted Drug (California) - Use only as directed.

Adverse Reactions: Reports of adverse reactions associated with oxytetracycline administration include injection site swelling, restlessness, ataxia, trembling, swelling of eyelids, ears, muzzle, anus and vulva (or scrotum and sheath in males), respiratory abnormalities (labored breathing, frothing at the mouth, collapse and possibly death. Some of these reactions may be attributed either to anaphylaxis (an allergic reaction) or to cardiovascular collapse of unknown cause.

Discussion:

Care of Sick Animals: The use of antibiotics in the management of diseases is based on an accurate diagnosis and an adequate course of treatment. When properly used in the treatment of diseases caused by susceptible organisms, most animals that have been treated with PENNOX™ 200 show a noticeable improvement within 24 to 48 hours. It is recommended that the diagnosis and treatment of animal diseases be carried out by a veterinarian. Since many diseases look alike but require different types of treatment, the use of professional veterinary and laboratory services can reduce treatment time, cost and needless losses. Good housing, sanitation and nutrition are important in the maintenance of healthy animals, and are essential in the treatment of diseased animals.

Presentation: PENNOX™ 200 is available in 500 mL serum bottles, packed 12 bottles per case.

Compendium Code No.: 10450171 08/00

PENNOX™ 343 SOLUBLE POWDER

PennField **Water Medication**

Oxytetracycline HCl Soluble Powder

ANADA No.: 200-026

Active Ingredient(s): Each 4.78 oz packet contains 102.4 grams of oxytetracycline HCl and will make:

512 gallons (1,938 L) containing 200 mg oxytetracycline HCl per gallon.
256 gallons (969 L) containing 400 mg oxytetracycline HCl per gallon.
128 gallons (484 L) containing 800 mg oxytetracycline HCl per gallon.
Each 23.9 oz packet contains 512 grams of oxytetracycline HCl and will make:
2,560 gallon (9,690 L) containing 200 mg oxytetracycline HCl per gallon.
1,280 gallons (4,845 L) containing 400 mg oxytetracycline HCl per gallon.
640 gallons (2,420 L) containing 800 mg oxytetracycline HCl per gallon.

Indications: A broad-spectrum antibiotic for control and treatment of specific diseases in poultry, cattle, swine and sheep.

Directions for Use: For the control and treatment of the following diseases caused by organisms susceptible to oxytetracycline.

Swine	Dosage
Bacterial enteritis caused by *Escherichia coli* and *Salmonella choleraesuis* Bacterial pneumonia caused by *Pasteurella multocida* For Breeding Swine: Leptospirosis (reducing the incidence of abortions and shedding of leptospira) caused by *Leptospira pomona*	Administer in the drinking water at a level of 10 mg oxytetracycline HCl per pound of body weight daily. Administer up to 5 days.
Calves, Beef Cattle and Non-Lactating Dairy Cattle	
Bacterial enteritis caused by *Escherichia coli* Bacterial pneumonia (shipping fever complex) caused by *Pasteurella multocida*	Administer in the drinking water at a level of 10 mg oxytetracycline HCl per pound of body weight daily. Administer up to 5 days.
Sheep	
Bacterial enteritis caused by *Escherichia coli* Bacterial pneumonia (shipping fever complex) caused by *Pasteurella multocida*	Administer in the drinking water at a level of 10 mg oxytetracycline HCl per pound of body weight daily. Administer up to 5 days.

The 4.78 oz packet will treat 10,240 pounds of swine, cattle or sheep at 10 mg/pound. The 23.9 oz packet will treat 51,200 pounds of swine, cattle or sheep at 10 mg/pound. Do not mix this product with milk or milk replacers. Administer one hour before or two hours after feeding milk or milk replacers.

Special Note: The concentration of drug required in medicated water must be adequate to compensate for variation in the age of the animal, feed consumption rate and the environmental temperature and humidity, each of which affects water consumption.

For the control of the following poultry diseases caused by organisms susceptible to oxytetracycline: Add the following amount to two gallons (4.78 oz packet), or ten gallons (23.9 oz packet) of stock solution when proportioner is set to meter at the rate of one ounce per gallon.

	Dosage	4.78 oz Packs/ 2 Gallons Stock Solution	23.9 oz packs/ 10 Gallons Stock Solution
Chickens			
Infectious synovitis caused by *Mycoplasma synoviae*	200-400 mg/gal	½-1	½-1
Chronic respiratory disease (CRD) and air-sac infection caused by *Mycoplasma gallisepticum* and *Escherichia coli*	400-800 mg/gal	1-2	1-2
Fowl cholera caused by *Pasteurella multocida*	400-800 mg/gal	1-2	1-2
Turkeys			
Hexamitiasis caused by *Hexamita meleagridis*	200-400 mg/gal	½-1	½-1
Infectious synovitis caused by *Mycoplasma synoviae*	400 mg/gal	1	1
Growing Turkeys - Complicating bacterial organisms associated with bluecomb (transmissible enteritis, coronaviral enteritis)	25 mg/lb body weight daily	varies with age and water consumption (1 pack will treat 4,096 pounds of turkeys)	varies with age and water consumption (1 pack will treat 20,480 pounds of turkeys)

Medicate continuously at the first clinical signs of disease and continue for 7 to 14 consecutive days. If improvement is not noted within 24 to 48 hours, consult a veterinarian or a diagnostic laboratory to determine diagnosis and advice on dosage.

Precaution(s): Recommended Storage: Store below 77°F (25°C).

Caution(s): Use as sole source of oxytetracycline. Not to be used for more than 14 consecutive days in chickens and turkeys or 5 consecutive days in cattle, swine or sheep. Prepare fresh solutions every 24 hours.

Do not administer this product with milk or milk replacers. Administer 1 hour before or 2 hours after feeding milk or milk replacers.

For use in drinking water only - Not for use in liquid feed supplements.

Warning(s): Do not administer to cattle or sheep within 5 days of slaughter. Zero day withdrawal in chickens, turkeys and swine. Do not administer to chickens or turkeys producing eggs for human consumption.

Livestock Drug—Not for human use. Keep out of reach of children.

Presentation: Available in 40 x 4.78 oz packets per pack and 24 x 23.9 oz packets per pack.

Compendium Code No.: 10450182 01/02

PENTASOL® POWDER Ⓒ

Delmarva **Euthanasia Agent**

Sodium Pentobarbital Powder (Non-Sterile)

ANADA No.: 200-071

Active Ingredient(s): When powder is reconstituted to 250 mL with water, each mL will contain 392 mg Sodium Pentobarbital.

Indications: For euthanasia of animals.

Dosage and Administration: Directions for Mixing: Add water slowly to between the 150 mL and 200 mL lines. After replacing cap, shake well to dissolve all of the powder. Fill to the 250 mL line only with more water. Do not fill above the 250 mL line.

Inject 1 mL for each 10 pounds of body weight (minimum 1 mL). Intravenous injection is preferred. Intraperitoneal or intracardiac injections may be made when intravenous injection is impractical, as in a very small dog, or cat, or in a comatose dog or cat with impaired vascular functions.

Precaution(s): Potency guaranteed for 120 days after reconstitution.

Caution(s): Federal law restricts this drug to use by or on the order of a licensed veterinarian.

For veterinary use only.

For animal euthanasia only.

Warning(s): Poison. Keep out of reach of children.

Must not be used for therapeutic purposes and must not be used in animals intended for food. If eye contact, flush with water and seek medical advice/attention.

Presentation: 250 mL (98 g) bottle (NDC-59079-103-25).

Compendium Code No.: 14260030 01893

PENTOTHAL® STERILE POWDER (VETERINARY) CIII

Abbott **General Anesthetic**

Sodium Thiopental for Injection

Active Ingredient(s):

Sodium thiopental .... 5.0 g

Indications: PENTOTHAL® (sodium thiopental) for Injection is recommended especially for minor surgery, reduction of fractures, physical examination, radiography and dentistry. Animals can be completely anesthetized with a single intravenous dose. Since the period of ataxia is short, the patient is able to leave the hospital or office without a prolonged delay.

This type of anesthesia is also useful in prolonged operations once the veterinarian develops the necessary technique for the several species, using intermittent or continuous injection.

It is also a valuable induction anesthetic in preparation for a volatile anesthetic which may be required for prolonged operations, particularly in large animals.

Dosage and Administration: PENTOTHAL® is intended for intravenous administration only.

Dogs:

Dosage: Range, 6.0 to 12.0 mg (1/10 to 1/5 gr.) per pound of body weight. The fatal dose is approximately twice the maximum recommended dose.[21]

For Anesthesia of Short Duration (8-10 minutes) which may be sufficient for X-ray, physical examination, and minor surgery, 6.0 to 7.5 mg (1/10 to 1/8 gr.)/lb.

For Anesthesia of Intermediate Duration (10-15 minutes) such as might be used for dentistry or reduction of fractures, 7.5 to 10 mg (1/8 to 1/6 gr.)/lb.

For Major Surgery requiring anesthesia of longer duration (longer than 15 minutes) induce anesthesia with 10 to 12 mg (1/6 to 1/5 gr.) per pound of body weight; about half the dose is given rapidly and the balance more slowly, administered over approximately 15 seconds.[1] Depth of anesthesia may be determined by the loss of pedal and eye reflexes. The first stage of anesthesia following the administration of sodium thiopental is commonly evidenced by a deep yawn followed very shortly by loss of reflexes.

Although the initial dose may be sufficient for an entire operation, the surgeon should be prepared to administer additional drug as needed. Some clinicians prefer to leave the needle in the vein. Any additional drug should be administered a little more slowly. As much as a third or more of the original dose may be required to produce the depth of anesthesia. Injections should not be at closer than 30 to 60-second intervals.

With Preanesthetic Agents. Preanesthetic agents (such as morphine or a tranquilizer) decrease the dosage requirements of sodium thiopental, provide for smoother induction and recovery, and may prolong the recovery period. Following morphine as a preanesthetic agent, the dose of this drug may be reduced as much as 40 to 50 percent; following a tranquilizer 10 to 25 percent.

The Urinary Bladder should be emptied immediately after anesthesia is induced, particularly when prolonged anesthesia is anticipated.

Cats:

PENTOTHAL® use and limitations for cats is similar to that detailed for dogs.[19] The usual dose range is 8 to 12 mg/lb intravenously.

Equines:

Dosage: For best results, the intravenous administration of a phenothiazine tranquilizer is recommended 10 to 20 minutes prior to the administration of sodium thiopental. Rapid injection of sodium thiopental is then recommended and the doses given are for this type of administration. Slower or repeated administration should be avoided. In the rare event that the animal fails to respond to the drug, the procedure should not be repeated in less than 24 hours.

With Preanesthetic Tranquilization, 2.7 to 5.9 mg (1/23 to 1/11 gr.) sodium thiopental per pound of body weight. An average of 3.75 mg (1/17 gr.) per pound of body weight is recommended.[11]

No restraint is necessary for the recovery period.

Without Preanesthetic Tranquilization, 4.0 to 7.0 mg (1/16 to 1/9 gr.) per pound of body weight. For an average horse (900 to 1100 lbs) the recommended dose is 4.5 to 5.0 mg (1/14 to 1/13 gr.)/lb. The largest dose level is recommended for smaller animals such as ponies. The smallest dose level is recommended for the larger draft horses and older debilitated animals.[15,16]

Restraint is recommended to reduce or eliminate struggling during recovery.[9]

Sodium thiopental is an effective and quick acting short-term general anesthetic for equines.[24] However, it is desirable either to apply restraint before the recovery period or to use a tranquilizer or sedative with this anesthetic agent to allow smooth recovery.

Ten to twenty minutes after the intravenous administration of a tranquilizer, (promazine hydrochloride), the rapid intravenous injection of sodium thiopental, in 20 to 40 mL sterile distilled water, will induce anesthesia easily and rapidly.[11] Surgical anesthesia ranges from 3 to 14 minutes, righting time from 15 to 120 minutes, and "restraint was not required and recovery was rapid and occurred without emergence excitement or struggling." Animals should not be stimulated to rise.

Sodium thiopental is particularly recommended for general anesthesia of short duration such as may be required for castration, point firing, dentistry, and minor surgery.[2,16,25]

PENTOTHAL® is the induction anesthetic of choice in preparation for a volatile anesthetic in prolonged operations required for major surgery.[1,12]

Bovine:

Dosage: In addition to individual variation in response to the anesthetic which cannot be always anticipated, there is a consistent difference in the response of nursing calves and of older animals, as pointed out below.

A. Animals 300 pounds or over

The recommended dose is 3.7 to 7.0 mg (1/17 to 1/9 gr.) per pound of body weight, depending on the depth of anesthesia required, administered rapidly. Rapid administration is defined as injecting the entire specified dose (10 to 30 mL) with a hypodermic syringe in one motion thrust. To deliver 5.0 mg/lb of body weight, using a 25% solution would require 2.0 mL for each 100 pounds of body weight.

Should additional drug be required (as in lighter weight animals) it should be injected more slowly, particularly in the obese animal, and the total amount should not exceed 10 mg (1/6 gr.) per pound of body weight. Nuttall[20] has reported one death from the rapid injection of 10 mg/lb.

When a phenothiazine tranquilizer is administered intravenously 10 to 15 minutes prior to the injection of sodium thiopental, the lower dose of this drug [3.7 to 4.5 mg (1/17 to 1/15 gr.)/lb] should be used. The anesthesia following the tranquilizer is more profound and the righting time is prolonged slightly.

B. Unweaned Calves

For unweaned calves, from which food has been withheld for 6 to 12 hours prior to anesthesia, no more than 3.0 mg (1/22 gr.) of PENTOTHAL® per pound is required for deep surgical anesthesia.

If a phenothiazine tranquilizer, is administered to such calves 10 to 20 minutes prior to anesthesia, the dose of sodium thiopental is reduced to 2.0 mg (1/32 gr.) per pound of body weight.[10]

This drug is an effective, quick-acting, short-term general anesthetic for the bovine. It is not necessary to provide restraint for the recovery period for the bovine. There is, however, a marked tendency for the bovine to regurgitate with resulting inhalation pneumonia and suffocation. Accordingly, the surgeon should be prepared to keep the trachea open. Lowering the head and endotracheal intubation are suggested means to help avoid mechanical suffocation. The response to this rapid intravenous drug is almost immediate. Within a few seconds the standing animal will fall and is ready for surgery. Surgical anesthesia usually lasts for 5 to 10 minutes. During this period respiration will appear shallow. There may be a slight reflex response to corneal and anal stimulation but no resistance to passive movement of the limbs. Righting time is usually 2 to 3 hours and uneventful.

This drug is particularly useful for operations of short duration such as laparotomies in calves, dehorning, hernial repair, other minor surgery, and induction anesthesia preceding the use of volatile anesthetics.

Henderson[7] used this drug successfully in operations on hundreds of cattle at doses of 4 to 5 mg per pound of body weight. He administered it rapidly in the jugular vein of the standing animal. Within seconds the animal would fall. It usually would remain in deep narcosis for 25 to 35 minutes and would not rise for 2 to 5 hours.

Ford[5] using 6 to 9 mg/kg, somewhat higher than the usually recommended dose, obtained deep surgical anesthesia in 8 to 14 seconds, apnea for 20 seconds to 2 minutes, followed by shallow but regular respiration. Recovery required 25 minutes to 5 hours.

Nuttall[20] produced deep surgical anesthesia, which lasted 30 to 60 minutes, immediately after the rapid intravenous injection of 3.0 mg/lb of drug to 10 unweaned but fasted calves. Nuttall further found that when a phenothiazine tranquilizer precedes the anesthetic, the dose of sodium thiopental to produce the same deep surgical anesthesia was reduced to 2.0 mg/lb.

When recovery is sufficiently apparent, it is helpful to roll the bovine up to rest on its sternum so that rumination and chewing of the cud may be resumed.

Ovine:

This preparation has been used successfully for experimental surgery in lambs weighing about 35 lbs each, at the rate of 4.5 to 6.75 mg/lb, depending on the depth of anesthesia desired.[23,26] Induction was rapid and without excitement; recovery was smooth and uneventful. About half of the maximum dose was infected rapidly in the jugular vein and thereafter continued more slowly — over a 30 to 60-second period — until the desired depth of anesthesia was achieved. For deep surgical anesthesia administration was continued until apnea was evident for about 15 seconds. (The practicing veterinary surgeon probably would not want to push anesthesia to this depth.) Apnea was followed by shallow but regular respiration, the absence of corneal reflex, and complete muscle relaxation.

Increased salivation and ruminal regurgitation in sheep, as in cattle, is a problem with general anesthesia and must be handled as in cattle.

Swine:

This preparation has been found to be a superior anesthetic for swine because of the ease of administration, rapid induction, and short smooth recovery period. It is indicated as the anesthetic of choice for this species.[18] As in other species, there is an inverse ratio between the dose level and the weight of the animal. The minimum anesthetic dose for healthy animals is shown in the following table:

Pounds of Body Weight	Dose	
	mg/lb	mL 5% (sol./lb)
10-50	5.0	0.1
50-100	4.5	0.09
100-200	4.0	0.08
200-300	3.5	0.07
300-400	3.0	0.06
400-600	2.5	0.05

Slightly over the dose, calculated from the above table, should be drawn into the syringe because an occasional animal may require slightly more. One-half the calculated dose is injected rapidly and the remainder more slowly until the desired anesthesia is obtained; caution should be used with unthrifty animals which may not require, and thus should not receive, the full calculated dose. Only a rare robust animal will require slightly more than the minimum calculated dose. Respiration should be watched, an occasional animal may require artificial respiration.

For large animals sodium thiopental is best administered through a small gauge needle into the ear vein while the animal is restrained with a regular swine holder or with a rope in the mouth.

Piglets and small swine may be placed conveniently in a trough in a supine position and injection made directly into the anterior vena cava.

This drug is a particularly useful anesthetic agent for such operations on swine as hernial repair, tumor (scirrhous cord) removal, tusk removal and similar oral surgery, castration, splenectomies, and lancing abscesses.

According to Muhrer,[18] the distinct advantages of this drug as an anesthetic agent for swine are:

1. There is less danger of injury to the surgeon or handlers.
2. It is more humane and places the operations on such farm animals on a high professional level.
3. It permits less commotion in the facilities in which the swine are housed.
4. It eliminates the need for physical restraint and handling of unruly animals which may be detrimental to the animal and may even interfere with the actual operation.
5. The drug is easily and quickly administered and thus a great time saver.
6. Once the desired depth of anesthesia is achieved, it is seldom necessary to supplement it with a volatile anesthetic or any other agent.

Precaution(s): Protect kits from freezing and extreme heat. Keep reconstituted solution in a cool place.

Contents of each kit should be completely reconstituted and used within 24 hours. Administer only clear solution.

Caution(s): Federal (U.S.A.) law restricts this drug to use by or on the order of a licensed veterinarian.

Each kit provides adequate medication for several patients.

Care must be taken that barbiturates are not injected perivascularly because soft tissue irritation can result. Care should also be taken that the barbiturate is not injected intra-arterially.

PENTOTHAL® has little effect upon blood pressure but may depress and slow respiration. In the rare cases of laryngeal spasm, an open air passage must be maintained. Overdosing may cause respiratory failure. In this event, artificial respiration and other respiratory stimulants should be used.

Additional care should be employed when anesthetizing anemic or hypovolemic animals, and animals with cardiac or respiratory problems. The following conditions may cause prolonged recovery after a barbiturate anesthetic: (1) liver pathology, (2) elevated urea nitrogen or electrolyte imbalance, and (3) hypothermic or malnourished animals following a prolonged surgical procedure. In general, barbiturates should not be employed for cesarean section because of respiratory depression to the fetus.

Preanesthetic agents, analgesics, some tranquilizers, corticosteroids, and sulfonamides[17] may potentiate the drug and thus reduce the amount necessary to induce a given depth of anesthesia.[22]

Since the placenta is not a protective barrier against sodium thiopental or any other barbiturate, the full anesthetic dose should not be used in pregnant animals. Light doses of this drug may be used as an induction agent in such cases.[3,13,14]

To reduce the chance of vomiting and excessive salivation, food should be withheld for 12 hours, when possible, prior to administration.

As with all general anesthetics, occasional hypersensitive animals will respond atypically to this drug.

During recovery from barbiturate anesthesia, it is suggested the animal be kept warm and undisturbed. If recovery is prolonged, the animal should be periodically turned over to decrease hyperstatic congestion. Food and water should be withheld until the animal is completely recovered from the anesthetic.

Discussion: The present interest in Veterinary PENTOTHAL® anesthesia has resulted from its safety, flexibility, smoothness, short action, and rapid elimination. The short, quiet recovery period with minimal side reactions adds to the advantages of this drug, making its use particularly valuable in veterinary surgery.[6]

PENTOTHAL® has advantages for both hospital and office use, especially for operative procedures of short duration. Intravenously, induction is prompt, anesthesia is of short duration and the animal recovers promptly with a short period of ataxia.

References: Available upon request.

Presentation: The water diluent in Veterinary PENTOTHAL® Kits is supplied in various size glass containers with various dosage sizes of PENTOTHAL®. Kits include all items needed for aseptic transfer of PENTOTHAL® powder from a squeeze bottle into the diluent container.

See following table for list of sizes available.

Veterinary PENTOTHAL® and Diluent Kits

List No.	Pentothal	Diluent	Reconstituted Concentration
8912	5.0 g	200 mL	2.5%
8913	5.0 g	100 mL	5.0%

® Registered trademark of Abbott Laboratories.

Distributed by: Merial.

Compendium Code No.: 10240070 06-9305/R3

PERCORTEN®-V ℞

Novartis **Corticosteroid Injection**

(desoxycorticosterone pivalate) Injectable Suspension

NADA No.: 141-029

Active Ingredient(s): Each mL contains:

Desoxycorticosterone pivalate (DOCP) .... 25 mg
Methylcellulose .... 10.5 mg
Sodium carboxymethylcellulose .... 3 mg
Polysorbate 80 .... 1 mg
Sodium chloride .... 8 mg
Thimerosal (preservative) 0.002%
In water for injection q.s.

Indications: For use as replacement therapy for the mineralocorticoid deficit in dogs with primary adrenocortical insufficiency.

Pharmacology: Description: The active ingredient in PERCORTEN®-V is desoxycorticosterone pivalate (DOCP). It is a mineralocorticoid hormone and an analog of desoxycorticosterone. It is white, odorless, and stable in air. It is practically insoluble in water, sparingly soluble in acetone, slightly soluble in methanol, ether and vegetable oils. The molecular weight is 414.58. It is designated chemically as 21 (2,2-dimethyl-1-oxopropoxy)-pregn-4-ene-3,20-dione. The empirical formula is $C_{26}H_{38}O_4$ and the structural formula is:

H_2C—O—C(=O)—$C(CH_3)_3$; H_3C; C=O; H_3C; O

PERCORTEN®-V is a white aqueous suspension. Each mL contains 25 mg desoxycorticosterone pivalate. Inactive ingredients are water for injection, methylcellulose, sodium carboxymethylcellulose, polysorbate 80, sodium chloride, and thimerosal.

Clinical Pharmacology: Desoxycorticosterone pivalate (DOCP), like other adrenocorticoid hormones, is thought to act by controlling the rate of synthesis of proteins. It reacts with receptor proteins in the cytoplasm to form a steroid-receptor complex. This complex moves into the nucleus, where it binds to chromatin that results in genetic transcription of cellular DNA to messenger RNA. The steroid hormones appear to induce transcription and synthesis of specific proteins, which produce the physiologic effects seen after administration.

DOCP is a long-acting ester of desoxycorticosterone acetate (DOCA), which is recognized as having the same qualitative effects as the natural mineralocorticoid hormone aldosterone.

The most important effect of DOCP is to increase the rate of renal tubular absorption of sodium. This effect is seen most intensely in the thick portion of the ascending limb of the loop of Henle. It also increases sodium absorption in the proximal convoluted tubule, but this effect is less important in sodium retention. Chloride follows the sodium out of the renal tubule.

Another important effect of DOCP is enhanced renal excretion of potassium. This effect is driven by the resorption of sodium which pulls potassium from the extracellular fluid into the renal tubules, thus promoting potassium excretion.

DOCP also acts to increase extracellular fluid volume. The enhanced retention of sodium, chloride and bicarbonate, creates an osmotic gradient that promotes water absorption from the renal tubules. The extracellular fluid volume is supported. This expands the blood volume and improves the venous return to the heart and cardiac output. The expanded blood volume and increased cardiac output may result in elevated blood pressure. PERCORTEN®-V prevents the life threatening hypotensive shock and pre-renal azotemia observed in animals suffering from hypoadrenocorticism.

The effects of PERCORTEN®-V on electrolytes and extracellular fluid volume are dependent on a functioning kidney. Animals suffering from hypovolemia, pre-renal azotemia, and inadequate tissue perfusion must be rehydrated with intravenous fluid (saline) therapy, before starting PERCORTEN®-V therapy. Primary renal disease should be ruled out before starting PERCORTEN®-V therapy.

DOCP is an insoluble ester of desoxycorticosterone. The crystals are injected intramuscularly as a microcrystalline depot where they slowly dissolve over time.

Dosage and Administration: Dosage:[1,2] In treating canine hypoadrenocorticism, PERCORTEN®-V replaces the mineralocorticoid hormones only. Glucocorticoid replacement must be supplied by small daily doses of glucocorticoid hormones (e.g., prednisone or prednisolone) (0.2 - 0.4 mg/kg/day).

Dosage requirements are variable and must be individualized on the basis of the response of the patient to therapy. Begin treatment with PERCORTEN®-V at a dose of 1.0 mg per pound of body weight every 25 days. In some patients the dose may be reduced. Serum sodium and potassium levels should be monitored to assure the animal is properly compensated. Most patients are well controlled with a dose range of 0.75 to 1.0 mg per pound of body weight, given every 21 to 30 days.

The well-controlled patient will have normal electrolytes at 14 days after administration or may exhibit slight hyponatremia and hyperkalemia. This needs no additional therapy as long as the patient is active and eating normally. Watch closely for depression, lethargy, vomiting or diarrhea which indicate a probable glucocorticoid deficiency.

At the end of the 25-day dosing interval, the patient should be clinically normal and have normal serum electrolytes. Alternatively, they may have slight hyponatremia and slight hyperkalemia. This constellation of signs indicate that the dosage and dosage interval should not be altered.

If the dog is not clinically normal or serum electrolytes are abnormal, then the dosage interval should be decreased 2-3 days.

Occasionally, dogs on PERCORTEN®-V therapy may develop polyuria and polydipsia (PU/PD). This usually indicates excess glucocorticoid but may also indicate a PERCORTEN®-V excess. It is prudent to begin by decreasing the glucocorticoid dose first. If the PU/PD persists, then decrease the dose of PERCORTEN®-V without changing the interval between doses.

Please note: Failure to administer glucocorticoids is the most common reason for treatment failure. Signs of glucocorticoid deficiency include; depression, lethargy, vomiting and diarrhea. Such signs should be treated with high doses of injectable glucocorticoids (prednisolone or dexamethasone), followed by continued oral therapy (0.2 - 0.4 mg/kg/day). Oral supplementation with salt (NaCl) is not necessary with animals receiving PERCORTEN®-V.

Guide to Maintenance Therapy:

Starting Dose:

DOCP 1 mg/lb every 25 days

Prednisone 0.2 - 0.4 mg/kg/day

Guides for Adjustment:

Clinical Problem/Solution:

Polyuria/Polydipsia:

- decrease prednisone dose first,
- then decrease DOCP dose,
- do not change DOCP interval

Depression, lethargy, vomiting or diarrhea:

- increase prednisone dose

Hyperkalemia, Hyponatremia:

- decrease DOCP interval 2-3 days

Administration: Before injection, shake the vial thoroughly to mix the microcrystals with the suspension vehicle. PERCORTEN®-V suspension is to be injected intramuscularly. Care should be used to prevent inadvertent intravenous injection, which may cause acute collapse and shock. Such animals should receive immediate therapy for shock with intravenous fluids and glucocorticoids.

Contraindication(s): Do not use this drug in pregnant dogs. Do not use in dogs suffering from congestive heart disease, severe renal disease or edema.

Precaution(s): Storage: Store at room temperature, preferably between 15° and 30°C (59° and 86°F). Protect from light. Protect from freezing.

Caution(s): Federal (U.S.A.) law restricts this drug to use by or on the order of a licensed veterinarian.

Some patients are more sensitive to the actions of PERCORTEN®-V and may exhibit side effects in an exaggerated degree. Some patients may show signs of hypernatremia or hypokalemia. The dosage of PERCORTEN®-V should be reduced in these patients.

Like other adrenocortical hormones, PERCORTEN®-V may cause severe side effects if dosage is too high or prolonged. It may cause polyuria, polydipsia, increased blood volume, edema and cardiac enlargement. Excessive weight gain may indicate fluid retention secondary to sodium retention. PERCORTEN®-V should be used with caution in patients with congestive heart disease, edema or renal disease.

Warning(s): Keep this and all drugs out of the reach of children. In case of human consumption, contact a physician or Poison Control Center immediately.

Adverse Reactions: The following adverse reactions have been reported following the use of PERCORTEN®-V: depression, polyuria, polydipsia, anorexia, skin and coat changes, diarrhea, vomiting, weakness, weight loss, incontinence, pain on injection and injection site abscess. Some of these effects may resolve with adjustments in dose or interval of PERCORTEN®-V or concomitant glucocorticoid medication.

Discussion: Case Management:[1,2] An accurate diagnosis of primary canine adrenocortical insufficiency is of paramount importance for treatment success and should be established before initiation of PERCORTEN®-V therapy. While hyponatremia and hyperkalemia are highly suggestive of adrenocortical insufficiency, they are not pathognomonic. A definitive diagnosis can only be made with an ACTH stimulation test. At diagnosis, classic cases of canine adrenocortical insufficiency may include clinical signs. Those signs are anorexia, lethargy, depression, weakness, vomiting and/or regurgitation, weight loss, diarrhea and collapse, serum sodium values less than 135 mEq/L, serum potassium greater than 6 mEq/L, sodium/potassium ratios below 25:1, plasma or serum cortisol concentration less than 4 μg/dl pre-and-post ACTH administration. Once the diagnosis is made, immediate therapy must be given to normalize electrolyte imbalance, correct hypovolemic shock and re-establish normal homeostasis. Such therapy should include, large volumes of intravenous physiologic saline, glucocorticoids (i.e., prednisolone, dexamethasone) at shock doses and PERCORTEN®-V. Once the acute crisis has passed, renal and cardiovascular function should return to normal. Then begin chronic lifelong therapy with PERCORTEN®-V and glucocorticoids.

Trial Data: Efficacy: PERCORTEN®-V given intramuscularly at the appropriate dose and interval, is effective in replacing the mineralocorticoid deficit in dogs suffering from primary hypoadrenocorticism.

Results of two 75-day clinical studies in dogs with primary hypoadrenocorticism have demonstrated the clinical efficacy of PERCORTEN®-V. Each dog received three doses of PERCORTEN®-V (on days 0, 25 and 50). The results are summarized below.

	Clinical Study Number	
	01	02
Number of Dogs	49	18
Average Diagnostic Values:		
Serum Sodium (mEq/L)	128.40	130.72
Serum Potassium (mEq/L)	7.28	7.47
Sodium/Potassium Ratio	18.09	17.86
ACTH Stimulation Test:		
Cortisol Resting (μg/dl)	0.28	0.68
Cortisol Post Stimulation (μg/dl)	0.27	1.34
Average PERCORTEN®-V Dose (mg/lb):		
Day 0	0.97	0.99
Day 25	0.96	0.99
Day 50	0.94	0.97
Concomitant Glucocorticoid (Pred)	47%	39%
Sodium/Potassium Ratios		
Day 0	25.18	26.42
Day 14	36.36	-
Day 25	29.64	-
Day 39	34.94	-
Day 50	30.33	.
Day 64	35.30	-
Day 75	30.32	30.59
% Efficacy Therapy	96%	100%

Safety:[3] In a laboratory study, the safety of PERCORTEN®-V, was established in five month old Beagle dogs. PERCORTEN®-V was administered IM to 24 Beagles at 0, 2.2, 6.6 or 11 mg/kg of body weight daily over a consecutive 3-day period every 28 days (equivalent to a cumulative monthly dosage of 0, 6.6, 19.8 or 33 mg/kg) for 6 months. This resulted in no mortality or any significant effects on body weight, food consumption, and ophthalmic observations at any dose level. However, polyuria and polydipsia were noted and creatinine concentration decreased (14-89 mg/dl) in the 1X, 3X and 5X groups. Histopathological changes were only observed in the kidneys when PERCORTEN®-V was administered at ≥ 6.6 mg/kg. The primary renal lesion consisted of glomerulonephropathy seen in all males at ≥ 6.6 mg/kg, in one female at 6.6 mg/kg, and in all females at 11 mg/kg. Other possible treatment-related lesions in the kidney, observed sporadically in the 6.6 and 11.0 mg/kg groups, were tubular hyperplasia, inflammation and tubular dilatation. Glomerulonephropathy may possibly be attributed to the pharmacological effects of the drug although there were no clinical measurements assessed in this study. In conclusion, PERCORTEN®-V was well tolerated, when administered at 2.2 mg/kg on three consecutive days in every 28-day period for six months.

References: Available upon request.

Presentation: 4 mL multiple-dose vials (1 vial per carton).

NAH/PER/VI/3 07/02

Compendium Code No.: 11310043

PERFORMAX™ RATION MAXIMIZER

Equicare **Large Animal Supplement**

Granular Feed Supplement

Guaranteed Analysis: Per 2 Oz.:

Crude Protein, minimum 15%
Crude Fat, minimum........ 15%
Crude Fiber, maximum........ 8%
Vitamin E, minimum........ 100 I.U.
Vitamin B_{12}, minimum .... 20 mcg
Riboflavin, minimum .... 20 mg
Pantothenic acid, minimum .... 30 mg
Thiamine, minimum........ 30 mg
Niacin, minimum .... 20 mg
Vitamin B_6, minimum........ 5.0 mcg
Folic acid, minimum........ 20 mg
Choline, minimum .... 100 mg
Biotin, minimum .... 0.5 mg
Ascorbic acid, minimum .... 30 mg
Saccharomyces cerevisiae .... 25 billion cells

Ingredients: Yeast culture product (YEA-SACC[1026]), soybean meal, vegetable fat, dextrose, heat stabilized flax meal, dl-α-tocopherol acetate, choline chloride, propionic acid, biotin, BHT/BHA, calcium pantothenate, thiamine mononitrate, ascorbic acid, riboflavin, folic acid, niacin, vitamin B_{12}, pyridoxine HCl.

The base ingredient in PERFORMAX™ Ration Maximizer is a live yeast culture. PERFORMAX™ Ration Maximizer also contains a complete profile of the B complex vitamins; antioxidant vitamins C and E; protein; and fats.

Indications: A granular feed supplement for all classes of horses containing B complex, vitamins E and C, calories and protein all in a yeast culture base.

Dosage and Administration: Feeding Instructions: Feed 2 to 4 ounces per day in regular grain ration (based on a 1100 pound adult horse).

Precaution(s): Store out of reach of children and animals. Keep in sealed container in a cool, dry place.

Presentation: 3.75 lbs (1.7 kg) (30 day supply), 8 lbs (3.6 kg) (64 day supply) and 20 lbs (9.07 kg) (160 day supply).

YEA-SACC is a registered trademark of Alltech, Inc.

Compendium Code No.: 14470110

PERFORMER® BORDE-VAC

AgriLabs **Bacterin**

Bordetella Bronchiseptica Bacterin, Extracted Cellular Antigens

U.S. Vet. Lic. No.: 462

Contents: This product contains the antigen listed above.

Contains thimerosal (merthiolate) as a preservative.

Indications: PERFORMER® Borde-Vac is recommended for use as an aid in the control of canine infectious tracheobronchitis (kennel cough) caused by the organism represented.

Directions: Shake well. Administer 1 mL to healthy dogs at 8 weeks of age. For initial vaccination, a second dose is required 2-4 weeks later. Administer by subcutaneous injection only. Annual revaccination with a single 1 mL dose is recommended.

Precaution(s): Store at 35°F-45°F (2°C-7°C). Do not freeze. Use entire contents when first opened.

Caution(s): In case of anaphylactoid reactions, epinephrine should be administered immediately. Transient local irritation at the site of injection, though rare, may occur subsequent to use of the product.

Use special caution when vaccinating miniature or small breed dogs.

Presentation: 1 dose with syringe, 25x1 dose vials, and 10 dose (10 mL) vial.

Manufactured by: Biocor Animal Health Inc., Omaha, NE 68134.

Compendium Code No.: 10581460 AL708-699 / AL7025-194

PERFORMER® EAR MITE KILLER

AgriLabs **Otic Parasiticide**

EPA Reg. No.: 769-583-53302

Active Ingredient(s):

Pyrethrins 0.15%
Piperonyl butoxide, technical* 1.00%
N-octyl bicycloheptene dicarboximide........ 0.50%
Di-n-propyl isocinchomeronate........ 1.00%
Inert ingredients 97.35%
Total 100.00%

*Equivalent to 0.80% of butylcarbityl 6-propylpiperonyl ether and 0.20% related compounds.

Contains aloe vera.

Indications: PERFORMER® EAR MITE KILLER works on cats, dogs, horses and rabbits on contact to kill and repel ear mites, flies, gnats, mosquitoes, fleas, ticks, lice and mange mites on exposed skin surfaces for 3-5 days.

Directions for Use: It is a violation of Federal Law to use this product in a manner inconsistent with its labeling.

Do not put treatment directly onto broken skin or an open wound. Treatment may be applied on a bandage.

Dogs, Puppies, Cats and Kittens:

To Kill and Repel Ear Mites: Clean ear to remove built-up wax and dirt. Gently dry ear with a cotton ball or soft cloth and apply a thin film of treatment. The treatment may be applied daily for 7 to 10 days.

To Kill Ticks: Make sure treatment covers ticks.

To Use as a Repellent: Spread treatment lightly on outer and inner surface of the outer ear and between the toes before animals enter infected area. Repeat daily as needed.

Horses and Foals:

To control Ticks, Gnats, Flies, Mosquitoes and Mange Mites: Before application remove dirt or debris by brushing or washing with a mild detergent. Allow to completely dry. Apply a light film to affected areas daily, massaging into the skin for 2 to 3 days. Then apply every 3 to 5 days.

Precautionary Statements: Hazards to Humans and Domestic Animals: Caution:

Human: Harmful if swallowed. Avoid inhaling vapors. Avoid contact with eyes. In case of contact, immediately flush eyes with plenty of water. Obtain medical attention if irritation persists. If swallowed, do not induce vomiting. Wash hands with soap and water after using.

Animals: Avoid contact with eyes. If in eyes, flush with water.

Environmental Hazards: This product is toxic to fish. Do not apply directly to water.

Physical or Chemical Hazards: None.

Storage and Disposal:

Storage: Store in a cool, dry area.

Disposal: Do not reuse the container. Wrap it and put it in the trash.

Warning(s): Do not use on meat or milk producing animals.

Keep out of reach of children.

Presentation: 6 fl. oz. containers.

Compendium Code No.: 10581470

PERFORMER®-FELINE 4

AgriLabs **Vaccine**

Feline Rhinotracheitis-Calici-Panleukopenia-Chlamydia Psittaci Vaccine, Modified Live Virus & Chlamydia

U.S. Vet. Lic. No.: 272

Contents: PERFORMER®-Feline 4 is a combination of modified live feline rhinotracheitis, calci and panleukopenia viruses and *Chlamydia psittaci.*

The product contains gentamicin and amphotericin B as preservatives.

Indications: The product is recommended for use in the vaccination of healthy cats against diseases caused by the organisms represented.

Dosage and Administration: Aseptically rehydrate the vial of desiccated antigens with the accompanying vial of virus vaccine. Shake well. Administer the entire contents (1 mL) subcutaneously to healthy cats.

The persistence of maternal antibody in kittens is known to interfere with the development of active immunity following vaccination. Ideally kittens should be vaccinated at or before nine (9) weeks of age with revaccination every three (3) to four (4) weeks until the animals are at least 12 to 13 weeks of age. Kittens from susceptible queens should be vaccinated at an earlier age. Adult cats should receive a 1 mL dose followed by a second dose three (3) to four (4) weeks later. Annual revaccination with a single 1 mL dose is recommended.

Precaution(s): Store at 35°-45°F (2°-7°C). Use entire contents when first rehydrated. Burn the container and all unused contents.

Caution(s): For veterinary use only.

Do not vaccinate pregnant queens.

An occasional animal may demonstrate a transient fever, and mild arthralgia and/or myalgia within the first week following vaccination. In case of anaphylactic reactions, epinephrine should be administered immediately.

Presentation: 1 dose with syringe.

Compendium Code No.: 10581480

PERFORMER®-SEVEN

AgriLabs **Bacterin-Vaccine**

Canine Distemper-Hepatitis-Parainfluenza-Parvovirus Vaccine, Modified Live Virus-Leptospira Bacterin

U.S. Vet. Lic. No.: 124

Description: PERFORMER®-Seven vaccine is a combination of highly antigenic, attenuated strains of Canine Distemper, Canine Parainfluenza, Canine Hepatitis and Parvovirus propagated in cell line tissue cultures. The accompanying liquid diluent is Parvovirus Vaccine-*Leptospira canicola-icterohaemorrhagiae* Bacterin. The CD Virus fraction has been proven safe and non-shedding when injected into susceptible dogs. The infectious Canine Hepatitis (CAV-1) fraction cross protects against respiratory disease caused by CAV-2.

Contains gentamicin and a fungistat as preservatives.

Indications: For the immunization of healthy, susceptible dogs against disease caused by canine distemper, hepatitis (canine adenovirus type 1), canine adenovirus type 2, parainfluenza, parvovirus, *Leptospira canicola* and *Leptospira icterohaemorrhagiae.*

Directions: The dry Distemper-Hepatitis-Parainfluenza Vaccine is rehydrated with 1 mL of liquid Parvovirus Vaccine-*Leptospira canicola-icterohaemorrhagiae* Bacterin. Shake well and use entire contents when first opened.

Instructions: Read the carton information carefully.

Always use care when handling the dog and provide proper restraint when vaccinating.

Prepare the vaccine by injecting the liquid diluent into the vial containing the vaccine cake.

Shake well. Remove the entire contents back into the syringe. Push out air trapped in the syringe.

To give subcutaneously, vaccinate under loose skin (back of neck or behind front limb) or give IM, or in the hind limb.

Do not vaccinate into blood vessels. If blood enters the syringe freely or when the plunger is pulled back slightly, choose another injection site.

Dosage: Using aseptic technique, inject 1 mL intramuscularly or subcutaneously. Repeat dosage in 3 to 4 weeks. Annual revaccination with a single dose is recommended. Puppies vaccinated before 9 weeks of age should be revaccinated at 3 to 4 week intervals until 14 to 16 weeks of age. Regardless of age all dogs should receive 2 doses of vaccine in order to insure adequate levels of immunity against canine parainfluenza and parvovirus.

Contraindication(s): Do not vaccinate pregnant animals.

Under no circumstances is this product recommended for use in ferrets or mink.

Precaution(s): Store out of direct sunlight at a temperature not over 45°F. Avoid freezing. Burn containers and all unused contents.

Caution(s): An occasional transitory corneal opacity may occur following administration of the vaccine. This will disappear without untoward effect on the animal. Protective immunity may not be established in all puppies vaccinated at less than 16 weeks of age because of maternal antibody interference. Anaphylactoid reactions may occur.

For use in dogs only.

Antidote(s): Administer epinephrine.

Presentation: 1 dose with syringe and 25 one dose vaccine vials.

One dose vials of Canine Adenovirus Type 2-Parvovirus Vaccine & L.C.I. Bacterin as diluent. Rehydrate to 1 mL.

Manufactured by: Boehringer Ingelheim Animal Health, Inc., St.Joseph, MO 64506.

Compendium Code No.: 10581490 22104-00

P

PERMECTRIN™ II

Aspen **Premise and Topical Insecticide**

EPA Reg. No.: 4691-108-40940

Active Ingredient(s):

Permethrin (3-phenoxyphenyl) methyl (±)-cis, trans-3-(2,2-dichloroethenyl)-2, 2-dimethylcyclopropanecarboxylate* 10.00%

Inert Ingredients** 90.00%

*cis/trans ratio: Min. 35% (±) cis, and max. 65% (±) trans isomers.

**contains petroleum distillates.

Contains 0.75 lb permethrin per gallon.

Indications: For use on horses, beef and dairy cattle, swine, sheep, poultry and dogs and their premises to kill flies, fleas, lice, mites and ticks including deer ticks (carrier of Lyme disease) and as an aid in control of cockroaches, mosquitoes and spiders.

Dosage and Administration: It is a violation of Federal law to use this product in a manner inconsistent with its labeling.

Mix PERMECTRIN™ II and apply the use-diluted material to animals and pest breeding or resting surfaces at the rates shown on accompanying chart. These dilutions and rates will provide most efficient pest control under conditions of heavy pressure when good contact is achieved. Timing and frequency of application should be based on pest populations reaching nuisance levels, but accompanying manure removal and sanitation practices should precede sprays. Do not spray feed, food, or water. Retreat as needed but not more often than once every two weeks. Wash udders thoroughly before milking.

Pests on Farm Premises (Barns, Dairies, Loafing Sheds, Milking Parlors, Feedlots, Stables, Paddocks, Poultry and Livestock Housing):

Pests: Houseflies, stableflies, lesser houseflies, and other manure breeding flies, fleas, lice, mites, ticks, including deer tick (carrier of Lyme disease). Aids in control of cockroaches, mosquitoes and spiders.

Permectrin II Dilutions For Use: Mix 1 qt in 25 gal; 8 oz in 6.25 gal; 1⅓ oz (40 cc) in 1 gal of water.**

How to Apply: Spray all surfaces to run-off with diluted emulsion using 1 gal per 750 sq ft.

Permectrin II Dilutions For Use: Use undiluted in mist blower. In power fogger, use 1 qt in 25 gal; 1⅓ oz (40 cc) in 1 gal of oil or water.**

How to Apply: Mist or fog 4 oz per 1000 sq ft.

Pests on Large Animals (Dairy or Beef Cattle and Horses)

Pests: Faceflies, hornflies, horseflies.

Permectrin II Dilutions For Use: Mix 1 qt in 20 gal; 8 oz in 5 gal, 1.6 oz (48 cc) in 1 gal oil* to charge backrubbers.

How to Apply: Animals self apply.

Recharge backrubber or oiler as needed.

Pests: Faceflies, hornflies, horseflies, stableflies, mosquitoes, lice, mites, ticks, including deer tick (carrier of Lyme disease).

Permectrin II Dilutions For Use: Mix 1 qt in 200 gal; 8 oz in 50 gal; ½ oz (15 cc) in 3 gal of water.

How to Apply: Spray to thoroughly cover entire animal. For Lice or Mites, a second treatment is recommended 14-21 days later.

Pests: Ear ticks, faceflies, hornflies.

Permectrin II Dilutions For Use: Mix 2 oz (60 cc) in 1 gal oil* or water for spot application.

How to Apply: Apply ½ oz per ear or 2-4 oz on face or 12-16 oz along the backline.

Pests on Swine, Sheep, Poultry and Dogs (Do not ship swine for slaughter within 5 days of last treatment.)

Pests: Mange mites.

Permectrin II Dilutions For Use: Mix 1 qt in 100 gal; 8 oz in 25 gal; 1 oz (30 cc) in 3 gal of water.

How to Apply: Spray or dip animals. Retreat after 14 days spraying walls and floor and replace bedding to kill late hatching, developing stages.

Pests: Blowflies, mosquitoes, hog lice, fleas, ticks, including deer tick (carrier of Lyme disease).

Permectrin II Dilutions For Use: Mix 1 qt in 100 gal; 8 oz in 25 gal; 1 oz (30 cc) in 3 gal of water.

How to Apply: Spray, paint, or dip to apply 1 pint per dog, pig or sheep, especially around ears.

Pests: Poultry mites.

Permectrin II Dilutions For Use: Mix 1 qt in 50 gal; 8 oz in 12.5 gal; 2 oz (60 cc) in 3 gal of water.

How to Apply: Spray ½ oz per bird, or 1 gal per 100 birds, directed toward vent area. Spray cages.

*Mineral oil or non-irritating organic oil. **1 oz is equivalent to 2 tablespoons or 30 cc.

Contraindication(s): Do not use on sick, old, or debilitated animals. Do not use this product on puppies less than 3 months old.

Precaution(s): Do not contaminate water, food, or feed by storage or disposal.

Keep container sealed when not in use. Protect from freezing.

In case of spill on floor or paved surfaces, soak up with sand, earth or synthetic absorbent. Remove to chemical waste area and dispose of in accordance with state and local regulations.

Pesticide Disposal: Wastes resulting from the use of this product may be disposed of on site or at an approved waste disposal facility.

Container Disposal: Do not reuse container. Triple rinse (or equivalent). Then offer for recycling or reconditioning, or puncture and dispose of in a sanitary landfill, or incinerate, or if allowed by state and local authorities, by burning. If burned, stay out of smoke.

Environmental Hazards: This pesticide is extremely toxic to fish. Use with care when applying to areas adjacent to any body of water. For terrestrial uses, do not apply directly to water, or to areas where surface water is present or to intertidal areas below the mean high water mark. Do not apply directly to water. Do not contaminate water by cleaning of equipment or disposal of wastes. Apply this product only as specified on the label.

Physical or Chemical Hazards: Do not use or store near heat or open flame.

Caution(s): Precautionary Statements - Hazards to Humans

May be harmful if swallowed, inhaled or absorbed through skin. Avoid breathing spray mist. Avoid contact with skin, eyes or clothing.

Warning(s): Statement of Practical Treatment:

If Swallowed: Call a physician or Poison Control Center immediately. Do not induce vomiting. Vomiting may cause aspiration pneumonia.

If on Skin: Remove contaminated clothing and wash affected areas with soap and water.

If in Eyes: Flush with plenty of water. Call a physician immediately.

If Inhaled: Remove victim to fresh air. Apply artificial respiration if indicated.

Limitation of Warranty: Buyer assumes all risks of use, handling and storage of the product not in strict accordance with label directions. Any implied warranty of merchantability or fitness for a particular use is excluded. Liability for any incidental or consequential damage or loss is specifically excluded at all times. Seller will not accept liability for more than product replacement.

Keep out of reach of children.

Presentation: 8 ounce (236.56 mL) and 1 quart (946 mL) containers.

Compendium Code No.: 14750610

PERMECTRIN™ II

Boehringer Ingelheim **Premise and Topical Insecticide**

Permethrin Insecticide Spray

EPA Reg. No.: 4691-108

Active Ingredient(s):

Permethrin (CAS No. 52645-53-1) 10.0%

Other Ingredients* 90.0%

Total 100.0%

*Contains petroleum distillates.

Contains 0.75 lb permethrin per gallon.

Indications: Use only on dogs and their premises, horses, beef and dairy cattle, swine, sheep and poultry, and their premises. Kills flies, fleas, lice, mites and ticks including deer ticks (carrier of Lyme disease) and aids in the control of cockroaches, mosquitoes and spiders.

Directions for Use: It is a violation of Federal law to use this product in a manner inconsistent with its labeling.

Mix PERMECTRIN™ II and apply the use-diluted material to animals and pest breeding or resting surfaces at the rates shown on accompanying chart. These dilutions and rates will provide most efficient pest control under conditions of heavy pressure when good contact is achieved. Timing and frequency of applications should be based on pest populations reaching nuisance levels, but accompanying manure removal and sanitation practices should precede sprays. Do not spray feed, food or water. Do not repeat treatment for 2 weeks. Wash udders thoroughly before milking. Consult a veterinarian before using this product on debilitated, aged, medicated, pregnant or nursing animals.

Read directions before using.

Pests	PERMECTRIN™ II Dilutions for Use	How to Apply
Pests on Farm Premises (Barns, Dairies, Loafing Sheds, Milking Parlors, Feedlots, Stables, Paddocks, Poultry and Livestock Housing)		
Houseflies, stableflies, lesser houseflies and other manure breeding flies, fleas, lice, mites, ticks, including deer ticks (carrier of Lyme disease). Aids in control of cockroaches, mosquitoes and spiders	Mix 1 qt in 25 gal; 8 oz in 6.25 gal; 1⅓ oz (40 cc) in 1 gal of water.**	Spray all surfaces to run-off with diluted emulsion using 1 gal per 750 sq ft.
	Use undiluted in mist blower. In power fogger, use 1 qt in 25 gal; 1⅓ oz (40 cc) in 1 gal of oil or water.**	Mist or fog 4 oz per 1000 sq ft.
Pests on Large Animals (Dairy or Beef Cattle and Horses)		
Faceflies, hornflies, horseflies	Mix 1 qt in 20 gal; 8 oz in 5 gal; 1.6 oz (48 cc) in 1 gal oil* to charge backrubs.	Animals self apply. Recharge backrub or oiler as needed.
Faceflies, hornflies, horseflies, stableflies, mosquitoes, lice, mites, ticks, including deer ticks (carrier of Lyme disease)	Mix 1 qt in 200 gal; 8 oz in 50 gal; ½ oz (15 cc) in 3 gal of water.	Spray to thoroughly cover entire animal. For lice or mites, a second treatment is recommended 14-21 days later.
Ear ticks, faceflies, hornflies	Mix 2 oz (60 cc) in 1 gal oil* or water for spot application.	Apply ½ oz per ear or 2-4 oz on face or 12-16 oz along the backline.
Pests on Swine, Sheep, Poultry and Dogs		
Mange mites	Mix 1 qt in 100 gal; 8 oz in 25 gal; 1 oz (30 cc) in 3 gal of water.	Spray or dip animals. Retreat after 14 days spraying walls and floor and replace bedding to kill late hatching, developing stages. Do not reapply product for 2 weeks.
Blowflies, mosquitoes, hog lice, fleas, ticks, including deer ticks (carrier of Lyme disease)	Mix 1 qt in 100 gal; 8 oz in 25 gal; 1 oz (30 cc) in 3 gal of water.	Spray, paint, or dip to apply 1 pint per dog, pig, or sheep, especially around ears. Do not reapply product for 2 weeks.
Poultry mites	Mix 1 qt in 50 gal; 8 oz in 12.5 gal; 2 oz (60 cc) in 3 gal of water.	Spray ½ oz per bird, or 1 gal per 100 birds, directed toward vent area. Spray cages.

*Mineral oil or non-irritating organic oil.

**1 oz is equivalent to 2 tablespoons or 30 cc.

Contraindication(s): Do not use this product on dogs under 12 weeks old.

Precautionary Statements: Hazards to Humans:

Caution: May be harmful if swallowed, inhaled or absorbed through skin. Avoid breathing spray mist. Avoid contact with skin, eyes or clothing.

Hazards to Domestic Animals:

Caution: Sensitivities may occur after using any pesticide product for pets. If signs of sensitivity occur, bathe your pet with mild soap and rinse with large amounts of water. If signs continue, consult a veterinarian immediately.

First Aid:

If Swallowed — Call a physician or Poison Control Center immediately. Do not induce vomiting. Vomiting may cause aspiration pneumonia.

If on Skin — Remove contaminated clothing and wash affected areas with soap and water.

If in Eyes — Flush eyes with plenty of water. Call a physician immediately.

If Inhaled — Remove victim to fresh air. Apply artificial respiration if indicated.

Environmental Hazards: This pesticide is extremely toxic to fish. Use with care when applying to areas adjacent to any body of water. For terrestrial uses, do not apply directly to water, or to areas where surface water is present or to intertidal areas below the mean high water mark. Do not contaminate water by cleaning of equipment or disposal of wastes. Apply this product only as specified on the label.

Physical or Chemical Hazards: Do not use or store near heat or open flame.

Storage and Disposal: Do not contaminate water, food or feed by storage or disposal.

Keep container sealed when not in use. Protect from freezing.

In case of spill on floor or paved surfaces, soak up with sand, earth or synthetic absorbent. Remove to chemical waste area and dispose of in accordance with state and local regulations.

Pesticide Disposal: Wastes resulting from the use of this product may be disposed of on site or at an approved waste disposal facility.

Container Disposal: Do not reuse container. Triple rinse (or equivalent). Then offer for recycling or reconditioning, or puncture and dispose of in a sanitary landfill, or incineration, or if allowed by state and local authorities, by burning. If burned, stay out of smoke.

Warning(s): Do not ship swine for slaughter within 5 days of last treatment.

Keep out of reach of children.

Disclaimer: Warranty and Limitations of Damages: Seller warrants that this material conforms to its chemical description and is reasonably fit for the purposes stated on the label when used in accordance with directions under normal conditions of use and Buyer assumes the risk of any use contrary to such directions. Seller makes no other express or implied warranty, including any other express or implied warranty of Fitness or of Merchantability, and no agent of Seller is authorized to do so except in writing and with specific reference to this warranty. In no event shall Seller's liability for any breach of warranty exceed the purchase price of the material as to which a claim is made.

Presentation: 8 fl oz (237 mL) and 1 quart (946 mL) containers.

Compendium Code No.: 10280871 BI 4014-3 9/99

PERMECTRIN™ CDS POUR-ON

Boehringer Ingelheim **Premise and Topical Insecticide**

Pour-On Insecticide-Synergized Formula

EPA Reg. No.: 4691-121

Active Ingredient(s):

Permethrin (CAS No. 52645-53-1) 7.4%
Piperonyl Butoxide Technical (CAS No. 51-03-6) 7.4%
Other Ingredients* 85.2%
Total 100.0%

* Contains petroleum distillates.

Indications: Can be applied topically to livestock and their premises.

Controls lice, horn and face flies, and aids in the control of ticks on beef and lactating dairy cattle.

Controls lice, horn, stable, deer and face flies, eye gnats and ticks on horses.

Controls sheep keds and lice on sheep.

Directions for Use: It is a violation of Federal law to use this product in a manner inconsistent with its labeling.

Important: This is a highly concentrated formulation. Use only with an accurate measuring container or applicator.

Except for Back Rubber/Ready to Use - No dilution necessary.

Apply to: Lactating and Non-lactating Dairy Cattle, Beef Cattle and Calves.

Target Pests	Application Instructions
Lice, Horn Flies, Face Flies. Aids in control of Horse Flies, Stable Flies, House Flies, Mosquitoes, Black Flies and Ticks. Controls Horn Flies up to 6 weeks after application.	Dosage: For moderate fly control apply 1.5 mL per 100 lbs body wt of animal, up to a maximum of 15 mL. For lice and severe horn fly control apply 2.0 mL per 100 lbs body wt of animal, up to a maximum of 20 mL. Pour-On: Pour correct dose along back and down face. Ready-To-Use Spray: Use undiluted in a mist sprayer to apply correct dose. Apply directly to neck, face, back, legs and ears. Back Rubber Use: Mix 64 mL (2.1 oz) per gallon of mineral oil. Keep rubbing device charged. Results improved by daily forced use.

For cattle and sheep, repeat treatment as needed, but not more than once every two weeks. For optimum lice control, two treatments at a 14-day interval are recommended.

Apply to: Horses and Foals.

Target Pests	Application Instructions
Stable Flies, Deer Flies, Horn Flies, Face Flies, House Flies, Eye Gnats, Lice and Ticks. Aids in control of Horse Flies, Mosquitoes and Black Flies.	Pour-On: Do not use this application method on foals. After riding or exercise, pour 8 mL to 16 mL per animal along back and down the face of Mature horses, being careful to avoid the eyes. Repeat as necessary. Wipe-On: Apply 8 mL to 16 mL. Dampen an applicator mitt, cloth or toweling (turkish). Rub over hair with special attention to the legs, shoulders, neck and facial areas where flies tend to congregate. Avoid the eyes. Repeat treatment as necessary. Ready-To-Use Spray: Use after riding or exercising. Apply 8 mL to 16 mL undiluted in a mist sprayer per animal. Apply directly to ticks. Repeat as necessary.

Apply to: Sheep and Lambs.

Target Pests	Application Instructions
Sheep Keds and Lice	Pour-On: Pour-On: Pour along the back. Apply 1 mL per 50 lb body weight of animal, up to maximum of 12 mL for any one animal. For optimum control, all animals in the flock should be treated after shearing.

Apply to: Horse, Beef, Dairy, Swine, Sheep and Poultry Premises, Animal Hospital Pens and Kennels and "Outside" Meat Processing Premises.

Target Pests	Application Instructions
House Flies, Stable Flies, Face Flies, Gnats, Mosquitoes, Black Flies, Fleas, Little House Flies (*Fannia* spp.). Aids in control of Cockroaches, Ants, Spiders and Crickets.	Ready-To-Use Spot or Premise Spray: Use undiluted in a mist sprayer. Apply directly to surface to leave a residual insecticidal coating, paying particular attention to areas where insects crawl or alight. 500 mL will treat approximately 7,200 square feet.

Special Note: PERMECTRIN™ CDS Pour-On is not effective in controlling cattle grubs.

PERMECTRIN™ CDS Pour-On is an oil-base, ready-to-use product that may leave an oily appearance on the hair coat of some animals.

PERMECTRIN™ CDS Pour-On should be used in an integrated pest management system which may involve repeat treatments and the use of other pest control practices.

Precautionary Statements: Hazards to Humans and Domestic Animals:

Caution: Harmful if absorbed through the skin. Avoid contact with skin, eyes, or clothing. Avoid breathing vapor or spray mist. Prolonged or frequently repeated skin contact may cause allergic reactions in some individuals. Remove contaminated clothing and wash contaminated clothing before reuse. Wash thoroughly with soap and water after handling.

First Aid:

If on Skin: Wash with plenty of soap and water. Get medical attention.

Environmental Hazards: This pesticide is extremely toxic to fish and other aquatic invertebrates. Do not add directly to water. Do not contaminate water when disposing of equipment washwaters.

Physical or Chemical Hazards: Do not use or store near heat or open flame.

Storage and Disposal: Do not contaminate water, food or feed by storage or disposal.

Storage: Keep container sealed when not in use. Do not store near food or feed.

Pesticide Disposal: Waste resulting from the use of this product may be disposed of on site or at an approved waste disposal facility.

Container Disposal: Triple rinse (or equivalent). Then offer for recycling or reconditioning, or puncture and dispose of in a sanitary landfill or incineration, or, if allowed by State and local authorities, by burning. If burned, stay out of smoke.

Warning(s): Keep out of reach of children.

Disclaimer: Warranty and Limitation of Damages: Seller warrants that this material conforms to its chemical description and is reasonably fit for the purposes stated on the label when used in accordance with directions under normal conditions of use and Buyer assumes the risk of any use contrary to such directions. Seller makes no other express or implied warranty, including any other express or implied warranty of Fitness or of Merchantability, and no agent of Seller is authorized to do so except in writing and with a specific reference to this warranty. In no event shall Seller's liability for any breach of warranty exceed the purchase price of the material as to which a claim is made.

Presentation: 1 pint (473 mL), 64 fl oz (1.8925 liters), and 2.5 U.S. gallons (9.5 liters) containers.

Compendium Code No.: 10280851 BI 4083-9R-2 4/00

PERMECTRIN™ FLY & LOUSE DUST

Boehringer Ingelheim **Topical Insecticide**

EPA Reg. No.: 4691-110

Active Ingredient(s):

Permethrin (CAS # 52645-53-1) 0.25%
Other Ingredients 99.75%
100.00%

Indications: For control of horn flies and lice on beef and dairy cattle. As an aid in reducing face fly population on beef and dairy cattle. Control of lice on swine. For control of Northern fowl mites on poultry.

Use in dust bags, shaker can, or mechanical dust applicator.

P

Directions for Use: It is a violation of federal law to use this product in a manner inconsistent with its labeling.

Beef and Dairy Cattle:

Horn Flies, Lice, Face Flies: Place contents of this package in any commercially available dust bag, suspend bags in areas frequently by cattle or in gateways or lanes through which the animals pass daily for water, feed or minerals. Bags may also be suspended in loafing sheds or in front of protected mineral feeders. For lactating dairy cows, bags may be suspended in the exit through which cows leave the milking barn. In all cases, the bags should be adjusted so that the bottom of the bag will hang four to six inches below the topline of the cattle. For reduction of face flies, the bags must be located so the animals will be forced to use them daily and hung at a height to insure that the faces of the cattle will be dusted.

Horn Flies, Lice — Direct Application: Apply 2.0 ounces of dust per animal by shaker can over the head, neck, shoulders, back and tailhead. Repeat as necessary.

Swine:

Lice on Swine — Direct Application: Apply not more than 1 oz* (3 level tablespoonfuls) per head as a uniform coat to the head, shoulders and back by use of a shaker can or suitable mechanical dust applicator. Repeat as necessary, but not more often than once every ten days.

In severe infestations, both individual animals and the bedding may be treated as directed above.

Poultry:

For Northern Fowl Mites — Direct Application: Apply not more than 1 lb/100 birds, directing dust to thoroughly cover vent area.

*Note: 1 oz of this material equals approximately three level tablespoonfuls.

Precautionary Statements: Hazards to Humans and Domestic Animals:

Caution: Harmful if inhaled. Avoid contact with skin and eyes. Avoid breathing dust. Wash thoroughly with soap and water after handling and before eating or smoking. Avoid contamination of feed and foodstuffs.

Statement of Practical Treatment: In case of eye contact, immediately flush eyes with plenty of water. Get medical attention if discomfort persists.

Environmental Hazards: This pesticide is toxic to fish. Do not apply directly to water, or to areas where surface water is present or to intertidal areas below the mean high water mark. Use this product only as specified on the label. Do not contaminate water by cleaning of equipment or disposal of wastes.

Physical or Chemical Hazards: Do not use or store near heat or open flame.

Storage and Disposal: Do not contaminate water, food or feed by storage or disposal. Open as needed. Keep container sealed when not in use. Do not reuse container. Completely empty bag into application equipment. Then dispose of empty bag in a sanitary landfill or by incineration, or, if allowed by State and local authorities, by burning. If burned, stay out of smoke.

Wastes resulting from the use of this product may be disposed of on site or at an approved waste disposal facility.

Warning(s): Do not ship swine for slaughter within 5 days of last treatment.

Keep out of reach of children.

Disclaimer: Warranty and Limitation of Damages: Seller warrants that this material conforms to its chemical description and is reasonably fit for the purposes stated on the label when used in accordance with directions under normal conditions of use and Buyer assumes the risk of any use contrary to such directions. Seller makes no other express or implied warranty, including any other express or implied warranty of Fitness or of Merchantability, and no agent of Seller is authorized to do so except in writing and with specific reference to this warranty. In no event shall Seller's liability for any breach of warranty exceed the purchase price of the material as to which a claim is made.

Presentation: 2 x 12½ lb and 4 x 12½ lb.

Dust Bag Kit: 1-dust bag with hanger bar and rope. 1-12½ lb dust refill cartridge.

U.S. Patent No. 4,024,163

Compendium Code No.: 10280860

PERMECTRIN™ POUR-ON

Boehringer Ingelheim **Topical Insecticide**

Insecticide

EPA Reg. No.: 28293-182-4691

Active Ingredient(s):

Permethrin (3-phenoxyphenyl) methyl (±) cis, trans-3-(2,2-dichloroethenyl)-2,2-dimethylcyclopropanecarboxylate* 1.0%

Inert Ingredients** 99.0%

Total 100.0%

*cis/trans ratio: Min. 35% (±) cis and max. 65% (±) trans

**Contains petroleum distillates

Indications: Kills lice, horn flies, and face flies on beef cattle, all dairy cattle, calves, and sheep.

Aids in control of horse flies, stable flies, mosquitoes, black flies, ticks on beef cattle, all dairy cattle, calves, and sheep.

Kills keds on sheep.

Directions for Use: It is a violation of Federal law to use this product in a manner inconsistent with its labeling.

Ready to use — No dilution necessary.

Application Instructions: Pour along back line and down face. Apply ½ fl oz per 100 lbs body weight of animal, up to a maximum of 5 fl oz for any one animal to kill lice, horn flies and face flies. Aids in the insecticidal control of horse flies, stable flies, mosquitoes, black flies and ticks on lactating and non-lactating diary cattle, beef cattle, calves and sheep. For Keds on sheep, pour along back line over neck, shoulders and rump. Apply ¼ fl oz per 50 lbs body weight of animal, up to a maximum of 3 fl oz for any one animal.

Repeat treatment as needed, but not more than once every two weeks. For optimum insecticidal effectiveness against lice, a double treatment at 14-day intervals is recommended.

Note: This product is not effective for grub control on cattle.

Precautionary Statements: Hazards to Humans and Domestic Animals:

Caution: Avoid contact with eyes.

Statement of Practical Treatment:

If in eyes: Immediately flush eyes with plenty of water. Get medical attention if discomfort persists.

If swallowed: Call a physician immediately. Do not induce vomiting unless advised by a physician.

Note to Physician: Solvent presents aspiration hazard. Gastric lavage is indicated if material was taken internally.

Environmental Hazards: This pesticide is extremely toxic to fish. Use with care when applying to areas adjacent to any body of water. Do not add directly to water. Do not contaminate water by cleaning of equipment or disposal of wastes. Apply this product only as specified on this label.

Physical or Chemical Hazards: Do not use or store near heat or open flame.

Storage and Disposal: Do not contaminate water, food or feed by storage or disposal.

Storage — Keep container sealed when not in use. Do not store near food or feed.

Pesticide Disposal — Wastes resulting from the use of this product may be disposed of on site or at an approved waste disposal facility.

Container Disposal — Triple rinse (or equivalent). Then offer for recycling or reconditioning, or puncture and dispose of in a sanitary landfill or incineration, or if allowed by State and local authorities, by burning. If burned, stay out of smoke.

Containers One Gallon and Under — Do not reuse empty container. Rinse thoroughly, wrap in several layers of newspaper and place in trash.

Warning(s): Keep out of reach of children.

Presentation: 1 gallon (3.785 liters) and 5 gallon (18.925 liters) containers.

Compendium Code No.: 10280880

PERMETHRIN 0.25% DUST

AgriLabs **Topical Insecticide**

EPA Reg. No.: 28293-126-53302

Active Ingredient(s):

Permethrin [(3-phenoxyphenyl) methyl (±) cis, trans-3-(2,2-dichloroethenyl)-2,2-dimethylcyclopropanecarboxylate]* 0.25%

Inert ingredients 99.75%

Total 100.00%

*Cis/trans ratio: Min. 35% (±) cis and max. 65% (±) trans.

Indications: To control horn flies, lice, and face flies on beef and dairy cattle and horses.

To control lice on swine.

Dosage and Administration: It is a violation of federal law to use the product in a manner inconsistent with its labeling.

Beef and Dairy Cattle and Horses: Can be used in dust bags, shaker cans and mechanical dust applicators.

Horn flies, lice and face flies: Place the contents of the package in any commercially available dust bag; suspend the bag in areas frequented by cattle or in gateways or lanes through which the animals must pass each day for water, feed, or minerals. The bags may also be placed in loafing sheds or in front of mineral feeders. For dairy cows, the bags may be suspended in the exit through which the cows leave the milking barn. The bags should hang four (4) to six (6) inches below the backline of the cattle. For reduction of face flies, the bags must be located so that the animals will be forced to use them daily, and hung at a height such that the face is dusted.

Horn flies and lice (direct application): Apply 2 oz. of dust per animal by shaker can, over the head, neck, shoulders and back, and tailhead. Repeat as necessary.

Horses: Dust horse for horn flies with a shaker can or dust glove along the back, neck and legs.

Swine: Lice on swine (direct application): Apply only 1 oz. per head as a uniform coat to the head, shoulder and back, by the use of a shaker can or suitable mechanical dust applicator. Repeat as necessary, but not more often than once every 10 days. In severe infestations, both animals and bedding may be treated.

Precaution(s):

Storage: Store in a cool, dry place. Do not contaminate feed or foodstuffs by storage or disposal.

Pesticide Disposal: Wastes resulting from the use of this product may be disposed of on site or at an approved waste disposal facility.

Container Disposal: Completely empty the container into the application equipment. Then dispose of the empty container in a sanitary landfill or by incineration, or, if allowed by state and local authorities, by burning. If burned, stay out of smoke.

Caution(s): Keep out of the reach of children.

Precautionary Statements:

Hazards to Humans and Domestic Animals: Harmful if swallowed. Avoid inhaling dust. Avoid contact with the eyes and skin. Wash thoroughly with soap and water after handling. Avoid contamination of feed and foodstuffs.

Statement of Practical Treatment:

If in eyes: Flush with plenty of water. Get medical attention if irritation persists.

If on skin: Wash with plenty of soap and water. Get medical attention if irritation persists.

Physical and Chemical Hazards: Do not use or store near heat or open flame.

Environmental Hazards: This product is toxic to fish. Do not apply directly to water. Do not contaminate water by the cleaning of equipment or the disposal of wastes.

Warning(s): Do not ship swine for slaughter within five (5) days of treatment.

Warranty and limitation of damages: Seller warrants that his material conforms to its chemical description and is reasonably fit for the purposes stated on the label when used in accordance with directions under normal conditions of use and the buyer assumes the risk of any use contrary to such directions. Seller makes no other express or implied warranty, including any other express or implied warranty of fitness or merchantability, and no agent of seller is authorized to do so except in writing and with specific reference to this warranty. In no event shall seller's liability for any breach of warranty exceed the purchase price of the material as to which a claim is made.

Presentation: 12 x 2 lb., 12½ lb. dust bag kits, and 2 x 12½ lb. refills.

Compendium Code No.: 10580810

PERMETHRIN 10%

Durvet **Premise and Topical Insecticide**

Oil Base Concentrate

EPA Reg. No.: 67517-80-12281

Active Ingredient(s):

Permethrin 10.0%

Other Ingredients* 90.0%

Total 100.0%

Cis/trans ratio: Max. 65% (±) trans and Min. 35% (±) cis.

*Contains Petroleum Distillate.

Contains 0.75 lbs. of Permethrin per gallon.

Indications: A long lasting livestock and premise spray that provides knockdown, broad spectrum insecticidal effectiveness and excellent residual activity for up to 28 days.

Kills Lessor Meal Worms (Darkling Beetle), Poultry Lice, Fowl Mites, Bed Bugs, Horn Flies, House Flies, Fleas, Ticks, and numerous other insects as listed in Directions for Use.

For use outdoors and in homes and non-food/feed areas of poultry houses, dairies, cattle barns, milking parlors, horse barns, swine houses, commercial buildings, institutions,

P

warehouses, theatres, office buildings, schools, motels, hotels, restaurants, food/feed processing establishments, hospitals, and kennels.

For agricultural, commercial/industrial use only.

Directions for Use: It is a violation of Federal law to use this product in a manner inconsistent with its labeling.

Read entire label before each use.

Keep container sealed when not in use. Protect from freezing. Shake or stir product thoroughly before using or reusing diluted emulsion.

To prepare dilutions, the concentrate should first be stirred or agitated well. Add the required amount of concentrate to water and blend thoroughly. Do not hold dilutions for more than 24 hours.

For maximum effectiveness, a combination of localized application and space treatment is recommended. Remove pets, birds and cover fish aquariums before spraying.

For initial clean up of severe insect infestation, dilute at a rate of (1) part concentrate in 19 parts water (6.7 fluid ounces per gallon) (0.5%).

For normal infestation dilute (1) part concentration in 100 parts water (1.33 ounces per gallon) (8 teaspoons per gallon) (0.1%).

Indoor Use Areas: Do not use in food/feed area of food/feed handling establishments, restaurants or other areas where food/feed is commercially prepared or processed. Do not use in serving areas while food is exposed or facility is in operation. Serving areas are areas where prepared foods are served such as dining rooms, but excluding areas where foods may be prepared or held. In the home, all food processing surfaces and utensils should be covered during treatment or thoroughly washed before use. Exposed food/feed should be covered or removed.

Non Food/Feed Areas:

Include (but not limited to) garbage rooms, lavatories, floor drains (to sewers), entries and vestibules, offices, locker rooms, machine rooms, boiler rooms, garages, mop closets and storage (after canning or bottling): Bakeries, Beverage Plants, Canneries, Flour Mills, Food Processing Plants, Grain Elevators, Granaries, Hospitals (non-occupied areas), Hotels, Motels, Industrial Installations, Kennels, Meat Packing Plants, Homes, Office Buildings, Railroad Cars, Restaurants, Schools, Ships' Holds, Supermarkets, Truck Trailers, Warehouses.

Do not apply to classrooms when in use. Do not apply this product in occupied patient rooms or in any rooms while occupied by the elderly or infirm.

Use in Federally Inspected Meat and Poultry Plants: Acceptable as a residual pesticide for use in the inedible product areas of official establishments operating under the Federal meat, poultry, shell egg grading, and egg products inspection programs. This product must be used in a manner that precludes entry into edible product areas through open windows, ventilating systems, etc.

As a Surface Spray to Control: Cockroaches, Waterbugs, Palmetto Bugs, Ants, Silverfish, Beetles, Mites, Weevils, Fireboats, Spiders, Crickets, Millipedes, Centipedes, Sowbugs, Pillbugs, Clover Mites, Cheese Mites, Granary Weevils, Rice Weevils, Confused Flour Beetles, Sawtoothed Grain Beetles, Red Rust Flour Beetles, Cigarette Beetles, Drugstore Beetles, Meal Worms, Grain Mites and Cadelle. Use a good sprayer and adjust to deliver a coarse wet spray. Direct the spray into hiding places, cracks and crevices, under pallets, around containers of stored foods (metal or glass), around the base of machinery, and behind shelves and drawers. Spray bookcases for silverfish. Spray ant trails, nests and points of entry. If surface application only is to be used, spray floors, walls and other surfaces applying at a rate of (1) gallon to 750 square feet of surface.

To Control: Fleas and Ticks (adult and larvae), thoroughly spray infested areas, pet beds, resting quarters, nearby cracks and crevices, along and behind baseboards, moldings, window and door frames, and localized areas of floor and floor covering. Fresh bedding should be placed in animal quarters following treatment. Apply with mechanical or compressed air equipment (non-thermal) adjusted to deliver a fine mist. Close doors and windows and shut off ventilating system. For rapid control of house flies, fruit flies, gnats, mosquitoes, skipper flies, wasps, hornets, bees, black flies, angoumois grain moths and tobacco moths, direct spray at an upward angle distributing it uniformly through the entire areas at a rate of (1) ounce per 1000 cubic feet of space. Keep area closed for at least 10 minutes. Vacate areas after treatment and ventilate and sweep up dead insects before occupying.

For rapid kill of exposed or accessible stages of other insects named on this label: Apply using conventional mechanical or compressed air equipment (non-thermal), following directions for space spraying. Apply the above dilutions at a rate of (1) ounce per 1000 cubic feet of space.

Outdoor Use Areas:

Application Sites: Corrals, Feedlots, Gardens, Parks, Homes, Drive-In Theatres, Drive-In Restaurants, Golf Courses, Playgrounds, Recreational Areas, Swine Lots, Urban Areas, Zoos.

For Temporary Reduction of Annoyance Flies, Gnats, Mosquitoes: In drive-in restaurants, drive-in theatres, golf course, urban areas, parks, playgrounds and other recreational areas. Dilute (1) part concentrate in 40 parts water (3.2 fluid ounces per gallon of water) (0.25%). Direct the spray into tall grass, shrubbery and around lawns, where these pests may hover or rest. Apply while the air is still and avoid wetting foliage. Application should be made prior to occupancy. Repeat as necessary.

In the treatment of corrals, feedlots, swine lots and zoos, cover any exposed water, drinking fountains and animal feed before application. Fill the area with mist and direct the spray into tall grass, shrubbery and around lawns where the above pests may hover or rest. Apply while the air is still and avoid wetting foliage. In zoos, prevent exposure of reptiles to the product. Repeat as necessary. Not to be used within 100 feet (30 meters) of lakes and streams.

Animals and Animal Premise Use:

Application Sites: Cattle Barns, Swine Houses, Milk Rooms, Kennels, Poultry Houses, Horse Barns, Dairies, Milking Parlors, Feedlots, Stables, Paddocks.

For initial clean up of severe insect infestation, dilute at a rate of (1) part concentrate in 19 parts water (6.7 ounces per gallon) (0.5%). For normal infestations dilute (1) part concentrate in 100 parts water (1.33 ounces per gallon) (8 teaspoonsful per gallon) (0.1%).

Pests on Farm Premises (Barns, Dairies, Loafing Sheds, Milking Parlors, Feedlots, Stables, Paddocks Poultry and Livestock Housing):

Horse Flies, Stable Flies, lesser Houseflies and other manure breeding flies, Fleas, Lice, Mites, Ticks, including Deer Tick (carrier of Lyme disease). Aids in control of Cockroaches, Mosquitoes and Spiders: Dilute 8 oz. in 6.25 gal. water or 1 pt. in 12½ gal. water or 1 qt. in 25 gal. water. Spray walls and surfaces thoroughly, but do not allow run-off to occur, about 1 gallon per 750-1000 sq. ft. Treat no more often than once every 2 weeks. Do not contaminate animal's feed or water by spray. Do not use in milk rooms. Animals should be removed from area prior to spraying.

Pests on Dog Premises (Kennels, Dog Houses, Runs and Yards):

Fleas, Flies, Ticks, Lice and Mange Mites (adult and larvae): Dilute 8 oz. in 6.25 gal. water or 1 pt. in 12½ gal. water or 1 qt. in 25 gal. water. Thoroughly wet pest breeding or resting areas, but do not allow runoff to occur. Most efficient pest control is accomplished when heavy pressure and good contact is achieved. Timing and frequency of applications should be based on pest populations reaching nuisance levels, but accompanying manure removal and sanitation practices should precede sprays. Do not spray feed, food or water. Repeat as needed but not more often than once every two weeks.

Pests in Cattle Barns, Horse Barns, Swine Houses, Kennels, Milking Parlors, Milk Rooms, Dairies, Poultry Houses, Feedlots, Stables and Paddocks:

Flies, Mosquitoes and Gnats: Dilute 8 oz. in 6.25 gal. water or 1 pt. in 12½ gal. water or 1 qt. in 25 gal. water.

Fog or Fine Mist: Apply, directing the spray toward the ceiling and upper corners until the area is filled with mist. Use about 2 ounces per 1000 cubic feet of space. For best results, close doors and windows before spraying and keep closed for ten to fifteen minutes. Animals should be removed from area prior to spraying. Ventilate before reoccupying. Repeat treatment as necessary.

Pests on Large Animals (Dairy or Beef Cattle, Horses, Sheep and Goats):

Face Flies, Horn Flies, Ear Ticks: Dilute 8 oz. in 5 gal. oil or 1 pt. in 10 gal. oil or 1 qt. in 20 gal. oil.

Back Rubber: Recharge backrubber as needed. Spray lactating dairy cows only after milking is completed.

Face Flies, Horn Flies, Stableflies, Mosquitoes, Lice, Mites, Ticks, including Deer Tick (carrier of Lyme disease): Dilute 8 oz. in 50 gal. water or 1 pt. in 100 gal. water or 1 qt. in 200 gal. water. Spray to thoroughly cover entire animal. For Lice or Mites, a second treatment is recommended 14-21 days later. Spray lactating dairy cows only after milking is completed.

Hornflies, Faceflies, Stableflies, Ear Ticks: Dilute 2 oz. in 1 gal. water or 1 pt. in 2½ gal. water. Spot Treatment Low Pressure Spray: Apply ½ oz. per ear or 2-4 oz. on face or 12-16 oz. along the backline.

Pests on Swine And Poultry:

Mange Mites: Dilute 8 oz. in 25 gal. water or 1 pt. in 50 gal. water or 1 qt. in 100 gal. water. Spray, dip or sponge animals. Retreat after 14 days, spraying walls and floor space and bedding to kill late hatching, developing stages.

Blowflies, Flies, Mosquitoes, Hog Lice, Fleas, Ticks, including Deer Ticks (carrier of Lyme disease): Dilute 8 oz. in 25 gal. water or 1 pt. in 50 gal. water or 1 qt. in 100 gal. water. Spray, dip or sponge to apply 1 pint per pig, especially around ears.

Poultry Mites, Northern Fowl Mites and Lice: Dilute 8 oz. in 12½ gal. water or 1 pt. in 25 gal. water or 1 qt. in 50 gal. water. Spray at the rate of ½ oz. per bird, or 1 gal. per 100 birds, with a fine mist. Spray roosts, walls and nests or cages.

Pests on Dogs (Do not use on puppies under twelve weeks of age):

Fleas, Ticks, including Deer Tick (carrier of Lyme disease), Lice and Mange: Dilute 8 oz. in 12½ gal. water or 1 pt. in 25 gal. water or 1 qt. in 50 gal. water. Thoroughly wet the animal by dipping, sponging or spraying. Allow animal to dry in a warm place without rinsing or toweling. Gives long lasting protection against reinfestation and applications at intervals of two to three weeks. Do not reapply more often than once every two weeks.

Hose-End Sprayer: To control listed insects, shake well before applying. Connect nozzle to hose, remove bottle cap, insert diptube and screw bottle onto nozzle. Turn on water at the tap. When ready to treat, place finger over the hole on right side of nozzle and the liquid will mix automatically at the proper ratio. Apply to surfaces in dairies, barns, feedlots, stables, poultry houses, swine and livestock housing to control House Flies, Stable Flies and other manure breeding flies. Also aids in control of Cockroaches, Ants, Spiders, Mosquitoes, Crickets and Face Flies. Walk and spray at a steady pace. Spray walls and surfaces thoroughly, but do not allow to run-off. Treat no more often than once every two weeks. Do not contaminate animals feed or water by spray.

Contraindication(s): Do not use on cats. Do not use on puppies under twelve weeks of age.

Precautionary Statements: Hazards to Humans and Domestic Animals. Caution.

Hazards to Humans: Harmful if swallowed or absorbed through the skin. Avoid contact with eyes, skin or clothing. Wash thoroughly after handling. Remove and wash clothing before reuse. Avoid contamination of food and feed. A respiratory protection device is recommended for general protection when applying in a non-ventilated space indoors as a space spray or fogger. Use one of the following Mine Safety and Health Administration (MSHA)/National Institute for Occupational Safety and Health (NIOSH) air purifying respirator types with approval number prefixes such as TC-23C, TC21C, TC19C, TC13F and TC14G.

Hazards to Domestic Animals: Use only on dogs. Do not use on cats. Harmful if swallowed. Avoid contact with eyes or mucous membranes. Consult a veterinarian before using this product on debilitated, aged, pregnant or nursing animals. Sensitivities may occur after using any pesticide product for pets. If signs of sensitivity occur bathe your pet with mild soap and rinse with large amounts of water. If signs continue, consult a veterinarian immediately. Certain medications can interact with pesticides. Consult a veterinarian before using on medicated animals. Do not use on puppies under twelve weeks of age.

First Aid:

If Swallowed: Contact a Physician or Poison Control Center immediately. Drink one or two glasses of water and induce vomiting by touching back of throat with finger. Do not induce vomiting or give anything by mouth to an unconscious person.

If Inhaled: Remove person to fresh air. Apply artificial respiration if indicated.

If on Skin: Remove contaminated clothing and wash affected areas with plenty of soap and water.

If in Eyes: Flush eyes with plenty of water. Call a physician if irritation persists.

Note to Physician: This product contains petroleum solvents. Vomiting may cause aspiration pneumonia.

Environmental Hazards: This pesticide is extremely toxic to fish. Do not apply directly to water, to areas where surface water is present or to intertidal areas below the mean high water mark. Drift and runoff from treated areas may be hazardous to aquatic organisms in treated areas. Do not contaminate water when disposing of equipment washwater/dip solution. This product is highly toxic to bees exposed to direct treatment on blooming crops or weeds while bees are actively visiting the treatment area.

Physical Hazards: Do not use or store near heat or open flame. Do not use this product in or on electrical equipment due to the possibility of shock hazard.

Storage and Disposal: Do not contaminate water, food or feed by storage or disposal.

Pesticide Storage and Spill Procedures: Store upright at room temperature. Avoid exposure to extreme temperatures. In case of spill or leakage, soak up with an absorbent material such as sand, sawdust, earth, fuller's earth, etc.

Pesticide Disposal: Pesticide, spray mixture or rinse water that cannot be used according to label instructions must be disposed of at or by an approved waste disposal facility.

Container Disposal: Triple rinse (or equivalent). Then offer for recycling or reconditioning or puncture and dispose of in a sanitary landfill, or by incineration, or if allowed by State and local authorities, by burning. If burned, stay out of smoke.

Warning(s): Do not ship swine for slaughter within 5 days of last treatment.

Keep out of reach of children.

Disclaimer: Notice of Warranty: Manufacturer makes no warranty of merchantability, fitness for any particular purpose, or otherwise, expressed or implied concerning this product or its uses which extend beyond the use of the product under normal conditions in accord with the statements made on this label.
Presentation: Available in 8 fl oz (236.56 mL), 16 fl oz (473.12 mL), 32 fl oz (946.25 mL) and 1 gallon (3.785 L).
Compendium Code No.: 10841281 12/98

PETABLES™ CLEAN AND HEAL POVIDONE IODINE BATH

A.A.H. **Antiseptic Shampoo**

Grooming Aids-Antiseptic, Germ Killing Cleansing Shampoo

Ingredient(s): USP Purified Water, Povidone Iodine, Hydroxyethylcellulose, Ammonium Lauryl Sulfate, Aloe Vera, Sodium Phosphate Dibasic Anhydrous, Panthenyl Hydroxyproplyl Steardimonium Chloride, Citric Acid.
Indications: PETABLES™ Clean and Heal Povidone Iodine Bath is a safe, rich, cleansing shampoo. It's 0.2% titratable iodine formula cleanses and kills or prevents the growth or regrowth of micro-organisms such as bacteria and fungi. It is gentle enough to use on a regular basis when needed. Clean and Heal contains conditioning and moisturizing ingredients, along with the healing properties of aloe vera.

For dogs and puppies.

Cleans contaminated superficial wounds. Gentle and painless. Non-staining.

Directions for Use: Wet your pet's skin thoroughly and apply approximately 1 to 2 ounces (depending on the size of the animal). PETABLES™ Clean and Heal Shampoo will work into a rich lather. Allow to remain on skin and coat for at least 1 minute before rinsing. Use on a regular basis until condition improves.
Precaution(s): Store in a cool area.
Caution(s): If irritation persists or worsens, discontinue use and consult your veterinarian. Avoid contact with eyes. If contact occurs, flush the eyes with copious amounts of water.

For animal use only.

Warning(s): Keep out of reach of children and pets.
Presentation: 16 fl oz (473 mL).
Compendium Code No.: 11180130

PETABLES™ FOAMING SILK BATH

A.A.H. **Antidermatosis Shampoo**

Grooming Aids-Soothing Luxury Shampoo

Ingredient(s): PETABLES™ Foaming Silk Bath is a rich, cleansing shampoo formulated with USP Purified Water, Sodium Lauryl Sulfate, Glycerin, Lauramidopropyl Betaine, Coco Diethanolamide, Disodium Ricinoleamide, MEA Sulfosuccinte, Colloidal Oatmeal, Panthequat, Polyquaternium 10, Diazolidinyl Urea and Iodopropynyl Butylcalbamate, Artificial Fragrance, Vitamin A Palmitate, Vitamin E Acetate, Aloe Vera and Citric Acid.
Indications: PETABLES™ Foaming Silk Bath helps restore moisture and resiliency to dry itchy skin and coat. It is vitamin enriched to reduce the effects of environmental stresses from heat, cold, humidity and harsh shampoos which can strip the skin and coat of natural protective oils.

Aloe vera provides additional healing and astringent action.

Cleanses and moisturizes. Relieves itching and irritation. Restores resiliency to skin and coat.

For dogs and cats.

Directions for Use: Wet your pet's skin thoroughly and apply approximately 1 to 2 ounces (depending on the size of the animal). Foaming Silk will quickly work into a rich lather. Allow to remain on skin and coat for at least 1 minute before rinsing. The thick lather will rinse easily. Use Foaming Silk every two weeks or as often as needed.

PETABLES™ Foaming Silk Bath is so gentle that you may use it as often as needed.

Precaution(s): Store in a cool area.
Caution(s): In case of irritation, discontinue use. Avoid contact with eyes. If contact occurs, flush the eyes with copious amounts of water.

For animal use only.

Warning(s): Keep out of reach of children and pets.
Presentation: 16 fl oz (473 mL).
Compendium Code No.: 11180140

PET-CAL™

Pfizer Animal Health **Small Animal Dietary Supplement**

A Palatable Calcium-Phosphorus-Vitamin D Preparation for Dogs and Cats

Guaranteed Analysis: per tablet: (All values are minimum quantities unless otherwise stated)

Crude Protein (minimum)	4.0%
Crude Fat (minimum)	1.0%
Crude Fiber (maximum)	1.0%
Moisture (maximum)	4.0%
Minerals:	
Calcium (minimum)	17.5%
(maximum)	21.0%
Phosphorus	14.0%
Salt (minimum)	0.10%
(maximum)	0.60%
Chloride	0.10%
Magnesium	0.02%
Vitamins:	
Vitamin D	400 IU

Ingredients: Dicalcium phosphate, malted milk, corn syrup, soy flour, spray-dried whey, nonfat milk powder, wheat flour, dried buttermilk, brewers dried yeast, magnesium stearate, corn oil, tricalcium phosphate, vitamin D_3 supplement.

Indications: PET-CAL™ tablets are recommended as a daily supplement for dogs and cats where appropriate to provide a dietary source of calcium, phosphorous, and Vitamin D.
Directions for Use:

Dogs and cats—1 tablet per 20 lb of body weight daily.

Administer by hand just prior to feeding, or crumble and mix with food.

Precaution(s): Keep bottle tightly closed to preserve freshness.
Caution(s): Keep out of reach of children.
Presentation: Bottles of 60 and 180 tablets.
Compendium Code No.: 36901241 85-8060-04 / 85-8061-04

PET CARE CANINE 7-ULTRA

Durvet **Bacterin-Vaccine**

Canine Distemper-Adenovirus Type 2-Parainfluenza-Parvovirus Vaccine, Modified Live and Killed Virus, Leptospira Bacterin

U.S. Vet. Lic. No.: 462
Contents: This product contains the antigens listed above. The Adenovirus and Leptospira fractions are inactivated. The remaining virus fractions are live, and attenuated to assure safety.

This product contains gentamicin and amphotericin B as preservatives.

Indications: CANINE 7-ULTRA is recommended for use in the vaccination of healthy dogs against disease caused by Canine Distemper, Infectious Canine Hepatitis, Canine Parvovirus, *Leptospira canicola* and *L. icterohaemorrhagiae* and respiratory disease caused by Canine Adenovirus Type 2 and Parainfluenza.
Directions: Aseptically rehydrate vial of desiccated antigens by injecting the liquid product into the vial containing the vaccine cake. Shake well. Remove the entire contents back into the syringe. Push out any air trapped in the syringe. Administer entire contents (1 mL) intramuscularly or subcutaneously. To give subcutaneously, vaccinate under loose skin (back of neck). To give intramuscularly, vaccinate in large muscle of hind limb. Do not vaccinate into blood vessels. If blood enters the syringe, choose another injection site.

Persistence of maternal origin antibodies in puppies should receive consideration in determining vaccination programs. Ideally, puppies should be vaccinated at 9 weeks of age with revaccination every 2-4 weeks until at least 18 weeks of age. Dogs vaccinated after 18 weeks of age should receive a 1 mL dose followed by a second dose 2-4 weeks later. Annual revaccination with a single 1 mL dose is recommended.

Precaution(s): Store at 35°F-45°F (2°C-7°C). Do not freeze. Use entire contents when first rehydrated. Burn these containers, including syringe and needle.
Caution(s): Do not vaccinate pregnant bitches. In case of anaphylactoid reactions, epinephrine should be administered immediately.

For use in dogs only.

Presentation: 1 dose.
Produced by: Biocor Animal Health Inc., Omaha, NE 68134 U.S.A.
Compendium Code No.: 10842010 12/00

PET CARE CANINE KENNEL COUGH VACCINE

Durvet **Bacterin**

Bordetella Bronchiseptica Bacterin, Extracted Cellular Antigens

U.S. Vet. Lic. No.: 462
Description: CANINE KENNEL COUGH VACCINE is a nonadjuvanted antigenic extract prepared from the cells of *Bordetella bronchiseptica.*

This product contains thimerosal (merthiolate) as a preservative.

Indications: CANINE KENNEL COUGH VACCINE is recommended for use as an aid in the control of canine infectious tracheobronchitis (kennel cough) caused by the organism represented.
Directions: Shake well. Aseptically remove entire contents into the syringe. Push out any air trapped in the syringe. Administer entire contents (1 mL) subcutaneously under loose skin (back of neck) to healthy dogs at least 8 weeks of age. Do not vaccinate into blood vessels. If blood enters the syringe, choose another injection site. For initial vaccination, a second dose is required 2-4 weeks later. This product should be administered by subcutaneous injection only. Annual revaccination with a single 1 mL dose is recommended.
Precaution(s): Store at 35°F-45°F (2°C-7°C). Do not freeze.

Use entire contents when first opened. Care should be taken to avoid microbial contamination of the product.

Caution(s): In case of anaphylactoid reactions, epinephrine should be administered immediately. Transient local irritation at the site of injection, though rare, may occur subsequent to use of this product.

Use special caution when vaccinating miniature or small breed dogs.

For use in dogs only.

Discussion: The effect of persisting *B. bronchiseptica* maternal antibody on the immune response in puppies to this bacterin has not been determined. Puppies from bitches immune to the organism usually have low antibody titers that are dissipated by 4-6 weeks of age. Although kennel cough is considered a disease of complex etiology, it can be reproduced by challenge with *B. bronchiseptica* alone. A close association and/or confinement of dogs facilitates spread of the disease syndrome. Antibiotic therapy has been shown to be generally unsuccessful in reducing or eliminating *B. bronchiseptica* infection in dogs.
Presentation: 1 dose - 1 mL.
Manufactured by: Biocor Animal Health Inc., Omaha, NE 68134
Compendium Code No.: 10841300 DV7001-999

PET CARE CANINE PARVO-ULTRA

Durvet **Vaccine**

Parvovirus Vaccine, Modified Live Virus

U.S. Vet. Lic. No.: 462
Contents: This product contains the antigen listed above.

This product contains gentamicin, amphotericin B and thimerosal as preservatives.

Indications: CANINE PARVO-ULTRA is recommended for use in the vaccination of healthy dogs against disease caused by Canine Parvovirus.
Directions: Shake well. Aseptically remove entire contents into the syringe. Push out any air trapped in the syringe. Administer entire contents (1 mL) subcutaneously or intramuscularly. To give subcutaneously, vaccinate under loose skin (back of neck). To give intramuscularly, vaccinate in large muscle of hind limb. Do not vaccinate into blood vessels. If blood enters the syringe, choose another injection site.

Persistence of maternal origin antibodies in puppies should receive consideration in determining vaccination programs. Ideally, puppies should be vaccinated at 9 weeks of age with revaccination every 2-4 weeks until at least 18 weeks of age. Dogs vaccinated after 18 weeks of age should receive a 1 mL dose followed by a second dose 2-4 weeks later. Annual revaccination with a single 1 mL dose is recommended.

Precaution(s): Store at 35°F-45°F (2°C-7°C). Do not freeze. Use entire contents when first rehydrated. Burn this container, including syringe and needle.
Caution(s): Do not vaccinate pregnant bitches. In case of anaphylactoid reactions, epinephrine should be administered immediately.

For use in dogs only.

Presentation: 1 dose (1 mL).
Produced by: Biocor Animal Health Inc., Omaha, NE 68134 U.S.A.
Compendium Code No.: 10842020 12/00

PET CARE EAR MITE LOTION & REPELLENT

Durvet **Parasiticide-Topical**

EPA Reg. No.: 769-583-12281

Active Ingredient(s):

Pyrethrins 0.15%
*Piperonyl Butoxide, technical 1.00%
N-octyl bicycloheptene dicarboximide 0.50%
Di-n-propyl isocinchomeronate 1.00%
Inert ingredients: 97.35%
Total 100.0%

*Equivalent to 0.80% butylcarbityl 6-propylpiperonyl ether and 0.20% of related compounds.

Indications: Recommended as a topical insecticide and repellent for dogs, cats, and horses. Kills on contact and repels ear mites, flies, mosquitoes, gnats, fleas, ticks, lice, and mange mites for 3 to 5 days.

Dosage and Administration: Dogs-puppies-cats-kittens:

It is a violation of Federal law to use this product in a manner inconsistent with its labeling.

Do not put treatment directly on broken skin or an open wound. Treatment may be applied on a bandage.

To kill and repel ear mites: Clean ear to remove built-up wax and dirt. Gently dry ear with a cotton ball or soft cloth and apply a thin film of treatment. The treatment may be applied daily for 7 to 10 days.

To kill ticks: Make sure treatment covers ticks.

To use as a repellent: Spread treatment lightly on outer and inner surface of the outer ear and between the toes before animals enter infested area. Repeat daily as needed.

Horses-foals: To control ticks, gnats, flies, mosquitoes and mange mites: Before application remove dirt or debris by brushing or washing with a mild detergent. Allow to completely dry. Apply a light film to affected areas daily, massaging into the skin for 2 to 3 days. Then apply every 3 to 5 days as needed.

Precaution(s): Storage: Store in a cool, dry area.

Disposal: Do not reuse empty container. Wrap container and put in trash collection.

Environmental hazards: This product is toxic to fish. Do not apply directly to water.

Physical or chemical hazards: None.

Caution(s): Precautionary statements:

Caution: Hazards to humans and domestic animals.

Human: Harmful if swallowed. Avoid breathing vapors. Avoid contact with eyes. In case of contact, immediately flush eyes with plenty of water. Obtain medical attention if irritation persists. If swallowed, do not induce vomiting. Wash hands with soap and water after using.

Animals: Avoid contact with eyes. If in eyes, flush with water. Do not use on meat or milk producing animals.

Warning(s): Do not use on meat or milk producing animals.

Keep out of reach of children.

Presentation: 6 oz.

Compendium Code No.: 10841310

PET CARE EAR MITE SOLUTION

Durvet **Otic Parasiticide**

EPA Reg. No.: 28293-42-12281

Active Ingredient(s):

Rotenone 0.12%
Cube Resins 0.16%
Inert Ingredients 99.72%

Indications: EAR MITE SOLUTION is used to kill ear mites on dogs, cats and rabbits.

Directions for Use: It is a violation of Federal Law to use this product in a manner inconsistent with its labeling.

Read entire label before each use.

Use only on dogs, cats, or rabbits.

Diagnosis: Ear mites usually induce the formation of a dry, dark brown, waxy exudate with crusts in the ears of dogs, cats, and rabbits. Ear mites may be detected by placing some of the ear exudate on a dark surface and carefully watching for the movement of tiny white specks away from the exudate. Inflamed, watery, or blocked ear canals indicate a more serious condition which requires the services of a veterinarian.

While holding the pet firmly, fill each ear canal half full with EAR MITE SOLUTION and massage the base of the ear to ensure that the insecticidal action penetrates the ear wax. Repeat the treatment every other day until the condition is relieved. Improvement is usually noted after two applications.

Precautionary Statements: Hazards to Humans and Domestic Animals:

Caution: Harmful if swallowed. Avoid breathing vapors. Avoid contact with the skin. Do not use on puppies or kittens under twelve (12) weeks of age. Not for use in animals intended for food. Consult a veterinarian before using this product on debilitated, aged, pregnant or nursing animals or animals on medication. Sensitivities may occur after using any pesticide product for pets. If signs of sensitivity occur, bathe your pet with mild soap and rinse with large amounts of water. If signs continue, consult a veterinarian immediately.

Statement of Practical Treatment/First Aid:

If Swallowed: Drink one or two glasses of water and induce vomiting by sticking a finger in the back of the throat. Repeat until the fluid is clear. Call a physician immediately. Do not induce vomiting or give anything by mouth to an unconscious person.

If on Skin: Wash immediately with soap and water.

If in Eyes: Flush with water for 15 minutes. See a physician.

Environmental Hazards: Do not contaminate water when disposing of equipment washwaters.

Storage and Disposal:

Storage: Store in the original container in a locked storage area.

Disposal: Do not reuse the container. Rinse thoroughly, and securely wrap the original container in several layers of newspaper and discard in the trash.

Warning(s): Keep out of reach of children.

Presentation: 4 fl oz.

Compendium Code No.: 10840731 9/98

PET CARE FAST KILL FLEA & TICK SPRAY FOR DOGS & CATS

Durvet **Parasiticide Spray**

EPA Reg. No.: 9468-31-12281

Active Ingredient(s):

Pyrethrins 0.15%
Piperonyl butoxide, technical* 1.50%
(N-octyl bicycloheptene dicarboximide) 0.5%
(Di-n-propyl isocinchomeronate) 0.50%
Inert Ingredients** 97.35%
Total 100.00%

*Equivalent to 1.2% (butylcarbityl) (6-propylpiperonyl) ether and 0.3% related compounds.

**Inert Ingredients include a grooming and conditioning agent to ease combing and brushing of coat to remove dead fleas, ticks and lice.

Indications: Controls and kills fleas, ticks and lice on dogs, cats, and horses, and for temporarily repelling gnats, mosquitoes and biting flies.

Directions for Use: It is a violation of Federal Law to use this product in a manner inconsistent with its labeling.

Read entire label before each use.

Use only on dogs, cats or horses.

Use only in a well ventilated area. Remove birds and cover aquariums before spraying. Remove safety cap and insert sprayer.

Cats and Dogs: Cover animal's eyes with hand and with a firm fast stroke, to get a proper spray mist, spray head, ears, and chest until damp. With finger tips, rub into face and around mouth, nose and eyes. Then spray neck, middle, and hind quarters, finishing legs last. For best penetration of spray to the skin, direct spray against the natural lay of the hair. On long-haired dogs rub your hands against the lay of the hair, spraying the ruffled hair directly behind the hand. Make sure spray thoroughly wets ticks. Repeat every 5 days if needed. Do not use on puppies or kittens under 12 weeks old.

Pet Sleeping Quarters: Spray around baseboards, windows, door frames, wall cracks and local area of floors. If mosquitoes, gnats or flies are present, spray lightly into the air. Repeat as needed. The bedding should be sprayed and then replaced with fresh bedding for best results.

Horses: To control stable flies, horse flies, deer flies and face flies apply to face, legs, flanks, topline and other body areas commonly attacked by these flies. Repeat treatment as needed.

Precautionary Statements: Hazards to Humans and Domestic Animals:

Humans: Harmful if swallowed or inhaled. Avoid breathing spray mist. Avoid contact with skin or eyes. Avoid contamination of feed or foodstuffs. Wash hands with soap and water after using.

Animals: Avoid contact with animal's eyes. Consult a veterinarian before using this product on debilitated, aged, pregnant, nursing or animals on medication. Sensitivities may occur after using any pesticide product for pets. If signs of sensitivity occur bathe your pet with mild soap and rinse with large amounts of water. If signs continue, consult a veterinarian immediately.

First Aid:

If Swallowed: Do not induce vomiting. Contains petroleum distillate - vomiting may cause aspiration pneumonia. Call a physician, veterinarian or Poison Control Center immediately.

If in Eyes: Hold eyelids open and flush with a steady, gentle stream of water for 15 minutes. Get medical attention.

If on Skin: Wash with soap and water. Get medical attention if irritation persists.

Environmental Hazards: This product is toxic to aquatic organisms. Do not apply directly to water. Do not contaminate water when disposing of equipment washwaters.

Physical or Chemical Hazards: Flammable: Keep away from heat or open flame. Do not use this product in or on electrical equipment due to possibility of shock hazard.

Storage and Disposal: Do not contaminate food or foodstuffs by storage or disposal. Do not reuse empty container. Wrap empty container and put in trash collection.

Warning(s): Not for use on animals to be used as a source for food or feed.

Keep out of reach of children.

Presentation: 16 oz and 32 oz.

Compendium Code No.: 10841842 2/01

PET CARE FELINE 3-C VACCINE

Durvet **Vaccine**

Feline Rhinotracheitis-Calici-Panleukopenia-Chlamydia Psittaci Vaccine, Modified Live Virus and Chlamydia

U.S. Vet. Lic. No.: 462

Contents: FELINE 3-C VACCINE is a combination of modified live Feline Rhinotracheitis, Calici and Panleukopenia viruses and *Chlamydia psittaci*.

This product contains gentamicin and amphotericin B as preservatives.

Indications: Recommended for use in the vaccination of healthy cats against disease caused by the organisms represented.

Directions: Aseptically rehydrate vial of desiccated antigens by injecting the liquid product into the vial containing the vaccine cake. Shake well. Remove the entire contents back into the syringe. Push out air trapped in the syringe. Administer entire contents (1 mL) subcutaneously under loose skin (back of neck). Do not vaccinate into blood vessels. If blood enters the syringe, choose another injection site.

Persistence of maternal origin antibody in kittens is known to interfere with development of active immunity following vaccination. Ideally, kittens should be vaccinated at 9 weeks of age with revaccination 3-4 weeks later. Adult cats should receive a 1 mL dose followed by a second dose 3-4 weeks later. Annual revaccination with a single 1 mL dose is recommended.

Precaution(s): Store at 35°F-45°F (2°C-7°C). Do not freeze. Use entire contents when first rehydrated. Burn these containers, including syringe and needle.

Caution(s): Do not vaccinate pregnant queens. An occasional animal may demonstrate a transient fever, and mild arthralgia and/or myalgia within the first week following vaccination. In case of anaphylactoid reactions, epinephrine should be administered immediately.

For use in cats only.

Presentation: 1 dose.

Produced by: Biocor Animal Health Inc., Omaha, NE 68134 U.S.A.

Compendium Code No.: 10840811 5/99

PET CARE FELINE 3 VACCINE

Durvet **Vaccine**

Feline Rhinotracheitis-Calici-Panleukopenia Vaccine, Modified Live and Killed Virus

U.S. Vet. Lic. No.: 462

Contents: FELINE 3 VACCINE is a combination of modified live Feline Rhinotracheitis and Calici viruses with inactivated Panleukopenia virus vaccine. All fractions are subjected to tests for potency and safety prior to release for market.

This product contains gentamicin and amphotericin B as preservatives.

Indications: Recommended for use in the vaccination of healthy cats against disease caused by the organisms represented.

Directions: Aseptically rehydrate vial of desiccated antigens by injecting the liquid product into the vial containing the vaccine cake. Shake well. Remove the entire contents back into the syringe. Push out air trapped in the syringe. Administer entire contents (1 mL) subcutaneously under loose skin (back of neck). Do not vaccinate into blood vessels. If blood enters the syringe, choose another injection site.

Persistence of maternal origin antibody in kittens is known to interfere with development of active immunity following vaccination. Present indications are that Rhinotracheitis and Calicivirus antibodies of maternal origin endure in kittens for approximately 8 weeks. Panleukopenia antibody somewhat longer - up to 13 weeks. Ideally, kittens should be vaccinated at 9 weeks of age with revaccination 3-4 weeks later. Adult cats should receive a 1 mL dose followed by a second dose 3-4 weeks later. Annual revaccination with a single 1 mL dose is recommended.

Precaution(s): Store at 35°F-45°F (2°C-7°C). Do not freeze. Use entire contents when first rehydrated. Burn these containers, including syringe and needle.

Caution(s): Do not vaccinate pregnant queens. An occasional animal may demonstrate a transient fever, and mild arthralgia and/or myalgia within the first week following vaccination. In case of anaphylactoid reactions, epinephrine should be administered immediately. For use in cats only.

Presentation: 1 dose.

Produced by: Biocor Animal Health Inc., Omaha, NE 68134 U.S.A.

Compendium Code No.: 10840801 9/01

PET CARE HOUSE & CARPET POWDER

Durvet **Household Insecticide**

EPA Reg. No.: 45087-55-12281

Active Ingredient(s):

Pyrethrin	0.15%
Piperonyl Butoxide, Technical**	1.50%
Inert Ingredients:	99.35%
Total	100.00%

**Equivalent to 1.2% (butylcarbityl) (6-propylpiperonyl) ether and 0.3% related compounds.

Contains Pyrenone®.

Indications: Kills fleas and ticks that live and breed in carpets. For use in homes, vacation cabins, basements, pet sleeping quarters and storage areas.

Directions for Use: It is a violation of Federal law to use this product in a manner inconsistent with its labeling.

Directions: Shake well before using. Punch plastic seal. For use on carpets, hold upside down and shake powder evenly across surface. Brush lightly with a broom to allow powder to penetrate carpet fibers. Wait 60 minutes, then vacuum. For severe problems or where ticks are known to be hiding, wait 2-3 hours before vacuuming. If powder adheres to a spot, brush it out and vacuum immediately. Apply to dry surfaces only. Do not allow powder to become wet. For use on upholstery, remove all loose cushions. Sprinkle along creases, in corners. Brush gently, wait 60 minutes, vacuum. Sprinkle along underside of furniture. Do not use on exposed fabric: may cause staining. Remove bag from vacuum cleaner. Wrap securely in several layers of newspaper and discard in trash.

Test hidden surface or upholstery before cleaning. If texture or color is affected, do not use. Clean carpet after using this product. Treat pets with a registered flea and tick control powder prior to re-entry into treated area.

Precautionary Statements: Hazards to Humans and Domestic Animals.

Caution: Harmful if swallowed. Avoid breathing of dust and contact with eyes, skin or clothing. Wash hands with soap and water after handling and before eating or smoking. For eyes, flush with plenty of water. If irritation persists get medical attention. Do not contaminate feed, water or foodstuffs. Do not use in food serving areas while food is exposed. Keep children and pets away from treated carpet and upholstered furniture until the treated areas have been vacuumed and any visible powder removed.

Statement of Practical Treatment:

If Swallowed: Call a physician or Poison Control Center immediately. Induce vomiting by giving victim 1 or 2 glasses of water and touching back of throat with finger. Never give anything by mouth to an unconscious person.

If in Eyes: Flush eyes with plenty of water. Get medical attention if irritation persists.

If on Skin: Wash with soap and warm water.

If Inhaled: Remove victim to fresh air. Apply artificial respiration if indicated. Give nothing by mouth to an unconscious person.

Storage and Disposal: Do not contaminate water, food, or feed by storage or disposal.

Storage: Store in original container in an area inaccessible to children and pets and away from heat and sunlight. Avoid exposure to moisture.

Disposal: do not reuse empty container. Wrap container in several layers of newspaper before discarding in trash.

Warning(s): Keep out of reach of children.

Presentation: 20 oz. (567 g). Treats three carpets 12x14 (504 sq. ft.).

® Pyrenone - Registered Trademark of Roussel Uclaf Corporation.

Compendium Code No.: 10841341 3/96

P

PET CARE IGR-HOUSE & CARPET SPRAY

Durvet **Household Insecticide**

Insect Growth Regulator

EPA Reg. No.: 1021-1622-12281

Active Ingredient(s):

2-[1-Methyl-2-(4-phenoxyphenoxy) ethoxy] pyridine	0.015%
Tetramethrin [(1-Cyclohexene-1,2-dicarboximido) methyl, 2,2-dimethyl-3-(2-methylpropenyl) cyclopropanecarboxylate	0.400%
3-Phenoxybenzyl-(1RS, 3RS; 1RS 3SR)-2,2-dimethyl-3-(2-methylprop-1-enyl) cyclopropanecarboxylate	0.300%
Inert Ingredients:	99.285%
Total	100.000%

Contains Nylar®.

Indications: Kills adult and preadult fleas. Kills ticks.

Directions for Use: It is a violation of Federal law to use this product in a manner inconsistent with its labeling.

For indoor use only.

IGR HOUSE & CARPET SPRAY kills fleas and ticks. It contains a unique combination of ingredients that kills both adult and preadult fleas. Even kills fleas before they grow up to bite. Nylar®, a unique ingredient in this flea spray, continues to kill fleas for 120 days (4 months) by preventing their development into adult biting stage. It reaches fleas hidden in carpets, rugs, drapes, upholstery, pet bedding, floor cracks. Protects your home from reinfestation and flea buildup, your pets and family from bites. One treatment with this spray gives continuous flea protection for 120 days. Leaves no objectional odor or sticky mess and, used as directed, does not stain furnishings.

Fleas and Ticks: Shake well. Hold can 2 or 3 feet from surfaces to be treated. Be sure to apply uniformly using a sweeping motion to carpets, rugs, drapes and all surfaces of upholstered furniture. Be sure to treat pet bedding as this is a primary hiding place for fleas. No need to remove pet bedding after treatment. Do not treat pets. Use a registered flea control product on your pets in conjunction with this treatment. Repeat as necessary. Avoid wetting furniture and carpeting. A fine mist or spray applied uniformly is all that is necessary to kill fleas and ticks.

Precautionary Statements: Hazards to Humans and Domestic Animals:

Caution: Harmful if swallowed or absorbed through skin. Contains petroleum distillate. Do not induce vomiting because of aspiration pneumonia hazard. Do not breathe vapors or spray mist. Avoid contact with skin or eyes. In case of contact, flush with plenty of water. Wash with soap and warm water after use. Obtain medical attention if irritation persists. Avoid contamination of food or feedstuffs.

Do not use in commercial food processing, preparation, food storage or serving areas. In the home, all food processing surfaces and utensils should be covered during treatment, or thoroughly washed before use. Exposed food should be covered or removed.

Remove pets, birds, and cover fish aquariums before spraying.

Statement of Practical Treatment:

If Swallowed: Call a physician or Poison Control Center immediately. Do not induce vomiting because of aspiration pneumonia hazard.

If in Eyes: Flush with plenty of water. Get medical attention if irritation persists.

If on Skin or Clothing: Remove contaminated clothing and wash before reuse. Wash skin with soap and warm water. Get medical attention if irritation persists.

If Inhaled: Remove victim to fresh air. Apply artificial respiration if indicated.

Physical or Chemical Hazards: Contents under pressure. Keep away from heat, sparks, and open flame. Do not puncture or incinerate container. Exposure to temperatures above 130°F may cause bursting.

Storage and Disposal:

Storage: Store in a cool, dry place inaccessible to children. Keep container closed.

Disposal: Do not reuse empty container. Wrap container in several layers of newspaper and discard in trash.

Warning(s): Keep out of reach of children.

Presentation: 16 oz (454 g).

® Nylar - Registered trademark of McLaughlin Gormley King Co.

Compendium Code No.: 10841351 4/96

PET CARE INDOOR PREMISE SPRAY

Durvet **Household Insecticide**

EPA Reg. No.: 45087-31-12281

Active Ingredient(s):

Chlorpyrifos (0,0 diethyl 0-(3,5,6 Trichloro-2-Pyridyl) Phosphorothioate)	0.50%
Inert ingredients:	99.5%
Total	100%

Contains Dursban†.

Indications: Premise, kennel, spot carpet treatment for control of fleas and ticks. Also kills ants, cockroaches, crickets, silverfish, and spiders. Kills flea larvae.

Directions for Use: It is a violation of Federal law to use this product in a manner inconsistent with its labeling.

For control of fleas, ticks, cockroaches and other insect pests, thoroughly apply as a spray for spot treatment to infested areas: pet beds, kennel runs and resting quarters; nearby cracks and crevices; along and behind baseboards, window and door frames and localized areas of floor and floor covering where these pests may be present. Old bedding of pets should be removed and replaced with clean, fresh bedding after treatment of pet area. Repeat treatment in two weeks or as often as needed. Do not treat pets with this product. Use Pet Care Flea and Tick Spray for Dogs or Pet Care Flea and Tick Spray for Cats for pest control on pets.

Contraindication(s): Do not treat dogs or cats with this product.

Precautionary Statements: Hazards to Humans: Avoid contact with eyes, skin and clothing. Avoid breathing vapors or spray mist. Keep away from food, feedstuffs and domestic water supplies. Wash thoroughly after handling.

Statement of Practical Treatment:

If Inhaled: Remove victim to fresh air. Apply artificial respiration if necessary.

If Swallowed: Call a physician or Poison Control Center. Drink 1 to 2 glasses of water and induce vomiting by touching back of throat with finger. Do not induce vomiting or give anything by mouth to an unconscious person.

If on Skin: In case of contact, remove contaminated clothing and immediately wash skin with plenty of soap and water.

If in Eyes: Flush eyes with plenty of water.

Note to Physician: Chlorpyrifos is a cholinesterase inhibitor. Treat symptomatically. Atropine by injection is the preferable antidote. Oximes such as 2-PAM may or may not be therapeutic, but it is recommended they not be used in place of atropine.

Physical or Chemical Hazards:

Environmental Hazards: PET CARE INDOOR PREMISE SPRAY is toxic to fish, birds and other wildlife. Do not contaminate water by cleaning of equipment or disposal of wastes.

Storage and Disposal:

Storage: Store in original container in locked storage area around 32 degrees F. Do not use or store near heat or open flame.

Disposal: Wrap original container in several layers of newspaper and discard in trash. Do not reuse container or sprayer. Rinse thoroughly before discarding in trash.
Warning(s): Keep out of reach of children.
Presentation: 16 fl. oz. (472 mL).
† Dursban is Registered TM of DowElanco Co.
Compendium Code No.: 10841371 3/96

PET CARE LIQUID WORMER

Durvet **Parasiticide-Oral**
Pyrantel pamoate
ANADA No.: 200-028
Active Ingredient(s): 2.27 mg of pyrantel base as pyrantel pamoate per mL.
Indications: To prevent reinfestation of *Toxocara canis* in puppies and adult dogs and in lactating bitches after whelping. For the removal of large roundworms (ascarids), *Toxocara canis* and *Toxascaris leonina,* and hookworms, *Ancylostoma caninum* and *Uncinaria stenocephala*, in dogs. The presence of these parasites should be confirmed by laboratory fecal examination. Consult your veterinarian for assistance in the diagnosis, treatment, and control of parasitism.
Directions for Use: Shake well before use.

For maximum control and prevention of reinfestation, it is recommended that puppies be treated at 2, 3, 4, 6, 8, and 10 weeks of age. Lactating bitches should be treated 2-3 weeks after whelping. Adult dogs kept in heavily contaminated quarters may be treated at monthly intervals to prevent *T. canis* reinfestation. Administer one full teaspoonful (5 mL) for each 5 lb of body weight.

For the removal of large roundworms (ascarids) and hookworms, put one full teaspoonful (5 mL) for each 5 lb of dog's body weight in the animal's food bowl. To assure proper dosage, weigh animal prior to treatment. Dogs usually find this wormer very palatable and will lick the dose from the bowl willingly. If there is reluctance to accept the dose, mix in a small quantity of dog food to encourage consumption. It is not necessary to withhold food from your dog prior to treatment.

The presence of large roundworms (ascarids) and hookworms should be confirmed by laboratory fecal examination. It is recommended that dogs maintained under conditions of constant exposure to worm infestation should have a follow-up fecal exam within 2 to 4 weeks after first treatment.

If your dog looks or acts sick, consult your veterinarian before treatment.
Precaution(s): Recommended Storage: Store below 86°F (30°C).
Warning(s): Keep out of reach of children.
Presentation: 2 fl oz (60 mL).
Compendium Code No.: 10841381 11/98

PET CARE LIQUID WORMER 2X

Durvet **Parasiticide-Oral**
Double Strength (pyrantel pamoate)
ANADA No.: 200-028
Active Ingredient(s): Each mL contains 4.54 mg of pyrantel base as pyrantel pamoate.
Indications: LIQUID WORMER 2X suspension is a highly palatable formulation intended as a single treatment for the removal of large roundworms *(Toxocara canis* and *Toxascaris leonina)* and hookworms *(Ancylostoma caninum* and *Uncinaria stenocephala)* in dogs and puppies.

LIQUID WORMER 2X suspension may also be used to prevent reinfestation of *Toxocara canis* in puppies and adult dogs and in lactating bitches after whelping.
Pharmacology: LIQUID WORMER 2X is a suspension of pyrantel pamoate in a palatable caramel-flavored vehicle.

Pyrantel pamoate is a compound belonging to a family classified chemically as tetrahydropyrimidines. It is a yellow, water-insoluble crystalline salt of the tetrahydropyrimidine base and pamoic acid containing 34.7% base activity. The chemical structure and name are given below:

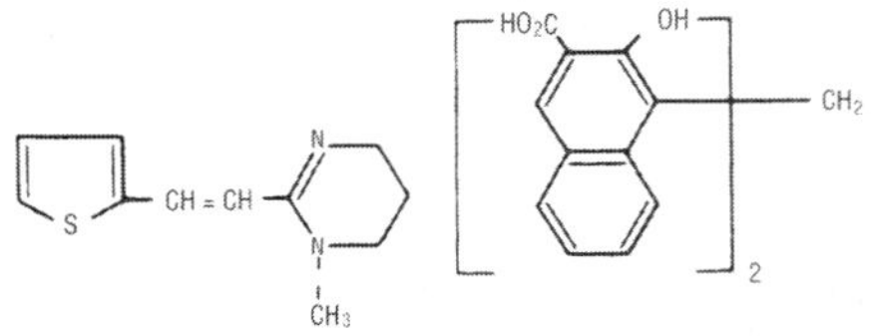

(E)-1,4,5,6-Tetrahydro-1-methyl-2-[2-(2-thienyl) vinyl] pyrimidine 4,4' methylenebis [3-hydroxy-2-naphthoate] (1:1)
Dosage and Administration: Shake well before use.

Administer one full teaspoon (5 mL) for each 10 pounds of body weight (2.27 mg base per lb of body weight). Although most dogs have been observed to find this formulation very palatable and willingly consume it undiluted, it may be necessary to mix a small quantity of formulation in the dog's normal ration to encourage consumption. Fasting prior to or after treatment is not necessary. For maximum control and prevention of reinfestation, it is recommended that puppies be treated at 2, 3, 4, 6, 8, and 10 weeks of age. Lactating bitches should be treated 2-3 weeks after whelping. Adult dogs kept in heavily contaminated quarters may be treated at monthly intervals to prevent *T. canis* reinfestation.

The presence of large roundworms (ascarids) and hookworms should be confirmed by laboratory fecal examination. It is recommended that dogs maintained under conditions of constant exposure to worm infestation should have a follow-up fecal exam within 2 to 4 weeks after first treatment.

Consult your veterinarian for assistance in the diagnosis, treatment, and control of parasitism.
Precaution(s): Recommended Storage: Store below 86°F (30°C).
Caution(s): This product is a suspension and as such will separate. To insure uniform resuspension and to achieve proper dosage, it is extremely important that the product be shaken thoroughly before every use.

For animal use only.
Warning(s): Keep out of reach of children.
Toxicology: Safety: One of the most outstanding and significant features of LIQUID WORMER 2X is its wide margin of therapeutic safety in dogs. The acute oral LD_{50} of pyrantel pamoate administered in gelatin capsules to female and male dogs is greater than 314 mg base per pound of body weight, which indicates a therapeutic index in excess of 138x the recommended dosage. In subacute and chronic studies, no significant morphological abnormalities could be attributed to LIQUID WORMER 2X when administered to dogs at daily dose rates of up to 94 mg base per pound of body weight (40x) for periods of 19, 30, and 90 days. Clinical studies conducted in a wide variety of geographic locations using more than 40 different breeds of dogs showed no drug-induced toxic effects. Included in these studies were nursing pups, weaned pups, adults, pregnant bitches, and males at stud. Additional data have demonstrated the safe use of LIQUID WORMER 2X (pyrantel pamoate) in (1) dogs having heartworm infections and/or receiving medication for heartworms, (2) dogs exposed to organophosphate flea collars or flea/tick dip treatments, and (3) dogs undergoing concurrent treatment or medication at the time of worming such as immunization and antibacterial treatment.
Trial Data: Efficacy: Critical (worm count) studies in dogs demonstrated that LIQUID WORMER 2X at the recommended dosage is highly efficacious against *T. leonina* (99%), *T. canis* (85%), *A. caninum* (97%), and *U. stenocephala* (94%).
Presentation: 2 fl oz (60 mL) and 8 fl oz (237 mL).
Compendium Code No.: 10841391 11/98

PET CARE LITTER, KENNEL AND STALL ODOR CONTROL POWDER

Durvet **Deodorant Product**
Indications: Helps to eliminate manure, and ammonia odors in stalls, kennels, kitty litter, dog runs and pens.

Completely biodegradable, environmentally safe - Non-toxic.
Directions for Use:

Stalls: Spread LITTER, KENNEL AND STALL POWDER evenly on any type of bedding to extend the life of its use. Use approximately one pound per stall every ten (10) days.

Litter Boxes: Sprinkle LITTER, KENNEL AND STALL POWDER evenly over bottom of litter box at every litter change. May also be used over the top of existing litter to extend the life of the litter.

Kennels, Dog Runs and Pens: Sprinkle LITTER, KENNEL AND STALL POWDER evenly over the surface area to be deodorized.

Use one pound (1/2 shaker) per 12 foot by 12 foot area. Retreat area approximately every 10 days.
Presentation: 2 lb. (0.91 kg).
Compendium Code No.: 10841400

PET CARE PUPPY 5-ULTRA

Durvet **Vaccine**
Canine Distemper-Adenovirus Type 2-Parainfluenza-Parvovirus Vaccine, Modified Live and Killed Virus
U.S. Vet. Lic. No.: 462
Contents: This product contains the antigens listed above. The Adenovirus fraction is inactivated. The remaining virus fractions are live, and attenuated to assure safety.

This product contains gentamicin and amphotericin B as preservatives.
Indications: PUPPY 5-ULTRA is recommended for use in the vaccination of healthy dogs against disease caused by Canine Distemper, Infectious Canine Hepatitis, Canine Parvovirus and respiratory disease caused by Canine Adenovirus Type 2 and Parainfluenza.
Directions: Aseptically rehydrate vial of desiccated antigens by injecting the liquid product into the vial containing the vaccine cake. Shake well. Remove the entire contents back into the syringe. Push out any air trapped in the syringe. Administer entire contents (1 mL) intramuscularly or subcutaneously. To give subcutaneously, vaccinate under loose skin (back of neck). To give intramuscularly, vaccinate in large muscle of hind limb. Do not vaccinate into blood vessels. If blood enters the syringe, choose another injection site.

Persistence of maternal origin antibodies in puppies should receive consideration in determining vaccination programs. Ideally, puppies should be vaccinated at 9 weeks of age with revaccination every 2-4 weeks until at least 18 weeks of age. Dogs vaccinated after 18 weeks of age should receive a 1 mL dose followed by a second dose 2-4 weeks later. Annual revaccination with a single 1 mL dose is recommended.
Precaution(s): Store at 35°F-45°F (2°C-7°C). Do not freeze. Use entire contents when first rehydrated. Burn these containers, including syringe and needle.
Caution(s): Do not vaccinate pregnant bitches. In case of anaphylactoid reactions, epinephrine should be administered immediately.

For use in dogs only.
Presentation: 1 dose.
Produced by: Biocor Animal Health Inc., Omaha, NE 68134 U.S.A.
Compendium Code No.: 10842030 12/00

PETCHEK® ANTI FIV ANTIBODY TEST KIT

Idexx Labs. **FIV Test**
U.S. Vet. Lic. No.: 313
Description: Feline immunodeficiency virus antibody test kit.
Components: Reagents:

Reagents	Volume
1. FIV Ag coated immunoassay strips	2 Plates
2. FIV Ag: Horseradish Peroxidase (HRPO) Conjugate in buffer with protein stabilizers. Preserved with Gentamicin	10 mL
3. Positive Control. Anti-FIV antibody positive serum. Contains a preservative.	1 mL
4. Negative Control. Anti-FIV antibody negative serum. Contains a preservative.	1 mL
5. TMB Concentrate.	25 mL
6. TMB Diluent. Citrate-phosphate buffer containing hydrogen peroxide. Contains a preservative.	25 mL
7. Wash Solution (10x). Preserved with Gentamicin.	100 mL
8. Stop Solution.	25 mL

Materials Required But Not Provided:
1. 96-well plate (EIA) Reader capable of reading absorbance at 650 nm.
2. Precision Pipets: 0.100, 0.050 mL or multiple delivery pipeting devices.
3. Disposable pipet tips.
4. Distilled or deionized water.
5. Device for the delivery and aspiration of wash solution.
6. A vacuum source and a trap for retaining the aspirate.

Indications: PETCHEK® Anti-FIV is an enzyme immunoassay for the detection of antibody to feline immunodeficiency virus (FIV) in feline serum or plasma.

Test Principles: PETCHEK® Anti-FIV is an enzyme immunoassay designed to detect the presence of antibody to FIV in feline serum or plasma. A microtitration format has been devised in which FIV antigens are coated on 12-well strips, and conjugated to the enzyme horseradish peroxidase (HRPO) to form an FIV:HRPO conjugate.

The test sample and FIV conjugate are incubated in the FIV coated microassay wells. Antibody specific for FIV (if present) will bind to both the coated FIV antigens and the FIV:HRPO conjugate, thus forming specific immune complexes.

Unbound components are washed away and an enzyme substrate (H_2O_2)/chromogen solution (tetramethylbenzidine, TMB) is added. Subsequent color development is proportional to the amount of specific antibody present in the sample.

Test Procedure: All reagents must come to room temperature before use. Reagents should be mixed by gentle swirling or vortexing.

Specimen Information:

1. Serum or Plasma, either fresh, previously frozen or stored at 2°-7°C (36°-45°F), may be used in this test. Serum or plasma may be stored for up to 7 days at 2°-7°C. For longer storage, sample should be frozen (-20°C or colder).
2. Care should be taken to ensure that serum and plasma samples are cell-free. Hemolyzed samples may be used. However highly-hemolyzed samples may yield a high background.
3. EDTA, heparin or citrate in plasma will not affect results.
4. Previously frozen or older samples must be centrifuged before use.

Preparation of Wash Solution: Occasionally, salt crystals may form in the Wash Concentrate upon storage. If this occurs, allow concentrate to come to room temperature and mix by swirling to redissolve crystals before preparing the wash solution.

Dilute Wash Concentrate 10 fold with distilled or deionized water (e.g. 3 mL of Wash Concentrate plus 27 mL of water for each strip to be assayed). Diluted wash may be stored at room temperature for a period of up to one week. Do not store diluted wash solution in direct sunlight.

Assay Protocol:

1. Obtain antigen-coated strip(s) and record the control and sample positions on a PetChek worksheet. Each control and sample requires a separate well.
2. Dispense 0.05 mL of Negative Control (NC) into the first two wells.
3. Dispense 0.05 mL of Positive Control (PC) into the next two wells.
4. Dispense 0.05 mL of serum or plasma sample into appropriate test well(s).
5. Dispense 1 drop (0.05 mL) of FIV:HRPO Conjugate into each well. Mix by gently tapping the side of the plate 3-5 times.
6. Incubate for 30 minutes at room temperature.
7. Aspirate liquid contents of all wells into an appropriate waste reservoir.
8. Wash each well five times with approximately 0.30 mL of diluted wash solution. Aspirate liquid contents of all wells following each wash. Following the final wash aspiration, gently but firmly, tap residual wash fluid from wells onto absorbent paper. Avoid plate drying between washes and prior to addition of reagents.
9. Dispense 1 drop (0.05 mL) of TMB Diluent Solution into each well followed by 1 drop (0.05 mL) of TMB Concentrate into each well. Mix gently by tapping. NOTE: Equal volumes of TMB Diluent and TMB Substrate may be premixed. Dispense 2 drops (0.10 mL) of the premixed reagent into each well.
10. Incubate for 15 minutes at room temp.
11. Dispense 2 drops (0.10 mL) Stop Solution into each well to stop the enzymatic reaction.
12. Blank reader on air.
13. Measure and record absorbance values at 650 nm, A(650), for samples and controls.

Results: For the assay to be valid, the difference between the positive control mean and the negative control mean ($PC\bar{x}$ - $NC\bar{x}$) should be greater than 0.25. In addition, the negative control mean absorbance should be less than or equal to 0.15. For invalid tests, technique may be suspect, and the assay should be repeated.

The presence or absence of antibody to FIV is determined by relating the A(650) value of the sample to the positive control mean. The positive control has been standardized and represents significant antibody levels to FIV in serum or plasma. The relative level of antibody in the sample can be determined by calculating the sample to positive (S/P) ratio. (See Calculations.) If this ratio is less than 0.5, the sample is classified as negative. S/P ratios equal to or greater than 0.5 indicate the presence of antibody to FIV.

Test Interpretation: Interpretation of Results: Samples with S/P ratios of less than 0.5 are classified as negative. Samples with S/P ratios equal to or greater than 0.5 should be considered reactive and should be retested. Samples that repeat as reactive should be considered positive and indicate exposure to FIV.

Calculations:

1. Calculation of Negative Control Mean ($NC\bar{x}$):

$$\frac{\text{Well NC1 A(650)} + \text{Well NC2 A(650)}}{2} = NC\bar{x}$$

Example:

$$\frac{0.050 + 0.056}{2} = \frac{0.106}{2} = 0.053$$

2. Calculation of Positive Control Mean ($PC\bar{x}$):

$$\frac{\text{Well PC1 A(650)} + \text{Well PC2 A(650)}}{2} = PC\bar{x}$$

Example:

$$\frac{0.56 + 0.52}{2} = \frac{1.08}{2} = 0.54$$

3. Calculation of S/P Ratio:

$$\frac{\text{Sample} - NC\bar{x}}{PC\bar{x} - NC\bar{x}} = S/P$$

Example: Sample A(650) = 1.23:

$$\frac{1.23 - 0.053}{0.54 - 0.053} = \frac{1.177}{0.487} = 2.42$$

Storage: Store all reagents at 2°-7°C (36°-45°F). Bring to room temperature 15°-30°C (59°-86°F) prior to use, and return to 2°-7°C following use.

Caution(s): Handle all biological materials as though capable of transmitting FIV.

FIV antigen used to prepare the test strips and conjugate has been chemically inactivated. However, strips should be handled as if capable of transmitting FIV.

Do not pipet by mouth.

There should be no eating, drinking or smoking where specimens or kit reagents are being handled.

Do not expose TMB solutions to strong light or any oxidizing agents.

All wastes should be properly decontaminated prior to disposal.

Care should be taken to prevent contamination of kit components.

Do not use test kit past expiration date. Do not intermix components from kits with different serial numbers.

Optimal results will be obtained by strict adherence to this protocol. Careful pipeting and washing throughout this procedure are necessary to maintain precision and accuracy.

References: Available upon request.

Presentation: Two plate kit.

Compendium Code No.: 11160381

PETCHEK® FeLV

Idexx Labs. **FeLV Test**

U.S. Vet. Lic. No.: 313

Description: This feline leukemia virus antigen test kit is an enzyme immunoassay.

Components:

Reagents	Volume	
	1 plate	5 plate
1. Anti-FeLV Coated Wells	8 x 12 wells	40 x 12 wells
2. Anti-FeLV Horseradish Peroxidase Conjugate preserved with gentamicin	25 mL	25 mL
3. Positive Control preserved with gentamicin	2 mL	2 mL
4. Negative Control preserved with gentamicin	2 mL	2 mL
5. TMB Concentrate	25 mL	25 mL
6. TMB Diluent	25 mL	25 mL
7. Wash Concentrate (10X) - preserved with gentamicin	100 mL	100 mL
8. Stop Solution	25 mL	25 mL
A. Solution A - Sample Diluent preserved with gentamicin (for confirmatory protocol)	0.5 mL	0.5 mL
B. Solution B - Neutralizing Reagent preserved with gentamicin (for confirmatory protocol)	0.5 mL	0.5 mL

Materials Required but Not Provided:

1. Distilled or deionized water.
2. Wash bottle.

Other Components Provided:

1. Sample pretreatment tubes (for confirmatory protocol).

Other Components Provided (1 plate kit only):

1. Precision Pipet.
2. Disposable pipet tips.
3. 10 μL Capillary Pipets (for confirmatory protocol).

Use of Precision Pipet to Dispense 50 μL: Place disposable pipet tip on pipet. Depress button on pipet, place tip in sample and release button slowly to pull up sample. Depress button completely to dispense the entire 50 μL sample volume from the pipet tip to the well.

Indications: To screen for and confirm the presence of feline leukemia virus antigen (FeLV) in feline serum or plasma. Whole blood samples may be used in the Screening Protocol, but serum or plasma must be used in the confirmatory protocol.

Test Principles: This test kit uses monoclonal antibodies specific for FeLV p27. These antibodies are coated on microtiter wells which are arranged in 12-well strips.

In the screening protocol, samples are incubated in the test wells with antibodies conjugated to Horseradish Peroxidase (HRPO). Any FeLV antigen in the sample will bind with both the antibody coated on the test well and with the Antibody:HRPO Conjugate. Unbound materials are washed from the wells, then substrate and chromogen are added. Subsequent color development is proportional to the amount of FeLV group-specific antigen (p27) present in the test sample.

However, in the screening protocol, it is possible that samples which contain non-FeLV material (such as feline anti-mouse antibodies) will react with the test kit.

For this reason, any positive results should be checked with the confirmatory protocol.

The confirmatory protocol checks the accuracy of positive results obtained on the screening protocol.

The confirmatory protocol is identical to the screening protocol except for the addition of a sample pretreatment step. A sample screened as positive is pretreated with neutralizing antibody (polyclonal). Antigen, if present in the serum or plasma, will react with the polyclonal antibodies, complexing the available binding sites. This treated sample is then transferred to a test well and assayed per the confirmatory protocol. Since most of the binding sites on the antigen are already complexed, the sample will produce substantially reduced absorbance values. For comparison, the sample is also treated with a non-reactive diluent and assayed concurrently with the neutralized sample. The sample is considered positive if the neutralizing antibody reduces color formation by 50% or greater as compared to the sample treated with non-reactive diluent.

Test Procedure: All reagents must come to room temperature before use. Reagents should be mixed by gentle swirling or vortexing.

Specimen Information:

1. Serum or plasma, either fresh, previously frozen or stored at 2°-7°C (36°-45°F), may be used in this test. Serum or plasma may be stored for up to 7 days at 2°-7°C. For longer storage, sample should be frozen (-20°C or colder).
2. Whole blood may be used only in the Screening Protocol. Whole blood must be anticoagulated with EDTA, heparin or citrate and may be used either fresh or after refrigeration 2°-7°C (36°-45°F) for up to one week.
3. Care should be taken to ensure that serum and plasma samples are cell-free. Hemolyzed samples may be used. However highly-hemolyzed samples may yield a high background.
4. EDTA, heparin or citrate in plasma will not affect results.
5. Previously frozen or older samples must be centrifuged before use.

Preparation of Wash Solution: Occasionally, salt crystals may form in the Wash Concentrate upon storage. If this occurs, allow concentrate to come to room temperature and mix by swirling to redissolve crystals before preparing wash solution.

Dilute Wash Concentrate 10 fold with distilled or deionized water (e.g. 3 mL of Wash Concentrate plus 27 mL of water for each strip to be assayed). Diluted wash may be stored at room temperature for a period of up to one week. Do not store diluted wash solution in direct sunlight.

Screening Protocol:

1. Count the number of samples to be tested plus two wells for the positive and negative

controls. Remove the required number of test wells from the bag and place in the rack provided. Leave the test wells attached to one another in a strip. Record the positions of samples and controls on a worksheet.

2. Add 1 drop (50 μL) of Positive Control to the first test well and 1 drop (50 μL) of Negative Control into the second test well.
3. Using precision pipet and a separate pipet tip for each sample, add 50 μL serum, plasma or whole blood sample to appropriate test wells.
4. Add 1 drop (50 μL) of Anti-FeLV:HRPO Conjugate to each test well. Tap the side of the rack gently to mix.
5. Incubate for 5 minutes at room temperature.
6. Discard the fluid from the test wells by inverting into a suitable receptacle, then strike firmly onto absorbent paper. Wash wells with a forceful stream of diluted wash solution from a wash bottle. Completely fit all wells and discard the fluid. Strike wells onto absorbent paper after each wash, taking care to discard all fluid. Repeat 5 times. After the final wash, strike wells on absorbent paper until no additional fluid can be removed from the wells. Note: Wells cannot be over washed.
7. Add 1 drop (50 μL) of TMB Diluent followed by 1 drop (50 μL) of TMB Concentrate to each test well. Tap to mix. Incubate for 5 minutes at room temperature.
8. Add 1 drop (50 μL) of Stop Solution to each test well. Mix by tapping to terminate the reaction. Color will be stable for 15 minutes.
9. Read result visually. A spectrophotometer will provide inaccurate interpretation for this test procedure.

Results (Screening Protocol): For the test to be valid, the Positive Control must develop a distinct blue color. Negative Control must be clear or very lightly colored. For invalid tests, technique may be suspect and the assay should be repeated.

Confirmatory Protocol:

1. Remove the required number of test wells from the bag and place in the rack provided. Allow one well for the Negative Control. Note that both the Positive Control and each sample require two test wells for the confirmatory assay: one for the portion treated with Sample Diluent (Solution A), the other for the portion treated with Neutralizing Reagent (Solution B). Record the positions of samples and controls on a worksheet.
2. Place an equal number of pretreatment tubes into the rack to match the layout of positive controls and samples on the worksheet.
3. Add 1 drop (50 μL) of the Positive Control into each of two clean pretreatment tubes. Designate one pretreatment tube as "A", the other pretreatment tube as "B".
4. Using precision pipet and a separate pipet tip for each sample, add 50 μL of each plasma or serum sample to be confirmed into each of two clean pretreatment tubes (do not use whole blood in this protocol). Designate one pretreatment tube as "A", the other pretreatment tube as "B".
5. To each "A" tube add 10 μL of Solution A, mixing each tube after addition of Solution A by pipetting the sample in and out 5-10 times. Use a separate capillary pipet for each sample.
6. To each "B" tube add 10 μL of Solution B, mixing each tube after addition of Solution B by pipetting the sample in and out 5-10 times. Use a separate capillary pipet for each sample.
7. Incubate for 5 minutes at room temperature.
8. Review sample positions on the worksheet.
9. Dispense 1 drop (50 μL) of Negative Control into the first test well. Transfer 50 μL of the Positive Control treated with Solution A into the second test well. Transfer 50 μL of the Positive Control treated with Solution B into the third test well.
10. For each sample, transfer 50 μL of Solution A treated portion (pretreatment tube "A") into one test well; transfer 50 μL of Solution B treated portion (pretreatment tube "B") into a consecutive test well. Use precision pipet and separate pipet tips. Continue until all samples have been transferred from the pretreatment tubes to the test wells.
11. Add 1 drop (50 μL) of Anti-FeLV:HRPO Conjugate to each test well. Mix by gentle tapping. Incubate for 5 minutes at room temperature.
12. Discard the fluid from the test wells by inverting into a suitable receptacle, then strike firmly onto absorbent paper. Wash wells with a forceful stream of diluted wash solution from a wash bottle. Completely fill all wells and discard the fluid. Strike wells onto absorbent paper after each wash, taking care to discard all fluid. Repeat 5 times. After the final wash, strike wells on absorbent paper until no additional fluid can be removed from the wells. Note: Wells cannot be over washed.
13. Add 1 drop (50 μL) of TMB Diluent followed by 1 drop (50 μL) of TMB Concentrate into each test well. Mix gently by tapping.
14. Incubate for 5 minutes at room temperature.
15. Add 1 drop (50 μL) of Stop Solution to each test well. Mix by tapping to terminate the reaction.
16. Read result visually.

Results (Confirmatory Protocol): For the confirmatory test to be valid, the Negative Control must be clear or very lightly colored. The Solution A treated portion of the Positive Control must develop a distinct blue color and the Solution B treated portion of the Positive Control should have less than half of the color of Solution A treated portion. For invalid tests, technique may be suspect and the assay should be repeated.

Test Interpretation:

Screening Protocol: Compare the sample color to the Negative Control color. If the sample color is less than or equal to the Negative Control color, then the sample is classified as negative for FeLV p27 antigen.

If a sample has more color than the Negative Control, the sample is classified as reactive to p27 antigen and should be retested using the confirmatory protocol.

Confirmatory Protocol:

1. If the Solution A treated sample has less or equal color than the Negative Control, the sample is classified as negative, nonrepeatable reactive for FeLV p27 antigen.
2. If the Solution A treated sample has more color than the negative control, the sample is classified as repeatably reactive and the neutralization of the Solution B treated sample must be assessed. Complete the classification by following paragraphs a, b and c below.
   a. If the Solution A treated sample has less or equal color than the Solution A treated portion of the positive control but the Solution B treated sample has not been neutralized at least 50% (Solution B treated sample has more than half of the color of the Solution A treated sample), the sample is classified as a negative, nonconfirming sample.
   b. If the Solution A treated sample has more color than the Solution A treated portion of the Positive Control and the Solution B treated sample has not been neutralized at least 50% (Solution B treated sample has more than half of the color of the Solution A treated sample), then retest the sample diluted 1:11 in sample diluent Solution A (e.g. 10 μL sample + 100 μL of sample diluent Solution A). Retest following the Confirmatory Protocol.
   c. If the Solution A treated sample has more color than the Negative Control and the Solution B treated sample has been neutralized at least 50% (Solution B treated sample has less than half the color of the Solution A treated sample), the sample is confirmed positive for FeLV p27 antigen. Note: Due to the nature of FeLV infection, cats yielding positive results should be retested in 3 to 4 weeks.

Storage: Store all reagents at 2°-7°C (36°-45°F). Bring to room temperature 15°-30°C (59°-86°F) prior to use, and return to 2°-7°C following use.

Caution(s): Handle all biological materials as though capable of transmitting FeLV.

The Positive Control contains chemically inactivated FeLV. However, do not assume complete inactivation.

Do not pipet by mouth.

There should be no eating, drinking, or smoking where specimens or kit reagents are being handled.

Do not expose TMB Solutions to strong light or any oxidizing agents.

All wastes should be properly decontaminated prior to disposal.

Care should be taken to prevent contamination of kit components.

Do not use test kit past expiration date. Do not intermix components from kits with different serial numbers.

Optimal results will be obtained by strict adherence to this protocol. Careful pipetting and washing throughout this procedure are necessary to maintain precision and accuracy.

For veterinary use only.

References: Available upon request.

Presentation: 5 plates per kit.

PETCHEK® FeLV is an Idexx registered trademark.

Compendium Code No.: 11160393

PETCHEK® FIV Ag

Idexx Labs. **FIV Test**

U.S. Vet. Lic. No.: 313

Description: This feline immunodeficiency virus antigen test kit is an enzyme-linked immunoabsorbent assay (ELISA).

Components: Reagents:

1. Anti-FIV Coated Plate (8 strips).
2. Anti-FIV:Horseradish Peroxidase (HRPO) Conjugate. In buffer with protein stabilizers.
3. Positive Control. Inactivated and lyophilized FIV antigen.
4. Negative Control. Sample non-reactive for FIV antigen in buffer with protein stabilizers.
5. Sample Treatment Solution. In buffer with protein stabilizers.
6. TMB Concentrate.
7. TMB Diluent. Citrate-phosphate buffer containing hydrogen peroxide.
8. Wash Concentrate. (10x) Preserved with gentamicin.
9. Stop Solution.
10. Solution A, Sample Diluent in buffer with protein stabilizers (see Confirmatory Protocol).
11. Solution B, Neutralizing Reagent. Anti-FIV polyclonal antibodies in buffer with protein stabilizers (see Confirmatory Protocol).
12. Sample incubation tubes (see Confirmatory Protocol).

Materials Required But Not Provided:

1. 96 well plate (EIA) reader capable of reading absorbance at 650 nm.
2. Precision pipettes: 0.02, 0.04, 0.05, 0.20 mL or multiple delivery pipetting devices.
3. Disposable pipette tips.
4. Distilled or deionized water.
5. Device for the delivery and aspiration of wash solution.
6. A vacuum source and a trap for retaining the aspirate.

Indications: For the detection of feline immunodeficiency virus (FIV) antigen in tissue culture and laboratory samples.

Test Principles: PETCHEK® FIV Ag is an enzyme immunoassay designed to detect the presence of FIV p26 antigen in tissue culture and laboratory samples. A microtitration format has been devised in which monoclonal antibodies specific for the FIV group-associated antigen (p26) are coated on 12-well microtiter strips. Following addition and incubation of the test sample, FIV antigen (if present) forms a specific complex with the immobilized monoclonal antibodies. Following a wash procedure, horseradish peroxidase conjugated anti-FIV p26 monoclonal antibodies are added and bind to FIV antigen attached to the immobilized monoclonal antibodies. In the final step of the assay, unbound conjugate is washed away and enzyme substrate (hydrogen peroxide) and a chromogen (tetramethylbenzidine, TMB) are added. Subsequent color development is proportional to the amount of FIV p26 antigen present in the sample.

P

The sensitivity of the assay is not markedly affected by the media used to contain the FIV. A moderate variation (< 30%) may be observed and a selection of recommended sample diluents have been included (see Recommendations for Sample Preparation). The test utilizes the absorbance value of the Negative Control supplied with the kit for calculation of the assay cutoff. An Experimental Negative Control sample representing the diluent or media used to contain the FIV should be tested and compared to results obtained for the kit Negative Control to determine reagent compatibility (see Results section).

The confirmatory procedure is identical to the testing protocol except for the addition of a sample neutralization step. A sample initially testing positive is pretreated with neutralizing polyclonal antibodies. The polyclonal antibodies react with the antigen (if present) and block available binding sites. The treated sample will produce a substantially reduced absorbance value when assayed by the confirmatory protocol because most of the binding sites on the FIV antigen are complexed by the polyclonal antibodies. For comparison, the sample is also treated when a diluent non-reactive to FIV and assayed concurrently with the neutralized sample. The sample is confirmed positive if the neutralizing antibodies reduce color formation by 50% or greater as compared to the sample treated with diluent.

Test Procedure:

Specimen Information: Samples from tissue culture or laboratory preparations of purified or partially purified virus may be used in this test. FIV can be propagated in Crandell feline kidney (Crfk) cells or uninfected feline peripheral blood lymphocyte (PBL) cells. The length of time required for FIV antigen positive samples to productively infect tissue culture media and produce a detectable level of antigen was found to vary from 0.5 to 14 days.

Recommendations for Sample Preparation: Optimal assay performance is obtained for dilutions of FIV in Dulbecco's Modified Eagle's Medium supplemented with 5% fetal bovine serum,. Minimum Essential Medium Eagle, fetal bovine serum, and phosphate buffered saline (PBS). Antigen dilutions prepared in SPF cat plasma, 10% bovine serum albumin (BSA), Dulbecco's Modified Eagle's Medium, NCTC 135 Medium, Basal Medium Eagle and 0.1M Tris (pH 7.5) containing 0.1 M NaCl generated absorbance values 15-30% less than the above diluents. Extremes of pH and ionic strength will affect assay results. The suggested pH range of test media is pH 6.0 to pH 10.0 at salt levels ranging from 0.02 to 1.0 M. Samples obtained from tissue culture should be centrifuged (13,000g for 15 minutes) to remove cells before testing.

Preparation of Wash Solution: Dilute Wash Concentrate 10 fold with distilled/deionized water (e.g. 5 mL of Wash Concentrate plus 45 mL of water for each assay strip).

Occasionally, salt crystals may form in the Wash Concentrate upon storage. If this occurs, allow concentrate to come to room temperature and mix by swirling to redissolve crystals before preparing wash solution.

Preparation of Positive Control: The Positive Control is reconstituted by adding 4.0 mL deionized water to the Positive Control vial. This should then be held at room temperature for 15 minutes and fully solubilized by gentle vortexing.

Allow reagents to come to room temperature before use. Reagents should be mixed by gentle swirling or vortexing.

Assay Protocol/Screening:

Note: The Negative Control (NC) supplied with the kit must be run to calculate the assay cutoff and validate individual assays as described in the Results section. In addition, a negative control sample from a known uninfected tissue culture fluid or laboratory specimen representing the diluent media that the FIV is contained in must be assayed. Specifications for the Experimental Negative Control (ENC) assay result are described in the Results section.

Sample Treatment Solution is used to control non-specific reactions in test samples. This solution is added to the test sample and control wells prior to the addition of sample and controls (see Assay Protocol). Components of the Sample Treatment Solution have been incorporated in the confirmatory reagents supplied with the kit. Sample Treatment Solution should not be added to assay wells containing these kit reagents (see Assay Protocol Confirmatory Test).

1. Obtain strips and record sample positions on a laboratory worksheet. Each test requires one positive and two kit negative control wells, and one Experimental Negative Control (ENC) well.
2. Dispense 20 μL of Sample Treatment Solution into each control well and into each sample well.
3. Dispense 200 μL of the kit Negative Control (NC) into the two designated wells.
4. Dispense 200 μL of the reconstituted Positive Control (PC) into the designated well.
5. Dispense 200 μL of the ENC into the designated well.
6. Dispense 200 μL of sample into each sample well. Mix by gently tapping plate 3-5 times.
7. Incubate 2 hours at room temperature. Start timing at the end of step 6.
8. Aspirate liquid contents of all wells into an appropriate waste container.
9. Wash each well five times with approximately 300 μL of diluted wash solution. Aspirate liquid contents of all wells following each wash. Following the final aspiration, gently but firmly tap residual wash fluid from wells into absorbent paper. Avoid plate drying between washes and prior to addition of reagents.
10. Dispense four drops (200 μL) of anti-FIV:HRPO Conjugate into each well.
11. Incubate for 30 minutes at room temperature.
12. Aspirate and wash five times as in Steps 8 and 9.
13. Dispense 2 drops (100 μL) of TMB Diluent into each well.
    Dispense 2 drops (100 μL) of TMB Concentrate into each well. Mix by gently tapping.
    Note: Equal volumes of TMB Diluent and TMB Concentrate may be premixed. Dispense 4 drops (200 μL) of the premixed reagent into each well.
14. Incubate for 30 minutes at room temperature.
15. Dispense 1 drop (50 μL) of Stop Solution into each well to stop the enzymatic reaction.
16. Blank reader on air.
17. Measure and record absorbance values at 650 nm [A(650)].
18. Calculate results (refer to the Calculations section for examples).
    a. Calculate the Negative Control Mean:
    $$\text{Negative Control Mean} = \frac{A(650)NC\#1 + A(650)NC\#2}{2}$$
    b. Calculate the P-N:
    P-N = A(650) Positive Control - Negative Control Mean
    c. Calculate the Assay Cutoff:
    Assay Cutoff = Negative Control Mean + 0.150

Results: For the assay to be valid, the difference between the Positive Control and the Negative Control Mean (P-N) must be greater than or equal to 0.500. In addition, the Negative Control Mean must be less than or equal to 0.250. For invalid tests, technique may be suspect and the assay should be repeated.

The presence or absence of FIV p26 antigen is determined by relating the A(650) value of the unknown sample to the assay cutoff.

The A(650) of the Experimental Negative Control sample would be +/- 0.100 absorbance units of the Negative Control Mean. If this is not found, technique or the diluent media may be suspect and the assay should be repeated.

Confirmatory Test:

Note: Each sample is treated individually with Sample Diluent (Solution A) and Neutralizing Reagent (Solution B) to determine specific neutralization. The Positive Control (PC) is treated with Solution A and Solution B and tested to validate the neutralization procedure.

Sample Incubation Protocol:

1. Record control and sample positions on laboratory worksheet. Allow one well for the Negative Control (NC). Both the PC and each sample require two wells for the confirmatory assay: one for the portion treated with Sample Diluent (Solution A), the other for the portion treated with Neutralizing Reagent (Solution B).
2. Place appropriate number of incubation tubes into a test tube rack to match the layout of controls and samples on the laboratory worksheet.
3. Dispense 200 μL of the PC into each of two clean incubation tubes. Designate one aliquot as "A", the other aliquot as "B".
4. Dispense 200 μL of each sample to be confirmed into each of two clean incubation tubes. Designate one aliquot as "A", the other aliquot as "B".
5. To each "A" tube add 40 μL of Solution A, mixing the contents of each tube subsequent to addition of Solution A by pipetting the sample in and out of the tip 5-10 times. Change pipette tip after each sample.
6. To each "B" tube add 40 μL of Solution B, mixing the contents of each tube after addition of Solution B by pipetting the sample in and out of the tip 5-10 times. Change pipette tip after each sample.
7. Incubate for 15 minutes at room temperature.

Assay Protocol/Confirmatory Test:

Note: The NC supplied with the kit is assayed separately to calculate the Confirmatory Test Assay Cutoff and to validate the test as described in the Results/Confirmatory Test section. The ENC is not used in the Confirmatory Test.

1. Obtain antibody coated strip(s), assemble into strip holder, and review sample positions on the laboratory worksheet.
2. Dispense 20 μL of Sample Treatment Solution into the well assigned for the NC, then add 200 μL of NC.
   Note: The Sample Treatment Solution is not used with samples treated with Solution A or Solution B. Components of the Sample Treatment Solution have been incorporated in these reagents.
3. Dispense 200 μL of the Aliquot A PC into the second well.
4. Dispense 200 μL of the Aliquot B PC into the third well.
5. For each sample, dispense 200 μL of Aliquot A into one well; dispense 200 μL of Aliquot B into a consecutive well. Continue until all samples have been added.
6. Incubate 2 hours at room temperature. Start timing at the end of Step 5.
7. Aspirate liquid contents of all wells into an appropriate waste container.
8. Wash each well five times with approximately 300 μL of diluted wash solution. Aspirate liquid contents of all wells following each wash. Following the final aspiration, gently but firmly tap residual wash fluid from wells onto absorbent paper. Avoid plate drying between washes and prior to addition of reagents.
9. Dispense 4 drops (200 μL) of anti-FIV:HRPO Conjugate into each well.
10. Incubate for 30 minutes at room temperature.
11. Aspirate and wash 5 times as in Steps 7 and 8.
12. Dispense 2 drops (100 μL) of TMB Diluent into each well.
    Dispense 2 drops (100 μL) of TMB Concentrate into each well.
    Mix by gently tapping.
    Note: Equal volumes of TMB Diluent and TMB Concentrate may be premixed. Dispense 4 drops (200 μL) of the premixed reagent into each well.
13. Incubate for 30 minutes at room temperature.
14. Dispense 1 drop (50 μL) of Stop Solution into each well to stop the enzymatic reaction.
15. Blank reader on air.
16. Measure and record absorbance values at 650 nm [A(650)].
17. Calculate results (refer to Calculations section for examples).
    a. Calculate the P-N:
    P-N = A(650) Aliquot A PC - A(650) NC
    b. Calculate the Cutoff:
    Assay Cutoff = A(650) NC + 0.125
    c. Calculate % Neutralization for the PC:
    $$\%\ \text{Neutralization} = \frac{(A(650)\ \text{Aliquot A PC} - A(650)\ \text{Aliquot B PC})}{A(650)\ \text{Aliquot A PC}} \times 100$$
    d. Calculate % Neutralization for each sample where the A(650) for the Solution A treated portion is greater than or equal to the cutoff calculated for the Confirmatory Test:
    $$\%\ \text{Neutralization} = \frac{(A(650)\ \text{Aliquot A sample} - A(650)\ \text{Aliquot B sample})}{A(650)\ \text{Aliquot A sample}} \times 100$$

Results/Confirmatory Test: For the assay to be valid, P-N should be greater than or equal to 0.500, the NC absorbance must be less than or equal to 0.250, and the PC must have a % Neutralization greater than 50%. For invalid tests, technique may be suspect and the assay should be repeated.

Test Interpretation:

Screening: If the A(650) of the sample is less than the cutoff, the sample is classified as Negative for FIV p26 antigen. If the A(650) of the sample is greater than or equal to the cutoff, the sample is classified as reactive for FIV p26 antigen and should be retested using the Confirmatory Test.

Confirmatory Test: Assay results are interpreted in the following manner.

1. A(650) Aliquot A sample is less than Confirmatory Test Cutoff: Sample is Negative, nonrepeatably reactive, % Neutralization is not calculated.
2. A(650) Aliquot A sample is greater than or equal to Confirmatory Test Cutoff: Sample is Repeatably Reactive, % Neutralization is calculated.
   a. % Neutralization is greater than or equal to 50%: Sample is confirmed Positive.
   b. % Neutralization is less than 50%, and A(650) Aliquot A sample less than 2.0: Sample is Negative, nonconfirming sample.
   c. % Neutralization is less than 50%, and A(650) Aliquot A sample is greater than or equal to 2.0: Sample is diluted 1:10 in NC (e.g. 25 μL + 225 μL NC) and retested by the Confirmatory Protocol.

Calculations:

1. Calculation of P-N:
   Screening:
   NC#1 = 0.063
   NC#2 = 0.069
   $$\text{NC Mean} = \frac{0.063 + 0.069}{2} = 0.066$$
   P-N = A(650)PC - NC Mean
   Example:
   PC = 0.675
   NC Mean = 0.066
   P-N = 0.675 - 0.066 = 0.609
   Confirmatory:
   P-N = A(650) Solution A treated PC - A(650) NC (Confirmatory)
   Example:
   Solution A Treated PC = 0.675
   Negative Control = 0.066
   P-N = 0.675 - 0.066 - 0.609
2. Calculation of Cutoff:
   Screening:
   Cutoff = Negative Control Mean + 0.150
   Example:
   Negative Control Mean = 0.066
   Cutoff = 0.066+ 0.150 = 0.216
   Confirmatory:
   Cutoff = Negative Control A(650)+ 0.125
   Example:
   Negative Control = 0.066
   Cutoff = 0.066+ 0.125 = 0.191
3. Comparison of Sample to Cutoff:
   Screening:
   a. Sample 1 A(650) = 0.070
   Cutoff = 0.216, sample less than cutoff; therefore

Negative for FIV p26
b. Sample 2 A(650) = 0.341
Cutoff = 0.216, sample greater than cutoff; therefore
Reactive for FIV p26

Confirmatory: Calculate as for screening protocol, but use Solution A treated portion of sample for comparisons to Confirmatory Test Cutoff.

4. Calculation of % Neutralization:

$$\% \text{ Neutralization} = \frac{\text{(A(650) Aliquot A sample} - \text{A(650) Aliquot B sample)}}{\text{A(650) Aliquot A sample}} \times 100$$

Example:
A(650) Aliquot A sample = 0.341
A(650) Aliquot B sample = 0.069

$$\% \text{ Neutralization} = \frac{(0.341 - 0.069)}{0.341} \times 100 = 79.7\%$$

Precaution(s): Store all reagents at 2 to 7°C. Allow reagents to come to room temperature (15 to 30°C) prior to use, and return to 2 to 7°C following use.

Caution(s): Handle all biological materials as though capable of transmitting FIV. All wastes should be properly decontaminated prior to disposal.

The Positive Control contains chemically inactivated FIV antigen. However, this should be handled as if capable of transmitting FIV.

Optimal results will be obtained by strict adherence to this protocol. Careful pipetting and washing throughout this procedure are necessary to maintain precision and accuracy.

Do not expose TMB solutions to strong light or any oxidizing agents.

Care should be taken to prevent contamination of kit components. There should be no eating, drinking or smoking where specimens or kit reagents are being handled.

Do not use test kit past expiration date. Do not intermix components from different kit serials.

Do not pipette by mouth.

Discussion: The feline immunodeficiency virus [formerly feline T-lymphotropic lentivirus (FTLV)] is a recently described feline-specific retrovirus than can produce chronic immunodeficiency-like disorders in cats.[1] The FIV agent has a strong tropism for feline T-lymphocyte cells. The cytopathic effect exhibited following infection of these cells may be responsible for the immunosuppressive nature of the virus. Viral particle morphology and the Mg^{+2} requirement of the viral reverse transcriptase are characteristic of lentiviruses. The virus is distinct from previously reported feline retroviruses and represents the initial description of a feline-specific lentivirus.

The predominant group-associated antigen of FIV (p26) can be used to detect and monitor growth of the virus in tissue culture fluids. The FIV Ag ELISA is a qualitative and quantitative test for the direct detection of the FIV p26 antigen. The assay can be used to demonstrate the presence of virus in media following culturing of lymphocytes from feline blood or tissue extracts. The FIV Ag ELISA is several times more sensitive than the assay of viral reverse transcriptase (RT) activity.

References:

1. Pedersen, N.C., Ho, E.W., Brown, M.L., Yamamoto, J.K., Isolation of T-Lymphotropic Virus from Domestic Cats with an Immunodeficiency-Like Syndrome. Science 235:790-793, 1987.

Presentation: 1 plate (8 strips) per kit.
Compendium Code No.: 11160401

PETCHEK® HTWM PF

Idexx Labs. **Heartworm Test**

U.S. Vet. Lic. No.: 313

Description: PETCHEK® Canine Heartworm Antigen Test is an enzyme immunoassay for the detection of *Dirofilaria immitis* antigen in canine or feline serum or plasma.

Components:

Components	Volume
1. Anti-Heartworm Coated Wells	192 wells
2. Anti-Heartworm: HRPO conjugate (horseradish peroxidase) preserved with gentamicin	20 mL
3. TMB Diluent	25 mL
4. TMB Concentrate	25 mL
5. HTWM Positive Control *D immitis* antigen positive serum	4 mL
6. HTWM Negative Control serum free of *D immitis* antigen	4 mL
7. Wash Concentrate preserved with gentamicin	100 mL
8. Stop Solution	25 mL

Additional Components Provided:
1. Precision pipet capable of dispensing 0.1 mL (100 µl) of sample.
2. Disposable pipet tips.
3. Well Holder.

Materials Required but not Provided:
1. Distilled or deionized water.
2. Wash bottle

Items Required for Laboratory Protocol only
1. 96-well plate EIA spectrophotometer, capable of reading absorbance at 650 nm.
2. Device for the delivery and aspiration of wash solution.

Test Principles: PetChek® Heartworm Antigen is an enzyme immunoassay designed to detect the presence of circulating antigen from adult *D immitis* in serum or plasma. A microtitration format has been devised in which antibodies to *D immitis* antigen are coated on test wells. Upon incubation of the sample in the coated test well, antigen in the sample forms complexes with the coated antibodies.

Following the removal of the sample, an enzyme conjugated monoclonal antibody is added and binds to antigen captured in the well. In the final step of the assay, unbound conjugate is washed away and enzyme substrate (hydrogen peroxide) and a chromogen (tetramethylbenzadine, TMB) are added. Subsequent color development is proportional to the amount of antigen present in the sample.

Test Procedure: Sample information: Serum or plasma may be used in this test. Serum or plasma (e.g., Heparin, EDTA) may be stored for up to 7 days at 2°-7°C (36°-45°F). Highly hemolyzed samples should not be used, however moderately hemolyzed or lipemic samples will not affect results. For longer storage, the sample should be frozen (-20°C or colder).

Use of precision pipet to dispense 100 µl: Place disposable pipet tip on pipet. Depress button on pipet, place tip in sample and release button slowly to pull up sample. Depress button to dispense sample in well.

Preparation of Wash Solution: Dilute Wash Concentrate 10 fold (1:10) with distilled/deionized water (e.g. 5 mL of Wash Concentrate plus 45 mL of water for each 12 wells). Salt crystals may form in the Wash Concentrate upon storage. If salt crystals form, allow the concentrate to come to room temperature and mix by swirling to redissolve the crystals before preparing the wash solution.

Test Procedure: Allow reagents to come to room temperature before use.

Mix reagents by gentle vortexing.

Note: Two assay procedures are provided: Procedure #1 is for in-clinic use. Results are read visually. Procedure #2 is for laboratory use and requires washing equipment and a spectrophotometer. Alternative testing procedures are provided for the convenience of the user. The sensitivity and specificity of these assay procedures are equivalent.

Procedure #1: In-Clinic Protocol:
1. Count the number of samples to be tested plus two wells for the positive and negative controls. Remove the required number of wells from the bag and place them in the holder provided. Leave the wells attached to one another in a strip. Record the positions of samples and controls on a worksheet.
2. Add 2 drops of Positive Control to the first well and 2 drops Negative Control to the second well.
3. Using precision pipet provided in kit and a separate pipet tip for each sample, add 100 µL of serum or plasma to appropriate wells. Incubate sample in well for 5 minutes.
4. Discard the fluid from the wells by inverting. Slap firmly onto absorbent paper to remove all fluid.
5. Add 2 drops of HRPO Conjugate solution to each well. Wait 5 minutes.
6. Discard the fluid from the wells by inverting. Slap firmly onto absorbent paper to remove all fluid. Wash wells with a forceful stream of diluted wash solution by completely filling each well and discarding the fluid. Slap wells onto absorbent paper after each wash. Repeat for a total of 5 wash cycles.
7. Add 1 drop of TMB Diluent followed by 1 drop of TMB Concentrate to each well. Tap the side of the rack gently to mix. Wait 5 minutes.
8. Add 1 drop of Stop Solution to each well. Mix by tapping gently. Read result visually. Color will be stable for 15 minutes.

Procedure #2: Laboratory Protocol:
1. Count the number of samples to be tested plus two wells for the positive and negative controls. Remove the required number of wells from the bag and place them in the rack provided. Leave the wells attached to one another in a strip. Record the positions of samples and controls on a worksheet.
2. Add 2 drops (100 µL) of Positive Control to the first well and 2 drops (100 µL) Negative Control to the second well.
3. Using a precision pipet and a separate pipet tip for each sample, add 100 µL of serum or plasma to appropriate wells.
4. Incubate sample for 30 minutes at room temperature. Aspirate and discard the contents of all wells.
5. Wash each well 5 times with approximately 0.30 mL of diluted wash solution. Aspirate the contents of all wells following each wash. Following the final wash, firmly tap residual wash fluid from wells onto absorbent paper. Avoid drying between washes and prior to the addition of reagents.
6. Add 3 drops (100 µL) of HRPO Conjugate solution to each well. Incubate 30 minutes at room temperature.
7. Wash as in Step 5 above.
8. Add 1 drop (50 µL) of TMB Diluent followed by 1 drop (50 µL) of TMB Concentrate to each well. Tap the side of the rack gently to mix. Incubate for 10 minutes at room temperature.
9. Add 1 drop (50 µL) of Stop Solution to each well.
10. Blank spectrophotometer on air.
11. Measure and record the absorbance values at 650 nm for the samples and controls.
12. Calculate results:
    a. Calculate the P-N: P-N = A(650) Positive Control - A(650) Negative Control
    b. Calculate the cutoff: Cutoff = A(650) Negative Control +0.05

Test Interpretation: Procedure #1: In-Clinic Protocol:

A sample is considered positive if it has more color than the negative control. For the assay to be valid, the positive control must develop a distinct blue color. The negative control must be clear or very lightly colored.

All positive samples that have not been run in duplicate should be retested. If duplicate samples or repeat testing yield inconsistent results, repeat test.

Procedure #2: Laboratory Protocol: For the assay to be valid, the P-N should be greater than 0.150. In addition the negative control absorbance value should be less than or equal to 0.150. For invalid tests, technique may be suspect and the assay should be repeated.

Interpretation of Results:

If the A(650) of the sample is less than the cutoff, the sample is negative.

If the A(650) of the sample is greater than or equal to the cutoff, the sample is positive.

All positive samples that have not been run in duplicate should be retested. If duplicate samples or repeat testing yield inconsistent results, repeat test.

Caution(s):
1. Do not expose TMB solutions to direct sunlight or any oxidizing agents.
2. Store all reagents at 2°-7°C (36°-45°F). Allow reagents to come to room temperature before use.
3. Care should be taken to prevent contamination of kit components.
4. Do not use test kit past expiration date. Do not intermix components from different kit serial numbers.
5. Optimal results will be obtained by strict adherence to this procedure. Careful pipeting and washing technique throughout this procedure are necessary to maintain precision and accuracy.

Warning(s): For veterinary use only.

Discussion: Heartworm disease, caused by the filarial nematode *Dirofilaria immitis (D immitis)*, has a worldwide distribution. The insect vector for *D immitis* is the mosquito. Adult worms reach a size of 8-14 inches in length and ⅛ inch in diameter. They inhabit the blood and vascular tissues especially the heart and adjacent blood vessels. *D immitis* often interferes with heart function and the circulation of blood, and it may damage other vital organs.

Fertile female worms release microfilariae into the circulation, and microscopic detection of the larval stage in the blood is the most common method of diagnosis of heartworm disease. The accuracy and sensitivity of microscopic diagnostic methods is limited by several factors. First, *D immitis* infections may occur without subsequent production of microfilariae. These occult infections may be caused by immune-mediated or drug induced worm sterility, as well as single sex, prepatent or ectopic infections. In addition, the presence of morphologically similar microfilariae (*Dipetalonema reconditum*) may result in misdiagnosis. Furthermore, microfilarial counts are influenced by the diurnal rhythm of microfilariae, the volume of blood examined and the skill of the examiner.

Accurate diagnosis of heartworm infections is important. Inappropriate administration of heartworm preventives to an infected animal may result in severe or fatal reaction. Failure to eliminate adult worms can result in impaired heart function and circulation, and progressive deterioration of other organs and vascular tissues. However, proper treatment of adult worms in the early stages of infection can result in a complete recovery.

Presentation: 192 wells per kit.
Compendium Code No.: 11160411

PET-F.A. LIQUID®

Pfizer Animal Health — **Small Animal Dietary Supplement**

A Liquid Fatty Acid Supplement for Dogs and Cats

Guaranteed Analysis: per pump (1.9 mL): (All values are minimum quantities unless otherwise stated)

Crude Fat (minimum) 95.0%
Linoleic Acid (minimum) 60.0%
Moisture (maximum) 2.0%
Minerals:
Salt (minimum) 0.00%
(maximum) 0.02%
Zinc .... 3.4 mg
Vitamins:
Vitamin A .... 380 IU
Vitamin D .... 38 IU
Vitamin E .... 3.8 IU

Ingredients: Safflower oil, cod liver oil, colloidal silicon, lecithin, glyceryl monooleate, zinc sulfate heptahydrate, water, vitamin E acetate, methylparaben, propylparaben, vitamin A palmitate, vitamin D supplement.

Indications: PET-F.A. LIQUID® is a nutritional supplement of essential fatty acid, Vitamins A, D, and E, and the mineral zinc.

Directions for Use:

Dogs and cats—Administer once daily according to the following schedule:

Body Weight	Dose*
Under 15 lb	1 pump
15-30 lb	2 pumps
31-50 lb	3 pumps
51 lb and over	4 pumps

*(1 pump = 1.9 mL)

PET-F.A. LIQUID® should be mixed with or poured over food. Quantity should be adjusted according to the size of the pet.

Caution(s): Shake well before each use. Keep out of reach of children.
Presentation: 8 fl oz (236.6 mL) bottles with pump.
Compendium Code No.: 36901250 — 85-8105-05

PET-FORM®

Vet-A-Mix — **Small Animal Dietary Supplement**

Tasty chewable vitamin-mineral supplement

Guaranteed Analysis: per Tablet:
(All values are minimum quantities unless otherwise stated.)
Minerals:
Calcium (min.) 8.3%
(max.) 10.0%
Phosphorus 4.4%
Iron .... 6 mg
Zinc .... 2.5 mg
Manganese .... 1 mg
Copper .... 0.375 mg
Cobalt .... 0.125 mg
Iodine .... 0.1 mg
Vitamins and Others:
Choline chloride .... 20 mg
Niacin .... 10 mg
Vitamin E .... 2 IU
Thiamine mononitrate .... 1 mg
Riboflavin .... 1 mg
Vitamin A .... 1500 IU
D-Pantothenic Acid .... 0.5 mg
Pyridoxine hydrochloride .... 0.1 mg
Folic acid .... 0.05 mg
Vitamin D_3 .... 150 IU
Vitamin B_{12} .... 3 mcg

Ingredients: Brewers dried yeast, Extracted glandular meal (pork), Dicalcium phosphate, Calcium carbonate, Animal liver meal (pork), Glycerin, Cellulose powder, Silicon dioxide, Lactose, Choline chloride, Gelatin, DL-methionine, Soybean oil, Ferrous fumarate, Niacin, Dextrose, Vitamin A palmitate, DL-alpha tocopheryl acetate, Thiamine mononitrate, Manganese sulfate, Zinc oxide, Vitamin B_{12} supplement, Copper sulfate, Povidone, Potassium phosphate, Riboflavin, D-pantothenic acid, Cholecalciferol, Cobalt sulfate, Folic acid, Ethylenediamine dihydriodide, Pyridoxine hydrochloride.

Indications: Use as a dietary supplement for dogs and cats.

Dosage and Administration: Administration: Feed free choice, from the hand or crumble and mix into the food.

Dosage:
Dogs - Small breeds, ½ to 1 tablet. Medium breeds, 1 tablet. Large breeds, 2 to 4 tablets.
Cats - All breeds and sizes, 1 tablet.

Precaution(s): Store at room temperature. Protect from light. Avoid excessive heat (40°C or 104°F).
Warning(s): Keep out of reach of children.
Presentation: Bottles of 50, 150, and 500 tablets.
Compendium Code No.: 10500221 — 0399

PET GUARD™ GEL

Virbac — **External Parasiticide**

EPA Reg. No.: 2382-92
Active Ingredient(s):
Pyrethrins 0.10%
Piperonyl butoxide*, technical 1.00%
N-octyl bicycloheptene dicarboximide 0.50%
Butoxypolypropylene glycol 10.00%
Inert ingredients 88.40%
Total 100.00%

*Equivalent to 0.80% (butylcarbityl) (6-propylpiperonyl) ether and 0.20% related compounds.

Indications: A combination insecticide-repellent designed to protect dogs and cats from flies, mosquitoes and gnats.

Directions for Use: It is a violation of federal law to use the product in a manner inconsistent with its labeling.

Application: PET GUARD™ Gel is a ready-to-use wipe-on product. Lift the nozzle cap and apply a squeezing pressure to the bottle for flow of the product onto the palm of the hand or desired area, then rub it into the coat. PET GUARD™ Gel imparts a high gloss to the coat when rubbed in or brushed out leaving no other visible signs of treatment. It is adaptable for treating difficult areas, such as the face or ears and will not blister, remove or discolor hair. Avoid the pet's eyes during application.

Precautionary Statements: Hazards to Humans and Domestic Animals: Animal remedy - Not for human use. For external use only. Avoid getting into the eyes or mucous membranes. Discontinue use if irritation develops. Harmful if swallowed.

Statement of Practical Treatment: If eye exposure occurs, flush eyes with plenty of water. Get medical attention if irritation persists.

Physical or Chemical Hazards: Flammable. Keep away from heat or open flame.

Storage and Disposal:
Storage: Flammable. Keep away from heat or open flame.
Disposal: Do not re-use the empty container. Wrap the container and put it in the trash.

Warning(s): Keep out of the reach of children.
Presentation: 4 fl. oz. and 8 fl. oz. containers.
Compendium Code No.: 10230391

PETLAC™ POWDER

Pet-Ag — **Milk Replacer**

Milk Food Specifically Formulated For All Pets

Guaranteed Analysis:
Crude Protein, min. 23%
Crude Fat, min. 30%
Crude Fiber, max. 0%
Moisture, max. 3%
Ash, max. 8%

Ingredients: Whey protein concentrate, Whey, Animal and vegetable fat, Lecithin, Calcium carbonate, Dicalcium phosphate, Silico aluminate, DL-methionine, Preserved with BHA, Propyl Gallate and citric acid, Mono- and diglycerides, Choline chloride, Ferrous sulfate, Magnesium sulfate, Zinc sulfate, Manganese Sulfate, Folic acid, Ascorbic acid, Vitamin B_{12}, d-calcium pantothenate, Niacin, Pyridoxine hydrochloride, Riboflavin, Thiamine hydrochloride, Vitamin A, Vitamin D_3, Vitamin E, Artificial flavors.

Indications: Milk food specifically formulated for all pets. Fortified for pregnant and nursing pets. Easy to digest supplement for ill and convalescent pets. All milk protein. Maximizes show pet potential.

For use in rabbits, puppies, kittens and ferrets.

Dosage and Administration: Use as milk food: Mix 1 part PETLAC™ with 2 parts room temperature water. Feed 5 mL of liquid per 120 g body weight, 3 times per day. Weigh the pet to assure accurate feeding.

Use as a supplement: Feed ill or stressed pets 10 g of PETLAC™ per kg body weight. Fortify pet feed with 5 g of PETLAC™ per kg of body weight.

Caution(s): This product is intended for intermittent or supplemental feeding only.
Presentation: 21 g (¾ oz) and 300 g.
Compendium Code No.: 10970370 — 522 02/01 / 521FR 100

PETROMALT®

Virbac — **Laxative**

Active Ingredient(s): PETROMALT® is an emulsion of liquid petrolatum (44%), malt extract, glycerine, acacia and thiamine HCl - 1 mg per ounce.

Indications: An intestinal lubricant and laxative for kittens and puppies.

Dosage and Administration: Give a one-inch ribbon of PETROMALT® once a day until symptoms disappear. Thereafter, give a one-inch ribbon once or twice a week for prevention.

For kittens and pups over four (4) weeks of age, give a half-inch ribbon once or twice a week.

PETROMALT® should be given between meals, either by placing it on the animals nose or on its front paws where it can be licked off.

PETROMALT® should not be mixed with food or given close to mealtime.

Note: A veterinarian may give specific directions. Follow the professional advice closely.

Precaution(s): Store at room temperature.
Caution(s): Keep out of the reach of children. For veterinary use only.
Presentation: 56.7 g tube and 92 g pump.
Compendium Code No.: 10230400

PETROTECH 25™

Alpha Tech Pet — **Petroleum Remover**

25% Concentrate

Indications: Oil and petroleum contaminant remover for use fur and feather bearing animals.

Directions for Use: This product is designed specifically for removal of oil, grease, diesel fuel, gasoline and kerosene from fur and feather bearing animals, whether they be contaminated wildlife or household pets. Frequency and repetition of the following treatment steps are dependant largely on the type of contaminant and the depth of its penetration.

For most applications the product may be diluted to a 10% end-use solution. To make a 10% end-use solution simply mix 1 bottle of PETROTECH 25™ (25% concentrate) with 5 quarts of water.

Apply product (in the 10% end-use solution) with a moist towel or rag to the surface of the area being treated. Using a medium bristle brush and/or rag, gently spread and agitate the concentrate into the area vigorously. PETROTECH will mix with the petroleum contaminant becoming a golden-brown color.

Add water as needed to the product by moistening a rag and gently scrubbing with the brush if the stain persists.

Rinse well. At this point, the petroleum contaminant should be loosened, if not completely removed. If the stain persists, repeat the steps above with more concentrate (a 6-25% end-use solution). Brush or scrub the area directly before any large amount of water is added.

Precaution(s): PETROTECH 25™ is a spill mitigation agent listed on the EPA National Contingency Plan. Material is not hazardous under RCRA 40 CFR 261. In the event of a spill, flush spill area with amounts of water until material dissipates. Product may be disposed of in a conventional non-hazardous manner. Non-flammable.

Warning(s): Keep out of reach of children. Use as directed. If ingested, swallow large amounts of water (single dose ingestion is relatively harmless, no chronic symptoms are likely). Consult a physician if symptoms or discomfort persist. If splashed into eyes, rinse thoroughly with water.

Presentation: ½ gallons (1 to a case).

Compendium Code No.: 10140050

PET-TABS®

Pfizer Animal Health **Small Animal Dietary Supplement**

Guaranteed Analysis: per tablet: (All values are minimum quantities unless otherwise stated)

Minerals:	
Calcium (minimum)	2.5%
(maximum)	3.5%
Phosphorus	2.5%
Potassium	0.4%
Salt (minimum)	0.1%
(maximum)	0.6%
Chloride	0.1%
Magnesium	0.15%
Iron	3.0 mg
Copper	0.1 mg
Manganese	0.25 mg
Zinc	1.4 mg
Vitamins:	
Vitamin A	1,000 IU
Vitamin D	100 IU
Vitamin E	2 IU
Thiamine	0.81 mg
Riboflavin	1.0 mg
Niacin	10.0 mg
Pyridoxine	0.1 mg
Vitamin B_{12}	0.5 mcg

Ingredients: Wheat germ, kaolin, corn syrup, pork liver meal, dicalcium phosphate, sucrose, lactose, safflower oil, gelatin, corn starch, stearic acid, niacinamide, hydrolyzed vegetable protein, iron oxide and peptone, magnesium stearate, dl-alpha tocopheryl acetate, vitamin A acetate, zinc oxide, riboflavin, thiamine mononitrate, pyridoxine hydrochloride, cyanocobalamin, manganese sulfate, copper acetate monohydrate, vitamin D_3 supplement, cobalt sulfate.

Indications: A palatable vitamin-mineral supplement for dogs.

Directions for Use:

Puppies and dogs under 10 lb—1/2 tablet daily.

Dogs over 10 lb—1 tablet daily.

PET-TABS® are made with a special taste appeal. Administer by hand just prior to feeding, or crumble and mix with food.

Precaution(s): Keep bottle tightly closed to preserve freshness.

Caution(s): Keep out of reach of children.

Presentation: Bottles of 60, 180 and 500 tablets.

Compendium Code No.: 36901260 85-8083-09

PET-TABS®/F.A. GRANULES

Pfizer Animal Health **Small Animal Dietary Supplement**

A Palatable Dietary Supplement for Dogs and Cats

Guaranteed Analysis: per 10 grams (1 tablespoon): (All values are minimum quantities unless otherwise stated)

Linoleic Acid (minimum)	4.5%
Minerals:	
Calcium (minimum)	1.0%
(maximum)	1.5%
Phosphorus	1.0%
Potassium	0.7%
Salt (minimum)	0.5%
(maximum)	1.0%
Chloride	0.4%
Magnesium	0.1%
Iron	2.3 mg
Copper	0.04 mg
Manganese	0.06 mg
Zinc	10.0 mg
Iodine	0.05 mg
Vitamins:	
Vitamin A	1,000 IU
Vitamin D	100 IU
Vitamin E	2 IU
Thiamine	0.81 mg
Riboflavin	1.0 mg
Niacin	10.0 mg
Pyridoxine	0.08 mg
Vitamin B_{12}	0.2 mcg

Ingredients: Wheat germ, spray-dried whey, corn syrup, pork liver meal, kaolin, sucrose, dicalcium phosphate, menhaden fish oil, safflower oil, soybean oil, zinc gluconate, niacinamide, hydrolyzed vegetable protein, dl-alpha tocopheryl acetate, iron oxide and peptone, copper gluconate, vitamin A acetate, magnesium stearate, riboflavin, thiamine mononitrate, lactose, pyridoxine hydrochloride, cyanocobalamin, manganese sulfate, vitamin D_3 supplement, cobalt sulfate, potassium iodide.

Indications: An aid in the improvement and maintenance of healthy skin and coat.

Directions for Use:

Dogs—1 tablespoon for approximately each 30 lb of body weight or 1 teaspoon for each 10 lb of body weight daily.

Cats—½-1 tablespoon daily.

PET-TABS®/F.A. Granules may be mixed with or sprinkled on food. Quantity should be adjusted according to size and condition of animal.

Precaution(s): Keep container tightly closed to preserve freshness.

Store at controlled room temperature 15°-30°C (59°-86°F)

Presentation: PET-TABS®/F.A. Granules are supplied in bulk canisters containing 1 lb 6.9 oz (650 g) and 1,500 g.

Compendium Code No.: 36901290 50-8102-09

PET-TABS® JR.

Pfizer Animal Health **Small Animal Dietary Supplement**

Guaranteed Analysis: per tablet: (All values are minimum quantities unless otherwise stated)

Crude Protein (minimum)	23.5%
Crude Fat (minimum)	3.5%
Crude Fiber (maximum)	3.0%
Moisture (maximum)	10.0%
Minerals:	
Calcium (minimum)	3.0%
(maximum)	4.0%
Phosphorus	3.0%
Potassium	0.5%
Salt (minimum)	0.30%
(maximum)	0.80%
Chloride	0.25%
Magnesium	0.10%
Iron	1.13 mg
Copper	0.03 mg
Manganese	0.03 mg
Zinc	0.75 mg
Iodine	0.02 mg
Vitamins:	
Vitamin A	500 IU
Vitamin D	50 IU
Vitamin E	1 IU
Thiamine	0.41 mg
Riboflavin	0.5 mg
Niacin	5.0 mg
Pyridoxine	0.04 mg
Vitamin B_{12}	0.1 mcg

Ingredients: Wheat germ, kaolin, corn syrup, liver meal, dicalcium phosphate, fish meal, sucrose, lactose, safflower oil, gelatin, corn starch, stearic acid, niacinamide, hydrolyzed vegetable protein, dl-alpha tocopheryl acetate, iron oxide and peptone, magnesium stearate, vitamin A acetate, zinc oxide, riboflavin, thiamine mononitrate, cobalt sulfate, potassium iodide, pyridoxine hydrochloride, cyanocobalamin, manganese sulfate, vitamin D_3 supplement, copper acetate monohydrate.

Indications: A palatable vitamin-mineral supplement for puppies and toy breeds.

Directions for Use:

Puppies and dogs under 10 lb—1 tablet daily.

Dogs over 10 lb—2 tablets daily.

PET-TABS® Jr. tablets may be given by hand just prior to feeding, or crumble and mix with food.

Precaution(s): Keep bottle tightly closed to preserve freshness.

Caution(s): Keep out of reach of children.

Presentation: Bottles of 50 tablets and trial size bottles of 14 tablets.

Compendium Code No.: 36901270 85-8087-07

PET-TABS® PLUS

Pfizer Animal Health **Small Animal Dietary Supplement**

High Potency Nutritional Supplement for Special Vitamin-Mineral Needs

Guaranteed Analysis: per tablet: (All values are minimum quantities unless otherwise stated)

Minerals:	
Calcium (minimum)	2.5%
(maximum)	3.5%
Phosphorus	2.5%
Potassium	0.4%
Salt (minimum)	1.1%
(maximum)	1.6%
Chloride	0.7%
Magnesium	0.15%
Iron	3.0 mg
Copper	0.1 mg
Manganese	0.25 mg
Zinc	1.4 mg
Vitamins:	
Vitamin A	1,500 IU
Vitamin D	150 IU
Vitamin E	15 IU
Thiamine	0.24 mg
Riboflavin	0.65 mg
Pantothenic Acid	0.68 mg
Niacin	3.4 mg
Pyridoxine	0.24 mg
Folic Acid	0.05 mg
Vitamin B_{12}	7.0 mcg
Choline	40.0 mg

Ingredients: Wheat germ, kaolin, corn syrup, pork liver meal, dicalcium phosphate, sorbitol, choline chloride, sucrose, dl-alpha tocopheryl acetate, safflower oil, gelatin, hydrolyzed vegetable protein, ascorbic acid, stearic acid, cyanocobalamin, iron oxide and peptone, magnesium stearate, vitamin A acetate, niacinamide, zinc oxide, pyridoxine hydrochloride, calcium pantothenate, riboflavin, lactose, thiamine mononitrate, phytonadione (vitamin K1), vitamin D_3, manganese sulfate, copper acetate monohydrate, cobalt sulfate, folic acid, d-biotin.

Indications: PET-TABS® Plus is designed for use in dogs with special dietary needs.
Directions for Use:
Dogs under 20 lb—½ tablet daily.
Dogs over 20 lb—1 tablet daily.
PET-TABS® Plus is made with special taste appeal. Administer by hand prior to feeding, or crumble and mix with food.
Precaution(s): Keep bottle tightly closed to preserve freshness.
Caution(s): Keep out of reach of children.
Presentation: Bottles of 60, 180, and 365 tablets.
Compendium Code No.: 36901280 85-8107-08

PET-TINIC®

Pfizer Animal Health **Small Animal Dietary Supplement**

Guaranteed Analysis: per teaspoon (5 mL/6.385 g): (All values are minimum quantities unless otherwise stated.)
Moisture (maximum) 42%
Minerals:
Iron . . . . . 12.5 mg
Copper . . . . . 0.2 mg
Vitamins:
Thiamine . . . . . 2.0 mg
Riboflavin . . . . . 1.0 mg
Niacin . . . . . 10.0 mg
Vitamin B_6 . . . . . 1.0 mg
Vitamin B_{12} . . . . . 2.1 mcg

Ingredients: Corn syrup, water, sucrose, glycerin, beef liver paste, iron proteinate, sodium citrate, caramel color, citric acid, niacinamide, potassium sorbate, cyanocobalamin, thiamine hydrochloride, pyridoxine hydrochloride, riboflavin, cupric sulfate, natural anise flavor, sodium hydroxide.
Indications: A palatable liquid vitamin-mineral supplement for dogs and cats.
Dosage and Administration: Dosage for diet supplement:
Dogs and Cats: Approximately ½ teaspoon (2½ mL) per 25 lb of body weight twice a day.
Palatable drops may be placed directly into pet's mouth or poured over food.
Precaution(s): Store at controlled room temperature 15°-30°C (59°-86°F).
Caution(s): For animal use only.
Presentation: 1 fl oz (30 mL) amber glass bottles with dropper in dispensing boxes and 4 fl oz (120 mL) amber glass bottles.
Compendium Code No.: 36901300 85-8044-03, 85-8045-06

PET VITES

Vetus **Small Animal Dietary Supplement**

Guaranteed Analysis: Per Tablet: (All values are minimum quantities unless otherwise stated):
Crude Protein (minimum) 15.3%
Crude Fat (minimum) 8.5%
Crude Fiber (maximum) 20.4%
Moisture (maximum) 9.3%
Minerals:
Calcium
minimum 7.0%
maximum 8.4%
Phosphorus 5.5%
Potassium 0.2%
Sodium
minimum 0.15%
maximum 0.22%
Chloride 0.4%
Magnesium 0.04%
Iron . . . . . 2.25 mg
Manganese . . . . . 0.06 mg
Zinc . . . . . 1.5 mg
Iodine . . . . . 0.05 mg
Cobalt . . . . . 0.003 mg
Vitamins:
Vitamin A . . . . . 1000 IU
Vitamin D_3 . . . . . 100 IU
Vitamin E . . . . . 2 IU
Thiamine (B_1) . . . . . 0.089 mg
Riboflavin (B_2) . . . . . 1.0 mg
Niacinamide (B_3) . . . . . 10.0 mg
Pyridoxine (B_6) . . . . . 0.08 mg
Vitamin B_{12} . . . . . 0.2 mcg
Essential Fatty Acid:
Linoleic Acid . . . . . 30.0 mg

Ingredients: DiCalcium phosphate, Microcrystalline cellulose, Wheat germ meal, Animal livers' meal, Fish meal, Dextrose, Caramel color, Stearic Acid, Sorbitol, Safflower oil, Hydrolyzed soy protein, Magnesium Stearate, Corn starch, Silicon dioxide, Beef flavor, Iron oxide, Potassium chloride, Sodium chloride, Niacinamide, Ferrous sulfate, Zinc oxide, Vitamin A supplement, Riboflavin supplement, Thiamine monohydrate, Manganese sulfate, Vitamin D_3 supplement, Pyridoxine hydrochloride, Calcium iodide, Vitamin B_{12} supplement, Cobalt sulfate.
Indications: PET VITES are recommended for dogs and cats for the prevention of vitamin and mineral deficiencies.
Directions: PET VITES are made with a special taste appeal to dogs and cats. Administer by hand just prior to feeding or crumble and mix with food. Warm tablet in hand prior to feeding to bring out full flavor.
Usage:
Dogs under 10 pounds - ½ Tablet daily.
Dogs over 10 pounds - 1 Tablet daily.
Puppies under 10 lbs. - 1 Tablet daily.
Puppies over 10 lbs. - 2 Tablets daily.
For sick, convalescing, pregnant, or nursing dogs - 2 Tablets daily.
Cats - ½ Tablet daily, depending on size and condition.
Precaution(s): Keep product at controlled room temperature. Do not expose to excessive heat or moisture.
Caution(s): For veterinary use only.
Warning(s): Keep out of reach of children.
Presentation: 60 and 360 (NDC: 47611-512-22) tablets.
Distributed by: Burns Veterinary Supply, Inc., Westbury, NY. 11590
Compendium Code No.: 14440721

PET VITES O.F.A. CHEWABLE TABLETS

Vetus **Small Animal Dietary Supplement**

Microencapsulated Omega Fatty Acids with Fat Soluble Vitamins, Zinc and Amino Acids
Composition: Each PET VITES O.F.A. CHEWABLE TABLET Contains:
Omega Fatty Acids:
Microencapsulated Marine Lipid . . . . . 270 mg
Vegetable Oils . . . . . 57 mg
Total Fatty Acids . . . . . 327 mg
Vitamins:
Vitamin A . . . . . 1500 IU
Vitamin D_3 . . . . . 300 IU
Vitamin E . . . . . 25 IU
Choline . . . . . 1550 mcg
Inositol . . . . . 1100 mcg
Minerals:
Zinc . . . . . 2 mg

Proteins: Includes the following amino acids: Alanine, Arginine, Aspartic acid, Cysteine, Cystine, Glutamic acid, Glycine, Histidine, Hydroxyproline, Isoleucine, Leucine, Lysine, Methionine, Phenylalanine, Proline, Serine, Threonine, Tyrosine, Tryptophan, and Valine.
Ingredients: Whey, Microencapsulated Marine Lipid, Dried Brewers Yeast, Vegetable Oil, Vitamin E Supplement, Zinc Sulfate, Choline Chloride, Vitamin A Acetate, Inositol, Vitamin D_3 Supplement.
Indications: PET VITES O.F.A. CHEWABLE TABLETS for small and medium dogs are a supplemental source for Omega Fatty Acids, Vitamins A, D_3, and E, Choline, Inositol, and Zinc, which are beneficial in dogs for the maintenance of healthy skin and coat.
Dosage and Administration: For diet supplementation.
Dogs under 10 lbs: ½ to 1 Tablet Daily
Dogs 10 lbs and over: 1 to 2 Tablets Daily
Caution(s): For animal use only.
Warning(s): Keep out of reach of children.
Presentation: 60 Tablets (NDC 47611-510-09).
Distributed by: Burns Veterinary Supply, Inc.
Compendium Code No.: 14440920 Rev. 8-00

P.G. 600® ESTRUS CONTROL

Intervet **PMSG-HCG**

NADA No.: 140-856
Active Ingredient(s): P.G. 600® is a combination of serum gonadotropin (Pregnant Mare Serum Gonadotropin or PMSG) and chorionic gonadotropin (Human Chorionic Gonadotropin or hCG) for use in prepuberal gilts (gilts that have not yet exhibited their first estrus) and in sows at weaning. It is supplied in freeze-dried form with sterile diluent for reconstitution.
P.G. 600® is available in two package sizes:
Single Dose Vials — When reconstituted, each single dose vial (5 mL) of P.G. 600® contains:
Serum Gonadotropin (PMSG) . . . . . 400 I.U.
Chorionic Gonadotropin (hCG) . . . . . 200 I.U.
(equivalent to 200 USP Units chorionic gonadotropin)
Five Dose Vials — When reconstituted, the five dose vial (25 mL) of P.G. 600® contains:
Serum Gonadotropin (PMSG) . . . . . 2,000 I.U.
Chorionic Gonadotropin (hCG) . . . . . 1,000 I.U.
(equivalent to 1,000 USP Units chorionic gonadotropin)
Indications:
Prepuberal Gilts: P.G. 600® is indicated for induction of fertile estrus (heat) in healthy prepuberal (non-cycling) gilts over five and one-half months of age and weighing at least 85 kg (187 lb.).
Sows at Weaning: P.G. 600® is indicated for induction of estrus in healthy weaned sows experiencing delayed return to estrus.
Pharmacology: In gilts, the action of serum gonadotropin is similar to the action of Follicle-Stimulating Hormone (FSH), which is produced by the animals' anterior pituitary gland. It stimulates the follicles of the ovaries to produce mature ova (eggs), and it promotes the outward signs of estrus (heat).
The action of chorionic gonadotropin in gilts and sows is similar to the action of Luteinizing Hormone (LH), which is also produced by the animals' anterior pituitary gland. It causes the release of mature ova from the follicles of the ovaries (ovulation), and it promotes the formation of corpora lutea, which are necessary for the maintenance of pregnancy once the gilt has become pregnant.
The combination of serum gonadotropin and chorionic gonadotropin in P.G. 600® induces fertile estrus in most prepuberal gilts and weaned sows three to seven days after administration (Schilling and Cerne, 1972; Britt et al., 1986; Bates et al., 1991). The animals may then be mated, or in the case of gilts, mating may be delayed until the second estrus after treatment.
Dosage and Administration: One dose (5 mL) of reconstituted P.G. 600®, containing 400 I.U. serum gonadotropin (PMSG) and 200 I.U chorionic gonadotropin (hCG), should be injected into the gilt or sow's neck behind the ear.
Prepuberal gilts should be injected when they are selected for addition to the breeding herd. Sows should be injected at weaning during periods of delayed return to estrus.
Directions for Use:
Single Dose Vials: Using a sterile syringe and a sterile 0.90 x 38 mm (20 G x 1½") hypodermic needle, transfer the contents of one vial of sterile diluent (5 mL) into one vial of freeze-dried powder. Shake gently to dissolve the powder. Inject the contents of the vial into the gilt or sow's neck behind the ear.
Five Dose Vials: Using a sterile syringe and a sterile 0.90 x 38 mm (20 G x 1½") hypodermic needle, transfer approximately 5 mL of the sterile diluent into the vial of freeze-dried powder. Shake gently to dissolve the powder. Transfer the dissolved product back into the vial of diluent and shake gently to mix. Inject one dose (5 mL) into the gilt or sow's neck behind the ear.
Note: P.G. 600® is intended as a management tool to improve reproductive efficiency in swine

P

production operations. To obtain maximum benefit from this product, estrus detection and other aspects of reproductive management must be adequate. If you are in doubt about the adequacy of your breeding program, consult your veterinarian.

Precaution(s): Store at or below room temperature, 77°F (25°C).

Once reconstituted, P.G. 600® should be used immediately. Unused solution should be disposed of properly and not stored for future use.

Spent hypodermic needles and syringes generated as a result of the use of this product must be disposed of properly in accordance with all applicable Federal, State and local regulations.

Caution(s): Treatment will not induce estrus in gilts that have already reached puberty (begun to cycle). Gilts that are less than five and one-half months of age or that weight less than 85 kg (187 lb.) may not be mature enough to continue normal estrus cycles or maintain a normal pregnancy to full term after treatment.

Treatment will not induce estrus in sows that are returning to estrus normally three to seven days after weaning. Delayed return to estrus is most prevalent after the first litter; the effectiveness of P.G. 600® has not been established after later litters. Delayed return to estrus often occurs during periods of adverse environmental conditions, and sows mated under such conditions may farrow smaller than normal litters.

For animal use only.

Discussion: Gilts normally reach puberty (begin experiencing normal estrous cycles and exhibiting regular estrus or heat) at any time between six and eight months of age, although some gilts will not have exhibited their first estrus at ten months of age. Age at first estrus influenced by several factors including breed type, season of the year, environmental conditions, and management practice (Hurtgen, 1986).

Sows normally exhibit estrus three to seven days after weaning their litters; however, some otherwise healthy sows may not exhibit estrus for 30 days or more after weaning (Dial and Britt, 1986). The causes of delayed return to estrus in healthy sows are poorly understood, but probably include season of the year (so-called seasonal anestrus; Hurtgen, 1979), adverse environmental conditions, such as high ambient temperatures (Love. 1978), and the number of previous litters, because the condition is more prevalent after the first litter than after later litters (Hurtgen, 1986).

References: Available upon request.

Presentation: P.G. 600® is available in two package sizes:

Single Dose Vials — Five vials containing white freeze-dried powder, plus five vials containing sterile diluent.

Five Dose Vials — One vial containing white freeze-dried powder, and one vial containing sterile diluent.

Compendium Code No.: 11061040

PHD 22.5

Bio-Tek **Disinfectant**

Cleaner-Disinfectant-Deodorant

EPA No.: 11725-8

Active Ingredient(s):

para-tertiary-Amylphenol	10.0%
ortho-Benzyl-para-Chlorophenol	6.5%
ortho-Phenylphenol	6.0%
	77.5%
Total	100.0%

Indications: PHD 22.5 is a synthetic detergent with wide spectrum kill of gram positive and gram negative microorganisms, provides good cleaning and disinfecting in one operation, non-flammable and non-volatile in use dilutions and excellent solubility.

**After this products use as a disinfectant, it will biodegrade in sewage systems and/or the environment.

The PHD 22.5 foaming detergent system has been especially formulated to provide cleaning, wetting and penetration of soils and organic matter and easy rinsing of surfaces. Good foam is obtained at ½ oz per gallon of water (1:256) to provide prolonged contact time.

PHD 22.5 at ½ ounce per gallon of water (1:256) provides residual control of odor causing bacteria in the presence of moisture.

PHD 22.5 is recommended for use when used as directed on ceramic and glazed tile surfaces, stainless steel, aluminum, chrome, galvanized metal, glass, and other non-porous surfaces such as treated wood, polyethylene, polypropylene, PVC (polyvinyl chloride), polystyrene, vinyl, fiberglass, viton, ethylene propylene, nitrile, acrylic and polyurethane.

PHD 22.5 at ½ oz per gallon of water (1:256) is suited for disinfecting and cleaning all environmental surfaces of hospitals, medical research centers, health care facilities, schools, animal care facilities and research centers, laboratories, veterinary facilities, zoos, kennels and swine operations. In poultry and turkey barns, breeder and laying operations, poultry house grow-out operations, hatcheries -- in hatchers and setters, humidifying systems and ceiling fans, live haul equipment, chick busses, transfer trucks, trays, coop washing, polyethylene chick boxes, foot pans and feed bins.

Toxicity tests required by the U.S. Environmental Protection Agency for PHD 22.5 Cleaner-Disinfectant-Deodorant have been done in conformity with the FDA and EPA Good Laboratory Practice Regulations.

Proven effective as a disinfectant by the following tests: A.O.A.C. (use dilution test method) in conformance with the 14th Edition 1984. All dilutions at 1:256. The following organisms tested at 1000 ppm water hardness as calcium carbonate and 10% horse serum (as organic soil): *Enterobacter aerogenes* ATCC #13048, *Klebsiella pneumoniae* ATCC #4352, *Mycobacterium bovis* (BCG) ATCC #35743 A.O.A.C. tuberculocidal test, *Staphylococcus aureus*, Methicillin resistant ATCC #25923, *Staphylococcus aureus* ATCC #6538, *Salmonella paratyphi B* ATCC #9281, *Salmonella typhimurium* ATCC #13311, *Salmonella schottmeulleri* ATCC #8759, *Streptococcus pyogenes* ATCC #19615, *Shigella sonnei* ATCC #25931.

+The following viruses tested in accordance with U.S. Environmental Protection Agency Pesticide Assessment Guidelines on inanimate environmental surfaces. Tested at 1000 ppm water hardness as calcium carbonate and 10% horse serum (as organic soil): Human Immunodeficiency Virus, HTLV-IIIB strain of HIV-1 (Aids virus), vaccinia virus ATCC #VR-325, human adenovirus ATCC #VR-5.

PHD 22.5 has also been tested according to A.O.A.C. use dilution test methods and proven effective as a disinfectant against the following organisms at 500 ppm water hardness as calcium carbonate and 5% horse serum (as organic soil): *Trichophyton mentagrophytes* ATCC #9533 A.O.A.C. fungicidal test, *Salmonella choleraesius* ATCC #10708, *Pseudomonas aeruginosa* ATCC #15442, *Escherichia coli* ATCC #11229.

All tests were in conformance with the 14th Edition 1984. All dilutions were tested at 1:256.

+The following viruses tested in accordance with U.S. Environmental Protection Agency Pesticide Assessment Guidelines on inanimate environmental surfaces. Tested at 500 ppm water hardness as calcium carbonate and 5% serum (as organic soil): Herpes simplex Type 1, human influenza A/Hong Kong virus.

Other Claims: Conductive: PHD 22.5 has been tested by Hood Patterson-Dewar, Electrical Testing Engineers, for its effect on conductive flooring. The method used conforms to the specifications known as NFPA Standard No. 56A, published by the National Fire Protection Association, Second Edition, 1987. PHD 22.5 meets the requirement of NFPA 56A.

Directions for Use: It is a violation of Federal law to use this product in a manner inconsistent with its labeling.

General Use Directions: PHD 22.5 is effective against all organisms listed at 500 ppm water hardness and 5% organic soil. Note: PHD 22.5 is also effective against a number of organisms (identified **above/below) under the more stringent conditions of 1000 ppm water hardness and 10% organic soil.

1. To clean, disinfect and deodorize walls, floors, tables, drinking fountains, sinks, refrigerators, stoves, restroom fixtures, and garbage cans: Remove gross filth and heavy soil with a preliminary cleaning step prior to the application of PHD 22.5. Apply solution of ½ oz of PHD 22.5 per gallon of water (1:256) with a sponge, mop, mechanical spray device or foaming apparatus, making sure that all surfaces are wetted thoroughly. Allow surface to remain wet for 10 minutes.
2. To clean and disinfect such articles as combs, brushes, razors, scissors, and rubber goods: Wipe articles clean and soak for 10 minutes in a solution containing ½ oz of PHD 22.5 per gallon of water (1:256).
3. To disinfect fabrics such as sheets, linens, aprons and uniforms: First rinse to remove gross filth or heavy soil, then soak for 10 minutes in a solution containing ½ oz of PHD 22.5 per gallon of water (1:256).
4. To clean gross filth or heavy soil on environmental surfaces prior to disinfection, use ½ oz of PHD 22.5 per gallon of water (1:256).
5. PHD 22.5 is an effective tuberculocide against *Mycobacterium bovis* in 10 minutes at 20°C when used on hard, non-porous inanimate environmental surfaces. Follow above directions, including removal of gross filth or heavy soil prior to application of PHD 22.5.

Directions for use in poultry house and farm premise: Do not use in milking stalls, milking parlors, or milk houses.

1. Remove all poultry, animals, and feed from the premises.
2. Remove all trucks, coops, crates, water troughs and feed racks.
3. Remove all gross soil, litter, manure, droppings from animals and poultry from floors, walls and surfaces of barns, pens, stalls, chutes, and other facilities and fixtures occupied or traversed by animals and poultry.
4. Thoroughly clean and saturate all surfaces with a solution of ½ oz of PHD 22.5 per gallon of water (1:256), using conventional spraying methods.
5. Allow to remain in contact for at least ten minutes.
6. Immerse halters, ropes and other types of equipment used in handling and restraining animals, forks, shovels, scrapers used for removing litter and manure, in a solution of PHD 22.5 at ½ oz per gallon of water (1:256). Allow to remain in contact for 10 minutes.
7. Thoroughly scrub treated feed racks, troughs, automatic feeders, fountains, waterers, and mangers with a solution of PHD 22.5 at ½ oz per gallon of water (1:256). Rinse with potable water before reuse.
8. Ventilate buildings, coops and other closed spaces. Do not house poultry or livestock or employ equipment until treatment has been absorbed, set or dried.

PHD 22.5 is recommended for use in fogging (wet misting) operations as an adjunct either preceding or following regular cleaning and disinfecting procedures. The recommended dilution is ½ oz per gallon of water (1:256). Set the automatic timer on the Bio-Tek Fogger, for 3 minutes for 1,000 cu ft - leave the room. Allow at least 2 hours before entering area that has been fogged. All food and food packaging items must be removed or carefully protected. Treated food contact surfaces must be thoroughly scrubbed with PHD 22.5 at ½ oz per gallon (1:256) and rinsed with potable water prior to re-use.

Precautionary Statements:

Hazards to Humans and Domestic Animals: Danger. Corrosive. Causes eye and skin damage or skin irritation. Do not get in eyes, on skin, or on clothing. Wear goggles or face shield and rubber gloves when handling. Harmful or fatal if swallowed.

Statement of Practical Treatment:

First Aid: In case of contact, immediately flush eyes or skin with plenty of water. For eyes, call a physician. Remove and wash contaminated clothing before reuse. If swallowed, drink promptly large quantities of water. Avoid alcohol and call a physician.

Note to Physician: Probable mucosal damage may contraindicate the use of gastric lavage. Measures against circulatory shock, respiratory depression and convulsion may be needed.

Storage and Disposal:

Pesticide Disposal: Pesticide wastes are acutely hazardous. Improper disposal of excess pesticide, spray mixture, or rinsate is a violation of Federal Law. If these wastes cannot be disposed of by use according to label instructions, contact your State Pesticide or Environmental Control Agency, or the Hazardous Waste representative at the nearest EPA Regional Office for guidance. Do not contaminate water, food or feed by storage or disposal.

Container Disposal: Triple rinse (or equivalent). Then offer for recycling or reconditioning, or puncture and dispose of in a sanitary landfill, or by incineration, or, if allowed by state and local authorities, by burning. If burned, stay out of smoke.

Warning(s): Keep out of reach of children.

Presentation: 4x1 U.S. gallon cases and 5 gallon drums.

Compendium Code No.: 13700020

PHENO-TEK II

Bio-Tek **Disinfectant**

Disinfectant-Cleaner-Deodorant

EPA Reg. No.: 11725-11

Active Ingredient(s):

para-tertiary-Amylphenol	8.44%
ortho-benzyl-para-chlorophenol	5.49%
ortho-Phenylphenol	5.07%
Inert Ingredients:	81.00%
Total:	100.00%

Indications: Description: PHENO-TEK II is a synthetic detergent/disinfectant with wide spectrum kill of gram positive and gram negative microorganisms. It provides good cleaning and disinfecting in one operation, is non-flammable and non-volatile in use dilution, and provides excellent solubility.

The PHENO-TEK II detergent system has been especially formulated to provide cleaning, wetting and penetration of soils and organic matter and easy rinsing of surfaces. Good foam is obtained at ½ oz. per gallon of water (1:256) to provide prolonged contact time.

PHENO-TEK II at ½ oz. per gallon water (1:256) provides residual control of odor causing bacteria in the presence of moisture.

P

PHENO-TEK II is recommended for use when used as directed on ceramic and glazed tile surfaces, stainless steel, aluminum, chrome, galvanized metal, glass, and other non-porous surfaces such as treated wood, polyethylene, polypropylene, (PVC) polyvinyl chloride), polystyrene, vinyl, fiberglass, viton, ethylene propylene, nitrile, acrylic and polyurethane.

PHENO-TEK II at ½ oz. per gallon water (1:256) is suited for disinfecting and cleaning all hard, non-porous environmental surfaces on side paneling. It is ideally suited for use in Swine Operations, in Poultry and Turkey Barns, Breeder and Laying Operations, Poultry House Grow-Out Operations, Hatcheries -- in hatchers and setters, humidifying systems and ceiling fans, live haul equipment, chick buses, transfer trucks, coop washing, polyethylene chick boxes, foot pans and feed bins.

PHENO-TEK II is recommended for use in fogging (wet misting) operations as an adjunct either preceding or following regular cleaning and disinfecting procedures. The recommended dilution is ½ oz. per gallon water (1:256). Fog for 3 minutes per 2,000 cu. ft.—leave the room. Allow at least 2 hours before entering area that has been fogged. All food and food packaging items must be removed or carefully protected. Treated food contact surfaces must be thoroughly scrubbed with PHENO-TEK II at ½ oz. per gallon water (1:256) and rinsed with potable water prior to reuse.

Toxicity tests required by the U.S. Environmental Protection Agency for PHENO-TEK II Cleaner-Disinfectant-Deodorant have been done in conformance with FDA and EPA Good Laboratory Practice Regulations.

Directions for Use: It is a violation of Federal Law to use this product in a manner inconsistent with its labeling.

Do not apply this product in a way that will contact workers or other persons, either directly or through drift. Only protected handlers may be in the area during application. Following application as a low or high pressure spray, do not enter or allow others to enter the treated areas until sprays have dried. Thoroughly ventilate entire closed area after fogging applications. Do not enter, allow other persons to enter, house livestock, or use equipment in the treated area until ventilation is complete and any liquid has been absorbed, set, or dried. For entry into fogged areas before ventilation is complete and the fog has completely dissipated, all persons must wear the PPE, including a full face respirator, required in the precautionary section of this labeling for applicators and other handlers.

General Use Directions:

1. To clean, disinfect and deodorize walls, floors, tables, drinking fountains, sinks, refrigerators, stoves, restroom fixtures, and garbage cans: Remove gross filth and heavy soil with a preliminary cleaning step prior to application of PHENO-TEK II. Apply a solution of ½ oz. per gallon water (1:256) with a sponge, mop, mechanical spray device or foaming apparatus, making sure that all surfaces are wetted thoroughly. Allow surface to remain wet for 10 minutes.
2. To clean, disinfect such articles as combs, brushes, razors, scissors, and rubber goods: Wipe articles clean and soak for 10 minutes in a solution containing ½ oz. PHENO-TEK 11 per gallon water (1:256).
3. To clean gross filth or heavy soil on environmental surfaces prior to disinfection, use ½ oz. PHENO-TEK II per gallon water (1:256).

Directions For Use In Poultry House and Farm Premise: Do not use in milking stalls, milking parlors, or milk houses.

1. Remove all poultry, livestock, and feed from the premises.
2. Remove all trucks, coops, crates, water troughs and feed racks.
3. Remove all gross soil, litter, manure, droppings, from livestock and poultry from floors, walls and surfaces of barns, pens, stalls, chutes and other facilities and fixtures occupied or traversed by animals and poultry.
4. Thoroughly clean and saturate all surfaces with a solution of ½ oz. PHENO-TEK II per gallon of water (1:256) using conventional spraying methods.
5. Allow to remain in contact for at least 10 minutes.
6. Immerse halters, ropes, and other types of equipment used in handling and restraining livestock, forks, shovels, scrapers used for removing litter and manure in a solution of PHENO-TEK II at ½ oz. per gallon of water (1:256). Allow to remain in contact for 10 minutes.
7. Thoroughly scrub treated feed racks, troughs, automatic feeders, fountains, waterers, and mangers with a solution of PHENO-TEK II at ½ oz. per gallon of water (1:256). Rinse with potable water before reuse.
8. Ventilate buildings, coops, and other closed spaces. Do not house poultry or livestock or employ equipment until treatment has been absorbed, set, or dried.

Precautionary Statements: Hazards to Human and Domestic Animals: Danger. Corrosive. Causes irreversible eye damage and skin burns. Do not get in eyes, on skin, or on clothing. Wear goggles or face shield, protective clothing, and chemical resistant rubber gloves when handling. Harmful if swallowed. Wash thoroughly with soap and water after handling and before eating, drinking, or using tobacco. Remove contaminated clothing and wash before reuse.

Personal Protective Equipment (PPE): Applicators and other handlers must wear:

- Long sleeve shirt and long pants, socks plus shoes, chemical resistant gloves. In addition, for applicators and other handlers exposed to fog during fogging applications, and until fog has dissipated and the enclosed area has been thoroughly ventilated, must wear:

- A full face respirator with a canister or cartridge approved for pesticides (MSHA/NIOSH approval number prefix TC-14G)

Environmental Hazards: Do not discharge effluent containing this product into lakes, ponds, streams, estuaries, oceans, or other waters unless in accordance with the requirements of a National Pollutant Discharge Elimination System (NPDES) permit and the permitting authority has been notified in writing prior to discharge. Do not discharge effluent containing this product to sewer systems without previously notifying the local sewage treatment plant authority. For guidance, contact your State Water Board or Regional Office of the EPA.

Statement of Practical Treatment:

If On Skin: Wash with plenty of soap and water. Get medical attention.

If In Eyes: Hold eyelids open and flush with a steady stream of water for 15 minutes. Get medical attention.

If Swallowed: Call a physician immediately. Drink promptly a large quantity of milk, egg whites, gelatin solution, or, if these are not available, large quantities of water. Never induce vomiting or give anything by mouth to an unconscious person. Avoid alcohol.

Note To Physician: Probable mucosal damage may contraindicate the use of gastric lavage. Measures against circulatory shock, respiratory depression convulsion may be needed.

Storage and Disposal:

Pesticide Disposal: Pesticide wastes are acutely hazardous. Improper disposal of excess pesticide, spray mixture, or rinsate is a violation of Federal Law. If these wastes cannot be disposed of by use according to label instructions, contact your State Pesticide or Environmental Control Agency, or the Hazardous Waste representative at the nearest EPA Regional Office for guidance. Do not contaminate water, food, or feed by storage or disposal.

Container Disposal: Triple rinse (or equivalent). The offer for recycling or reconditioning, or puncture and dispose of in a sanitary landfill, or by incineration, or, if allowed by State and local authorities, by burning. If burned, stay out of smoke.

Warning(s): Keep out of reach of children.

Discussion: Staphylocidal, Salmonellacidal, Pseudomonacidal, Virucidal†.

Proven effective as a disinfectant by the following tests: AOAC (use dilution test method) in conformance with the 14th Edition, 1984. All dilutions at 1:256. The following organisms tested at 400 ppm water hardness as calcium carbonate and 5% animal serum as organic soil: *Aspergillus fumigatis* ATCC# 24547, *Escherichia coli* ATCC# 11229, *Pasteurella anatis* ATCC# 43329, *Pseudomonas aeruginosa* ATCC# 15442, *Salmonella choleraesuis* ATCC# 10708, *Salmonella enteritidis* ATCC# 13076, *Staphylococcus aureus* ATCC# 6538.

†The following viruses tested in accordance with U.S. Environmental Protection Agency Pesticide Assessment Guidelines on inanimate environmental surfaces. Tested in 400 ppm water hardness as calcium carbonate and 5% animal serum (as organic soil): All dilutions at 1:256: Avian influenza virus (AI), Avian laryngotracheitis virus (LT), Transmissible gastroenteritis virus (TGE).

Conductive: PHENO-TEK II has been tested by Hood Patterson-Dewar, Electrical Testing Engineers, its effect on conductive flooring. The method used conforms to the specifications known NFPA Standard No. 56A, published by the National Fire Protection Association, Second Edition, 1987. PHENO-TEK II meets the requirement of NFPA 56A.

Presentation: 4x1 gallon cases and 55 gallon drums.

Compendium Code No.: 13700030

PHENYLBUTAZONE 20% INJECTION ℞

Vet Tek **Phenylbutazone-Injection**

(Phenylbutazone)

ANADA No.: 200-126

Active Ingredient(s): Each mL contains:

Phenylbutazone . . . . 200 mg
Benzyl Alcohol (as preservative) . . . . 10.45 mg
Water for Injection . . . . q.s.

Sodium hydroxide to adjust pH to 9.5 to 10.0

Indications: For relief of inflammatory conditions associated with the musculoskeletal system in horses.

Pharmacology: Description: PHENYLBUTAZONE 20% INJECTION (phenylbutazone) is a synthetic, nonhormonal anti-inflammatory, antipyretic compound useful in the management of inflammatory conditions. The apparent analgesic effect is probably related mainly to the compound's anti-inflammatory properties.

Chemically, phenylbutazone is 4-butyl-1,2-diphenyl-3,5-pyrazolidinedione. It is a pyrazolon derivative entirely unrelated to the steroid hormones, and has the following structural formula:

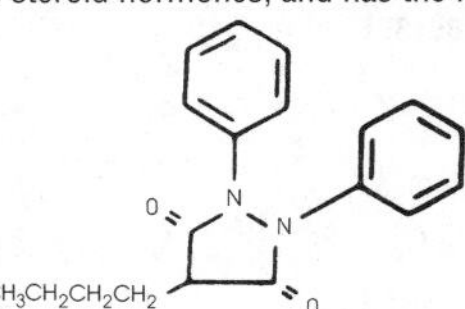

Background Pharmacology: Kuzell,[1,2,3] Payne,[4] Fleming,[5] and Denko[6] demonstrated clinical effectiveness of phenylbutazone in acute rheumatism, gout, gouty arthritis, and various other rheumatoid disorders in man. Anti-rheumatic and anti-inflammatory activity has been well established by Fabre,[7] Domenjoz,[8] Wilhelmi,[9] and Yourish.[10]

Camberos[14] reported favorable results with phenylbutazone following intermittent treatment of Thoroughbred horses for arthritis and chronic arthrosis (e.g., osteoarthritis of medial and distal bones of the hock, arthritis of stifle and hip, arthrosis of the spine, chronic hip pains, chronic pain in trapezius muscles, and generalized arthritis). Results were less favorable in cases of traumatism, muscle rupture, strains and inflammations of the third phalanx. Sutter[15] reported favorable response in chronic equine arthritis, fair results in a severely bruised mare, and poor results in two cases where the condition was limited to the third phalanx.

Dosage and Administration: Horses:

Intravenously: 1 to 2 g per 1,000 lbs of body weight (5 to 10 mL/1,000 lbs daily. Injection should be given slowly and with care. Limit intravenous administration to a maximum of 5 successive days, which may be followed by oral phenylbutazone dosage forms.

Guidelines to Successful Therapy:

1. Use a relatively high dose for the first 48 hours, then reduce gradually to a maintenance dose. Maintain lowest dose capable of producing desired clinical response.
2. Response to phenylbutazone therapy is prompt, usually occurring within 24 hours. If no significant clinical response is evident after 5 days, reevaluate diagnosis and therapeutic approach.
3. In animals, phenylbutazone is largely metabolized in 8 hours. It is recommended that a third of the daily dose be administered at 8 hour intervals. Reduce dosage as symptoms regress. In some cases, treatment may be given only when symptoms appear with no need for continuous medication. If long-term therapy is planned, oral administration is suggested.
4. Many chronic conditions will respond to phenylbutazone therapy, but discontinuance of treatment may result in recurrence of symptoms.

Contraindication(s): Treated animals should not be slaughtered for food purposes. Parenteral injections should be made intravenously only; do not inject subcutaneously or intramuscularly. Use with caution in patients who have a history of drug allergy.

Precaution(s): Store in a refrigerator between 2°C and 8°C (36°F and 46°F).

Caution(s): Federal law restricts this drug to use by or on the order of a licensed veterinarian.

Stop medication at the first sign of gastrointestinal upset, jaundice, or blood dyscrasia. Authenticated cases of agranulocytosis associated with the drug have occurred in man; fatal reactions, although rare, have been reported in dogs after long-term therapy. To guard against this possibility, conduct routine blood counts at Weekly intervals during the early phase of therapy and at intervals of two weeks thereafter. Any significant fall in the total white count, relative decrease in granulocytes, or black or tarry stools, should be regarded as a signal for immediate cessation of therapy and institution of appropriate countermeasures.

In the treatment of inflammatory conditions associated with infections, specific anti-infective therapy is required. For horses only.

Warning(s): Not for use in horses intended for food. Keep out of reach of children.

References: Available upon request.

Presentation: 100 mL vials (NDC 60270-049-10).

Manufactured by: Phoenix Scientific, Inc., St. Joseph, MO 64503.

Compendium Code No.: 14200141 Iss. 8-95

PHENYLBUTAZONE INJECTION 20% ℞

Aspen **Phenylbutazone**

ANADA No.: 200-126

Active Ingredient(s): Each mL contains 200 mg of phenylbutazone, 10.45 mg of benzyl alcohol as preservative, sodium hydroxide to adjust pH to 9.5 to 10.0, and water for injection, q.s.

Indications: For relief of inflammatory conditions associated with the musculoskeletal system in horses.

Pharmacology: Description: Phenylbutazone is a synthetic, nonhormonal anti-inflammatory, antipyretic compound useful in the management of inflammatory conditions. The apparent analgesic effect is probably related mainly to the compound's anti-inflammatory properties.

Chemically, phenylbutazone is 4-butyl-1,2-diphenyl- 3,5-pyrazolidinedione. It is a pyrazolon derivative entirely unrelated to the steroid hormones, and has the following structural formula:

Mol. Wt. 308.38

Phenylbutazone is a white crystalline solid, slightly soluble in water, and soluble in some organic solvents. It has no odor and a slightly bitter taste.

Background Pharmacology: Kuzell,[1,2,3] Payne,[4] Fleming,[5] and Denko[6] demonstrated clinical effectiveness of phenylbutazone in acute rheumatism, gout, gouty arthritis, and various other rheumatoid disorders in man. Anti-rheumatic and anti-inflammatory activity has been well established by Fabre, Domenjoz,[8] Wilhelmi,[9] and Yourish.[10]

Liberman[11] reported on the effective use of phenylbutazone in the treatment of painful conditions of the musculoskeletal system in dogs; including posterior paralysis associated with invertebral disc syndrome, painful fractures, arthritis, and painful injuries to the limbs and joints. Joshua[12] observed objective movement without toxicity following long-term therapy of two aged arthritic dogs. Ogilvie and Sutter[13] reported rapid response to phenylbutazone therapy in a review of 19 clinical cases including posterior paralysis, posterior weakness, arthritis rheumatism and other conditions associated with lameness and musculoskeletal weakness.

Camberos[14] reported favorable results with phenylbutazone following intermittent treatment of Thoroughbred horses for arthritis and chronic arthrosis (e.g., osteoarthritis of medial and distal bones of the hock, arthritis of the stifle and hip, arthrosis of the spine, chronic hip pains, chronic pain in trapezius muscles, and generalized arthritis). Results were less favorable in cases of traumatism, muscle rupture, strains and inflammations of the third phalanx. Sutter reported favorable response in chronic equine arthritis, fair results in a severely bruised mare, and poor results in two cases where the condition was limited to the third phalanx.

Dosage and Administration: Horses: Intravenously: 1 to 2 g per 1,000 lbs of body weight (5 to 10 mL/1,000 lbs) daily. Injection should be given slowly and with care. Limit intravenous administration to a maximum of 5 successive days, which may be followed by oral phenylbutazone dosage forms.

Response to phenylbutazone is usually prompt. If there is no significant clinical effect in 5 days, a re-evaluation of the diagnosis and treatment should be made.

Guidelines to Successful Therapy:

1. Use a relatively high dose for the first 48 hours, then reduce gradually to a maintenance dose. Maintain lowest dose capable of producing desired clinical response.
2. Response to phenylbutazone therapy is prompt, usually occurring within 24 hours. If no significant clinical response is evident after 5 days, reevaluate diagnosis and therapeutic approach.
3. In animals, phenylbutazone is largely metabolized in 8 hours. It is recommended that a third of the daily dosage be administered at 8 hour intervals. Reduce dosage as symptoms regress. In some cases, treatment may be given only when symptoms appear with no need for continuous medication. If long-term therapy is planned, oral administration is suggested.
4. Many chronic conditions will respond to phenylbutazone therapy, but discontinuance of treatment may result in recurrence of symptoms.

Contraindication(s): Parenteral injections should be made intravenously only; do not inject subcutaneously or intramuscularly.

Use with caution in patients who have a history of drug allergy.

Precaution(s): Store in a refrigerator between 2°C and 8°C (36°F and 46°F).

Caution(s): Federal law restricts this drug to use by or on the order of a licensed veterinarian.

Stop medication at the first sign of gastrointestinal upset, jaundice, or blood dyscrasia. Authenticated cases of agranulocytosis associated with the drug have occurred in man; fatal reactions, although rare, have been reported in dogs after long-term therapy. To guard against this possibility, conduct routine blood counts at weekly intervals during the early phase of therapy and at intervals of two weeks thereafter. Any significant fall in the total white count, relative decrease in granulocytes, or black or tarry stools, should be regarded as a signal for immediate cessation of therapy and institution of appropriate countermeasures.

In the treatment of inflammatory conditions associated with infections, specific anti-infective therapy is required.

Warning(s): Not for use in horses intended for food.

For horses only.

Side Effects: Oral doses of phenylbutazone higher than those recommended have been shown to produce intestinal ulcerative lesions. Necrotizing phlebitis in the portal vein has been observed in horses receiving high doses for extended periods of time.

References: Available upon request.

Presentation: 100 mL vials.

Manufactured by: Phoenix Scientific, Inc., St. Joseph, MO 64506

Compendium Code No.: 14750620 600043

PHENYLBUTAZONE INJECTION 20% ℞

RXV **Phenylbutazone-Injection**

(Phenylbutazone)

ANADA No.: 200-126

Active Ingredient(s): Each mL contains:

Phenylbutazone	200 mg
Benzyl Alcohol (as preservative)	10.45 mg
Sodium hydroxide to adjust pH to 9.5 to 10.0	
Water For Injection	q.s.

Indications: For relief of inflammatory conditions associated with the musculoskeletal system in horses.

Dosage and Administration: Intravenous dosage (not for subcutaneous or intramuscular use):

Horses: 1 to 2 g per 1,000 lb body weight (5 to 10 mL/1,000 lb) daily.

See package insert for additional information.

Precaution(s): Store in a refrigerator between 2°C and 8°C (36°F-46°F).

Caution(s): Federal law restricts this drug to use by or on the order of a licensed veterinarian.

For horses only.

Keep out of reach of children.

Warning(s): Not for use in horses intended for food.

Presentation: 100 mL, 12 per case.

Compendium Code No.: 10910110

PHENYLBUTAZONE INJECTION 200 MG/ML ℞

Butler **Phenylbutazone**

ANADA No.: 200-126

Active Ingredient(s): Each mL contains:

Phenylbutazone	200 mg
Benzyl Alcohol (as preservative)	10.45 mg
Water for Injection	q.s.
Sodium Hydroxide to adjust pH to 9.5 to 10.0	

Indications: For relief of inflammatory conditions associated with the musculoskeletal system in horses.

Pharmacology: Description: PHENYLBUTAZONE INJECTION 200 MG/ML (phenylbutazone) is a synthetic, nonhormonal anti-inflammatory, antipyretic compound useful in the management of inflammatory conditions. The apparent analgesic effect is probably related mainly to the compound's anti-inflammatory properties.

Chemically, phenylbutazone is 4-butyl-1,2-diphenyl-3,5-pyrazolidinedione. It is a pyrazolon derivative entirely unrelated to the steroid hormones, and has the following structural formula:

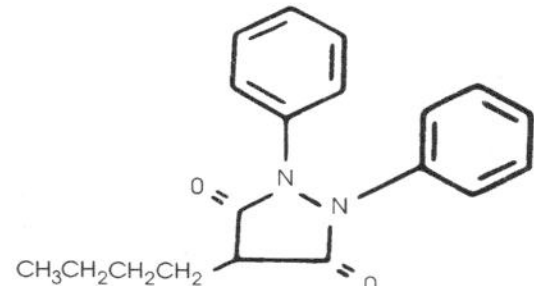

Background Pharmacology: Kuzell,[1,2,3] Payne,[4] Fleming,[5] and Denko[6] demonstrated clinical effectiveness of phenylbutazone in acute rheumatism, gout, gouty arthritis, and various other rheumatoid disorders in man. Anti-rheumatic and anti-inflammatory activity has been well established by Fabre,[7] Domenjoz,[8] Wilhelmi,[9] and Yourish.[10]

Lieberman[11] reported on the effective use of phenylbutazone in the treatment of conditions of the musculoskeletal system in dogs, including posterior paralysis associated with intervertebral disc syndrome, fracture, arthritis and injuries to the limbs and joints. Joshua[12] observed objective improvement without toxicity following long-term therapy of two aged arthritic dogs. Ogilvie and Sutter[13] reported rapid response to phenylbutazone therapy in a review of 19 clinical cases including posterior paralysis, posterior weakness, arthritis, rheumatism and other conditions associated with lameness and musculoskeletal weakness.

Camberos[14] reported favorable results with phenylbutazone following intermittent treatment of Thoroughbred horses for arthritis and chronic arthrosis (e.g., osteoarthritis of medial and distal bones of the hock, arthritis of stifle and hip, arthrosis of the spine, chronic hip pains, chronic pain in trapezius muscles, and generalized arthritis). Results were less favorable in cases of traumatism, muscle rupture, strains and inflammations of the third phalanx. Sutter[15] reported favorable response in chronic equine arthritis, fair results in a severely bruised mare, and poor results in two cases where the condition was limited to the third phalanx.

Dosage and Administration: Horses:

Intravenously: 1 to 2 g per 1,000 lbs of body weight (5 to 10 mL/1,000 lbs) daily. Injection should be given slowly and with care. Limit intravenous administration to a maximum of 5 successive days, which may be followed by oral phenylbutazone dosage forms.

Guidelines To Successful Therapy:

1. Use a relatively high dose for the first 48 hours, then reduce gradually to a maintenance dose. Maintain lowest dose capable of producing desired clinical response.
2. Response to phenylbutazone therapy is prompt, usually occurring within 24 hours. If no significant clinical response is evident after 5 days, reevaluate diagnosis and therapeutic approach.
3. In animals, phenylbutazone is largely metabolized in 8 hours. It is recommended that a third of the daily dose be administered at 8 hour intervals. Reduce dosage as symptoms regress. In some cases, treatment may be given only when symptoms appear with no need for continuous medication. If long-term therapy is planned, oral administration is suggested.
4. Many chronic conditions will respond to phenylbutazone therapy, but discontinuance of treatment may result in recurrence of symptoms.

Contraindication(s): Parenteral injections should be made intravenously only; do not inject subcutaneously or intramuscularly.

Use with caution in patients who have a history of drug allergy.

Precaution(s): Store in a refrigerator between 2°C and 8°C (36°F and 46°F).

Caution(s): Federal law restricts this drug to use by or on the order of a licensed veterinarian.

Stop medication at the first sign of gastrointestinal upset, jaundice, or blood dyscrasia. Authenticated cases of agranulocytosis associated with the drug have occurred in man; fatal reactions, although rare, have been reported in dogs after long-term therapy. To guard against this possibility, conduct routine blood counts at weekly intervals during the early phase of therapy and at intervals of two weeks thereafter. Any significant fall in the total white count, relative decrease in granulocytes, or black or tarry stools, should be regarded as a signal for immediate cessation of therapy and institution of appropriate countermeasures.

In the treatment of inflammatory conditions associated with infections, specific anti-infective therapy is required.

For horses only.

Warning(s): Not for use in horses intended for food.

Keep out of reach of children.

References: Available upon request.

Presentation: 100 mL vials, 200 mg/mL (NDC 11695-3571-1).

Manufactured by: Phoenix Scientific, Inc., St. Joseph, MO 64506.

Compendium Code No.: 10821421 Iss. 8-95

P

PHENYLBUTAZONE TABLETS (Dogs) ℞

RXV **Phenylbutazone-Oral**

NADA No.: 049-187

Active Ingredient(s): Each tablet contains:

Phenylbutazone .... 100 mg

A nonhormonal anti-inflammatory agent.

Indications: Phenylbutazone is indicated for the treatment of inflammatory conditions of the musculoskeletal system in dogs.

Dosage and Administration: Orally: 20 mg per pound of body weight (100 mg/5 lbs.) a day in three (3) divided doses, but not to exceed 800 mg a day, regardless of body weight.

Contraindication(s): Phenylbutazone should not be administered to patients with serious hepatic, renal or cardiac pathology, or those with a history of blood dyscrasia.

Precaution(s): Use with caution in patients with a history of drug allergy. Stop medication at the first sign of gastro-intestinal upset, jaundice or blood dyscrasia. To guard against this possibility, conduct routine blood counts at not more than seven day intervals during the early course of therapy. Any significant fall in the total white count, relative decrease in granulocytes or black or tarry stool should be regarded as a signal for immediate cessation of therapy and institution of appropriate treatment. When treating inflammatory conditions associated with infection, specific anti-infective therapy is required. Response to phenylbutazone therapy is prompt, usually occurring within 24 hours. If a significant clinical response is not evident after five days of therapy, re-evaluate the diagnosis and therapeutic regimen.

Caution(s): Federal law restricts this drug to use by or on the order of a licensed veterinarian.

Keep out of the reach of children.

Warning(s): For dogs only.

Presentation: 100 and 1,000 tablet containers.

Compendium Code No.: 10910120

PHENYLBUTAZONE TABLETS (Dogs) ℞

Vedco **Phenylbutazone-Oral**

NADA No.: 049-187

Active Ingredient(s): Each tablet contains:

Phenylbutazone .... 100 mg

A nonhormonal anti-inflammatory agent.

Indications: Phenylbutazone is indicated for the treatment of inflammatory conditions of the musculoskeletal system in dogs.

Dosage and Administration: Orally: 20 mg per pound of body weight (100 mg/5 lbs.) a day in three (3) divided doses, but not to exceed 800 mg a day, regardless of body weight.

Contraindication(s): Phenylbutazone should not be administered to patients with serious hepatic, renal or cardiac pathology, or those with a history of blood dyscrasia.

Caution(s): Federal law restricts this drug to use by or on the order of a licensed veterinarian.

Use with caution in patients with a history of drug allergy. Stop medication at the first sign of gastro-intestinal upset, jaundice or blood dyscrasia. To guard against this possibility, conduct routine blood counts at not more than seven day intervals during the early course of therapy. Any significant fall in the total white count, relative decrease in granulocytes or black or tarry stool should be regarded as a signal for immediate cessation of therapy and institution of appropriate treatment. When treating inflammatory conditions associated with infection, specific anti-infective therapy is required. Response to phenylbutazone therapy is prompt, usually occurring within 24 hours. If a significant clinical response is not evident after five days of therapy, re-evaluate the diagnosis and therapeutic regimen.

For dogs only.

Warning(s): Keep out of reach of children.

Presentation: 500 and 1,000 tablet containers.

Compendium Code No.: 10941671

PHENYLBUTAZONE TABLETS, USP ℞

Vet Tek **Phenylbutazone-Oral**

Anti-inflammatory

NADA No.: 091 -818

Active Ingredient(s): Each tablet contains 1 g of phenylbutazone.

Indications: Phenylbutazone is for the relief of inflammatory conditions associated with the musculoskeletal system in horses.

Pharmacology: Phenylbutazone chemically is 4-butyl-1, 2 diphenyl-3, 5-pyrazolidinedione.

$C_{19}H_{20}N_2O_2$

Mol. Wt. 308.38

Background Pharmacology: Phenylbutazone was first synthesized in 1948 and introduced into human medicine in 1949. Kuzell (1), (2), (3), Payne, (4), Fleming, (5) and Denko, (6) demonstrated the clinical effectiveness of phenylbutazone in gout, gouty arthritis, acute arthritis, acute rheumatism and various other rheumatoid disorders in humans. Fabre (7), Domenjoz, (8), Wilhelmi, (9) and Yourish, (10), have established the anti-rheumatic and anti-inflammatory activity of phenylbutazone. It is entirely unrelated to the steroid hormones.

Toxicity of phenylbutazone has been investigated in rats and mice (11), and dogs (12).

Phenylbutazone has been used by Camberos (13), in thoroughbred horses. Favorable results were reported in cases of traumatism, muscle rupture, strains and inflammations of the third phalanx. Results were not as favorable in the periodic treatment of osteoarthritis of the stifle and hip, arthrosis of the trapezious muscles and general arthritis. Sutter, (14) reported a favorable response in chronic equine arthritis of long duration, fair results in severely bruised mare and poor results in two cases where the condition was limited to the third phalanx.

Dosage and Administration: For Horses Only: Orally 1 to 2 tablets per 500 pounds of body weight, but not to exceed 4 g per animal daily. Use high dose for the first 48 hours, then gradually reduce to a maintenance dose.

Contraindication(s): Use with caution in patients who have history of drug allergy.

Precaution(s): Store at controlled room temperature, 20° to 25°C (68° to 77°F).

Dispense in tight, child resistant containers.

Caution(s): Federal law restricts this drug to use by or on the order of a licensed veterinarian.

In the treatment of inflammatory conditions associated with infections, specific anti-infective therapy should be used concurrently.

For oral use in horses only.

Keep out of reach of children.

Warning(s): Not for horses intended for food.

References: Available upon request.

Presentation: Tablets containing 1 gram of phenylbutazone are supplied in bottles of 100 tablets.

Manufactured by: Phoenix Scientific, Inc., St. Joseph, MO 64503

Compendium Code No.: 14200150 Iss. 01-00

PHENYLBUTAZONE TABLETS, USP 100 MG ℞

Butler **Phenylbutazone-Oral**

Anti-Inflammatory

NADA No.: 094-170

Active Ingredient(s): Each tablet contains:

Phenylbutazone, USP .... 100 mg

Indications: For relief of inflammatory conditions associated with the musculoskeletal system in dogs.

Pharmacology: Description: Phenylbutazone is a synthetic, non-hormonal anti-inflammatory compound useful in the management of inflammatory conditions. The apparent analgesic effect is probably related to the compound's anti-inflammatory properties.

Chemically, Phenylbutazone is 4-butyl-1,2-diphenyl-3,5-pyrazolidinedione. It is a pyrazolon derivative, entirely unrelated to the Steroid hormones, and has the following structural formula:

Background Pharmacology: Kuzell[1,2,3], Payne[4], Fleming[5], and Denko[6], demonstrated clinical effectiveness of Phenylbutazone in acute rheumatism, gout, gouty, arthritis, and various other rheumatoid disorders in man. Anti-inflammatory activity has been well established by Fabre[7], Domenjoz[8], Wilhelmi[9], and Yourish[10].

Lieberman[11] reported on the effective use of phenylbutazone in the treatment of painful conditions of the musculoskeletal system in dogs. Joshua[12] observed objective improvement without toxicity following long term therapy of two aged arthritic dogs. Ogilvie and Sutter[13] reported rapid response to phenylbutazone therapy in a review of 19 clinical cases including arthritis, rheumatism, and other conditions associated with lameness and musculoskeletal weakness. Camberos[14] reported favorable results with phenylbutazone following intermittent treatment of Thoroughbred horses for arthritis and chronic arthrosis (e.g., osteoarthritis of medial, and distal bones of the hock, arthritis of stifle and hip, arthrosis of the spine, chronic hip pains, chronic pain in trapezius muscles, and generalized arthritis). Results were less favorable in cases of traumatism, muscle rupture, strains, and inflammations of the third phalanx. Sutter[15] reported favorable response in chronic equine arthritis, fair results in a severely bruised mare, and poor results in two cases where the condition was limited to the third phalanx.

Dosage and Administration: Orally — 20 mg per lb of body weight (100 mg/5 lb) in three divided doses daily. Maximum dose is 800 mg per day regardless of weight. Use a relatively high dose for the first 48 hours, then reduce gradually to a maintenance dose. Maintain lowest dose capable of producing desired clinical response.

Guidelines to Successful Therapy:

1. Response to Phenylbutazone therapy is prompt, usually occurring within 24 hours. If no significant clinical response is evident after 5 days, re-evalutate diagnosis and therapeutic approach.
2. In animals, Phenylbutazone is largely metabolized in 8 hours. It is recommended that a third of the daily dose be administered at 8 hour intervals. Reduce dosage as symptoms regress. In some cases, treatment may be given only when symptoms appear with no need for continuous medication. If long term therapy is planned, oral administration is suggested.
3. In many cases, tablets may be crushed and given with feed.
4. Many chronic conditions will respond to Phenylbutazone therapy, but discontinuance of treatment may result in recurrence of symptoms.
5. The duration of treatment will depend upon the degree of severity of the condition and generally ranges from 6 to 14 days with retreatment given only to control recurring symptoms. If there is no improvement in 5 days, discontinue treatment.

Contraindication(s): Animals showing evidence of cardiac, hepatic, or renal damage or a history of blood dyscrasia, or those with signs or history of anemia.

Precaution(s): Store at controlled room temperature, 20° to 25°C (68° to 77°F).

Dispense in a tight container with child-resistant closure.

Caution(s): Federal (U.S.A.) law restricts this drug to use by or on the order of a licensed veterinarian.

Stop medication at first sign of gastrointestinal upset, jaundice, or blood dyscrasia. Authenticated cases of agranulocytosis associated with the drug have occurred in man; fatal reactions, although rare, have been reported in dogs after long-term therapy. To guard against this possibility, conduct routine blood counts at weekly intervals during the early phase of therapy and at intervals of two weeks thereafter. Any significant fall in the total white count, relative decrease in granulocytes, or black or tarry stools, should be regarded as a signal for immediate cessation of therapy and institution of appropriate counter measures.

In the treatment of inflammatory conditions associated with infections, specific anti-infective therapy is required.

For oral use in dogs only.

Warning(s): Keep out of reach of children.

References: Available upon request.

Presentation: PHENYLBUTAZONE TABLETS, USP 100 MG are supplied in bottles of 500 and 1000 (NDC 11695-3563-26) tablets.

Manufactured by: Phoenix Scientific, Inc., St. Joseph, MO 64503.

Compendium Code No.: 10821432 Rev. 4/00

PHENYLBUTAZONE TABLETS, USP 1 GRAM ℞

Butler **Phenylbutazone-Oral**

NADA No.: 048-647

Active Ingredient(s): Each tablet contains:

Phenylbutazone, U.S.P. .... 1 gram

Plus excipients.

Indications: Phenylbutazone is for the relief of inflammatory conditions associated with the musculoskeletal system in horses.

A non-hormonal anti-inflammatory agent.

Pharmacology: Description and Pharmacology: Phenylbutazone chemically is 4-butyl-1, 2-diphenyl-3, 5-pyrazolidinedione. It has the following structural formula:

$C_{19}H_{20}N_2O_2$
Mol. Wt. 308.38

Phenylbutazone was first synthesized in 1948 and introduced into human medicine in 1949, Kuzell[1,2,3], Payne[4], Fleming[5], and Denko[6], demonstrated the clinical effectiveness of phenylbutazone in gout, gouty arthritis, acute arthritis, acute rheumatism and various other rheumatoid disorders in humans. Fabre[7], Domenjoz[8], Wilhelmi[9], and Yourish[10], have established the anti-rheumatic and anti-inflammatory activity of phenylbutazone. It is entirely unrelated to the steroid hormones.

Toxicity of phenylbutazone has been investigated in rats and mice[11], Ogilvie and Sutter[12], have also made a study on the chronic toxicity of phenylbutazone in dogs. They have shown that dogs receiving 10 mg and 100 mg per kg body weight, per day for 90 days, maintain good appetites, excrete normal feces, gain weight and maintain a normal blood picture. They also report no abnormal macroscopic or microscopic changes in sacrificed animals which could have been attributed to the drug.

Phenylbutazone has been used by Camberos[13] in thoroughbred horses. Favorable results were reported in cases of traumatism, muscle rupture, strains and inflammations of the third phalanx. Results were not as favorable in the periodic treatment of osteo-arthritis of medial and distal bones of the hock, arthritis of the stifle and hip, arthrosis of the trapezious muscles, and generalized arthritis. Sutter[14] reported a favorable response in chronic equine arthritis of long duration, fair results in a severely bruised mare, and poor results in two cases where the condition was limited to the third phalanx.

Dosage and Administration: For horses only.

Horses: Orally - 1 to 2 tablets per 500 lb body weight. Do not exceed 4 grams daily. Reduce dosage as symptoms regress. Intermittent treatment given only when symptoms appear may be indicated.

Contraindication(s): Use with caution in patients who have a history of drug allergy.

Precaution(s): Storage: Store at controlled room temperature between 15°-30°C (59°-86°F). Keep container tightly closed when not in use.

Caution(s): Federal law restricts this drug to use by or on the order of a licensed veterinarian.

In the treatment of inflammatory conditions associated with infections, specific anti-infective therapy should be used concurrently.

For animal use only.

Warning(s): Not for use in horses intended for food.

Keep out of reach of children.

References: Available upon request.

Presentation: Available in 1 g tablets - 100 tablets per bottle (NDC 11695-2196-1).

Manufactured by: First Priority, Inc., Elgin, IL 60123-1146.

Compendium Code No.: 10821441

PHENYLBUTE® INJECTION 20% ℞

Phoenix Pharmaceutical **Phenylbutazone**

(Phenylbutazone)

ANADA No.: 200-126

Active Ingredient(s): Each mL contains:

Phenylbutazone .... 200 mg
Benzyl Alcohol (as preservative) .... 10.45 mg
Water for Injection .... q.s.

Sodium Hydroxide to adjust pH to 9.5 to 10.0

Indications: For relief of inflammatory conditions associated with the musculoskeletal system in horses.

Pharmacology: Description: PHENYLBUTE® Injection 20% (phenylbutazone) is a synthetic, nonhormonal anti-inflammatory, antipyretic compound useful in the management of inflammatory conditions. The apparent analgesic effect is probably related mainly to the compound's anti-inflammatory properties.

Chemically, phenylbutazone is 4-butyl-1,2-diphenyl-3,5-pyrazolidinedione. It is a pyrazolon derivative entirely unrelated to the steroid hormones, and has the following structural formula:

Background Pharmacology: Kuzell,[1,2,3] Payne,[4] Fleming,[5] and Denko[6] demonstrated clinical effectiveness of phenylbutazone in acute rheumatism, gout, gouty arthritis, and various other rheumatoid disorders in man. Anti-rheumatic and anti-inflammatory activity has been well established by Fabre,[7] Domenjoz,[8] Wilhelmi,[9] and Yourish.[10]

Camberos[14] reported favorable results with phenylbutazone following intermittent treatment of Thoroughbred horses for arthritis and chronic arthrosis (e.g., osteoarthritis of medial and distal bones of the hock, arthritis of stifle and hip, arthrosis of the spine, chronic hip pains, chronic pain in trapezius muscles, and generalized arthritis). Results were less favorable in cases of traumatism, muscle rupture, strains and inflammations of the third phalanx. Sutter[15] reported favorable response in chronic equine arthritis, fair results in a severely bruised mare, and poor results in two cases where the condition was limited to the third phalanx.

Dosage and Administration: Horses:

Intravenously: 1 to 2 g per 1,000 lbs of body weight (5 to 10 mL/1,000 lbs) daily. Injection should be given slowly and with care. Limit intravenous administration to a maximum of 5 successive days, which may be followed by oral phenylbutazone dosage forms.

Guidelines To Successful Therapy:

1. Use a relatively high dose for the first 48 hours, then reduce gradually to a maintenance dose. Maintain lowest dose capable of producing desired clinical response.
2. Response to phenylbutazone therapy is prompt, usually occurring within 24 hours. If no significant clinical response is evident after 5 days, reevaluate diagnosis and therapeutic approach.
3. In animals, phenylbutazone is largely metabolized in 8 hours. It is recommended that a third of the daily dose be administered at 8 hour intervals. Reduce dosage as symptoms regress. In some cases, treatment may be given only when symptoms appear with no need for continuous medication. If long-term therapy is planned, oral administration is suggested.
4. Many chronic conditions will respond to phenylbutazone therapy, but discontinuance of treatment may result in recurrence of symptoms.

Contraindication(s): Treated animals should not be slaughtered for food purposes. Parenteral injections should be made intravenously only; do not inject subcutaneously or intramuscularly. Use with caution in patients who have a history of drug allergy.

Precaution(s): Store in a refrigerator between 2°C and 8°C (36°F and 46°F).

Caution(s): Federal law restricts this drug to use by or on the order of a licensed veterinarian.

Stop medication at the first sign of gastrointestinal upset, jaundice, or blood dyscrasia. Authenticated cases of agranulocytosis associated with the drug have occurred in man; fatal reactions, although rare, have been reported in dogs after long-term therapy. To guard against this possibility, conduct routine blood counts at weekly intervals during the early phase of therapy and at intervals of two weeks thereafter. Any significant fall in the total white count, relative decrease in granulocytes, or black or tarry stools, should be regarded as a signal for immediate cessation of therapy and institution of appropriate countermeasures.

In the treatment of inflammatory conditions associated with infections, specific anti-infective therapy is required.

For horses only.

Warning(s): Not for use in horses intended for food.

Keep out of reach of children.

References: Available upon request.

Presentation: 100 mL vials (NDC 57319-339-05).

Manufactured by: Phoenix Scientific, Inc., St. Joseph, MO 64503.

Compendium Code No.: 12560632 Rev. 8-01

PHENYLBUTE® PASTE ℞

Phoenix Pharmaceutical **Phenylbutazone-Oral**

Phenylbutazone

NADA No.: 116-087

Active Ingredient(s): Each 1 g marking on the plunger contains:

Phenylbutazone .... 1 g

Indications: For the relief of inflammatory conditions associated with the musculoskeletal system in horses.

Pharmacology: Phenylbutazone is a synthetic, nonhormonal anti-inflammatory, antipyretic compound useful in the management of inflammatory conditions. The apparent analgesic effect is probably related mainly to the compound's anti-inflammatory properties.

Chemically, phenylbutazone is 4-butyl-1,2-diphenyl-3,5-pyrazolidinedione. It is a pyrazolone derivative, entirely unrelated to the steroid hormones, and has the following structural formula:

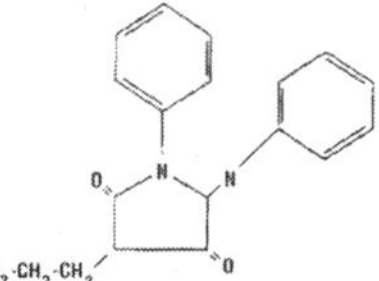

Dosage and Administration: Orally - 1 to 2 g of phenylbutazone per 500 lb of body weight, but not to exceed 4 g daily. Oral cavity should be empty. Deposit paste on back of tongue by depressing plunger that has been previously set to deliver the correct dose.

Guidelines to Successful Therapy:

1. Use a relatively high dose for the first 48 hours, then reduce gradually to maintenance dose. Maintain lowest dose capable of producing desired clinical response.
2. Response to PHENYLBUTE® therapy is prompt, usually occurring within 24 hours. If no significant clinical response is evident after 5 days, re-evaluate diagnosis and therapeutic approach.
3. When administering PHENYLBUTE® Paste, the oral cavity should be empty. Deposit paste on back of tongue by depressing plunger that has been previously set to deliver the correct dose.
4. Many chronic conditions will respond to PHENYLBUTE® therapy, but discontinuance of treatment may result in recurrence of symptoms.

Contraindication(s): Use with caution in patients who have a history of drug allergy.

Precaution(s): Storage: Store at 15°-30°C (59°-86°F).

Caution(s): Federal (U.S.A.) law restricts this drug to use by or on the order of a licensed veterinarian.

Stop medication at the first sign of gastro-intestinal upset, jaundice, or blood dyscrasia. Authenticated cases of agranulocytosis associated with the drug have occurred in man; fatal reactions, although rare, have been reported in dogs after long-term therapy. To guard against this possibility, conduct routine blood counts at weekly intervals during the early phase of therapy and at intervals of 2 weeks thereafter. Any significant fall in the total white count, relative decrease in granulocytes, or black or tarry stools, should be regarded as a signal for immediate cessation of therapy and institution of appropriate counter measures.

In the treatment of inflammatory conditions associated with infectious, specific anti-infective therapy is required.

Veterinary—For horses only.

Warning(s): Not for use in horses intended for food.

Keep out of reach of children.

Presentation: 12 g syringes (NDC 57319-377-60).

Manufactured by: Schering-Plough Animal Health Corp., Union, NJ 07083

Compendium Code No.: 12560641 3/01

PHENYLBUTE® TABLETS 100 MG ℞

Phoenix Pharmaceutical **Phenylbutazone-Oral**

(Phenylbutazone Tablets, USP) 100 mg Anti-inflammatory

NADA No.: 094-170

Active Ingredient(s): Each tablet contains:

Phenylbutazone, USP .... 100 mg

Indications: For relief of inflammatory conditions associated with the musculoskeletal system in dogs.

Pharmacology:

Description: Phenylbutazone is a synthetic, non-hormonal anti-inflammatory compound useful in the management of inflammatory conditions. The apparent analgesic effect is probably related to the compound's anti-inflammatory properties.

Chemically, Phenylbutazone is 4-butyl-1,2-diphenyl-3,5-pyrazolidinedione. It is a pyrazolon derivative, entirely unrelated to the Steroid hormones, and has the following structural formula:

$CH_3-CH_2-CH_2-CH_2$

Background Pharmacology: Kuzell, (1,2,3) Payne, (4) Fleming, (5) and Denko, (6) demonstrated clinical effectiveness of Phenylbutazone in acute rheumatism, gout, gouty, arthritis, and various other rheumatoid disorders in man. Anti-inflammatory activity has been well established by Fabre, (7), Domenjoz, (8) Wilhelmi, (9) and Yourish, (10).

Lieberman (11) reported on the effective use of phenylbutazone in the treatment of painful conditions of the musculoskeletal system in dogs. Joshua (12) observed objective improvement without toxicity following long term therapy of two aged arthritic dogs. Ogilvie and Sutter (13) reported rapid response to phenylbutazone therapy in a review of 19 clinical cases including arthritis, rheumatism, and other conditions associated with lameness and musculoskeletal weakness. Camberos (14) reported favorable results with phenylbutazone following intermittent treatment of Thoroughbred horses for arthritis and chronic arthrosis (e.g., osteoarthritis of medial, and distal bones of the hock, arthritis of stifle and hip, arthrosis of the spine, chronic hip pains, chronic pain in trapezius muscles, and generalized arthritis). Results were less favorable in cases of traumatism, muscle rupture, strains, and inflammations of the third phalanx. Sutter (15) reported favorable response in chronic equine arthritis, fair results in a severely bruised mare, and poor results in two cases where the condition was limited to the third phalanx.

Dosage and Administration: Orally — 20 mg per lb of body weight (100 mg/5 lb) in three divided doses daily. Maximum dose is 800 mg per day regardless of weight. Use a relatively high dose for the first 48 hours, then reduce gradually to a maintenance dose. Maintain lowest dose capable of producing desired clinical response.

Guidelines to Successful Therapy:

1. Response to Phenylbutazone therapy is prompt, usually occurring within 24 hours. If no significant clinical response is evident after 5 days, re-evalutate diagnosis and therapeutic approach.
2. In animals, Phenylbutazone is largely metabolized in 8 hours. It is recommended that a third of the daily dose be administered at 8 hour intervals. Reduce dosage as symptoms regress. In some cases, treatment may be given only when symptoms appear with no need for continuous medication. If long term therapy is planned, oral administration is suggested.
3. In many cases, tablets may be crushed and given with feed.
4. Many chronic conditions will respond to Phenylbutazone therapy, but discontinuance of treatment may result in recurrence of symptoms.
5. The duration of treatment will depend upon the degree of severity of the condition and generally ranges from 6 to 14 days with retreatment given only to control recurring symptoms. If there is no improvement in 5 days, discontinue treatment.

Contraindication(s): Animals showing evidence of cardiac, hepatic, or renal damage or a history of blood dyscrasia, or those with signs or history of anemia.

Precaution(s): Store at controlled room temperature, 20° to 25°C (68° to 77°F).

Dispense in a tight container with child-resistant closure.

Caution(s): Federal (U.S.A.) law restricts this drug to use by or on the order of a licensed veterinarian.

Stop medication at first sign of gastrointestinal upset, jaundice, or blood dyscrasia. Authenticated cases of agranulocytosis associated with the drug have occurred in man; fatal reactions, although rare, have been reported in dogs after long-term therapy. To guard against this possibility, conduct routine blood counts at weekly intervals during the early phase of therapy and at intervals of two weeks thereafter. Any significant fall in the total white count, relative decrease in granulocytes, or black or tarry stools, should be regarded as a signal for immediate cessation of therapy and institution of appropriate counter measures.

In the treatment of inflammatory conditions associated with infections, specific anti-infective therapy is required. For oral use in dogs only. Keep out of reach of children.

References: Available upon request.

Presentation: PHENYLBUTE® Tablets (Phenylbutazone Tablets, USP) 100 mg are supplied in bottles of 1000 tablets.

Manufactured by: Phoenix Scientific, Inc.

Compendium Code No.: 12560661

PHENYLBUTE® TABLETS 200 MG ℞

Phoenix Pharmaceutical **Phenylbutazone-Oral**

(Phenylbutazone Tablets, USP) 200 mg Anti-Inflammatory

NADA No.: 094-170

Active Ingredient(s): Each tablet contains:

Phenylbutazone, USP.......... 200 mg

Indications: For relief of inflammatory conditions associated with the musculoskeletal system in dogs.

Pharmacology: Description: Phenylbutazone is a synthetic, non-hormonal anti-inflammatory compound useful in the management of inflammatory conditions. The apparent analgesic effect is probably related to the compound's anti-inflammatory properties.

Chemically, Phenylbutazone is 4-butyl-1,2-diphenyl-3,5-pyrazolidinedione. It is a pyrazolon derivative, entirely unrelated to the Steroid hormones, and has the following structural formula:

$CH_3-CH_2-CH_2-CH_2$

Background Pharmacology: Kuzell,[1,2,3] Payne,[4] Fleming,[5] and Denko,[6] demonstrated clinical effectiveness of Phenylbutazone in acute rheumatism, gout, gouty, arthritis, and various other rheumatoid disorders in man. Anti-inflammatory activity has been well established by Fabre,[7] Domenjoz,[8] Wilhelmi,[9] and Yourish,[10].

Lieberman[11] reported on the effective use of phenylbutazone in the treatment of painful conditions of the musculoskeletal system in dogs. Joshua[12] observed objective improvement without toxicity following long term therapy of two aged arthritic dogs. Ogilvie and Sutter[13] reported rapid response to phenylbutazone therapy in a review of 19 clinical cases including arthritis, rheumatism, and other conditions associated with lameness and musculoskeletal weakness. Camberos[14] reported favorable results with phenylbutazone following intermittent treatment of Thoroughbred horses for arthritis and chronic arthrosis (e.g., osteoarthritis of medial, and distal bones of the hock, arthritis of stifle and hip, arthrosis of the spine, chronic hip pains, chronic pain in trapezius muscles, and generalized arthritis). Results were less favorable in cases of traumatism, muscle rupture, strains, and inflammations of the third phalanx. Sutter[15] reported favorable response in chronic equine arthritis, fair results in a severely bruised mare, and poor results in two cases where the condition was limited to the third phalanx.

Dosage and Administration: Orally — 20 mg per lb of body weight (200 mg/10 lb) in three divided doses daily. Maximum dose is 800 mg per day regardless of weight. Use a relatively high dose for the first 48 hours, then reduce gradually to a maintenance dose. Maintain lowest dose capable of producing desired clinical response.

Guidelines to Successful Therapy:

1. Response to Phenylbutazone therapy is prompt, usually occurring within 24 hours. If no significant clinical response is evident after 5 days, re-evalutate diagnosis and therapeutic approach.
2. In animals, Phenylbutazone is largely metabolized in 8 hours. It is recommended that a third of the daily dose be administered at 8 hour intervals. Reduce dosage as symptoms regress. In some cases, treatment may be given only when symptoms appear with no need for continuous medication. If long term therapy is planned, oral administration is suggested.
3. In many cases, tablets may be crushed and given with feed.
4. Many chronic conditions will respond to Phenylbutazone therapy, but discontinuance of treatment may result in recurrence of symptoms.
5. The duration of treatment will depend upon the degree of severity of the condition and generally ranges from 6 to 14 days with retreatment given only to control recurring symptoms. If there is no improvement in 5 days, discontinue treatment.

Contraindication(s): Animals showing evidence of cardiac, hepatic, or renal damage or a history of blood dyscrasia, or those with signs or history of anemia.

Precaution(s): Store at controlled room temperature, 20° to 25°C (68° to 77°F).

Dispense in a tight container with child-resistant closure.

Caution(s): Federal (U.S.A.) law restricts this drug to use by or on the order of a licensed veterinarian.

Stop medication at first sign of gastrointestinal upset, jaundice, or blood dyscrasia. Authenticated cases of agranulocytosis associated with the drug have occurred in man; fatal reactions, although rare, have been reported in dogs after long-term therapy. To guard against this possibility, conduct routine blood counts at weekly intervals during the early phase of therapy and at intervals of two weeks thereafter. Any significant fall in the total white count, relative decrease in granulocytes, or black or tarry stools, should be regarded as a signal for immediate cessation of therapy and institution of appropriate counter measures.

In the treatment of inflammatory conditions associated with infections, specific anti-infective therapy is required.

For oral use in dogs only.

Warning(s): Keep out of reach of children.

References: Available upon request.

Presentation: PHENYLBUTE® Tablets, 200 mg are supplied in bottles of 500 tablets (NDC 57319-452-15).

Manufactured by: Phoenix Scientific, Inc.

Compendium Code No.: 12561140 Iss. 02-01

PHENYLBUTE® TABLETS 1 GRAM ℞

Phoenix Pharmaceutical **Phenylbutazone-Oral**

(Phenylbutazone Tablets, USP) 1 gram Anti-inflammatory

NADA No.: 091 -818

Active Ingredient(s): Each tablet contains:

Phenylbutazone.......... 1 gram

Indications: Phenylbutazone is for the relief of inflammatory conditions associated with the musculoskeletal system in horses.

Pharmacology: Phenylbutazone chemically is 4-butyl-1, 2 diphenyl-3, 5-pyrazolidinedione.

$C_{19}H_{20}N_2O_2$

Mol. Wt. 308.38

Background Pharmacology: Phenylbutazone was first synthesized in 1948 and introduced into human medicine in 1949. Kuzell,[1,2,3] Payne,[4] Fleming,[5] and Denko,[6] demonstrated the clinical effectiveness of phenylbutazone in gout, gouty arthritis, acute arthritis, acute rheumatism and various other rheumatoid disorders in humans. Fabre,[7] Domenjoz,[8] Wilhelmi,[9] and Yourish,[10] have established the anti-rheumatic and anti-inflammatory activity of phenylbutazone. It is entirely unrelated to the steroid hormones.

Toxicity of phenylbutazone has been investigated in rats and mice[11] and dogs[12].

Phenylbutazone has been used by Camberos[13] in thoroughbred horses. Favorable results were reported in cases of traumatism, muscle rupture, strains and inflammations of the third phalanx. Results were not as favorable in the periodic treatment of osteoarthritis of the stifle and hip, arthrosis of the trapezious muscles and general arthritis. Sutter,[14] reported a favorable response in chronic equine arthritis of long duration, fair results in severely bruised mare and poor results in two cases where the condition was limited to the third phalanx.

Dosage and Administration: For Horses Only: Orally 1 to 2 tablets per 500 pounds of body weight, but not to exceed 4 g per animal daily. Use high dose for the first 48 hours, then gradually reduce to a maintenance dose.

Contraindication(s): Use with caution in patients who have history of drug allergy.

Precaution(s): Store at controlled room temperature, 20° to 25°C (68° to 77°F).

Dispense in tight, child resistant containers.

Caution(s): Federal law restricts this drug to use by or on the order of a licensed veterinarian.

In the treatment of inflammatory conditions associated with infections, specific anti-infective therapy should be used concurrently.

For oral use in horses only.

Warning(s): Not for use in horses intended for food.

Keep out of reach of children.

References: Available upon request.

Presentation: Tablets containing 1 gram of phenylbutazone are supplied in bottles of 100 tablets (NDC 57319-422-13).

Manufactured by: Phoenix Scientific, Inc.

Compendium Code No.: 12560651 Rev. 7-01

PHENYLZONE® PASTE ℞

Schering-Plough **Phenylbutazone-Oral**

(phenylbutazone) Anti-inflammatory—Antipyretic compound

NADA No.: 116-087

Active Ingredient(s): Each syringe contains:

Phenylbutazone .... 6 g or 12 g

Indications: For the relief of inflammatory conditions associated with the musculoskeletal system in horses.

Pharmacology: PHENYLZONE® is a synthetic, nonhormonal, anti-inflammatory, antipyretic compound useful in the management of inflammatory conditions. The apparent analgesic effect is probably related mainly to the compound's anti-inflammatory properties.

Chemically, PHENYLZONE® is 4-butyl-1,2-diphenyl-3,5-pyrazolidine-dione. It is a pyrazolone derivative, entirely unrelated to the steroid hormones.

Dosage and Administration: Orally - 1 to 2 g of phenylbutazone per 500 lbs. of body weight, but not to exceed 4 g a day. Use a relatively high dose for the first 48 hours, then reduce it gradually to a maintenance dose. Maintain the lowest dose capable of producing the desired clinical response.

Guidelines To Successful Therapy:

1. Use a relatively high dose for the first 48 hours, then reduce it gradually to a maintenance dose. Maintain lowest dose capable of producing desired clinical response.
2. The response to PHENYLZONE® therapy is prompt, usually occurring within 24 hours. If a significant clinical response is not evident after five (5) days, re-evaluate the diagnosis and therapeutic approach.
3. When administering PHENYLZONE® Paste, the oral cavity should be empty. Deposit the paste on the back of the tongue by depressing the plunger that has been previously set to deliver the correct dose.
4. Many chronic conditions will respond to PHENYLZONE® therapy, but discontinuance of treatment may result in the recurrence of symptoms.

Contraindication(s): Use with caution in patients who have a history of drug allergy.

Precaution(s): Stop medication at the first sign of gastro-intestinal upset, jaundice, or blood dyscrasia. Authenticated cases of agranulocytosis associated with the drug have occurred in man; fatal reactions, although rare have been reported in dogs after long-term therapy. To guard against this possibility, conduct routine blood counts at weekly intervals during the early phase of therapy and at intervals of two weeks thereafter. Any significant fall in the total white count, relative decrease in granulocytes, or black or tarry stools, should be regarded as a signal for immediate cessation of therapy and institution of the appropriate counter measures.

In the treatment of inflammatory conditions associated with infections, specific anti-infective therapy is required.

Caution(s): Federal (USA) law restricts this drug to use by or on the order of a licensed veterinarian. Keep out of the reach of children.

Warning(s): Not for use in horses intended for food.

Presentation: Syringes containing 6 g and 12 g of phenylbutazone.

Compendium Code No.: 10471470

PHF-VAX® ℞

Schering-Plough **Bacterin**

Ehrlichia risticii Bacterin

U.S. Vet. Lic. No.: 165A

Active Ingredient(s): *Ehrlichia risticii* bacterin.

Preservative: Gentamicin.

Indications: PHF-VAX® is recommended for use in healthy equines in the control and prevention of equine monocytic ehrlichiosis (Potomac horse fever) caused by *E. risticii* infection.

Dosage and Administration: 1 mL injected intramuscularly in the healthy equine. Repeat in three (3) to four (4) weeks. Administer a single 1 mL booster dose annually. A 1 mL booster dose every six (6) months is recommended in endemic areas. Vaccination of foals may be initiated after three (3) months of age.

Precaution(s): Store at 2-7°C (35-45°F). Do not freeze. Shake well before use.

Caution(s): Federal law restricts this drug to use by or on the order of a licensed veterinarian.

Transient local reactions may occur at the injection site. If an allergic response occurs, administer epinephrine or its equivalent.

Warning(s): Do not vaccinate within 21 days before slaughter.

Presentation: Box of 10 x 1 mL single dose vials and 10 doses (10 mL).

Compendium Code No.: 10471481

P.H.M. BAC® 1

AgriLabs **Bacterial Vaccine**

Pasteurella Haemolytica-Multocida Vaccine, Avirulent Live Culture

U.S. Vet. Lic. No.: 286

Contents: This product contains the antigens listed above.

This product contains streptomycin as a preservative.

Indications: For use in the vaccination of healthy cattle against respiratory disease caused by *Pasteurella haemolytica* and *Pasteurella multocida*.

Directions: Aseptically rehydrate vial of desiccated product with accompanying vial of diluent. Shake well. Administer 2 mL intramuscularly to healthy cattle. Annual revaccination with a single 2 mL dose is recommended.

Precaution(s): Store in the dark, 35°F-45°F (2°C-7°C). Do not freeze. Use entire contents when first rehydrated. Care should be taken to avoid chemical or microbial contamination of the product. Burn these containers and all unused contents.

Caution(s): In case of anaphylactoid reactions, epinephrine should be administered immediately.

For veterinary use only.

Warning(s): Do not vaccinate within 21 days before slaughter.

Presentation: 10 doses (20 mL) and 50 doses (100 mL).

Manufactured by: Intervet Inc., Millsboro, DE 19966.

Compendium Code No.: 10580792 7971001 / 7975001

PHOS-AID

Butler **Phosphorus-Injectable**

NDC No.: 11695-1232-5

Active Ingredient(s): Each mL contains:

Sodium salt of 4-dimethylamino-2-methyl-phenyl phosphinic acid .... 200 mg
Propylene glycol .... 100 mg
Phenylethanol .... 6.0 mg
Sodium sulfite .... 2.0 mg
Water for Injection .... q.s.

pH adjusted with sodium carbonate.

Indications: For parenteral use as a supplemental source of nutritional phosphorus while the ration is being corrected in areas where feeding rations are inadequate to supply all phosphorus needs for cattle.

Dosage and Administration: Injectable phosphorus may be administered by intravenous or deep intramuscular injection. Divide high intramuscular dosage between two injection sites. Dosage range is 1 mL per 50 to 100 lbs of body weight. Dose range in cattle is 10 to 20 mL. Two injections are sufficient if the ration deficiency is immediately corrected.

Precaution(s): Store at temperatures between 2°C-30°C (36°F-86°F).

Warning(s): For animal use only. Keep out of reach of children.

Presentation: 100 mL sterile vials.

Compendium Code No.: 10821450

PHOS-AID SOLUTION ℞

Neogen **Phosphorus-Injectable**

Injectable Phosphorus-Sterile Solution

Active Ingredient(s): Each mL contains:

Sodium Salt of 4-dimethylamino-2 methyl-phenyl phosphinic Acid .... 200 mg
Propylene glycol .... 100 mg
Phenylethanol .... 6.0 mg
Sodium Sulfite .... 2.0 mg
Water for injection .... q.s.

pH adjusted with sodium carbonate.

Indications: For parenteral use as a supplemental source of nutritional phosphorus while the ration is being corrected in areas where feeding rations are inadequate to supply all phosphorus needs for cattle.

Dosage and Administration: Injectable phosphorus may be administered by intravenous or deep intramuscular injection. Divide high intramuscular dosages between two injection sites. Dosage range is 1 mL per 50 to 100 lbs of body weight. Dose range in cattle is 10 to 20 mL. Two injections are usually sufficient if the ration deficiency is immediately corrected.

Precaution(s): Store at temperature between 2°-30°C (36°-86°F).

Caution(s): Federal law restricts this drug to use by or on the order of a licensed veterinarian.

For animal use only.

Warning(s): Keep out of reach of children.

Presentation: 12 x 100 mL amber glass vials per carton (NDC: 59051-9070-5).

Manufactured by: Omega Laboratories, Montreal, Quebec, H3M 3E4.

Compendium Code No.: 14910092 L567-0201

PHOS-K™ GEL

PRN Pharmacal **Mineral Supplement**

Active Ingredient(s): Each 300 mL tube contains:

Monosodium Phosphate .... 32 grams
Trisodium Phosphate .... 32 grams
Total Phosphorus (Min. 4.3%)
Potassium Chloride .... 9 grams
Potassium (Min. 1.6%)

Ingredients: Monosodium phosphate, trisodium phosphate, potassium chloride, propylene glycol, methylparaben, propylparaben, water, in a rapidly absorbing base.

Indications: A phosphorus and potassium nutritional supplement for cattle.

Directions for Use:

1. Hold the head of the cow in a normal to slightly elevated position.
2. Place tube in cow's mouth directly over the tongue.
3. The product is carefully and quickly pressed out of the 300 mL tube.
4. Hold the cow's mouth closed and allow time to swallow.
5. Administer the entire 300 mL tube for each dose.

Precaution(s): Store at room temperature.

Caution(s): When administering PHOS-K™ GEL use extreme care to prevent injury to cow's oral membranes. Do not allow the cow to chew on the tip of the tube which can result in mouth lacerations. Supplement may cause irritation to eyes and skin.

Warning(s): Keep out of reach of children. For livestock use only.

Presentation: 300 mL (10 oz) tube.

Compendium Code No.: 10900120

PHOS P 200 ℞

Phoenix Pharmaceutical **Phosphorus-Injectable**

Injectable Phosphorus Sterile Solution

Active Ingredient(s): Each mL contains:

Sodium salt of 4-dimethylamino-2-methy-phenyl phosphinic acid .... 200 mg
Propylene glycol .... 100 mg
Phenylethanol .... 6.0 mg
Sodium sulfite .... 2.0 mg
Water for Injection .... q.s.

pH adjusted with sodium carbonate.

Indications: For parenteral use as a supplemental source of nutritional phosphorus while the ration is being corrected in areas where feeding rations are inadequate to supply all phosphorus needs for cattle.

Dosage and Administration: Injectable phosphorus may be administered by intravenous or deep intramuscular injection. Divide high intramuscular dosages between two injection sites. Dosage

P

range is 1 mL per 50 to 100 lbs of body weight. Dose range in cattle is 10 to 20 mL. Two injections are sufficient if the ration deficiency is immediately corrected.
Precaution(s): Store at temperatures between 2°-30°C (36°-86°F).
Caution(s): Federal law restricts this drug to use by or on the order of a licensed veterinarian.
For animal use only.
Warning(s): Keep out of reach of children.
Presentation: 100 mL (NDC 57319-356-05).
Compendium Code No.: 12560671 1099

PHOSPHAID INJECTION ℞

Vedco **Phosphorus-Injectable**
Active Ingredient(s): Each mL of injectable phosphorus solution contains:
Sodium salt of 4-dimethylamino-2-methyl-phenyl phosphinic acid . . . 200 mg
Propylene Glycol . . . 100 mg
Phenylethanol . . . 6.0 mg
Sodium sulfite . . . 2.0 mg
Water for injection . . . qs
pH adjusted with sodium carbonate.
Indications: For parenteral use as a supplemental source of nutritional phosphorus while the ration is being corrected in areas where feeding rations are inadequately to supply all phosphorus needs for cattle.
Dosage and Administration: Injectable phosphorus may be administered by intravenous or deep intramuscular injection. Divide high intramuscular dosages between two injection sites. Dosage range is 1 mL per 50 to 100 lbs of body weight. Dose range in cattle is 10 to 20 mL. Two injections are sufficient if the ration deficiency is corrected immediately.
Precaution(s): Store at temperatures between 2-30°C (36-86°F).
Caution(s): Federal law restricts this drug to use by or on the order of a licensed veterinarian.
Warning(s): For animal use only. Keep out of reach of children.
Presentation: 100 mL.
Compendium Code No.: 10941680

PHYSIOLOGICAL SALINE SOLUTION ℞

Butler **Saline Solution**
Active Ingredient(s): Each 100 mL of sterile aqueous solution contains:
Sodium chloride . . . 0.9 g
Milliequivalents per liter:
Cations:
Sodium . . . 154 mEq/L
Anions:
Chloride . . . 154 mEq/L
Total osmolarity is 308 mOsm/L.
Indications: For use in replacement therapy of sodium chloride and water which may become depleted in many diseases. Because the solution is isotonic with body fluids, it may also be used as a solvent or diluent for antibiotics and other pharmaceuticals and biologicals, and for washing mucous membranes and other tissue surfaces.
Dosage and Administration: Warm the solution to body temperature and administer slowly by intravenous or subcutaneous injection. The amount and rate of administration must be judged by the veterinarian in relation to the condition being treated and the clinical response of the animal, being careful to avoid overhydration. When used as a solvent or diluent for pharmaceuticals and biologicals, follow the manufacturer's directions.
Precaution(s): Store at a controlled room temperature between 15° and 30°C (59°-86°F).
Caution(s): Federal law restricts this drug to use by or on the order of a licensed veterinarian.
The product does not contain preservatives. Use the entire contents when first opened. Discard any unused solution. For veterinary use only. Keep out of the reach of children.
Presentation: 250 mL, 500 mL and 1,000 mL containers.
Compendium Code No.: 10821460

PIC-M-UP™

AgriPharm **Large Animal Dietary Supplement**
Nutritional Concentrate
Guaranteed Analysis:
Crude Protein, not less than . . . 9.0%
Crude Fat, not less than . . . 0.25%
Crude Fiber, not more than . . . 1.0%
Crude Ash, not more than . . . 4.0%
Ingredients:
Nutrients: Dextrose, dried skimmed milk, dried whey, enzymatic hydrolysates of yeast, sodium caseinate, soy protein, glycine, dl-methionine and corn starch.
Vitamins: Vitamin A (as acetate and palmitate), vitamin D_9, vitamin E, riboflavin (vitamin B_2), d-pantothenic acid (vitamin B_9), niacin (vitamin B_9), menadione dimethylpyrimidinolbisulphite (source of vitamin K), folic acid, thiamine mononitrate (vitamin B_1), d-biotin, pyridoxine hydrochloride (vitamin B_6), cyanocobalamin (vitamin B_{12}).
Electrolytes: Sodium chloride, potassium chloride, sodium bicarbonate and potassium phosphate.
Trace Minerals: Prozeinates of zinc, cobalt, manganese, iron, and copper.
Indications: PIC-M-UP™ is a source of amino acids, energy, vitamins and electrolytes. It is designed for oral use in cattle and calves.
Directions: Give 1 pound per 500-1000 pounds body weight. Suspend product in at least 2 quarts of lukewarm water and administer through a stomach tube or as a drench. Repeat as indicated. Consult your veterinarian concerning correct drenching procedure. Prepare fresh solution daily.
Presentation: 20 pounds.
Compendium Code No.: 14570830

PIG-95

Skylabs **Large Animal Dietary Supplement**
Active Ingredient(s):
Iron (Fe) . . . 1.0% (avg.)
Glycine . . . 11.5% (avg.)
Salt (NaCl) . . . 1.5% (avg.)
Potassium (K) . . . 1.2% (avg.)
Citric Acid . . . 1.7% (avg.)
Dextrose . . . 72.9% (avg.)
Vitamin A . . . 4,166.56 U.S.P. units (142.5 g) (act.)
Vitamin D_3 . . . 16250 IC units (act.)
Vitamin E . . . 8.3 I.U. (act.)
Vitamin K . . . 16.25 mg (act.)
Vitamin B_{12} . . . 0.0325 mg (act.)
Riboflavin . . . 16.25 mg (act.)
Ingredients: Dextrose, glycine, citric acid, potassium chloride, ascorbic acid, sodium chloride, ferrous sulfate, vitamin A acetate, d-activated animal sterol, dl-alpha-tocopherol acetate, vitamin B_{12} supplement, menadione sodium bisulfite complex, riboflavin, artificial flavors and colors.
Indications: A water soluble iron, electrolyte, and vitamin supplement designed to complement sows' and gilts' milk.
Dosage and Administration: Add one (1) packet (142.5 g) to 7.75 L of drinking water and use free choice from birth to 21 days of age, as a source of drinking water for piglets.
Presentation: 142.5 g.
Compendium Code No.: 10920011

PIGEON POX VACCINE

ASL **Vaccine**
Pigeon Pox Vaccine, Live Virus
U.S. Vet. Lic. No.: 226
Description: PIGEON POX VACCINE is prepared from a strain of Pigeon Pox Virus that has the ability to give good takes and immunity in chickens four weeks of age or older when applied by the wing-web method. The vial of dried virus material contains stabilized Pigeon Pox Virus blended and ready for use according to the following directions.
Gentamicin is added as a bacteriostatic agent.
Indications: This vaccine is recommended for the vaccination of healthy broilers and roasters at four weeks of age against Fowl Pox. Chickens that are kept for laying purposes should be vaccinated with Fowl Pox Vaccine before they come into production.
Dosage and Administration: Preparation of the Vaccine: Do not open and mix the vaccine until ready to begin vaccination. Use the vaccine immediately after mixing.

1. Tear off the aluminum seal from the vial containing the dried vaccine.
2. Lift off the rubber stopper.
3. Remove the aluminum seal from the vial of diluent.
4. Pour a small amount of diluent into the vial of dried vaccine.
5. Put back the rubber stopper and shake.
6. Pour the partly dissolved vaccine into the bottle containing the rest of the diluent.
7. Replace the rubber stopper and shake vigorously until all of the material is dissolved.

The vaccine is now ready for use by the following method. For the best results, be sure to follow the directions carefully.
Wing-Web Application:

1. Rehydrate the vaccine as directed above. Do not break off any of the needles on the applicator.
2. Hold the chicken and spread the underside of one wing outward.
3. Dip the applicator into the vaccine bottle, wetting both needles.
4. Pierce the web of the exposed wing with the charged applicator.
5. Redip the applicator in the vaccine vial and proceed to the next chicken.
6. Avoid hitting blood vessels, bones and the wing muscle.
7. Be careful not to touch any part of the chicken with the vaccine except the area to be inoculated.
8. Examine and record takes within 7 to 10 days following vaccination. A normal take shows a slight swelling and scab formation at the site of vaccination. Takes generally disappear in 2 weeks following vaccination.

Contraindication(s): Chickens to be vaccinated should be free of all diseases, including the latent form of chronic respiratory disease (CRD), clinical coccidiosis, blackhead, parasite infestations, etc. and maintained under good environmental conditions.
Precaution(s): Store vaccine in refrigerator under 45°F (7—C). Use entire contents of each vial when first opened. Burn containers and all unused contents.
Caution(s): Consult your poultry pathologist for further recommendations based on conditions existing in a designated area at any given time.
Chickens should not be placed on contaminated premises. Exposure should be avoided immediately following vaccination, because it takes up to 10 days to develop resistance.
All susceptible chickens on the same premises should be vaccinated at the same time. If this is not possible, then strict isolation and separate caretakers should be employed for non-vaccinated units. Efforts should be taken to reduce stress conditions at the time the vaccine is administered.
Notice: All American Scientific Laboratories, Inc. vaccines released for sale meet the requirements of the licensing authority (U.S. Department of Agriculture) in regard to safety, purity, potency and the capacity to immunize normal, susceptible chickens.
The capacity of the vaccine to produce satisfactory results depends on many factors, including, but not limited to, conditions of storage and handling by the user, administration of the vaccine, health and responsiveness of individual animals and the degree of field exposure. Therefore, the directions for use should be followed carefully.
The use of this vaccine is subject to applicable state and federal laws and regulations.
Warning(s): Do not vaccinate within 21 days before slaughter.
Discussion: Vaccination Programs: Many factors must be considered in determining the proper vaccination program for a particular farm or poultry operation. To be fully effective, the vaccine must be administered to healthy receptive chickens held in a proper environment under good management. In addition, the response may be modified by the age of the chickens and their immune status. Seldom does one vaccination under field conditions produce complete protection for all individuals in a given flock. The amount of protection required will vary with the type of operation and the degree of exposure that a flock is likely to encounter. For these reasons, a program of periodic revaccination may be required.
Presentation: Wing-web use: 10 x 1,000 dose vials (NDC 0138-5111-01).
Compendium Code No.: 11020271 0077R4

PIGEON POX VACCINE (Chickens and Turkeys)

L.A.H.I. (New Jersey) **Vaccine**
Pigeon Pox Vaccine, Live Virus
U.S. Vet. Lic. No.: 196
Active Ingredient(s): This product is a live virus vaccine of chicken embryo origin for the prevention of fowl pox in poults as well as growing birds.
Contains neomycin as a preservative.
This vaccine was carefully produced and passed all tests in accordance with the U.S. Government requirements.

Indications: This product is used for initial vaccination and revaccination of chickens for the prevention of fowl pox. This product can be used for chickens and turkeys in production.

Vaccination is recommended in six-week-old or older chickens by the wing-web method.

Turkeys at six weeks of age, or older, are vaccinated by the thigh method.

Dosage and Administration: Preparation of Vaccine: The active agent of the vaccine is supplied in a dried form in the bottle labeled "Vaccine". Open the bottle by removing the aluminum tear seal and rubber stopper. Open the diluent and pour a small quantity of diluent into the bottle of vaccine, replace the stopper and shake well. Pour the mixture back into the bottle containing the remainder of the diluent and shake mixture vigorously. Do not open or mix the vaccine until ready to use.

Method of Vaccination: In chickens, vaccination is accomplished by dipping a double needle or a single needle in the mixed vaccine and piercing the "web of the wing" from the underside. Do not apply through feathers, muscle or bone. The applicator must be redipped between each application.

In turkeys, vaccination is accomplished by applying the vaccine in the thigh. For this purpose, a few feathers are removed from the inner side of the thigh. The vaccine is brushed into the resulting follicles. The brush must be redipped after each application.

Birds from the flock should be examined for evidence of a "take" to insure that the vaccine was applied properly.

The evidence of a successful vaccination in chickens will appear at the point of vaccination in from 7 to 10 days after vaccination. Brownish, black scabs will be found on both the under and upper surfaces of the web of the wing through which the needle vaccinator was thrust on the feather follicles where vaccine was applied in the turkeys.

Contraindication(s): Vaccinate only healthy chickens and turkeys.

Precaution(s): Keep vaccine in the dark between 2-7°C (35-45°F).

Use entire contents when first opened. Burn this container and all unused contents.

Caution(s): When administered to susceptible birds, a mild form of the disease results which stimulates immunity.

No vaccine confers immediate protection against Fowl Pox. While immunity begins to develop immediately, it takes 2 to 3 weeks for birds to establish maximum immunity to Fowl Pox following vaccination, during which time they should not be placed in contaminated premises nor otherwise exposed to Fowl Pox.

All susceptible birds on any farm should be vaccinated at the same time. If this is not possible, individual lots may be vaccinated if strict isolation and separate caretakers are provided for the vaccinated and unvaccinated lots of birds.

It is imperative that the user of this product comply with the indications for use, contraindication, cautions and methods of vaccination stated on the direction sheet packed with the product. The vaccine must be prepared and administered as directed to obtain best results.

Warning(s): Do not vaccinate within 21 days before slaughter.

Care should be taken to avoid contaminating your hands, eyes and clothing with the vaccine.

For veterinary use only.

Presentation: 500 and 1,000 doses.

Compendium Code No.: 10080352

PILIGUARD® E. COLI-1

Schering-Plough **Bacterin**

Escherichia coli Bacterin, Bovine Isolate

U.S. Vet. Lic. No.: 165A

Active Ingredient(s): *Escherichia coli* bacterin, bovine isolate.

Preservatives: Formaldehyde and gentamicin.

Indications: For use in healthy pregnant heifers and cows to aid in the control of neonatal calf diarrhea caused by enterotoxigenic *E. coli* organisms.

Dosage and Administration: Shake well. Inject 2 mL intramuscularly in the neck three (3) weeks to six (6) months prior to calving.

Precaution(s): Store at 2-7°C (35-45°F). Do not freeze. Use entire contents when first opened.

Caution(s): For deep intramuscular injection only. Subcutaneous use may lead to development of granulomas which may persist for several weeks. Transient local reactions may occur at the injection site. If an allergic response occurs, administer epinephrine or its equivalent.

Warning(s): Do not vaccinate within 60 days before slaughter.

Use extreme caution with any oil emulsion vaccine to avoid injecting a finger or hand. Accidental injection can cause serious local reaction. Contact a physician immediately if accidental injection occurs.

Presentation: 20 mL (10 dose) and 100 mL (50 dose) vials.

Compendium Code No.: 10471510

PILIGUARD® PINKEYE-1

Durvet **Bacterin**

Moraxella Bovis Bacterin-Trivalent

U.S. Vet. Lic. No.: 165A

Contents: This product contains chemically-inactivated cultures of *Moraxella bovis* isolates referred to by Schering-Plough as Strains Epp 63, Fla 64 and SAH 38 in an oil emulsion adjuvant.

Preservative: Gentamicin.

Indications: For use in healthy cattle to aid in the prevention of pinkeye associated with infection by *Moraxella bovis* strains expressing pili similar to those expressed by isolates referred to by Schering-Plough as Strains Epp 63, Fla 64 and SAH 38.

Dosage and Administration: Shake well before use. The vaccine may be warmed to room temperature prior to injection. Inject 2 mL subcutaneously or intramuscularly into the neck 3 to 6 weeks prior to onset of pinkeye season. Annual revaccination is recommended.

Precaution(s): Store at 2-7°C (35-45°F), do not freeze. Use entire contents when first opened.

Caution(s): For veterinary use only. Use may occasionally lead to development of granulomas which may persist for several weeks. Transient local reaction may occur at the injection site. If anaphylaxis occurs administer epinephrine.

Extreme caution should be used when injecting any oil emulsion vaccine to avoid injecting your own finger or hand. Accidental injection can cause serious local reaction. Contact a physician immediately if accidental injection occurs.

Warning(s): Do not vaccinate within 60 days prior to slaughter.

Presentation: 10 dose (20 mL) (NDC 0061-1151-09) and 50 dose (100 mL) (NDC 0061-1151-10) vials.

PILIGUARD® is a registered trademark of Schering-Plough Animal Health

Manufactured by: Schering-Plough Animal Health Corporation, Omaha, Nebraska 68103.

Compendium Code No.: 10841851 9/95

PILIGUARD® PINKEYE-1

Schering-Plough **Bacterin**

Moraxella bovis Bacterin

U.S. Vet. Lic. No.: 165A

Active Ingredient(s): *Moraxella bovis* bacterin.

Preservatives: Formaldehyde and gentamicin.

Indications: PILIGUARD® Pinkeye-1 is recommended for use in healthy cattle to aid in the control and prevention of pinkeye caused by *Moraxella bovis*.

Dosage and Administration: Inject 2.0 mL intramuscularly three (3) to six (6) weeks prior to the onset of the pinkeye season. An annual booster dose is recommended.

Precaution(s): Store at 2-7°C (35-45°F). Do not freeze. Shake well before each use. Use the entire contents when first opened.

Caution(s): Transient local reactions may occur at the injection site. If an allergic response occurs, administer epinephrine or its equivalent.

Warning(s): Do not vaccinate within 60 days before slaughter.

Extreme caution should be used when injecting any oil emulsion vaccine to avoid injecting a finger or hand. Accidental injection can cause a serious local reaction. Contact a physician immediately if accidental injection occurs.

Presentation: 10 doses (20 mL) and 50 doses (100 mL).

Compendium Code No.: 10471531

PILIGUARD® PINKEYE + 7

Schering-Plough **Bacterin-Toxoid**

Clostridium Chauvoei-Septicum-Novyi-Sordellii-Perfringens Types C & D-Moraxella Bovis Bacterin-Toxoid

U.S. Vet. Lic. No.: 165A

Contents: This product contains the antigens listed above.

Preservative: Gentamicin.

Indications: PILIGUARD® Pinkeye + 7 is recommended for the vaccination of healthy susceptible cattle as an aid in the control of pinkeye caused by *Moraxella bovis* strains expressing pili similar to those expressed by isolates referred to by Schering-Plough as strains EPP 63, FLA 64 and SAH 38, and against diseases caused by *Clostridium chauvoei, C. septicum, C. novyi* Type B, *C. sordellii, C. perfringens* Types C and D. Immunity is also provided against the beta and epsilon toxins of an additional clostridial organism, *C. perfringens* Type B. This immunity is derived from the combination of the Type C (beta) and Type D (epsilon) fractions.

Dosage and Administration: Using aseptic technique, inject cattle subcutaneously with 5 mL. Repeat in 3-4 weeks and annually prior to periods of extreme risk or parturition. For C. novyi, revaccinate every 5-6 months. Animals vaccinated under 3 months of age should be revaccinated at weaning or at 4-6 months of age.

Precaution(s): Store at 2° to 7°C (35° to 45°F). Do not freeze. Shake well before use. Use the entire contents when first opened.

Caution(s): For veterinary use only.

Transient local reactions may occur at the injection site. The incidence and severity of reactions may be higher in calves under 3 months of age. If allergic response occurs, administer epinephrine.

Warning(s): Do not vaccinate within 21 days of slaughter.

Presentation: 10 doses (50 mL) (NDC-0061-0865-05) and 50 doses (250 mL).

Compendium Code No.: 10471521 P13800-11

PINKEYE-3

Aspen **Bacterin**

Moraxella bovis Bacterin

U.S. Vet. Lic. No.: 165A

Contents: Contains chemically inactivated cultures of *Moraxella bovis*, strains Epp 63, Fla 64, and SAH 38 in an oil emulsion adjuvant.

Indications: Recommended for use in healthy cattle to aid in the control and prevention of pinkeye caused by *Moraxella bovis*.

Dosage and Administration: Shake well. Inject 2 mL intramuscularly or subcutaneously 3 to 6 weeks prior to the onset of pinkeye season. An annual booster is recommended.

No minimum vaccination age. Vaccinate as early as one week.

Precaution(s): Refrigerate at 35°-45°F.

Warning(s): Do not vaccinate within 21 days before slaughter.

Discussion: True 1-shot season-long pinkeye protection.

No need to collect and work cattle twice.

Exclusive 3-strain protection against *Moraxella bovis* (EPP 63, FLA 64 and SAH 38).

Better protection as these 3 strains were selected as their pili were the most cross-reactive with the pili of the 60 field isolates studied.

Presentation: 10 dose (20 mL) vial, and 50 dose (100 mL) vial.

Compendium Code No.: 14750630

PINKEYE SHIELD™ XT4

Novartis Animal Vaccines **Bacterin**

Moraxella Bovis Bacterin

U.S. Vet. Lic. No.: 303

Composition: This bacterin contains inactivated cultures of *Moraxella bovis* adjuvanted with Xtend III®. Contains penicillin, streptomycin, and thimerosal as preservatives.

Indications: For use in healthy cattle as an aid in the prevention and control of ocular lesions caused by *Moraxella bovis*.

Dosage and Administration: Shake well before using. Administer 2 mL intramuscularly. Revaccinate annually.

Precaution(s): Store in the dark at 35°-45°F (2°-7°C). Do not freeze. Use entire contents when first opened.

Caution(s): Transient swelling may occur at the site of injection. Anaphylactic reactions may occur following the use of this biological. Symptomatic treatment: Epinephrine.

For veterinary use only.

Warning(s): Do not vaccinate within 60 days prior to slaughter.

Discussion: Infectious bovine keratoconjunctivitis (pinkeye, IBK) is an economically important cattle disease with worldwide distribution. One of its causes is a bacteria, *Moraxella bovis*, that is easily transmitted from animal to animal by flies that feed on eye secretions of infected animals. Clinical signs of pinkeye include sensitivity to light, lacrimation, conjunctivitis, corneal opacity, and corneal ulcers, which may affect one or both eyes. Most affected animals will recover within 3-4 weeks, but some animals will be permanently blinded. Pinkeye by itself is not a fatal disease, but it may indirectly cause death if an affected animal is blinded to the extent that it is unable to find food or water. Pinkeye affects 10 million calves annually. A study showed a 17 lb loss when one eye was affected and up to a 65 lb loss when both eyes were involved.[4] This study suggests that Q Pili are specific and necessary for colonization of bovine corneal epithelium. I Pili enable maintenance of an established infection.[5]

Pinkeye is a seasonal disease, with most cases being seen in late spring, summer, and early fall. This coincides with the time of year having the most sunlight exposure. The ultraviolet light in sunlight acts on the *M bovis* organisms to make them more virulent.

All ages of cattle can be affected by pinkeye if they have not developed immunity, but the disease is most common in calves. After an animal is infected it develops fairly solid immunity. Recovered animals may carry and shed the bacteria in their lacrimal secretions for more than one year, which explains how the disease can be carried over in a herd from year to year. First symptoms of the disease are lacrimation or tearing and light sensitivity which progress to corneal cloudiness and corneal ulcers. In severe cases the eyeball may rupture or abscess causing complete and irreversible blindness.

Other diseases that can cause conjunctivitis, such as Infectious Bovine Rhinotracheitis (IBR) other bacteria and some strains of *Mycoplasma,* can be confused with pinkeye. These agents may coinfect the animal along with *Moraxella bovis* making the disease more difficult to control.

If affected animals are detected early and treated aggressively, they will usually recover with minimal or no permanent eye damage, however, treatment is expensive and time-consuming. Animals that have had pinkeye often lag behind the rest of the herd in performance. For this reason Novartis Animal Vaccines, Inc. has developed PINKEYE SHIELD™ XT4, a bacterin that is administered to animals to aid in the prevention of the disease. Animals should receive a 2 mL intramuscular dose, which produces immunity against the devastating effects of pinkeye caused by *Moraxella bovis.*

Trial Data: PINKEYE SHIELD™ XT4 Host Animal Study - Average Daily Score:

	Vaccinates (N=18)	Controls (N=18)
Average per Animal	1.52	4.16
Average per Eye	0.76	2.08

p=0.005 Very significant.

Animals were observed daily for a total of 7 days. Eye lesions were graded on a scale of 0-6, with 0 being normal and 6 being severe lesions with blindness. PINKEYE SHIELD™ XT4 vaccinates showed very significant levels of protection following challenge with virulent *Moraxella bovis* organisms.

References: Available upon request.

Presentation: Available in 10 dose (20 mL) and 50 dose (100 mL) bottles.

Compendium Code No.: 11140293

PINNACLE™ I.N.

Fort Dodge **Vaccine**

Streptococcus Equi Vaccine, Live Culture

U.S. Vet. Lic. No.: 112

Contents: This product contains the antigens listed above.

Indications: For the vaccination of healthy horses as an aid in the prevention of disease caused by *Streptococcus equi.*

Dosage and Administration: Aseptically rehydrate with the entire contents of the accompanying sterile diluent. Instill the entire rehydrated vaccine into one nostril using a syringe with applicator tip. Administer a second dose 2 to 3 weeks later. Annual revaccination is recommended.

InfoVax-ID® System: The InfoVax-ID® System provides a simple and effective method of recording pertinent information on the vaccines administered to animals in a veterinary practice.

For vaccines requiring reconstitution, remove label from both vials and affix both labels to the animal's medical chart.

Using the InfoVax-ID® System:

1. Grasp the lower right hand corner of the tab at the arrow marked "Peel Here" between your thumb and forefinger.
2. Pull steadily at a slight upward angle until the top portion of the label is separated from the vial.
3. Place the label on the animal's medical chart. Press down on the label to ensure adhesion.

Precaution(s): Store in the dark at 2° to 7°C (35° to 45°F). Avoid freezing. Shake well after rehydration. Use entire contents when first opened. Burn container and all unused contents.

Caution(s): In the absence of a veterinarian-client-patient relationship, Federal law prohibits the relabeling, repackaging, resale, or redistribution of the individual contents of this package. (9 CFR 112.6)

This product contains live bacteria and is designed for intranasal use only. Disinfect hands and equipment after use. Contamination of the user's hands or equipment with reconstituted vaccine could lead to infections if proper disinfection practices are not followed prior to procedures that require asepsis. Injection equipment used to reconstitute or administer PINNACLE™ I.N. should not be reused, and should be disposed of appropriately. In case of anaphylactoid reaction, administer epinephrine. After administration a small number of horses may experience non-contagious transitory upper respiratory signs including nasal discharge and lymphadenectasis. Purpura hemorrhagica may be seen in hypersensitive individuals following exposure to streptococcal proteins.

Do not administer by any route other than intranasal.

Warning(s): Do not vaccinate within 30 days before slaughter.

Presentation: 10 doses (10 x 2.5 mL vials of vaccine plus 10 x 2.5 mL vials of diluent), featuring the InfoVax-ID® System.

U.S. Patent No. 5,183,659
U.S. Patent Pending
U.S. Pat. No. 5,704,648 (InfoVax-ID® System)

Compendium Code No.: 10031451 1393E

PIPA-TABS ℞

Vet-A-Mix **Parasiticide-Oral**

Active Ingredient(s): Each tablet contains either:

Piperazine base (equivalent to 94.4 mg piperazine dihydrochloride) .... 50 mg
Piperazine base (equivalent to 472 mg piperazine dihydrochloride) .... 250 mg

Indications: For the treatment and control of ascarids; *Toxocara canis* in dogs and *Toxascaris leonina* in cats.

Dosage and Administration: The recommended piperazine dosage for dogs and cats is 25 mg piperazine base per pound of body weight.

PIPA-TABS, 50 mg: The initial dose is one (1) tablet per 2 lbs. of body weight.

PIPA-TABS, 250 mg: The initial dose is one (1) tablet per 10 lbs. of body weight.

A second dose should be administered after 10 days.

In heavily infested animals, a third dose should be given after another 10-day rest period. In thin and undernourished animals, the dosage should be reduced to one-third (8 to 10 mg per pound of body weight) and given over a three day period.

Dogs and cats may be wormed at six (6) to eight (8) weeks of age.

Precaution(s): Although piperazine is a drug with a high degree of safety, an occasional animal may show nausea, vomiting or muscular tremors. Such side effects are usually associated with overdosage, therefore, the recommended dosage should be followed carefully. Animals with known kidney pathology should be treated only by a veterinarian.

Caution(s): Federal law restricts this drug to use by or on the order of a licensed veterinarian.

Consult a veterinarian before using in severely debilitated animals.

Keep out of the reach of children.

Presentation: Bottles of 500 tablets.

Compendium Code No.: 10500230

PIPERAZINE-17 MEDICATED

Durvet **Parasiticide-Oral**

Active Ingredient(s): Each 100 cc contains 17 grams of Piperazine base. Color, flavoring, and preservative added.

Indications: A wormer for use in drinking water for the control of large roundworms *(Toxocara canis and Toxascaris leonina)* in dogs and cats, and large roundworms or Ascarids *(Parascaris equorum),* strongyles *(Strongylus vulgaris)* and small strongyles and pinworms *(Oxyuris equi)* in horses.

Directions:

Dogs and Cats - Give 1 mL (15 drops) PIPERAZINE-17 for each 6 pounds of body weight. Dose the dog and cat individually or give in milk, water or food. Repeat treatment in 30 days or when necessary.

Horses: (non-food producing) Give 1 fluid ounce PIPERAZINE-17 for each 100 pounds of body weight. Give the full dose with a dose syringe. If feed administration is preferred, give bran mash with a small amount of PIPERAZINE-17 for 2 or 3 feedings, then give full dose in bran mash. Repeat treatment in 30 days or when necessary.

Precaution(s): Store out of direct sunlight and above freezing temperatures.

Caution(s): Although Piperazine is a drug with a wide margin of safety, occasionally an animal may show nausea, vomiting, or muscular tremors. Such side effects are usually associated with over-dosage. Therefore, recommended dosage should be followed carefully. Animals with known kidney pathology should be treated only by a veterinarian.

Consult your veterinarian for assistance in the diagnosis, treatment and control of parasitism.

For oral animal use only.

For veterinary use only.

Warning(s): Keep out of reach of children.

Not for human consumption.

Presentation: 8 fl oz (237 mL) (NDC 30798-254-28), 16 fl oz (1 pt) (473 mL) (NDC 30798-254-31), and 1 gallon (3.785 L) (NDC 30798-254-35).

Compendium Code No.: 10842040 Rev. 11-00/5-00

PIPOVAX®

Schering-Plough **Vaccine**

Pigeon Pox Vaccine, Live Virus

U.S. Vet. Lic. No.: 165A

Active Ingredient(s): PIPOVAX® is a live virus vaccine of chicken embryo origin containing a pigeon pox virus selected for its mild characteristics as well as its ability to stimulate strong protection against fowl pox in chickens. The vaccine contains gentamicin as a preservative.

Indications: For the vaccination of healthy chickens six weeks of age or older, as an aid in preventing fowl pox through vaccination by the wing-web method.

Dosage and Administration:

When to Vaccinate: Six (6) weeks of age or older.

Vaccination Program: The development of a durable, strong protection depends upon the use of an effective vaccination program as well as many circumstances such as administration techniques, environment and flock health at the time of vaccination. Also, the immune response to one (1) vaccination under field conditions is seldom complete for all animals within a given flock. Even when vaccination is successful, the protection stimulated in individual animals against different diseases may not be life-long. Therefore, under certain circumstances revaccination may be necessary.

Preparation of the Vaccine:

1. Do not open and mix the vaccine until ready for use.
2. Mix only one (1) vial at a time and use the entire contents within two (2) hours.
3. Remove the tear-off aluminum seal and stopper from the vial containing the dried vaccine.
4. Remove the tear-off aluminum seal and stopper from the bottle containing the diluent.
5. Hold the diluent bottle firmly in an upright position and insert the vaccine vial on the adapter of the diluent bottle. The neck of the vaccine vial should snap into position and should be seated securely on the adapter on the diluent bottle.
6. Invert the two (2) containers so that the vaccine vial is on the bottom and allow the diluent to flow into the vaccine vial. If the diluent does not flow freely, squeeze the bottle gently and the diluent will flow into the vaccine vial. The vaccine vial should be completely filled with diluent to prevent excess foaming.
7. Hold the joined containers by the ends and shake vigorously until the vaccine plug is completely dissolved.
8. Return the joined containers to their original position (diluent bottle on the bottom). Allow the vaccine to flow into the diluent bottle. If the vaccine does not flow into the diluent bottle, tap or squeeze the diluent bottle gently and release to draw the vaccine into the diluent bottle. Be sure that all of the product is removed from the vaccine vial.
9. Remove the vaccine vial and adapter from the neck of the diluent bottle.
10. The vaccine is now ready for use.

How to Vaccinate: Vaccination is accomplished by dipping the needle applicator into the mixed vaccine and piercing the webbed portion of the underside of the wing. Avoid piercing through feathers which may wipe off the vaccine, and avoid hitting the wing muscle or bone to minimize reaction. The applicator is designed to pick up the proper amount of vaccine on the needle, which is deposited in the tissues when the wing is pierced. Redip the applicator in the vaccine before each application. Excess vaccine adhering to the applicator should be removed by touching the applicator to the side of the vaccine vial.

Examine for Takes: Examine the birds for takes six (6) to eight (8) days following vaccination. A positive take, showing that the vaccination was successful, is indicated by swelling of the skin or scab formation at the point of inoculation. The absence of takes may mean that birds were immune before vaccination or that improper vaccination methods were used. Protection will normally develop within about 10 to 14 days after vaccination. Swelling and scabs will disappear two (2) to three (3) weeks following vaccination.

Records: Keep a record of the vaccine type, quantity, serial number, expiration date, and place of purchase; the date and time of vaccination; the number, age, breed, and location of the birds; the names of operators performing the vaccination; and any observed reactions.

Precaution(s): Store at 35° to 45° F (2° to 7°C).

Caution(s): For veterinary use only.

1. Vaccinate healthy birds only. Although disease may not be evident, coccidiosis, chronic respiratory disease, mycoplasma infection, lymphoid leukosis, infectious bursal disease, Marek's disease, or other disease conditions may cause serious complications or reduce protection.
2. All birds within a house should be vaccinated on the same day. Isolate other susceptible birds on the premises from the birds being vaccinated.
3. In outbreak situations, vaccinate healthy birds first, progressing toward outbreak areas in order to vaccinate diseased birds last.
4. Do not spill or spatter the vaccine. Use the entire contents of the vial when first opened. Burn the empty bottles, caps, and all unused vaccine and accessories.
5. Do not dilute the vaccine or otherwise stretch the dosage.
6. Wash hands thoroughly after using the vaccine.

Warning(s): Do not vaccinate within 21 days before slaughter.

Presentation: Supplied in 10 x 1,000 dose units (combo pak) with diluent and applicator.

Compendium Code No.: 10471540

PIRSUE® STERILE SOLUTION ℞

Pharmacia & Upjohn **Mastitis Therapy**

brand of pirlimycin hydrochloride

NADA No.: 141-036

Active Ingredient(s): Each 10 mL Plastet® Disposable Syringe contains:

Pirlimycin free base equivalents .... 50 mg
Aqueous vehicle .... q.s.

Indications: PIRSUE® Sterile Solution (pirlimycin hydrochloride) is indicated for the treatment of clinical and subclinical mastitis in lactating dairy cattle. PIRSUE® Sterile Solution has been proven effective only against *Staphylococcus* species such as *Staphylococcus aureus* and *Streptococcus* species such as *Streptococcus agalactiae*, *Streptococcus dysgalactiae* and *Streptococcus uberis*. Cows with systemic clinical signs caused by mastitis should receive other appropriate therapy under the direction of a licensed veterinarian.

Pharmacology: Description: Pirlimycin hydrochloride is a lincosaminide antibiotic.

Chemical Structure of Pirlimycin Hydrochloride:

Chemical Name of Pirlimycin Hydrochloride: Methyl(2S-Cis)-7-chloro-6,7,8-trideoxy-6[[(4-ethyl-2-piperidinyl)carbonyl]amino]-1-thio-L-threo-α-D-*galacto*-octopyranoside hydrochloride hydrate.

PIRSUE® Sterile Solution is a clear solution.

Microbiology: Pirlimycin is a lincosaminide antibiotic which has activity against gram-positive mastitis pathogens. Pirlimycin functions by binding to the 50s ribosomal subunit of bacterial ribonucleic acid (RNA) which interferes with protein synthesis within the bacteria. Pirlimycin has demonstrated *in vitro* and clinical activity against staphylococcal organisms such as *Staphylococcus aureus* and streptococcal organisms such as *Streptococcus agalactiae*, *Streptococcus dysgalactiae* and *Streptococcus uberis*. These organisms are associated with clinical and subclinical mastitis in lactating dairy cattle. Thornsberry et al 1993 and Watts and Salmon 1997[1,2] demonstrated that a significant percentage of all staphylococcal organisms produce β-lactamase. These percentages range from 21.6% for *Staphylococcus aureus* to 84% for *Staphylococcus epidermidis*. Thornsberry et al 1993 reported that β-lactamase activity has no bearing on the activity of pirlimycin since β-lactamase activity has no activity on lincosaminide antibiotics.

Table 1. Minimum Inhibitory Concentrations of Pirlimycin Against Staphylococcal and Streptococcal Isolates.

Organism	MIC Values (μg/mL)
Staphylococcus aureus	0.25-0.50
*Staphylococcus epidermidis**	0.5
*Staphylococcus chromogenes**	0.5
*Staphylococcus hyicus**	1.0
*Staphylococcus xylosus**	1.0
Streptococcus agalactiae	0.0625-0.125
Streptococcus dysgalactiae	≤0.0625
Streptococcus uberis	≤0.0625
*Streptococcus bovis**	0.25
*Enterococcus faecalis**	2.0

*The clinical significance of this *in vitro* data in cattle is not known.

Utilizing MIC data from the gram-positive mastitis pathogens and milk residue data from cows treated with 50 mg of pirlimycin administered twice at a 24-hour interval, MIC breakpoints were determined.[1] Organisms with MIC values less than or equal to 2 μg/mL are susceptible and those organisms greater than or equal to 4 μg/mL are resistant. A 2 microgram disk for pirlimycin was found to be optimal. Using procedures from the National Committee of Clinical Laboratory Standards, zones of inhibition for the gram-positive mastitis pathogens were determined.[3] Zone diameter interpretive standards are presented in the following table.

Antimicrobial Agent	Code	Disk Potency	Zone Diameter Interpretive Standards (mm)		Control Zone Diameter Limit (mm)		
			Resistant	Susceptible	*S. aureus*	*E. coli*	*P. aeruginosa*
Pirlimycin	PRL-2	2 μg	≤ 12 mm	≥ 13 mm	ATCC 25923 15-19	ATCC 25922 —	ATCC 27853 —

Dosage and Administration: Dosage: Infuse one (1) syringe into each infected quarter. Repeat this treatment once after a 24-hour interval.

Directions for Using the Flexi-Tube® System: The Flexi-Tube® is designed to provide the choice of either insertion of the full cannula as has traditionally been practiced, or insertion of no more than ⅛ inch of the cannula, as reported by Eberhart, R.J., et. al. 1987. Current Concepts of Bovine Mastitis, 3rd Edition, National Mastitis Council, Arlington, VA.

a. Full insertion: Remove the white end cap by pulling straight up. Gently insert the full cannula into the teat canal; carefully infuse the product.
b. Partial insertion: Remove both the white end cap and the red cannula by pushing sideways as shown. Gently insert the exposed white tip into the teat canal; carefully infuse the product.

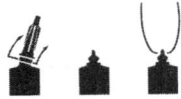

Administration:

Treatment: Wash teats thoroughly with warm water containing a suitable dairy antiseptic. Dry the teats thoroughly. Milk out the udder completely. Using an alcohol pad provided, wipe off the end of the affected teat using a separate pad for each teat. Choose the desired insertion length (full or partial) and insert tip into teat canal; push plunger to dispense entire contents, massage the quarter to distribute the solution into the milk cistern.

Reinfection: After successful treatment, reinfection may occur unless good herd management, sanitation and mechanical safety measures are practiced. Affected cows should be watched carefully to detect recurrence of infection and possible spread to other animals.

Precaution(s): Storage Conditions: Store at controlled room temperature 20° to 25°C (68° to 77°F). [see USP]. Store plastets in carton until used.

Discard empty container; do not re-use.

Caution(s): Federal (USA) law restricts this drug to use by or on the order of a licensed veterinarian.

For intramammary infusion in lactating cows only.

For use in animals only. Not for human use.

Restricted Drug — Use only as directed (California).

Warning(s): Residue Warnings

1. Milk taken from animals during treatment and for 36 hours after the last treatment must not be used for food.
2. Treated animals must not be slaughtered for 9 days following the last treatment.
3. Use of this product in a manner other than indicated under Dosage might result in violative residues.

Keep out of reach of children.

Trial Data: Efficacy: The efficacy of pirlimycin was demonstrated in a field dose response study in lactating dairy cattle with clinical mastitis. Cows with abnormal milk (clots, flakes) and with or without udder clinical signs (swelling, redness, or soreness) were enrolled. These cows were treated in the affected quarter(s). The decision to treat was based solely on the presence of clinical mastitis regardless of the mastitis pathogen isolated or the pre-treatment somatic cell count. In this study, three university investigators enrolled 486 cows from 39 herds. Cows were treated with 50, 100 or 200 mg of pirlimycin twice at a 24-hour interval. A non-treated control group was included.

In this study, an individual quarter was cured if it had normal milk, absence of udder clinical signs, and the milk was negative for any mastitis pathogen at 10 days post-treatment. If no bacteria were isolated pre-treatment, a decrease in somatic cell count was required. A cow was cured if all enrolled quarters in that cow were cured. In this study, all three treatment levels had significantly greater cow cure rates than the non-treated control. From this study, the dose of 50 mg of pirlimycin per quarter administered twice at a 24-hour interval was determined to be the effective dose for the treatment of clinical mastitis. PIRSUE® Sterile Solution administered at this dose is indicated for the treatment of clinical and subclinical mastitis in lactating dairy cattle. PIRSUE® Sterile Solution has been proven effective against *Staphylococcus* species such as *Staphylococcus aureus* (including β-lactamase producing strains) and *Streptococcus* species such as *Streptococcus agalactiae*, *Streptococcus dysgalactiae* and *Streptococcus uberis*.

Animal Safety: Two pivotal studies addressing target animal safety indicate that the formulation is safe and non-irritating to the bovine. Clinical safety observations were also made during the clinical efficacy study. No udder irritation was noted due to udder infusion with this product during these studies.

Milk Residue Depletion: The established tolerance of pirlimycin in milk is 0.40 ppm. A milk residue depletion study was conducted. Normal cows were infused with 50 mg of pirlimycin twice at a 24-hour interval into all four quarters. As a result of this study, milk taken from cows during treatment and for 36 hours following treatment must not be used for food and must be discarded.

Effect on Milk Manufacturing Starter Cultures: A study was conducted to examine the effect of varying concentrations of pirlimycin in milk on the growth of bacterial starter cultures used to produce fermented milk products. Pirlimycin did not adversely affect bacterial starter cultures used for the production of fermented milk products at concentrations found following normal label use including proper milk discard periods. Violative levels of pirlimycin (>0.40 ppm) can adversely affect the growth of bacterial starter cultures.

References: Available upon request.

Presentation: PIRSUE® Sterile Solution is available in cartons containing 1 unbroken package of 12—10 mL Plastet® Disposable Syringes with 12 individually wrapped 70% isopropyl alcohol pads (NDC 0009-7688-04) and in pails containing 12 unbroken packages of 12—10 mL Plastet® Disposable Syringes with 144 individually wrapped 70% isopropyl alcohol pads (NDC 0009-7688-05).

Compendium Code No.: 10490441 817 565 002

PLASMA CALF IgG MIDLAND QUICK TEST KIT™

Midland BioProducts **IgG Test**

Description: A qualitative test of immunity levels to determine the health and value of your calf.

Contents: Each kit contains: cassette, 0.2 mL pipette, dilution vial, and instructions.

Indications: The PLASMA CALF IgG MIDLAND QUICK TEST KIT™ is designed to detect immunoglobulin G (IgG) in newborn calves, in a rapid test format, without the use of elaborate laboratory equipment.

Test Principles: The PLASMA CALF IgG MIDLAND QUICK TEST KIT™ consists of a 4 mm strip enclosed in a plastic cassette, incorporating both complexing and detection reagents. Using the pipette provided, sample is transferred to the dilution vial and mixed.

A portion of the diluted sample is then transferred to the sample well of the cassette. If bovine IgG is greater than 10 mg/mL, it complexes with a complexing agent in the cassette. The complex then migrates through the test strip and bypasses the immobilized detection line (position "T") but reacts with the immobilized control line (position "C") causing a single red colored line to develop. However, if the bovine IgG is less than 10 mg/mL, it will not complex with complexing agent. The free complexing reagent will migrate through the test strip and react with both the immobilized "T" and "C" lines causing the development of two red lines. Excess sample will be absorbed in an upper filter.

As noted above, regardless of the concentration of the IgG sample, a line should develop at the "C" position. This has been incorporated into the cassette as a control mechanism. If no line is observed at the "C" position, then the test should be considered invalid and should be repeated with a new, unused kit. If the same results are obtained in the repeated test, contact Midland BioProducts at 1.800.370.6367.

Test Procedure:

Step 1: Sample Collection: Collection supplies are not included with the kit. Contact a veterinarian for proper collection technique.

1. Label the collection tube with calf number, date, time of collection, etc.
2. Collect approximately 2 mL of whole blood in collection tube using a collection needle and holder. Alternately, whole blood may be collected with a syringe and needle, then gently expelled into the collection tube.
3. Allow the whole blood to clot at room temperature for 30-90 minutes. Clotting may be accelerated by placing a wooden applicator stick into the collection tube with the whole blood. Optional: After clotting, centrifugation at 1,000xg for 10 minutes will aid the separation of the sample from the clot.
4. After clotting, the sample (which is the liquid portion) will be visible.
5. Sample may be stored refrigerated, in the collection tube with the clot for 4-7 days. Clots should not be frozen. If sample is drawn off the clot, it may be stored in a tightly sealed container for weeks in a refrigerator or freezer.

Step 2: Procedure

1. Obtain sample (see Sample Collection).
2. Remove the cassette from the foil pouch by tearing at the notched end.
3. Discard the foil pouch and desiccant.
4. Label or otherwise identify the cassette so that each sample can be associated with its cassette.
5. Using a clean pipette from the pouch provided with the kit, completely depress the bulb, which will allow the sample to be drawn into the pipette.
   The pipette will not be completely full.
   Quickly releasing the bulb increases the likelihood that air will be drawn into the pipette which may affect the accuracy of the test.
6. Remove the cap from the dilution vial and transfer the sample into it. Rinse the pipette by repeatedly drawing up and expressing its contents into the dilution vial.
7. Recap the dilution vial and invert several times to thoroughly mix the sample. Avoid shaking. Shaking will harm the sample and possibly affect the accuracy of the test device.
8. Once the sample is thoroughly mixed, remove the cap from the dilution vial. Using the pipette from step 6, completely depress the bulb and submerge the pipette into the dilution vial. Gently release the bulb, which will allow the diluted sample to be drawn into the pipette.
9. Express two to four drops of the diluted sample into the sample well of the cassette, making sure that it is on a level surface.
10. Allow the test to proceed for 20 minutes, then read the results. For accuracy, do not read results after 40 minutes.

Test Interpretation:

Step 3: Interpretation of Test Results

A. IgG levels less than 10 mg/mL Indicated by Two lines; One at the "T" position and One at the "C" position. Even a faint line at the "T" position indicates less than 10 mg/mL IgG.

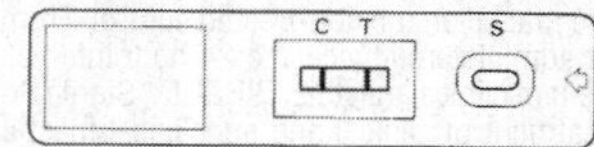

Low to marginal IgG Results

B. IgG levels equal to or greater than 10 mg/mL Indicated by One line at the "C" position.

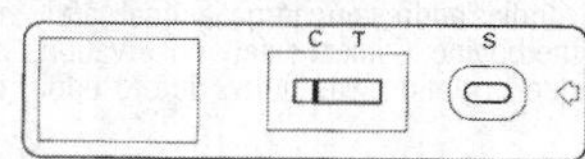

Satisfactory to High IgG Results

Storage: Room temperature.

Do not freeze the dilution vial.

Do not remove the cassette from the foil pouch until ready for use. Even though the foil pouch includes a desiccant packet, exposure to high humidity conditions should be minimized.

Caution(s): Do not use components past expiration date and do not mix components from kits with different lot numbers.

The dilution vial in this kit contains sodium azide. Sodium azide may react with lead or copper plumbing to form highly explosive metal azides. On disposal, flush with a large volume of water to prevent azide build-up. For further information, refer to the manual issued by the Centers for Disease Control.

Do not ingest desiccant.

Dispose of all kit components in an appropriate manner.

Discussion: Failure of Passive Transfer (FPT): Calves are born virtually devoid of any detectable level of immunoglobulin G (IgG). The neonatal calf's immunity to infectious agents relies on the ingestion and absorption of maternal IgG from colostrum in mother's milk. This process, termed passive transfer, is a critical determinant of calf health.[6] Failure of passive transfer (FPT) may occur as a result of inadequate suckling, poor absorption of IgG, low levels of IgG in colostrum, or environmental stress. Despite a number of studies that have shown an increased risk of morbidity and mortality in FPT calves,[1,2,3,4] its prevalence in the field remains high. In fact, it is not uncommon to find herds with 40% of calves in this classification.[5]

The calf's ability to absorb IgG is optimal at birth and progressively declines in absorptive efficiency. The highest rate of absorption occurs during the first 4 hours followed by a gradual slowing until 12 hours. From 12 to 24 hours there is a substantial decline in absorption. Estimated closure time for IgG is approximately 24 hours.[8]

A number of studies have identified the specific concentrations of IgG that indicate adequate passive transfer.[5,6,7] Serum IgG concentrations of less than 10 mg/mL are considered to show FPT, while serum IgG concentrations above 10 mg/mL are considered to have an adequate level of immunity.

The rapid identification of calves with adequate IgG levels can be used to assess management and husbandry practices. In addition, if low IgG levels are detected, intervention strategies may be developed in conjunction with your health professional to optimize calf health and farm productivity.

References: Available upon request.

Presentation: Kits are packaged and sold in the following sizes: Packages of 6, 12, and 24.

U.S. Patent 6,245,577

Compendium Code No.: 15010012 9014 rev. 4

PLASMA FOAL IgG MIDLAND QUICK TEST KIT™

Midland BioProducts **IgG Test**

Description: A qualitative test of immunity levels to determine the health and value of newborn foals.

Contents: Contents for 4 mg/mL (400 mg/dL) kit and the 8 mg/m L (800 mg/dL) kit:

Each kit contains: cassette, 0.2 mL pipette, dilution vial, and instructions.

Indications: The PLASMA FOAL IgG MIDLAND QUICK TEST KIT™ is designed to detect immunoglobulin G (IgG) concentrations from 0 to 7 day old foals, in a rapid test format without elaborate laboratory equipment.

Test Procedure:

Step 1: Sample Collection: Collection supplies are not included with the kit. Contact your veterinarian for proper collection technique.

1. Label the collection tube with foal no., date, age, etc.
2. Collect approximately 2 mL of serum in a collection tube using a collection needle and holder. Alternately, serum may be collected with a syringe and needle, then gently expelled into the collection tube.
3. After clotting, centrifugation at 1,000xg for 10 minutes will aid the separation of the sample from the clot. Optional: Allow the serum sample to clot at room temperature for 30-90 minutes. Accelerate clotting by placing a wooden applicator stick into the collection tube with the serum. After clotting, the sample (which is the liquid portion) will be visible.
4. Sample may be stored refrigerated, in the collection tube with the clot for 4-7 days. Clots should not be frozen. If sample is drawn off the clot, it may be stored in a tightly sealed container for weeks in a refrigerator or freezer.

Step 2: Procedure

1. Obtain the foal plasma sample (see "Sample Collection").
2. Next, in the foil pouch, remove the Cassette from the foil pouch by tearing at the notched end on the side of the pouch. Discard the Cassette foil pouch and the desiccant inside the pouch.
3. Label or otherwise identify the Cassette so that each foal plasma sample can be associated with its Cassette.
4. In the kit, take the dilution vial and remove the seal and septum (cap) from the dilution vial.
5. Using a clean pipette provided with the kit, completely depress the bulb, and put the pipette in the foal plasma sample. Release the bulb, which will allow the sample to be drawn into the pipette. Note: The pipette will not be completely full. Quickly releasing the bulb increases the likelihood that air will be drawn into the pipette which may effect the accuracy of the test.
6. Transfer the foal plasma sample in the pipette to the dilution vial. Rinse the pipette by repeatedly drawing up and expressing its contents back into the dilution vial.
7. Put the septum (cap) on the dilution vial and invert several times to thoroughly mix the sample. Avoid shaking.
8. Once the sample is thoroughly mixed, remove the septum from the dilution vial. Using the pipette from step 5 and 6, completely depress the bulb and submerge the pipette into the diluted sample in the dilution vial. Gently release the bulb, which will allow the diluted sample to be drawn into the pipette.
9. Express 2 to 4 drops of the diluted sample into the sample well of the Cassette (marked "S"), making sure that the Cassette is on a level surface. Allow the test to proceed for 20 minutes, then read the results. For accuracy, do not read the results before 20 minutes or after 40 minutes.

Test Interpretation:

Step 3: Interpretation of Test Results

Example of PLASMA FOAL IgG MIDLAND QUICK TEST KIT™ cassette results (Control = "C", Test = "T" and Sample = "S"):

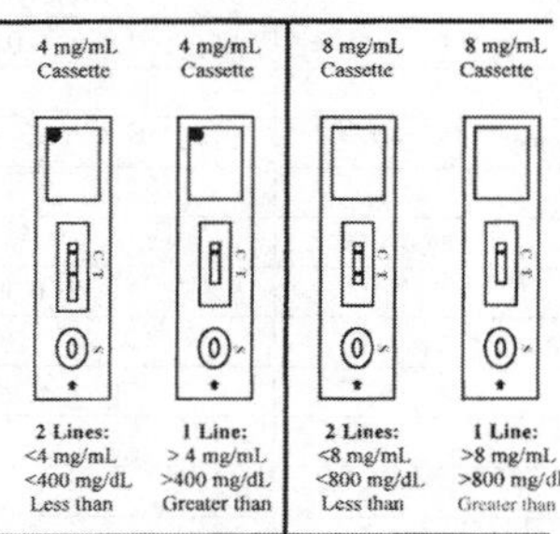

Storage: Avoid prolonged temperature and humidity extremes.

Do not remove the cassette from the foil pouch until ready for use.

Even though the foil pouch includes a desiccant packet, exposure to high humidity conditions should be minimized.

If the buffer in the dilution vial freezes, thaw before using.

Caution(s): Do not use components past expiration date and do not mix components from kits from different lot numbers.

The dilution vial in this kit contains sodium azide. Sodium azide may react with lead or copper plumbing to form highly explosive metal azides. On disposal, flush with a large volume of water to prevent azide build-up. For further information, refer to the manual issued by the Centers for Disease Control.

Do not ingest the desiccant or the buffer solution.

Dispose of all kit components in an appropriate manner.

Discussion: Failure of Passive Transfer (FPT): Foals are born virtually devoid of any detectable level of immunoglobulin G (IgG). The neonatal foal's immunity to infectious agent relies on the ingestion and absorption of maternal IgG from colostrum in mother's milk. This process, termed passive transfer, is a critical determinant of foal health. Failure of passive transfer (FPT) may occur as a result of inadequate suckling, poor absorption of IgG, low levels of IgG in colostrum, or environmental stress.[2] FPT in foals has been estimated to be as high as 24%.[3] As a result, the foal is at a greater risk of developing severe respiratory illness, diarrhea and other septicemic illnesses.[3,4,5,6]

The foal's ability to absorb IgG is optimal at birth and progressively declines in absorptive efficiency. The highest rate of absorption occurs during the first 12 hours. From 12 to 24 hours there is a substantial decline in absorption. Estimated closure time for IgG is approximately 24 hours.[3,7]

Studies have identified the specific concentrations of IgG that indicate adequate passive transfer.[6,7,8] Serum IgG concentrations less than 4 mg/mL (400 mg/dL) are considered to show FPT. While serum IgG concentrations between 4 mg/mL (400 mg/dL) and 8 mg/mL (800 mg/dL) may have an adequate level of immunity, they are considered to have partial failure of passive transfer (PFPT). Serum IgG concentrations above 8 mg/mL (800 mg/dL) are considered to have an adequate level of immunity.

The rapid identification of foals with adequate IgG levels can be used to assess management and husbandry practices. In addition, if low IgG levels are detected, intervention strategies may be developed in conjunction with your health professional to optimize foal health and farm productivity.

Presentation: Kits are packaged and sold in the following sizes:
4 mg/mL (400 mg/dL): Packages of 6, 12 and 24 tests.
8 mg/mL (800 mg/dL): Packages of 6, 12 and 24 tests.

Patent Pending

Compendium Code No.: 15010040 9048 rev.0

PLASMUNE J

Lake Immunogenics **Equine Plasma**

Normal Equine Plasma

Contents: Each single dose bag contains approximately 950 mL of normal plasma equine plasma with Na. Citrate as an anticoagulant, derived from healthy horses with no A or Q r.b.c. factors and no serum r.b.c. antibodies. All donor horse are negative to EIA and EVA. There is no preservative added.

Indications: For intravenous use in cases of fluid volume loss, plasma component loss, or whenever plasma replacement is necessary.

Dosage and Administration: Keep frozen until used. Thaw rapidly not exceeding 120°F. Administer by filtered intravenous infusion until fluid volume loss or plasma component loss has been corrected. Discard the unused portion. In case of a reaction, marked most often by tenesmus and hyperventilation, slow the speed of administration. If this does not abate the signs, stop administration until the signs abate, then continue administration at a slower rate. If signs persist, suspend administration, treat with antihistamines and anti-inflammatory agents. Administration may be attempted again after treatment to relieve adverse response has been successful.

Caution(s): Each serial is tested for negative for aerobic bacteria, anaerobic bacteria, and fungi. However, the transmission of viral disease is possible with the administration of any untreated blood product. This is a rare occurrence.

For veterinary use only.

Presentation: 950 mL.

Compendium Code No.: 11190021

PLAZVAX®

Schering-Plough **Vaccine**

Anaplasmosis Vaccine, Killed

U.S. Vet. Lic. No.: 107

Contents: An emulsion vaccine containing concentrated, inactivated *Anaplasma marginale* antigens and an adjuvant suspended in 10% oil.

Indications: For the vaccination of normal healthy cattle as an aid in the prevention of anaplasmosis caused by *A marginale.*

Dosage and Administration: Shake well before use. Inject 1 mL subcutaneously using aseptic technique. Repeat in 3 to 4 weeks. Revaccinate annually or prior to time of stress or exposure with a single 1 mL dose.

Precaution(s): Store at 2°-7°C (35°-45°F). Protect from freezing. Use entire contents when first opened.

Caution(s): For use by or under the supervision of a licensed veterinarian.

This product has been tested under laboratory conditions and shown to meet all Federal standards for safety and ability to immunize normal healthy animals. This level of performance may be affected by conditions such as stress, weather, nutrition, disease, parasitism, other treatments, individual idiosyncrasies or impaired immunological competency. These factors should be considered by the user when evaluating product performance or freedom from reactions.

Anaphylactic reactions may occur following use.

Antidote(s): Epinephrine, followed by supportive therapy.

Warning(s): Do not vaccinate within 60 days of slaughter.

To the Physician: Accidental self-injection with this oil-based product can cause intense vascular spasm, which may, for example, result in the loss of a digit. Expert prompt surgical attention is required and may necessitate early incision and irrigation of the injected area, especially where there is involvement of muscle, nerves, tendon sheaths or joint capsules.

For veterinary use only.

Presentation: 25 dose (25 mL) vial.

Compendium Code No.: 10471550

PLEASCENT® PUPPY

Thornell **Deodorant Product**

Indications: For accidents while house-breaking.

Stops odors. Eliminates many stains from puppy urine and feces in rugs, floors, bedding, upholstery.

Directions:

Application. For a fine spray use a quick, short squeeze with bottle upright or slightly tipped. For a stream use a sustained squeeze.

Odor. If recent, blot urine or remove the fecal matter. Treat soiled area. If deeply imbedded, area must be thoroughly saturated. In each case PLEASCENT® Puppy must come in contact with the source of the odor to be completely effective. Let air dry.

Stains. Rub area thoroughly with a sponge or cloth saturated with PLEASCENT® Puppy. Blot with clean cloth. Let dry and vacuum. This is a quality stain remover, however, not all stains can be removed with a single agent.

Always spot test before using.

Warning(s): Safe: nontoxic, nonirritating and biodegradable.

However, as with all chemicals keep out of reach of children.

Presentation: 3.75 oz (106 grams).

Compendium Code No.: 11210060

PLEUROGUARD® 4

Pfizer Animal Health **Bacterin**

Actinobacillus Pleuropneumoniae-Bordetella Bronchiseptica-Erysipelothrix Rhusiopathiae-Pasteurella Multocida Bacterin

U.S. Vet. Lic. No.: 189

Description: PLEUROGUARD® 4 contains chemically inactivated cultures of 4 sero-types of *A. pleuropneumoniae* (serotypes 1, 3, 4, and 5), *B. bronchiseptica, E. rhusio-pathiae,* and *P. multocida* combined with a sterile adjuvant to enhance the immune response.

Indications: PLEUROGUARD® 4 is for vaccination of healthy swine as an aid in preventing respiratory disease caused by *Actinobacillus pleuropneumoniae,* and disease caused by *Bordetella bronchiseptica, Erysipelothrix rhusiopathiae,* and *Pasteurella multocida.*

Directions:

1. General Directions: Shake well. Aseptically administer 3 mL intramuscularly or subcutaneously.
2. Primary Vaccination: Healthy pigs should receive a single 3-mL dose at weaning, followed by a second dose 2-3 weeks later. Caution: Field trials have shown that transient lethargy, anorexia, and vomiting may occur in some pigs immediately after inoculation. Healthy, pregnant swine should receive 2 doses at least 2 weeks apart with the second dose administered 2 weeks before farrowing.
3. Revaccination: For sows, revaccination with a single dose is recommended before each subsequent farrowing. Semiannual revaccination with a single dose is recommended for boars.
4. Good animal husbandry and herd health management practices should be employed.

Precaution(s): Store at 2°-7°C. Prolonged exposure to higher temperatures may adversely affect potency. Do not freeze.

Use entire contents when first opened.

Sterilized needles and syringes should be used to administer this vaccine.

Caution(s): Transient local reactions may occur after administration.

As with many vaccines, anaphylaxis may occur after use. Initial antidote of epinephrine is recommended and should be followed with appropriate supportive therapy.

This product has been shown to be efficacious in healthy animals. A protective immune response may not be elicited if animals are incubating an infectious disease, are malnourished or parasitized, are stressed due to shipment or environmental conditions, are otherwise immunocompromised, or the vaccine is not administered in accordance with label directions.

Warning(s): Do not vaccinate within 21 days before slaughter.

For use in swine only.

For veterinary use only.

Discussion: Disease Description: *A. pleuropneumoniae* infection results in acute and chronic forms of swine respiratory disease. Acute disease can cause death within 3 hours after experimental infection. Affected pigs may become cyanotic, show severe respiratory distress characterized by open mouth breathing, and express a blood-tinged nasal discharge. Animals often remain in a sitting posture. Extensive pleural hemorrhages occur with death resulting from cardiac and circulatory failure. Chronic disease may be subclinical and is characterized by an intermittent cough, deteriorating performance, and an extended finishing period. Pathology typically consists of bilateral fibrino-purulent bronchopneumonia with fibrinous pleuritis. Marked variation in virulence occurs between serotypes.

B. bronchiseptica is a principal cause of atrophic rhinitis in swine. Particularly in young pigs, the disease is characterized by acute rhinitis followed by chronic atrophy of the turbinate bones. Impairment of the turbinate filtering system predisposes the animal to respiratory infections, including pneumonia, and is associated with reduced rate of gain and an extended finishing period. In combined infections, *B. bronchiseptica* and *P. multocida* have been shown to cause atrophic rhinitis lesions of greater severity than in cases where either agent functions alone.[1,2]

E. rhusiopathiae infection in swine (swine erysipelas) has a variety of manifestations. These include acute septicemia, skin discoloration characterized by hyperemic or necrotic diamond-shaped lesions, chronic arthritis, and vegetative endocarditis.

Trial Data: Safety and Efficacy: Chemical inactivation renders PLEUROGUARD® 4 incapable of causing infectious disease. Temporary induration and moderate swelling may be observed at the injection site.

Efficacy of the *A. pleuropneumoniae* fraction in PLEUROGUARD® 4 was established in rigorous challenge-of-immunity tests. Vaccinates received 2 subcutaneous doses administered 2 weeks apart. Respective test groups were challenged with virulent A. pleuro-pneumoniae serotypes 1, 3, 4, and 5 (Table 1). For serotype 1, two tests were conducted. A market weight challenge was administered to 1 group 120 days after primary vaccination, and a short-term challenge was administered to a second group 42 days after primary vaccination. For serotype 3, challenge was administered 38 days after primary vaccination. For serotypes 4 and 5, challenge was administered 49 and 28 days after primary vaccination, respectively. In each test, all pigs were

P

necropsied and evaluated for lung disease either after death or termination of the test at 6-12 days postchallenge.

Results are shown in Table 1. All vaccinates seroconverted to each of the *A. pleuropneumoniae* serotypes tested. Vaccinated pigs demonstrated a high level of protection against a severe challenge that produced lung lesions in 97% of the controls.

Table 1. Results of *A. pleuropneumoniae* Vaccination and Challenge in Preweaned Pigs

Test No.	Serotype & Procedure	Test Groups	Postvaccination Seroconversion	Percent Protected from Lung Lesions
1	type 1 challenge (market weight)	19 vaccinates	100	74 (14/19)
		5 controls	-	0 (0/5)
2	type 1 challenge	19 vaccinates	100	84 (16/19)
		4 controls	-	25 (1/4)
3	type 3 challenge	25 vaccinates	100	76 (19/25)
		6 controls	-	0 (0/6)
4	type 4 challenge	21 vaccinates	100	95 (20/21)
		5 controls	-	0 (0/5)
5	type 5 challenge, seronegative pigs	20 vaccinates	100	95 (19/20)
		5 controls	-	0 (0/5)
6	type 5 challenge, seropositive pigs*	20 vaccinates	-	90 (18/20)
		5 controls	-	0 (0/5)

* Test animals had maternally derived antibodies

The market weight challenge for serotype 1 demonstrated that vaccination provided substantial protection over the course of the feeding period, even against severe challenge.

One of the challenge-of-immunity tests (test 6) was designed to evaluate the effects of vaccination and challenge in pigs with maternal immunity. (Prevaccination geometric mean titers for *A. pleuropneumoniae* were 1:31 in vaccinates and 1:45 in controls.) Postchallenge, all controls developed lung lesions, indicating that passive immunity may be of limited benefit in the face of a severe challenge. Ninety percent of the vaccinates were protected against lung lesions, underscoring the value of active immunization. After administration of vaccine, pigs developed a 2-fold increase in the geometric mean serologic titer (Table 2), demonstrating that vaccination can produce active immunity in pigs carrying maternal antibodies.

Table 2. Serologic Values in Maternally Immune Pigs After *A. pleuropneumoniae* Vaccination and Challenge

No. & Group	Geometric Mean Serum Agglutination Titers*			
	Pre Vacc.	Post 1st Vacc.	Post 2nd Vacc.	Post Challenge
20 vaccinates	31	69	64	66
5 controls	-	-	45	78

* Expressed as the reciprocal of end point dilutions.

The *B. bronchiseptica* fraction has been evaluated in challenge-of-immunity tests in susceptible 12-week-old pigs. Results are shown in Table 3, and indicate that the most effective vaccination program requires vaccination of both sows and pigs.

Table 3. Results of Challenge After Vaccination with *B. bronchiseptica* Bacterin

No. Animals	Vaccination Status	% Incidence of Turbinate Atrophy
25	nonvaccinated pigs from nonvaccinated sows	96
35	nonvaccinated pigs from vaccinated sows	60
23	vaccinated pigs from nonvaccinated sows	39
40	vaccinated pigs from vaccinated sows	20

P

Efficacy of the *E. rhusiopathiae* fraction was demonstrated in a controlled challenge-of-immunity test. A single subcutaneous dose administered to seronegative test pigs protected them from challenge with *E. rhusiopathiae* administered 2 weeks postvaccination. All controls were clinically affected with signs of erysipelas after the same challenge.

References: Available upon request.

Presentation: 35 dose vials.

Compendium Code No.: 36900530

75-4597-07

PLEXADOL™ SHAMPOO

Butler **Antidermatosis Shampoo**

Active Ingredient(s):

Nonylphenoxypoly (ethyleneoxy) ethanol-iodine complex 8.75%
(Yielding 1.75% titratable iodine.)

Inert ingredients: Linear alcohol ethoxylate sulfates, coco diethanolamides, ethoxylated linear alcohols, deionized water, buffering agents.

Indications: A mild form of complexed iodine incorporated into a high sudsing shampoo base for the cleaning and grooming of dogs, cats, and horses. Iodine is a recognized antimicrobial showing a broad-spectrum antiseptic action against gram-negative and gram-positive bacteria, as well as fungi.

Dosage and Administration: For external use only.

1. Wet the hair or coat with warm water at room temperature.
2. Apply the shampoo and work into a rich lather. Continue to massage the lather into the coat for a minimum of five (5) minutes.
3. Rewet the hair or coat and again massage into a rich lather.
4. Rinse the animal with clear water to remove the shampoo.

Precaution(s): Keep from freezing.

Caution(s): Harmful if swallowed. Avoid contact with the eyes. In case of contact with eyes, flush with copious amounts of water. Contact a physician. Avoid contamination of feed and foodstuffs. Keep out of the reach of children.

Presentation: 8 oz. and 1 gallon containers.

Compendium Code No.: 10821470

PLEXAMINO® BOLUS

Bimeda **Large Animal Dietary Supplement**

Guaranteed Analysis:

	Per Bolus	Per Pound
Crude Protein, min.	10.0 g	28.90%
Calcium (Ca), min.	5.0 g	14.50%
Calcium (Ca), max.	6.0 g	17.40%
Phosphorus (P), min.	1.0 g	3.00%
Salt (Nacl), min.	2.0 g	5.50%
Salt (Nacl), max.	2.3 g	6.60%
Sodium (Na), min.	778.0 mg	2.20%
Potassium (K), min.	500.5 mg	1.40%
Magnesium (Mg), min.	7.3 mg	0.02%
Sulfur (S), min.	379.0 mg	1.10%
Cobalt (Co), min.	3.3 mg	0.01%
Copper (Cu), min.	7.4 mg	0.02%
Iron (Fe), min.	598.6 g	1.70%
Manganese (Mn), min.	8.7 mg	0.02%
Zinc (Zn), min.	90.0 mg	0.20%

Ingredients: L-Lysine, DL-Methionine, Meat Protein Isolate, Dicalcium Phosphate, Calcium Carbonate, Ferrous Sulfate, Sodium Chloride, Potassium Chloride, Magnesium Sulfate, Zinc Oxide, Copper Sulfate, Manganese Sulfate, Cobalt Sulfate, Dextrose, Microcrystalline cellulose, magnesium stearate.

Indications: A supplemental nutritive bolus that provides protein, and trace elements, minerals and carbohydrates for horses, cattle, sheep and swine.

Directions for Use: Administer orally 1 to 4 boluses for each 250 pounds of body weight per day. Bolus should be lubricated with mineral oil or petroleum jelly and administered with the aid of a balling gun. Boluses may also be crushed and top dressed on feed or given as a drench.

Precaution(s): Keep container tightly closed when not in use. Store in a cool, dry place.

Caution(s): For animal use only.

Warning(s): Keep out of reach of children.

Presentation: 50 boluses (34.5 g/bolus).

PLEXAMINO® is a registered trademark of Bimeda, Inc.

Compendium Code No.: 13990031

Iss. 06-01

PLEX-SOL C

Vet-A-Mix **Small Animal Dietary Supplement**

(Concentrated vitamin complex)-Water Dispersible

Guaranteed Analysis: Per Kilogram

Vitamin A . . . . 2,000,000 IU
Vitamin D_3 . . . . 250,000 IU
Vitamin E . . . . 5,000 IU
Vitamin C (Ascorbic Acid) . . . . 40,000 mg
Menadione (K_3 from Menadione sodium bisulfite) . . . . 2,000 mg
Niacin . . . . 10,000 mg
D-Pantothenic acid . . . . 2,500 mg
Riboflavin . . . . 2,500 mg
Thiamine Mononitrate . . . . 1,000 mg
Pyridoxine hydrochloride . . . . 1,000 mg
Vitamin B_{12} . . . . 10 mg
Folic acid . . . . 500 mg

Ingredients: Dextrose, sucrose, vitamin B_{12} supplement, ascorbic acid, niacin supplement, vitamin E supplement, magnesium sulfate, sodium sulfate, menadione sodium bisulfite complex, vitamin A supplement, calcium pantothenate, folic acid, riboflavin supplement, thiamine mononitrate, pyridoxine hydrochloride, vitamin D_3 supplement, and BHT (a preservative).

Indications: For use as a dietary and supportive supplement in horses, cattle, swine, poultry, dogs, cats, pet birds and laboratory animals such as rats, guinea pigs, hamsters and monkeys.

Dosage and Administration:

For Mixing in the Daily Ration: For prevention of vitamin deficiencies, mix 3 grams in each 1.5 kilograms (500 g per 550 lb) of diet.

For Mixing in the Drinking Water: For prevention of vitamin deficiencies, mix one gram in each liter (500 g per 125 gallons) of water.

To insure freshness, prepare a water/vitamin mixture every day.

The enclosed teaspoon measure contains 3.0 grams when level full.

For therapeusis, double the above dosages.

Precaution(s): Keep container closed when not in use. Do not store at temperatures exceeding 80°F (27°C).

Caution(s): When using PLEX-SOL C as a nutritional dietary supplement, other food sources of the vitamins contained in PLEX-SOL C should be considered.

Warning(s): Keep out of reach of children.

Presentation: 500 g bottles.

Compendium Code No.: 10500241

1198

PM-ONEVAX™

Schering-Plough **Vaccine**

Pasteurella multocida Vaccine, Avirulent Live Culture, Avian Isolate

U.S. Vet. Lic. No.: 165A

Active Ingredient(s): *Pasteurella multocida* vaccine, avirulent live culture, avian isolate.

The seed culture used to make the vaccine has been laboratory tested for protection against challenge with the P1059 (USDA challenge) strain of *P. multocida*.

Indications: For vaccinating healthy breeder and market turkeys six weeks of age or older as an aid in the prevention of fowl cholera due to *P. multocida*.

Dosage and Administration:

When to Vaccinate: Best results are obtained when the vaccine is administered initially to turkeys six (6) to eight (8) weeks of age and repeated every four (4) to six (6) weeks thereafter as necessary according to exposure conditions.

Vaccination Program: The development of a durable, strong protection to fowl cholera depends upon the use of an effective vaccination program as well as many other circumstances such as administration techniques, environment ,and flock health at the time of vaccination. Also, the immune response to one (1) vaccination under field conditions is seldom complete for all animals within a given flock. Even when vaccination is successful, the protection stimulated in individual birds against different diseases may not be life long. Therefore, a program of periodic revaccination is necessary.

Preparation of the Vaccine:

1. Assemble the vaccine and equipment needed to vaccinate the entire flock at one time.
2. Do not open and rehydrate the vaccine until ready for use.
3. Remove the tear-off aluminum seal from the vaccine vial without disturbing the rubber stopper.
4. Use cool, clean, nonchlorinated tap water to which powdered milk has been added as directed under How to Vaccinate.
5. Remove the rubber stopper from the vaccine vial and rehydrate the vaccine by filling the vial about half-full with tap water (milk added).
6. Reseat the stopper and shake to thoroughly dissolve the vaccine.

How to Vaccinate: Do not mix the vaccine into the drinking water until ready for use. Drinking water for vaccination should be mixed with powdered milk to prevent possible inactivation from chlorine or other water additives and also to stabilize the vaccine bacteria. The powdered milk should be added to the water at the rate of one (1) heaped teaspoon per 3 U.S. gallons or 2.5 imperial gallons (3 g per 11 L); or one (1) heaped cupful per 80 U.S. gallons or 66 imperial gallons (90 g per 300 L).

Use only clean waterers and equipment free of disinfectants or sanitizers. All water must be withheld from the birds for at least two (2) hours prior to vaccination to ensure that all of the turkeys drink. Mix the rehydrated vaccine in the quantity of drinking water (milk added) which will be consumed by thirsty turkeys in approximately two (2) hours.

The following schedule is a general guideline for the amount of water to use with the vaccine. These amounts will vary depending upon the individual management conditions, climate, age and sex of the birds.

Age	Sex	Climate	Amount of water for each 1,000 doses		
			U.S. Gallons	Imperial Gallons	Liters
6-8 weeks	Toms	Hot	25	21	95
6-8 weeks	Hens	Hot	20	17	76
6-8 weeks	Toms	Cold	13	11	49
6-8 weeks	Hens	Cold	10	8	38
10-14 weeks	Toms	Hot	35	29	133
10-14 weeks	Hens	Hot	27	22	103
10-14 weeks	Toms	Cold	18	15	68
10-14 weeks	Hens	Cold	14	12	53

Another helpful guideline for daily water consumption is one (1) U.S. gallon or 0.8 imperial gallon (3.8 L) of water per week of age per 100 poults; figure 40% of this amount. This 40% is about a 3-hour supply for the flock.

Distribute 1,000 doses of the vaccine in water as used by 1,000 turkeys, or 2,500 doses of the vaccine in water as used by 2,500 turkeys. Provide ample watering space so that all of the turkeys can drink easily. Do not administer through water lines with a proportioner or medication tank.

Records: Keep a record of the vaccine type, quantity, serial number, expiration date, and place of purchase; the date and time of vaccination; the number, age, breed, and location of the birds; the names of operators performing the vaccination and any observed reactions.

Contraindication(s): Turkeys must be healthy and free of environmental or physical stress at the time of vaccination. Initial vaccination with this vaccine should not be conducted in turkeys older than 12 weeks of age. Do not use this vaccine within two weeks before or two weeks after vaccinating turkeys with a live virus Newcastle vaccine.

Precaution(s): Store at 35° to 45°F (2° to 7°C).

Caution(s): For veterinary use only.

1. To avoid interference with the development of protection, turkeys to be vaccinated should not be given any antibiotic and/or sulfonamide medication, used in the prevention or treatment of fowl cholera for three days before and five days after vaccination.
2. Vaccinate healthy birds only. Coccidiosis, respiratory disease, mycoplasma infection, or other disease conditions may cause serious complications or reduce protection. Vaccinated flocks should be watched closely and medicated as necessary to control more severe reactions. Avoid exposing birds other than turkeys to the vaccine.
3. All birds within a flock should be vaccinated on the same day. Isolate other susceptible birds on the premises from the birds being vaccinated.
4. In outbreak situations, vaccinate healthy birds first progressing toward outbreak areas in order to vaccinate diseased birds last. Vaccination in the face of an acute outbreak is not recommended. Under these conditions, use an effective fowl cholera treatment, wait at least three days or until the outbreak subsides and then vaccinate.
5. Do not spill or spatter the vaccine. Burn the empty bottles, caps and all unused vaccine and accessories. Use the entire contents of the vial when first opened.
6. Wash hands thoroughly after using the vaccine.
7. Do not dilute the vaccine or otherwise stretch the dosage.

Warning(s): Do not vaccinate within 21 days before slaughter.

Presentation: Supplied lyophilized in 10 x 1,000 and 10 x 2,500 dose unit packs.

Compendium Code No.: 10471570

PM-ONEVAX®-C

Schering-Plough **Vaccine**

Pasteurella Multocida Vaccine, Avirulent Live Culture, Avian Isolate

U.S. Vet. Lic. No.: 165A

Contents: PM-ONEVAX®-C vaccine is a live bacterial vaccine containing the mild avirulent PM-1 strain of *Pasteurella multocida* in a freeze-dried preparation sealed under vacuum. The vaccine strain has been shown to offer protection as an aid in the prevention of fowl cholera in chickens and turkeys. The seed culture used to make this vaccine has been laboratory tested for protection in chickens against challenge with the X-73 (Type 1) strain of *P. multocida* and in turkeys against challenge with the P1059 (Type 3) strain of *P. multocida*.

Indications: Chickens: Use by wing-web stab to vaccinate chickens 10-12 weeks of age and again at 18-20 weeks of age as an aid in the prevention of pasteurellosis (fowl cholera) due to *P. multocida* Type 1.

Turkeys: Use by wing-web stab to vaccinate turkey breeders 15 weeks of age or older as an aid in the prevention of pasteurellosis (fowl cholera) due to *P. multocida* Type 3.

Dosage and Administration: When to Vaccinate:

Chickens: Use by wing-web stab to vaccinate chickens 10-12 weeks of age and again at 18-20 weeks of age as an aid in the prevention of pasteurellosis (fowl cholera) due to *P. multocida* Type 1. There should be at least 6 weeks and not more than 10 weeks between vaccinations.

Turkeys: Use by wing-web stab to vaccinate turkey breeders 15 weeks of age or older as an aid in the prevention of pasteurellosis (fowl cholera) due to *P. multocida* Type 3. Birds should initially be wing-web vaccinated at 15-18 weeks of age and again 8 weeks later. Turkey breeders must be vaccinated at least twice with live fowl cholera vaccine via oral route prior to wing-web vaccination. The interval between the last oral vaccination and the first wing-web vaccination should not exceed 6 weeks. Additional wing-web vaccination every 6-8 weeks throughout the life of the bird may be required in areas of endemic exposure to fowl cholera.

Your Vaccination Program: The development of a durable, strong protection to this disease depends upon the use of an effective vaccination program as well as many circumstances such as administration techniques, environment, and flock health at the time of vaccination. Also the immune response to one vaccination under field conditions is seldom complete for all animals within a given flock. Even when vaccination is successful, the protection stimulated in individual animals against different diseases may not be life long. Therefore, a program of periodic revaccination may be necessary.

Preparation of the Vaccine:

1. Do not open and mix the vaccine until ready for use.
2. Mix only one vial at a time and use entire contents within 2 hours.
3. Remove the tear-off aluminum seal and stopper from the vial containing the dried vaccine.
4. Remove the tear-off aluminum seal and stopper from the bottle containing the diluent.
5. Hold the diluent bottle firmly in an upright position and insert the shorter end of the transfer tube. Still holding the diluent bottle in an upright position, insert the neck of the vaccine vial over the longer end of the transfer tube. The vaccine vial should snap into position, connecting the two vials securely.
6. Invert the two containers so that the vaccine vial is on the bottom and allow the diluent to flow into the vaccine vial. If the diluent does not flow freely, squeeze the diluent bottle gently and the diluent will flow into the vaccine vial. The vaccine vial should be completely filled with diluent to prevent excess foaming.
7. Hold the joined containers by the ends and shake vigorously until the vaccine plug is completely dissolved.
8. Return the joined containers to their original position (diluent bottle on the bottom). Allow the vaccine to flow into the diluent bottle. If the vaccine does not flow into the diluent bottle, tap or squeeze the diluent bottle gently and release to draw the vaccine into the diluent bottle. Be sure all the product is removed from the vaccine vial.
9. Remove the vaccine vial and transfer tube from the neck of the diluent bottle.
10. The vaccine is now ready for use.
11. Wash hands thoroughly after mixing the vaccine.

How to Vaccinate: Vaccination is accomplished by dipping the needle applicator into the mixed vaccine and piercing the webbed portion of the underside of the wing. Avoid piercing through feathers which may wipe off the vaccine, and avoid hitting the wing muscle or bone to minimize reaction. The applicator is designed to pick up the proper amount of vaccine on the needles, which is deposited in the tissues when the wing is pierced. Redip the applicator in the vaccine before each application. Excess vaccine adhering to the applicator should be removed by touching the applicator to the inside of the vial.

Reactions:

Examination for Takes: Normally, no overall clinical reaction is observed. At 5 to 10 days following vaccination, a swelling of the skin (subcutaneous granuloma) will develop on the wing-web at the point of inoculation. The absence of this local reaction may mean that improper vaccination methods were used. Examination for these "takes" at 7 days post-vaccination may be used to assure that the proper vaccination has been conducted. Protection will normally develop within 14 days after vaccination.

Records: Keep a record of vaccine type, quantity, serial number, expiration date, and place of purchase; the date and time of vaccination; the number, age, breed, and location of the birds; names of operators performing the vaccination, and any observed reactions.

Contraindication(s): Chickens: Initial vaccination in chickens over 12 weeks of age may be undesirable because larger granulomas may develop at the site of inoculation and this may result in the downgrading of carcasses at slaughter.

Turkeys: Use of this vaccine in turkeys which have not been orally prevaccinated may cause severe post-vaccination reactions, including lameness and death.

Precaution(s): Store at 2° to 7°C (35° to 45°F).

Do not spill or spatter the vaccine. Use entire contents of the vial when first opened. Burn empty bottles, caps and all unused vaccine and accessories.

Caution(s):

1. For veterinary use only.
2. Vaccinate only healthy birds. Although disease may not be evident, disease conditions may cause serious complications or reduce protection.
3. Avoid vaccinating birds during weather-induced stress periods and 7 days prior to and 7 days after moving and handling. To avoid interference with development of protection, birds to be vaccinated should not be given any antibiotic and/or sulfonamide medication used in the prevention or treatment of fowl cholera for 3 days before and 5 days after vaccination.
4. All birds within a flock should be vaccinated on the same day. Isolate other susceptible birds on the premises from the birds being vaccinated.
5. In outbreak situations, vaccinate healthy birds first, progressing toward outbreak areas in order to vaccinate diseased birds last.
6. Wash hands thoroughly after using the vaccine.
7. Do not dilute the vaccine or otherwise stretch the dosage.

Warning(s): Do not vaccinate within 21 days of slaughter.

Avoid contact of open wounds or inoculation of vaccinating personnel with the vaccine since this might cause a bacterial infection. If this occurs, consult a physician immediately to obtain proper treatment. The vaccine organism, as with any *Pasteurella multocida* strain, may accidently act as a human pathogen and precautions should be taken to avoid exposure.

Presentation: Supplied lyophilized in 10 x 1,000 dose unit packs (NDC 0138-0878-01).

Compendium Code No.: 10471561

PNEUMABORT-K®+1b

Fort Dodge **Vaccine**

Equine Rhinopneumonitis Vaccine, Killed Virus

U.S. Vet. Lic. No.: 112

Composition: PNEUMABORT-K®+1b is a killed virus vaccine of EHV 1p and 1b (equine rhinopneumonitis virus) which has been chemically inactivated with formalin, and combined with a specially prepared oil adjuvant. PNEUMABORT-K®+1b is grown and prepared on an equine cell line substrate.

Thimerosal, neomycin, polymyxin B and amphotericin B added as preservatives.

Indications: For vaccination of healthy horses as an aid in the prevention of respiratory disease caused by the EHV 1p and EHV 1b viruses as well as for use in pregnant mares as an aid in the prevention of abortion due to EHV 1 infections. Horses incubating other infections or suffering from malnutrition, parasitism or other diseases and conditions subjecting them to stress are poor subjects for immunization and may not develop or maintain a serviceable immune response.

Dosage and Administration: For pregnant mares, aseptically administer one 2 mL dose intramuscularly during the 5th, 7th and 9th months of pregnancy. Revaccinate annually at the 5th, 7th and 9th months of pregnancy.

For young horses, administer one 2 mL dose intramuscularly followed by a second 2 mL dose 3 to 4 weeks later. Revaccinate with a single 2 mL dose 6 months after the second primary dose and annually thereafter. To insure proper placement and retention of the vaccine, inject deep into the heavy muscles of the hindquarter. Mild exercise to promote absorption is recommended for one week after injection.

Maiden and barren mares kept in barn- or pasture-contact with vaccinated pregnant mares should be vaccinated on the same schedule as the pregnant mares with which they are in contact. Mares more than five months pregnant at the time of arrival on a farm should be vaccinated upon arrival and at two-month intervals until foaling.

Pregnant mares that are in contact with mares that have aborted equine herpesvirus 1 infected fetuses should be vaccinated. Such vaccination may provide immunity for those mares in the group which are not incubating an abortigenic infection at the time of vaccination.

General Information: A short duration of serviceable immunity occurs after herpesvirus 1 infection or vaccination. It is necessary to maintain as high a level of immunity as possible to aid in protection against upper respiratory tract infection, and spread of field strains of virus to pregnant mares. Pregnant mares require the highest possible level of protection against infection after the fifth month of pregnancy; this should be maintained throughout pregnancy.

The vaccine is a killed virus preparation, and may be administered at any time to horses or mares that may be moved from the premises, or that may be exposed to infection.

Precaution(s): Store in dark at 2° to 7°C (35° to 45°F). Avoid freezing. Shake vigorously to assure uniform suspension of the vaccine.

Caution(s): When used according to instructions, local or systemic reactions rarely occur. An occasional local swelling or induration at the site of injection may be encountered. In case of anaphylactoid reaction, administer epinephrine.

Warning(s): Do not vaccinate within 60 days before slaughter.

For veterinary use only.

Presentation: 25 x 2 mL prefilled syringes (25 doses), 20 mL (10 doses), 12 x 1 dose (syringe pouch pack) and 10 dose vials.

Compendium Code No.: 10031460 2885A

PNEUMOSUIS® III

Pfizer Animal Health **Bacterin**

Actinobacillus Pleuropneumoniae Bacterin

U.S. Vet. Lic. No.: 189

Contents: PNEUMOSUIS® III consists of killed, standardized cultures of *A. pleuropneumoniae* with an aluminum hydroxide adjuvant.

Indications: For use in healthy swine as an aid in preventing disease caused by *Actinobacillus pleuropneumoniae* serotypes 1, 5, and 7.

Directions: Shake well. Aseptically administer 2 mL subcutaneously or intramuscularly. Healthy sows and gilts should receive 2 doses administered at 4 and 2 weeks before farrowing. Revaccination with a single dose 3 weeks before subsequent farrowings is recommended. Healthy pigs should receive a single 2-mL dose at weaning, followed by a second dose 3-4 weeks later.

Precaution(s): Store at 2°-7°C. Do not freeze. Use entire contents when first opened.

Caution(s): As with many vaccines, anaphylaxis may occur after use. Initial antidote of epinephrine is recommended and should be followed with appropriate supportive therapy.

Warning(s): Do not vaccinate within 21 days before slaughter.

For use in swine only.

For veterinary use only.

Presentation: 50 dose (100 mL) vials.

Compendium Code No.: 36900180 85-4186-01

PNEU PAC®

Schering-Plough **Bacterin**

Actinobacillus pleuropneumoniae Bacterin, Serotypes 1, 5 and 7

U.S. Vet. Lic. No.: 165A

Active Ingredient(s): This bacterin contains inactivated *Haemophilus pleuropneumoniae* organisms (serotypes 1, 5 and 7). It is adjuvanted with emulsified paraffin.

Prepared from young cultures of *Haemophilus pleuropneumoniae* organisms. Chemically inactivated. Contains polymyxin B sulfate as a preservative.

Indications: For the immunization of healthy swine over four weeks of age against pneumonia caused by *Haemophilus pleuropneumoniae* organisms. This bacterin has been shown to protect susceptible swine against intranasal challenge with virulent serotypes 1, 5 and 7 *Haemophilus pleuropneumoniae* organisms.

Dosage and Administration: Shake well and occasionally during use. Administer 2 mL intramuscularly of subcutaneously in the lower flank or immediately behind the ear. Use sterile syringes and needles. Repeat in 21 to 28 days. This repeat dose is essential for maximum immune response. If losses occur in older swine administer a third injection. Annual revaccination of breeding swine is recommended.

Precaution(s): Use the entire contents when first opened. Store at not over 45°F (7°C). Keep from freezing.

Caution(s): Vaccination, especially repeated injections can result in anaphylaxis.

Antidote(s): Administer epinephrine.

Warning(s): Do not vaccinate within 60 days of slaughter.

Presentation: 50 dose (100 mL) and 125 dose (250 mL) plastic vials.

Compendium Code No.: 10471580

PNEU PAC®-ER

Schering-Plough **Bacterin**

Actinobacillus pleuropneumoniae-Erysipelothrix rhusiopathiae Bacterin

U.S. Vet. Lic. No.: 165A

Active Ingredient(s): This bacterin contains inactivated *Haemophilus pleuropneumoniae* (serotypes 1, 5 and 7) and *Erysipelothrix rhusiopathiae* organisms. It is adjuvanted with emulsified paraffin-Emulsigen™.

Prepared from cultures of *Haemophilus pleuropneumoniae* and *Erysipelothrix rhusiopathiae* organisms.

Preservatives: Gentamicin, polymyxin B, neomycin.

Indications: For the immunization of healthy swine over four weeks of age against pneumonia caused by *Haemophilus pleuropneumoniae* and erysipelas caused by *Erysipelothrix rhusiopathiae* organisms. This bacterin has been shown to protect susceptible swine against intranasal challenge with virulent HPP serotype(s) 1, 5 and 7.

Dosage and Administration: Shake well. Administer 2 mL intramuscularly immediately behind the ear in swine four (4) weeks of age or older using aseptic technique. Repeat in 21 to 28 days. If losses occur in older swine administer a third injection. Annual revaccination of breeding swine is recommended.

Precaution(s): Store at 2-7°C (35-45°F). Do not freeze. Use the entire contents when first opened.

Caution(s): Transient local reactions may be observed at the injection site. If an allergic response occurs, administer epinephrine or its equivalent.

Warning(s): Do not vaccinate within 60 days of slaughter.

Presentation: 50 dose (100 mL) and 125 dose (250 mL) plastic vials.

Compendium Code No.: 10471590

PNEU PARAPAC®+ER

Schering-Plough **Bacterin**

Actinobacillus pleuropneumoniae-Erysipelothrix rhusiopathiae-Haemophilus parasuis Bacterin

U.S. Vet. Lic. No.: 165A

Contents: Contains chemically-inactivated cultures of *A pleuropneumoniae* Serotypes 1, 5 and 7, *H parasuis* and *E rhusiopathiae.*

Preservatives: Gentamicin, polymyxin B and amphotericin B.

Indications: For use in healthy swine four weeks of age or older for prevention of Glasser's disease caused by *H parasuis,* pneumonia caused by *A pleuropneumoniae* serotypes 1, 5 and 7, and erysipelas caused by *E rhusiopathiae.*

Dosage and Administration: Shake well. Using aseptic technique, inject swine four weeks of age or older subcutaneously with 3 mL. Repeat in 21 to 28 days. If losses due *A pleuropneumoniae* occur in older swine, administer a third injection of a Schering-Plough bacterin containing *Actinobacillus pleuropneumoniae* at that time. Annual revaccination of breeding swine is recommended.

Precaution(s): Store at 2° to 7°C (35° to 45°F). Do not freeze. Use entire contents when first opened.

Caution(s): Transient local reaction may occur at the injection site. If anaphylaxis occurs administer epinephrine.

Antidote(s): Epinephrine.

Warning(s): Do not vaccinate within 60 days prior to slaughter.

For veterinary use only.

Extreme caution should be used when injecting any oil emulsion vaccine to avoid injecting your own finger or hand. Accidental injection can cause serious local reaction. Contact a physician immediately if accidental injection occurs.

Presentation: 35 dose (105 mL) and 75 dose (225 mL) vials.

Compendium Code No.: 10471611

POLY-BAC B® 3

Texas Vet Lab **Bacterin-Toxoid**

Haemophilus Somnus-Pasteurella Haemolytica-Multocida Bacterin-Toxoid

U.S. Vet. Lic. No.: 290

Contents: This product contains the antigens listed above.

Indications: For use in stocker and feeder calves as an aid in the prevention of respiratory disease associated with *Haemophilus somnus, Pasteurella haemolytica* A1 and *Pasteurella multocida* A3.

Dosage and Administration: Instructions: Shake well and aseptically inject 2 mL subcutaneously in the side of the neck. Give a second dose 14 days after the first on the opposite side of the neck.

Precaution(s): Do not contaminate with dirt or chemicals. Use sterile equipment and adequately clean and disinfect bottle cap prior to each entry. Use entire contents when opened. Store at 2 to 7°C. Do not use if emulsion is broken as indicated by separation at the bottom of bottle.

Caution(s): May cause local swelling. Do not inject into muscle, may cause carcass trim. In case of anaphylactoid reaction, treat symptomatically.

For veterinary use only.

Warning(s): Do not vaccinate within 60 days of slaughter.

Presentation: 50 doses (100 mL) and 100 doses (200 mL) bottles.

Compendium Code No.: 11080051

POLY-BAC B® 7

Texas Vet Lab **Bacterin-Toxoid-Vaccine**

Bovine Rhinotracheitis-Virus Diarrhea Vaccine-Haemophilus Somnus-Pasteurella Haemolytica-Multocida Salmonella Typhimurium Bacterin-Toxoid, Killed Virus

U.S. Vet. Lic. No.: 290

Contents: This product contains the antigens listed above.

Indications: For use in healthy stocker and feeder calves as an aid in the prevention of respiratory disease associated with infectious Bovine Rhinotracheitis, Bovine Viral Diarrhea, *Haemophilus somnus, Pasteurella haemolytica* A1, *Pasteurella haemolytica* A6 and *Pasteurella multocida* A3 and salmonellosis caused by *Salmonella typhimurium.*

Dosage and Administration: Instructions: Shake well and aseptically inject 2 mL subcutaneously in the side of the neck. Give a second dose 14 days after the first on the opposite side of the neck. If severe exposure to IBR and/or BVD is anticipated, consideration should be given to revaccination with modified live IBR and/or BVD vaccine.

Precaution(s): Do not contaminate with dirt or chemicals or other biologics. Use sterile equipment and adequately clean and disinfect bottle cap prior to each entry. Use entire contents when opened. Store at 2 to 7°C. Do not use if emulsion is broken as indicated by separation at the bottom of bottle.

Caution(s): May cause local swelling. Do not inject into muscle, may cause carcass trim. In case of anaphylactoid reaction, treat symptomatically.

For veterinary use only.

Warning(s): Do not vaccinate within 60 days of slaughter.

Presentation: 50 dose (100 mL) and 100 dose (200 mL) bottles.

Compendium Code No.: 11080060

POLY-BAC B® SOMNUS

Texas Vet Lab **Bacterin-Toxoid**

Haemophilus Somnus-Pasteurella Haemolytica-Multocida-Salmonella Typhimurium Bacterin-Toxoid

U.S. Vet. Lic. No.: 290

Contents: This product contains the antigens listed above.

Indications: For use in stocker and feeder calves as an aid in the prevention of respiratory disease associated with *Haemophilus somnus, Pasteurella haemolytica* A1 and *Pasteurella multocida* A3 and salmonellosis caused by *Salmonella typhimurium.*

Dosage and Administration: Instructions: Shake well and aseptically inject 2 mL subcutaneously in the side of the neck. Give a second dose 14 days after the first on the opposite side of the neck.

Precaution(s): Do not contaminate with dirt or chemicals. Use sterile equipment and adequately clean and disinfect bottle cap prior to each entry. Use entire contents when opened. Store at 2 to 7°C. Do not use if emulsion is broken as indicated by separation at the bottom of bottle.

Caution(s): May cause local swelling. Do not inject into muscle, may cause carcass trim. In case of anaphylactoid reaction, treat symptomatically.

For veterinary use only.

Warning(s): Do not vaccinate within 60 days of slaughter.

Presentation: 50 dose (100 mL) and 100 dose (200 mL) bottles.

Compendium Code No.: 11080070

POLYBRON® B_1

ASL **Vaccine**

Newcastle-Bronchitis Vaccine, B_1 Type, B_1 Strain, Mass. & Conn. Types, Live Virus

U.S. Vet. Lic. No.: 226

Description: POLYBRON® B_1 is formulated from carefully selected strains of infectious bronchitis viruses of Mass. and Conn. types (Polybron®) and the B_1 strain of Newcastle virus. The viruses are grown under exacting standards of quality control in eggs produced by healthy chickens in closely supervised flocks.

Gentamicin is added as a preservative.

Indications: For the vaccination of chickens against Newcastle disease and infectious Bronchitis (Mass. and Conn. types).

This vaccine is recommended for initial vaccination at 4 weeks of age by intraocular or drinking water methods of application.

POLYBRON® B_1 offers high levels of protection with mild respiratory reaction, i.e. mild rates, helps stimulate susceptible chickens to develop immunity.

Dosage and Administration: Rehydration of the Vaccine (for intraocular use): Do not open and mix the vaccine until ready to begin vaccination. Use the vaccine immediately after mixing.

1. Tear off the aluminum seal from the vial containing the dried vaccine.
2. Lift off the rubber stopper.
3. Remove plastic applicator.
4. Pour a small amount of diluent into the vial of dried vaccine.
5. Replace the rubber stopper and shake.
6. Pour the partly dissolved vaccine into the bottle containing the rest of the diluent.
7. Insert plastic applicator and shake vigorously until all the material is dissolved.

The vaccine is now ready for use by the following method. For the best results, be sure to follow the directions carefully.

Intraocular Administration: For chickens four weeks of age or older.

Place one full drop of vaccine into the open eye. Do not release the chicken until after it has swallowed.

Rehydration of the Vaccine (for drinking water use): Do not open and mix the vaccine until ready to begin vaccination. Use vaccine immediately after mixing.

1. Tear off the aluminum seal from the vial containing the dried vaccine.
2. Lift off the rubber stopper.
3. Carefully pour clean, cool, non-chlorinated water into the vaccine vial until the vial is approximately two-thirds full.
4. Replace the rubber stopper and shake vigorously until all the material is dissolved.
5. The vaccine is now ready for drinking water use in accordance with directions below. For best results be sure to follow directions carefully.

Drinking Water Administration: For chickens four weeks of age or older.

1. Remove all medications, sanitizers, and disinfectants from the drinking water, preferably 72 hours before vaccinating, and for 24 hours following vaccination.
2. Provide enough watering space so that at least two-thirds of the chickens can drink at one time.
3. Scrub waterers thoroughly and rinse with fresh, clean water.
4. Withhold water for 2 hours before vaccinating to stimulate thirst.
5. Rehydrate the vaccine as directed above.
6. Add the rehydrated vaccine to clean, cool, non-chlorinated water and mix in accordance with the following chart:

Age of Chickens	For each 1,000 doses add to this amount of water
4-8 weeks	5 gal. (19 L)
Over 8 weeks	10 gal. (38 L)

7. Distribute the solution, as prepared above, among the waterers provided for the chickens. Avoid placing the waterers in direct sunlight.
8. Provide no other drinking water until all of the vaccine treated water has been consumed.

Precaution(s): Store vaccine in refrigerator under 45°F (7°C). Use entire contents of each vial when first opened. Burn containers and all unused contents.

Caution(s): Only vaccinate healthy chickens.

Consult your poultry pathologist for further recommendations based on conditions existing in your area at any given time.

The vaccination program for replacement pullets should not be started after chickens are 16 weeks of age.

Chickens should not be placed on contaminated premises. Exposure should be avoided immediately after vaccination because it takes up to 10 days to develop resistance.

All susceptible chickens on the same premises should be vaccinated at the same time. If this is not possible, then strict isolation and separate caretakers should be employed for non-vaccinated units. Efforts should be taken to reduce stressful conditions at the time the vaccine is administered.

Notice: All Schering-Plough Animal Health vaccines released for sale meet the requirements of the licensing authority (U.S. Department of Agriculture) in regard to safety, purity, potency and the capacity to immunize normal, susceptible chickens.

The capacity of this vaccine to produce satisfactory results depends upon many factors including, but not limited to, conditions of storage and handling by the user, administration of the vaccine, health and responsiveness of individual animals and the degree of field exposure. Therefore, directions for use should be followed carefully.

The use of this vaccine is subject to applicable state and federal laws and regulations.

Warning(s): Do not vaccinate within 21 days before slaughter.

Newcastle Disease virus can cause inflammation of the eyelids of humans, lasting two or three days. The user should avoid contaminating hands, eyes and clothing with this vaccine.

Discussion: Vaccination Programs: Many factors must be considered in determining the proper vaccination program for a particular farm or poultry operation. To be fully effective, the vaccine must be administered to healthy receptive chickens held in a proper environment under good management. In addition, the response may be modified by the age of the chickens and their immune status. Seldom does one vaccination under field conditions produce complete protection for all individuals in a given flock. The amount of protection required will vary with the type of operation and the degree of exposure that a flock is likely to encounter. For these reasons, a program of periodic revaccination may be required.

Presentation: Intraocular or drinking water use: 10 x 1,000 dose vials (NDC 0138-5112-01). Drinking water use: 10 x 2,500 dose (NDC 0138-5112-05) and 10 x 10,000 dose vials (NDC 0138-5112-02).

Compendium Code No.: 11020281 0029R9 / 0028R2 / 0031R4

POLYBRON® N-63

ASL **Vaccine**

Newcastle Bronchitis Vaccine, B_1 Type, LaSota Strain, Mass. & Conn. Types, Live Virus

U.S. Vet. Lic. No.: 226

Description: POLYBRON® N-63 is formulated from carefully selected strains of infectious bronchitis viruses of Mass. and Conn. types (Polybron®), and the LaSota Strain of Newcastle virus. The viruses are grown under exacting standards of quality control in eggs produced by healthy chickens in closely supervised flocks.

Gentamicin is added as a preservative.

Indications: POLYBRON® N-63 is recommended for initial vaccination of chickens, broilers and replacement chickens, by intraocular or drinking water methods of application against Newcastle disease and infectious bronchitis (Mass. and Conn. types) 4 weeks of age or older.

POLYBRON® N-63 offers high levels of protection with mild respiratory reaction, i.e. snicking, helps stimulate susceptible chickens to develop immunity.

Dosage and Administration: Read full directions below carefully.

Rehydration of the Vaccine (for intraocular use):

Do not open and mix the vaccine until ready to begin vaccination. Use vaccine immediately after mixing.

1. Tear off the aluminum seal from the vial containing the dried vaccine.
2. Lift off the rubber stopper.
3. Remove the plastic screw-cap and applicator insert from the polyethylene bottle of diluent.
4. Pour a small amount of diluent into vial of dried vaccine.
5. Put back the rubber stopper and shake.
6. Pour the partly dissolved vaccine into the bottle containing the rest of the diluent.
7. Replace the plastic applicator insert and screw-cap and shake vigorously until all material is dissolved. Use applicator insert for intraocular administration.

The vaccine is now ready for use by the following method.

Intraocular Administration: For chickens 4 weeks of age or older.

Place one full drop of vaccine into the open eye. Do not release the chicken until after it has swallowed.

Rehydration of the Vaccine (for drinking water use):

Do not open and mix the vaccine until ready to begin vaccination. Use vaccine immediately after mixing.

1. Tear off the aluminum seal from the vial containing the dried vaccine.
2. Lift off the rubber stopper.
3. Carefully pour clean, cool, non-chlorinated water into the vaccine vial until the vial is approximately two-thirds full.
4. Put back the rubber stopper and shake vigorously until all the material is dissolved.
5. The vaccine is now ready for drinking water use in accordance with directions below. For best results be sure to follow directions carefully.

Drinking Water Administration:

1. Remove all medications, sanitizers, and disinfectants from the drinking water, preferably 72 hours before vaccinating, and for 24 hours following vaccination.
2. Provide enough watering space so that at least two-thirds of the chickens can drink at one time.
3. Scrub waterers thoroughly and rinse with fresh, clean water.
4. Withhold water for 2 hours before vaccinating to stimulate thirst.
5. Rehydrate the vaccine as directed above.
6. Add rehydrated vaccine to clean, cool, non-chlorinated water and mix in accordance with the following chart:

Age of Chickens	1,000 Doses added to this amount of water
4 to 8 weeks	5 gal. (18.9 L)
8 weeks or older	10 gal. (37.9 L)

7. Distribute the vaccine solution, as prepared above, among the waterers provided for the chickens. Avoid placing waterers in direct sunlight.
8. Provide no other drinking water until all the vaccine treated water has been consumed.

Precaution(s): Store vaccine in refrigerator under 45°F (7°C). Use entire contents of each vial when first opened. Burn containers and all unused contents.

Caution(s): Only vaccinate healthy chickens.

Consult your poultry pathologist for further recommendations based on conditions existing in your area at any given time.

Different vaccines should not be mixing for single application.

The vaccination program for replacement pullets should not be started after chickens are 15 weeks of age.

Chickens should not be placed on contaminated premises. Exposure should be avoided immediately following vaccination because it takes up to 10 days to develop resistance.

All susceptible chickens on the premises should be vaccinated at the same time. If this is not possible, then strict isolation and separate caretakers should be employed for non-vaccinated units. Efforts should be taken to reduce stress conditions at the time the vaccine is administered.

Notice: All Schering-Plough Animal Health vaccines released for sale meet the requirements of the licensing authority (U.S. Department of Agriculture) in regard to safety, purity, potency and the capacity to immunize normal, susceptible chickens.

The capacity of this vaccine to produce satisfactory results depends on many factors including, but not limited to, conditions of storage and handling by the user, administration of the vaccine, health and responsiveness of individual animals and degree of field exposure. Therefore, directions for use should be followed carefully.

The use of this vaccine is subject to applicable state and federal laws and regulations.

Warning(s): Do not vaccinate within 21 days before slaughter.

Newcastle Disease virus can cause inflammation of the eyelids of humans, lasting two or three days. The user should avoid contaminating hands, eyes or clothing with this vaccine.

Discussion: Vaccination Programs: Many factors must be considered in determining the proper vaccination program for a particular farm or poultry operation. To be fully effective, the vaccine must be administered to healthy receptive chickens held in a proper environment under good management. In addition, the response may be modified by the age of the chickens and their immune status. Seldom does one vaccination under field conditions produce complete protection for all individuals in a given flock. The amount of protection required will vary with the type of operation and the degree of exposure that a flock is likely to encounter. For these reasons, a program of periodic revaccination may be required.

Presentation: Intraocular or drinking water use: 10 x 1,000 dose vials (NDC 0138-5113-01). Drinking water use: 10 x 2,500 dose (NDC 0138-5113-04) and 10 x 10,000 dose vials (NDC 0138-5113-02).

Compendium Code No.: 11020291 0049R4 / 0048 / 0160R4

POLYDINE™ SPRAY

First Priority **Disinfectant**

Broad Spectrum Topical Antiseptic Microbicide

Active Ingredient(s): This product contains polydine complex yielding 1% titratable iodine.

Indications: POLYDINE™ Spray aids in the treatment and prevention of bacterial and fungal skin infections common to animals. Kills gram-negative and gram-positive bacteria, fungi, viruses, protozoa, and yeasts. Film-forming, virtually non-irritating and non-staining to skin, hair, and natural fabrics. Mild enough for everyday use.

Directions: Apply full strength as often as needed (two or three times daily). Wet area thoroughly with POLYDINE™ Spray to insure complete coverage and penetration, but avoid pooling. May be covered with bandage if necessary.

Precaution(s): Avoid storing at excessive heat.

Caution(s): Avoid contact with eyes. May be harmful if swallowed. In case of deep or puncture wounds or serious burns, consult a veterinarian. If irritation or infection persists or increases, discontinue use and consult a veterinarian.

For animal use only.

Warning(s): Keep out of reach of children.

Presentation: 8 fl oz (240 mL), 16 fl oz (473 mL) with trigger sprayer and 1 gallon (3.785 L).

POLYDINE is a trademark of First Priority, Inc.

Compendium Code No.: 11390632 Rev. 2-97

POLYFLEX® ℞

Fort Dodge **Ampicillin Injection**

(Ampicillin for Injectable Suspension, Veterinary) for Aqueous Injection

NADA No.: 055-030

Active Ingredient(s): Each vial contains:

Ampicillin . . . . 10 g or 25 g

Indications: POLYFLEX® has proved effective in the treatment of many infections previously beyond the spectrum of penicillin therapy. This drug is particularly indicated in the treatment of the following infections caused by susceptible strains of organisms:

Dogs and Cats:

Respiratory tract infections: Upper respiratory infections, tonsillitis and bronchopneumonia due to hemolytic streptococci, *Staphylococcus aureus, Escherichia coli, Proteus mirabilis*, and *Pasteurella* spp.

Urinary tract infections due to *Proteus mirabilis, Escherichia coli, Staphylococcus* spp., hemolytic streptococci and *Enterococcus* spp.

Gastrointestinal infections due to *Enterococcus* spp., *Staphylococcus* spp. and *Escherichia coli*.

Skin, soft-tissue and post-surgical infections: Abscesses, pustular dermatitis, cellulitis and infections of the anal gland, due to *Escherichia coli, Proteus mirabilis*, hemolytic streptococci, *Staphylococcus* spp. and *Pasteurella* spp.

Cattle and calves including non-ruminating (veal calves):

Respiratory tract infections: Bacterial pneumonia (shipping fever, calf pneumonia, and bovine pneumonia) caused by *Aerobacter* spp., *Klebsiella* spp., *Staphylococcus* spp., *Streptococcus* spp., *Pasteurella multocida* and *E. coli* susceptible to ampicillin trihydrate.

Pharmacology:

Description: POLYFLEX® (ampicillin for injectable suspension, veterinary) is a broad-spectrum penicillin which has bactericidal activity against a wide range of common gram-positive and gram-negative bacteria.

Action: The antimicrobial action of ampicillin is bactericidal, and only a small percentage of the antibiotic is serum-bound. Peak serum levels in dogs and cats are reached approximately one-half hour following subcutaneous or intramuscular injection, and in cattle 1 hour to 2 hours following intramuscular injection.

In vitro studies have demonstrated sensitivity of the following organisms to ampicillin: gram-positive bacteria - alpha- and beta-hemolytic streptococci, staphylococci (non-penicillinase-producing), *Bacillus anthracis* and most strains of enterococci and clostridia; gram-negative bacteria - *Proteus mirabilis, E. coli* and many strains of Salmonella and *Pasteurella multocida*.

The drug does not resist destruction by penicillinase and, hence, is not effective against strains of staphylococci resistant to penicillin G. Susceptibility tests should be conducted to estimate the *in vitro* susceptibility of bacterial isolates to ampicillin.

Dosage and Administration:

Dosage:

The dosage of POLYFLEX® will vary according to the animal being treated, the severity of the infection and the animal's response.

Dogs and Cats - The recommended dose for dogs or cats is 3 mg/lb of body weight administered twice daily by subcutaneous or intramuscular injection.

Cattle and calves including non-ruminating (veal calves) - From 2 mg to 5 mg/lb of body weight once daily by intramuscular injection. Do not treat for more than 7 days.

In all species, 3 days treatment is usually adequate, but treatment should be continued for 48 to 72 hours after the animal has become afebrile or asymptomatic.

Directions for use:

The multiple-dose dry-filled vials should be reconstituted to the desired concentration by adding the required amount of sterile water for injection, USP, according to label directions.

After reconstitution this product is stable for 12 months under refrigeration or for 1 month at 25°C and will be white to pale yellow in color.

At the time of reconstitution the vial should be dated and the concentration noted on the label.

Contraindication(s): A history of allergic reactions to penicillin, cephalosporins or their analogues should be considered a contraindication for the use of this agent.

Precaution(s): Store at controlled room temperature 15° to 30°C (59° to 86°F).

Because it is a derivative of 6-aminopenicillanic acid, POLYFLEX® has the potential for producing allergic reactions. If they should occur, POLYFLEX® should be discontinued and the subject treated with the usual agents (antihistamines, pressor amines, corticosteroids).

Caution(s): Federal law restricts this drug to use by or on the order of a licensed veterinarian.

Warning(s): Do not treat for more than 7 days.

Milk from treated cows must not be used for food during treatment, or for 48 hours (4 milkings) after the last treatment.

Treated animals must not be slaughtered for food during treatment, or for 144 hours (6 days) after the last treatment.

Presentation: POLYFLEX® (ampicillin for injectable suspension, veterinary).

For aqueous injection - Vials containing 10 g and 25 g ampicillin activity as ampicillin trihydrate.

NDC 0856-2717-52 - 10 g vial

NDC 0856-2717-53 - 25 g vial

Compendium Code No.: 10031471 4470H

POLYLITES IV

Butler **Electrolytes-Oral**

Active Ingredient(s): Contains: Sodium chloride, sodium citrate, potassium chloride, calcium lactate, magnesium citrate and dextrose.

Indications: For oral administration to cattle as a source of supplemental electrolytes during periods of stress, such as during and immediately following shipping; during disease and convalescence, when the animal's normal intake of feed and water is reduced.

Dosage and Administration: For oral use, dissolve in the drinking water at the rate of 8 oz. in approximately 20 gallons of drinking water.

Directions for Intravenous Use: For making parenteral solutions - representing in mEq/L: Na^+ 140, K^+ 10, Ca^{++} 5, Mg^{++} 3, Cl^- 103, HCO_3^- (after metabolic conversion) 55, in 5% dextrose solution - dissolve aseptically in 4,000 mL of water for injection in a clean container suitable for heat sterilization (or 8-500 mL serum bottles). Stopper loosely and boil for at least 30 minutes or autoclave for 20 minutes at 15 lbs. p.s.i. (250°F). Seal the stoppers and allow the bottles to cool at room temperature. Use promptly.

Note: If turbid, the solution becomes clear on boiling or standing a few minutes.

Large animals receive intravenously up to 4,000 mL (approx. 1 gallon) of the finished solution as indicated by the degree of dehydration. The treatment may be repeated according to clinical judgment.

Precaution(s): Store at room temperature and protect from light.

Avoid excessive heat (104°F).

Caution(s): For veterinarians only.

Keep out of the reach of children.

Presentation: 8 oz. containers.

Compendium Code No.: 10821480

POLYMAG™ BOLUS

Butler **Antacid-Laxative**

Active Ingredient(s): Each bolus contains:

Magnesium Hydroxide . . . . 90 gr.

With Other Ingredients: dl-methionine, yeast autolysate, ginger, capsicum, cobalt sulfate, FD&C color, pharmaceutic aids, excipients, q.s.

Indications: A mild laxative and antacid for oral use in mild digestive upsets in cattle.

Dosage and Administration: Orally 2 to 4 boluses, depending upon size and condition of animal. Repeat as necessary. Allow access to clean, fresh drinking water at all times.

Precaution(s): Store at room temperature.

Protect from heat and moisture.

Warning(s): For animal use only.

Not for human use.

Keep out of reach of children.

Presentation: 50 boluses.

Compendium Code No.: 10821500

POLYMUNE™

V.D.I. **Plasma**

Normal Plasma, Equine Origin

U.S. Vet. Lic. No.: 360

Active Ingredient(s): Normal plasma, equine origin. The plasma does not contain preservatives, and the donors used have been found free of hemolysins and agglutinins against 32 of the main antigens in blood groups A, C, D, K, P, Q and U. Donors have also tested negative for EIA, EVA, dourine, piroplasmosis, brucellosis, glanders, Potomac horse fever and Lyme disease.

Indications: Normal equine plasma can be administered in the following situations:

1. Intravenously to foals with hypogammaglobulinemia.
2. Intravenously to horses of any age with hypoproteinemia and/or hypovolemia.

Dosage and Administration: Only for use in horses by a licensed veterinarian.

The plasma should be kept frozen until required. It should be thawed using only warm water and then warmed to body temperature. Plasma can be damaged by thawing in microwaves. Administer by slow filtered intravenous infusion.

The dosage is based on systemic immunoglobulin G levels of plasma recipients, verified by immunodiffusion or equivalent testing before and after administration, or based upon experience resulting from past testing in similar circumstances. The usual dose is from 1 to 2 L, but caution should be taken to avoid volume overload.

Caution(s): The product is frozen immediately after collection and is not pasteurized. The transmission of viral diseases is possible with the administration of any blood product, as is the development of serum sickness, but these are rare occurrences using plasma in equidae.

Side Effects: Complications are very infrequent, but may include mild reactions such as tachypnea and trembling. If these symptoms become severe and also include sweating and excessive shaking, it is advisable to slow the rate of administration or to stop and restart in 5-10 minutes. If the symptoms recur or persist, discontinue administration.
Discussion: High levels of antibodies are maintained by immunization against: *E. coli* (J5) and *Salmonella typhimurium* (endotoxemia), *Rhodococcus equi, Clostridium botulinum* types B and C, rhinopneumonitis, encephalitis, tetanus, strangles and rotavirus infections.
Presentation: 950 mL bags.
Compendium Code No.: 11280080

POLYMUNE-J™

V.D.I. **Plasma**

Escherichia coli Plasma, Equine Origin
CA Vet. Biol. Lic. No.: 100
Active Ingredient(s): The plasma does not contain preservatives, and the donors used have been found free of hemolysins and agglutinins against 32 of the main antigens in blood groups A, C, D, K, B, Q and U. Donors have also tested negative for EIA, EVA, dourine, piroplasmosis, brucellosis, glanders, Potomac horse fever and Lyme disease.
Indications: *E. coli* (J-5) plasma can be administered to modulate the immune response to endotoxic shock associated with gram-negative infections.
Dosage and Administration: The plasma should be kept frozen until required. It should be thawed using only warm water and then warmed to body temperature. Administer by slow filtered intravenous infusion. Do not mix with anything or transfer into another container. The usual dosage for a foal is 1-2 L and in an adult 2-4 L.
Caution(s): The product is frozen immediately after collection and is not pasteurized. The transmission of viral diseases is possible with the administration of any blood product, but this is a rare occurrence using plasma in horses.
For use in horses only by a licensed veterinarian.
Side Effects: Complications are infrequent but may include mild reactions such as tachypnea and trembling. If these symptoms become severe and also include sweating and shaking, it is advisable to slow the rate of administration or stop and restart in 5-10 minutes. If the symptoms persist, discontinue the use of the product.
Presentation: 950 mL bags.
Compendium Code No.: 11280070

POLYMUNE™ PLUS

V.D.I. **Plasma**

Normal Plasma, Equine Origin
U.S. Vet. Lic. No.: 360
Active Ingredient(s): Normal plasma, equine origin containing an IgG level of 2,600 mg/dL. The plasma does not contain preservatives, and donors used have been found free of hemolysins and agglutinins against 32 of the main antigens in blood groups A, C, D, K, P, Q and U. Donors have also tested negative for EIA, EVA, dourine, piroplasmosis, brucellosis, glanders, Potomac horse fever and Lyme disease.
Indications: Normal equine plasma can be administered in the following situations:
1. Intravenously to foals with hypogammaglobulinemia.
2. Intravenously to horses of any age with hypoproteinemia and/or hypovolemia.

Dosage and Administration: Only for use in horses by a licensed veterinarian.
The plasma should be kept frozen until required. It should be thawed using only warm water and then warmed to body temperature. Plasma can be damaged by thawing in microwaves. Administer by slow filtered intravenous infusion.
The dosage is based on systemic immunoglobulin G levels of plasma recipients, verified by immunodiffusion or equivalent testing before and after administration, or based upon experience resulting from past testing in similar circumstances. The usual dose is from 600-1,000 mL, but caution should be taken to avoid volume overload.
Caution(s): The product is frozen immediately after collection and is not pasteurized. The transmission of viral diseases is possible with the administration of any blood product, as is the development of serum sickness, but these are rare occurrences using plasma in equidae.
Side Effects: Complications are very infrequent, but may include mild reactions such as tachypnea and trembling. If these symptoms become severe and also include sweating and excessive shaking, it is advisable to slow the rate of administration or to stop and restart in 5-10 minutes. If the symptoms recur or persist, discontinue administration.
Discussion: High levels of antibodies are maintained by immunization against: *E. coli* (J5) and *Salmonella typhimurium* (endotoxemia), *Rhodococcus equi, Clostridium botulinum* types B and C, rhinopneumonitis, encephalitis, tetanus, strangles and rotavirus infections.
Presentation: 600 mL and 950 mL bags.
Compendium Code No.: 11280090

POLYOTIC® SOLUBLE POWDER

Fort Dodge **Water Medication**

Tetracycline Hydrochloride-Antibiotic
NADA No.: 065-269
Active Ingredient(s): This packet contains 10 grams of Polyotic tetracycline hydrochloride (25 g/lb).
Indications: For veterinary use in drinking water.
Calves: Control and treatment of bacterial enteritis (scours) caused by *Escherichia coli* and bacterial pneumonia associated with *Pasteurella* spp., *Actinobacillus pleuropneumoniae* (*Haemophilus* spp.) and *Klebsiella* spp. susceptible to tetracycline hydrochloride.
Swine: Control and treatment of bacterial enteritis (scours) caused by *Escherichia coli* and bacterial pneumonia associated with *Pasteurella* spp., *Actinobacillus pleuropneumoniae* (*Haemophilus* spp.) and *Klebsiella* spp. susceptible to tetracycline hydrochloride.
Dosage and Administration: Dosage:
Calves: 10 mg/lb body weight daily (1 packet will treat five 200-lb calves). Administer 3 to 5 days.
Swine: 10 mg/lb body weight daily (1 packet will treat ten 100-lb pigs). Administer 3 to 5 days.
Administration: As a generalization, these animals will consume approximately 1 gallon per 100 lbs body weight per day. At this rate, solutions containing 1 gram of tetracycline hydrochloride per gallon (1 packet per 10 gallons), as the only source of water, will provide the proper dose. However, variations in age and environmental temperature affect water consumption, and the concentration of the solution should be adjusted appropriately to compensate for the variation observed in individual situations. Alternatively, the Soluble Powder may be administered to calves as a drench to provide 10 mg tetracycline hydrochloride per pound body weight daily in divided doses.
General Note on Dosage: If no improvement is noted in 3-5 days, consult a veterinarian.
Precaution(s): Store at controlled room temperature, 15° to 30°C (59° to 86°F).
Caution(s): Prepare fresh solutions daily. Administer at this rate in the total water consumed over a full 24-hour period.
Warning(s):
Calves: Do not administer this product with milk or milk replacers. Administer 1 hour before or 2 hours after feeding milk or milk replacers. Do not administer to calves within 4 days of slaughter. Use as sole source of tetracyclines.
A withdrawal period has not been established for this product in pre-ruminating calves. Do not use in calves to be processed for veal.
Swine: Do not administer this product with milk or milk replacers. Administer 1 hour before or 2 hours after feeding milk or milk replacers. Do not administer to swine within 7 days of slaughter. Use as sole source of tetracycline.
Presentation: 6.4 oz (181.4 g) packets.
Manufactured by: PM Resources, Inc., Bridgeton, MO 63044
Compendium Code No.: 10032631 6651B

POLYOX® POWDER

Bimeda **Antacid-Laxative**

Active Ingredient(s): Each package contains:
Magnesium hydroxide. . . . . 106 g
Other Ingredients: Cobalt sulfate, african ginger, capsicum, yeast autolysate, DL-methionine, color, and other inert ingredients.
Indications: A mild laxative and antacid for use in digestive upsets in cattle.
Dosage and Administration: Cattle: Give one-half (½) to one (1) package (6 to 12 oz.), diluted in one (1) gallon of water by a stomach tube, depending upon the size and condition of the animal. Repeat as necessary.
Warning(s): For animal use only. Not for human use. Keep out of reach of children.
Presentation: 12 oz. (340 g) pouch.
Compendium Code No.: 13990340

POLYOX® II BOLUS

AgriPharm **Antacid-Laxative**

Active Ingredient(s): Each Bolus Contains:
Magnesium hydroxide. . . . . 90 gr
Other Ingredients: DL-Methionine; Yeast Autolysate; Ginger; Capsicum; Cobalt Sulfate; color; other inert ingredients.
Indications: A mild laxative and antacid indicated for use in mild digestive upsets in cattle.
Directions: Dosage: Administer orally, 2 to 4 boluses, depending upon the size and condition of the animal. Repeat as indicated.
Warning(s): For animal use only. Not for human use. Keep out of reach of children.
Presentation: 50 boluses per jar.
®POLYOX is a Registered Trademark of Bimeda, Inc.
Compendium Code No.: 14571230 Iss. 06-00

POLYOX® II BOLUS

Bimeda **Antacid-Laxative**

Active Ingredient(s): Each bolus contains:
Magnesium hydroxide. . . . . 90 gr.
Other Ingredients: DL-methionine, yeast autolysate, ginger, capsicum, cobalt sulfate, color, and other inert ingredients.
Indications: A mild laxative and antacid indicated for use in mild digestive upsets in cattle.
Dosage and Administration: Administer orally, two (2) to four (4) boluses, depending upon the size and condition of the animal. Repeat as indicated.
Warning(s): For animal use only. Not for human use. Keep out of reach of children.
Presentation: 50 boluses per jar.
Compendium Code No.: 13990330

POLY SERUM®

Novartis Animal Vaccines **Antiserum**

Actinomyces pyogenes-Escherichia coli-Pasteurella haemolytica-Pasteurella multocida-Salmonella typhimurium Antiserum, Bovine Origin
U.S. Vet. Lic. No.: 303
Composition: The antiserum is prepared from the blood of cattle hyperimmunized with *Actinomyces pyogenes, Escherichia coli, Pasteurella haemolytica, Pasteurella multocida*, and *Salmonella typhimurium*.
The antiserum contains phenol and thimerosal as preservatives.
Indications: For use as an aid in the prevention and treatment of enteric and respiratory conditions in cattle and sheep caused by *Actinomyces pyogenes, Escherichia coli, Pasteurella haemolytica, Pasteurella multocida* and *Salmonella typhimurium*.
Dosage and Administration: Shake well before using. Administer the following doses subcutaneously or intramuscularly:

	Prevention	Treatment
Calves (as soon after birth as possible)*	20-40 mL	40-100 mL
Cattle	50-75 mL	75-150 mL
Sheep	10-15 mL	20-40 mL

*In several locations, not more than 15 mL per site.
The recommended dose for treatment is to be administered at 12-24 hour intervals until improvement is noted.
Precaution(s): Store in the dark at 35°-45°F (2°-7°C). Do not freeze. Use the entire contents when first opened.
Caution(s): Anaphylactic reactions may occur following the use of the product. Symptomatic treatment: Epinephrine. For veterinary use only.
Warning(s): Do not vaccinate within 21 days of slaughter.
Discussion: Infectious enteritis (scours) and pneumonia are the two most common causes of death in calves of less than one month of age. Calf scours is the number one killer of calves of less than 10 days of age, while pneumonia causes most of the deaths in calves between three and sixteen weeks of age.
Neonatal Diarrhea (scours or enteritis): Despite advances in sanitation, vaccinations, and antibiotics, baby calf scours caused by *Escherichia coli* (colibacillosis) is still the number one killer of newborn calves. It causes 50% of deaths in newborn dairy calves and 75% of deaths in beef calves.

Preventing calf scours requires management of the cow, the environment, and the calves. Immunizing the cow with a bacterin can be very beneficial, but a heifer or young cow's immune capacity may not be developed enough to provide her calf with adequate protection through colostrum and milk antibodies. Treatment of *E. coli* scours can be costly, time-consuming, and may be too late. *Salmonella typhimurium* can be a contributing factor to *E. coli* scours or may cause severe diarrhea by itself. *Salmonella typhimurium* scours are most commonly seen on dairy farms or calf-raising operations. The disease usually does not occur in calves of less than two weeks of age. However, it has been reported in beef calves on pasture and in calves less than one week old. The disease can also progress to a septicemia (blood infection) causing meningitis, arthritis, or pneumonia. Calves that survive Salmonella infections are commonly "poor-doers".

Calf Pneumonia: Pneumonia may occur suddenly in young, normal calves and commonly occurs in calves stressed by scours. The most commonly isolated bacteria associated with calf pneumonia are *Pasteurella haemolytica, Pasteurella multocida*, and *Actinomyces pyogenes.* As with calf scours, prevention of pneumonia in calves requires management of the cow, the environment, and the calf. *Pasteurella haemolytica* and *Pasteurella multocida* are the most common bacterial causes of pneumonia in calves, especially when animals are kept in enclosed crowded conditions where ventilation is inadequate and humidity is high. *A. pyogenes* is a secondary invader found in chronic pneumonia cases. Cows may provide inadequate levels of protection against Pasteurella and Actinomyces in their colostrum and milk. This leaves the young calf susceptible to these infectious agents. Signs of calf pneumonia include rapid breathing, a cough, and nasal discharge. Body temperature may be elevated above the normal 101°F to 103°F or higher. Affected calves are frequently depressed and have poor appetites. Once signs appear, treatment may be too late or the calf may suffer permanent damage to its respiratory system.

Presentation: Available in 250 mL bottles.

Compendium Code No.: 11140303

PORCINE ECOLIZER® 3

Novartis Animal Vaccines **Antiserum**

Escherichia coli Antiserum, Equine Origin

U.S. Vet. Lic. No.: 303

Composition: This antiserum is prepared from the blood of horses hyperimmunized with K88, K99, and 987P piliated *Escherichia coli.* Contains oxytetracycline, phenol, and thimerosal as preservatives.

Indications: For use in newborn piglets as an aid in the prevention of colibacillosis caused by K88, K99, and 987P piliated *Escherichia coli*.

Dosage and Administration: Shake well before using. Administer 2 mL orally to piglets less than 12 hours old. Slowly syringe toward the back of the piglet's mouth. Colostrum should be fed to each piglet.

Precaution(s): Store in the dark at 35°-45°F (2°-7°C). Do not freeze. Use entire contents when first opened.

Caution(s): Anaphylactic reactions may occur following the use of this biological. Symptomatic treatment: Epinephrine.

Warning(s): Do not administer within 21 days prior to slaughter.

Discussion: Despite advances in sanitation, vaccination and antibiotics, baby pig scours caused by *Escherichia coli* (colibacillosis) is still the number one problem in the farrowing house. Colibacillosis accounts for 42% of all death losses nationwide in growing pigs. Approximately 22.5% of all pigs farrowed are infected with colibacillosis.

Preventing baby pig scours requires careful management of the sow, the environment, and the piglets. The problem is two-fold. First, a gilt's immune capacity is not developed enough to provide adequate piglet protection through colostrum and milk antibodies. The second problem stems from litter size. A sow normally farrows a large number of offspring. The first eight or so piglets farrowed absorb all the passive immunity a sow has to offer through her colostrum. Subsequent piglets don't receive enough colostrum protection and may become colostrum deprived.

The colostrum deprived piglets become very susceptible to colibacillosis unless they receive passive antibody protection from another source. Once infected, the colostrum deprived piglets shed enteropathogenic *E. coli* organisms into the environment. Even the colostrum protected piglet's immunity is overcome and the entire litter breaks with scours.

Trial Data: PORCINE ECOLIZER® 3 Challenge Trial (37% less death loss):

	% Mortality			Avg. Total Clinical Score			Avg. Daily Weight Gain (lbs)		
	K99	K88	987P	K99	K88	987P	K99	K88	987P
Controls	48	60	32	18.6	19.0	13.5	+0.11	+0.02	+0.22
Ecolizer Treatment	0	18	11	0.78	7.0	7.5	+0.36	+0.25	+0.26

Efficacy Study: Following severe challenges in 3 groups of piglets (K88, K99, 987P), the average death loss in the treatment groups was only 9% compared to 46% in controls. The treatment groups also showed twice the weight gain with average daily weight gains of .29 lbs compared to only .11 lbs in the control groups (data on file with USDA).

Presentation: Available in a 50 dose (100 mL) bottle and 100 dose (200 mL) pump bottle.

Compendium Code No.: 11140312

PORCINE ECOLIZER® 3+C

Novartis Animal Vaccines **Antibodies**

Clostridium perfringens Type C Antitoxin-Escherichia coli Antiserum, Equine Origin

U.S. Vet. Lic. No.: 303

Composition: This product contains antibodies against *Clostridium perfringens* Type C and K88, K99, and 987P piliated *Escherichia coli.* Contains oxytetracycline, phenol, and thimerosal as preservatives.

Indications: For use in newborn piglets as an aid in the prevention of disease caused by *Clostridium perfringens* Type C and K88, K99 and 987P piliated *Escherichia coli.*

Dosage and Administration:

100 mL bottle: Shake well before using. Administer 2 mL orally to piglets less than 6 hours old. Slowly syringe toward the back of the piglet's mouth. Colostrum should be fed to each piglet.

200 mL bottle: Shake well before using. Insert dispenser into bottle. Place dispenser extender on nozzle. Administer 2 mL (1 pump stroke) orally to piglets less than 6 hours old. Slowly dispense toward the back of the piglet's mouth. Colostrum should be fed to each piglet.

Precaution(s): Store in the dark at 35°-45°F (2°-7°C). Do not freeze. Use entire contents when first opened.

Caution(s): Anaphylactic reactions may occur following the use of this biological. Symptomatic treatment: Epinephrine.

Warning(s): Do not administer within 21 days prior to slaughter.

Discussion: Despite advances in sanitation, vaccination and antibiotics, baby pig scours caused by *Escherichia coli* (colibacillosis) is still the number one problem in the farrowing house. Colibacillosis accounts for 42% of all death losses nationwide in growing pigs. Approximately 22.5% of all pigs farrowed are infected with colibacillosis.

Preventing baby pig scours requires careful management of the sow, the environment, and the piglets. The problem is two-fold. First, a gilt's immune capacity is not developed enough to provide adequate piglet protection through colostrum and milk antibodies. The second problem stems from litter size. A sow normally farrows a large number of offspring. The first eight or so piglets farrowed absorb all the passive immunity a sow has to offer through her colostrum. Subsequent piglets don't receive enough colostrum protection and may become colostrum deprived.

The colostrum deprived piglets become very susceptible to colibacillosis unless they receive passive antibody protection from another source. Once infected, the colostrum deprived piglets shed enteropathogenic *E. coli* organisms into the environment. Even the colostrum protected piglet's immunity is overcome and the entire litter breaks with scours.

Type C enterotoxemia is caused by an intestinal overgrowth of *Clostridium perfringens* Type C which produces primarily beta and some alpha exotoxins. *Clostridium perfringens* Type C is widely distributed in the soil and is a common inhabitant of the intestinal tract. It multiplies rapidly in the small intestine when conditions are suitable.

Piglets from one to ten days old may be found dead without previously showing symptoms. Symptoms seen in affected animals include abdominal pain, diarrhea (sometimes blood-tinged), depression, and cessation of nursing.

Engorgement with milk is considered a predisposing factor for enterotoxemia. It is believed that a large intake of milk may slow the digestive process, allowing the clostridial bacteria time to multiply. In addition, the proteolytic enzyme trypsin, which can inactivate the beta toxin, may not be present in adequate concentrations under these circumstances. It is usually the healthy, vigorous offspring of high-producing mothers which are affected by the disease.

Postmortem lesions vary according to the predominating type of exotoxin. If alpha toxin predominates, there will be extensive hemorrhage in the jejunum and ileum as well as in the mesenteric and intestinal lymph nodes. There will be blood-stained contents in the lower small intestine and the colon. If beta toxin predominates, there will be necrosis of the jejunum and ileum and peritonitis. Petechial hemorrhages will be found on the spleen, heart, thymus, and serosal surfaces.

Trial Data: *Clostridium perfringens* Type C Antitoxin (oral administration) *Clostridium perfringens* Type C Challenge:

Test Group	% Mortality	
Treatments	13%	2/15
Controls	77%	10/13

Porcine Ecolizer® 3 Challenge Trial (37% less death loss):

	% Mortality			Avg. Total Clinical Score			Avg. Daily Weight Gain (lbs)		
	K99	K88	987P	K99	K88	987P	K99	K88	987P
Controls	48	60	32	18.6	19.0	13.5	+0.11	+0.02	+0.22
Ecolizer Treatment	0	18	11	0.78	7.0	7.5	+0.36	+0.25	+0.26

Efficacy Study: Following severe challenges in 3 groups of piglets (K88, K99, 987P), the average death loss in the treatment groups was only 9% compared to 46% in controls. The treatment groups also showed twice the weight gain with average daily weight gains of .29 lbs compared to only .11 lbs in the control groups (data on file with USDA).

Presentation: Available in 50 dose (100 mL) bottles and 100 dose (200 mL) pump bottles.

Compendium Code No.: 11140322

PORCINE MAXIMIZER™

Novartis Animal Vaccines **Large Animal Dietary Supplement**

Active Ingredient(s): A mixture of four fatty acids.

Indications: Oxidation of fatty acids is an important source of energy in newborn piglets. MAXIMIZER™ provides an additional supply of these fatty acids, which translate to not only more pigs, but also heavier pigs at weaning.

Dosage and Administration: Piglets receive 4 mL of MAXIMIZER™ orally within the first 24 hours after birth. This is easily accomplished by incorporating it into routine newborn piglet processing.

Discussion: Newborn piglets are born with very low energy reserves; consequently, they are very susceptible to the effects of even short-term starvation. Anything that affects the piglet's delicate energy balance, whether by decreasing available energy supplies (i.e. poor-milking sows, large litters) or by increasing energy expenditures (i.e. cold ambient temperature), will produce adverse consequences in relationship to piglet survivability and well-being. In addition to the deaths directly attributable to starvation, piglets with a low energy intake quickly become weak and are likely to die from factors such as chilling and being crushed by the sow. All-in-all, these factors combine to produce a very significant profit loss to the average swine producer.

Fatty acid oxidation is an important source of energy for the piglet, and MAXIMIZER™ provides this additional energy. Providing this extra energy is essential to give newborn piglets the best possible start.

Trial Data: To demonstrate the effectiveness of MAXIMIZER™, 319 piglets were divided into two group, controls (not treated) and MAXIMIZER™-treated piglets. These two groups were further subdivided on the basis of birth weight into low-, medium- and high-birth weight groups. Both control and treated piglets were put back with their dams and held under similar conditions to avoid other variables that might affect the results. Piglets were raised to weaning (approximately 21 days of age) and then compared for differences in survivability and weaning weights.

Table 1: Relative Survival of controls versus pigs treated with MAXIMIZER™:

Birth Wt. (lbs.)	Total Pigs Evaluated	Percent survived to weaning		MAXIMIZER™ Difference
		Control	MAXIMIZER™	
<3.11	103	73	80	+7%
3.11-3.70	109	85	88	+3%
>3.70	107	92	95	+3%
All weights	319	83	88	+5%

Table 1 shows the increased survival rates obtained by treating piglets with 4 mL of MAXIMIZER™ after birth. The highest increase, 7%, was seen in the group of piglets with the lowest birth weights, but even the group with the highest birth weights showed a 3% increase in survival. The overall increase when comparing all piglets was 5%.

Table 2: Weaning weights of control versus treated pigs in various birth-weight classes:

Birth Wt. (lbs.)	# Pigs	Control Weight Lbs.	# Pigs	MAXIMIZER™ Weight Lbs.	MAXIMIZER™ Advantage (lbs.)
<3.11	38	9.68	41	10.03	+0.35
3.11-3.70	50	11.13	44	11.88	+0.75
>3.70	45	11.74	55	12.60	+0.86
All weights	133	10.92	140	11.62	+0.70 (P=.02)

Table 2 shows the increase in 21-day weaning weights in piglets treated with MAXIMIZER™. Although this increase was highest in the piglets with the heaviest birth weights, even the lightest pigs showed an advantage. As a whole, piglets in the treated group had a weight gain of 0.70 lbs. more than the control group.

Presentation: Available in 60 dose (240 mL) pump bottles and 960 dose (3,840 mL) jugs.

Compendium Code No.: 11140332

PORCINE PILI SHIELD™

Novartis Animal Vaccines **Bacterin**

Escherichia coli Bacterin

U.S. Vet. Lic. No.: 303

Composition: The bacterin contains all the antigens from four selected strains of *E. coli* bearing K99, K88, 987P and F41 pili. The inactivated cultures are blended to provide a broad spectrum of protection, and adjuvanted with aluminum hydroxide.

Indications: For use in healthy pregnant swine for the prevention of diseases in baby piglets caused by *Escherichia coli.*

Dosage and Administration: Administer two (2) 2 mL doses deep intramuscularly behind the ear to pregnant swine approximately five (5) and two (2) weeks prior to farrowing for maximum transfer of maternal antibodies. Revaccinate with one (1) dose, two (2) weeks before each subsequent farrowing to maintain high levels of immunity.

Precaution(s): Store at 35°-45°F (2°-7°C). Do not freeze. Use the entire contents when first opened.

Caution(s): It is essential that baby pigs receive colostrum at birth to ensure immunity. Anaphylactic reactions may occur following the use of the product. Symptomatic treatment: Epinephrine.

Warning(s): Do not vaccinate within 21 days prior to slaughter.

Discussion: Enteric colibacillosis (EC) (scours in baby pigs caused by *Escherichia coli)* is the number one killer of piglets, accounting for 42% of all death losses nationwide. Approximately 22.5% of all young pigs are infected with *E. coli.*

EC occurs typically in pigs from two to three hours of age until weaning. Pigs die from rapid dehydration resulting from the loss of body fluids in the lumen of the intestines. When death occurs quickly, the only marked post-mortem changes are a greatly expanded volume of fluid in the intestines and scours. (In very acute cases, pronounced diarrhea may not be evident because most of the fluids may be retained in the lumen of the intestines.)

Prevention of EC in pigs can be achieved by vaccination of the sow or gilt prior to farrowing and by maintaining a warm and clean environment for the baby pigs. Timely vaccination of the sow with PORCINE PILI SHIELD™ to produce the maximum output of maternal antibodies in the colostrum and milk is critical in the prevention of enteric colibacillosis. As baby pigs ingest these antibodies from both the colostrum and milk of the sow, there is a steady flow of these antibodies through their gastrointestinal tracts which will block *E. coli's* pilus attachments to the intestinal mucosa and prevent their replication.

Trial Data: PORCINE PILI SHIELD™ Challenge Trial:

	% Mortality			
	K99	K88	987P	F41
Unvaccinated Controls	49%	62%	57%	33%
PORCINE PILI SHIELD™ Vaccinates	0%	0%	14%	9%

	Average daily clinical score			
	K99	K88	987P	F41
Unvaccinated Controls	2.64	19.6	4.8	11.8
PORCINE PILI SHIELD™ Vaccinates	0.21	0.6	2.4	3.0

	Average daily weight gain			
	K99	K88	987P	F41
Unvaccinated Controls	+0.12	+0.07	-0.04	+0.15
PORCINE PILI SHIELD™ Vaccinates	+0.43	+0.33	+0.26	+0.25

Thirty (30) gilts were vaccinated with PORCINE PILI SHIELD™ - two 2 mL doses - five and two weeks prior to farrowing. Their 225 piglets were taken at farrowing and separated into four groups. Each group was challenged orally with one of the four strains (K99, K88, 987P, and F41) of virulent *E. coli.* Twenty-nine (29) gilts were not vaccinated and their 199 piglets were used as controls and challenged in the same way as the vaccinates. Each group was observed over a four-day period.

1. The average number of deaths (% mortality) in the control group was 50.25% whereas only 5.75% of the piglets from vaccinated gilts died.
2. The severity of symptoms associated with enteric colibacillosis (average daily clinical score) averaged 9.71 for the controls, contrasted with an average score of 1.55 for the protected piglets.
3. The average daily weight gain for the controls was 0.095 lbs./day compared with 0.318 lbs./day for the protected piglets.

In summary, the study showed that the piglet group which received colostrum from vaccinated gilts experienced approximately ⅑ the death losses, ⅙ the severity of clinical symptoms and 3⅓ times the daily weight gain when compared to the control piglets.

Presentation: Available in 10 dose (20 mL) or 50 dose (100 mL) bottles.

Compendium Code No.: 11140342

PORCINE PILI SHIELD™+C

Novartis Animal Vaccines **Bacterin-Toxoid**

Clostridium perfringens Type C-Escherichia coli Bacterin-Toxoid

U.S. Vet. Lic. No.: 303

Composition: PORCINE PILI SHIELD™+C is inactivated using a special process which retains maximum antigenicity.

This product contains inactivated cultures of *Clostridium perfringens* Type C and K88, K99, 987P and F41 piliated *Escherichia coli* adjuvanted with aluminum hydroxide. Contains amphotericin B, penicillin, streptomycin and thimerosal as preservatives.

Indications: For use in healthy pregnant swine as an aid in the prevention and control of diseases in piglets caused by *Clostridium perfringens* Type C and K88, K99, 987P and F41 piliated *Escherichia coli.*

Dosage and Administration: Shake well before using. Administer 2 mL intramuscularly 5 and 2 weeks prior to farrowing. Revaccinate prior to each subsequent farrowing.

Precaution(s): Store in the dark at 35°-45°F (2°-7°C). Do not freeze. Use entire contents when first opened.

Caution(s): Anaphylactic reactions may occur following the use of this biological. Symptomatic treatment: Epinephrine.

For veterinary use only.

Warning(s): Do not vaccinate within 21 days prior to slaughter.

Discussion: Colibacillosis (scours in baby pigs caused by *Escherichia coli)* is the number one killer of piglets, accounting for 42% of all death losses nationwide.

Colibacillosis occurs typically in pigs from two to three hours of age until weaning. Pigs die from rapid dehydration resulting from loss of body fluids into the intestines. In very acute cases, pronounced diarrhea may not be evident because most of the fluids are still retained in the lumen of the intestines.

Clostridium perfringens Type C enterotoxemia occurs in piglets during the first weeks of life, with death occurring 2-48 hours after the onset of symptoms. Death may occur as early as 8 hours after birth.

Pathogenic clostridia are found as normal flora of the intestinal tracts of domestic animals. These organisms can proliferate rapidly and secrete a potent necrotizing toxin. Clinical signs in the piglet are depression, dehydration, and diarrhea that is often bloody. Pathological signs are hemorrhagic or necrotizing enteritis principally affecting the jejunum.

Vaccination of the sow with PORCINE PILI SHIELD™+C will produce protective maternal antibodies in the colostrum and milk which are so critical in the prevention of colibacillosis and enterotoxemia caused by Type C. As baby pigs ingest these antibodies from the colostrum and milk of the sow, there is a steady flow of the antibodies through their gastrointestinal tracts which will block *E. coli's* pilus attachments to the intestinal mucosa and prevent their replication and will protect against both the bacteria and the toxin of *Clostridium perfringens* Type C.

Trial Data: *Clostridium perfringens* Type C Trial Data: Eighty-three percent of piglets from vaccinated gilts survived challenge with *Clostridium perfringens* Type C toxin. In contrast, none of the piglets from nonvaccinated gilts survived challenge, indicating the effectiveness of vaccinating the dam in the prevention of enterotoxemia caused by *Cl. perfringens* Type C.

E. coli Trial Data: Two hundred twenty-five piglets from 30 vaccinated gilts were taken at farrowing and separated into four groups. Each group was challenged orally with one of four strains (K99, K88, 987P or F41) of *E. coli.* One hundred ninety-nine piglets from 29 nonvaccinated gilts were used as controls and challenged in the same way as the vaccinates. Each group was observed over a four-day period.

In summary, piglets from vaccinated gilts experienced an average of approximately only 11% of the death losses, only 17% of the severity of clinical symptoms and 333% increase in the daily weight gain when compared to control piglets. Results such as these indicate the bottom line value of using PORCINE PILI SHIELD™+C. Data on file at USDA.

Presentation: Available in 10 dose (20 mL) (F169) and 50 dose (100 mL) (F168) bottles.

Compendium Code No.: 11140352

PORIDON™

Neogen **Parasiticide-Topical**

Equine Insecticidal Pour-On

EPA Reg. No.: 72726-1

Active Ingredient(s):

Permethrin (3-phenoxyphenyl) methyl (±)-cis, trans-3-(2,2-dichloroethenyl)-2,2-dimethylcyclopropanecarboxylate† 1.84%
Piperonyl Butoxide, Technical‡ 10.00%
Inert Ingredients 88.16%
100.00%

† cis/trans ratio: Max. 55% (±) cis and Min. 45% (±) trans

‡ Equivalent to 8.0% (Butycarbityl) (6-propylpiperonyl) ether and 2.0% related compounds

Indications: For use on horses. Aids in the control of house flies, stable flies, horn flies, face flies, horse flies, deer flies, mosquitoes, gnats, lice and ticks.

Directions for Use: Shake well.

Apply approximately 2-4 oz per animal. Start by pouring a line bead from the poll, along the neck and continue posteriorly down the back parallel with the spinal column. Or apply as a wipe-on. If used as a wipe, apply with a clean absorbent cloth or sponge to animal's hair. Reapply as needed. Do not apply with bare hands. It is a violation of Federal Law to use this product in a manner inconsistent with its labeling.

Precautionary Statements: Hazards to Humans & Domestic Animals:

Warning: Harmful if swallowed, inhaled or comes in contact with skin. Avoid breathing vapors. Causes eye and skin irritation. Do not get in eyes or on skin or on clothing. Wash thoroughly with soap and water after handling. Remove contaminated clothing and wash before reuse. Wear goggles or safety glasses. In case of contact, flush with plenty of water. Get medical attention if irritation persists.

Statement of Practical Treatment:

If swallowed: Call physician or poison control center. Drink 1 or 2 glasses of water and induce vomiting by touching back of throat with finger. Do not induce vomiting or give anything by mouth to an unconscious person.

If in eyes: Flush with plenty of water. Get attention if irritation persists.

Environmental Hazards: Do not add directly to water. Do not contaminate water by cleaning of equipment or disposal of wastes.

Physical & Chemical Hazards: Flammable. Keep away from heat and open flame.

Storage and Disposal: Store in cool dry area away from heat or open flame. Do not contaminate water, food or feed by storage or disposal. Do not reuse empty container. Wrap container and put in trash.

Warning(s): Do not use on horses intended for food.

Keep out of reach of children.

Disclaimer: Limited Warranty: Neogen Corporation makes no warranty concerning uses which extend beyond the use of the product under normal conditions in accord with the statements made on the label. Neogen Corporation shall not be liable for (1) any consequential, incidental or special damages related in any way to this product or its uses, or (2) any damages related in any way to resistance to insecticides.

Presentation: 16 fl oz (473 mL) bottle.

Compendium Code No.: 14910481 2001

POSILAC 1 STEP®

Monsanto **Anabolic Agent**

(sometribove zinc suspension)

NADA No.: 140-872

Active Ingredient(s): Description: POSILAC 1 STEP® (sterile sometribove zinc suspension) is a sterile, prolonged-release injectable formulation of a recombinant DNA-derived bovine somatotropin analogue in ready to use, single-dose syringes each containing 500 mg of sometribove zinc.

Indications: POSILAC 1 STEP® is for use in healthy lactating dairy cows to increase the production of marketable milk.

Dosage and Administration: Dosage: Inject one syringe of POSILAC 1 STEP® every 14 days beginning during the 9th and 10th week after calving and continuing until the end of lactation.

Administration: Allow syringes to warm to room temperature (15° to 30°C; 59° to 86°F) before use.

Inject POSILAC 1 STEP® subcutaneously (under the skin). Recommended injection sites are in the neck area, in the postscapular region (behind the shoulder) or in the depression on either side of the tailhead. Alternate between the cow's left and right side on consecutive injections. The injection site should be free of surface debris. Inject entire contents of the syringe subcutaneously. Do not reuse syringes.

Inject directly into the deepest depressions on either side of the tailhead. Care should be taken to avoid the bone, muscles, tendons and ligaments of the tail and the rectal and anal muscles. Do not inject into the caudal tail fold. These structures to avoid can be located quickly by raising the tail.

Gather skin and inject between skin and muscle layers.

Precaution(s): Storage: Store under refrigeration (2° to 8°C; 36° to 46°F). Do not freeze. Avoid prolonged exposure to excessively high temperature and sunlight to prevent a decrease in product activity. Expiration dates are stated on the syringe and carton labeling.

Environmental Safety: Used syringes with pre-attached needles should be placed in a leak-resistant, puncture-resistant container for disposal in accordance with applicable Federal, state, and local regulations.

Caution(s): Use in lactating dairy cattle only.

Safety to replacement bulls from dairy cows injected with POSILAC 1 STEP® (sterile sometribove zinc suspension) has not been established.

To minimize injection site blemishes on the carcass at time of slaughter, avoid injections of POSILAC 1 STEP® within 2 weeks of expected slaughter.

Nutritional Management: Feed intake increases over several weeks after initiating the use of POSILAC 1 STEP®. The increase occurs earlier for first calf heifers than for second lactation or older cows. Use of POSILAC 1 STEP® may reduce the amount of body condition that is normally regained during lactation. This effect is more pronounced for second lactation or older cows. Voluntary feed intake may be increased and body condition decreased during both the dry period and subsequent early lactation.

Cows should be fed diets formulated to meet or exceed the nutritional requirements recommended by the National Research Council. Milk yield, stage of lactation, and body condition should be considered when making dietary changes. The feeding program should be managed to optimize milk yield and to have cows in appropriate body condition particularly during late lactation and the dry period. Increasing the energy density of diets fed to POSILAC-treated cows is normally not required. In general, sudden dietary changes should be avoided.

Reproduction: Use of POSILAC 1 STEP® may result in reduced pregnancy rates in injected cows and an increase in days open for first calf heifers. Cows injected with POSILAC 1 STEP® may have small decreases in gestation length and birth weight of calves. Also, the incidence of retained placenta may be higher. The use of POSILAC 1 STEP® should be preceded by implementation of a comprehensive and ongoing herd reproductive health program.

Mastitis: Cows injected with POSILAC 1 STEP® are at an increased risk for clinical mastitis (visibly abnormal milk). The number of cows affected with clinical mastitis and the number of cases per cow may increase. In addition, the risk of subclinical mastitis (milk not visibly abnormal) is increased. In some herds, the use of POSILAC 1 STEP® has been associated with increases in somatic cell counts. Mastitis management practices should be thoroughly evaluated prior to initiating the use of POSILAC 1 STEP®.

General Health: Use of POSILAC 1 STEP® is associated with an increased frequency of use of medication in cows for mastitis and other health problems.

P

Cows injected with POSILAC 1 STEP® may experience periods of increased body temperature unrelated to illness. To minimize this effect, take appropriate measures during periods of high environmental temperature to reduce heat stress. Care should be taken to differentiate increased body temperature due to the use of POSILAC 1 STEP® from an increased body temperature that may occur due to illness.

Use of POSILAC 1 STEP® may result in an increase in digestive disorders such as indigestion, bloat, and diarrhea.

There may be an increase in the number of cows experiencing periods of "off-feed" (reduced feed intake) during the use of POSILAC 1 STEP®.

Studies indicated that cows injected with POSILAC 1 STEP® had increased numbers of enlarged hocks and lesions (e.g., lacerations, enlargements, calluses) of the knee (carpal region), and second lactation or older cows had more disorders of the foot region. However, results of these studies did not indicate that the use of POSILAC 1 STEP® increased lameness.

Injection Site Reactions: A mild transient swelling of 3-5 cm (1-2 inches) in diameter may occur at the injection site beginning about 3 days after injection and may persist for up to 6 weeks following injection. Larger swellings may occur in cows injected in the neck region compared to the postscapular region (behind the shoulder) or in the depression on either side of the tailhead. Some cows may experience swellings up to 10 cm (4 inches) in diameter that remain permanent but are not associated with animal health problems. However, if permanent blemishes are objectionable to the user, administration of the product to the particular animal should be discontinued. Use of POSILAC 1 STEP® in cows in which injection site swellings repeatedly open and drain should be discontinued.

Udder Edema: POSILAC 1 STEP® is approved for use beginning during the 9th or 10th week of lactation. Initiation of use in later lactation has been associated with increased risk of udder edema.

Additional Veterinary Information: Care should be taken to differentiate increased body temperature due to the use of POSILAC 1 STEP® from an increased body temperature that may occur due to illness.

Use of POSILAC 1 STEP® has been associated with reductions in hemoglobin and hematocrit values during treatment.

Additional Information: When using the tailhead injection site, do not inject into the caudal tail fold which is the site of official USDA tuberculosis testing. Failure to avoid the caudal tail fold could hinder or invalidate official USDA tuberculosis testing. The caudal tail fold and other structures to avoid can be located quickly by raising the tail.

Milk production response during each 14 day injection period is cyclic and will be greatest during the middle of each period.

Warning(s): No milk discard or preslaughter withdrawal period is required.

Human Warnings: Avoid prolonged or repeated contact of POSILAC 1 STEP® with eyes and skin. POSILAC 1 STEP® is a protein. Frequent skin contact with proteins in general may produce an allergic skin reaction in some people. Always wash hands and skin exposed to POSILAC 1 STEP® with soap and water after handling. Clothing soiled with the product should be laundered before reuse. Not for human use. Keep out of reach of children.

Presentation: Single-dose syringes in 25 and 100 pack cartons.

POSILAC 1 STEP® is a registered trademark of Monsanto Technology LLC

Compendium Code No.: 11360003 40 360 5

POTASSIJECT ℞

Vetus **Fluid Therapy**

Composition: Each mL of sterile solution contains: potassium chloride, 2 mEq (149 mg). May contain HCl for pH adjustment. 4 mOsmol/mL (calc.).

Indications: For the treatment of potassium deficiency states when oral replacement is not feasible.

Dosage and Administration: For I.V. use. Must be diluted to appropriate strength with water or other suitable fluid prior to administration.

Precaution(s): Store between 15°C and 30°C (59°F-86°F).

Caution(s): Federal law restricts this drug to use by or on the order of a licensed veterinarian.

Concentrate - Must be diluted before use. Discard unused portion. For animal use only.

Presentation: 10 mL and 20 mL single dose vials.

Compendium Code No.: 14440731

POTASSIUM CHLORIDE ℞

Butler **Fluid Therapy**

NDC No.: 11695-3540-0

Active Ingredient(s): Each mL of sterile aqueous solution contains: Potassium chloride, 2 mEq (149 mg). May contain HCl for pH adjustment. 4 mOsmol/mL (calc).

Indications: For the treatment of potassium deficiency states when oral replacement is not feasible.

Dosage and Administration: This concentrate must be diluted to appropriate strength with water or other suitable fluid prior to administration. Dilute 10 mL (single dose) and administer I.V. Discard unused portion.

Precaution(s): Store between 15°C and 30°C (59°F-86°F).

Caution(s): Federal law restricts this drug to use by or on the order of a licensed veterinarian.

Warning(s): For animal use only.

Presentation: 10 mL.

Compendium Code No.: 10821510

POTASSIUM CHLORIDE ℞

Phoenix Pharmaceutical **Fluid Therapy**

Inj. Concentrate, USP (2 mEq/mL)

Active Ingredient(s): Composition: Each mL of sterile aqueous solution contains: Potassium chloride 2 mEq (149 mg). May contain HCl for pH adjustment 4 mOsmol/mL (calc).

Indications: For the treatment of potassium deficiency states when oral replacement is not feasible.

Dosage and Administration: For intravenous use. Must be diluted to the appropriate strength with water or another suitable fluid prior to administration.

Precaution(s): Store between 15°C and 30°C (59°F-86°F). Discard unused portion.

Caution(s): Federal law restricts this drug to use by or on the order of a licensed veterinarian. For animal use only.

Warning(s): Keep out of reach of children.

Presentation: 10 mL (NDC 57319-297-02) and 20 mL (NDC 57319-297-26) single dose vials.

Manufactured by: Phoenix Scientific, Inc., St. Joseph MO 64503.

Compendium Code No.: 12560682 Rev. 11-01 / Rev. 7-00

POTASSIUM CHLORIDE ℞

Vedco **Fluid Therapy**

Concentrate, USP (2 mEq/mL)

Active Ingredient(s): Each mL of sterile aqueous solution contains: potassium chloride, 2 mEq (149 mg). May contain HCl for pH adjustment 4 mOsmol/mL (calc).

Indications: For the treatment of potassium deficiency states when oral replacement is not feasible.

Dosage and Administration: For I.V. use. Must be diluted to appropriate strength with water or other suitable fluid prior to administration.

Precaution(s): Store between 15°C-30°C (59°F-86°F).

Caution(s): Federal law restricts this drug to use by or on the order of a licensed veterinarian.

This concentrate must be diluted before use. For animal use only. Discard unused portion.

Presentation: 10 mL.

Compendium Code No.: 10941690

POTASSIUM GEL ℞

Butler **Potassium-Oral**

Potassium Gluconate

Active Ingredient(s): Each 2.34 g (½ teaspoon) contains 2 mEq (468 mg) of potassium gluconate in a palatable base.

Indications: For use as a supplement in potassium deficient states in cats and dogs.

Dosage and Administration: Dosage: The suggested dosage of POTASSIUM GEL for adult cats and dogs is 2.34 g (½ teaspoon) per 10 lbs (4.5 kg) body weight twice daily. Dosage may be adjusted to satisfy patient's need.

Administration: POTASSIUM GEL is highly palatable. To initiate interest in taste, place small amount on the animal's nose or on the roof of its mouth. Gel may be placed on the paw after initial interest has been established.

Precaution(s): Store at controlled room temperature 15°-30°C (59°-86°F).

Caution(s): Federal law restricts this drug to use by or on the order of a licensed veterinarian.

Use with caution in the presence of cardiac disease, particularly in digitized patients or in the presence of renal disease.

Do not administer in diseases where high potassium levels may be encountered, such as severe renal insufficiency or adrenal insufficiency.

For animal use only.

Warning(s): Keep out of reach of children.

Presentation: 5 oz (142 g) tube.

Manufactured by: Corwood Laboratories, Hauppage, NY 11788.

Compendium Code No.: 10821990 L517-0601

POTASSIUM POWDER ℞

Butler **Mineral Supplement**

Potassium Gluconate

Active Ingredient(s): Each 0.65 g (¼ level teaspoonful) contains:

Potassium gluconate .... 2 mEq (468 mg)

In a palatable protein base.

Indications: For use as a supplement in potassium deficient states in cats and dogs.

Dosage and Administration: The suggested dose of POTASSIUM POWDER for adult cats and dogs is 0.65 g (¼ level teaspoonful) per 10 lb (4.5 kg) body weight twice daily with food. Dosage may be adjusted to satisfy patient's need.

Precaution(s): Store at controlled room temperature 15°-30°C (59°-86°F).

Caution(s): Federal law restricts this drug to use by or on the order of a licensed veterinarian.

Do not administer in diseases where high potassium levels may be encountered, such as severe renal insufficiency or adrenal insufficiency.

Use with caution in the presence of cardiac disease, particularly in digitalized patients or in the presence of renal disease.

Warning(s): For animal use only.

Keep out of reach of children.

Presentation: 4 oz.

Compendium Code No.: 10821520

POTASSIUM TABLETS ℞

Butler **Potassium-Oral**

Potassium Gluconate

Active Ingredient(s): Each Tablet Contains:

Potassium Gluconate .... 2 mEq (468mg)

Indications: For use as a supplement in potassium deficient states in cats and dogs.

Dosage and Administration: The suggested dose of POTASSIUM TABLETS for adult cats and dogs is one (1) tablet per 10 lb. (4.5 kg) body weight twice daily. Dosage may be adjusted to satisfy patient's need.

Precaution(s): Store at controlled room temperature 15°-30°C (69°-86°F).

Caution(s): Federal law restricts this drug to use by or on the order of a licensed veterinarian.

Use with caution in the presence of cardiac disease, particularly in digitalized patients or in the presence of renal disease.

Keep out of reach of children.

For animal use only.

Warning(s): Do not administer in diseases where high potassium levels may be encountered, such as severe renal insufficiency or adrenal insufficiency.

Presentation: 100 tablets.

Compendium Code No.: 10821530

POTOMACGUARD®

Fort Dodge **Bacterin**

Ehrlichia Risticii Bacterin

U.S. Vet. Lic. No.: 112

Composition: POTOMACGUARD® consists of inactivated *Ehrlichia risticii* organisms.

The MetaStim® adjuvant is added to enhance the immune response and to promote the proper rate of vaccine absorption following inoculation.

Formalin, neomycin, polymyxin B and amphotericin B added as preservatives.

Indications: For intramuscular vaccination of healthy horses as an aid in the prevention of Potomac Horse Fever.

Dosage and Administration: Horses, inject one 1 mL dose intramuscularly using aseptic technique. Administer a second 1 mL dose 3 to 4 weeks after the first dose. Revaccinate annually using one 1 mL dose. To insure proper placement of the vaccine, inject deep into the heavy muscles of the hindquarter. Mild daily exercise to promote absorption is recommended for one week after injection.

Precaution(s): Store in dark at 2° to 7°C (35° to 45°F). Avoid freezing. Shake well.

Caution(s): In some instances, transient local reactions may occur at the injection site. In case of anaphylactoid reaction, administer epinephrine.

Warning(s): Do not vaccinate within 60 days before slaughter.

For veterinary use only.

Presentation: Package of 12 x 1 mL prefilled disposable plastic syringes with needles (12 doses), package of 25 x 1 mL prefilled disposable plastic syringes with needles (25 doses) and 10 mL (10 dose) vials.

Compendium Code No.: 10031481 2665B

POTOMACGUARD® EWT

Fort Dodge **Bacterin-Toxoid**

Encephalomyelitis Vaccine, Eastern and Western, Killed Virus-Ehrlichia Risticii-Tetanus Bacterin-Toxoid

U.S. Vet. Lic. No.: 112

Composition: POTOMACGUARD® EWT consists of inactivated *ehrlichia risticii* organisms, equine encephalomyelitis virus Eastern and Western and tetanus.

The MetaStim™ adjuvant is added to enhance the immune response and to promote the proper rate of vaccine absorption following inoculation.

The *ehrlichia risticii* and encephalomyelitis virus fractions are grown and prepared in stable equine cell line substrates. This highly refined process further eliminates foreign protein material commonly associated with reactions in the horse and yields a more consistently pure vaccine. These components are inactivated, standardized and combined with tetanus toxoid, which has been refined and concentrated.

Formalin, thimerosal, neomycin, polymyxin B and amphotericin B added as preservatives.

Indications: For vaccination of healthy horses as an aid in the prevention of Potomac Horse Fever, Eastern and Western encephalomyelitis and tetanus.

Dosage and Administration: Horses, inject one 1 mL dose intramuscularly using aseptic technique. Administer a second 1 mL dose 3 to 4 weeks after the first dose. Revaccinate annually using one 1 mL dose. To insure proper placement of the vaccine, inject deep into the heavy muscles of the hindquarter. Mild daily exercise to promote absorption is recommended for one week after injection.

Precaution(s): Store in dark at 2° to 7°C (35° to 45°F). Avoid freezing. Shake well.

Caution(s): When used according to instructions, it is unusual for reactions to appear, other than those expected with any vaccination of horses; for example, occasional temporary local swelling. In case of anaphylactoid reaction, administer epinephrine.

Warning(s): Do not vaccinate within 60 days before slaughter.

For veterinary use only.

Presentation: Package of 12 x 1 mL prefilled disposable plastic syringes with needles (12 doses), 25 x 1 dose (prefilled syringe) and 10 dose vials.

Compendium Code No.: 10031490 2671C

POTOMAC SHIELD™

Novartis Animal Vaccines **Bacterin**

Ehrlichia Risticii Bacterin

U.S. Vet. Lic. No.: 303

Composition: This bacterin contains inactivated cultures of *Ehrlichia risticii.* Contains thimerosal as a preservative.

Indications: For use in healthy horses as an aid in the prevention of Potomac Horse Fever (Equine Monocytic Ehrlichiosis) caused by *Ehrlichia risticii.*

Dosage and Administration: Shake well before using. Administer 1 mL intramuscularly at 1 year of age or older. Repeat in 2-3 weeks. Revaccinate annually with a 1 mL dose.

Precaution(s): Store in the dark at 2°-7°C (35°-45°F). Do not freeze. Use entire contents when first opened.

Caution(s): Transient swelling may occur at the site of injection. Anaphylactic reactions may occur following the use of this biological. Symptomatic treatment: Epinephrine.

For veterinary use only.

Warning(s): Do not vaccinate within 21 days prior to slaughter.

Presentation: 10 dose (10 mL) bottle.

Manufactured by: Protatek International, Inc., St. Paul, MN 55114.

Compendium Code No.: 11140750 F261

POULT PAK

Alpharma **Water Additive**

With Antioxidants and Trace Minerals

Ingredient(s): Potassium chloride, sodium chloride, niacinamide, vitamin E supplement, ascorbic acid stabilized, sodium citrate, d-calcium pantothenic acid, vitamin A supplement, vitamin D_3 supplement, menadione sodium bisulfite complex, riboflavin, biotin supplement, vitamin B_{12} supplement, pyridoxine HCl, thiamine HCl, magnesium sulfate, folic acid, ferrous sulfate, copper sulfate, zinc sulfate, manganese sulfate, cobalt sulfate, calcium lactate, potassium sulfate, magnesium carbonate, ethylenediamine dihydriodide.

Guaranteed analysis per pound:

Vitamin A	4,500,000 IU
Vitamin D_3	3,000,000 IU
Vitamin E	15,000 IU
Vitamin B_{12}	10 mg
Biotin	50 mg
Riboflavin	3,000 mg
Niacinamide	30,000 mg
MSB Complex	4,000 mg
Folic Acid	420 mg
Thiamine HCl	2,000 mg
Pyridoxine HCl	2,000 mg
Ascorbic acid (Supplied by Stabilized C)	10,000 mg
d-Calcium Pantothenate Acid	12,500 mg

Indications: Water soluble vitamin mixture for use in turkey drinking water as an aid in getting poults off to a good start, during periods of reduced feed intake and during extreme conditions.

Directions: Use 4 oz (1 pack) POULT PAK in 128 gallons of water for starting poults or during periods of reduced feed intake. 8 oz (2 packs) POULT PAK can be used in 128 gallons of water during extreme conditions.

Precaution(s): Store in cool, dry place.

Caution(s): For oral animal use only.

Not for human use.

Keep out of reach of children.

Presentation: 4 oz (113.4 g) packets.

Compendium Code No.: 10220521 AHF-038 0005

POULVAC® CHICK-N-POX™

Fort Dodge **Vaccine**

Fowl Pox Vaccine, Live Virus

U.S. Vet. Lic. No.: 112

Contents: This product contains the antigen listed above.

Contains gentamicin and amphotericin B as preservatives.

Indications: Fort Dodge Animal Health, Inc., POULVAC® CHICK-N-POX™ brand of Fowl Pox Vaccine, is recommended for wing-web stab of healthy chickens one day of age or older against fowl pox.

Dosage and Administration: Read in full, follow directions carefully.

When to Vaccinate: Vaccination may be performed as early as 1 day of age. If chicks are vaccinated against fowl pox at 1 day of age and premises have a history of heavy challenge, revaccination after 7 weeks of age is recommended. Birds vaccinated at 7 weeks of age or older may require only one vaccination.

Directions:

1. Rehydrate 1 vial of vaccine with 1 vial of diluent.
2. Remove aluminum seal and rubber stopper from vaccine vial and diluent vial. Avoid contamination of the stopper and vial contents.
3. Pour approximately one-half the diluent into the vaccine vial. Replace stopper and shake gently until contents are dissolved.
4. Pour all the reconstituted vaccine back into the remaining diluent in the diluent bottle. Replace diluent stopper and gently mix. The vaccine is then ready for use.
5. Hold individual bird and spread wing with the underside facing upwards.
6. Dip the vaccinator tool into the vaccine, wetting both needles.

7. Stick the needles through the web of the wing, avoiding blood vessels, bones, and the wing muscle. The vaccine should not touch feathers, the head of the birds, or the skin except at the site of vaccination.

How Takes Appear: The usual take consists of some swelling at the site of the puncture as early as the fourth day following vaccination. The swelling increases during the next five days until a scab is formed. Revaccinate birds that do not show takes.

Records: Keep a record of vaccine serial number and expiration date; date of receipt and date of vaccination; where vaccination takes place; and any reactions observed.

Precaution(s): Store this vaccine at not over 45°F (7°C).

Use entire contents when vial is first opened.

Burn vaccine container and all unused contents.

Do not expose vaccine to either direct sunlight or extreme heat during vaccination.

This vaccine is nonreturnable.

Caution(s): Vaccinate healthy chickens only.

This product should be stored, transported, and administered in accordance with the instructions and directions.

The use of this vaccine is subject to state laws, wherever applicable.

Warning(s): Do not vaccinate within 21 days before slaughter. For veterinary use only.

Presentation: 10 x 1,000 doses.

Compendium Code No.: 10031501 10960B

POULVAC® CORYZA ABC IC3

Fort Dodge **Bacterin**

Haemophilus Paragallinarum Bacterin

U.S. Vet. Lic. No.: 112

Contents: POULVAC® Coryza ABC contains adjuvanted, inactivated cultures of strains representing *Haemophilus paragallinarum* serovars A, B, and C.

Indications: For the vaccination of healthy chickens as an aid in the prevention of clinical signs associated with *Haemophilus paragallinarum* caused by serovars A, B, and C.

Dosage and Administration: Inject 0.5 mL (0.5 cc) subcutaneously (in the lower neck region) or intramuscularly using aseptic technique. Vaccinate only healthy chickens 8 weeks of age or older. Revaccinate at least 3 weeks following initial vaccination and no less than 4 weeks prior to onset of lay.

Precaution(s): Store in the dark at 36° to 45°F (2° to 7°C). Do not freeze. Warm to 72°F (22°C) and shake well before using. Use entire contents when first opened.

Warning(s): Do not vaccinate within 42 days before slaughter.

In case of accidental human injection seek immediate medical attention.

For veterinary use only.

Presentation: 1,000 doses (500 mL).

Compendium Code No.: 10031510 10211B

POULVAC® MAREK RISPENS CVI+HVT

Fort Dodge **Vaccine**

Marek's Disease Vaccine, Serotypes 1 and 3, Live Virus

U.S. Vet. Lic. No.: 112

Contents: This product contains the antigen listed above.

Contains gentamicin as a preservative.

Indications: This product is recommended for the subcutaneous vaccination of healthy one-day-old chicks or the *in ovo* vaccination of 18 to 19 day-old embryonated chicken eggs, to aid in the prevention of very virulent Marek's disease. Use only the Fort Dodge Animal Health sterile diluent included.

Dosage and Administration: Read in full, follow directions carefully.

Directions for Subcutaneous Administration:

1. Vaccinate healthy one-day-old chicks only.
2. Avoid early exposure of chicks to Marek's disease, to allow for development of protection.
3. The exact amount of diluent is provided for each shipment of vaccine. Use Fort Dodge Animal Health diluent only. Store diluent at not over 80°F (27°C).
4. Wear protective clothing when withdrawing vaccine from liquid-nitrogen refrigerator; protect hands with gloves, wear long sleeves, and use a face mask or goggles.
5. Before opening liquid-nitrogen refrigerator, prepare a clean, wide-mouthed container with a capacity of 1 to 5 gallons (3.8-19 liters). Half-fill this container with water 80°F (27°C).
6. When withdrawing a cane of vials from the liquid-nitrogen refrigerator, expose only the vial to be used immediately. When removing a vial from the cane, hold palm of gloved hand away from face and body. Dilute only 1 vial at a time. Immediately replace cane with remaining vials into the canister in the liquid-nitrogen refrigerator.
7. Place the vial into prepared container half-filled with water 80°F (27°C). The frozen material thaws rapidly. When thawed, towel-dry vial.
8. The vials are pre-scored below the gold band. Before snapping off the top portion, wrap vial with a cloth, holding the top part away from face and body.
9. For subcutaneous route of vaccination, use 200 mLs of diluent per 1,000 doses of vaccine.
10. Using a sterile mixing syringe with a 1½-inch (3.8 cm) 18-gauge needle, draw up a small amount of diluent. Then draw the contents from the vaccine vial into the syringe and swirl gently. Insert needle into diluent bottle and slowly expel contents of syringe. Mix well by gently swirling the bottle. Withdraw a small amount of the reconstituted vaccine and use to rinse each vial injecting the rinses back into reconstituted vaccine. The vaccine is ready for use.
11. While vaccinating, maintain the diluted vaccine (in the diluent bottle) at 70° to 80°F (21° to 27°C). If the temperature cannot be held as low as 80°F (27°C), place the diluent bottle containing the diluted vaccine in an ice bath.
12. For vaccination, an automatic syringe with 22- to 20-gauge needles, ⅜- to ½-inch (0.95 to 1.27 cm) long, is recommended. Make certain that all equipment is sterilized and change needles frequently.
13. Inject each chick subcutaneously with 0.2 mL of the vaccine.
14. After diluting, use the vaccine within 2 hours. Do not save any vaccine that has been diluted. Burn vaccine containers and all unused contents.

Directions for use with Embrex Inovoject® Egg Injection System:

1. Vaccinate using the *in ovo* route of vaccination in 18 to 19 day-old healthy embryonated chicken eggs only.
2. The exact amount of diluent is provided for each shipment of vaccine. Use Fort Dodge Animal Health diluent only. Store diluent at not over 80°F (27°C).
3. Sanitize the Inovoject® Egg Injection System in accordance with the procedures described in the Inovoject® operator's manual.
4. Wear protective clothing when withdrawing vaccine from liquid-nitrogen refrigerator; protect hands with gloves, wear long sleeves, and use a face mask or goggles.
5. Before opening liquid-nitrogen refrigerator, prepare a clean, wide-mouthed container with a capacity of 1 to 5 gallons (3.8-19 liters). Half-fill this container with water at 80°F (27°C).
6. When withdrawing a cane of vials from the liquid-nitrogen refrigerator, expose only the vials to be used immediately. When removing a vial from the cane, hold palm of gloved hand away from face and body. Dilute only 4 vials at a time. Immediately replace the cane with remaining vials into the canister in the liquid-nitrogen refrigerator.
7. Place the vials into a prepared container half-filled with water 80°F (27°C). The frozen material thaws rapidly. When thawed, towel-dry vial.
8. The vials are pre-scored below the gold band. Before snapping off the top portion, wrap the vial with a cloth, holding the top part away from face and body.
9. For *in ovo* route of vaccination, use 100 mLs diluent per 1,000 doses of vaccine. For example: 4,000 doses of vaccine - 400 mL diluent.
10. Using 4 sterile mixing syringes with a 1½-inch (3.8 cm) 18-gauge needle, draw up a small amount of diluent into each syringe. Then draw the contents from one vaccine vial into the syringe and swirl gently. Repeat this step with the other 3 syringes. Insert needle into diluent container and slowly expel contents of syringe. Repeat this step with the other 3 syringes. Mix well by gently swirling the container. Withdraw a small amount of the reconstituted vaccine and use to rinse each vial injecting the rinses back into reconstituted vaccine. The vaccine is ready for use.
11. While vaccinating, maintain the diluted vaccine (in the diluent container) at 70° to 80°F (21° to 27°C). If the temperature cannot be held as low as 80°F (27°C), place the diluent container containing the diluted vaccine in an ice bath.
12. Carefully read and follow the Inovoject® operator's manual before initiating vaccination. Failure to follow instructions for Inovoject® operation may result in personal injury and/or embryonic morbidity and mortality.
13. The Inovoject® Egg Injection machine is equipped with an automatic injection system which utilizes a 20-gauge needle and deposits the vaccine about 1-inch deep into the egg.
14. Inject each egg *in ovo* with 0.1 mL of the vaccine solution.
15. After diluting, use the vaccine solution within 2 hours. Do not save any vaccine that has been diluted. Burn all unused material.

Records: Keep a record of vaccine serial number and expiration date; date of receipt and date of vaccination; where vaccination takes place; and any reactions observed.

Precaution(s): Store in liquid nitrogen. Dilute before using. Use entire contents of vial when first opened.

Burn vaccine container and all unused contents.

This product is nonreturnable.

Caution(s): This product should be stored, transported, and administered in accordance with the instructions and directions.

The use of this vaccine is subject to state laws, wherever applicable.

Combining this product with other biological products is not recommended.

Warning(s): Do not vaccinate within 21 days before slaughter.

Take all precautionary measures, including the use of gloves and face shield or goggles, to avoid potential hazards of handling liquid nitrogen and the possibility of explosion of glass vials as they are taken from the liquid-nitrogen refrigerator or canister or holding cane, or as they are placed in the thawing container. When removing the vial from the cane, hold palm of the gloved hand away from face and body.

Only vaccines, diluents etc., that have been approved by Embrex and are labeled appropriately for *in ovo* use can be used in the Inovoject® Egg Injection System.

Before using this vaccine, be certain to read directions.

For veterinary use only.

Disclaimer: Having cautioned the user concerning the handling of liquid nitrogen and the possibility of explosion of glass ampules as they are removed from the nitrogen or holding cane, or when placed in the thawing container, and having no control over the safety measures taken other than cautioning against possible dangers, Fort Dodge Animal Health shall not be responsible for personal injury and/or property damage resulting from said handling and/or the possibility of explosion.

Presentation: 5 x 1,000 doses and 5 x 2,000 doses.

Inovoject is a registered trademark of Embrex, Inc.

Compendium Code No.: 10031521 10835C

POULVAC® SE

Fort Dodge **Bacterin**

Salmonella Enteritidis Bacterin

U.S. Vet. Lic. No.: 112

Contents: A bacterin containing phage types 4, 8 and 13a.

Indications: For subcutaneous administration to healthy 12 week-old chickens as an aid in the reduction of *Salmonella enteritidis* colonization of the internal organs, including the reproductive tract and intestines.

Dosage and Administration: Inject 0.3 mL (0.3 cc) subcutaneously using aseptic technique. Vaccinate only healthy birds. Administer two separate doses 3 to 4 weeks apart.

Precaution(s): Store in the dark at 36° to 45°F (2° to 7°C). Do not freeze. Warm to 65° to 85°F (18° to 29°C) and shake well before using.

Use entire contents when first opened.

Warning(s): Do not vaccinate within 21 days before slaughter.

In case of accidental human injection seek immediate medical attention.

For veterinary use only.

Presentation: 1,000 doses (300 mL).

Compendium Code No.: 10031530 15072D

POULVAC® SE-ND-IB

Fort Dodge **Bacterin-Vaccine**

Newcastle-Bronchitis Vaccine-Salmonella Enteritidis Bacterin, Mass. Type, Killed Virus

U.S. Vet. Lic. No.: 112

Contents: An inactivated vaccine containing *Salmonella enteritidis*, phage types 4, 8 and 13a, infectious bronchitis virus and Newcastle disease virus.

Contains gentamicin as a preservative.

Indications: It is recommended for subcutaneous administration to healthy 12 week-old chickens as an aid in the reduction of *Salmonella enteritidis* colonization of the internal organs, including the reproductive tract and intestines, and as an aid in the prevention of the signs and lesions associated with Newcastle disease and infectious bronchitis.

Dosage and Administration: Inject 0.3 mL (0.3 cc) subcutaneously using aseptic technique. Vaccinate only healthy birds. Administer two separate doses 3 to 4 weeks apart.
Precaution(s): Store in the dark at 36° to 45°F (2° to 7°C). Do not freeze. Warm to 65° to 85°F (18° to 29°C) and shake well before using. Use entire contents when first opened.
Warning(s): Do not vaccinate within 21 days before slaughter.
In case of accidental human injection seek immediate medical attention.
For veterinary use only.
Presentation: 1,000 doses (300 mL).
Compendium Code No.: 10031540 15542C

POVIDERM MEDICAL SCRUB

Vetus **Surgical Scrub**
NDC No.: 47611-201-90
Active Ingredient(s):
Povidone-iodine.................................... 7.5% (titratable iodine 0.75%)
Indications: For use as an antiseptic skin cleanser for pre-surgical prepping and post-surgical cleaning, for use as an antiseptic hand scrub prior to surgery or examination, for use as an aid in the prevention and treatment of skin infections in cuts, scratches, abrasions and burns, and in the treatment of bacterial and fungal skin infections in animals. Non-staining to skin, hair and natural fabrics.
Dosage and Administration: Add water to a small quantity of the scrub and work into a lather. Cleanse the area and rinse thoroughly with clean water.
Precaution(s): Avoid storing at excessive heat.
Caution(s): For external use only.
May be harmful if swallowed. Avoid contact with the eyes.
If infection or irritation persists, discontinue use and consult a veterinarian.
For veterinary use only.
Keep out of the reach of children.
Presentation: 1 gallon containers.
Compendium Code No.: 14440740

POVIDERM MEDICATED SHAMPOO

Vetus **Antidermatosis Shampoo**
Active Ingredient(s):
Povidone-iodine.. 5% (titratable iodine 0.5%)
Indications: A nonirritating shampoo for use as an aid in the treatment of bacterial and fungal skin infection in dogs, cats, horses, cattle and swine. Non-staining to skin, hair and natural fabrics.
Dosage and Administration: Wet the animal with water and apply a sufficient amount of the shampoo to work into a lather. Allow the lather to remain on the animal for three (3) minutes and rinse thoroughly. Repeat once a day or as needed.
Precaution(s): Avoid storing at excessive heat.
Caution(s): For external use only.
May be harmful if swallowed. Avoid contact with the eyes.
If infection or irritation persists, discontinue use and consult a veterinarian.
For veterinary use only.
Keep out of the reach of children.
Presentation: 8 oz. bottles and 1 gallon containers.
Compendium Code No.: 14440750

POVIDERM SOLUTION

Vetus **Topical Antibacterial**
NDC No.: 47611-202-90
Active Ingredient(s):
Povidone-iodine...................................... 10% (titratable iodine 1.0%)
Indications: A nonirritating topical antiseptic for use on dogs, cats, horses, cattle and swine, effective against gram-negative and gram-positive bacteria, fungi, viruses, protozoa and yeasts. Film-forming for continued protection, non-staining to skin, hair and natural fabrics.
Dosage and Administration: Apply full-strength to the affected area once a day or as needed. Wet the area thoroughly to ensure complete coverage and penetration. Avoid pooling. May be covered with a bandage if necessary.
Precaution(s): Avoid storing at excessive heat.
Caution(s): For external use only.
May be harmful if swallowed. Avoid contact with the eyes.
If infection persists, discontinue use and consult a veterinarian.
For veterinary use only.
Keep out of the reach of children.
Presentation: 1 gallon containers.
Compendium Code No.: 14440760

POVIDINE

AgriPharm **Topical Antibacterial**
Active Ingredient(s): 10% polyvinyl pyrrolidone-iodine complex (titratable iodine 1.0%).
Indications: Antiseptic-microbicide.
Dosage and Administration: For minor wounds and infections, apply directly to affected area full strength. May be covered with gauze or adhesive bandage.
Precaution(s): Avoid storage in excessive heat.
Caution(s): In case of deep or puncture wounds or serious burns, consult veterinarian. If redness, irritation, swelling or pain persists or increases, or if infection occurs, discontinue use and consult a veterinarian.
Virtually non-irritating, film-forming, non-staining to skin, fur and natural fibers.
Avoid contact with eyes.
For animal use only.
Keep out of the reach of children.
Presentation: 0.946 L (1 quart), 12 per case and 3.785 L (1 gallon), 4 per case.
Compendium Code No.: 14570840

POVIDINE 0.75% SCRUB

AgriPharm **Surgical Scrub**
Active Ingredient(s): Povidone-Iodine Scrub is equivalent to 0.75% titratable iodine.
Indications: An antibacterial, non-irritating surgical scrub for pre-operative and post-operative scrubbing or washing by hospital personnel and for general use in the physician's office.
Dosage and Administration: Wet hands with water, pour approximately 5 mL of POVIDINE SCRUB in palm of hand. Lather thoroughly. Add enough water to make a lather. Rinse thoroughly under potable water.
For Pre-Operative Use: Place approximately 5 mL of POVIDINE SCRUB into hands, rubbing with potable water. Scrub with brush around nails, under nails, and in nail and cuticle areas. Scrub entire hand and arm up to elbow creases for five (5) minutes. Rinse and repeat.
Precaution(s): Avoid storing in excessive heat. Store at temperatures between 50°-85°F.
Caution(s): For external use only. For animal use only. Keep out of reach of children.
Presentation: 3.785 L (1 gallon), 4 per case.
Compendium Code No.: 14570850

POVIDINE™ BOLUS

Butler **Disinfectant**
NDC No.: 11695-3301-2
Active Ingredient(s): Each bolus contains: 250 mg available iodine as the polyvinylpyrrolidone-iodine complex in a urea base.
Indications: For disinfecting and cleaning wounds, and for topical disinfection
Dosage and Administration: Uses: To prepare a solution of active iodine for disinfecting and cleaning wounds, and for topical disinfection: Dissolve one bolus in 50 to 100 mL of clean water. Apply this solution as a soak or cleanse area with the solution on gauze.
Precaution(s): Do not store over 30°C. (86°F).
Warning(s): For topical use only. For veterinary use only. Livestock drug.
Keep out of reach of children.
Presentation: 50 boluses.
Compendium Code No.: 10821540

POVIDONE IODINE OINTMENT

First Priority **Topical Wound Dressing**
Topical Antiseptic & Wound Protectant-Water Resistant Formula
Active Ingredient(s): Povidone-iodine (1% titratable iodine).
Contains lanolin as an emollient and protectant.
Indications: Antibacterial and antifungal ointment for wounds, cuts, abrasions. Water-resistant formula adheres to wound to provide long lasting protection even in harsh weather.
Directions: Apply to wound after cleansing and drying. Apply as needed to maintain coverage. May bandage if necessary.
Precaution(s): Storage: Store at controlled room temperature between 15°-30°C (59°-86°F). Keep container tightly closed when not in use.
Caution(s): For veterinary use only. For deep or puncture wounds, use as directed by veterinarian.
Warning(s): Keep out of reach of children.
Presentation: 4 oz (113.3 g) (NDC# 58829-121-04) and 1 lb (453.6 g) (NDC# 58829-121-16).
Compendium Code No.: 11390642 Rev. 4-99 / Rev. 07-01

POVIDONE IODINE SCRUB

First Priority **Surgical Scrub**
Active Ingredient(s): POVIDONE IODINE SCRUB is equivalent to 0.75% titratable iodine.
Indications: A germicidal cleanser for pre-operative and post-operative skin washing, and shampoo for bacterial and fungal skin infections in animals. Used routinely, it also helps prevent infection in cuts, scratches, abrasions, and burns. Non-staining to skin, hair, and natural fabrics.
Precaution(s): Storage: Store at controlled room temperature between 15°-30°C (59°-86°F). Keep container tightly closed when not in use. Avoid storing at excessive heat.
Caution(s): In case of deep or puncture wounds or serious burns, consult a veterinarian. If irritation or infection persists, discontinue use and consult a veterinarian.
For animal use only. For veterinary use only.
Warning(s): Keep out of reach of children.
Presentation: 32 fl oz (960 mL) (NDC# 58829-110-32) and 1 gallon (3.785 L) (NDC# 58829-110-01).
Compendium Code No.: 11390653 Iss. 1-98 / Rev. 07-01

POVIDONE IODINE SHAMPOO

First Priority **Antidermatosis Shampoo**
Active Ingredient(s): Povidone Iodine (Titratable Iodine 0.5%).
Indications: POVIDONE IODINE SHAMPOO aids in the treatment and prevention of fungal and bacterial skin infections in animals. Mild formulation for every day use.
Directions for Use: Shake well. Wet animal with water. Apply one to two ounces of POVIDONE IODINE SHAMPOO to the entire body. Work into a rich lather and rinse thoroughly. Repeat application and rinse again for maximum effectiveness.
Precaution(s): Storage: Store at controlled room temperature between 15°-30°C (59°-86°F). Keep container tightly closed when not in use. Avoid storing at excessive heat.
Caution(s): For external use only. Do not use with other topical medications or pesticides. If infection or irritation persists, discontinue use and consult a veterinarian. For animal use only.
Warning(s): Keep out of reach of children.
Presentation: 8 fl oz (240 mL), 16 fl oz (473 mL) (NDC# 58829-130-16), 32 fl oz (960 mL) (NDC# 58829-130-32) and 1 gallon (3.785 L) (NDC# 58829-130-01).
Compendium Code No.: 11390663 Rev. 01-02 / Iss. 2-99 / Rev. 3-97

POVIDONE IODINE SHAMPOO

Vedco **Antidermatosis Shampoo**
Active Ingredient(s): Povidone iodine (titratable iodine 0.5%).
Indications: POVIDONE IODINE SHAMPOO aids in the treatment of fungal and bacterial skin infections in animals. Mild formulation for daily use.
Directions: Shake well. Wet animal with water. Apply one to two ounces of POVIDONE IODINE SHAMPOO to the entire body. Work into a rich lather and rinse thoroughly. Repeat application and rinse again for maximum effectiveness.
Precaution(s): Avoid storing at excessive heat.
Caution(s): For external use only. Do not use with other topical medications or pesticides. If infection or irritation persists, discontinue use and consult a veterinarian.
For animal use only. Sold to veterinarians only.
Warning(s): Keep out of reach of children.
Presentation: 16 oz.
Compendium Code No.: 10941700

POVIDONE IODINE SOLUTION

First Priority — **Topical Antibacterial**

Antiseptic Microbicide

Active Ingredient(s): POVIDONE IODINE SOLUTION is equivalent to 1.0% Titratable Iodine.

Indications: Kills gram-negative and gram-positive bacteria, fungi, viruses, protozoa, and yeasts. Film-forming, virtually non-irritating and non-staining to skin, hair, and natural fabrics.

Directions for Use: Apply full-strength as often as needed. Wet area thoroughly to ensure complete coverage and penetration, but avoid "pooling". May be covered with bandage if necessary.

Precaution(s): Storage: Store at controlled room temperature between 15°-30°C (59°-86°F). Keep container tightly closed when not in use. Avoid storing at excessive heat.

Caution(s): Avoid contact with eyes. May be harmful if swallowed. If infection or irritation persists, discontinue use and consult a veterinarian. For animal use only.

Warning(s): Keep out of reach of children.

Presentation: 32 fl oz (960 mL) (NDC# 58829-120-32) and 1 gallon (3.785 L) (NDC# 58829-120-01).

Compendium Code No.: 11390673 Iss. 08-01 / Rev. 06-01

POVIDONE-IODINE SOLUTION 10%

Equicare — **Antiseptic**

Titratable iodine 1.0%

Active Ingredient(s): Povidone-iodine 10%.

Indications: An aid in the prevention and treatment of fungal and bacterial skin infections.

For use on horses, cattle, swine, dogs and cats.

This product is film-forming, virtually non-irritating and non-staining to skin, hair and natural fabrics.

Directions for Use: Apply full-strength as often as needed. Wet area thoroughly to insure complete coverage and penetration but avoid "pooling". May be covered with bandage if necessary.

Precaution(s): Avoid storing at excessive heat.

Caution(s): For external use only. Avoid contact with eyes. If infection or irritation persists, discontinue use and consult a veterinarian.

Warning(s): Keep out of reach of children. May be harmful if swallowed.

Presentation: 32 oz and 3.785 L (1 gallon).

Compendium Code No.: 14470121

POVIDONE-IODINE SURGICAL SCRUB 7 1/2%

Equicare — **Surgical Scrub**

Titratable iodine 0.75%

Active Ingredient(s): Povidone-iodine 7.5%.

Indications: A cleanser for preoperative and postoperative skin washing. Used routinely, it also aids in the prevention of infection in cuts, scratches, abrasions, and burns. Non-staining to skin, hair and natural fabrics.

For use on horses, cattle, swine, dogs and cats.

Directions for Use: Add water to approximately one tablespoon of scrub. Work mixture into a rich lather. Cleanse specific area thoroughly. Rinse with clean water.

Precaution(s): Avoid storing at excessive heat.

Caution(s): For external use only. In case of deep or puncture wounds or serious burns, consult a veterinarian. If irritation or infection persists, discontinue use and consult a veterinarian.

Presentation: 32 oz and 3.785 L (1 gallon).

Compendium Code No.: 14470131

POVIDONE SCRUB

Butler — **Surgical Scrub**

Active Ingredient(s):

Povidone-iodine (titrable iodine 0.75%) 7.5%

Indications: A germicidal cleanser for pre-operative and postoperative skin washing, and a shampoo for bacterial and fungal skin infections in animals. Used routinely, it also helps to prevent infection in cuts, scratches, abrasions, and burns. Nonstaining to skin, hair, and natural fabrics.

Dosage and Administration: For pre-operative washing by the veterinary surgeon and operating personnel:

1. Wet hands with water and pour approximately 5 mL (1 teaspoonful) of POVIDONE SCRUB on the palm of the hand and spread over both hands. Without adding more water, scrub in the usual manner. Use a brush if necessary to clean under fingernails. Add a small amount of water and continue to scrub developing copious amounts of suds. Rinse thoroughly under running water.
2. Complete the procedure by scrubbing with another 5 mL of POVIDONE SCRUB in the same manner. Use the proper technique of rinsing and drying following washing.

For pre-operative and postoperative prepping of animals after the surgical area is shaved, wet with water and apply surgical scrub (1 to 2 mL to cover an area of 20 to 30 sq. in.). Develop a lather and scrub thoroughly. Rinse with a sterile gauze pad and water. Repeat a second time. The surgical area should then be painted with iodine and allowed to dry.

Precaution(s): Avoid storing at excessive heat.

Caution(s): For veterinary use only.

In case of deep or puncture wounds or serious burns, consult a veterinarian. If irritation or infection persists, discontinue use of the product and consult a veterinarian.

Presentation: 1 gallon containers.

Compendium Code No.: 10821550

POVIDONE SHAMPOO 5%

Butler — **Antidermatosis Shampoo**

Active Ingredient(s):

Povidone-iodine 5%

Indications: POVIDONE SHAMPOO 5% is nonstaining and nonirritating and aids in the treatment of bacterial and fungal skin infections common to animals.

Dosage and Administration: Shake gently. Wet the animal with water and apply a sufficient amount of shampoo to work into a rich lather. For maximum effectiveness, allow the lather to remain on the animal for three (3) minutes. Rinse thoroughly. Repeat once a day or as needed.

Precaution(s): Avoid storing at excessive heat.

Caution(s): For veterinary use only.

For external use only. Avoid contact with the eyes.

Keep out of the reach of children. If infection or irritation persists, discontinue use of the product and consult a veterinarian.

Do not use in conjunction with other medications or pesticides.

Presentation: 8 fl. oz. and 1 gallon containers.

Compendium Code No.: 10821560

POVIDONE SOLUTION

Butler — **Antiseptic**

Active Ingredient(s): Povidone-iodine (titratable iodine 1.0%).

Indications: Kills gram-negative and gram-positive bacteria, fungi, viruses, protozoa, and yeasts. Film-forming, virtually nonirritating and nonstaining to skin, hair, and natural fabrics.

Dosage and Administration: Apply full strength as often as needed. Wet the area thoroughly to ensure complete coverage and penetration, but avoid pooling. May be covered with a bandage if necessary.

Precaution(s): Avoid storing at excessive heat.

Caution(s): For veterinary use only. Avoid contact with the eyes.

Keep out of the reach of children.

May be harmful if swallowed. If infection or irritation persists, discontinue use of the product and consult a veterinarian.

Presentation: 1 gallon containers.

Compendium Code No.: 10821571

POWER PUNCH™

Vets Plus — **Dietary Supplement**

Cattle Drench Formula - High Potency Complete Nutrient Balancer

Guaranteed Analysis: (min. per ounce):

Protein	1.54%
Lipid	2.50%
Fiber	0.05%
Vitamin A	20,000 IU
Vitamin B_{12}	33 mcg
Vitamin D_3	10,000 IU
Vitamin E	200 IU
Niacin	50.00 mg
Riboflavin	3,333.00 mcg
Iron	7.20 ppm
Zinc	1,000.00 ppm
Selenium	0.1 mg
L-Tryptophan	0.57 mg
L-Valine	4.18 mg
L-Alanine	4.15 mg
L-Arginine	4.19 mg
L-Aspartate	6.15 mg
L-Glutamine	8.80 mg
L-Histidine	1.61 mg
L-Isoleucine	3.02 mg
L-Leucine	3.02 mg
L-Lysine	4.78 mg
L-Methionine	1.43 mg
L-Phenylalanine	3.17 mg
L-Proline	3.39 mg
L-Serine	2.86 mg
L-Threonine	2.69 mg
L-Tyrosine	2.10 mg

Ingredients: Cane Molasses, Dextrose, Ascorbic Acid (Vitamin C), d-Calcium Pantothenate, Vitamin A Acetate, D-Activated Animal Sterol (Vitamin D_3), DL-alpha-Tocopheryl Acetate (Vitamin E), Cyanocobalamin (Vitamin B_{12}), Choline Bitartrate, Folic Acid, Riboflavin, Lactic Acid, Methylparaben, Propylene Glycol, Sodium Selenite, Beef Peptone, Pyridoxine Hydrochloride (Vitamin B_6), Niacinamide, Caramel Flavor, *Lactobacillus acidophilus* DDS-1 fermentation product, *Lactobacillus acidophilus* fermentation product, *Lactobacillus plantarum* fermentation product, *Lactobacillus fermentum* fermentation product, *Lactobacillus casei* fermentation product, *Enterococcus faecium* fermentation product, Silica, and Preservative.

Indications: Administer to cattle when calving, weaning, vaccinating, handling, weather changes, shipping or post antibiotic treatment. POWER PUNCH™ provides the natural elements needed to boost energy, stimulate appetite, and aid in digestion.

Dosage and Administration: Provide 1 ounce per 100 pounds of body weight up to a maximum of 6 ounces per dose. Administer no more than three doses per day. If conditions do not improve, consult your veterinarian.

Feeding Directions: Shake or mix well before using. Administer orally using a drench gun. Hold the head of the animal in a slightly elevated position and carefully place nozzle into back of the mouth between the cheek and teeth. Administer recommended dosage. Do not give to animals that are unable to swallow. You may also top dress or add to water, milk, or milk replacer, if desired.

Precaution(s): Keep in a cool dry place. Avoid freezing.

Caution(s): Keep out of the reach of children. Not for human use. Animal use only.

Presentation: 12x1-quart bottles per case, 4x1 gallon (3.8 liter) containers per case, 5-gallon pails, and 15 gallon drums.

Compendium Code No.: 10730130

POWER SHOWER SPRAY™

SSI Corp. — **Hoof Product**

Indications: For use in power shower spray units.

Aids in the treatment and prevention of footwarts.

Directions: Power Shower Directions: Use Power Shower every milking. Set the proportioner solution rate at 1:50 for at least 10 to 14 days or until control of footwarts is achieved. Then solution rate may be reduced to a maintenance rate of 1:100.

If, while using the maintenance rate, an increase of footwarts occurs, return the solution rate setting to 1:50 until control is again achieved.

Precaution(s): Keep from freezing.

Caution(s): Eye irritant. In case of contact, flush for 15 minutes. If irritation persists, call a physician.

Warning(s): Keep out of the reach of children.

Presentation: 5 gallon, 30 gallon and 55 gallon containers.

Compendium Code No.: 14930110

POX BLEN®

Merial Select **Vaccine**

Pigeon Pox Vaccine, Live Virus

U.S. Vet. Lic. No.: 279

Contents: This product contains the antigen listed above.

Contains Gentamicin as a bacteriostatic agent.

Notice: Merial Select's vaccines have met the requirements of the USDA in regard to safety, purity, potency, and the capability to protect susceptible chickens. This vaccine has been tested by the Master Seed immunogenicity test for efficacy.

Indications: This vaccine is recommended for the vaccination of chickens between four and 16 weeks of age by wing web stab as an aid in the prevention of infectious fowl pox.

This vaccine is recommended for the protection of healthy chickens. It is essential that the chickens be maintained under good environmental conditions and that exposure to disease viruses be reduced as much as possible.

Dosage and Administration: Wing Web Method:

1. Pull up on the plastic tear-flip-up top to remove the aluminum seal from the bottle containing the vaccine. Carefully pry up one edge of the rubber stopper to permit air to replace the vacuum in the bottle, then remove the stopper.
2. Remove the aluminum seal from the bottle containing the diluent, and transfer the entire contents to the bottle containing the vaccine. Replace the stopper and shake the contents vigorously until the vaccine is evenly suspended.
3. To apply the vaccine, dip the two-pronged applicator supplied in the package into the vaccine and stab into the webbed portion of the wing from the underside. Avoid stabbing through feathers which may wipe off the vaccine.
4. The applicator is designed to carry the proper amount of vaccine in the grooves of the needles. The needles should be touched briefly to the inner lip of the bottle before withdrawing to avoid wasting vaccine which may drop from the needles. Dip the applicator before each application.

Check for Takes: At about seven to ten days after vaccination, the birds may be examined for takes. A good take reaction, indicating that a satisfactory vaccination was done, shows swelling of the skin with scab formation at the point of vaccination. The scabs will fall off about two to three weeks following vaccination. Good immunity to fowl pox is established two to three weeks after vaccination.

If good takes are not seen, it may mean that the birds were immune to fowl pox, that the vaccination job was poor, or that the vaccine used had lost its potency through extended storage or mishandling.

Precaution(s): Store vaccine at 35-45°F (2-7°C). Do not freeze. Use entire vial contents when first opened. Burn this container and all unused contents.

This vaccine is non-returnable.

Caution(s): Do not vaccinate diseased chickens.

Vaccinate all chickens on the premises at one time.

Administer a minimum of one dose per chicken.

Avoid stress conditions during and following vaccination.

Do not place chickens in contaminated facilities.

Exposure to disease must be minimized as much as possible.

For veterinary use only.

The capability of this vaccine to produce satisfactory results depends upon many factors, including — but not limited to — conditions of storage and handling by the user, administration of the vaccine, health and responsiveness of individual chickens, and degree of field exposure. Therefore, directions for use should be followed carefully. The use of this vaccine is subject to applicable state and federal laws and regulations.

Warning(s): Do not vaccinate within 21 days of slaughter.

Presentation: POX BLEN® is supplied with a diluent for rehydration to 10 mL (25 x 1,000 doses).

A bottle of liquid diluent is provided with each package of vaccine.

Compendium Code No.: 11050392 PL-1M 0100

POXIMUNE®

Biomune **Vaccine**

Fowl Pox Vaccine, Live Virus

U.S. Vet. Lic. No.: 368

Contents: POXIMUNE® contains live fowl pox virus vaccine for the vaccination of chickens as an aid in the prevention of fowl pox.

Contains gentamicin and amphotericin B as preservatives.

Indications: Administer by wing web to healthy, susceptible chickens at least eight weeks of age but at least four weeks prior to the start of egg production as an aid in the prevention of fowl pox due to fowl pox virus.

Dosage and Administration: Remove seal and stopper from vaccine vial and diluent vial. Pour entire contents of diluent vial into vaccine vial, insert stopper, and shake well. The vaccine is ready for use and should be used within one hour. Hold each individual bird and spread the wing with the underside facing up. Dip the applicator into the vaccine so that the grooves fill with liquid and deliver 0.01 mL per bird. Insert the double-pronged applicator into the web portion of the wing avoiding blood vessels, muscle, and bone. Seven to ten days after vaccination, observe several chickens for evidence of "takes" that include swelling and/or scab formation at the site of injection.

Precaution(s): Federal regulations prohibit repackaging or sale of the contents of this package in fractional units. Do not accept if seal is broken.

Store vaccine at 35-45°F (2-7°(C).

Use entire contents immediately after rehydrating. Burn containers and all unused contents.

Caution(s): All birds on a farm should be vaccinated at one time.

Warning(s): Do not vaccinate within 21 days of slaughter.

Presentation: 10 x 1000 doses.

Compendium Code No.: 11290400 670

POXIMUNE® AE

Biomune **Vaccine**

Avian Encephalomyelitis-Fowl Pox Vaccine, Live Virus

U.S. Vet. Lic. No.: 368

Contents: POXIMUNE® AE contains live fowl pox virus vaccine and live avian encephalomyelitis virus vaccine for the vaccination of chickens as an aid in the prevention of fowl pox and avian encephalomyelitis.

Contains gentamicin and amphotericin B as preservatives.

Indications: Administer by wing web to healthy, susceptible chickens at least eight weeks of age but at least four weeks prior to the start of egg production as an aid in the prevention of fowl pox due to fowl pox virus and avian encephalomyelitis due to avian encephalomyelitis virus.

Dosage and Administration: Remove seal and stopper from vaccine vial and diluent vial. Pour entire contents of diluent vial into vaccine vial, insert stopper, and shake well. The vaccine is ready for use and should be used within one hour. Hold each individual bird and spread the wing with the underside facing up. Dip the applicator into the vaccine so that the grooves fill with liquid and deliver 0.01 mL per bird. Insert the double-pronged applicator into the web portion of the wing avoiding blood vessels, muscle, and bone. Seven to ten days after vaccination, observe several chickens for evidence of "takes" that include swelling and/or scab formation at the site of injection.

Precaution(s): Federal regulations prohibit repackaging or sale of the contents of this package in fractional units. Do not accept if seal is broken.

Store vaccine at 35-45°F (2-7°C).

Use entire contents immediately after rehydrating. Burn containers and all unused contents.

Caution(s): All birds on a farm should be vaccinated at one time.

Warning(s): Do not vaccinate within 21 days of slaughter.

Presentation: 10 x 1000 doses.

Compendium Code No.: 11290410 678

POXIMUNE® C

Biomune **Vaccine**

Canary Pox Vaccine, Modified Live Virus

U.S. Vet. Lic. No.: 368

Contents: POXIMUNE® C is a modified live virus vaccine that when administered to susceptible canaries confers immunity to canary pox disease. The vaccine is supplied in lyophilized (freeze-dried) form and is supplied with diluent and a single needle vaccinator for the wing web application.

Indications: POXIMUNE® C is indicated for the immunization of canaries against canary pox virus infection. All susceptible birds on the same premises should be vaccinated at the same time. Young birds may be vaccinated at weaning age. Booster vaccinations are recommended every 6 to 12 months (depending on the disease risk) and four weeks prior to laying or vector season. Vaccination in the face of a disease outbreak is also indicated and has been demonstrated to control the outbreak and stop mortality in those birds not yet showing clinical symptoms.

Dosage and Administration: Immediately prior to administration the desiccated vaccine is dissolved with the diluent supplied. The single needle vaccinator is dipped into the mixed vaccine to completely fill the groove of the needle with the proper vaccine dose. Vaccination is accomplished by piercing the needle through the underneath surface of the wing-web which should be devoid of feathers. The administration should be a slow, steady motion (not a quick poke) to ensure release of the entire vaccine dose from the needle groove onto the epithelial tissue. See package insert for complete information.

Post-Vaccination: Following wing-web vaccination, typical cutaneous pox lesions should develop locally (at the site of inoculation) which correlate with immunity or "take" of the vaccine. At about 7-10 days post vaccination, the wing-web should be examined for a satisfactory "take" reaction characterized by a focal point of swelling, inflammation or scab formation at the site of inoculation. Revaccination is recommended if a "take" reaction is not evident. Although immunity begins to develop immediately following vaccination, three (3) to four (4) weeks are required to establish maximum immunity.

Precaution(s): Store in the dark at 35°-45°F.

Use the entire contents when first opened. Burn the container and all unused contents.

Caution(s): Vaccinate healthy birds only. Do not rehydrate the vaccine until ready for use because the rehydrated vaccine virus is rapidly perishable.

For veterinary use only.

Warning(s): Do not vaccinate within four (4) weeks of onset of egg production or during egg production.

Discussion: The vaccine is used to protect canaries against canary pox disease, a highly infectious and fatal disease in canaries commonly spread by mosquitoes or direct contact between birds. Clinical expression of the disease varies from an acute respiratory form to a chronic form with skin lesions around the eyes, beak or feet. Mortality rates are devastating and can reach 100%.

Presentation: 1 x 10 dose vials of vaccine, 1 x 10 dose vials of diluent, wing-web vaccinators;
10 x 10 dose vials of vaccine, 10 x 10 dose vials of diluent, wing-web vaccinators.

Compendium Code No.: 11290252

POXINE®

Fort Dodge **Vaccine**

Fowl Pox Vaccine, Live Virus

U.S. Vet. Lic. No.: 112

Contents: This product contains the antigen listed above.

Contains gentamicin as a preservative.

Indications: POXINE® is recommended for vaccination against fowl pox in healthy chickens 6 weeks of age or older and in healthy turkeys 8 weeks of age or older.

Directions: Read in full, follow directions carefully.

When to Vaccinate:

Chickens: Vaccination with POXINE® is to be performed when chickens are at least 6 weeks of age and at least 1 month before they come into production. This vaccine is also recommended for the revaccination, at 12 weeks of age, of chickens that have been vaccinated at an age earlier than 6 weeks with another vaccine for the prevention of fowl pox.

Turkeys: Fowl-pox vaccination of turkeys is recommended in most areas because of the frequent and widespread occurrence of the disease. It is a common practice to vaccinate poults when they are transferred from the brooder house to other quarters or the range (usually at 8 weeks of age). It is recommended that the vaccination of turkeys for market be avoided during the last 8 weeks prior to marketing.

1. Rehydrate 1 vial of vaccine with 1 vial of diluent.
2. Remove aluminum seal and rubber stopper from the vaccine vial and diluent vial. Avoid contamination of the stopper and vials contents.
3. Pour approximately one-half the diluent into the vaccine vial. Replace stopper and shake gently until contents are dissolved.
4. Pour all the reconstituted vaccine back into the remaining diluent in the diluent bottle. Replace diluent stopper and gently mix. The vaccine is then ready for use.
5. Hold individual bird and spread wing with the underside facing upwards.
6. Dip the vaccinator tool into the vaccine, wetting both needles.
7. Stick the needles through the web of the wing, avoiding blood vessels, bones, and wing muscles. The vaccine should not touch the feathers, the head of the birds, or the skin except at the site of vaccination.

How Takes Appear: The usual take consists of some swelling at the site of the puncture as

P

early as the fourth day following vaccination. The swelling increases during the next five days until a scab is formed. Revaccinate birds that do not show takes.

Records: Keep a record of vaccine serial number and expiration date; date of receipt and date of vaccination; where vaccination takes place; and any reactions observed.

Precaution(s): Store this vaccine at not over 45°F (7°C).

Use entire contents of vial when first opened.

Burn this container and all unused contents.

Do not expose the vaccine to either direct sunlight or extreme heat during vaccination.

This vaccine is nonreturnable.

Caution(s): Vaccinate healthy chickens or turkeys only.

This product should be stored, transported, and administered in accordance with the instructions and directions.

The use of this vaccine is subject to state laws, wherever applicable.

Warning(s): Do not vaccinate within 21 days before slaughter. For veterinary use only.

Presentation: 10 x 1,000 doses.

Compendium Code No.: 10031551 10950B

PP-1 SPECIAL BLEND

AgriPharm **Large Animal Dietary Supplement**

Guaranteed Analysis: Represented as total colony forming units 20 x 10^9 colony forming units per pound, equivalent to approximately 4.4 x 10^7 colony forming units per gram.

Ingredients: Vegetable oil, dextrose, dried egg, sorbitan monostearate, *Lactobacillus acidophilus, Bifidobacterium thermophilum, Bifidobacterium longum, Streptococcus faecium*, lactase enzymes.

Indications: This product contains porcine host specific lactic acid producing bacteria to provide an oral source of these bacteria. These bacteria were selected for their ability to be compatible in a wide range of gut conditions.

Dosage and Administration: Administer orally on the back of tongue.

Usage Rate: 3-4 grams per piglet.

Precaution(s): Store product in a cool place. Refrigeration recommended for extended storage period.

Presentation: 60 g and 300 g packages.

Compendium Code No.: 14570860

PP-VAC®

Intervet **Vaccine**

Pigeon Pox Vaccine, Live Virus

U.S. Vet. Lic. No.: 286

Description: PP-VAC®, a live virus vaccine, is prepared from a proven strain of pigeon pox virus which was selected for its mildness and its protective characteristics against fowl pox in chickens. The virus has been propagated in SPF (Specific Pathogen Free) substrates. The immunizing capability of this vaccine has also been proven by the Master Seed Immunogenicity Test.

This vaccine contains gentamicin as a preservative.

Quality tested for purity, potency, and safety.

Indications: PP-VAC® is indicated for immunization of healthy chickens 6 to 18 weeks of age against fowl pox via wing-weg stick method.

Dosage and Administration: Preparation of Vaccine: Do not open and mix the vaccine until ready to begin vaccination. Use vaccine immediately after mixing.

1. Remove the tear-off seal and stopper from the vial containing vaccine and vial containing diluent.
2. Pour one-half of diluent from diluent vial into vial of vaccine. Insert the rubber stopper and shake until resuspended.
3. Pour resuspended vaccine into diluent vial. Add rubber stopper and shake well. Vaccine is now ready for use.

Wing-Web Administration:

1. Vaccine is applied to the web of the wing. Use the enclosed two-pronged applicator.
2. Vaccinate by dipping the applicator into the vaccine mixture and stabbing the webbed portion of the wing from beneath. Avoid feathered areas of the web.
3. At about 7 to 10 days after vaccination, a few chickens should be examined for takes. A good take reaction, indicating that a satisfactory vaccination job was done, shows swelling of the skin at the point of vaccination with scab formation. The scabs will fall off about 2 to 3 weeks following vaccination. Good immunity is established 2 to 3 weeks after vaccination.

Records: Keep a record of vaccine, quantity, serial number, expiration date and place of purchase; the date and time of vaccination; the number, age, breed and locations of chickens; names of operators performing the vaccination and any observed reactions.

Precaution(s): Store vaccine between 2 and 7°C (35 and 45°F).

Do not spill or splash the vaccine.

Use entire contents when first opened.

Burn containers and all unused contents.

This product is non-returnable.

Caution(s): Vaccinate only healthy chickens. Although disease may not be evident, coccidiosis, mycoplasma infection, Marek's disease and other disease conditions may cause complications or reduce immunity.

All susceptible chickens on the same premises should be vaccinated at the same time.

Efforts should be taken to reduce stress conditions at the time of vaccination and during the reaction period.

Do not dilute the vaccine or otherwise stretch the dosage.

For veterinary use only.

Notice: This vaccine has undergone rigid potency, safety and purity tests, and meets Intervet America Inc. and USDA requirements. It is designed to stimulate effective immunity when used as directed, but the user must be advised that the response to the product depends upon many factors, including, but not limited to, conditions of storage and handling by the user, administration of the vaccine, health and responsiveness of individual chickens and the degree of field exposure. Therefore, directions should be followed carefully.

This product is not hazardous when used according to directions supplied. A material safety data sheet (MSDS) is available upon request. This and any other consumer information can be obtained by calling Intervet Customer Service at 1-800-441-8272 or 1-302-934-8051.

The use of this vaccine is subject to applicable federal and local laws and regulations.

Use only as directed.

Warning(s): Do not vaccinate within 21 days of slaughter or 28 days prior to onset and during egg production.

Presentation: 10 x 1,000 doses for wing-web administration with 10 x 10 mL sterile diluent.

Compendium Code No.: 11061201 01306 AL111

PRE-CONDITIONING/RECEIVING FORMULA GEL

Durvet **Large Animal Dietary Supplement**

Ingredient(s): Dried *Lactobacillus acidophilus* fermentation product, dried *L. fermentum* fermentation product, dried *L. plantarum* fermentation product, dried *Streptococcus faecium* fermentation product, dried *L. casei* fermentation product, vegetable oils, sucrose, silicon dioxide, vitamin A propionate, vitamin A palmitate, d-activated animal sterol (source of vitamin D_3), dl-alpha tocopheryl acetate (source of vitamin E), dl-methionine, glycine, l-Lysine, sodium bicarbonate, potassium chloride, artificial color, polysorbate 80, preserved with ethoxyquin.

Minimum Contents of 300 mL Dose:

Sodium (from sodium bicarbonate)	445 mg - 2.9%
Potassium chloride	750 mg - 5.0%
Vitamin A	200,000 I.U.
Vitamin D_3	40,000 I.U.
Vitamin E	100 I.U.
dl-methionine	250 mg - 1.6%
Glycine	250 mg - 1.6%
l-Lysine	250 mg - 1.6%
Lactic Acid Bacteria	15 billion CFU

Guaranteed total viable Lactic Acid Bacteria: One billion Colony Forming Units (CFU) per mL.

Indications: A pre-conditioning and receiving formula gel containing vitamins, amino acids, minerals, sodium bicarbonate and live naturally occurring micro-organisms for cattle, sheep and goats.

Dosage and Administration: Administer orally onto the back of the tongue. Each full pull (3 clicks) of the trigger delivers 15 mL of gel.

Cattle over 400 lbs.	15 mL
Cattle under 400 lbs.	10 mL
Feeder Lambs	10 mL
Adult Sheep and Goats	10 mL
Newborn Calves	10 mL
Veal Calves	10 mL

Precaution(s): Keep cool.

Caution(s): For animal use only. Not for human use.

Not a drug.

Warning(s): Keep out of reach of children.

No withdrawal time.

Presentation: 80 mL and 300 mL.

Patent pending.

Compendium Code No.: 10841411 10/92

PREDEF® 2X ℞

Pharmacia & Upjohn **Steroidal Anti-inflammatory**

Isoflupredone acetate sterile aqueous suspension

NADA No.: 011-789

Active Ingredient(s): Each mL of PREDEF® 2X Sterile Aqueous Suspension contains 2 mg of isoflupredone acetate; also 4.5 mg sodium citrate hydrous; 120 mg polyethylene glycol 3350; 1 mg povidone; 0.201 mg myristyl-gamma-picolinium chloride added as preservative. When necessary, pH was adjusted with hydrochloric acid and/or sodium hydroxide.

Indications: It is for intramuscular or intrasynovial injection in animals and is indicated in situations requiring glucocorticoid, anti-inflammatory, and/or supportive effect.

Bovine Ketosis: PREDEF® 2X Sterile Aqueous Suspension, by its gluconeogenic and glycogen deposition activity, is an effective and valuable treatment for the endocrine and metabolic imbalance of primary bovine ketosis. The stresses of parturition and high milk production predispose the dairy cow to this condition. This adrenal steroid causes a prompt physiological effect, with blood glucose levels returning to normal or above within 8 to 24 hours following injection. There is a decrease in circulating eosinophils, followed by a reduction in blood and urine ketones. Usually the general attitude of the cow is much improved, appetite returns, and milk production rises to previous levels within 3 to 5 days. In secondary bovine ketosis, where the condition is complicated by pneumonia, mastitis, endometritis, traumatic gastritis, etc, PREDEF® 2X should be used concurrently with proper local and parenteral antibacterial therapy, infusion solutions, and other accepted treatments for the primary conditions.

Musculoskeletal Conditions: As with other adrenal steroids, this preparation has been found useful in alleviating the pain and lameness associated with generalized and acute localized arthritic conditions in large animals. PREDEF® 2X has been used successfully to treat laminitis, rheumatoid and traumatic arthritis, osteoarthritis, periostitis, tendinitis, tenosynovitis, bursitis, and myositis. Generalized muscular soreness, stiffness, depression, and anorexia resulting from overwork, shipping, unusual physical exertion, etc, respond promptly. Remission of symptoms may be permanent, or symptoms may recur, depending on the cause and extent of structural degeneration.

Allergic Reactions: PREDEF® 2X is especially beneficial in treating acute hypersensitivity reactions resulting from treatment with a sensitizing drug or exposure to other allergenic agents. Usual manifestations are anaphylactoid reactions and urticaria. Less severe allergic manifestations, such as atopic and contact dermatitis, summer eczema, and conjunctivitis, may also be treated. Response is usually rapid and complete, although in severe cases with extensive lesions, more prolonged adrenocorticoid therapy and other appropriate treatment may be indicated.

Overwhelming Infections with Severe Toxicity: In animals moribund from overwhelmingly severe infections for which specific antibacterial therapy is available (eg, critical pneumonia, peritonitis, endometritis, septic mastitis), intensive PREDEF® 2X therapy may aid in correcting the circulatory defect by counteracting the responsible inflammatory changes, thereby permitting the antibacterial agent to exert its full effect. As supportive therapy, this steroid combats the stress and improves the general attitude of the animal being treated. All necessary procedures for the establishment of a bacterial diagnosis should be carried out whenever possible before institution of therapy. PREDEF® 2X Sterile Aqueous Suspension therapy in the presence of infection should be administered for the shortest possible time compatible with maintenance of an adequate response, and antibacterial therapy should be continued for at least three days after the hormone has been withdrawn. Combined hormone and antibacterial therapy does not obviate the need for indicated surgical treatment.

Shock: PREDEF® 2X is indicated in adrenal failure and shocklike states occurring in association with severe injury or other trauma, emergency surgery, anaphylactoid reactions, and elective surgery in poor surgical risks. It is recommended as an adjuvant to standard methods of combating shock, including use of plasma expanders. Because of interrelated physiologic activities, beneficial effects may not be exhibited until all such procedures have been employed.

Other Indications: Exhaustion following surgery or dystocia, retained placenta, inflammatory ocular conditions, snakebite, and other stress conditions are also indications for use. Its employment in the treatment of these conditions is recommended as a supportive measure to standard procedures and time-honored treatments will give comfort to the animal and hasten complete recovery.

PREDEF® 2X has been found useful as supportive therapy in the treatment of the stress associated with parturient paresis ie, milk fever. It should be given intramuscularly, before or after the administration of the calcium infusion solutions commonly employed in treating the disease. PREDEF® 2X is not to be added to the infusion solutions.

Pharmacology: Metabolic and Hormonal Effects: PREDEF® 2X, a potent corticosteroid developed in the Research Laboratories of The Upjohn Company, has greater glucocorticoid activity than an equal quantity of prednisolone.

The glucocorticoid activity of PREDEF® 2X is approximately 10 times that of prednisolone, 50 times that of hydrocortisone, and 67 times that of cortisone as measured by liver glycogen deposition in rats. The gluconeogenic activity is borne out by its hyperglycemic effect in both normal and ketotic cattle.

Dosage and Administration: PREDEF® 2X Sterile Aqueous Suspension is administered by deep intramuscular injection for systemic effect, or into joint cavity, tendon sheath, or bursa for local effect.

Cattle: The usual intramuscular dose for cattle is 10 to 20 mg, according to the size of the animal and severity of the condition. This dose may be repeated in 12 to 24 hours if indicated.

Ketosis studies have demonstrated that relatively high initial doses of corticoids produce a more prompt recovery with a lower incidence of relapse than when relatively low doses are used, even when these are repeated. Response of ketosis to PREDEF® 2X therapy parallels that derived with prednisolone. PREDEF® 2X is 10 times more glucogenic than prednisolone. Thus, 10 mg of isoflupredone acetate therapeutically equals 100 mg of prednisolone.

In the event of poor response or relapse, diagnosis should be reconfirmed by re-examining the animal for complications (ie, pneumonia, metritis, traumatic gastritis, mastitis).

Horses: The usual intramuscular dose for horses is 5 to 20 mg repeated as necessary. The usual intrasynovial dose in joint inflammation, tendinitis, or bursitis is 5 to 20 mg or more, depending on the size of the cavity to be injected.

Swine: The usual intramuscular dose for swine is 5 mg for a 300 pound animal. The dose for larger or smaller pigs is proportional to the weight of the animal.

Precaution(s): Store at controlled room temperature 20° to 25°C (68° to 77°F) [see USP].

Caution(s): Federal (USA) law restricts this drug to use by or on the order of a licensed veterinarian.

PREDEF® 2X Sterile Aqueous Suspension exerts an inhibitory influence on the mechanisms and the tissue changes associated with inflammation. Vascular permeability is decreased, exudation diminished, and migration of the inflammatory cells markedly inhibited. In addition, systemic manifestations such as fever and signs of toxemia may also be suppressed. While certain aspects of this alteration of the inflammatory reaction may be beneficial, the suppression of inflammation may mask the signs of infection and tend to facilitate spread of microorganisms. However, in infections characterized by overwhelming toxicity, PREDEF® 2X therapy in conjunction with appropriate antibacterial therapy is effective in reducing mortality and morbidity. Without concurrent use of an antibiotic to which the invader-organism is sensitive, injudicious use of the adrenal hormones in animals with infections can be hazardous. As with other corticoids, continued or prolonged use is discouraged.

While no sodium retention nor potassium depletion has been observed at the doses recommended in animals receiving 9-fluoroprednisolone acetate, as with all corticoids, animals should be under close observation for possible untoward effects. If symptoms of hypopotassemia should occur, corticoid therapy should be discontinued and 5% solution of potassium chloride administered by continuous intravenous drip.

For use in animals only.

Warning(s): Animals intended for human consumption should not be slaughtered within 7 days of last treatment. A withdrawal period has not been established for this product in preruminating calves. Do not use in calves to be processed for veal. Not for human use.

Clinical and experimental data have demonstrated that corticosteroids administered orally or parenterally to animals may induce the first stage of parturition when administered during the last trimester of pregnancy and may precipitate premature parturition followed by dystocia, fetal death, retained placenta, and metritis.

Additionally, corticosteroids administered to dogs, rabbits, and rodents during pregnancy have resulted in cleft palate in offspring. Corticosteroids administered to dogs during pregnancy have also resulted in other congenital anomalies, including deformed forelegs, phocomelia, and anasarca.

Presentation: PREDEF® 2X Sterile Aqueous Suspension, 2 mg per mL, is available in 10 mL vials, NDC 0009-0620-01 and 100 mL vials, NDC 0009-0620-08.

Compendium Code No.: 10490451 810 880 111/810 880 311

PREDICT-A-FOAL

V.D.I. **Foaling Test**

Mare Foaling Predictor Kit

U.S. Vet. Lic. No.: 360

Components: Collection vial, reagent solution, test tubes, indicator test strips, comparison chart.

Indications: Measures levels of calcium and magnesium in the mare's secretions/milk. As the foaling time nears, these levels begin to rise considerably.

Test Principles: 5 indicator squares that are impregnated with special chemicals placed on a plastic strip. Each square contains a different amount of chemical in it (to indicate degrees ranging from low to very high) which react according to the levels in the mare's milk/secretions. As the squares on the test strip change color, this correlates with the chart supplied with the kit offering the probability of the mare foaling within the next 12 hours.

Test Procedure: Secretions are expressed into a collection vial.

1. Gently clean the udder with a clean cloth and warm water - no soap. Begin at the top and work down to the nipples, rinsing the cloth as needed. Be sure to clean in the "cleavage" between the halves of the udder. When cleaned, allow to completely air dry. Gently dab the ends of the teats with a clean, dry cloth to remove any contaminating material before beginning to sample. This process gets the mare accustomed to having her udder touched (no small feat with many maiden mares!), encourages the milk to "let down" (be released from the upper part of the udder into the collecting system of the teats) and relaxes the mare.
2. Place the thumb and first one or two fingers around the areas of the udder just above where the teat begins and compress gently but not too tightly. This helps to bring the milk or other secretions down.
3. Return to the junction of the upper teat with the udder, with your thumb and first one or two fingers again, compressing as tightly as you can this time. In one smooth motion, without letting up on the pressure, slip your hand down the full length of the teat and express the milk. Be careful not to pull the teat toward you - keep it perpendicular to the ground. Allow the first few "squirts" to go to the ground - you will often have fine particles of dirt or skin contaminating the initial sample even with washing the udder.
4. Repeat step #3, collecting the milk into the container.

Reagent solution is then added to a test tube to a marked line, and 0.6 cc of mare's milk/secretion is added to this.

The test tube is gently inverted to mix the milk with reagent, and a test strip is then dipped into the test tube. After waiting exactly one minute, the test strip, which has five boxes on it, is examined for any color changes.

Interpretation of Results: Results are read as follows: No change, 1 percent chance of foaling; one box changed, 1 percent chance; two boxes, 10 percent; three boxes, 40 percent; four boxes, 80 percent; and five boxes 90 percent chance of imminent foaling.

Precaution(s): Store in a cool, dry place. Can be used next foaling season.

Presentation: 15 tests.

Compendium Code No.: 11280100

PREDNISTAB® ℞

Phoenix Pharmaceutical **Corticosteroid-Oral**

(Brand of Prednisolone, USP) 5 mg

NADA No.: 140-921

Active Ingredient(s): Each Tablet Contains:

Prednisolone, USP .... 5 mg

Indications: PREDNISTAB® is intended for use in dogs. The indications for PREDNISTAB® are the same as those for other anti-inflammatory steroids and comprise the various collagen, dermal, allergic, ocular, otic, and musculoskeletal conditions known to be responsive to the anti-inflammatory corticosteroids. Representative of the conditions in which the use of steroid therapy and the benefits to be derived therefrom have had repeated confirmation in the veterinary literature are: (1) dermal conditions, such as nonspecific eczema, summer dermatitis, and burns; (2) allergic manifestations, such as acute urticaria, allergic dermatitis, drug and serum reactions, bronchial asthma, and pollen sensitivities; (3) ocular conditions, such as iritis, iridocyclitis, secondary glaucoma, uveitis, and chorioretinitis; (4) otic conditions, such as otitis externa; (5) musculoskeletal conditions, such as myositis, rheumatoid arthritis, osteoarthritis, and bursitis; (6) various chronic or recurrent diseases of unknown etiology such as ulcerative colitis and nephrosis.

In acute adrenal insufficiency, prednisolone may be effective because of its ability to correct the defect in carbohydrate metabolism and relieve the impaired diuretic response to water, characteristic of primary or secondary adrenal insufficiency. However, because this agent lacks significant mineralocorticoid activity, hydrocortisone sodium succinate, hydrocortisone, or cortisone should be used when salt retention is indicated.

Pharmacology: Description: Prednisolone, like methylprednisolone, is a potent anti-inflammatory steroid. Prednisolone, 11,17,21-trihydroxypregna-1,4-diene-3,20-dione, is a synthetic dehydrogenated analogue of cortisone. Prednisolone and methylprednisolone have a greater anti-inflammatory potency and less tendency to induce sodium and water retention than the older corticoids, cortisone and hydrocortisone. The relative anti-inflammatory potency for hydrocortisone is 1.0; cortisone is 0.8; prednisolone is 4 and methylprednisolone is 5. The relative sodium retaining potency for hydrocortisone is 4; prednisolone is 3 and methylprednisolone is 2.[1,2]

Dosage and Administration: Dosage: 2.5 mg per 10 lb (4.5 kg) body weight per day. Average total daily oral doses for dogs are as follows:

5 to 20 lb (2 to 9 kg) body weight	1.25 to 5 mg
20 to 40 lb (9 to 18 kg) body weight	5 to 10 mg
40 to 80 lb (18 to 36 kg) body weight	10 to 20 mg
80 to 160 lb (38 to 72 kg) body weight	20 to 40 mg

The total daily dose should be given in divided doses, 6 to 10 hours apart.

Administration: The keystone of satisfactory therapeutic management with PREDNISTAB® prednisolone tablets, as with other steroid predecessors, is individualization of dosage in reference to the severity of the disease, the anticipated duration of steroid therapy, and the animal patient's threshold or tolerance for steroid excess. The prime objective of steroid therapy should be to achieve a satisfactory degree of control with a minimum effective daily dose.

The dosage recommendations are suggested average total daily doses and are intended as guides. As with other orally administered corticosteroids, the total daily dose of prednisolone should be given in equally divided doses. The initial suppressive dose level is continued until a satisfactory clinical response is obtained, a period usually of 2 to 7 days in the case of musculoskeletal diseases, allergic conditions affecting the skin or respiratory tract, and ocular inflammatory diseases. If a satisfactory response is not obtained in 7 days, reevaluation of the case to confirm the original diagnosis should be made. As soon as a satisfactory clinical response is obtained, the daily dose should be reduced gradually, either to termination of treatment in the case of acute conditions (e.g., seasonal asthma, dermatitis, acute ocular inflammations) or to the minimal effective maintenance dose level in the case of chronic conditions (e.g., rheumatoid arthritis). In chronic conditions, and in rheumatoid arthritis especially, it is important that the reduction in dosage from initial to maintenance dose levels be accomplished slowly. The maintenance dose level should be adjusted from time to time as required by fluctuation in the activity of the disease and the animal's general status. Accumulated experience has shown that the long-term benefits to be gained from continued steroid maintenance are probably greater the lower the maintenance dose level. In rheumatoid arthritis in particular, maintenance steroid therapy should be at the lowest possible level.

Important: In the therapeutic management of animal patients with chronic diseases such as rheumatoid arthritis, prednisolone should be regarded as a highly valuable adjunct, to be used in conjunction with, but not as replacement for, standard therapeutic measures.

Contraindication(s): Do not use in viral infections. Prednisolone, like methylprednisolone, is contraindicated in animals with peptic ulcer, corneal ulcer, and Cushingoid syndrome. The presence of diabetes, osteoporosis, predisposition to thrombophlebitis, hypertension, congestive heart failure, renal insufficiency, and active tuberculosis necessitates carefully controlled use. Some of the above conditions occur only rarely in dogs but should be kept in mind.

Precaution(s): Storage: Store at controlled room temperature 15°-30°C (59°-86°F).

Caution(s): Federal law restricts this drug to use by or on the order of a licensed veterinarian.

Because of its inhibitory effect on fibroplasia, prednisolone may mask the signs of infection and enhance dissemination of the infecting organism. Hence, all animal patients receiving prednisolone should be watched for any evidence of intercurrent infection. Should infection occur, it must be brought under control by use of appropriate antibacterial measures, or administration of prednisolone should be discontinued.

Prednisolone, like methylprednisolone and other adrenocortical steroids, is a potent therapeutic agent influencing the biochemical behavior of most, if not all, tissues of the body. Because this anti-inflammatory steroid manifests little sodium-retaining activity, the usual early sign of cortisone or hydrocortisone overdosage (i.e., increase in body weight due to fluid retention) is not a reliable index of overdosage. Hence, recommended dose levels should not be exceeded, and all animal patients receiving prednisolone should be under close medical supervision. All precautions pertinent to the use of methylprednisolone apply to prednisolone. Moreover, the veterinarian should endeavor to keep informed of current studies of corticosteroids as they are reported in the veterinary literature.

Use of corticosteroids, depending on dose, duration and specific steroid, may result in inhibition of endogenous steroid production following drug withdrawal. In patients presently receiving or recently withdrawn from systemic corticosteroid treatments, therapy with a rapid-acting corticosteroid should be considered only in unusually stressful situations.

For oral use in dogs only.

For animal use only.

Warning(s): Not for human use. Clinical and experimental data have demonstrated that corticosteroids administered orally or by injection to animals may induce the first stage of parturition if used during the last trimester of pregnancy and may precipitate premature parturition followed by dystocia, fetal death, retained placenta, and metritis.

Additionally, corticosteroids administered to dogs, rabbits, and rodents during pregnancy have resulted in cleft palate in offspring. Corticosteroids administered to dogs during pregnancy have also resulted in other congenital anomalies including deformed forelegs, phocomelia, and anasarca.

Keep out of reach of children.

Adverse Reactions: Prednisolone is similar to methylprednisolone in regard to the kinds of side effects and metabolic alterations to be anticipated when treatment is intensive or prolonged. In animal patients with diabetes mellitus, use of prednisolone may be associated with an increase in the insulin requirement. Negative nitrogen balance may occur, particularly in animals that require protracted maintenance therapy; measures to counteract persistent nitrogen loss include a high protein intake and the administration, when indicated, of a suitable anabolic agent. Excessive loss of potassium, like excessive retention of sodium, is not likely to be induced by effective maintenance doses of prednisolone. However, these effects should be kept in mind and the usual regulatory measures employed as indicated. Ecchymotic manifestations in dogs may occur. If such reactions do occur and are serious, reduction in dose or discontinuance of prednisolone therapy may be indicated.

Side effects, such as SAP and SALT enzyme elevations, weight loss, anorexia, polydipsia and polyuria have occurred following the use of synthetic corticosteroids in dogs. Vomiting and diarrhea (occasionally bloody) have also been observed. Cushing's syndrome in dogs has been reported in association with prolonged or repeated steroid therapy.

Since prednisolone, like methylprednisolone, suppresses endogenous adrenocortical activity, it is highly important that the animal patient receiving prednisolone be under careful observation, not only during the course of treatment but for some time after treatment is terminated. Adequate adrenocortical supportive therapy with cortisone or hydrocortisone, and including ACTH, must be employed promptly if the animal is subjected to any unusual stress such as surgery, trauma, or severe infection.

References: Available upon request.

Presentation: PREDNISTAB® is available as 5 mg compressed quarter-scored tablets in bottles of 1000 (NDC 57319-441-16).

Manufactured by: Vet-A-Mix, Shenandoah, IA 51601.

Compendium Code No.: 12560692 Rev. 05-02

PREDNISTAB® ℞

Vedco **Corticosteroid-Oral**

5 mg Prednisolone, USP

NADA No.: 140-921

NDC No.: 50989-163-53

Active Ingredient(s): Each tablet contains:

Prednisolone, U.S.P. .... 5 mg

Indications: PREDNISTAB® is intended for oral use in dogs only. The indications for PREDNISTAB® are the same as those for other anti-inflammatory steroids and comprise the various collagen, dermal, allergic, ocular, otic, and musculoskeletal conditions known to be responsive to the anti-inflammatory corticosteroids. Representative of the conditions in which the use of steroid therapy and the benefits to be derived therefrom have had repeated confirmation in the veterinary literature are: (1) dermal conditions, such as nonspecific eczema, summer dermatitis, and burns; (2) allergic manifestations, such as acute urticaria, allergic dermatitis, drug and serum reactions, bronchial asthma, and pollen sensitivities; (3) ocular conditions, such as iritis, iridocyclitis, secondary glaucoma, uveitis, and chorioretinitis; (4) otic conditions, such as otitis externa; (5) musculoskeletal conditions, such as myositis, rheumatoid arthritis, osteo-arthritis, and bursitis; (6) various chronic or recurrent diseases of unknown etiology such as ulcerative colitis and nephrosis.

In acute adrenal insufficiency, prednisolone may be effective because of its ability to correct the defect in carbohydrate metabolism and relieve the impaired diuretic response to water, characteristic of primary or secondary adrenal insufficiency. However, because this agent lacks significant mineralocorticoid activity, hydrocortisone sodium succinate, hydrocortisone, or cortisone should be used when salt retention is indicated.

Pharmacology: Prednisolone, like methylprednisolone, is a potent anti-inflammatory steroid. Prednisolone, 11,17,21-trihydroxypregna-1,4-diene-3,20-dione, is a synthetic dehydrogenated analogue of cortisone. Prednisolone and methylprednisolone have a greater anti-inflammatory potency and have less tendency to induce sodium and water retention than the older corticoids, cortisone and hydrocortisone. The relative anti-inflammatory potency for hydrocortisone is 1.0, cortisone is 0.8, prednisolone is 4 and methylprednisolone is 5. The relative sodium retaining potency for hydrocortisone is 4, prednisolone is 3 and methylprednisolone is 2.[1,2]

Dosage and Administration: The average total daily oral doses for dogs are as follows:

Body Weight	Daily Dosage
5-15 lbs. (2-7 kg)	2.5 mg
15-40 lbs. (7-18 kg)	2.5 to 5 mg
40-80 lbs. (18-36 kg)	5 to 10 mg

The total daily dose should be given in divided doses, 6-10 hours apart.

The keystone of satisfactory therapeutic management with PREDNISTAB® prednisolone tablets is the individualization of dosage with reference to the severity of the disease, the anticipated duration of steroid therapy, and the animal patient's threshold or tolerance for steroid excess. The prime objective of steroid therapy should be to achieve a satisfactory degree of control with a minimum effective daily dose.

The dosage recommendations are suggested average total daily doses and are intended as guides. As with other orally administered corticosteroids, the total daily dose of prednisolone should be given in equally divided doses. The initial suppressive dose level is continued until a satisfactory clinical response is obtained, usually a period of two (2) to seven (7) days in the case of musculoskeletal diseases, allergic conditions affecting the skin or respiratory tract, and ocular inflammatory diseases. If a satisfactory response is not obtained in seven (7) days, re-evaluation of the case to confirm the original diagnosis should be made. As soon as a satisfactory clinical response is obtained, the daily dose should be reduced gradually, either to the termination of treatment in the case of acute conditions (e.g., seasonal asthma, dermatitis, acute ocular inflammations) or to the minimal effective maintenance dose level in the case of chronic conditions (e.g., rheumatoid arthritis). In chronic conditions, and in rheumatoid arthritis especially, it is important that the reduction in dosage from the initial to maintenance dose levels be accomplished slowly. The maintenance dose level should be adjusted from time to time as required by fluctuations in the activity of the disease and the animal's general status. Accumulated experience has shown that the long-term benefits to be gained from continued steroid maintenance are probably greater the lower the maintenance dose level. In rheumatoid arthritis in particular, maintenance steroid therapy should be at the lowest possible level.

Important: In the therapeutic management of animal patients with chronic diseases such as rheumatoid arthritis, prednisolone should be regarded as a highly valuable adjunct, to be used in conjunction with, but not as replacement for, standard therapeutic measures.

Contraindication(s): Do not use in viral infections. Prednisolone, like methylprednisolone, is contraindicated in animals with peptic ulcer, corneal ulcer, and Cushing's syndrome. The presence of diabetes, osteoporosis, predisposition to thrombophlebitis, hypertension, congestive heart failure, renal insufficiency, and active tuberculosis necessitates carefully controlled use. Some of the above conditions occur only rarely in dogs, but should be kept in mind.

Precaution(s): Store at a controlled room temperature of 15° to 30°C (59° to 86°F).

Prednisolone, like methylprednisolone and other adrenocortical steroids, is a potent therapeutic agent influencing the biochemical behavior of most, if not all, tissues of the body. Because this anti-inflammatory steroid manifests little sodium-retaining activity, the usual early sign of cortisone or hydrocortisone overdosage (i.e., increase in body weight due to fluid retention) is not a reliable index of overdosage. Hence, the recommended dose levels should not be exceeded, and all animal patients receiving prednisolone should be under close medical supervision. All precautions pertinent to the use of methylprednisolone apply to prednisolone. Moreover, the veterinarian should endeavor to keep informed of current studies of corticosteroids as they are reported in the veterinary literature.

The use of corticosteroids, depending upon the dose, duration and specific steroid, may result in the inhibition of endogenous steroid production following drug withdrawal. In patients presently receiving or recently withdrawn from systemic corticosteroid treatments, therapy with a rapid-acting corticosteroid should be considered only in unusually stressful situations.

Caution(s): Federal law restricts this drug to use by or on the order of a licensed veterinarian.

Because of its inhibitory effect on fibroplasia, prednisolone may mask the signs of infection and enhance dissemination of the infecting organism. Hence, all animal patients receiving prednisolone should be watched for any evidence of intercurrent infection. Should infection occur, it must be brought under control by the use of appropriate antibacterial measures, or the administration of prednisolone should be discontinued.

Keep out of the reach of children.

Warning(s): Not for human use. Clinical and experimental data have demonstrated that corticosteroids administered orally or parenterally to animals may induce the first stage of parturition if used during the last trimester of pregnancy and may precipitate premature parturition followed by dystocia, fetal death, retained placenta, and metritis.

Additionally, corticosteroids administered to dogs, rabbits, and rodents during pregnancy have resulted in cleft palate in offspring. Corticosteroids administered to dogs during pregnancy have also resulted in other congenital anomalies, including deformed forelegs, phocomelia, and anasarca.

Side Effects: Prednisolone is similar to methylprednisolone with regard to the kinds of side effects and metabolic alterations to be anticipated when the treatment is intensive or prolonged. In animal patients with diabetes mellitus, the use of prednisolone may be associated with an increase in the insulin requirement. Negative nitrogen balance may occur, particularly in animals that require protracted maintenance therapy; measures to counteract persistent nitrogen loss include a high protein intake and the administration, when indicated, of a suitable anabolic agent. Excessive loss of potassium, like excessive retention of sodium, is not likely to be induced by effective maintenance doses of prednisolone. However, these effects should be kept in mind and the usual regulatory measures employed as indicated. Ecchymotic manifestations in dogs may occur. If such reactions do occur and are serious, a reduction in the dose or discontinuance of prednisolone therapy may be indicated.

Side effects, such as SAP and SALT enzyme elevations, weight loss, anorexia, polydipsia and polyuria have occurred following the use of synthetic corticosteroids in dogs. Vomiting and diarrhea (occasionally bloody) have also been observed. Cushing's syndrome in dogs has been reported in association with prolonged or repeated steroid therapy.

Since prednisolone, like methylprednisolone, suppresses endogenous adrenocortical activity, it is very important that the animal patient receiving prednisolone be under careful observation, not only during the course of treatment, but for some time after the treatment is terminated. Adequate adrenocortical supportive therapy with cortisone or hydrocortisone, and including ACTH, must be promptly employed if the animal is subjected to any unusual stress such as surgery, trauma, or severe infection.

References: Available upon request.

Presentation: Bottles of 1,000 tablets.

Compendium Code No.: 10941710

PREDNISTAB® ℞

Vet-A-Mix **Corticosteroid-Oral**

Prednisolone, USP

NADA No.: 140-921

Active Ingredient(s): Each compressed quarter-scored tablet contains:

Prednisolone, USP .... 5 mg or 20 mg

Indications: PREDNISTAB® is intended for use in dogs. The indications for PREDNISTAB® are the same as those for other anti-inflammatory steroids and comprise the various collagen, dermal, allergic, ocular, otic, and musculoskeletal conditions known to be responsive to the anti-inflammatory corticosteroids. Representative of the conditions in which the use of steroid therapy and the benefits to be derived therefrom have had repeated confirmation in the veterinary literature are: (1) dermal conditions, such as nonspecific eczema, summer dermatitis, and burns; (2) allergic manifestations, such as acute urticaria, allergic dermatitis, drug and serum reactions, bronchial asthma, and pollen sensitivities; (3) ocular conditions, such as iritis, iridocyclitis, secondary glaucoma, uveitis, and chorioretinitis; (4) otic conditions, such as otitis externa; (5) musculoskeletal conditions, such as myositis, rheumatoid arthritis, osteoarthritis, and bursitis; (6) various chronic or recurrent diseases of unknown etiology such as ulcerative colitis and nephrosis.

In acute adrenal insufficiency, prednisolone may be effective because of its ability to correct the defect in carbohydrate metabolism and relieve the impaired diuretic response to water, characteristic of primary or secondary adrenal insufficiency. However, because this agent lacks significant mineralocorticoid activity, hydrocortisone sodium succinate, hydrocortisone, or cortisone should be used when salt retention is indicated.

Pharmacology: Description: Prednisolone, like methylprednisolone, is a potent anti-inflammatory steroid. Prednisolone, 11,17,21-trihydroxypregna-1,4-diene-3,20-dione, is a synthetic dehydrogenated analogue of cortisone. Prednisolone and methylprednisolone have a greater anti-inflammatory potency and less tendency to induce sodium and water retention than the older corticoids, cortisone and hydrocortisone. The relative anti-inflammatory potency for hydrocortisone is 1.0; cortisone is 0.8; prednisolone is 4 and methylprednisolone is 5. The relative sodium retaining potency for hydrocortisone is 4; prednisolone is 3 and methylprednisolone is 2.[1,2]

Dosage and Administration: Dosage: 2.5 mg per 10 lb (4.5 kg) body weight per day. Average total daily oral doses for dogs are as follows:

5 to 20 lb (2 to 9 kg) body weight .... 1.25 to 5 mg
20 to 40 lb (9 to 18 kg) body weight .... 5 to 10 mg
40 to 80 lb (18 to 36 kg) body weight .... 10 to 20 mg
80 to 160 lb (36 to 73 kg) body weight .... 20 to 40 mg

The total daily dose should be given in divided doses, 6 to 10 hours apart.

Administration: The keystone of satisfactory therapeutic management with prednisolone tablets, as with other steroid predecessors, is individualization of dosage in reference to the severity of the disease, the anticipated duration of steroid therapy, and the animal patient's threshold or tolerance for steroid excess. The prime objective of steroid therapy should be to achieve a satisfactory degree of control with a minimum effective daily dose.

The dosage recommendations are suggested average total daily doses and are intended as guides. As with other orally administered corticosteroids, the total daily dose of prednisolone should be given in equally divided doses. The initial suppressive dose level is continued until a satisfactory clinical response is obtained, a period usually of 2 to 7 days in the case of musculoskeletal diseases, allergic conditions affecting the skin or respiratory tract, and ocular inflammatory diseases. If a satisfactory response is not obtained in 7 days, reevaluation of the case to confirm the original diagnosis should be made. As soon as a satisfactory clinical response is obtained, the daily dose should be reduced gradually, either to termination of treatment in the case of acute conditions (e.g., seasonal asthma, dermatitis, acute ocular inflammations) or to the minimal effective maintenance dose level in the case of chronic conditions (e.g., rheumatoid arthritis). In chronic conditions, and in rheumatoid arthritis especially, it is important that the reduction in dosage from initial to maintenance dose levels be accomplished slowly. The maintenance dose level should be adjusted from time to time as required by fluctuation in the activity of the disease and the animal's general status. Accumulated experience has shown that the long-term benefits to be gained from continued steroid maintenance are probably greater the lower the maintenance dose level. In rheumatoid arthritis in particular, maintenance steroid therapy should be at the lowest possible level.

Important: In the therapeutic management of animal patients with chronic diseases such as rheumatoid arthritis, prednisolone should be regarded as a highly valuable adjunct, to be used in conjunction with, but not as a replacement for, standard therapeutic measures.

Contraindication(s): Do not use in viral infections. Prednisolone, like methylprednisolone, is contraindicated in animals with peptic ulcer, corneal ulcer, and Cushingoid syndrome. The presence of diabetes, osteoporosis, predisposition to thrombophlebitis, hypertension, congestive heart failure, renal insufficiency, and active tuberculosis necessitates carefully controlled use. Some of the above conditions occur only rarely in dogs, but should be kept in mind.

Precaution(s): Store at controlled room temperature 15°-30°C (59°-86°F).

Caution(s): Federal law restricts this drug to use by or on the order of a licensed veterinarian.

Because of its inhibitory effect on fibroplasia, prednisolone may mask the signs of infection and enhance dissemination of the infecting organism. Hence, all animal patients receiving prednisolone should be watched for evidence of intercurrent infection. Should infection occur, it must be brought under control by use of appropriate antibacterial measures, or administration of prednisolone should be discontinued.

Prednisolone, like methylprednisolone and other adrenocortical steroids, is a potent therapeutic agent influencing the biochemical behavior of most, if not all, tissues of the body. Because this anti-inflammatory steroid manifests little sodium-retaining activity, the usual early sign of cortisone or hydrocortisone overdosage (i.e., increase in body weight due to fluid retention) is not a reliable index of overdosage. Hence, recommended dose levels should not be exceeded, and all animal patients receiving prednisolone should be under close medical supervision. All precautions pertinent to the use of methylprednisolone apply to prednisolone. Moreover, the veterinarian should endeavor to keep informed of current studies of corticosteroids as they are reported in the veterinary literature.

Use of corticosteroids, depending on dose, duration and specific steroid, may result in inhibition of endogenous steroid production following drug withdrawal. In patients presently receiving or recently withdrawn from systemic corticosteroid treatments, therapy with a rapid-acting corticosteroid should be considered in unusually stressful situations.

For oral use in dogs only.

Warning(s): Not for human use. Clinical and experimental data have demonstrated that corticosteroids administered orally or by injection to animals may induce the first stage of parturition if used during the last trimester of pregnancy and may precipitate premature parturition followed by dystocia, fetal death, retained placenta, and metritis.

Additionally, corticosteroids administered to dogs, rabbits, and rodents during pregnancy have resulted in cleft palate in offspring. Corticosteroids administered to dogs during pregnancy have also resulted in other congenital anomalies, including deformed forelegs, phocomelia, and anasarca.

Adverse Reactions: Prednisolone is similar to methylprednisolone in regard to kinds of side effects and metabolic alterations to be anticipated when treatment is intensive or prolonged. In animal patients with diabetes mellitus, use of prednisolone may be associated with an increase in the insulin requirement. Negative nitrogen balance may occur, particularly in animals that require protracted maintenance therapy; measures to counteract persistent nitrogen loss include a high protein intake and the administration, when indicated, of a suitable anabolic agent. Excessive loss of potassium, like excessive retention of sodium, is not likely to be induced by effective maintenance doses of prednisolone. However, these effects should be kept in mind and the usual regulatory measures employed as indicated. Ecchymotic manifestations in dogs may occur. If such reactions do occur and are serious, reduction in dose or discontinuance of prednisolone therapy may be indicated.

Side effects, such as SAP and SALT enzyme elevations, weight loss, anorexia, polydipsia and polyuria have occurred following the use of synthetic corticosteroids in dogs. Vomiting and diarrhea (occasionally bloody) have also been observed. Cushing's syndrome in dogs has been reported in association with prolonged or repeated steroid therapy.

Since prednisolone, like methylprednisolone, suppresses endogenous adrenocortical activity, it is highly important that the animal patient receiving prednisolone be under careful observation, not only during the course of treatment, but for some time after treatment is terminated. Adequate adrenocortical supportive therapy with cortisone or hydrocortisone, and including ACTH, must be employed promptly if the animal is subjected to any unusual stress such as surgery, trauma, or severe infection.

References: Available upon request.

Presentation: PREDNISTAB® is available as 5 mg compressed quarter-scored tablets in bottles of 1000 and 20 mg compressed quarter-scored tablets in bottles of 500.

Compendium Code No.: 10500251

0198

PREDNISTAB® ℞

Vetus — **Corticosteroid-Oral**

(5 mg Prednisolone, USP)

NADA No.: 140-921

Active Ingredient(s): Each Tablet Contains:

Prednisolone, USP .... 5 mg

Indications: PREDNISTAB® is intended for use in dogs. The indications for PREDNISTAB® are the same as those for other anti-inflammatory steroids and comprise the various collagen, dermal, allergic, ocular, otic, and musculoskeletal conditions known to be responsive to the anti-inflammatory corticosteroids. Representative of the conditions in which the use of steroid therapy and the benefits to be derived therefrom have had repeated confirmation in the veterinary literature are: (1) dermal conditions, such as nonspecific eczema, summer dermatitis, and burns; (2) allergic manifestations, such as acute urticaria, allergic dermatitis, drug and serum reactions, bronchial asthma, and pollen sensitivities; (3) ocular conditions, such as iritis, iridocyclitis, secondary glaucoma, uveitis, and chorioretinitis; (4) otic conditions, such as otitis externa; (5) musculoskeletal conditions, such as myositis, rheumatoid arthritis, osteoarthritis, and bursitis; (6) various chronic or recurrent diseases of unknown etiology such as ulcerative colitis and nephrosis.

In acute adrenal insufficiency, prednisolone may be effective because of its ability to correct the defect in carbohydrate metabolism and relieve the impaired diuretic response to water, characteristic of primary or secondary adrenal insufficiency. However, because this agent lacks significant mineralocorticoid activity, hydrocortisone sodium succinate, hydrocortisone, or cortisone should be used when salt retention is indicated.

Pharmacology: Description: Prednisolone, like methylprednisolone, is a potent anti-inflammatory steroid. Prednisolone, 11,17,21-trihydroxypregna-1,4-diene-3,20-dione, is a synthetic dehydrogenated analogue of cortisone. Prednisolone and methylprednisolone have a greater anti-inflammatory potency and less tendency to induce sodium and water retention than the older corticoids, cortisone and hydrocortisone. The relative anti-inflammatory potency for hydrocortisone is 1.0; cortisone is 0.8; prednisolone is 4 and methylprednisolone is 5. The relative sodium retaining potency for hydrocortisone is 4; prednisolone is 3 and methylprednisolone is 2.[1,2]

Dosage and Administration: Dosage: 2.5 mg per 10 lb (4.5 kg) body weight per day. Average total daily oral doses for dogs are as follows:

5 to 20 lb (2 to 9 kg) body weight.................................... 1.25 to 5 mg
20 to 40 lb (9 to 18 kg) body weight.................................... 5 to 10 mg
40 to 80 lb (18 to 36 kg) body weight.................................... 10 to 20 mg
80 to 160 lb (36 to 73 kg) body weight.................................... 20 to 40 mg

The total daily dose should be given in divided doses, 6 to 10 hours apart.

Administration: The keystone of satisfactory therapeutic management with prednisolone tablets, as with other steroid predecessors, is individualization of dosage in reference to the severity of the disease, the anticipated duration of steroid therapy, and the animal patient's threshold or tolerance for steroid excess. The prime objective of steroid therapy should be to achieve a satisfactory degree of control with a minimum effective daily dose.

The dosage recommendations are suggested average total daily doses and are intended as guides. As with other orally administered corticosteroids, the total daily dose of prednisolone should be given in equally divided doses. The initial suppressive dose level is continued until a satisfactory clinical response is obtained, a period usually of 2 to 7 days in the case of musculoskeletal diseases, allergic conditions affecting the skin or respiratory tract, and ocular inflammatory diseases. If a satisfactory response is not obtained in 7 days, reevaluation of the case to confirm the original diagnosis should be made. As soon as a satisfactory clinical response is obtained, the daily dose should be reduced gradually, either to termination of treatment in the case of acute conditions (e.g., seasonal asthma, dermatitis, acute ocular inflammations) or to the minimal effective maintenance dose level in the case of chronic conditions (e.g., rheumatoid arthritis). In chronic conditions, and in rheumatoid arthritis especially, it is important that the reduction in dosage from initial to maintenance dose levels be accomplished slowly. The maintenance dose level should be adjusted from time to time as required by fluctuation in the activity of the disease and the animal's general status. Accumulated experience has shown that the long-term benefits to be gained from continued steroid maintenance are probably greater the lower the maintenance dose level. In rheumatoid arthritis in particular, maintenance steroid therapy should be at the lowest possible level.

Important: In the therapeutic management of animal patients with chronic diseases such as rheumatoid arthritis, prednisolone should be regarded as a highly valuable adjunct, to be used in conjunction with, but not as a replacement for, standard therapeutic measures.

Contraindication(s): Do not use in viral infections. Prednisolone, like methylprednisolone, is contraindicated in animals with peptic ulcer, corneal ulcer, and Cushingoid syndrome. The presence of diabetes, osteoporosis, predisposition to thrombophlebitis, hypertension, congestive heart failure, renal insufficiency, and active tuberculosis necessitates carefully controlled use. Some of the above conditions occur only rarely in dogs, but should be kept in mind.

Precaution(s): Store at controlled room temperature 15°-30°C (59°-86°F).

Caution(s): Federal law restricts this drug to use by or on the order of a licensed veterinarian.

Because of its inhibitory effect on fibroplasia, prednisolone may mask the signs of infection and enhance dissemination of the infecting organism. Hence, all animal patients receiving prednisolone should be watched for evidence of intercurrent infection. Should infection occur, it must be brought under control by use of appropriate antibacterial measures, or administration of prednisolone should be discontinued.

Prednisolone, like methylprednisolone and other adrenocortical steroids, is a potent therapeutic agent influencing the biochemical behavior of most, if not all, tissues of the body. Because this anti-inflammatory steroid manifests little sodium-retaining activity, the usual early sign of cortisone or hydrocortisone overdosage (i.e., increase in body weight due to fluid retention) is not a reliable index of overdosage. Hence, recommended dose levels should not be exceeded, and all animal patients receiving prednisolone should be under close medical supervision. All precautions pertinent to the use of methylprednisolone apply to prednisolone. Moreover, the veterinarian should endeavor to keep informed of current studies of corticosteroids as they are reported in the veterinary literature.

Use of corticosteroids, depending on dose, duration and specific steroid, may result in inhibition of endogenous steroid production following drug withdrawal. In patients presently receiving or recently withdrawn from systemic corticosteroid treatments, therapy with a rapid-acting corticosteroid should be considered in unusually stressful situations.

For oral use in dogs only.

Warning(s): Not for human use. Clinical and experimental data have demonstrated that corticosteroids administered orally or by injection to animals may induce the first stage of parturition if used during the last trimester of pregnancy and may precipitate premature parturition followed by dystocia, fetal death, retained placenta, and metritis.

Additionally, corticosteroids administered to dogs, rabbits, and rodents during pregnancy have resulted in cleft palate in offspring. Corticosteroids administered to dogs during pregnancy have also resulted in other congenital anomalies, including deformed forelegs, phocomelia, and anasarca.

Keep out of reach of children.

Adverse Reactions: Prednisolone is similar to methylprednisolone in regard to kinds of side effects and metabolic alterations to be anticipated when treatment is intensive or prolonged. In animal patients with diabetes mellitus, use of prednisolone may be associated with an increase in the insulin requirement. Negative nitrogen balance may occur, particularly in animals that require protracted maintenance therapy; measures to counteract persistent nitrogen loss include a high protein intake and the administration, when indicated, of a suitable anabolic agent. Excessive loss of potassium, like excessive retention of sodium, is not likely to be induced by effective maintenance doses of prednisolone. However, these effects should be kept in mind and the usual regulatory measures employed as indicated. Ecchymotic manifestations in dogs may occur. If such reactions do occur and are serious, reduction in dose or discontinuance of prednisolone therapy may be indicated.

Side effects, such as SAP and SALT enzyme elevations, weight loss, anorexia, polydipsia and polyuria have occurred following the use of synthetic corticosteroids in dogs. Vomiting and diarrhea (occasionally bloody) have also been observed. Cushing's syndrome in dogs has been reported in association with prolonged or repeated steroid therapy.

Since prednisolone, like methylprednisolone, suppresses endogenous adrenocortical activity, it is highly important that the animal patient receiving prednisolone be under careful observation, not only during the course of treatment, but for some time after treatment is terminated. Adequate adrenocortical supportive therapy with cortisone or hydrocortisone, and including ACTH, must be employed promptly if the animal is subjected to any unusual stress such as surgery, trauma, or severe infection.

References: Available upon request.

Presentation: PREDNISTAB® is available as 5 mg compressed quarter-scored tablets in bottles of 1000 (NDC 47611-859-10).

Manufactured by: Vet-A-Mix, Shenandoah, IA 51601.

Distributed by: Burns Veterinary Supply, Inc., Westbury, NY 11590.

Compendium Code No.: 14440930 0901

PREEMPT™

Milk Specialties **Microorganisms**

Defined Competitive Exclusion Culture

NADA No.: 141-101

Active Ingredient(s): Anaerobic bacterial culture.

Inactive Ingredient: Skim milk.

Reconstitution Powder: Sodium carbonate, casein peptone, potassium phosphate, di-potassium phosphate, yeast extract, arginine, serine, glucose, cysteine, sodium lactate, and succinic acid.

One dose contains at least 1 X 10^7 CFU/chick (normal gut bacteria).

Indications: For the early establishment of intestinal microflora in chickens to reduce *Salmonella* colonization.

Pharmacology: Description: PREEMPT™ is a laboratory stabilized and characterized bacterial culture originally derived from the ceca of adult healthy chickens. PREEMPT™ is stored as frozen pellets and prepared by reconstituting the pellets in a protective solution prepared using reconstitution powder.

Mechanism of Action: Administration of PREEMPT™ provides chicks with the bacteria needed to establish a normal gut microflora at a time when they are vulnerable to infection with *Salmonella* bacteria. Normal gut bacteria (PREEMPT™) are sprayed onto the chicks. Through normal preening, the bacteria establish themselves within the chick intestinal tract and provide protection from the establishment of *Salmonella.* Protection occurs through a competitive exclusion process.

Dosage and Administration:

Preparation and Administration: Clean all equipment to come in contact with reconstituted PREEMPT™. Do not use chemical disinfectants.

Prepare reconstitution media before removing PREEMPT™ foil packages from storage. Add one 2000 dose package of reconstitution powder to 490 mL of deionized water in a 1 L container. Mix gently or stir until all solids are dissolved. Add one 5000 dose package of reconstitution powder to 1250 mL of deionized water in a 2 L container. Mix gently or stir until all solids are dissolved.

Remove one 2000 or 5000 dose PREEMPT™ foil package from storage. Open package and pour the frozen pellets into the prepared reconstitution media. Mix gently or stir until suspension is homogeneous.

Allow the reconstituted PREEMPT™ to stand at room temperature for approximately 45 minutes. Use the reconstituted PREEMPT™ within 5 hours.

Reconstituted PREEMPT™ is administered as a topical spray via a spray box. See spray box manual for instructions on proper use.

Twenty-five (25) mL of reconstituted PREEMPT™ is sprayed onto each tray of 100 chicks (approximately 0.25 mL/chick).

Expose chicks to light for at least 5 minutes after spray treatment to encourage preening.

Clean and rinse spray box thoroughly after each use.

For Optimal Results: Administer to chicks as soon as possible after hatch, preferably less than one day of age.

Chicks must be given access to feed and water as soon as possible after treatment.

Preening, and thus PREEMPT™ uptake, is encouraged by moving chicks from darkness prior to treatment, into moderately bright light following treatment.

Stacking of trays immediately after spraying is not recommended since it creates a semi-dark situation which discourages preening.

Chicks must be dry and free from disease at time of treatment.

PREEMPT™ should be used as part of a comprehensive *Salmonella* control program covering the hatchery, the growout facility, and the processing plant.

Dosage: When mixed per instructions, each package will treat 2000 or 5000 chicks. One dose of PREEMPT™ contains at least 1 X 10^7 CFU/chick.

Precaution(s): Storage Conditions: PREEMPT™ must be stored at approximately -70°C (dry ice temperature). Do not refreeze thawed packages. Do not use if thawing of product has occurred during storage.

Reconstitution powder should be stored refrigerated.

Disposal: Dispose of unused PREEMPT™ by incineration or by inactivation with one part household bleach (5% NaOCl) to nine parts resuspended PREEMPT™. The empty foil package should be treated with bleach or autoclaved and disposed of in a sanitary landfill.

Caution(s): Do not administer antibiotics to PREEMPT™ treated chicks. The efficacy of PREEMPT™ is reduced by antibiotics. Exposure of chicks to antibiotics at the hatchery or use of antibiotics in the starter feed impairs establishment of the PREEMPT™ culture. Administration of therapeutic levels of antibiotics during growout may eliminate the PREEMPT™ bacteria along with other intestinal bacteria and create an environment open to colonization with *Salmonella*. PREEMPT™ is a live bacterial culture and should remain in a restricted area. The area should be regularly sanitized with bleach or disinfectant. Materials exposed to PREEMPT™ should be properly discarded or sanitized. This product is a preventive treatment and does not reduce *Salmonella* in birds with preexisting *Salmonella* colonization.

Warning(s): Administer PREEMPT™ in a well-ventilated area. Respiratory masks and protective eyewear are strongly recommended due to potentially irritating reconstitution powder components. Respiratory masks should be capable of excluding bacteria and personnel should be trained in their use. Gloves and laboratory coats are also recommended.

Although PREEMPT™ consists of non-pathogenic bacteria, prolonged or direct exposure of the eyes or respiratory passages to PREEMPT™ is not recommended. Care should be taken to avoid contamination of eyes, hands, clothing, and respiratory passages with PREEMPT™. People with known allergies or asthma should take extra precautions to avoid exposure to this product.

The material safety data sheet (MSDS) provides occupational safety information. For a copy of the MSDS or to report adverse reactions attributable to exposure to this product, call 1-888-772-5825.

Not for human use. Keep out of reach of children.

Adverse Reactions: No adverse reactions have been observed in association with the use of PREEMPT™ in pre-approval/investigational studies.

Presentation: 2000-dose pouches, 40 per box.
5000-dose pouches, 20 per box.

PREEMPT™ is a TM of MS BioScience, Inc.

Compendium Code No.: 10850100 3/00

PREEMPT™

MS BioScience **Microorganisms**

Defined Competitive Exclusion Culture

NADA No.: 141-101

Active Ingredient(s): Anaerobic bacterial culture.

Inactive Ingredient: Skim milk.

Reconstitution Powder: Sodium carbonate, casein peptone, potassium phosphate, di-potassium phosphate, yeast extract, arginine, serine, glucose, cysteine, sodium lactate, and succinic acid.

One dose contains at least 1 X 10^7 CFU/chick (normal gut bacteria).

Indications: For the early establishment of intestinal microflora in chickens to reduce *Salmonella* colonization.

Pharmacology: Description: PREEMPT™ is a laboratory stabilized and characterized bacterial culture originally derived from the ceca of adult healthy chickens. PREEMPT™ is stored as frozen pellets and prepared by reconstituting the pellets in a protective solution prepared using reconstitution powder.

Mechanism of Action: Administration of PREEMPT™ provides chicks with the bacteria needed to establish a normal gut microflora at a time when they are vulnerable to infection with *Salmonella* bacteria. Normal gut bacteria (PREEMPT™) are sprayed onto the chicks. Through normal preening, the bacteria establish themselves within the chick intestinal tract and provide protection from the establishment of *Salmonella.* Protection occurs through a competitive exclusion process.

Dosage and Administration:

Preparation and Administration: Clean all equipment to come in contact with reconstituted PREEMPT™. Do not use chemical disinfectants.

Prepare reconstitution media before removing PREEMPT™ foil packages from storage. Add one 2000 dose package of reconstitution powder to 490 mL of deionized water in a 1 L container. Mix gently or stir until all solids are dissolved. Add one 5000 dose package of reconstitution powder to 1250 mL of deionized water in a 2 L container. Mix gently or stir until all solids are dissolved.

Remove one 2000 or 5000 dose PREEMPT™ foil package from storage. Open package and pour the frozen pellets into the prepared reconstitution media. Mix gently or stir until suspension is homogeneous.

Allow the reconstituted PREEMPT™ to stand at room temperature for approximately 45 minutes. Use the reconstituted PREEMPT™ within 5 hours.

Reconstituted PREEMPT™ is administered as a topical spray via a spray box. See spray box manual for instructions on proper use.

Twenty-five (25) mL of reconstituted PREEMPT™ is sprayed onto each tray of 100 chicks (approximately 0.25 mL/chick).

Expose chicks to light for at least 5 minutes after spray treatment to encourage preening.

Clean and rinse spray box thoroughly after each use.

For Optimal Results: Administer to chicks as soon as possible after hatch, preferably less than one day of age.

Chicks must be given access to feed and water as soon as possible after treatment.

Preening, and thus PREEMPT™ uptake, is encouraged by moving chicks from darkness prior to treatment, into moderately bright light following treatment.

Stacking of trays immediately after spraying is not recommended since it creates a semi-dark situation which discourages preening.

Chicks must be dry and free from disease at time of treatment.

PREEMPT™ should be used as part of a comprehensive *Salmonella* control program covering the hatchery, the growout facility, and the processing plant.

Dosage: When mixed per instructions, each package will treat 2000 or 5000 chicks. One dose of PREEMPT™ contains at least 1 X 10^7 CFU/chick.

Precaution(s): Storage Conditions: PREEMPT™ must be stored at approximately -70°C (dry ice temperature). Do not refreeze thawed packages. Do not use if thawing of product has occurred during storage.

Reconstitution powder should be stored refrigerated.

Disposal: Dispose of unused PREEMPT™ by incineration or by inactivation with one part household bleach (5% NaOCl) to nine parts resuspended PREEMPT™. The empty foil package should be treated with bleach or autoclaved and disposed of in a sanitary landfill.

Caution(s): Do not administer antibiotics to PREEMPT™ treated chicks. The efficacy of PREEMPT™ is reduced by antibiotics. Exposure of chicks to antibiotics at the hatchery or use of antibiotics in the starter feed impairs establishment of the PREEMPT™ culture. Administration of therapeutic levels of antibiotics during growout may eliminate the PREEMPT™ bacteria along with other intestinal bacteria and create an environment open to colonization with *Salmonella*. PREEMPT™ is a live bacterial culture and should remain in a restricted area. The area should be regularly sanitized with bleach or disinfectant. Materials exposed to PREEMPT™ should be properly discarded or sanitized. This product is a preventive treatment and does not reduce *Salmonella* in birds with preexisting *Salmonella* colonization.

Warning(s): Administer PREEMPT™ in a well-ventilated area. Respiratory masks and protective eyewear are strongly recommended due to potentially irritating reconstitution powder components. Respiratory masks should be capable of excluding bacteria and personnel should be trained in their use. Gloves and laboratory coats are also recommended.

Although PREEMPT™ consists of non-pathogenic bacteria, prolonged or direct exposure of the eyes or respiratory passages to PREEMPT™ is not recommended. Care should be taken to avoid contamination of eyes, hands, clothing, and respiratory passages with PREEMPT™. People with known allergies or asthma should take extra precautions to avoid exposure to this product.

The material safety data sheet (MSDS) provides occupational safety information. For a copy of the MSDS or to report adverse reactions attributable to exposure to this product, call 1-888-772-5825.

Not for human use. Keep out of reach of children.

Adverse Reactions: No adverse reactions have been observed in association with the use of PREEMPT™ in pre-approval/investigational studies.

Presentation: 2000-dose pouches, 40 per box.
5000-dose pouches, 20 per box.

PREEMPT™ is a TM of MS BioScience, Inc.

Compendium Code No.: 10650000 3/00

PREFARROW SHIELD™ 9

Novartis Animal Vaccines **Bacterin-Toxoid**

Bordetella Bronchiseptica-Clostridium Perfringens Type C-Erysipelothrix Rhusiopathiae-Escherichia Coli-Pasteurella Multocida Bacterin-Toxoid

U.S. Vet. Lic. No.: 303

Composition: This bacterin contains inactivated cultures of *Bordetella bronchiseptica, Clostridium perfringens* Type C, *Erysipelothrix rhusiopathiae,* K88, K99, 987P, and F41 piliated *Escherichia coli, Pasteurella multocida* Type A, and toxigenic *Pasteurella multocida* Type D adjuvanted with aluminum hydroxide.

Indications: For use in healthy, pregnant swine as an aid in the prevention and control of disease in piglets caused by *Bordetella bronchiseptica, Clostridium perfringens* Type C, *Erysipelothrix rhusiopathiae,* K88, K99, 987P, and F41 piliated *Escherichia coli,* and the toxin of *Pasteurella multocida* Types A and D.

Dosage and Administration: Shake well before using. Administer 5 mL intramuscularly 5 and 2 weeks prior to farrowing. Piglets from vaccinated dams should be vaccinated with Rhini Shield™ TX4 (Bordetella Bronchiseptica-Erysipelothrix Rhusiopathiae-Pasteurella Multocida Bacterin-Toxoid) according to the label instructions.

Precaution(s): Store in the dark at 35°-45°F (2°-7°C). Do not freeze. Use entire contents when first opened.

Caution(s): It is essential that newborn pigs receive colostrum from the vaccinated dam. Anaphylactic reactions may occur following the use of this biological. Symptomatic treatment: Epinephrine.

For veterinary use only.

Warning(s): Do not vaccinate within 21 days prior to slaughter.

Discussion: Technical Disease Information:

Erysipelas: Erysipelas in swine is caused by a bacterium, *Erysipelothrix rhusiopathiae.* Pigs become infected most commonly from ingesting the organism, although it may also enter the body through skin wounds. The source of the infection is usually other carrier pigs or wild animals such as rodents and birds.

Clinical signs of erysipelas in swine can be acute, subacute, or chronic. In the acute form, animals show signs of systemic disease. They lie around and are reluctant to rise. If forced to rise, they will stand with their legs tucked under their bodies. Affected pigs are off feed and have fevers of 104°-108°F. Pregnant sows may abort. Raised red skin lesions ("diamond skin" lesions) often appear within 2-3 days, and animals that develop severe skin lesions usually die.

Subacute erysipelas includes many of the same symptoms, but they are less severe, sometimes to the point of being unnoticed.

Chronic erysipelas may follow cases of acute or subacute erysipelas, or it may show up in pigs that have had no previous signs of illness. Pigs with chronic erysipelas usually show signs of arthritis due to degenerative changes in the joints. The valves of the heart may also be affected, in which case the animals will show signs of heart disease such as shortness of breath. Perhaps the major economic losses are in animals infected with the chronic form of the disease because of high treatment costs, retarded growth, arthritic conditions, and poor performance in feeder pigs.

The pathogen is spread via the oral route, and many swine are carriers of the organism. It has been estimated that up to 30% of clinically normal swine have erysipelas-infected tonsils.

Swine of all ages are susceptible to erysipelas. As a group, animals less than one month of age are less affected due to maternal protection from their immunized dams. However, newborn or young pigs are very susceptible to erysipelas if maternal protection is not in place. Animals older than 3 years of age are usually resistant to infection because of subclinical exposure or from vaccination programs.

Bordetella bronchiseptica: Bordetella bronchiseptica has long been established as a primary cause of atrophic rhinitis (AR) and pneumonia. In the case of AR, *B. bronchiseptica* may act as a primary invader and, depending on the virulence of the strain, may act alone or may compromise the nasal epithelium so that secondary *Pasteurella* organisms can invade and cause more extensive damage.

The most common clinical signs of AR are sneezing, snuffling, rubbing the nose, black tear streaks from the eye and excessive nasal discharge.

A more severe clinical situation associated with *B. bronchiseptica* is bronchopneumonia. This can occur in piglets as young as three to five days of age and is considered a primary infection. The clinical signs of *B. bronchiseptica* bronchopneumonia are coughing and labored breathing. Morbidity and mortality can be high.

Pasteurella multocida: Pasteurella multocida is another important cause of pneumonia and atrophic rhinitis in swine. It is found worldwide, and it is a common inhabitant of the respiratory tract of healthy animals. It can affect animals of any age.

P. multocida is divided into two types, A and D. Type A is a common cause of pneumonia. Its importance is as a secondary invader. Lungs damaged by other causes such as poor air quality, ascarid (roundworm) migrations, or other infectious agents, can be invaded by *Pasteurella,* which causes further lung damage and culminates in a severe pneumonia. These animals will show typical pneumonia symptoms-coughing, shortness of breath, labored breathing ("thumping"), and fevers up to 107°F. If not treated in the early stages, many animals become chronic cases. Death losses, while typically low, may be high in some cases.

Toxin-producing strains of *P. multocida* Type D are an important cause of atrophic rhinitis. The bacteria colonize the nasal turbinates, then release a toxin which causes damage to the tissues and results in the typical signs of AR-sneezing, snuffling, teary eyes and crooked snouts. An important feature with Type D is that it can infect older pigs and cause severe AR, whereas piglets normally have to be infected with *B. bronchiseptica* within a few days after birth in order to develop AR.

Nasal turbinates damaged by AR are not able to do an effective job of filtering the air the pig breathes, allowing more bacteria access to the lungs. This, in turn, makes it more likely that the pig will develop severe pneumonia.

Escherichia coli: Enteric colibacillosis (EC) (scours in baby pigs caused by *Escherichia coli)* is the number one killer of piglets, accounting for 42% of all death losses nationwide. Approximately 22.5% of all young pigs are infected with *E. coli.*

EC occurs typically in pigs from two to three hours of age until weaning. Pigs die from rapid dehydration resulting from loss of body fluids into the lumen of the intestines. When death occurs quickly, the only marked post-mortem signs are a greatly expanded volume of fluid in the intestines. In very acute cases pronounced diarrhea may not be evident because most of the fluids may be retained in the lumen of the intestines.

Clostridium perfringens Type C: *Clostridium perfringens* Type C enterotoxemia occurs in piglets during the first weeks of life, with death occurring 2-48 hours after the onset of symptoms. Death may occur as early as 8 hours after birth.

Pathogenic clostridia are found as normal flora of the intestinal tracts of domestic animals. These organisms can proliferate rapidly and secrete a potent necrotizing toxin. Piglets from one to ten days old may be found dead without previously showing symptoms. Symptoms seen in affected animals include abdominal pain, diarrhea (sometime blood-tinged), depression, and cessation of nursing.

Postmortem lesions vary according to the predominating type of exotoxin. If alpha toxin predominates, there will be extensive hemorrhage in the jejunum and ileum as well as in the mesenteric and intestinal lymph nodes. There will be bloodstained contents in the lower small intestine and the colon. If beta toxin predominates, there will be necrosis of the jejunum and ileum and peritonitis. Petechial hemorrhages will be found on the spleen, heart, thymus, and serosal surfaces.

Trial Data: *Escherichia coli* Challenge Trial Data: Two hundred twenty-five piglets from 30 vaccinated gilts were taken at farrowing and separated into four groups. Each group was challenged orally with one of four strains (K99, K88, 987P or F41) of *E. coli.* One hundred ninety-nine piglets from 29 nonvaccinated gilts were used as controls and challenged in the same way as the vaccinates. Each group was observed over a four-day period.

In summary, piglets from vaccinated gilts experienced an average of approximately only 11% of the death losses, only 17% of the severity of clinical symptoms and 333% increase in the daily weight gain when compared to control piglets.

Clostridium perfringens Type C Trial Data: Eighty-three percent of piglets from vaccinated gilts survived challenge with *Clostridium perfringens* Type C toxin. In contrast, none of the piglets from nonvaccinated gilts survived challenge, indicating the effectiveness of vaccinating the dam in the prevention of enterotoxemia caused by *Cl. perfringens* Type C.

Bordetella bronchiseptica Challenge Study: The mortality rate in piglets from the vaccinate group was almost six times lower than that in the control (unvaccinated) group. In addition, vaccinate group piglets showed a statistically significant reduction in the degree of atrophic rhinitis as measured by nasal turbinate atrophy scores.

Pasteurella multocida Type D Challenge Study: Piglets in the control group showed nearly eight times more atrophic rhinitis, as measured by nasal turbinate atrophy scores, than piglets from the vaccinate group. Also, vaccinate group piglets showed a statistically significant increase in weight gained during the duration of the study.

Presentation: Available in 10 dose (50 mL), 20 dose (100 mL), and 50 dose (250 mL) bottles.

Compendium Code No.: 11140682 MP-F223-JUNE01

PREFARROW STREP SHIELD®

Novartis Animal Vaccines **Bacterin**

Streptococcus Suis Bacterin

U.S. Vet. Lic. No.: 303

Composition: This bacterin contains inactivated cultures of *Streptococcus suis* adjuvanted with aluminum hydroxide. Contains penicillin, streptomycin, and thimerosal as preservatives.

Indications: For use in healthy swine as an aid in the prevention and control of diseases caused by *Streptococcus suis* serotype 2.

Dosage and Administration: Shake well before using. Administer 2 mL intramuscularly to sows and gilts 5 and 2 weeks prior to each farrowing to provide passive protection in the newborn pigs. Administer 2 mL intramuscularly to piglets at 3 and 5 weeks of age for active immunization.

Precaution(s): Store in the dark at 35°-45°F (2°-7°C). Do not freeze. Use entire contents when first opened.

Caution(s): It is essential that newborn pigs receive colostrum from the vaccinated dam to insure passive immunity. Anaphylactic reactions may occur following the use of this biological. Symptomatic treatment: Epinephrine.

For veterinary use only.

Warning(s): Do not vaccinate within 21 days prior to slaughter.

Discussion: Diagnosticians and practitioners recognize *Streptococcus suis* as a primary cause of meningitis and septicemia in the post-weaning pig. It has also been associated with pneumonia, arthritis, and rhinitis in pigs and with abortion and infertility in sows and gilts.

Strep suis is generally introduced into a herd by a healthy carrier pig. *Strep suis* can persist on the tonsils of healthy carrier pigs without causing disease. It can also persist in pigs receiving penicillin-medicated feed for up to 512 days. Sows and gilts infect their own piglets at the time of farrowing via the respiratory route. Infected piglets can then develop disease or infect susceptible pigs when mixed at the time of weaning. Although *Strep suis* infection generally occurs at the time of farrowing, disease may not occur until the time of weaning, a period of high stress. Disease from *Strep suis* appears more often in swine confinement operations and during the fall to spring months.

Clinical signs of *Strep suis* can include the central nervous system (incoordination, paralysis, paddling, opisthotonos, tremors and convulsions), pneumonia, arthritis, septicemia and polyserositis in young pigs. Blindness, deafness and laminitis can also be seen. Septicemia and arthritis in the absence of meningitis are less striking and may go undetected. Disease in the adult is generally limited to female reproductive problems.

Diagnosis of *Strep suis* infections should consider clinical signs, gross and histological post-mortem changes, bacterial culture, and a differential diagnosis. *Strep suis* must be differentiated from *Haemophilus parasuis*, pseudorabies, *Mycoplasma*, other *Streptococci*, and toxicities that cause central nervous system signs.

Treatment of *Strep suis* infections in individual sick animals is not rewarding, especially if the central nervous signs are present. Ampicillin and penicillin are the injectable drugs of choice in the disease.

Presentation: Available in 50 dose (100 mL) and 125 dose (250 mL) bottles.

Compendium Code No.: 11140363

PREFERENCE™ STAIN & ODOR REMOVER

Virbac **Deodorant Product**

Indications: Removes stains and odors from carpets and upholstery on contact.

Directions:

Stain: Test for color-fastness on an inconspicuous area. Remove as much solid waste as possible. Apply PREFERENCE™ Stain & Odor Remover directly and liberally to the stain. Use a brush handle or fingertips to agitate. Blot with a damp, clean white cloth until stain is lifted. Repeat if necessary.

Odor: After stain removal, saturate the area, allowing PREFERENCE™ Stain & Odor Remover to soak into any padding. Allow to dry. If odor persists, repeat. Not intended for use on wool carpet or wool fabrics. Pet stains contain certain acids which could result in permanent fiber discoloration.

Presentation: 16 fl oz (473 mL).

Compendium Code No.: 10230410

PREGGUARD™ FP 9

Pfizer Animal Health **Bacterin-Vaccine**

Bovine Rhinotracheitis-Virus Diarrhea-Parainfluenza$_3$, Modified Live Virus-Campylobacter Fetus-Leptospira Canicola-Grippotyphosa-Hardjo-Icterohaemorrhagiae-Pomona Bacterin

U.S. Vet. Lic. No.: 189

Description: The freeze-dried vaccine is a preparation of modified live virus (MLV) strains of IBR, BVD, and PI$_3$ propagated on an established cell line. The *Campylobacter* bacterin is an inactivated suspension of *C. fetus.* It is combined with an inactivated *Leptospira* bacterin prepared from whole cultures of the agents indicated. The *Campylobacter-Leptospira* bacterin is supplied as a diluent for the IBR-BVD-PI$_3$ vaccine.

Contains gentamicin as preservative.

Indications: PREGGUARD™ FP 9 is for vaccination of healthy cows and heifers prior to breeding as an aid in preventing abortion caused by infectious bovine rhinotracheitis (IBR, bovine herpesvirus Type 1) virus; persistent infection caused by bovine virus diarrhea (BVD) virus Types 1 and 2 fetal infection; respiratory disease caused by IBR, BVD Types 1 and 2, and parainfluenza$_3$ (PI$_3$) virus; campylobacteriosis (vibriosis) caused by *Campylobacter fetus;* and leptospirosis caused by *Leptospira canicola, L. grippotyphosa, L. hardjo, L. icterohaemorrhagiae,* and *L. pomona.*

Directions:

1. General Directions: Vaccination of healthy, non-pregnant cattle is recommended. Aseptically rehydrate the freeze-dried vaccine (Bovi-Shield™ 3) with the liquid bacterin provided (Vibrio/Leptoferm-5™), shake well, and administer 2 mL intramuscularly. In accordance with Beef Quality Assurance guidelines, this product should be administered in the muscular region of the neck.
2. Primary Vaccination: Administer a single 2 mL dose to all breeding cows and heifers approximately 1 month prior to breeding or being added to the herd, followed 2-4 weeks later by a single dose of Vibrio/Leptoferm-5™.
3. Revaccination: Annual revaccination with a single dose of PREGGUARD™ FP 9 is recommended.
4. Good animal husbandry and herd health management practices should be employed.

Precaution(s): Store at 2°-7°C. Prolonged exposure to higher temperatures and/or direct sunlight may adversely affect potency. Do not freeze.

Use entire contents when first opened.

Sterilized syringes and needles should be used to administer this vaccine. Do not sterilize with chemicals because traces of disinfectant may inactivate the vaccine.

Burn containers and all unused contents.

Caution(s): Do not use in pregnant cows (abortions can result) or in calves nursing pregnant cows. Do not vaccinate neonatal calves.

Vaccination of stressed animals should be delayed.

Occasional hypersensitivity reactions may occur up to 18 hours post-vaccination. Owners should be advised to observe animals during this period. While this event appears to be rare overall, dairy cattle may be affected more frequently than other cattle. Animals affected may display excessive salivation, incoordination, and/or dyspnea. Animals displaying such signs should be treated immediately with epinephrine or equivalent. In non-responsive animals, other modes of treatment should be considered.

As with many vaccines, anaphylaxis may occur after use. Initial antidote of epinephrine is recommended and should be followed with appropriate supportive therapy.

This product has been shown to be efficacious in healthy animals. A protective immune response may not be elicited if animals are incubating an infectious disease, are malnourished or parasitized, are stressed due to shipment or environmental conditions, are otherwise immunocompromised, or the vaccine is not administered in accordance with label directions.

For veterinary use only.

Warning(s): Do not vaccinate within 21 days before slaughter.

Discussion: Disease Description: IBR, BVD, and PI$_3$ viruses are commonly associated with respiratory disease and/or reproductive failure in cattle. IBR virus infection is characterized by high temperature, excessive nasal discharge, conjunctivitis and ocular discharge, inflamed nose ("red nose"), increased rate of respiration, coughing, loss of appetite, and depression. Cattle infected during pregnancy may abort.

BVD virus may be transmitted in nasal secretions, saliva, blood, feces, and/or urine, and by direct contact with contaminated objects; it invades through the nose and mouth and replicates systemically. Infection during pregnancy may result in abortion, fetal resorption, or congenital malformation of the fetus. Moreover, if susceptible cows are infected with non-cytopathic BVD virus during the first trimester of pregnancy, their calves may be born persistently infected with the virus. Exposure of those calves to certain virulent cytopathic BVD virus strains may precipitate BVD-mucosal disease. Clinical signs of BVD include loss of appetite, ulcerations in the mouth, profuse salivation, elevated temperature, diarrhea, dehydration, and lameness.

PI$_3$ virus usually localizes in the upper respiratory tract, causing elevated temperature and moderate nasal and ocular discharge. Although clinical signs typically are mild, PI$_3$ infection weakens respiratory tissues. Invasion and replication of other pathogens, particularly *Pasteurella* spp., is thereby facilitated and may result in pneumonia.

Campylobacteriosis (vibriosis) is an insidious venereal disease of cattle. The *Campylobacter* organism infects the cow's genital tract causing early embryonic death. The disease is characterized by infertility, repeat breeding, and a prolonged calving season.

Leptospirosis may be caused by several serovars of *Leptospira*, of which *L. canicola, L. grippotyphosa, L. hardjo, L. icterohaemorrhagiae,* and *L. pomona* are the most common affecting cattle. *Leptospira* localize in the kidneys, are shed in the urine, and cause anaemia, bloody urine, fever, loss of appetite, and prostration in calves. Signs are usually subclinical in adult cattle. Infected pregnant cows, however, often abort, and dairy cows may exhibit a marked decrease in milk production. *Leptospira* spp. are known zoonotic pathogens.

Trial Data: Safety and Efficacy: The cell lines on which the modified live virus fractions are produced have been extensively tested to ensure freedom from adventitious agents. In the case of the BVD fraction, susceptible calves inoculated intranasally with a field dose, or parenterally with 10 times the field dose remained clinically normal. The immunizing agents in the *Campylobacter-Leptospira* bacterin have been rendered non-infective by means of inactivation.

Separate challenge-of-immunity tests for the modified live virus fractions were conducted in accordance with federal regulations. All vaccinated calves remained clinically normal following challenge that produced typical signs of disease in non-vaccinated control calves.

Immunogenicity of the *Campylobacter* and *Leptospira* fractions were confirmed by challenge-of-immunity or serologic tests.

The effectiveness of PREGGUARD™ FP 9 in preventing IBR-induced abortion was demonstrated by vaccinating susceptible heifers approximately 1 month prior to breeding. The vaccinated heifers, along with a group of non-vaccinated controls, were challenged with virulent IBR virus (Cooper strain) at approximately 190 days post-breeding. Results are summarized in the following table.

Group	No. of Pregnant Heifers	No. of Abortions[3,4]	Percent of Abortions[4]
Vaccinates[1]	20	1/20[3]	5.0%
Vaccinates[2]	20	0/20	0.0%
Controls	11	10/11[4]	91.0%[4]

[1] Vaccination with a single dose 1 month prior to breeding. Seronegative heifers with no history of vaccination with any product containing IBR or BVD vaccine viruses were selected for use in the efficacy studies.

[2] Vaccination with 2 doses at 5 months and 1 month prior to breeding.

[3] One stillbirth (IBR positive). Nineteen of 20 normal.

[4] Nine abortions (IBR positive). One calf appeared healthy at birth, subsequently became ill (IBR positive). One of 11 animals normal.

Similar study designs were used to demonstrate the effectiveness of the BVD fraction contained in PREGGUARD™ FP 9 in preventing fetal infections associated with both Types 1 and 2 BVD. In these studies, vaccinated heifers, along with a group of non-vaccinated control heifers, were challenged with virulent strains of BVD virus when fetal ages ranged from approximately 73-98 days. Results of these studies are summarized in the following table.

Group	Challenge	No. of Heifers Challenged	Viremia Heifers[3]	No. of Calves Evaluated	Calves BVD Positive[4]
Vaccinates[1]	BVD1	19	0/19 (0.0%)	19	1/19 (5.3%)
Vaccinates[2]	BVD1	19	0/19 (0.0%)	19	0/19 (0.0%)
Controls	BVD1	10	9/10 (90.0%)	10	7/10 (70.0%)
Vaccinates[1]	BVD2	20	1/20 (5.0%)	18	6/18 (33.3%)
Vaccinates[2]	BVD2	20	1/20 (5.0%)	19	7/19 (36.8%)
Controls	BVD2	10	9/10 (90.0%)	10	9/10 (90.0%)

[1] Vaccination with a single dose 1 month prior to breeding. Seronegative heifers with no history of vaccination with any product containing IBR or BVD vaccine viruses were selected for use in the efficacy studies.

[2] Vaccination with 2 doses at 5 months and 1 month prior to breeding.

[3] Virus isolations performed on whole blood samples collected on days 0, 2, 4, 6, 8, 10, and 14 post-challenge of heifers.

[4] Whole blood collected from calves on the day of calving and prior to nursing (pre-colostral) was tested for BVD virus. Full-thickness ear notch and skin sample biopsies were tested by immunocytochemistry evaluation for the presence of BVD virus. If any sample was determined to be positive, the fetus was considered persistently infected with BVD virus.

Presentation: 10 dose and 25 dose vials.

Compendium Code No.: 36900621 75-4658-03

PRE-GOLD® GERMICIDAL PRE-MILKING TEAT DIP (ACTIVATOR)

Alcide **Teat Dip**

Active Ingredient(s): 0.64% Orthophosphoric Acid.

Indications: An aid in reducing the spread of organisms which may cause mastitis.

For use only with Pre-Gold® Base.

Directions for Use: Measure equal volumes of Pre-Gold® base and PRE-GOLD® activator into a clean dip cup/container and mix until the color is uniform throughout. Do not dilute. Mix only enough product for one milking of the herd. Dip cups should be washed after each milking.

Application: If teats are visibly dirty, wash and dry teats with a single service towel prior to dipping. Before each cow is milked, dip the teats as far up as possible. Leave PRE-GOLD® Teat Dip on teats for at least 15-30 seconds. Wipe teats dry using a single service towel before milking.

Always use freshly mixed, full strength PRE-GOLD® Teat Dip. If product in dip cup becomes visibly dirty, discard contents and fill with fresh PRE-GOLD® Teat Dip. PRE-GOLD® Teat Dip may be diluted with water and safely flushed down drain.

Note 1: If teat irritation occurs, discontinue use until irritation subsides. Consult your veterinarian and milking equipment service personnel if irritation persists.

Note 2: The gold color in the mixed product fades with time. At higher temperatures the fading is more rapid. However, this will not affect the efficacy of the product.

Note 3: PRE-GOLD® is to be used as a pre-dip only. Recommended post dips include UDDERgold® Plus and 4XLA® Germicidal Teat Dips.
Caution(s): For external use only. Not for use in sanitizing dairy equipment. Do not mix with any other teat dip or other product. Avoid contact with food. Avoid contact with eyes. If contact occurs, flush eyes with large quantities of water. See a physician if irritation develops.
Storage and Disposal: Store at room temperature. Protect from heat and freezing. Always store away from continuous artificial light or direct sunlight.
Disposal: Unused teat dip may be diluted with water and flushed down drain. Do not reuse containers. Empty containers should be thoroughly rinsed with water and taken to a recycling center.
Avoid freezing: If product is exposed to freezing temperatures, components must be mixed thoroughly prior to use.
Warning(s): Keep out of the reach of children.
Disclaimer: Distributor's and Alcide's liability on any claim, whether in negligence or any other tort or in contract or otherwise, with respect to products delivered hereunder, shall not exceed the purchase price of the products sold or, if Distributor and Alcide shall so elect, buyer shall be entitled only to replacement of product. In no event shall Distributor and Alcide be liable for buyer's incidental or consequential damages.
Presentation: Available in 1, 5, 15 and 55 gallon sizes.
European Patent 565,134
Foreign Patents Issued and Pending
PRE-GOLD® is a registered trademark of Alcide Corporation.
Distributed by: Universal Marketing Services, 5545 Avenida de los Robles, Visalia, CA 93291.
Compendium Code No.: 14760060 L8210A Rev. 01 11-98

PRE-GOLD® GERMICIDAL PRE-MILKING TEAT DIP (BASE)

Alcide **Teat Dip**

Active Ingredient(s): 0.64% Sodium Chlorite.
Indications: An aid in reducing the spread of organisms which may cause mastitis.
For use only with Pre-Gold® Activator.
Directions for Use: Measure equal volumes of PRE-GOLD® base and Pre-Gold® activator into a clean dip cup/container and mix until the color is uniform throughout. Do not dilute. Mix only enough product for one milking of the herd. Dip cups should be washed after each milking.
Application: If teats are visibly dirty, wash and dry teats with a single service towel prior to dipping. Before each cow is milked, dip the teats as far up as possible. Leave PRE-GOLD® Teat Dip on teats for at least 15-30 seconds. Wipe teats dry using a single service towel before milking.
Always use freshly mixed, full strength PRE-GOLD® Teat Dip. If product in dip cup becomes visibly dirty, discard contents and fill with fresh PRE-GOLD® Teat Dip. PRE-GOLD® Teat Dip may be diluted with water and safely flushed down drain.
Note 1: If teat irritation occurs, discontinue use until irritation subsides. Consult your veterinarian and milking equipment service personnel if irritation persists.
Note 2: The gold color in the mixed product fades with time. At higher temperatures the fading is more rapid. However, this will not affect the efficacy of the product.
Note 3: PRE-GOLD® is to be used as a pre-dip only. Recommended post dips include UDDERgold® and 4XLA® Germicidal Teat Dips.
Caution(s): For external use only. Not for use in sanitizing dairy equipment. Do not mix with any other teat dip or other product. Avoid contact with food. Avoid contact with eyes. If contact occurs, flush eyes with large quantities of water. See a physician if irritation develops.
Storage and Disposal: Store at room temperature. Protect from heat and freezing. Always store away from continuous artificial light or direct sunlight.
Disposal: Unused teat dip may be diluted with water and flushed down drain. Do not reuse containers. Empty containers should be thoroughly rinsed with water and taken to a recycling center.
Avoid freezing: If product is exposed to freezing temperatures, components must be mixed thoroughly prior to use.
Warning(s): Keep out of the reach of children.
Disclaimer: Distributor's and Alcide's liability on any claim, whether in negligence or any other tort or in contract or otherwise, with respect to products delivered hereunder, shall not exceed the purchase price of the products sold or, if Distributor and Alcide shall so elect, buyer shall be entitled only to replacement of product. In no event shall Distributor and Alcide be liable for buyer's incidental or consequential damages.
Presentation: Available in 1, 5, 15 and 55 gallon sizes.
European Patent 565,134
Foreign Patents Issued and Pending
PRE-GOLD® is a registered trademark of Alcide Corporation.
Distributed by: Universal Marketing Services, 5545 Avenida de los Robles, Visalia, CA 93291.
Compendium Code No.: 14760070 L8210B Rev. 01 11-98

PRESPONSE® HM

Fort Dodge **Bacterin-Toxoid**

Pasteurella Multocida Bacterial Extract-Pasteurella Haemolytica Toxoid
U.S. Vet. Lic. No.: 112
Contents: This product contains the antigens listed above.
Thimerosal added as preservative.
Indications: For vaccination of healthy dairy or beef cattle seven months of age or older as an aid in the prevention of pneumonic pasteurellosis by stimulating immunity to *P. multocida* and *P. haemolytica*.
Dosage and Administration: Dose: Cattle, inject one 2 mL dose intramuscularly using aseptic technique. Although only a single dose is necessary to confer active immunity, a booster dose is recommended whenever subsequent stress is likely. Healthy cattle should be vaccinated at a minimum of 14 days prior to shipping or exposure to stress which may precipitate infectious conditions.
Precaution(s): Store in dark at 2° to 7°C (35° to 45°F). Shake well. Do not freeze. Use entire contents when first opened.
Caution(s): Transient injection site reactions may occur in a small percentage of vaccinates. In case of anaphylactoid reaction, administer epinephrine.
Warning(s): Do not vaccinate within 21 days before slaughter.
For veterinary use only.
Presentation: 10 dose (20 mL) and 50 dose (100 mL) vials.
U.S. Patent Nos. 4,957,739; 5,165,924; 5,336,491 and 5,378,615.
Compendium Code No.: 10031571 3767C

PRESPONSE® SQ

Fort Dodge **Toxoid**

Pasteurella Haemolytica Toxoid, Adjuvanted
U.S. Vet. Lic. No.: 112
Contents: This product contains the antigen listed above.
Thimerosal added as a preservative.
Indications: For vaccination of healthy dairy or beef cattle three months of age or older as an aid in the prevention of pneumonic pasteurellosis by stimulating immunity to *P. haemolytica*.
Dosage and Administration: Cattle, inject one 2 mL dose subcutaneously in the neck area anterior to the shoulder using aseptic technique. Healthy cattle should be vaccinated a minimum of 14 days prior to shipping or exposure to stress which may precipitate infectious conditions. Although only a single dose is necessary to confer active immunity, a booster dose is recommended whenever subsequent stress is likely.
Precaution(s): Store in dark at 2° to 7°C (35° to 45°F). Do not freeze. Shake well. Use entire contents when first opened.
Caution(s): In case of anaphylactoid reaction, administer epinephrine.
Warning(s): Do not vaccinate within 21 days before slaughter.
For veterinary use only.
Presentation: 10 dose (20 mL) and 50 dose (100 mL) vials.
U.S. Patent Nos. 4,957,739; 5,165,924; 5,336,491 and 5,378,615.
Compendium Code No.: 10031582 0846D

PRESTIGE® WITH HAVLOGEN®*

Intervet **Vaccine**

Equine Rhinopneumonitis Vaccine, Killed Virus
U.S. Vet. Lic. No.: 286
Description: A combination of inactivated, purified, concentrated, adjuvanted equine tissue culture origin Equine Herpesvirus EHV-1 and EHV-4.
Neomycin, polymyxin B, nystatin and thimerosal added as preservatives.
Indications: For vaccination of healthy horses against respiratory diseases caused by Equine Herpesvirus.
Dosage and Administration: For primary immunization, aseptically inject 1 mL intramuscularly. Repeat the dose in 4 to 6 weeks. A 1 mL dose should be administered annually and at any time epidemic conditions exist or are reported and exposure is imminent.
Precaution(s): Store at 35° to 45°F (2° to 7°C). Shake well before using. Use entire contents when first opened.
Caution(s): Local reactions may occur if this product is given subcutaneously. Inject deep into the muscle only. Anaphylactoid reactions may occur.
For use in animals only.
Antidote(s): Epinephrine.
Warning(s): Do not vaccinate within 21 days before slaughter.
Presentation: 1 dose (1 mL) syringe with separate sterile needle and 10 dose (10 mL) vial.
*Adjuvant—U.S. Patent Nos. 3,790,665 and 3,919,411.
Compendium Code No.: 11061290

PRESTIGE® II WITH HAVLOGEN®*

Intervet **Vaccine**

Equine Rhinopneumonitis-Influenza Vaccine, Killed Virus
U.S. Vet. Lic. No.: 286
Description: A combination of inactivated, purified, concentrated, adjuvanted, tissue culture origin Equine Herpesvirus EHV-1 and EHV-4 and Equine Influenza Virus subtypes A1 and A2 including KY93 strain. Intervet serological data suggest cross protection against certain U.S. and European Strains, including Prague 56, KY 63, KY 81 and 87, Fountainbleau 79 and Berlin 84 and 89.**
Neomycin, polymyxin B, nystatin and thimerosal added as preservatives.
Indications: For vaccination of healthy horses against respiratory disease caused by Equine Herpesvirus and Equine Influenza Virus.
Dosage and Administration: For primary immunization, aseptically inject 1 mL intramuscularly and repeat the dose in 4 to 6 weeks. A 1 mL dose should be administered annually and at any time epidemic conditions exist or are reported and exposure is imminent.
Precaution(s): Store at 35° to 45°F (2° to 7°C). Shake well before using. Use entire contents when first opened.
Caution(s): Local reactions may occur if this product is given subcutaneously. Inject deep into the muscle only. Anaphylactoid reactions may occur.
For use in animals only.
Antidote(s): Epinephrine.
Warning(s): Do not vaccinate within 21 days before slaughter.
References: **Available upon request.
Presentation: 1 dose (1 mL), 10 dose (10 x 1 mL) syringes with separate sterile needle and 10 doses (10 mL).
*Adjuvant—Intervet's Proprietary Technology
Compendium Code No.: 11061270

PRESTIGE® V WITH HAVLOGEN®*

Intervet **Toxoid-Vaccine**

Encephalomyelitis-Rhinopneumonitis-Influenza Vaccine, Eastern and Western, Killed Virus-Tetanus Toxoid
U.S. Vet. Lic. No.: 286
Description: A combination of inactivated, purified, concentrated, adjuvanted, tissue culture origin Equine Encephalomyelitis Virus, Eastern and Western, Equine Herpesvirus EHV-1 and EHV-4, Equine Influenza Virus subtypes A1 and A2 including KY93 strain, and Tetanus Toxoid. Intervet serological data suggest Influenza cross protection against certain U.S. and European strains, including Prague 56, Detroit 91, Miami 63, Kentucky 93, 94, 95 and 96, Suffolk 89, Kildare 89 and 92, Austria 92, Switzerland 93, New Market/1/93, and /2/93, Berlin 94, Italy 96 and Meath 96.**
Neomycin, polymyxin B, nystatin and thimerosal added as preservatives.
Indications: For vaccination of healthy horses against Eastern and Western Encephalomyelitis, Equine Influenza Virus and Tetanus, and as an aid in the prevention of respiratory disease caused by Equine Herpesvirus and Equine Influenza Virus.
Dosage and Administration: For primary immunization aseptically inject 1 mL intramuscularly

P

and repeat the dose in 3 to 4 weeks. A 1 mL dose should be administered annually and at any time epidemic conditions exist or are reported and exposure is imminent.
Precaution(s): Store at 35° to 45°F (2° to 7°C). Shake well before using. Use entire contents when first opened.
Caution(s): Local reactions may occur if this product is given subcutaneously. Inject deep into the muscle only. Anaphylactoid reactions may occur.
For use in animals only.
Antidote(s): Epinephrine.
Warning(s): Do not vaccinate within 21 days before slaughter.
References: **Available upon request.
Presentation: 1 dose (1 mL) and 10 dose (10 x 1 mL) syringes with separate sterile needle.
*Adjuvant—Intervet's Proprietary Technology
Compendium Code No.: 11061280

PRESTIGE® V + VEE WITH HAVLOGEN®

Intervet — **Toxoid-Vaccine**

Encephalomyelitis-Rhinopneumonitis-Influenza Vaccine, Eastern, Western & Venezuelan Equine Encephalomyelitis (Sleeping Sickness)-Tetanus Toxoid
U.S. Vet. Lic. No.: 286
Description: A combination of inactivated, purified, concentrated, adjuvanted, tissue culture origin, Equine Encephalomyelitis Virus, Eastern, Western, and Venezuelan, Equine Herpesvirus EHV-1 and EHV-4, Equine Influenza Virus subtypes A1 and A2 including KY 93 strain and Tetanus Toxoid. Intervet serological data suggest Influenza cross protection against certain U.S. and European strains, including Kentucky 93, 94, 95 and 96, Suffolk 89, Kildare 89 and 92, Austria 92, Switzerland 93, New Market 1/93 and 2/93, Berlin 94, Italy 96 and Meath 96.
Neomycin, polymyxin B, nystatin and thimerosal added as preservatives.
Indications: For vaccination of healthy horses against Eastern, Western and Venezuelan Encephalomyelitis, Equine Influenza Virus and Tetanus, and as an aid in the prevention of respiratory disease caused by Equine Herpesvirus and Equine Influenza Virus.
Dosage and Administration: For primary immunization, aseptically inject 1 mL intramuscularly and repeat the dose in 3 to 4 weeks. A 1 mL dose should be administered annually and at any time epidemic conditions exist or are reported and exposure is imminent.
Precaution(s): Store at 35° to 45°F (2° to 7°C). Shake well before using. Use entire contents when first opened.
Caution(s): Local reactions may occur if this product is given subcutaneously. Inject deep into the muscle only. Anaphylactoid reactions may occur.
Antidote(s): Epinephrine.
Warning(s): Do not vaccinate within 21 days before slaughter.
Presentation: 10 x 1 mL (1 dose) sterile syringes per box, individually printed plastic bag with needle and 10 x 1 mL (10 dose) vials.
Compendium Code No.: 11062550 — 71004840, R.1

PREVAIL MYCOPLEX™

Aspen — **Bacterin**

Mycoplasma hyopneumoniae Bacterin
U.S. Vet. Lic. No.: 165A
Composition: Prepared from cultures of the organisms listed.
Preservatives: Ampicillin, gentamicin, and thimerosal.
Indications: Recommended for use as an aid in the prevention of pneumonia caused by *Mycoplasma hyopneumoniae* infection in swine.
Dosage and Administration: Using aseptic technique, inject 1 mL subcutaneously at 7-10 days of age or older. Revaccinate with 1 mL 2 weeks after initial vaccination. Revaccinate with a single 1 mL dose annually.
Precaution(s): Store at 2°-7°C (35°-45°F). Do not freeze. Use entire contents when first opened.
Caution(s): Transient local swelling may occur at the injection site. If allergic response occurs, administer epinephrine.
Warning(s): Do not vaccinate within 60 days before slaughter.
Extreme caution should be used when injecting any oil emulsion vaccine to avoid injecting your own finger or hand. Accidental injection can cause serious local reaction. Contact a physician immediately if accidental injection occurs.
For veterinary use only.
Presentation: 100 dose (100 mL) and 250 dose (250 mL) vials.
Manufactured by: Schering-Plough Animal Health Corp.
Compendium Code No.: 14750640

P

PREVAIL™ PARA PLEURO BAC+3DT

Aspen — **Bacterin**

Actinobacillus Pleuropneumoniae-Bordetella Bronchiseptica-Erysipelothrix Rhusiopathiae-Haemophilus Parasuis-Pasteurella Multocida Bacterin
U.S. Vet. Lic. No.: 303
Composition: This bacterin contains inactivated cultures of *Actinobacillus pleuropneumoniae* serotypes 1, 5, and 7, *Bordetella bronchiseptica, Erysipelothrix rhusiopathiae, Haemophilus parasuis*, and *Pasteurella multocida* Type A adjuvanted with aluminum hydroxide. Contains penicillin and streptomycin as preservatives.
Indications: For use in healthy swine as an aid in the prevention and control of disease caused by *Actinobacillus pleuropneumoniae* serotypes 1, 5, and 7, *Bordetella bronchiseptica, Erysipelothrix rhusiopathiae, Haemophilus parasuis*, and *Pasteurella multocida* Type A.
Dosage and Administration: Shake well before using. This product is designed for use in feeder pigs from sows previously vaccinated with Prevail™ Borde-Ery-Past (*Bordetella Bronchiseptica-Erysipelothrix Rhusiopathiae-Pasteurella Multocida* Bacterin). Administer 5 mL intramuscularly at 7 weeks of age or older. Revaccinate in 2-3 weeks.
Precaution(s): Store in the dark at 35°-45°F(2°-7°C). Do not freeze. Use entire contents when first opened.
Caution(s): Anaphylactic reactions may occur following the use of this biological. Symptomatic treatment: Epinephrine.
Warning(s): Do not vaccinate within 21 days prior to slaughter.
Presentation: 10 dose (50 mL) and 50 dose (250 mL) vials.
Compendium Code No.: 14750650

PREVAIL™ PARVOPLEX 6-WAY+E

Aspen — **Bacterin-Vaccine**

Parvovirus Vaccine, Killed Virus-Erysipelothrix Rhusiopathiae-Leptospira Canicola-Grippotyphosa-Hardjo-Icterohaemorrhagiae-Pomona Bacterin
U.S. Vet. Lic. No.: 303
Composition: This product contains inactivated cultures of porcine parvovirus, *Erysipelothrix rhusiopathiae, Leptospira canicola, grippotyphosa, hardjo, icterohaemorrhagiae*, and *pomona* adjuvanted with aluminum hydroxide. Contains amphotericin B, penicillin, streptomycin, and thimerosal as preservatives.
Indications: For use in healthy swine as an aid in the prevention and control of disease caused by porcine parvovirus, *Erysipelothrix rhusiopathiae, Leptospira canicola, grippotyphosa, hardjo, icterohaemorrhagiae*, and *pomona*.
Dosage and Administration: Shake well before using. Administer 5 mL intramuscularly to gilts and sows 4-6 weeks prior to breeding. Repeat in 3-4 weeks. Revaccinate with a single dose 4-6 weeks prior to each subsequent breeding. Vaccinate boars semiannually.
Precaution(s): Store in the dark at 35°-45°F (2°-7°C). Do not freeze. Use entire contents when first opened.
Caution(s): Anaphylactic reactions may occur following the use of this biological. Symptomatic treatment: Epinephrine.
Warning(s): Do not vaccinate within 21 days prior to slaughter.
Presentation: 10 dose (50 mL) and 50 dose (250 mL) vials.
Compendium Code No.: 14750660

PRE-VENT 6™

AgriLabs — **Bacterin**

Campylobacter fetus-Leptospira canicola-grippotyphosa-hardjo-icterohaemorrhagiae-pomona Bacterin
U.S. Vet. Lic. No.: 272
Active Ingredient(s): *Campylobacter fetus, Leptospira canicola, L. grippotyphosa, L. hardjo, L. icterohaemorrhagiae* and *L. pomona* bacterin.
Indications: For the protection of healthy cattle against infection caused by *Vibrio (Campylobacter) fetus* and leptospirosis caused by *Leptospira canicola, L. grippotyphosa, L. hardjo, L. icterohaemorrhagiae* and *L. pomona.*
Dosage and Administration: Inject 2 mL intramuscularly or subcutaneously to cows two (2) to four (4) weeks prior to breeding. Revaccinate prior to each breeding to maintain high levels of immunity.
Precaution(s): Store at 35-45°F (2-7°C). Do not freeze.
Caution(s): Use the entire contents when first opened. Anaphylactic reactions may occur with this biological. Symptomatic treatment: Epinephrine.
Warning(s): Do not vaccinate within 21 days of slaughter.
Presentation: 20 mL (10 dose) and 100 mL (50 dose) vials.
Compendium Code No.: 10580820

PREVENTEF® FLEA AND TICK COLLAR FOR CATS

Virbac — **Parasiticide Collar**

EPA Reg. No.: 2382-95
Active Ingredient(s):

Diazinon [0,0-diethyl 0-(2-isopropyl-6-methyl-4-pyrimidinyl) phosphorothioate]	11.0%
Inert Ingredients*	89.0%
Total	100.0%

*Includes 5% unsaturated fatty acids as a grooming aid.
Indications: A flea and tick collar for cats with EFA* that kills fleas and ticks for 5 months.
*Slow release coat conditioner helps enhance texture, manageability and luster.
Directions for Use: It is a violation of Federal Law to use this collar in a manner inconsistent with its labelling.
Place PREVENTEF® collar around the cat's neck, adjust for proper fit and buckle in place. Cut off and dispose of excess length. The collar must be worn loosely so that two fingers can be placed between collar and cat's neck. If collar is worn too tightly, it may produce neck irritation. Activity against fleas starts within 24 hours, reaches maximum effectiveness in 3-4 days and continues as long as the collar is worn (up to 150 days). Ticks are relatively harder to kill and die more slowly. Activity against ticks will occur within a few days and will continue killing and controlling ticks for up to 150 days. Fleas and ticks present in the animal's environment that may reappear on the cat will be killed and controlled by the action of the collar. Replace collar when effectiveness diminishes. Collar is not affected by normal wetting such as rainfall; however, it is suggested the collar be removed before bathing.
This PREVENTEF® collar contains Essential Fatty Acids necessary for healthy skin and hair. Unsaturated fatty acids released from the collar are rapidly absorbed to help maintain a lustrous, manageable coat.
Precautionary Statements: Hazards to Humans and Domestic Animals: This collar is intended for use as an insecticide generator and is not to be taken internally by man or animal. Not intended for use on humans. The insecticide in this collar is a cholinesterase inhibitor. Do not allow children to handle or play with this collar. May cause contact sensitization following repeated contact with skin in susceptible individuals. Avoid repeated contact with skin. If sensitization reactions result, contact a physician.
Note to Physicians/Veterinarians: Diazinon is an organophosphate insecticide. If symptoms of cholinesterase inhibition are present, atropine sulfate by injection is antidotal. 2-PAM is also antidotal and may be administered, but only in conjunction with atropine.
Do not use other cholinesterase-inhibiting drugs, pesticides or chemicals on cat while collar is worn. Some cats and humans may be sensitive to this collar. Remove at first sign of irritation or adverse reaction. Do not use on sick or convalescing animals. Do not use on Persian cats.
Disposal: Do not reuse empty pouch or box. Wrap pouch or box and put in trash collection. When discarding used collar, wrap in newspaper and place in trash collection.
Presentation: One 0.67 oz (19.0 g) collar.
Compendium Code No.: 10230420

PREVENTEF® FLEA AND TICK COLLAR FOR DOGS

Virbac — **Parasiticide Collar**

EPA Reg. No.: 2382-97
Active Ingredient(s):

Diazinon [0,0-diethyl 0-(2-isopropyl-6-methyl-4-pyrimidinyl) phosphorothioate]	11.0%
Inert Ingredients*	89.0%
Total	100.0%

*Includes 5% unsaturated fatty acids as a grooming aid.

Indications: A flea and tick collar for dogs with EFA* that kills fleas and ticks for 5 months.
*Slow release coat conditioner helps enhance texture, manageability and luster.
Directions for Use: It is a violation of Federal Law to use this collar in a manner inconsistent with its labelling.

Place PREVENTEF® collar around the dog's neck, adjust for proper fit and buckle in place. Cut off and dispose of excess length. The collar must be worn loosely so that two fingers can be placed between collar and dog's neck. If collar is worn too tightly, it may produce neck irritation. Activity against fleas starts within 24 hours, reaches maximum effectiveness in 3-4 days and continues as long as the collar is worn (up to 150 days). Ticks are relatively harder to kill and die more slowly. Activity against ticks will occur within a few days and will continue killing and controlling ticks for up to 150 days. For unusually large breeds, collar aids in tick control in the head and neck area for up to 2 months. Fleas and ticks present in the animal's environment that may reappear on the dog will be killed and controlled by the action of the collar. Replace collar when effectiveness diminishes. Collar is not affected by normal wetting such as rainfall; however, it is suggested the collar be removed before bathing.

This PREVENTEF® collar contains Essential Fatty Acids necessary for healthy skin and hair. Unsaturated fatty acids released from the collar are rapidly absorbed to help maintain a lustrous, manageable coat.

Precautionary Statements: Hazards to Humans and Domestic Animals: This collar is intended for use as an insecticide generator and is not to be taken internally by man or animal. Not intended for use on humans. The insecticide in this collar is a cholinesterase inhibitor. Do not allow children to handle or play with this collar. May cause contact sensitization following repeated contact with skin in susceptible individuals. Avoid repeated contact with skin. If sensitization reactions result, contact a physician.

Note to Physicians/Veterinarians: This product contains a cholinesterase inhibitor. Atropine sulfate and 2-PAM are antidotal only if signs of cholinesterase inhibition are present.

Do not use other cholinesterase-inhibiting drugs, pesticides or chemicals on dog while collar is worn. Some dogs and humans may be sensitive to this collar. Remove at first sign of irritation or adverse reaction. Do not use on sick or convalescing animals. Do not use on puppies less than 5 weeks of age.

Disposal: Do not reuse empty pouch or box. Wrap pouch or box and put in trash collection. When discarding used collar, wrap in newspaper and place in trash collection.
Presentation: One 1.44 oz (41.0 g) collar.
Compendium Code No.: 10230430

PREVENTIC® COLLAR FOR DOGS

Virbac **Parasiticide Collar**
Antiparasitic
EPA Reg. No.: 2382-104
Active Ingredient(s):

Amitraz: N'-(2,4-dimethylphenyl)-N-[[2,4-dimethylphenyl)-imino]methyl]-N-methylmethanimidamide 9.0%
Inert Ingredients.......... 91.0%

Indications: Tick collar for dogs. Kills ticks for 3 months.
Directions for Use: Read entire label directions before each use.

It is a violation of Federal Law to use this collar in a manner inconsistent with its labeling.

Place the PREVENTIC® collar around the dog's neck, buckle and adjust for proper fit. Cut off and dispose of excess length. Do not allow dogs to play with cut-off excess. The collar must be worn tightly enough to contact skin and so that the dog cannot remove it. Activity against ticks starts within 24 hours and continues as long as the collar is worn (up to 90 days). Ticks present in the dog's environment that may reappear on the dog will not attach and will be killed in less than 24 hours. Replace collar when effectiveness diminishes. The effectiveness of the collar is not diminished by normal wetting such as rainfall, however, it is suggested that the collar be removed before bathing. The active ingredient is not an insecticide. Therefore, use other means for the control of fleas.

Contraindication(s): Use only on dogs. Do not use on cats.
Precautionary Statements: Hazard to Humans and Domestic Animals:

Caution: This collar is intended for use as an acaricide generator and is not to be taken internally by man or animal. Not intended for use on humans. Do not allow children to handle or play with this collar.

Harmful if absorbed through skin. Causes moderate eye irritation. Avoid contact with skin, eyes or clothing. Some humans may develop skin irritation through contact with collared pet. Wash thoroughly with soap and water after handling.

Do not use on puppies less than 12 weeks old. Consult a veterinarian before using on debilitated, aged, medicated, pregnant or nursing animals. Do not treat collared dogs with other monoamine oxidase inhibitors, or with tricyclic antidepressants, selective serotonin reuptake inhibitors or pressor agents. Some dogs may be sensitive to this collar. Remove at first sign of irritation or adverse reaction, bathe dog with a non-pesticidal shampoo and rinse with large amounts of water. If signs continue, consult a veterinarian immediately. There is a risk of collar breakage and ingestion if collar is worn by unattended dogs that play by mouthing each other in the neck area. If collar is missing from a dog, search for, retrieve and recover the entire collar. Immediately consult a veterinarian if dog is depressed.

Note to Veterinarian: If a dog ingests a PREVENTIC® collar and exhibits intoxication (primary sign is severe depression), induce vomiting, administer non-oily laxative, activated charcoal and enema. Provide supportive therapy until collar fragments are voided. If dog cannot be roused, Yohimbine, 0.1 mg/kg by intravenous injection is antidotal. Repeat as needed.

Disposal: Do not reuse empty pouch, box or collar. Wrap in newspaper and put in trash collection.
Warning(s): Keep out of reach of children.

For veterinary use only.

Presentation: One 25" collar - Net. wt. 0.97 oz (27.5 g).
Compendium Code No.: 10230441

PREVENTIC® PLUS TICK AND FLEA IGR COLLAR FOR DOGS

Virbac **Parasiticide Collar**
Antiparasitic
EPA Reg. No.: 2382-170
Active Ingredient(s):

Pyriproxyfen.......... 0.5%
Amitraz.......... 9.0%
Inert Ingredients.......... 90.5%
Total.......... 100%

Indications: Tick and flea IGR collar for dogs. Kills and detaches ticks for 3 months. Nylar® IGR sterilizes fleas and kills flea eggs for 3 months.

Directions for Use: Read entire label directions before each use. Use only on dogs.

It is a violation of Federal Law to use this collar in a manner inconsistent with its labeling.

Place the collar around the dog's neck, adjust for proper fit and buckle in place. Cut off and dispose of excess length. Do not allow dogs to play with cut-off excess. The collar must be worn tightly enough to contact skin and so the dog cannot remove it.

Contraindication(s): Do not use on cats.

Do not use on puppies less than 12 weeks.

Precautionary Statements: Hazards to Humans and Domestic Animals: Caution:

Hazards to Humans: Not intended for use on humans. Do not allow children to handle or play with this collar. Harmful if absorbed through skin. Causes moderate eye irritation. Avoid contact with skin, eyes or clothing. Some humans may develop skin irritation through contact with collared pet. Remove collar, shampoo pet and consult physician if irritation persists. Wash thoroughly with soap and water after handling.

Hazards to Pets: Do not use on puppies less than 12 weeks old. Consult a veterinarian before using on debilitated, aged, medicated, pregnant or nursing animals. Do not treat collared dogs with other monoamine oxidase inhibitors, tricyclic antidepressants, selective serotonin reuptake inhibitors or pressor agents. Remove at first sign of irritation or adverse reaction, bathe dog with a non-pesticidal shampoo and rinse with large amounts of water. If signs continue, consult a veterinarian immediately. There is a risk of collar breakage and ingestion if collar is worn by unattended dogs that play by mouthing each other in the neck area. If collar is missing from a dog, search for, retrieve and recover the entire collar. Immediately consult a veterinarian if dog is depressed.

Note to Veterinarian: If a dog ingests a PREVENTIC® PLUS collar and exhibits intoxication (primary sign is severe depression), induce vomiting, administer non-oily laxative, activated charcoal and enema. Provide supportive therapy until collar fragments are voided. If dog cannot be roused, Yohimbine, 0.1 mg/kg by intravenous injection is antidotal. Repeat as needed. Temporary and reversible hyperglycemia was observed when the product was tested at 5 times the recommended dose.

Storage and Disposal: Store in a cool, dry place.

Disposal: Do not reuse empty pouch or box. Wrap pouch and put in trash collection. When discarding cut off end and used collar, wrap in newspaper and place in trash collection.

Warning(s): Keep out of reach of children.
Discussion: The two active ingredients in this collar have different and complementary functions. The IGR (synthetic flea hormone), pyriproxyfen (Nylar®), sterilizes all fleas that jump on the pet (even new fleas before they start laying eggs) and kills all flea eggs. Pyriproxyfen is continuously released from the collar, spreads over the pet in the natural oils of the haircoat and skin and adheres tightly to hair and skin to provide more than 3 months of continuous flea ovisterilant efficacy. This breaks the flea's life cycle by preventing the development of new fleas in the environment that would normally reinfest the pet. This ovicidal activity of pyriproxyfen starts immediately, reaches 100% effectiveness within 3-4 days and continues at 100% effectiveness as long as the collar is worn. The second active, amitraz, also spreads over the pet in the oil of its skin and haircoat where its activity starts within 24 hours to detach and kill existing ticks on the pet. Amitraz continues to prevent attachment and feeding and kills new ticks that may climb onto the pet for up to 90 days. The collar and its active ingredients are not affected by normal wetting such as rainfall, however, it is suggested the collar be removed before bathing. This collar should be replaced when new ticks are seen to persist on the pet. For optimal efficacy for tick control and flea prevention you should replace the collar every 3 months.

Presentation: One Amitraz-Pyriproxyfen Collar - Net Wt. 0.97 oz (27.5 g).
Nylar® is a registered trademark of McLaughlin Gormley King Company.
Compendium Code No.: 10230680

260443-1

PRIBUTAZONE™ TABLETS ℞

First Priority **Phenylbutazone-Oral**
NADA No.: 048-647
Active Ingredient(s): Each tablet contains:

Phenylbutazone, U.S.P. .... 1 gram
Plus excipients.

Indications: Phenylbutazone is for the relief of inflammatory conditions associated with the musculoskeletal system in horses.

A non-hormonal anti-inflammatory agent.

Pharmacology: Phenylbutazone chemically is 4-butyl-1, 2-diphenyl-3, 5-pyrazolidinedione. It has the following structural formula:

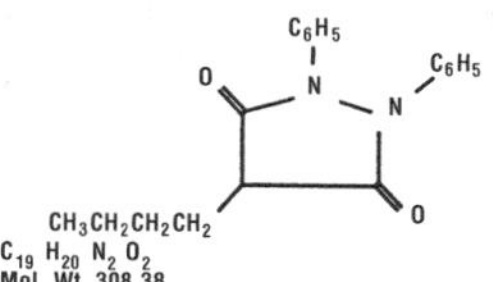

Phenylbutazone was first synthesized in 1948 and introduced into human medicine in 1949. Kuzell[1,2,3], Payne[4], Fleming[5], and Denko[6], demonstrated the clinical effectiveness of phenylbutazone in gout, gouty arthritis, acute arthritis, acute rheumatism and various other rheumatoid disorders in humans. Fabre[7], Domenjoz[8], Wilhelmi[9], and Yourish[10], have established the anti-rheumatic and anti-inflammatory activity of phenylbutazone. It is entirely unrelated to the steroid hormones.

Toxicity of phenylbutazone has been investigated in rats and mice[11], Ogilvie and Sutter[12], have also made a study on the chronic toxicity of phenylbutazone in dogs. They have shown that dogs receiving 10 mg and 100 mg per kg body weight, per day for 90 days, maintain good appetites, excrete normal feces, gain weight and maintain a normal blood picture. They also report no abnormal macroscopic or microscopic changes in sacrificed animals which could have been attributed to the drug.

Phenylbutazone has been used by Camberos[13] in thoroughbred horses. Favorable results were reported in cases of traumatism, muscle rupture, strains and inflammations of the third phalanx. Results were not as favorable in the periodic treatment of osteo-arthritis of medial and distal bones of the hock, arthritis of the stifle and hip, arthrosis of the trapezious muscles, and generalized arthritis. Sutter[14] reported a favorable response in chronic equine arthritis of long duration, fair results in a severely bruised mare, and poor results in two cases where the condition was limited to the third phalanx.

Dosage and Administration: For horses only.

Horses: Orally - 1 to 2 tablets per 500 lb body weight. Do not exceed 4 grams daily. Reduce dosage as symptoms regress. Intermittent treatment given only when symptoms appear may be indicated.

Contraindication(s): Use with caution in patients who have a history of drug allergy.

P

Precaution(s): Storage: Store at controlled room temperature between 15°-30°C (59°-86°F). Keep container tightly closed when not in use.

Caution(s): Federal law restricts this drug to use by or on the order of a licensed veterinarian.

In the treatment of inflammatory conditions associated with infections, specific anti-infective therapy should be used concurrently.

For animal use only.

Warning(s): Not for use in horses intended for food.

Keep out of reach of children.

References: Available upon request.

Presentation: Available in 1 g tablets - 100 tablets per bottle (NDC# 58829-313-10).

Compendium Code No.: 11390870 Iss. 06-02

PRIMEVAC IBD-3®

Intervet **Vaccine**

Bursal Disease Vaccine, Live Virus, Standard and Variant

U.S. Vet. Lic. No.: 286

Description: PRIMEVAC IBD-3®, a live lyophilized vaccine, contains three strains of infectious bursal disease (IBD) virus - Standard, Delaware and GLS. The vaccine is prepared using SPF substrates.

This vaccine contains gentamicin as a preservative.

Quality tested for purity, potency, and safety.

Indications: PRIMEVAC IBD-3® is indicated for revaccinating healthy 8 weeks of age or older breeder replacement pullets via the drinking water that have been previously primed with a standard IBDV vaccine. This will provide optimal priming for Standard, Delaware variant, and GLS infectious bursal disease viruses.

Warning: Use of this product in chickens that are under eight weeks of age and unvaccinated may result in bursal lesions and immunosuppression.

Dosage and Administration: Vaccination Program: Immune status, general health, and field exposure to IBD virus must be assessed to develop an effective program. Immunological priming of breeder replacement chickens can be accomplished by early vaccination at 2 to 4 weeks of age with an intermediate live vaccine (i.e. Clonevac-D78®) and subsequent use of PRIMEVAC IBD-3® at 8-12 weeks of age. Inactivated IBD vaccine would then be used at 16 to 20 weeks of age.

Preparation of Vaccine:

For Drinking Water Use: Do not open and mix the vaccine until ready to begin vaccination. Use vaccine immediately after mixing.

1. Remove the tear-off seal and stopper from the vial containing the freeze dried vaccine.
2. Carefully pour clean, cool, non-chlorinated tap water into the vial until the vial is approximately two-thirds full.
3. Insert the rubber stopper and shake vigorously until all material is dissolved.
4. The vaccine is now ready for use in accordance with the directions below. For the best results, be sure to follow directions carefully!
5. Do not use any disinfectants in the drinking water for 48 hours before vaccinating and for 24 hours after vaccination.
6. Withhold the water from the chickens until they are thirsty. Withholding periods will vary from 2 to 12 hours according to the age of chickens and climatic conditions.
7. Scrub waterers and rinse thoroughly with fresh, clean water. Do not use disinfectants for cleaning the waterers.
8. Rehydrate the vaccine as directed above.
9. Mix the rehydrated vaccine with clean, cool, non-chlorinated tap water in accordance with the following chart:

Age of Chickens	Water Per 1,000 Doses Vaccines
8 weeks or older	16 gal. (64 liters)

As an aid in preserving the virus, 3.2 ounces (85 mL) of non-fat powdered milk may be added with each 10 gallons of water used for mixing the vaccine. Add the dried milk first and mix until dissolved. Then add the rehydrated vaccine from the vial and mix thoroughly.

10. Distribute the vaccine solution, as prepared above, among the waterers provided for the chickens. Avoid placing waterers in direct sunlight.
11. Provide no other drinking water until all the vaccine-water solution has been consumed.

P

Records: Keep a record of vaccine quantity, serial number, expiration date and place of purchase; the date and time of vaccination; the number, age, breed and locations of chickens; names of operators performing the vaccination and any observed reactions.

Precaution(s): Store vaccine between 2 and 7°C (35 and 45°F).

Do not spill or splash the vaccine.

Use entire contents when first opened.

Burn containers and all unused contents.

This product is non-returnable.

Caution(s): Use only in localities where permitted and on premises with a history of infectious bursal disease.

Chickens must have been previously vaccinated with a live IBD vaccine.

It is recommended that serological tests be conducted to confirm the presence of IBD antibody in flock before use of this vaccine.

Vaccinate only healthy birds. Although disease may not be evident, coccidiosis, Mycoplasma infection, Marek's disease, and other disease conditions may cause complications or reduce immunity.

All chickens on the same premises should be vaccinated at the same time.

Efforts should be taken to reduce stress conditions at the time of vaccination and during the reaction period.

Do not dilute the vaccine or otherwise stretch the dosage.

For veterinary use only.

Use of this vaccine is subject to applicable local, state and federal laws and regulations.

Do not use on premises where unvaccinated birds (IBD) are present. Spread to unvaccinated birds will cause typical lesions resulting in immunosuppression or death.

Notice: This vaccine has undergone rigid potency, safety and purity tests, and meets Intervet Inc. and USDA requirements. PRIMEVAC IBD-3® is designed to stimulate effective immunity when used as directed. The user must be advised that the response to the product depends upon many factors, including, but not limited to, conditions of storage and handling by the user, administration of the vaccine, health and responsiveness of individual chickens, and the degree of field exposure. Therefore, directions should be followed carefully.

This product is not hazardous when used according to directions supplied. A material safety data sheet (MSDS) is available upon request. This and any other consumer information can be obtained by calling Intervet Customer Service at 1-800-441-8272 or 1-302-934-8051.

Use only as directed.

Warning(s): Do not vaccinate within 21 days before slaughter.

Presentation: 10 x 1,000 dose vials for drinking water use.

U.S. Patent Nos. 4,530,831, 5,064,646

Compendium Code No.: 11061301 24102 AL141

PRIMIDONE ℞

Butler **Anticonvulsant**

NADA No.: 117-689

Active Ingredient(s): Each tablet contains 250 mg of primidone.

Indications: For use in dogs only to treat:

Idiopathic epilepsy: Archibald[6] has reported on the use of primidone in treatment of idiopathic epilepsy in dogs previously treated with other anticonvulsants without success. In this experience, primidone was found to be an effective agent completely controlling the convulsions in most of the case studies and reducing the number and severity of seizures in the remaining small percentage.

Epileptiform convulsions: Clinically, these convulsions are similar to those of true epilepsy. Primidone may be useful as symptomatic treatment of these convulsions of unknown etiology.

Viral encephalitis, distemper, hardpad disease which occurs as a clinically recognizable lesion in certain entities in dogs: Primidone provides an effective means of controlling convulsions associated with infectious neuropathies such as viral encephalitis, distemper or hardpad disease. Supplementation of therapy with primidone is recommended as soon as a diagnosis is made. Oliver and Hoerlin (1965), reported that primidone has been the most effective agent in the dog for the control of seizures associated with post-distemper convulsions. Clinical experience has revealed that once the seizure of a dog cannot be controlled with primidone, none of the other anticonvulsants is likely to do any better.[7] However, it must be borne in mind that primidone does not correct the primary causes of these disorders, but is a valuable adjunct to therapy, making control of seizures possible without hypnosis or interference with proper nutrition.

Primidone has not proved useful in the treatment of chorea.

Pharmacology: Primidone 5-ethyldihydro-5-phenyl-4, 6 (1H, 5H)-pyrimidinedione is a white crystalline substance and is a pyrimidine derivative. Studies of chronic administration of primidone indicate it can metabolize into two active metabolites, phenobarbital and phenylethylmalonamide (PEMA).[1,2,3]

Although primidone is less potent than phenobarbital as a general CNS depressant, primidone is more potent than phenobarbital in the protection of animals against maximal seizures induced by both electroshock and pentylenetetrazole.[4,5,10] As indicated above, primidone may undergo a somewhat complex metabolism involving the production of phenobarbital, and the practitioner should take this into consideration if administering other drugs such as anti-epileptics concurrently.

Primidone acts upon the central nervous system to raise the seizure threshold, hence its value as an anticonvulsant, whether the seizure is induced electrically or is a symptom of a primary disease process.

Dosage and Administration: Usual daily dosage - 25 mg/lb. of body weight (55 mg/kg).

Tablets may be administered whole or crushed and mixed with food. When convulsions are frequent, the dosage should be divided and administered at intervals. When convulsions occur only every few days, or less often, the daily dosage should be given at one time.[10]

The initial dose of primidone is gradually increased until an optimum control of convulsions is achieved, and the dosage level necessary to establish this effect is usually maintained. Reduction in dosage should be made gradually and never be discontinued abruptly.

Caution(s): Federal law restricts this drug to use by or on the order of a licensed veterinarian.

Keep out of the reach of children.

Do not use in feline species, as PRIMIDONE appears to have a specific neurotoxicity in cats.

In long term therapy using primidone there is the possibility of serum alkaline phosphatase (SAP) elevation to slightly above normal. When primidone therapy is discontinue the SAP should return to normal unless the elevation was caused by other abnormal conditions, such as bone disease, healing fractures or pregnancy.

For use in dogs only.

Side Effects: Primidone is well tolerated at the effective therapeutic levels. Side reactions such as staggering and drowsiness occur infrequently and usually disappear with an adjustment in dosage.

Several investigators have successfully treated megaloblastic anemia associated with long-term primidone use with folic acid, vitamin B_{12} and iron.[8,9]

References: Available upon request.

Presentation: Bottles of 100 and 1,000 tablets.

Compendium Code No.: 10821580

PRIMIDONE ℞

Fort Dodge **Anticonvulsant**

NADA No.: 009-392

Active Ingredient(s): Each tablet contains 50 mg or 250 mg of primidone.

Indications: Use only in dogs to treat:

Idiopathic Epilepsy: Archibald has reported on the use of primidone in the treatment of idiopathic epilepsy in dogs previously treated with other anticonvulsants without success. In his experience primidone was found to be an effective agent completely controlling the convulsions in most of the cases studied and reducing the number and severity of seizures in the remaining small percentage.

According to Chappel, effective control of convulsions has been achieved on daily dosages ranging from 30 to 40 mg/kg of body weight (or approximately 0.15 g to 0.2 g of primidone per 10 lb). As optimum therapeutic effect was obtained, dosage was gradually reduced to maintenance level, and in some cases, therapy was eventually discontinued.

Epileptiform Convulsions: Clinically, these convulsions are similar to those of true epilepsy. Primidone may be useful as a symptomatic treatment of these convulsions of unknown etiology.

Virus Encephalitis, Distemper and Hard Pad Disease Which Occurs as a Clinically Recognizable Lesion in Certain Entities in Dogs: Primidone provides an effective means of controlling convulsions associated with infectious neuropathies such as virus encephalitis, distemper and hard pad disease which occurs as a clinically recognizable lesion in certain entities in dogs. Supplementation of therapy with primidone is recommended as soon as diagnosis is made.

This is particularly important in distemper, since early protection against convulsions may help to promote recovery. However, it must be borne in mind that PRIMIDONE does not correct the primary cause of these disorders, but is a valuable adjunct to therapy, making possible control of seizures without hypnosis or interference with proper nutrition.

Primidone has not proved useful in the treatment of chorea.

Pharmacology:

Description: Primidone [5-ethyldihydro-5-phenyl-4,6 (1*H*, 5*H*)-pyrimidinedione] is a white crystalline substance. This pyrimidine derivative was discovered in 1949 by Bogue and Carrington, in their search for an anticonvulsant less toxic than those available at that time. These investigators demonstrated the protective action of primidone against both electrically and chemically induced convulsions in laboratory animals, a property also confirmed by Goodman, Swinyard, Brown, Schiffman, *et al.*

Subsequent trials have further substantiated the effectiveness of primidone and its high margin of safety in both dogs and man. No apparent gastrointestinal irritation has been noted. Abortion did not occur in pregnant bitches receiving high therapeutic doses of primidone.

In some cases, improvement in behavior pattern has been observed during primidone therapy, the animals being more alert and easier to manage. Weight gains have been reported.

Actions: Primidone acts upon the central nervous system to raise the seizure threshold, hence its value as an anticonvulsant, whether the seizure is induced electrically or is a symptom of a primary disease process.

Dosage and Administration:

Usual Daily Dosage - 55 mg/kg (25 mg/lb) of body weight.

Tablets may be administered whole, or crushed and mixed with food.

When convulsions are frequent, the daily dosage should be divided and administered at intervals. When convulsions occur only every few days, or less often, daily dosage should be given at one time.

Reduction in dosage should always be made gradually and treatment should never be discontinued abruptly.

The initial dose of PRIMIDONE is gradually increased until optimum control of convulsions is achieved and the dosage level necessary to establish this effect is usually maintained. In severe cases, certain workers have found it necessary to utilize higher dosages than those recommended for idiopathic epilepsy and epileptiform convulsions.

Precaution(s): Store at controlled room temperature 15° to 30°C (59° to 86°F).

Caution(s): Federal law restricts this drug to use by or on the order of a licensed veterinarian.

For use only in dogs.

Do not use in feline species. Primidone is not recommended for use in the cat, because it appears to have, as do many other compounds, a specific neurotoxicity for this species.

In long term therapy using primidone there is the possibility of serum alkaline phosphatase (SAP) elevation to slightly above normal. When primidone therapy is discontinued SAP should return to normal unless the elevation was caused by other abnormal conditions, such as bone disease, healing fractures or pregnancy.

Toxicology: In dogs receiving dosages well above effective therapeutic levels, for instance, in excess of 200 mg/kg of body weight, postmortem examinations showed no untoward pathologic effects on the alimentary canal, liver, kidneys, spleen, brain or endocrine glands.

Adverse Reactions: PRIMIDONE is well tolerated at effective therapeutic levels. Side reactions such as staggering and drowsiness occur infrequently and usually disappear with adjustment in dosage.

Potential side effects of primidone are polydipsia, polyuria and polyphagia.

Hepatic dysfunction has been reported in a small percentage of dogs maintained on chronic primidone therapy, alone or in combination with other primary anticonvulsants (phenytoin and phenobarbital).

Biochemical monitoring (including measurements of serum gamma glutaryl transferase activity, bile acid concentration and BSP retention) of patients prior to commencement of and at regular intervals during primidone therapy may identify early hepatic injury or intercurrent hepatic disease, which may be indications for dosage adjustments to the minimum required to control seizures. The risk of potential hepatotoxicity appears to be small relative to the risk associated with intractable seizures and may be an idiosyncratic reaction related to individual susceptibility to the drug.

The activity of drug metabolizing enzymes can be inhibited by certain compounds, such as chloramphenicol. Concurrent administration of chloramphenicol and primidone (or the other primary anticonvulsants) may result in accumulation of the anticonvulsant drug and clinical signs of toxicity (sedation, ataxia, prolonged anesthesia).

One reported case of laboratory-confirmed megaloblastic anemia was successfully treated with folic acid, vitamin B_{12} and iron.

Presentation:

50 mg: Bottles of 500 (NDC 0856-0082-01).

250 mg: Bottles of 100 (NDC 0856-0081-01) and 1000 tablets (NDC 0856-0081-02).

Compendium Code No.: 10031590 0810E

PRIMIDONE 250 MG TABLETS ℞

Vedco **Anticonvulsant**

NADA No.: 030-137

Active Ingredient(s): Each tablet contains:

Primidone .... 250 mg

Indications: For the control of convulsions associated with true epilepsy, epileptiform seizures, virus encephalitis, distemper, and hardpad disease which occurs as a clinically recognizable lesion in certain entities in dogs.

Dosage and Administration: Usual daily dosage: 25 mg/lb. of body weight. The tablets may be administered whole or crushed and mixed with food. When convulsions are frequent, the daily dosage should be divided and administered at intervals.

Precaution(s): Store at a controlled room temperature between 59-86°F (15-30°C).

Caution(s): Federal law restricts this drug to use by or on the order of a licensed veterinarian.

Keep the container closed, away from pets and out of the reach of children.

Presentation: 100 and 1,000 tablet containers.

Compendium Code No.: 10941720

PRIMITABS ℞

Vetus **Anticonvulsant**

NDC No.: 47611-251-01/47611-251-10

Active Ingredient(s): Each PRIMITAB tablet contains:

Primidone .... 250 mg

Indications: For use in dogs to treat:

Idiopathic epilepsy: Archibald has reported on the use of primidone in the treatment of idiopathic epilepsy in dogs previously treated with other anticonvulsants without success. Primidone was found to be an effective agent completely controlling the convulsions in most of the cases studied and reducing the number and severity of seizures in the remaining small percentage.

Epileptiform convulsions: Clinically, these convulsions are similar to those of true epilepsy. Primidone may be useful as a symptomatic treatment of these convulsions of unknown etiology.

Virus encephalitis, distemper, hardpad disease which occurs as a clinically recognizable lesion in certain entities in dogs: Primidone provides an effective means of controlling convulsions associated with infectious neuropathies such as virus encephalitis, distemper or hardpad disease. Supplementation of therapy with primidone is recommended when the diagnosis is made. Oliver and Hoerlin (1965), reported that primidone has been the most effective agent in the dog for the control of seizures associated with post distemper convulsions. Clinical experience has revealed that when the seizure of a dog cannot be controlled with primidone, none of the other anticonvulsants is likely to control it either.

However, primidone does not correct the primary causes of these disorders, but is an adjunct to therapy, making possible control of seizures without hypnosis or interference with proper nutrition.

The initial dose of primidone is gradually increased until the optimum control of convulsions is achieved, and the dosage level necessary to establish this effect is usually maintained.

Primidone has not proven useful in the treatment of chorea.

Pharmacology: Primidone 5-ethyldihydro-5-phenyl-4,6 (1H,-5H)-pyrimidinedione is a white crystalline substance, and is a pyrimidine derivative. Studies of the chronic administration of primidone indicate it can metabolize into two active metabolites, phenobarbital and phenylethylmalonamide (PEMA).

Although primidone is less potent than phenobarbital as a general CNS depressant, primidone is more potent than phenobarbital in the protection of animals against maximal seizures induced by both electroshock and pentylenetetrazole.

As indicated above, primidone may undergo a somewhat complex metabolism involving the production of phenobarbital and the practitioner should take this into consideration if administering other drugs such as other antiepileptics concurrently.

Primidone acts upon the central nervous system to raise the seizure threshold, hence its value as an anticonvulsant, whether the seizure is induced electrically or is a symptom of a primary disease process.

Dosage and Administration:

Usual daily dose: 25 mg/lb. of body weight (55 mg/kg of body weight). The tablets may be administered whole, or crushed and mixed with food. When convulsions are frequent, the dose should be divided and administered at intervals. When convulsions occur every few days, or less often, a daily dose should be given at one time.

A reduction in the dose should be made gradually and the treatment should never be discontinued abruptly.

Caution(s): Federal law restricts this drug to use by or on the order of a licensed veterinarian.

Do not use in the feline species. Primidone has a specific neurotoxicity in cats.

In long term therapy using primidone there is the possibility of serum alkaline phosphatase (SAP) elevation to slightly above normal. When primidone therapy is discontinued the SAP should return to normal unless the elevation was caused by other abnormal conditions, such as bone disease, healing fractures or pregnancy.

Keep out of the reach of children.

Side Effects: Primidone is tolerated at effective therapeutic levels. Side reactions such as staggering and drowsiness occur infrequently and usually disappear with an adjustment in the dosage.

The potential side effects of primidone are polydipsia, polyuria and polyphagia.

Hepatic dysfunction has been reported in a small percentage of dogs maintained on chronic primidone therapy, alone or in combination with other primary anticonvulsants (phenytoin and phenobarbital).

Biochemical monitoring (including measurements of serum gamma glutaryl transferase activity, bile acid concentration, and BSP retention) of patients prior to the commencement of and at regular intervals during primidone therapy may identify early hepatic injury or intercurrent hepatic disease, which may be indications for dosage adjustments to the minimum required to control seizures. The risk of potential hepatotoxicity appear to be small relative to the risk associated with intractable seizures, and may be an idiosyncratic reaction related to individual susceptibility to the drug.

The activity of drug metabolizing enzymes can be inhibited by certain compounds, such as chloramphenicol. Concurrent administration of chloramphenicol and primidone (or the other primary anticonvulsants) may result in an accumulation of the anticonvulsant drug and clinical signs of toxicity (sedation, ataxia, prolonged anesthesia).

Several investigators successfully treated megaloblastic anemia associated with long-term primidone with folic acid, vitamin B_{12} and iron.

Presentation: Bottles of 100 and 1,000 tablets.

Compendium Code No.: 14440770

PRIMOR® ℞

Pfizer Animal Health **Potentiated Sulfa**

(sulfadimethoxine/ormetoprim) Tablets

NADA No.: 100-929

Active Ingredient(s):

PRIMOR® 120: 100 mg sulfadimethoxine/20 mg ormetoprim.

PRIMOR® 240: 200 mg sulfadimethoxine/40 mg ormetoprim.

PRIMOR® 600: 500 mg sulfadimethoxine/100 mg ormetoprim.

PRIMOR® 1200: 1000 mg sulfadimethoxine/200 mg ormetoprim.

Indications: PRIMOR® is for the treatment of skin and soft tissue infections (wounds and abscesses) in dogs caused by strains of *Staphylococcus aureus* and *Escherichia coli* and urinary tract infections caused by *Escherichia coli, Staphylococcus* spp., and *Proteus mirabilis* susceptible to sulfadimethoxine/ormetoprim.

Pharmacology: Description: PRIMOR® is an antimicrobial drug containing sulfadimethoxine and ormetoprim in a 5 to 1 ratio. The combination of these 2 compounds results in the potentiation of sulfadimethoxine, providing increased efficacy, a broadened spectrum of activity to include some sulfonamide-resistant organisms, and reduction in the rate of resistance development.

Sulfadimethoxine is a white, almost tasteless and odorless powder. Chemically, it is N[1]-(2,6-dimethoxy-4-pyrimidinyl)-sulfanilamide. The structural formula is:

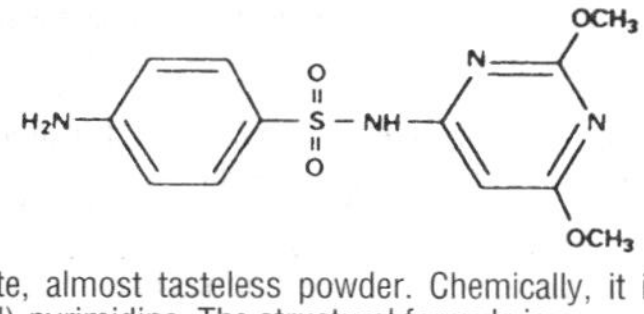

Ormetoprim is a white, almost tasteless powder. Chemically, it is 2,4-diamino-5-(4,5-dimethoxy-2-methylbenzyl)-pyrimidine. The structural formula is:

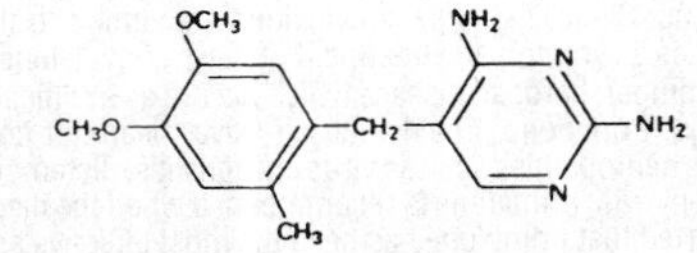

Clinical Pharmacology: Sulfadimethoxine is not acetylated in the dog, as in most other animals, and is excreted predominantly as the unchanged drug.[3] Sulfadimethoxine has a relatively high solubility at the pH normally occurring in the kidney, precluding the possibility of precipitation and crystalluria. Slow renal excretion results from a high degree of tubular reabsorption. Plasma protein binding is very high, providing a blood reservoir of the drug. Thus sulfadimethoxine maintains higher blood levels than most other long-acting sulfonamides. Single, comparatively low doses of sulfadimethoxine give rapid and sustained therapeutic blood levels.[4]

The systemically active sulfonamides, which include sulfadimethoxine, are bacteriostatic agents. Sulfonamides competitively inhibit bacterial synthesis of folic acid (pteroylglutamic acid) from para-aminobenzoic acid. Mammalian cells are capable of utilizing folic acid in the presence of sulfonamides.

Ormetoprim, like other diaminopyrimidines, inhibits the reduction of dihydrofolic acid to tetrahydrofolic acid by bacterial cells. Sulfadimethoxine/ormetoprim thus blocks 2 sequential steps of the folic acid metabolism of bacteria, depriving them of folate coenzymes. Potentiated sulfonamides have been shown to exhibit bactericidal as well as bacteriostatic action.

Microbiology: Sulfadimethoxine is a low-dosage, rapidly absorbed, long-acting sulfonamide effective for the treatment of a wide range of bacterial infections commonly encountered in dogs. Sulfadimethoxine has been demonstrated under laboratory and field conditions to be effective against a variety of gram-positive and gram-negative, aerobic and anaerobic organisms belonging to the genera *Streptococcus, Klebsiella, Proteus, Shigella, Staphylococcus, Escherichia, Salmonella,* and *Clostridium.*[1,2] Most strains of these organisms were found to be susceptible to PRIMOR® *in vitro,* but the *in vivo* significance has not been determined for some canine isolates.

Ormetoprim potentiates the activity of sulfadimethoxine. The *in vitro* antibacterial spectrum and activity of the 2 compounds are very similar. On a molar basis, ormetoprim is more active than sulfadimethoxine. Sulfadimethoxine/ormetoprim shows enhanced *in vitro* and *in vivo* activity (potentiation) over that of either compound used alone. *In vitro,* the potentiation results in a reduction of the minimum inhibitory concentration of each drug, and an increase in activity against sulfonamide-resistant organisms, such as *Streptococcus, Staphylococcus, Corynebacterium, Escherichia, Klebsiella, Proteus, Brucella, Bordetella,* and *Clostridium.*[1] The susceptibility of organisms to PRIMOR® Tablets should be determined using a potentiated sulfonamide sensitivity disc such as sulfamethoxazole and trimethoprim (BBL® Sensi-Disc® SXT*). Specimens for susceptibility testing should be collected prior to initiation of therapy.

Dosage and Administration: Administer an initial oral dose of 25 mg/lb (55 mg/kg) of body weight on the first day of treatment. Administer subsequent daily doses at the rate of 12.5 mg/lb (27.5 mg/kg) of body weight. Continue treatment for at least 2 days after remission of clinical signs. Do not extend treatment for more than 21 consecutive days. Suggested dosage schedules follow:

	Body Weight (lb) Up To	No. of Tablets First Day	No. of Tablets Subsequent Days
PRIMOR® 120	5	1	½
	10	2	1
	15	3	1½
PRIMOR® 240	10	1	½
	20	2	1
	30	3	1½
PRIMOR® 600	25	1	½
	50	2	1
PRIMOR® 1200	50	1	½
	100	2	1

P

For optimal therapeutic effect: (1) the drug must be given early in the course of the disease; (2) therapeutically effective levels must be maintained in the body throughout the treatment period; (3) treatment should continue for at least 2 days after remission of clinical signs; and (4) the causative bacterial agents must be sensitive to the drug.

Contraindication(s): PRIMOR® should not be used in dogs showing marked liver parenchymal damage, blood dyscrasias, or in those with a history of sulfonamide hypersensitivity.

Precaution(s): Storage: Store at controlled room temperature 15°-30°C (59°-86°F).

Caution(s): Federal law restricts this drug to use by or on the order of a licensed veterinarian.

Individual animal hypersensitivity may result in local or generalized reactions. Anaphylactoid reactions, although rare, may also occur.

Decreased water consumption and aciduria enhance the probability of the formation of sulfonamide crystals in the urine. Monitoring urine samples for crystal formation is recommended from animals with acid urine receiving the drug. As with any sulfonamide therapy, make certain dogs maintain adequate water intake. If dogs show no improvement within 2 or 3 days, reevaluate the diagnosis.

Antidote(s): Epinephrine for anaphylactoid reactions.

Warning(s): Not for human use. For use in dogs only.

Keep out of reach of children.

Toxicology: Toxicity and Safety:[1] Toxicity data for PRIMOR® indicates that the drug is safe when used at the recommended dosage.

Following oral administration of PRIMOR® to dogs at 27.5 mg/kg/day (12.5 mg/lb/day) for 8 weeks, no changes were noted in hematology, blood chemistry, urinalysis, gross pathology, and histopathology, except for elevated serum cholesterol, increased thyroid and liver weights, enlarged basophilic cells in the pituitary, and mild follicular thyroid hyperplasia. These changes are known to be associated with prolonged administration of sulfonamides to dogs and have been shown to be reversible.

Safety in breeding dogs has not been established.

Adverse Reactions: Conditions reported following use of sulfonamides or potentiated sulfonamides include polyarthritis, urticaria, facial swelling, fever, hemolytic anemia, polydypsia, polyuria, hepatitis, vomiting, anorexia, diarrhea, and neurologic disorders. In rare instances, neurologic signs including behavioral changes, ataxia, seizures, aggression, and hyperexcitability have been reported. Keratitis sicca, possibly due to prolonged use of sulfonamides, has been reported.

Trial Data: In an experimentally induced, controlled soft tissue infection study in dogs, the therapeutic efficacy of PRIMOR® was significantly greater than the 2 individual components when administered separately, providing clear evidence of the potentiation of sulfadimethoxine by ormetoprim in the target species.[1]

Blood Levels:[1] Therapeutically effective blood levels of both sulfadimethoxine and ormetoprim are obtained and maintained in dogs when using the recommended PRIMOR® dosing regimen of 25 mg/lb on day one and of 12.5 mg/lb on following days. Blood levels of sulfadimethoxine and ormetoprim were studied in 2 male and 2 female dogs. The initial drug dose was administered at zero hours. Blood samples were taken at 11 intervals, 6 of which are reported in Table 1. A second dose of PRIMOR® was administered immediately following the 24-hour blood samples and blood values were determined 2 hours later (26 hours from the initial dose).

Table 1: Blood levels (mcg/mL) obtained with administration of a 25 mg/lb dose of PRIMOR® followed with a 12.5 mg/lb dose at 24 hours:

Sample	2 hr	8 hr	24 hr*	26 hr	32 hr	48 hr
Sulfadimethoxine	23.00	41.00	39.00	60.00	67.00	36.00
Ormetoprim	1.04	0.55	0.09	1.08	0.44	0.03

*Sample collected before administration of the second dose.

References: Available upon request.

Presentation: PRIMOR® is available as scored tablets for the following potencies: 120 mg, 240 mg, 600 mg, and 1200 mg.

PRIMOR® 120 - 100 and 1,000 tablet bottles.
PRIMOR® 240 - 50 and 100 tablet bottles.
PRIMOR® 600 - 100 and 250 tablet bottles.
PRIMOR® 1200 - 100 tablet bottles.

*BBL® and Sensi-Disc® are registered trademarks owned by Becton, Dickinson and Company, Paramus, New Jersey.

Compendium Code No.: 36901320 75-8438-06

PRIMUCELL FIP®

Pfizer Animal Health **Vaccine**

Feline Infectious Peritonitis Vaccine, Modified Live Virus

U.S. Vet. Lic. No.: 189

Description: PRIMUCELL FIP® contains an attenuated, temperature-sensitive (TS) strain of FIP virus propagated on an established feline cell line. The vaccine is freeze-dried to preserve stability.

Contains gentamicin as preservative.

Indications: PRIMUCELL FIP® is for intranasal (IN) vaccination of healthy cats 16 weeks of age or older as an aid in preventing feline infectious peritonitis caused by feline infectious peritonitis virus (FIPV).

Cats vaccinated IN with PRIMUCELL FIP® develop a protective immune response and do not become hypersensitized. This practical benefit may be attributed to the temperature-sensitive PRIMUCELL FIP® vaccine strain, which replicates in the upper respiratory tract, but does not spread systemically at 39°C, the cat's body temperature.

Directions:

1. General Directions: Vaccination of healthy cats is recommended. Aseptically rehydrate the freeze-dried vaccine with the sterile diluent provided. Mix well. Use dropper to inoculate entire volume into nasal passages (½ volume into each nasal passage). Cats may sneeze or shake their heads at the time of administration.
2. Primary Vaccination: Healthy cats 16 weeks of age or older should receive 2 IN doses administered 3-4 weeks apart.
3. Revaccination: Annual revaccination with a single dose is recommended.

Precaution(s): Store at 2°-7°C. Prolonged exposure to higher temperatures and/or direct sunlight may adversely affect potency. Do not freeze.

Use entire contents when first opened.

Burn containers and all unused contents.

Caution(s): Droppers should be used to administer this vaccine.

As with many vaccines, anaphylaxis may occur after use. Initial antidote of epinephrine is recommended and should be followed with appropriate supportive therapy.

This product has been shown to be efficacious in healthy animals. A protective immune response may not be elicited if animals are incubating an infectious disease, are malnourished or parasitized, are stressed due to shipment or environmental conditions, are otherwise immunocompromised, or the vaccine is not administered in accordance with label directions.

Warning(s): For use in cats only.

For veterinary use only.

Discussion: Disease Description: FIP is a complex disease of cats caused by FIPV, a coronavirus related to transmissible gastroenteritis virus (TGEV) of pigs, enteric coronavirus of dogs, and respiratory coronavirus of humans.[1]

Although scientists do not completely understand its pathogenesis, they believe that FIP is an immune-mediated disease. FIPV first multiplies in epithelial cells of the upper respiratory tract and intestine.[2] Clinically apparent FIP occurs after the virus crosses the mucosal barrier and spreads throughout the cat in infected macrophages and monocytes.

Primary FIP may be mild, consisting of fever and a slight nasal and ocular discharge. While most cats with the primary form of FIP recover, others become chronically infected carriers. Secondary FIP may develop following primary infection and appears in 2 forms: (1) Effusive or wet form, characterized by peritonitis and pleuritis with ascites and pleural effusion, and (2) Noneffusive or dry form, characterized by granulomatous inflammation of various organs and little or no exudate.[3,4] Both forms may appear together.

Once clinical symptoms occur, FIP usually takes a fatal course. The most commonly diagnosed clinical manifestation is accumulation of fluid within the peritoneal cavity with progressive, painless enlargement of the abdomen. Infected animals also may experience difficult breathing, have an elevated temperature, appear depressed, and lose weight. Other clinical symptoms, such as ocular involvement, disseminated intravascular coagulation, and renal involvement, are observed occasionally.[5] Exudate obtained from body cavities by paracentesis appears pale yellow or golden in color and is relatively clear. Hemograms of cats with FIP typically indicate a stress response. There may be a mild to moderate anemia and leukocytosis attributed to an increased percentage of neutrophils.

FIP most frequently occurs in young cats between the ages of 6 months and 2 years of age. Incidence of disease is also higher in older cats, between 11 and 15 years of age.

Trial Data: Safety and Efficacy: Comprehensive tests were conducted to demonstrate the safety of PRIMUCELL FIP®.

In these tests, PRIMUCELL FIP® did not cause illness in cats when administered intranasally. It did not cause illness in cats infected with feline leukemia, in cats exposed to feline enteric coronavirus, in dexamethasone-immunosuppressed cats, in nonvaccinated cats that survived FIP challenge, or in kittens.

PRIMUCELL FIP® did not interfere with the development of an antibody response to any of the following feline vaccine antigens: feline leukemia virus, feline rhinotracheitis virus, feline calicivirus, feline panleukopenia virus, and *Chlamydia psittaci*. Conversely, none of these vaccine antigens interfered with the immunogenicity of PRIMUCELL FIP®.

Efficacy of PRIMUCELL FIP® also was demonstrated in a series of tests.

In the first of 2 immunogenicity studies, 20 seronegative cats were vaccinated with a 2-dose primary regimen (given 3 weeks apart). All vaccinates developed FIPV antibody titers, and 17 of the 20 (85%) survived an FIPV challenge that caused FIP in 12 of 12 (100%) nonvaccinated controls. Ten of the 12 controls died. Sixteen of the 17 (94%) vaccinated cats that survived the first challenge survived a second challenge, which caused FIP in 4 of 6 nonvaccinated controls.

In the second immunogenicity study, 20 of 20 seronegative cats developed FIPV antibody titers after primary vaccination with 2 doses given 3 weeks apart. Fifteen of 20 (75%) vaccinates were protected against a challenge of immunity in which 7 of 10 (70%) nonvaccinated control cats died of FIP. All but 1 of the surviving vaccinated cats from the first challenge survived a second challenge, which killed 6 of 6 nonvaccinated controls.

In addition to protecting against homologous challenge, PRIMUCELL FIP® also protected cats against a heterologous challenge strain (WSU-1146). Clinical FIP symptoms of vaccinated cats were significantly lower (P) than symptoms of control cats following WSU-1146 challenge. Eight of 10 (80%) vaccinated cats survived a challenge of immunity with the WSU-1146 strain of FIP in which 3 of 5 (60%) non-vaccinated controls died of FIP.

References: Available upon request.

Presentation: Cartons of 25 1-dose vials.

Compendium Code No.: 36901330 75-4643-05

PRISM™ 4

Fort Dodge **Vaccine**

Bovine Rhinotracheitis-Virus Diarrhea-Parainfluenza-3-Respiratory Syncytial Virus Vaccine, Modified Live and Killed Virus

U.S. Vet. Lic. No.: 112

Contents: This product contains modified live IBR, PI-3 and BRSV and inactivated BVD (Types I and II).

Thimerosal, neomycin and polymyxin B added as preservatives.

Indications: For vaccination of healthy cattle as an aid in the prevention of disease caused by bovine rhinotracheitis, bovine virus diarrhea (Types I and II), bovine parainfluenza-3 and bovine respiratory syncytial viruses.

Dosage and Administration: Aseptically rehydrate with the accompanying diluent. Cattle, inject one 2 mL dose subcutaneously or intramuscularly using aseptic technique. Cattle should be revaccinated at 14 to 28 days with a 2 mL booster dose of Triangle® 1 + Type II BVD, Killed Virus vaccine. Annual revaccination is recommended. Protect animals from exposure for at least 14 days after vaccination. Calves vaccinated under six months of age should be revaccinated at six months of age.

Precaution(s): Store in dark at 2° to 7°C (35° to 45°F). Avoid freezing. Shake well. Use entire contents when first opened. Burn container and all unused contents.

Caution(s): Do not use in pregnant cows or in calves nursing pregnant cows. A small percentage of animals may show transient mild injection site swelling. In case of anaphylactoid reaction, administer epinephrine.

Warning(s): Do not vaccinate within 21 days before slaughter.

For veterinary use only.

Presentation: One vial vaccine, one vial diluent. 10 doses (rehydrate to 20 mL) and one vial vaccine, one vial diluent. 50 doses (rehydrate to 100 mL).

U.S. Patent Nos. 5,733,555 — 5,958,423

Compendium Code No.: 10031600 2575B

PRISM™ 9

Fort Dodge **Bacterin-Vaccine**

Bovine Rhinotracheitis-Virus Diarrhea-Parainfluenza-3-Respiratory Syncytial Virus Vaccine, Modified Live and Killed Virus-Leptospira Canicola-Grippotyphosa-Hardjo-Icterohaemorrhagiae-Pomona Bacterin

U.S. Vet. Lic. No.: 112

Contents: This product contains modified live IBR, PI-3 and BRSV, inactivated BVD (Types I and II), and a 5 way Leptospira bacterin.

Thimerosal, neomycin and polymyxin B added as preservatives.

Indications: For vaccination of healthy cattle as an aid in the prevention of disease caused by bovine rhinotracheitis, bovine virus diarrhea (Types I and II), bovine parainfluenza-3, bovine respiratory syncytial virus and *L. canicola, L. grippotyphosa, L. hardjo, L. icterohaemorrhagiae* and *L. pomona*.

Dosage and Administration: Aseptically rehydrate with the accompanying diluent.

Cattle, inject one 2 mL dose subcutaneously or intramuscularly using aseptic technique. Cattle should be revaccinated at 14 to 28 days with a 2 mL booster dose of Triangle® 1 + Type II BVD, Killed Virus vaccine. Annual revaccination is recommended. Calves vaccinated under six months of age should be revaccinated at six months of age. Protect animals from exposure for at least 14 days after the last dose of vaccine.

Precaution(s): Store in dark at 2° to 7°C (35° to 45°F). Avoid freezing. Shake well. Use entire contents when first opened. Burn container and all unused contents.

Caution(s): Do not use in pregnant cows or in calves nursing pregnant cows. A small percentage of animals may show transient mild injection site swelling. In case of anaphylactoid reaction, administer epinephrine.

Warning(s): Do not vaccinate within 21 days before slaughter.

For veterinary use only.

Presentation: One vial vaccine, one vial diluent. 10 doses (rehydrate to 20 mL) and one vial vaccine, one vial diluent. 50 doses (rehydrate to 100 mL).

U.S. Patent No. 5,733,555 — 5,958,423

Compendium Code No.: 10031610 2695D

PRIVASAN™ ANTISEPTIC OINTMENT

First Priority **Topical Wound Dressing**

ANADA No.: 200-301

Active Ingredient(s): 1% chlorhexidine acetate in a hydrophilic ointment base which contains 10% stearyl alcohol.

Indications: Dogs, Cats and Horses - For use as a topical antiseptic ointment for surface wounds.

Dosage and Administration: Suggested Usage:

Dogs, Cats and Horses - Carefully cleanse the wound area and apply daily.

Precaution(s): Storage: Store at controlled room temperature between 15°-30°C (59°-86°F). Keep container tightly closed when not in use. Protect from freezing.

Caution(s): In case of deep or puncture wounds or serious burns, consult veterinarian. If redness, irritation or swelling persists or increases, discontinue use and consult veterinarian.

For animal use only.

Warning(s): Not to be used on horses intended for use as food.

Keep out of reach of children.

Presentation: 1 oz tube, 7 oz (198 g) jar (NDC# 58829-288-07) and 1 lb (453.6 g) jar (NDC# 58829-288-16).

Compendium Code No.: 11390830 Rev. 11-01 / Rev. 08-01

PRIVERMECTIN™ DRENCH FOR SHEEP

First Priority **Parasiticide-Oral**

(ivermectin) 0.08% Solution

ANADA No.: 200-327

Active Ingredient(s): PRIVERMECTIN™ (ivermectin) Drench for Sheep is a liquid, administered orally for sheep, consisting of an 0.08% solution of ivermectin.

Indications: PRIVERMECTIN™ (ivermectin) Drench for Sheep is indicated for the effective treatment of gastrointestinal roundworms (including *Haemonchus contortus)*, lungworms and nasal bots in sheep.

When used as recommended, it provides effective control of the parasites listed in the table. PRIVERMECTIN™ Drench for Sheep kills these parasites:

Gastrointestinal roundworms	Adults	Larvae (4th stage)
Haemonchus contortus	X	X
Haemonchus placei	X	
Ostertagia circumcincta	X	X
Trichostrongylus axei	X	X
Trichostrongylus colubriformis	X	X
Cooperia curticei	X	X
Cooperia oncophora	X	
Oesophagostomum columbianum	X	X
Oesophagostomum venulosum	X	
Nematodirus battus	X	X
Nematodirus spathiger	X	X
Strongyloides papillosus	X	
Chabertia ovina	X	
Trichuris ovis	X	
Lungworms:		
Dictyocaulus filaria	X	X
Nasal bots:		
Oestrus ovis	(all larval stages)	

Pharmacology: Formulation: PRIVERMECTIN™ (ivermectin) Drench for Sheep is an 0.08% w/v pale amber colored solution of ivermectin.

Ivermectin is derived from the avermectins, a family of highly active, broad spectrum, antiparasitic agents which are produced from fermentation products of *Streptomyces avermitilis*.

Mode of Action: The avermectin family of compounds, of which ivermectin is a member, kills certain parasitic nematodes (roundworms) and arthropods. The action is unique and not shared by other antiparasitic agents and involves a chemical that serves as a signal from one nerve cell to another, or from a nerve cell to a muscle cell. This chemical, a neurotransmitter, is called *gamma* aminobutyric acid or GABA. In roundworms, ivermectin stimulates the release of GABA from nerve endings and enhances binding of GAGA to special receptors at nerve functions, thus interrupting nerve impulses - thereby paralyzing and killing the parasite.

The enhancement of the GABA effect in arthropods resembles that in roundworms except that nerve impulses are interrupted between the nerve ending and the muscle cell. Again, this leads to paralysis and death in most species. Ivermectin has no measurable effect against flukes or tapeworms, presumably because they do not have GABA as a nerve impulse transmitter. Recommended doses of ivermectin have a wide safety margin in livestock. The principal peripheral neurotransmitter in mammals, acetylcholine, is unaffected by ivermectin. Ivermectin does not readily penetrate the central nervous system of mammals where GABA functions as a neurotransmitter.

Dosage and Administration: Dosing: PRIVERMECTIN™ (ivermectin) Drench for Sheep is formulated only for administration to sheep; do not use in other species. The recommended dose level is 3 mL of PRIVERMECTIN™ (ivermectin) Drench for Sheep, containing 2400 mcg ivermectin, which is sufficient to treat 26 pounds of body weight.

Dosage: PRIVERMECTIN™ (ivermectin) Drench for Sheep should only be administered orally at the recommended dose level of 200 mcg ivermectin per kilogram of body weight. Three mL of PRIVERMECTIN™ (ivermectin) Drench for Sheep contains sufficient ivermectin to treat 26 pounds of body weight.

Volume	Sheep Body Weight Dosed
3 mL	26 lbs
6 mL	52 lbs
9 mL	78 lbs
12 mL	104 lbs
15 mL	130 lbs
18 mL	156 lbs
21 mL	182 lbs
24 mL	208 lbs
27 mL	234 lbs
30 mL	260 lbs

To avoid underdosing, it is important to get the dose according to the weight of the heaviest sheep in a group (ewes, lambs or rams), not the average weight. Several of the largest sheep should be weighed, judgment by the eye can be deceiving.

Administration: Any standard drenching equipment, or any equipment which provides a consistent dose volume, can be used. Dose rates and equipment should be checked before drenching commences. Be sure the head is properly positioned for each sheep to receive the full dose.

PRIVERMECTIN™ (ivermectin) Drench for Sheep is readily accepted by sheep, but

P

inconsequential coughing may be observed in some animals during and for several minutes after drenching. If slobbering occurs, the dose may be lost, and that sheep should be redosed.

Frequency of Dosing: Resistant parasites are a particular problem for sheep.

Please consult your veterinarian, county extension office or animal health supplier for the control program recommended in your area.

Safety: PRIVERMECTIN™ (ivermectin) Drench for Sheep has been demonstrated to have a wide safety margin at the recommended dose level and may be used in sheep of all ages. Ewes may be treated at any stage of pregnancy.

Acceptability: Coughing may be observed in some animals during and for several minutes following drenching.

Precaution(s): Stability: PRIVERMECTIN™ (ivermectin) Drench for Sheep is stable for 24 months when stored under normal conditions. Protect from light.

Environmental Safety: Studies indicate that when ivermectin comes in contact with the soil, it readily and tightly binds to the soil and becomes inactive over time. Free ivermectin may adversely affect fish and certain waterborn organisms on which they feed. Do not permit water runoff from feedlots to enter lakes, streams, or ground water. Do not contaminate water by direct application or by the improper disposal of drug containers. Spills of PRIVERMECTIN™ (ivermectin) Drench for Sheep should be contained and soaked up with absorbent towels or into loose soils. Gloves should be worn to prevent skin exposure. All the collected material (contaminated towels and soil), as well as all used drug containers, should be placed in an impervious film bag (plastic) and disposed of by incineration or in an approved landfill.

This product is not to be used parenterally. Protect from light. Store at controlled room temperature between 15°-30°C (59°-86°F). Keep container tightly closed when not in use.

Caution(s): PRIVERMECTIN™ (ivermectin) Drench for Sheep has been formulated for use in sheep only. This product should not be used in other animal species as severe adverse reactions, including fatalities in dogs, may result.

Keep this and all drugs out of the reach of children.

Human Safety: When used as recommended in sheep, PRIVERMECTIN™ (ivermectin) Drench for Sheep does not pose a hazard to human health. As a routine precaution, it is advisable to wash hands after use. As with all drugs, the product should be kept out of reach of children. Refrain from smoking and eating when handling. Contact with skin and eyes should be avoided, but protective clothing is not required.

Warning(s): Sheep must not be treated within 11 days of slaughter for human consumption.

Discussion: Discovered and developed by scientists from Merck Sharp and Dohme Research Laboratories, ivermectin is a unique chemical entity. As such, the chances of cross-resistance in parasites that have developed resistance to other wormers is highly unlikely. Additionally, its convenience broad spectrum efficacy, and wide therapeutic index make PRIVERMECTIN™ (ivermectin) Drench for Sheep an exceptionally valuable product for parasite control in sheep.

Presentation: PRIVERMECTIN™ (ivermectin) Drench for Sheep is available in a convenient pack size: The 32.46 fl oz (960 mL) pack contains sufficient solution to treat 83 sheep averaging 100 lbs. The packs are high-density polyethylene containers, colored opaque white, with screw caps and tamper-evident seals. They are shipped in cardboard cartons as follows: 4 x 960 mL containers per case.

Compendium Code No.: 11390860 Iss. 02-02

PRIVERMECTIN™ EQUINE ORAL LIQUID ℞

First Priority **Parasiticide-Oral**

(ivermectin) 10 mg/mL

ANADA No.: 200-321

Active Ingredient(s): PRIVERMECTIN™ Equine Oral Liquid is a clear, ready-to-use solution with each mL containing 1% ivermectin (10 mg), 0.2 mL propylene glycol, 80 mg polysorbate 80, 9 mg sodium phosphate monobasic monohydrate, 1.3 mg sodium phosphate dibasic anhydrous, 1 mg butylated hydroxytoluene, 0.1 mg disodium edetate, 3% benzyl alcohol and purified water q.s. ad 100%.

Indications: PRIVERMECTIN™ Equine Oral Liquid is indicated for the effective treatment and control of the following parasites or parasitic conditions in horses:

Large Strongyles: *Strongylus vulgaris* (adults and arterial larval stages), *S. edentatus* (adults and tissue stages), *S. equinus* (adults), *Triodontophorus* spp (adults).

Small Strongyles - including those resistant to some benzimidazole class compounds (adults and fourth-stage larvae): *Cyathostomum* spp, *Cylicocyclus* spp, *Cylicostephanus* spp, *Cylicodontophorus* spp.

Pinworms (adults and fourth-stage larvae): *Oxyuris equi.*

Ascarids (adults and third- and fourth-stage larvae): *Parascaris equorum.*

Hairworms (adults): *Trichostrongylus axei.*

Largemouth Stomach Worms (adults): *Habronema muscae.*

Bots (oral and gastric stages): *Gastrophilus* spp.

Lungworms (adults and fourth-stage larvae): *Dictyocaulus arnfieldi.*

Intestinal Threadworms (adults): *Strongyloides westeri.*

Summer Sores caused by *Habronema* and *Draschia* spp cutaneous third-stage larvae.

Dermatitis caused by neck threadworm microfilariae, *Onchocerca* sp.

Pharmacology: Ivermectin is derived from the avermectins, a family of potent, broad-spectrum antiparasitic agents, which are isolated from fermentation of *Streptomyces avermitilis.*

Mode of Action: Ivermectin, one of the avermectins, kills certain parasitic roundworms and ectoparasites such as mites and lice. The avermectins are different in their action from other antiparasitic agents. This action involves a chemical that serves as a signal from one nerve cell to another, or from a nerve cell to a muscle cell. This chemical, a neurotransmitter, is called gammaaminobutyric acid or GABA. In roundworms, ivermectin stimulates the release of GABA from nerve endings and enhances binding of GABA to special receptors at nerve junctions, thus interrupting nerve impulses - thereby paralyzing and killing the parasite.

The enhancement of the GABA effect in arthropods such as mites and lice resembles that in roundworms except that nerve impulses are interrupted between the nerve ending and the muscle cell. Again, this leads to paralysis and death.

The principle peripheral neurotransmitter in mammals, acetylcholine, is unaffected by ivermectin. Ivermectin does not readily penetrate the central nervous system of mammals where GABA functions as a neurotransmitter.

Dosage and Administration: Dosage: PRIVERMECTIN™ Equine Oral Liquid for Horses is formulated for administration by stomach tube (nasogastric intubation) or as an oral drench. The recommended dose is 200 mcg of ivermectin per kilogram (91 mcg/lb) of bodyweight. Each mL contains sufficient ivermectin to treat 110 lb (50 kg) of body weight: 10 mL will treat an 1100 lb (500 kg) horse.

Administration: Use a calibrated dosing syringe inserted into the bottle to measure the appropriate dose, or pour the PRIVERMECTIN™ Equine Oral Liquid into a graduated cylinder for dose measurement. Use a clean syringe if accessing the bottle to avoid contaminating the remaining product.

Administration by stomach tube (gravity or positive flow): The recommended dose can be used undiluted or diluted up to 40 times with clean tepid water (see Notes to Veterinarian). Use tepid water to flush any drug remaining in the tube into the horse's stomach.

Administration by drench: For administration by this method, an undiluted dose is usually preferred. Clear the horse's mouth of any food material, elevate the horse's head, and using a syringe, deposit the appropriate dose in the back of the mouth. In order to avoid unnecessary coughing or the potential for material to enter the trachea and lungs, do not use excessive pressure (squirting), do not use a large (diluted) dose volume, and do not deposit the dose in the laryngeal area. Increased dose rejection may occur if the dose is deposited in the buccal space. Keep the horse's head elevated and observe the horse to insure the dose is retained.

Suggested Parasite Control Program: All horses should be included in a regular parasite control program with particular attention being paid to mares, foals and yearlings. Foals should be treated initially at 6 to 8 weeks of age, and routine treatment repeated as appropriate. PRIVERMECTIN™ Equine Oral Liquid effectively controls gastrointestinal nematodes and bots in horses. Regular treatment will reduce the chances of verminous arteritis and colic caused by *S. vulgaris.* With its broad spectrum, PRIVERMECTIN™ Equine Oral Liquid is well suited to be the major product in a parasite control program.

Precaution(s): Storage: Store in a tightly closed container at room temperature (between 15-30°C, 59-86°F). Protect PRIVERMECTIN™ Equine Oral Liquid (undiluted or diluted) from light.

Environmental Safety: Studies indicate that when ivermectin comes in contact with the soil, it readily and tightly binds to the soil and becomes inactive over time. Free ivermectin may adversely affect fish and certain water-borne organisms on which they feed. Do not contaminate lakes, streams, or ground water by direct application or by improper disposal of drug containers. Dispose of drug container in an approved landfill or by incineration.

Caution(s): Federal (U.S.A.) law restricts this drug to use by or on the order of a licensed veterinarian.

PRIVERMECTIN™ Equine Oral Liquid has been formulated specifically for use in horses only. This product should not be used in other animal species as severe adverse reactions, including fatalities in dogs may result.

Notes to Veterinarian: Swelling and itching reactions after treatment with PRIVERMECTIN™ Equine Oral Liquid have occurred in horses carrying heavy infections of neck threadworm microfilariae, *Onchocerca* sp. These reactions were most likely the result of microfilariae dying in large numbers. Symptomatic treatment may be advisable.

Healing of summer sores involving extensive tissue changes may require other therapy in conjunction with PRIVERMECTIN™ Equine Oral Liquid. Reinfection, and measures for its prevention, should also be considered.

Special consideration should be given to the effects or potential for injury from handling, restraint and placement of the tube during administration by stomach tube.

PRIVERMECTIN™ Equine Oral Liquid should be administered by drench if the risks associated with tubing are of concern. Due to the consequences of improper administration (also see Dosage and Administration), PRIVERMECTIN™ Equine Oral Liquid is intended for use by a veterinarian only and is not recommended for dispensing.

PRIVERMECTIN™ Equine Oral Liquid in 1 to 20 and 1 to 40 dilutions with tap water has been shown to be stable for 72 hours under the conditions recommended for the product (i.e., at room temperature, in a tightly closed container, protected from light). The diluted product does not promote the growth of common organisms. However, prolonged storage of the diluted product cannot be recommended, as the effects of possible contaminants and interactions with untested materials are unknown.

For veterinary use only.

Warning(s): Do not use in horses intended for food purposes.

Refrain from smoking and eating when handling. Wash hands after use. Avoid contact with eyes. Keep this and all drugs out of the reach of children.

Toxicology: Safety: PRIVERMECTIN™ Equine Oral Liquid may be used in horses of all ages including mares at any stage of pregnancy. Stallions may be treated without adversely affecting their fertility. These horses have been treated with no adverse effects other than those noted under Notes to Veterinarian.

Discussion: PRIVERMECTIN™ Equine Oral Liquid (ivermectin) for Horses has been formulated for professional administration by stomach tube or oral drench. One low-volume dose is effective against important internal parasites, including the arterial stages of *Strongylus vulgaris,* and bots.

Ivermectin is a potent antiparasitic agent whose chemical structure is different from those of other antiparasitic agents. Its convenience, broad-spectrum efficacy and safety margin make PRIVERMECTIN™ Equine Oral Liquid an ideal parasite control product for horses.

Presentation: PRIVERMECTIN™ Equine Oral Liquid is available in a 100 mL plastic bottle. Each bottle contains sufficient ivermectin to treat 10-500 kg (1100 lb) horses. Contents may be poured into a graduated cylinder for dose measurement. Alternatively, a clean syringe may be inserted directly into the bottle to draw off the appropriate dose (NDC# 58829-294-10).

PRIVERMECTIN™ is a registered trademark of First Priority, Inc.

Compendium Code No.: 11390821 Iss. 09-01

PRN HI-ENERGY SUPPLEMENT™

PRN Pharmacal **Large Animal Dietary Supplement**

Active Ingredient(s): Each tube contains: Amino Acids 44 mg, Thiamine 32 mg, Riboflavin 8 mg, Pyridoxine HCl 16 mg, Niacinamide 80 mg, D-Calcium Pantothenate 48 mg, Liver 3 grams, Iron Citrate 240 mg, Vitamin B12 400 mcg, q.s. Propylene Glycol.

Indications: PRN HI-ENERGY SUPPLEMENT™ is a nutritional product supplying additional propylene glycol, amino acids, vitamins and iron suggested for animals that have reduced or restricted food intake.

Directions for Use: For cattle and horses, give ½ to 1 tube twice daily. If in doubt, consult veterinarian.

1. Hold the head of the animal in a normal to slightly elevated position.
2. Place tube in animal's mouth directly over the tongue.
3. The product is carefully and quickly pressed out of the 10 oz tube.
4. Hold the animal's mouth closed and allow time to swallow.

Caution(s): Use extreme care to prevent injury to the animal's mouth and throat tissue when administering PRN HI-ENERGY SUPPLEMENT™. Do not allow the animal to chew on the tip of the tube which can result in mouth laceration. Do not administer to animals with open sores in the mouth or throat. Supplement may cause irritation to eyes and skin. For livestock use only.

Warning(s): Keep out of reach of children.

For veterinarian use only.

Presentation: 300 mL (10 oz) tube.

Compendium Code No.: 10900130

PRN HIGH POTENCY CALCIUM GEL®

PRN Pharmacal **Calcium-Oral**

Guaranteed Analysis:

Calcium Chloride .... 470 mg per mL (350 mg/g)
Calcium (from calcium chloride) .... Min. 11.8%, Max. 14.16%

Each tube contains: A solution of calcium chloride in a specially prepared patent pending pharmaceutical elegant base.

Ingredients: Calcium chloride, ethylcellulose.

Indications: PRN HIGH POTENCY CALCIUM GEL® is a supplemental source of nutritional calcium used before, during and after calving.

A mineral supplement for dairy and beef cattle.

Directions for Use: Give one tube within 24 hours prior to calving.

Give another tube within 24 hours after calving.

1. Hold the head of the cow in a normal to slightly elevated position.
2. Place tube in cow's mouth directly over the tongue.
3. The product is carefully and quickly pressed out of the 300 mL tube.
4. Hold the cow's mouth closed and allow time to swallow.

Caution(s): Use extreme care to prevent injury to the cow's mouth and throat tissue when administering PRN HIGH POTENCY CALCIUM GEL®. Do not allow the cow to chew on the tip of the tube which can result in mouth laceration. Do not administer to cows with open sores in the mouth or throat. Gel may cause irritation to eyes and skin.

Contact with eyes, wounds, or prolonged contact with skin can cause irritation. Flush with warn water if exposed.

Warning(s): Keep out of reach of children For veterinary use only.

Presentation: 300 mL (390 g) tube.

Compendium Code No.: 10900140

PRO 35™ TEARLESS SHAMPOO

Tomlyn **Grooming Shampoo**

Active Ingredient(s): Sodium laureth sulfate (CAS 9004-83-4), Alkyl polyglycoside, Cocamidopropyl betaine (CAS 61789-40-0), Cocamide DEA (CAS 61791-31-9), Water (Cas 7732-18-5).

Indications: A grooming shampoo for use on puppies, kittens and ferrets over four weeks of age.

Directions for Use: Just add water.

Add 1 gallon of water to about 3½ fl oz of PRO 35™. This single 1 gallon bottle will make 35 gallons of rich, easy-to-rinse shampoo.

Wet animal thoroughly with warm water. Work PRO 35™ into coat until lather is produced. Rinse thoroughly with warm water. Towel dry. Keep pet in a warm environment free from drafts until dry.

Precaution(s): Store at room temperature.

Caution(s): For external animal use only. Keep out of reach of children and pets.

Presentation: 4 x 1 gallon (128 fl oz - 3.79 L) bottle.

Compendium Code No.: 11220200 679-2

PRO-BAC-C

AgriLabs **Feed Medication**

Medicated

Active Ingredient(s):

Lasalocid (as lasalocid sodium) .... 6,400 grams/ton

Guaranteed Analysis:

Vitamin A, Min. .... 2,800,000 I.U./lb.
Vitamin D3, Min. .... 1,640,000 I.U./lb.
Vitamin E, Min. .... 988 I.U./lb.
Vitamin B12 Min. .... 8,250 mcg/lb.
Thiamine, Min. .... 823 mg/lb.
Ascorbic Acid (Vit. C), Min. .... 3,200 mg/lb.
Niacin, Min. .... 4,940 mg/lb.
Folic Acid, Min. .... 210 mg/lb.
Choline Bitartrate, Min. .... 4,116 mg/lb.

Guaranteed Microbial Analysis: *CFU (Colony-Forming Units):

Lactic Acid Bacteria** .... 1.35×10^{10} CFU*/lb.
Live Cell Yeast .... 9.0×10^{10} CFU*/lb.

***Lactobacillus acidophilus*
***Lactobacillus casei*
***Entercococcus faecium*
***Bifidobacterium thermophilum*

PRO-BAC-C Medicated contains a source of live (viable) naturally occurring microorganisms.

Ingredients: Vitamin A acetate, d-activated animal sterol (source of vitamin D3 activity), dl-alpha tocopheryl acetate (source of vitamin E), vitamin B12 supplement, niacin supplement, choline bitartrate, folic acid, thiamine mononitrate, ascorbic acid, dextrose, dried *saccharomyces cerevisiae* fermentation product, dried *lactobacillus acidophilus* fermentation product, dried *lactobacillus casei* fermentation product, dried *entercoccus faecium* fermentation product, dried *bifidobacteriumthermophilum* fermentation product, dried *aspergillus oryzae* fermentation extract and sodium silico aluminate.

Indications: For the control of coccidiosis caused by *Eimeria bovis* and *Eimeria zuernii*.

Directions: Feeding Directions:

(Small measure enclosed approximates ⅛ oz. Cup measure enclosed approximates 6 oz.)

Dairy Calves: Add PRO-BAC-C Medicated to the milk replacer liquid at the rate of ⅛ ounce twice daily for a 110 lb. (50 kg.) calf to provide 50 mg. of lasalocid. Increase or decrease proportionately based on calf size to provide 1 mg. lasalocid per kg. of calf body weight. Do not use in combination with other sources of lasalocid.

Contraindication(s): Do not feed to horses.

Precaution(s): Store in a cool, dry place.

Caution(s): The safety of lasalocid in unapproved species has not been established; do not allow horses or other equines access to lasalocid as ingestion may be fatal. Feeding undiluted, mixing errors or inadequate mixing (recirculation or agitation of liquid supplements) resulting in excessive concentrations of lasalocid could be fatal.

For veterinary animal use only.

Warning(s): A withdrawal period has not been established for this product in pre-ruminating cattle. Do not use in calves to be processed for veal. Keep out of reach of children.

Presentation: 5 lbs, 15 lbs and 35 lbs.

Compendium Code No.: 10581340

PROBIOCIN® ORAL GEL FOR PETS

Chr. Hansen **Small Animal Dietary Supplement**

Contents: Contains a source of live (viable), naturally occurring microorganisms.

Guarantee: Lactic acid bacteria*, not less than 10 million CFU**/g.

**Enterococcus faecium, Lactobacillus acidophilus, Lactobacillus casei, Lactobacillus plantarum*

**Colony Forming Units

Ingredients: Vegetable oil, corn starch, sucrose, silicon dioxide, dried *Enterococcus faecium* fermentation product, dried *Lactobacillus acidophilus* fermentation product, dried *Lactobacillus casei* fermentation product, dried *Lactobacillus plantarum* fermentation product, polysorbate 80, sodium silico aluminate, and ethoxyquin, as a preservative.

Indications: This product is intended for use as a source of *Enterococcus faecium, Lactobacillus acidophilus, Lactobacillus casei,* and *Lactobacillus plantarum* in pets.

Dosage and Administration: Administer orally according to the schedule below:

Age	Dosage*
Newborns	1 g at birth
Post-weaning	1 g/10 lb of body weight, following therapy or digestive upset

*Repeat as needed.

Precaution(s): Store in a cool, dry area for maximum stability.

Caution(s): This product is intended as a stabilized source of the microorganisms listed only.

Buyer assumes all responsibility for use, storage and handling of this product. Chr. Hansen BioSystems makes no other claims or warranties expressed or implied, and will not be responsible for consequential or incidental damages.

Presentation: 15 g.

Compendium Code No.: 13110000

PROBIOS® BOVINE ONE ORAL GEL FOR RUMINANTS

Chr. Hansen **Large Animal Dietary Supplement**

Contents: Contains a source of live (viable), naturally occurring microorganisms.

Guarantee: Lactic acid bacteria*, not less than 10 million CFU**/g.

**Enterococcus faecium, Lactobacillus acidophilus, Lactobacillus casei, Lactobacillus plantarum*

**Colony Forming Units

Ingredients: Vegetable oil, corn starch, sucrose, silicon dioxide, dried *Enterococcus faecium* fermentation product, dried *Lactobacillus acidophilus* fermentation product, dried *Lactobacillus casei* fermentation product, dried *Lactobacillus plantarum* fermentation product, polysorbate 80, sodium silico aluminate, certified color, and ethoxyquin, as a preservative.

Indications: This product is intended for use as a source of *Enterococcus faecium, Lactobacillus acidophilus, Lactobacillus casei,* and *Lactobacillus plantarum* in cattle, sheep and goats.

Dosage and Administration: Administer orally according to the schedule below:

Animal	Age	Dosage*
Beef	Newborns	5 g at birth
	Calves	Under 400 lb, 10 g Over 400 lb, 15 g
	Incoming Feedlot/Stockers	Under 400 lb, 10 g Over 400 lb, 15 g
	Hospital	15 g first and last day of therapy
Dairy	Calves	5 g at birth
	Heifers	Under 400 lb, 10 g Over 400 lb, 15 g
	Cows	30 g at freshening
	Hospital	15 g first and last day of therapy
Sheep/Goats	Newborns	5 g at birth

*Repeat as needed.

Precaution(s): Store in a cool, dry area for maximum stability.

Caution(s): This product is intended as a stabilized source of the microorganisms listed only.

Buyer assumes all responsibility for use, storage and handling of this product. Chr. Hansen BioSystems makes no other claims or warranties expressed or implied, and will not be responsible for consequential or incidental damages.

Presentation: 60 g and 300 g.

Compendium Code No.: 13110010

PROBIOS® DISPERSIBLE POWDER

Chr. Hansen **Dietary Supplement**

Contents: Contains a source of live (viable), naturally occurring microorganisms.

Guarantee: Lactic acid bacteria*, not less than 10 million CFU**/g.

**Enterococcus faecium, Lactobacillus acidophilus, Lactobacillus casei, Lactobacillus plantarum*

**Colony Forming Units

Ingredients: Sucrose, dried whey, sodium silico aluminate, dried *Enterococcus faecium* fermentation product, dried *Lactobacillus acidophilus* fermentation product, dried *Lactobacillus casei* fermentation product, dried *Lactobacillus plantarum* fermentation product and sodium thiosulfate.

Indications: This product is intended for use as a source of *Enterococcus faecium, Lactobacillus acidophilus, Lactobacillus casei,* and *Lactobacillus plantarum* in cattle, swine, horses, sheep, goats, and pets.

Dosage and Administration: Administer orally according to the schedule below:

Animal	Age	Dosage*
Beef	Calves	5 g/head/day with fluids
Dairy	Calves	5 g/head/day with fluids
Swine	Nursery	2 g/head/day in milk replacer
Equine	Foals	5 g/head/day in milk replacer
	Horses-Adult	5 g/head/day in ration
Sheep/Goats		5 g/head/day in milk replacer
Pets		1-5 g

*Repeat as needed.

P

Precaution(s): Store in a cool, dry area for maximum stability.
Caution(s): This product is intended as a stabilized source of the microorganisms listed only.
Buyer assumes all responsibility for use, storage and handling of this product. Chr. Hansen BioSystems makes no other claims or warranties expressed or implied, and will not be responsible for consequential or incidental damages.
Presentation: 240 g, 2.27 kg (5 lb), and 11.34 kg (25 lb).
Compendium Code No.: 13110020

PROBIOS® EQUINE ONE ORAL GEL

Chr. Hansen **Equine Dietary Supplement**

Contents: Contains a source of live (viable), naturally occurring microorganisms.
Guarantee: Lactic acid bacteria*, not less than 10 million CFU**/g.
**Enterococcus faecium, Lactobacillus acidophilus, Lactobacillus casei, Lactobacillus plantarum*
**Colony Forming Units
Ingredients: Vegetable oil, corn starch, sucrose, silicon dioxide, dried *Enterococcus faecium* fermentation product, dried *Lactobacillus acidophilus* fermentation product, dried *Lactobacillus casei* fermentation product, dried *Lactobacillus plantarum* fermentation product, polysorbate 80, sodium silico aluminate, and ethoxyquin, as a preservative.
Indications: This product is intended for use as a source of *Enterococcus faecium, Lactobacillus acidophilus, Lactobacillus casei,* and *Lactobacillus plantarum* in horses.
Dosage and Administration: Administer orally according to the schedule below:

Age	Dosage*
Foals	10 g at birth and day 4
Horses-Adult	15 g at foaling, following therapy or during training, transport or digestive upset

*Repeat as needed.
Precaution(s): Store in a cool, dry area for maximum stability.
Caution(s): This product is intended as a stabilized source of the microorganisms listed only.
Buyer assumes all responsibility for use, storage and handling of this product. Chr. Hansen BioSystems makes no other claims or warranties expressed or implied, and will not be responsible for consequential or incidental damages.
Presentation: 30 g.
Compendium Code No.: 13110030

PROBIOS® FEED GRANULES

Chr. Hansen **Large Animal Dietary Supplement**

Contents: Contains a source of live (viable), naturally occurring microorganisms.
Guarantee: Lactic acid bacteria*, not less than 10 million CFU**/g.
**Enterococcus faecium, Lactobacillus acidophilus, Lactobacillus casei, Lactobacillus plantarum*
**Colony Forming Units
Ingredients: Calcium carbonate, sodium silico aluminate, dried *Enterococcus faecium* fermentation product, dried *Lactobacillus acidophilus* fermentation product, dried *Lactobacillus casei* fermentation product, and dried *Lactobacillus plantarum* fermentation product.
Indications: This product is intended for use as a source of *Enterococcus faecium, Lactobacillus acidophilus, Lactobacillus casei,* and *Lactobacillus plantarum* in cattle, swine, horses, sheep and goats.
Dosage and Administration: Administer orally according to the schedule below:

Animal	Age	Dosage*
Beef	Calves	5 g/head/day in starter ration
	Incoming Feedlot/Stocker/Hospital	10 g/head/day in ration
Dairy	Heifers	5 g/head/day in ration
	Cows	5 g/head/day pre-freshening through peak lactation
	Hospital	10 g/head/day
Swine	Sows	10 g/head/day two weeks prior to farrowing and during
	Starter/grower	5 g/head/day in ration
Equine	Foals	5 g/head/day in ration
	Horses-Adult	5 g/head/day in ration
Sheep/Goats		5 g/head/day in starter ration

*Repeat as needed.
Precaution(s): Store in a cool, dry area for maximum stability. Avoid leaving bag open for extended period of time.
Caution(s): This product is intended as a stabilized source of the microorganisms listed only.
Buyer assumes all responsibility for use, storage and handling of this product. Chr. Hansen BioSystems makes no other claims or warranties expressed or implied, and will not be responsible for consequential or incidental damages.
Presentation: 2.27 kg (5 lb) and 22.7 kg (50 lb).
Compendium Code No.: 13110040

PROBIOS® MICROBIAL CALF PAC

Chr. Hansen **Large Animal Dietary Supplement**

Contents: Contains a source of live (viable), naturally occurring microorganisms.
Guarantee: Lactic acid bacteria*, not less than 420 million CFU**/g.
**Lactobacillus acidophilus, Bifidobacterium bifidum, Bacillus licheniformis, Bacillus subtilis, Lactobacillus lactis*
**Colony Forming Units
Indications: This product is intended for use as a source of *Lactobacillus acidophilus, Bifidobacterium bifidum, Bacillus licheniformis, Bacillus subtilis,* and *Lactobacillus lactis* in beef and dairy calves.
Directions:

Animal	Age	Dosage*
Beef	Calves	3 g/head/day
Dairy	Calves	3 g/head/day

PROBIOS® Microbial Calf Pac can be added to milk replacer, mixed with fluids or top-dressed.
*Repeat as needed.
1 teaspoon holds approximately 3 g.
1 tablespoon holds approximately 9 g.
Precaution(s): Keep cool and dry.
Presentation: 1,500 g. A scoop is enclosed.
Compendium Code No.: 13110050

PROBIOS® ORAL BOLUSES FOR RUMINANTS

Chr. Hansen **Large Animal Dietary Supplement**

Contents: Contains a source of live (viable), naturally occurring microorganisms.
Guarantee: Lactic acid bacteria*, not less than 7 million CFU**/g.
**Enterococcus faecium, Lactobacillus acidophilus, Lactobacillus casei, Lactobacillus plantarum*
**Colony Forming Units
Ingredients: Lactose, microcrystalline cellulose, dried *Enterococcus faecium* fermentation product, dried *Lactobacillus acidophilus* fermentation product, dried *Lactobacillus casei* fermentation product, and dried *Lactobacillus plantarum* fermentation product, modified cellulose gum, magnesium stearate and sodium silico aluminate.
Indications: This product is intended for use as a source of *Enterococcus faecium, Lactobacillus acidophilus, Lactobacillus casei,* and *Lactobacillus plantarum* in cattle, sheep and goats.
Dosage and Administration: Administer orally according to the schedule below:

Animal	Dosage*	
	1⁄4 oz (7 g) Bolus	1⁄2 oz (14 g) Bolus
Dairy/Beef		
Newborns	1 bolus at birth	
Calves		
Under 400 lb	1 bolus	1⁄2 bolus
Over 400 lb	2 boluses	1 bolus
Cows, At freshening	4 boluses	2 boluses
Sheep/Goats	1 bolus	1⁄2 bolus

*Repeat as needed.
Precaution(s): Store in a cool, dry area for maximum stability.
Caution(s): This product is intended as a stabilized source of the microorganisms listed only.
Buyer assumes all responsibility for use, storage and handling of this product. Chr. Hansen BioSystems makes no other claims or warranties expressed or implied, and will not be responsible for consequential or incidental damages.
Presentation: 50 boluses.
Compendium Code No.: 13110060

PROBIOS® ORAL SUSPENSION FOR SWINE

Chr. Hansen **Large Animal Dietary Supplement**

Contents: Contains a source of live (viable), naturally occurring microorganisms.
Guarantee: Lactic acid bacteria*, not less than 5 million CFU**/mL.
**Enterococcus faecium, Lactobacillus acidophilus, Lactobacillus casei, Lactobacillus plantarum*
**Colony Forming Units
Ingredients: Vegetable oil, corn starch, sucrose, silicon dioxide, dried *Enterococcus faecium* fermentation product, dried *Lactobacillus acidophilus* fermentation product, dried *Lactobacillus casei* fermentation product, dried *Lactobacillus plantarum* fermentation product, polysorbate 80, sodium silico aluminate, and ethoxyquin, as a preservative.
Indications: This product is intended for use as a source of *Enterococcus faecium, Lactobacillus acidophilus, Lactobacillus casei,* and *Lactobacillus plantarum* in swine.
Dosage and Administration: Administer orally according to the schedule below:

Age	Dosage*
Nursery	2 g (one full pump) at birth

*Repeat as needed.
Precaution(s): Shake well.
Store in a cool, dry area for maximum stability.
Caution(s): This product is intended as a stabilized source of the microorganisms listed only.
Buyer assumes all responsibility for use, storage and handling of this product. Chr. Hansen BioSystems makes no other claims or warranties expressed or implied, and will not be responsible for consequential or incidental damages.
Presentation: 100 doses [215 mL (8 oz)].
Compendium Code No.: 13110070

PROBIOS® PLUS NATURAL E BOVINE ONE ORAL GEL FOR RUMINANTS

Chr. Hansen **Large Animal Dietary Supplement**

Contents: Contains a source of live (viable), naturally occurring microorganisms and a natural source of vitamin E.
Guarantee: Lactic acid bacteria*, not less than 10 million CFU**/g; Vitamin E, 50 IU/g.
**Enterococcus faecium, Lactobacillus acidophilus, Lactobacillus casei, Lactobacillus plantarum*
**Colony Forming Units
Ingredients: Vegetable oil, vitamin E supplement, sucrose, silicon dioxide, corn starch, dried *Enterococcus faecium* fermentation product, dried *Lactobacillus acidophilus* fermentation product, dried *Lactobacillus casei* fermentation product, dried *Lactobacillus plantarum* fermentation product, polysorbate 80, sodium silico aluminate, and ethoxyquin, as a preservative.
Indications: This product is intended for use as a source of *Enterococcus faecium, Lactobacillus acidophilus, Lactobacillus casei,* and *Lactobacillus plantarum* in beef and dairy cattle.

Dosage and Administration: Administer orally according to the schedule below:

Animal	Age	Dosage*
Beef	Newborns	5 g at birth
	Calves	Under 400 lb, 10 g Over 400 lb, 15 g
	Incoming Feedlot/Stockers	Under 400 lb, 10 g Over 400 lb, 15 g
	Hospital	15 g first and last day of therapy
Dairy	Calves	5 g at birth
	Heifers	Under 400 lb, 10 g Over 400 lb, 15 g
	Cows	30 g at freshening
	Hospital	15 g first and last day of therapy

*Repeat as needed.

Precaution(s): Store in a cool, dry area for maximum stability.

Caution(s): This product is intended as a stabilized source of the microorganisms listed only.

Buyer assumes all responsibility for use, storage and handling of this product. Chr. Hansen BioSystems makes no other claims or warranties expressed or implied, and will not be responsible for consequential or incidental damages.

Presentation: 60 g and 300 g.

Compendium Code No.: 13110080

PROBIOS® TC

Chr. Hansen **Large Animal Dietary Supplement**

Contents: Contains a source of live (viable), naturally occurring microorganisms.

Guarantee:

Total Bacteria[1], not less than 2.5 Billion CFU[2]/g.

Total Yeast Cells[3], not less than 2.5 Billion CFU/g.

Total Viable Yeast Cells, not less than 1.0 Billion CFU/g.

[1]Two Strains of *Enterococcus faecium,* EF301 and EF273

[2]Colony Forming Units

[3]*Saccharomyces cerevisiae*

Ingredients: Calcium Carbonate, Dried *Saccharomyces Cerevisiae* Fermentation Product, Dried *Enterococcus Faecium* Fermentation Product, and Sodium Silico Aluminate.

Indications: This product is intended for transition cows as a stabilized source of *Enterococcus faecium* and *Saccharomyces cerevisiae* only.

Directions: Feed PROBIOS® TC at a rate of 2 grams per head per day from 21 days pre-calving to 60 days post-calving or until peak dry matter intake.

Precaution(s): Storage and Handling: Store in a cool, dry area for maximum stability. Avoid leaving bag open for extended periods of time.

Disclaimer: Buyer assumes all responsibility for use, storage and handling of this product. Chr. Hansen BioSystems makes no other claims or warranties expressed or implied, and will not be responsible for consequential or incidental damages.

Presentation: 25 lb (11.34 kg) bag.

Compendium Code No.: 13110090 ADV089

PROBIOTIC PLUS E FOR CALVES

Vets Plus **Large Animal Dietary Supplement**

Guaranteed Analysis: (min) per bolus:

Vitamin E . . . . . . 100 IU
Lactic Acid Bacteria . . . . . . not less than 70 million CFU

Lactobacillus acidophilus, Lactobacillus plantarum, Lactobacillus casei, Enterococcus faecium, Lactobacillus acidophilus DDS-1.

Ingredients: Maltodextrin, Lactose, Corn Starch, Fructo-oligosaccharides, d-Alpha Tocopheryl Acetate (Source of Natural Vitamin E), Dried *Lactobacillus acidophilus* Fermentation Product, Dried *Lactobacillus plantarum* Fermentation Product, Dried *Lactobacillus acidophilus* DDS-1 Fermentation Product, Dried *Enterococcus faecium* Fermentation Product, Dried *Lactobacillus casei* Fermentation Product, Silicon Dioxide, and Magnesium Stearate.

Indications: Microbial boluses with natural vitamin E for calves. Contains a source of live (viable) naturally occurring microorganisms with prebiotic FOS.

Dosage and Administration:

Dairy/Beef:

Newborns at birth . . . . . . 1 bolus
Calves under 400 lb. . . . . . . 1 bolus
Calves over 400 lb. . . . . . . 2 boluses
Cows at freshening . . . . . . 4 boluses
Sheep/Goats: . . . . . . 1 bolus

Repeat as needed.

Precaution(s): Storage and Handling: Store in a cool, dry area for maximum stability. This product is intended as a stabilized source of *Lactobacillus acidophilus, Lactobacillus plantarum, Lactobacillus acidophilus* DDS-1, *Enterococcus faecium* and *Lactobacillus casei* only.

Keep lid tightly closed.

Caution(s): Keep out of reach of children.

For animal use only.

Disclaimer: Buyer assumes all responsibility for use, storage and handling of this product. Vets Plus Inc. makes no other claims or warranties expressed or implied, and will not be responsible for consequential or incidental damages.

Presentation: 50 boluses ¼ oz. (7 g) each.

Compendium Code No.: 10730200

PROBIOTIC PLUS E FOR CATTLE

Vets Plus **Large Animal Dietary Supplement**

Guaranteed Analysis: (min) per bolus:

Vitamin E . . . . . . 200 IU
Lactic Acid Bacteria . . . . . . not less than 140 million CFU

Lactobacillus acidophilus, Lactobacillus plantarum, Lactobacillus casei, Enterococcus faecium, Lactobacillus acidophilus DDS-1.

Ingredients: Maltodextrin, Lactose, Corn Starch, Fructo-oligosaccharides, d-Alpha Tocopheryl Acetate (Source of Natural Vitamin E), Dried *Lactobacillus acidophilus* Fermentation Product, Dried *Lactobacillus plantarum* Fermentation Product, Dried *Lactobacillus acidophilus* DDS-1 Fermentation Product, Dried *Enterococcus faecium* Fermentation Product, Dried *Lactobacillus casei* Fermentation Product, Silicon Dioxide, and Magnesium Stearate.

Indications: Microbial boluses with natural vitamin E for cattle. Contains a source of live (viable) naturally occurring microorganisms with prebiotic FOS.

Dosage and Administration:

Dairy/Beef:

Calves under 400 lb. . . . . . . ½ bolus
Calves over 400 lb. . . . . . . 1 bolus
Cows at freshening . . . . . . 2 boluses
Sheep/Goats: . . . . . . ½ bolus

Repeat as needed.

Precaution(s): Storage and Handling: Store in a cool, dry area for maximum stability. This product is intended as a stabilized source of *Lactobacillus acidophilus, Lactobacillus plantarum, Lactobacillus acidophilus* DDS-1, *Enterococcus faecium* and *Lactobacillus casei* only.

Keep lid tightly closed.

Caution(s): Keep out of reach of children.

For animal use only.

Disclaimer: Buyer assumes all responsibility for use, storage and handling of this product. Vets Plus Inc. makes no other claims or warranties expressed or implied, and will not be responsible for consequential or incidental damages.

Presentation: 50 boluses ½ oz. (14 g) each.

Compendium Code No.: 10730210

PROBIOTIC POWER™

Vets Plus **Dietary Supplement**

Guaranteed Analysis: (min. per lb.):

Vitamin A . . . . . . 2,800,000 IU
Vitamin D_3. . . . . . 1,200,000 IU
Vitamin E . . . . . . 1,000 IU
Vitamin B_{12} . . . . . . 5,000 mcg
Vitamin B_6. . . . . . 250 mg
Vitamin C . . . . . . 1,000 mg
Niacin . . . . . . 6,000 mg
Choline . . . . . . 5,000 mg
d-Pantothenic Acid . . . . . . 2,000 mg
Riboflavin . . . . . . 500 mg
Folic Acid . . . . . . 150 mg
Lactic Acid Bacteria. . . . . . 60 Billion CFU

(Lactobacillus acidophilus, Lactobacillus plantarum, Lactobacillus fermentum, Lactobacillus casei, Enterococcus faecium, Lactobacillus acidophilus DDS-1)

Ingredients: Ascorbic Acid (Vitamin C), d-Calcium Pantothenate, Vitamin A Acetate, d-Activated Animal Sterol (Vitamin D_3), DL-alpha-Tocopheryl Acetate, (Vitamin E), Cyanocobalamin (Vitamin B_{12}), Choline Bitartrate, Folic Acid, Riboflavin, Pyridoxine Hydrochloride (Vitamin B_6), Niacinamide, *Lactobacillus acidophilus, Lactobacillus plantarum, Lactobacillus fermentum, Lactobacillus casei, Enterococcus faecium, Lactobacillus acidophilus* DDS-1, Silica, and Dextrose.

Indications: Administer to any animal during diet change, birth, weaning, shipping, or weather change. PROBIOTIC POWER™ provides Lactic Acid Bacteria, including *Lactobacillus acidophilus* DDS-1 and vitamins to stimulate appetite and strengthen the immune system.

A concentrated source of live (viable) naturally occurring microorganisms.

Directions for Use: Add to TMR, top dress or mix into ground feed, water, milk or milk replacer.

Dosage:

Cattle: . . . . . . 1 lb/ton of feed
Lactating . . . . . . 4 g/head/day
Stockers . . . . . . 4 g/head/day
Feedlot
0 - 4 days . . . . . . 4 g/head/day
4 - finish. . . . . . 2 g/head/day
Calves
Newborn and purchased. . . . . . 4 g/head/day
Milk/Milk replacer . . . . . . 1 g/head/day
Swine:. . . . . . 1 lb/ton of feed
Birth. . . . . . 1 g/head/day
Purchased (for three days) . . . . . . 1 g/head/day
Weaning to market. . . . . . 2 g/head/day
Sows and gilts . . . . . . 2 g/head/day
Lactating Sows . . . . . . 2 g/head/day
Suckling/Weaned pigs (3-9 weeks) . . . . . . 13 g/gallon of water
Grower/Finisher (weaning to market). . . . . . 7 g/gallon of water
Gestation/lactation. . . . . . 7 g/gallon of water

Add through water system at rates equal to one gallon/128 gallons drinking water.

Unused portion of stock solution should be refrigerated and used within 24 hours.

Sheep:. . . . . . 1 lb/ton of feed
Horse:
Foals
Birth . . . . . . 4 g/head/day
After birth . . . . . . 1 g/head/day
Adult
Maintenance . . . . . . 2 g/head/day
Breeding and Performance . . . . . . 4 g/head/day
Cats and Dogs: . . . . . . 2 g/head/day
Exotic Animals:
Birth. . . . . . 1 g/head/day
Under 50 lbs . . . . . . 1 g/head/day
Over 50 lbs . . . . . . 2 g/head/day

In severe stress conditions the dose may be doubled.

Scoop provided equals 1 gram and 4 grams.

One Tablespoon equals 10 grams.

Precaution(s): Keep in cool, dry place.

Caution(s): Keep out of the reach of children.

For animal use only.

Presentation: 6x5 lb. (2.27 kg) pails per case and 25 lb. pail.

Compendium Code No.: 10730140

PRO-BUTE™ INJECTION ℞

AgriLabs **Phenylbutazone-Injection**

Active Ingredient(s): Each mL of sterile aqueous solution contains:

Phenylbutazone .... 200 mg
Benzyl alcohol 1.5%

Sodium hydroxide used to adjust pH. Purified water, U.S.P.

Indications: A nonhormonal anti-inflammatory agent for horses only.

Dosage and Administration: For intravenous use only.

Horses: 5 to 10 mL (1 to 2 g) per 1,000 lbs. per day. Limit to five (5) consecutive days.

Precaution(s): Store the product in a cool place (46° to 59°F), or alternatively store in a refrigerator.

Caution(s): Federal law restricts this drug to use by or on the order of a licensed veterinarian.

Warning(s): Not for use in horses intended for food.

Presentation: 100 mL sterile multiple dose vials (NDC #864-1026-11).

Compendium Code No.: 10581670

PRO-BUTE™ TABLETS 1 GRAM ℞

AgriLabs **Non-Steroidal Anti-Inflammatory**

(phenylbutazone) 1 gram per Tablet

NADA No.: 099-618

Active Ingredient(s): Each tablet contains: Phenylbutazone (4-butyl-1, 2-diphenyl-3,5-pyrazolidinedione) 1 gram; inert ingredients (as excipients) - q.s.

Indications: PRO-BUTE™ (phenylbutazone) Tablets have non-hormonal anti-inflammatory properties in the management of musculoskeletal conditions in horses, such as generalized arthritis.

Dosage and Administration: Horses: 2 to 4 mg per lb of body weight (equivalent to 1 to 2 grams per 500 lb of body weight) or 2 to 4 PRO-BUTE™ Tablets, 1 g for 1000 lb of body weight per day.

Do not exceed 4 grams per animal per day. As symptoms regress, reduce dosage 25% to 50% of initial dose as needed to control symptoms. If there is no improvement in 5 days discontinue treatment. Infective conditions should be treated concurrently with the proper anti-infectives. Response to treatment is variable, as is also the tolerance for the drug. Withdrawal of the drug may be followed by reappearance of symptoms, after which it may be given intermittently to control symptoms. The drug is symptomatic in action and not curative.

Recommendations: Use up to the maximum recommended dose for the first 48 hours. As symptoms regress, reduce dosage 25% to 50% of the initial "loading dose" as needed to control symptoms.

Because of the more rapid metabolism in animals, administer PRO-BUTE™ Tablets in 3 divided daily doses (at 8-hour intervals) to maintain therapeutic blood level. Response to PRO-BUTE™ Tablet treatment usually occurs within 24 hours after the initial dose. If no response is evident after 5 days of dosing, treatment should be discontinued.

While many chronic conditions, such as chronic osteoarthritis, will respond to PRO-BUTE™ Tablet therapy, no permanent cure can be effected owing to the advance tissue changes. In such cases discontinuance of treatment often will result in recurrence of symptoms. However, intermittent therapy may be extremely valuable to alleviate symptoms of chronic inflammatory lesions.

Contraindication(s): Animals showing evidence of cardiac, hepatic, or renal damage or a history of blood dyscrasia, or those with signs or history of anemia.

Precaution(s): Store at controlled room temperature, 59°-86°F (15°-30°C).

Caution(s): Federal (U.S.A.) law restricts this drug to use by or on the order of a licensed veterinarian.

Stop medication at first sign of gastrointestinal upset, blood dyscrasia, jaundice, or black or tarry stools. Agranulocytosis associated with the drug has occurred in man and was reversible upon discontinuance of treatment. Fatal reactions, although rare, have been reported in dogs after long-term therapy. Routine blood counts should be made at weekly intervals during the early phase of therapy and thereafter at intervals of two weeks. A significant fall in total white count, or a relative decrease in granulocytes, or black or tarry stools indicate that therapy with PRO-BUTE™ Tablets, 1 gram should be immediately discontinued. In the treatment of inflammatory conditions associated with infection specific anti-infective therapy is required. Caution should be observed when administering to patients with a history of drug allergy.

Warning(s): Treated animals should not be used for food purposes.

Keep out of the reach of children. For use in animals only.

Trial Data: Description: The clinical effectiveness of phenylbutazone in acute rheumatism, gout, gouty arthritis, and various other rheumatoid disorders in man was demonstrated by Kuzell[1,2,3], Payne[4], Fleming[5], and Denko[6]. Anti-inflammatory activity has been well-established by Fabre[7], Domenjoz[8], Wilhelmi[9], and Yourish[10]. The effective use of phenylbutazone in the treatment of painful conditions of the musculoskeletal system in dogs, including arthritis and painful injuries to the limbs and joints has been reported by Lieberman[11]. Joshua[12] observed objective improvement without toxicity following long-term therapy of two aged arthritic dogs. Ogilvie and Sutter[13] reported rapid response to phenylbutazone therapy in a review of 19 clinical cases including posterior weakness, arthritis, rheumatism, and other conditions associated with lameness and musculoskeletal weakness.

Favorable results have been reported by Camberos[14] following intermittent treatment of horses in generalized arthritis, chronic pain in trapezius muscles, osteoarthritis of the medial and distal bones of the hock, chronic hip pains, arthritis of stifle and hip, arthrosis of the spine.

In cases of traumatism, muscle rupture, inflammation of the third phalanx, and strains, results were less favorable. Sutter[15] reported favorable response to chronic equine arthritis.

References: Available upon request.

Presentation: Bottles of 100 tablets.

Compendium Code No.: 10581680 445114L-01-9909

PROCAL™ POWDER ℞

Butler **Large Animal Dietary Supplement**

Active Ingredient(s): Contains per pound:

Torula yeast (food grade)* .... 113.4 g
Dried skim milk* .... 113.4 g
Sodium propionate .... 113.4 g
Sodium bicarbonate .... 56.7 g
Protein hydrolysate* (from casein) .... 25.0 g
Potassium chloride .... 720 mg
Magnesium citrate soluble .... 454 mg
Calcium lactate (from monohydrate) .... 920 mg

*Yielding total nitrogen 19 g, of which 1.1 g is amino nitrogen.

Indications: A source of amino acids, electrolytes and minerals for use in sick, convalescent or anorectic cattle. Supplies carbohydrate in a form (propionate) readily converted to blood sugar by ruminants. Provides a rich nutrient media to aid in the restoration of normal bacterial flora in the rumen. It also acts as a buffering agent to aid in the stabilization of gastric pH.

Dosage and Administration: The usual dose is 1 lb. per 1,000 lbs. of body weight, once a day, administered through a stomach tube or as a drench. Suspend PROCAL™ Powder in at least one-half (½) gallon of water before administering.

Precaution(s): Store in a cool, dry place. Keep tightly closed.

Caution(s): Federal (USA) law restricts this drug to use by or on the order of a licensed veterinarian. For veterinarian use only. Keep out of the reach of children.

Presentation: 16 oz. (1 lb.) containers.

Compendium Code No.: 10821590

PRODIGY® WITH HAVLOGEN®*

Intervet **Vaccine**

Equine Rhinopneumonitis Vaccine, Killed Virus

U.S. Vet. Lic. No.: 286

Description: An inactivated, purified, concentrated, adjuvanted, tissue culture origin Equine Herpesvirus EHV-1 vaccine.

Preservatives: Neomycin, Polymixin B, Nystatin and Thimerosal.

Indications: For vaccination of healthy horses 6 months of age or older, as an aid in the prevention of abortion and respiratory disease associated with Equine Herpesvirus 1 infection.

Dosage and Administration: For pregnant mares administer a 2 mL dose intramuscularly in the 5th, 7th and 9th months of pregnancy. Three doses are essential for primary immunization. Maiden and barren mares housed or pastured with pregnant mares should be vaccinated on the same schedule. For primary immunization against respiratory disease administer three 2 mL doses intramuscularly at 4 to 6 week intervals. A 2 mL booster dose should be administered annually and at any time epidemic conditions exist or are reported and exposure is imminent.

Precaution(s): Store at 35° to 45°F (2° to 7°C). Shake well before using. Use entire contents when first opened.

Caution(s): Local reactions may occur if this product is given subcutaneously. Inject deep in the muscle only. Anaphylactoid reactions may occur. For use in animals only.

Antidote(s): Epinephrine.

Warning(s): Do not vaccinate within 21 days before slaughter.

Presentation: 1 dose (2 mL) syringe with separate sterile needle and 10 dose (20 mL) vial.

*Adjuvant—U.S. Patent Nos. 3,790,665 and 3,919,411.

Compendium Code No.: 11061310

PRODINE OINTMENT

Phoenix Pharmaceutical **Topical Antibacterial**

Topical Antiseptic and Wound Protectant

Active Ingredient(s): Povidone-iodine (1% titratable iodine).

Contains lanolin as an emollient and protectant.

Indications: An antibacterial and antifungal ointment for wounds, cuts, and abrasions.

The water-resistant formula adheres to wounds to provide long lasting protection even in harsh weather.

Directions: Apply to wound after cleansing and drying. Apply as needed to maintain coverage. May bandage if necessary.

Caution(s): For veterinary use only. For deep or puncture wounds, use as directed by a veterinarian. For animal use only.

Warning(s): Keep out of reach of children.

Presentation: 16 oz (1 lb) (NDC 57319-294-27).

Compendium Code No.: 12560701 Rev. 7-00

PRODINE SCRUB

Phoenix Pharmaceutical **Surgical Scrub**

Antiseptic Microbial Skin Cleanser

Active Ingredient(s): Povidone-Iodine (0.75% Titratable).

Indications: A germicidal cleanser for pre-operative and post-operative skin washing. Used routinely, it also helps prevent infection in cuts, scratches, abrasions, and burns. Non-irritating and non-staining to skin, hair and natural fabrics.

Directions: Wet hands or skin area with water. Add approximately one 1 teaspoon Scrub and work into a rich lather. Scrub thoroughly for three minutes. Rinse thoroughly.

Contraindication(s): Do not use on animals that are allergic or sensitive to iodine.

Precaution(s): Avoid storing at excessive heat.

Caution(s): For external use only. Avoid contact with eyes.

If redness, swelling or irritation occurs discontinue use and consult a veterinarian.

For animal use only.

Warning(s): Keep out of reach of children.

Presentation: 1 gallon (3.785 L) containers (NDC 57319-327-09).

Compendium Code No.: 12560711 Rev. 08-00

PRODINE SOLUTION

Phoenix Pharmaceutical **Topical Antibacterial**

Antiseptic Microbicide

Active Ingredient(s): Povidone-Iodine (1.0% Titratable).

Indications: Kills gram-negative and gram-positive bacteria, fungi, viruses, protozoa, and yeasts. Film forming, virtually non-irritating and non-staining to skin, hair and natural fabrics.

Directions: Apply full-strength as often as needed. Wet the area thoroughly to ensure complete coverage and penetration, but avoid "pooling". May be covered with bandage if necessary.

Contraindication(s): Do not use on animals that are allergic or sensitive to iodine.

Precaution(s): Avoid storing at excessive heat.

Caution(s): For external use only.

Avoid contact with eyes.

May be harmful if swallowed.

If redness, swelling or irritation occurs, discontinue use and consult a veterinarian.

In case of deep or puncture wounds or serious burns consult a veterinarian.

Warning(s): Keep out of reach of children.

Presentation: 1 gallon (3.785 L) containers (NDC 57319-328-29).

Compendium Code No.: 12560721 Iss. 10-98

PRODUMEC™ INJECTION FOR CATTLE AND SWINE

TradeWinds **Parasiticide Injection**

(ivermectin) 1% Sterile Solution

NADA No.: 128-409

Active Ingredient(s): PRODUMEC™ Injection is a clear, ready-to-use, sterile solution containing 1% ivermectin, 40% glycerol formal, and propylene glycol, q.s. ad 100%.

Indications: A parasiticide for the treatment and control of internal and external parasites in cattle and swine.

Cattle: PRODUMEC™ Injection is indicated for the effective treatment and control of the following harmful species of gastrointestinal roundworms, lungworms, grubs, sucking lice, and mange mites in cattle:

Gastrointestinal Roundworms (adults and fourth-stage larvae): *Ostertagia ostertagi* (including inhibited *O. ostertagi), O. lyrata, Haemonchus placei, Trichostrongylus axei, T. colubriformis, Cooperia oncophora, C. punctata, C. pectinata, Oesophagostomum radiatum, Bunostomum phlebotomum, Nematodirus helvetianus* (adults only), *N. spathiger* (adults only).

Lungworms (adults and fourth-stage larvae): *Dictyocaulus viviparus.*

Cattle Grubs (parasitic stages): *Hypoderma bovis, H. lineatum.*

Sucking Lice: *Linognathus vituli, Haematopinus eurysternus, Solenopotes capillatus.*

Mites (scabies): *Psoroptes ovis* (syn. *P. communis* var. *bovis), Sarcoptes scabiei* var. *bovis.*

Persistent activity: PRODUMEC™ Injection has been proved to effectively control infections and to protect cattle from re-infection with *Dictyocaulus viviparus* for 28 days and *Ostertagia ostertagi* for 21 days after treatment; *Oesophagostomum radiatum, Haemonchus placei, Trichostrongylus axei, Cooperia punctata,* and *Cooperia oncophora* for 14 days after treatment.

Swine: PRODUMEC™ Injection is indicated for the effective treatment and control of the following harmful species of gastrointestinal roundworms, lungworms, lice, and mange mites in swine:

Gastrointestinal Roundworms:

Large roundworm: *Ascaris suum* (adults and fourth-stage larvae).

Red stomach worm: *Hyostrongylus rubidus* (adults and fourth-stage larvae).

Nodular worm: *Oesophagostomum* spp (adults and fourth-stage larvae).

Threadworm: *Strongyloides ransomi* (adults).

Somatic Roundworm Larvae:

Threadworm: *Strongyloides ransomi* (somatic larvae).

Sows must be treated at least seven days before farrowing to prevent infection in piglets.

Lungworms:

Metastrongylus spp (adults).

Lice:

Haematopinus suis.

Mange Mites:

Sarcoptes scabiei var. *suis.*

Reindeer: For the treatment and control of warbles *(Oedemagena tarandi)* in reindeer (see Special Minor Use section under Dosage and Administration).

American Bison: For the treatment and control of grubs *(Hypoderma bovis)* in American bison (see Special Minor Use section under Dosage and Administration).

Pharmacology: Product Description: Ivermectin is derived from the avermectins, a family of potent, broad-spectrum antiparasitic agents isolated from fermentation of *Streptomyces avermitilis.*

Mode of Action: Ivermectin is a member of the macrocyclic lactone class of endectocides which have a unique mode of action. Compounds of the class bind selectively and with high affinity to glutamate-gated chloride ion channels which occur in invertebrate nerve and muscle cells. This leads to an increase in the permeability of the cell membrane to chloride ions with hyperpolarization of the nerve or muscle cell, resulting in paralysis and death of the parasite. Compounds of this class may also interact with other ligand-gated chloride channels, such as those gated by the neurotransmitter gamma-aminobutyric acid (GABA).

The safety margin for compounds of this class is attributable to the fact that mammals do not have glutamate-gated chloride channels, the macrocyclic lactones have a low affinity for other mammalian ligand-gated chloride channels and they do not readily cross the blood-brain barrier.

Dosage and Administration: Dosage:

Cattle: PRODUMEC™ Injection should be given only by subcutaneous injection under the loose skin in front of or behind the shoulder at the recommended dose level of 200 mcg ivermectin per kilogram of body weight. Each mL of PRODUMEC™ contains 10 mg of ivermectin, sufficient to treat 110 lb (50 kg) of body weight (maximum 10 mL per injection site).

Body Weight (lb)	Dose Volume (mL)
220	2
330	3
440	4
550	5
660	6
770	7
990	9
1100	10

Swine: PRODUMEC™ Injection should be given only by subcutaneous injection in the neck of swine at the recommended dose level of 300 mcg of ivermectin per kilogram (2.2 lb) of body weight. Each mL of PRODUMEC™ contains 10 mg of ivermectin, sufficient to treat 75 lb of body weight.

	Body Weight (lb)	Dose Volume (mL)
Growing Pigs	19	¼
	38	½
	75	1
	150	2
Breeding animals (Sows, Gilts, and Boars)	225	3
	300	4
	375	5
	450	6

Administration:

Cattle: PRODUMEC™ Injection is to be given subcutaneously only, to reduce risk of potentially fatal clostridial infection of the injection site. Animals should be appropriately restrained to achieve the proper route of administration. Use of a 16-gauge ½" to ¾" needle is suggested. Inject under the loose skin in front of or behind the shoulder (see illustration).

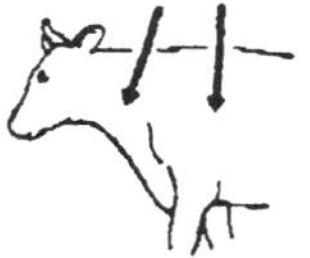

When using the 200 or 500 mL pack size, use only automatic syringe equipment.

Use sterile equipment and sanitize the injection site by applying a suitable disinfectant. Clean, properly disinfected needles should be used to reduce the potential for injection site infection.

No special handling or protective clothing is necessary.

Swine: PRODUMEC™ (ivermectin) Injection is to be given subcutaneously in the neck. Animals should be appropriately restrained to achieve the proper route of administration. Use of a 16- or 18-gauge needle is suggested for sows and boars, while an 18- or 20-gauge needle may be appropriate for young animals. Inject under the skin, immediately behind the ear (see illustration).

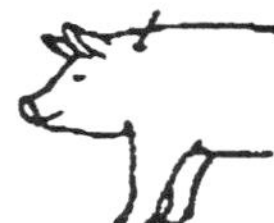

When using the 200 or 500 mL pack size, use only automatic syringe equipment. As with any injection, sterile equipment should be used. The injection site should be cleaned and disinfected with alcohol before injection. The rubber stopper should also be disinfected with alcohol to prevent contamination of the contents. Mild and transient pain reactions may be seen in some swine following subcutaneous administration.

Recommended Treatment Program:

Swine: At the time of initiating any parasite control program, it is important to treat all breeding animals in the herd. After the initial treatment, use PRODUMEC™ Injection regularly as follows:

Breeding Animals:

Sows: Treat prior to farrowing, preferably 7-14 days before, to minimize infection of piglets.

Gilts: Treat 7-14 days prior to breeding. Treat 7-14 days prior to farrowing.

Boars: Frequency and need for treatments are dependent upon exposure.

Treat at least two times a year.

Feeder Pigs (Weaners/Growers/Finishers): All weaner/feeder pigs should be treated before placement in clean quarters.

Pigs exposed to contaminated soil or pasture may need retreatment if reinfection occurs.

Note:

1. PRODUMEC™ Injection has a persistent drug level sufficient to control mite infestations throughout the egg to adult life cycle. However, since the ivermectin effect is not immediate, care must be taken to prevent reinfestation from exposure to untreated animals or contaminated facilities. Generally, pigs should not be moved to clean quarters or exposed to uninfested pigs for approximately one week after treatment. Sows should be treated at least one week before farrowing to minimize transfer of mites to newborn baby pigs.
2. Louse eggs are unaffected by PRODUMEC™ Injection and may require up to three weeks to hatch. Louse infestations developing from hatching eggs may require retreatment.
3. Consult a veterinarian for aid in the diagnosis and control of internal and external parasites of swine.

Special Minor Use:

Reindeer: For the treatment and control of warbles *(Oedemagena tarandi)* in reindeer, inject 200 micrograms ivermectin per kilogram of body weight, subcutaneously. Follow use directions for cattle as described under Administration.

American Bison: For the treatment and control of grubs *(Hypoderma bovis)* in American bison, inject 200 micrograms ivermectin per kilogram of body weight, subcutaneously. Follow use directions for cattle as described under Administration.

Consult your veterinarian for assistance in the diagnosis, treatment and control of parasitism.

Precaution(s): Protect product from light.

Environmental Safety: Studies indicate that when ivermectin comes in contact with the soil, it readily and tightly binds to the soil and becomes inactive over time. Free ivermectin may adversely affect fish and certain water-borne organisms on which they feed. Do not permit water runoff from feedlots or production sites to enter lakes, streams, or ponds. Do not contaminate water by direct application or by the improper disposal of drug containers. Dispose of containers in an approved landfill or by incineration.

Caution(s): Transitory discomfort has been observed in some cattle following subcutaneous administration. A low incidence of soft tissue swelling at the injection site has been observed. These reactions have disappeared without treatment. For cattle, divide doses greater than 10 mL between two injection sites to reduce occasional discomfort or site reaction.

Use sterile equipment and sanitize the injection site by applying a suitable disinfectant. Clean, properly disinfected needles should be used to reduce the potential for injection site infections.

Observe cattle for injection site reactions. Reactions may be due to clostridial infection and should be aggressively treated with appropriate antibiotics. If injection site infections are suspected, consult your veterinarian.

This product is not for intravenous or intramuscular use.

PRODUMEC™ Injection for Cattle and Swine has been developed specifically for use in cattle, swine, reindeer and American bison only. The product should not be used in other animal species as severe adverse reactions, including fatalities in dogs, may result.

Warning(s): Residue Information: Do not treat cattle within 35 days of slaughter. Because a withdrawal time in milk has not been established, do not use in female dairy cattle of breeding age.

Do not treat swine within 18 days of slaughter.

Do not treat reindeer or bisons within 8 weeks (56 days) of slaughter.

Not for use in humans.

Keep this and all drugs out of the reach of children.

Discussion: PRODUMEC™ (ivermectin) is an injectable parasiticide for cattle and swine. One low-volume dose effectively treats and controls the following internal and external parasites that may impair the health of cattle and swine: gastrointestinal roundworms (including inhibited *Ostertagia ostertagi* in cattle), lungworms, grubs, sucking lice, and mange mites of cattle; and gastrointestinal roundworms, lungworms, lice and mange mites of swine. Discovered and developed by scientists from Merck Research Laboratories, ivermectin is a novel chemical entity.

Its convenience, broad-spectrum efficacy, and safety margin make PRODUMEC™ Injection a unique product for parasite control of cattle and swine.

PRODUMEC™ Injection is formulated to deliver the recommended dose level of 200 mcg ivermectin/kilogram of body weight in cattle when given subcutaneously at the rate of 1 mL/110 lb (50 kg). In swine, PRODUMEC™ Injection is formulated to deliver the recommended dose level of 300 mcg ivermectin/kilogram body weight when given subcutaneously in the neck at the rate of 1 mL per 75 lb (33 kg).

When to Treat Cattle with Grubs: PRODUMEC™ effectively controls all stages of cattle grubs. However, proper timing of treatment is important. For most effective results, cattle should be treated as soon as possible after the end of the heel fly (warble fly) season. Destruction of *Hypoderma* larvae (cattle grubs) at the period when these grubs are in vital areas may cause undesirable host-parasite reactions including the possibility of fatalities. Killing *Hypoderma lineatum* when it is in the tissue surrounding the esophagus (gullet) may cause salivation and bloat, killing *H. bovis* when it is in the vertebral canal may cause staggering or paralysis. These reactions are not specific to treatment with PRODUMEC™, but can occur with any successful treatment of grubs. Cattle should be treated either before or after these stages of grub development. Consult your veterinarian concerning the proper time for treatment.

Cattle treated with PRODUMEC™ after the end of the heel fly season may be retreated with PRODUMEC™ during the winter for internal parasites, mange mites, or sucking lice without danger of grub-related reactions. A planned parasite control program is recommended.

Presentation: PRODUMEC™ Injection for Cattle and Swine is available in two ready-to-use pack sizes:

The 200 mL pack is a soft, collapsible pack designed for use with automatic syringe equipment. Each pack contains sufficient solution to treat 40 head of 550 lb (250 kg) cattle or 400 head of 38 lb (17.3 kg) swine.

The 500 mL pack is a soft, collapsible pack designed for use with automatic syringe equipment. Each pack contains sufficient solution to treat 100 head of 550 lb (250 kg) cattle or 1000 head of 38 lb (17.3 kg) swine.

U.S. Pat. 4,199,569 and 4,853,372

PRODUMEC is a trademark licensed to TradeWinds.

Compendium Code No.: 12610080 9335400

PRODUMEC™ POUR-ON FOR CATTLE

TradeWinds **Parasiticide-Topical**

(ivermectin) 5 mg/mL-Parasiticide

NADA No.: 140-841

Active Ingredient(s): Contains 5 mg ivermectin/mL.

Indications: A parasiticide for the treatment and control of external parasites of cattle.

PRODUMEC™ Pour-On applied at the recommended dose level of 500 mcg/kg is indicated for the effective control of these parasites.

Gastrointestinal Roundworms: *Ostertagia ostertagi* (including inhibited stage) (adults and L_4), *Haemonchus placei* (adults and L_4), *Trichostrongylus axei* (adults and L_4), *T. colubriformis* (adults and L_4), *Cooperia* spp. (adults and L_4), *Strongyloides papillosus* (adults), *Oesophagostomum radiatum* (adults and L_4), *Trichuris* spp. (adults).

Lungworms: *Dictyocaulus viviparus* (adults and L_4).

Cattle Grubs (parasitic stages): *Hypoderma bovis, H. lineatum.*

Mites: *Sarcoptes scabiei* var. *bovis.*

Lice: *Linognathus vituli, Haematopinus eurysternus, Damalinia bovis, Solenopotes capillatus.*

Horn Flies: *Haematobia irritans.*

Persistent Activity: PRODUMEC™ Pour-On has been proved to effectively control infections and to protect cattle from re-infection with *Ostertagia ostertagi, Oesophagostomum radiatum, Haemonchus placei, Trichostrongylus axei, Cooperia punctata* and *Cooperia oncophora* for 14 days after treatment.

Pharmacology: Mode of Action: Ivermectin is a member of the macrocyclic lactone class of endectocides which have a unique mode of action. Compounds of the class bind selectively and with high affinity to glutamate-gated chloride ion channels which occur in invertebrate nerve and muscle cells.

This leads to an increase in the permeability of the cell membrane to chloride ions with hyperpolarizatoin of the nerve or muscle cell, resulting in paralysis and death of the parasite. Compounds of this class may also interact with other ligand-gated chloride channels, such as those gated by the neurotransmitter gamma-aminobutyric acid (GABA).

The safety margin for compounds of this class is attributable to the fact that mammals do not have glutamate-gated chloride channels, the macrocyclic lactones have a low affinity for other mammalian ligand-gated chloride channels and they do not readily cross the blood-brain barrier.

Dosage and Administration: Dosage: The dose rate is 1 mL for each 22 lb of body weight. The formulation should be applied along the topline in a narrow strip from the withers to the tailhead.

Administration:

Collapsible Pack (84.5 fl oz/2.5 L Pack and 169 fl oz/5 L Pack):

Connect the applicator gun to the collapsible pack as follows:

Attach the open end of the draw-off tubing to the dosing equipment. (Because of the solvents used in the formulation, only the Protector Drench Gun from Instrument Supplies Limited, or equivalent, is recommended. Other applicators may exhibit compatibility problems resulting in locking, incorrect dosage or leakage.)

Replace the shipping cap with the draw-off cap and tighten down. Attach draw-off tubing to the draw-off cap.

Gently prime the applicator gun, checking for leaks.

Follow the manufacturer's directions for adjusting the dose.

When the interval between uses of the applicator gun is expected to exceed 12 hours, disconnect the gun and draw-off tubing from the product container and empty the product from the gun and tubing back into the product container. To prevent removal of special lubricants from the Protector Drench Gun, the gun and tubing must not be washed.

Treatment of Cattle for Horn Flies: PRODUMEC™ Pour-On controls horn flies *(Haematobia irritans)* for up to 28 days after dosing. For best results PRODUMEC™ Pour-On should be part of a parasite control program for both internal and external parasites based on the epidemiology of these parasites. Consult your veterinarian or an entomologist for the most effective timing of applications.

Consult your veterinarian for assistance in the diagnosis, treatment and control of parasitism.

Precaution(s): Flammable! Keep away from heat, sparks, open flame, and other sources of ignition.

Store away from excessive heat (104°F/40°C) and protect from light.

Use only in well-ventilated areas or outdoors.

Close container tightly when not in use.

Cloudiness in the formulation may occur when PRODUMEC™ (ivermectin) Pour-On is stored at temperatures below 32°F. Allowing to warm at room temperature will restore the normal appearance without affecting efficacy.

Environmental Safety: Studies indicate that when ivermectin comes in contact with the soil, it readily and tightly binds to the soil and becomes inactive over time. Free ivermectin may adversely affect fish or certain water-borne organisms on which they feed. Do not permit cattle to enter lakes, streams or ponds for at least six hours after treatment. Do not contaminate water by direct application or by the improper disposal of drug containers. Dispose of containers in an approved landfill or by incineration.

Caution(s): Cattle should not be treated when hair or hide is wet since reduced efficacy may be experienced.

Do not use when rain is expected to wet cattle within six hours after treatment.

This product is for application to skin surface only. Do not give orally or parenterally.

Antiparasitic activity of ivermectin will be impaired if the formulation is applied to areas of the skin with mange scabs or lesions, or with dermatoses or adherent materials, e.g., caked mud or manure.

Ivermectin has been associated with adverse reactions in sensitive dogs; therefore, PRODUMEC™ Pour-On is not recommended for use in species other than cattle.

Warning(s): Residue Information: Cattle must not be treated within 48 days of slaughter for human consumption. Because a withdrawal time in milk has not been established, do not use in female dairy cattle of breeding age.

Not for use in humans.

Keep this and all drugs out of reach of children.

The Material Safety Data Sheet (MSDS) contains more detailed occupational safety information. To report adverse effects, obtain an MSDS or for assistance, contact TradeWinds at 1-877-734-7565.

This product should not be applied to self or others because it may be irritating to human skin and eyes and absorbed through the skin. To minimize accidental skin contact, the user should wear a long-sleeved shirt and rubber gloves. If accidental skin contact occurs, wash immediately with soap and water. If accidental eye exposure occurs, flush eyes immediately with water and seek medical attention.

Discussion: PRODUMEC™ Pour-On delivers internal and external parasite control in one convenient low-volume application. Discovered and developed by scientists from Merck Research Laboratories, PRODUMEC™ Pour-On contains ivermectin, a unique chemical entity.

When to Treat Cattle with Grubs: PRODUMEC™ Pour-On effectively controls all stages of cattle grubs. However, proper timing of treatment is important. For the most effective results, cattle should be treated as soon as possible after the end of the heel fly (warble fly) season. While this is not peculiar to ivermectin, destruction of *Hypoderma* larvae (cattle grubs) at the period when these grubs are in vital areas may cause undesirable host-parasite reactions. Killing *Hypoderma lineatum* when it is in the esophageal tissues may cause bloat; killing *H. bovis* when it is in the vertebral canal may cause staggering or paralysis. Cattle should be treated either before or after these stages of grub development.

Cattle treated with PRODUMEC™ Pour-On at the end of the fly season may be re-treated with PRODUMEC™ during the winter without danger of grub-related reactions. For further information and advice on a planned parasite control program, consult your veterinarian.

Trial Data: Animal Safety: Studies conducted in the U.S.A. have demonstrated the safety margin for ivermectin. Based on plasma levels, the topically applied formulation is expected to be at least as well tolerated by breeding animals as is the subcutaneous formulation which had no effect on breeding performance.

Presentation: PRODUMEC™ Pour-On is available in an 84.5 fl oz/2.5 L or 169 oz/5 L collapsible pack intended for use with appropriate automatic dosing equipment.

PRODUMEC is a trademark licensed to TradeWinds.

U.S. Pat 4,199,569 and 4,853,372

Compendium Code No.: 12610090 9336500

PROFLOK® AE ELISA KIT

Synbiotics **ELISA Test**

Avian Encephalomyelitis Antibody Test Kit

U.S. Vet. Lic. No.: 350

Reagents:

a) 1 AE antigen coated plate.
b) 10 µL AE Positive Control Serum.
c) 10 µL Normal Control Serum (NCS).
d) 100 µL Goat anti-Chicken IgG (H+L) Peroxidase Conjugate Solution.
e) 40 mL Dilution Buffer.
f) 10 mL ABTS-Hydrogen Peroxide Substrate Solution.
g) 2.5 mL 5X Stop Solution, 5% SDS (dilute [1:5] with laboratory grade water).
h) 20 mL 20X Wash Solution (dilute [1:20] with laboratory grade water).

Equipment and Materials Required but not Provided:

a) High precision pipette (i.e. 1-20 microliter pipette).
b) 0.2 mL, 1.0 mL and 5.0 mL pipettes.
c) 8 or 12 channel pipette (or transplating device) and pipette tips.
d) 2 graduated cylinders (50 mL).
e) 1 mL and 5 mL borosilicate glass test tubes.
f) Uncoated low binding 96 well plates (i.e. Nunc catalog #269620).
g) Laboratory grade (Distilled or R.O.) water.
h) 96 well plate reading spectrophotometer with 405-410 nm filter.
i) Plate washing apparatus.
j) Waste container with bleach or other oxidizing agent.

Indications: The PROFLOK® AE ELISA Kit is a rapid serologic test for the detection of AE antibody in chicken serum samples.

Test Principles: Avian encephalomyelitis (AE) is an infectious virus disease of poultry[2], primarily affecting young chickens, that is characterized by ataxia and tremors.[1] AE is caused by a picornavirus that is egg-transmitted from infected hen to chick, or horizontally transmitted between infected and susceptible birds.[1,2]

The assay is designed to measure AE antibody bound to AE antigen coated plates. The principle of the test is as follows: Serum obtained from chickens exposed to Avian encephalomyelitis contains specific anti-AE antibodies. Serum, diluted in Dilution Buffer, is added to an AE antigen coated plate. Specific AE antibody in the serum forms an antibody-antigen complex with the AE antigen bound to the plate. After washing the plate, an affinity purified goat anti-chicken IgG (H+L) peroxidase conjugate is added to each well. The antibody-antigen complex remaining from the previous step reacts with the conjugate. After a brief incubation period, the unreacted conjugate is removed by a second wash step. Substrate, which contains a chromagen (ABTS), is added to each well. Chromagen color change (from clear to green-blue) occurs in the presence of the peroxidase enzyme. The relative intensity of color developed in 15 minutes (compared to controls) is directly proportional to the level of AE antibody in the serum. After the substrate has incubated, Stop Solution is added to each well to terminate the reaction and the plate is read using an ELISA plate reader at 405-410 nm.

Test Procedure:

Sample Collection: For routine serologic flock monitoring, it is suggested that at least 30 or more sera per flock be randomly collected at standard time intervals (i.e. every four weeks). Proper sample collection procedures, serum harvest and serum sample storage (4°C for up to four days or -20°C for longer periods) are needed to provide reliable test results.

Sample Dilution Procedure: Dilute serum samples using Dilution Buffer in a clean, uncoated 96 well microtiter plate. Frozen serum samples should be completely thawed and thoroughly mixed before diluting. Set up samples and controls as shown in Figure 1.

Preparation of the Serum Dilution Plate:

a) Add 300 μL Dilution Buffer to each well of an uncoated 96 well microtiter plate. This plate is referred to as the serum dilution plate.

b) Add 6 μL unknown serum per well as per Figure 1 (producing a 1:50 dilution). Start with well A4 and end with well H9 (moving left to right, row by row of wells). For example, wells 1 through 30 contain the diluted sera of flock 1, wells 31-60 contain the diluted sera of flock 2, etc.

c) Add 6 μL of Normal Control Serum (producing a 1:50 dilution) to wells A2, H10 and H12.

d) Aspirate and remove any liquid in dilution plate wells A1, A3 and H11.

e) Allow all diluted serums to equilibrate in Dilution Buffer for 5 minutes before transferring to an AE antigen coated ELISA plate.

f) Diluted serum should be tested within 24 hours.

This dilution format provides adequate quantities of diluted serum samples to conduct four additional ProFLOK® ELISA tests (i.e. IBD, REO, IBV or NDV) using the same serum dilution plate.

Preparation of AE Positive Control: An AE Positive Control Serum has been provided with this kit. Dilute the appropriate volume of AE Positive Control Serum with Dilution Buffer (1:50) in a clean, glass test tube. For example, dilute 6 μL of positive control serum in 300 μL Dilution Buffer. Mix well. 150 μL of diluted AE Positive Control is needed per ELISA plate.

Preparation of Conjugate Solution: The horseradish peroxidase conjugated anti-chicken IgG (H+L) is supplied in 50% glycerol. Dilute 100 μL stock conjugate in 10 mL Dilution Buffer (1:100 dilution). Mix well. This 10 mL preparation will supply sufficient conjugate for one 96 well ELISA plate.

Preparation of 1X Wash Solution: Dilute 20 mL concentrated Wash Solution in 380 mL laboratory grade (distilled or R.O.) water (1:20). Mix well. Approximately 400 mL Wash Solution is needed for each 96 well ELISA plate.

Preparation of the Substrate Solution: The Substrate Solution is ready to use. Each plate will require approximately 10 mL substrate solution. For example, 10 plates requires 100 mL substrate. For best results, the substrate solution must be equilibrated to room temperature before use.

Preparation of 1X Stop Solution: Dilute 2.5 mL concentrated Stop Solution in 10 mL laboratory grade (distilled or R.O.) water (1:5). Mix well. Approximately 12.5 mL Stop Solution is needed for each 96 well ELISA plate.

Note: Storage of 5X Stop Solution at refrigerated temperatures may cause the formation of a white solid. This does not affect product performance. Warm at room temperature or 37°C to dissolve before use.

Figure 1.

	1	2	3	4	5	6	7	8	9	10	11	12
A	+	−	+	1	2	3	4	5	6	7	8	9
B	10	11	12	13	14	15	16	17	18	19	20	21
C	22	23	24	25	26	27	28	29	30	31	32	33
D	34	35	36	37	38	39	40	41	42	43	44	45
E	46	47	48	49	50	51	52	53	54	55	56	57
F	58	59	60	61	62	63	64	65	66	67	68	69
G	70	71	72	73	74	75	76	77	78	79	80	81
H	82	83	84	85	86	87	88	89	90	−	+	−

ELISA Test Procedure:

Preparing the Test Plate:

a) Remove an AE antigen test plate from the protective bag and label according to serum dilution plate identification.

b) Add 50 μL Dilution Buffer to all wells on the test plate.

c) Add 50 μL diluted Positive Control Serum to wells A1, A3 and H11. Discard pipette tip.

d) Using an 8 or 12 channel pipette transfer 50 μL/well of each of the diluted serum samples and Normal Control Serum samples from the serum dilution plate to the corresponding wells of the AE coated test plate (yields a 1:100 dilution). Discard pipette tips after each row of sample is transferred. Transfer of samples to the ELISA plate should be done as quickly as possible.

e) Incubate plate for 30 minutes at room temperature.

Wash Procedure:

f) Tap out liquid from each well into an appropriate vessel containing bleach or other decontamination agent.

g) Using an 8 or 12 channel pipette (or comparable automatic washing device), fill each well with approximately 300 μL Wash Solution. Allow to soak in wells for 3 minutes; then discard contents into an appropriate waste container (waste container should contain bleach solution). Tap inverted plate to ensure that all residual liquid is removed. Repeat wash procedure 2 more times.

Note: The wash procedure is a very critical step in any ELISA procedure. Please follow the above steps as directed.

Addition of Anti-Chicken IgG Peroxidase Conjugate, Substrate and Stop Solution:

h) Using an 8 or 12 channel pipette (or transplating device) dispense 100 μL diluted conjugate (prepared as described above) into each assay well. Discard pipette tips.

i) Incubate for 30 minutes at room temperature.

j) Wash as in steps f and g above.

k) Using an 8 or 12 channel pipette (or transplating device) dispense 100 μL Substrate Solution into each test well. Discard pipette tips.

l) Incubate 15 minutes at room temperature.

m) Using an 8 or 12 channel pipette (or transplating device) add 100 μL diluted Stop Solution (prepared as described above) to each test well.

n) Allow bubbles to dissipate before reading plate.

Manual Processing of Data:

a) Read the plate using an ELISA plate reader set at 405-410 nm. Be sure to blank the reader as directed. If a Flow Multiscan reader is used, the reader should be blanked using an empty microtiter plate. If a Bio-tek or Dynatech reader is used, the machine may be blanked with air.

b) Calculate the average Positive Control Serum absorbance (Optical Density [O.D.]) using the absorbance values of wells A1, A3 and H11. Calculate the average Normal Control Serum (NCS) absorbance using values obtained from wells A2, H10 and H12. Record both averages.

c) Subtract the average negative (NCS) absorbance from the average positive absorbance. The difference is the Corrected Positive Control.

d) Calculate a sample to positive (Sp) ratio by subtracting the average negative control absorbance from each sample absorbance. The difference is divided by the corrected positive control. Use the following equation format:

$$SP = \frac{\text{(Sample Absorbance)} - \text{(Average Normal Control Absorbance)}}{\text{Corrected Positive Control Absorbance}}$$

e) An AE ELISA titer can be calculated by the following suggested equation:

$\text{Log}_{10}\ \text{Titer} = (0.717 \times \text{Log}_{10}\ \text{Sp}) + 3.906$

Titer = Antilog of Log_{10} Titer

Example:

1. Example Positive Control Absorbance:
   0.585, 0.610, 0.590
   Average = (0.585 + 0.610 + 0.590) / 3 = 0.595
2. Example Normal Controls:
   0.078, 0.067, 0.057
   Average = (0.078 + 0.067 + 0.057) / 3 = 0.067
3. Corrected Positive Control:
   (0.595) - (0.067) = 0.528
4. Example Sp value calculation:
   Absorbance of sample = 0.560
   (0.560) - (0.067) / 0.528 = 0.934
5. Example of Calculation of titer using the Sp from above:
   Log_{10} Titer = 0.717 X (Log_{10} 0.934) + 3.906
   Titer = Antilog 3.88
   Titer = 7669

Test Interpretation: Results:

Assay Control Values: Valid AE ELISA results are obtained when the average optical density (O.D.) value of the Normal Control Serum is less than 0.200 and the Corrected Positive Control value range is between 0.250 and 0.900. If either of these values are out of range, the AE test results should be considered invalid and the samples should be retested. Samples testing with an Sp value of less than or equal to 0.300 will receive a 0 titer value and are considered negative for AE antibody.

Under optimal conditions* the suggested O.D. value ranges of 0.060 to 0.130 for AE Normal Control Serum and 0.350 to 0.900 for AE Positive Control Serum should be strived for to ensure the most consistent laboratory test results. Please note that tests with O.D. values which do not fall within the suggested O.D. ranges above does not constitute an invalid test.

*Optimal conditions are at room temperature [70 to 75°F (21 to 24°C)]. Higher room temperatures may result in slightly higher O.D. values.

Interpretation of Results: The AE ELISA titer values obtained represent a comparison of the AE antibody level within each field chicken serum tested and the AE ELISA kit positive and normal control sera. Therefore, it is important to first determine that the AE ELISA positive and normal control sera values obtained are valid as detailed above in the "Assay Control Values" section of this pamphlet before AE ELISA results are interpreted.

A "0" AE ELISA titer represents a chicken serum sample that contains an extremely low to insignificant AE antibody level compared to the AE ELISA kit positive and normal control sera.

An AE ELISA titer value above "0" indicates only that a chicken serum sample contains a significant and ELISA-detectable AE antibody level compared to the AE ELISA kit positive and normal control sera. However, these titers do not imply or ensure "protection" nor provide serologic differentiation between an AE vaccine response or an AE field infection.

Optimal AE vaccine administration practices and "protective" flock AE titer target values must be determined by each AE ELISA kit user by comparing flock pre- and post-vaccination AE ELISA results [i.e. coefficient of variation (%CV) and geometric titer (GMT) values] with flock performance parameters (i.e. morbidity, mortality, flock body weight gain or uniformity) over time.

Storage: Store all reagents provided in the kit at 2-7°C. Reagents should not be frozen.

Caution(s): To the Users of Reagents and AE Antigen Coated Plates:

a) Handle all reagents and samples as biohazardous material.

b) Keep all reagents away from skin and eyes. If exposure should occur, immediately flush affected areas with cold water.

c) Wash solution, control sera, test plates, field samples and all other test kit reagents should be properly decontaminated with bleach or other strong oxidizing agent before disposal.

d) Take special care not to contaminate any of the test reagents with serum or bacterial agents.

e) Humidity indicators are supplied with each plate. If any of the indicators exhibit a pink color, the plate may be compromised in some way; decontaminate (i.e. wash the plate with bleach solution) and dispose of the plate.

f) The best results are achieved by following the protocols as they are described above, using good, safe laboratory techniques.

g) Do not use this kit after the expiration date.

h) Never pipette by mouth.

Allow all reagents to come to room temperature before starting.

References: Available upon request.

Presentation: 900 tests.

Compendium Code No.: 11150170

P

PROFLOK® AE-IBD-IBV-NDV-REO ELISA KIT

Synbiotics **ELISA Test**

Avian Encephalomyelitis-Bronchitis-Bursal Disease-Newcastle Disease-Reovirus Antibody Test Kit

U.S. Vet. Lic. No.: 350

Reagents:

a) 1 antigen coated plate (AE, IBD, IBV, NDV or REO).
b) 10 µL Positive Control Serum (AE, IBD, IBV, NDV or REO).
c) 10 µL Normal Control Serum (NCS)*.
d) 100 µL Goat anti-Chicken IgG (H+L) Peroxidase Conjugate Solution*.
e) 40 mL Dilution Buffer*.
f) 10 mL ABTS-Hydrogen Peroxide Substrate Solution*.
g) 2.5 mL 5X Stop Solution, 5% SDS (dilute [1:5] with laboratory grade water)*.
h) 20 mL 20X Wash Solution (dilute [1:20] with laboratory grade water)*.
*Reagents can be used with all antigen coated plates in the kit.

Equipment and Materials Required but not Provided:

a) High precision pipette (i.e. 1-20 microliter pipette).
b) 0.2 mL, 1.0 mL and 5.0 mL pipettes.
c) 8 or 12 channel pipette (or transplating device) and pipette tips.
d) 2 graduated cylinders (50 mL).
e) 1 mL and 5 mL borosilicate glass test tubes.
f) Uncoated low binding 96 well plates (i.e. Nunc catalog #269620).
g) Laboratory grade (Distilled or R.O.) water.
h) 96 well plate reading spectrophotometer with 405-410 nm filter.
i) Plate washing apparatus.
j) Waste container with bleach or other oxidizing agent.

Indications: The PROFLOK® ELISA Kit is a rapid serologic test for the detection of antibody in chicken serum samples. It was developed primarily to aid in the detection of pre- and post-vaccination antibody levels in chickens.

Test Principles: This ELISA kit contains a combination of five different antibody detection products. The kit includes antigen coated plates for the detection of antibody to Avian Encephalomyelitis (AE), Infectious Bursal Disease Virus (IBD), Infectious Bronchitis Virus (IBV), Newcastle Disease Virus (NDV) and Avian Reovirus (REO). The kit includes the antigen coated plates, two for each agent, and five positive control vials, one per agent, and the reagents necessary to run ten test plates.

The assay is designed to measure antibody bound to antigen coated plates. The principle of the test is as follows: Serum obtained from chickens exposed to antigens contains specific antibodies. Serum, diluted in Dilution Buffer, is added to an antigen coated plate. Specific antibody in the serum forms an antibody-antigen complex with the antigen bound to the plate. After washing the plate, an affinity purified goat anti-chicken IgG (H+L) peroxidase conjugate is added to each well. The antibody-antigen complex remaining from the previous step binds with the conjugate. After a brief incubation period, the unbound conjugate is removed by a second wash step. Substrate, which contains a chromagen (ABTS), is added to each well. Chromagen color change (from clear to green-blue) occurs in the presence of the peroxidase enzyme. The relative intensity of color developed in 15 minutes (compared to controls) is directly proportional to the level of antibody in the serum. After the substrate has incubated, Stop Solution is added to each well to terminate the reaction and the plate is read using an ELISA plate reader at 405-410 nm.

Test Procedure:

Sample Collection: For routine serologic flock monitoring, it is suggested that at least 30 or more sera per flock be randomly collected at standard time intervals (i.e. every four weeks). Proper sample collection procedures, serum harvest and serum sample storage (4°C for up to four days or -20°C for longer periods) are needed to provide reliable test results. Test only good quality serum (i.e. avoid bacterial contamination, heavy hemolysis or clotted fat).

Sample Dilution Procedure: Dilute serum samples using Dilution Buffer in a clean, uncoated 96 well microtiter plate. Frozen serum samples should be completely thawed and thoroughly mixed before diluting. Set up samples and controls as shown in Figure 1.

Preparation of the Serum Dilution Plate:

a) Add 300 µL Dilution Buffer to each well of an uncoated 96 well microtiter plate. This plate is referred to as the serum dilution plate.
b) Add 6 µL unknown serum per well as per Figure 1 (producing a 1:50 dilution). Start with well A4 and end with well H9 (moving left to right, row by row of wells). For example, wells 1 through 30 contain the diluted sera of flock 1, wells 31-60 contain the diluted sera of flock 2, etc.
c) Add 6 µL of Normal Control Serum (producing a 1:50 dilution) to wells A2, H10 and H12.
d) Aspirate and remove any liquid in dilution plate wells A1, A3 and H11.
e) Allow all diluted serums to equilibrate in Dilution Buffer for 5 minutes before transferring to an antigen coated ELISA plate.
f) Diluted serum should be tested within 24 hours.

This dilution format provides adequate quantities of diluted serum samples to conduct five additional ProFLOK® ELISA tests (i.e. REO, NDV, IBV, IBD and AE) using the same serum dilution plate.

Preparation of Positive Control (prepare for each antigen coated plate): A Positive Control Serum for each agent has been provided with this kit. Dilute the appropriate volume of the appropriate Positive Control Serum with Dilution Buffer (1:50) in a clean, glass test tube. For example, dilute 6 µL of positive control serum in 300 µL Dilution Buffer. Mix well. 150 µL of diluted Positive Control is needed per ELISA plate.

Preparation of Conjugate Solution: The horseradish peroxidase conjugated anti-chicken IgG (H+L) is supplied in 50% glycerol. Dilute 100 µL stock conjugate in 10 mL Dilution Buffer (1:100 dilution). Mix well. This 10 mL preparation will supply sufficient conjugate for one 96 well ELISA plate.

Preparation of 1X Wash Solution: Dilute 20 mL concentrated Wash Solution in 380 mL laboratory grade (distilled or R.O.) water (1:20). Mix well. Approximately 400 mL Wash Solution is needed for each 96 well ELISA plate.

Preparation of the Substrate Solution: The Substrate Solution is ready to use. Each plate will require approximately 10 mL substrate solution. For best results, the substrate solution must be equilibrated to room temperature before use.

Preparation of 1X Stop Solution: Dilute 2.5 mL concentrated Stop Solution in 10 mL laboratory grade (distilled or R.O.) water (1:5). Mix well. Approximately 12.5 mL Stop Solution is needed for each 96 well ELISA plate.

Note: Storage of 5X Stop Solution at refrigerated temperatures may cause the formation of a white solid. This does not affect product performance. Warm at room temperature or 37°C to dissolve before use.

Figure 1.

ELISA Test Procedure:

Preparing the Test Plate:

a) Remove an antigen coated test plate from the protective bag and label according to dilution plate identification.
b) Add 50 µL Dilution Buffer to all wells on the test plate.
c) Add 50 µL diluted Positive Control Serum to wells A1, A3 and H11. Discard pipette tip.

Note: Be sure that positive control sample is appropriate for antigen coated plate being used (i.e. IBD Positive Control is used with IBD antigen coated plate).

d) Using an 8 or 12 channel pipette transfer 50 µL/well of each of the diluted serum samples and Normal Control Serum samples from the dilution plate to the corresponding wells of the coated test plate (yields a 1:100 dilution). Discard pipette tips after each row of sample is transferred. Transfer of samples to the ELISA plate should be done as quickly as possible.
e) Incubate plate for 30 minutes at room temperature.

Wash Procedure:

f) Tap out liquid from each well into an appropriate vessel containing bleach or other decontamination agent.
g) Using an 8 or 12 channel pipette (or comparable automatic washing device), fill each well with approximately 300 µL Wash Solution. Allow to soak in wells for 3 minutes; then discard contents into an appropriate waste container (waste container should contain bleach solution). Tap inverted plate to ensure that all residual liquid is removed. Repeat wash procedure 2 more times.

Note: The wash procedure is a very critical step in any ELISA procedure. Please follow the above steps as directed.

Addition of Anti-Chicken IgG Peroxidase Conjugate, Substrate and Stop Solution:

h) Using an 8 or 12 channel pipette (or transplating device) dispense 100 µL diluted conjugate (prepared as described above) into each assay well. Discard pipette tips.
i) Incubate for 30 minutes at room temperature.
j) Wash as in steps f and g above.
k) Using an 8 or 12 channel pipette (or transplating device) dispense 100 µL Substrate Solution into each test well. Discard pipette tips.
l) Incubate 15 minutes at room temperature.
m) Using an 8 or 12 channel pipette (or transplating device) add 100 µL diluted Stop Solution (prepared as described above) to each test well.
n) Allow bubbles to dissipate before reading plate.

Manual Processing of Data:

a) Read the plate using an ELISA plate reader set at 405-410 nm. Be sure to blank the reader as directed. If a Flow Multiscan reader is used, the reader should be blanked using an empty microtiter plate. If a Bio-tek or Dynatech reader is used, the machine may be blanked with air.
b) Calculate the average Positive Control Serum absorbance (Optical Density [O.D.]) using the absorbance values of wells A1, A3 and H11. Calculate the average Normal Control Serum (NCS) absorbance using values obtained from wells A2, H10 and H12. Record both averages.
c) Subtract the average normal control absorbance from the average positive absorbance. The difference is the Corrected Positive Control.
d) Calculate a sample to positive (Sp) ratio by subtracting the average normal control absorbance from each sample absorbance. The difference is divided by the corrected positive control. Use the following equation format:

$$SP = \frac{\text{(Sample Absorbance)} - \text{(Average Normal Control Absorbance)}}{\text{Corrected Positive Control Absorbance}}$$

Titer Calculations: When a sample produces and Sp value above the Sp threshold (see Results section) a titer is calculated using the following titer calculation:

Log_{10} Titer = (a x Log_{10}Sp) + b

Titer = antilog [(a x Log_{10}Sp) + b]

Values for the slope (a) and the offset (b) are listed below:

ELISA Test	a	b
IBD	1.172	3.614
IBV	1.642	3.568
NDV	1.464	3.740
REO	1.077	3.460
AE	0.717	3.906

An IBD ELISA titer calculation is illustrated below:

Log_{10} Titer = (1.172 X Log_{10}Sp) + 3.614

Titer = Antilog of Log_{10} Titer

Example:

1. Example Positive Control Absorbance:
   0.585, 0.610, 0.590
   Average = (0.585 + 0.610 + 0.590) / 3 = 0.595
2. Example Normal Controls:
   0.110, 0.102, 0.112
   Average = (0.110 + 0.102 + 0.112) / 3 = 0.108
3. Corrected Positive Control:
   (0.595) - (0.108) = 0.487
4. Example Sp value calculation:
   Absorbance of sample = 0.560
   (0.560) - (0.108) / 0.487 = 0.928

5. Example of Calculation of titer using the Sp from above:
   Log_{10} Titer = 1.172 X (Log_{10} 0.928) + 3.614
   Titer = Antilog 3.57
   Titer = 3767

Test Interpretation: Results:

Assay Control Values: Valid ELISA results are obtained when the average optical density (O.D.) value of the Normal Control Serum is less than 0.250 for IBD, IBV, NDV and REO and less than 0.200 for AE and the Corrected Positive Control value range for all five agents is between 0.250 and 0.900. If either of these values are out of range, the test results should be considered invalid and the samples should be retested.

SP Threshold: When calculating antibody titers, and Sp threshold is used to separate ELISA negative samples from ELISA positive samples. Samples with an Sp value equal to or less than the Sp threshold are assigned a zero titer and considered ELISA negative. Samples with an Sp value above the Sp threshold are considered ELISA positive and titers are calculated. The Sp threshold for each ELISA included in this kit is listed below:

ELISA Test	Sp Threshold	Lowest Reported Titer
IBD	0.180	554
IBV	0.150	165
NDV	0.150	98
REO	0.150	376
AE	0.300	3397

Interpretation of Results: The ELISA titer values obtained represent a comparison of the antibody level within each field chicken serum tested and the ELISA kit positive and normal control sera. Therefore, it is important to first determine that the ELISA positive and normal control sera values obtained are valid as detailed above in the "Assay Control Values" section of this pamphlet before ELISA results are interpreted.

A "0" ELISA titer represents a chicken serum sample that contains an extremely low to insignificant antibody level compared to the ELISA kit positive and normal control sera.

An ELISA titer value above "0" indicates only that a chicken serum sample contains a significant and ELISA-detectable antibody level compared to the ELISA kit positive and normal control sera. However, these titers do not imply or ensure "protection" nor provide serologic differentiation between a vaccine response or field infection.

Optimal vaccine administration practices and "protective" flock titer target values must be determined by each AE ELISA kit user by comparing flock pre- and post-vaccination ELISA results [i.e. coefficient of variation (%CV) and geometric mean titer (GMT) values] with flock performance parameters (i.e. morbidity, mortality, flock body weight gain or uniformity) over time.

Storage: Store all reagents provided in the kit at 2-7°C. Reagents should not be frozen.

Caution(s): To the Users of Reagents and Antigen Coated Plates:

a) Handle all reagents and samples as biohazardous material.
b) Keep all reagents away from skin and eyes. If exposure should occur, immediately flush affected areas with cold water.
c) Wash solution, control sera, test plates, field samples and all other test kit reagents should be properly decontaminated with bleach or other strong oxidizing agent before disposal.
d) Take special care not to contaminate any of the test reagents with serum or bacterial agents.
e) Humidity indicators are supplied with each plate. If any of the indicators exhibit a pink color, the plate may be compromised in some way; decontaminate (i.e. wash the plate with bleach solution) and dispose of the plate.
f) The best results are achieved by following the protocols as they are described above, using good, safe laboratory techniques.
g) Do not use this kit after the expiration date.
h) Never pipette by mouth.

Allow all reagents to come to room temperature before starting.

References: Available upon request.

Presentation: 900 tests.

Compendium Code No.: 11150180

PROFLOK® AIV ELISA KIT

Synbiotics **ELISA Test**

Avian Influenza Virus Antibody Test Kit

U.S. Vet. Lic. No.: 350

Reagents:

a) 1 AIV antigen coated plate.
b) 10 µL AIV Positive Control Serum.
c) 10 µL Normal Control Serum.
d) 100 µL Goat anti-Chicken IgG (H+L) Peroxidase Conjugate Solution.
e) 40 mL Dilution Buffer.
f) 10 mL ABTS-Hydrogen Peroxide Substrate Solution.
g) 2.5 mL 5X Stop Solution, 5% SDS (dilute [1:5] with laboratory grade water).
h) 20 mL 20X Wash Solution (dilute [1:20] with laboratory grade water).

Equipment and Materials Required but not Provided:

a) High precision pipette (i.e. 1-20 microliter pipette).
b) 0.2 mL, 1.0 mL and 5.0 mL pipettes.
c) 8 or 12 channel pipette (or transplating device) and pipette tips.
d) 2 graduated cylinders (50 mL).
e) 1 mL and 5 mL borosilicate glass test tubes.
f) Uncoated low binding 96 well plates (i.e. Nunc catalog #269620).
g) Laboratory grade (Distilled or R.O.) water.
h) 96 well plate reading spectrophotometer with 405-410 nm filter.
i) Plate washing apparatus.
j) Waste container with bleach or other oxidizing agent.

Indications: The PROFLOK® AIV ELISA Kit is a rapid and specific presumptive screening test for the detection of antibody to AIV in chicken serum samples. It was designed for screening large numbers of chicken sera from numerous flocks; however, additional conventional AIV serologic testing [i.e. agar gel precipitin (AGP), hemagglutination-inhibition (HI) test and neuraminidase-inhibition (NI)][1,4] and virus isolation techniques are needed to confirm AIV negative and AIV-infected chicken flocks.

Test Principles: Avian Influenza Virus (AIV), also known as Fowl Plague, is a viral disease of domestic and wild birds that is characterized by a full range of responses from almost no signs of the disease to very high mortality. The causal orthomyxoviruses are type A influenza viruses. There are 14 known serologically distinct subtypes based on surface hemagglutinins and 9 based on neuraminidases.[3] Subtypes H5 and H7 are associated with significant to catastrophic losses. Disease signs range from only a slight decrease in egg production to a highly fatal fulminating infection. Signs of infection may include respiratory problems, edema of the head and face and diarrhea. The most severe lesions arc generally characterized as congestive and hemorrhagic.[3]

The assay is designed to measure AIV antibody bound to AIV antigen coated plates. The principle of the test is as follows: Serum obtained from chickens exposed to AIV antigens contains specific anti-AIV antibodies. Serum, diluted in Dilution Buffer, is added to an AIV antigen coated plate. Specific AIV antibody in the serum forms an antibody-antigen complex with the AIV antigen bound to the plate. After washing the plate, an affinity purified goat anti-chicken IgG (H+L) peroxidase conjugate is added to each well. The antibody-antigen complex remaining from the previous step binds with the conjugate. After a brief incubation period, the unbound conjugate is removed by a second wash step. Substrate, which contains a chromagen (ABTS), is added to each well. Chromagen color change (from clear to green-blue) occurs in the presence of the peroxidase enzyme. The relative intensity of color developed in 15 minutes (compared to controls) is directly proportional to the level of AIV antibody in the serum. After the substrate has incubated, Stop Solution is added to each well to terminate the reaction and the plate is read using an ELISA plate reader at 405-410 nm.

Test Procedure:

Sample Collection: For routine serologic flock monitoring, it is suggested that at least 30 or more sera per flock be randomly collected at standard time intervals (i.e. every four weeks). Proper sample collection procedures, serum harvest and serum sample storage (4°C for up to four days or -20°C for longer periods) are needed to provide reliable test results. To achieve better specificity and to minimize possible false positive reactions, serum samples that are contaminated with bacteria or are very fatty should be excluded from testing.

Sample Dilution Procedure: Dilute serum samples using Dilution Buffer in a clean, uncoated 96 well microtiter plate. Frozen serum samples should be completely thawed and thoroughly mixed before diluting. Set up samples and controls as shown in Figure 1.

Preparation of the Serum Dilution Plate:

a) Add 300 µL Dilution Buffer to each well of an uncoated 96 well microtiter plate. This plate is referred to as the serum dilution plate.
b) Add 6 µL unknown serum per well as per Figure 1 (producing a 1:50 dilution). Start with well A4 and end with well H9 (moving left to right, row by row of wells). For example, wells 1 through 30 contain the diluted sera of flock 1, wells 31-60 contain the diluted sera of flock 2, etc.
c) Add 6 µL of Normal Control Serum (producing a 1:50 dilution) to wells A2, H10 and H12.
d) Aspirate and remove any liquid in dilution plate wells A1, A3 and H11.
e) Allow all diluted serums to equilibrate in Dilution Buffer for 5 minutes before transferring to an AIV antigen coated ELISA plate.
f) Diluted serum should be tested within 24 hours.

This dilution format provides adequate quantities of diluted serum samples to conduct four additional ProFLOK® ELISA tests (i.e. IBD, IBV, ILT and REO) using the same serum dilution plate.

Preparation of AIV Positive Control: An AIV Positive Control Serum has been provided with this kit. Dilute the appropriate volume of AIV Positive Control Serum with Dilution Buffer (1:50) in a clean, glass test tube. For example, dilute 6 µL of positive control serum in 300 µL Dilution Buffer. Mix well. 150 µL of diluted AIV Positive Control is needed per ELISA plate.

Preparation of Conjugate Solution: The horseradish peroxidase conjugated anti-chicken IgG (H+L) is supplied in 50% glycerol. Dilute 100 µL stock conjugate in 10 mL Dilution Buffer (1:100 dilution). Mix well. This 10 mL preparation will supply sufficient conjugate for one 96 well ELISA plate.

Preparation of 1X Wash Solution: Dilute 20 mL concentrated Wash Solution in 380 mL laboratory grade (distilled or R.O.) water (1:20). Mix well. Approximately 400 mL Wash Solution is needed for each 96 well ELISA plate.

Preparation of the Substrate Solution: The Substrate Solution is ready to use. Each plate will require approximately 10 mL substrate solution. For best results, the substrate solution must be equilibrated to room temperature before use.

Preparation of 1X Stop Solution: Dilute 2.5 mL concentrated Stop Solution in 10 mL laboratory grade (distilled or R.O.) water (1:5). Mix well. Approximately 12.5 mL Stop Solution is needed for each 96 well ELISA plate.

Note: Storage of 5X Stop Solution at refrigerated temperatures may cause the formation of a white solid. This does not affect product performance. Warm at room temperature or 37°C to dissolve before use.

Figure 1.

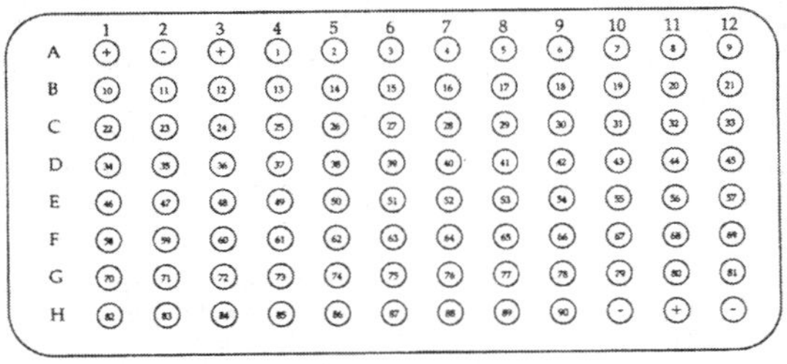

	1	2	3	4	5	6	7	8	9	10	11	12
A	+	-	+	1	2	3	4	5	6	7	8	9
B	10	11	12	13	14	15	16	17	18	19	20	21
C	22	23	24	25	26	27	28	29	30	31	32	33
D	34	35	36	37	38	39	40	41	42	43	44	45
E	46	47	48	49	50	51	52	53	54	55	56	57
F	58	59	60	61	62	63	64	65	66	67	68	69
G	70	71	72	73	74	75	76	77	78	79	80	81
H	82	83	84	85	86	87	88	89	90	-	+	-

ELISA Test Procedure:

Preparing the Test Plate:

a) Remove an AIV antigen test plate from the protective bag and label according to serum dilution plate identification.
b) Add 50 µL Dilution Buffer to all wells on the test plate.
c) Add 50 µL diluted Positive Control Serum to wells A1, A3 and H11. Discard pipette tip.
d) Using an 8 or 12 channel pipette transfer 50 µL/well of each of the diluted serum samples and Normal Control Serum samples from the serum dilution plate to the corresponding wells of the AIV coated test plate (yields a 1:100 dilution). Discard pipette tips after each row of sample is transferred. Transfer of samples to the ELISA plate should be done as quickly as possible.
e) Incubate plate for 30 minutes at room temperature.

Wash Procedure:

f) Tap out liquid from each well into an appropriate vessel containing bleach or other decontamination agent.
g) Using an 8 or 12 channel pipette (or comparable automatic washing device), fill each well with approximately 300 µL Wash Solution. Allow to soak in wells for 3 minutes; then discard contents into an appropriate waste container (waste container should contain bleach

solution). Tap inverted plate to ensure that all residual liquid is removed. Repeat wash procedure 2 more times.

Note: The wash procedure is a very critical step in any ELISA procedure. Please follow the above steps as directed.

Addition of Anti-Chicken IgG Peroxidase Conjugate, Substrate and Stop Solution:

h) Using an 8 or 12 channel pipette (or transplating device) dispense 100 µL diluted conjugate (prepared as described above) into each assay well. Discard pipette tips.

i) Incubate for 30 minutes at room temperature.

j) Wash as in steps f and g above.

k) Using an 8 or 12 channel pipette (or transplating device) dispense 100 µL Substrate Solution into each test well. Discard pipette tips.

l) Incubate 15 minutes at room temperature.

m) Using an 8 or 12 channel pipette (or transplating device) add 100 µL diluted Stop Solution (prepared as described above) to each test well.

n) Allow bubbles to dissipate before reading plate.

Manual Processing of Data:

a) Read the plate using an ELISA plate reader set at 405-410 nm. Be sure to blank the reader as directed. If a Flow Multiscan reader is used, the reader should be blanked using an empty microtiter plate. If a Bio-tek or Dynatech reader is used, the machine may be blanked with air.

b) Calculate the average Positive Control Serum absorbance (Optical Density [O.D.]) using the absorbance values of wells A1, A3 and H11. Calculate the average Normal Control Serum absorbance using values obtained from wells A2, H10 and H12. Record both averages.

c) Subtract the average normal control absorbance from the average positive absorbance. The difference is the Corrected Positive Control.

d) Calculate a sample to positive (Sp) ratio by subtracting the average normal control absorbance from each sample absorbance. The difference is divided by the corrected positive control. Use the following equation format:

$$SP = \frac{\text{(Sample Absorbance)} - \text{(Average Normal Control Absorbance)}}{\text{Corrected Positive Control Absorbance}}$$

e) An AIV ELISA titer can be calculated by the following suggested equation:

$\text{Log}_{10}\ \text{Titer} = (1.464 \times \text{Log}_{10}\ \text{Sp}) + 3.197$

Titer = Antilog of Log_{10} Titer

Example:

1. Example Positive Control Absorbance:
   0.585, 0.610, 0.590
   Average = (0.585 + 0.610 + 0.590) / 3 = 0.595
2. Example Normal Controls:
   0.078, 0.067, 0.057
   Average = (0.078 + 0.067 + 0.057) / 3 = 0.067
3. Corrected Positive Control:
   (0.595) - (0.067) = 0.528
4. Example Sp value calculation:
   Absorbance of sample = 0.560
   (0.560) - (0.067) / 0.528 = 0.934
5. Example of Calculation of titer using the Sp from above:
   Log_{10} Titer = 1.464 X (Log_{10} 0.934) + 3.197
   Titer = Antilog 3.15
   Titer = 1413

Test Interpretation: Results:

Assay Control Values: Valid AIV ELISA results are obtained when the average optical density (O.D.) value of the Normal Control Serum is less than 0.200 and the Corrected Positive Control value range is between 0.250 and 0.900. If either of these values are out of range, the AIV test results should be considered invalid and the samples should be retested. Samples testing with an Sp value of less than or equal to 0.299 will receive a 0 titer value and are considered negative for AIV antibody.

Under optimal conditions* the suggested O.D. value ranges of 0.050 to 0.095 for AIV Normal Control Serum and 0.400 to 1.00 for AIV Positive Control Serum should be strived for to ensure the most consistent laboratory test results. Please note that tests with O.D. values which do not fall within the suggested O.D. ranges above does not constitute an invalid test.

*Optimal conditions are at room temperature [70 to 75°F (21 to 24°C)]. Higher room temperatures may result in slightly higher OD values.

Interpretation of Results: The AIV Sp ratio values and/or ELISA titer values obtained for sera should be interpreted using the following value ranges:

Sample to Positive (Sp) Value	AIV ELISA Titer Range	AIV Presumed Antibody Status
Less than 0.300	0	Non-Reactive[a]
0.300 to 0.499	270 to 569	Suspect[b,c]
Greater or equal to 0.5	570 or greater	Positive[c]

a. Non-reactive. Serum samples with an AIV Sp ratio value of less than 0.300 receive a "0" titer value and are presumed non-reactive for AIV antibody. However, a variety of factors, such as possible AIV strain variations that may exhibit atypical biological and/or antigenic properties,[3] prevalence of an AIV strain within a flock and timing and randomness of serum sample collection procedures could result in an AIV-infected chicken flock yielding AIV non-reactive ELISA results. It is therefore recommended that each chicken flock only be considered to be AIV non-reactive after (a) each flock has been adequately sampled and repeatedly tested several times and has yielded negative AIV ELISA results each time and (b) each flock has been adequately sampled and repeatedly tested by standard conventional serologic tests (AGP, HI and NI) and AIV virus isolation techniques[1,2] and has yielded AIV non-reactive serologic and virus isolation results each time.

b. Suspect. Presumed AIV antibody suspect denotes the ELISA Sp value range within which AIV ELISA and conventional (AGP, HI and NI) test data may suggest but may not conclusively detect AIV antibody within a sample. The suspect range represents a "suspect" or "gray" area in which AIV ELISA results may or may not be supported by conventional serologic (AGP, HI and NI) test results. It is highly recommended that additional conventional serologic tests and AIV virus isolation techniques[1,2] be conducted on serum and collected from AIV ELISA suspect chicken flocks, as recommended in parts a and c, to confirm whether each flock is an AIV non-reactive or AIV positive-infected flock.

c. Positive. Additional conventional serologic testing (AGP, HI and NI) and virus isolation of samples collected from presumed AIV ELISA antibody suspect and positive chicken flocks, using standard techniques,[1,2] are needed to obtain a confirmed positive diagnosis of AIV infection within a chicken flock. Samples may yield false positive results if the serum tested is fatty or highly contaminated with bacteria or debris. Please exclude poor quality serum samples from the ELISA analysis.

*All positive samples and/or results should be submitted to the National Veterinary Services Lab for H and N titration

*U.S. Customers Only

Storage: Store all reagents provided in the kit at 2-7°C. Reagents should not be frozen.

Caution(s): To the Users of Reagents and AIV Antigen Coated Plates:

a) Handle all reagents and samples as biohazardous material.

b) Keep all reagents away from skin and eyes. If exposure should occur, immediately flush affected areas with cold water.

c) Wash solution, control sera, test plates, field samples and all other test kit reagents should be properly decontaminated with bleach or other strong oxidizing agent before disposal.

d) Take special care not to contaminate any of the test reagents with serum or bacterial agents.

e) Humidity indicators are supplied with each plate. If any of the indicators exhibit a pink color, the plate may be compromised in some way; decontaminate (i.e. wash the plate with bleach solution) and dispose of the plate.

f) The best results are achieved by following the protocols as they are described above, using good, safe laboratory techniques.

g) Do not use this kit after the expiration date.

h) Never pipette by mouth.

Allow all reagents to come to room temperature before starting.

References: Available upon request.

Presentation: 900 tests.

Compendium Code No.: 11150190

PROFLOK® ALV ANTIGEN TEST KIT

Synbiotics **ELISA Test**

Avian Leukosis Virus Antigen Test Kit

U.S. Vet. Lic. No.: 350

Reagents:

a) 1 p27 antibody coated plate.

b) 300 µL ALV Positive Control.

c) 300 µL Negative Control.

d) 200 µL Rabbit anti-p27 Peroxidase Conjugate Solution.

e) 10 mL Dilution Buffer.

f) 10 mL ABTS-Hydrogen Peroxide Substrate Solution.

g) 3 mL 5X Stop Solution (dilute [1:5] with laboratory grade water).

h) 20 mL 20X Wash Solution (dilute [1:20] with laboratory grade water).

Equipment and Materials Required:

a) High precision pipette (i.e. 50-200 microliter pipette).

b) 1 mL and 5 mL pipettes.

c) 8 or 12 channel pipette (or transplating device).

d) 2 graduated cylinders (50 mL).

e) Laboratory grade (Distilled or R.O.) water.

f) 96 well plate reading spectrophotometer with 405-410 nm filter.

g) Plate washing apparatus.

h) Waste container with bleach or other oxidizing agent.

Indications: The PROFLOK® Avian Leukosis Virus (ALV) Antigen Test Kit offers a rapid method for the detection of ALV p27 antigen in chicken serum and egg albumin.

Test Principles: Lymphoid leukosis, caused by Avian Leukosis Virus (ALV) is an insidious but economically important disease of chickens.[2] ALV infection may be associated with lymphoid leukosis tumors, decreased egg production and increased nonspecific mortality.[2] ALV is transmitted vertically from hen to chick through the egg and horizontally from bird to bird by direct or indirect contact.[1,4]

The PROFLOK® ALV Antigen Test Kit is designed to measure antigen bound to anti-p27 antibody coated microtiter plates. The principle of this test is as follows: Samples collected from chickens infected with ALV contain specific ALV antigens, including p27. Serum or egg albumin samples are added to an anti-p27 antibody-coated plate. Specific antigen in the sample forms an antibody-antigen complex with the anti-p27 antibody bound to the plate. After washing the plate, an affinity purified rabbit anti-p27 peroxidase conjugate is added to each well. The antibody-antigen complex remaining from the previous step reacts with the conjugate. After a brief incubation period the unreacted conjugate is removed by a second wash step. Substrate, which contains a chromagen (ABTS), is added to each well. Chromagen color change (from clear to green-blue) occurs in the presence of the peroxidase enzyme. The relative intensity of color developed in 15 minutes (compared to controls) is directly proportional to the quantity of p27 antigen in the sample. After the substrate has incubated, Stop Solution is added to each well to terminate the reaction. The plate is read using an ELISA reader with a 405-410 nm filter and a sample to positive (Sp) value is calculated for each sample tested.

Test Procedure:

Sample Collection: For routine serologic flock monitoring, it is suggested that at least 30 or more sera or egg albumin samples per flock be randomly collected at standard time intervals (i.e. every four weeks). Proper sample collection procedures, serum harvest and serum sample storage (4°C for up to four days or -20°C for longer periods) are needed to provide reliable test results.

Sample Dilution Procedure: Serum or egg albumin samples may be added directly to the antibody coated plate without dilution. Frozen samples should be completely thawed and thoroughly mixed. Set up samples and controls as shown in Figure 1.

Preparation of Controls: An ALV Positive Control and a Negative Control have been provided with this kit in ready-to-use form. Allow the ALV Positive and Negative Control samples to equilibrate to room temperature.

Note: No dilution of the ALV positive and negative controls is needed.

Preparation of Conjugate Solution: A horseradish peroxidase conjugated rabbit anti-p27 antibody is supplied in 50% glycerol. Dilute 200 µL of the conjugate solution in 10 mL Dilution Buffer (1:50 dilution). Mix well. This 10 mL preparation will supply sufficient conjugate for one 96 well ELISA plate.

Preparation of 1X Wash Solution: Dilute 20 mL concentrated Wash Solution in 380 mL laboratory grade (distilled or R.O.) water (1:20). Mix well. Approximately 400 mL Wash Solution is needed for each 96 well ELISA plate.

Preparation of the Substrate Solution: Determine the total number of plates needed to assay the samples. Each plate will require approximately 10 mL of substrate solution. For example, 10 plates requires 100 mL substrate. For best results, the substrate solution must be equilibrated to room temperature before use.

Preparation of 1X Stop Solution: Dilute 2.5 mL concentrated Stop Solution in 10 mL laboratory

P

grade (distilled or R.O.) water. Mix well. Approximately 10 mL Stop Solution is needed for each 96 well ELISA plate.

Note: Storage of 5X Stop Solution at refrigerated temperatures may cause the formation of a white solid. This does not affect product performance. Warm at room temperature or 37°C to dissolve before use.

Figure 1.

	1	2	3	4	5	6	7	8	9	10	11	12
A	+	-	+	1	2	3	4	5	6	7	8	9
B	10	11	12	13	14	15	16	17	18	19	20	21
C	22	23	24	25	26	27	28	29	30	31	32	33
D	34	35	36	37	38	39	40	41	42	43	44	45
E	46	47	48	49	50	51	52	53	54	55	56	57
F	58	59	60	61	62	63	64	65	66	67	68	69
G	70	71	72	73	74	75	76	77	78	79	80	81
H	82	83	84	85	86	87	88	89	90	-	+	-

ELISA Test Procedure:

Preparing the Test Plate:

a) Remove an anti-p27 antibody coated test plate from the protective bag and label according.

b) Directly add 10 µL Negative Control to wells A2, H10 and H12. Do not dilute. Discard pipette tip.

c) Directly add 100 µL Positive Control to wells A1, A3 and H11. Do not dilute. Discard pipette tip.

d) Add approximately 100 µL unknown sample (or two drops of egg albumin) per well as per Figure 1. Start with well A4 and end with well H9 (moving left to right, row by row of wells). For example, wells 1 through 30 contain the samples of flock 1, wells 31-60 contain the samples of flock 2, etc.

e) Incubate plate for 30 minutes at room temperature.

Wash Procedure:

f) Vigorously tap out liquid from each well into an appropriate decontamination vessel containing bleach or other agent for decontamination.

g) Using an 8 or 12 channel pipette (or comparable automatic washing device), fill each well with approximately 300 µL of 1X Wash Solution. Allow to soak in the wells for 3 minutes; then discard contents into the decontamination vessel. Tap inverted plate to ensure that all residual liquid is removed. Repeat wash procedure 2 more times.

Note: The wash procedure is a very critical step in any ELISA procedure. Please follow the above steps as directed.

Addition of Anti-p27 Peroxidase Conjugate, Substrate, and Stop Solution:

h) Using an 8 or 12 channel pipette (or transplating device) dispense 100 µL diluted conjugate (prepared as described above) into each assay well. Discard pipette tips.

i) Incubate for 30 minutes at room temperature.

j) Wash as in steps f and g above.

k) Using an 8 or 12 channel pipette (or transplating device) dispense 100 µL Substrate Solution into each test well. Discard pipette tips.

l) Incubate 15 minutes at room temperature.

m) Using an 8 or 12 channel pipette (or transplating device) add 100 µL diluted Stop Solution to each test well.

n) Allow bubbles to dissipate before reading plate.

Manual Processing of Data:

a) Read the plate using an ELISA plate reader set at 405-410 nm. Be sure to blank the reader as directed. If a Flow Multiscan reader is used it should be blanked using an empty microtiter plate. If a Bio-tek or Dynatech reader is used, the machine may be blanked with air.

b) Calculate the average Positive Control absorbance [Optical Density (O.D.)] using the absorbance values of wells A1, A3 and H11. Calculate the average Negative Control absorbance using the absorbance values obtained from wells A2, H10 and H12. Record both averages.

c) Subtract the average negative absorbance from the average positive absorbance. The difference is the Corrected Positive Control (CPC).

d) Calculate a sample to positive (Sp) ratio by subtracting the average normal control absorbance from each sample absorbance. The difference is divided by the corrected positive control. Use the following equation format:

$$SP = \frac{\text{(Sample Absorbance)} - \text{(Average Negative Control Absorbance)}}{\text{Corrected Positive Control (CPC) Absorbance}}$$

e) Approximate picogram per mL concentration of p27 antigen per sample can be calculated by the following suggested equation:

$\text{Log [p27] pg/mL} = (1.224 \times \text{Log}_{10}\text{ Sp}) + 3.860$

$\text{[p27] pg/mL} = \text{Antilog of Log}_{10}\text{ p27}$

Example:

1. Example Positive Control Absorbances:
   .585, .610, .590
   Average = (.585 + .610 + .590) / 3 = .595
2. Example Negative Controls:
   .078, .067, .057
   Average = (.078 + .067 + .057) / 3 = .067
3. Corrected Positive Control (CPC):
   (.595) - (.067) = .528
4. Example Sp value calculation:
   Absorbance of sample = .560
   (.560) - (.067) / .528 = .934
5. Example of calculation of [p27] using the Sp value from above.
   $\text{Log}_{10}\text{ [p27] pg/mL} = 1.224 \times (\text{Log}_{10}\ 0.934) + 3.860$
   [p27] pg/mL = Antilog 3.82
   [p27] = 6,607 pg/mL

Test Interpretation:

Assay Control Values: Valid ALV ELISA results are obtained when the average optical density (O.D.) value of the Negative Control is less than 0.250 and the Corrected Positive Control value range is between 0.150 and 1.200. If either of these values are out of range, the ALV test results should be considered invalid and the samples should be retested. Samples testing with an Sp value of less than 0.199 will receive a 0 titer value and are considered negative for p-27 antibody.

Under optimal conditions* the suggested O.D. value ranges of 0.06 to 0.20 for ALV Negative Control and 0.50 to 1.00 for ALV Positive Control should be strived for to ensure the most consistent laboratory test results. Please note that tests with O.D. values which do not fall within the suggested O.D. ranges above does not constitute an invalid test.

*Optimal conditions are at room temperature [70 to 75°F (21 to 24°C)]. Higher room temperatures may result in slightly higher O.D. values.

Interpretation of Results: Sp values reported by this system represent comparisons of the unknown antigen level of the sample to the positive control antigen. Therefore, it is important to first determine that the ALV ELISA positive and negative control values obtained are valid as detailed above in the "Assay Control Values" section of this pamphlet before ALV ELISA results are interpreted.

A "0" ALV ELISA value represents a chicken serum sample that contains an extremely low to insignificant p-27 antigen level compared to the ALV ELISA kit positive and negative controls.

An ALV ELISA value above "0" indicates only that a chicken serum sample contains a significant and ELISA-detectable p-27 level compared to the ALV ELISA kit positive and negative controls. However, these values do not imply or ensure "protection" nor provide serologic differentiation between an ALV vaccine response or an ALV field infection. Note: An Sp value of 0.199 equates to a calculated 1000 picograms p27 antigen per mL by the Lowry Protein Assay[3].

Storage: Store all reagents provided in the kit at 2-10°C.

Caution(s): To the Users of Reagents and Coated Plates:

a) Handle all reagents and samples as biohazardous material.

b) Keep all of the reagents away from your skin and eyes. If exposure should occur, immediately flush affected areas with cold water.

c) Wash solution, control samples, test plates, field samples and all other test kit reagents should be properly decontaminated with bleach or other strong oxidizing agent before disposal.

d) Take special care not to contaminate test reagents.

e) Humidity indicators are supplied with each plate. If any of the indicators exhibit a pink color, the plate may be compromised in some way; decontaminate (i.e. wash the plate with bleach solution) and dispose of the plate.

f) The best results are achieved by following the protocols as they are described above, using safe laboratory techniques.

g) Do not use this kit after the expiration date.

h) Never pipette by mouth.

Allow all reagents to come to room temperature before starting.

References: Available upon request.

Presentation: 900 tests.

Compendium Code No.: 11150200

PROFLOK® BA-T ELISA KIT

Synbiotics **ELISA Test**

Bordetella avium Antibody Test Kit (Turkey)

U.S. Vet. Lic. No.: 350

Reagents:

a) 1 BA-T antigen coated plate.

b) 10 µL BA-T Positive Control Serum.

c) 10 µL Normal Control Serum (NCS).

d) 100 µL Goat anti-Turkey IgG (H+L) Peroxidase Conjugate Solution.

e) 40 mL Dilution Buffer.

f) 10 mL ABTS-Hydrogen Peroxide Substrate Solution.

g) 2.5 mL 5X Stop Solution (dilute [1:5] with laboratory grade water).

h) 20 mL 20X Wash Solution (dilute [1:20] with laboratory grade water).

Equipment and Materials Required:

a) High precision pipette (i.e. 1-20 microliter pipette).

b) 0.2 mL, 1.0 mL and 5.0 mL pipettes.

c) 8 or 12 channel pipette (or transplating device).

d) 2 graduated cylinders (50 mL).

e) 5 mL borosilicate glass test tubes.

f) Uncoated low binding 96 well plates (i.e. Nunc catalog #269620).

g) Laboratory grade (Distilled or R.O.) water.

h) 96 well plate reading spectrophotometer with 405-410 nm filter.

i) Plate washing apparatus.

Indications: The PROFLOK® BA-T ELISA Kit is a rapid serologic test for the detection of BA antibody in turkey serum samples. The BA-T ELISA was developed to aid in the detection of pre and post vaccination BA antibody levels in turkeys and as a presumptive serodiagnosis of BA field infection.

Test Principles: *Bordetella avium* (BA) is the causative agent of bordetellosis which is commonly referred to as turkey coryza.[1] Bordetellosis is a highly contagious disease of the upper respiratory tract of turkeys characterized by abrupt onset of sneezing, oculonasal discharge, stunted growth and predisposition to other infectious disease.[2] High morbidity and low mortality has been reported.[3]

The assay is designed to measure BA antibody bound to BA antigen coated plates. The principle of the test is as follows: Serum obtained from turkeys exposed to *Bordetella avium* contains specific anti-BA antibodies. Serum, diluted in Dilution Buffer, is added to an BA antigen coated plate. Specific BA antibody in the serum forms an antibody-antigen complex with the BA antigen bound to the plate. After washing the plate, an affinity purified goat anti-turkey IgG (H+L) peroxidase conjugate is added to each well. The antibody-antigen complex remaining from the previous step reacts with the conjugate. After a brief incubation period, the unreacted conjugate is removed by a second wash step. Substrate, which contains a chromagen (ABTS), is added to each well. Chromagen color change (from clear to green-blue) occurs in the presence of the peroxidase enzyme. The relative intensity of color developed in 15 minutes (compared to controls) is directly proportional to the level of BA antibody in the serum. After the substrate has incubated, Stop Solution is added to each well to terminate the reaction and the plate is read using an ELISA plate reader at 405-410 nm.

Test Procedure:

Sample Collection: For routine serologic flock monitoring, it is suggested that at least 30 or more sera per flock be randomly collected at standard time intervals (i.e. every four weeks). Proper sample collection procedures, serum harvest and serum sample storage (4°C for up to four days or -20°C for longer periods) are needed to provide reliable test results.

Sample Dilution Procedure: Dilute serum samples using Dilution Buffer in a clean, uncoated 96 well microtiter plate. Set up samples and controls as shown in Figure 1.

Preparation of the Serum Dilution Plate:

a) Add 300 µL Dilution Buffer to each well of an uncoated 96 well microtiter plate. This plate is referred to as the serum dilution plate. Label serum dilution plate.

P

b) Add 6 µL unknown serum per well as per Figure 1 (producing a 1:50 dilution). Start with well A4 and end with well H9 (moving left to right, row by row of wells). For example, wells 1 through 30 contain the diluted sera of flock 1, wells 31-60 contain the diluted sera of flock 2, etc.

c) Add 6 µL of Normal Control Serum (producing a 1:50 dilution) to wells A2, H10 and H12.

d) Aspirate and remove any liquid in dilution plate wells A1, A3 and H11.

e) Allow all diluted serums to equilibrate in Dilution Buffer for 5 minutes before transferring to an BA antigen coated ELISA plate.

f) Diluted serum should be tested within 24 hours.

This dilution format provides adequate quantities of diluted serum samples to conduct four additional ProFLOK® ELISA tests (i.e. MG, MS, MM, NDV or HE) using the same serum dilution plate.

Preparation of Controls: A BA-T Positive Control Serum has been provided with this kit. Dilute the appropriate volume of BA-T Positive Control Serum with Dilution Buffer (1:50) in a clean, glass test tube. For example, dilute 6 µL of Positive Control Serum in 300 µL Dilution Buffer. Mix well. 150 µL of diluted BA-T Positive Control is needed per ELISA plate.

Preparation of Conjugate Solution: The horseradish peroxidase conjugated anti-turkey IgG (H+L) is supplied in 50% glycerol. Dilute 100 µL stock conjugate in 10 mL Dilution Buffer (1:100 dilution). Mix well. This 10 mL preparation will supply sufficient conjugate for one 96 well ELISA plate.

Preparation of 1X Wash Solution: Dilute 20 mL concentrated Wash Solution in 380 mL laboratory grade (distilled or R.O.) water (1:20). Mix well. Approximately 400 mL Wash Solution is needed for each 96 well ELISA plate.

Preparation of the Substrate Solution: The Substrate Solution is ready to use. Each plate will require approximately 10 mL Substrate Solution. For best results, the substrate solution must be equilibrated to room temperature before use.

Preparation of 1X Stop Solution: Dilute 2.5 mL concentrated Stop Solution in 10 mL laboratory grade (distilled or R.O.) water (1:5). Mix well. Approximately 12.5 mL Stop Solution is needed for each 96 well ELISA plate.

Note: Storage of 5X Stop Solution at refrigerated temperatures may cause the formation of a white solid. This does not affect product performance. Warm at room temperature or 37°C to dissolve before use.

Figure 1.

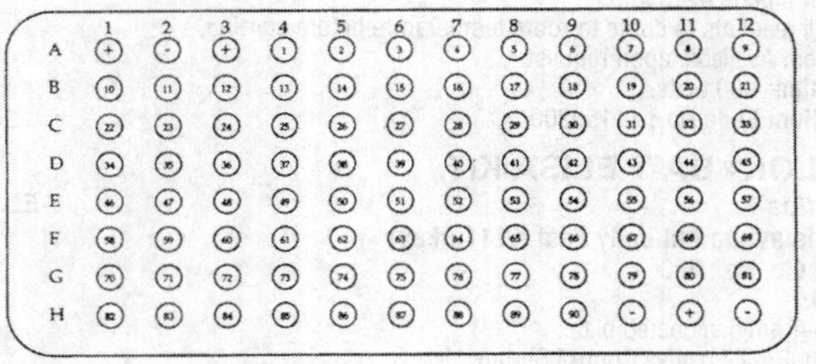

ELISA Test Procedure:

Preparing the Test Plate:

a) Remove a BA antigen coated test plate from the protective bag and label according to serum dilution plate identification.

b) Add 50 µL Dilution Buffer to all wells on the test plate.

c) Add 50 µL diluted Positive Control Serum to wells A1, A3 and H11. Discard pipette tip.

d) Using an 8 or 12 channel pipette transfer 50 µL/well of each of the diluted serum samples and Normal Control Serum samples from the dilution plate to the corresponding wells of the BA coated test plate. Discard pipette tips after each row of sample is transferred. Transfer of samples to the ELISA plate should be done as quickly as possible.

e) Incubate plate for 30 minutes at room temperature.

Wash Procedure:

f) Tap out liquid from each well into an appropriate vessel containing bleach or other decontamination agent.

g) Using an 8 or 12 channel pipette (or comparable automatic washing device), fill each well with approximately 300 µL Wash Solution. Allow to soak in wells for 3 minutes; then discard contents into an appropriate waste container (waste container should contain bleach solution). Tap inverted plate to ensure that all residual liquid is removed. Repeat wash procedure 2 more times.

Note: The wash procedure is a very critical step in any ELISA procedure. Please follow the above steps as directed.

Addition of Anti-Turkey IgG Peroxidase Conjugate, Substrate and Stop Solution:

h) Using an 8 or 12 channel pipette (or transplating device) dispense 100 µL diluted conjugate (prepared as described above) into each assay well. Discard pipette tips.

i) Incubate for 30 minutes at room temperature.

j) Wash as in steps f and g above.

k) Using an 8 or 12 channel pipette (or transplating device) dispense 100 µL Substrate Solution into each test well. Discard pipette tips.

l) Incubate 15 minutes at room temperature.

m) Using an 8 or 12 channel pipette (or transplating device) add 100 µL Stop Solution to each test well.

n) Allow bubbles to dissipate before reading plate.

Manual Processing of Data:

a) Read the plate using an ELISA plate reader set at 405-410 nm. Be sure to blank the reader as directed. If a Flow Multiscan reader is used, the reader should be blanked using an empty microtiter plate. If a Bio-tek or Dynatech reader is used, the machine may be blanked with air.

b) Calculate the average Positive Control Serum absorbance (Optical Density [O.D.]) using the absorbance values of wells A1, A3 and H11. Calculate the average Normal Control Serum absorbance using values obtained from wells A2, H10 and H12. Record both averages.

c) Subtract the average Normal Control absorbance from the average Positive Control absorbance. The difference is the Corrected Positive Control.

d) Calculate a sample to positive (Sp) ratio by subtracting the average Normal Control absorbance from each sample absorbance. The difference is divided by the Corrected Positive Control. Use the following equation format:

$$SP = \frac{\text{(Sample Absorbance)} - \text{(Average Normal Control Absorbance)}}{\text{Corrected Positive Control Absorbance}}$$

e) A BA-T ELISA titer can be calculated by the following suggested equation:

Log_{10} Titer = (1.464 X Log_{10} Sp) + 3.197

Titer = Antilog of Log_{10} Titer

Example:

1. Example Positive Control Absorbance:
   0.585, 0.610, 0.590
   Average = (0.585 + 0.610 + 0.590) / 3 = 0.595
2. Example Normal Control Absorbance:
   0.078, 0.067, 0.057
   Average = (0.078 + 0.067 + 0.057) / 3 = 0.067
3. Corrected Positive Control:
   (0.595) - (0.067) = 0.528
4. Example Sp value calculation:
   Absorbance of sample = 0.560
   (0.560) - (0.067) / 0.528 = 0.934
5. Example of Calculation of titer using the Sp from above:
   Log_{10} Titer = 1.464 X (Log_{10} 0.934) + 3.197
   Titer = Antilog 3.15
   Titer = 1424

Test Interpretation: Results:

Assay Control Values: Valid BA-T ELISA results are obtained when the average optical density (O.D.) value of the Normal Control Serum is less than 0.250 and the Corrected Positive Control value range is between 0.350 and 1.000. If either of these values are out of range, the BA test results should be considered invalid and the samples should be retested. Samples testing with an Sp value of less than or equal to 0.299 will receive a 0 titer value and are considered negative for BA antibody.

Under optimal conditions* the suggested O.D. value ranges of 0.055 to 0.085 for BA Normal Control Serum and 0.400 to 0.800 for BA Positive Control Serum should be strived for to ensure the most consistent laboratory test results.

*Optimal conditions are at room temperature [70 to 75°F (21 to 24°C)]. Higher room temperatures may result in slightly higher O.D. values.

Interpretation of Results: The BA-T ELISA titer values obtained represent a comparison of the BA antibody level within each field turkey serum tested and the BA-T ELISA kit positive and normal control sera. Therefore, it is important to first determine that the BA-T ELISA positive and normal control sera values obtained are valid as detailed above in the "Assay Control Values" section of this pamphlet before BA-T ELISA results are interpreted.

A "0" BA-T ELISA titer represents a turkey serum sample that contains an extremely low to insignificant BA antibody level compared to the BA-T ELISA kit positive and normal control sera.

A BA-T ELISA titer value above "0" indicates only that a turkey serum sample contains a significant and ELISA-detectable BA antibody level compared to the BA-T ELISA kit positive and normal control sera. However, these titers do not imply or ensure "protection" nor provide serologic differentiation between a BA vaccine response or BA field infection.

Optimal BA vaccine administration practices and "protective" flock BA titer target values must be determined by each BA-T ELISA kit user by comparing flock pre- and post-vaccination BA-T ELISA results [i.e. coefficient of variation (%CV) and geometric mean titer (GMT) values] with flock performance parameters (i.e. morbidity, mortality, flock body weight gain or uniformity) over time.

Storage: Store all reagents provided in the kit at 2-10°C.

Caution(s): To the Users of Reagents and BA Antigen Coated Plates:

a) Handle all reagents and samples as biohazardous material.

b) Keep all reagents away from skin and eyes. If exposure should occur, immediately flush affected areas with cold water.

c) Wash solution, control sera, test plates, field samples and all other test kit reagents should be properly decontaminated with bleach or other strong oxidizing agent before disposal.

d) Take special care not to contaminate any of the test reagents with serum or bacterial agents.

e) Humidity indicators are supplied with each plate. If any of the indicators exhibit a pink color, the plate may be compromised in some way; decontaminate (i.e. wash the plate with bleach solution) and dispose of the plate.

f) The best results are achieved by following the protocols as they are described above, using good, safe laboratory techniques.

g) Do not use this kit after the expiration date.

h) Never pipette by mouth.

Allow all reagents to come to room temperature before starting.

References: Available upon request.

Presentation: 900 tests.

Compendium Code No.: 11150210

PROFLOK® CAV ELISA KIT

Synbiotics **ELISA Test**

Chicken Anemia Virus Antibody Test Kit

U.S. Vet. Lic. No.: 350

Reagents: Reagents Required To Perform 90 Tests:

a) 1 CAV antigen coated plate

b) 10 µL CAV Positive Control Serum

c) 10 µL Normal Control Serum

d) 10 mL Goat anti-Chicken IgG (H+L) Biotin Conjugate Solution

e) 100 µL HRP Streptavidin Solution

f) 40 mL Dilution Buffer

g) 10 mL ABTS-Hydrogen Peroxide Substrate Solution

h) 2.5 mL 5X Stop Solution, 5% SDS (dilute [1:5] with laboratory grade water)

i) 15 mL 20X Wash Solution (dilute [1:20] with laboratory grade water)

Equipment and Materials Required but Not Provided:

a) High precision pipette (i.e. 1-20 microliter pipette)

b) 0.2 mL, 1.0 mL and 5.0 mL pipettes

c) 8 or 12 channel pipette (or transplating device) and pipette tips

d) 2 graduated cylinders (50 mL)

e) 1 mL or 5 mL borosilicate glass test tubes

f) Uncoated low binding 96 well plates (i.e. Nunc catalog #269620)

g) Laboratory grade (Distilled or R.O.) water

h) 96 well plate reading spectrophotometer with 405-410 nm filter

i) Plate washing apparatus

j) Waste container with bleach or other oxidizing agent

Indications: The assay is designed to measure CAV antibody bound to CAV antigen coated plates.

Test Principles: Chicken Anemia Virus (CAV) is an etiological agent that can cause serious immunosuppression in young chickens.[1,2] Typically, horizontal transmission to chicks occurs at about 5 weeks of age and comes from the feces of vertically infected birds. Flocks infected through vertical transmission can experience mortality of up to 60% by 23 weeks of age.[3,4] CAV has been shown to produce marked aplastic anemia, subcutaneous and muscular hemorrhages, aplasia of bone marrow, gangrenous dermatitis, and atrophy of all lymphoid organs in susceptible chicks.[1,2]

CAV infection is usually diagnosed by isolating the virus or by detecting serum antibody to CAV by ELISA, IFA, or VN. IFA and VN tests require the continuous passage of the virus which makes them cumbersome for use in large serologic surveys.[4,5,6,7] ELISA does have several distinct advantages over other detection methods. It requires no microscopic examination, it is generally more sensitive than immunofluorescence and it is designed for automated systems. These advantages make it suitable for testing large numbers of serum samples and for investigating the epidemiology of CAV in chickens.[4,5,6,7]

The principle of the test is as follows: Serum obtained from chickens exposed to CAV antigens contains specific anti-CAV antibodies. Serum, diluted in Dilution Buffer, is added to a CAV antigen coated plate. Specific CAV antibody in the serum forms an antibody-antigen complex with the CAV antigen bound to the plate. After washing the plate, an affinity purified goat anti-chicken IgG (H+L) biotin conjugate is added to each well. After a brief incubation period, the unbound biotin conjugate is removed by a second wash step. Next, an HRP-Streptavidin conjugate is added to each well. The HRP-Streptavidin conjugate binds to the biotin labeled antibody-antigen complex remaining from the previous step. After another brief incubation period, the unbound HRP-Streptavidin is removed by a third wash step. Substrate, which contains a chromagen (ABTS), is added to each well. Chromagen color change (from clear to green-blue) occurs in the presence of the peroxidase enzyme. The relative intensity of color developed in 15 minutes (compared to controls) is directly proportional to the level of CAV antibody in the serum. After the substrate has incubated, Stop Solution is added to each well to terminate the reaction and the plate is read using an ELISA plate reader at 405-410 nm.

Test Procedure:

Sample Collection: For routine serologic flock monitoring, it is suggested that at least 30 or more sera per flock be randomly collected at standard time intervals (i.e. every four weeks). Proper sample collection procedures, serum harvest and serum sample storage (4°C for up to four days or -20°C for longer periods) are needed to provide reliable test results. To achieve better specificity and to minimize possible false positive reactions, serum samples that are contaminated with bacteria or are very fatty should be excluded from testing.

Sample Dilution Procedure: Dilute serum samples using Dilution Buffer in a clean, uncoated 96 well microtiter plate. Frozen serum samples should be completely thawed and thoroughly mixed before diluting. Set up samples and controls as shown in Figure 1.

Preparation of the Serum Dilution Plate:

a) Add 300 μL Dilution Buffer to each well of an uncoated 96 well microtiter plate. This plate is referred to as the serum dilution plate.
b) Add 6 μL unknown serum per well as per Figure 1 (producing a 1:50 dilution). Start with well A4 and end with well H9 (moving left to right, row by row of wells). For example, wells 1 through 30 contain the diluted sera of flock 1, wells 31-60 contain the diluted sera of flock 2, etc.
c) Add 6 μL of Normal Control Serum (producing a 1:50 dilution) to wells A2, H10 and H12.
d) Aspirate and remove any liquid in dilution plate wells Al, A3 and H11.
e) Allow all diluted serums to equilibrate in Dilution Buffer for 5 minutes before transferring to a CAV antigen coated ELISA plate.
f) Diluted serum should be tested within 24 hours.

This dilution format provides adequate quantities of diluted serum samples to conduct four additional ProFlok® ELISA tests (i.e. IBD, IBV, NDV and REO) using the same serum dilution plate.

Preparation of CAV Positive Control: A CAV Positive Control Serum has been provided with this kit. Dilute the appropriate volume of CAV Positive Control Serum with Dilution Buffer (1:50) in a clean, glass test tube. For example, dilute 6 μL of positive control serum in 300 μL Dilution Buffer. Mix well. 150 μL of diluted CAV Positive Control is needed per ELISA plate.

Preparation of Biotin Conjugate Solution: The Biotin conjugated anti-chicken IgG (H+L) is supplied in a ready-to-use form. No dilution of the Biotin Conjugate is necessary. Each plate will require approximately 10 mL of Biotin Conjugate Solution.

Preparation of HRP-Streptavidin Solution: Dilute 100 μL of the stock HRP-Streptavidin Solution in 10 mL of Dilution Buffer (1:100 dilution). Mix well. This 10 mL preparation will supply sufficient volume for one CAV ELISA plate.

Preparation of 1X Wash Solution: Dilute 15 mL concentrated Wash Solution in 285 mL laboratory grade (distilled or R.O.) water (1:20). Mix well. Approximately 300 mL Wash Solution is needed for each CAV ELISA plate.

Preparation of the Substrate Solution: The Substrate Solution is ready to use. Each plate will require approximately 10 mL substrate solution. For best results, the substrate solution must be equilibrated to room temperature before use.

Preparation of 1X Stop Solution: Dilute 2.5 mL concentrated Stop Solution in 10 mL laboratory grade (distilled or R.O.) water (1:5). Mix well. Approximately 10 mL Stop Solution is needed for each CAV ELISA plate.

Note: Storage of 5X Stop Solution at refrigerated temperatures causes the formation of a white solid. This does not affect product performance. Warm at room temperature or 37°C to dissolve before use.

Figure 1.

	1	2	3	4	5	6	7	8	9	10	11	12
A	+	-	+	1	2	3	4	5	6	7	8	9
B	10	11	12	13	14	15	16	17	18	19	20	21
C	22	23	24	25	26	27	28	29	30	31	32	33
D	34	35	36	37	38	39	40	41	42	43	44	45
E	46	47	48	49	50	51	52	53	54	55	56	57
F	58	59	60	61	62	63	64	65	66	67	68	69
G	70	71	72	73	74	75	76	77	78	79	80	81
H	82	83	84	85	86	87	88	89	90	-	+	-

ELISA Test Procedure:

Preparing the Test Plate:

a) Remove a CAV antigen coated test plate from the protective bag and label according to serum dilution plate identification.
b) Add 50 μL Dilution Buffer to all wells on the test plate.
c) Add 50 μL diluted CAV Positive Control Serum to wells A1, A3 and H11. Discard pipette tip.
d) Using an 8 or 12 channel pipette transfer 50 μL/well of each of the diluted serum samples and Normal Control Serum samples from the serum dilution plate to the corresponding wells of the CAV coated test plate (yields a 1:100 dilution). Discard pipette tips after each row of sample is transferred. Transfer of samples to the ELISA plate should be done as quickly as possible.
e) Incubate plate for 30 minutes at room temperature.

Wash Procedure:

f) Tap out liquid from each well into an appropriate vessel containing bleach or other decontamination agent.
g) Using an 8 or 12 channel pipette (or comparable automatic washing device), fill each well with approximately 300 μL Wash Solution. Allow to soak in wells for 3 minutes; then discard contents into an appropriate waste container (waste container should contain bleach solution). Tap inverted plate to ensure that all residual liquid is removed. Repeat wash procedure 2 more times.

Note: The wash procedure is a very critical step in any ELISA procedure. Please follow the above steps as directed.

Addition of Anti-Chicken IgG Biotin Conjugate, HRP-Streptavidin, Substrate and Stop Solution:

h) Using an 8 or 12 channel pipette (or transplating device) dispense 100 μL biotin conjugate (prepared as described above) into each assay well. Discard pipette tips.
i) Incubate for 30 minutes at room temperature.
j) Wash as in steps f and g above.
k) Using an 8 or 12 channel pipette (or transplating device) dispense 100 μL diluted HRP-Streptavidin (prepared as described above) into each assay well. Discard pipette tips.
l) Incubate for 30 minutes at room temperature.
m) Wash as in steps f and g above.
n) Using an 8 or 12 channel pipette (or transplating device) dispense 100 μL Substrate Solution into each test well. Discard pipette tips.
o) Incubate 15 minutes at room temperature.
p) Using an 8 or 12 channel pipette (or transplating device) add 100 μL diluted Stop Solution (prepared as described above) to each test well.
q) Allow bubbles to dissipate before reading plate.

Manual Processing of Data:

a) Read the plate using an ELISA plate reader set at 405-410 nm. Be sure to blank the reader as directed.
b) Calculate the average Positive Control Serum absorbance (Optical Density [O.D.]) using the absorbance values of wells A1, A3 and H11. Calculate the average Normal Control Serum absorbance using values obtained from wells A2, H10 and H12. Record both averages.
c) Subtract the average normal control absorbance from the average positive absorbance. The difference is the Corrected Positive Control.
d) Calculate a sample to positive (Sp) ratio by subtracting the average normal control absorbance from each sample absorbance. The difference is divided by the corrected positive control. Use the following equation format:

$$SP = \frac{(\text{Sample Absorbance}) - (\text{Average Negative Control Absorbance})}{\text{Corrected Positive Control (CPC) Absorbance}}$$

e) A CAV ELISA titer can be calculated by the following suggested equation:

$\text{Log}_{10}\ \text{Titer} = (1.009 \text{ X } \text{Log}_{10}\ \text{Sp}) + 3.628$

$\text{Titer} = \text{Antilog of } \text{Log}_{10}\ \text{Titer}$

Example:

1. Example Positive Control Absorbance:
   0.585, 0.610, 0.590
   Average = (0.585 + 0.610 + 0.590) / 3 = 0.595
2. Example Normal Controls:
   0.078, 0.067, 0.057
   Average = (0.078 + 0.067 + 0.057) / 3 = 0.067
3. Corrected Positive Control:
   (0.595) - (0.067) = 0.528
4. Example Sp value calculation:
   Absorbance of sample = 0.560
   (0.560) (0.067) / 0.528 = 0.934
5. Example of Calculation of titer using the Sp from above:
   $\text{Log}_{10}\ \text{Titer} = 1.009 \text{ X } (\text{Log}_{10}\ 0.934) + 3.628$
   Titer = Antilog 3.598
   Titer = 3964

Test Interpretation: Results:

Assay Control Values: Valid CAV ELISA results are obtained when the average optical density (O.D.) value of the Normal Control Serum is less than 0.200 and the Corrected Positive Control value range is between 0.250 and 0.900. If either of these values are out of range, the CAV test results should be considered invalid and the samples should be retested. Samples testing with an Sp value of less than or equal to 0.349 will receive a 0 titer value and are considered nonreactive for CAV antibody.

Under optimal conditions* the suggested O.D. value ranges of 0.075 to 0.150 for CAV Normal Control Serum and 0.400 to 1.00 for CAV Positive Control Serum should be strived for to ensure the most consistent laboratory test results. Please note that tests with O.D. values which do not fall within the suggested O.D. ranges above does not constitute an invalid test.

*Optimal conditions are at room temperature [70 to 75°F (21 to 24°C)]. Higher room temperatures may result in slightly higher OD values.

Interpretation of Results: The CAV ELISA titer values obtained represent a comparison of the CAV antibody level within each field chicken serum tested and the CAV ELISA kit positive and normal control sera. Therefore, it is important to first determine that the CAV ELISA positive and normal control sera values obtained are valid as detailed above in the "Assay Control Values" section before CAV ELISA results are interpreted.

A "0" CAV ELISA titer represents a chicken serum sample that contains an extremely low to insignificant CAV antibody level compared to the CAV ELISA kit positive and normal control sera.

A CAV ELISA titer value above "0" indicates only that a chicken serum sample contains a significant and ELISA-detectable CAV antibody level compared to the CAV ELISA kit positive and normal control sera. However, titers do not imply or ensure "protection" nor provide serologic differentiation between a CAV vaccine response or field infection.

Optimal CAV vaccine administration practices and "protective" flock CAV titer target values must be determined by each CAV ELISA kit user by comparing flock pre- and post-vaccination CAV ELISA results [i.e. coefficient of variation (%CV) and geometric mean titer (GMT) values] with flock performance parameters (i.e. morbidity, mortality, flock body weight gain or uniformity) over time.

Storage: Store all reagents provided in the kit at 2-7°C. Reagents should not be frozen.
Caution(s): To the Users of Reagents and CAV Antigen Coated Plates:

a) Handle all reagents and samples as biohazardous material.
b) Keep all reagents away from skin and eyes. If exposure should occur, immediately flush affected areas with cold water.
c) Wash solution, control sera, test plates, field samples and all other test kit reagents should be properly decontaminated with bleach or other strong oxidizing agent before disposal.
d) Take special care not to contaminate any of the test reagents with serum or bacterial agents.
e) Humidity indicators are supplied with each plate. If any of the indicators exhibit a pink color, the plate may be compromised in some way; decontaminate (i.e. wash the plate with bleach solution) and dispose of the plate.
f) The best results are achieved by following the protocols as they are described, using good, safe laboratory techniques.
g) Do not use this kit after the expiration date.
h) Never pipette by mouth.

Allow all reagents to come to room temperature before starting.
References: Available upon request.
Presentation: 90 test kit.
Compendium Code No.: 11150520 L-277-01

PROFLOK® HEV-T ELISA KIT

Synbiotics **ELISA Test**
Hemorrhagic Enteritis Antibody Test Kit (Turkey)
U.S. Vet. Lic. No.: 350
Reagents:

a) 1 HE-T antigen coated plate.
b) 10 µL HE-T Positive Control Serum.
c) 10 µL Normal Control Serum (NCS).
d) 100 µL Goat anti-Turkey IgG (H+L) Peroxidase Conjugate Solution.
e) 40 mL Dilution Buffer.
f) 10 mL ABTS-Hydrogen Peroxide Substrate System.
g) 2.5 mL 5X Stop Solution (dilute [1:5] with laboratory grade water).
h) 20 mL 20X Wash Solution (dilute [1:20] with laboratory grade water).

Equipment and Materials Required:

a) High precision pipette (i.e. 1-20 microliter pipette).
b) 0.2 mL, 1.0 mL, and 5.0 mL pipettes.
c) 8 or 12 channel pipette (or transplating device).
d) 2 graduated cylinders (50 mL).
e) 5 mL borosilicate glass test tubes.
f) Uncoated low binding 96 well plates (i.e. Nunc Catalog #269620).
g) Laboratory grade (Distilled or R.O.) water.
h) 96 well plate reading spectrophotometer with 405-410 nm filter.
i) Plate washing apparatus.

Indications: The PROFLOK® HEV-T ELISA Kit is a rapid serologic test for the detection of HE antibody in turkey serum samples. It was developed primarily to aid in detection of pre- and post-vaccination HE antibody levels in turkeys.

Test Principles: Hemorrhagic Enteritis is an acute disease of 4-week-old or older turkeys characterized by depression, bloody droppings and variable but often high mortality.[1,3] In addition, HE appears to play a role in triggering or exacerbating colibacillosis or other infections within affected turkey flocks.[2]

The assay is designed to measure HE antibody bound to HE antigen coated plates. The principle of the test is as follows: Serum obtained from turkeys exposed to HE antigens contains specific anti-HE antibodies. Serum, diluted in Dilution Buffer, is added to an HE antigen coated plate. Specific HE antibody in the serum forms an antibody-antigen complex with the HE antigen bound to the plate. After washing the plate, an affinity purified goat anti-turkey IgG (H+L) peroxidase conjugate is added to each well. The antibody-antigen complex remaining from the previous step reacts with the conjugate. After a brief incubation period, the unreacted conjugate is removed by a second wash step. Substrate, which contains a chromagen (ABTS), is added to each well. Chromagen color change (from clear to green-blue) occurs in the presence of the peroxidase enzyme. The relative intensity of color developed in 15 minutes (compared to controls) is directly proportional to the level of HE antibody in the serum. After the substrate has incubated, Stop Solution is added to each well to terminate the reaction and the plate is read using an ELISA plate reader at 405-410 nm.

Test Procedure:

Sample Collection: For routine serologic flock monitoring, it is suggested that at least 30 or more sera per flock be randomly collected at standard time intervals (i.e. every four weeks). Proper sample collection procedures, serum harvest and serum sample storage (4°C for up to four days or -20°C for longer periods) are needed to provide reliable test results.

Sample Dilution Procedure: Dilute serum samples using Dilution Buffer in a clean, uncoated 96 well microtiter plate is recommended. Set up samples and controls as shown in Figure 1.

Preparation of the Serum Dilution Plate:

a) Add 300 µL Dilution Buffer to each well of an uncoated 96 well microtiter plate. This plate is referred to as the serum dilution plate.
b) Add 6 µL unknown serum per well as per Figure 1 (producing a 1:50 dilution). Start with well A4 and end with well H9 (moving left to right, row by row of wells). For example, wells 1 through 30 contain the diluted sera of flock 1, wells 31-60 contain the diluted sera of flock 2, etc.
c) Add 6 µL of Normal Control Serum (producing a 1:50 dilution) to wells A2, H10 and H12.
d) Aspirate and remove any liquid in dilution plate wells A1, A3 and H11.
e) Allow all diluted serums to equilibrate in Dilution Buffer for 5 minutes before transferring to an HE-T antigen coated ELISA plate.
f) Diluted serum should be tested within 24 hours.

This dilution format provides adequate quantities of diluted serum samples to conduct four additional ProFLOK® ELISA tests (i.e. MG, MS, MM and NDV) using the same serum dilution plate.

Preparation of HE-T Positive Control: An HE-T Positive Control Serum has been provided with this kit. Dilute the appropriate volume of HE-T Positive Control Serum with Dilution Buffer (1:50) in a clean, glass tube. For example, dilute 6 µL of positive control serum in 300 µL Dilution Buffer. Mix well. 150 µL of HE-T Positive Control is needed per ELISA plate.

Preparation of Conjugate Solution: The horseradish peroxidase conjugated anti-turkey IgG (H+L) is supplied in 50% glycerol. Dilute 100 µL stock conjugate in 10 mL Dilution Buffer (1:100 dilution). Mix well. This 10 mL preparation will supply sufficient conjugate for one 96 well ELISA plate.

Preparation of 1X Wash Solution: Dilute 20 mL concentrated Wash Solution in 380 mL laboratory grade (distilled or R.O.) water (1:20). Mix well. Approximately 400 mL Wash Solution is needed for each 96 well ELISA plate.

Preparation of the Substrate Solution: The Substrate Solution is ready to use. Each plate will require approximately 10 mL substrate solution. For best results, the substrate solution must be equilibrated to room temperature before use.

Preparation of 1X Stop Solution: Dilute 2.5 mL concentrated Stop Solution in 10 mL laboratory grade (distilled or R.O.) water (1:5). Mix well. Approximately 12.5 mL Stop Solution is needed for each 96 well ELISA plate.

Note: Storage of 5X Stop Solution at refrigerated temperatures may cause the formation of a white solid. This does not affect product performance. Warm at room temperature or 37°C to dissolve before use.

Figure 1.

	1	2	3	4	5	6	7	8	9	10	11	12
A	+	-	+	1	2	3	4	5	6	7	8	9
B	10	11	12	13	14	15	16	17	18	19	20	21
C	22	23	24	25	26	27	28	29	30	31	32	33
D	34	35	36	37	38	39	40	41	42	43	44	45
E	46	47	48	49	50	51	52	53	54	55	56	57
F	58	59	60	61	62	63	64	65	66	67	68	69
G	70	71	72	73	74	75	76	77	78	79	80	81
H	82	83	84	85	86	87	88	89	90	-	+	-

ELISA Test Procedure:
Preparing the Test Plate:

a) Remove an HE-T antigen coated test plate from the protective bag and label according to serum dilution plate identification.
b) Add 50 µL Dilution Buffer to all wells on the test plate.
c) Add 50 µL diluted HE-T Positive Control Serum to wells A1, A3 and H11. Discard pipette tip.
d) Using an 8 or 12 channel pipette, transfer 50 µL/well of each of the diluted serum samples and Normal Control Serum samples from the dilution plate to the corresponding wells of the HE-T antigen test plate. Discard pipette tips after each row of sample is transferred. Transfer of samples to the ELISA plate should be done as quickly as possible.
e) Incubate plate for 30 minutes at room temperature.

Wash Procedure:

f) Tap out liquid from each well into an appropriate decontamination vessel containing bleach or other decontamination agent.
g) Using an 8 or 12 channel pipette (or comparable automatic washing device), fill each well with approximately 300 µL Wash Solution. Allow to soak in the wells for 3 minutes; then discard contents into an appropriate waste container (waste container should contain bleach solution). Tap inverted plate to ensure that all residual liquid is removed. Repeat wash procedure 2 more times.

Note: The wash procedure is a very critical step in any ELISA procedure. Please follow the above steps as directed.

Addition of Anti-Turkey IgG Peroxidase Conjugate, Substrate and Stop Solution:

h) Using an 8 or 12 channel pipette (or transplating device) dispense 100 µL diluted conjugate (prepared as described above) into each assay well. Discard pipette tips.
i) Incubate for 30 minutes at room temperature.
j) Wash as in steps f and g above.
k) Using an 8 or 12 channel pipette (or transplating device) dispense 100 µL Substrate Solution into each test well. Discard pipette tips.
l) Incubate 15 minutes at room temperature.
m) Using an 8 or 12 channel pipette (or transplating device) add 100 µL Stop Solution to each test well.
n) Allow bubbles to dissipate before reading plate.

Manual Processing of Data:

a) Read the plate using an ELISA plate reader set at 405-410 nm. Be sure to blank the reader as directed. If a Flow Multiscan reader is used, the reader should be blanked using an empty microtiter plate. If a Bio-tek or Dynatech reader is used, the machine may be blanked with air.
b) Calculate the average Positive Control Serum absorbance [Optical Density (O.D.)] using the absorbance values of wells A1, A3 and H11. Calculate the average Normal Control Serum absorbance using values obtained from wells A2, H10 and H12. Record both averages.
c) Subtract the average normal control absorbance from the average positive absorbance. The difference is the Corrected Positive Control.
d) Calculate a sample to positive (Sp) ratio by subtracting the average negative control absorbance from each sample absorbance. The difference is divided by the corrected positive control. Use the following equation format:

$$SP = \frac{\text{(Sample Absorbance)} - \text{(Avg. Normal Control Absorbance)}}{\text{Corrected Positive Control Absorbance}}$$

e) An HE-T ELISA titer can be calculated by the following suggested equation:

$\text{Log}_{10}\text{ Titer} = (1.464 \text{ X Log}_{10}\text{ Sp}) + 3.197$
Titer = Antilog of Log_{10} Titer

Example:

1. Example Positive Control Absorbances:
   0.585, 0.610, 0.590
   Average = (0.585 + 0.610 + 0.590) / 3 = 0.595
2. Example Normal Control Absorbance:
   0.078, 0.067, 0.057
   Average = (0.078 + 0.067 + 0.057) / 3 = 0.067
3. Corrected Positive Control:
   (0.595) - (0.067) = 0.528
4. Example Sp value calculation:
   (0.560) - (0.067) / 0.528 = 0.934
5. Example of calculation of titer using the Sp from above:
   $\text{Log}_{10}\text{ Titer} = 1.464 \text{ X } (\text{Log}_{10}\text{ } 0.934) + 3.197$
   Titer = Antilog 3.154
   Titer = 1424

Test Interpretation: Results:

Assay Control Values: Valid HE-T ELISA results are obtained when the average optical density (O.D.) value of the Normal Control Serum is less than 0.200 and the Corrected Positive Control value range is between 0.250 and 0.900. If either of these values are out of range, the HE-T test results should be considered invalid and the samples should be retested. Samples testing with an Sp value of less than or equal to 0.200 will receive a 0 titer value and are considered negative for HE antibody.

Under optimal conditions* the suggested OD value ranges of 0.070 to 0.160 for HE Normal Control Serum and 0.350 to 0.850 for HE Positive Control Serum should be strived for to ensure the most consistent laboratory test results. Please note that tests with O.D. values which do not fall within the suggested O.D. ranges above does not constitute an invalid test.

*Optimal conditions are at room temperature [70 to 75°F (21 to 24°C)]. Higher room temperatures may result in slightly higher OD values.

Interpretation of Results: The HE-T ELISA titer values obtained represent a comparison of the HE antibody level within each field turkey serum tested and the HE-T ELISA kit positive and normal control sera. Therefore, it is important to first determine that the HE-T ELISA positive and normal control sera values obtained are valid as detailed above in the "Assay Control Values" section of this pamphlet before HE-T ELISA results are interpreted.

A "0" HE-T ELISA titer represents a turkey serum sample that contains an extremely low to insignificant HE-T antibody level compared to the HE-T ELISA kit positive and normal control sera.

An HE-T ELISA titer value above "0" indicates only that a turkey serum sample contains a significant and ELISA-detectable HE antibody level compared to the HE-T ELISA kit positive and normal control sera. However, these titers do not imply or ensure "protection" nor provide serologic differentiation between an HE vaccine virus response or HE field virus infection.

Optimal HE vaccine administration practices and "protective" flock HE-T titer target values must be determined by each HE-T ELISA kit user by comparing flock pre- and post-vaccination HE-T ELISA results [i.e. coefficient of variation (%CV) and geometric mean titer (GMT) values] with flock performance parameters (i.e. morbidity, mortality, flock body weight gain or uniformity) over time.

Storage: Store all reagents provided in the kit at 2-7°C.

Caution(s): To the Users of Reagents and HE Antigen Coated Plates:

a) Handle all reagents and samples as biohazardous material.
b) Keep all the reagents away from skin and eyes. If exposure should occur, immediately flush affected areas with cold water.
c) Wash solution, control sera, test plates, field samples and all other test kit reagents should be properly decontaminated with bleach or other strong oxidizing agent before disposal.
d) Take special care not to contaminate test reagents with serum or bacterial agents.
e) Humidity indicators are supplied with each plate. If any of the indicators exhibit a pink color, the plate may be compromised in some way; decontaminate (i.e. wash the plate with bleach solution) and dispose of the plate.
f) The best results are achieved by following the protocols as they are described above, using good, safe laboratory techniques.
g) Do not use this kit after the expiration date.
h) Never pipette by mouth.

Allow all reagents to come to room temperature before starting.

References: Available upon request.

Presentation: 900 tests.

Compendium Code No.: 11150221

PROFLOK® IBD ELISA KIT

Synbiotics **ELISA Test**

Infectious Bursal Disease Antibody Test Kit

U.S. Vet. Lic. No.: 350

Reagents:

a) 1 IBD antigen coated plate.
b) 10 µL IBD Positive Control Serum.
c) 10 µL Normal Control Serum.
d) 100 µL Goat anti-Chicken IgG (H+L) Peroxidase Conjugate Solution.
e) 40 mL Dilution Buffer.
f) 10 mL ABTS-Hydrogen Peroxide Substrate Solution.
g) 2.5 mL 5X Stop Solution (dilute [1:5] with laboratory grade water).
h) 20 mL 20X Wash Solution (dilute [1:20] with laboratory grade water).

Equipment and Materials Required:

a) High precision pipette (i.e. 1-20 microliter pipette).
b) 0.2 mL, 1.0 mL and 5.0 mL pipettes.
c) 8 or 12 channel pipette (or transplating device).
d) 2 graduated cylinders (50 mL).
e) 1 mL and 5 mL borosilicate glass test tubes.
f) Uncoated low binding 96 well plates (i.e. Nunc catalog #269620).
g) Laboratory grade (Distilled or R.O.) water.
h) 96 well plate reading spectrophotometer with 405-410 nm filter.
i) Plate washing apparatus.

Indications: The PROFLOK® IBD ELISA Kit is a rapid serologic test for the detection of IBD antibody in chicken serum samples. It was developed primarily to aid in the detection of pre- and post-vaccination IBD antibody levels in chickens.

Test Principles: Infectious Bursal Disease (IBD) was first described by Cosgrove in 1962.[1] IBD is one of the most economically important diseases that affects commercial chickens. High levels of maternal antibody against IBD, passed from the hen to the chick, provide young chickens with passive protection against field varieties of IBD. Antibody against IBD in hen or chick sera has previously been measured by the enzyme linked immunoassay (ELISA).[2]

The assay is designed to measure IBD antibody bound to IBD antigen coated plates. The principle of the test is as follows: Serum obtained from chickens exposed to IBD antigens contains specific anti-IBD antibodies. Serum, diluted in Dilution Buffer, is added to an IBD antigen coated plate. Specific IBD antibody in the serum forms an antibody-antigen complex with the IBD antigen bound to the plate. After washing the plate, an affinity purified goat anti-chicken IgG (H+L) peroxidase conjugate is added to each well. The antibody-antigen complex remaining from the previous step binds with the conjugate. After a brief incubation period, the unbound conjugate is removed by a second wash step. Substrate, which contains a chromagen (ABTS), is added to each well. Chromagen color change (from clear to green-blue) occurs in the presence of the peroxidase enzyme. The relative intensity of color developed in 15 minutes (compared to controls) is directly proportional to the level of IBD antibody in the serum. After the substrate has incubated, Stop Solution is added to each well to terminate the reaction and the plate is read using an ELISA plate reader at 405-410 nm.

Test Procedure:

Sample Collection: For routine serologic flock monitoring, it is suggested that at least 30 or more sera per flock be randomly collected at standard time intervals (i.e. every four weeks). Proper sample collection procedures, serum harvest and serum sample storage (4°C for up to four days or -20°C for longer periods) are needed to provide reliable test results.

Sample Dilution Procedure: Dilute serum samples using Dilution Buffer in a clean, uncoated 96 well microtiter plate. Set up samples and controls as shown in Figure 1.

Preparation of the Serum Dilution Plate:

a) Add 300 µL Dilution Buffer to each well of an uncoated 96 well microtiter plate. This plate is referred to as the serum dilution plate.
b) Add 6 µL unknown serum per well as per Figure 1 (producing a 1:50 dilution). Start with well A4 and end with well H9 (moving left to right, row by row of wells). For example, wells 1 through 30 contain the diluted sera of flock 1, wells 31-60 contain the diluted sera of flock 2, etc.
c) Add 6 µL of Normal Control Serum (producing a 1:50 dilution) to wells A2, H10 and H12.
d) Aspirate and remove any liquid in dilution plate wells A1, A3 and H11.
e) Allow all diluted serums to equilibrate in Dilution Buffer for 5 minutes before transferring to an IBD antigen coated ELISA plate.
f) Diluted serum should be tested within 24 hours.

This dilution format provides adequate quantities of diluted serum samples to conduct four additional ProFLOK® ELISA tests (i.e. REO, NDV, IBV, and ILT) using the same serum dilution plate.

Preparation of IBD Positive Control: An IBD Positive Control Serum has been provided with this kit. Dilute the appropriate volume of IBD Positive Control Serum with Dilution Buffer (1:50) in a clean, glass test tube. For example, dilute 6 µL of positive control serum in 300 µL Dilution Buffer. Mix well. 150 µL of IBD Positive Control is needed per ELISA plate.

Preparation of Conjugate Solution: The horseradish peroxidase conjugated anti-chicken IgG (H+L) is supplied in 50% glycerol. Dilute 100 µL stock conjugate in 10 mL Dilution Buffer (1:100 dilution). Mix well. This 10 mL preparation will supply sufficient conjugate for one 96 well ELISA plate.

Preparation of 1X Wash Solution: Dilute 20 mL concentrated Wash Solution in 380 mL laboratory grade (distilled or R.O.) water (1:20). Mix well. Approximately 400 mL Wash Solution is needed for each 96 well ELISA plate.

Preparation of the Substrate Solution: The Substrate Solution is ready to use. Each plate will require approximately 10 mL substrate solution. For best results, the substrate solution must be equilibrated to room temperature before use.

Preparation of 1X Stop Solution: Dilute 2.5 mL concentrated Stop Solution in 10 mL laboratory grade (distilled or R.O.) water (1:5). Mix well. Approximately 12.5 mL Stop Solution is needed for each 96 well ELISA plate.

Note: Storage of 5X Stop Solution at refrigerated temperatures may cause the formation of a white solid. This does not affect product performance. Warm at room temperature or 37°C to dissolve before use.

Figure 1.

	1	2	3	4	5	6	7	8	9	10	11	12
A	+	-	+	1	2	3	4	5	6	7	8	9
B	10	11	12	13	14	15	16	17	18	19	20	21
C	22	23	24	25	26	27	28	29	30	31	32	33
D	34	35	36	37	38	39	40	41	42	43	44	45
E	46	47	48	49	50	51	52	53	54	55	56	57
F	58	59	60	61	62	63	64	65	66	67	68	69
G	70	71	72	73	74	75	76	77	78	79	80	81
H	82	83	84	85	86	87	88	89	90	-	+	-

ELISA Test Procedure:

Preparing the Test Plate:

a) Remove an IBD antigen coated test plate from the protective bag and label according to dilution plate identification.
b) Add 50 µL Dilution Buffer to all wells on the test plate.
c) Add 50 µL diluted Positive Control Serum to wells A1, A3 and H11. Discard pipette tip.
d) Using an 8 or 12 channel pipette transfer 50 µL/well of each of the diluted serum samples and Normal Control Serum samples from the dilution plate to the corresponding wells of the IBD coated test plate. Discard pipette tips after each row of sample is transferred. Transfer of samples to the ELISA plate should be done as quickly as possible.
e) Incubate plate for 30 minutes at room temperature.

Wash Procedure:

f) Tap out liquid from each well into an appropriate vessel containing bleach or other decontamination agent.
g) Using an 8 or 12 channel pipette (or comparable automatic washing device), fill each well with approximately 300 µL Wash Solution. Allow to soak in wells for 3 minutes; then discard contents into an appropriate waste container (waste container should contain bleach solution). Tap inverted plate to ensure that all residual liquid is removed. Repeat wash procedure 2 more times.

Note: The wash procedure is a very critical step in any ELISA procedure. Please follow the above steps as directed.

Addition of Anti-Chicken IgG Peroxidase Conjugate, Substrate and Stop Solution:

h) Using an 8 or 12 channel pipette (or transplating device) dispense 100 µL diluted conjugate (prepared as described above) into each assay well. Discard pipette tips.
i) Incubate for 30 minutes at room temperature.
j) Wash as in steps f and g above.
k) Using an 8 or 12 channel pipette (or transplating device) dispense 100 µL Substrate Solution into each test well. Discard pipette tips.
l) Incubate 15 minutes at room temperature.
m) Using an 8 or 12 channel pipette (or transplating device) add 100 µL diluted Stop Solution (prepared as described above) to each test well.
n) Allow bubbles to dissipate before reading plate.

Manual Processing of Data:

a) Read the plate using an ELISA plate reader set at 405-410 nm. Be sure to blank the reader as directed. If a Flow Multiscan reader is used, the reader should be blanked using an empty microtiter plate. If a Bio-tek or Dynatech reader is used, the machine may be blanked with air.

b) Calculate the average Positive Control Serum absorbance (Optical Density [O.D.]) using the absorbance values of wells A1, A3 and H11. Calculate the average Normal Control Serum absorbance using values obtained from wells A2, H10 and H12. Record both averages.

c) Subtract the average normal control absorbance from the average positive absorbance. The difference is the Corrected Positive Control.

d) Calculate a sample to positive (Sp) ratio by subtracting the average normal control absorbance from each sample absorbance. The difference is divided by the corrected positive control. Use the following equation format:

$$SP = \frac{\text{(Sample Absorbance)} - \text{(Avg Normal Control Absorbance)}}{\text{Corrected Positive Control Absorbance}}$$

e) An IBD ELISA titer can be calculated by the following suggested equation:

Log_{10} Titer = (1.172 X Log_{10} Sp) + 3.614

Titer = Antilog of Log_{10} Titer

Example:

1. Example Positive Control Absorbance:
   0.585, 0.610, 0.590
   Average = (0.585 + 0.610 + 0.590) / 3 = 0.595
2. Example Normal Controls:
   0.110, 0.102, 0.112
   Average = (0.110 + 0.102 + 0.112) / 3 = 0.108
3. Corrected Positive Control:
   (0.595) - (0.108) = 0.487
4. Example Sp value calculation:
   Absorbance of sample = 0.560
   (0.560) - (0.108) / 0.487 = 0.928
5. Example of Calculation of titer using the Sp from above:
   Log_{10} Titer = 1.172 X (Log_{10} 0.928) + 3.614
   Titer = Antilog 3.57
   Titer = 3767

Test Interpretation: Results:

Assay Control Values: Valid IBD ELISA results are obtained when the average optical density (O.D.) value of the Normal Control Serum is less than 0.250 and the Corrected Positive Control value range is between 0.250 and 0.900. If either of these values are out of range, the IBD test results should be considered invalid and the samples should be retested. Samples testing with an Sp value of less than or equal to 0.180 will receive a 0 titer value and are considered negative for IBD antibody.

Under optimal conditions*, the suggested O.D. value ranges of 0.100 to 0.160 for IBD Normal Control Serum and 0.400 to 0.850 for IBD Positive Control Serum should be strived for to ensure the most consistent laboratory test results. Please note that tests with O.D. values which do not fall within the suggested O.D. ranges above does not constitute an invalid test.

*Optimal conditions are at room temperature [70 to 75°F (21 to 24°C)]. Higher room temperatures may result in slightly higher OD values.

Interpretation of Results: The IBD ELISA titer values obtained represent a comparison of the IBD antibody level within each field chicken serum tested and the IBD ELISA kit positive and normal control sera. Therefore, it is important to first determine that the IBD ELISA positive and normal control sera values obtained are valid as detailed above in the "Assay Control Values" section of this pamphlet before IBD ELISA results are interpreted.

A "0" IBD ELISA titer represents a chicken serum sample that contains an extremely low to insignificant IBD antibody level compared to the IBD ELISA kit positive and normal control sera.

An IBD ELISA titer value above "0" indicates only that a chicken serum sample contains a significant and ELISA-detectable IBD antibody level compared to the IBD ELISA kit positive and normal control sera. However, these titers do not imply or ensure "protection" nor provide serologic differentiation between an IBD vaccine virus response or IBD field virus infection.

Optimal IBD vaccine administration practices and "protective" flock IBD titer target values must be determined by each IBD ELISA kit user by comparing flock pre- and post-vaccination IBD ELISA results [i.e. coefficient of variation (%CV) and geometric titer (GMT) values] with flock performance parameters (i.e. morbidity, mortality, flock body weight gain or uniformity) over time.

Storage: Store all reagents provided in the kit at 2-10°C.

Caution(s): To the Users of Reagents and IBD Antigen Coated Plates:

a) Handle all reagents and samples as biohazardous material.

b) Keep all reagents away from skin and eyes. If exposure should occur, immediately flush affected areas with cold water.

c) Wash solution, control sera, test plates, field samples and all other test kit reagents should be properly decontaminated with bleach or other strong oxidizing agent before disposal.

d) Take special care not to contaminate any of the test reagents with serum or bacterial agents.

e) Humidity indicators are supplied with each plate. If any of the indicators exhibit a pink color, the plate may be compromised in some way; decontaminate (i.e. wash the plate with bleach solution) and dispose of the plate.

f) The best results are achieved by following the protocols as they are described above, using good, safe laboratory techniques.

g) Do not use this kit after the expiration date.

h) Never pipette by mouth.

Allow all reagents to come to room temperature before starting.

References: Available upon request.

Presentation: 900 tests.

Compendium Code No.: 11150230

PROFLOK® IBV ELISA KIT

Synbiotics **ELISA Test**

Infectious Bronchitis Virus Antibody Test Kit

U.S. Vet. Lic. No.: 350

Reagents:

a) 1 IBV antigen coated plate.

b) 10 µL IBV Positive Control Serum.

c) 10 µL Normal Control Serum (NCS).

d) 100 µL Goat anti-Chicken IgG (H+L) Peroxidase Conjugate Solution.

e) 40 mL Dilution Buffer.

f) 10 mL ABTS-Hydrogen Peroxide Substrate Solution.

g) 2.5 mL 5X Stop Solution (dilute [1:5] with laboratory grade water).

h) 20 mL 20X Wash Solution (dilute [1:20] with laboratory grade water).

Equipment and Materials Required:

a) High precision pipette (i.e. 1-20 microliter pipette).

b) 0.2 mL, 1.0 mL and 5.0 mL pipettes.

c) 8 or 12 channel pipette (or transplating device).

d) 2 graduated cylinders (50 mL).

e) 5 mL borosilicate glass test tubes.

f) Uncoated low binding 96 well plates (i.e. Nunc catalog #269620).

g) Laboratory grade (Distilled or R.O.) water.

h) 96 well plate reading spectrophotometer with 405-410 nm filter.

i) Plate washing apparatus.

Indications: The PROFLOK® IBV ELISA Kit is a rapid serologic test for the detection of IBV antibody in chicken serum samples. It was developed primarily to aid in the detection of pre- and post-vaccination IBV antibody levels in chickens.

Test Principles: Infectious Bronchitis Disease (IBV) produces a highly contagious disease in chickens. The disease has been associated with respiratory infections (in young chickens), nephrosis, and loss of egg production and egg quality (in layers).[1]

The assay is designed to measure IBV antibody bound to IBV antigen coated plates. The principle of the test is as follows: Serum obtained from chickens exposed to IBV antigens contains specific anti-IBV antibodies. Serum, diluted in Dilution Buffer, is added to an IBV antigen coated plate. Specific IBV antibody in the serum forms an antibody-antigen complex with the IBV antigen bound to the plate. After washing the plate, an affinity purified goat anti-chicken IgG (H+L) peroxidase conjugate is added to each well. The antibody-antigen complex remaining from the previous step binds with the conjugate. After a brief incubation period, the unbound conjugate is removed by a second wash step. Substrate, which contains a chromagen (ABTS), is added to each well. Chromagen color change (from clear to green-blue) occurs in the presence of the peroxidase enzyme. The relative intensity of color developed in 15 minutes (compared to controls) is directly proportional to the level of IBV antibody in the serum. After the substrate has incubated, Stop Solution is added to each well to terminate the reaction and the plate is read using an ELISA plate reader at 405-410 nm.

Test Procedure:

Sample Collection: For routine serologic flock monitoring, it is suggested that at least 30 or more sera per flock be randomly collected at standard time intervals (i.e. every four weeks). Proper sample collection procedures, serum harvest and serum sample storage (4°C for up to four days or -20°C for longer periods) are needed to provide reliable test results.

Sample Dilution Procedure: Dilute serum samples using Dilution Buffer in a clean, uncoated 96 well microtiter plate. Set up samples and controls as shown in Figure 1.

Preparation of the Serum Dilution Plate:

a) Add 300 µL Dilution Buffer to each well of an uncoated 96 well microtiter plate. This plate is referred to as the serum dilution plate.

b) Add 6 µL unknown serum per well as per Figure 1 (producing a 1:50 dilution). Start with well A4 and end with well H9 (moving left to right, row by row of wells). For example, wells 1 through 30 contain the diluted sera of flock 1, wells 31-60 contain the diluted sera of flock 2, etc.

c) Add 6 µL of Normal Control Serum (producing a 1:50 dilution) to wells A2, H10 and H12.

d) Aspirate and remove any liquid in dilution plate wells A1, A3 and H11.

e) Allow all diluted serums to equilibrate in Dilution Buffer for 5 minutes before transferring to an IBV antigen coated ELISA plate.

f) Diluted serum should be tested within 24 hours.

This dilution format provides adequate quantities of diluted serum samples to conduct four additional ProFLOK® ELISA tests (i.e. REO, NDV, IBD and ILT) using the same serum dilution plate.

Preparation of IBV Positive Control: An IBV Positive Control Serum has been provided with this kit. Dilute the appropriate volume of IBV Positive Control Serum with Dilution Buffer (1:50) in a clean, glass test tube. For example, dilute 6 µL of Positive Control serum in 300 µL Dilution Buffer. Mix well. 150 µL of IBV Positive Control is needed per ELISA plate.

Preparation of Conjugate Solution: The horseradish peroxidase conjugated anti-chicken IgG (H+L) is supplied in 50% glycerol. Dilute 100 µL stock conjugate in 10 mL Dilution Buffer (1:100 dilution). Mix well. This 10 mL preparation will supply sufficient conjugate for one 96 well ELISA plate.

Preparation of 1X Wash Solution: Dilute 20 mL concentrated Wash Solution in 380 mL laboratory grade (distilled or R.O.) water (1:20). Mix well. Approximately 400 mL Wash Solution is needed for each 96 well ELISA plate.

Preparation of the Substrate Solution: The Substrate Solution is ready to use. Each plate will require approximately 10 mL substrate solution. For best results, the substrate solution must be equilibrated to room temperature before use.

Preparation of 1X Stop Solution: Dilute 2.5 mL concentrated Stop Solution in 10 mL laboratory grade (distilled or R.O.) water (1:5). Mix well. Approximately 12.5 mL Stop Solution is needed for each 96 well ELISA plate.

Note: Storage of 5X Stop Solution at refrigerated temperatures may cause the formation of a white solid. This does not affect product performance. Warm at room temperature or 37°C to dissolve before use.

Figure 1.

	1	2	3	4	5	6	7	8	9	10	11	12
A	+	-	+	1	2	3	4	5	6	7	8	9
B	10	11	12	13	14	15	16	17	18	19	20	21
C	22	23	24	25	26	27	28	29	30	31	32	33
D	34	35	36	37	38	39	40	41	42	43	44	45
E	46	47	48	49	50	51	52	53	54	55	56	57
F	58	59	60	61	62	63	64	65	66	67	68	69
G	70	71	72	73	74	75	76	77	78	79	80	81
H	82	83	84	85	86	87	88	89	90	-	+	-

ELISA Test Procedure:

Preparing the Test Plate:

a) Remove an IBV antigen coated test plate from the protective bag and label according to dilution plate identification.

b) Add 50 µL Dilution Buffer to all wells on the test plate.

c) Add 50 µL diluted IBV Positive Control Serum to wells A1, A3 and H11. Discard pipette tip.

d) Using an 8 or 12 channel pipette transfer 50 µL/well of each of the diluted serum samples and Normal Control Serum samples from the dilution plate to the corresponding wells of the IBV coated test plate. Discard pipette tips after each row of sample is transferred. Transfer of samples to the ELISA plate should be done as quickly as possible.

e) Incubate plate for 30 minutes at room temperature.

Wash Procedure:

f) Tap out liquid from each well into an appropriate vessel containing bleach or other decontamination agent.

g) Using an 8 or 12 channel pipette (or comparable automatic washing device), fill each well with approximately 300 µL Wash Solution. Allow to soak in wells for 3 minutes; then discard contents into an appropriate waste container (waste container should contain bleach solution). Tap inverted plate to ensure that all residual liquid is removed. Repeat wash procedure 2 more times.

Note: The wash procedure is a very critical step in any ELISA procedure. Please follow the above steps as directed.

Addition of Anti-Chicken IgG Peroxidase Conjugate, Substrate and Stop Solution:

h) Using an 8 or 12 channel pipette (or transplating device) dispense 100 µL diluted conjugate (prepared as described above) into each assay well. Discard pipette tips.

i) Incubate for 30 minutes at room temperature.

j) Wash as in steps f and g above.

k) Using an 8 or 12 channel pipette (or transplating device) dispense 100 µL Substrate Solution into each test well. Discard pipette tips.

l) Incubate 15 minutes at room temperature.

m) Using an 8 or 12 channel pipette (or transplating device) add 100 µL diluted Stop Solution (prepared as described above) to each test well.

n) Allow bubbles to dissipate before reading plate.

Manual Processing of Data:

a) Read the plate using an ELISA plate reader set at 405-410 nm. Be sure to blank the reader as directed. If a Flow Multiscan reader is used, the reader should be blanked using an empty microtiter plate. If a Bio-tek or Dynatech reader is used, the machine may be blanked with air.

b) Calculate the average Positive Control Serum absorbance (Optical Density [O.D.]) using the absorbance values of wells A1, A3 and H11. Calculate the average Normal Control Serum absorbance using values obtained from wells A2, H10 and H12. Record both averages.

c) Subtract the average normal control absorbance from the average positive absorbance. The difference is the Corrected Positive Control.

d) Calculate a sample to positive (Sp) ratio by subtracting the average normal control absorbance from each sample absorbance. The difference is divided by the corrected positive control. Use the following equation format:

$$SP = \frac{\text{(Sample Absorbance)} - \text{(Average Normal Control Absorbance)}}{\text{Corrected Positive Control Absorbance}}$$

e) An IBV ELISA titer can be calculated by the following suggested equation:

Log_{10} Titer = (1.642 X Log_{10} Sp) + 3.568

Titer = Antilog of Log_{10} Titer

Example:

1. Example Positive Control Absorbance:
   0.585, 0.610, 0.590
   Average = (0.585 + 0.610 + 0.590) / 3 = 0.595
2. Example Normal Controls:
   0.110, 0.102, 0.112
   Average = (0.110 + 0.102 + 0.112) / 3 = 0.108
3. Corrected Positive Control:
   (0.595) - (0.108) = 0.487
4. Example Sp value calculation:
   Absorbance of sample = 0.560
   (0.560) - (0.108) / 0.487 = 0.928
5. Example of Calculation of titer using the Sp from above:
   Log_{10} Titer = 1.642 X (Log_{10} 0.928) + 3.568
   Titer = Antilog 3.51
   Titer = 3271

Test Interpretation: Results:

Assay Control Values: Valid IBV ELISA results are obtained when the average optical density (O.D.) value of the Normal Control Serum is less than 0.250 and the Corrected Positive Control value range is between 0.250 and 0.900. If either of these values are out of range, the IBV test results should be considered invalid and the samples should be retested. Samples testing with an Sp value of less than or equal to 0.150 will receive a 0 titer value and are considered negative for IBV antibody.

Under optimal conditions*, the suggested O.D. value ranges of 0.080 to 0.150 for IBV Normal Control Serum and 0.400 to 0.850 for IBV Positive Control Serum should be strived for to ensure the most consistent laboratory test results. Please note that a plate with O.D. values which do not fall within the suggested O.D. ranges above does not constitute an invalid test.

*Optimal conditions are at room temperature [70 to 75°F (21 to 24°C)]. Higher room temperatures may result in slightly higher O.D. values.

Interpretation of Results: The IBV ELISA titer values obtained represent a comparison of the IBV antibody level within each field chicken serum tested and the IBV ELISA kit positive and normal control sera. Therefore, it is important to first determine that the IBV ELISA positive and normal control sera values obtained are valid as detailed above in the "Assay Control Values" section of this pamphlet before IBV ELISA results are interpreted.

A "0" IBV ELISA titer represents a chicken serum sample that contains an extremely low to insignificant IBV antibody level compared to the IBV ELISA kit positive and normal control sera. Non-specific absorbance will vary from test to test and may interfere with sensitivity if it is too high (above 0.250). Birds receiving agents other than IBV, in oil emulsions may exhibit low level titers to IBV (i.e. titers <600).

An IBV ELISA titer value above "0" indicates only that a chicken serum sample contains a significant and ELISA-detectable IBV antibody level compared to the IBV ELISA kit positive and normal control sera. However, these titers do not imply or ensure "protection" nor provide serologic differentiation between an IBV vaccine virus response or IBV field infection.

Optimal IBV vaccine administration practices and "protective" flock IBV titer target values must be determined by each IBV ELISA kit user by comparing flock pre- and post-vaccination IBV ELISA results [i.e. coefficient of variation (%CV) and geometric titer (GMT) values] with flock performance parameters (i.e. morbidity, mortality, flock body weight gain or uniformity) over time.

Storage: Store all reagents provided in the kit at 2-10°C.

Caution(s): To the Users of Reagents and IBV Antigen Coated Plates:

a) Handle all reagents and samples as biohazardous material.

b) Keep all reagents away from skin and eyes. If exposure should occur, immediately flush affected areas with cold water.

c) Wash solution, control sera, test plates, field samples and all other test kit reagents should be properly decontaminated with bleach or other strong oxidizing agent before disposal.

d) Take special care not to contaminate any of the test reagents with serum or bacterial agents.

e) Humidity indicators are supplied with each plate. If any of the indicators exhibit a pink color, the plate may be compromised in some way; decontaminate (i.e. wash the plate with bleach solution) and dispose of the plate.

f) The best results are achieved by following the protocols as they are described above, using good, safe laboratory techniques.

g) Do not use this kit after the expiration date.

h) Never pipette by mouth.

Allow all reagents to come to room temperature before starting.

References: Available upon request.

Presentation: 900 tests.

Compendium Code No.: 11150240

PROFLOK® ILT ELISA KIT

Synbiotics **ELISA Test**

Fowl Laryngotracheitis Antibody Test Kit

U.S. Vet. Lic. No.: 350

Reagents:

a) 1 LT antigen coated plate.

b) 10 µL LT Positive Control Serum.

c) 10 µL Normal Control Serum (NCS).

d) 100 µL Goat anti-Chicken IgG (H+L) Peroxidase Conjugate Solution.

e) 40 mL Dilution Buffer.

f) 10 mL ABTS-Hydrogen Peroxide Substrate Solution.

g) 2.5 mL 5X Stop Solution (dilute [1:5] with laboratory grade water).

h) 20 mL 20X Wash Solution (dilute [1:20] with laboratory grade water).

Equipment and Materials Required:

a) High precision pipette (i.e. 1-20 microliter pipette).

b) 0.2 mL, 1.0 mL and 5.0 mL pipettes.

c) 8 or 12 channel pipette (or transplating device).

d) 2 graduated cylinders (50 mL).

e) 1 mL or 5 mL borosilicate glass test tubes.

f) Uncoated low binding 96 well plates (i.e. Nunc catalog #269620).

g) Laboratory grade (Distilled or R.O.) water.

h) 96 well plate reading spectrophotometer with 405-410 nm filter.

i) Plate washing apparatus.

Indications: The PROFLOK® ILT ELISA Kit is a rapid serologic test for the detection of LT antibody in chicken serum samples. It was developed primarily to aid in the detection of pre- and post-vaccination LT antibody levels in chickens.

Test Principles: Laryngotracheitis (LT) is an acute disease of chickens characterized by coughing, gasping and expectoration of bloody exudate.[1] LT is often associated with high morbidity, mortality and egg production losses.[2] LT is a serious, worldwide disease problem in highly concentrated poultry producing areas.[1]

The assay is designed to measure LT antibody bound to LT antigen coated plates. The principle of the test is as follows: Serum obtained from chickens exposed to LT antigens contains specific anti-LT antibodies. Serum, diluted in Dilution Buffer, is added to an LT antigen coated plate. Specific LT antibody in the serum forms an antibody-antigen complex with the LT antigen bound to the plate. After washing the plate, an affinity purified goat anti-chicken IgG (H+L) peroxidase conjugate is added to each well. The antibody-antigen complex remaining from the previous step binds with the conjugate. After a brief incubation period, the unbound conjugate is removed by a second wash step. Substrate, which contains a chromagen (ABTS), is added to each well. Chromagen color change (from clear to green-blue) occurs in the presence of the peroxidase enzyme. The relative intensity of color developed in 15 minutes (compared to controls) is directly proportional to the level of LT antibody in the serum. After the substrate has incubated, Stop Solution is added to each well to terminate the reaction and the plate is read using an ELISA plate reader at 405-410 nm.

Test Procedure:

Sample Collection: For routine serologic flock monitoring, it is suggested that at least 30 or more sera per flock be randomly collected at standard time intervals (i.e. every four weeks). Proper sample collection procedures, serum harvest and serum sample storage (4°C for up to four days or -20°C for longer periods) are needed to provide reliable test results.

Sample Dilution Procedure: Dilute serum samples using Dilution Buffer in a clean, uncoated 96 well microtiter plate. Set up samples and controls as shown in Figure 1.

Preparation of the Serum Dilution Plate:

a) Add 300 µL Dilution Buffer to each well of an uncoated 96 well microtiter plate. This plate is referred to as the serum dilution plate.

b) Add 6 µL unknown serum per well as per Figure 1 (producing a 1:50 dilution). Start with well A4 and end with well H9 (moving left to right, row by row of wells). For example, wells 1 through 30 contain the diluted sera of flock 1, wells 31-60 contain the diluted sera of flock 2, etc.

c) Add 6 µL of Normal Control Serum (producing a 1:50 dilution) to wells A2, H10 and H12.

d) Aspirate and remove any liquid in dilution plate wells A1, A3 and H11.

e) Allow all diluted serums to equilibrate in Dilution Buffer for 5 minutes before transferring to an LT antigen coated ELISA plate.

f) Diluted serum should be tested within 24 hours.

This dilution format provides adequate quantities of diluted serum samples to conduct four additional ProFLOK® ELISA tests (i.e. REO, NDV, IBD and IBV) using the same serum dilution plate.

Preparation of LT Positive Control: An LT Positive Control Serum has been provided with this kit. Dilute the appropriate volume of LT Positive Control Serum with Dilution Buffer (1:50) in a clean, glass test tube. For example, dilute 6 µL of Positive Control serum in 300 µL Dilution Buffer. Mix well. 150 µL of LT Positive Control is needed per ELISA plate.

Preparation of Conjugate Solution: The horseradish peroxidase conjugated anti-chicken IgG (H+L) is supplied in 50% glycerol. Dilute 100 µL stock conjugate in 10 mL Dilution Buffer (1:100 dilution). Mix well. This 10 mL preparation will supply sufficient conjugate for one 96 well ELISA plate.

Preparation of 1X Wash Solution: Dilute 20 mL concentrated Wash Solution in 380 mL laboratory grade (distilled or R.O.) water (1:20). Mix well. Approximately 400 mL Wash Solution is needed for each 96 well ELISA plate.

Preparation of the Substrate Solution: The Substrate Solution is ready to use. Each plate will require approximately 10 mL substrate solution. For best results, the substrate solution must be equilibrated to room temperature before use.

Preparation of 1X Stop Solution: Dilute 2.5 mL concentrated Stop Solution in 10 mL laboratory grade (distilled or R.O.) water (1:5). Mix well. Approximately 12.5 mL Stop Solution is needed for each 96 well ELISA plate.

Note: Storage of 5X Stop Solution at refrigerated temperatures may cause the formation of a white solid. This does not affect product performance. Warm at room temperature or 37°C to dissolve before use.

Figure 1.

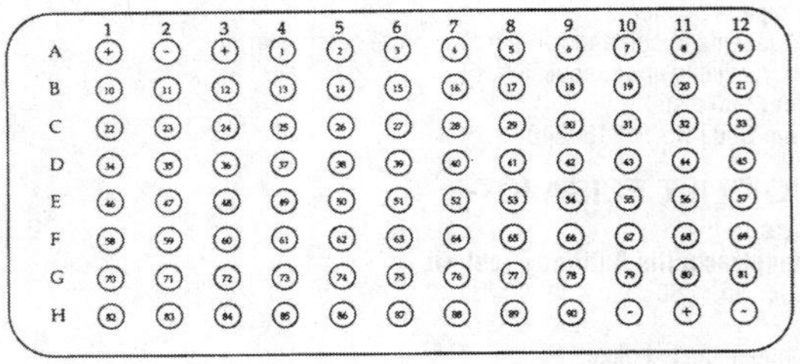

ELISA Test Procedure:

Preparing the Test Plate:

a) Remove an LT antigen coated test plate from the protective bag and label according to dilution plate identification.

b) Add 50 μL Dilution Buffer to all wells on the test plate.

c) Add 50 μL diluted LT Positive Control Serum to wells A1, A3 and H11. Discard pipette tip.

d) Using an 8 or 12 channel pipette transfer 50 μL/well of each of the diluted serum samples and Normal Control Serum samples from the dilution plate to the corresponding wells of the LT coated test plate. Discard pipette tips after each row of sample is transferred. Transfer of samples to the ELISA plate should be done as quickly as possible.

e) Incubate plate for 30 minutes at room temperature.

Wash Procedure:

f) Tap out liquid from each well into an appropriate vessel containing bleach or other decontamination agent.

g) Using an 8 or 12 channel pipette (or comparable automatic washing device), fill each well with approximately 300 μL Wash Solution. Allow to soak in wells for 3 minutes; then discard contents into an appropriate waste container (waste container should contain bleach solution). Tap inverted plate to ensure that all residual liquid is removed. Repeat wash procedure 2 more times.

Note: The wash procedure is a very critical step in any ELISA procedure. Please follow the above steps as directed.

Addition of Anti-Chicken IgG Peroxidase Conjugate, Substrate and Stop Solution:

h) Using an 8 or 12 channel pipette (or transplating device) dispense 100 μL diluted conjugate (prepared as described above) into each assay well. Discard pipette tips.

i) Incubate for 30 minutes at room temperature.

j) Wash as in steps f and g above.

k) Using an 8 or 12 channel pipette (or transplating device) dispense 100 μL Substrate Solution into each test well. Discard pipette tips.

l) Incubate 15 minutes at room temperature.

m) Using an 8 or 12 channel pipette (or transplating device) add 100 μL diluted Stop Solution (prepared as described above) to each test well.

n) Allow bubbles to dissipate before reading plate.

Manual Processing of Data:

a) Read the plate using an ELISA plate reader set at 405-410 nm. Be sure to blank the reader as directed. If a Flow Multiscan reader is used, the reader should be blanked using an empty microtiter plate. If a Bio-tek or Dynatech reader is used, the machine may be blanked with air.

b) Calculate the average Positive Control Serum absorbance (Optical Density [O.D.]) using the absorbance values of wells A1, A3 and H11. Calculate the average Normal Control Serum absorbance using values obtained from wells A2, H10 and H12. Record both averages.

c) Subtract the average normal control absorbance from the average positive control absorbance. The difference is the Corrected Positive Control.

d) Calculate a sample to positive (Sp) ratio by subtracting the average normal control absorbance from each sample absorbance. The difference is divided by the corrected positive control. Use the following equation format:

$$SP = \frac{\text{(Sample Absorbance)} - \text{(Average Normal Control Absorbance)}}{\text{Corrected Positive Control Absorbance}}$$

e) An LT ELISA titer can be calculated by the following suggested equation:

Log_{10} Titer = (1.450 X Log_{10} Sp) + 3.726

Titer = Antilog of Log_{10} Titer

Example:

1. Example Positive Control Absorbance:
   0.585, 0.610, 0.590
   Average = (0.585 + 0.610 + 0.590) / 3 = 0.595
2. Example Normal Controls:
   0.078, 0.067, 0.057
   Average = (0.078 + 0.067 + 0.057) / 3 = 0.067
3. Corrected Positive Control:
   (0.595) - (0.067) = 0.528
4. Example Sp value calculation:
   Absorbance of sample = 0.560
   (0.560) - (0.067) / 0.528 = 0.934
5. Example of calculation of titer using the Sp from above:
   Log_{10} Titer = 1.450 X (Log_{10} 0.934) + 3.726
   Titer = Antilog 3.68
   Titer = 4820

Test Interpretation: Results:

Assay Control Values: Valid LT ELISA results are obtained when the average optical density (O.D.) value of the Normal Control Serum is less than 0.200 and the Corrected Positive Control value range is between 0.250 and 0.900. If either of these values are out of range, the LT test results should be considered invalid and the samples should be retested. Samples testing with an Sp value of less than or equal to 0.150 will receive a 0 titer value and are considered negative for LT antibody.

Under optimal conditions* the suggested O.D. value ranges of 0.060 to 0.080 for LT Normal Control Serum and 0.400 to 0.750 for LT Positive Control Serum should be strived for to ensure the most consistent laboratory test results. Please note that a plate with O.D. values which do not fall within the suggested O.D. ranges above does not constitute an invalid test.

*Optimal conditions are at room temperature [70 to 75°F (21 to 24°C)]. Higher room temperatures may result in slightly higher O.D. values.

Interpretation of Results: The LT ELISA titer values obtained represent a comparison of the LT antibody level within each field chicken serum tested and the LT ELISA kit positive and normal control sera. Therefore, it is important to first determine that the LT ELISA positive and normal control sera values obtained are valid as detailed above in the "Assay Control Values" section of this pamphlet before LT ELISA results are interpreted.

A "0" LT ELISA titer represents a chicken serum sample that contains an extremely low to insignificant LT antibody level compared to the LT ELISA kit positive and normal control sera.

An LT ELISA titer value above "0" indicates only that a chicken serum sample contains a significant and ELISA-detectable LT antibody level compared to the LT ELISA kit positive and normal control sera. However, these titers do not imply or ensure "protection" nor provide serologic differentiation between an LT vaccine response or LT field infection.

Optimal LT vaccine administration practices and "protective" flock LT titer target values must be determined by each LT ELISA kit user by comparing flock pre- and post-vaccination LT ELISA results [i.e. coefficient of variation (%CV) and geometric mean titer (GMT) values] with flock performance parameters (i.e. morbidity, mortality, flock body weight gain or uniformity) over time.

Storage: Store all reagents provided in the kit at 2-7°C.

Caution(s): To the Users of Reagents and LT Antigen Coated Plates:

a) Handle all reagents and samples as biohazardous material.

b) Keep all reagents away from skin and eyes. If exposure should occur, immediately flush affected areas with cold water.

c) Wash solution, control sera, test plates, field samples and all other test kit reagents should be properly decontaminated with bleach or other strong oxidizing agent before disposal.

d) Take special care not to contaminate any of the test reagents with serum or bacterial agents.

e) Humidity indicators are supplied with each plate. If any of the indicators exhibit a pink color, the plate may be compromised in some way; decontaminate (i.e. wash the plate with bleach solution) and dispose of the plate.

f) The best results are achieved by following the protocols as they are described above, using good, safe laboratory techniques.

g) Do not use this kit after the expiration date.

h) Never pipette by mouth.

Allow all reagents to come to room temperature before starting.

References: Available upon request.

Presentation: 900 tests.

Compendium Code No.: 11150251

PROFLOK® MG ELISA KIT

Synbiotics **ELISA Test**

Mycoplasma gallisepticum Antibody Test Kit

U.S. Vet. Lic. No.: 350

Reagents:

a) 1 MG antigen coated plate.

b) 10 μL MG Positive Control Serum.

c) 10 μL Normal Control Serum.

d) 100 μL Goat anti-Chicken IgG (H+L) Peroxidase Conjugate Solution.

e) 40 mL Dilution Buffer.

f) 10 mL ABTS-Hydrogen Peroxide Substrate Solution.

g) 2.5 mL 5X Stop Solution (dilute [1:5] with laboratory grade water).

h) 20 mL 20X Wash Solution (dilute [1:20] with laboratory grade water).

Equipment and Materials Required:

a) High precision pipette (i.e. 1-20 microliter pipette).

b) 0.2 mL, 1.0 mL and 5.0 mL pipettes.

c) 8 or 12 channel pipette (or transplating device).

d) 2 graduated cylinders (50 mL).

e) 1 mL or 5 mL borosilicate glass test tubes.

f) Uncoated low binding 96 well plates (i.e. Nunc catalog #269620).

g) Laboratory grade (Distilled or R.O.) water.

h) 96 well plate reading spectrophotometer with 405-410 nm filter.

i) Plate washing apparatus.

Indications: The PROFLOK® MG ELISA Kit is a rapid and specific presumptive screening test for the detection of antibody to most conventional MG strains in chicken serum samples. It was designed for screening large numbers of chicken sera from numerous flocks; however, additional conventional MG serologic testing [i.e. serum plate agglutination (SPA) and hemagglutination-inhibition (HI) test] and culture techniques are needed to confirm MG negative and MG-infected chicken flocks.

Test Principles: *Mycoplasma gallisepticum* (MG) infection of chickens is associated with airsacculitis, reduced feed conversion and egg production efficiency, and increased condemnation at slaughter.[1] MG infection is one of the costliest disease problems confronting the poultry industry.[2]

The assay is designed to measure MG antibody bound to MG antigen coated plates. The principle of the test is as follows: Serum obtained from chickens exposed to MG antigens contains specific anti-MG antibodies. Serum, diluted in Dilution Buffer, is added to an MG antigen coated plate. Specific MG antibody in the serum forms an antibody-antigen complex with the MG antigen bound to the plate. After washing the plate, an affinity purified goat anti-chicken IgG (H+L) peroxidase conjugate is added to each well. The antibody-antigen complex remaining from the previous step binds with the conjugate. After a brief incubation period, the unbound conjugate is removed by a second wash step. Substrate, which contains a chromagen (ABTS), is added to each well. Chromagen color change (from clear to green-blue) occurs in the presence of the peroxidase enzyme. The relative intensity of color developed in 15 minutes (compared to controls) is directly proportional to the level of MG antibody in the serum. After the substrate has incubated, Stop Solution is added to each well to terminate the reaction and the plate is read using an ELISA plate reader at 405-410 nm.

Test Procedure:

Sample Collection: For routine serologic flock monitoring, it is suggested that at least 30 or more sera per flock be randomly collected at standard time intervals (i.e. every four weeks). Proper sample collection procedures, serum harvest and serum sample storage (4°C for up to four days or -20°C for longer periods) are needed to provide reliable test results.

Sample Dilution Procedure: Dilute serum samples using Dilution Buffer in a clean, uncoated 96 well microtiter plate. Set up samples and controls as shown in Figure 1.

Preparation of the Serum Dilution Plate:

a) Add 300 µL Dilution Buffer to each well of an uncoated 96 well microtiter plate. This plate is referred to as the serum dilution plate.
b) Add 6 µL unknown serum per well as per Figure 1 (producing a 1:50 dilution). Start with well A4 and end with well H9 (moving left to right, row by row of wells). For example, wells 1 through 30 contain the diluted sera of flock 1, wells 31-60 contain the diluted sera of flock 2, etc.
c) Add 6 µL of Normal Control Serum (producing a 1:50 dilution) to wells A2, H10 and H12.
d) Aspirate and remove any liquid in dilution plate wells A1, A3 and H11.
e) Allow all diluted serums to equilibrate in Dilution Buffer for 5 minutes before transferring to an MG antigen coated ELISA plate.
f) Diluted serum should be tested within 24 hours.

This dilution format provides adequate quantities of diluted serum samples to conduct four additional ProFLOK® ELISA tests (i.e. MS, IBD, IBV and REO) using the same serum dilution plate.

Preparation of MG Positive Control: An MG Positive Control Serum has been provided with this kit. Dilute the appropriate volume of MG Positive Control Serum with Dilution Buffer (1:50) in a clean, glass test tube. For example, dilute 6 µL of positive control serum in 300 µL Dilution Buffer. Mix well. 150 µL of MG Positive Control is needed per ELISA plate.

Preparation of Conjugate Solution: The horseradish peroxidase conjugated anti-chicken IgG (H+L) is supplied in 50% glycerol. Dilute 100 µL stock conjugate in 10 mL Dilution Buffer (1:100 dilution). Mix well. This 10 mL preparation will supply sufficient conjugate for one 96 well ELISA plate.

Preparation of 1X Wash Solution: Dilute 20 mL concentrated Wash Solution in 380 mL laboratory grade (distilled or R.O.) water (1:20). Mix well. Approximately 400 mL Wash Solution is needed for each 96 well ELISA plate.

Preparation of the Substrate Solution: The Substrate Solution is ready to use. Each plate will require approximately 10 mL substrate solution. For best results, the substrate solution must be equilibrated to room temperature before use.

Preparation of 1X Stop Solution: Dilute 2.5 mL concentrated Stop Solution in 10 mL laboratory grade (distilled or R.O.) water (1:5). Mix well. Approximately 12.5 mL Stop Solution is needed for each 96 well ELISA plate.

Note: Storage of 5X Stop Solution at refrigerated temperatures may cause the formation of a white solid. This does not affect product performance. Warm at room temperature or 37°C to dissolve before use.

Figure 1.

	1	2	3	4	5	6	7	8	9	10	11	12
A	+	-	+	1	2	3	4	5	6	7	8	9
B	10	11	12	13	14	15	16	17	18	19	20	21
C	22	23	24	25	26	27	28	29	30	31	32	33
D	34	35	36	37	38	39	40	41	42	43	44	45
E	46	47	48	49	50	51	52	53	54	55	56	57
F	58	59	60	61	62	63	64	65	66	67	68	69
G	70	71	72	73	74	75	76	77	78	79	80	81
H	82	83	84	85	86	87	88	89	90	-	+	-

ELISA Test Procedure:

Preparing the Test Plate:

a) Remove an MG antigen coated test plate from the protective bag and label according to dilution plate identification.
b) Add 50 µL Dilution Buffer to all wells on the test plate.
c) Add 50 µL diluted MG Positive Control Serum to wells A1, A3 and H11. Discard pipette tip.
d) Using an 8 or 12 channel pipette transfer 50 µL/well of each of the diluted serum samples and Normal Control Serum samples from the dilution plate to the corresponding wells of the MG coated test plate. Discard pipette tips after each row of sample is transferred. Transfer of samples to the ELISA plate should be done as quickly as possible.
e) Incubate plate for 30 minutes at room temperature.

Wash Procedure:

f) Tap out liquid from each well into an appropriate vessel containing bleach or other decontamination agent.
g) Using an 8 or 12 channel pipette (or comparable automatic washing device), fill each well with approximately 300 µL Wash Solution. Allow to soak in wells for 3 minutes; then discard contents into an appropriate waste container (waste container should contain bleach solution). Tap inverted plate to ensure that all residual liquid is removed. Repeat wash procedure 2 more times.

Note: The wash procedure is a very critical step in any ELISA procedure. Please follow the above steps as directed.

Addition of Anti-Chicken IgG Peroxidase Conjugate, Substrate and Stop Solution:

h) Using an 8 or 12 channel pipette (or transplating device) dispense 100 µL diluted conjugate (prepared as described above) into each assay well. Discard pipette tips.
i) Incubate for 30 minutes at room temperature.
j) Wash as in steps f and g above.
k) Using an 8 or 12 channel pipette (or transplating device) dispense 100 µL Substrate Solution into each test well. Discard pipette tips.
l) Incubate 15 minutes at room temperature.
m) Using an 8 or 12 channel pipette (or transplating device) add 100 µL diluted Stop Solution (prepared as described above) to each test well.
n) Allow bubbles to dissipate before reading plate.

Manual Processing of Data:

a) Read the plate using an ELISA plate reader set at 405-410 nm. Be sure to blank the reader as directed. If a Flow Multiscan reader is used, the reader should be blanked using an empty microtiter plate. If a Bio-tek or Dynatech reader is used, the machine may be blanked with air.
b) Calculate the average Positive Control Serum absorbance (Optical Density [O.D.]) using the absorbance values of wells A1, A3 and H11. Calculate the average Normal Control Serum absorbance using values obtained from wells A2, H10 and H12. Record both averages.
c) Subtract the average normal control absorbance from the average positive absorbance. The difference is the Corrected Positive Control.
d) Calculate a sample to positive (Sp) ratio by subtracting the average normal control absorbance from each sample absorbance. The difference is divided by the corrected positive control. Use the following equation format:

$$SP = \frac{\text{(Sample Absorbance)} - \text{(Average Normal Control Absorbance)}}{\text{Corrected Positive Control Absorbance}}$$

e) An MG ELISA titer can be calculated by the following suggested equation:

Log_{10} Titer = (1.464 X Log_{10} Sp) + 3.197

Titer = Antilog of Log_{10} Titer

Example:

1. Example Positive Control Absorbance:
   0.585, 0.610, 0.590
   Average = (0.585 + 0.610 + 0.590) / 3 = 0.595
2. Example Normal Controls:
   0.110, 0.102, 0.112
   Average = (0.110 + 0.102 + 0.112) / 3 = 0.108
3. Corrected Positive Control:
   (0.595) - (0.108) = 0.487
4. Example Sp value calculation:
   Absorbance of sample = 0.560
   (0.560) - (0.108) / 0.487 = 0.928
5. Example of Calculation of titer using the Sp from above:
   Log_{10} Titer = 1.464 X (Log_{10} 0.934) + 3.197
   Titer = Antilog 3.15
   Titer = 1413

Test Interpretation: Results:

Assay Control Values: Valid MG ELISA results are obtained when the average optical density (O.D.) value of the Normal Control Serum is less than 0.200 and the Corrected Positive Control value range is between 0.250 and 0.900. If either of these values are out of range, the MG test results should be considered invalid and the samples should be retested. Samples testing with an Sp value of less than or equal to 0.199 will receive a 0 titer value and are considered negative for MG antibody.

Under optimal conditions* the suggested O.D. value ranges of 0.060 to 0.120 for MG Normal Control Serum and 0.350 to 0.750 for MG Positive Control Serum should be strived for to ensure the most consistent laboratory test results. Please note that tests with O.D. values which do not fall within the suggested O.D. ranges above does not constitute an invalid test.

*Optimal conditions are at room temperature [70 to 75°F (21 to 24°C)]. Higher room temperatures may result in slightly higher O.D. values.

Interpretation of Results: The MG Sp ratio values and/or ELISA titer values obtained for sera should be interpreted using the following value ranges:

Sample to Positive (Sp) Value	MG ELISA Titer Range	MG Presumed Antibody Status
Less than 0.200	0	Negative[a]
0.200 to 0.599	149 to 743	Probable[b,c]
Greater or equal to 0.6	744 or greater	Positive[c]

a. Negative. Serum samples with an MG Sp ratio value of less than 0.200 receive a "0" titer value and are presumed negative for MG antibody. However, a variety of factors, such as possible MG strain variations that may exhibit atypical biological and/or antigenic properties,[1] prevalence of an MG strain within a flock and timing and randomness of serum sample collection procedures could result in an MG-infected chicken flock yielding MG-negative ELISA results. It is therefore recommended that each chicken flock only be considered to be MG negative after (a) each flock has been adequately sampled and repeatedly tested several times and has yielded negative MG ELISA results each time and (b) each flock has been adequately sampled and repeatedly tested by standard conventional serologic tests (SPA and HI) and MG culture techniques[3] and has yielded MG negative serologic and culture results each time.

b. Probable. Presumed MG antibody probable denotes the ELISA Sp value range within which MG ELISA and conventional (SPA and HI) test data may suggest but may not conclusively detect MG antibody within a sample. The probable range represents a "suspect" or "gray" area in which MG ELISA results may or may not be supported by conventional serologic (SPA and HI) test results. It is highly recommended that additional conventional serologic tests and MG culture techniques[3] be conducted on serum and culture samples collected from MG ELISA probable chicken flocks, as recommended in parts a and c, to confirm whether each flock is an MG negative or MG positive-infected flock.

c. Positive. Additional conventional serologic testing (SPA and HI) and culturing of samples collected from presumed MG ELISA antibody probable and positive chicken flocks, using standard techniques,[3] are needed to obtain a confirmed positive diagnosis of MG infection within a chicken flock.

Storage: Store all reagents provided in the kit at 2-10°C.

Caution(s): To the Users of Reagents and MG Antigen Coated Plates:

a) Handle all reagents and samples as biohazardous material.
b) Keep all reagents away from skin and eyes. If exposure should occur, immediately flush affected areas with cold water.
c) Wash solution, control sera, test plates, field samples and all other test kit reagents should be properly decontaminated with bleach or other strong oxidizing agent before disposal.
d) Take special care not to contaminate any of the test reagents with serum or bacterial agents.
e) Humidity indicators are supplied with each plate. If any of the indicators exhibit a pink color, the plate may be compromised in some way; decontaminate (i.e. wash the plate with bleach solution) and dispose of the plate.
f) The best results are achieved by following the protocols as they are described above, using good, safe laboratory techniques.
g) Do not use this kit after the expiration date.
h) Never pipette by mouth.

Allow all reagents to come to room temperature before starting.

References: Available upon request.

Presentation: 900 tests.

Compendium Code No.: 11150260

PROFLOK® MG-MS ELISA KIT

Synbiotics **ELISA Test**

Mycoplasma gallisepticum-synoviae Antibody Test Kit

U.S. Vet. Lic. No.: 350

Reagents:

a) 1 antigen coated plate (MG or MS).
b) 10 µL Positive Control Serum (MG or MS).
c) 10 µL Normal Control Serum (NCS)*.
d) 100 µL Goat anti-Chicken IgG (H+L) Peroxidase Conjugate Solution*.
e) 40 mL Dilution Buffer*.
f) 10 mL ABTS-Hydrogen Peroxide Substrate Solution*.
g) 2.5 mL 5X Stop Solution, 5% SDS (dilute [1:5] with laboratory grade water)*.
h) 20 mL 20X Wash Solution (dilute [1:20] with laboratory grade water)*.
*Reagents can be used with either antigen coated plates in the kit.

Equipment and Materials Required but not Provided:

a) High precision pipette (i.e. 1-20 microliter pipette).
b) 0.2 mL, 1.0 mL and 5.0 mL pipettes.
c) 8 or 12 channel pipette (or transplating device).
d) 2 graduated cylinders (50 mL).
e) 1 mL or 5 mL borosilicate glass test tubes.
f) Uncoated low binding 96 well plates (i.e. Nunc catalog #269620).
g) Laboratory grade (Distilled or R.O.) water.
h) 96 well plate reading spectrophotometer with 405-410 nm filter.
i) Plate washing apparatus.

Indications: The PROFLOK® ELISA Kit is a rapid and specific presumptive screening test for the detection of antibody to most conventional MG and MS strains in chicken serum samples. It was designed for screening large numbers of chicken sera from numerous flocks; however, additional conventional MG and MS serologic testing [i.e. serum plate agglutination (SPA) and hemagglutination-inhibition (HI) test] and culture techniques are needed to confirm MG and MS negative and MG or MS infected chicken flocks.

Test Principles: This ELISA kit contains a combination of two different antibody detection products. The kit includes antigen coated plates for the detection of antibody to *Mycoplasma gallisepticum* (MG) and plates for the detection of antibody to *Mycoplasma synoviae* (MS). The kit includes five antigen coated plates for each of the two agents and two positive control vials, one per agent, and the reagents necessary to run ten test plates.

The assay is designed to measure antibody bound to antigen coated plates. The principle of the test is as follows: Serum obtained from chickens exposed to MG or MS antigens contains specific MG or MS antibodies. Serum, diluted in Dilution Buffer, is added to an antigen coated plate. Specific antibody in the serum forms an antibody-antigen complex with the antigen bound to the plate. After washing the plate, an affinity purified goat anti-chicken IgG (H+L) peroxidase conjugate is added to each well. The antibody-antigen complex remaining from the previous step binds with the conjugate. After a brief incubation period, the unbound conjugate is removed by a second wash step. Substrate, which contains a chromagen (ABTS), is added to each well. Chromagen color change (from clear to green-blue) occurs in the presence of the peroxidase enzyme. The relative intensity of color developed in 15 minutes (compared to controls) is directly proportional to the level of antibody in the serum. After the substrate has incubated, Stop Solution is added to each well to terminate the reaction and the plate is read using an ELISA plate reader at 405-410 nm.

Test Procedure:

Sample Collection: For routine serologic flock monitoring, it is suggested that at least 30 or more sera per flock be randomly collected at standard time intervals (i.e. every four weeks). Proper sample collection procedures, serum harvest and serum sample storage (4°C for up to four days or -20°C for longer periods) are needed to provide reliable test results. Tests only good quality serum (i.e. avoid bacterial contamination, heavy hemolysis or clotted fat.

Sample Dilution Procedure: Dilute serum samples using Dilution Buffer in a clean, uncoated 96 well microtiter plate. Frozen serum samples should be completely thawed and thoroughly mixed before diluting. Set up samples and controls as shown in Figure 1.

Preparation of the Serum Dilution Plate:

a) Add 300 µL Dilution Buffer to each well of an uncoated 96 well microtiter plate. This plate is referred to as the serum dilution plate.
b) Add 6 µL unknown serum per well as per Figure 1 (producing a 1:50 dilution). Start with well A4 and end with well H9 (moving left to right, row by row of wells). For example, wells 1 through 30 contain the diluted sera of flock 1, wells 31-60 contain the diluted sera of flock 2, etc.
c) Add 6 µL of Normal Control Serum (producing a 1:50 dilution) to wells A2, H10 and H12.
d) Aspirate and remove any liquid in dilution plate wells A1, A3 and H11.
e) Allow all diluted serums to equilibrate in Dilution Buffer for 5 minutes before transferring to an antigen coated ELISA plate.
f) Diluted serum should be tested within 24 hours.

This dilution format provides adequate quantities of diluted serum samples to conduct three additional ProFLOK® ELISA tests (i.e. REO, NDV, IBV, IBD or AE) using the same serum dilution plate.

Preparation of Positive Control: A Positive Control Serum for each agent has been provided with this kit. Dilute the appropriate volume of the appropriate Positive Control Serum with Dilution Buffer (1:50) in a clean, glass test tube. For example, dilute 6 µL of positive control serum in 300 µL Dilution Buffer. Mix well. 150 µL of diluted Positive Control is needed per ELISA plate.

Preparation of Conjugate Solution: The horseradish peroxidase conjugated anti-chicken IgG (H+L) is supplied in 50% glycerol. Dilute 100 µL stock conjugate in 10 mL Dilution Buffer (1:100 dilution). Mix well. This 10 mL preparation will supply sufficient conjugate for one 96 well ELISA plate.

Preparation of 1X Wash Solution: Dilute 20 mL concentrated Wash Solution in 380 mL laboratory grade (distilled or R.O.) water (1:20). Mix well. Approximately 400 mL Wash Solution is needed for each 96 well ELISA plate.

Preparation of the Substrate Solution: The Substrate Solution is ready to use. Each plate will require approximately 10 mL substrate solution. For best results, the substrate solution must be equilibrated to room temperature before use.

Preparation of 1X Stop Solution: Dilute 2.5 mL concentrated Stop Solution in 10 mL laboratory grade (distilled or R.O.) water (1:5). Mix well. Approximately 12.5 mL Stop Solution is needed for each 96 well ELISA plate.

Note: Storage of 5X Stop Solution at refrigerated temperatures may cause the formation of a white solid. This does not affect product performance. Warm at room temperature or 37°C to dissolve before use.

Figure 1.

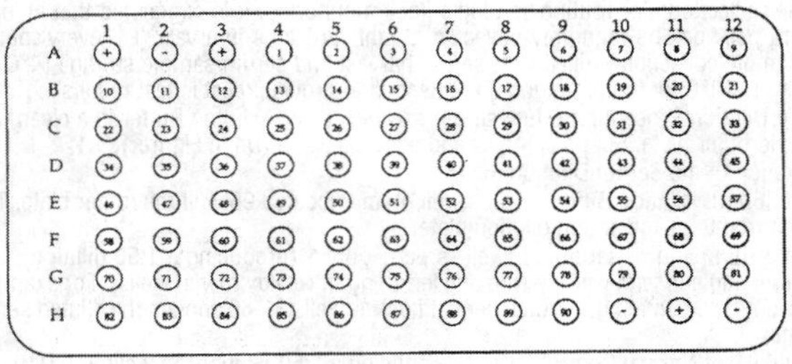

ELISA Test Procedure:

Preparing the Test Plate:

a) Remove an antigen coated test plate from the protective bag and label according to dilution plate identification.
b) Add 50 µL Dilution Buffer to all wells on the test plate.
c) Add 50 µL diluted Positive Control Serum to wells A1, A3 and H11. Discard pipette tip.

Note: Be sure that positive control sample is appropriate for antigen coated plate being used (i.e. MG Positive Control is added to MG antigen coated plate).

d) Using an 8 or 12 channel pipette transfer 50 µL/well of each of the diluted serum samples and Normal Control Serum samples from the dilution plate to the corresponding wells of the coated test plate (yields a 1:100 dilution). Discard pipette tips after each row of sample is transferred. Transfer of samples to the ELISA plate should be done as quickly as possible.
e) Incubate plate for 30 minutes at room temperature.

Wash Procedure:

f) Tap out liquid from each well into an appropriate vessel containing bleach or other decontamination agent.
g) Using an 8 or 12 channel pipette (or comparable automatic washing device), fill each well with approximately 300 µL Wash Solution. Allow to soak in wells for 3 minutes; then discard contents into an appropriate waste container (waste container should contain bleach solution). Tap inverted plate to ensure that all residual liquid is removed. Repeat wash procedure 2 more times.

Note: The wash procedure is a very critical step in any ELISA procedure. Please follow the above steps as directed.

Addition of Anti-Chicken IgG Peroxidase Conjugate, Substrate and Stop Solution:

h) Using an 8 or 12 channel pipette (or transplating device) dispense 100 µL diluted conjugate (prepared as described above) into each assay well. Discard pipette tips.
i) Incubate for 30 minutes at room temperature.
j) Wash as in steps f and g above.
k) Using an 8 or 12 channel pipette (or transplating device) dispense 100 µL Substrate Solution into each test well. Discard pipette tips.
l) Incubate 15 minutes at room temperature.
m) Using an 8 or 12 channel pipette (or transplating device) add 100 µL diluted Stop Solution (prepared as described above) to each test well.
n) Allow bubbles to dissipate before reading plate.

Manual Processing of Data:

a) Read the plate using an ELISA plate reader set at 405-410 nm. Be sure to blank the reader as directed. If a Flow Multiscan reader is used, the reader should be blanked using an empty microtiter plate. If a Bio-tek or Dynatech reader is used, the machine may be blanked with air.
b) Calculate the average Positive Control Serum absorbance (Optical Density [O.D.]) using the absorbance values of wells A1, A3 and H11. Calculate the average Normal Control Serum absorbance using values obtained from wells A2, H10 and H12. Record both averages.
c) Subtract the average normal control absorbance from the average positive absorbance. The difference is the Corrected Positive Control.
d) Calculate a sample to positive (Sp) ratio by subtracting the average normal control absorbance from each sample absorbance. The difference is divided by the corrected positive control. Use the following equation format:

$$SP = \frac{\text{(Sample Absorbance)} - \text{(Average Normal Control Absorbance)}}{\text{Corrected Positive Control Absorbance}}$$

e) An ELISA titer for MG or MS can be calculated by the following suggested equation:

Log_{10} Titer = (1.464 X Log_{10} Sp) + 3.197
Titer = Antilog of Log_{10} Titer

Example:

1. Example Positive Control Absorbance:
   0.585, 0.610, 0.590
   Average = (0.585 + 0.610 + 0.590) / 3 = 0.595
2. Example Normal Controls:
   0.078, 0.067, 0.057
   Average = (0.078 + 0.067 + 0.057) / 3 = 0.067
3. Corrected Positive Control:
   (0.595) - (0.067) = 0.528
4. Example Sp value calculation:
   Absorbance of sample = 0.560
   (0.560) - (0.067) / 0.528 = 0.934
5. Example of Calculation of titer using the Sp from above:
   Log_{10} Titer = 1.464 X (Log_{10} 0.934) + 3.197
   Titer = Antilog 3.15
   Titer = 1413

Test Interpretation: Results:

Assay Control Values: Valid ELISA results are obtained when the average optical density (O.D.) value of the Normal Control Serum is less than 0.200 for MG or MS and the Corrected Positive Control value range for both agents is between 0.250 and 0.900. If either of these values are out of range, the test results should be considered invalid and the samples should be retested.

Interpretation of Results: The MG ELISA Sp ratio values and/or ELISA titer values obtained for sera should be interpreted using the following value ranges:

Sample to Positive (Sp) Value	MG ELISA Titer Range	MG Presumed Antibody Status
Less than 0.200	0	Negative[a]
0.200 to 0.599	149 to 743	Suspect[b,c]
Greater or equal to 0.6	744 or greater	Positive[c]

The MS ELISA Sp ratio values and/or ELISA titer values obtained for sera should be interpreted using the following value ranges:

Sample to Positive (Sp) Value	MS ELISA Titer Range	MS Presumed Antibody Status
Less than 0.300	0	Negative[a]
0.300 to 0.599	270 to 743	Suspect[b,c]
Greater or equal to 0.6	744 or greater	Positive[c]

a. Negative. Serum samples with an MG Sp ratio value of less than 0.200 or an MS Sp ratio of less than 0.300 receive a "0" titer value and are presumed negative for antibody. However, a variety of factors, such as possible strain variations that may exhibit atypical biological and/or antigenic properties,[1,2] prevalence of a strain within a flock and timing and randomness of serum sample collection procedures could result in an infected chicken flock yielding negative ELISA results. It is therefore recommended that each chicken flock only be considered to be negative after (a) each flock has been adequately sampled and repeatedly tested several times and has yielded negative ELISA results each time and (b) each flock has been adequately sampled and repeatedly tested by standard conventional serologic tests (SPA and HI) and MG or MS culture techniques[2,3] and has yielded negative serologic and culture results each time.

b. Suspect. Presumed antibody suspect denotes the ELISA Sp value range within which ELISA and conventional (SPA and HI) test data may suggest but may not conclusively detect antibody within a sample. The suspect range represents a "suspect" or "gray" area in which ELISA results may or may not be supported by conventional serologic (SPA and HI) test results. It is highly recommended that additional conventional serologic tests and MG or MS culture techniques[3,4] be conducted on serum and culture samples collected from MG or MS ELISA probable chicken flocks, as recommended in parts a and c, to confirm whether each flock is a negative or positive-infected flock.

c. Positive. Additional conventional serologic testing (SPA and HI) and culturing of samples collected from presumed MG or MS ELISA antibody suspect and positive chicken flocks, using standard techniques,[3,4] are needed to obtain a confirmed positive diagnosis of MG or MS infection within a chicken flock.

Storage: Store all reagents provided in the kit at 2-7°C. Reagents should not be frozen.

Caution(s): To the Users of Reagents and Antigen Coated Plates:

a) Handle all reagents and samples as biohazardous material.

b) Keep all reagents away from skin and eyes. If exposure should occur, immediately flush affected areas with cold water.

c) Wash solution, control sera, test plates, field samples and all other test kit reagents should be properly decontaminated with bleach or other strong oxidizing agent before disposal.

d) Take special care not to contaminate any of the test reagents with serum or bacterial agents.

e) Humidity indicators are supplied with each plate. If any of the indicators exhibit a pink color, the plate may be compromised in some way; decontaminate (i.e. wash the plate with bleach solution) and dispose of the plate.

f) The best results are achieved by following the protocols as they are described above, using good, safe laboratory techniques.

g) Do not use this kit after the expiration date.

h) Never pipette by mouth.

Allow all reagents to come to room temperature before starting.

References: Available upon request.

Presentation: 900 tests.

Compendium Code No.: 11150270

PROFLOK® MG-T ELISA KIT

Synbiotics **ELISA Test**

Mycoplasma gallisepticum Antibody Test Kit (Turkey)

U.S. Vet. Lic. No.: 350

Reagents:

a) 1 MG-T antigen coated plate.

b) 10 µL MG-T Positive Control Serum.

c) 10 µL Normal Control Serum.

d) 100 µL Goat anti-Turkey IgG (H+L) Peroxidase Conjugate Solution.

e) 40 mL Dilution Buffer.

f) 10 mL ABTS-Hydrogen Peroxide Substrate Solution.

g) 2.5 mL 5X Stop Solution (dilute [1:5] with laboratory grade water).

h) 20 mL 20X Wash Solution (dilute [1:20] with laboratory grade water).

Equipment and Materials Required:

a) High precision pipette (i.e. 1-20 microliter pipette).

b) 0.2 mL, 1.0 mL and 5.0 mL pipettes.

c) 8 or 12 channel pipette (or transplating device).

d) 2 graduated cylinders (50 mL).

e) 5 mL borosilicate glass test tubes.

f) Uncoated low binding 96 well plates (i.e. Nunc catalog #269620).

g) Laboratory grade (Distilled or R.O.) water.

h) 96 well plate reading spectrophotometer with 405-410 nm filter.

i) Plate washing apparatus.

Indications: The PROFLOK® MG-T ELISA Kit is a rapid and presumptive serologic screening test for the detection of antibody to most conventional MG strains (i.e. S-6, R-Strain etc.) in turkey serum samples. It was designed for screening large numbers of turkey sera from numerous flocks; however, additional conventional MG serologic testing [i.e. serum plate agglutination (SPA) and hemagglutination-inhibition (HI) test] and culture techniques are needed to confirm MG negative and MG-infected turkey flocks.

Test Principles: *Mycoplasma gallisepticum* (MG) infection of turkeys is characterized by respiratory rales, coughing, nasal discharge and sinusitis.[4] MG infection is associated with reduced feed and egg production efficiency, increased medication costs and increased condemnation.[4]

The assay is designed to measure MG antibody bound to MG antigen coated plates. The principle of the test is as follows: Serum obtained from turkeys exposed to MG antigens contains specific anti-MG antibodies. Serum, diluted in Dilution Buffer, is added to an MG antigen coated plate. Specific MG antibody in the serum forms an antibody-antigen complex with the MG antigen bound to the plate. After washing the plate, an affinity purified goat anti-turkey IgG (H+L) peroxidase conjugate is added to each well. The antibody-antigen complex remaining from the previous step binds with the conjugate. After a brief incubation period, the unbound conjugate is removed by a second wash step. Substrate, which contains a chromagen (ABTS), is added to each well. Chromagen color change (from clear to green-blue) occurs in the presence of the peroxidase enzyme. The relative intensity of color developed in 15 minutes (compared to controls) is directly proportional to the level of MG antibody in the serum. After the substrate has incubated, Stop Solution is added to each well to terminate the reaction and the plate is read using an ELISA plate reader at 405-410 nm.

Test Procedure:

Sample Collection: For routine serologic flock monitoring, it is suggested that at least 30 or more sera per flock be randomly collected at standard time intervals (i.e. every four weeks). Proper sample collection procedures, serum harvest and serum sample storage (4°C for up to four days or -20°C for longer periods) are needed to provide reliable test results.

Sample Dilution Procedure: Dilute serum samples using Dilution Buffer in a clean, uncoated 96 well microtiter plate. Set up samples and controls as shown in Figure 1.

Preparation of the Serum Dilution Plate:

a) Add 300 µL Dilution Buffer to each well of an uncoated 96 well microtiter plate. This plate is referred to as the serum dilution plate.

b) Add 6 µL unknown serum per well as per Figure 1 (producing a 1:50 dilution). Start with well A4 and end with well H9 (moving left to right, row by row of wells). For example, wells 1 through 30 contain the diluted sera of flock 1, wells 31-60 contain the diluted sera of flock 2, etc.

c) Add 6 µL of Normal Control Serum (producing a 1:50 dilution) to wells A2, H10 and H12.

d) Aspirate and remove any liquid in dilution plate wells A1, A3 and H11.

e) Allow all diluted serums to equilibrate in Dilution Buffer for 5 minutes before transferring to an MG antigen coated ELISA plate.

f) Diluted serum should be tested within 24 hours.

This dilution format provides adequate quantities of diluted serum samples to conduct four additional ProFLOK® ELISA tests (i.e. MS, MM, NDV and HE) using the same serum dilution plate.

Preparation of MG-T Positive Control: An MG-T Positive Control Serum has been provided with this kit. Dilute the appropriate volume of MG-T Positive Control Serum with Dilution Buffer (1:50) in a clean, glass test tube. For example, dilute 6 µL of positive control serum in 300 µL Dilution Buffer. Mix well. 150 µL of MG-T Positive Control is needed per ELISA plate.

Preparation of Conjugate Solution: The horseradish peroxidase conjugated anti-turkey IgG (H+L) is supplied in 50% glycerol. Dilute 100 µL stock conjugate in 10 mL Dilution Buffer (1:100 dilution). Mix well. This 10 mL preparation will supply sufficient conjugate for one 96 well ELISA plate.

Preparation of 1X Wash Solution: Dilute 20 mL concentrated Wash Solution in 380 mL laboratory grade (distilled or R.O.) water (1:20). Mix well. Approximately 400 mL Wash Solution is needed for each 96 well ELISA plate.

Preparation of the Substrate Solution: The Substrate Solution is ready to use. Each plate will require approximately 10 mL substrate solution. For best results, the substrate solution must be equilibrated to room temperature before use.

Preparation of 1X Stop Solution: Dilute 2.5 mL concentrated Stop Solution in 10 mL laboratory grade (distilled or R.O.) water (1:5). Mix well. Approximately 12.5 mL Stop Solution is needed for each 96 well ELISA plate.

Note: Storage of 5X Stop Solution at refrigerated temperatures may cause the formation of a white solid. This does not affect product performance. Warm at room temperature or 37°C to dissolve before use.

Figure 1.

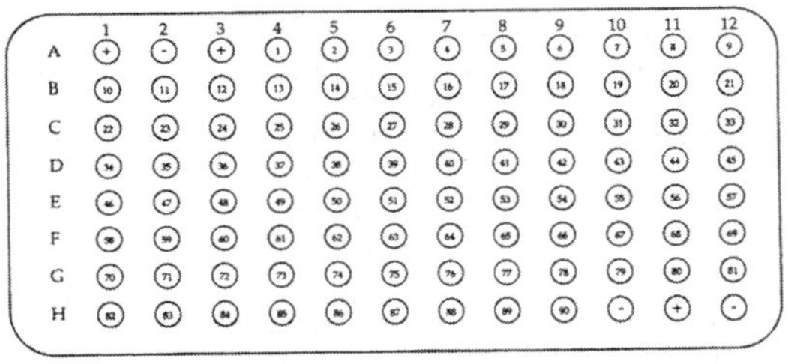

	1	2	3	4	5	6	7	8	9	10	11	12
A	+	-	+	1	2	3	4	5	6	7	8	9
B	10	11	12	13	14	15	16	17	18	19	20	21
C	22	23	24	25	26	27	28	29	30	31	32	33
D	34	35	36	37	38	39	40	41	42	43	44	45
E	46	47	48	49	50	51	52	53	54	55	56	57
F	58	59	60	61	62	63	64	65	66	67	68	69
G	70	71	72	73	74	75	76	77	78	79	80	81
H	82	83	84	85	86	87	88	89	90	-	+	-

ELISA Test Procedure:

Preparing the Test Plate:

a) Remove an MG-T test plate from the protective bag and label according to dilution plate identification.

b) Add 50 µL Dilution Buffer to all wells on the test plate.

c) Add 50 µL diluted MG-T Positive Control Serum to wells A1, A3 and H11. Discard pipette tip.

d) Using an 8 or 12 channel pipette transfer 50 µL/well of each of the diluted serum samples and Normal Control Serum samples from the dilution plate to the corresponding wells of the MG coated test plate. Discard pipette tips after each row of sample is transferred. Transfer of samples to the ELISA plate should be done as quickly as possible.

e) Incubate plate for 30 minutes at room temperature.

Wash Procedure:

f) Tap out liquid from each well into an appropriate vessel containing bleach or other decontamination agent.

g) Using an 8 or 12 channel pipette (or comparable automatic washing device), fill each well with approximately 300 µL Wash Solution. Allow to soak in wells for 3 minutes; then discard contents into an appropriate waste container (waste container should contain bleach solution). Tap inverted plate to ensure that all residual liquid is removed. Repeat wash procedure 2 more times.

Note: The wash procedure is a very critical step in any ELISA procedure. Please follow the above steps as directed.

Addition of Anti-Turkey IgG Peroxidase Conjugate, Substrate and Stop Solution:

h) Using an 8 or 12 channel pipette (or transplating device) dispense 100 µL diluted conjugate (prepared as described above) into each assay well. Discard pipette tips.

i) Incubate for 30 minutes at room temperature.

j) Wash as in steps f and g above.

k) Using an 8 or 12 channel pipette (or transplating device), dispense 100 µL Substrate Solution into each test well. Discard pipette tips.
l) Incubate 15 minutes at room temperature.
m) Using an 8 or 12 channel pipette (or transplating device), add 100 µL diluted Stop Solution (prepared as described above) to each test well.
n) Allow bubbles to dissipate before reading plate.

Manual Processing of Data:
a) Read the plate using an ELISA plate reader set at 405-410 nm. Be sure to blank the reader as directed. If a Flow Multiscan reader is used, the reader should be blanked using an empty microtiter plate. If a Bio-tek or Dynatech reader is used, the machine may be blanked with air.
b) Calculate the average Positive Control Serum absorbance (Optical Density [O.D.]) using the absorbance values of wells A1, A3 and H11. Calculate the average Normal Control Serum absorbance using values obtained from wells A2, H10 and H12. Record both averages.
c) Subtract the average normal control absorbance from the average positive absorbance. The difference is the Corrected Positive Control.
d) Calculate a sample to positive (Sp) ratio by subtracting the average normal control absorbance from each sample absorbance. The difference is divided by the Corrected Positive Control. Use the following equation format:

$$SP = \frac{\text{(Sample Absorbance)} - \text{(Average Normal Control Absorbance)}}{\text{Corrected Positive Control Absorbance}}$$

e) An MG-T ELISA titer can be calculated by the following suggested equation:
$\text{Log}_{10}\ \text{Titer} = (1.464 \times \text{Log}_{10}\ \text{Sp}) + 3.197$
Titer = Antilog of Log_{10} Titer

Example:
1. Example Positive Control Absorbance:
 0.585, 0.610, 0.590
 Average = (0.585 + 0.610 + 0.590) / 3 = 0.595
2. Example Normal Controls:
 0.082, 0.085, 0.079
 Average = (0.082 + 0.085 + 0.079) / 3 = 0.082
3. Corrected Positive Control:
 (0.595) - (0.082) = 0.513
4. Example Sp value calculation:
 Absorbance of sample = 0.560
 (0.560) - (0.082) / 0.513 = 0.931
5. Example of Calculation of titer using the Sp from above:
 Log_{10} Titer = 1.464 X (Log_{10} 0.931) + 3.197
 Titer = Antilog 3.15
 Titer = 1413

Test Interpretation: Results:

Assay Control Values: Valid MG-T ELISA results are obtained when the average optical density (O.D.) value of the Normal Control Serum is less than 0.200 and the Corrected Positive Control value range is between 0.250 and 0.900. If either of these values are out of range, the MG test results should be considered invalid and the samples should be retested. Samples testing with an Sp value of less than or equal to 0.299 will receive a 0 titer value and are considered negative for MG antibody.

Under optimal conditions* the suggested O.D. value ranges of 0.05 to 0.08 for MG-T Normal Control Serum and 0.40 to 0.80 for MG-T Positive Control Serum should be strived for to ensure the most consistent laboratory test results. Please note that tests with O.D. values which do not fall within the suggested O.D. ranges above does not constitute an invalid test.

*Optimal conditions are at room temperature [70 to 75°F (21 to 24°C)]. Higher room temperatures may result in slightly higher O.D. values.

Interpretation of Results: The MG-T Sp ratio values and/or ELISA titer values obtained for sera should be interpreted using the following value ranges:

Sample to Positive (Sp) Value	MG ELISA Titer Range	MG Presumed Antibody Status
Less than 0.300	0	Negative[a]
0.300 to 0.599	270 to 743	Probable[b,c]
Greater or equal to 0.6	744 or greater	Positive[c]

a. Negative. Serum samples with an MG-T Sp ratio value of less than 0.300 receive a "0" titer value and are presumed negative for MG antibody. However, a variety of factors, such as the biological and antigenic properties of various *Mycoplasma gallisepticum* isolates,[1,3] onset and stage of infection, prevalence of an MG isolate infection within a flock and timing and randomness of serum sample collection procedures could result in an MG-infected turkey flock yielding MG-negative ELISA results. It is therefore recommended that each turkey flock only be considered to be MG negative after (a) each flock has been adequately sampled and repeatedly tested several times and has yielded negative MG ELISA results each time and (b) each flock has been adequately sampled and repeatedly tested by standard conventional serologic tests (SPA and HI) and MG culture techniques[2] and has yielded MG negative serologic and culture results each time.

b. Probable. Presumed MG antibody probable denotes the ELISA Sp value range within which MG-T ELISA and conventional (SPA and HI) test data may suggest but may not conclusively detect MG antibody within a sample. The probable range represents a "suspect" or "gray" area in which MG-T ELISA results may or may not be supported by conventional serologic (SPA and HI) test results. It is highly recommended that additional conventional serologic tests and MG culture techniques[2] be conducted on serum and culture samples collected from MG-T ELISA probable turkey flocks, as recommended in parts a and c, to confirm whether each flock is an MG negative or MG positive-infected flock.

c. Positive. Additional conventional serologic testing (SPA and HI) and culturing of samples collected from presumed MG-T ELISA antibody probable and positive turkey flocks, using standard techniques,[2] are needed to obtain a confirmed positive diagnosis of MG infection within a turkey flock.

Storage: Store all reagents provided in the kit at 2-7°C.

Caution(s): To the Users of Reagents and MG Antigen Coated Plates:
a) Handle all reagents and samples as biohazardous material.
b) Keep all reagents away from skin and eyes. If exposure should occur, immediately flush affected areas with cold water.
c) Wash solution, control sera, test plates, field samples and all other test kit reagents should be properly decontaminated with bleach or other strong oxidizing agent before disposal.
d) Take special care not to contaminate any of the test reagents with serum or bacterial agents.
e) Humidity indicators are supplied with each plate. If any of the indicators exhibit a pink color, the plate may be compromised in some way; decontaminate (i.e. wash the plate with bleach solution) and dispose of the plate.
f) The best results are achieved by following the protocols as they are described above, using good, safe laboratory techniques.
g) Do not use this kit after the expiration date.
h) Never pipette by mouth.

Allow all reagents to come to room temperature before starting.

References: Available upon request.

Presentation: 900 tests.

Compendium Code No.: 11150280

PROFLOK® MM-T ELISA KIT

Synbiotics **ELISA Test**

Mycoplasma meleagridis Antibody Test Kit (Turkey)

U.S. Vet. Lic. No.: 350

Reagents:
a) 1 MM-T antigen coated plate.
b) 10 µL MM-T Positive Control Serum.
c) 10 µL Normal Control Serum.
d) 100 µL Goat anti-Turkey IgG (H+L) Peroxidase Conjugate Solution.
e) 40 mL Dilution Buffer.
f) 10 mL ABTS-Hydrogen Peroxide Substrate Solution.
g) 2.5 mL 5X Stop Solution (dilute [1:5] with laboratory grade water).
h) 20 mL 20X Wash Solution (dilute [1:20] with laboratory grade water).

Equipment and Materials Required:
a) High precision pipette (i.e. 1-20 microliter pipette).
b) 0.2 mL, 1.0 mL and 5.0 mL pipettes.
c) 8 or 12 channel pipette (or transplating device).
d) 2 graduated cylinders (50 mL).
e) 5 mL borosilicate glass test tubes.
f) Uncoated low binding 96 well plates (i.e. Nunc catalog #269620).
g) Laboratory grade (Distilled or R.O.) water.
h) 96 well plate reading spectrophotometer with 405-410 nm filter.
i) Plate washing apparatus.

Indications: The PROFLOK® MM-T ELISA Kit is a rapid and presumptive serologic screening test for the detection of antibody to most conventional MM strains in turkey serum samples. It was designed for screening large numbers of turkey sera from numerous flocks; however, additional conventional MM serologic testing [i.e. serum plate agglutination (SPA) and hemagglutination-inhibition (HI) test] and culture techniques are needed to confirm MM negative and MM-infected turkey flocks.

Test Principles: *Mycoplasma meleagridis* (MM) infection of turkeys is the etiological agent of an egg-transmitted disease of turkeys characterized by decreased hatchability, skeletal abnormalities, reduced growth performance and airsacculitis in the progeny.

The assay is designed to measure MM antibody bound to MM antigen coated plates. The principle of the test is as follows: Serum obtained from turkeys exposed to MM antigens contains specific anti-MM antibodies. Serum, diluted in Dilution Buffer, is added to an MM antigen coated plate. Specific MM antibody in the serum forms an antibody-antigen complex with the MM antigen bound to the plate. After washing the plate, an affinity purified goat anti-turkey IgG (H+L) peroxidase conjugate is added to each well. The antibody-antigen complex remaining from the previous step binds with the conjugate. After a brief incubation period, the unbound conjugate is removed by a second wash step. Substrate, which contains a chromagen (ABTS), is added to each well. Chromagen color change (from clear to green-blue) occurs in the presence of the peroxidase enzyme. The relative intensity of color developed in 15 minutes (compared to controls) is directly proportional to the level of MM antibody in the serum. After the substrate has incubated, Stop Solution is added to each well to terminate the reaction and the plate is read using an ELISA plate reader at 405-410 nm.

Test Procedure:

Sample Collection: For routine serologic flock monitoring, it is suggested that at least 30 or more sera per flock be randomly collected at standard time intervals (i.e. every four weeks). Proper sample collection procedures, serum harvest and serum sample storage (4°C for up to four days or -20°C for longer periods) are needed to provide reliable test results.

Sample Dilution Procedure: Dilute serum samples using Dilution Buffer in a clean, uncoated 96 well microtiter plate. Set up samples and controls as shown in Figure 1.

Preparation of the Serum Dilution Plate:
a) Add 300 µL Dilution Buffer to each well of an uncoated 96 well microtiter plate. This plate is referred to as the serum dilution plate. Label serum dilution plate.
b) Add 6 µL unknown serum per well as per Figure 1 (producing a 1:50 dilution). Start with well A4 and end with well H9 (moving left to right, row by row of wells). For example, wells 1 through 30 contain the diluted sera of flock 1, wells 31-60 contain the diluted sera of flock 2, etc.
c) Add 6 µL of Normal Control Serum (producing a 1:50 dilution) to wells A2, H10 and H12.
d) Aspirate and remove any liquid in dilution plate wells A1, A3 and H11.
e) Allow all diluted serums to equilibrate in Dilution Buffer for 5 minutes before transferring to an MM antigen coated ELISA plate.
f) Diluted serum should be tested within 24 hours.

This dilution format provides adequate quantities of diluted serum samples to conduct four additional ProFLOK® ELISA tests (i.e. MS, MG, NDV and HE) using the same serum dilution plate.

Preparation of MM-T Positive Control: An MM-T Positive Control Serum has been provided with this kit. Dilute the appropriate volume of MM-T Positive Control Serum with Dilution Buffer (1:50) in a clean, glass test tube. For example, dilute 6 µL of positive control serum in 300 µL Dilution Buffer. Mix well. 150 µL of MM-T Positive Control is needed per ELISA plate.

Preparation of Conjugate Solution: The horseradish peroxidase conjugated anti-turkey IgG (H+L) is supplied in 50% glycerol. Dilute 100 µL stock conjugate in 10 mL Dilution Buffer (1:100 dilution). Mix well. This 10 mL preparation will supply sufficient conjugate for one 96 well ELISA plate.

Preparation of 1X Wash Solution: Dilute 20 mL concentrated Wash Solution in 380 mL laboratory grade (distilled or R.O.) water (1:20). Mix well. Approximately 400 mL diluted Wash Solution is needed for each 96 well ELISA plate.

Preparation of the Substrate Solution: The Substrate Solution is ready to use. Each plate will require approximately 10 mL substrate solution. For best results, the substrate solution must be equilibrated to room temperature before use.

Preparation of 1X Stop Solution: Dilute 2.5 mL concentrated Stop Solution in 10 mL laboratory grade (distilled or R.O.) water (1:5). Mix well. Approximately 12.5 mL diluted Stop Solution is needed for each 96 well ELISA plate.

Note: Storage of 5X Stop Solution at refrigerated temperatures may cause the formation of a white solid. This does not affect product performance. Warm at room temperature or 37°C to dissolve before use.

Figure 1.

	1	2	3	4	5	6	7	8	9	10	11	12
A	+	-	+	1	2	3	4	5	6	7	8	9
B	10	11	12	13	14	15	16	17	18	19	20	21
C	22	23	24	25	26	27	28	29	30	31	32	33
D	34	35	36	37	38	39	40	41	42	43	44	45
E	46	47	48	49	50	51	52	53	54	55	56	57
F	58	59	60	61	62	63	64	65	66	67	68	69
G	70	71	72	73	74	75	76	77	78	79	80	81
H	82	83	84	85	86	87	88	89	90	-	+	-

ELISA Test Procedure:

Preparing the Test Plate:

a) Remove an MM-T test plate from the protective bag and label according to dilution plate identification.

b) Add 50 µL Dilution Buffer to all wells on the test plate.

c) Add 50 µL diluted MM-T Positive Control Serum to wells A1, A3 and H11. Discard pipette tip.

d) Using an 8 or 12 channel pipette transfer 50 µL/well of each of the diluted serum samples and Normal Control Serum samples from the dilution plate to the corresponding wells of the MM coated test plate. Discard pipette tips after each row of sample is transferred. Transfer of samples to the ELISA plate should be done as quickly as possible.

e) Incubate plate for 30 minutes at room temperature.

Wash Procedure:

f) Tap out liquid from each well into an appropriate vessel containing bleach or other decontamination agent.

g) Using an 8 or 12 channel pipette (or comparable automatic washing device), fill each well with approximately 300 µL Wash Solution. Allow to soak in wells for 3 minutes; then discard contents into an appropriate waste container (waste container should contain bleach solution). Tap inverted plate to ensure that all residual liquid is removed. Repeat wash procedure 2 more times.

Note: The wash procedure is a very critical step in any ELISA procedure. Please follow the above steps as directed.

Addition of Anti-Turkey IgG Peroxidase Conjugate, Substrate and Stop Solution:

h) Using an 8 or 12 channel pipette (or transplating device) dispense 100 µL diluted conjugate (prepared as described above) into each assay well. Discard pipette tips.

i) Incubate for 30 minutes at room temperature.

j) Wash as in steps f and g above.

k) Using an 8 or 12 channel pipette (or transplating device), dispense 100 µL Substrate Solution into each test well. Discard pipette tips.

l) Incubate 15 minutes at room temperature.

m) Using an 8 or 12 channel pipette (or transplating device), add 100 µL diluted Stop Solution (prepared as described above) to each test well.

n) Allow bubbles to dissipate before reading plate.

Manual Processing of Data:

a) Read the plate using an ELISA plate reader set at 405-410 nm. Be sure to blank the reader as directed. If a Flow Multiscan reader is used, the reader should be blanked using an empty microtiter plate. If a Bio-tek or Dynatech reader is used, the machine may be blanked with air.

b) Calculate the average Positive Control Serum absorbance (Optical Density [O.D.]) using the absorbance values of wells A1, A3 and H11. Calculate the average Normal Control Serum absorbance using values obtained from wells A2, H10 and H12. Record both averages.

c) Subtract the average normal control absorbance from the average positive control absorbance. The difference is the Corrected Positive Control.

d) Calculate a sample to positive (Sp) ratio by subtracting the average normal control absorbance from each sample absorbance. The difference is divided by the Corrected Positive Control. Use the following equation format:

$$SP = \frac{\text{(Sample Absorbance)} - \text{(Average Normal Control Absorbance)}}{\text{Corrected Positive Control Absorbance}}$$

e) An MM-T ELISA titer can be calculated by the following suggested equation:

$\text{Log}_{10}\ \text{Titer} = (1.464 \times \text{Log}_{10}\ \text{Sp}) + 3.197$

Titer = Antilog of Log_{10} Titer

Example:

1. Example Positive Control Absorbance:
   0.585, 0.610, 0.590
   Average = (0.585 + 0.610 + 0.590) / 3 = 0.595
2. Example Normal Controls:
   0.082, 0.085, 0.079
   Average = (0.082 + 0.085 + 0.079) / 3 = 0.082
3. Corrected Positive Control:
   (0.595) - (0.082) = 0.513
4. Example Sp value calculation:
   Absorbance of sample = 0.560
   (0.560) - (0.082) / 0.513 = 0.931
5. Example of calculation of titer using the Sp from above:
   Log_{10} Titer = 1.464 X (Log_{10} 0.931) + 3.197
   Titer = Antilog 3.15
   Titer = 1413

Test Interpretation: Results:

Assay Control Values: Valid MM-T ELISA results are obtained when the average optical density (O.D.) value of the Normal Control Serum is less than 0.200 and the Corrected Positive Control value range is between 0.250 and 0.900. If either of these values are out of range, the MM test results should be considered invalid and the samples should be retested. Samples testing with an Sp value of less than or equal to 0.299 will receive a 0 titer value and are considered negative for MM antibody.

Under optimal conditions* the suggested O.D. value ranges of 0.045 to 0.095 for MM-T Normal Control Serum and 0.350 to 0.800 for MM-T Positive Control Serum should be strived for to ensure the most consistent laboratory test results. Please note that a plate with O.D. values which do not fall within the suggested O.D. ranges above does not constitute an invalid test.

*Optimal conditions are at room temperature [70 to 75°F (21 to 24°C)]. Higher room temperatures may result in slightly higher O.D. values.

Interpretation of Results: The MM-T Sp ratio values and/or ELISA titer values obtained for sera should be interpreted using the following value ranges:

Sample to Positive (Sp) Value	MM ELISA Titer Range	MM Presumed Antibody Status
Less than 0.300	0	Negative[a]
0.300 to 0.599	270 to 743	Probable[b,c]
Greater or equal to 0.6	744 or greater	Positive[c]

a. Negative. Serum samples with an MM-T Sp ratio value of less than 0.300 receive a "0" titer value and are presumed negative for MM antibody. However, a variety of factors, such as the biological and antigenic properties of various *Mycoplasma meleagridis* strains,[1,2] prevalence of an MM strain within a flock and timing and randomness of serum sample collection procedures could result in an MM-infected turkey flock yielding MM-negative ELISA results. It is therefore recommended that each turkey flock only be considered to be MM negative after (a) each flock has been adequately sampled and repeatedly tested several times and has yielded negative MM ELISA results each time and (b) each flock has been adequately sampled and repeatedly tested by standard conventional serologic tests (SPA and HI) and MM culture techniques[2] and has yielded MM negative serologic and culture results each time.

b. Probable. Presumed MM antibody probable denotes the ELISA Sp value range within which MM-T ELISA and conventional (SPA and HI) test data may suggest but may not conclusively detect MM antibody within a sample. The probable range represents a "suspect" or "gray" area in which MM-T ELISA results may or may not be supported by conventional serologic (SPA and HI) test results. It is highly recommended that additional conventional serologic tests and MM culture techniques[2] be conducted on serum and culture samples collected from MM-T ELISA probable turkey flocks, as recommended in parts a and c, to confirm whether each flock is an MM negative or MM positive-infected flock.

c. Positive. Additional conventional serologic testing (SPA and HI) and culturing of samples collected from presumed MM-T ELISA antibody probable and positive turkey flocks, using standard techniques,[2] are needed to obtain a confirmed positive diagnosis of MM infection within a turkey flock.

Storage: Store all reagents provided in the kit at 2-10°C.

Caution(s): To the Users of Reagents and MM Antigen Coated Plates:

a) Handle all reagents and samples as biohazardous material.

b) Keep all reagents away from skin and eyes. If exposure should occur, immediately flush affected areas with cold water.

c) Wash solution, control sera, test plates, field samples and all other test kit reagents should be properly decontaminated with bleach or other strong oxidizing agent before disposal.

d) Take special care not to contaminate any of the test reagents with serum or bacterial agents.

e) Humidity indicators are supplied with each plate. If any of the indicators exhibit a pink color, the plate may be compromised in some way; decontaminate (i.e. wash the plate with bleach solution) and dispose of the plate.

f) The best results are achieved by following the protocols as they are described above, using good, safe laboratory techniques.

g) Do not use this kit after the expiration date.

h) Never pipette by mouth.

Allow all reagents to come to room temperature before starting.

References: Available upon request.

Presentation: 900 tests.

Compendium Code No.: 11150290

PROFLOK® MS ELISA KIT

Synbiotics **ELISA Test**

Mycoplasma synoviae Antibody Test Kit

U.S. Vet. Lic. No.: 350

Reagents:

a) 1 MS antigen coated plate.

b) 10 µL MS Positive Control Serum.

c) 10 µL Normal Control Serum.

d) 100 µL Goat anti-Chicken IgG (H+L) Peroxidase Conjugate Solution.

e) 40 mL Dilution Buffer.

f) 10 mL ABTS-Hydrogen Peroxide Substrate Solution.

g) 2.5 mL 5X Stop Solution (dilute [1:5] with laboratory grade water).

h) 20 mL 20X Wash Solution (dilute [1:20] with laboratory grade water).

Equipment and Materials Required:

a) High precision pipette (i.e. 1-20 microliter pipette).

b) 0.2 mL, 1.0 mL and 5.0 mL pipettes.

c) 8 or 12 channel pipette (or transplating device).

d) 2 graduated cylinders (50 mL).

e) 5 mL borosilicate glass test tubes.

f) Uncoated low binding 96 well plates (i.e. Nunc catalog #269620).

g) Laboratory grade (Distilled or R.O.) water.

h) 96 well plate reading spectrophotometer with 405-410 nm filter.

i) Plate washing apparatus.

Indications: The PROFLOK® MS ELISA Kit is a rapid and specific presumptive screening test for the detection of antibody to most conventional MS strains in chicken serum samples. It was designed for screening large numbers of chicken sera from numerous flocks; however, additional conventional MS serologic testing [i.e. serum plate agglutination (SPA) and hemagglutination-inhibition (HI) test] and culture techniques are needed to confirm MS-negative and MS-infected chicken flocks.

Test Principles: *Mycoplasma synoviae* (MS) infection of chickens is associated with acute to chronic infectious synovitis, airsacculitis and increased condemnation losses.[1,3] MS may be vertically transmitted from infected hens to progeny or horizontally transmitted via the respiratory tract.[1,3]

The assay is designed to measure MS antibody bound to MS antigen coated plates. The principle of the test is as follows: Serum obtained from chickens exposed to MS antigens contains specific anti-MS antibodies. Serum, diluted in Dilution Buffer, is added to an MS antigen coated plate. Specific MS antibody in the serum forms an antibody-antigen complex with the MS antigen bound to the plate. After washing the plate, an affinity purified goat anti-chicken IgG (H+L) peroxidase conjugate is added to each well. The antibody-antigen complex remaining from the previous step binds with the conjugate. After a brief incubation period, the unbound conjugate is removed by a second wash step. Substrate, which contains a chromagen (ABTS), is added to each well. Chromagen color change (from clear to green-blue) occurs in the presence of the peroxidase enzyme. The relative intensity of color developed in 15 minutes (compared to controls) is directly proportional to the level of MS antibody in the serum. After the substrate has incubated, Stop Solution is added to each well to terminate the reaction and the plate is read using an ELISA plate reader at 405-410 nm.

Test Procedure:

Sample Collection: For routine serologic flock monitoring, it is suggested that at least 30 or more sera per flock be randomly collected at standard time intervals (i.e. every four weeks). Proper sample collection procedures, serum harvest and serum sample storage (4°C for up to four days or -20°C for longer periods) are needed to provide reliable test results.

Sample Dilution Procedure: Dilute serum samples using Dilution Buffer in a clean, uncoated 96 well microtiter plate. Set up samples and controls as shown in Figure 1.

Preparation of the Serum Dilution Plate:

a) Add 300 μL Dilution Buffer to each well of an uncoated 96 well microtiter plate. This plate is referred to as the serum dilution plate.
b) Add 6 μL unknown serum per well as per Figure 1 (producing a 1:50 dilution). Start with well A4 and end with well H9 (moving left to right, row by row of wells). For example, wells 1 through 30 contain the diluted sera of flock 1, wells 31-60 contain the diluted sera of flock 2, etc.
c) Add 6 μL of Normal Control Serum (producing a 1:50 dilution) to wells A2, H10 and H12.
d) Aspirate and remove any liquid in dilution plate wells A1, A3 and H11.
e) Allow all diluted serums to equilibrate in Dilution Buffer for 5 minutes before transferring to an MS antigen coated ELISA plate.
f) Diluted serum should be tested within 24 hours.

This dilution format provides adequate quantities of diluted serum samples to conduct four additional ProFLOK® ELISA tests (i.e. MG, IBD, IBV and REO) using the same serum dilution plate.

Preparation of MS Positive Control: An MS Positive Control Serum has been provided with this kit. Dilute the appropriate volume of MS Positive Control Serum with Dilution Buffer (1:50) in a clean, glass test tube. For example, dilute 6 μL of Positive Control Serum in 300 μL Dilution Buffer. Mix well. 150 μL of MS Positive Control Serum is needed per ELISA plate.

Preparation of Conjugate Solution: The horseradish peroxidase conjugated anti-chicken IgG (H+L) is supplied in 50% glycerol. Dilute 100 μL stock conjugate in 10 mL Dilution Buffer (1:100 dilution). Mix well. This 10 mL preparation will supply sufficient conjugate for one 96 well ELISA plate.

Preparation of 1X Wash Solution: Dilute 20 mL concentrated Wash Solution in 380 mL laboratory grade (distilled or R.O.) water (1:20). Mix well. Approximately 400 mL diluted Wash Solution is needed for each 96 well ELISA plate.

Preparation of the Substrate Solution: The Substrate Solution is ready to use. Each plate will require approximately 10 mL substrate solution. For best results, the substrate solution must be equilibrated to room temperature before use.

Preparation of 1X Stop Solution: Dilute 2.5 mL concentrated Stop Solution in 10 mL laboratory grade (distilled or R.O.) water (1:5). Mix well. Approximately 12.5 mL diluted Stop Solution is needed for each 96 well ELISA plate.

Note: Storage of 5X Stop Solution at refrigerated temperatures may cause the formation of a white solid. This does not affect product performance. Warm at room temperature or 37°C to dissolve before use.

Figure 1.

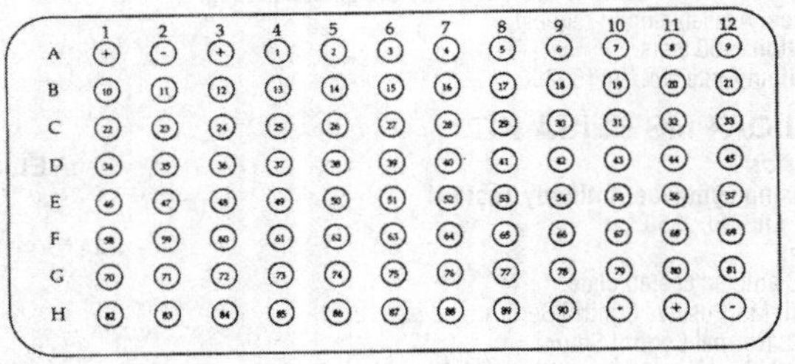

	1	2	3	4	5	6	7	8	9	10	11	12
A	+	-	+	1	2	3	4	5	6	7	8	9
B	10	11	12	13	14	15	16	17	18	19	20	21
C	22	23	24	25	26	27	28	29	30	31	32	33
D	34	35	36	37	38	39	40	41	42	43	44	45
E	46	47	48	49	50	51	52	53	54	55	56	57
F	58	59	60	61	62	63	64	65	66	67	68	69
G	70	71	72	73	74	75	76	77	78	79	80	81
H	82	83	84	85	86	87	88	89	90	-	+	-

ELISA Test Procedure:

Preparing the Test Plate:

a) Remove an MS antigen coated test plate from the protective bag and label according to dilution plate identification.
b) Add 50 μL Dilution Buffer to all wells on the test plate.
c) Add 50 μL diluted MS Positive Control Serum to wells A1, A3 and H11. Discard pipette tip.
d) Using an 8 or 12 channel pipette transfer 50 μL/well of each of the diluted serum samples and Normal Control Serum samples from the dilution plate to the corresponding wells of the MS coated test plate. Discard pipette tips after each row of sample is transferred. Transfer of samples to the ELISA plate should be done as quickly as possible.
e) Incubate plate for 30 minutes at room temperature.

Wash Procedure:

f) Tap out liquid from each well into an appropriate vessel containing bleach or other decontamination agent.
g) Using an 8 or 12 channel pipette (or comparable automatic washing device), fill each well with approximately 300 μL Wash Solution. Allow to soak in wells for 3 minutes; then discard contents into an appropriate waste container (waste container should contain bleach solution). Tap inverted plate to ensure that all residual liquid is removed. Repeat wash procedure 2 more times.

Note: The wash procedure is a very critical step in any ELISA procedure. Please follow the above steps as directed.

Addition of Anti-Chicken IgG Peroxidase Conjugate, Substrate and Stop Solution:

h) Using an 8 or 12 channel pipette (or transplating device) dispense 100 μL diluted conjugate (prepared as described above) into each assay well. Discard pipette tips.
i) Incubate for 30 minutes at room temperature.
j) Wash as in steps f and g above.
k) Using an 8 or 12 channel pipette (or transplating device) dispense 100 μL Substrate Solution into each test well. Discard pipette tips.
l) Incubate 15 minutes at room temperature.
m) Using an 8 or 12 channel pipette (or transplating device) add 100 μL diluted Stop Solution (prepared as described above) to each test well.
n) Allow bubbles to dissipate before reading plate.

Manual Processing of Data:

a) Read the plate using an ELISA plate reader set at 405-410 nm. Be sure to blank the reader as directed. If a Flow Multiscan reader is used, the reader should be blanked using an empty microtiter plate. If a Bio-tek or Dynatech reader is used, the machine may be blanked with air.
b) Calculate the average Positive Control Serum absorbance (Optical Density [O.D.]) using the absorbance values of wells A1, A3 and H11. Calculate the average Normal Control Serum absorbance using values obtained from wells A2, H10 and H12. Record both averages.
c) Subtract the average normal control absorbance from the average positive absorbance. The difference is the Corrected Positive Control.
d) Calculate a sample to positive (Sp) ratio by subtracting the average normal control absorbance from each sample absorbance. The difference is divided by the Corrected Positive Control. Use the following equation format:

$$SP = \frac{\text{(Sample Absorbance)} - \text{(Average Normal Control Absorbance)}}{\text{Corrected Positive Control Absorbance}}$$

e) An MS ELISA titer can be calculated by the following suggested equation:

Log_{10} Titer = (1.464 X Log_{10} Sp) + 3.197

Titer = Antilog of Log_{10} Titer

Example:

1. Example Positive Control Absorbance:
   0.585, 0.610, 0.590
   Average = (0.585 + 0.610 + 0.590) / 3 = 0.595
2. Example Normal Controls:
   0.078, 0.067, 0.057
   Average = (0.078 + 0.067 + 0.057) / 3 = 0.067
3. Corrected Positive Control:
   (0.595) - (0.067) = 0.528
4. Example Sp value calculation:
   Absorbance of sample = 0.560
   (0.560) - (0.067) / 0.528 = 0.934
5. Example of calculation of titer using the Sp from above:
   Log_{10} Titer = 1.464 X (Log_{10} 0.934) + 3.197
   Titer = Antilog 3.15
   Titer = 1413

Test Interpretation: Results:

Assay Control Values: Valid MS ELISA results are obtained when the average optical density (O.D.) value of the Normal Control Serum is less than 0.200 and the Corrected Positive Control value range is between 0.250 and 0.900. If either of these values are out of range, the MS test results should be considered invalid and the samples should be retested. Samples testing with an Sp value of less than or equal to 0.299 will receive a 0 titer value and are considered negative for MS antibody.

Under optimal conditions* the suggested O.D. value ranges of 0.050 to 0.100 for MS Normal Control Serum and 0.400 to 0.850 for MS Positive Control Serum should be strived for to ensure the most consistent laboratory test results. Please note that tests with O.D. values which do not fall within the suggested O.D. ranges above does not constitute an invalid test.

*Optimal conditions are at room temperature [70 to 75°F (21 to 24°C)]. Higher room temperatures may result in slightly higher O.D. values.

Interpretation of Results: The MS Sp ratio values and/or ELISA titer values obtained for sera should be interpreted using the following value ranges:

Sample to Positive (Sp) Value	MS ELISA Titer Range	MS Presumed Antibody Status
Less than 0.300	0	Negative[a]
0.300 to 0.599	270 to 743	Probable[b,c]
Greater or equal to 0.6	744 or greater	Positive[c]

a. Negative. Serum samples with an MS Sp ratio value of less than 0.300 receive a "0" titer value and are presumed negative for MS antibody. However, a variety of factors, such as possible MS strain variations that may exhibit atypical biological and/or antigenic properties,[1,2] prevalence of an MS strain within a flock and timing and randomness of serum sample collection procedures could result in an MS-infected chicken flock yielding MS-negative ELISA results. It is therefore recommended that each chicken flock only be considered to be MS negative after (a) each flock has been adequately sampled and repeatedly tested several times and has yielded negative MS ELISA results each time and (b) each flock has been adequately sampled and repeatedly tested by standard conventional serologic tests (SPA and HI) and MS culture techniques[2] and has yielded MS negative serologic and culture results each time.

b. Probable. Presumed MS antibody probable denotes the ELISA Sp value range within which MS ELISA and conventional (SPA and HI) test data may suggest but may not conclusively detect MS antibody within a sample. The probable range represents a "suspect" or "gray" area in which MS ELISA results may or may not be supported by conventional serologic (SPA and HI) test results. It is highly recommended that additional conventional serologic tests and MS culture techniques[3] be conducted on serum and culture samples collected from MS ELISA probable chicken flocks, as recommended in parts a and c, to confirm whether each flock is an MS negative or MS positive-infected flock.

c. Positive. Additional conventional serologic testing (SPA and HI) and culturing of samples collected from presumed MS ELISA antibody probable and positive chicken flocks, using standard techniques,[3] are needed to obtain a confirmed positive diagnosis of MS infection within a chicken flock.

Storage: Store all reagents provided in the kit at 2-10°C.

Caution(s): To the Users of Reagents and MS Antigen Coated Plates:

a) Handle all reagents and samples as biohazardous material.
b) Keep all reagents away from skin and eyes. If exposure should occur, immediately flush affected areas with cold water.
c) Wash solution, control sera, test plates, field samples and all other test kit reagents should be properly decontaminated with bleach or other strong oxidizing agent before disposal.
d) Take special care not to contaminate any of the test reagents with serum or bacterial agents.
e) Humidity indicators are supplied with each plate. If any of the indicators exhibit a pink color, the plate may be compromised in some way; decontaminate (i.e. wash the plate with bleach solution) and dispose of the plate.

f) The best results are achieved by following the protocols as they are described above, using good, safe laboratory techniques.
g) Do not use this kit after the expiration date.
h) Never pipette by mouth.
Allow all reagents to come to room temperature before starting.

References: Available upon request.
Presentation: 900 tests.
Compendium Code No.: 11150300

PROFLOK® MS-T ELISA KIT

Synbiotics **ELISA Test**

Mycoplasma synoviae Antibody Test Kit (Turkey)
U.S. Vet. Lic. No.: 350

Reagents:
a) 1 MS-T antigen coated plate.
b) 10 μL MS-T Positive Control Serum.
c) 10 μL Normal Control Serum.
d) 100 μL Goat anti-Turkey IgG (H+L) Peroxidase Conjugate Solution.
e) 40 mL Dilution Buffer.
f) 10 mL ABTS-Hydrogen Peroxide Substrate Solution.
g) 2.5 mL 5X Stop Solution (dilute [1:5] with laboratory grade water).
h) 20 mL 20X Wash Solution (dilute [1:20] with laboratory grade water).

Equipment and Materials Required:
a) High precision pipette (i.e. 1-20 microliter pipette).
b) 0.2 mL, 1.0 mL and 5.0 mL pipettes.
c) 8 or 12 channel pipette (or transplating device).
d) 2 graduated cylinders (50 mL).
e) 5 mL borosilicate glass test tubes.
f) Uncoated low binding 96 well plates (i.e. Nunc catalog #269620).
g) Laboratory grade (Distilled or R.O.) water.
h) 96 well plate reading spectrophotometer with 405-410 nm filter.
i) Plate washing apparatus.

Indications: The PROFLOK® MS-T ELISA Kit is a rapid and presumptive serologic screening test for the detection of antibody to most conventional MS strains (i.e. WVU-1853) in turkey serum samples. It was designed for screening large numbers of turkey sera from numerous flocks; however, additional conventional MS serologic testing [i.e. serum plate agglutination (SPA) and hemagglutination-inhibition (HI) test] and culture techniques are needed to confirm MS negative and MS-infected turkey flocks.

Test Principles: *Mycoplasma synoviae* (MS) infection of turkeys is associated with acute to chronic infectious synovitis, airsacculitis and increased condemnation losses.[1,2] MS may be vertically transmitted from infected hens to progeny or horizontally transmitted via the respiratory tract.[1,2]

The assay is designed to measure MS antibody bound to MS antigen coated plates. The principle of the test is as follows: Serum obtained from turkeys exposed to MS antigens contains specific anti-MS antibodies. Serum, diluted in Dilution Buffer, is added to an MS antigen coated plate. Specific MS antibody in the serum forms an antibody-antigen complex with the MS antigen bound to the plate. After washing the plate, an affinity purified goat anti-turkey IgG (H+L) peroxidase conjugate is added to each well. The antibody-antigen complex remaining from the previous step binds with the conjugate. After a brief incubation period, the unbound conjugate is removed by a second wash step. Substrate, which contains a chromagen (ABTS), is added to each well. Chromagen color change (from clear to green-blue) occurs in the presence of the peroxidase enzyme. The relative intensity of color developed in 15 minutes (compared to controls) is directly proportional to the level of MS antibody in the serum. After the substrate has incubated, Stop Solution is added to each well to terminate the reaction and the plate is read using an ELISA plate reader at 405-410 nm.

Test Procedure:

Sample Collection: For routine serologic flock monitoring, it is suggested that at least 30 or more sera per flock be randomly collected at standard time intervals (i.e. every four weeks). Proper sample collection procedures, serum harvest and serum sample storage (4°C for up to four days or -20°C for longer periods) are needed to provide reliable test results.

Sample Dilution Procedure: Dilute serum samples using Dilution Buffer in a clean, uncoated 96 well microtiter plate. Set up samples and controls as shown in Figure 1.

Preparation of the Serum Dilution Plate:
a) Add 300 μL Dilution Buffer to each well of an uncoated 96 well microtiter plate. This plate is referred to as the serum dilution plate. Label serum dilution plate.
b) Add 6 μL unknown serum per well as per Figure 1 (producing a 1:50 dilution). Start with well A4 and end with well H9 (moving left to right, row by row of wells). For example, wells 1 through 30 contain the diluted sera of flock 1, wells 31-60 contain the diluted sera of flock 2, etc.
c) Add 6 μL of Normal Control Serum (producing a 1:50 dilution) to wells A2, H10 and H12.
d) Aspirate and remove any liquid in dilution plate wells A1, A3 and H11.
e) Allow all diluted serums to equilibrate in Dilution Buffer for 5 minutes before transferring to an MS antigen coated ELISA plate.
f) Diluted serum should be tested within 24 hours.

This dilution format provides adequate quantities of diluted serum samples to conduct four additional ProFLOK® ELISA tests (i.e. MG, MM, NDV and HE) using the same serum dilution plate.

Preparation of MS-T Positive Control: An MS-T Positive Control Serum has been provided with this kit. Dilute the appropriate volume of MS-T Positive Control Serum with Dilution Buffer (1:50) in a clean, glass test tube. For example, dilute 6 μL of positive control serum in 300 μL Dilution Buffer. Mix well. 150 μL of MS-T Positive Control is needed per ELISA plate.

Preparation of Conjugate Solution: The horseradish peroxidase conjugated anti-turkey IgG (H+L) is supplied in 50% glycerol. Dilute 100 μL stock conjugate in 10 mL Dilution Buffer (1:100 dilution). Mix well. This 10 mL preparation will supply sufficient conjugate for one 96 well ELISA plate.

Preparation of 1X Wash Solution: Dilute 20 mL concentrated Wash Solution in 380 mL laboratory grade (distilled or R.O.) water (1:20). Mix well. Approximately 400 mL diluted Wash Solution is needed for each 96 well ELISA plate.

Preparation of the Substrate Solution: The Substrate Solution is ready to use. Each plate will require approximately 10 mL substrate solution. For best results, the substrate solution must be equilibrated to room temperature before use.

Preparation of 1X Stop Solution: Dilute 2.5 mL concentrated Stop Solution in 10 mL laboratory grade (distilled or R.O.) water (1:5). Mix well. Approximately 12.5 mL diluted Stop Solution is needed for each 96 well ELISA plate.

Note: Storage of 5X Stop Solution at refrigerated temperatures may cause the formation of a white solid. This does not affect product performance. Warm at room temperature or 37°C to dissolve before use.

Figure 1.

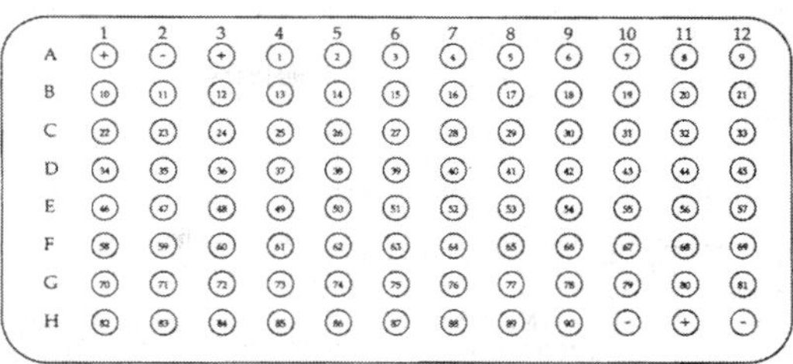

ELISA Test Procedure:

Preparing the Test Plate:
a) Remove an MS-T test plate from the protective bag and label according to dilution plate identification.
b) Add 50 μL Dilution Buffer to all wells on the test plate.
c) Add 50 μL diluted MS-T Positive Control Serum to wells A1, A3 and H11. Discard pipette tip.
d) Using an 8 or 12 channel pipette transfer 50 μL/well of each of the diluted serum samples and Normal Control Serum samples from the dilution plate to the corresponding wells of the MS coated test plate. Discard pipette tips after each row of sample is transferred. Transfer of samples to the ELISA plate should be done as quickly as possible.
e) Incubate plate for 30 minutes at room temperature.

Wash Procedure:
f) Tap out liquid from each well into an appropriate vessel containing bleach or other decontamination agent.
g) Using an 8 or 12 channel pipette (or comparable automatic washing device), fill each well with approximately 300 μL Wash Solution. Allow to soak in wells for 3 minutes; then discard contents into an appropriate waste container (waste container should contain bleach solution). Tap inverted plate to ensure that all residual liquid is removed. Repeat wash procedure 2 more times.

Note: The wash procedure is a very critical step in any ELISA procedure. Please follow the above steps as directed.

Addition of Anti-Turkey IgG Peroxidase Conjugate, Substrate and Stop Solution:
h) Using an 8 or 12 channel pipette (or transplating device), dispense 100 μL diluted conjugate (prepared as described above) into each assay well. Discard pipette tips.
i) Incubate for 30 minutes at room temperature.
j) Wash as in steps f and g above.
k) Using an 8 or 12 channel pipette (or transplating device), dispense 100 μL Substrate Solution into each test well. Discard pipette tips.
l) Incubate 15 minutes at room temperature.
m) Using an 8 or 12 channel pipette (or transplating device) add 100 μL diluted Stop Solution (prepared as described above) to each test well.
n) Allow bubbles to dissipate before reading plate.

Manual Processing of Data:
a) Read the plate using an ELISA plate reader set at 405-410 nm. Be sure to blank the reader as directed. If a Flow Multiscan reader is used, the reader should be blanked using an empty microtiter plate. If a Bio-tek or Dynatech reader is used, the machine may be blanked with air.
b) Calculate the average Positive Control Serum absorbance (Optical Density [O.D.]) using the absorbance values of wells A1, A3 and H11. Calculate the average Normal Control Serum absorbance using values obtained from wells A2, H10 and H12. Record both averages.
c) Subtract the average normal control absorbance from the average positive absorbance. The difference is the Corrected Positive Control.
d) Calculate a sample to positive (Sp) ratio by subtracting the average normal control absorbance from each sample absorbance. The difference is divided by the Corrected Positive Control. Use the following equation format:

$$SP = \frac{\text{(Sample Absorbance)} - \text{(Average Normal Control Absorbance)}}{\text{Corrected Positive Control Absorbance}}$$

e) An MS-T ELISA titer can be calculated by the following suggested equation:
Log_{10} Titer = (1.464 X Log_{10} Sp) + 3.197
Titer = Antilog of Log_{10} Titer

Example:
1. Example Positive Control Absorbance:
0.585, 0.610, 0.590
Average = (0.585 + 0.610 + 0.590) / 3 = 0.595
2. Example Normal Controls:
0.082, 0.085, 0.079
Average = (0.082 + 0.085 + 0.079) / 3 = 0.082
3. Corrected Positive Control:
(0.595) - (0.082) = 0.513
4. Example Sp value calculation:
Absorbance of sample = 0.560
(0.560) - (0.082) / 0.513 = 0.931
5. Example of calculation of titer using the Sp from above:
Log_{10} Titer = 1.464 X (Log_{10} 0.931) + 3.197
Titer = Antilog 3.15
Titer = 1413

Test Interpretation: Results:

Assay Control Values: Valid MS-T ELISA results are obtained when the average optical density (O.D.) value of the Normal Control Serum is less than 0.200 and the Corrected Positive Control value range is between 0.250 and 0.900. If either of these values are out of range, the MS test results should be considered invalid and the samples should be retested. Samples testing with an Sp value of less than or equal to 0.299 will receive a 0 titer value and are considered negative for MS antibody.

P

Under optimal conditions* the suggested O.D. value ranges of 0.060 to 0.120 for MS-T Normal Control Serum and 0.400 to 0.800 for MS-T Positive Control Serum should be strived for to ensure the most consistent laboratory test results. Please note that tests with O.D. values which do not fall within the suggested O.D. ranges above does not constitute an invalid test.

*Optimal conditions are at room temperature [70 to 75°F (21 to 24°C)]. Higher room temperatures may result in slightly higher O.D. values.

Interpretation of Results: The MS-T Sp ratio values and/or ELISA titer values obtained for sera should be interpreted using the following value ranges:

Sample to Positive (Sp) Value	MS ELISA Titer Range	MS Presumed Antibody Status
Less than 0.300	0	Negative[a]
0.300 to 0.599	270 to 743	Probable[b,c]
Greater or equal to 0.6	744 or greater	Positive[c]

a. Negative. Serum samples with an MS-T Sp ratio value of less than 0.300 receive a "0" titer value and are presumed negative for MS antibody. However, a variety of factors, such as possible MS strain variations that may exhibit atypical biological and/or antigenic properties,[1,2] prevalence of an MS strain within a flock and timing and randomness of serum sample collection procedures could result in an MS-infected turkey flock yielding MS-negative ELISA results. It is therefore recommended that each turkey flock only be considered to be MS negative after (a) each flock has been adequately sampled and repeatedly tested several times and has yielded negative MS-T ELISA results each time and (b) each flock has been adequately sampled and repeatedly tested by standard conventional serologic tests (SPA and HI) and MS culture techniques[2] and has yielded MS negative serologic and culture results each time.

b. Probable. Presumed MS antibody probable denotes the ELISA Sp value range within which MS-T ELISA and conventional (SPA and HI) test data may suggest but may not conclusively detect MS antibody within a sample. The probable range represents a "suspect" or "gray" area in which MS-T ELISA results may or may not be supported by conventional serologic (SPA and HI) test results. It is highly recommended that additional conventional serologic tests and MS culture techniques[2] be conducted on serum and culture samples collected from MS-T ELISA probable turkey flocks, as recommended in parts a and c, to confirm whether each flock is an MS negative or MS positive-infected flock.

c. Positive. Additional conventional serologic testing (SPA and HI) and culturing of samples collected from presumed MS-T ELISA antibody probable and positive turkey flocks, using standard techniques,[2] are needed to obtain a confirmed positive diagnosis of MS infection within a turkey flock.

Storage: Store all reagents provided in the kit at 2-10°C.

Caution(s): To the Users of Reagents and MS Antigen Coated Plates:

a) Handle all reagents and samples as biohazardous material.
b) Keep all reagents away from skin and eyes. If exposure should occur, immediately flush affected areas with cold water.
c) Wash solution, control sera, test plates, field samples and all other test kit reagents should be properly decontaminated with bleach or other strong oxidizing agent before disposal.
d) Take special care not to contaminate any of the test reagents with serum or bacterial agents.
e) Humidity indicators are supplied with each plate. If any of the indicators exhibit a pink color, the plate may be compromised in some way; decontaminate (i.e. wash the plate with bleach solution) and dispose of the plate.
f) The best results are achieved by following the protocols as they are described above, using good, safe laboratory techniques.
g) Do not use this kit after the expiration date.
h) Never pipette by mouth.

Allow all reagents to come to room temperature before starting.

References: Available upon request.

Presentation: 900 tests.

Compendium Code No.: 11150310

PROFLOK® NDV+ ELISA KIT

Synbiotics **ELISA Test**

Newcastle Disease Antibody Test Kit

U.S. Vet. Lic. No.: 350

Reagents:

a) 1 NDV antigen coated plate.
b) 10 μL NDV Positive Control Serum.
c) 10 μL Normal Control Serum (NCS).
d) 100 μL Goat anti-Chicken IgG (H+L) Peroxidase Conjugate Solution.
e) 40 mL Dilution Buffer.
f) 10 mL ABTS-Hydrogen Peroxide Substrate Solution.
g) 2.5 mL 5X Stop Solution (dilute [1:5] with laboratory grade water).
h) 20 mL 20X Wash Solution (dilute [1:20] with laboratory grade water).

Equipment and Materials Required:

a) High precision pipette (i.e. 1-20 microliter pipette).
b) 0.2 mL, 1.0 mL and 5.0 mL pipettes.
c) 8 or 12 channel pipette (or transplating device).
d) 2 graduated cylinders (50 mL).
e) Uncoated low binding 96 well plates (i.e. Nunc catalog #269620).
f) Laboratory grade (Distilled or R.O.) water.
g) 96 well plate reading spectrophotometer with 405-410 nm filter.
h) Plate washing apparatus.

Indications: The PROFLOK® NDV+ ELISA Kit is a rapid serologic test for the detection of NDV antibody in chicken serum samples. The PROFLOK® NDV ELISA test was developed primarily to aid in the detection of pre- and post-vaccination NDV antibody levels in chickens.

Test Principles: Newcastle Disease Virus (NDV) causes a range of disease states from mild respiratory disease to severe diarrhea and death. The severity of the disease is determined by the infecting strain of NDV. Highly pathogenic strains (Velogenic NDV) can cause swelling of the tissues around the eyes, diarrhea and death within 8 days after exposure.[1,2] Moderately pathogenic strains (Mesogenic NDV) produce acute respiratory tract infections and reductions in egg production.[3] Milder strains (Lentogenic NDV) produce an inapparent respiratory infection. Assessment of antibody levels in the bird to the NDV group antigen by Enzyme Linked Immunoabsorbent Assay (ELISA) has been previously described by Snyder and coworkers.[4]

The assay is designed to measure NDV antibody bound to NDV antigen coated plates. The principle of the test is as follows: Serum obtained from chickens exposed to Newcastle Disease Virus contains specific anti-NDV antibodies. Serum, diluted in Dilution Buffer, is added to an NDV antigen coated plate. Specific NDV antibody in the serum forms an antibody-antigen complex with the NDV antigen bound to the plate. After washing the plate, an affinity purified goat anti-chicken IgG (H+L) peroxidase conjugate is added to each well. The antibody-antigen complex remaining from the previous step binds with the conjugate. After a brief incubation period, the unbound conjugate is removed by a second wash step. Substrate, which contains a chromagen (ABTS), is added to each well. Chromagen color change (from clear to green-blue) occurs in the presence of the peroxidase enzyme. The relative intensity of color developed in 15 minutes (compared to controls) is directly proportional to the level of NDV antibody in the serum. After the substrate has incubated, Stop Solution is added to each well to terminate the reaction and the plate is read using an ELISA plate reader at 405-410 nm.

Test Procedure:

Sample Collection: For routine serologic flock monitoring, it is suggested that at least 30 or more sera per flock be randomly collected at standard time intervals (i.e. every four weeks). Proper sample collection procedures, serum harvest and serum sample storage (4°C for up to four days or -20°C for longer periods) are needed to provide reliable test results.

Sample Dilution Procedure: Dilute serum samples using Dilution Buffer in a clean, uncoated 96 well microtiter plate. Set up samples and controls as shown in Figure 1.

Preparation of the Serum Dilution Plate:

a) Add 300 μL Dilution Buffer to each well of an uncoated 96 well microtiter plate. This plate is referred to as the serum dilution plate.
b) Add 6 μL unknown serum per well as per Figure 1 (producing a 1:50 dilution). Start with well A4 and end with well H9 (moving left to right, row by row of wells). For example, wells 1 through 30 contain the diluted sera of flock 1, wells 31-60 contain the diluted sera of flock 2, etc.
c) Add 6 μL of Normal Control Serum (producing a 1:50 dilution) to wells A2, H10 and H12.
d) Aspirate and remove any liquid in dilution plate wells A1, A3 and H11.
e) Allow all diluted serums to equilibrate in Dilution Buffer for 5 minutes before transferring to an NDV antigen coated ELISA plate.
f) Diluted serum should be tested within 24 hours.

This dilution format provides adequate quantities of diluted serum samples to conduct four additional ProFLOK® ELISA tests (i.e. IBD, REO, IBV and ILT) using the same serum dilution plate.

Preparation of NDV Positive Control: An NDV Positive Control Serum has been provided with this kit. Dilute the appropriate volume of NDV Positive Control Serum with Dilution Buffer (1:50) in clean, separate 5 mL test tubes. For example, dilute 6 μL of positive control serum in 300 μL Dilution Buffer. Mix well. 150 μL of NDV Positive Control is needed per ELISA plate.

Preparation of Conjugate Solution: The horseradish peroxidase conjugated anti-chicken IgG (H+L) is supplied in 50% glycerol. Dilute 100 μL stock conjugate in 10 mL Dilution Buffer (1:100 dilution). Mix well. This 10 mL preparation will supply sufficient conjugate for one 96 well ELISA plate.

Preparation of 1X Wash Solution: Dilute 20 mL concentrated Wash Solution in 380 mL laboratory grade (distilled or R.O.) water (1:20). Mix well. Approximately 400 mL Wash Solution is needed for each 96 well ELISA plate.

Preparation of the Substrate Solution: Determine the total number of plates needed to assay the samples. Each plate will require approximately 10 mL substrate solution. For example, 10 plates requires 100 mL substrate. For best results, the substrate solution must be equilibrated to room temperature before use.

Preparation of 1X Stop Solution: Dilute 2.5 mL concentrated Stop Solution in 10 mL laboratory grade (distilled or R.O.) water (1:5). Mix well. Approximately 12.5 mL Stop Solution is needed for each 96 well ELISA plate.

Note: Storage of 5X Stop Solution at refrigerated temperatures may cause the formation of a white solid. This does not affect product performance. Warm at room temperature or 37°C to dissolve before use.

Figure 1.

	1	2	3	4	5	6	7	8	9	10	11	12
A	+	-	+	1	2	3	4	5	6	7	8	9
B	10	11	12	13	14	15	16	17	18	19	20	21
C	22	23	24	25	26	27	28	29	30	31	32	33
D	34	35	36	37	38	39	40	41	42	43	44	45
E	46	47	48	49	50	51	52	53	54	55	56	57
F	58	59	60	61	62	63	64	65	66	67	68	69
G	70	71	72	73	74	75	76	77	78	79	80	81
H	82	83	84	85	86	87	88	89	90	-	+	-

ELISA Test Procedure:

Preparing the Test Plate:

a) Remove an NDV antigen coated test plate from the protective bag and label according to dilution plate identification.
b) Add 50 μL Dilution Buffer to all wells on the test plate.
c) Add 50 μL diluted NDV Positive Control Serum to wells A1, A3 and H11. Discard pipette tip.
d) Using an 8 or 12 channel pipette transfer 50 μL/well of each of the diluted serum samples and Normal Control Serum samples from the dilution plate to the corresponding wells of the NDV coated test plate. Discard pipette tips after each row of sample is transferred. Transfer of samples to the ELISA plate should be done as quickly as possible.
e) Incubate plate for 30 minutes at room temperature.

Wash Procedure:

f) Tap out liquid from each well into an appropriate vessel containing bleach or other decontamination agent.
g) Using an 8 or 12 channel pipette (or comparable automatic washing device), fill each well with approximately 300 μL Wash Solution. Allow to soak in wells for 3 minutes; then discard contents into an appropriate waste container (waste container should contain bleach solution). Tap inverted plate to ensure that all residual liquid is removed. Repeat wash procedure 2 more times.

Note: The wash procedure is a very critical step in any ELISA procedure. Please follow the above steps as directed.

Addition of Anti-Chicken IgG Peroxidase Conjugate, Substrate and Stop Solution:

h) Using an 8 or 12 channel pipette (or transplating device) dispense 100 μL diluted conjugate (prepared as described above) into each assay well. Discard pipette tips.
i) Incubate for 30 minutes at room temperature.
j) Wash as in steps f and g above.

P

k) Using an 8 or 12 channel pipette (or transplating device) dispense 100 µL Substrate Solution into each test well. Discard pipette tips.

l) Incubate 15 minutes at room temperature.

m) Using an 8 or 12 channel pipette (or transplating device) add 100 µL diluted Stop Solution to each test well.

n) Allow bubbles to dissipate before reading plate.

Manual Processing of Data:

a) Read the plate using an ELISA plate reader set at 405-410 nm. Be sure to blank the reader as directed. If a Flow Multiscan reader is used, the reader should be blanked using an empty microtiter plate. If a Bio-tek or Dynatech reader is used, the machine may be blanked with air.

b) Calculate the average Positive Control Serum absorbance (Optical Density [O.D.]) using the absorbance values of wells A1, A3 and H11. Calculate the average Normal Control Serum absorbance using values obtained from wells A2, H10 and H12. Record both averages.

c) Subtract the average normal control absorbance from the average positive absorbance. The difference is the Corrected Positive Control (CPC).

d) Calculate a sample to positive (Sp) ratio by subtracting the average normal control absorbance from each sample absorbance. The difference is divided by the corrected positive control. Use the following equation format:

$$SP = \frac{\text{(Sample Absorbance)} - \text{(Avg. Normal Control Absorbance)}}{\text{Corrected Positive Control (CPC) Absorbance}}$$

e) An NDV ELISA titer can be calculated by the following suggested equation:

Log_{10} Titer = (1.464 X Log_{10}Sp) + 3.740

Titer = Antilog of Log_{10} Titer

Example:

1. Example Positive Control Absorbance:
   0.585, 0.610, 0.590
   Average = (0.585 + 0.610 + 0.590) / 3 = 0.595
2. Example Normal Controls:
   0.078, 0.067, 0.057
   Average = (0.078 + 0.067 + 0.057) / 3 = 0.067
3. Corrected Positive Control (CPC):
   (0.595) - (0.067) = 0.528
4. Example Sp value calculation:
   Absorbance of sample = 0.560
   (0.560) - (0.067) / 0.528 = 0.934
5. Example of Calculation of titer using the Sp from above:
   Log_{10} Titer = 1.464 X (Log_{10} 0.934) + 3.740
   Titer = Antilog 3.70
   Titer = 4973

Test Interpretation: Results:

Assay Control Values: Valid NDV ELISA results are obtained when the average optical density (O.D.) value of the Normal Control Serum is less than 0.250 and the Corrected Positive Control (CPC) value range is between 0.250 and 0.900. If either of these values are out of range, the NDV test results should be considered invalid and the samples should be retested. Samples testing with an Sp value of less than or equal to 0.150 will receive a 0 titer value and are considered negative for NDV antibody.

Under optimal conditions* the suggested O.D. value ranges of 0.060 to 0.08 for NDV Normal Control Serum and 0.40 to 0.800 for NDV Positive Control Serum should be strived for to ensure the most consistent laboratory test results. Please note that tests with O.D. values which do not fall within the suggested O.D. ranges above does not constitute an invalid test.

*Optimal conditions are at room temperature [70 to 75°F (21 to 24°C)]. Higher room temperatures may result in slightly higher OD values.

Interpretation of Results: The NDV ELISA titer values obtained represent a comparison of the NDV antibody level within each field chicken serum tested and the NDV ELISA kit positive and normal control sera. Therefore, it is important to first determine that the NDV ELISA positive and normal control sera values obtained are valid as detailed above in the "Assay Control Values" section of this pamphlet before NDV ELISA results are interpreted.

A "0" NDV ELISA titer represents a chicken serum sample that contains an extremely low to insignificant NDV antibody level compared to the NDV ELISA kit positive and normal control sera.

An NDV ELISA titer value above "0" indicates only that a chicken serum sample contains a significant and ELISA-detectable NDV antibody level compared to the NDV ELISA kit positive and normal control sera. However, these titers do not imply or ensure "protection" nor provide serologic differentiation between an NDV vaccine response or NDV field infection.

Optimal NDV vaccine administration practices and "protective" flock NDV titer target values must be determined by each NDV ELISA kit user by comparing flock pre- and post-vaccination NDV ELISA results [i.e. coefficient of variation (%CV) and geometric titer (GMT) values] with flock performance parameters (i.e. morbidity, mortality, flock body weight gain or uniformity) over time.

Storage: Store all reagents provided in the kit at 2-10°C.

Caution(s): To the Users of Reagents and NDV Antigen Coated Plates:

a) Handle all reagents and samples as biohazardous material.

b) Keep all reagents away from skin and eyes. If exposure should occur, immediately flush affected areas with cold water.

c) Wash solution, control sera, test plates, field samples and all other test kit reagents should be properly decontaminated with bleach or other strong oxidizing agent before disposal.

d) Take special care not to contaminate any of the test reagents with serum or bacterial agents.

e) Humidity indicators are supplied with each plate. If any of the indicators exhibit a pink color, the plate may be compromised in some way; decontaminate (i.e. wash the plate with bleach solution) and dispose of the plate.

f) The best results are achieved by following the protocols as they are described above, using good, safe laboratory techniques.

g) Do not use this kit after the expiration date.

h) Never pipette by mouth.

Allow all reagents to come to room temperature before starting.

References: Available upon request.

Presentation: 900 tests.

Compendium Code No.: 11150321

PROFLOK® NDV-T ELISA KIT

Synbiotics — **ELISA Test**

Newcastle Disease Antibody Test Kit (Turkey)

U.S. Vet. Lic. No.: 350

Reagents:

a) 1 NDV-T antigen coated plate.

b) 10 µL NDV-T Positive Control Serum.

c) 10 µL Normal Control Serum.

d) 100 µL Goat anti-Turkey IgG (H+L) Peroxidase Conjugate Solution.

e) 40 mL Dilution Buffer.

f) 10 mL ABTS-Hydrogen Peroxide Substrate Solution.

g) 2.5 mL 5X Stop Solution (dilute [1:5] with laboratory grade water).

h) 20 mL 20X Wash Solution (dilute [1:20] with laboratory grade water).

Equipment and Materials Required:

a) High precision pipette (i.e. 1-20 microliter pipette).

b) 0.2 mL, 1.0 mL and 5.0 mL pipettes.

c) 8 or 12 channel pipette (or transplating device).

d) 2 graduated cylinders (50 mL).

e) 5 mL borosilicate glass test tubes.

f) Uncoated low binding 96 well plates (i.e. Nunc catalog #269620).

g) Laboratory grade (Distilled or R.O.) water.

h) 96 well plate reading spectrophotometer with 405-410 nm filter.

i) Plate washing apparatus.

Indications: The PROFLOK® NDV-T ELISA Kit is a rapid serologic test for the detection of NDV antibody in turkey serum samples. It was developed primarily to aid in the detection of pre- and post-vaccination NDV antibody levels in turkeys.

Test Principles: Newcastle Disease is an economically important disease of domestic turkeys. Clinical signs associated with Newcastle disease virus (NDV) infection vary from mild, subclinical infection to fulminating disease with high mortality.[1]

The assay is designed to measure turkey NDV antibody bound to NDV antigen coated plates. The principle of the test is as follows: Serum obtained from turkeys exposed to Newcastle Disease Virus contains specific anti-NDV antibodies. Serum, diluted in Dilution Buffer, is added to an NDV antigen coated plate. Specific NDV antibody in the serum forms an antibody-antigen complex with the NDV antigen bound to the plate. After washing the plate, an affinity purified goat anti-turkey IgG (H+L) peroxidase conjugate is added to each well. The antibody-antigen complex remaining from the previous step binds with the conjugate. After a brief incubation period, the unbound conjugate is removed by a second wash step. Substrate, which contains a chromagen (ABTS), is added to each well. Chromagen color change (from clear to green-blue) occurs in the presence of the peroxidase enzyme. The relative intensity of color developed in 15 minutes (compared to controls) is directly proportional to the level of NDV antibody in the serum. After the substrate has incubated, Stop Solution is added to each well to terminate the reaction and the plate is read using an ELISA plate reader at 405-410 nm.

Test Procedure:

Sample Collection: For routine serologic flock monitoring, it is suggested that at least 30 or more sera per flock be randomly collected at standard time intervals (i.e. every four weeks). Proper sample collection procedures, serum harvest and serum sample storage (4°C for up to four days or -20°C for longer periods) are needed to provide reliable test results.

Sample Dilution Procedure: Dilute serum samples using Dilution Buffer in a clean, uncoated 96 well microtiter plate. Set up samples and controls as shown in Figure 1.

Preparation of the Serum Dilution Plate:

a) Add 300 µL Dilution Buffer to each well of an uncoated 96 well microtiter plate. This plate is referred to as the serum dilution plate.

b) Add 6 µL unknown serum per well as per Figure 1 (producing a 1:50 dilution). Start with well A4 and end with well H9 (moving left to right, row by row of wells). For example, wells 1 through 30 contain the diluted sera of flock 1, wells 31-60 contain the diluted sera of flock 2, etc.

c) Add 6 µL of Normal Control Serum (producing a 1:50 dilution) to wells A2, H10 and H12.

d) Aspirate and remove any liquid in dilution plate wells A1, A3 and H11.

e) Allow all diluted serums to equilibrate in Dilution Buffer for 5 minutes before transferring to an NDV-T antigen coated ELISA plate.

f) Diluted serum should be tested within 24 hours.

This dilution format provides adequate quantities of diluted serum samples to conduct four additional ProFLOK® ELISA tests (i.e. MG, MS, MM and HE) using the same serum dilution plate.

Preparation of NDV-T Positive Control: An NDV-T Positive Control Serum has been provided with this kit. Dilute the appropriate volume of NDV-T Positive Control Serum with Dilution Buffer (1:50) in clean, glass test tube. For example, dilute 6 µL of positive control serum in 300 µL Dilution Buffer. Mix well. 150 µL of NDV-T Positive Control is needed per ELISA plate.

Preparation of Conjugate Solution: The horseradish peroxidase conjugated anti-turkey IgG (H+L) is supplied in 50% glycerol. Dilute 100 µL stock conjugate in 10 mL Dilution Buffer (1:100 dilution). Mix well. This 10 mL preparation will supply sufficient conjugate for one 96 well ELISA plate.

Preparation of 1X Wash Solution: Dilute 20 mL concentrated Wash Solution in 380 mL laboratory grade (distilled or R.O.) water (1:20). Mix well. Approximately 400 mL Wash Solution is needed for each 96 well ELISA plate.

Preparation of the Substrate Solution: The Substrate Solution is ready to use. Each plate will require approximately 10 mL substrate solution. For best results, the substrate solution must be equilibrated to room temperature before use.

Preparation of 1X Stop Solution: Dilute 2.5 mL concentrated Stop Solution in 10 mL laboratory grade (distilled or R.O.) water (1:5). Mix well. Approximately 12.5 mL Stop Solution is needed for each 96 well ELISA plate.

Note: Storage of 5X Stop Solution at refrigerated temperatures may cause the formation of a white solid. This does not affect product performance. Warm at room temperature or 37°C to dissolve before use.

Figure 1.

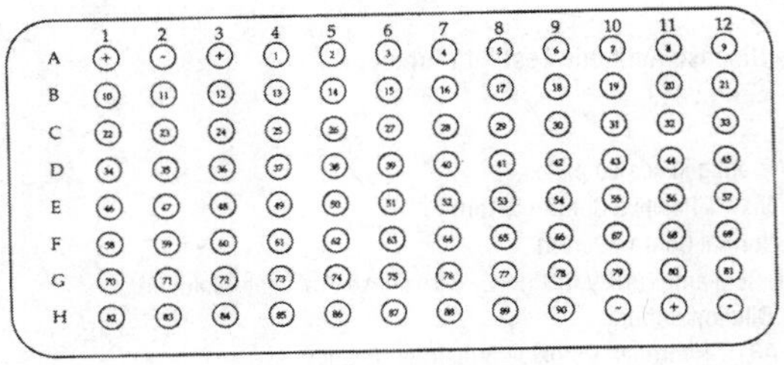

ELISA Test Procedure:

Preparing the Test Plate:

a) Remove an NDV-T antigen coated test plate from the protective bag and label according to dilution plate identification.
b) Add 50 μL Dilution Buffer to all wells on the test plate.
c) Add 50 μL diluted NDV-T Positive Control Serum to wells A1, A3 and H11. Discard pipette tip.
d) Using an 8 or 12 channel pipette transfer 50 μL/well of each of the diluted serum samples and Normal Control Serum samples from the dilution plate to the corresponding wells of the NDV-T antigen test plate. Discard pipette tips after each row of sample is transferred. Transfer of samples to the ELISA plate should be done as quickly as possible.
e) Incubate plate for 30 minutes at room temperature.

Wash Procedure:

f) Tap out liquid from each well into an appropriate vessel containing bleach or other decontamination agent.
g) Using an 8 or 12 channel pipette (or comparable automatic washing device), fill each well with approximately 300 μL Wash Solution. Allow to soak in wells for 3 minutes; then discard contents into an appropriate waste container (waste container should contain bleach solution). Tap inverted plate to ensure that all residual liquid is removed. Repeat wash procedure 2 more times.

Note: The wash procedure is a very critical step in any ELISA procedure. Please follow the above steps as directed.

Addition of Anti-Turkey IgG Peroxidase Conjugate, Substrate and Stop Solution:

h) Using an 8 or 12 channel pipette (or transplating device) dispense 100 μL diluted conjugate (prepared as described above) into each assay well. Discard pipette tips.
i) Incubate for 30 minutes at room temperature.
j) Wash as in steps f and g above.
k) Using an 8 or 12 channel pipette (or transplating device) dispense 100 μL Substrate Solution into each test well. Discard pipette tips.
l) Incubate 15 minutes at room temperature.
m) Using an 8 or 12 channel pipette (or transplating device) add 100 μL diluted Stop Solution to each test well.
n) Allow bubbles to dissipate before reading plate.

Manual Processing of Data:

a) Read the plate using an ELISA plate reader set at 405-410 nm. Be sure to blank the reader as directed. If a Flow Multiscan reader is used, the reader should be blanked using an empty microtiter plate. If a Bio-tek or Dynatech reader is used, the machine may be blanked with air.
b) Calculate the average Positive Control Serum absorbance (Optical Density [O.D.]) using the absorbance values of wells A1, A3 and H11. Calculate the average Normal Control Serum absorbance using values obtained from wells A2, H10 and H12. Record both averages.
c) Subtract the average normal control absorbance from the average positive absorbance. The difference is the Corrected Positive Control.
d) Calculate a sample to positive (Sp) ratio by subtracting the average normal control absorbance from each sample absorbance. The difference is divided by the corrected positive control. Use the following equation format:

$$SP = \frac{\text{(Sample Absorbance)} - \text{(Avg Normal Control Absorbance)}}{\text{Corrected Positive Control Absorbance}}$$

e) An NDV-T ELISA titer can be calculated by the following suggested equation:

$\text{Log}_{10}\ \text{Titer} = (0.717\ \text{X}\ \text{Log}_{10}\text{Sp}) + 3.906$

Titer = Antilog of Log_{10} Titer

Example:

1. Example Positive Control Absorbance:
   0.585, 0.610, 0.590
   Average = (0.585 + 0.610 + 0.590) / 3 = 0.595
2. Example Normal Controls:
   0.078, 0.067, 0.057
   Average = (0.078 + 0.067 + 0.057) / 3 = 0.067
3. Corrected Positive Control (CPC):
   (0.595) - (0.067) = 0.528
4. Example Sp value calculation:
   Absorbance of sample = 0.560
   (0.560) - (0.067) / 0.528 = 0.934
5. Example of Calculation of titer using the Sp from above:
   Log_{10} Titer = 0.717 X (Log_{10} 0.934) + 3.906
   Titer = Antilog 3.80
   Titer = 7586

Test Interpretation: Results:

Assay Control Values: Valid NDV-T ELISA results are obtained when the average optical density (O.D.) value of the Normal Control Serum is less than 0.200 and the Corrected Positive Control value range is between 0.250 and 0.900. If either of these values are out of range, the NDV-T test results should be considered invalid and the samples should be retested. Samples testing with an Sp value of less than or equal to 0.150 will receive a 0 titer value and are considered negative for NDV antibody.

Under optimal conditions*, the suggested O.D. value ranges of 0.060 to 0.120 for NDV-T Normal Control Serum and 0.350 to 0.750 for NDV-T Positive Control Serum should be strived for to ensure the most consistent laboratory test results. Please note that tests with O.D. values which do not fall within the suggested O.D. ranges above does not constitute an invalid test.

*Optimal conditions are at room temperature [70 to 75°F (21 to 24°C)]. Higher room temperatures may result in slightly higher OD values.

Interpretation of Results: The NDV-T ELISA titer values obtained represent a comparison of the NDV antibody level within each field turkey serum tested and the NDV-T ELISA kit positive and normal control sera. Therefore, it is important to first determine that the NDV-T ELISA positive and normal control sera values obtained are valid as detailed above in the "Assay Control Values" section of this pamphlet before NDV-T ELISA results are interpreted.

A "0" NDV-T ELISA titer represents a turkey serum sample that contains an extremely low to insignificant NDV-T antibody level compared to the NDV-T ELISA kit positive and normal control sera.

An NDV-T ELISA titer value above "0" indicates only that a turkey serum sample contains a significant and ELISA-detectable NDV antibody level compared to the NDV-T ELISA kit positive and normal control sera. However, these titers do not imply or ensure "protection" nor provide serologic differentiation between an NDV vaccine response or NDV field infection.

Optimal NDV vaccine administration practices and "protective" flock NDV-T titer target values must be determined by each NDV-T ELISA kit user by comparing flock pre- and post-vaccination NDV-T ELISA results [i.e. coefficient of variation (%CV) and geometric titer (GMT) values] with flock performance parameters (i.e. morbidity, mortality, flock body weight gain or uniformity) over time.

Storage: Store all reagents provided in the kit at 2-10°C.

Caution(s): To the Users of Reagents and NDV Antigen Coated Plates:

a) Handle all reagents and samples as biohazardous material.
b) Keep all reagents away from skin and eyes. If exposure should occur, immediately flush affected areas with cold water.
c) Wash solution, control sera, test plates, field samples and all other test kit reagents should be properly decontaminated with bleach or other strong oxidizing agent before disposal.
d) Take special care not to contaminate any of the test reagents with serum or bacterial agents.
e) Humidity indicators are supplied with each plate. If any of the indicators exhibit a pink color, the plate may be compromised in some way; decontaminate (i.e. wash the plate with bleach solution) and dispose of the plate.
f) The best results are achieved by following the protocols as they are described above, using good, safe laboratory techniques.
g) Do not use this kit after the expiration date.
h) Never pipette by mouth.

Allow all reagents to come to room temperature before starting.

References: Available upon request.

Presentation: 900 tests.

Compendium Code No.: 11150330

PROFLOK® PLUS ALV-J ELISA KIT

Synbiotics **ELISA Test**

Avian Leukosis Virus Subgroup J Antibody Test Kit

U.S. Vet. Lic. No.: 350

Reagents: Reagents Required to Perform 90 Tests:

a) 1 ALV-J antigen coated plate
b) 10 μL ALV-J Positive Control Serum
c) 10 μL Normal Control Serum
d) 100 μL Goat anti-Chicken IgG (H+L) Peroxidase Conjugate Solution
e) 40 mL Dilution Buffer
f) 10 mL ABTS-Hydrogen Peroxide Substrate Solution
g) 2.5 mL 5X Stop Solution, 5% SDS (dilute [1:5] with laboratory grade water)
h) 20 mL 20X Wash Solution (dilute [1:20] with laboratory grade water)

Equipment and Materials Required but Not Provided:

a) High precision pipette (i.e. 1-20 microliter pipette)
b) 0.2 mL, 1.0 mL and 5.0 mL pipettes
c) 8 or 12 channel pipette (or transplating device) and pipette tips
d) 2 graduated cylinders (50 mL)
e) 1 mL or 5 mL borosilicate glass test tubes
f) Uncoated low binding 96 well plates
g) Laboratory grade (Distilled or R.O.) water
h) 96 well plate reading spectrophotometer with 405-410 nm filter
i) Plate washing apparatus
j) Waste container with bleach or other oxidizing agent

Indications: The PROFLOK® PLUS ALV-J ELISA Kit is a rapid and specific presumptive screening test for the detection of antibody to ALV-J in chicken serum samples.[4] It was designed for screening large numbers of chicken sera from numerous flocks; however, additional conventional ALV-J testing [i.e. virus neutralization] and virus isolation techniques are suggested to confirm ALV-J negative and ALV-J infected chickens.

Test Principles: Avian Leukosis Virus subgroup J (ALV-J) is a recently discovered member of the avian leukosis-sarcoma group of retroviruses.[1] It induces myelocytic myeloid leukosis (ML) and has a tropism for the cells of the myeloid rather than lymphoid lineage.[2] The virus has unique envelope properties and nucleotide sequence analysis has shown that the gp85 domain of the subgroup J virus has about 40% identity with corresponding regions of the other ALV subgroups.[3]

Among the ALV-J encoded proteins, the virus envelope gp85 protein contains targets for neutralizing antibodies as well as regions that may be important in interactions with the host receptor. The gp85 protein is highly immunogenic and is specific for ALV-J.[3] A recombinant gp85 protein is used in the ELISA for the detection of ALV-J specific antibodies.

The assay is designed to measure ALV-J specific antibody bound to ALV-J antigen coated plates. The principle of the test is as follows: Serum obtained from chickens exposed to ALV-J virus contains specific anti-ALV-J antibodies. Serum, diluted in Dilution Buffer, is added to an ALV-J antigen coated plate. Specific ALV-J antibody in the serum forms an antibody-antigen complex with the ALV-J antigen bound to the plate. After washing the plate, an affinity purified goat anti-chicken IgG (H+L) peroxidase conjugate is added to each well. The antibody-antigen complex remaining from the previous step binds with the conjugate. After a brief incubation period, the unbound conjugate is removed by a second wash step. Substrate, which contains a chromagen (ABTS), is added to each well. Chromagen color change (from clear to green-blue) occurs in the presence of the peroxidase enzyme. The relative intensity of color developed in 15 minutes (compared to controls) is directly proportional to the level of ALV-J antibody in the serum. After the substrate has incubated, Stop Solution is added to each well to terminate the reaction and the plate is read using an ELISA plate reader at 405-410 nm.

Test Procedure:

Sample Collection: For routine serologic flock monitoring, it is suggested that at least 30 or more sera per flock be randomly collected at standard time intervals (i.e. every four weeks).

Proper sample collection procedures, serum harvest and serum sample storage (4°C for up to four days or -20°C for longer periods) are needed to provide reliable test results. To achieve better specificity and to minimize possible false positive reactions, serum samples that are contaminated with bacteria or are very fatty should be excluded from testing.

Sample Dilution Procedure: Dilute serum samples using Dilution Buffer in a clean, uncoated 96 well microtiter plate. Frozen serum samples should be completely thawed and thoroughly mixed before diluting. Set up samples and controls as shown in Figure 1 below.

Preparation of the Serum Dilution Plate:

a) Add 300 μL Dilution Buffer to each well of an uncoated 96 well microtiter plate. This plate is referred to as the serum dilution plate.
b) Add 6 μL unknown serum per well as per Figure 1 (producing a 1:50 dilution). Start with well A4 and end with well H9 (moving left to right, row by row of wells). For example, wells 1 through 30 contain the diluted sera of flock 1, wells 31-60 contain the diluted sera of flock 2, etc.
c) Add 6 μL of Normal Control Serum (producing a 1:50 dilution) to wells A2, H10 and H12.
d) Aspirate and remove any liquid in dilution plate wells A1, A3 and H11.
e) Allow all diluted serums to equilibrate in Dilution Buffer for 5 minutes before transferring to an ALV-J antigen coated ELISA plate.
f) Diluted serum should be tested within 24 hours.

This dilution format provides adequate quantities of diluted serum samples to conduct four additional ProFlok® ELISA tests (i.e. IBD, IBV, NDV and REO) using the same serum dilution plate.

Preparation of ALV-J Positive Control: An ALV-J Positive Control Serum has been provided with this kit. Dilute the appropriate volume of ALV-J Positive Control Serum with Dilution Buffer (1:50) in a clean, glass test tube. For example, dilute 6 μL of positive control serum in 300 μL Dilution Buffer. Mix well. 150 μL of diluted ALV-J Positive Control is needed per ELISA plate.

Preparation of Conjugate Solution: The horseradish peroxidase conjugated anti-chicken IgG (H+L) is supplied in 50% glycerol. Dilute 100 μL stock conjugate in 10 mL Dilution Buffer (1:100 dilution). Mix well. This 10 mL preparation will supply sufficient conjugate for one 96 well ELISA plate.

Preparation of 1X Wash Solution: Dilute 20 mL concentrated Wash Solution in 380 mL laboratory grade (distilled or R.O.) water (1:20). Mix well. Approximately 400 mL Wash Solution is needed for each 96 well ELISA plate.

Preparation of the Substrate Solution: The Substrate Solution is ready to use. Each plate will require approximately 10 mL substrate solution. For best results, the substrate solution must be equilibrated to room temperature before use.

Preparation of 1X Stop Solution: Dilute 2.5 mL concentrated Stop Solution in 10 mL laboratory grade (distilled or R.O.) water (1:5). Mix well. Approximately 12.5 mL Stop Solution is needed for each 96 well ELISA plate.

Note: Storage of 5X Stop Solution at refrigerated temperatures may cause the formation of a white solid. This does not affect product performance. Warm at room temperature or 37°C to dissolve before use.

Figure 1.

	1	2	3	4	5	6	7	8	9	10	11	12
A	+	-	+	1	2	3	4	5	6	7	8	9
B	10	11	12	13	14	15	16	17	18	19	20	21
C	22	23	24	25	26	27	28	29	30	31	32	33
D	34	35	36	37	38	39	40	41	42	43	44	45
E	46	47	48	49	50	51	52	53	54	55	56	57
F	58	59	60	61	62	63	64	65	66	67	68	69
G	70	71	72	73	74	75	76	77	78	79	80	81
H	82	83	84	85	86	87	88	89	90	-	+	-

ELISA Test Procedure:

Preparing the Test Plate:

a) Remove an ALV-J antigen coated test plate from the protective bag and label according to serum dilution plate identification.
b) Add 50 μL Dilution Buffer to all wells on the test plate.
c) Add 50 μL diluted ALV-J Positive Control Serum to wells A1, A3 and H11. Discard pipette tip.
d) Using an 8 or 12 channel pipette transfer 50 μL/well of each of the diluted serum samples and Normal Control Serum samples from the serum dilution plate to the corresponding wells of the ALV-J coated test plate (yields a 1:100 dilution). Discard pipette tips after each row of sample is transferred. Transfer of samples to the ELISA plate should be done as quickly as possible.
e) Incubate plate for 30 minutes at room temperature.

Wash Procedure:

f) Tap out liquid from each well into an appropriate vessel containing bleach or other decontamination agent.
g) Using an 8 or 12 channel pipette (or comparable automatic washing device), fill each well with approximately 300 μL Wash Solution. Allow to soak in wells for 3 minutes; then discard contents into an appropriate waste container (waste container should contain bleach solution). Tap inverted plate to ensure that all residual liquid is removed. Repeat wash procedure 2 more times.

Note: The wash procedure is a very critical step in any ELISA procedure. Please follow the above steps as directed.

Addition of Anti-Chicken IgG Peroxidase Conjugate, Substrate and Stop Solution:

h) Using an 8 or 12 channel pipette (or transplating device) dispense 100 μL diluted conjugate (prepared as described above) into each assay well. Discard pipette tips.
i) Incubate for 30 minutes at room temperature.
j) Wash as in steps f and g above.
k) Using an 8 or 12 channel pipette (or transplating device) dispense 100 μL Substrate Solution into each test well. Discard pipette tips.
l) Incubate 15 minutes at room temperature.
m) Using an 8 or 12 channel pipette (or transplating device) add 100 μL diluted Stop Solution (prepared as described above) to each test well.
n) Allow bubbles to dissipate before reading plate.

Manual Processing of Data:

a) Read the plate using an ELISA plate reader set at 405-410 nm. Be sure to blank the reader as directed.
b) Calculate the average Positive Control Serum absorbance (Optical Density [O.D.]) using the absorbance values of wells A1, A3 and H11. Calculate the average Normal Control Serum absorbance using values obtained from wells A2, H10 and H12. Record both averages.
c) Subtract the average normal control absorbance from the average positive absorbance. The difference is the Corrected Positive Control.
d) Calculate a sample to positive (Sp) ratio by subtracting the average normal control absorbance from each sample absorbance. The difference is divided by the corrected positive control. Use the following equation format:

$$SP = \frac{\text{(Sample O.D.)} - \text{(Avg. Normal Control O.D.)}}{\text{Corrected Positive Control O.D.}}$$

e) An ALV-J ELISA titer can be calculated by the following suggested equation:
$\text{Log}_{10}\ \text{Titer} = (1.224 \times \text{Log}_{10}\ \text{Sp}) + 3.860$
Titer = Antilog of Log_{10} Titer

Example:

1. Example Positive Control Absorbance:
0.585, 0.610, 0.590
Average = (0.585 + 0.610 + 0.590) / 3 = 0.595
2. Example Normal Controls:
0.078, 0.067, 0.057
Average = (0.078 + 0.067 + 0.057) / 3 = 0.067
3. Corrected Positive Control:
(0.595 - 0.067) = 0.528
4. Example Sp value calculation:
Absorbance of sample = 0.560
(0.560) - (0.067) / 0.528 = 0.934
5. Example of Calculation of titer using the Sp from above:
$\text{Log}_{10}\ \text{Titer} = 1.224 \times (\text{Log}_{10}\ 0.934) + 3.860$
Titer = Antilog 3.82
Titer = 6664

Test Interpretation: Results:

Assay Control Values: Valid ALV-J ELISA results are obtained when the average optical density (O.D.) value of the Normal Control Serum is less than 0.200 and the Corrected Positive Control value range is between 0.250 and 0.900. If either of these values are out of range, the ALV-J test results should be considered invalid and the samples should be retested. Samples testing with an Sp value of less than or equal to 0.399 will receive a 0 titer value and are considered non-reactive for ALV-J antibody.

Under optimal conditions* the suggested O.D. value ranges of 0.050 to 0.095 for ALV-J Normal Control Serum and 0.400 to 1.00 for ALV-J Positive Control Serum should be strived for to ensure the most consistent laboratory test results. Please note that tests with O.D. values which do not fall within the suggested O.D. ranges above does not constitute an invalid test.

*Optimal conditions are at room temperature [70 to 75°F (21 to 24°C)]. Higher room temperatures may result is slightly higher O.D. values.

Interpretation of Results: The ALV-J ELISA titer values obtained represent a comparison of the ALV-J antibody level within each chicken serum tested and the ALV-J ELISA kit positive and normal control sera. Therefore, it is important to first determine that the ALV-J ELISA positive and normal control sera values obtained are valid as detailed above in the "Assay Control Values" section before ALV-J ELISA results are interpreted.

A â0" ALV-J ELISA titer represents a chicken serum sample that contains an extremely low to insignificant ALV-J antibody level compared to the ALV-J ELISA kit positive and normal control sera.

An ALV-J ELISA titer value above "0" indicates only that a chicken serum sample contains a significant and ELISA-detectable ALV-J antibody level compared to the ALV-J ELISA kit positive and normal control sera. However, these titers do not imply or ensure "protection" nor provide serologic differentiation between a vaccine response or ALV-J infection.

Storage: Store all reagents provided in the kit at 2-7°C. Reagents should not be frozen.

Caution(s): To the Users of Reagents and ALV-J Antigen Coated Plates:

a) Handle all reagents and samples as biohazardous material.
b) Keep all reagents away from skin and eyes. If exposure should occur, immediately flush affected areas with cold water.
c) Wash solution, control sera, test plates, field samples and all other test kit reagents should be properly decontaminated with bleach or other strong oxidizing agent before disposal.
d) Take special care not to contaminate any of the test reagents with serum or bacterial agents.
e) Humidity indicators are supplied with each plate. If any of the indicators exhibit a pink color, the plate may be compromised in some way; decontaminate (i.e. wash the plate with bleach solution) and dispose of the plate.
f) The best results are achieved by following the protocols as they are described, using good, safe laboratory techniques.
g) Do not use this kit after the expiration date.
h) Never pipette by mouth.

Allow all reagents to come to room temperature before starting.

References: Available upon request.

Presentation: 90 test kit.

Compendium Code No.: 11150530

L-343-01

PROFLOK® PLUS IBD ELISA KIT

Synbiotics **ELISA Test**

Infectious Bursal Disease Antibody Test Kit

U.S. Vet. Lic. No.: 350

Reagents:

a) 1 IBD antigen coated plate
b) 10 μL IBD Positive Control Serum
c) 10 μL Normal Control Serum
d) 100 μL Goat anti-Chicken IgG (H+L) Peroxidase Conjugate Solution
e) 40 mL Dilution Buffer
f) 10 mL ABTS-Hydrogen Peroxide Substrate Solution
g) 2.5 mL 5X Stop Solution (dilute [1:5] with laboratory grade water)
h) 20 mL 20X Wash Solution (dilute [1:20] with laboratory grade water)

Equipment and Materials Required:

a) High precision pipette (i.e. 1-20 microliter pipette)
b) 0.2 mL, 1.0 mL and 5.0 mL pipettes
c) 8 or 12 channel pipette (or transplating device)
d) 2 graduated cylinders (50 mL)
e) 1 mL and 5 mL borosilicate glass test tubes

P

f) Uncoated low binding 96 well plates
g) Laboratory grade (Distilled or R.O.) water
h) 96 well plate reading spectrophotometer with 405-410 nm filter
i) Plate washing apparatus

Indications: The PROFLOK® Plus IBD ELISA Kit is a rapid serologic test for the detection of IBD antibody in chicken serum samples. It was developed primarily to aid in the detection of pre and post-vaccination IBD antibody levels in chickens.

Test Principles: Infectious Bursal Disease (IBD) was first described by Cosgrove in 1962.[1] IBD is one of the most economically important diseases that affects commercial chickens.[2] The ELISA procedure has been widely adapted for IBD serology and provides a rapid, quantifiable, sensitive and reproducible test.[3] The PROFLOK® Plus IBD ELISA specifically detects IBD antibody and demonstrates excellent correlation with the Virus Neutralization (VN) test. It shows broad reactivity to both classic and variant strains of IBD virus.[4]

The assay is designed to measure IBD antibody bound to IBD antigen coated plates. The principle of the test is as follows: Serum obtained from chickens exposed to IBD antigens contains specific anti-IBD antibodies. Serum, diluted in Dilution Buffer, is added to an IBD antigen coated plate. Specific IBD antibody in the serum forms an antibody-antigen complex with the IBD antigen bound to the plate. After washing the plate, an affinity purified goat anti-chicken IgG (H+L) peroxidase conjugate is added to each well. The antibody-antigen complex remaining from the previous step binds with the conjugate. After a brief incubation period, the unbound conjugate is removed by a second wash step. Substrate, which contains a chromagen (ABTS), is added to each well. Chromagen color change (from clear to green-blue) occurs in the presence of the peroxidase enzyme. The relative intensity of color developed in 15 minutes (compared to controls) is directly proportional to the level of IBD antibody in the serum. After the substrate has incubated, Stop Solution is added to each well to terminate the reaction and the plate is read using an ELISA plate reader at 405-410 nm.

Sample Collection: For routine serologic flock monitoring, it is suggested that at least 30 or more sera per flock be randomly collected at standard time intervals (i.e. every four weeks). Proper sample collection procedures, serum harvest and serum sample storage (4°C for up to four days or -20°C for longer periods) are needed to provide reliable test results.

Test Procedure:

Sample Dilution Procedure: Dilute serum samples using Dilution Buffer in a clean, uncoated 96 well microtiter plate. Set up samples and controls as shown in Figure 1.

Preparation of the Serum Dilution Plate:

a) Add 300 μL Dilution Buffer to each well of an uncoated 96 well microtiter plate. This plate is referred to as the serum dilution plate.
b) Add 6 μL unknown serum per well as per Figure 1 (producing a 1:50 dilution). Start with well A4 and end with well H9 (moving left to right, row by row of wells). For example, wells 1 through 30 contain the diluted sera of flock 1, wells 31-60 contain the diluted sera of flock 2, etc.
c) Add 6 μL of Normal Control Serum (producing a 1:50 dilution) to wells A2, H10 and H12.
d) Aspirate and remove any liquid in dilution plate wells A1, A3 and H11.
e) Allow all diluted serums to equilibrate in Dilution Buffer for 5 minutes before transferring to an IBD antigen coated ELISA plate.
f) Diluted serum should be tested within 24 hours.

This dilution format provides adequate quantities of diluted serum samples to conduct four additional ProFLOK® ELISA tests (i.e. REO, NDV, IBV and AE) using the same serum dilution plate.

Preparation of IBD Positive Control: An IBD Positive Control Serum has been provided with this kit. Dilute the appropriate volume of IBD Positive Control Serum with Dilution Buffer (1:50) in a clean, glass test tube. For example, dilute 6 μL of positive control serum in 300 μL Dilution Buffer. Mix well. 150 μL of IBD Positive Control is needed per ELISA plate.

Preparation of Conjugate Solution: The horseradish peroxidase conjugated anti-chicken IgG (H+L) is supplied in 50% glycerol. Dilute 100 μL stock conjugate in 10 mL Dilution Buffer (1:100 dilution). Mix well. This 10 mL preparation will supply sufficient conjugate for one 96 well ELISA plate.

Preparation of 1X Wash Solution: Dilute 20 mL concentrated Wash Solution in 380 mL laboratory grade (distilled or R.O.) water (1:20). Mix well. Approximately 400 mL Wash Solution is needed for each 96 well ELISA plate.

Preparation of the Substrate Solution: The Substrate Solution is ready to use. Each plate will require approximately 10 mL substrate solution. For best results, the substrate solution must be equilibrated to room temperature before use.

Preparation of 1X Stop Solution: Dilute 2.5 mL concentrated Stop Solution in 8 mL laboratory grade (distilled or R.O.) water (1:5). Mix well. Approximately 10 mL Stop Solution is needed for each 96 well ELISA plate.

Note: Storage of 5X Stop Solution at refrigerated temperatures may cause the formation of a white solid. This does not affect product performance. Warm at room temperature or 37°C to dissolve before use.

Figure 1

	1	2	3	4	5	6	7	8	9	10	11	12
A	+	-	+	1	2	3	4	5	6	7	8	9
B	10	11	12	13	14	15	16	17	18	19	20	21
C	22	23	24	25	26	27	28	29	30	31	32	33
D	34	35	36	37	38	39	40	41	42	43	44	45
E	46	47	48	49	50	51	52	53	54	55	56	57
F	58	59	60	61	62	63	64	65	66	67	68	69
G	70	71	72	73	74	75	76	77	78	79	80	81
H	82	83	84	85	86	87	88	89	90	-	+	-

ELISA Test Procedure:

Preparing the Test Plate:

a) Remove an IBD antigen coated test plate from the protective bag and label according to dilution plate identification.
b) Add 50 μL Dilution Buffer to all wells on the test plate.
c) Add 50 μL diluted Positive Control Serum to wells A1, A3 and H11. Discard pipette tip.
d) Using an 8 or 12 channel pipette transfer 50 μL/well of each of the diluted serum samples and Normal Control Serum samples from the serum dilution plate to the corresponding wells of the IBD coated test plate. Discard pipette tips after each row of sample is transferred. Transfer of samples to the ELISA plate should be done as quickly as possible.
e) Incubate plate for 30 minutes at room temperature.

Wash Procedure:

f) Tap out liquid from each well into an appropriate vessel containing bleach or other decontamination agent.
g) Using an 8 or 12 channel pipette (or comparable automatic washing device), fill each well with approximately 300 μL Wash Solution. Allow to soak in wells for 3 minutes; then discard contents into an appropriate waste container (waste container should contain bleach solution). Tap inverted plate to ensure that all residual liquid is removed. Repeat wash procedure 2 more times.

Note: The wash procedure is a very critical step in any ELISA procedure. Please follow the above steps as directed.

Addition of Anti-Chicken IgG Peroxidase Conjugate, Substrate and Stop Solution:

h) Using an 8 or 12 channel pipette (or transplating device) dispense 100 μL diluted conjugate (prepared as described above) into each assay well. Discard pipette tips.
i) Incubate for 30 minutes at room temperature.
j) Wash as in steps f and g above.
k) Using an 8 or 12 channel pipette (or transplating device) dispense 100 μL Substrate Solution into each test well. Discard pipette tips.
l) Incubate 15 minutes at room temperature.
m) Using an 8 or 12 channel pipette (or transplating device) add 100 μL diluted Stop Solution (prepared as described above) to each test well.
n) Allow bubbles to dissipate before reading plate.

Manual Processing of Data:

a) Read the plate using an ELISA plate reader set at 405-410 nm.
b) Calculate the average Positive Control Serum absorbance (Optical Density [O.D.]) using the absorbance values of wells A1, A3 and H11. Calculate the average Normal Control Serum absorbance using values obtained from wells A2, H10 and H12. Record both averages.
c) Subtract the average normal control absorbance from the average positive absorbance. The difference is the Corrected Positive Control.
d) Calculate a sample to positive (Sp) ratio by subtracting the average normal control absorbance from each sample absorbance. The difference is divided by the corrected positive control. Use the following equation format:

$$SP = \frac{\text{(Sample Absorbance)} - \text{(Average Normal Control Absorbance)}}{\text{Corrected Positive Control Absorbance}}$$

e) An IBD ELISA titer can be calculated by the following suggested equation:

Log_{10} Titer = (1.172 X Log_{10} Sp) + 3.614

Titer = Antilog of Log_{10} Titer

Example:

1. Example Positive Control Absorbance:
   0.585, 0.610, 0.590
   Average = (0.585 + 0.610 + 0.590) / 3 = 0.595
2. Example Normal Controls:
   0.110, 0.102, 0.112
   Average = (0.110 + 0.102 + 0.112) / 3 = 0.108
3. Corrected Positive Control:
   (0.595) - (0.108) = 0.487
4. Example Sp value calculation:
   Absorbance of sample = 0.560
   (0.560) - (0.108) / 0.487 = 0.928
5. Example of Calculation of titer using the Sp from above:
   Log_{10} Titer = 1.172 X (Log_{10} 0.928) + 3.614
   Titer = Antilog 3.57
   Titer = 3767

Interpretation of Results: Results:

Assay Control Values: Valid IBD ELISA results are obtained when the average optical density (O.D.) value of the Normal Control Serum is less than 0.250 and the Corrected Positive Control value range is between 0.250 and 0.900. If either of these values are out of range, the IBD test results should be considered invalid and the samples should be retested. Samples testing with an Sp value of less than or equal to 0.299 will receive a 0 titer value.

Under optimal conditions*, the suggested O.D. value ranges of 0.080 to 0.200 for IBD Normal Control Serum and 0.400 to 0.850 for IBD Positive Control Serum should be strived for to ensure the most consistent laboratory test results. Please note that tests with O.D. values which do not fall within the suggested O.D. ranges above does not constitute an invalid test.

*Optimal conditions are at room temperature [70 to 75°F (21 to 24°C)]. Higher room temperatures may result in slightly higher OD values.

The IBD ELISA titer values obtained represent a comparison of the IBD antibody level within each field chicken serum tested and the IBD ELISA kit positive and non reactive sera. Therefore, it is important to first determine that the IBD ELISA positive and normal control sera values obtained are valid as detailed above in the "Assay Control Values" section of this pamphlet before IBD ELISA results are interpreted.

A "0" IBD ELISA titer represents a chicken serum sample that contains an extremely low to insignificant IBD antibody level.

An IBD ELISA titer value above "0" indicates only that a chicken serum sample contains a significant and ELISA-detectable IBD antibody level compared to the IBD ELISA kit positive and normal control sera. However, these titers do not imply or ensure "protection" nor provide serologic differentiation between an IBD vaccine response or IBD field infection.

Optimal IBD vaccine administration practices and "protective" flock IBD titer target values must be determined by each IBD ELISA kit user by comparing flock pre- and post-vaccination IBD ELISA results [i.e. coefficient of variation (%CV) and geometric titer (GMT) values] with flock performance parameters (i.e. morbidity, mortality, flock body weight gain or uniformity) over time.

Storage: Store all reagents provided in the kit at 2-10°C.

Caution(s): To the Users of Reagents and IBD Antigen Coated Plates:

a) Handle all reagents and samples as biohazardous material.
b) Keep all reagents away from skin and eyes. If exposure should occur, immediately flush affected areas with cold water.
c) Wash solution, control sera, test plates, field samples and all other test kit reagents should be properly decontaminated with bleach or other strong oxidizing agent before disposal.
d) Take special care not to contaminate any of the test reagents with serum or bacterial agents.
e) Humidity indicators are supplied with each plate. If any of the indicators exhibit a pink color,

the plate may be compromised in some way; decontaminate (i.e. wash the plate with bleach solution) and dispose of the plate.

f) The best results are achieved by following the protocols as they are described above, using good, safe laboratory techniques.

g) Do not use this kit after the expiration date.

h) Never pipette by mouth.

Allow all reagents to come to room temperature before starting.

References: Available upon request.

Presentation: 900 tests.

Compendium Code No.: 11150340

PROFLOK® PM ELISA KIT

Synbiotics **ELISA Test**

Pasteurella multocida Antibody Test Kit

U.S. Vet. Lic. No.: 350

Reagents:

a) 1 PM antigen coated plate.

b) 10 µL PM Positive Control Serum.

c) 10 µL Normal Control Serum (NCS).

d) 100 µL Goat anti-Chicken IgG (H+L) Peroxidase Conjugate Solution.

e) 40 mL Dilution Buffer.

f) 10 mL ABTS-Hydrogen Peroxide Substrate Solution.

g) 2.5 mL 5X Stop Solution 5% SDS (dilute [1:5] with laboratory grade water).

h) 20 mL 20X Wash Solution (dilute [1:20] with laboratory grade water).

Equipment and Materials Required:

a) High precision pipette (i.e. 1-20 microliter pipette).

b) 0.2 mL, 1.0 mL and 5.0 mL pipettes.

c) 8 or 12 channel pipette (or transplating device).

d) 2 graduated cylinders (50 mL).

e) Uncoated low binding 96 well plates (i.e. Nunc catalog #269620).

f) Laboratory grade (Distilled or R.O.) water.

g) 96 well plate reading spectrophotometer with 405-410 nm filter.

h) Plate washing apparatus.

Indications: The PROFLOK® PM ELISA Kit is a rapid serologic test for the detection of PM antibody in chicken serum samples. The PROFLOK® PM ELISA test was developed primarily to aid in the serodiagnosis of Fowl Cholera and the detection of pre- and post-vaccination PM antibody levels in chickens.

Test Principles: *Pasteurella multocida* (PM) is the causative agent of fowl cholera, a contagious septicemic disease of domestic poultry and wild birds that is often associated with high morbidity and mortality.[1]

The assay is designed to measure PM antibody bound to PM antigen coated plates. The principle of the test is as follows: Serum obtained from chickens exposed to *Pasteurella multocida* contains specific anti-PM antibodies. Serum, diluted in Dilution Buffer, is added to a PM antigen coated plate. Specific PM antibody in the serum forms an antibody-antigen complex with the PM antigen bound to the plate. After washing the plate, an affinity purified goat anti-chicken IgG (H+L) peroxidase conjugate is added to each well. The antibody-antigen complex remaining from the previous step reacts with the conjugate. After a brief incubation period, the unreacted conjugate is removed by a second wash step. Substrate, which contains a chromagen (ABTS), is added to each well. Chromagen color change (from clear to green-blue) occurs in the presence of the peroxidase enzyme. The relative intensity of color developed in 15 minutes (compared to controls) is directly proportional to the level of PM antibody in the serum. After the substrate has incubated, Stop Solution is added to each well to terminate the reaction and the plate is read using an ELISA plate reader at 405-410 nm.

Test Procedure:

Sample Collection: For routine serologic flock monitoring, it is suggested that at least 30 or more sera per flock be randomly collected at standard time intervals (i.e. every four weeks). Proper sample collection procedures, serum harvest and serum sample storage (4°C for up to four days or -20°C for longer periods) are needed to provide reliable test results.

Sample Dilution Procedure: Dilute serum samples using Dilution Buffer in a clean, uncoated 96 well microtiter plate. Frozen serum samples should be completely thawed and thoroughly mixed before diluting. Set up samples and controls as shown in Figure 1.

Preparation of the Serum Dilution Plate:

a) Add 300 µL Dilution Buffer to each well of an uncoated 96 well microtiter plate. This plate is referred to as the serum dilution plate.

b) Add 6 µL unknown serum per well as per Figure 1 (producing a 1:50 dilution). Start with well A4 and end with well H9 (moving left to right, row by row of wells). For example, wells 1 through 30 contain the diluted sera of flock 1, wells 31-60 contain the diluted sera of flock 2, etc.

c) Add 6 µL of Normal Control Serum (producing a 1:50 dilution) to wells A2, H10 and H12.

d) Aspirate and remove any liquid in dilution plate wells A1, A3 and H11.

e) Allow all diluted serums to equilibrate in Dilution Buffer for 5 minutes before transferring to a PM antigen coated ELISA plate.

f) Diluted serum should be tested within 24 hours.

This dilution format provides adequate quantities of diluted serum samples to conduct four additional ProFLOK® ELISA tests (i.e. IBD, REO, IBV or NDV) using the same serum dilution plate.

Preparation of Controls: A PM Positive Control Serum has been provided with this kit. Dilute the appropriate volume of PM Positive Control Serum with Dilution Buffer (1:50) in a clean, glass test tube. For example, dilute 6 µL of postivie control serum in 300 µL Dilution Buffer. Mix well. 150 µL of diluted control is needed per ELISA plate.

Preparation of Conjugate Solution: The horseradish peroxidase conjugated anti-chicken IgG (H+L) is supplied in 50% glycerol. Dilute 100 µL stock conjugate in 10 mL Dilution Buffer (1:100 dilution). Mix well. This 10 mL preparation will supply sufficient conjugate for one 96 well ELISA plate.

Preparation of 1X Wash Solution: Dilute 20 mL concentrated Wash Solution in 380 mL laboratory grade (distilled or R.O.) water (1:20). Mix well. Approximately 400 mL Wash Solution is needed for each 96 well ELISA plate.

Preparation of the Substrate Solution: The Substrate Solution is ready to use. Each plate will require approximately 10 mL substrate solution. For example, 10 plates requires 100 mL substrate. For best results, the substrate solution must be equilibrated to room temperature before use.

Preparation of 1X Stop Solution: Dilute 2.5 mL concentrated Stop Solution in 10 mL laboratory grade (distilled or R.O.) water (1:5). Mix well. Approximately 12.5 mL Stop Solution is needed for each 96 well ELISA plate.

Note: Storage of 5X Stop Solution at refrigerated temperatures may cause the formation of a white solid. This does not affect product performance. Warm at room temperature or 37°C to dissolve before use.

Figure 1.

	1	2	3	4	5	6	7	8	9	10	11	12
A	+	-	+	1	2	3	4	5	6	7	8	9
B	10	11	12	13	14	15	16	17	18	19	20	21
C	22	23	24	25	26	27	28	29	30	31	32	33
D	34	35	36	37	38	39	40	41	42	43	44	45
E	46	47	48	49	50	51	52	53	54	55	56	57
F	58	59	60	61	62	63	64	65	66	67	68	69
G	70	71	72	73	74	75	76	77	78	79	80	81
H	82	83	84	85	86	87	88	89	90	-	+	-

ELISA Test Procedure:

Preparing the Test Plate:

a) Remove a PM antigen coated test plate from the protective bag and label according to dilution plate identification.

b) Add 50 µL Dilution Buffer to all wells on the test plate.

c) Add 50 µL diluted Positive Control Serum to wells A1, A3 and H11. Discard pipette tip.

d) Using an 8 or 12 channel pipette transfer 50 µL/well of each of the diluted serum samples from the dilution plate to the corresponding wells of the PM coated test plate (yields a 1:100 dilution). Discard pipette tips after each transfer. Transfer of samples to the ELISA plate should be done as quickly as possible.

e) Incubate plate for 30 minutes at room temperature.

Wash Procedure:

f) Tap out liquid from each well into an appropriate vessel containing bleach or other decontamination agent.

g) Using an 8 or 12 channel pipette (or comparable automatic washing device), fill each well with approximately 300 µL Wash Solution. Allow to soak in wells for 3 minutes; then discard contents into an appropriate waste container (waste container should contain bleach solution). Tap inverted plate to ensure that all residual liquid is removed. Repeat wash procedure 2 more times.

Note: The wash procedure is a very critical step in any ELISA procedure. Please follow the above steps as directed.

Addition of Anti-Chicken IgG Peroxidase Conjugate, Substrate and Stop Solution:

h) Using an 8 or 12 channel pipette (or transplating device) dispense 100 µL diluted conjugate (prepared as described above) into each assay well. Discard pipette tips.

i) Incubate for 30 minutes at room temperature.

j) Wash as in steps f and g above.

k) Using an 8 or 12 channel pipette (or transplating device) dispense 100 µL Substrate Solution into each test well. Discard pipette tips.

l) Incubate 15 minutes at room temperature.

m) Using an 8 or 12 channel pipette (or transplating device) add 100 µL Stop Solution to each test well.

n) Allow bubbles to dissipate before reading plate.

Manual Processing of Data:

a) Read the plate using an ELISA plate reader set at 405-410 nm. Be sure to blank the reader as directed. If a Flow Multiscan reader is used, the reader should be blanked using an empty microtiter plate. If a Bio-Tek or Dynatech reader is used, the machine may be blanked with air.

b) Calculate the average Positive Control Serum absorbance (Optical Density [O.D.]) using the absorbance values of wells A1, A3 and H11. Calculate the average Normal Control Serum (NCS) absorbance using values obtained from wells A2, H10 and H12. Record both averages.

c) Subtract the average negative (NCS) absorbance from the average positive absorbance. The difference is the Corrected Positive Control (CPC).

d) Calculate a sample to positive (Sp) ratio by subtracting the average negative control absorbance from each sample absorbance. The difference is divided by the corrected positive control. Use the following equation format:

$$SP = \frac{\text{(Sample Absorbance)} - \text{(Avg. Normal Control Absorbance)}}{\text{Corrected Positive Control (CPC) Absorbance}}$$

e) A PM ELISA titer can be calculated by the following suggested equation:

Log_{10} Titer = (1.464 X Log_{10} Sp) + 3.197

Titer = Antilog of Log_{10} Titer

Example:

1. Example Positive Control Absorbance:
   0.585, 0.610, 0.590
   Average = (0.585 + 0.610 + 0.590) / 3 = 0.595
2. Example Normal Controls:
   0.078, 0.067, 0.057
   Average = (0.078 + 0.067 + 0.057) / 3 = 0.067
3. Corrected Positive Control (CPC):
   (0.595) - (0.067) = 0.528
4. Example Sp value calculation:
   Absorbance of sample = 0.560
   (0.560) - (0.067) / 0.528 = 0.934
5. Example of Calculation of titer using the Sp from above:
   Log_{10} Titer = 1.464 X (Log_{10} 0.934) + 3.197
   Titer = Antilog 3.15
   Titer = 1413

Test Interpretation: Results:

Assay Control Values: Valid PM ELISA results are obtained when the average optical density (O.D.) value of the Normal Control Serum is less than 0.200 and the Corrected Positive Control (CPC) value range is between 0.250 and 0.900. If either of these values are out of range, the PM test results should be considered invalid and the samples should be retested. Samples testing with an Sp value of less than or equal to 0.199 will receive a 0 titer value and are considered negative for PM antibody.

Under optimal conditions* the suggested O.D. value ranges of 0.060 to 0.080 for PM Normal Control Serum and 0.400 to 0.750 for PM Positive Control Serum should be strived for to ensure the most consistent laboratory test results.

*Optimal conditions are at room temperature [70 to 75°F (21 to 24°C)]. Higher room temperatures may result in slightly higher OD values.

Interpretation of Results: The PM ELISA titer values obtained represent a comparison of the PM antibody level within each field chicken serum tested and the PM ELISA kit positive and normal control sera. Therefore, it is important to first determine that the PM ELISA positive and normal control sera values obtained are valid as detailed above in the "Assay Control Values" section of this pamphlet before PM ELISA results are interpreted.

A "0" PM ELISA titer represents a chicken serum sample that contains an extremely low to insignificant PM antibody level compared to the PM ELISA kit positive and normal control sera.

A PM ELISA titer value above "0" indicates only that a chicken serum sample contains a significant and ELISA-detectable PM antibody level compared to the PM ELISA kit positive and normal control sera. However, these titers do not imply or ensure "protection" nor provide serologic differentiation between a PM vaccine virus response or PM field infection.

Optimal PM vaccine administration practices and "protective" flock PM titer target values must be determined by each PM ELISA kit user by comparing flock pre- and post-vaccination PM ELISA results [i.e. coefficient of variation (%CV) and geometric titer values] with flock performance parameters (i.e. morbidity, mortality, flock body weight gain or uniformity) over time.

Storage: Store all reagents provided in the kit at 2-10°C.

Caution(s): To the Users of Reagents and PM Antigen Coated Plates:

a) Handle all reagents and samples as biohazardous material.
b) Keep all reagents away from skin and eyes. If exposure should occur, immediately flush affected areas with cold water.
c) Wash solution, control sera, test plates, field samples and all other test kit reagents should be properly decontaminated with bleach or other strong oxidizing agent before disposal.
d) Take special care not to contaminate any of the test reagents with serum or bacterial agents.
e) Humidity indicators are supplied with each plate. If any of the indicators exhibit a pink color, the plate may be compromised in some way; decontaminate (i.e. wash the plate with bleach solution) and dispose of the plate.
f) The best results are achieved by following the protocols as they are described above, using good, safe laboratory techniques.
g) Do not use this kit after the expiration date.
h) Never pipette by mouth.

Allow all reagents to come to room temperature before starting.

References: Available upon request.

Presentation: 900 tests.

Compendium Code No.: 11150350

PROFLOK® PM-T ELISA KIT

Synbiotics **ELISA Test**

Pasteurella multocida Antibody Test Kit (Turkey)

U.S. Vet. Lic. No.: 350

Reagents:

a) 1 T-PM antigen coated plate.
b) 10 μL T-PM Positive Control Serum.
c) 10 μL Normal Control Serum (NCS).
d) 100 μL Goat anti-Turkey IgG (H+L) Peroxidase Conjugate Solution.
e) 40 mL Dilution Buffer.
f) 10 mL ABTS-Hydrogen Peroxide Substrate Solution.
g) 2.5 mL 5X Stop Solution (dilute [1:5] with laboratory grade water).
h) 20 mL 20X Wash Solution (dilute [1:20] with laboratory grade water).

Equipment and Materials Required:

a) High precision pipette (i.e. 1-20 microliter pipette).
b) 0.2 mL, 1.0 mL and 5.0 mL pipettes.
c) 8 or 12 channel pipette (or transplating device).
d) 2 graduated cylinders (50 mL).
e) 5 mL borosilicate glass test tubes.
f) Uncoated low binding 96 well plates (i.e. Nunc catalog #269620).
g) Laboratory grade (Distilled or R.O.) water.
h) 96 well plate reading spectrophotometer with 405-410 nm filter.
i) Plate washing apparatus.

Indications: The PROFLOK® PM-T ELISA Kit is a rapid serologic test for the detection of PM antibody (Serotypes 1, 3 and 4) in turkey serum samples. It was developed primarily to aid in the detection of pre- and post-vaccination PM antibody levels in turkeys with commercially available PM vaccines (Serotypes 1, 3 and 4).

Test Principles: *Pasteurella multocida* (PM) is the causative agent of fowl cholera, a contagious septicemic disease of domestic poultry and wild birds that is often associated with high morbidity and mortality.[1]

The assay is designed to measure PM antibody bound to T-PM antigen coated plates. The principle of the test is as follows: Serum obtained from turkeys exposed to *Pasteurella multocida* contains specific anti-PM antibodies. Serum, diluted in Dilution Buffer, is added to a T-PM antigen coated plate. Specific PM antibody in the serum forms an antibody-antigen complex with the T-PM antigen bound to the plate. After washing the plate, an affinity purified goat anti-turkey IgG (H+L) peroxidase conjugate is added to each well. The antibody-antigen complex remaining from the previous step reacts with the conjugate. After a brief incubation period, the unreacted conjugate is removed by a second wash step. Substrate, which contains a chromagen (ABTS), is added to each well. Chromagen color change (from clear to green-blue) occurs in the presence of the peroxidase enzyme. The relative intensity of color developed in 15 minutes (compared to controls) is directly proportional to the level of PM antibody in the serum. After the substrate has incubated, Stop Solution is added to each well to terminate the reaction and the plate is read using an ELISA plate reader at 405-410 nm.

Test Procedure:

Sample Collection: For routine serologic flock monitoring, it is suggested that at least 30 or more sera per flock be randomly collected at standard time intervals (i.e. every four weeks). Proper sample collection procedures, serum harvest and serum sample storage (4°C for up to four days or -20°C for longer periods) are needed to provide reliable test results.

Sample Dilution Procedure: Dilute serum samples using Dilution Buffer in a clean, uncoated 96 well microtiter plate. Set up samples and controls as shown in Figure 1.

Preparation of the Serum Dilution Plate:

a) Add 300 μL Dilution Buffer to each well of an uncoated 96 well microtiter plate. This plate is referred to as the serum dilution plate. Label the dilution plate.
b) Add 6 μL unknown serum per well as per Figure 1 (producing a 1:50 dilution). Start with well A4 and end with well H9 (moving left to right, row by row of wells). For example, wells 1 through 30 contain the diluted sera of flock 1, wells 31-60 contain the diluted sera of flock 2, etc.
c) Add 6 μL of Normal Control Serum (producing a 1:50 dilution) to wells A2, H10 and H12.
d) Aspirate and remove any liquid in dilution plate wells A1, A3 and H11.
e) Allow all diluted serums to equilibrate in Dilution Buffer for 5 minutes before transferring to a PM antigen coated ELISA plate.
f) Diluted serum should be tested within 24 hours.

This dilution format provides adequate quantities of diluted serum samples to conduct four additional turkey ProFLOK® ELISA tests (i.e. MG, MS, MM, HE or NDV) using the same serum dilution plate.

Preparation of T-PM Positive Control: A T-PM Positive Control Serum has been provided with this kit. Dilute the appropriate volume of T-PM Positive Control Serum with Dilution Buffer (1:50) in a clean, separate 5 mL test tube. For example, dilute 6 μL of Positive Control serum in 300 μL Dilution Buffer. Mix well. 150 μL of diluted T-PM Positive Control is needed per ELISA plate.

Preparation of Conjugate Solution: The horseradish peroxidase conjugated anti-turkey IgG (H+L) is supplied in 50% glycerol. Dilute 100 μL stock conjugate in 10 mL Dilution Buffer (1:100 dilution). Mix well. This 10 mL preparation will supply sufficient conjugate for one 96 well ELISA plate.

Preparation of 1X Wash Solution: Dilute 20 mL concentrated Wash Solution in 380 mL laboratory grade (distilled or R.O.) water (1:20). Mix well. Approximately 400 mL Wash Solution is needed for each 96 well ELISA plate.

Preparation of the Substrate Solution: The substrate solution is ready to use. Each plate will require approximately 10 mL substrate solution. For best results, the substrate solution must be equilibrated to room temperature before use.

Preparation of 1X Stop Solution: Dilute 2.5 mL concentrated Stop Solution in 10 mL laboratory grade (distilled or R.O.) water (1:5). Mix well. Approximately 12.5 mL diluted Stop Solution is needed for each 96 well ELISA plate.

Note: Storage of 5X Stop Solution at refrigerated temperatures may cause the formation of a white solid. This does not affect product performance. Warm at room temperature or 37°C to dissolve before use.

Figure 1.

	1	2	3	4	5	6	7	8	9	10	11	12
A	+	-	+	1	2	3	4	5	6	7	8	9
B	10	11	12	13	14	15	16	17	18	19	20	21
C	22	23	24	25	26	27	28	29	30	31	32	33
D	34	35	36	37	38	39	40	41	42	43	44	45
E	46	47	48	49	50	51	52	53	54	55	56	57
F	58	59	60	61	62	63	64	65	66	67	68	69
G	70	71	72	73	74	75	76	77	78	79	80	81
H	82	83	84	85	86	87	88	89	90	-	+	-

ELISA Test Procedure:

Preparing the Test Plate:

a) Remove a T-PM antigen test plate from the protective bag and label according to dilution plate identification.
b) Add 50 μL Dilution Buffer to all wells on the test plate.
c) Add 50 μL diluted T-PM Positive Control Serum to wells A1, A3 and H11. Discard pipette tip.
d) Using an 8 or 12 channel pipette transfer 50 μL/well of each of the diluted serum samples and Normal Control Serum samples from the serum dilution plate to the corresponding wells of the PM coated test plate. Discard pipette tips after each row of sample is transferred. Transfer of samples to the ELISA plate should be done as quickly as possible.
e) Incubate plate for 30 minutes at room temperature.

Wash Procedure:

f) Tap out liquid from each well into an appropriate vessel containing bleach or other decontamination agent.
g) Using an 8 or 12 channel pipette (or comparable automatic washing device), fill each well with approximately 300 μL Wash Solution. Allow to soak in wells for 3 minutes; then discard contents into an appropriate waste container (waste container should contain bleach solution). Tap inverted plate to ensure that all residual liquid is removed. Repeat wash procedure 2 more times.

Note: The wash procedure is a very critical step in any ELISA procedure. Please follow the above steps as directed.

Addition of Anti-Turkey IgG Peroxidase Conjugate, Substrate and Stop Solution:

h) Using an 8 or 12 channel pipette (or transplating device) dispense 100 μL diluted conjugate (prepared as described above) into each assay well. Discard pipette tips.
i) Incubate for 30 minutes at room temperature.
j) Wash as in steps f and g above.
k) Using an 8 or 12 channel pipette (or transplating device) dispense 100 μL Substrate Solution into each test well. Discard pipette tips.
l) Incubate 15 minutes at room temperature.
m) Using an 8 or 12 channel pipette (or transplating device) add 100 μL diluted Stop Solution to each test well.
n) Allow bubbles to dissipate before reading plate.

Manual Processing of Data:

a) Read the plate using an ELISA plate reader set at 405-410 nm. Be sure to blank the reader as directed. If a Flow Multiscan reader is used, the reader should be blanked using an empty microtiter plate. If a Bio-tek or Dynatech reader is used, the machine may be blanked with air.
b) Calculate the average Positive Control Serum absorbance (Optical Density [O.D.]) using the absorbance values of wells A1, A3 and H11. Calculate the average Normal Control Serum absorbance using values obtained from wells A2, H10 and H12. Record both averages.
c) Subtract the average normal control absorbance from the average positive absorbance. The difference is the Corrected Positive Control.
d) Calculate a sample to positive (Sp) ratio by subtracting the average normal control

absorbance from each sample absorbance. The difference is divided by the corrected positive control. Use the following equation format:

$$SP = \frac{(\text{Sample Absorbance}) - (\text{Average Normal Control Absorbance})}{\text{Corrected Positive Control Absorbance}}$$

e) A T-PM ELISA titer can be calculated by the following suggested equation:
Log_{10} Titer = (1.464 X Log_{10} Sp) + 3.197
Titer = Antilog of Log_{10} Titer
Example:
1. Example Positive Control Absorbance:
   0.585, 0.610, 0.590
   Average = (0.585 + 0.610 + 0.590) / 3 = 0.595
2. Example Normal Controls:
   0.078, 0.067, 0.057
   Average = (0.078 + 0.067 + 0.057) / 3 = 0.067
3. Corrected Positive Control:
   (0.595) - (0.067) = 0.528
4. Example Sp value calculation:
   Absorbance of sample = 0.560
   (0.560) - (0.067) / 0.528 = 0.934
5. Example of Calculation of titer using the Sp from above:
   Log_{10} Titer = 1.464 X (Log_{10} 0.934) + 3.197
   Titer = Antilog 3.15
   Titer = 1424

Test Interpretation: Results:

Assay Control Values: Valid T-PM ELISA results are obtained when the average optical density (O.D.) value of the Normal Control Serum is less than 0.250 and the Corrected Positive Control value range is between 0.250 and 0.900. If either of these values are out of range, the T-PM test results should be considered invalid and the samples should be retested. Samples testing with an Sp value of less than or equal to 0.199 will receive a 0 titer value and are considered negative for PM antibody.

Under optimal conditions* the suggested O.D. value ranges of 0.060 to 0.095 for PM Normal Control Serum and 0.400 to 0.850 for T-PM Positive Control Serum should be strived for to ensure the most consistent laboratory test results. Please note that a plate with O.D. values which do not fall within the suggested O.D. ranges above does not constitute an invalid test.

*Optimal conditions are at room temperature [70 to 75°F (21 to 24°C)]. Higher room temperatures may result in slightly higher O.D. values.

Interpretation of Results: The T-PM ELISA titer values obtained represent a comparison of the PM antibody level within each field turkey serum tested and the T-PM ELISA kit positive and normal control sera. Therefore, it is important to first determine that the T-PM ELISA positive and normal control sera values obtained are valid as detailed above in the "Assay Control Values" section of this pamphlet before T-PM ELISA results are interpreted.

A "0" T-PM ELISA titer represents a turkey serum sample that contains an extremely low to insignificant PM antibody level compared to the T-PM ELISA kit positive and normal control sera.

A T-PM ELISA titer value above "0" indicates only that a turkey serum sample contains a significant and ELISA-detectable PM antibody level compared to the T-PM ELISA kit positive and normal control sera. However, these titers do not imply or ensure "protection" nor provide serologic differentiation between a PM vaccine response or PM field infection.

Optimal PM vaccine administration practices and "protective" flock T-PM titer target values must be determined by each T-PM ELISA kit user by comparing flock pre- and post-vaccination T-PM ELISA results [i.e. coefficient of variation (%CV) and geometric titer (GMT) values] with flock performance parameters (i.e. morbidity, mortality, flock body weight gain or uniformity) over time.

Storage: Store all reagents provided in the kit at 2-10°C.

Caution(s): To the Users of Reagents and PM Antigen Coated Plates:
a) Handle all reagents and samples as biohazardous material.
b) Keep all reagents away from skin and eyes. If exposure should occur, immediately flush affected areas with cold water.
c) Wash solution, control sera, test plates, field samples and all other test kit reagents should be properly decontaminated with bleach or other strong oxidizing agent before disposal.
d) Take special care not to contaminate any of the test reagents with serum or bacterial agents.
e) Humidity indicators are supplied with each plate. If any of the indicators exhibit a pink color, the plate may be compromised in some way; decontaminate (i.e. wash the plate with bleach solution) and dispose of the plate.
f) The best results are achieved by following the protocols as they are described above, using good, safe laboratory techniques.
g) Do not use this kit after the expiration date.
h) Never pipette by mouth.

Allow all reagents to come to room temperature before starting.

References: Available upon request.
Presentation: 900 tests.
Compendium Code No.: 11150371

PROFLOK® REO ELISA KIT

Synbiotics **ELISA Test**

Avian Reovirus Antibody Test Kit
U.S. Vet. Lic. No.: 350

Reagents:
a) 1 REO antigen coated plate.
b) 10 µL REO Positive Control Serum.
c) 10 µL Normal Control Serum (NCS).
d) 100 µL Goat anti-Chicken IgG (H+L) Peroxidase Conjugate Solution.
e) 40 mL Dilution Buffer.
f) 10 mL ABTS-Hydrogen Peroxide Substrate Solution.
g) 2.5 mL 5X Stop Solution (dilute [1:5] with laboratory grade water).
h) 20 mL 20X Wash Solution (dilute [1:20] with laboratory grade water).

Equipment and Materials Required:
a) High precision pipette (i.e. 1-20 microliter pipette).
b) 0.2 mL, 1.0 mL and 5.0 mL pipettes.
c) 8 or 12 channel pipette (or transplating device).
d) 2 graduated cylinders (50 mL).
e) Uncoated low binding 96 well plates (i.e. Nunc catalog #269620).
f) Laboratory grade (Distilled or R.O.) water.
g) 96 well plate reading spectrophotometer with 405-410 nm filter.
h) Plate washing apparatus.

Indications: The PROFLOK® REO ELISA Kit is a rapid serologic test for the detection of REO antibody in chicken serum samples. The PROFLOK® REO ELISA test was developed primarily to aid in the detection of pre- and post-vaccination REO antibody levels in chickens.

Test Principles: Reovirus has been isolated from chickens with arthritis (Tenosynovitis), diarrhea and growth retardation.[1] Chickens and turkeys have been found to be susceptible to Reovirus derived viral arthritis.[1] The disease is most common in 5 to 7 week old broiler chickens, but can occur in older birds. The infection causes inflammation of the synovial membrane and tendon sheath. Determination of group specific antibody to viral antigens by Enzyme Linked Immunosorbent Assay (ELISA) has been previously described by Snyder and coworkers.[2]

The assay is designed to measure REO antibody bound to REO antigen coated plates. The principle of the test is as follows: Serum obtained from chickens exposed to Avian Reovirus contains specific anti-REO antibodies. Serum, diluted in Dilution Buffer, is added to a REO antigen coated plate. Specific REO antibody in the serum forms an antibody-antigen complex with the REO antigen bound to the plate. After washing the plate, an affinity purified goat anti-chicken IgG (H+L) peroxidase conjugate is added to each well. The antibody-antigen complex remaining from the previous step binds with the conjugate. After a brief incubation period, the unbound conjugate is removed by a second wash step. Substrate, which contains a chromagen (ABTS), is added to each well. Chromagen color change (from clear to green-blue) occurs in the presence of the peroxidase enzyme. The relative intensity of color developed in 15 minutes (compared to controls) is directly proportional to the level of REO antibody in the serum. After the substrate has incubated, Stop Solution is added to each well to terminate the reaction and the plate is read using an ELISA plate reader at 405-410 nm.

Test Procedure:

Sample Collection: For routine serologic flock monitoring, it is suggested that at least 30 or more sera per flock be randomly collected at standard time intervals (i.e. every four weeks). Proper sample collection procedures, serum harvest and serum sample storage (4°C for up to four days or -20°C for longer periods) are needed to provide reliable test results.

Sample Dilution Procedure: Dilute serum samples using Dilution Buffer in a clean, uncoated 96 well microtiter plate. Set up samples and controls as shown in Figure 1.

Preparation of the Serum Dilution Plate:
a) Add 300 µL Dilution Buffer to each well of an uncoated 96 well microtiter plate. This plate is referred to as the serum dilution plate.
b) Add 6 µL unknown serum per well as per Figure 1 (producing a 1:50 dilution). Start with well A4 and end with well H9 (moving left to right, row by row of wells). For example, wells 1 through 30 contain the diluted sera of flock 1, wells 31-60 contain the diluted sera of flock 2, etc.
c) Add 6 µL of Normal Control Serum (producing a 1:50 dilution) to wells A2, H10 and H12.
d) Aspirate and remove any liquid in dilution plate wells A1, A3 and H11.
e) Allow all diluted serums to equilibrate in Dilution Buffer for 5 minutes before transferring to a REO antigen coated ELISA plate.
f) Diluted serum should be tested within 24 hours.

This dilution format provides adequate quantities of diluted serum samples to conduct four additional ProFLOK® ELISA tests (i.e. IBD, NDV, IBV and ILT) using the same serum dilution plate.

Preparation of REO Positive Control: A REO Positive Control Serum has been provided with this kit. Dilute the appropriate volume of REO Positive Control Serum with Dilution Buffer (1:50) in clean, separate 5 mL test tubes. For example, dilute 6 µL of positive control serum in 300 µL Dilution Buffer. Mix well. 150 µL of REO Positive Control is needed per ELISA plate.

Preparation of Conjugate Solution: The horseradish peroxidase conjugated anti-chicken IgG (H+L) is supplied in 50% glycerol. Dilute 100 µL stock conjugate in 10 mL Dilution Buffer (1:100 dilution). Mix well. This 10 mL preparation will supply sufficient conjugate for one 96 well ELISA plate.

Preparation of 1X Wash Solution: Dilute 20 mL concentrated Wash Solution in 380 mL laboratory grade (distilled or R.O.) water (1:20). Mix well. Approximately 400 mL Wash Solution is needed for each 96 well ELISA plate.

Preparation of the Substrate Solution: Determine the total number of plates needed to assay the samples. Each plate will require approximately 10 mL substrate solution. For example, 10 plates requires 100 mL substrate. For best results, the substrate solution must be equilibrated to room temperature before use.

Preparation of 1X Stop Solution: Dilute 2.5 mL concentrated Stop Solution in 10 mL laboratory grade (distilled or R.O.) water (1:5). Mix well. Approximately 12.5 mL Stop Solution is needed for each 96 well ELISA plate.

Note: Storage of 5X Stop Solution at refrigerated temperatures may cause the formation of a white solid. This does not affect product performance. Warm at room temperature or 37°C to dissolve before use.

Figure 1.

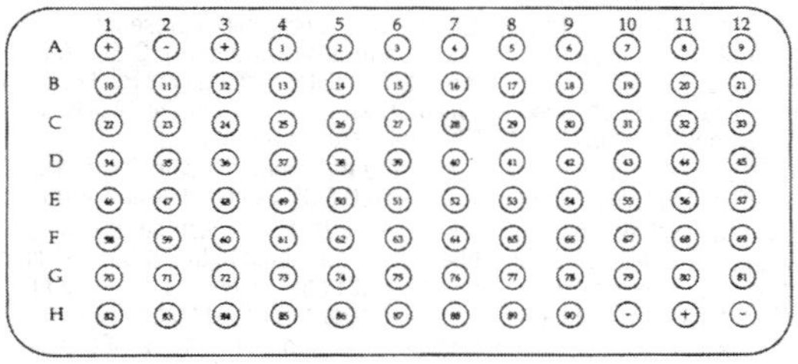

	1	2	3	4	5	6	7	8	9	10	11	12
A	+	-	+	1	2	3	4	5	6	7	8	9
B	10	11	12	13	14	15	16	17	18	19	20	21
C	22	23	24	25	26	27	28	29	30	31	32	33
D	34	35	36	37	38	39	40	41	42	43	44	45
E	46	47	48	49	50	51	52	53	54	55	56	57
F	58	59	60	61	62	63	64	65	66	67	68	69
G	70	71	72	73	74	75	76	77	78	79	80	81
H	82	83	84	85	86	87	88	89	90	-	+	-

ELISA Test Procedure:

Preparing the Test Plate:
a) Remove a REO antigen coated test plate from the protective bag and label according to dilution plate identification.
b) Add 50 µL Dilution Buffer to all wells on the test plate.
c) Add 50 µL diluted REO Positive Control Serum to wells A1, A3 and H11. Discard pipette tip.
d) Using an 8 or 12 channel pipette, transfer 50 µL/well of each of the diluted serum samples and Normal Control Serum samples from the dilution plate to the corresponding wells of the REO coated test plate. Discard pipette tips after each row of sample is transferred. Transfer of samples to the ELISA plate should be done as quickly as possible.
e) Incubate plate for 30 minutes at room temperature.

Wash Procedure:
f) Tap out liquid from each well into an appropriate vessel containing bleach or other decontamination agent.

g) Using an 8 or 12 channel pipette (or comparable automatic washing device), fill each well with approximately 300 μL Wash Solution. Allow to soak in wells for 3 minutes; then discard contents into an appropriate waste container (waste container should contain bleach solution). Tap inverted plate to ensure that all residual liquid is removed. Repeat wash procedure 2 more times.

Note: The wash procedure is a very critical step in any ELISA procedure. Please follow the above steps as directed.

Addition of Anti-Chicken IgG Peroxidase Conjugate, Substrate and Stop Solution:

h) Using an 8 or 12 channel pipette (or transplating device) dispense 100 μL diluted conjugate (prepared as described above) into each assay well. Discard pipette tips.

i) Incubate for 30 minutes at room temperature.

j) Wash as in steps f and g above.

k) Using an 8 or 12 channel pipette (or transplating device) dispense 100 μL Substrate Solution into each test well. Discard pipette tips.

l) Incubate 15 minutes at room temperature.

m) Using an 8 or 12 channel pipette (or transplating device) add 100 μL diluted Stop Solution to each test well.

n) Allow bubbles to dissipate before reading plate.

Manual Processing of Data:

a) Read the plate using an ELISA plate reader set at 405-410 nm. Be sure to blank the reader as directed. If a Flow Multiscan reader is used, the reader should be blanked using an empty microtiter plate. If a Bio-tek or Dynatech reader is used, the machine may be blanked with air.

b) Calculate the average Positive Control Serum absorbance (Optical Density [O.D.]) using the absorbance values of wells A1, A3 and H11. Calculate the average Normal Control Serum absorbance using values obtained from wells A2, H10 and H12. Record both averages.

c) Subtract the average normal control absorbance from the average positive absorbance. The difference is the Corrected Positive Control (CPC).

d) Calculate a sample to positive (Sp) ratio by subtracting the average normal control absorbance from each sample absorbance. The difference is divided by the corrected positive control. Use the following equation format:

$$SP = \frac{\text{(Sample Absorb)} - \text{(Avg Normal Control Absorb)}}{\text{Corrected Positive Control (CPC) Absorbance}}$$

e) A REO ELISA titer can be calculated by the following suggested equation:

$\text{Log}_{10}\ \text{Titer} = (1.077 \times \text{Log}_{10}\text{Sp}) + 3.460$

Titer = Antilog of Log_{10} Titer

Example:

1. Example Positive Control Absorbance:
   0.585, 0.610, 0.590
   Average = (0.585 + 0.610 + 0.590) / 3 = 0.595
2. Example Normal Controls:
   0.078, 0.067, 0.057
   Average = (0.078 + 0.067 + 0.057) / 3 = 0.067
3. Corrected Positive Control (CPC):
   (0.595) - (0.067) = 0.528
4. Example Sp value calculation:
   Absorbance of sample = 0.560
   (0.560) - (0.067) / 0.528 = 0.934
5. Example of Calculation of titer using the Sp from above:
   $\text{Log}_{10}\ \text{Titer} = 1.077 \times (\text{Log}_{10}\ 0.934) + 3.460$
   Titer = Antilog 3.43
   Titer = 2680

Test Interpretation: Results:

Assay Control Values: Valid REO ELISA results are obtained when the average optical density (O.D.) value of the Normal Control Serum is less than 0.250 and the Corrected Positive Control (CPC) value range is between 0.250 and 0.900. If either of these values are out of range, the REO test results should be considered invalid and the samples should be retested. Samples testing with an Sp value of less than or equal to 0.150 will receive a 0 titer value and are considered negative for REO antibody.

Under optimal conditions* the suggested O.D. value ranges of 0.060 to 0.080 for REO Normal Control Serum and 0.400 to 0.800 for REO Positive Control Serum should be strived for to ensure the most consistent laboratory test results. Please note that tests with O.D. values which do not fall within the suggested O.D. ranges above does not constitute an invalid test.

*Optimal conditions are at room temperature [70 to 75°F (21 to 24°C)]. Higher room temperatures may result in slightly higher OD values.

Interpretation of Results: The REO ELISA titer values obtained represent a comparison of the REO antibody level within each field chicken serum tested and the REO ELISA kit positive and normal control sera. Therefore, it is important to first determine that the REO ELISA positive and normal control sera values obtained are valid as detailed above in the "Assay Control Values" section of this pamphlet before REO ELISA results are interpreted.

A "0" REO ELISA titer represents a chicken serum sample that contains an extremely low to insignificant REO antibody level compared to the REO ELISA kit positive and normal control sera.

A REO ELISA titer value above "0" indicates only that a chicken serum sample contains a significant and ELISA-detectable REO antibody level compared to the REO ELISA kit positive and normal control sera. However, these titers do not imply or ensure "protection" nor provide serologic differentiation between a REO vaccine response or REO field infection.

Optimal REO vaccine administration practices and "protective" flock REO titer target values must be determined by each REO ELISA kit user by comparing flock pre- and post-vaccination REO ELISA results [i.e. coefficient of variation (%CV) and geometric mean titer (GMT) values] with flock performance parameters (i.e. morbidity, mortality, flock body weight gain or uniformity) over time.

Storage: Store all reagents provided in the kit at 2-7°C.

Caution(s): To the Users of Reagents and REO Antigen Coated Plates:

a) Handle all reagents and samples as biohazardous material.

b) Keep all reagents away from skin and eyes. If exposure should occur, immediately flush affected areas with cold water.

c) Wash solution, control sera, test plates, field samples and all other test kit reagents should be properly decontaminated with bleach or other strong oxidizing agent before disposal.

d) Take special care not to contaminate any of the test reagents with serum or bacterial agents.

e) Humidity indicators are supplied with each plate. If any of the indicators exhibit a pink color, the plate may be compromised in some way; decontaminate (i.e. wash the plate with bleach solution) and dispose of the plate.

f) The best results are achieved by following the protocols as they are described above, using good, safe laboratory techniques.

g) Do not use this kit after the expiration date.

h) Never pipette by mouth.

Allow all reagents to come to room temperature before starting.

References: Available upon request.

Presentation: 900 tests.

Compendium Code No.: 11150360

PROGARD®-5

Intervet **Vaccine**

Canine Distemper-Adenovirus Type 2-Parainfluenza-Parvovirus Vaccine, Modified Live Virus

U.S. Vet. Lic. No.: 286

Contents: PROGARD®-5 is a modified live virus vaccine containing attenuated strains of canine distemper virus, adenovirus type 2, parainfluenza virus and parvovirus grown in the Pro-Cell Stable Cell Line™. PROGARD®-5 is presented in a desiccated, single dose form with sterile diluent provided for reconstitution.

The attenuated distemper virus strain used in PROGARD®-5 is the Onderstepoort strain. The parvovirus component is patented* CPV Strain 154® which is an attenuated parvovirus strain of canine origin. The unique InterTek™ production process has made it possible to produce PROGARD®-5 with high titered CPV and CDV components which are highly immunogenic.

The Manhattan strain of adenovirus type 2 in PROGARD®-5 confers protection against canine infectious hepatitis caused by CAV-1 as well as infectious tracheobronchitis caused by CAV-2. Use of the Manhattan strain of CAV-2 provides dual protection without the adverse reactions associated with CAV-1, such as corneal edema ("blue eye").

Contains gentamicin as a preservative.

Indications: PROGARD®-5 is for the vaccination of healthy dogs against canine distemper virus infection, canine infectious hepatitis caused by CAV-1, canine respiratory infection caused by CAV-2, canine parainfluenza virus infection and canine parvovirus infection.

Dosage and Administration: Aseptically reconstitute desiccated vaccine vial with sterile diluent provided and administer 1 mL by subcutaneous or intramuscular route. Initial vaccination of healthy dogs may be given as early as 6 weeks of age with booster injections administered every 3-4 weeks until 12 weeks of age. Dogs over 12 weeks of age should initially receive 2 doses 3-4 weeks apart. Annual revaccination with a single dose is recommended.

Precaution(s): Recommended storage temperature 35-45°F (2-7°C).

Shake well before use.

Use contents promptly once reconstituted.

Non-chemically sterilized needles and syringes should be used for administration of vaccine.

Burn this container and all unused contents.

Caution(s): Avoid vaccinating pregnant bitches.

Administration of epinephrine may be indicated in the event of an anaphylactic reaction.

Only healthy animals should be vaccinated. Animals incubating any disease, or animals stressed due to shipping, malnutrition or parasitism may not achieve or maintain an adequate immune response.

This product is not hazardous when used according to directions supplied. A material safety data sheet (MSDS) is available upon request. This and any other consumer information can be obtained by calling Intervet's Customer Service Department at 1-800-441-8272.

For use in dogs only.

Trial Data: Safety and Efficacy: The safety, efficacy and compatibility of each of the components of PROGARD®-5 have been demonstrated to meet or exceed the standards set forth by the U.S.D.A. Extensive safety testing has demonstrated that CPV Strain 154® is safe when given to puppies as young as 4 weeks of age. In challenge studies, CPV Strain 154® prevented virulent CPV infection and subsequent lymphopenia and excretion of virulent CPV in 100% of the vaccinates. Severe clinical signs and lymphopenia, accompanied by excretion of virulent CPV, were present in 100% of the control dogs. Severity of challenge was evident in the control dogs for both CPV and CDV challenge studies. Clinical signs of CPV and CDV infections were prevented in 100% of the vaccinates.

Presentation: Cartons of 25 - 1 dose desiccated vaccine vials and 25 - 1 dose sterile diluent vials. Packaged in recyclable plastic containers.

* U.S. Patent No. 4,810,494

Compendium Code No.: 11061340

PROGARD®-6

Intervet **Vaccine**

Canine Distemper-Adenovirus Type 2-Coronavirus-Parainfluenza-Parvovirus Vaccine, Modified Live and Killed Virus

U.S. Vet. Lic. No.: 286

Contents: PROGARD®-6 is a modified live virus vaccine containing attenuated strains of canine distemper virus, adenovirus type 2, parainfluenza virus and parvovirus grown in the Pro-Cell Stable Cell Line™. PROGARD®-6 is presented in a desiccated form with inactivated canine coronavirus as the diluent.

The attenuated distemper virus strain used in PROGARD®-6 is the Onderstepoort strain. The parvovirus component is patented* CPV Strain 154® which is an attenuated parvovirus strain of canine origin. The unique InterTek™ production process has made it possible to produce PROGARD®-6 with high titered CPV and CDV components which are highly immunogenic.

The Manhattan strain of adenovirus type 2 in PROGARD®-6 confers protection against canine infectious hepatitis caused by CAV-1 as well as infectious tracheobronchitis caused by CAV-2. The use of the Manhattan strain of CAV-2 provides dual protection without the adverse reactions associated with CAV-1, such as corneal edema ("blue eye").

Contains gentamicin as a preservative.

Indications: PROGARD®-6 is for the vaccination of healthy dogs against canine distemper virus, canine infectious hepatitis caused by CAV-1, canine respiratory infection caused by CAV-2, canine parainfluenza virus, canine parvovirus, and canine coronavirus.

Dosage and Administration: Aseptically reconstitute the desiccated vaccine vial with the canine coronavirus diluent provided and administer 1 mL by the subcutaneous route. Initial vaccination of healthy dogs may be given as early as 6 weeks of age with booster injections administered every 3-4 weeks until 12 weeks of age. Dogs over 12 weeks of age should receive 2 doses 3-4 weeks apart. Annual revaccination with a single dose is recommended.

Precaution(s): Recommended storage temperature 35-45°F (2-7°C). Do not freeze. Shake well before use. Use contents promptly once reconstituted. Non-chemically sterilized needles and syringes should be used for administration of vaccine. Burn this container and all unused contents.

Caution(s): Avoid vaccinating pregnant bitches. Administration of epinephrine may be indicated in the event of an anaphylactic reaction. Only healthy animals should be vaccinated. Animals incubating any disease, or animals stressed due to shipping, malnutrition or parasitism may not achieve or maintain an adequate immune response. This product is not hazardous when used according to directions supplied. A material safety data sheet (MSDS) is available upon request. This and any other consumer information can be obtained by calling Intervet's Customer Service Department at 1-800-441-8272.

For use in dogs only.

Trial Data: Safety and Efficacy: The safety, efficacy and compatibility of each of the components of PROGARD®-6 have been demonstrated to meet or exceed the standards set forth by the U.S.D.A. Extensive safety testing has demonstrated that CPV Strain 154® and the CDV components are safe when given to puppies as young as 4 weeks of age. In challenge studies, CPV Strain 154® prevented virulent CPV infection and subsequent lymphopenia and excretion of virulent CPV in 100% of the vaccinates. Severe clinical signs and lymphopenia, accompanied by excretion of virulent CPV, were present in 100% of the control dogs. Severity of challenge was evident in the control dogs for both CPV and CDV challenge studies. Clinical signs of CPV and CDV infections were prevented in 100% of the vaccinates.

Presentation: Cartons of 25-1 dose desiccated vaccine vials and 25-1 dose inactivated canine coronavirus vials as diluent. Packaged in recyclable plastic containers.

U.S. Patent No. 4,810,494

Compendium Code No.: 11061350

PROGARD®-7

Intervet **Bacterin-Vaccine**

Canine Distemper-Adenovirus Type 2-Parainfluenza-Parvovirus Vaccine, Modified Live Virus, Leptospira Bacterin

U.S. Vet. Lic. No.: 286

Contents: PROGARD®-7 is a modified live virus vaccine containing attenuated strains of canine distemper virus, adenovirus type 2, parainfluenza virus and parvovirus grown in the Pro-Cell Stable Cell Line™. PROGARD®-7 is presented in a desiccated form with an inactivated *Leptospira canicola* and *Leptospira icterohaemorrhagiae* bacterin as the diluent.

The attenuated distemper virus strain used in PROGARD®-7 is the Onderstepoort strain. The parvovirus component is patented* CPV Strain 154® which is an attenuated parvovirus strain of canine origin. The unique InterTek™ production process has made it possible to produce PROGARD®-7 with high titered CPV and CDV components which are highly immunogenic.

The Manhattan strain of adenovirus type 2 in PROGARD®-7 confers protection against canine infectious hepatitis caused by CAV-1 as well as infectious tracheobronchitis caused by CAV-2. Use of the Manhattan strain of CAV-2 provides dual protection without the adverse reactions associated with CAV-1, such as corneal edema ("blue eye").

Contains gentamicin as a preservative.

Indications: PROGARD®-7 is for vaccination of healthy dogs against canine distemper virus infection, canine infectious hepatitis caused by CAV-1, canine respiratory infection caused by CAV-2, canine parainfluenza virus infection, canine parvovirus infection and leptospirosis caused by *L. canicola* and *L. icterohaemorrhagiae.*

Dosage and Administration: Aseptically reconstitute the desiccated vaccine vial with the Leptospira spp bacterin provided and administer 1 mL by subcutaneous or intramuscular route. Initial vaccination of healthy dogs may be given as early as 6 weeks of age with booster injections administered every 3-4 weeks until 12 weeks of age. Dogs over 12 weeks of age should receive 2 doses 3-4 weeks apart. Annual revaccination with a single dose is recommended.

Precaution(s): Recommended storage temperature 35-45°F (2-7°C). Do not freeze.

Shake well before use.

Use contents promptly once reconstituted.

Non-chemically sterilized needles and syringes should be used for administration of vaccine.

Burn this container and all unused contents.

Caution(s): Avoid vaccinating pregnant bitches.

Administration of epinephrine may be indicated in the event of an anaphylactic reaction.

Only healthy animals should be vaccinated. Animals incubating any disease, or animals stressed due to shipping, malnutrition or parasitism may not achieve or maintain an adequate immune response.

This product is not hazardous when used according to directions supplied. A material safety data sheet (MSDS) is available upon request. This and any other consumer information can be obtained by calling Intervet's Customer Service Department at 1-800-441-8272.

For use in dogs only.

Trial Data: Safety and Efficacy: The safety, efficacy and compatibility of each of the components of PROGARD®-7 have been demonstrated to meet or exceed the standards set forth by the U.S.D.A. Extensive safety testing has demonstrated that CPV Strain 154® is safe when given to puppies as young as 4 weeks of age. In challenge studies, CPV Strain 154® prevented virulent CPV infection and subsequent lymphopenia and excretion of virulent CPV in 100% of the vaccinates. Severe clinical signs and lymphopenia, accompanied by excretion of virulent CPV, were present in 100% of the control dogs. Severity of challenge was evident in the control dogs for both CPV and CDV challenge studies. Clinical signs of CPV and CDV infections were prevented in 100% of the vaccinates.

Presentation: Cartons of 25 - 1 dose desiccated vaccine vials and 25 - 1 dose Leptospira canicola and Leptospira icterohaemorrhagiae combined bacterin vials as diluent. Packaged in recyclable plastic containers.

* U.S. Patent No. 4,810,494

Compendium Code No.: 11061360

PROGARD®-8

Intervet **Bacterin-Vaccine**

Canine Distemper-Adenovirus Type 2-Coronavirus-Parainfluenza-Parvovirus Vaccine, Modified Live and Killed Virus-Leptospira Bacterin

U.S. Vet. Lic. No.: 286

Contents: PROGARD®-8 is a modified live virus vaccine containing attenuated strains of canine distemper virus, adenovirus type 2, parainfluenza virus and parvovirus grown in the Pro-Cell Stable Cell Line™. PROGARD®-8 is presented in a desiccated form with inactivated canine coronavirus-Leptospira canicola and Leptospira icterohaemorrhagiae bacterin as the diluent.

The attenuated distemper virus strain used in PROGARD®-8 is the Onderstepoort strain. The parvovirus component is patented* CPV Strain 154® which is an attenuated parvovirus strain of canine origin. The unique InterTek™ production process has made it possible to produce PROGARD®-8 with high titered CPV and CDV components which are highly immunogenic.

The Manhattan strain of adenovirus type 2 in PROGARD®-8 confers protection against canine infectious hepatitis caused by CAV-1 as well as infectious tracheobronchitis caused by CAV-2. The use of the Manhattan strain of CAV-2 provides dual protection without the adverse reactions associated with CAV-1, such as corneal edema ("blue eye").

Contains gentamicin as a preservative.

Indications: PROGARD®-8 is for the vaccination of healthy dogs against canine distemper virus, canine infectious hepatitis caused by CAV-1, canine respiratory infection caused by CAV-2, canine parainfluenza virus, canine parvovirus, canine coronavirus, and leptospirosis caused by *L. canicola* and *L. icterohaemorrhagiae.*

Dosage and Administration: Aseptically reconstitute the desiccated vaccine vial with the canine coronavirus-Leptospira spp bacterin provided and administer 1 mL by the subcutaneous route. Initial vaccination of healthy dogs may be given as early as 6 weeks of age with booster injections administered every 3-4 weeks until 12 weeks of age. Dogs over 12 weeks of age should receive 2 doses 3-4 weeks apart. Annual revaccination with a single dose is recommended.

Precaution(s): Recommended storage temperature 35-45°F (2-7°C). Do not freeze. Shake well before use. Use contents promptly once reconstituted. Non-chemically sterilized needles and syringes should be used for administration of vaccine. Burn this container and all unused contents.

Caution(s): Avoid vaccinating pregnant bitches. Administration of epinephrine may be indicated in the event of an anaphylactic reaction. Only healthy animals should be vaccinated. Animals incubating any disease, or animals stressed due to shipping, malnutrition or parasitism may not achieve or maintain an adequate immune response. This product is not hazardous when used according to directions supplied. A material safety data sheet (MSDS) is available upon request. This and any other consumer information can be obtained by calling Intervet's Customer Service Department at 1-800-441-8272.

For use in dogs only.

Trial Data: Safety and Efficacy: The safety, efficacy and compatibility of each of the components of PROGARD®-8 have been demonstrated to meet or exceed the standards set forth by the U.S.D.A. Extensive safety testing has demonstrated that CPV Strain 154® and the CDV components are safe when given to puppies as young as 4 weeks of age. In challenge studies, CPV Strain 154® prevented virulent CPV infection and subsequent lymphopenia and excretion of virulent CPV in 100% of the vaccinates. Severe clinical signs and lymphopenia, accompanied by excretion of virulent CPV, were present in 100% of the control dogs. Severity of challenge was evident in the control dogs for both CPV and CDV challenge studies. Clinical signs of CPV and CDV infections were prevented in 100% of the vaccinates.

Presentation: Cartons of 25-1 dose desiccated vaccine vials and 25-1 dose inactivated canine coronavirus-Leptospira canicola and Leptospira icterohaemorrhagiae combined bacterin vials as diluent. Packaged in recyclable plastic containers.

U.S. Patent No. 4,810,494

Compendium Code No.: 11061370

PROGARD®-CPv

Intervet **Vaccine**

Canine Parvovirus Vaccine, Modified Live Virus

U.S. Vet. Lic. No.: 286

Contents: PROGARD®-CPv is a modified live virus vaccine containing an attenuated strain of parvovirus grown in the Pro-Cell Stable Cell Line™. PROGARD®-CPv is presented in a ready to use liquid form.

The parvovirus strain in PROGARD®-CPv is an attenuated strain of canine origin. This patented* CPV Strain 154® is grown using Intervet's InterTek™ production process. This process produces parvovirus at a high titer which is highly immunogenic.

Contains gentamicin as a preservative.

Indications: PROGARD®-CPv is for vaccination of healthy dogs against canine parvovirus infection.

Dosage and Administration: Aseptically administer 1 mL subcutaneously or intramuscularly. Initial vaccination of healthy dogs may be given as early as 4 weeks of age with booster injections administered every 3 to 4 weeks until 12 weeks of age. Dogs over 12 weeks of age should initially receive 2 doses 3-4 weeks apart. Annual revaccination with a single dose is recommended.

Precaution(s): Recommended storage temperature 35-45°F (2-7°C).

Use entire contents when first opened.

Non-chemically sterilized needles and syringes should be used for administration of vaccine.

Burn this container and all unused contents.

Caution(s): Avoid vaccinating pregnant bitches.

Administration of epinephrine may be indicated in the event of an anaphylactic reaction.

Only healthy animals should be vaccinated. Animals incubating any disease, or animals stressed due to shipping, malnutrition or parasitism may not achieve or maintain an adequate immune response.

This product is not hazardous when used according to directions supplied. A material safety data sheet (MSDS) is available upon request. This and any other consumer information can be obtained by calling Intervet's Customer Service Department at 1-800-441-8272.

For use in dogs only.

Trial Data: Safety and Efficacy: The safety and efficacy of PROGARD®-CPv have been demonstrated to meet or exceed the standards set forth by the U.S.D.A. Extensive safety testing has demonstrated that CPV Strain 154® is safe when given to puppies as young as 4 weeks of age. Field trials conducted in puppies as young as 4 weeks of age demonstrated PROGARD®-CPv was virtually 100% reaction-free. In challenge studies, CPV Strain 154® prevented virulent CPV infection and subsequent lymphopenia and excretion of virulent CPV in 100% of the vaccinates. Severe clinical signs and lymphopenia, accompanied by excretion of virulent CPV, were present in 100% of the control dogs. In contrast, clinical signs of CPV infection were prevented in 100% of the vaccinates.

Presentation: 10 dose vials (5-10 dose vials per carton). Packaged in recyclable plastic containers.

* U.S. Patent No. 4,810,494

Compendium Code No.: 11061380

PROGARD®-CPv+CvK

Intervet **Vaccine**

Canine Coronavirus-Parvovirus Vaccine, Modified Live and Killed Virus

U.S. Vet. Lic. No.: 286

Contents: PROGARD®-CPv+CvK contains attenuated canine parvovirus grown in the Pro-Cell Stable Cell Line™ and inactivated canine coronavirus. PROGARD®-CPv+CvK is presented in a desiccated form with inactivated canine coronavirus as the diluent.

The parvovirus component used in PROGARD®-CPv+CvK is patented* CPV Strain 154® which is an attenuated parvovirus strain of canine origin. The unique InterTek™ production process has made it possible to produce PROGARD®-CPv+CvK with a high titered CPV component which is highly immunogenic.

Contains gentamicin as a preservative.

P

Indications: PROGARD®-CPv+CvK is for the vaccination of healthy dogs against canine parvovirus and canine coronavirus.

Dosage and Administration: Aseptically reconstitute the desiccated vaccine vial with the canine coronavirus diluent provided and administer 1 mL by the subcutaneous route. Initial vaccination of healthy dogs may be given as early as 6 weeks of age with booster injections administered every 3-4 weeks until 12 weeks of age. Dogs over 12 weeks of age should receive 2 doses 3-4 weeks apart. Annual revaccination with a single dose is recommended.

Precaution(s): Recommended storage temperature 35-45°F (2-7°C). Do not freeze. Shake well before use. Use entire contents promptly once reconstituted. Non-chemically sterilized needles and syringes should be used for administration of vaccine. Burn this container and all unused contents.

Caution(s): Avoid vaccinating pregnant bitches. Administration of epinephrine may be indicated in the event of an anaphylactic reaction. Only healthy animals should be vaccinated. Animals incubating any disease, or animals stressed due to shipping, malnutrition or parasitism may not achieve or maintain an adequate immune response. This product is not hazardous when used according to directions supplied. A material safety data sheet (MSDS) is available upon request. This and any other consumer information can be obtained by calling Intervet's Customer Service Department at 1-800-441-8272.

For use in dogs only.

Trial Data: Safety and Efficacy: The safety, efficacy and compatibility of each of the components of PROGARD®-CPv+CvK have been demonstrated to meet or exceed the standards set forth by the U.S.D.A. Extensive safety testing has demonstrated that CPV Strain 154® is safe when given to puppies as young as 4 weeks of age. In challenge studies, CPV Strain 154® prevented virulent CPV infection and subsequent lymphopenia and excretion of virulent CPV in 100% of the vaccinates. Severe clinical signs and lymphopenia, accompanied by excretion of virulent CPV, were present in 100% of the control dogs.

Presentation: Cartons of 25-1 dose desiccated vaccine vials and 25-1 dose inactivated canine coronavirus vials as diluent. Packaged in recyclable plastic containers.

U.S. Patent No. 4,810,494

Compendium Code No.: 11061390

PROGARD®-CvK

Intervet **Vaccine**

Canine Coronavirus Vaccine, Killed Virus

U.S. Vet. Lic. No.: 286

Contents: PROGARD®-CvK is an inactivated virus vaccine presented in a ready to use liquid form.

Note: Virus grown in the Pro-Cell Stable Cell Line™ to provide uniform, highly consistent growth and harvest, free from adventitious agents.

Contains gentamicin as a preservative.

Indications: For vaccination of healthy dogs against canine coronavirus disease.

Dosage and Administration: Shake well before use. Aseptically administer 1 mL subcutaneously or intramuscularly to dogs as early as 6 weeks of age, revaccinate every 2-3 weeks until 12 weeks of age. Vaccinate dogs over 12 weeks of age including those vaccinated under 12 weeks with one dose followed by a booster dose 2-4 weeks later. Revaccinate annually with a single dose.

Precaution(s): Recommended storage temperature 35-45°F (2-7°C). Do not freeze.

Shake well before use.

Use entire contents when opened.

Non-chemically sterilized needles and syringes should be used for administration of vaccine. Burn this container and all unused contents.

Caution(s): Administration of epinephrine may be indicated in the event of an anaphylactic reaction.

Only healthy animals should be vaccinated. Animals incubating disease or stressed due to shipping, malnutrition or parasitism may not achieve or maintain an adequate immune response.

This product is not hazardous when used according to directions supplied. A material safety data sheet (MSDS) is available upon request. This and any other consumer information can be obtained by calling Intervet's Customer Service Department at 1-800-441-8272.

For use in dogs only.

Presentation: 10 dose vials (5-10 dose vials per carton).

Packaged in recyclable plastic containers.

Compendium Code No.: 11061400

PROGARD®-KC

Intervet **Vaccine**

Canine Parainfluenza-Bordetella Bronchiseptica Vaccine, Modified Live Virus, Avirulent Live Culture

U.S. Vet. Lic. No.: 286

Contents: PROGARD®-KC is a modified live intranasal vaccine containing attenuated canine parainfluenza virus and *Bordetella bronchiseptica* avirulent live culture. PROGARD®-KC is presented in a desiccated form with sterile diluent provided for reconstitution.

Note: Virus grown in the Pro-Cell Stable Cell Line™ to provide uniform, highly consistent growth and harvest, free from adventitious agents.

Indications: PROGARD®-KC is for vaccination of healthy, susceptible puppies and dogs for prevention of canine infectious tracheobronchitis ("kennel cough") due to canine parainfluenza virus and *B. bronchiseptica*.

Dosage and Administration: Aseptically reconstitute the desiccated vaccine with the sterile diluent provided. Remove the needle and administer 0.4 mL into one nostril. Because of the small dose volume, an applicator tip is not required for administration of the vaccine. Healthy puppies three weeks of age or older and dogs should be vaccinated at least 72 hours prior to confinement or when risk of canine infectious tracheobronchitis ("kennel cough") may exist. Revaccinate annually.

Precaution(s): Recommended storage temperature 35-45°F (2-7°C).

Shake well before use.

Use contents promptly once reconstituted.

Non-chemically sterilized needles and syringes should be used for administration of vaccine. Burn this container and all unused contents.

Caution(s): Administration of epinephrine may be indicated in the event of an anaphylactic reaction.

Only healthy animals should be vaccinated. Animals incubating any disease, or animals stressed due to shipping, malnutrition or parasitism may not achieve or maintain an adequate immune response.

This product is not hazardous when used according to directions supplied. A material safety data sheet (MSDS) is available upon request. This and any other consumer information can be obtained by calling Intervet's Customer Service Department at 1-800-441-8272.

For use in dogs only.

Discussion: Canine infectious tracheobronchitis (ITB), also known as "kennel cough" is an acute, highly contagious respiratory disorder of multifactorial etiology. *B. bronchiseptica* and canine parainfluenza virus are the most common bacterial and viral agents, respectively, associated with canine ITB[1]. Because these organisms are transmitted via the aerosol route, dogs in close confinement, such as in kennels, hospitals or pet stores, are at greatest risk for infection. Puppies are particularly susceptible as maternal immunity is thought to be short-lived[1].

PROGARD®-KC contains avirulent strains of *B. bronchiseptica* and canine parainfluenza virus for intranasal administration. Vaccination with PROGARD®-KC stimulates rapid, local immunity in the respiratory tract, thereby inhibiting infection at the port of entry as well as preventing clinical signs. Protection against *B. bronchiseptica* after vaccination with PROGARD®-KC occurs by 72 hours post-vaccination. In addition to local immunity, PROGARD®-KC also stimulates systemic immunity within 3 weeks of intranasal administration. The small volume (0.4 mL) and one nostril application of PROGARD®-KC provides for ease in vaccination, particularly in small breeds of young puppies.

Trial Data: Safety Data: Extensive internal and field safety studies have demonstrated that PROGARD®-KC is safe in puppies as young as two weeks of age and in pregnant bitches. Four hundred fifty-nine (459) two week old puppies were vaccinated with PROGARD®-KC and observed 14-21 days post-vaccination. Of the two week old puppies, only one puppy developed any clinical signs which may have been attributed to the vaccine. This one puppy exhibited mucopurulent nasal discharge on day 10 post-vaccination and recovered uneventfully. One hundred-five (105) bitches were vaccinated during the first, second or third trimester of pregnancy. No adverse effects were observed in the bitches or the puppies born subsequently. PROGARD®-KC was demonstrated to be 99.7% reaction-free when administered to 1289 dogs of various ages, breed and sex.

Efficacy Data: Challenge studies were conducted to evaluate the efficacy of PROGARD®-KC in three week old puppies. Puppies vaccinated with PROGARD®-KC were protected against virulent canine parainfluenza virus challenge. Clinical signs and viral shedding were present in the control puppies, but were prevented in the vaccinates. PROGARD®-KC also provided protection against virulent *B. bronchiseptica* as demonstrated by significant reduction in clinical signs of ITB in the vaccinates as compared to control puppies. Additional studies evaluating the onset of immunity demonstrated protection against *B. bronchiseptica* 72 hours after vaccination with PROGARD®-KC.

References: Available upon request.

Presentation: Cartons of 25-1 dose desiccated vaccine vials and 25-1 dose sterile diluent vials.

Cartons of 1-10 dose desiccated vaccine vial and 1-10 dose sterile diluent vial.

Packaged in recyclable plastic containers.

Compendium Code No.: 11061410

PROGARD®-KC PLUS

Intervet **Vaccine**

Canine Adenovirus Type 2-Parainfluenza-Bordetella Bronchiseptica Vaccine, Modified Live Virus, Avirulent Live Culture

U.S. Vet. Lic. No.: 286

Contents: PROGARD®-KC PLUS is a modified live intranasal vaccine containing attenuated canine adenovirus type 2, parainfluenza virus and *Bordetella bronchiseptica* avirulent live culture. PROGARD®-KC PLUS is presented in a desiccated form with sterile diluent provided for reconstitution.

Indications: PROGARD®-KC PLUS is for vaccination of healthy dogs and puppies three weeks of age or older for prevention of canine infectious tracheobronchitis ("kennel cough") due to canine adenovirus type 2, parainfluenza virus and *B. bronchiseptica*.

Dosage and Administration: Aseptically reconstitute the desiccated vaccine with the sterile diluent provided. Remove the needle and administer 0.4 mL into one nostril. Because of the small dose volume, an applicator tip is not required for administration of the vaccine. Healthy puppies three weeks of age or older and dogs should be vaccinated prior to confinement or when risk of canine infectious tracheobronchitis ("kennel cough") may exist. Revaccinate annually.

Precaution(s): Recommended storage temperature 35-45°F (2-7°C). Shake well before use. Use contents promptly once reconstituted. Non-chemically sterilized needles and syringes should be used for administration of vaccine. Burn this container and all unused contents.

Caution(s): Administration of epinephrine may be indicated in the event of an anaphylactic reaction. Only healthy animals should be vaccinated. Animals incubating any disease, or animals stressed due to shipping, malnutrition or parasitism may not achieve or maintain an adequate immune response. This product is not hazardous when used according to directions supplied. A material safety data sheet (MSDS) is available upon request. This and any other consumer information can be obtained by calling Intervet's Customer Service Department at 1-800-441-8272. For use in dogs only.

Discussion: Canine infectious tracheobronchitis (ITB), also known as "kennel cough" is an acute, highly contagious respiratory disorder of multifactorial etiology. *B. bronchiseptica*, canine parainfluenza virus and canine adenovirus type 2 are the most common bacterial and viral agents, respectively, associated with ITB[1]. Because these organisms are transmitted via the aerosol route, dogs in close confinement, such as in kennels, hospitals or pet stores, are at greatest risk for infection. Puppies are particularly susceptible as maternal immunity is thought to be short-lived.[1]

PROGARD®-KC PLUS contains avirulent strains of *B. bronchiseptica*, canine adenovirus type 2 and canine parainfluenza virus for intranasal administration. Vaccination with PROGARD®-KC PLUS stimulates rapid, local immunity in the respiratory tract, thereby inhibiting infection at the port of entry as well as preventing clinical signs. In addition to local immunity, PROGARD®-KC PLUS also stimulates systemic immunity within three weeks of intranasal administration. The small volume (0.4 mL) and one nostril application of PROGARD®-KC PLUS provide for ease in vaccination, particularly in small breeds of young puppies.

Trial Data: Safety Data: Extensive internal and field safety studies have demonstrated that PROGARD®-KC PLUS is safe in puppies as young as two weeks of age and in pregnant bitches. Three hundred thirty-one (331) two-week-old puppies were vaccinated with PROGARD®-KC PLUS and observed 14 days post-vaccination. One hundred ninety (190) bitches were vaccinated during the first, second or third trimester of pregnancy. No adverse effects were observed in the bitches or the puppies born subsequently. PROGARD®-KC PLUS was demonstrated to be 99.9% reaction-free when administered to 1,702 dogs of various ages, breed, and sex.

Efficacy Data: Challenge studies were conducted to evaluate the efficacy of PROGARD®-KC PLUS in 3-week-old puppies. Puppies vaccinated with PROGARD®-KC PLUS were protected against virulent canine adenovirus type 2, parainfluenza virus and *B. bronchiseptica* challenges.

References: Available upon request.

Presentation: Cartons of 25x1-dose desiccated vaccine vials and 25x1-dose sterile diluent vials.

Cartons of 1x10-dose desiccated vaccine vial and 1x10-dose sterile diluent vial.

Packaged in recyclable plastic containers.

Compendium Code No.: 11061420

PROGARD® PUPPY-DPv

Intervet **Vaccine**

Canine Distemper-Parvovirus Vaccine, Modified Live Virus

U.S. Vet. Lic. No.: 286

Contents: PROGARD® Puppy-DPv is a modified live virus vaccine containing attenuated strains of canine distemper virus and parvovirus grown in the Pro-Cell Stable Cell Line™. PROGARD® Puppy-DPv is presented in a desiccated, single dose form with sterile diluent provided for reconstitution.

The attenuated distemper virus strain used in PROGARD® Puppy-DPv is the Onderstepoort strain. The parvovirus component is patented* CPV Strain 154® which is an attenuated parvovirus strain of canine origin. The InterTek™ production process has made it possible to produce PROGARD® Puppy-DPv with high titered CPV and CDV components which are highly immunogenic.

Contains gentamicin as a preservative.

Indications: PROGARD® Puppy-DPv is for vaccination of healthy dogs against canine distemper virus infection and canine parvovirus infection.

Dosage and Administration: Aseptically reconstitute the desiccated vaccine vial with the sterile diluent provided and administer 1 mL by subcutaneous or intramuscular route. Initial vaccination of healthy dogs may be given as early as 4 weeks of age with booster injections administered every 3-4 weeks until 12 weeks of age. Dogs over 12 weeks of age should initially receive 2 doses 3-4 weeks apart. Annual revaccination with a single dose is recommended.

Precaution(s): Recommended storage temperature 35-45°F (2-7°C).

Shake well before use.

Use contents promptly once reconstituted.

Non-chemically sterilized needles and syringes should be used for administration of vaccine.

Burn this container and all unused contents.

Caution(s): Avoid vaccinating pregnant bitches.

Administration of epinephrine may be indicated in the event of an anaphylactic reaction.

Only healthy animals should be vaccinated. Animals incubating any disease, or animals stressed due to shipping, malnutrition or parasitism may not achieve or maintain an adequate immune response.

This product is not hazardous when used according to directions supplied. A material safety data sheet (MSDS) is available upon request. This and any other consumer information can be obtained by calling Intervet's Customer Service Department at 1-800-441-8272.

For use in dogs only.

Trial Data: Safety and Efficacy: The safety, efficacy and compatibility of each of the components of PROGARD® Puppy-DPv have been demonstrated to meet or exceed the standards set forth by the U.S.D.A. Extensive safety testing has demonstrated that CPV Strain 154® is safe when given to puppies as young as 4 weeks of age.

In challenge studies, CPV Strain 154® prevented virulent CPV infection and subsequent lymphopenia and excretion of virulent CPV in 100% of the vaccinates. Severe clinical signs and lymphopenia, accompanied by excretion of virulent CPV, were present in 100% of the control dogs. Severity of challenge was evident in the control dogs for both CPV and CDV challenge studies. Clinical signs of CPV and CDV infections were prevented in 100% of the vaccinates.

Presentation: Cartons of 25 - 1 dose desiccated vaccine vials and 25 - 1 dose sterile diluent vials. Packaged in recyclable plastic containers.

* U.S. Patent No. 4,810,494

Compendium Code No.: 11061320

PROGARD® PUPPY-DPv+CvK

Intervet **Vaccine**

Canine Distemper-Coronavirus-Parvovirus Vaccine, Modified Live and Killed Virus

U.S. Vet. Lic. No.: 286

Contents: PROGARD® Puppy-DPv+CvK is a modified live virus vaccine containing attenuated strains of canine distemper virus and parvovirus grown in the Pro-Cell Stable Cell Line™. PROGARD® Puppy-DPv+CvK is presented in a desiccated form with inactivated canine coronavirus as the diluent.

The attenuated distemper virus strain used in PROGARD® Puppy-DPv+CvK is the Onderstepoort strain. The parvovirus component is patented* CPV Strain 154® which is an attenuated parvovirus strain of canine origin. The unique InterTek™ production process has made it possible to produce PROGARD® Puppy-DPv+CvK with a high titered CPV and CDV components which are highly immunogenic.

Contains gentamicin as a preservative.

Indications: PROGARD® Puppy-DPv+CvK is for the vaccination of healthy dogs against canine distemper virus, canine parvovirus and canine coronavirus.

Dosage and Administration: Aseptically reconstitute the desiccated vaccine vial with the canine coronavirus diluent provided and administer 1 mL by the subcutaneous route. Initial vaccination of healthy dogs may be given as early as 6 weeks of age with booster injections administered every 3-4 weeks until 12 weeks of age. Dogs over 12 weeks of age should receive 2 doses 3-4 weeks apart. Annual revaccination with a single dose is recommended.

Precaution(s): Recommended storage temperature 35-45°F (2-7°C). Do not freeze. Shake well before use. Use contents promptly once reconstituted. Non-chemically sterilized needles and syringes should be used for administration of vaccine. Burn this container and all unused contents.

Caution(s): Avoid vaccinating pregnant bitches. Administration of epinephrine may be indicated in the event of an anaphylactic reaction. Only healthy animals should be vaccinated. Animals incubating any disease, or animals stressed due to shipping, malnutrition or parasitism may not achieve or maintain an adequate immune response. This product is not hazardous when used according to directions supplied. A material safety data sheet (MSDS) is available upon request. This and any other consumer information can be obtained by calling Intervet's Customer Service Department at 1-800-441-8272.

For use in dogs only.

Trial Data: Safety and Efficacy: The safety, efficacy and compatibility of each of the components of PROGARD® Puppy-DPv+CvK have been demonstrated to meet or exceed the standards set forth by the U.S.D.A. Extensive safety testing has demonstrated that CPV Strain 154® and CDV components are safe when given to puppies as young as 4 weeks of age. In challenge studies, CPV Strain 154® prevented virulent CPV infection and subsequent lymphopenia and excretion of virulent CPV in 100% of the vaccinates. Severe clinical signs and lymphopenia, accompanied by excretion of virulent CPV, were present in 100% of the control dogs. Severity of challenge was evident in the control dogs for both CPV and CDV challenge studies. Clinical signs of CPV and CDV infections were prevented in 100% of the vaccinates.

Presentation: Cartons of 25-1 dose desiccated vaccine vials and 25-1 dose inactivated canine coronavirus vials as diluent. Packaged in recyclable plastic containers.

U.S. Patent No. 4,810,494

Compendium Code No.: 11061330

PRO-GEN® 20%

Fleming **Feed Additive**

Arsanilic Acid (90 Grams Per Pound)-Type A Medicated Article

NADA No.: 008-019

Active Ingredient(s): Arsanilic Acid 20% (90 grams per pound).

Inactive Ingredients: Rice hulls, calcium carbonate, and mineral oil.

With exclusive Lectra-Guard® anti-static treatment.

Indications: For use only in manufacturing medicated feeds for swine, chickens, and turkeys. Must be thoroughly mixed in feeds before use.

For increased rate of weight gain and improved feed efficiency in growing swine, and aid in control of swine dysentery (hemorrhagic enteritis, bloody dysentery). For growth promotion, feed efficiency, and improving pigmentation in growing chickens and turkeys.

Directions for Use:

Note: To secure even distribution, mix the required amount of PRO-GEN® 20% in a small quantity of feed ingredients. Add this mixture to the remainder of the batch of ingredients and mix thoroughly. Use as follows:

Indications For Use	Use Level of Arsanilic Acid	Pounds of PRO-GEN® 20% Per Ton of Complete Feed
Swine		
For increased rate of weight gain and improved feed efficiency in growing swine.	0.005-0.01% (45-90 grams per ton of complete feed). Feed continuously.	0.5-1 0
Aid in control of swine dysentery (hemorrhagic enteritis, bloody dysentery).	0.01% (90 grams per ton of complete feed). Feed continuously.	1.0
Chickens and Turkeys		
For growth promotion, feed efficiency, and improving pigmentation in growing chickens and turkeys.	0.01% (90 grams per ton of complete feed). Feed continuously.	1.0

Caution(s): Swine, chickens, and turkeys must have adequate drinking water at all times. Use as the sole source of organic arsenic.

Warning(s): Withdraw 5 days prior to slaughter.

For animal use only. Not for human consumption. Keep out of the reach of children.

Avoid breathing dust. Use toxic dust respirator which is MSHA/NIOSH approved against dust with TWA not less than 0.05 mg/m. Avoid contact with skin, eyes, and clothing. Wash immediately and thoroughly after handling.

If swallowed, call a physician, poison control center, or hospital immediately. Induce vomiting by giving Ipecac syrup as directed.

Presentation: 50 pound (22.7 kg) multi-wall paper bags.

"PRO-GEN®" and "Lectra-Guard®" are registered trademarks of Fleming Laboratories, Inc.

Compendium Code No.: 10120010

PRO-GEN® 100%

Fleming **Feed Medication**

Arsanilic Acid 99.5%-Type A Medicated Article

NADA No.: 008-019

Active Ingredient(s): Arsanilic Acid 99.5% (451 g/lb).

With exclusive Lectra-Guard® anti-static treatment.

Indications: For manufacturing use only to formulate medicated feed premixes for swine, chickens and turkeys.

a. Chickens and Turkeys: For growth promotion and feed efficiency; improving pigmentation.

b. Swine: For increased weight gain and improved feed efficiency in growing swine. As an aid in control of swine dysentery at 0.01% level.

Dosage and Administration:

a. Chickens and Turkeys: 0.01% (90 g/ton).

b. Swine: 0.005-0.01% (45-90 g/ton).

Caution(s): Swine, chickens and turkeys must have adequate drinking water at all times. Use as the sole source of organic arsenic.

Warning(s): Withdraw 5 days prior to slaughter.

For animal use only. Not for human consumption. Keep out of reach of children.

Avoid breathing dust. Use toxic dust respirator which is NIOSH/MSHA approved against dust with TWA not less than 0.05 mg/m. Avoid contact with skin, eyes and clothing. Wash immediately and thoroughly after handling.

If swallowed, call a physician, poison control center, or hospital immediately. Induce vomiting by giving Ipecac syrup as directed.

Presentation: 50 kg (110 lb) (NDC 15565-550-31).

"PRO-GEN®" and "Lectra-Guard®" are registered trademarks of Fleming Laboratories, Inc.

Compendium Code No.: 10120000

PROGRAM® 6 MONTH INJECTABLE FOR CATS ℞

Novartis **Flea Control**

(Lufenuron)

NADA No.: 141-105

Active Ingredient(s): Lufenuron.

Indications: PROGRAM® 6 Month Injectable for Cats is indicated for use in cats, six weeks of age and older, for the control of flea populations.

Lufenuron controls flea populations by preventing the development of flea eggs and does not kill adult fleas. Concurrent use of insecticides may be necessary for adequate control of adult fleas.

Pharmacology: Description: PROGRAM® (lufenuron) 6 Month Injectable for Cats is available in two syringe sizes for subcutaneous administration to cats and kittens according to their weight. (See Dosage.) Each preloaded syringe is formulated to provide 4.54 mg/pound (10 mg/kg) body weight of lufenuron. The active ingredient of PROGRAM® 6 Month Injectable for Cats is lufenuron, a benzoylphenyl-urea derivative with the following chemical composition: N-[2,5-dichloro-4-(1,1,2,3,3,3,-hexafluoropropoxy)-phenylaminocarbonyl]-2,6-difluorobenzamide. Benzoylphenyl-urea compounds, including lufenuron, are classified as insect development inhibitors (IDIs).

Mode of Action: Lufenuron, the active ingredient of PROGRAM® 6 Month Injectable for Cats, is an insect development inhibitor which breaks the flea life cycle by inhibiting egg development. Lufenuron's mode of action is interference with chitin synthesis, polymerization and deposition. Lufenuron has no effect on adult fleas.

After biting a lufenuron-treated cat, the female flea ingests a blood meal containing lufenuron which is subsequently deposited in her eggs. Lufenuron prevents flea eggs from hatching and developing into adults and thus controls flea populations by breaking the life cycle. (See Efficacy.)

Dosage and Administration: Dosage: PROGRAM® 6 Month Injectable for Cats is injected subcutaneously once every six months at the recommended minimum dosage of 4.54 mg lufenuron per pound (10 mg/kg) of body weight.

Recommended Dosage Schedule:

Body Weight	Syringe Size	Lufenuron Dose
Up to 8.8 lbs (4.0 kg)	Small (0.4 mL)	40 mg
8.9 lbs to 17.6 lbs (4.1 to 8.0 kg)	Large (0.8 mL)	80 mg

Administration: Administer PROGRAM® 6 Month Injectable for Cats subcutaneously using standard injection technique. Before administration, shake well to thoroughly mix the sterile suspension. Remove the needle guard and subcutaneously inject the entire contents of the syringe. Do not inject intramuscularly. The empty syringe should be disposed of in an approved manner.

To ensure the greatest benefits from the use of PROGRAM® 6 Month Injectable for Cats, it is important to treat all cats within a household. All dogs within the household should be treated with lufenuron tablets. Untreated dogs and cats may develop infestations which could reduce the overall flea control within a household.

Do not administer this product to dogs.

Contraindication(s): Do not use in dogs. A severe local reaction may occur in dogs that is not seen in cats.

Precaution(s): PROGRAM® 6 Month Injectable for Cats should be stored at room temperature between 59° and 86°F (15-30°C).

Caution(s): U.S. Federal law restricts this drug to use by or on the order of a licensed veterinarian.

The safety of PROGRAM® 6 Month Injectable for Cats in reproducing animals has not been established.

PROGRAM® 6 Month Injectable for Cats breaks the flea life cycle by inhibiting egg development. However, pre-existing flea populations may continue to develop and emerge after treatment with PROGRAM® 6 Month Injectable for Cats. Based on results of clinical studies, this emergence generally occurs during the first 30-60 days. Therefore, noticeable control may not be observed until several weeks after dosing when a pre-existing infestation is present. Cooler geographic areas may have longer lag periods due to a prolonged flea life cycle. Insecticides may be used concurrently depending on the severity of the infestation.

Adverse Reactions: The following adverse reactions were observed in clinical field trials with PROGRAM® 6 Month Injectable for Cats: pain on injection, injection site lumps/granulomas, vomiting, listlessness/lethargy and anorexia.

Histologic examination of one cat's injection site lump showed evidence of inflammation surrounding an area of necrosis with marked proliferation of fibrous connective tissue. In another cat, granulamatous inflammation was noted which included non-pleomorphic fibrocytes and fibroplasia.

Trial Data: Efficacy: Laboratory and clinical trials have shown that PROGRAM® 6 Month Injectable for Cats is a safe, effective and convenient method to control flea populations. A single dose provides long-lasting control for a full 6 months.

In laboratory studies, PROGRAM® 6 Month Injectable for Cats provided a cumulative percent control of egg development of 94.8% and 97.7% beginning 14 days post-treatment through six months post-treatment in the dose titration and dose confirmation studies, respectively. There was a 2-3 week "induction phase" in these studies before significant effects on flea reproduction were seen.

PROGRAM® 6 Month Injectable for Cats was effective in controlling flea populations when administered to 183 pet cats in a clinical setting. At study initiation, treated cats averaged 45 fleas per cat. Six months post-injection these cats averaged 11.4 fleas per cat.

Safety: PROGRAM® 6 Month Injectable for Cats has been used and tested safely in over sixteen breeds of cats, including females, males and kittens. In well-controlled clinical trials, 294 cats were treated with lufenuron. PROGRAM® 6 Month Injectable for Cats has also been safely used in cats receiving frequently used veterinary products such as vaccines, anthelmintics, antibiotics, steroids and insecticides.

The acute toxicity of injectable lufenuron was evaluated by administering 100 mg/kg bw, 10x the recommended 10 mg/kg bw dose rate, to adult cats. The potential cumulative toxicity of 1x and 3x the 10 mg/kg six month use rate of lufenuron injectable in 2 week old kittens was evaluated over a two month period. Other than injection site reactions (see below), no clinical signs of toxicity were reported in these studies.

Cumulative toxicity of injectable lufenuron in 2 month old cats was evaluated by administering 1, 3, or 5x the six-month dose three times during the 6 month study. This equates to cumulative doses of 3X, 9X, and 15X, respectively. Other than injection site reactions (see below), no clinical signs of toxicity were reported in these studies. Heinz body inclusions were present in all the control and treated cats, however, erythrocytes in the 50 mg/kg (15X cumulative dose) group had slightly elevated levels of Heinz bodies at 3-6 months.

The following injection site reactions were noted in these laboratory studies. Transient, minor discomfort was noted in some kittens and cats upon injection. Small raised areas at the injection sites, presumed to be deposits of lufenuron, were seen immediately after administration and persisted in some cases for the duration of the studies. This response at the injection site correlated microscopically with acute to granulomatous inflammation and fibrosis. Older injection sites showed less inflammation which indicates these effects may resolve with time. No neoplastic transformations were found. (See Adverse Reactions).

Presentation: PROGRAM® 6 Month Injectable for Cats is available in 0.4 mL and 0.8 mL unit dose syringes, formulated according to the weight of the cat. Unit dose packs are available in packages of 10 syringes per carton.

Compendium Code No.: 11310050

P

PROGRAM® FLAVOR TABS®

Flea Control

Novartis

(Lufenuron)

NADA No.: 141-035

Active Ingredient(s): Description: PROGRAM® Flavor Tabs® are available in two sizes (90.0 mg, 204.9 mg lufenuron) of tablets for oral administration to cats and kittens according to their weight (see Dosage section).

PROGRAM® Flavor Tabs® are available in four sizes (45.0 mg, 90.0 mg, 204.9 mg, 409.8 mg lufenuron) for oral administration to dogs and puppies according to their weight (see Dosage section).

Indications: The once-a-month flavored tablet that controls flea populations on cats.

PROGRAM® Flavor Tabs® are indicated for use in cats and kittens, six weeks of age and older, for the control of flea populations.

The flavored once-a-month tablet that prevents and controls flea populations in dogs.

PROGRAM® Flavor Tabs® are labeled for use in dogs and puppies, six weeks of age and older, for the prevention and control of flea populations.

Lufenuron controls flea populations by preventing the development of flea eggs and does not kill adult fleas. Concurrent use of insecticides may be necessary for adequate control of adult fleas.

Pharmacology: The active ingredient of PROGRAM® Flavor Tabs® is lufenuron, a benzoylphenylurea derivative with the following chemical composition: N-[2,5-dichloro-4-(1,1,2,3,3,3,-hexafluoropropoxy)-phenylaminocarbonyl]-2,6-difluorobenzamide. Benzoylphenylurea compounds, including lufenuron, are classified as insect development inhibitors (IDIs).

As an insect development inhibitor, PROGRAM® Flavor Tabs® does not kill adult fleas, but effectively and safely controls flea populations on your pet through a mode of action which breaks the flea's life cycle at the egg stage.

Dosage and Administration: Administration:

Cats: To ensure adequate absorption, always administer PROGRAM® Flavor Tabs® in conjunction with a normal meal.

Be certain the cat consumes the entire tablet or tablets. The tablets can be broken prior to direct dosing for ease of administration to small cats and kittens. As an alternative to direct dosing, the tablets can be broken and mixed into wet food. In multiple cat households, each cat should be treated separately to achieve adequate dosing. Watch the cat closely following dosing to be sure the entire dose has been consumed. If it is not entirely consumed, redose once with the full recommended dose as soon as possible.

PROGRAM® Flavor Tabs® must be administered monthly, preferably on the same date each month in conjunction with a normal meal. Treatment with PROGRAM® Flavor Tabs® may begin at any time of year. Treatment should continue until the end of "flea season." If there is a risk of exposure to fleas year-round, then treatment should continue the entire year without interruption. Ask your veterinarian for details concerning your geographic area and the most effective treatment schedule for your cat.

Dogs: To ensure adequate absorption, always administer PROGRAM® Flavor Tabs® to dogs immediately after or in conjunction with a normal meal.

Be certain the dog consumes the entire tablet or tablets. As an alternative to direct dosing tablets may be offered in food. Watch the dog closely following dosing to be sure the entire dose has been consumed. If it is not entirely consumed, redose once with the full recommended dose as soon as possible.

PROGRAM® Flavor Tabs® must be administered monthly, preferably on the same date each month in conjunction with a normal meal. Treatment with PROGRAM® Flavor Tabs® may begin at any time of year. In geographic areas where flea infestations are seasonal, the treatment schedule should begin several weeks prior to the expected onset of infestations. Treatments should continue until the end of "flea season." If there is risk of exposure to fleas year-round, then treatment should continue the entire year without interruption. Ask your veterinarian for details concerning your geographic area and the most effective treatment schedule for your pet.

To maximize benefits from the use of PROGRAM® Flavor Tabs®, it is important to treat all cats and dogs within a household. All cats within the household should be treated with lufenuron suspension or tablets. All dogs within the household should be treated with lufenuron tablets. Fleas can reproduce on untreated dogs and cats and allow infestations to persist.

Dosage:

Cats: PROGRAM® Flavor Tabs® are given orally, once a month, at the recommended minimum dosage of 13.6 mg lufenuron per pound (30 mg/kg) of body weight.

Recommended Dosage Schedule

Body Weight	Dose	Lufenuron Per Tablet
Up to 6 lbs.	One Tablet	90.0 mg
7 to 15 lbs.	One Tablet	204.9 mg

Cats over 15 lbs. are provided the appropriate combination of tablets.

Once-A-Month: PROGRAM® Flavor Tabs® will safely and effectively control flea infestations only if administered in conjunction with a normal meal on a monthly dosing schedule. To help you remember the monthly dosing, use the enclosed reminder stickers on the appropriate dates on your calendar.

Dogs: PROGRAM® Flavor Tabs® are given orally, once a month, at the recommended minimum dosage of 4.5 mg lufenuron per pound (10 mg/kg) of body weight.

Recommended Dosage Schedule

Body Weight	Dose	Lufenuron Per Tablet
Up to 10 lbs.	One tablet	45.0 mg
11 to 20 lbs.	One tablet	90.0 mg
21 to 45 lbs.	One tablet	204.9 mg
46 to 90 lbs.	One tablet	409.8 mg

Dogs over 90 lbs. should receive the appropriate combination of tablets.

Once-A-Month: PROGRAM® Flavor Tabs® will safely and effectively control flea infestations only if administered in conjunction with a normal meal on a monthly dosing schedule. To help you remember the monthly dosing, use the enclosed reminder stickers on the appropriate dates on your calendar.

Precaution(s): Storage Conditions: PROGRAM® Flavor Tabs® should be stored at room temperature between 59° and 86°F (15-30°C).

Caution(s): PROGRAM® Flavor Tabs® have no effect on adult fleas, but act to immediately break the flea life cycle by preventing eggs from developing into adults. However, pre-existing immature fleas in the pet's environment may continue to develop and emerge as adults after treatment with PROGRAM® Flavor Tabs®. Based on results of clinical studies, this emergence generally occurs during the first 30-60 days. Therefore, if your pet already has a flea infestation before starting PROGRAM® Flavor Tabs®, noticeable results may not be observed until several weeks after dosing. In cooler climates, immature fleas may take longer to complete the life cycle and emerge as adults. To speed control, traditional products that kill adult fleas may be used temporarily with PROGRAM® Flavor Tabs®, depending on the severity of the infestation.

If a treated cat comes in contact with a flea-infested environment, adult fleas may infest the treated animal. However, these adult fleas are unable to reproduce and will soon die off. Depending on the number of adult fleas, the temporary use of conventional adulticidal insecticides may be used to control these adult fleas. Your veterinarian can recommend the most effective treatment plan for your pet.

If a PROGRAM® Flavor Tabs® treated dog comes in contact with a flea-infested environment, adult fleas may infest the treated animal. However, these adult fleas will be unable to reproduce. Depending on the number of adult fleas, the temporary use of conventional adulticidal insecticides may be used to control these adult fleas. Your veterinarian can recommend the most effective treatment plan for your pet.

To ensure that your pet gets the greatest benefit from PROGRAM® Flavor Tabs®, you must administer the dose (tablet or tablets) once a month in conjunction with a normal meal. If you miss the 30-day interval, give PROGRAM® Flavor Tabs® immediately and resume your monthly dosing schedule. It is important to treat all cats and dogs within the household. All cats within the household should be treated with lufenuron suspension or tablets. All dogs within the household should be treated with lufenuron tablets. Fleas can reproduce on untreated dogs and cats and allow infestations to persist.

The active ingredient in PROGRAM® Flavor Tabs® is excreted in high concentrations in the milk, however, no resulting adverse effects have been recognized.

Warning(s): Keep out of reach of children.

Adverse Reactions: The following adverse reactions have been reported in cats after giving PROGRAM®: vomiting, depression/lethargy, anorexia (loss of appetite), diarrhea, hyperactivity, dyspnea (labored breathing), pruritus (itchy skin), and skin eruptions (rash).

The following adverse reactions have been reported in dogs after giving PROGRAM®: vomiting, depression/lethargy, pruritus (itchy, scratchy skin), urticaria (wheals, hives), diarrhea, anorexia (loss of appetite), and skin congestion (red skin).

Discussion: Flea Infestations on Cats and Dogs: Although other flea species may be found on cats and dogs, the cat flea *(Ctenocephalides felis)* is the predominant flea associated with infestations on cats and dogs in the United States. In addition to the common nuisance irritations associated with infestations, fleas can be responsible for medical problems in your pet such as flea allergy dermatitis (FAD), a skin reaction to flea bites. Also, fleas transmit other parasites, including tapeworms. Controlling flea infestations is important to your pet's health while also reducing the major and minor annoyances associated with these parasites.

Lufenuron, the active ingredient of PROGRAM® Flavor Tabs® does not kill adult fleas, but effectively breaks the flea's life cycle by inhibiting egg development. The following diagram illustrates the flea's life cycle and where PROGRAM® Flavor Tabs® acts to break this cycle.

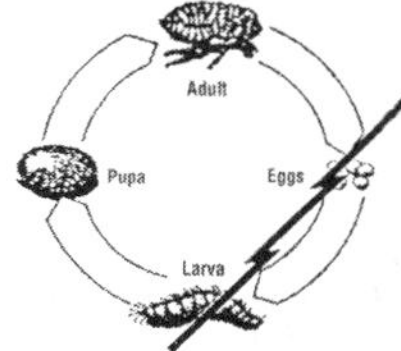

Fleas can be a problem because they reproduce so rapidly. A single female flea may produce up to 2,000 eggs over her lifetime. Eggs hatch and can develop into adults within only three weeks. Adult female fleas feed by ingesting blood from your pet and subsequently lay eggs which drop off your pet's coat. Within days, larvae hatch from the eggs and live undetected in your pet's surroundings, such as the carpet, bedding, and other protected areas. Flea larvae spin a cocoon, and when appropriately stimulated, a young adult flea emerges and jumps onto your pet to continue the life cycle. After biting a PROGRAM® Flavor Tabs® treated pet, the female flea ingests lufenuron which is deposited in her eggs. Lufenuron prevents these flea eggs from developing into mature adults. This safe and convenient approach to flea control effectively breaks the flea's life cycle and controls flea populations.

Presentation: Cats: PROGRAM® Flavor Tabs® are available in two tablet sizes (see Dosage section), formulated according to the weight of the cat. Each tablet size is available in color-coded packages of 6 tablets each.

Dogs: PROGRAM® Flavor Tabs® are available in four tablet sizes (see Dosage section), formulated according to the weight of the dog. Each tablet size is available in color-coded packages of six tablets each.

Compendium Code No.: 11310082 NAH/PRO-FT/PI/1 7/98

PROGRAM® SUSPENSION

Novartis **Flea Control**

Lufenuron

NADA No.: 141-026

Active Ingredient(s): PROGRAM® Suspension is available in two sizes of packs for oral administration to cats and kittens according to their weight (see Dosage and Administration section). Each unit dose pack is formulated to provide 13.6 mg/pound (30 mg/kg) of body weight of lufenuron.

Indications: PROGRAM® Suspension is labeled for use in cats and kittens, six weeks of age and older, for the control of flea populations.

Pharmacology: The active ingredient of PROGRAM® Suspension is lufenuron, a benzoylphenylurea derivative with the following chemical composition: N-[2,5-dichloro-4-(1,1,2,3,3,3,-hexafluoropropoxy)-phenylaminocarbonyl]-2,6-difluorobenzamide. Benzoylphenyl-urea compounds, including lufenuron, are classified as insect development inhibitors (IDIs).

As an insect development inhibitor, PROGRAM® does not kill adult fleas, but effectively and safely controls flea populations on your pet through a mode of action which breaks the flea's life cycle at the egg stage.

Dosage and Administration: PROGRAM® Suspension is given orally by mixing into food, once a month, at the recommended minimum dosage of 13.6 mg lufenuron per pound (30 mg/kg) of body weight.

Recommended Dosage Schedule:

Body Weight	Pack Per Month	Lufenuron Per Pack	Pack Color
Up to 10 lbs	1 Small	135 mg	Orange
11 to 20 lbs	1 Large	270 mg	Green

Cats over 20 lbs are provided the appropriate combination of packs.

To ensure adequate absorption, always administer PROGRAM® Suspension to cats in conjunction with a normal meal.

PROGRAM® Suspension is administered by mixing into food. If the dose is not entirely consumed, redose once with the full recommended dose as soon as possible. In multiple cat households, each cat should be treated separately to ensure adequate dosing.

PROGRAM® Suspension must be administered monthly, preferably on the same date each month in conjunction with a normal meal. To help you remember the monthly dosing, use the enclosed reminder stickers on the appropriate dates on your calendar. Treatment with PROGRAM® Suspension may begin at any time of year. Treatment should continue until the end of "flea season". If there is risk of exposure to fleas year-round, then treatment should continue the entire year without interruption. Ask your veterinarian for details concerning your geographic area and the most effective treatment schedule for your pet.

To maximize benefits from the use of PROGRAM® Suspension, it is important to treat all cats within a household. All dogs within the household should be treated with Program® Tablets. Fleas can reproduce on untreated cats and dogs and allow infestations to persist.

Mix the entire contents of the appropriate size PROGRAM® Suspension pack(s) with about two tablespoons of the cat's food. Since PROGRAM® Suspension is a liquid, it mixes easily with wet food. You can make it a special treat for your cat by mixing it with your cat's favorite wet food.

Observe the cat closely to ensure the entire dose has been consumed and then provide its normal meal. Always administer PROGRAM® to cats in conjunction with a normal meal as food is important for complete absorption of PROGRAM®. If your cat does not consume its meal following administration of PROGRAM®, try withholding the cat's food the night before to ensure it eats a meal with PROGRAM®.

Some cats have special dietary needs, so be sure to consult your veterinarian before giving your cat any new foods or before withholding food overnight.

Precaution(s): Storage Conditions: PROGRAM® Suspension should be stored at room temperature between 59° and 86°F (15-30°C).

Caution(s): PROGRAM® Suspension has no effect on adult fleas but acts to immediately break the flea life cycle by preventing eggs from developing into adults. However, pre-existing immature fleas in the cat's environment may continue to develop and emerge as adults after treatment with PROGRAM® Suspension. Based on results of clinical studies, this emergence generally occurs during the first 30-60 days. Therefore, if your pet already has a flea infestation before starting PROGRAM®, noticeable results may not be observed until several weeks after dosing. In cooler climates, immature fleas may take longer to complete the life cycle and emerge as adults. To speed control, traditional products that kill adult fleas may be used temporarily with PROGRAM®, depending on the severity of the infestation.

If a PROGRAM®-treated cat comes in contact with a flea-infested environment, adult fleas may infest the treated animal. However, these adult fleas will be unable to reproduce and will soon die off. Depending on the number of adult fleas, the temporary use of conventional adulticidal insecticides may be used to control these adult fleas. Your veterinarian can recommend the most effective treatment plan for your pet.

To ensure that your pet gets the greatest benefit from PROGRAM® Suspension, you must administer the dose once a month in conjunction with a normal meal. If you miss the 30-day interval, give PROGRAM® Suspension to your cat immediately and resume your monthly dosing schedule. It is important to treat all cats within the household. All dogs within the household should be treated with Program® Tablets.

Fleas can reproduce on untreated dogs and cats and allow infestations to persist.

The active ingredient in PROGRAM® is excreted in high concentrations in the milk, however, no resulting adverse effects have been recognized.

Warning(s): Keep out of the reach of children.

Side Effects: The following adverse reactions have been reported in cats after giving PROGRAM®: vomiting, depression/lethargy, anorexia (loss of appetite), diarrhea, dyspnea (labored breathing), pruritus (itchy, scratchy skin), and skin disorder.

Discussion: Flea Infestations on Cats: Although other flea species may be found on cats, the cat flea *(Ctenocephalides felis)* is the predominant flea associated with infestations on cats in the United States. In addition to the common nuisance irritations associated with infestations, fleas can be responsible for medical problems in your pet such as miliary dermatitis, a skin reaction to flea bites. Also, fleas transmit other parasites, including tapeworms. Controlling flea infestations is important to your pet's health while also reducing the major and minor annoyances associated with these parasites.

Lufenuron, the active ingredient of PROGRAM® Suspension does not kill adult fleas but effectively breaks the flea's life cycle by inhibiting egg development.

Life Cycle of the Flea: Fleas can be a problem because they reproduce so rapidly. A single female flea may produce up to 2,000 eggs over her lifetime. Eggs hatch and can develop into adults within only three weeks. Adult female fleas feed by ingesting blood from your cat and subsequently lay eggs which drop off your cat's coat. Within days, larvae hatch from the eggs and live undetected in your cat's surroundings such as the carpet, bedding, and other protected areas. Flea larvae spin a cocoon, and when appropriately stimulated, a young adult flea emerges and jumps onto your cat to continue the life cycle. After biting a PROGRAM®-treated cat, the female flea ingests lufenuron which is deposited in her eggs. Lufenuron prevents these eggs from hatching or developing into mature adults. This safe and convenient approach to flea control effectively breaks the flea's life cycle and controls flea populations.

Presentation: PROGRAM® Suspension is available in two pack sizes (see Dosage and Administration section), formulated and color-coded according to the weight of the cat. Both pack sizes are available in color-coded packages of 6 packs per carton.

Compendium Code No.: 11310071 NAH/PRO-S/PI/1 6/97

PROHEART® 6 ℞

Fort Dodge **Parasiticide Injection**

(moxidectin) Sustained Release Injectable for Dogs

NADA No.: 141-189

Active Ingredient(s): Description: PROHEART® 6 (moxidectin) Sustained Release Injectable consists of two separate vials. Vial 1 contains 10% moxidectin sterile microspheres and Vial 2 contains a specifically formulated sterile vehicle for constitution with Vial 1. No other diluent should be used. A clear or translucent appearance of the vehicle is normal. Each mL of constituted drug product contains 3.4 mg moxidectin, 3.1% glyceryl tristearate, 2.4% hydroxypropyl methylcellulose, 0.87% sodium chloride, 0.17% methylparaben, 0.02% propylparaben and 0.001% butylated hydroxytoluene. Hydrochloric acid is used to adjust pH.

Indications: PROHEART® 6 is indicated for use in dogs six months of age and older for the prevention of heartworm disease caused by *Dirofilaria immitis*.

PROHEART® 6 is indicated for the treatment of existing larval and adult hookworm *(Ancylostoma caninum* and *Uncinaria stenocephala)* infections.

Pharmacology: Moxidectin is a semi-synthetic methoxime derivative of nemadectin which is a fermentation product of *Streptomyces cyaneogriseus* subsp *noncyanogenus*. Moxidectin is a pentacyclic 16-membered lactone macrolide.

Moxidectin has activity resulting in paralysis and death of affected parasites. The stage of the canine heartworm affected at the recommended dose rate of 0.17 mg moxidectin/kg body weight

P

is the tissue larval stage. The larval and adult stages of the canine hookworms, *Ancylostoma caninum* and *Uncinaria stenocephala*, are susceptible.

Following injection with PROHEART® 6, peak moxidectin blood levels will be observed approximately 7-14 days after treatment. At the end of the six month dosing interval, residual drug concentrations are negligible. Accordingly, little or no drug accumulation is expected to occur with repeated administrations.

Dosage and Administration: Frequency of Treatment: PROHEART® 6 prevents infection by *D. immitis* for six months. It should be administered within one month of the dog's first exposure to mosquitoes. Follow-up treatments may be given every six months if the dog has continued exposure to mosquitoes. When replacing another heartworm preventive product, PROHEART® 6 should be given within one month of the last dose of the former medication.

PROHEART® 6 eliminates the larval and adult stages of *A. caninum* and *U. stenocephala* present at the time of treatment. However, persistent effectiveness has not been established for this indication. Re-infection with *A. caninum* and *U. stenocephala* may occur sooner than 6 months.

Dose: The recommended subcutaneous dose is 0.05 mL of the constituted suspension/kg body weight (0.0227 mL/lb.). This amount of suspension will provide 0.17 mg moxidectin/kg bodyweight (0.0773 mg/lb.). To ensure accurate dosing, calculate each dose based on the dog's weight at the time of treatment. Do not overdose growing puppies in anticipation of their expected adult weight. The following dosage chart may be used as a guide.

Dosage Chart:

Dog Wt.		Dose Volume
lb.	kg	mL/Dog
11	5	0.25
22	10	0.50
33	15	0.75
44	20	1.00
55	25	1.25
66	30	1.50
77	35	1.75
88	40	2.00
99	45	2.25
110	50	2.50
121	55	2.75
132	60	3.00

Injection Technique: The two-part sustained release product must be mixed at least 30 minutes prior to the intended time of use (See Constitution Procedures for initial mixing instructions). Once constituted, swirl the bottle gently before every use to uniformly re-suspend the microspheres. Withdraw 0.05 mL of suspension/kg body weight into an appropriately sized syringe fitted with an 18G or 20G hypodermic needle. Dose promptly after drawing into dosing syringe. If administration is delayed, gently roll the dosing syringe prior to injection to maintain a uniform suspension and accurate dosing.

Using aseptic technique, inject the product subcutaneously in the left or right side of the dorsum of the neck cranial to the scapula. No more than 3 mL should be administered in a single site. The location(s) of each injection (left or right side) should be noted so that prior injection sites can be identified and the next injection can be administered on the opposite side.

Constitution Procedures: The two-part PROHEART® 6 product must be mixed at least 30 minutes prior to the intended time of use.

Items needed to constitute PROHEART® 6: Microspheres (vial 1); Sterile 20 mL syringe for transfer; Enclosed vent needle (25G); Transfer needle (18G or 20G); Vehicle (vial 2).

Constitution of the 20 mL vial product:

1. Shake the microsphere vial to break up any aggregates prior to constitution.
2. Using an 18G or 20G needle and sterile syringe withdraw 17.0 mL of the unique vehicle from the vial. There is more vehicle supplied than the 17.0 mL required.
3. Insert the enclosed 25G vent needle into the microsphere vial.
4. Slowly transfer the vehicle into the microsphere vial through the stopper using the transfer needle and syringe.
5. Once the vehicle has been added, remove the vent and transfer needles from the microsphere vial. Discard unused vehicle and needles.
6. Shake the microsphere vial vigorously until a thoroughly mixed suspension is produced.
7. Record the time and date of mixing on the microsphere vial.
8. Allow suspension to stand for at least 30 minutes to allow large air bubbles to dissipate.
9. Before every use, gently swirl the mixture to achieve uniform suspension. The microspheres and vehicle will gradually separate on standing.
10. Use a 1 mL or 3 mL syringe and an 18G or 20G needle for dosing. Dose promptly after drawing into dosing syringe. If administration is delayed, gently roll the dosing syringe prior to injection to maintain a uniform suspension and accurate dosing.
11. Refrigerate the unused product. The constituted product remains stable for 4 weeks in a refrigerator. Avoid direct sunlight.

Contraindication(s): PROHEART® 6 is contraindicated in animals previously found to be hypersensitive to this drug.

Precaution(s): Storage Information: Store the unconstituted product at or below 25°C (77°F). Do not expose to light for extended periods of time. After constitution, the product is stable for 4 weeks stored under refrigeration at 2° to 8°C (36° to 46°F).

Caution(s): Federal (U.S.A.) law restricts this drug to use by or on the order of a licensed veterinarian.

Use with caution in sick, debilitated or underweight animals (see Safety).

PROHEART® 6 should not be used more frequently than every 6 months.

The safety and effectiveness of PROHEART® 6 has not been evaluated in dogs less than 6 months of age.

Prior to administration of PROHEART® 6, dogs should be tested for existing heartworm infections. At the discretion of the veterinarian, infected dogs should be treated to remove adult heartworms. PROHEART® 6 is not effective against adult *D. immitis* and, while the number of circulating microfilariae may decrease following treatment, PROHEART® 6 is not effective for microfilariae clearance.

No adverse reactions were observed in dogs with patent heartworm infections when PROHEART® 6 was administered at three times the labeled dose. Higher doses were not tested.

Warning(s): Human Warnings: Not for human use. Keep this and all drugs out of the reach of children.

May be slightly irritating to the eyes. May cause slight irritation to the upper respiratory tract if inhaled. May be harmful if swallowed. If contact with the eyes occurs, rinse thoroughly with water for 15 minutes and seek medical attention immediately. If accidental ingestion occurs, contact a Poison Control Center or a physician immediately. The material safety data sheet (MSDS) contains more detailed occupational safety information.

Adverse Reactions: In field studies, the following adverse reactions were observed in approximately 1% of 280 dogs treated with PROHEART® 6: vomiting, diarrhea, listlessness, weight loss, seizures, injection site pruritus, and elevated body temperature.

Post-Approval Experience: Although not all adverse reactions are reported, the following reactions are based on voluntary post-approval drug experience reporting: anaphylaxis/toid reactions, depression/lethargy, urticaria, and head/facial edema. As with anaphylaxis/toid reactions resulting from the use of other injectable products, standard therapeutic intervention should be initiated immediately.

To report suspected adverse reactions or to obtain technical assistance, call (800) 533-8536.

Trial Data: Animal Safety:

General Safety: PROHEART® 6 has been safely administered to a wide variety of healthy dogs six months of age and older, including a wide variety of breeds, pregnant and lactating females, breeding males, and ivermectin-sensitive collies. However, in clinical studies, two geriatric dogs with a history of weight loss after the initial PROHEART® 6 injection died within a month of the second 6 month injection. A third dog who was underweight for its age and breed and who had a history of congenital problems experienced lethargy following the initial injection of PROHEART® 6. The dog never recovered and died 3 months later (see Cautions).

PROHEART® 6 administered at 3 times the recommended dose in dogs with patent heartworm infections and up to 5 times the recommended dose in ivermectin-sensitive collies did not cause any adverse reactions. PROHEART® 6 administered at 3 times the recommended dose did not adversely effect the reproductive performance of male or female dogs. PROHEART® 6 administered up to 5 times the recommended dose in 7-8 month old puppies did not cause any systemic adverse effects.

In well controlled clinical studies, PROHEART® 6 was safely used in conjunction with a variety of veterinary products including vaccines, anthelmintics, antiparasitics, antibiotics, analgesics, steroids, non-steroidal anti-inflammatory drugs (NSAIDs), anesthetics and flea control products.

Injection Site Reactions: Injection site observations were recorded during effectiveness and safety studies. In clinical studies, PROHEART® 6 was administered at six-month intervals to client-owned dogs under field conditions. There were no reports of injection site reactions in these field studies and evaluations of the injection sites revealed no abnormalities.

In a laboratory safety study, PROHEART® 6 was administered at 1, 3 and 5 times the recommended dose to 7-8 month old puppies. Injection sites were clipped to facilitate observation. Slight swelling/edema at the injection site was observed in some dogs from all treated groups. These injection site reactions appeared as quickly as 8 hours post injection and lasted up to 3 weeks. A three-year repeated injection study was conducted to evaluate the safety of up to 6 injections of PROHEART® 6 administered at the recommended dose (0.17 mg/kg) every 6 months. Mild erythema and localized deep subcuticular thickening were seen in dogs that received four injections in the same area on the neck and in one dog that received two injections in the same area on the neck. Microscopic evaluation on the injection sites from all dogs 6 months after the last injection consistently showed mild granulomatous panniculitis with microvacuolation. The only adverse reaction seen that was not related to the injection site was weight loss in one dog.

Some dogs treated with PROHEART® 6 in laboratory effectiveness studies developed transient, localized inflammatory injection site reactions. These injection site reactions were visible grossly for up to 3 weeks after injection. Histologically, well-defined granulomas were observed in some dogs at approximately 5 months after injection.

Presentation: PROHEART® 6 is available in the following two package sizes.

1. 5-Pack
   NDC 0856-3670-25 - 20 mL vial product:
   5 - 10% moxidectin sterile microspheres - 598 mg/vial
   5 - Sterile vehicle - 17 mL vial
2. 10-Pack
   NDC 0856-3670-29 - 20 mL vial product:
   10 - 10% moxidectin sterile microspheres - 598 mg/vial
   10 - Sterile vehicle -17 mL vial

U.S. Patent No. 4,916,154 and 6,340,671

Compendium Code No.: 10032692 3670B

PROHEART® TABLETS ℞

Fort Dodge **Parasiticide-Oral**

Moxidectin-Heartworm Prevention Tablets for Dogs

NADA No.: 141-051

Active Ingredient(s): Each tablet contains either:

Moxidectin . . . . 30 μg, 68 μg or 136 μg

Indications: PROHEART® (moxidectin) heartworm prevention tablets are indicated for once-a-month use in dogs to prevent infections by the canine heartworm, *Dirofilaria immitis*, and the subsequent development of canine heartworm disease.

Pharmacology: Description: Each PROHEART® heartworm prevention tablet is formulated to provide 1.36 μg moxidectin/lb body weight (3 μg/kg). Moxidectin is a semi-synthetic methoxime derivative of nemadectin which is a fermentation product of *Streptomyces cyaneogriseus* subsp *non-cyanogenus*. Moxidectin is a pentacyclic 16-membered lactone macrolide.

Moxidectin has activity resulting in paralysis and death of affected parasites. The stage of the canine heartworm affected at the recommended dose rate of 3 μg/kg body weight is the tissue larval (L3) stage. There is no effect against the adult heartworm at this dose rate.

Dosage and Administration: Administer tablets orally at one-month intervals during the time when the intermediate host (the mosquito) is present. Dosing should start within one month after the first exposure to mosquitoes and should continue at monthly intervals until one month after the last exposure to mosquitoes. To establish a routine, it is recommended that the same day or date be used each month to administer the tablet to the dog.

PROHEART® (moxidectin) is recommended for dogs eight weeks of age and older. The recommended minimum dose rate is 1.36 μg moxidectin/lb (3 μg/kg) body weight which is achieved by using tablets as follows:

Dog Weight	Tablets per Month	Tablet Weight	Moxidectin per tablet
Up 10 22 lbs.	1	182 mg	30 μg
23 to 50 lbs.	1	412 mg	68 μg
51 to 100 lbs.	1	824 mg	136 μg

Dogs weighing over 100 pounds should be given the appropriate combination of these tablets. For example, a dog weighing 120 pounds should be given one large tablet containing 136 μg moxidectin and one small tablet containing 30 μg moxidectin each month.

The whole dosage should be swallowed. This may be achieved by manually placing the tablet(s) over the back of the tongue or by wrapping the tablet(s) in the dog's food. The dog should be

P

observed closely for several minutes to insure that the dosage has been swallowed. If it is thought that the entire dosage has not been swallowed, the dog should be redosed.

After administering the proper dose, as stated above, return the card with the remaining tablets to the package to protect the product from both moisture and light.

Precaution(s): Store at room temperature up to 25°C (77°F). Do not store at temperatures greater than 25°C or expose to light for extended periods of time.

Caution(s): Federal law restricts this drug to use by or on the order of a licensed veterinarian.

PROHEART® heartworm prevention tablets should only be used in dogs testing negative for the presence of heartworm infection. Infected dogs should be treated to remove adult heartworms and microfilaria prior to initiating treatment with PROHEART® tablets.

A complete heartworm disease prevention program includes a periodic physical examination and a test for the presence of adult heartworm by a licensed veterinarian. All dogs not currently on an approved heartworm prevention program should be tested for the presence of adult heartworms before using PROHEART® heartworm prevention tablets.

If replacing another preventative medication, the first dosage of PROHEART® heartworm prevention tablets must be administered within one month of cessation of the original program.

If a dosage of PROHEART® heartworm prevention tablets is forgotten for a period of less than 1 month (not more than 1 full month), give the full dosage immediately and then revert to the regular dosing routine. If a dosage is forgotten by a period exceeding one month (more than two months have passed since the last dose), a test for the presence of adult heartworms should be performed before re-establishing the monthly dosing routine. A follow-up test within the next year is also recommended.

Hypersensitivity reactions have not been observed in trials where animals were administered moxidectin up to five times the recommended dose level. Transient inappetence, decreased motor activity, and increased respiration were observed in microfilaria-positive animals administered moxidectin at 10 times the recommended dose level. Consult a veterinarian immediately if any adverse reaction is suspected.

Warning(s):

Human Warning: Keep this and all drugs out of reach of children. In case of human consumption, contact a Poison Control Center or a physician immediately.

Toxicology:

Target Animal Safety: PROHEART® heartworm prevention tablets have been safely administered to a wide variety of dog breeds.

The target animal safety testing program for PROHEART® heartworm prevention tablets includes field tests at the recommended dose level, tests with sensitive collie dogs, tests with dogs known to have patent heartworm infections, reproductive studies with breeding bitches and stud dogs, and safety studies with puppies eight weeks of age. These studies showed that PROHEART® tablets were safe at the recommended dose level, at three times the recommended dose level in the breeding safety studies, at five times the recommended dose level in the collie and patent heartworm infection safety studies, and up to 10 times the recommended dose in puppies eight weeks of age. Mild signs of depression, ataxia and salivation were seen in one collie dog at 30 times the recommended dose.

As part of the field-testing program, PROHEART® tablets were safely used in conjunction with a variety of veterinary products commonly used with dogs. These products included vitamins and nutritional supplements, steroid and antibiotic medications, shampoos, dips, and other ectoparasite treatments.

Moxidectin was fed to dogs daily for a period of one year to determine the safety of the product in the target species. When fed at levels in excess of 300 times the recommended monthly dose, moxidectin was determined to be safe for dogs.

Adverse Reactions: The following adverse reactions may be observed following the use of PROHEART® (moxidectin): lethargy, vomiting, ataxia, anorexia, diarrhea, nervousness, weakness, increased thirst, and itching.

Presentation: PROHEART® (moxidectin) Heartworm Prevention Tablets — Packs containing 6 tablets each are packaged 10 packs per display carton.

NDC 0856-8851-01 — 30 µg per tablet
NDC 0856-8852-01 — 68 µg per tablet
NDC 0856-8853-01 — 136 µg per tablet

Packaged by: Sharp, Conshohocken, PA 19428 U.S. Patent No. 4,916,154
Compendium Code No.: 10031654 8850C

PROHIBIT® SOLUBLE DRENCH POWDER

AgriLabs **Parasiticide-Oral**

(Levamisole Hydrochloride) Soluble Drench Powder-Anthelmintic

NADA No.: 200-225

Active Ingredient(s): Each packet contains 46.8 g of levamisole hydrochloride activity.

Each bottle contains 544.5 g of levamisole hydrochloride activity.

Indications: PROHIBIT® (levamisole hydrochloride) is a broad-spectrum anthelmintic and is effect against the following nematode infections in cattle and sheep:

Stomach Worms: *(Haemonchus, Trichostrongylus, Ostertagia).*

Intestinal Worms: *(Trichostrongylus, Cooperia, Nematodirus, Bunostomum, Oesophagostomum) [Chabertia* - sheep only].

Lungworms: *(Dictyocaulus).*

Dosage and Administration:

Cattle:

Standard Drench Solution: Place the contents of the packet in a 1 quart (32 fl. oz.) container, fill with water, swirl until dissolved. Administer as a single drench dose according to the following table:

Weight	Drench Dosage	Packet Will Treat
200 lb.	½ fl. oz.	64 head
400 lb.	1 fl. oz.	32 head
600 lb.	1½ fl. oz.	21 head
800 lb.	2 fl. oz.	16 head

Concentrated Drench Solution: For use with automatic syringe. Place the contents of the packet in a standard household measuring container and add water to the 8¾ fl. oz. level; or use the measuring container available from your supplier and add water to the mark. Swirl until dissolved. Give 2 mL (milliliter) per 100 lb. body weight. Refer to the table above for the number of cattle the packet will treat.

Sheep:

Standard Drench Solution: Place the contents of the packet in a 1 gallon (128 fl. oz.) container, fill with water, swirl until dissolved. Administer as a single drench dose according to the following table:

Weight	Drench Dosage	Packet Will Treat
50 lb.	½ fl. oz.	256 head
100 lb.	1 fl. oz.	128 head
150 lb.	1 ½ fl. oz.	84 head
200 lb.	2 fl. oz.	64 head

Concentrated Drench Solution: For use with automatic syringe. Place the contents of the packet in a standard household measuring container and add water to the 17½ fl. oz. level. Swirl until dissolved. Give 2 mL per 50 lb. body weight. Refer to the table above for the number of sheep the packet will treat.

Bottle: When ready to deworm cattle or sheep, add water to the powder in the bottle up to the 3 L mark. Swirl to mix thoroughly before using. If there is any solution left over, it may be stored for up to three (3) months in the tightly capped bottle. Shake well before using.

Administer as a single drench dose as follows:

Weight	Drench Dosage	Bottle will Treat
Cattle: 2 mL per 100 lbs. of body weight.		
100 lbs.	2 mL	1,500 head
300 lbs.	6 mL	500 head
500 lbs.	10 mL	300 head
700 lbs.	14 mL	214 head
1,000 lbs.	20 mL	150 head
Sheep: 1 mL per 50 lbs. of body weight.		
50 lbs.	1 mL	3,000 head
100 lbs.	2 mL	1,500 head
150 lbs.	3 mL	1,000 head
200 lbs.	4 mL	750 head

Note: Careful weight estimates are essential for the proper performance of this product.

Cattle and sheep maintained under conditions of constant helminth exposure may require retreatment within two to four weeks after the first treatment.

Consult a veterinarian for assistance in the diagnosis, treatment and control of parasitism.

Precaution(s): Store between 15-30°C (59-86°F).

Prepare solutions as needed. However, excess solutions may be stored in clean closed containers up to 90 days without loss of anthelmintic activity.

Caution(s): Muzzle foam may be observed. However, the reaction will disappear with a few hours. If this condition persists, a veterinarian should be consulted. Follow recommended dosage carefully. Consult veterinarian before using in severely debilitated animals.

For oral use in cattle and sheep. For animal use only.

Warning(s): Do not administer to cattle within 48 hours of slaughter for food. Do not administer to sheep within 72 hours of slaughter for food. To prevent residues in milk, do not administer to dairy animals of breeding age. Keep out of reach of children.

Presentation: 30 x 1.8 oz (52 g) packets and 21.34 oz. (1.3 lb.) (605 g) bottles.

Compendium Code No.: 10580831 Iss. 0998

PROIN™ 50 CHEWABLE TABLETS ℞

PRN Pharmacal **Adrenergic**

Active Ingredient(s): Each tablet contains: Phenylpropanolamine HCl 50 mg.

Indications: A supplemental product for urinary incontinence in dogs.

Dosage and Administration: 1 to 2 mg/kg every 12 hours by mouth.

Precaution(s): Store at controlled room temperature.

Caution(s): Federal law restricts this drug to use by or on the order of a licensed veterinarian.

May cause excitability and restlessness.

Warning(s): For animal use only. Keep out of reach of children.

Presentation: 60 tablets.

Manufactured by: Pegasus Laboratories.

Compendium Code No.: 10900150

PROIN™ DROPS ℞

PRN Pharmacal **Adrenergic**

Active Ingredient(s): Contains: 25 mg/mL phenylpropanolamine HCl.

Indications: A supplemental product for urinary incontinence in dogs.

Dosage and Administration: 1 to 2 mg/kg every 12 hours by mouth.

Use as directed by veterinarian. Mix well with canine's food.

Precaution(s): Store at controlled room temperature. Do not refrigerate.

Caution(s): Federal law restricts this drug to use by or on the order of a licensed veterinarian.

May cause excitability and restlessness.

Warning(s): Keep out of reach of children. For animal use only.

Presentation: 2 fl oz.

Manufactured by: Pegasus Laboratories.

Compendium Code No.: 10900160

PROLATE®/LINTOX®-HD

Wellmark **Topical Insecticide**

Insecticidal spray and backrubber for livestock with phosmet

EPA Reg. No.: 2724-262

Active Ingredient(s):

Phosmet (CAS #732-11-6) 11.75%
Other Ingredients*: 88.25%
Total 100.00%

* Contains petroleum distillates.

Contains 1 lb active ingredient per gallon.

Indications: For the control of horn flies, lice, mange, and ticks on cattle.

For the control of lice and mange on swine.

Directions for Use: It is a violation of Federal Law to use this product in a manner inconsistent with its labeling.

Stir thoroughly. Apply fresh mixture as high pressure spray, taking care to wet skin, not just hair. Apply to point of run-off.

P

Dilute as shown in tables below:

Beef and Non-Lactating Dairy Cattle Spray:

To Control	Dilution Rate: One gallon of product in gallons of water:	One quart of product in gallons of water:
Cattle Ticks, Southern Cattle Ticks	240	60
Horn Flies	200	50
Lice	150	38
Sarcoptic Mange Winter Ticks, Lone Star Ticks, Gulf Coast Ear Ticks	100	25

Cattle Backrubber:

	Dilution Rate
To Control Horn Flies	One gallon of product in 50 gallons of fuel oil or other suitable carrier
Charge backrubber device or soak sack or cloth, as required. Retreat backrubber as needed.	

Swine Spray:

	Dilution Rate	
To Control Lice, Sarcoptic Mange	One gallon of product in 100 gallons of water	One quart of product in 25 gallons of water

In cattle, repeat treatment as necessary, but not more often than every 7 to 10 days. Treatment for lice, ticks, sarcoptic mange, and horn flies may be made any time of the year except when cattle grub larvae are in the gullet or spinal canal. Consult your veterinarian, extension live stock specialist, or extension entomologist regarding timing of treatment.

Contraindication(s): Cattle:

PROLATE®/LINTOX®-HD is a cholinesterase inhibitor. Do not use this product on animals simultaneously or within a few days before or after treatment with or exposure to cholinesterase inhibiting drugs, pesticides, or chemicals. Atropine is antidotal. Consult veterinarian at first sign of adverse reaction.

Do not treat sick, convalescent, stressed, or animals less than 3 months old.

Swine:

PROLATE®/LINTOX®-HD is a cholinesterase inhibitor. Do not use this product on animals simultaneously or within a few days before or after treatment with or exposure to cholinesterase inhibiting drugs, pesticides, or chemicals. Atropine is antidotal. Consult veterinarian at first sign of adverse reaction.

Do not treat sick, convalescent, or stressed animals. Do not apply directly to suckling pigs.

In swine, single applications for lice and sarcoptic mange control are usually effective; however, should a second application be necessary, it may be made 14 days following first treatment.

Precautionary Statements: Hazards to Humans and Domestic Animals:

Danger: Corrosive. Causes irreversible eye damage. May be fatal if swallowed. Harmful if absorbed through skin. Causes eye and skin irritation. Do not get in eyes, on skin, or on clothing. Wash thoroughly with soap and water after handling. Avoid breathing spray mist. Applicators must wear protective eyeware (goggles, face shield, or safety glasses), long-sleeved shirt, long pants, elbow length waterproof gloves, waterproof apron, and unlined waterproof boots. Remove contaminated clothing and wash clothing before reuse.

First Aid:

If in Eyes: Hold eyelids open and flush with a steady gentle stream of water for 15 minutes. Get medical attention.

If Swallowed: Call a physician or Poison Control Center immediately. Do not induce vomiting. Do not give anything by mouth to an unconscious person. Avoid alcohol.

If on Skin: Remove contaminated clothing. Wash promptly with plenty of soap and water.

If Spray Mist is Inhaled: Remove individual to fresh air. Apply artificial respiration, if indicated.

Note to Physician/Veterinarian: Probable mucosal damage may contraindicate the use of gastric lavage. PROLATE®/LINTOX®-HD is an organophosphate insecticide and a cholinesterase inhibitor. If signs of cholinesterase inhibition are present, atropine is antidotal. 2-PAM is also antidotal and may be administered in conjunction with atropine. If ingested, do not induce vomiting. May present aspiration hazard. Usual symptoms of organophosphate poisoning in humans include: headache, blurred vision, weakness, nausea, discomfort in the chest, vomiting, abdominal cramps, diarrhea, salivation, sweating, pin-point pupils. Usual symptoms of poisoning in animals include: salivation, labored breathing, gastrointestinal disturbance, tremors, staggering, and pin-point pupils.

Environmental Hazards: This pesticide is extremely toxic to fish. Do not apply directly to water, or to areas where surface water is present, or to intertidal areas below the mean high water mark. Do not contaminate water by cleaning of equipment or disposal of equipment washwaters. Drift or runoff from treated areas may be hazardous to aquatic organisms in neighboring areas.

Physical or Chemical Hazards: Do not use or store near heat or open flame. Protect from temperatures below 20°F.

Storage and Disposal: Do not contaminate water, food, or feed by storage or disposal.

Pesticide Disposal: Pesticide wastes are acutely hazardous. Improper disposal of excess pesticide, spray mixture, or rinsate is a violation of Federal Law. If these wastes cannot be disposed of by use according to label instructions, contact your State Pesticide or Environmental Control Agency or the Hazardous Waste Representative at the nearest EPA Regional Office for guidance.

Container Disposal: Triple rinse (or equivalent). Then offer for recycling or reconditioning, or puncture and dispose of in a sanitary landfill, or by other procedures approved by state and local authorities.

Warning(s): Cattle may be slaughtered 3 days after a treatment.

Do not treat non-lactating dairy cattle within 28 days of freshening. If freshening should occur within the 28 day period after treatment, that milk must not be used as human food.

Swine may be slaughtered one day after treatment.

Keep out of reach of children.

Disclaimer: Seller makes no warranty, express or implied, concerning the use of this product other than indicated on the label. Buyer assumes all risk of use and handling of this material when such use and handling are contrary to label instructions.

Presentation: 32 oz and 1 gallon.

PROLATE® is a registered trademark of Zeneca Ag Products.

LINTOX-HD® is a registered trademark of Wellmark International.

Compendium Code No.: 10930021

PROLYME®

Intervet **Bacterial Extract**

Borrelia Burgdorferi Bacterial Extract Subunit

U.S. Vet. Lic. No.: 286

Contents: PROLYME® is a purified extract of *Borrelia burgdorferi* comprised of outer surface protein A (OspA) and is adjuvanted to elicit a maximal immune response. This OspA antigen induces protection against disease caused by *B. burgdorferi* infection.

Indications: PROLYME® is for the vaccination of healthy puppies and dogs to prevent disease caused by *B. burgdorferi* infection. Vaccination with PROLYME® is highly effective in reducing the transmission of infective *B. burgdorferi* from the tick to the dog.

Dosage and Administration: Aseptically administer 1 mL by the subcutaneous route. Vaccinate healthy dogs 4 weeks of age or older with two doses 3-4 weeks apart. Annual revaccination with a single dose is recommended.

Precaution(s): Recommended storage temperature 35-45°F (2-7°C). Do not freeze. Shake well before use. Non-chemically sterilized needles and syringes should be used for administration of vaccine.

Caution(s): Administration of epinephrine may be indicated in the event of an anaphylactic reaction. Only healthy animals should be vaccinated. Animals incubating any disease, or animals stressed due to shipping, malnutrition or parasitism may not achieve or maintain an adequate immune response. This product is not hazardous when used according to directions supplied. A material safety data sheet (MSDS) is available upon request. This and any other consumer information can be obtained by calling Intervet's Customer Service Department at 1-800-441-8272.

For use in dogs only.

Discussion: *B. burgdorferi* is the causative agent of Lyme borreliosis or "Lyme disease." Initially recognized as a cause of arthritis in humans, *B. burgdorferi* has also been demonstrated to induce clinical disease in dogs. The most common clinical signs of canine borreliosis are fever, lameness and joint pain. Transmission occurs primarily through hard-shelled ticks, such as those in the genus *Ixodes*. Vaccination with an OspA vaccine is effective in preventing *B. burgdorferi* infection, in addition to preventing clinical signs.[1] It appears that OspA vaccinates induce an immune response that takes effect within the tick vector, thereby preventing *B. burgdorferi* from even entering the host.[1] Also, use of OspA vaccines has been preferred because of the potential risk of immune-mediated reactions arising from the use of whole cell bacterins.[1,2,3]

Trial Data: Safety Data: PROLYME® may be safely administered to healthy dogs or puppies as young as 4 weeks of age. Safety studies using multiple vaccinations did not induce any adverse effects regardless of *Borrelia* serological status.

Efficacy Data: PROLYME® has been demonstrated in natural tick challenge studies one year post-vaccination to protect against disease caused by *B. burgdorferi* infection and clinical signs, such as lameness, fever, depression, decreased appetite and lymphadenopathy. Furthermore, no clinical signs were observed in these dogs during the six month observation period after the one year post-vaccination challenge. Studies have shown that vaccination with PROLYME® is highly effective in reducing the transmission of infective *B. burgdorferi* from the tick to the dog. PROLYME® has also been demonstrated to induce borreliacidal (neutralizing) antibodies against *B. burgdorferi* isolates obtained from various endemic geographic regions of the U.S.

References: Available upon request.

Presentation: Cartons of 50-1 dose (1 mL) vaccine vials and cartons of 5-10 dose (10 mL) vaccine vials.

Compendium Code No.: 11061430

PROMACE® ℞

Fort Dodge **Tranquilizer**

(acepromazine maleate injectable and tablets, USP)

NADA No.: 015-030 (Injection)/032-702 (Tablets)

Active Ingredient(s): Each mL contains 10 mg PROMACE® (acepromazine maleate, USP). (Also contains sodium citrate 0.36%, citric acid 0.075%, benzyl alcohol 1% and Water for Injection, USP).

Each light orange tablet contains 5 mg of PROMACE® (acepromazine maleate, USP).

Each orange tablet contains 10 mg of PROMACE®.

Each yellow tablet contains 25 mg of PROMACE®.

Indications:

Dogs and Cats: PROMACE® Injectable and Tablets can be used as an aid in controlling intractable animals during examination, treatment, grooming, x-ray and minor surgical procedures; to alleviate itching as a result of skin irritation; as an antiemetic to control vomiting associated with motion sickness.

PROMACE® Injectable is particularly useful as a preanesthetic agent (1) to enhance and prolong the effects of barbiturates, thus reducing the requirements for general anesthesia; (2) as an adjunct to surgery under local anesthesia.

Horses: PROMACE® Injectable can be used as an aid in controlling fractious animals during examination, treatment, loading and transportation. Particularly useful when used in conjunction with local anesthesia for firing, castration, neurectomy, removal of skin tumors, ocular surgery and applying casts.

Pharmacology:

Description: PROMACE® (acepromazine maleate, USP), a potent neuroleptic agent with a low order of toxicity, is of particular value in the tranquilization of dogs, cats and horses. Its rapid action and lack of hypnotic effect are added advantages. According to Baker,[1] the scope of possible applications for this compound in veterinary practice is only limited by the imagination of the practitioner.

Chemistry: Acepromazine [10-[3-(dimethylamino) propyl] phenothiazin-2-yl-methyl ketone] Maleate, USP has the following chemical structure:

S; N; $COCH_3$; $CH_2–CH_2–CH_2–N(CH_3)_2$ • CH–C(=O)–OH ‖ CH–C(=O)–OH

Actions: PROMACE® has a depressant effect on the central nervous system and, therefore, causes sedation, muscular relaxation and a reduction in spontaneous activity. It acts rapidly, exerting a prompt and pronounced calming effect.

Dosage and Administration: The dosage should be individualized, depending upon the degree of tranquilization required. As a general rule, the dosage requirement in mg/lb of body weight decreases as the weight of the animal increases.

PROMACE® Injectable (acepromazine maleate injection, USP):

May be given intravenously, intramuscularly or subcutaneously. The following schedule may be used as a guide to IV, IM or SC injections:

Dogs: 0.25-0.5 mg/lb of body weight

Cats: 0.5-1 mg/lb of body weight

Horses: 2-4 mg/100 lb of body weight

IV doses should be administered slowly, and a period of at least 15 minutes should be allowed for the drug to take full effect.

PROMACE® Tablets (acepromazine maleate tablets, USP):

Dogs: 0.25-1 mg/lb of body weight. Dosage may be repeated as required.

Cats: 0.5-1 mg/lb of body weight. Dosage may be repeated as required.

Contraindication(s): Phenothiazines may potentiate the toxicity of organophosphates and the activity of procaine hydrochloride. Therefore, do not use PROMACE® (acepromazine maleate) to control tremors associated with organic phosphate poisoning. Do not use in conjunction with organophosphorus vermifuges or ectoparasiticides, including flea collars. Do not use with procaine hydrochloride.

Precaution(s): Store at controlled room temperature 15° to 30°C (59° to 86°F).

Caution(s): Federal law restricts this drug to use by or on the order of a licensed veterinarian.

Tranquilizers are potent central nervous system depressants and they can cause marked sedation with suppression of the sympathetic nervous system.

Tranquilizers can produce prolonged depression or motor restlessness when given in excessive amounts or when given to sensitive animals.

Tranquilizers are additive in action to the actions of other depressants and will potentiate general anesthesia. Tranquilizers should be administered in smaller doses and with greater care during general anesthesia and also to animals exhibiting symptoms of stress, debilitation, cardiac disease, sympathetic blockade, hypovolemia or shock. PROMACE®, like other phenothiazine derivatives, is detoxified in the liver; therefore, it should be used with caution in animals with a previous history of liver dysfunction or leukopenia.

Hypotension can occur after rapid intravenous injection causing cardiovascular collapse.

Epinephrine is contraindicated for treatment of acute hypotension produced by phenothiazine-derivative tranquilizers since further depression of blood pressure can occur. Other pressor amines, such as norepinephrine or phenylephrine, are the drugs of choice.

In horses, paralysis of the retractor penis muscle has been associated with the use of phenothiazine-derivative tranquilizers. Such cases have occurred following the use of PROMACE®. This risk should be duly considered prior to the administration of PROMACE® to male horses (castrated and uncastrated). When given, the dosage should be carefully limited to the minimum necessary for the desired effect. At the time of tranquilization, it is not possible to differentiate between reversible protrusion of the penis (a normal clinical sign of narcosis) and the irreversible paralysis of the retractor muscle. The cause of this side reaction has not been determined. It has been postulated that such paralysis may occur when a tranquilizer is used in conjunction with testosterone (or in stallions).

Accidental intracarotid injection in horses can produce clinical signs ranging from disorientation to convulsive seizures and death.

A few rare but serious occurrences of idiosyncratic reactions to Acepromazine may occur in dogs following oral or parenteral administration. These potentially serious adverse reactions include behavioral disorders in dogs such as aggression, biting/chewing, and nervousness.

Warning(s): Not for use in animals intended for food.

Toxicology: Acute and chronic toxicity studies have shown a very low order of toxicity.

Acute toxicity: The LD_{50} dose of PROMACE® in mice was determined by means of a probit transformation with the following results:[2]

Intravenous route — 61.37 mg/kg

Oral route — 256.8 mg/kg

Subcutaneous route — 130.5 mg/kg

Chronic toxicity: Tests[3] in rats revealed no deleterious effects on renal or hepatic function or on hemopoietic activity. In several groups of two male and two female beagle hounds treated for six months with daily oral doses of 20 to 40 mg/kg, no untoward effects were encountered. Hematologic studies and urinalysis gave values within normal limits. Another group of four dogs, given gradually increasing oral doses up to a level of 220 mg/kg daily and reaching a total daily dose of 2.2 g per dog, showed some signs of pulmonary edema and hyperemia of the internal organs, but no animal died.

When administered intramuscularly, PROMACE® causes a brief sensation of stinging comparable with that observed with other phenothiazine tranquilizers.

Trial Data: Clinical Data: Controlled clinical studies in the United States and Canada have demonstrated the effectiveness and safety of PROMACE® as a tranquilizer.

Good to excellent results were reported[1,4,5] in dogs, cats and horses given PROMACE® Injectable for restraint during examination, treatment and minor surgery and for preanesthetic sedation. In dogs, the drug reportedly[4] helps control convulsions associated with distemper.

In both dogs and cats, good to excellent results were obtained[4] when PROMACE® Tablets were used to control nervousness, excessive vocalization, neurotic and excitable behavior, vomiting associated with motion sickness, coughing and itching caused by dermatitis.

In horses, Bauman[6] had good results using the drug as an aid in the control of painful spasms due to colic.

Other practitioners[7,8] found the drug useful as a preanesthetic sedative for nervous or aggressive horses, but it had to be administered while the animals were quiet and not in an excited state. In a trial[9] on more than 200 horses with a wide variety of disorders, PROMACE® Injectable proved to be both effective and safe.

References: Available upon request.

Presentation: NDC 0856-3020-01 — 10 mg/mL — 50 mL vial
NDC 0856-0040-01 — 5 mg — bottles of 100
NDC 0856-0070-01 — 10 mg — bottles of 100
NDC 0856-0070-02 — 10 mg — bottles of 500
NDC 0856-0100-01 — 25 mg — bottles of 100
NDC 0856-0100-02 — 25 mg — bottles of 500

Manufactured by: Fort Dodge Animal Health, Fort Dodge, Iowa 50501 USA (Injection); Ayerst Laboratories, Inc., Rouses Point, NY 12979 (Tablets)

Compendium Code No.: 10031661 1000G

PROMECTIN B™ POUR-ON

Vedco **Parasiticide-Topical**

(ivermectin) Pour-On for Cattle

ANADA No.: 200-219

Active Ingredient(s): Contains 5 mg ivermectin/mL.

Indications: PROMECTIN B™ (ivermectin) Pour-On applied at the recommended dose level of 500 mcg/kg is indicated for the effective control of these parasites:

Gastrointestinal Roundworms: *Ostertagia ostertagi* (including inhibited stage) (adults and L_4), *Haemonchus placei* (adults and L_4), *Trichostrongylus axei* (adults and L_4), *T. colubriformis* (adults and L_4), *Cooperia* spp (adults and L_4), *Strongyloides papillosus* (adults), *Oesophagostomum radiatum* (adults and L_4), *Trichuris* spp (adults).

Lungworms: *Dictyocaulus viviparus* (adults and L_4).

Cattle Grubs (parasitic stages): *Hypoderma bovis, H. lineatum.*

Mites: *Sarcoptes scabiei var. bovis.*

Lice: *Linognathus vituli, Haematopinus eurysternus, Damalinia bovis, Solenopotes capillatus.*

Horn Flies: *Haematobia irritans.*

Pharmacology: Mode of Action: Ivermectin as a member of the avermectin family kills certain parasitic roundworms and ectoparasites, such as mites, lice, horn flies and other insects. Its action is unique to the avermectin class of antiparasitic agents. This action involves a chemical that serves as a signal from one nerve cell to another, or from a nerve cell to a muscle cell. This chemical, a neurotransmitter, is called gamma-aminobutyric acid or GABA.

In roundworms, ivermectin stimulates the release of GABA from nerve endings and enhances binding of GABA to special receptors at nerve junctions, thus interrupting nerve impulses — thereby paralyzing and killing the parasite.

The enhancement of the GABA effect in arthropods such as mites, lice, and horn flies resembles that in roundworms except that nerve impulses are interrupted between the nerve ending and the muscle cell. Again, this leads to paralysis and death.

Ivermectin has no measurable effect against flukes or tapeworms, presumably because they do not have GABA as a nerve impulse transmitter.

The principal peripheral neurotransmitter in mammals, acetylcholine, is unaffected by ivermectin. Ivermectin does not readily penetrate the central nervous system of mammals where GABA functions as a neurotransmitter.

Dosage and Administration:

Treatment for Cattle for Horn Flies: PROMECTIN B™ (ivermectin) Pour-On controls horn flies *(Haematobia irritans)* for up to 28 days after dosing. For best results, PROMECTIN B™ (ivermectin) Pour-On should be part of a parasite control program for both internal and external parasites based on the epidemiology of these parasites. Consult a veterinarian or an entomologist for the most effective timing of applications.

Dosage: The dose rate is 1 mL for each 22 lb of body weight. The formulation should be applied along the topline in a narrow strip extending from the withers to the tailhead.

Administration:

Dispensing Cap (250 mL, 500 mL and 1 L bottles): The enclosed dispensing cap is graduated in 5 mL increments. Each 5 mL will treat 110 lbs body weight. When body weight is between markings, use the next higher increment.

Attach the dispensing cap to the bottle.

Select the correct dose rate by rotating the adjuster top in either direction to position the dose indicator to the appropriate level.

Hold the bottle upright and gently squeeze it to deliver a slight excess of the required dose as indicated by the calibration lines.

By releasing the pressure, the dose automatically adjusts to the correct level. Tilt the bottle to deliver the dose. The off (stop) position will close the system between dosing.

Applicator Gun* (3.785 L bottle, 5 L backpack and 25 L carboy): Because of the solvents used in PROMECTIN B™ (ivermectin) Pour-On, only the PROMECTIN B ™ (ivermectin) applicator gun from Simcro Tech Limited, or equivalent, is recommended. Other applicators may exhibit compatibility problems, resulting in locking, incorrect dosage or leakage.

Remove the draw-off cap and backpack strap from the indentation in the back of the bottle and refer to the diagram to fit the strap to the bottle.

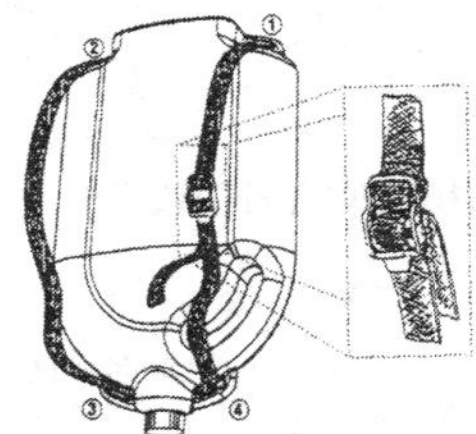

Thread the strap through the bottle eyelet number 1, then 2, 3, and 4, taking care to follow the diagram when connecting the strap to the buckle.

The strap is adjustable by lifting the tab on the buckle.

Slide one of the coil springs over one end of the draw-off tubing. Attach that end of the draw-off tubing to the stem on the applicator gun and slide the spring up to the connection. Slide the second coil spring over the other end of the draw-off tubing and connect that end to the cap that has the stem. Slide the spring to the connection. Replace the shipping cap with the cap having the draw-off tubing attached. Tighten this draw-off cap to the bottle. Invert the bottle and use as a backpack (for 5 L backpack).

Follow the applicator gun manufacturer's directions for priming the gun, adjusting the dose, and care of the applicator gun following use.

Weight	Dose
220 lb (100 kg)	10 mL
330 lb (150 kg)	15 mL
440 lb (200 kg)	20 mL
550 lb (250 kg)	25 mL
660 lb (300 kg)	30 mL
770 lb (350 kg)	35 mL
880 lb (400 kg)	40 mL
990 lb (450 kg)	45 mL
1100 lb (500 kg)	50 mL

P

*Additional Applicator Guns and Draw Tubes may be purchased from your local retail dealer or through Phoenix Scientific, Inc.

When to Treat Cattle with Grubs: PROMECTIN B™ (ivermectin) Pour-On effectively controls all stages of cattle grubs. However, proper timing of treatment is important. For the most effective results, cattle should be treated as soon as possible after the end of the heel fly (warble fly) season. While this is not peculiar to ivermectin, destruction of *Hypoderma* larvae (cattle grubs) at the period when these grubs are in vital areas may cause undesirable host-parasite reactions. Killing *Hypoderma lineatum* when it is in the esophageal tissues may cause bloat; killing *H. bovis* when it is in the vertebral canal may cause staggering or paralysis. Cattle should be treated either before or after these stages of grub development.

Cattle treated with PROMECTIN B™ (ivermectin) Pour-On at the end of the fly season may be re-treated with PROMECTIN B™ (ivermectin) during the winter without danger of grub-related reactions. For further information and advice on a planned parasite control program, consult a veterinarian.

Consult a veterinarian for assistance in the diagnosis, treatment and control of parasitism.

Precaution(s): Flammable! Keep away from heat, sparks, open flame, and other sources of ignition.

Store between 15°-30°C (59°-86°F).

Store away from excessive heat (104°F/40°C) and protect from light.

Use only in well-ventilated areas or outdoors.

Close container tightly when not in use.

Cloudiness in the formulation may occur when PROMECTIN B™ (ivermectin) Pour-On is stored at temperatures below 32°F. Allowing to warm at room temperature will restore the normal appearance without affecting efficacy.

Environmental Safety: Studies indicate that when ivermectin comes in contact with the soil, it readily and tightly binds to the soil and becomes inactive over time. Free ivermectin may adversely affect fish or certain water-borne organisms on which they feed. Do not permit cattle to enter lakes, streams or ponds for at least six hours after treatment. Do not contaminate water by direct application or by the improper disposal of drug containers. Dispose of containers in an approved landfill or by incineration.

Caution(s): Cattle should not be treated when hair or hide is wet since reduced efficacy may be experienced.

Do not use when rain is expected to wet cattle within six hours after treatment.

This product is for application to skin surface only. Do not give orally or parenterally.

Antiparasitic activity of ivermectin will be impaired if the formulation is applied to areas of the skin with mange scabs or lesions, or with dermatoses or adherent materials, e.g., caked mud or manure.

Ivermectin has been associated with adverse reactions in sensitive dogs; therefore, PROMECTIN B™ (ivermectin) Pour-On is not recommended for use in species other than cattle.

This product should not be applied to self or others because it may be irritating to human skin and eyes and absorbed through the skin. To minimize accidental skin contact, the user should wear a long-sleeved shirt and rubber gloves. If accidental skin contact occurs, wash immediately with soap and water. If accidental eye exposure occurs, flush eyes immediately with water and seek medical attention.

Warning(s): Residue Warning: Cattle must not be treated within 48 days of slaughter for human consumption. Because a withdrawal time in milk has not been established, do not use on female dairy cattle of breeding age.

Not for use in humans.

Keep this and all drugs out of the reach of children.

Toxicology: Safety: Studies conducted in the U.S.A. have demonstrated the safety margin for ivermectin. Based on plasma levels, the topically applied formulation is expected to be at least as well tolerated by breeding animals as is the subcutaneous formulation which had no effect on breeding performance.

Discussion: PROMECTIN B™ (ivermectin) Pour-On delivers internal and external parasite control in one convenient low-volume application. Ivermectin is a potent antiparasitic agent whose chemical structure is different from those of other antiparasitic agents.

Presentation: PROMECTIN B™ (ivermectin) Pour-On is available in a 250 mL (8.5 fl oz) bottle (NDC 50989-487-25), a 500 mL (16.9 fl oz) bottle (NDC 50989-487-16), a 1 L (33.8 fl oz) bottle for use with the dispensing cap provided (NDC 50989-487-12), or in a 3.785 L (1 gal) bottle (NDC 50989-487-29), a 5 L (169 fl oz) backpack (NDC 50989-487-32) or a 25 L carboy (NDC 50989-487-59) for use with the appropriate automatic dosing applicator.

Manufactured by: Phoenix Scientific, Inc., St. Joseph, MO 64503.

Compendium Code No.: 10942270 Rev. 7-00 / Rev. 7-00 / Iss. 8-98 / Rev. 7-99 / Iss. 10-99 / Iss. 4-00

P

PROMECTIN E™ LIQUID FOR HORSES ℞

Vedco **Parasiticide-Oral**

(ivermectin) 10 mg/mL

ANADA No.: 200-202

Active Ingredient(s): PROMECTIN E ™ (ivermectin) Liquid is a clear, ready-to-use solution with each mL containing 1% ivermectin (10 mg), 0.2 mL propylene glycol, 80 mg polysorbate 80, 9 mg sodium phosphate monobasic monohydrate, 1.3 mg sodium phosphate dibasic anhydrous, 1 mg butylated hydroxytoluene, 0.1 mg disodium edetate, 3% benzyl alcohol and water for injection q.s. ad 100%.

Indications: PROMECTIN E™ Liquid is indicated for the effective treatment and control of the following parasites or parasitic conditions in horses:

Large Strongyles: *Strongylus vulgaris* (adults and arterial larval stages), *S. edentatus* (adults and tissue stages), *S. equinus* (adults), *Triodontophorus* spp (adults).

Small Strongyles - including those resistant to some benzimidazole class compounds (adults and fourth-stage larvae): *Cyathostomum* spp, *Cylicocyclus* spp, *Cylicostephanus* spp, *Cylicodontophorus* spp.

Pinworms (adults and fourth-stage larvae): *Oxyuris equi.*

Ascarids (adults and third- and fourth-stage larvae): *Parascaris equorum.*

Hairworms (adults): *Trichostrongylus axei.*

Large-mouth Stomach Worms (adults): *Habronema muscae.*

Bots (oral and gastric stages): *Gasterophilus* spp.

Lungworms (adults and fourth-stage larvae): *Dictyocaulus arnfieldi.*

Intestinal Threadworms (adults): *Strongyloides westeri.*

Summer Sores caused by *Habronema* and *Draschia* spp cutaneous third-stage larvae.

Dermatitis caused by neck thread-worm microfilariae, *Onchocerca* sp.

Pharmacology: Product Description: Ivermectin is derived from the avermectins, a family of potent, broad-spectrum antiparasitic agents, which are isolated from fermentation of *Streptomyces avermitilis.*

Mode of Action: Ivermectin, one of the avermectins, kills certain parasitic roundworms and ectoparasites such as mites and lice. The avermectins are different in their action from other antiparasitic agents. This action involves a chemical that serves as a signal from one nerve cell to another, or from a nerve cell to a muscle cell. This chemical, a neurotransmitter, is called gamma-aminobutyric acid or GABA.

In roundworms, ivermectin stimulates the release of GABA from nerve endings and enhances binding of GABA to special receptors at nerve junctions, thus interrupting nerve impulses - thereby paralyzing and killing the parasite.

The enhancement of the GABA effect in arthropods such as mites and lice resembles that in roundworms except that nerve impulses are interrupted between the nerve ending and the muscle cell. Again, this leads to paralysis and death.

The principal peripheral neurotransmitter in mammals, acetylcholine, is unaffected by ivermectin. Ivermectin does not readily penetrate the central nervous system of mammals where GABA functions as a neurotransmitter.

Dosage and Administration: Dosage: PROMECTIN E™ (ivermectin) Liquid for Horses is formulated for administration by stomach tube (nasogastric intubation) or as an oral drench. The recommended dose is 200 mcg of ivermectin per kilogram (91 mcg/lb) of body weight. Each mL contains sufficient ivermectin to treat 110 lb (50 kg) of body weight: 10 mL will treat an 1100 lb (500 kg) horse.

Administration: Use a calibrated dosing syringe inserted into the bottle to measure the appropriate dose, or pour the PROMECTIN E™ (ivermectin) Liquid into a graduated cylinder for dose measurement. Use a clean syringe if accessing the bottle to avoid contaminating the remaining product.

Administration by stomach tube (gravity or positive flow): The recommended dose can be used undiluted or diluted up to 40 times with clean tepid water (see Notes to Veterinarian). Use tepid water to flush any drug remaining in the tube into the horse's stomach.

Administration by drench: For administration by this method, an undiluted dose is usually preferred. Clear the horse's mouth of any food material, elevate the horse's head, and using a syringe, deposit the appropriate dose in the back of the mouth. In order to avoid unnecessary coughing or the potential for material to enter the trachea and lungs, do not use excessive pressure (squirting), do not use a large (diluted) dose volume, and do not deposit the dose in the laryngeal area. Increased dose rejection may occur if the dose is deposited in the buccal space. Keep the horse's head elevated and observe the horse to insure the dose is retained.

Suggested Parasite Control Program: All horses should be included in a regular parasite control program with particular attention being paid to mares, foals and yearlings. Foals should be treated initially at 6 to 8 weeks of age, and routine treatment repeated as appropriate. PROMECTIN E™ (ivermectin) effectively controls gastrointestinal nematodes and bots in horses. Regular treatment will reduce the chances of verminous arteritis and colic caused by *S. vulgaris.* With its broad spectrum, PROMECTIN E™ (ivermectin) is well suited to be the major product in a parasite control program.

Precaution(s): Store in a tightly closed container at room temperature.

Protect PROMECTIN E™ (ivermectin) Liquid (undiluted or diluted) from light.

Environmental Safety: Studies indicate that when ivermectin comes in contact with the soil, it readily and tightly binds to the soil and becomes inactive over time. Free ivermectin may adversely affect fish and certain water-borne organisms on which they feed. Do not contaminate lakes, streams, or ground water by direct application or by improper disposal of drug containers. Dispose of drug container in an approved landfill or by incineration.

Caution(s): Federal (U.S.A.) law restricts this drug to use by or on the order of a licensed veterinarian.

Notes to Veterinarian: Swelling and itching reactions after treatment with PROMECTIN E™ (ivermectin) have occurred in horses carrying heavy infections of neck threadworm microfilariae, *Onchocerca* sp. These reactions were most likely the result of microfilariae dying in large numbers. Symptomatic treatment may be advisable.

Healing of summer sores involving extensive tissue changes may require other therapy in conjunction with PROMECTIN E™ (ivermectin). Reinfection, and measures for its prevention, should also be considered.

Special consideration should be given to the effects or potential for injury from handling, restraint, and placement of the tube during administration by stomach tube. PROMECTIN E™ (ivermectin) Liquid should be administered by drench if the risks associated with tubing are of concern. Due to the consequences of improper administration (also see Dosage and Administration), PROMECTIN E™ (ivermectin) Liquid is intended for use by a veterinarian only and is not recommended for dispensing.

PROMECTIN E™ (ivermectin) Liquid in 1 to 20 and 1 to 40 dilutions with tap water has been shown to be stable for 72 hours under the conditions recommended for the product (i.e., at room temperature, in a tightly closed container, protected from light). The diluted product does not promote the growth of common organisms. However, prolonged storage of the diluted product cannot be recommended, as the effects of possible contaminants and interactions with untested materials are unknown.

PROMECTIN E™ (ivermectin) Liquid has been formulated specifically for use in horses only. This product should not be used in other animal species as severe adverse reactions, including fatalities in dogs, may result.

Refrain from smoking and eating when handling. Wash hands after use. Avoid contact with eyes.

For veterinary use only.

Warning(s): Residue Warning: Do not use in horses intended for food purposes.

Keep this and all drugs out of the reach of children.

Toxicology: Safety: PROMECTIN E™ (ivermectin) Liquid may be used in horses of all ages including mares at any stage of pregnancy. Stallions may be treated without adversely affecting their fertility. These horses have been treated with no adverse effects other than those noted under Notes to Veterinarian.

Discussion: PROMECTIN E™ (ivermectin) Liquid for Horses has been formulated for professional administration by stomach tube or oral drench. One low-volume dose is effective against important internal parasites, including the arterial stages of *Strongylus vulgaris,* and bots.

Ivermectin is a potent antiparasitic agent whose chemical structure is different from those of other antiparasitic agents. Its convenience, broad-spectrum efficiency and safety margin make PROMECTIN E™ (ivermectin) Liquid an ideal parasite control product for horses.

Presentation: PROMECTIN E™ (ivermectin) Liquid for Horses is available in a 100 mL (NDC 50989-4884-12) or 200 mL (NDC 50989-484-34) plastic bottle. The 100 mL bottle contains sufficient ivermectin to treat 10-500 kg (1100 lb) horses. The 200 mL bottle contains sufficient ivermectin to treat 20-500 kg (1100 lb) horses. Contents may be poured into a graduated cylinder for dose measurement. Alternatively, a clean syringe may be inserted directly into the bottle to draw off the appropriate dose.

Manufactured by: Phoenix Scientific, Inc., St. Joseph, MO 64503.

Compendium Code No.: 10942280 Iss. 6-98 / Rev. 6-00

PROMECTIN E™ PASTE

Vedco **Parasiticide-Oral**

(ivermectin Paste 1.87%) Anthelmintic & Boticide

ANADA No.: 200-286

Active Ingredient(s):

Ivermectin 1.87%

Indications: Consult a veterinarian for assistance in the diagnosis, treatment, and control of parasitism. PROMECTIN E™ (ivermectin) Paste provides effective control of the following parasites in horses:

Large Strongyles (adults) - *Strongylus vulgaris* (also early forms in blood vessels), *S. edentatus* (also tissue stages), *S. equinus, Triodontophorus* spp.; Small Strongyles including those resistant to some benzimidazole class compounds (adults and fourth-stage larvae) - *Cyathostomum* spp, *Cylicocyclus* spp, *Cylicostephanus* spp, *Cylicodontophorus* spp; Pinworms (adults and fourth-stage larvae) - *Oxyuris equi*; Ascarids (adults and third- and fourth-stage larvae) - *Parascaris equorum;* Hairworms (adults) *Trichostrongylus axei;* Large-mouth Stomach Worms (adults) - *Habronema muscae;* Bots (oral and gastric stages) - *Gastrophilus* spp; Lungworms (adults and fourth-stage larvae) - *Dictyocaulus arnfieldi;* Intestinal Threadworms (adults) - *Strongyloides westeri;* Summer Sores caused by *Habronema* and *Draschia* spp cutaneous third-stage larvae; Dermatitis caused by neck threadworm microfilariae, *Onchocerca* sp.

Dosage and Administration: The syringe contains sufficient paste to treat one 1250 lb horse at the recommended dose rate of 91 mcg PROMECTIN E™ (ivermectin) per lb (200 mcg/kg) body weight. Each weight marking on the syringe plunger delivers enough paste to treat 250 lb body weight.

(1) While holding plunger, turn the knurled ring on the plunger to the right so the side nearest the barrel is at the prescribed weight marking. (2) Make sure that the horse's mouth contains no feed. (3) Remove the cover from the tip of the syringe. (4) Insert the syringe tip into the horse's mouth at the space between the teeth (5) Depress the plunger as far as it will go, depositing paste on the back of the tongue. (6) Immediately raise the horse's head for a few seconds after dosing.

Parasite Control Program: All horses should be included in a regular parasite control program with particular attention being paid to mares, foals and yearlings. Foals should be treated initially at 6 to 8 weeks of age, and routine treatment repeated as appropriate. Consult a veterinarian for a control program to meet your specific needs. PROMECTIN E™ (ivermectin) Paste effectively controls gastrointestinal nematodes and bots of horses. Regular treatment will reduce the chances of verminous arteritis caused by *S vulgaris*.

Precaution(s): Store at controlled room temperature, 20° to 25°C (68° to 77°F).

Do not contaminate ground or surface water. Dispose of the PROMECTIN E™ (ivermectin) Paste syringe in an approved landfill or by incineration.

Caution(s): PROMECTIN E™ (ivermectin) Paste has been formulated specifically for use in horses only. This product should not be used in other animal species as severe adverse reactions, including fatalities in dogs, may result. Refrain from smoking and eating when handling. Wash hands after use. Avoid contact with eyes. Ivermectin and excreted ivermectin residues may adversely affect aquatic organisms.

Note to User: Swelling and itching reactions after treatment with PROMECTIN E™ (ivermectin) Paste have occurred in horses carrying heavy infections of neck threadworm *(Onchocerca* sp.) microfilariae. These reactions were most likely the result of microfilariae dying in large numbers. Symptomatic treatment may be advisable. Consult a veterinarian should any such reactions occur. Healing of summer sores involving extensive tissue changes may require other appropriate therapy in conjunction with treatment with PROMECTIN E™ (ivermectin) Paste. Reinfection, and measures for its prevention, should also be considered. Consult a veterinarian if the condition does not improve.

For oral use in horses only.

Warning(s): Residue Warning: Do not use in horses intended for food purposes.

Keep this and all drugs out of the reach of children.

Toxicology: Safety - PROMECTIN E™ (ivermectin) Paste may be used in horses of all ages, including mares at any stage of pregnancy. Stallions may be treated without adversely affecting their fertility.

Discussion: Product Advantages: Broad-spectrum Control — PROMECTIN E™ (ivermectin) Paste kills important internal parasites, including bots and the arterial stages of *Strongylus vulgaris*, with a single dose. PROMECTIN E™ (ivermectin) Paste is a potent antiparasitic agent that is neither a benzimidazole nor an organophosphate.

Presentation: 6.08 g (0.21 oz) syringe (NDC 50989-612-14).

Compendium Code No.: 10942290 Iss. 3/00

PROMECTIN™ INJECTION FOR CATTLE AND SWINE

Vedco **Parasiticide Injection**

1% Sterile Solution (ivermectin)

ANADA No.: 200-228

Active Ingredient(s): PROMECTIN™ Injection is a clear, ready-to-use, sterile solution containing 1% ivermectin, 40% glycerol formal, 1.5% benzyl alcohol (preservative), and propylene glycol, q.s. ad 100%. It is formulated to deliver the recommended dose level of 200 mcg ivermectin/kilogram of body weight in cattle when given subcutaneously at the rate of 1 mL/110 lb (50 kg).

In swine, PROMECTIN™ Injection is formulated to deliver the recommended dose level of 300 mcg ivermectin/kilogram body weight when given subcutaneously in the neck at the rate of 1 mL/75 lb (33 kg).

Indications: A parasiticide for the treatment and control of internal and external parasites of cattle and swine.

Cattle: PROMECTIN™ Injection is indicated for the effective treatment and control of the following harmful species of gastrointestinal roundworms, lungworms, grubs, sucking lice, and mange mites in cattle:

Gastrointestinal Roundworms (adults and fourth-stage larvae): *Ostertagia ostertagi* (including inhibited *O. ostertagi*), *O. lyrata, Haemonchus placei, Trichostrongylus axei, T. colubriformis, Cooperia oncophora, C. punctata, C. pectinata, Oesophagostomum radiatum, Bunostomum phlebotomum, Nematodirus helvetianus* (adults only), *N. spathiger* (adults only).

Lungworms (adults and fourth-stage larvae): *Dictyocaulus viviparus*.

Cattle Grubs (parasitic stages): *Hypoderma bovis, H. lineatum*.

Sucking Lice: *Linognathus vituli, Haematopinus eurysternus, Solenopotes capillatus*.

Mites (scabies): *Psoroptes ovis* (syn. *P. communis* var. *bovis*), *Sarcoptes scabiei var. bovis*.

Persistent Activity: PROMECTIN™ Injection has been proved to effectively control infections and to protect cattle from reinfection with *Dictyocaulus viviparus* for 21 days after treatment; *Ostertagia ostertagi* for 21 days after treatment; *Oesophagostomum radiatum, Haemonchus placei, Trichostrongylus axei, Cooperia punctata*, and *Cooperia oncophora* for 14 days after treatment.

Swine: PROMECTIN™ Injection is indicated for the effective treatment and control of the following harmful species of gastrointestinal roundworms, lungworms, lice, and mange mites in swine:

Gastrointestinal Roundworms (adults and fourth-stage larvae): Large roundworm: *Ascaris suum.*

Red stomach worm: *Hyostrongylus rubidus*.

Nodular worm: *Oesophagostomum* spp.

Threadworm: *Strongyloides ransomi* (adults only).

Somatic Roundworm Larvae:

Threadworm: *Strongyloides ransomi* (somatic larvae).

Sows must be treated at least seven days before farrowing to prevent infection in piglets.

Lungworms: *Metastrongylus* spp (adults).

Lice: *Haematopinus suis*.

Mange Mites: *Sarcoptes scabiei* var. *suis*.

Reindeer: For the treatment and control of warbles *(Oedemagena tarandi)* in reindeer (see Special Minor Use section under "Dosage and Administration").

American Bison: For the treatment and control of grubs *(Hypoderma bovis)* in American bison (see Special Minor Use section under "Dosage and Administration").

Pharmacology: Product Description: Ivermectin is derived from the avermectins, a family of potent, broad-spectrum antiparasitic agents isolated from fermentation of *Streptomyces avermitilis*.

Mode of Action: Ivermectin is a member of the macrocyclic lactone class of endectocides which have a unique mode of action. Compounds of the class bind selectively and with high affinity to glutamate-gated chloride ion channels which occur in invertebrate nerve and muscle cells. This leads to an increase in the permeability of the cell membrane to chloride ions with hyperpolarization of the nerve or muscle cell, resulting in paralysis and death of the parasite. Compounds of this class may also interact with other ligand-gated chloride channels, such as those gated by the neurotransmitter gamma-aminobutyric acid (GABA).

The wide margin of safety is attributable to the fact that mammals do not have glutamate-gated chloride channels, the macrocyclic lactones have a low affinity for other mammalian ligand-gated chloride channels and they do not readily cross the blood-brain barrier.

Dosage and Administration: Dosage:

Cattle: PROMECTIN™ Injection should be given only by subcutaneous injection under the loose skin in front of or behind the shoulder at the recommended dose level of 200 mcg ivermectin per kilogram of body weight. Each mL of PROMECTIN™ contains 10 mg of ivermectin, sufficient to treat 110 lb (50 kg) of body weight (maximum 10 mL per injection site).

Body Weight (lb)	Dose (mL)
220	2
330	3
440	4
550	5
660	6
770	7
880	8
990	9
1100	10

Swine: PROMECTIN™ Injection should be given only by subcutaneous injection in the neck of swine at the recommended dose level of 300 mcg of ivermectin per kilogram (2.2 lb) of body weight. Each mL of PROMECTIN™ contains 10 mg of ivermectin, sufficient to treat 75 lb of body weight.

	Body Weight (lb)	Dose (mL)
Growing Pigs	19	1/4
	38	1/2
	75	1
	150	2
Breeding Animals (Sows, Gilts, and Boars)	225	3
	300	4
	375	5
	450	6

Administration:

Cattle: PROMECTIN™ Injection is to be given subcutaneously only, to reduce risk of potentially fatal clostridial infection of the injection site. Animals should be appropriately restrained to achieve the proper route of administration. Use of a 16-gauge ½ to ¾" needle is suggested. Inject under the loose skin in front of or behind the shoulder (see illustration).

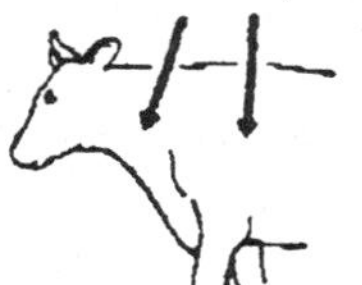

Any single-dose syringe or standard automatic syringe equipment may be used with the 50 mL package size. When using the 200 mL or 500 mL package size, use only automatic syringe equipment.

Use sterile equipment and sanitize the injection site by applying a suitable disinfectant. Clean, properly disinfected needles should be used to reduce the potential for injection site infection. No special handling or protective clothing is necessary.

Swine: PROMECTIN™ (ivermectin) Injection is to be given subcutaneously in the neck. Animals should be appropriately restrained to achieve the proper route of administration. Use of a 16- or

P

18-gauge needle is suggested for sows and boars, while an 18- or 20-gauge needle may be appropriate for young animals. Inject under the skin, immediately behind the ear (see illustration).

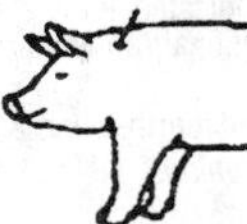

Any single-dose syringe or standard automatic syringe equipment may be used with the 50 mL package size. When using the 200 mL or 500 mL package size, use only automatic syringe equipment. As with any injection, sterile equipment should be used. The injection site should be cleaned and disinfected with alcohol before injection. The rubber stopper should also be disinfected with alcohol to prevent contamination of the contents. Mild and transient pain reactions may be seen in some swine following subcutaneous administration.

Recommended Treatment Program:

Swine: At the time of initiating any parasite control program, it is important to treat all breeding animals in the herd. After the initial treatment, use PROMECTIN™ (ivermectin) Injection regularly as follows:

Breeding Animals:

Sows: Treat prior to farrowing, preferably 7-14 days before, to minimize infection of piglets.

Gilts: Treat 7-14 days prior to breeding. Treat 7-14 days prior to farrowing.

Boars: Frequency and need for treatments are dependent upon exposure. Treat at least two times a year.

Feeder Pigs (Weaners/Growers/Finishers): All weaner/feeder pigs should be treated before placement in clean quarters.

Pigs exposed to contaminated soil or pasture may need retreatment if reinfection occurs.

Note:

1. PROMECTIN™ Injection has a persistent drug level sufficient to control mite infestations throughout the egg to adult life cycle. However, since the ivermectin effect is not immediate, care must be taken to prevent reinfestation from exposure to untreated animals or contaminated facilities. Generally, pigs should not be moved to clean quarters or exposed to uninfested pigs for approximately one week after treatment. Sows should be treated at least one week before farrowing to minimize transfer of mites to newborn baby pigs.
2. Louse eggs are unaffected by PROMECTIN™ Injection and may require up to three weeks to hatch. Louse infestations developing from hatching eggs may require retreatment.
3. Consult a veterinarian for aid in the diagnosis and control of internal and external parasites of swine.

Special Minor Use:

Reindeer: For the treatment and control of warbles *(Oedemagena tarandi)* in reindeer, inject 200 micrograms ivermectin per kilogram of body weight, subcutaneously. Follow use directions for cattle as described under Dosage and Administration.

American Bison: For the treatment and control of grubs *(Hypoderma bovis)* in American Bison, inject 200 micrograms ivermectin per kilogram of body weight, subcutaneously. Follow use directions for cattle as described under Dosage and Administration.

Consult a veterinarian for assistance in the diagnosis, treatment and control of parasitism.

Contraindication(s): PROMECTIN™ Injection for Cattle and Swine has been developed specifically for use in cattle, swine, reindeer and American bison only. This product should not be used in other animal species as severe adverse reactions, including fatalities in dogs, may result.

Precaution(s): Store between 15°C-30°C (59°F-86°F).

Protect product from light.

Use sterile equipment and sanitize the injection site by applying a suitable disinfectant. Clean, properly disinfected needles should be used to reduce the potential for injection site infections.

Environmental Safety: Studies indicate that when ivermectin comes in contact with the soil, it readily and tightly binds to the soil and becomes inactive over time. Free ivermectin may adversely affect fish and certain water-borne organisms on which they feed. Do not permit water runoff from feedlots or production sites to enter lakes, streams, or ponds. Do not contaminate water by direct application or by the improper disposal of drug containers. Dispose of containers in an approved landfill or by incineration.

Caution(s): Transitory discomfort has been observed in some cattle following subcutaneous administration. A low incidence of soft tissue swelling at the injection site has been observed. These reactions have disappeared without treatment. For cattle, divide doses greater than 10 mL between two injection sites to reduce occasional discomfort or site reaction.

Observe cattle for injection site reactions. Reactions may be due to clostridial infection and should be aggressively treated with appropriate antibiotics. If injection site infections are suspected, consult a veterinarian.

This product is not for intravenous or intramuscular use.

Warning(s): Residue Warning: Do not treat cattle within 35 days of slaughter. Because a withdrawal time in milk has not been established, do not use in female dairy cattle of breeding age.

Do not treat swine within 18 days of slaughter.

Do not treat reindeer or American bison within 8 weeks (56 days) of slaughter.

Keep this and all drugs out of the reach of children.

Not for use in humans.

Discussion: PROMECTIN™ (ivermectin) Injection is an injectable parasiticide for cattle and swine. One low-volume dose effectively treats and controls the following internal and external parasites that may impair the health of cattle and swine: gastrointestinal roundworms (including inhibited *Ostertagia ostertagi* in cattle), lungworms, grubs, sucking lice, and mange mites of cattle; and gastrointestinal roundworms, lungworms, lice, and mange mites of swine.

When to Treat Cattle with Grubs: PROMECTIN™ Injection effectively controls all stages of cattle grubs. However, proper timing of treatment is important. For most effective results, cattle should be treated as soon as possible after the end of the heel fly (warble fly) season.

Destruction of *Hypoderma* larvae (cattle grubs) at the period when these grubs are in vital areas may cause undesirable host-parasite reactions including the possibility of fatalities. Killing *Hypoderma lineatum* when it is in the tissue surrounding the esophagus (gullet) may cause salivation and bloat; killing *H. bovis* when it is in the vertebral canal may cause staggering or paralysis. These reactions are not specific to treatment with PROMECTIN™ Injection, but can occur with any successful treatment of grubs. Cattle should be treated either before or after these stages of grub development. Consult a veterinarian concerning the proper time for treatment.

Cattle treated with PROMECTIN™ Injection after the end of the heel fly season may be retreated with PROMECTIN™ Injection during the winter for internal parasites, mange mites, or sucking lice without danger of grub-related reactions. A planned parasite control program is recommended.

Presentation: PROMECTIN™ Injection for Cattle and Swine is available in three ready-to-use sizes:

The 50 mL bottle (NDC 50989-619-11) contains sufficient solution to treat 10 head of 550 lb (250 kg) cattle or 100 head of 38 lb (17.3 kg) swine.

The 200 mL bottle (NDC 50989-615-34) contains sufficient solution to treat 40 head of 550 lb (250 kg) cattle or 400 head of 38 lb (17.3 kg) swine. Use automatic syringe equipment only.

The 500 mL bottle (NDC 50989-615-16) contains sufficient solution to treat 100 head of 550 lb (250 kg) cattle or 1000 head of 38 lb (17.3 kg) swine. Use automatic syringe equipment only.

Manufactured by: Phoenix Scientific, Inc., St. Joseph, MO 64503.

Compendium Code No.: 10942300 Rev. 3-01 / Iss. 01-01 / Iss. 01-01

PROMYCIN™ 100

Phoenix Pharmaceutical **Oxytetracycline Injection**

(Oxytetracycline Hydrochloride Injection) 100 mg/mL-Sterile Antibiotic

ANADA No.: 200-068

Active Ingredient(s): Each mL contains:

Oxytetracycline base (as HCl) .... 100 mg
Magnesium Chloride•$6H_2O$ .... 5.76% w/v
Water for Injection .... 17% v/v
Propylene Glycol .... q.s.

With Sodium Formaldehyde Sulfoxylate, 1.3% w/v as a preservative and Monoethanolamine for pH adjustment.

Indications: A great many of the pathogens involved in cattle diseases are known to be susceptible to Oxytetracycline Hydrochloride therapy. Many strains of organisms, however, have shown resistance to Oxytetracycline. In the case of certain coliforms, *streptococci* and *staphylococci*, it may be advisable to conduct culture and sensitivity testing to determine susceptibility of the infecting organism to Oxytetracycline. In this manner, the likelihood of successful treatment with PROMYCIN™ 100 (Oxytetracycline Hydrochloride Injection) solution can be determined in advance.

Diseases for Which PROMYCIN™ 100 (Oxytetracycline Hydrochloride Injection) is Indicated: The use of PROMYCIN™ 100 (Oxytetracycline Hydrochloride Injection) is indicated in beef cattle, beef calves, non-lactating dairy cattle and dairy calves for treatment of the following disease conditions caused by one or more of the Oxytetracycline sensitive pathogens listed as follows:

Disease	Causative Organism(s) Which Show Sensitivity to PROMYCIN™ 100 (Oxytetracycline HCl Infection)
Bacterial Pneumonia and Shipping Fever Complex Associated with *Pasteurella* spp	*Pasteurella* spp
Bacterial Enteritis (scours)	*Escherichia coli*
Necrotic Pododermatitis (foot rot)	*Fusobacterium necrophorum*
Calf Diphtheria	*Fusobacterium necrophorum*
Wooden Tongue	*Actinobacillus lignieresii*
Wound Infections; Acute Metritis; Traumatic Injury	Caused by oxytetracycline-susceptible strains of streptococcal and staphylococcal organisms.

Pharmacology: Description: PROMYCIN™ 100 (Oxytetracycline Hydrochloride Injection) is a sterile ready-to-use preparation containing 100 mg/mL Oxytetracycline HCl for administration of the broad spectrum antibiotic, Oxytetracycline, by injection.

Antibiotic Action of Oxytetracycline: Oxytetracycline is effective against a wide range of gram-negative and gram-positive organisms that are pathogenic for cattle. The antibiotic is primarily bacteriostatic in effect, and is believed to exert its antimicrobial action by the inhibition of microbial protein synthesis. The antibiotic activity of Oxytetracycline is not appreciably diminished in the presence of body fluids, serum or exudates. Since the drugs in the tetracycline class have similar antimicrobial spectra, organisms can develop cross resistance among them. Oxytetracycline is concentrated by the liver in the bile and excreted in the urine and feces at high concentrations and in a biologically active form.

Dosage and Administration: Recommended Daily Dosages: Treat at the first clinical signs of disease.

The intravenous injection of 3 to 5 mg of Oxytetracycline Hydrochloride per pound of body weight per day (3 to 5 mL per 100 lbs body weight) is the recommended dosage.

Severe foot-rot and the severe forms of the indicated diseases should be treated with 5 mg per pound of body weight. Surgical procedures may be indicated in some forms of foot-rot or other conditions.

In disease treatment, the daily dose of PROMYCIN™ 100 (Oxytetracycline Hydrochloride Injection) should be continued 24 to 48 hours following remission of disease symptoms; however, not to exceed a total of 4 consecutive days.

Directions for Making an Intravenous Injection in Cattle:

Equipment Recommended:

1. Choke rope - a rope or cord about 5 feet long, with a loop in one end, to be used as a tourniquet.
2. Syringe and needles; gravity flow intravenous set.
3. Use new, very sharp hypodermic needles, 16-gauge, 1½ to 2 inches long. Dull needles will not work. Extra needles should be available in case the one being used becomes clogged.
4. Scissors or clippers.
5. 70% rubbing alcohol compound or other equally effective antiseptic for disinfecting the skin.
6. The medication to be given.

Preparation of Equipment: Thoroughly clean the needles, syringe and intravenous set and disinfect them by boiling in water for twenty minutes or by immersing in a suitable chemical disinfectant such as 70% alcohol for a period of not less than 30 minutes. Warm the bottle of medication to approximately body temperature and keep warm until used.

It is recommended that the correct dose be diluted in water for injection, sodium chloride injection or other suitable vehicle immediately prior to administration. Doses up to 50 mL may be diluted in 250 mL. Larger doses may be diluted in 500 mL of one of the diluents. Adverse reactions may be minimized and the drug dose can be better regulated by this method of administration.

Avoid touching the needle with the hands at all times.

In case of the syringe method of administration, disinfect the vial cap by wiping with 70% alcohol or other suitable antiseptic. Touching a sterile needle only by the hub, attach it to the syringe and push the plunger down the barrel to empty it of air. Puncture the rubber cap of the vial and withdraw the plunger upward in the syringe to draw up a volume of PROMYCIN™ 100 (Oxytetracycline Hydrochloride Injection), 100 mg/mL of about 5 mL more than is needed for injection. Withdraw from the vial and, pointing the needle upward, remove all air bubbles from the syringe by pushing the plunger upward to the volume required.

If the injection cannot be made immediately, the tip of the needle may be covered with cotton soaked in 70% alcohol to prevent contamination.

Preparation of the Animal for Injection:

1. Approximate location of vein. The jugular vein runs in the jugular groove on each side of the neck from the angle of the jaw to just above the brisket and slightly above and to the side of the windpipe.
2. Method of restraint - A stanchion or chute is ideal for restraining the animal. With a halter, rope or cattle leader (nose tongs), pull the animal's head around the side of the stanchion, cattle chute or post in such a manner to form a bow in the neck, then snub the head securely to prevent movement. By forming the bow in the neck, the outside curvature of the bow tends to expose the jugular vein and make it easily accessible. Caution: Avoid a tight rope or halter around the throat or upper neck which might impede blood flow. Animals that are down present no problem so far as restraint is concerned.
3. Clip hair in area where injection is to be made (over the vein in the upper third of the neck). Clean and disinfect the skin with alcohol or other suitable antiseptic.

Dosage for Injection: Refer to the table below for proper dosage according to body weight of the animal.

Weight of Animals, Lbs (Beef Cattle, Beef Calves, Non-Lactating Dairy Cattle, Dairy Calves)	Milligrams of Oxytetracycline Hydrochloride per 100 lbs of Body Weight Per Day	Daily Dosage of PROMYCIN™ 100 (Oxytetracycline Hydrochloride Injection) (mL)
50 lbs	300-500 mg	1.5-2.5 mL
100 lbs	300-500 mg	3-5 mL
200 lbs	300-500 mg	6-10 mL
300 lbs	300-500 mg	9-15 mL
400 lbs	300-500 mg	12-20 mL
500 lbs	300-500 mg	15-25 mL
600 lbs	300-500 mg	18-30 mL
800 lbs	300-500 mg	24-40 mL
1000 lbs	300-500 mg	30-50 mL
1200 lbs	300-500 mg	36-60 mL
1400 lbs	300-500 mg	42-70 mL

Caution: If no improvement is noted within 24 to 48 hours consult a veterinarian.

For intravenous use only.

Entering the Vein and Making the Injection:

1. Raise the vein. This is accomplished by tying the choke rope tight around the neck, close to the shoulder. The rope should be tied in such a way that it will not come loose and so that it can be untied quickly by pulling the loose end. In thick-necked animals, a block of wood placed in the jugular groove between the rope and the hide will help considerably in applying the desired pressure at the right point. The vein is a soft flexible tube through which blood flows back to the heart. Under ordinary conditions it cannot be seen or felt with the fingers. When the flow of blood is blocked at the base of the neck by the choke rope, the vein becomes enlarged and rigid because of the back pressure. If the choke rope is sufficiently tight, the vein stands out and can be easily seen and felt in thick-necked animals. As a further check in identifying the vein, tap it with the fingers in front of the choke rope. Pulsations that can be seen or felt with the fingers in front of the point being tapped will confirm the fact that the vein is properly distended. It is impossible to put the needle into the vein unless it is distended. Experienced operators are able to raise the vein simply by hand pressure, but the use of a choke rope is more certain.
2. Inserting the needle. This involves three distinct steps. First, insert the needle through the hide. Second, insert the needle into the vein. This may require two or three attempts before the vein is entered. The vein has a tendency to roll away from the point of the needle, especially if the needle is not sharp. The vein can be steadied with the thumb and finger of one hand. With the other hand, the needle point is placed directly over the vein, slanting it so that its direction is along the length of the vein, either toward the head or toward the heart. Properly positioned this way, a quick thrust of the needle will be followed by a spurt of blood through the needle, which indicates that the vein has been entered. Third, once in the vein, the needle should be inserted along the length of the vein all the way to the hub, exercising caution to see that the needle does not penetrate the opposite side of the vein. Continuous steady flow of blood through the needle indicates that the needle is still in the vein. If blood does not flow continuously, the needle is out of the vein (or clogged) and another attempt must be made. If difficulty is encountered, it may be advisable to use the vein on the other side of the neck.
3. While the needle is being placed in proper position in the vein, an assistant should get the medication ready so that the injection can be started without delay after the vein has been entered. Remove the rubber stopper from the bottle of intravenous solution, connect the intravenous tube to the neck of the bottle, invert the bottle and allow some of the solution to run through the tube to eliminate all air bubbles.
4. Making the injection. With needle in proper position as indicated by continuous flow of blood, release the choke rope by a quick pull on the free end. This is essential - the medication cannot flow into the vein while the vein is blocked. Immediately connect the intravenous tube to the needle, and raise the bottle. The solution will flow by gravity. Rapid injection may occasionally produce shock. Administer slowly. The animal should be observed at all times during the injection in order not to give the solution too fast. This may be determined by watching the respiration of the animal and feeling or listening to the heart beat. If the heart beat and respiration increase markedly, the rate of injection should be immediately stopped by pinching the tube until the animal recovers approximately to its previous respiration or heart beat rate, when the injection can be resumed at a slower rate. The rate of flow can be controlled by pinching the tube between the thumb and forefinger or by raising and lowering the bottle.

   Bubbles entering the bottle through the air tube or valve indicate the rate at which the medication is flowing. If the flow should stop, this means the needle has slipped out of the vein (or is clogged) and the operation will have to be repeated. If using the syringe technique, pull back gently on the plunger: if blood flows into the syringe, the needle is in proper position. Depress the plunger slowly. If there is any resistance to the depression of the plunger, stop and repeat insertion procedure. The resistance indicates that either the needle is clogged or it has slipped out of the vein. With either method of administration, syringe or gravity flow, watch for any swelling under the skin near the needle, which would indicate that the medication is not going into the vein. Should this occur, it is best to try the vein on the opposite side of the neck. Sudden movement of the animal, especially twisting of the neck or raising or lowering the head, may sometimes cause the needle to slip out of the vein. To prevent this, tape the needle hub to the skin of the neck to hold the needle in position. Whenever there is any doubt as to the position of the needle, this should be checked in the following manner: Pinch off the intravenous tube to stop flow, disconnect the tube from the needle and re-apply pressure to the vein. Free flow of blood through the needle indicates that it is in proper position and the injection can then be continued. If using the syringe, gently pull back on the plunger. Blood should flow into the syringe.
5. Removing the needle. When the injection is complete, remove needle with a straight pull. Then apply pressure over area of injection momentarily to control any bleeding through needle puncture, using cotton soaked in alcohol or other suitable antiseptic.

Instructions for Care of Sick Animals: The use of antibiotics, as with most medications used in the management of diseases, is based on accurate diagnosis and adequate treatment. When properly used in the treatment of diseases caused by oxytetracycline susceptible organisms, animals usually show a noticeable improvement within 24 to 48 hours. If improvement does not occur within this period of time, the diagnosis and treatment of animal diseases should be carried out by a veterinarian. The use of professional veterinary and laboratory services can reduce treatment costs, time and needless losses. Good management, housing, sanitation and nutrition are essential in the care of animals and in the successful treatment of disease.

Contraindication(s): Because bacteriostatic drugs interfere with the bactericidal action of Penicillin, do not give Oxytetracycline Hydrochloride in conjunction with Penicillin.

Precaution(s): Store between 15°C and 30°C (59°-86°F).

Note: Solution may darken on storage but potency remains unaffected.

Caution(s): Rapid intravenous administration may result in animal collapse. Oxytetracycline should be administered intravenously slowly over a period of at least 5 minutes.

If no improvement occurs within 24 to 48 hours, consult a veterinarian. Do not use the drug for more than 4 consecutive days. Use beyond 4 days or doses higher than maximum recommended dose may result in antibiotic tissue residues beyond the withdrawal period.

The improper or accidental injection of the drug outside of the vein will cause local tissue irritation manifested by temporary swelling and discoloration at the injection site.

Shortly after injection, treated animals may have a transient hemoglobinuria (darkened urine).

Consult with your veterinarian prior to administering this product in order to determine the proper treatment required in the event of an adverse reaction. At the first sign of any adverse reaction, discontinue use of product and seek the advice of your veterinarian. Some of the reactions may be attributed either to anaphylaxis (an allergic reaction) or to cardiovascular collapse of unknown cause.

As with other antibiotics, use of this drug may result in over-growth of nonsusceptible organisms. If any unusual symptoms occur or in the absence of a favorable response following treatment, discontinue use immediately and call a veterinarian.

For use in beef cattle, beef calves, non-lactating dairy cattle and dairy calves only.

For use in animals only.

Restricted Drug (California) - Use only as directed.

Warning(s): Discontinue treatment with PROMYCIN™ 100 (Oxytetracycline Hydrochloride Injection) at least 22 days prior to slaughter of the animal. Not for use in lactating dairy animals.

A withdrawal period has not been established for this product in pre-ruminating calves. Do not use in calves to be processed for veal.

Keep out of reach of children.

Adverse Reactions: Reports of adverse reactions associated with oxytetracycline administration include injection site swelling, restlessness, ataxia, trembling, swelling of eyelids, ears, muzzle, anus and vulva (or scrotum and sheath in males), respiratory abnormalities (labored breathing), frothing at the mouth, collapse and possibly death. Some of these reactions may be attributed either to anaphylaxis (an allergic reaction) or to cardiovascular collapse of unknown cause.

Presentation: PROMYCIN™ 100 (Oxytetracycline Hydrochloride Injection) is available in 500 mL multidose vials containing 100 mg Oxytetracycline Hydrochloride per mL (NDC 57319-119-07).

Manufactured by: Phoenix Scientific, Inc.

Compendium Code No.: 12560732 Rev. 8-01

PROPACK-EXP

Durvet **Water Additive**

Guaranteed Analysis:

Vitamin A (Min %)	8,168,400 IU/lb
Vitamin D_3 (Min %)	1,662,898 IU/lb
Vitamin E (Min %)	8,165 IU/lb
Sodium (Min %)	65%
(Max %)	70%
Potassium (Min %)	20%

Ingredients: Sodium chloride, potassium chloride, dextrose, calcium gluconate, citric acid, horse radish, sodium bicarbonate, vitamin A supplement, vitamin E (A tocopherol), vitamin B_3 (niacin), vitamin B_5 (D-calcium pantothenate), menadione sodium bisulfite complex (source of vitamin K_3 activity), vanillin, vitamin H (biotin), vitamin C (ascorbic acid), vitamin D_3 supplement, sodium aluminosilicate, vitamin B_6 (pyridoxine HCl), vitamin B_{12} supplement, vitamin B_1 (thiamin HCl), vitamin B_9 (folic acid), vitamin B_2 riboflavin), sodium saccharin, amyl butyrate, benzyl acetate, copper sulfate, ethyl butyrate, gamma undecalactone, propylene glycol, silicon dioxide, xanthan gum.

Indications: Vitamin and mineral supplement aromatized from plant extract for all swine, poultry and cattle.

Directions: Shake well. Dilute before usage.

Swine, Poultry and Cattle:

Drinking water: 1 cup (8 ounces/50 grams) of PROPACK-EXP per 256 gallons (1,000 liters) of drinking water.

Dilution: Mix half cup (4 ounces/125 grams) per gallon (4 liters) of stock solution with a proportioner set at 1:128. For best result use lukewarm water for stock solution.

Note:

1. Feeding Vitamins other than Vitamins A, D, E to ruminants older than three months of age may not have a beneficial effect.
2. The final dilution can be obtained from the manufacturer.
3. When animals are facing high environmental temperature consumption of final product should be limited to quantity of normal water consumption.

Length of Supplementation: 7 to 15 days.

Precaution(s): Protect from light. Store in a cool, dry place.

Caution(s): Not for injection.

Presentation: 5 oz, 4.4 lb, 11 lb (5 kg) and 22 lb (10 kg).

Manufactured by: Nutrapro Inc., 1905 Lamoureux, Suite 202, St. Hyacinthe, Québec, J2S 8B1, Canada.

Compendium Code No.: 10842070

PROPOFLO™ ℞

Abbott **General Anesthetic**

Anesthetic Injection

NADA No.: 141-098

Active Ingredient(s): Each mL contains 10 mg propofol.

Indications: PROPOFLO™ is an anesthetic injection for use in dogs as follows:

1. For induction of anesthesia.
2. For maintenance of general anesthesia for up to 20 minutes.
3. For induction of general anesthesia where maintenance is provided by inhalant anesthetics.

Pharmacology: Description: PROPOFLO™ Injection is a sterile, nonpyrogenic emulsion containing 10 mg/mL of propofol suitable for intravenous administration. Propofol is chemically described as 2, 6-diisopropylphenol and has a molecular weight of 178.27. Propofol is very slightly soluble in water and is therefore formulated as a white, oil-in-water emulsion. In addition to the active component, propofol, the formulation also contains soybean oil (100 mg/mL), glycerol (22.5 mg/mL), and egg lecithin (12 mg/mL), with sodium hydroxide to adjust the pH. The propofol emulsion is isotonic and has a pH of 7-8.5.

Clinical Pharmacology: Propofol injection is an intravenous sedative hypnotic agent for use in the induction and maintenance of anesthesia. Intravenous injection of propofol in the dog is followed by extensive metabolism of propofol in the liver to inactive conjugates which are excreted in the urine. Elimination form the central compartment occurs rapidly, with an initial elimination phase of less than 10 minutes.[1]

Induction of anesthesia will usually be observed within 75-120 seconds after the beginning of propofol administration. The duration of anesthesia following the recommended induction doses averages 6.7 minutes in premedicated and unpremedicated animals.

Recommended maintenance doses for anesthesia in unpremedicated animals, animals premedicated with acepromazine, and animals premedicated with a combination of agents results in anesthesia lasting an average of 3.68, 3.80 and 5.43 minutes, respectively, after each maintenance dose.

Recovery from propofol is rapid; full standing recovery is generally observed within 20 minutes. The use of certain premedicant combinations (e.g., acepromazine/oxymorphone) may result in prolonged recovery. Recovery may be delayed in Sighthounds.

Dosage and Administration: Shake the vial thoroughly before opening.

Parenteral drug products should be inspected visually for particulate matter and discoloration prior to administration, whenever solution and container permit. Propofol is a white stable emulsion; do not use if there is evidence of separation of the phases.

Propofol contains no antimicrobial preservatives. Strict aseptic techniques must always be maintained during handling since the vehicle is capable of supporting the rapid growth of microorganisms. Failure to follow aseptic handling procedures may result in microbial contamination causing fever, infection/sepsis, and/or other life-threatening illness. Do not use if contamination is suspected.

Once propofol has been opened, vial contents should be drawn into sterile syringes; each syringe should be prepared for single patient use only. Unused product should be discarded within 6 hours.

The emulsion should not be mixed with other therapeutic agents prior to administration. Administer by intravenous injection only.

Induction of General Anesthesia: For induction, propofol injection should be titrated against the response of the patient over 30-60 seconds or until clinical signs show the onset of anesthesia. Rapid injection of propofol (≤5 seconds) may be associated with an increased incidence of apnea.[2]

The average propofol induction dose rates for healthy dogs given propofol alone, or when propofol is preceded by a premedicant, are indicated in the table below. The table is for guidance only. The dose and rate should be based upon patient response.

Induction Dosage Guidelines:

Preanesthetic	Propofol Induction Dose	Propofol Rate of Administration		
	mg/kg	Seconds	mg/kg/min	mL/kg/min
None	5.5	40-60	5.5-8.3	0.55-0.83
Acepromazine	3.7	30-50	4.4-7.4	0.44-0.74
Acepromazine / Oxymorphone	2.6	30-50	3.1-5.2	0.31-0.52

Propofol doses and rates for the above premedicants were based upon the following average dosages. These doses may be lower than the label directions for their use as a single medication.[3,4]

	Dose (mg/kg)	Routes
Acepromazine	0.060	IM, SC, IV
Oxymorphone	0.090	IM, SC, IV
Xylazine	0.33	IM, SC

The use of these drugs as preanesthetics markedly reduces propofol requirements. As with other sedative hypnotic agents, the amount of opioid and/or α-2 agonist premedication will influence the response of the patient to an induction dose of propofol.

In the presence of premedication, the dose of propofol may be reduced with increasing age of the animal. The dose of propofol should always be titrated against the response of the patient.

During induction, additional low doses of propofol, similar to those used for maintenance with propofol, may be administered to facilitate intubation or the transition to inhalant maintenance anesthesia.

Maintenance of General Anesthesia:

A. Intermittent Propofol Injections: Anesthesia can be maintained by administering propofol in intermittent IV injections. Clinical response will be determined by the amount and the frequency of maintenance injections. The following table is provided for guidance:

Maintenance Dosage Guidelines:

Preanesthetic	Propofol Maintenance Dose	Rate of Administration		
	mg/kg	Seconds	mg/kg/min	mL/kg/min
None	2.2	10-30	4.4-13.2	0.44-1.32
Acepromazine	1.6	10-30	3.2-9.6	0.32-0.96
Acepromazine / Oxymorphone	1.8	10-30	3.6-10.8	0.36-1.08

Repeated maintenance doses of propofol do not result in increased recovery times or dosing intervals, indicating that the anesthetic effects of propofol are not cumulative.

B. Maintenance by Inhalant Anesthetics: Due to the rapid metabolism of propofol, additional low doses of propofol, similar to those used for maintenance with propofol, may be required to complete the transition to inhalant maintenance anesthesia.

Clinical trials using propofol have shown that it may be necessary to use a higher initial concentration of the inhalant anesthetic halothane than is usually required following induction using barbiturate anesthetics, due to rapid recovery from propofol.[5]

Compatibilities: PROPOFLO™ has been used in association with atropine, glycopyrrolate, acepromazine, xylazine, oxymorphone, halothane and isoflurane. No pharmacological incompatibility has been observed.

Contraindication(s): Propofol injection is contraindicated in dogs with a known hypersensitivity to propofol or its components, or when general anesthesia or sedation are contraindicated.

Precaution(s): Propofol undergoes oxidative degradation in the presence of oxygen and is therefore packaged under nitrogen to eliminate this degradation path. Store between 4 and 22°C (40°-72°F). Do not store below 4°C (40°F). Protect from light. Shake well before use.

Caution(s): Federal law restricts this drug to use by or on the order of a licensed veterinarian.

Rapid single or repeat bolus administration may cause undesirable cardiorespiratory depression including hypotension, apnea and oxygen desaturation.

When using propofol, patients should be continuously monitored and facilities for the maintenance of a patent airway, artificial ventilation, and oxygen supplementation must be immediately available.

Also observe the following:

1. Propofol contains no antimicrobial preservatives. Strict aseptic techniques must always be maintained during handling since the vehicle is capable of supporting the rapid growth of microorganisms. Failure to follow aseptic handling procedures may result in microbial contamination causing fever, infection/sepsis, and/or other life-threatening illness. Do not use if contamination is suspected.

   Once propofol has been opened, vial contents should be drawn into sterile syringes; each syringe should be prepared for single patient use only. Unused product should be discarded within 6 hours.
2. Anesthesia effects: Careful monitoring of the patient is necessary when using propofol as a maintenance anesthetic due to the possibility of rapid arousal. Apnea may occur following maintenance doses of propofol.

   Following induction, additional propofol may be needed to complete the transition to inhalant maintenance anesthesia due to rapid recovery from propofol. Doses administered during the transition to inhalant anesthesia may result in apnea.

   Propofol has also been used during inhalant maintenance anesthesia to increase anesthetic depth. Propofol used during inhalant maintenance may result in apnea.
3. Physiological effects: Mild hypotension may occur during propofol anesthesia.
4. Premedicants: Premedicants may increase the anesthesia or sedative effect of propofol and result in more pronounced changes in systolic, diastolic and mean arterial blood pressures.
5. Breeding animals: The use of propofol in pregnant and breeding dogs has not been evaluated. Propofol crosses the placenta and, as with other general anesthetic agents, the administration of propofol may be associated with neonatal depression.
6. Neonates: Propofol has not been evaluated in dogs less than 10 weeks of age.
7. Compromised or debilitated dogs: Doses may need adjustment for geriatric or debilitated patients. The administration of propofol to patients with renal failure and/or hepatic failure has not been evaluated. As with other anesthetic agents, caution should be exercised in dogs with cardiac, respiratory, renal or hepatic impairment, or in hypovolemic or debilitated dogs. Geriatric dogs may require less propofol for induction of anesthesia (see Dosage and Administration).
8. Sighthounds: Propofol induction and maintenance produced satisfactory anesthesia and recoveries in sighthounds. In the clinical study, a total of 27 sighthounds were induced with propofol, 6 of which were maintained on propofol. Induction doses were similar in sighthounds compared to other animals, however, recoveries were delayed.
9. Cardiac arrhythmias: In one study, propofol increased myocardial sensitivity to the development of epinephrine-induced ventricular arrhythmias in a manner similar to other anesthetics.[6] in the clinical study, transient ventricular arrhythmias associated with propofol were observed in 2 of 145 animals induced and maintained on propofol.
10. Concurrent medication: No significant adverse interactions with commonly used drugs have been observed.
11. Perivascular administration: Perivascular administration does not produce local tissue reaction.

For animal use only.

Warning(s): Human User Safety: Not for human use. Keep out of the reach of children.

Rare cases of self-administration have been reported, including fatalities. Propofol should be managed to prevent the risk of diversion, through such measures as restriction of access and the use of drug accountability procedures appropriate to the clinical setting.

Exercise caution to avoid accidental self-injection. Overdose is likely to cause cardiorespiratory depression (such as hypotension, bradycardia and/or apnea). Remove the individual from the source of exposure and seek medical attention. Respiratory depression should be treated by artificial ventilation and oxygen.

Hypersensitivity reactions to propofol, including anaphylaxis, may occur in some individuals who are also allergic to muscle relaxants.[7]

Avoid inhalation and direct contact of this product with skin, eyes, and clothes. In case of contact, eyes and skin should be liberally flushed with water for 15 minutes. Consult a physician if irritation persists.

The Material Safety Data Sheet (MSDS) contains more detailed occupational safety information.

Overdose: Rapid administration or accidental overdosage of propofol may cause cardiopulmonary depression. Respiratory arrest (apnea) may be observed. In cases of respiratory depression, stop drug administration, establish a patent airway, and initiate assisted or controlled ventilation with pure oxygen. Cardiovascular depression should be treated with plasma expanders, pressor agents, antiarrhythmic agents or other techniques as appropriate for the observed abnormality.

Side Effects: The primary side effect of propofol is respiratory depression as evidenced by tachypnea and apnea. Tachypnea and apnea were observed in 43 and 26% of the cases in the clinical trial, respectively. All cases of apnea resumed normal breathing spontaneously, or responded satisfactorily to oxygen supplementation and/or controlled ventilation.

Other transient side effects are observed infrequently or rarely:

Respiratory: labored breathing

Cardiovascular: hypotension, bradycardia, tachycardia, membrane cyanosis, arrhythmias

Musculoskeletal: fasciculations, tenseness, paddling, movements

Central Nervous System: excitation, opisthotonus, seizures, excessive depression

Gastrointestinal: emesis, retching, salivation

References: Available upon request.

Presentation: PROPOFLO™ is supplied in 5 mL and cartons of five-20 mL vials containing 200 mg per vial, 10 mg propofol per mL.

Compendium Code No.: 10240081 1342071A R896 Reference 06-9805/R1

P

PROPYLENE GLYCOL

AgriLabs **Acetonemia Preparation**

Active Ingredient(s): Contains propylene glycol.
Indications: An aid in the treatment of bovine ketosis (acetonemia).
Dosage and Administration: Administer orally.
Cows: 8 oz. twice a day for four (4) days.
Caution(s): Keep out of the reach of children.
Presentation: 1 gallon (3.785 L) containers.
Compendium Code No.: 10580840

PROPYLENE GLYCOL

AgriPharm **Acetonemia Preparation**

Active Ingredient(s): Propylene glycol.
Indications: For use as an aid in the treatment and prevention of bovine ketosis (acetonemia).
Dosage and Administration: For use mixed with feed or as a drench.
Prevention:
Dairy cattle . . . . . 6-8 fl. oz./head/day
Begin two (2) weeks before calving and continue for six (6) weeks after calving.
Treatment:
Dairy cattle . . . . . 6-16 fl. oz./head/day
Dosage dependant upon severity, to be given for 10 days.
PROPYLENE GLYCOL is very palatable and up to 10% in feed is acceptable to dairy cows. PROPYLENE GLYCOL does not destroy rumen micro-organisms or leave undesirable residues after oxidation.
Caution(s): For animal use only. Keep out of the reach of children.
Before administering PROPYLENE GLYCOL to cows suffering from milk fever, mastitis or metritus, consult a veterinarian.
Presentation: 1 gallon containers.
Compendium Code No.: 14570870

PROPYLENE GLYCOL

Aspen **Acetonemia Preparation**

Prevention/Treatment of Ketosis
Active Ingredient(s):
Propylene Glycol 100%
Indications: For use as an aid in the prevention and treatment of ketosis (Acetonemia) in dairy cattle.
Dosage and Administration: As an aid in the prevention of ketosis in dairy cattle, feed at the rate of 0.25 lbs per day at calving and continue for 8 weeks. Mix with feed or use as a drench.
Consult veterinarian if condition does not respond.
Precaution(s): Store between 2°-30°C (36°-86°F).
Warning(s): For animal use only.
Keep out of reach of children.
Presentation: 1 gal (3.785 L).
Compendium Code No.: 14750680

PROPYLENE GLYCOL

Centaur **Acetonemia Preparation**

Active Ingredient(s): Propylene glycol, feed grade.
Indications: An aid in the treatment and prevention of bovine ketosis (acetonemia).
Dosage and Administration:
Prevention: As an aid in prevention of acetonemia (ketosis) in dairy cattle, give 6 to 8 fluid ounces per head per day, beginning 2 weeks before calving and continuing for 6 weeks after calving.
Treatment: As an aid in treatment of acetonemia (ketosis) in dairy cattle, give 6 to 16 fluid ounces (dependant of severity) per head per day for 10 days. Use as drench or mix with feed.
When administering PROPYLENE GLYCOL to cows suffering from milk fever, mastitis or metritis, consult your veterinarian.
Caution(s): PROPYLENE GLYCOL is very palatable and up to 10% in feed is acceptable to dairy cows. Propylene glycol does not destroy rumen micro-organisms or leave undesirable residues after oxidation.
For animal use only.
Warning(s): Keep out of reach of children.
Presentation: 1 pint (16 fl oz) 473 mL and 1 gallon (128 fl oz) 3.785 L containers.
Compendium Code No.: 14880260

PROPYLENE GLYCOL

Durvet **Acetonemia Preparation**

Propylene Glycol, U.S.P.
Active Ingredient(s):
Propylene Glycol 100%
Indications: For use as an aid in prevention and treatment of Ketosis (Acetonemia) in dairy cattle.
Directions for Use: For use mixed with feed or as a drench.
Prevention: Dairy Cattle: 6-8 fl oz/head/day
Begin 2 weeks before calving and continue for 6 weeks after calving.
Treatment: Dairy Cattle: 6-16 fl oz/head/day
Dosage dependant upon severity, to be given for 10 days.
Consult veterinarian if condition does not respond.
Precaution(s): Storage: Store at controlled room temperature between 2°-30°C (36°-86°F). Keep container tightly closed when not in use.
Caution(s): For animal use only.
Livestock drug.
Warning(s): Keep out of reach of children.
Disclaimer: Seller makes no warranty of any kind whether in accordance with directions or not.
Presentation: 1 gallon (3.785 L) container (NDC 30798-012-35).
Compendium Code No.: 10841421 Rev. 2-02

PROPYLENE GLYCOL ℞

Vedco **Acetonemia Preparation**

Active Ingredient(s): Contains propylene glycol.
Indications: For the prevention and treatment of ketosis in dairy cattle. Consult a veterinarian.
Dosage and Administration: As an aid in the prevention of ketosis in dairy cattle, feed at the rate of 0.25 lbs. per head per day at calving and continue for six (6) weeks. Mix with feed or use as a drench.
Seller makes no warranty of any kind whether in accordance with directions or not.
Caution(s): Federal law restricts this drug to use by or on the order of a licensed veterinarian.
Keep out of the reach of children. For veterinary use only.
Presentation: 1 gallon containers.
Compendium Code No.: 10941730

PROPYLENE GLYCOL U.S.P.

Dominion **Acetonemia Preparation**

Active Ingredient(s):
Propylene Glycol USP 100%
Indications: As an aid in the treatment of acetonemia (ketosis) of cattle.
Dosage and Administration: Administer in the drinking water, in the grain ration, or as a drench.
Mild Cases: 120 mL morning and evening.
Severe Cases: 240 mL morning and evening.
Repeat as required.
Caution(s): Keep out of reach of children.
Presentation: 4 liter jug; 4 jugs/carton.
Compendium Code No.: 15080050

PROPYLENE GLYCOL (U.S.P.)

First Priority **Acetonemia Preparation**

Active Ingredient(s):
Propylene Glycol 100%
Indications: For use as an aid in prevention and treatment of Ketosis (Acetonemia) in dairy cattle.
Directions for Use: For use mixed with feed or as a drench.
Prevention:
Dairy Cattle . . . . . 6-8 fl oz/head/day
Begin 2 weeks before calving and continue for 6 weeks after calving.
Treatment:
Dairy Cattle . . . . . 6-16 fl oz/head/day
Dosage dependant upon severity, to be given for 10 days.
Consult veterinarian if condition does not respond.
Precaution(s): Storage: Store at 15°-30°C (59°-86°F). Keep bottle tightly closed.
Caution(s): For animal use only.
Warning(s): Keep out of reach of children.
Disclaimer: Seller makes no warranty of any kind whether in accordance with directions or not.
Presentation: 1 gallon (3.785 L) (NDC# 58829-235-01).
Compendium Code No.: 11390681 Rev. 06-01

PROPYLENE GLYCOL (U.S.P.)

Phoenix Pharmaceutical **Acetonemia Preparation**

Active Ingredient(s): Contents:
Propylene Glycol 100%
Indications: For use as an aid in prevention and treatment of Ketosis (Acetonemia) in dairy cattle.
Dosage and Administration: For use mixed with feed or as a drench.
Prevention:
Dairy Cattle . . . . . 6-8 fl oz/head/day
Begin 2 weeks before calving and continue for 6 weeks after calving.
Treatment:
Dairy Cattle . . . . . 6-16 fl oz/head/day
Dosage dependant upon severity, to be given for 10 days.
Consult veterinarian if condition does not respond.
Precaution(s): Store at 2°C-30°C (36°F-86°F). Keep bottle tightly closed.
Caution(s): For animal use only.
Livestock drug.
Warning(s): Keep out of reach of children.
Disclaimer: Seller makes no warranty of any kind whether in accordance with directions or not.
Presentation: 1 gallon (3.785 L) container (NDC 57319-413-09).
Compendium Code No.: 12561101 Rev. 09-00

PROPYLENE GLYCOL, USP

Vet Tek **Acetonemia Preparation**

Active Ingredient(s): Contains:
Propylene glycol 100%
(Provides 5.7 calories per gram.)
Indications: For the prevention and treatment of acetonemia (ketosis) in dairy cattle.
Directions for Use:
As a liquid source of energy for new cattle and calves when they are off feed. Drench at the rate of 1.5 oz. per 100 lbs. of body weight, 1.5 oz. proves 243 calories.
As an aid in the prevention of acetonemia (ketosis) in dairy cattle. Depending upon past history of severity of ketosis and upon size (breed), feed at the rate of 0.25 to 0.50 lbs. (4 to 8 fl. oz.) of PROPYLENE GLYCOL per head per day beginning two weeks before freshening. Continue feeding for 6 weeks after freshening. Mix with feed or use as a drench.
As a treatment for acetonemia (ketosis) in dairy cattle: Depending upon the severity of ketosis, feed at the rate of 0.25 to 1 lb. (4 to 16 fl. ozs.) of PROPYLENE GLYCOL per head per day for 10 days. Mix with feed or use as a drench.
Precaution(s): Store between 2°-30°C (36°-86°F).
Caution(s): Notice: Some cows may not respond to treatment as a result of complicating factors, such as milk fever, hardware, etc. These conditions must be treated in conjunction with the acetonemia. Consult your veterinarian if in doubt.
For animal use only.
Warning(s): Keep out of reach of children.
Presentation: 1 gallon (3.785 L) (NDC 60270-329-35).
Compendium Code No.: 14200290 Iss. 6-99

PRORAB®-1

Intervet **Vaccine**

Rabies Vaccine, Killed Virus

U.S. Vet. Lic. No.: 286

Contents: PRORAB®-1 is an inactivated virus vaccine produced form the Pasteur-RIV/PTA/78 rabies virus strain grown on the Pro-Cell Stable Cell Line™. PRORAB®-1 contains an adjuvant to enhance long-lasting immunity and is presented in a ready to use liquid form.

Contains thimerosal, neomycin and polymyxin B as preservatives.

Indications: For vaccination of healthy dogs, cats and sheep against rabies.

Dosage and Administration: Dogs and Cats—Aseptically administer 1 mL subcutaneously or intramuscularly. Primary vaccination is recommended at 3 months of age or older. Annual revaccination with a single dose is recommended. Sheep—Aseptically administer 2 mL intramuscularly. Primary vaccination is recommended at 3 months of age or older. Annual revaccination with a single dose is recommended.

Precaution(s): Recommended storage temperature 35-45°F (2-7°C). Do not freeze.

Shake well before use.

Use entire contents when first opened.

Non-chemically sterilized needles and syringes should be used for administration of vaccine.

Burn this container and all unused contents.

Caution(s): Administration of epinephrine may be indicated in the event of an anaphylactic reaction.

Only healthy animals should be vaccinated. Animals incubating disease or stressed due to shipping, malnutrition or parasitism may not achieve or maintain an adequate immune response.

This product is not hazardous when used according to directions supplied. A material safety data sheet (MSDS) is available upon request. This and any other consumer information can be obtained by calling Intervet's Customer Service Department at 1-800-441-8272.

Warning(s): Do not vaccinate food producing animals within 21 days of slaughter.

Trial Data: Safety and Efficacy: The safety and efficacy of PRORAB®-1 have been established in extensive studies conducted in accordance with U.S.D.A. regulations.

Presentation: 10 dose vials (5-10 dose vials per carton). Packaged in recyclable plastic containers.

Compendium Code No.: 11061440

PROSEL-300

Durvet **Water Additive**

Guaranteed Analysis:

Vitamin E supplement min. (15,420 IU/lb) . . . . 34,000 IU/kg (128,520 IU/gal)

Added Selenium: Actual 224 mg/lb or 495 oz/kg

Ingredients: Ethylic alcohol, vitamin E (A tocopherol), apple pomace dried, ethoxyquin as a preservative, sodium benzoate, sodium selenite, xanthan gum, methylparaben.

Indications: Vitamin and mineral supplement aromatized from plant extract for swine, poultry and cattle.

Liquid vitamin E and selenium for all poultry, swine and cattle.

Directions: Shake well. Dilute before usage.

Swine:

Drinking water: 1 cup (8 ounces or 250 mL) of PROSEL-300 in 256 gallons (1,000 liters) of drinking water in a proportioner at 1:128. Use ½ cup (4 ounces or 125 mL) of PROSEL-300 in 4 liters of stock/solution. For best results use lukewarm water for stock solution.

Poultry:

Drinking water: 1 cup (8 ounces or 250 mL) of PROSEL-300 in 256 gallons (1,000 liters) of drinking water.

Dilution: Mix half to ½ cup (4 ounces or 125 mL) of PROSEL-300 per 1 gallon (4 liters) of stock solution with a proportioner set at 1:128. For best results use lukewarm water for stock solution.

All Beef Cattle:

Drinking water: Half cup (4 ounces or 125 mL) of PROSEL-300 in 256 gallons (1,000 liters) of drinking water.

Dilution: Mix 2 ounces (60 mL) of PROSEL-300 per 1 gallon (4 liters) of stock solution with a proportioner set at 1:128. For best results use lukewarm water for stock solution.

Length of Supplementation: 7 to 15 days.

Note:

1. Do not use in association with any other feed containing supplemental selenium.
2. The final dilution can be obtained from the manufacturer.
3. When animals are facing high environmental temperature consumption of final product should be limited to quantity of normal water consumption.

Precaution(s): Protect from light. Store in cool, dry place.

Caution(s): Not for injection.

The selenium content of the feed should not exceed 0.3 ppm.

The viscosity of this product may vary inversely with the temperature at 74°F. 1.0 gram = 1 mL.

Directions for use must be carefully followed.

Presentation: 0.5 gallon and 1 gallon (3.78 L).

Manufactured by: Nutrapro Inc., 1905 Lamoureux, Suite 202, St. Hyacinthe, Québec, J2S 8B1, Canada.

Compendium Code No.: 10842080

PROSTAMATE™ ℞

Aspen **Prostaglandin**

(dinoprost tromethamine injection) Sterile Solution

ANADA No.: 200-253

Active Ingredient(s): This product contains the naturally occurring prostaglandin F2 alpha (dinoprost) as the tromethamine salt. Each mL contains dinoprost tromethamine equivalent to 5 mg dinoprost: also, benzyl alcohol, 9.45 mg added as preservative. When necessary, pH was adjusted with sodium hydroxide and/or hydrochloric acid. Dinoprost tromethamine is a white or slightly off-white crystalline powder that is readily soluble in water at room temperature in concentrations to at least 200 mg/mL.

Indications: For intramuscular use for estrus synchronization, treatment of unobserved (silent) estrus and pyometra (chronic endometritis) in cattle; for abortion of feedlot and other non-lactating cattle; for parturition induction in swine; and for controlling the timing of estrus in estrous cycling mares and clinically anestrous mares that have a corpus luteum.

Cattle: PROSTAMATE™ Sterile Solution is indicated as a luteolytic agent.

PROSTAMATE™ is effective only in those cattle having a corpus luteum, i.e., those which ovulated at least five days prior to treatment. Future reproductive performance of animals that are not cycling will be unaffected by injection of PROSTAMATE™.

Swine: For intramuscular use for parturition induction in swine. PROSTAMATE™ Sterile Solution is indicated for parturition induction in swine when injected within 3 days of normal predicted farrowing.

Mares: PROSTAMATE™ Sterile Solution is indicated for its luteolytic effect in mares. This luteolytic effect can be utilized to control the timing of estrus in estrous cycling and clinically anestrous mares that have a corpus luteum.

Pharmacology:

General Biologic Activity: Prostaglandins occur in nearly all mammalian tissues. Prostaglandins, especially PGE's and PGF's, have been shown, in certain species, to 1) increase at time of parturition in amniotic fluid, maternal placenta, myometrium, and blood, 2) stimulate myometrial activity, and 3) to induce either abortion or parturition. Prostaglandins, especially PGF2α, have been shown to 1) increase in the uterus and blood to levels similar to levels achieved by exogenous administration which elicited luteolysis, 2) be capable of crossing from the uterine vein to the ovarian artery (sheep), 3) be related to IUD induced luteal regression (sheep), and 4) be capable of regressing the corpus luteum of most mammalian species studied to date. Prostaglandins have been reported to result in release of pituitary tropic hormones. Data suggest prostaglandins, especially PGE's and PGF's, may be involved in the process of ovulation and gamete transport. Also PGF2α has been reported to cause increase in blood pressure, bronchoconstriction, and smooth muscle stimulation in certain species.

Metabolism: A number of metabolism studies have been done in laboratory animals. The metabolism of tritium labeled dinoprost (^{3}H PGF2 alpha) in the rat and in the monkey was similar. Although quantitative differences were observed, qualitatively similar metabolites were produced. A study demonstrated that equimolar doses of ^{3}H PGF2 alpha Tham and ^{3}H PGF2 alpha free acid administered intravenously to rats demonstrated no significant differences in blood concentration of dinoprost. An interesting observation in the above study was that the radioactive dose of ^{3}H PGF2 alpha rapidly distributed in tissues and dissipated in tissues with almost the same curve as it did in the serum. The half-life of dinoprost in bovine blood has been reported to be on the order of minutes. A complete study on the distribution of decline of ^{3}H PGF2 alpha Tham in the tissue of rats was well correlated with the work done in the cow. Cattle serum collected during 24 hours after doses of 0 to 250 mg dinoprost have been assayed by RIA for dinoprost and the 15-keto metabolites. These data support previous reports that dinoprost has a half-life of minutes. Dinoprost is a natural prostaglandin. All systems associated with dinoprost metabolism exist in the body; therefore, no new metabolic, transport, excretory, binding or other systems need be established by the body to metabolize injected dinoprost.

Dosage and Administration:

Cattle: PROSTAMATE™ Sterile Solution is supplied at a concentration of 5 mg dinoprost per mL. PROSTAMATE™ is luteolytic in cattle at 25 mg (5 mL) administered intramuscularly. As with any multidose vial, practice aseptic techniques in withdrawing each dose. Adequately clean and disinfect the vial closure prior to entry with a sterile needle.

Instructions for Use:

1. For Intramuscular Use for Estrus Synchronization in Beef Cattle and Non-Lactating Dairy Heifers. PROSTAMATE™ is used to control the timing of estrus and ovulation in estrous cycling cattle that have a corpus luteum.

   Inject a dose of 5 mL PROSTAMATE™ (25 mg PGF2α) intramuscularly either once or twice at a 10 to 12 day interval.

   With the single injection, cattle should be bred at the usual time relative to estrus. With the two injections cattle can be bred after the second injection either at the usual time relative to detected estrus or at about 80 hours after the second injection of PROSTAMATE™.

   Estrus is expected to occur 1 to 5 days after injection if a corpus luteum was present. Cattle that do not become pregnant to breeding at estrus on days 1 to 5 after injection will be expected to return to estrus in about 18 to 24 days.

2. For Intramuscular Use for Unobserved (Silent) Estrus in Lactating Dairy Cows with a Corpus Luteum. Inject a dose of 5 mL PROSTAMATE™ (25 mg PGF2α) intramuscularly. Breed cows as they are detected in estrus. If estrus has not been observed by 80 hours after injection, breed at 80 hours. If the cow returns to estrus breed at the usual time relative to estrus.

Management Considerations: Many factors contribute to success and failure of reproduction management, and these factors are important also when time of breeding is to be regulated with PROSTAMATE™ Sterile Solution. Some of these factors are:

a. Cattle must be ready to breed-they must have a corpus luteum and be healthy;
b. Nutritional status must be adequate as this has a direct effect on conception and the initiation of estrus in heifers or return of estrous cycles in cows following calving;
c. Physical facilities must be adequate to allow cattle handling without being detrimental to the animal;
d. Estrus must be detected accurately if timed A1 is not employed;
e. Semen of high fertility must be used;
f. Semen must be inseminated properly.

A successful breeding program can employ PROSTAMATE™ effectively, but a poorly managed breeding program will continue to be poor when PROSTAMATE™ is employed unless other management deficiencies are remedied first.

Cattle expressing estrus following PROSTAMATE™ are receptive to breeding by a bull. Using bulls to breed large numbers of cattle in heat following PROSTAMATE™ will require proper management of bulls and cattle.

3. For Intramuscular Use for Treatment of Pyometra (chronic endometritis) in Cattle. Inject a dose of 5 mL PROSTAMATE™ (25 mg PGF2α) intramuscularly. In studies conducted with dinoprost tromethamine sterile solution, pyometra was defined as presence of a corpus luteum in the ovary and uterine horns containing fluid but not a conceptus based on palpation *per rectum*. Return to normal was defined as evacuation of fluid and return of the uterine horn size to 40 mm or less based on palpation *per rectum* at 14 and 28 days. Most cattle that recovered in response to PROSTAMATE™ recovered within 14 days after injection. After 14 days, recovery rate of treated cattle was no different than that of non-treated cattle.

4. For Intramuscular Use for Abortion of Feedlot and Other Non-Lactating Cattle. PROSTAMATE™ is indicated for its abortifacient effect in feedlot and other non-lactating cattle during the first 100 days of gestation. Inject a dose of 25 mg intramuscularly. Cattle that abort will abort within 35 days of injection.

   Commercial cattle were palpated *per rectum* for pregnancy in six feedlots. The percent of pregnant cattle in each feedlot less than 100 days of gestation ranged between 26 and 84; 80% or more of the pregnant cattle were less than 150 days of gestation. The abortion rates following injection of dinoprost tromethamine sterile solution increased with increasing doses up to about 25 mg. As examples, the abortion rates, over 7 feedlots on the dose titration study, were 22%, 50%, 71%, 90% and 78% for cattle up to 100 days of gestation when injected IM with dinoprost tromethamine sterile solution doses of 0, 1 (5 mg), 2 (10 mg), 4 (20 mg) and 8 (40 mg) mL, respectively. The statistical predicted relative abortion rate based on the dose titration data, was about 93% for the 5 mL (25 mg) dinoprost tromethamine sterile solution dose for cattle injected up to 100 days of gestation.

Swine: PROSTAMATE™ Sterile Solution will induce parturition in swine at 10 mg (2 mL) when injected intramuscularly.

As with any multidose vial, practice aseptic techniques in withdrawing each dose. Adequately clean and disinfect the vial closure prior to entry with a sterile needle.

Instructions for Use: The response to treatment varies by individual animals with a mean interval from administration of 2 mL PROSTAMATE™ (10 mg dinoprost) to parturition of approximately 30 hours. This can be employed to control the time of farrowing in sows and gilts in late gestation.

Management Considerations: Several factors must be considered for the successful use of PROSTAMATE™ Sterile Solution for parturition induction in swine. The product must be administered at a relatively specific time (treatment earlier than 3 days prior to normal predicted farrowing may result in increased piglet mortality). It is important that adequate records be maintained on (1) the average length of gestation period for the animals on a specific location, and (2) the breeding and projected farrowing dates for each animal. This information is essential to determine the appropriate time for administration of PROSTAMATE™.

Mares:

1. Evaluate the reproductive status of the mare.
2. Administer a single intramuscular injection of 1 mg per 100 lbs (45.5 kg) body weight which is usually 1 mL to 2 mL PROSTAMATE™ Sterile Solution.
3. Observe for signs of estrus by means of daily teasing with a stallion, and evaluate follicular changes on the ovary by palpation of the ovary *per rectum.*
4. Some clinically anestrous mares will not express estrus but will develop a follicle which will ovulate. These mares may become pregnant if inseminated at the appropriate time relative to rupture of the follicle.
5. Breed mares in estrus in a manner consistent with normal management.

Dinoprost tromethamine is administered once as a single intramuscular injection of 1 mg per 100 lbs (45.5 kg) body weight which is usually 1 mL to 2 mL of PROSTAMATE™ containing 5 mg dinoprost as the tromethamine salt per milliliter.

Instructions for Use: PROSTAMATE™ Sterile Solution is indicated for its luteolytic effect in mares. This luteolytic effect can be utilized to control the timing of estrus in estrous cycling and clinically anestrous mares that have a corpus luteum in the following circumstances:

1. Controlling Time of Estrus of Estrous Cycling Mares: Mares treated with PROSTAMATE™ during diestrus (4 or more days after ovulation) will return to estrus within 2 to 4 days in most cases and ovulate 8 to 12 days after treatment. This procedure may be utilized as an aid to scheduling the use of stallions.
2. Difficult-to-Breed Mares: In extended diestrus there is failure to exhibit regular estrous cycles which is different from true anestrus. Many mares described as anestrus during the breeding season have serum progesterone levels consistent with the presence of a functional corpus luteum.

   A proportion of "barren", maiden, and lactating mares do not exhibit regular estrous cycles and may be in extended diestrus. Following abortion, early fetal death and resorption, or as a result of "pseudopregnancy", there may be serum progesterone levels consistent with a functional corpus luteum.

   Treatment of such mares with PROSTAMATE™ usually results in regression of the corpus luteum followed by estrus and/or ovulation. In one study with 122 Standardbred and Thoroughbred mares in clinical anestrus for an average of 58 days and treated during the breeding season, behavioral estrus was detected in 81 percent at an average time of 3.7 days after injection with 5 mg dinoprost tromethamine sterile solution; ovulation occurred an average of 7.0 days after treatment. Of those mares bred, 59% were pregnant following an average of 1.4 services during that estrus.

   Treatment of "anestrous" mares which abort subsequent to 36 days of pregnancy may not result in return to estrus due to presence of functional endometrial cups.

Precaution(s): Store at controlled room temperature 20° to 25°C (68° to 77°F).

Caution(s): Federal (USA) law restricts this drug to use by or on the order of a licensed veterinarian.

Cattle: Do not administer to pregnant cattle unless abortion is desired.

Do not administer intravenously (I.V.), as this route might potentiate adverse reactions.

Cattle administered a progestogen would be expected to have a reduced response to PROSTAMATE™ Sterile Solution.

Aggressive antibiotic therapy should be employed at the first sign of infection at the injection site whether localized or diffuse. As with all parenteral products careful aseptic techniques should be employed to decrease the possibility of post injection bacterial infections.

Swine: Do not administer to sows and/or gilts prior to 3 days of normal predicted farrowing, as increased number of stillborn and postnatal mortality may result.

Mares: PROSTAMATE™ Sterile Solution is ineffective when administered prior to day-5 after ovulation.

Pregnancy status should be determined prior to treatment, since PROSTAMATE™ has been reported to induce abortion and parturition when sufficient doses were administered.

Mares should not be treated if they suffer from either acute or subacute disorders of the vascular system, gastrointestinal tract, respiratory system, or reproductive tract.

Do not administer by intravenous route.

Nonsteroidal anti-inflammatory drugs (i.e., indomethacin) may inhibit prostaglandin synthesis, therefore these drugs should not be administered concurrently.

Warning(s):

Cattle: No milk discard or preslaughter drug withdrawal period is required for labeled uses.

Swine: No preslaughter drug withdrawal period is required for labeled uses.

Mares: Not for use in horses intended for food.

Not for human use.

Women of child-bearing age, asthmatics, and persons with bronchial and other respiratory problems should exercise extreme caution when handling this product. In the early stages, women may be unaware of their pregnancies. Dinoprost tromethamine is readily absorbed through the skin and can cause abortion and/or bronchiospasms. Direct contact with the skin should, therefore, be avoided. Accidental spillage on the skin should be washed off immediately with soap and water.

Use of this product in excess of the approved dose may result in drug residues.

For use in animals only.

Restricted drug-Use only as directed (California).

Keep out of reach of children.

Toxicology: Safety and Toxicity:

Laboratory Animals: Dinoprost was non-teratogenic in rats when administered orally at 1.25, 3.2, 10.0 and 20.0 mg/kg/day from day 6th-15th of gestation or when administered subcutaneously at 0.5 and 1.0 mg/kg/day on gestation days 6, 7 and 8 or 9, 10 and 11 or 12, 13 and 14. Dinoprost was non-teratogenic in the rabbit when administered either subcutaneously at doses of 0.5 and 1.0 mg/kg/day on gestation days 6, 7 and 8 or 9, 10 and 11 or 12, 13 and 14 or 15, 16 and 17 or orally at doses of 0.01, 0.1 and 1.0 mg/kg/day on days 6-18 or 5.0 mg/kg/day on days 8-18 of gestation. A slight and marked embryo lethal effect was observed in dams given 1.0 and 5.0 mg/kg/day respectively. This was due to the expected luteolytic properties of the drug.

A 14-day continuous intravenous infusion study in rats at 20 mg PGF2α per kg body weight indicated prostaglandins of the F series could induce bone deposition. However, such bone changes were not observed in monkeys similarly administered dinoprost tromethamine sterile solution at 15 mg PGF2α per kg body weight for 14 days.

Cattle: In cattle, evaluation was made of clinical observations, clinical chemistry, hematology, urinalysis, organ weights, and gross plus microscopic measurements following treatment with various doses up to 250 mg dinoprost administered twice intramuscularly at a 10 day interval or doses of 25 mg administered daily for 10 days. There was no unequivocal effect of dinoprost on the hematology or clinical chemistry parameters measured. Clinically, a slight transitory increase in heart rate was detected. Rectal temperature was elevated about 1.5°F through the 6th hour after injection with 250 mg dinoprost, but had returned to baseline at 24 hours after injection. No dinoprost associated gross lesions were detected. There was no evidence of toxicological effects. Thus, dinoprost had a safety factor of at least 10X on injection (25 mg luteolytic dose vs. 250 mg safe dose), based on studies conducted with cattle. At luteolytic doses, dinoprost had no effect on progeny. If given to a pregnant cow, it may cause abortion; the dose required for abortion varies considerably with the stage of gestation.

Induction of abortion in feedlot cattle at stages of gestation up to 100 days of gestation did not result in dystocia, retained placenta or death of heifers in the field studies. The smallness of the fetus at this early stage of gestation should not lead to complications at abortion. However, induction of parturition or abortion with any exogenous compound may precipitate dystocia, fetal death, retained placenta and/or metritis, especially at latter stages of gestation.

Swine: In pigs, evaluation was made of clinical observations, food consumption, clinical pathologic determinations, body weight changes, urinalysis, organ weights, and gross and microscopic observations following treatment with single doses of 10, 30, 50 and 100 mg dinoprost administered intramuscularly. The results indicated no treatment related effects from dinoprost treatment that were deleterious to the health of the animals or to their offspring.

Mares: Dinoprost tromethamine was administered to adult mares (weighing 320 to 485 kg; 2 to 20 years old), at the rates of 0, 100, 200, 400, and 800 mg per mare per day for 8 days. Route of administration for each dose group was both intramuscularly (2 mares) and subcutaneously (2 mares). Changes were detected in all treated groups for clinical (reduced sensitivity to pain; locomotor incoordination; hypergastromotility; sweating; hyperthermia; labored respiration), blood chemistry (elevated cholesterol, total bilirubin, LDH, and glucose), and hematology (decreased eosinophils; increased hemoglobin, hematocrit, and erythrocytes) measurements. The effects in the 100 mg dose, and to a lesser extent, the 200 mg dose groups were transient in nature, lasting for a few minutes to several hours. Mares did not appear to sustain adverse effects following termination of the side effects.

Mares treated with either 400 mg or 800 mg exhibited more profound symptoms. The excessive hyperstimulation of the gastrointestinal tract caused a protracted diarrhea, slight electrolyte imbalance (decreased sodium and potassium), dehydration, gastrointestinal irritation, and slight liver malfunction (elevated SGOT, SGPT at 800 mg only). Heart rate was increased but pH of the urine was decreased. Other measurements evaluated in the study remained within normal limits. No mortality occurred in any of the groups. No apparent differences were observed between the intramuscular and subcutaneous routes of administration. Luteolytic doses of dinoprost tromethamine are on the order of 5 to 10 mg administered on one day, therefore, dinoprost tromethamine sterile solution was demonstrated to have a wide margin of safety. Thus, the 100 mg dose gave a safety margin of 10 to 20X for a single injection or 80 to 160X for the 8 daily injections.

Additional studies investigated the effects in the mare of single intramuscular doses of 0, 0.25, 1.0, 2.5, 3.0, 5.0, and 10.0 mg dinoprost tromethamine. Heart rate, respiration rate, rectal temperature, and sweating were measured at 0, 0.25, 0.50, 0.75, 1.0, 1.5, 2.0, 3.0, 4.0, 5.0, and 6.0 hr. after injection. Neither heart rate nor respiration rates were significantly altered ($P > 0.05$) when compared to contemporary control values. Sweating was observed for 0 of 9, 2 of 9, 7 of 9, 9 of 9, and 8 of 9 mares injected with 0.25, 1.0, 2.5, 3.0, 5.0, or 10.0 mg dinoprost tromethamine, respectively. Sweating was temporary in all cases and was mild for doses of 3.0 mg or less but was extensive (beads of sweat over the entire body and dripping) for the 10 mg dose. Sweating after the 5.0 mg dose was intermediate between that seen for mares treated with 3.0 and 10.0 mg. Sweating began within 15 minutes after injection and ceased by 45 to 60 minutes after injection. Rectal temperature was decreased during the interval 0.5 until 1.0, 3 to 4, or 5 hours after injection for 0.25 and 1.0 mg, 2.5 and 3.0, or 5.0 and 10.0 mg dose groups, respectively. Average rectal temperature during the periods of decreased temperature was on the order of 97.5 to 99.6, with the greatest decreases observed in the 10 mg dose group.

Adverse Reactions:

Cattle:

1. The most frequently observed side effect is increased rectal temperature at a 5X or 10X overdose. However, rectal temperature change has been transient in all cases observed and has not been detrimental to the animal.
2. Limited salivation has been reported in some instances.
3. Intravenous administration might increase heart rate.
4. Localized post injection bacterial infections that may become generalized have been reported. In rare instances such infections have terminated fatally. See Cautions.

Swine: The most frequently observed side effects were erythema and pruritus, slight incoordination, nesting behavior, itching, urination, defecation, abdominal muscle spasms, tail movements, hyperpnea or dyspnea, increased vocalization, salivation, and at the 100 mg (10X) dose only, vomition. These side effects are transitory, lasting from 10 minutes to 3 hours, and were not detrimental to the health of the animal.

Mares: The most frequently observed side effects are sweating and decreased rectal temperature. However, these have been transient in all cases observed and have not been detrimental to the animal. Other reactions seen have been increase in heart rate, increase in respiration rate, some abdominal discomfort, locomotor incoordination, and lying down. These effects are usually seen within 15 minutes of injection and disappear within one hour. Mares usually continue to eat during the period of expression of side effects. One anaphylactic reaction of several hundred mares treated with dinoprost tromethamine sterile solution was reported but was not confirmed.

Presentation: PROSTAMATE™ Sterile Solution is available in 30 mL vials.

Manufactured by: Phoenix Scientific, Inc.

Compendium Code No.: 14750690

PROSTAMATE™ ℞

Butler **Prostaglandin**

(Dinoprost Tromethamine Injection) Sterile Solution

ANADA No.: 200-253

Active Ingredient(s): This product contains the naturally occurring prostaglandin F2 alpha (dinoprost) as the tromethamine salt. Each mL contains dinoprost tromethamine equivalent to 5 mg dinoprost: also, benzyl alcohol, 9.45 mg added as preservative. When necessary, pH was adjusted with sodium hydroxide and/or hydrochloric acid. Dinoprost tromethamine is a white or slightly off-white crystalline powder that is readily soluble in water at room temperature in concentrations to at least 200 mg/mL.

Indications: For intramuscular use for estrus synchronization, treatment of unobserved (silent) estrus and pyometra (chronic endometritis) in cattle; for abortion of feedlot and other non-lactating cattle; for parturition induction in swine; and for controlling the timing of estrus in estrous cycling mares and clinically anestrous mares that have a corpus luteum.

Cattle: PROSTAMATE™ Sterile Solution is indicated as a luteolytic agent.

PROSTAMATE™ is effective only in those cattle having a corpus luteum, i.e., those which ovulated at least five days prior to treatment. Future reproductive performance of animals that are not cycling will be unaffected by injection of PROSTAMATE™.

Swine: For intramuscular use for parturition induction in swine. PROSTAMATE™ Sterile Solution is indicated for parturition induction in swine when injected within 3 days of normal predicted farrowing.

Mares: PROSTAMATE™ Sterile Solution is indicated for its luteolytic effect in mares. This luteolytic effect can be utilized to control the timing of estrus in estrous cycling and clinically anestrous mares that have a corpus luteum.

Pharmacology:

General Biologic Activity: Prostaglandins occur in nearly all mammalian tissues. Prostaglandins, especially PGE's and PGF's, have been shown, in certain species, to 1) increase at time of parturition in amniotic fluid, maternal placenta, myometrium, and blood, 2) stimulate myometrial activity, and 3) to induce either abortion or parturition. Prostaglandins, especially PGF2α, have been shown to 1) increase in the uterus and blood to levels similar to levels achieved by exogenous administration which elicited luteolysis, 2) be capable of crossing from the uterine vein to the ovarian artery (sheep), 3) be related to IUD induced luteal regression (sheep), and 4) be capable of regressing the corpus luteum of most mammalian species studied to date. Prostaglandins have been reported to result in release of pituitary tropic hormones. Data suggest prostaglandins, especially PGE's and PGF's, may be involved in the process of ovulation and gamete transport. Also PGF2α has been reported to cause increase in blood pressure, bronchoconstriction, and smooth muscle stimulation in certain species.

Metabolism: A number of metabolism studies have been done in laboratory animals. The metabolism of tritium labeled dinoprost (^{3}H PGF2 alpha) in the rat and in the monkey was similar. Although quantitative differences were observed, qualitatively similar metabolites were produced. A study demonstrated that equimolar doses of ^{3}H PGF2 alpha Tham and ^{3}H PGF2 alpha free acid administered intravenously to rats demonstrated no significant differences in blood concentration of dinoprost. An interesting observation in the above study was that the radioactive dose of ^{3}H PGF2 alpha rapidly distributed in tissues and dissipated in tissues with almost the same curve as it did in the serum. The half-life of dinoprost in bovine blood has been reported to be on the order of minutes. A complete study on the distribution of decline of ^{3}H PGF2 alpha Tham in the tissue of rats was well correlated with the work done in the cow. Cattle serum collected during 24 hours after doses of 0 to 250 mg dinoprost have been assayed by RIA for dinoprost and the 15-keto metabolites. These data support previous reports that dinoprost has a half-life of minutes. Dinoprost is a natural prostaglandin. All systems associated with dinoprost metabolism exist in the body; therefore, no new metabolic, transport, excretory, binding or other systems need be established by the body to metabolize injected dinoprost.

Dosage and Administration:

Cattle: PROSTAMATE™ Sterile Solution is supplied at a concentration of 5 mg dinoprost per mL. PROSTAMATE™ is luteolytic in cattle at 25 mg (5 mL) administered intramuscularly. As with any multidose vial, practice aseptic techniques in withdrawing each dose. Adequately clean and disinfect the vial closure prior to entry with a sterile needle.

Instructions for Use:

1. For Intramuscular Use for Estrus Synchronization in Beef Cattle and Non-Lactating Dairy Heifers. PROSTAMATE™ is used to control the timing of estrus and ovulation in estrous cycling cattle that have a corpus luteum.

   Inject a dose of 5 mL PROSTAMATE™ (25 mg PGF2α) intramuscularly either once or twice at a 10 to 12 day interval.

   With the single injection, cattle should be bred at the usual time relative to estrus. With the two injections cattle can be bred after the second injection either at the usual time relative to detected estrus or at about 80 hours after the second injection of PROSTAMATE™.

   Estrus is expected to occur 1 to 5 days after injection if a corpus luteum was present. Cattle that do not become pregnant to breeding at estrus on days 1 to 5 after injection will be expected to return to estrus in about 18 to 24 days.
2. For Intramuscular Use for Unobserved (Silent) Estrus in Lactating Dairy Cows with a Corpus Luteum. Inject a dose of 5 mL PROSTAMATE™ (25 mg PGF2α) intramuscularly. Breed cows as they are detected in estrus. If estrus has not been observed by 80 hours after injection, breed at 80 hours. If the cow returns to estrus breed at the usual time relative to estrus.

Management Considerations: Many factors contribute to success and failure of reproduction management, and these factors are important also when time of breeding is to be regulated with PROSTAMATE™ Sterile Solution. Some of these factors are:

a. Cattle must be ready to breed-they must have a corpus luteum and be healthy;
b. Nutritional status must be adequate as this has a direct effect on conception and the initiation of estrus in heifers or return of estrous cycles in cows following calving;
c. Physical facilities must be adequate to allow cattle handling without being detrimental to the animal;
d. Estrus must be detected accurately if timed A1 is not employed;
e. Semen of high fertility must be used;
f. Semen must be inseminated properly.

A successful breeding program can employ PROSTAMATE™ effectively, but a poorly managed breeding program will continue to be poor when PROSTAMATE™ is employed unless other management deficiencies are remedied first.

Cattle expressing estrus following PROSTAMATE™ are receptive to breeding by a bull. Using bulls to breed large numbers of cattle in heat following PROSTAMATE™ will require proper management of bulls and cattle.

3. For Intramuscular Use for Treatment of Pyometra (chronic endometritis) in Cattle. Inject a dose of 5 mL PROSTAMATE™ (25 mg PGF2α) intramuscularly. In studies conducted with dinoprost tromethamine sterile solution, pyometra was defined as presence of a corpus luteum in the ovary and uterine horns containing fluid but not a conceptus based on palpation *per rectum*. Return to normal was defined as evacuation of fluid and return of the uterine horn size to 40 mm or less based on palpation *per rectum* at 14 and 28 days. Most cattle that recovered in response to PROSTAMATE™ recovered within 14 days after injection. After 14 days, recovery rate of treated cattle was no different than that of non-treated cattle.
4. For Intramuscular Use for Abortion of Feedlot and Other Non-Lactating Cattle. PROSTAMATE™ is indicated for its abortifacient effect in feedlot and other non-lactating cattle during the first 100 days of gestation. Inject a dose of 25 mg intramuscularly. Cattle that abort will abort within 35 days of injection.

   Commercial cattle were palpated *per rectum* for pregnancy in six feedlots. The percent of pregnant cattle in each feedlot less than 100 days of gestation ranged between 26 and 84; 80% or more of the pregnant cattle were less than 150 days of gestation. The abortion rates following injection of dinoprost tromethamine sterile solution increased with increasing doses up to about 25 mg. As examples, the abortion rates, over 7 feedlots on the dose titration study, were 22%, 50%, 71%, 90% and 78% for cattle up to 100 days of gestation when injected IM with dinoprost tromethamine sterile solution doses of 0, 1 (5 mg), 2 (10 mg), 4 (20 mg) and 8 (40 mg) mL, respectively. The statistical predicted relative abortion rate based on the dose titration data, was about 93% for the 5 mL (25 mg) dinoprost tromethamine sterile solution dose for cattle injected up to 100 days of gestation.

Swine: PROSTAMATE™ Sterile Solution will induce parturition in swine at 10 mg (2 mL) when injected intramuscularly.

As with any multidose vial, practice aseptic techniques in withdrawing each dose. Adequately clean and disinfect the vial closure prior to entry with a sterile needle.

Instructions for Use: The response to treatment varies by individual animals with a mean interval from administration of 2 mL PROSTAMATE™ (10 mg dinoprost) to parturition of approximately 30 hours. This can be employed to control the time of farrowing in sows and gilts in late gestation.

Management Considerations: Several factors must be considered for the successful use of PROSTAMATE™ Sterile Solution for parturition induction in swine. The product must be administered at a relatively specific time (treatment earlier than 3 days prior to normal predicted farrowing may result in increased piglet mortality). It is important that adequate records be maintained on (1) the average length of gestation period for the animals on a specific location, and (2) the breeding and projected farrowing dates for each animal. This information is essential to determine the appropriate time for administration of PROSTAMATE™.

Mares:

1. Evaluate the reproductive status of the mare.
2. Administer a single intramuscular injection of 1 mg per 100 lbs (45.5 kg) body weight which is usually 1 mL to 2 mL PROSTAMATE™ Sterile Solution.
3. Observe for signs of estrus by means of daily teasing with a stallion, and evaluate follicular changes on the ovary by palpation of the ovary *per rectum*.
4. Some clinically anestrous mares will not express estrus but will develop a follicle which will ovulate. These mares may become pregnant if inseminated at the appropriate time relative to rupture of the follicle.
5. Breed mares in estrus in a manner consistent with normal management.

Dinoprost tromethamine is administered once as a single intramuscular injection of 1 mg per 100 lbs (45.5 kg) body weight which is usually 1 mL to 2 mL of PROSTAMATE™ containing 5 mg dinoprost as the tromethamine salt per milliliter.

Instructions for Use: PROSTAMATE™ Sterile Solution is indicated for its luteolytic effect in mares. This luteolytic effect can be utilized to control the timing of estrus in estrous cycling and clinically anestrous mares that have a corpus luteum in the following circumstances:

1. Controlling Time of Estrus of Estrous Cycling Mares: Mares treated with PROSTAMATE™ during diestrus (4 or more days after ovulation) will return to estrus within 2 to 4 days in most cases and ovulate 8 to 12 days after treatment. This procedure may be utilized as an aid to scheduling the use of stallions.
2. Difficult-to-Breed Mares: In extended diestrus there is failure to exhibit regular estrous cycles which is different from true anestrus. Many mares described as anestrus during the breeding season have serum progesterone levels consistent with the presence of a functional corpus luteum.

   A proportion of "barren", maiden, and lactating mares do not exhibit regular estrous cycles and may be in extended diestrus. Following abortion, early fetal death and resorption, or as a result of "pseudopregnancy", there may be serum progesterone levels consistent with a functional corpus luteum.

   Treatment of such mares with PROSTAMATE™ usually results in regression of the corpus luteum followed by estrus and/or ovulation. In one study with 122 Standardbred and Thoroughbred mares in clinical anestrus for an average of 58 days and treated during the breeding season, behavioral estrus was detected in 81 percent at an average time of 3.7 days after injection with 5 mg dinoprost tromethamine sterile solution; ovulation occurred an average of 7.0 days after treatment. Of those mares bred, 59% were pregnant following an average of 1.4 services during that estrus.

   Treatment of "anestrous" mares which abort subsequent to 36 days of pregnancy may not result in return to estrus due to presence of functional endometrial cups.

Precaution(s): Store at controlled room temperature 20° to 25°C (68° to 77°F).

Caution(s): Federal (USA) law restricts this drug to use by or on the order of a licensed veterinarian.

Cattle: Do not administer to pregnant cattle unless abortion is desired.

Do not administer intravenously (I.V.), as this route might potentiate adverse reactions.

Cattle administered a progestogen would be expected to have a reduced response to PROSTAMATE™ Sterile Solution.

Aggressive antibiotic therapy should be employed at the first sign of infection at the injection site whether localized or diffuse. As with all parenteral products careful aseptic techniques should be employed to decrease the possibility of post injection bacterial infections.

Swine: Do not administer to sows and/or gilts prior to 3 days of normal predicted farrowing, as increased number of stillborn and postnatal mortality may result.

Mares: PROSTAMATE™ Sterile Solution is ineffective when administered prior to day-5 after ovulation.

Pregnancy status should be determined prior to treatment, since PROSTAMATE™ has been reported to induce abortion and parturition when sufficient doses were administered.

Mares should not be treated if they suffer from either acute or subacute disorders of the vascular system, gastrointestinal tract, respiratory system, or reproductive tract.

Do not administer by intravenous route.

Nonsteroidal anti-inflammatory drugs (i.e., indomethacin) may inhibit prostaglandin synthesis, therefore these drugs should not be administered concurrently.

Warning(s):

Cattle: No milk discard or preslaughter drug withdrawal period is required for labeled uses.

Swine: No preslaughter drug withdrawal period is required for labeled uses.

Mares: Not for use in horses intended for food.

Not for human use.

Women of child-bearing age, asthmatics, and persons with bronchial and other respiratory problems should exercise extreme caution when handling this product. In the early stages, women may be unaware of their pregnancies. Dinoprost tromethamine is readily absorbed through the skin and can cause abortion and/or bronchiospasms. Direct contact with the skin should, therefore, be avoided. Accidental spillage on the skin should be washed off immediately with soap and water.

Use of this product in excess of the approved dose may result in drug residues.

For use in animals only.

Keep out of reach of children.

Toxicology: Safety and Toxicity:

Laboratory Animals: Dinoprost was non-teratogenic in rats when administered orally at 1.25, 3.2, 10.0 and 20.0 mg/kg/day from day 6th-15th of gestation or when administered subcutaneously at 0.5 and 1.0 mg/kg/day on gestation days 6, 7 and 8 or 9, 10 and 11 or 12, 13 and 14. Dinoprost was non-teratogenic in the rabbit when administered either subcutaneously at doses of 0.5 and 1.0 mg/kg/day on gestation days 6, 7 and 8 or 9, 10 and 11 or 12, 13 and 14 or 15, 16 and 17 or orally at doses of 0.01, 0.1 and 1.0 mg/kg/day on days 6-18 or 5.0 mg/kg/day on days 8-18 of gestation. A slight and marked embryo lethal effect was observed in dams given 1.0 and 5.0 mg/kg/day respectively. This was due to the expected luteolytic properties of the drug.

A 14-day continuous intravenous infusion study in rats at 20 mg PGF2α per kg body weight indicated prostaglandins of the F series could induce bone deposition. However, such bone changes were not observed in monkeys similarly administered dinoprost tromethamine sterile solution at 15 mg PGF2α per kg body weight for 14 days.

Cattle: In cattle, evaluation was made of clinical observations, clinical chemistry, hematology, urinalysis, organ weights, and gross plus microscopic measurements following treatment with various doses up to 250 mg dinoprost administered twice intramuscularly at a 10 day interval or doses of 25 mg administered daily for 10 days. There was no unequivocal effect of dinoprost on the hematology or clinical chemistry parameters measured. Clinically, a slight transitory increase in heart rate was detected. Rectal temperature was elevated about 1.5°F through the 6th hour after injection with 250 mg dinoprost, but had returned to baseline at 24 hours after injection. No dinoprost associated gross lesions were detected. There was no evidence of toxicological effects. Thus, dinoprost had a safety factor of at least 10X on injection (25 mg luteolytic dose vs. 250 mg safe dose), based on studies conducted with cattle. At luteolytic doses, dinoprost had no effect on progeny. If given to a pregnant cow, it may cause abortion; the dose required for abortion varies considerably with the stage of gestation.

Induction of abortion in feedlot cattle at stages of gestation up to 100 days of gestation did not result in dystocia, retained placenta or death of heifers in the field studies. The smallness of the fetus at this early stage of gestation should not lead to complications at abortion. However, induction of parturition or abortion with any exogenous compound may precipitate dystocia, fetal death, retained placenta and/or metritis, especially at latter stages of gestation.

Swine: In pigs, evaluation was made of clinical observations, food consumption, clinical pathologic determinations, body weight changes, urinalysis, organ weights, and gross and microscopic observations following treatment with single doses of 10, 30, 50 and 100 mg dinoprost administered intramuscularly. The results indicated no treatment related effects from dinoprost treatment that were deleterious to the health of the animals or to their offspring.

Mares: Dinoprost tromethamine was administered to adult mares (weighing 320 to 485 kg; 2 to 20 years old), at the rates of 0, 100, 200, 400, and 800 mg per mare per day for 8 days. Route of administration for each dose group was both intramuscularly (2 mares) and subcutaneously (2 mares). Changes were detected in all treated groups for clinical (reduced sensitivity to pain; locomotor incoordination; hypergastromotility; sweating; hyperthermia; labored respiration), blood chemistry (elevated cholesterol, total bilirubin, LDH, and glucose), and hematology (decreased eosinophils; increased hemoglobin, hematocrit, and erythrocytes) measurements. The effects in the 100 mg dose, and to a lesser extent, the 200 mg dose groups were transient in nature, lasting for a few minutes to several hours. Mares did not appear to sustain adverse effects following termination of the side effects.

Mares treated with either 400 mg or 800 mg exhibited more profound symptoms. The excessive hyperstimulation of the gastrointestinal tract caused a protracted diarrhea, slight electrolyte imbalance (decreased sodium and potassium), dehydration, gastrointestinal irritation, and slight liver malfunction (elevated SGOT, SGPT at 800 mg only). Heart rate was increased but pH of the urine was decreased. Other measurements evaluated in the study remained within normal limits. No mortality occurred in any of the groups. No apparent differences were observed between the intramuscular and subcutaneous routes of administration. Luteolytic doses of dinoprost tromethamine are on the order of 5 to 10 mg administered on one day, therefore, dinoprost tromethamine sterile solution was demonstrated to have a wide margin of safety. Thus, the 100 mg dose gave a safety margin of 10 to 20X for a single injection or 80 to 160X for the 8 daily injections.

Additional studies investigated the effects in the mare of single intramuscular doses of 0, 0.25, 1.0, 2.5, 3.0, 5.0, and 10.0 mg dinoprost tromethamine. Heart rate, respiration rate, rectal temperature, and sweating were measured at 0, 0.25, 0.50, 0.75, 1.0, 1.5, 2.0, 3.0, 4.0, 5.0, and 6.0 hr. after injection. Neither heart rate nor respiration rates were significantly altered ($P > 0.05$) when compared to contemporary control values. Sweating was observed for 0 of 9, 2 of 9, 7 of 9, 9 of 9, and 8 of 9 mares injected with 0.25, 1.0, 2.5, 3.0, 5.0, or 10.0 mg dinoprost tromethamine, respectively. Sweating was temporary in all cases and was mild for doses of 3.0 mg or less but was extensive (beads of sweat over the entire body and dripping) for the 10 mg dose. Sweating after the 5.0 mg dose was intermediate between that seen for mares treated with 3.0 and 10.0 mg. Sweating began within 15 minutes after injection and ceased by 45 to 60 minutes after injection. Rectal temperature was decreased during the interval 0.5 until 1.0, 3 to 4, or 5 hours after injection for 0.25 and 1.0 mg, 2.5 and 3.0, or 5.0 and 10.0 mg dose groups, respectively. Average rectal temperature during the periods of decreased temperature was on the order of 97.5 to 99.6, with the greatest decreases observed in the 10 mg dose group.

Adverse Reactions:

Cattle:

1. The most frequently observed side effect is increased rectal temperature at a 5X or 10X overdose. However, rectal temperature change has been transient in all cases observed and has not been detrimental to the animal.
2. Limited salivation has been reported in some instances.
3. Intravenous administration might increase heart rate.
4. Localized post injection bacterial infections that may become generalized have been reported. In rare instances such infections have terminated fatally. See Cautions.

Swine: The most frequently observed side effects were erythema and pruritus, slight incoordination, nesting behavior, itching, urination, defecation, abdominal muscle spasms, tail movements, hyperpnea or dyspnea, increased vocalization, salivation, and at the 100 mg (10X) dose only, vomition. These side effects are transitory, lasting from 10 minutes to 3 hours, and were not detrimental to the health of the animal.

Mares: The most frequently observed side effects are sweating and decreased rectal temperature. However, these have been transient in all cases observed and have not been detrimental to the animal. Other reactions seen have been increase in heart rate, increase in respiration rate, some abdominal discomfort, locomotor incoordination, and lying down. These effects are usually seen within 15 minutes of injection and disappear within one hour. Mares usually continue to eat during the period of expression of side effects. One anaphylactic reaction of several hundred mares treated with dinoprost tromethamine sterile solution was reported but was not confirmed.

Presentation: PROSTAMATE™ Sterile Solution is available in 30 mL vials (NDC 11695-3580-5).

Manufactured by: Phoenix Scientific, Inc., St. Joseph, MO 64503

Compendium Code No.: 10821600 Iss. 2-00

PROSTAMATE® ℞

Phoenix Pharmaceutical **Prostaglandin**

(dinoprost tromethamine injection) Sterile Solution

ANADA No.: 200-253

Active Ingredient(s): This product contains the naturally occurring prostaglandin F2 alpha (dinoprost) as the tromethamine salt. Each mL contains dinoprost tromethamine equivalent to 5 mg dinoprost: also, benzyl alcohol, 9.45 mg added as preservative. When necessary, pH was adjusted with sodium hydroxide and/or hydrochloric acid. Dinoprost tromethamine is a white or slightly off-white crystalline powder that is readily soluble in water at room temperature in concentrations to at least 200 mg/mL.

Indications: For intramuscular use for estrus synchronization, treatment of unobserved (silent) estrus and pyometra (chronic endometritis) in cattle; for abortion of feedlot and other non-lactating cattle; for parturition induction in swine; and for controlling the timing of estrus in estrous cycling mares and clinically anestrous mares that have a corpus luteum.

Cattle: PROSTAMATE® Sterile Solution is indicated as a luteolytic agent.

PROSTAMATE® is effective only in those cattle having a corpus luteum, i.e., those which ovulated at least five days prior to treatment. Future reproductive performance of animals that are not cycling will be unaffected by injection of PROSTAMATE®.

Swine: For intramuscular use for parturition induction in swine. PROSTAMATE® Sterile Solution is indicated for parturition induction in swine when injected within 3 days of normal predicted farrowing.

Mares: PROSTAMATE® Sterile Solution is indicated for its luteolytic effect in mares. This luteolytic effect can be utilized to control the timing of estrus in estrous cycling and clinically anestrous mares that have a corpus luteum.

Pharmacology: General Biologic Activity: Prostaglandins occur in nearly all mammalian tissues. Prostaglandins, especially PGE's and PGF's, have been shown, in certain species, to 1) increase at time of parturition in amniotic fluid, maternal placenta, myometrium, and blood, 2) stimulate myometrial activity, and 3) to induce either abortion or parturition. Prostaglandins, especially PGF2α, have been shown to 1) increase in the uterus and blood to levels similar to levels achieved by exogenous administration which elicited luteolysis, 2) be capable of crossing from the uterine vein to the ovarian artery (sheep), 3) be related to IUD induced luteal regression (sheep), and 4) be capable of regressing the corpus luteum of most mammalian species studied to date. Prostaglandins have been reported to result in release of pituitary tropic hormones. Data suggest prostaglandins, especially PGE's and PGF's, may be involved in the process of ovulation and gamete transport. Also PGF2α has been reported to cause increase in blood pressure, bronchoconstriction, and smooth muscle stimulation in certain species.

Metabolism: A number of metabolism studies have been done in laboratory animals. The metabolism of tritium labeled dinoprost (^{3}H PGF2 alpha) in the rat and in the monkey was similar. Although quantitative differences were observed, qualitatively similar metabolites were produced. A study demonstrated that equimolar doses of ^{3}H PGF2 alpha Tham and ^{3}H PGF2 alpha free acid administered intravenously to rats demonstrated no significant differences in blood concentration of dinoprost. An interesting observation in the above study was that the radioactive dose of ^{3}H PGF2 alpha rapidly distributed in tissues and dissipated in tissues with almost the same curve as it did in the serum. The half-life of dinoprost in bovine blood has been reported to be on the order of minutes. A complete study on the distribution of decline of ^{3}H PGF2 alpha Tham in the tissue of rats was well correlated with the work done in the cow. Cattle serum collected during 24 hours after doses of 0 to 250 mg dinoprost have been assayed by RIA for dinoprost and the 15-keto metabolites. These data support previous reports that dinoprost has a half-life of minutes. Dinoprost is a natural prostaglandin. All systems associated with dinoprost metabolism exist in the body; therefore, no new metabolic, transport, excretory, binding or other systems need be established by the body to metabolize injected dinoprost.

Dosage and Administration:

Cattle: PROSTAMATE® Sterile Solution is supplied at a concentration of 5 mg dinoprost per mL. PROSTAMATE® is luteolytic in cattle at 25 mg (5 mL) administered intramuscularly. As with any multidose vial, practice aseptic techniques in withdrawing each dose. Adequately clean and disinfect the vial closure prior to entry with a sterile needle.

Instructions for Use:

1. For Intramuscular Use for Estrus Synchronization in Beef Cattle and Non-Lactating Dairy Heifers. PROSTAMATE® is used to control the timing of estrus and ovulation in estrous cycling cattle that have a corpus luteum.

   Inject a dose of 5 mL PROSTAMATE® (25 mg PGF2α) intramuscularly either once or twice at a 10 to 12 day interval.

   With the single injection, cattle should be bred at the usual time relative to estrus. With the two injections cattle can be bred after the second injection either at the usual time relative to detected estrus or at about 80 hours after the second injection of PROSTAMATE®.

   Estrus is expected to occur 1 to 5 days after injection if a corpus luteum was present. Cattle that do not become pregnant to breeding at estrus on days 1 to 5 after injection will be expected to return to estrus in about 18 to 24 days.
2. For Intramuscular Use for Unobserved (Silent) Estrus in Lactating Dairy Cows with a Corpus Luteum. Inject a dose of 5 mL PROSTAMATE® (25 mg PGF2α) intramuscularly. Breed cows as they are detected in estrus. If estrus has not been observed by 80 hours after injection, breed at 80 hours. If the cow returns to estrus breed at the usual time relative to estrus.

Management Considerations: Many factors contribute to success and failure of reproduction management, and these factors are important also when time of breeding is to be regulated with PROSTAMATE® Sterile Solution. Some of these factors are:

a. Cattle must be ready to breed-they must have a corpus luteum and be healthy;
b. Nutritional status must be adequate as this has a direct effect on conception and the initiation of estrus in heifers or return of estrous cycles in cows following calving;
c. Physical facilities must be adequate to allow cattle handling without being detrimental to the animal;
d. Estrus must be detected accurately if timed A1 is not employed;
e. Semen of high fertility must be used;
f. Semen must be inseminated properly.

P

A successful breeding program can employ PROSTAMATE® effectively, but a poorly managed breeding program will continue to be poor when PROSTAMATE® is employed unless other management deficiencies are remedied first.

Cattle expressing estrus following PROSTAMATE® are receptive to breeding by a bull. Using bulls to breed large numbers of cattle in heat following PROSTAMATE® will require proper management of bulls and cattle.

3. For Intramuscular Use for Treatment of Pyometra (chronic endometritis) in Cattle. Inject a dose of 5 mL PROSTAMATE® (25 mg PGF2α) intramuscularly. In studies conducted with dinoprost tromethamine sterile solution, pyometra was defined as presence of a corpus luteum in the ovary and uterine horns containing fluid but not a conceptus based on palpation *per rectum.* Return to normal was defined as evacuation of fluid and return of the uterine horn size to 40 mm or less based on palpation *per rectum* at 14 and 28 days. Most cattle that recovered in response to PROSTAMATE® recovered within 14 days after injection. After 14 days, recovery rate of treated cattle was no different than that of non-treated cattle.
4. For Intramuscular Use for Abortion of Feedlot and Other Non-Lactating Cattle. PROSTAMATE® is indicated for its abortifacient effect in feedlot and other non-lactating cattle during the first 100 days of gestation. Inject a dose of 25 mg intramuscularly. Cattle that abort will abort within 35 days of injection.

   Commercial cattle were palpated *per rectum* for pregnancy in six feedlots. The percent of pregnant cattle in each feedlot less than 100 days of gestation ranged between 26 and 84; 80% or more of the pregnant cattle were less than 150 days of gestation. The abortion rates following injection of dinoprost tromethamine sterile solution increased with increasing doses up to about 25 mg. As examples, the abortion rates, over 7 feedlots on the dose titration study, were 22%, 50%, 71%, 90% and 78% for cattle up to 100 days of gestation when injected IM with dinoprost tromethamine sterile solution doses of 0, 1 (5 mg), 2 (10 mg), 4 (20 mg) and 8 (40 mg) mL, respectively. The statistical predicted relative abortion rate based on the dose titration data, was about 93% for the 5 mL (25 mg) dinoprost tromethamine sterile solution dose for cattle injected up to 100 days of gestation.

Swine: PROSTAMATE® Sterile Solution will induce parturition in swine at 10 mg (2 mL) when injected intramuscularly.

As with any multidose vial, practice aseptic techniques in withdrawing each dose. Adequately clean and disinfect the vial closure prior to entry with a sterile needle.

Instructions for Use: The response to treatment varies by individual animals with a mean interval from administration of 2 mL PROSTAMATE® (10 mg dinoprost) to parturition of approximately 30 hours. This can be employed to control the time of farrowing in sows and gilts in late gestation.

Management Considerations: Several factors must be considered for the successful use of PROSTAMATE® Sterile Solution for parturition induction in swine. The product must be administered at a relatively specific time (treatment earlier than 3 days prior to normal predicted farrowing may result in increased piglet mortality). It is important that adequate records be maintained on (1) the average length of gestation period for the animals on a specific location, and (2) the breeding and projected farrowing dates for each animal. This information is essential to determine the appropriate time for administration of PROSTAMATE®.

Mares:

1. Evaluate the reproductive status of the mare.
2. Administer a single intramuscular injection of 1 mg per 100 lbs (45.5 kg) body weight which is usually 1 mL to 2 mL PROSTAMATE® Sterile Solution.
3. Observe for signs of estrus by means of daily teasing with a stallion, and evaluate follicular changes on the ovary by palpation of the ovary *per rectum*.
4. Some clinically anestrous mares will not express estrus but will develop a follicle which will ovulate. These mares may become pregnant if inseminated at the appropriate time relative to rupture of the follicle.
5. Breed mares in estrus in a manner consistent with normal management.

Dinoprost tromethamine is administered once as a single intramuscular injection of 1 mg per 100 lbs (45.5 kg) body weight which is usually 1 mL to 2 mL of PROSTAMATE® containing 5 mg dinoprost as the tromethamine salt per milliliter.

Instructions for Use: PROSTAMATE® Sterile Solution is indicated for its luteolytic effect in mares. This luteolytic effect can be utilized to control the timing of estrus in estrous cycling and clinically anestrous mares that have a corpus luteum in the following circumstances:

1. Controlling Time of Estrus of Estrous Cycling Mares: Mares treated with PROSTAMATE® during diestrus (4 or more days after ovulation) will return to estrus within 2 to 4 days in most cases and ovulate 8 to 12 days after treatment. This procedure may be utilized as an aid to scheduling the use of stallions.
2. Difficult-to-Breed Mares: In extended diestrus there is failure to exhibit regular estrous cycles which is different from true anestrus. Many mares described as anestrus during the breeding season have serum progesterone levels consistent with the presence of a functional corpus luteum.

   A proportion of "barren", maiden, and lactating mares do not exhibit regular estrous cycles and may be in extended diestrus. Following abortion, early fetal death and resorption, or as a result of "pseudopregnancy", there may be serum progesterone levels consistent with a functional corpus luteum.

   Treatment of such mares with PROSTAMATE® usually results in regression of the corpus luteum followed by estrus and/or ovulation. In one study with 122 Standardbred and Thoroughbred mares in clinical anestrus for an average of 58 days and treated during the breeding season, behavioral estrus was detected in 81 percent at an average time of 3.7 days after injection with 5 mg dinoprost tromethamine sterile solution; ovulation occurred an average of 7.0 days after treatment. Of those mares bred, 59% were pregnant following an average of 1.4 services during that estrus.

   Treatment of "anestrous" mares which abort subsequent to 36 days of pregnancy may not result in return to estrus due to presence of functional endometrial cups.

Precaution(s): Storage Conditions: Store at controlled room temperature 20° to 25°C (68° to 77°F).

Caution(s): Federal (USA) law restricts this drug to use by or on the order of a licensed veterinarian.

Cattle: Do not administer to pregnant cattle unless abortion is desired.

Do not administer intravenously (I.V.), as this route might potentiate adverse reactions.

Cattle administered a progestogen would be expected to have a reduced response to PROSTAMATE® Sterile Solution.

Aggressive antibiotic therapy should be employed at the first sign of infection at the injection site whether localized or diffuse. As with all parenteral products careful aseptic techniques should be employed to decrease the possibility of post injection bacterial infections.

Swine: Do not administer to sows and/or gilts prior to 3 days of normal predicted farrowing, as increased number of stillborn and postnatal mortality may result.

Mares: PROSTAMATE® Sterile Solution is ineffective when administered prior to day-5 after ovulation.

Pregnancy status should be determined prior to treatment, since PROSTAMATE® has been reported to induce abortion and parturition when sufficient doses were administered.

Mares should not be treated if they suffer from either acute or subacute disorders of the vascular system, gastrointestinal tract, respiratory system, or reproductive tract.

Do not administer by intravenous route.

Nonsteroidal anti-inflammatory drugs (i.e., indomethacin) may inhibit prostaglandin synthesis, therefore these drugs should not be administered concurrently.

Restricted Drug-Use only as directed (California).

For use in animals only.

Warning(s):

Cattle: No milk discard or preslaughter drug withdrawal period is required for labeled uses.

Swine: No preslaughter drug withdrawal period is required for labeled uses.

Mares: Not for use in horses intended for food.

Not for human use.

Women of child-bearing age, asthmatics, and persons with bronchial and other respiratory problems should exercise extreme caution when handling this product. In the early stages, women may be unaware of their pregnancies. Dinoprost tromethamine is readily absorbed through the skin and can cause abortion and/or bronchiospasms. Direct contact with the skin should, therefore, be avoided. Accidental spillage on the skin should be washed off immediately with soap and water.

Use of this product in excess of the approved dose may result in drug residues.

Keep out of reach of children.

Toxicology: Safety and Toxicity:

Laboratory Animals: Dinoprost was non-teratogenic in rats when administered orally at 1.25, 3.2, 10.0 and 20.0 mg/kg/day from day 6th-15th of gestation or when administered subcutaneously at 0.5 and 1.0 mg/kg/day on gestation days 6, 7 and 8 or 9, 10 and 11 or 12, 13 and 14. Dinoprost was non-teratogenic in the rabbit when administered either subcutaneously at doses of 0.5 and 1.0 mg/kg/day on gestation days 6, 7 and 8 or 9, 10 and 11 or 12, 13 and 14 or 15, 16 and 17 or orally at doses of 0.01, 0.1 and 1.0 mg/kg/day on days 6-18 or 5.0 mg/kg/day on days 8-18 of gestation. A slight and marked embryo lethal effect was observed in dams given 1.0 and 5.0 mg/kg/day respectively. This was due to the expected luteolytic properties of the drug.

A 14-day continuous intravenous infusion study in rats at 20 mg PGF2α per kg body weight indicated prostaglandins of the F series could induce bone deposition. However, such bone changes were not observed in monkeys similarly administered dinoprost tromethamine sterile solution at 15 mg PGF2α per kg body weight for 14 days.

Cattle: In cattle, evaluation was made of clinical observations, clinical chemistry, hematology, urinalysis, organ weights, and gross plus microscopic measurements following treatment with various doses up to 250 mg dinoprost administered twice intramuscularly at a 10 day interval or doses of 25 mg administered daily for 10 days. There was no unequivocal effect of dinoprost on the hematology or clinical chemistry parameters measured. Clinically, a slight transitory increase in heart rate was detected. Rectal temperature was elevated about 1.5°F through the 6th hour after injection with 250 mg dinoprost, but had returned to baseline at 24 hours after injection. No dinoprost associated gross lesions were detected. There was no evidence of toxicological effects. Thus, dinoprost had a safety factor of at least 10X on injection (25 mg luteolytic dose vs. 250 mg safe dose), based on studies conducted with cattle. At luteolytic doses, dinoprost had no effect on progeny. If given to a pregnant cow, it may cause abortion; the dose required for abortion varies considerably with the stage of gestation.

Induction of abortion in feedlot cattle at stages of gestation up to 100 days of gestation did not result in dystocia, retained placenta or death of heifers in the field studies. The smallness of the fetus at this early stage of gestation should not lead to complications at abortion. However, induction of parturition or abortion with any exogenous compound may precipitate dystocia, fetal death, retained placenta and/or metritis, especially at latter stages of gestation.

Swine: In pigs, evaluation was made of clinical observations, food consumption, clinical pathologic determinations, body weight changes, urinalysis, organ weights, and gross and microscopic observations following treatment with single doses of 10, 30, 50 and 100 mg dinoprost administered intramuscularly. The results indicated no treatment related effects from dinoprost treatment that were deleterious to the health of the animals or to their offspring.

Mares: Dinoprost tromethamine was administered to adult mares (weighing 320 to 485 kg; 2 to 20 years old), at the rates of 0, 100, 200, 400, and 800 mg per mare per day for 8 days. Route of administration for each dose group was both intramuscularly (2 mares) and subcutaneously (2 mares). Changes were detected in all treated groups for clinical (reduced sensitivity to pain; locomotor incoordination; hypergastromotility; sweating; hyperthermia; labored respiration), blood chemistry (elevated cholesterol, total bilirubin, LDH, and glucose), and hematology (decreased eosinophils; increased hemoglobin, hematocrit, and erythrocytes) measurements. The effects in the 100 mg dose, and to a lesser extent, the 200 mg dose groups were transient in nature, lasting for a few minutes to several hours. Mares did not appear to sustain adverse effects following termination of the side effects.

Mares treated with either 400 mg or 800 mg exhibited more profound symptoms. The excessive hyperstimulation of the gastrointestinal tract caused a protracted diarrhea, slight electrolyte imbalance (decreased sodium and potassium), dehydration, gastrointestinal irritation, and slight liver malfunction (elevated SGOT, SGPT at 800 mg only). Heart rate was increased but pH of the urine was decreased. Other measurements evaluated in the study remained within normal limits. No mortality occurred in any of the groups. No apparent differences were observed between the intramuscular and subcutaneous routes of administration. Luteolytic doses of dinoprost tromethamine are on the order of 5 to 10 mg administered on one day, therefore, dinoprost tromethamine sterile solution was demonstrated to have a wide margin of safety. Thus, the 100 mg dose gave a safety margin of 10 to 20X for a single injection or 80 to 160X for the 8 daily injections.

Additional studies investigated the effects in the mare of single intramuscular doses of 0, 0.25, 1.0, 2.5, 3.0, 5.0, and 10.0 mg dinoprost tromethamine. Heart rate, respiration rate, rectal temperature, and sweating were measured at 0, 0.25, 0.50, 0.75, 1.0, 1.5, 2.0, 3.0, 4.0, 5.0, and 6.0 hr. after injection. Neither heart rate nor respiration rates were significantly altered ($P > 0.05$) when compared to contemporary control values. Sweating was observed for 0 of 9, 2 of 9, 7 of 9, 9 of 9, and 8 of 9 mares injected with 0.25, 1.0, 2.5, 3.0, 5.0, or 10.0 mg dinoprost tromethamine, respectively. Sweating was temporary in all cases and was mild for doses of 3.0 mg or less but was extensive (beads of sweat over the entire body and dripping) for the 10 mg dose. Sweating after the 5.0 mg dose was intermediate between that seen for mares treated with 3.0 and 10.0 mg. Sweating began within 15 minutes after injection and ceased by 45 to 60 minutes after injection. Rectal temperature was decreased during the interval 0.5 until 1.0, 3 to 4, or 5 hours after injection for 0.25 and 1.0 mg, 2.5 and 3.0, or 5.0 and 10.0 mg dose groups, respectively. Average rectal temperature during the periods of decreased temperature was on the order of 97.5 to 99.6, with the greatest decreases observed in the 10 mg dose group.

Adverse Reactions:

Cattle:

1. The most frequently observed side effect is increased rectal temperature at a 5X or 10X overdose. However, rectal temperature change has been transient in all cases observed and has not been detrimental to the animal.
2. Limited salivation has been reported in some instances.
3. Intravenous administration might increase heart rate.
4. Localized post injection bacterial infections that may become generalized have been reported. In rare instances such infections have terminated fatally. See Cautions.

Swine: The most frequently observed side effects were erythema and pruritus, slight incoordination, nesting behavior, itching, urination, defecation, abdominal muscle spasms, tail movements, hyperpnea or dyspnea, increased vocalization, salivation, and at the 100 mg (10X) dose only, vomition. These side effects are transitory, lasting from 10 minutes to 3 hours, and were not detrimental to the health of the animal.

Mares: The most frequently observed side effects are sweating and decreased rectal temperature. However, these have been transient in all cases observed and have not been detrimental to the animal. Other reactions seen have been increase in heart rate, increase in respiration rate, some abdominal discomfort, locomotor incoordination, and lying down. These effects are usually seen within 15 minutes of injection and disappear within one hour. Mares usually continue to eat during the period of expression of side effects. One anaphylactic reaction of several hundred mares treated with dinoprost tromethamine sterile solution was reported but was not confirmed.

Presentation: PROSTAMATE® Sterile Solution is available in 30 mL vials (NDC 57319-433-03).

Manufactured by: Phoenix Scientific, Inc., St. Joseph, MO 64503.

Compendium Code No.: 12560742 Rev. 10-01

PROSTAMATE™ ℞

RXV **Prostaglandin**

(dinoprost tromethamine injection) Sterile Solution

ANADA No.: 200-253

Active Ingredient(s): This product contains the naturally occurring prostaglandin F2 alpha (dinoprost) as the tromethamine salt. Each mL contains dinoprost tromethamine equivalent to 5 mg dinoprost: also, benzyl alcohol, 9.45 mg added as preservative. When necessary, pH was adjusted with sodium hydroxide and/or hydrochloric acid. Dinoprost tromethamine is a white or slightly off-white crystalline powder that is readily soluble in water at room temperature in concentrations to at least 200 mg/mL.

Indications: For intramuscular use for estrus synchronization, treatment of unobserved (silent) estrus and pyometra (chronic endometritis) in cattle; for abortion of feedlot and other non-lactating cattle; for parturition induction in swine; and for controlling the timing of estrus in estrous cycling mares and clinically anestrous mares that have a corpus luteum.

Cattle: PROSTAMATE™ Sterile Solution is indicated as a luteolytic agent.

PROSTAMATE™ is effective only in those cattle having a corpus luteum, i.e., those which ovulated at least five days prior to treatment. Future reproductive performance of animals that are not cycling will be unaffected by injection of PROSTAMATE™.

Swine: For intramuscular use for parturition induction in swine. PROSTAMATE™ Sterile Solution is indicated for parturition induction in swine when injected within 3 days of normal predicted farrowing.

Mares: PROSTAMATE™ Sterile Solution is indicated for its luteolytic effect in mares. This luteolytic effect can be utilized to control the timing of estrus in estrous cycling and clinically anestrous mares that have a corpus luteum.

Pharmacology:

General Biologic Activity: Prostaglandins occur in nearly all mammalian tissues. Prostaglandins, especially PGE's and PGF's, have been shown, in certain species, to 1) increase at time of parturition in amniotic fluid, maternal placenta, myometrium, and blood, 2) stimulate myometrial activity, and 3) to induce either abortion or parturition. Prostaglandins, especially PGF2α, have been shown to 1) increase in the uterus and blood to levels similar to levels achieved by exogenous administration which elicited luteolysis, 2) be capable of crossing from the uterine vein to the ovarian artery (sheep), 3) be related to IUD induced luteal regression (sheep), and 4) be capable of regressing the corpus luteum of most mammalian species studied to date. Prostaglandins have been reported to result in release of pituitary tropic hormones. Data suggest prostaglandins, especially PGE's and PGF's, may be involved in the process of ovulation and gamete transport. Also PGF2α has been reported to cause increase in blood pressure, bronchoconstriction, and smooth muscle stimulation in certain species.

Metabolism: A number of metabolism studies have been done in laboratory animals. The metabolism of tritium labeled dinoprost (^{3}H PGF2 alpha) in the rat and in the monkey was similar. Although quantitative differences were observed, qualitatively similar metabolites were produced. A study demonstrated that equimolar doses of ^{3}H PGF2 alpha Tham and ^{3}H PGF2 alpha free acid administered intravenously to rats demonstrated no significant differences in blood concentration of dinoprost. An interesting observation in the above study was that the radioactive dose of ^{3}H PGF2 alpha rapidly distributed in tissues and dissipated in tissues with almost the same curve as it did in the serum. The half-life of dinoprost in bovine blood has been reported to be on the order of minutes. A complete study on the distribution of decline of ^{3}H PGF2 alpha Tham in the tissue of rats was well correlated with the work done in the cow. Cattle serum collected during 24 hours after doses of 0 to 250 mg dinoprost have been assayed by RIA for dinoprost and the 15-keto metabolites. These data support previous reports that dinoprost has a half-life of minutes. Dinoprost is a natural prostaglandin. All systems associated with dinoprost metabolism exist in the body; therefore, no new metabolic, transport, excretory, binding or other systems need be established by the body to metabolize injected dinoprost.

Dosage and Administration:

Cattle: PROSTAMATE™ Sterile Solution is supplied at a concentration of 5 mg dinoprost per mL. PROSTAMATE™ is luteolytic in cattle at 25 mg (5 mL) administered intramuscularly. As with any multidose vial, practice aseptic techniques in withdrawing each dose. Adequately clean and disinfect the vial closure prior to entry with a sterile needle.

Instructions for Use:

1. For Intramuscular Use for Estrus Synchronization in Beef Cattle and Non-Lactating Dairy Heifers. PROSTAMATE™ is used to control the timing of estrus and ovulation in estrous cycling cattle that have a corpus luteum.

   Inject a dose of 5 mL PROSTAMATE™ (25 mg PGF2α) intramuscularly either once or twice at a 10 to 12 day interval.

   With the single injection, cattle should be bred at the usual time relative to estrus. With the two injections cattle can be bred after the second injection either at the usual time relative to detected estrus or at about 80 hours after the second injection of PROSTAMATE™.

   Estrus is expected to occur 1 to 5 days after injection if a corpus luteum was present. Cattle that do not become pregnant to breeding at estrus on days 1 to 5 after injection will be expected to return to estrus in about 18 to 24 days.
2. For Intramuscular Use for Unobserved (Silent) Estrus in Lactating Dairy Cows with a Corpus Luteum. Inject a dose of 5 mL PROSTAMATE™ (25 mg PGF2α) intramuscularly. Breed cows as they are detected in estrus. If estrus has not been observed by 80 hours after injection, breed at 80 hours. If the cow returns to estrus breed at the usual time relative to estrus.

Management Considerations: Many factors contribute to success and failure of reproduction management, and these factors are important also when time of breeding is to be regulated with PROSTAMATE™ Sterile Solution. Some of these factors are:

a. Cattle must be ready to breed-they must have a corpus luteum and be healthy;
b. Nutritional status must be adequate as this has a direct effect on conception and the initiation of estrus in heifers or return of estrous cycles in cows following calving;
c. Physical facilities must be adequate to allow cattle handling without being detrimental to the animal;
d. Estrus must be detected accurately if timed A1 is not employed;
e. Semen of high fertility must be used;
f. Semen must be inseminated properly.

A successful breeding program can employ PROSTAMATE™ effectively, but a poorly managed breeding program will continue to be poor when PROSTAMATE™ is employed unless other management deficiencies are remedied first.

Cattle expressing estrus following PROSTAMATE™ are receptive to breeding by a bull. Using bulls to breed large numbers of cattle in heat following PROSTAMATE™ will require proper management of bulls and cattle.

3. For Intramuscular Use for Treatment of Pyometra (chronic endometritis) in Cattle. Inject a dose of 5 mL PROSTAMATE™ (25 mg PGF2α) intramuscularly. In studies conducted with dinoprost tromethamine sterile solution, pyometra was defined as presence of a corpus luteum in the ovary and uterine horns containing fluid but not a conceptus based on palpation *per rectum*. Return to normal was defined as evacuation of fluid and return of the uterine horn size to 40 mm or less based on palpation *per rectum* at 14 and 28 days. Most cattle that recovered in response to PROSTAMATE™ recovered within 14 days after injection. After 14 days, recovery rate of treated cattle was no different than that of non-treated cattle.
4. For Intramuscular Use for Abortion of Feedlot and Other Non-Lactating Cattle. PROSTAMATE™ is indicated for its abortifacient effect in feedlot and other non-lactating cattle during the first 100 days of gestation. Inject a dose of 25 mg intramuscularly. Cattle that abort will abort within 35 days of injection.

   Commercial cattle were palpated *per rectum* for pregnancy in six feedlots. The percent of pregnant cattle in each feedlot less than 100 days of gestation ranged between 26 and 84; 80% or more of the pregnant cattle were less than 150 days of gestation. The abortion rates following injection of dinoprost tromethamine sterile solution increased with increasing doses up to about 25 mg. As examples, the abortion rates, over 7 feedlots on the dose titration study, were 22%, 50%, 71%, 90% and 78% for cattle up to 100 days of gestation when injected IM with dinoprost tromethamine sterile solution doses of 0, 1 (5 mg), 2 (10 mg), 4 (20 mg) and 8 (40 mg) mL, respectively. The statistical predicted relative abortion rate based on the dose titration data, was about 93% for the 5 mL (25 mg) dinoprost tromethamine sterile solution dose for cattle injected up to 100 days of gestation.

Swine: PROSTAMATE™ Sterile Solution will induce parturition in swine at 10 mg (2 mL) when injected intramuscularly.

As with any multidose vial, practice aseptic techniques in withdrawing each dose. Adequately clean and disinfect the vial closure prior to entry with a sterile needle.

Instructions for Use: The response to treatment varies by individual animals with a mean interval from administration of 2 mL PROSTAMATE™ (10 mg dinoprost) to parturition of approximately 30 hours. This can be employed to control the time of farrowing in sows and gilts in late gestation.

Management Considerations: Several factors must be considered for the successful use of PROSTAMATE™ Sterile Solution for parturition induction in swine. The product must be administered at a relatively specific time (treatment earlier than 3 days prior to normal predicted farrowing may result in increased piglet mortality). It is important that adequate records be maintained on (1) the average length of gestation period for the animals on a specific location, and (2) the breeding and projected farrowing dates for each animal. This information is essential to determine the appropriate time for administration of PROSTAMATE™.

Mares:

1. Evaluate the reproductive status of the mare.
2. Administer a single intramuscular injection of 1 mg per 100 lbs (45.5 kg) body weight which is usually 1 mL to 2 mL PROSTAMATE™ Sterile Solution.
3. Observe for signs of estrus by means of daily teasing with a stallion, and evaluate follicular changes on the ovary by palpation of the ovary *per rectum*.
4. Some clinically anestrous mares will not express estrus but will develop a follicle which will ovulate. These mares may become pregnant if inseminated at the appropriate time relative to rupture of the follicle.
5. Breed mares in estrus in a manner consistent with normal management.

Dinoprost tromethamine is administered once as a single intramuscular injection of 1 mg per 100 lbs (45.5 kg) body weight which is usually 1 mL to 2 mL of PROSTAMATE™ containing 5 mg dinoprost as the tromethamine salt per milliliter.

Instructions for Use: PROSTAMATE™ Sterile Solution is indicated for its luteolytic effect in mares. This luteolytic effect can be utilized to control the timing of estrus in estrous cycling and clinically anestrous mares that have a corpus luteum in the following circumstances:

1. Controlling Time of Estrus of Estrous Cycling Mares: Mares treated with PROSTAMATE™ during diestrus (4 or more days after ovulation) will return to estrus within 2 to 4 days in most cases and ovulate 8 to 12 days after treatment. This procedure may be utilized as an aid to scheduling the use of stallions.
2. Difficult-to-Breed Mares: In extended diestrus there is failure to exhibit regular estrous cycles which is different from true anestrus. Many mares described as anestrus during the breeding season have serum progesterone levels consistent with the presence of a functional corpus luteum.

   A proportion of "barren", maiden, and lactating mares do not exhibit regular estrous cycles and may be in extended diestrus. Following abortion, early fetal death and resorption, or as a result of "pseudopregnancy", there may be serum progesterone levels consistent with a functional corpus luteum.

   Treatment of such mares with PROSTAMATE™ usually results in regression of the corpus luteum followed by estrus and/or ovulation. In one study with 122 Standardbred and Thoroughbred mares in clinical anestrus for an average of 58 days and treated during the breeding season, behavioral estrus was detected in 81 percent at an average time of 3.7 days after injection with 5 mg dinoprost tromethamine sterile solution; ovulation occurred an average of 7.0 days after treatment. Of those mares bred, 59% were pregnant following an average of 1.4 services during that estrus.

   Treatment of "anestrous" mares which abort subsequent to 36 days of pregnancy may not result in return to estrus due to presence of functional endometrial cups.

Precaution(s): Store at controlled room temperature 20°-25°C (68°-77°F).

Caution(s): Federal (USA) law restricts this drug to use by or on the order of a licensed veterinarian.

Cattle: Do not administer to pregnant cattle unless abortion is desired.

Do not administer intravenously (I.V.), as this route might potentiate adverse reactions.

Cattle administered a progestogen would be expected to have a reduced response to PROSTAMATE™ Sterile Solution.

Aggressive antibiotic therapy should be employed at the first sign of infection at the injection site whether localized or diffuse. As with all parenteral products careful aseptic techniques should be employed to decrease the possibility of post injection bacterial infections.

Swine: Do not administer to sows and/or gilts prior to 3 days of normal predicted farrowing, as increased number of stillborn and postnatal mortality may result.

Mares: PROSTAMATE™ Sterile Solution is ineffective when administered prior to day-5 after ovulation.

Pregnancy status should be determined prior to treatment, since PROSTAMATE™ has been reported to induce abortion and parturition when sufficient doses were administered.

Mares should not be treated if they suffer from either acute or subacute disorders of the vascular system, gastrointestinal tract, respiratory system, or reproductive tract.

Do not administer by intravenous route.

Nonsteroidal anti-inflammatory drugs (i.e., indomethacin) may inhibit prostaglandin synthesis, therefore these drugs should not be administered concurrently.

Warning(s):

Cattle: No milk discard or preslaughter drug withdrawal period is required for labeled uses.

Swine: No preslaughter drug withdrawal period is required for labeled uses.

Mares: Not for use in horses intended for food.

Not for human use.

Women of child-bearing age, asthmatics, and persons with bronchial and other respiratory problems should exercise extreme caution when handling this product. In the early stages, women may be unaware of their pregnancies. Dinoprost tromethamine is readily absorbed through the skin and can cause abortion and/or bronchiospasms. Direct contact with the skin should, therefore, be avoided. Accidental spillage on the skin should be washed off immediately with soap and water.

Use of this product in excess of the approved dose may result in drug residues.

For use in animals only.

Restricted drug-Use only as directed (California).

Keep out of reach of children.

Toxicology: Safety and Toxicity:

Laboratory Animals: Dinoprost was non-teratogenic in rats when administered orally at 1.25, 3.2, 10.0 and 20.0 mg/kg/day from day 6th-15th of gestation or when administered subcutaneously at 0.5 and 1.0 mg/kg/day on gestation days 6, 7 and 8 or 9, 10 and 11 or 12, 13 and 14. Dinoprost was non-teratogenic in the rabbit when administered either subcutaneously at doses of 0.5 and 1.0 mg/kg/day on gestation days 6, 7 and 8 or 9, 10 and 11 or 12, 13 and 14 or 15, 16 and 17 or orally at doses of 0.01, 0.1 and 1.0 mg/kg/day on days 6-18 or 5.0 mg/kg/day on days 8-18 of gestation. A slight and marked embryo lethal effect was observed in dams given 1.0 and 5.0 mg/kg/day respectively. This was due to the expected luteolytic properties of the drug.

A 14-day continuous intravenous infusion study in rats at 20 mg PGF2α per kg body weight indicated prostaglandins of the F series could induce bone deposition. However, such bone changes were not observed in monkeys similarly administered dinoprost tromethamine sterile solution at 15 mg PGF2α per kg body weight for 14 days.

Cattle: In cattle, evaluation was made of clinical observations, clinical chemistry, hematology, urinalysis, organ weights, and gross plus microscopic measurements following treatment with various doses up to 250 mg dinoprost administered twice intramuscularly at a 10 day interval or doses of 25 mg administered daily for 10 days. There was no unequivocal effect of dinoprost on the hematology or clinical chemistry parameters measured. Clinically, a slight transitory increase in heart rate was detected. Rectal temperature was elevated about 1.5°F through the 6th hour after injection with 250 mg dinoprost, but had returned to baseline at 24 hours after injection. No dinoprost associated gross lesions were detected. There was no evidence of toxicological effects. Thus, dinoprost had a safety factor of at least 10X on injection (25 mg luteolytic dose vs. 250 mg safe dose), based on studies conducted with cattle. At luteolytic doses, dinoprost had no effect on progeny. If given to a pregnant cow, it may cause abortion; the dose required for abortion varies considerably with the stage of gestation.

Induction of abortion in feedlot cattle at stages of gestation up to 100 days of gestation did not result in dystocia, retained placenta or death of heifers in the field studies. The smallness of the fetus at this early stage of gestation should not lead to complications at abortion. However, induction of parturition or abortion with any exogenous compound may precipitate dystocia, fetal death, retained placenta and/or metritis, especially at latter stages of gestation.

Swine: In pigs, evaluation was made of clinical observations, food consumption, clinical pathologic determinations, body weight changes, urinalysis, organ weights, and gross and microscopic observations following treatment with single doses of 10, 30, 50 and 100 mg dinoprost administered intramuscularly. The results indicated no treatment related effects from dinoprost treatment that were deleterious to the health of the animals or to their offspring.

Mares: Dinoprost tromethamine was administered to adult mares (weighing 320 to 485 kg; 2 to 20 years old), at the rates of 0, 100, 200, 400, and 800 mg per mare per day for 8 days. Route of administration for each dose group was both intramuscularly (2 mares) and subcutaneously (2 mares). Changes were detected in all treated groups for clinical (reduced sensitivity to pain; locomotor incoordination; hypergastromotility; sweating; hyperthermia; labored respiration), blood chemistry (elevated cholesterol, total bilirubin, LDH, and glucose), and hematology (decreased eosinophils; increased hemoglobin, hematocrit, and erythrocytes) measurements. The effects in the 100 mg dose, and to a lesser extent, the 200 mg dose groups were transient in nature, lasting for a few minutes to several hours. Mares did not appear to sustain adverse effects following termination of the side effects.

Mares treated with either 400 mg or 800 mg exhibited more profound symptoms. The excessive hyperstimulation of the gastrointestinal tract caused a protracted diarrhea, slight electrolyte imbalance (decreased sodium and potassium), dehydration, gastrointestinal irritation, and slight liver malfunction (elevated SGOT, SGPT at 800 mg only). Heart rate was increased but pH of the urine was decreased. Other measurements evaluated in the study remained within normal limits. No mortality occurred in any of the groups. No apparent differences were observed between the intramuscular and subcutaneous routes of administration. Luteolytic doses of dinoprost tromethamine are on the order of 5 to 10 mg administered on one day, therefore, dinoprost tromethamine sterile solution was demonstrated to have a wide margin of safety. Thus, the 100 mg dose gave a safety margin of 10 to 20X for a single injection or 80 to 160X for the 8 daily injections.

Additional studies investigated the effects in the mare of single intramuscular doses of 0, 0.25, 1.0, 2.5, 3.0, 5.0, and 10.0 mg dinoprost tromethamine. Heart rate, respiration rate, rectal temperature, and sweating were measured at 0, 0.25, 0.50, 0.75, 1.0, 1.5, 2.0, 3.0, 4.0, 5.0, and 6.0 hr. after injection. Neither heart rate nor respiration rates were significantly altered ($P > 0.05$) when compared to contemporary control values. Sweating was observed for 0 of 9, 2 of 9, 7 of 9, 9 of 9, and 8 of 9 mares injected with 0.25, 1.0, 2.5, 3.0, 5.0, or 10.0 mg dinoprost tromethamine, respectively. Sweating was temporary in all cases and was mild for doses of 3.0 mg or less but was extensive (beads of sweat over the entire body and dripping) for the 10 mg dose. Sweating after the 5.0 mg dose was intermediate between that seen for mares treated with 3.0 and 10.0 mg. Sweating began within 15 minutes after injection and ceased by 45 to 60 minutes after injection. Rectal temperature was decreased during the interval 0.5 until 1.0, 3 to 4, or 5 hours after injection for 0.25 and 1.0 mg, 2.5 and 3.0, or 5.0 and 10.0 mg dose groups, respectively. Average rectal temperature during the periods of decreased temperature was on the order of 97.5 to 99.6, with the greatest decreases observed in the 10 mg dose group.

Adverse Reactions:

Cattle:

1. The most frequently observed side effect is increased rectal temperature at a 5X or 10X overdose. However, rectal temperature change has been transient in all cases observed and has not been detrimental to the animal.
2. Limited salivation has been reported in some instances.
3. Intravenous administration might increase heart rate.
4. Localized post injection bacterial infections that may become generalized have been reported. In rare instances such infections have terminated fatally. See Cautions.

Swine: The most frequently observed side effects were erythema and pruritus, slight incoordination, nesting behavior, itching, urination, defecation, abdominal muscle spasms, tail movements, hyperpnea or dyspnea, increased vocalization, salivation, and at the 100 mg (10X) dose only, vomition. These side effects are transitory, lasting from 10 minutes to 3 hours, and were not detrimental to the health of the animal.

Mares: The most frequently observed side effects are sweating and decreased rectal temperature. However, these have been transient in all cases observed and have not been detrimental to the animal. Other reactions seen have been increase in heart rate, increase in respiration rate, some abdominal discomfort, locomotor incoordination, and lying down. These effects are usually seen within 15 minutes of injection and disappear within one hour. Mares usually continue to eat during the period of expression of side effects. One anaphylactic reaction of several hundred mares treated with dinoprost tromethamine sterile solution was reported but was not confirmed.

Presentation: PROSTAMATE™ Sterile Solution is available in 10 and 30 mL vials.

Manufactured by: Phoenix Scientific, Inc.

Compendium Code No.: 10910130

PROSTAMATE™ ℞

Vedco **Prostaglandin**

(dinoprost tromethamine injection) Sterile Solution

ANADA No.: 200-253

Active Ingredient(s): Description: This product contains the naturally occurring prostaglandin F2 alpha (dinoprost) as the tromethamine salt. Each mL contains dinoprost tromethamine equivalent to 5 mg dinoprost: also, benzyl alcohol, 9.45 mg added as preservative. When necessary, pH was adjusted with sodium hydroxide and/or hydrochloric acid. Dinoprost tromethamine is a white or slightly off-white crystalline powder that is readily soluble in water at room temperature in concentrations to at least 200 mg/mL.

Indications: For intramuscular use for estrus synchronization, treatment of unobserved (silent) estrus and pyometra (chronic endometritis) in cattle; for abortion of feedlot and other non-lactating cattle; for parturition induction in swine; and for controlling the timing of estrus in estrous cycling mares and clinically anestrous mares that have a corpus luteum.

Cattle: PROSTAMATE™ Sterile Solution is indicated as a luteolytic agent.

PROSTAMATE™ is effective only in those cattle having a corpus luteum, i.e., those which ovulated at least five days prior to treatment. Future reproductive performance of animals that are not cycling will be unaffected by injection of PROSTAMATE™.

Swine: For intramuscular use for parturition induction in swine. PROSTAMATE™ Sterile Solution is indicated for parturition induction in swine when injected within 3 days of normal predicted farrowing.

Mares: PROSTAMATE™ Sterile Solution is indicated for its luteolytic effect in mares. This luteolytic effect can be utilized to control the timing of estrus in estrous cycling and clinically anestrous mares that have a corpus luteum.

Pharmacology: General Biologic Activity: Prostaglandins occur in nearly all mammalian tissues. Prostaglandins, especially PGE's and PGF's, have been shown, in certain species, to 1) increase at time of parturition in amniotic fluid, maternal placenta, myometrium, and blood, 2) stimulate myometrial activity, and 3) to induce either abortion or parturition. Prostaglandins, especially PGF2α, have been shown to 1) increase in the uterus and blood to levels similar to levels achieved by exogenous administration which elicited luteolysis, 2) be capable of crossing from the uterine vein to the ovarian artery (sheep), 3) be related to IUD induced luteal regression (sheep), and 4) be capable of regressing the corpus luteum of most mammalian species studied to date. Prostaglandins have been reported to result in release of pituitary tropic hormones. Data suggest prostaglandins, especially PGE's and PGF's, may be involved in the process of ovulation and gamete transport. Also PGF2α has been reported to cause increase in blood pressure, bronchoconstriction, and smooth muscle stimulation in certain species.

Metabolism: A number of metabolism studies have been done in laboratory animals. The metabolism of tritium labeled dinoprost (^{3}H PGF2 alpha) in the rat and in the monkey was similar. Although quantitative differences were observed, qualitatively similar metabolites were produced. A study demonstrated that equimolar doses of ^{3}H PGF2 alpha Tham and ^{3}H PGF2 alpha free acid administered intravenously to rats demonstrated no significant differences in blood concentration of dinoprost. An interesting observation in the above study was that the radioactive dose of ^{3}H PGF2 alpha rapidly distributed in tissues and dissipated in tissues with almost the same curve as it did in the serum. The half-life of dinoprost in bovine blood has been reported to be on the order of minutes. A complete study on the distribution of decline of ^{3}H PGF2 alpha Tham in the tissue of rats was well correlated with the work done in the cow. Cattle serum collected during 24 hours after doses of 0 to 250 mg dinoprost have been assayed by RIA for dinoprost and the 15-keto metabolites. These data support previous reports that dinoprost has a half-life of minutes. Dinoprost is a natural prostaglandin. All systems associated with dinoprost metabolism exist in the body; therefore, no new metabolic, transport, excretory, binding or other systems need be established by the body to metabolize injected dinoprost.

Dosage and Administration:

Cattle: PROSTAMATE™ Sterile Solution is supplied at a concentration of 5 mg dinoprost per mL. PROSTAMATE™ is luteolytic in cattle at 25 mg (5 mL) administered intramuscularly. As with any multidose vial, practice aseptic techniques in withdrawing each dose. Adequately clean and disinfect the vial closure prior to entry with a sterile needle.

Instructions for Use:

1. For Intramuscular Use for Estrus Synchronization in Beef Cattle and Non-Lactating Dairy Heifers: PROSTAMATE™ is used to control the timing of estrus and ovulation in estrous cycling cattle that have a corpus luteum.

   Inject a dose of 5 mL PROSTAMATE™ (25 mg PGF2α) intramuscularly either once or twice at a 10 to 12 day interval.

   With the single injection, cattle should be bred at the usual time relative to estrus. With the two injections cattle can be bred after the second injection either at the usual time relative to detected estrus or at about 80 hours after the second injection of PROSTAMATE™.

   Estrus is expected to occur 1 to 5 days after injection if a corpus luteum was present. Cattle that do not become pregnant to breeding at estrus on days 1 to 5 after injection will be expected to return to estrus in about 18 to 24 days.

2. For Intramuscular Use for Unobserved (Silent) Estrus in Lactating Dairy Cows with a Corpus Luteum: Inject a dose of 5 mL PROSTAMATE™ (25 mg PGF2α) intramuscularly. Breed cows as they are detected in estrus. If estrus has not been observed by 80 hours after injection, breed at 80 hours. If the cow returns to estrus breed at the usual time relative to estrus.

Management Considerations: Many factors contribute to success and failure of reproduction management, and these factors are important also when time of breeding is to be regulated with PROSTAMATE™ Sterile Solution. Some of these factors are:

a. Cattle must be ready to breed-they must have a corpus luteum and be healthy;
b. Nutritional status must be adequate as this has a direct effect on conception and the initiation of estrus in heifers or return of estrous cycles in cows following calving;
c. Physical facilities must be adequate to allow cattle handling without being detrimental to the animal;
d. Estrus must be detected accurately if timed A1 is not employed;
e. Semen of high fertility must be used;
f. Semen must be inseminated properly.

A successful breeding program can employ PROSTAMATE™ effectively, but a poorly managed breeding program will continue to be poor when PROSTAMATE™ is employed unless other management deficiencies are remedied first.

Cattle expressing estrus following PROSTAMATE™ are receptive to breeding by a bull. Using bulls to breed large numbers of cattle in heat following PROSTAMATE™ will require proper management of bulls and cattle.

3. For Intramuscular Use for Treatment of Pyometra (chronic endometritis) in Cattle: Inject a dose of 5 mL PROSTAMATE™ (25 mg PGF2α) intramuscularly. In studies conducted with dinoprost tromethamine sterile solution, pyometra was defined as presence of a corpus luteum in the ovary and uterine horns containing fluid but not a conceptus based on palpation *per rectum*. Return to normal was defined as evacuation of fluid and return of the uterine horn size to 40 mm or less based on palpation *per rectum* at 14 and 28 days. Most cattle that recovered in response to PROSTAMATE™ recovered within 14 days after injection. After 14 days, recovery rate of treated cattle was no different than that of non-treated cattle.

4. For Intramuscular Use for Abortion of Feedlot and Other Non-Lactating Cattle: PROSTAMATE™ is indicated for its abortifacient effect in feedlot and other non-lactating cattle during the first 100 days of gestation. Inject a dose of 25 mg intramuscularly. Cattle that abort will abort within 35 days of injection.

   Commercial cattle were palpated *per rectum* for pregnancy in six feedlots. The percent of pregnant cattle in each feedlot less than 100 days of gestation ranged between 26 and 84; 80% or more of the pregnant cattle were less than 150 days of gestation. The abortion rates following injection of dinoprost tromethamine sterile solution increased with increasing doses up to about 25 mg. As examples, the abortion rates, over 7 feedlots on the dose titration study, were 22%, 50%, 71%, 90% and 78% for cattle up to 100 days of gestation when injected IM with dinoprost tromethamine sterile solution doses of 0, 1 (5 mg), 2 (10 mg), 4 (20 mg) and 8 (40 mg) mL, respectively. The statistical predicted relative abortion rate based on the dose titration data, was about 93% for the 5 mL (25 mg) dinoprost tromethamine sterile solution dose for cattle injected up to 100 days of gestation.

Swine: PROSTAMATE™ Sterile Solution will induce parturition in swine at 10 mg (2 mL) when injected intramuscularly.

As with any multidose vial, practice aseptic techniques in withdrawing each dose. Adequately clean and disinfect the vial closure prior to entry with a sterile needle.

Instructions for Use: The response to treatment varies by individual animals with a mean interval from administration of 2 mL PROSTAMATE™ (10 mg dinoprost) to parturition of approximately 30 hours. This can be employed to control the time of farrowing in sows and gilts in late gestation.

Management Considerations: Several factors must be considered for the successful use of PROSTAMATE™ Sterile Solution for parturition induction in swine. The product must be administered at a relatively specific time (treatment earlier than 3 days prior to normal predicted farrowing may result in increased piglet mortality). It is important that adequate records be maintained on (1) the average length of gestation period for the animals on a specific location, and (2) the breeding and projected farrowing dates for each animal. This information is essential to determine the appropriate time for administration of PROSTAMATE™.

Mares:

1. Evaluate the reproductive status of the mare.
2. Administer a single intramuscular injection of 1 mg per 100 lbs (45.5 kg) body weight which is usually 1 mL to 2 mL PROSTAMATE™ Sterile Solution.
3. Observe for signs of estrus by means of daily teasing with a stallion, and evaluate follicular changes on the ovary by palpation of the ovary *per rectum*.
4. Some clinically anestrous mares will not express estrus but will develop a follicle which will ovulate. These mares may become pregnant if inseminated at the appropriate time relative to rupture of the follicle.
5. Breed mares in estrus in a manner consistent with normal management.

Dinoprost tromethamine is administered once as a single intramuscular injection of 1 mg per 100 lbs (45.5 kg) body weight which is usually 1 mL to 2 mL of PROSTAMATE™ containing 5 mg dinoprost as the tromethamine salt per milliliter.

Instructions for Use: PROSTAMATE™ Sterile Solution is indicated for its luteolytic effect in mares. This luteolytic effect can be utilized to control the timing of estrus in estrous cycling and clinically anestrous mares that have a corpus luteum in the following circumstances:

1. Controlling Time of Estrus of Estrous Cycling Mares: Mares treated with PROSTAMATE™ during diestrus (4 or more days after ovulation) will return to estrus within 2 to 4 days in most cases and ovulate 8 to 12 days after treatment. This procedure may be utilized as an aid to scheduling the use of stallions.
2. Difficult-to-Breed Mares: In extended diestrus there is failure to exhibit regular estrous cycles which is different from true anestrus. Many mares described as anestrus during the breeding season have serum progesterone levels consistent with the presence of a functional corpus luteum.

   A proportion of "barren", maiden, and lactating mares do not exhibit regular estrous cycles and may be in extended diestrus. Following abortion, early fetal death and resorption, or as a result of "pseudopregnancy", there may be serum progesterone levels consistent with a functional corpus luteum.

   Treatment of such mares with PROSTAMATE™ usually results in regression of the corpus luteum followed by estrus and/or ovulation. In one study with 122 Standardbred and Thoroughbred mares in clinical anestrus for an average of 58 days and treated during the breeding season, behavioral estrus was detected in 81 percent at an average time of 3.7 days after injection with 5 mg dinoprost tromethamine sterile solution; ovulation occurred an average of 7.0 days after treatment. Of those mares bred, 59% were pregnant following an average of 1.4 services during that estrus.

   Treatment of "anestrous" mares which abort subsequent to 36 days of pregnancy may not result in return to estrus due to presence of functional endometrial cups.

Precaution(s): Storage Conditions: Store at controlled room temperature 20° to 25°C (68° to 77°F).

Caution(s): Federal (USA) law restricts this drug to use by or on the order of a licensed veterinarian.

Cattle: Do not administer to pregnant cattle unless abortion is desired.

Do not administer intravenously (I.V.), as this route might potentiate adverse reactions.

Cattle administered a progestogen would be expected to have a reduced response to PROSTAMATE™ Sterile Solution.

Aggressive antibiotic therapy should be employed at the first sign of infection at the injection site whether localized or diffuse. As with all parenteral products careful aseptic techniques should be employed to decrease the possibility of post injection bacterial infections.

Swine: Do not administer to sows and/or gilts prior to 3 days of normal predicted farrowing, as increased number of stillborn and postnatal mortality may result.

Mares: PROSTAMATE™ Sterile Solution is ineffective when administered prior to day-5 after ovulation.

Pregnancy status should be determined prior to treatment, since PROSTAMATE™ has been reported to induce abortion and parturition when sufficient doses were administered.

Mares should not be treated if they suffer from either acute or subacute disorders of the vascular system, gastrointestinal tract, respiratory system, or reproductive tract.

Do not administer by intravenous route.

Nonsteroidal anti-inflammatory drugs (i.e., indomethacin) may inhibit prostaglandin synthesis, therefore these drugs should not be administered concurrently.

Restricted Drug-Use only as directed (California).

For use in animals only.

Warning(s):

Cattle: No milk discard or preslaughter drug withdrawal period is required for labeled uses.

Swine: No preslaughter drug withdrawal period is required for labeled uses.

Mares: Not for use in horses intended for food.

Not for human use.

Women of child-bearing age, asthmatics, and persons with bronchial and other respiratory problems should exercise extreme caution when handling this product. In the early stages, women may be unaware of their pregnancies. Dinoprost tromethamine is readily absorbed through the skin and can cause abortion and/or bronchiospasms. Direct contact with the skin should, therefore, be avoided. Accidental spillage on the skin should be washed off immediately with soap and water.

Use of this product in excess of the approved dose may result in drug residues.

Keep out of reach of children.

Toxicology: Safety and Toxicity:

Laboratory Animals: Dinoprost was non-teratogenic in rats when administered orally at 1.25, 3.2, 10.0 and 20.0 mg/kg/day from day 6th-15th of gestation or when administered subcutaneously at 0.5 and 1.0 mg/kg/day on gestation days 6, 7 and 8 or 9, 10 and 11 or 12, 13 and 14. Dinoprost was non-teratogenic in the rabbit when administered either subcutaneously at doses of 0.5 and 1.0 mg/kg/day on gestation days 6, 7 and 8 or 9, 10 and 11 or 12, 13 and 14 or 15, 16 and 17 or orally at doses of 0.01, 0.1 and 1.0 mg/kg/day on days 6-18 or 5.0 mg/kg/day on days 8-18 of gestation. A slight and marked embryo lethal effect was observed in dams given 1.0 and 5.0 mg/kg/day respectively. This was due to the expected luteolytic properties of the drug.

A 14-day continuous intravenous infusion study in rats at 20 mg PGF2α per kg body weight indicated prostaglandins of the F series could induce bone deposition. However, such bone changes were not observed in monkeys similarly administered dinoprost tromethamine sterile solution at 15 mg PGF2α per kg body weight for 14 days.

Cattle: In cattle, evaluation was made of clinical observations, clinical chemistry, hematology, urinalysis, organ weights, and gross plus microscopic measurements following treatment with various doses up to 250 mg dinoprost administered twice intramuscularly at a 10 day interval or doses of 25 mg administered daily for 10 days. There was no unequivocal effect of dinoprost on the hematology or clinical chemistry parameters measured. Clinically, a slight transitory increase in heart rate was detected. Rectal temperature was elevated about 1.5°F through the 6th hour after injection with 250 mg dinoprost, but had returned to baseline at 24 hours after injection. No dinoprost associated gross lesions were detected. There was no evidence of toxicological effects. Thus, dinoprost had a safety factor of at least 10X on injection (25 mg luteolytic dose vs. 250 mg safe dose), based on studies conducted with cattle. At luteolytic doses, dinoprost had no effect on progeny. If given to a pregnant cow, it may cause abortion; the dose required for abortion varies considerably with the stage of gestation.

Induction of abortion in feedlot cattle at stages of gestation up to 100 days of gestation did not result in dystocia, retained placenta or death of heifers in the field studies. The smallness of the fetus at this early stage of gestation should not lead to complications at abortion. However, induction of parturition or abortion with any exogenous compound may precipitate dystocia, fetal death, retained placenta and/or metritis, especially at latter stages of gestation.

Swine: In pigs, evaluation was made of clinical observations, food consumption, clinical pathologic determinations, body weight changes, urinalysis, organ weights, and gross and microscopic observations following treatment with single doses of 10, 30, 50 and 100 mg dinoprost administered intramuscularly. The results indicated no treatment related effects from dinoprost treatment that were deleterious to the health of the animals or to their offspring.

Mares: Dinoprost tromethamine was administered to adult mares (weighing 320 to 485 kg; 2 to 20 years old), at the rates of 0, 100, 200, 400, and 800 mg per mare per day for 8 days. Route of administration for each dose group was both intramuscularly (2 mares) and subcutaneously (2 mares). Changes were detected in all treated groups for clinical (reduced sensitivity to pain; locomotor incoordination; hypergastromotility; sweating; hyperthermia; labored respiration), blood chemistry (elevated cholesterol, total bilirubin, LDH, and glucose), and hematology (decreased eosinophils; increased hemoglobin, hematocrit, and erythrocytes) measurements. The effects in the 100 mg dose, and to a lesser extent, the 200 mg dose groups were transient in nature, lasting for a few minutes to several hours. Mares did not appear to sustain adverse effects following termination of the side effects.

Mares treated with either 400 mg or 800 mg exhibited more profound symptoms. The excessive hyperstimulation of the gastrointestinal tract caused a protracted diarrhea, slight electrolyte imbalance (decreased sodium and potassium), dehydration, gastrointestinal irritation, and slight liver malfunction (elevated SGOT, SGPT at 800 mg only). Heart rate was increased but pH of the urine was decreased. Other measurements evaluated in the study remained within normal limits. No mortality occurred in any of the groups. No apparent differences were observed between the intramuscular and subcutaneous routes of administration. Luteolytic doses of dinoprost tromethamine are on the order of 5 to 10 mg administered on one day, therefore, dinoprost tromethamine sterile solution was demonstrated to have a wide margin of safety. Thus, the 100 mg dose gave a safety margin of 10 to 20X for a single injection or 80 to 160X for the 8 daily injections.

Additional studies investigated the effects in the mare of single intramuscular doses of 0, 0.25, 1.0, 2.5, 3.0, 5.0, and 10.0 mg dinoprost tromethamine. Heart rate, respiration rate, rectal temperature, and sweating were measured at 0, 0.25, 0.50, 0.75, 1.0, 1.5, 2.0, 3.0, 4.0, 5.0, and 6.0 hr. after injection. Neither heart rate nor respiration rates were significantly altered ($P > 0.05$) when compared to contemporary control values. Sweating was observed for 0 of 9, 2 of 9, 7 of 9, 9 of 9, and 8 of 9 mares injected with 0.25, 1.0, 2.5, 3.0, 5.0, or 10.0 mg dinoprost tromethamine, respectively. Sweating was temporary in all cases and was mild for doses of 3.0 mg or less but was extensive (beads of sweat over the entire body and dripping) for the 10 mg dose. Sweating after the 5.0 mg dose was intermediate between that seen for mares treated with 3.0 and 10.0 mg. Sweating began within 15 minutes after injection and ceased by 45 to 60 minutes after injection. Rectal temperature was decreased during the interval 0.5 until 1.0, 3 to 4, or 5 hours after injection for 0.25 and 1.0 mg, 2.5 and 3.0, or 5.0 and 10.0 mg dose groups, respectively. Average rectal temperature during the periods of decreased temperature was on the order of 97.5 to 99.6, with the greatest decreases observed in the 10 mg dose group.

Adverse Reactions:

Cattle:

1. The most frequently observed side effect is increased rectal temperature at a 5X or 10X overdose. However, rectal temperature change has been transient in all cases observed and has not been detrimental to the animal.
2. Limited salivation has been reported in some instances.
3. Intravenous administration might increase heart rate.
4. Localized post injection bacterial infections that may become generalized have been reported. In rare instances such infections have terminated fatally. See Cautions.

Swine: The most frequently observed side effects were erythema and pruritus, slight incoordination, nesting behavior, itching, urination, defecation, abdominal muscle spasms, tail movements, hyperpnea or dyspnea, increased vocalization, salivation, and at the 100 mg (10X) dose only, vomition. These side effects are transitory, lasting from 10 minutes to 3 hours, and were not detrimental to the health of the animal.

Mares: The most frequently observed side effects are sweating and decreased rectal temperature. However, these have been transient in all cases observed and have not been detrimental to the animal. Other reactions seen have been increase in heart rate, increase in respiration rate, some abdominal discomfort, locomotor incoordination, and lying down. These effects are usually seen within 15 minutes of injection and disappear within one hour. Mares usually continue to eat during the period of expression of side effects. One anaphylactic reaction of several hundred mares treated with dinoprost tromethamine sterile solution was reported but was not confirmed.

Presentation: PROSTAMATE™ Sterile Solution is available in 30 mL vials (NDC 50989-413-10).
Manufactured by: Phoenix Scientific, Inc., St. Joseph, MO 64503.
Compendium Code No.: 10942310 Rev. 2-00

PROSTAMATE™ ℞

Vet Tek **Prostaglandin**

(dinoprost tromethamine injection) Sterile Solution

ANADA No.: 200-253

Active Ingredient(s): This product contains the naturally occurring prostaglandin F2 alpha (dinoprost) as the tromethamine salt. Each mL contains dinoprost tromethamine equivalent to 5 mg dinoprost: also, benzyl alcohol, 9.45 mg added as preservative. When necessary, pH was adjusted with sodium hydroxide and/or hydrochloric acid. Dinoprost tromethamine is a white or slightly off-white crystalline powder that is readily soluble in water at room temperature in concentrations to at least 200 mg/mL.

P

Indications: For intramuscular use for estrus synchronization, treatment of unobserved (silent) estrus and pyometra (chronic endometritis) in cattle; for abortion of feedlot and other non-lactating cattle; for parturition induction in swine; and for controlling the timing of estrus in estrous cycling mares and clinically anestrous mares that have a corpus luteum.

Cattle: PROSTAMATE™ Sterile Solution is indicated as a luteolytic agent.

PROSTAMATE™ is effective only in those cattle having a corpus luteum, i.e., those which ovulated at least five days prior to treatment. Future reproductive performance of animals that are not cycling will be unaffected by injection of PROSTAMATE™.

Swine: For intramuscular use for parturition induction in swine. PROSTAMATE™ Sterile Solution is indicated for parturition induction in swine when injected within 3 days of normal predicted farrowing.

Mares: PROSTAMATE™ Sterile Solution is indicated for its luteolytic effect in mares. This luteolytic effect can be utilized to control the timing of estrus in estrous cycling and clinically anestrous mares that have a corpus luteum.

Pharmacology: General Biologic Activity: Prostaglandins occur in nearly all mammalian tissues. Prostaglandins, especially PGE's and PGF's, have been shown, in certain species, to 1) increase at time of parturition in amniotic fluid, maternal placenta, myometrium, and blood, 2) stimulate myometrial activity, and 3) to induce either abortion or parturition. Prostaglandins, especially PGF2α, have been shown to 1) increase in the uterus and blood to levels similar to levels achieved by exogenous administration which elicited luteolysis, 2) be capable of crossing from the uterine vein to the ovarian artery (sheep), 3) be related to IUD induced luteal regression (sheep), and 4) be capable of regressing the corpus luteum of most mammalian species studied to date. Prostaglandins have been reported to result in release of pituitary tropic hormones. Data suggest prostaglandins, especially PGE's and PGF's, may be involved in the process of ovulation and gamete transport. Also PGF2α have been reported to cause increase in blood pressure, bronchoconstriction, and smooth muscle stimulation in certain species.

Metabolism: A number of metabolism studies have been done in laboratory animals. The metabolism of tritium labeled dinoprost (^{3}H PGF2 alpha) in the rat and in the monkey was similar. Although quantitative differences were observed, qualitatively similar metabolites were produced. A study demonstrated that equimolar doses of ^{3}H PGF2 alpha Tham and ^{3}H PGF2 alpha free acid administered intravenously to rats demonstrated no significant differences in blood concentration of dinoprost. An interesting observation in the above study was that the radioactive dose of ^{3}H PGF2 alpha rapidly distributed in tissues and dissipated in tissues with almost the same curve as it did in the serum. The half-life of dinoprost in bovine blood has been reported to be on the order of minutes. A complete study on the distribution of decline of ^{3}H PGF2 alpha Tham in the tissue of rats was well correlated with the work done in the cow. Cattle serum collected during 24 hours after doses of 0 to 250 mg dinoprost have been assayed by RIA for dinoprost and the 15-keto metabolites. These data support previous reports that dinoprost has a half-life of minutes. Dinoprost is a natural prostaglandin. All systems associated with dinoprost metabolism exist in the body; therefore, no new metabolic, transport, excretory, binding or other systems need be established by the body to metabolize injected dinoprost.

Dosage and Administration:

Cattle: PROSTAMATE™ Sterile Solution is supplied at a concentration of 5 mg dinoprost per mL. PROSTAMATE™ is luteolytic in cattle at 25 mg (5 mL) administered intramuscularly. As with any multidose vial, practice aseptic techniques in withdrawing each dose. Adequately clean and disinfect the vial closure prior to entry with a sterile needle.

Instructions for Use:

1. For Intramuscular Use for Estrus Synchronization in Beef Cattle and Non-Lactating Dairy Heifers. PROSTAMATE™ is used to control the timing of estrus and ovulation in estrous cycling cattle that have a corpus luteum.
   Inject a dose of 5 mL PROSTAMATE™ (25 mg PGF2α) intramuscularly either once or twice at a 10 to 12 day interval.
   With the single injection, cattle should be bred at the usual time relative to estrus. With the two injections cattle can be bred after the second injection either at the usual time relative to detected estrus or at about 80 hours after the second injection of PROSTAMATE™.
   Estrus is expected to occur 1 to 5 days after injection if a corpus luteum was present. Cattle that do not become pregnant to breeding at estrus on days 1 to 5 after injection will be expected to return to estrus in about 18 to 24 days.
2. For Intramuscular Use for Unobserved (Silent) Estrus in Lactating Dairy Cows with a Corpus Luteum. Inject a dose of 5 mL PROSTAMATE™ (25 mg PGF2α) intramuscularly. Breed cows as they are detected in estrus. If estrus has not been observed by 80 hours after injection, breed at 80 hours. If the cow returns to estrus breed at the usual time relative to estrus.

Management Considerations: Many factors contribute to success and failure of reproduction management, and these factors are important also when time of breeding is to be regulated with PROSTAMATE™ Sterile Solution. Some of these factors are:

a. Cattle must be ready to breed-they must have a corpus luteum and be healthy;
b. Nutritional status must be adequate as this has a direct effect on conception and the initiation of estrus in heifers or return of estrous cycles in cows following calving;
c. Physical facilities must be adequate to allow cattle handling without being detrimental to the animal;
d. Estrus must be detected accurately if timed A1 is not employed;
e. Semen of high fertility must be used;
f. Semen must be inseminated properly.

A successful breeding program can employ PROSTAMATE™ effectively, but a poorly managed breeding program will continue to be poor when PROSTAMATE™ is employed unless other management deficiencies are remedied first.

Cattle expressing estrus following PROSTAMATE™ are receptive to breeding by a bull. Using bulls to breed large numbers of cattle in heat following PROSTAMATE™ will require proper management of bulls and cattle.

3. For Intramuscular Use for Treatment of Pyometra (chronic endometritis) in Cattle. Inject a dose of 5 mL PROSTAMATE™ (25 mg PGF2α) intramuscularly. In studies conducted with dinoprost tromethamine sterile solution, pyometra was defined as presence of a corpus luteum in the ovary and uterine horns containing fluid but not a conceptus based on palpation *per rectum*. Return to normal was defined as evacuation of fluid and return of the uterine horn size to 40 mm or less based on palpation *per rectum* at 14 and 28 days. Most cattle that recovered in response to PROSTAMATE™ recovered within 14 days after injection. After 14 days, recovery rate of treated cattle was no different than that of non-treated cattle.
4. For Intramuscular Use for Abortion of Feedlot and Other Non-Lactating Cattle. PROSTAMATE™ is indicated for its abortifacient effect in feedlot and other non-lactating cattle during the first 100 days of gestation. Inject a dose of 25 mg intramuscularly. Cattle that abort will abort within 35 days of injection.
   Commercial cattle were palpated *per rectum* for pregnancy in six feedlots. The percent of pregnant cattle in each feedlot less than 100 days of gestation ranged between 26 and 84; 80% or more of the pregnant cattle were less than 150 days of gestation. The abortion rates following injection of dinoprost tromethamine sterile solution increased with increasing doses up to about 25 mg. As examples, the abortion rates, over 7 feedlots on the dose titration study, were 22%, 50%, 71%, 90% and 78% for cattle up to 100 days of gestation when injected IM with dinoprost tromethamine sterile solution doses of 0.1 (5 mg), 2 (10 mg), 4 (20 mg) and 8 (40 mg) mL, respectively. The statistical predicted relative abortion rate based on the dose titration data, was about 93% for the 5 mL (25 mg) dinoprost tromethamine sterile solution dose for cattle injected up to 100 days of gestation.

Swine: PROSTAMATE™ Sterile Solution will induce parturition in swine at 10 mg (2 mL) when injected intramuscularly.

As with any multidose vial, practice aseptic techniques in withdrawing each dose. Adequately clean and disinfect the vial closure prior to entry with a sterile needle.

Instructions for Use: The response to treatment varies by individual animals with a mean interval from administration of 2 mL PROSTAMATE™ (10 mg dinoprost) to parturition of approximately 30 hours. This can be employed to control the time of farrowing in sows and gilts in late gestation.

Management Considerations: Several factors must be considered for the successful use of PROSTAMATE™ Sterile Solution for parturition induction in swine. The product must be administered at a relatively specific time (treatment earlier than 3 days prior to normal predicted farrowing may result in increased piglet mortality). It is important that adequate records be maintained on (1) the average length of gestation period for the animals on a specific location, and (2) the breeding and projected farrowing dates for each animal. This information is essential to determine the appropriate time for administration of PROSTAMATE™.

Mares:

1. Evaluate the reproductive status of the mare.
2. Administer a single intramuscular injection of 1 mg per 100 lbs (45.5 kg) body weight which is usually 1 mL to 2 mL PROSTAMATE™ Sterile Solution.
3. Observe for signs of estrus by means of daily teasing with a stallion, and evaluate follicular changes on the ovary by palpation of the ovary *per rectum*.
4. Some clinically anestrous mares will not express estrus but will develop a follicle which will ovulate. These mares may become pregnant if inseminated at the appropriate time relative to rupture of the follicle.
5. Breed mares in estrus in a manner consistent with normal management.

Dinoprost tromethamine is administered once as a single intramuscular injection of 1 mg per

100 lbs (45.5 kg) body weight which is usually 1 mL to 2 mL of PROSTAMATE™ containing 5 mg dinoprost as the tromethamine salt per milliliter.

Instructions for Use: PROSTAMATE™ Sterile Solution is indicated for its luteolytic effect in mares. This luteolytic effect can be utilized to control the timing of estrus in estrous cycling and clinically anestrous mares that have a corpus luteum in the following circumstances:

1. Controlling Time of Estrus of Estrous Cycling Mares: Mares treated with PROSTAMATE™ during diestrus (4 or more days after ovulation) will return to estrus within 2 to 4 days in most cases and ovulate 8 to 12 days after treatment. This procedure may be utilized as an aid to scheduling the use of stallions.
2. Difficult-to-Breed Mares: In extended diestrus there is failure to exhibit regular estrous cycles which is different from true anestrus. Many mares described as anestrus during the breeding season have serum progesterone levels consistent with the presence of a functional corpus luteum.

   A proportion of "barren", maiden, and lactating mares do not exhibit regular estrous cycles and may be in extended diestrus. Following abortion, early fetal death and resorption, or as a result of "pseudopregnancy", there may be serum progesterone levels consistent with a functional corpus luteum.

   Treatment of such mares with PROSTAMATE™ usually results in regression of the corpus luteum followed by estrus and/or ovulation. In one study with 122 Standardbred and Thoroughbred mares in clinical anestrus for an average of 58 days and treated during the breeding season, behavioral estrus was detected in 81 percent at an average time of 3.7 days after injection with 5 mg dinoprost tromethamine sterile solution; ovulation occurred an average of 7.0 days after treatment. Of those mares bred, 59% were pregnant following an average of 1.4 services during that estrus.

   Treatment of "anestrous" mares which abort subsequent to 36 days of pregnancy may not result in return to estrus due to presence of functional endometrial cups.

Precaution(s): Storage Conditions: Store at controlled room temperature 20° to 25°C (68° to 77°F).

Caution(s): Federal (USA) law restricts this drug to use by or on the order of a licensed veterinarian.

Cattle: Do not administer to pregnant cattle unless abortion is desired.

Do not administer intravenously (I.V.), as this route might potentiate adverse reactions.

Cattle administered a progestogen would be expected to have a reduced response to PROSTAMATE™ Sterile Solution.

Aggressive antibiotic therapy should be employed at the first sign of infection at the injection site whether localized or diffuse. As with all parenteral products careful aseptic techniques should be employed to decrease the possibility of post injection bacterial infections.

Swine: Do not administer to sows and/or gilts prior to 3 days of normal predicted farrowing, as increased number of stillborn and postnatal mortality may result.

Mares: PROSTAMATE™ Sterile Solution is ineffective when administered prior to day-5 after ovulation.

Pregnancy status should be determined prior to treatment, since PROSTAMATE™ has been reported to induce abortion and parturition when sufficient doses were administered.

Mares should not be treated if they suffer from either acute or subacute disorders of the vascular system, gastrointestinal tract, respiratory system, or reproductive tract.

Do not administer by intravenous route.

Nonsteroidal anti-inflammatory drugs (i.e., indomethacin) may inhibit prostaglandin synthesis, therefore these drugs should not be administered concurrently.

For use in animals only.

Restricted drug-Use only as directed (California).

Warning(s):

Cattle: No milk discard or preslaughter drug withdrawal period is required for labeled uses.

Swine: No preslaughter drug withdrawal period is required for labeled uses.

Mares: Not for use in horses intended for food.

Not for human use.

Women of child-bearing age, asthmatics, and persons with bronchial and other respiratory problems should exercise extreme caution when handling this product. In the early stages, women may be unaware of their pregnancies. Dinoprost tromethamine is readily absorbed through the skin and can cause abortion and/or bronchiospasms. Direct contact with the skin should, therefore, be avoided. Accidental spillage on the skin should be washed off immediately with soap and water.

Use of this product in excess of the approved dose may result in drug residues.

Keep out of reach of children.

Toxicology: Safety and Toxicity:

Laboratory Animals: Dinoprost was non-teratogenic in rats when administered orally at 1.25, 3.2, 10.0 and 20.0 mg/kg/day from day 6th-15th of gestation or when administered subcutaneously at 0.5 and 1.0 mg/kg/day on gestation days 6, 7 and 8 or 9, 10 and 11 or 12, 13 and 14. Dinoprost was non-teratogenic in the rabbit when administered either subcutaneously at doses of 0.5 and 1.0 mg/kg/day on gestation days 6, 7 and 8 or 9, 10 and 11 or 12, 13 and 14 or 15, 16 and 17 or orally at doses of 0.01, 0.1 and 1.0 mg/kg/day on days 6-18 or 5.0 mg/kg/day on days 8-18 of gestation. A slight and marked embryo lethal effect was observed in dams given 1.0 and 5.0 mg/kg/day respectively. This was due to the expected luteolytic properties of the drug.

A 14-day continuous intravenous infusion study in rats at 20 mg PGF2α per kg body weight indicated prostaglandins of the F series could induce bone deposition. However, such bone changes were not observed in monkeys similarly administered dinoprost tromethamine sterile solution at 15 mg PGF2α per kg body weight for 14 days.

Cattle: In cattle, evaluation was made of clinical observations, clinical chemistry, hematology, urinalysis, organ weights, and gross plus microscopic measurements following treatment with various doses up to 250 mg dinoprost administered twice intramuscularly at a 10 day interval or doses of 25 mg administered daily for 10 days. There was no unequivocal effect of dinoprost on the hematology or clinical chemistry parameters measured. Clinically, a slight transitory increase in heart rate was detected. Rectal temperature was elevated about 1.5°F through the 6th hour after injection with 250 mg dinoprost, but had returned to baseline at 24 hours after injection. No dinoprost associated gross lesions were detected. There was no evidence of toxicological effects. Thus, dinoprost had a safety factor of at least 10X on injection (25 mg luteolytic dose vs. 250 mg safe dose), based on studies conducted with cattle. At luteolytic doses, dinoprost had no effect on progeny. If given to a pregnant cow, it may cause abortion; the dose required for abortion varies considerably with the stage of gestation.

Induction of abortion in feedlot cattle at stages of gestation up to 100 days of gestation did not result in dystocia, retained placenta or death of heifers in the field studies. The smallness of the fetus at this early stage of gestation should not lead to complications at abortion. However, induction of parturition or abortion with any exogenous compound may precipitate dystocia, fetal death, retained placenta and/or metritis, especially at latter stages of gestation.

Swine: In pigs, evaluation was made of clinical observations, food consumption, clinical pathologic determinations, body weight changes, urinalysis, organ weights, and gross and microscopic observations following treatment with single doses of 10, 30, 50 and 100 mg dinoprost administered intramuscularly. The results indicated no treatment related effects from dinoprost treatment that were deleterious to the health of the animals or to their offspring.

Mares: Dinoprost tromethamine was administered to adult mares (weighing 320 to 485 kg; 2 to 20 years old), at the rates of 0, 100, 200, 400, and 800 mg per mare per day for 8 days. Route of administration for each dose group was both intramuscularly (2 mares) and subcutaneously (2 mares). Changes were detected in all treated groups for clinical (reduced sensitivity to pain; locomotor incoordination; hypergastromotility; sweating; hyperthermia; labored respiration), blood chemistry (elevated cholesterol, total bilirubin, LDH, and glucose), and hematology (decreased eosinophils; increased hemoglobin, hematocrit, and erythrocytes) measurements. The effects in the 100 mg dose, and to a lesser extent, the 200 mg dose groups were transient in nature, lasting for a few minutes to several hours. Mares did not appear to sustain adverse effects following termination of the side effects.

Mares treated with either 400 mg or 800 mg exhibited more profound symptoms. The excessive hyperstimulation of the gastrointestinal tract caused a protracted diarrhea, slight electrolyte imbalance (decreased sodium and potassium), dehydration, gastrointestinal irritation, and slight liver malfunction (elevated SGOT, SGPT at 800 mg only). Heart rate was increased but pH of the urine was decreased. Other measurements evaluated in the study remained within normal limits. No mortality occurred in any of the groups. No apparent differences were observed between the intramuscular and subcutaneous routes of administration. Luteolytic doses of dinoprost tromethamine are on the order of 5 to 10 mg administered on one day, therefore, dinoprost tromethamine sterile solution was demonstrated to have a wide margin of safety. Thus, the 100 mg dose gave a safety margin of 10 to 20X for a single injection or 80 to 160X for the 8 daily injections.

Additional studies investigated the effects in the mare of single intramuscular doses of 0, 0.25, 1.0, 2.5, 3.0, 5.0, and 10.0 mg dinoprost tromethamine. Heart rate, respiration rate, rectal temperature, and sweating were measured at 0, 0.25, 0.50, 0.75, 1.0, 1.5, 2.0, 3.0, 4.0, 5.0, and 6.0 hr. after injection. Neither heart rate nor respiration rates were significantly altered ($P > 0.05$) when compared to contemporary control values. Sweating was observed for 0 of 9, 2 of 9, 7 of 9, 9 of 9, and 8 of 9 mares injected with 0.25, 1.0, 2.5, 3.0, 5.0, or 10.0 mg dinoprost tromethamine, respectively. Sweating was temporary in all cases and was mild for doses of 3.0 mg or less but was extensive (beads of sweat over the entire body and dripping) for the 10 mg dose. Sweating after the 5.0 mg dose was intermediate between that seen for mares treated with 3.0 and 10.0 mg. Sweating began within 15 minutes after injection and ceased by 45 to 60 minutes after injection. Rectal temperature was decreased during the interval 0.5 until 1.0, 3 to 4, or 5 hours after injection for 0.25 and 1.0 mg, 2.5 and 3.0, or 5.0 and 10.0 mg dose groups, respectively. Average rectal temperature during the periods of decreased temperature was on the order of 97.5 to 99.6, with the greatest decreases observed in the 10 mg dose group.

Adverse Reactions:

Cattle:

1. The most frequently observed side effect is increased rectal temperature at a 5X or 10X overdose. However, rectal temperature change has been transient in all cases observed and has not been detrimental to the animal.
2. Limited salivation has been reported in some instances.
3. Intravenous administration might increase heart rate.
4. Localized post injection bacterial infections that may become generalized have been reported. In rare instances such infections have terminated fatally. See Cautions.

Swine: The most frequently observed side effects were erythema and pruritus, slight incoordination, nesting behavior, itching, urination, defecation, abdominal muscle spasms, tail movements, hyperpnea or dyspnea, increased vocalization, salivation, and at the 100 mg (10X) dose only, vomition. These side effects are transitory, lasting from 10 minutes to 3 hours, and were not detrimental to the health of the animal.

Mares: The most frequently observed side effects are sweating and decreased rectal temperature. However, these have been transient in all cases observed and have not been detrimental to the animal. Other reactions seen have been increase in heart rate, increase in respiration rate, some abdominal discomfort, locomotor incoordination, and lying down. These effects are usually seen within 15 minutes of injection and disappear within one hour. Mares usually continue to eat during the period of expression of side effects. One anaphylactic reaction of several hundred mares treated with dinoprost tromethamine sterile solution was reported but was not confirmed.

Presentation: PROSTAMATE™ Sterile Solution is available in 30 mL vials (NDC 60270-809-03).

Manufactured by: Phoenix Scientific, Inc.

Compendium Code No.: 14200162 Rev. 2-00

PROSTAMATE® ℞

Vetus **Prostaglandin**

(dinoprost tromethamine injection) Sterile Solution

ANADA No.: 200-253

Active Ingredient(s): This product contains the naturally occurring prostaglandin F2 alpha (dinoprost) as the tromethamine salt. Each mL contains dinoprost tromethamine equivalent to 5 mg dinoprost: also, benzyl alcohol, 9.45 mg added as preservative. When necessary, pH was adjusted with sodium hydroxide and/or hydrochloric acid. Dinoprost tromethamine is a white or slightly off-white crystalline powder that is readily soluble in water at room temperature in concentrations to at least 200 mg/mL.

Indications: For intramuscular use for estrus synchronization, treatment of unobserved (silent) estrus and pyometra (chronic endometritis) in cattle; for abortion of feedlot and other non-lactating cattle; for parturition induction in swine; and for controlling the timing of estrus in estrous cycling mares and clinically anestrous mares that have a corpus luteum.

Cattle: PROSTAMATE® Sterile Solution is indicated as a luteolytic agent.

PROSTAMATE® is effective only in those cattle having a corpus luteum, i.e., those which ovulated at least five days prior to treatment. Future reproductive performance of animals that are not cycling will be unaffected by injection of PROSTAMATE®.

Swine: For intramuscular use for parturition induction in swine. PROSTAMATE® Sterile Solution is indicated for parturition induction in swine when injected within 3 days of normal predicted farrowing.

Mares: PROSTAMATE® Sterile Solution is indicated for its luteolytic effect in mares. This luteolytic effect can be utilized to control the timing of estrus in estrous cycling and clinically anestrous mares that have a corpus luteum.

Pharmacology: General Biologic Activity: Prostaglandins occur in nearly all mammalian tissues. Prostaglandins, especially PGE's and PGF's, have been shown, in certain species, to 1) increase at time of parturition in amniotic fluid, maternal placenta, myometrium, and blood, 2) stimulate myometrial activity, and 3) to induce either abortion or parturition. Prostaglandins, especially PGF2α, have been shown to 1) increase in the uterus and blood to levels similar to levels achieved by exogenous administration which elicited luteolysis, 2) be capable of crossing from the uterine vein to the ovarian artery (sheep), 3) be related to IUD induced luteal regression (sheep), and 4) be capable of regressing the corpus luteum of most mammalian species studied to date. Prostaglandins have been reported to result in release of pituitary tropic hormones. Data suggest prostaglandins, especially PGE's and PGF's, may be involved in the process of ovulation and gamete transport. Also PGF2α have been reported to cause increase in blood pressure, bronchoconstriction, and smooth muscle stimulation in certain species.

Metabolism: A number of metabolism studies have been done in laboratory animals. The metabolism of tritium labeled dinoprost (^{3}H PGF2 alpha) in the rat and in the monkey was similar. Although quantitative differences were observed, qualitatively similar metabolites were produced. A study demonstrated that equimolar doses of ^{3}H PGF2 alpha Tham and ^{3}H PGF2 alpha free acid administered intravenously to rats demonstrated no significant differences in blood concentration of dinoprost. An interesting observation in the above study was that the radioactive dose of ^{3}H PGF2 alpha rapidly distributed in tissues and dissipated in tissues with almost the same curve as it did in the serum. The half-life of dinoprost in bovine blood has been reported to be on the order of minutes. A complete study on the distribution of decline of ^{3}H PGF2 alpha Tham in the tissue of rats was well correlated with the work done in the cow. Cattle serum collected during 24 hours after doses of 0 to 250 mg dinoprost have been assayed by RIA for dinoprost and the 15-keto metabolites. These data support previous reports that dinoprost has a half-life of minutes. Dinoprost is a natural prostaglandin. All systems associated with dinoprost metabolism exist in the body; therefore, no new metabolic, transport, excretory, binding or other systems need be established by the body to metabolize injected dinoprost.

Dosage and Administration: Cattle: PROSTAMATE® Sterile Solution is supplied at a concentration of 5 mg dinoprost per mL. PROSTAMATE® is luteolytic in cattle at 25 mg (5 mL) administered intramuscularly. As with any multidose vial, practice aseptic techniques in withdrawing each dose. Adequately clean and disinfect the vial closure prior to entry with a sterile needle.

Instructions for Use:

1. For Intramuscular Use for Estrus Synchronization in Beef Cattle and Non-Lactating Dairy Heifers. PROSTAMATE® is used to control the timing of estrus and ovulation in estrous cycling cattle that have a corpus luteum.

   Inject a dose of 5 mL PROSTAMATE® (25 mg PGF2α) intramuscularly either once or twice at a 10 to 12 day interval.

   With the single injection, cattle should be bred at the usual time relative to estrus. With the two injections cattle can be bred after the second injection either at the usual time relative to detected estrus or at about 80 hours after the second injection of PROSTAMATE®.

   Estrus is expected to occur 1 to 5 days after injection if a corpus luteum was present. Cattle that do not become pregnant to breeding at estrus on days 1 to 5 after injection will be expected to return to estrus in about 18 to 24 days.
2. For Intramuscular Use for Unobserved (Silent) Estrus in Lactating Dairy Cows with a Corpus Luteum. Inject a dose of 5 mL PROSTAMATE® (25 mg PGF2α) intramuscularly. Breed cows as they are detected in estrus. If estrus has not been observed by 80 hours after injection, breed at 80 hours. If the cow returns to estrus breed at the usual time relative to estrus.

Management Considerations: Many factors contribute to success and failure of reproduction management, and these factors are important also when time of breeding is to be regulated with PROSTAMATE® Sterile Solution. Some of these factors are:

a. Cattle must be ready to breed-they must have a corpus luteum and be healthy;
b. Nutritional status must be adequate as this has a direct effect on conception and the initiation of estrus in heifers or return of estrous cycles in cows following calving;
c. Physical facilities must be adequate to allow cattle handling without being detrimental to the animal;
d. Estrus must be detected accurately if timed A1 is not employed;
e. Semen of high fertility must be used;
f. Semen must be inseminated properly.

A successful breeding program can employ PROSTAMATE® effectively, but a poorly managed breeding program will continue to be poor when PROSTAMATE® is employed unless other management deficiencies are remedied first.

Cattle expressing estrus following PROSTAMATE® are receptive to breeding by a bull. Using bulls to breed large numbers of cattle in heat following PROSTAMATE® will require proper management of bulls and cattle.

3. For Intramuscular Use for Treatment of Pyometra (chronic endometritis) in Cattle. Inject a dose of 5 mL PROSTAMATE® (25 mg PGF2α) intramuscularly. In studies conducted with dinoprost tromethamine sterile solution, pyometra was defined as presence of a corpus luteum in the ovary and uterine horns containing fluid but not a conceptus based on palpation *per rectum.* Return to normal was defined as evacuation of fluid and return of the uterine horn size to 40 mm or less based on palpation *per rectum* at 14 and 28 days. Most cattle that recovered in response to PROSTAMATE® recovered within 14 days after injection. After 14 days, recovery rate of treated cattle was no different than that of non-treated cattle.
4. For Intramuscular Use for Abortion of Feedlot and Other Non-Lactating Cattle. PROSTAMATE® is indicated for its abortifacient effect in feedlot and other non-lactating cattle during the first 100 days of gestation. Inject a dose of 25 mg intramuscularly. Cattle that abort will abort within 35 days of injection.

   Commercial cattle were palpated *per rectum* for pregnancy in six feedlots. The percent of pregnant cattle in each feedlot less than 100 days of gestation ranged between 26 and 84; 80% or more of the pregnant cattle were less than 150 days of gestation. The abortion rates following injection of dinoprost tromethamine sterile solution increased with increasing doses up to about 25 mg. As examples, the abortion rates, over 7 feedlots on the dose titration study, were 22%, 50%, 71%, 90% and 78% for cattle up to 100 days of gestation when injected IM with dinoprost tromethamine sterile solution doses of 0, 1 (5 mg), 2 (10 mg), 4 (20 mg) and 8 (40 mg) mL, respectively. The statistical predicted relative abortion rate based on the dose titration data, was about 93% for the 5 mL (25 mg) dinoprost tromethamine sterile solution dose for cattle injected up to 100 days of gestation.

Swine: PROSTAMATE® Sterile Solution will induce parturition in swine at 10 mg (2 mL) when injected intramuscularly.

As with any multidose vial, practice aseptic techniques in withdrawing each dose. Adequately clean and disinfect the vial closure prior to entry with a sterile needle.

Instructions for Use: The response to treatment varies by individual animals with a mean interval from administration of 2 mL PROSTAMATE® (10 mg dinoprost) to parturition of approximately 30 hours. This can be employed to control the time of farrowing in sows and gilts in late gestation.

Management Considerations: Several factors must be considered for the successful use of PROSTAMATE® Sterile Solution for parturition induction in swine. The product must be administered at a relatively specific time (treatment earlier than 3 days prior to normal predicted farrowing may result in increased piglet mortality). It is important that adequate records be maintained on (1) the average length of gestation period for the animals on a specific location, and (2) the breeding and projected farrowing dates for each animal. This information is essential to determine the appropriate time for administration of PROSTAMATE®.

Mares:

1. Evaluate the reproductive status of the mare.
2. Administer a single intramuscular injection of 1 mg per 100 lbs (45.5 kg) body weight which is usually 1 mL to 2 mL PROSTAMATE® Sterile Solution.
3. Observe for signs of estrus by means of daily teasing with a stallion, and evaluate follicular changes on the ovary by palpation of the ovary *per rectum.*
4. Some clinically anestrous mares will not express estrus but will develop a follicle which will ovulate. These mares may become pregnant if inseminated at the appropriate time relative to rupture of the follicle.
5. Breed mares in estrus in a manner consistent with normal management.

Dinoprost tromethamine is administered once as a single intramuscular injection of 1 mg per 100 lbs (45.5 kg) body weight which is usually 1 mL to 2 mL of PROSTAMATE® containing 5 mg dinoprost as the tromethamine salt per milliliter.

Instructions for Use: PROSTAMATE® Sterile Solution is indicated for its luteolytic effect in mares. This luteolytic effect can be utilized to control the timing of estrus in estrous cycling and clinically anestrous mares that have a corpus luteum in the following circumstances:

1. Controlling Time of Estrus of Estrous Cycling Mares: Mares treated with PROSTAMATE® during diestrus (4 or more days after ovulation) will return to estrus within 2 to 4 days in most cases and ovulate 8 to 12 days after treatment. This procedure may be utilized as an aid to scheduling the use of stallions.
2. Difficult-to-Breed Mares: In extended diestrus there is failure to exhibit regular estrous cycles which is different from true anestrus. Many mares described as anestrus during the breeding season have serum progesterone levels consistent with the presence of a functional corpus luteum.

   A proportion of "barren", maiden, and lactating mares do not exhibit regular estrous cycles and may be in extended diestrus. Following abortion, early fetal death and resorption, or as a result of "pseudopregnancy", there may be serum progesterone levels consistent with a functional corpus luteum.

   Treatment of such mares with PROSTAMATE® usually results in regression of the corpus luteum followed by estrus and/or ovulation. In one study with 122 Standardbred and Thoroughbred mares in clinical anestrus for an average of 58 days and treated during the breeding season, behavioral estrus was detected in 81 percent at an average time of 3.7 days after injection with 5 mg dinoprost tromethamine sterile solution; ovulation occurred an average of 7.0 days after treatment. Of those mares bred, 59% were pregnant following an average of 1.4 services during that estrus.

   Treatment of "anestrous" mares which abort subsequent to 36 days of pregnancy may not result in return to estrus due to presence of functional endometrial cups.

Precaution(s): Storage Conditions: Store at controlled room temperature 20° to 25°C (68° to 77°F).

Caution(s): Federal (USA) law restricts this drug to use by or on the order of a licensed veterinarian.

Cattle: Do not administer to pregnant cattle unless abortion is desired.

Do not administer intravenously (I.V.), as this route might potentiate adverse reactions.

Cattle administered a progestogen would be expected to have a reduced response to PROSTAMATE® Sterile Solution.

Aggressive antibiotic therapy should be employed at the first sign of infection at the injection site whether localized or diffuse. As with all parenteral products careful aseptic techniques should be employed to decrease the possibility of post injection bacterial infections.

Swine: Do not administer to sows and/or gilts prior to 3 days of normal predicted farrowing, as increased number of stillborn and postnatal mortality may result.

Mares: PROSTAMATE® Sterile Solution is ineffective when administered prior to day-5 after ovulation.

Pregnancy status should be determined prior to treatment, since PROSTAMATE® has been reported to induce abortion and parturition when sufficient doses were administered.

Mares should not be treated if they suffer from either acute or subacute disorders of the vascular system, gastrointestinal tract, respiratory system, or reproductive tract.

Do not administer by intravenous route.

Nonsteroidal anti-inflammatory drugs (i.e., indomethacin) may inhibit prostaglandin synthesis, therefore these drugs should not be administered concurrently.

Restricted Drug - Use only as directed (California).

For use in animals only.

Warning(s): Important:

Cattle: No milk discard or preslaughter drug withdrawal period is required for labeled uses.

Swine: No preslaughter drug withdrawal period is required for labeled uses.

Mares: Not for use in horses intended for food.

Not for human use.

Women of child-bearing age, asthmatics, and persons with bronchial and other respiratory problems should exercise extreme caution when handling this product. In the early stages, women may be unaware of their pregnancies. Dinoprost tromethamine is readily absorbed through the skin and can cause abortion and/or bronchiospasms. Direct contact with the skin should, therefore, be avoided. Accidental spillage on the skin should be washed off immediately with soap and water.

Use of this product in excess of the approved dose may result in drug residues.

Keep out of reach of children.

Toxicology: Safety and Toxicity:

Laboratory Animals: Dinoprost was non-teratogenic in rats when administered orally at 1.25, 3.2, 10.0 and 20.0 mg/kg/day from day 6th-15th of gestation or when administered subcutaneously at 0.5 and 1.0 mg/kg/day on gestation days 6, 7 and 8 or 9, 10 and 11 or 12, 13 and 14. Dinoprost was non-teratogenic in the rabbit when administered either subcutaneously at doses of 0.5 and 1.0 mg/kg/day on gestation days 6, 7 and 8 or 9, 10 and 11 or 12, 13 and 14 or 15, 16 and 17 or orally at doses of 0.01, 0.1 and 1.0 mg/kg/day on days 6-18 or 5.0 mg/kg/day on days 8-18 of gestation. A slight and marked embryo lethal effect was observed in dams given 1.0 and 5.0 mg/kg/day respectively. This was due to the expected luteolytic properties of the drug.

A 14-day continuous intravenous infusion study in rats at 20 mg PGF2α per kg body weight indicated prostaglandins of the F series could induce bone deposition. However, such bone changes were not observed in monkeys similarly administered dinoprost tromethamine sterile solution at 15 mg PGF2α per kg body weight for 14 days.

Cattle: In cattle, evaluation was made of clinical observations, clinical chemistry, hematology, urinalysis, organ weights, and gross plus microscopic measurements following treatment with various doses up to 250 mg dinoprost administered twice intramuscularly at a 10 day interval or doses of 25 mg administered daily for 10 days. There was no unequivocal effect of dinoprost on the hematology or clinical chemistry parameters measured. Clinically, a slight transitory increase in heart rate was detected. Rectal temperature was elevated about 1.5°F through the 6th hour after injection with 250 mg dinoprost, but had returned to baseline at 24 hours after injection. No dinoprost associated gross lesions were detected. There was no evidence of toxicological effects. Thus, dinoprost had a safety factor of at least 10X on injection (25 mg luteolytic dose vs. 250 mg safe dose), based on studies conducted with cattle. At luteolytic doses, dinoprost had no effect on progeny. If given to a pregnant cow, it may cause abortion; the dose required for abortion varies considerably with the stage of gestation.

Induction of abortion in feedlot cattle at stages of gestation up to 100 days of gestation did not result in dystocia, retained placenta or death of heifers in the field studies. The smallness of the fetus at this early stage of gestation should not lead to complications at abortion. However, induction of parturition or abortion with any exogenous compound may precipitate dystocia, fetal death, retained placenta and/or metritis, especially at latter stages of gestation.

Swine: In pigs, evaluation was made of clinical observations, food consumption, clinical pathologic determinations, body weight changes, urinalysis, organ weights, and gross and microscopic observations following treatment with single doses of 10, 30, 50 and 100 mg dinoprost administered intramuscularly. The results indicated no treatment related effects from dinoprost treatment that were deleterious to the health of the animals or to their offspring.

Mares: Dinoprost tromethamine was administered to adult mares (weighing 320 to 485 kg; 2 to 20 years old), at the rates of 0, 100, 200, 400, and 800 mg per mare per day for 8 days. Route of administration for each dose group was both intramuscularly (2 mares) and subcutaneously (2 mares). Changes were detected in all treated groups for clinical (reduced sensitivity to pain; locomotor incoordination; hypergastromotility; sweating; hyperthermia; labored respiration), blood chemistry (elevated cholesterol, total bilirubin, LDH, and glucose), and hematology (decreased eosinophils; increased hemoglobin, hematocrit, and erythrocytes) measurements. The effects in the 100 mg dose, and to a lesser extent, the 200 mg dose groups were transient in nature, lasting for a few minutes to several hours. Mares did not appear to sustain adverse effects following termination of the side effects.

Mares treated with either 400 mg or 800 mg exhibited more profound symptoms. The excessive hyperstimulation of the gastrointestinal tract caused a protracted diarrhea, slight electrolyte imbalance (decreased sodium and potassium), dehydration, gastrointestinal irritation, and slight liver malfunction (elevated SGOT, SGPT at 800 mg only). Heart rate was increased but pH of the urine was decreased. Other measurements evaluated in the study remained within normal limits. No mortality occurred in any of the groups. No apparent differences were observed between the intramuscular and subcutaneous routes of administration. Luteolytic doses of dinoprost tromethamine are on the order of 5 to 10 mg administered on one day, therefore, dinoprost tromethamine sterile solution was demonstrated to have a wide margin of safety. Thus, the 100 mg dose gave a safety margin of 10 to 20X for a single injection or 80 to 160X for the 8 daily injections.

Additional studies investigated the effects in the mare of single intramuscular doses of 0, 0.25, 1.0, 2.5, 3.0, 5.0, and 10.0 mg dinoprost tromethamine. Heart rate, respiration rate, rectal temperature, and sweating were measured at 0, 0.25, 0.50, 0.75, 1.0, 1.5, 2.0, 3.0, 4.0, 5.0, and 6.0 hr. after injection. Neither heart rate nor respiration rates were significantly altered ($P > 0.05$) when compared to contemporary control values. Sweating was observed for 0 of 9, 2 of 9, 7 of 9, 9 of 9, and 8 of 9 mares injected with 0.25, 1.0, 2.5, 3.0, 5.0, or 10.0 mg dinoprost tromethamine, respectively. Sweating was temporary in all cases and was mild for doses of 3.0 mg or less but was extensive (beads of sweat over the entire body and dripping) for the 10 mg dose. Sweating after the 5.0 mg dose was intermediate between that seen for mares treated with 3.0 and 10.0 mg. Sweating began within 15 minutes after injection and ceased by 45 to 60 minutes after injection. Rectal temperature was decreased during the interval 0.5 until 1.0, 3 to 4, or 5 hours after injection for 0.25 and 1.0 mg, 2.5 and 3.0, or 5.0 and 10.0 mg dose groups, respectively. Average rectal temperature during the periods of decreased temperature was on the order of 97.5 to 99.6, with the greatest decreases observed in the 10 mg dose group.

Adverse Reactions: Cattle:

1. The most frequently observed side effect is increased rectal temperature at a 5X or 10X overdose. However, rectal temperature change has been transient in all cases observed and has not been detrimental to the animal.
2. Limited salivation has been reported in some instances.
3. Intravenous administration might increase heart rate.
4. Localized post injection bacterial infections that may become generalized have been reported. In rare instances such infections have terminated fatally. See Cautions.

Swine: The most frequently observed side effects were erythema and pruritus, slight incoordination, nesting behavior, itching, urination, defecation, abdominal muscle spasms, tail movements, hyperpnea or dyspnea, increased vocalization, salivation, and at the 100 mg (10X) dose only, vomition. These side effects are transitory, lasting from 10 minutes to 3 hours, and were not detrimental to the health of the animal.

Mares: The most frequently observed side effects are sweating and decreased rectal temperature. However, these have been transient in all cases observed and have not been detrimental to the animal. Other reactions seen have been increase in heart rate, increase in respiration rate, some abdominal discomfort, locomotor incoordination, and lying down. These effects are usually seen within 15 minutes of injection and disappear within one hour. Mares usually continue to eat during the period of expression of side effects. One anaphylactic reaction of several hundred mares treated with dinoprost tromethamine sterile solution was reported but was not confirmed.

Presentation: PROSTAMATE® Sterile Solution is available in 30 mL glass vials (NDC: 47611-780-75).

Manufactured by: Phoenix Scientific, Inc., St. Joseph, MO 64503.

Distributed by: Burns Veterinary Supply, Inc., Westbury, NY 11590.

Compendium Code No.: 14441061 Iss. 5-02

PROSYSTEM® CE

Intervet **Bacterin-Toxoid**

Clostridium Perfringens Type C-Escherichia Coli Bacterin-Toxoid

U.S. Vet. Lic. No.: 286

Contents: A purified, adjuvanted product containing four major *E. coli* antigens (K88, K99, F41 and 987P), and *C. perfringens* type C toxoid.

Contains thimerosal and polymyxin B as preservatives.

Indications: For use in healthy pregnant swine as an aid in the prevention of colibacillosis and enterotoxemia in their nursing piglets.

Dosage and Administration: When used alone, shake well and administer one 2 mL intramuscularly or subcutaneously to healthy pregnant swine at 5 weeks and again at 1-2 weeks before farrowing. In subsequent farrowings, administer one dose 2 weeks before farrowing.

When packaged with ProSystem® Rota or ProSystem® TGE/Rota refer to insert for full directions.

Precaution(s): Store in the dark at not over 45°F (7°C). Do not freeze. Use entire contents when first opened; do not save partial contents.

Caution(s): Use only in healthy pregnant swine.

If allergic reaction occurs, treat with epinephrine.

For veterinary use only.

Warning(s): Do not vaccinate within 21 days of slaughter.

Presentation: 50 dose (100 mL) vials.

Compendium Code No.: 11061531

PROSYSTEM® PILIMUNE

Intervet **Bacterin**

Escherichia Coli Bacterin

U.S. Vet. Lic. No.: 286

Contents: A purified, adjuvanted product containing *E. coli* pilus antigens: K88, K99, F41 and 987P.

Contains thimerosal and polymyxin B as preservatives.

Indications: For use in healthy swine or cattle as an aid in the prevention of colibacillosis in their nursing young.

Dosage and Administration: When used alone, shake well and administer one 2 mL dose intramuscularly or subcutaneously to healthy pregnant swine or cattle at 5 weeks and again at 2 weeks before parturition. In subsequent pregnancies, administer one dose 2 weeks before parturition.

If packaged with ProSystem® TGE/Rota or ProSystem® Rota refer to insert for complete directions.

Precaution(s): Store in the dark at not over 45°F (7°C). Do not freeze. Use entire contents when first opened; do not save partial contents.

Caution(s): Use only in healthy animals.

If allergic reaction occurs, treat with epinephrine.

For veterinary use only.

Warning(s): Do not vaccinate within 21 days of slaughter.

Presentation: 50 dose (100 mL) vials.

Compendium Code No.: 11061521

PROSYSTEM® RCE

Intervet **Bacterin-Toxoid-Vaccine**

Porcine Rotavirus Vaccine, Modified Live Virus-Clostridium Perfringens Type C-Escherichia Coli Bacterin-Toxoid

U.S. Vet. Lic. No.: 286

Contents: Contains two major Rotavirus serotypes, four major *E. coli* pilus antigens (K88, K99, F41 and 987P) and *C. perfringens* type C toxoid.

Contains gentamicin, polymyxin B and thimerosal as preservatives.

Indications: For use in healthy pregnant swine as an aid in the prevention of rotaviral diarrhea, enterotoxemia and colibacillosis in their nursing piglets.

Dosage and Administration: Shake bacterin-toxoid well and restore accompanying vial of desiccated virus vaccine with 10-15 mL bacterin-toxoid and then transfer rehydrated vaccine to plastic bacterin bottle. Shake well, immediately inject a 2 mL dose intramuscularly into healthy pregnant swine at 5 weeks and again at 2 weeks before farrowing. In subsequent farrowings, inject one 2 mL dose 2 weeks before farrowing.

Precaution(s): Store in the dark at not over 45°F (7°C). Do not freeze. Use immediately after restoration; do not save partial contents; burn both containers and all unused contents.

Caution(s): Use only in healthy pregnant swine. If allergic reaction occurs, treat with epinephrine.

For veterinary use only.

Warning(s): Do not vaccinate within 21 days of slaughter.

Presentation: 10 doses (20 mL) and 25 doses (50 mL).

Compendium Code No.: 11061511

PROSYSTEM® ROTA

Intervet **Vaccine**

Porcine Rotavirus Vaccine, Modified Live Virus

U.S. Vet. Lic. No.: 286

Contents: Porcine Rotavirus Vaccine is a modified live virus vaccine containing 2 modified live G serotypes 5 and 4 of Serogroup A rotavirus, which have been modified so that they do not cause disease in baby pigs, feeder pigs or pregnant swine.

Contains gentamicin as preservative.

Indications: The vaccine is recommended as an aid in the prevention of rotaviral disease in young pigs. Rotavirus is one cause of viral gastroenteritis characterized by vomiting, watery diarrhea, dehydration and death in young pigs; therefore, the clinical signs may be identical to those of TGE. The disease is very common in both nursing and weaned pigs, and all swine herds so far examined show serologic evidence of its presence.

Dosage and Administration: Dosage Guidelines: Follow directions carefully.

Each baby pig should receive, before weaning, at least two doses of PROSYSTEM® Rota vaccine. One oral dose and one intramuscular dose about 7-10 days pre-weaning.

Reconstitute the dried vaccine with sterile diluent provided. Use 50 mL for the 50-dose size. Reconstitute the 50-dose vaccine vial with 10-15 mL sterile diluent and then return the liquid vaccine to the remainder of the diluent in the plastic 50 mL diluent vial. The 50 doses of vaccine can then be administered with either automatic syringe or a plastic oral dosing bottle.

Inoculate each pig orally with 1 mL of the reconstituted PROSYSTEM® Rota vaccine and inject one dose intramuscularly. Do not return the pig to the sow for at least 30 minutes after oral vaccination. Always wash oral vaccine dispensers thoroughly with soap and water and rinse thoroughly with clean water before addition of vaccine.

It is recommended that pregnant sows and gilts always be vaccinated with ProSystem® TGE/Rota (Porcine Rotavirus-Transmissible Gastroenteritis vaccine) (as directed) prior to farrowing. This should result in increased levels of milk antibody and protection of nursing pigs. Since pigs lose their passive milk protection when they are weaned, it is necessary to actively immunize them by oral and intramuscular vaccination prior to weaning.

Precaution(s): Store in the dark at not over 45°F (7°C). Do not freeze. Use vaccine immediately after reconstitution. Always use clean syringes and dispensers without chemical residues, which can destroy the vaccine. Use entire contents when first opened. Burn the container and all unused contents.

Caution(s): Use vaccine in healthy animals only.

If allergic reaction follow use of this product, treat with epinephrine. If diarrhea persists after use of the vaccine, additional diagnostic work may be warranted.

Although this product has been shown to be efficacious, some animals may be unable to develop or maintain an adequate immune response following vaccination if they are incubating any infectious disease, are malnourished or parasitized, or stressed due to shipment or adverse environmental conditions.

For veterinary use only.

Warning(s): Do not vaccinate within 21 days of slaughter.

Trial Data: Efficacy of the rotavirus vaccine has been demonstrated in both pregnant sows and baby pigs. Oral and intramuscular vaccination of nursing pigs induces active immunity and will protect them against post-weaning rotavirus-induced scours. Laboratory confirmation of the cause of baby pig diarrhea is recommended since other viral, bacterial and coccidial agents can cause similar disease signs.

Presentation: 25 doses (50 mL) and 50 doses (100 mL).

Compendium Code No.: 11061471 761198-01

PROSYSTEM® TGE

Intervet **Vaccine**

Transmissible Gastroenteritis Vaccine, Modified Live Virus

U.S. Vet. Lic. No.: 286

Contents: Transmissible Gastroenteritis (TGE) vaccine consists of a unique strain of TGE virus which has been modified so that it does not cause disease in newborn pigs, which are most susceptible to the natural disease. The vaccine contains the modified or attenuated virus in the dried state in order to preserve its potency and it must be reconstituted with the diluent provided immediately prior to use.

Contains gentamicin as preservative.

Indications: Experimental results indicate that sows as well as their baby pigs can be protected from TGE if the sow is fed the vaccine during the later stages of pregnancy. It is well known that feeding virulent TGE virus to pregnant sows a few weeks before farrowing will provide a good immunity to TGE for both the sow and her nursing piglets. Oral immunization provides more effective antibodies associated with the immunoglobulin. A fraction in the sow's milk, thus providing more effective immunity to TGE for the sow's nursing piglets. Baby pigs, however, will become susceptible to TGE after weaning. Therefore, active immunization of the baby pigs before weaning is recommended and oral administration of TGE vaccine is effective for baby pigs nursing either immune or non-immune sows. The virus used in this vaccine has been shown to be safe in both laboratory and field trials in swine. However, due to the nature of TGE immunity in piglets nursing immune sows, any condition in the sow resulting in reduction or cessation of milk flow can seriously impair immunity in her piglets. For this reason, active immunization of baby pigs is desirable.

The vaccine also has been shown to be safe for feeder pigs, boars and pregnant sows or gilts.

Dosage and Administration: Dosage Guidelines: Follow directions carefully. Two vaccination programs may be used.

Intramuscular (Injection) vaccination method: to be used for sows and gilts having significant virulent TGE exposure within the prior 12 months.

1. Reconstitute PROSYSTEM® TGE virus vaccine with sterile diluent: shake well.
2. Inject pregnant sow or gilt with 2.0 mL intramuscularly at 5 weeks and again at 2 weeks before each farrowing.

Oral and intramuscular (Oral) vaccination method: to be used for sows and gilts not previously exposed to virulent TGE.

1. For initial use, each pregnant sow or gilt must receive at least 2 oral and 1 intramuscular dosings of PROSYSTEM® TGE virus vaccine before farrowing.
   a. 5 weeks before farrowing - 1 oral dose PROSYSTEM® TGE
   b. 3 weeks before farrowing - 1 oral dose PROSYSTEM® TGE
   c. 1 week before farrowing - 1 intramuscular dose of PROSYSTEM® TGE
2. Subsequent farrowings - 2 weeks before farrowing administer 1 oral dose and 1 intramuscular dose of PROSYSTEM® TGE.

Baby Pig Vaccination: Orally vaccinate each baby pig at 1 to 3 days of age with one-fifth the sow dose. A second dose may be given 2 to 4 days later. Reconstitute the dried vaccine with sterile diluent provided. Add 5 mL cool milk to the 20 mL vial. Inoculate each pig orally with 0.5 mL of the vaccine-milk mixture using a syringe and spraying or dropping the inoculum into the back of the throat area. Do not return pigs to the sow for at least 30 minutes after oral vaccination.

For best TGE protection: sows and gilts which have never been exposed to virulent TGE virus, along with their baby pigs, should be vaccinated following the oral vaccination guidelines - refer to the five-step method for sow and gilt oral vaccination. Transfer the desired number of doses to skim milk (prepared by adding one pound dried milk solids to 2½ gallons clean cool water) or into cool pasteurized milk at a ratio of one dose per quart. Add clean ground grain to the vaccine-milk mixture until thickened and immediately feed to sow. Solid feed should be withheld overnight prior to vaccination in order to facilitate vaccine consumption and efficacy.

Recommended Methods for Oral Vaccination of Swine:

Step 1: Pour approximately 2 to 2½ gallons of cool water into a large plastic bucket. Add 5 - 10 cups of dry milk (any type of dry milk for human consumption is acceptable). Do not use hot water - it will destroy the vaccine.

Step 2: Stir milk mixture well. Drywall paddles attached to ½" drill make mixing easier.

Step 3: Remove metal ring and stopper. Reconstitute vaccine with diluent or milk; add reconstituted vaccine to milk, and stir.

Step 4: Slowly add 40 lbs. of clean ground corn to the milk/vaccine mixture. Stir continuously, using an electric ½" drill and drywall paddle, until mixture thickens and drill pulls down. There should be no run-off seen. Mixing procedure takes approximately 3 minutes.

Step 5: Feed to pregnant sows and gilts in one of two ways:

1. Feed sows individually with approximately 4 lbs. of milk/vaccine/corn mixture.
2. Spread milk/vaccine/corn mixture in a row onto concrete, feeding 10 sows at a time.

Precaution(s): Store in dark at not over 45°F. (7°C.). Do not freeze.

Use vaccine immediately after reconstitution. Use entire contents when first opened. Burn this container and all unused contents.

Caution(s): Do not use commercial milk replacers or complete rations to prepare oral vaccine mixture, as they may adversely affect vaccine potency.

Do not pour vaccine-milk mixture on top of ground corn, as sows may not receive sufficient vaccine.

Use vaccine in healthy animals only.

If allergic reaction follows use of this product, treat with epinephrine.

Conditions which interfere with lactation adversely affect immunity in baby pigs.

Although this product has been shown to be efficacious, some animals may be unable to develop or maintain an adequate immune response following vaccination if they are incubating any infectious disease, are malnourished or parasitized, or stressed due to shipment or adverse environmental conditions.

For highly TGE-susceptible (seronegative) sows and gilts, always use oral TGE vaccination program.

For veterinary use only

Warning(s): Do not vaccinate within 21 days of slaughter.

Presentation: 10 sow doses/50 piglet doses (20 mL).

Compendium Code No.: 11061461 760-01

PROSYSTEM® TG-EMUNE® ROTA WITH IMUGEN® II

Intervet **Vaccine**

Porcine Rotavirus-Transmissible Gastroenteritis Vaccine, Killed Virus

U.S. Vet. Lic. No.: 286

Contents: This product contains the antigens listed above.

Contains gentamicin as a preservative.

Indications: For the immunization of healthy sows, gilts and their litters against disease caused by transmissible gastroenteritis virus and porcine rotaviruses types 1 and 2.

Dosage and Administration:

Sows and Gilts: Give 5 mL intramuscularly 6 and 2 weeks before farrowing. Vaccinate the piglets with 1 mL intraperitoneally at 3-10 days of age.

Gilts should be given one 5 mL dose prior to introduction into TGE-positive breeding herds.

Precaution(s): Store at 2° to 7°C (35°-45°F). Use entire contents when first opened.

Caution(s): In case of anaphylactoid reaction administer epinephrine.

For veterinary use only.

Warning(s): Do not vaccinate within 60 days before slaughter.

Presentation: 20 adult dose (100 mL) vial.

Compendium Code No.: 11062041 7372001

PROSYSTEM® TG-EMUNE® WITH IMUGEN® II

Intervet **Vaccine**

Transmissible Gastroenteritis Vaccine, Killed Virus

U.S. Vet. Lic. No.: 286

Contents: This product contains the antigen listed above.

Contains gentamicin as a preservative.

Indications: For the immunization of healthy sows, gilts and their litters against diarrhea caused by Transmissible Gastroenteritis virus.

Dosage and Administration: Shake well.

Sows and Gilts: Give 5 mL intramuscularly 6 and 2 weeks before farrowing. Vaccinate the piglets with 1 mL intraperitoneally at 3-10 days of age.

Gilts should be given one 5 mL dose prior to introduction into TGE-positive breeding herds.

Precaution(s): Store at 2° to 7°C (35°-45°F). Use entire contents when first opened.

Caution(s): In case of anaphylactoid reaction administer epinephrine.

For veterinary use only.

Warning(s): Do not vaccinate within 60 days before slaughter.

Presentation: 20 adult dose (100 mL) vial.

Compendium Code No.: 11062051 7362001

PROSYSTEM® TGE/ROTA

Intervet **Vaccine**

Porcine Rotavirus-Transmissible Gastroenteritis Vaccine, Modified Live Virus

U.S. Vet. Lic. No.: 286

Contents: Porcine Rotavirus-Transmissible Gastroenteritis vaccine is a modified live virus vaccine containing three unique virus strains:

1. Rotavirus (2 modified live G serotypes 5 and 4 of Serogroup A rotavirus).
2. TGE (transmissible gastroenteritis).

All three viruses have been modified so that they do not cause disease in feeder pigs and pregnant swine.

Contains gentamicin as preservative.

Indications: The vaccine is recommended for use in healthy pregnant swine as an aid in the prevention of rotaviral diarrhea and TGE in their nursing piglets. Both diseases produce identical clinical signs, occasional vomition and profuse watery diarrhea, in young pigs. Laboratory confirmation of the cause of baby pig diarrhea is recommended since other viral, bacterial and coccidial agents also can cause similar disease signs.

Dosage and Administration: Dosage Guidelines: Follow directions carefully. Two vaccination programs may be used.

Intramuscular (Injection) vaccination method: To be used for sows and gilts having significant virulent TGE exposure within the prior 12 months.

1. Reconstitute PROSYSTEM® TGE/Rota virus vaccine with sterile diluent, shake well.
2. Inject pregnant sow or gilt with 2.0 mL intramuscularly at 5 weeks and again at 2 weeks before each farrowing.

Oral and intramuscular (oral) vaccination method: To be used for sows and gilts not previously exposed to virulent TGE.

1. For initial use, each pregnant sow or gilt must receive at least 2 oral and 1 intramuscular dosings of PROSYSTEM® TGE/Rota virus vaccine before farrowing.
   a. 5 weeks before farrowing - 1 oral dose PROSYSTEM® TGE/Rota.
   b. 3 weeks before farrowing - 1 oral dose PROSYSTEM® TGE/Rota.
   c. 1 week before farrowing - 1 intramuscular dose of PROSYSTEM® TGE/Rota.
2. Subsequent farrowings - 2 weeks before farrowing administer 1 oral dose and 1 intramuscular dose of PROSYSTEM® TGE/Rota.

Recommended Methods for Oral Vaccination of Swine:

Step 1: Pour approximately 2 to 2½ gallons of cool water into a large plastic bucket. Add 5 - 10 cups of dry milk (any type of dry milk for human consumption is acceptable). Do not use hot water - it will destroy the vaccine.

Step 2: Stir milk mixture well. Drywall paddles attached to ½" drill make mixing easier.

Step 3: Remove metal ring and stopper. Reconstitute vaccine with diluent or milk; add reconstituted vaccine to milk, and stir.

Step 4: Slowly add 40 lbs. of clean ground corn to the milk/vaccine mixture. Stir continuously, using an electric ½" drill and drywall paddle, until mixture thickens and drill pulls down. There should be no run-off seen. Mixing procedure takes approximately 3 minutes.

Step 5: Feed to pregnant sows and gilts in one of two ways:

1. Feed sows individually with approximately 4 lbs. of milk/vaccine/corn mixture.
2. Spread milk/vaccine/corn mixture in a row onto concrete, feeding 10 sows at a time.

For best TGE protection: Sows and gilts which have never been exposed to virulent TGE virus, along with their baby pigs, should be vaccinated following the oral vaccination guidelines - refer to the five-step method for sow and gilt oral vaccination. Transfer the desired number of doses to skim milk (prepared by adding one pound dried milk solids to 2½ gallons clean cool water) or into cool pasteurized milk at a ratio of one dose per quart. Add clean ground grain to the vaccine-milk mixture until thickened and immediately feed to sow. Solid feed should be withheld overnight prior to vaccination in order to facilitate vaccine consumption and efficacy.

Precaution(s): Store in the dark at not over 45°F (7°C). Do not freeze. Use vaccine immediately after reconstitution. Use entire contents when first opened. Burn the container and all unused contents.

Caution(s): Do not use commercial milk replacers or complete rations to prepare oral vaccine mixture, as they may adversely affect vaccine potency. Do not pour vaccine-milk mixture on top of ground corn, as sows may not receive sufficient vaccine.

Conditions which interfere with lactation adversely affect immunity in baby pigs.

Use vaccine in healthy, pregnant swine only.

If allergic reaction follows use of this product, treat with epinephrine.

Although this product has been shown to be efficacious, some animals may be unable to develop or maintain an adequate immune response following vaccination if they are incubating any infectious disease, are malnourished or parasitized, or stressed due to shipment or adverse environmental conditions.

For highly TGE-susceptible (seronegative) sows and gilts, always use oral TGE vaccination program.

Do not use for the vaccination of baby pigs.

For veterinary use only.

Warning(s): Do not vaccinate within 21 days of slaughter.

Trial Data: Efficacy of the TGE virus component as a monovalent vaccine has shown for pregnant swine and baby pigs by oral vaccination. Efficacy of rotavirus without the TGE component has been demonstrated in both pregnant sows and baby pigs. Pregnant sows, when vaccinated with the Rotavirus-TGE vaccine, subsequently develop high persisting levels of antibody in their milk, thereby aiding in the control of diarrhea in their nursing pigs. Pigs are protected by receiving colostral and milk antibodies from vaccinated dams, therefore it is mandatory that sows and gilts are lactating and baby pigs are nursing adequately.

Presentation: 10 dose (20 mL) vial.

Compendium Code No.: 11061481 762-01

PROSYSTEM® TREC

Intervet **Bacterin-Toxoid-Vaccine**

Porcine Rotavirus-Transmissible Gastroenteritis Vaccine, Modified Live Virus-Clostridium Perfringens Type C-Escherichia Coli Bacterin-Toxoid

U.S. Vet. Lic. No.: 286

Contents: The Rotavirus-TGE vaccine (ProSystem® TGE/Rota) contains 2 major serotypes of modified live Rotavirus and a modified live TGE virus in desiccated form. The bacterin-toxoid diluent (ProSystem® CE) is a purified, adjuvanted liquid product containing four major *E coli* pilus antigens - K88, K99, F41 and 987P, and *C. perfringens* type C toxoid. Each serial of ProSystem® CE bacterin-toxoid is demonstrated to be compatible (non-viricidal) with ProSystem® TGE/Rota virus vaccine and therefore can be used as a diluent when packaged with the viral vaccine.

Contains gentamicin, polymyxin and thimerosal as preservatives.

Indications: Porcine Rotavirus-Transmissible Gastroenteritis vaccine and *Clostridium perfringens* type C-*Escherichia coli* bacterin-toxoid are used for the vaccination of healthy pregnant swine, to provide passive protection to their nursing pigs against disease caused by eight pathogens:

1. Rotavirus (2 modified live G serotypes 5 and 4 of Serogroup A rotavirus).
2. TGE (transmissible gastroenteritis).
3. Colibacillosis *(Escherichia coli* pilus antigens K88, K99, F41 and 987P).
4. Enterotoxemia *(Clostridium perfringens* type C).

These etiologic agents are the most important causes of neonatal porcine diarrhea. They often occur in combination with each other causing increased morbidity and mortality. Furthermore, several of these diseases may produce similar clinical signs in baby pigs; therefore, it is desirable to provide broad spectrum protection to nursing pigs. Laboratory confirmation of the cause of baby pig diarrhea is recommended since other viral, bacterial and coccidial agents also can cause similar disease signs.

Dosage and Administration: Dosage Guidelines: Follow directions carefully. Two vaccination programs may be used.

Intramuscular (Injection) vaccination method: To be used for sows and gilts having significant virulent TGE exposure within the prior 12 months.

1. Reconstitute ProSystem® TGE/Rota virus vaccine with ProSystem® CE bacterin-toxoid diluent, shake bacterin-toxoid well before and after addition to the virus vaccine.
2. Inject pregnant sow or gilt with 2.0 mL intramuscularly at 5 weeks and again at 2 weeks before each farrowing.

Oral and intramuscular (oral) vaccination method: To be used for sows and gilts not previously exposed to virulent TGE.

1. For initial use, each pregnant sow or gilt must receive at least 2 oral and 1 intramuscular dosings of ProSystem® TGE/Rota virus vaccine and 2 doses of ProSystem® CE bacterin-toxoid before farrowing. Refer to the five-step method for oral vaccination, as shown below, using desiccated viral vaccine.
   a. 5 weeks before farrowing - 1 oral dose ProSystem® TGE/Rota and 1 intramuscular dose of ProSystem® CE bacterin-toxoid.
   b. 3 weeks before farrowing - 1 oral dose ProSystem® TGE/Rota.
   c. 1 week before farrowing - 1 intramuscular dose of ProSystem® TGE/Rota rehydrated with ProSystem® CE bacterin-toxoid.
2. Subsequent farrowings - 2 weeks before farrowing, administer 1 oral dose of ProSystem® TGE/Rota and 1 intramuscular dose of ProSystem® TGE/Rota rehydrated with ProSystem® CE bacterin-toxoid.

For combination injection, reconstitute ProSystem® TGE/Rota dried vaccine with the accompanying ProSystem® CE bacterin-toxoid diluent. Shake well before use. If the bacterin-toxoid is given separately (e.g., at the time of oral vaccination with ProSystem® TGE/Rota), the 2.0 mL dose can be injected either intramuscularly or subcutaneously.

Recommended Methods for Oral Vaccination of Swine:

Step 1: Pour approximately 2 to 2½ gallons of cool water into a large plastic bucket. Add 5 - 10 cups of dry milk (any type of dry milk for human consumption is acceptable). Do not use hot water - it will destroy the vaccine.

Step 2: Stir milk mixture well. Drywall paddles attached to ½" drill make mixing easier.

Step 3: Remove metal ring and stopper. Reconstitute vaccine with milk mixture; add reconstituted vaccine to milk, and stir. (The bacterin-toxoid packaged in combination with viral vaccine must always be injected).

Step 4: Slowly add 40 lbs. of clean ground corn to the milk/vaccine mixture. Stir continuously, using an electric ½" drill and drywall paddle, until mixture thickens and drill pulls down. There should be no run-off seen. Mixing procedure takes approximately 3 minutes.

Step 5: Feed to pregnant sows and gilts in one of two ways:

1. Feed sows individually with approximately 4 lbs. of milk/vaccine/corn mixture.
2. Spread milk/vaccine/corn mixture in a row onto concrete, feeding 10 sows at a time.

For best TGE protection, sows and gilts which have never been exposed to virulent TGE virus should be vaccinated following the oral vaccination guidelines (above) and their baby pigs should be orally vaccinated with ProSystem® TGE (Transmissible Gastroenteritis vaccine).

Precaution(s): Store in the dark at not over 45°F (7°C). Do not freeze. Use vaccine immediately after reconstitution. Use entire contents when first opened. Burn the container and all unused contents.

Caution(s): Use in healthy pregnant swine only.

Conditions which interfere with lactation adversely affect immunity in baby pigs.

If allergic reaction follows use of this product, treat with epinephrine.

Although this product has been shown to be efficacious, some animals may be unable to develop or maintain an adequate immune response following vaccination if they are incubating any infectious disease, are malnourished or parasitized, or stressed due to shipment or adverse environmental conditions.

For highly TGE-susceptible (seronegative) sows and gilts, always use oral TGE vaccination program.

For veterinary use only.

Warning(s): Do not vaccinate within 21 days of slaughter.

Trial Data: Safety and efficacy of the modified live rotaviruses and TGE have been demonstrated. The Rotavirus-TGE vaccine, rehydrated with the bacterin-toxoid, and the bacterin-toxoid alone have been evaluated for safety in pregnant swine as well as in laboratory animals. No adverse reactions were observed. Baby pigs are protected from disease caused by these agents by receiving colostral and milk antibodies from vaccinated dams. Therefore, it is mandatory that sows and gilts are lactating and baby pigs are nursing adequately.

Presentation: One 10 dose (20 mL) vial of each ProSystem® TGE/Rota and ProSystem® CE.

Compendium Code No.: 11061491 762708-01

PROTECTA-PAD®

Evsco **Topical Product**

Active Ingredient(s): Skin emollients.

Indications: Restores lost moisture to dry cracked pads.

PROTECTA-PAD® is an aid in the care and repair of dry, calloused pads of working and hunting dogs. PROTECTA-PAD® softens calloused areas and increases the pliability of the pad, while maintaining the resiliency consistent with normal healthy tissue. May be applied to elbow joint callouses caused by sleeping on rugs and hard surfaces.

Dosage and Administration: Apply as needed. Work PROTECTA-PAD® thoroughly into cracks and crevices of pad and elbow or other calloused areas.

Warning(s): For veterinary use only. Keep out of reach of children.

Presentation: 4 oz (113.4 g) jar.

Compendium Code No.: 10050310

PROTECTA-PAD®

Tomlyn **Topical Product**

Active Ingredient(s): Skin emollients.

Indications: PROTECTA-PAD® is specially compounded as an aid in the care and repair of dry, calloused pads of working and hunting dogs. PROTECTA-PAD® softens calloused areas and increases the pliability of the pad, while maintaining the resiliency consistent with normal healthy tissue. May be applied to elbow joint callouses caused by sleeping on rugs and hard surfaces.

Directions: Apply as needed. Work PROTECTA-PAD® thoroughly into cracks and crevices of pad and elbow or other calloused areas.

Precaution(s): Store at room temperature.

Caution(s): For animal use only.

Keep out of reach of children.

Presentation: 12 x 4 oz (113.4 g).

Compendium Code No.: 11220210 020-1

PRO'TECT™ HE

Brinton **Vaccine**

Hemorrhagic Enteritis Vaccine, Live Virus

U.S. Vet. Lic. No.: 343

Active Ingredient(s): Hemorrhagic enteritis vaccine, live, avirulent cell culture grown virus.

Indications: PRO'TECT™ HE is a live virus vaccine containing an avirulent strain of hemorrhagic enteritis virus which is immunogenic for turkeys when administered via drinking water to healthy poults that are between four and six weeks of age.

Dosage and Administration: How to Vaccinate:

1. Vaccinate only healthy poults free from environmental or physical stress.
2. Use only clean water tanks, lines, and fountains free of disinfectants or sanitizers. To ensure PRO'TECT™ HE stability, stabilizer or powdered milk can be flushed through the drinking system a minimum of two (2) hours prior to vaccination. (Use 1 lb. of stabilizer per 100 gallons of water.)
3. Administer PRO'TECT™ HE at day's first light. Calculate the quantity of water that will be consumed in four (4) hours by the number of turkeys to be vaccinated. Average four (4) hour water consumption for 1,000 turkeys at four (4) weeks of age is 16 gallons, at five (5) weeks of age is 20 gallons, and at six (6) weeks of age is 24 gallons.
4. Stabilizer (or powdered milk) should be added to the amount of water calculated (in #3 above) approximately 30 minutes prior to adding the PRO'TECT™ HE. (Use 1 lb. stabilizer per 100 gallons of water).
5. Do not thaw the vaccine until ready for use. Thaw the number of doses needed by placing the vaccine bottles in cold water. As soon as they are thawed, tip each bottle back and forth to ensure that the contents are thoroughly mixed.
6. Tear off the aluminum seal and remove the rubber stopper. Pour contents into a tank containing stabilized water.

7. The contents of tank should be thoroughly mixed for several minutes and remixed at frequent intervals during vaccine administration.
8. Provide ample watering space so that all of the turkeys have easy water access. PRO'TECT™ HE should be consumed in approximately four (4) hours.

Precaution(s): Keep frozen until ready for use.
Caution(s): Use the entire contents when first opened.
Burn the container and all unused contents. Do not re-use or refreeze open bottles.
Warning(s): Do not vaccinate within 21 days before slaughter.
Presentation: Available in cartons containing 10,000 doses. Choice of 2x5,000 dose vials or 10x1,000 dose vials.
Compendium Code No.: 11250000

PROTEOSEPTIC BOLUS

Vedco **Uterine Bolus**
NDC No.: 50989-359-49
Active Ingredient(s): Each bolus contains:
Urea .... 13.4 g
Indications: For use as an antiseptic and proteolytic aid in beef and dairy cattle and sheep.
Dosage and Administration: For intra-uterine or topical use only. Insert boluses into the uterus or dissolve in one (1) pint of warm water to make a flush.
Cattle .... 2-4 boluses
Sheep .... ½ to 1 bolus
For topical application, dissolve four (4) boluses in one (1) pint of warm water and thoroughly flush the wound. Repeat the treatment in 24 to 48 hours if necessary.
Precaution(s): Store in a cool, dry place. Keep the container tightly closed when not in use.
Caution(s): Do not administer orally.
Strict cleanliness must be observed to prevent the introduction of further infections. Thoroughly cleanse the hands and arms of the operator and external genital parts of the animal with soap and water before inserting the boluses or flush.
Do not use in deep or puncture wounds or for serious burns.
For animal use only. Keep out of the reach of children.
Presentation: 50 boluses.
Compendium Code No.: 10941740

PROTEX®-3

Intervet **Vaccine**
Feline Rhinotracheitis-Calici-Panleukopenia Vaccine, Modified Live Virus
U.S. Vet. Lic. No.: 286
Contents: PROTEX®-3 is a modified live virus vaccine containing attenuated strains of feline rhinotracheitis virus, calicivirus and panleukopenia virus grown in the Pro-Cell Stable Cell Line™. PROTEX®-3 is presented in a desiccated, single dose form with sterile diluent provided for reconstitution.
Contains gentamicin as a preservative.
Indications: PROTEX®-3 is for vaccination of healthy cats against feline viral rhinotracheitis, feline calicivirus and feline panleukopenia.
Dosage and Administration: Aseptically reconstitute the desiccated vaccine vial with the sterile diluent provided and administer 1 mL by subcutaneous or intramuscular route. Vaccinate healthy cats 8 weeks of age or older with two doses 3-4 weeks apart. Cats less than 12 weeks of age should be revaccinated at 3-4 week intervals until 12-16 weeks of age. Annual revaccination with a single dose is recommended.
Precaution(s): Recommended storage temperature 35-45°F (2-7°C).
Shake well before use.
Use contents promptly once reconstituted.
Non-chemically sterilized needles and syringes should be used for administration of vaccine.
Burn this container and all unused contents.
Caution(s): Do not vaccinate pregnant queens.
Administration of epinephrine may be indicated in the event of an anaphylactic reaction.
Only healthy animals should be vaccinated. Animals incubating any disease, or animals stressed due to shipping, malnutrition or parasitism may not achieve or maintain an adequate immune response.
This product is not hazardous when used according to directions supplied. A material safety data sheet (MSDS) is available upon request. This and any other consumer information can be obtained by calling Intervet's Customer Service Department at 1-800-441-8272.
For use in cats only.
Trial Data: Safety and Efficacy: The safety and efficacy of PROTEX®-3 have been demonstrated to meet or exceed the standards set forth by the U.S.D.A. Field safety trials conducted in kittens as young as 6 weeks of age demonstrated PROTEX®-3 was virtually reaction-free.
Presentation: Cartons of 25 - 1 dose desiccated vaccine vials and 25 - 1 dose sterile diluent vials. Packaged in recyclable plastic containers.
Compendium Code No.: 11061590

PROTEX®-4

Intervet **Vaccine**
Feline Rhinotracheitis-Calici-Panleukopenia-Chlamydia Psittaci Vaccine, Modified Live Virus and Chlamydia
U.S. Vet. Lic. No.: 286
Contents: PROTEX®-4 is a modified live virus vaccine containing attenuated strains of feline rhinotracheitis virus, calicivirus, panleukopenia virus and *Chlamydia psittaci* grown in the Pro-Cell Stable Cell Line™. PROTEX®-4 is presented in a desiccated form with sterile diluent provided for reconstitution. Contains gentamicin as a preservative.
Indications: PROTEX®-4 is for vaccination of healthy cats against disease caused by feline rhinotracheitis virus, feline calicivirus, feline panleukopenia, and *C. psittaci*.
Dosage and Administration: Aseptically reconstitute the desiccated vaccine with the sterile diluent provided and administer 1 mL by subcutaneous route. Vaccinate healthy kittens eight weeks of age or older with two doses 3-4 weeks apart. Cats less than 12 weeks of age should be revaccinated at 3-4 week intervals until 12-16 weeks of age. Annual revaccination with a single dose is recommended.
Precaution(s): Recommended storage temperature 35-45°F (2-7°C). Shake well before use. Use contents promptly once reconstituted. Non-chemically sterilized needles and syringes should be used for administration of vaccine. Burn this container and all unused contents.
Caution(s): Do not vaccinate pregnant queens. Administration of epinephrine may be indicated in the event of an anaphylactic reaction. Only healthy animals should be vaccinated. Animals incubating any disease, or animals stressed due to shipping, malnutrition or parasitism may not achieve or maintain an adequate immune response. This product is not hazardous when used according to directions supplied. A material safety data sheet (MSDS) is available upon request. This and any other consumer information can be obtained by calling Intervet's Customer Service Department at 1-800-441-8272. For use in cats only.
Presentation: Cartons of 25x1-dose desiccated vaccine vials and 25x1-dose sterile diluent vials. Packaged in recyclable plastic containers.
Compendium Code No.: 11061600

PROTEX®-Bb

Intervet **Vaccine**
Bordetella Bronchiseptica Vaccine, Avirulent Live Culture
U.S. Vet. Lic. No.: 286
Contents: PROTEX®-Bb is an intranasal vaccine containing an avirulent live culture of *Bordetella bronchiseptica*. PROTEX®-Bb is presented in a desiccated form with sterile diluent provided for reconstitution.
Indications: PROTEX®-Bb is for vaccination of healthy kittens and cats for prevention of disease caused by *B. bronchiseptica*.
Dosage and Administration: Aseptically reconstitute the desiccated vaccine with the sterile diluent provided. Remove the needle and administer 0.2 mL intranasally. Healthy kittens 8 weeks of age or older should be vaccinated prior to confinement or when risk of exposure to *B. bronchiseptica* may exist.
Precaution(s): Recommended storage temperature 35-45°F (2-7°C).
Shake well before use. Use contents promptly once reconstituted.
Non-chemically sterilized syringes should be used for administration of vaccine.
Burn this container and all unused contents.
Caution(s): Administration of epinephrine may be indicated in the event of an anaphylactic reaction.
Only healthy animals should be vaccinated. Animals incubating any disease, or animals stressed due to shipping, malnutrition or parasitism may not achieve or maintain an adequate immune response.
This product is not hazardous when used according to directions supplied. A material safety data sheet (MSDS) is available upon request. This and any other consumer information can be obtained by calling Intervet's Customer Service Department at 1-800-441-8272.
For use in cats only.
Discussion: Research has demonstrated that *B. bronchiseptica* acts as a primary or secondary pathogen in feline respiratory disease. Traditionally, feline herpesvirus (FHV) and feline calicivirus (FCV) have been implicated as the most common agents associated with feline upper respiratory infection (URI). However, studies have shown that *B. bronchiseptica* may be the sole infectious agent in feline URI.[1,2] Clinical signs associated with *B. bronchiseptica* infection may include fever, sneezing, nasal discharge, coughing and submandibular lymphadenopathy. In some cases, the infection progresses to pneumonia. Research regarding interspecies transmission has demonstrated isolates from cats and dogs housed in the same location were similar if not identical.[3] Because *B. bronchiseptica* is transmitted by the aerosol route, animals in close confinement such as in catteries, boarding facilities, hospitals or pet stores or cats from multi-cat households are at greatest risk for infection.
Efficacy Data: Challenge studies have shown that kittens vaccinated at 4 weeks of age with PROTEX®-Bb were protected against disease when challenged 3 weeks post-vaccination. Further studies to establish duration of immunity have not yet been completed. Studies to evaluate the onset of immunity have demonstrated protection against *B. bronchiseptica* 72 hours after vaccination in 8 week old kittens.
References: Available upon request.
Presentation: Cartons of 25-1 dose desiccated vaccine vials and 25-1 dose sterile diluent vials.
Packaged in recyclable plastic containers. * U.S. Patent No. 5,595,744
Compendium Code No.: 11061610

PROTEX®-FeLV

Intervet **Vaccine**
Feline Leukemia Vaccine, Killed Virus
U.S. Vet. Lic. No.: 286
Contents: This product contains the antigen listed above.
Contains gentamicin as a preservative.
Indications: For vaccination of healthy cats as an aid in prevention of disease associated with feline leukemia virus infection.
Directions: Aseptically administer 1 mL by the subcutaneous route to cats as early as 9 weeks of age with booster injections every 2-3 weeks until 12 weeks of age. Cats over 12 weeks of age should receive 2 doses 2-3 weeks apart. Revaccinate annually with a single dose.
Precaution(s): Store at 35-45°F (2-7°C). Use entire contents when first opened.
Caution(s): In case of anaphylactoid reaction, administer epinephrine.
For cats only. For veterinary use only.
Presentation: 50 x 1 dose (1 mL) and 5 x 10 dose (10 mL) vials.
Compendium Code No.: 11062560

PROTICALL® INSECTICIDE FOR DOGS

Schering-Plough **Topical Insecticide**
EPA Reg. No.: 773-73
Active Ingredient(s):
Permethrin† 65%
Other Ingredients 35%
Total .... 100% wt/wt.
†cis/trans ratio: Max 55% (±) cis and min. 45% (±) trans, CAS #52645-53-1.
Indications: For use on dogs and puppies.
Kills and Repels:
Fleas: Up to 4 weeks.
Deer Ticks *(Ixodes scapularis)*: Up to 4 weeks.*
Brown Dog Ticks *(Rhipicephalus sanguineus)*: Up to 4 weeks.*
American Dog Ticks *(Dermacentor variabilis)*: 2 to 3 weeks.
Lone Star Ticks *(Amblyomma americanum)*: 2 to 3 weeks.
Mosquitoes *(Aedes Aegypti)*: Up to 4 weeks.
Dog Lice *(Trichodectes canis)*: Up to 4 weeks.
Mites *(Cheyletiella yasguri)*: Up to 4 weeks.
* 3 to 4 weeks for extra large dogs.
Directions for Use: It is a violation of Federal Law to use this product in a manner inconsistent with its labeling. Read entire label completely before using.

Do not use on cats. May be toxic and potentially fatal if applied to or ingested by cats. Do not use this product in or on electrical equipment due to the possibility of shock hazard. PROTICALL® Insecticide for Dogs may be used on puppies as young as 4 weeks of age.

How to Apply:

1. Remove tubes along perforations.
2. Hold tube in upright position.
3. Point tip of tube up and away from user's face and body.
4. Cut across tip where indicated.
5. Part dog's hair between the shoulder blades.
6. Invert tube over dog.
7. Squeeze the tube firmly and apply the amount of solution to the skin of the dog's back between the shoulder blades. For large and extra large dogs, another application of the solution to the dog's skin directly in front of the base of the tail is also required. See "Recommended Dosing" guidelines.
8. When application is complete, follow Pesticide Disposal under "Storage and Disposal" section.

Recommended Dosing: Follow the appropriate instructions based on the pet's weight.

Puppies and Small Dogs:

Dosage for Puppies and Small Dogs weighing 33 lbs (15 kg) or less: Apply 1 (one) cc (1 tube) of PROTICALL® Insecticide solution to the skin of the dog's back between the shoulder blades.

Large Dogs:

Dosage for Large Dogs Weighing 33-65 lbs (15-29 kg): Apply 1 cc (1 tube) of PROTICALL® Insecticide solution to the skin of the dog's back and 1 cc (1 tube) to the skin of the dog's back directly in front of the base of the tail.

Extra Large Dogs:

Dosage for Extra Large Dogs weighing 66 lbs (30 kg) or more: Apply 2 cc (2 tubes) of PROTICALL® Insecticide solution to the skin of the dog's back and 2 cc (2 tubes) to the skin of the dog's back directly in front of the base of the tail.

Consult your veterinarian or entomologist for program recommendations.

PROTICALL® Insecticide may become less effective if dog is frequently bathed or gets wet. Repeat applications may be made as necessary, but do not apply at intervals less than 7 days.

Contraindication(s): Do not use on cats. May be harmful if applied to or ingested by cats.

Precautionary Statements: Hazards to Humans and Domestic Animals:

Caution: Harmful if swallowed or absorbed through the skin. Causes moderate eye irritation. Avoid contact with skin, eyes or clothing. Wash thoroughly with soap and water after handling. Do not use on cats. Cats which actively groom or engage in close physical contact with recently treated dogs may be at risk of serious harmful effect. Do not use this product in households with both dogs and cats. Consult a veterinarian before using this product on debilitated, aged, or medicated animals. Consult a veterinarian before using on dogs with known organ dysfunction. Sensitivities may occur after using any pesticide product for pet. If signs of sensitivity occur, bathe your pet with mild soap and rinse with large amount of water. If signs continue, consult a veterinarian immediately.

Adverse Reactions: Some animals may be sensitive to ingredients in this product. Reported reactions in dogs have included skin sensitivity, increased itchiness, redness and rash. Hair discoloration or hair loss at the application site may occur. Dogs may also show lethargy. Observe the dog following treatment. If sensitivity to PROTICALL® Insecticide for Dogs occurs, discontinue use and bathe the dog. Seek veterinary advice.

First Aid:

If on Skin: Take off contaminated clothing. Rinse skin immediately with plenty of water for 15-20 minutes. Call a poison control center or doctor for treatment advice.

If in Eyes: Hold eye open and rinse slowly and gently with water for 15-20 minutes. Remove contact lenses, if present, after the first 5 minutes, then continue rinsing eye. Call a physician if irritation persists.

If Swallowed: Call a poison control center or doctor immediately for treatment advice. Have person sip a glass of water if able to swallow. Do not induce vomiting unless told to do so by the poison control center or doctor. Do not induce vomiting or give anything by mouth to an unconscious person.

Hot Line Number: Have the product container or label with you when calling a poison control center or doctor, or going for treatment. You may also contact the Rocky Mountain Poison Center at 1-303-595-4869 for emergency medical treatment information.

Environmental Hazards: This product is extremely toxic to fish. Do not add directly to water. Do not contaminate water by cleaning of equipment or disposal of equipment washwaters.

Physical or Chemical Hazards: Do not use or store near heat or open flame.

Storage and Disposal: Do not contaminate water, food or feed by storage or disposal.

Storage: Store in cool, dry place. Protect from freezing.

Pesticide Disposal: Securely wrap original container in several layers of newspaper and discard in trash. Container Disposal: Do not reuse empty container. Wrap container and put in trash.

Warning(s): Keep out of reach of children.

Disclaimer: Notice of Warranty: Schering-Plough Animal Health Corp. makes no warranty of merchantability, fitness for any particular purpose or otherwise expressed or implied concerning this product or its uses which extend beyond the use of the product under normal conditions in accord with the statements made on the label.

Discussion: PROTICALL® Insecticide for Dogs is an effective and easy to use product. PROTICALL® Insecticide greater than 92% control of fleas within 3 days of application. As with all flea and tick control products, PROTICALL® Insecticide should be used as part of a control program aimed at reducing flea populations in the dog's environment (bedding, carpets, kennel, yard). Sold only through veterinary clinics.

Presentation: Six 1 cc applicators, box of 12.

® PROTICALL is a registered trademark of Schering-Plough Animal Health Corporation.

U.S. Patent Nos. 5,344,018 and 5,236,954.

Compendium Code No.: 10471651 20783532 Rev. 1/01

PROTOBOLIC™ BOLUS IMPROVED

Butler **Large Animal Dietary Supplement**

Active Ingredient(s): Each bolus contains:

Protein (not less than) ... 12.0 g

Containing these amino acids: Arginine*, histidine*, isoleucine*, leucine*, lysine*, methionine*, phenylalanine*, threonine*, tryptophan*, valine*, alanine, aspartic acid, cysteine, glutamic acid, glycine, proline, serine, and tyrosine.

*Essential amino acids.

Dicalcium phosphate • $2H_2O$ ... 5.0 g
Brewer's yeast ... 3.5 g
Dextrose • H_2O ... 2.5 g
Iron sulfate • H_2O ... 2.0 g
Sodium chloride ... 2.0 g
Potassium chloride ... 1.0 g
Magnesium sulfate • $7H_2O$ ... 750.0 mg
Zinc oxide ... 125.0 mg
Copper sulfate • $5H_2O$ ... 30.0 mg
Manganese sulfate ... 30.0 mg
Cobalt sulfate • H_2O ... 10.0 mg
Vitamin A ... 10,000 U.S.P. units
Vitamin D_3 ... 1,000 U.S.P. units

Indications: For use as a supplemental source of protein, vitamins and minerals for cattle, horses, sheep and swine.

Dosage and Administration: Administer one (1) to four (4) boluses orally for each 250 pounds of body weight per day, depending upon the condition of the animal and the individual need for supplementation. Boluses should be lubricated with mineral oil or petroleum jelly before administering with a balling gun. Alternatively, the boluses may be crushed and mixed with the feed or given as a drench.

Precaution(s): Keep the lid tightly closed when not in use and store in a cool, dry place. Do not store at temperatures above 30°C (86°F).

Caution(s): For veterinary use only. Keep out of the reach of children.

Presentation: Boxes of 50 boluses.

Compendium Code No.: 10821610

PROUD FLESH POWDER

First Priority **Topical Wound Dressing**

Ingredient(s): Copper Sulfate, $5H_2O$, Parachlorometaxylenol, Corn Starch.

Indications: An aid in the treatment of slow healing wounds. Priority Care PROUD FLESH POWDER helps retard excessive granulation tissue.

Directions for Use: Thoroughly cleanse the affected area. Rinse with warm water and pat dry. Dust evenly with generous amounts of Priority Care PROUD FLESH POWDER often enough to keep the injured tissue dry. May be applied under a bandage. Repeat treatment as necessary.

Caution(s): For external use only. Not for use in deep or puncture wounds. If irritation develops, discontinue use and consult your veterinarian. Use only as directed. For animal use only.

Warning(s): Not for use on animals intended for food. Keep out of reach of children.

Presentation: 6 oz (170 g) (NDC# 58829-189-06).

Compendium Code No.: 11390691 Rev. 09-01

PROUDSOFF™

Creative Science **Topical Wound Dressing**

Proud Flesh Ointment

Active Ingredient(s): Contains: Cupric sulfate, 49%, Special base, 51%.

Indications: For the control and removal of proud flesh from horses, cattle, sheep and goats.

Directions: Cover entire area affected by proud flesh with a thin coating of PROUDSOFF™ once daily. Dead tissue and debris from the previous use must be removed before each application. This can be done with cotton or a soft gauze. Do not wash the lesion. Discontinue use when all proud flesh has been removed. Do not use on wounds that do not contain proud flesh.

Contraindication(s): Do not use on dogs, cats or other household pets.

Precaution(s): Store in a cool, dry place.

Caution(s): For animal use only.

Note: If swelling or irritation increases or persists after using the product for several days, discontinue its use. Consult a veterinarian.

Warning(s): Not for use in animals intended for food use.

Avoid contact with eyes and with normal tissue. Wash hands thoroughly with soap and water after applying the product to animals. Keep out of reach of children.

Presentation: 3 oz (85 g) container.

Compendium Code No.: 13760021

PRO VAC® 2 ACL™

Fort Dodge **Vaccine**

Bursal Disease-Reovirus Vaccine, Killed Virus

U.S. Vet. Lic. No.: 112

Contents: This product contains the antigens listed above.

Gentamicin and amphotericin B added as preservatives.

Indications: For the revaccination of healthy chickens as an aid in the prevention of the signs and lesions associated with infectious bursal disease caused by standard and variant strains and avian reovirus infections which cause malabsorption syndrome.

Progeny of vaccinates are aided in the prevention of signs and lesions associated with infectious bursal disease via maternal antibodies.

Dosage and Administration: Inject 0.5 mL (0.5 cc) intramuscularly or subcutaneously (in the lower neck region) using aseptic technique. Vaccinate only healthy birds. For primed birds, a single dose between 16 and 22 weeks (approximately 4 weeks prior to lay) is indicated.

Precaution(s): Store in the dark at 36° to 45°F (2° to 7°C). Do not freeze. Warm to 72°F (22°C) and shake well before using. Use entire contents when first opened.

Warning(s): Do not vaccinate within 42 days before slaughter.

In case of accidental human injection seek immediate medical attention.

For veterinary use only.

Presentation: 1,000 doses (500 mL).

Compendium Code No.: 10031621 10091B

PRO VAC® 3 ACL™

Fort Dodge **Vaccine**

Bursal Disease-Newcastle Disease-Bronchitis Vaccine, Mass. Type, Killed Virus

U.S. Vet. Lic. No.: 112

Contents: This product contains the antigens listed above.

Gentamicin added as a preservative.

Indications: For the revaccination of healthy chickens as an aid in the prevention of the signs associated with infectious bursal disease, Newcastle disease and infectious bronchitis, Massachusetts type. Progeny of vaccinates are aided in the prevention of signs and lesions associated with infectious bursal disease and Newcastle disease.

Dosage and Administration: Inject 0.5 mL (0.5 cc) intramuscularly or subcutaneously (in the lower neck region) using aseptic technique. Vaccinate only healthy birds. For primed birds, a single dose between 16 and 22 weeks (approximately 4 weeks prior to lay) is indicated.

Precaution(s): Store in the dark at 36° to 45°F (2° to 7°C). Do not freeze. Warm to 72°F (22°C) and shake well before using. Use entire contents when first opened.
Warning(s): Do not vaccinate within 42 days before slaughter.
In case of accidental human injection seek immediate medical attention.
For veterinary use only.
Presentation: 1,000 doses (500 mL).
Compendium Code No.: 10031631 10131C

PRO VAC® 4 ACL™

Fort Dodge **Vaccine**

Bursal Disease-Newcastle Disease-Bronchitis-Reovirus Vaccine, Mass. Type, Killed Virus

U.S. Vet. Lic. No.: 112
Contents: This product contains the antigens listed above.
Gentamicin and amphotericin B added as preservatives.
Indications: For the revaccination of healthy chickens as an aid in the prevention of the signs and lesions associated with infectious bursal disease caused by standard and variant strains, Newcastle disease, infectious bronchitis, Massachusetts type and avian reovirus infections which cause malabsorption syndrome. Progeny of vaccinates are aided in the prevention of signs and lesions associated with infectious bursal disease caused by standard and variant strains, Newcastle disease and reovirus disease via maternal antibodies.
Dosage and Administration: Inject 0.5 mL (0.5 cc) intramuscularly or subcutaneously (in the lower neck region) using aseptic technique. Vaccinate only healthy birds. For primed birds, a single dose between 16 and 22 weeks (approximately 4 weeks prior to lay) is indicated.
Precaution(s): Store in the dark at 36° to 45°F (2° to 7°C). Do not freeze. Warm to 72°F (22°C) and shake well before using. Use entire contents when first opened.
Warning(s): Do not vaccinate within 42 days before slaughter.
In case of accidental human injection seek immediate medical attention.
For veterinary use only.
Presentation: 1,000 doses (500 mL).
Compendium Code No.: 10031641 10151B

PROVAC ND/IBD/REO ACL™

Fort Dodge **Vaccine**

Bursal Disease-Newcastle Disease-Reovirus Vaccine, Killed Virus

U.S. Vet. Lic. No.: 112
Contents: This product contains the antigens listed above.
Gentamicin and amphotericin B added as preservatives.
Indications: For revaccination of healthy chickens as an aid in the prevention of the signs associated with infectious bursal disease caused by standard and variant strains, Newcastle disease and avian reovirus infections which cause malabsorption syndrome. Progeny of vaccinates are aided in the prevention of signs and lesions associated with infectious bursal disease caused by standard and variant strains, Newcastle disease and reovirus disease via maternal antibodies.
Dosage and Administration: Inject 0.5 mL (0.5 cc) subcutaneously (in the lower neck region) or intramuscularly using aseptic technique. Vaccinate only healthy birds. For primed birds, a single dose between 16 and 22 weeks (approximately 4 weeks prior to lay) is indicated.
Precaution(s): Store in the dark at 36° to 45°F (2° to 7°C). Do not freeze. Warm to 72°F (22°C) and shake well before using. Use entire contents when first opened.
Warning(s): Do not vaccinate within 42 days before slaughter.
In case of accidental human injection seek immediate medical attention.
For veterinary use only.
Presentation: 1,000 doses (500 mL).
Compendium Code No.: 10031680 15001B

PROZAP® AQUEOUS FLY SPRAY

Loveland **Premise and Topical Insecticide**

EPA Reg. No.: 34704-247-36208
Active Ingredient(s):

Pyrethrins	0.1%
Piperonyl Butoxide, Technical*	1.0%
Inert Ingredients:	98.9%
Total	100.0%

*Equivalent to 0.8% (butylcarbityl) (6-propylpiperonyl) ether and 0.2% related compounds.
Indications: For use in homes and farms to control fleas, Brown Dog ticks, horn flies, house flies, mosquitoes, gnats, stable flies, deer flies and lice. Recommended for use on cattle and horses, and for use in kennels.
Directions for Use: It is a violation of Federal law to use this product in a manner inconsistent with its labeling.
To Control Fleas and Brown Dog Ticks: Thoroughly spray infested areas, pet beds, resting quarters, nearby cracks and crevices, along and behind baseboards, moulding, window and door frames, and localized areas of floor and floor covering. Fresh bedding should be placed in animal quarters following treatment. Concurrent treatment of animals with an approved insecticide is recommended. Repeat the treatment as needed.
On Animals:
To protect cattle and horses from Horn Flies, House Flies, Mosquitoes and Gnats: Apply a light mist sufficient to wet the surface of the hair.
To control Stable Flies, Horse Flies and Deer Flies: Apply at a rate of two (2) ounces per adult cow or horse sufficient to wet the hair thoroughly. Repeat treatment daily or at intervals necessary to give continued protection.
To Control Blood-Sucking Lice: Apply to the infested areas of the animal using a stiff brush to get the spray to the base of the hair. Repeat every two (2) to three (3) weeks if required.
Precautionary Statements: Hazards to Humans and Domestic Animals:
Caution: Harmful if swallowed, inhaled, or absorbed through skin. Avoid breathing vapors or spray mist. Avoid contact with skin, eyes or clothing. Wash thoroughly with soap and water after handling. Remove contaminated clothing and wash clothing before reuse.
The use of this product in food processing establishments should be confined to time periods when the plant is not in operation. Food should be removed or covered during treatment. All food processing surfaces should be removed or covered during treatment. All food processing surfaces should be covered during treatment or thoroughly cleaned with an effective cleaning compound and rinsed with potable water before reuse.
Vacate treated area and ventilate before reoccupying.
Remove pets, birds and cover fish aquaria before spraying.
Do not transport under 32°F.
Statement of Practical Treatment:
If Swallowed: Call a physician or Poison Control Center. Drink one (1) or two (2) glasses of water and induce vomiting by touching back of throat with finger. If person is unconscious, do not give anything by mouth and do not induce vomiting. If On Skin: Wash with plenty of soap and water. Get medical attention if irritation persists. If Inhaled: Remove victim to fresh air. If not breathing, give artificial respiration, preferably mouth-to-mouth. Get medical attention. If In Eyes: Flush with plenty of water. Call a physician if irritation persists.
Environmental Hazards: This product is toxic to fish. For terrestrial uses, do not directly to water, to areas where surface water is present or to intertidal areas below the mean high water mark. Do not contaminate water by cleaning of equipment or disposal of equipment washwaters.
Storage and Disposal: Do not contaminate water, food or feed by storage or disposal.
Pesticide Storage: Do not store under conditions which might adversely affect the container or its ability to function properly. Do not store below temperature of 32°F. Store in safe manner. Store in original container only. Store in cool, dry place. Keep container tightly closed when not in use. Reduce stacking height where local conditions can affect package strength. Personnel should use clothing and equipment consistent with good pesticide handling.
Pesticide Disposal: Pesticide, spray mixture or rinse water that cannot be used according to label instructions must be disposed of according to applicable Federal, state or local procedures.
Container Disposal: Metal: Triple rinse (or equivalent). Then offer for recycling or reconditioning, or puncture and dispose of in a sanitary landfill, or by other procedures approved by state and local authorities. Plastic: Triple rinse (or equivalent). Then offer for recycling or reconditioning, or puncture and dispose of in a sanitary landfill, or by incineration, or, if allowed by state and local authorities, by burning. If burned, stay out of smoke.
Household Use Disposal: Do not reuse empty container. Securely wrap original container in several layers of newspaper and discard in trash.
Warning(s): Keep out of reach of children.
Disclaimer: Except as expressly provided herein, neither Loveland nor seller makes any warranties, guarantees, or representations of any kind, either by usage of trade, statutory or otherwise, with regard to the product sold, including, but not limited to merchantability, fitness for a particular purpose, use or eligibility of the product for any particular trade usage.
Unintended consequences may result because of, but not limited to, such factors as presence of other materials, or the manner of use or application, all of which are beyond the control of Loveland Industries, Inc. or seller. In no case shall seller be liable for consequential, special, or indirect damages resulting from the use or handling of this product. All such risks shall be assumed by the buyer or user.
Applicator's or grower's exclusive remedy against Loveland Industries, Inc. or seller for any cause of action relating to the product is a claim for damages, and in no event shall damages or any other recovery exceed the purchase price of the product in respect of which such claim is made.
Presentation: 1 gallon (3.78 L) and 2½ gallon plastic containers.
Compendium Code No.: 10860210

PROZAP® BEEF & DAIRY SPRAY RTU

Loveland **Premise and Topical Insecticide**

EPA Reg. No.: 2393-480-36208
Active Ingredient(s):

2,2-Dichlorovinyl Dimethyl Phosphate*	0.92%
Related Compounds*	0.08%
Inert Ingredients**:	99.00%
Total	100.00%

*Equivalent to 1% Vapona® Insecticide
**Contains petroleum distillates
Indications: Ready-to-use for control of face flies, hornflies, stable flies, houseflies, gnats and mosquitoes attacking beef and dairy cattle.
For use in foggers, mist sprayers and hand sprayers.
Directions for Use: It is a violation of Federal Law to use this product in a manner inconsistent with its labeling.
Restrictions:
Do not contaminate water or foodstuffs. Do not contaminate milk or milk equipment. Do not apply in areas where animals have received direct application of DDVP within eight (8) hours. Care should be taken that the spray does not come in direct contact with lactating dairy cow's teats unless they are washed with an approved cleansing solution and dried before milking. Brahman and Brahman cross cattle should not be treated as they may show hypersensitivity to organic phosphates. Do not apply to calves under six months of age. Do not contaminate food crops. Do not use in edible products areas of food processing plants, restaurants or other areas here food is commercially prepared or processed. Do not use in serving areas while food is exposed. Food should be removed and food handling equipment covered during application, or thoroughly cleaned before using. Do not treat food processing areas or food processing plants while in operation. Thoroughly wash food contact surfaces with soap and water if they become contaminated by application of this product.
Applications:
Cattle (Beef and Dairy): To Control Hornflies, Houseflies, Stable Flies, Face Flies): Apply one (1) to two (2) fluid ounces of PROZAP® Beef & Dairy Spray RTU per animal as a mist spray daily with hand or automatic sprayer. Apply spray so as to wet the hair. Cover the animal with spray with particular attention to the back, flanks, legs and shoulders. Do not use in excess of two (2) fluid ounces per adult animal. Apply proportionately less to small animals. Do not soak the skin or wet the hides.
Fogging Outdoors: To Control Flies, Gnats and Mosquitoes: Outdoor fogging with this product should be limited to use by or under the direction of trained personnel. Apply five (5) to ten (10) pints per acre (0.05 to 0.1 pounds actual dichlorvos) as a dense fog when wind is calm. Do not contaminate food crops. Avoid wetting foliage as plant injury may occur.
Fogging Indoors: To Control Flies, Gnats and Mosquitoes: Indoor fogging in food processing plants, restaurants and warehouses is limited to application by pest control operators. Households should be treated by a pest control operator. Do not use this solution for fogging areas where animals have received direct application within eight (8) hours. Do not contaminate water, feed or foodstuffs, milk or milking utensils. Before applying, reduce air movement as much as possible by closing doors, windows and other openings. Eliminate ignition sources such as pilot lights, fires and open flames. Disconnect electrical power. Fog for one (1) to five (5) seconds per 1,000 cubic feet, but use no more then one gallon per 64,000 cubic feet. Do not fog into or near an open flame. Occupants should vacate premises before treatment and should not reoccupy the premises until it has been ventilated. Leave treated area closed for at least 15 to 30 minutes and then open windows and doors to ventilate.
Animal Buildings (Horse Barns, Dairy Barns, Shelter Sheds, Milk Sheds): To Control Flies, Gnats, Mosquitoes, Roaches, Fleas, Ants, Sowbugs, Brown Dog Ticks, Spiders and Silverfish:

Apply as a coarse wet spray using one (1) pint per 1,000 square feet. Spiders and Silverfish: Apply as a coarse wet spray using one (1) pint per 1,000 square feet. Treat around doorways, feed storage rooms, alleyways and windowsills. For control of Fly Maggots in maggot breeding areas, apply at the rate of one (1) to two (2) pints per 100 square feet.

In treating dog kennels, apply to outside dog runways, windowsills and ledges. For control of Fleas and Brown Dog Ticks, increase dosage to one (1) quart per 1,000 square feet. Treat infested area, baseboards, cracks, walls and doors. Do not allow children in treated areas until dry. Do not use this product on dogs. Use an approved product registered for direct application to dogs.

Precautionary Statements: Hazards to Humans and Domestic Animals:

Warning: May be fatal if swallowed, inhaled, or absorbed through skin or eyes. Rapidly absorbed through skin and eyes. Do not get into eyes, on skin or on clothing. Do not breathe vapor or spray mist. Wash thoroughly with soap and water after handling and before eating or smoking. Do not contaminate feed, water, foodstuffs, milk or milking utensils. Wear clean, natural rubber gloves, protective clothing, and goggles, faceshield or equivalent. Wear a pesticide respirator jointly approved by MSHA (Mine Safety and Health Administration) and NIOSH (National Institute for Occupational Safety and Health) under the provisions of 30 CFR Part 11. Wear impervious footwear or protective covers as shoes, boots and other articles made of leather or similar porous materials may be dangerously contaminated. Wash contaminated clothing with soap and hot water before reuse.

Statement of Practical Treatment:

If Swallowed: Call a physician or Poison Control Center immediately. Do not induce vomiting. Vomiting may cause aspiration pneumonia. If Inhaled: Remove victim to fresh air. Apply respiration if indicated. If On Skin: Wash contaminated skin with soap and water. Launder contaminated clothing in detergent and hot water before reuse. If In Eyes: Flush eyes with plenty of water. Get medical attention immediately. Note to Physician: Empty stomach if material was taken internally. Gastric lavage may be indicated. If symptoms of cholinesterase inhibition are present, atropine is antidotal. 2-PAM is also antidotal and may be administered in conjunction with atropine.

Environmental Hazards: This product is toxic to fish, birds and other wildlife. For terrestrial uses, do not apply directly to water, or to areas where surface water is present or to intertidal areas below the mean high water mark. Do not contaminate water by cleaning of equipment or disposal of wastes.

Physical or Chemical Hazards: Do not use or store near heat or open flame.

Storage and Disposal: Do not contaminate water, food or feed by storage or disposal.

Storage: Do not use or store near heat or open flame. Keep product upright in original container, tightly closed. High temperatures may shorten shelf life of product.

Pesticide Disposal: Wastes resulting from the use of this product may be disposed of on site or at an approved waste disposal facility.

Container Disposal: Metal: Triple rinse (or equivalent). Then offer for recycling or reconditioning, or puncture and dispose of in a sanitary landfill, or by other procedures approved by state and local authorities. Plastic: Triple rinse (or equivalent). Then offer for recycling or reconditioning, or puncture and dispose of in a sanitary landfill, or by incineration, or, if allowed by state and local authorities, by burning. If burned, stay out of smoke.

Warning(s): Keep out of the reach of children.

Disclaimer: Except as expressly provided herein, neither Loveland nor seller makes any warranties, guarantees, or representations of any kind, either by usage of trade, statutory or otherwise, with regard to the product sold, including, but not limited to merchantability, fitness for a particular purpose, use or eligibility of the product for any particular trade usage.

Unintended consequences may result because of, but not limited to, such factors as presence of other materials, or the manner of use or application, all of which are beyond the control of Loveland Industries, Inc. or seller. In no case shall seller be liable for consequential, special, or indirect damages resulting from the use or handling of this product. All such risks shall be assumed by the buyer or user.

Applicator's or grower's exclusive remedy against Loveland Industries, Inc. or seller for any cause of action relating to the product is a claim for damages, and in no event shall damages or any other recovery exceed the purchase price of the product in respect of which such claim is made.

Presentation: 1 gallon (3.78 L).

® Vapona is a registered trademark of Fermenta Animal Health Co.

Compendium Code No.: 10860220

PROZAP® DAIRY & FEEDLOT INSECTICIDE CONCENTRATE

Loveland **Premise and Topical Insecticide**

with Vapona®

EPA Reg. No.: 34704-603-36208

Active Ingredient(s):

Dichlorvos: 2,2-Dichlorovinyl dimethyl phosphate*	22.0%
Related Compounds*	1.7%
Inert Ingredients**:	76.3%
Total	100.0%

*Equivalent to 23.7% dichlorvos and related compounds

**This product contains Aliphatic petroleum hydrocarbons.

Contains 2 lbs Vapona® Insecticide per gallon.

Indications: A dairy and livestock emulsible spray for control of face flies and certain other livestock pests.

Applications: This product is a specially prepared animal insecticide for use in the control of certain insects attacking livestock (face flies, house flies, horn flies, stable flies, mosquitoes and gnats).

Directions for Use: It is a violation of Federal law to use this product in a manner inconsistent with its labeling.

Mixing Directions:

1% Solution: Mix 5⅓ fluid ounces (10⅔ tablespoons) concentrate with 1 gallon water (1 quart to 6¼ gallons).

0.5% solution: Mix 2⅔ fluid ounces (5⅓ tablespoons) concentrate with 1 gallon water (1 quart to 12½ gallons).

Recommendations:

Beef and Dairy Cattle: Flies (House flies, Horn flies, Stable flies, Face flies) and Mosquitoes. Apply 1 to 2 ounces of 1% solution per animal as a mist spray daily with a hand or automatic sprayer. Spray to thoroughly cover all parts of the animal, including the legs but do not wet the skin. Do not apply in excess of 2 fluid ounces per animal per day.

Face Fly: For maximum face fly control, add 1 to 2 cups of sugar to each gallon of 1% solution.

Cattle Feed Lots, Stock Yards, Holding Pens and Corrals: Flies, Mosquitoes and Gnats. Apply at the rate of 4⅔ gallons 0.5% solution per acre with a mist blower or other suitable equipment as an overall application. The mist spray should be directed over the entire area. Particular attention should be given to areas where flies congregate on fences, spillage areas around feed bunks and walls of buildings. Animals may be present during treatment. Avoid direct application to exposed feed and water. For baited solutions dissolve one pound of sugar per 5 to 10 gallons of water before adding the Vapona® concentrate.

Animal Buildings (Dairy Barns, Milk Sheds, Shelter Sheds and Horse Barns): For control of flies, gnats and mosquitoes. Before applying reduce air movement as much as possible by closing doors, windows and other openings.

Surface Spray: Apply 1 quart of 0.5% solution or 1 pint of 1% solution as a coarse wet spray per 1000 sq. ft. For milk sheds, stables, livestock barns, loafing sheds, pig pens and outdoor areas, treat around doorways, feed storage rooms, alleyways and window sills. In Poultry Houses apply to manure, window sills, outside of penned enclosures and on floors of feed and storage rooms. Also controls roaches, fleas, ants, sowbugs and brown dog ticks. Repeat as necessary. Do not treat animals or humans.

Fog or Mist: Use 1 quart of 0.5% solution or 1 pint of 1% solution per 8000 cubic feet of space. Animals can be left in buildings provided they have not received a direct application within eight hours.

Fly Maggots: In maggot breeding areas on garbage dumps and manure piles. Dilute 1 to 2 pints of 1% Vapona® in equal parts of diesel fuel and apply 1 to 2 quarts of the 0.5% solution per 100 square feet.

Precautionary Statements: Hazards to Humans and Domestic Animals:

Danger. This product is poisonous if swallowed, inhaled, or absorbed through the skin or eyes. Do not get on skin or eyes. Do not breathe fumes. Avoid exposure to fumes.

Personal Protective Equipment: Wear coveralls worn over long-sleeved shirt and long pants, socks, chemical resistant footwear, waterproof gloves and protective eyewear. Wear a respirator with either an organic vapor removing cartridge with a prefilter approved for pesticides (MSHA/NIOSH approval number prefix TC-23C), or a canister approved for pesticides (MSHA/NIOSH approval number prefix TC-14G); and a chemical resistant apron when mixing or loading. Keep all unprotected persons out of operational area.

In case of contact, wash immediately with soap and water. Wash hands, arms and face thoroughly with soap and water before eating or smoking. Wash all contaminated clothing with soap and hot water before reuse.

Statement of Practical Treatment:

If Swallowed: Call a physician or Poison Control Center. Drink 1 or 2 glasses of water and induce vomiting by touching back of throat with finger, or, if available, by administering syrup of ipecac. Do not induce vomiting or give anything by mouth to an unconscious person.

If on Skin: If the material has been spilled on the skin, immediately remove patient from the vicinity of the insecticide, remove all contaminated clothing, and wash skin with soap and running water.

If in Eyes: Wash immediately with running water for at least 10 minutes. Get medical attention immediately.

If Inhaled: Remove victim to fresh air immediately. Apply artificial respiration if indicated. Get medical attention.

Atropine is the emergency antidote for Vaponafi Insecticide poisoning. Consult your physician about obtaining an adequate supply of 1-100-grain atropine tablets for emergency use. Call a physician immediately in all cases of suspected poisoning.

If Warning Symptoms Appear: Administer two 1-100-grain atropine tablets immediately. Never administer atropine unless warning symptoms appear. (See Warning Symptoms below). Keep patient prone and quiet. Start artificial respiration immediately if patient is not breathing. Transport the patient immediately to the nearest physician.

Note to Physicians:

Warning Symptoms: Symptoms include weakness, headache, tightness in chest, blurred vision, non-reactive pin-point pupils, salivation, sweating, nausea, vomiting, diarrhea and abdominal cramps.

Treatment: Atropine is the specific therapeutic antagonist of choice against parasympathetic nervous stimulation. If there are signs of parasympathetic stimulation, atropine sulfate should be injected at 10 minute intervals, in doses of 1 to 2 milligrams, until complete atropinization has occurred. Morphine is contraindicated. Clear chest and postural drainage. Observe patient continuously for 48 hours. Repeated exposure to cholinesterase inhibitors may without warning cause prolonged susceptibility to very small doses of any cholinesterase regeneration has been allowed as determined by blood test.

Environmental Hazards: This product is toxic to fish and wildlife. Do not apply directly to water or to areas where surface waters are present or to intertidal area below the mean high water mark. Do not contaminate water when disposing of equipment washwaters.

Storage and Disposal: Do not contaminate water, feed or foodstuffs, milk or milking utensils.

Prohibitions: Do not contaminate water, food or feed by storage or disposal. Open dumping is prohibited. Do not reuse empty container. Do not store under conditions which might adversely affect the container or its ability to function properly.

Storage: Do not store below temperature of 0°F. Store in a safe manner. Store in original container only. Store in a cool, dry place. Keep container tightly closed when not in use. Reduce stacking height where local conditions can affect package strength. Personnel should use clothing and equipment listed under Danger when handling open containers.

Spilled Material: Block or dike to prevent spreading of spill. Cover with absorbent materials such as lime, clay or sawdust. Scoop and sweep into a disposal container. Wash area with strong lye solutions, absorb and place into a disposal container.

Pesticide Disposal: Pesticide wastes are acutely hazardous. Improper disposal of excess pesticide, spray mixture, or rinsate is a violation of Federal Law. If these wastes cannot be disposed of by use according to label instructions, contact your State Pesticide or Environmental Control Agency, or the Hazardous Waste representative at the nearest EPA Regional Office for guidance.

Container Disposal: Metal: Triple rinse (or equivalent). Then offer for recycling or reconditioning, or puncture and dispose of in a sanitary landfill, or by other procedures approved by state and local authorities. Plastic: Triple rinse (or equivalent). Then offer for recycling or reconditioning, or puncture and dispose of in a sanitary landfill, or by incineration, or, if allowed by state and local authorities, by burning. If burned, stay out of smoke.

Precautions in Using: This product and the diluted emulsion are poisonous. Therefore, precautions must be observed while handling them. (See antidote and warnings on this label).

Store the concentrate in a safe place. Children and animals must not be able to reach or handle the concentrate or diluted emulsion. It is recommended that only the amount of diluted emulsion be prepared from the concentrate that will be used immediately.

Mix the concentrate into water outdoors or in a well ventilated room. Wash off the outside of the container of concentrate in running water before storing away. Wash after handling.

Not for use or storage in or around the home. Do not contaminate feed, water or foodstuffs. Do not make direct application to livestock more frequently than once per day.

Warning(s): Keep out of reach of children.

For agricultural/commercial uses only.

Disclaimer: Notice: Loveland Industries, Inc. warrants that this product conforms to the chemical description on the label thereof and is reasonable fit for the purposes stated on such label only when used in accordance with the directions under normal use conditions. It is impossible to eliminate all risks inherently associated with the use of this product. Animal injury, ineffectiveness, or other unintended consequences may result because of such factors as weather conditions, presence of other materials, or the manner of use or application, all of which are beyond the control of Loveland Industries, Inc. In no case shall Loveland Industries, Inc. be liable for consequential, special or indirect damages resulting from the use or handling of this product. All such risks shall be assumed by the buyer.

Except as expressly provided herein, Loveland Industries, Inc. makes no warranties, guarantees, or representations of any kind, either expressed or implied, or by usage of trade, statutory, or otherwise, with regard to the product sold, including, but not limited to, merchantability, fitness for a particular purpose, use or eligibility of the product for any particular trake usage. Buyer's or user's exclusive remedy, and Loveland Industries, Inc.'s total liability, shall be for damages not exceeding the cost of the product.

Presentation: 1 gallon.

® Vapona is a registered trademark of Shell Chemical Company

Compendium Code No.: 10860231

PROZAP® DRYCIDE®

Loveland **Topical Insecticide**

EPA Reg. No.: 28293-126-36208

Active Ingredient(s):

Permethrin* 0.25%
Inert Ingredients** 99.75%
Total 100%

*[3-(Phenoxyphenyl) methyl (±) cis-trans-3-(2,2-dichloroethenyl)-2,2-dimethylcyclo-propanecarboxylate]

Cis-trans ratio: Max 65% (±) trans and 35% (±) cis

Indications: Insecticide dust for livestock and pets.

Directions for Use: It is a violation of Federal law to use this product in a manner inconsistent with its labeling.

Swine: Lice on swine direct application: Apply only 1 ounce per head as a uniform coat to the head, shoulder and back by use of a shaker can or suitable mechanical dust applicator. Repeat as necessary but not more than once every 10 days. In severe infestation, both animals and the bedding may be treated.

Beef and Dairy Cattle: Horn Flies, Lice application: Apply 2 ounces of dust per animal by shaker can. Repeat as necessary.

Horses: Dust horses for Hornflies with shaker can or dust glove along back, neck and legs.

Poultry: To control Northern Fowl Mites, apply 1 lb per 100 birds. Ensure thorough treatment of vent area.

Pets: To control Fleas, Ticks and Lice on cats and dogs, dust animal thoroughly, working the dust into the hair down to the skin. Pay close attention to legs and feet. Use ½ oz on animals 20 pounds and under and 1 oz on pets over 20 pounds. Avoid getting dust in pet's eyes. Repeat treatment as needed. Dust sleeping area including bedding and cracks and crevices.

Precautionary Statements: Hazards to Humans and Domestic Animals:

Caution: Harmful if swallowed, inhaled. Avoid breathing dust. Avoid contact with eyes and skin. Wash thoroughly with soap and water after handling. Avoid contamination of feed and foodstuffs.

Statement of Practical Treatment:

If in eyes: Flush eyes with plenty of water. Get medical attention if irritation persists.

If on skin: Wash with plenty of soap and water. Get medical attention if irritation persists.

Physical and Chemical Hazards: Do not use or store near heat or open flame.

Environmental Hazards: This product is toxic to fish. Do not apply directly to water, or to areas where surface water is present or to intertidal areas below the mean high water mark. Do not contaminate water by cleaning of equipment or disposal of wastes.

Storage and Disposal:

Storage: Store in cool, dry place. Do not contaminate feed or foodstuffs by storage or disposal.

Pesticide Disposal: Wastes resulting from the use of this product may be disposed of on site or at an approved waste disposal facility.

Container Disposal: Completely empty container into application equipment. Then dispose of empty container in a sanitary landfill or by incineration, or, if allowed by state and local authorities, by burning. If burned, stay out of smoke.

Warning(s): Swine: Do not ship animals for slaughter within 5 days of treatment.

Keep out of reach of children.

Disclaimer: Except as expressly provided herein, neither Loveland nor seller makes any warranties, guarantees, or representations of any kind, either by usage of trade, statutory or otherwise, with regard to the product sold, including, but not limited to merchantability, fitness for a particular purpose, use or eligibility of the product for any particular trade usage.

Unintended consequences may result because of, but not limited to, such factors as presence of other materials, or the manner of use or application, all of which are beyond the control of Loveland Industries, Inc. or seller. In no case shall seller be liable for consequential, special, or indirect damages resulting from the use or handling of this product. All such risks shall be assumed by the buyer or user.

Applicator's or grower's exclusive remedy against Loveland Industries, Inc. or seller for any cause of action relating to the product is a claim for damages, and in no event shall damages or any other recovery exceed the purchase price of the product in respect of which such claim is made.

Presentation: 20 lb (9.09 kg) containers.

Compendium Code No.: 10860240

PROZAP® DUST'R™

Loveland **Premise and Topical Insecticide**

EPA Reg. No.: 2393-393-36208

Active Ingredient(s):

Tetrachlorvinphos: 2-chloro-1-(2,4,5-trichlorophenyl) vinyl dimethyl phosphate 3%
Inert Ingredients: 97%
Total 100%

Indications: A ready-to-use insecticide to control hornflies and lice and aid in the control of face flies on beef cattle and dairy cattle and to control lice on swine and Northern fowl mites, chicken mites and lice on or around poultry.

Directions for Use: It is a violation of Federal law to use this product in a manner inconsistent with its labeling.

PROZAP® DUST'R™ is a ready-to-use insecticide dust which can be applied by hand or thorough the use of self-treating dust bags. There is no withholding period from last application to slaughter.

Animal	Insect	
Beef Cattle Dairy Cattle	Horn Flies Face Flies Lice	Hand Dusting: Apply approximately 2 oz of dust by shaker can, rotary duster or by spoon to the upper portions of the back, neck and poll and to the face as an aid in the control of face flies. Rub in lightly to carry the dust beneath the hair. Repeat as necessary. Self-Treating Dust Bag: Forced Use: Put PROZAP® DUST'R™ in cotton cloth or double burlap bags or use pre-packed weatherproof cattle dust bags and hang in barn door exits or alleyways leading from animal buildings, salt or mineral blocks, or watering holes. Protect cloth or burlap bags from weather. Free Choice Use: Use the same dust bags as above but place in loafing sheds, holding pens, feedlots, near watering holes or other areas where cattle gather. The free choice use aids in the control of lice.
Swine	Lice	Hand Dusting: Apply 3 to 4 oz of dust by conventional hand or powder duster to each animal with special attention given to the neck and around the ears. Repeat as necessary but not more often than once every 14 days. In severe infestations, both individual animals and bedding may be treated. One lb of 3% dust should be applied per 150 sq. ft. of bedding.

Poultry:

Type Housing	Applications	Remarks
Wire cages	1 lb/300 birds Plunger, rotary type duster or shaker can duster.	For individual treatment direct dust to vent and fluff area. Group treatment may be preferred. Dust should reach skin. Do not repeat more often then every 14 days. Wire rungs and corners should also be treated.

Note: For Northern Fowl Mites on roosters, thorough individual application of the dust will assure long-lasting control and reduce reinfestation of breeding flocks.

Floor Management	Applications	Remarks
Litter	1 lb/100 sq. ft. Plunger or rotary type duster.	Treat evenly and thoroughly. Also treat roosts, cracks and crevices where pests may hide.
Dust box	2 lbs/100 birds	Use box about 2 ft. by 2 ft. by 1 ft. deep.
Roost paint	1 lb/100 ft. Make thick slurry by mixing 1 lb of dust with 1 pt. of water, continually stirring.	Treat roosts thoroughly, particularly the cracks and crevices.

Precautionary Statements: Hazard to Humans and Domestic Animals:

Caution: Harmful if swallowed, inhaled or absorbed through skin. Avoid breathing dust. Do not get in eyes, on skin, or on clothing. If the material gets into the eyes, wash with plenty of water; if irritation persists, see a physician. Wash thoroughly with soap and water after handling and before eating or smoking. Avoid contamination of feed and foodstuffs. Do not apply in dwellings. Wear long-sleeved shirt and pants; chemical-resistant gloves; shoes and socks.

Environmental Hazards: This pesticide is toxic to fish. Drift and runoff may be hazardous to aquatic organisms in adjacent areas. For terrestrial uses, do not apply directly to water, or to areas where surface water is present or to intertidal areas below the mean high water mark. Do not contaminate water when disposing of equipment washwater.

This product is highly toxic to bees exposed to direct treatment on blooming crops or weeds. Do not apply this product or allow it to drift to blooming crops or weeds if bees are visiting the treatment area.

Storage and Disposal: Do not contaminate water, food or feed by storage or disposal.

Storage: Store product in original container, tightly closed. High temperatures may shorten shelf life of product. Do not reuse container.

Pesticide Disposal: Wastes resulting from the use of this product may be disposed of on site or at an approved waste disposal facility.

Container Disposal: Completely empty bag into application equipment. Then dispose of empty bag in a sanitary landfill or by incineration, or, if allowed by State and local authorities, by burning. If burned, stay out of smoke.

Warning(s): Keep out of reach of children.

Disclaimer: Except as expressly provided herein, neither Loveland nor seller makes any warranties, guarantees, or representation of any kind, either express or implied, or by usage of trade, statutory or otherwise, with regard to the product sold, including, but not limited to merchantability, fitness for a particular purpose, use or eligibility of the product for any particular trade usage.

Unintended consequences may result because of, but not limited to, such factors as presence of other materials, or the manner of use or application, all of which are beyond the control of Loveland Industries, Inc. or seller. In no case shall seller be liable for consequential, special, or indirect damages resulting from the use or handling of this product. All such risks shall be assumed by the buyer or user.

Applicator's or grower's exclusive remedy against Loveland Industries, Inc. or seller for any cause of action relating to the product is a claim for damages, and in no event shall damages or any other recovery exceed the purchase price of the product in respect of which such claim is made.

Presentation: 12.50 pound (5.68 kg) container.

Compendium Code No.: 10860251

PROZAP® GARDEN & POULTRY DUST

Loveland **Premise and Topical Insecticide**

EPA Reg. No.: 2393-375-36208

Active Ingredient(s):

Carbaryl (1-Naphthyl methylcarbamate) 5%
Inert Ingredients*: 95%
Total 100%

Indications: An insecticidal dust for use against certain insects attacking poultry, dogs and cats as directed.

Directions for Use: It is a violation of Federal law to use this product in a manner inconsistent with its labeling.

Chickens, Turkeys, Ducks, Geese, Game Birds such as Partridges and Pheasants, and Pigeons:

Litter Treatment: Apply one (1) pound per 40 square feet to control Northern fowl mite, chicken mite, lice and bed bugs. Use a scoop and scatter by hand or apply by hand duster. Avoid contamination of nests, eggs, feeding and watering troughs.

Hand Application to Birds: Use one (1) pound to treat 100 birds by means of a shaker can, squeeze bottle or hand duster to control Northern fowl mite, chicken mite, lice and fleas. Direct dust to vent and fluff areas. Repeat in four (4) weeks if necessary. Hand application to birds for chicken mite and fleas is a supplement to litter treatment for control of these pests.

Poultry Houses: Apply 25 pounds per 1,000 square feet. Apply thoroughly to floors, roosts and interior surfaces. Do not apply directly to eggs or nest litter. Do not contaminate feed or drinking water.

Dogs and Cats: Against brown dog tick and fleas, rub in skin and apply in sleeping quarters weekly.

Contraindication(s): Do not treat kittens or puppies under four (4) weeks old. Do not use on pregnant dogs.

Precautionary Statements: Hazards to Humans and Domestic Animals:

Caution: May be harmful if swallowed. Avoid breathing dust. Avoid contact with eyes, skin or clothing. Wash thoroughly after handling. Take shower after work. Change contaminated clothing daily. Wear regular long-sleeved clothing. Avoid contamination of feed and foodstuffs. Do not feed treated vines or trash to meat or dairy animals.

Note for Physicians: Carbaryl is a moderate reversible, cholinesterase inhibitor. Atropine is antidotal.

Environmental Hazards: This pesticide is extremely toxic to aquatic and estuarine invertebrates. For terrestrial uses, do not apply directly to water, or to areas where surface water is present or to intertidal areas below the mean high water mark. Do not contaminate water by cleaning of equipment or disposal of wastes.

This product is highly toxic to bees exposed to direct treatment or residues on blooming crops or weeds. Do not apply this product or allow it to drift to blooming crops or weeds if bees are visiting the treatment area.

Storage and Disposal: Do not contaminate water, food or feed by storage or disposal.

Storage: Store in original container only, preferably in a locked area. Keep container tightly closed when not in use. Store in a cool, dry place. High temperatures may shorten shelf life of product. Do not use food or drink containers for mixing or storage.

Pesticide Disposal: Securely wrap original container in several layers of newspaper and discard in trash.

Container Disposal: Do not reuse empty container. Wrap container and put in trash.

Warning(s): Chickens, Turkeys, Ducks, Geese, Game Birds such as Partridges and Pheasants and Pigeons: Do not apply within seven (7) days of slaughter.

Poultry Houses: Do not house birds in treated houses within seven (7) days of slaughter.

Keep out of reach of children.

Disclaimer: Except as expressly provided herein, neither Loveland nor seller makes any warranties, guarantees, or representation of any kind, either express or implied, or by usage of trade, statutory or otherwise, with regard to the product sold, including, but not limited to merchantability, fitness for a particular purpose, use or eligibility of the product for any particular trade usage.

Unintended consequences may result because of, but not limited to, such factors as presence of other materials, or the manner of use or application, all of which are beyond the control of Loveland Industries, Inc. or seller. In no case shall seller be liable for consequential, special, or indirect damages resulting from the use or handling of this product. All such risks shall be assumed by the buyer or user.

Applicator's or grower's exclusive remedy against Loveland Industries, Inc. or seller for any cause of action relating to the product is a claim for damages, and in no event shall damages or any other recovery exceed the purchase price of the product in respect of which such claim is made.

Presentation: 2 pounds (908 g) containers.

Compendium Code No.: 10860270

PROZAP® INSECTRIN® DUST

Loveland **Topical Insecticide**

General Purpose Livestock and Poultry Dust

EPA Reg. No.: 28293-126-36208

Active Ingredient(s):

Permethrin-(3-phenoxyphenyl) methyl (±) cis, trans-3-(2,2-dichloroethenyl)-2,2-dimethylcyclopropanecarboxylate* 0.25%

Inert Ingredients: 99.75%

Total 100.00%

*Cis/trans ratio: Min. 35% (±) cis, Max. 65% (±) cis

Indications:

Swine: Lice.

Beef and Dairy Cattle and Horses: Horn flies, lice, face flies.

Poultry: To control Northern fowl mites.

Pets: To control fleas, ticks and lice on cats and dogs.

Directions for Use: It is a violation of Federal law to use this product in a manner inconsistent with its labeling.

Swine: Lice on Swine Direction Application: Apply only one (1) ounce per head as a uniform coat to the head, shoulder and back by use of a shaker can or suitable mechanical dust applicator. Repeat as necessary but not more often than once every 10 days. In severe infestation, both animals and the bedding may be treated.

Beef and Dairy Cattle and Horses: Can be used in dust bags, shaker can and mechanical dust applicator.

Horn Flies, Lice, Face Flies: Place contents of this package in any commercially available dust bag, suspend bag in areas frequented by cattle or in gateways or lanes through which the animals must pass daily for water, feed, or minerals. Bags may also be placed in loafing sheds or in front of mineral feeders. For dairy cows, bags may be suspended in the exit through which the cows leave the milking barn. The bags should hand 4 to 6 inches below the back line of the cattle. For reduction of face flies, bags must be located so animals will be forced to use them daily and hung at a height so that the face is dusted.

Horn Flies, Lice Direct Application: Apply 2 oz. of dust per animal by shaker can over head, neck, shoulders and back and tailhead. Repeat as necessary.

Horses: Dust horse for hornflies with shaker can or dust glove along back, neck and legs.

Poultry: To control Northern fowl mites, apply at a rate of one (1) pound per 100 birds. Ensure thorough treatment of vent area.

Pets: To control fleas, ticks and lice on cats and dogs, dust animals thoroughly, working the dust into the hair down to the skin. Pay close attention to legs and feet. Use ½ ounce on animals 20 pounds and under and one (1) ounce on pets over 20 pounds. Avoid getting dust in pet's eyes. Repeat treatment as needed. Dust sleeping area including bedding and cracks and crevices.

Precautionary Statements: Hazards to Humans and Domestic Animals:

Caution: Harmful if swallowed, inhaled. Avoid breathing dust. Avoid contact with eyes and skin. Wash thoroughly with soap and water after handling. Avoid contamination of feed and foodstuffs.

Statement of Practical Treatment:

If in Eyes: Flush with plenty of water. Get medical attention if irritation persists.

If on Skin: Wash with plenty of soap and water. Get medical attention if irritation persists.

Physical and Chemical Hazards: Do not use or store near heat or open flame.

Environmental Hazards: This product is toxic to fish. Do not apply directly to water, or to areas where surface water is present or to intertidal areas below the mean high water mark. Do not contaminate water by cleaning of equipment or disposal of wastes.

Storage and Disposal:

Storage: Store in a cool, dry place. Do not contaminate feed or foodstuffs by storage or disposal.

Pesticide Disposal: Wastes resulting from the use of this product may be disposed of on site or at an approved waste disposal facility.

Container Disposal: Completely empty container into application equipment. Then dispose of empty container in a sanitary landfill or by incineration, or, if allowed by State and local authorities, by burning. If burned, stay out of smoke.

Disclaimer: Except as expressly provided herein, neither Loveland nor seller makes any warranties, guarantees, or representation of any kind, either express or implied, or by usage of trade, statutory or otherwise, with regard to the product sold, including, but not limited to merchantability, fitness for a particular purpose, use or eligibility of the product for any particular trade usage.

Unintended consequences may result because of, but not limited to, such factors as presence of other materials, or the manner of use or application, all of which are beyond the control of Loveland Industries, Inc. or seller. In no case shall seller be liable for consequential, special, or indirect damages resulting from the use or handling of this product. All such risks shall be assumed by the buyer or user.

Applicator's or grower's exclusive remedy against Loveland Industries, Inc. or seller for any cause of action relating to the product is a claim for damages, and in no event shall damages or any other recovery exceed the purchase price of the product in respect of which such claim is made.

Warning(s): Swine: Do not ship animals for slaughter within 5 days of treatment.

Keep out of reach of children.

Presentation: 2 pounds (908 g) and 12.50 pounds (5.68 kg) containers.

Compendium Code No.: 10860280

PROZAP® INSECTRIN® X

Loveland **Premise and Topical Insecticide**

EPA Reg. No.: 28293-128-36208

Active Ingredient(s):

Permethrin* 10.0%

Inert Ingredients:** 90.0%

Total 100.0%

*[(3-Phenoxyphenyl) methyl (±)-cis-trans-3-(2,2-dichloroethenyl)-2,2-dimethylcyclopropanecarboxylate]

Cis-trans ratio: Max. 65% (±) trans and 35% (±) cis

**Contains petroleum distillates.

Contains 0.75 lbs of permethrin per gallon

Indications: Emulsifiable concentrate / repellent livestock and premise spray.

A long lasting livestock and premise spray that provides knockdown, broad spectrum insecticidal effectiveness, and excellent residual activity for up to 28 days.

Kills poultry lice, fowl mites, bed bugs, horn flies, house flies, fleas ticks, and numerous other insects as listed below.

For use outdoors and in homes and non-food areas of poultry houses, dairies, cattle barns, milking parlors, horse barns, swine houses, kennels, commercial buildings, institutions, and others.

Recommended for agricultural / commercial use.

Directions for Use: It is a violation of Federal law to use this product in a manner inconsistent with its labeling.

Keep container sealed when not in use. Protect from freezing. Shake or stir product thoroughly before using or reusing diluted emulsion. To prepare dilutions, the concentrate should first be stirred or agitated well. Add the required amount of concentrate to water and blend thoroughly. Do not hold dilutions for more than 24 hours. For maximum effectiveness, a combination of localized application and space treatment is recommended. Remove pets, birds and cover fish aquariums before spraying.

For initial clean up of severe insect infestation, dilute at a rate of one (1) part concentrate in 19 parts water (6.7 fluid ounces per gallon) (0.5%).

For normal infestations, dilute one (1) part concentrate in 100 parts water (1.33 ounces per gallon) 98 teaspoonsful per gallon) (0.1%).

Indoor Use Areas: Do not use in feed area of feed handling establishments or other area where feed is commercially prepared or processed. Exposed feed should be covered or removed.

Non Feed Areas: Include (but not limited to) kennels.

As a Surface Spray to Control: Cockroaches, Waterbugs, Palmetto Bugs, Ants, Silverfish, Beetles, Mites, Weevils. Use a good sprayer and adjust to deliver a coarse wet spray. Direct the spray into hiding places, cracks and crevices, under pallets, around container of stored foods, and behind shelves and drawers. If surface application only is to be used, spray floors, walls and other surfaces applying at a rate of one (1) gallon to 750 square feet of surface.

To Control: Fleas and Ticks (adult and larvae), thoroughly spray infested areas, pet beds, resting quarters nearby cracks and crevices, along and behind baseboards, moldings, window and door frames, and localized areas of floor and floor covering. Fresh bedding should be placed in animal quarters following treatment. Apply with mechanical or compressed air equipment (non-thermal) adjusted to deliver a fine mist. Close doors and windows and shut off ventilating systems. For rapid control of house flies, fruit flies, gnats, mosquitoes, skipper flies, wasps, hornets, bees, blackflies, angoumois grain moths and tobacco moths, direct spray at an upward angle distributing it uniformly through the entire area at a rate of one (1) ounces per 1,000 cubic feet of space. Keep area closed for at least 10 minutes. Vacate areas after treatment and ventilate and sweep up dead insects before occupying.

For rapid kill of exposed or accessible stages of other insects named on this label: Apply using conventional mechanical or compressed air equipment (non-thermal), following directions for space spraying. Apply the above dilutions at a rate of one (1) ounce per 1,000 cubic feet of space.

Outdoor Use Areas: Corrals, Feedlots, Swine Lots, Zoos.

For Temporary Reduction of Annoyance Flies, Gnats, Mosquitoes: In the treatment of corrals, feedlots, swine lots and zoos, cover any exposed water, drinking fountains and animal feed before application. Fill the area with mist and direct the spray into tall grass, shrubbery and around lawns, where these pests may hover or rest. Apply while the air is still and avoid wetting foliage. In zoos, prevent exposure of reptiles to the product. Repeat as necessary.

Animals and Animal Premise Use: Cattle Barns, Swine Houses, Milk Rooms, Kennels, Poultry Houses, Horse Barns, Dairies, Milking Parlors, Feedlots, Stables, Paddocks. For initial clean-up of severe insect infestation, dilute at a rate of one (1) part concentrate in 19 parts water (6.7 ounces per gallon) (0.5%). For normal infestations dilute one (1) part concentrate in 100 parts water (1.33 ounces per gallon) (8 teaspoonsful per gallon) (0.1%).

Reference Chart:

Pests	Dilutions (Mix Well)	How to Apply
Pests on Farm Premises (Barns, Dairies, Loafing Sheds, Milking Parlors, Feedlots, Stables, Paddocks, Poultry and Livestock Housing)		
Horseflies, Stableflies, lesser Houseflies and other manure breeding flies, Fleas, Lice, Mites, Ticks, including Deer tick (carrier of Lyme disease). Aids in control of Cockroaches, Mosquitoes and Spiders	Dilute 8 ounces in 6.25 gallons water Dilute 1 pint in 12.5 gallons water Dilute 1 quart in 25 gallons water	Spray walls and surfaces to the point of run-off, about one (1) gallon per 750-1,000 square feet. Treat no more often than once every two (2) weeks. Do not contaminate animal's feed or water by spray. Do not use in milk rooms.
Pests on Dog Premises (Kennels, Dog Houses, Runs and Yards)		
Fleas, Flies, Ticks, Lice and Mange Mites (adult and larvae)	Dilute 8 ounces in 6.25 gallons water Dilute 1 pint in 12.5 gallons water Dilute 1 quart in 25 gallons water	Thoroughly wet pest breeding or resting areas to run-off. Most efficient pest control is accomplished when heavy pressure and good contact is achieved. Timing and frequency of applications should be based on pest populations reaching nuisance levels, but accompanying manure removal and sanitation practices should precede sprays. Do not spray feed, food or water. Repeat as needed but not more often than once every two weeks.
Pests in Cattle Barns, Horse Barns, Swine Houses, Kennels, Milking Parlors, Milk Rooms, Dairies, Poultry Houses, Feedlots, Stables and Paddocks		
Flies, Mosquitoes and Gnats	Dilute 8 ounces in 6.25 gallons water Dilute 1 pint in 12.5 gallons water Dilute 1 quart in 25 gallons water	Fog or Fine Mist: Apply directing the spray toward the ceiling and upper corners until the area is filled with mist. Use about two (2) ounces per 1,000 cubic feet of space. For best results, close doors and windows before spraying and keep closed for ten to fifteen minutes. Vacate the treated area and ventilate before reoccupying. Repeat treatment as necessary.
Pests on Large Animals (Dairy or Beef Cattle, Horses, Sheep and Goats)		
Faceflies, Hornflies, Horseflies, Ear Ticks	Dilute 8 ounces in 5 gallons oil Dilute 1 pint in 10 gallons oil Dilute 1 quart in 20 gallons oil	Backrubber: Recharge backrubber as needed. Spray lactating dairy cows only after milking is completed.
Faceflies, Hornflies, Stableflies, Mosquitoes, Lice, Mites, Ticks [including Deer tick (carrier of Lyme disease)]	Dilute 8 ounces in 50 gallons water Dilute 1 pint in 100 gallons water Dilute 1 quart in 200 gallons water	Spray to thoroughly cover entire animal. For Lice or Mites: A second treatment is recommended 14-21 days later. Spray lactating dairy cows only after milking is completed.
Hornflies, Faceflies, Stableflies, Ear Ticks	Dilute 2 ounces in 1 gallon water Dilute 1 pint in 2.5 gallons water	Spot Treatment - Low Pressure Spray: Apply 0.5 ounce per ear or 2 to 4 ounces on face or 12 to 16 ounces along the backline.
Pests on Swine and Poultry		
Mange Mites	Dilute 8 ounces in 25 gallons water Dilute 1 pint in 50 gallons water Dilute 1 quart in 100 gallons water	Spray, dip or sponge animals. Retreat after 14 days, spraying walls and floor space and bedding to kill late hatching, developing stages.
Blowflies, Flies, Mosquitoes, Hog Lice, Fleas, Ticks [including Deer tick (carrier of Lyme disease)]	Dilute 8 ounces in 25 gallons water Dilute 1 pint in 50 gallons water Dilute 1 quart in 100 gallons water	Spray, dip or sponge to apply one (1) pint per pig, especially around ears.
Poultry Mites, Northern Fowl Mites and Lice	Dilute 8 ounces in 12.5 gallons water Dilute 1 pint in 25 gallons water Dilute 1 quart in 50 gallons water	Spray at the rate of 0.5 ounces per bird, or 1 gallon per 100 birds, with a fine mist. Spray roosts, walls and nests or cages.
Pests on Dogs (do not treat puppies less than four weeks old)		
Fleas, Ticks [including Deer tick (carrier of Lyme disease)], Lice and Mange	Dilute 8 ounces in 12.5 gallons water Dilute 1 pint in 25 gallons water Dilute 1 quart in 50 gallons water	Thoroughly wet the animal by dipping, sponging or spraying. Allow animal to dry in a warm place without rinsing to toweling. Gives long-lasting protection against reinfestation and applications at intervals of two to three weeks. Repeat applications as necessary.

Hose-End Sprayer: To control listed insects, shake well before applying. Connect nozzle to hose; remove bottle cap, insert diptube and screw bottle onto nozzle. Turn on water at the tap. When ready to treat, place finger over the hole on right side of nozzle and the liquid will mix automatically at the proper ratio. Apply to surfaces in dairies, barns, feedlots, stables, poultry houses, swine and livestock housing: to control House Flies, Stable Flies and other manure breeding flies. Also aids in control of Cockroaches, Ants, Spiders, Mosquitoes, Crickets and Face Flies. Walk and spray at a steady pace. Spray walls and surfaces to the point of run-off. Treat no more often than once every two weeks. Do not contaminate animals' feed or water by spray.

Precautionary Statements: Hazards to Humans and Domestic Animals:

Caution: Harmful if swallowed or absorbed through the skin. Avoid contact with eyes, skin and clothing. Wash thoroughly after handling. Remove and wash clothing before reuse. Avoid contamination of food and feed. Full-faced gas mask with canister is recommended for general protection when applying indoors as a space spray or fogger.

Environmental Hazards: This pesticide is extremely toxic to fish. Do not apply directly to water, to areas where surface water is present or to intertidal areas below the mean high water mark. Drift and runoff from treated areas may be hazardous to aquatic organisms in treated areas. Do not contaminate water when disposing of equipment washwater/dip solution. This product is highly toxic to bees exposed to direct treatment on blooming crops or weeds while bees are actively visiting the treatment area.

Physical Hazards: Do not use or store near heat or open flame. Do not use this product in or on electrical equipment due to the possibility of shock hazard.

Statement of Practical Treatment:

If Swallowed: Call a physician or Poison Control Center immediately. Drink one or two glasses of water and induce vomiting by touching back of the throat with finger. Do not induce vomiting or give anything by mouth to an unconscious person. If Inhaled: Remove person to fresh air. Apply artificial respiration if indicated. If on Skin: Remove contaminated clothing and wash affected areas with plenty of soap and water. If in Eyes: Flush eyes with plenty of water. Call a physician if irritation persists. Note to Physician: This product contains petroleum solvents. Vomiting may cause aspiration pneumonia.

Storage and Disposal: Do not contaminate water, food or feed by storage or disposal.

Pesticide Storage and Spill Procedure: Store upright at room temperature. Avoid exposure to extreme temperatures. In case of spill or leakage, soak up with an absorbent material such as sand, sawdust, earth, fuller's earth, etc.

Pesticide Disposal: Pesticide, spray mixture or rinse water that cannot be used according to label instructions must be disposed of at or by an approved waste disposal facility.

Container Disposal: For containers one (1) gallon or over: Triple rinse (or equivalent). Then offer for recycling or reconditioning, or puncture and dispose of in a sanitary landfill, or incineration. or, by other procedures approved by state and local authorities. For containers under one (1) gallon: Do not reuse container. Wrap container in several layers of newspaper and discard in trash.

Warning(s): Do not ship swine for slaughter within five (5) days of last treatment.

Keep out of reach of children.

Disclaimer: Except as expressly provided herein, neither Loveland nor seller makes any warranties, guarantees, or representation of any kind, either by usage of trade, statutory or otherwise, with regard to the product sold, including, but not limited to merchantability, fitness for a particular purpose, use or eligibility of the product for any particular trade usage.

Unintended consequences may result because of, but not limited to, such factors as presence of other materials, or the manner of use or application, all of which are beyond the control of Loveland Industries, Inc. or seller. In no case shall seller be liable for consequential, special, or indirect damages resulting from the use or handling of this product. All such risks shall be assumed by the buyer or user.

Applicator's or grower's exclusive remedy against Loveland Industries, Inc. or seller for any cause of action relating to the product is a claim for damages, and in no event shall damages or any other recovery exceed the purchase price of the product in respect of which such claim is made.

Presentation: 8 oz.

Compendium Code No.: 10860291

PROZAP® IVERMECTIN POUR-ON

Loveland **Parasiticide-Topical**

Ivermectin

ANADA No.: 200-219

Active Ingredient(s): 5 mg ivermectin per mL.

Indications: PROZAP® (ivermectin) Pour-On applied at the recommended dose level of 500 mcg/kg is indicated for the effective control of these parasites.

Gastrointestinal Roundworms: *Ostertagia ostertagi* (including inhibited stage) (adults and L_4), *Haemonchus placei* (adults and L_4), *Trichostrongylus axei* (adults and L_4), *T. colubriformis* (adults and L_4), *Cooperia* spp (adults and L_4), *Strongyloides papillosus* (adults), *Oesophagostomum radiatum* (adults and L_4), *Trichuris* spp (adults).

Lungworms: *Dictyocaulus viviparus* (adults and L_4).

Cattle Grubs (parasitic stages): *Hypoderma bovis, H. lineatum.*

Mites: *Sarcoptes scabiei* var. *bovis.*

Lice: *Linognathus vituli, Haematopinus eurysternus, Damalinia bovis, Solenopotes capillatus.*

Horn Flies: *Haematobia irritans.*

Pharmacology: Mode of Action: Ivermectin as a member of the avermectin family kills certain parasitic roundworms and ectoparasites, such as mites, lice, horn flies and other insects. Its action is unique to the avermectin class of antiparasitic agents. This action involves a chemical that serves as a signal from one nerve cell to another, or from a nerve cell to a muscle cell. This chemical, a neurotransmitter, is called gamma-aminobutyric acid or GABA.

In roundworms, ivermectin stimulates the release of GABA from nerve endings and enhances binding of GABA to special receptors at nerve junctions, thus interrupting nerve impulses - thereby paralyzing and killing the parasite.

The enhancement of the GABA effect in arthropods such as mites, lice, and horn flies resembles that in roundworms except that nerve impulses are interrupted between the nerve ending and the muscle cell. Again, this leads to paralysis and death.

Ivermectin has no measurable effect against flukes or tapeworms, presumably because they do not have GABA as a nerve impulse transmitter.

The principal peripheral neurotransmitter in mammals, acetylcholine, is unaffected by ivermectin. Ivermectin does not readily penetrate the central nervous system of mammals where GABA functions as a neurotransmitter.

Dosage and Administration:

Treatment for Cattle for Horn Flies: PROZAP® (ivermectin) Pour-On controls horn flies *(Haematobia irritans)* for up to 28 days after dosing. For best results PROZAP® (ivermectin) Pour-On should be part of a parasite control program for both internal and external parasites based on the epidemiology of these parasites. Consult your veterinarian or an entomologist for the most effective timing of applications.

Dosage: The dose rate is 1 mL for each 22 lbs of body weight. The formulation should be applied along the topline in a narrow strip extending from the withers to the tailhead.

Administration:

Measuring Cup (250 mL, 500 mL and 1 L bottles): The enclosed measuring cup is graduated in 5 mL increments. Each 5 mL will treat 110 lbs body weight. When body weight is between markings, use the next higher increment.

Applicator Gun* (3.785 L bottle): Because of the solvents used in PROZAP® (ivermectin) Pour-On, only the Prozap® Applicator Gun from Simcro Tech Limited, or equivalent, is recommended. Other applicators may exhibit compatibility problems, resulting in locking, incorrect dosage or leakage.

Insert the brass end of the draw tube into the larger hole on the back side of the cap with the stem.

Slide one of the coil springs over one end of the draw-off tubing. Attach that end of the draw-off tubing to the stem on the applicator gun and slide the spring up to the connection. Slide the other soil spring over the other end of the draw-off tubing and connect that end to the cap that has the stem. Slide the spring to the connection. Replace the shipping cap with the cap having the draw-off tubing and draw tube attached. Tighten this draw-off cap to the bottle.

Follow the applicator gun manufacturer's directions for priming the gun, adjusting the dose, and care of the applicator gun following use.

Weight	Dose
220 lb (100 kg)	10 mL
330 lb (150 kg)	15 mL
440 lb (200 kg)	20 mL
550 lb (250 kg)	25 mL
660 lb (300 kg)	30 mL
770 lb (350 kg)	35 mL
880 lb (400 kg)	40 mL
990 lb (450 kg)	45 mL
1100 lb (500 kg)	50 mL

*Additional Applicator Guns and Draw Tubes may be purchased from your local retail dealer or through Loveland Industries, Inc.

When to Treat Cattle with Grubs: PROZAP® (ivermectin) Pour-On effectively controls all stages of cattle grubs. However, proper timing of treatment is important. For the most effective results, cattle should be treated as soon as possible after the end of the heel fly (warble fly) season. While this is not peculiar to ivermectin, destruction of *Hypoderma* larvae (cattle grubs) at the period when these grubs are in vital areas may cause undesirable host-parasite reactions. Killing *Hypoderma lineatum* when it is in the esophageal tissues may cause bloat; killing *H. bovis* when it is in the vertebral canal may cause staggering or paralysis. Cattle should be treated either before or after these stages of grub development.

Cattle treated with PROZAP® (ivermectin) Pour-On at the end of the fly season may be re-treated with PROZAP® (ivermectin) Pour-On during the winter without danger of grub-related reactions. For further information and advice on a planned parasite control program, consult your veterinarian.

Safety: Studies conducted in the U.S.A. have demonstrated the safety margin for ivermectin. Based on plasma levels, the topically applied formulation is expected to be at least as well tolerated by breeding animals as is the subcutaneous formulation, which had no effect on breeding performance.

Consult your veterinarian for assistance in the diagnosis, treatment and control of parasitism.

Precaution(s): Flammable! Keep away from heat, sparks, open flame and other sources of ignition.

Store at controlled room temperature 15° to 30°C (59° to 86°F).

Store away from excessive heat (104°F/40°C) and protect from light.

Use only in well-ventilated areas or outdoors.

Close container tightly when not in use.

Cloudiness in the formulation may occur when PROZAP® (ivermectin) Pour-On is stored at temperatures below 32°F. Allowing to warm at room temperature will restore the normal appearance without affecting efficacy.

Environmental Safety: Studies indicate that when ivermectin comes in contact with the soil, it readily and tightly binds to the soil and becomes inactive over time. Free ivermectin may adversely affect fish or certain water-borne organisms on which they feed. Do not permit cattle to enter lakes, streams or ponds for at least six hours after treatment. Do not contaminate water by direct application or by the improper disposal of drug containers. Dispose of containers in an approved landfill or by incineration.

Caution(s): Cattle should not be treated when hair or hide is wet since reduced efficacy may be experienced.

Do not use when rain is expected to wet cattle within six hours after treatment.

This product is for application to skin surface only. Do not give orally or parenterally.

Anti-parasitic activity of ivermectin will be impaired if the formulation is applied to areas of the skin with mange scabs or lesions, or with dermatoses or adherent materials, e.g., caked mud or manure.

Ivermectin has been associated with adverse reaction in sensitive dogs; therefore, PROZAP® (ivermectin) Pour-On is not recommended for use in species other than cattle.

Warning(s): Cattle must not be treated within 48 days of slaughter for human consumption. Because a withdrawal time in milk has not been established, do not use on female dairy cattle of breeding age.

Not for use in humans.

This product should not be applied to self or others because it may be irritating to human skin and eyes and absorbed through the skin. To minimize accidental skin contact, the user should wear a long-sleeved shirt and rubber gloves. If accidental skin contact occurs, wash immediately with soap and water. If accidental eye exposure occurs, flush eyes immediately with water and seek medical attention.

Keep this and all drugs out of the reach of children.

Presentation: PROZAP® (ivermectin) Pour-On is available in a 250 mL (8.5 fl oz) bottle, a 500 mL (16.9 fl oz) bottle, a 1 L (33.8 fl oz) bottle for use with appropriate automatic dosing applicator.

Compendium Code No.: 10860300

PROZAP® LD-44Z

Loveland **Premise Insecticide**

Farm Insect Fogger

EPA Reg. No.: 499-323-36208

Active Ingredient(s):

Pyrethrins 0.5%
*Piperonyl Butoxide, Technical 4.0%
Inert Ingredients: 95.5%
Total 100.0%

*Equivalent to 3.2% (butylcarbityl) (6-propylpiperonyl) ether and 0.8% related compounds.

Indications: For use in and around, but not limited to, beef cattle operations, catteries, dairy farms (including milk house, milk parlor, loafing sheds, and holding lot), farms, hog operations, horse barns and stables, kennels and poultry operations.

This product kills and repels flies, ants, clover mites, cluster flies, centipedes, cockroaches, crickets, deer flies, face flies, fleas, fruit flies, gnats, hornets, horn flies, horse flies, house flies, lice, millipedes, mosquitoes, mud daubers, small flying moths, sow bugs, spiders, stable flies and wasps.

Directions for Use: It is a violation of Federal Law to use this product in a manner inconsistent with its labeling.

Dairy Farm Use: Milking Parlor and Milk Room: Close all windows and doors. Direct fog upward and in all directions at a rate of 1 to 3 seconds per 1,000 cu. ft. Keep room closed for 15 minutes after treatment. Open and ventilate before reoccupying. Cover milking utensils and milk to prevent contamination from spray and dead falling insects.

Animal Use: From approximately 2 foot distance, thoroughly spray entire animal as it is being released to pasture. Do not spray directly toward animal's eyes. Spot treat withers, shoulders and back where saliva accumulates from head tossing.

Stanchion Barn Use: Walk behind animals and direct spray over backs allowing 1 second per animal. For most effective results, apply each morning.

Beef Cattle Operations: In barns, close all windows and doors. Spray at the rate of 1 to 2 seconds per 1,000 cu. ft. Keep area closed for 15 minutes following application. Ventilate area after treatment is complete. If area cannot be closed, double the dosage. Repeat application daily or as necessary.

Horse Barns and Stables: Close all windows and doors. Spray at a rate of 1 to 2 seconds per 1,000 cu. ft. Keep area closed for 15 minutes following application. Ventilate area after treatment is complete. If area cannot be closed, double the dosage. For animal application, lightly mist over the backs of horses and ponies from a distance of at least two feet. Repeat application daily or as necessary.

Poultry Operations: Use only in empty poultry houses (when birds are not present). Close all windows and doors. Spray at the rate of 1 to 2 seconds per 1,000 cu. ft. Keep area closed for 15 minutes following application. Ventilate area after treatment is complete. If area cannot be closed, double the dosage. Treat daily or as necessary.

Hog Operations: In hog houses, close all windows and doors. Spray at the rate of 1 to 2 seconds per 1,000 cu. ft. Keep area closed for 15 minutes after application. Ventilate the area after treatment is complete. If area cannot be closed, double the dosage. For animal application, direct spray over backs and spray for 1 to 2 seconds per hog. Do not spray directly toward animal's face or eyes. Repeat application daily or as necessary.

Mud Dauber and Wasp Nests: Spray mist directly on insects and their nests from approximately 2 ft. distance. Contacted insects will fly away from fog. Applications should be made in late evening when insects are at rest. Spray into hiding and breeding places contacting as many insects as possible.

Fleas: General Volumetric Treatment: Hold aerosol 36" above floor and direct spray toward floor and lower walls at a rate of 10 seconds per 100 sq. ft. making sure that all floor areas are contacted. Change litter before application. Keep area closed for 15 minutes. Remove animals before spraying. Open and ventilate before reoccupying. Repeat treatment after 7 days or as necessary.

Kennels and Catteries: Remove animals before spraying. Ventilate after treatment is complete.

Outdoor Ground Application: Flies, Gnats and Mosquitoes in open areas near building and in campgrounds. Best results are obtained when wind speed is five (5) MPH or less. Apply at a rate of 60-80 seconds per acre. Spray in wide swaths across area to be treated. Allow spray drift to penetrate dense foliage. Repeat treatment as necessary.

Contraindication(s): Do not spray sick animals.

Precautionary Statements: Hazards to Humans and Domestic Animals:

Caution: Harmful if swallowed or absorbed through skin. Do not remain in treated area and ventilate the area after treatment is completed. Avoid breathing of vapor. Avoid contact with skin, eyes, or clothing. Wash thoroughly after using and before smoking or eating. Do not contaminate water, food, or foodstuffs. Remove all pets and birds. Cover fish tanks or remove before spraying.

Statement of Practical Treatment:

If swallowed: Call a physician or Poison Control Center immediately. Gastric lavage is indicated if material was taken internally. Do not induce vomiting. Vomiting may cause aspiration pneumonia. If inhaled: Remove patient to fresh air. Apply artificial respiration if indicated. If on skin: Remove contaminated clothing and wash affected skin areas with soap and water. Get medical attention if irritation persists. If in eyes: Flush eyes with plenty of water. Get medical attention if irritation persists.

Environmental Hazards: This product is toxic to fish, birds, and other wildlife. Do not apply directly to water, or to areas where surface water is present or to intertidal areas below the mean high water mark. Apply this product only as specified on the label.

Physical or Chemical Hazards: Flammable. Contents under pressure. Keep away from heat, sparks, and open flame. Do not puncture or incinerate container. Exposure to temperatures above 130°F may cause bursting. Do not spray on plastic, painted, or varnished surfaces or directly onto any electronic equipment such as radios, televisions, computers, etc.

Storage and Disposal: Do not contaminate water, food or feed by storage or disposal.

Storage: Store in a cool area away from heat or open flame.

Pesticide Disposal: Waste resulting from the use of this product may be disposed of on site or at an approved waste disposal facility.

Container Disposal: Replace cap and discard empty container in trash, landfill, or by other approved state and local procedures. Do not incinerate or puncture.

For best results product should be used when can temperature is above 60°F, store at room temperature until a temperature above 60°F is reached.

Warning(s): Not for use in Federally inspected meat and poultry plants. Contains no CFC's or other ozone depleting substances. Federal regulations prohibit CFC propellants in aerosols.

Keep out of reach of children.

Presentation: 20 oz and 25 oz containers.

Compendium Code No.: 10860310

PROZAP® RESIDUAL INSECT SPRAY 2EC

Loveland **Premise Insecticide**

Organophosphate Insecticide

EPA Reg. No.: 2393-377-36208

Active Ingredient(s):

Dimethoate: 0,0-Dimethyl S-methylcarbamoylmethyl phosphorodithioate 23.4%
Inert Ingredients*: 76.6%
Total 100.00%

*This product contains xylene-range aromatics

(1 gallon contains 2 pounds dimethoate)

Indications: Controls houseflies and maggots in dairy barns, hog pens, calf barns, poultry and other farm buildings.

Controls flies up to 8 weeks.

Directions for Use: It is a violation of Federal law to use this product in a manner inconsistent with its labeling.

P

Houseflies: For localized housefly control, apply as a spray containing ½ pint of PROZAP® Residual Insect Spray 2EC in 5 quarts of water with a knapsack or similar type sprayer to areas frequented by flies, such as doorways, around windows, etc. Repeat applications should be made when necessary. Good sanitation is a necessary part of any effective fly control program. Maggot Sprays: For the control of housefly maggots, mix ½ pint of PROZAP® Residual Insect Spray 2EC in 5 quarts of water and apply as a coarse spray or with a sprinkling can to fly-breeding areas, such as poultry droppings in caged-layer houses, garbage dumps and manure piles. Repeat application as additional manure or garbage is added. Residual Wall Sprays: For the control of houseflies including resistant-strains in dairy barns, hog pens, calf barns, poultry houses and other farm buildings, apply a 1% residual spray to the ceilings, walls, stanchions, etc. Prepare the spray by mixing ½ pint of PROZAP® Residual Insect Spray 2EC in 1½ gallons of water. Thoroughly wet all fly resting areas to the point of runoff. One gallon of spray will cover 500 to 1,000 square feet of surface. Repeat applications should be made when necessary. Remove all animals from buildings when applying residual wall spray. PROZAP® Residual Insect Spray 2EC is acceptable for use as a residual-type insecticide in and around federally inspected meat packing plants except where meat food products are produced or handled.

PROZAP® Residual Insect Spray 2EC controls flies up to 8 weeks or longer.

General Outside Use: For the control of houseflies around homes and recreation areas, garbage cans, animal quarters, food-processing plants. warehouses, loading docks and refuse areas: thoroughly spray exposed surfaces such as walls, fences, garbage and refuse containers with ½ pint of PROZAP® Residual Insect Spray 2EC in 1½ gallons of water. Repeat applications should be made when necessary.

Precautionary Statements: Hazards to Humans and Domestic Animals:

Warning: Vapor harmful - Harmful or fatal if swallowed.

Concentrated material causes eye irritation.

Avoid breathing vapor or spray mist. Avoid contact with skin or eyes. Use only with adequate ventilation. Do not contaminate food. Do not use in homes. Rinse spills on outside of container after use. Do not contaminate feed and foodstuffs, drinking fountains, litter and feed troughs. Do not use in milk-processing rooms, including milk houses and milk storage rooms.

Aerial Application: Automatic flagging devices should be used whenever feasible. If human flaggers are employed, they must wear the protective clothing and respirator specified on this label.

Personal Protective Equipment: Some materials that are chemical-resistant to this product are listed below. If you want more options, follow the instructions for category F an the EPA resistance category selection chart.

Applicators and other handlers must wear: coveralls over short-sleeved shirt and short pants, chemical-resistant gloves, such as barrier laminate, butyl rubber, nitrite rubber or viton, chemical-resistant footwear plus socks, protective eyewear and chemical-resistant headgear for overhead exposure. For exposures in enclosed areas, a respirator with either an organic vapor-removing cartridge with a prefilter approved for pesticides (MSHA/NIOSH approval number prefix TC-23C), or a canister approved for pesticides (MSHA/NIOSH approval number prefix TC-14G). For exposure outdoors, a dust/mist filtering respirator (MSHA/NIOSH approved number prefix TC-21C). Discard clothing and other absorbent materials that have been drenched or heavily contaminated with this product's concentrate. Do not reuse them. Follow manufacturer's instructions for cleaning and maintaining PPE. If no such instructions for washables, use detergent and hot water. Keep and wash PPE separately from other laundry.

Engineering controls statements: When handlers use closed systems, enclosed cabs, or aircraft in a manner that meets with requirements listed in the Worker Protection Standard (WPS) for agricultural pesticides [40 CFR 170.240 (d) (4-6)], the handler PPE requirements may be reduced modified as specified in the WPS.

User Safety Recommendations: Users should:

Wash hands before eating, drinking, chewing gum, using tobacco or using the toilet.

Remove clothing immediately if pesticide gets inside. Then wash thoroughly and put on clean clothing.

Remove PPE immediately after handling this product. Wash the outside of gloves before removing. As soon as possible, wash thoroughly and change into clean clothing.

Environmental Hazards: This pesticide is toxic to wildlife and aquatic invertebrates. For terrestrial uses, do not apply directly to water, or to areas where surface water is present or to intertidal areas below the mean high water mark. Do not contaminate water by cleaning equipment or disposal of wastes. This pesticide is highly toxic to bees exposed to direct treatment or residues on blooming crops or weeds. Do not apply this product or allow it to drift to blooming crops or weeds if bees are visiting the treatment area.

Chemical Hazards: Combustible. Do not use, pour, spill or store near heat or open flame.

Do not apply this product in a way that will contact workers or other persons, either directly or through drift. Only protected handlers may be in the area during application.

For any requirements specific to your State or Tribe, consult the agency responsible for pesticide regulation.

Agricultural Use Requirements:

Use this product only in accordance with its labeling and with the Worker Protection Standard, 40 CFR part 170. This Standard contains requirements for the protection of agricultural workers on farms, forests, nurseries, and greenhouses, and handlers of agricultural pesticides. It contains requirements for training, decontamination, notification and emergency assistance. It also contains specific instructions and exceptions pertaining to the statements on this label about personal protective equipment (PPE), and restricted-entry interval. The requirements in this box only apply to uses of this product that are covered by the Worker Protection Standard. Do not enter or allow worker entry into treated areas during the restricted entry interval (REI) of 48 hours. PPE required for early entry to treated areas that is permitted under the Worker Protection Standard and that involves contact with anything that has been treated, such as plants, soil, or water, is: coveralls over short-sleeved shirt and short pants, chemical-resistant gloves, such as barrier laminate, butyl rubber, nitrile rubber or viton, chemical-resistant footwear plus socks, protective eyewear and chemical-resistant headgear for overhead exposure.

Non-Agricultural Use Requirements:

The requirements in this box apply to uses of this product that are not within the scope of the Worker Protection Standard for agricultural pesticides (40 CFR Part 170). The WPS applies when this product is used to produce agricultural plants on farms, forests, nurseries or greenhouses.

Keep children and pets out of the treated area until sprays have dried.

Statement of Practical Treatment:

If Swallowed: Call a physician or Poison Control Center immediately. Gastric lavage is usually indicated. Do not induce vomiting. Vomiting may cause aspiration pneumonia. Do not induce vomiting or give substances by mouth to an unconscious person.

If Inhaled: Remove victim to fresh air. Assist respiration if indicated.

If on Skin: Promptly wash contaminated skin with soap and water.

If in Eyes: Immediately flush eyes with plenty of water. Get medical attention if irritation persists.

Note to Physicians: This product may cause cholinesterase inhibition. Atropine is antidotal.

Storage and Disposal: Do not contaminate water, food or feed by storage or disposal.

Storage: Do not store near heat or open flame. Do not store below 40°F. Mix as needed, do not store diluted material.

Pesticide Disposal: Pesticide wastes are acutely hazardous. Improper disposal of excess pesticide, spray mixture, or rinsate is a violation of Federal Law. If these wastes cannot be disposed of by use according to label instructions, contact your State Pesticide or Environmental Control Agency, or the Hazardous Waste representative at the nearest EPA Regional Office for guidance. Container Disposal: Metal: Triple rinse (or equivalent). Then offer for recycling or reconditioning, or puncture and dispose of in a sanitary landfill, or by other procedures approved by state and local authorities. Plastic: Triple rinse (or equivalent). Then offer for recycling or reconditioning, or puncture and dispose of in a sanitary landfill, or incineration, or, if allowed by state and local authorities, by burning. If burned, stay out of smoke.

Disclaimer: Except as expressly provided herein, neither Loveland nor seller makes any warranties, guarantees, or representation of any kind, either express or implied, or by usage of trade, statutory or otherwise, with regard to the product sold, including, but not limited to merchantability, fitness for a particular purpose, use or eligibility of the product for any particular trade usage.

Unintended consequences may result because of, but not limited to, such factors as presence of other materials, or the manner of use or application, all of which are beyond the control of Loveland Industries, Inc. or seller. In no case shall seller be liable for consequential, special, or indirect damages resulting from the use or handling of this product. All such risks shall be assumed by the buyer or user.

Applicator's or grower's exclusive remedy against Loveland Industries, Inc. or seller for any cause of action relating to the product is a claim for damages, or in no event shall damages or any other recovery exceed the purchase price of the product in respect of which such claim is made.

Presentation: 1 gallon (3.78 L).

Compendium Code No.: 10860330

PROZAP® VIP INSECT SPRAY

Loveland **Premise and Topical Insecticide**

EPA Reg. No.: 2393-382-36208

Active Ingredient(s):

2,2-Dichlorovinyl Dimethyl Phosphate*	0.92%
Related Compounds*	0.08%
Technical piperonyl butoxide**	0.10%
Pyrethrins	0.01%
Inert Ingredients***:	98.89%
Total	100.00%

*Equivalent to 1.0% of Vapona® Insecticide

**Equivalent to 0.08% (Butylcarbityl) (6-propylpiperonyl) ether and 0.02% related compounds.

***Contains petroleum distillates.

Indications: For insect control in horse barns, dairy barns, shelter sheds, milk sheds, outdoor areas and poultry houses.

This ready-to-use solution is intended for the control of insects, face flies, houseflies, gnats, hornflies, fleas, mosquitoes, stable flies, ticks and wasps attacking livestock.

Directions for Use: It is a violation of Federal laws to use this product in a manner inconsistent with its labeling.

Restrictions: Do not contaminate water or foodstuffs. Do not contaminate milk or milk equipment. Do not apply in areas where animals have received direct application of DDVP within eight (8) hours. Care should be taken that the spray does not come into direct contact with the lactating dairy cow's teats unless they are washed with an approved cleansing solution and dried before milking. Brahman and Brahman cross cattle should not be treated as they may show hypersensitivity to organophosphates. Do not apply to calves under six months of age.

Applications:

Cattle (Beef and Dairy) to control Hornflies, Houseflies, Stable Flies, Face Flies: Apply one (1) to two (2) fluid ounces of PROZAP® VIP Insect Spray per animal as a mist spray daily with hand or automatic sprayer. Apply spray so as to wet the air. Cover the animal with spray with particular attention given to the back, flanks, legs and shoulders. Do not use in excess of two (2) ounces per adult animal per day. Apply proportionately less to smaller animals. Do not soak the skin or wet the hides.

For Fogging: Control of Flies, Gnats and Mosquitoes in animal buildings (Horse Barns, Dairy Barns, Shelters): Use one (1) pint of PROZAP® VIP Insect Spray per 8,000 cu. ft. Before applying, reduce air movements as much as possible by closing doors, windows, and other openings. Eliminate potential ignition sources such as pilot lights, open flames, sparks, etc. Do not contaminate water, feed or foodstuffs, milk or milking utensils. Do not use this solution for fogging purposes in areas where animals have received direct applications within eight (8) hours. Do not remain in treated areas and ventilate the area after treatment is complete. Remove animals prior to treatment.

Animal Buildings (Horse Barns, Dairy Barns, Shelter Sheds), Milk Sheds, Outdoor Areas: To control Flies, Gnats, Mosquitoes, Roaches, Fleas, Ants, Sowbugs, Brown Dog Ticks, Wasps, Flying Moths and other small flying insects, Cockroaches, Spiders and Silverfish: Apply PROZAP® VIP Insect Spray as a coarse, wet spray at the rate of one (1) pint per 1,000 sq. ft. for milk sheds, stables, livestock barns, loafing sheds, pig pens, and outdoor areas, treat around doorways, feed storage rooms, alleyways and window sills. Do not contaminate milk or milking utensils. For control of Fly Maggots in Maggot breeding areas, apply at the rate of one (1) to two (2) pints per 100 sq. ft. For Cockroaches and Silverfish, spray in cracks, crevices and other hiding places. For Ants, spray trails and places where ants enter premises. For Brown Dog Ticks and Fleas, spray floor areas, cracks, crevices and sleeping quarters of animals. Bedding should be allowed to dry thoroughly before use or replaced with fresh bedding. As many insects as possible should be hit with the spray. Do not use this product on dogs. Use an approved product registered for direct application to dogs.

In Poultry Houses: For Fly control: Apply as a coarse wet spray to manure, window sills, outside of penned enclosures and on the floor of feed storage rooms.

For Outdoor Use: To control Flies, Gnats and Mosquitoes: Use one (1) pint per 1,000 sq. ft. as a coarse wet spray to treat: Picnic Grounds, Loading Docks, Outdoor Latrines, Parking Areas, Refuse Areas, Around Service Stations, Open-Air Drive-Ins, Outdoor Ice Cream Stands, Garbage Collection and Disposal Areas. Avoid contact with desirable plants as plant injury or loss may occur.

In Treating Dog Kennels: Apply to outside dog runways, window sills and ledges. For control of fleas and brown dog ticks, increase the dose to one (1) quart of PROZAP® VIP Insect Spray per 1,000 sq. ft. Treat infested areas, baseboards, cracks, walls, doors. Do not allow children in treated areas until dry. Do not use this product on dogs. Use an approved product registered for direct application to dogs.

Precautionary Statements: Hazards to Humans and Domestic Animals:

Warning: May be fatal if swallowed, inhaled, or absorbed through skin or eyes. Rapidly absorbed through skin and eyes. Do not get into eyes, on skin or on clothing. Do not breathe vapor or spray mist. Wash thoroughly with soap and water after handling and before eating or smoking. Do not contaminate feed, water, foodstuffs, milk or milking utensils.

Wear clean rubber gloves, protective clothing, and goggles, faceshield or equivalent. Wear a pesticide respirator jointly approved by the National Institute for Occupational Safety and Health (NIOSH) or the Mining Safety and Health Administration (MSHA) when applying indoors as a space spray or fog. Wear impervious footwear or protective covers as shoes, boots and other articles made of leather or similar porous materials may be dangerously contaminated.

Statement of Practical Treatment:

If Swallowed: Call a physician or Poison Control Center immediately. Do not induce vomiting. Vomiting may cause aspiration pneumonia. If Inhaled: Remove victim to fresh air. Apply respiration if indicated. If On Skin: Wash contaminated skin with soap and water. Launder contaminated clothing in detergent and hot water before reuse. If In Eyes: Flush eyes with plenty of water. Get medical attention immediately. Note to Physician: Empty stomach if material was taken internally. Gastric lavage may be indicated. If symptoms of cholinesterase inhibition are present, atropine by injection is antidotal. 2-PAM is also antidotal and may be administered in conjunction with atropine.

Environmental Hazards: This product is toxic to fish, birds and other wildlife. For terrestrial uses, do not apply directly to water, or to areas where surface water is present or to intertidal areas below the mean high water mark. Do not contaminate water when disposing of equipment washwaters.

Storage and Disposal: Do not contaminate water, food or feed by storage or disposal.

Do not use or store near heat or an open flame. Keep the product in an upright position in the original container, tightly closed. High temperatures may shorten the shelf life of the product.

Pesticide Disposal: Wastes resulting from the use of the product may be disposed of on site or at an approved waste disposal facility.

Container Disposal: Triple rinse (or equivalent). Then offer for recycling or reconditioning, or puncture and dispose of in a sanitary landfill, or by incineration, or if allowed by state and local authorities, by burning. If burned, stay out of smoke.

Warning(s): Keep out of reach of children.

Disclaimer: Except as expressly provided herein, neither Loveland nor seller makes any warranties, guarantees, or representation of any kind, either by usage of trade, statutory or otherwise, with regard to the product sold, including, but not limited to merchantability, fitness for a particular purpose, use or eligibility of the product for any particular trade usage.

Unintended consequences may result because of, but not limited to, such factors as presence of other materials, or the manner of use or application, all of which are beyond the control of Loveland Industries, Inc. or seller. In no case shall seller be liable for consequential, special, or indirect damages resulting from the use or handling of this product. All such risks shall be assumed by the buyer or user.

Applicator's or grower's exclusive remedy against Loveland Industries, Inc. or seller for any cause of action relating to the product is a claim for damages, and in no event shall damages or any other recovery exceed the purchase price of the product in respect of which such claim is made.

Presentation: 1 gallon (3.78 L).

Compendium Code No.: 10860340

PROZAP® ZIPCIDE®

Loveland **Topical Insecticide**

EPA Reg. No.: 2393-385-36208

Active Ingredient(s):

Coumaphos: 0,0-diethyl 0-(3-chloro-4-methyl-2-oxo-2H-1-benzopyran-7-yl) phosphorothioate 1%

Inert Ingredients: 99%

Total 100%

Indications: For control of horn flies and lice on beef and dairy cattle and lice on swine.

Directions for Use: It is a violation of Federal law to use this product in a manner inconsistent with its labeling.

Recommended Applications: Hold container at a distance from the area to be treated that will permit even distribution of the dust. Keep lid closed when container is not in use.

Animal	Parasite	Remarks
Cattle (Dairy and Beef)	Hornflies/lice	Direct Application: Apply not more than 2 oz*/animal. Dust evenly over the head, neck, shoulders, back and tailhead. Repeat as necessary but not more often than every 10 days. No interval is required between treatment and use of meat or milk as food.
Swine	Lice	Direct Application: Apply not more than 1 oz*/animal as a uniform coat to the shoulders and back. Repeat as necessary but not more than once every 10 days. No interval is required between treatment and use of meat or milk as food. Bedding Treatment: Apply 2 oz* uniformly over each 30 square feet of fresh, dry bedding. Repeat as necessary, but not more than once every 10 days. Direct Application and Bedding Treatment: In severe infestations, both individual animals and the bedding may be treated as directed above.

*Note: 1 oz of this material equals approximately three level tablespoons.

Restrictions: For external insecticidal use on above specified animals only. Avoid contamination of feed troughs, water and water utensils. Provide thorough ventilation while dusting.

Contraindication(s): Do not apply to sick, stressed or convalescent animals.

Precautionary Statements: Hazards to Humans and Domestic Animals:

Caution: Harmful if swallowed, inhaled or absorbed through skin. Avoid breathing dusts. Avoid contact with eyes, skin and clothing. Wash thoroughly with soap and warm water after handling. Do not contaminate feed or food.

Statement of Practical Treatment:

If swallowed: Call a physician or Poison Control Center immediately. Drink one or two glasses of water and induce vomiting by touching back of throat with finger. Repeat until vomit fluid is clear. Do not induce vomiting or give anything by mouth to an unconscious person.

If inhaled: Remove victim to fresh air. Apply artificial respiration if indicated. Get medical attention of victim displays signs of poisoning.

If on skin: Remove contaminated clothing and wash affected areas with soap and water.

If in eyes: Flush eyes with plenty of water. Call a physician immediately.

To Physician: Prolonged or repeated exposure will result in cholinesterase depression. Atropine sulfate by injection is antidotal. 2-PAM is also antidotal, and may be administered in conjunction with atropine.

Environmental Hazards: This pesticide is toxic to birds, fish and aquatic invertebrates. For terrestrial uses, do not apply directly to water, or to areas where surface water is present or to intertidal areas below the mean high water mark. Do not contaminate water when disposing of equipment washwater or rinsate.

Storage and Disposal: Do not contaminate water, food or feed by storage or disposal.

Storage: Keep product in original container. Keep container tightly closed. High temperatures may shorten shelf life of product.

Pesticide Disposal: Wastes resulting from the use of this product may be disposed of on site or at an approved waste disposal facility.

Container Disposal: Do not reuse empty container. Discard empty container in trash.

Warning(s): Keep out of reach of children.

Disclaimer: Except as expressly provided herein, neither Loveland nor seller makes any warranties, guarantees, or representation of any kind, either express or implied, or by usage of trade, statutory or otherwise, with regard to the product sold, including, but not limited to merchantability, fitness for a particular purpose, use or eligibility of the product for any particular trade usage.

Unintended consequences may result because of, but not limited to, such factors as presence of other materials, or the manner of use or application, all of which are beyond the control of Loveland Industries, Inc. or seller. In no case shall seller be liable for consequential, special, or indirect damages resulting from the use or handling of this product. All such risks shall be assumed by the buyer or user.

Applicator's or grower's exclusive remedy against Loveland Industries, Inc. or seller for any cause of action relating to the product is a claim for damages, and in no event shall damages or any other recovery exceed the purchase price of the product in respect of which such claim is made.

Presentation: 2 pounds (908 g) containers.

® Co-Ral is a registered trademark of the parent company of Farbenfabriken Bayer, GmbH, Leverkusen.

Compendium Code No.: 10860350

PRROMISE®*

Intervet **Vaccine**

Porcine Reproductive & Respiratory Syndrome Vaccine, Reproductive Form, Killed Virus

U.S. Vet. Lic. No.: 286

Contents: This product contains the antigens listed above. This product is adjuvanted with Spur®** to enhance the immune response.

Contains neomycin as a preservative.

Indications: For use as an aid in the reduction of losses at farrowing due to the reproductive form of the disease caused by Porcine Reproductive and Respiratory Syndrome Virus (PRRS) in healthy female breeding age swine.

Dosage and Administration: Shake well before using. Administer two 2 mL doses intramuscularly using aseptic technique. Administer the first 2 mL dose 5-8 weeks after breeding and the second 2 mL dose 14-28 days later. Repeat the 2 dose vaccination schedule on subsequent breedings.

Precaution(s): Store at 35° to 45°F (2° to 7°C). Use entire contents when first opened. Burn the container and all unused contents.

Caution(s): Allergic reactions may follow the use of products of this nature.

For use in animals only.

Antidote(s): Epinephrine.

Warning(s): Do not vaccinate within 21 days of slaughter.

Presentation: 50 dose (100 mL) vials.

*U.S. Patent Nos. 5,587,164 and 5,510,258

**Adjuvant—Intervet's proprietary technology.

Compendium Code No.: 11062221 7255001

PR-VAC®

Pfizer Animal Health **Vaccine**

Pseudorabies Vaccine, Modified Live Virus

U.S. Vet. Lic. No.: 189

Description: PR-VAC® is a preparation of naturally attenuated pseudorabies virus grown on an established porcine cell line and is packaged in freeze-dried form.

Contains gentamicin as preservative.

Indications: PR-VAC® is for vaccination of healthy swine 3 days of age or older as an aid in the prevention of pseudorabies (Aujeszky's disease, mad itch, infectious bulbar paralysis) caused by pseudorabies virus (PRV).

Directions:

1. General Directions: Aseptically rehydrate the freeze-dried vaccine with the sterile diluent provided, shake well, and administer 2 mL intramuscularly.
2. Primary Vaccination: Pigs nursing nonimmune dams should be vaccinated at any time after 3 days of age. Pigs nursing immune dams should be vaccinated when maternal antibody levels have declined, generally when pigs are 8-12 weeks of age. In an emergency situation where exposure is imminent, it may be desirable to immediately vaccinate all swine on the premises.
3. Revaccination: Semiannual revaccination with a single dose is recommended for animals retained for breeding. Boars may be revaccinated at any time. Sows should be revaccinated before breeding.

Precaution(s): Store at 2°-7°C. Prolonged exposure to higher temperatures and/or direct sunlight may adversely affect potency. Do not freeze.

Use entire contents when first opened.

Sterilized syringes and needles should be used to administer this vaccine. Do not sterilize with chemicals because traces of disinfectant may inactivate the vaccine.

Burn containers and all unused contents.

Caution(s): Vaccination with PR-VAC® produces an antibody response to pseudorabies, thereby rendering swine positive to a serum neutralization (SN) test. Vaccinated swine can be differentiated from infected swine using a USDA-approved differential pseudorabies test, Pseudorabies Virus gp1 Antibody Test Kit, provided the animals have received a Pfizer Animal Health PRV vaccine. Distribution of this vaccine is limited to authorized recipients designated by proper state officials and under such conditions as these officials may require.

As with many vaccines, anaphylaxis may occur after use. Initial antidote of epinephrine is recommended and should be followed with appropriate supportive therapy.

This product has been shown to be efficacious in healthy animals. A protective immune response may not be elicited if animals are incubating an infectious disease, are malnourished

P

or parasitized, are stressed due to shipment or environmental conditions, are otherwise immunocompromised, or the vaccine is not administered in accordance with label directions.
Warning(s): Do not vaccinate within 21 days before slaughter.
For use in swine only. Not for use in any other animal.
For veterinary use only.
Discussion: Disease Description: Pseudorabies is an acute infectious disease caused by a herpesvirus. Swine are most commonly affected although pseudorabies has a broad host range that includes dogs, rodents, and several species of farm animals. Human beings are apparently not susceptible. The disease is generally more severe in younger animals. Signs may include vomiting, diarrhea, pyrexia, and CNS disturbances progressing to paralysis and death. Older swine may have acute or subclinical infection. Abortions, stillbirths, and mummified fetuses may occur in affected sows.
Trial Data: Safety and Efficacy: PR-VAC® has demonstrated a high degree of safety and efficacy in extensive experimental and field use. In one immunogenicity test, a single dose protected all 23 susceptible pigs from a virulent challenge that affected all 9 controls. Shedding of virulent virus from exposed swine was reduced by prior vaccination, thus limiting the probability of disease transmission. Extensive clinical experience with the vaccine has shown it to be safe in pigs 3 days of age or older.
Presentation: 5 dose, 25 dose, and 50 dose vials.
Compendium Code No.: 36900500 75-4601-00

PR-VAC®-KILLED

Pfizer Animal Health **Vaccine**
Pseudorabies Vaccine, Killed Virus
U.S. Vet. Lic. No.: 189
Description: PR-VAC®-KILLED is prepared by growing a pseudorabies virus strain on a porcine cell line. The vaccine is inactivated and contains a sterile adjuvant to enhance the immune response.
Contains gentamicin as preservative.
Indications: PR-VAC®-KILLED is for vaccination of healthy swine as an aid in the prevention of pseudorabies (Aujeszky's disease, mad itch, infectious bulbar paralysis) caused by pseudorabies virus (PRV).
Directions:
1. General Directions: For use in swine only! Not for use in any other animal. Shake well. Administer 2 mL intramuscularly.
2. Primary Vaccination: Administer a single 2-mL dose at weaning. Pigs nursing immune dams should be vaccinated when maternal antibody levels have declined, generally when pigs are 8-12 weeks of age. Boars may be vaccinated at any time, and pregnant sows may be vaccinated.
3. Revaccination: Semiannual revaccination with a single dose is recommended for animals retained for breeding.

Precaution(s): Store at 2°-7°C. Prolonged exposure to higher temperatures may adversely affect potency. Do not freeze.
Use entire contents when first opened.
Caution(s): Vaccination with PR-VAC®-KILLED produces an antibody response to pseudorabies, thereby rendering swine positive to a serum neutralization (SN) test. Vaccinated swine can be differentiated from infected swine using a USDA-approved differential pseudorabies test, Pseudorabies Virus gpI Antibody Test Kit, provided the animals have received a Pfizer Animal Health PRV vaccine. Distribution of this vaccine is limited to authorized recipients designated by proper state officials and under such conditions as these officials may require.
As with many vaccines, anaphylaxis may occur after use. Initial antidote of epinephrine is recommended and should be followed with appropriate supportive therapy.
This product has been shown to be efficacious in healthy animals. A protective immune response may not be elicited if animals are incubating an infectious disease, are malnourished or parasitized, are stressed due to shipment or environmental conditions, are otherwise immunocompromised, or the vaccine is not administered in accordance with label directions.
For use in swine only.
For veterinary use only.
Warning(s): Do not vaccinate within 21 days before slaughter.
Discussion: Disease Description: Pseudorabies is an acute infectious disease caused by a herpesvirus. Swine are most commonly affected although pseudorabies has a broad host range that includes dogs, rodents, and several species of farm animals. Human beings are apparently not susceptible. The disease is generally more severe in younger animals. Signs may include vomiting, diarrhea, pyrexia, and CNS disturbances progressing to paralysis and death. Older swine may have acute or subclinical infection. Abortions, stillbirths, and mummified fetuses may occur in affected sows.
Trial Data: Safety and Efficacy: An inactivated product, PR-VAC®-KILLED poses no danger of shed or spread of vaccine virus from vaccinated to susceptible contact animals. Developmental studies have shown that vaccination with PR-VAC®-KILLED prevents clinical pseudorabies following exposure to virulent virus.
Presentation: 25 dose vials.
Compendium Code No.: 36901820 75-4615-12

PR-VAC PLUS®

Pfizer Animal Health **Vaccine**
Pseudorabies Vaccine, Modified Live Virus
U.S. Vet. Lic. No.: 189
Description: PR-VAC PLUS® is a freeze-dried preparation of naturally attenuated pseudorabies virus grown on an established porcine cell line. A sterile diluent containing Amphigen®, a unique oil adjuvant to enhance the immune response, is used to rehydrate the freeze-dried vaccine.
Contains gentamicin as preservative.
Indications: PR-VAC PLUS® is for vaccination of healthy swine 3 weeks of age or older as an aid in the prevention of pseudorabies (Aujeszky's disease) caused by pseudorabies virus (PRV).
Directions:
1. General Directions: Vaccination of healthy swine is recommended. Shake diluent before use. Aseptically rehydrate the freeze-dried vaccine with accompanying adjuvant-containing sterile diluent, shake well, and administer 2 mL intramuscularly.
2. Primary Vaccination: Administer a single 2-mL dose to pigs 3 weeks of age or older. In piglets nursing immune sows, vaccinate when maternal antibody has declined, at approximately 8-12 weeks of age.
3. Revaccination: Semiannual revaccination is recommended for animals retained for breeding. Sows may be safely revaccinated at greater than 40 days gestation.

Precaution(s): Store at 2°-7°C. Prolonged exposure to higher temperatures may adversely affect potency. Do not freeze.
Use entire contents when first opened.
Sterilized syringes and needles should be used to administer this vaccine. Do not sterilize with chemicals because traces of disinfectant may inactivate the vaccine.
Burn containers and all unused contents.
Caution(s): Vaccination with PR-VAC PLUS® produces an antibody response to pseudorabies, thereby rendering swine positive to a serum neutralization (SN) test. Vaccinated swine can be differentiated from infected swine using a USDA-approved differential pseudorabies test, Pseudorabies Virus gp1 Antibody Test Kit, provided the animals have received a Pfizer PRV vaccine. Distribution of this vaccine is limited to authorized recipients designated by proper state officials and under such conditions as these officials may require.
As with many vaccines, anaphylaxis may occur after use. Initial antidote of epinephrine is recommended and should be followed with appropriate supportive therapy.
This product has been shown to be efficacious in healthy animals. A protective immune response may not be elicited if animals are incubating an infectious disease, are malnourished or parasitized, are stressed due to shipment or environmental conditions, are otherwise immunocompromised, or the vaccine is not administered in accordance with label directions.
Warning(s): Do not vaccinate within 21 days before slaughter.
For use in swine only.
For veterinary use only.
Discussion: Disease Description: Pseudorabies is an acute infectious disease caused by a herpesvirus. Swine are most commonly affected although pseudorabies has a broad host range that includes dogs, rodents, and several species of farm animals. Human beings apparently are not susceptible. The disease is generally more severe in younger animals. Signs may include vomiting, diarrhea, pyrexia, and CNS disturbances progressing to paralysis and death. Older swine may have acute or subclinical infection. Abortions, stillbirths, and mummified fetuses may occur in affected sows.
Trial Data: Safety and Efficacy: In field safety trials, PR-VAC PLUS® has been shown to be safe in weaning-age pigs (3 weeks of age or older) and in pregnant females greater than 40 days gestation. When given to sows prior to day 40 of gestation, a small reduction in farrowing rate was observed (97.76%) as compared to PR-Vac® (99.62%).
Efficacy of PR-VAC PLUS® was demonstrated in challenge-of-immunity studies. In one challenge-of-immunity test, a single dose of PR-VAC PLUS® protected 21 of 22 pigs from clinical signs of disease in a challenge that caused severe disease or death in 9 of 10 control pigs. Virus shed after challenge was detected in only 4 of 22 vaccinated pigs, compared to 10 of 10 control pigs. Mean body temperatures at the peak of the febrile response (5 days postchallenge) were 103.2°F for the vaccinated group, compared to 105.5°F for the control group.
Presentation: 10-dose, 25-dose and 50-dose vials.
Compendium Code No.: 36900510 75-4008-03

PRV-BEGONIA WITH DILUVAC FORTE®

Intervet **Vaccine**
Pseudorabies Vaccine, Modified Live Virus
U.S. Vet. Lic. No.: 286
Description: PRV-BEGONIA WITH DILUVAC FORTE® contains a modified live pseudorabies virus (PRV) which is gI⁻ antigen deleted (a marker vaccine) and tk⁻. The virus has been modified so that it does not cause disease in baby pigs, feeder pigs, or adult swine, including females in all stages of pregnancy.
Contains neomycin, polymyxin B and thimerosal as preservatives.
Indications: The vaccine is recommended for use in healthy swine 3 days of age or older for the prevention of pseudorabies (Aujeszky's disease), and when administered by injection (IM), as an aid in the prevention of the respiratory form of the disease.
Dosage and Administration: Dosage Guidelines: Follow directions carefully.
Rehydrate vaccine with 5-10 mL of the diluent provided, shake well, and transfer the rehydrated vaccine into the diluent bottle. Shake well and administer.
Inject a single 2.0 mL dose intramuscularly using aseptic technique or administer a single 2.0 mL dose intranasally (1.0 mL per nostril). This vaccine may be given to seronegative pigs 3 days of age or older. Pigs nursing immune dams should be revaccinated when maternal antibody levels will allow active immunization. Semi-annual revaccination of animals kept for breeding stock is recommended. Sows may be vaccinated at any stage of pregnancy.
Precaution(s): Store in the dark at not over 45°F (7°C). Do not freeze. Use immediately after reconstitution; do not save partial contents. Burn containers and all unused product.
Caution(s): Use only in healthy swine. If allergic reaction occurs, treat with epinephrine.
Note: Pigs vaccinated with this product can be serologically differentiated from pigs naturally infected with PRV by a USDA-licensed Pseudorabies Virus gpI Antibody Test Kit.
For veterinary use only.
Warning(s): Do not vaccinate within 21 days of slaughter.
Trial Data: Efficacy of PRV-BEGONIA WITH DILUVAC FORTE® has been demonstrated by the vaccination of 3 day old pigs on seronegative sows by intramuscular and intransal routes. Efficacy was confirmed at two ages: 1) in young pigs, preventing central nervous system signs and death, and 2) in growing pigs, against the respiratory form of the disease.
Discussion: Pseudorabies is characterized primarily by weakness, central nervous system signs and sudden death in baby pigs; fever, depression, inappetance and respiratory signs in growing pigs; and reproductive failures (abortions) in pregnant females. The disease affects swine of all ages and is most devastating in the young pig.
Presentation: 50 doses (100 mL) and 250 doses (500 mL).
U.S. Patent Nos. RE33772, 5,650,155, 5,667,784.
Compendium Code No.: 11062650 Rev. 719-03

PRV/MARKER GOLD®

SyntroVet **Vaccine**
Pseudorabies Vaccine, Modified Live Virus, Bioengineered gI and gX Deletions
U.S. Vet. Lic. No.: 165A
Description: PRV/MARKER GOLD® vaccine is a genetically designed, live virus vaccine. Specific genetic modifications have been made in the vaccine virus to optimize safety and efficacy, and to allow serologic differentiation based on either gI or gX deletions.
Contains gentamicin as a preservative.
Indications: This vaccine is for the immunization of healthy pigs 3 days of age or older against pseudorabies (Aujeszky's disease), including the respiratory form of the disease.
Dosage and Administration: For use in swine only.
Aseptically transfer 40-50 mL of sterile diluent from the large diluent vial to the smaller vial containing lyophilized vaccine. After rehydration is complete, aseptically transfer the rehydrated vaccine back to the large diluent vial. Administer 2 mL intramuscularly or intranasally.
Pigs nursing non-immune dams may be safely and effectively vaccinated at 3 days of age or older. Pigs nursing immune dams should be vaccinated when maternal antibody levels will allow

P

active immunization. Semi-annual revaccination is recommended for pigs retained for breeding. Sows may be safely vaccinated at any stage of pregnancy.
Precaution(s): Store at 35°-45°F (2°-7°C). Use entire contents without delay after rehydration. Burn container and all unused contents.
Caution(s): Anaphylactoid reactions may occur.
Note: Vaccination with PRV/MARKER GOLD® vaccine will yield seropositive results in non-differentiating SN, ELISA and latex agglutination tests. Distribution is limited to individuals designated by authorized officials, under such conditions as these authorities may require.
Antidote(s): Epinephrine.
Warning(s): Do not vaccinate within 21 days of slaughter.
Presentation: 25 dose (50 mL), 50 dose (100 mL), 100 dose (200 mL) multiple dose vials, and 12 x 100 dose (200 mL) Multi-Pack.
Compendium Code No.: 11170022

PRV/MARKER GOLD®-MAXIVAC® FLU

SyntroVet **Bacterin**
Pseudorabies-Swine Influenza Vaccine, Modified Live and Killed Virus
U.S. Vet. Lic. No.: 165A
Contents: PRV/MARKER GOLD®-MAXIVAC® FLU is an adjuvanted combination vaccine for the immunization of healthy swine against pseudorabies (Aujeszky's disease) and swine influenza. Specific genetic modifications have been engineered into the modified live pseudorabies virus to optimize safety and efficacy, and to allow serologic differentiation based on either gI or gX deletions. An inactivated, highly immunogenic type A, subtype H1N1 swine influenza virus isolate is also included in the vaccine.
Contains gentamicin and thimerosal as preservatives.
Indications: For the immunization of healthy pigs of weaning age or older against pseudorabies (including the respiratory form of the disease) and swine influenza.
Dosage and Administration: For use in swine only. Shake the adjuvanted MaxiVac® FLU vaccine fraction and aseptically rehydrate the lyophilized PRV/Marker Gold® vaccine fraction. Administer 2 mL intramuscularly. Pigs nursing nonimmune dams may be safely and effectively vaccinated at weaning. Pigs nursing immune dams should be vaccinated when maternal antibody levels will allow active immunization. For primary immunization, pigs should be revaccinated with a second dose of swine influenza vaccine (MaxiVac® FLU) in 3-4 weeks. Sows may be safely vaccinated at any stage of pregnancy. The swine influenza fraction has been shown to provide immunity for at least three months following vaccination.
Precaution(s): Store at 35°-45°F (2°-7°C). Use entire contents without delay after rehydration. Burn containers and all unused contents.
Caution(s): Anaphylactoid reactions may occur.
Note: Vaccination with PRV/MARKER GOLD®-MAXIVAC® FLU will yield seropositive results in nondifferentiating SN, ELISA and latex agglutination tests. Distribution is limited to individuals designated by authorized officials, under such conditions as these authorities may require.
Antidote(s): Epinephrine.
Warning(s): Do not vaccinate within 21 days of slaughter.
Presentation: 10 dose (20 mL) and 50 dose (100 mL) vials.
Compendium Code No.: 11170031 P19202-10

PSD COMPLEX II

PRN Pharmacal **Small Animal Dietary Supplement**
Active Ingredient(s): Each tablet contains:

Complex calcium phosphates	1,000 mg
supplying calcium	166 mg
supplying phosphorus	210 mg
Vitamin A Acetate	2,000 I.U.
Vitamin D_3	500 I.U.

Indications: A calcium and phosphorus nutritional supplement for puppies of all breeds.
Dosage and Administration:

15 to 30 lbs	2 tablets daily
30 to 60 lbs	3 tablets daily
60 to 100 lbs	4 tablets daily

or as directed by a veterinarian.
Presentation: 60 tablets.
Compendium Code No.: 10900170

PSITTIMUNE® APV

Biomune **Vaccine**
Avian Polyomavirus Vaccine, Killed Virus
U.S. Vet. Lic. No.: 368
Contents: Avian Polyomavirus Vaccine is an inactivated viral vaccine prepared from an antigenic isolate of avian polyomavirus. The vaccine contains a virus that is carefully inactivated (killed) to maintain its antigenicity and an adjuvant for enhanced response to vaccination.
This vaccine contains gentamicin and amphotericin B as preservatives.
Indications: The vaccine is intended for use as an aid in the prevention of avian polyomavirus infection in psittacine birds. Only healthy birds should be vaccinated.
Dosage and Administration: Birds weighing 200 grams or greater should receive a 0.5 mL dose and birds weighing less than 200 grams should receive a 0.25 mL dose. Young birds should not be initially vaccinated before 5 weeks of age. To complete primary immunization a second dose must be given at two to three weeks following the initial vaccination. Annual revaccination is recommended. Susceptible breeders should be vaccinated prior to the laying season. Product performance has been evaluated in selected but not all psittacine species.
The vaccine should be warmed to room temperature (72°-75°F) before use. It is essential to shake the vaccine before and during use since the vaccine quickly settles. Shake the bottle of vaccine well before removing each dose with a syringe and needle.
Using aseptic technique, the vaccine should be subcutaneously administered with a 26 gauge needle at caudal end of the breast muscle avoiding the keel. The direction may be toward or away from the head depending on personal preference. Care should be taken not to inject the vaccine into muscle tissue or internal organs or intradermally. Administer the second vaccination on the contralateral side two to three weeks later.
Precaution(s): Store in the dark at 35° to 45°F (2° - 7°C). Do not freeze.
Use entire contents when first opened.
Caution(s): Because the polyomavirus in this vaccine is killed, there is no risk of causing polyomavirus infection with use of the vaccine. However, if a bird has recently been infected with polyomavirus but is not yet exhibiting clinical signs, vaccination will not prevent the progression of disease.
For veterinary use only.
Side Effects: A transient loss of appetite (1-3 days) may be seen following the use of this product. This vaccine may cause post-vaccination tissue reactions including discoloration or thickening of skin or granuloma formation at the site of injection. Certain individual birds may be more sensitive to these types of reactions. Changes should resolve without treatment within 6-8 weeks later. Reactions may also be aggravated by improper vaccination technique. Further complications may result from the stress and handling of birds associated with the vaccination procedure.
Discussion: Disease Description: Polyomavirus infection is one of the leading causes of death in young psittacine birds. Infections in young birds are usually rapidly fatal. Adult birds are also susceptible to polyomavirus infection, and although they seldom suffer clinical illness, they are the source of amplification of polyomavirus within an aviary leading to exposure of neonates in the nursery.
In the budgerigar, the disease is called budgerigar fledgling disease. Clinical signs in acute infections may include abdominal distention, hemorrhage under the skin, reduced formation of down and contour feathers, and neurological signs characterized by ataxia and tremors of the head and neck. Birds that survive infection may exhibit feather abnormalities characterized by dystrophic primary and tail feathers, lack of downfeathers, and lack of filoplumes on the head and neck.
In nonbudgerigar psittacine birds peracute death with no premonitory signs is the most common clinical finding. Acute infection is characterized by death following a period of clinical changes that include depression, anorexia, delayed crop emptying, regurgitation, diarrhea, dehydration, bleeding under the skin, and polyuria. Birds that survive several days after the onset of clinical signs can develop yellowish urates indicative of liver damage. Chronic disease progression typified by weight loss, intermittent anorexia, polyuria, poor feather development, and recurrent bacterial and fungal infections have also been described. In latently infected breeder birds, the virus has been shown to cause decreased egg hatchability, embryonic death, and increased mortality.
Presentation: 10 dose vials.
Patent No. 5,747,045
Compendium Code No.: 11290001 116

PSITTIMUNE® PDV

Biomune **Vaccine**
Pacheco's Disease Vaccine, Inactivated Virus, Oil Emulsion
U.S. Vet. Lic. No.: 368
Contents: PSITTIMUNE® PDV is an inactivated virus vaccine adjuvinated in an oil emulsion for long acting immunity. The vaccine is used for the protection of selected psittacine birds against the infectious and fatal Pacheco's disease.
The vaccine has been carefully produced and has undergone purity, sterility, safety, efficacy and potency tests to meet Biomune's requirements and USDA regulations.
Indications: PSITTIMUNE® PDV is indicated for the vaccination of selected psittacine species to aid in the prevention of disease caused by Pacheco's virus infection.
Dosage and Administration: Allow the vaccine to reach ambient temperature, 65°-75°F, and shake well before and periodically during use. Vaccination is accomplished by using a syringe and a 21 to 23 gauge needle to administer 0.25 cc of the vaccine subcutaneously in smaller psittacines under 100 grams and either subcutaneously or intramuscularly in larger psittacines. The intramuscular injection site should be in the pectoral muscle mass being careful not to inject into a blood vessel or strike the breastbone. Aseptic technique should be followed using alcohol to clean the injection site and a new sterile syringe and needle between each bird.
See the package insert for complete information.
Precaution(s): Store in a refrigerator at 35°-45°F. Use the entire contents when first opened.
Caution(s): Vaccinate only healthy birds.
Oil emulsion vaccines may cause post-vaccination tissue reactions including swelling or granuloma formation at the site of injection. Certain cockatoo species may be more sensitive to these types of reactions. Such reactions may also be aggravated by improper vaccination technique. Further complications may result from the stress of handling birds associated with the vaccination procedure.
For veterinary use only.
Warning(s): Vaccinations should be completed at least four (4) weeks prior to the onset of egg production.
Discussion: The product is derived from an immunogenic psittacine herpesvirus and contains a virus isolated from a recent Pacheco's disease outbreak. Laboratory studies demonstrate that Biomune's vaccine virus has a broader antigenic spectrum than the classic Simpson-Hanley virus isolated in 1975. The vaccine virus is completely inactivated so there is no risk of introducing the disease into a bird collection by its use.
Presentation: 1 x 10 dose vials.
Compendium Code No.: 11290262

PT BLEN®

Merial Select **Vaccine**
Avian Encephalomyelitis-Pigeon Pox Vaccine, Live Virus
U.S. Vet. Lic. No.: 279
Contents: This vaccine contains live avian encephalomyelitis and fowl pox viruses.
Contains Gentamicin as a bacteriostatic agent.
Notice: Merial Select's vaccines have met the requirements of the USDA in regard to safety, purity, and potency. This vaccine has been tested by the Master Seed immunogenicity test for efficacy.
Indications: This vaccine is for the vaccination of commercial layer or breeder replacements pullets between ten weeks of age and four weeks before production by wing web stab as an aid in the prevention of avian encephalomyelitis and fowl pox. It is essential that the chickens be maintained under good environmental conditions and that exposure to disease viruses be reduced as much as possible.
Dosage and Administration: Wing Web Method:
1. Pull up on the plastic tear-flip-up top to remove the aluminum seal from the bottle containing the vaccine. Carefully pry up one edge of the rubber stopper to permit air to replace the vacuum in the bottle, then remove the stopper.
2. Remove the aluminum seal from the bottle containing the diluent, and transfer the entire contents to the bottle containing the vaccine. Replace the stopper and shake the contents vigorously until the vaccine is evenly suspended.
3. To apply the vaccine, dip the two-pronged applicator supplied in the package into the vaccine and stab into the webbed portion of the wing from the underside. Avoid stabbing through feathers which may wipe off the vaccine.
4. The applicator is designed to carry the proper amount of vaccine in the grooves of the needles. The needles should be touched briefly to the inner lip of the bottle before

withdrawing to avoid wasting vaccine which may drop from the needles. Dip the applicator before each application.

Check for Takes: At about seven to ten days after vaccination, the birds may be examined for takes. A good take reaction, indicating that a satisfactory vaccination was done, shows swelling of the skin with scab formation at the point of vaccination. The scabs will fall off about two to three weeks following vaccination. Good immunity to fowl pox is established two to three weeks after vaccination. Immunity to avian encephalomyelitis is established three to four weeks after the vaccination.

If good takes are not seen, it may mean that the birds were immune to fowl pox, that the vaccination job was poor, or that the vaccine used had lost its potency through extended storage or mishandling.

Precaution(s): Store vaccine at 35-45°F (2-7°C). Do not freeze. Use entire contents within four hours of opening. Burn this container and all unused contents.

This vaccine is non-returnable.

Caution(s): Do not vaccinate diseased chickens.

Vaccinate all chickens on the premises at one time.

Administer a minimum of one dose per chicken.

Avoid stress conditions during and following vaccination.

Do not place chickens in contaminated facilities.

Exposure to disease must be minimized as much as possible. For veterinary use only.

The capability of this vaccine to produce satisfactory results depends upon many factors, including — but not limited to — conditions of storage and handling by the user, administration of the vaccine, health and responsiveness of individual chickens, and degree of field exposure. Therefore, directions for use should be followed carefully. The use of this vaccine is subject to applicable state and federal laws and regulations.

Warning(s): Do not vaccinate within 21 days of slaughter.

Presentation: PT BLEN® is supplied with a diluent for rehydration to 10 mL for the 25 x 1,000 dose size.

Compendium Code No.: 11050402 PL-1M 0801

PULLORUM ANTIGEN (POLYVALENT)

L.A.H.I. (New Jersey) **Salmonella Test**

U.S. Vet. Lic. No.: 196

Description: PULLORUM ANTIGEN, stained antigen polyvalent type is designed for use in the rapid whole blood test for the detection of pullorum disease and fowl typhoid. When it is added to blood samples of the birds, it reacts to produce a clumping with the blood of an infected bird.

Antigens: This product consists of 50 per cent standard U.S. strains and 50 per cent Canadian variant strains of *Salmonella pullorum.*

The antigen is harmless because the organisms in it are killed and cannot spread the disease.

This antigen was carefully produced and passed all tests in accordance with the U.S. Government requirements.

Indications: Pullorum disease is caused by bacteria known to scientists as *Salmonella pullorum.* This bacterial infection endures in the ovaries of the laying female. The disease is transmitted from mother to chick through the incubated egg. If the egg hatches, the chick is already infected when it leaves the shell. Through the droppings other chicks become quickly infected, until the disease spreads through the brood as a devastating plague.

The one and only effective control measure for *Pullorum* disease is the elimination of infected breeders. This involves blood testing, so that *Pullorum* "carriers" may be detected and removed from the breeding flocks.

Test Procedure:

1. Shake the antigen well.
2. Place a drop of the stained antigen on a test plate with the dropper syringe contained in the bottle.
3. Draw blood from the bird by lancing the vein under the wing.
4. Using a wire loop, also supplied with every package, lift a loopful of blood from the wing of the bird, and add it to the stained antigen already on the test plate.
5. Mix with the Stained Antigen by stirring with the wire loop, followed by rotating the plate.
6. A clumping of the mixture within two minutes will appear in the case of a positive reactor. If there is not clumping, the reaction is negative, and the bird is passed as *Pullorum*-free.
7. Immediately remove a reactor from the flock.
8. Rinse and dry the loop between tests to prevent contamination of one sample with another.

P

Storage: Keep product in the dark, between 2-7°C (35-45°F). Avoid freezing.

Caution(s): It is imperative that the buyer or user of this product comply with the indications for use stated here. The product must be prepared and used as directed to obtain best results.

Consult your poultry pathologist regarding an adequate testing program for your flocks.

When testing birds, it is best to do the test in a shaded place; this is, out of the direct sunlight and place where there is a minimum of dust. Rinse and dry the loop between tests in order to prevent contamination of one sample with another.

Warning(s): Care should be taken to avoid contaminating hands, eyes and clothing with the material. For veterinary use only.

Presentation: 1,000 tests - 50 mL.

Compendium Code No.: 10080372

PULLORUM STAINED ANTIGEN

Fort Dodge **Salmonella Test**

Pullorum Stained Antigen, K Polyvalent

U.S. Vet. Lic. No.: 112

Indications: For pullorum-typhoid testing: PULLORUM STAINED ANTIGEN, K polyvalent, is used to detect infection caused by both standard and variant strains of *Salmonella pullorum, Salmonella gallinarum,* and certain other specific members of the Salmonella group in chickens.

Test Procedure:

Equipment Necessary for Testing: Antigen, testing plate, thermometer, bleeding needle, blood loop (standardized), small glass of water for rinsing loop, disinfectant, a pail of water, soft cloths or chamois skin, and a device to hold birds individually (or in groups of 10 or less) while waiting for the reaction to develop, are necessary equipment for testing.

Handling the Birds: Handle the birds carefully. Use chutes or catching coops to help catch the birds; do not chase or excite them. Birds should be held on tables or in coops until test is completed.

Testing:

1. Test in groups of 6 or more birds — conveniently as many as there are squares across the testing plate. Test surface should be between 70°F and 80°F (21°C and 26°C). Mix antigen and place a drop (0.05 cc) on a testing square.
2. Pluck feathers from elbow region on underside of wing. Puncture blue vein with bleeding needle, and lift a fresh non-clotting drop with blood loop (0.02 cc).
3. Transfer blood to testing square, stirring into antigen with loop, making a smear 1 inch in diameter. Rotate test plate in a circular motion to thoroughly mix the antigen and blood and to facilitate agglutination. Read test (see explanation below). Release bird if no reaction occurs. Retest partial or suspicious agglutinations. Isolate birds showing positive reactions.
4. Between birds: Rinse loop in clean water and dry by touching it to a piece of clean blotting paper.

Follow Up: In flocks showing positive reactions or suspicious agglutinations, it is desirable to examine representative birds bacteriologically to determine the presence or absence of *Salmonella pullorum.*

Pointers on Testing:

1. Perform the test out of direct sunlight in a dust-free area.
2. Maintain 70° to 80°F (21° to 26°C) temperature on testing surface. A lower temperature may affect accuracy of results.
3. Correct proportions are important: a loopful (0.02 cc) of blood to 1 drop (0.05 cc) of antigen.
4. On completion of testing, remove reacting birds from premises and burn litter. Then disinfect house and equipment with a suitable disinfectant.

Blood Testing Problems: Faulty technique, improper interpretation, unsuitable equipment, or defective antigen may cause erroneous results in the usually reliable agglutination test.

Occasionally, large numbers of positive reactors of a previously tested flock may be the result of one or more of the following:

1. Contaminated premises may infect other birds.
2. Vaccination with vaccine containing *Salmonella gallinarum,* or certain other strains of Salmonella may agglutinate the antigen. Do not test flocks for pullorum or typhoid within a 60-day period after vaccinating for fowl typhoid.
3. All positive reactors may not have been removed in previous tests.

Things to Avoid: Deteriorated antigen may give false readings. Before testing, check a drop of antigen, without blood, on the plate for spontaneous agglutination. Excessive evaporation, high temperatures, or incorrectly interpreting late powder or marginal flocculation as positive reactions may also lead to false readings. Delay in reading tests causes errors; Tests should not be read after 2 minutes. Testers should use care, not speed; for the number of birds tested is less important than maximum accuracy.

Cleansing the Testing Surface: Clean plate with clear water. Hot water may coagulate blood, making it difficult to remove. Soaps, disinfectants, or cleaning compounds may leave a residue which may affect subsequent tests. Grease on plate may prevent blood-antigen mixture from spreading properly; It may be removed with soap, after which plate must be thoroughly rinsed. After cleansing, polish plate with clean cloth, leaving no blood or lint.

Interpretation of Results: Reading the Tests: Positive reactions are indicated by a clumping of the antigen in well-developed, blue-colored clusters surrounded by clear spaces easily seen against a white background. The greater the agglutination ability of the blood, the more rapid the clumping and the larger the clumps. A lesser reaction shows small, but clearly visible clumps surrounded by spaces only partially clear. A fine, barely visible granulation sometimes occurs and there may be a fine marginal flocculation just before the smear dries. These should be regarded as negative. Reactions which occur after 2 minutes should not be considered positive.

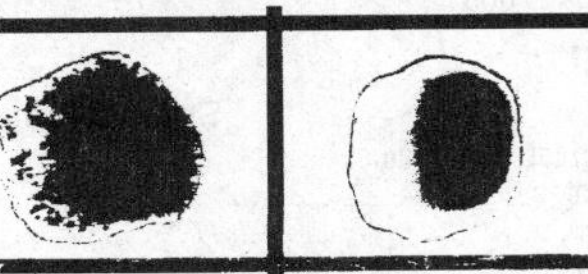

Biological reactions may vary between clear-cut positive and negative. A reactor should show clumping as at left. At right, a typical negative test.

When interpreting reactions in the test, several factors, such as flock history, should be considered. The judgment of a professional flock manager should always be exercised before birds are condemned.

Storage: Store in the dark at not over 45°F (7°C). Do not freeze. Shake gently before use.

This product is nonreturnable.

Presentation: 500 tests (25 mL).

Compendium Code No.: 10031691 10010A

PULMO-GUARD™ PH-M

Boehringer Ingelheim **Bacterin-Toxoid**

Pasteurella Haemolytica-Multocida Bacterin-Toxoid

U.S. Vet. Lic. No.: 315

Contents: This product contains a toxoid as well as cell associated antigens from multiple isolates of *Pasteurella haemolytica* Type A-1.

Indications: For use in cattle, 30 days of age or older, as an aid in the prevention of respiratory disease due to *P. haemolytica* and *P. multocida.*

Dosage and Administration: Shake well. Inject 2 mL IM or Sub Q in the neck. Repeat in 14-28 days. Annual revaccination is recommended.

Precaution(s): Store below 45°F (7°C). Do not freeze. Use entire contents when first opened.

Caution(s): Epinephrine should be on hand in case of anaphylaxis. Delayed and intermediate hypersensitivity reactions should be treated symptomatically. Hypersensitivity reactions, including delayed hypersensitivity, or death may occur with a biological product and can cause reduced milk production in lactating dairy cattle. Following subcutaneous use, persistent swelling may occur at the injection site.

Warning(s): Do not vaccinate within 60 days of slaughter.

Presentation: 10 doses (20 mL) and 50 doses (100 mL).

Manufactured by: American Animal Health, Inc., Grand Prairie, TX 75052-7610.

Compendium Code No.: 10280901 BI 4023-1R-1 5/02

PULMO-GUARD™ PHM-1

Boehringer Ingelheim **Bacterin-Toxoid**

Pasteurella Haemolytica-Multocida Bacterin-Toxoid

U.S. Vet. Lic. No.: 315

Composition: This product contains toxoids (leukotoxoids) and cell-associated antigens from multiple isolates of *P. haemolytica* Type A-1 fractions, and cell-associated and soluble antigens from *P. multocida.*

Indications: Recommended for the vaccination of healthy, susceptible cattle as an aid in the prevention of respiratory disease caused by *Pasteurella haemolytica* and *Pasteurella multocida.*

Dosage and Administration: Using aseptic technique, inject 2 mL subcutaneously in front of the shoulder and midway of the neck, away from the suprascapular lymph node. Although only a single dose is necessary to confer active immunity, a booster dose is recommended 21 days prior to subsequent stress.

Precaution(s): Store between 35-45°F (2-7°C). Do not freeze. Shake well before using. Use entire contents when first opened.

Caution(s): Anaphylactoid reactions can occur. Hypersensitivity reactions, including delayed hypersensitivity or death, may occur with a biological product and can cause reduced milk production in lactating dairy cattle. Persistent swelling may occur at the injection site.

Antidote(s): Epinephrine.

Warning(s): Do not vaccinate within 60 days before slaughter.

Presentation: 10 doses (20 mL) and 50 doses (100 mL).

Manufactured by: American Animal Health, Inc.

Compendium Code No.: 10280920 BI 4054-1 1/00

PULMOTIL® 90

Elanco **Feed Medication**

Tilmicosin-Type A Medicated Article

NADA No.: 141-064

Active Ingredient(s):

Tilmicosin (as tilmicosin phosphate) . . . . 90.7 g/lb (200 g/kg)

Inert ingredients: ground corn cobs.

Indications: PULMOTIL® is indicated for the control of swine respiratory disease associated with *Actinobacillus pleuropneumoniae* and *Pasteurella multocida*.

Pharmacology: Oral dosing of tilmicosin phosphate at 181 to 363 g/ton of feed results in serum tilmicosin levels which do not correlate with efficacy. Lung concentrations of tilmicosin are significantly higher than serum. Lung levels are achieved within 2 days after beginning feeding and plateau by 4 days. Swine alveolar macrophages have been shown *in vitro* to concentrate large amounts of tilmicosin; these cells may serve as an important reservoir in lung tissue.

Description: PULMOTIL® is a formulation of the antibiotic tilmicosin. Tilmicosin is produced semi-synthetically and is in the macrolide class of antibiotics. Each kilogram of Type A Medicated Article contains 200 grams (0.44 lbs) of tilmicosin adsorbed onto ground corn cobs.

Activity: Tilmicosin has an *in vitro** antibacterial spectrum that is predominantly Gram-positive with activity against certain Gram-negative microorganisms. Activity against several mycoplasma species has also been detected.

Microorganism	MIC (μg/mL)
Actinobacillus pleuropneumoniae	16
Pasteurella multocida	8
Mycoplasma hyopneumoniae	0.5
Escherichia coli	>64.0
Salmonella choleraesuis	>64.0
Streptococcus suis	>64.0

*The clinical significance of these *in vitro* data in swine has not been demonstrated.

Directions: Feeding Directions: PULMOTIL® is to be fed continuously at 181 grams to 363 grams tilmicosin per ton (200 ppm to 400 ppm) of Type C medicated feed as the sole ration for a 21-day period, beginning approximately 7 days before an anticipated disease outbreak.

Important: Must be thoroughly mixed in feeds before use.

Do not feed undiluted.

Mixing: Thoroughly mix PULMOTIL® Type A medicated article with feed to provide a Type B medicated feed containing up to 36,300 grams tilmicosin per ton or to provides complete Type C medicated feed containing 181 to 363 g tilmicosin per ton. Do not use in concentrates or feeds containing bentonite. Bentonite in feeds may affect the efficacy of tilmicosin.

Starting concentration of PULMOTIL® Type A Medicated Article	Amount of Type A Medicated Article to add per ton	Resulting concentration in Type B Medicated Feed	
grams per pound	pounds	grams per ton	grams per pound
90.7	400	36,300	18.1
	300	27,200	13.6
	200	18,100	9.05

Starting concentration of PULMOTIL® Type A Medicated Article	Amount of Type A Medicated Article to add per ton	Resulting concentration in Type C Medicated Feed
grams per pound	pounds	grams per ton
90.7	4	363
	3	272
	2	181

Precaution(s): Avoid moisture and excessive heat (40° C).

Not to be used after the date printed on the bag.

Avoid inhalation, oral exposure, and direct contact with skin or eyes. Operators mixing and handing PULMOTIL® 90 should use protective clothing, impervious gloves, goggles, and a NIOSH-approved dust mask. Wash thoroughly with soap and water after handling. If accidental eye contact occurs, immediately rinse thoroughly with water. If irritation persists, seek medical attention. Not for human consumption. Keep out of reach of children. The Material Safety Data Sheet contains more detailed occupational safety information. To report adverse effects in users, to obtain more information, or to obtain a material safety data sheet, call 1-800-428-4441.

Caution(s): Federal law limits this drug to use under the professional supervision of a licensed veterinarian. Animal feed bearing or containing this veterinary feed directive drug shall be fed to animals only by or upon a lawful veterinary feed directive issued by a licensed veterinarian in the course of the veterinarians professional practice.

Do not allow horses or other equine access to feeds containing tilmicosin. The safety of tilmicosin has not been established in pregnant swine or swine intended for breeding purposes.

For use in swine feeds only.

Warning(s): Feeds containing PULMOTIL® must be withdrawn 7 days prior to slaughter.

Toxicology: The cardiovascular system is the target of toxicity in laboratory and domestic animals given tilmicosin by oral or parenteral routes. Primary cardiac effects are increased heart rate (tachycardia) and decreased contractility (negative inotropy). Given orally, the median lethal dose is 800 mg/kg in fasted rats and 2250 mg/kg in non-fasted rats. No compound-related lesions were found at necropsy. Results of genetic toxicology studies were all negative. Results of teratology and reproduction studies in rats were all negative. The no effect level in dogs after daily oral doses for up to one year is 4 mg/kg of body weight.

Tilmicosin was included in the diet of 18 adult horses for a period of 14 days at dose levels of 400, 1200, and 2000 ppm. Some horses at both the low and high dose levels demonstrated gastrointestinal disturbance with more severe colic evident at the higher levels. One horse died after consuming the 2000 ppm diet.

Adverse Reactions: No adverse toxicological effects were observed in swine given rations containing 2000 ppm tilmicosin for 42 days and 4000 ppm for 21 days.

Presentation: 10 kg (22 lb) bag.

PULMOTIL® is a trademark of Eli Lilly and Company.

Compendium Code No.: 10310092 BG6004DEAMB (I-JAN-01)

PUPPY DROPS™

Tomlyn **Small Animal Dietary Supplement**

Guaranteed Analysis: Per 1 mL:

Vitamin A (min) . . . . 8145 I.U.
Vitamin D_3 (min) . . . . 8121 I.U.
Vitamin E (min) . . . . 1.71 I.U.
Thiamine (Vit B_1) (min) . . . . 1.8 mg
Riboflavin (Vit B_2) (min) . . . . 0.54 mg
Pyridoxine (Vit B_6) (min) . . . . 0.9 mg
Cyanocobalamin (Vit B_{12}) (min) . . . . 0.42 mcg
Menadione (Vit K) (min) . . . . 5.0 mcg
Niacinamide (min) . . . . 8.1 mg
D-Panthenol (min) . . . . 3.4 mg
Iron (min) (0.27%) . . . . 2.7 mg
Copper (min) (0.004%) . . . . 44.0 mcg

Ingredients: Water, sugar, sorbitol, polysorbate 80, liver extract, gelatin by-products, ferric ammonium citrate (source of iron), niacinamide, vitamin A palmitate, d-panthenol, thiamine HCl (vit. B_1), citric acid (preservative), alpha tocopheryl acetate (vit. E), saccharin sodium, pyridoxine HCl (vit. B_6); sodium benzoate and methylparaben (preservatives), riboflavin 5 phosphate sodium (source of vit. B_2), vitamin D_3 supplement, copper sulfate, BHA (preservative), menadione sodium bisulfite complex, (source of vit. K), cyanocobalamin (Vit. B_{12}).

Indications: A vitamin supplement with liver and iron for use in puppies.

Dosage and Administration: To Supplement Diet: Give puppies ½ dropperful per 10 lbs of body weight twice daily. Give adult dogs one dropperful 2-3 times daily. This mixture is water dispersible and may be given by dropping directly on the tongue or mixed with food or milk.

(1 dropperful = 1 mL)

Precaution(s): Store at room temperature.

Caution(s): For veterinary use only.

Keep out of reach of children.

Presentation: 12 x 1 fl oz (29.6 mL).

Compendium Code No.: 11220221 603-1 4

PUPPY FORMULA

Vet Solutions **Milk Replacer**

Guaranteed Analysis:

Crude Protein (min) 22%
Crude Protein from milk sources (min) 22%
Crude Fat (min) 23%
Crude Fiber (max) 0.25%
Moisture 7%
Ash 6.5%
Sodium 0.65%
Calcium 1.15%
Phosphorus 0.85%
Iron . . . . 90 mg/kg
Manganese . . . . 48 mg/kg
Zinc . . . . 110 mg/kg
Selenium . . . . 0.3 mg/kg
Vitamin A . . . . 15,000 IU/kg
Vitamin D_3 . . . . 2,000 IU/kg
Vitamin E . . . . 100 IU/kg
Thiamine . . . . 12 mg/kg
Riboflavin . . . . 20 mg/kg
Niacin . . . . 50 mg/kg
Vitamin B_{12} . . . . 50 μg/kg
Biotin . . . . 250 μg/kg
Ascorbic Acid . . . . 100 mg/kg

Additionally Contains:

Colostrum . . . . 25 mg/kg
Eicosapentaenoic acid (EPA) . . . . 68 mg/kg
Decosahexaenoic acid (DHA) . . . . 268 mg/kg

Ingredients: Dried whey/whey product, homogenized and spray-dried animal/vegetable fat containing BHA and BHT, dried skimmed milk, corn syrup solids, dextroglucose, lecithin, L-lysine, DL-methionine, L-threonine, calcium formate, citric acid, phosphoric acid, dicalcium phosphate, Vitamin A, Vitamin D_3, Vitamin E, menadione sodium bisulphite, thiamin hydrochloride, riboflavin, niacinamide, pyridoxine hydrochloride, sodium ascorbate, choline chloride, folic acid, D-biotin, Vitamin B_{12}, iron sulphate, zinc sulphate, manganous sulphate, magnesium oxide, sodium chloride, copper sulphate, ethylene diamine dihydroiodide, cobalt sulphate, sodium selenite, silica dioxide, fish oil, flavor and aroma agents, dry colostrum.

Indications: Mother's milk replacer for puppies and food supplement for adult dogs containing Colostrum and Docosahexaenoic acid (DHA).

Vet Solutions PUPPY FORMULA is a nutritionally complete milk replacer to be fed as a nutritional supplement when the supply of bitch's milk is inadequate or as the sole ration for orphan puppies. When indicated, PUPPY FORMULA may be used to fortify the ration of bitches to help meet the increased nutritional requirements in late gestation and early lactation. Whenever possible puppies should receive colostrum (bitch's first milk) for the first 2 days, since this supplies antibodies essential to disease resistance in early life.

Dosage and Administration: Mixing Instructions: Prepare enough PUPPY FORMULA, with the enclosed measuring scoop, for use in a 24-hour period. Add 1 scoop (1 Tbsp.) per 2 scoops (1 ounce) of warm water. Stir or mix until smooth.

Feeding Instructions: Reconstituted PUPPY FORMULA solution should be fed at body temperature. Use of a nurser bottle is recommended. Feed puppies at least 2 tablespoons (30 mL) per 4 ounces (113 g) of body weight daily. Divide the daily feeding amount into equal portions for each feeding. For the first 4 days of feeding PUPPY FORMULA, the daily amount should be divided into 6 to 8 feedings. The number of feedings can then be gradually reduced to 4 per day (dividing the daily volumes into 4 equal parts). Puppies should be allowed to consume as much formula as they want during each feeding. Stool consistency provides a measure of the appropriate feeding level. If diarrhea develops, reduce the concentration of the solution (i.e. maintain water level but reduce the level of PUPPY FORMULA by 10-20% until stool consistency returns to normal). Should diarrhea persist, consult a veterinarian for advice.

Cleanliness of feeding equipment (nursing bottle/bowl) is extremely important. Always wash with hot, soapy water, rinse and dry well after each use.

Weaning Puppies: When puppies are old enough to lap, begin offering reconstituted formula in a shallow bowl. Wean puppies between 4-6 weeks of age. Mix equal parts of PUPPY FORMULA and weaning cereal or puppy food and add enough water to make a soupy gruel. Gradually increase the proportion of puppy food until puppy is on solid food. Ensure a source of clean water is always available.

Pregnant and lactating bitches: Feed 2 teaspoons (4 g) per 5 lbs. (2.2 kg) body weight until 2 weeks after whelping.

Growing Puppies, Show Dogs and Convalescing Dogs: Supplement regular ration with 1 teaspoons (2 g) of PUPPY FORMULA per 5 lbs. (2.2 kg) body weight daily.

Precaution(s): Storage: Moisture and high temperature will degrade PUPPY FORMULA. Store sealed container at controlled room temperature. May be stored indefinitely in the freezer. Do not mix more than will be consumed within 24 hours. Reconstituted PUPPY FORMULA should be refrigerated.

Presentation: 8 oz and 400 g (14.1 oz).

Compendium Code No.: 10610200 010701

PURALUBE® VET OPHTHALMIC OINTMENT

Pharmaderm **Ophthalmic Preparation**

Petrolatum Ophthalmic Ointment, Sterile Ocular Lubricant

Active Ingredient(s): Contains: White petrolatum and light mineral oil.

Indications: For the use as a protectant against further irritation, or to relieve dryness of the eye.

Directions: Pull down the lower lid of the affected eye and apply a small amount (one-fourth inch) of ointment to the inside of the eyelid.

Precaution(s): Keep tightly closed.

Store at room temperature.

Caution(s): If condition persists or increases discontinue use and consult veterinarian. Keep container tightly closed. To avoid contamination do not touch tip of container to any surface. Replace cap after using. Please note cap/closure has tamper indicative feature. Do not use if previously opened.

Warning(s): Keep out of reach of children.

Presentation: 3.5 g (⅛ oz) sterile tamper proof tubes.

Compendium Code No.: 10880020

PURALUBE® VET TEARS

Pharmaderm **Ophthalmic Solution**

Lubricant Eye Drops

Active Ingredient(s): Polyvinyl alcohol 1.4 %; Inactive: Edetate disodium, potassium chloride and sodium chloride, preserved with benzalkonium chloride in purified water, USP.

Indications: For use as a lubricant to prevent further irritation or to relieve dryness of the eye.

Directions: Instill 1 or 2 drops in the affected eye(s) as needed.

Precaution(s): Keep container tightly closed.

Caution(s): In case of accidental ingestion, seek professional assistance or contact a Poison Control Center immediately.

Tamper Evident — Do not use if cap band imprinted "Sterile Solution" is missing or damaged.

Warning(s): To avoid contamination, do not touch tip of container to any surface. Replace cap after using. If continued redness or irritation of the eye is evident or if the condition worsens or persists for more than 72 hours, discontinue use and consult a veterinarian. If solution changes color or becomes cloudy, do not use.

Keep this and all drugs out of the reach of children.

Presentation: 15 mL (½ oz) dropper bottle.

Compendium Code No.: 10880030

PUREVAX™ FELINE 3

Merial **Vaccine**

Feline Rhinotracheitis-Calici-Panleukopenia Vaccine, Modified Live Virus

U.S. Vet. Lic. No.: 298

Description: PUREVAX™ Feline 3 contains a lyophilized suspension of modified live feline rhinotracheitis, calici, and panleukopenia viruses, each propagated in a stable cell line, plus sterile water diluent. Safety and immunogenicity of this product have been demonstrated by vaccination and challenge tests in susceptible cats.

Contains gentamicin as a preservative.

Indications: PUREVAX™ Feline 3 is recommended for the vaccination of healthy cats 6 weeks of age or older for prevention of disease due to feline rhinotracheitis, calici, and panleukopenia viruses.

Dosage and Administration: Reconstitute the lyophilized vaccine with accompanying liquid diluent and aseptically inject 1 mL (1 dose) subcutaneously or intramuscularly into healthy cats. For primary vaccination, revaccinate with a second 1 mL dose 3 to 4 weeks later. Cats younger than 12 weeks of age should be revaccinated with a single 1 mL dose every 3 to 4 weeks, the last dose given at or over 12 weeks of age. Revaccinate annually with a single 1 mL dose.

Precaution(s): Store at 2-7°C (35-45°F). Use immediately after reconstitution. Do not use chemicals to sterilize syringes and needles. Burn the container and all unused contents.

Caution(s): Do not vaccinate pregnant cats. In rare instances, administration of vaccines may cause lethargy, fever, and inflammatory or hypersensitivity types of reactions. Treatment may include antihistamines, anti-inflammatories, and/or epinephrine.

For veterinary use only.

Presentation: Contains 25 doses: 25 x 1 dose, lyophilized and 25 x 1 mL, sterile water.

Sold to veterinarians only.

PUREVAX is a trademark of Merial.

Compendium Code No.: 11110501 RM503R4

PUREVAX™ FELINE 3 + LEUCAT®

Merial **Vaccine**

Feline Leukemia-Rhinotracheitis-Calici-Panleukopenia Vaccine, Modified Live and Killed Virus

U.S. Vet. Lic. No.: 298

Description: PUREVAX™ FELINE 3 + LEUCAT® contains a lyophilized suspension of modified live feline rhinotracheitis, calici, and panleukopenia viruses propagated in stable cell lines, plus a liquid suspension of inactivated feline leukemia virus propagated in a continuously infected lymphoid cell line which expresses subgroups A, B, and C. PUREVAX™ FELINE 3 + LEUCAT® stimulates serum neutralizing antibodies against the whole virus as well as viral components including gp70. Safety and immunogenicity of this product have been demonstrated by vaccination and challenge tests in susceptible cats.

Contains gentamicin and amphotericin B as preservatives.

Indications: PUREVAX™ FELINE 3 + LEUCAT® is recommended for the vaccination of healthy cats 8 weeks of age or older for prevention of disease due to feline rhinotracheitis, calici, and panleukopenia viruses and as an aid in the prevention of disease due to feline leukemia virus.

Dosage and Administration: Reconstitute the lyophilized vaccine with accompanying liquid diluent and aseptically inject 1 mL (1 dose) subcutaneously into healthy cats. For primary vaccination, revaccinate with a second 1 mL dose 3 to 4 weeks later. Cats younger than 12 weeks of age should be revaccinated with a single 1 mL dose every 3 to 4 weeks, the last dose given at or over 12 weeks of age. Revaccinate annually with a single 1 mL dose. Diagnostic testing for FeLV prior to vaccination is recommended.

Precaution(s): Store at 2-7°C (35-45°F). Do not freeze. Use immediately after reconstitution. Do not use chemicals to sterilize syringes and needles. Burn the container and all unused contents.

Caution(s): Do not vaccinate pregnant cats. In rare instances, administration of vaccines may cause lethargy, fever, and inflammatory or hypersensitivity types of reactions. Treatment may include antihistamines, anti-inflammatories, and/or epinephrine.

For veterinary use only.

Presentation: Contains 25 doses: 25 x 1 dose, lyophilized and 25 x 1 dose (1 mL), liquid.

Sold to veterinarians only.

PUREVAX and LEUCAT are trademarks of Merial.

Compendium Code No.: 11110511 RM310R5

PUREVAX™ FELINE 3/RABIES

Merial **Vaccine**

Feline Rhinotracheitis-Calici-Panleukopenia-Rabies Vaccine, Modified Live Virus, Canarypox Vector

U.S. Vet. Lic. No.: 298

Description: PUREVAX™ Feline 3/Rabies contains a nonadjuvanted lyophilized suspension of modified live feline rhinotracheitis, calici, and panleukopenia viruses; recombinant vectored rabies vaccine; plus a sterile water diluent. A canarypox vector has been modified, using recombinant technology, to produce expression of desired antigens capable of stimulating a protective immune response to rabies. Safety and immunogenicity of this product have been demonstrated by vaccination and challenge studies in susceptible cats.

Contains gentamicin as a preservative.

Indications: PUREVAX™ Feline 3/Rabies is recommended for the vaccination of healthy cats 8 weeks of age or older for prevention of disease due to feline rhinotracheitis, calici, panleukopenia, and rabies virus.

Dosage and Administration: Reconstitute the lyophilized vaccine with accompanying liquid diluent and aseptically inject 1 mL (1 dose) subcutaneously into healthy cats. For primary vaccination for all antigens except rabies, which requires only 1 dose at 8 weeks of age or older, revaccinate with a second 1 mL dose of this product or PureVax™ Feline 3, 3 to 4 weeks later. Cats younger than 12 weeks of age should be revaccinated with a single 1 mL dose every 3 to 4 weeks, the last dose given at or over 12 weeks of age. Revaccinate annually with a single 1 mL dose.

Precaution(s): Store at 2-7°C (35-45°F). Use immediately after reconstitution. Do not use chemicals to sterilize syringes and needles. Burn the container and all unused contents.

Caution(s): Do not vaccinate pregnant cats. In rare instances, administration of vaccines may cause lethargy, fever, and inflammatory or hypersensitivity types of reactions. Treatment may include antihistamines, anti-inflammatories, and/or epinephrine.

For veterinary use only.

Presentation: Contains 25 doses: 25 x 1 dose lyophilized, 25 x 1 mL sterile water.

Sold to veterinarians only.

PUREVAX is a trademark of Merial.

Compendium Code No.: 11110522 RM820R5

PUREVAX™ FELINE 3/RABIES + LEUCAT®

Merial **Vaccine**

Feline Leukemia-Rhinotracheitis-Calici-Panleukopenia-Rabies Vaccine, Modified Live Virus and Killed Virus, Canarypox Vector

U.S. Vet. Lic. No.: 298

Description: PUREVAX™ FELINE 3/RABIES + LEUCAT® contains a nonadjuvanted lyophilized suspension of modified live feline rhinotracheitis, calici, and panleukopenia viruses; recombinant vectored rabies vaccine; plus a liquid suspension of inactivated feline leukemia virus. FeLV is propagated in a continuously infected lymphoid cell line which expresses subgroups A, B, and C. The FeLV component stimulates serum neutralizing antibodies against the whole virus as well as viral components including gp70. A canarypox vector has been modified, using recombinant technology, to produce expression of desired antigens capable of stimulating a protective immune response to rabies. Safety and immunogenicity of this product have been demonstrated by vaccination and challenge studies in susceptible cats.

Contains gentamicin and amphotericin B as preservatives.

Indications: PUREVAX™ FELINE 3/RABIES + LEUCAT® is recommended for the vaccination of healthy cats 8 weeks of age or older for prevention of disease due to feline rhinotracheitis, calici, panleukopenia, and rabies viruses and as an aid in the prevention of disease due to feline leukemia virus.

Dosage and Administration: Reconstitute the lyophilized vaccine with accompanying liquid diluent and aseptically inject 1 mL (1 dose) subcutaneously into healthy cats. For primary vaccination for all antigens except rabies, which requires only 1 dose at 8 weeks of age or older, revaccinate with a second 1 mL dose of this product or PureVax™ Feline 3 + Leucat®, 3 to 4 weeks later. Cats younger than 12 weeks of age should be revaccinated with a single 1 mL dose every 3 to 4 weeks, the last dose given at or over 12 weeks of age. Revaccinate annually with a single 1 mL dose.

Precaution(s): Store at 2-7°C (35-45°F). Do not freeze. Use immediately after reconstitution. Do not use chemicals to sterilize syringes and needles. Burn the container and all unused contents.
Caution(s): Do not vaccinate pregnant cats. In rare instances, administration of vaccines may cause lethargy, fever, and inflammatory or hypersensitivity types of reactions. Treatment may include antihistamines, anti-inflammatories, and/or epinephrine.

For veterinary use only.

Presentation: Contains 25 doses: 25 x 1 dose lyophilized, 25 x 1 dose (1 mL) liquid.
Sold to veterinarians only.
PUREVAX and LEUCAT are trademarks of Merial.
Compendium Code No.: 11110532 RM840R5

PUREVAX™ FELINE 4

Merial **Vaccine**

Feline Rhinotracheitis-Calici-Panleukopenia-Chlamydia Psittaci Vaccine, Modified Live Virus and Chlamydia

U.S. Vet. Lic. No.: 298

Description: PUREVAX™ Feline 4 contains a lyophilized suspension of modified live feline rhinotracheitis, calici, and panleukopenia viruses and *Chlamydia psittaci*, each propagated in a stable cell line, plus sterile water diluent. Safety and immunogenicity of this product have been demonstrated by vaccination and challenge tests in susceptible cats.

Contains gentamicin as a preservative.

Indications: PUREVAX™ Feline 4 is recommended for the vaccination of healthy cats 6 weeks of age and older for prevention of disease due to feline rhinotracheitis, calici, and panleukopenia viruses and as an aid in the reduction of disease due to *Chlamydia psittaci*.
Dosage and Administration: Reconstitute the lyophilized vaccine with accompanying liquid diluent and aseptically inject 1 mL (1 dose) subcutaneously or intramuscularly into healthy cats. For primary vaccination, revaccinate with a second 1 mL dose 3 to 4 weeks later. Cats younger than 12 weeks of age should be revaccinated with a single 1 mL dose every 3 to 4 weeks, the last dose given at or over 12 weeks of age. Revaccinate annually with a single 1 mL dose.
Precaution(s): Store at 2-7°C (35-45°F). Use immediately after reconstitution. Do not use chemicals to sterilize syringes and needles. Burn the container and all unused contents.
Caution(s): Do not vaccinate pregnant cats. In rare instances, administration of vaccines may cause lethargy, fever, and inflammatory or hypersensitivity types of reactions. Treatment may include antihistamines, anti-inflammatories, and/or epinephrine.

For veterinary use only.

Presentation: Contains 25 doses: 25 x 1 dose, lyophilized and 25 x 1 mL, sterile water.
Sold to veterinarians only.
PUREVAX is a trademark of Merial.
Compendium Code No.: 11110541 RM504R4

PUREVAX™ FELINE 4 + LEUCAT®

Merial **Vaccine**

Feline Leukemia-Rhinotracheitis-Calici-Panleukopenia-Chlamydia Psittaci Vaccine, Modified Live Virus and Chlamydia and Killed Virus

U.S. Vet. Lic. No.: 298

Description: PUREVAX™ FELINE 4 + LEUCAT® contains a lyophilized suspension of modified live feline rhinotracheitis, calici, and panleukopenia viruses and *Chlamydia psittaci* propagated in stable cell lines, plus a liquid suspension of inactivated feline leukemia virus propagated in a continuously infected lymphoid cell line which expresses subgroups A, B, and C. PUREVAX™ FELINE 4 + LEUCAT® stimulates serum neutralizing antibodies against the whole virus as well as viral components including gp70. Safety and immunogenicity of this product have been demonstrated by vaccination and challenge tests in susceptible cats.

Contains gentamicin and amphotericin B as preservatives.

Indications: PUREVAX™ FELINE 4 + LEUCAT® is recommended for the vaccination of healthy cats 8 weeks of age or older for prevention of disease due to feline rhinotracheitis, calici, and panleukopenia viruses; and as an aid in the prevention of disease due to feline leukemia virus and the reduction of disease due to *Chlamydia psittaci*.
Dosage and Administration: Reconstitute the lyophilized vaccine with accompanying liquid diluent and aseptically inject 1 mL (1 dose) subcutaneously into healthy cats. For primary vaccination, revaccinate with a second 1 mL dose 3 to 4 weeks later. Cats younger than 12 weeks of age should be revaccinated with a single 1 mL dose every 3 to 4 weeks, the last dose given at or over 12 weeks of age. Revaccinate annually with a single 1 mL dose. Diagnostic testing for FeLV prior to vaccination is recommended.
Precaution(s): Store at 2-7°C (35-45°F). Do not freeze. Use immediately after reconstitution. Do not use chemicals to sterilize syringes and needles. Burn the container and all unused contents.
Caution(s): Do not vaccinate pregnant cats. In rare instances, administration of vaccines may cause lethargy, fever, and inflammatory or hypersensitivity types of reactions. Treatment may include antihistamines, anti-inflammatories, and/or epinephrine.

For veterinary use only.

Presentation: Contains 25 doses: 25 x 1 dose, lyophilized and 25 x 1 dose (1 mL), liquid.
Sold to veterinarians only.
PUREVAX and LEUCAT are trademarks of Merial.
Compendium Code No.: 11110551 RM321R5

PUREVAX™ FELINE 4/RABIES

Merial **Vaccine**

Feline Rhinotracheitis-Calici-Panleukopenia-Chlamydia Psittaci-Rabies Vaccine, Modified Live Virus and Chlamydia, Canarypox Vector

U.S. Vet. Lic. No.: 298

Description: PUREVAX™ Feline 4/Rabies contains a nonadjuvanted lyophilized suspension of modified live feline rhinotracheitis, calici, and panleukopenia viruses and *Chlamydia psittaci;* recombinant vectored rabies vaccine; plus a sterile water diluent. A canarypox vector has been modified, using recombinant technology, to produce expression of desired antigens capable of stimulating a protective immune response to rabies. Safety and immunogenicity of this product have been demonstrated by vaccination and challenge studies in susceptible cats.

Contains gentamicin as a preservative.

Indications: PUREVAX™ Feline 4/Rabies is recommended for the vaccination of healthy cats 8 weeks of age and older for prevention of disease due to feline rhinotracheitis, calici, panleukopenia, and rabies viruses and as an aid in the reduction of disease due to *Chlamydia psittaci*.
Dosage and Administration: Reconstitute the lyophilized vaccine with accompanying liquid diluent and aseptically inject 1 mL (1 dose) subcutaneously into healthy cats. For primary vaccination for all antigens except rabies, which requires only 1 dose at 8 weeks of age or older, revaccinate with a second 1 mL dose of this product or PureVax™ Feline 4, 3 to 4 weeks later. Cats younger than 12 weeks of age should be revaccinated with a single 1 mL dose every 3 to 4 weeks, the last dose given at or over 12 weeks of age. Revaccinate annually with a single 1 mL dose.
Precaution(s): Store at 2-7°C (35-45°F). Use entire contents immediately after reconstitution. Do not use chemicals to sterilize syringes and needles. Burn the container and all unused contents.
Caution(s): Do not vaccinate pregnant cats. In rare instances, administration of vaccines may cause lethargy, fever, and inflammatory or hypersensitivity types of reactions. Treatment may include antihistamines, anti-inflammatories, and/or epinephrine.

For veterinary use only.

Presentation: Contains 25 doses: 25 x 1 dose lyophilized, 25 x 1 dose (1 mL) sterile water.
Sold to veterinarians only.
PUREVAX is a trademark of Merial.
Compendium Code No.: 11110562 RM830R5

PUREVAX™ FELINE 4/RABIES + LEUCAT®

Merial **Vaccine**

Feline Leukemia-Rhinotracheitis-Calici-Panleukopenia-Chlamydia Psittaci-Rabies Vaccine, Modified Live and Chlamydia and Killed Virus, Canarypox Vector

U.S. Vet. Lic. No.: 298

Description: PUREVAX™ FELINE 4/RABIES + LEUCAT® contains a nonadjuvanted lyophilized suspension of modified live feline rhinotracheitis, calici, and panleukopenia viruses and *Chlamydia psittaci;* recombinant vectored rabies vaccine; plus a liquid suspension of inactivated feline leukemia virus. FeLV is propagated in a continuously infected lymphoid cell line which expresses subgroups A, B, and C. The FeLV component stimulates serum neutralizing antibodies against the whole virus as well as viral components including gp70. A canarypox vector has been modified, using recombinant technology, to produce expression of desired antigens capable of stimulating a protective immune response to rabies. Safety and immunogenicity of this product have been demonstrated by vaccination and challenge studies in susceptible cats.

Contains gentamicin and amphotericin B as preservatives.

Indications: PUREVAX™ FELINE 4/RABIES + LEUCAT® is recommended for the vaccination of healthy cats 8 weeks of age and older for prevention of disease due to feline rhinotracheitis, calici, panleukopenia, and rabies viruses, and as an aid in the prevention of disease due to feline leukemia virus and the reduction of disease due to *Chlamydia psittaci*.
Dosage and Administration: Reconstitute the lyophilized vaccine with accompanying liquid diluent and aseptically inject 1 mL (1 dose) subcutaneously into healthy cats. For primary vaccination for all antigens except rabies, which requires only 1 dose at 8 weeks of age or older, revaccinate with a second 1 mL dose of this product or PureVax™ Feline 4 + Leucat®, 3 to 4 weeks later. Cats younger than 12 weeks of age should be revaccinated with a single 1 mL dose every 3 to 4 weeks, the last dose given at or over 12 weeks of age. Revaccinate annually with a single 1 mL dose.
Precaution(s): Store at 2-7°C (35-45°F). Do not freeze. Use entire contents immediately after reconstitution. Do not use chemicals to sterilize syringes and needles. Burn the container and all unused contents.
Caution(s): Do not vaccinate pregnant cats. In rare instances, administration of vaccines may cause lethargy, fever, and inflammatory or hypersensitivity types of reactions. Treatment may include antihistamines, anti-inflammatories, and/or epinephrine.

For veterinary use only.

Presentation: Contains 25 doses: 25 x 1 dose lyophilized, 25 x 1 dose (1 mL) liquid.
Sold to veterinarians only.
PUREVAX and LEUCAT are trademarks of Merial.
Compendium Code No.: 11110572 RM850R5

PUREVAX™ FELINE RABIES

Merial **Vaccine**

Rabies Vaccine, Live Canarypox Vector

U.S. Vet. Lic. No.: 298

Description: PUREVAX™ Feline Rabies contains a nonadjuvanted lyophilized suspension of a recombinant vectored rabies vaccine plus a sterile water diluent. A canarypox vector has been modified, using recombinant technology, to produce expression of desired antigens capable of stimulating a protective immune response to rabies. Safety and immunogenicity of this product have been demonstrated by vaccination and challenge studies in susceptible cats.

Contains gentamicin as a preservative.

Indications: PUREVAX™ Feline Rabies is recommended for the vaccination of healthy cats 8 weeks of age or older for prevention of disease due to rabies virus.
Dosage and Administration: Reconstitute the lyophilized vaccine with accompanying liquid diluent and aseptically inject 1 mL (1 dose) subcutaneously into healthy cats. Revaccinate annually with a single 1 mL dose.
Precaution(s): Store at 2-7°C (35-45°F). Use immediately after reconstitution. Do not use chemicals to sterilize syringes and needles. Burn the container and all unused contents.
Caution(s): It is generally recommended to avoid vaccination of pregnant cats. In rare instances, administration of vaccines may cause lethargy, fever, and inflammatory or hypersensitivity types of reactions. Treatment may include antihistamines, anti-inflammatories, and/or epinephrine.

For veterinary use only.

Presentation: Contains 25 doses: 25 x 1 dose lyophilized, 25 x 1 mL sterile water.
Sold to veterinarians only.
PUREVAX is a trademark of Merial.
Compendium Code No.: 11110582 RM860R7

PUREVAX™ FERRET DISTEMPER

Merial **Vaccine**

Distemper Vaccine, Live Canarypox Vector

U.S. Vet. Lic. No.: 298

Description: PUREVAX™ Ferret Distemper is a lyophilized vaccine of a recombinant canarypox vector expressing the HA and F glycoproteins of canine distemper virus. Safety and immunogenicity of this product have been demonstrated by vaccination and challenge tests in susceptible ferrets.

Contains gentamicin as a preservative.

Indications: PUREVAX™ Ferret Distemper is recommended for the vaccination of healthy ferrets 8 weeks of age and older for prevention of disease due to canine distemper virus.
Dosage and Administration: Reconstitute the lyophilized vaccine with accompanying liquid diluent and aseptically inject 1 mL (1 dose) subcutaneously into healthy ferrets 8 weeks of age

and older. Primary vaccination requires two additional 1 mL doses at 3 week intervals. Revaccinate annually with a single 1 mL dose.

Precaution(s): Store at 2-7°C (35-45°F). Use immediately after reconstitution. Do not use chemicals to sterilize syringes and needles. Burn container and all unused contents.

Caution(s): It is generally recommended to avoid vaccination of pregnant ferrets. Administration of vaccines may cause lethargy, fever, and inflammatory or hypersensitivity types of reactions. Treatment may include antihistamines, anti-inflammatories, and/or epinephrine.

For veterinary use only.

Presentation: Contains 10 doses: 10 x 1 dose, lyophilized and 10 x 1 mL, sterile water.

PUREVAX is a trademark of Merial.

Compendium Code No.: 11110830 RM985R2

PUREVAX™ LEUCAT®

Merial **Vaccine**

Feline Leukemia Vaccine, Killed Virus

U.S. Vet. Lic. No.: 298

Description: PUREVAX™ LEUCAT® contains a liquid suspension of inactivated feline leukemia virus propagated in a continuously infected lymphoid cell line which expresses subgroups A, B and C. The safety of this product is ensured through virus inactivation, purification and concentration to eliminate tissue culture components. PUREVAX™ LEUCAT® stimulates serum neutralizing antibodies against the whole virus as well as viral components including gp70. Safety and immunogenicity of this product have been demonstrated by vaccination and challenge tests in susceptible cats.

Contains gentamicin and amphotericin B as preservatives.

Indications: PUREVAX™ LEUCAT® is recommended for the vaccination of healthy cats 8 weeks of age or older and as an aid in the prevention of disease due to feline leukemia virus.

Dosage and Administration: Aseptically inject 1 mL (1 dose) subcutaneously into healthy cats. For primary vaccination, revaccinate with a second 1 mL dose 3 to 4 weeks later. Revaccinate annually with a single 1 mL dose. Diagnostic testing for FeLV prior to vaccination is recommended.

Precaution(s): Store at 2-7°C (35-45°F). Do not freeze. Do not use chemicals to sterilize syringes and needles.

Caution(s): In rare instances, administration of vaccines may cause lethargy, fever, and inflammatory or hypersensitivity types of reactions. Treatment may include antihistamines, anti-inflammatories, and/or epinephrine. For veterinary use only.

Presentation: 50 x 1 dose (1 mL), liquid.

Sold to veterinarians only.

PUREVAX and LEUCAT are trademarks of Merial.

Compendium Code No.: 11110593 RM500R5

PURPLE LOTION

Vedco **Topical Wound Dressing**

Active Ingredient(s): Contains: Isopropyl alcohol (73.4%), propylene glycol, glycerin, urea, sodium propionate, furfural, gentian violet, and acriflavine.

Indications: A germicidal, fungicidal, antiseptic, and protective wound dressing for use as an aid in the treatment of minor cuts, galls, scratches, and wound infections.

Dosage and Administration: Shake well before using. Remove pus and exudate from the infected area and apply the product freely with the dauber or a piece of gauze. Apply an amount sufficient to cover the wound. One (1) application is usually sufficient. May be repeated once or twice a day in severe cases.

Caution(s): PURPLE LOTION will stain. Avoid contact with hands and clothing.

Contains isopropyl alcohol, a flammable liquid. Do not use the product near an open flame.

In case of deep or puncture wounds or serious burns, consult a veterinarian. If redness, irritation, or swelling persists or increases, discontinue use of the product and consult a veterinarian.

Hazardous livestock remedy. Sold to veterinarians only.

Keep out of the reach of children. For external veterinary use only.

Warning(s): Not for use on horses intended for food use.

Presentation: 4 fl. oz. (118 mL) containers.

Compendium Code No.: 10941750

P

PURPLE LOTION WOUND DRESSING

Durvet **Topical Wound Dressing**

Topical Antiseptic

Active Ingredient(s): Contains Isopropyl Alcohol (73.4% v/v), Propylene Glycol, Glycerine, Urea, Sodium Propionate, Furfural, Methyl Violet and Acriflavine.

Indications: A germicidal, fungicidal, antiseptic and protective wound dressing for use in the treatment of minor cuts, scratches and superficial abrasions.

Directions: Remove pus and exudate from infected area. When spraying hold container approximately 6 inches from area to be treated. Spray an amount sufficient to cover wound. One application is usually sufficient. May be repeated once or twice daily on severe cases.

Precaution(s): Flammable. Do not expose to heat or store at a temperature above 120°F. Do not use near an open flame. Store in a cool place.

Caution(s): In case of deep or puncture wounds or serious burns, consult veterinarian. If redness, irritation, or swelling persists or increases, discontinue use and consult veterinarian. Keep away from eyes or mucous membranes.

Hazardous- Livestock remedy. Not for human use.

The following statement is made in compliance with the State of California Agricultural Code: Livestock remedy—Not for human use. For external veterinary use only.

Warning(s): For horses not intended for food use. Keep out of reach of children.

Presentation: 4 fl. oz. (¼ pt) and 16 fl. oz. (1 pt).

Compendium Code No.: 10841431 Rev. 10-94 / Rev. 2-94

PURPLE LOTION WOUND DRESSING

First Priority **Topical Wound Dressing**

Topical Antiseptic

Ingredient(s): Isopropyl Alcohol (73.4% v/v), Propylene Glycol, Glycerin, Urea, Sodium Propionate, Furfural, Gentian Violet and Acriflavine.

Indications: PURPLE LOTION WOUND DRESSING is a quick-drying, penetrating antiseptic treatment for superficial wounds and minor cuts and abrasions. Germicidal and fungicidal.

Directions for Use:

4 fl oz with Dauber: Thoroughly cleanse the area to be treated with soap and water or warm water to which a reliable disinfectant has been added. The use of hydrogen peroxide may aid the cleansing of conditions involving pus formation. PURPLE LOTION WOUND DRESSING should be applied freely in the morning and evening for several days until condition has been relieved.

16 fl oz with Sprayer: Remove pus and exudate from infected area. When spraying hold container approximately 6 inches from area to be treated. Spray an amount sufficient to cover wound. One application is usually sufficient. May be repeated once or twice daily on severe cases.

Contraindication(s): Do not use on cats.

Precaution(s): Storage: Store at controlled room temperature between 15°-30°C (59°-86°F). Keep container tightly closed when not in use. Flammable. Do not expose to heat or store at a temperature above 120°F. Do not use near an open flame.

Caution(s): Use only as directed. Avoid contact with eyes and mucous membranes. Avoid inhaling. Do not apply to large areas of broken skin. In case of deep or puncture wounds or serious burns, or if redness, rash, irritation, or swelling persist or increase, consult veterinarian. Not for prolonged use.

Hazardous - Livestock remedy. Not for human use.

The following statement is made in compliance with the State of California Agricultural Code: Livestock Remedy - For animal use only.

Warning(s): For horses not intended for food purposes.

Wash treated udder and teat parts of dairy animals thoroughly before each milking to prevent contamination of milk. Keep out of reach of children.

Presentation: 4 fl oz (120 mL) with dauber (NDC# 58829-321-04) and 16 fl oz (473 mL) with sprayer (NDC# 58829-307-16).

Compendium Code No.: 11390801 Iss. 11-01 / Rev. 07-01

PURPLE SPRAY

AgriPharm **Marker**

Ingredient(s): Water, propylene glycol, benzalkonium chloride, ethylene dianime tetra-acetate, and methyl violet.

Indications: Suitable for use as a marker, laboratory indicator, and reagent.

Precaution(s): Protect from freezing.

Warning(s): For veterinary use only. Keep out of reach of children.

Presentation: 473 mL (16 fl oz).

Compendium Code No.: 14570880

PURRGE™ DROPS

PPI **Laxative**

Laxative and Lubricant for Hairball Removal

Active Ingredient(s): Contains: Liquid petrolatum, malt syrup, cod liver oil, dl-alpha tocopherol acetate in a special palatable base.

Indications: For oral use as a laxative in dogs and cats, and for hairball removal for cats.

Dosage and Administration: Suggested dosage: Suggested dosage: Cats—For hair balls—2 to 5 mL for 2 or 3 days then 1 to 2 mL 2 or 3 times a week. Laxative—1 to 2 mL 2 or 3 times a week.

Dogs—as a laxative—2 to 5 mL 2 or 3 times a week.

Caution(s): Keep out of reach of children.

Presentation: 60 mL with calibrated dropper for easy dosing.

Distributed by: The Triton Group, St. Louis, MO 63103

Compendium Code No.: 12270030

P-VAC™

United **Bacterin**

Pseudomonas aeruginosa Bacterin

U.S. Vet. Lic. No.: 245

Active Ingredient(s): An inactivated vaccine which contains *Pseudomonas aeruginosa* serotypes 5, 6 and 7-8 (IATS).

Indications: P-VAC™ is for use as an aid in the prevention of Pseudomonas pneumonia in healthy, susceptible mink.

Dosage and Administration: Use sharp, sterile needles and sterile syringes. Inject 1 mL under the loose skin of the armpit of mink of at least six (6) weeks of age. For a proper suspension, shake before and occasionally during use. Revaccinate all adults at the time of kit vaccination.

Precaution(s): Store at 35-45°F (2-7°C).

Caution(s): Use the entire contents when the container is first opened.

Consult a veterinarian or United Vaccines Inc. before using the vaccine in mink on a farm where disease exists or has occurred in the last 18 months, or for an alternate vaccinating schedule.

Presentation: 100 dose, 250 dose and 500 dose vials.

Compendium Code No.: 11040101

PVP IODINE

Western Chemical **Disinfectant**

Active Ingredient(s): 10% solution of polyvinylpyrrolidone iodine complex.

Indications: Fish egg disinfectant for salmon and trout species.

Dosage and Administration: Use at 50 ppm during water hardening and 100 ppm after water hardening.

Presentation: 4x1 gallon case, 5 gallon bucket, 15, 30 and 55 gallon drums.

Compendium Code No.: 10210010

PVP IODINE OINTMENT

Vedco **Topical Antibacterial**

Active Ingredient(s): Contains:

Polyvinylpyrrolidone-iodine complex (1.0% titratable iodine) 10%

Indications: A topical antiseptic cream for use on horses, cattle, swine, and sheep to aid in the treatment of foot rot, sores, minor cut, bruises, abrasions, and burns. The cream base contains emolients and moisturizers which aid in the restoration of the skin's natural moisture balance.

Dosage and Administration: Cleanse the wound or area to be treated and apply PVP IODINE OINTMENT at full strength, repeating as necessary to maintain the characteristic iodine color on the skin. The PVP IODINE OINTMENT color indicates its germ-killing activity is still present.

Note: When used on or near the teats or udders of dairy animals, the teats and udders should be thoroughly washed before the next milking to prevent contamination of milk.

Precaution(s): Store in a cool place.
Caution(s): Keep out of the reach of children. In case of accidental ingestion, seek professional assistance or contact a poison control center immediately. For external veterinary use only.

Not for use on serious burns, in body cavities, or in deep or puncture wounds. If redness, irritation, swelling, or an infection occurs, discontinue use and consult a veterinarian. Do not apply to the eyes, mucous membranes, or large areas of abraded skin.
Presentation: 1 lb. (16 oz.) containers.
Compendium Code No.: 10941760

PYOBEN® GEL ℞

Virbac **Antidermatosis Gel**

NDC No.: 51311-014-30
Active Ingredient(s): PYOBEN® Gel contains 5% micronized benzoyl peroxide in a water base gel containing docusate sodium, edetate disodium, poloxamer 182, carbomer-940, propylene glycol, silicon dioxide and purified water. May also contain citric acid and/or sodium hydroxide to adjust pH.
Indications: PYOBEN® Gel is a topical water base preparation for use in treating superficial microbial infections. Benzoyl peroxide is an oxidizing agent which possesses antibacterial and keratolytic properties.

Benzoyl peroxide is an antibacterial agent and causes drying and peeling.

PYOBEN® Gel is indicated in dog and cat skin conditions responsive to topical, antimicrobial and/or keratolytic agents.
Dosage and Administration: PYOBEN® Gel should be applied to the affected areas once or twice a day after cleansing the area.
Contraindication(s): Contraindicated in patients hypersensitive to any of the components in the formulation.
Precaution(s): Store at a controlled room temperature (59° to 86°F).
Caution(s): Federal law (USA) restricts this drug to use by or on the order of a licensed veterinarian.

For external use only on dogs and cats. Avoid contact with the eyes or mucous membranes. If irritation develops, decrease frequency of use or discontinue use.

Contact dermatitis has been reported in humans but not in dogs.

Important: As benzoyl peroxide is a potent oxidizing agent, it will bleach many fabrics i.e. carpets, upholstery, etc. Advise clients to keep pets away from all fabric during therapy.

Depending upon the severity of the condition, concomitant systemic antibiotic therapy may be indicated.
Presentation: 30 g (1 oz.) plastic tubes.
Compendium Code No.: 10230460

PYOBEN® SHAMPOO ℞

Virbac **Antidermatosis Shampoo**
with Spherulites®

Ingredient(s): Benzoyl peroxide 3% in a shampoo base containing water, sodium C14-C16 olefin sulfonate, Spherulites, glycerin, citric acid, carbomer 940 and chitosanide. Chitosanide and glycerin are present in encapsulated (Spherulites) and free forms. Urea is present in encapsulated form.
Indications: PYOBEN® Shampoo is an antimicrobial, keratolytic and follicular flushing shampoo specifically formulated for the topical treatment of deep cutaneous infection in dogs and cats.

PYOBEN® Shampoo is an antimicrobial, keratolytic and follicular flushing shampoo for use on dogs and cats of any age.
Directions: Shake well before use. Wet the coat with warm water and apply sufficient shampoo to create a rich lather. Massage PYOBEN® into wet coat, lather freely. Rinse and repeat. Allow to remain on hair for 5 to 10 minutes, then rinse thoroughly with clean water.

Frequency of use: initially two to three times a week for four weeks, then reducing to once a week, or as directed by your veterinarian.
Caution(s): Federal Law (USA) restricts this drug to use by or on the order of a licensed veterinarian. For external use only on dogs and cats. Avoid contact with eyes or mucous membranes. If condition persists or does not improve in 7 days, consult your veterinarian. Wash hands and exposed skin after using. May bleach colored fabric.

Available through licensed veterinarians only.
Warning(s): Keep out of reach of children.
Discussion: PYOBEN® contains Spherulites, an exclusive and patented encapsulation system developed by Virbac to provide slow release of ingredients long after the shampoo is rinsed off.

PYOBEN® also contains Chitosanide, a natural biopolymer creating a protective film on the skin and hair.
Presentation: 8 fl oz (237 mL) containers.
Compendium Code No.: 10230470

PYRAMID® 4+PRESPONSE® SQ

Fort Dodge **Toxoid-Vaccine**

Bovine Rhinotracheitis-Virus Diarrhea-Parainfluenza-3-Respiratory Syncytial Virus Vaccine, Modified Live Virus-Pasteurella Haemolytica Toxoid
U.S. Vet. Lic. No.: 112
Contents: This product contains the antigens listed above.

Thimerosal, neomycin and polymyxin B added as preservatives.
Indications: For vaccination of healthy dairy or beef cattle as an aid in the prevention of disease caused by bovine rhinotracheitis, bovine virus diarrhea, bovine parainfluenza-3, bovine respiratory syncytial virus and *P. haemolytica.*
Dosage and Administration: Aseptically rehydrate with the accompanying diluent. Cattle, inject one 2 mL dose subcutaneously using aseptic technique. Protect animals from exposure for at least 14 days after vaccination. Calves vaccinated under 6 months of age should be revaccinated at 6 months of age. Healthy cattle should be vaccinated a minimum of 14 days prior to shipping or exposure to stress which may precipitate infectious conditions.

For viral fractions, annual revaccination with Pyramid® MLV4 is recommended. For *Pasteurella haemolytica*, although only a single dose is necessary to confer immunity, a booster dose with Presponse® SQ is recommended whenever subsequent stress is likely.
Contraindication(s): Do not use in pregnant cows or in calves nursing pregnant cows.
Precaution(s): Store in dark at 2° to 7°C (35° to 45°F). Avoid freezing. Shake well. Use entire contents when first opened. Burn container and all unused contents.
Caution(s): A small percentage of animals may show transient mild injection site swelling. In case of anaphylactoid reaction, administer epinephrine.
Warning(s): Do not vaccinate within 21 days before slaughter.

For veterinary use only.
Presentation: 10 dose virus vaccine vials with one vial toxoid diluent to rehydrate to 20 mL. 50 dose virus vaccine vials with one vial toxoid diluent to rehydrate to 100 mL.
U.S. Pat. Nos. 4,957,739; 5,165,924; 5,336,491; 5,378,615 and 5,733,555.
Compendium Code No.: 10031711 2157F

PYRAMID® 8

Fort Dodge **Bacterin-Vaccine**

Bovine Rhinotracheitis-Virus Diarrhea-Parainfluenza-3 Vaccine, Modified Live Virus-Leptospira Canicola-Grippotyphosa-Hardjo-Icterohaemorrhagiae-Pomona Bacterin
U.S. Vet. Lic. No.: 112
Contents: This product contains the antigens listed above.

Thimerosal, neomycin and polymyxin B added as preservatives.
Indications: For vaccination of healthy cattle as an aid in the prevention of disease caused by bovine rhinotracheitis, bovine virus diarrhea, bovine parainfluenza-3, *Leptospira canicola, L. grippotyphosa, L. hardjo, L. icterohaemorrhagiae* and *L. pomona.*
Dosage and Administration: Aseptically rehydrate with the accompanying diluent. Cattle, inject one 2 mL dose subcutaneously or intramuscularly using aseptic technique. Annual revaccination is recommended. Protect animals from exposure for at least 14 days after vaccination. Calves vaccinated under six months of age should be revaccinated at six months of age.
Precaution(s): Store in dark at 2° to 7°C (35° to 45°F). Avoid freezing. Shake well. Use entire contents when first opened. Burn container and all unused contents.
Caution(s): Do not use in pregnant cows or in calves nursing pregnant cows. A small percentage of animals may show transient mild injection site swelling. In case of anaphylactoid reaction, administer epinephrine.
Warning(s): Do not vaccinate within 21 days before slaughter.

For veterinary use only.
Presentation: One vial vaccine, one vial diluent. 10 doses (rehydrate to 20 mL) and one vial vaccine, one vial diluent. 50 doses (rehydrate to 100 mL). Patent Pending
Compendium Code No.: 10031731 2075D

PYRAMID® 9

Fort Dodge **Bacterin-Vaccine**

Bovine Rhinotracheitis-Virus Diarrhea-Parainfluenza-3-Respiratory Syncytial Virus Vaccine, Modified Live Virus-Leptospira Canicola-Grippotyphosa-Hardjo-Icterohaemorrhagiae-Pomona Bacterin
U.S. Vet. Lic. No.: 112
Contents: This product contains the antigens listed above.

Thimerosal, neomycin and polymyxin B added as preservatives.
Indications: For vaccination of healthy cattle as an aid in the prevention of disease caused by bovine rhinotracheitis, bovine virus diarrhea, bovine parainfluenza-3, bovine respiratory syncytial virus, *Leptospira canicola, L. grippotyphosa, L. hardjo, L. icterohaemorrhagiae* and *L. pomona.*
Dosage and Administration: Aseptically rehydrate with the accompanying diluent. Cattle, inject one 2 mL dose subcutaneously or intramuscularly using aseptic technique. Annual revaccination is recommended. Protect animals from exposure for at least 14 days after vaccination. Calves vaccinated under six months of age should be revaccinated at six months of age.
Precaution(s): Store in dark at 2° to 7°C (35° to 45°F). Avoid freezing. Shake well. Use entire contents when first opened. Burn container and all unused contents.
Caution(s): Do not use in pregnant cows or in calves nursing pregnant cows. A small percentage of animals may show transient mild injection site swelling. In case of anaphylactoid reaction, administer epinephrine.
Warning(s): Do not vaccinate within 21 days before slaughter. For veterinary use only.
Presentation: One vial vaccine, one vial diluent. 5 doses (rehydrate to 10 mL), one vial vaccine, one vial diluent. 10 doses (rehydrate to 20 mL) and one vial vaccine, one vial diluent. 50 doses (rehydrate to 100 mL). U.S. Patent Nos. 5,733,555 — 5,958,423
Compendium Code No.: 10031720 2163C

PYRAMID® IBR

Fort Dodge **Vaccine**

Bovine Rhinotracheitis Vaccine, Modified Live Virus
U.S. Vet. Lic. No.: 112
Contents: This product contains the antigen listed above.

Thimerosal, neomycin and polymyxin B added as preservatives.
Indications: For vaccination of healthy cattle 6 months of age or older as an aid in the prevention of disease caused by bovine rhinotracheitis virus.
Dosage and Administration: Aseptically rehydrate with the accompanying diluent. Cattle, inject one 2 mL dose subcutaneously or intramuscularly using aseptic technique. Annual revaccination is recommended. Protect animals from exposure for at least 14 days after the last dose of vaccine.
Precaution(s): Store in dark at 2° to 7°C (35° to 45°F). Avoid freezing. Shake well. Use entire contents when first opened. Burn container and all unused contents.
Caution(s): Do not use in pregnant cows or in calves nursing pregnant cows. A small percentage of animals may show transient mild injection site swelling. In case of anaphylactoid reaction, administer epinephrine.
Warning(s): Do not vaccinate within 21 days before slaughter. For veterinary use only.
Presentation: 10 dose vial of vaccine with one vial diluent (Rehydrate to 20 mL) and 50 dose vial of vaccine with one vial diluent (Rehydrate to 100 mL). Patent Pending
Compendium Code No.: 10031741 2067A

PYRAMID® IBR+LEPTO

Fort Dodge **Bacterin-Vaccine**

Bovine Rhinotracheitis Vaccine, Modified Live Virus-Leptospira Canicola-Grippotyphosa-Hardjo-Icterohaemorrhagiae-Pomona Bacterin
U.S. Vet. Lic. No.: 112
Contents: This product contains the antigens listed above.

Thimerosal, neomycin and polymyxin B added as preservatives.
Indications: For vaccination of healthy cattle as an aid in the prevention of disease caused by bovine rhinotracheitis, *Leptospira canicola, L. grippotyphosa, L. hardjo, L. icterohaemorrhagiae* and *L. pomona.*
Dosage and Administration: Aseptically rehydrate with the accompanying diluent. Cattle, inject one 2 mL dose subcutaneously or intramuscularly using aseptic technique. Annual revaccination

is recommended. Protect animals from exposure for at least 14 days after vaccination. Calves vaccinated under six months of age should be revaccinated at six months of age.

Precaution(s): Store in dark at 2° to 7°C (35° to 45°F). Avoid freezing. Shake well. Use entire contents when first opened. Burn container and all unused contents.

Caution(s): Do not use in pregnant cows or in calves nursing pregnant cows. A small percentage of animals may show transient mild injection site swelling. In case of anaphylactoid reaction, administer epinephrine.

Warning(s): Do not vaccinate within 21 days before slaughter.

For veterinary use only.

Presentation: One vial vaccine, one vial diluent. 10 doses (rehydrate to 20 mL) and one vial vaccine, one vial diluent. 50 doses (rehydrate to 100 mL).

Patent Pending

Compendium Code No.: 10031751 2086D

PYRAMID® MLV 3

Fort Dodge **Vaccine**

Bovine Rhinotracheitis-Virus Diarrhea-Parainfluenza-3 Vaccine, Modified Live Virus

U.S. Vet. Lic. No.: 112

Contents: This product contains the antigens listed above.

Thimerosal, neomycin and polymyxin B added as preservatives.

Indications: For vaccination of healthy cattle as an aid in the prevention of disease caused by bovine rhinotracheitis, bovine virus diarrhea and bovine parainfluenza-3.

Dosage and Administration: Aseptically rehydrate with the accompanying diluent. Cattle, inject one 2 mL dose subcutaneously or intramuscularly using aseptic technique. Annual revaccination is recommended. Protect animals from exposure for at least 14 days after vaccination. Calves vaccinated under 6 months of age should be revaccinated at 6 months of age.

Precaution(s): Store in dark at 2° to 7°C (35° to 45°F). Avoid freezing. Shake well. Use entire contents when first opened. Burn container and all unused contents.

Caution(s): Do not use in pregnant cows or in calves nursing pregnant cows. A small percentage of animals may show transient mild injection site swelling. In case of anaphylactoid reaction, administer epinephrine.

Warning(s): Do not vaccinate within 21 days before slaughter.

For veterinary use only.

Presentation: 10 dose vial of vaccine with one vial diluent (Rehydrate to 20 mL).
50 dose vial of vaccine with one vial diluent (Rehydrate to 100 mL).

U.S. Patent No. 5,733,555

Compendium Code No.: 10031761 2035B

PYRAMID® MLV 4

Fort Dodge **Vaccine**

Bovine Rhinotracheitis-Virus Diarrhea-Parainfluenza-3-Respiratory Syncytial Virus Vaccine, Modified Live Virus

U.S. Vet. Lic. No.: 112

Contents: This product contains the antigens listed above.

Thimerosal, neomycin and polymyxin B added as preservatives.

Indications: For vaccination of healthy cattle as an aid in the prevention of disease caused by bovine rhinotracheitis, bovine virus diarrhea, bovine parainfluenza-3 and bovine respiratory syncytial virus.

Dosage and Administration: Aseptically rehydrate with the accompanying diluent. Cattle, inject one 2 mL dose subcutaneously or intramuscularly using aseptic technique. Annual revaccination is recommended. Protect animals from exposure for at least 14 days after vaccination. Calves vaccinated under 6 months of age should be revaccinated at 6 months of age.

Precaution(s): Store in dark at 2° to 7°C (35° to 45°F). Avoid freezing. Shake well. Use entire contents when first opened. Burn container and all unused contents.

Caution(s): Do not use in pregnant cows or in calves nursing pregnant cows. A small percentage of animals may show transient mild injection site swelling. In case of anaphylactoid reaction, administer epinephrine.

Warning(s): Do not vaccinate within 21 days before slaughter.

For veterinary use only.

Presentation: 10 dose vial of vaccine with one vial diluent (Rehydrate to 20 mL).
50 dose vial of vaccine with one vial diluent (Rehydrate to 100 mL).

U.S. Patent No. 5,733,555

Compendium Code No.: 10031771 1915C

PYRETHRIN PLUS

Durvet **Premise and Topical Insecticide**

EPA Reg. No.: 47000-33-12281

Active Ingredient(s):

Pyrethrins	0.1%
Technical Piperonyl Butoxide**	1.0%
Inert Ingredients*	98.9%

*Contains petroleum distillates.

**Equivalent to 0.80% of (butylcarbityl) (6-propylpiperonyl) ether and 0.20% of related compounds.

Indications: For the protection of dairy animals from biting flies and the control of houseflies in barns and milk houses.

Protects against hornflies, stableflies, houseflies, gnats, mosquitoes and blood sucking lice.

A temporary treatment to relieve cattle from annoyance caused by face flies.

Directions for Use: It is a violation of Federal law to use this product in a manner inconsistent with its labeling.

To protect dairy stock from hornflies, houseflies, stableflies, gnats and mosquitoes, spray after cattle enter the barn using 1 to 2 ounces per head, not to exceed 2 ounces per animal, per day. The spray should be applied as a light mist primarily to envelop or hit the flies as they attempt to leave the cows.

For blood-sucking lice on cattle, apply the spray lightly to infested areas, not over 2 ounces per animal, and use a stiff brush on such areas to get the spray to the base of the hair. Treatment for lice should not be repeated more than once every three weeks.

Space treatment in barns, houses and milk parlors for effective control of flies. Direct mist toward the upper portions of the enclosure, filling the air with fine spray particles, using approximately 2 ounces of material for each 1,000 cubic feet of space. Whenever possible, keep doors and windows closed for 10 minutes after application.

Face fly spray: Apply to face of animal in morning while stanchioned, just before releasing to pasture. Use a spray which produces large wetting droplets. Apply sufficient material to wet the face of the animal, but do not exceed 1.5 ounces per animal. Repeat daily, or as necessary.

Precautionary Statements: Hazards to Humans and Domestic Animals: Harmful if swallowed. Do not induce vomiting. Contact physician. If in eyes, flush with water and contact physician. If on the skin or clothing, remove clothing. Wash skin with soap and water. Avoid contamination of milk and milk handling equipment.

Statement of Practical Treatment:

If Swallowed: Call a physician or Poison Control Center. Do not induce vomiting. This product contains petroleum solvent Aspiration may be a hazard. Call a physician at once.

Inhaled: Remove to fresh air. Use artificial respiration if needed. Contact a physician.

In Eyes: In case of contact, immediately flush eyes with plenty of water. Get medical attention if irritation persists.

On Skin: Wash with soap and water immediately. Get medical attention if irritation persists.

Environmental Hazards: The product is toxic to fish. Keep out of water. Do not contaminate water by the cleaning of equipment or the disposal of wastes. Apply this product only as specified on the label.

Physical and Chemical Hazards: Do not use, pour, spill, or store near heat or open flame.

Storage and Disposal:

Prohibitions: Do not contaminate water, food, or feed by storage or disposal.

Pesticide disposal: Wastes resulting from the use of this product may be disposed of on site or at an approved waste disposal facility.

Container: Triple rinse (or equivalent). Then offer for recycling or reconditioning, or puncture and dispose of in a sanitary landfill, or incineration, or, if allowed by state and local authorities, by burning. If burned, stay out of smoke.

Warning(s): Keep out of reach of children.

Disclaimer: Notice- Seller's guarantee shall be limited to the terms of the label and subject thereto the buyer assumes any risk to persons or property arising out of use or handling and accepts the product on these conditions.

Presentation: 2.5 gallons.

Compendium Code No.: 10841441 9-96

PYRETHRIN PLUS SHAMPOO

Vedco **Parasiticide Shampoo**

EPA Reg. No.: 28293-140-44084

Active Ingredient(s):

Pyrethrins	0.15%
Piperonyl butoxide, technical*	1.50%
N-octyl bicycloheptene dicarboximide	0.50%
Inert ingredients	97.85%
Total	100.00%

*Equivalent to 1.20% (butylcarbityl) (6-propylpiperonyl) ether and 0.3% related compounds.

The product contains a protein base surfactant.

Indications: For use on dogs and cats to control fleas, lice and ticks.

Removes loose dandruff, dirt and scales. Leaves the coat soft and shining.

Directions for Use: It is a violation of federal law to use the product in a manner inconsistent with its labeling.

Thoroughly wet the entire animal with warm water. Apply enough shampoo to produce a lather.

Dilute one (1) part concentrate with two (2) parts water and apply as indicated below.

For the best effects on fleas, lice and ticks, allow the lather to remain on the animals for approximately five (5) minutes before rinsing.

Rinse thoroughly with warm water. May be repeated once or twice a week.

Precautionary Statements: Hazards to Humans and Domestic Animals: Harmful if swallowed. Avoid contact with the eyes. In case of contact, immediately flush the eyes with plenty of water. Get medical attention if irritation persists.

For external use on animals only.

Storage and Disposal:

Storage: Store in the original container in a cool, locked storage area.

Disposal: Do not re-use the empty container. Rinse thoroughly before discarding it in the trash. Securely wrap the original container in several layers of newspaper and discard it in the trash.

Warning(s): Keep out of reach of children.

Presentation: 6 oz, 12 oz and 1 gallon containers.

Compendium Code No.: 10941781

PYRETHRINS DIP AND SPRAY

Davis **Parasiticide Dip**

EPA Reg. No.: 50591-3

Active Ingredient(s):

Pyrethrins	3.0%
Piperonyl butoxide, technical*	30.0%
Petroleum distillate	12.0%
Inert ingredients	55.0%
Total	100.0%

*Equivalent to 24% (butylcarbityl)(6-propylpiperonyl) ether and 6% related compounds.

Indications: Davis PYRETHRINS DIP AND SPRAY is an ultra concentrated pyrethrin dip that kills fleas, ticks, and lice on dogs and cats (puppies and kittens over six weeks of age).

Dosage and Administration: It is a violation of federal law to use the product in a manner inconsistent with its labeling.

Shake well before using. To prepare dilutions, the concentrate should first be stirred or agitated well. Add the required amount of concentrate to the water and blend thoroughly.

To kill fleas and ticks on dogs and cats and to obtain protection against re-infestation, follow these steps:

1. Dilute ½ oz. (1 tbsp.) of the concentrate per one (1) gallon of water. For severe flea infestations, dilute 1 oz. (2 tbsp.) of the concentrate per one (1) gallon of water.
2. Apply directly to the animal by dipping or spraying. Dip or spray until the animal's skin is wet. Do not rinse.

To control fleas and ticks in the animal's environment, follow these steps:

1. Dilute 4 oz. of the concentrate per one (1) gallon of water.
2. Thoroughly spray the infested areas, pet beds, resting quarters, nearby cracks and crevices, along and behind baseboards, moldings, window and door frames and localized areas of floor and floor coverings. Fresh bedding should be placed in the animal quarters following treatment.

Precaution(s): Do not re-use the empty container. Wrap the container in several layers of newspaper and discard it in the trash. Do not use or store near heat or an open flame.

Caution(s): Keep out of the reach of children.

Precautionary Statements:

Hazards to Humans: Harmful if swallowed. Do not get in the eyes. Wash hands thoroughly after each use and before eating or smoking.

Hazards to Domestic Animals: Do not apply directly to or on the eyes, mouth or genitals of pets. Do not treat or cause exposure to kittens or puppies of less than four weeks of age.

Statement of Practical Treatment:

If swallowed: Contact a physician or poison control center immediately. Do not induce vomiting. The product contains petroleum distillate. Vomiting may cause aspiration pneumonia.

If in eyes or on skin: Flush the affected areas with plenty of water. Contact a physician if irritation persists.

Environmental Hazards: The product is toxic to fish. Do not dispose of in lakes, streams or open ponds.

Warning(s): Buyer assumes all risks of use, storage or handling of the material not in strict accordance given on the label.

Presentation: 16 oz. and 1 gallon containers.

Compendium Code No.: 11410341

PZI VET® ℞

Idexx Pharm. **Insulin**

(Protamine Zinc Insulin)

Active Ingredient(s): PZI VET® insulin is a white to off-white sterile injectable suspension that contains 40 International Units (U) of insulin per milliliter. It is formulated within a pH range of 7.1 to 7.4. Inactive ingredients include phenol, glycerin, dibasic sodium phosphate, and sterile water for injection.

Indications: PZI VET® insulin is indicated for the reduction of hyperglycemia and hyperglycemia-associated clinical signs in cats with diabetes mellitus.

Pharmacology: Description PZI VET® insulin is composed of a mixture of 90% beef and 10% pork insulin. Species differences in insulin structure occur due to amino acid substitutions. Feline insulin differs from bovine insulin by one amino acid and from porcine insulin by four amino acids.[1,2]

The insulin is complexed with protamine zinc to form a microcrystalline suspension that results in prolonged dissolution, delivery and an extended duration of effect.[3,4]

Dosage and Administration: PZI VET® insulin should be administered subcutaneously. Dosage regimens of PZI VET® insulin will vary among patients. The recommended starting dose is 0.1-0.3 U per pound of body weight (0.22-0.6 U/kg) every 12 to 24 hours. This dose should be adjusted based on changes in blood glucose levels and resolution of clinical signs. Further adjustments in dosage may be necessary with changes in the cat's diet, body weight, or concomitant medication, or if the cat develops concurrent infection, inflammation, neoplasia, or an additional endocrine or other medical disorder.[5]

The time course of action of all insulin types may vary within and between individual patients. The duration also depends on the site of injection, concurrent secretion of insulin antagonistic hormones and the cat's hydration status and physical activity level.

The vial should be gently rolled to re-suspend the insulin before each use. Do not shake. PZI VET® insulin should appear uniformly cloudy or milky after re-suspending. Do not use if a pellet of white material remains at the bottom of the vial after re-suspending. Do not use if clumps are apparent after re-suspending.

Drug Interactions: Insulin requirements may be increased by medications with hyperglycemic activity, most notably glucocorticoids and progestagens.[8,9] Insulin requirements may be decreased by medications with antidiabetic activity, such as oral hypoglycemic drugs, or antihyperglycemic drugs.

Contraindication(s): PZI VET® insulin is contraindicated during episodes of hypoglycemia and in cats sensitive to protamine zinc insulin or any other ingredients in PZI VET® insulin.

Precaution(s): Storage Conditions: Store at 2°-8°C (36°-46°F). Do not freeze. Do not expose to direct sunlight.

Caution(s): Federal (USA) law restricts this drug to use by or on the order of a licensed veterinarian.

Any change in insulin should be made cautiously and only under a veterinarian's supervision. Changes in insulin strength, manufacturer, type, species (animal, human) or method of manufacture (rDNA versus animal-source insulin) may result in the need for a change in dosage.

Use PZI VET® with U-40 syringes only. Use of a syringe other than a U-40 syringe will result in incorrect dosing.

General: Hypoglycemia, hypokalemia, hypophosphatemia and allergic reactions are among the clinical adverse effects associated with the use of insulin.[5,6] Care should be taken in dosing cats with inappetence or vomiting.

Hypoglycemic reaction may be associated with the administration of PZI VET® (see Warnings). Common causes for hypoglycemia include excessive doses of insulin, failure to eat, overlap of insulin activity in cats treated twice daily, strenuous exercise, correction of obesity or other insulin antagonistic disorders, concomitant use of oral antidiabetic drugs, discontinuation of insulin antagonistic drugs, and reversion to a noninsulin-dependent state.[5,7]

Mixing and Diluting of Insulins: Diluting PZI VET® insulin or mixing it with other insulins is not recommended.

For animal use only.

Warning(s): Keep out of reach of children.

Human safety: Contact your physician immediately in case of accidental injection with this insulin product.

Animal safety: Use of this product, even at established doses, has been associated with hypoglycemia. An animal with signs of hypoglycemia should be treated immediately. Glucose should be given orally or intravenously as dictated by clinical signs. Insulin should be temporarily withheld and, subsequently, the dosage should be adjusted, if indicated.

Adverse Reactions: Hypoglycemia with and without associated clinical signs (lethargy, shakiness, and seizures) may be observed after treatment with PZI VET®. To report adverse reactions, call 1-800-374-8006.

References: Available upon request.

Presentation: 10 mL multiple dose vials, each mL containing 40 U protamine zinc insulin.

PZI VET is a trademark of Idexx Pharmaceuticals, Inc.

Compendium Code No.: 15070030 3-490-1611

P

P

Disclaimer
Every effort has been made to ensure the accuracy of the information published. However, it remains the responsibility of the readers to familiarize themselves with the product information contained on the product label or package insert.
Inclusion or omission of products does not imply endorsement or criticism by the Publisher or anyone involved in the publication. Inclusion does not imply product availability and/or product registration. The Publisher, Editorial Team and all those involved in the production of this book cannot be held responsible for publication errors or any consequence that could result from the use of published information.

Q

QUADRITOP™ CREAM ℞

Vetus **Topical Antimicrobial-Antifungal-Corticosteroid**

Nystatin-Neomycin Sulfate-Thiostrepton-Triamcinolone Acetonide Cream Veterinary

ANADA No.: 200-245

Active Ingredient(s): Description: Nystatin-Neomycin Sulfate-Thiostrepton-Triamcinolone Acetonide Cream combines nystatin, neomycin sulfate, thiostrepton, and triamcinolone acetonide.

Each gram contains:

Nystatin	100,000 units
Neomycin sulfate equivalent to neomycin base	2.5 mg
Thiostrepton	2500 units
Triamcinolone acetonide	1.0 mg

in an aqueous. nonirritating vanishing cream base with cetearyl alcohol (and) ceteareth-20, ethylenediamine hydrochloride, methyl paraben, propyl paraben, propylene glycol, sorbitol solution, titanium dioxide, sodium citrate, citric acid, white petrolatum, glyceryl monostearste, polyethylene glycol monostearate, sorbic acid and simethicone.

Indications: Nystatin-Neomycin Sultate-Thiostrepton-Triamcinolone Acetonide Cream is indicated in the management of dermatologic disorders in dogs and cats, characterized by inflammation and dry or exudative dermatitis, particularly those caused, complicated or threatened by bacterial or candidal *(Candida albicans)* infections. It is also of value in eczematous dermatitis; contact dermatitis, and seborrheic dermatitis, and as an adjunct in the treatment of dermatitis due to parasitic infestation.

Pharmacology: Actions: By virtue of its four active ingredients, Nystatin-Neomycin Sulfate-Thiostrepton-Triamcinolone Acetonide Cream provides four basic therapeutic effects: antiinflammatory, antipruritic, antifungal and antibacterial. Triamcinolone Acetonide is a potent synthetic corticosteroid providing rapid and prolonged symptomatic relief on topical administration. Inflammation, edema, and pruritus promptly subside, and lesions are permitted to heal. Nystatin is the first well tolerated antifungal agent antibiotic of dependable efficacy for the treatment of cutaneous infections caused by *Candida albicans* (Monilia). Nystatin is fungistatic *in vitro* against a variety of yeast and yeast like fungi including many fungi pathogenic to animals. No appreciable activity is exhibited against bacteria. Thiostrepton has a high order of activity against gram positive organisms, including many which are resistant to other antibiotics; neomycin exerts antimicrobial action against a wide range of gram-positive and gram negative bacteria. Together they provide comprehensive therapy against those organisms responsible for most superficial bacterial infections.

Dosage and Administration: Frequency of administration is dependent on the severity of the condition. For mild inflammation, application may range from once daily to once a week; for severe conditions Nystatin-Neomycin Sulfate-Thiostrepton-Triamcinolone Acetonide Cream may be applied as often as 2 to 3 times daily, if necessary. Frequency of treatment may be decreased as improvement occurs.

Clean affected areas, removing any encrusted discharge or exudate. Apply Nystatin-Neomycin Sulfate-Thiostrepton-Triamcinolone Acetonide Cream sparingly in a thin film.

Contraindication(s): Nystatin-Neomycin Sulfate-Thiostrepton-Triamcinolone Acetonide Cream should not be used ophthalmically.

Caution(s): Federal law restricts this drug to use by or on the order of a licensed veterinarian.

Nystatin-Neomycin Sulfate-Thiostrepton-Triamcinolone Acetonide Cream is not intended for the treatment of deep abscesses or deep seated infections such as inflammation of the lymphatic vessels. Parenteral antibiotic therapy is indicated in these infections.

Nystatin-Neomycin Sulfate-Thiostrepton-Triamcinolone Acetonide Cream has been extremely well tolerated. The occurrence of systemic reactions is rarely a problem with topical administration.

Sensitivity to neomycin may occur. If redness, irritation or swelling persists or increases, discontinue use. Do not use if pus is present since the drug may allow the infection to spread.

Avoid ingestion. Oral or parenteral use of corticosteroids, depending on dose, duration and specific steroids, may result in inhibition of endogenous steroid production following drug withdrawal.

Warning(s): Nystatin-Neomycin-Sulfate-Thiostrepton-Triamcinolone Acetonide Cream is indicated for use in dogs and cats only. Not for use in animals which are raised for food.

Absorption of triamcinolone acetonide through topical application and by licking may occur. Therefore animals should be observed closely for signs of polydipsia, polyuria, and increased weight gain particularly when the preparation is used over large areas or for extended periods of time.

Clinical and experimental data have demonstrated that corticosteroids administered orally or by injection to animals may induce the first stage of parturition if used during the last trimester of pregnancy and may precipitate premature parturition followed by dystocia, fetal death, retained placenta and metritis.

Additionally, corticosteroids administered to dogs, rabbits and rodents during pregnancy have resulted in cleft palate in offspring. Corticosteroids administered to dogs during pregnancy have also resulted in other congenital anomalies including deformed forelegs, phocomelia and anasarca.

Side Effects: SAP and SGPT (ALT) enzyme elevation, polydipsia and polyuria have occurred following parenteral or systemic use of synthetic corticosteroids in dogs. Vomiting and diarrhea (occasionally bloody) have been observed in dogs. Cushing's syndrome in dogs has been reported in association with prolonged or repeated steroid therapy.

Presentation: Nystatin-Neomycin Sulfate-Thiostrepton-Triamcinolone Acetonide Cream is supplied in 7.5 gram and 15 gram tubes.

Manufactured by: Med-Pharmex, Inc., Pomona, CA 91767

Compendium Code No.: 14440790

April 1999

QUADRITOP™ OINTMENT

Vetus **Topical Antimicrobial-Antifungal-Corticosteroid**

Nystatin-Neomycin Sulfate-Thiostrepton-Triamcinolone Acetonide Ointment

NADA No.: 140-810

Active Ingredient(s): QUADRITOP™ Ointment is a combination of nystatin, neomycin sulfate, thiostrepton and triamcinolone acetonide in a nonirritating vehicle, a polyethylene and mineral oil gel base.

Each mL contains:

Nystatin	100,000 units
Neomycin sulfate (equivalent to neomycin base)	2.5 mg
Thiostrepton	2,500 units
Triamcinolone acetonide	1.0 mg

Indications: QUADRITOP™ Ointment is useful in the treatment of acute and chronic otitis of varied etiologies, in interdigital cysts in cats and dogs, and in anal gland infections in dogs.

The preparation is also indicated in the management of dermatologic disorders characterized by inflammation and dry or exudative dermatitis, particularly those caused, complicated, or threatened by bacterial or candidal *(Candida albicans)* infections.

It is also indicated in eczematous dermatitis, contact dermatitis, and seborrheic dermatitis, and for use as an adjunct in the treatment of dermatitis due to parasitic infection.

Pharmacology: The ointment provides four therapeutic effects including anti-inflammatory, antipruritic, antifungal and antibacterial. Triamcinolone acetonide is a synthetic corticosteroid providing rapid and prolonged symptomatic relief upon topical administration. Inflammation, edema and pruritus subside and lesions are permitted to heal. Nystatin is the first well-tolerated antifungal antibiotic of dependable efficacy for the treatment of cutaneous infection caused by *Candida albicans* (monilia).

Nystatin is fungistatic *in vitro* against a variety of yeast and yeast-like fungi including many fungi pathogenic to animals. Activity is not exhibited against bacteria.

Thiostrepton has activity against gram-positive organisms, including many which are resistant to other antibiotics, neomycin exerts antimicrobial action against a wide range of gram-positive and gram-negative bacterial. Together they provide comprehensive therapy against organisms responsible for most superficial bacterial infections.

Dosage and Administration: The frequency of administration depends upon the severity of the condition.

For mild inflammations, the application may range from once a day to once a week.

For severe conditions QUADRITOP™ Ointment may be applied two (2) to three (3) times a day, if necessary. The frequency of the treatment may be decreased as improvement occurs.

Wear gloves during the administration of the ointment or wash hands immediately after the application.

Otitis: Clean the ear canal of impacted cerumen. Inspect the canal and remove any foreign bodies such as grass lawns, ticks, etc. Instill three (3) to five (5) drops of QUADRITOP™ Ointment. Preliminary use of a local anesthetic such as Proparacaine Hydrochloride Ophthalmic Solution may be advisable.

Infected anal glands, cystic areas, etc.: Drain the gland or cyst and then fill it with QUADRITOP™ Ointment.

Other dermatologic disorders: Clean the affected areas, removing any encrusted discharge or exudate. Apply thiostrepton-traimcinolone acetonide ointment sparingly in a thin film.

Precaution(s):

7.5 mL, 15 mL and 30 mL tubes: Store at room temperature and avoid excessive heat (104°F).

240 mL bottle: Do not store above 86°F.

Caution(s): QUADRITOP™ Ointment is not intended for the treatment of deep abscesses or deep-seated infections such as inflammation of the lymphatic vessels. Parenteral antibiotic therapy is indicated in these infections.

QUADRITOP™ Ointment (nystatin-neomycin sulfate-thiostrepton-triamcinolone acetonide ointment) has been well-tolerated. Cutaneous reactions attributable to its use have been rare. The occurrence of systemic reaction is rarely a problem with topical administration.

There is evidence that corticosteroids can be absorbed after topical application and cause systemic effects. Therefore, an animal receiving QUADRITOP™ Ointment therapy should be observed closely for signs such as polydipsia, polyuria, and increased weight gain. QUADRITOP™ Ointment is not generally recommended for the treatment of deep or puncture wounds, or serious burns.

Sensitivity to neomycin may occur. If redness, irritation or swelling persists or increases, discontinue use. Do not use if pus is present since the drug may allow the infection to spread.

Keep out of the reach of children.

Avoid ingestion.

Oral or parental use of corticosteroids (depending upon the dose, the duration of use, and the specific steroid) may result in the inhibition of endogenous steroid production following drug withdrawal.

Before instilling any medication into the ear, examine the external ear canal thoroughly so that the tympanic membrane is not ruptured, avoiding the possibility of transmitting an infection into the middle ear as well as damaging the cochlea or vestibular apparatus from prolonged contact.

If hearing or vestibular dysfunction is noted during the course of treatment, discontinue the use of QUADRITOP™ Ointment.

Warning(s): Clinical and experimental data have demonstrated that corticosteroids administered orally or by injection to animals may induce the first stage of parturition if used during the last trimester of pregnancy and may precipitate premature parturition followed by dystocia, fetal death, retained placenta and metritis.

Corticosteroids administered to dogs, rabbits, and rodents during pregnancy have resulted in cleft palate in the offspring.

In dogs, other congenital anomalies have resulted including deformed forelegs, phocomelia and anasarca.

Side Effects: SAP and SGPT (ALT) enzyme elevations, polydipsia and polyuria, vomiting, and diarrhea (occasionally bloody) have been observed following the parenteral or systemic use of synthetic corticosteroids in dogs.

Cushing's syndrome has been reported in association with prolonged or repeated steroid therapy in dogs. Temporary hearing loss has been reported in conjunction with treatment of otitis with products containing corticosteroids. However, regression usually occurs following withdrawal of the drug. If hearing dysfunction is noted during the course of treatment with QUADRITOP™ Ointment, discontinue its use.

Presentation: QUADRITOP™ Ointment is supplied in ¼ fl. oz. (7.5 mL) tubes, ¼ fl. oz. (7.5 mL) tubes x 144 units, ½ fl. oz. (15 mL) tubes, ½ fl. oz. (15 mL) tubes x 72 units, 1 fl. oz. (30 mL) tubes and a 8 fl. oz. (240 mL) tube applicator bottle.

Compendium Code No.: 14440800

QUARTERMASTER® ℞

Pharmacia & Upjohn **Mastitis Therapy**

penicillin-dihydrostreptomycin in oil

NADA No.: 055-028

Active Ingredient(s): Each 10 mL Plastet® Disposable Syringe contains 1,000,000 units of Procaine Penicillin G micronized, and 1 gram of Dihydrostreptomycin base, as Dihydrostreptomycin Sulfate, in an extended action base consisting of 1% w/v Hydrogenated Peanut Oil, 3% w/v Aluminum Monostearate, and Peanut Oil, q.s.

Manufactured by a non-sterilizing process.

Indications: For intramammary use to reduce the frequency of existing infection and to prevent new infections with *Staphylococcus aureus* in dry cows.

Pharmacology: Action: Infusion of antibiotics at the start of the drying off period has the following advantages: (1) it is active against existing infections; (2) it is prophylactic against new infections, during the time when cattle are likely to become infected[1]; (3) the antibiotic remains in the udder for a sufficiently long period to accomplish the intended objective and is not diluted with milk, as is the case in lactation therapy; (4) the danger of drug residues in the milk is reduced.

Antibiotic control is to be considered an adjunct to good herd hygiene management and milking management. Detailed field studies in England and the United States have demonstrated that a program consisting of treatment, at the time of drying off, with a highly effective antibiotic preparation in a slow-release base, and routine dipping of teats after each milking with an effective disinfectant, markedly reduces the incidence of all udder infections at calving.[2,3,4]

It has recently been recommended that a disinfectant teat dip be used on unmilked cows, or at least be used for 10 days before parturition[5], to reduce the bacterial challenge to the depleted levels of antibiotic in the teat as freshening is approached.[6]

When the herd infection level has been reduced, or when herds are not heavily infected initially, it may be desirable to be selective in treating dry quarters.[7]

Directions for Use:

Directions for Using the Flexi-Tube® System: The Flexi-Tube® is designed to provide the choice of either insertion of the full cannula, as has traditionally been practiced, or insertion of no more than 1/8 inch of the cannula, as recommended by the National Mastitis Council.

a. Full Insertion: Remove the white end cap by pulling straight up as shown. Gently insert the full cannula into the teat canal; carefully infuse the product.

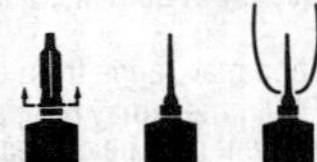

b. Partial Insertion: Remove both the white end cap and the red cannula by pushing sideways as shown. Gently insert the exposed white tip into the teat canal; carefully infuse the product.

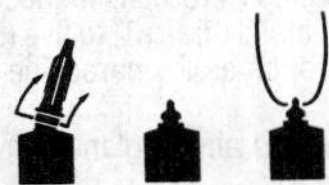

At the last milking prior to drying off, completely milk out cow. Warm the syringe containing QUARTERMASTER® Suspension to body temperature; choose the desired insertion length (full or partial) and insert tip into teat canal; slowly infuse the entire contents. Instill the contents of one syringe into each quarter. Discard the syringe after use. Treated teats should then be dipped into an effective teat dip. The teat or quarter should not be manipulated again until the cow freshens. To achieve and maintain a lower frequency of infection, proper dipping of teats during lactation is recommended.

Shake vigorously for 10 seconds immediately before using.

Precaution(s): Storage Conditions: Store at controlled room temperature 20° to 25°C (68° to 77°F) [see USP].

Caution(s): Federal law restricts this drug to use by or on the order of a licensed veterinarian.

Warning(s): For udder instillation upon drying off only. Not to be used within six (6) weeks of freshening. Not for use in lactating cows. Milk taken from animals within 96 hours (8 milkings) after calving must not be used for food. Animals infused with this product must not be slaughtered for food within 60 days from time of infusion nor within 96 hours after calving.

Attention Doctor: It is your responsibility to inform your clients of the warnings stated above so as to avoid adulteration of meat or milk and possible prosecution under Federal law.

References: Available upon request.

Presentation: QUARTERMASTER® Suspension is supplied in packers containing 12-10 mL (.33 fl oz) Plastet® Disposable Syringes with 12 convenient single-use isopropyl alcohol pads (NDC 0009-3267-03).

Manufactured by: West Agro, Inc., Hamilton, NY 13346.

QUARTERMASTER is a Trademark of West Agro, Inc.

Compendium Code No.: 10490461 817 005 001

QUATCIDE

Bio-Tek **Disinfectant**

Disinfectant-Sanitizer, Virucide*-Mildewstat (on hard inanimate surfaces)

EPA Reg. No.: 10324-94-11725

Active Ingredient(s):

n-Alkyl (60% C_{14}, 30% C_{16}, 5% C_{12}, 5% C_{18}) dimethyl benzyl ammonium chloride	10.0%
n-Alkyl (68% C_{12}, 32% C_{14}) dimethyl ethylbenzyl ammonium chloride	10.0%
Inert Ingredients:	80.0%
Total:	100.0%

Directions for Use: It is a violation of Federal Law to use this product in a manner inconsistent with its labeling.

This product is not to be used as a terminal sterilant/high level disinfectant on any surface or instrument that (1) is introduced directly into the human body, either into or in contact with the bloodstream or normally sterile areas of the body or (2) contacts intact mucous membranes but which does not ordinarily penetrate the blood barrier or otherwise enter normally sterile areas of the body. This product may be used to preclean or decontaminate critical or semi-critical medical devices prior to sterilization or high level disinfection.

Solution is designed specifically for hospitals, food processing plants, dairies, restaurants, bars, animal quarters, poultry and turkey farms, hatcheries, kennels and institutions where disinfection, sanitation, and deodorization is of prime importance. When used as directed, solution is formulated to disinfect pre-cleaned inanimate, hard surfaces such as walls, floors, sink tops, tables, chairs telephones, and bed frames.

This product deodorizes those areas which generally are hard to keep fresh smelling, such as garbage storage areas, empty garbage bins and cans, pet areas and any other areas which are prone to odors caused by microorganism. In addition, this product will sanitize previously cleaned and rinsed non-porous food contact surfaces such as tanks, chopping blocks, counter tops, drinking glasses and eating utensils. This product can also be used to sanitize previously cleaned food grade eggs in shell egg and egg product processing plants.

Disinfection: To disinfect pre-cleaned, inanimate, hard surfaces apply this product with a mop, cloth, sponge or mechanical sprayer so as to wet all surfaces thoroughly. Allow to remain wet for 10 minutes, then remove excess liquid. For disinfection, a pre-cleaning step is required. Prepare a fresh solution for each use.

Dilution Rates:

General Disinfection: Add 1½ ounces of this product per 5 gallons of water for disinfection against *Staphylococcus aureus, Salmonella choleraesuis, Listeria monocytogenes.*

Hospital Disinfection: Add 1¾ ounces of this product per 5 gallons of water for disinfection against *Pseudomonas aeruginosa.*

Other Uses: For disinfection of pre-cleaned surgical instruments, barber tools and dental equipment, simply submerge instruments into solution containing ¾ ounce of this product per gallon of water for 10 minutes.

For disinfection of pre-cleaned poultry equipment (brooders. watering founts, feeding equipment and incubators), animal quarters and kennels, apply a solution of 1¾ ounces of this product per 5 gallons of water. Small utensils should be immersed in this solution. Prior to disinfection, all poultry, other animals and their feeds must be removed from the premise. This includes emptying all troughs, racks and other feeding and watering appliances. Remove all litter and droppings from floors, walls and other surfaces occupied or traversed by poultry or other animals.

After disinfection, ventilate building, coops, and other closed spaces. Do not house poultry or other animals or employ equipment until treatment has been absorbed, set or dried. After treatment, thoroughly scrub treated feed racks, troughs, automatic feeders, fountains, and waterers with soap or detergent and rinse with potable water before reuse. All treated equipment that will contact feed or drinking water must be rinsed with potable water before reuse.

Sanitation: Recommended for use in restaurants, dairies, food processing plants, and bars. When used as directed, this product is an effective sanitizer against *Escherichia coli* and *Staphylococcus aureus.* Remove all gross food particles and soil from areas which are to be sanitized with a good detergent, pre-flush, pre-soak or pre-scrape treatment. Rinse with a potable water rinse.

To sanitize pre-cleaned and potable water-rinsed, non-porous food contact surfaces prepare a 200 ppm active quaternary solution by adding ½ ounce of this product to 4 gallons of water, 1¼ ounces to 10 gallons of water or 2½ ounces to 20 gallons of water.

To sanitize immobile items such as tanks, chopping blocks and counter tops, flood the area with a 200 ppm active quaternary solution for at least 60 seconds, making sure to wet all surfaces completely. Remove, drain the use solution from the surface, and air dry. Prepare a fresh solution daily or more frequently as soil is apparent.

To sanitize mobile items such as drinking glasses and eating utensils, immerse in a 200 ppm active quaternary solution for at least 60 seconds, making sure to immerse completely. Remove, drain the used solution from the surface and air dry. Prepare a fresh solution daily or more frequently as soil is apparent.

Efficacy tests have demonstrated that this product is an effective bactericide and virucide in the presence of organic soil (5% blood serum).

To sanitize mobile items such as drinking glasses and eating utensils, immerse in a 200 ppm active quaternary solution for at least 60 seconds, making sure to immerse completely. Remove, drain the used solution from the surface and air dry. Prepare a fresh solution daily or more frequently as soil is apparent. When used for sanitization of previously cleaned food equipment or food contact items, limit the active quaternary to 200 ppm. No potable water rinse is required. This product in an effective sanitizer when diluted in water to 750 ppm hardness. ($CaCO_3$).

To sanitize previously cleaned food grade eggs in shell egg and egg product processing plants, spray with a solution of ½ ounce of this product in 4 gallons of warm water (200 ppm active quaternary solution) The solution should be warmer than the eggs, but not to exceed 130°F. Wet eggs thoroughly and allow to drain. Eggs sanitized with this product shall be subjected to potable water rinse only if they are broken immediately for use in the manufacture of egg products. Eggs should be dry before casing or breaking. The solution should not be reused for sanitizing eggs.

Virucidal Activity: This product, when used on environmental, inanimate hard surfaces at 1¾ ounces per 5 gallons of water exhibits effective virucidal activity against Influenza A2/Japan (representative of the common flu virus). Herpes Simplex Type 1, (causative agent of fever blisters), Vaccinia virus (representative of the pox virus group), Avian influenza A/Turkey/Wisconsin (causative agent of an acute avian lower respiratory tract infection) Newcastle disease virus and Laryngotracheitis Virus.

At 2.5 oz. per 5 gallons in the presence of 5% blood serum and 400 ppm of hardness for a 2 minute contact time this product was found to be effective against HIV-1 (AIDS Virus).

Special Instructions for Cleaning and Decontamination Against HIV-1 on Surface/Objects Soiled with Blood/Body Fluids.

Effective against HIV on pre-cleaned environmental surfaces/objects previously soiled with blood/body fluids in health care settings or other settings in which there is an expected likelihood of soiling of inanimate surfaces/objects with blood or body fluids, and in which the surfaces/objects likely to be soiled with blood or body fluids can be associated with the potential for transmission of human immunodeficiency virus Type 1 (HIV-1) (associated with AIDS).

Personal Protection: Specific barrier protection items to be used when handling items soiled with blood or body fluids are disposable latex gloves, gowns, masks, or eye coverings.

Cleaning Procedure: Blood and other body fluids must be thoroughly cleaned from surfaces and objects before application of the disinfectant.

Disposal of Infectious Materials: Blood and other body fluids should be autoclaved and disposed of according to federal, state and local regulations for infectious waste disposal.

Contact Time: Leave surfaces wet for 2 minutes. This contact time will not control other common type of viruses and bacteria.

Deodorization: To deodorize, apply this product as indicated under the heading General Disinfection.

Mildewstat: To control mold and mildew on pre-cleaned, hard, nonporous surfaces add 1½ ounces of this product per 5 gallons of water. Apply solution with a cloth, mop or sponge making sure to wet all surfaces completely. Let air dry. Prepare a fresh solution for each use. Repeat application at weekly intervals or when mildew growth appears.

Precautionary Statements: Hazards to Humans and Domestic Animals:

Danger: Corrosive. Causes irreversible eye damage and skin burns. Do not get in eyes, on skin or on clothing. Wear goggles or face shield and rubber gloves when handling. May be fatal if swallowed. Remove contaminated clothing and wash clothing before reuse. Wash thoroughly with soap and water after handling and before eating, drinking or using tobacco.

Statement of Practical Treatment:

If on Skin: Wash with plenty of soap and water. Get medical attention.

If in Eyes: Hold eyelids open and flush with a steady, gentle stream of water for 15 minutes. Get medical attention.

If Swallowed: Call a physician or Poison Control Center. Drink 1 or 2 glasses of water and induce vomiting by touching the back of the throat with finger. If person is unconscious, do not give anything by mouth and do not induce vomiting.

Storage and Disposal: Do not contaminate water, food or feed by storage or disposal. Open dumping is prohibited. Store only in original container. Do not reuse empty container. Keep this product under locked storage sufficient to make it inaccessible to children or persons unfamiliar with its proper use.

Pesticide Disposal: Pesticide wastes are acutely hazardous. Improper disposal of excess pesticide, spray mixture or rinsate is a violation of federal law. If these wastes cannot be disposed of by use according to label instructions, contact your State Pesticide or Environmental Control Agency, or the Hazardous Waste Representative at the nearest EPA Regional Office for guidance.

Container Disposal:

Larger than 1 gallon - Triple rinse (or equivalent). Then offer for recycling or reconditioning, or puncture and dispose of in a sanitary landfill, or by other procedures approved by state and local authorities. In addition, plastic containers may be disposed of by incineration, of if allowed by state and local authorities, by burning. If burned, stay out of smoke.

1 gallon and smaller - Do not reuse empty container. Wrap container and put in trash.

Warning(s): Keep out of reach of children.

Presentation: 4 x 1 gallon containers per case and 55 gallon drums.

Compendium Code No.: 13700050

QUATRACON-2X™

Boehringer Ingelheim **Antiserum**

Actinomyces Pyogenes-Escherichia Coli-Pasteurella Multocida-Salmonella Typhimurium Antibody, Bovine Origin

U.S. Vet. Lic. No.: 124

Composition: The concentrated serum is prepared from the blood of cattle hyperimmunized with *Actinomyces pyogenes, Pasteurella multocida,* Carter's Serotype A, *Escherichia coli* serotype 78:K80:NM, and *Salmonella typhimurium.*

Contains 0.2% cresol as a preservative.

Indications: This product is recommended for the prophylaxis and treatment of disease caused by *Actinomyces pyogenes, Pasteurella multocida, Escherichia coli,* and *Salmonella typhimurium* in cattle.

Dosage and Administration: Shake well before using.

Prophylactic: 15 mL per 50 lbs. body weight administered subcutaneously as soon as possible after birth.

Therapeutic: 30 mL per 50 lbs. body weight, repeat each 12 to 24 hours (depending upon condition of the animal) until improvement is satisfactory.

Precaution(s): Store out of direct sunlight at a temperature between 35-45°F (2-7°C). Avoid freezing. Use entire contents when first opened.

Caution(s): Do not vaccinate with bovine virus diarrhea vaccine, bovine rhinotracheitis vaccine, or bovine parainfluenza$_3$ vaccine or *Haemophilus somnus* or *Pasteurella haemolytica* bacterin within 21 days after use of this serum. Anaphylactoid reactions may occur.

Antidote(s): Epinephrine.

Warning(s): Do not vaccinate within 21 days before slaughter.

Presentation: 250 mL vials.

Compendium Code No.: 10280931 BI 1137-3 2/01

QUATROL

Bio-Tek **Disinfectant**

Cleaner, Disinfectant, Detergent, Fungicide (against Pathogenic fungi), Deodorizer, Sanitizer, Virucide*, Mildewstat (on hard inanimate surfaces)

EPA Reg. No.: 10324-56-11725

Active Ingredient(s):

n-Alkyl (60% C_{14}, 30% C_{16}, 5% C_{12}, 5% C_{18}) dimethyl benzyl ammonium chloride	6.25%
n-Alkyl (68% C_{12}, 32% C_{14}) dimethyl ethylbenzyl ammonium chloride	6.25%
Inert Ingredients:	87.50%
Total	100.00%

Directions for Use: It is a violation of Federal Law to use this product in a manner inconsistent with its labeling.

This product is not to be used as a terminal sterilant/high level disinfectant on any surface or instrument that (1) is introduced directly into the human body, either into or in contact with the bloodstream or normally sterile areas of the body, or (2) contacts intact mucous membranes but which does not ordinarily penetrate the blood barrier or otherwise enter normally sterile areas of the body. This product may be used to preclean or decontaminate critical or semi-critical medical devices prior to sterilization or high level disinfection.

This detergent/disinfectant has been designed specifically for hospitals, nursing homes, schools, food processing plants, food service establishments and other institutions where housekeeping is of prime importance.

Disinfection: To disinfect hard inanimate surfaces (such as walls, floors, table tops) add ½ oz detergent/disinfectant per gallon of water. Apply solution with mop, cloth, sponge or mechanical sprayer so as to wet all surfaces thoroughly. Allow to remain wet for 10 minutes and then let air dry. To disinfect toilet bowls, flush toilet, add ½ oz detergent/disinfectant directly to the bowl water. Swab the bowl completely using a scrub brush or toilet mop making sure to get under the rim. Let stand for 10 minutes and flush.

For heavily soiled areas, a pre-cleaning step is required. Prepare a fresh solution for each use.

Mildewstat: Controls the growth of mold and mildew on pre-cleaned hard non-porous surfaces (such as floors, walls, table tops) add ½ oz of this product per gallon of water. Apply solution with a cloth, mop or sponge making sure to wet all surfaces completely. Let air dry. Prepare a fresh solution for each use. Repeat application at weekly intervals or when mildew growth reappears.

Sanitization: To sanitize previously cleaned and rinsed non-porous food contact surfaces, prepare 200 ppm active quaternary solution by adding 1 oz to 5 gallons of water. When used for sanitization of previously cleaned food equipment or food contact items limit active quaternaries — to 200 ppm. At this level no potable water rinse is required.

To sanitize immobile items (such as tanks, chopping blocks, counter tops) flood the area with 200 ppm solution or apply with a cloth or sponge making sure to wet all surfaces completely for at least 60 seconds. Let air dry. Prepare a fresh solution for each use.

To sanitize mobile items (such as drinking glasses, eating utensils), immerse in 200 ppm solution for at least 60 seconds making sure to immerse completely. Remove and let air dry. Prepare a fresh solution daily or more frequently as soil is apparent.

It is an effective sanitizer when diluted in water up to 600 ppm hardness ($CaCO_3$).

Disinfection: At ½ oz per gallon dilution, this product exhibits effective disinfectant activity against the following - *Brevibacterium ammoniagenes; Enterobacter aerogenes; Escherichia coli; Klebsiella pneumoniae; Pseudomonas aeruginosa,* PRD-10; *Salmonella choleraesuis; Salmonella schottmuelleri; Shigella dysenteriae; Staphylococcus aureus; Streptococcus faecalis; Streptococcus salivarius.*

At this level the product is also fungicidal against the pathogenic fungi: *Trichophyton mentagrophytes.*

Virucidal* Activity: The product when used on environmental inanimate hard surfaces at ½ oz per gallon of water exhibits effective virucidal* activity against Influenza A2/Japan (representative of the common flu virus), Herpes simplex, Type 1 (causative agent of fever blisters) and Vaccinia Virus (representative of the pox virus group). Efficacy tests have demonstrated that this product is an effective bactericide, fungicide and virucide* in the presence of organic soil (5% blood serum).

At 1.5 ounces per 2 gallons in the presence of 5% blood serum and 400 ppm of hardness for a 2 minute contact time this product was found to be effective against HIV-1 (AIDS Virus).

Special Instructions for Cleaning and Decontamination Against HIV-1 on Surfaces/Objects Soiled with Blood/Body Fluids:

Effective against HIV on pre-cleaned environmental surfaces/objects previously soiled with blood/body fluids in health care settings or other settings in which there is an expected likelihood of soiling of inanimate surfaces/objects with blood or body fluids, and in which the surfaces/objects likely to be soiled with blood or body fluids can be associated with the potential for transmission of human immunodeficiency virus Type 1 (HIV-1) (associated with AIDS).

Personal Protection: Specific barrier protection items to be used when handling items soiled with blood or body fluids are disposable latex gloves, gowns, masks, or eye coverings.

Cleaning Procedure: Blood and other body fluids must be thoroughly cleaned from surfaces and objects before application of the disinfectant.

Disposal of Infectious Materials: Blood and other body fluids should be autoclaved and disposed of according to federal, state and local regulations for infectious waste disposal.

Contact Time: Leave surfaces wet for 2 minutes. This contact time will not control other common type of viruses and bacteria.

Mold and Mildewstat: This product controls the growth of mold and mildew and the odors they cause on hard non-porous inanimate surfaces.

This product is a phosphate free detergent/disinfectant which provides effective cleaning, deodorizing, disinfection, and sanitization. It been designed specifically for hospitals, nursing homes, schools, food processing plants, and other institutions where housekeeping is of prime importance in controlling the hazard of cross contamination.

This product when diluted at the rate of ½ ounces per gallon of water is an effective disinfectant against the organism *Pseudomonas aeruginosa* and meets all requirements for hospital use. When used as directed, it is formulated to disinfect inanimate hard surfaces such as walls, floors, sink tops, toilet bowls, tables, chairs and telephones, and bed frames. For larger areas such as operating rooms, patient care facilities and restrooms, the product is designed to provide both general cleaning and disinfecting.

In addition, this product deodorizes those areas which generally are hard to keep fresh smelling, such as garbage storage areas, empty garbage bins and cans, toilet bowls, and any other areas which are prone to odors caused by microorganisms.

Precautionary Statements: Hazard to Humans and Domestic Animals:

Danger: Keep out of reach of children. Corrosive. Causes severe eye and skin damage. Do not get in eyes, skin or on clothing. Wash thoroughly with soap and water after handling. Harmful if swallowed. Wear goggles or face shield and rubber gloves when handling. Avoid contamination of food. Remove and wash contaminated clothing.

Statement of Practical Treatment: In case of contact, immediately flush eyes or skin with plenty of water for at least 15 minutes. For eyes, call a physician. Remove and wash all contaminated clothing before reuse. If swallowed, drink promptly a large quantity of water. Call a physician.

Note to Physician: Probable mucosal damage may contraindicate the use of gastric lavage.

Storage and Disposal: Do not contaminate water, food or feed by storage or disposal. Open dumping is prohibited. Store only in original container. Do not reuse empty container. Keep this product under locked storage sufficient to make it inaccessible to children or persons unfamiliar with its proper use.

Container Disposal: Larger than 1 gal - Do not reuse empty container. Wrap container and put in trash.

Presentation: 4 x 1 gallon containers per case and 55 gallon drums.

Compendium Code No.: 13700060 QT12.5-04/02

QUATSAN

Bio-Tek **Disinfectant**

Odorless-Concentrated Liquid Sanitizer-Disinfectant-Deodorizer-Sanitizer-Virucidal*

EPA Reg. No.: 2311-11-11725

Active Ingredient(s):

n-Alkyl (60% C_{14}, 30% C_{16}, 5% C_{18}) dimethyl benzyl ammonium chlorides	5%
n-Alkyl (68% C_{12}, 32% C_{14}) dimethyl ethylbenzyl ammonium chlorides	5%
Inert Ingredients:	90%
Total	100%

Directions for Use: QUATSAN is a concentrate and should be diluted before using.

Hospitals: For floors, walls and other hard surfaces. In Nursing Homes, institutions, as well as sink tops, garbage pails, telephones and restrooms, use 3½ ounces per 5 gallons of water. Apply with cloth, mop, or sponge. At this level effective against *Pseudomonas aeruginosa* PRD-10. For heavily soiled or contaminated areas, a precleaning step is recommended.

Cold Disinfection: For disinfection of previously cleaned surgical instruments, barber tools and dental equipment, simply submerge instruments into solution containing 1½ ounces per gallon of water for 10 minutes.

General: For sanitizing and disinfecting floors, walls and inanimate hard surfaces. For schools, homes, locker rooms, garbage pails, sink tops, corridors, classrooms, offices and shower stalls: Apply solution with mop or cloth. Sanitize with 1 ounce to 4 gallons of water. Disinfect with 3 ounces to 5 gallons of water. Kills *Staphylococcus aureus* and *Salmonella choleraesuis.* For heavily soiled or contaminated areas, a pre-cleaning step is recommended.

Restaurant and Bar Rinse: Dishes, glassware, silverware, cooking utensils wash with soap or synthetic detergent, rinse thoroughly and immerse in a sanitized solution containing 1 ounce to 4 gallons of water. No terminal potable water rinse required.

*This product when used on environmental inanimate, hard surfaces at 3½ ounces per 5 gallons of water is effective against influenza A2, Herpes Simplex, Adenovirus type 5 and Vaccinia Viruses.

Food Processing Equipment: For sanitization of previously cleaned food processing equipment and food utensils dilute 1 ounce per 4 gallons water to provide 200 ppm of active quaternaries. At this level no potable water rinse is required.

Dairies: To sanitize dairy equipment such as tanks, lines, pails, and milk cans, first clean and rinse the equipment thoroughly. Then apply sanitizing solution containing 1 ounce to 4 gallons of water (200 ppm). At this level no potable water rinse is required. Follow recommendations of local Health Board.

Room Fogging: To minimize the danger of cross-contamination from environmental surfaces apply solution as a fog as described below, before applying standard routine terminal cleaning and disinfecting practices.

1. Remove all human, animal and plant life from room.
2. Open closet doors and drawers.
3. Set up 34" revolving platform in center of room.

Q

4. Mount Jet Fog-Master Tri-Jet Model or other fogging device delivering equivalent spray at 3 RPM.
5. Fill sprayer reservoir with 1.5 oz to 1 gallon water to produce 1150 ppm active ingredients.
6. Set sprayer mechanism to deliver 1 gallon of solution.
7. Fog for 15 minutes for an average 2100 cu. ft. room. For different room sizes, vary spray time proportionately to ensure complete wetting of exposed surfaces.
8. Wait 2 hours before entering room after treatment.
9. Rinse fogging equipment thoroughly with clear water following use.

Precautionary Statements: Danger: Keep out of reach of children. Corrosive. Causes severe eye and skin damage. Do not get in eyes or skin or on clothing. Protect eyes and skin when handling concentrate. Harmful if swallowed. Avoid contamination of food.

First Aid: In case of contact, immediately flush eyes or skin with plenty of water for at least 15 minutes. For eyes, call a physician. Remove and wash all contaminated clothing before reuse. If swallowed, drink milk, egg whites, gelatin solution or if these are not available, drink large quantities of water. Call a physician.

Note to Physician: Probable mucosal damage may contraindicate use of gastric lavage. Measures against circulatory shock, respiratory depression and convulsion may be needed.

Storage and Disposal: Do not contaminate water, food or feed by storage or disposal. Open dumping is prohibited. Do not reuse empty container.

Pesticide Disposal: Pesticides that cannot be used or chemically reprocessed should be disposed of in a landfill approved for pesticide or buried in a safe place.

Container Disposal: Triple rinse (or equivalent) and dispose in an incinerator or landfill approved for pesticide containers, or bury in a safe place.

Do not reuse empty container. Rinse thoroughly with water before discarding or returning to drum reconditioner.

Presentation: 4 x 1 gallon containers per case and 55 gallon drums.

Compendium Code No.: 13700070

QUEST® 2% EQUINE ORAL GEL

Fort Dodge **Parasiticide-Oral**

Dewormer & Boticide

NADA No.: 141-087

Active Ingredient(s): Contains 20 mg moxidectin/mL (2.0% w/v).

Indications: QUEST® (moxidectin) 2% Equine Oral Gel when administered at the recommended dose level of 0.4 mg moxidectin/kg (2.2 lb) body weight is effective in the treatment and control of the following stages of gastrointestinal and subcutaneous parasites of horses and ponies:

Large strongyles: *Strongylus vulgaris* - (adults and L_4/L_5 arterial stages); *Strongylus edentatus* - (adults and tissue stages); *Triodontophorus brevicauda* - (adults); *Triodontophorus serratus* - (adults).

Small strongyles: *Cyathostomum* spp. - (adults); *Cylicocyclus* spp. - (adults); *Cylicostephanus* spp. - (adults); *Gyalocephalus capitatus* - (adults); Undifferentiated lumenal larvae.

Encysted cyathostomes: Late L_3 and L_4 mucosal cyathostome larvae.

Ascarids: *Parascaris equorum* - (adults and L_4 larval stages).

Pin worms: *Oxyuris equi* - (adults and L_4 larval stages).

Hair worms: *Trichostrongylus axei* - (adults).

Large-mouth stomach worms: *Habronema muscae* - (adults).

Horse stomach bots: *Gasterophilus intestinalis* - (2nd and 3rd instars); *Gasterophilus nasalis* - (3rd instars).

Neck Threadworms: *Onchocerca cervicalis* - (microfilariae).

One administration of the recommended dose rate of QUEST® (moxidectin) 2% Equine Oral Gel also suppresses strongyle egg production through 84 days.

QUEST® is indicated for use in horses and ponies, including breeding mares and stallions, and foals four months of age and older.

Pharmacology: Mode of Action: QUEST® 2% Equine Oral Gel acts by interfering with chloride channel-mediated neurotransmission in the parasite. This results in paralysis and elimination of the parasite. Moxidectin is safe for use in horses and ponies because it does not have the same injurious effect on the mammalian nervous system.

Q

Dosage and Administration: QUEST® (moxidectin) 2% Equine Oral Gel is specially formulated as a palatable gel which is easily administered to horses and ponies.

QUEST® Gel is packaged in ready-to-use Sure-Dial™ syringes. The syringe is calibrated in 50-pound increments, up to 1150 pounds. This enables the administration of the recommended dose level of 0.4 mg moxidectin/kg body weight by choosing a setting consistent with the animal's weight.

How To Set the Dose: Since the dose is based on the weight of the animal, you need to use a scale or weight tape to find each animal's weight before treating with QUEST® Gel. Once the weight is known, set the dose for each horse or pony as follows.

1. Hold the syringe with the capped end pointing to the left and so that you can see the weight measurements and tick marks (small black lines). Each tick mark relates to 50 lbs. of body weight.
2. Turn the green dial ring until the left side of the ring lines up with the weight of the animal.

How to Give QUEST® Gel to a Horse or Pony:

1. Make sure there is no feed in the animal's mouth.
2. Remove the cap from the end of the syringe. Save the cap for reuse.
3. Place the tip of the syringe inside the animal's mouth at the space between the teeth.
4. Gently push the plunger until it stops, depositing the gel on the back of the tongue.
5. Remove the syringe from the animal's mouth and raise the animal's head slightly to make sure it swallows the gel.
6. Replace the syringe cap.

Treating a Second Horse or Pony With the Same Syringe: If the first animal you treat weighs less than 1150 lbs., there will be gel left in the syringe. You can use this gel to treat other horses or ponies. To set the next dose, add the weight of the animal you want to treat to the dose setting already on the syringe. For example, if the syringe was first used to treat a 250 lb. animal, the green dial ring is set on 250 lbs. To treat a 500 lb. animal next, move the green dial ring to the 750 lb. marking (250+500=750). You need more than one syringe to treat horses weighing more than 1150 lbs.

Sure-Dial™ Syringe:

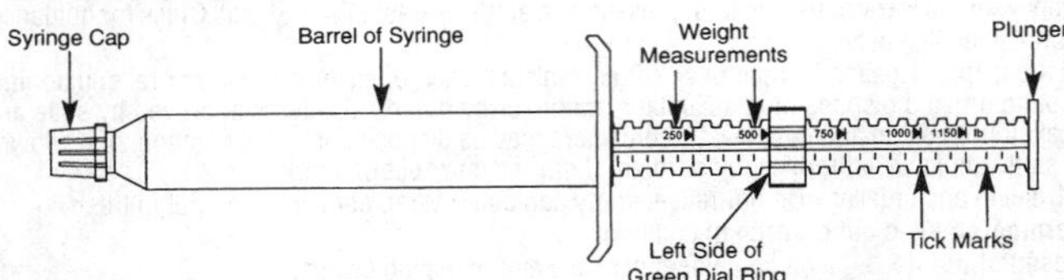

Each syringe of QUEST® 2% Equine Oral Gel may be used to treat more than one animal especially when dosing foals, ponies and growing and lighter breeds of horses. The table below will help estimate the number of horses or ponies the contents of each syringe will treat.

	Ponies			Light Horses			Heavy Horses		
	Weight		Treated Animals	Weight		Treated Animals	Weight		Treated Animals
Age	(lbs)	(kg)	(per syringe)	(lbs)	(kg)	(per syringe)	(lbs)	(kg)	(per syringe)
4 months	150	(68)	7	250	(113)	4	350	(159)	3
8 months	200	(91)	5	350	(159)	3	550	(249)	2
Mature	450	(204)	2	850	(386)	1	1100+	(499+)	1

Precaution(s): Store at or near room temperature 15° to 30°C (59° to 86°F). Avoid freezing. If frozen, thaw completely before use. Store partially-used syringes with the cap tightly secured.

Environmental Safety: Care should be taken to avoid the release of significant volumes of moxidectin into either ground or free-running water since moxidectin may be injurious to aquatic life. Sure-Dial™ syringes and their contents should be disposed of in an approved landfill or by incineration.

Caution(s): QUEST® 2% Equine Oral Gel has been formulated specifically for use in horses and ponies only. This product should not be used in other animal species as severe adverse reactions, including fatalities in dogs, may result.

Warning(s): Extreme caution should be used when administering the product to foals, young and miniature horses, as overdosage may result in serious adverse reactions. Do not use in horses or ponies intended for food.

Human Warning: Do not ingest. If swallowed, induce vomiting. Wash hands and contaminated skin with soap and water. If accidental contact with eyes occurs, flush repeatedly with water. If irritation or any other symptom attributable to exposure to this product persists, consult your physician. Keep this and all drugs out of reach of children.

Toxicology: Animal Safety: QUEST® (moxidectin) 2% Equine Oral Gel can be safely administered at the recommended dose of 0.4 mg moxidectin/kg body weight to horses and ponies of all breeds at least 4 months of age or older. Transient depression, ataxia and recumbency may be seen when very young or debilitated animals are treated. In these instances, supportive care may be advisable. Reproductive safety studies demonstrate a wide margin of safety when the product is used in the treatment of estrual and pregnant mares and breeding stallions.

To report adverse drug reactions or to obtain a copy of the Material Safety Data Sheet (MSDS) call (800)477-1365.

Discussion: Strategic Protection Programs: Consult your veterinarian for assistance in the diagnosis, treatment, and control of parasitism. For best control of parasites, all horses and ponies should be included in a strategic treatment program, with particular attention given to high performance animals, brood mares, stallions and foals. In foals, initial treatment is recommended at 4 months of age, after which they should be included in a recurrent treatment program. Because QUEST® provides effective control of the mucosal stages of small strongyles (encysted cyathostomes), it is useful in reducing the frequency of treatment required for successful strategic equine parasite control. A veterinarian can assist in preparing the best program for your needs.

QUEST® 2% Equine Oral Gel when used at the recommended dose rate suppresses strongyle egg production through 84 days following a single oral administration. This residual strongyle control reduces pasture contamination and provides a period of protection from reinfection for horses and ponies maintained on the same pasture.

Presentation: QUEST® 2% Equine Oral Gel is available in one syringe applicator size. Each Sure-Dial™ syringe contains 0.4 oz (11.3 g) of QUEST® 2% Equine Oral Gel which is sufficient to treat a single horse weighing up to 1150 lb, or two or more lighter animals with a combined body weight of up to 1150 lb. Also available in 50-pack cartons.

NDC 0856-7441-03 - 0.4 oz (11.3 g) syringe.

QUEST® is a registered trademark of American Cyanamid Company.

U.S. Patent No. 4,916,154

Compendium Code No.: 10031783 7440I

QUICKBAYT™

Fly Bait

Bayer

For Pest Management Professionals, Livestock Producers And Commercial Use Only.

ACTIVE INGREDIENT:

Imidacloprid,
1-[(6-Chloro-3-pyridinyl)methyl]-
N nitro-2-imidazolidinimine 0.50%
Z-9-Tricosene 0.10%
OTHER INGREDIENTS 99.40%
100.00%

STOP-Read the label before use.

Keep out of reach of children.

CAUTION

PRECAUTIONARY STATEMENTS

HAZARDS TO HUMANS AND DOMESTIC ANIMALS

See below for First Aid statement.

CAUTION: Harmful if swallowed, absorbed through skin, or inhaled. Avoid contact with eyes, skin or clothing. Wash thoroughly with soap and water after handling and before eating, drinking or using tobacco.

FIRST AID	
If swallowed:	• Call a poison control center or doctor immediately for treatment advice. • Have person sip a glass of water if able to swallow. • Do not induce vomiting unless told to by a poison control center or doctor. • Do not give anything to an unconscious person.
If on skin:	• Take off contaminated clothing. • Rinse skin immediately with plenty of water for 15 to 20 minutes. • Call a poison control center or doctor for treatment advice.
If inhaled:	• Move person to fresh air. • If person is not breathing, call 911 or an ambulance, then give artificial respiration, preferably mouth-to-mouth if possible. • Call a poison control center or doctor for further treatment advice.
If in eyes:	• Hold eye open and rinse slowly and gently with water for 15 to 20 minutes. Remove contact lenses, if present, after the first 5 minutes, then continue rinsing eye. • Call a poison control center or doctor for treatment advice.
Have the product container or label with you when calling a poison control center or doctor or going for treatment. For emergency medical treatment call 1-877-258-2280. For product information call 1-800-633-3796.	
Note to Physician: No specific antidote is available. Treat the patient symptomatically.	

ENVIRONMENTAL HAZARDS

This product is highly toxic to aquatic invertebrates. Do not apply directly to water, or to areas where surface water is present or to intertidal areas below the mean high water mark. Do not contaminate water when disposing of equipment washwaters or rinsate. This product is highly toxic to bees exposed to direct treatment or residues on blooming crops or weeds. Do not apply this product or allow it to drift to blooming crops or weeds if bees are visiting the treatment area. This chemical has properties and characteristics associated with chemicals detected in groundwater. The use of this chemical in areas where soils are permeable, particularly where the water table is shallow, may result in groundwater contamination.

STORAGE AND DISPOSAL	
Do not contaminate water, food or feed by storage or disposal.	
Storage	• Store in a cool, dry place and in such a manner as to prevent cross contamination with other pesticides, fertilizers, food, or feed. • Store in original containers and out of the reach of children, preferably in a locked storage area. • Handle and open container in a manner as to prevent spillage.
Pesticide Disposal	• Wastes resulting from the use of this product may be disposed of on site or at an approved waste disposal facility.
Container Disposal	• Completely empty container. • Dispose of container at an approved waste disposal facility or by incineration if allowed by state and local authorities. • Do not use container in connection with food, feed, or drinking water.
Spills	• If the container is leaking or material is spilled, carefully sweep up spilled bait and wash exposed area. • In spill or leak incidents, keep unauthorized people away.

PRO FACTS	
• Fast acting. • Ready-to-use scatter bait or paint-on application. • Contains a specially formulated mixture of attractants. • Controls flies resistant to organophosphates and carbamates.	
QUICKBAYT™ FLY BAIT	• Ready-to-use bait containing 0.5% imidacloprid. • Contains the attractant Muscalure®. • Contains Bitrex® bittering agent to help prevent ingestion by animals, children and pets.
CONTROLS	Flies.
WHERE TO APPLY	• Around the outside of structures or partially enclosed or protected areas. • In and around agricultural production facilities. • Around the outside of commercial facilities.
MIXING INFORMATION	• Ready-to-use scatter bait. • Paint-on application: Mix the fly bait with water.
HOW TO APPLY	• Scatter application. • Place in any fly bait station. • Paint-on application.
COVERAGE	5.7 to 6.3 oz/1000 sq ft
RE-APPLY	Re-apply every 7 days as needed.
QUESTIONS??	For questions or comments, call toll-free 1-800-633-3796 or visit us online at www.quickbayt.com.

DIRECTIONS FOR USE	
It is a violation of Federal law to use this product in a manner inconsistent with its labeling. IMPORTANT: Read entire label and Conditions of Sale before using this product.	
FLY MANAGEMENT	
WHERE TO APPLY	• For use only around the outside of commercial facilities like canneries, dairy, meat and poultry processing plants, beverage plants, food processing plants, restaurants, bakeries, supermarkets, warehouses, dumpsters, grease pits, recycling areas, loading docks. • For use only around the outside of agricultural production facilities like broiler houses, feedlots, livestock housing structures, and horse stables. • For use only around the outside of and in walkways of caged layer houses. Place bait in areas inaccessible to animals. • In horse stables, apply bait only in fly bait stations. Place bait stations in areas inaccessible to animals.
USE RATE	• 5.7 to 6.3 oz/1000 sq ft (scatter bait and bait station).
HOW TO APPLY	Apply the bait in many locations. Avoid cool or windy locations because flies prefer warm sites for resting. Time applications to begin at the start of the season before fly populations have reached their peak. • **Scatter application:** Scatter the bait directly from the container onto dry level surfaces so that the individual granules lie near each other without forming small piles. • **Bait stations:** Place in any fly bait station. Use 1 bait station to cover approximately 250 sq ft, and add up to 1.6 oz of bait per station. Secure bait stations at least 4 feet above the ground. Bait stations should be inaccessible to food-producing animals, children and pets. • **Paint-on application:** Mix 1.5 oz bait with 1 fl oz warm water (3 lbs bait in 1 quart water) and stir thoroughly. Let stand for about 15 minutes until a paste consistency suitable for painting has formed. Apply the paste with a brush to surfaces where flies rest avoiding surfaces that are dusty.
RESTRICTIONS 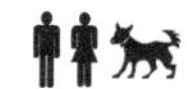	• Do not place bait in areas accessible to food producing animals, children and pets. • Do not allow bait to come into contact with food or water. • Do not apply to milking equipment. • Do not apply inside food processing plants, restaurants or other commercial facilities.
MANAGEMENT TIPS	
For Best Results: Use the bait as part of an overall Integrated Pest Management program. • Use proper sanitation and manure management. • Use along with dilutable sprays like TEMPO® • Use environmental controls, such as proper light management. • Consult with Cooperative Extension.	

CONDITIONS OF SALE:

THE DIRECTIONS ON THIS LABEL WERE DETERMINED THROUGH RESEARCH TO BE APPROPRIATE FOR THE CORRECT USE OF THIS PRODUCT. THIS PRODUCT HAS BEEN TESTED UNDER DIFFERENT ENVIRONMENTAL CONDITIONS BOTH INDOORS AND OUTDOORS SIMILAR TO THOSE THAT ARE ORDINARY AND CUSTOMARY WHERE THE PRODUCT IS TO BE USED. INSUFFICIENT CONTROL OF PESTS OR PLANT INJURY MAY RESULT FROM THE OCCURRENCE OF EXTRAORDINARY OR UNUSUAL CONDITIONS, OR FROM FAILURE TO FOLLOW LABEL DIRECTIONS. IN ADDITION, FAILURE TO FOLLOW LABEL DIRECTIONS MAY CAUSE INJURY TO ANIMALS, MAN, AND DAMAGE TO THE ENVIRONMENT. BAYER OFFERS, AND THE BUYER ACCEPTS AND USES, THIS PRODUCT SUBJECT TO THE CONDITIONS THAT EXTRAORDINARY OR UNUSUAL ENVIRONMENTAL CONDITIONS, OR FAILURE TO FOLLOW LABEL DIRECTIONS ARE BEYOND THE CONTROL OF BAYER AND ARE, THEREFORE, THE RESPONSIBILITY OF THE BUYER.

EPA Reg. No. 3125-573-11556

EPA Establishment No. 7319-NL-1

SUPPLIED:

Code 08731635-066399 — 5 Pounds (2.25 kg)

Code 08731627-064599 — 40 Pounds (18 kg)

Manufactured for Bayer Corporation, Agriculture Division, Animal Health, Shawnee Mission, Kansas 66201 U.S.A.

Made in Holland R.0

Compendium Code No.: 10400430

QUICKHIT™ FOR DAIRY CATTLE

SSI Corp. **Topical Product**

Active Ingredient(s):

Zinc (Zn) 0.35%
Copper (Cu) 0.2%
Sulfur (S) 6.39%
Inert 93.06%

Indications: Aids in the treatment and control of footwarts (Papillomatous Digital Dermatitis) in dairy cattle.

Contains no antibiotics, easy to use — no mixing.

Directions: Use as a direct topical spray or drench to aid in the treatment of footwarts (Papillomatous Digital Dermatitis). Clean affected area beforehand as well as possible. Use full strength. Spray or drench to the point of runoff twice daily (morning milking and evening milking). Improvement should be noted in four to six applications. Continue spraying until problem is resolved.

For severe cases wrapping may be necessary. Soak a cotton ball or gauze in QUICKHIT™, apply to affect area then wrap. Remove wrap after three days and inspect.

Follow treatment with a prevention program using HoofPro+®, Rotational Zinc™, MagSalt™ or E-Z-Copper™.

Precaution(s): Keep from freezing.
Caution(s): Eye irritant. In case of eye contact, flush for 15 minutes. If irritation persists, call a physician.
Warning(s): Keep out of the reach of children.
Presentation: 1 and 2.5 gallon containers.
Compendium Code No.: 14930041

QUICK SHIELD™ INTRANASAL IBR-PI$_3$

Novartis Animal Vaccines **Vaccine**

Bovine Rhinotracheitis-Parainfluenza$_3$ Virus Vaccine, Modified Live Virus

U.S. Vet. Lic. No.: 303
Composition: This vaccine contains modified live IBR and PI$_3$ viruses propagated on an established bovine cell line. Contained gentamicin as a preservative.
Indications: For use in healthy nonpregnant cattle as an aid in the prevention of disease caused by infectious bovine rhinotracheitis and parainfluenza Type 3 viruses.
Dosage and Administration: Aseptically rehydrate with diluent supplied. Shake well before using. Administer 2 mL intranasally. Revaccinate annually.
Precaution(s): Store in the dark at 35°-45°F (2°-7°C). Do not freeze. Needles and syringes should not be sterilized with chemicals. Use entire contents when first opened. Burn this container and any unused contents.
Caution(s): Do not use in pregnant cows or calves nursing pregnant cows. Anaphylactic reactions may occur following the use of this biological. Symptomatic treatment: Epinephrine.
For veterinary use only.
Warning(s): Do not vaccinate within 21 days prior to slaughter.
Presentation: 10 dose (20 mL) and 50 dose (100 mL) bottles.
Compendium Code No.: 11140760 F107 / F105B

QUICK-START™

Vedco **Dietary Supplement**

Guaranteed Analysis:

	Per Fl Oz	Per Pound (W/W)
Crude Protein not more than	3.0%	3.0%
Crude Fat not less than	50.0%	45.0%
Vitamin A	50.0 IU	7,245.0 IU
Vitamin D$_3$	38.0 IU	565.0 IU
Vitamin E	3.0 IU	43.4 IU
Thiamine (vit B$_1$)	0.13 mg	1.88 mg
Riboflavin (vit B$_2$)	0.17 mg	2.46 mg
Pyridoxine (vit B$_6$)	0.20 mg	2.90 mg
Ascorbic acid (vit C)	6.0 mg	86.9 mg
Niacin	2.0 mg	29.0 mg
D-Pantothenic Acid	0.42 mg	6.0 mg
Folic Acid	0.04 mg	0.58 mg
Omega 3 Fatty Acids	1200.0 mg	17,380.0 mg

Ingredients: Vegetable oil, sucrose, fructose, malto dextrins, non fat dry milk solids, vegetable gums, egg white solids, glycerine, citrus pectin, sodium benzoate, vitamin A acetate, cholecalciferol (vitamin D$_3$), dl-alpha tocopheryl acetate (vitamin E), ascorbic acid (vitamin C), niacinamide, calcium pantothenate, pyridoxine hydrochloride, riboflavin, thiamine mononitrate, folic acid.
Energy: 180 kcal per fl oz.
Indications: A high calorie concentrate with essential vitamin supplementation.
Dosage and Administration:
Dogs and Cats Maintenance (administer with dose syringe):
5-10 lbs body weight .... 5 mL twice daily
10-30 lbs body weight .... 10 mL twice daily
30 lbs or more .... 15 mL twice daily
Calves (200-400 lbs): ½ tube twice daily for two days.
Cows: One tube daily for two days.
Foals: ½ tube daily for two days.
Horses: One tube morning and evening.
Precaution(s): Store in a cool, dry place.
Warning(s): For veterinary use only. Keep out of reach of children.
Presentation: 60 mL dose syringe and 300 mL (10 fl oz) tube.
Compendium Code No.: 10941790

QUIKCHEK™ B.U.N. REAGENT STRIPS

Centaur **Reagent Strips**

Description: B.U.N. Reagent Strips are a reagent strip for the determination of blood urea nitrogen. A semi-permeable membrane is employed. Each strip is stable and ready to use when removed from the storage vial.
Indications: B.U.N Reagent Strips are a one minute test for blood urea nitrogen in whole blood, serum or heparinized plasma.
Test Procedure: Specimen Collection and Preparation: B.U.N. Reagent strips are intended for use with whole blood, serum or heparinized plasma only.
Specifications:
1. Range: 10-100 mg/dl
2. Specimen: whole blood, serum or heparinized plasma
3. Sample Volume: 50-100 µL (1 drop)
4. Reaction Time: 1 minute
5. Storage: room temperature only

Whole blood with fluoride as a preservative should be avoided. Hematocrits greater than 55% can cause lower results.
If patient is severely dehydrated use serum or plasma only.
Test Interpretation: Normal Value for B.U.N.:
Canine: 10-20 mg/dl
Feline: 10-30 mg/dl
Equine: 10-25 mg/dl
Proper timing is critical for this technique.
1. Apply 1 large drop (50-100 µL) of sample to the pad.
2. Wait 30 seconds.
3. Wipe sample off with a tissue. Use moderate pressure evenly on the reagent pad area. Remove all excess sample.
4. Wait an additional 30 seconds.
5. Compare color of the pad with the color chart to obtain B.U.N. value.

Storage: Reagent strips should be stored in the vial in a cool, dry place at room temperature. Avoid excessive humidity, temperature extremes, and direct sunlight. The vial should be stored tightly capped with the desiccant. Remove desired number of strips and recap immediately. Do not handle reagent pad area. Do not refrigerate.
Caution(s): B.U.N. Reagent strips are for *in-vitro* diagnostic use.
Presentation: B.U.N. Reagent strips are available in kits of 25 tests.
Compendium Code No.: 14880060

QUIKCHEK™ GLUCOSE REAGENT STRIPS

Centaur **Reagent Strips**

Description: Glucose Reagent strips are a disposable plastic reagent strip for the determination of glucose. A semi-permeable membrane is employed to serve as a barrier to prevent blood cells from entering into the reagent pad area. Each strip is stable and ready to use when removed from the storage vial.
Indications: Glucose Reagent Strips are a one minute test for glucose in whole blood, serum or heparinized plasma.
Test Procedure: Specimen Collection and Preparation: Glucose Reagent Strips are intended for use with serum, heparinized plasma, or whole blood. Blood glucose undergoes glycolysis rapidly after drawing. To prevent loss due to glycolysis use blood samples immediately.
Specifications:
1. Range: 50-400 mg/dl
2. Specimen: Serum, heparinized plasma or whole blood
3. Sample Volume: 50-100 µL
4. Reaction Time: 60 seconds
5. Storage: Room temperature below 30°C (86°F)

Whole blood with fluoride as a preservative should be avoided. Hematocrits greater than 55% can cause lower results.
Proper timing is critical for this technique.
1. Apply 1 large drop (50-100 µL) of sample to the pad.
2. Wait 30 seconds.
3. Wipe sample off with a tissue. Use moderate pressure evenly on the reagent pad area. Remove all excess sample.
4. Wait an additional 30 seconds.
5. Compare color of the pad with the color chart to obtain glucose value.

Storage: Reagent strips should be stored in the vial in a cool, dry place at room temperature below 30°C (86°F). Avoid excessive humidity, temperature extremes, and direct sunlight. The vial should be stored tightly capped with the desiccant. Remove desired number of strips and recap immediately. Do not handle reagent pad area.
Caution(s): Glucose strips are for *in-vitro* diagnostic use.
Presentation: Glucose reagent strips are available in vials of 25 strips.
Compendium Code No.: 14880070

QUIKCHEK™ SERUM CREATININE ASSAY

Centaur **Serum Chemistry**

Components: This creatinine test kit contains two reagent bottles, pipets and disposable vials with caps.
Indications: A 5 minute assay for the determination of creatinine in serum or plasma.
Test Procedure: Specimen Collection and Preparation: Non-hemolyzed serum or plasma must be used. Sample should be at room temperature.
Specifications:
1. Range: 0-10 mg/dl
2. Specimen: Serum or Plasma
3. Sample Volume: 50-100 µL (1 drop)
4. Reaction Time: 5 minutes
5. Storage: Room Temperature

Do not use whole blood or severely hemolyzed serum or plasma.
Test Procedure:
1. Put 2 drops of solution #1 into a vial.
2. Add 5 drops of solution #2 into the same vial and swirl.
3. Add 4 drops of sample (300 µL) of serum or plasma into the vial, swirl to mix.
4. Wait for 5 minutes.
5. Compare color developed in the vial to the color chart for the creatinine value of the sample.

Test Interpretation: Normal Value for Serum Creatinine:
Canine: 1.0-2.0 mg/dl Feline: 1.0-2.0 mg/dl Equine: 1.0-2.0 mg/dl
Storage: Test kit should be stored at room temperature out of reach of children.
Caution(s): This creatinine assays is for *in-vitro* use only. Do not refrigerate reagent bottles. Test kit should be stored out of reach of children.
Presentation: Serum Creatinine test is available in kits of 25 tests.
Compendium Code No.: 14880090

QUIKCLEAN™ WATERLESS SHAMPOO

Fort Dodge **Grooming Product**

Contents: QUIKCLEAN™ Waterless Shampoo contains conditioners and lanolin. Contains no harsh chemicals, leaves no irritating residue, is pH balanced and mild.
Indications: A shampoo without wetting or rinsing, when bathing is not practical. For use on dogs, cats and horses.
Directions for Use: Wet the hair of the area to be cleaned thoroughly with QUIKCLEAN™ Waterless Shampoo and massage well until a light cleansing foam appears. Use a sponge on the face. Dry with a soft, absorbent towel - then simply brush, comb or blow dry.
Discussion: A few of the many uses for QUIKCLEAN™ Waterless Shampoo: To remove stains; between bathings; for cold weather cleaning; to spot clean and deodorize; after surgery; soiling mishaps/manure stains; when caring for kittens, puppies and foals; for old or sick pets.
QUIKCLEAN™ Waterless Shampoo has been specifically developed for quick drying - no water or rinsing needed.
Presentation: 8 fl oz (236 mL) and 32 fl oz (946 mL) bottles with sprayer.
Compendium Code No.: 10031790 13102A

R

RABBIT EAR MITICIDE

Farnam **Otic Parasiticide**

EPA Reg. No.: 270-168

Active Ingredient(s):

Pyrethrins 0.05%
Technical Piperonyl Butoxide* 0.50%
Inert Ingredients. 99.45%

*Equivalent to 0.4% (butylcarbityl) (6 propylpiperonyl) ether and 0.1% related compounds.

Indications: For the treatment of ear mites (*Otodectes cynotis)* in rabbits, dogs and cats.

Directions for Use: It is a violation of Federal law to use this product in a manner inconsistent with its labeling.

Hold pet securely. Cleanse ear thoroughly. Fill outer ear canal half full with RABBIT EAR MITICIDE. Massage base of the ear to distribute solution into ear wax. Repeat every other day until condition is relieved. Symptoms should improve in 4 to 6 days. Continue treatment for 12 days. Since ear mites occasionally are found on other parts of the body, reinfestation may occur unless a suitable dip or other full-body treatment is used.

Precautionary Statements: Hazards to Humans and Domestic Animals:

Caution: Harmful if swallowed. Avoid contact with eyes. In case of eye contact, flush with plenty of water. Consult a physician if irritation persists (humans). Avoid contamination of foodstuffs or utensils. For animals, discontinue use if irritation develops.

Storage and Disposal: Do not contaminate water, food or feed by storage or disposal.

Storage: Keep away from heat.

Disposal: Do not reuse empty container. Wrap and put in trash collection.

Warning(s): Keep out of reach of children.

For veterinary use only.

Discussion: Ear mites normally cause a dry, dark brown, waxy exudate with crusts in the ears of rabbits, dogs and cats. Mites are easily observed by placing some of the ear wax on a dark surface and watching closely for moving white specks. Do not injure the delicate tissue of the ear. Inflamed, watery or blocked ear canals indicate a more serious condition which requires special treatment.

Presentation: 4 fl oz (118 mL) plastic bottle with dropper cap.

Compendium Code No.: 10000750 9CC3

RABDOMUN® VACCINE

Schering-Plough **Vaccine**

Rabies Vaccine, Killed Virus

U.S. Vet. Lic. No.: 189

Contents: The vaccine is prepared from cell-culture grown, chemically-inactivated rabies virus. The seed virus is a highly immunogenic, fixed strain of rabies virus which originated from Louis Pasteur's original isolate in 1882. The inactivated virus is formulated with a highly purified adjuvant and is packaged in liquid form.

Contains gentamicin as a preservative.

Indications: RABDOMUN® is for vaccination of healthy dogs, cats, cattle and sheep as an aid in preventing rabies.

Directions:

Dogs and Cats:

1. General Directions: Shake well. Aseptically administer 1 mL subcutaneously. Dogs may be vaccinated intramuscularly or subcutaneously.
2. Primary Vaccination: Administer a single 1 mL dose at 3 months of age or older to healthy dogs and cats. A repeat dose should be administered 1 year later.
3. Revaccination: Subsequent revaccination every 3 years with a single dose is recommended.

Cattle and Sheep:

1. General Directions: Shake well. Aseptically administer 2 mL intramuscularly.
2. Primary Vaccination: Administer a single 2 mL dose at 3 months of age or older to healthy cattle and sheep. A repeat dose should be administered 1 year later.
3. Revaccination: Annual revaccination with a single dose is recommended.

Precaution(s): Store at 2°-7°C. Prolonged exposure to higher temperatures may adversely affect potency. Do not freeze. Use entire contents when first opened.

Sterilized syringes and needles should be used to administer this vaccine.

Caution(s): As with any vaccine, anaphylaxis may occur after use. Initial antidote of epinephrine is recommended and should be followed with appropriate supportive therapy.

This product has been tested under laboratory conditions and shown to meet all Federal Standards for safety and ability to immunize normal healthy animals. This level of performance may be affected by conditions of use such as stress, weather, nutrition, disease, parasitism, other treatments, individual idiosyncrasies or impaired immunological competency. These factors should be considered by the user when evaluating product performance or freedom from reactions.

Restricted to use by or under the direction of a licensed veterinarian.

For use in dogs, cats, cattle and sheep only.

For veterinary use only.

Warning(s): Do not vaccinate within 21 days before slaughter.

Discussion: Disease Description: Rabies is a worldwide, high mortality disease affecting mammalian species. Wild animals are common vectors of the disease and the major source of transmission to humans and domestic animals. Despite successful attempts to reduce the incidence of rabies, recent published reports indicate that in the U.S. more than 30,000 people undergo treatment every year for possible exposure.[1] Domestic animals are the major source of exposure for humans. Since 1980, the most commonly reported rabid domestic animals have been cats, cattle and dogs. In 1990, a total of 4,881 cases of animal rabies were reported to the Center for Disease Control by all 50 states, the District of Columbia and Puerto Rico.[2] Susceptibility to rabies varies according to pet species. Rabies is not a treatable disease and suspect pets are usually quarantined until a clinical diagnosis is made, at which time they are destroyed.

The route of infection can be oral, respiratory, or parenteral. Following injection, a paralytic syndrome ensues, emerging as either the "furious" or "dumb" form. "Furious rabies" is characterized by unusual aggression, "dumb rabies" by lethargy and a desire to avoid contact. Respiratory failure is the immediate cause of death.

Trial Data: Safety and Efficacy: Because RABDOMUN® is produced on an established cell line, it has safety advantages over inactivated brain-origin rabies vaccines. Tissue-origin vaccines contain extraneous protein in addition to rabies antigen that can lead to autoimmune disease.

The established cell line used in RABDOMUN® has been extensively tested for freedom from contaminating agents. In addition, use of an established cell line yields a vaccine of consistent potency from serial to serial. RABDOMUN® has proven to be uniformly safe in experimental tests, and no significant adverse reactions were reported in extensive clinical trials of the vaccine.

A duration of immunity study, conducted in accordance with federal regulation and under U.S. Department of Agriculture direction, demonstrated that a 1 mL dose met federal guidelines for protection of dogs and cats against virulent challenge administered 3 years after vaccination. Cattle and sheep were likewise protected one year after receiving a 2 mL dose of RABDOMUN®.

References: Available upon request.

Presentation: 5 x 10 dose (10 mL) vials/box (NDC 0061-5152-02).

Manufactured by: Pfizer Animal Health.

Compendium Code No.: 10471671 4077A

RABDOMUN® 1 VACCINE

Schering-Plough **Vaccine**

Rabies Vaccine, Killed Virus

U.S. Vet. Lic. No.: 189

Active Ingredient(s): The vaccine is prepared form cell-culture grown, chemically-inactivated rabies virus.

The seed virus is a highly immunogenic, fixed strain of rabies virus which originated from Louis Pasteur's original isolate in 1882.

The inactivated virus is formulated with a highly purified adjuvant and is packaged in liquid form.

The vaccine contains gentamicin as a preservative.

Indications: RABDOMUN® 1 is used for the vaccination of healthy dogs and cats as an aid in the prevention of rabies.

Dosage and Administration:

1. General Directions: Shake well. Aseptically administer 1 mL subcutaneously. Dogs may be vaccinated intramuscularly or subcutaneously.
2. Primary Vaccination: Healthy dogs and cats should receive a single dose at three (3) months of age or older. A repeat dose should be administered one (1) year later.
3. Revaccination: Annual revaccination with a single dose is recommended.

Precaution(s): Store at 2°-7°C. Prolonged exposure to higher temperatures may adversely affect potency. Do not freeze.

Caution(s):

1. Use the entire contents when first opened.
2. As with any vaccine, anaphylactic reactions may occur after use. An initial antidote of epinephrine is recommended and should be followed with appropriate supportive therapy.
3. The product has been tested under laboratory conditions and shown to meet all federal standards for safety and ability to immunize normal healthy animals. The level of performance may be affected by conditions of use such as stress, weather, nutrition, disease, parasitism, other treatments, individual idiosyncrasies or impaired immunological competency. These factors should be considered by the user when evaluating product performance or freedom from reaction.
4. Restricted to use by or under the direction of a licensed veterinarian.

Discussion: Rabies is a worldwide, high mortality disease affecting mammalian species. Wild animals are common vectors of the disease and the major source of transmission to humans and domestic animals. Despite successful attempts to reduce the incidence of rabies, recent published reports indicate that in the U.S. more than 30,000 people undergo treatment every year for possible exposure.[1] Domestic animals are the major source of exposure for humans. Since 1980, the most commonly reported of rabies in domestic animals have been cats, cattle and dogs.

In 1980, a total of 4,881 cases of animal rabies were reported to the Center for Disease Control by all 50 states, the District of Columbia and Puerto Rico.[2] Susceptibility to rabies varies according to pet species. Rabies is not a treatable disease and suspect pets are usually quarantined until a clinical diagnosis is made, at which time they are destroyed.

The route of infection can be oral, respiratory, or parenteral. Following injection, a paralytic syndrome ensues, emerging as either the "furious" or "dumb" form. "Furious rabies" is characterized by unusual aggression, "dumb rabies" by lethargy and a desire to avoid contact. Respiratory failure is the immediate cause of death.

Trial Data: Because RABDOMUN® 1 is produced on an established cell line, it has safety advantages over inactivated brain-origin rabies vaccines. Tissue-origin vaccines contain extraneous protein in addition to rabies antigen that can lead to autoimmune disease.

The established cell line used in RABDOMUN® 1 has been extensively tested for freedom from contaminating agents. In addition, use of an established cell line yields a vaccine of consistent potency from serial to serial. RABDOMUN® 1 has proven to be uniformly safe in experimental tests, and significant adverse reactions were not reported in extensive clinical trials of the vaccine.

A duration of immunity study, conducted in accordance with federal regulation and under U.S. Department of Agriculture direction, demonstrated that a 1 mL dose met federal guidelines for protection of dogs and cats against virulent challenge administered more than a year after vaccination.

References: Available upon request.

Presentation: 5 x 10 dose (10 mL) vials/box.

Compendium Code No.: 10471661

RABON® 3% DUST

AgriLabs **Topical Insecticide**

A Ready-To-Use Insecticide Dust

EPA Reg. No.: 34704-266-53302

Active Ingredient(s): By Wt.

Tetrachlorvinphos: 2-chloro-1-(2,4,5-trichlorophenyl) vinyl dimethyl phosphate 3.00%
Inert Ingredients 97.00%
Total 100.00%

Indications: To control horn flies and lice and aid in the control of face flies on beef cattle, dairy cattle and to control lice on swine.

Directions for Use: It is a violation of Federal Law to use this product in a manner inconsistent with its labeling. Take time. Observe all label directions.

Applications: This product is a ready-to-use insecticide dust which can be applied by hand or through the use of self treating dust bags. Do not apply with bare hands. Wear long-sleeved shirt and pants; chemical resistant gloves; shoes and socks.

Beef Cattle, Dairy Cattle: Horn flies, face flies, lice:

Hand Dusting: Apply approximately 2 oz. of dust by shaker can, rotary duster or by spoon to the upper portions of the back, neck and poll, and to the face as an aid in the control of face flies. Rub in lightly to carry the dust beneath the hair. Repeat as necessary.

R

Self-Treating Dust Bag:

Forced Use - Put dust in cotton cloth or double burlap bags or use pre-packed weather-proof cattle dust bags and hang in barn door exits or alleyways leading from animal buildings, salt or mineral blocks, or watering holes. Protect cloth or burlap bags from weather.

Free Choice Use - Use the same dust bags as above but place in loafing sheds, holding pens, feedlots, near watering holes or other areas where cattle gather daily. The free choice aids in the control of lice.

Swine: Lice:

Hand Dusting - Apply 3-4 oz. of dust by conventional hand or power duster to each animal with special attention given to the neck and around the ears. Repeat as necessary but not more often than once every 14 days. In severe infestations, both individual animals and bedding may be treated. One lb. of 3% dust should be applied per 150 sq. ft. of bedding.

Precautionary Statements: Hazards to Humans and Domestic Animals:

Caution: Harmful if swallowed. Do not breathe dust. Do not get in eyes, on skin, or on clothing. Wash thoroughly with soap and water after handling and before eating or smoking.

Environmental Hazards: This product is toxic to fish. Drift and runoff may be hazardous to aquatic organisms in adjacent areas. For terrestrial uses, do not apply directly to water, or to areas where surface water is present or to intertidal areas below the mean high water mark. Do not contaminate water when disposing of equipment washwaters.

This product is highly toxic to bees exposed to direct treatment on blooming crops or weeds. Do not apply this product or allow it to drift to blooming crops or weeds if bees are visiting the treatment area.

Statement of Practical Treatment:

If swallowed - Call a physician or Poison Control Center immediately. Drink one or two glasses of water and induce vomiting by touching the back of throat with a finger. Do not induce vomiting or give anything by mouth to an unconscious or convulsing person.

If inhaled - Remove victim to fresh air. Apply artificial respiration if indicated.

If on skin - Remove contaminated clothing and wash affected areas with soap and water.

If in eyes - Flush eyes with plenty of water. Call a physician if irritation persists.

Storage and Disposal:

Prohibitions: Do not contaminate water, food or feed by storage or disposal.

Storage: Store in a cool, dry place in original container.

Pesticide Disposal: Wastes resulting from the use of this product may be disposed of on site or at an approved waste disposal facility.

Container Disposal: Completely empty bag into application equipment. Then dispose of empty bag in a sanitary landfill or by incineration, or, if allowed by State and local authorities, by burning. If burned, stay out of smoke.

Warning(s): There is no withholding period from last application to slaughter.

Keep out of reach of children.

Disclaimer: Notice of Warranty: Manufacturer and seller warrants that this product conforms to the chemical description on the label thereof and is reasonably fit for the purposes stated on such label only when used in accordance with the directions under normal use conditions. It is impossible to eliminate all risks inherently associated with the use of this product. Livestock injury, ineffectiveness, or other unintended consequences may result because of such factors as weather conditions, presence of other materials, or the manner of use or application, all of which are beyond the control of the manufacturer or seller. In no case shall manufacturer or seller be liable for consequential, special or indirect damages resulting from the use or handling of this product. All such risks shall be assumed by the buyer.

Except as expressly provided herein, manufacturer and seller makes no warranties, guarantees, or representations of any kind, either expressed or implied, or by usage of trade, statutory or otherwise, with regard to the product sold, including, but not limited to, merchantability, fitness for a particular purpose, use or eligibility of the product for any particular trade usage, buyers or user's exclusive remedy, and manufacturer's or seller's total liability, shall be for damages not exceeding the cost of the product.

Presentation: 12½ pounds (5.67 kg).

U.S. Patent No. 3777716

Compendium Code No.: 10580860

RABON® 7.76 ORAL LARVICIDE PREMIX

Boehringer Ingelheim **Feed Medication**

EPA Reg. No.: 4691-134

Active Ingredient(s): **By Weight**

Tetrachlorvinphos: (CAS #22248-79-9) 7.76%*

Other Ingredients 92.24%**

Total 100.00%

* RABON® Insecticide - Contains 35 grams of RABON® per pound.

**Refers only to ingredients which are not larvicidal.

R

Indications: To prevent the development of horn flies, face flies, house flies and stable flies in the manure of treated cattle; house flies in the manure of treated swine, house flies and stables flies in the manure of treated horses and house flies in the manure of treated mink.

Directions for Use: It is a violation of Federal law to use this product in a manner inconsistent with its labeling.

Rations containing this product may be fed up to slaughter and to lactating dairy cows without withholding the milk from market during or after treatment.

Start feeding RABON® larvicidal feeds early in the spring before flies begin to appear and continue feeding throughout the summer and into the fall until cold weather restricts fly activity.

When fed, this product passes through the digestive system into the animal's manure where it kills fly larvae on contact shortly after fly eggs hatch.

It prevents the development of fly larvae in the manure of treated animals, but it is not effective against existing adult flies.

In some cases, supplemental fly control measures may be needed in and around cattle lots and barns to control adult house flies and stable flies which can breed not only in manure but in other decaying vegetable matter or silage on the premises.

In order to achieve optimum fly control, this product should be used in conjunction with other good management and sanitation practices.

This product will mix uniformly in feeds when standard mixing procedures are followed. Thus, usual problems that are common to all feed preparation and which cause stratification, such as excessive freefall or excessive handling, are to be avoided. It is recommended that appropriate preblending techniques be employed to ensure adequate distribution throughout the feed mix. The premix should be preblended with ground grain, protein supplements, mineral mixes, etc. before being added to roughages, such as chopped hay or silage. Mixing time should be adequate to ensure uniform dispersion. Optimum performance can be ensured only if this product is dispersed uniformly with the feedstuff at the recommended level. Common feed mixing equipment (i.e. vertical mixers, horizontal blenders, mixer/feeder truck) may be used to prepare formulated feeds.

General Precautions and Restrictions: Do not apply this product in a way that will contact workers or other persons, either directly or through drift. Only protected handlers may be in the area during application. Feeds prepared with this product should not be pelleted nor be mixed with feeds containing predominantly pellets. Further, this product should not be mixed in liquid feed supplements.

Application Instructions: This product may be fed to cows, swine, and mink up to slaughter and to lactating cows.

Cattle: In a Concentrate Feed - Roughage Fed Separately:

This product can be used to prepare concentrate feeds that will provide 70 mg of RABON® per 100 pounds of body weight daily.

To prepare a larvicidal concentrate feed, mix this product according to the amount of concentrate to be fed per animal per day. Use the following table as a guide for determining the proper mixing rate.

Mixing Guide:

Pounds of Concentrate Consumed per Animal per Day	RABON® in the Concentrate		Pounds of RABON® 7.76 Oral Larvicide Premix per Ton of Concentrate
	mg/lb	%	
0.5	1584	0.35	90.0
1.0	792	0.18	45.0
1.5	528	0.12	30.0
2.0	396	0.087	22.5
5.0	159	0.035	9.0
10.0	79	0.018	4.5
15.0	53	0.012	3.0
20.0	39	0.0087	2.3
25.0	32	0.0069	1.8
30.0	26	0.0059	1.5

Feed the appropriate larvicidal concentrate to cattle weighing between 400 and 1200 pounds. For larger cattle weighing between 1200 and 1700 pounds, increase the amount of premix per ton of concentrate to 1½ times that indicated.

Cattle: In a Complete Ration - No Other Roughage Fed:

This product can be used to prepare rations that contain 26.4 mg of RABON® per pound of complete ration.

To prepare a larvicidal ration, mix 1.5 pounds of this product per ton of complete mixed ration containing both grain and roughage.

Full-feed this larvicidal ration to feeder cattle weighing from 400 to 1400 pounds or to dairy cattle at a rate to sustain milk production, but not less than 2.6 pounds of the ration per 100 pounds of body weight daily.

Swine:

All swine should be treated.

Pigs (weaners to market weight): Mix 1.3 pounds of this product per ton of meal type feed and offer free choice. This is equivalent to 22.7 mg of RABON® per pound of feed.

Sows, Boars and Breeding Gilts: Mix 2.6 pounds of this product per ton of meal-type feed and offer 4 to 6 pounds of feed per animal per day. This is equivalent to 45.4 mg of RABON® per pound of feed.

Horses: In a Concentrate Feed:

This product can be used to prepare concentrate feeds that will provide 70 mg of RABON® per 100 pounds of body weight daily. All horses in the stable area should be treated.

To prepare a larvicidal concentrate feed, mix this product according to the amount of concentrate to be fed per animal per day. Use the following as a guide for determining the proper mixing rate.

Mixing Guide:

Pounds of Concentrate Consumed per Horse per Day	Pounds of RABON® 7.76 Oral Larvicide Premix per Ton of Concentrate			
	250 lb. Horse	500 lb. Horse	1000 lb. Horse	2000 lb. Horse
2.5	4.0	8.0	16.0	32.0
5.0	2.0	4.0	8.0	16.0
10.0	1.0	2.0	4.0	8.0
15.0	0.7	1.4	2.7	5.4

As a Topdressing: Add this product daily to the grain or concentrate portion of the horse's diet to provide 70 mg of RABON® per 100 pounds of body weight. This is equivalent to the following: ½ tablespoon for a 250 lb. animal; 1 level tablespoon for a 500 lb. animal; 2 level tablespoons (8.8 g) for a 1000 lb. animal or 4 tablespoons for a 2000 lb. animal.

All horses in the stable area should be treated.

Mink:

When fed to mink, RABON® passes through the digestive system into the droppings where fly larvae are killed on contact shortly after the fly eggs hatch. This product can be mixed in mink feeds to prevent the development of house flies but should not be used as the sole method of control. It is recommended that appropriate preblending techniques be employed when mixing to assure an adequate distribution of RABON® throughout the feed mix. Preblend with soybean meal, alfalfa meal, mineral mix, etc. before being added to other ingredients. Common feed mixing equipment (i.e.: vertical mixers, horizontal blenders) may be used to prepare formulated feeds.

Add this product to the total feed at a rate that will ensure that each animal will consume 3 mg of RABON® per kg of body weight (1-2 mg/pound) per day. Use the following table as a guide.

Mixing Guide for Mink:

Food Consumption (lbs.) Daily Per Animal	Amount of RABON® 7.76 to Mix in Food		
	500 lb.	1000 lb.	2000 lb
0.10	318 grams	1.4 lbs.	2.8 lbs.
0.25	114 grams	227 grams	1.0 lbs.
0.33	90 grams	180 grams	360 grams
0.50	59 grams	118 grams	236 grams
0.75	40 grams	80 grams	160 grams
1.00	35 grams	70 grams	140 grams

Start feeding Mink larvicidal feeds early in the spring before flies begin to appear and continue feeding throughout the summer until cold weather restricts fly activity. Supplemental adult fly control measures may be needed in and around the animal facilities and feed building to control adult flies, especially house flies that can breed in many kinds of organic matter.

In order to achieve optimum fly control this product should be used in conjunction with other good management and sanitation practices.

Precautionary Statements: Hazards to Humans and Domestic Animals:

Caution: Harmful if swallowed or absorbed through the skin. Causes moderate eye irritation. Avoid contact with eyes, skin or clothing. Prolonged or frequently repeated skin contact may cause allergic reaction in some individuals.

Personal Protective Equipment: Mixers and Handlers must wear:

- long-sleeved shirt and pants
- shoes and socks
- chemical resistant gloves

User Safety Requirements: Follow manufacturer's instructions for cleaning/maintaining PPE. If no such instructions for washables, use detergent and hot water. Keep and wash PPE separately from other laundry.

User Safety Recommendations:

Users should wash hands before eating, drinking, chewing gum, using tobacco or using the toilet.

Users should remove clothing immediately if pesticide gets inside. Then wash thoroughly and put on clean clothing.

Users should remove PPE immediately after handling this product. Wash the outside of gloves before removing. As soon as possible, wash thoroughly and change into clean clothing.

First Aid:

If Swallowed: Call a physician or Poison Control Center. Drink 1 or 2 glasses of water and induce vomiting by touching back of throat with finger, or if available, by administering syrup of ipecac. If person is unconscious, do not give anything by mouth and do not induce vomiting.

If On Skin: Wash with plenty of water. Get medical attention.

If In Eyes: Flush eyes with plenty of water. Call a physician if irritation persists.

Environmental Hazards: This pesticide is toxic to fish. Do not contaminate water when disposing of equipment wash water.

Storage and Disposal: Do not contaminate water, food or feed by storage or disposal.

Storage: Store in a dry place in original container.

Container Disposal: Completely empty bag into mixing equipment. Then dispose of empty bag in a sanitary landfill or by incineration or if allowed by State and local authorities by burning. If burned, stay out of smoke. Wastes resulting from the use of this product may be disposed of on site or at an approved waste disposal facility.

Warning(s): This product is not to be used on horses destined for slaughter.

Keep out of reach of children.

Disclaimer: Warranty and Limitation of Damages: Seller warrants that this material conforms to its chemical description and is reasonably fit for the purposes stated on the label when used in accordance with directions under normal conditions of use and Buyer assumes the risk of any use contrary to such directions. Seller makes no other express or implied warranty, including any other express or implied warranty of Fitness or of Merchantability, and no agent of Seller is authorized to do so except in writing and with specific reference to this warranty. In no event shall Seller's liability for any breach of warranty exceed the purchase price of the material as to which a claim is made.

Presentation: 40 lb. bags.

Compendium Code No.: 10280951

RABON® 50% WP

Boehringer Ingelheim **Premise and Topical Insecticide**

EPA Reg. No.: 4691-128

Active Ingredient(s):

	By Weight
2-chloro-1-(2,4,5-trichlorophenyl) vinyl dimethyl phosphate	50.0%
Inert ingredients	50.0%
Total	100.0%

Indications: An organophosphate insecticide for use on beef cattle, swine, poultry, premises, poultry litter and fly breeding areas to kill and control lice, ticks, litter beetles, mites, face flies, horn flies, house flies, and maggots on or around livestock, poultry and animal buildings.

Directions for Use: It is a violation of federal law to use the product in a manner inconsistent with its labeling.

RABON® 50% WP is suitable for use in conventional power or low pressure knapsack sprayers. Occasional agitation is recommended to prevent undue settling of the suspension. Follow the use directions for the proper percent solution needed for a specific insect and areas or types of wall surfaces. Refer to premise use directions for the quantity of insecticide needed to make the percent solution recommended.

Livestock Use Directions: There is not a withholding period from last application to slaughter.

Beef cattle: For horn flies and lice, dilute 4 lbs. in 75 gallons of water. For lone star ticks, dilute 4 lbs. in 50 gallons of water. Apply as a coarse spray. Use between one-half (½) and one (1) gallon of diluted spray per animal depending upon the size and hair coat.

Swine: For lice, dilute 4 lbs. in 50 gallons of water. Apply as a coarse spray using one (1) to two (2) quarts of diluted spray per head to thoroughly wet the animal. Repeat in two (2) weeks if necessary.

Poultry Use Directions: For lice and mites:

Wire cages: Dilute 4 lbs. in 50 gallons of water. Apply directly to birds (1 gallon of diluted spray per 100 birds). Spray vent and fluff areas from below. Repeat when necessary. Do not repeat more than once every 14 days. For individual bird treatment, apply one (1) ounce of diluted spray per bird.

Note: For maximum lasting control of the northern fowl mite, penetration of the feathers around the vent areas is absolutely essential. Use a power sprayer at 100-125 psi at no less than the recommended pressure. More attention must be given each individual bird when using low-pressure equipment. Treat roosters carefully and thoroughly to avoid re-infestation in breeding flocks.

Floor management dust boxes: Use 50% WP as a dry dust. Mix evenly throughout the top layer of the box contents using 2.5 oz. per 50 birds (approximately 1 tbsp. per nest box).

Floor management roost paint: Dilute 4 lbs. in 25 gallons of water. Treat with a brush or spray thoroughly, particularly cracks and crevices using 1 pt. of diluted spray per 100 ft.

For litter beetles: Floor management litter, dilute 4 lbs. in 50 gallons of water. Apply 1-2 gallons of diluted spray per 100 sq. ft. evenly for penetration to litter surface. Also apply thoroughly to walls, roost, cracks, crevices, interior. 50% WP can also be used as a dry dust for this purpose. Treat evenly and thoroughly using ¾ oz. per 100 sq. ft. Use a rotary, mechanical or electrostatic duster. Use a face mask when applying.

For fowl ticks (blue bugs) in all types of housing, dilute 4 lbs. in 25 gallons of water. Apply one (1) gallon of diluted spray per 100-150 sq. ft. thoroughly to walls, ceiling, floor cracks, and crevices with a power sprayer.

Premise Use Directions:

For flies in dairy barns, poultry houses, swine barns and other animal buildings, dilute 4 lbs. in 12½ gallons of water for dry white washed wood or concrete block surfaces, one (1) gallon of diluted spray per 500 sq. ft.; 4 lbs. in 25 gallons of water for unpainted wood or painted concrete block surfaces, one (1) gallon of diluted spray per 500 sq. ft.; or 4 lbs. in 25 gallons of water for masonite or galvanized sheet metal surfaces, one-half (½) gallon of diluted spray per 500 sq. ft.

For maggots in poultry droppings, manure piles, garbage piles and under feed troughs, dilute 4 lbs. in 25 gallons of water. Apply one (1) gallon of diluted spray per 100 sq. ft. Penetrate the problem area the first time - repeat every 7-10 days thereafter.

For ticks in campgrounds, backyards, picnic areas, recreational parks and other outdoor living areas, dilute 4 lbs. in 50 gallons of water. Spray the infested areas thoroughly (approximately 25 gallons of diluted spray per acre). Spray along foot paths and roadsides leading to such areas.

Precautionary Statements:

Hazards to Humans: Harmful if swallowed. Avoid inhaling spray mist and dust. Do not get in eyes, on skin, or on clothing. Wash thoroughly with soap and water after handling and before eating or smoking. Avoid the contamination of feed and foodstuffs. Do not apply in dwellings.

Statement of Practical Treatment:

If swallowed, drink one or two glasses of water and induce vomiting by touching the back of the throat with a finger. Repeat until the vomit fluid is clear. Call a physician immediately. Do not induce vomiting or give anything by mouth to an unconscious person.

If inhaled, remove victim to fresh air. Apply respiration if indicated.

If on skin, remove contaminated clothing and wash the affected areas with soap and water.

If in eyes, flush eyes for at least 15 minutes with water. Call a physician if irritation persists.

Environmental Hazards: The product is toxic to fish. Keep out of lakes, streams or ponds. Do not contaminate water by the cleaning of equipment or the disposal of wastes. Apply the product only as specified on the label.

Storage and Disposal: Do not contaminate water, food or feed by storage or disposal.

Storage: Store in a dry place in the original container.

Container Disposal: Completely empty the bag into the application equipment. Then dispose of the empty bag in a sanitary landfill or by incineration, or, if allowed by state and local authorities, by burning. If burned, stay out of smoke.

Pesticide Disposal: Wastes resulting from the use of the product may be disposed of on-site or at an approved waste disposal facility.

Warning(s): Keep out of the reach of children.

Disclaimer: Warranty and limitation of damages: Seller warrants that this material conforms to its chemical description and is reasonably fit for the purposes stated on the label when used in accordance with directions under normal conditions of use and buyer assumes the risk of any use contrary to such directions. Seller makes no other express or implied warranty, including any other express or implied warranty of fitness or of merchantability and no agent of seller is authorized to do so except in writing and with specific reference to this warranty. In no event shall seller's liability for any breach of warranty exceed the purchase price of the material as to which a claim is made.

Presentation: Available in 4 lb. bags or in a case of 6 x 4 lbs.

Compendium Code No.: 10280941

RABON® 97.3 ORAL LARVICIDE PREMIX

Boehringer Ingelheim **Feed Medication**

EPA Reg. No.: 4691-133

Active Ingredient(s):

	By Weight
Tetrachlorvinphos (CAS No. 22248-79-9)	97.3%*
Other Ingredients:	2.7%
Total:	100.0%

*RABON® Insecticide—442 grams per pound

Indications: For use in cattle feeds to prevent the development of horn flies, face flies, house flies and stable flies in the manure of treated cattle.

Directions for Use: It is a violation of Federal law to use this product in a manner inconsistent with its labeling.

This product is specifically prepared granulated material designed for use in cattle feeds. RABON® 97.3 Oral Larvicide prevents the development of fly larvae in the manure of treated cattle. When used as directed, it will aid in the control of horn flies, face flies, house flies and stable flies which develop in cattle manure.

This product can be used in complete feeds, concentrates, protein supplements, mineral supplements or liquid feed supplements provided recommended guidelines are followed. RABON® larvicidal rations may be fed to breeding cattle, lactating dairy cattle or growing finishing cattle, either in dry lot or on pasture.

Application Restrictions: Do not apply this product in a way that will contact workers or other persons, either directly or through drift. Only protected handlers may be in the area during application. Feeds prepared using this product should not be pelleted unless tests are conducted to assure adequate RABON® levels after pelleting. Do not mix this product with feeds containing predominantly pellets due to particle size differences and potential segregation.

Precautionary Statements: Hazards to Humans and Domestic Animals:

Caution: Harmful if swallowed or absorbed through the skin. Causes moderate eye irritation. Avoid contact with eyes, skin or clothing. Prolonged or frequent contact may cause allergic reaction in some individuals. Wash thoroughly with soap and water after handling.

Personal Protective Equipment: Handlers must wear:

Long sleeved shirt and pants

Shoes and socks

Chemical resistant gloves

User Safety Requirements: Follow manufacturer's instructions for cleaning/maintaining PPE. If no such instructions for washables, use detergent and hot water. Keep and wash PPE separately from other laundry.

User Safety Recommendations:

Wash hands before eating, drinking, chewing gum, using tobacco or using the toilet.

Remove clothing immediately if pesticide gets inside. Then wash thoroughly and put on clean clothing.

Remove PPE immediately after handling this product. Wash the outside of gloves before removing. As soon as possible, wash thoroughly and change into clean clothing.

First Aid:

If Swallowed: Call a physician or Poison Control Center. Drink 1 or 2 glasses of water and induce vomiting or if available by administering syrup of ipecac. If person is unconscious, do not give anything by mouth and do not induce vomiting.

R

If On Skin: Wash with plenty of soap and water. Get medical attention if irritation persists.

If In Eyes: Flush eyes with plenty of water. Call a physician if irritation persists.

Note to Physicians and Veterinarians:

Poisoning Symptoms: Symptoms include weakness, headache, tightness in chest, blurred vision, non-reactive pinpoint pupils, salivation, sweating, nausea, vomiting, diarrhea, and abdominal cramps.

Treatment: Tetrachlorvinphos is an organophosphate insecticide. If symptoms of cholinesterase inhibition are present, atropine sulfate by injection is antidotal. 2-PAM is also antidotal and maybe administered, but only in conjunction with atropine. Atropine is antidotal only if symptoms of cholinesterase inhibition are present.

Do not use this product on animals simultaneously or within a few days before or after treatment with cholinesterase inhibiting drugs, pesticides, or chemicals.

Environmental Hazards: This pesticide is toxic to fish. Do not contaminate water when disposing of equipment wash waters.

Storage and Disposal: Do not contaminate water, food or feed by storage or disposal.

Storage: Store in a dry place in original container.

Container Disposal: Completely empty liner by shaking and tapping sides and bottom to loosen clinging particles. Empty residue into mixing equipment. Then offer for recycling or reconditioning, or puncture and dispose of with liner in a sanitary landfill or by incineration, if allowed by State and local authorities. If burned, stay out of smoke.

Pesticide Disposal: Wastes resulting from the use of this product maybe disposed of on-site or at an approved waste disposal facility.

Warning(s): Keep out of reach of children.

Disclaimer: Warranty and Limitation of Damages: Seller warrants that this material conforms to its chemical description and is reasonably fit for the purposes stated on the label when used in accordance with directions under normal conditions of use and Buyer assumes the risk of any use contrary to such directions. Seller makes no other express or implied warranty, including any other express or implied warranty of Fitness or of Merchantability, and no agent of Seller is authorized to do so except in writing and with a specific reference to this warranty. In no event shall Seller's liability for any breach of warranty exceed the purchase price of the material as to which a claim is made.

Presentation: 100 lbs (45.4 kg).

Compendium Code No.: 10281230 658001L-01-9911

RABVAC™ 1

Fort Dodge **Vaccine**

Rabies Vaccine, Killed Virus

U.S. Vet. Lic. No.: 112

Contents: This product contains the antigen listed above.

Contains gentamicin as a preservative.

Indications: RABVAC™ 1 is a killed virus vaccine for the vaccination of healthy dogs and cats against rabies. This vaccine meets the one year duration of immunity requirements for dogs and cats.

Dosage and Administration: Dogs and Cats: Inject one 1 mL dose subcutaneously or at one site in the thigh intramuscularly at 3 months of age or older. Revaccinate one year later and annually thereafter.

InfoVax-ID® System: The InfoVax-ID® System provides a simple and effective method of recording pertinent information on the vaccines administered to animals in a veterinary practice.

For vaccines requiring reconstitution, remove label from both vials and affix both labels to the animal's medical chart.

Using the InfoVax-ID® System:

1. Grasp the lower right hand corner of the tab at the arrow marked "Peel Here" between your thumb and forefinger.
2. Pull steadily at a slight upward angle until the top portion of the label is separated from the vial.
3. Place the label on the animal's medical chart. Press down on the label to ensure adhesion.

Precaution(s): Store between 2° and 7°C (35° and 45°F). Do not freeze. Shake well before use.

Caution(s): This product is restricted for use by or under the supervision of a veterinarian.

In the absence of a veterinarian-client-patient relationship, Federal law prohibits the relabeling, repackaging, resale, or redistribution of the individual contents of this package. (9 CFR 112.6)

The use of a biological may produce anaphylaxis and/or other inflammatory immune-mediated hypersensitivity reactions. Antidote: Epinephrine, corticosteroids, and antihistamines may all be indicated depending on the nature and severity of the reaction.

A local reaction may occur at the injection site following subcutaneous administration.

Warning(s): For use in dogs and cats only.

For veterinary use only.

Presentation: Boxes of 50 x 1 mL single dose vials and 10 x 10 mL multiple dose vials, featuring the InfoVax-ID® System.

U.S. Pat. No. 5,704,648 (InfoVax-ID® System)

Compendium Code No.: 10031801 E12136A

RABVAC™ 3

Fort Dodge **Vaccine**

Rabies Vaccine, Killed Virus

U.S. Vet. Lic. No.: 112

Contents: This product contains the antigen listed above.

Contains gentamicin as a preservative.

Indications: RABVAC™ 3 is a killed virus vaccine for the vaccination of healthy dogs, cats and horses against rabies. This vaccine meets the three year duration of immunity requirements for dogs and cats, and one year duration of immunity for horses.

Dosage and Administration: Dogs and Cats: Inject one 1 mL dose subcutaneously or at one site in the thigh intramuscularly.

Vaccinate dogs and cats 3 months of age or older with one dose. Revaccinate with a repeat dose one year later. Revaccinate both dogs and cats every 3 years.

Horses: Inject one 2 mL dose intramuscularly.

Note: Two 1 mL vials must be used.

Vaccinate horses 3 months of age or older. Revaccinate with one 2 mL dose one year later. Annual revaccination with one 2 mL dose is required.

InfoVax-ID® System: The InfoVax-ID® System provides a simple and effective method of recording pertinent information on the vaccines administered to animals in a veterinary practice.

For vaccines requiring reconstitution, remove label from both vials and affix both labels to the animal's medical chart.

Using the InfoVax-ID® System:

1. Grasp the lower right hand corner of the tab at the arrow marked "Peel Here" between your thumb and forefinger.
2. Pull steadily at a slight upward angle until the top portion of the label is separated from the vial.
3. Place the label on the animal's medical chart. Press down on the label to ensure adhesion.

Precaution(s): Store between 2° and 7°C (35° and 45°F). Do not freeze. Shake well before use.

Caution(s): This product is restricted for use by or under the supervision of a veterinarian.

In the absence of a veterinarian-client-patient relationship, Federal law prohibits the relabeling, repackaging, resale, or redistribution of the individual contents of this package. (9 CFR 112.6)

Transitory fever, lethargy, lack of appetite and injection site swelling or pain may occur following vaccination. These signs can last one or more days. They are normally self-limiting. The use of a biological product can be associated with rare life threatening events. One example: Anaphylaxis. Antidote: Epinephrine. Depending upon severity, other therapeutic interventions may be indicated.

Warning(s): Do not vaccinate horses within 21 days before slaughter.

For use in dogs, cats and horses only.

For veterinary use only.

Presentation: Boxes of 50 x 1 mL single dose vials and 10 x 10 mL multiple dose vials, featuring the InfoVax-ID® System.

U.S. Pat. No. 5,704,648 (InfoVax-ID® System)

Compendium Code No.: 10031811 12156E

RALGRO® IMPLANTS (Cattle)

Schering-Plough **Implant**

Beef Cattle Implants

NADA No.: 038-233

Active Ingredient(s): Each implant contains 36 mg zeranol (three pellets, each containing 12 mg zeranol).

Zeranol, the active drug in RALGRO®, is a derivative of resorcylic acid lactone fermentation product.

Indications: Used to increase the rate of weight gain and improve feed conversion in suckling beef calves, including replacement heifers between one month of age and weaning, weaned beef calves, growing beef cattle, feedlot steers and feedlot heifers.

Dosage and Administration: The dose for all classes of beef cattle is 36 mg (three 12 mg pellets). The implant site is subcutaneous, between the skin and cartilage on the back side of the ear and below the midline of the ear. The implant must not be placed closer to the head than the edge of the auricular cartilage ring furthest from the head. The location for insertion of the needle is a point toward the tip of the ear and at least a needle length away from the intended deposition site. Care should be taken to avoid injuring the major blood vessels or cartilage of the ear. Squeeze the trigger of the Ralogun® to deliver a full dose of RALGRO®. Keep the trigger depressed while withdrawing the needle to be sure that the RALGRO® implants stay in place.

Caution(s): Do not use in bulls intended for reproduction or dairy animals.

Do not use before one month of age or after weaning in heifers intended for reproduction.

Edema of the vulva and udder, teat elongation, rectal and vaginal prolapse, and signs of estrus may occur when heifers are implanted. Delayed testicular development may occur in young males. To avoid difficulty in castration, young males should be castrated at the time of implanting.

Discussion: Zeranol acts by stimulating the pituitary gland in the brain to produce more of its own natural growth hormone, somatotropin. Maximum response will be attained with good quality stock, free from parasites, disease and on a good plane of nutrition.

Zeranol is an anabolic agent that has a positive influence on the dynamic state of protein metabolism in the animal. Studies indicate that one mode of action of zeranol is stimulation of the pituitary gland to produce increased amounts of somatotrophin. Implanted animals can be expected to gain 10% faster and improve feed conversion 8% over nonimplanted animals.

Presentation: 24 doses per cartridge and 10 x 10 dose strips (100 doses).

Compendium Code No.: 10471681

RALGRO® IMPLANTS (Lamb)

Schering-Plough **Implant**

Feedlot Lamb Implants

NADA No.: 038-233

Active Ingredient(s): Each implant contains 12 mg zeranol (one pellet, each containing 12 mg zeranol).

Zeranol, the active drug in RALGRO®, is a derivative of resorcylic acid lactone fermentation product.

Indications: Used to increase the rate of weight gain and improve feed conversion of feedlot lambs.

Dosage and Administration: The dose for feedlot lambs is 12 mg (one 12 mg pellet). The implant site is subcutaneous, between the skin and cartilage on the back side of the ear and below the midline of the ear. The location for insertion of the needle is a point toward the tip of the ear and at least a needle length away from the intended deposition site. Care should be taken to avoid injuring the major blood vessels or cartilage of the ear. Squeeze the trigger of the Ralogun® implant device to deliver a full dose of RALGRO®. Keep the trigger depressed while withdrawing the needle to be sure that RALGRO® implants stay in place.

Caution(s): Under certain management conditions, especially creep fed lambs implanted at an early age, there have been occasional reports of vaginal and/or rectal prolapse, after implanting.

Warning(s): Not for use in animals intended for breeding purposes.

Do not implant feedlot lambs within 40 days of slaughter.

Trial Data: Zeranol is an anabolic agent that has a positive influence on the dynamic state of protein metabolism in the animal. Studies indicate that one mode of action of zeranol is stimulation of the pituitary gland to produce increased amounts of somatotrophin. Implanted animals can be expected to gain 12% faster and improve feed conversion 10% over nonimplanted animals.

Presentation: 24 doses per cartridge.

Compendium Code No.: 10471690

RALGRO® MAGNUM™ IMPLANTS

Schering-Plough **Implant**

Implants for steers

NADA No.: 038-233

Active Ingredient(s): Zeranol, 72 mg.

RALGRO® MAGNUM™ pellets each contain 12 mg of zeranol. Six pellets are required for a 72 mg dose.

A single pull of the Dur-A-Tract® injector trigger delivers the proper 72 mg dose (six-12 mg pellets per chamber).

Manufactured by a non-sterilizing process.

Indications: RALGRO® MAGNUM™ implant is an anabolic agent that increases rate of weight gain and improves feed efficiency in steers fed in confinement for slaughter.

Dosage and Administration: Directions for Using RALGRO® MAGNUM™ Implants in Strip Cartridges with the Dur-A-Tract® Pellet Injector.

Step 1: Each chamber of the plastic strip cartridge contains a full dose of RALGRO® MAGNUM™ Implant. Insert the strip cartridge into the bottom of the Dur-A-Tract® Implanter with the open end of the inverted V pointing down and the arrow on the top of the cartridge pointing to the front (needle portion) of the implanter until the top wing is flush with the upper surface of the injector. To ensure proper seating, check window on the side of the implanter to ensure the pellet chamber is aligned with the plunger.

Step 2: Always use sharp needle. A dull needle tears tissue and makes proper implanting difficult.

Step 3: After appropriately restraining the animal to allow access to the ear, cleanse the skin at the implant needle puncture site.

Step 4: The implant site is subcutaneous, between the skin and the cartilage on the back of the ear and below the midline of the ear. The implant must not be placed closer to the head than the edge of the auricular cartilage ring farthest from the head. The location for insertion of the needle is a point toward the tip of the ear and at least a needle length away from the intended deposition site.

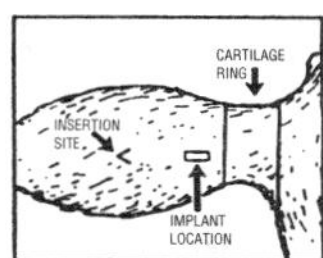

Step 5: Care should be taken to avoid injuring the major blood vessels or cartilage of the ear. Squeeze the trigger of the Dur-A-Tract® Implanter to deliver a full dose of RALGRO® MAGNUM™ Implant. Keep trigger depressed while withdrawing the needle to be sure that RALGRO® MAGNUM™ implants stay in place.

Step 6: Wipe needle with cotton or gauze moistened with alcohol or other suitable disinfectant. Do not dip needle in solution because solution clinging to inside of needle will cause plugging of needle.

Step 7: Depress the advancement mechanism fully to ensure that the strip cartridge has advanced. Check in the window on the side of the Dur-A-Tract® Implanter to ensure that the next dose of RALGRO® MAGNUM™ implant is properly aligned with the plunger and is ready to be delivered.

Precaution(s): RALGRO® MAGNUM™ pellets are stable when stored at room temperature (15°-30°C) conditions.

Caution(s): Restricted drug (California), use only as directed.

Warning(s): Do not attempt to salvage implant site for human or animal food. Implant pellets in the ear only. Any other location is in violation of Federal law.

Trial Data: Note: In a clinical study evaluating several test doses of zeranol implants for feed efficiency (including 36 mg, 48 mg, and 72 mg doses), the 48 mg and 72 mg doses were shown to be superior to the 36 mg dose, but the 72 mg dose was not shown to be superior for feed efficiency to the 48 mg dose.

Presentation: Ten 10-dose strips (100 doses). Implant needle enclosed.

Compendium Code No.: 10471700

RALLY™-20 ℞

Vedco — **Antihistamine**

(Tripelennamine Hydrochloride Injection) 20 mg/mL

ANADA No.: 200-162

Active Ingredient(s): Each mL contains:

Tripelennamine hydrochloride USP . . . . 20 mg

Indications: For use in cattle and horses in conditions in which antihistaminic therapy may be expected to lead to alleviation of some signs of disease.

Pharmacology: Tripelennamine hydrochloride is a white, crystalline material which is stable, nonhygroscopic, and readily soluble in water.

Tripelennamine hydrochloride is characterized by its capacity to antagonize many of the pharmacologic effects of histamine.

Dosage and Administration: Warm the solution to near body temperature.

Using aseptic precautions, administer intravenously or intramuscularly as specified below. Intramuscular injections should be made into the heavy musculature of the hind leg or cervical area.

The doses specified below may be repeated in 6 to 12 hours if necessary.

Cattle: Administer intravenously or intramuscularly at a dose of 0.5 mg per lb of body weight (2.5 mL for each 100 lbs of body weight). For a more rapid onset of action, the intravenous route of administration is recommended.

Horses: Administer intramuscularly only at a dose of 0.5 mg per lb of body weight (2.5 mL for each 100 lbs of body weight).

Precaution(s): Protect from light. Store between 15°C and 30°C (59°F-86°F). Avoid excessive heat (104°F).

Caution(s): Federal law restricts this drug to use by or on the order of a licensed veterinarian.

Central nervous system stimulation in the form of hyperexcitability, nervousness, and muscle tremors lasting up to 20 minutes have been noted in horses, particularly following intravenous administration; therefore, only the intramuscular route of administration should be used in horses.

Overdosage of tripelennamine hydrochloride may give rise to excitement, ataxia, and convulsions.

Depression of the central nervous system and incoordination may occur when the drug is used at therapeutic dose levels.

Disturbances in gastrointestinal function may occur in some instances.

While poisonous snake bites have been treated with antihistaminic drugs, other conjunctive therapy is required because of toxic reactions associated with the protein complex of venom.

Warning(s): Do not use in horses intended for food purposes.

Milk that has been taken during treatment and for 24 hours (two milkings) after the last treatment must not be used for food.

Treated cattle must not be slaughtered for food during treatment and for four days following the last treatment.

A withdrawal period has not been established for this product in pre-ruminating calves. Do not use in calves to be processed for veal.

For animal use only.

Keep out of reach of children.

Presentation: RALLY™-20 (Tripelennamine Hydrochloride Injection) is supplied in 250 mL and 500 mL multiple dose vials.

Compendium Code No.: 10941800

RAM EPIDIDYMITIS BACTERIN

Colorado Serum — **Bacterin**

Ram Epididymitis Bacterin

U.S. Vet. Lic. No.: 188

Active Ingredient(s): An inactivated aqueous culture of an isolate from the epididymis of an infected ram. The bacterin is adsorbed with aluminum hydroxide.

Contains thimerosal as a preservative.

Indications: For vaccinating rams to stimulate resistance to ram epididymitis.

Dosage and Administration: Inject 2 mL subcutaneously. The loose skin behind the shoulder or at the side of the neck are suggested sites. Repeat the dose in 30-60 days. Ram lambs at weaning age and mature rams may be vaccinated. Annual revaccination is recommended.

Precaution(s): Shake well before using. Store in the dark at temperatures not over 7°C. Do not freeze.

Caution(s): Anaphylactic reactions sometimes follow administration of products of this nature. If noted, administer adrenaline or an equivalent drug.

Use the entire contents when first opened.

For veterinary use only.

Warning(s): Do not vaccinate within 21 days before slaughter.

Presentation: 10 dose (20 mL) vials.

Compendium Code No.: 11010290

RAPID JOHNE'S TEST

ImmuCell — **Johne's Disease Test**

U.S. Vet. Lic. No.: 327

Contents: Reagents and materials:

1) One vial 0.25 mL *Mycobacterium paratuberculosis* antigen, labelled vial #1.
2) One vial 0.40 mL bovine serum positive control, labelled vial #2.
3) 10 agarose gel immunodiffusion plates, (10 tests, 10 controls).

Indications: The ImmuCell AGID test has been designed specifically to aid in the differential diagnosis of cattle with clinical Johne's disease. The test is subject to the limitations and sensitivity stated in the section "Limitations of the Test".

Test Principle: The agarose gel immunodiffusion (AGID) test is a reliable, easy-to-use method for the detection of serum antibodies to *Mycobacterium paratuberculosis,* the causative agent of Johne's disease.

The test relies on the diffusion of two components in an agarose gel matrix. The two components are 1) a protoplasmic extract of *M. paratuberculosis* and 2) positive control or serum sample containing circulating antibodies to *M. Paratuberculosis.* When these two components combine under the proper conditions, an antibody-antigen precipitate will form in the gel and eventually appear as a diffuse or precipitin line depending upon the relative concentration of the two reactants. This precipitin line will usually form within 24-48 hours after the introduction of sample and antigen into the gel. The presence of a precipitin band, regardless of intensity, is considered a positive result. The absence, however, of a precipitin line at the end of incubation does not mean the animal is free of the disease. A negative test result may be due to serum antibody levels which are insufficient to cause immune precipitation in the gel, a condition commonly referred to as antigen excess. It is recommended that fecal culture be performed in all cases where a negative AGID test is observed in animals with apparent clinical symptoms.

Test Procedure:

1. Remove the agar gel plate from the tray.
2. Remove the lid from the plate and place the plate on a smooth, level surface. Be careful not to scratch the bottom of the plate as scratches within the test area may be misinterpreted as positive test reactions.
3. The triangular pattern of wells on the plate should be positioned so that the smallest well is located at the top of the triangle. This well is the antigen well. The remaining large wells at the bottom of the triangle should be marked "S" and "C" (sample and control).
4. Into the antigen well carefully dispense 20 µL of the antigen from vial "1". Place the pipette directly into the well, thereby preventing accidental discharge of fluid onto the gel surface. Improper filling of the well may effect the test results.
5. The control serum provided with the kit is assurance that the test components are working properly. A positive control should be run with every test. Carefully dispense (as in step #4) 35 µL of positive control serum from vial #2 into the well marked "C".
6. Dispense 35 µL of serum from a suspect animal into the well marked "S".
7. Following the addition of antigen, positive control and sample to the appropriate wells, the plate lid should be replaced firmly to prevent dehydration of the gel during incubation.
8. Allow the plate to incubate on a level surface at room temperature for 48 hours. The plate should be located in an area that is free from significant temperature variations and accidental movement.
9. Upon completion of the 48-hour period, the plate(s) are ready to observe for the presence of precipitin lines.
10. Carefully wipe the bottom of the plate with a soft cloth or paper towel to remove any smudges, fingerprints, etc., giving special attention to the center area (test area) of the plate.
11. Remove the lid from the plate and hold the plate between the fingertips in order to avoid smudging the previously cleaned plate bottom.

The results are sometimes easier to observe when backlighting, such as with a desk lamp. When using a light source such as a desk lamp, hold the test plate approximately six (6) inches from a dark background with illumination directed from the side of the plate. Look for a white precipitin band similar to the one generated by the positive control.

Specimen collection: The best results are obtained using fresh bovine serum taken in the proper manner. Slight hemolysis does not interfere with the performance of the test.

The presence of a positive AGID test in addition to the observation of clinical signs of Johne's disease (diarrhea, rapid weight loss) indicates an animal with high probability of Johne's infection. The absence of a precipitin line or "negative result" cannot be interpreted as a negative test result. This is due to the sensitivity limits of the agarose gel test. It is recommended that a "negative" result be followed-up by a fecal culture. During the course of Johne's disease there are usually fluctuations in the serum antibody titer. This variation in titer may result in intense precipitin band(s). The use of backlighting will enhance the visibility of weaker reactions.

Limitations of the test: The test is not intended to be used as a screening tool. The detection of subclinical animals, although desirable, is not a salient feature of the test.

The test is intended to be used as a differential diagnostic tool in the presence of clinical symptoms (e.g., diarrhea and rapid weight loss). In the presence of clinical signs, the RAPID JOHNE'S TEST has a 85% sensitivity rate.

A negative result cannot be interpreted as a true negative and fecal culture is recommended. Although 97 culture negative cows have been tested and found to give a negative AGID reaction, the possibility that infections with organisms other than *M. paratuberculosis* could yield a positive result cannot be ruled out. Asymptomatic animals which test positive in the RAPID JOHNE'S TEST should therefore be evaluated by fecal culture to confirm *M. paratuberculosis* infection.

Precaution(s):

1. Do not use reagents beyond the expiration date.
2. Gently swirl both the positive control and antigen vials to ensure proper mixing of the contents.
3. Do not freeze the gel plates, they will be useless.
4. Be certain that the gel plate covers are securely fastened to the plate bottoms to prevent dehydration of the gel.
5. Avoid placing the plates on surfaces that can mar or scratch the plate bottoms, scratched plate bottoms could interfere with the detection of precipitin lines.
6. Dispose of the kit components in the proper manner through autoclaving or the use of bio-bags. Do not use the kit components if a positive control reaction is not visible after 48 hours of incubation.
7. Wash and/or disinfect the hands thoroughly after use, handle the *M. paratuberculosis* antigen (vial #1) with precautions appropriate to infective material.
8. Store in a refrigerator at 35-45°F (4-7°C).
9. Store the positive control and antigen frozen after the first use.

Warning(s): The manufacturer makes only an express warranty which is limited to the statement that the product will function as described in the package insert. The express warranty shall not apply if the product has not been used or operated in accordance with the manufacturer's printed instruction, or if it has been used for any purposes other than those described in the printed instructions. The diagnostic test kit is sold as is, with the stated functional limitations in the package insert regarding sensitivity, specific and intended uses, please read the instructions before using.

User Quality Control:

Positive control serum should be used with each test. Failure of the control serum to show a distinctly visible precipitin line at 48 hours indicates either component failure or inappropriate use of the components such as accidental over or underfilling of the wells.

Discussion: Johne's disease is a slow-developing often chronic "wasting" disease of ruminant animals which is caused by the bacterium *Mycobacterium paratuberculosis*.[1] Passed by fecal-oral transmission from animals that are either acutely ill or asymptomatic shedders, *M. paratuberculosis* organisms are highly resistant to environmental degradation and can remain viable in manure and stagnant water for more than a year.[2] Identification of animals with clinical or subclinical disease is therefore important in controlling the spread of infection.

In the United States, Johne's disease has its greatest economic impact in cattle where estimated losses in weight gain and milk production among infected herds is significant.[3]

Symptoms of the disease in cattle include severe weight loss which may or may not be accompanied by persistent diarrhea. When present, diarrhea associated with Johne's disease is characteristically profuse, uniform in consistency and generally free of blood and mucous. Periodic weight loss in the presence of a normal appetite and body temperature are early clinical features of the disease which may precede diarrhea.

Efforts to control Johne's, a largely untreatable disease, have focused on detection of symptomatic and asymptomatic animals shedding infectious bacteria. Segregation or removal of shedding animals from the herd can prevent the spread of the bacteria to those animals at greatest risk of infection such as calves and breeding age heifers.[4] The most reliable methods for detecting Johne's infections include histopathological examination of intestinal tissue through biopsy or bacteriological culturing of suspect stool. Fecal culture on selective bacteriological media is the most common diagnostic procedure used in screening exposed or suspect animals, however, the 8-12 weeks required for bacterial growth makes culturing impractical for confirming clinical cases.

An alternative to fecal culture is the agar gel immunodiffusion (AGID) test which has been shown to be a reliable means of detecting paratuberculosis in cattle with clinical disease. A recent study of 50 cows with symptoms of weight loss and/or persistent diarrhea indicated that 98% animals fecal culture and/or necropsy positive for *M. paratuberculosis* were successfully identified by serological AGID testing.[5]

References: Available upon request.

Presentation: 10 test kit.

Compendium Code No.: 11200021

R

RAPIDVET™-D

DMS Laboratories **Dermatophyte Test**

Description: Screening system for veterinary dermatophytes.

Components: Test Reagents and/or Materials:

1. 25 tubes with blue caps containing the selective RAPIDVET™-D reaction substrate.
2. 25 labels for identifying reaction tubes.

Materials Required but not Provided:

1. Sterile scalpel.
2. Sterile forceps, scissors or nail clipper (optional).

Indications: RAPIDVET™-D is for use as part of the differential diagnosis of dermatological conditions in companion animals: dogs, cats, rabbits and horses. It is especially designed to provide a statistically significant indication of the involvement, or absence, of dermatophytes as a causal factor of the underlying condition. Since RAPIDVET™-D employs a proprietary formulation designed for the detection of only those fungi that cause clinical complications in the noted animal species, the product should not be used for other animal species or for humans. Likewise, RAPIDVET™-D is not designed for testing for the presence of viable but relatively dormant dermatophytes superficially present on the fur of asymptomatic animals which, while frequently present, are not a causal factor in any underlying condition.

Test Principles: In the late 1960's and early 1970's Taplin and colleagues formulated a culture medium for dermatophyte identification and ancillary growth that improved the earlier work of Sabouraud. Specific nutrients in the medium promoted the growth of dermatophytes, while selective antibiotics inhibited the growth of nonpathogenic saprophytic mycetes and bacteria. The alkaline metabolites produced by the Microsporum, Trichophyton and Epidermophyton genera that selectively grow on that medium cause a distinctive and discernible color change in the pH indicator, Phenol Red, contained in the medium (Table 1).

Table 1. Frequency of Dermatophytes in Companion Animals:

	Dogs	Cats	Horses	Rabbits
M. canis	++++	++++	+	+
M. gypseum	+++	+	+++	+++
M. audouinii	+			+
M. distortum	+	+	+	
T. mentagrophytes	+	+	+	++++
T. verrucosum	+		+	
T. equinum	+		++++	
T. rubrum	+			
T. gallinae	+			
T. schoenleinii	+	+	+	+

+ = reported
++ = occasional
+++ = common
++++ = frequent

RAPIDVET™-D is a further improvement of this work to focus on the specific needs of the veterinary practice. It is used by the clinician to rapidly determine, within acceptable statistical limits rather than with absolute certainty, the likelihood of dermatophyte involvement. This has been accomplished by evolution of a proprietary formulation of a reaction substrate to address the specific needs involved.

RAPIDVET™-D is a selective, differential reaction substrate that enables the target organisms to metabolize various nutrients and produce substances that cause the pH indicator to change color within a specified time span. It also suppresses, within the same time span, the metabolism of other organisms that would normally cause the pH indicator to change color. Thus, a color change, or absence thereof, within the indicated time span, can statistically be considered an indication of the presence or absence of dermatophytes in the sample.

Test Procedure: Specimen Collection and Inoculation: The site of sampling must be inspected to ensure that it has not been treated with medicaments that could affect the result. If necessary, clean the site carefully so as not to destroy the viability of any dermatophytes collected. It is sometimes necessary to clean the site to reduce bacterial and/or saprophytic contamination. If so, cleaning should be limited to gentle use of a pad soaked in 70% alcohol.

To collect the specimen, use a sterile scalpel to take scales and/or hair from the border of obvious lesions. In some instances, use of forceps may be more convenient for removal of hair. If a hair sample is utilized, that portion of the hair more than 2 cm (0.8 inch) from the skin should be clipped off and discarded. If the nail area is infected, clippings from the nail edges can be used as the sample.

Place the sample on the surface of the reaction substrate without cutting or pushing into it. Close the tube, but not completely since moisture buildup in the tube is to be avoided. Label the tube with the patient's name and date using the labels provided. The tube is maintained at room temperature for the duration of the test period. Note: Room temperature means 22-25°C (72-77°F).

Test Interpretation: Results: Periodically examine the reaction substrate in each tube for 72 hours, starting after 24 hours. Any change in color from yellow to red, even in only a region of the reaction substrate, is interpreted as positive for the presence of dermatophytes. However, the degree of red will intensify with time and the area of color will spread with time. The test period is deemed terminated at the end of 72 hours and the tube should be discarded in an environmentally correct manner.

Storage: In order to meet the needs of the veterinary practice, RAPIDVET™-D has been designed to be stable at room temperature (away from direct sunlight) for 20 months. Shelf life can be extended to 36 months by refrigeration at 2-8°C (36-46°F). If refrigeration is used, the tube(s) to be used should be brought to room temperature before use. In any event, freezing and/or overheating must be avoided. The expiration date on the box is that corresponding to refrigerated storage.

Caution(s): The following precautions are necessary requisites for obtaining results in 72 hours.

Sample must be properly collected from the edge of the lesion where the organism is most active.

RAPIDVET™-D reaction tubes must be at room temperature (22-25°C/72-77°F) immediately before and during the entire period of use.

Sample must be placed on the surface of the reaction substrate. Results may not be reliable if sample is pressed below the surface of the reaction substrate.

The tubes must be loosely capped to avoid moisture buildup which can slow the reaction.

Discussion: Performance Characteristics: When used to test samples from 820 dogs, 369 cats and 492 horses having suspected dermatophyte lesions, RAPIDVET™-D produced positive results on 510 samples, or 30.3%, of which 494 were confirmed to be positive by reference methodology conducted by a specialist in dermatophyte infections. Thus, the false positive rate can be considered to be 3.3%. The remaining 1171 samples, or 69.7% produced negative results of which 1150 were confirmed to be negative by reference methodology conducted by a specialist in dermatophyte infections. Thus, the false negative rate can be considered to be 1.8%.

The overall accuracy can be considered to be 97.7% and not materially different by species tested.

Limitations of the Assay:

1. RAPIDVET™-D is only for *in vitro* diagnostic use on samples taken from symptomatic dogs, cats, rabbits and horses.
2. RAPIDVET™-D is intended for use by the clinician who wants to obtain a result that is highly likely to be clinically significant. It is not intended for use by a microbiologist who wants a conclusive result.
3. While it is possible for a practiced eye to determine the identity of the dermatophyte involved by maintaining the tube for an extended period of time, until colony growth is noted, and then examining the colonies with comparison to pictorial representations in standard reference works, this is not the intended use of this product.

References: Available upon request.

Presentation: 25 tests.

RAPIDVET is a trademark of DMS Laboratories, Inc.
Made in Italy by Agrolabo S.p.A.
DMS 11025, December 1996

Compendium Code No.: 14810030

RAPIDVET™-H (CANINE DEA 1.1)

DMS Laboratories **Blood Group Test**

Blood Group Determination Assay

Components: Reagents and Materials: This test kit contains the reagents and materials listed below. Store upright.

Auto-Agglutination Saline Screen Card. This card has 3 visually defined wells and is packaged in a sealed polyethylene sleeve.

Agglutination Test Cards. Each card has 3 visually defined wells identified as "DEA 1.1 Positive Control", "DEA 1.1 Negative Control" and "Patient Test". The cards are packaged individually in sealed polyethylene sleeves each containing a small desiccant bag. Store at room temperature or in a refrigerator (2-7°C).

1 Bottle Diluent. The clear plastic bottle contains 0.02 mol/L phosphate buffered saline (PBS) at pH 7.4. The dropping tip accurately dispenses 40 μL. Refrigerate (2-7°C).

1 Bottle Positive Control. The white plastic bottle contains a biological material. The dropping tip accurately dispenses 40 μL. Refrigerate (2-7°C).

1 Bottle Negative Control. The white plastic bottle contains a biological material. The dropping tip accurately dispenses 40 μL. Refrigerate (2-7°C).

Pipettes and Stirrers. Each polyethylene bag contains 2 plastic pipettes and 4 stirrers.

Materials Required But Not Provided: None.

Reagent Preparation: None.

Quality Control: All reagents and materials incorporated into this kit have been quality controlled by standard testing procedures using a routine quality control program during manufacture.

Indications: RAPIDVET™-H (Canine DEA 1.1) is intended for use to classify dogs as DEA 1.1 positive or negative.

For *in vitro* use.

Test Principles: Principle and Explanation of the Assay: The RAPIDVET™-H (Canine DEA 1.1) assay is based on the agglutination reaction that occurs when an erythrocyte which contains a DEA 1.1 antigen on its surface membrane interacts with a murine monoclonal antibody proven specific to DEA 1.1 which is lyophilized on the Test Card. The monoclonal antibody is reconstituted with a diluent to form an antiserum, and is thoroughly mixed with whole blood from the patient. All DEA 1.1 positive erythrocytes react with the antiserum causing agglutination. The antiserum is completely nonreactive with all DEA 1.1 negative erythrocytes. The results are visually identified.

Test Procedure:

1. Draw blood from the patient into a syringe or lavender tube coated with or containing EDTA as an anticoagulant. The assay requires only 100 μL whole blood but the tube or syringe should be full so that there is a proper concentration of EDTA. If the type is not to be determined immediately, nutrients such as CPDA should not be added.
2. Remove the Auto-Agglutination Saline Screen Card from its plastic sleeve and place the card on a flat surface.
3. Write the name/number of the dog and the testing date on the Auto-Agglutination Saline Screen Card adjacent to the well to be used.
4. Dispense 1 drop of diluent (40 μL) from the dropping bottle into the well to be used.
5. Aspirate a small amount of patient sample into the pipette and release 1 drop (50 μL) into the well. Using a stirrer, spread and mix the materials within the entirety of this well for about 10 seconds, pressing downward firmly. (See Note 1 for correct use of the pipette.)
6. A small percentage of ill dogs and of healthy dogs auto-agglutinate. If agglutination is observed, stop the test and perform normal cell washing procedures before proceeding. After the materials on the card have dried, replace the card in its plastic sleeve for future use.
7. Remove the Test Card from its plastic sleeve. Save the plastic sleeve and set aside the desiccant bags.
8. Write the name/number of the dog and the testing date on the card.
9. Place the Test Card on a flat surface.
10. Dispense 1 drop of diluent (40 μL) from the dropping bottle into each well. The diluent assists in reconstitution of the lyophilized material in the control and patient well.
11. Gently swirl the bottles containing the control and the patient sample to resuspend any solid material.
12. Unscrew the top of the control bottle and place it on table in front of the Test Card. Place the cap behind the respective bottle.
13. Dispense 1 drop (40 μL) Positive Control into the well marked "DEA 1.1 Positive Control". Using a new stirrer, spread and mix the materials within the entirety of the well for about 10 seconds. Stir firmly with downward pressure on the card to reconstitute the lyophilized material.
14. Dispense 1 drop (40 μL) Negative Control into the well marked "DEA 1.1 Negative Control". Using a new stirrer, spread and mix the materials within the entirety of the well for about 10 seconds. Stir firmly with downward pressure on the card to reconstitute the lyophilized material.
15. Aspirate a small amount of patient sample into a pipette and release 1 drop (50 μL) into the well marked "Patient Test". Using a new stirrer, and pressing downward firmly, spread and mix the materials within the entirety of the well for about 10 seconds.
16. Rock the card with a transaxial motion for 2 minutes, being sure that the materials are mixing and "rotating" within each well. Be careful not to cross-contaminate.
17. Set the card at a 10° angle to allow excess blood to run to the bottom of the wells. Placing the top of the card on the desiccant bag will accomplish this.
18. Read the results and note the wells where gross agglutination has occurred.
19. After the materials on the card have dried, replace the card in its plastic sleeve for a permanent record.
20. Before replacing the control bottles in the box, tap the bottom of each bottle firmly on the table to cause residual liquid in the dropper tip to fall back into the bottle. Store upright. (See Note 2 below for further explanation.)

Procedure Note 1: Use of the pipette: Hold the plastic tube between thumb and forefinger near the flat, sealed end, squeeze tightly and do not release pressure. Hold the specimen tube vertically and place the open end of the plastic tube below the surface of the specimen. Release finger pressure to draw up the sample.

Next, hold the pipette in a perpendicular position directly over the well to which the sample is to be delivered. Squeeze gently and allow one free drop to fall into the well (50 μL). The pipette is designed to expel slightly in excess of 50 μL to compensate for a small amount of specimen retained by the stirrer.

Use each pipette only once, then discard. Under no circumstance should the pipette be used more than once as cross-contamination can occur causing inaccurate test results.

Procedure Note 2: At times, due to improper handling (see "20" above) fibrin filaments may form in the tip of the control bottle. The diameter of the bore of the tip is such that it is unlikely that an available pin or needle will penetrate the bore. The tip of the dropper bottle can be removed and a pipette used to dispense 50 μL of the control.

Test Interpretation: Results: If the assay was run correctly, visible, gross agglutination should have occurred in the well marked "DEA 1.1 Positive Control".

If the patient sample shows gross agglutination in the well marked "Patient Test" and there is no auto-agglutination, the patient is DEA 1.1 positive. If no agglutination is visible in the well marked "Patient Test", the patient is DEA 1.1 negative.

Any fine, granular appearance developing after 2 minutes should be disregarded in determining the results. The speed of agglutination and the size of the clumps of cells of a DEA 1.1 positive patient may differ from that of the positive control. Unlike humans, an individual animal may possess more than one primary blood type. In such case, the red cells will carry antigens for each such type. Such an animal will carry less DEA 1.1 antigens than an animal that has only DEA 1.1 as a primary blood type.

If the patient is anemic, the pattern of agglutination may be in the form of discrete, small aggregations each like the head of a large pin rather than gross agglutination.

Limitations of the Procedure:

1. Be careful to replace the cap to the bottle from which it was removed. Failure to do so will cross-contaminate controls and provide inaccurate results.
2. To obtain accurate results it is essential that correct procedure be followed.
3. Always use a new dispensing pipette for each specimen and a new stirrer for each well. Reusing any device will cause cross-contamination and inaccurate results.
4. Always run the controls on each Test Card even if testing several patients and using several Test Cards. The controls are used as evidence that the assay has been performed correctly, to provide comparison results and to create a proper permanent record.
5. The stability of the individual components of the kit varies. Store the components as indicated on the labels. Do not use any component beyond the indicated expiration date. Use of expired materials may cause unreliable results.
6. The diluent is provided in a bottle with a screw cap to minimize inadvertent bacterial or other contamination. Diluent from other sources in the laboratory should not be utilized.
7. The physical integrity of the patient sample is critical to correct results.
8. Always draw a full syringe or lavender tube containing EDTA. Less blood will cause too high a concentration of EDTA in the specimen to be tested.

Known Interfering Substances: None.

Trouble Shooting Guide:

Problem	Possible Cause	Corrective Action
No agglutination in "DEA 1.1 Positive Control" well	a) active material settled out b) forgot to use diluent to reconstitute lyophilized material c) did not use downward pressure in stirring to reconstitute lyophilized material	a) swirl bottle as per Procedure Step #11 b) see Procedure Step #10 c) see Procedure Step #13
No reaction in "Patient Test" well for an animal said to be DEA 1:1 positive by another methodology	a) see (a), (b) and(c) above b) inadequate amount of blood relative to EDTA in sample draw c) use of packed cells instead of whole blood as a sample d) the other methodology is not accurate	a) see (a), (b) and (c) above b) see Procedure Step #1 and Limitations of the Procedure #8 c) dilute sample 1:1 with saline and re-run
Agglutination in "DEA 1.1 Negative Control" well	a) cross-contamination via multiple use of a stirrer b) reading result after two minutes	a) see Procedure Step #14 and Limitations of the Procedure #3 b) see Results re granularity forming after two minutes
Unable to dispense controls	Fibrin filaments in snout of top of control bottle due to improper storage	See Procedure Step #20 and Procedure Note #2. Unscrew top and use extra pipette
Agglutination exists in "Patient Test" well but is of a different character than that in "DEA 1.1 Positive Control" well	This is normal	See Results

Storage: Storage and Stability:

1. The Auto-Agglutination Saline Screen Card can be kept at room temperature and is stable indefinitely if stored in its polyethylene sleeve away from direct sunlight.
2. The Agglutination Test Cards are stable at room temperature (20-25°C) for a period of 19 months from date of manufacture. Each Test Card has an imprinted expiration date. Storage in a refrigerator (2-7°C) does not materially lengthen the period of stability but has no detrimental effect on the assay and protects against unexpected, or even unknown, variations in room temperature outside of this range. It is not necessary to bring the Test Card to room temperature prior to use.
3. The diluent is stable for 18 months from the date of manufacture if refrigerated (2-7°C). Each bottle of diluent is labeled with an expiration date.
4. The controls are stable for up to 6 months from date of preparation if refrigerated (2-7°C). When shipped, the controls have a 5 month shelf life. Each control is labeled with an expiration date.

Note: Each RAPIDVET™-H (Canine DEA 1.1) test kit is imprinted with an expiration date which represents the date of expiration of the shortest dated component in the kit. While some components may have later individual expiration dates, their use with other components from other kits is not recommended.

Disposal: Dispose of all biological materials, pipettes and stirrers in a safe and approved manner.

Caution(s): Caveat: A certain number of canine patients exhibit auto-agglutination of varying degrees due to serum factors that cause agglutination of the patient's own red cells. If a patient exhibits this under test conditions, it will not be possible to definitively type this patient without separating the serum and serially washing the remaining red cells before performing the test. RAPIDVET™-H (Canine DEA 1.1) provides a separate reaction card for use to screen for such patients.

Discussion: Intended Use: As the practice of veterinary transfusion medicine has undergone tremendous growth in recent years, the importance of identifying blood types has increased.[1,2]

While it is broadly true that dogs do not possess isoantibodies to incompatible blood groups and thus will generally tolerate well an initial incompatible transfusion, sound practice of veterinary medicine dictates that transfusions be avoided. The half life of the transfused incompatible cells will be quite short and, thus, the intended therapeutic result may not even be attained. Also, the potential future needs of the canine patient must be considered. Antibodies resulting from a transfusion of incompatible blood[3-7] may form in only 5 to 7 days and will have long-term viability. This eliminates the option of using incompatible blood in a future emergency situation.

In addition, antibodies developed in bitches by sensitization resulting from transfusion of incompatible blood groups must be of special concern to breeders. Since antibodies are present in the colostrum, bitches with isoantibodies to a given blood type should not be bred to a sire possessing that blood group if they are expected to nurse the resulting puppies.[4] The nursing puppies will develop isoerythrolysis and may be susceptible to disease or even die due to hemolytic anemia.[4,8-10]

Eight specific antigens have been identified on the surface of the canine erythrocytes.[1,3] The internationally accepted canine blood group system, the "DEA" (Dog Erythrocyte Antigen), is based on these antigens. It currently characterizes eight common blood groups, the antigens DEA 1.1, 1.2, 3, 4, 5, 6, 7, and 8.

DEA 1.1 and 1.2 are the most significant blood factors in the dog. Both are highly antigenic but DEA 1.1 is the primary lytic factor in canine transfusion medicine.[1,4,11-14,22-24] Although all of the blood group antigens are capable of stimulating formation of isoantibodies, DEA 1.1 has the greatest stimulation potential. Thus most reactions resulting from the transfusion of incompatible cells occur when DEA 1.1 positive blood is given to a DEA 1.1 negative recipient.[4] Clinically significant reactions to DEA 1.2 may occur but are less severe than reactions to DEA 1.1. DEA 7 may be a factor in transfusion reactions, but since it is a cold agglutin and a naturally occurring isoantibody, it is considered to have very low clinical significance. The remaining antigens are considered to cause clinically insignificant transfusion problems.[4]

Ideally, all transfused blood would be DEA 1.1 and DEA 1.2 negative. Certain breeds such as the Greyhounds are particularly suitable as blood donors because of a low frequency of DEA 1.1, DEA 1.2 and DEA 7 antigens. However, until the concept of the canine blood bank is widely accepted with blood readily available from commercial sources, transfusion from dogs that are present in the area at the time of need will remain the norm.

It is estimated that 40% of all dogs are DEA 1.1 positive.[3] Because a number of dogs auto-agglutinate and because a very anemic dog may give equivocal results, typing prior to an urgent need for the information is indicated. Identifying a particular dog as DEA 1.1 positive or negative at birth greatly simplifies future decision making. A DEA 1.1 positive dog can receive both DEA 1.1 positive and negative blood. A dog that is DEA 1.1 negative should not receive DEA 1.1 positive blood.

Performance Characteristics: A total of 145 canine erythrocyte samples, 127 of which were randomly chosen, were tested utilizing both a canine anti-DEA 1.1 antiserum and the RAPIDVET™-H (Canine DEA 1.1) assay. The results were identical: 91 samples were DEA 1.1 positive and 54 were DEA 1.1 negative. Nine of these samples were tested multiple times (from 2 to 5) over a period of several days with consistent results thus proving the reproducibility of the assay.

References: Available upon request.

Presentation: The 2 card test kit contains sufficient reagents and materials to determine the blood group of 2 dogs when run individually. The 5 card test kit contains sufficient reagents and materials to determine the blood group of 5 dogs when run individually. The 20 card test kit contains sufficient reagents and materials to determine the blood group of 20 dogs when run individually.

RAPIDVET is a trademark of DMS Laboratories, Inc.

Manufactured under license from: Kansas State University and dms/agrolabo products ag, Neuhausen am Rheinfall, Switzerland.

Manufactured by: Agrolabo S.p.A., Strada Statale 26, Regione Poarello, 10090 Romano Canavese (TO), Italy.

Compendium Code No.: 14810041 06/2002 CUS

RAPIDVET™-H (FELINE)

DMS Laboratories **Blood Group Test**

Blood Group Determination Assay

Components: Reagents and Materials: This test kit contains the reagents and materials listed below. Store upright.

Agglutination Test Cards. Each card has 3 visually defined wells. This includes one well identified as "Auto-Agglutination Saline Screen" and two wells identified as "Patient Test" one Type A and one Type B. The cards are packaged individually in sealed polyethylene sleeves each containing a desiccant bag. The cards must be stored in a refrigerator at 2-7°C.

1 Bottle Diluent. The clear plastic bottle contains 0.02 mol/L phosphate buffered saline (PBS) at pH 7.4. The dropping tip accurately dispenses 40 µL. Refrigerate (2-7°C).

Pipettes and Stirrers. Each polyethylene bag contains 2 plastic pipettes and 3 stirrers.

Materials Required But Not Provided: None.

Reagent Preparation: None.

Quality Control: All reagents and materials incorporated into this kit have been quality controlled by standard testing procedures using a routine quality control program during manufacture.

Indications: RAPIDVET-H™ (Feline) is intended for use to classify cats as blood group Type A, Type B, or Type AB.

For *in vitro* use.

Test Principles: Principle and Explanation of the Assay: The RAPIDVET-H™ (Feline) assay is based on the agglutination reaction that occurs when an erythrocyte which contains either a Type A, Type B or a Type AB antigen on its surface membrane interacts with a lyophilized antisera specific to the particular antigen. The material lyophilized on the Test Card is not easily visible.

Type A erythrocytes are characterized by the $NeuGc_2G_{D3}$ form glycolipid antigen on its surface membrane.[12] RAPIDVET-H™ (Feline) uses a murine monoclonal antibody proven specific to this antigen lyophilized on the test card. The antibody molecule gives it the ability to cross-link and agglutinate antigens specific to Type A blood.

Type B erythrocytes are characterized by the $NeuAc_2G_{D3}$ form of neuraminic acid present in the ganglioside and lack the NeuGc present on Type A erythrocytes.[13] The binding specificity of this form with a lectin, *Triticum vulgaris,* has been established.[14] The RAPIDVET™-H (Feline) uses the *Triticum vulgaris* lectin to detect the presence of Type B blood.

In both cases, the antisera lyophilized on a Test Card is reconstituted and well mixed with whole blood from the patient. All Type A erythrocytes react with their specific antiserum causing agglutination; all Type B erythrocytes react similarly; all Type AB erythrocytes react with both antisera causing agglutination in all cases. The results are visually identified. The characteristics of the agglutination in the "A" wells and in the "B" wells differs significantly because of the different nature of the antisera used.

Test Procedure:

1. Draw blood from the patient into a syringe or tube coated with or containing EDTA as an anticoagulant. The assay requires only 150 µL whole blood but the tube should be full or the syringe should be filled so that there is a proper concentration of EDTA. If the type is not to be determined immediately, nutrients such as CPDA should not be added.
2. Remove the Test Card from its plastic sleeve. Save the plastic sleeve and set aside the desiccant bag.
3. Write the name/number of the cat and the testing date on the card.
4. Place the Test Card on a flat surface.
5. Dispense 1 drop of diluent (40 µL) from the dropping bottle into the well marked "Auto-Agglutination Saline Screen".
6. Aspirate a small amount of patient sample into the pipette and release 1 drop (50 µL) into the well marked "Auto-Agglutination Saline Screen". Using a stirrer, spread and mix the materials within the entirety of this well for about 10 seconds, pressing downward firmly. (See Note 1 for correct use of the pipette.)
7. A small percentage of ill cats and of healthy cats auto-agglutinate. If agglutination is observed, stop the test and perform normal cell washing procedures before proceeding.
8. Dispense 1 drop of diluent (40 µL) from the dropping bottle into each remaining well to be used. The diluent assists in the reconstitution of the lyophilized material.
9. Gently swirl the tube containing the patient sample to resuspend any solid material.
10. Aspirate a small amount of patient sample into the pipette and release 1 drop (50 µL) into each of the 2 wells marked "Patient Test". Using a stirrer, spread and mix the materials within the entirety of one of the wells for about 10 seconds, pressing downward firmly. Take a new stirrer and similarly spread and mix the materials within the entirety of the other well for about 10 seconds.
11. (New) Add a second drop of diluent to the well marked "Type A". Do not stir the well with a stirrer.
12. Rock the card with a transaxial motion for 2 minutes, being sure that the materials are mixing and "rotating" within each well. Be careful not to cross-contaminate.
13. Set the card at a 10-20° angle to allow excess blood to run to the bottom of the wells. Placing the top of the card on the desiccant bag will accomplish this.
14. Read the results and note the wells where agglutination has occurred.
15. After the materials on the card have dried, replace the card in its plastic sleeve for a permanent record.

Procedure Note 1: Use of the pipette: Hold the plastic tube between thumb and forefinger near the flat, sealed end, squeeze tightly and do not release pressure. Hold the specimen tube vertically and place the open end of the plastic tube below the surface of the specimen. Release finger pressure to draw up the sample.

Next, hold the pipette in a perpendicular position directly over the well to which the sample is to be delivered. Squeeze gently and allow one free drop to fall into the well (50 µL). Each pipette is designed to expel slightly in excess of 50 µL to compensate for a small amount of specimen retained by the stirrer.

Repeat for the second well.

Use each pipette for only one patient sample, then discard. Under no circumstance should the pipette be used for more than one sample as cross-contamination will occur, and the test results will be inaccurate.

Test Interpretation: Results: If the assay was run correctly, visible agglutination should have occurred in at least one of the wells marked "Patient Test".

If the patient sample shows agglutination in the well marked Type A, the cat tested has blood group A. If the patient sample shows agglutination in the well marked Type B, the cat tested has blood group B. If the patient sample shows agglutination in both patient wells, the cat tested has blood group AB.

Any fine, granular appearance developing after 2 minutes should be disregarded in determining the results. The character of the agglutination in the Type B well is different from that in the Type A well. Agglutination in the Type B well usually includes a small number of large, amoebic globs. The agglutination in the Type A well will usually be in the form of a large number of discrete, small aggregations, each like the head of a small pin.

If the patient is very anemic, and if the patient is Type A, the antigen sites may become saturated with bound antibody preventing cross-linking and agglutination. This is due to stearic hindrance of the anti-A antibody. If the patient has a low PCV, or if there is no reaction in the patient wells but the optional controls, if used, run normally, run the test without using PBS in the patient wells.

Limitations of the Procedure:

1. To obtain accurate results it is essential that correct procedure be followed.
2. Always use a new dispensing pipette for each specimen and a new stirrer for each well. Reusing any device will cause cross-contamination and inaccurate results.
3. The stability of the individual components of the kit varies. Store the components as indicated on the labels. Do not use any component beyond the indicated expiration date. Use of expired materials may cause unreliable results.
4. The diluent is provided in a bottle with a screw cap to minimize inadvertent bacterial or other contamination. Diluent from other sources in the laboratory should not be utilized.
5. The physical integrity of the patient sample is critical to correct results.
6. Always draw a full syringe or tube containing EDTA. Less blood will cause too high a concentration of EDTA in the specimen to be tested.

Known Interfering Substances: None.

Trouble Shooting Guide:

Problem	Possible Cause	Corrective Action
No agglutination in "Patient Test" wells	a) active material settled out	a) swirl tube as per Procedure Step #9
	b) forgot to use diluent to reconstitute lyophilized material	b) see Procedure Step #8
	c) did not use downward pressure in stirring to reconstitute lyophilized material	c) see Procedure Step #10
	d) inadequate amount of blood relative to EDTA in sample draw	d) see Procedure Step #1 and Limitations of the Procedure #6
	e) use of packed cells instead of whole blood as a sample	e) dilute sample 1.1 with saline and re-run
Character of agglutination in Type B well differs from that in Type A well	This is normal	See Results

Storage: Storage and Stability:

1. The Agglutination Test Cards are stable for a period of 18 months from date of manufacture

if refrigerated. Each Test Card is labeled with an expiration date. It is not necessary to bring the Test Card to room temperature prior to use.

2. The diluent is stable for 18 months from the date of manufacture if refrigerated (2-7°C). Each bottle of diluent is labeled with an expiration date.
3. If the test is run properly, at least one of the wells labeled "Patient Test" will agglutinate. Thus, the test is self-controlled.

Note: Each RAPIDVET™-H (Feline) test kit is imprinted with an expiration date which represents the date of expiration of the shortest dated component in the kit. While some components may have later individual expiration dates, their use with other components from other kits is not recommended.

Disposal: Dispose of all biological materials, pipettes and stirrers in a safe and approved manner.

Caution(s): Caveat: A certain number of feline patients exhibit auto-agglutination of varying degrees due to serum factors that cause agglutination of the patient's own red cells. If a patient exhibits this under test conditions, it will not be possible to definitively type this patient without separating the serum and serially washing the remaining red cells before performing the test. RAPIDVET™-H (Feline) provides a well for use to screen for such patients.

Discussion: Description and Intended Use: As the practice of veterinary transfusion medicine has undergone tremendous growth in recent years, the importance of identifying blood groups in cats has increased. In particular, the demand for identifying blood groups is on the rise, because only by predetermining the blood type of a blood transfusion recipient can potentially fatal transfusion mistakes be avoided.[1]

One blood group system consisting of two antigens expressed either alone or in combination has been described in cats: Type A, Type B and Type AB.[1-4] The antigens are unrelated to human A B O antigens and are defined by feline alloimmune sera. Blood group incidence varies among breeds. Blood groups in cats are inherited as simple autosomal traits, with Type A being dominant over Type B. Most cats possess the A antigen, and about one-third of those have naturally occurring, low-titered, anti-B antibody. Type B cats all have a naturally occurring, highly titered anti-A antibody. A recent survey in the United States showed that the percentage of cats with the B antigen varied depending on the breed.[3] Those breeds with high frequency of Type B blood are noted below:

Breed	Frequency of B Type (%)
Abyssinian	14
Birman	16
British SH	40
Cornish Rex	34
Devon Rex	41
Japanese Bobtail	16
Persian	14
Scottish Fold	18
Somali	17
Sphynx	19

Type AB cats are rare and since such cats have both A and B antigens on the erythrocyte membrane, they do not have or develop anti-A or anti-B antibodies.

Blood typing of cats is important in veterinary medical practice to prevent transfusion reactions[1-8,15-16] in cats with A or B erythrocytes. Cats with B erythrocytes exhibit an immediate and catastrophic systemic anaphylactic reaction (hypotension, bradycardia, apnea, urination, defecation, vomiting, and severe neurological depression) and hemolytic signs (hemoglobinemia and hemoglobinuria) when transfused with Type A blood because of their natural high-titered anti-A antibody. Those cats with A erythrocytes and natural low-titered anti-B antibody will exhibit only a mild reaction when transfused with the B blood, but even this can make a difference in recovery rates in a medical situation since the transfused erythrocytes have a short life span. Other cats with A erythrocytes will not exhibit a reaction when first transfused with Type B blood but will, as a result, develop mode rate titers of anti-B antibody that will result in a serious reaction upon a subsequent incompatible transfusion.

Blood group determinations in cats is also important in making breeding decisions and in understanding medical problems in kittens. Neonatal isoerythrolysis can occur when there is blood group incompatibility between maternal and fetal blood.[1-4,9-12,15-16] Because of the naturally occurring highly titered anti-A antibodies in Type B cats, neonatal isoerythrolysis can occur in Type A kittens resulting from a mating of a Type B queen with a Type A male. The maternal anti-type A antibody occurs in the colostrum where it can be absorbed by the newborn kitten, and consequently, destroy its erythrocytes. Clinically, the kittens can seem normal at birth, but develop signs after nursing, fade and die within the first days of life. Determining the blood groups of the queen and the tom prior to mating, coupled with appropriate genetic counseling, can minimize neonatal isoerythrolysis.

Performance Characteristics: A total of 2116 feline erythrocyte samples were tested on the RAPIDVET™-H (Feline) assay utilizing the anti-A monoclonal antibody. Of these, 2075 were Type A, 31 were Type B and 10 were determined to be Type AB. The results conform to results obtained by cross-matching with known antisera and by other reference methods.

References: Available upon request.

Presentation: When run individually, the 2 card test kit contains sufficient reagents and materials to determine the blood group of 2 cats, the 5 card test kit contains sufficient reagents and materials to determine the blood group of 5 cats, and the 15 card test kit contains sufficient reagents and materials to determine the blood group of 15 cats.

RAPIDVET is a trademark of DMS Laboratories, Inc.

U.S. Patent No. 5,143,826

Manufactured under license from: Kansas State University and dms/agrolabo products ag, Neuhausen am Rheinfall, Switzerland.

Manufactured by: Agrolabo S.p.A., Strada Statale 26, Regione Poarello, 10090 Romano Canavese (TO), Italy.

Compendium Code No.: 14810053 06/2002 FUS-E U-M

RAPIDVET™ PLASM-EX™

DMS Laboratories **Plasma Extender**

Colloidal plasma extender in physiologic electrolyte solution with a pH of 7.4

Active Ingredient(s): Each 250 mL contains:

Oxypolygelatin .... 13.75 g
Sodium Bicarbonate .... 0.63 g
Sodium Chloride .... 1.46 g
Edetate Disodium .... 0.05 g
Calcium Chloride .... 0.02 g

Millequivalents per 250 mL:

Sodium .... 36.25 mEq
Chloride .... 25.00 mEq
Calcium .... 0.25 mEq
Hydrogen Carbonate .... 7.50 mEq

Function of the individual components of RAPIDVET™ PLASM-EX™

Component	Function
Ionic Oxypolygelatin	Colloidal substitute for plasma protein
Ionic Chloride	Physiological chloride content of plasma
Ionic Hydrogen Bicarbonate	Physiological buffer substance of blood
Ionic Sodium	Counter ions to the ionic chloride, the ionic bicarbonate and the anionic groups of oxypolygelatin
Ionic Calcium*	

* The virtual elimination of Ca ions assures miscibility of oxypolygelatin with citrated blood, streptokinase and Kabikinase® preparations, and usage with other drugs such as digitalis.

To ensure broad applicability, pharmacologically active ingredients have been omitted in formulating RAPIDVET™ PLASM-EX™. Apart from the colloid which serves as the essential component, the solution contains only the additives required for adjustment of physiological balance and to maintain a physiologically buffered pH.

Indications: RAPIDVET™ PLASM-EX™, a colloidal plasma extender, is intended for use in companion animals to reestablish and maintain circulatory equilibrium in the presence of actual or incipient circulatory disturbances. The purpose is to provide tissue perfusion only until such time that the plasma deficit can be adequately compensated for by endogenous restitution or by other therapeutic measures. Therefore, the attending clinician need not alter the type, quantity and frequency of the initial infusion because of undue concern about any possible intermediate or long term side effects.

These actual or incipient circulatory disturbances include: Shock due to loss of blood (hemorrhagic shock); Traumatic shock (hypovolemia without loss of blood); Burns; Septic shock; Shock prevention (before, during and after surgery); Shock prevention in geriatric dentistry; and Parvovirus stabilization of COP.

RAPIDVET™ PLASM-EX™ can also be used for expansion of blood volume in the exchange unit of dialyzers or oxygenators in extracorporeal circulation and in thrombotic or other states where hemodilution is indicated.

Dosage and Administration: For intravenous use only. The quantity, rate and duration of infusion must be determined for each patient individually. Administer contents or such lesser amount as determined by a veterinarian. For bolus pressure infusion 250 mL can be given to dogs in 10-15 minutes in emergency situations. Normally, administer a maximum of 3 mL to 5 mL/kg (2.72 mL/lb), over the first 15 minutes; then continue administration at a slower rate as needed with a total volume of 10 mL to 20 mL/kg per dose and prior to status review. The volume effect lasts approximately 4 hours. The amount infused, if no additional loss of fluid has occurred, should not exceed 500-750 mL (actual amount used based on weight) during a 24 hour period.

Contraindication(s): The use of any plasma extender is contraindicated in animals with known coagulation disorders if fresh frozen plasma is available or in animals with preexisting severe cardiac pulmonary or renal insufficiency. Use of this product is contraindicated in animals with known gelatin allergy or hyperproteinemia.

Stability: RAPIDVET™ PLASM-EX™ remains stable at room temperature for at least 4 years, and under extreme conditions (e.g. when carried in an automobile) for at least 1 year.

Alternate freezing and thawing does not affect the quality of RAPIDVET™ PLASM-EX™, if the contents of the bottle are rehomogenized by shaking before opening.

Caution(s): For veterinary intravenous use in non-food animals.

Adverse Reactions: There are no major side effects reported in the literature related to the use of this or similar purified and buffered oxypolygelatin plasma extenders in companion animals, however possible anaphylactoid reactions during and after infusion must always be considered as possible, if rare, events. Individual human patients with pronounced pathological signs of tissue breakdown (e.g. tumor patients) have been reported to have occasionally developed transient urticaria after oxypolygelatin infusions, but such reaction subsided within ½-3 hours without affecting the patient's general condition. This reaction is likely to have arisen from the incompatibility occasionally seen with infusion of any foreign protein.

As with any plasma extender, over administration can result in acute pulmonary edema and hypervolemia. Drug interactions must always be considered.

References: Available upon request.

Presentation: 250 mL.

RAPIDVET and PLASM-EX are trademarks of DMS Laboratories, Inc.
Kabikinase is a registered trademark of Pharmacia & Upjohn Company.

Compendium Code No.: 14810020

RAPINOVET™ ANESTHETIC INJECTION ℞

Schering-Plough **General Anesthetic**

Propofol

NADA No.: 141-070

Active Ingredient(s): Each mL contains 10 mg propofol.

Indications: Emulsion for intravenous use in dogs and cats.

RAPINOVET™ (propofol) is an anesthetic injection for use in dogs and cats as follows:

1. As a single injection to provide general anesthesia for short procedures.
2. For induction and maintenance of general anesthesia using incremental doses to effect.
3. For induction of general anesthesia where maintenance is provided by inhalant anesthetics.

Induction of anesthesia will usually be observed within 30-60 seconds after the end of administration (administration should take 60-90 seconds). The doses for induction and maintenance vary depending upon species, and preanesthetics. The duration of anesthesia varies depending upon species, dose and preanesthetics.

In dogs, the duration of anesthesia following the recommended induction dose (5.5-7.0 mg/kg without premedication) is generally 5-7 minutes. The duration of anesthesia after maintenance doses varies from 2-6 minutes following 1.1 mg/kg to 6-10 minutes following 3.3 mg/kg. Full standing recovery is generally observed within 10-20 minutes after the end of anesthesia, regardless of the duration of anesthesia. Recovery may be delayed in sighthounds or if preanesthetics are administered.

In cats, the duration of anesthesia following the recommended induction dose (8.0-13.2 mg/kg without premedication) is generally 5-12 minutes. The duration of anesthesia after maintenance doses varies from 5-7 minutes following 1.1 mg/kg to 12-18 minutes following 4.4 mg/kg. Full standing recovery is generally observed within 30-45 minutes after the end of anesthesia, regardless of the duration of anesthesia. Recovery may be delayed if preanesthetics are administered.

Pharmacology: RAPINOVET™ (propofol) injection is a sterile, nonpyrogenic emulsion suitable containing 10 mg/mL of propofol suitable for intravenous administration. Propofol is chemically described as 2,6-diisopropylphenol and has a molecular weight of 178.28. Propofol is very slightly soluble in water and is therefore formulated as a white, oil-in-water emulsion. In addition to the active component, propofol, the formulation also contains soybean oil (100 mg/mL), glycerol (22.5 mg/mL), and egg lecithin (12 mg/mL), with sodium hydroxide to adjust the pH. The propofol emulsion is isotonic and has a pH of 7-8.5.

Clinical Pharmacology: After a single dose, propofol blood level profiles are characterized by a rapid distribution phase and a rapid elimination phase. The liver is the main site of metabolism with the major portion of metabolites being excreted in urine. No change in pharmacokinetics occurs after multiple daily dosing in dogs. Concomitant medication may affect the pharmacokinetics of either propofol or other medications.[1]

In dogs, RAPINOVET™ injection has been used in association with acepromazine, atropine, glycopyrrolate, halothane, isoflurane, medetomidine, oxymorphone, and xylazine. No pharmacological incompatibility has been encountered.

In cats, RAPINOVET™ injection has been used in association with acepromazine, atropine, glycopyrrolate, butorphanol, oxymorphone, xylazine, and halothane. No pharmacological incompatibility has been encountered.

Dosage and Administration: Shake the ampule thoroughly before opening.

RAPINOVET™ injection contains no antimicrobial preservatives. Strict aseptic techniques must always be maintained during handling since the vehicle is capable of supporting the rapid growth of microorganisms. Failure to follow aseptic handling procedures may result in microbial contamination causing fever, infection/sepsis, and/or other life-threatening illness. Do not use if contamination is suspected.

RAPINOVET™ injection should be prepared for use just prior to initiation of each individual anesthetic procedure. The ampule neck surface should be disinfected using 70% isopropyl alcohol. The entire contents of the ampule should be drawn into sterile syringes immediately after ampules are opened. Administration should commence promptly and be completed within 6 hours after the ampules are opened. Any unused product should be discarded within 6 hours.

Administer by intravenous injection only.

The emulsion should not be mixed with other therapeutic agents or injected into containers of infusion fluids prior to administration.

Induction of General Anesthesia: For induction, RAPINOVET™ injection should be titrated against the response of the patient over approximately 60 to 90 seconds or until clinical signs show the onset of anesthesia.

If RAPINOVET™ is injected too slowly (greater than 90 seconds), an inadequate plane of anesthesia can occur. If this occurs, an additional low dose (1.1 mg/kg) of propofol may be administered to facilitate intubation or the transition to inhalant maintenance anesthesia.

The average induction dose ranges and dosage rates for healthy dogs given propofol alone, or when propofol is preceded by a premedicant, are indicated in the following table (the table is for guidance only; in practice, the dose should be based upon patient response):

Preanesthetic	Induction Dosage Guidelines for Dogs				
	Propofol Induction Dose		Propofol Rate of Administration		
	mg/kg	mg/lb	seconds	mg/kg/min	mL/kg/min
None	5.5-7.0	2.5-3.2	60-90	3.7-7.0	0.37-0.70
Acepromazine	4.0-4.4	1.8-2.0	60-90	2.7-4.4	0.27-0.44
Xylazine	2.2-3.3	1.0-1.5	60-90	1.5-3.3	0.15-0.33
Oxymorphone	2.2-3.3	1.0-1.5	60-90	1.5-3.3	0.15-0.33
Medetomidine	2.2-2.8	1.0-1.3	60-90	1.5-2.8	0.15-0.28

The required dosage of tranquilizers, sedatives, or analgesics administered as preanesthetic medications (listed below) may be lower than the label directions for their use as a single medication.[1]

Acepromazine	0.03-0.1 mg/kg	IM, SC, IV
Xylazine	0.25-0.5 mg/kg	IV
Xylazine	0.5-1.0 mg/kg	IM, SC
Oxymorphone	0.1-0.2 mg/kg	IM, SC, IV
Medetomidine	5.0-10.0 μg/kg	IM

The use of the drugs listed above as preanesthetics for dogs markedly reduces propofol requirements. As with other sedative hypnotic agents, the amount of phenothiazine, opioid, and/or alpha$_2$-agonist premedication will influence the response of the patient to an induction dose of RAPINOVET™ injection. The induction dose will also be influenced by the interval between the administration of premedication and induction, and by the rate of administration of propofol.

The average induction dose ranges and dosage rates for healthy cats given propofol alone, or when propofol is preceded by a premedicant, are indicated in the following table (the table is for guidance only; in practice, the dose should be based upon patient response):

R

Preanesthetic	Induction Dosage Guidelines for Cats				
	Propofol Induction Dose		Propofol Rate of Administration		
	mg/kg	mg/lb	seconds	mg/kg/min	mL/kg/min
None	8.0-13.2	3.6-6.0	60-90	5.3-13.2	0.53-1.32
Acepromazine	8.0-13.2	3.6-6.0	60-90	5.3-13.2	0.53-1.32
Butorphanol	8.0-13.2	3.6-6.0	60-90	5.3-13.2	0.53-1.32
Oxymorphone	8.0-13.2	3.6-6.0	60-90	5.3-13.2	0.53-1.32
Xylazine	7.0-12.0	3.2-5.5	60-90	4.7-12.0	0.47-1.20

The required dosage of tranquilizers, sedatives, or analgesics administered as preanesthetic medications (listed below) may be lower than the label directions for their use as a single medication.[1,8,9]

Acepromazine	0.03-0.1 mg/kg	IM, SC, IV
Butorphanol	0.1-0.4	mg/kg
Oxymorphone	0.1-0.4 mg/kg	IM, SC, IV
Xylazine	0.25-0.5 mg/kg	IV
Xylazine	0.5-1.0 mg/kg	IM, SC

The use of the drugs listed above as preanesthetics for cats may reduce propofol requirements. As with other sedative hypnotic agents, the amount of phenothiazine, opioid, and/or alpha$_2$-agonist premedication will influence the response of the patient to an induction dose of RAPINOVET™ injection. The induction dose will also be influenced by the interval between the administration of premeditation and induction, and by the rate of administration of propofol.

Maintenance of General Anesthesia:

A. Intermittent Propofol Injections: Anesthesia can be maintained by administering propofol in intermittent IV injections. Clinical response will be determined by the amount, the rate of administration, and the frequency of maintenance injections. The following tables is provided for guidance:

Preanesthetic	Maintenance Dosage Guidelines for Dogs				
	Propofol Maintenance Dose		Propofol Rate of Administration		
	mg/kg	mg/lb	seconds	mg/kg/min	mL/kg/min
None	1.1-3.3	0.5-1.5	30-60	1.1-3.3	0.11-0.33
Acepromazine	1.1	0.5	30-60	1.1-2.2	0.11-0.22
Xylazine	1.1	0.5	30-60	1.1-2.2	0.11-0.22
Oxymorphone	1.1	0.5	30-60	1.1-2.2	0.11-0.22
Medetomidine	1.1	0.5	30-60	1.1-2.2	0.11-0.22

Repeated maintenance doses of propofol do not result in increased recovery times, indicating that the anesthetic effects of propofol are not cumulative in dogs.

Preanesthetic	Maintenance Dosage Guidelines for Cats				
	Propofol Maintenance Dose		Propofol Rate of Administration		
	mg/kg	mg/lb	seconds	mg/kg/min	mL/kg/min
None	1.1-4.4	0.5-2.0	30-60	1.1-4.4	0.11-0.44
Acepromazine	1.1-4.4	0.5-2.0	30-60	1.1-4.4	0.11-0.44
Butorphanol	1.1-4.4	0.5-2.0	30-60	1.1-4.4	0.11-0.44
Oxymorphone	1.1-4.4	0.5-2.0	30-60	1.1-4.4	0.11-0.44
Xylazine	1.1-2.2	0.5-1.0	30-60	1.1-2.2	0.11-0.22
Acepromazine/Butorphanol	1.1-3.3	0.5-1.5	30-60	1.1-3.3	0.11-0.33
Acepromazine/Oxymorphone	1 1-3.3	0.5-1.5	30-60	1.1-3.3	0.11-0.33

Repeated maintenance doses of propofol may result in slightly increased recovery times, indicating that the anesthetic effects of propofol may be cumulative in cats.

B. Maintenance by Inhalant Anesthetics: Clinical trials using propofol have shown that it may be necessary to use a higher initial concentration of the inhalant anesthetic than is usually required following induction using barbiturate anesthetics, due to rapid recovery from RAPINOVET™.

Compatibilities: RAPINOVET™ has been used in association with atropine, acepromazine, xylazine, glycopyrrolate, oxymorphone, halothane, and isoflurane. No pharmacological incompatibility has been encountered.[2]

Contraindication(s): RAPINOVET™ injection is contraindicated in dogs and cats with a known hypersensitivity to propofol or its components, or when general anesthesia or sedation are contraindicated.

Precaution(s): Store between 4°-22°C (40°-72°F). Do not freeze. Protect from light. Shake well before use. Discard opened ampule with care. Within 6 hours after opening, any withdrawn unused product should be discarded safely.

Caution(s): Federal law restricts this drug to use by or on the order of a licensed veterinarian.

1. When using RAPINOVET™ injection, patients should be continuously monitored, and facilities for the maintenance of a patent airway, artificial ventilation, and oxygen supplementation must be immediately available. The clinical use of propofol without available supplemental oxygen and artificial ventilation has not been adequately evaluated and is not recommended.
2. Anesthesia effects: Careful monitoring of the patient is necessary when using RAPINOVET™ injection as a maintenance anesthetic due to the possibility of rapid arousal. Apnea may occur following maintenance doses of RAPINOVET™ injection.
   Following induction, additional RAPINOVET™ injection at the lower maintenance dose may be needed to complete the transition to inhalant maintenance anesthesia due to rapid recovery from propofol. Doses administered during the transition to inhalant anesthesia or during inhalant maintenance anesthesia may result in apnea.
3. Physiological effects: During induction of anesthesia, mild hypotension and increased heart rate may occur when RAPINOVET™ injection is used alone.
4. Premedicants: Premedicants may increase the anesthesia or sedative effect of RAPINOVET™ injection and result in more pronounced changes in systolic, diastolic, and mean arterial blood pressures. The use of ketamine (an approved compound for restraint in cats) is not recommended as a preanesthetic prior to propofol due to an increased number of patients experiencing apnea.
5. Breeding Animals: Adequate data concerning the safe use of RAPINOVET™ injection in pregnant, lactating, and breeding dogs and cats have not been obtained. Propofol crosses the placenta, and as with other general anesthetic agents, the administration of propofol may be associated with neonatal depression.
6. Puppies and Kittens: The use of propofol has not been evaluated in puppies or kittens.
7. Compromised or debilitated dogs and cats: Doses may need adjustment for geriatric or debilitated patients. The administration of RAPINOVET™ injection to patients with renal failure and/or hepatic failure has not been evaluated. As with other anesthetic agents, caution should be exercised in dogs or cats with cardiac, respiratory, renal or hepatic impairment, or in hypovolemic or debilitated dogs and cats.
8. Sighthounds: RAPINOVET™ injection induction followed by inhalant anesthetic agents produced satisfactory anesthesia and recovery times in sighthounds. Propofol alone in 6 greyhounds and 7 non-greyhounds showed satisfactory but longer recovery times in the greyhounds (averages of 47 and 18 minutes, respectively).[2] In a propofol pharmacokinetics study, greyhounds had higher propofol levels in plasma, a lower volume of distribution, slower total body clearance rates and longer recovery times than did mixed-breed dogs. The elimination half life was similar in both groups.[3]
9. Arrhythmogenicity: In one study in dogs, propofol increased myocardial sensitivity to the development of epinephrine-induced ventricular arrhythmias in a manner similar to other anesthetics.[4]
10. Consecutive day treatment: Heinz bodies increased dramatically in cats following repeat administration of propofol on consecutive days and were associated with decreases in RBC count and hematocrit. Large numbers of Heinz bodies can lead to hemolytic anemia.[5,6] In one study in cats, treatment with propofol once a day for 3 days led to a marked increase in Heinz bodies. Treatment for 5 or more consecutive days resulted in generalized malaise and/or facial edema; clinical signs of illness resolved within 24-48 hours after cessation of propofol.
11. Concurrent Medication: No significant adverse interactions with commonly used drugs have been observed.

12. Perivascular Administration: Perivascular administration does not produce local tissue reaction.

Warning(s): Induction of anesthesia with RAPINOVET™ is frequently associated with apnea and respiratory depression. Hypotension and oxygen desaturation can occur also, especially following rapid bolus administration. Apnea is observed less frequently following maintenance doses of RAPINOVET™ when given as the sole maintenance agent, or when a maintenance dose is administered during inhalant anesthesia.

When using RAPINOVET™ injection, patients should be continuously monitored, and facilities for the maintenance of a patent airway, artificial ventilation, and oxygen supplementation must be immediately available. The clinical use of propofol without available supplemental oxygen and artificial ventilation has not been adequately evaluated and is not recommended.

Human User Safety: Not for human use. Keep out of reach of children.

RAPINOVET™ injection should be managed to prevent the risk of diversion, through such measures as restriction of access and the use of drug accountability procedures appropriate to the clinical setting. Rare cases of self-administration of propofol have been reported, including dose-related fatalities.

Preventive care should be taken to avoid self-administration; for example, use of a guarded needle until the moment of injection is recommended. Symptoms of self-administration may include cardiovascular and/or respiratory depression. Anaphylaxis to propofol may occur during its first use, especially in patients with a history of drug allergy.[7] In the event of accidental self-administration, seek medical attention immediately.

Contact of this product with skin, eyes, and clothes should be avoided. If contact occurs, skin and eyes should be liberally flushed with water for 15 minutes. If irritation develops and continues, consult a physician.

Initial arousal following propofol anesthesia can be extremely rapid. Caution should be used at this time in manipulations involving the mouth, such as removing an endotracheal tube.

The material safety data sheet (MSDS) contains more detailed occupational safety information. For customer service, and/or a copy of the MSDS, call 800-770-8878. To report adverse effects, call 800-224-5318.

For use in animals only.

Overdose: Rapid administration or accidental overdosage of RAPINOVET™ injection may cause neurologic and cardiopulmonary depression. Respiratory arrest (apnea) may be observed. In cases of respiratory depression, stop drug administration, establish a patent airway, and initiate assisted or controlled ventilation with oxygen. Cardiovascular depression should be treated with plasma expanders, pressor agents, antiarrhythmic agents, or other techniques as appropriate for the observed abnormality.

In feline safety studies using healthy cats and elevated doses of propofol, unexplained decreases in albumin, globulin, and total protein values were noted. Increases in bile acids and triglycerides were also noted and were probably due to the lipid content of the drug formulation. These transient changes were not clinically significant in healthy cats.

Side Effects: The primary side effect of RAPINOVET™ injection in dogs is respiratory depression and apnea. Apnea was observed in 20% of the dog cases in the clinical trial. Apnea was observed in 1.4% of the cat cases in the clinical trial. All apnea cases responded satisfactorily to oxygen supplementation and/or controlled ventilation.

Apnea lasting less than 1 minute in healthy dogs or cats may cause no harm. Animals breathing atmospheric air that become apneic may show signs of cerebral damage after 2 minutes. Animals breathing 100% oxygen that become apneic may not show signs of cerebral damage for 5-8 minutes. Ventricular arrhythmias may occur secondary to hypoxia induced by apnea.

The primary side effect of RAPINOVET™ injection in cats is paddling during recovery. Paddling was observed in 11% of the cat cases in the clinical trial.

Other transient side effects in dogs or cats are observed infrequently or rarely:

Respiratory: panting, reverse sneezing, cyanosis.

Musculoskeletal: paddling during recovery, tremors, tenseness, movements, fasciculations

Cardiovascular: bradycardia, hypotension, cyanosis, tachycardia, premature ventricular contractions

Central Nervous System: excitation, opisthotonus, seizure

Injection Site: pain during injection

Gastrointestinal: emesis/retching

Other: rubbing at face or nose during recovery, vocalization during recovery, chewing or licking the injection site during recovery

References: Available upon request.

Presentation: RAPINOVET™ injection is supplied in cartons of five-20 mL ampules containing 10 mg propofol per mL.

Compendium Code No.: 10471710

RAVAP® E.C.

Boehringer Ingelheim **Premise and Topical Insecticide**

Livestock, Poultry & Premise Insecticide Spray

EPA Reg. No.: 4691-136

Active Ingredient(s): By Weight

Tetrachlorvinphos (CAS# 22248-79-9)* 23.0%
Dichlorvos (CAS# 62-73-7)** 5.3%
Related Compounds** 0.4%
Other Ingredients*** 71.3%
Total 100.0%

*Rabon® Insecticide. **Equivalent to 5.7% W. Vapona® Insecticide.

***Other ingredients include Xylene. Contains Rabon® and Vapona® Insecticides.

This product contains the toxic inert ingredient phenol.

Indications: Use as a beef cattle, lactating dairy cattle spray, a back rub or face rub for cattle, on caged chickens, on chicken litter, as a roost paint, on poultry buildings and as a residual surface spray or larvicide.

Directions for Use: It is a violation of Federal Law to use this product in a manner inconsistent with its labeling. Read the entire label prior to use.

For agricultural/commerical use only. Not for sale for any other uses.

This product is suitable for use in conventional power or low pressure knapsack sprayers and in livestock backrubbers. Follow the use directions for the proper dilution needed for specific insect control. Must be diluted in water except for backrubber use.

Kennel Use Directions:

Use	Insect	Dilution•RAVAP® in Water	Remarks
Residual Surface Spray — Kennels	Ticks, Fleas	1 gal. in 50 gal. or 5 oz. in 2 gal.	Apply 1 gal. of dilution/500-1000 sq. ft. Thoroughly treat infested kennel and outside runways.

Livestock Use Directions: Do not make direct application to livestock more frequently than once per day.

Use	Insect	Dilution•RAVAP® In Water	Remarks
Livestock Spray (Beef Cattle)	Horn Flies, Lice, including Tail Lice, and aids in control of Face Flies	1 gal. in 75 gal. or 5 oz. in 3 gal.	Dilute in water as indicated and spray directly on the animal only to the point of runoff. Use between ½ to 1 gallon of diluted spray solution per animal depending on size and hair coat. Do not treat more often than every 10 days. Do not apply to calves under six months of age. Brahman and Brahman-cross cattle should not be treated as they may show hypersensitivity to organophosphate pesticides. Do not apply in combination with other dermal organophosphate pesticides (e.g. trichlorfon). There is no withholding period from last application to slaughter.
	Horn Flies, Lone Star Ticks	1 gal. in 200 gal. or 2 oz. in 3 gal.	Apply as above. For severe tick infestations, dilution may be increased to 1 gallon in 50 gallons of water.
Livestock Spray (Lactating Dairy Cattle)	Horn Flies, Lice, Lone Star Ticks, and aids in control of Face Flies	1 gal. in 200 gal. or 2 oz. in 3 gal.	Dilute in water as indicated. Direct spray to cover thoroughly with up to ½ gallon of the dilution per animal. Repeat as necessary. Do not apply to calves under six months of age. No milk discard is required. Care should be taken that the spray does not come in direct contact with the lactating dairy cow's teats unless they are washed with an approved cleansing solution and dried before milking. Apply the spray at least 20 minutes prior to milking or after milking has been completed.

Backrubber Use Directions:

Use	Insect	Dilution•RAVAP® In Oil	Remarks
Backrubber or Facerubber (Beef and Dairy Cattle)	Horn Flies, and aids in control of Face Flies	1 gal. in 25 gal. or 5 oz. in 1 gal.	Mix with any approved backrubber base oil. Pour diluted solution into oil reservoir of mechanical rubbing devices or pour one gallon per 20 linear feet on burlap or rope backrubbers. Keep backrubber or facerubber charged.

Poultry Use Directions:

Use	Insect	Dilution•RAVAP® In Water	Remarks
Caged Chickens	Lice & Mites	1 gal. in 50 gal. or 5 oz. in 2 gal.	Apply 1 gal. of dilution/100 birds under high pressure (no less than 100-125 psi) to the vent and fluff areas from below. Repeat when necessary; however, not more often than every 14 days. For individual bird treatment, apply 1 ounce of dilution per bird.
Chickens on Litter	Lice & Mites	1 gal. in 50 gal. or 5 oz. in 2 gal.	Apply 1-2 gal. of dilution/1000 sq. ft. evenly with penetration of litter surface. Also apply thoroughly to walls, roosts, cracks and crevices. Spray birds as above. Treat roosters carefully to avoid reinfestation of breeding flocks.
Roost Paint	Lice & Mites	1 gal. in 25 gal. or 5 oz. in 1 gal.	Apply 1 pt. of dilution/100 ft. of roost area with brush or spray.
Poultry Buildings	Fowl Tick (Blue Bug)	1 gal. in 25 gal. or 5 oz. in 1 gal.	Apply 1 gal. of dilution/100-150 sq. ft. to thoroughly cover walls, ceilings, floors, cracks and crevices using high pressure spray.

Premise Use Directions for Poultry and Livestock Facilities:

Use	Insect	Dilution•RAVAP® In Water	Remarks
Residual Surface Spray	Flies, Gnats, Litter Beetles, Mosquitoes, Spiders, Wasps	1 gal. in 25 gal. or 5 oz. in 1 gal.	Apply 1 gal. of dilution/500-1000 sq. ft. Thoroughly cover walls, ceilings or other areas where pests rest or congregate in dairy barns, horse barns, poultry houses, swine buildings, livestock sheds and other farm buildings. Extreme infestations may necessitate increasing the diluted spray to one gallon per 12½ gal. or 10 oz. per 1 gal. of water.
Larvicide	Maggots (fly larvae)	1 gal. in 25 gal. or 5 oz. in 1 gal.	Apply 1 gal. of dilution/100 sq. ft. of droppings as a coarse spray. Repeat at 7-10 day intervals until droppings begin to cone up, then treat only "hot spots" (small areas found to have large number of maggots). Do not spray manure where runoff to soil or water can occur. Do not spray animals directly with this concentration.

Precautionary Statements: Hazards to Humans and Domestic Animals: Danger. Corrosive, causes eye damage and skin irritation. Do not get in eyes (including animals), on skin or on clothing. Wear goggles or face shield and chemical resistant glove and shoes, long-sleeved shirt, pants and socks when handling. This product may cause skin sensitization in certain individuals.

Harmful if inhaled. Avoid breathing spray mist.

Harmful or fatal if swallowed. Wash thoroughly after using and before smoking or eating. Avoid contamination of food.

Statement of Practical Treatment:

If swallowed — Call a physician or Poison Control Center immediately. If possible, vomiting should be induced under medical supervision. Drink 1 or 2 glasses of water and induce vomiting by touching back of throat with finger. Do not induce vomiting or give anything by mouth to an unconscious person.

If inhaled — Remove victim to fresh air. Apply respiration if necessary.

If on skin — Remove contaminated clothing and wash skin immediately with soap and water.

If in eyes — Flush eyes with plenty of water. Call a physician immediately.

Note to physician — If signs of cholinesterase inhibition are observed, atropine by injection is antidotal and may be administered in conjunction with 2-PAM (Pralidoxime Chloride). The product may cause aspiration pneumonia. Gastric lavage may be indicated if product was taken internally.

Environmental Hazards: This product is toxic to fish, birds and other wildlife. Drift and runoff may be hazardous to aquatic organisms in adjacent areas. Do not apply directly to water, or to areas where surface water is present or to intertidal areas below the mean high water mark. Do not contaminate water when disposing of equipment washwater.

Physical and Chemical Hazards: Do not use, pour, spill or store near heat or open flame. Do not use with thermal foggers or heat-generating devices.

Storage and Disposal: Do not contaminate water, food or feed by storage or disposal.

Pesticide Storage — Store in original container only. Store at temperatures above 32°F. Do not store above 120°F for an extended period of time. Do not store diluted product.

Pesticide Disposal — Pesticide wastes are acutely toxic. Improper disposal of excess pesticide, spray mixture, or rinsate is a violation of Federal Law. If these wastes cannot be disposed of by use according to label instructions, contact a State Pesticide or Environmental Control Agency, or the Hazardous Waste representative at the nearest EPA Regional Office for guidance.

Container Disposal — Triple rinse (or equivalent). Then offer for recycling or reconditioning or puncture and dispose of in a sanitary landfill, or by other approved State and local procedures.

Warning(s): Keep out of reach of children.

Disclaimer: Notice of Warranty: Boehringer Ingelheim Vetmedica, Inc., makes no warranty of merchantability, fitness for any particular purpose, or otherwise, expressed or implied concerning this product or its uses which extend beyond the use of the product under normal conditions in accord with the statements made on the label.

Presentation: 1 quart (946 mL), 1 gallon (3.785 L) and 5 gallon (19 L) containers.

Compendium Code No.: 10280962 BI 6275-2 12/99

REASHURE™ CHOLINE

Balchem **Dietary Supplement**

Rumen Stable Encapsulated Choline

Guaranteed Analysis: 25% Choline, Minimum.

Ingredients: Hydrogenated Vegetable Oil, Choline Chloride, Roughage Products, Iron, Emulsifier.

Indications: REASHURE™ choline has been proven under field conditions to successfully deliver choline to dairy cows.

Directions: Suggested feeding: REASHURE™ choline should be fed to close-up dry cows and to fresh and early lactation cows. A suggested minimal feeding time period is from 2-3 weeks pre-calving through 30 to 50 days into lactation.

Each cow should be fed 2 ounces of REASHURE™ choline per day throughout the entire feeding period.

Precaution(s): Storage and Handling:

REASHURE™ choline should be stored in a dry environment at temperatures below 120°F (49°C). As with other encapsulates, this product performs best when not subjected to extreme conditions.

After opening, the bags should be closed tightly and stored in a dry area.

REASHURE™ choline can be mixed in with the Total Mixed Ration (TMR) or top-dressed. When added to the TMR, REASHURE™ choline should be added at the same time as other mineral and vitamin supplements.

Presentation: 25 lbs. (11.3 kg) bag. U.S. Patent #5,190,775

Compendium Code No.: 10640000

R

RECOMBITEK® C4

Merial **Vaccine**

Canine Distemper-Adenovirus Type 2-Parainfluenza-Parvovirus Vaccine, Modified Live Virus, Canarypox Vector

U.S. Vet. Lic. No.: 298

Description: RECOMBITEK® C4 contains a lyophilized suspension of a recombinant canarypox vector expressing the HA and F glycoproteins of canine distemper virus; modified live adenovirus type 2, parainfluenza virus, and parvovirus; plus sterile water diluent. Safety and immunogenicity of this product have been demonstrated by vaccination and challenge tests in susceptible dogs.

Contains gentamicin as a preservative.

Indications: RECOMBITEK® C4 is recommended for the vaccination of healthy dogs 6 weeks of age and older for prevention of disease due to canine distemper virus, canine parvovirus, canine adenovirus type 1 (canine hepatitis), canine adenovirus type 2 (canine respiratory disease complex), and canine parainfluenza virus.

Dosage and Administration: Reconstitute the lyophilized vaccine with accompanying liquid diluent and aseptically inject 1 mL (1 dose) subcutaneously or intramuscularly into healthy dogs. For primary vaccination, revaccinate with a second 1 mL dose 2 to 3 weeks later. Dogs younger than 12 weeks of age should be revaccinated with a single 1 mL dose every 2 to 3 weeks, the last dose given at or over 12 weeks of age. Revaccinate annually with a single 1 mL dose.

Precaution(s): Store at 2-7°C (35-45°F). Use immediately after reconstitution. Do not use chemicals to sterilize syringes and needles. Burn container and all unused contents.

Caution(s): It is generally recommended to avoid vaccination of pregnant dogs. In rare instances, administration of vaccines may cause lethargy, fever, and inflammatory or hypersensitivity types of reactions. Treatment may include antihistamines, anti-inflammatories, and/or epinephrine.

For veterinary use only.

Presentation: Contains 25 doses: 25 x 1 dose lyophilized, 25 x 1 mL sterile water.

Sold to veterinarians only.

RECOMBITEK is a registered trademark of Merial.

Compendium Code No.: 11110602 RM515R8

RECOMBITEK® C4/CV

Merial **Vaccine**

Canine Distemper-Adenovirus Type 2-Coronavirus-Parainfluenza-Parvovirus Vaccine, Modified Live Virus, Canarypox Vector

U.S. Vet. Lic. No.: 298

Description: RECOMBITEK® C4/CV contains a lyophilized suspension of a recombinant canarypox vector expressing the HA and F glycoproteins of canine distemper virus; modified live adenovirus type 2, parainfluenza virus, parvovirus, and coronavirus; plus sterile water diluent. Safety and immunogenicity of this product have been demonstrated by vaccination and challenge tests in susceptible dogs.

Contains gentamicin as a preservative.

Indications: RECOMBITEK® C4/CV is recommended for the vaccination of healthy dogs 6 weeks of age and older for prevention of disease due to canine distemper virus, canine parvovirus, canine coronavirus, canine adenovirus type 1 (canine hepatitis), canine adenovirus type 2 (canine respiratory disease complex), and canine parainfluenza virus.

Dosage and Administration: Reconstitute the lyophilized vaccine with accompanying liquid diluent and aseptically inject 1 mL (1 dose) subcutaneously or intramuscularly into healthy dogs. For primary vaccination, revaccinate with a second 1 mL dose 2 to 3 weeks later. Dogs younger than 12 weeks of age should be revaccinated with a single 1 mL dose every 2 to 3 weeks, the last dose given at or over 12 weeks of age. Revaccinate annually with a single 1 mL dose.

Precaution(s): Store at 2-7°C (35-45°F). Use immediately after reconstitution. Do not use chemicals to sterilize syringes and needles. Burn container and all unused contents.

Caution(s): It is generally recommended to avoid vaccination of pregnant dogs. In rare instances, administration of vaccines may cause lethargy, fever, and inflammatory or hypersensitivity types of reactions. Treatment may include antihistamines, anti-inflammatories, and/or epinephrine.

For veterinary use only.

Presentation: Contains 25 doses: 25 x 1 dose lyophilized, 25 x 1 mL sterile water.

Sold to veterinarians only.

RECOMBITEK is a registered trademark of Merial.

Compendium Code No.: 11110622 RM545R8

RECOMBITEK® C6

Merial **Bacterin-Vaccine**

Canine Distemper-Adenovirus Type 2-Parainfluenza-Parvovirus Vaccine, Modified Live Virus, Canarypox Vector-Leptospira Bacterin

U.S. Vet. Lic. No.: 298

Descriptions: RECOMBITEK® C6 contains a lyophilized suspension of a recombinant canarypox vector expressing the HA and F glycoproteins of canine distemper virus; modified live adenovirus type 2, parainfluenza virus, parvovirus; and a liquid suspension of inactivated cultures of *Leptospira canicola* and *L. icterohaemorrhagiae*. Safety and immunogenicity of this product have been demonstrated by vaccination and challenge tests in susceptible dogs.

Contains gentamicin as a preservative.

Indications: RECOMBITEK® C6 is recommended for the vaccination of healthy dogs 6 weeks of age and older for prevention of disease due to canine distemper virus, canine parvovirus, canine adenovirus type 1 (canine hepatitis), canine adenovirus type 2 (canine respiratory disease complex), canine parainfluenza virus, and the bacteria *L. canicola* and *L. icterohaemorrhagiae*.

Dosage and Administration: Reconstitute the lyophilized vaccine with accompanying liquid diluent and aseptically inject 1 mL (1 dose) subcutaneously or intramuscularly into healthy dogs. For primary vaccination, revaccinate with a second 1 mL dose 2 to 3 weeks later. Dogs younger than 12 weeks of age should be revaccinated with a single 1 mL dose every 2 to 3 weeks, the last dose given at or over 12 weeks of age. Revaccinate annually with a single 1 mL dose.

Precaution(s): Store at 2-7°C (35-45°F). Do not freeze. Use immediately after reconstitution. Do not use chemicals to sterilize syringes and needles. Burn container and all unused contents.

Caution(s): It is generally recommended to avoid vaccination of pregnant dogs. In rare instances, administration of vaccines may cause lethargy, fever, and inflammatory or hypersensitivity types of reactions. Treatment may include antihistamines, anti-inflammatories, and/or epinephrine.

For veterinary use only.

Presentation: Contains 25 doses: 25 x 1 dose lyophilized, 25 x 1 dose (1 mL) liquid.

Sold to veterinarians only.

RECOMBITEK is a registered trademark Merial.

Compendium Code No.: 11110642 RM525R7

RECOMBITEK® C6/CV

Merial **Bacterin-Vaccine**

Canine Distemper-Adenovirus Type 2-Coronavirus-Parainfluenza-Parvovirus Vaccine, Modified Live Virus, Canarypox Vector-Leptospira Bacterin

U.S. Vet. Lic. No.: 298

Description: RECOMBITEK® C6/CV contains a lyophilized suspension of a recombinant canarypox vector expressing the HA and F glycoproteins of canine distemper virus; modified live adenovirus type 2, parainfluenza virus, parvovirus, and coronavirus; and a liquid suspension of *Leptospira canicola* and *L. icterohaemorrhagiae*. Safety and immunogenicity of this product have been demonstrated by vaccination and challenge tests in susceptible dogs.

Contains gentamicin as a preservative.

Indications: RECOMBITEK® C6/CV is recommended for the vaccination of healthy dogs 6 weeks of age and older for prevention of disease due to canine distemper virus, canine parvovirus, canine coronavirus, canine adenovirus type 1 (canine hepatitis), canine adenovirus type 2 (canine respiratory disease complex), canine parainfluenza virus, and the bacteria *L. canicola* and *L. icterohaemorrhagiae*.

Dosage and Administration: Reconstitute the lyophilized vaccine with accompanying liquid diluent and aseptically inject 1 mL (1 dose) subcutaneously or intramuscularly into healthy dogs. For primary vaccination, revaccinate with a second 1 mL dose 2 to 3 weeks later. Dogs younger than 12 weeks of age should be revaccinated with a single 1 mL dose every 2 to 3 weeks, the last dose given at or over 12 weeks of age. Revaccinate annually with a single 1 mL dose.

Precaution(s): Store at 2-7°C (35-45°F). Do not freeze. Use immediately after reconstitution. Do not use chemicals to sterilize syringes and needles. Burn container and all unused contents.

Caution(s): It is generally recommended to avoid vaccination of pregnant dogs. In rare instances, administration of vaccines may cause lethargy, fever, and inflammatory or hypersensitivity types of reactions. Treatment may include antihistamines, anti-inflammatories, and/or epinephrine.

For veterinary use only.

Presentation: Contains 25 doses: 25 x 1 dose lyophilized, 25 x 1 dose (1 mL) liquid.

Sold to veterinarians only.

RECOMBITEK is a registered trademark of Merial.

Compendium Code No.: 11110652 RM555R7

RECOMBITEK® CANINE CORONA-MLV

Merial **Vaccine**

Canine Coronavirus Vaccine, Modified Live Virus

U.S. Vet. Lic. No.: 298

Description: RECOMBITEK® Canine Corona-MLV contains a lyophilized suspension of modified live canine coronavirus propagated in a stable cell line plus sterile water diluent. Safety and immunogenicity of this vaccine have been demonstrated by vaccination and challenge tests in susceptible dogs.

Contains gentamicin as a preservative.

Indications: RECOMBITEK® Canine Corona-MLV is recommended for the vaccination of healthy dogs 6 weeks of age and older for prevention of disease due to canine coronavirus.

Dosage and Administration: Reconstitute the lyophilized vaccine with accompanying liquid diluent and aseptically inject 1 mL (1 dose) subcutaneously or intramuscularly into healthy dogs. For primary vaccination, revaccinate with a second 1 mL dose 2 to 3 weeks later. Dogs less than 12 weeks of age should be revaccinated with a single 1 mL dose every 2 to 3 weeks, the last dose given at or over 12 weeks of age. Revaccinate annually with a single 1 mL dose.

Precaution(s): Store at 2-7°C (35-45°F). Use immediately after reconstitution. Do not use chemicals to sterilize syringes and needles. Burn container and all unused contents.

Caution(s): It is generally recommended to avoid vaccination of pregnant dogs. In rare instances, administration of vaccines may cause lethargy, fever, and inflammatory or hypersensitivity types of reactions. Treatment may include antihistamines, anti-inflammatories, and/or epinephrine.

For veterinary use only.

Presentation: Contains 25 doses: 25 x 1 dose, lyophilized and 25 x 1 mL, sterile water.

Sold to veterinarians only.

RECOMBITEK is a registered trademark of Merial.

Compendium Code No.: 11110012 RM530R6

RECOMBITEK® CANINE PARVO

Merial **Vaccine**

Parvovirus Vaccine, Modified Live Virus

U.S. Vet. Lic. No.: 298

Description: RECOMBITEK® Canine Parvo contains canine parvovirus, propagated in a stable cell line. Safety and efficacy of this product have been demonstrated by vaccination and challenge tests.

Contains gentamicin as a preservative.

Indications: RECOMBITEK® Canine Parvo is recommended for the vaccination of healthy dogs 6 weeks of age and older for prevention of disease due to canine parvovirus.

Dosage and Administration: Aseptically inject 1 mL (1 dose) subcutaneously or intramuscularly into healthy dogs. For primary vaccination, revaccinate with a second 1 mL dose 2 to 3 weeks later. Dogs younger than 12 weeks of age should be revaccinated with a single 1 mL dose every 2 to 3 weeks, the last dose given at or over 12 weeks of age. Revaccinate annually with a single 1 mL dose.

Precaution(s): Store at 2-7°C (35-45°F). Do not use chemicals to sterilize syringes and needles. Burn container and all unused contents.

Caution(s): It is generally recommended to avoid vaccination of pregnant dogs. In rare instances, administration of vaccines may cause lethargy, fever, and inflammatory or hypersensitivity types of reactions. Treatment may include antihistamines, anti-inflammatories, and/or epinephrine.

For veterinary use only.

Presentation: 50 x 1 dose (1 mL).

Sold to veterinarians only.

RECOMBITEK is a registered trademark of Merial.

Compendium Code No.: 11110023 RM511R7

RECOMBITEK® CANINE PARVO+CORONA-MLV

Merial **Vaccine**

Canine Coronavirus-Parvovirus Vaccine, Modified Live Virus

U.S. Vet. Lic. No.: 298

Description: RECOMBITEK® Canine Parvo+Corona-MLV contains a lyophilized suspension of modified live canine coronavirus plus a liquid suspension canine parvovirus, each propagated in a stable cell line. Safety and efficacy of this product have been demonstrated by vaccination and challenge tests.

Contains gentamicin as a preservative.

Indications: RECOMBITEK® Canine Parvo+Corona-MLV is recommended for the vaccination of healthy dogs 6 weeks of age and older for prevention of disease due to canine coronavirus and canine parvovirus.

Dosage and Administration: Reconstitute the lyophilized vaccine with accompanying liquid diluent and aseptically inject 1 mL (1 dose) subcutaneously or intramuscularly into healthy dogs. For primary vaccination, revaccinate with a second 1 mL dose 2 to 3 weeks later. Dogs younger than 12 weeks of age should be revaccinated with a single 1 mL dose every 2 to 3 weeks, the last dose given at or over 12 weeks of age. Revaccinate annually with a single 1 mL dose.

Precaution(s): Store at 2-7°C (35-45°F). Use immediately after reconstitution. Do not use chemicals to sterilize syringes and needles. Burn container and all unused contents.

Caution(s): It is generally recommended to avoid vaccination of pregnant dogs. In rare instances, administration of vaccines may cause lethargy, fever, and inflammatory or hypersensitivity types of reactions. Treatment may include antihistamines, anti-inflammatories, and/or epinephrine.

For veterinary use only.

Presentation: Contains 25 doses: 25 x 1 dose, lyophilized and 25 x 1 dose (1 mL), liquid.

Sold to veterinarians only.

RECOMBITEK is a registered trademark of Merial.

Compendium Code No.: 11110032 RM512R6

RECOMBITEK® LYME

Merial **Bacterin**

Borrelia Burgdorferi Bacterial Extract

U.S. Vet. Lic. No.: 298

Description: RECOMBITEK® Lyme is a liquid suspension of inactivated, purified outer surface protein (OspA) of *Borrelia burgdorferi* derived from a bacterial recombinant vector.

Contains gentamicin as a preservative.

Indications: RECOMBITEK® Lyme is recommended for the vaccination of healthy dogs 9 weeks of age and older as an aid in the reduction of disease associated with infection by *Borrelia burgdorferi*.

Dosage and Administration: Aseptically inject 1 mL (1 dose) subcutaneously into healthy dogs. For primary vaccination, revaccinate with a second 1 mL dose 2 to 3 weeks later. Revaccinate annually with a single 1 mL dose.

Precaution(s): Store at 2-7°C (35-45°F). Do not freeze. Do not use chemicals to sterilize syringes and needles.

Caution(s): In rare instances administration of vaccines may cause lethargy, fever, and inflammatory or hypersensitivity types of reactions. Treatment may include antihistamines, anti-inflammatories, and/or epinephrine.

For veterinary use only.

Presentation: 20 x 1 dose (1 mL) and 50 x 1 dose (1 mL) vials.

Sold to veterinarians only.

RECOMBITEK is a registered trademark of Merial.

Compendium Code No.: 11110663 RM501R6 / RM502R1

RE-COVR® INJECTION ℞

Fort Dodge **Antihistamine**

Tripelennamine Hydrochloride Injection

ANADA No.: 200-162

Active Ingredient(s): Description: Tripelennamine hydrochloride is a white, crystalline material which is stable, nonhygroscopic, and readily soluble in water. It is supplied in multiple dose vials containing 20 mg of tripelennamine hydrochloride U.S.P. per mL.

Indications: For use in cattle and horses in conditions in which antihistaminic therapy may be expected to lead to alleviation of some signs of disease.

Pharmacology: Action: Tripelennamine hydrochloride is characterized by its capacity to antagonize many of the pharmacologic effects of histamine.

Dosage and Administration: Warm the solution to near body temperature. Using aseptic precautions, administer intravenously or intramuscularly as specified below. Intramuscular injections should be made into the heavy musculature of the hind leg or cervical area.

The doses specified below may be repeated in 6 to 12 hours if necessary.

Cattle - Administer intravenously or intramuscularly at a dose of 0.5 mg per lb of body weight (2.5 mL for each 100 lbs of body weight). For a more rapid onset of action, the intravenous route of administration is recommended.

Horses - Administer intramuscularly only at a dose of 0.5 mg per lb of body weight (2.5 mL for each 100 lbs of body weight).

Precaution(s): Protect from light. Store between 15°C and 30°C (59°F-86°F. Avoid excessive heat (104°F).

Caution(s): Federal law restricts this drug to use by or on the order of a licensed veterinarian.

Central nervous system stimulation in the form of hyperexcitability, nervousness and muscle tremors lasting up to 20 minutes have been noted in horses, particularly following intravenous administration; therefore, only the intramuscular route of administration should be used in horses.

Overdosage of tripelennamine hydrochloride may give rise to excitement, ataxia and convulsions.

Depression of the central nervous system and incoordination may occur when the drug is used at therapeutic dose levels.

Disturbances in gastrointestinal function may occur in some instances.

While poisonous snake bites have been treated with antihistaminic drugs, other conjunctive therapy is required because of toxic reactions associated with the protein complex of venom.

Warning(s): Do not use in horses intended for food purposes.

Milk that has been taken during treatment and for 24 hours (two milkings) after the last treatment must not be used for food.

Treated cattle must not be slaughtered for food during treatment and for four days following the last treatment.

A withdrawal period has not been established for this product in pre-ruminating calves. Do not use in calves to be processed for veal.

Presentation: RE-COVR® Injection (tripelennamine hydrochloride injection) is supplied in 100 mL, 250 mL and 500 mL multiple dose vials.

NDC 53501-659-04 — 100 mL.
NDC 53501-659-05 — 250 mL.
NDC 53501-659-10 — 500 mL.

Manufactured by: Phoenix Scientific, Inc., St. Joseph, MO 64506

Compendium Code No.: 10031821 12720A

RED ALERT

Neogen **Dietary Supplement**

Multi-Vitamin Supplement

Ingredients: Each ounce contains:

Vitamin A	39,000 I.U.
Vitamin D_3	7,800 I.U.
Vitamin E	23 I.U.
Folic Acid	3000 mcg
Biotin	25 mcg
Vitamin B_{12}	11 mcg
Niacin	280 mg
Choline bitartrate	200 mg
Ferric ammonium citrate	100 mg
Thiamine mononitrate B_1	78 mg
Inositol	66 mg
Riboflavin B_2	31 mg
Pantothenic acid	19 mg
Pyridoxine HCL B_6	11 mg

Methyl paraben, propylparaben, artificial flavor, sodium saccharin, FD&C red #40, dextrose.

Indications: A water-dispersible blend of vitamins for horses and dogs.

R

Dosage and Administration: Dosage orally:
Horses: 1 fluid ounce 1 or 2 times daily.
Dogs: 1 tablespoon 1 or 2 times daily. Small Animals: Dose proportionately.
Caution(s): For veterinary use only.
Warning(s): Keep out of reach of children.
Presentation: 128 fl oz (1 gallon) 3.785 L (NDC: 59051-9137-9).
Compendium Code No.: 14910391 L417-0501

RED CELL®

Horse Health **Equine Dietary Supplement**

Yucca Flavored Vitamin-Iron-Mineral Supplement for Horses

Guaranteed Analysis:

		Each lb. Contains Not Less Than:	Each Fluid Ounce Contains:
Iron (Fe)	9,400 ppm	4,250.0 mg	300 mg
Copper (Cu)	1,100 ppm	500.0 mg	36 mg
Cobalt (Co)	60 ppm	28.0 mg	2 mg
Potassium (K)	0.31%	1,400.0 mg	100 mg
Sulfur (S) 0.9%	0.78%	3,550.0 mg	250 mg
Magnesium (Mg)	0.06%	280.0 mg	20 mg
Manganese (Mn)	1,200 ppm	540.0 mg	39 mg
Zinc (Zn)	3,400 ppm	1,540.0 mg	110 mg
Iodine (I)	8 ppm	3.6 mg	0.25 mg
Selenium (Se)	20 ppm	9.0 mg	0.65 mg
Vitamin A		356,923.0 I.U.	25,000 I.U.
Vitamin D-3		49,969.0 I.U.	3,500 I.U.
Vitamin E		500.0 I.U.	35 I.U.
Vitamin B12		1,680 mcg	120 mcg
Thiamine		428.0 mg	30 mg
Riboflavin		356.0 mg	25 mg
Vitamin B6		114.0 mg	8 mg
Menadione		35.0 mg	2.5 mg
Folic Acid		100.0 mg	7 mg
Biotin		0.285 mg	0.020 mg
Choline		2,855 mg	200 mg
d-Pantothenic Acid		685.0 mg	48 mg

Ingredients: Water, Ferric Sulfate, Ammonium Hydroxide, Citric Acid, Choline Chloride, Zinc Sulfate, Sorbitol, Magnesium Sulfate, Potassium Chloride, Vitamin E, Vitamin A Acetate, D-activated Animal Sterol irradiated (source of Vitamin D-3), Copper Sulfate, Xanthan Gum, Manganese Sulfate, Thiamine Hydrochloride, d-Calcium Pantothenate, Sodium Saccharin, Riboflavin, Pyridoxine Hydrochloride, Folic Acid, Cobalt Sulfate, Menadione Sodium Bisulfite complex (source of Vitamin K), Sodium Benzoate, Niacinamide, Sodium Bicarbonate, Biotin, Sodium Selenite, Kelp Extract, Yucca Schidigera Extract, Dried Meat Solubles, Liver Concentrate, Ethylenedediamine Dihydriodide, Vitamin B-12 Supplement, Artificial Cherry Flavoring, FD&C Red #40 and Potassium Sorbate (as preservative).
Indications: RED CELL® is a palatable yucca-flavoured Vitamin-Iron-Mineral feed supplement for horses formulated to provide supplemental vitamins and minerals that may be lacking or are in insufficient quantities in a horse's regular feed.
Directions: Feeding Directions:
Horses in training: Feed 2 fluid ounces of RED CELL® daily.
Horses not in training: Feed 1 fluid ounce of RED CELL® daily.
Feed RED CELL® by mixing into daily feed ration or orally with a dose syringe.
Important: Intake of supplemental selenium should not exceed 0.3 ppm on a complete ration basis.
Precaution(s): Store in a cool, dry place. Shake well before using. Keep from freezing. Close container after each use. Store in area inaccessible to children and animals.
Caution(s): Follow label directions. The addition to feed of higher levels of this premix containing selenium is not permitted. Excessive amounts of selenium may be toxic. This product should not be fed to copper sensitive animals, such as sheep.
For animal use only.
Warning(s): Keep out of reach of children.
Presentation: 946 mL (1 quart) [Net weight: 1.02 kg (2.25 lbs)], 1 gallon, 5 gallon and 15 gallon drums.
Compendium Code No.: 15000041

R

REDGLO®

Equicare **Equine Dietary Supplement**

Guaranteed Analysis:

Contains not less than:	Per Lb:	Per Fl Oz:
Methionine	0.294%	0.294%
Iron, min.	5,675 ppm	5,675 ppm
Selenium (SE)	7 ppm	7 ppm
Vitamin A	479,880 I.U.	36,000 I.U.
Vitamin D_3	95,976 I.U.	7,200 I.U.
Vitamin E	300 I.U.	22.5 I.U.
Vitamin B_{12}	1.5 mg	0.11 mg
Riboflavin	373 mg	28 mg
d-Pantothenic Acid	213 mg	16 mg
Thiamine	1,000 mg	75 mg
Niacin	3,732 mg	280 mg
Vitamin B_6	133 mg	10 mg
Folic Acid	40 mg	3 mg
Choline	3,066 mg	230 mg
Biotin	0.33 mg	0.025 mg
Inositol	866 mg	65 mg

Ingredients: Water, sugar, alcohol, Ferric Ammonium Citrate, Choline Chloride, Polysorbate 80, Niacinamide, Sodium Carboxymethyl Cellulose, Dried Meat Solubles, Natural and Artificial Flavors, Citric Acid, Yeast Extract, DL-Methionine, Liver Powder, Thiamine Mononitrate, Inositol, Vitamin E Supplement, Riboflavin, Vitamin A and D Blend, Methyl Paraben, d-Pantothenic Acid, p-Aminobenzoic Acid, Pyridoxine Hydrochloride, Propyl Paraben, Folic Acid, Artificial colors, Menadione Sodium Bisulfite Complex, d-Biotin, Sodium Selenite, and Vitamin B_{12} Supplement.
Indications: A liquid multi-vitamin supplement for horses. Enriched with iron.
Dosage and Administration: For horses in training, feed two ounces of REDGLO® once or twice daily. For horses not in training, feed one ounce daily. Mix into daily feed ration or feed orally by syringe.
Caution(s): Follow label directions. The addition to feed of higher levels of this supplement containing selenium is not permitted. Overdosing may be toxic.
Warning(s): If accidental ingestion should occur, consult a physician immediately.
For animal use only.
Keep out of reach of children.
Presentation: 32 oz and 3.785 (1 gallon).
Compendium Code No.: 14470141

REDUCINE® ABSORBENT FOR HORSES

Equicare **Counterirritant**

Active Ingredient(s):
Iodine, resublimed . . . . . 2.5% w/w
Potassium iodide . . . . . 2.5% w/w
Pinetar . . . . . 47.5% w/w
Indications: A counter-irritant ointment for use as an aid in the temporary relief of minor muscle stiffness and soreness caused by over exertion.
Dosage and Administration: Stir well before using. Do not apply too much REDUCINE® Absorbent at a time; enough to dampen the skin is sufficient. Clip the hair from the part to be treated and rub REDUCINE® Absorbent in well, either by hand or with a small stiff brush. Repeat the treatment on succeeding days until the skin shows signs of cracking or scaling. As soon as this is noticed stop the applications and leave the part entirely alone. Do not use oil or lard as is customary after blistering. If very lame, the animal should be turned out in a paddock, or led about by hand for half an hour twice a day. If not, it should be exercised gently every day, but in no case should it be allowed to stand all day in a stable. For ease of application, warm REDUCINE® Absorbent, if necessary. REDUCINE® Absorbent does not cause scars or blemishes.
Precaution(s): Store in a cool and dry place.
Caution(s): For external use only. Avoid contact with the eyes and mucous membranes. Do not use on cats.
Keep this and all medicines out of the reach of children. For veterinary use only.
Warning(s): Do not use on horses intended for food.
Presentation: 454 g (16.0 oz. = 1 lb.).
* REDUCINE is a registered trademark of Reducine Co.
Compendium Code No.: 14470150

REDUCINE® POULTICE

Equicare **Poultice**

Ingredient(s): Kaolin, water, bentonite, glycerine, boric acid, ferrous sulfate, and aloe vera with artificial peppermint fragrance added.
Indications: A poultice for use on horse's knees, tendons, and ankles.
REDUCINE® Poultice is for use as a tightener and for temporary relief of inflammation and soreness. REDUCINE® Poultice is also recommended as a hoof packing to aid in drawing out soreness and moisturizing the hoof.
Directions for Use: Clean all medication, chemicals and foreign matter from the area to be treated. Apply a layer of REDUCINE® up to ¼ inch thick over the area to be treated. Wrap the preparation with plastic or moist brown paper. Cover with cotton bandage. REDUCINE® is easily removed with water.
Notice: Due to varying temperature changes and REDUCINE®'s high moisture content, occasional liquid may accumulate on the surface. This is no way affects the quality of the product. Use this liquid as a starter to moisturize the horse's leg or pour it off.
Presentation: 6 lbs (2.72 kg) and 24 lbs.
Compendium Code No.: 14470171

REFRESH® IODINE TEAT DIP (1.00%)

Metz **Teat Dip**

Post Milking Teat Dip (1% Iodine)

Active Ingredient(s):
Iodine . . . . . 1.00% w/w
(Provides 1.00% titratable iodine. Equivalent to 10,000 parts per million titratable iodine.)
Glycerine 10.0%
Minimum pH 4.0
Indications: An aid in controlling the spread of bacteria that may cause mastitis.
Directions for Use:
As a Post-Dip: Immediately after milker is removed, dip or spray the teats with undiluted product. If the cow will be returned to a below freezing temperature environment allow the teat dip to dry before discharging her from the milking area. Immediately before the next milking wash and/or pre-dip the teats and udder.
Caution(s): Do not use for cleaning or sanitizing milking equipment.
Warning(s): Harmful if swallowed. If swallowed, drink large quantities of milk or water and induce vomiting. Call a physician immediately. Will irritate eyes and mucous membranes. Flush gently with large amounts of water and see a physician immediately.
Avoid contact with food. Keep out of the reach of children.
Presentation: 5 gallon, 15 gallon, 30 gallon, and 55 gallon.
Patent No 5 534,266 and patent pending Patent No. 5720984
Compendium Code No.: 10190080

REGRESSIN®-V

Bioniche Animal Health (formerly Vetrepharm) **Immunostimulant**

Mycobacterium Cell Wall Fraction Immunostimulant

U.S. Vet. Lic. No.: 289
Active Ingredient(s): The mycobacteriaceae have been known for many years to have antitumor activity. REGRESSIN®-V is an emulsion of cell wall fractions which have been modified to reduce their toxic and allergic effect, but retain their antitumor activity. REGRESSIN®-V stimulates the activation of macrophages and thymic lymphocytes which kill tumor cells. REGRESSIN®-V

contains procaine hydrochloride 0.2% w/v (which exhibits local analgesic properties) and green tracking dye solution 0.1% w/v (which helps indicate the infiltration of the injected tumor mass or area).

Indications: REGRESSIN®-V is recommended for the immunotherapy of mixed mammary tumor and mammary adenocarcinoma in dogs and equine sarcoid in horses. Although REGRESSIN®-V is administered by intratumoral injection, the response is generalized, and untreated sites frequently undergo regression. Prognosis should be guarded in advanced malignant disease with metastases, as remissions will be less frequent. Remissions cannot be guaranteed as each tumor will vary in its response.

Dosage and Administration: REGRESSIN®-V is administered only by intratumoral injection. The entire tumor and a small region of adjacent and underlying tissue must be thoroughly infiltrated using no larger than a 20 gauge needle. Injection without careful infiltration of the tumor may not be effective. It is important to mix the emulsion thoroughly and inject the tumor as quickly as possible because the emulsion may begin to separate soon after mixing. The tumor tissue may be very firm and excessive pressure on the syringe plunger may be required to infiltrate the tumor. The injection may produce pain in some animals; anesthetics or additional analgesics may be used. Dosage varies with tumor size, but 1 mL should be considered a minimum dose.

Dogs: REGRESSIN®-V proved to be effective against mixed mammary tumors and mammary adenocaricinomas in dogs, but was not effective against liposarcomas in dogs. Canine mammary tumors may be treated once, two (2) to four (4) weeks prior to surgery. Whereas surgical removal of mammary tumors produces a desireable cosmetic result, tumor-free survivals is not significantly improved. On the other hand, dogs treated with mycobacterium cell wall fractions, prior to surgery, experience significantly extended mean tumor-free survival time, and a significantly greater number of dogs survive free of tumor.[4] REGRESSIN®-V is well-tolerated by aged dogs with chronic cardiovascular and renal disease. This makes immunotherapy without surgery an attractive method of treatment for those patients who are poor surgical risks. Treatment should be repeated every one (1) to three (3) weeks. Tumors that fail to respond after four (4) treatments should be considered refractory and therapy discontinued. Eighty-eight percent of dogs treated with immunotherapy only were free of tumor two (2) years later. Individual doses range from 1 to 30 mL (average about 2.5 mL). The average cumulative dose is about 10 mL.

Horses: Equine sarcoid is very responsive to immunotherapy with mycobacterium cell wall fractions.[5] Large, pedunculated sarcoids should be debulked by partial excision prior to therapy. REGRESSIN®-V is safe for use in pregnant mares. Treatment should be repeated every one (1) to three (3) weeks. Tumors that fail to respond after four (4) treatments should be considered refractory and therapy discontinued. Ninety-four (94) percent of horses treated were free of tumor two (2) years later. Individual doses range from 1 to 60 mL (average about 10 mL). The average cumulative dose is about 10 mL.

Contraindication(s): Immunotherapy may not be effective in animals receiving concurrent immunosuppressive therapies. Avoid the use of corticosteroids or ACTH where possible.

Precaution(s): Store at 2-7°C in a refrigerator, but do not freeze. The emulsion separates on standing. Resuspend by shaking or rotating the vial between the hands until the emulsion has a homogeneous "milky" appearance. If necessary, REGRESSIN®-V may be heated to 65°C to facilitate suspension.

Caution(s): The inflammatory response with edema and malaise occasionally is severe after the initial treatment. Therapy should be discontinued until the reaction has subsided. This product contains procaine hydrochloride and should not be used in performance horses within 96 hours of the event.

Warning(s): Do not use in food producing animals.

Side Effects: Mild fever, drowsiness and an increased metabolic rate leading to decreased appetite may occur for one to two days following a REGRESSIN®-V injection. These are all normal responses to the release of cytokines.[1,2,3] An elevated body temperature enhances the immune function by stimulating lymphocyte activity,[2] and thus should not be considered an adverse side effect. Local inflammation which is sensitive to the touch occurs fairly often, but it usually is not bothersome to the patient. Necrosis with suppuration may occur in regressing tumors and clients should be informed that the tumor may drain for several weeks. Tumors may be aspirated with a sterile syringe and needle to help prevent drainage. If drainage develops, it often may be stopped by application of astringents such as silver nitrate and styptic powders.

References: Available upon request.

Presentation: 10 mL vials.

Compendium Code No.: 11070051

REGU-MATE® SOLUTION ℞

Intervet **Progestin**

(Altrenogest)* Solution 0.22% Oral Progestin

NADA No.: 131-310

Active Ingredient(s): Each mL of REGU-MATE® (altrenogest) Solution 0.22% contains 2.2 mg of altrenogest in an oil solution.

Indications: REGU-MATE® (altrenogest) Solution 0.22% is indicated to suppress estrus in mares.

Suppression of estrus allows for a predictable occurrence of estrus following drug withdrawal. This facilitates the attainment of regular cyclicity during the transition from winter anestrus to the physiological breeding season. Suppression of estrus will also facilitate management of prolonged estrus conditions. Suppression of estrus may be used to facilitate scheduled breeding during the physiological breeding season.

Pharmacology: REGU-MATE® (altrenogest) Solution 0.22% contains the active synthetic progestin, altrenogest. The chemical name is 17α-allyl-17β-hydroxyestra-4,9,11-trien-3-one. The CAS Registry Number is 850-52-2. The chemical structure is:

REGU-MATE® (altrenogest) Solution 0.22% produces a progestational effect in mares.

Dosage and Administration: While wearing protective gloves, administer orally at the rate of 1 mL per 110 pounds body weight (0.044 mg/kg) to be given one dose daily for 15 consecutive days. Administer directly on the posteriodorsal surface of the mare's tongue using a dose syringe or suitable plastic syringe. The drug may also be administered on the usual grain ration.

Dosage Chart:

Approximate Weight In Pounds	Dose in mL
770	7
880	8
990	9
1100	10
1210	11
1320	12

Which Mares Will Respond to REGU-MATE® (altrenogest) Solution 0.22%: Extensive clinical trials have demonstrated that estrus will be suppressed in approximately 95% of the mares within three days; however, the post-treatment response depended on the level of ovarian activity when treatment was initiated. Estrus in mares exhibiting regular estrus cycles during the breeding season will be suppressed during treatment; these mares return to estrus four to five days following treatment and continue to cycle normally. Mares in winter anestrus with small follicles continued in anestrus and failed to exhibit normal estrus following withdrawal.

Response in mares in the transition phase between winter anestrus and the summer breeding season depended on the degree of follicular activity. Mares with inactive ovaries and small follicles failed to respond with normal cycles post-treatment, whereas a higher proportion of mares with ovarian follicles 20 mm or greater in diameter exhibited normal estrus cycles post-treatment. REGU-MATE® (altrenogest) Solution 0.22% was very effective for suppressing the prolonged estrus behavior frequently observed in mares during the transition period (February, March and April). In addition, a high proportion of these mares responded with regular estrus cycles post-treatment.

Contraindication(s): REGU-MATE® (altrenogest) Solution 0.22% is contraindicated for use in mares having a previous or current history of uterine inflammation (i.e., acute, subacute, or chronic endometritis). Natural or synthetic gestagen therapy may exacerbate existing low-grade or "smoldering" uterine inflammation into a fulminating uterine infection in some instances.

Precaution(s): Store at room temperature.

Reclose tightly.

Caution(s): Federal law restricts this drug to use by or on the order of a licensed veterinarian.

Keep this and all medication out of the reach of children.

Various synthetic progestins, including altrenogest, when administer to rats during the embryogenic stage of pregnancy at doses manyfold greater than the recommended equine dose caused fetal anomalies, specifically masculinization of the female genitalia.

Warning(s): Do not use in horses intended for food.

Caution for Handlers: Skin contact must be avoided as REGU-MATE® (altrenogest) Solution 0.22% is readily absorbed through unbroken skin. Protective gloves must be worn by all persons handling this product. Pregnant women or women who suspect they are pregnant should not handle REGU-MATE® (altrenogest) Solution 0.22%. Women of child bearing age should exercise extreme caution when handling this product. Accidental absorption could lead to a disruption of the menstrual cycle or prolongation of pregnancy. Direct contact with the skin should therefore be avoided. Accidental spillage on the skin should be washed off immediately with soap and water.

Information for Handlers: REGU-MATE® (altrenogest) Solution 0.22% is readily absorbed by the skin. Skin contact must be avoided; protective gloves must be worn when handling this product.

Effects of Overexposure: There has been no human use of this specific product. The information contained in this section is extrapolated from data available on other products of the same pharmacological class that have been used in humans. Effects anticipated are due to the progestational activity of altrenogest.

Acute effects after a single exposure are possible; however, continued daily exposure has the potential for more untoward effects such as disruption of the menstrual cycle, uterine or abdominal cramping, increased or decreased uterine bleeding, prolongation of pregnancy and headaches. The oil base may also cause complications if swallowed.

In addition, the list of people who should not handle this product (see below) is based upon the known effects of progestins used in humans on a chronic basis.

People who should not handle this product.

1. Women who are or suspect they are pregnant.
2. Anyone with thrombophlebitis or thromboembolic disorders or with a history of these events.
3. Anyone with cerebral-vascular or coronary-artery disease.
4. Women with known or suspected carcinoma of the breast.
5. People with known or suspected estrogen-dependent neoplasia.
6. Women with undiagnosed vaginal bleeding.
7. People with benign or malignant tumors which developed during the use of oral contraceptives or other estrogen-containing products.
8. Anyone with liver dysfunction or disease.

Accidental Exposure: Altrenogest is readily absorbed from contact with the skin. In addition, this oil based product can penetrate porous gloves. Altrenogest should not penetrate intact rubber or impervious gloves; however, if there is leakage (i.e., pinhole, spillage, etc.), the contaminated area covered by such occlusive materials may have increased absorption. The following measures are recommended in case of accidental exposure.

Skin Exposure: Wash immediately with soap and water.

Eye Exposure: Immediately flush with plenty of water for 15 minutes. Get medical attention.

If swallowed: Do not induce vomiting. REGU-MATE® (altrenogest) Solution 0.22% contains an oil. Call a physician. Vomiting should be supervised by a physician because of possible pulmonary damage via aspiration of the oil base. If possible bring the container and labeling to the physician.

For oral use in horses only.

For veterinary use only.

Discussion: Specific Uses for REGU-MATE® (altrenogest) Solution 0.22%: Suppression of estrus to:

1. Facilitate attainment of regular cycles during the transition period from winter anestrus to the physiological breeding season.

   To facilitate attainment of regular cycles during the transition phase, mares should be examined to determine the degree of ovarian activity. Estrus in mares with inactive ovaries (no follicles greater than 20 mm in diameter) will be suppressed but these mares may not begin regular cycles following treatment. However, mares with active ovaries (follicles greater than 20 mm in diameter) frequently respond with regular post-treatment estrus cycles.
2. Facilitate management of the mare exhibiting prolonged estrus during the transition period. Estrus will be suppressed in mares exhibiting prolonged behavioral estrus either early or late during the transition period. Again, the post-treatment response depends on the level

R

of ovarian activity. The mares with greater ovarian activity initiate regular cycles and conceive sooner than the inactive mares. REGU-MATE® (altrenogest) Solution 0.22% may be administered early in the transition period to suppress estrus in mares with inactive ovaries to aid in the management of these mares or to mares later in the transition period with active ovaries to prepare and schedule the mare for breeding.

3. Permit scheduled breeding of mares during the physiological breeding season. To permit scheduled breeding, mares which are regularly cycling or which have active ovarian function should be given REGU-MATE® Solution 0.22% daily for 15 consecutive days beginning 20 days before the date of the planned estrus.

   Ovulation will occur 5 to 7 days following the onset of estrus as expected for non-treated mares. Breeding should follow usual procedures for mares in estrus. Mares may be regulated and scheduled either individually or in groups.

Trial Data: A 3-year well controlled reproductive safety study was conducted in 27 pregnant mares, and compared with 24 untreated control mares. Treated mares received 2 mL altrenogest/110 lb body weight (2x dosage recommended for estrus suppression) from day 20 to day 325 of gestation. This study provided the following data:

1. In filly offspring (all ages) of treated mares, clitoral size was increased.
2. Filly offspring from treated mares had shorter interval from Feb. 1 to first ovulation than fillies from their untreated mare counterparts.
3. There were no significant differences in reproductive performance between treated and untreated animals (mares and their respective offspring) measuring the following parameters:
   - interval from Feb. 1 to first ovulation, in mares only.
   - mean interovulatory interval from first to second cycle and second to third cycle, mares only.
   - follicle size, mares only.
   - at 50 days gestation, pregnancy rate in treated mares was 81.8% (9/11) and untreated mares was 100% (4/4).
   - after 3 cycles, 11/12 treated mares were pregnant (91.7%) and 4/4 untreated mares were pregnant (100%).
   - colt offspring of treated and control mares reached puberty at approximately the same age (82 and 84 weeks respectively.)
   - stallion offspring from treated and control mares showed no differences in seminal volume, spermatozoal concentration, spermatazoal motility, and total sperm per ejaculate.
   - stallion offspring from treated and control mares showed no difference in sexual behavior.
   - testicular characteristics (scrotal width, testis weight, parenchymal weight, epididymal weight and height, testicular height, width and length) were the same between stallion offspring of treated and control mares.

References: Available upon request.
Presentation: Available in 150 mL and 1000 mL plastic bottles.
* US Patents 3,453,267; 3,478,067; 3,484,462 REGU-MATE Reg TM of Roussel Uclaf
Manufactured by: DPT Laboratories
Compendium Code No.: 11061630

RELIANT® 3

Merial **Vaccine**

Bovine Rhinotracheitis-Virus Diarrhea-Parainfluenza$_3$ Vaccine, Modified Live Virus
U.S. Vet. Lic. No.: 298
Contents: This product contains the antigens listed above.
Contains gentamicin and nystatin as preservatives.
Indications: For the vaccination of healthy cattle (weaned calves, feedlot cattle, yearlings) as an aid in the prevention of disease due to IBR, BVD, and PI$_3$.
Dosage and Administration: Shake well before using. Aseptically reconstitute the lyophilized vaccine with the accompanying diluent and inject 2 mL (1 dose) intramuscularly or subcutaneously. Calves vaccinated under 6 months of age should be revaccinated after reaching 6 months of age. Revaccinate with a single 2 mL dose annually or prior to times of stress or exposure.
Precaution(s): Store at 2-7°C (35-45°F). Do not freeze. Do not expose to heat or direct sunlight. Use entire contents when first opened. Burn the container and all unused contents. Do not use chemicals to sterilize syringes and needles.
Caution(s): Do not vaccinate pregnant cows or calves nursing pregnant cows.
In rare instances, administration of vaccines may cause lethargy, fever, and inflammatory or hypersensitivity types of reactions. Treatment may include antihistamines, anti-inflammatories, and/or epinephrine. For veterinary use only.
Warning(s): Do not vaccinate within 21 days prior to slaughter.
Presentation: 10 dose (20 mL) and 50 dose (100 mL) vials.
RELIANT is a registered trademark of Merial.
Compendium Code No.: 11110672 RM071R7 / RM075R6

RELIANT® 4

Merial **Vaccine**

Bovine Rhinotracheitis-Virus Diarrhea-Parainfluenza$_3$-Respiratory Syncytial Virus Vaccine, Modified Live and Killed Virus
U.S. Vet. Lic. No.: 298
Contents: This product contains the antigens listed above.
Contains gentamicin and nystatin as preservatives.
Indications: For the vaccination of healthy cattle (weaned calves, feedlot cattle, yearlings) as an aid in the prevention of disease due to IBR, BVD, PI$_3$, and BRSV.
Dosage and Administration: Shake well before using. Aseptically reconstitute the lyophilized vaccine with the accompanying diluent and inject 2 mL (1 dose) intramuscularly or subcutaneously. For primary vaccination, revaccinate with a second 2 mL dose 2 to 4 weeks later. Calves vaccinated under 6 months of age should be revaccinated after reaching 6 months of age. Revaccinate with a single 2 mL dose annually or prior to times of stress or exposure.
Precaution(s): Store at 2-7°C (35-45°F). Do not freeze. Do not expose to heat or direct sunlight. Use entire contents when first opened. Burn the container and all unused contents. Do not use chemicals to sterilize syringes and needles.
Caution(s): Do not vaccinate pregnant cows or calves nursing pregnant cows.
In rare instances, administration of vaccines may cause lethargy, fever, and inflammatory or hypersensitivity types of reactions. Treatment may include antihistamines, anti-inflammatories, and/or epinephrine. For veterinary use only.
Warning(s): Do not vaccinate within 21 days prior to slaughter.
Presentation: 10 dose (20 mL) and 50 dose (100 mL) vials.
RELIANT is a registered trademark of Merial.
Compendium Code No.: 11110682 RM121R6 / RM125R5

RELIANT® 8

Merial **Vaccine**

Bovine Rhinotracheitis-Virus Diarrhea-Parainfluenza$_3$ Vaccine-Leptospira Canicola-Grippotyphosa-Hardjo-Icterohaemorrhagiae-Pomona Bacterin, Modified Live Virus
U.S. Vet. Lic. No.: 298
Contents: This product contains the antigens listed above.
Contains gentamicin and nystatin as preservatives.
Indications: For the vaccination of healthy cattle (calves, open cows, open heifers) as an aid in the prevention of disease due to IBR, BVD, PI$_3$, *L. canicola, L. grippotyphosa, L. hardjo, L. icterohaemorrhagiae,* and *L. pomona.*
Dosage and Administration: Shake well before using. Aseptically reconstitute the lyophilized vaccine with the accompanying diluent and inject 2 mL (1 dose) intramuscularly. For primary vaccination, revaccinate with a second 2 mL dose 2 to 4 weeks later. Calves vaccinated under 6 months of age should be revaccinated after reaching 6 months of age. Revaccinate with a single 2 mL dose annually or prior to times of stress or exposure.
Precaution(s): Store at 2-7°C (35-45°F). Do not freeze. Do not expose to heat or direct sunlight. Use entire contents when first opened. Burn the container and all unused contents. Do not use chemicals to sterilize syringes and needles.
Caution(s): Do not vaccinate pregnant cows or calves nursing pregnant cows.
In rare instances, administration of vaccines may cause lethargy, fever and inflammatory or hypersensitivity types of reactions. Treatment may include antihistamines, anti-inflammatories, and/or epinephrine.
For veterinary use only.
Warning(s): Do not vaccinate within 21 days prior to slaughter.
Presentation: 10 dose (20 mL) and 50 dose (100 mL) vials.
RELIANT is a registered trademark of Merial.
Compendium Code No.: 11110692 RM021R6 / RM025R6

RELIANT® IBR

Merial **Vaccine**

Bovine Rhinotracheitis Vaccine, Modified Live Virus
U.S. Vet. Lic. No.: 298
Contents: This product contains the antigen listed above.
Contains gentamicin and nystatin as preservatives.
Indications: For the vaccination of healthy cattle (weaned calves, feedlot cattle, yearlings) as an aid in the prevention of disease due to IBR.
Dosage and Administration: Shake well before using. Aseptically reconstitute the lyophilized vaccine with the accompanying diluent and inject 2 mL (1 dose) intramuscularly or subcutaneously. Calves vaccinated under 6 months of age should be revaccinated after reaching 6 months of age. Revaccinate with a single 2 mL dose annually or prior to times of stress or exposure.
Precaution(s): Store at 2-7°C (35-45°F). Do not freeze. Do not expose to heat or direct sunlight. Use entire contents when first opened. Burn the container and all unused contents. Do not use chemicals to sterilize syringes and needles.
Caution(s): Do not vaccinate pregnant cows or calves nursing pregnant cows.
In rare instances, administration of vaccines may cause lethargy, fever, and inflammatory or hypersensitivity types of reactions. Treatment may include antihistamines, anti-inflammatories, and/or epinephrine.
For veterinary use only.
Warning(s): Do not vaccinate within 21 days prior to slaughter.
Presentation: 10 dose (20 mL) and 50 dose (100 mL) vials.
RELIANT is a registered trademark of Merial.
Compendium Code No.: 11110702 RM051R7 / RM055R6

RELIANT® IBR/BVD

Merial **Vaccine**

Bovine Rhinotracheitis-Virus Diarrhea Vaccine, Modified Live Virus
U.S. Vet. Lic. No.: 298
Contents: This product contains the antigens listed above.
Contains gentamicin and nystatin as preservatives.
Indications: For the vaccination of healthy cattle (weaned calves, feedlot cattle, yearlings) as an aid in the prevention of disease due to IBR and BVD.
Dosage and Administration: Shake well before using. Aseptically reconstitute the lyophilized vaccine with the accompanying liquid diluent and inject 2 mL (1 dose) intramuscularly or subcutaneously. Calves vaccinated under 6 months of age should be revaccinated after reaching 6 months of age. Revaccinate with a single 2 mL dose annually or prior to times of stress or exposure.
Precaution(s): Store at 2-7°C (35-45°F). Do not freeze. Do not expose to heat or direct sunlight. Use entire contents when first opened. Burn the container and all unused contents. Do not use chemicals to sterilize syringes and needles.
Caution(s): Do not vaccinate pregnant cows or calves nursing pregnant cows.
In rare instances, administration of vaccines may cause lethargy, fever, and inflammatory or hypersensitivity types of reactions. Treatment may include antihistamines, anti-inflammatories, and/or epinephrine.
For veterinary use only.
Warning(s): Do not vaccinate within 21 days prior to slaughter.
Presentation: 10 dose (20 mL) vials.
RELIANT is a registered trademark of Merial.
Compendium Code No.: 11110712 RM081R7

RELIANT® IBR/LEPTO

Merial **Bacterin-Vaccine**

Bovine Rhinotracheitis Vaccine, Modified Live Virus-Leptospira Pomona Bacterin
U.S. Vet. Lic. No.: 298
Contents: This product contains the antigens listed above.
Contains gentamicin and nystatin as preservatives.
Indications: For the vaccination of healthy cattle (open cows, open heifers, weaned calves, feedlot cattle, yearlings) as an aid in the prevention of disease due to IBR and *L. pomona.*
Dosage and Administration: Shake well before using. Aseptically reconstitute the lyophilized vaccine with the accompanying diluent and inject 2 mL (1 dose) intramuscularly. Calves vaccinated under 6 months of age should be revaccinated after reaching 6 months of age. Revaccinate with a single 2 mL dose annually or prior to times of stress or exposure.

Precaution(s): Store at 2-7°C (35-45°F). Do not freeze. Do not expose to heat or direct sunlight. Use entire contents when first opened. Burn the container and all unused contents. Do not use chemicals to sterilize syringes and needles.

Caution(s): Do not vaccinate pregnant cows or calves nursing pregnant cows.

In rare instances, administration of vaccines may cause lethargy, fever, and inflammatory or hypersensitivity types of reactions. Treatment may include antihistamines, anti-inflammatories, and/or epinephrine.

For veterinary use only.

Warning(s): Do not vaccinate within 21 days prior to slaughter.

Presentation: 10 dose (20 mL) and 50 dose (100 mL) vials.

RELIANT is a registered trademark of Merial.

Compendium Code No.: 11110732 RM091R6 / RM095R5

RELIANT® PLUS BVD-K (DUAL IBR™)

Merial **Vaccine**

Bovine Rhinotracheitis-Virus Diarrhea-Parainfluenza$_3$-Respiratory Syncytial Virus Vaccine, Modified Live and Killed Virus

U.S. Vet. Lic. No.: 298

Contents: This product contains the antigens listed above.

Contains gentamicin and nystatin as preservatives.

Indications: For the vaccination of healthy cattle (weaned calves, feedlot cattle, yearlings) as an aid in the prevention of disease due to IBR, BVD, PI$_3$, and BRSV.

Dosage and Administration: Shake well before using. Aseptically reconstitute the lyophilized vaccine with the accompanying diluent and inject 2 mL (1 dose) intramuscularly or subcutaneously. For primary vaccination, revaccinate with a second 2 mL dose 2 to 4 weeks later. Calves vaccinated under 6 months of age should be revaccinated after reaching 6 months of age. Revaccinate with a single 2 mL dose annually or prior to times of stress or exposure.

Precaution(s): Store at 2-7°C (35-45°F). Do not freeze. Do not expose to heat or direct sunlight. Use entire contents when first opened. Burn the container and all unused contents. Do not use chemicals to sterilize syringes and needles.

Caution(s): Do not vaccinate pregnant cows or calves nursing pregnant cows.

In rare instances, administration of vaccines may cause lethargy, fever, and inflammatory or hypersensitivity types of reactions. Treatment may include antihistamines, anti-inflammatories, and/or epinephrine.

For veterinary use only.

Warning(s): Do not vaccinate within 21 days prior to slaughter.

Presentation: 10 dose (20 mL) and 50 dose (100 mL) vials.

RELIANT and DUAL IBR are trademarks of Merial.

Compendium Code No.: 11110860 RM171R7 / RM175R6

RELIANT® PLUS (DUAL IBR™)

Merial **Vaccine**

Bovine Rhinotracheitis-Virus Diarrhea-Parainfluenza$_3$-Respiratory Syncytial Virus Vaccine, Modified Live and Killed Virus

U.S. Vet. Lic. No.: 298

Contents: This product contains the antigens listed above.

Contains gentamicin and nystatin as preservatives.

Indications: For the vaccination of healthy cattle (weaned calves, feedlot cattle, yearlings) as an aid in the prevention of disease due to IBR, BVD, PI$_3$, and BRSV.

Dosage and Administration: Shake well before using. Aseptically reconstitute the lyophilized vaccine with the accompanying diluent and inject 2 mL (1 dose) intramuscularly or subcutaneously. For primary vaccination, revaccinate with a second 2 mL dose 2 to 4 weeks later. Calves vaccinated under 6 months of age should be revaccinated after reaching 6 months of age. Revaccinate with a single 2 mL dose annually or prior to times of stress or exposure.

Precaution(s): Store at 2-7°C (35-45°F). Do not freeze. Do not expose to heat or direct sunlight. Use entire contents when first opened. Burn the container and all unused contents. Do not use chemicals to sterilize syringes and needles.

Caution(s): Do not vaccinate pregnant cows or calves nursing pregnant cows.

In rare instances, administration of vaccines may cause lethargy, fever, and inflammatory or hypersensitivity types of reactions. Treatment may include antihistamines, anti-inflammatories, and/or epinephrine.

For veterinary use only.

Warning(s): Do not vaccinate within 21 days prior to slaughter.

Presentation: 10 dose (20 mL) and 50 dose (100 mL) vials.

RELIANT, and DUAL IBR are trademarks of Merial.

Compendium Code No.: 11110252 RM151R6 / RM155R5

RELIEF® CREME RINSE

DVM **Antidermatosis Rinse**

Active Ingredient(s): Pramoxine hydrochloride 1%.

Indications: For the temporary relief of itching and flaking caused by seborrheic dermatitis.

Product Description: RELIEF® Creme Rinse has been formulated with pramoxine HCl and colloidal ointment. Relief is complemented with omega-6 fatty acids for dermal renourishing and is delivered in a quaternary-based, anti-static vehicle containing moisturizers, emollients and coat conditioners.

Directions for Use: Shake well before use. First, shampoo pet and rinse thoroughly. Then, while pet is still wet, apply RELIEF® Creme Rinse evenly over haircoat and rub in well. RELIEF® Creme Rinse may be used as a leave-on conditioner or lightly rinsed after 5-10 minutes of contact time. May be used as often as necessary, or as directed by your veterinarian.

Precaution(s): Store at room temperature.

Caution(s): For topical use on animals only. If redness or irritation persists or increases, discontinue use unless directed by your veterinarian. Do not use in eyes or nose. If contact occurs, rinse thoroughly with water.

Warning(s): Keep out of reach of children.

Presentation: 8 fl oz (237 mL) (NDC 47203-940-08), 12 fl oz (355 mL) (NDC 47203-940-12) and 1 gallon (3.78 L) (NDC 47203-940-28).

Compendium Code No.: 11420481 Rev 0499

RELIEF! FLY OINTMENT

Davis **Topical Insecticide**

EPA Reg. No.: 2781-9-50591

Active Ingredient(s): Pyrethrins I and II 0.2%, piperonyl butoxide tech. 0.5% (equiv. to 0.4% (butylcarbityl) 6-propylpiperonyl) ether and 0.1% of related compounds). Di-n-propyl isocinchomeronate 1.0%. Inert Ingredients: 98.3%

Indications: For use on dogs and horses.

For wounds and sores.

Repels house flies, stable flies, face flies, horn flies.

Kills on contact, effective for hours.

Directions for Use: For Dogs and Horses.

To treat superficial wounds, abrasions, sores and scratches apply enough ointment to completely cover the affected area. Use daily.

It is a violation of Federal Law to use this product in a manner inconsistent with its labeling.

Precautionary Statements: Hazard to Humans and Domestic Animals: Not for human use. Wash hands after using.

Environmental Hazards: This product is toxic to fish. Keep out of lakes, streams, or ponds. Do not apply where runoff is likely to occur. Do not contaminate water by cleaning of equipment or disposal of wastes.

Storage and Disposal: Do not reuse empty container. Wrap container and put it in trash collection.

Warning(s): Do not use on horses to be used for human consumption. Keep out of reach of children.

Presentation: 2 oz (56.5 g).

Compendium Code No.: 11410350

RELIEF® SHAMPOO

DVM **Antidermatosis Shampoo**

Active Ingredient(s): Pramoxine hydrochloride 1%.

Indications: For use as a cleansing shampoo and for temporary relief of itching and flaking caused by seborrheic dermatitis.

Product Description: RELIEF® Shampoo has been formulated with pramoxine HCl and colloidal oatmeal. Relief is complemented with omega-6 fatty acids for dermal renourishing and is delivered in a soap-free, cosmetically pleasing, cleansing system for high luster and manageability.

Directions for Use: Shake well before use. Wet coat thoroughly. Apply sufficient amount of RELIEF® Shampoo to lather well into haircoat. Contact with the skin is important. When entire coat is treated, allow to stand for 5-10 minutes. Then rinse thoroughly with water. RELIEF® Shampoo may be used as often as necessary, or as directed by your veterinarian.

Precaution(s): Store at room temperature.

Caution(s): For topical use on animals only. If redness or irritation persists or increases, discontinue use unless directed by your veterinarian. Do not use in eyes or nose. If contact occurs, rinse thoroughly with water.

Warning(s): Keep out of reach of children.

Presentation: 8 fl oz (237 mL) (NDC 47203-900-08), 12 fl oz (355 mL) (NDC 47203-900-12) and 1 gallon (3.78 L) (NDC 47203-900-28).

Compendium Code No.: 11420491 Rev 0499

RELIEF® SPRAY

DVM **Antidermatosis Spray**

Active Ingredient(s): Pramoxine hydrochloride 1%.

Indications: For temporary relief of itching and flaking caused by seborrheic dermatitis. For topical use on dogs and cats.

Product Description: RELIEF® Spray has been formulated with colloidal oatmeal and pramoxine hydrochloride HCl. Relief is complemented with omega-6 fatty acids for dermal renourishing and is delivered in a hydrating medium containing moisturizers and coat conditioners.

Directions for Use: Shake well before use. Spray affected, itchy areas of pet's skin. Rub in well. If necessary, part haircoat so that RELIEF® Spray makes direct contact with the skin. Rub in well and groom with a brush. Be sure to push down on sprayer with sufficient pressure so as to obtain a fine mist.

RELIEF® Spray may be used daily, or as directed by your veterinarian.

Precaution(s): Store at room temperature.

Caution(s): If redness or irritation persists or increases, discontinue use unless directed by your veterinarian. do not use in eyes or nose. If contact occurs, rinse thoroughly with water.

Warning(s): Keep out of reach of children.

Presentation: 8 fl oz (237 mL) (NDC 47203-950-08).

Compendium Code No.: 11420501 Rev 0499

R

RENAKARE™ ℞

Neogen **Potassium-Oral**

Potassium Gluconate

Active Ingredient(s): Each tablet contains:

Potassium Gluconate . . . . 2 mEq (468 mg)

Each 0.65 g (¼ teaspoon) of powder contains:

Potassium Gluconate . . . . 2 mEq (468 mg)

In a palatable protein base.

Each 2.34 g (½ teaspoon) of gel contains:

Potassium Gluconate . . . . 2 mEq (468 mg)

In a palatable protein base.

Indications: For use as a supplement in potassium deficient states in cats and dogs.

Dosage and Administration: The suggested dosage of RENAKARE™ for adult dogs and cats is:

Tablets: One (1) tablet per 10 lb (4.5 kg) body weight twice daily.

Powder: 0.65 g (¼ level teaspoon) per 10 lb (4.5 kg) body weight twice daily with food.

Gel: 2.34 g (½ teaspoon) per 10 lbs (4.5 kg) body weight twice daily.

Administration: (Gel) RENAKARE™ Gel is highly palatable. To initiate interest in taste, place small amount on the animal's nose or on the roof of its mouth. Gel may be placed on the paw after initial interest has been established.

Dosage may be adjusted to satisfy patient's need.

Precaution(s): Store at controlled room temperature between 15°-30°C (59°-86°F).

Caution(s): Federal law restricts this drug to use by or on the order of a licensed veterinarian.

Use with caution in the presence of cardiac disease, particularly in digitized patients or in the presence of renal disease.

For animal use only.

Warning(s): Do not administer in diseases where high potassium levels may be encountered, such as severe renal insufficiency or adrenal insufficiency.

Keep out of reach of children.

Presentation: Plastic bottles containing: 100 tablets, 12 per case (NDC: 59051-9074-5).
Plastic bottles containing: 4 oz (113 g) powder, 12 per case (NDC: 59051-9075-1).
Plastic tubes containing: 5 oz (142 g) gel, 12 per case (NDC: 59051-9076-6).

Manufactured by: Tabs Limited, St. Joseph, MO 64501 (Tablets and Powder).
Corwood Laboratories, Hauppage, NY 11788 (Gel).

Compendium Code No.: 14910102 0501 / 0501 / L517-0601

RENOGEN

Novartis (Aqua Health) **Bacterial Vaccine**

Arthrobacter Vaccine, Live Culture

U.S. Vet. Lic. No.: 335

Contents: This vaccine is presented as a lyophilized live culture of a microorganism that shares common antigenic determinants with *Renibacterium salmoninarum*, and is to be resuspended with sterile diluent before use.

A sterile diluent (0.9% Sodium Chloride) for the resuspension of lyophilized culture of the live microorganism *Arthrobacter* sp. *nov.*, sharing common antigenic determinants with *Renibacterium salmoninarum.* The final formulation of ready to use RENOGEN is a suspension of live microorganism in diluent.

Indications: As an aid in the prevention of Bacterial Kidney Disease caused by *Renibacterium salmoninarum* in healthy salmonids 10 g or larger.

Directions for Use:

A. Resuspension of lyophilized culture

1. Flip off the red cap on the vial of RENOGEN lyophilized culture.
2. Using the hypodermic syringe provided, puncture the rubber septum of the RENOGEN vial and withdraw 2 cc of air from the vial into the syringe. Evacuate the syringe.
3. Using the hypodermic syringe provided, withdraw 2 cc of sterile diluent from the addition port of the diluent bag.
4. Inject the withdrawn sterile diluent into the vial of RENOGEN and shake the vial until the culture is completely dissolved and resuspended in the diluent.

B. Final formulation of ready-to-use RENOGEN vaccine

1. Insert the hypodermic syringe into the vial of resuspended RENOGEN, invert the vial, and withdraw all of the culture into the syringe.
2. Inject the contents of the syringe into the diluent bag through the addition port. Shake the bag well to ensure complete mixing of the components.
3. Discard the hypodermic syringe in a secure manner to prevent injury. Do not reuse.
4. Remove the product transfer kit from its sterile package. Tear the tab from the spike port of the diluent bag and insert the spike of the transfer kit into the port.
5. Attach the opposite end of the transfer kit to the injection gun.

Dosage and Administration: To use, fish are anaesthetized until immobilized, and are then injected with 0.1 mL of the vaccine intra-peritoneally along the midline, one fin length ahead of the pelvic fins.

Additional Information: Due to the relationship between water temperature and onset of immunity, it is recommended that a minimum period of 400 degree days (number of days multiplied by the mean water temperature for each day in °C during period) is allowed before exposure to disease occurs.

Precaution(s): Use entire contents within 4 hours of resuspension of the culture. Shake well before using.

Store package at 2-7°C (35-45°F). Protect from light. Do not freeze.

Live microorganism. Any unused vaccine, used containers, and hypodermic syringes should be disposed of by burning.

Caution(s): Vaccinate healthy fish only.

It is recommended that antimicrobial drugs not be administered 14 days before or after vaccination. It is recommended that oxytetracycline not be administered 6 weeks before or after vaccination.

Diagnostic kits which employ the use of polyclonal antiserum against *Renibacterium salmoninarum* should not be used to screen fish vaccinated with this product for at least 4 weeks after vaccination, since kidney samples from vaccinated fish will yield positive test results.

If accidental injection of the operator occurs, the operator should discontinue activity immediately and seek medical advice immediately.

For veterinary use only.

Warning(s): Do not vaccinate within 60 days of slaughter.

Presentation: One (1) 5 cc glass vial of lyophilized culture, one (1) intravenous bag containing 1,000 mL of sterile diluent, and one (1) 3 cc sterile hypodermic syringe.

Produced For: Mr. J. Zinn., Aqua Health USA Inc., Buhl, Idaho 83316

Compendium Code No.: 14970121 L-33-1 / L-34-1

R

REN-O-SAL® TABLETS

Fort Dodge **Water Medication**

Active Ingredient(s):

Roxarsone (3-nitro-4-hydroxyphenylarsonic acid) . . . . 36 mg

Inactive ingredients: Ammonium and sodium phenolsulfonates and boric acid.

Indications: For increased rate of weight gain, improved feed efficiency and improved pigmentation for growing chickens and growing turkeys. An aid in preventing coccidiosis due to *Eimeria tenella* in flocks of chickens during growing period.

Dosage and Administration:

For increased rate of weight gain, improved feed efficiency and improved pigmentation for growing chickens and growing turkeys: Dissolve 2 tablets in every U.S. gallon (3.8 liters) of drinking water and stir well. Prepare fresh solution at time of use. Do not prepare solutions in galvanized or rusty containers as a loss of product potency may occur. This mixture provides 0.002% roxarsone in water. Give continuously through growing period.

As an aid in preventing coccidiosis due to *Eimeria tenella* in flocks of growing chickens: Dissolve 8 tablets in every U.S. gallon (3.8 liters) of drinking water and give for not more than 10 consecutive days. Prepare fresh solution at time of use. Do not prepare solutions in galvanized or rusty containers as a loss of product potency may occur. This mixture provides 0.008% roxarsone in water. May be repeated after 5 days off medication.

Precaution(s): Store in a dry place. Keep closed.

Caution(s): Keep out of reach of children.

In case of coccidiosis, chickens must consume enough medicated water to provide a therapeutic dose. Poultry should have access to drinking water at all times. Overdosage or the lack of water intake may result in weakness or paralysis of the legs.

Use as the sole source of organic arsenic.

Poison-Arsenic.

Hazardous. Not for human use.

Antidote(s): If swallowed, call a physician, poison control center, or hospital immediately. Induce vomiting by giving Ipecac Syrup as directed.

Warning(s): Withdraw 5 days before slaughter.

Presentation: 100 tablets (NDC 53501-047-01), 250 tablets (NDC 53501-047-02), 1,000 tablets (NDC 53501-047-03) and 10,000 tablets (NDC 53501-047-04).

Compendium Code No.: 10031831 12485A

REOGUARD L

Merial Select **Vaccine**

Tenosynovitis Vaccine, Modified Live Virus

U.S. Vet. Lic. No.: 279

Contents: This product contains the mild 1133 strain of avian reovirus.

Contains Streptomycin Sulfate and Penicillin as bacteriostatic agents and Amphotericin B as a fungistatic agent.

Notice: Merial Select's vaccines have met the requirements of the USDA in regard to safety, purity, potency, and the capability to protect susceptible chickens. This vaccine has been tested by the Master Seed immunogenicity test for efficacy.

Indications: It is recommended for the vaccination of healthy chickens two weeks of age or older by drinking water as an aid in the prevention of tenosynovitis (viral arthritis).

This vaccine is recommended for the protection of healthy chickens. It is essential that the chickens be maintained under good environmental conditions and that exposure to disease viruses be reduced as much as possible.

Dosage and Administration: Read fully directions carefully.

Drinking Water Vaccination Using Pouring Application: Drinking water vaccination is recommended for healthy chickens two weeks of age or older.

1. Remove all medications, sanitizers and disinfectants from the drinking water 72 hours (three days) prior to vaccination.
2. Provide sufficient waterers so that all the chickens can drink at one time. Shut off water supply and allow chickens to consume all the water in the lines.
3. Raise water lines above the chickens' heads. Clean and rinse the waterers thoroughly.
4. Withhold all water from the chickens for a minimum of two hours in warm weather to four hours in cool weather prior to vaccination to stimulate thirst. Withdrawal time should be reduced if half-house brooding is in process.
5. Do not open or mix vaccine until ready to vaccinate.
6. Drinking water for vaccine delivery should contain one ounce (29 gram) of non-fat dry milk per gallon (3.8 liters) of non-chlorinated water, or should contain milk product based stabilizer prepared according to the manufacturer's instructions.
7. Reconstitute the vaccine in 3 gallons (11 liters) of milk-water during cool weather or 4 gallons (15 liters) of milk-water during warm weather for each 1,000 doses.
8. Distribute vaccine solution among waterers. Avoid direct sunlight.
9. Lower waterers and allow the chickens to drink freely. Add the remaining vaccine solution to the water lines as the chickens drink.
10. Do not provide additional drinking water until all the vaccine is consumed.

Drinking Water Vaccination Using Proportioner Application: Drinking water vaccination is recommended for healthy chickens seven two weeks of age or older. Set proportioner to deliver one ounce (30 mL) of vaccine concentrate per one gallon (3.8 liters) of water.

1. Remove all medications. sanitizers and disinfectants from the drinking water 72 hours (three days) prior to vaccination.
2. Clean all containers, hoses and waterers prior to vaccination.
3. Withhold all water from the chickens for a minimum of two hours in warm weather to four hours in cool weather prior to vaccination to stimulate thirst. Withdrawal time should be reduced if halfhouse brooding is in process.
4. Do not open or mix vaccine until ready to vaccinate.
5. Calculate to supply vaccine solution at a rate of 3 gallons (11 liters) per 1,000 chickens in cool weather and 4 gallons (15 liters) per 1,000 chickens in warm weather. The age of the chickens should be considered when calculating water supply. Always use non-chlorinated water when vaccinating chickens.
   Example:
   5,000 chickens in cool weather x 3 gallons (11 liters) = 15 gallons (55 liters).
   5,000 chickens in warm weather x 4 gallons (15 liters) = 20 gallons (75 liters).
6. Prepare vaccine stock solution as follows:
   a. Determine the quantity of vaccine concentrate required by multiplying one ounce (30 mL) x gallons of water needed for vaccine/drinking water.
      Example:
      For 5,000 chickens: 15 gallons x 1 ounce (30 mL) = 15 ounces (450 mL).
   b. Add 3 ounces (85 gm) of non-fat dry milk per 16 ounces (480 mL) of cool water, or use a commercial milk product based stabilizer according to the manufacturer's instructions. For 5,000 chickens add 2.5 ounces (75 gm) non-fat dry milk to the 15 ounces (450 mL) of water.
   c. Reconstitute the dried vaccine with the milk solution. Rinse the vaccine vial to remove all the vaccine.
7. Insert proportioner hose into the vaccine stock solution and start water flow. Continue until all solution has been consumed before changing water supply to direct flow.
8. Do not medicate or use disinfectants for 24 hours after vaccination.

Precaution(s): Store vaccine at 35-45°F (2-7°C). Do not freeze. Use entire vial contents when first opened. Burn the container and all unused contents.

This vaccine is non-returnable.

Caution(s): Do not vaccinate diseased chickens.

Vaccinate all chickens on the premises at one time.

Administer a minimum of one dose per chicken.

Avoid stress conditions during and following vaccination.

Do not place chickens in contaminated facilities.

Exposure to disease must be minimized as much as possible.

For veterinary use only.

The capability of this vaccine to produce satisfactory results depends upon many factors, including — but not limited to — conditions of storage and handling by the user, administration of the vaccine, health and responsiveness of individual chickens, and degree of field exposure. Therefore, directions for use should be followed carefully. The use of this vaccine is subject to applicable state and federal laws and regulations.

Warning(s): Do not vaccinate within 21 days of slaughter.

Presentation: Supplied in 5000 dose vials, 10 vials per pack.

Compendium Code No.: 11050421 5M 0699

REOMUNE® 2

Biomune **Vaccine**

Avian Reovirus Vaccine, Killed Virus

U.S. Vet. Lic. No.: 368

Contents: This vaccine contains antigenic viruses which are inactivated and suspended in an oil emulsion.

Contains gentamicin and amphotericin B as preservatives.

Indications: The vaccine is indicated for use in chickens against disease caused by avian reovirus. Breeder vaccination provides maternal antibody to progeny of breeder hens for the prevention of tenosynovitis and malabsorption caused by reovirus.

A prime with live tenosynovitis vaccine is recommended at least four weeks in advance of administration of the killed vaccine.

Dosage and Administration: Vaccinate chickens at least 18 weeks of age with 0.5 mL (½ cc) per bird. The vaccine is to be administered by the subcutaneous route in the back of the neck, midway between the head and the body, in a direction away from the head. Do not inject into muscle or vertebrae.

Precaution(s): Do not freeze. Store in the dark at 35°-45°F (2°-7°C). Warm to room temperature and shake before using and during use. Use entire contents when first opened.

This product is non-returnable.

Caution(s): Notice: This vaccine has undergone rigid potency, safety and purity tests, and meets Biomune and USDA requirements. However, the user is advised that response to vaccination depends on numerous factors, including, but not limited to, storage, handling, aseptic administration technique, and the health and responsiveness of individual chickens.

Due to the stress of handling or moving birds, vaccination of hens in lay may result in a drop in egg production.

This vaccine should be stored, transported and administered in accordance with the instructions and directions.

For veterinary use only.

Warning(s): Do not vaccinate within 42 days before slaughter.

This product contains an oil based adjuvant; accidental injection of this vaccine into a human may cause a serious localized reaction. Seek expert medical attention immediately.

Presentation: 1,000 dose (500 mL) bottle.

Compendium Code No.: 11290440 May 3, 1999

REOMUNE® 3

Biomune **Vaccine**

Avian Reovirus Vaccine, Standard and SS412 Types, Killed Virus

U.S. Vet. Lic. No.: 368

Contents: REOMUNE® 3 is an inactivated oil emulsion vaccine containing three avian reoviruses including strain S1133 (a tenosynovitis pathotype), strain 2408 (a malabsorption pathotype) and strain SS412 (a distinct serotype from the S1133 standard type reoviruses and a causative agent of proventriculitis and malabsorption in broilers). All reoviruses contained in REOMUNE® 3 are of chicken embryo origin.

The vaccine has undergone rigid potency, safety and purity tests and meets Biomune and USDA requirements.

Indications: The vaccine is indicated for use in healthy replacement chickens and breeder hens against diseases caused by avian reoviruses. Breeder vaccination provides maternal antibody to the progeny for the prevention of early exposure to tenosynovitis (viral arthritis) and malabsorption which includes feed passage and proventriculitis.

Dosage and Administration: A prime with live infectious tenosynovitis vaccine is recommended at least four (4) weeks in advance of administration of the killed vaccine.

Vaccinate chickens with 0.5 mL per bird. The vaccine is to be administered by the subcutaneous route in the back of the neck, midway between the head and the body, in a direction away from the head. Do not inject into muscle or vertebrae.

Refer to the product label for specific use directions and precautions.

Precaution(s): Store the vaccine at 35°-45°F (2°-7°C). Do not freeze.

Warning(s): Do not vaccinate with oil emulsion vaccine within 42 days before slaughter.

Avoid injection of the vaccine into a human. Should accidental injection of a human occur, seek medical attention immediately since a serious localized reaction may result.

Presentation: 1,000 dose (500 mL) bottle.

Compendium Code No.: 11290272

REOMUNE® SS412

Biomune **Vaccine**

Avian Reovirus Vaccine, Killed Virus

U.S. Vet. Lic. No.: 368

Contents: This vaccine contains reovirus SS412 type which is inactivated and suspended in an oil emulsion.

Indications: The vaccine is indicated for use in healthy breeder replacement chickens and breeder hens against malabsorption caused by avian reovirus of the SS412 type. Breeder vaccination provides maternal antibody to progeny of breeder hens for the prevention of malabsorption caused by early exposure to reovirus SS412 type.

A prime of tenosynovitis vaccine is recommended at least four weeks in advance of administration of the killed vaccine.

Dosage and Administration: Vaccinate chickens at least 18 weeks of age with 0.5 mL (½ cc) per bird. The vaccine is to be administered by the subcutaneous route in the back of the neck, midway between the head and the body, in a direction away from the head. Do not inject into muscle or vertebrae.

Precaution(s): Do not freeze. Store in the dark at 35°-45°F (2°-7°C). Warm to room temperature and shake before using and during use. Use entire contents when first opened.

This product is non-returnable.

Caution(s): Notice: This vaccine has undergone rigid potency, safety and purity tests, and meets Biomune and USDA requirements. However, the user is advised that response to vaccination depends on numerous factors, including, but not limited to, storage, handling, aseptic administration technique, and the health and responsiveness of individual chickens.

This vaccine should be stored, transported and administered in accordance with the instructions and directions.

For veterinary use only.

Warning(s): Do not vaccinate with oil emulsion vaccine within 42 days before slaughter. Due to the stress of handling or moving birds, vaccination of hens in lay may result in a drop in egg production.

This product contains an oil based adjuvant; accidental injection of this vaccine into a human may cause a serious localized reaction. Seek expert medical attention immediately.

Presentation: 1,000 dose (500 mL) bottle.

Compendium Code No.: 11290450 March 2, 2000

REPEL-X® INSECTICIDE & REPELLENT

Farnam **Parasiticide-Topical**

EPA Reg. No.: 270-294

Active Ingredient(s):

Pyrethrins	0.05%
Piperonyl Butoxide*, Technical	0.50%
Permethrin**	0.10%
Inert Ingredients	99.35%
Total	100.00%

*Equivalent to 0.4% (butylcarbityl) (6-propylpiperonyl) ether and 0.1% of related compounds.

**(3-phenoxyphenyl) methyl (±) cis/trans 3-(2,2-dichloroethenyl) 2,2-dimethyl cyclopropane carboxylate.

cis/trans ratio: min. 35% (±) cis and max. 65% (±) trans.

Indications: Ready to use insecticide and repellent for use on horses and their premises. Kills and repels six fly species, ticks, gnats, mosquitoes.

Directions for Use: It is a violation of Federal law to use this product in a manner inconsistent with labeling.

Use: For horses use full strength. This non-oily insecticide repellent may be applied with a trigger spray applicator or as a wipe. Kills and repels horse flies, stable flies, horn flies, house flies, face flies, deer flies, mosquitoes, fleas chiggers, gnats, lice and ticks.

Directions for Wipe-On Use: Thoroughly brush horse to remove excess dirt and dust. Extremely dirty horses should be shampooed, rinsed and allowed to dry before applying wipe. Use a sponge or clean soft cloth or mitt. Apply liberally over areas to be protected. Pay special attention to legs, belly, shoulders, neck, and facial areas. Avoid eyes and mucous membranes.

Directions for Trigger Spray Use: Remove excess dirt and dust. Apply light spray mist to coat while brushing lightly against lay of the hair. Avoid spray in eyes and mucous membranes. Apply with sponge or cloth to those areas.

To Kill and Repel Flying Insects in Animal Quarters: Spray in areas where insects congregate. Direct spray to contact insects for rapid knockdown and kill. Spray around outside of door facings and screen to render area unattractive to insects. This helps to repel insects and prevent entrance into building.

Precautionary Statements: Hazards to Humans and Domestic Animals:

Caution: For animal use only. Not for use on humans. Harmful if swallowed, inhaled, or absorbed through skin. Avoid breathing spray mist. Avoid contact with eyes, skin or clothing. Wash thoroughly with soap and water after handling. Remove contaminated clothing and wash before reuse.

First Aid:

If Swallowed: Drink 1 or 2 glasses of water and induce vomiting by touching back of throat with finger. Repeat until vomit fluid is clear. Do not induce vomiting or give anything by mouth to an unconscious person. Call a physician or Poison Control Center immediately.

If Inhaled: Remove affected person to fresh air. Apply artificial respiration if indicated. Get medical attention if irritation persists.

If in Eyes: Immediately flush eyes with plenty of water. Get medical attention if irritation persists.

If on Skin: Remove contaminated clothing and wash affected areas with soap and water. Get medical attention if irritation persists.

Environmental Hazards: This product is toxic to fish. Do not apply directly to water. Do not contaminate water when disposing of equipment washwaters.

Physical and Chemical Hazards: Do not use this product in or on electrical equipment due to the possibility of shock hazard.

Storage and Disposal:

Storage: Store in a cool, dry place. Do not store near heat or open flame.

Disposal: Securely wrap original container in several layers of newspaper and discard in trash.

Container Disposal: Do not use empty container. Wrap container and put in trash.

Warning(s): Keep out of reach of children.

Disclaimer: Buyer assumes all risk of use, storage or handling of this product not in strict accordance with directions given herein.

Presentation: 32 fl oz (.946 L) refill and sprayer and 1 gallon.

Compendium Code No.: 10000291

REPEL-X® LOTION

Farnam **Insect Repellent**

EPA Reg. No.: 270-253

Active Ingredient(s):

Cypermethrin [(±)-a-cyano-(3-phenoxyphenyl) methyl (±)cis, trans, 3-(2,2-dichloroethenyl)-2,2-dimethylcyclopropanecarboxylate]	0.15%
Pyrethrins	0.20%
Piperonyl Butoxide Technical*	1.63%
Di-n-propyl isocinchomeronate	0.50%
Butoxy Polypropylene Glycol	4.85%
Inert Ingredients:**	92.67%

*Equivalent to 1.30% (butylcarbityl) (6-propylpiperonyl) ether and 0.33% of related compounds. **Contains Petroleum Distillates.

Indications: Fly repellent for horses and ponies.

Directions for Use: It is a violation of Federal law to use this product in a manner inconsistent with its labeling.

To protect horses from House Flies, Face Flies, Horn Flies, Stable Flies, Black Flies, Horse Flies, Deer Flies, Lice and Ticks, and from biting gnats such as Punkies and No-see-ums. Thoroughly brush the horse's coat prior to application to remove loose dirt and debris. For best results, shampoo and rinse, wait until coat is completely dry and apply REPEL-X® Lotion. Using protective gloves or mitt, apply a light film to spot treat areas of the horse where flies gather. May be applied around superficial wounds and abrasions. Avoid direct application to eyes, nose and mouth.

Repeat application as necessary but no more often than once every 5 to 7 days. Wash hands with soap and water after use.

Precautionary Statements: Hazards to Humans and Domestic Animals:

Caution: For animal use only. Not for use on humans. Harmful if absorbed through skin or inhaled. Contact with this product may cause transitory tingling sensation. Avoid contact with skin, eyes or clothing. Avoid breathing vapors. Wash thoroughly with soap and water after handling. Remove contaminated clothing and wash before reuse.

Statement of Practical Treatment:

If on Skin: Wash with plenty of soap and water. Get medical attention.

If Inhaled: Remove victim to fresh air. If not breathing, give artificial respiration, preferably mouth-to-mouth. Get medical attention.

If in Eyes: Flush with plenty of water. Call a physician if irritation persists.

If Swallowed: Call a physician or Poison Control Center. Drink 1 or 2 glasses of water and induce vomiting by touching back of throat with finger. Do not induce vomiting or give anything by mouth to an unconscious person.

Environmental Hazards: This product is toxic to fish. Do not apply directly to water. Do not contaminate water when disposing of equipment washwaters.

Storage and Disposal: Do not contaminate water, food or feed by storage or disposal.

Storage: Store in a cool, dry place inaccessible to children and pets.

Disposal: Securely wrap original container in several layers of newspaper and discard in trash.

Warning(s): Not for use on horses intended for human consumption.

Keep out of reach of children.

Presentation: 8 fl oz (240 mL).

Compendium Code No.: 10000301

REPEL-X®p EMULSIFIABLE FLY SPRAY

Farnam **Parasiticide-Topical**

EPA Reg. No.: 270-150

Active Ingredient(s):

Pyrethrins	0.40%
*Piperonyl Butoxide, Technical	1.00%
Inert Ingredients	98.60%
	100.00%

Contains petroleum distillate.

* Equivalent to 0.8% (butylcarbityl) (6-propylpiperonyl) ether and 0.20% of related compounds.

Indications: REPEL-X®p Emulsifiable Fly Spray provides economical fly protection for horses and ponies. Repels and kills horn, house, stable, horse, and deer flies (tabanids), gnats, mosquitoes and ticks - including deer ticks which may transmit Lyme Disease.

Directions for Use: It is a violation of Federal law to use this product in a manner inconsistent with its labeling.

For use only on horses and ponies.

Shake well before using.

Mix REPEL-X®p Emulsifiable Fly Spray with water at proper dilution. First put the required amount into sprayer or mixing container. Then add water according to directions and mix thoroughly before using.

Important: Mix fresh solution before each use. Apply with pressure sprayer or you can sponge it on horses. Make sure animal's coat is thoroughly wet. Use approximately 8 oz. for each animal depending on size of horse or pony. Avoid getting solution into the animal's eyes.

Horses: To protect horses from horn flies, house flies, gnats and mosquitoes apply at a 1 to 7 dilution. Each pint of concentrate makes a gallon of finished spray. Repeat application every 3 to 4 days, or as often as needed. Where horse flies, deer flies (tabanids), stable flies, ticks, or Deer Ticks, that may transmit Lyme Disease, are a problem, apply a 1 to 4 dilution and repeat as often as needed.

(After long-standing non-use, mix contents by inverting several times.)

Precautionary Statements: Hazards to Humans and Domestic Animals:

Caution: For animal use only. Not for use on humans. Harmful if swallowed. Avoid contamination of food and feeds.

Statement of Practical Treatment:

If Swallowed: Do not induce vomiting due to aspiration hazard. Contains petroleum distillate. Contact a physician or Poison Control Center immediately.

If on Skin: Wash with plenty of soap and water.

If in Eyes: Immediately flush eyes with plenty of water. Consult a physician if irritation persists.

Environmental Hazards: This product is toxic to fish. Keep out of lakes, streams or ponds. Do not contaminate water when disposing of equipment washwaters.

Physical Hazards: Do not use or store near heat or open flame.

Storage and Disposal:

Storage: Store in a cool, dry place inaccessible to children and pets.

Disposal: Do not reuse empty container. Wrap container and put in trash.

Warning(s): Do not use on horses intended for human consumption.

Keep out of reach of children.

Presentation: 16 fl oz, 32 fl oz and 128 fl oz (3.785 L).

Compendium Code No.: 10000311

ReproCHEK™

Synbiotics **Pregnancy Test**

Canine Pregnancy Test Kit

U.S. Vet. Lic. No.: 312

Kit Contents:

Antibody Coated Wells	48 wells
Bottle A - Conjugate Diluent	2.5 mL
Bottle B - Conjugate	2.5 mL
Bottle C - Negative Control	1.5 mL
Bottle D - Positive Control	1.5 mL
Bottle E - 10X Wash Solution	100 mL
Bottle F - Chromogenic Substrate	10 mL

Microwell Holder

50 µL pipet; disposable pipet tips

Additional material required:

Deionized or distilled water

Squirt bottles (2); Timer

Optional: Microwell plate reader

Indications: For the detection of the canine hormone relaxin.

Test Principles: The ReproCHEK™ test kit is a microwell immunoassay for determining pregnancy in dogs. The plastic wells are coated with polyclonal anti-relaxin antibodies. A second antibody, highly specific to relaxin, is labeled with the enzyme horseradish peroxidase (HRP). The sample to be tested is placed directly into the coated well containing diluted HRP-antibody conjugate. Relaxin present in the sample will bind to the well and the HRP-antibody conjugate at the same time. The free HRP-antibody conjugate is washed away and a chromogenic substrate is added. The development of a blue color greater than the blue color of the negative control indicates the presence of relaxin in the sample. Absence of color indicates no relaxin in the sample.

ReproCHEK™ test results can be obtained in 15 minutes. The test kit contains a Positive Control and a Negative Control which must be included each time the test is performed. Visual comparison of the color of sample to the Negative Control will allow accurate detection of the presence of relaxin in the sample. If desired, test results may be determined by the use of a microwell plate reader.

Test Procedure:

Sample Information: 50 µL of plasma or whole blood is required. Serum and EDTA anti-coagulated samples must not be used. Samples may be stored at 2°-7°C up to 48 hours. Plasma samples may be kept frozen for longer storage. Severely hemolyzed or lipemic samples may produce background color. When in doubt, obtain a better quality sample.

Preparation of Wash Solution: Allow 10X Wash Concentrate to come to room temperature. Mix gently by inversion. Dilute wash concentrate 10-fold (1 part concentrate to 9 parts distilled water), mix and place in a wash bottle.

A. Preparation:

1. Calculate required number of wells:

- 1 well for Negative Control
- 1 well for Positive Control
- 1 well for each sample

Note: No more than 10 samples should be tested at one time.

Remove required number of wells.

Leave wells attached to each other.

Place wells in well holder.

Note: If a microwell plate reader will be used to read the results, leave the appropriate space empty so that the plate reader will blank on air.

B. Conjugate:

2. Add 1 drop Reagent A - Conjugate Diluent (White Cap) into each well.

Add 1 drop Reagent B - Conjugate (Blue Cap) into each well.

C. Sample Addition:

3. Controls

Add 2 drops Bottle C - Negative Control (Grey Cap) into the first well.

Add 2 drops Bottle D - Positive Control (Red Cap) into the second well.

Samples

Add 50 µL of sample into the next well following the controls.

For each additional sample, add 50 µL to subsequent wells. Use a separate pipette tip for each sample.

Wait 10 minutes. (Tap side of well holder for the first 15 seconds of the 10 minute incubation period. Be careful not to splash reagents.)

D. Blot and Wash:

4. Discard fluid from wells into sink or appropriate container.

Invert holder and blot firmly onto a paper towel to remove final drops.

5. Flush wells vigorously.

Wash by vigorously filling the wells to overflowing with diluted wash solution (See Section Preparation of Wash Solution for preparation).

Direct a forceful stream into each well. (Oversplashing will not contaminate adjacent wells).

Shake out excess wash solution.

Repeat wash cycle 5 times. Wash wells 2 more times with distilled or deionized water to remove bubbles.

Blot against a paper towel to dry wells.

E. Develop:

6. Add 3 drops of Bottle F - Chromogenic Substrate (Green Cap) into each well.

Wait 5 minutes. (Tap side of well holder for the first 15 seconds of the 5 minute incubation period. Be careful not to splash reagents.)

Read results at exactly 5 minutes.

Interpretation of Results:

A. Controls—For a valid test, the Positive Control must produce a distinct blue color and the Negative Control should be clear to light blue in color. If color does not develop in the Positive Control well or if there is distinct blue color development in the Negative Control well, results are invalid and the test should be repeated.

Evaluation of Test Wells in a valid test—Samples producing distinct blue color are Positive for relaxin.

Samples producing no color or blue color of less intensity than the blue color of the Negative Control are Negative for relaxin.

After the test is completed, the sample well can be detached and held alongside the Negative Control well against a white background for easier visual inspection.

If desired, results may be read on a microwell plate reader using an air blank. For single wavelength readers, set the wavelength of the plate reader at 630 nm. For plate readers with dual wavelength capability, set the test wavelength at 630 nm and reference wavelength at 450 nm or 490 nm. Samples producing at Optical Density equal to or less than the optical density of the Negative Control are Negative for relaxin. Samples producing an optical density greater than the optical density of the Negative Control are Positive for relaxin.

Controls:

Negative Control should be clear to light blue color.

Positive Control should be distinctly blue.

Note: If controls appear different than above the test is invalid and must be repeated.

Samples:

Positive samples will produce blue color darker than the color of the Negative Control. When read on a plate reader, Positive samples will produce an optical density greater than the optical density of the Negative Control (see "Evaluation of Test Wells").

Negative samples will produce no color or blue color of less intensity then the blue color of the Negative Control. When read on a plate reader, Negative samples will produce an optical density equal to or less than the optical density of the Negative Control (see "Evaluation of Test Wells").

Good Techniques:

Kit Positive and Negative Controls must be performed in each test to ensure accurate interpretation of sample results.

Plasma or anticoagulated whole blood may be used as a sample; however do not use serum or EDTA anticoagulated samples.

Hemolyzed and lipemic samples may be used; however, severely hemolyzed and/or lipemic samples may produce blue background color. When in doubt, obtain a better quality sample.

Washing is a very important step. Microwells cannot be overwashed. Underwashing may result in non-specific blue color development in the negative control and sample wells.

Prolonged incubation for more than 5 minutes in Step 6 may result in non-specific color development.

Do not use the test kit past the expiration date and do not intermix components from different serial numbers.

Storage and Stability: Store the test kit and unused diluted wash solution at 2°-7°C (36°-45°F). Do not freeze. Reagents are stable until expiration date provided they have been stored properly.

Allow kit to come to room temperature before use.

Caution(s):

1. Allow kit to come to room temperature (21°-25°C; 70°-78°F) prior to use.
2. Use separate pipet tip for each sample.
3. It is not recommended to test more than 10 samples per run.
4. Do not expose kit to direct sunlight.
5. Do not use expired reagents or mix from different kit lots.
6. Follow instructions exactly. Improper washing or contamination of reagents may produce nonspecific color development.
7. For veterinary use only.

Discussion: Synbiotics' ReproCHEK™ Canine Pregnancy Test Kit uses highly purified and specific antibodies to detect the presence of the hormone relaxin in canine whole blood or plasma. The presence of significant amounts of relaxin indicates pregnancy. The ReproCHEK™ test offers an early, inexpensive and reliable means of determining the success or failure of a planned mating or unwanted exposure. The ReproCHEK™ test may also be used to detect a sudden decrease in relaxin levels to indicate that spontaneous abortion has occurred.

How soon can ReproCHEK™ detect pregnancy in the bitch? Research confirms that relaxin rises to detectable levels as a result of fertilized egg implantation. Implantation occurs in the normal bitch, assuming fertilization has occurred, 26-31 days after the LH surge. This window is due to biological variables such as ova maturation and time of fertilization. The canine fertile period is commonly accepted as 4-7 days after the LH surge. Because of varied breeding strategies and different "counting" methods used to determine whelping dates, there is potential for confusion when the reference point is the date(s) of breeding. (These dates may or may not correspond to the bitch's actual estrous cycle/fertile period and the day that fertilization actually occurs.) In general, if the bitch was bred at the appropriate time in her estrous cycle, pregnancy can be determined 22-27 days post breeding (26-31 days post-LH surge).

In Figure A, the day of the last breeding is indicated as Day 0. Assuming that fertilization occurred on the day of the last breeding, implantation of the fertilized ovum and the corresponding increase in relaxin concentration to a detectable level would occur 22 to 27 days after the last breeding. In instances where early breeding occurred, testing 22 days post breeding would be too early (i.e., before implantation). Pregnancy is a possibility in early breeding as sperm cells can survive for a period of time in the uterus. In this instance retesting one week later (29 days post breeding) would provide sufficient time for a fertilized egg to implant resulting in the increase of relaxin concentration to a level detectable by the ReproCHEK™ test. If there is confusion or uncertainty regarding fertile periods and the timing of breeding, it is recommended that a negative test be confirmed 1 week following the first test (carried out 22-27 days post breeding) to ensure that sufficient time has passed for implantation of the fertilized egg to have occurred.

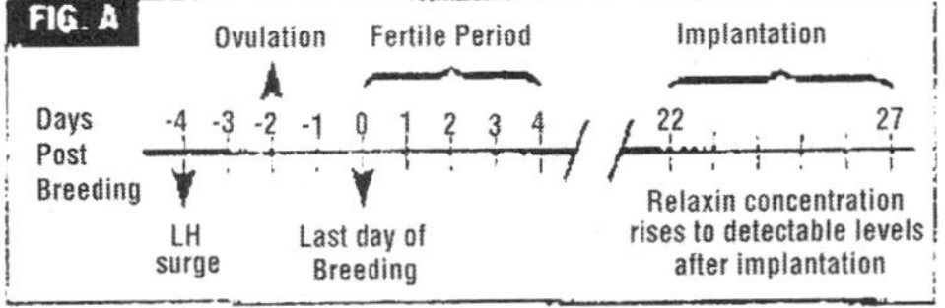

Presentation: 16-46 tests/kit.

Compendium Code No.: 11150380

REPROCYC® PRRS-PLE

Boehringer Ingelheim **Bacterin-Vaccine**

Porcine Reproductive and Respiratory Syndrome-Parvovirus Vaccine, Reproductive Form, Modified Live and Killed Virus-Erysipelothrix Rhusiopathiae-Leptospira Canicola-Grippotyphosa-Hardjo-Icterohaemorrhagiae- Pomona Bacterin

U.S. Vet. Lic. No.: 319

Contents: This product contains the antigens listed above.

Contains amphotericin B, neomycin, penicillin, streptomycin and thimerosal as preservatives.

Indications: Recommended for the vaccination of healthy, susceptible sows and gilts, as an aid in the reduction of disease associated with Porcine Reproductive and Respiratory Syndrome Virus, reproductive form, and as an aid in the prevention and control of disease caused by porcine parvovirus, *Erysipelothrix rhusiopathiae* and *Leptospira canicola-grippotyphosa-hardjo-ictero-haemorrhagiae-pomona*.

Dosage and Administration: Shake well and use immediately. Vaccinate healthy sows and gilts intramuscularly with a single 5 mL dose of REPROCYC® PRRS-PLE 4-6 weeks prior to breeding. Revaccinate with ReproCyc® PLE (parvovirus/*Leptospira*/erysipelas vaccine) 3-4 weeks following initial vaccination. Revaccinate with a single dose of REPROCYC® PRRS-PLE vaccine prior to subsequent breedings and only vaccinate gilts and sows in PRRS-positive herds.

Precaution(s): Store out of direct sunlight in the outer carton. Store at 35-45°F (2-7°C). Do not freeze. Use entire contents when first opened.

Caution(s): Anaphylactoid reactions may occur.

For veterinary use only.

Antidote(s): Administer epinephrine.

Warning(s): Do not vaccinate within 21 days before slaughter.

Presentation: 20 dose (100 mL) vials.

Compendium Code No.: 10280981 BIN 76-01-01-01 5/98

REPROMUNE™ 4

Biomune **Vaccine**

Bursal Disease-Newcastle Disease-Bronchitis-Reovirus Vaccine, Mass. Type, Killed Virus

U.S. Vet. Lic. No.: 368

Contents: REPROMUNE™ 4 is an inactivated oil emulsion vaccine containing infectious bursal disease virus, Newcastle disease virus, infectious bronchitis viruses of the Mass. serotype (Holland strain and Mass. M41) and two reoviruses strain S1133 (a tenosynovitis pathotype) and strain 2408 (a malabsorption pathotype).

Indications: The vaccine is indicated for use in healthy breeder replacement chickens and breeder hens against diseases caused by infectious bursal disease virus, Newcastle disease virus, infectious bronchitis virus and reovirus. Breeder vaccination provides maternal antibody to progeny of breeder hens for prevention of early exposure to bursal disease, tenosynovitis (viral arthritis) and malabsorption syndrome.

Dosage and Administration: Optimum results with REPROMUNE™ 4 require that chickens are adequately primed with live infectious bursal disease vaccine, tenosynovitis vaccine and bronchitis vaccine of the Mass. type at least four weeks in advance of administration of the inactivated vaccine.

Vaccinate chickens with 0.5 mL (½ cc) per bird. The vaccine is to be administered by the subcutaneous route in the back of the neck, midway between the head and the body and in a direction away from the head. Do not inject into muscle or vertebrae.

Precaution(s): Store the vaccine at 35°-45°F (2°-7°C). Do not freeze.

Caution(s): This vaccine has undergone rigid potency, safety and purity tests and meets Biomune and USDA requirements.

Warning(s): Do not vaccinate with oil emulsion vaccine within 42 days before slaughter. Avoid injection of this vaccine into a human. Should accidental injection of a human occur, seek expert medical attention immediately since a serious localized reaction may result.

Presentation: 1000 dose (500 mL) bottles.

Compendium Code No.: 11290281

REPROMUNE™ IBD

Biomune **Vaccine**

Bursal Disease Vaccine, Killed Virus

U.S. Vet. Lic. No.: 368

Contents: REPROMUNE™ IBD is an inactivated oil emulsion vaccine containing infectious bursal disease virus.

Indications: The vaccine is indicated for use in healthy replacement chickens and breeder hens against disease caused by infectious bursal disease virus. Breeder vaccination provides maternal antibody to progeny of breeder hens for prevention of early exposure to bursal disease.

Dosage and Administration: A prime with live infectious bursal disease vaccine is recommended at least four weeks in advance of administration of the inactivated vaccine.

Vaccinate chickens with 0.5 mL (½ cc) per bird. The vaccine is to be administered by the subcutaneous route in the back of the neck, midway between the head and the body and in a direction away from the head. Do not inject into muscle or vertebrae.

Precaution(s): Store the vaccine at 35°-45°F (2°-7°C). Do not freeze.

Caution(s): This vaccine has undergone rigid potency, safety and purity tests and meets Biomune and USDA requirements.

Warning(s): Do not vaccinate with oil emulsion vaccine within 42 days before slaughter. Avoid injection of this vaccine into a human. Should accidental injection of a human occur, seek expert medical attention immediately since a serious localized reaction may result.

Presentation: 1000 dose (500 mL) bottles.

Compendium Code No.: 11290321

REPROMUNE™ IBD/ND

Biomune **Vaccine**

Bursal Disease-Newcastle Disease Vaccine, Killed Virus

U.S. Vet. Lic. No.: 368

Contents: REPROMUNE™ IBD/ND is an inactivated oil emulsion vaccine containing Newcastle disease and infectious bursal disease viruses.

Indications: The vaccine is indicated for use in healthy replacement chickens and breeder hens against disease. Breeder vaccination provides maternal antibody to progeny of breeder hens for the prevention of early exposure to bursal disease.

Dosage and Administration: A prime with live infectious bursal disease vaccine is recommended at least four weeks in advance of administration of the inactivated vaccine.

Vaccinate chickens with 0.5 mL (½ cc) per bird. The vaccine is to be administered by the subcutaneous route in the back of the neck, midway between the head and the body and in a direction away from the head. Do not inject into muscle or vertebrae.

Precaution(s): Store the vaccine at 35°-45°F (2°-7°C). Do not freeze.

Caution(s): This vaccine has undergone rigid potency, safety and purity tests and meets Biomune and USDA requirements.

Warning(s): Do not vaccinate with oil emulsion vaccine within 42 days before slaughter. Avoid injection of this vaccine into a human. Should accidental injection of a human occur, seek expert medical attention immediately since a serious localized reaction may result.

Presentation: 1000 dose (500 mL) bottles.

Compendium Code No.: 11290301

REPROMUNE™ IBD/ND/IB

Biomune **Vaccine**

Bursal Disease-Newcastle Disease-Bronchitis Vaccine, Mass. Type, Killed Virus

U.S. Vet. Lic. No.: 368

Contents: REPROMUNE™ IBD/ND/IB is an inactivated oil emulsion vaccine containing bursal disease virus, Newcastle disease virus and two infectious bronchitis viruses of the Mass. serotype, (Holland strain and Mass. M41).

Indications: The vaccine is indicated for use in healthy chickens prior to the onset of egg production against diseases caused by infectious bursal disease virus, Newcastle disease virus and infectious bronchitis virus. One dose of REPROMUNE™ IBD/ND/IB provides uniform and high serological titers eliminating the need for use of live Newcastle-bronchitis vaccines during lay.

Dosage and Administration: Breeder vaccination provides maternal antibody to progeny for prevention of early exposure to bursal disease.

A prime with live infectious bursal disease vaccine and bronchitis vaccine of the Mass. type is recommended at least four weeks in advance of administration of the inactivated vaccine.

Revaccination during molt is recommended.

Vaccinate chickens with 0.5 mL (½ cc) per bird. The vaccine is to be administered by the subcutaneous route in the back of the neck, midway between the head and the body and in a direction away from the head. Do not inject into muscle or vertebrae.

Precaution(s): Store the vaccine at 35°-45°F (2°-7°C). Do not freeze.

Caution(s): This vaccine is thoroughly tested before sale and meets the requirements of Biomune and the U.S. Department of Agriculture.

Warning(s): Do not vaccinate with oil emulsion vaccine within 42 days before slaughter. Avoid injection of this vaccine into a human. Should accidental injection of a human occur, seek expert medical attention immediately since a serious localized reaction may result.

Presentation: 1000 dose (500 mL) bottles.

Compendium Code No.: 11290291

REPROMUNE IBD/ND/REO™

Biomune **Vaccine**

Bursal Disease-Newcastle Disease-Reovirus Vaccine, Killed Virus

U.S. Vet. Lic. No.: 368

Contents: This vaccine contains antigenic viruses which are inactivated and suspended in an oil emulsion.

Contains gentamicin and amphotericin B as preservatives.

Indications: The vaccine is indicated for use in breeder hens against diseases caused by Newcastle disease virus, infectious bursal disease virus and avian reovirus. Breeder vaccination provides maternal antibody to progeny of breeder hens for the prevention of bursal disease caused by infectious bursal disease virus and tenosynovitis and maladsorption caused by reovirus.

A prime with live infectious bursal disease vaccine and tenosynovitis vaccine is recommended at least four weeks in advance of administration of the killed vaccine.

Dosage and Administration: Vaccinate chickens at least 18 weeks of age with 0.5 mL (½ cc) per bird. The vaccine is to be administered by the subcutaneous route in the back of the neck, midway between the head and the body, in a direction away from the head. Do not inject into muscle or vertebrae.

Precaution(s): Do not freeze. Store in the dark at 35°-45°F (2°-7°C). Warm to room temperature and shake before using and during use. Use entire contents when first opened.

This product is non-returnable.

Caution(s): Notice: This vaccine has undergone rigid potency, safety and purity tests and meets Biomune and USDA requirements. However, the user is advised that response to vaccination depends on numerous factors, including, but not limited to, storage, handling, aseptic administration technique and the health and responsiveness of individual chickens.

Due to the stress of handling or moving birds, vaccination of hens in lay may result in a drop in egg production.

This vaccine should be stored, transported and administered in accordance with the instructions and directions.

For veterinary use only.

Warning(s): Do not vaccinate with oil emulsion vaccine within 42 days before slaughter.

This product contains an oil based adjuvant; accidental injection of this vaccine into a human may cause a serious localized reaction. Seek expert medical attention immediately.

Presentation: 1,000 dose (500 mL) bottle.

Compendium Code No.: 11290460 June 2, 1998

REPROMUNE™ IBD/REO

Biomune **Vaccine**

Bursal Disease-Reovirus Vaccine, Killed Virus

U.S. Vet. Lic. No.: 368

Contents: REPROMUNE™ IBD/REO is an inactivated oil emulsion vaccine containing infectious bursal disease virus and two reoviruses including strain S1133 (a tenosynovitis pathotype) and strain 2408 (a malabsorption pathotype).

All viruses in REPROMUNE™ IBD/REO are non-cloned isolates produced from SPF chicken eggs.

Indications: The vaccine is indicated for use in healthy breeder replacement chickens and breeder hens against diseases caused by infectious bursal disease and reoviruses. Breeder vaccination provides maternal antibody to progeny of breeder hens for the prevention of early exposure to bursal disease, tenosynovitis (viral arthritis) and malabsorption syndrome.

Dosage and Administration: Optimum results with REPROMUNE™ IBD/REO require that chickens are adequately primed with live infectious bursal disease vaccine and tenosynovitis vaccine at least four weeks in advance of administration of the inactivated vaccine.

Vaccinate chickens with 0.5 mL (½ cc) per bird. The vaccine is to be administered by the subcutaneous route in the back of the neck, midway between the head and the body, in a direction away from the head. Do not inject into muscle or vertebrae.

Precaution(s): Store the vaccine at 35°-45°F (2°-7°C). Do not freeze.

Caution(s): This vaccine has undergone rigid potency, safety and purity tests and meets Biomune and USDA requirements.

Warning(s): Do not vaccinate with oil-emulsion vaccine within 42 days before slaughter. Avoid injection of this vaccine into a human. Should accidental injection of a human occur, seek expert medical attention immediately since a serious localized reaction may result.

Presentation: 1,000 dose (500 mL) bottles.

Compendium Code No.: 11290311

RESICHLOR™ LEAVE-ON CONDITIONER ℞

Virbac **Antidermatosis Conditioner**

Active Ingredient(s): Chlorhexidine gluconate 2% in a luxuriant conditioning base containing water, cetyl alcohol, stearyl alcohol, stearalkonium chloride, dimethyl stearamine, lactic acid, tetrasodium EDTA, methylchloroisothiazolinone, methylisothiazolinone, fragrance, FD&C blue #1, FD&C yellow #5.

Indications: Specially formulated for dermatological conditions where an antifungal, antiseptic and antimicrobial conditioner may be beneficial.

Dosage and Administration: Shake well before using.

After shampooing (or wetting) the hair coat, apply an adequate amount to cover entire hair coat along back of animal. Massage well into the skin and hair coat. Apply more as needed. (Amount will vary according to size of animal and length of hair coat.) May be used in localized areas or between shampoos.

Precaution(s): Store at controlled room temperature 59°-86°F.

Caution(s): Federal Law (USA) restricts this drug to use by or on the order of a licensed veterinarian. For external use on dogs and cats only. Avoid contact with eyes or mucous membranes. Consult a veterinarian before using on debilitated animal. If condition persists, or no improvement in 21 days, consult your veterinarian. Wash hands and exposed skin after using.

Keep out of reach of children.

Presentation: 8 fl oz, 16 fl oz and 1 gallon (3.79 L).

Compendium Code No.: 10230490 250215-01

RESICORT® LEAVE-ON CONDITIONER ℞

Virbac **Topical Antipruritic**

NDC No.: 51311-072-08

Active Ingredient(s): Hydrocortisone 1% in a conditioning base containing water, sorbitan stearate, stearyl alcohol, sodium lauryl sulfate, cocphosphatidyl PG-Dimonium chloride, cetrimonium chloride, glycerin, dimethicone, triethanolamine, carbomer, cetyl alcohol, methylparaben, fragrance, DMDM hydantoin, FD & C yellow #5, FD & C red #40. May also contain citric acid.

Indications: Specifically formulated to relieve inflammation and pruritis associated with corticosteroid-responsive dermatoses.

Dosage and Administration: Shake well before using.

After shampooing (or wetting) the hair coat, apply an adequate amount to cover entire hair coat along back of animal. Massage well into the skin and hair coat. Apply more as needed. (Amount will vary according to size of animal and length of hair coat.) May be used in localized areas or between shampoos.

Precaution(s): Store at controlled room temperature 59°-86°F.

Caution(s): Federal law (USA) restricts this drug to use by or on the order of a licensed veterinarian. For external use on dogs and cats only. Avoid contact with eyes or mucous membranes. Consult a veterinarian before using on debilitated animal. If condition persists, or no improvement in 14 days, consult your veterinarian.

Warning(s): Keep out of the reach of children.

Presentation: 8 fl oz and 16 fl oz.

Compendium Code No.: 10230500

RESIHIST® LEAVE-ON CONDITIONER ℞

Virbac **Topical Antipruritic**

NDC No.: 51311-073-08

Active Ingredient(s): Diphenhydramine hydrochloride 2% in a conditioning base containing water, cetyl alcohol, stearyl alcohol, steryalkonium chloride, dimethyl stearamine, lactic acid, tetrasodium EDTA, DMDM hydantoin, fragrance, sodium hydroxide, D & C red #33.

Indications: Specifically formulated to provide temporary relief of itching associated with sensitive, allergic skin.

Dosage and Administration: Shake well before using.

After shampooing (or wetting) the hair coat, apply an adequate amount to cover entire hair coat along back of animal. Massage well into the skin and hair coat. Apply more as needed. (Amount will vary according to size of animal and length of hair coat.) May be used in localized areas or between shampoos.

Precaution(s): Store at controlled room temperature 59°-86°F.

Caution(s): Federal law (USA) restricts this drug to use by or on the order of a licensed veterinarian. For external use on dogs and cats only. Avoid contact with eyes or mucous membranes. Consult a veterinarian before using on debilitated animal. If condition persists, or no improvement in 7 days, consult your veterinarian.

Warning(s): Keep out of the reach of children.

Presentation: 8 fl oz and 16 fl oz.

Compendium Code No.: 10230510

RESIPROX™ LEAVE-ON CONDITIONER ℞

Virbac **Antidermatosis Conditioner**

Pramoxine HCl Leave-On Conditioner

Active Ingredient(s): Pramoxine HCl 1.5% in a conditioning base containing water, cetyl alcohol, stearyl alcohol, stearalkonium chloride, dimethyl stearamine, lactic acid, colloidal oatmeal, triethanolamine, hydroxyethylcellulose, dimethicone, DMDM hydantoin, fragrance, FD&C yellow #5.

Indications: RESIPROX™ Leave-On Conditioner is recommended to provide temporary relief of dry, itchy, irritated skin. For use on dogs and cats.

This product does not leave any oily or sticky residue on the hair coat.

Dosage and Administration: Shake well before using.

After shampooing (or wetting) the hair coat, apply an adequate amount to cover entire hair coat along back of animal. Massage well into the skin and hair coat. Apply more as needed. (Amount will vary according to size of animal and length of hair coat.) May be used in localized areas or between shampoos. Apply only to wet hair coat. May be used daily or as directed by veterinarian.

Precaution(s): Store at controlled room temperature 59°-86°F.

Caution(s): Federal Law (USA) restricts this drug to use by or on the order of a licensed veterinarian. For external use only on dogs and cats. Avoid contact with eyes and mucous membranes. Wash hands and exposed skin after using. If undue skin irritation develops or increases, discontinue use and consult a veterinarian.

Warning(s): Keep out of reach of children.

Presentation: 8 fl oz (237 mL).

Compendium Code No.: 10230520

RESISOOTHE® LEAVE-ON CONDITIONER

Virbac **Grooming Aid**

Active Ingredient(s): Colloidal oatmeal conditioning base containing water, cetyl alcohol, stearyl alcohol, steryalkonium chloride, dimethyl stearamine, glycerin, lactic acid, tetrasodium EDTA, DMDM hydantoin, sunflower oil, tocopherol, fragrance.

Indications: Specifically formulated to relieve dry, irritated, itchy skin. The unique formula imparts a high sheen to the hair coat and leaves it more manageable.

Dosage and Administration: Shake well before using.

After shampooing (or wetting) the hair coat, apply an adequate amount to cover entire hair coat along back of animal. Massage well into the skin and hair coat. Apply more as needed.

(Amount will vary according to size of animal and length of hair coat.) May be used in localized areas or between shampoos. Apply only to a wet hair coat.

Caution(s): For external use on dogs and cats only. Avoid contact with eyes or mucous membranes.

Warning(s): Keep out of the reach of children.

Presentation: 8 fl oz, 16 fl oz and 1 gallon.

Compendium Code No.: 10230530

RESIST™ 7

AgriPharm **Bacterin-Toxoid**

Clostridium Chauvoei-Septicum-Novyi-Sordellii-Perfringens Types C & D Bacterin- Toxoid

U.S. Vet. Lic. No.: 124

Composition: Prepared from cultures of the organisms listed. Alum precipitated.

Indications: Recommended for the vaccination of healthy, susceptible cattle and sheep against disease caused by *Clostridium chauvoei, Cl. septicum, Cl. novyi, Cl. sordellii* and *Cl. perfringens* Types C and D. Although *Clostridium perfringens* Type B is not a significant problem in the U.S.A., immunity may be provided against the beta and epsilon toxins elaborated by *Clostridium perfringens* Type B. This immunity is derived from the combination of Type C (beta) and Type D (epsilon) fractions.

Dosage and Administration:

Cattle: Using aseptic technique, inject 5 mL subcutaneously. Repeat in 21 to 28 days and once annually.

Sheep: Using aseptic technique, inject 2.5 mL subcutaneously. Repeat in 21 to 28 days and once annually.

Precaution(s): Store out of direct sunlight at a temperature between 35-45°F (2-7°). Avoid freezing. Shake well before using. Use entire contents when first opened.

Caution(s): Anaphylactoid reactions may occur.

Antidote(s): Administer epinephrine.

Warning(s): Do not vaccinate within 21 days before slaughter.

Animal inoculation only.

Presentation: 10 cattle doses or 20 sheep doses (50 mL), 50 cattle doses or 100 sheep doses (250 mL), and 200 cattle doses or 400 sheep doses (1,000 mL).

Manufactured by: Boehringer Ingelheim Vetmedica, Inc. St. Joseph, Missouri 64506, U.S.A.

Compendium Code No.: 14571240

RESIST™ 7HS

AgriPharm **Bacterin-Toxoid**

Clostridium Chauvoei-Septicum-Novyi-Sordellii-Perfringens Types C & D-Haemophilus Somnus Bacterin-Toxoid

U.S. Vet. Lic. No.: 124

Composition: Prepared from cultures of the organisms listed. Alum precipitated.

Indications: Recommended for the vaccination of healthy, susceptible cattle against diseases caused by *Clostridium chauvoei, Cl. septicum, Cl. novyi, Cl. sordellii, Cl. perfringens* Types C and D and *Haemophilus somnus.* Although *Clostridium perfringens* Type B is not a significant problem in the U.S.A., immunity may be provided against the beta and epsilon toxins elaborated by *Clostridium perfringens* Type B. This immunity is derived from the combination of Type C (beta) and Type D (epsilon) fractions.

Dosage and Administration: Using aseptic technique, inject 5 mL subcutaneously. Repeat in 21 to 28 days and once annually.

Precaution(s): Store out of direct sunlight at a temperature between 35-45°F (2-7°). Avoid freezing. Shake well before using. Use entire contents when first opened.

Caution(s): Transient swelling at the injection site may occur. Anaphylactoid reactions may occur.

Antidote(s): Administer epinephrine.

Warning(s): Do not vaccinate within 21 days before slaughter.

Animal inoculation only.

Presentation: 10 doses (50 mL), 50 doses (250 mL), and 200 doses (500 mL).

Manufactured by: Boehringer Ingelheim Vetmedica, Inc. St. Joseph, Missouri 64506, U.S.A.

Compendium Code No.: 14571260

RESIST™ 8

AgriPharm **Bacterin-Toxoid**

Clostridium Chauvoei-Septicum-Haemolyticum-Novyi-Sordellii-Perfringens Types C & D Bacterin-Toxoid

U.S. Vet. Lic. No.: 124

Composition: This product contains the antigens listed above.

Indications: Recommended for the vaccination of healthy, susceptible cattle and sheep against diseases caused by *Clostridium chauvoei, Cl. septicum, Cl. haemolyticum, Cl. novyi, Cl. sordellii* and *Cl. perfringens* Types C and D. Although *Clostridium perfringens* Type B is not a significant problem in the U.S.A., immunity may be provided against the beta and epsilon toxins elaborated by *Clostridium perfringens* Type B. This immunity is derived from the combination of Type C (beta) and Type D (epsilon) fractions.

Dosage and Administration:

Cattle: Using aseptic technique, inject 5 mL subcutaneously. Repeat in 21 to 28 days and once annually.

Sheep: Using aseptic technique, inject 2.5 mL subcutaneously. Repeat in 21 to 28 days and once annually.

Precaution(s): Store out of direct sunlight at a temperature between 35-45°F (2-7°C). Avoid freezing. Shake well before using. Use entire contents when first opened.

Caution(s): Anaphylactoid reactions may occur.

Antidote(s): Epinephrine.

Warning(s): Do not vaccinate within 21 days before slaughter.

Presentation: 10 cattle doses or 20 sheep doses (50 mL) and 50 cattle doses or 100 sheep doses (250 mL).

Manufactured by: Boehringer Ingelheim Vetmedica, Inc. St. Joseph, Missouri 64506, U.S.A.

Compendium Code No.: 14571250

RESIZOLE™ LEAVE-ON CONDITIONER ℞

Virbac **Antidermatosis Conditioner**

Miconazole 2% Leave-On Conditioner

Active Ingredient(s): Miconazole 2% in a conditioning base containing water, cetyl alcohol, stearyl alcohol, stearalkonium chloride, dimethyl stearamine, lactic acid, dimethicone, hydroxyethylcellulose, DMDM hydantoin, fragrance, FD&C blue #1, FD&C red #4.

Indications: RESIZOLE™ Leave-On Conditioner is recommended for dermatologic conditions responsive to miconazole in dogs and cats.

This product does not leave any oily or sticky residue on the hair coat.

Dosage and Administration: Shake well before using.

After shampooing (or wetting) the hair coat, apply an adequate amount to cover entire hair coat along back of animal. Massage well into the skin and hair coat. Apply more as needed. (Amount will vary according to size of animal and length of hair coat.) May be used in localized areas or between shampoos. Apply only to wet hair coat. May be used 2 or 3 times a week or as directed by veterinarian.

Precaution(s): Store at controlled room temperature 59°-86°F.

Caution(s): Federal Law (USA) restricts this drug to use by or on the order of a licensed veterinarian. For external use only on dogs and cats. Avoid contact with eyes and mucous membranes. Wash hands and exposed skin after using. If condition persists or undue skin irritation develops or increases, discontinue use and consult a veterinarian.

Warning(s): Keep out of reach of children.

Presentation: 8 fl oz (237 mL).

Compendium Code No.: 10230540

RESORB®

Pfizer Animal Health **Electrolytes-Oral**

Oral Hydration, Electrolyte Product

NADA No.: 125-961

Active Ingredient(s): RE-SORB® formula contains the following ingredients:

Sodium chloride	8.82 grams
Potassium phosphate	4.2 grams
Citric acid, anhydrous	0.5 grams
Potassium citrate	0.12 grams
Aminoacetic acid (glycine)	6.36 grams
Glucose	44 grams

Osmolarity of the reconstituted solution is approximately 315 mOsm/kg. The pH of the reconstituted solution is approximately 4.3.

Indications: RE-SORB® is a readily absorbed source of fluids and electrolytes. It is a convenient and effective means of increasing absorption of water, energy sources, and electrolytes. RE-SORB® is indicated for use in the control of dehydration associated with diarrhea (scours) in calves, including veal calves. RE-SORB® may be used by the livestock owner as an early treatment at the first signs of scouring. It may also be used as follow-up treatment for the dehydrated calf following intravenous fluid therapy.

RE-SORB®, because of its ready source of fluid and electrolytes, makes it an ideal first feed (upon arrival) for newly purchased or severely stressed calves.

Pharmacology: Action: Oral glucose/glycine compounds have been used with excellent success to treat dehydration accompanying human cholera for many years.[1-3] The rationale for oral rehydration therapy is based upon the active absorption of glucose and glycine when given orally to scouring animals. Their absorption is linked to the simultaneous absorption of sodium and water. This principle has been verified in scouring animals.[4]

E. coli produces scours by secreting toxins in the small intestine. These toxins, while causing profuse secretion of water and electrolytes, have no effect on glucose/glycine absorption in the calf.[5] When RE-SORB® is administered, the glucose/glycine along with the water and sodium are absorbed resulting in a net gain in water thereby correcting the dehydration.

In diarrhea caused by viruses, the disease process causes a flattening of the intestinal mucosa which reduces digestion and absorption of milk. The undigested milk passes into the colon where bacterial fermentation results in additional diarrhea.[6] The replacement of milk with RE-SORB® for 2 days followed by a gradual re-introduction of milk mixed with RE-SORB®, provides an opportunity for the gastrointestinal mucosa to rest.

Since RE-SORB® is readily absorbed, it provides the livestock owner with an ideal first feed for the stressed or newly purchased calf. It is widely believed that it is often beneficial to starve or only provide half of the initial feeding of milk to newly purchased calves to reduce stress on the gastrointestinal system. RE-SORB® may be given as the initial feeding following by a 50:50 mixture of RE-SORB® and milk at the second feeding to reduce stress on the gastrointestinal tract.

Dosage and Administration:

Mixing Directions: Add the contents of 1 packet (both sides) to 2 quarts of warm water. Stir until dissolved.

Scouring Calves: Feed 2 quarts of RE-SORB® solution made up as directed, twice daily for 2 days (4 feedings). No milk or milk replacer should be fed during this period. For the next 4 feedings (days 3 and 4), use 1 quart of RE-SORB® solution mixed together with 1 quart of milk or milk replacer. Thereafter, feed as normal.

Newly Purchased Calves: Feed 2 quarts of RE-SORB® solution made up as directed instead of milk as the first feed upon arrival. For the next scheduled feeding, use 1 quart of RE-SORB® solution mixed together with 1 quart of milk or milk replacer. Thereafter, feed as normal.

Precaution(s): Storage: Store at controlled room temperature 15°-30°C (59°-86°F).

Caution(s): RE-SORB® should not be used in animals with severe dehydration (down, comatose, or in a state of shock). Such animals need intravenous fluids since oral therapy in these cases is too slow. A veterinarian should be consulted in such severely scouring calves or in cases requiring antibacterial therapy.

Antibacterial therapy is often indicated in bacterial scours due to *E. coli* and/or Salmonella. RE-SORB® does not contain antibacterial agents.

Adequate colostrum intake during the first 12 hours is essential for healthy, vigorous calves.

RE-SORB® is not nutritionally complete if administered by itself for long periods of time. It should not be administered beyond the recommended treatment period without the addition of milk or milk replacer.

Warning(s): For use in calves only.

Discussion: The 3 main causes of calf scours and resulting dehydration are bacteria *(E. coli* and Salmonella, etc.), viruses, and nutritional factors. In all cases, there is a loss of water and electrolytes due to the scours, which can lead to severe dehydration and death. Generally, whatever the cause of the scours, dehydration is the main cause of death. When fecal loss of water exceeds the water intake, dehydration occurs. This can be corrected with administration of either oral or intravenous fluids. In the severely dehydrated calf, intravenous administration is the route of choice.

Oral rehydration is of particular value as it permits the livestock owner to start rehydration therapy at the initial signs of scours which, in many cases, will reduce the severity of the condition. RE-SORB® also provides the owner with a practical method of following up intravenous therapy.

References: Available upon request.

Presentation: RE-SORB® is supplied in boxes containing 12 packets (double-sided) and in buckets containing 72 packets (double-sided).

U.S. Patent No. 4,164,568

Compendium Code No.: 36900190 75-8112-07

RESPIMUNE™

Biomune **Vaccine**

Newcastle Disease Vaccine, B1 Type, Lasota Strain, Live Virus

U.S. Vet. Lic. No.: 368

Description: This vaccine contains Newcastle Disease Virus, B1 Type, Lasota strain, grown in specific pathogen free (SPF) chicken embryos.

Contains gentamicin as a preservative.

Warranty: This vaccine was thoroughly tested before sale and meets the requirements of the U.S. Department of Agriculture.

Indications: This vaccine is recommended for vaccination of healthy chickens at two weeks of age or older using drinking water, coarse spray or intraocular routes of administration. Revaccination is recommended at 4 weeks and 16 weeks of age. Chickens should be maintained under good environmental conditions and exposure to disease should be reduced as much as possible.

The application of this vaccine to two-week-old chickens will aid in the prevention of Newcastle disease.

Dosage and Administration: For drinking water, coarse spray or intraocular use.

Directions for Drinking Water Application:

1. Do not open or rehydrate the vaccine until ready to vaccinate.
2. Do not use any medications, sanitizers or disinfectants in the drinking water for 48 hours before vaccination and for 24 hours after vaccination.
3. Prior to administration of the vaccine, withhold water from the chickens for 2 hours in warm weather and up to 4 hours in cool weather to stimulate thirst. Be careful in hot weather.
4. Thoroughly rinse water lines or waterers with fresh, clean water. Do not use disinfectants for cleaning water lines or waterers.
5. Rehydrate the vaccine as follows:
   Note: As an aid in preserving the vaccine, 30 mL (1 ounce) of rehydrated non-fat powdered milk may be added to each 3.8 liter (1 gallon of clean, cool, non-chlorinated water used for rehydrating and mixing the vaccine.
   a. Remove the seal and stopper from the vial containing the freeze-dried vaccine.
   b. Carefully pour the milk/water into the vaccine vial until the vial is approximately two-thirds full.
   c. Insert the stopper and shake vigorously until all material is rehydrated.
   d. Rinse vaccine vial to remove all vaccine and add to the vaccine solution to be administered.
6. Mix rehydrated vaccine with milk/water in accordance with the chart below:

Age of Chickens	Water per 1000 Doses of Vaccine	
2 to 3 weeks	6 gallons	22.8 Liters
4 to 7 weeks	12 gallons	45.6 Liters
8 weeks or older	16 gallons	60.8 Liters

7. Distribute the vaccine into the proportioner or among the waterers provided for the chickens. Avoid placing vaccine in direct sunlight.
8. Provide no other drinking water until all the vaccine-water solution has been consumed.

Directions for Coarse Spray Application:

1. Remove the seal and stopper from the vial containing the freeze-dried vaccine.
2. Carefully pour clean, non-chlorinated water into the vaccine vial until the vial is approximately two-thirds full.
3. Insert the stopper and shake vigorously until all material is rehydrated.
4. Pour the rehydrated vaccine into the clean reservoir of the sprayer and dilute further by using 350 mL (or the volume necessary to spray vaccinate 1,000 birds with the sprayer being used) of clean, cool non-chlorinated water for each 1,000 doses of vaccine. For coarse spray administration the droplet size should be greater than or equal to 80 microns.
5. Prior to spraying, reduce air movement in the house by shutting off all fans. Fans should remain on the lowest setting for approximately 10-15 minutes after spraying. Care should be taken so that the chickens are not heat stressed.
6. Spray chickens at the rate of 1,000 per minute while walking slowly through the house. Aim the spray just above the heads of the chickens.
7. Use the sprayer for vaccination purposes only. Clean thoroughly after each use.
8. Avoid direct contact with the vaccine solution. Individual(s) spraying chickens should wear face masks and goggles.

Directions for Intraocular Application:

1. Remove the aluminum seal and rubber stopper from the vial containing the freeze-dried vaccine and pour part of the diluent into the vial.
2. Insert the rubber stopper and shake well until all material is rehydrated. Pour the rehydrated vaccine back into the remaining diluent in the diluent vial and mix.
3. Place the dropper tip on the diluent vial. The vaccine is now ready for intraocular administration as stated below.
4. Hold the bird on its side and allow one drop of the mixed vaccine to fall into the open eye.
5. Hold the bird until the drop of vaccine disappears. Care must be taken to avoid injury to the eye with the dropper tip.

Precaution(s): Store the vaccine at 35°-45°F (2°-7°C).

Do not open and mix the vaccine until ready to begin vaccination.

Use entire contents of vial immediately after mixing.

Burn the container and all unused contents.

This vaccine is not returnable to the manufacturer.

Caution(s): Do not dilute or otherwise extend the dosage.

Vaccinate all chickens on the premises at the same time.

Vaccinate only healthy chickens.

Warning(s): Do not vaccinate within 21 days of slaughter.

Newcastle disease virus may cause redness or inflammation of the eyelids of humans. Avoid contact with eyes, hands and clothing. Wear goggles and mask while mixing and administering vaccine.

Presentation: 10 x 1,000 doses, 10 x 2,000 doses, 10 x 2,500 doses, 10 x 5,000 doses, 10 x 10,000 doses and 10 x 25,000 doses.

Compendium Code No.: 11290470 February 13, 2002

RESPIRAGEN™ SERUM ANTIBODIES

Colorado Serum **Antiserum**

Corynebacterium pyogenes-Pasteurella haemolytica-multocida Antiserum, Bovine and Porcine Isolates, Bovine Origin

U.S. Vet. Lic. No.: 188

Active Ingredient(s): Prepared from the blood of cattle hyperimmunized against *Corynebacterium pyogenes, Pasteurella haemolytica,* and *Pasteurella multocida* isolated from cattle, which have also received repeated injections of virus fluids of bovine rhinotracheitis, bovine virus diarrhea and parainfluenza-3.

Contains phenol and thimerosal as preservatives.

Indications: For use in cattle, sheep and swine for the prevention and as an aid in the treatment of pasteurellosis and complications of diphtheroid infections associated with the organisms named in the formulation.

Dosage and Administration: RESPIRAGEN™ is indicated whenever diphtheroid infection is present in combination with pasteurellosis in cattle, sheep and swine. The products can also be used by administering the recommended doses a few days prior to shipping animals as a preconditioning procedure. The response is almost immediate, lasting for approximately two (2) to three (3) weeks.

Cattle should not be vaccinated for bovine rhinotracheitis, virus diarrhea or parainfluenza-3 for 21 days after the administration of RESPIRAGEN™.

Injections may be subcutaneous or intramuscular.

For prevention:

Calves: 20 mL to 40 mL, as soon after birth as possible.

Cattle: 50 mL to 75 mL.

Sheep and Swine: 10 mL to 15 mL.

For treatment:

Calves: 40 mL to 100 mL.

Cattle: 75 mL to 150 mL.

Sheep and Swine: 20 mL to 40 mL.

The dosage may be repeated according to the judgment of the user.

Injections may be subcutaneous or intramuscular. Multiple sites may be used when injecting large doses.

Precaution(s): Store in the dark at 2-7°C.

Sterilize needles and syringes by boiling in clean water.

Caution(s): Anaphylactic reactions sometimes follow administration of products of this nature. If noted, administer adrenaline or an equivalent drug.

Use the entire contents when the bottle is first opened.

For veterinary use only.

Warning(s): Do not vaccinate within 21 days before slaughter.

Needle punctures and tissue damage may result in condemnation of carcasses.

Because of the viral antibodies in RESPIRAGEN™, cattle should not be vaccinated with IBR, BVD, or PI_3 vaccines, or any other combination thereof for at least 21 days after injection of the antiserum.

Discussion: Cattle bred and raised in the mountains of the western United States are injected with increasingly large doses of cultures of *Corynebacterium pyogenes, Pasteurella haemolytica* and *Pasteurella multocida*, bovine and porcine isolates, and with virus fluids of bovine rhinotracheitis, bovine virus diarrhea, and parainfluenza-3. Antiserum is processed from the blood of these animals.

The terms shipping fever and hemorrhagic septicemia have been commonly used to describe an infectious febrile disease that develops when animals are moved through concentrating areas from ranges and other customary environment. The syndrome is now recognized as a highly complex involvement of the respiratory tract in which viruses as well as bacteria play an important part. The disease is not seasonal but may be more frequently observed in the fall as cattle move from summer ranges. Show cattle may also become affected as they travel the circuit.

The symptoms that are usually observed are a dull, tired appearance, loss of appetite, chilling, and a soft cough. Temperatures may run to 105°F, or higher. Sometimes an increase in temperature precedes all other symptoms. Affected animals become gaunt. Respiration quickens as the disease progresses and a watery discharge from the nose and eyes and an encrusted muzzle may be noted. Outright deaths are significant although the major losses are economic coming from a drastic loss of weight, chronic disease development, and the inability of the animals to regain efficient utilization of feed.

The exact cause or causes of infection associated with the shipping fever syndrome have not been fully determined but it is known that when virus infections are complicated with pasteurellosis the death loss increases substantially. Stress lowering the animal's natural defense against diarrhea, is also an important factor.

Presentation: 100 mL and 250 mL vials.

Compendium Code No.: 11010300

RESPISHIELD™ 4

Merial **Vaccine**

Bovine Rhinotracheitis-Virus Diarrhea-Parainfluenza$_3$-Respiratory Syncytial Virus Vaccine, Killed Virus

U.S. Vet. Lic. No.: 298

Contents: This product contains the antigens listed above.

Contains gentamicin and nystatin as preservatives.

Indications: For the vaccination of healthy cattle (calves, heifers, cows) as an aid in the prevention of disease due to IBR, BVD, PI_3, and BRSV.

Dosage and Administration: Shake well before using. Inject 5 mL (1 dose) intramuscularly or subcutaneously. For primary vaccination, revaccinate with a second 5 mL dose 2 to 4 weeks later. Calves vaccinated under 6 months of age should be revaccinated after reaching 6 months of age. Revaccinate with a single 5 mL dose annually or prior to times of stress or exposure.

Precaution(s): Store at 2-7°C (35-45°F). Do not freeze. Do not expose to heat or direct sunlight. Use entire contents when first opened. Do not use chemicals to sterilize syringes and needles.

Caution(s): In rare instances, administration of vaccines may cause lethargy, fever and

R

inflammatory or hypersensitivity types of reactions. Treatment may include antihistamines, anti-inflammatories, and/or epinephrine.

For veterinary use only.

Warning(s): Do not vaccinate within 21 days prior to slaughter.

Presentation: 10 dose (50 mL) and 50 dose (250 mL) vials.

RESPISHIELD is a trademark of Merial.

Compendium Code No.: 11110752 RM821R4 / RM825R5

RESPISHIELD™ 4 L5

Merial **Bacterin-Vaccine**

Bovine Rhinotracheitis-Virus Diarrhea-Parainfluenza$_3$-Respiratory Syncytial Virus Vaccine-Leptospira Canicola-Grippotyphosa-Hardjo-Icterohaemorrhagiae-Pomona Bacterin, Killed Virus

U.S. Vet. Lic. No.: 298

Contents: This product contains the antigens listed above.

Contains gentamicin and nystatin as preservatives.

Indications: For the vaccination of healthy cattle (calves, heifers, cows) as an aid in prevention of disease due to IBR, BVD, PI$_3$, BRSV, *L. canicola, L. grippotyphosa, L. hardjo, L. icterohaemorrhagiae*, and *L. pomona.*

Dosage and Administration: Shake well before using. Inject 5 mL (1 dose) intramuscularly or subcutaneously. For primary vaccination, revaccinate with a second 5 mL dose 2 to 4 weeks later. Calves vaccinated under 6 months of age should be revaccinated after reaching 6 months of age. Revaccinate with a single 5 mL dose annually or prior to the time of stress or exposure.

Precaution(s): Store at 2-7°C (35-45°F). Do not freeze. Do not expose to heat or direct sunlight. Use entire contents when first opened. Do not use chemicals to sterilize syringes and needles.

Caution(s): In rare instances, administration of vaccines may cause lethargy, fever and inflammatory or hypersensitivity types of reactions. Treatment may include antihistamines, anti-inflammatories, and/or epinephrine.

For veterinary use only.

Warning(s): Do not vaccinate within 21 days prior to slaughter.

Presentation: 10 dose (50 mL) and 50 dose (250 mL) vials.

RESPISHIELD is a trademark of Merial.

Compendium Code No.: 11110762 RM831R4 / RM835R6

RESPISURE®

Pfizer Animal Health **Bacterin**

Mycoplasma Hyopneumoniae Bacterin

U.S. Vet. Lic. No.: 189

Description: RESPISURE® contains a chemically inactivated whole cell culture of *M. hyopneumoniae*, coupled with an oil adjuvant, Amphigen®, to enhance and prolong the immune response without causing detectable tissue damage at the injection site.

Indications: RESPISURE® is for vaccination of healthy swine as an aid in the prevention of chronic pneumonia caused by *Mycoplasma hyopneumoniae.*

Directions:

1. General Directions: For best results, vaccination of all swine in a herd is recommended. Shake well. Aseptically administer two 2-mL doses intramuscularly, at least 2 weeks apart.
2. Primary Vaccination: Administer a single 2-mL dose to pigs at approximately 1 week of age with a booster dose 2 weeks later. Pregnant swine may be safely vaccinated at 6 weeks and 2 weeks prior to farrowing.
3. Revaccination: Dams should be revaccinated 2 weeks before farrowing. Boars should be revaccinated semiannually.

Precaution(s): Store at 2°-7°C. Prolonged exposure to higher temperatures may adversely affect potency. Do not freeze.

Use entire contents when first opened.

Sterilized syringes and needles should be used to administer this vaccine.

Caution(s): As with any vaccine, anaphylaxis may occur after use. Initial antidote of epinephrine is recommended and should be followed with appropriate supportive therapy.

This product has been shown to be efficacious in healthy animals. A protective immune response may not be elicited if animals are incubating an infectious disease, are malnourished or parasitized, are stressed due to shipment or environmental conditions, are otherwise immunocompromised, or the vaccine is not administered in accordance with label directions.

For use in swine only.

Warning(s): Do not vaccinate within 21 days before slaughter.

For veterinary use only.

Discussion: Disease Description: Mycoplasmal pneumonia of swine (MPS), or enzootic pneumonia, is a widespread, chronic disease characterized by coughing, growth retardation, and reduced feed efficiency. The etiologic agent is *M. hyopneumoniae*; however, the naturally occurring disease often results from a combination of bacterial and mycoplasmal infections.

MPS causes considerable economic loss in all areas where swine are raised. Surveys conducted at various locations throughout the world indicate that lesions typical of those seen with MPS occur in 30% to 80% of slaughter-weight swine. Because mycoplasmal lesions may resolve before hogs reach slaughter weight, the actual incidence may be higher. The prevalence of *M. hyopneumoniae* infection in chronic swine pneumonia has been reported to range from 25%[1] to 93%.[2] Research indicates that MPS infections can add up to 30 days to market and increase feed consumption by 0.75 lb per lb of weight gain.

Pigs of all ages are susceptible to MPS, but the disease is most common in growing and finishing swine. Current evidence indicates the *M. hyopneumoniae* is transmitted by aerosol or direct contact with respiratory tract secretions from infected swine. In some cases, transmission has been attributed to carrier pigs, but other evidence demonstrates that transmission among penmates can occur once a few pigs are infected.[3-4] Transmission from sow to pig during lactation is possible.[5] Once established, MPS occurs year after year in affected herds, varying in severity with such environmental factors as season, ventilation, and concentration of swine.

Clinical signs of MPS include a chronic nonproductive cough continuing for weeks or months, unthrifty appearance, and retarded growth, even though the appetites of infected swine remain normal. Stunting may occur, resulting in considerable variation in size among affected pigs. Death loss associated with secondary bacterial infection and stress may occur at 4-6 months of age.

M. hyopneumoniae causes a loss of ciliary motility in the bronchial passages. Eventually the cilia are destroyed, resulting in a reduction in natural defense in the upper respiratory tract and increased susceptibility to secondary infection with bacterial agents such as *Pasteurella multocida, Haemophilus parasuis, Actinobacillus pleuropneumoniae,* and *Bordetella bronchiseptica.* Swine lungworm and roundworm larvae infections may also increase the severity of MPS.

Trial Data: Safety and Efficacy: Chemical inactivation renders RESPISURE® incapable of causing infectious disease. Necropsy data from in-house clinical trials showed that tissue damage occurred at only 6 (1.87%) of 320 injection sites, and none of the reactions were larger than 1 cm in diameter. The oil-base adjuvant in RESPISURE® does not produce the major tissue damage sometimes associated with conventional oil adjuvants.

Efficacy of RESPISURE® was evaluated in rigorous challenge-of-immunity studies. In repeated studies, RESPISURE® vaccinates had between 72% and 92% less lung involvement caused by homologous and heterologous challenge strains of *M. hyopneumoniae* than controls. In 2 such tests, vaccinates received 2 intramuscular doses of bacterin, the first at 1 week of age, the second at 3 weeks. One week after the second vaccination, 1 group of vaccinated and nonvaccinated control pigs were challenged intranasally with a homologous strain of *M. hyopneumoniae* culture, the second group with a heterologous strain. About 3 weeks after challenge, all pigs were necropsied and individual lungs were evaluated for lung damage and gross lesions characteristic of *M. hyopneumoniae* infection and scored according to a system devised by Goodwin and Whittlestone.[6] Results are presented in Figures 1 and 2.

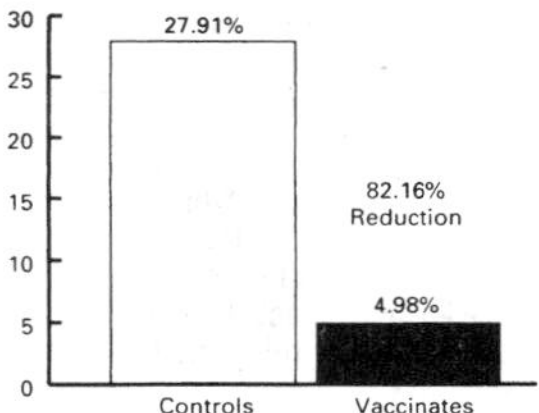

Figure 1. Mean percentage of lung damage following challenge with homologous *M. hyopneumoniae.*

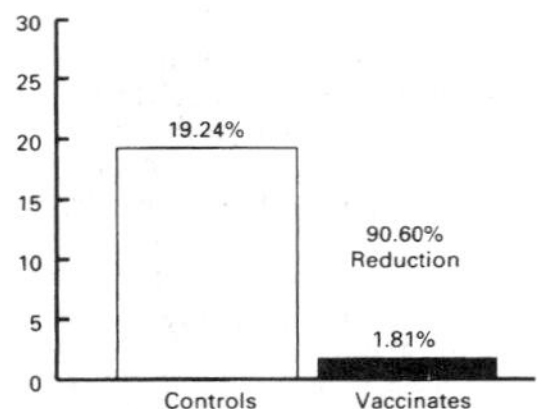

Figure 2. Mean percentage of lung damage following challenge with heterologous *M. hyopneumoniae.*

In pigs challenged with the homologous strain, the mean percentage of lung damage was 4.98% in vaccinates and 27.91% in controls (an 82.16% reduction in lung damage in vaccinates when compared to controls). Mean lung damage score for pigs challenged with the heterologous strain was 1.81% for vaccinates and 19.24% for controls (a 90.6% reduction in lung damage in vaccinates when compared to controls).

In an independent challenge-of-immunity study conducted at Iowa State University, pigs vaccinated at approximately 6 weeks and again at 8 weeks of age with RESPISURE® showed evidence of less severe *M. hyopneumoniae* infection (1.9% mean percentage of lung damage) than nonvaccinated control pigs (7.9% mean percentage of lung damage), a 75.91% reduction in lung damage in vaccinates when compared to controls ($p = <0.01$). Vaccinates also had fewer lung lobes with lesions (6 of 9 vaccinates had lesions in 12 of 63 lobes) than controls (8 of 8 had lesions in 35 of 56 lobes), and the lesions were less severe.

Evaluation of lung tissue and lesions by fluorescent antibody (FA) testing revealed that 7 of 8 control pigs and 3 of 9 vaccinates were positive for *M. hyopneumoniae.* Based on a system rating the intensity of infection in lung lobes as measured by immunofluorescence from 1-4, the severity of vaccinates' infections (average 0.18) was 71% less than that of controls (average 0.63) (Figure 3).

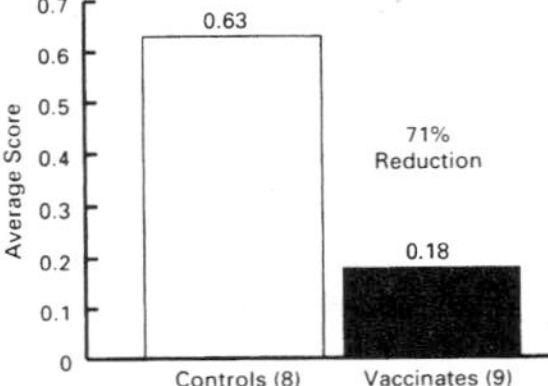

Figure 3. Severity of lung infection as measured by immunofluorescence following challenge with *M. hyopneumoniae* (0=no infection).

References: Available upon request.

Presentation: 50 dose (100 mL), 250 dose (500 mL), and 500 dose (1,000 mL) vials.

Compendium Code No.: 36900370 75-4589-00

RESPISURE 1 ONE®

Pfizer Animal Health **Bacterin**

Mycoplasma Hyopneumoniae Bacterin

U.S. Vet. Lic. No.: 189

Description: RESPISURE 1 ONE® is a liquid preparation of a chemically inactivated whole cell culture of *M. hyopneumoniae*, coupled with a unique oil adjuvant Amphigen® to enhance and prolong the immune response without causing detectable tissue damage at the injection site.

Indications: RESPISURE 1 ONE® is for vaccination of healthy swine 1 week of age or older as an aid in preventing chronic pneumonia caused by *Mycoplasma hyopneumoniae* for a period of 25 weeks following vaccination.

Directions:

1. General Directions: Shake well. Aseptically administer 2 mL intramuscularly.
2. Primary Vaccination: Administer a single 2 mL dose to healthy swine 1 week of age or older.
3. Revaccination: Semiannual revaccination with a single dose is recommended.
4. Good animal husbandry and herd health management practices should be employed.

Precaution(s): Store at 2°-7°C. Prolonged exposure to higher temperatures may adversely affect potency. Do not freeze.

Use entire contents when first opened.

Sterilized syringes and needles should be used to administer this vaccine.

R

Caution(s): As with many vaccines, anaphylaxis may occur after use. Initial antidote of epinephrine is recommended and should be followed with appropriate supportive therapy.

This product has been shown to be efficacious in healthy animals. A protective immune response may not be elicited if animals are incubating an infectious disease, are malnourished or parasitized, are stressed due to shipment or environmental conditions, are otherwise immunocompromised, or the vaccine is not administered in accordance with label directions.

For use in swine only

For veterinary use only

Warning(s): Do not vaccinate within 21 days before slaughter.

Discussion: Disease Description: Mycoplasmal pneumonia of swine (MPS) or enzootic pneumonia is a widespread, chronic disease characterized by coughing, growth retardation, and reduced feed efficiency. The etiologic agent is *M. hyopneumoniae;* however, the naturally occurring disease often results from a combination of bacterial and mycoplasmal infections.

MPS causes considerable economic loss in all areas where swine are raised. Surveys conducted at various locations throughout the world indicate that lesions typical of those seen with MPS occur in 30%-80% of slaughter-weight swine. Because mycoplasmal lesions may resolve before hogs reach slaughter weight, the actual incidence may be higher. The prevalence of *M. hyopneumoniae* infection in chronic swine pneumonia has been reported to range from 25%[1]-93%.[2] Pigs of all ages are susceptible to MPS, but the disease is most common in growing and finishing swine. Current evidence indicates that *M. hyopneumoniae* is transmitted by aerosol or direct contact with respiratory tract secretions from infected swine. Transmission from sow to pig during lactation is possible.[3] Once established, MPS occurs year after year in infected herds, varying in severity with such environmental factors as season, ventilation, and concentration of swine.

Clinical signs of MPS include a chronic, nonproductive cough continuing for weeks or months, unthrifty appearance, and retarded growth, even though the appetites of infected swine remain normal. Stunting may occur, resulting in considerable variation in size among affected pigs. Death loss associated with secondary bacterial infection and stress may occur.

M. hyopneumoniae causes a loss of ciliary motility in the bronchial passages. Eventually the cilia are destroyed, resulting in reduction in natural defense in the upper respiratory tract and increased susceptibility to secondary infection with bacterial agents such as *Pasteurella multocida, Haemophilus parasuis, Actinobacillus pleuropneumoniae,* and *Bordetella bronchiseptica.* Swine lungworm and roundworm larvae infections may also increase the severity of MPS.

Trial Data: Safety and Efficacy: In clinical studies conducted by Pfizer Animal Health, RESPISURE 1 ONE® has been shown to be safe and free from significant adverse reactions when administered according to label directions. Chemical inactivation renders RESPISURE 1 ONE® incapable of causing infectious disease. The oil-base adjuvant in RESPISURE 1 ONE® does not produce the major tissue damage sometimes associated with conventional oil adjuvants.

Efficacy of RESPISURE 1 ONE® was demonstrated in host animal studies conducted by Pfizer; duration-of-immunity studies demonstrated efficacy up to 25 weeks after a single vaccination in pigs as young as 1 week of age. In all of these duration-of-immunity studies, pigs vaccinated with RESPISURE 1 ONE®, followed by challenge, had significantly lower lung lesion scores than pigs vaccinated with a placebo.

Duration-of-immunity studies: The purpose of the 7 studies below in Table 1 was to demonstrate protection against challenge with virulent *M. hyopneumoniae* 8, 18, 23 or 25 weeks after a single vaccination with RESPISURE 1 ONE® in 1-, 3- or 8-week-old pigs. All pigs were necropsied and lung lesion scores determined (percent of total lung with lesions[4]). In all cases pigs vaccinated with RESPISURE 1 ONE® had significantly lower lung lesion scores than pigs vaccinated with a placebo.

Table 1.

Study	Treatment	No. of Pigs	Vaccination (age in wks)	Challenge (wks after vacc)	Challenge (age in wks)	% Lung Lesion
1	Placebo	22	3	8	11	2.7[a]
	RESPISURE 1 ONE®	24	3	8	11	0.1[b]
2	Placebo	20	3	18	21	13.2[a]
	RESPISURE 1 ONE®	19	3	18	21	5.5[b]
3	Placebo	18	8	8	16	10.3[a]
	RESPISURE 1 ONE®	20	8	8	16	0.5[b]
4	Placebo	21	8	18	26	9.6[a]
	RESPISURE 1 ONE®	20	8	18	26	0.9[b]
5	Placebo	19	3	23	26	9.0[a]
	RESPISURE 1 ONE®	22	3	23	26	2.1[b]
6	Placebo	26*	1	25	26	4.5[a]
	RESPISURE 1 ONE®	22*	1	25	26	2.0[b]
7	Placebo	24	1	25	26	5.9[a]
	RESPISURE 1 ONE®	20	1	25	26	0.3[b]

[a,b] Within each study group, values with different superscripts are statistically significant vs. placebo ($p \leq 0.05$).

* Pigs were serologically positive for *M. hyopneumoniae.*

References: Available upon request.

Presentation: 15 dose (30 mL), 250 dose (500 mL), and 500 dose (1000 mL) bottles.

Compendium Code No.: 36900341

75-5001-05

RESPISURE 1 ONE®/ER BAC PLUS®

Pfizer Animal Health **Bacterin**

Erysipelothrix Rhusiopathiae-Mycoplasma Hyopneumoniae Bacterin

U.S. Vet. Lic. No.: 189

Description: RESPISURE-ONE®/ER BAC PLUS® is a liquid preparation of a chemically inactivated whole cell culture of *Mycoplasma hyopneumoniae* and a serum-free, clarified *Erysipelothrix rhusiopathiae* culture, plus Amphigen®, a unique oil-in-water adjuvant to enhance the immune response.

Indications: RESPISURE-ONE®/ER BAC PLUS® is for vaccination of healthy swine 3 weeks of age or older as an aid in preventing erysipelas caused by *E. rhusiopathiae* for a period of 20 weeks and respiratory disease caused by *M. hyopneumoniae* for a period of 23 weeks.

Directions:

1. General Directions: Vaccination of all pigs on the premises is recommended to enhance herd immunity. Shake well. Aseptically administer 2 mL intramuscularly.
2. Primary Vaccination: Administer a single 2 mL dose to healthy swine 3 weeks of age or older, followed by a single dose of ER Bac Plus® approximately 3 weeks later. In young pigs, vaccinate after maternally derived antibodies to *E. rhusiopathiae* have declined.
3. Revaccination: Semiannual revaccination with a single dose is recommended.
4. Good animal husbandry and herd health management practices should be employed.

Precaution(s): Store at 2°-7°C. Prolonged exposure to higher temperatures may adversely affect potency. Do not freeze.

Use entire contents when first opened or rehydrated.

Sterilized syringes and needles should be used to administer this vaccine.

Caution(s): As with many vaccines, anaphylaxis may occur after use. Initial antidote of epinephrine is recommended and should be followed with appropriate supportive therapy.

This product has been shown to be efficacious in healthy animals. A protective immune response may not be elicited if animals are incubating an infectious disease, are malnourished or parasitized, are stressed due to shipment or environmental conditions, are otherwise immunocompromised, or the vaccine is not administered in accordance with label directions.

For use in swine only.

For veterinary use only.

Warning(s): Do not vaccinate within 21 days before slaughter.

Discussion: Disease Description: Mycoplasmal pneumonia of swine (MPS), or enzootic pneumonia, is a widespread, chronic disease characterized by coughing, growth retardation, and reduced feed efficiency. The etiologic agent is *M. hyopneumoniae;* however, the naturally occurring disease often results from a combination of bacterial and mycoplasmal infections.

MPS causes considerable economic loss in all areas where swine are raised. Surveys conducted at various locations throughout the world indicate that lesions typical of those seen with MPS occur in 30%-80% of slaughter-weight swine. Because mycoplasmal lesions may resolve before hogs reach slaughter weight, the actual incidence may be higher. The prevalence of *M. hyopneumoniae* infection in chronic swine pneumonia has been reported to range from 25%[1]-93%.[2] Pigs of all ages are susceptible to MPS, but the disease is most common in growing and finishing swine. Current evidence indicates that *M. hyopneumoniae* is transmitted by aerosol or direct contact with respiratory tract secretions from infected swine. Transmission from sow to pig during lactation is possible.[3] Once established, MPS occurs year after year in infected herds, varying in severity with such environmental factors as season, ventilation, and concentration of swine.

Clinical signs of MPS include a chronic, nonproductive cough continuing for weeks or months, unthrifty appearance, and retarded growth, even though the appetites of infected swine remain normal. Stunting may occur, resulting in considerable variation in size among affected pigs. Death loss associated with secondary bacterial infection and stress may occur.

M. hyopneumoniae causes a loss of ciliary motility in the bronchial passages. Eventually the cilia are destroyed, resulting in reduction in natural defense in the upper respiratory tract and increased susceptibility to secondary infection with bacterial agents such as *Pasteurella multocida, Haemophilus parasuis, Actinobacillus pleuropneumoniae,* and *Bordetella bronchiseptica.* Swine lungworm and roundworm larvae infections may also increase the severity of MPS.

Erysipelas is caused by the bacterium *E. rhusiopathiae* and has been identified as a pathogen in swine since 1878. The disease is worldwide in distribution and is of economic importance throughout Europe, Asia, Australia, and North and South America. Swine 3 months through 3 years of age are most susceptible to erysipelas; outbreaks are usually more severe in herds on soil and during periods of wet weather. Erysipelas can take one of several forms or a combination of the following forms. Acute erysipelas is a general infection by *E. rhusiopathiae* in the bloodstream. This form often causes sudden death. Abortion may result in sows infected during pregnancy. Skin erysipelas manifests as diamond-shaped patches of swollen, purple skin on a pig's body, especially the belly and thighs. If the tips of the ears and tail are affected, tissues may die and slough. Arthritic erysipelas is a chronic disease occurring in pigs that have survived acute erysipelas. Affected pigs often have swollen and stiff joints. They do not gain weight efficiently, and their carcasses are often trimmed or condemned by inspectors at packing houses. Cardiac erysipelas usually occurs in older pigs raised on farms where the chronic form exists. Cardiac erysipelas may result in growths on the heart valves altering the normal flow of blood.[4]

Trial Data: Safety and Efficacy: The safety of RESPISURE-ONE®/ER BAC PLUS® was demonstrated in 3 field safety studies conducted in 3 different geographic locations. Nine hundred and six pigs were vaccinated at approximately 3 and 6 weeks of age. No injection site reactions or serious systemic reactions were observed following vaccination.

The efficacy of RESPISURE-ONE®/ER BAC PLUS® as an aid in preventing pneumonia caused by *M. hyopnuemoniae* was demonstrated in host animal challenge studies conducted by Pfizer. Duration-of-immunity studies demonstrated protection against challenge with virulent *M. hyopneumoniae* up to 23 weeks after a single vaccination in pigs as young as 3 weeks of age. In all studies, vaccinated pigs had significantly lower lung lesion scores than pigs receiving a placebo.

Table 1. *Mycoplasma hyopneumoniae* Efficacy Studies:

Study	Treatment	No. of Pigs	Vaccination (age in weeks)	Challenge (wks after vacc)	Challenge (age in wks)	% Lung Lesion
1	Placebo	23	3	7	10	9.9[a]
	RESPISURE 1 ONE®/ ER BAC PLUS®	24	3	7	10	1.8[b]
2	Placebo	20	3	18	21	13.2[a]
	RespiSure 1 One®	19	3	18	21	5.5[b]
3	Placebo	19	3	23	26	9.0[a]
	RespiSure 1 One®	22	3	23	26	2.1[b]

[a,b] Within each study group, values with different superscripts are statistically significant vs. placebo ($p \leq 0.05$).

Host animal studies were also conducted to demonstrate the efficacy of RESPISURE-ONE®/ER BAC PLUS® in preventing disease caused by *E. rhusiopathiae.* Pigs were vaccinated at approximately 3 and 6 weeks of age and challenged at either 4 or 20 weeks post-second vaccination. Pigs were monitored daily for rectal temperature and for clinical signs of disease. In both studies, vaccination provided significant protection from challenge.

R

Table 2. *Erysipelothrix rhusiopathiae* Efficacy Studies:

Study	Treatment	No. of Pigs	Challenge (wks after vacc)	Percent of animals with clinical signs of disease
1	Placebo	10	4	100
	RESPISURE-ONE®/ ER BAC PLUS®	19	4	0
2	Placebo	10	20	90
	ER Bac Plus®	20	20	25

References: Available upon request.
Presentation: 50 dose (100 mL), 250 dose (500 mL) and 500 dose (1,000 mL) vials.
Compendium Code No.: 36902010 75-0270-00

RESPOMUNE™ 2

Biocor **Vaccine**

Feline Rhinotracheitis-Calici Vaccine, Modified Live Virus
U.S. Vet. Lic. No.: 462
Contents: This product contains the antigens listed above.
This product contains gentamicin and amphotericin B as preservatives.
Indications: RESPOMUNE™ 2 is recommended for use in the vaccination of healthy cats against disease caused by feline viral rhinotracheitis and calicivirus.
Directions: Aseptically rehydrate vial of desiccated virus with the accompanying vial of diluent. Shake well. Administer entire contents (1 mL) subcutaneously.
Persistence of maternal origin antibody in kittens is known to interfere with development of active immunity following vaccination. Present indications are that rhinotracheitis and calicivirus antibodies of maternal origin endure in kittens for approximately 8 weeks. Ideally kittens should be vaccinated at 9 weeks of age with revaccination 3-4 weeks later. Previously unvaccinated cats should receive a 1 mL dose followed by a second dose 3-4 weeks later. Annual revaccination with a single 1 mL dose is recommended.
Contraindication(s): Do not vaccinate pregnant queens.
Precaution(s): Store at 35°F-45°F (2°C-7°C). Do not freeze. Use entire contents when first rehydrated. Burn these containers and all unused contents.
Caution(s): An occasional animal may demonstrate a transient fever, and mild arthralgia and/or myalgia within the first week following vaccination. In case of anaphylactoid reactions, epinephrine should be administered immediately.
For use in cats only.
Presentation: Code 68611B - 25 x 1 dose (1 mL) vials with diluent.
™ trademark of Biocor Animal Health Inc.
Compendium Code No.: 13940270 BAH3525-401

RESPOMUNE®-CP

Biocor **Vaccine**

Feline Rhinotracheitis-Calici-Panleukopenia Vaccine, Modified Live and Killed Virus
U.S. Vet. Lic. No.: 462
Contents: RESPOMUNE®-CP is a combination of modified live Feline Rhinotracheitis and Calici viruses with inactivated Panleukopenia virus vaccine. All fractions are subjected to tests for potency and safety prior to release for market.
This product contains gentamicin and amphotericin B as preservatives.
Indications: Recommended for use in the vaccination of healthy cats against disease caused by the organisms represented.
Dosage and Administration: Aseptically rehydrate vial of desiccated virus with the accompanying vial of killed virus fluid. Shake well. Administer entire contents (1 mL) SC.
Persistence of maternal origin antibody in kittens is known to interfere with development of active immunity following vaccination. Present indications are that Rhinotracheitis and Calicivirus antibodies of maternal origin endure in kittens for approximately 8 weeks. Panleukopenia antibody somewhat longer - up to 13 weeks. Ideally kittens should be vaccinated at 9 weeks of age with revaccination 3-4 weeks later. Adult cats should receive a 1 mL dose followed by a second dose 3-4 weeks later. Annual revaccination with a single 1 mL dose is recommended.
Precaution(s): Store at 35°F-45°F (2°C-7°C). Do not freeze. Use entire contents when first rehydrated. Burn these containers and all unused contents.
Caution(s): Do not vaccinate pregnant queens. An occasional animal may demonstrate a transient fever, and mild arthralgia and/or myalgia within the first week following vaccination. In case of anaphylactoid reactions, epinephrine should be administered immediately.
For veterinary use only.
Presentation: Code 68811B - 25 x 1 dose (1 mL) vials with diluent.
® Registered trademark of Biocor Animal Health Inc. U.S.A.
Compendium Code No.: 13940141

RESPOND

Jorgensen **Calcium-Oral**

Active Ingredient(s): Guaranteed mineral content:
Calcium . . . . . 53 g (11.9%)
Magnesium . . . . . 5.54 g (1.24%)
Cobalt. . . . . 0.028 g (0.006%)
Contents: Water, calcium chloride, calcium sulfate, magnesium chloride, hydrated magnesium, aluminum silicates, sodium chloride and cobalt sulfate.
Indications: A calcium and trace mineral supplement for use in the prevention of low blood calcium in the periparturient dairy cow.
Dosage and Administration: Consult a veterinarian before use.
One (1) tube can be given immediately before or after calving, then repeated 12-16 hours later. After regular intravenous treatment, one (1) tube is given 2-3 hours later and again in 12-16 hours.
Dosing: Load the cartridge into a standard dosing gun and remove the protective end cap. Place the nozzle near the back of the oral cavity and empty the tube contents, allowing the cow to swallow.
Caution(s): Exposure to humans can cause irritation to the eyes or open wounds. Flush with warm water if exposed.
Animal Caution: The cow must have a swallowing reflex and normal motility for the product to be effective. The nozzle should be placed near the back of the mouth. Extra care should be taken not to puncture the pharyngeal wall. If a puncture occurs, cease administration and contact a veterinarian.
Presentation: 447 g tube.
Compendium Code No.: 11520130

RESPONSE®

Westfalia•Surge **Udder Wash**

High Detergency-Iodine Based Udder Wash
Active Ingredient(s):
Nonylphenoxypoly (ethyleneoxy) ethanol iodine complex
(provides 1.0% of titratable iodine) 8.2%
Indications: High detergency - iodine based udder wash.
Directions for Use: Prepare an udder wash solution by adding 1 oz (30 mL) of RESPONSE® for each 5 U.S. gallons (19 L) of warm 100-110°F (38-43°C) water. Use a clean single service paper towel for each cow. Soak the towel in the udder wash solution and wash and massage the udder and teats. Never reuse towel or dip used towel back into solution. Thoroughly dry udder and teats with a second single service paper towel. Automatic metering devices used to inject udder wash directly into water should be checked with a test kit to ensure proper proportioning. Solution strength should have a minimum of 12 ppm titratable iodine.
Contraindication(s): Do not use as a teat dip.
Precaution(s): Store RESPONSE® in a cool, dry place. Keep from freezing. If frozen, thaw completely and mix well prior to use. Keep containers closed to prevent contamination.
Warning(s): Danger: Keep out of reach of children. Concentrated product can cause eye damage and skin irritation.
General Chemical Warnings: Always read label directions completely before using product. Always exercise caution when handling any chemicals, avoid contact with eyes, skin and clothing. Never dispense any chemical product from its original container into another container for storage or resale. Never mix two or more products together. Mixing of products could result in release of toxic gases and/or render product ineffective for recommended use application. Always use product in ventilated area. Avoid inhaling vapors or fumes. Always use product according to recommendations for particular application. Never exceed recommended usage without consulting trained personnel.
Protect eyes when handling. Do not get in eyes or on clothing. Harmful if swallowed. Avoid contamination of food.
First Aid:
Eyes: In case of contact with eyes, flush immediately with plenty of water for at least 15 minutes. Call a physician.
Internal: Do not take internally. If swallowed drink promptly large quantities of water. Avoid alcohol. Call a physician.
Presentation: Contact the company for container sizes available.
RESPONSE® is a Registered Trademark of Westfalia•Surge, Inc.
Compendium Code No.: 10020121

RESPONSE II™

Westfalia•Surge **Udder Wash**

High Detergency-Iodine Based Udder Wash
Active Ingredient(s):
Nonylphenoxypoly (ethyleneoxy) ethanol iodine complex
(provides 1.75% of titratable iodine) 13.75%
Indications: High detergency - iodine based udder wash.
Directions for Use: Prepare an udder wash solution by adding 1 oz (30 mL) of RESPONSE II™ for each 10 U.S. gallons (38 L) of warm 100-110°F (38-43°C) water. Use a clean towel in the udder wash solution and wash and massage the udder and teats. Never reuse towel or dip used towel back into solution. Thoroughly dry udder and teats with a second single service paper towel. Automatic metering devices used to inject udder wash directly into water should be checked with a test kit to ensure proper proportioning. Solution strength should have a minimum of 12 ppm titratable iodine. If a concentration of 25 ppm is desired, diluted to a proportion of 1 oz (30 mL) of RESPONSE II™ per 5 gallons (19 L) of water.
Contraindication(s): Do not use as a teat dip.
Precaution(s): Store RESPONSE II™ in a cool, dry place. Keep from freezing. If frozen, thaw completely and mix well prior to use. Keep containers closed to prevent contamination.
Warning(s): Keep out of reach of children.
General Chemical Warnings: Always read label directions completely before using product. Always exercise caution when handling any chemicals, avoid contact with eyes, skin and clothing. Never dispense any chemical product from its original container into another container for storage or resale. Never mix two or more products together. Mixing of products could result in release of toxic gases and/or render product ineffective for recommended use application. Always use product in ventilated area. Avoid inhaling vapors or fumes. Always use product according to recommendations for particular application. Never exceed recommended usage without consulting trained personnel.
Danger: Corrosive. Concentrated product causes eye damage and skin irritation.
Contains phosphoric acid. Protect eyes when handling. Do not get in eyes, on skin, or on clothing. Harmful if swallowed. Avoid contamination of food.
First Aid:
Eyes: In case of contact with eyes, flush immediately with plenty of water for at least 15 minutes. Call a physician.
Skin: Wash promptly. If irritation persists, get medical attention.
Internal: If swallowed, rinse mouth, then drink promptly large quantities of water. Avoid alcohol. Call a physician. Never give anything by mouth to an unconscious person.
Presentation: Contact the company for container sizes available.
Compendium Code No.: 10020111

RESPROMUNE® 4

AgriLabs **Vaccine**

Bovine Rhinotracheitis-Virus Diarrhea-Parainfluenza 3-Respiratory Syncytial Virus Vaccine, Killed Virus
U.S. Vet. Lic. No.: 462
Composition: RESPROMUNE® 4 is an inactivated, multivalent immunogen containing the Cooper strain of IBR; New York and Singer strains of BVD; PI_3 and BRSV.
This product contains gentamicin and amphotericin B as preservatives and is adjuvanted with aluminum hydroxide and *Haemophilus somnus* cultures.
Indications: For use in the vaccination of healthy cattle against disease caused by the organisms represented.
Directions: Shake well. Administer 5 mL intramuscularly or subcutaneously. For initial vaccination, a second dose is required 2-4 weeks later.
RESPROMUNE® 4 may be safely used in pregnant cows at any stage of gestation or very young calves nursing pregnant cows. Calves vaccinated before 6 months of age should be revaccinated

R

at 6 months of age followed by a second dose 2-4 weeks later. Annual revaccination with a single 5 mL dose is recommended.

Precaution(s): Store at 35°F-45°F (2°C-7°C). Do not freeze. Use entire contents when first opened.

Caution(s): In case of anaphylactoid reactions, epinephrine should be administered immediately.

For veterinary use only.

Warning(s): Do not vaccinate within 21 days before slaughter.

Presentation: 10 dose (50 mL) and 50 dose (250 mL) vials.

Manufactured by: Biocor Animal Health Inc., Omaha, NE 68134 U.S.A.

Compendium Code No.: 10581370 AL 1378-499 / AL 1379-499

RESPROMUNE® 4 I-B-P+BRSV

AgriLabs **Vaccine**

Bovine Rhinotracheitis-Virus Diarrhea-Parainfluenza 3-Respiratory Syncytial Virus Vaccine, Killed Virus

U.S. Vet. Lic. No.: 303

Composition: This vaccine contains an IBR virus, a cytopathic Type 1 BVD virus, a noncytopathic Type 2 BVD virus, a PI_3 virus, and a BRS virus propagated on an established bovine cell line. The vaccine is chemically inactivated and adjuvanted with oil. Contains amphotericin B, penicillin, streptomycin, and thimerosal as preservatives.

Indications: For use in healthy cattle as an aid in the prevention of disease caused by infectious bovine rhinotracheitis, bovine virus diarrhea Type 1, bovine virus diarrhea Type 2, parainfluenza Type 3, and bovine respiratory syncytial viruses.

Dosage and Administration: Shake well before using. Administer 5 mL intramuscularly or subcutaneously. Revaccinate in 4-5 weeks. This vaccine may be administered to pregnant animals at any stage of gestation. Vaccinate dairy cows during the dry off period. Revaccinate annually.

Precaution(s): Store in the dark at 35°-45°F (2°-7°C). Do not freeze. Use entire contents when first opened.

Caution(s): Transient swelling may occur at the site of injection. Anaphylactic reactions may occur following the use of this biological. Symptomatic treatment: Epinephrine.

For veterinary use only.

Warning(s): Do not vaccinate within 60 days prior to slaughter.

Presentation: 10 dose (50 mL) and 50 dose (250 mL) vials.

Manufactured by: Agri Lab Biologicals, Inc., St. Joseph, MO 64503

Compendium Code No.: 10580911 AL 198 / AL 199

RESPROMUNE® 4+SOMNUMUNE® (I.M.)

AgriLabs **Bacterin-Vaccine**

Bovine Rhinotracheitis-Virus Diarrhea-Parainfluenza 3-Respiratory Syncytial Virus Vaccine, Killed Virus-Haemophilus Somnus Bacterin

U.S. Vet. Lic. No.: 303

Composition: This product contains an IBR virus, a cytopathic BVD virus, a noncytopathic BVD virus, a PI_3 virus, and a BRS virus propagated on an established bovine cell line and cultures of *Haemophilus somnus.* The product is chemically inactivated and adjuvanted with oil. Contains amphotericin B, penicillin, streptomycin, and thimerosal as preservatives.

Indications: For use in healthy cattle as an aid in the prevention of disease caused by infectious bovine rhinotracheitis, bovine virus diarrhea, parainfluenza Type 3, and bovine respiratory syncytial viruses and *Haemophilus somnus.*

Dosage and Administration: Shake well before using. Administer 5 mL intramuscularly at 3 months of age or older. Revaccinate in 4-5 weeks. This vaccine may be administered to pregnant animals at any stage of gestation. Vaccinate dairy cows during the dry off period. Revaccinate annually.

Precaution(s): Store in the dark at 35°-45°F (2°-7°C). Do not freeze. Use entire contents when first opened.

Caution(s): Transient swelling may occur at the site of injection. Anaphylactic reactions may occur following the use of this biological. Symptomatic treatment: Epinephrine.

For veterinary use only.

Warning(s): Do not vaccinate within 60 days prior to slaughter.

Presentation: 10 dose (50 mL) and 50 dose (250 mL) vials.

Manufactured by: Agri Lab Biologicals, Inc., St. Joseph, MO 64503

Compendium Code No.: 10580901 AL 202

R

RESPROMUNE® 4+SOMNUMUNE® (I.M., S.C.)

AgriLabs **Bacterin-Vaccine**

Bovine Rhinotracheitis-Virus Diarrhea-Parainfluenza 3-Respiratory Syncytial Virus Vaccine, Killed Virus-Haemophilus Somnus Bacterin

U.S. Vet. Lic. No.: 462

Composition: RESPROMUNE® 4+SOMNUMUNE® is an inactivated, multivalent immunogen containing the Cooper strain of IBR; New York and Singer strains of BVD; PI_3 and BRSV in combination with *Haemophilus somnus.*

This product contains gentamicin and amphotericin B as preservatives.

Indications: For use in the vaccination of healthy cattle against disease caused by the organisms represented.

Directions: Shake well. Administer 5 mL intramuscularly or subcutaneously. For initial vaccination, a second dose is required 2-4 weeks later.

RESPROMUNE® 4+SOMNUMUNE® may be safely used in pregnant cows at any stage of gestation or very young calves nursing pregnant cows. Calves vaccinated before 6 months of age should be revaccinated at 6 months of age followed by a second dose 2-4 weeks later. Annual revaccination with a single 5 mL dose is recommended.

Precaution(s): Store at 35°F-45°F (2°C-7°C). Do not freeze. Use entire contents when first opened.

Caution(s): In case of anaphylactoid reactions, epinephrine should be administered immediately.

For veterinary use only.

Warning(s): Do not vaccinate within 21 days before slaughter.

Presentation: 10 dose (50 mL) and 50 dose (250 mL) vials.

Manufactured by: Biocor Animal Health Inc., Omaha, NE 68134 U.S.A.

Compendium Code No.: 10581380 AL 1398-499 / AL 1399-499

RESPROMUNE® 5+VL5

AgriLabs **Bacterin-Vaccine**

Bovine Rhinotracheitis-Virus Diarrhea-Parainfluenza 3-Respiratory Syncytial Virus Vaccine, Killed Virus-Campylobacter Fetus-Leptospira Canicola-Grippotyphosa-Hardjo-Icterohaemorrhagiae-Pomona Bacterin

U.S. Vet. Lic. No.: 303

Composition: This product contains an IBR virus, a cytopathic Type 1 BVD virus, a noncytopathic Type 2 BVD virus, a PI_3 virus, and a BRS virus propagated on an established bovine cell line and cultures of *Campylobacter fetus, Leptospira canicola, grippotyphosa, hardjo, icterohaemorrhagiae* and *pomona.* The product is chemically inactivated and adjuvanted with oil. Contains amphotericin B, gentamicin, and thimerosal as preservatives.

Indications: For use in healthy breeding cattle as an aid in the prevention of disease caused by infectious bovine rhinotracheitis, bovine virus diarrhea Type 1, bovine virus diarrhea Type 2, parainfluenza Type 3, and bovine respiratory syncytial viruses and *Campylobacter fetus, Leptospira canicola, grippotyphosa, hardjo, icterohaemorrhagiae,* and *pomona.*

Dosage and Administration: Shake well before using. Administer 5 mL intramuscularly 2-4 weeks prior to breeding. Revaccinate with ResProMune® 5 IBP+BRSV (Bovine Rhinotracheitis-Virus Diarrhea-Parainfluenza 3-Respiratory Syncytial Virus Vaccine) in 4-5 weeks. Revaccinate annually.

Precaution(s): Store in the dark at 35°-45°F (2°-7°C). Do not freeze. Use entire contents when first opened.

Caution(s): Transient swelling may occur at the site of injection. Milk reduction and transient depression may be observed in lactating dairy cows for 3-6 days following vaccination. Anaphylactic reactions may occur following the use of this biological. Symptomatic treatment: Epinephrine.

For veterinary use only.

Warning(s): Do not vaccinate within 60 days prior to slaughter.

Presentation: 10 dose (50 mL) and 50 dose (250 mL) vials.

Manufactured by: Agri Lab Biologicals, Inc., St. Joseph, MO 64503

Compendium Code No.: 10580881 AL 153 / AL 154

RESPROMUNE® 8

AgriLabs **Bacterin-Vaccine**

Bovine Rhinotracheitis-Virus Diarrhea-Parainfluenza 3 Vaccine, Killed Virus-Leptospira Canicola-Grippotyphosa-Hardjo-Icterohaemorrhagiae-Pomona Bacterin

U.S. Vet. Lic. No.: 462

Composition: RESPROMUNE® 8 is an inactivated, multivalent immunogen containing the Cooper strain of IBR; New York and Singer strains of BVD; and PI_3 in combination with the Leptospira serovars represented.

This product contains gentamicin and amphotericin B as preservatives and is adjuvanted with aluminum hydroxide and *Haemophilus somnus* cultures.

Indications: For use in the vaccination of healthy cattle against disease caused by the organisms represented.

Directions: Shake well. Administer 5 mL intramuscularly or subcutaneously. For initial vaccination, a second dose is required 2-4 weeks later.

RESPROMUNE® 8 may be safely used in pregnant cows at any stage of gestation or very young calves nursing pregnant cows. Calves vaccinated before 6 months of age should be revaccinated at 6 months of age followed by a second dose 2-4 weeks later. Annual revaccination with a single 5 mL dose is recommended.

Precaution(s): Store at 35°F-45°F (2°C-7°C). Do not freeze. Use entire contents when first opened.

Caution(s): In case of anaphylactoid reactions, epinephrine should be administered immediately.

For veterinary use only.

Warning(s): Do not vaccinate within 21 days before slaughter.

Presentation: 50 mL (10 dose) and 250 mL (50 dose) vials.

Manufactured by: Biocor Animal Health Inc., Omaha, NE 68134 U.S.A.

Compendium Code No.: 10580921 AL 1358-499 / AL 1359-499

RESPROMUNE™ 9

AgriLabs **Bacterin-Vaccine**

Bovine Rhinotracheitis-Virus Diarrhea-Parainfluenza 3-Respiratory Syncytial Virus Vaccine-Leptospira canicola-grippotyphosa-hardjo-icterohaemorrhagiae-pomona Bacterin, Killed Virus

U.S. Vet. Lic. No.: 272

Active Ingredient(s): RESPROMUNE™ 9 is an inactivated, multivalent immunogen containing bovine rhinotracheitis (IBR), virus diarrhea (BVD), parainfluenza-3 (PI_3), respiratory syncytial virus (BRSV) vaccine and *Leptospira canicola, L. grippotyphosa, L. hardjo, L. icterohaemorrhagiae* and *L. pomona.*

The product contains gentamicin and amphotericin B as preservatives and is adjuvanted with aluminum hydroxide and *Haemophilus somnus* cultures.

Indications: RESPROMUNE™ 9 is for use in the vaccination of healthy cattle against diseases caused by IBR, BVD, PI_3 and BRSV viruses, and the Leptospira serovars represented.

Dosage and Administration: Shake well. Administer 5 mL intramuscularly or subcutaneously to healthy cattle of any age. For initial immunization, a second dose is required two (2) to four (4) weeks later.

RESPROMUNE™ 9 may be safely used in pregnant cows at any stage of gestation or in very young animals nursing pregnant cows. Calves vaccinated before six (6) months of age should be revaccinated at six (6) months of age or older followed by a second dose two (2) to four (4) weeks later. Annual revaccination with a single 5 mL dose is recommended.

Precaution(s): Store at 35°-45°F (2°-7°C). Do not freeze.

Caution(s): Use the entire contents when first opened. In case of anaphylactic reactions, epinephrine should be administered immediately.

Warning(s): Do not vaccinate within 21 days before slaughter.

Presentation: 50 mL (10 dose) and 250 mL (50 dose) vials.

Compendium Code No.: 10580930

RESPROMUNE™ 10

AgriLabs **Bacterin-Vaccine**

Bovine Rhinotracheitis-Virus Diarrhea-Parainfluenza 3-Respiratory Syncytial Virus Vaccine, Killed Virus-Haemophilus somnus-Leptospira canicola-grippotyphosa-hardjo-icterohaemorrhagiae-pomona Bacterin

U.S. Vet. Lic. No.: 272

Active Ingredient(s): RESPROMUNE™ 10 is an inactivated, multivalent immunogen containing bovine rhinotracheitis (IBR), virus diarrhea (BVD), parainfluenza-3 (PI_3), respiratory syncytial virus (BRSV) vaccine and *Haemophilus somnus* and *Leptospira canicola, L. grippotyphosa, L. hardjo, L. icterohaemorrhagiae* and *L. pomona.*

The product contains gentamicin and amphotericin B as preservatives.

Indications: RESPROMUNE™ 10 is recommended for use in the vaccination of healthy cattle against disease caused by IBR, BVD, PI_3 and BRSV viruses, and *H. somnus* the Leptospira serovars represented.

Dosage and Administration: Shake well. Administer 5 mL intramuscularly or subcutaneously to healthy cattle. For initial immunization, a second dose is required two (2) to four (4) weeks later.

RESPROMUNE™ 10 may be safely used in pregnant cows at any stage of gestation or in very young animals nursing pregnant cows. Calves vaccinated before six (6) months of age should be revaccinated at six (6) months of age or older followed by a second dose two (2) to four (4) weeks later. Annual revaccination with a single 5 mL dose is recommended.

Precaution(s): Store at 35°-45°F (2°-7°C). Do not freeze.

Caution(s): Use the entire contents when first opened. In case of anaphylactic reactions, epinephrine should be administered immediately.

Warning(s): Do not vaccinate within 21 days before slaughter.

Presentation: 50 mL (10 dose) and 250 mL (50 dose) vials.

Compendium Code No.: 10580891

RESVAC® 4/SOMUBAC®

Pfizer Animal Health **Bacterin-Vaccine**

Bovine Rhinotracheitis-Virus Diarrhea-Parainfluenza$_3$-Respiratory Syncytial Virus Vaccine, Modified Live Virus-Haemophilus somnus Bacterin

U.S. Vet. Lic. No.: 189

Description: RESVAC® 4/SOMUBAC® consists of a standardized combination of freeze-dried, attenuated strains of IBR, BVD, PI_3, and BRSV viruses propagated in stable cell lines; accompanied by liquid, inactivated, standardized *Haemophilus somnus* bacterin diluent. Somubac® is prepared from selected strains of *Haemophilus somnus* which are grown serum-free in an environmentally controlled fermentation system and inactivated in such a manner as to maintain their immunogenic integrity. The bacterin is adjuvanted with aluminum hydroxide. The vaccine viruses are produced under the precisely controlled conditions of Pfizer Animal Health's Frozen Stable Cell Bank™ system. The use of this special cell system in producing Resvac® 4 ensures freedom from potentially harmful adventitious agents. The vaccine viruses are blended with a special stabilizer and presented in freeze-dried form. The product is tested for purity, safety, potency, and efficacy in accordance with the regulations of the United States Department of Agriculture.

Contains polymyxin B and neomycin as preservatives.

Indications: RESVAC® 4/SOMUBAC® is for vaccination of healthy, nonpregnant cattle as an aid in preventing infectious bovine rhinotracheitis caused by infectious bovine rhinotracheitis (IBR) virus, bovine viral diarrhea caused by bovine viral diarrhea (BVD) virus, and disease caused by parainfluenza-3 (PI_3) virus, bovine respiratory syncytial virus (BRSV), and *Haemophilus somnus.*

Directions:

1. General Directions: Vaccination of healthy, nonpregnant cattle is recommended. Aseptically rehydrate the freeze-dried vaccine with the liquid bacterin provided, shake well, and administer 2 mL intramuscularly. In accordance with Beef Quality Assurance guidelines, this product should be administered in the muscular region of the neck.
2. Primary Vaccination: Administer a single 2-mL dose to healthy, nonpregnant cattle 3 months of age or older, followed by a second dose of Resvac® BRSV/Somubac® 2-4 weeks later.
3. Revaccination: Annual revaccination with a single dose is recommended. Calves with maternal antibodies may not develop or maintain satisfactory levels of immunity; therefore, calves vaccinated before 6 months of age should be revaccinated at 6 months of age or at weaning.
4. Good animal husbandry and herd health management practices should be employed.

Precaution(s): Store at 2°-7°C. Prolonged exposure to higher temperatures and/or direct sunlight may adversely affect potency. Do not freeze.

Use entire contents when first opened.

Sterilized syringes and needles should be used to administer this vaccine. Do not sterilize with chemicals because traces of disinfectant may inactivate the vaccine.

Burn containers and all unused contents.

Caution(s): Do not use in pregnant cows (abortions can result) or in calves nursing pregnant cows.

As with many vaccines, anaphylaxis may occur after use. Initial antidote of epinephrine is recommended and should be followed with appropriate supportive therapy.

This product has been shown to be efficacious in healthy animals. A protective immune response may not be elicited if animals are incubating an infectious disease, are malnourished or parasitized, are stressed due to shipment or environmental conditions, are otherwise immunocompromised, or the vaccine is not administered in accordance with label directions.

Warning(s): Do not vaccinate within 21 days before slaughter.

For veterinary use only.

Discussion: Disease Description: IBR, commonly known as "red nose" disease, is a mild to very acute inflammation of the upper respiratory tract in cattle. Infection with IBR virus may result in the following syndromes: a respiratory form, abortion, encephalitis, conjunctivitis, enteritis, and genital infections.

BVD infection can cause a variety of clinical signs in cattle, including fever, mild to severe leukopenia, lacrimation, corneal opacity, various respiratory related signs, mucosal disease, diarrhea, and abortion. Subclinical infection is common and may predispose animals to subsequent respiratory or enteric disease.

Parainfluenza is an upper respiratory infection in cattle characterized by fever, mild leukopenia, serous nasal discharge, coughing, and lacrimation. The causative virus, PI_3, is often isolated and recognized as a predisposing infection in shipping fever and as a complicating entity in outbreaks of pasteurellosis, IBR, BVD, and BRSV disease. The infection may be mild or inapparent or frequently may be concurrent with other bacterial and viral agents.

Laboratory diagnosis of BRSV has proven difficult, and only recently has it gained recognition as an important component of the bovine respiratory disease complex. As a causative agent, the virus is a pathogen of the lower respiratory tract with characteristic clinical signs of serous nasal discharge, coughing, lacrimation, and pyrexia. Subclinical infections can occur and have been shown to predispose cattle to secondary bacterial infections. Based on antibody prevalence, approximately ⅔ of all herds, both beef and dairy, have been exposed. Exacerbation of clinical signs has been documented when concurrent BRSV and BVD or IBR infection exists.

Diseases associated with *Haemophilus somnus* are widespread and occur sporadically in beef and dairy cattle populations. Several disease manifestations are observed. In the respiratory form, the infected animal develops an acute fibrinous pneumonia and pleuritis. The disease may become septicemic, with the involvement of most tissues and organs. A temperature response from 106°-108°F is common. If death does not occur, the animal becomes a poor weight gainer, and may develop other signs such as arthritis, knuckling, and a dry, hacking cough. Another disease manifestation resulting from septicemia is infectious thromboembolic meningoencephalitis (TEME), which can occur without any obvious respiratory involvement. The septicemia may lead to vasculitis and thrombosis, and disease can be expressed in several syndromes. Many times the first sign of the disease is finding dead cattle. Early signs are stiffness, listlessness, and high temperatures. Circling may occur with abnormal eye movements, along with muscular tremors due to CNS involvement. Death occurs in a few hours in acute cases.

Haemophilus somnus has also been incriminated in reproductive disorders of beef and dairy cattle.

Trial Data: Experimental studies have shown that transmission of the vaccinal BVD virus from 27 vaccinated cattle to 9 susceptible contact controls (including 4 pregnant cows) did not occur.

Purity—The master seed viruses were purified using the latest available procedures to assure the highest degree of purity. The master cell stocks were prepared and pretested for use in vaccine production. The master cell stocks and master seed viruses were found to be negative for bacteria, fungi, mycoplasma, and adventitious viruses.

Safety and Efficacy: Studies in cattle show RESVAC® 4/SOMUBAC® to be safe and free from untoward reactions. This product was field tested in thousands of cattle by practicing veterinarians. No undesirable effects attributable to the product were noted. Vaccination/challenge studies in cattle showed each fraction contained in Resvac® 4 to be effective as an aid in the prevention of disease caused by IBR, BVD, PI_3 and BRSV viruses. Cattle vaccinated with Somubac® were protected against challenge with a highly virulent strain of *Haemophilus somnus.* Antigen interference studies in cattle show each fraction of the RESVAC® 4/SOMUBAC® combination to be compatible.

Presentation: 10 dose and 50 dose vials.

Compendium Code No.: 36900200

75-4308-05

RESVAC® BRSV/SOMUBAC®

Pfizer Animal Health **Bacterin-Vaccine**

Bovine Respiratory Syncytial Virus Vaccine, Modified Live Virus-Haemophilus Somnus Bacterin

U.S. Vet. Lic. No.: 189

Description: RESVAC® BRSV/SOMUBAC® consists of a standardized, freeze-dried, attenuated strain of BRSV propagated in a stable cell line; accompanied by liquid, inactivated, standardized *Haemophilus somnus* bacterin diluent. Somubac® is prepared from selected strains of *Haemophilus somnus* which are grown serum-free in an environmentally controlled fermentation system and inactivated in such a manner as to maintain their immunogenic integrity. The bacterin is adjuvanted with aluminum hydroxide. The vaccine virus is produced under the precisely controlled conditions of Pfizer Animal Health's Frozen Stable Cell Bank™ system. The use of this special cell system in producing Resvac® BRSV ensures freedom from potentially harmful adventitious agents. The vaccine virus is blended with a special stabilizer and presented in freeze-dried form. The product is tested for purity, safety, potency, and efficacy in accordance with the regulations of the United States Department of Agriculture.

Contains polymyxin B and neomycin as preservatives.

Indications: RESVAC® BRSV/SOMUBAC® is for vaccination of healthy cattle as an aid in preventing disease caused by bovine respiratory syncytial virus (BRSV) and *Haemophilus somnus.*

Directions:

1. General Directions: Vaccination of healthy cattle is recommended. Aseptically rehydrate the freeze-dried vaccine with the liquid bacterin provided, shake well, and administer 2 mL intramuscularly. In accordance with Beef Quality Assurance guidelines, this product should be administered in the muscular region of the neck.
2. Primary Vaccination: Administer a single 2-mL dose to healthy cattle 3 months of age or older, followed by a second dose 2-4 weeks later.
3. Revaccination: Annual revaccination with a single dose is recommended. Calves with maternal antibodies may not develop or maintain satisfactory levels of immunity; therefore, calves vaccinated before 6 months of age should be revaccinated at 6 months of age or at weaning.
4. Good animal husbandry and herd health management practices should be employed.

Precaution(s): Store at 2°-7°C. Prolonged exposure to higher temperatures and/or direct sunlight may adversely affect potency. Do not freeze.

Use entire contents when first opened.

Sterilized syringes and needles should be used to administer this vaccine. Do not sterilize with chemicals because traces of disinfectant may inactivate the vaccine.

Burn containers and all unused contents.

Caution(s): Safety of this vaccine for use in pregnant cattle has not been established.

As with many vaccines, anaphylaxis may occur after use. Initial antidote of epinephrine is recommended and should be followed with appropriate supportive therapy.

This product has been shown to be efficacious in healthy animals. A protective immune response may not be elicited if animals are incubating an infectious disease, are malnourished or parasitized, are stressed due to shipment or environmental conditions, are otherwise immunocompromised, or the vaccine is not administered in accordance with label directions.

Warning(s): Do not vaccinate within 21 days before slaughter.

For veterinary use only.

Discussion: Disease Description: Laboratory diagnosis of BRSV has proven difficult, and only recently has it gained recognition as an important component of the bovine respiratory disease complex. As a causative agent, the virus is a pathogen of the lower respiratory tract with characteristic clinical signs of serous nasal discharge, coughing, lacrimation, and pyrexia. Subclinical infections can occur and have been shown to predispose cattle to secondary bacterial infections. Based on antibody prevalence, approximately ⅔ of all herds, both beef and dairy, have been exposed. Exacerbation of clinical signs has been documented when concurrent BRSV and BVD or IBR infection exists.

Diseases associated with *Haemophilus somnus* are widespread and occur sporadically in beef and dairy cattle populations. Several disease manifestations are observed. In the respiratory form, the infected animal develops an acute fibrinous pneumonia and pleuritis. The disease may become septicemic, with the involvement of most tissues and organs. A temperature response

R

from 106°-108°F is common. If death does not occur, the animal becomes a poor weight gainer, and may develop other signs such as arthritis, knuckling, and a dry, hacking cough.

Another disease manifestation resulting from septicemia is infectious thromboembolic meningoencephalitis (TEME), which can occur without any obvious respiratory involvement. The septicemia may lead to vasculitis and thrombosis, and disease can be expressed in several syndromes. Many times the first sign of the disease is finding dead cattle. Early signs are stiffness, listlessness, and high temperatures. Circling may occur with abnormal eye movements, along with muscular tremors due to CNS involvement. Death occurs in a few hours in acute cases.

Haemophilus somnus has also been incriminated in reproductive disorders of beef and dairy cattle.

Trial Data: Purity—The master seed virus was purified using the latest available procedures to assure the highest degree of purity. The master cell stock was prepared and pretested for use in vaccine production. The master cell stock and master seed virus were found to be negative for bacteria, fungi, mycoplasma, and adventitious viruses.

Safety and Efficacy: Studies in cattle show RESVAC® BRSV/SOMUBAC® to be safe and free from untoward reactions. This product was field tested in hundreds of cattle by practicing veterinarians. No undesirable effects attributable to the product were noted. Vaccination/challenge studies in cattle showed Resvac® BRSV to be effective as an aid in the prevention of disease caused BRSV. Cattle vaccinated with Somubac® were protected against challenge with a highly virulent strain of *Haemophilus somnus.* Antigen interference studies in cattle show each fraction of the RESVAC® BRSV/SOMUBAC® combination to be compatible.

Presentation: 1 x 10 dose or 1 x 50 dose vials with diluent.

75-4314-05

Compendium Code No.: 36900210

REVALOR®-200

Intervet **Implant**

(trenbolone acetate and estradiol)

NADA No.: 140-992

Active Ingredient(s): Description: REVALOR®-200 (trenbolone acetate, CAS Registry Number 10161-34-9, and estradiol, CAS Registry Number 50-28-2) is an implant containing 200 mg of trenbolone acetate and 20 mg estradiol. Each implant consists of 10 small yellow pellets. Ten implants are provided in a cartridge.

Manufactured by a non-sterilizing process.

Indications: This product contains trenbolone acetate and estradiol in a slow-release delivery system which increases rate of weight gain and improves feed efficiency in steers and heifers fed in confinement for slaughter.

Note: REVALOR®-200 is not better for increased average daily gain or improved feed efficiency than Revalor®-H (140 mg trenbolone acetate/14 mg estradiol) in heifers fed in confinement for slaughter.

Studies have demonstrated that the administration of REVALOR®-200 can result in decreased marbling scores when compared to non-implanted steers.

Dosage and Administration: Dosage Form: One implant containing 200 mg trenbolone acetate and 20 mg estradiol is administered to each animal. The 10 pellets which make up the dosage of REVALOR®-200 are contained in one division of the multiple dose cartridge. Ten doses are in each cartridge. The cartridge is designed to be used with a special implant gun.

Route of Administration: The implant is placed under the skin on the posterior aspect of the ear by means of a special implanter available from Intervet, Inc.

With the animal suitably restrained, the skin on the outer surface of the ear should be cleaned. The implant is then administered by the method shown in the diagram below.

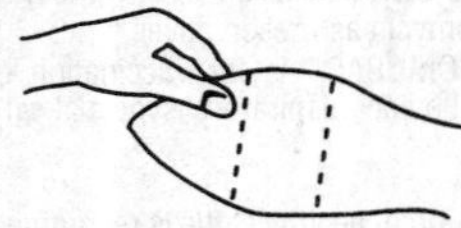

Fig. 1 - Ear of Bovine Ready for Implantation

Site of Implantation: After appropriately restraining the animal to allow access to the ear, cleanse the skin at the implant needle puncture site. It is subcutaneous between the skin and cartilage on the back of the ear and below the midline of the ear.

The implant must not be placed closer to the head than the edge of the cartilage ring farthest from the head.

The location of insertion of the needle is a point toward the tip of the ear and at least a needle length away from the intended deposition site. Care should be taken to avoid injuring the major blood vessels or cartilage of the ear.

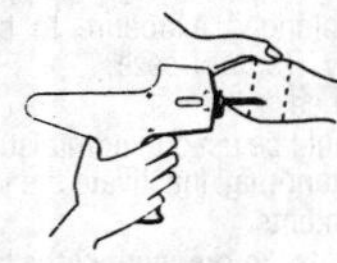

Fig. 2 - Rear View of the Bovine Ear Showing the Site for Insertion of the Implanter Needle.

Method of Use:

1. Do not remove the cap of the cartridge containing the implants.
2. Place the cartridge (with the capped end to the front) into slot at the top of the implanter magazine.
3. Gently push the cartridge into the slot until it clicks into place.
4. The implanter is then ready for use.
5. Take the ear of the animal firmly with the free hand (in the manner shown in Fig. 1). Then insert the needle into the subcutaneous tissue at the point indicated (in Fig. 2).
6. After inserting the needle to its full extent, squeeze the trigger gradually. Allow the pellets of the implant to be deposited in a single row.
7. Withdraw the implanter. This will advance the cartridge one groove in the magazine and the next implant is now ready for use.
8. When all the implants have been administered, the cartridge will fall out the bottom of the magazine and may be replaced by a new one.
9. To change the needle, loosen the needle locking nut and replace the needle. Tighten the nut finger tight and implanter is ready for use.

Precaution(s): Storage Conditions: Store in a refrigerator (2-8°C; 36-47°F) and protect from sunlight. Use before the expiration date printed on the cartridge.

Caution(s): For animal treatment only.

Implant pellets in the ear only. Any other location is in violation of Federal Law.

Warning(s): Not to be used in animals intended for subsequent breeding, or in dairy animals.

Not for use in humans.

Do not attempt salvage of implanted site for human or animal food.

Presentation: Box of 10 x 10 cartridge implants.

Compendium Code No.: 11062571 482220-A

REVALOR®-G

Intervet **Implant**

(trenbolone acetate and estradiol)

NADA No.: 140-897

Active Ingredient(s): REVALOR®-G is an implant containing 40 mg of trenbolone acetate and 8 mg estradiol.

Indications: Increases rate of weight gain in pasture cattle (slaughter, stocker and feeder steers and heifers.) in a slow-release delivery system.

Dosage and Administration: Dosage Form: One implant containing 40 mg trenbolone acetate and 8 mg estradiol is administered to each animal. The 2 pellets which make up the dosage of REVALOR®-G are contained in one division of the multiple dose cartridge. Ten doses are in each cartridge. The cartridge is designed to be used with a special implant gun.

Route of Administration: The implant is placed under the skin on the posterior aspect of the ear by means of a special implanter available from Intervet Inc. With the animal suitably restrained, the skin on the outer surface of the ear should be cleaned. The implant is then administered by the method shown in the diagram below.

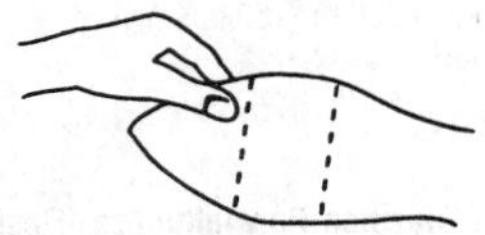

Fig. 1 - Ear of Bovine Ready for Implantation

Site of Implantation: After appropriately restraining the animal to allow access to the ear, cleanse the skin at the implant needle puncture site. It is subcutaneous between the skin and cartilage on the back side of the ear and below the midline of the ear. The implant must not be placed closer to the head than the edge of the cartilage ring farthest from the head. The location of insertion of the needle is a point toward the tip of the ear and at least a needle length away from the intended deposition site. Care should be taken to avoid injuring the major blood vessels or cartilage of the ear.

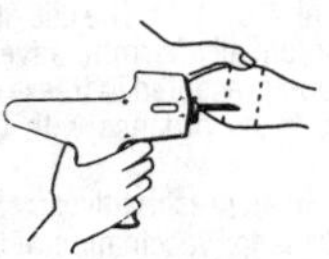

Fig. 2 - Rear View of the Bovine Ear Showing the Site for Insertion of the Implanter Needle.

Method of Use:

1. Do not remove the cap of the cartridge containing the implants.
2. Place the cartridge (with the capped end to the front) into slot at the top of the implanter magazine.
3. Gently push the cartridge into the slot until it clicks into place.
4. The implanter is then ready for use.
5. Take the ear of the animal firmly with the free hand in the manner shown in Fig. 1. Then insert the needle into the subcutaneous tissue at the point indicated in Fig. 2.
6. After inserting the needle to its full extent, squeeze the trigger gradually. Allow the pellets of the implant to be deposited in a single row.
7. Withdraw the implanter. This will advance the cartridge one groove in the magazine and the next implant is now ready for use.
8. When all the implants have been administered, the cartridge will fall out of the bottom of the magazine and may be replaced by a new one.
9. To change the needle, loosen the needle locking nut and replace the needle. Tighten the nut finger tight and the implanter is ready for use.

Precaution(s): Storage Conditions: Store in refrigerator (2-8°C; 36-47°F) and protect from sunlight. Use before the expiration date printed on the cartridge.

Warning(s): Not to be used in animals intended for subsequent breeding, or in dairy animals. For animal treatment only. Not for use in humans. Implant pellets in the ear only. Any other location may result in violation of Federal Law. Do not attempt salvage of implanted site for human or animal food.

Presentation: Box of 10 x 10 cartridge implants. Each implant consists of 2 small yellow pellets. Ten implants are provided in a cartridge.

Compendium Code No.: 11061641 781200-B

REVALOR®-H

Intervet **Implant**

(trenbolone acetate and estradiol)

NADA No.: 140-992

Active Ingredient(s): REVALOR®-H is an implant containing 140 mg of trenbolone acetate and 14 mg of estradiol.

Manufactured by a non-sterilizing process.

Indications: Increases rate of weight gain and improved feed efficiency in a slow-release delivery system. For heifers fed in confinement for slaughter.

Note: Studies have demonstrated that the administration of REVALOR®-H can result in decreased marbling scores when compared to non-implanted heifers.

Dosage and Administration: Dosage Form: One implant containing 140 mg trenbolone acetate and 14 mg estradiol is administered to each animal. The 7 pellets which make up the dosage of REVALOR®-H are contained in one division of the multiple dose cartridge. Ten doses are in each cartridge. The cartridge is designed to be used with a special implant gun.

Route of Administration: The implant is placed under the skin on the posterior aspect of the ear by means of a special implanter available from Intervet Inc.

With the animal suitably restrained, the skin on the outer surface of the ear should be cleaned. The implant is then administered by the method shown in the diagram below.

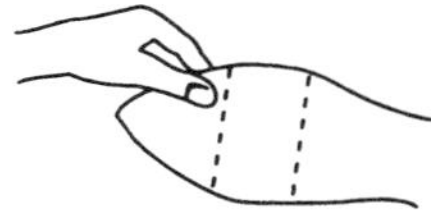

Fig. 1 - Ear of Bovine Ready for implantation

Site of Implantation: After appropriately restraining the animal to allow access to the ear, cleanse the skin at the implant needle puncture site. It is subcutaneous between the skin and cartilage on the back of the ear and below the midline of the ear.

The implant must not be placed closer to the head than the edge of the cartilage ring farthest from the head. The location of insertion of the needle is a point toward the tip of the ear and at least a needle length away from the intended deposition site. Care should be taken to avoid injuring the major blood vessels or cartilage of the ear.

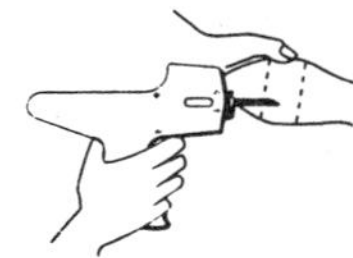

Fig. 2 - Rear View of the Bovine Ear Showing the Site for Insertion of the Implanter Needle.

Method of Use:

1. Do not remove the cap of the cartridge containing the implants.
2. Place the cartridge (with the capped end to the front) into slot at the top of the implanter magazine.
3. Gently push the cartridge into the slot until it clicks into place.
4. The implanter is then ready for use.
5. Take the ear of the animal firmly with the free hand in the manner shown in Fig. 1. Then insert the needle into the subcutaneous tissue at the point indicated in Fig. 2.
6. After inserting the needle to its full extent, squeeze the trigger gradually. Allow the pellets of the implant to be deposited in a single row.
7. Withdraw the implanter. This will advance the cartridge one groove in the magazine and the next implant is now ready for use.
8. When all the implants have been administered, the cartridge will discharge out the bottom of the magazine and may be replaced by a new one.
9. To change the needle, loosen the needle locking nut and replace the needle. Tighten the nut finger tight and implanter is ready for use.

Precaution(s): Storage Conditions: Store in a refrigerator (2-8°C; 36-47°F) and protect from sunlight. Use before the expiration date printed on the box and on the cartridge.

Warning(s): Not to be used in animals intended for subsequent breeding, or in dairy animals. For animal treatment only. Not for use in humans. Implant pellets in the ear only. Any other location is in violation of Federal Law. Do not attempt salvage of implanted site for human or animal food.

Presentation: Box of 10 x 10 cartridge implants. Each implant consists of 7 small yellow pellets. Ten implants are provided in a cartridge.

Compendium Code No.: 11061651 781000-B

REVALOR®-IH

Intervet **Implant**

(trenbolone acetate and estradiol)

NADA No.: 140-992

Active Ingredient(s): Description: REVALOR®-IH is an implant containing 80 mg of trenbolone acetate and 8 mg of estradiol. Each implant consists of 4 small yellow pallets. Ten implants are provided in a cartridge.

Manufactured by a non-sterilizing process.

Indications: Increases rate of weight gain in a slow-release delivery system.

For heifers fed in confinement for slaughter.

Dosage and Administration: Dosage Form: One implant containing 80 mg trenbolone acetate and 8 mg estradiol is administered to each animal. The 4 pellets which make up the dosage of REVALOR®-IH are contained in one division of the multiple dose cartridge. Ten doses are in each cartridge. The cartridge is designed to be used with a special implant gun.

Route of Administration: The implant is placed under the skin on the posterior aspect of the ear by means of a special implanter available from Intervet, Inc.

With the animal suitably restrained, the skin on the outer surface of the ear should be cleaned. The implant is then administered by the method shown in the diagram below.

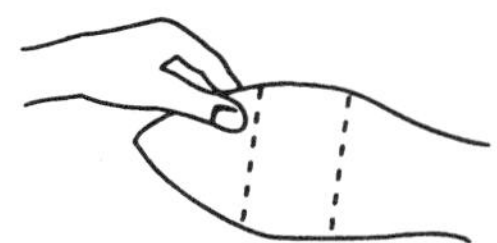

Fig. 1 - Ear of Bovine Ready for Implantation

Site of Implantation: After appropriately restraining the animal to allow access to the ear, cleanse the skin at the implant needle puncture site. It is subcutaneous between the skin and cartilage on the back of the ear and below the midline of the ear.

The implant must not be placed closer to the head than the edge of the cartilage ring farthest from the head.

The location of insertion of the needle is a point toward the tip of the ear and at least a needle length away from the intended deposition site. Care should be taken to avoid injuring the major blood vessels or cartilage of the ear.

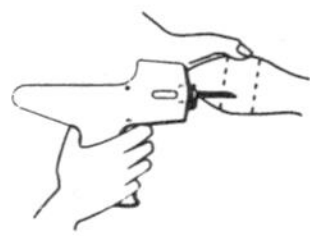

Fig. 2 - Rear View of the Bovine Ear Showing the Site for Insertion of the Implanter Needle.

Method of Use:

1. Do not remove the cap of the cartridge containing the implants.
2. Place the cartridge (with the capped end to the front) into slot at the top of the implanter magazine.
3. Gently push the cartridge into the slot until it clicks into place.
4. The implanter is then ready for use.
5. Take the ear of the animal firmly with the free hand in the manner shown in Fig. 1. Then insert the needle into the subcutaneous tissue at the point indicated in Fig. 2.
6. After inserting the needle to its full extent, squeeze the trigger gradually. Allow the pellets of the implant to be deposited in a single row.
7. Withdraw the implanter. This will advance the cartridge one groove in the magazine and the next implant is now ready for use.
8. When all the implants have been administered, the cartridge will discharge out the bottom of the magazine and may be replaced by a new one.
9. To change the needle, loosen the needle locking nut and replace the needle. Tighten the nut finger tight and implanter is ready for use.

Precaution(s): Storage Conditions: Store in refrigerator (2-8°C; 36-47°F) and protect from sunlight. Use before the expiration date printed on the cartridge.

Caution(s): For animal treatment only. Implant pellets in the ear only, any other location is in violation of Federal Law.

Warning(s): Not to be used in animals intended for subsequent breeding, or in dairy animals.

Not for use in humans.

Do not attempt salvage of implanted site for human or animal food.

Trial Data: Note: Studies have demonstrated that the administration of REVALOR®-IH can result in decreased marbling scores when compared to non-implanted heifers.

Presentation: Box of 10 x 10 cartridge implants.

Compendium Code No.: 11062580

REVALOR®-IS

Intervet **Implant**

(trenbolone acetate and estradiol)

NADA No.: 140-897

Active Ingredient(s): Description: REVALOR®-IS (trenbolone acetate and estradiol) is an implant containing 80 mg of trenbolone acetate and 16 mg estradiol. Each implant consists of 4 small yellow pellets. Ten implants are provided in a cartridge.

Manufactured by a non-sterilizing process.

Indications: Increases rate of weight gain and improves feed efficiency in a slow-release delivery system.

For steers fed in confinement for slaughter.

Dosage and Administration: Dosage Form: One implant containing 80 mg trenbolone acetate and 16 mg estradiol is administered to each animal. The 4 pellets which make up the dosage of REVALOR®-IS are contained in one division of the multiple dose cartridge. Ten doses are in each cartridge. The cartridge is designed to be used with a special implant gun.

Route of Administration: The implant is placed under the skin on the posterior aspect of the ear by means of a special implanter available from Intervet, Inc.

With the animal suitably restrained, the skin on the outer surface of the ear should be cleaned. The implant is then administered by the method shown in the diagram below.

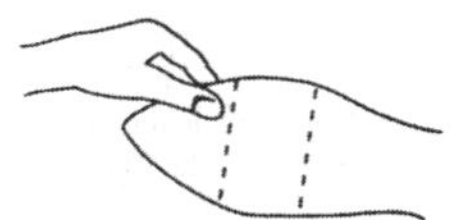

Fig. 1 - Ear of Bovine Ready for Implantation

Site of Implantation: After appropriately restraining the animal to allow access to the ear, cleanse the skin at the implant needle puncture site. It is subcutaneous, between the skin and cartilage on the back side of the ear and below the midline of the ear.

The implant must not be placed closer to the head than the edge of the cartilage ring farthest from the head.

The location of insertion of the needle is a point toward the tip of the ear and at least a needle length away from the intended deposition site. Care should be taken to avoid injuring the major blood vessels or cartilage of the ear.

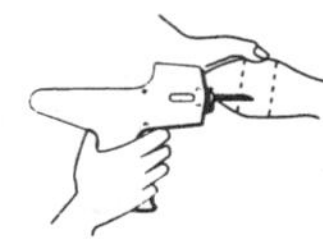

Fig. 2 - Rear View of the Bovine Ear Showing the Site for Insertion of the Implanter Needle.

Method of Use:

1. Do not remove the cap of the cartridge containing the implants.
2. Place the cartridge (with the capped end to the front) into slot at the top of the implanter magazine.
3. Gently push the cartridge into the slot until it clicks into place.
4. The implanter is then ready to use.
5. Take the ear of the animal firmly with the free hand in the manner shown in Fig. 1. Then insert the needle into the subcutaneous tissue at the point indicated in Fig. 2.
6. After inserting the needle to its full extent, squeeze the trigger gradually. Allow the pellets of the implant to be deposited in a single row.
7. Withdraw the implanter. This will advance the cartridge one groove in the magazine and the next implant is now ready for use.

R

8. When all the implants have been administered, the cartridge will discharge out of the bottom of the magazine and may be replaced by a new one.
9. To change the needle, loosen the needle locking nut and replace the needle. Tighten the nut finger tight and the implanter is ready to use.

Precaution(s): Storage Conditions: Store in a refrigerator (2-8°C; 36-47°F) and protect from sunlight. Use before the expiration date printed on the box and on the cartridge.

Caution(s): For animal treatment only. Implant pellets in the ear only, any other location is in violation of Federal Law.

Warning(s): Not to be used in animals intended for subsequent breeding, or in dairy animals.

Not for use in humans.

Do not attempt salvage of implanted site for human or animal food.

Trial Data: Note: Studies have demonstrated that the administration of REVALOR®-IS can result in decreased marbling scores when compared to non-implanted steers.

Presentation: Box of 10 x 10 cartridge implants.

Compendium Code No.: 11062590

REVALOR®-S

Intervet **Implant**

(trenbolone acetate and estradiol)

NADA No.: 140-897

Active Ingredient(s): REVALOR®-S (trenbolone acetate and estradiol) is an implant containing 120 mg of trenbolone acetate and 24 mg estradiol.

Manufactured by a non-sterilizing process.

Indications: Increases rate of weight gain and improves feed efficiency in a slow-release delivery system for steers fed in confinement for slaughter.

Note: Studies have demonstrated that the administration of REVALOR®-S can result in decreased marbling scores when compared to non-implanted steers.

Dosage and Administration: Dosage Form: One implant containing 120 mg trenbolone acetate and 24 mg estradiol is administered to each animal. The 6 pellets which make up the dosage of REVALOR®-S are contained in one division of the multiple dose cartridge. Ten doses are in each cartridge. The cartridge is designed to be used with a special implant gun.

Route of Administration: The implant is placed under the skin on the posterior aspect of the ear by means of a special implanter available from Intervet Inc. With the animal suitably restrained, the skin on the outer surface of the ear should be cleaned. The implant is then administered by the method shown in the diagram below.

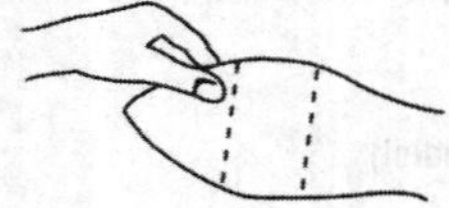

Fig. 1 - Ear of Bovine Ready for Implantation

Site of Implantation: After appropriately restraining the animal to allow access to the ear, cleanse the skin at the implant needle puncture site. It is subcutaneous, between the skin and cartilage on the back side of the ear and below the midline of the ear. The implant must not be placed closer to the head than the edge of the cartilage ring farthest from the head. The location of insertion of the needle is a point toward the tip of the ear and at least a needle length away from the intended deposition site. Care should be taken to avoid injuring the major blood vessels or cartilage of the ear.

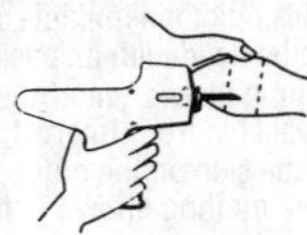

Fig. 2 - Rear View of the Bovine Ear Showing the Site for Insertion of the Implanter Needle.

Method of Use:

1. Do not remove the cap of the cartridge containing the implants.
2. Place the cartridge (with the capped end to the front) into slot at the top of the implanter magazine.
3. Gently push the cartridge into the slot until it clicks into place.
4. The implanter is then ready for use.
5. Take the ear of the animal firmly with the free hand in the manner shown in Fig. 1. Then insert the needle into the subcutaneous tissue at the point indicated in Fig. 2.
6. After inserting the needle to its full extent, squeeze the trigger gradually. Allow the pellets of the implant will be deposited in a single row.
7. Withdraw the implanter. This will advance the cartridge one groove in the magazine and the next implant is now ready for use.
8. When all the implants have been administered, the cartridge will fall out of the bottom of the magazine and may be replaced by a new one.
9. To change the needle, loosen the needle locking nut and replace the needle. Tighten the nut finger tight and the implanter is ready for use.

Precaution(s): Storage Conditions: Store in a refrigerator (2-8°C; 36-47°F) and protect from sunlight. Use before the expiration date printed on the box and on the cartridge.

Warning(s): Not to be used in animals intended for subsequent breeding, or in dairy animals. For animal treatment only. Not for use in humans. Implant pellets in the ear only. Any other location is in violation of Federal Law. Do not attempt salvage of implanted site for human or animal food.

Presentation: Box of 10 x 10 cartridge implants. Each implant consists of 6 small yellow pellets. Ten implants are provided in a cartridge.

Compendium Code No.: 11061661 780900-B

REVITILYTE™

Vets Plus **Electrolytes-Oral**

Oral Electrolyte Supplement

Active Ingredient(s):

Dextrose	59.35 g
Starch	15.00 g
Sodium Bicarbonate	12.71 g
Glycine	3.54 g
Sodium Chloride	3.31 g
Potassium Chloride	2.81 g
Tri-Calcium Phosphate	1.28 g
Guaranteed Analysis* (Min)	Per Pouch
Sodium	184.2 mEq/L
Dextrose	174.3 mEq/L
Bicarbonate	110.2 mEq/L
Chloride	45.7 mEq/L
Potassium	38.0 mEq/L
Glycine	24.9 mEq/L

*When reconstituted as directed.

Indications: A ready to mix powder that provides a concentrated source of electrolytes and nutrients.

Dosage and Administration: One pouch per calf, twice daily for two consecutive days.

Also for piglets, swine, poultry, cattle, lambs, sheep, kids, goats, foals and companion animals.

Precaution(s): Keep in a cool, dry place.

Caution(s): Animal use only.

Warning(s): Keep out of the reach of children.

Presentation: 3.5 oz. (100 g) per pouch - 16 pouches per case.

Compendium Code No.: 10730151

REVITILYTE-EQ™

Horses Prefer **Electrolytes-Oral**

Guaranteed Analysis: (Minimum per lb.):

Calcium, min.	0.25%
Calcium, max.	0.75%
Salt (NaCl), min.	68.00%
Salt (NaCl), max.	70.00%
Potassium, min.	11.00%
Magnesium, min.	0.40%

Ingredients: Salt (Sodium Chloride), Potassium Chloride, Magnesium Sulfate, Tricalcium Phosphate, Dextrose, Glycine, and Apple Flavor.

Indications: Suggested Use: REVITILYTE-EQ™ is formulated to supplement horses to provide additional electrolyte salts that may be lost by dehydration.

Directions: May be administered in horse's drinking water or feed.

In water: 2 ounces per 10 gallons of fresh drinking water. Do not allow any other source of drinking water.

In feed: 2 ounces in the horse's daily feed in place of regular salt.

One 1-ounce scoop included.

Precaution(s): Store in a cool dry place.

Caution(s): For animal use only.

Warning(s): Keep out of reach of children.

Presentation: 1 lb and 5 lbs.

Compendium Code No.: 36950041

REVITILYTE-GELLING™

Vets Plus **Electrolytes-Oral**

Oral Electrolyte Supplement With Thickening Agent

Active Ingredient(s):

Dextrose	45.00 g
Starch	15.00 g
Sodium Bicarbonate	12.71 g
Glycine	3.54 g
Sodium Chloride	3.31 g
Potassium Chloride	2.81 g
Tri-Calcium Phosphate	1.28 g
Guaranteed Analysis* (Min)	Per Pouch
Dextrose	220.1 mEq/L
Sodium	184.2 mEq/L
Bicarbonate	110.2 mEq/L
Chloride	45.7 mEq/L
Potassium	38.0 mEq/L
Glycine	24.9 mEq/L

*When reconstituted as directed.

Indications: When mixed with water, provides a concentrated nutritional supplement for calves containing dextrose in a readily available form fortified with a thickening agent to slow fluid loss.

Dosage and Administration: One pouch per calf, twice daily for two consecutive days.

Also for piglets, swine, poultry, cattle, lambs, sheep, kids, goats, foals and companion animals.

Precaution(s): Keep in a cool, dry place.

Caution(s): Keep out of the reach of children.

Animal use only.

Presentation: 3.5 oz. (100 g) per pouch - 16 pouches per case.

Compendium Code No.: 10730160

REVITILYTE-PLUS™

Vets Plus **Large Animal Dietary Supplement**

Guaranteed Analysis: (Per lb.):

Vitamin A	10,000,000 IU
Vitamin D_3	1,000,000 IU
Vitamin E	2,000 IU
Vitamin K	1,000 mg
Riboflavin	500 mg
d-Calcium Pantothenate	6,000 mg
Thiamine	250 mg
Niacinamide	250 mg
Potassium	13,620 mg
Lactic Acid Bacteria	1 billion CFU

(Lactobacillus acidophilus DDS-1, *Lactobacillus acidophilus, Lactobacillus casei, Lactobacillus fermentum, Lactobacillus plantarum, Enterococcus faecium).*

Ingredients: Vitamin A acetate, d-Activated animal sterol (vitamin D_3), DL-alpha-tocopheryl acetate (vitamin E), riboflavin, niacinamide, d-Calcium pantothenate, thiamine hydrochloride, menadione sodium bisulfite (vitamin K), potassium chloride, sodium chloride, *Lactobacillus acidophilus* DDS-1, *Lactobacillus acidophilus, Lactobacillus casei, Lactobacillus fermentum, Lactobacillus plantarum, Enterococcus faecium,* dextrose, and zeothix silica.

Indications: Administer to any species during ration change, disease conditions, weaning, shipping, or weather change. REVITILYTE-PLUS™ provides electrolytes, vitamins, and live (viable) naturally occurring microorganisms to stimulate the digestive system and appetite.

Dosage and Administration:

Cattle & Swine: Mix 1 rounded scoop of REVITILYTE-PLUS™ in 128 gallons of water, milk, or milk replacer and give for 3 to 5 days. Repeat as needed.

Auto-proportioner - make stock solution of 1 rounded scoop of REVITILYTE-PLUS™ in one gallon of water. Set the proportioner to deliver 1 ounce of solution per gallon of water. Mix fresh stock solution daily.

Feed - Mix 1 lb./ton of complete feed.

Poultry: Mix 1 level scoop of REVITILYTE-PLUS™ in 128 gallons of water and administer for 3-5 days. Repeat as needed.

Auto-proportioner - make stock solution of 1 level scoop of REVITILYTE-PLUS™ in one gallon of water. Set proportioner to deliver 1 ounce per gallon of drinking water. Mix fresh stock solution daily.

Scoop provided approximately equals 4 ounces when rounded and 3 ounces when level.

Feeding Directions: Mix REVITILYTE-PLUS™ with milk, milk replacer or water. Can also be added to ground feed or TMR mix. Provide access to fresh clean drinking water. If conditions do not improve, consult your veterinarian.

Precaution(s): Keep in cool, dry place.

Caution(s): Keep out of the reach of children.

For animal use only.

Presentation: 25 lbs. (11.53 kg).

Compendium Code No.: 10730170

REVOLUTION® ℞

Pfizer Animal Health **Parasiticide-Topical**

(selamectin)

NADA No.: 141-152

Active Ingredient(s):

Selamectin . . . . 60 or 120 mg/mL

Description: REVOLUTION® (selamectin) Topical Parasiticide is available as a colorless to yellow, ready to use solution in single dose tubes for topical (dermal) treatment of dogs and cats six weeks of age and older. The content of each tube is formulated to provide a minimum of 2.7 mg/lb (6 mg/kg) of body weight of selamectin. The chemical composition of selamectin is (5Z, 25S)-25-cyclohexyl-4'-*O*-de(2,6-dideoxy-3-*O*-methyl-α-L-*arabino*-hexopyranosyl)-5-de-methoxy-25-de(1-methylpropyl)-22, 23-dihydro-5-hydroxyiminoavermectin A_{1a}.

Indications: REVOLUTION® is recommended for use in dogs and cats six weeks of age or older for the following parasites and indications:

Dogs: REVOLUTION® kills adult fleas and prevents flea eggs from hatching for one month and is indicated for the prevention and control of flea infestations *(Ctenocephalides felis)*, prevention of heartworm disease caused by *Dirofilaria immitis*, and the treatment and control of ear mite *(Otodectes cynotis)* infestations. REVOLUTION® also is indicated for the treatment and control of sarcoptic mange *(Sarcoptes scabiei)* and for the control of tick infestations due to *(Dermacentor variabilis)*.

Cats: REVOLUTION® kills adult fleas and prevents flea eggs from hatching for one month and is indicated for the prevention and control of flea infestations *(Ctenocephalides felis)*, prevention of heartworm disease caused by *Dirofilaria immitis*, and the treatment and control of ear mite *(Otodectes cynotis)* infestations. REVOLUTION® also is indicated for the treatment and control of roundworm *(Toxocara cati)* and intestinal hookworm *(Ancylostoma tubaeforme)* infections in cats.

Dosage and Administration:

Dosage: The recommended minimum dose is 2.7 mg selamectin per pound (6 mg/kg) of body weight.

Administer the entire contents of a single dose tube (or two tubes used in combination for dogs weighing over 85 pounds) of REVOLUTION® topically in accordance with the following tables. (See Administration for the recommended treatment intervals.)

Cats (lb)	Package color	mg per tube	Potency (mg/mL)	Administered volume (mL)
Up to 5	Mauve	15 mg	60	0.25
5.1-15	Blue	45 mg	60	0.75

For cats over 15 lbs use the appropriate combination of tubes.

Dogs (lb)	Package color	mg per tube	Potency (mg/mL)	Administered volume (mL)
Up to 5	Mauve	15 mg	60	0.25
5.1-10	Purple	30 mg	120	0.25
10.1-20	Brown	60 mg	120	0.5
20.1-40	Red	120 mg	120	1.0
40.1-85	Teal	240 mg	120	2.0
85.1-130	Plum	120 mg + 240 mg*	120	3.0

*Two tubes used in combination.

For dogs over 130 lbs use the appropriate combination of tubes.

Recommended for use in animals 6 weeks of age and older.

Administration: Firmly depress the cap to puncture the seal on the REVOLUTION® tube; then remove the cap to administer the product.

Part the hair on the back of the animal at the base of the neck in front of the shoulder blades until the skin is visible. Place the tip of the tube on the skin, release the hair and squeeze the tube to empty its entire contents directly onto the skin in one spot. Do not massage the product into the skin. Due to alcohol content, do not apply to broken skin. Avoid contact between the product and fingers. Do not apply when the hair coat is wet. Bathing or shampooing the animal 2 or more hours after treatment will not reduce the effectiveness of REVOLUTION®. Stiff hair, clumping of hair, hair discoloration, or a slight powdery residue may be observed at the treatment site in some animals. These effects are temporary and do not affect the safety or effectiveness of the product. Discard empty tubes in your ordinary household refuse.

Flea Control in Dogs and Cats: For the prevention and control of flea infestations, REVOLUTION® should be administered at monthly intervals throughout the flea season, starting one month before fleas become active. In controlled laboratory studies >98% of fleas were killed within 36 hours. Results of clinical field studies using REVOLUTION® monthly demonstrated >90% control of flea infestations within 30 days of the first dose. Dogs and cats treated with REVOLUTION™, including® those with pre-existing flea allergy dermatitis showed improvement in clinical signs associated with fleas as a direct result of eliminating the fleas from the animals and their environment.

If the dog or cat is already infested with fleas when the first dose of REVOLUTION® is administered, adult fleas on the animal are killed and no viable fleas hatch from eggs after the first administration. However, an environmental infestation of fleas may persist for a short time after beginning treatment with REVOLUTION® because of the emergence of adult fleas from pupae.

Heartworm Prevention in Dogs and Cats: For the prevention of heartworm disease, REVOLUTION® must be administered on a monthly basis. REVOLUTION® may be administered year-round or at least within one month after the animal's first exposure to mosquitoes and monthly thereafter until the end of the mosquito season. The final dose must be given within one month after the last exposure to mosquitoes. If a dose is missed and a monthly interval between dosing is exceeded then immediate administration of REVOLUTION® and resumption of monthly dosing will minimize the opportunity for the development of adult heartworms. When replacing another heartworm preventive product in a heartworm disease prevention program, the first dose of REVOLUTION® must be given within a month of the last dose of the former medication.

At the discretion of the veterinarian, cats ≥6 months of age may be tested to determine the presence of existing heartworm infections before beginning treatment with REVOLUTION®. Cats already infected with adult heartworms can safely be given REVOLUTION® monthly to prevent further infections.

Ear Mite Treatment in Dogs and Cats: For the treatment of ear mite *(O. cynotis)* infestations in dogs and cats, REVOLUTION® should be administered once as a single topical dose. A second monthly dose may be required in some dogs. Monthly use of REVOLUTION® will control any subsequent ear mite infestations. In the clinical field trials ears were not cleaned, and many animals still had debris in their ears after the second dose. Cleansing of the infested ears is recommended to remove the debris.

Sarcoptic Mange Treatment in Dogs: For the treatment of sarcoptic mange *(S. scabiei)* in dogs, REVOLUTION® should be administered once as a single topical dose. A second monthly dose may be required in some dogs. Monthly use of REVOLUTION® will control any subsequent sarcoptic mange mite infestations. Because of the difficulty in finding sarcoptic mange mites on skin scrapings, effectiveness assessments also were based on resolution of clinical signs. Resolution of the pruritus associated with the mite infestations was observed in approximately 50% of the dogs 30 days after the first treatment and in approximately 90% of the dogs 30 days after the second monthly treatment.

Tick Control in Dogs: For the control of tick *(Dermacentor variabilis)* infestations in dogs, REVOLUTION® should be administered on a monthly basis. In heavy tick infestations, complete efficacy may not be achieved after the first dose. In these cases, one additional dose may be administered two weeks after the previous dose, with monthly dosing continued thereafter.

Nematode Treatment in Cats: For the treatment of intestinal hookworm *(A. tubaeforme)* and roundworm *(T. cati)* infections, REVOLUTION® should be applied once as a single topical dose.

Precaution(s): Storage Conditions: Store below 30°C (86°F).

Caution(s): U.S. Federal law restricts this drug to use by or on the order of a licensed veterinarian.

Use with caution in sick, debilitated or underweight animals (see Safety).

Prior to administration of REVOLUTION®, dogs should be tested for existing heartworm infections. At the discretion of the veterinarian, infected dogs should be treated to remove adult heartworms. REVOLUTION® is not effective against adult *D. immitis* and, while the number of circulating microfilariae may decrease following treatment, REVOLUTION® is not effective for microfilariae clearance.

Hypersensitivity reactions have not been observed in dogs with patent heartworm infections administered three times the recommended dose of REVOLUTION®. Higher doses were not tested.

Warning(s): Not for human use. Keep out of the reach of children.

In humans, REVOLUTION® may be irritating to skin and eyes. Reactions such as hives, itching and skin redness have been reported in humans in rare instances. REVOLUTION® contains isopropyl alcohol and the preservative butylated hydroxytoluene (BHT). Wash hands after use and wash off any product in contact with the skin immediately with soap and water. If contact with eyes occurs, then flush eyes copiously with water. In case of ingestion by a human, contact a physician immediately. The material safety data sheet (MSDS) provides more detailed occupational safety information. For a copy of the MSDS or to report adverse reactions attributable to exposure to this product, call 1-800-366-5288.

Flammable—Keep away from heat, sparks, open flames or other sources of ignition.

Adverse Reactions: Pre-approval clinical trials: Following treatment with REVOLUTION®, transient localized alopecia with or without inflammation at or near the site of application was observed in approximately 1% of 691 treated cats. Other signs observed rarely (≤0.5% of 1743 treated cats and dogs) included vomiting, loose stool or diarrhea with or without blood, anorexia, lethargy, salivation, tachypnea, and muscle tremors.

Post-approval experience: In addition to the aforementioned clinical signs that were reported in pre-approval clinical trials, there have been reports of pruritus, urticaria and erythema. There have also been rare reports of seizures and ataxia in dogs.

Trial Data: Safety: REVOLUTION® has been tested safe in over 100 different pure and mixed breeds of healthy dogs and over 15 different pure and mixed breeds of healthy cats, including pregnant and lactating females, breeding males and females, puppies and kittens six weeks of age and older, and avermectin-sensitive collies. However, a kitten, estimated to be 5-6 weeks old (0.3 kg), died 8½ hours after receiving a single treatment of REVOLUTION® at the recommended dosage. The kitten displayed clinical signs which included muscle spasms, salivation and neurological signs. The kitten was a stray with an unknown history and was malnourished and underweight (see Cautions).

Dogs: In safety studies REVOLUTION® was administered at 1, 3, 5, and 10 times the recommended dose to 6 week old puppies, and no adverse reactions were observed. The safety of REVOLUTION® administered orally also was tested in case of accidental oral ingestion. Oral administration of REVOLUTION® at the recommended topical dose in 5 to 8 month old beagles did not cause any adverse reactions. In a pre-clinical study selamectin was dosed orally to ivermectin-sensitive collies. Oral administration of 2.5, 10, and 15 mg/kg in this dose escalating study did not cause any adverse reactions; however, eight hours after receiving 5 mg/kg orally, one avermectin-sensitive collie became ataxic for several hours, but did not show any other adverse reactions after receiving subsequent doses of 10 and 15 mg/kg orally. In a topical safety study conducted with avermectin-sensitive collies at 1, 3 and 5 times the recommended dose of REVOLUTION®, salivation was observed in all treatment groups, including the vehicle control. REVOLUTION® also was administered at 3 times the recommended dose to heartworm infected dogs, and no adverse effects were observed.

Cats: In safety studies, REVOLUTION® was applied at 1, 3, 5, and 10 times the recommended dose to six week old kittens. No adverse reactions were observed. The safety of REVOLUTION® administered orally also was tested in case of accidental oral ingestion. Oral administration of the recommended topical dose of REVOLUTION® to cats caused salivation and intermittent vomiting. REVOLUTION® also was applied at 4 times the recommended dose to patent heartworm infected cats, and no adverse reactions were observed.

In well-controlled clinical studies, REVOLUTION® was used safely in animals receiving other frequently used veterinary products such as vaccines, anthelmintics, antiparasitics, antibiotics, steroids, collars, shampoos and dips.

Presentation: Available in six separate dose strengths for dogs and cats of different weights (see Dosage). REVOLUTION® for puppies and kittens is available in cartons containing 3 single dose tubes. REVOLUTION® for cats and dogs is available in cartons containing 3 or 6 single dose tubes. REVOLUTION® for dogs weighing more than 85 lbs is available in cartons containing 6 or 12 single dose tubes.

Compendium Code No.: 36901341 69-9876-00-1

RFD® LIQUID WORMER

Pfizer Animal Health **Parasiticide-Oral**

(pyrantel pamoate)

NADA No.: 100-237

Active Ingredient(s): 2.27 mg of pyrantel base as pyrantel pamoate per mL.

Indications: For the removal of large roundworms *(Toxocara canis* and *Toxascaris leonina)* and hookworms *(Ancylostoma caninum* and *Uncinaria stenocephala)* in dogs and puppies. The presence of these parasites should be confirmed by laboratory fecal exam. Consult your veterinarian for assistance in the diagnosis, treatment and control of parasitism.

RFD® Liquid Wormer may also be used to prevent reinfestation of *T. canis* in puppies and adult dogs and in lactating bitches after whelping.

Directions for Use: Administer 1 teaspoon (5 mL) for each 5 lb of body weight. To assure proper dosage, weigh animal prior to treatment. It is not necessary to withhold food prior to treatment. Dogs usually find this dewormer very palatable and will lick the dose from the bowl willingly. If there is reluctance to accept the dose, mix in a small quantity of dog food to encourage consumption. It is recommended that dogs maintained under conditions of constant exposure to worm infestation should have a follow-up fecal exam within 2-4 weeks after first treatment. If your dog looks or acts sick, consult your veterinarian before treatment.

For maximum control and prevention of reinfestation, it is recommended that puppies be treated at 2, 3, 4, 6, 8 and 10 weeks of age. Lactating bitches should be treated 2-3 weeks after whelping. Adult dogs kept in heavily contaminated quarters may be treated at monthly intervals to prevent *T. canis* reinfestation.

Precaution(s): Recommended Storage: Store below 30°C (86°F).

Shake well before use.

Caution(s): Keep out of reach of children.

Presentation: 2 fl oz (60 mL) bottle.

Compendium Code No.: 36901850 85-7985-00

RHINICELL®

Novartis Animal Vaccines **Vaccine**

Bordetella bronchiseptica Vaccine, Avirulent Live Culture

U.S. Vet. Lic. No.: 303

Composition: The vaccine contains a highly antigenic, avirulent live culture of *Bordetella bronchiseptica.* It is produced in a specially designed media to maintain a guaranteed potency of 10 million viable *Bordetella bronchiseptica* per mL for at least two years when used and stored properly. Initial protection is induced when the vaccine colonizes the turbinate structures during the first 24 hours after administration. Pathogenic *Bordetella bronchiseptica* strains are then unable to infect the turbinates that are colonized by the vaccine organisms.

Indications: For use as an aid in the prevention and control of diseases caused by *Bordetella bronchiseptica.*

Dosage and Administration: Shake well before using. Inoculate sows and gilts intramuscularly with two (2) 2 mL doses five (5) and two (2) weeks prior to farrowing. Revaccinate during each pregnancy to maintain high levels of immunity. Administer 1 mL (½ mL into each nostril) intranasally into piglets one (1) day of age.

Precaution(s): Store at 35°-45°F in the dark. Do not freeze. Use the entire contents immediately after opening if possible. Unused portions may be used within seven days only if refrigerated. Needles and syringes should not be sterilized with chemicals.

Caution(s): Do not use the vaccine in the presence of antibiotics effective against *Bordetella bronchiseptica.*

Warning(s): Do not vaccinate within 21 days before slaughter.

Presentation: Available in 30 mL (30 piglet doses, 15 sow doses) or 100 mL (100 piglet doses, 50 sow doses) bottles.

Compendium Code No.: 11140382

RHINICELL®+E

Novartis Animal Vaccines **Vaccine**

Bordetella bronchiseptica-Erysipelothrix rhusiopathiae Vaccine, Avirulent Live Culture

R

U.S. Vet. Lic. No.: 303

Composition: RHINICELL®+E combination vaccine contains highly antigenic, avirulent live cultures of *Bordetella bronchiseptica* and *Erysipelothrix rhusiopathiae.*

Indications: For use in swine as an aid in the prevention and control of diseases caused by *Bordetella bronchiseptica* and *Erysipelothrix rhusiopathiae.*

Dosage and Administration: Aseptically rehydrate Erycell™ with the supplied RHINICELL® and shake well before using.

Sows and Gilts: Inoculate two (2) 2 mL doses intramuscularly (I.M.) five (5) and two (2) weeks prior to farrowing. Revaccinate during each pregnancy to maintain high levels of immunity.

Piglets: Administer 1 mL (0.5 mL/nostril) intranasally (I.N.) into piglets one (1) to three (3) days of age.

Precaution(s): Store between 35°-45°F (2°-7°C). Do not freeze. Needles and syringes should be sterilized by boiling. Do not use chemical sterilization as traces of chemicals may inactivate the vaccine. Use the entire contents without delay after rehydration. Burn the containers and any unused contents.

Caution(s): Do not use the vaccine in the presence of antibiotics effective against *Bordetella bronchiseptica* and *Erysipelothrix rhusiopathiae.* Anaphylactic reactions may occur with the vaccine. Symptomatic treatment: Epinephrine.

Warning(s): Do not vaccinate within 21 days of slaughter.

Discussion: Atrophic rhinitis: The primary pathogen of atrophic rhinitis is a small gram-negative bacterium, *Bordetella bronchiseptica.* Infections may be intensified by other predisposing factors such as the presence of other microorganisms *(Pasteurella* sp., *Pseudomonas* sp., *Klebsiella* sp., *Streptococcus suis, H. parasuis,* etc.) and environmental factors including poor management and sanitation practices.

The vaccine strain of avirulent *Bordetella bronchiseptica* protects the piglet in two ways. Initial protection is given the newborn because of the attachment of the live vaccine strain to the nasal tissues and cilia after intranasal application. The organisms begin to grow, producing microcolonies which spread over the tissues. Subsequent attachment of environmental pathogenic strains is inhibited because the "vaccine strain" has taken up the available attachment sites (competitive inhibition). Because the pathogens cannot attach, they are processed through the animal's normal lines of defense and eliminated from the body. After the vaccine strain is established in the nasal tissues of the vaccinated animal, secretory antibodies are produced in response to the antigens, providing the second line of protection. The combination results in solid protection against atrophic rhinitis in young piglets which carries through to market weight.

Erysipelas: Swine erysipelas is an infectious disease caused by *Erysipelothrix rhusiopathiae.* The gram-positive rod-shaped organism is found worldwide. The disease manifests itself in one of three forms: acute, subacute, or chronic. The acute form is most frequently characterized by sudden death or septicemia with fevers up to 108°F. The subacute form is less severe and is characterized by diamond-shaped raised skin lesions. The chronic form follows the acute or subacute form and may include arthritis or subclinical infections.

The pathogen is spread via the oral route, and many swine are carriers of the organism. It has been estimated that up to 30% of clinically normal swine have positive tonsils.

Swine of all ages are susceptible to erysipelas. As a group, animals less than one month of age are less affected due to maternal protection from their immunized dams. However, newborn or young pigs are very susceptible to erysipelas if maternal protection is not in place. Animals older than three years of age are usually resistant to infection because of subclinical exposure or from vaccination programs.

Generally, the most susceptible group of swine to the disease are animals recently weaned. Maternal protection drops off to low levels at about five to eight weeks of age. If the piglets are not actively immunized prior to that time, little protection is afforded.

The newborn piglets will benefit from their immunized mothers by receiving maternal antibodies passed through the colostrum. Intranasal vaccination of the neonatal piglet produces an immediate protective local cell mediated immune response which enables the piglet to start producing its own protective antibody as the maternal protection wanes. Intranasal administration of RHINICELL®+E overrides any potential interference caused by the presence of maternal antibodies, thus stimulating the piglet's immune system to produce antibodies. The result is active protection when the maternal antibodies no longer provide protection to the animal.

The vaccine strain of *Erysipelothrix rhusiopathiae* colonizes the piglet without causing disease. The piglet's immune system is stimulated by the avirulent vaccine strain to produce specific antibody that will protect the piglet from pathogenic organisms.

Trial Data: Sow/gilt and baby piglet vaccination study:*

Sow Vaccination	Piglet Vaccination	Mortality	% Normal Temp.	% Protection (Absence from clinical symptoms)
2 mL I.M. prior to farrowing	1.0 mL I.M.	0%	100%	95%
None	None	97%	3%	3%
None	1.0 mL I.N.	0%	94%	100%

*Vaccinated with RHINICELL®+E, challenged with *Erysipelothrix rhusiopathiae.*

Summary:

1. Newborn piglets are susceptible to *E. rhusiopathiae* and *B. bronchiseptica* infections.
2. Immunized dams transfer passive protection against *E. rhusiopathiae* and *B. bronchiseptica* to nursing piglets.
3. Piglets born to immunized dams are actively immunized when vaccinated intranasally at birth with an avirulent *B. bronchiseptica-Erysipelothrix rhusiopathiae* vaccine. Maternal antibodies did not interfere with immunity.

Since both *Bordetella bronchiseptica* and *Erysipelothrix rhusiopathiae* are live microorganisms, precaution must be taken in the use of antibiotics during the vaccination regimen. The following lists the antibiotic sensitivity results for each microorganism. The work was completed *in vitro,* so results may vary in the live pig.

Bordetella bronchiseptica is susceptible to sulfonamides, gentamycin, neomycin, kanamycin, tetracycline, and erythromycin. It is resistant to ampicillin, bacitracin, furadantin, streptomycin, and penicillin.

Erysipelothrix rhusiopathiae is susceptible to penicillin, tetracycline, tylosin, and erythromycin. It is resistant to streptomycin, dihydrostreptomycin, bacitracin, polymyxin B, and sulfonamides.

Maximum effectiveness of the vaccine may be prevented if used in conjunction with antibiotics to which it is susceptible.

Two safety tests were also conducted on the combination product:

1. Extensive field trial safety testing of the product was completed in swine of mixed breeds and various ages without observations of any untoward or adverse reactions. This study was conducted under the supervision of approved veterinary investigators.
2. Exaggerated dose safety testing of the product was completed in one day old baby piglets. The piglets received six times the concentration of vaccine that they would normally receive and again untoward or adverse reactions were not noted by the independent, qualified veterinarian conducting the study.

References: Available upon request.

Presentation: Available in 30 mL bottles (30 piglet doses, 15 sow doses).

Compendium Code No.: 11140392

RHINI SHIELD™ TX4

Novartis Animal Vaccines **Bacterin-Toxoid**

Bordetella bronchiseptica-Erysipelothrix rhusiopathiae-Pasteurella multocida Bacterin-Toxoid

U.S. Vet. Lic. No.: 303

Contents: This bacterin contains inactivated cultures of *Bordetella bronchiseptica, Erysipelothrix rhusiopathiae, Pasteurella multocida* Type A, and toxigenic *Pasteurella multocida* Type D adjuvanted with aluminum hydroxide. Contains penicillin and streptomycin as preservatives.

Indications: For use in healthy swine as an aid in the prevention and control of atrophic rhinitis caused by *Bordetella bronchiseptica* or the toxin of *Pasteurella multocida* Types A and D, erysipelas caused by *Erysipelothrix rhusiopathiae,* and pneumonia caused by *Pasteurella multocida* Type A.

Dosage and Administration: Shake well before using. Administer intramuscularly or subcutaneously. Four doses must be given (two gilt/sow doses and two piglet doses). Vaccinate gilts and sows with a 5 mL dose at 5 and 2 weeks prior to farrowing. Vaccinate piglets from vaccinated dams with a 1 mL dose at 7-10 days of age and a 2 mL dose 2 weeks later.

Precaution(s): Store in the dark at 35°-45°F (2°-7°C). Do not freeze. Use entire contents when first opened.

Caution(s): Anaphylactic reactions may occur following the use of this biological. Symptomatic treatment: Epinephrine.

Warning(s): Do not vaccinate within 21 days prior to slaughter.

For veterinary use only.

Discussion: Erysipelas: *Erysipelothrix rhusiopathiae* causes swine erysipelas (SE-diamond skin disease). Many apparently normal animals can carry and shed the organism. SE is divided into three general classifications - peracute, subacute, and chronic. The peracute septicemic form may be seen as sudden death, fever, lameness, and depression. The subacute form is a milder manifestation of the peracute case. The chronic form will most often appear as lameness and bacterial growths in the heart.

Bordetella bronchiseptica: *Bordetella bronchiseptica* is a primary cause of atrophic rhinitis (AR) and pneumonia. In the case of AR, *B. bronchiseptica* may act as a primary invader or may compromise the nasal epithelliam so that secondary *Pasteurella* organisms can invade and cause more extensive damage.

The clinical signs of AR are sneezing, snuffling, rubbing the nose, black tear streaks from the eye, and excessive nasal discharge.

A more severe clinical situation associated with *B. bronchiseptica* is bronchopneumonia. This can occur in piglets as young as three to five days of age and is considered a primary infection.

Pasteurella multocida: *P. multocida* is divided into two types. Type A is a common cause of secondary pneumonia. Lungs damaged by other causes can be invaded by *Pasteurella*, which causes severe pneumonia. Death losses may be high in some cases.

Toxin-producing strains of *P. multocida* Type D are an important cause of atrophic rhinitis. The bacteria release a toxin which results in the typical signs of AR - sneezing, sniffling, teary eyes, and crooked snouts. Type D can infect older pigs and cause severe AR, whereas piglets normally have to be infected with *B. bronchiseptica* within a few days after birth to develop AR.

Nasal turbinates damaged by AR cannot do an effective job of filtering the air, allowing more bacteria into the lungs. This makes it more likely that the pig will develop severe pneumonia.

Presentation: Available in 50 mL and 100 mL bottles.

Compendium Code No.: 11140372

RHINOGEN® BPE

Intervet **Bacterin-Toxoid**

Bordetella Bronchiseptica-Erysipelothrix Rhusiopathiae-Pasteurella Multocida Bacterin-Toxoid

U.S. Vet. Lic. No.: 286

Contents: A chemically inactivated, adjuvanted culture of *Bordetella bronchiseptica, Erysipelothrix rhusiopathiae* and *Pasteurella multocida* non-toxigenic type A and toxigenic type D.

Contains gentamicin and thimerosal as preservatives.

Indications: For use in healthy swine as an aid in the prevention of atrophic rhinitis and pneumonia caused by *B. bronchiseptica* and *P. multocida* non-toxigenic type A and toxigenic types A and D, and erysipelas caused by *Erysipelothrix rhusiopathiae*.

Dosage and Administration: Shake well, inject intramuscularly or subcutaneously.

Sows and Gilts: One 2 mL dose at 5 weeks and 2 weeks prefarrowing; one 2 mL dose at 1-2 weeks before subsequent farrowings.

Baby Pigs: One 1 mL dose at 5-7 days of age; one 1 mL dose at 23-28 days of age.

Feeder Pig Vaccination: One 1 mL dose at weaning (3 weeks of age); one 1 mL dose 3 weeks later.

Boars: One 2 mL dose annually.

Precaution(s): Store in the dark at not over 45°F (7°C). Do not freeze. Use entire contents when first opened; do not save partial contents.

Caution(s): Use only in healthy swine.

If allergic reaction occurs, treat with epinephrine. Transient local swelling may occur at site of injection.

Not to be used as a diluent for viral products.

For veterinary use only.

Warning(s): Do not vaccinate within 21 days of slaughter.

Presentation: 50 sow/100 piglet dose (100 mL) vials.

Compendium Code No.: 11061541 7125001

RHINOGEN® CTE 5000

Intervet **Bacterin-Toxoid**

Bordetella Bronchiseptica-Erysipelothrix Rhusiopathiae-Pasteurella Multocida Bacterin-Toxoid

U.S. Vet. Lic. No.: 286

Contents: This product contains the antigens listed above.

Contains gentamicin as a preservative.

Indications: For use as an aid in the prevention of atrophic rhinitis caused by *B. bronchiseptica* and the toxin of *P. multocida* serotypes A and D. Also aids in the prevention of erysipelas caused by *E. rhusiopathiae*.

Dosage and Administration: Both sows and gilts and their piglets must be vaccinated as follows:

Sows and gilts: 2 mL I.M. Give 2 doses at least 2 weeks apart with the second dose administered 2 weeks before farrowing. Revaccinate before each subsequent farrowing.

Piglets: 2 mL S.C. at 7-10 days of age or prior to weaning. Repeat with a second dose in 2-3 weeks.

Breeding stock: Vaccinate all new breeding stock with 2 doses given at least 2 weeks apart with first dose given at 6 months of age or prior to introduction into herd. Revaccinate boars with a single dose annually.

Precaution(s): Store at 2° to 7°C (35° to 45°F). Do not freeze. Shake well. Use entire contents when first opened.

Caution(s): For the vaccination of healthy swine.

In case of anaphylactoid reaction administer epinephrine.

For veterinary use only.

Warning(s): Do not vaccinate within 21 days before slaughter.

Presentation: 50 dose (100 mL) vials.

Compendium Code No.: 11061681 7755001

RHINOGEN® CTSE

Intervet **Bacterin-Toxoid**

Bordetella Bronchiseptica-Erysipelothrix Rhusiopathiae-Pasteurella Multocida-Streptococcus Suis Bacterin-Toxoid

U.S. Vet. Lic. No.: 286

Contents: This product contains the antigens listed above.

Contains gentamicin as preservative.

Indications: The bacterin-toxoid will serve as an aid in the prevention of atrophic rhinitis caused by *Bordetella bronchiseptica* and the toxin of *Pasteurella multocida* serotypes A and D. It will also serve as an aid in the prevention of arthritis and meningitis caused by *Streptococcus suis* and erysipelas caused by *Erysipelothrix rhusiopathiae*.

Dosage and Administration: Both sows and gilts and their piglets must be vaccinated as follows:

Sows and gilts: 2 mL I.M. Give two doses at least 2 weeks apart with the second dose administered 2 weeks before farrowing. Revaccinate before each subsequent farrowing.

Piglets: 2 mL S.C. at 7-10 days of age or prior to weaning. Repeat with a second dose in 2-3 weeks.

Precaution(s): Store at 2° to 7°C (35° to 45°F). Do not freeze. Shake well. Use entire contents when first opened.

Caution(s): In case of anaphylactoid reaction administer epinephrine.

For veterinary use only.

Warning(s): Do not vaccinate within 21 days before slaughter.

Presentation: 50 dose (100 mL) vial.

Compendium Code No.: 11061691 7745001

RHINOMUNE®

Pfizer Animal Health **Vaccine**

Equine Rhinopneumonitis Vaccine, Modified Live Virus

U.S. Vet. Lic. No.: 189

Description: RHINOMUNE® is prepared by growing an attenuated strain of EHV-1 on an equine cell line and is packaged in freeze-dried form. The sterile diluent is used to rehydrate the freeze-dried component.

Contains gentamicin as preservative.

Indications: RHINOMUNE® is for vaccination of healthy horses 3 months of age or older as an aid in preventing respiratory disease caused by equine herpesvirus type 1 (EHV-1).

Directions:

1. General Directions: Vaccination of all horses on the premises is recommended to enhance herd immunity. Aseptically rehydrate the freeze-dried vaccine with the sterile diluent provided, shake well, and administer 1 mL intramuscularly. Appropriate preparation of the inoculation site is advised to prevent introduction of bacterial contaminants.
2. Primary Vaccination: Healthy horses 3 months of age or older should receive 2 doses administered 3-4 weeks apart. Foals should be vaccinated when maternal antibodies have declined, generally at 3 months of age. If vaccinated earlier, foals should receive the 2-dose series after reaching 3 months of age. Pregnant mares should be vaccinated after the second month of pregnancy.
3. Revaccination: Revaccination every 3 months with a single dose is recommended.[1]
4. Good animal husbandry and herd health management practices should be employed.

Precaution(s): Store at 2°-7°C. Prolonged exposure to higher temperatures and/or direct sunlight may adversely affect potency. Do not freeze.

Use entire contents when first opened.

Sterilized syringes and needles should be used to administer this vaccine. Do not sterilize with chemicals because traces of disinfectant may inactivate the vaccine.

Burn containers and all unused contents.

Caution(s): As with many vaccines, anaphylaxis may occur after use. Initial antidote of epinephrine is recommended and should be followed with appropriate supportive therapy.

This product has been shown to be efficacious in healthy animals. A protective immune response may not be elicited if animals are incubating an infectious disease, are malnourished or parasitized, are stressed due to shipment or environmental conditions, are otherwise immunocompromised, or the vaccine is not administered in accordance with label directions.

Warning(s): Do not vaccinate within 21 days before slaughter.

For veterinary use only.

Discussion: Disease Description: Primary infection with EHV-1 causes an acute respiratory disease characterized by nasal discharge, coughing, labored breathing, fever, slight loss of appetite, and depression. Annual outbreaks may occur among foals in areas with a large equine population. Clinical signs, occasionally persisting as long as 7 days, are generally more severe in young horses, and may be exacerbated by strenuous activity. Subclinical reinfection may also occur, with latent carriers the probable reservoir of EHV-1. Immunity following natural infection typically endures for 3-9 months and is usually enhanced by subclinical or mild reinfection.

Trial Data: Safety and Efficacy: In extensive laboratory and field tests, no adverse reactions were reported in vaccinated horses, including young, susceptible foals and pregnant mares. Mares vaccinated after the second month of pregnancy remained clinically normal and delivered live, healthy foals. In challenge-of-immunity tests, vaccinated horses remained clinically normal after challenge with EHV-1 that produced typical signs of respiratory disease in nonvaccinated horses.

References: Available upon request.

Presentation: 1 dose and 5 dose vials.

Compendium Code No.: 36901360 75-4842-06

R

RHINOPAN®-4

Biocor **Vaccine**

Feline Rhinotracheitis-Calici-Panleukopenia-Chlamydia Psittaci Vaccine, Modified Live Virus and Chlamydia

U.S. Vet. Lic. No.: 462

Contents: RHINOPAN®-4 is a combination of modified live Feline Rhinotracheitis, Calici and Panleukopenia viruses and *Chlamydia psittaci*.

This product contains gentamicin and amphotericin B as preservatives.

Indications: Recommended for use in the vaccination of healthy cats against the disease caused by the organisms represented.

Directions: Aseptically rehydrate vial of desiccated antigens with the accompanying vial of virus vaccine. Shake well. Administer entire contents (1 mL) SC.

Persistence of maternal origin antibody in kittens is known to interfere with development of active immunity following vaccination. Ideally kittens should be vaccinated at 9 weeks of age with revaccination 3-4 weeks later. Adult cats should receive a 1 mL dose followed by a second dose 3-4 weeks later. Annual revaccination with a single 1 mL dose is recommended.

Precaution(s): Store at 35°F-45°F (2°C-7°C). Do not freeze. Use entire contents when first rehydrated. Burn these containers and all unused contents.

Caution(s): Do not vaccinate pregnant queens. An occasional animal may demonstrate a transient fever, and mild arthralgia and/or myalgia within the first week following vaccination. In case of anaphylactoid reactions, epinephrine should be administered immediately.

For veterinary use only.

Presentation: Code 69111B - 25 x 1 dose (1 mL) vials with diluent.

Compendium Code No.: 13940153 BAH4225-1098

RHINOPAN®-MLV

Biocor **Vaccine**

Feline Rhinotracheitis-Calici-Panleukopenia Vaccine, Modified Live Virus

U.S. Vet. Lic. No.: 462

Contents: RHINOPAN®-MLV is a combination of modified live Feline Rhinotracheitis, Calici and Panleukopenia viruses. The live viruses contained have been attenuated to assure safety upon administration.

This product contains gentamicin and amphotericin B as preservatives.

Indications: Recommended for use in the vaccination of healthy cats against disease caused by the organisms represented.

Dosage and Administration: Aseptically rehydrate vial of desiccated virus with the accompanying vial of liquid vaccine. Shake well. Administer entire contents (1 mL) SC.

Persistence of maternal origin antibody in kittens should receive consideration in determining vaccination programs. Ideally kittens should be vaccinated at 9 weeks of age with revaccination 3-4 weeks later. Adult cats should receive a 1 mL dose followed by a second dose 3-4 weeks later. Annual revaccination with a single 1 mL dose is recommended.

Precaution(s): Store at 35°F-45°F (2°C-7°C). Do not freeze. Use entire contents when first rehydrated. Burn these containers and all unused contents.

Caution(s): Do not vaccinate pregnant queens. An occasional animal may demonstrate a transient fever, and mild arthralgia and/or myalgia within the first week following vaccination. In case of anaphylactoid reactions, epinephrine should be administered immediately.

For veterinary use only.

Presentation: Code 69011B - 25 x 1 dose (1 mL) vials with diluent.

® Registered trademark of Biocor Animal Health Inc. U.S.A.

Compendium Code No.: 13940161

RHODOCOCCUS EQUI ANTIBODY

Lake Immunogenics **Antibodies**

Rhodococcus Equi Antibody, Equine Origin

U.S. Vet. Lic. No.: 318

Contents: Each single dose bag contains plasma as a source of *Rhodococcus equi* antibodies with sodium citrate as an anticoagulant derived from healthy horses with no A or Q r.b.c. factors and no A or Q serum r.b.c. antibodies. All donor horses are negative to EIA and EVA.

Indications: For intravenous use in the prevention of pneumonia associated with *Rhodococcus equi* infection in the equine neonate.

Dosage and Administration: The dose is 10 mL/lb body weight. The average 45 kg foal should receive one 950 mL unit between 2-3 weeks of age.

Caution(s): The possibility of transmission of viral disease is possible with the administration of any blood product. This is a rare occurrence.

Thaw quickly not exceeding 120°F. Administer by filtered intravenous infusion. Discard the unused portion. In case of a reaction, marked most often by tenesmus and hyperventilation, slow the speed of administration. If this does not abate the signs, stop administration until signs abate, and continue at a slower rate. If signs persist suspend administration and treat with histamine blockers and anti-inflammatory agents. Administration may be attempted again after treatment to relieve the adverse response has been successful.

Discussion: Research has shown the administration of *Rhodococcus equi* antibodies prior to exposure may be beneficial in the prevention of pneumonia caused by *Rhodococcus equi*. The primary incidence of this disease occurs between 6-12 weeks of age, but in endemic areas if exposure and environmental conditions favoring exposure are present, a second dose may be necessary for foals up to 16 weeks of age. This product has been conditionally licensed. Studies to determine efficacy are underway and as of yet, satisfactory potency has not been established.

Presentation: 950 mL.

Compendium Code No.: 11190030

RHODOCOCCUS EQUI ANTIBODY

V.D.I. **Plasma**

Rhodococcus Equi Antibody, Equine Origin

U.S. Vet. Lic. No.: 360

Contents: The plasma contains no preservatives, and donors used have been found free of hemolysins and agglutinins against 32 of the main antigens in blood groups A, C, D, K, P, Q and U. Donors have also tested negative for EIA, EVA, dourine, piroplasmosis, brucellosis and glanders.

Indications: This product can be administered in the following situation: For prophylactic administration to foals less than 6 months of age against respiratory disease associated with *Rhodococcus equi*.

Dosage and Administration: Dosage:

1. One initial dose is recommended for foals less than 2 months of age.
2. A second dose may be administered 4-6 weeks later, based upon experience with similar circumstances of the endemic area.

Administration: The plasma should be kept frozen until required. It should be thawed using only warm water and then warmed to body temperature. Plasma can be damaged by thawing in very hot water or by microwaves. Administer directly from the bag by slow filtered intravenous infusion. Do not add anything to the product. Caution should be taken to avoid volume overload.

Caution(s): Only for use in horses by a licensed veterinarian.

This product license is conditional.

Efficacy and potency test studies are in progress.

This product is frozen immediately after collection and is not pasteurized or otherwise treated. The transmission of infectious diseases is possible with the administration of any blood product.

Administer through a sterile blood administration set with filter.

Side Effects: Complications are very infrequent but may include mild reactions such as tachypnea and trembling. If these symptoms become severe and include sweating and excessive shaking, it is advisable to slow the rate of administration or to stop and restart in 5-10 minutes. If the symptoms recur or persist, discontinue administration.

Presentation: 950 mL bags.

Compendium Code No.: 11280110

RIMADYL® CAPLETS ℞

Pfizer Animal Health **Non-Steroidal Anti-Inflammatory**

(carprofen)

NADA No.: 141-053

Active Ingredient(s): RIMADYL® caplets are scored, and contain 25 mg, 75 mg, or 100 mg of carprofen per caplet.

Indications: RIMADYL® is indicated for the relief of pain and inflammation associated with osteoarthritis and for the control of postoperative pain associated with soft tissue and orthopedic surgeries in dogs.

Pharmacology: Description: RIMADYL® (carprofen) is a non-steroidal anti-inflammatory drug (NSAID) of the propionic acid class that includes ibuprofen, naproxen, and ketoprofen. Carprofen is the nonproprietary designation for a substituted carbazole, 6-chloro-α-methyl-9H-carbazole-2-acetic acid. The empirical formula is $C_{15}H_{12}ClNO_2$ and the molecular weight 273.72. The chemical structure of carprofen is:

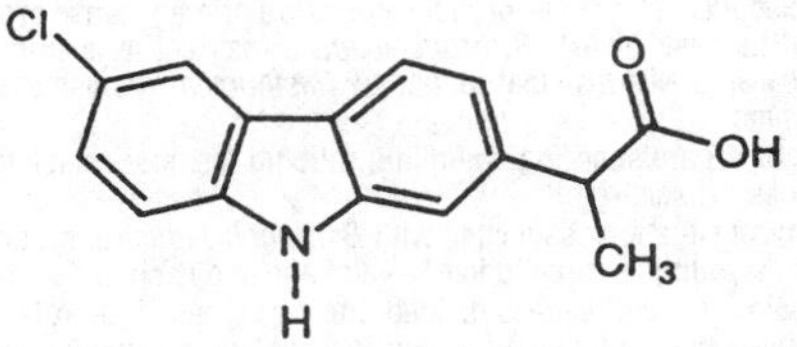

Carprofen is a white, crystalline compound. It is freely soluble in ethanol, but practically insoluble in water at 25°C.

Clinical Pharmacology: Carprofen is a non-narcotic, non-steroidal anti-inflammatory agent with characteristic analgesic and antipyretic activity approximately equipotent to indomethacin in animal models.[1]

The mechanism of action of carprofen, like that of other NSAIDs, is believed to be associated with the inhibition of cyclooxygenase activity. Two unique cyclooxygenases have been described in mammals.[2] The constitutive cyclooxygenase, COX-1, synthesizes prostaglandins necessary for normal gastrointestinal and renal function. The inducible cyclooxygenase, COX-2, generates prostaglandins involved in inflammation. Inhibition of COX-1 is thought to be associated with gastrointestinal and renal toxicity while inhibition of COX-2 provides anti-inflammatory activity. The specificity of a particular NSAID for COX-2 versus COX-1 may vary from species to species.[3] In an *in vitro* study using canine cell cultures, carprofen demonstrated selective inhibition of COX-2 versus COX-1.[4] Clinical relevance of these data has not been shown. Carprofen has also been shown to inhibit the release of several prostaglandins in two inflammatory cell systems: rat polymorphonuclear leukocytes (PMN) and human rheumatoid synovial cells, indicating inhibition of acute (PMN system) and chronic (synovial cell system) inflammatory reactions.[1]

Several studies have demonstrated that carprofen has modulatory effects on both humoral and cellular immune responses.[5-9] Data also indicate that carprofen inhibits the production of osteoclast-activating factor (OAF), PGE_1, and PGE_2 by its inhibitory effects on prostaglandin biosynthesis.[1]

Based upon comparison with data obtained from intravenous administration, carprofen is rapidly and nearly completely absorbed (more than 90% bioavailable) when administered orally.[10] Peak blood plasma concentrations are achieved in 1-3 hours after oral administration of 1, 5, and 25 mg/kg to dogs. The mean terminal half-life of carprofen is approximately 8 hours (range 4.5-9.8 hours) after single oral doses varying from 1-35 mg/kg of body weight. After a 100 mg single intravenous bolus dose, the mean elimination half-life was approximately 11.7 hours in the dog. RIMADYL® is more than 99% bound to plasma protein and exhibits a very small volume of distribution.

Carprofen is eliminated in the dog primarily by biotransformation in the liver followed by rapid excretion of the resulting metabolites (the ester glucuronide of carprofen and the ether glucuronides of 2 phenolic metabolites, 7-hydroxy carprofen and 8-hydroxy carprofen) in the feces (70-80%) and urine (10-20%). Some enterohepatic circulation of the drug is observed.

Dosage and Administration: Always provide Client Information Sheet with prescription. The recommended dosage for oral administration to dogs is 2 mg/lb (4.4 mg/kg) of body weight daily. The total daily dose may be administered as 2 mg/lb of body weight once daily or divided and administered as 1 mg/lb (2.2 mg/kg) twice daily. For the control of postoperative pain, administer approximately 2 hours before the procedure. Caplets are scored and dosage should be calculated in half-caplet increments.

Contraindication(s): RIMADYL® should not be used in dogs exhibiting previous hypersensitivity to carprofen or other NSAIDs.

Precaution(s): Storage: Store at controlled room temperature 15°-30°C (59°-86°F).

Caution(s): Federal law restricts this drug to use by or on the order of a licensed veterinarian.

As a class, cyclooxygenase inhibitory NSAIDs may be associated with gastrointestinal and renal toxicity. Effects may result from decreased prostaglandin production and inhibition of the enzyme cyclooxygenase which is responsible for the formation of prostaglandins from arachidonic acid.[11-14] When NSAIDs inhibit prostaglandins that cause inflammation they may also inhibit those prostaglandins which maintain normal homeostatic function. These anti-prostaglandin effects may result in clinically significant disease in patients with underlying or pre-existing disease more often than in healthy patients.[12,14] NSAID therapy could unmask occult disease which has previously been undiagnosed due to the absence of apparent clinical signs. Patients with underlying renal disease for example, may experience exacerbation or decompensation of their renal disease while on NSAID therapy.[11-14] The use of parenteral fluids during surgery should be considered to reduce the potential risk of renal complications when using NSAIDs perioperatively.

Carprofen is an NSAID, and as with others in that class, adverse reactions may occur with its use. The most frequently reported effects have been gastrointestinal signs. Events involving suspected renal, hematologic, neurologic, dermatologic, and hepatic effects have also been reported. Patients at greatest risk for renal toxicity are those that are dehydrated, on concomitant diuretic therapy, or those with renal, cardiovascular, and/or hepatic dysfunction. Concurrent administration of potentially nephrotoxic drugs should be approached cautiously, with appropriate monitoring. Since many NSAIDs possess the potential to induce gastrointestinal ulceration, concomitant use of RIMADYL® with other anti-inflammatory drugs, such as corticosteroids and NSAIDS, should be avoided or very closely monitored. Sensitivity to drug-associated adverse events varies with the individual patient. For example, RIMADYL® treatment was not associated with renal toxicity or gastrointestinal ulceration in well-controlled safety studies of up to ten times the dose in dogs.

RIMADYL® is not recommended for use in dogs with bleeding disorders (e.g., Von Willebrand's disease), as safety has not been established in dogs with these disorders. The safe use of RIMADYL® in animals less than 6 weeks of age, pregnant dogs, dogs used for breeding purposes, or in lactating bitches has not been established. Studies to determine the activity of RIMADYL® when administered concomitantly with other protein-bound or similarly metabolized drugs have not been conducted. Drug compatibility should be monitored closely in patients requiring additional therapy. Such drugs commonly used include cardiac, anticonvulsant and behavioral medications. It has been suggested that treatment with carprofen may reduce the level of inhalant anesthetics needed.[15]

If additional pain medication is warranted after administration of the total daily dose of RIMADYL®, alternative analgesia should be considered. The use of another NSAID is not recommended.

Warning(s): Keep out of reach of children. Not for human use. Consult a physician in cases of accidental ingestion by humans. For use in dogs only. Do not use in cats.

All dogs should undergo a thorough history and physical examination before initiation of NSAID therapy. Appropriate laboratory tests to establish hematological and serum biochemical baseline data prior to, and periodically during, administration of any NSAID should be considered. Owners should be advised to observe for signs of potential drug toxicity (see Information for Dog Owners and Adverse Reactions).

For oral use in dogs only.

Adverse Reactions: During investigational studies of osteoarthritis with twice daily administration of 1 mg/lb, no clinically significant adverse reactions were reported. Some clinical signs were observed during field studies (n=297) which were similar for carprofen- and placebo-treated dogs. Incidences of the following were observed in both groups: vomiting (4%), diarrhea (4%), changes in appetite (3%), lethargy (1.4%), behavioral changes (1%), and constipation (0.3%). The product vehicle served as control.

There were no serious adverse events reported during clinical field studies of osteoarthritis with once daily administration of 2 mg/lb. The following categories of abnormal health observations were reported. The product vehicle served as control.

Percentage of Dogs with Abnormal Health Observations Reported in Osteoarthritis Field Study (2 mg/lb once daily)		
Observation	RIMADYL® (n=129)	Placebo (n=132)
Inappetance	1.6	1.5
Vomiting	3.1	3.8
Diarrhea/Soft stool	3.1	4.5
Behavior change	0.8	0.8
Dermatitis	0.8	0.8
PU/PD	0.8	—
SAP increase	7.8	8.3
ALT increase	5.4	4.5
AST increase	2.3	0.8
BUN increase	3.1	1.5
Bilirubinuria	16.3	12.1
Ketonuria	14.7	9.1

Clinical pathology parameters listed represent reports of increases from pre-treatment values; medical judgement is necessary to determine clinical relevance.

During investigational studies of surgical pain for the caplet formulation, no clinically significant adverse reactions were reported. The product vehicle served as control.

Percentage of Dogs with Abnormal Health Observations Reported in Surgical Pain Field Studies with Caplets (2 mg/lb once daily)		
Observation*	RIMADYL® (n=148)	Placebo (n=149)
Vomiting	10.1	13.4
Diarrhea/soft stool	6.1	6.0
Ocular disease	2.7	0
Inappetance	1.4	0
Dermatitis/skin lesion	2.0	1.3
Dysrhythmia	0.7	0
Apnea	1.4	0
Oral/periodontal disease	1.4	0
Pyrexia	0.7	1.3
Urinary tract disease	1.4	1.3
Wound drainage	1.4	0

* A single dog may have experienced more than one occurrence of an event.

Post-Approval Experience: Although not all adverse reactions are reported, the following adverse reactions are based on voluntary post-approval adverse drug experience reporting. The categories of adverse reactions are listed in decreasing order of frequency by body system.

Gastrointestinal: Vomiting, diarrhea, constipation, inappetence, melena, hematemesis, gastrointestinal ulceration, gastrointestinal bleeding, pancreatitis.

Hepatic: Inappetence, vomiting, jaundice, acute hepatic toxicity, hepatic enzyme elevation, abnormal liver function test(s), hyperbilirubinemia, bilirubinuria, hypoalbuminemia. Approximately one-fourth of hepatic reports were in Labrador Retrievers.

Neurologic: Ataxia, paresis, paralysis, seizures, vestibular signs, disorientation.

Urinary: Hematuria, polyuria, polydipsia, urinary incontinence, urinary tract infection, azotemia, acute renal failure, tubular abnormalities including acute tubular necrosis, renal tubular acidosis, glucosuria.

Behavioral: Sedation, lethargy, hyperactivity, restlessness, aggressiveness.

Hematologic: Immune-mediated hemolytic anemia, immune-mediated thrombocytopenia, blood loss anemia, epistaxis.

Dermatologic: Pruritus, increased shedding, alopecia, pyotraumatic moist dermatitis (hot spots), necrotizing panniculitis/vasculitis, ventral ecchymosis.

Immunologic or hypersensitivity: Facial swelling, hives, erythema.

In rare situations, death has been associated with some of the adverse reactions listed above.

To report a suspected adverse reaction call 1-800-366-5288.

For a copy of the Material Safety Data Sheet (MSDS) or to report adverse reactions call Pfizer Animal Health at 1-800-366-5288.

Trial Data: Effectiveness: Confirmation of the effectiveness of RIMADYL® for the relief of pain and inflammation associated with osteoarthritis, and for the control of postoperative pain associated with soft tissue and orthopedic surgeries was demonstrated in 5 placebo-controlled, masked studies examining the anti-inflammatory and analgesic effectiveness of RIMADYL® caplets in various breeds of dogs.

Separate placebo-controlled, masked, multicenter field studies confirmed the anti-inflammatory and analgesic effectiveness of RIMADYL® caplets when dosed at 2 mg/lb once daily or when divided and administered at 1 mg/lb twice daily. In these two field studies, dogs diagnosed with osteoarthritis showed statistically significant overall improvement based on lameness evaluations by the veterinarian and owner observations when administered RIMADYL® at labeled doses.

Separate placebo-controlled, masked, multicenter field studies confirmed the effectiveness of RIMADYL® caplets for the control of postoperative pain when dosed at 2 mg/lb once daily in various breeds of dogs. In these studies, dogs presented for ovariohysterectomy, cruciate repair and aural surgeries were administered RIMADYL® preoperatively and for a maximum of 3 days (soft tissue) or 4 days (orthopedic) postoperatively. In general, dogs administered RIMADYL® showed statistically significant improvement in pain scores compared to controls.

Animal Safety Studies: Laboratory studies in unanesthetized dogs and clinical field studies have demonstrated that RIMADYL® is well tolerated in dogs after oral administration.

In target animal safety studies, RIMADYL® was administered orally to healthy Beagle dogs at 1, 3, and 5 mg/lb twice daily (1, 3 and 5 times the recommended total daily dose) for 42 consecutive days with no significant adverse reactions. Serum albumin for a single female dog receiving 5 mg/lb twice daily decreased to 2.1 g/dL after 2 weeks of treatment, returned to the pre-treatment value (2.6 g/dL) after 4 weeks of treatment, and was 2.3 g/dL at the final 6-week evaluation. Over the 6-week treatment period, black or bloody stools were observed in 1 dog (1 incident) treated with 1 mg/lb twice daily and in 1 dog (2 incidents) treated with 3 mg/lb twice daily. Redness of the colonic mucosa was observed in 1 male that received 3 mg/lb twice daily.

Two of 8 dogs receiving 10 mg/lb orally twice daily (10 times the recommended total daily dose) for 14 days exhibited hypoalbuminemia. The mean albumin level in the dogs receiving this dose was lower (2.38 g/dL) than each of 2 placebo control groups (2.88 and 2.93 g/dL, respectively). Three incidents of black or bloody stool were observed in 1 dog. Five of 8 dogs exhibited reddened areas of duodenal mucosa on gross pathologic examination. Histologic examination of these areas revealed no evidence of ulceration, but did show minimal congestion of the lamina propria in 2 of the 5 dogs.

In separate safety studies lasting 13 and 52 weeks, respectively, dogs were administered orally up to 11.4 mg/lb/day (5.7 times the recommended total daily dose of 2 mg/lb) of carprofen. In both studies, the drug was well tolerated clinically by all of the animals. No gross or histologic changes were seen in any of the treated animals. In both studies, dogs receiving the highest doses had average increases in serum L-alanine aminotransferase (ALT) of approximately 20 IU.

In the 52 week study, minor dermatologic changes occurred in dogs in each of the treatment groups but not in the control dogs. The changes were described as slight redness or rash and were diagnosed as non-specific dermatitis. The possibility exists that these mild lesions were treatment related, but no dose relationship was observed.

Clinical field studies were conducted with 549 dogs of different breeds at the recommended doses for 14 days (297 dogs were included in a study evaluating 1 mg/lb twice daily and 252 dogs were included in a separate study evaluating 2 mg/lb once daily). In both studies the drug was clinically well tolerated and the incidence of clinical adverse reactions for RIMADYL®-treated animals was no higher than placebo-treated animals (placebo contained inactive ingredients found in RIMADYL®). For animals receiving 1 mg/lb twice daily, the mean post-treatment serum ALT values were 11 IU greater and 9 IU less than pre-treatment values for dogs receiving RIMADYL® and placebo, respectively. Differences were not statistically significant. For animals receiving 2 mg/lb once daily, the mean post-treatment serum ALT values were 4.5 IU greater and 0.9 IU less than pre-treatment values for dogs receiving RIMADYL® and placebo, respectively. In the latter study, 3 RIMADYL®-treated dogs developed a 3-fold or greater increase in (ALT) and/or (AST) during the course of therapy. One placebo-treated dog had a greater than 2-fold increase in ALT. None of these animals showed clinical signs associated with laboratory value changes. Changes in clinical laboratory values (hematology and clinical chemistry) were not considered clinically significant. The 1 mg/lb twice daily course of therapy was repeated as needed at 2-week intervals in 244 dogs, some for as long as 5 years.

Clinical field studies were conducted in 297 dogs of different breeds undergoing orthopedic or soft tissue surgery. Dogs were administered 2 mg/lb of RIMADYL® two hours prior to surgery then once daily, as needed for 2 days (soft tissue surgery) or 3 days (orthopedic surgery). RIMADYL® was well tolerated when used in conjunction with a variety of anesthetic-related drugs. The type and severity of abnormal health observations in RIMADYL®- and placebo-treated animals were approximately equal and few in number (see Adverse Reactions). The most frequent abnormal health observation was vomiting and was observed at approximately the same frequency in RIMADYL®- and placebo-treated animals. Changes in clinicopathologic indices of hematopoetic, renal, hepatic, and clotting function were not clinically significant. The mean post-treatment serum ALT values were 7.3 IU and 2.5 IU less than pre-treatment values for dogs receiving RIMADYL® and placebo, respectively. The mean post-treatment AST values were 3.1 IU less for dogs receiving RIMADYL® and 0.2 IU greater for dogs receiving placebo.

Discussion: Information for Dog Owners: RIMADYL®, like other drugs of its class, is not free from adverse reactions. Owners should be advised of the potential for adverse reactions and be informed of the clinical signs associated with drug intolerance. Adverse reactions may include decreased appetite, vomiting, diarrhea, dark or tarry stools, increased water consumption, increased urination, pale gums due to anemia, yellowing of gums, skin or white of the eye due to jaundice, lethargy, incoordination, seizure, or behavioral changes. Serious adverse reactions associated with this drug class can occur without warning and in rare situations result in death (see Adverse Reactions). Owners should be advised to discontinue RIMADYL® therapy and contact their veterinarian immediately if signs of intolerance are observed. The vast majority of patients with drug related adverse reactions have recovered when the signs are recognized, the drug is withdrawn, and veterinary care, if appropriate, is initiated. Owners should be advised of the importance of periodic follow up for all dogs during administration of any NSAID.

References: Available upon request.

Presentation: Each caplet size is packaged in bottles containing 14, 60, or 180 caplets.

Compendium Code No.: 36901372 75-8600-04

RIMADYL® CHEWABLE TABLETS ℞

Pfizer Animal Health **Non-Steroidal Anti-Inflammatory**

(carprofen)

NADA No.: 141-111

Active Ingredient(s): RIMADYL® Chewable Tablets are scored, and contain 25 mg, 75 mg, or 100 mg of carprofen per tablet.

Indications: RIMADYL® is indicated for the relief of pain and inflammation associated with osteoarthritis in dogs.

Pharmacology: Description: RIMADYL® (carprofen) is a non-steroidal anti-inflammatory drug (NSAID) of the propionic acid class that includes ibuprofen, naproxen, and ketoprofen. Carprofen is the non-proprietary designation for a substituted carbazole, 6-chloro-α-methyl-9H-carbazole-2-acetic acid. The empirical formula is $C_{15}H_{12}ClNO_2$ and the molecular weight 273.72.

The chemical structure of carprofen is:

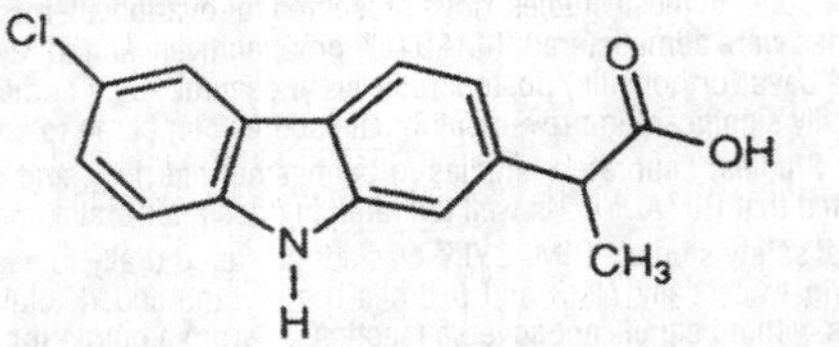

Carprofen is a white, crystalline compound. It is freely soluble in ethanol, but practically insoluble in water at 25°C.

Clinical Pharmacology: Carprofen is a non-narcotic, non-steroidal anti-inflammatory agent with characteristic analgesic and antipyretic activity approximately equipotent to indomethacin in animal models.[1]

The mechanism of action of carprofen, like that of other NSAIDs, is believed to be associated with the inhibition of cyclooxygenase activity. Two unique cyclooxygenases have been described in mammals.[2] The constitutive cyclooxygenase, COX-1, synthesizes prostaglandins necessary for normal gastrointestinal and renal function. The inducible cyclooxygenase, COX-2, generates prostaglandins involved in inflammation. Inhibition of COX-1 is thought to be associated with gastrointestinal and renal toxicity while inhibition of COX-2 provides anti-inflammatory activity. The specificity of a particular NSAID for COX-2 versus COX-1 may vary from species to species.[3] In an *in vitro* study using canine cell cultures, carprofen demonstrated selective inhibition of COX-2 versus COX-1.[4] Clinical relevance of these data has not been shown. Carprofen has also been shown to inhibit the release of several prostaglandins in two inflammatory cell systems: rat polymorphonuclear leukocytes (PMN) and human rheumatoid synovial cells, indicating inhibition of acute (PMN system) and chronic (synovial cell system) inflammatory reactions.[1]

Several studies have demonstrated that carprofen has modulatory effects on both humoral and cellular immune responses.[5-9] Data also indicate that carprofen inhibits the production of osteoclast-activating factor (OAF), PGE_1, and PGE_2 by its inhibitory effect in prostaglandin biosynthesis.[1]

Based upon comparison with data obtained from intravenous administration, carprofen is rapidly and nearly completely absorbed (more than 90% bioavailable) when administered orally.[10] Peak blood plasma concentrations are achieved in 1-3 hours after oral administration of 1, 5, and 25 mg/kg to dogs. The mean terminal half-life of carprofen is approximately 8 hours (range 4.5-9.8 hours) after single oral doses varying from 1-35 mg/kg of body weight.

After a 100 mg single intravenous bolus dose, the mean elimination half-life was approximately 11.7 hours in the dog. RIMADYL® is more than 99% bound to plasma protein and exhibits a very small volume of distribution.

Carprofen is eliminated in the dog primarily by biotransformation in the liver followed by rapid excretion of the resulting metabolites (the ester glucuronide of carprofen and the ether glucuronides of 2 phenolic metabolites, 7-hydroxy carprofen and 8-hydroxy carprofen) in the feces (70-80%) and urine (10-20%). Some enterohepatic circulation of the drug is observed.

Dosage and Administration: The recommended dosage for oral administration to dogs is 2 mg/lb of body weight daily. The total daily dose may be administered as 2 mg/lb of body weight once daily or divided and administered as 1 mg/lb twice daily. RIMADYL® Chewable Tablets are scored and dosage should be calculated in half-tablet increments. Tablets can be halved by placing the tablet on a hard surface and pressing down on both sides of the score. RIMADYL® Chewable Tablets are palatable and willingly consumed by most dogs when offered by the owner. Therefore, they may be fed by hand or placed on food. Care should be taken to ensure that the dog consumes the complete dose.

Contraindication(s): RIMADYL® should not be used in dogs exhibiting previous hypersensitivity to carprofen or other NSAIDs.

Do not use in cats.

Precaution(s): Storage: Store at controlled room temperature 15°-30°C (59°-86°F).

Caution(s): Federal law restricts this drug to use by or on the order of a licensed veterinarian.

As a class, cyclooxygenase inhibitory NSAIDs may be associated with gastrointestinal and renal toxicity. Effects may result from decreased prostaglandin production and inhibition of the enzyme cyclooxygenase which is responsible for the formation of prostaglandins from arachidonic acid.[11-14] When NSAIDs inhibit prostaglandins that cause inflammation they may also inhibit those prostaglandins which maintain normal homeostatic function. These anti-prostaglandin effects may result in clinically significant disease in patients with underlying or pre-existing disease more often than in healthy patients.[12,14] NSAID therapy could unmask occult disease which has previously been undiagnosed due to the absence of apparent clinical signs. Patients with underlying renal disease for example, may experience exacerbation or decompensation of their renal disease while on NSAID therapy.[11-14]

R

Carprofen is an NSAID, and as with others in that class, adverse reactions may occur with its use. The most frequently reported effects have been gastrointestinal signs. Events involving suspected renal, hematologic, neurologic, dermatologic, and hepatic effects have also been reported. Patients at greatest risk for renal toxicity are those that are dehydrated, on concomitant diuretic therapy, or those with renal, cardiovascular, and/or hepatic dysfunction. Since many NSAIDs possess the potential to induce gastrointestinal ulceration, concomitant use of RIMADYL® with other anti-inflammatory drugs, such as corticosteroids and NSAIDs, should be avoided or very closely monitored. Sensitivity to drug-associated adverse reactions varies with the individual patient. For example, RIMADYL® treatment was not associated with renal toxicity or gastrointestinal ulceration in well-controlled safety studies of up to ten times the dose in dogs.

RIMADYL® is not recommended for use in dogs with bleeding disorders (e.g., Von Willebrand's disease), as safety has not been established in dogs with these disorders. The safe use of RIMADYL® in pregnant dogs, dogs used for breeding purposes, or in lactating bitches has not been established. Studies to determine the activity of RIMADYL® when administered concomitantly with other protein-bound or similarly metabolized drugs have not been conducted. Drug compatibility should be monitored closely in patients requiring additional therapy.

Due to the palatable nature of RIMADYL® Chewable Tablets, store out of reach of dogs in a secured location. Severe adverse reactions may occur if large quantities of tablets are ingested. If you suspect your dog has consumed RIMADYL® Chewable Tablets above the labeled dose, please call your veterinarian for immediate assistance and notify Pfizer Animal Health (1-800-366-5288).

Information for Dog Owners: RIMADYL®, like other drugs of its class, is not free from adverse reactions. Owners should be advised of the potential for adverse reactions and be informed of the clinical signs associated with drug intolerance. Adverse reactions may include decreased appetite, vomiting, diarrhea, dark or tarry stools, increased water consumption, increased urination, pale gums due to anemia, yellowing of gums, skin or white of the eye due to jaundice, lethargy, incoordination, seizure, or behavioral changes. Serious adverse reactions associated with this drug class can occur without warning and in rare situations result in death (see Adverse Reactions). Owners should be advised to discontinue RIMADYL® therapy and contact their veterinarian immediately if signs of intolerance are observed. The vast majority of patients with drug related adverse reactions have recovered when the signs are recognized, the drug is withdrawn, and veterinary care, if appropriate, is initiated. Owners should be advised of the importance of periodic follow up for all dogs during administration of any NSAID.

For use in dogs only.

All dogs should undergo a thorough history and physical examination before initiation of NSAID therapy. Appropriate laboratory tests to establish hematological and serum biochemical baseline data prior to, and periodically during, administration of any NSAID should be considered. Owners should be advised to observe for signs of potential drug toxicity (see Information for Dog Owners and Adverse Reactions).

For oral use in dogs only.

Warning(s): Keep out of reach of children. Not for human use. Consult a physician in cases of accidental ingestion by humans.

Adverse Reactions: During investigational studies for the caplet formulation with twice daily administration of 1 mg/lb, no clinically significant adverse reactions were reported. Some clinical signs were observed during field studies (n=297) which were similar for carprofen caplet- and placebo-treated dogs. Incidences of the following were observed in both groups: vomiting (4%), diarrhea (4%), changes in appetite (3%), lethargy (1.4%), behavioral changes (1%), and constipation (0.3%). The product vehicle served as control.

There were no serious adverse events reported during clinical field studies with once daily administration of 2 mg/lb. The following categories of abnormal health observations were reported. The product vehicle served as control.

Percentage of Dogs with Abnormal Health Observations Reported in Clinical Field Study (2 mg/lb once daily):

Observation	RIMADYL® (n=129)	Placebo (n=132)
Inappetence	1.6	1.5
Vomiting	3.1	3.8
Diarrhea/Soft stool	3.1	4.5
Behavior change	0.8	0.8
Dermatitis	0.8	0.8
PU/PD	0.8	—
SAP increase	7.8	8.3
ALT increase	5.4	4.5
AST increase	2.3	0.8
BUN increase	3.1	1.5
Bilirubinuria	16.3	12.1
Ketonuria	14.7	9.1

Clinical pathology parameters listed represent reports of increases from pre-treatment values; the use of clinical judgement is necessary to determine clinical relevance. During investigational studies for the chewable tablet formulation, gastrointestinal signs were observed in some dogs. These signs included vomiting and soft stools.

Post-Approval Experience: Although not all adverse reactions are reported, the following adverse reactions are based on voluntary post-approval adverse drug experience reporting. The categories of adverse reactions are listed in decreasing order of frequency by body system.

Gastrointestinal: Vomiting, diarrhea, constipation, inappetence, melena, hematemesis, gastrointestinal ulceration, gastrointestinal bleeding, pancreatitis.

Hepatic: Inappetence, vomiting, jaundice, acute hepatic toxicity, hepatic enzyme elevation, abnormal liver function test(s), hyperbilirubinemia, bilirubinuria, hypoalbuminemia. Approximately one-fourth of hepatic reports were in Labrador Retrievers.

Neurologic: Ataxia, paresis, paralysis, seizures, vestibular signs, disorientation.

Urinary: Hematuria, polyuria, polydipsia, urinary incontinence, urinary tract infection, azotemia, acute renal failure, tubular abnormalities including acute tubular necrosis, renal tubular acidosis, glucosuria.

Behavioral: Sedation, lethargy, hyperactivity, restlessness, aggressiveness.

Hematologic: Immune-mediated hemolytic anemia, immune-mediated thrombocytopenia, blood loss anemia, epistaxis.

Dermatologic: Pruritus, increased shedding, alopecia, pyotraumatic moist dermatitis (hot spots), necrotizing panniculitis/vasculitis, ventral ecchymosis.

Immunologic or hypersensitivity: Facial swelling, hives, erythema.

In rare situations, death has been associated with some of the adverse reactions listed above.

To report a suspected adverse reaction call 1-800-366-5288.

For a copy of the Material Safety Data Sheet (MSDS) or to report adverse reactions call Pfizer Animal Health at 1-800-366-5288.

Trial Data: Palatability: A controlled palatability study was conducted which demonstrated that RIMADYL® Chewable Tablets were readily accepted and consumed on first offering by a majority of dogs.

Effectiveness: Separate placebo-controlled, masked, multicenter field studies confirmed the anti-inflammatory and analgesic effectiveness of RIMADYL® in various breeds of dogs when dosed at 2 mg/lb of body weight once daily or when divided and administered at 1 mg/lb twice daily.

In these two field studies, dogs diagnosed with osteoarthritis showed significant improvement in lameness based on masked owner and veterinarian evaluations when administered at the labeled dosages.

Animal Safety Studies: Laboratory studies and clinical field trials have demonstrated that RIMADYL® is well tolerated in dogs after oral administration.

In target animal safety studies, RIMADYL® was administered orally to healthy Beagle dogs at 1, 3, and 5 mg/lb twice daily (1, 3 and 5 times the recommended total daily dose) for 42 consecutive days with no significant adverse reactions. Serum albumin for a single female dog receiving 5 mg/lb twice daily decreased to 2.1 g/dL after 2 weeks of treatment, returned to the pre-treatment value (2.6 g/dL) after 4 weeks of treatment, and was 2.3 g/dL at the final 6-week evaluation. Over the 6-week treatment period, black or bloody stools were observed in 1 dog (1 incident) treated with 1 mg/lb twice daily and in 1 dog (2 incidents) treated with 3 mg/lb twice daily. Redness of the colonic mucosa was observed in 1 male that received 3 mg/lb twice daily.

Two of 8 dogs receiving 10 mg/lb orally twice daily (10 times the recommended total daily dose) for 14 days exhibited hypoalbuminemia. The mean albumin level in the dogs receiving this dose was lower (2.38 g/dL) than each of 2 placebo control groups (2.88 and 2.93 g/dL, respectively). Three incidents of black or bloody stool were observed in 1 dog. Five of 8 dogs exhibited reddened areas of duodenal mucosa on gross pathologic examination.

Histologic examination of these areas revealed no evidence of ulceration, but did show minimal congestion of the lamina propria in 2 of the 5 dogs.

In separate safety studies lasting 13 and 52 weeks, respectively, dogs were administered orally up to 11.4 mg/lb/day (5.7 times the recommended total daily dose of 2 mg/lb) of carprofen. In both studies, the drug was well tolerated clinically by all of the animals. No gross or histologic changes were seen in any of the treated animals. In both studies, dogs receiving the highest doses had average increases in serum L-alanine aminotransferase (ALT) of approximately 20 IU.

In the 52-week study, minor dermatologic changes occurred in dogs in each of the treatment groups but not in the control dogs. The changes were described as slight redness or rash and were diagnosed as non-specific dermatitis. The possibility exists that these mild lesions were treatment related, but no dose relationship was observed.

Clinical field studies were conducted with 549 dogs of different breeds at the recommended doses for 14 days (297 dogs were included in a study evaluating 1 mg/lb twice daily and 252 dogs were included in a separate study evaluating 2 mg/lb once daily). In both studies the drug was clinically well tolerated and the incidence of clinical adverse reactions for RIMADYL®-treated animals was no higher than placebo-treated animals (placebo contained inactive ingredients found in RIMADYL®). For animals receiving 1 mg/lb twice daily, the mean post-treatment serum ALT values were 11 IU greater and 9 IU less than pre-treatment values for dogs receiving RIMADYL® and placebo, respectively. Differences were not statistically significant. For animals receiving 2 mg/lb once daily, the mean post-treatment serum ALT values were 4.5 IU greater and 0.9 IU less than pre-treatment values for dogs receiving RIMADYL® and placebo, respectively. In the latter study, 3 RIMADYL®-treated dogs developed a 3-fold or greater increase in (ALT) and/or (AST) during the course of therapy. One placebo-treated dog had a greater than 2-fold increase in ALT. None of these animals showed clinical signs associated with the laboratory value changes. Changes in clinical laboratory values (hematology and clinical chemistry) were not considered clinically significant. The 1 mg/lb twice daily course of therapy was repeated as needed at 2-week intervals in 244 dogs, some for as long as 5 years.

References: Available upon request.

Presentation: Each tablet size is packaged in bottles containing 14, 60, or 180 tablets.

Compendium Code No.: 36901381 75-8501-05

RIS-MA™

Intervet **Vaccine**

Marek's Disease Vaccine, Serotypes 1 & 3, Live Virus

U.S. Vet. Lic. No.: 286

Contents: RIS-MA™ is a frozen vaccine that contains the CVI 988 strain of chicken herpesvirus, and the FC-126 strain of turkey herpesvirus. The CVI 988 strain was specially selected for its immunogenicity and has been used extensively in Europe with excellent results.

This vaccine contains Gentamicin as a preservative.

Indications: RIS-MA™ is recommended for vaccination of healthy one-day-old chickens by subcutaneous injection to aid in the prevention of very virulent Marek's disease. The viruses will infect chickens even though they may possess maternal antibodies to Marek's disease virus (MDV).

Dosage and Administration: Preparation of Vaccine:

Caution: Read warning advice on handling vaccine ampule. Sterilize vaccinating equipment by boiling in water for 30 minutes or by autoclaving (20 minutes at 121°C). Do not use chemical disinfectants.

1. Use 1,000 doses of vaccine with 200 mL sterile diluent per 1,000 chickens.
2. Before withdrawing vaccine from liquid nitrogen canister, protect hands with gloves, wear long sleeves and use a face mask or goggles. It is possible an accident could occur with either the liquid nitrogen or the ampules of vaccine. When removing an ampule from the cane, hold palm of gloved hand away from body and face.
3. When withdrawing a cane of ampules from canister in liquid nitrogen refrigerator, expose only the ampule to be used immediately. We recommend handling only one ampule at a time. After removing the ampule from the cane, the remaining ampules should be replaced immediately in the canister of the liquid nitrogen refrigerator.
4. The contents of the ampule are thawed rapidly by immersing in water at room temperature. Shake ampule to disperse contents. Then break ampule at its neck and immediately proceed as below. 1,000 doses of RIS-MA™ is added for each 200 mL of diluent. Caution: Ampules have been known to explode on sudden temperature changes. Do not thaw in hot or ice cold water.
5. Draw contents of ampule into a sterile 10 mL syringe, mounted with an 18-gauge needle.
6. Dilute immediately by filling the syringe slowly with a portion of the diluent. Important: The diluent should be at room temperature (60°-80°F) at time of mixing.
7. The contents of the filled syringe are then added to remaining diluent. It is important that this be done slowly. Slowly empty the syringe, allowing the vaccine to run down the side of the diluent container. Gently swirl the container as the vaccine is being mixed. Withdraw a portion of the diluent with the syringe to flush ampule. Inject the washing back into the diluent container. Remove the syringe.
8. Fill the previously sterilized automatic syringe according to the manufacturer's recommendations and set the dose at 0.2 mL.
9. The vaccine is now ready for use.

Method of Vaccination: Subcutaneous Administration:

1. Hold the chicken by the back of the neck just below the head. The loose skin in the area is raised by gently pinching with the thumb and forefinger. Insert the needle beneath the skin in a downward direction away from the head. Inject 0.2 mL per chicken.
2. Avoid hitting the muscles and bones in the neck.
3. Entire contents of container must be used within 1 hour after mixing or be discarded according to caution statement No. 9.
4. After reconstitution, the vaccine should be kept cool and swirled frequently - every 5 minutes.

Records: Keep a record of vaccine, quantity, serial number, expiration date, and place of purchase; the date and time of vaccination; the number, age, breed, and locations of chickens; names of operators performing the vaccination and any observed reactions.

Precaution(s): Important: Storage Conditions:

Ampules - Store in liquid nitrogen container.

Diluent - Store at room temperature.

Container - Store liquid nitrogen container securely in upright position in a dry, well-ventilated area and away from incubator intakes and chicken boxes.

Safety Precautions: Liquid nitrogen container and vaccine should be handled only by properly trained personnel who are thoroughly conversant with the Union Carbide publication and instruction booklet regarding the use of, precautions and safe practices for liquefied atmospheric gases (particularly liquid nitrogen).

When removing ampule cane, handling frozen ampules, or adding liquid nitrogen, wear long sleeves, a plastic face shield and gloves to protect the skin from contact with the liquid nitrogen. All storage and handling of the liquid nitrogen container must be in a dry, ventilated area. Do not inhale liquid nitrogen vapors. If drowsiness occurs, get fresh air quickly; then ventilate entire area. If breathing difficulty occurs, apply artificial respiration. If any of these difficulties persist or there is a loss of consciousness, summon a physician immediately.

Care should be exercised to prevent contaminating your hands, eyes and clothing with the vaccine.

Caution(s): Good management practices are recommended to reduce exposure to Marek's disease for at least three weeks following vaccination. Directions should be followed carefully.

1. Do not mix any substance, not approved by Intervet Inc., with this vaccine.
2. Store vaccine in liquid nitrogen at a temperature below -150°C.
3. Gloves and visor should be worn when handling liquid nitrogen.
4. Once thawed, the product should not be refrozen.
5. Do not dilute or otherwise stretch the dosage of this vaccine.
6. Once mixed with diluent, the vaccine should be swirled frequently, every 5 minutes.
7. Once mixed with diluent, the vaccine should be used within 1 hour.
8. Only healthy chickens should be vaccinated.
9. Burn this container and all unused contents.
10. For veterinary use only.
11. Read the above directions carefully.

Notice: This vaccine has undergone rigid potency, safety and purity tests, and meets Intervet Inc. and USDA requirements. It is designed to stimulate effective immunity when used as directed, but the user must be advised that the response to the product depends upon many factors, including, but not limited to, conditions of storage and handling by the user, administration of the vaccine, health and responsiveness of the individual chickens, and the degree of field exposure.

This product is not hazardous when used according to directions supplied. A material safety data sheet (MSDS) is available upon request. This and any other consumer information can be obtained by calling Intervet Inc. Customer Service at 1-800-441-8272 or 1-302-934-8051.

The use of this vaccine is subject to applicable local and federal laws and regulations.

Warning(s): Do not vaccinate within 21 days before slaughter.

Presentation: One 1,000-dose ampule and 200 mL of sterile diluent for subcutaneous injection.

RIS-MA™ is packaged in two separate units. One is an ampule containing 1,000 doses of frozen, live, cell-associated, turkey and chicken herpesvirus. The second is a container of sterile diluent. The ampules are inserted in metal canes and shipped in a liquid nitrogen container. The diluent is packaged in separate containers and is used at the rate of 200 mL of diluent per 1,000 doses of vaccine.

Compendium Code No.: 11061720

RIS-MA-SB™

Intervet **Vaccine**

Marek's Disease Vaccine, Serotypes 1, 2 & 3, Live Virus

U.S. Vet. Lic. No.: 286

Contents: RIS-MA™ is a frozen vaccine that contains the CVI 988 strain of chicken herpesvirus, and the FC-126 strain of turkey herpesvirus, and the SB-1 strain of chicken herpesvirus. The CVI 988 strain was specially selected for its immunogenicity and has been used extensively in Europe with excellent results.

This vaccine contains Gentamicin as a preservative.

Indications: RIS-MA-SB™ is recommended for vaccination of healthy one-day-old chickens by subcutaneous injection to aid in the prevention of very virulent Marek's disease. The viruses will infect chickens even though they may possess maternal antibodies to Marek's disease virus (MDV).

Dosage and Administration: Preparation of Vaccine:

Caution: Read warning advice on handling vaccine ampule. Sterilize vaccinating equipment by boiling in water for 30 minutes or by autoclaving (20 minutes at 121°C). Do not use chemical disinfectants.

1. Use 1,000 doses of vaccine with 200 mL sterile diluent per 1,000 chickens.
2. Before withdrawing vaccine from liquid nitrogen canister, protect hands with gloves, wear long sleeves and use a face mask or goggles. It is possible an accident could occur with either the liquid nitrogen or the ampules of vaccine. When removing an ampule from the cane, hold palm of gloved hand away from body and face.
3. When withdrawing a cane of ampules from canister in liquid nitrogen refrigerator, expose only the ampule to be used immediately. We recommend handling only one ampule at a time. After removing the ampule from the cane, the remaining ampules should be replaced immediately in the canister of the liquid nitrogen refrigerator.
4. The contents of the ampule are thawed rapidly by immersing in water at room temperature. Shake ampule to disperse contents. Then break ampule at its neck and immediately proceed as below. 1,000 doses of RIS-MA-SB™ is added for each 200 mL of diluent. Caution: Ampules have been known to explode on sudden temperature changes. Do not thaw in hot or ice cold water.
5. Draw contents of ampule into a sterile 10 mL syringe, mounted with an 18-gauge needle.
6. Dilute immediately by filling the syringe slowly with a portion of the diluent. Important: The diluent should be at room temperature (60°-80°F) at time of mixing.
7. The contents of the filled syringe are then added to remaining diluent. It is important that this be done slowly. Slowly empty the syringe, allowing the vaccine to run down the side of the diluent container. Gently swirl the container as the vaccine is being mixed. Withdraw a portion of the diluent with the syringe to flush ampule. Inject the washing back into the diluent container. Remove the syringe.
8. Fill the previously sterilized automatic syringe according to the manufacturer's recommendations and set the dose at 0.2 mL.
9. The vaccine is now ready for use.

Method of Vaccination: Subcutaneous Administration:

1. Hold the chicken by the back of the neck just below the head. The loose skin in the area is raised by gently pinching with the thumb and forefinger. Insert the needle beneath the skin in a downward direction away from the head. Inject 0.2 mL per chicken.
2. Avoid hitting the muscles and bones in the neck.
3. Entire contents of container must be used within 1 hour after mixing or be discarded according to caution statement No. 10.
4. After reconstitution, the vaccine should be kept cool and swirled frequently - every 5 minutes.

Records: Keep a record of vaccine, quantity, serial number, expiration date, and place of purchase; the date and time of vaccination; the number, age, breed, and locations of chickens; names of operators performing the vaccination and any observed reactions.

Precaution(s): Important: Storage Conditions:

Ampules - Store in liquid nitrogen container.

Diluent - Store at room temperature.

Container - Store liquid nitrogen container securely in upright position in a dry, well-ventilated area and away from incubator intakes and chicken boxes.

Safety Precautions: Liquid nitrogen container and vaccine should be handled only by properly trained personnel who are thoroughly conversant with the Union Carbide publication and instruction booklet regarding the use of, precautions and safe practices for liquefied atmospheric gases (particularly liquid nitrogen).

When removing ampule cane, handling frozen ampules, or adding liquid nitrogen, wear long sleeves, a plastic face shield and gloves to protect the skin from contact with the liquid nitrogen. All storage and handling of the liquid nitrogen container must be in a dry, ventilated area. Do not inhale liquid nitrogen vapors. If drowsiness occurs, get fresh air quickly; then ventilate entire area. If breathing difficulty occurs, apply artificial respiration. If any of these difficulties persist or there is a loss of consciousness, summon a physician immediately.

Care should be exercised to prevent contaminating your hands, eyes and clothing with the vaccine.

Caution(s): Good management practices are recommended to reduce exposure to Marek's disease for at least three weeks following vaccination. Directions should be followed carefully.

1. Do not mix any substance, not approved by Intervet Inc., with this vaccine.
2. Store vaccine in liquid nitrogen at a temperature below -150°C.
3. Gloves and visor should be worn when handling liquid nitrogen.
4. Once thawed, the product should not be refrozen.
5. Do not dilute or otherwise stretch the dosage of this vaccine.
6. Once mixed with diluent, the vaccine should be swirled frequently, every 5 minutes.
7. Once mixed with diluent, the vaccine should be used within 1 hour.
8. Only healthy chickens should be vaccinated.
9. Serotype 2 strains of chicken herpesvirus have been shown to allow for the development of lymphoid leukosis under certain circumstances in certain types of chickens.
10. Burn this container and all unused contents.
11. For veterinary use only.
12. Read the above directions carefully.

Notice: This vaccine has undergone rigid potency, safety and purity tests, and meets Intervet Inc. and USDA requirements. It is designed to stimulate effective immunity when used as directed, but the user must be advised that the response to the product depends upon many factors, including, but not limited to, conditions of storage and handling by the user, administration of the vaccine, health and responsiveness of the individual chickens, and the degree of field exposure.

This product is not hazardous when used according to directions supplied. A material safety data sheet (MSDS) is available upon request. This and any other consumer information can be obtained by calling Intervet Inc. Customer Service at 1-800-441-8272 or 1-302-934-8051.

The use of this vaccine is subject to applicable local and federal laws and regulations.

Warning(s): Do not vaccinate within 21 days before slaughter.

Presentation: One 1,000-dose ampule and 200 mL of sterile diluent for subcutaneous injection.

RIS-MA-SB™ is packaged in two separate units. One is an ampule containing 1,000 doses of frozen, live, cell-associated, turkey and both chicken herpesviruses. The second is a container of sterile diluent. The ampules are inserted in metal canes and shipped in a liquid nitrogen container. The diluent is packaged in separate containers and is used at the rate of 200 mL of diluent per 1,000 doses of vaccine.

Compendium Code No.: 11061710

RISMAVAC®

Intervet **Vaccine**

Marek's Disease Vaccine, Serotype 1, Live Virus

U.S. Vet. Lic. No.: 286

Description: RISMAVAC® is a frozen, cell associated, live virus vaccine that contains the low passage CVI 988 strain of chicken herpesvirus.

This vaccine contains Gentamicin as a preservative.

Quality tested for purity, potency, and safety.

Indications: RISMAVAC® is recommended for vaccination of healthy one-day-old chickens by subcutaneous injection or 18-day-old chicken embryos by the *in ovo* route to aid in the prevention of very virulent Marek's disease.

Dosage and Administration: Preparation of Vaccine:

Caution: Read "Safety Precautions" advice on handling vaccine ampule. Sterilize vaccinating equipment by boiling in water for 30 minutes or by autoclaving (20 minutes at 250°F or 121°C). Do not use chemical disinfectants.

1. Use 1,000 doses of vaccine with 200 mL sterile diluent per 1,000 chickens when administering vaccine by the subcutaneous route. Use 1,000 doses of vaccine with 100 mL sterile diluent per 1,000 chicken embryos to administer one 0.10 mL dose per chicken embryo or use 50 mL sterile diluent per 1,000 chicken embryos to administer one 0.05 mL dose per chicken embryo.
2. Before withdrawing vaccine from liquid nitrogen canister, protect hands with gloves, wear long sleeves and use a face mask or goggles. It is possible an accident could occur with either the liquid nitrogen or the ampules of vaccine. When removing an ampule from the cane, hold palm of gloved hand away from body and face.
3. When withdrawing a cane of ampules from canister in liquid nitrogen container, expose only the ampule to be used immediately. We recommend handling only one ampule at a time. After removing the ampule from the cane, the remaining ampules should be replaced immediately in the canister of the liquid nitrogen container.
4. The contents of the ampule are thawed rapidly by immersing in water at room temperature. Shake ampule to disperse contents. Then break ampule at its neck and immediately proceed as below. Dilute the vaccine with diluent for administration. 1,000 doses of vaccine is added for each 50, 100, 200 mL of diluent. Caution: Ampules have been known to explode on sudden temperature changes. Do not thaw in hot or ice cold water.
5. Draw contents of ampule into a sterile 10 mL syringe, mounted with an 18-gauge needle.
6. Dilute immediately by filling the syringe slowly with a portion of the diluent. Important: The diluent should be at room temperature (60°-80°F or 16°-27°C) at time of mixing.
7. The contents of the filled syringe are then added to remaining diluent. It is important that this be done slowly. Slowly empty the syringe, allowing the vaccine to run down the side of the diluent container. Gently agitate the container as the vaccine is being mixed. Withdraw a portion of the diluent with the syringe to flush ampule. Remove the remaining diluent from the ampule and inject gently into the diluent container. Remove the syringe.
8. Fill the previously sterilized automatic syringe or egg inoculation machine according to the manufacturer's recommendations.
9. The vaccine is now ready for use.

Method of Vaccination:

Subcutaneous Administration:

1. Hold the chicken by the back of the neck just below the head. The loose skin in the area is raised by gently pinching with the thumb and forefinger. Insert the needle beneath the skin in a downward direction away from the head. Inject 0.2 mL per chicken.
2. Avoid hitting the muscles and bones in the neck.
3. Entire contents of container must be used within 1 hour after mixing or be discarded according to Precaution(s).
4. After reconstitution, the vaccine should be kept cool and gently agitated frequently.

In Ovo Administration:

1. Inoculate each 18-day-old chicken embryo with a full dose (0.05 mL or 0.10 mL).
2. Entire contents of container must be used within 1 hour after mixing or be discarded according to Precaution(s).
3. After reconstitution, the vaccine should be kept cool and gently agitated frequently.

Records: Keep a record of vaccine, quantity, serial number, expiration date, and place of purchase; the date and time of vaccination; the number, age, breed, and locations of chickens; names of operators performing the vaccination and any observed reactions.

Precaution(s): Important: Storage Conditions:

Ampules - Store in liquid nitrogen container.

Diluent - Store at room temperature.

Container - Store liquid nitrogen container securely in upright position in a dry, well-ventilated area and away from incubator intakes and chicken boxes.

Safety Precautions: Liquid nitrogen container and vaccine should be handled only by properly trained personnel who are thoroughly conversant with the Union Carbide publication and instruction booklet regarding the use of, precautions for, and safe practices for liquefied atmospheric gases (particularly liquid nitrogen).

When removing ampule cane, handling frozen ampules, or adding liquid nitrogen, wear long sleeves, a plastic face shield and gloves to protect the skin from contact with the liquid nitrogen. All storage and handling of the liquid nitrogen container must be in a dry, ventilated area. Do not inhale liquid nitrogen vapors. If drowsiness occurs, get fresh air quickly; then ventilate entire area. If breathing difficulty occurs, apply artificial respiration. If any of these difficulties persist or there is a loss of consciousness, summon a physician immediately.

Care should be exercised to prevent contaminating your hands, eyes and clothing with the vaccine.

Do not mix any substance, not approved by Intervet Inc., with this vaccine.

Store vaccine in liquid nitrogen at a temperature below - 238°F or -150°C.

Gloves and visor should be worn when handling liquid nitrogen.

Once thawed, the product should not be refrozen.

Once mixed with diluent, the vaccine should be gently agitated frequently.

Once mixed with diluent, the vaccine should be used within 1 hour.

Burn the container and all unused contents.

This product is non-returnable.

Caution(s): It is recommended that good management practices be followed to reduce exposure to Marek's disease for at least three weeks following vaccination.

Do not dilute or otherwise stretch the dosage of this vaccine.

Only healthy chickens or chicken embryos should be vaccinated.

For veterinary use only.

Read the directions carefully.

Notice: This vaccine has undergone rigid potency, safety and purity tests, and meets Intervet Inc. and USDA requirements. It is designed to stimulate effective immunity when used as directed, but the user must be advised that the response to the product depends upon many factors, including, but not limited to, conditions of storage and handling by the user, administration of the vaccine, health and responsiveness of the individual chickens, and the degree of field exposure.

This product is not hazardous when used according to directions supplied. A material safety data sheet (MSDS) is available upon request. This and any other consumer information can be obtained by calling Intervet Inc. Customer Service at 1-800-441-8272 or 1-302-934-8051.

The use of this vaccine is subject to applicable local and federal laws and regulations.

Use only as directed.

Warning(s): Do not vaccinate within 21 days before slaughter.

Presentation: 1 x 1,000 dose ampule with 200 mL sterile diluent per 1,000 doses.

RISMAVAC® is packaged in 1,000 dose glass ampules and supplied with diluent packaged in a separate container. The vaccine ampules are inserted in metal canes, stored and shipped in a liquid nitrogen container.

Compendium Code No.: 11061741 Rev. 27603 AL163

RITTER'S TICK AND FLEA POWDER

Ritter **Parasiticide Powder**

EPA Reg. No.: 49784-3-47256

Active Ingredient(s):

Carbaryl (1-napthyl n-methylcarbamate) . . . 12.50%
Methoxychlor, technical . . . 0.25%
(Equivalent to 0.22% 2,2 bis (p-methoxyphenyl)-1,1,1-trichloroethane and 0.03% other isomers and related compounds.)
Inactive ingredients . . . 87.25%
Total . . . 100.00%

Indications: For the control of ticks and fleas on dogs and cats.

Directions for Use: It is a violation of federal law to use the product in a manner inconsistent with its labeling.

Read entire label before each use.

Consult a veterinarian before using this product on debilitated, aged, pregnant, nursing, or animals on medication. Do not use on kittens or puppies under 12 weeks of age. Use product only outside or in well-ventilated area. This product should not be applied by children. Wearing household latex or rubber gloves, dust entire animal avoiding pet's eyes, nose, mouth and genital areas. Rub or brush pet's hair to work dust down to the skin being sure to include ears, legs, feet and between the toes. Repeat application at one to three week intervals if necessary.

Precautionary Statements: Hazards to Humans and Domestic Animals: Caution.

Humans: May be harmful if swallowed. Avoid inhaling dust. Avoid contact with the skin, eyes or clothing.

Animals: Carbaryl is a cholinesterase inhibitor. Do not use this product on animals simultaneously or within 30 days before or after treatment with or exposure to other cholinesterase inhibiting drugs, pesticides or chemicals. Consult a veterinarian at the first sign of any adverse reaction. Atropine is antidotal.

Some sensitivities may occur after using any pesticide product for pets. If signs of sensitivity occur, bathe your pet with mild soap and rinse with large amounts of water. If signs continue, consult a veterinarian immediately.

First Aid:

If Swallowed: Call a physician, veterinarian or poison control center immediately. Drink one or two glasses of water and induce vomiting by touching the back of the throat with finger. Repeat until vomit fluid is clear. Do not induce vomiting or give anything by mouth to an unconscious person.

If in Eyes: Flush with plenty of water. See a physician if irritation persists.

If on Skin: Remove contaminated clothing and wash affected areas with soap and water.

Environmental Hazards: This pesticide is extremely toxic to aquatic invertebrates. Do not apply directly to water. Do not contaminate water by cleaning of equipment or disposal of wastes.

This product is highly toxic to bees exposed to direct treatment or residues on blooming crops or weeds. Do not apply this product or allow it to drift to blooming crops or weeds if bees are visiting the treatment areas.

User Safety Requirements: Wear long-sleeved shirt, long pants, shoes plus socks and household latex or rubber gloves when applying this product.

Change clothing as soon as possible after use.

Wash the outside of gloves before removing. As with any pesticide product, wash hand thoroughly immediately after handling and before eating, smoking or using the toilet.

Storage and Disposal: Do not contaminate water, food or feed by storage or disposal.

Storage: Do not store product under conditions of excessive moisture or humidity.

Product Disposal: Securely wrap original container in several layers of newspaper and discard in trash.

Container Disposal: Do not reuse container. Discard container in trash.

Warning(s): Keep out of the reach of children.

Presentation: 226.6 g (8 oz) containers.

Compendium Code No.: 13710000

ROBAMOX®-V ORAL SUSPENSION ℞

Fort Dodge — **brand of amoxicillin**

NADA No.: 065-495

Active Ingredient(s): Each 15 mL bottle contains 0.75 g of amoxicillin activity.

After reconstitution with the required amount of water, each mL will contain 50 mg of amoxicillin as the trihydrate.

Inactive Ingredients: Cherry flavor, colloidal silicon dioxide, FD&C Red #40, polyoxyethylene-polyoxypropylene glycol, sodium benzoate, sodium citrate, sodium saccharin, and sucrose.

Indications: ROBAMOX®-V (amoxicillin) for oral suspension is indicated in the treatment of the following infections in dogs when caused by susceptible strains of organisms:

Bacterial Dermatitis due to *Staphylococcus aureus, Streptococcus* spp., *Staphylococcus* spp., and *E. coli.*

Soft Tissue Infections (abscesses, wounds, lacerations) due to *Staphylococcus aureus, Streptococcus* spp., *E. coli, Proteus mirabilis,* and *Staphylococcus* spp.

As is true with all antibiotic therapy, appropriate *in vitro* cultures and sensitivities should be conducted prior to treatment.

Pharmacology: Description: ROBAMOX®-V (amoxicillin) is a broad spectrum, semisynthetic antibiotic which provides bactericidal activity against a wide range of common gram-positive and gram-negative pathogens. Amoxicillin chemically is D-(-)a-amino-p-hydroxybenzyl penicillin trihydrate.

Action: Amoxicillin has bactericidal activity against susceptible organisms similar to that of ampicillin. It acts by inhibiting the biosynthesis of bacterial cell wall mucopeptide. Most strains of the following gram-positive and gram-negative bacteria have demonstrated susceptibility to amoxicillin, both *in vitro* and *in vivo:* non-penicillinase-producing staphylococci, alpha- and beta-hemolytic streptococci, *Streptococcus faecalis, Escherichia coli,* and *Proteus mirabilis.* Amoxicillin does not resist destruction by penicillinase; therefore, it is not effective against penicillinase-producing bacteria, particularly resistant staphylococci. Most strains of Enterobacter and Klebsiella and all strains of Pseudomonas are resistant.

Amoxicillin may be given without regard to meals because it is stable in gastric acid. It is rapidly absorbed following oral administration and diffuses readily into most body fluids and tissues. It diffuses poorly into the brain and spinal fluid except when the meninges are inflamed. Most of amoxicillin is excreted in the urine unchanged.

Dosage and Administration: The recommended dosage is 5 mg per pound of body weight administered twice daily for 5 to 7 days. Continue for 48 hours after all symptoms have subsided. If no improvement is noted in 5 days, the diagnosis should be reconsidered and therapy changed.

Directions for Mixing Oral Suspension: Add sufficient water to the bottle as indicated in the table below and shake vigorously. Each mL of suspension will contain 50 mg of amoxicillin as the trihydrate.

Bottle Size	Amount of Water to Add for Reconstitution
15 mL	11 mL

Note: When stored at room temperature or in refrigerator, discard unused portion of reconstituted suspension after 14 days.

Contraindication(s): Use of amoxicillin is contraindicated in animals with a history of an allergic reaction to penicillin.

Caution(s): Federal law restricts this drug to use by or on the order of a licensed veterinarian.

Until adequate reproductive studies are accomplished, ROBAMOX®-V (amoxicillin) for oral suspension should not be used in pregnant or breeding animals.

Warning(s): For use in dogs only.

Adverse Reactions: Amoxicillin is a semisynthetic penicillin and, therefore, has the potential for producing allergic reactions. Epinephrine and/or steroids should be administered if an allergic reaction occurs.

Presentation: ROBAMOX®-V (amoxicillin) for oral suspension is supplied in bottles of 15 mL (NDC 0856-7180-78).

Manufactured by: Teva Pharmaceuticals USA, Sellersville, PA 18960

Compendium Code No.: 10031840 5120D

ROBAMOX®-V TABLETS ℞

Fort Dodge — **Amoxicillin Oral**

NADA No.: 141-005

Active Ingredient(s): Each tablet contains either:

Amoxicillin . . . . 50 mg, 100 mg, 200 mg, or 400 mg

Inactive Ingredients: Dibasic calcium phosphate, magnesium stearate, microcrystalline cellulose, and sodium starch glycolate.

Indications: ROBAMOX®-V (amoxicillin) Tablets are indicated in the treatment of the following infections in dogs when caused by susceptible strains of organisms:

Bacterial Dermatitis due to *Staphylococcus aureus, Streptococcus* spp., *Staphylococcus* spp., and *E. coli.*

Soft Tissue Infections (abscesses, wounds, lacerations) due to *Staphylococcus aureus, Streptococcus* spp., *E. coli, Proteus mirabilis* and *Staphylococcus* spp.

As is true with all antibiotic therapy, appropriate *in vitro* cultures and sensitivities should be conducted prior to treatment.

Pharmacology: Description: ROBAMOX®-V (amoxicillin) is a broad spectrum, semisynthetic antibiotic which provides bactericidal activity against a wide range of common gram-positive and gram-negative pathogens. Amoxicillin chemically is D-(-)a-amino-p-hydroxybenzyl penicillin trihydrate.

Action: Amoxicillin has bactericidal activity against susceptible organisms similar to that of ampicillin. It acts by inhibiting the biosynthesis of bacterial cell wall mucopeptide. Most strains of the following gram-positive and gram-negative bacteria have demonstrated susceptibility to amoxicillin, both *in vitro* and *in vivo:* non-penicillinase-producing staphylococci, alpha- and beta-hemolytic streptococci, *Streptococcus faecalis, Escherichia coli* and *Proteus mirabilis.* Amoxicillin does not resist destruction by penicillinase; therefore, it is not effective against penicillinase-producing bacteria, particularly resistant staphylococci. Most strains of *Enterobacter* and *Klebsiella* and all strains of *Pseudomonas* are resistant.

Amoxicillin may be given without regard to meals because it is stable in gastric acid. It is rapidly absorbed following oral administration and diffuses readily into most body fluids and tissues. It diffuses poorly into the brain and spinal fluid except when the meninges are inflamed. Most of amoxicillin is excreted in the urine unchanged.

Dosage and Administration: The recommended dosage is 5 mg per pound of body weight administered twice daily for 5 to 7 days or 48 hours after all symptoms have subsided. If no improvement is noted in 5 days, the diagnosis should be reconsidered and therapy changed.

Contraindication(s): Use of amoxicillin is contraindicated in animals with a history of an allergic reaction to penicillin.

Caution(s): Federal law restricts this drug to use by or on the order of a licensed veterinarian.

Does not meet USP water content specification.

Until adequate reproductive studies are accomplished, ROBAMOX®-V (amoxicillin) Tablets should not be used in pregnant or breeding animals.

Warning(s): For use in dogs only.

Adverse Reactions: Amoxicillin is a semisynthetic penicillin and, therefore, has the potential for producing allergic reactions. Epinephrine and/or steroids should be administered if an allergic reaction occurs.

Presentation: ROBAMOX®-V (amoxicillin) Tablets are supplied in 50 mg (NDC 0856-7131-70), 100 mg (NDC 0856-7141-70), 200 mg (NDC 0856-7151-70) and 400 mg (NDC 0856-7171-70) concentrations in bottles of 500 tablets.

Manufactured by: Teva Pharmaceuticals USA, Sellersville, PA 18960

Compendium Code No.: 10031850 5240F

ROBAXIN®-V ℞

Fort Dodge — **Muscle Relaxant**

brand of Methocarbamol

NADA No.: 038-838 (Injection)/045-715 (Tablets)

Active Ingredient(s): Each mL contains 100 mg of methocarbamol in sterile 50 percent aqueous solution of polyethylene glycol-300. pH adjusted, when necessary, with hydrochloric acid and/or sodium hydroxide.

Each tablet contains:

Methocarbamol. . . . . 500 mg

Indications:

Dogs and Cats, oral and intravenous — ROBAXIN®-V is indicated as an adjunct to therapy of acute inflammatory and traumatic conditions of the skeletal muscle and to reduce muscular spasms. The efficacy of both tablets and injectable in the treatment of acute skeletal muscle hyperactivity secondary to the following conditions has been demonstrated:

1. Intervertebral disc syndrome, compressive myelitis, spinal cord injury where cord remains intact.
2. Traumatism causing muscular and ligamentous sprains and strains.
3. Myositis, fibrositis, bursitis, synovitis.
4. Muscular spasm prior to or following surgical procedures.
5. Miscellaneous conditions: Tablets — To maintain therapeutic benefits of the injectable form in strychnine poisoning and tetanus.

Horses, intravenous — As an adjunct to therapy of acute inflammatory and traumatic conditions of the skeletal muscle to reduce muscular spasms, and effect striated muscle relaxation. The efficacy in the treatment of acute skeletal muscle hyperactivity secondary to the following conditions has been demonstrated:

1. Trauma, muscular and ligamentous sprains and strains.
2. Myositis, fibrositis, bursitis and synovitis.
3. Tying up syndrome.
4. Muscular spasm prior to or following surgical procedures.
5. Maintenance of muscle relaxation in tetanus.

ROBAXIN®-V can be used concurrently with adrenal corticosteroids and other medications usually employed in these cases without untoward effects.

Pharmacology: Description: ROBAXIN®-V (methocarbamol) is a potent skeletal muscle relaxant which has an unusually selective action on the central nervous system, specifically on the internuncial neurons of the spinal cord. This specific action results in a diminution of skeletal muscle hyperactivity without concomitant alteration in normal muscle tone. It is long-acting and essentially non-toxic, and has proved effective in a wide range of disorders involving acute muscle spasm.

Methocarbamol has the following structural formula:

3-(2-methoxyphenoxyl)-1,2-propanediol 1-carbamate, or methocarbamol

Animal studies have shown that methocarbamol acts primarily on the internuncial neurons of the spinal cord. It exerts a prolonged blocking effect on polysynaptic reflex pathways at dosages which do not significantly alter transmission through monosynaptic reflex arcs and interrupts abnormal impulses from areas of disturbed muscle. It has no direct action on the contractile mechanism of striated muscle, the motor end-plate or the nerve fiber.

Methocarbamol affords a marked protective action against the effects of strychnine in rats, cats and dogs. It prevents both convulsions and death when administered prior to strychnine in the rodent. In dogs and cats, it promptly controls the classical and severe symptoms of strychnine poisoning. Methocarbamol is more potent than mephenesin or mephenesin carbamate in blocking convulsions induced with pentylenetetrazol or electroshock.

Signs of central nervous system depression are produced by large doses of methocarbamol. Included are loss of righting reflex, prostration and ataxia. Also indicative of CNS depression is the finding that methocarbamol potentiates barbiturate hypnosis in mice.

The results of acute and subchronic studies emphasize that methocarbamol is relatively non-toxic. It does not significantly alter hematologic or biochemical values. Similarly, gross and microscopic tissue examinations revealed no significant findings attributable to it.

Dosage and Administration:

Injectable — This preparation is for intravenous administration and may be given undiluted directly into a vein. Dosage and frequency of injection should be based on the severity of symptoms and on the therapeutic response noted.

ROBAXIN®-V is compatible with general anesthetics, causing no depression of vital body functions or no prolonging of anesthesia. However, specific studies using the injectable form have shown that additional muscle relaxation does occur and the anesthetic dosage may be reduced.

Dogs and Cats: For relief of moderate conditions, a dose of ⅕ mL/lb (20 mg/lb) body weight may be adequate.

An initial dose of ¼ to 1 mL/lb body weight is suggested for controlling the severe effects of strychnine and tetanus. Additional amounts may be needed for relieving residual effects and for preventing the recurrence of symptoms.

A total cumulative dose of 150 mg/lb body weight should not be exceeded. Administer rapidly half the estimated dose, pause until the animal starts to relax, then continue administration to effect. When satisfactory muscular relaxation is achieved, it can usually be maintained with tablets.

Horses: Give drug to effect: moderate conditions, a dose of 2 to 10 mg/lb; for severe conditions (tetanus), a dose of 10 to 25 mg/lb.

Tablets — Dogs and Cats: Dosage and frequency of administration should be based on the severity of symptoms and on the therapeutic response noted. The usual canine and feline dose of ROBAXIN®-V is 60 mg/lb body weight in divided doses followed by 30 or 60 mg/lb body weight each following day. The total dose should be divided into two or three equal doses (given at twelve or eight hour intervals respectively).

Due to the nature of the conditions for which ROBAXIN®-V therapy is recommended, it is important that an accurate diagnosis is made. If no response is evident within five days of the initiation of treatment, the diagnosis should be redetermined.

Recommended Dosage Schedule for Tablets: Load dose — 1st day, 60 mg/lb; maintenance dose — 2nd day, 30 mg to 60 mg/lb.

Wt. of Dog	1st Day Load Dose	2nd Day Maintenance Dose
12½ lbs	½ tablet t.i.d.	¼ to ½ tablet t.i.d.
25 lbs	1 tablet t.i.d.	½ to 1 tablet t.i.d.
50 lbs	2 tablets t.i.d.	1 to 2 tablets t.i.d.

Contraindication(s): Although rat studies have indicated no adverse effects on the pregnant female, fetus or neonate, ROBAXIN®-V should not be used during pregnancy unless in the judgment of the veterinarian the potential benefits outweigh the possible hazards.

ROBAXIN®-V Injectable should not be administered to patients with known or suspected renal pathology. This caution is necessary because of the presence of polyethylene glycol-300 in the vehicle. A much larger amount of polyethylene glycol 300 than is present in recommended doses of ROBAXIN®-V Injectable is known to have increased pre-existing acidosis and urea retention in humans with renal impairment. Although the amount present in this preparation is well within the limits of safety, caution dictates this contraindication.

R

Methocarbamol is contraindicated in patients hypersensitive to the ingredients.

Precaution(s): Store at controlled room temperature 15° to 30°C (59° to 86°F).

Caution(s): Federal law restricts this drug to use by or on the order of a licensed veterinarian.

As with any drug administered intravenously, careful attention must be given to the dose and the rate of injection.

In dogs and cats, the rate should not exceed 2 mL per minute. Since ROBAXIN®-V Injectable is hypertonic, vascular extravasation must be avoided. A recumbent position will reduce the likelihood of side reactions.

In the horse, the most effective response is achieved by injecting rapidly through a 15- or 17-gauge needle.

Blood aspirated into the syringe does not mix with the hypertonic solution. This phenomenon occurs with many other intravenous preparations. The blood may be safely injected with the methocarbamol or the injection may be stopped when the plunger reaches the blood.

Warning(s): Not to be used in horses intended for food.

Toxicology: Toxicity studies have shown ROBAXIN®-V to be well tolerated at doses of 400 mg/kg divided in two daily doses given 5 days a week for 26 weeks. The usual treatment during clinical trials did not exceed 14 to 21 days.

Adverse Reactions: Side effects following administration of injectable methocarbamol are seldom encountered. Excessive salivation, emesis, muscular weakness and ataxia have been noted in both dogs and cats. These effects were prompt in appearance and were generally of short duration. Their incidence was closely related to administration of large doses and/or to a rapid rate of injection. They may serve, therefore, as indicators of overdosage, particularly when methocarbamol is administered at a slow rate.

Presentation: ROBAXIN®-V Injectable (methocarbamol) is supplied in 100 mL vials (NDC 0856-7411-09).

ROBAXIN®-V (methocarbamol) 500 mg. White scored tablets in bottles of 100 (NDC 0856-7417-63) and 500 (NDC 0856-7417-70).

Manufactured by: Elkins-Sinn, Inc., Cherry Hill, NJ 08003 (Injection); Whitehall-Robins, Richmond, VA 23220 (Tablets)

Compendium Code No.: 10031862 5250C

ROBENZ®

Alpharma **Feed Medication**

Robenidine Hydrochloride-Type A Medicated Article-Coccidiostat

NADA No.: 048-486

Active Ingredient(s):

Robenidine hydrochloride . . . . . . 6.6% (30 g/lb)

Carrier: Soybean feed, solvent extracted; Soybean meal, solvent extracted.

Indications: As an aid in the prevention of coccidiosis caused by *Eimeria mivati, E. brunetti, E. tenella, E. acervulina, E. maxima* and *E. necatrix* in broiler chickens only.

Directions: Mix 1 pound of ROBENZ® Type A Medicated Article in one ton of feed to provide 0.0033% concentration in feed.

Limitations: Feed continuously as the sole ration. Do not use in feeds containing bentonite.

Caution(s): Type C feeds containing ROBENZ® robenidine hydrochloride must be fed within 50 days from the date of manufacture.

Note: Manufacture of Type B or C feeds from this product requires a Medicated Feed License Application approved by FDA.

Labels for feeds containing ROBENZ® must contain appropriate indications, limitations and warnings as well as required feed ingredient information.

For use in manufacturing medicated feeds only.

Warning(s): Do not feed to chickens producing eggs for food. Withdraw 5 days prior to slaughter.

Presentation: 50 lb (22.68 kg) bag.

Compendium Code No.: 10220542 AHG-030 0103

ROBINUL®-V ℞

Fort Dodge **Anticholinergic**

brand of Glycopyrrolate Injectable

NADA No.: 101-777

Active Ingredient(s): Each 1 mL contains:

Glycopyrrolate . . . . . . 0.2 mg
Benzyl alcohol (preservative) 0.9%
Water for injection, USP . . . . . . q.s.

pH adjusted, when necessary, with hydrochloric acid and/or sodium hydroxide.

Indications: ROBINUL®-V (glycopyrrolate) is indicated as a preanesthetic anticholinergic agent in dogs and cats.

In dogs it reduces salivary, tracheobronchial and pharyngeal secretions, reduces the volume and free acidity of gastric secretion, and blocks cardiac vagal inhibitory reflexes during induction of anesthesia and intubation.

In cats it reduces salivary and pharyngeal secretions.

Pharmacology: ROBINUL®-V (glycopyrrolate) is a synthetic anticholinergic agent. It is a quaternary ammonium compound with the following chemical structure:

ROBINUL®-V is a clear colorless liquid.

Glycopyrrolate, like other anticholinergic agents, inhibits the action of acetylcholine on structures innervated by post-ganglionic cholinergic nerves and on smooth muscles that respond to acetylcholine that lack cholinergic innervation. In the dog it diminishes the volume and free acidity of gastric secretions and reduces intestinal motility. It diminishes and controls excessive pharyngeal, tracheal and bronchial secretions and has a longer lasting effect than atropine. In the cat it controls excessive salivation and pharyngeal secretions.

In anesthetized dogs intravenous doses of 0.0023 to 0.0045 mg/lb markedly reduced intestinal tone and moderately inhibited amplitude of intestinal contraction but had essentially no effect on respirations, periodic arterial blood pressure or cardiac rate. These doses of glycopyrrolate reduced bradycardia, hypertension and the intestinal hyperactivity resulting from peripheral vagal stimulation.

In dog studies glycopyrrolate antagonized muscarinic symptoms (e.g., bronchorrhea, bronchospasm, bradycardia and intestinal hypermotility) induced by cholinergic drugs such as the anticholinesterases, affording the same protection as atropine against bradycardia.

The intestinal hyperactivity and copious salivation produced by a subcutaneous dose of methacholine chloride, 0.5 mg/kg, were suppressed by glycopyrrolate in intravenous doses as low as 0.0045 mg/lb in the dog.

In a study[1] glycopyrrolate at 0.004 and 0.008 mg/lb had a longer lasting effect and more smooth-muscle relaxation, with little adverse cardiovascular effect when compared to atropine at 0.02 mg/lb. Glycopyrrolate was effective in preventing aspiration of gastric secretions and the resulting pulmonary complications, not only by producing a higher pH of gastric secretions but in the reduction of intestinal smooth-muscle activity and thus the likelihood of regurgitation.

The polar ammonium moiety of glycopyrrolate limits its passage across the lipid membranes such as the blood-brain barrier in contrast to the belladonna alkaloids which are non-polar tertiary amines.

In a cat study, ^{14}C-labeled glycopyrrolate was administered intramuscularly at doses ranging from 0.018 to 0.024 mg/kg (0.008 to 0.011 mg/lb). Peak blood levels of radioactivity were detected at 15 minutes following injections. Blood levels of radioactivity declined slowly during a 48-hour period with the drug being excreted approximately equally between urinary and fecal excretion routes.

In dog studies peak effect occurred approximately 30 to 45 minutes after subcutaneous or intramuscular administration. The vagal blocking effect persisted for two to three hours and the antisialagogue effect persisted for up to seven hours, periods longer than for atropine. With intravenous injection the onset of action was generally evident within one minute.

Dosage and Administration: For intramuscular, intravenous or subcutaneous use in dogs and intramuscular use in cats.

Dogs: ROBINUL®-V may be administered intravenously, intramuscularly or subcutaneously at the rate of 5 micrograms/lb body weight (0.25 mL per 10 lbs body weight).

Cats: ROBINUL®-V may be administered intramuscularly at the rate of 5 micrograms/lb body weight (0.25 mL per 10 lbs body weight). For maximum anticholinergic effect administer ROBINUL®-V 15 minutes prior to anesthetic administration in cats.

Contraindication(s): There are no absolute contraindications to the use of ROBINUL®-V in conjunction with anesthesia except known hypersensitivity to glycopyrrolate.

Precaution(s): Store at controlled room temperature 15° to 30°C (59° to 86°F).

Caution(s): Federal law restricts this drug to use by or on the order of a licensed veterinarian.

Reproduction studies in rats and rabbits revealed no teratogenic effects from glycopyrrolate; however, the anticholinergic action in this agent resulted in diminished rates of conception and of survival at weaning in rats in a dose-related manner. Reproduction studies have not been conducted on glycopyrrolate in dogs and cats. Therefore, ROBINUL®-V should not be administered to pregnant bitches or queens. The excretion of ROBINUL®-V may be prolonged in animals with impaired renal function or impaired gastrointestinal function.

For preanesthetic use in dogs and cats only.

Toxicology: Acute and chronic toxicity studies have shown glycopyrrolate to have a low order of toxicity.

In the dog the LD_{50} for intravenous administration is 25 mg/kg and daily intravenous doses of either 0.4 or 2 mg/kg five days per week for four consecutive weeks revealed no signs of toxicity. The oral feeding of high levels (27 mg/kg) of glycopyrrolate for seven weeks produced no signs of toxicity in the dog.

In the cat the LD_{50} for intramuscular administration is 283 mg/kg. In a ten-week study cats received daily intramuscular doses of 0.01, 0.03 and 0.05 mg/kg. No changes considered to be related to glycopyrrolate were seen in food consumption, hematology, biochemical, urinalysis or gross pathology. Histopathology showed slight to moderate proliferation of intrahepatic bile ducts at the 0.05 mg/kg/day dose level.

Side Effects: Mild mydriasis, xerostomia and tachycardia may be seen with ROBINUL®-V. These are extensions of the fundamental pharmacological action of anticholinergics.

References: Available upon request.

Presentation: ROBINUL®-V (glycopyrrolate) is supplied in 20 mL vials (0.2 mg/mL) (NDC 0856-7895-83).

Manufactured by: Elkins-Sinn, Inc., Cherry Hill, NJ 08003

Compendium Code No.: 10031880 5070C

ROCADYNE

Rochester Midland **Disinfectant**

Disinfectant

EPA Reg. No.: 4959-15-527

Active Ingredient(s):

Iodine* 1.75%
Inert Ingredients 98.25%
Total 100.00%

*From alpha-(p-nonylphenyl)-omega-hydroxypoly (oxyethylene)-iodine complex

Indications: ROCADYNE is a concentrated broad spectrum iodophor for use as a one-step cleaner-disinfectant and no-rinse sanitizer in: veterinary clinics, poultry and livestock drinking water, sanitizing commercial eggs, egg processing plants, dairy and poultry farms, meat and poultry plants, food processing plants, kennels, pet shops and zoos, hand sanitizing in food plants and animal handling facilities.

For industrial, institutional and agricultural use.

Not for residential use.

Directions for Use: It is a violation of Federal law to use this product in a manner inconsistent with its labeling.

The color of a ROCADYNE solution is proportional to the titratable iodine concentration. Prepare a fresh solution daily, or when there is a noticeable change in its rich amber color, or more often if the solution becomes diluted or soiled.

Used as directed ROCADYNE is effective in hard water (up to 400 ppm as CACO3) and in 5% organic serum load against the following viruses, bacteria and pathogenic fungi: Polio 1*, Vaccinia*, Herpes Simplex Type 1*, Influenza A2/Japan 305*, and Canine Parvovirus*; bactericidal against *Salmonella cholerasuis, Staphylococcus aureus, Pseudortanas aeruginosa, and E. Coli;* is fungicidal against *Trichophylon mentagropfrytes* (the athlete's foot fungus).

On pre-cleaned food contact surfaces ROCADYNE is effective against *Salmonella choleraesuis, Listeria monocytocytogenes* and *Escherichia coli,* 0157:H7, Hemorrhagic.

Used as directed ROCADYNE is tuberculocidal when used in hard water (up to 400 ppm as CACO3) on pre-cleaned surfaces at 20°C for a contact time of 10 minutes. Prepare a solution of 3 ounces ROCADYNE to 5 gallons water (provides 75 ppm titratable iodine).

One-Step Cleaning and Disinfecting:

Prior to Use in Veterinary Clinics, Animal Handling Facilities, Farm Premises, Kennels, Pet Shops and Zoos: Remove all animals and feeds from premises, vehicles and enclosures. Remove all litter and manure from floors, walls and all surfaces to be treated. Empty all troughs, racks and other feeding and watering appliances. Then proceed as directed below.

To Clean and Disinfect: Before applying disinfecting solution, food products and packaging materials must be removed from the room or carefully protected. Remove heavy soil deposits before applying the disinfecting solution. Using a solution of 3 ounces ROCADYNE per 5 gallons of warm water (68°F, 20°C or warmer), immerse objects in disinfecting solution, or apply solution with a mop, sponge or brush. Where appropriate, use a mechanical sprayer to produce coarse spray. Allow a 10 minute contact time with disinfecting solution. For efficacy against Canine Parvovirus, allow a 120 minute contact time; surface must remain wet. All food contact surfaces must be rinsed with potable water before reuse. Floors, walls and all other non-food contact surfaces may drain dry without rinsing. Note: When mixing ROCADYNE with cold water (as low as 41°F, 5°C), increase use to 6 oz. per 5 gallons water.

Before Rehousing Animals: Ventilate buildings, vehicles and other closed spaces. Do not house animals or use equipment until treatment absorbs, sets or dries. Thoroughly rinse all treated feed racks, mangers, troughs, automatic feeders, fountains and waterers with potable water before reuse.

Shoe Bath: Routine use of shoe bath sanitizers helps reduce the spread of disease causing organisms between poultry houses, farrowing houses, hog barns and other livestock buildings. Use 3 ounces of ROCADYNE per 1 gallon of water. Place sanitizing solution in shallow plastic or stainless steel pans inside all entrances to poultry and livestock buildings. Scrape shoes outside doorway and stand in shoe bath for 30 seconds before entering building. Replace shoe bath daily or more often if solution becomes soiled.

Cleaning Milking Equipment and Bulk Tanks: Immediately after milking, flush milking equipment and utensils with lukewarm (100°F, 38°C) water to wash out all milk. Take apart milking machines and immerse air hoses, inflations, metal parts (except pulsator) and utensils in a solution containing 1 ounce of ROCADYNE per 5 gallons of water . Brush all parts thoroughly. Drain completely, rinse with water and allow to air dry. After emptying bulk tanks, flush tanks thoroughly with 100°F (38°C) water to wash out all milk. Brush tanks thoroughly with a solution containing 1 ounce ROCADYNE per 5 gallons of water. Allow wash solution to drain, rinse with water and air dry.

Sanitizing Milking Machines and Bulk Tanks: Before each milking, flush assembled milking machines and empty bulk tanks with a solution containing 1 ounce of ROCADYNE per 5 gallons of water. Allow a 1 minute contact time. Drain thoroughly and air dry before use.

Removal of Milkstone and Hard Water Deposits: Yellow color may appear on equipment after the first use of ROCADYNE. This may indicate the presence of milkstone or hard water deposits. Remove these deposits by applying a solution containing equal parts of ROCADYNE and lukewarm water. Wait 2-3 minutes, brush and then rinse with potable water. Daily use of ROCADYNE will help prevent the formation of milkstone and hard water deposits.

Sanitizing Poultry and Livestock Drinking Water: Add 1 ounce of ROCADYNE per 10 gallons of drinking water. Regular use of this product in drinking water reduces the buildup of slime and mineral deposits in watering equipment. Do not use this product together with other water treatments such as medications.

Sanitizing Previously Cleaned Food Contact Surfaces: Sanitize previously cleaned and rinsed hard, non-porous surfaces such as glass, metal, plastic and porcelain with a solution containing 1 ounce of ROCADYNE per 5 gallons of water. Immerse equipment with sanitizing solution and allow 1 minute of contact time. Drain solution from equipment; do not rinse. ROCADYNE used at 1 ounce per 5 gallons of water contains 25 ppm titratable iodine and does not require a final rinse with potable water in accordance with Federal Food Additive Regulation 178.1010.

Sanitizing Food-Grade Egg Shells: Coarse spray previously cleaned food-grade eggs shells with a solution containing 1 ounce of ROCADYNE per 5 gallons of water. Solution temperature should be warmer than the eggs, but not to exceed 130°F (53°C). Wet eggs thoroughly for 1 minute and allow to drain. A final potable water rinse is not required. Eggs should be reasonably dry before casing or breaking. Do not reuse solution to sanitize eggs.

Hand Sanitizing: Thoroughly wash and rinse hands before sanitizing. Dip or rinse hands in a solution containing 1 ounce of ROCADYNE per 5 gallons of water. ROCADYNE may be injected directly into wash or rinse water at a rate of 1 ounce per 5 gallons of water. A final potable water rinse is not required.

Deodorizing: ROCADYNE destroys many odors as it sanitizes and disinfects. For general deodorant applications (garbage pails, refuse containers, etc.), swab surface to be treated with a solution containing 1 ounce of ROCADYNE per gallon of water. Allow treated surface to drain and air dry.

Use Dilution Table:

ROCADYNE/Water=	Titratable Iodine
1 oz to 10 gal.	12.5 ppm
1 oz to 5 gal.	25 ppm
3 oz to 5 gal.	75 ppm
1 oz to 1 gal.	125 ppm
6 oz to 5 gal.	150 ppm

Precautionary Statements: Hazards to Humans and Domestic Animals:

Danger: Corrosive. Causes irreversible eye damage. Harmful if swallowed. Do not get in eyes or on clothing. Avoid contact with skin. Wear goggles or face shield. Wash thoroughly with soap and water after handling. Remove contaminated clothing and wash before reuse.

Environmental Hazards: This product is toxic to fish and aquatic organisms. Do not contaminate water by cleaning of equipment or disposal of wastes. Do not discharge effluent containing this product into lakes, streams, ponds, estuaries, oceans or other water unless in accordance with the requirements of a National Pollutant Discharge Elimination System (NPDES) permit and the permitting authority has been notified in writing prior to discharge. Do not discharge effluent containing this product to sewer systems without previously notifying the local sewage treatment plant authority. For guidance contact your State Water Board or Regional Office of the EPA.

First Aid:

If in Eyes: Hold eye open and rinse slowly and gently with water for 15-20 minutes. Remove contact lenses, if present, after first 5 minutes. Then continue rinsing. Call a poison control center or doctor for treatment advice.

If on Skin: Take off contaminated clothing. Rinse skin immediately with plenty of water for 15-20 minutes. Call a poison control center or doctor for treatment advice.

If Swallowed: Call a poison control center or doctor for treatment advice. Have the person sip a glass of water if able to swallow. Do not induce vomiting unless told to do so by the poison control center or doctor. Do not give anything by mouth to an unconscious person.

If Inhaled: Move person to fresh air. If person is not breathing call 911 or an ambulance, then give artificial respiration, preferably mouth-to-mouth, if possible. Call a poison control center or doctor for treatment advice.

Note to Physician: Probable mucosal damage may contraindicate the use of gastric lavage. Measures against circulatory shock, respiratory depression and convulsions may be needed.

Storage and Disposal: Keep container closed when not in use. Do not store below 25°F or above 100°F for extended periods.

Prohibitions: Do not contaminate water, food or feed by storage or disposal. Open dumping is prohibited.

Pesticide Disposal: Pesticide wastes are acutely hazardous. Improper disposal of excess pesticide, spray mixture or rinsate is a violation of Federal law. If these wastes cannot be disposed of by use according to label instructions, contact your State Pesticide or Environmental Control Agency, or the Hazardous Waste representative at the nearest EPA Regional Office for guidance.

Container Disposal: Triple rinse (or equivalent). Then offer for recycling or reconditioning or puncture and dispose of in a sanitary landfill, or incinerate, or, if allowed by State and local authorities, burn container. If burned, stay out of smoke.

Warning(s): Keep out of reach of children.

Presentation: 4 x 1 gallon containers/case, 5 gallon pails and 55 gallon (208.2 liter) drums.

Compendium Code No.: 13690112 Rev. 3/20/01

ROCCAL®-D PLUS

Pharmacia & Upjohn **Disinfectant**

Veterinary and Animal Care Disinfectant

EPA Reg. No.: 65020-12-1023

Active Ingredient(s):

Didecyl dimethyl ammonium chloride 9.2%
Alkyl (C_{12}, 61%; C_{14}, 23%; C_{16}, 11%; C_{18}, 2.5%; C_8 & C_{10}, 2.5%) dimethyl benzyl ammonium chloride 9.2%
Alkyl (C_{12}, 40%; C_{14}, 50%; C_{16}, 10%) dimethyl benzyl ammonium chloride 4.6%
bis-n-tributyltin oxide 1.0%
Inert Ingredients: 76.0%

Indications: Bactericide, fungicide, virucide for veterinary, laboratory animal, kennel and animal breeder facilities.

Effective in 400 ppm hard water as ($CaCO_3$). Disinfects in 5% organic soil load.

ROCCAL®-D PLUS is a complete, chemically balanced disinfectant providing clear use solutions even in hard water.

It is also a residual bacteriostat and inhibits bacterial growth on moist surfaces and contains rust corrosion inhibitors.

It deodorizes by killing most microorganisms that cause offensive odors.

Directions for Use: In veterinary clinics, animal care facilities, animal research centers, animal breeding facilities, kennels and animal quarantine areas.

It is a violation of Federal Law to use this product in a manner inconsistent with its labeling. ROCCAL®-D Plus is a one-step germicide, fungicide, soapless cleaner and deodorant effective in the presence of organic soil (5% serum). It is non-selective and when used as directed, will not harm tile, terrazo, resilient flooring, concrete, painted or varnished wood, glass or metals.

To clean and disinfect hard surfaces, use ½ fluid ounce of ROCCAL®-D Plus per gallon of water. Apply by immersion, flushing solution over treated surfaces with a mop, sponge, cloth or bowl mop to thoroughly wet surfaces. Prepare fresh solutions daily or when solution becomes visibly dirty.

To clean badly soiled areas, use up to 1½ fluid ounce per gallon of water.

To disinfect, allow treated surfaces to remain moist for at least 10 minutes before wiping or rinsing.

To control mold and mildew growth on previously cleaned, hard nonporous surfaces, use ½ fluid ounce per gallon. Allow to dry without wiping. Reapply as new growth appears.

Boot Bath: Use 1 fluid ounce per gallon in boot baths. Change solution daily and anytime it becomes visibly soiled. Use a nylon bristled brush to clean soils from boots.

Disinfecting Vans, Trucks and Farm Vehicles: Clean and rinse vehicles and disinfect with ½ fluid ounce per gallon ROCCAL®-D Plus. If desired, rinse after 10 minutes contact or leave unrinsed.

Do not use ROCCAL®-D Plus on vaccination equipment, needles or diluent bottles as the residual germicide may render the vaccines ineffective.

ROCCAL®-D Plus should not be mixed with other cleaning or disinfecting compounds or products. Broad spectrum germicidal action in hard water and under soil load conditions: At ½ fluid ounce per gallon (1:256) in official AOAC Use Dilution and Fungicidal Tests, ROCCAL®-D Plus is effective in water up to 400 ppm hardness (as $CaCO_3$) and an organic soil load of 5% serum against the following organisms.

Bacteria: *Pseudomonas aeruginosa* ATCC 15442, *Salmonella choleraesuis* ATCC 10708, *Enterobacter aerogenes* ATCC 63809, *Pasteurella multocida* ATCC 7707, *Shigella dysenteriae* ATCC 13313, *Klebsiella pneumoniae* ATCC 4352, *Enterococcus faecium* ATCC 6569, *Salmonella gallinarum* ATCC 9184, *Serratia marcescens* ATCC 264, *Bordetella avium* ATCC 35086, *Streptococcus agalactiae* ATCC 27916, *Mycoplasma gallisepticum* ATCC 15302, *Mycoplasma gallinarum* ATCC 19708, *Actinomyces pyogenes* ATCC 19411, *Actinobacillus pleuropneumoniae* ATCC 27088, *Corynebacterium pseudotuberculosis* ATCC 19410, *Rhodococcus equi* ATCC 6939, *Streptococcus equi var. zooepidemicus* ATCC 43079, *Staphylococcus aureus* ATCC 6538, *Salmonella enteriditis* ATCC 4931, *Streptococcus pyogenes* ATCC 9547, *Salmonella pullorum* ATCC 9120, *Escherichia coli* ATCC 11229, *Alcaligenes faecalis* ATCC 8748, *Shigella sonnei* ATCC 29930, *Salmonella typhosa* ATCC 6539, *Proteus morganii* ATCC 25830, *Proteus mirabilis* ATCC 25933, *Mycoplasma iners* ATCC 19705, *Mycoplasma hypopneumoniae* ATCC 25934, *Bordetella bronchiseptica* ATCC 19395, *Streptococcus equi var. equi* ATCC 33398.

Fungi: *Aspergillus fumigatus* ATCC 10894, *Trichophyton mentagrophytes var. interdigitale* ATCC 9533, *Candida albicans* ATCC 18804.

Viruses: Using accepted virus propagation and hard surface test methods, ROCCAL®-D Plus is effective at 1:256 in 400 ppm hard water and 5% serum against the following viruses: Avian laryngotracheitis ATCC VR-783, canine parvovirus ATCC VR-953, infectious bronchitis ATCC VR-22, transmissible gastroenteritis ATCC VR-763, *Mycoplasma gallisepticum* ATCC 15302, infectious bursal disease (Gumboro) ATCC VR-478, canine distemper onderstepoort strain, equine herpesvirus ATCC VR-700, feline infectious peritonitis strain, DF-2, swine PRRS virus, reference stain, NVSL, Newcastle's disease ATCC VR-109, parainfluenza ATCC VR281, pseudorabies ATCC VR-135, avian influenza ATCC VR-798, canine herpesvirus ATCC VR-552, equine influenza A ATCC VR-297, porcine parvovirus ATCC VR-742, vesicular stomatitus virus, Indiana.

Precautionary Statements: Hazards to Humans and Domestic Animals:

Corrosive: Causes severe eye and skin damage. Do not get into eyes, on skin or clothing. Wear goggles or face shield and rubber gloves when handling the concentrate. Harmful or fatal if swallowed. Avoid contamination of food. Wash thoroughly with soap and water after handling.

Environmental Hazards: This product is toxic to fish. Do not discharge effluent containing this product into lakes, streams, ponds, estuaries, oceans or other waters unless in accordance with the requirements of a National Pollutant Discharge Elimination System (NPDES) permit and the permitting authority has been notified in writing prior to discharge. Do not discharge effluent containing this product to sewer systems without previously notifying the local sewage treatment plant authority. For guidance contact your State Water Board or Regional Office of the EPA.

Physical and Chemical Hazards: Do not use or store near heat or open flame.

Statement of Practical Treatment: In case of contact, immediately flush eyes or skin with plenty of water for at least 15 minutes. For eyes, call a physician. Remove and wash contaminated clothing before reuse. If ingested, drink promptly a large quantity of raw egg whites, gelatin solution, or if these are not available, drink a large quantity of water. Avoid alcohol. Call a physician immediately.

Note to Physician: Probable mucosal damage may contraindicate the use of gastric lavage.

Storage and Disposal: Store only in tightly closed original container in a secure area inaccessible to children. Do not contaminate water, food or feed by storage and disposal. Disposal: Pesticide wastes are acutely hazardous. Improper disposal of excess pesticide spray mixture, or rinsate is a violation of Federal Law. If these wastes cannot be disposed of by use according to label instructions, contact your State Pesticide or Environmental Control Agency, or the hazardous waste representative at the nearest EPA Regional Office for guidance.

Do not reuse empty container. Rinse container thoroughly before discarding in trash.

Warning(s): Danger. Keep out of reach of children.

Presentation: 1 gallon (NDC 0009-7308-01) and 5 gallons (NDC 0009-7308-05).

Compendium Code No.: 10490472 816 538 002

ROFENAID® 40

Alpharma **Feed Medication**

Sulfadimethoxine & Ormetoprim-Type A Medicated Article (medicated premix)-Antibacterial-Anticoccidiocidal

NADA No.: 040-209

Active Ingredient(s): Sulfadimethoxine 113.5 grams per pound (25%), and ormetoprim 68.1 grams per pound (15%) in a carrier suitable for incorporation in feed.

Indications:

Broiler and replacement (breeder and layer) chickens: As an aid in the prevention of coccidiosis caused by *Eimeria tenella, E. necatrix, E. acervulina, E. maxima, E. brunetti* and *E. mivati;* as an aid in the prevention of bacterial infections caused by *H. gallinarum* (infectious coryza), *E. coli* (colibacillosis) and *P. multocida* (fowl cholera).

Turkeys: As an aid in the prevention of coccidiosis caused by *E. adenoeides, E. gallopavonis,* and *E. meleagrimitis;* for the prevention of bacterial infections caused by *P. multocida* (fowl cholera).

Ducks:

As an aid in the control of *P. multocida* (fowl cholera) in ducks including breeding ducks.

As an aid in the control of E. coli, *Riemerella anatipestifer* (strains 2, 3 & 4) and severe challenge of *P. multocida* (fowl cholera).

Chukar Partridges: For the prevention of coccidiosis caused by *E. kofoidi* and *E. legionensis.*

Directions: Use Directions:

Broiler and replacement (breeder and layer) chickens: As an aid in the prevention of coccidiosis caused by *Eimeria tenella, E. necatrix, E. acervulina, E. maxima, E. brunetti* and *E. mivati;* as an aid in the prevention of bacterial infections caused by *H. gallinarum* (infectious coryza), *E. coli* (colibacillosis) and *P. multocida* (fowl cholera).

Add 1 lb of ROFENAID® 40 to one ton of feed to provide 0.02% (0.0125% sulfadimethoxine and 0.0075% ormetoprim) concentration in feed.

Limitations: Feed continuously as the sole ration.

Turkeys: As an aid in the prevention of coccidiosis caused by *E. adenoeides, E. gallopavonis,* and *E. meleagrimitis;* for the prevention of bacterial infections caused by *P. multocida* (fowl cholera).

Add ½ lb of ROFENAID® 40 to one ton of feed to provide 0.01% (0.00625% sulfadimethoxine and 0.00375% ormetoprim) concentration in feed.

Limitations: Feed continuously as the sole ration.

Ducks:

As an aid in the control of *P. multocida* (fowl cholera) in ducks including breeding ducks.

Add 2 lbs of ROFENAID® 40 to one ton of feed to provide 0.04% (0.025% sulfadimethoxine and 0.015% ormetoprim) concentration in feed.

As an aid in the control of E. coli, *Riemerella anatipestifer* (strains 2, 3 & 4) and severe challenge of *P. multocida* (fowl cholera).

Add 4 lbs of ROFENAID® 40 to one ton of feed to provide 0.08% (0.050% sulfadimethoxine and 0.030% ormetoprim) concentration in feed.

Limitations: Feed for 7 days as the sole ration.

The safety of feeding ROFENAID® at levels higher than 0.04% in breeding ducks has not been established.

Chukar Partridges: For the prevention of coccidiosis caused by *E. kofoidi* and *E. legionensis.*

Add 1 lb of ROFENAID® 40 to one ton of feed to provide 0.02% (0.0125% sulfadimethoxine and 0.0075% ormetoprim) concentration in feed.

Limitations: Feed continuously as the sole ration to young birds up to 8 weeks of age.

The safety of feeding ROFENAID® to breeding stock has not been established.

Caution(s): For control of duck disease, medication should be started at the first signs of infection.

Note: Manufacture of Type B or C feeds from this product requires a Medicated Feed License Application approved by FDA.

Labels for feeds containing ROFENAID® 40 must contain appropriate indications, limitations and warnings as well as required feed ingredient information.

For use in broiler, replacement (breeder and layer) chickens, turkeys, ducks and chukar partridges only.

For use in manufacturing medicated feeds only.

Warning(s): Do not feed to turkeys and ducks producing eggs for food. Withdraw 5 days prior to slaughter for broiler and replacement chickens, turkeys, and ducks.

Do not feed to chickens over 16 weeks (112 days) of age.

Presentation: 50 lb (22.68 kg) bag.

Compendium Code No.: 10220552 770302 0103

ROLL-ON™ FLY REPELLENT

Farnam **Insect Repellent**

EPA Reg. No.: 270-107

Active Ingredient(s):

Pyrethrins 0.40%
Piperonyl Butoxide Technical* 1.00%
Di-n-propyl isocinchomeronate 1.00%
N-octyl bicycloheptene dicarboximide 0.40%
Inert Ingredients: 97.20%

*Equivalent to 0.80% (butylcarbityl) (6-propylpiperonyl) ether and 0.20% related compounds.

Indications: Fly repellent for horses, ponies and dogs. Repels house flies, stable flies, face flies, and horn flies from sensitive areas of the face and head and also from wounds. Kills on contact.

Directions for Use: Read entire label before each use.

Use only on horses, ponies or dogs.

It is a violation of Federal law to use this product in a manner inconsistent with its labeling. Shake well before using. Remove cap from bottle. Apply around animal's nose, eyes, ears, mouth; also around wounds and other surface lesions. Do not put solution directly in animal's eyes, mouth or wounds. Reapply everyday. Replace cap after use.

Precautionary Statements: Hazards to Humans and Domestic Animals:

Caution: Harmful if swallowed. For animal use only. Do not use on animals under 12 weeks. Consult a veterinarian before using this product on debilitated, aged, medicated, pregnant or nursing animals. Not for human use. Wash hands after using. Sensitivities may occur after using any pesticide product for pets. If signs of sensitivity occur, bathe your pet with mild soap and rinse with large amounts of water. If signs continue, consult a veterinarian immediately.

First Aid: If swallowed do not induce vomiting. Call a Physician or Poison Control Center immediately.

Environmental Hazards: This product is toxic to fish. Keep out of lakes, streams and ponds. Do not apply where runoff is likely to occur. Do not contaminate water by cleaning of equipment or disposal of wastes. Apply this product only as directed on the label.

Storage and Disposal:

Storage: Store in original container in a cool place inaccessible to children and pets.

Disposal: Dispose of container by wrapping in several layers of newspaper and discard in trash.

Warning(s): Do not use on horses intended for human consumption.

Keep out of reach of children.

Presentation: 2 fl. oz (59 mL) bottle.

Compendium Code No.: 10000320

ROMET® 30

Alpharma **Feed Medication**

Sulfadimethoxine & Ormetoprim-Type A Medicated Article (medicated premix)-Antibacterial

NADA No.: 125-933

Active Ingredient(s): Sulfadimethoxine 113.5 grams per pound (25%), ormetoprim 22.7 grams per pound (5%) in a carrier suitable for incorporation in feeds.

Indications: For the control of furunculosis in salmonids (trout and salmon) caused by *Aeromonas salmonicida* and of enteric septicemia of catfish caused by *Edwardsiella ictaluri* strains susceptible to the sulfadimethoxine and ormetoprim combination.

Dosage and Administration: Administer medicated feed daily for five consecutive days to provide approximately 50 mg of active ingredients per kg (23 mg/lb) of live body weight of fish per day.

Preparation of medicated feeds: Establish the weight of fish to be treated and calculate the amount of feed needed per day according to fish size and water temperature. Calculate the amount of ROMET® 30 required for medicating the feed at the rate of 16.7 g of ROMET® 30 per 100 kg (7.6 g of ROMET® 30/100 lb) of fish body weight per day.

Medication of feed before pelletizing or extruding: Thoroughly mix the calculated amount of ROMET® 30 into the mash feed prior to pelletizing or extruding. Refer to the dosage table below for recommended levels of use.

Feed Intake of Fish as Percent (%) of Body Weight	lbs of ROMET® 30 per Ton of Feed
1	33.30
2	16.70
3	11.10
4	8.33
5	6.66
6	5.55

Medication of feed after pelletizing: Prepare a liquid slurry by suspending ROMET® 30 in edible vegetable oil or 5% gelatin solution. Coat the pelleted fish feed with the slurry, which should be constantly agitated to ensure uniform suspension of the ROMET® 30 during addition. As a general rule, one gallon of vegetable oil or gelatin solution is required to coat 200 lbs of pellets. For example, to medicate 6666 lb of fish for one day, with a 3% body weight feed intake, mix 1.1 lbs of ROMET® 30 with one gallon of vegetable oil to prepare a slurry to be used for coating 200 lbs of pellets. Pellets may be placed in a cement mixer (if fifty lbs or more are to be coated) or spread on plastic or a smooth concrete surface for the coating process. The pellets should be mixed constantly but gently while the slurry is being slowly added to insure even distribution without undue pellet breakage. The coated pellets are then spread out and allowed to air dry for several hours. Rebag and store under proper feed storage conditions.

Caution(s): If fish show no improvement within 2 to 3 days, or if signs of disease reappear after termination of treatment, reevaluate management practices, diagnosis of outbreak, and establish susceptibility of the bacterial isolate(s) to the drug.

Labels for feeds containing ROMET® 30 must contain appropriate indications, limitations and warnings as well as required feed ingredient information.

For use in manufacturing medicated feeds only.

Warning(s): Withdraw 42 days in salmonids and 3 days in catfish before slaughter or release as stocker fish.

Presentation: 50 lb (22.68 kg) bag.

Compendium Code No.: 10220563 770301 0103

ROTAMUNE® WITH IMUGEN® II

Intervet **Vaccine**

Porcine Rotavirus Vaccine, Killed Virus

U.S. Vet. Lic. No.: 286

Contents: This product contains the antigen listed above.

Contains gentamicin as a preservative.

Indications: Use: For the immunization of healthy sows, gilts and their litters against disease caused by porcine rotaviruses types 1 and 2.

Directions: Shake well. Sows and Gilts: Give 5 mL intramuscularly 6 and 2 weeks before farrowing. Vaccinate the piglets with 1 mL intraperitoneally at 3-10 days of age.

Gilts should be given one 5 mL dose prior to introduction into breeding herds.

Precaution(s): Store at 2° to 7°C (35°-45°F). Use entire contents when first opened.

Caution(s): In case of anaphylactoid reaction administer epinephrine.

For veterinary use only.

Warning(s): Do not vaccinate within 60 days before slaughter.

Presentation: 20 adult doses (100 mL).

Compendium Code No.: 11061750

ROTATIONAL ZINC™

SSI Corp. **Hoof Product**

Active Ingredient(s):

Zinc (Zn) 1.43%
Sulfur (S) 3.28%
Inert 95.29%

Indications: Aids in the treatment and prevention of footwarts (papillomatous digital dermatitis) on dairy cattle.

Directions: ROTATIONAL ZINC™ can be applied two ways:

Spraying for Prevention (Preferred Method): Use as a direct topical spray by mixing one (1) part ROTATIONAL ZINC™ to three (3) parts water. Clean feet beforehand. Spray all animals, all feet, or at least the back feet, four to five milkings straight. ROTATIONAL ZINC™ can be used in your rotation program every third to fourth week.

Foot Baths (Optional Method): Mix one (1) quart of ROTATIONAL ZINC™ to fifty (50) gallons of water. Change every 150 head. Foot bath may need to be cleaned and redosed more often than every 150 head depending on environment and hygiene conditions. When using foot baths a product rotation is best. Products such as SSI's HoofPro+® and MagSalt™ as well as traditional products work well in rotation with ROTATIONAL ZINC™. Footbaths require careful management. If not properly managed results are reduced significantly.

Precaution(s): Keep from freezing.

Caution(s): Eye irritant. In case of eye contact, flush for 15 minutes. If irritation persists, call a physician.

Warning(s): Keep out of the reach of children.

Discussion: ROTATIONAL ZINC™ is specifically formulated to be used in a rotational program of product for the prevention of papillomatous digital dermatitis (footwarts). ROTATIONAL ZINC™ can be used in your prevention program with SSI's HoofPro+® and MagSalt™ as well as E-Z Copper™. A regularly scheduled preventative maintenance program for all animals should be implemented, as risk of reoccurrence of footwarts is likely.

For treatment of active lesions use SSI's QuickHit™ as an aid in the treatment of footwarts.

Presentation: 2.5, 5 and 30 gallon drums.

Compendium Code No.: 14930051

ROTECTIN™ 1 PASTE 1.87%

Farnam **Parasiticide-Oral**

Anthelmintic and Boticide

Active Ingredient(s): The paste contains:

Ivermectin. 1.87%

Indications: ROTECTIN™ 1 (ivermectin) Paste provides effective control of the following parasites in horses: Large Strongyles (adults) *Strongylus vulgaris* (also early forms in blood vessels), *S edentatus* (also tissue stages), *S equinus*, *Triodontophorus* spp; Small Strongyles including those resistant to some benzimidazole class compounds (adults and fourth-stage larvae) - *Cyathostomum* spp, *Cylicocyclus* spp, *Cylicostephanus* spp, *Cylicodontophorus* spp; Pinworms (adults and fourth-stage larvae) - *Oxyuris equi*; Ascarids (adults and third- and fourth-stage larvae) - *Parascaris equorum*; Hairworms (adults) - *Trichostrongylus axei*; Large-mouth Stomach Worms (adults) - *Habronema muscae*; Bots (oral and gastric stages) - *Gasterophilus* spp; Lungworms (adults and fourth-stage larvae) - *Dictyocaulus arnfieldi*; Intestinal Threadworms (adults) - *Strongyloides westeri*; Summer Sores caused by *Habronema* and *Draschia* spp cutaneous third-stage larvae; Dermatitis caused by neck threadworm microfilariae, Onchocerca sp.

Dosage and Administration: This syringe contains sufficient paste to treat one 1250 lb horse at the recommended dose rate of 91 mcg ivermectin per lb (200 mcg/kg) body weight. Each weight marking on the syringe plunger delivers enough paste to treat 250 lb body weight. (1) While holding plunger, turn the knurled ring on the plunger ¼ turn to the left and slide it so the side nearest the barrel is at the prescribed weight marking. (2) Lock the ring in place by making a ¼ turn to the right. (3) Make sure that horse's mouth contains no feed. (4) Remove the cover from the tip of the syringe. (5) Insert the syringe tip into the horse's mouth at the space between the teeth. (6) Depress the plunger as far as it will go, depositing paste on the back of the tongue. (7) Immediately raise the horse's head for a few seconds after dosing.

Contraindication(s): ROTECTIN™ 1 (ivermectin) Paste has been formulated specifically for use in horses only. This product should not be used in other animal species as severe adverse reactions, including fatalities in dogs, may result.

Caution(s): For oral use in horses only.

Consult your veterinarian for assistance in the diagnosis, treatment, and control of parasitism.

Swelling and itching reactions after treatment with ROTECTIN™ 1 (ivermectin) Paste have occurred in horses carrying heavy infections of neck threadworm (*Onchocerca* sp) microfilariae. These reactions were most likely the result of microfilariae dying in large numbers. Symptomatic treatment may be advisable. Consult your veterinarian should any such reactions occur. Healing of summer sores involving extensive tissue changes may require other appropriate therapy in conjunction with treatment with ROTECTIN™ 1 (ivermectin) Paste. Reinfection, and measures for its prevention, should also be considered. Consult your veterinarian if the condition does not improve.

Warning(s): Do not use in horses intended for food purposes.

Refrain from smoking and eating when handling. Wash hands after use. Avoid contact with eyes. Keep this and all drugs out of the reach of children.

Ivermectin and excreted ivermectin residues may adversely affect aquatic organisms. Do not contaminate ground or surface water. Dispose of the syringe in an approved landfill or by incineration.

Discussion: Parasite Control Program: All horses should be included in a regular parasite control program with particular attention being paid to mares, foals and yearlings. Foals should be treated initially at 6 to 8 weeks of age, and routine treatment repeated as appropriate. Consult your veterinarian for a control program to meet your specific needs. ROTECTIN™ 1 Paste effectively controls gastrointestinal nematodes and bots of horses. Regular treatment will reduce the chances of verminous arteritis caused by *S vulgaris*.

Product Advantages: Broad-spectrum Control - ROTECTIN™ 1 Paste kills important internal parasites, including bots and the arterial stages of *Strongylus vulgaris*, with a single dose. ROTECTIN™ 1 Paste is a potent anti-parasitic agent that is neither a benzimidazole nor an organophosphate.

Safety - ROTECTIN™ 1 (ivermectin) Paste may be used in horses of all ages, including mares at any stage of pregnancy. Stallions may be treated without adversely affecting their fertility.

Presentation: 0.21 oz (6.08 g) tube.

Distributed by: TRC Animal Health.

Compendium Code No.: 10000331

ROTECTIN™ 2 PASTE

Farnam **Parasiticide-Oral**

Equine Anthelmintic

NADA No.: 129-831

Active Ingredient(s): Each milliliter contains 180 milligrams pyrantel base as pyrantel pamoate.

Indications: For the removal and control of mature infections of large strongyles *(Strongylus vulgaris, S edentatus, S equinus)*; small strongyles; pinworms *(Oxyuris equi)*; and large roundworms *(Parascaris equorum)* in horses and ponies.

Dosage and Administration: Contents will treat up to 1200 lb body weight.

Administer as a single oral dose of 3 milligrams pyrantel base per pound of body weight. The syringe has four weight mark increments. Each weight mark indicates the recommended dose for 300 pounds of body weight.

Body Weight Range	Volume	mg Pyrantel Base
up to 300 lb	¼ syringe (5 mL)	900 mg
301 to 600 lb	½ syringe(10 mL)	1800 mg
601 to 900 lb	¾ syringe (15 mL)	2700 mg
901 to 1200 lb	1 full syringe (20 mL)	3600 mg

Note: Position screw-gauge over appropriate mark on plunger.

For maximum control of parasitism, it is recommended that foals (2-8 months of age) be dosed every 4 weeks. To minimize the potential source of infection that the mare may pose to the foal, the mare should be treated 1 month prior to anticipated foaling date followed by retreatment 10 days to 2 weeks after birth of foal. Horses and ponies over 8 months of age should be routinely dosed every 6 weeks.

It is recommended that severely debilitated animals not be treated with this preparation.

Precaution(s): Store at room temperature, 59°-86°F (15°-30°C).

Caution(s): For oral use in horses only.

Consult your veterinarian for assistance in the diagnosis, treatment, and control of parasitism.

Warning(s): Not for use in horses intended for food. Keep out of reach of children.

For animal use only.

Presentation: 23.6 g (20 mL) tube.

Distributed by: TRC Animal Health.

Compendium Code No.: 10000340

ROTENONE SHAMPOO

Goodwinol **Parasiticide Shampoo**

Active Ingredient(s): Rotenone and benzocaine.

Indications: Shampoo/conditioner that combats body mites in cats, and helps to prevent the recurrence of mange of dogs.

Dosage and Administration: Wet the hair of the pet with warm water. Apply 1-2 oz. of shampoo. Lather thoroughly adding more water if needed. Leave on for 10 minutes. Rinse well and dry. Apply once a week.

Presentation: Available in 8 oz, ½ gallon and 1 gallon containers.

Compendium Code No.: 14380010

R-PEN

Alpharma **Water Medication**

Antibiotic-Non-sterile

ANADA No.: 200-106

Active Ingredient(s): 0.384 billion units penicillin G potassium or 0.500 billion units, nonsterile.

Indications: For treatment of erysipelas in turkeys (caused by *Erysipelothrix rhusiopathiae)*.

Dosage and Administration: Administer orally at a dosage of 1,500,000 units of penicillin per gallon (3.8 liter) of drinking water for 5 consecutive days.

Directions: Combine contents of entire package and approximately 1.5 pints of water in a glass or plastic container. Stir to dissolve. Allow the concentrated solution to stand until the foam disappears.

Automatic Watering System:

For 0.384 B.U. pack: Pour the concentrated solution into a glass or plastic container, then add enough water to make two gallons (7.6 liters) of solution (this amount of solution will medicate 256 gallons [969 liters] of drinking water). The automatic waterer should be adjusted to deliver one ounce (30 mL) of stock solution per gallon (3.8 liters) of drinking water. In automatic watering systems, prepare fresh solution every 12 hours.

For 0.500 B.U. pack: Pour the concentrated solution into a glass or plastic container, then add enough water to make 2.6 gallons (9.9 liters) of solution. [This amount of solution will medicate 333 gallons (1260 liters) of drinking water.] The automatic waterer should be adjusted to deliver one ounce (30 mL) of stock solution per gallon (3.8 liters) of drinking water. In automatic watering systems, prepare fresh solution every 12 hours.

Gravity Flow Watering Systems:

For 0.384 B.U. pack: Pour the concentrated solution into enough water to make 256 gallons (969 liters) of drinking water. In gravity flow watering systems, prepare fresh solution every 12 hours.

For 0.500 B.U. pack: Pour the concentrated solution into enough water to make 333 gallons (1260 liters) of drinking water. In gravity flow watering systems, prepare fresh solution every 12 hours.

Drinking water prepared as directed above will contain 1,500,000 units of penicillin G per gallon (3.8 liters).

Precaution(s): Store at room temperature; avoid excessive heat (104°F or 40°C).

Caution(s): For best results, the treatment should be started at the first sign of infection. If improvement is not noted after 3 to 4 days of treatment, consult a poultry pathologist or veterinarian.

For oral use in turkeys only.

Restricted drug - Use only as directed (CA).

Warning(s): Treated turkeys must not be slaughtered for food during treatment and for one day after last treatment.

Do not use in turkeys producing eggs for human consumption.

Keep this and all other medications out of reach of children.

Presentation: R-PEN is packaged in 10 unbreakable, foil packs per durable plastic pail in a 0.384 B.U. size, and 8 packs in a 0.500 B.U. size.

Compendium Code No.: 10220532 AHF-052-0008

RUBEOLA VIRUS IMMUNOMODULATOR

Eudaemonic **Equine Immunomodulator**

U.S. Vet. Lic. No.: 385

Active Ingredient(s): An inactivated rubeola virus combined with histamine phosphate in physiological saline. Contains phenol as a preservative. Each 2 mL dose contains 0.1 mcg of neomycin.

Indications: RVI acts to modify the immune and inflammatory responses to alleviate chronic myofascial inflammation (myositis) and its associated problems in the equine.

Dosage and Administration: Inject 2 mL subcutaneously in the neck once a day regardless of weight or age for three (3) to six (6) days or until the desired clinical condition is observed. In severe cases, a daily injection may be required until the horse recovers. Maintenance doses and frequency will depend upon the individual animal but may vary from one (1) dose every other day to one (1) dose a week or even every two (2) weeks. Care should be exercised to ensure that the injection is delivered subcutaneously.

Precaution(s): Store at 35°-45°F (2°-7°C). Protect from freezing.

Caution(s): Rare transient local reactions may occur at the injection site but should subside within 24 hours. For veterinary use only.

Warning(s): Not for use in horses intended for food.

Discussion: T-lymphocytes, including suppressor T-cells, significantly modulate the immune response. Unfortunately these cells are very sensitive to insult, whether from stress, dietary changes, infection, or environmental toxins. These suppressor T-cells function by controlling B-cells (the antibody producers), cytotoxic cells, and helper T-cells from over-responding to insults. Unless controlled, this over response could result in an immune response to auto or self antigens. Evidence indicates an auto immune component to chronic myofascial inflammation and myositis. Studies reflect a decrease in suppressor T-cell function, although not necessarily a decrease in the absolute number of T-cells. RVI acts by specifically modulating suppressor T-cell function in a controlled fashion to allow re-establishment of the normal balance between various subpopulations of T- and B-lymphocytes. This will aid in the healing process leading to the decrease or elimination of myofascial inflammation in the affected animals.

References: Available upon request.

Presentation: 12 x 12 mL six dose vials.

* U.S. Patent No. 4,705,685

Compendium Code No.: 14040010

RUMALAX™ BOLUS

AgriLabs **Antacid-Laxative**

Active Ingredient(s): Each bolus contains:

Magnesium oxide . . . . 27 g (416 grains)

Also contains capsicum, ginger, methyl salicylate and other inert ingredients.

Indications: For oral administration as an aid in the treatment of digestive disturbances requiring an antacid or mild laxative in cattle.

Dosage and Administration: Two (2) to four (4) boluses depending on the size and condition of the animal. Three (3) boluses are equivalent to one (1) quart of milk of magnesia.

Lubricate the boluses with mineral oil or other nonirritating lubricants before administering.

Precaution(s): Store in a cool, dry place.

Caution(s): Keep out of the reach of children. For animal use only.

Presentation: Boxes of 50 boluses.

Compendium Code No.: 10580940

RUMATEL®

Phibro **Feed Medication**

(morantel tartrate) Medicated Premix-88 Cattle Anthelmintic

NADA No.: 092-444

Active Ingredient(s):

Morantel tartrate . . . . 19.4% (88 g per pound)

Other Ingredients: Roughage products, calcium carbonate, sodium aluminosilicate, and mineral oil.

Moisture: Not more than 8%.

Screen analysis: Not more than 10% on 20 U.S. Standard sieve mesh; not more than 15% through 100 U.S. Standard sieve mesh.

Indications: For the removal and control of mature gastro-intestinal nematode infections of cattle including stomach worms *(Haemonchus* spp., *Ostertagia* spp., *Trichostrongylus* spp.), worms of the small intestine *(Cooperia* spp., *Trichostrongylus* spp., *Nematodirus* spp.) and worms of the large intestine *(Oesophagostomum radiatum)*.

Directions: For use in the manufacture of medicated beef and dairy cattle feeds.

Mixing and Use Directions: The following are examples in the approved range (0.44-4.4 g/lb.):

Lbs. feed per 100 lbs. of body weight	Lbs. Premix	Lbs. non-medicated feed	Resulting concentration (grams/lb.)
1.0	10	1,990	0.44
0.4	25	1,975	1.10
0.2	50	1,950	2.20
0.1	100	1,900	4.40

Directions for Use of Medicated Ration: Use as a single therapeutic treatment. Medicated feed is to be fed at the rate of 0.44 g of morantel tartrate per 100 lbs. of body weight. The medicated feed mix should be consumed within six (6) hours. May be fed as the sole ration or mixed with one (1) to two (2) parts of complete feed or as a top dress. When used as a top dress the medication as well as the underlying feed should be evenly distributed. Withhold feed overnight prior to treatment to ensure the ration will be readily consumed. Group cattle by size for optimum efficacy. Fresh water should be available at all times. When all medicated feed is consumed, resume normal feeding. Conditions of constant worm exposure may require retreatment within two (2) to four (4) weeks. Consult your veterinarian for assistance in the diagnosis, treatment and control of parasitism.

Note: Form FD-1900 is required to manufacture animal feeds from type A medicated articles containing morantel tartrate.

Precaution(s): Precautions such as the following should be considered: dust masks or respirators and protective clothing should be worn; dust-arresting equipment and adequate ventilation should be utilized; personal hygiene should be observed; wash before eating or leaving a work site; be alert for signs of allergic reactions - seek prompt medical treatment if such reactions are suspected.

Caution(s): Certain components of animal feeds, including medicated premixes, possess properties that may be a potential health hazard or a source of personal discomfort to certain individuals who are exposed to them. Human exposure should, therefore, be minimized by observing the general industry standards for occupational health and safety.

Consult a veterinarian before using in severely debilitated animals.

Do not mix in feeds containing bentonite.

Milk discard is not required following use in dairy cattle.

Warning(s): Do not treat animals within 14 days of slaughter.

Discussion: RUMATEL® is a broad-spectrum anthelmintic that eliminates the major internal nematode parasites of cattle. RUMATEL® may be administered to lactating dairy cattle without milk withdrawal. Thus, dairy cattle may be treated with RUMATEL® at any time during their production cycle, whether dry, pregnant, or lactating. RUMATEL®, when administered during safety trials at twenty times the recommended dose level, produced no adverse reactions. Animal reproductive performance was unaffected by RUMATEL® treatment. RUMATEL® may be simultaneously administered with vaccines, injectable pharmaceuticals, implants, sprays, or dips without concern of increased cholinesterase inhibition.

Presentation: Available in 25 pound bags.

RUMATEL is a registered trademark of Phibro Animal Health, for morantel tartrate.

Compendium Code No.: 36930131

RUMEN BOLUSES

Durvet — **Antacid-Laxative**

NDC No.: 30798-013-69

Active Ingredient(s): Each bolus contains:

Magnesium oxide .... 276 grs (17.9 g)

(Equivalent to magnesium hydroxide, 400 grs).

In a flavored base, with artificial color added.

Indications: For oral administration to ruminants as an aid in the treatment of digestive disturbances requiring an antacid or a mild laxative in cattle.

Dosage and Administration: One and one-half (1½) RUMEN BOLUSES are equivalent to one (1) pint of milk of magnesia.

Give two (2) to four (4) boluses orally to ruminants, depending upon the size and the condition of the animal. Lubricate the boluses and administer with a balling gun.

Precaution(s): Store at a controlled room temperature between 59°-86°F (15° and 30°C).

Keep tightly closed when not in use.

Caution(s): Avoid frequent or continued use. Keep out of the reach of children.

For animal use only.

Presentation: 50 boluses.

Compendium Code No.: 10841450

RUMEN-EZE

Vet-A-Mix — **Bloat Preparation**

Active Ingredient(s): RUMEN-EZE is an emulsion containing vegetable oil, emulsifiers and preservatives.

Indications: RUMEN-EZE is intended for use as an aid in the treatment of frothy bloat in cattle and sheep.

Dosage and Administration: Shake well before using.

Administer the contents of the special dosing container orally as a drench to relieve bloat in average size mature cattle. Young cattle and sheep should receive 6-12 fluid ounces as the severity of the condition indicates.

Caution(s): Keep out of the reach of children.

Presentation: 12 fl. oz. dosing bottle.

Compendium Code No.: 10500260

RUMENSIN® 80

Elanco — **Feed Additive**

Monensin Premix, USP-Type A Medicated Article

NADA No.: 095-735

Active Ingredient(s): Monensin Granulated, USP, 80 g monensin activity per pound.

Indications:

I. Feedlot Cattle:

A. For improved feed efficiency (cattle fed in confinement for slaughter).

B. For the prevention and control of coccidiosis due to *Eimeria bovis* and *Eimeria zuernii.*

II. Pasture Cattle (Slaughter, stocker, feeder, dairy and beef replacement heifers):

A. For increased rate of weight gain.

B. For the prevention and control of coccidiosis due to *Eimeria bovis* and *Eimeria zuernii.*

III. Mature Reproducing Beef Cows:

A. For improved feed efficiency when receiving supplemental feed.

B. For the prevention and control of coccidiosis due to *Eimeria bovis* and *Eimeria zuernii.*

IV. Goats:

A. For the prevention of coccidiosis caused by *Eimeria crandallis*, *Eimeria christenseni*, and *Eimeria ninakohlyakimovae* in goats maintained in confinement.

V. Calves (excluding veal calves):

A. For the prevention and control of coccidiosis caused by *Eimeria bovis* and *Eimeria zuernii.*

Directions for Use: Read all directions carefully before mixing and feeding.

Do not feed undiluted.

I. Feedlot Cattle:

A. For improved feed efficiency. Feeding Directions: Thoroughly mix RUMENSIN® 80 to make one ton of complete feed that provides 5 to 30 g/ton monensin on a 90% dry matter basis (Table 1). Feed complete feed (5 to 30 g/ton) continuously to growing finishing beef cattle to provide not less than 50 nor more than 360 mg monensin activity per head per day.

B. For the prevention and control of coccidiosis due to *Eimeria bovis* and *Eimeria zuernii.* Feeding Directions: Feed continuously at the rate of 0.14 to 0.42 mg per pound body weight per day, depending upon severity of challenge, up to a maximum of 360 mg of monensin per head per day.

II. Pasture Cattle (slaughter, stocker, and feeder, dairy and beef replacement heifers):

A. For increased rate of weight gain. Feeding Directions: Feed at the rate of not less than 50 nor more than 200 mg per head per day in not less than one pound of Type C Medicated Feed; or after the 5th day, feed at the rate of 400 mg per head per day every other day in not less than 2 pounds of Type C Medicated Feed. The monensin activity in the pasture Type C Medicated Feed must be between 25 and 400 grams per ton. During the first 5 days, cattle should receive no more than 100 mg per day contained in not less than 1 pound of feed. Do not self feed.

B. For the prevention and control of coccidiosis due to *Eimeria bovis* and *Eimeria zuernii.* Feeding Directions: Feed at a rate to provide 0.14 to 0.42 mg per pound body weight per day depending upon severity of challenge up to a maximum of 200 mg per head per day. During the first 5 days, cattle should receive no more than 100 mg per day contained in not less than 1 pound of feed.

C. Free-Choice (Self-Fed) Supplements: Free-choice supplements must be formulated to provide not less than 50 nor more than 200 mg monensin per head per day (manufacturers of Type C free-choice feeds from this product require a Medicated Feed License Applications approved by the FDA).

III. Mature Reproducing Beef Cows (on pasture or in dry lot):

A. For improved feed efficiency when receiving supplemental feed. Feeding Directions: Feed 50 to 200 mg per head per day. Blend into a minimum of 1 pound of Type C Medicated Feed and either hand feed or mix into the total ration. Feed (other than the Type C Medicated Feed containing RUMENSIN®) can be restricted to 95% (of normal requirements) when 50 mg of monensin activity is fed, and to 90% at 200 mg. Cows on pasture or in dry lot must receive a minimum of 1 pound of Type C Medicated Feed per head per day. Additionally, a minimum of 16 pounds (air-dry basis) of roughage such as silage, haylage, ammoniated straw, hay or equivalent feedstuffs should be fed in order to meet NRC recommendations for mature reproducing beef cows to gain 0.25 to 0.75 pounds per head per day. Standing, dried winter range forage may not be of adequate quality to result in improved efficiency when supplemented with RUMENSIN®. During the first 5 days, pastured cattle should receive no more than 100 mg per day contained in not less than 1 pound of feed. Do not self feed.

B. For the prevention and control of coccidiosis due to *Eimeria bovis* and *Eimeria zuernii.* Feeding Directions: Feed at a rate to provide 0.14 to 0.42 mg per pound body weight per day depending upon severity of challenge up to a maximum of 200 mg per head per day. During the first 5 days, pastured cattle should receive no more than 100 mg per day contained in not less than 1 pound of feed.

IV. Goats

A. For prevention of coccidiosis. Feeding Directions: Feed complete feed (20 g/ton) continuously to goats as the sole ration. Feed only to goats maintained in confinement.

V. Calves (excluding veal calves):

A. For the prevention and control of coccidiosis due to *Eimeria bovis* and *Eimeria zuernii.* Feed at a rate of 0.14 to 1.00 mg per pound of body weight per day, depending upon severity of challenge, up to a maximum of 200 mg of monensin per head per day.

VI. Type B or C Medicated Feed Mixing Directions (Dry and Liquid)

A. Dry or Liquid

Thoroughly mix the following amounts of RUMENSIN® 80 to make one ton of Type B or C Medicated Feed to provide the levels shown in Table 1. Dry Only - An Intermediate blending step should be performed to insure an adequate mix.

B. Liquid Limitations

1. The supplement pH must be between 4.3-7.1.
2. Stored liquid Type B Medicated Feeds containing RUMENSIN®: Recirculate or agitate liquid Type B Medicated Feeds daily even when no Type B feed is used and immediately prior to use for no less than 10 minutes moving no less than 10% of the contents from the bottom of the tank.

Table 1. Mixing Directions:

Amount of RUMENSIN® 80 per ton		Monensin Activity in Medicated Feed	
lbs	grams	grams/ton	mg/lb feed
0.06	27	5	2.5
0.25	113	20	10
0.37	168	30	15
5.0	2268	400	200
15.0	6804	1200	600

Precaution(s): Avoid moisture and excessive heat. Not to be used after date printed at top of bag.

When mixing and handling RUMENSIN® 80, use protective clothing, impervious gloves and a dust mask. Operators should wash thoroughly with soap and water after handling. If accidental eye contact occurs, immediately rinse with water.

Caution(s): Do not allow horses or other equines access to feeds containing RUMENSIN®. Ingestion of RUMENSIN® by horses has been fatal. RUMENSIN® medicated feed is intended for use in cattle or in goats. Consumption by unapproved species may result in toxic reactions. Feeding undiluted or mixing errors resulting in high concentrations of RUMENSIN® has been fatal to cattle and could be fatal to goats. Must be thoroughly mixed in feeds before use. Do not exceed the levels of RUMENSIN® recommended in the feeding directions as reduced average daily gains may result.

For animal use only.

Inadequate mixing (recirculation or agitation) of RUMENSIN® Liquid Type B or C Medicated Feeds has resulted in increased RUMENSIN® concentrations which have been fatal to cattle and could be fatal to goats.

Warning(s): Do not feed to lactating dairy cows. Do not feed to lactating goats. A withdrawal time has not been established for pre-ruminating calves. Do not use in calves to be processed for veal.

Presentation: 50 lb (22.68 kg) bag.

RUMENSIN® is a trademark of Eli Lilly and Company.

Compendium Code No.: 10310101 — BG 1383 AMB

RUMEN YEAST CAPS PLUS

TechMix — **Large Animal Dietary Supplement**

Guaranteed Analysis:

Live Cell Count, Minimum .... 30 Billion CFU*/bolus capsule

*CFU (Colony-Forming Units)

Ingredients: Dried *Saccaromyces cervisiae* fermentation product, dried *Aspergillus oryzae* fermentation extract, dried *Aspergillus niger* fermentation product, dried *Bacillus subtilis* fermentation product, dried *Lactobacillus acidophilus* fermentation product, dried *Lactobacillus lactis* fermentation product, dried *Lactobacillus casei* fermentation product, dried *Streptococcus diacetylactis* fermentation product, dried *Streptococcus faecium* fermentation product, dried *Bifidobacterium bifidum* fermentation product, niacin supplement, vitamin B_{12} supplement, riboflavin supplement, thiamin mononitrate, pyridoxine hydrochloride, dried whey, sodium silico aluminate, soybean oil, and natural and artificial flavors added.

Indications: Viable yeast cultures in capsule form with supplemental microbial cultures specifically designed for use in beef and dairy cattle.

Dosage and Administration: Dairy Cows: Administer one capsule daily for two to three days in

R

succession following calving or freshening or whenever feed or dry matter intake drops below normal as a result of hot weather or environmental changes.

Feedlot Cattle, Stockers and Yearlings: Administer one capsule daily for two to three days in succession after arrival in the feedlot or whenever feed or dry matter intake drops below normal as a result of hot weather or environmental changes.

Precaution(s): Store in a cool, dry place out of direct sunlight.

Caution(s): Cattle exhibiting elevated body temperatures or consuming less than 85-90 percent of their normal dry matter intake should be treated and fed as directed by a veterinarian and/or nutritionist.

Warning(s): RUMEN YEAST CAPS PLUS are only intended for use as a source of supplemental yeast and microbial cultures. No other additional claims or warranties are implied by the manufacturer.

Livestock product.

Keep out of reach of children.

Discussion: By providing supplemental yeast cultures, RUMEN YEAST CAPS PLUS help activate and maintain yeast fermentation activity essential for normal rumen function. The capsules facilitate a convenient and easy way to provide yeast fortification to the cow or feedlot calf that may have gone off feed.

Presentation: 12x25 capsule jars/case - 0.7 oz (20 grams) each.

Compendium Code No.: 11440110

RUMINANT LACTOBAC GEL

Vedco **Large Animal Dietary Supplement**

Active Ingredient(s): Contains: Dried *Lactobacillus acidophilus* fermentation product, dried *L. fermentum* fermentation product, dried *L. plantarum* fermentation product, dried *Streptococcus faecium* fermentation product, dried *L. casei* fermentation product, vegetable oil, sucrose, silicon dioxide, vitamins (A, D_3, E), dl-methionine, glycine, l-lysine, sodium bicarbonate, potassium chloride, artificial color, polysorbate 80, TBHQ and ethoxyquin.

Each 15 g contains:

Vitamin A	2,000,000 I.U.
Vitamin D_3	40,000 I.U.
Vitamin E	100 I.U.
dL-Methionine	250 mg
Glycine	250 mg
L-Lysine	250 mg
Potassium chloride	750 mg
Sodium bicarbonate	1,650 mg

The guaranteed total viable lactic producing bacteria is 1 billion colony forming units (CFU) per gram, 15 billion CFU per full 15 g dose.

Indications: A cartridge (syringe) delivery system containing a probiotic gel with high density viable Lactobacillus culture, minerals, vitamins and amino acids for oral administration to animals facing adverse conditions.

A supplemental source of live (viable), natural occurring lactic acid bacteria.

Dosage and Administration: Administer orally on the back of the tongue.

Veal Calves	10 g
Cattle under 400 lbs.	10 g
Cattle over 400 lbs.	15 g
Feeder Lambs	10 g
Adult Sheep and Goats	10 g
New Born Calves	10 g

Presentation: 30 mL and 300 mL tubes.

Compendium Code No.: 10941811

RUMINANT LACTOBACILLUS GEL

First Priority **Large Animal Dietary Supplement**

Guaranteed Analysis: (per 15 g):

Vitamin A	200,000 IU
Vitamin D_3	40,000 IU
Vitamin E	100 IU
Sodium Bicarbonate	1,650 mg
Potassium Chloride	750 mg
DL-Methionine	250 mg
Glycine	250 mg
L-Lysine	250 mg

Guaranteed total viable lactic producing bacteria: One billion colony forming units (CFU) per gram, fifteen (15) billion CFR per full 15 gram dose.

Ingredients: Dried *Lactobacillus acidophilus* Fermentation Product, Dried *L. fermentum* Fermentation Product, Dried *L. plantarum* Fermentation Product, Dried *Streptococcus faecium* Fermentation Product, Dried *L. casei* Fermentation Product, Vegetable Oil, Sucrose, Silicon Dioxide, Vitamins (A, D_3, E), DL-methionine, Glycine, L-Lysine, Sodium Bicarbonate, Potassium Chloride, Artificial Color, Polysorbate 80, TBHQ and Ethoxyquin.

Indications: Contains vitamins, amino acids, minerals, sodium bicarbonate and live naturally occurring micro-organisms for cattle, sheep, goats, lambs and calves.

Directions for Use: Administer orally on back of tongue.

80 mL Syringe: Each mark on the plunger is equivalent to 5 mL (5 g) of product.

300 mL Tube: Each full pull (3 clicks) of the trigger delivers 15 mL of gel.

Cattle Over 400 lb Body Weight	15 mL
Cattle Under 400 lb Body Weight	10 mL
Feeder Lambs	10 mL
Adult Sheep and Goats	10 mL
Newborn Calves	10 mL
Veal Calves	10 mL

Precaution(s): Storage: Store at controlled room temperature between 15°-30°C (59°-86°F). Keep container tightly closed when not in use.

Caution(s): For animal use only.

Warning(s): Keep out of reach of children.

Presentation: 80 mL syringe (NDC# 58829-318-80) and 300 mL tube (NDC# 58829-318-30).

Compendium Code No.: 11390840 Iss. 04-02

RXV-PP-1 (PORCINE PROBIOTIC PASTE)

AgriPharm **Large Animal Dietary Supplement**

Guaranteed Analysis: Represented as total colony forming units 20 x 10^9 colony forming units per pound, equivalent to approximately 4.4 x 10^7 colony forming units per gram.

Ingredients: Vegetable oil, dextrose, dried egg, sorbitan monostearate, *Lactobacillus acidophilus, Bifidobacterium thermophilum, Bifidobacterium longum, Streptococcus faecium,* lactase enzymes.

Indications: This product contains porcine host specific lactic acid producing bacteria to provide an oral source of these bacteria. These bacteria were selected for their ability to be compatible in a wide range of gut conditions.

Dosage and Administration: Administer orally on the back of tongue.

Usage Rate: 3-4 grams per piglet.

Precaution(s): Store product in a cool place. Refrigeration recommended for extended storage period.

Presentation: 60 g and 300 g packages.

Compendium Code No.: 14570890

S

SABER™ EXTRA INSECTICIDE EAR TAGS

Schering-Plough **Insecticide Ear Tags**

EPA Reg. No.: 773-75

Active Ingredient(s):

Lambdacyhalothrin: [1 α-(S), 3 α (Z)]-(±)-cyano-(3-phenoxyphenyl) methyl 3-(2-chloro-3,3,3-trifluoro-1-propenyl)-2,2-dimethylcyclopropanecarboxylate 10%
Piperonyl Butoxide Technical* 13%
Other Ingredients 77%
Total 100%

*Equivalent to Min. 10.4% (butylcarbityl) (6-propylpiperonyl) ether and 2.6% related compounds.

Indications: For up to 5 months control of horn flies and up to 4 months control of face flies on beef and non-lactating dairy cattle and calves.

Directions for Use: It is a violation of Federal law to use this product in a manner inconsistent with its labeling. The labeling must be in the possession of the user at the time of pesticide application. Avoid contamination of feed or foodstuffs.

1. Place male button onto pin until it projects through the tip.
2. Dip tag button into disinfectant solution.
3. Press female tag under the clip by depressing lever.
4. Apply through ear between second and third rib, halfway between ear tip and head.

For optimum control and to minimize development of insect resistance, use two tags per animal (one in each ear). All animals in the herd should be tagged. Apply when flies first appear in the spring. Replace as necessary. Apply with Allflex® Tagging System. Tags remain effective up to 5 months. Remove tags in the fall.

Continual exposure of horn flies to a single class of insecticides (e.g., pyrethroids or organophosphates) may lead to the development of resistance to that class of insecticides. In order to reduce the possibility of horn flies developing resistance, it is important to rotate the class of insecticide used and/or the method of horn fly control on a seasonal basis. For advice concerning current control practices with relation to specific local conditions, consult resources in resistive management programs and/or your Cooperative Agricultural Extension Service.

Precautionary Statements: Hazards to Humans and Domestic Animals:

Caution: Harmful if swallowed, inhaled, or absorbed through the skin. Avoid contact with skin, eyes, or clothing. Wear rubber or non-permeable protective gloves when applying or removing tags. Avoid breathing vapor. Remove contaminated clothing and wash before reuse. Wash thoroughly with soap and water after handling and before eating, drinking, or using tobacco.

First Aid:

If on Skin or Clothing: Take off contaminated clothing. Rinse skin immediately with plenty of water for 15-20 minutes. Call a poison control center or doctor for treatment advice.

If Inhaled: Move person to fresh air. If person is not breathing, call 911 or an ambulance, then give artificial respiration, preferably mouth-to-mouth if possible. Call a poison control center or doctor for further treatment advice.

If Swallowed: Call a poison control center or doctor immediately for treatment advice. Have person sip a glass of water if able to swallow. Do not induce vomiting unless told to do so by the poison control center or doctor. Do not induce vomiting or give anything by mouth to an unconscious person.

Hotline Number: Have the product container or label with you when calling the poison control center or doctor or going for treatment. You may also contact the Rocky Mountain Poison Center at 1-303-595-4869 for emergency medical treatment information.

Environmental Hazards: Do not apply to any body of water. Do not contaminate water by disposal of used tags. This product is toxic to fish.

Storage and Disposal: Do not contaminate water, food, or feed by storage or disposal.

Storage: Store in cool place away from direct sunlight. Pesticide Disposal: Remove tags before slaughter. Tags may be disposed of on site or at an approved waste disposal facility.

Container Disposal: Dispose of empty bag in a sanitary landfill or by incineration, or, if allowed by State and local authorities, by burning. If burned, stay out of smoke.

Warning(s): Remove tags before slaughter.

Keep out of reach of children.

Disclaimer: Notice of Warranty: Schering-Plough Animal Health Corp. makes no warranty of merchantability, fitness for any particular purpose, or otherwise, expressed or implied concerning this product or its uses which extend beyond the use of the product under normal conditions in accordance with the statements on the label.

Presentation: 20 x 9.5 g tags and buttons per case (NDC 0061-5019-02).

®Allflex is a registered trademark of Allflex USA, Inc.

U.S. Patent No. 4,953,313
Patent 4,581,834

Compendium Code No.: 10471731 Rev. 3/01

SABER™ POUR-ON INSECTICIDE

Schering-Plough **Topical Insecticide**

EPA Reg. No.: 773-74

Active Ingredient(s): % [W/W]

Lambdacyhalothrin: [1 α(S), 3 α (Z)]-(±)-cyano (3-phenoxyphenyl)-methyl-3-(2-chloro-3,3,3-trifluoro-1-propenyl)-2,2-dimethylcyclopropanecarboxylate 1.0%
Inert Ingredients 99.0%
Total 100.0%

Indications: A pour-on insecticide for control of horn flies and lice on beef cattle and calves.

Directions for Use: It is a violation of Federal law to use this product in a manner inconsistent with its labeling.

Ready to Use: No dilution necessary. May be used with automatic dosing system.

Do not apply to lactating or dry dairy cows. Do not apply this product to face of beef cattle or calves.

Apply To	Target Insects	Dosage
Beef Cattle and Calves	Lice, Horn Flies	Apply product down the backline at the rate of 10 mL (1⁄3 fl oz) per head for cattle weighing less than 600 lb. or at a rate of 15 mL (1⁄2 fl oz) per head for cattle weighing more than 600 lb.

Repeat treatment as needed, however, do not apply more than once every 2 weeks and do not apply more often than four times within any 6-month period. For reduction of sucking lice, two treatments at a 14-day interval are recommended.

Special Note: SABER™ Pour-On is not recommended for use on veal calves. SABER™ Pour-On is not effective in controlling cattle grubs. Therefore, this product can be used on cattle at any time of the year without fear of host-parasite reactions commonly associated with grub treatment products. SABER™ Pour-On should be used in an integrated pest management system which may involve repeat treatments and the use of other pest control practices. Continual exposure of horn flies to a single class of insecticide (e.g. pyrethroids or organophosphates) may lead to the development of resistance to that class of insecticide. In order to reduce the possibility of horn flies developing resistance, it is important to rotate, on a seasonal basis, the class of insecticide used and/or the method of horn fly control. For advice concerning current control practices with relation to specific local conditions, consult resources in resistance management programs and your Cooperative Agricultural Extension Service.

Precautionary Statements: Hazards to Humans and Domestic Animals:

Caution: Harmful if swallowed, absorbed through the skin or inhaled. Causes moderate eye irritation. Avoid breathing vapors or spray mist. Avoid contact with skin, eyes or clothing. Remove contaminated clothing and wash before re-use. Wash thoroughly with soap and water after handling. Avoid contact with eyes. Wear rubber or non-permeable protective gloves when applying this product. Data indicate this product to be a contact allergenic. Do not apply product to face of cattle.

First Aid:

If inhaled: Move person to fresh air. If person is not breathing, call 911 or an ambulance, then give artificial respiration, preferably mouth-to-mouth, if possible. Call a poison control center or doctor for further treatment advice.

If on skin or clothing: Take off contaminated clothing. Rinse skin immediately with plenty of water for 15-20 minutes. Call a poison control center or doctor for treatment advice.

If in eyes: Hold eye open and rinse slowly and gently with water for 15-20 minutes. Remove contact lenses, if present, after the first 5 minutes, then continue rinsing eye. Call a poison control center or doctor for treatment advice.

If swallowed: Call a poison control center or doctor immediately for treatment advice. Have person sip a glass of water if able to swallow. Do not induce vomiting unless told to do so by the poison control center or doctor. Do not give anything by mouth to an unconscious person.

Hotline Number: Have the product container or label with you when calling a poison control center or doctor, or going for treatment. You may also contact the Rocky Mountain Poison Center 303-595-4869 for emergency medical treatment information.

Environmental Hazards: This pesticide is extremely toxic to fish. Use with care when applying in areas adjacent to any body of water. Do not add directly to water. Do not contaminate water by cleaning of equipment or disposal of rinse water. Apply this product only as specified on the label.

Physical or Chemical Hazards: Do not use or store near heat or open flame.

Storage and Disposal: Do not contaminate water, food or feed by storage or disposal.

Storage: Keep container sealed when not in use. Do not store near food or feed.

Pesticide Disposal: Wastes resulting from the use of this product may be disposed of on site or at an approved waste disposal facility.

Container Disposal: Triple rinse (or equivalent). Then offer for recycling or reconditioning or puncture and dispose of in a sanitary landfill or incineration, or, if allowed by State and local authorities, by burning. If burned, stay out of smoke.

Warning(s): Do not apply to lactating or dry dairy cows. SABER™ Pour-On is not recommended for use on veal calves.

Keep out of reach of children.

Disclaimer: Notice of Warranty: Schering-Plough Animal Health Corporation makes no warranty of merchantability, fitness for any particular purpose or otherwise expressed or implied concerning this product or its uses which extend beyond the use of this product under normal conditions in accord with the statements made on the label.

Presentation: 30 fl oz (900 mL) in a Squeeze 'N' Measure™ bottle (NDC 0061-5062-01) and 1 U.S. gallon (3.785 L) (NDC 0061-5062-04).

Compendium Code No.: 10471742 Rev. 8/99, Rev. 1/01 / Rev. 4/00, Rev. 1/01

SACOX® 60

Intervet **Feed Medication**

Salinomycin Sodium-Type A Medicated Article

ANADA No.: 200-075

Active Ingredient(s): Salinomycin equivalent to 60 grams salinomycin sodium activity per pound.

Ingredients: Calcium carbonate, mineral oil, calcium silicate and silicon dioxide.

Medicated Premix: Sixty (60) grams salinomycin sodium activity per pound.

Indications: For the prevention of coccidiosis caused by *Eimeria tenella, E. necatrix, E. acervulina, E. maxima, E. brunetti* and *E. mivati.*

For use in broiler chickens only.

Dosage and Administration: SACOX 60® can be used to provide concentrations of salinomycin ranging from 40 to 60 g/ton. The dosage should be adjusted to meet the severity of the coccidial challenge, which varies with environmental and management conditions.

Mixing Directions: Thoroughly mix the correct amount of the premix according to the directions below with an amount of non-medicated feed to provide the level of salinomycin per ton of feed.

Salinomycin Sodium Activity (grams per ton)	Amount of SACOX® Premix Per Ton of Feed
40	11 ounces
45	12 ounces
50	13.5 ounces
55	14.5 ounces
60	1 pound

Important: Must be thoroughly mixed in feeds before use. Not for use with pellet binders.

Feeding Directions: Feed continuously as the only ration.

Precaution(s): Store in a cool, dry place.

Caution(s): May be fatal if accidentally fed to adult turkeys or to horses.

Warning(s): No withdrawal required. Do not feed to laying chickens.

When mixing and handling SACOX 60® Premix, use protective clothing, impervious gloves, eye protection and an approved dust respirator. Operators should wash thoroughly with soap and water after handling. If accidental eye contact occurs, immediately rinse thoroughly with water.

Presentation: 50 lbs (22.68 kg).

Compendium Code No.: 11061761 385856A

SA-ELISA II (EIA TEST KIT)

Centaur **EIA Test**

Equine Infectious Anemia Antibody Test

U.S. Vet. Lic. No.: 320

Contents: Reagents: Except for the PBS Wash Concentrate, all materials are provided ready-to use.

Materials Provided

1. Microplate wells, coated with synthetic EIAV antigen and recombinant core antigen.
2. Conjugate, of both synthetic EIAV antigen and recombinant core antigen and horseradish peroxidase in phosphate buffered saline with 10% fetal bovine serum (contains 0.02% thimerosal as a preservative).
3. Substrate A, TMB (Tetramethylbenzidine) Peroxidase Substrate.
4. Substrate B, Hydrogen Peroxide, 0.02% in citric acid buffer.
5. PBS (Phosphate Buffered Saline) Wash Concentrate (contains 0.4% thimerosal as a preservative). Must be diluted prior to use (see Preliminary Steps, number 4).
6. Positive Control Serum (contains 0.1% thimerosal as a preservative).
7. Negative Control Serum (contains 0.1% thimerosal as a preservative).
8. Stop Solution (contains 1.0 M phosphoric acid).

Materials Required But Not Provided

1. Graduated cylinder for dilution of PBS Wash Solution.
2. Wash bottle or microplate wash system.
3. Micropipettor (50 microliter) and disposable tips.
4. Optional microplate reader.

Indications: Synthetic antigen enzyme-linked immunosorbent assay.

Test Principles: In the SA-ELISA II test, the wells of the microplate are coated with a synthetic peptide antigen which is chemically identical to a section of an EIAV envelope protein and a recombinant core antigen. The antigens contain multiple epitopes of EIAV which bind antibody present in the serum specimen.

A sample of serum is added to a well and after an incubation period, the well is washed and a conjugate of both the synthetic antigen and the recombinant core antigen and horseradish peroxidase is added. Upon completion of a second incubation period, the well is again washed and TMB (tetramethylbenzidine) as a substrate is added to the well.

If antibodies are present in the test specimen, color develops in the well. If antibodies are not present, no color or only minimal color develops. Positive and negative control sera are included with each group of serum specimens to provide representative color development.

Sample Collection: Specimen Collection and Preparation: Horse serum is recommended for use with the SA-ELISA II test kit. Whole blood may be collected by venipuncture and the serum fraction separated by centrifugation for 10 minutes at approximately 2500 rpm. Serum separators may be used. Anticoagulants are not recommended.

Specimens may be stored at refrigerator temperature (2 to 7°C) for five days. If longer storage is needed, specimens should be frozen at -20°C. Repeated freezing and thawing should be avoided. Frozen samples should thaw at room temperature and should be mixed by gentle inversion before testing begins.

Test Procedure: Assay Methods: Preliminary Steps

1. Remove the SA-ELISA II test kit from the refrigerator about one hour before use to allow reagents and microplate wells to come to room temperature.
2. Use a single microplate well for each serum specimen, Positive Control Serum and Negative Control Serum. Return the remainder of microplate wells in the plate to the storage bag with the desiccant and return the wells to the refrigerator.
3. Identify and record a well location for each control and serum specimen. Alternatively, identification may be written directly on the side of the well.
4. Dilute the 30 mL PBS Wash Concentrate with 570 mL distilled water. Mix thoroughly to ensure that the Wash Concentrate is completely solubilized. Other volumes may be used for convenience. The dilution of one part PBS concentrate with 19 parts distilled water must be maintained. Label the diluted PBS Wash Solution with an expiration of 30 days from the date of dilution. Do not use the Wash Solution after that date. Store diluted PBS Wash Solution at 2 to 7°C.
5. Washing the wells is a critical step in the assay procedure and should be done with care and diligence. Where the Testing Procedure requires the wells to be washed, the contents of the wells should be discarded and the wells completely filled with PBS Wash Solution. After all wells have been filled, empty the wells over a suitable container and immediately tap the inverted wells vigorously on absorbent material to remove any residual wash solution. It is important to maintain the plate in an inverted position during the interval between emptying and tapping the wells. Each well should be washed five times as indicated below (see Testing Procedure).

Testing Procedure

1. Add 50 microliters of control or serum specimen to the appropriate well. Use a new pipette tip for each sample.
2. Gently tap the side of the microplate to dislodge any trapped air bubbles. Incubate the uncovered wells at room temperature (23 to 29°C) for fifteen (15) minutes.
3. At the end of the incubation period, invert the well strip and discard the serum. Wash wells five (5) times with diluted PBS Wash Solution as described above. The washing operation must be done with care to minimize the possibility of nonspecific reactions or cross contamination of wells.
4. Add one drop (0.05 mL) Conjugate to each microplate well. Incubate at room temperature for fifteen (15) minutes.
5. Wash wells five (5) times with diluted PBS Wash Solution. Add one drop (0.05 mL) of Substrate A to each test microwell and then add one drop (0.05 mL) of substrate B to each well.
6. Incubate for fifteen (15) minutes to allow for blue color development.
7. Add one drop (0.05 mL) Stop Solution to each well. The blue color will now become yellow. The use of a white background facilitates the observation of color. Alternatively, the microplate may be read spectrophotometrically at 450 nm.

Quality Control: The Positive Control Serum produces an intense color in the assay. When read spectrophotometrically with the spectrophotometer blanked on air, the Positive Control Serum should yield an O.D. of 0.5 to 2.0. If color development in the Positive Control Serum is weak or appears to be less than usual to the experienced worker, the assay should be repeated. A lack of color development in the Positive Control Serum could be due to the use of expired reagents or wells. The Negative Control Serum produces either no color or only a faint tint. When read spectrophotometrically, the Negative Control Serum should yield an O.D. of 0.0 to 0.15. The presence of color could be due to cross contamination during the test procedure.

Interpretation of Results: Results: For visual determination, any test well yielding color development greater than the Negative Control Serum should be considered positive for antibodies to EIAV. Wells which visually show color development equal to or less than the Negative Control Serum should be considered to contain serum specimens which are free of detectable antibody to EIAV.

For spectrophotometric determination, blank the spectrophotometer on air. Add 0.05 OD to the negative control value to establish the test cutoff value. Specimen wells with values above the cutoff should be considered positive for antibodies to EIAV. Specimen wells with values equal to or below the cutoff should be considered negative for antibodies to EIAV. It Is recommended that any positive ELISA evaluation be confirmed using the agar gel immunodiffusion (AGID) test. Discrepant samples should be retested and sent to the National Veterinary Services Laboratory for confirmation before being reported as positive.

Storage: Storage and Stability: All materials provided in the test kit should be stored at 2 to 7°C. Wells of the microplate should be stored with the desiccant in the bag provided. After dilution, PBS Wash Solution should again be stored at 2 to 7°C.

Important! Warm reagents to room temperature (23 to 29°C) prior to each use. Materials should not be used after the expiration date shown on the package label.

Caution(s):

1. Do not mix reagents or microplate wells of one kit with those of another kit.
2. For veterinary use only and for sale only to USDA/APHIS approved laboratories.

Warning(s): Extreme care must be taken in washing microplate wells to avoid cross contamination of adjacent wells which could cause false results.

Discussion: Summary and Explanation: The SA-ELISA II kit utilizes synthetic envelope antigen and a recombinant core antigen in an enzyme-linked immunosorbent assay (ELISA) for the qualitative determination of antibodies to Equine Infectious Anemia Virus (EIAV) in horse serum. The synthetic viral peptide antigen and recombinant core antigen are coated onto the microwells and conjugated to horseradish peroxidase. In field trails, the results of testing by the EIAV antibody test show a high correlation with the agar gel immunodiffusion test of Coggins (1). Because there is no cure and no effective vaccine for EIAV, disease control measures are limited to the identification and isolation of infected animals (2,3). The SA-ELISA II antibody test provides a rapid and reliable method for the detection of EIAV antibodies.

Technical Services: If you have any questions regarding the use of this test, please call the manufacturer, Viral Antigens, Inc. technical services in the USA at (901) 382-8716.

References: Available upon request.

Presentation: 96 wells.

Manufactured by: Viral Antigens, Memphis, TN 38134 USA

Compendium Code No.: 14880120 09/99 V2111

SAFE4HOURS™ MEDICAL FORMULA

Safe4Hours **Skin Protector**

Antimicrobial Skin Sanitizer

Active Ingredient(s): Triclosan 1%.

Indications: SAFE4HOURS™ Medical Formula contains no alcohol, waxes or silicones. The base of SAFE4HOURS™ is its patent pending polymer delivery system. This unique delivery system, will not wash off, maintains a persistent kill of a broad spectrum of bacteria, is non-occlusive, helps reduce the risk of cross-contamination, moisturizes dry irritated skin, contains no dyes or fragrances, and will stay bonded to the skin for up to four hours.

Directions: For optimal protection, wash and dry hands thoroughly. Next, apply 0.7 mL (approximately dime-size) of SAFE4HOURS™ Medical Formula wherever protection is required. Work evenly into both sides of hands, paying close attention to cuticles and skin under the fingernails. It will take approximately 20-30 seconds for the product to dry. Reapply every four hours.

Discussion: SAFE4HOURS™ Medical Formula Antimicrobial Skin Sanitizer is a proprietary cross polymer formulation that benefits health care professionals by:

1. Reduces Occupational Hand Disease (OHD).
2. Persistent Antimicrobial Activity.
3. Encourages Healthy Skin to Withstand Environmental Irritants.

Mandated hand washing protocols are a major cause of OHD and the number 2 cause of occupational disease in the workplace. Independent studies have proven that SAFE4HOURS™ helps reduce OHD. In addition producing agents including: *Streptococcus pyogenes, Staphylococcus epidermidis, Staphylococcus aureus* (MRSA), *Enterococcus faecalis* (MDR/VRE).

Presentation: 2 fl oz (57 mL), 4 fl oz (113 mL), 8 fl oz (236 mL), 16 fl oz (473 mL), and 1 liter.

Compendium Code No.: 10560001

SAFECIDE® IC

Schering-Plough **Premise Insecticide**

EPA Reg. No.: 66986-1-45860

Active Ingredient(s):

Orthoboric Acid	99.0%
Inert Ingredients	1.0%
Total	100.0%

Indications: For darkling and lesser mealworm beetle, hide beetle and fly control in poultry houses. (Adults and Larvae). For the control of fire ants.**

Dosage and Administration: It is a violation of Federal law to use this product in a manner inconsistent with its labeling.

For poultry houses in which birds are grown on litter:

Dry Application: Prior to application of SAFECIDE® Brand IC, remove birds. Apply dust uniformly to floor of poultry house or to old litter with a fertilizer or seed spreader, at the rate of 1-2 pounds per 100 square feet, in bands along feeder lines. Then introduce birds. Reapply after each grow-out, if needed, in the sequence outlined above.

For poultry houses in which birds are grown in cages (layer or high rise 'pit type' houses):

Dry Application: Prior to application of SAFECIDE® Brand IC, remove birds. Apply at the rate of 1-2 pounds for each 100 square feet of treated surface. Using appropriate equipment, thoroughly dust side walls, top plates, posts, and framing. Dust into cracks and crevices around insulation. Then, introduce birds. Reapply after each grow-out, if needed, in the sequence outlined above. However, if facility is washed down and sanitized using standard cleaning and disinfecting procedures, SAFECIDE® Brand IC must be reapplied to continue beetle control. SAFECIDE® Brand IC can be applied directly to manure for fly control.

Wet Application: Prior to the application of SAFECIDE® Brand IC to top levels of layer house, remove birds. Mix dust at the rate of 1-2 pounds per three gallons of water. Apply at the rate of three gallons of mix for each 100 square feet of treated surface. Using appropriate pressure spray equipment, saturate side walls, top plates, posts, and framing. Spray mix into cracks and crevices around insulation. Do not expose birds to spray. Reapply after each grow-out, if needed, in the sequence outlined above. However, if facility is washed down and sanitized using standard cleaning and disinfecting procedures, SAFECIDE® Brand IC must be reapplied to continue beetle control. SAFECIDE® Brand IC can be applied directly to manure for fly control.

For the control of fire ants**:

Methods of Application: Apply SAFECIDE® Brand IC when ants are actively foraging. This is usually when soil temperatures are above 60°F. Avoid application when the soil is wet. Heavy rainfall within 2 to 3 hours of application may reduce effectiveness. In cases where reinfestation occurs or when very large mounds remain active, retreatment may be desirable after 2 to 3 weeks. Do not apply to pasture, rangeland or other areas which may be grazed by cattle, sheep or other domestic animal.

Mound Application: Apply 1 to 2 cups of SAFECIDE® Brand IC per mound uniformly distributing material 3 to 4 feet around the base of the mound. Do not contaminate kitchen utensils by use or storage of product.

Precaution(s): Do not contaminate water, food, or feed by storage or disposal.

Storage: Store in a dry place. Do not store where children or animals may gain access.

Pesticide Disposal: Wastes resulting from the use of this product may be disposed of on site or at an approved waste disposal facility.

Container Disposal: Completely empty bag into application equipment. Then dispose of empty bag in a sanitary landfill or by incineration, or, if allowed by State and local authorities, by burning. If burned, stay out of smoke.

Environmental Hazards: For terrestrial uses, do not apply directly to water, or to areas where surface water is present, or to intertidal areas below the mean high water mark. Do not contaminate water when disposing of equipment washwaters or rinsate.

Caution(s): Hazards to Humans and Domestic Animals:

Precautionary Statements: Harmful if swallowed or absorbed through the skin. Causes eye irritation. Avoid contact with skin, eyes or clothing. Wash thoroughly with soap and water after handling.

Applicators and other handlers of this product must wear a dust mask or dust/mist filtering respirator and protective gloves for all application methods described on the label.

Warning(s): Statement of Practical Treatment:

If Swallowed: Call a physician or Poison Control Center.

If in Eyes: Flush eyes with plenty of water. Call a physician if irritation persists.

If on Skin: Wash with plenty of soap and water. Get medical attention.

**Not for use in California. Keep out of reach of children.

Presentation: 50 pounds.

® Registered trademark of: Parasitix Corporation.

Compendium Code No.: 10741760

SAFE-GUARD® 20% DEWORMER TYPE A MEDICATED ARTICLE

Intervet **Parasiticide-Oral**

Fenbendazole

NADA No.: 131-675

Active Ingredient(s): Fenbendazole 200 grams per kilogram (90.7 grams per pound).

Inert Ingredients: Roughage products or roughage products and calcium carbonate; and mineral oil or soybean oil.

Indications:

Zoo and Wildlife Animals: For the removal and control of: Internal parasites in hoofed zoo and wildlife animals (see dosage section for specific parasites, animal species and required doses).

Cattle: Dairy and Beef Cattle: For the removal and control of:

Lungworms: *(Dictyocaulus viviparus)*.

Stomach worms: Barberpole worms *(Haemonchus contortus)*, brown stomach worms *(Ostertagia oastertagi)*, small stomach worms *(Trichostrongylus axei)*.

Intestinal worms: Hookworms *(Bunostomum phlebotomum)*, thread-necked intestinal worms *(Nematodirus helvetianus)*, small intestinal worms *(Cooperia punctata* and *C. oncophora)*.

Bankrupt worms: *(Trichostrongylus colubriformis)*.

Nodular worms: *(Oesophagostomum radiatum)*.

Swine: Growing pigs, gilts, pregnant sows, and boars: For the removal and control of:

Lungworms: *(Metastrongylus apri, Metastrongylus pudendotectus)*.

Gastrointestinal worms: Adult and larvae (L_3, L_4 stages, liver, lung, intestinal forms); large roundworms *(Ascaris suum)*; nodular worms *(Oesophagostomum dentatum, O quadrispinulatum)*; small stomach worms *(Hyostrongylus rubidus)*; adult and larvae stages (L_2, L_3, L_4 stages - intestinal mucosal forms); *(Trichuris suis)*.

Kidney worms: Adult and larvae *(Stephanurus dentatus)*.

Dosage and Administration: Zoo and Wildlife Animals:

Dose/Dosage Regimens:

Host Animal	Recommended Treatment for	mg Fenbendazole/kg Body Wt./Day x Days of Treatment
Bighorn Sheep *(Ovis canadensis canadensis)*	lungworms *(Protostrongylus* spp.)	10 mg x 3
Feral Swine *(Sus scrofa)*	kidney worms *(Stephanurus dentatus)*, round worms *(Ascaris suum)*, nodular worms *(Oesophagostomum dentatum)*	3 mg x 3
Ruminants - subfamily antilopinae: Persian gazelles *(Gazella subgutturosa subgutturosa)* Addra gazelle *(Gazella dama ruficollis)* Slenderhorn Gazelle *(Gazella leptoceros)* Kenya impala *(Aepyceros melampus rendilis)* Roosevelt's gazelle *(Gazella granti roosevelti)* Indian blackbuck *(Antilope cervicapra)* Mhorr gazelle *(Gazella dama mhorr)* Thomson's gazelles *(Gazella thomsoni thomsoni)* Ruminants - subfamily hippotraginae: Addax *(Addax nasomasculatus)* Angolan roan antelope *(Hippotragus equinus cottoni)* Fringed-ear oryx *(Oryx gazella callotis)* Arabian oryx *(Oryx leucoryx)* Ruminants - subfamily caprinae: Armenian mouflon *(Ovis orientalis gmelini)* Russian saiga *(Saiga tatarica)*	small stomach worms: *(Trichostrongylus* spp.), thread-necked intestinal worms: *(Nematodirus* spp.), barberpole worms: *(Haemonchus* spp.), whipworms *(Trichuris* spp.)	2.5 mg x 3

It is recommended that the user exercise judgmental expertise as needed for retreatment within six (6) weeks. This would depend upon the conditions of continued exposure to parasites, condition of treated animals, and ambient temperatures.

General Mixing Directions: SAFE-GUARD® 20% Type A Medicated Article must be mixed according to directions and at correct concentrations based upon the species to be treated. It is recommended that SAFE-GUARD® 20% Type A Medicated Article be diluted before addition to the final feed. The correct proportions of premix and feed ingredients should be established for blending into the complete feed. This premix and feed ingredient combination should be thoroughly and uniformly mixed with the complete feed.

SAFE-GUARD® 20% Type A Medicated Article can be fed to adult and young animals either in a mash or pelleted feed. No prior withdrawal of feed or water is necessary.

Cattle: Dairy and Beef Cattle:

Dosage Regimen: 5 mg fenbendazole per kg body weight in a one (1) day treatment (2.27 mg fenbendazole per pound).

Example of Mixing and Feeding Rates for SAFE-GUARD® 20% Type A Medicated Article: For a one (1) day treatment, mix the following quantities of SAFE-GUARD® 20% Type A Medicated Article into the daily ration according to body weight and number of cattle per pen.

Amount of SAFE-GUARD® 20% Type A Medicated Article for:

Body Weight		10 Cattle		20 Cattle		100 Cattle	
lbs	kg	g	lbs	g	lbs	g	lbs
200	90.7	23	0.05	46	0.10	230	0.5
400	181.4	46	0.10	92	0.20	460	1.0
600	272.2	69	0.15	138	0.30	690	1.5
800	362.9	92	0.20	184	0.40	920	2.0
1000	453.6	114	0.25	228	0.50	1140	2.5
1400	635.0	160	0.35	320	0.70	1600	3.5

Feed as the sole ration for one (1) day. No prior withdrawal of feed or water necessary. When feed containing SAFE-GUARD® has been fed for 1 day and blended according to the above rates based on weight and number of cattle treated, a total intake of 2.27 mg fenbendazole per pound of body weight is assured. Cattle feed containing SAFE-GUARD® can be fed pelleted or as meal.

Under conditions of continued exposure to parasites, retreatment may be needed after 4-6 weeks.

General Mixing Directions: It is recommended that SAFE-GUARD® 20% Type A Medicated Article be diluted before addition to the final feed. A dilution of one part of SAFE-GUARD® 20% Type A Medicated Article and nine parts of grain carrier is the suggested working premix. The working premix is then blended with the complete feed mixture. Thoroughly mix both working premix and complete feed to ensure complete and uniform distribution of the SAFE-GUARD® 20% Type A Medicated Article.

Swine: Growing pigs, gilts, pregnant sows, and boars:

Dosage Regimen: 9 mg fenbendazole per kg body weight (4.08 mg fenbendazole per pound) to be fed as the sole ration over a period of 3 to 12 days.

Example of Mixing and Feeding Rates for SAFE-GUARD® 20% Type A Medicated Article:

Average daily feed consumption		Amount of SAFE-GUARD® 20% Type A Medicated Article added to each ton of swine feed based on weight and average feed consumption.					
		Treatment Period					
Pig. Wt. (lbs)	lbs of Feed	3 Days		6 Days		12 Days	
		lbs	Grams	lbs	Grams	lbs	Grams
30	2.25	0.40	182	0.20	91	0.10	46
50	3.20	0.47	213	0.24	107	0.12	54
75	4.25	0.53	241	0.27	121	0.14	61
100	5.30	0.57	258	0.29	129	0.15	65
150	6.80	0.66	301	0.33	151	0.17	76
200	8.00	0.75	341	0.38	171	0.19	86

Feed as the sole ration for three (3) to twelve (12) consecutive days. No prior withdrawal of feed or water necessary. When feed containing SAFE-GUARD® has been blended according to the above rates based on pig weight and average daily feed consumption, and is then fed for 3-12 days, a total intake of 9 mg fenbendazole per kilogram body weight (4.08 mg fenbendazole per pound) is assured. Swine feeds containing SAFE-GUARD® can be fed pelleted or as meal.

General Mixing Directions: It is recommended that SAFE-GUARD® 20% Type A Medicated Article be diluted before addition to the final feed. A dilution of one part of SAFE-GUARD® 20% Type A Medicated Article and nine parts of grain carrier is the suggested working premix. The working premix is then blended with the complete feed mixture. Thoroughly mix both working premix and complete feed to ensure complete and uniform distribution of the SAFE-GUARD® 20% Type A Medicated Article.

Contraindication(s): Animal Safety: No contraindications for the use of fenbendazole in a zoo environment have been established. Administration to breeding and pregnant ruminants at 2 to 22 times the recommended dose has had no apparent adverse effect.

There are no known contraindications to the use of the drug in cattle. For dairy cattle, there is no milk withdrawal period.

Warning(s): Zoo and Wildlife Animals: Do not use 14 days before or during the hunting season.

Cattle: Dairy and Beef Cattle: Cattle must not be slaughtered within 13 days following last treatment.

Swine: Growing pigs, gilts, pregnant sows, and boars: There is no pre-slaughter withdrawal as SAFE-GUARD® can be fed to day of slaughter.

Keep this and all drugs out of the reach of children. Not for use in humans. The Material Safety Data Sheet (MSDS) contains more detailed occupational safety information. To report adverse effects, obtain an MSDS, or for assistance contact Hoechst Roussel Vet National Service Center at 1-800-247-4838.

For use in manufactured feeds only.

Consult your veterinarian for assistance in the diagnosis, treatment, and control of parasitism.

Presentation: 25 pounds (11.34 kg).

SAFE-GUARD Reg TM Hoechst Celanese Corporation

Compendium Code No.: 11061800

SAFE-GUARD® BEEF & DAIRY CATTLE DEWORMER

Intervent **Parasiticide-Oral**

(fenbendazole) Suspension 10%-100 mg/mL

NADA No.: 128-620

Active Ingredient(s): Each mL contains 100 mg of fenbendazole.

Indications: Beef and Dairy Cattle: For the removal and control of:

Lungworm: *(Dictyocaulus viviparus)*.

Stomach worm (adults): *Ostertagia ostertagi* (Brown stomach worm).

Stomach worm (adults and 4th stage larvae): *Haemonchus contortus/placei* (barberpole worm), *Trichostrongylus axei* (small stomach worm). Intestinal worm (adults and 4th stage larvae): *Bunostomum phlebotomum* (hookworm), *Nematodirus helvetianus* (thread-necked intestinal worm), *Cooperia puncata* and *C. oncophora* (small intestinal worm), *Trichostrongylus colubriformis* (bankrupt worm), *Oesophagostomum radiatum* (nodular worm).

Dosage and Administration: Beef and Dairy Cattle - 5 mg/kg (2.3 mg/lb.) for the removal and control of:

Lungworm: *(Dictyocaulus viviparus)*.

Stomach worm (adults): *Ostertagia ostertagi* (Brown stomach worm).

Stomach worm (adults and 4th stage larvae): *Haemonchus contortus/placei* (barberpole worm), *Trichostrongylus axei* (small stomach worm). Intestinal worm (adults and 4th stage larvae): *Bunostomum phlebotomum* (hookworm), *Nematodirus helvetianus* (thread-necked intestinal worm), *Cooperia puncata* and *C. oncophora* (small intestinal worm), *Trichostrongylus colubriformis* (bankrupt worm), *Oesophagostomum radiatum* (nodular worm).

Directions: Determine the proper dose according to estimated body weight. Administer orally. The recommended dose of 5 mg/kg is achieved when 2.3 mL of the drug are given for each 100 lb. body weight.

Examples:

Dose (5 mg/kg)	Cattle Weight
2.3 mL	100 lb.
4.6 mL	200 lb.
6.9 mL	300 lb.
9.2 mL	400 lb.
11.5 mL	500 lb.
23.0 mL	1000 lb.
34.5 mL	1500 lb.

Under conditions of continued exposure to parasites, retreatment may be needed after 4-6 weeks.

Consult your veterinarian for assistance in the diagnosis, treatment and control of parasitism.

Contraindication(s): There are no known contraindications to the use of the drug in cattle.

Precaution(s): Store at or below 25°C (77°F). Protect from freezing. Shake well before use.

Warning(s): Residue Warning: Cattle must not be slaughtered within 8 days following treatment.

For dairy cattle, there is no milk withdrawal period.

Keep this and all medication out of the reach of children.

Presentation: 1000 mL (33.8 fl oz) and 1 gallon (3785 mL) bottles.

Manufactured by: DPT Laboratories, San Antonio, TX 78215.

Compendium Code No.: 11061881 697510-A/697515-A / 697935-A/697938-A

SAFE-GUARD® BEEF AND DAIRY CATTLE DEWORMER (290 G)

Intervet **Parasiticide-Oral**

(Fenbendazole) 10%

NADA No.: 132-872

Active Ingredient(s):

Fenbendazole .... 100 mg/g

Indications: For the removal and control of: Lungworm: *(Dictyocaulus viviparus)*. Stomach worms: Barberpole worm *(Haemonchus contortus/placei)*, Brown stomach worm *(Ostertagia ostertagi)*, Small stomach worm *(Trichostrongylus axei)*. Intestinal worms: Hookworm *(Bunostomum phlebotomum)*, Thread-necked intestinal worm *(Nematodirus helvetianus)*, Small intestinal worms *(Cooperia punctata* and *C. oncophora)*, Bankrupt worm *(Trichostrongylus colubriformis)*, Nodular worm *(Oesophagostomum radiatum)*.

Dosage and Administration: To be used only with Safe-Guard® dosing equipment.

S

Treats 58 animals of 220 lbs each.

This cartridge is intended for use only with the dispensing gun designed for this product.

To prepare dispensing gun for administration of paste:

1. Turn plunger rod so that notches face up and retract rod fully.
2. Insert cartridge and ring into gun handle until flush with rubber gasket. Turn cartridge and ring clockwise to secure cartridge to gun.
3. Push plunger rod forward until firm contact is made with cartridge plunger.
4. Turn plunger rod so that notches face downward.
5. Remove cap from cartridge.
6. Depress trigger until paste has been ejected. Discard ejected paste. This is to insure a full initial dose.
7. One full depression of trigger delivers one dose for a 220 lb animal.
8. Insert nozzle through the interdental space and deposit paste on back of the tongue by depressing the trigger for the appropriate number of depressions as determined from the table in the dosage section.

Dosage: SAFE-GUARD® (fenbendazole) Paste is given orally to beef and dairy cattle. The dose is 5 mg fenbendazole/kg (2.3 mg/lb) or 5 g SAFE-GUARD® (fenbendazole) Paste per 220 lb body weight (100 kg). Each full depression of the dispensing gun trigger delivers approximately 5 g SAFE-GUARD® (fenbendazole) Paste.

Administer according to the following table:

Cattle Weight	No. of Depressions	One Tube Will Treat
220 lb	1	58 head
440 lb	2	29 head
660 lb	3	19 head
880 lb	4	14 head
1,100 lb	5	11 head
1,540 lb	7	8 head

Do not underdose.

Under conditions of continued exposure to parasites, retreatment may be needed after 4-6 weeks.

Contraindication(s): There are no known contraindications to the use of the drug in cattle. In dairy cattle, there is no milk withdrawal period.

Precaution(s): Store at or below 25°C (77°F).

Warning(s): Cattle must not be slaughtered within 8 days following last treatment.

Keep this and all medication out of the reach of children.

Consult your veterinarian for assistance in the diagnosis, treatment and control of parasitism.

Presentation: 290 g (10.2 oz) cartridges. Starter kit also available containing 2 tubes of 290 g paste and one application gun and hook.

SAFE-GUARD Reg TM Hoechst Celanese Corporation

Manufactured by: DPT Laboratories

Compendium Code No.: 11061851

SAFE-GUARD® EQUINE DEWORMER (25 g)

Intervet **Parasiticide-Oral**

(fenbendazole) 25 g Paste 10% (100 mg/g)

NADA No.: 120-648

Active Ingredient(s): Each gram of SAFE-GUARD® (fenbendazole) Paste 10% contains 100 mg of fenbendazole and is flavored with artificial apple-cinnamon liquid.

Indications: SAFE-GUARD® (fenbendazole) Paste 10% is indicated for the control of large strongyles *(Strongylus edentatus, S. equinus, S. vulgaris)*, encysted early third stage (hypobiotic), late third stage and fourth stage cyathostome larvae, small strongyles, pinworms *(Oxyuris equi)*, ascarids *(Parascaris equorum)*, and arteritis caused by fourth stage larvae of *Strongylus vulgaris* in horses.

SAFE-GUARD® (fenbendazole) Paste 10% is approved for use concomitantly with an approved form of trichlorfon. Trichlorfon is approved for the treatment of stomach bots *(Gasterophilus* spp.) in horses. Refer to the manufacturer's label for directions for use and cautions for trichlorfon.

Pharmacology: SAFE-GUARD® (fenbendazole) Paste 10% contains the active anthelmintic, fenbendazole. The chemical name of fenbendazole is methyl 5-(phenylthio)-2- benzimidazole carbamate.

The chemical structure is:

H N NHCOOCH₃ S N

Actions: The antiparasitic action of SAFE-GUARD® (fenbendazole) Paste 10% is believed to be due to the inhibition of energy metabolism in the parasite.

Dosage and Administration: SAFE-GUARD® (fenbendazole) Paste 10% is administered orally at a rate of 2.3 mg/lb (5 mg/kg) for the control of large strongylus, small strongyles, and pinworms. One syringe will deworm a 1,100 lb horse. For foals and weanlings (less than 18 months of age) where ascarids are a common problem, the recommended dose is 4.6 mg/lb (10 mg/kg); one syringe will deworm a 550 lb horse.

For control of encysted early third stage (hypobiotic), late third stage and fourth stage cyathostome larvae, and fourth stage larvae of *Strongylus vulgaris*, the recommended dose is 4.6 mg/lb (10 mg/kg) daily for 5 consecutive days; administer one syringe for each 550 lbs body weight per day.

Directions for Use:

1. Determine the weight of the horse.
2. Remove syringe tip.
3. Turn the dial ring until the edge of the ring nearest the tip lines up with zero.
4. Depress plunger to advance paste to tip.
5. Now set the dial ring at the graduation nearest the weight of the horse (do not underdose).
6. Horse's mouth must be free of food.
7. Insert nozzle of syringe through the interdental space and deposit the paste on the back of the tongue by depressing the plunger.

Retreatment Recommendations:

Internal Parasites: Regular deworming at intervals of six to eight weeks may be required due to the possibility of reinfection.

Migrating Tissue Parasites: In the case of 4th stage larvae of *Strongylus vulgaris*, treatment and retreatment should be based on the life cycle and the epidemiology. Treatment should be initiated in the spring and repeated in the fall after a six month interval.

Optimum Deworming Program for Control of *S. vulgaris:* Optimum reduction of *S. vulgaris* infections is achieved by reducing the infectivity of the pastures. When horses are running on pasture, in temperate North America, maximum pasture infectivity occurs in October-December. If horses are removed from those pastures in January, pasture infectivity will decline to zero by July 1. Egg production of *S. vulgaris* is minimal from January through April, peaking in August and declining to minimal values in December.

Recommended Deworming Program: *December 1, February 1, April 1, June 1, August 1, October 1.

The April 1st and October 1st treatments are the recommended periods when the 5 day treatment regimen for the control of the migrating larvae of *S. vulgaris* should be performed.

*For other areas in the world, retreatment periods for the migrating larvae of *S. vulgaris* may be different; consult with your veterinarian.

Contraindication(s): There are no known contraindications for the use of SAFE-GUARD® (fenbendazole) Paste 10% in horses.

Precaution(s): Store at or below 25°C (77°F).

Caution(s): When using SAFE-GUARD® (fenbendazole) Paste 10% concomitantly with trichlorfon, refer to the manufacturer's labels for use and cautions for trichlorfon.

Consult your veterinarian for assistance in the diagnosis, treatment and control of parasitism.

For use in animals only.

Warning(s): Do not use in horses intended for food.

Keep this and all medication out of the reach of children.

Side Effects: Side effects associated with SAFE-GUARD® (fenbendazole) Paste 10% could not be established in well-controlled safety studies in horses with single doses as high as 454 mg/lb (1,000 mg/kg) and 15 consecutive daily doses of 22.7 mg/lb (50 mg/kg). Particularly with higher doses, the lethal action of fenbendazole may cause the release of antigens by the dying parasites. This phenomenon may result in either a local or systemic hypersensitive reaction. As with any drug, these reactions should be treated symptomatically.

SAFE-GUARD® (fenbendazole) Paste 10% has been evaluated for safely in pregnant mares during all stages of gestation with doses as high as 11.4 mg/lb (25 mg/kg) and in stallions with doses as high as 11.4 mg/lb (25 mg/kg). No adverse effects on reproductivity were detected. The recommended dose for control of 4th stage larvae of *Strongylus vulgaris,* 4.6 mg/lb (10 mg/kg) daily for 5 consecutive days, has not been evaluated for safety in stallions or pregnant mares.

Presentation: SAFE-GUARD® (fenbendazole) Paste 10% Equine Dewormer is supplied in 25 g (0.88 oz) syringes.

Manufactured by: DPT Laboratories, San Antonio, TX 78215.

Compendium Code No.: 11061861 409804-D/698630-C

SAFE-GUARD® HORSE AND CATTLE DEWORMER (92 g)

Intervet **Parasiticide-Oral**

(fenbendazole) Paste 10% (100 mg/g)

NADA No.: 120-648 (horse)/132-872 (cattle)

Active Ingredient(s): Each gram of SAFE-GUARD® Paste 10% contains 100 mg of fenbendazole and is flavored with artificial apple-cinnamon liquid.

Indications: Horse: SAFE-GUARD® Paste 10% is indicated for the control of large strongyles *(Strongylus edentatus, S. equinus, S. vulgaris),* encysted early 3rd stage (hypobiotic), late 3rd stage and 4th stage cysthostome larvae, small strongyles, pinworms *(Oxyuris equi),* ascarids *(Parascaris equorum),* and arteritis caused by 4th stage larvae of *Strongylus vulgaris* in horses.

SAFE-GUARD® Paste 10% is approved for use concomitantly with an approved form of trichlorfon. Trichlorfon is approved for the treatment of stomach bots *(Gasterophilus* spp) in horses. Refer to the manufacturer's label for directions for use and cautions for trichlorfon.

Beef and Dairy Cattle: SAFE-GUARD® Paste 10% is indicated for the removal and control of: Lungworm *(Dictyocaulus viviparus);* Stomach worms: *(Haemonchus contortus, Ostertagia ostertagi, Trichostrongylus axei);* Intestinal worms *(Bunostomum phlebotomum, Nematodirus helvetianus, Cooperia punctata* and *C. oncophora, Trichostrongylus colubriformis, Oesophagostomum radiatum).*

Pharmacology: SAFE-GUARD® (fenbendazole) Paste 10% contains the active anthelmintic, fenbendazole. The chemical name of fenbendazole is methyl 5-(phenyl-thio)-2- benzimidazole carbamate.

The CAS Registry Number is 43210-67-9.

The chemical structure is:

Actions: The antiparasitic action of SAFE-GUARD® Paste 10% is believed to be due to the inhibition of energy metabolism in the parasite.

Dosage and Administration: Treats 8 animals of 500 lbs each.

Horse: SAFE-GUARD® Paste 10% is administered orally at a rate of 2.3 mg/lb (5 mg/kg) for the control of large strongyles, small strongyles, and pinworms. Each mark on the plunger rod corresponds to a dose of 5 mg/kg (2.3 mg/lb) for 250 lbs body weight.

For foals and weanlings (less than 18 months of age) where ascarids are a common problem, the recommended dose is 4.6 mg/lb (10 mg/kg) or two marks will deworm a 250 lb horse.

For control of 4th stage larvae of *Strongylus vulgaris,* the recommended dose is 4.6 mg/lb (10 mg/kg) daily for 5 consecutive days; administer two marks for each 250 lbs body weight per day.

Retreatment Recommendations for Horses:

Internal Parasites: Regular deworming at intervals of six to eight weeks may be required due to the possibility of reinfection.

Migrating Tissue Parasites: In the case of 4th stage larvae of *Strongylus vulgaris,* treatment and retreatment should be based on the life cycle and the epidemiology. Treatment should be initiated in the spring and repeated in the fall after a six-month interval.

Optimum Deworming Program for control of *S. vulgaris:* Optimum reduction of *S. vulgaris* infections is achieved by reducing the infectivity of the pastures. When horses are running on pasture, in temperate North America, maximum pasture infectivity occurs in October-December. If horses are removed from those pastures in January, pasture infectivity will decline to zero by July 1. Egg production of *S. vulgaris* is minimal from January through April, peaking in August and declining to minimal values in December.

Recommended Deworming Program: *December 1, February 1, April 1, June 1, August 1, October 1.

The April 1 and October 1 treatments are the recommended periods when the 5 day treatment regimen for the control of the migrating larvae of *S. vulgaris* should be performed.

*For other areas in the world, retreatment periods for the migrating larvae of *S. vulgaris* may be different; consult with your veterinarian.

Beef and Dairy Cattle: SAFE-GUARD® Paste 10% is administered orally at a rate of 2.3 mg/lb (5 mg/kg) or 11.5 g SAFE-GUARD® (fenbendazole) Paste for 500 lb body weight (227 kg). Under conditions of continuous exposure to parasites, retreatment may be needed after 4-6 weeks.

Directions for Use:

1. Determine the weight of the animal.
2. Remove the syringe tip.
3. Turn the dial ring until the edge of the ring nearest the tip lines up with zero.
4. Fully depress plunger and discard expelled paste. Syringe is ready for dosing.
5. Each mark on the plunger rod corresponds to a dose of 5 mg/kg (2.3 mg/lb) for 250 lbs body weight. Dial the ring edge nearest the tip back by one mark for each 250 lbs body weight (do not underdose).
   Examples:
   250 lbs: 1 mark
   500 lbs: 2 marks
   750 lbs: 3 marks
   1000 lbs: 4 marks
   1500 lbs: 6 marks
6. Animal's mouth should be free of food. Insert nozzle of syringe through the interdental space and deposit the paste on the back of the tongue by depressing the plunger.
7. Repeat steps 1, 5 and 6 for each additional animal.

Contraindication(s): There are no known contraindications for the use of SAFE-GUARD® Paste 10% in horses or cattle.

Precaution(s): Store at or below 25°C (77°F).

Caution(s): When using SAFE-GUARD® (fenbendazole) Paste 10% concomitantly with trichlorfon, refer to the manufacturer's labels for use and cautions for trichlorfon.

Consult your veterinarian for assistance in the diagnosis, treatment and control of parasitism.

Warning(s): Do not use in horses intended for food.

Cattle must not be slaughtered within 8 days following last treatment.

In dairy cattle, there is no milk withdrawal period.

Keep this and all medication out of the reach of children.

Side Effects: Horse: Side effects associated with SAFE-GUARD® Paste 10% could not be established in well-controlled safety studies in horses with single doses as high as 454 mg/lb (1,000 mg/kg) and 15 consecutive daily doses of 22.7 mg/lb (50 mg/kg). At higher dose levels, the lethal action of fenbendazole may cause the release of antigens by the dying parasites. This phenomenon may result in either a local or systemic hypersensitive reaction varying in severity from itching or a rash to increased respiration and collapse. A veterinarian should be consulted if this type of reaction is suspected.

SAFE-GUARD® Paste 10% has been evaluated for safety in pregnant mares during all stages of gestation with doses as high as 11.4 mg/lb (25 mg/kg) and in stallions with doses as high as 11.4 mg/lb (25 mg/kg). No adverse effects on reproductivity were detected. The recommended dose for control of 4th stage larvae of *Strongylus vulgaris,* 4.6 mg/lb (10 mg/kg) daily for 5 consecutive days, has not been evaluated for safety in stallions or pregnant mares.

Presentation: SAFE-GUARD® Paste 10% Horse and Cattle Dewormer is supplied in 92 gram (3.2 oz) syringes, 12 syringes per carton.

Manufactured by: DPT Laboratories, San Antonio, TX 78215.

Compendium Code No.: 11061871

SAFE-GUARD® MEDICATED DEWORMER FOR BEEF & DAIRY CATTLE, & SWINE

Intervet **Parasiticide-Oral**

0.5% (fenbendazole) Alfalfa-Based Pellets

Active Ingredient(s):

Fenbendazole .... 0.5% (2.27 g/lb)

Guaranteed Analysis

Crude Protein .... (min.) 15%
Crude Fat .... (min.) 1%
Crude Fiber .... (max.) 30%
Moisture Content .... (max.) 13%
Ash Content .... (max.) 15%

Inert Ingredients: Dehydrated Alfalfa Meal, Roughage Products, Calcium Carbonate, Mineral Oil.

Indications: Cattle: Dairy and beef cattle:

For the removal and control of:

Lungworms: *(Dictyocaulus viviparus).*

Stomach worms: Barberpole worms *(Haemonchus contortus),* brown stomach worms *(Ostertagia ostertagi),* small stomach worms *(Trichostrongylus axei).*

Intestinal worms: Hookworms *(Bunostomum phlebotomum),* thread-necked intestinal worms *(Nematodirus helvetianus),* small intestinal worms *(Cooperia punctata* and *C. oncophora),* Bankrupt worms *(Trichostrongylus colubriformis),* Nodular worms *(Oesophagostomum radiatum).*

Swine: Growing pigs, gilts, pregnant sows, and boars:

For the removal and control of:

Lungworms: *(Metastrongylus apri, Metastrongylus pudendotectus).*

Gastrointestinal worms: Adult and larvae (L_3, L_4 stages, liver, lung, intestinal forms) large roundworms *(Ascaris suum);* nodular worms *(Oesophagostomum dentatum, O. quadrispinulatum);* small stomach worms *(Hyostrongylus rubidus);* whipworms, adult and larvae (L_2, L_3, L_4 stages - intestinal mucosal forms, *(Trichuris suis).*

Kidney worms: Adult and larvae *(Stephanurus dentatus).*

Dosage and Administration: Dairy and Beef Cattle Dosage: 5 mg fenbendazole per kg body weight in a one (1) day treatment (2.27 mg fenbendazole per pound of body weight).

Examples of Feeding Rates for SAFE-GUARD® 0.5% (fenbendazole) Alfalfa-Based Pellets for Cattle:

Body Weight (lbs)	SAFE-GUARD® 0.5% Pellets
200	0.2 lbs
500	0.5 lbs
1000	1.0 lbs

Feed for one (1) day. No prior withdrawal of feed or water necessary. When feed containing SAFE-GUARD® has been fed for 1 day according to the above rates, a total intake of 2.27 mg fenbendazole per pound of body weight is assured.

Under conditions of continued exposure to parasites, retreatment may be needed after 4-6 weeks.

Swine Dosage: 4.08 mg fenbendazole per lb body weight (9 mg fenbendazole per kg body weight) to be fed as the sole ration over a period of 3 to 12 consecutive days. Following are examples of feeding rates based on pig weight and average daily feed consumption:

Examples of Feeding Rates For SAFE-GUARD® 0.5% (fenbendazole) Alfalfa-Based Pellets for Swine:

Pig Wt. (lbs)	Avg. Daily Feed Intake (lbs/hd/day)	Treatment Period		
		3 Days-1 lb SAFE-GUARD® 0.5% Pellets in:	6 Days-1 lb SAFE-GUARD® 0.5% Pellets in:	12 Days-1 lb SAFE-GUARD® 0.5% Pellets in:
30	2.25	125 lbs of feed treats 18 pigs	250 lbs of feed treats 18 pigs	375 lbs of feed treats 18 pigs
50	3.20	105 lbs of feed treats 11 pigs	210 lbs of feed treats 11 pigs	315 lbs of feed treats 11 pigs
75	4.25	90 lbs of feed treats 7 pigs	180 lbs of feed treats 7 pigs	270 lbs of feed treats 7 pigs
100	5.30	80 lbs of feed treats 5 pigs	160 lbs of feed treats 5 pigs	240 lbs of feed treats 5 pigs

Caution(s): Consult your veterinarian for assistance in the diagnosis, treatment, and control of parasitism.

Warning(s): Residue Warning: Cattle must not be slaughtered within 13 days following last treatment. For dairy cattle, there is no milk withdrawal period.

There is no pre-slaughter withdrawal period for swine as SAFE-GUARD® can be fed to day of slaughter.

Keep this and all drugs out of the reach of children. Not for use in humans.

Presentation: 10 lb (4.54 kg).

Compendium Code No.: 11061771 580210-C

SAFE-GUARD® MEDICATED DEWORMER FOR BEEF & DAIRY CATTLE (FLAKED MEAL)

Intervet **Parasiticide-Oral**

(1.96% fenbendazole) Type B Medicated Feed

Active Ingredient(s):

Fenbendazole . . . . 19.6 grams per kilogram (8.9 grams per pound)

Other Ingredients: Rice Hulls, Calcium Carbonate and Mineral Oil.

Guaranteed Analysis:

Calcium (Ca) . . . . (min) 19.0%
Calcium (Ca) . . . . (max) 22.5%

Indications: For the removal and control of:

Lungworm: *(Dictyocaulus viviparus).*

Stomach worms: Barberpole worm *(Haemonchus contortus)*, Brown Stomach worm *(Ostertagia ostertagi)*, Small stomach worm *(Trichostrongylus axei).*

Intestinal worms: Hookworm *(Bunostomum phlebotomum)*, Thread-necked intestinal worm *(Nematodirus helvetianus)*, Small intestinal worms *(Cooperia punctata* and *C oncophora).*

Bankrupt worm: *(Trichostrongylus colubriformis).*

Nodular worm: *(Oesophagostomum radiatum).*

Dosage and Administration: Dairy Cattle and Beef Cattle Dosage: 5 mg fenbendazole per kg body weight in one (1) day treatment (2.27 mg fenbendazole per pound).

Example of Mixing and Feeding Rate: For a one (1) day treatment, add the SAFE-GUARD® Dewormer to the daily ration at the rate of 0.25 pounds per 1,000 pounds of body weight (one [1] scoop per 1,350 pounds body weight).

The package treats 98,000 pounds of cattle.

Weight of Cattle	No. Head Treated per Package
500 lbs	196
1000 lbs	98
1500 lbs	65

Feed for one (1) day. No prior withdrawal of feed or water necessary. When feed containing SAFE-GUARD® has been fed for 1 day and blended according to the above rates based on weight and number of cattle treated, a total intake of 2.27 mg fenbendazole per pound of body weight is assured.

Under conditions of continued exposure to parasites, retreatment may be needed after 4-6 weeks.

General Use Directions: SAFE-GUARD® Dewormer must be spread uniformly on top of the daily ration. Sufficient bunk space must be available so all animals can eat at the same time to insure uniform consumption. All cattle must be eating normally to insure that each animal consumes an adequate amount. SAFE-GUARD® Dewormer can also be uniformly blended with the complete ration at the feed mill.

Contraindication(s): There are no known contraindications to the use of the drug in cattle.

For dairy cattle, there is no milk withdrawal period.

Precaution(s): Store at room temperature.

Caution(s): Consult your veterinarian for assistance in the diagnosis, treatment, and control of parasitism.

Must be mixed before feeding according to directions and permitted claims.

For use in manufactured feeds only.

Warning(s): Cattle must not be slaughtered within 13 days following last treatment. For dairy cattle, there is no milk withdrawal period.

Presentation: 25 pounds (11.35 kg) (scoop included).

Compendium Code No.: 11061781 585300-B

SAFE-GUARD® MEDICATED DEWORMER FOR BEEF & DAIRY CATTLE (SOFT MINI PELLETS)

Intervet **Parasiticide-Oral**

(1.96% fenbendazole) Type B Medicated Feed

Active Ingredient(s):

Fenbendazole . . . . 19.6 grams per kilogram (8.9 grams per pound)

Other Ingredients: Forage Products, Mineral Oil and preserved with Propionic Acid.

Guaranteed Analysis:

Crude Protein . . . . (min.) 14.00%
Crude Fat . . . . (min.) 1.50%
Crude Fiber. . . . . (max.) 25.00%

Indications: For the removal and control of:

Lungworm: *(Dictyocaulus viviparus).*

Stomach worms: Barberpole worm *(Haemonchus contortus)*, Brown Stomach worm *(Ostertagia ostertagi)*, Small stomach worm *(Trichostrongylus axei).*

Intestinal worms: Hookworm *(Bunostomum phlebotomum)*, Thread-necked intestinal worm *(Nematodirus helvetianus)*, Small intestinal worms *(Cooperia punctata* and *C. oncophora).*

Bankrupt worm: *(Trichostrongylus colubriformis).*

Nodular worm: *(Oesophagostomum radiatum).*

Dosage and Administration: Dairy Cattle and Beef Cattle Dosage: 5 mg fenbendazole per kg body weight in one (1) day treatment (2.27 mg fenbendazole per pound).

Example of Mixing and Feeding Rate: For a one (1) day treatment, add the SAFE-GUARD® Dewormer to the daily ration at the rate of 0.25 pounds per 1,000 pounds of body weight (one [1] scoop per 1,350 pounds body weight).

The package treats 98,000 pounds of cattle.

Weight of Cattle	No. Head Treated per Package
500 lbs	196
1000 lbs	98
1500 lbs	65

Feed for one (1) day. No prior withdrawal of feed or water necessary. When feed containing SAFE-GUARD® has been fed for 1 day and blended according to the above rates based on weight and number of cattle treated, a total intake of 2.27 mg fenbendazole per pound of body weight is assured.

Under conditions of continued exposure to parasites, retreatment may be needed after 4-6 weeks.

General Use Directions: SAFE-GUARD® Dewormer must be spread uniformly on top of the daily ration. Sufficient bunk space must be available so all animals can eat at the same time to ensure uniform consumption. All cattle must be eating normally to ensure that each animal consumes an adequate amount. SAFE-GUARD® Dewormer can also be uniformly blended with the complete ration at the feed mill.

Contraindication(s): There are no known contraindications to the use of the drug in cattle.

For dairy cattle, there is no milk withdrawal period.

Precaution(s): Store at room temperature.

Caution(s): Consult your veterinarian for assistance in the diagnosis, treatment, and control of parasitism.

Must be mixed before feeding according to directions and permitted claims.

For use in manufactured feeds only.

Warning(s): Cattle must not be slaughtered within 13 days following last treatment. For dairy cattle, there is no milk withdrawal period.

Presentation: 25 pounds (11.35 kg) (scoop included).

Compendium Code No.: 11061791 585302-B/585303-B

SAFE-GUARD® MEDICATED DEWORMER FOR BEEF CATTLE (20% PROTEIN BLOCK)

Intervet **Parasiticide-Oral**

(fenbendazole)

Active Ingredient(s):

Fenbendazole . . . . 750 mg/lb

Guaranteed Analysis:

Crude Protein . . . . (Min) 20.00%
Crude Fat . . . . (Min) 1.00%
Crude Fiber . . . . (Max) 12.00%
Calcium (Ca). . . . . (Min) 2.00%
Calcium (Ca). . . . . (Max) 3.00%
Phosphorus (P) . . . . (Min) 0.85%
Salt (NaCl). . . . . (Min) 13.50%
Salt (NaCl). . . . . (Max) 16.00%
Magnesium (Mg) . . . . (Min) 0.60%
Cobalt (Co) . . . . (Min) 3 ppm
Copper (Cu) . . . . (Min) 200 ppm
Fluorine (F) . . . . (Max) 100 ppm
Iodine (I). . . . . (Min) 20 ppm
Manganese (Mn). . . . . (Min) 500 ppm
Zinc (Zn). . . . . (Min) 800 ppm
Vitamin A . . . . (Min) 20,000 IU/lb
Vitamin D_3. . . . . (Min) 5,000 IU/lb

Ingredients: Cottonseed Meal, Dehydrated Alfalfa Meal, Salt, Cane Molasses, Rice Hulls, Calcium Carbonate, Magnesium Limestone, Defluorinated Phosphate, Hemicellulose Extract, Bentonite, Vitamin A Supplement, Potassium Sulfate, Magnesium Sulfate, Iron Sulfate, Cobalt Sulfate, Manganese Oxide, Manganese Sulfate, Mineral Oil, Dicalcium Phosphate, Monocalcium Phosphate, Magnesium Oxide, Vitamin D_3 Supplement, Calcium Iodate, Copper Sulfate, Zinc Oxide, Zinc Sulfate.

Indications: For the removal and control of:

Lungworm: *(Dictyocaulus viviparus).*

Stomach worms: Barberpole worm *(Haemonchus contortus)*, Brown stomach worm *(Ostertagia ostertagi)* and Small stomach worm *(Trichostrongylus axei).*

Intestinal worms: Hookworm *(Bunostomum phlebotomum)*, Thread-necked intestinal worm *(Nematodirus helvetianus)*, Small intestinal worms *(Cooperia punctata* and *C. oncophora)*, Bankrupt worm *(Trichostrongylus colubriformis)*, Nodular worm *(Oesophagostomum radiatum).*

Dosage and Administration: 1.67 mg fenbendazole per kg of body weight per day for three (3) days. The total dose for the three (3) day period of 5 mg fenbendazole per kg of body weight (2.27 mg fenbendazole per lb).

Feeding Directions: Adequate forage must be available at all times to cattle receiving supplemental block feeding. SAFE-GUARD® (fenbendazole) 20% Protein Deworming Block (Medicated) is designed for deworming pastured cattle by feeding these medicated blocks for three (3) days only as the sole source of salt. It is essential to establish full cattle adaptation to supplemental block feeding prior to treating cattle with SAFE-GUARD® 20% Protein Deworming Block (Medicated). Cattle behavior and per capita consumption must be established by feeding nonmedicated 20% Protein Blocks prior to medicated block treatment. Adaptation to block feed intake for medicated treatment may take twelve (12) to nineteen (19) days of prior exposure to unmedicated feed blocks depending on consumption rates and environmental conditions. When cattle block consumption of 0.1 lb (1.6 oz) per 100 lbs of body weight (or 1.0 lb for mature cattle) per day is attained for several days on the nonmedicated 20% Protein Block, the three (3) day medicated treatment with SAFE-GUARD® 20% Protein Deworming Blocks (Medicated) may begin.

For effective treatment, the cattle must consume an average of 0.1 lbs of SAFE-GUARD® 20% Protein Blocks (Medicated) per 100 lbs of body weight each day for the three (3) days of treatment. This is equivalent to an average of one (1) lb per head per day to mature cattle for the three days of treatment in order to provide a total dose of 2.27 mg fenbendazole per lb of body weight.

To commence deworming treatment, replace the nonmedicated blocks with SAFE- GUARD® 20% Protein Deworming Blocks (Medicated). Place these medicated blocks at the same locations where cattle have demonstrated adequate per capita block intake (0.1 lbs per 100 lbs of body weight per day).

Daily treatment (to be continued for three [3] days):

Cattle Body Weight (lbs)	Average Block Intake (lb/head/day)	No. of Head per Block*
500	1/2	16
750	3/4	11
Mature Cattle	1	8

*Number of head fully treated by each block when consumed in three (3) days.

Following the three (3) day treatment any remaining SAFE-GUARD® 20% Protein Deworming Blocks (Medicated) should be removed from the pasture, and cattle may be returned to their normal supplemental feeding program. Remaining blocks, or portions of blocks, can be utilized for retreatment purposes if used prior to the expiration date.

It is essential that good block feeding husbandry practices be followed at all times. Block feeding techniques include, but are not limited to, a variety of practices. Blocks should be first located in those areas where cattle are seen to browse or loaf. It may be desirable to relocate unconsumed blocks to locations where obvious block consumption is identified. Increased consumption may often be obtained by moving feeding stations into shaded or loafing areas, closer to water sources, increasing the number of blocks available to the animals or combinations of these practices. Decreased consumption may often be obtained by the reverse of the above practices.

Under conditions of continuous exposure to parasites, retreatment may be needed after 6 to 8 weeks.

Caution(s): Consult your veterinarian for assistance in the diagnosis, treatment and control of parasitism.

Warning(s): Cattle must not be slaughtered within 16 days following last treatment.

Presentation: 25 lb (11.34 kg) blocks.

SAFE-GUARD® is a registered trademark of Intervet Inc.

Manufactured by: Sweetlix LLC, Salt Lake City, UT 84111.

Compendium Code No.: 11061811

SAFE-GUARD® MEDICATED DEWORMER FOR BEEF CATTLE (EN-PRO-AL® MOLASSES BLOCK)

Intervet **Parasiticide-Oral**

(fenbendazole)

NADA No.: 139-189

Active Ingredient(s):

Fenbendazole . . . . . 750 mg/lb

Guaranteed Analysis:

Crude Protein . . . . . (min) 4.75%
Crude Fat . . . . . (min) 0.10%
Crude Fiber . . . . . (max) 2.00%
Calcium (Ca) . . . . . (min) 0.80%
Calcium (Ca) . . . . . (max) 1.00%
Phosphorus (P) . . . . . (min) 0.07%
Salt (NaCl) . . . . . (min) 16.00%
Salt (NaCl) . . . . . (max) 18.50%
Magnesium (Mg) . . . . . (min) 3.00%
Flourine (F) . . . . . (max) 0.0002%
Ash Content . . . . . (max) 38.00%

Ingredients: Cane molasses, salt, cottonseed meal, magnesium oxide, deflourinated phosphate, rice hulls, calcium carbonate, manganese oxide, zinc oxide, iron oxide, mineral oil, manganese sulfate, iron sulfate, ethylenediamine dihydriodide, magnesium sulfate, potassium sulfate, copper sulfate, cobalt carbonate, copper oxide, zinc sulfate, and cobalt sulfate.

Indications: Drug Claim: For the removal and control of:

Lungworm: *(Dictyocaulus viviparus)*.

Stomach worms: Barberpole worm *(Haemonchus contortus)*, Brown stomach worm *(Ostertagia ostertagi)*, Small stomach worm *(Trichostrongylus axei)*.

Intestinal worms: Hookworm *(Bunostomum phlebotomum)*, Thread-necked intestinal worm *(Nematodirus helvetianus)*, Small intestinal worms *(Cooperia punctata* and *C. oncophora)*, Bankrupt worm *(Trichostrongylus colubriformis)*, Nodular worm *(Oesophagostomum radiatum)*.

Dosage and Administration: 1.67 mg fenbendazole per kg body weight per day for three (3) days. Total dose for the three day period of 5 mg fenbendazole per kg of body weight (2.27 mg fenbendazole per pound).

Feeding Directions: Adequate forage must be available at all times to cattle receiving supplemental block feeding.

SAFE-GUARD® (fenbendazole) EN-PRO-AL® Molasses Deworming Supplement Block (Medicated) is designed for deworming pastured cattle by feeding these medicated blocks for three (3) days only as the sole source of salt.

It is essential to establish full cattle adaptation to supplemental block feeding prior to treating cattle with SAFE-GUARD® EN-PRO-AL® Molasses Deworming Block (Medicated). Cattle behavior and per capita consumption must be established by feeding nonmedicated EN-PRO-AL® blocks prior to medicated block treatment. Adaptation to block feed intake for medicated treatment may take twelve (12) to nineteen (19) days prior exposure to unmedicated feed blocks depending on consumption rates and environmental conditions. When cattle block consumption of 0.1 pounds (1.6 ounces) per 100 pounds of body weight (or 1.0 pound for mature cattle) per day is attained for several days on the nonmedicated EN-PRO-AL® Block, the three (3) day medicated treatment with SAFE-GUARD® EN-PRO-AL® Molasses Deworming Supplement Block (Medicated) may begin.

For effective treatment, the cattle must consume an average of 0.1 pounds of SAFE-GUARD® EN-PRO-AL® Molasses Deworming Supplement Block (Medicated) per 100 pounds of body weight each day for three (3) days of treatment. This is equivalent to an average of one (1) pound per head per day to mature cattle for three days of treatment in order to provide a total dose of 2.27 mg fenbendazole per pound of body weight.

To commence deworming treatment, replace the nonmedicated blocks with SAFE-GUARD® EN-PRO-AL® Molasses Deworming Supplement Blocks (Medicated). Place these medicated blocks at the same locations where cattle have demonstrated adequate per capita block intake (0.1 pounds per 100 pounds of body weight per day).

Daily Treatment (To Be Continued for Three (3) Days Only):

Cattle Body Weight (pounds)	Average Block Intake (lb/head/day)	Number of Head per Block*
500	1/2	16
750	3/4	11
Mature Cattle	1	8

*Number of head fully treated by each block when consumed in three (3) days.

Following the three (3) day treatment any remaining SAFE-GUARD® EN-PRO-AL® Molasses Deworming Supplement Blocks (Medicated) should be removed from the pasture, and cattle may be returned to their normal supplemental feeding program. Remaining blocks, or portions of blocks, can be utilized for treatment purposes if used prior to expiration date.

It is essential that good block feeding husbandry practices be followed at all times. Block feeding techniques include, but are not limited to, a variety of practices. Blocks should be first located in those areas where cattle are seen to browse or loaf. It may be desirable to relocate unconsumed blocks to locations where obvious block consumption is identified. Increased consumption may often be obtained by moving feeding stations into shaded or loafing areas, closer to water source, increasing the number of blocks available to the animals or combinations of these practices. Decreased consumption may often be obtained by the reverse of the above practices.

Under conditions of continuous exposure to parasites, retreatment may be needed after 6 to 8 weeks.

Caution(s): Consult your veterinarian for assistance in the diagnosis, treatment and control of parasitism.

Warning(s): Cattle must not be slaughtered within 11 days following last treatment.

Presentation: 25 lb (11.34 kg) blocks.

EN-PRO-AL is a registered trademark of Sweetlix LLC.

Compendium Code No.: 11061891 780125-B

SAFE-GUARD® MEDICATED DEWORMER FOR SWINE (EZ SCOOP®)

Intervet **Parasiticide-Oral**

(fenbendazole) Type B Medicated Feed

Active Ingredient(s):

Fenbendazole . . . . . 1.8% (8.172 g/lb)

Guaranteed Analysis:

Calcium (Ca) . . . . . (min) 20.0%
Calcium (Ca) . . . . . (max) 24.0%

Other Ingredients: Rice Hulls, Calcium Carbonate and Mineral Oil.

Indications: 3 to 12 Day Treatment Regimen for the Removal of:

Lungworms: *(Metastrongylus apri, M. pudendotectus)*.

Gastrointestinal Worms: Adult and larvae (L_3, L_4 stages -liver, lung, intestinal forms) large roundworms *(Ascaris suum)*, nodular worms *(Oesophagostomum dentatum, O. quadrispinulatum)*, small stomach worms *(Hyostrongylus rubidus)*, adult and larvae (L_2, L_3, L_4 stages-intestinal mucosal forms) whipworms *(Trichuris suis)*.

Kidneyworms: Adult and larvae *(Stephanurus dentatus)*.

Directions for Use: Dosage Regimen: 9 mg fenbendazole per kg body weight (4.08 mg fenbendazole per lb body weight) over a period of 3 to 12 days.

SAFE-GUARD® EZ SCOOP® premix should be mixed to a concentration of 10 to 300 grams fenbendazole per ton of feed prior to feeding.

For Group Feeding (Pigs, Gilts, Sows or Boars):

Examples of Mixing and Feeding Rates for SAFE-GUARD® EZ SCOOP® Premix:

Pounds of SAFE-GUARD® EZ SCOOP® premix per ton of swine feed based on pig weight and average daily feed consumption:							
Pig Wt. (lbs)	Average daily feed consumption (lbs)	Treatment Period					
		3 days		6 days		12 days	
		lbs premix	Treats approximately:	lbs premix	Treats approximately:	lbs premix	Treats approximately:
50	3.20	5.2	208 pigs	2.6	104 pigs	1.3	52 pigs
75	4.25	5.8	156 pigs	2.9	78 pigs	1.5	39 pigs
100	5.30	6.2	125 pigs	3.1	62 pigs	1.6	31 pigs
150	6.80	7.3	98 pigs	3.7	49 pigs	1.8	24 pigs
200	8.00	8.3	83 pigs	4.1	41 pigs	2.1	20 pigs

For Individual 400 lb Sow Feeding: Mix 1 level scoop (1.07 ounces) of SAFE-GUARD® EZ SCOOP® premix into 4 to 6 lbs of an individual 400 lb sow's daily ration and feed once daily for 3 consecutive days.

Precaution(s): Store at or below 25°C (77°F).

Caution(s): Consult your veterinarian for assistance in the diagnosis, treatment and control of parasitism.

Warning(s): There is no pre-slaughter withdrawal period as SAFE-GUARD® EZ SCOOP® can be fed to day of slaughter.

Presentation: 10 lb (4.54 kg) and 20 lb (9.08 kg) (2 x 10 lb) pails (scoop included).

The name EZ SCOOP is a registered trademark of North American Nutrition.

Compendium Code No.: 11061831 584410-B / 884430-B

SAL BAC®

Biomune **Bacterin**

Salmonella typhimurium Bacterin

U.S. Vet. Lic. No.: 368

Contents: SAL BAC® is an inactivated bacterial vaccine adjuvanted with aluminum hydroxide. It also contains a patented biological adjuvant (U.S. Patent No. 4,789,544) which acts as an immune enhancer to ensure the level of response to vaccination and provide long-lasting immunity. The bacterin contains three antigenic strains of *Salmonella typhimurium*, the most common species of Salmonella identified in cases of Paratyphoid in pigeons. Paratyphoid (Salmonellosis) is a devastating and fatal disease of pigeons. Clinical expression of the disease varies from a septicemic form displaying diarrhea, depression and nervous disorders to an articular form characterized by swelling of joints, dropped wings or lameness.

Indications: SAL BAC® is indicated for use an aid in the prevention of paratyphoid infection attributed to *Salmonella typhimurium* in pigeons.

Dosage and Administration: Young birds may be vaccinated at weaning age. Two vaccinations are recommended 3-4 weeks apart. Vaccinations should be completed at least 2-3 weeks prior to racing or showing or the onset of egg production. Thereafter, boosters are recommended semi-annually to annually depending on risk of infection.

Vaccination is accomplished by using a syringe and small gauge needle to inject 0.5 mL of bacterin subcutaneously at the base of the neck and midline at the level of the shoulders in the direction away from the head and toward the base of the neck. Withdraw slightly on the syringe plunger prior to injection to ensure that delivery of bacterin is not into a blood vessel. Caution should be taken to administer this product at shoulder level and not higher up on the back of the neck to avoid an extensive venous plexus present in pigeons. Aseptic technique should be followed using alcohol to clean the injection site and a new sterile syringe and needle between each bird.

Precaution(s): Shake well before using and use entire contents when first opened. Multidose vials should be discarded after initial use regardless of the remaining contents in the vial. Store in a refrigerator at 35°-45°F.

Caution(s): Vaccinate only healthy birds. In case of anaphylactic reaction administer epinephrine or atropine sulfate.

This bacterin has been carefully produced and has undergone purity, sterility, safety, efficacy and potency tests to meet Biomune requirements and USDA regulations.

Warning(s): Do not vaccinate within 21 days of slaughter.

Presentation: 50 dose and 100 dose vials.

Compendium Code No.: 11290330

SALINE 0.9% SOLUTION ℞

Vetus **Saline Solution**

Active Ingredient(s): Each 100 mL of sterile aqueous solution contains:

Sodium Chloride .... 0.9 g

Millequivalents per liter:

Cations:

Sodium .... 154 mEq/L

Anions:

Chloride .... 154 mEq/L

Total osmolarity is 308 milliosmoles per liter.

Indications: For use in replacement therapy of sodium, chloride and water which may become depleted in many diseases. Because this solution is isotonic with body fluids, it may also be used as a solvent or diluent, for antibiotics and other pharmaceuticals and biologicals where compatible, and for washing mucous membranes and other tissue surfaces.

Dosage and Administration: Warm to body temperature and administer slowly by intravenous or subcutaneous injection. The amount and rate of administration must be judged by the veterinarian in relation to the condition being treated and the clinical response of the animal, being careful to avoid overhydration. When used as a solvent or diluent for pharmaceuticals and biologicals, follow the manufacturer's directions.

Precaution(s): Store at a controlled room temperature between 15°-30°C (59°-86°F).

Caution(s): Federal law restricts this drug to use by or on the order of a licensed veterinarian.

This product contains no preservatives. Use entire contents when fist opened. Discard any unused solution.

Warning(s): For animal use only. Keep out of the reach of children.

Presentation: 250 mL and 1,000 mL vials.

Compendium Code No.: 14440810

SALINE SOLUTION ℞

Vedco **Saline Solution**

Active Ingredient(s): Each 100 mL contains:

Sodium chloride .... 0.9 g

Cations:

Sodium .... 154 mEq/L

Anions:

Chloride .... 154 mEq/L

Total osmolarity is 308 milliosmoles per liter.

The product does not contain preservatives.

Indications: For use in replacement therapy of sodium chloride and water which may become depleted in many diseases. Because the solution is isotonic with body fluids, it may also be used as a solvent or diluent for antibiotics and other pharmaceuticals or biologicals, and for washing mucous membranes and other tissue surfaces.

Dosage and Administration: Warm to body temperature and administer slowly by intravenous or subcutaneous injection. The amount and rate of administration must be judged by the veterinarian in relation to the condition being treated and the clinical response of the animal, being careful to avoid overhydration. When used as a solvent or diluent for pharmaceuticals or biologicals, follow the manufacturer's directions.

Precaution(s): Store at a controlled room temperature between 59-86°F (15-30°C).

Caution(s): Federal law restricts this drug to use by or on the order of a licensed veterinarian.

Keep out of the reach of children.

Use the entire contents when first opened. Discard any unused solution.

Presentation: 250 mL, 500 mL and 1,000 mL containers.

Compendium Code No.: 10941820

SALINE 0.9% SOLUTION ℞

AgriLabs **Saline Solution**

Contents: (grams/100 mL):

Sodium Chloride 0.9%

Water for injection (sterile, nonpyrogenic) .... q.s.

Contains no preservatives.

Indications: For the correction of electrolyte depletion and dehydration of cattle, swine, sheep, goats, horses, dogs and cats.

Dosage and Administration: 5-10 mL per pound of body weight, 3 times daily for 3 days, intravenously. Administer slowly using sterile equipment. Stop if adverse symptoms develop.

Precaution(s): Store at 22°C-28°C.

Caution(s): Federal law restricts this drug to use by or on the order of a licensed veterinarian.

Utilize aseptic technique by swabbing closure with 70% alcohol before entering container with sterile equipment.

Avoid contamination of product.

Use promptly once opened and discard unused portion.

Warning(s): For animal use only. Keep away from children.

Presentation: 250 mL, 500 mL, and 1000 mL.

Compendium Code No.: 10581690

SALINE SOLUTION 0.9% ℞

Phoenix Pharmaceutical **Saline Solution**

Active Ingredient(s): Composition: Each 100 mL of sterile aqueous solution contains:

Sodium Chloride .... 0.9 g

Milliequivalents per liter:

Cations:

Sodium .... 154 mEq/L

Anions:

Chloride .... 154 mEq/L

Total osmolarity is 308 milliosmoles per liter.

This product contains no preservatives.

Indications: For use in replacement therapy of sodium, chloride and water which may become depleted in many diseases. Because the solution is isotonic with body fluids, it may also be used as a solvent or diluent, for antibiotics and other pharmaceuticals and biologicals where compatible, and for washing mucous membranes and other tissue surfaces.

Dosage and Administration: Warm to body temperature and administer slowly by intravenous or subcutaneous injection. The amount and rate of administration must be judged by a veterinarian in relation to the condition being treated and the clinical response of the animal, being careful to avoid overhydration. When used as a solvent or diluent for pharmaceuticals and biologicals, follow the manufacturer's directions.

Precaution(s): Store between 15°C and 30°C (59°F-86°F).

Use entire contents when first opened. Discard any unused solution.

Caution(s): Federal law restricts this drug to use by or on the order of a licensed veterinarian.

For animal use only.

Warning(s): Keep out of reach of children.

Presentation: 250 mL (NDC 57319-077-06), 500 mL (NDC 57319-077-07) and 1000 mL (NDC 57319-077-08) vials.

Manufactured by: Phoenix Scientific, Inc., St. Joseph, MO 64503.

Compendium Code No.: 12560752 Rev. 7-01 / Rev. 6-01

SALIX™ ℞

Intervet **Diuretic**

(furosemide)

NADA No.: 034-478

Active Ingredient(s): Parenteral:

SALIX™ Injection 5%: Each mL contains: 50 mg furosemide as a diethanolamine salt preserved and stabilized with myristyl-gamma-picolinium chloride 0.02%, EDTA sodium 0.1%, sodium sulfite 0.1% with sodium chloride 0.2% in distilled water, pH adjusted with sodium hydroxide.

SALIX™ Tablets:

12.5 mg tablets: Each tablet contains 12.5 mg of furosemide: 4-chloro-N-furfuryl-5-sulfamoylanthranilic acid.

50 mg (scored) tablets: Each tablet contains 50.0 mg of furosemide: 4-chloro-N-furfuryl-5-sulfamoylanthranilic acid.

Indications: A diuretic-saluretic for prompt relief of edema.

Dogs, Cats and Horses: SALIX™ is an effective diuretic possessing a wide therapeutic range. Pharmacologically it promotes the rapid removal of abnormally retained extracellular fluids. The rationale for the efficacious use of diuretic therapy is determined by the clinical pathology producing the edema. SALIX™ is indicated for the treatment of edema (pulmonary congestion, ascites) associated with cardiac insufficiency and acute non-inflammatory tissue edema.

The continued use of heart stimulants, such as digitalis or its glycosides, is indicated in cases of edema involving cardiac insufficiency.

Cattle: SALIX™ is indicated for the treatment of physiological parturient edema of the mammary gland and associated structures.

Pharmacology: Description: SALIX™ (furosemide) is a chemically distinct diuretic and saluretic pharmacodynamically characterized by the following:

1. A high degree of efficacy, low-inherent toxicity and a high therapeutic index.
2. A rapid onset of action of comparatively short duration.[1,2]
3. Pharmacological action in the functional area of the nephron, i.e., proximal and distal tubules and the ascending limb of the loop of Henle.[2,3,4]
4. A dose-response relationship and a ratio of minimum to maximum effective dose range greater than tenfold.[1,2]
5. It may be administered orally or parenterally. It is readily absorbed from the intestinal tract and well tolerated.

The intravenous route produces the most rapid diuretic response.

The CAS Registry Number is 54-31-9.

SALIX™, a diuretic, is an anthranilic acid derivative with the following structural formula:

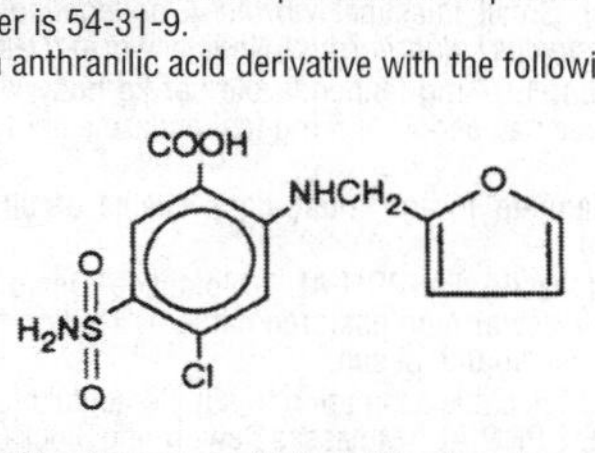

Generic name: Furosemide (except in United Kingdom-furosemide). Chemical name: 4-chloro-N-furfuryl-5-sulfamoylanthranilic acid.

Actions: The therapeutic efficacy of SALIX™ is from the activity of the intact and unaltered molecule throughout the nephron, inhibiting the reabsorption of sodium not only in the proximal and distal tubule but also in the ascending limb of the loop of Henle. The prompt onset of action is a result of the drug's rapid absorption and a poor lipid solubility. The low lipid solubility and a rapid renal excretion minimize the possibility of its accumulation in tissues and organs or crystalluria. SALIX™ has no inhibitory effect on carbonic anhydrase or aldosterone activity in the distal tubule. The drug possesses diuretic activity in presence of either acidosis or alkalosis.[1,2,3,4,5,6,7]

Dosage and Administration: The usual dosage of SALIX™ is 1 to 2 mg/lb body weight (approximately 2.5 to 5 mg/kg). The lower dosage is suggested for cats. Administer once or twice daily at 6 to 8 hour intervals either orally, intravenously or intramuscularly. A prompt diuresis usually ensues from the initial treatment. Diuresis may be initiated by the parenteral administration of SALIX™ Injection and then maintained by oral administration.

The dosage should be adjusted to the individual's response. In severe edematous or refractory cases, the dose may be doubled or increased by increments of 1 mg per pound body weight.

The established effective dose should be administered once or twice daily. The daily schedule of administration can be timed to control the period of micturition for the convenience of the client or veterinarian. Mobilization of the edema may be most efficiently and safely accomplished by utilizing an intermittent daily dosage schedule, i.e., every other day or 2 to 4 consecutive days weekly.

Diuretic therapy should be discontinued after reduction of the edema, or maintained after determining a carefully programmed dosage schedule to prevent recurrence of edema. For long-term treatment, the dose can generally be lowered after the edema has once been reduced. Re-examination and consultations with client will enhance the establishment of a satisfactorily programmed dosage schedule. Clinical examination and serum BUN, CO_2 and electrolyte determinations should be performed during the early period of therapy and periodically thereafter, especially in refractory cases. Abnormalities should be corrected or the drug temporarily withdrawn.

Dosage:

Oral:

Dog and Cat: One-half to one 50 mg scored tablet per 25 pounds body weight.

One 12.5 mg tablet per 5 to 10 pounds body weight.

Administer once or twice daily, permitting a 6 to 8 hour interval between treatments. In refractory or severe edematous cases, the dosage may be doubled or increased by increments of 1 mg per pound body weight as recommended in preceding paragraphs "Dosage and Administration".

Parenteral:

Dog and Cat: Administer intramuscularly or intravenously ¼ to ½ mL per 10 pounds body weight.

Administer once or twice daily, permitting a 6 to 8 hour interval between treatments. In refractory or severe edematous cases, the dosage may be doubled or increased by increments of 1 mg per pound body weight as recommended in preceding paragraphs, "Dosage and Administration".

Horse: The individual dose is 250 to 500 mg (5 to 10 mL) administered intramuscularly or intravenously once or twice daily at 6 to 8 hour intervals until desired results are achieved. The veterinarian should evaluate the degree of edema present and adjust dosage schedule accordingly. Do not use in horses intended for food.

Cattle: The individual dose administered intramuscularly or intravenously is 500 mg (10 mL) once daily or 250 mg (5 mL) twice daily at 12 hour intervals. Treatment not to exceed 48 hours postparturition.

Milk taken from animals during treatment and for 48 hours (four milkings) after the last treatment must not be used for food. Cattle must not be slaughtered for food within 48 hours following last treatment.

Contraindication(s): SALIX™ is a highly effective diuretic-saluretic which if given in excessive amounts may result in dehydration and electrolyte imbalance. Therefore, the dosage and schedule may have to be adjusted to the patient's needs. The animal should be observed for early signs of electrolyte imbalance and corrective measures administered. Early signs of electrolyte imbalance are: increased thirst, lethargy, drowsiness or restlessness, fatigue, oliguria, gastro-intestinal disturbances and tachycardia. Special attention should be given to potassium levels. SALIX™ may lower serum calcium levels and cause tetany in rare cases of animals having an existing hypocalcemic tendency.[10,11,12,13,14]

Although diabetes mellitus is a rarely reported disease in animals, active or latent diabetes mellitus may on rare occasions be exacerbated by SALIX™. While it has not been reported in animals, the use of high doses of salicylates, as in rheumatic diseases, in conjunction with SALIX™ may result in salicylate toxicity because of competition for renal excretory sites.

Transient loss of auditory capacity has been experimentally produced in cats following intravenous injection of excessive doses of SALIX™ at a very rapid rate.[15,16,17]

Electrolyte balance should be monitored prior to surgery in patients receiving SALIX™. Imbalances must be corrected by administration of suitable fluid therapy.

SALIX™ is contraindicated in anuria. Therapy should be discontinued in cases of progressive renal disease if increasing azotemia and oliguria occur during the treatment. Sudden alterations of fluid and electrolyte imbalance in an animal with cirrhosis may precipitate hepatic coma, therefore, observation during period of therapy is necessary. In hepatic coma and in states of electrolyte depletion, therapy should not be instituted until the basic condition is improved or corrected. Potassium supplementation may be necessary in cases routinely treated with potassium-depleting steroids.

Precaution(s): SALIX™ Injection 5%: Store between 59° and 86°F. Protect from freezing.

SALIX™ Tablets: Store at or below 25°C (77°F). Do not use if bottle closure seal is broken.

Caution(s): Federal law restricts this drug to use by or on the order of a licensed veterinarian.

SALIX™ is a highly effective diuretic and if given in excessive amounts, as with any diuretic, may lead to excessive diuresis that could result in electrolyte imbalance, dehydration and reduction of plasma volume, enhancing the risk of circulatory collapse, thrombosis, and embolism. Therefore, the animal should be observed for early signs of fluid depletion with electrolyte imbalance, and corrective measures administered. Excessive loss of potassium in patients receiving digitalis or its glycosides may precipitate digitalis toxicity. Caution should be exercised in animals administered potassium-depleting steroids.

It is important to correct potassium deficiency with dietary supplementation. Caution should be exercised in prescribing enteric-coated potassium tablets.

There have been several reports in human literature, published and unpublished, concerning non-specific small-bowel lesions consisting of stenosis, with or without ulceration, associated with the administration of enteric-coated thiazides with potassium salts. These lesions may occur with enteric-coated potassium tablets alone or when they are used with non-enteric-coated thiazides, or certain other oral diuretics. These small-bowel lesions may have caused obstruction, hemorrhage, and perforation. Surgery was frequently required and deaths have occurred. Available information tends to implicate enteric-coated potassium salts, although lesions of this type also occur spontaneously. Therefore, coated potassium containing formulations should be administered only when indicated, and should be discontinued immediately if abdominal pain, distension, nausea, vomiting, or gastro-intestinal bleeding occurs.

Human patients with known sulfonamide sensitivity may show allergic reactions to SALIX™; however, these reactions have not been reported in animals.

Sulfonamide diuretics have been reported to decrease arterial responsiveness to pressor amines and to enhance the effect of tubocurarine. Caution should be exercised in administering curare or its derivatives to patients undergoing therapy with SALIX™ and it is advisable to discontinue SALIX™ for one day prior to any elective surgery.

For veterinary use only.

Warning(s): Cattle: Milk taken from animals during treatment and for 48 hours (four milkings) after the last treatment must not be used for food. Cattle must not be slaughtered for food within 48 hours following last treatment.

Horses: Do not use in horses intended for food.

Keep this and all medication out of the reach of children.

Toxicology: Acute Toxicity: The following table illustrates low acute toxicity of SALIX™ in three different species. (Two values indicate two different studies.)

LD_{50} of SALIX™ in mg/kg body weight:

Species	Oral	Intravenous
Mouse	1,050-1,500	308
Rat	2,650-4,600*	680
Dog	>1,000 and >4,640	>300 and >464

*Note: The lower value for the rat oral LD_{50} was obtained in a group of fasted animals; the higher figure is from a study performed in fed rats.

Toxic doses lead to convulsions, ataxia, paralysis and collapse. Animals surviving toxic dosages may become dehydrated and depleted of electrolytes due to the massive diuresis and saluresis.

Chronic Toxicity: Chronic toxicity studies with SALIX™ were done in a one-year study in rats and dogs. In a one-year study in rats, renal tubular degeneration occurred with all doses higher than 50 mg/kg. A six-month study in dogs revealed calcification and scarring of the renal parenchyma at all doses above 10 mg/kg.

Reproductive Studies: Reproductive studies were conducted in mice, rats and rabbits. Only in rabbits administered high doses (equivalent to 10 to 25 times the recommended average dose of 2 mg/kg for dogs, cats, horses and cattle) of furosemide during the second trimester period did unexplained maternal deaths and abortions occur. The administration of SALIX™ is not recommended during the second trimester of pregnancy.

References: Available upon request.

Presentation: SALIX™ Injection 5%: Available in 50 mL multidose vials.
SALIX™ Tablets:
12.5 mg Tablets: Available in bottles of 500 tablets.
50 mg Tablets: Available in bottles of 500 tablets.

SALIX™ Injection 5%:

Manufactured by: Akorn Inc., Decatur, IL 62522.

SALIX™ Tablets 12.5 mg and 50 mg:

Manufactured by: Patheon Inc., Don Mills, Ontario, M3B 1Y6, Canada.

Lasix® is a registered trademark of Hoechst AG.

Compendium Code No.: 11060811 746150-A

SALMONELLA DUBLIN-TYPHIMURIUM BACTERIN

Colorado Serum **Bacterin**

Salmonella dublin-typhimurium Bacterin, Bovine Isolates

U.S. Vet. Lic. No.: 188

Active Ingredient(s): Formalin killed, aluminum hydroxide adsorbed cultures of *Salmonella dublin* and *Salmonella typhimurium,* bovine isolates.

Contains thimerosal as a preservative.

Indications: For the vaccination of healthy cattle to induce resistance to salmonella infections caused by the micro-organisms named.

Dosage and Administration: In areas where salmonella infections have been a problem, adult cattle, pregnant cows and new born calves should all be given two (2) injections of 2 mL each at an interval of 14-21 days. Boost immunity in pregnant cows with an annual 2 mL injection. Vaccinate adult cattle prior to placing on feed and pregnant cows four (4) to six (6) weeks before calving time. Newborn calves should be left on cows for seven (7) days at which time the bacterin can be administered.

All injections should be subcutaneous.

Precaution(s): Shake well. Each dose must have a proportionate share of the precipitate for a proper response. Store in the dark at 2-7°C. Do not freeze.

Caution(s): Anaphylactic reactions sometimes follow administration of products of this nature. If noted, administer adrenaline or an equivalent drug.

Use the entire contents when the bottle is first opened.

For veterinary use only.

Warning(s): Do not vaccinate within 21 days before slaughter.

Presentation: 10 dose (20 mL) and 50 dose (100 mL) vials.

Compendium Code No.: 11010310

SALMO SHIELD® 2

Novartis Animal Vaccines **Bacterin**

Salmonella choleraesuis-typhimurium Bacterin

U.S. Vet. Lic. No.: 303

Composition: The bacterin contains whole inactivated cultures of *Salmonella choleraesuis,* var. *kunzendorf* and *Salmonella typhimurium,* adjuvanted with aluminum hydroxide.

Indications: For use in healthy swine as an aid in the prevention and control of diseases caused by *Salmonella choleraesuis* and *Salmonella typhimurium.*

Dosage and Administration: Shake well before and during use. Administer two (2) 2 mL doses intramuscularly or subcutaneously to pregnant sows and gilts approximately five (5) and two (2) weeks prior to farrowing. Administer a 2 mL dose to piglets at weaning. Repeat in two (2) to four (4) weeks.

Precaution(s): Store at 35°-45°F (2°-7°C). Do not freeze. Use the entire contents when first opened.

Caution(s): Anaphylactic reactions may occur with the product. Symptomatic treatment: Epinephrine.

Warning(s): Do not vaccinate within 21 days prior to slaughter.

Discussion: Swine salmonellosis is the fourth most costly disease in swine. Swine salmonellosis is caused primarily by two organisms: *Salmonella choleraesuis* and *S. typhimurium. S. choleraesuis* primarily causes septicemia, characterized by pneumonia, liver abscesses, and enteritis. *S. typhimurium* causes a severe enteritis. Although not new, these two diseases are difficult to diagnose and have been ignored or overlooked in their importance by producers and veterinarians. Losses in swine due to salmonellosis in the United States are estimated to be between $20 million and $100 million annually.

S. choleraesuis is the second most commonly isolated of all salmonellas in the U.S. While host-adapted to swine, *S. choleraesuis* is an uncommon, but extremely deadly pathogen of humans. *S. choleraesuis* is transmitted directly from pig to pig, and does not spread easily to other species, or to the environment. The organism persists in the tonsils and intestines of carrier hogs, much like human typhoid fever carriers. Confinement swine production, especially in crowded conditions, favors the spread of *S. choleraesuis.*

S. typhimurium affects a wide range of hosts, including humans. It is the most common cause of Salmonella food poisoning. In swine, it causes fever, vomiting, and diarrhea. *S. typhimurium* is often carried by rats, and is transmitted by fecal contamination of feed and water.

Salmonella usually causes disease as a single organism infection. However, it could be complicated with other bacterial or viral disease. *Salmonella choleraesuis* and *S. typhimurium* account for over 90% of salmonellosis in swine. Producers and veterinarians should always keep in mind the incidence and importance of salmonellosis in swine.

Presentation: Available in 50 dose (100 mL) bottles.

Compendium Code No.: 11140402

SALMO SHIELD® LIVE

Novartis Animal Vaccines **Vaccine**

Salmonella Choleraesuis Vaccine, Avirulent Live Culture

U.S. Vet. Lic. No.: 303

Composition: This vaccine contains an avirulent live culture of *Salmonella choleraesuis*.

Indications: For use in healthy swine as an aid in the prevention and control of salmonellosis caused by *Salmonella choleraesuis*.

Dosage and Administration: Aseptically rehydrate with diluent supplied. Shake well before using. Administer 1 mL intramuscularly at 3 weeks of age or older.

Precaution(s): Store in the dark at 35°-45°F (2°-7°C). Do not freeze. Needles and syringes should not be sterilized with chemicals. Use entire contents when first opened. Burn the container and any unused contents.

Caution(s): Anaphylactic reactions may occur following the use of this biological. Symptomatic treatment: Epinephrine.

For veterinary use only.

Warning(s): Do not vaccinate within 21 days prior to slaughter.

Discussion: Swine salmonellosis is the fourth most costly disease of swine. Swine salmonellosis is primarily caused by one organism, *Salmonella choleraesuis. S. choleraesuis* causes septicemia, characterized by pneumonia, liver abscesses, and enteritis. Although not new, this disease is difficult to diagnose and has been ignored or overlooked in its importance by producers and veterinarians. Losses in swine due to salmonellosis in the United States are estimated to be between $20 and $100 million annually.

S. choleraesuis is the most commonly isolated of all *Salmonella* in the U.S swine herds. While host-adapted to swine, *S. choleraesuis* is an uncommon but extremely deadly pathogen of humans. Human salmonellosis has recently been of great concern to consumers and the meat industry. *S. choleraesuis* is transmitted directly from pig to pig, and does not spread easily to other species, or to the environment.

The organism persists in the tonsils and intestines of carrier hogs, much like human typhoid fever carriers. Confinement swine production, especially in crowded conditions, favors the spread of *S. choleraesuis*.

Salmonella usually causes disease as a single organism infection. However, it can be complicated with other bacterial or viral diseases. *Salmonella choleraesuis* accounts for approximately 60% of salmonellosis in swine. Producers and veterinarians should always keep in mind the incidence and importance of salmonellosis in swine.

Trial Data: Mortality Rates:

Test Group	No. Dead/Total	% Mortality
Vaccinates	0/23	0
Controls	10/21	48

P=0.0001

Weight Gain:

Test Group*	Average Total Gain
Vaccinates	26.7 lbs.
Controls	11.6 lbs.

P=0.0008

*Pigs that died during the observation period are not included in weight gain calculations.

Clinical Scores Data:

Test Group	Average Clinical Score Per Pig
Vaccinates	1.1
Controls	140.1

P=0.00

Reisolation of *S. choleraesuis* Organisms at Necropsy:

Test Group	Mean No. of Reisolations Per Pig
Vaccinates	0.04
Controls	1.05

P=0.0024

A total of forty four (44) animals, 23 vaccinates and 21 controls, were used in the SALMO SHIELD® LIVE Host Animal Vaccination/Challenge Efficacy Trial study. Vaccinate and control groups were segregated until the day of challenge to prevent vaccine strain exposure to the control animals. Each animal in the vaccine group received a single, 1 mL intramuscular dose of SALMO SHIELD® LIVE at approximately 3 weeks of age.

Vaccinate and control groups were commingled and intranasally challenged at approximately 6 weeks of age with a virulent strain of *Salmonella choleraesuis*. Pigs were observed once daily for clinical signs of salmonellosis and mortality for 28 days post challenge. Pigs that died during the observation period were necropsied and cultured for *S. choleraesuis*. All surviving pigs were euthanized on day 28 post challenge and cultured for *S. choleraesuis* organisms.

Presentation: Available in 30 dose (30 mL) bottles.

Compendium Code No.: 11140422

SALMO SHIELD® T

Novartis Animal Vaccines **Bacterin**

Salmonella typhimurium Bacterin

U.S. Vet. Lic. No.: 303

Composition: The bacterin contains whole inactivated cultures of *Salmonella typhimurium*, adjuvanted with aluminum hydroxide.

Indications: For use in healthy cattle as an aid in the prevention and control of diseases caused by *Salmonella typhimurium*.

Dosage and Administration: Shake well before and during use. Administer a 2 mL dose intramuscularly or subcutaneously to adult cattle, pregnant cows and newborn calves over seven (7) days of age. Repeat in two (2) to four (4) weeks. Pregnant cows should be vaccinated four (4) to six (6) weeks before calving and given an annual 2 mL booster injection.

Precaution(s): Store at 35°-45°F (2°-7°C). Do not freeze. Use the entire contents when first opened.

Caution(s): Anaphylactic reactions may occur following the use of the product. Symptomatic treatment: Epinephrine.

Warning(s): Do not vaccinate within 21 days prior to slaughter.

Discussion: *Salmonella typhimurium* affects a wide range of hosts, including humans, and is the most common cause of *Salmonella* food poisoning. The bacteria produce a potent endotoxin, and this endotoxin is what causes the various symptoms.

In cattle, *S. typhimurium* causes an acute to chronic disease characterized by fever, depression, anorexia, weakness, and a foul-smelling diarrhea. The stool is watery, brownish in color, and often contains pieces of sloughed intestinal mucosa and fresh blood. Later, the organism may localize in joints and cause arthritis, or cause ischemic necrosis of the extremities (ears, tail, etc.) due to disruption of blood flow. In acute cases, death may occur within one to two days. Mortality rates average 5-10%, but may reach 75% in severe cases.

The bacteria are picked up either by ingestion or through the navel in newborn calves. They are spread either directly from carrier animals or indirectly through contaminated feed, water, and bedding. Studies have shown that *S. typhimurium* can survive on or in soil for 200 to 300 days. Calves may secrete the organism in saliva, and it can also be shed in manure, milk and urine from carrier animals.

Calves are more susceptible than adults, but stress factors such as parturition, parasitism, bad weather, poor nutrition, and transportation may trigger the disease in older animals.

The disease may mimic BVD or coccidiosis, but can be distinguished by culturing the bacteria from infected animals. Postmortem lesions include enlarged mesenteric lymph nodes and pseudomembranes lining the gut. The ileum, cecum and colon are the primary areas affected, but severe cases may also involve the duodenum and jejunum.

The treatment of affected animals is limited to antibiotics and supportive therapy. Prevention of the disease, the preferred route, includes eliminating carrier animals and contaminated fomites, and vaccination.

References: Available upon request.

Presentation: Available in 50 dose (100 mL) bottle.

Compendium Code No.: 11140432

SALMO SHIELD® TD

Novartis Animal Vaccines **Bacterin**

Salmonella dublin-typhimurium Bacterin

U.S. Vet. Lic. No.: 303

Composition: This bacterin contains inactivated cultures of *Salmonella dublin,* and *typhimurium* adjuvanted with aluminum hydroxide. Contains penicillin and streptomycin as preservatives.

Indications: For use in healthy cattle as an aid in the prevention and control of disease caused by *Salmonella dublin* and *typhimurium.*

Dosage and Administration: Shake well before using. Administer 2 mL intramuscularly or subcutaneously. Repeat in 2-4 weeks. Revaccinate annually.

Precaution(s): Store in the dark at 35°-45°F (2°-7°C). Do not freeze. Use entire contents when first opened.

Caution(s): Transient swelling may occur at the site of injection. Milk reduction and transient depression may be observed in lactating dairy cows 3-6 days following vaccination. Anaphylactic reactions may occur following the use of this biological. Symptomatic treatment: Epinephrine.

For veterinary use only.

Warning(s): Do not vaccinate within 21 days prior to slaughter.

Discussion: *Salmonella typhimurium: Salmonella typhimurium* affects a wide range of hosts, including humans, and is the most common cause of *Salmonella* food poisoning. The bacteria produce a potent endotoxin, and this endotoxin is what causes the various symptoms.

In cattle *S. typhimurium* causes an acute to chronic disease characterized by fever, depression, anorexia, weakness, and foul-smelling diarrhea. The stool is watery, brownish in color, and often contains pieces of sloughed intestinal mucosa and fresh blood. Later, the organism may localize in joints and cause arthritis, or cause ischemic necrosis of the extremities (ears, tail, etc.) due to disruption of blood flow. In acute cases, death may occur within 1-2 days. Mortality rates average 5-10% but may reach 75% in severe cases.

The bacteria are picked up either by ingestion or through the navel in newborn calves. They are spread either directly from carrier animals or indirectly through contaminated feed, water, and bedding. Studies have shown that *S. typhimurium* can survive on or in soil for 200 or 300 days. Calves may secrete the organism in saliva, and it can also be shed in manure, milk and urine from carrier animals.

Calves are more susceptible than adults, but stress factors such as parturition, parasitism, bad weather, poor nutrition, and transportation may trigger the disease in older animals.

Salmonella dublin: Salmonella dublin is another of the common causes of salmonellosis in cattle and it is found throughout the world. In the United States, it is more common in the West, but severe outbreaks have been seen in the Midwest and as far east as North Carolina. It is fairly well host-adapted to cattle, but can cause severe disease with high mortality rates in humans.

Clinical syndromes seen in cattle include septicemia, acute enteritis and chronic enteritis. Septicemia is more often seen in young calves and occurs when the organisms are able to escape from the gastrointestinal (GI) tract into the bloodstream. Signs include depression, fever and death, with or without diarrhea. Nervous system signs may also be seen, as can polyarthritis, pneumonia and dry gangrene of the extremities (ears, tail and feet). Acute enteritis shows symptoms of fever (which may disappear when the diarrhea begins), severe watery diarrhea that often contains blood, and pain and straining with defecation. The diarrhea is foul-smelling and contains much mucus and intestinal debris. In less acute cases, there may only be a mild fever, soft feces and lack of appetite. In chronic enteritis, animals will show persistent diarrhea and emaciation. Survivors of the disease will often be unthrifty for their lifetimes, due to permanent damage to the intestinal tract. In pregnant cows, abortion is often seen, either as part of a disease syndrome or as the only observed symptom. *S. dublin* is one of the major causes of abortion in cattle.

Salmonella dublin tends to be endemic on some farms, with morbidity rates above 50% and mortality rates approaching 100% unless animals are aggressively treated very early. Animals pick up the bacteria orally from feed or water that has been contaminated with infected manure. The bacteria may also be present in animal-origin feedstuffs that have been improperly processed. *Salmonella* can survive for months in wet, warm environments. They can also survive freezing, but are rapidly killed by heat and sunlight. They are also inactivated by most of the commonly-used disinfectants; thus, cleanliness is an important factor in limiting the spread of the infection.

One of the main reasons *Salmonella dublin* is such a serious strain is its tendency to produce long-term carriers. The bacteria localize in the gall bladder, mesenteric lymph nodes and sometimes the tonsils, from which they are intermittently shed into the manure of clinically normal carrier animals. Carrier cows can also shed the organism into their milk. Calves rarely become carriers, but adult animals can harbor *Salmonella dublin* for years - unlike *S. typhimurium,* with which long-term carriers are uncommon.

The disease usually requires some triggering stress factor such as weaning, movement or parturition. In addition, animals infested with liver flukes seem to be more susceptible and develop more severe disease. Both calves and adult animals are equally affected, and the severity of the disease depends on such things as the dose size of the bacteria, the immune status of the exposed animals, and any previous exposure to the bacteria. In addition, the severity in calves depends on the amount of protective maternal antibody that the calf has gotten from its dam. The disease is more common under intense husbandry where the bacteria spread easily from animal to animal.

Once in the animal's body, bacteria multiply in the gut and produce endotoxins that cause gut damage. If the bacteria remain localized in the gut, the animal develops only enteritis. However, they often penetrate into the lymph nodes from which they enter the liver and bloodstream, resulting in septicemia. As mentioned earlier, many animals may become carriers. These carriers usually cannot be cleared up with antibiotics, since the bacteria tend to localize inside cells where antibiotics cannot easily reach.

This disease is diagnosed by culturing the bacteria, usually at necropsy. The mesenteric lymph nodes will be enlarged and possibly hemorrhagic. The lower jejunum, ileum, cecum and colon are the areas of intestine affected, and will appear necrotic, often with hemorrhagic areas. Diseases that can be confused with salmonellosis include *E. coli* septicemia, Bovine Viral Diarrhea (BVD), coccidiosis and some types of poisoning.

Treatment of affected animals is limited to antibiotics and supportive therapy, which are often ineffective. Prevention of salmonellosis, the preferred route, includes keeping infected animals out of a herd (often hard to do because of clinically normal carriers), and limiting disease spread within a herd. This includes segregating affected animals, disinfecting areas where sick animals have been housed, and vaccinating to raise the immune level of the herd.

References: Available upon request.
Presentation: 50 doses (100 mL bottle) (F171).
Compendium Code No.: 11140443

SALMO VAC

AgriPharm — **Bacterin**

Salmonella Dublin-Typhimurium Bacterin
U.S. Vet. Lic. No.: 303
Composition: This bacterin contains inactivated cultures of *Salmonella dublin* and *typhimurium* adjuvanted with aluminum hydroxide. Contains penicillin and streptomycin as preservatives.
Indications: For use in healthy cattle as an aid in the prevention and control of disease caused by *Salmonella dublin* and *typhimurium.*
Dosage and Administration: Shake well before using. Administer 2 mL intramuscularly or subcutaneously. Revaccinate in 2-4 weeks. Vaccinate dairy cows during the dry off period. Revaccinate annually.
Precaution(s): Store in the dark at 35°-45°F (2°-7°C). Do not freeze. Use entire contents when first opened.
Caution(s): Transient swelling may occur at the site of injection. Anaphylactic reactions may occur following the use of this biological. Symptomatic treatment: Epinephrine.
Warning(s): Do not vaccinate within 21 days prior to slaughter.
For animal use only. Keep out of reach of children.
Presentation: 50 doses (100 mL).
Produced by: Advance Biologics, Inc.
Compendium Code No.: 14570900

SALMUNE™

Biomune — **Vaccine**

Salmonella Typhimurium Vaccine, Live Culture
U.S. Vet. Lic. No.: 368
Contents: This vaccine contains a live avirulent strain of *Salmonella typhimurium* and is recommended for initial vaccination of day-old, healthy, susceptible chickens.
Indications: The vaccine will provide protection of internal organs, intestines and ceca against colonization by *Salmonella typhimurium, Salmonella heidelberg, Salmonella hadar, Salmonella kentucky* and *Salmonella enteritidis.*
Dosage and Administration: This vaccine is recommended for initial vaccination of healthy chickens at day of age using coarse spray or drinking water. If water vaccination is used, a second water vaccination is required at 7 days of age.

Directions for Administration by Spray Application: The spray application of this vaccine to chickens at day of age will provide protection through at least 7 weeks of age. If chickens are to be maintained past 7 weeks of age, a repeat vaccination is recommended.

Directions for Spray Use at the Hatchery:

1. Do not use gentamicin or ceftiofur antibiotics in ovo or at day of age, such as in Marek's vaccine, since they will interfere with vaccination.
2. Use cool, sterile, nonchlorinated water that contains no anti-microbials to reconstitute the vaccine. Do not use any other type of diluent to reconstitute the vaccine.
3. Reconstitute the vaccine at a rate of 70 mL vaccine per 1,000 chicks.
4. To each box of 100 chicks, administer 7 mL of vaccine by spraying approximately 12 inches above the box using a coarse spray nozzle.
5. Although this vaccine is not known to cause a human safety problem, it is advised to take precautions, such as wearing a mask and gloves, to avoid direct contact with the vaccine.
6. Take care to administer a full dose to each chick.
7. Ensure chicks are dry before administering this vaccine. Allow chicks to dry after vaccine administration and avoid chilling.

Directions for Administration by Drinking Water: Drinking water application of this vaccine at day of age and repeated at 7 days of age will provide protection through at least 7 weeks of age. If chickens are to be maintained past 7 weeks of age, a repeat vaccination is recommended.

Directions for Drinking Water Use:

1. Do not use gentamicin or ceftiofur antibiotics in ovo or at day of age, such as in Marek's vaccine, since they will interfere with vaccination. Discontinue water medication, sanitizers, and disinfectants 72 hours before vaccination. Do not resume any medication, sanitizers, or disinfectants in the water for 72 hours after all vaccine water has been consumed. The waterers should be thoroughly cleaned and rinsed before use. Do not use disinfecting solutions during cleaning as the disinfectant residue may destroy the vaccine. Drinking containers must be free of all disinfecting solutions and medicants prior to vaccination.
2. For repeat vaccination, deprive the birds of water for up to two hours prior to vaccination.
3. Tear off the seal from the vial containing the dried vaccine and remove the stopper.
4. Use clean, nonchlorinated water for rehydration of the dried vaccine. Do not use any other type of diluent to reconstitute the vaccine. Allow 2.7 mL for each day-old chick and 5 mL for each seven day-old chick.

Mix as follows:

Water For Day-Old Chicks Per 1,000 Doses		Water For 7 Day-Old Chicks Per 1,000 Doses	
0.7 gallons (90 oz.)	2.7 Liters	1.3 gallons	5.0 Liters

5. Provide enough waterers so that all birds may have an opportunity to drink the vaccine-treated water.
6. Do not resume watering until water containing vaccine has been consumed.
7. Take care to administer a full dose to each chick.

Precaution(s): Store the vaccine at 35-45°F (2-7°C).
Use entire contents of vial immediately after mixing.
Do not dilute or otherwise extend the dosage.
Burn empty bottles and unused vaccine.
Caution(s): Exposure to *salmonella* in the hatchery prior to vaccination may colonize the chick and may interfere with vaccination.
Use of antibiotics within 72 hours prior to or after vaccination may interfere with vaccination.
Avoid stress conditions during and following vaccination.
This vaccine is not returnable to the manufacturer.
Warning(s): Do not vaccinate within 28 days of slaughter.
Presentation: 10 x 1000 doses, 10 x 2000 doses, 10 x 2500 doses, 10 x 5000 doses, 10 x 8000 doses, and 10 x 10,000 doses.
This vaccine is sold under a commercial licensing agreement with Lohmann Animal Health GmBH & Co., Cuxhaven, Germany.
Patent pending.
Compendium Code No.: 11290420 211R

SANDCLEAR™

Farnam — **Laxative**

Guaranteed Analysis:
Crude Protein (min.) 4.5%
Crude Fat (min.) 1.5%
Crude Fiber (max.) 5.0%
Ash (max.) 3.5%
Ingredients: Psyllium seed husk, natural and artificial flavors.
Indications: SANDCLEAR™ contains 99% psyllium seed husk, a natural soluble fiber that increases feed ration bulk. Includes apple and molasses flavoring.
Psyllium contains more soluble fiber than oat bran and wheat bran combined. There is 80% soluble fiber in psyllium, while oat bran contains less than 15% soluble fiber and wheat bran contains 10%.
Dosage and Administration: For average size (1,000 lb.) adult horse - mix in one to two scoops of SANDCLEAR™ with daily grain ration for one full week (7 days) out of every month. Feed less to ponies, yearlings and foals; more to larger horses and draft breeds.
(One scoop = 3.75 oz.)
Warning(s): For animal use only.
Presentation: 1.36 kg (3 lb.), 10 lb, 20 lb and 50 lb containers.
Compendium Code No.: 10000351

SAND-PASTURE FORMULA™

Horses Prefer — **Laxative**

Dietary Fiber Supplement
Guaranteed Analysis: (Minimum per lb.)
Biotin 1.4%
Ingredients: Psyllium Seed Husk, Wheat Middling, Biotin, Apply Flavor and Soy Oil.
Indications: Suggested Use: SAND-PASTURE FORMULA™ is a carefully formulated dietary fiber supplement containing psyllium seed husk. SAND-PASTURE FORMULA™ may be used on horses grazing short pastures and those consuming sand and dirt.
Directions: Mix with daily feed.
Adults Horses: (1,000 lb.): 1-2 scoops for 7 consecutive days every month.
Feed one scoop to ponies and up three scoops to heavy breeds.
Provide access to water at all times.
One 3-ounce scoop included.
Precaution(s): Store in a cool dry place.
Caution(s): Contact your veterinarian if horses show symptoms of colic.
For animal use only.
Warning(s): Keep out of reach of children.
Presentation: 5 lbs.
Compendium Code No.: 36950051

SARCOCYSTIS NEURONA VACCINE

Fort Dodge — **Protozoal Vaccine**

Sarcocystis Neurona Vaccine, Killed Protozoa
U.S. Vet. Lic. No.: 112
Contents: This product contains the antigens listed above.
Thimerosal, neomycin and polymyxin B added as preservatives
Indications: For vaccination of healthy horses as an aid in the prevention of neurologic disease (Equine Protozoal Myeloencephalitis) caused by subsequent exposure to the protozoan *Sarcocystis neurona.*
This product license is conditional. Efficacy and potency test studies are in progress.
Dosage and Administration: Dose: Horses, inject one 1 mL dose intramuscularly using aseptic technique. Administer a second 1 mL dose 3 to 6 weeks after the first dose. A 1 mL booster dose should be given annually. Mild exercise to promote absorption is recommended for one week after injection.
Precaution(s): Store in dark at 2° to 7°C (35° to 45°F). Avoid freezing. Use entire contents when first opened.
Caution(s): Successful field safety tests have included both seropositive and seronegative horses. Due to the prolonged incubation period and pathogenesis of *S. neurona* infection, vaccination of healthy horses infected with *S. neurona* may not prevent further progression of *S. neurona* infection or clinical signs of EPM.
In some instances, transient local reactions may occur at the injection site. In case of anaphylactoid reaction, administer epinephrine.
Warning(s): Do not vaccinate within 21 days before slaughter.
For veterinary use only.
Presentation: 10 doses (10 mL).
Patent Pending
Compendium Code No.: 10032680 3643F

S

SAV-A-CAF® FINISHER IRON

IntAgra **Iron-Oral**

Guaranteed Analysis:

Iron	6,000 mg/lb	410 mg/fl oz	1.32%
Copper	300 mg/lb	20 mg/fl oz	0.066%
Maximum Moisture			80.5%

Ingredients: Ferrous Proteinate, Copper Proteinate, Dried Torula Yeast, Guar Gum, Artificial Flavoring, Water.

Indications: SAV-A-CAF® Finisher Iron is a non-staining chelated iron plus copper oral supplement for veal calves.

Directions: Shake well just before using.

Feeding wholesale entire barn: Mixing 3 fluid ounces of Finisher Iron to 100 lbs of dry feed will furnish about 28 ppm (parts per million) of iron.

Product may thicken from evaporation. If so, recondition with distilled water and shake well.

Precaution(s): Store and use at room temperature.

Caution(s): Not for human use.

Warning(s): Keep out of reach of children.

Presentation: 1 gallon (net weight 9 lbs).

Compendium Code No.: 14900010 Rev. 5.00

SAV-A-CAF® STARTER IRON

IntAgra **Iron-Oral**

Guaranteed Analysis:

Iron	18,000 mg/lb	50 mg/cc	3.96%
Copper	1,800 mg/lb	5 mg/cc	0.396%
Maximum Moisture			49.1%

Ingredients: Ferrous Proteinate, Copper Proteinate, Dried Torula Yeast, Guar Gum, Artificial Flavoring, Water.

Indications: SAV-A-CAF® Starter Iron is a non-staining chelated iron plus copper-oral supplement for veal calves.

Directions: Shake well just before using.

Every fluid ounce of Full Strength Starter Iron contains 1500 mg of Iron (from ferrous sulfate and 150 mg of Copper (from Copper Sulfate). Mixing 3 fluid ounces of Starter Iron to 100 lbs of dry feed will furnish approximately 100 ppm (parts per million) of Iron.

Product may thicken from evaporation. If so, recondition with distilled water and shake well.

Precaution(s): Store and use at room temperature.

Caution(s): Not for human use.

Warning(s): Keep out of reach of children.

Presentation: 1 gallon (net weight 10 lbs).

Compendium Code No.: 14900020 Rev. 5.00

SAV-A-PIG® ORAL IRON

IntAgra **Iron-Oral**

Guaranteed Analysis:

Iron	50 mg/cc	18,000 mg/lb	3.95%
Copper	5 mg/cc	1,800 mg/lb	0.396%
Maximum Moisture			49.1%

Ingredients: Ferrous Proteinate, Copper Proteinate, Dried Torula Yeast, Guar Gum, Artificial Flavoring, Water.

Indications: SAV-A-PIG® Oral Iron is a chelated oral supplement for suckling pigs.

Directions: Always shake just before reusing.

Colostrum: Vital for newborn piglets. It allows the sow to pass on antibodies to help piglets ward off infection and disease. They should nurse immediately; test within 15 minutes of birth and definitely within 2 hours. Colostrum must be absorbed by pigs for first 6-8 hours, and piglets should be active and nursing well before giving Oral Iron.

Timing: For best results, give 2 cc (one pump) from 12 hours to 24 hours after farrowing. Before dosing be sure all piglets are nursing, especially small weak pigs.

For best efficiency, many do their entire processing routine (clip eye teeth, apply iodine to navel, etc.) within the 12 to 24 hour time slot.

If you wait until after 24 hours, pigs will be less likely to absorb iron due to "gut closure". After this, giving Oral Iron is still worthwhile, it is just not quite as efficient.

In most cases, one pump is all they need. Fastest growing piglets may require a second pump at 7-10 days.

Proper Oral Administration: While holding pig's head parallel to floor, carefully insert pump dispenser spout just inside mouth of pig, slightly above center of tongue. Do not force product down throat (inhalation of any foreign matter into lungs may cause pneumonia or suffocation).

Push plunger just once for each pig. Each stroke gives 2 cc, with 100 mg of Iron and 10 cc of Copper.

Precaution(s): Store and use at room temperature.

Housekeeping: Pump will perform best if you rinse it clean after use, and re-seal container with cap. Product may thicken from evaporation. Restore consistency with distilled water and shake well.

Warning(s): Not for human use.

Keep out of reach of children.

Side Effects: Possible Side Effects: Oral Iron is designed to make iron easily available to the pig. Unfortunately, as iron becomes more available to the pig, it also becomes more available to bacteria present in the digestive tract.

Certain strains of intestinal bacteria can multiply to a pathological level in the presence of iron and produce toxins. These can cause vomiting, scouring, or even death if left untreated for too long.

These instances are rare, but may occur. Watch pigs carefully after using the supplement it may be necessary to follow the iron treatment with an appropriate scours treatment. We suggest you consult a veterinarian.

Presentation: Bulk only.

Compendium Code No.: 14900031

SB-1 FROZEN

Intervet **Vaccine**

Monovalent Marek's Disease Vaccine, Serotype 2, Live Virus (strain SB-1)

U.S. Vet. Lic. No.: 286

Contents: SB-1 monovalent Marek's disease vaccine consists of a live chicken herpesvirus and is derived from the serotype 2 Marek's disease virus (strain SB-1).

The vaccine contains gentamicin and amphotericin B as preservatives.

Notice: This vaccine has undergone rigid safety, purity and potency tests to meet USDA and Intervet Inc. standards. The use of this vaccine is subject to state laws, where applicable.

Indications: Marek's disease vaccines are recommended for vaccination of healthy one-day-old chicks through subcutaneous route.

Dosage and Administration: Read the instructions fully. Instructions must be followed exactly for best results. Prevent exposure to Marek's disease for at least two weeks.

1. Know and follow all precautions and safety practices for handling liquid nitrogen.
2. Before withdrawing vaccine from liquid nitrogen, protect hands with gloves, wear long sleeves and protect face with a plastic face shield or wear protective goggles.
3. Remove from the liquid nitrogen only the ampules that are going to be used immediately. Match the dosage size of the vaccine ampules and diluent bottle. Move quickly but carefully.

1000 doses of vaccine - 200 mL diluent

2000 to 9000 doses of vaccine - 400 mL to 1800 mL diluent

4. Place the ampule(s) in a clean large container of lukewarm water (75-85°F) to thaw ampule(s) quickly. Gentle agitation promotes rapid thawing and evenly distributes the vaccine in the ampule. Thaw the entire contents.
5. Mix vaccine with the room temperature diluent immediately after thawing. Remove closure from top of diluent bottle. Draw vaccine from the ampule into the sterile disposable mixing syringe.
6. Gently agitate syringe and expel contents into the diluent bottle. Rinse the ampule once with the diluted vaccine.
7. Place the diluted vaccine into an ice bath. Agitate as needed to ensure uniform suspension of the cells.
8. For subcutaneous vaccination, set sterilized automatic syringe to 0.2 mL per dose. Syringe, needles and accessory equipment should be sterilized by autoclaving or boiling.
9. For administering the vaccine subcutaneously, use a short (3/8" or 1/2"), 20 gauge needle to prevent injury to chicks. @NUM2 = 10. Vaccinate only healthy chicks at one day of age. Inject 0.2 mL (two-tenths of a milliliter) subcutaneously into the back of the neck.
11. Keep accurate records of chicks or eggs, vaccine serial numbers, vaccinator and doses used. Be sure to note unusual circumstances that occur before, during, or after vaccinating which may affect the level of immunity.

Precaution(s): Marek's disease vaccines, produced by Intervet, Inc. contain cell associated virus in live chicken cells. The cells and virus particles are very fragile and require careful handling to prevent damage and to preserve them intact to be used as a vaccine in chicks.

Make all preparations in advance and follow directions carefully.

Thaw vaccine immediately before use.

Make sure all personnel handling and/or using vaccine understand the importance of following these instructions completely.

Storage Conditions:

Vaccine Ampule - Store in liquid nitrogen.

Diluent - Store at room temperature. Chill after concentrated vaccine has been added as well as during use.

Burn all discarded containers and unused contents.

Caution(s): Combining this product with other biological products is not recommended.

This product should be stored, transported and administered in accordance with the instructions and directions.

For subcutaneous injection in one-day old chicks only.

Warning(s): Do not vaccinate within 21 days before slaughter.

Presentation: SB-1 is available in 1,000 dose size units.

Compendium Code No.: 11061901

SB-VAC®

Intervet **Vaccine**

Marek's Disease Vaccine, Live Chicken Herpesvirus, Cell Associated

U.S. Vet. Lic. No.: 286

Active Ingredient(s): SB-VAC® is of chicken tissue culture origin using SPF (Specific Pathogen Free) eggs. The product contains the SB-1 strain of chicken herpesvirus and is used for the prevention of Marek's disease in chickens. It is packaged in two separate units. One is an ample containing 1,000 doses of frozen live cell associated chicken herpesvirus and the other is a bottle of sterile diluent. The ampules are inserted in metal canes and shipped in a liquid nitrogen (LN) container. The diluent is packaged in separate cartons in bottles of 200 mL, 1,200 mL or 1,600 mL. The vaccine may contain either neomycin or gentamicin in an individual ampule as a preservative.

Indications: The vaccine is recommended for use in healthy one day old chickens. When used in combination with the live turkey herpesvirus (HVT) form of Marek's Disease Vaccine optimal protection is achieved. The virus will infect chickens even though they may be carrying maternal antibodies to Marek's disease herpesvius (MDHV).

Dosage and Administration: Preparation of Vaccine:

Caution: Read the safety precaution advice on handling the vaccine ampule. Sterilize vaccinating equipment by boiling in water for 30 minutes or by autoclaving (20 minutes at 121°C). Do not use chemical disinfectants.

1. Use the contents of one (1) ampule with 200 mL of sterile diluent per 1,000 chickens.
2. Before withdrawing the vaccine from the liquid nitrogen canister, protect the hands with gloves, wear long sleeves and use a face mask or goggles. It is possible that an accident could occur with either the liquid nitrogen or the ampules of vaccine. When removing an ampule from the cane, hold the palm of the gloved hand away from the body and the face.
3. When withdrawing a cane of ampules from the canister in the liquid nitrogen refrigerator, expose only the ampule to be used immediately. We recommend handling only one (1) ampule at a time. After removing the ampule from the cane, the remaining ampules should be replaced immediately in the canister of the liquid nitrogen refrigerator.
4. The contents of the ampule are thawed rapidly by immersing it in water at room temperature. Shake the ampule to disperse the contents. Then break the ampule at its neck and immediately proceed. One (1) ampule of SB-VAC® is added to the 200 mL bottle of diluent, six (6) to the 1,200 mL bottle and eight (8) to the 1,600 mL bottle. Caution: Ampules have been known to explode on sudden temperature changes. Do not thaw in hot or ice cold water.

5. Draw the contents of the ampule into a sterile 5 or 10 mL syringe, mounted with an 18-gauge needle.
6. Dilute immediately by filling the syringe slowly with a portion of the diluent. Important: The diluent should be at room temperature (15°-25°C) at the time of mixing.
7. The contents of the filled syringe are then added to the remaining diluent. It is important that this be done slowly. Slowly empty the syringe, allowing the vaccine to run down the side of the bottle. Gently shake the bottle as the vaccine is being mixed. Withdraw a portion of the diluent with the syringe to flush the ampule. Inject the washing back into the diluent bottle. Remove the syringe.
8. When used in combination with the live turkey herpesvirus form of Marek's disease vaccine, add the contents of the two (2) separate vaccine ampules into 200 mL of diluent.
9. Fill the previously sterilized automatic syringe according to the manufacturer's recommendations and set the dose for 0.20 mL.
10. The vaccine is now ready for use.

Method of Vaccination: Subcutaneous administration:

1. Hold the chicken by the back of the neck just below the head. The loose skin in the area is raised by gently pinching with a thumb and forefinger. Insert the needle beneath the skin in a downward direction away from the head. Inject 0.20 mL per chicken. The bottle of vaccine should be kept in an ice bath and swirled frequently.
2. Avoid hitting the muscles and bones in the neck.
3. The entire contents of the bottle must be used within one (1) hour after mixing or discarded.

Records: Keep a record of vaccine, quantity, serial number, expiration date, and place of purchase; the date and time of vaccination; the number, age, breed, and locations of chickens; names of operators performing the vaccination and any observed reactions.

Precaution(s):

Ampules: Store in the liquid nitrogen container.

Diluent: Store at room temperature.

Container: Store the liquid nitrogen container securely in an upright position in a dry, well ventilated area and away from incubator intakes and chicken boxes.

Safety Precautions: The liquid nitrogen container and the vaccine should be handled only by properly trained personnel who are thoroughly conversant with the Union Carbide publication and instruction booklet regarding the use of, precautions and safe practices for liquified atmospheric gases (particularly nitrogen).

When removing the ampule cane, handling the frozen ampules, or adding the liquid nitrogen, wear long sleeves, a plastic face shield and gloves to protect the skin from contact with the liquid nitrogen. All storage and handling of the liquid nitrogen container must be in a dry, ventilated area. Do not inhale liquid nitrogen vapors. If drowsiness occurs, get fresh air quickly; then ventilate the entire area. If breathing difficulty occurs, apply artificial respiration. If any of these difficulties persist or there is a loss of consciousness, summon a physician immediately. Care should be exercised to prevent contaminating the hands, eyes and clothing with the vaccine.

Use only as directed. Store vaccines in liquid nitrogen. The product is not returnable.

Caution(s): Good management practices are recommended to reduce exposure to MDHV for at least three weeks following vaccination. Therefore, directions should be followed carefully.

1. Do not mix any substance, other than HVT vaccine, with the vaccine. The vaccine is recommended for use only in combination with HVT type Marek's vaccine.
2. The SB-1 strain has been shown to allow for the development of lymphoid leukosis under certain circumstances in certain types of chickens.
3. Gloves and a visor should be worn when handling liquid nitrogen.
4. Read the directions carefully.
5. Only healthy chickens should be vaccinated.
6. Store the vaccine in liquid nitrogen at a temperature below -150°C.
7. Once diluted the vaccine should be used within one hour and the unused vaccine discarded into disinfectant or burned.
8. Once thawed, the product should not be refrozen.

Warning(s): Do not vaccinate within 21 days before slaughter.

Discussion: The vaccine has undergone rigid potency, safety and purity tests, and meets Intervet America Inc. and USDA requirements. It is designed to stimulate effective immunity when used as directed, but the user must be advised that the response to the product depends upon many factors, including, but not limited to, conditions of storage and handling by the user, administration of the vaccine, health and responsiveness of the individual chickens, and the degree of field exposure.

The use of the vaccine is subject to applicable federal and local laws and regulations.

Presentation: 1 x 1,000 dose ampule with 1 x 200 mL bottle of diluent.
6 x 1,000 dose ampules with 1 x 1,200 mL bottle of diluent.
8 x 1,000 dose ampules with 1 x 1,600 mL bottle of diluent.

Compendium Code No.: 11061910

SCARLET OIL

First Priority **Topical Wound Dressing**

Wound Dressing

Ingredient(s): Mineral Oil, Isopropyl Alcohol, Methyl Salicylate, Benzyl Alcohol, Pine Oil, Eucalyptus Oil, Parachlorometaxylenol, and Biebrich Scarlet Red.

Indications: For use as a dressing for simple wounds, cuts and abrasions on horses and mules.

Directions for Use: Clean the affected area, clipping hair if necessary. Direct spray at the site to be treated. Hold container 4 to 6 inches from animal. Apply freely as an open wound treatment or wrap with a clean bandage. Treatment may be applied once or twice daily.

Precaution(s): Storage: Store at controlled room temperature between 15°-30°C (59°-86°F). Keep container tightly closed when not in use.

Caution(s): Use only as directed. Avoid contact with eyes and mucous membranes. Do not apply to large areas of broken skin. In case of deep or puncture wounds or serious burns consult a veterinarian. If redness, irritation, or swelling persists or increases, discontinue use and consult a veterinarian.

For animal use only.

Warning(s): Not for use on animals intended for food.

Keep out of reach of children.

Presentation: 16 fl oz (473 mL) (NDC# 58829-259-16) and 1 gallon (3.785 L) (NDC# 58829-259-01).

Compendium Code No.: 11390703 Rev. 10-01 / Rev. 07-01

SCARLET OIL

Vedco **Topical Wound Dressing**

Active Ingredient(s): Contains: Mineral oil, isopropyl alcohol (32.1% v/v), pine oil, benzyl alcohol (2.4% v/v), oil of eucalyptus, methyl salicylate, parachlorometaxylenol, biebrich scarlet.

Indications: An external application for superficial lacerations, wire cuts, burns and surface wounds of horses and mules.

Dosage and Administration: Apply freely with a dauber or gauze to the affected parts. May be used under a bandage if desired. The treatment may be repeated once or twice a day as indicated.

Caution(s): Keep out of the reach of children. For external veterinary use only.

In case of deep, or puncture wounds or serious burns or if redness, irritation, or swelling persists or increases, consult a veterinarian. Keep away from the eyes or mucous membranes. Avoid inhaling. A combustible liquid, do not use near an open flame.

Warning(s): For horses and mules not intended for food use.

Presentation: 4 oz., 16 oz. and 1 gallon containers.

Compendium Code No.: 10941830

SCARLET OIL PUMP SPRAY

Dominion **Topical Wound Dressing**

Active Ingredient(s): Contents: Each mL contains:

Menthol	7.5 mg
Phenol	7.5 mg
Oil of Camphor	7.5 mg
Oil of Eucalyptus	7.5 mg
Oil of Pine	7.5 mg
Oil of Thyme	2.8 mg
Peru Balsam	1.5 mg
Biebrich Scarlet Red	100 ppm

Indications: Dressing for treatment of superficial cuts, wounds, and burns of horses and mules.

Directions: Shake well before using!

Remove pump cap from the top of the container. Direct spray at the site to be treated. Hold the container 10 to 15 cm from the animal and press down on the valve to spray. Apply the spray freely and use it as an open wound treatment or under bandage. The treatment may be repeated once or twice daily as indicated.

Caution(s): In case of deep or puncture wounds or serious burns consult a veterinarian. If redness, irritation, or swelling persists or increases, discontinue use and consult a veterinarian. Keep out of reach of children.

Presentation: 500 mL bottle; 12 bottles/carton.

Compendium Code No.: 15080060

SCARLET OIL SMEAR

First Priority **Topical Wound Dressing**

Ingredient(s): Mineral Oil, Methyl Salicylate, Eucalyptus Oil, Pine Oil, Phenol, Menthol, Colloidial Silica, Biebrich Scarlet Red.

Indications: For use on horses as an antiseptic dressing for superficial wounds, cuts, abrasions, and minor burns.

Directions for Use: Apply freely with a dauber or gauze to lacerations. SCARLET OIL SMEAR may be used under a bandage if desired. Apply once daily until healed. Read caution and contraindication statements before using.

Contraindication(s): Do not use on cats. Do not apply to large areas of broken skin. Do not use on dairy animals.

Precaution(s): Storage: Store at controlled room temperature between 15°-30°C (59°-86°F). Keep container tightly closed when not in use.

Caution(s): Use only as directed. In case of deep or puncture wounds or serious burns, consult a veterinarian. If redness, irritation or swelling continues or increases, discontinue use and consult a veterinarian. Avoid contact with eyes and mucous membranes.

For animal use only.

For external veterinary use only.

Warning(s): Not for use on food producing animals.

Keep out of reach of children.

Presentation: 3.75 fl oz (111 mL) with dauber (NDC# 58829-320-04).

Compendium Code No.: 11390850 Iss. 11-01

SCARLET OIL WITH ALOE VERA

Life Science **Topical Wound Dressing**

Topical Antiseptic

Active Ingredient(s): Contains: Biebrich scarlet, aloe vera, parachlorometaxylenol, mineral oil, pine oil, benzyl alcohol, oil of eucalyptus, methyl salicylate, and isopropyl alcohol.

Indications: A nondrying, oleaginous dressing for use as an aid in the treatment of cuts, wounds, abrasions, or burns on horses.

Directions: First clean and dry affected areas to be treated. Then apply generously with dauber or spray directly onto lesion.

Repeat applications twice daily until healing takes place.

Caution(s): In case of deep or puncture wounds or serious burns, or if redness, irritation, or swelling persists or increases, consult a veterinarian. Keep away from eyes or mucous membranes. Avoid inhaling.

For external use only.

For animal use only.

Warning(s): Not for use on horses intended for food use.

SCARLET OIL will stain. Avoid contact with hands and clothing.

Keep out of reach of children.

Presentation: 1 pint (473 mL) with sprayer and 1 gallon (3.785 L).

Compendium Code No.: 10870151

SCARLET OIL WOUND DRESSING

AgriPharm **Topical Wound Dressing**

Active Ingredient(s): Contains: Mineral oil, isopropyl alcohol, (30%), pine oil, benzyl alcohol (3.0% w/w), oil of eucalyptus, methyl salicylate, parachlorometaxylenol, biebrich scarlet.

Indications: Topical antiseptic. A nondrying, oleaginous dressing for use as an aid in the treatment of cuts, wounds, abrasions and burns.

Dosage and Administration: Remove pus and exudate from the infected area. When spraying hold the container approximately five (5) inches from the area to be treated. Spray an amount sufficient to cover the wound. One (1) application is usually sufficient. May be repeated once or twice a day on severe cases.

Precaution(s): Store in a cool place. Store at 35°-86°F (2°-30°C).

A combustible liquid, do not use near an open flame.

Caution(s): For external veterinary use only.

Hazardous: Livestock remedy. Not for human use. Keep out of the reach of children.

For use on horses or mules not intended for human food.

In case of deep, or puncture wounds or serious burns or if redness, irritation, or swelling persists or increases, consult a veterinarian. Keep away from eyes and mucous membranes. Avoid inhaling.

Presentation: 16 oz. containers.

Compendium Code No.: 14570910

SCARLET OIL WOUND DRESSING

Durvet **Topical Wound Dressing**

Topical Antiseptic

Active Ingredient(s): Contains: Mineral Oil, Isopropyl Alcohol, Pine Oil, Benzyl Alcohol, Oil of Eucalyptus, Methyl Salicylate and Scarlet Red.

Indications: A non drying, oleaginous dressing for use as an aid in the treatment of cuts, wounds, abrasions and burns.

Directions: Remove pus and exudate from infected area. When spraying hold container approximately 5 inches from area to be treated. Spray an amount sufficient to cover wound. One application is usually sufficient. May be repeated once or twice daily.

Precaution(s): Storage: Store at 2°C to 30°C (35°F to 86°F). Store in a cool place.

Flammable. Keep away from fire or flame.

A combustible liquid, do not use near open flame.

Caution(s): In case of deep, or puncture wounds or serious burns or if redness, irritation, or swelling persists or increases, consult a veterinarian. Keep away from eyes or mucous membranes. Avoid inhaling.

Hazardous: Livestock remedy, not for human use.

The following statement is made in compliance with the State of California Agricultural Code: Livestock remedy—Not for human use.

For external use only.

For animal use only.

Warning(s): For use on horses or mules not intended for human food.

Keep out of reach of children.

Presentation: 16 oz (473 mL) (1 pt).

Compendium Code No.: 10841461 5-95

SCARLEX® SCARLET OIL

Farnam **Topical Wound Dressing**

NDC No.: 17135-314-01

Active Ingredient(s): Biebrich scarlet red, p-chloro-m-xylenol, methyl salicylate, oil of eucalyptus, pine oil, benzyl alcohol 3.075%, mineral oil, and propellants 40%.

Indications: A soothing, slow-drying antiseptic dressing for minor skin lesions, surface wounds, cuts and burns. Indicated also for superficial dermatitis. Contains 500 applications.

Dosage and Administration: Shake well: Remove protective cap. Point nozzle opening toward wound or affected area to be treated. Spray from a distance of 2 to 4 inches. Release spray by pressing valve stem down for just an instant. A one second application over area to be treated provides an adequate dosage. The application should be repeated once a day until healing takes place. Whenever possible clean and dry area to be treated before applying. Do not use on exceedingly large areas or in deep wounds.

Precaution(s): Danger. Extremely Flammable. Do not spray near sparks, heat or open flames. Vapors will accumulate readily and may ignite explosively. Keep area ventilated during use and until all vapors are gone. Do not smoke. Extinguish all flames, pilot lights and heaters. Turn off stoves, electric tools and appliances, and any other sources of ignition.

Contents are under pressure. Avoid prolonged exposure to sunlight or heat from radiators, stoves, hot water and other heat sources that may cause bursting. Do not puncture, incinerate, burn or store above 120°F. Do not discard the empty can in home garbage compactor.

Caution(s): For external use only. In case of deep or puncture wounds or serious burns, consult a veterinarian. If redness, irritation, or swelling persists or increases, discontinue use of the product and consult a veterinarian. Avoid contact with eyes and mucous membranes. The product is to be used on non-food producing animals only.

Warning(s): The vapor is harmful. Use with adequate ventilation. Avoid continuous inhalation of vapor and spray mist.

This product is to be used on non-food producing animals only.

Discussion: Farnam SCARLEX® provides scarlet oil dressing in a pressurized spray bomb, with p-chloro-m-xylenol added. P-chloro-m-xylenol is both a germicide and fungicide, and many times more powerful than phenol, yet is non-irritating to skin tissue.

Presentation: 142 g (5 oz) can.

Compendium Code No.: 10000360

SCHIRMER TEAR TEST

S

Schering-Plough **Schirmer Tear Test**

Description: The Schirmer Tear Test (STT) is indicated to measure the rate of tear production.

Indications: It should be used in the evaluation of conjunctivitis to diagnose tear deficiency as a contributing factor to ocular surface diseases including: Keratoconjunctivitis sicca (KCS), pigmentary keratitis, indolent corneal ulcers, exposure keratitis, and others. In addition, it should be used to assess lacrimal gland function prior to cataract surgery.

Test Procedure: The tear test is performed with standardized sterile 5x35mm strips. In veterinary species, the test is performed for 60 seconds. The standardized test (Schirmer I) should be performed before instillation of any topical medication or manipulation of the eyelids. Topical anesthesia is not used to perform the standardized STT. Avoid touching the ocular end of the strip with fingers. Although copious discharge present on the surface of the eye may be removed with a gauze sponge prior to performing the STT, it is not necessary to do so.

Hook the rounded notched end of the sterile strip over the juncture of the temporal and middle thirds of the lower lid margin. Note the time. The eyelids can be held shut, or the patient can be allowed to keep its eyes open and blink freely during the Schirmer test. After 60 seconds have elapsed, remove the strip and immediately measure the length of the moistened area. Immediate evaluation is important because, as with all Schirmer tear test strips, the tear front will continue advancing a few millimeters after it has been removed from the eye. Visualization of the length of wetting of the paper strip is aided by a blue dye that advances with the tear front. A millimeter scale is printed on each strip.

The result should be recorded on the patient's chart. An example may be as follows: Schirmer tear test: right 10 mm/min; left 5 mm/min. If the entire strip is wetted within 1 minute, this should be noted on the chart. If the test strip is dislodged from the lids prior to 60 seconds, a new paper strip should be used, and the test repeated. If the test is prematurely interrupted, for instance in a non-compliant patient, it is valid to repeat the test without an interval of time delay between tests.

Test Interpretation: Normal Values: The normal range for the STT varies among species. Normal ranges for common veterinary species are listed below.

Dog: 19.8 ± 5.3 mm/minute

Cat: 16.9 ± 5.7 mm/minute

Horse: 24.8 ± 4.8 mm/minute

Rabbit: 15.3 ± 3.0 mm/minute

Interpretation of Abnormal Values: Excessive wetting suggest epiphora and should prompt further investigation of painful corneal condition such as corneal ulcer.

Interpretation of below normal wetting requires consideration of several factors. An STT value <5 mm/min. is sufficient clinical evidence to diagnose KCS in dogs and cats. The normal physiologic response to ocular inflammation or irritation is increased tearing; therefore, when signs of ocular surface inflammation are seen in the presence of a moderately low STT, i.e., between 5-10 mm/min. animals are also typically diagnosed as having KCS. Assessment of a borderline tear deficiency, 10-15 mm/min. in dogs, should take into consideration any abnormal eyelid anatomy which would contribute to excessive tear evaporation and subsequent exposure keratitis. With a borderline STT value, clinical signs of KCS ocular surface lesions can develop in dogs with additive factors which contribute to ocular drying or infection such as: exophthalmos, lagophthalmos, ectropion, a floppy lid-glove apposition (megalofissure), distichia and chronic pyoderma. Cats usually have correct anatomical apposition of the lids and globe, and are usually asymptomatic with a STT >5 mm/min.

Administration of anti-cholinergic drugs, such as atropine, can temporarily suppress tear secretion and cause decreased STT value. Sympathetic stimulation associated with fear or excitement can also cause transient decreases in the STT, and is a common cause of low STT values in cats. When the diagnosis is uncertain, several measurements may be made on repeated visits and averaged to enhance the accuracy of this test.

Caution(s): The Schirmer Tear Tests are intended for single patient use only. Contents are sterile if package is unopened and undamaged. Do not use if package has been previously opened.

References: Available upon request.

Presentation: Box of 10 envelopes, 5 pair strips per envelope.

Compendium Code No.: 10471770

SCORE®

Intervet **Bacterin-Toxoid**

Bordetella Bronchiseptica-Erysipelothrix Rhusiopathiae-Pasteurella Multocida Bacterin-Toxoid

U.S. Vet. Lic. No.: 286

Contents: Inactivated cultures of *B. bronchiseptica* and *E. rhusiopathiae* and toxoids of toxigenic strains of *P. multocida* capsular serotype A and *P. multocida* capsular serotype D.

Contains gentamicin as a preservative.

Indications: For the protection of healthy sows and gilts and their litters against atrophic rhinitis caused by *B. bronchiseptica* and the toxin of *P. multocida* serotypes A and D. This product is also an aid in the prevention of erysipelas in the sow herd caused by *E. rhusiopathiae*.

Directions: Sows and gilts and their piglets must be vaccinated as follows:

Sows and gilts: 2 mL intramuscularly (IM). Give 2 doses at least 2 weeks apart with the second dose administered 2 weeks before farrowing. Revaccinate before each subsequent farrowing.

Pigs: 2 mL subcutaneously (SQ) at 7-10 days of age or prior to weaning. Repeat with a second dose in 2-3 weeks.

Breeding Stock: Vaccinate all new breeding stock with 2 doses given 2 weeks apart with the first dose given at 6 months of age or prior to introduction into the herd. Revaccinate boars with a single dose annually.

Precaution(s): Shake well. Use entire contents when first opened. Store at 2°-7°C (35°-45°F). Do not freeze.

Caution(s): In case of anaphylactoid reaction administer epinephrine.

For veterinary use only.

Warning(s): Do not vaccinate within 21 days before slaughter.

Presentation: 50 doses (100 mL).

Compendium Code No.: 11061920

SCOUR BOS™ 4

Novartis Animal Vaccines **Vaccine**

Bovine Rota-Coronavirus Vaccine, Killed Virus

U.S. Vet. Lic. No.: 303

Composition: This bacterin contains inactivated bovine rotavirus and bovine coronavirus adjuvanted with Xtend III®. Contains amphotericin B, penicillin, streptomycin, and thimerosal as preservatives.

Indications: For use in healthy pregnant cattle as an aid in the prevention and control of disease caused by bovine rotavirus and bovine coronavirus.

Dosage and Administration: Shake well before using. Administer 2 mL intramuscularly 8-10 weeks prior to calving. Repeat in 6 weeks. Revaccinate with one dose 8-10 weeks prior to each subsequent calving.

Precaution(s): Store in the dark at 35°-45°F (2°-7°C). Do not freeze. Use entire contents when first opened.

Caution(s): It is essential that calves receive colostrum from the vaccinated dam. Anaphylactic reactions may occur following the use of this biological. Symptomatic treatment: Epinephrine.

Warning(s): Do not vaccinate within 60 days prior to slaughter.

This product may cause persistent swelling at the site of injection.

For veterinary use only.

Discussion: Technical Disease Information: Coronavirus: Coronavirus causes one of the most severe viral diarrheas of neonatal calves. It may produce complete villus atrophy of the intestines. It is found worldwide and produces a severe diarrhea with dehydration and moderate mortality. A dual infection with rotavirus or *E. coli* can escalate the disease. Affected calves are extremely depressed but they often continue nursing. Coronavirus is also capable of infecting lung tissues and may produce respiratory signs. Calves most commonly affected with coronavirus diarrhea range in age from 5-21 days. Diarrhea usually lasts 4-5 days. Affected calves are the main source of infection to other calves, but evidence indicates that some recovered calves and cows will continue to carry virus and serve as long-term reservoirs for the virus.

Rotavirus: Bovine rotavirus diarrhea is found worldwide. Rotaviral diarrhea results from replication of the virus in villus enterocytes of the small intestine. Clinical signs range from mild to severe diarrhea, depending on the strain of virus. This diarrhea results in dehydration, depression and sometimes death. A high incidence of rotaviruses has been detected in scouring calves on both ranches and dairy farms and this occurs most frequently within the first two weeks of life. The severity of the disease is often worse in calves co-infected with other enteropathogens.

The most common G serotypes of group A rotaviruses affecting calves are G6 and G10. Three P serotypes (genotypes) have been identified in calves with diarrhea: P6 [1], P7 [5] and P8 [11]. Novartis' vaccine contains three field isolates of bovine rotavirus, group A, that encompass all of the common G and P types encountered in the United States. The virulent bovine rotavirus challenge used in this study also contained bovine rotavirus group A with G8 genotype. If G8 is emerging as a prevalent genotype, results from this study show protection to this type as well.

Treatment: Treatment for rotavirus and coronavirus enteritis consists of maintaining hydration and electrolyte balance through the use of fluids administered either orally or intravenously. It is important to maintain calves on milk, since electrolyte fluids alone cannot supply all the nutrition a calf requires. The use of appropriate antibiotics is also employed to control secondary bacterial infections.

Prevention: Preventing viral diarrhea requires careful management of the dam, the environment, and the calf. The most important step in the program is immunization of the dam with an effective vaccine. This will result in high levels of maternal antibodies that are passed to the calf in the colostrum that it receives after birth. SCOUR BOS™ 4 is the ideal vaccine because it provides heterologous coverage for multiple rotavirus and coronavirus serotypes. It requires two doses the first year; thereafter it requires only a single yearly vaccination to the cow prior to calving.

It is vital that herds are managed to insure that all calves receive adequate levels of colostrum within the first critical hours (0-6) after birth. On severely contaminated premises, it may also be necessary for dairy calves to continue receiving milk from vaccinated cows, free of Johne's disease, until they have passed the susceptible age.

Trial Data: Coronavirus Challenge:

Group	Geometric Mean Titers		Dehydration Difference	Depression Difference	Clinical Difference
	Calf Serum	Dam Colostrum			
Vaccinates	2.5X increase	4X increase	p = 0.0004	p = 0.0005	p = 0.0003
Controls	baseline	baseline	Extremely Significant		

Rotavirus Challenge:

Group	Geometric Mean Titers		Dehydration Difference	Depression Difference	Clinical Difference
	Calf Serum	Dam Colostrum			
Vaccinates	13X increase	7X increase	p = 0.0004	p = 0.0004	p = 0.001
Controls	baseline	baseline	Extremely Significant		

Presentation: Available in 10 dose (20 mL) and 50 dose (100 mL) bottles.

Compendium Code No.: 11140452 MP-F248-MAR00

SCOUR BOS™ 6

Novartis Animal Vaccines **Bacterin-Toxoid-Vaccine**

Bovine Coronavirus Vaccine, Killed Virus-Clostridium Perfringens Type C, Escherichia Coli Bacterin-Toxoid

U.S. Vet. Lic. No.: 303

Composition: This product contains inactivated cultures of bovine coronavirus, *Clostridium perfringens* Type C, and K99 piliated *Escherichia coli* adjuvanted with Xtend III®. Contains amphotericin B, penicillin, streptomycin, and thimerosal as preservatives.

Indications: For use in healthy pregnant cattle as an aid in the prevention and control of disease caused by bovine coronavirus, *Clostridium perfringens* Type C, and K99 piliated *Escherichia coli.*

Dosage and Administration: Shake well before using. Administer 2 mL intramuscularly 8-10 weeks prior to calving. Revaccinate with one dose 8-10 weeks prior to each subsequent calving.

Precaution(s): Store in the dark at 35°-45°F (2°-7°C). Do not freeze. Use entire contents when first opened.

Caution(s): It is essential that newborn calves receive colostrum from the vaccinated dam. Anaphylactic reactions may occur following the use of this biological. Symptomatic treatment: Epinephrine.

For veterinary use only.

Warning(s): Do not vaccinate within 60 days prior to slaughter.

This product may cause persistent swelling at the site of injection.

Discussion: Technical Disease Information: Coronavirus: Coronavirus causes one of the most severe viral diarrheas of neonatal calves. It may produce complete villus atrophy of the intestine. It is found worldwide and produces a severe diarrhea with dehydration and moderate mortality. A dual infection with rotavirus or *E. coli* can escalate the disease. Affected calves are extremely depressed but they often continue nursing. Coronavirus is also capable of infecting lung tissues and may produce respiratory signs. Calves most commonly affected with coronavirus diarrhea range in age from 5-21 days. Diarrhea usually lasts 4-5 days. Affected calves are the main source of infection to other calves, but evidence indicates that some recovered calves and cows will continue to carry virus and serve as long-term reservoirs for the virus.

Treatment: Treatment for coronavirus enteritis consists of maintaining hydration and electrolyte balance, through the use of fluids administered either orally or intravenously. It is important to maintain calves on milk, since electrolyte fluids alone cannot supply all the nutrition a calf requires. Antibiotic therapy is also usually incorporated to control secondary bacterial infections.

Escherichia coli: E. coli (colibacillosis) is primarily an enteric disease of calves from birth to 7 days of age. It may cause a severe diarrhea. Pathogenic *E. coli* are commonly found in the manure of healthy cows, which results in most calves being exposed shortly after birth. Unless the calf has received some type of protection immediately following birth, it is very susceptible to developing colibacillosis. The bacteria attach to the lining cells of the intestine by means of projections called pili. After attachment, the bacteria produce toxins which cause the intestine to secrete large amounts of fluid which results in diarrhea, dehydration and possible death.

Clostridium perfringens Type C: *Clostridium perfringens* Type C is commonly found in soil. It is also a common inhabitant of the intestinal tract in healthy animals. Engorgement with milk is often a predisposing factor. Type C enterotoxemia is caused by an overgrowth of these bacteria in the calf's intestine. This results in severe toxemia and high mortality rates. Calves may be found dead without showing any symptoms. They may show signs including bloating, abdominal pain, hemorrhagic diarrhea or extreme weakness.

Prevention: Preventing baby calf scours requires careful management of the dam, the environment, and the calf. The most important step in the program is immunization of the dam with an effective vaccine. This will result in high levels of maternal antibodies that are passed to the calf in the colostrum that it receives after birth. SCOUR BOS™ 6 is the ideal vaccine because it provides heterologous coverage for coronavirus, 4 types of *E. coli*, and *Clostridium perfringens* Type C with a single yearly vaccination to the cow.

It is vital that herds are managed to insure that all calves receive adequate levels of colostrum within the first critical hours (0-6) after birth. In severe outbreaks, it may also be necessary for dairy calves to continue receiving milk from vaccinated cows, free of Johne's disease, until they have passed the susceptible age.

Trial Data: *Cl. perfringens* Type C Antitoxin Titers:

Group (pooled samples)	Titer (AU/mL)
Dam's colostrum	≥ 50 < 100
Calf serum (3 days of age)	≥ 10
Calf serum (10 days of age)	≥ 10

E. coli Challenge:

Group	% Mortality	Avg. Clinical Score
Vaccinates	0%	1.5
Controls	70% p = 0.0002	82.9 p = 0.0000
	Extremely Significant	

Coronavirus Challenge:

Group	Geometric Mean Titers		Dehydration Difference	Depression Difference	Clinical Difference
	Calf Serum	Dam Colostrum			
Vaccinates	2.5X increase	4X increase	p = 0.0004	p = 0.0005	p = 0.0003
Controls	baseline	baseline	Extremely Significant		

Presentation: Available in 10 dose (20 mL) and 50 dose (100 mL) bottles.

Compendium Code No.: 11140462 MP-F241-APR00

SCOUR BOS™ 9

Novartis Animal Vaccines **Bacterin-Toxoid-Vaccine**

Bovine Rota-Coronavirus Vaccine, Killed Virus-Clostridium Perfringens Type C, Escherichia Coli Bacterin-Toxoid

U.S. Vet. Lic. No.: 303

Composition: This product contains inactivated cultures of bovine rotavirus, bovine coronavirus, *Clostridium perfringens* Type C, and K99 piliated *Escherichia coli* adjuvanted with Xtend III®. Contains amphotericin B, penicillin, streptomycin, and thimerosal as preservatives.

Indications: For use in healthy pregnant cattle as an aid in the prevention and control of disease caused by bovine rotavirus, bovine coronavirus, *Clostridium perfringens* Type C, and K99 piliated *Escherichia coli.*

Dosage and Administration: Shake well before using. Administer 2 mL intramuscularly 8-10 weeks prior to calving. Revaccinate with Scour Bos™ 4 (Bovine Rota-Coronavirus Vaccine) in 6 weeks. Revaccinate with one dose 8-10 weeks prior to each subsequent calving.

Precaution(s): Store in the dark at 35°-45°F (2°-7°C). Do not freeze. Use entire contents when first opened.

Caution(s): It is essential that newborn calves receive colostrum from the vaccinated dam. Anaphylactic reactions may occur following the use of this biological. Symptomatic treatment: Epinephrine.

For veterinary use only.

Warning(s): Do not vaccinate within 60 days prior to slaughter.

This product may cause persistent swelling at the site of injection.

Discussion: Technical Disease Information: Coronavirus: Coronavirus causes one of the most severe viral diarrheas of neonatal calves. It may produce complete villus atrophy of the intestine. It is found worldwide and produces a severe diarrhea with dehydration and moderate mortality. A dual infection with rotavirus or *E. coli* can escalate the disease. Affected calves are extremely depressed but they often continue nursing. Coronavirus is also capable of infecting lung tissues and may produce respiratory signs. Calves most commonly affected with coronavirus diarrhea range in age from 5-21 days. Diarrhea usually lasts 4-5 days. Affected calves are the main source of infection to other calves, but evidence indicates that some recovered calves and cows will continue to carry virus and serve as long-term reservoirs for the virus.

Rotavirus: Bovine rotavirus diarrhea is found worldwide. Rotaviral diarrhea results from replication of the virus in villus enterocytes of the small intestine. Clinical signs range from mild to severe diarrhea depending on the strain of virus. This diarrhea results in dehydration, depression and sometimes death. A high incidence of rotaviruses has been detected in scouring calves on both ranches and dairy farms, and this occurs most frequently within the first two weeks of life. The severity of the disease is often worse in calves co-infected with other enteropathogens.

The most common G serotypes of group A rotaviruses affecting calves are G6 and G10. Three P serotypes (genotypes) have been identified in calves with diarrhea: P6 [1], P7 [5] and P8 [11]. Novartis' vaccine contains three field isolates of bovine rotavirus, group A, that encompass all of the common G and P types encountered in the United States. The virulent bovine rotavirus challenge used in this study also contained bovine rotavirus group A with G8 genotype. If G8 is emerging as a prevalent genotype, results from this study show protection to this type as well.

Treatment: Treatment for rotavirus and coronavirus enteritis consists of maintaining hydration and electrolyte balance, through the use of fluids administered either orally or intravenously. It is important to maintain calves on milk, since electrolyte fluids alone cannot supply all the nutrition a calf requires. Antibiotic therapy is also usually incorporated to control secondary bacterial infections.

Escherichia coli: E. coli (colibacillosis) is primarily an enteric disease of calves from birth to 7 days of age. It may cause a severe diarrhea. Pathogenic *E. coli* are commonly found in the manure of healthy cows. This results in most calves being exposed shortly after birth. Unless the calf has received some type of protection, it is very susceptible to developing colibacillosis. The bacteria attach to the lining cells of the intestine by means of projections called pili. After attachment, the bacteria produce toxins which cause the intestine to secrete large amounts of fluid which results in diarrhea, dehydration and possible death.

Clostridium perfringens Type C: *Clostridium perfringens* Type C is commonly found in soil. It is also a common inhabitant of the intestinal tract in healthy animals. Engorgement with milk is often a predisposing factor. Type C enterotoxemia is caused by an overgrowth of these bacteria in the calf's intestine. This results in severe toxemia and high mortality rates. Calves may be found dead without showing any symptoms. They may show signs including bloating, abdominal pain, hemorrhagic diarrhea or extreme weakness.

Prevention: Preventing baby calf scours requires careful management of the dam, the environment, and the calf. The most important step in the program is immunization of the dam with an effective vaccine. This will result in high levels of maternal antibodies passed to the calf through the colostrum it receives after birth. SCOUR BOS™ 9 is the ideal vaccine because it

S

provides heterologous coverage for multiple rotavirus serotypes, coronavirus, 4 types of *E. coli*, and *Clostridium perfringens* Type C.

It is vital that herds are managed to insure that all calves receive adequate levels of colostrum within the first critical hours after birth. In severe outbreaks, it may also be necessary for dairy calves to continue receiving milk from vaccinated cows, free of Johne's disease, until they have passed the susceptible age.

Trial Data: *Cl. perfringens* Type C Antitoxin Titers:

Group (pooled samples)	Titer (AU/mL)
Dam's colostrum	≥ 50 < 100
Calf serum (3 days of age)	≥ 10
Calf serum (10 days of age)	≥ 10

E. coli Challenge:

Group	% Mortality	Avg. Clinical Score
Vaccinates	0%	1.5
Controls	70% p = 0.0002	82.9 p = 0.0000
	Extremely Significant	

Coronavirus Challenge:

Group	Geometric Mean Titers: Calf Serum	Geometric Mean Titers: Dam Colostrum	Dehydration Difference	Depression Difference	Clinical Difference
Vaccinates	2.5X increase	4X increase	p = 0.0004	p = 0.0005	p = 0.0003
Controls	baseline	baseline	Extremely Significant		

Rotavirus Challenge:

Group	Geometric Mean Titers: Calf Serum	Geometric Mean Titers: Dam Colostrum	Dehydration Difference	Depression Difference	Clinical Difference
Vaccinates	13X increase	7X increase	p = 0.0004	p = 0.0004	p = 0.001
Controls	baseline	baseline	Extremely Significant		

Presentation: Available in 10 dose (20 mL) and 50 dose (100 mL) bottles.
Compendium Code No.: 11140472 MP-F251-APR00

SCOURGUARD 3® (K)

Pfizer Animal Health **Bacterin-Toxoid-Vaccine**

Bovine Rota-Coronavirus Vaccine, Killed Virus-Escherichia Coli Bacterin

U.S. Vet. Lic. No.: 189

Description: SCOURGUARD 3® (K) is a liquid preparation of inactivated bovine rotavirus and coronavirus propagated on established cell lines and K99 *E. coli* bacterin adjuvanted to enhance the immune response.

Contains gentamicin as preservative.

Indications: SCOURGUARD 3® (K) is for vaccination of healthy, pregnant cows as an aid in passive maternal immunization of their calves against neonatal calf diarrhea caused by bovine rotavirus, bovine coronavirus, and enterotoxigenic strains of *Escherichia coli (E. coli)* having the K99 pili adherence factor.

Directions:

1. General Directions: Vaccination of healthy, pregnant cows is recommended. Shake well. Aseptically administer 2 mL intramuscularly (IM) only. In accordance with Beef Quality Assurance guidelines, this product should be administered in the muscular region of the neck.
2. Primary Vaccination: Administer 2 IM doses at least 2 weeks apart to pregnant cows, with the second dose given 2-3 weeks before calving. If cows have not calved within 40 days after receiving their last dose, revaccination with a single dose is recommended.
3. Revaccination: Revaccination with a single dose 2-3 weeks before each subsequent calving is recommended.
4. Good animal husbandry and herd health management practices should be employed.

Precaution(s): Store at 2°-7°C. Prolonged exposure to higher temperatures may adversely affect potency. Do not freeze.

Use entire contents when first opened.

Sterilized syringes and needles should be used to administer this vaccine.

Transient temperature increases may occur following vaccination.

Caution(s): As with many vaccines, anaphylaxis may occur after use. Initial antidote of epinephrine is recommended and should be followed with appropriate supportive therapy.

S

This product has been shown to be efficacious in healthy animals. A protective immune response may not be elicited if animals are incubating an infectious disease, are malnourished or parasitized, are stressed due to shipment or environmental conditions, are otherwise immunocompromised, or the vaccine is not administered in accordance with label directions.

Warning(s): Do not vaccinate within 21 days before slaughter.

For veterinary use only.

Discussion: Disease Description: Neonatal calf diarrhea is a disease of complex origin that can be caused by both viral and bacterial agents. Enterotoxigenic *E. coli*, rotavirus, and coronavirus are commonly isolated from scouring calves, often in combination with other bacteria or viruses.[1,2] Studies have shown that most enterotoxigenic *E. coli* strains isolated from scouring calves have K99 pili, antigenic structures which facilitate colonization of the gut lining.[3,4] Enterotoxins produced by those strains, combined with intestinal cell damage by rotavirus and coronavirus, cause secretion of body fluids and electrolytes into the gut. Such fluid loss produces a severe diarrhea, which results in dehydration, electrolyte imbalance, and metabolic acidosis. Incidence of calf diarrhea is most frequent and severe within the first 2 weeks of life.[2,5-7] Hence, a calf's primary source of protection is immediate consumption of colostrum containing high levels of maternal antibodies for effective passive immunization.[8-10]

Trial Data: Safety and Efficacy: No adverse postvaccination reactions, either local or systemic, were observed in over 1,600 vaccinated pregnant cows during product development.

For effective passive immunization, newborn calves must immediately consume and absorb adequate amounts of colostrum containing high levels (titers) of maternal antibodies. In efficacy studies of the rota-coronavirus vaccine, the effect of vaccination on colostrum and milk antibody titers, i.e., lactogenic immunity, was evaluated. Pregnant cattle were vaccinated with 2 doses, and colostrum/milk samples were collected on the day of calving and at weekly intervals after calving. Similar samples were also collected from nonvaccinated control cows. All samples were analyzed for antibody titers against rotavirus and coronavirus.

Results presented in Table 1 show that cows that calved within 40 days of vaccination had mean colostrum/milk virus-neutralizing (VN) antibody titers against rotavirus that were 45-fold higher than in nonvaccinated cows on the day of calving and were still 4-fold higher than in nonvaccinated cows at 24-29 days after calving. Vaccinated cows had mean VN antibody titers against coronavirus that were 3.5-fold higher than VN antibody titers of nonvaccinated cows on the day of calving.

Table 1. Mean Postcalving Colostrum/Milk Antibody Titers in SCOURGUARD 3® (K)-Vaccinated Cows and Nonvaccinated Cows

Test Group	Mean Colostrum/Milk VN Antibody Titers[1] at Days After Calving: 0	3-7	10-14	17-21	24-29
Rotavirus					
14 Vaccinated cows	4096	91	56	88	34
9 Nonvaccinated cows	91	8	11	11	8
Coronavirus					
14 Vaccinated cows	1024	104	44	34	21
9 Nonvaccinated cows	294	38	23	28	20

[1] Virus-neutralization antibody titers expressed as reciprocals of endpoint dilutions; geometric mean.

Efficacy of the *E. coli* K99 factor was demonstrated in a controlled challenge-of-immunity study. Pregnant cows that received 2 doses of bacterin provided maternal immunity which fully protected 80% of their calves from virulent challenge. The remaining 20% of calves in that group experienced transient diarrhea lasting less than 48 hours, with no deaths occurring. Conversely, 100% of calves from nonvaccinated cows experienced severe diarrhea resulting in a 58.8% death loss after challenge.

Serological studies indicated no immunologic interference among the viral and bacterial components of SCOURGUARD 3® (K). After administration of this product, antibody titers to each of the viral components were slightly higher than after administration of rota-coronavirus vaccine alone.

References: Available upon request.

Presentation: 10 dose and 50 dose vials.

Compendium Code No.: 36900630 75-4854-05

SCOURGUARD 3® (K)/C

Pfizer Animal Health **Bacterin-Toxoid-Vaccine**

Bovine Rota-Coronavirus Vaccine, Killed Virus-Clostridium Perfringens Type C-Escherichia Coli Bacterin-Toxoid

U.S. Vet. Lic. No.: 189

Description: SCOURGUARD 3® (K)/C contains a liquid preparation of inactivated bovine rotavirus and coronavirus propagated on established cell lines, a K99 *E. coli* bacterin, and *Cl. perfringens* type C toxoid. The vaccine is adjuvanted to enhance the immune response.

Contains gentamicin and merthiolate as preservatives.

Indications: SCOURGUARD 3® (K)/C is for vaccination of healthy, pregnant cows as an aid in passive maternal immunization of their calves against neonatal calf diarrhea caused by bovine rotavirus, bovine coronavirus, enterotoxigenic strains of *Escherichia coli (E. coli)* having the K99 pili adherence factor, and neonatal calf diarrhea caused by *Clostridium perfringens (Cl. perfringens)* type C (beta) toxin.

Directions:

1. General Directions: Vaccination of healthy, pregnant cows is recommended. Shake well. Aseptically administer 2 mL intramuscularly (IM) only. In accordance with Beef Quality Assurance guidelines, this product should be administered in the muscular region of the neck.
2. Primary Vaccination: Administer 2 IM doses at least 2 weeks apart to pregnant cows, with the second dose given 2-3 weeks before calving. If cows have not calved within 40 days after receiving their last dose, revaccination with a single dose is recommended.
3. Revaccination: Revaccination with a single dose 2-3 weeks before each subsequent calving is recommended.
4. Good animal husbandry and herd health management practices should be employed.

Precaution(s): Store at 2°-7°C. Prolonged exposure to higher temperatures may adversely affect potency. Do not freeze.

Use entire contents when first opened.

Sterilized syringes and needles should be used to administer this vaccine.

Transient temperature increases may occur following vaccination.

Caution(s): As with many vaccines, anaphylaxis may occur after use. Initial antidote of epinephrine is recommended and should be followed with appropriate supportive therapy.

This product has been shown to be efficacious in healthy animals. A protective immune response may not be elicited if animals are incubating an infectious disease, are malnourished or parasitized, are stressed due to shipment or environmental conditions, are otherwise immunocompromised, or the vaccine is not administered in accordance with label directions.

Warning(s): Do not vaccinate within 21 days before slaughter.

For veterinary use only.

Discussion: Disease Description: Neonatal calf diarrhea is a disease of complex origin that can be caused by both viral and bacterial agents. Enterotoxigenic *E. coli*, rotavirus, and coronavirus are commonly isolated from scouring calves, often in combination with other bacteria or viruses.[1,2] Studies have shown that most enterotoxigenic *E. coli* strains isolated from scouring calves have K99 pili, antigenic structures which facilitate colonization of the gut lining.[3,4] Enterotoxins produced by those strains, combined with intestinal cell damage by rotavirus and coronavirus, cause secretion of body fluids and electrolytes into the gut. Such fluid loss produces a severe diarrhea, which results in dehydration, electrolyte imbalance, and metabolic acidosis. Incidence of calf diarrhea is most frequent and severe within the first 2 weeks of life.[5,6] Hence, a calf's primary source of protection is immediate consumption of colostrum containing high levels of maternal antibodies for effective passive immunization.[7,8]

In cattle, infection with *Cl. perfringens* type C causes severe enteritis, dysentery, and toxemia, as well as high mortality in calves. It can also cause enterotoxemia in adult cattle.

Trial Data: Safety and Efficacy: Immunogenicity tests measuring antibody levels were conducted for all components of SCOURGUARD 3® (K)/C. Serological response to vaccination in pregnant test cows was compared to that in nonvaccinated control cows. Table 1 shows antibody response in both colostrum and calf serum to *Cl. perfringens* type C toxoid, when administered as part of the combined vaccine (containing all the antigens in SCOURGUARD 3® (K)/C).

Table 1. Geometric Mean Antibody Response in Colostrum and Calf Serum to *Cl. perfringens* Type C (beta) Toxoid in a Polyvalent Vaccine

Test Group and Sample	Serologic Value*
Group 1 (Vaccinates)	
Colostral Ab	>37.0
Calf serum Ab (3 days)	>17.7
Calf serum Ab (30 days)	8.6
Group 2 (Nonvaccinates)	
Colostral Ab	<0.70
Calf serum Ab (3 days)	<0.73
Calf serum Ab (30 days)	0.53

* Geometric mean levels are antitoxin levels expressed in international units (IU) of antitoxin/mL for both colostrum and calf serum.

The protective level of type C antitoxin for cattle has not been determined experimentally, but a level of 0.10 to 0.15 IU/mL for both colostrum and serum has been determined to be protective in sheep,[9] and that level is generally considered protective in cattle as well. Type C antitoxin levels in colostrum and calf serum far exceeding the 0.15 IU/mL level occurred following vaccination, even when calves were born as many as 117 days after the cow received her last vaccine dose.

In immunogenicity studies of the rota-coronavirus vaccine component, the effect of vaccination on colostrum and milk antibody levels was evaluated. Colostrum samples were collected from vaccinated cows on the day of calving. Milk samples were collected from cows at various intervals after calving. Similar samples were collected from nonvaccinated control cows. All samples were tested for antibody levels against rotavirus and coronavirus.

Results presented in Table 2 show antibody levels in both colostrum and milk to rotavirus and coronavirus components of the combined vaccine, which contained all the antigens in SCOURGUARD 3® (K)/C. The geometric mean antibody levels to rotavirus and coronavirus were significantly greater in vaccinates than in nonvaccinates.

Table 2. Mean Antibody Response in Colostrum and Milk to Rotavirus and Coronavirus in a Polyvalent Vaccine

Test Group and Sample	Immunizing Agent and Serological Value	
	Rotavirus	Coronavirus
Group 1 (Vaccinates: N=14)		
Colostral Ab	4096	1024
Milk Ab (3-7 days)	91	104
Milk Ab (24-29 days)	34	21
Group 2 (Nonvaccinates: N=9)		
Colostral Ab	91	294
Milk Ab (3-7 days)	8	38
Milk Ab (24-29 days)	8	20

* Reciprocal geometric mean titers.

Efficacy of the *E. coli* K99 factor was demonstrated in a controlled challenge-of-immunity study. Pregnant cows that received 2 doses of bacterin provided maternal immunity which fully protected 80% of their calves from virulent challenge. The remaining 20% of calves in that group experienced transient diarrhea lasting less than 48 hours, with no deaths occurring. Conversely, 100% of calves from nonvaccinated cows experienced severe diarrhea resulting in a 58.8% death loss after challenge.

References: Available upon request.
Presentation: 10 dose and 50 dose vials.
Compendium Code No.: 36900640 75-4858-04

SCOURMUNE®

Schering-Plough **Bacterin**
Escherichia coli Bacterin
U.S. Vet. Lic. No.: 165A
Active Ingredient(s): *Escherichia coli* bacterin. Contains pili types K88, K99, 987P and type 1, aluminum hydroxide adsorbed.

Preservatives: Formaldehyde and gentamicin.

Indications: This product is recommended for use in healthy pregnant gilts and sows to aid in the control of neonatal pig diarrhea caused by *E. coli* expressing pili types K88, K99, 987P and type 1.
Dosage and Administration: Shake well before each use and administer using normal aseptic techniques.

First farrowing: Two (2) doses are necessary for immunization.

First dose: Inject 2 mL subcutaneously into healthy pregnant swine six (6) to seven (7) weeks prior to farrowing.

Second dose: Inject 2 mL subcutaneously three (3) to four (4) weeks following the first dose.

Subsequent farrowing: A single 2 mL dose should be administered two (2) to three (3) weeks prior to each subsequent farrowing.

Precaution(s): Store at 2-7°C (35-45°F). Do not freeze. Use the entire contents when first opened.
Caution(s): Transient local reactions may be observed at the injection site. If an allergic response occurs, administer epinephrine or its equivalent.
Warning(s): Do not vaccinate within 21 days before slaughter.
Presentation: 25 dose (50 mL) vials.
Compendium Code No.: 10471780

SCOURMUNE®-C

Schering-Plough **Bacterin-Toxoid**
Clostridium perfringens Type C-Escherichia coli Bacterin-Toxoid
U.S. Vet. Lic. No.: 165A
Active Ingredient(s): *Clostridium perfringens* type C, *Escherichia coli** bacterin-toxoid.

*Contains pili types K88, K99, 987P and type 1.

Preservatives: Formaldehyde and gentamicin.

Indications: This product is recommended for use in healthy pregnant gilts and sows to aid in the control of colibacillosis by *E. coli* expressing pili types K88, K99, 987P and type 1 and enterotoxemia caused by *Cl. perfringens* type C.
Dosage and Administration: Two (2) doses are necessary for immunization. Shake well before each use and administer using normal aseptic techniques.

First dose: Inject 2 mL subcutaneously into healthy pregnant swine six (6) to seven (7) weeks prior to farrowing.

Second dose: Inject 2 mL subcutaneously three (3) to four (4) weeks following the first dose.

Subsequent farrowing: A single 2 mL dose should be administered two (2) to three (3) weeks prior to each subsequent farrowing.

Precaution(s): Store at 2-7°C (35-45°F). Do not freeze. Use the entire contents when first opened.
Caution(s): Do not use intramuscularly. Transient local reactions may be observed at the injection site. If an allergic response occurs, administer epinephrine or its equivalent.
Warning(s): Do not vaccinate within 21 days before slaughter.
Presentation: 10 dose (20 mL) and 25 dose (50 mL) vials.
Compendium Code No.: 10471791

SCOURMUNE®-CR

Schering-Plough **Bacterin-Toxoid-Vaccine**
Porcine Rotavirus Vaccine, Killed Virus-Clostridium perfringens Type C-Escherichia coli Bacterin-Toxoid
U.S. Vet. Lic. No.: 165A
Active Ingredient(s): Porcine rotavirus vaccine (killed virus) *Clostridium perfringens* type C, *Escherichia coli* bacterin-toxoid.

Preservative: Gentamicin.

Indications: SCOURMUNE®-CR is recommended for use in healthy pregnant gilts and sows to aid in the prevention and control of baby pig diarrhea caused by porcine rotavirus and enterotoxigenic *E. coli* expressing pili types K88, K99, 987P and type 1 and enterotoxemia caused by *Cl. perfringens* type C.
Dosage and Administration: Two (2) doses prior to each farrowing are required.

First dose: 2 mL intramuscularly (I.M.) six (6) to seven (7) weeks prior to farrowing.

Second dose: 2 mL I.M. three (3) to four (4) weeks following the first dose.

Precaution(s): Store at 2-7°C (35-45°F). Do not freeze. Use entire contents when first opened.
Caution(s): Transient local reactions may be observed at the injection site. If an allergic reaction occurs, administer epinephrine or its equivalent.
Warning(s): Do not vaccinate within 60 days before slaughter.
Presentation: 10 dose (20 mL) and 25 dose (50 mL) vials.
Compendium Code No.: 10471800

SCOUR VAC™ 2K

Durvet **Vaccine**
Bovine Rota-Coronavirus Vaccine, Killed Virus
U.S. Vet. Lic. No.: 303
Composition: This vaccine contains inactivated bovine rotavirus and bovine coronavirus adjuvanted with oil. Contains amphotericin B, penicillin, streptomycin, and thimerosal as preservatives.
Indications: For use in healthy pregnant cattle as an aid in the prevention and control of disease in calves caused by bovine rotavirus and bovine coronavirus.
Dosage and Administration: Shake well before using. Administer 2 mL intramuscularly 8-10 weeks prior to calving. Repeat in 6 weeks. Revaccinate with one dose 8-10 weeks prior to each subsequent calving.
Precaution(s): Store in the dark at 35°-45°F. (2°-7°C). Do not freeze. Use entire contents when first opened.
Caution(s): It is essential that newborn calves receive colostrum from the vaccinated dam. This product may cause persistent swelling at the site of injection. Anaphylactic reactions may occur following the use of this biological. Symptomatic treatment: Epinephrine.
Warning(s): Do not vaccinate within 60 days prior to slaughter.
Presentation: 10 doses (20 mL) and 50 doses (100 mL).
Manufactured by: Advance Biologics, Inc., Freeman SD 57029.
Compendium Code No.: 10841871 9/00

SCOUR VAC™ 3K+C

Durvet **Bacterin-Toxoid-Vaccine**
Bovine Rota-Coronavirus Vaccine, Killed Virus-Clostridium Perfringens Type C-Escherichia Coli Bacterin-Toxoid
U.S. Vet. Lic. No.: 303
Composition: This product contains inactivated bovine rotavirus, bovine coronavirus, *Clostridium perfringens* Type C, and K99 piliated *Escherichia coli* adjuvanted with oil. Contains amphotericin B, penicillin, streptomycin, and thimerosal as preservatives.
Indications: For use in healthy pregnant cattle as an aid in the prevention and control of disease in calves caused by bovine rotavirus, bovine coronavirus, *Clostridium perfringens* Type C, and K99 piliated *Escherichia coli.*
Dosage and Administration: Shake well before using. Administer 2 mL intramuscularly 8-10 weeks prior to calving. Revaccinate with Scour Vac™ 2K (Bovine Rota-Coronavirus Vaccine) in 6 weeks. Revaccinate with one dose 8-10 weeks prior to each subsequent calving.
Precaution(s): Store in the dark at 35°-45°F. (2°-7°C). Do not freeze. Use entire contents when first opened.
Caution(s): It is essential that newborn calves receive colostrum from the vaccinated dam. This product may cause persistent swelling at the site of injection. Anaphylactic reactions may occur following the use of this biological. Symptomatic treatment: Epinephrine.
Warning(s): Do not vaccinate within 60 days prior to slaughter.
Presentation: 10 doses (20 mL) and 50 doses (100 mL).
Manufactured by: Advance Biologics, Inc., Freeman SD 57029.
Compendium Code No.: 10841881 9/00

SCOUR VAC™ 4

AgriLabs **Vaccine**
Bovine Rota-Coronavirus Vaccine, Killed Virus
U.S. Vet. Lic. No.: 303
Composition: This vaccine contains inactivated bovine rotavirus and bovine coronavirus adjuvanted with oil. Contains amphotericin B, penicillin, streptomycin, and thimerosal as preservatives.
Indications: For use in healthy pregnant cattle as an aid in the prevention and control of disease in calves caused by bovine rotavirus and bovine coronavirus.
Dosage and Administration: Shake well before using. Administer 2 mL intramuscularly 8-10

weeks prior to calving. Repeat in 6 weeks. Revaccinate with one dose 8-10 weeks prior to each subsequent calving.

Precaution(s): Store in the dark at 35°-45°F (2°-7°C). Do not freeze. Use entire contents when first opened.

Caution(s): It is essential that newborn calves receive colostrum from the vaccinated dam. Anaphylactic reactions may occur following the use of this biological. Symptomatic treatment: Epinephrine.

For veterinary use only.

Warning(s): Do not vaccinate within 60 days prior to slaughter.

This product may cause persistent swelling at the site of injection.

Presentation: 10 dose (20 mL) and 50 dose (100 mL) vials.

Manufactured by: Agri Lab Biologicals, Inc., St. Joseph, MO 64503

Compendium Code No.: 10581390 AL 248 / AL 249

SCOUR VAC™ 9

AgriLabs **Bacterin-Toxoid-Vaccine**

Bovine Rota-Coronavirus Vaccine, Killed Virus-Clostridium Perfringens Type C-Escherichia Coli Bacterin-Toxoid

U.S. Vet. Lic. No.: 303

Composition: This product contains inactivated cultures of bovine rotavirus, bovine coronavirus, *Clostridium perfringens* Type C, and K99 piliated *Escherichia coli* adjuvanted with oil. Contains amphotericin B, penicillin, streptomycin, and thimerosal as preservatives.

Indications: For use in healthy pregnant cattle as an aid in the prevention and control of disease in calves caused by bovine rotavirus, bovine coronavirus, *Clostridium perfringens* Type C, and K99 piliated *Escherichia coli.*

Dosage and Administration: Shake well before using. Administer 2 mL intramuscularly 8-10 weeks prior to calving. Revaccinate with Scour Vac™ 4 (Bovine Rota-Coronavirus Vaccine) in 6 weeks. Revaccinate with one dose 8-10 weeks prior to each subsequent calving.

Precaution(s): Store in the dark at 35°-45°F (2°-7°C). Do not freeze. Use entire contents when first opened.

Caution(s): It is essential that newborn calves receive colostrum from the vaccinated dam. Anaphylactic reactions may occur following the use of this biological. Symptomatic treatment: Epinephrine.

For veterinary use only.

Warning(s): Do not vaccinate within 60 days prior to slaughter.

This product may cause persistent swelling at the site of injection.

Presentation: 10 dose (20 mL) and 50 dose (100 mL) vials.

Manufactured by: Agri Lab Biologicals, Inc., St. Joseph, MO 64503

Compendium Code No.: 10581400 AL 251

SCOUR VAC™ E COLI + C

AgriLabs **Bacterin-Toxoid**

Clostridium Perfringens Type C-Escherichia Coli Bacterin-Toxoid

U.S. Vet. Lic. No.: 303

Composition: This product contains inactivated cultures of *Clostridium perfringens* Type C and K99 piliated *Escherichia coli* adjuvanted with oil. Contains thimerosal as a preservative.

Indications: For use in healthy pregnant cattle as an aid in the prevention and control of enterotoxemia in calves caused by *Clostridium perfringens* Type C and colibacillosis in calves caused by K99 piliated *Escherichia coli.*

Dosage and Administration: Shake well before using. Administer 1 mL intramuscularly 1-3 months prior to calving. Vaccinate dairy cows during the dry off period. Revaccinate prior to each subsequent calving.

Precaution(s): Store in the dark at 35°-45°F (2°-7°C). Do not freeze. Use entire contents when first opened.

Caution(s): It is essential that calves receive colostrum from the vaccinated dam. Anaphylactic reactions may occur following the use of this biological. Symptomatic treatment: Epinephrine.

For veterinary use only.

Warning(s): Do not vaccinate within 60 days prior to slaughter.

This product may cause persistent swelling at the site of injection.

Presentation: 20 dose (20 mL) and 100 dose (100 mL) vials.

Manufactured by: Agri Lab Biologicals, Inc., St. Joseph, MO 64503

Compendium Code No.: 10581410 AL 246 / AL 247

SCRATCHEX® 30 DAY FLEA & TICK TREATMENT (30 LBS. & UNDER)

S

Combe **Flea Control**

EPA Reg. No.: 28293-293-4306

Active Ingredient(s):

Permethrin (CAS #52645-53-1) 45.0%
Other Ingredients 55.0%

Indications: Kills fleas before they lay eggs.

Kills and repels the deer tick which may carry Lyme Disease.

Directions for Use: Read entire label before each use.

It is a violation of Federal law to use this product in a manner inconsistent with its labeling.

This product contains three monthly dosages, each 1 mL, for Dogs and Puppies 30 pounds and under. Apply the full contents of a single applicator tube between the dog's shoulder blades.

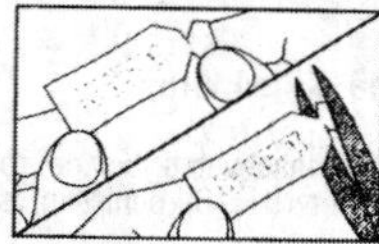

1. Remove applicator tube from package and hold in an upright position.
2. Twist or cut off top of applicator tube.

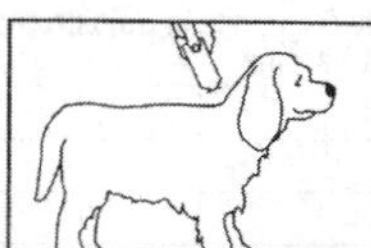

3. Position the tip of the applicator tube on the dog's back between the shoulder blades and squeeze out the entire contents of the applicator tube.

Reapply every 30 days.

Contraindication(s): Do not use on puppies less than six months old.

Precautionary Statements: Hazards to Humans and Domestic Animals:

Caution: Humans Causes eye irritation. Avoid contact with eyes or clothing. Wash thoroughly with soap and water after handling. Animals Do not use on cats. Do not use on puppies less than six months old. Consult a veterinarian before using this product on debilitated, aged, pregnant or nursing animals, or animals on medication. Sensitivities may occur after using any pesticide product for pets. If signs of sensitivity occur; bathe your pet with mild soap and rinse with large amounts of water. If signs continue, consult a veterinarian immediately.

Environmental Hazards: This product is toxic to fish. Do not add directly to water. Do not contaminate water when disposing of product or packaging.

First Aid:

If in Eyes: Flush with plenty of water. Call a physician if irritation persists.

As with all flea and tick products, this product is most effective when used as part of a total program aimed at reducing fleas and ticks in your pet's environment. Be sure to treat the animal's bedding and the areas it frequents with products registered for these uses.

Storage and Disposal: Do not contaminate water, food or feed by storage and disposal. Store in a cool, dry place. Do not reuse empty tube. Wrap and discard in trash.

Warning(s): Keep out of reach of children.

Presentation: 3 tubes, 1 mL (0.03 fl oz) each, 3 mL (0.09 fl oz) total.

Compendium Code No.: 10290000

SCRATCHEX® 30 DAY FLEA & TICK TREATMENT (OVER 30 LBS.)

Combe **Flea Control**

EPA Reg. No.: 28293-293-4306

Active Ingredient(s):

Permethrin (CAS #52645-53-1) 45.0%
Other Ingredients 55.0%

Indications: Kills fleas before they lay eggs.

Kills and repels the deer tick which may carry Lyme Disease.

Directions for Use: Read entire label before each use.

It is a violation of Federal law to use this product in a manner inconsistent with its labeling.

This product contains three monthly dosages, each 2 mL, for Dogs and Puppies over 30 pounds and under. Apply one-half of the applicator tube's contents between the dog's shoulder blades, the second one-half of the applicator tube's contents to the base of the dog's tail.

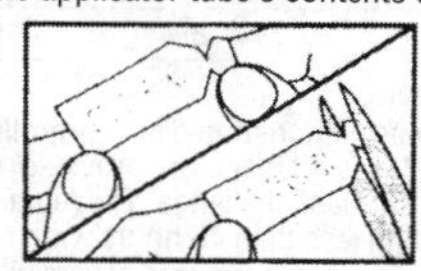

1. Remove applicator tube from package and hold in an upright position.
2. Twist or cut off top of applicator tube.

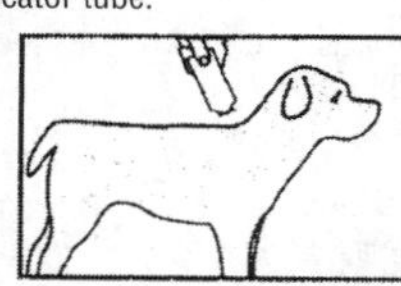

3. Position the tip of the applicator tube on the dog's back between the shoulder blades and squeeze out one-half of the contents of the applicator tube.

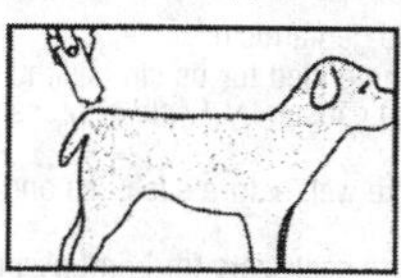

4. Next, position the tip of the applicator tube at the base of the tail and squeeze out the remaining contents on the base of the tail.

Reapply every 30 days.

Contraindication(s): Do not use on puppies less than six months old.

Precautionary Statements: Hazards to Humans and Domestic Animals:

Caution: Humans Causes eye irritation. Avoid contact with eyes or clothing. Wash thoroughly with soap and water after handling. Animals Do not use on cats. Do not use on puppies less than six months old. Consult a veterinarian before using this product on debilitated, aged, pregnant or nursing animals, or animals on medication. Sensitivities may occur after using any pesticide product for pets. If signs of sensitivity occur; bathe your pet with mild soap and rinse with large amounts of water. If signs continue, consult a veterinarian immediately.

Environmental Hazards: This product is toxic to fish. Do not add directly to water. Do not contaminate water when disposing of product or packaging.

First Aid:

If in Eyes: Flush with plenty of water. Call a physician if irritation persists.

As with all flea and tick products, this product is most effective when used as part of a total program aimed at reducing fleas and ticks in your pet's environment. Be sure to treat the animal's bedding and the areas it frequents with products registered for these uses.

Storage and Disposal: Do not contaminate water, food or feed by storage and disposal. Store in a cool, dry place. Do not reuse empty tube. Wrap and discard in trash.

Warning(s): Keep out of reach of children.

Presentation: 3 tubes, 2 mL (0.06 fl oz) each, 6 mL (0.18 fl oz) total.

Compendium Code No.: 10290010

SCRATCHEX® FLEA & TICK COLLAR FOR CATS

Combe **Parasiticide Collar**

EPA Reg. No.: 4306-16

Active Ingredient(s):

Chlorpyrifos [0,0-diethyl 0-(3,5,6-trichloro-2-pyridyl) phosphorothioate] 3%
Inert ingredients 97%
Total 100%

Indications: SCRATCHEX® Flea & Tick Collar for Cats with Dursban® insecticide provides 11 month flea killing and six month protection against ticks on cats of all sizes.

The collar will reach its maximum effectiveness within two to three days after placing it on the cat and will continue to protect the cat against fleas for 11 months and ticks for six months. Ticks are only occasional and usually temporary pests of cats.

Dosage and Administration: It is a violation of federal law to use the product in a manner inconsistent with its labeling.

Place the collar around the cat's neck, buckle and adjust it for proper fit. Cut off close to the buckle and dispose of the excess length. The collar must be worn loosely so that two fingers may be placed between the collar and the cat's neck. If the collar is worn too tightly, it may produce neck irritation. Fleas and ticks present in the cat's environment that may re-appear on the pet will be killed by the action of the collar. The collar's effectiveness is not diminished by normal wetting such as rainfall. Use only one (1) collar on an animal at a time.

Precaution(s):

Storage: Store in the original unopened container away from children.

Disposal: Do not re-use the empty box, pouch, or collar. Wrap it in newspaper and put it in the trash collection.

Caution(s): Precautionary Statements:

Hazards to Humans and Domestic Animals: Do not open the protective pouch until ready to use. The collar is intended for use as an insecticide generator and is not to be taken internally by man or animals. Not intended for use by humans. Do not allow children to play with the collar. Wash hands with soap and water after handling the collar. Do not use on sick or debilitated animals or cats under 12 weeks of age.

Do not use other cholinesterase inhibiting insecticides on the animal while wearing the collar. Some cats may be sensitive to the collar. Remove at the first sign of irritation or adverse reaction (muscular tremor, salivation, vomiting and/or diarrhea).

The insecticide in the collar is a cholinesterase inhibitor.

Antidote(s): Note to Physician/Veterinarian: Atropine only by injection is antidotal. Use only if symptoms of cholinesterase inhibition are present.

Presentation: One 0.46 oz. collar.

* Dursban is a registered trademark of DowElanco.

Compendium Code No.: 10290020

SCRATCHEX® FLEA & TICK COLLAR FOR DOGS

Combe **Parasiticide Collar**

EPA Reg. No.: 4306-15

Active Ingredient(s):

Chlorpyrifos [0,0-diethyl 0-(3,5,6-trichloro-2-pyridyl) phosphorothioate] 8%
Inert ingredients 92%
Total 100%

Indications: SCRATCHEX® Flea & Tick Collar for Dogs with Dursban® insecticide provides 12 month flea killing and seven month protection against ticks on dogs of all sizes.

The collar will reach its maximum effectiveness within two to three days after placing it on the dog and will continue to protect the dog against fleas for up to 12 months and ticks for up to seven months.

Dosage and Administration: It is a violation of federal law to use the product in a manner inconsistent with its labeling.

Place the collar around the dog's neck, buckle and adjust it for proper fit. Cut off close to the buckle and dispose of the excess length. The collar must be worn loosely so that two fingers may be placed between the collar and the dog's neck. If the collar is worn too tightly, it may produce neck irritation. Fleas and ticks present in the dog's environment that may re-appear on the pet will be killed by the action of the collar. The collar's effectiveness is not diminished by normal wetting such as rainfall. Use only one (1) collar on an animal at a time.

Precaution(s):

Storage: Store in the original unopened container away from children.

Disposal: Do not re-use the empty box, pouch, or collar. Wrap it in newspaper and put it in the trash collection.

Caution(s): Precautionary Statements:

Hazards to Humans and Domestic Animals: Do not open the protective pouch until ready to use. The collar is intended for use as an insecticide generator and is not to be taken internally by man or animals. Not intended for use by humans. Do not allow children to play with the collar. Wash hands with soap and water after handling the collar. Do not use on sick or debilitated animals or dogs under 12 weeks of age.

Do not use other cholinesterase inhibiting insecticides on the animal while wearing the collar. Some dogs may be sensitive to the collar. Remove at the first sign of irritation or adverse reaction (muscular tremor, salivation, vomiting and/or diarrhea).

The insecticide in the collar is a cholinesterase inhibitor.

Antidote(s): Note to Physician/Veterinarian: Atropine only by injection is antidotal. Use only if symptoms of cholinesterase inhibition are present.

Presentation: One 1.1 oz. collar.

* Dursban is a registered trademark of DowElanco.

Compendium Code No.: 10290030

SCRATCHEX® FLEA & TICK POWDER

Combe **Parasiticide Powder**

EPA Reg. No.: 4306-10

Active Ingredient(s):

Pyrethrins 0.067%
Piperonyl butoxide, technical* 0.134%
N-octyl bicycloheptene dicarboximide** 0.224%
Carbaryl (1-napthyl n-methylcarbamate) 5.000%
Inert ingredients 94.575%
Total 100.000%

*Equivalent to 0.107% (butycarbityl) (6-propylpiperonyl) ether and 0.027% other related compounds.

**MGK 264 insecticide synergist.

Indications: The double-insecticide formula of SCRATCHEX® Powder kills fleas, ticks and lice and helps prevent re-infestation.

Dosage and Administration: It is a violation of federal law to use the product in a manner inconsistent with its labeling.

To kill fleas and ticks on dogs and cats, dust the powder liberally over the animal by shaking or squeezing the powder from the container. Begin at the head and work backwards, being sure to work the powder down to the skin. Treat the feet and legs. Dust the pet's sleeping area or bedding. Repeat as necessary for control.

Precaution(s):

Storage: Store in a cool, dry place.

Disposal: Do not re-use the empty container. Wrap the container in several layers of newspaper and put it in the trash collection.

Caution(s): Keep out of the reach of children.

Precautionary Statements:

Hazards to Humans and Domestic Animals: Harmful if swallowed. Do not inhale dust. Avoid contact with the eyes. In case of contact, immediately flush the eyes or skin with plenty of water. Get medical attention if irritation persists. Do not use on pregnant dogs or cats, or on kittens or puppies under four weeks of age. Wash hands after use.

Presentation: 3.75 oz. squeeze bottle

Compendium Code No.: 10290040

SCRATCHEX® FLEA & TICK SHAMPOO

Combe **Parasiticide Shampoo**

EPA Reg. No.: 4306-7

Active Ingredient(s):

Pyrethrins 0.072%
Piperonyl butoxide, technical 0.144%
N-octyl bicycloheptene dicarboximide 0.240%
Inert ingredients 99.544%
Total 100.000%

Indications: SCRATCHEX® Flea & Tick Shampoo for dogs and cats has been specially formulated to kill fleas and ticks on contact and to condition the coat also. Thick, rich SCRATCHEX® Shampoo deep-cleans and deodorizes.

Directions for Use: It is a violation of federal law to use the product in a manner inconsistent with its labeling.

Wet the dog or cat's hair thoroughly with warm water. Starting with the head, rub the shampoo into the coat. Work backwards until the coat is completely covered with lather. Allow the lather to remain on the animal for five (5) minutes. Rinse thoroughly and towel dry.

It is recommended that the pet's bedding or sleeping quarters be treated for fleas, ticks, lices, or chiggers with a spray registered for such use.

Precautionary Statements: Hazards to Humans and Domestic Animals: Causes eye irritation. Do not get into the eyes. In case of contact, immediately flush the eyes with plenty of water. Get medical attention if irritation persists.

Storage and Disposal:

Storage: Store in a cool, dry place.

Disposal: Do not re-use the empty container. Wrap the container and put it in the trash collection.

Warning(s): Keep out of the reach of children.

Presentation: 8 fl oz (236 mL) and 12 fl oz (354 mL) bottles.

Compendium Code No.: 10290051

SCRATCHEX® FLEA & TICK SPRAY

Combe **Parasiticide Spray**

EPA Reg. No.: 4306-11

Active Ingredient(s):

Pyrethrins 0.056%
Permethrin [*3-phenoxyphenyl methyl (±) cis-trans-3-(2, 2-dichloroethenyl) 2, 2-dimethylcyclopropanecarboxylate] 0.050%
Related compounds 0.004%
Inert ingredients 99.890%
Total ingredients 100.000%

*cis-trans isomer ration: Min. 35% (±) cis, Max. 65% (±) trans.

Indications: SCRATCHEX® Flea & Tick Spray has been formulated to kill fleas for up to 14 days and ticks for up to four days on dogs, and fleas and ticks for up to nine days on cats. Safe for use on both dogs and cats, it can also be used safely on the pet's bedding, furniture and carpets to prevent re-infestation. Kills ticks that can spread Lyme disease.

Directions for Use: It is a violation of Federal law to use the product in a manner inconsistent with its labeling.

Shake the container well before using. Hold the container upright during use. Spray the animal from a distance of 8-12 inches. Start spraying at the tail, moving the dispenser rapidly and making sure the animal's entire body is covered, including the legs and under the body. Fluff the hair while spraying so that the spray penetrates to the skin. The spray should wet the ticks thoroughly. Repeat as needed. Use in the pet's sleeping area or on bedding, walls, furniture, floors and carpeting to control re-infestation.

Precautionary Statements: Hazards to Humans and Domestic Animals: Harmful if swallowed. Avoid inhaling vapors. Do not spray in the eyes, face, or on genitalia. Do not use on nursing puppies or kittens under three months of age. Avoid contact with the skin or clothing.

Statement of Practical Treatment:

If swallowed: Call a physician or poison control center.

If in eyes: Flush with plenty of water. Get medical attention if irritation persists.

If on skin: Wash with soap and warm water. Get medical attention if irritation persists.

If inhaled: Remove the victim to fresh air and call a physician if effects occur.

Physical or Chemical Hazards: Contents under pressure. Do not use or store near heat or open flame. Do not incinerate the container. Exposure to temperatures above 130°F may cause bursting.

Storage and Disposal:

Storage: Store in a cool area away from heat and open flame.

Disposal: Do not re-use the empty container. Wrap the original container in several layers of newspapers and discard it in the trash.

Warning(s): Keep out of the reach of children.

Presentation: 7 fl oz (207 mL) bottle.

Compendium Code No.: 10290061

SCRATCHEX® SUPER SPRAY™

Combe **Parasiticide Spray**

with Fenoxycarb Insect Growth Regulator

EPA Reg. No.: 56493-85-4306

Active Ingredient(s):

Fenoxycarb [ethyl(2-(4-phenoxyphenoxy)ethyl]carbamate] 0.10%
d-trans-chrysanthemum monocarboxylic acid ester of
d-2-allayl-4-hydroxy-3-methyl-2-cyclopenten-1-one 0.10%
Permethrin [(3-phenoxyphenyl)methyl (±) cis-trans-3-
2,2-dichloroethenyl) 2,2-dimethyl cyclopropanecarboxylate)* 0.15%
Piperonyl butoxide, technical** 0.50%
N-octyl bicycloheptene dicarboximide 1.00%
Di-n-propyl isocinchomeronate*** 0.20%
Inert Ingredients 97.95%

*cis/trans isomer ratio: min. 35% (±) cis; max. 65% (±) trans.

**Equivalent to 0.4% (butylcarbityl) (6-propylpiperonyl) ether and 0.1% related compounds.

***MGK 326, insect repellent.

Indications: Kills fleas, flea eggs, and ticks and repels fleas and ticks on dogs and cats.

Directions for Use: Read entire label before each use.

Use only on dogs and cats.

It is a violation of Federal law to use this product in a manner inconsistent with its labeling. Shake well before using. For Dogs, Cats: Cover animal's eyes with hand and with a firm, fast stroke, to get proper spray mist, spray head, ears and chest. With fingertips, rub into face around mouth, nose and eyes. Then spray the neck, middle and hind quarters, finishing with legs last. Apply spray until animal is uniformly damp. Animal should not be soaked or sprayed to the point of run off. For best penetration, spray against natural lay of the hair. On a heavily coated animal, rub your hand against the lay of the hair, spraying the ruffled hair directly behind your hand. Make sure spray thoroughly wets attached ticks. Repeat every 7 days as necessary. Allow spray to dry before allowing cats to groom themselves. Wash hands thoroughly with soap and water after treating pet. Use this product in a well ventilated area. This product is not a cholinesterase inhibitor.

Precautionary Statements: Hazards to Humans and Domestic Animals:

Caution: Harmful if swallowed. Use in a well ventilated area. Avoid contact with eyes. Wash thoroughly with soap and water after handling. Do not use on dogs or cats under 12 weeks of age. Consult a veterinarian before using this product on debilitated, aged, medicated, pregnant or nursing animals. Sensitivities may occur after using any pesticide product for pets. If signs of sensitivity occur, bathe your pet with mild soap and rinse with large amounts of water. If signs continue, consult a veterinarian immediately.

First Aid:

If Swallowed: Call a physician or Poison Control Center. Drink 1 or 2 glasses of water and induce vomiting by touching back of throat with finger. Do not induce vomiting or give anything by mouth to an unconscious person.

If in Eyes: Hold eyelids open and flush with a steady, gentle stream of water. Call a physician if irritation persists.

Physical or Chemical Hazards: Flammable: Keep away from heat and open flame.

Environmental Hazards: This product is toxic to aquatic organisms. Do not apply directly to water. Do not contaminate water when disposing of equipment wash waters.

Storage and Disposal:

Storage: Store in a cool, dry place, away from children. Store above freezing (32°F) and protect from high temperatures.

Disposal: Do not reuse empty container. Rinse thoroughly before discarding. Securely wrap original container in several layers of newspaper and discard in trash.

Warning(s): Keep out of reach of children.

Presentation: 7 fl oz (207 mL).

Compendium Code No.: 10290080

SCREWWORM EAR TICK AEROSOL

Durvet **Parasiticide Spray**

EPA Reg. No.: 4691-122-12281

Active Ingredient(s):

Permethrin (CAS No. 52645-53-1) 0.50%
Other Ingredients 99.50%
Total 100.00%

Indications: A screwworm and ear tick spray that controls insect pests on beef cattle, dairy cattle, sheep, goats, hogs and horses.

For use on wounds to kill and repel flies and fly maggots. Controls ear ticks on livestock. Kills and repels flies on livestock.

Directions for Use: It is a violation of Federal law to use this product in a manner inconsistent with its labeling.

Shake well before using.

Remove protective cap, hold container upright and spray from a distance of 12 to 15 inches except where stated otherwise. Remove birds and cover fish aquaria before spraying.

Directions for Use on Livestock:

To kill and control screwworms, fleece worms (wool maggots) and other blow fly maggots in and around superficial wounds: Spray wounds thoroughly allowing spray to penetrate into pockets made by maggots. Apply over discharge around wound to prevent reinfestation. Treat at five to seven day intervals until wound is healed.

To protect wounds from flies: For castration, de-horning, docking, branding, wire and shear cut wounds, spray directly onto the wound and on surrounding area. Treat navels of newborn animals. Apply to drainage are below wound to prevent fly infestations. Repeat at five to seven day intervals until wounds are healed. Bacterial infections of wounds should be prevented or treated with supplemental disinfectants or appropriate antibiotic therapy.

To kill ear ticks: For spinose ear ticks: Spray downward directly into animal's ear. Retreat as necessary. For Gulf Coast ear ticks: Spray directly onto ticks or outer surface of animal's ear. Retreat as necessary.

To protect beef cattle, dairy cattle, goats, sheep, hogs and horses from attacks of stable flies, horse flies, deer flies, face flies, house flies, horn flies, mosquitoes and gnats. Spray about 3 seconds on each side being careful to spray back, withers and forelegs thoroughly. To protect from face flies, spray the face and head, but do not spray into eyes. Repeat treatment when flies are troublesome.

To control blood sucking lice: Apply to the infested areas of the animal using a stiff brush to get the spray to the base of the hair. Repeat every 3 weeks if required.

To control poultry lice: Spray roosts, walls and nests or cages thoroughly. This should be followed by spraying over the birds with a fine mist.

Precautionary Statements: Hazards to Humans and Domestic Animals:

Caution: Harmful if swallowed, absorbed through the skin, or inhaled. Causes moderate eye irritation. Avoid breathing vapor or spray mist. Avoid contact with skin, eyes, or clothing. Wash thoroughly with soap and water after handling and before smoking or eating. Remove contaminated clothing and wash before reuse.

Avoid contamination of feed and foodstuffs. Remove pets and birds and cover fish aquaria before space spraying or surface applications. This product is not for use on humans. Vacate room after treatment and ventilate before reoccupying. Do not allow children or pets in contact treated areas until surfaces are dry.

First Aid:

If Swallowed: Call a physician or Poison Control Center. Drink 1 or 2 glasses of water and induce vomiting by touching back of throat with finger. If person is unconscious, do not give anything by mouth and do not induce vomiting.

If on Skin: Wash with plenty of soap and water. Get medical attention if irritation persists.

If in Eyes: Flush eyes with plenty of water. Contact a physician if irritation persists.

If Inhaled: Remove victim to fresh air. If not breathing, give artificial respiration, preferably mouth to mouth. Get medical attention.

Environmental Hazards: This product is toxic to fish. Do not apply directly to water.

Physical Chemical Hazards: Contents under pressure. Do not use or store near heat or open flame. Do not puncture or incinerate container. Exposure to temperatures above 130°F may cause bursting.

Storage and Disposal: Store in a cool, dry area. Do not transport or store below 32°F. Replace cap, wrap container in several layers of newspaper. Discard in trash. Do not incinerate or puncture.

Warning(s): For swine: Do not ship animals for slaughter within 5 days of last treatment.

Keep out of reach of children.

Disclaimer: Notice of Warranty: Durvet, Inc. makes no warranty of merchantability, fitness for any particular purpose, or otherwise expressed or implied concerning this product or its uses which extend beyond the use of the product under normal conditions in accord with the statements made on the label.

Presentation: 10 oz.

Compendium Code No.: 10841891 1/01

SDM INJECTION

Phoenix Pharmaceutical **Sulfadimethoxine**

(Sulfadimethoxine Injection - 40%) Antibacterial

ANADA No.: 200-177

Active Ingredient(s): Each mL contains 400 mg sulfadimethoxine compounded with 20% propylene glycol, 1% benzyl alcohol (preservative), 0.1 mg disodium edetate, 1 mg sodium formaldehyde sulfoxylate, and pH adjusted with sodium hydroxide.

Indications: Cattle: SDM INJECTION (sulfadimethoxine) is indicated for the treatment of bovine respiratory disease complex (shipping fever complex) and bacterial pneumonia associated with *Pasteurella* spp sensitive to sulfadimethoxine; necrotic pododermatitis (foot rot) and calf diphtheria caused by *Fusobacterium necrophorum (Sphaerophorus necrophorus)*, sensitive to sulfadimethoxine.

Pharmacology: SDM INJECTION (sulfadimethoxine) is a low-dosage, rapidly absorbed, long-acting sulfonamide, effective for the treatment of shipping fever complex, bacterial pneumonia, calf diphtheria and foot rot in cattle.

Sulfadimethoxine is a white, almost tasteless and odorless compound. Chemically, it is N^1-(2,6-dimethoxy-4-pyrimidinyl) sulfanilamide. The structural formula is:

Actions: Sulfadimethoxine has been demonstrated clinically or in the laboratory to be effective against a variety of organisms, such as *streptococci, klebsiella, proteus, shigella, staphylococci, escherichia,* and *salmonella*.[1,2]

The systemic sulfonamides which include sulfadimethoxine are bacteriostatic agents. Sulfonamides competitively inhibit bacterial synthesis of folic acid (pteroylglutamic acid) from para-aminobenzoic acid. Mammalian cells are capable of utilizing folic acid in the presence of sulfonamides.

The tissue distribution of sulfadimethoxine, as with all sulfonamides, is a function of plasma levels, degree of plasma protein binding, and subsequent passive distribution in the tissues of the lipid-soluble un-ionized form. The relative amounts are determined by both its pKa and by the pH of each tissue. Therefore, levels tend to be higher in less acid tissue and body fluids or those diseased tissues having high concentrations of leucocytes.[2]

Slow renal excretion results from a high degree of tubular reabsorption,[3] and plasma protein binding is very high, providing a blood reservoir of the drug. Thus, sulfadimethoxine maintains higher blood levels than most other long-acting sulfonamides. Single, comparatively low doses of sulfadimethoxine give rapid and sustained therapeutic blood levels.[1]

To assure successful sulfonamide therapy (1) the drug must be given early in the course of the disease, and it must produce a high sulfonamide level in the body rapidly after administration, (2) therapeutically effective sulfonamide levels must be maintained in the body throughout the treatment period, (3) treatment should continue for a short period of time after the clinical signs have disappeared, and (4) the causative organisms must be sensitive to this class of drugs.

Dosage and Administration: SDM INJECTION (sulfadimethoxine) must be administered only by the intravenous route in cattle. Cattle should receive 1 mL of SDM INJECTION (sulfadimethoxine) per 16 pounds of body weight (55 mg/kg) as an initial dose, followed by 0.5 mL per 16 pounds of body weight (27.5 mg/kg) every 24 hours thereafter. Sulfadimethoxine Boluses may be utilized for maintenance therapy in cattle. Representative weights and doses are indicated in the following table:

Animal Weight	Initial Dose 25 mg/lb (55 mg/kg)	Subsequent Daily Doses 12.5 mg/lb (27.5 mg/kg)
250 lb (113.6 kg)	15.6 mL	7.8 mL
500 lb (227.2 kg)	31.2 mL	15.6 mL
750 lb (340.9 kg)	46.9 mL	23.5 mL
1000 lb (454.5 kg)	62.5 mL	31.3 mL

Length of treatment depends on the clinical response. In most cases treatment for 3 to 5 days is adequate. Treatment should be continued until the animal is asymptomatic for 48 hours.

Directions for Intravenous Injection:

Equipment needed:

1. A nose lead and/or halter sufficiently strong enough to effectively restrain or hold the animal's head steady so that the intravenous injection can be made with ease.
2. Hypodermic needles, 16 or 18 gauge and 2 inches long. Only new, sharp and sterile hypodermic needles should be used. Dull needles should be discarded. Extra needles should always be available in case the needles being used should become clogged.
3. Hypodermic syringes, 40 or 50 mL sterile disposable or reusable glass syringes should be available.
4. Alcohol (70%) or equally effective antiseptic for disinfecting the skin.

Preparation of the equipment: Glass syringes and regular hypodermic needles should be thoroughly cleaned and washed. Following this, the needles and syringes should be immersed in boiling water for 30 minutes prior to each injection. Regular hypodermic needles should not be used more than 3-4 times as repeated skin puncturing and boiling of the needles causes them to become quite dull. Disposable hypodermic needles and syringes should not be used more than once.

Restraint of animal: The cow should preferably be in a stanchion for maximum restraint. If this is not possible, the animal should be restrained in a manner to prevent excessive movement. A nose lead should be applied and the animal's head turned sidewise to stretch the skin and tense the muscles of the neck region.

Locating the jugular vein: Once the animal has been restrained (as above), you will notice a long depression of the skin from below the angle of the jaw to just above the shoulder. This is known as the jugular furrow or jugular groove. The jugular vein is located just under the jugular groove.

Preparation of SDM INJECTION (sulfadimethoxine) for injection: The rubber cap of the bottle should be thoroughly cleaned with 70% alcohol or another satisfactory antiseptic. The correct amount of SDM INJECTION (sulfadimethoxine) for treatment should be calculated (see dosage directions) and that amount withdrawn into a syringe. One or two syringefuls of air should be injected into the bottle first to make withdrawing the drug easier. SDM INJECTION (sulfadimethoxine) should preferably be at room temperature when filling syringes and when injecting intravenously.

Entering the vein: The skin of the injection area should be clean and free of dirt. Cotton saturated with 70% alcohol (or suitable antiseptic) should be used to wipe the injection site.

Apply pressure over the jugular vein close to the shoulder. This will reduce the flow of blood to the heart and cause the jugular vein to bulge or enlarge (See Figure 1) When the jugular vein has been "raised", insert the hypodermic needle at a 45 degree angle through the skin just underneath the jugular vein. The beveled edge of the hypodermic needles should be up.

After the skin has been punctured, the point of the needle should be directed toward the side of the vein and pushed into the center of the vein (See Figure 2). When the needle is in the center of the vein, there will be a free flow of blood back through the needle. Release external pressure when you are sure the needle is within the vein.

Injecting the SDM INJECTION (sulfadimethoxine): After the needle has been accurately inserted into the jugular vein, firmly attach the syringe containing SDM INJECTION (sulfadimethoxine) to the inserted hypodermic needle. Caution, be sure syringe is free of air. Exert firm pressure on the plunger of the syringe to inject the SDM INJECTION (sulfadimethoxine) while the barrel is held firmly. The injection should be made moderately slow - never rapidly.

If the animal moves, causing resistance in pushing the plunger of the syringe, or if a bubble of the drug is noted under the skin, the needle is no longer within the vein. The needle should be repositioned.

When the injection is completed, quickly withdraw the syringe and needle with a quick pull and apply light pressure over the injection site with alcohol and cotton to minimize bleeding from the puncture site.

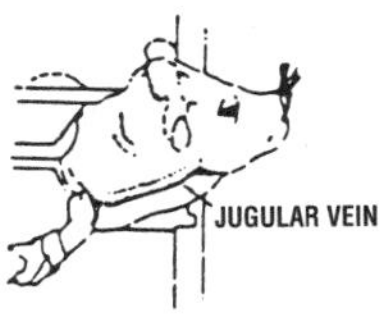

JUGULAR VEIN

Fig. 1

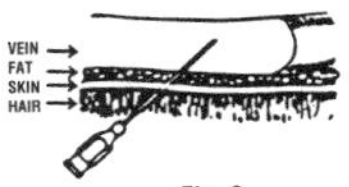

VEIN FAT SKIN HAIR

Fig. 2

Precaution(s): Store at room temperature between (15° and 30°C (59° and 86°F). Should crystallization occur at cold temperatures, crystals will dissolve either by storing at room temperature for several days or by heating the vial in warm water. Crystallization and redissolution do not impair the efficacy of the product.

Caution(s): During treatment period, make certain that animals maintain adequate water intake.

If animals show no improvement within 2 or 3 days, consult a veterinarian.

Tissue damage may result from perivascular infiltration.

Limitations: Sulfadimethoxine is not effective in viral or rickettsial infections, and as with any anti-bacterial agent, occasional failures in therapy may occur due to resistant microorganisms. The usual precautions in sulfonamide therapy should be observed.

Warning(s): Milk taken from animals during treatment and for 60 hours (5 milkings) after the latest treatment must not be used for food. Do not administer within 5 days of slaughter. A withdrawal period has not yet been established for this product in pre-ruminating calves.

Do not use calves to be processed for veal.

For intravenous use only in cattle.

Restricted drug, Use only as directed - Not for human use (California).

For animal use only. Keep out of the reach of children.

Toxicology: Toxicity and Safety: Data regarding acute (LD_{50}) and chronic toxicities of sulfadimethoxine indicate the drug is safe. The LD_{50} in mice is greater than 2 g/kg body weight when administered intraperitoneally and greater than 16 g/kg when administered orally. In dogs receiving massive single oral doses of 3.2 g/kg body weight, diarrhea was the only adverse effect observed. Dogs given 160 mg/kg body weight orally daily for 13 weeks showed no signs of toxicity.

In cattle sulfadimethoxine has been shown to be safe through extensive clinical use with other dosage forms. In addition, studies with intravenous administration of SDM INJECTION have demonstrated that hemolysis of erythrocytes does not occur by this route of administration. Sulfadimethoxine has a relatively high solubility at the pH normally occurring in the kidney, precluding the possibility of precipitation and crystalluria.

References: Available upon request.

Presentation: 250 mL bottles (NDC 57319-374-06).

Manufactured by: Phoenix Scientific, Inc.

Compendium Code No.: 12560761 Rev. 6-00

SDM POWDER

Bimeda **Water Medication**

Sulfadimethoxine Soluble Powder-Antibacterial

ANADA No.: 200-031

Active Ingredient(s): Each packet contains 3.34 oz (94.6 g) Sulfadimethoxine in the form of the soluble sodium salt and disodium edetate.

Indications: For Broiler and Replacement Chickens Only: Use for the treatment of disease outbreaks of coccidiosis, fowl cholera, and infectious coryza.

For Meat-producing Turkeys Only: Use for the treatment of disease outbreaks of coccidiosis and fowl cholera.

For Dairy Calves, Dairy Heifers, and Beef Cattle: Use for the treatment of shipping fever complex, bacterial pneumonia, calf diphtheria, and foot rot.

Dosage and Administration:

Species	Concentration	Use Directions
Chickens	0.05%	Contents of packet to 50 gallons of water.
Turkeys	0.025%	Contents of packet to 100 gallons of water.

Automatic Proportioners: To make stock solution, add contents of 5 packets to 2 gallons of water for chickens and to 4 gallons of water for turkeys. Set proportioner to feed at rate of 1 fl oz of stock solution per gallon of water.

Treatment Period: 6 consecutive days.

Dairy Calves, Dairy Heifers and Beef Cattle:

Dosage: 25 mg/lb first day followed by 12.5 mg/lb/day for 4 days.

Sulfadimethoxine in Water:

		Water Consumption	
	Amount of Stock Solution for Cattle*	(Summer) 1 gallon/** 100 lb body weight	(Winter) 1 gallon/** 150 lb body weight
First Day Add	1 quart	10 gallons	7 gallons
	2 quarts	20 gallons	14 gallons
	1 gallon	40 gallons	28 gallons
Next 4 Days Add	1 quart	20 gallons	14 gallons
	2 quarts	40 gallons	28 gallons
	1 gallon	80 gallons	56 gallons

*Note: Make a cattle stock solution by adding 1 packet of Sulfadimethoxine Soluble Powder to 1 gallon of water.

*Twenty fl oz of cattle stock solution will medicate one-600 lb animal initially or two-600 lb animals on maintenance dose. Contents of packet will medicate six-600 lb animals initially or twelve-600 lb animals on maintenance dose.

**This dosage recommendation is based on a water consumption of 1 gallon per 100 lb of body weight per day, the expected water consumption rate for summer. Water consumption during cold months (winter) may drop markedly (30-40%). Accordingly, adjustments must be made in the dilution rates to compensate for this and insure proper drug intake.

For treatment of individual cattle, Sulfadimethoxine Soluble Powder stock solution for cattle may be given as a drench. Administer using same mg/lb dosage as outlined above.

Treatment Period: 5 consecutive days

Caution(s): Chickens and Turkeys: If animals show no improvement within 5 days, discontinue treatment and re-evaluate diagnosis. Prepare a fresh stock solution daily. Handle the recommended dilutions (chickens 0.05% and turkeys 0.025%) as regular drinking water. Administer as sole source of drinking water and sulfonamide medication.

Chickens and turkeys that have survived fowl cholera outbreaks should not be kept for replacements or breeders.

Cattle: During treatment period, make certain that animals maintain adequate water intake.

If animals show no improvement within 2 or 3 days, re-evaluate diagnosis. Treatment should not be continued beyond 5 days.

Restricted Drug (California)—Use only as directed.

Warning(s): Chickens and Turkeys: Withdraw 5 days before slaughter. Do not administer to chickens over 16 weeks (112 days) of age or to turkeys over 24 weeks (168 days) of age.

Cattle: Withdraw 7 days before slaughter. For dairy calves, dairy heifers and beef cattle only. A withdrawal period has not been established for this product in pre-ruminating calves. Do not use in calves to be processed for veal.

Not for human use.

Presentation: 107 g (3.77 oz) packet.

Manufactured by: Bimeda, Inc., Le Sueur, MN 56058.

Compendium Code No.: 13990600 8SDM005-401

S

SDM SOLUTION

Phoenix Pharmaceutical **Water Medication**

(Sulfadimethoxine 12.5% Oral Solution) Antibacterial

ANADA No.: 200-192

Active Ingredient(s): Each fluid ounce contains 3.75 g sulfadimethoxine solubilized with sodium hydroxide.

Indications:

Broiler and Replacement Chickens: Use for the treatment of disease outbreaks of coccidiosis, fowl cholera, and infectious coryza.

Meat Producing Turkeys: Use for the treatment of disease outbreaks of coccidiosis and fowl cholera.

Dairy Calves, Dairy Heifers and Beef Cattle: Use in the treatment of shipping fever complex, bacterial pneumonia, calf diphtheria, and foot rot.

Dosage and Administration: Prepare a fresh stock solution daily.

Species	Concentration	Use Directions
Chickens	0.05%	Add 1 fl oz* to 2 gallons of drinking water -or- 25 fl oz to 50 gallons of drinking water
Turkeys	0.025%	Add 1 fl oz* to 4 gallons of drinking water -or- 25 fl oz to 100 gallons of drinking water

Automatic Proportioners** Stock Solution — To make 2 gallons of Stock Solution use:

Chickens	1 gal Sulfadimethoxine 12.5% Drinking Water Solution Concentrate - plus - 1 gal of water
Turkeys	2 qts Sulfadimethoxine 12.5% Drinking Water Solution Concentrate - plus - 6 qts of water

Treatment Period: 6 consecutive days.

Dairy Calves, Dairy Heifers and Beef Cattle:

Dosage: 25 mg/lb first day followed by 12.5 mg/lb/day for 4 days.

		Sulfadimethoxine in Water	
		Water Consumption	
		(Summer) 1 gallon/† 100 lb b.w.	(Winter) 1 gallon/† 150 lb b.w.
First Day Add:	1 pint (16 fl oz) to:	25 gallons	16 gallons
	1 quart (32 fl oz) to:	50 gallons	33 gallons
	1 gallon (128 fl oz) to:	200 gallons	127 gallons
Next 4 Days Add:	1 pint (16 fl oz) to:	50 gallons	33 gallons
	1 quart (32 fl oz) to:	100 gallons	66 gallons
	1 gallon (128 fl oz) to:	400 gallons	266 gallons

†This dosage recommendation is based on a water consumption of 1 gallon per 100 lb of body weight per day, the expected water consumption rate for summer. Water consumption during cold months (winter) may drop markedly (30-40%). Accordingly, adjustments in drug concentration in drinking water must be made to insure proper drug intake.

For individual treatment of cattle, Sulfadimethoxine 12.5% Drinking Water Solution may be given as a drench. Administer using same mg/lb dose as outlined above. Four fluid ounces will medicate one-600 lb animal initially or two-600 lb animals on maintenance dose.

Treatment Period: 5 consecutive days.

*1 fl oz Sulfadimethoxine 12.5% Drinking Water Solution = 30 mL or 2 tablespoonfuls.

**Set proportioner to a feed rate of 1 fl oz of Sulfadimethoxine Stock Solution per gallon of water.

Precaution(s): Store at room temperature; if freezing occurs, thaw before using. Protect from light; direct sunlight may cause discoloration. Freezing or discoloration does not affect potency.

Caution(s):

Chickens and Turkeys: If animals show no improvement within 5 days, discontinue treatment and re-evaluate diagnosis. Handle the recommended dilutions (chickens 0.05% and turkeys 0.025%) as regular drinking water. Administer as sole source of drinking water and sulfonamide medication.

Chickens and turkeys that have survived fowl cholera outbreaks should not be kept for replacements or breeders.

Cattle: During treatment period, make certain that animals maintain adequate water intake. If animals show no improvement within 2 or 3 days, re-evaluate diagnosis. Treatment should not be continued beyond 5 days. For use in animals only.

Restricted drug (California)-Use only as directed. Not for human use.

Warning(s):

Chickens and Turkeys: Withdraw 5 days before slaughter.

Do not administer to chickens over 16 weeks (112 days) of age or to turkeys over 24 weeks (168 days) of age.

Cattle: Withdraw 7 days before slaughter. For dairy calves, dairy heifers and beef cattle only. A withdrawal period has not been established for this product in pre-ruminating calves. Do not use in calves to be processed for veal. Keep out of reach of children.

Presentation: 3.785 L (1 gal) (128 fl oz) containers (NDC 57319-375-09).

Compendium Code No.: 12560771 Rev. 6-98

SDT-GUARD™

Boehringer Ingelheim **Bacterin**

Salmonella Dublin-Typhimurium Bacterin

U.S. Vet. Lic. No.: 315

Contents: This product contains the antigens listed above.

Indications: For use in healthy cattle as an aid in the prevention of Salmonellosis caused by *Salmonella dublin* and *Salmonella typhimurium.*

Dosage and Administration: Shake well. Inject 2 mL IM or Sub Q in the middle of the neck. Repeat in 14 to 28 days. Annual revaccination is recommended.

Precaution(s): Store below 45°F (7°C). Do not freeze. Use entire contents when first opened.

Caution(s): Persistent swelling may occur at the injection site, particularly following subcutaneous administration. Epinephrine should be on hand in case of anaphylaxis. Delayed and intermediate hypersensitivity reactions should be treated symptomatically. Hypersensitivity reactions, including delayed hypersensitivity, or death may occur with a biological product. This product can cause reduced milk production in lactating dairy cattle.

Warning(s): Do not vaccinate within 60 days of slaughter.

Presentation: 50 doses (100 mL).

Manufactured by: American Animal Health, Inc., Grand Prairie, TX 75052-7610

Compendium Code No.: 10280991 BI 4028-1R-1 1/01

SEBALYT® SHAMPOO

DVM **Antidermatosis Shampoo**

All Purpose Antiseborrheic Antibacterial Cleansing Formulation

Active Ingredient(s): Sulfur 2%, salicylic acid 2% and triclosan 0.5%.

Indications: To relieve scaling and related symptoms of seborrhea and other non-specific dermatoses on dogs and cats.

Product Description: SEBALYT® is a soap-free, antibacterial, antiseborrheic, keratolytic formulation in a pH-adjusted shampoo base. The formulation is complemented with protein coat conditioners for manageability and high luster.

Directions for Use: Shake well before use. Wet coat thoroughly. Apply and lather. Shampoo over entire body, allowing for 5-10 minutes of contact time. Rinse thoroughly. Repeat as necessary, or as directed by veterinarian.

Precaution(s): Store at room temperature.

Caution(s): For topical use only. Avoid contact with eyes. If contact occurs, rinse thoroughly with water. If irritation develops, discontinue and consult your veterinarian.

Warning(s): Keep out of reach of children.

Presentation: 8 fl oz (237 mL) (NDC 47203-350-08), 12 fl oz (355 mL) (NDC 47203-350-12) and 1 gallon (3.78 L) (NDC 47203-350-28).

Compendium Code No.: 11420511 Rev 0597

SEBOLUX® SHAMPOO

Virbac **Antidermatosis Shampoo**

with Spherulites®

Ingredient(s): Contains: Solubilized sulfur (equivalent to 2% elemental sulfur) and 2% salicylic acid in a shampoo base containing water, sodium lauryl sulfate, lauryl glucoside, Spherulites, glycerin, chitosanide, lauramide DEA, sodium hydroxide and fragrance. Chitosanide, glycerin, salicylic acid and sulfur are present in encapsulated (Spherulites) and free forms. Urea is present in encapsulated form.

Indications: SEBOLUX® is a unique antiseborrheic, keratoplastic and antiseptic shampoo. It removes scales and crusts associated with seborrhea and other nonspecific dermatoses while leaving the skin clean and the coat soft and lustrous.

SEBOLUX® is an antiseborrheic, keratoplastic and antiseptic shampoo for use on dogs and cats of any age.

Directions: Shake well before use. Wet the coat with warm water and apply sufficient shampoo to create a rich lather. Massage SEBOLUX® into wet coat, lather freely. Rinse and repeat. Allow to remain on hair for 5 to 10 minutes, then rinse thoroughly with clean water.

Frequency of use: initially two to three times a week for four weeks, then reducing to once a week, or as directed by your veterinarian.

Caution(s): For topical use only. Avoid contact with eyes. In case of contact, flush eyes with water and seek medical attention if irritation persists.

Available through licensed veterinarians only.

Warning(s): Keep out of reach of children.

Discussion: SEBOLUX® contains Spherulites, an exclusive and patented encapsulation system developed by Virbac to provide slow release of ingredients long after the shampoo is rinsed off.

SEBOLUX® also contains Chitosanide, a natural biopolymer creating a protective film on the skin and hair.

Presentation: 8 oz (237 mL), 16 oz (473 mL), and 1 gallon (3.79 L) containers.

Compendium Code No.: 10230550

SEBORX™ SHAMPOO

DVM **Antidermatosis Shampoo**

Antiseborrheic Antiseptic Formulation

Active Ingredient(s): Salicylic acid 3%, solubilized sulfur 2% and triclosan 0.5%.

Indications: To relieve symptoms of seborrheic dermatitis and other non-specific dermatoses in dogs and cats. May also be used as a general cleansing antiseptic shampoo.

SEBORx™ Shampoo has been formulated for the relief of scaling and mild infection associated with canine and feline seborrheic dermatitis. SEBORx™ Shampoo is a concentrated antiseptic, antiseborrheic, keratolytic formulation in a high lathering shampoo base. The formulation is complemented with omega-6 fatty acids for their dermal renourishing effects and supplemented with protein coat conditioners for coat manageability and high luster.

Directions for Use: Shake well before use. Wet coat thoroughly with warm water. Apply sufficient SEBORx™ Shampoo to affected areas and lather in well. Then lather entire coat. Allow lather to remain 5-10 minutes. Contact time with skin is important for optimal benefits. Rinse thoroughly. Repeat if necessary, or as directed by a veterinarian.

Precaution(s): Store at room temperature.

Caution(s): For topical use only on dogs and cats. Avoid contact with eyes.

Warning(s): Keep out of reach of children.

Presentation: 8 fl oz (237 mL) (NDC 47203-365-08), 12 fl oz (355 mL) (NDC 47203-365-12), and 1 gallon (3.78 L) (NDC 47203-365-28).

Compendium Code No.: 11420523 Rev 0199 / Rev 0200

SEDAZINE® ℞

Fort Dodge **Analgesic-Sedative**

(Xylazine) 100 mg/mL Injectable

ANADA No.: 200-088

Active Ingredient(s): Each mL contains 100 mg SEDAZINE® (xylazine, base equivalent), 0.9 mg methylparaben, 0.1 mg propylparaben, water for injection; citric acid and sodium citrate for pH adjustment to 5.5 ± 0.3.

Xylazine hydrochloride (Equivalent to 10% base) 11.4%

Inert Ingredients: 88.6%

100.0%

Indications: SEDAZINE® (xylazine) should be used in horses and *Cervidae* (Fallow Deer, Mule Deer, Sika Deer, White-Tailed Deer and Elk) when it is desirable to produce a state of sedation accompanied by a shorter period of analgesia.

Horses: SEDAZINE® (xylazine) has been used successfully as follows:

1. Diagnostic procedures—oral and ophthalmic examinations, abdominal palpation, rectal palpation, vaginal examination, catheterization of the bladder and radiographic examinations.
2. Orthopedic procedures, such as application of casting materials and splints.
3. Dental procedures.
4. Minor surgical procedures of short duration such as debridement, removal of cutaneous neoplasms and suturing of lacerations.
5. To calm and facilitate handling of fractious animals.

S

6. Therapeutic medication for sedation and relief of pain following injury or surgery.
7. Major surgical procedures:
   a. When used as a preanesthetic to general anesthesia.
   b. When used in conjunction with local anesthetics.

Cervidae: SEDAZINE® (xylazine) may be used for the following:

1. To calm and facilitate the handling of fractious animals.
2. Diagnostic procedures.
3. Minor surgical procedures.
4. Therapeutic medication for sedation and relief of pain following injury or surgery.
5. As a preanesthetic to local anesthesia. SEDAZINE® (xylazine) at the recommended dosages can be used in conjunction with local anesthetics, such as procaine or lidocaine.

Pharmacology: SEDAZINE® (xylazine), a non-narcotic compound, is a sedative and analgesic as well as muscle relaxant. Its sedative and analgesic activity is related to central nervous system depression. Its muscle relaxant effect is based on inhibition of the intraneural transmission of impulses in the central nervous system. The principal pharmacological activities develop within 10 to 15 minutes after intramuscular injection in horses and *Cervidae,* and within 3 to 5 minutes following intravenous administration in horses.

A sleeplike state, the depth of which is dose-dependent, is usually maintained for 1 to 2 hours, while analgesia lasts from 15 to 30 minutes. The centrally-acting muscle relaxant effect causes relaxation of the skeletal musculature, complementing sedation and analgesia.

In horses and *Cervidae* under the influence of SEDAZINE® (xylazine), the respiratory rate is reduced as in natural sleep. Following treatment with SEDAZINE® (xylazine), the heart rate is decreased and a transient change in the conductivity of the cardiac muscle may occur, as evidenced by a partial atrioventricular block. This resembles the atrioventricular block often observed in normal horses.[1,2,3,4] Partial A-V block may occasionally occur following intramuscular injection of SEDAZINE® (xylazine). When given intravenously in horses, the incidence of partial A-V block is higher. Intravenous administration causes a transient rise in blood pressure in horses, followed by a slight decrease.

SEDAZINE® (xylazine) has no effect on blood clotting time or other hematologic parameters.

Dosage and Administration: Horses:

1. Dosage:
   Intravenously—0.5 mL/100 lbs body weight (0.5 mg/lb)
   Intramuscularly—1.0 mL/100 lbs body weight (1.0 mg/lb)
   Following injection of SEDAZINE® (xylazine), the animal should be allowed to rest quietly until the full effect has been reached.
   These dosages produce sedation which is usually maintained for 1 to 2 hours, and analgesia which lasts for 15 to 30 minutes.
2. Preanesthetic to Local Anesthesia: SEDAZINE® (xylazine) at the recommended dosages can be used in conjunction with local anesthetics, such as procaine or lidocaine.
3. Preanesthetic to General Anesthesia: SEDAZINE® (xylazine) at the recommended dosage rates produces an additive effect to central nervous system depressants such as pentobarbital sodium, thiopental sodium and thiamylal sodium. Therefore, the dosage of such compounds should be reduced and administered to the desired effect. In general, only ⅓ to ½ of the calculated dosage of the barbiturates will be needed to produce a surgical plane of anesthesia. Post-anesthetic or emergence excitement has not been observed in animals preanesthetized with SEDAZINE® (xylazine).
   SEDAZINE® (xylazine) has been used successfully as a preanesthetic agent for pentobarbital sodium, thiopental sodium, thiamylal sodium, nitrous oxide, ether, halothane, glyceryl guaiacolate and methoxyflurane anesthesia.

Cervidae: Administer intramuscularly, either by hand syringe or syringe dart, in the heavy muscles of the croup or shoulder.

Dosage Range:
Fallow Deer *(Dama dama)*—2.0 to 4.0 mL/100 lbs body weight (2.0 to 4.0 mg/lb)
Mule Deer *(Odocoileus hemionus)*—1.0 to 2.0 mL/100 lbs body weight (1.0 to 2.0 mg/lb)
Sika Deer *(Cervus nippon)*—1.0 to 2.0 mL/100 lbs body weight (1.0 to 2.0 mg/lb)
White-Tailed Deer *(Odocoileus virginianus)*—1.0 to 2.0 mL/100 lbs body weight (1.0 to 2.0 mg/lb)
Elk *(Cervus canadensis)*—0.25 to 0.5 mL/100 lbs body weight (0.25 to 0.5 mg/lb)

Following injection of SEDAZINE® (xylazine), the animal should be allowed to rest quietly until the full effect has been reached.

These dosages produce sedation which is usually maintained for 1 to 2 hours and analgesia which lasts for 15 to 30 minutes.

Precaution(s): Store at controlled room temperature (15° to 30°C or 59° to 86°F).

Caution(s): Federal law restricts this drug to use by or on the order of a licensed veterinarian.

Careful consideration should be given before administering to horses and *Cervidae* with significantly depressed respiration, severe pathologic heart disease, advanced liver or kidney disease, severe endotoxic or traumatic shock and stress conditions such as extreme heat, cold, high altitude or fatigue.

Do not use SEDAZINE® (xylazine) in conjunction with tranquilizers.

Analgesic effect is variable, and depth should be carefully assayed prior to surgical or clinical procedures. Variability of analgesia occurs most frequently at the distal extremities of horses and *Cervidae.* In spite of sedation, the practitioner and handlers should proceed with caution since defence reactions may not be diminished.

Horses: Since an additive effect results from the use of SEDAZINE® (xylazine) and the barbiturate compounds, it should be used with caution with these central nervous system depressants. Products known to produce respiratory depression or apnea, such as thiamylal sodium, should be given at a reduced dosage and, when injected intravenously, should be administered slowly. When intravenous administration of SEDAZINE® (xylazine) is desired, avoid perivascular injection in order to achieve the desired effect. Studies have shown negligible evidence of tissue irritation, however, following perivascular injection of xylazine.

Intracarotid arterial injection should be avoided. As with many compounds, including tranquilizers, immediate violent seizures followed by collapse may result from inadvertent administration into the carotid artery. Although the reaction with SEDAZINE® (xylazine) is usually transient and recovery may be rapid and complete, special care should be taken to assure that the needle is in the jugular vein rather than the carotid artery.

Bradycardia and an arrhythmia in the form of incomplete atrioventricular block have been reported following SEDAZINE® (xylazine) administration. Although clinically the importance of this effect is questioned,[1,2,3,4] a standard dose of atropine given prior to or following xylazine will greatly decrease the incidence.

Sedation for transport is most successful if actual transportation is begun after the full effect of the drug has been reached and the animal's stability is maintained while standing. In addition, it should be noted that animals under the influence of xylazine can be aroused by noise or other stimuli and this may increase the risk of injury.

Cervidae: As in all ruminants, it is preferable to administer SEDAZINE® (xylazine) to fasted *Cervidae* as a safeguard against aspiration of food material into the lungs and/or bloat during deep sedation.

Care should be taken to administer SEDAZINE® (xylazine) in the heavy muscles of the croup or shoulder. Injections given subcutaneously, intraperitoneally or into fat deposits will give unpredictable results.

Intra-arterial injection should be avoided, as with many compounds, including tranquilizers, immediate violent seizures followed by collapse may result from inadvertent administration into an artery.

The animal should not be disturbed during induction or until the full effect of the drug has been reached which is usually 10 to 15 minutes following injection.

The usual time to initial effect of the drug is 2 to 5 minutes. The administrator of the drug should be fully cognizant of this interval prior to administration of drug to free-ranging deer or elk, especially at night or in heavily wooded areas.

If the animal has been underdosed (faulty injection or miscalculation on weight) it is advisable to wait for one hour before administering a second dose.

Adequate ventilation—especially in cages or crates—is mandatory; keep head and neck in position to insure patent air passage and to prevent aspiration of stomach contents.

During sedation, animals should be prevented from assuming lateral recumbency. A sternal recumbent position is desirable.

While under the effects of SEDAZINE® (xylazine), the animal should be protected from extreme hot or cold environments.

Efforts should be made to prevent patient from rising until almost complete recovery is attained.

The transportation of *Cervidae* given SEDAZINE® (xylazine) should be carefully monitored to prevent excessive struggling, injury or death.

Hyperthermic reactions may occur, especially if the subject is in a highly excited state when the drug is administered. Hosing the head and entire body with cold water has usually proven to be an effective deterrent.

The safety of SEDAZINE® (xylazine) has not been demonstrated in pregnant *Cervidae.* Avoid use during the breeding season.

Cervidae should be observed closely until all of the sedative effects of SEDAZINE® (xylazine) are gone.

Care should be taken at all times when administering SEDAZINE® (xylazine) to *Cervidae.* This is due to the method of administration (usually darting), the difficulty in estimating body weights and the accepted theory that wild animals are more unpredictable in their response to sedatives and analgesics than the domesticated species.

Warning(s): This drug should not be administered to domestic food-producing animals. Not for use in horses intended for food.

Do not use in *Cervidae* less than 15 days before or during the hunting season.

Avoid accidental administration to humans. Should such exposure occur, notify a physician immediately. Artificial respiration may be indicated.

In *Cervidae,* occasional capture-associated deaths occur. Clinical trials reveal a mortality rate of approximately 3.5% attendant with the administration of xylazine.

Toxicology: Safety: SEDAZINE® (xylazine) is tolerated at 10 times the recommended dose in horses, and at doses above the recommended range in *Cervidae.* However, some elevated doses produced muscle tremors and long periods of sedation.

Side Effects: SEDAZINE® (xylazine), in horses and *Cervidae,* used at recommended dosage levels may occasionally cause slight muscle tremors, bradycardia with partial A-V heart block and a reduced respiratory rate. Movement in response to sharp auditory stimuli may be observed.

In horses, sweating, rarely profuse, has been reported following administration. In *Cervidae,* salivation, various vocalizations (bellowing, bleating, groaning, grunting, snoring) on expiration, audible grinding of molar teeth, protruding tongue and elevated temperatures have also been noted in some cases.

References: Available upon request.

Presentation: SEDAZINE® (xylazine) 100 mg/mL for intravenous or intramuscular use is available in 50 mL multiple dose vials (NDC 0856-8602-01).

Manufactured by: Phoenix Scientific, Inc., St. Joseph, MO 64506

Compendium Code No.: 10031891 8600F

SEE SPOT GO!™

Tomlyn **Deodorant Product**

Active Ingredient(s): Contains 2-Butoxyethanol and Isopropyl Alcohol.

Does not contain phosphates or fluorocarbons.

Indications: Veterinarian recommended for:

Stains and odors caused by puppy and kitten housebreaking.

Stains and odors associated with older or accident prone pets.

Litter box area, carpets, furniture, clothing, auto interiors.

Directions for Use: Carefully follow directions to avoid personal injury. Can should always be held upside down to spray. Blot up excess soil or liquid. Remove protective cap. Hold can upside down. Point opening in spray tip towards spot or stain. Depress the tab on the top of the spray tip to spray. Hold can at arm's length and avoid spraying toward any part of the body. It is not necessary to bend down to apply this product. To avoid splashback, do not spray at hard surfaces. Apply until spot or stain is well covered. Stain or spot will be gone in seconds. Certain stains may require additional applications. Wait until material is dry before reapplying to see if necessary.

Precaution(s): Contents under pressure.

Use in well ventilated area. Do not puncture or incinerate container. Do not expose to heat or store at temperatures above 120°F.

Caution(s): Check for colorfastness on an inconspicuous area. Do not oversaturate. If can is cold, product will foam but this will not interfere with the product's effectiveness. Not recommended for use on wool.

Contact with skin or eyes can cause irritation and permanent eye damage. Vapor may be harmful. Harmful if swallowed.

If sprayed on skin, wash with soap and water.

If sprayed in eyes, flush thoroughly with water for 15 minutes and see physician.

Warning(s): Keep out of reach of children.

Presentation: 14 oz (397 g) can.

Compendium Code No.: 11220370 015-2 3

SENTINEL® FLAVOR TABS® ℞

Novartis **Flea Control & Oral Parasiticide**

(milbemycin oxime/lufenuron)

NADA No.: 141-084

Active Ingredient(s): Description: SENTINEL® Flavor Tabs® are available in four tablet sizes in color-coded packages for oral administration to dogs and puppies according to their weight. (See Dosage Section.) Each tablet is formulated to provide a minimum of 0.23 mg/pound (0.5 mg/kg) of milbemycin oxime and 4.55 mg/pound (10 mg/kg) body weight of lufenuron.

Indications: SENTINEL® Flavor Tabs® are indicated for use in dogs and puppies, four weeks of age and older, and two pounds body weight or greater. SENTINEL® Flavor Tabs® are also indicated for the prevention of heartworm disease caused by *Dirofilaria immitis*, for the prevention and control of flea populations, the control of adult *Ancylostoma caninum* (hookworm), and the removal and control of adult *Toxocara canis* and *Toxascaris leonina* (roundworm) and *Trichuris vulpis* (whipworm) infections.

Lufenuron controls flea populations by preventing the development of flea eggs and does not kill adult fleas. Concurrent use of insecticides may be necessary for adequate control of adult fleas.

Pharmacology: Milbemycin oxime consists of the oxime derivatives of 5-didehydromilbemycins in the ratio of approximately 80% A_4 ($C_{32}H_{45}NO_7$, MW 555.71) and 20% A_3 ($C_{31}H_{43}NO_7$, MW 541.68). Milbemycin oxime is classified as a macrocyclic anthelmintic.

Lufenuron is a benzoylphenylurea derivative with the following chemical composition: N-[2,5-dichloro-4-(1,1,2,3,3,3, -hexafluoropropoxy)-phenylaminocarbonyl]-2,6-difluorobenzamide ($C_{17}H_8Cl_2F_8N_2O_3$, MW 511.15). Benzoylphenylurea compounds, including lufenuron, are classified as insect development inhibitors (IDIs).

Mode of Action: Milbemycin oxime, one active ingredient in SENTINEL® Flavor Tabs®, is a macrocyclic anthelmintic which is believed to act by interfering with invertebrate neurotransmission. Milbemycin oxime eliminates the tissue stage of heartworm larvae and the adult stage of hookworm *(Ancylostoma caninum)*, roundworm *(Toxocara canis* and *Toxascaris leonina)* and whipworm *(Trichuris vulpis)* infestations when administered orally according to the recommended dosage schedule.

Lufenuron, the other active ingredient in SENTINEL® Flavor Tabs®, is an insect development inhibitor which breaks the flea life cycle by inhibiting egg development. Lufenuron's mode of action is interference with chitin synthesis, polymerization and deposition. Lufenuron has no effect on the adult flea. After biting a lufenuron-treated dog, the female flea ingests a blood meal containing lufenuron which is subsequently deposited in her eggs. Lufenuron prevents most flea eggs from hatching or maturing into adults and thus prevents and controls flea populations by breaking the life cycle (See Efficacy).

Dosage and Administration: Dosage: SENTINEL® Flavor Tabs® are given orally, once a month, at the recommended minimum dosage of 0.23 mg/lb (0.5 mg/kg) milbemycin oxime and 4.55 mg/lb (10 mg/kg) lufenuron.

Recommended Dosage Schedule:

Body Weight	Milbemycin Oxime Per Tablet	Lufenuron Per Tablet
2 to 10 lbs.	2.3 mg	46 mg
11 to 25 lbs.	5.75 mg	115 mg
26 to 50 lbs.	11.5 mg	230 mg
51 to 100 lbs.	23.0 mg	460 mg

Dogs over 100 lbs are provided the appropriate combination of tablets.

Administration: To ensure adequate absorption, always administer SENTINEL® Flavor Tabs® to dogs immediately after or in conjunction with a normal meal.

SENTINEL® Flavor Tabs are palatable and most dogs will consume the tablet when offered by the owner. As an alternative to direct dosing, the tablets can be hidden in food. Be certain the dog consumes the entire tablet or tablets. Administer SENTINEL® Flavor Tabs® to dogs, immediately after or in conjunction with a normal meal. Food is essential for adequate absorption of lufenuron. Watch the dog closely following administration to be sure the entire dose has been consumed. If it is not entirely consumed, redose with the full recommended dose as soon as possible.

SENTINEL® Flavor Tabs® must be administered monthly, preferably on the same date each month. Treatment with SENTINEL® Flavor Tabs® may begin at any time of year. In geographic areas where mosquitoes and fleas are seasonal, the treatment schedule should begin one month prior to the expected onset and should continue until the end of "mosquito and flea season". In areas with year-round infestations, treatment should continue through the entire year without interruption.

To ensure the greatest flea control from the use of SENTINEL® Flavor Tabs®, it is important to treat all dogs and cats within a household for fleas. All cats within the household should be treated with lufenuron suspension, injectable or tablets because untreated dogs and cats may develop infestations which could reduce the overall flea control within a household (See Cautions).

If a dose is missed and a 30-day interval between dosing is exceeded, administer SENTINEL® Flavor Tabs® immediately and resume the monthly dosing schedule. If SENTINEL® Flavor Tabs® replace daily diethylcarbamazine (DEC) for heartworm prevention, the first dose must be given within 30 days after the last dose of DEC.

Precaution(s): Storage Conditions: Store in a dry place at controlled room temperature, between 59° and 86°F (15-30°C).

Caution(s): U.S. Federal law restricts this drug to use by or on the order of a licensed veterinarian.

Do not use in puppies less than four weeks of age and less than two pounds of body weight. Prior to administration of SENTINEL® Flavor Tabs®, dogs should be tested for existing heartworm infections. Infected dogs should be treated to remove adult heartworms and microfilariae prior to initiating treatment with SENTINEL® Flavor Tabs®. Mild, transient hypersensitivity reactions manifested as labored respiration, vomiting, salivation and lethargy, have been noted in some treated dogs carrying a high number of circulating microfilariae. These reactions are presumably caused by release of protein from dead or dying microfilariae.

SENTINEL® Flavor Tabs® immediately break the flea life cycle by inhibiting egg development. However, pre-existing flea populations may continue to develop and emerge after treatment with SENTINEL® Flavor Tabs®. Based on results of clinical studies, this emergence generally occurs during the first 30-60 days. Therefore, noticeable control may not be observed until several weeks after dosing when a pre-existing infestation is present. Cooler geographic areas may have longer lag periods due to a prolonged flea life cycle. The concurrent use of conventional insecticidal products may be employed depending on the severity of the infestation.

If a SENTINEL® Flavor Tabs®-treated dog comes in contact with a flea-infested environment, adult fleas may infest the treated animal. These adult fleas are unable to produce viable offspring. Depending on the severity of infestation, the temporary use of conventional adulticides in an integrated flea control program may be necessary to control these adult fleas.

Adequate flea control may not be achieved in dogs that have repeated exposure to flea infested animals or environments.

Adverse Reactions: The following adverse reactions have been reported in dogs after giving milbemycin oxime or lufenuron: vomiting, depression/lethargy, pruritus, urticaria, diarrhea, anorexia, skin congestion, ataxia, convulsions, hypersalivation and weakness.

Trial Data: Efficacy:

Milbemycin Oxime: Milbemycin oxime provided complete protection against heartworm infection in both controlled laboratory and clinical trials.

In laboratory studies, a single dose of milbemycin oxime at 0.5 mg/kg was effective in removing roundworm, hookworm and whipworm. In well-controlled clinical trials, milbemycin oxime was also effective in removing roundworms and whipworms and in controlling hookworms.

Lufenuron: Lufenuron provided 99% control of flea egg development for 32 days following a single dose of lufenuron at 10 mg/kg in studies using experimental flea infestations. In well-controlled clinical trials, when treatment with lufenuron tablets was initiated prior to the flea season, mean flea counts were lower in lufenuron-treated dogs versus placebo-treated dogs. After 6 monthly treatments, the mean number of fleas on lufenuron-treated dogs was approximately 4 compared to 230 on placebo-treated dogs.

When treatment was initiated during the flea season, lufenuron tablets were effective in controlling flea infestations on dogs that completed the study. The mean flea count per lufenuron-treated dog was approximately 74 prior to treatment but had decreased to 4 after six monthly doses of lufenuron. A topical adulticide was used in the first eight weeks of the study to kill the pre-existing adult fleas.

Safety:

Milbemycin Oxime: Milbemycin oxime has been tested safely in over 75 different breeds of dogs, including collies, pregnant females, breeding males and females, and puppies over two weeks of age. In well-controlled clinical field studies 786 dogs completed treatment with milbemycin oxime. Milbemycin oxime was used safely in animals receiving frequently used veterinary products such as vaccines, anthelmintics, antibiotics, steroids, flea collars, shampoos and dips.

Two studies in heartworm-infected dogs were conducted which demonstrated mild, transient hypersensitivity reactions in treated dogs with high microfilaremia counts (see Cautions for reactions observed). Safety studies in pregnant dogs demonstrated that high doses (1.5 mg/kg = 3X) of milbemycin oxime given in an exaggerated dosing regimen (daily from mating through weaning), resulted in measurable concentrations of the drug in milk. Puppies nursing these females which received exaggerated dosing regimens demonstrated milbemycin-related effects. These effects were directly attributable to the exaggerated experimental dosing regimen. The product is normally intended for once-a-month administration only. Subsequent studies included using 3X daily from mating to one week before weaning and demonstrated no effects on the pregnant females or their litters. A second study where pregnant females were dosed once at 3X the monthly use rate either before, on the day of or shortly after whelping resulted in no effects on the puppies.

Some nursing puppies, at 2, 4, and 6 weeks of age, given greatly exaggerated oral doses of milbemycin oxime (9.6 mg/kg = 19X) exhibited signs typified by tremors, vocalization and ataxia. These effects were all transient and puppies returned to normal within 24 to 48 hours. No effects were observed in puppies given the recommended dose of milbemycin oxime (0.5 mg/kg). This product has not been tested in dogs less than 2.2 pounds in body weight.

A rising-dose safety study conducted in rough coated collies, manifested a clinical reaction consisting of ataxia, pyrexia and periodic recumbency, in one of fourteen dogs treated with milbemycin oxime at 12.5 mg/kg (25X monthly use rate). Prior to receiving the 12.5 mg/kg dose (25X monthly use rate) on day 56 of the study, all animals had undergone an exaggerated dosing regimen consisting of 2.5 mg/kg milbemycin oxime (5X monthly use rate) on day 0, followed by 5.0 mg/kg (10X monthly use rate) on day 14 and 10.0 mg/kg (20X monthly use rate) on day 32. No adverse reactions were observed in any of the collies treated with this regimen up through the 10.0 mg/kg (20X monthly use rate) dose.

Lufenuron: Lufenuron tablets have been used and tested safely in over forty breeds of dogs, including pregnant females, breeding males and puppies over six weeks of age. In well-controlled clinical trials, 151 dogs completed treatment with lufenuron tablets. Lufenuron tablets were used safely in animals receiving frequently used veterinary products such as vaccines, anthelmintics, antibiotics and steroids. In a ten-month study, doses up to 10X the recommended dose rate of 10 mg/kg caused no overt toxicity. A single dose of 200 mg/kg (20X the recommended dose rate) had no marked effect on adult dogs, but caused decreased activity and appetite in eight week old puppies. Mean body weights of male and female puppies were higher in treated versus control group at the end of the study. In specifically designed target animal safety studies, lufenuron tablets were tested with concurrent administration of flea adulticides containing carbaryl, permethrin, chlorpyriphos and cythioate. No toxicity resulted from these combinations. Lufenuron tablets did not cause cholinesterase inhibition nor did they enhance cholinesterase inhibition caused by exposure to organophosphates.

Four reproductive safety studies were conducted in breeding dogs with lufenuron tablets: two laboratory and two well-controlled clinical studies. In one of the laboratory studies, where lufenuron was administered to beagle dogs at doses equivalent to 90X (3X daily) the monthly recommended dose of 10 mg/kg, the ratio of gravid females to females mated was 8/8 or 100% in the control group and 6/9 or 67% in the lufenuron-treated group. The mean number of pups per litter was two animals higher in the treated versus control groups and the mean birth weights of pups from treated bitches in this study was lower than control groups. These pups grew at a similar rate to control pups. There was a higher incidence of four clinical signs in the lufenuron-treated versus control group: nasal discharge, pulmonary congestion, diarrhea/dehydration and sluggishness. The incidence of these signs was transient and decreasing by the end of lactation. Results from three additional reproductive safety studies, one laboratory and two clinical field studies evaluating eleven breeds of dogs, did not demonstrate any adverse findings for the reproductive parameters measured including fertility, pup birth weights and pup clinical signs after administration of lufenuron up to 5X the recommended monthly use rate.

Data from analysis of milk from lactating animals treated with lufenuron tablets at 2X and 6X the recommended monthly use rate, demonstrates that lufenuron concentrates in the milk of these dogs. The average milk:blood concentration ratio was approximately 60 (i.e., 60X higher drug concentrations in the milk compared to drug levels in the blood of treated bitches). Nursing puppies averaged 8-9 times higher blood concentrations of lufenuron compared to their dams.

Presentation: SENTINEL® Flavor Tabs® are available in four tablet sizes, (see Dosage Section), formulated according to the weight of the dog. Each tablet size is available in color-coded packages of six tablets each, which are packaged 10 per display carton.

U.S. Patent No. 4,547,520

Compendium Code No.: 11310092 NAH/SENT-FCT/VI/2 6/00

S

SEPTI-LUBE™

Boehringer Ingelheim **Lubricant**

Active Ingredient(s): An artificially-perfumed lubricant with detergent properties.

Indications: SEPTI-LUBE™ can be used as a lubricant of operator's hands and arms in obstetrical work, vaginal examinations, and rectal examinations; may also be used as a lubricant for catheters, stomach tubes, etc.

Dosage and Administration: Wet hands and arms with water and then apply SEPTI-LUBE™ liberally, thoroughly covering the entire surface. When the hands and arms are contaminated with foreign matter, the first application of SEPTI-LUBE™ should be massaged into the skin thoroughly and then removed with warm water. This cleanses the hands and arms. While the arms are still wet, apply another coating of SEPTI-LUBE™ before beginning the examination. If additional lubrication is needed, more SEPTI-LUBE™ can be applied while the arms are wet.

Note: The skin surfaces must be free of ordinary soap to obtain all of the advantages of using SEPTI-LUBE™.

Precaution(s): Keep from freezing.

Caution(s): Keep out of the reach of children. In case skin irritation should develop when using this product, discontinue use.

Presentation: 1 gallon containers.

Compendium Code No.: 10281000

SEPTI-SERUM®

Immvac **Antiserum**

Salmonella typhimurium Antiserum, Equine Origin, Re-17 Derived Mutagenically

U.S. Vet. Lic. No.: 345

Active Ingredient(s): *Salmonella typhimurium* antiserum, equine origin, Re-17 derived mutagenically.

Indications: SEPTI-serum® is recommended to aid in the protection against the effects of endotoxemia subsequent to parvoviral enteritis in dogs.

Dosage and Administration: Shake well before use and warm to room temperature. Administer intravenously 2-4 mL/lb. of body weight to dogs eight (8) weeks of age or older with post-parvo enteritis. The antiserum should be diluted at least 1:1 with a sterile isotonic fluid solution and administered in not less than 30 minutes.

Precaution(s): Store at 35°-45°F (2°-7°C). Do not freeze.

Caution(s): Sales are restricted to licensed veterinarians.

Use the entire contents when first opened.

The product is intended for one time administration only.

If an anaphylactic reaction occurs, administer epinephrine.

For veterinary use only.

Presentation: 50 mL containers.

Compendium Code No.: 11260040

SERAMUNE® I.V.

Sera **Equine Serum**

Equine IgG

U.S. Vet. Lic. No.: 328

Contents: SERAMUNE® Equine IgG is a concentrated, sterile serum product which is passed through a filtration process and gamma irradiated to inactivate virus. All donor horses are EVA and EIA negative. All donor animals are tested negative for RBC A&Q antibodies.

Indications: For the treatment of complete or partial failure of passive transfer of immunity in neonatal foals.

Dosage and Administration: Administer 250 mL intravenously in no less than 30 minutes. Repeat as clinical conditions indicate, within first 120 hours of life. Product may be diluted.

Precaution(s): Store refrigerated at 2-7°C/36-45°F. Do not freeze. Once opened, use entire contents as directed above.

Caution(s): For use by or under the direction of a veterinarian.

As with any serum product, adverse reactions may occur. In case of reactions, stop treatment and administer epinephrine.

To reduce possible reactions, the following measures are suggested:

A. Warm solution to body temperature.
B. Dilute serum into one to two liters of lactated ringers.
C. Pre-medicate with flunixin meglumine (IV @ 1.1 mg/kg).
D. A blood transfusion administration kit that includes a blood filtration apparatus should be used for all intravenous administrations.
E. Administer slowly for the first three to five minutes. The foal should be observed at all times during the transfusion. If the heart rate and/or respiration increases markedly, treatment should be discontinued until such signs return to normal. If signs persist or return, treatment should be terminated.
F. The antidote for anaphylaxis is epinephrine.

Presentation: 1 dose (250 mL) bottle.

Compendium Code No.: 14980000

SERAMUNE® ORAL

Sera **Equine Serum**

Equine IgG

U.S. Vet. Lic. No.: 328

Contents: Equine serum origin. Thimerosal is used as a preservative.

Indications: For the treatment of failure of passive transfer in neonatal foals.

Dosage and Administration: Administer orally in two even amounts (150 mL each) 1-2 hours apart, within first 12 hours of life.

Precaution(s): Protect from direct sunlight. Store refrigerated at 2°-7°C/36°-45°F. Do not freeze. Once opened, use entire contents as directed above.

Caution(s): For use by or under the direction of a veterinarian.

As with any serum product, adverse reactions may occur. In case of reactions, stop treatment and administer epinephrine.

Presentation: 1 dose (300 mL) bottle.

Compendium Code No.: 14980010

SERELISA™ PARATB

Synbiotics **Mycobacterium Test Reagent**

Mycobacterium Paratuberculosis Antibody Test Kit

U.S. Vet. Lic. No.: 312

Kit Contents: Each SERELISA™ ParaTB kit contains the following:

Label	Description	Single Plate Size	Five Plate Size
P	Positive Control	1 vial; 5.0 mL	2 vials; 5.0 mL per vial
N	Negative Control	1 vial; 5.0 mL	2 vials; 5.0 mL per vial
C	Conjugate	1 vial; 10.0 mL	1 vial; 50.0 mL
SD	Sample Diluent	1 vial; 25.0 mL	1 vial; 125 mL
CS	Chromogenic Substrate	1 vial; 10.0 mL	1 vial; 50.0 mL
W	Wash Solution, 20X concentrate*	1 vial; 100 mL	2 vials; 200 mL per vial
S	Stop Solution	1 vial; 6 mL	1 vial; 30 mL
	Antigen Coated Microwells	1 plate (96 wells)	5 plates (96 wells each)
	Sample Dilution/Transfer Plates	1 each (96 wells)	5 each (96 wells each)

*See "Preparation of Wash Solution" for instructions on diluting 20X concentrate.

Required Materials and Reagents Not Supplied in the SERELISA™ ParaTB Test Kit: Distilled or deionized water; Adjustable or fixed pipettes calibrated to measure and deliver between 0-1000 µL; Graduated cylinders (100 mL and 1000 mL); Automatic washing device for microwell plates; Microplate reader, fitted with filters for bichromic reading at 450 and 630 nm. (It is possible to use a monochromatic reader with a 450 nm filter.)

Indications: For the detection of antibodies to *Mycobacterium* spp. in bovine serum or plasma.

Test Principles: The plastic wells are coated with purified *Mycobacterium avium* antigen. Protein G derived from *Streptococcus* sp. is conjugated to the enzyme HRP. The serum or plasma sample is incubated in the coated wells followed by incubation with the Protein G conjugate. Reactive antibodies to *Mycobacterium avium,* if present in the bovine sample are bound to the well and in turn bind the Protein G conjugate. Unbound enzyme-linked Protein G is washed away and a chromogenic substrate is added. The development of a distinctly blue color indicates the presence of reactive antibody to *Mycobacterium avium.* In the absence of *Mycobacterium* antibody, no color change will be observed. Note: Blue color in wells will become yellow upon addition of stop solution.

SERELISA™ ParaTB is highly specific, sensitive and simple to perform. Test results can be obtained in 75 minutes. The diagnostic kit contains a positive control and a negative control which should be included each time the assay is performed. Spectrophotometric comparison of the optical density of the sample to the Positive Control will allow accurate detection of the presence of *Mycobacterium* antibody in the sample.

Sample Collection: Sample Information: Ten µL of serum or plasma is required. Use only bovine samples for test specimens. Samples may be stored at 2°-7°C (35°-45°F) up to seven days. If longer storage is desired, samples may be stood at -20°C (-4°F). Severely hemolyzed or lipemic serum may produce background color. When in doubt, obtain a better quality sample.

Test Procedure:

Preparation of Wash Solution: Allow wash concentrate to come to room temperature, Mix gently by inversion. Dilute wash concentrate 20-fold (1 part concentrate to 19 parts distilled or deionized water in a graduated cylinder. Diluted wash solution may be stored at 2°-7°C (35°-45°F).

Read the entire direction insert before beginning test. Strictly follow the procedure described below. Negative and Positive kit controls must be tested for each test run and/or for every plate.

A. Preliminary Steps:
   1. Prepare sufficient wash solution by diluting the 20X Wash Solution (Reagent W) 1:20 in distilled or deionized water.
   2. Allow one well for Positive Control, one well for Negative Control and one well for each test sample.
   3. Map out location of samples and controls using a 96 well grid pattern (e.g. well A1 for Positive Control, A2 for Negative Control, followed by sample wells.

B. Sample Preparation and Transfer:
   1. Using an uncoated transfer plate, add 125 µL of Positive Control (Reagent P) into the appropriate well.
   2. Add 125 µL of Negative Control (Reagent N) into the appropriate well of the same transfer plate.
   3. Pipet 10 µL of each sample into the bottom of the appropriate well of the same transfer plate. Use a separate pipet tip for each sample.
   4. Pipet 250 µL of Sample Diluent (Reagent SD) to each well of the transfer plate in which sample had been placed. Do not touch samples with pipet tips. Proceed immediately to Step 5.
   5. Using an 8 or 12 channel transfer pipet and fresh pipet tips for each column, mix and transfer 100 µL of controls and diluted test samples column by column into corresponding *M. paratuberculosis* antigen coated wells.
   6. Incubate for 30 minutes at room temperature (20°-25°C; 68°-77°F).

C. Wash:
   1. Wash wells 5 times with diluted wash solution using an automated plate washer.
   2. Blot excess liquid from wells on paper towel after final wash.

D. Conjugate:
   1. Add 100 µL of Conjugate (Reagent C) into each well using an 8 or 12 channel net transfer pipet.
   2. Incubate for 30 minutes at room temperature (20°-25°C; 68°-77°F).

E. Wash:
   1. Wash wells 5 times with diluted wash solution using an automated plate washer
   2. Blot excess liquid from wells on paper towel after final wash.

F. Chromogenic Substrate:
   1. Add 100 µL of Chromogenic Substrate (Reagent CS) into each well using an 8 or 12 channel transfer pipet.
   2. Incubate for 10 minutes at room temperature (20°-25°C; 68°-77°F).

G. Stop Solution:
   1. Add 50 µL of Stop Solution (Reagent S) into each well using an 8 or 12 channel transfer pipet. Gently tap side of plate to mix for 5-10 seconds.

H. Read Results:
   1. Read results within 15 minutes of adding Stop Solution.
   2. Use a dual wavelength plate reader set at a test wavelength of 450 nm and a reference wavelength of 630 nm or a single wavelength plate reader set at 450 nm.

Interpretation of Results:

Results: Results are measured using a plate reader with a test wavelength of 450 nm and a reference wavelength of 630 nm.

1. For the test to be valid, the Optical Density (O.D.) of the Negative Control must be less than or equal to 30% of the O.D. of the Positive Control. If these criteria are not met, the test is not valid and should be repeated.
2. A sample is considered positive for *M. paratuberculosis* reactive antibody if the O.D. of the sample is ≥125% of the O.D. of the Positive Control.
3. A sample is considered negative for *M. paratuberculosis* reactive antibody if the sample is ≤75% or the O.D. of the Positive Control.
4. A sample is considered suspect for *M. paratuberculosis* reactive antibody if the O.D. of the sample is between 75% and 125% of the O.D. of the Positive Control. In the event of a suspect result, a new sample from the animal should be collected after 3 months and retested. Confirmation of infection using an antigen test such as fecal culture or PCR may be considered as well.

A. Controls: The Optical Density (O.D.) of the Negative Control must be ≤30% of the Positive Control. If not, results are invalid and the test should be repeated with critical attention paid to the washing steps.

B. Evaluation of Sample Wells:

O.D. readings ≤75% of the O.D. of the Positive Control indicates absence of reactive antibody to *M. paratuberculosis*.

O.D. readings ≥125% of the O.D. of the Positive Control indicates presence of reactive antibody to *M. paratuberculosis*.

O.D. readings between 75% and 125% of the O.D. of the Positive Control indicates that infection with *M. paratuberculosis* is suspected. Animals producing results falling in this range should be re-tested in 8-12 weeks for antibody or infection. Should be confirmed with an antigen test such as culture or PCR.

Storage: To ensure optimal performance of the SERELISA™ ParaTB test kit through expiry, store the kit (including any diluted wash solution) at 2°-7°C (35°-45°F). The kit must be used before the expiration date. Kit serials are made up of optimal combinations of reagents; do not mix reagents from different serials of SERELISA™ ParaTB.

Store test kit at 2°-7°C (35°-45°F). Allow kit to come to room temperature before use.

Caution(s): Adherence to good laboratory practice is essential for quality results.

Read direction insert completely before starting test.

Do not use reagents after the expiry date.

Do not mix or associate reagents from kits with different batch numbers.

Allow all reagents to warm to room temperature prior to use.

Avoid inter-sample contamination during sample collection, storage or transport. Change the pipette tips for each sample.

Do not mouth pipette.

Avoid contact with the Chromogenic Substrate (hydrogen peroxide and tetramethylbenzidine) and the Stop Solution (4N sulphuric acid).

Decontaminate all disposable materials used during handling of samples either by immersion for a minimum of 1 hour in a freshly prepared 5% sodium hypochlorite solution before discarding them, or by autoclaving them at 120°C for a minimum of 1 hour.

Take particular care during the following operations.

For veterinary use only.

Washing: Conform to the minimum number of wash cycles indicated. Make sure that all wells are filled, then fully emptied. Washings are performed continuously, without any waiting period between the different cycles, using an automatic washer for microtitration plates. Manual washes with either a wash bottle or a dispenser should be avoided.

Addition of Chromogenic Substrate: Avoid accidentally contaminating the solution with metallic ions, oxidizing agents or detergents. Make sure that all containers are clean. Do not use the same container or the same pipette tip for the conjugate and the substrate.

Reading: A bichromatic reading is recommended. If a monochromatic reader is used, ensure the cleanliness of the bottom of the wells prior to reading.

Good Techniques = Accurate Results:

Serum or plasma must be used as a sample.

Hemolyzed and lipemic samples may be used; however, severely hemolyzed and lipemic samples may produce background color. When in doubt, obtain a better quality sample.

Washing is the most important step. The automated plate washer used must be monitored for adequate vacuum pressure, efficient and even dispensing of wash solution and greater than 90% aspiration of well contents. To assess washer efficiency, duplicate sample wells can be assayed. Duplicate samples should not vary more than 10%.

Do not use the test kit past the expiration date and do not intermix components from different serials of SERELISA™ ParaTB.

Discussion: Johne's disease is caused by *Mycobacterium avium* subspecies paratuberculosis and is a chronic, contagious enteritis characterized by persistent and progressive diarrhea, weight loss, debilitation, and ultimately death. It can affect all ruminants with worldwide distribution. The organism is shed in large numbers in the feces of infected animals. Infection is acquired by ingestion of contaminated feed and water. Nursing calves are infected soon after birth from udders contaminated by feces, presence of organisms in colostrum or milk, or contaminated pens. The highest incidence of infection is in animals less than 2 years of age whereafter resistance is stronger. The organisms infect macrophages in the mucosa of the small intestine and associated lymph nodes. If not cleared by a cell-mediated immune response, the organisms continue to multiply causing a chronic enteritis leading to shedding of organisms in feces, evidence of wasting and clinical disease. Early infection can take from months to years to become measurable by culture of organisms in feces or a detectable rise in antibodies to *Mycobacterium*.

References: Available upon request.

Presentation: SERELISA™ ParaTB is available in a single plate and 5 plate kit size.

Compendium Code No.: 11150500 03-2800-0800

SERGEANT'S® FLEA-FREE BREEZE™

Sergeant's **Flea Control & Premise Insecticide**

Odor Control Plus Flea Control

EPA Reg. No.: 4758-177-2517

Active Ingredient(s):

Pyriproxyfen 2-[1-Methyl-2-(4-phenoxyphenoxy) ethoxyl] pyridine‡	0.020%
Permethrin*	0.200%
n-Octyl Bicycloheptene Dicarboximide†	1.000%
Inert Ingredients	98.780%
Total	100.000%

‡ Nylar® Insect Growth Regulator, † MGK 264 Synergist

*(3-phenoxyphenyl)methyl (±) cis/trans 3-(2,2-dichloroethenyl)-2,2-dimethyl cyclopropanecarboxylate.

Cis/trans ratio: 35% (±) cis and max. 65% (±) trans

Indications: Eliminates odors in pet bedding, carpets, rugs, upholstered furniture and other areas frequented by pets. Features a new patent pending deodorizing technology. Plus, FLEA-FREE BREEZE™ kills fleas, ticks, flea eggs, and larvae.

Directions for Use: It is a violation of Federal law to use this product in a manner inconsistent with its labeling. Remove pets, birds and cover fish aquariums before spraying. Do not allow children or pets to contact surface until spray is dried.

Kennels or Pet Sleeping Quarters: Apply thoroughly to infested areas such as pet beds and resting quarters, nearby cracks and crevices, along and behind baseboards, window and door sills, and localized areas of floor and floor covering where fleas, ticks and lice may be present. Old pet bedding should be removed and replaced with fresh bedding after treatment of pet areas. Do not spray surfaces where spotting, staining or discoloration would be objectionable.

Precautionary Statements:

Hazards to Humans and Domestic Animals: Warning: Causes skin irritation and substantial but temporary eye injury. Do not get in eyes, on skin, or on clothing. Wear face shield or goggles. Prolonged or frequently repeated exposure may cause allergic reactions in some individuals. Remove contaminated clothing and wash before reuse. Wash thoroughly with soap and water after handling.

Statement of Practical Treatment

If On Skin: Remove contaminated clothing and wash with plenty of soap and water. Get medical attention.

If In Eyes: Flush with plenty of water. Get medical attention.

If Swallowed: Call a Doctor or get medical attention. Drink promptly a large quantity of milk, egg whites, gelatin solution, or if these are not available, drink large quantities of water. Avoid alcohol.

Physical and Chemical Hazards: Do not use this product in or around electrical equipment due to the possibility of shock hazard. Do not allow product to freeze.

Storage and Disposal: Do not contaminate water, food or feed by storage or disposal. Storage: Do not use or store near heat or open flame. Store in a dry area inaccessible to children. Disposal: Do not reuse empty bottle. Rinse thoroughly before discarding in trash.

Warning(s): Keep out of reach of children.

Presentation: 24 fl. oz. (709.7 mL).

Nylar® is a Registered Trademark of the McLaughlin Gormley King Company.

Compendium Code No.: 10830260

SERGEANT'S® PRETECT® FLEA AND TICK CARPET POWDER

Sergeant's **Flea Control & Premise Insecticide**

EPA Reg. No.: 4758-175-2517

Active Ingredient(s):

Linalool	2.500%
Piperonyl Butoxide, Technical*	0.500%
Pyrethrins	0.075%
Nylar: 2-(1-methyl-2-(4-phenoxyphenoxy) ethoxy) pyridine**	0.020%
Other Ingredients:	96.905%
	100.000%

*Equivalent to 0.4% (Butylcarbityl)(6-propylpiperonyl) ether and 0.1% related compounds

**Nylar is a Registered Trademark of McLaughlin Gormley King

Indications: Controls flea reinfestation for up to 365 days.

Breaks flea life cycle.

Directions for Use: It is a violation of Federal law to use this product in a manner inconsistent with its labeling.

Shake well before using. One 16 ounce canister contains enough powder to treat 1 to 2 rooms (200-400 square feet). When using this product at the lower rate, allow the powder to remain in place for 24 hours before vacuuming. Apply powder more heavily to areas of flooring or furniture on which pets spend most of their time. Apply to dry surfaces only. Do not wet powder.

Carpets: Shake powder evenly across surface. Brush lightly with broom to force powder deep into carpet where fleas and their larvae exist. Wait at least 60 minutes before (lightly) vacuuming to remove visible surface powder. For maximum efficacy, delay vacuuming for up to 24 hours.

Upholstery: Remove loose cushions. Sprinkle along creases and into corners. Brush lightly to work powder into folds and creases. Vacuum to remove visible powder on surfaces. Do not use on exposed fabric without first testing on a hidden surface for effects on color (staining) or texture. If powder adheres to a spot, brush out and vacuum that area immediately.

When emptying vacuum bag after use, wrap contents of disposable bag in several layers of newspaper and discard in trash.

Treat pets with a registered flea and tick control product prior to re-entry.

Precautionary Statements:

Hazards to Humans and Domestic Animals: Caution: Causes moderate eye irritation. Avoid contact with eyes or clothing. Wash thoroughly with soap and water after handling and before eating or smoking. Do not contaminate feed, water or foodstuffs. Do not apply to food processing surfaces or use in food processing areas where food is exposed. Cover fish aquariums before use. Keep children and pets off treated carpet and upholstered furniture during treatment and while powder is still visible on their surfaces.

Statement of Practical Treatment

If In Eyes: Flush eyes with plenty of water. Get medical attention if irritation persists.

Storage and Disposal:

Storage: Store in a cool, dry area inaccessible to children and pets.

Disposal: Do not reuse empty container. Wrap container and put in trash collection.

Warning(s): Keep out of reach of children.

Presentation: 16 oz (453 g) canister.

This container is sold by weight, not by volume. You can be assured of proper weight even though some settling of contents normally occurs during transportation and handling.

Compendium Code No.: 10830141 RIVD

S

SERGEANT'S® PRETECT® FLEA AND TICK SHAMPOO FOR CATS AND KITTENS

Sergeant's **Parasiticide Shampoo**

EPA Reg. No.: 2382-164-2517

Active Ingredient(s):

Pyriproxyfen	0.01%
Pyrethrins*	0.15%
Piperonyl butoxide, technical*	1.50%
n-Octyl bicyclopheptene dicarboximide	0.50%
Other Ingredients:	97.84%
	100.00%

*Equivalent to 1.2% (butylcarbityl) (6-propylpiperonyl) ether and 0.3% related compounds

Indications: The dual synergized pyrethrins provide immediate killing of fleas and ticks on the pet. Pyriproxyfen, in this special formulation, is absorbed onto and sticks tightly to hair and skin, even after complete rinsing. This insect growth regulator, a synthetic flea hormone, sterilizes all fleas that jump onto the pet (even new fleas before they start laying eggs) and therefore kills all flea eggs. This action persists for 1 month and breaks the flea's life cycle by preventing the development of new fleas in the pet's environment and the build-up of reinfestation pressure.

Use only on cats.

Directions for Use: It is a violation of Federal Law to use this product in a manner inconsistent with its labeling.

Read entire label before each use.

Shake well before using. Wet the pet thoroughly with warm water. Apply product onto its back at the rate of approximately 1¼ tablespoon (8.5 g per kg) for cats and kittens. Massage well into the skin to obtain good lathering over the entire body. Allow lather to remain in contact for at least 10 minutes then rinse off. Allow pet to air dry or blow dry. To maintain effective flea life cycle control through IGR flea egg killing, repeat treatment at least once every month. Under conditions of flea reinfestation pressure from the environment, repeat treatment when new parasites are seen on the pet, but not more frequently than twice monthly on cats.

Precautionary Statements:

Hazards to Humans and Domestic Animals: Caution: Do not treat nursing kittens. Do not use on kittens under 6 months of age. Consult a veterinarian before treating pregnant, nursing, sick, aged, debilitated or medicated cats. Sensitivities may occur after using any pesticide product on pets. If signs of sensitivity occur, bathe pet with mild soap or a non-pesticidal shampoo and rinse with large quantities of water. If signs continue consult a veterinarian immediately. Wash hands with soap and water after using.

In case of emergency, call: 1-800-224-PETS.

Storage and Disposal:

Storage: Store in closed container in a cool dry area.

Disposal: Do not reuse empty container. Wrap container and put in trash

Warning(s): Keep out of reach of children.

Presentation: 12 fl oz (354 mL).

Nylar® is a registered trademark of McLaughlin Gormley King Company

±Patent pending

Compendium Code No.: 10830152 MAR Y21118

SERGEANT'S® PRETECT® FLEA AND TICK SHAMPOO FOR DOGS AND PUPPIES

Sergeant's **Parasiticide Shampoo**

EPA Reg. No.: 4758-182-2517

Active Ingredient(s):

Permethrin: (3-Phenoxyphenyl) methyl (±) cis, trans*-3-(2,2-dichloroethenyl)-2,2-dimethyl cyclopropane carboxylate	0.10%
Piperonyl butoxide, technical**	0.50%
Pyriproxyfen: 2-[1-Methyl-2-(4-phenoxyphenoxy)ethoxyl] pyridine***	0.01%
Other Ingredients:	99.39%

*cis/trans isomers ratio: min. 35% (±) cis and max. 65% (±) trans

**equivalent to 0.4% of (butylcarbityl) (6-propylpiperonyl) ether and 0.1% related compounds.

***Nylar® Insect Growth Regulator

Indications: PRETECT® Shampoo for Dogs & Puppies kills fleas and ticks while it cleans and deodorizes in one easy and convenient step. This rich, conditioning, non-staining formula contains a highly effective flea and tick killing ingredient combined with an insect growth regulator that sterilizes new fleas and kills their eggs for 30 days. Kills ticks that may carry lyme disease. pH balanced for dog's coat.

Use only on dogs.

Directions for Use: It is a violation of Federal Law to use this product in a manner inconsistent with its labeling.

Read entire label before each use.

Wet dog's coat thoroughly. Pour into the cup of your hand. Starting at the head and working back, work up a lather with this quick lathering formula, being sure that the lather is worked thoroughly into dog's coat down to the skin. Allow lather to stand five minutes, then rinse completely and towel dry. It should not be necessary to repeat the shampoo application unless the animal is excessively dirty. Kills fleas fast and begins to kill ticks within 1 or 2 days; reaching maximum effectiveness in 7 to 10 days. To maintain maximum effectiveness against both fleas and ticks, repeat (or reapply) every week.

Precautionary Statements:

Hazards to Humans and Domestic Animals: Caution: Harmful if inhaled. Avoid breathing vapors. Causes moderate eye irritation. Avoid contact with eyes or clothing. Prolonged or frequently repeated skin contact may cause reactions in some individuals. Wear protective rubber gloves when applying this product. Wash thoroughly with soap and water after handling. Do not use on dogs under 12 weeks. Consult a veterinarian before using this product on debilitated, aged, medicated, pregnant or nursing animals. Sensitivities may occur after using any pesticide product for pets. If signs of sensitivities occur bathe your pet with mild soap and rinse with large amounts of water. If signs continue, consult a veterinarian immediately.

First Aid:

If In Eyes: Flush with plenty of water. Call physician if irritation persists.

If Inhaled: Remove victim to fresh air and get medical attention.

In case of emergency, call: 1-877-937-3059.

Storage and Disposal: Store in cool, dry place. Do not reuse container. Rinse thoroughly before discarding in trash.

Warning(s): Keep out of reach of children.

Presentation: 12 fl oz (354 mL).

Nylar® is a registered trademark of McLaughlin Gormley King Co.

Compendium Code No.: 10830161 Y211411

SERGEANT'S® PRETECT® FLEA AND TICK SPRAY FOR CATS AND KITTENS

Sergeant's **Flea Control and Topical Parasiticide**

EPA Reg. No.: 4691-153-2517

Active Ingredient(s):

Pyriproxyfen: 2-[1-methyl-2-(4-phenoxyphenoxy) ethoxyl] pyridine	0.125%
d-trans-chrysanthemum monocarboxylic acid ester of d-2-allyl-4-hydroxy-3-methyl-2-cyclopenten-1-one	0.100%
Permethrin [(3-phenoxyphenyl) methyl(±) cis-trans-3-(2,2-dichloroethenyl) 2,2-dimethylcyclopropane carboxylate]*	0.150%
Piperonyl butoxide, technical**	0.500%
N-octyl bicycloheptene dicarboximide	1.000%
Di-n-propyl isocinchomeronate***	0.200%
Other Ingredients:	97.925%
	100.000%

*cis/trans isomer ratio: min. 35% (±) cis; max. 65% (±) trans

**Equivalent to 0.4% (butylcarbityl)(6-propylpiperonyl) ether and 0.1% related compounds

***MGK 326 Insect Repellent

Indications: This product kills flea eggs for 100 days and adult fleas for 14 days. It breaks the flea life cycle.

Use only on cats and kittens.

Directions for Use: It is a violation of Federal law to use this product in a manner inconsistent with its labeling. Read entire label before each use.

Shake well before using. For Cats and Kittens: Cover animal's eyes with hand and with a firm, fast stroke, to get proper spray mist, spray head, ears and chest. With fingertips, rub into face around mouth, nose and eyes. Then spray the neck, middle and hind quarters, finishing with legs last. Apply spray until animal is uniformly damp. Animal should not be soaked or sprayed to the point of run-off. For best penetration, spray against natural lay of the hair. On a heavily coated animal, rub your hand against the lay of the hair, spraying the ruffled hair directly behind your hand. Make sure spray thoroughly wets attached ticks. Repeat every 7 days, if necessary, for control of adult fleas. Allow spray to dry before allowing cats to groom themselves. Wash hands thoroughly with soap and water after treating pet. Use this product in a well ventilated area. Consult a veterinarian before using this product on debilitated, aged, medicated, pregnant or nursing animals.

Contraindication(s): Do not use on kittens under 6 weeks old.

Precautionary Statements:

Hazards To Humans: Caution: Causes moderate eye injury. Do not get in eyes or on clothing. Wash thoroughly with soap and water after handling.

Hazards to Animals: Caution: Sensitivities may occur after using any pesticide product for pets. If signs of sensitivity occur, bathe your pet with mild soap and rinse with large amounts of water. If signs continue, consult a veterinarian immediately.

First Aid:

If Swallowed: Call a physician or Poison Control Center. Drink 1 or 2 glasses of water and induce vomiting by touching back of throat with finger. Do not induce vomiting or give anything by mouth to an unconscious person.

If In Eyes: Hold eyelids open and flush with a steady, gentle stream of water. Call a physician if irritation persists.

Environmental Hazards: Do not apply directly to water. Do not contaminate water when disposing of equipment wash waters.

Physical or Chemical Hazards: Flammable. Keep away from heat and open flame.

In case of emergency, call: 1-800-224-PETS.

Storage and Disposal: Store in a cool, dry place away from children. Store above freezing (32°F) and protect from high temperatures. Do not reuse empty container. Rinse thoroughly before discarding. Securely wrap original container in several layers of newspaper and discard in trash.

Warning(s): Keep out of reach of children.

Presentation: 8 fl oz (236 mL).

Compendium Code No.: 10830171 RIVD Y209781

SERGEANT'S® PRETECT® FLEA AND TICK SPRAY FOR DOGS AND PUPPIES

Sergeant's **Flea Control & Topical Parasiticide**

EPA Reg. No.: 4691-153-2517

Active Ingredient(s):

Pyriproxyfen: 2-[1-methyl-2-(4-phenoxyphenoxy) ethoxyl] pyridine	0.125%
d-trans-chrysanthemum monocarboxylic acid ester of d-2-allyl-4-hydroxy-3-methyl-2-cyclopenten-1-one	0.100%
Permethrin [(3-phenoxyphenyl) methyl(±) cis-trans-3-(2,2-dichloroethenyl) 2,2-dimethylcyclopropane carboxylate]*	0.150%
Piperonyl butoxide, technical**	0.500%
N-octyl bicycloheptene dicarboximide	1.000%
Di-n-propyl isocinchomeronate***	0.200%
Other Ingredients:	97.925%
	100.000%

*cis/trans isomer ratio: min. 35% (±) cis; max. 65% (±) trans

**Equivalent to 0.4% (butylcarbityl)(6-propylpiperonyl) ether and 0.1% related compounds

***MGK 326 Insect Repellent

Indications: This product kills flea eggs for 100 days and adult fleas for 14 days. It breaks the flea life cycle.

Use only on dogs and puppies.

Directions for Use: It is a violation of Federal law to use this product in a manner inconsistent with its labeling. Read entire label before each use.

Shake well before using. For Dogs and Puppies: Cover animal's eyes with hand and with a firm,

S

fast stroke, to get proper spray mist, spray head, ears and chest. With fingertips, rub into face around mouth, nose and eyes. Then spray the neck, middle and hind quarters, finishing with legs last. Apply spray until animal is uniformly damp. Animal should not be soaked or sprayed to the point of run-off. For best penetration, spray against natural lay of the hair. On a heavily coated animal, rub your hand against the lay of the hair, spraying the ruffled hair directly behind your hand. Make sure spray thoroughly wets attached ticks. Repeat every 7 days, if necessary, for control of adult fleas. Wash hands thoroughly with soap and water after treating pet. Use this product in a well ventilated area. Consult a veterinarian before using this product on debilitated, aged, medicated, pregnant or nursing animals.

Contraindication(s): Do not use on puppies under 6 weeks old.

Precautionary Statements:

Hazards to Humans: Caution: Causes moderate eye injury. Do not get in eyes or on clothing. Wash thoroughly with soap and water after handling.

Hazards to Animals: Caution: Sensitivities may occur after using any pesticide product for pets. If signs of sensitivity occur, bathe your pet with mild soap and rinse with large amounts of water. If signs continue, consult a veterinarian immediately.

First Aid:

If Swallowed: Call a physician or Poison Control Center. Drink 1 or 2 glasses of water and induce vomiting by touching back of throat with finger. Do not induce vomiting or give anything by mouth to an unconscious person.

If In Eyes: Hold eyelids open and flush with a steady, gentle stream of water. Call a physician if irritation persists.

Environmental Hazards: Do not apply directly to water. Do not contaminate water when disposing of equipment wash waters.

Physical or Chemical Hazards: Flammable. Keep away from heat and open flame.

Storage and Disposal: Store in a cool, dry place away from children. Store above freezing (32°F) and protect from high temperatures. Do not reuse empty container. Rinse thoroughly before discarding. Securely wrap original container in several layers of newspaper and discard in trash.

Warning(s): Keep out of reach of children.

Presentation: 8 fl oz (236 mL).

Compendium Code No.: 10830181 RIVD Y209761

SERGEANT'S® PRETECT® HOUSEHOLD FLEA AND TICK SPRAY

Sergeant's **Flea Control & Premise Insecticide**

EPA Reg. No.: 4758-169-2517

Active Ingredient(s):

Linalool	1.000%
N-octyl bicycloheptene dicarboximide*	1.000%
Nylar: 2-[1-Methyl-2-(4-phenoxyphenoxy) ethoxy] pyridine	0.015%
Permethrin**	0.200%
Other Ingredients:	97.785%
	100.000%

*MGK 264 Insecticide Synergist

**(3-phenoxyphenyl) methyl (±) cis/trans-3-(2,2-dichloroethenyl)-2,2-dimethylcyclopropanecarboxylate. Cis/trans ratio: 35% (±) cis and max. 65% (±) trans

Indications: Kills adult and pre-adult fleas utilizing an Insect Growth Regulator (IGR) in conjunction with other ingredients to kill adult fleas and prevent pre-adult fleas from developing into biting adults.

Reaches the hiding places of the flea: rugs, carpets, drapes, pet bedding, upholstery and furniture.

Protects the household from a buildup of fleas and reinfestation by providing 210-day residual activity from a single treatment.

Also kills ticks, roaches, ants, lice, waterbugs, silverfish, crickets, spiders, centipedes and sowbugs.

Directions for Use: It is a violation of Federal law to use this product in a manner inconsistent with its labeling. Do not allow children or pets to contact treated surfaces until spray has dried.

Indoors: Thoroughly vacuum all carpeting, upholstered furniture, drapes, along baseboards, under furniture and in closets. Seal vacuum bag and dispose of in outdoor trash. Spray SERGEANT'S® PRETECT® Household Flea and Tick Spray from a distance of two to three feet from surface being treated. Apply with a smooth back-and-forth motion to carpets, drapes, rugs and upholstered furniture. Avoid wetting or saturating carpets or furniture. An evenly applied fine mist spray is sufficient. Do not spray wood furniture, floors or trim as water spotting may occur. Repeat treatment as necessary to eliminate fleas and ticks. Apply directly to exposed insects: roaches, ants, spiders, crickets, centipedes, waterbugs, silverfish and sowbugs.

Pet Bedding: Treat pet bedding and resting places. Apply a uniform spray to nearby cracks and crevices, along baseboards, window and door sills and localized areas where fleas, ticks or lice may be present as these are primary hiding places for these pests. Removal and replacement of pet bedding after treatment is not necessary.

Precautionary Statements:

Hazards to Humans and Domestic Animals: Caution: May be harmful if absorbed through skin. Causes moderate eye irritation. Avoid contact with eyes, skin, or clothing. Wash thoroughly with soap and water after handling. Remove pets, birds and cover fish aquariums before spraying. In the home, food processing surfaces should be covered before treatment or thoroughly washed before use. Do not apply while food processing, preparation or serving is underway.

Statement of Practical Treatment

If In Eyes: Flush eyes with plenty of water. Get medical attention it irritation persists.

If On Skin: Wash with plenty of soap and water. Get medical attention.

Physical or Chemical Hazards: Contents under pressure. Do not use or store near heat of open flame. Do not puncture or incinerate container. Exposure to temperatures above 130°F may cause bursting. Provide adequate ventilation during use. Do not use in or around electrical equipment due to possibility of shock hazard. Protect from freezing.

Storage and Disposal:

Storage: Store in a cool, dry area out of reach of children. Protect from freezing.

Disposal: Do not puncture or incinerate container. Wrap container in several layers of newspaper and dispose of in trash collection.

Warning(s): Keep out of reach of children.

Presentation: 12 oz (340 g).

Compendium Code No.: 10830191 MVV

SERGEANT'S® PRETECT® INDOOR FLEA AND TICK FOGGER

Sergeant's **Flea Control & Premise Insecticide**

EPA Reg. No.: 4758-165-2517

Active Ingredient(s):

Permethrin [(3-phenoxyphenyl) Methyl (±) cis/trans-3-(2,2-dichloroethenyl) 2,2-dimethylcyclopropanecarboxylate]*	0.50%
Linalool	1.00%
Piperonyl butoxide, technical**	0.50%
Nylar: 2-(1-methyl-2-(4-phenoxyphenoxy) ethoxy) pyridine	0.10%
Other Ingredients:	97.90%
	100.00%

*cis/trans isomer ratio: min. 35% (±) cis; max. 65% (±) trans

**Equivalent to 0.4% (butylcarbityl)(6-propylpiperonyl) ether and 0.1% related compounds

Indications: This product will kill fleas (adult and pre-adult), roaches, houseflies, ticks, ants, spiders, and mosquitoes.

Directions for Use: It is a violation of Federal law to use this product in a manner inconsistent with its labeling.

Do not use more than one fogger per room. Do not use in small, enclosed spaces such as closets, cabinets or under counters or tables. Do not use in a room 5 ft. x 5 ft. or smaller; instead, allow fog to enter from other rooms. Turn of all ignition sources such as pilot lights (shut off gas valves), other open flames or running electrical appliances that cycle oil and on (i.e., refrigerators, thermostats, etc.). Call your gas utility or management company if you need assistance with your pilot lights.

Cover or remove exposed foods, dishes and food handling equipment. All food processing surfaces should be covered immediately prior to treatment or thoroughly cleaned after treatment. Close doors and windows. Open cabinets and interior doors within the treatment area. Shut off fans and air conditioners. Shut off electrical equipment. Remove pets. Cover or remove fish tanks and bowls. Fogger should be placed on floor in the middle of the room. Place newspaper under the container to prevent marring surfaces. Use one 2 ounce container for each 2,000 cubic feet (approximately 15.5' x 16' x 8' room). To start fogging, press down the actuator tab to locked position. Keep at arm's length when activating. Point top of can away from face and eyes. Set in upright position and leave building at once. Leave undisturbed for 2 hours. Open doors and windows and allow to air for 1 hour. Do not use in food areas of food handling establishments, restaurants, or other areas where food is commercially prepared or served. Do not use in serving areas while food is exposed.

Precautionary Statements:

Hazards to Humans and Domestic Animals: Caution: Use only when area to be treated is vacated by humans and pets.

Harmful if absorbed through the skin. Causes moderate eye irritation. Avoid contact with skin, eyes, or clothing. Wash thoroughly with soap and water after handling. Do not apply directly to food, in the home, all food processing surfaces and utensils should be covered during treatment or thoroughly washed before reuse. Remove pets and birds and cover fish aquariums before spraying. Remove all motor vehicles before using in garages.

Statement of Practical Treatment:

If On Skin: Remove contaminated clothing and wash with plenty of soap and water. Get medical attention.

If In Eyes: Flush eyes with plenty of water. Obtain medical attention if irritation persists.

Physical or Chemical Hazards: Highly Flammable Ingredient

This product contains a highly flammable ingredient. It may cause a fire or explosion if not used properly. Follow the "Directions for Use" on this label very carefully.

Extremely flammable. Contents under pressure. Do not use or store near heat or open flame. Do not puncture or incinerate container. Exposure to temperatures above 130°F may cause bursting. Never throw container into fire or incinerator. Newspapers should be spread on the floor for several feet around area of release.

In case of emergency call: 1-800-224-PETS.

Storage and Disposal:

Storage: Store in a cool, dry area, away from heat or open flame.

Disposal: Do not reuse container. Wrap container and put in trash collection. Do not puncture or incinerate.

Warning(s): Keep out of reach of children.

Presentation: 2 oz (57 g).

Sergeant's is a registered trademark of ConAgra® Brands, Inc.

Compendium Code No.: 10830202 VVV

SERGEANT'S® PRETECT® SQUEEZE-ON FLEA AND TICK CONTROL FOR DOGS (UNDER 15 LBS)

Sergeant's **Flea Control & Topical Parasiticide**

EPA Reg. No.: 270-278-2517

Active Ingredient(s):

Permethrin: (3-phenoxyphenyl) methyl (±) cis, trans-3-(2,2-dichloroethenyl)-2,2-dimethylcyclopropanecarboxylate*	45.0%
Pyriproxyfen: 2-[1-methyl-2-(4-phenoxyphenoxy) ethyoxy] pyridine (Nylar®)	5.0%
Other Ingredients:	50.0%
Total	100.0%

*cis/trans ratio: Max 55% (±) cis and min 45% (±) trans

Nylar® is a registered trademark of McLaughlin Gormley King and Company.

Indications: PRETECT® Squeeze-On Flea and Tick Control for Dogs prevents eggs from fleas on treated dogs from developing into biting adults for up to 123 days.

This product breaks the flea life cycle, kills and repels ticks and also protects against blood feeding by mosquitoes.

Use only on dogs over 12 weeks of age.

Directions for Use: It is a violation of Federal law to use this product in a manner inconsistent with its labeling. Read entire label completely before using.

Do not get this product in your dog's eyes or mouth. Repeat applications may be made if necessary, but do not apply more often than once every 3 weeks, except to reapply after shampooing the dog.

For Dogs Weighing 15 Pounds or Less: Apply one tube (1.0 mL) of PRETECT® Squeeze-On Flea and Tick Control for Dogs solution as a spot or stripe to the dog's back between the shoulder blades.

How to Apply: Remove product tube from the package. Holding tube with notched end pointing up and away from face and body, cut off narrow end at notches. Invert tube over dog and use open end to part dog's hair. Squeeze tube firmly to apply all of the solution to the dog's skin. Wrap tube and put in trash.

Contraindication(s): Do not use on cats or animals other than dogs.

Do not use on puppies under 12 weeks of age.

Precautionary Statements: Hazards to Humans and Domestic Animals: Caution:

Hazards to Humans: Harmful if swallowed. Avoid contact with eyes or clothing. Causes moderate eye irritation. Wash thoroughly with soap and water after handling.

Hazards to Domestic Animals: For external use on dogs only. Consult a veterinarian before using this product on debilitated, aged, medicated, pregnant, or nursing dogs. Consult a veterinarian before using on dogs with known organ dysfunction.

Do not use on cats or animals other than dogs. Cats which actively groom or engage in close physical contact with recently treated dogs may be at risk of toxic exposure. Certain medications can interact with pesticides. It is advisable to consult a veterinarian before using this product with any other pesticide or drug.

First Aid:

If Swallowed: Call a physician or Poison Control Center. Drink 1 or 2 glasses of water and induce vomiting by touching back of throat with finger or, if available, by administration of syrup of ipecac. Do not induce vomiting or give anything by mouth to an unconscious person.

If In Eyes: Flush eyes with plenty of water. Call a physician if irritation persists.

Adverse Reactions: Some animals may be sensitive to ingredients in this product. Reactions in dogs may include skin sensitivity. Dogs may show lethargy, increased pruritis (itchiness), erythema (redness), rash and hair discoloration or hair loss at the application site. Observe the dog following treatment. Sensitivity may occur after using any pesticide product on pets. If signs of sensitivity occur, bathe your dog with a mild, non-insecticidal shampoo and rinse with large amounts of water. If signs continue, consult a veterinarian immediately.

Environmental Hazards: This product is extremely toxic to fish. Do not add directly to water. Do not contaminate water when disposing of product or packaging.

In case of emergency, call: 1-800-781-4738.

Storage and Disposal: Do not contaminate water, food or feed by storage or disposal.

Storage: Store in cool, dry place. Protect from freezing.

Pesticide Disposal: Securely wrap original container in several layers of newspaper and discard in trash.

Container Disposal: Do not reuse empty container. Wrap container and put in trash.

Warning(s): Keep out of reach of children.

Disclaimer: Notice of Warranty: Sergeant's Pet Products makes no warranty of merchantability, fitness for any particular purpose, or otherwise expressed or implied concerning this product or its uses which extend beyond the use of the product under normal conditions in accordance with the statements made on this label.

Discussion: PRETECT® Squeeze-On Flea and Tick Control for Dogs is an effective and easy to use product. PRETECT® Squeeze-On Flea and Tick Control for Dogs has demonstrated greater than 92% control of fleas within one day of application.

As with all flea and tick control products, PRETECT® Squeeze-On Flea and Tick Control for Dogs should be used as part of a program aimed at reducing flea populations in the dog's environment (bedding, carpets, kennel, yard). Consult your veterinarian, entomologist, or retailer for program recommendations.

Presentation: Three 1.0 mL applicators (0.034 fl oz) (3 month supply).

Patent Pending

Compendium Code No.: 10830222 RAAA

SERGEANT'S® PRETECT® SQUEEZE-ON FLEA AND TICK CONTROL FOR DOGS (15 TO 33 LBS)

Sergeant's **Flea Control & Topical Parasiticide**

EPA Reg. No.: 270-278-2517

Active Ingredient(s):

Permethrin: (3-phenoxyphenyl) methyl (±)-cis, trans-3-(2,2-dichloroethenyl)-2,2-dimethylcyclopropanecarboxylate* 45.0%
Pyriproxyfen: 2-[1-methyl-2-(4-phenoxyphenoxy) ethyoxy] pyridine (Nylar®) 5.0%
Other Ingredients: 50.0%
Total 100.0%

*cis/trans ratio: Max 55% (±) cis and min 45% (±) trans

Nylar® is a registered trademark of McLaughlin Gormley King and Company.

Indications: PRETECT® Squeeze-On Flea and Tick Control for Dogs prevents eggs from fleas on treated dogs from developing into biting adults for up to 123 days.

This product breaks the flea life cycle, kills and repels ticks and also protects against blood feeding by mosquitoes.

Use only on dogs over 12 weeks of age.

Directions for Use: It is a violation of Federal law to use this product in a manner inconsistent with its labeling. Read entire label completely before using.

Do not get this product in your dog's eyes or mouth. Repeat applications may be made if necessary, but do not apply more often than once every 3 weeks, except to reapply after shampooing the dog.

For Dogs Weighing 15 to 33 Pounds: Apply one tube (1.5 mL) of PRETECT® Squeeze-On Flea and Tick Control for Dogs solution as a spot or stripe to the dog's back between the shoulder blades.

How to Apply: Remove product tube from the package. Holding tube with notched end pointing up and away from face and body, cut off narrow end at notches. Invert tube over dog and use open end to part dog's hair. Squeeze tube firmly to apply all of the solution to the dog's skin. Wrap tube and put in trash.

Contraindication(s): Do not use on cats or animals other than dogs.

Do not use on puppies under 12 weeks of age.

Precautionary Statements: Hazards to Humans and Domestic Animals: Caution:

Hazards to Humans: Harmful if swallowed. Avoid contact with eyes or clothing. Causes moderate eye irritation. Wash thoroughly with soap and water after handling.

Hazards to Domestic Animals: For external use on dogs only. Consult a veterinarian before using this product on debilitated, aged, medicated, pregnant, or nursing dogs. Consult a veterinarian before using on dogs with known organ dysfunction.

Do not use on cats or animals other than dogs. Cats which actively groom or engage in close physical contact with recently treated dogs may be at risk of toxic exposure. Certain medications can interact with pesticides. It is advisable to consult a veterinarian before using this product with any other pesticide or drug.

First Aid:

If Swallowed: Call a physician or Poison Control Center. Drink 1 or 2 glasses of water and induce vomiting by touching back of throat with finger or, if available, by administration of syrup of ipecac. Do not induce vomiting or give anything by mouth to an unconscious person.

If In Eyes: Flush eyes with plenty of water. Call a physician if irritation persists.

Adverse Reactions: Some animals may be sensitive to ingredients in this product. Reactions in dogs may include skin sensitivity. Dogs may show lethargy, increased pruritis (itchiness), erythema (redness), rash and hair discoloration or hair loss at the application site. Observe the dog following treatment. Sensitivity may occur after using any pesticide product on pets. If signs of sensitivity occur, bathe your dog with a mild, non-insecticidal shampoo and rinse with large amounts of water. If signs continue, consult a veterinarian immediately.

Environmental Hazards: This product is extremely toxic to fish. Do not add directly to water. Do not contaminate water when disposing of product or packaging.

In case of emergency, call: 1-800-781-4738.

Storage and Disposal: Do not contaminate water, food or feed by storage or disposal.

Storage: Store in cool, dry place. Protect from freezing.

Pesticide Disposal: Securely wrap original container in several layers of newspaper and discard in trash.

Container Disposal: Do not reuse empty container. Wrap container and put in trash.

Warning(s): Keep out of reach of children.

Disclaimer: Notice of Warranty: Sergeant's Pet Products makes no warranty of merchantability, fitness for any particular purpose, or otherwise expressed or implied concerning this product or its uses which extend beyond the use of the product under normal conditions in accordance with the statements made on this label.

Discussion: PRETECT® Squeeze-On Flea and Tick Control for Dogs is an effective and easy to use product. PRETECT® Squeeze-On Flea and Tick Control for Dogs has demonstrated greater than 92% control of fleas within one day of application.

As with all flea and tick control products, PRETECT® Squeeze-On Flea and Tick Control for Dogs should be used as part of a program aimed at reducing flea populations in the dog's environment (bedding, carpets, kennel, yard). Consult your veterinarian, entomologist, or retailer for program recommendations.

Presentation: Three 1.5 mL applicators (0.1 fl oz) (3 month supply).

Patent Pending

Compendium Code No.: 10830232 RAAA

SERGEANT'S® PRETECT® SQUEEZE-ON FLEA AND TICK CONTROL FOR DOGS (UNDER 33 LBS)

Sergeant's **Flea Control & Topical Parasiticide**

EPA Reg. No.: 270-278-2517

Active Ingredient(s):

Permethrin: (3-phenoxyphenyl) methyl (±)-cis, trans-3-(2,2-dichloroethenyl)-2,2-dimethylcyclopropanecarboxylate* 45.0%
Pyriproxyfen: 2-[1-methyl-2-(4-phenoxyphenoxy) ethyoxy] pyridine (Nylar®) 5.0%
Other Ingredients: 50.0%
Total 100.0%

*cis/trans ratio: Max 55% (±) cis and min 45% (±) trans

Nylar® is a registered trademark of McLaughlin Gormley King Co.

Indications: PRETECT® Squeeze-On Flea and Tick Control for Dogs prevents eggs from fleas on treated dogs from developing into biting adults for up to 123 days.

This product breaks the flea life cycle, kills and repels mosquitoes, protects against blood feeding by mosquitoes (vector of Heartworm) up to 4 weeks, kill and repels ticks including Deer Ticks (vector of Lyme Disease) up to 4 weeks and Kill and repels Brown Dog Ticks and American Dog Ticks for up to 3 to 4 weeks.

Use only on dogs over 12 weeks of age.

Directions for Use: It is a violation of Federal law to use this product in a manner inconsistent with its labeling. Read entire label completely before using.

Do not get this product in your dog's eyes or mouth. Repeat applications may be made if necessary, but do not apply more often than once every 3 weeks, except to reapply after shampooing the dog.

For Dogs Weighing Less Than 33 Pounds: Apply one tube (1.5 cc) of PRETECT® Squeeze-On Flea and Tick Control for Dogs solution as a spot or stripe to the dog's back between the shoulder blades.

How to Apply: Remove product tube from the package. Holding tube with notched end pointing up and away from face and body, cut off narrow end at notches. Invert tube over dog and use open end to part dog's hair. Squeeze tube firmly to apply all of the solution to the dog's skin. Wrap tube and put in trash.

Contraindication(s): Do not use on cats or animals other than dogs.

Do not use on puppies under 12 weeks of age.

Precautionary Statements: Hazards to Humans and Domestic Animals: Caution:

Hazards to Humans: Harmful if swallowed. Avoid contact with eyes or clothing. Causes moderate eye irritation. Wash thoroughly with soap and water after handling.

Hazards to Domestic Animals: For external use on dogs only. Consult a veterinarian before using this product on debilitated, aged, medicated, pregnant, or nursing dogs. Consult a veterinarian before using on dogs with known organ dysfunction.

Do not use on cats or animals other than dogs. Cats which actively groom or engage in close physical contact with recently treated dogs may be at risk of toxic exposure. Certain medications can interact with pesticides. It is advisable to consult a veterinarian before using this product with any other pesticide or drug.

First Aid:

If Swallowed: Call a physician or Poison Control Center. Drink 1 or 2 glasses of water and induce vomiting by touching back of throat with finger or, if available, by administration of syrup of ipecac. Do not induce vomiting or give anything by mouth to an unconscious person.

If In Eyes: Flush eyes with plenty of water. Call a physician if irritation persists.

Adverse Reactions: Some animals may be sensitive to ingredients in this product. Reactions in dogs may include skin sensitivity. Dogs may show lethargy, increased pruritis (itchiness), erythema (redness), rash and hair discoloration or hair loss at the application site. Observe the dog following treatment. Sensitivity may occur after using any pesticide product on pets. If signs of sensitivity occur, bathe your dog with a mild, non-insecticidal shampoo and rinse with large amounts of water. If signs continue, consult a veterinarian immediately.

Environmental Hazards: This product is extremely toxic to fish. Do not add directly to water. Do not contaminate water when disposing of product or packaging.

In case of emergency, call: 1-800-228-5635, ext. 233.

Storage and Disposal: Do not contaminate water, food or feed by storage or disposal.

Storage: Store in cool, dry place. Protect from freezing.

Pesticide Disposal: Securely wrap original container in several layers of newspaper and discard in trash.

Container Disposal: Do not reuse empty container. Wrap container and put in trash.

Warning(s): Keep out of reach of children.

Disclaimer: Notice of Warranty: Sergeant's Pet Products makes no warranty of merchantability, fitness for any particular purpose, or otherwise expressed or implied concerning this product or its uses which extend beyond the use of the product under normal conditions in accordance with the statements made on this label.

Discussion: PRETECT® Squeeze-On Flea and Tick Control for Dogs is an effective and easy to use product. PRETECT® Squeeze-On Flea and Tick Control for Dogs has demonstrated greater than 92% control of fleas within one day of application.

As with all flea and tick control products, PRETECT® Squeeze-On Flea and Tick Control for Dogs should be used as part of a program aimed at reducing flea populations in the dog's environment (bedding, carpets, kennel, yard). Consult your veterinarian, entomologist, or retailer for program recommendations.

Presentation: Two 1.5 cc applicators (0.1 fl oz).

Patent Pending

Compendium Code No.: 10830242 RIVD P001050

SERGEANT'S® PRETECT® SQUEEZE-ON FLEA AND TICK CONTROL FOR DOGS (OVER 33 LBS)

Sergeant's **Flea Control & Topical Parasiticide**

EPA Reg. No.: 270-278-2517

Active Ingredient(s):

Permethrin: (3-phenoxyphenyl) methyl (±)-cis, trans-3-(2,2-dichloroethenyl)-2, 2-dimethylcyclopropanecarboxylate* 45.0%
Pyriproxyfen: 2-[1-methyl-2-(4-phenoxyphenoxy) ethyoxy] pyridine (Nylar®) 5.0%
Other Ingredients: 50.0%
Total 100.0%

*cis/trans ratio: Max 55% (±) cis and min 45% (±) trans

Nylar® is a registered trademark of McLaughlin Gormley King and Company.

Indications: PRETECT® Squeeze-On Flea and Tick Control for Dogs prevents eggs from fleas on treated dogs from developing into biting adults for up to 123 days.

This product breaks the flea life cycle, kills and repels ticks and also protects against blood feeding by mosquitoes.

Use only on dogs over 12 weeks of age.

Directions for Use: It is a violation of Federal law to use this product in a manner inconsistent with its labeling. Read entire label completely before using.

Do not get this product in your dog's eyes or mouth. Repeat applications may be made if necessary, but do not apply more often than once every 3 weeks, except to reapply after shampooing the dog.

For Dogs Weighing More Than 33 Pounds: Apply approximately half (1.5 mL) of the tube of PRETECT® Squeeze-On Flea and Tick Control for Dogs solution as a spot or stripe to the dog's back between the shoulder blades and apply the rest of the tube's contents (1.5 mL) as a spot or stripe to the dog's back directly in front of the base of the tail. Or apply the entire tube (3.0 mL) as a continuous stripe on the dog's back starting between the shoulder blades and ending directly in front of the base of the tail.

How to Apply: Remove product tube from the package. Holding tube with notched end pointing up and away from face and body, cut off narrow end at notches. Invert tube over dog and use open end to part dog's hair. Squeeze tube firmly to apply all of the solution to the dog's skin. Wrap tube and put in trash.

Contraindication(s): Do not use on cats or animals other than dogs.

Do not use on puppies under 12 weeks of age.

Precautionary Statements: Hazards to Humans and Domestic Animals: Caution:

Hazards to Humans: Harmful if swallowed. Avoid contact with eyes or clothing. Causes moderate eye irritation. Wash thoroughly with soap and water after handling.

Hazards to Domestic Animals: For external use on dogs only. Consult a veterinarian before using this product on debilitated, aged, medicated, pregnant, or nursing dogs. Consult a veterinarian before using on dogs with known organ dysfunction.

Do not use on cats or animals other than dogs. Cats which actively groom or engage in close physical contact with recently treated dogs may be at risk of toxic exposure. Certain medications can interact with pesticides. It is advisable to consult a veterinarian before using this product with any other pesticide or drug.

First Aid:

If Swallowed: Call a physician or Poison Control Center. Drink 1 or 2 glasses of water and induce vomiting by touching back of throat with finger or, if available, by administration of syrup of ipecac. Do not induce vomiting or give anything by mouth to an unconscious person.

If In Eyes: Flush eyes with plenty of water. Call a physician if irritation persists.

Adverse Reactions: Some animals may be sensitive to ingredients in this product. Reactions in dogs may include skin sensitivity. Dogs may show lethargy, increased pruritis (itchiness), erythema (redness), rash and hair discoloration or hair loss at the application site. Observe the dog following treatment. Sensitivity may occur after using any pesticide product on pets. If signs of sensitivity occur, bathe your dog with a mild, non-insecticidal shampoo and rinse with large amounts of water. If signs continue, consult a veterinarian immediately.

Environmental Hazards: This product is extremely toxic to fish. Do not add directly to water. Do not contaminate water when disposing of product or packaging.

S

In case of emergency, call: 1-800-781-4738.

Storage and Disposal: Do not contaminate water, food or feed by storage or disposal.

Storage: Store in cool, dry place. Protect from freezing.

Pesticide Disposal: Securely wrap original container in several layers of newspaper and discard in trash.

Container Disposal: Do not reuse empty container. Wrap container and put in trash.

Warning(s): Keep out of reach of children.

Disclaimer: Notice of Warranty: Sergeant's Pet Products makes no warranty of merchantability, fitness for any particular purpose, or otherwise expressed or implied concerning this product or its uses which extend beyond the use of the product under normal conditions in accordance with the statements made on this label.

Discussion: PRETECT® Squeeze-On Flea and Tick Control for Dogs is an effective and easy to use product. PRETECT® Squeeze-On Flea and Tick Control for Dogs has demonstrated greater than 92% control of fleas within one day of application.

As with all flea and tick control products, PRETECT® Squeeze-On Flea and Tick Control for Dogs should be used as part of a program aimed at reducing flea populations in the dog's environment (bedding, carpets, kennel, yard). Consult your veterinarian, entomologist, or retailer for program recommendations.

Presentation: Three 3.0 mL applicators (0.207 fl oz) (3 month supply).

Patent Pending

Compendium Code No.: 10830252 RAAA

SERGEANT'S® PRETECT® SQUEEZE-ON FLEA CONTROL FOR CATS

Sergeant's **Flea Control**

EPA Reg. No.: 270-308-2517

Active Ingredient(s):

Pyriproxyfen: 2-[1-methyl-2-(4-phenoxyphenoxy) ethoxy] pyridine (Nylar®) 5.3%
Other Ingredients: 94.7%
Total 100.0%

Nylar® is a registered trademark of McLaughlin Gormley King Company.

Indications: PRETECT® Squeeze-On Flea Control for Cats prevents eggs on treated cats from developing into biting adults for three months. It breaks the flea life cycle.

Use only on cats and kittens.

Directions for Use: It is a violation of Federal law to use this product in a manner inconsistent with its labeling. Read entire label completely before using. Do not get this product in your pet's eyes or mouth. Repeat applications may be made if necessary, but do not apply more often than once every 3 weeks. Do not use this product in or on electrical equipment due to the possibility of shock hazard.

How to Apply: Remove product tube from package. Holding tube with notched end pointing up and away from face and body, cut off narrow end at notches. While gently holding cat, invert tube over cat and use open end to part cat's hair, and apply product as a narrow stripe down cat's back from back of head to base of tail. Squeeze tube firmly to apply all of the solution directly to the cat's skin. Continue to gently restrain cat for a few seconds until product absorbs into cat's coat. Wrap tube and put in trash.

Contraindication(s): Do not use on kittens under 12 weeks of age.

Precautionary Statements: Hazards To Humans And Domestic Animals: Caution:

Hazards to Humans: Causes moderate eye irritation. Avoid contact with eyes or clothing. Wash thoroughly with soap and water after handling.

Hazards to Domestic Animals: For External Use Only. Do not use on cats under 12 weeks of age. Consult a veterinarian before using this product on debilitated, aged, pregnant, or nursing animals.

Sensitivities may occur after using any pesticide product for pets. If signs of sensitivity occur, bathe your pet with mild soap and rinse with large amounts of water. If signs continue, consult a veterinarian immediately.

Certain medications can interact with pesticides. Consult a veterinarian before using on medicated animals.

First Aid:

If Swallowed: Call a physician or Poison Control Center. Drink 1 or 2 glasses of water and induce vomiting by touching back of throat with finger, or, if available, by administering syrup of ipecac. If person is unconscious, do not give anything by mouth and do not induce vomiting.

If In Eyes: Flush eyes with plenty of water. Call a physician if irritation persists.

In case of emergency, call: 1-800-781-4713.

Storage and Disposal:

Storage: Store in a cool, dry place. Protect from freezing. Pesticide Disposal: Securely wrap on original container in several layers of newspaper and discard in trash.

Container Disposal: Do not reuse empty container. Wrap container and put in trash.

Warning(s): Keep out of reach of children.

Disclaimer: Notice of Warranty: Sergeant's Pet Products makes no warranty of merchantability, fitness for any particular purpose, or otherwise expressed or implied concerning this product or its uses which extend beyond the use of the product under normal conditions in accordance with the statements made on this label.

Discussion: PRETECT® Squeeze-On Flea Control for Cats is an effective and easy to use product.

As with all flea control products, PRETECT® Squeeze-On Flea Control for Cats should be used as part of a program aimed at reducing flea populations in the cat's environment (bedding, carpets, yard). For existing flea infestations, a premise treatment inducting an adulticide and larvacide should be used prior to treating your cat with PRETECT® Squeeze-On Flea Control for Cats. Consult your veterinarian or entomologist or retailer for program recommendations.

Presentation: Two 1.5 mL applicators (0.1 fl oz) (6 month supply).

Compendium Code No.: 10830211 RAAA

SERGEANT'S® VETSCRIPTION® ALOE EAR MITE TREATMENT

Sergeant's **Otic Parasiticide**

EPA Reg. No.: 68688-41-2517

Active Ingredient(s):

Pyrethrins 0.05%
*Piperonyl Butoxide, Technical 0.50%
Inert Ingredients: 99.45%

*Equivalent to 0.4% of Butylcarbityl 6-propylpiperonyl ether and a 0.10% of related compounds

Contains aloe vera and lanolin.

Indications: For the treatment of ear mite infestations in dogs and cats.

Directions for Use: It is a violation of Federal Law to use this product in a manner inconsistent with its labeling.

Read entire label before each use.

To Kill Ear Mites: Clean ears to remove build-up of wax and dirt. While firmly holding pet, fill ear canal with recommended number of drops in each ear. Massage base of ear to insure insecticidal action penetrates ear wax. Gently dry ear with a cotton ball, soft cloth, or cotton swab. This product may be applied daily for 7 to 10 days. Repeat treatment in two weeks if necessary.

Body Weight	Dosage
5-15 lbs	4-5 drops
15-30 lbs	5-10 drops
30 lbs & over	10-15 drops

If conditions for which this preparation is used persists or if irritation develops, discontinue use and consult a veterinarian.

This product may be applied daily for 7 to 10 days. Repeat treatment in two weeks if necessary. Do not use on puppies or kittens less than 12 weeks. Consult a veterinarian before using this product on debilitated, aged, pregnant or nursing animals or animals on medication.

Use only on dogs and cats.

In case of emergency call 1-800-224-PETS.

Precautionary Statements: Hazards to Humans and Domestic Animals: Caution:

Humans: Harmful if swallowed. Avoid breathing vapors. Avoid contact with eyes. In case of contact, immediately flush eyes with plenty of water. Obtain medical attention if irritation persists. If swallowed, do not induce vomiting. Wash hands with soap and water after using.

Animals: Avoid contact with eyes. If in eyes, flush with water. Do not use on meat or milk producing animals. Sensitivities may occur after using any pesticide product for pets. If signs of sensitivity occur, bathe your pet with mild soap and rinse with large amounts of water. If signs continue, consult a veterinarian immediately.

Statement of Practical Treatment:

If Swallowed: Call a physician or Poison Control Center. Do not induce vomiting because of aspiration hazard.

If On Skin: Wash immediately with soap and water.

If In Eyes: Flush with plenty of water. See a physician if irritation persists.

If Inhaled: Remove victim to fresh air.

Storage and Disposal:

Storage: Store in a cool, dry area away from heat or open flame.

Disposal: Do not reuse empty container. Wrap and put in trash.

Warning(s): Keep out of reach of children.

Presentation: 3 fl oz (88 mL) plastic squeeze bottle.

Compendium Code No.: 10830001 NVD YC09701

SERGEANT'S® VETSCRIPTION® HAIRBALL REMEDY

Sergeant's **Laxative**

Ingredient(s): An emulsion of liquid petrolatum 44%, malt syrup 47%, glycerine 7%, Acacia 2% and vitamin B_1 (thiamine HCl)-1 mg per oz.

Indications: Recommended as an aid to eliminate and prevent hairballs in cats.

Directions for Use:

To eliminate hairballs — For adult cats, feed a one-inch ribbon of VETSCRIPTION® Hairball Remedy daily until symptoms disappear. Give either from your finger or by placing on top of cat's front paw where it can be licked off.

To prevent hairballs — Feed adult cats a one-inch ribbon once or twice a week and brush frequently.

Use with kittens — For kittens over four weeks of age, feed a half-inch ribbon once or twice a week.

Precaution(s): Store at room temperature 59°-86°F (15°-30°C).

Caution(s): Symptoms of hairballs include constipation, straining during bowel movement, dry cough and vomiting after meals. If symptoms persist, consult a veterinarian.

Warning(s): Keep out of reach of children.

Presentation: 3.2 oz pump.

Compendium Code No.: 10830011

SERGEANT'S® VETSCRIPTION® SURE SHOT® LIQUID WORMER FOR CATS & KITTENS

Sergeant's **Parasiticide-Oral**

Active Ingredient(s): Piperazine (Diethylenediamine) - equivalent to 4.25 grams Piperazine Base per 100 cc. Fish flavor.

Indications: VETSCRIPTION® SURE SHOT® Liquid Wormer is a safe, effective wormer for cats and kittens. May be fed directly from a spoon or added to food. Effective against large round worms *(Toxocara canis, Toxocara cati,* and *Toxascaris leonina).*

Directions: Mix proper dosage with an amount of any palatable feed that will be consumed in one serving. If possible, confine treated cats or kittens for a day or two so that droppings can be collected and destroyed. Heavily infested animals may require a second treatment two weeks after the first. Administer ½ teaspoon per 5 lbs. of body weight.

Important: Do not worm a kitten under six weeks of age. Never worm a sick cat or kitten. Consult your veterinarian for assistance in the diagnosis, treatment, and control of parasitism.

Precaution(s): Avoid freezing.

Caution(s): Consult veterinarian before using in severely debilitated animals. Do not worm animal more than twice yearly except as advised by a veterinarian. This product is effective for those roundworm stages found in the intestine and does not remove migrating larval stages. Animals should be checked periodically by a veterinarian for presence of other parasites.

Warning(s): Keep out of reach of children and pets.

Presentation: 3.3 fl oz (100 mL).

Compendium Code No.: 10830270 OAR YC11191

SERGEANT'S® VETSCRIPTION® SURE SHOT® LIQUID WORMER FOR PUPPIES AND DOGS

Sergeant's **Parasiticide-Oral**

(pyrantel pamoate)

ANADA No.: 200-248

Active Ingredient(s): SURE SHOT® Liquid Wormer (pyrantel pamoate suspension 2.27 mg) is a suspension of pyrantel pamoate in a palatable vanilla-flavored vehicle. Each mL contains 2.27 mg of pyrantel base as pyrantel pamoate.

Indications: SURE SHOT® Liquid Wormer suspension is a highly palatable formulation intended as a single treatment for the removal of large roundworms *(Toxocara canis* and *Toxascaris leonina)* and hookworms *(Anclyostoma caninum* and *Uncinaria stenocephala)* in dogs and puppies. SURE SHOT® Liquid suspension may also be used to prevent reinfection of *Toxocara canis* in puppies and adult dogs and in lactating bitches after whelping. Consult your veterinarian for assistance in the diagnosis, treatment, and control of parasitism.

Pharmacology: Pyrantel pamoate is a compound belonging to a family classified chemically as tetrahydropyrimidines. It is a yellow, water-insoluble crystalline salt of the tetrahydropyrimidine base and pamoic acid containing 34.7% base activity. The chemical structure and name are given below.

(E)-1,4,5,6-Tetrahydro-1-methyl-2-[2-(2-thienyl) vinyl] pyrimidine 4,4' methylenebis [3-hydroxy-2-naphthoate](1:1)

Dosage and Administration: Administer one full teaspoon (5 mL) for each 5 pounds of body weight (2.27 mg base per lb of body weight). Although most dogs have been observed to find this formulation very palatable and willingly consume it undiluted, it may be necessary to mix a small quantity of formulation in the dog's normal ration to encourage consumption. Fasting prior to or after treatment is not necessary. For maximum control and prevention of reinfection, it is recommended that puppies be treated at 2, 3, 4, 6, 8, and 10 weeks of age. Lactating bitches should be treated 2-3 weeks after whelping. Adult dogs kept in heavily contaminated quarters may be treated at monthly intervals to prevent *T. canis* reinfection.

In case of emergency call 1-800-224-PETS.

Precaution(s): This product is a suspension and as such will separate. To insure uniform resuspension and to achieve proper dosage, it is extremely important that the product be shaken thoroughly before every use.

Recommended Storage: Store below 86°F (30°C).

Caution(s): For animal use only.

Warning(s): Keep out of reach of children.

Toxicology: Safety: One of the most outstanding and significant features of pyrantel pamoate is its wide margin of therapeutic safety in dogs. The acute oral LD_{50} of pyrantel pamoate administered in gelatin capsules to female and male dogs is greater than 314 mg base per pound of body weight, which indicates a therapeutic index in excess of 138 x the recommended dosage. In subacute and chronic studies, no significant morphological abnormalities could be attributed to pyrantel pamoate when administered to dogs at daily dose rates up to 94 mg base per pound of body weight (40 x) for periods of 19, 30, and 90 days. Clinical studies conducted in a wide variety of geographic locations using more than 40 different breeds of dogs showed no drug-induced toxic effects. Included in these studies were nursing pups, weaned pups, adults, pregnant bitches, and males at stud. Additional data have demonstrated the safe use of pyrantel pamoate in (1) dogs having heartworm infections and/or receiving medication for heartworm (2) dogs exposed to organophosphate flea collars or flea/tick dip treatments, and (3) dogs undergoing concurrent treatment or medication at the time of worming such as immunization and antibacterial treatment.

Trial Data: Efficacy: Critical (worm count) studies in dogs demonstrated that pyrantel pamoate at the recommended dosage is highly efficacious against *T. leonina* (99%), *T. canis* (85%), *A. caninum* (97%), and *U. stenocephala* (94%).

Presentation: 2 fl oz (60 mL) bottle.

Compendium Code No.: 10830021 Iss. 7-00

SERGEANT'S® VETSCRIPTION® VITAMINS FOR CATS & KITTENS

Sergeant's **Small Animal Dietary Supplement**

Guaranteed Analysis: Each VETSCRIPTION® Cat Vitamin contains (Minimum values unless otherwise stated):

Vitamin A	250.0 IU
Vitamin D	25.0 IU
Vitamin E	2.5 IU
Thiamine (B_1)	.25 mg
Riboflavin (B_2)	.2 mg
Vitamin B_6	.2 mg
Vitamin B_{12}	1.0 mcg
Niacinamide	3.0 mg
Choline	2.5 mg
Inositol	2.0 mg
Folic Acid	40.0 mcg
Taurine	50.0 mg
Pantothenic Acid	.25 mg
Omega 3 Fatty Acids*	5.0 mg

*Not recognized as an essential nutrient by the AAFCO cat food nutrient profiles

Ingredients: Brewers Yeast, Dried Whey, Taurine, Desiccated Liver, Lecithin, Fish Oil, Fennel Seed, Vitamin A Supplement, Vitamin D_3 Supplement, Vitamin E Supplement, Vitamin B_{12} Supplement, Riboflavin Supplement, Niacin Supplement, Calcium Pantothenate, Folic Acid, Pyridoxine Hydrochloride, Thiamine Mononitrate.

Indications: A palatable vitamin and mineral chewable supplement for cats and kittens.

An excellent source of vitamins, minerals, taurine and Omega 3 fatty acids that will keep your cat's skin healthy and coat luxurious.

Directions: Vitamins can be hand fed as a treat prior to feeding or crumbled and mixed with food.

For Cats and Kittens weighing less than 10 lbs.	1 tablet daily
For sick, convalescing, pregnant or nursing cats	2 tablets daily

Warning(s): Keep out of the reach of children and pets.

Presentation: 100 daily chewable tablets.

Compendium Code No.: 10830031 OAR P995117

SERGEANT'S® VETSCRIPTION® VITAMINS FOR DOGS

Sergeant's **Small Animal Dietary Supplement**

Guaranteed Analysis: Each VETSCRIPTION® Dog Vitamin contains (Minimum values unless otherwise stated):

Minerals:	
Calcium	100 mg
Phosphorus	10 mg
Potassium	10 mg
Iron	1 mg
Iodine	16 mcg
Copper	55 mcg
Manganese	60 mcg
Zinc	1.5 mg
Cobalt	14 mcg
Glutathione	4 mg
Vitamins:	
Vitamin A	1,000 IU
Vitamin D_3	100 IU
Vitamin E	2 IU
Thiamine (B_1)	810 mcg
Riboflavin (B_2)	1 mg
Pyridoxine (B_6)	82 mcg
Vitamin (B_{12})	0.2 mcg

Niacin .... 10 mg
Choline .... 7 mg
Inositol .... 6 mg
Essential Fatty Acid:
Linoleic Acid .... 30 mg

Ingredients: Brewers Dry Yeast, Dry Whey, Dicalcium Phosphate, Desiccated Liver, Lecithin, Flax Seed Meal, Fennel Powder, Yucca Powder, Zinc Oxide, Petonized Iron, Copper Acetate, Potassium Iodide, Cobalt Sulfate, Vitamin A Acetate, Cholecalciferol, d-Alpha Tocopheryl Acetate (Vitamin E), Niacin, Riboflavin, Thiamine, Mononitrate, Pyridoxine Hydrochloride, Vitamin B_{12}.

Indications: A palatable vitamin and mineral chewable supplement for dogs and puppies. Features a natural source of Omega fatty acids and antioxidants.

Directions: Vitamins can be given directly just prior to feeding or crumbled and mixed with food.
For Dogs and Puppies weighing less than 10 lbs. .... ½ tablet daily
For Dogs and Puppies weighing more than 10 lbs. .... 1 tablet daily
For sick, convalescing, pregnant or nursing dogs .... 2 tablets daily

Warning(s): Keep out of the reach of children and pets.

Presentation: 100 chewable tablets.

SERGEANT'S is a registered trademark of ConAgra® Brands, Inc.

Compendium Code No.: 10830041 CAA P995118

SERGEANT'S® VETSCRIPTION® WORM-AWAY® FOR CATS

Sergeant's **Parasiticide-Oral**

NADA No.: 092-710

Active Ingredient(s): Each capsule contains 140 mg piperazine (as citrate).

Indications: For the removal of large roundworms, *Toxocara canis* and *Toxascaris leonina*, in cats.

Directions: For kittens and cats weighing:
Animals one to five pounds .... 1 capsule
Animals six to ten pounds .... 2 capsules
Animals eleven to fifteen pounds .... 3 capsules
Animals sixteen to twenty pounds .... 4 capsules

Pull each capsule apart and empty contents into cat's food. To be sure the full dose is taken, mix it well with only one-half of his regular feeding. When cat has finished eating the dosed food, give balance of the meal. Repeat first dose 10 days later. Reinfection may occur - repeat treatment if indicated.

Caution(s): Consult a veterinarian before using in severely debilitated cats and for assistance in the diagnosis, treatment, and control of parasitism.

Warning(s): Keep out of reach of children.

Presentation: 12 capsules per bottle.

Compendium Code No.: 10830051 FDA P991118

SERGEANT'S® VETSCRIPTION® WORM-AWAY® FOR DOGS

Sergeant's **Parasiticide-Oral**

NADA No.: 092-709

Active Ingredient(s): Each capsule contains 140 mg piperazine (as citrate).

Indications: For the removal of large roundworms, *Toxocara canis* and *Toxascaris leonina*, in dogs.

Directions: For puppies and dogs weighing:
Animals one to five pounds .... 1 capsule
Animals six to ten pounds .... 2 capsules
Animals eleven to fifteen pounds .... 3 capsules
Animals sixteen to twenty pounds .... 4 capsules
Animals twenty-one to twenty-five pounds .... 5 capsules
Animals over twenty-five pounds .... 6 capsules

Pull each capsule apart and empty contents into dog's food. To be sure the full dose is taken, mix it well with only one-half of his regular feeding. When dog has finished eating the dosed food, give balance of the meal. Repeat first dose 10 days later. Reinfection may occur - repeat treatment if indicated.

Caution(s): Consult a veterinarian before using in severely debilitated dogs and for assistance in the diagnosis, treatment, and control of parasitism.

Warning(s): Keep out of reach of children.

Presentation: 12 capsules per bottle.

Compendium Code No.: 10830061 FDA P991119

SERPENS SPECIES BACTERIN

Hygieia **Bacterin**

Serpens Species Bacterin, Killed Bacterin

U.S. Vet. Lic. No.: 407

Description: SERPENS SPECIES BACTERIN contains killed cultures of an isolate of *Serpens* species bacteria. The original isolate was obtained from PDD lesions.

Inactivated culture with aluminum hydroxide adjuvant.

Indications: SERPENS SPECIES BACTERIN is indicated for the prevention of and as an aid in the treatment of Papillomatous Digital Dermatitis (PDD, hairy footwart, strawberry heel wart) in dairy cattle.

Field trials have shown that SERPENS SPECIES BACTERIN can prevent PDD in lesion-free animals, and aids in the treatment of lesions due to PDD in currently affected animals.

Directions:

1. General directions: Shake well before using. Administer 5.0 cc subcutaneously (under the skin) using clean technique.
2. Prevention:
   a. Primary Vaccination: Three doses initially, given at four week intervals (0, 4 & 8 weeks).
   b. Revaccination: Revaccinate with a single booster dose four months after the third dose and every four to six months thereafter.
3. Treatment:
   a. Primary Vaccination: In PDD-affected animals, administer three 5.0 cc doses subcutaneously at four week intervals (0, 4 & 8 weeks) in conjunction with appropriate management practices which may include footbaths or wraps.
   b. Revaccination: After healing, follow prevention guidelines with single booster doses of this vaccine every four to six months.

Precaution(s): Keep refrigerated at 35-45°F. Do not freeze.

Use entire contents when first opened.

Caution(s): Do not use in animals with signs of systemic disease. Administration should be under the supervision of a licensed veterinarian. Occasionally, anaphylactic or other adverse reactions may occur. If adverse reactions occur, appropriate therapy with epinephrine or other antianaphylactic drugs should be initiated immediately.

Any adverse reactions following vaccination should be immediately reported to the manufacturer.

Efficacy of this product has been proven on commercial dairies; however, response to any vaccine is dependent upon the environmental challenge and immune function of the animal.

This product contains no antibiotics, and requires no milk withdrawal period.

Warning(s): Do not vaccinate within 21 days before slaughter.

For veterinary use only.

Discussion: Disease Description: Papillomatous digital dermatitis is a chronic disease of the feet and lower legs of cattle. This disease is clinically manifested by skin lesions which may be ulcerative or proliferative in nature. The lesions are typically located near the skin/horn junctions of the digit and may result in severe lameness with secondary production and reproductive losses.

Trial Data: Safety: Extensive field trials have shown this product to be safe in all stages of lactation and gestation. No adverse systemic effects have been seen with this vaccine. A transient vaccine site reaction has been observed in some animals. This reaction consists of a mild, non-painful swelling of the skin at the injection site, which usually resolves within a few weeks.

Presentation: 250 cc (50 dose) vials.

Patent Pending

This product license is conditional pending the development of an acceptable potency test.

Compendium Code No.: 15060020

SEVOFLO™ ℞

Abbott **Inhalation Anesthetic**

(sevoflurane)

NADA No.: 141-103

Active Ingredient(s): Sevoflurane.

Indications: SEVOFLO™ is indicated for induction and maintenance of general anesthesia in dogs.

Pharmacology: Description: SEVOFLO™ (sevoflurane), a volatile liquid, is a halogenated general inhalation anesthetic drug. Its chemical name is fluoromethyl 2,2,2-trifluoromethyl) ethyl ether, and its structural formula is:

$$F_3C-CH(CF_3)-OCH_2F$$

(H–C bonded to F_3C above, F_3C below, and OCH_2F)

Sevoflurane Physical Constants are:
Molecular weight 200.05
Boiling point at 760 mm Hg .... 58.6°C
Specific gravity at 20°C .... 1.520-1.525 g/mL
Vapor pressure in mm Hg
at 20°C 157
at 25°C 197
at 36°C 317
Distribution Partition Coefficients at 37°C:
Blood/Gas 0.63-0.69
Water/Gas 0.36
Olive Oil/Gas 47-54
Brain/Gas 1.15
Mean Component/Gas Partition Coefficients at 25°C for Polymers Used Commonly in Medical Applications:
Conductive rubber 14.0
Butyl rubber 7.7
Polyvinyl chloride 17.4
Polyethylene 1.3

Sevoflurane is nonflammable and nonexplosive as defined by the requirements of International Electrotechnical Commission 601-2-13.

Sevoflurane is a clear, colorless, stable liquid containing no additives or chemical stabilizers. Sevoflurane is nonpungent. It is miscible with ethanol, ether, chloroform and petroleum benzene, and it is slightly soluble in water. Sevoflurane is stable when stored under normal room lighting condition according to instructions.

Clinical Pharmacology: Sevoflurane is an inhalational anesthetic agent for induction and maintenance of general anesthesia. The Minimum Alveolar Concentration (MAC) of sevoflurane as determined in 18 dogs is 2.36%.[2] MAC is defined as that alveolar concentration at which 50% of healthy patients fail to respond to noxious stimuli. Multiples of MAC are used as a guide for surgical levels of anesthetic, which are typically 1.3 to 1.5 times the MAC value. Because of the low solubility of sevoflurane in blood (blood/gas partition coefficient at 37°C = 0.63-0.69), a minimal amount of sevoflurane is required to be dissolved in the blood before the alveolar partial pressure is in equilibrium with the arterial partial pressure. During sevoflurane induction, there is a rapid increase in alveolar concentration toward the inspired concentration. Sevoflurane produces only modest increases in cerebral blood flow and metabolic rate, and has little or no ability to potentiate seizures.[3] Sevoflurane has a variable effect on heart rate, producing increases or decreases depending on experimental conditions.[4,5] Sevoflurane produces dose-dependent decreases in mean arterial pressure, cardiac output and myocardial contraction.[6] Among inhalation anesthetics, sevoflurane has low arrhythmogenic potential.[7] Sevoflurane is chemically stable. No discernible degradation occurs in the presence of strong acids or heat. Sevoflurane reacts through direct contact with CO_2 absorbents (soda lime and barium hydroxide lime) producing pentafluoroisopropenyl fluoromethyl ether (PIFE, $C_4H_2F_6O$), also known as Compound A, and trace amounts of pentafluoromethoxy isopropyl fluoromethyl ether (PMFE, $C_5H_6F_6O$), also known as Compound B.

Compound A: The production of degradants in the anesthesia circuit results from the extraction of the acidic proton in the presence of a strong base (KOH and/or NaOH) forming an alkene (Compound A) from sevoflurane. Compound A is produced when sevoflurane interacts with soda lime or barium hydroxide lime. Reaction with barium hydroxide lime results in a greater production of Compound A than does reaction with soda lime. Its concentration in a circle absorber system increases with increasing sevoflurane concentrations and with decreasing fresh gas flow rates. Sevoflurane degradation in soda lime has been shown to increase with temperature. Since the reaction of carbon dioxide with absorbents is exothermic, this temperature increase will be determined by the quantities of CO_2 absorbed, which in turn will depend on fresh gas flow in the anesthetic circle system, metabolic status of the patient and ventilation. Although Compound A is a dose-dependent nephrotoxin in rats, the mechanism of this renal toxicity is unknown. Two spontaneously breathing dogs under sevoflurane anesthesia showed increases

S

in concentrations of Compound A as the oxygen flow rate was decreased at hourly intervals, from 500 mL/min (36 and 18 ppm Compound A) to 250 mL/min (43 and 31 ppm) to 50 mL/min (61 and 48 ppm).[8]

Fluoride ion metabolite: Sevoflurane is metabolized to hexafluoroisopropanol (HFIP) with release of inorganic fluoride and CO_2. Fluoride ion concentrations are influenced by the duration of anesthesia and the concentration of sevoflurane. Once formed, HFIP is rapidly conjugated with glucuronic acid and eliminated as a urinary metabolite. No other metabolic pathways for sevoflurane have been identified. In humans, the fluoride ion half-life was prolonged in patients with renal impairment, but human clinical trials contained no reports of toxicity associated with elevated fluoride ion levels. In a study in which 4 dogs were exposed to 4% sevoflurane for 3 hours, maximum serum fluoride concentrations of 17.0-27.0 mcmole/L were observed after 3 hours of anesthesia. Serum fluoride fell quickly after anesthesia ended, and had returned to baseline by 24 hours post-anesthesia. In a safety study, eight healthy dogs were exposed to sevoflurane for 3 hours/day, 5 days/week for 2 weeks (total 30 hours exposure) at a flow rate of 500 mL/min in a semi-closed, rebreathing system with soda lime. Renal toxicity was not observed in the study evaluation of clinical signs, hematology, serum chemistry, urinalysis, or gross or microscopic pathology.

Dosage and Administration: Inspired Concentration: The delivered concentration of SEVOFLO™ should be known. Since the depth of anesthesia may be altered easily and rapidly, only vaporizers producing predictable percentage concentrations at sevoflurane should be used. Sevoflurane should be vaporized using a precision vaporizer specifically calibrated for sevoflurane. Sevoflurane contains no stabilizer. Nothing in the drug product alters calibration or operation of these vaporizers. The administration of general anesthesia must be individualized based on the patient's response.

Premedication: No specific premedication is either indicated or contraindicated with sevoflurane. The necessity for and choice of premedication is left to the discretion of the veterinarian. Preanesthetic doses for premedicants may be lower than the label directions for their use as a single medication.[1]

Induction: For mask induction using sevoflurane, inspired concentrations at 5 to 7% sevoflurane alone with oxygen are employed to induce surgical anesthesia in the healthy dog. These concentrations can be expected to produce surgical anesthesia in 3 to 14 minutes. The use of premedicants does not affect the concentration of sevoflurane required for induction.

Maintenance: SEVOFLO™ may be used for maintenance anesthesia following mask induction using sevoflurane or following injectable induction agents. The concentration of vapor necessary to maintain anesthesia is much less than that required to induce it. Surgical levels of anesthesia in the healthy dog may be maintained with inhaled concentrations of 3.7-4.0% sevoflurane in oxygen in the absence of premedication and 3.3-3.6% in the presence of premedication. The use of injectable induction agents without premedication has little effect on the concentrations of sevoflurane required for maintenance. Anesthetic regimens that include opioid, $alpha_2$- agonist benzodiazepine or phenothiazine premedication will allow the use of lower sevoflurane maintenance concentrations.

Drug Interactions: In the clinical trial, sevoflurane was used safely in dogs that received frequently used veterinary products including steroids and heartworm and flea preventative products.

Intravenous Anesthetics: Sevoflurane administration is compatible with barbiturates, propofol and other commonly used intravenous anesthetics.

Benzodiazepines and Opioids: Benzodiazepines and opioids would be expected to decrease the MAC of sevoflurane in the same manner as other inhalational anesthetics. Sevoflurane is compatible with benzodiazepines and opioids as commonly used in surgical practice.

Phenothiazines and $Alpha_2$- Agonists: Sevoflurane is compatible with phenothiazines and $alpha_2$- agonists as commonly used in surgical practice. In a laboratory study, the use of the acepromazine/oxymorphone/thiopental/sevoflurane anesthetic regimen resulted in prolonged recoveries in eight (of 8) dogs compared to recoveries from sevoflurane alone.

Contraindication(s): SEVOFLO™ is contraindicated in dogs with a known sensitivity to sevoflurane or other halogenated agents.

Precaution(s): Storage Conditions: Store at room temperature 15°C-30°C (59°F-86°F).

Caution(s): Federal law restricts this drug to use by or on the order of a licensed veterinarian.

Sevoflurane is a profound respiratory depressant. Respiration must be monitored closely in the dog and supported when necessary with supplemental oxygen and/or assisted ventilation. In cases of severe cardiopulmonary depression, discontinue drug administration, ensure the existence of a patent airway and initiate assisted or controlled ventilation with pure oxygen. Cardiovascular depression should be treated with plasma expanders, pressor agents, antiarrhythmic agents or other techniques as appropriate for the observed abnormality. Due to sevoflurane's low solubility in blood, increasing the concentration may result in rapid hemodynamic changes (dose dependent decreases in blood pressure) compared to other volatile anesthetics. Excessive decreases in blood pressure or respiratory depression may be corrected by decreasing or discontinuing the inspired concentration of sevoflurane.

Halogenated volatile anesthetics can react with desiccated carbon dioxide (CO_2) absorbents to produce carbon monoxide (CO) that may result in elevated carboxyhemoglobin levels in some patients. To prevent this reaction, sevoflurane should not be passed through desiccated soda lime or barium hydroxide lime. The use of some anesthetic regimens that include sevoflurane may result in bradycardia that is reversible with anticholinergics. Studies using sevoflurane anesthetic regimens that included atropine or glycopyrrolate as premedicants showed these anticholinergics to be compatible with sevoflurane in dogs. During the maintenance of anesthesia, increasing the concentration of sevoflurane produces dose dependent decreases in blood pressure. Due to sevoflurane's low solubility in blood, these hemodynamic changes may occur more rapidly than with other volatile anesthetics. Excessive decreases in blood pressure or respiratory depression may be related to depth of anesthesia and may be corrected by decreasing the inspired concentration of sevoflurane. The low solubility of sevoflurane also facilitates rapid elimination by the lungs. The use of sevoflurane in humans increases both the intensity and duration of neuromuscular blockade induced by nondepolarizing muscle relaxants. The use of sevoflurane with nondepolarizing muscle relaxants has not been evaluated in dogs.

Compromised or debilitated dogs: Doses may need adjustment for geriatric or debilitated dogs. Because clinical experience in administering sevoflurane to dogs with renal, hepatic and cardiovascular insufficiency is limited, its safety in these dogs has not been established.

Breeding dogs: The safety of sevoflurane in dogs used for breeding purposes, during pregnancy, or in lactating bitches, has not been evaluated.

Neonates: The safety at sevoflurane in young dogs (less than 12 weeks of age) has not been evaluated.

Warning(s): Human Safety: Not for human use. Keep out of reach of children.

Operating rooms and animal recovery areas should be provided with adequate ventilation to prevent the accumulation of anesthetic vapors. There is no specific work exposure limit established for sevoflurane. However, the National Institute for Occupational Safety and Health has recommended an 8 hour time-weighted average limit of 2 ppm for halogenated anesthetic agents in general. Direct exposure to eyes may result in mild irritation. If eye exposure occurs, flush with plenty of water for 15 minutes. Seek medical attention if irritation persists. Symptoms of human overexposure (inhalation) to sevoflurane vapors include respiratory depression, hypotension, bradycardia, shivering, nausea and headache. If these symptoms occur, remove the individual from the source of exposure and seek medical attention. The material safety data sheet (MSDS) contains more detailed occupational safety information. For customer service, adverse effects reporting, and/or a copy of the MSDS, call (888) 299-7416.

Adverse Reactions: The most frequently reported adverse reactions during maintenance anesthesia were hypotension, followed by tachypnea, muscle tenseness, excitation, apnea, muscle fasciculations and emesis. Infrequent adverse reactions include paddling, retching, salivation, cyanosis, premature ventricular contractions and excessive cardiopulmonary depression. Transient elevations in liver function tests and white blood cell count may occur with sevoflurane, as with the use of other halogenated anesthetic agents.

Trial Data: Clinical Effectiveness: The effectiveness of sevoflurane was investigated in a clinical study involving 196 dogs. Thirty dogs were mask-induced with sevoflurane using anesthetic regimens that included various premedicants. During the clinical study, one hundred sixty-six dogs received sevoflurane maintenance anesthesia as part of several anesthetic regimens that used injectable induction agents and various premedicants. The duration of anesthesia and the choice of anesthetic regimens were dependent upon the procedures that were performed. Duration of anesthesia ranged from 16 to 424 minutes among the individual dogs. Sevoflurane vaporizer concentrations during the first 30 minutes of maintenance anesthesia were similar among the various anesthetic regimens. The quality of maintenance anesthesia was considered good or excellent in 169 out of 196 dogs.

The table shows the average vaporizer concentrations and oxygen flow rates during the first 30 minutes for all sevoflurane maintenance anesthesia regimens:

Average Vaporizer Concentrations among Anesthetic Regimens	Average Vaporizer Concentrations among Individual Dogs	Average Oxygen Flow Rates among Anesthetic Regimens	Average Oxygen Flow Rates among Individual Dogs
3.31-3.63%	1.6-5.1%	0.97-1.31 L/minute	0.5-3.0 L/minute

During the clinical trial, when a barbiturate was used for induction, the times to extubation, sternal recumbency and standing recovery were longer for dogs that received anesthetic regimens containing two preanesthetics compared to regimens containing one proanesthetic. Recovery times were shorter when anesthetic regimens used sevoflurane or propofol for induction. The quality of recovery was considered good or excellent in 184 out of 196 dogs. Anesthetic regimen drug dosages, physiological responses, and the quality of induction, maintenance and recovery were comparable between 10 sighthounds and other breeds evaluated in the study. During the clinical study there was no indication of prolonged recovery times in the sighthounds.

References: Available upon request.

Presentation: SEVOFLO™ (sevoflurane) is packaged in amber colored bottles containing 250 mL sevoflurane, List 5458.

SEVOFLO™ is a trademark of Abbott Laboratories.

Compendium Code No.: 10240091 58-6696/R3 April 2, 2002

SHEEN II SHAMPOO

Butler **Parasiticide Shampoo**

EPA Reg. No.: 68077-1-6480

Active Ingredient(s):

Pyrethrins 0.10%
*Piperonyl Butoxide, Technical 1.00%
Inert Ingredients: 98.90%
100.00%

*Equivalent to 0.4% (butylcarbityl) (6-propylpiperonyl) ether and 0.1% of related compounds.

Indications: A shampoo for use on dogs and cats that kills fleas and ticks.

Directions for Use: As a shampoo to kill fleas and ticks, wet the pet's coat with warm water. Starting at the head, work shampoo thoroughly into the hair. Allow the lather to penetrate the fur for five minutes before rinsing. Dry with a towel. The pet will have a clear lustrous coat, free of fleas and ticks, Repeat every week if necessary.

Pet bedding and quarters should be treated simultaneously with an approved product.

Consult a veterinarian before using this product on debilitated, aged, pregnant, nursing or animals on medication. Sensitivities may occur after using any pesticide product for pets. If signs of sensitivity occur bathe your pet with mild soap and rinse with large amounts of water. If signs continue, consult a veterinarian immediately.

It is a violation of Federal law to use this product in a manner inconsistent with labeling.

Contraindication(s): Do not use on puppies or kittens under 12 weeks of age.

Precautionary Statements: Read entire label before each use.

Use only on dogs or cats.

Hazards to Humans and Domestic Animals:

Caution: Harmful if swallowed. Causes eye irritation. Avoid contact with skin, eyes or clothing. Wash thoroughly with soap and water after handling.

First Aid:

If Swallowed: Call a physician or Poison Control Center. Drink 1 or 2 glasses of water and induce vomiting by touching back of throat with finger. If person is unconscious, do not give anything by mouth and do not induce vomiting.

If On Skin: Wash with plenty of soap and water. Get medical attention if irritation persists.

If In Eyes: Flush eyes with plenty of water. Get medical attention if irritation persists.

Storage and Disposal: Store in a cool, dry place, inaccessible to children and pets. Do not reuse container. Wrap container in several layers of newspaper and discard in trash.

Disclaimer: Buyer assumes all risks of use, storage or handling of this material not in strict accordance with directions given herewith.

Presentation: 12 fl oz, 1 gallon and 2.5 gallon containers.

Compendium Code No.: 10821620

SHEEPPRO™ COPPER SUSPENSION

SSI Corp. **Hoof Product**

Active Ingredient(s):

Copper (Cu) 0.67%
Sulfur (S) 2.2%
Inert 97.13%

Indications: Copper Suspension specially formulated to aid in the treatment and prevention of foot rot and other foot problems in sheep and goats.

Directions for Use: Use as a topical spray to aid in the treatment of foot rot. Mix one (1) part SHEEPPRO™ to three (3) parts water. Clean affected area as well as possible before spraying. Spray affected area to point of run-off twice daily until condition improves. Severe cases may

S

require wrapping. Soak a cotton ball or gauze directly in the SHEEPPRO™, apply to affected area and wrap. Remove wrap after three days and inspect.

For use in foot baths to aid in prevention of foot rot mix one (1) quart of SHEEPPRO™ to fifty (50) gallons of water. Change and recharge the foot bath every 300 head. Foot bath may need to be cleaned and recharged depending upon environmental and hygienic conditions. When using foot baths product rotations is best. Products such as SSI's SheepPro™ Zinc Suspension as well as traditional foot care products work well in rotation with SHEEPPRO™ Copper Suspension. Foot baths require a high level of management. If not properly managed results are reduced significantly.

Do not allow sheep or goats to drink from foot bath solution. Will not stain wool. Does not cause hoof to discolor, become hard, brittle or shrink. Safe for humans and animals.

Precaution(s): Do not freeze.

Caution(s): Eye irritant. In case of eye contact, flush for 15 minutes. If irritation persists, call a physician.

Warning(s): Keep out of the reach of children.

Presentation: 1 and 2.5 gallon containers.

Compendium Code No.: 14930061

SHEEPPRO™ ZINC SUSPENSION

SSI Corp. **Hoof Product**

Active Ingredient(s):

Zinc (Zn) 1.43%
Sulfur (S) 3.25%
Inert 95.29%

Indications: Zinc Suspension specially formulated to aid in the treatment and prevention of foot rot and other foot problems in sheep and goats.

Directions for Use: Use as a topical spray to aid in the treatment of foot rot. Mix one (1) part SHEEPPRO™ to three (3) parts water. Clean affected area as well as possible before spraying. Spray affected area to point of run-off twice daily until condition improves. Severe cases may require wrapping. Soak a cotton ball or gauze directly in the SHEEPPRO™, apply to affected area and wrap. Remove wrap after three days and inspect.

For use in foot baths to aid in prevention of foot rot mix one (1) quart of SHEEPPRO™ to fifty (50) gallons of water. Change and recharge the foot bath every 150 head. Foot bath may need to be cleaned and recharged depending upon environmental and hygienic conditions. When using foot baths product rotations is best. Products such as SSI's SheepPro™ Copper Suspension as well as traditional foot care products work well in rotation with SHEEPPRO™ Zinc Suspension. Foot baths require a high level of management. If not properly managed results are reduced significantly.

Do not allow sheep or goats to drink from foot bath solution. Will not stain wool. Does not cause hoof to discolor, become hard, brittle or shrink. Safe for humans and animals.

Precaution(s): Do not freeze.

Caution(s): Eye irritant. In case of eye contact, flush for 15 minutes. If irritation persists, call a physician.

Warning(s): Keep out of the reach of children.

Presentation: 1 and 2.5 gallon containers.

Compendium Code No.: 14930071

SHIN-BAND

Dominion **Counterirritant**

Active Ingredient(s): Active ingredients include gum benzoin, camphor, Barbadoes aloes, rosin, Churchill's iodine. Other ingredients include gum myrrh, storax, methyl salicylate and isopropyl alcohol.

Indications: This product combines analgesic and antiseptic properties. It is recommended in the prevention and treatment of leg ailments in the horse. It helps to promote improved circulation in the hoof.

Dosage and Administration: For prevention of leg ailments, apply a small amount directly to each leg after workout or vigorous exercise. SHIN-BAND can be applied with a toothbrush dipped into the bottle, or pour into a small container and use a narrow paint brush. Brush should have soft bristles.

After applying, wrap horse's legs in normal fashion.

For the treatment of specific leg ailments, such as splints, big knee swelling, sore tendons or soft muscles, apply directly to affected area with a soft brush. Apply stable wrap in normal fashion.

For hoof related problems, paint a small amount of the product onto coronet band or apply directly to bottom of hoof with a soft brush.

Warning(s): Poison - For external use only. For veterinary use only.

Presentation: 250 mL bottle.

Compendium Code No.: 15080071

SHIN-O-GEL®

Hawthorne **Liniment**

Active Ingredient(s): Each 16 U.S. oz contains:

Alcohol .... 180.00 g
Ether .... 10.91 g
Menthol .... 5 g
Camphor .... 5 g

Indications: For use as an aid in the temporary relief of minor stiffness and soreness caused by overexertion. SHIN-O-GEL® keeps horses in training by helping prevent bucked shins and is made especially for younger horses with sore shins and inflammation of the cannon bone.

Dosage and Administration: Apply freely to shin bone only. Rub against and with hair. Next apply with hair only and wrap. Leave on leg at least 48 hours. Repeat if necessary. Leave SHIN-O-GEL® on leg while working or exercising. To remove pad and SHIN-O-GEL®, use warm, soapy water, pulling with hair.

Caution(s): Keep away from children.

Warning(s): Do not use on food animals.

Presentation: 16 U.S. oz.

Compendium Code No.: 10670080

SHOR-BRON D

ASL **Vaccine**

Bronchitis Vaccine, Delaware Type, Modified Live Virus

U.S. Vet. Lic. No.: 226

Description: SHOR-BRON D is formulated from a modified strain of Delaware Type Infectious Bronchitis Virus. The virus was received from the University of Delaware and was modified for high immunizing capability and milder reaction, i.e. snicking. The virus is grown under exacting standards of quality control in eggs produced by healthy chickens in closely supervised flocks.

Gentamicin is added as a preservative.

Indications: SHOR-BRON D is recommended for vaccination of chickens at two weeks of age or older by the drinking water method against Delaware Type Infectious Bronchitis Virus. The frequency of occurrence of the various types of infectious Bronchitis Viruses should be considered in planning a vaccination program.

Dosage and Administration: Read full directions below carefully.

Preparation of the Vaccine (for drinking water use):

Do not open and mix the vaccine until ready to begin vaccination. Use vaccine immediately after mixing.

The contents of the ampules are thawed rapidly by immersing in water at room temperature. Shake ampule to dispense contents. Then break ampule at its neck and immediately proceed as below.

Caution: Ampules have been known to explode on sudden temperature changes. Do not thaw in hot or cold water.

Draw contents of the ampule into a sterile 10 cc syringe. Dilute immediately by filling the syringe slowly from a portion of the water. The contents of the filled syringe are then added to the remaining water. The vaccine is ready for use.

Rehydrate Vaccine in Water According to the Following Table:

	1,000 Doses Added to this Amount of Water:	10,000 Doses Added to this Amount of Water:
Chickens 2-4 Weeks of Age	2.5 Gallons	25 Gallons
Chickens 4-8 Weeks of Age	5 Gallons	50 Gallons
Chickens Over 8 Weeks of Age	10 Gallons	100 Gallons

Drinking Water Administration:

1. Remove all medications, sanitizers, and disinfectants from the drinking water, preferably 72 hours before vaccinating and 24 hours following vaccination.
2. Provide enough watering space so that at least ⅔ of the chickens can drink at one time.
3. Scrub waterers thoroughly and rinse with fresh, clean water.
4. Withhold water for 2 hours before vaccinating to stimulate thirst.
5. Rehydrate the vaccine as directed above.
6. Add rehydrated vaccine to clean, cool non-chlorinated water and mix in accordance with the chart above.
7. Distribute the vaccine solution, as prepared above, among the waterers provided for the chickens. Avoid placing waterers in direct sunlight.
8. Provide no other drinking water until all the vaccine treated water has been consumed.

Precaution(s): Use entire contents when first opened. Burn container and all unused contents.

Store vaccine in liquid nitrogen.

Caution(s): Only vaccinate healthy chickens.

Consult your poultry pathologist for further recommendations based on conditions existing in your area at any given time.

The vaccination program for replacement pullets should not be started after chickens are 15 weeks of age.

Chickens should not be placed on contaminated premises. Exposure should be avoided immediately after vaccination, because it takes 21 days to develop resistance.

All susceptible chickens on the same premises should be vaccinated at the same time. If this is not possible, then strict isolation and separate caretakers should be employed for non-vaccinated units. Efforts should be taken to reduce stressful conditions at the time the vaccine is administered.

Notice: All Schering-Plough Animal Health vaccines released for sale meet the requirements of the licensing authority (U.S. Department of Agriculture) in regard to safety, purity, potency and the capacity to immunize normal, susceptible chickens.

The capacity of this vaccine to produce satisfactory results depends upon many factors including, but not limited to, conditions of storage and handling by the user, administration of the vaccine, health and responsiveness of individual animals and the degree of field exposure. Therefore, directions for use should be followed carefully.

The use of this vaccine is subject to applicable state and federal laws and regulations.

For mass administration only.

Warning(s): Do not vaccinate within 21 days before slaughter.

Discussion: Vaccination Programs: Many factors must be considered in determining the proper vaccination program for a particular farm. To be fully effective, the vaccine must be administered to healthy receptive chickens held in a proper environment under good management. In addition, the responses may be modified by the age of the chickens and their immune status. Seldom does one vaccination under field conditions produce complete protection for all individuals in a given flock. The amount of protection required will vary with the type of operation and the degree of exposure that a flock is likely to encounter. For these reasons, a program of periodic revaccination may be required.

Presentation: 1,000 and 10,000 dose ampules.

Compendium Code No.: 11020301

SHO SNO™ SHAMPOO

Tomlyn **Grooming Shampoo**

Active Ingredient(s): Water (CAS 7732-18-5), Sodium lauryl sulfate (CAS 151-21-3), Sodium laureth sulfate (CAS 1335-72-4), Cocoyl diethanolamide (CAS 61791-31-9), Sodium chloride (CAS 7647-14-4).

Contains reflectones and moisturizers, but contains no bleach nor other harsh chemicals.

Indications: A grooming shampoo for use on dogs with white coats.

Directions: Wet animal thoroughly. Apply Tomlyn's SHO SNO™ Shampoo and work into rich lather. Allow to remain on hair approximately two minutes. Application may be repeated if necessary. The entire animal may be bathed with this shampoo regardless of color.

Precaution(s): Store at room temperature.

Caution(s): For external animal use only.

Keep out of reach of children and pets.

Presentation: 12 x 12 fl oz (355 mL) and 4 x 1 gallon (128 fl oz - 3.79 L).

Compendium Code No.: 11220231

077-1 6

SHOW WINNER!™ CAT VITAMINS

Farnam **Small Animal Dietary Supplement**

Daily Chewable Cat Vitamins

Guaranteed Analysis: per tablet:

Fatty Acid:

Linoleic Acid, min.	22 mg

Minerals:

Calcium, min.	3.6% (40 mg)
Phosphorus, min.	1.4% (31 mg)
Potassium, min.	31 mcg
Magnesium, min.	30 mg
Iron, min.	5 mg
Copper, min.	200 mcg
Manganese, min.	200 mcg
Zinc, min.	300 mcg
Iodine, min.	100 mcg
Cobalt, min.	100 mcg

Vitamins:

Vitamin A, min.	1500 I.U.
Vitamin D, min.	150 I.U.
Vitamin E, min.	4 I.U.
Thiamin (B1), min.	810 mcg
Riboflavin, min.	1 mg
d-Pantothenic Acid, min.	1 mg
Niacin, min.	4 mg
Pyridoxine, min.	410 mcg
Choline, min.	50 mg
Taurine, min.	50 mg
Inositol, min.	10 mg

Ingredients: Whey, dried corn syrup, artificial flavoring, beef livers meal, stearic acid, sucrose, choline bitartrate, taurine, dried brewers yeast, calcium phosphate, magnesium stearate, fish protein concentrate, linoleic acid, soybean flour, malted milk, safflower oil, soy protein isolate, inositol, vitamin E supplement, ferrous fumerate, silicon dioxide, niacin supplement, vitamin A acetate, vitamin D3 supplement, d-calcium pantothenate, riboflavin supplement, thiamine mononitrate, pyridoxine hydrochloride, zinc gluconate, copper gluconate, manganese sulfate, cobalt sulfate, and potassium iodide.

Indications: Daily chewable cat vitamins with taurine and antioxidants.

Dosage and Administration: For Dietary Supplement:

Mature cats: 1 tablet daily.

Kittens: ¼ to 1 tablet daily.

For sick, convalescing, pregnant or nursing cats: 2 tablets daily.

Administer liver-flavored SHOW WINNER™ cat vitamins by hand prior to feeding or crumble and mix with food.

Warning(s): Keep out of reach of children.

Presentation: Bottles of 60 tablets.

Compendium Code No.: 10000920 0AA0

SHOW WINNER!™ DOG VITAMINS

Farnam **Small Animal Dietary Supplement**

Daily Chewable Dog Vitamins

Guaranteed Analysis: per tablet:

Fatty Acid:

Linoleic Acid, min.	30 mg

Minerals:

Calcium, min.	4.23% (151 mg)
Phosphorus, min.	3.30% (116.2 mg)
Potassium, min.	16 mcg
Magnesium, min.	230 mcg
Iron, min.	1 mg
Copper, min.	50 mcg
Manganese, min.	60 mcg
Zinc, min.	1.5 mg
Iodine, min.	52 mcg
Cobalt, min.	14 mcg

Vitamins:

Vitamin A, min.	1000 I.U.
Vitamin D, min.	100 I.U.
Vitamin E, min.	2 I.U.
Thiamin (B1), min.	810 mcg
Riboflavin, min.	1 mg
Niacin, min.	10 mg
Pyridoxine, min.	82 mcg
Vitamin B12, min.	0.2 mcg

Ingredients: Wheat germ meal, dried corn syrup, kaolin, beef livers meal, calcium phosphate, stearic acid, animal digest, sucrose, lactose, safflower oil, gelatin, linoleic acid, whey, silicon dioxide, corn starch, niacin supplement, vitamin E supplement, vitamin A acetate, zinc oxide, iron proteinate, riboflavin supplement, magnesium stearate, vitamin D3 supplement, pyridoxine hydrochloride, manganese sulfate, potassium iodide, copper sulfate monohydrate, cobalt sulfate, and vitamin B12 supplement.

Indications: Daily chewable dog vitamins with antioxidants.

Dosage and Administration: For Dietary Supplement:

Dogs under 10 lbs.: ½ tablet daily.

Dogs over 10 lbs.: 1 tablet daily.

Liver-flavored SHOW WINNER™ vitamin tablets with antioxidants provide a special taste appeal. Administer by hand prior to feeding or crumble and mix with food.

Warning(s): Keep out of reach of children.

Presentation: Bottles of 60 tablets, 180 tablets and 365 tablets.

Compendium Code No.: 10000930 0AA0 / 0BB0 / 0AA0

SHOW WINNER!™ KITTEN VITAMINS

Farnam **Small Animal Dietary Supplement**

Daily Chewable Kitten Vitamins

Guaranteed Analysis: per tablet:

Fatty Acid:

Linoleic Acid, min.	11 mg

Minerals:

Calcium, min.	3.6% (20 mg)
Phosphorus, min.	1.4% (15.5 mg)
Potassium, min.	15.5 mcg
Magnesium, min.	30 mg
Iron, min.	2.5 mg
Copper, min.	100 mcg
Manganese, min.	100 mcg
Zinc, min.	150 mcg
Iodine, min.	50 mcg
Cobalt, min.	50 mcg

Vitamins:

Vitamin A, min.	750 I.U.
Vitamin D, min.	75 I.U.
Vitamin E, min.	2 I.U.
Thiamin (B1), min.	405 mcg
Riboflavin, min.	0.5 mg
d-Pantothenic Acid, min.	0.5 mg
Niacin, min.	2 mg
Pyridoxine, min.	205 mcg
Choline, min.	25 mg
Taurine, min.	25 mg
Inositol, min.	5 mg

Ingredients: Whey, dried corn syrup, artificial flavoring, beef livers meal, stearic acid, sucrose, dried brewers yeast, magnesium stearate, fish protein concentrate, choline bitartrate, taurine, calcium phosphate, soybean flour, malted milk, safflower oil, soy protein isolate, linoleic acid, inositol, silicon dioxide, vitamin E supplement, ferrous fumerate, niacin supplement, vitamin A acetate, vitamin D3 supplement, d-calcium pantothenate, thiamine mononitrate, pyridoxine hydrochloride, zinc gluconate, copper gluconate, manganese sulfate, cobalt sulfate, potassium iodide, and riboflavin supplement.

Indications: Daily chewable kitten vitamins. Contains vitamins essential for proper bone and tooth formation.

Dosage and Administration: For Dietary Supplement:

Kittens: 1 tablet daily for every 5 lbs of body weight (tablet may be broken for smaller kittens).

Mature Cats: 2 tablets daily.

For sick, convalescing, pregnant or nursing cats and kittens: 2 tablets daily for every 5 lbs of body weight.

SHOW WINNER™ tablets are made with a special taste appeal. Administer by hand just prior to feeding or crumble and mix with food.

Warning(s): Keep out of reach of children.

Presentation: Bottles of 60 tablets.

Compendium Code No.: 10000940 0AA0

SHOW WINNER!™ OLDER DOG VITAMINS

Farnam **Small Animal Dietary Supplement**

Daily Chewable Older Dog Vitamins

Guaranteed Analysis: per tablet:

Fatty Acid:

Linoleic Acid, min.	30 mg

Minerals:

Calcium, min.	4.23% (151 mg)
Phosphorus, min	3.30% (116.2 mg)
Potassium, min.	16 mcg
Magnesium, min.	230 mcg
Iron, min.	1 mg
Copper, min.	50 mcg
Manganese, min.	60 mcg
Zinc, min.	1.5 mg
Iodine, min.	52 mcg
Cobalt, min.	14 mcg

Vitamins:

Vitamin A, min.	1500 I.U.
Vitamin D, min.	150 I.U.
Vitamin E, min.	15 I.U.
Thiamin (B1), min.	243 mcg
Riboflavin, min.	665 mg
d-Pantothenic Acid, min.	684 mg
Niacin, min.	3.4 mg
Pyridoxine, min.	247 mcg
Vitamin B12, min.	7 mcg
Choline, min.	50 mg
Biotin, min.	30 mcg
Ascorbic Acid, min.	10 mg
Phytonadione, min.	300 mcg

Ingredients: Whey, dried corn syrup, stearic acid, beef livers meal, calcium phosphate, artificial flavoring, lactose, choline bitartrate, wheat germ meal, linoleic acid, soy protein isolate, gelatin, magnesium stearate, corn starch, vitamin E supplement, kaolin, safflower oil, silicon dioxide, ascorbic acid, niacin supplement, vitamin A acetate, zinc oxide, vitamin D3 supplement, iron proteinate, d-calcium pantothenate, riboflavin supplement, phytonadione, pyridoxine hydrochloride, thiamine mononitrate, manganese sulfate, folic acid, potassium iodide, copper acetate monohydrate, biotin, cobalt sulfate, and vitamin B12 supplement.

SHOW WINNER!™ PUPPY VITAMINS

Indications: Daily chewable older dog vitamins. High potency antioxidant formula.
Dosage and Administration: For Dietary Supplement:

Dogs under 10 lbs.: 1/2 tablet daily.

Dogs over 10 lbs.: 1 tablet daily.

Liver-flavored SHOW WINNER™ vitamin tablets with antioxidants provide a special taste appeal. Administer by hand prior to feeding or crumble and mix with food.
Warning(s): Keep out of reach of children.
Presentation: Bottles of 60 tablets and 180 tablets.
Compendium Code No.: 10000950 0AA0 / 0BB0

SHOW WINNER!™ PUPPY VITAMINS

Farnam **Small Animal Dietary Supplement**

Daily Chewable Puppy Vitamins

Guaranteed Analysis: per tablet:

Fatty Acid:
Linoleic Acid, min. .... 15 mg

Minerals:
Calcium, min. .... 4.23% (75.5 mg)
Phosphorus, min. .... 3.30% (58.1 mg)
Potassium, min. .... 8 mcg
Magnesium, min. .... 115 mcg
Iron, min. .... 0.5 mg
Copper, min. .... 25 mcg
Manganese, min. .... 30 mcg
Zinc, min. .... 0.75 mg
Iodine, min. .... 26 mcg
Cobalt, min. .... 7 mcg

Vitamins:
Vitamin A, min. .... 500 I.U.
Vitamin D, min. .... 50 I.U.
Vitamin E, min. .... 1.0 I.U.
Thiamin (B1), min. .... 405 mcg
Riboflavin, min. .... 0.5 mg
Niacin, min. .... 5 mg
Pyridoxine, min. .... 41 mcg
Vitamin B12, min. .... 0.1 mcg

Ingredients: Whey, dried corn syrup, stearic acid, beef livers meal, artificial flavoring, lactose, calcium phosphate, wheat germ meal, gelatin, corn starch, soy protein isolate, silicon dioxide, safflower oil, linoleic acid, vitamin E supplement, magnesium stearate, niacin supplement, vitamin A acetate, zinc oxide, iron proteinate, riboflavin supplement, vitamin D3 supplement, pyridoxine hydrochloride, thiamine mononitrate, manganese sulfate, potassium iodide, copper acetate monohydrate, cobalt sulfate, and vitamin B12 supplement.
Indications: Daily chewable puppy vitamins with antioxidants. A great training aid or healthy snack for puppies.
Dosage and Administration: For Dietary Supplement:

Puppies under 10 lbs.: ½ tablet daily.

Puppies over 10 lbs.: 1 tablet daily.

Tablets are made with a special taste appeal. Administer by hand just prior to feeding or crumble and mix with food.
Warning(s): Keep out of reach of children.
Presentation: Bottles of 60 tablets.
Compendium Code No.: 10000960 0AA0

SHUR HOOF™

Horse Health **Hoof Product**

Hoof Dressing for Horses

Ingredient(s): Contains: Fish Oil, Pine Tar, Linseed Oil, Wheat Germ Oil, Neatsfoot Oil, Povidone Iodine and Venice Turpentine.
Indications: SHUR HOOF™ is a topical hoof dressing for horse's hoofs.
Directions: Wash the horse's hoof thoroughly. Apply SHUR HOOF™ Dressing with a brush and work well into the edge of the hair and frog. Use two or three times weekly. May be used more often if necessary.
Caution(s): Harmful or fatal if swallowed.

If swallowed, contact a physician or Poison Control Centre immediately.

For animal use only.
Warning(s): Keep out of reach of children.
Presentation: 32 oz with brush and 1 gallon (3.8 L).
Compendium Code No.: 15000051

S

SHURJETS

Jorgensen **Udder Product**

NADA No.: 010-481
Active Ingredient(s):
Salicylic acid .... 0.55 grains per unit

Inert Ingredients: Gum Arabic, dextrin and water. Each SHURJET contains salicylic acid in a special adhesive base which permits the slow release of the active ingredients.
Indications: For the removal of scar tissue and to promote a healthy growth of the skin in the teat canal of hard to milk cows when such hard milking is due to a thickening of the skin in the teat canal.
Dosage and Administration: Cleanse the teat thoroughly after the quarter has been milked. Then insert a SHURJET into the teat canal and rotate it until the medication has been removed from the SHURJET. Then immediately insert a second SHURJET, but do not rotate it - just leave it in the teat canal so that the medication may be slowly released. Remove before each milking. After milking, insert a new SHURJET and leave in the teat canal until next milking. Continue this treatment until the desired degree of relaxation is obtained, usually three (3) to six (6) SHURJETS are adequate.

Teat injuries are always serious and their correction is difficult. Therefore, should SHURJET fail to give the desired degree of relaxation in two (2) days, discuss the case again with a veterinarian before undertaking additional treatment.

After care: Usually the excessive tissue can be milked out of the teat canal readily. However, when there is a great deal of scar tissue to be removed, it may adhere to the canal as a membrane. This membrane is usually whitish in color and can be easily differentiated from the underlying healthy tissue. When the scar tissue adheres in the teat as a whitish membrane, it may be removed by grasping it with a pair of tweezers or forceps and exerting gentle, but steady pressure.
Caution(s): SHURJETS should only be used after injuries have healed. Do not use SHURJETS on recently injured teats.
Warning(s): Discard all milk while using SHURJETS and continue to do so for 48 hours after discontinuing their use.
Presentation: 6 units.
Compendium Code No.: 11520140

SILVER NITRATE STICK APPLICATORS

Vedco **Hemostatic**

Active Ingredient(s):
Silver nitrate 75%
Potassium nitrate 25%
Indications: An astringent applicator to be used as an aid in stopping capillary bleeding.
Dosage and Administration: Apply tipped end of the applicator directly onto the bleeding capillary.
Caution(s): Poison.
Presentation: 100-6" applicators packaged in a foil-lined pouch.
Compendium Code No.: 10941840

SINGLVAX®

Schering-Plough **Vaccine**

Newcastle Disease Vaccine, B_1 Type, LaSota Strain Live Virus

U.S. Vet. Lic. No.: 165A
Contents: Newcastle disease vaccine B_1 type, LaSota strain live virus. This vaccine contains gentamicin as a preservative.
Indications: For use in chickens 4 weeks of age or older as an aid in preventing Newcastle disease through vaccination by the water route (initial vaccination) and water or spray routes (revaccination). Birds vaccinated at a younger age should be revaccinated at 4 weeks of age.
Dosage and Administration:

Initial Vaccination: Water: 4 weeks to 16 weeks of age.

Birds vaccinated initially before 4 weeks of age should be revaccinated as below.

Water: 4 weeks of age or older

Spray: 4 weeks of age or older

Preparation of the Vaccine:

Assemble the vaccine and equipment needed to vaccinate the entire flock at one time.

Do not open and mix the vaccine until ready for use.

Remove the tear-off aluminum seal from the vaccine vial without disturbing the rubber stopper.

Use cool, clean, non-chlorinated tap water to which powdered milk has been added as directed under How to Vaccinate.

Holding vial submerged in a pail of water or under a running stream of water, lift the top of the rubber stopper so that the water (milk added) is sucked into the vial.

Reseat the stopper and shake the vial to thoroughly dissolve the vaccine.

How to Vaccinate:

Drinking Water Method:

Eliminate disinfectants from the lines 2 to 3 days prior to vaccination.

Flush lines with powdered or condensed milk the night before vaccination to tie up any remaining disinfectant. Use the equivalent of 2½ heaping cups of powdered milk (six 3.2 oz packs) per gallon of stock solution or 1 cup per 50 gallons when using a vaccination tank or direct pump system for non-chlorinated water. If drinking water is chlorinated, research has shown that amounts double those above are required to neutralize up to 5 ppm of chlorine.

Withhold Water

Nipples or Dry Cups: Raise water lines.

Troughs or bell drinkers: turn off water. Monitor the drinkers closely: as soon as you see the first dry drinkers, raise all drinkers. This is the start of the "off water" time. Withhold water for 1½ to 2 hours (weather dependent). The idea is to make the birds quite thirsty. Temperature, time of day, and experience with watching bird reactions will help fine-tune the water withholding time.

Water Requirements: Vaccine must be consumed in 1½ to 2 hours.

Rule of Thumb: Total daily water consumption for the flock at a given age, divided by 4, equals the amount of vaccine the birds will drink in 1½ to 2 hours.

Example: 16 day-old broilers at 70°F may drink about 16 to 18 gallons per day per 1,000 birds. Plan on 4 to 4½ oz of stock solution for each 1,000 birds to be vaccinated.

Example Water Requirements:

Each 5,000 Birds	U.S. Gallons	Imperial Gallons	Metric Liters
4 to 8 Weeks	25	20	100
Over 8 Weeks	50	40	200

The best vaccination results are usually achieved by vaccinating first thing in the morning, using stock volumes 1.5 to 2 times greater than the rule of thumb suggests (because the birds eat and drink more at this time of day).

Vaccination

Use non-chlorinated water for vaccination. If only chlorinated water is available, use double the powdered milk amounts indicated below to help inactivate the chlorine.

Step 1: Mix powdered milk (2½ heaping cups or six 3.2 oz packs), commercial vaccine stabilizer, or evaporated milk (ten 12 oz cans) per gallon of stock solution. Dilute the total doses for the house into the milky stock solution. Open the vials, dip them into the milky solution, put the stopper back in and shake to dissolve the cake. Rinse the vial 3 more times after emptying the contents into the stock solution to insure that all of the vaccine is rinsed out. Do not just drop the open vials into the stock bucket!

Step 2: Open the far end of the water line and flush the vaccine through until the milky water is flushed through the whole system. If through or bell drinkers are used, dump any water out of the drinkers before flushing the line.

Step 3: Lower the drinkers, and allow the proportioner or pump to operate until all of the vaccine solution has been used.

Step 4: Slowly walk the walls until vaccination is complete, encouraging all of the birds to get up and drink. Running the feed lines will also motivate the birds to get up and move around.

Step 5: Refill the stock bucket or vaccination tank with fresh water and flush water and flush the proportioner or pump.

Spray Method:

For revaccination method. Proper spray application of this vaccine is accomplished only through use of a clean sprayer. The droplet size of the spray is important: a fine mist (spray droplets of 5-20 microns) will produce a stronger immune response, but may also elicit strong reactions. A coarse spray (spray droplets of 30-50 microns) will produce less respiratory reaction, but also reduce immunity. Environmental conditions, bird strain and bird health will determine which droplet size is appropriate for your operation. Use the spray method only in houses that can be closed during vaccination and for 15 minutes thereafter. Cross wind, drafts or operating ventilation fans prevent effective application.

Rehydrate the vaccine according to the above instructions "Preparation of the Vaccine."

Further dilute each 5000 doses (150 mL) of vaccine to 500 mL using distilled water. Place the rehydrated vaccine in the sprayer container. Apply vaccine at the rate of 1 dose per square foot or one dose per bird, whichever is greater. Vaccine should be applied at the rate of 700 doses of vaccine per minute.

Records: Keep a record of vaccine type, quantity, serial number, expiration date, and place of purchase; the date and time of vaccination; the number, age, breed, and location of the birds; names of operators performing the vaccination and any observed reactions.

Precaution(s): Store at 2° to 7°C (35° to 45°F).

Do not dilute the vaccine beyond the recommended levels or otherwise stretch the dosage.

Do not spill or splatter the vaccine. Use entire contents of vial when first opened. Burn empty bottles, caps and all unused vaccine.

Wash hands thoroughly after using the vaccine.

Caution(s): Vaccinate only healthy birds.

Although disease may not be evident, coccidiosis, chronic respiratory disease, mycoplasma infection, lymphoid leukosis, infectious bursal disease, Marek's disease, or other disease conditions may cause serious complications or reduce protection.

All birds within a house should be vaccinated on the same day. Isolate other susceptible birds on the premises from the birds being vaccinated.

In outbreak situations, vaccinate healthy birds first progressing toward outbreak areas in order to vaccinate diseased birds last.

Warning(s): Do not vaccinate within 21 days before slaughter.

Newcastle virus occasionally causes inflammation of the eyelids in humans, lasting two or three days. Avoid contact of eyes with vaccine.

For veterinary use only.

Use protective goggles during vaccination to avoid eye contact with Newcastle vaccine.

Discussion: SINGLVAX® is a live virus vaccine of chicken embryo origin prepared from the ASL N-47 (LaSota strain, B_1 type Newcastle virus). This strain provides stronger, more durable immunity than the B_1 Newcastle strain while causing only a slightly increased reaction.

The increased strength and spreading potential of this virus render it especially desirable for use in areas of high Newcastle disease incidence and for revaccination of replacement birds prior to lay.

Vaccination Program: The development of a durable, strong protection against this disease depends upon the use of an effective vaccination program as well as many circumstances such as administration techniques, environment and flock health at time of vaccination. Also, the immune response to one vaccination under field conditions is seldom complete for all birds within a given flock. Even when vaccination is successful, the protection stimulated in individual animals against different diseases may not be life long. Therefore, a program of periodic revaccination may be necessary.

Presentation: 5000 dose vials.

Compendium Code No.: 10471820

SITEGUARD® G

Schering-Plough **Toxoid**

Clostridium perfringens Types C & D Toxoid

U.S. Vet. Lic. No.: 311

Contents: This toxoid contains fractions of *Clostridium perfringens* Types C and D.

Indications: For the vaccination of healthy cattle and sheep against diseases caused by *Clostridium perfringens* Types C and D.

Although *Clostridium perfringens* Type B is not a significant problem in the USA, immunity may be provided against the beta and epsilon toxins elaborated by *Cl. perfringens* Type B. This immunity is derived from the combination of Type C (beta) and Type D (epsilon) fractions.

Dosage and Administration: Shake well. Using aseptic technique, inject subcutaneously or intramuscularly. Cattle, 4 mL; sheep, 2 mL, repeated in 3 to 4 weeks. Revaccinate annually prior to periods of extreme risk or parturition.

Precaution(s): Store at 35°-45°F (2°-7°C). Protect from freezing. Use entire contents when first opened.

Caution(s): Anaphylactoid reactions may occur following use.

This product has been tested under laboratory conditions and shown to meet all Federal standards for safety and efficacy. This level of performance may be affected by conditions of use such as stress, weather, nutrition, disease, parasitism, other treatments, individual idiosyncrasies or impaired immunological competency. These factors should be considered by the user when evaluating product performance or freedom from reactions.

Local reactions may be observed following subcutaneous administration to cattle.

Antidote(s): Epinephrine.

Warning(s): Do not vaccinate within 21 days before slaughter.

For veterinary use only.

Presentation: 40 mL (10 cattle doses/20 sheep doses) and 200 mL (50 cattle doses/100 sheep doses) vials.

Manufactured by: Schering-Plough Animal Health Limited

Compendium Code No.: 10471831

SITEGUARD® MLG VACCINE

Schering-Plough **Bacterin-Toxoid**

Clostridium chauvoei-septicum-haemolyticum-novyi-sordellii-perfringens Types C & D Bacterin-Toxoid

U.S. Vet. Lic. No.: 107

Active Ingredient(s) A formalin-inactivated, alum-precipitated bacterin-toxoid prepared from highly toxigenic cultures and culture filtrates of *Clostridium chauvoei, Cl. septicum, Cl. sordellii, Cl. novyi* type B, *Cl. haemolyticum* (known elsewhere as *Cl. novyi* type D*) and *Cl. perfringens* types C and D.

All components of each serial of the final product are tested for potency using USDA-approved laboratory and/or host animal tests.

Indications: For the active immunization of healthy cattle and sheep against diseases caused by *Clostridium chauvoei, Cl. septicum, Cl. sordellii, Cl. novyi* type B, *Cl. haemolyticum* (known elsewhere as *Cl. novyi* type D), and *Cl. perfringens* types C & D.

Although *Cl. perfringens* type B is not a significant problem in the USA, immunity may be provided against the beta and epsilon toxins elaborated by *Cl. perfringens* type B. The immunity is derived from the combination of type C (beta) and type D (epsilon) fractions.

Dosage and Administration: Shake well. Using aseptic technique, inject subcutaneously or intramuscularly.

Dosage: 5 mL, repeated in 3-4 weeks. Revaccinate annually prior to periods of extreme risk, or parturition. For *Cl. novyi* and *Cl. haemolyticum*, revaccinate every 5-6 months. Animals vaccinated under three (3) months of age should be revaccinated at weaning or at 4-6 months of age.

Precaution(s): Store at 35°-45°F (2°-7°C). Protect from freezing.

The product has been tested under laboratory conditions and has met all Federal standards for safety and ability to immunize normal healthy animals. The level of performance may be affected by conditions of use such as stress, weather, nutrition, disease, parasitism, other treatments, individual idiosyncrasies or impaired immunological competency. These factors should be considered by the user when evaluating product performance or freedom from reactions.

Caution(s): Use the entire contents when first opened.

Anaphylactic reactions may occur following use.

Antidote(s): Epinephrine.

Warning(s): Do not vaccinate within 21 days before slaughter.

Discussion: * *Cl. novyi* and *Cl. haemolyticum* are generally indistinguishable without extensive biochemical tests. Macheak[1] has stated: *Cl. haemolyticum* and *Cl. novyi* should be regarded in the laboratory as one group since their morphologic and cultural characteristics are closely related. All strains of *Cl. novyi* appear to have two somatic antigens in common; one of these is shared with *Cl. haemolyticum.* European scientists have suggested that *Cl. haemolyticum* should be classified as *Cl. novyi* type D.

Siteguard® vaccines are Electroferm® products produced by an electronically-controlled deep culture process.

The specific toxoids and/or cellular antigens required for optimal disease protection are emphasized in the growth of Electroferm® cultures. These cultures are highly concentrated and when divided for the blending of combination vaccines make possible the production of low volume doses. Exacting procedures are employed in the blending process to ensure that each dose of combination vaccine contains an accurate amount of each component.

Clostridial organisms fall into groupings based on the primary site at which infection occurs. These sites are muscle, liver and the gastro-intestinal (GI) tract as shown below.

Primary Infection Sites of Clostridial Organisms of Most Concern in Cattle and Sheep:

Organism	Muscle	Liver	GI Tract
Cl. chauvoei	+		
Cl. septicum	+		
Cl. sordellii	+		
Cl. novyi type B		+	
Cl. novyi type D		+	
Cl. perfringens type B			+
Cl. perfringens type C			+
Cl. perfringens type D			+

Muscle Group: Highly resistant spores of the clostridial organisms whose primary infection site is the muscle *(Cl. chauvoei, Cl. septicum, Cl. sordellii)* are deposited there by the circulation following oral ingestion or contamination of wounds. Under localized anoxic conditions produced by injuries, bruises, etc., these spores vegetate and the resulting organisms multiply. These conditions commonly occur in feedlots and farms during handling, transportation, and animal interaction, i.e., butting and riding. Bacterial growth produces gangrenous myositis. Toxins released by the multiplying organisms and by destroyed cells enter the circulation, producing death through destructive effects on vital organs. Fatalities may occur suddenly, as early as 12 hours from onset of infection.

Liver Group: Spores of the clostridial organisms whose primary infection site is the liver *(Cl. novyi* types B and D) are latent residents of such tissue. These spores are acquired from the digestive tract following ingestion of contaminated plants, dust, feed, etc. Some form of liver damage is necessary for their activation and initiation of disease. Precipitating and predisposing factors include abscesses, chemicals, fatty changes, internal parasites, flukes, plant toxins, telangiectasis (sawdust liver) and bacterial hepatitis. The management programs of feedlots and production operations often produce these factors. Powerful toxins produced by the multiplying organisms cause death through destructive effects on vital organs and blood vessels. Fatalities may occur suddenly, as early as 24 hours after onset of infection.

Gastro-intestinal Group: *Cl. perfringens* types B, C, and D are normal inhabitants of the intestinal tract of cattle, sheep and swine. Under anoxic conditions caused by the ingestion of large quantities of concentrated feeds, sudden changes in diet, etc., these organisms multiply rapidly and release destructive toxins. In the very young, this frequently follows the ingestion of large quantities of rich milk. This condition often takes the form of a pure toxemia (enterotoxemia), with toxins being absorbed into the circulation from the intestine and producing destructive effects on vital organs and sudden death. It may in addition cause severe intestinal lesions, particularly in young animals (hemorrhagic enteritis, necrotic enteritis). The management programs of feeding and production operations often predispose animals to the condition.

References: Available upon request.

Presentation: 10 dose, 50 dose and 200 dose vials.

* SITEGUARD and Electroferm are registered trademarks of Schering-Plough Animal Health Corporation.

Compendium Code No.: 10471840

SK-SUREKILL® BRAND PYRETHRIN PLUS FLY SPRAY

IntAgra **Premise and Topical Insecticide**

Spray Insecticide with Vapona®

EPA Reg. No.: 4866-3

Active Ingredient(s):

Pyrethrins 0.05%

Technical Piperonyl Butoxide 0.10%

Consists of 0.08% (butylcarbityl) (6-propyl piperonyl) ether and 0.02% other related compounds.

Dichlorvos [2,2-dichlorovinyl dimethyl phosphate] (DDVP) (Vapona®) 0.465%

Related compounds 0.035%

S

Inert Ingredients: 98.35%
Total 100.00%

Contains petroleum distillates.

Indications: This is a dual-purpose formula designed to protect dairy and beef cattle from attacks of biting fleas in barns and out on the pasture, and also to function as an effective space spray for quick knockdown and kill of flies in barns.

Directions for Use: It is a violation of Federal law to use this product in a manner inconsistent with its labeling. Use this product safely. Read entire label before using.

Animal Spray: To protect animals against attacks of stable flies, horn flies, mosquitoes and gnats, apply just enough to wet ends of hairs but not enough to soak the hide. One or two ounces is enough to treat an adult cow. Apply once daily, preferably in morning, for protection during day. Repeat daily, or as necessary for continued protection.

Do not apply in excess of two fluid ounces per animal per day. Do not spray udders of lactating dairy animals. For milking dairy animals, apply 20 to 30 minutes before beginning to milk. Do not apply to animals under 6 months of age.

Space Spray for Barn Fly Control: To attain quick knockdown and kill of flies, gnats and mosquitoes in enclosed spaces, spray toward ceiling and corners until space is filled with light mist. Apply at rate of one to two ounces per 1000 cubic feet. Do not treat animals or humans. Do not contaminate water, feed or foodstuffs, milk or milking utensils. Do not use in areas where animals have received direct application within 8 hours.

Remove animals prior to treatment. For best results, close all windows and doors prior to spraying and keep them closed for 10 to 15 minutes after spraying. When used in enclosed areas, do not remain in treated areas after spraying. Ventilate before reentering.

Precautionary Statements:

Caution: Hazards to Humans and Domestic Animals: Harmful if swallowed, inhaled or absorbed through the skin. Avoid inhalation of vapor or spray mist. Avoid contact with skin, eyes, and clothing. Wash thoroughly with soap and water after handling and before eating or smoking. Wear NIOSH or OSHA approved respirator when applying indoors as space spray or fog.

Do not contaminate water, feed, or foodstuffs. Do not use in food areas of food handling establishments, restaurants or other areas where food is commercially prepared or processed. Do not use in serving areas while food is exposed or facility is in operation.

Do not apply to animals under 6 months of age. Brahman or Brahman Cross cattle should not be treated, as they may show hypersensitivity to organophosphates.

Environmental Hazards: This product is toxic to fish, birds and other wildlife. Do not contaminate water when disposing of equipment washwaters.

Physical or Chemical Hazards: Do not use, pour, spill or store near heat or flame.

Statement of Practical Treatment:

If swallowed: Call a physician or Poison Control Center immediately. Do not induce vomiting; vomiting may cause aspiration pneumonia.

Gastric lavage is indicated if material was taken internally.

If inhaled: Remove victim to fresh air. Apply artificial respiration if indicated.

If on skin: Remove contaminated clothing. Wash affected areas with soap and water.

If in eyes: Flush eyes with plenty of water. Get medical attention if irritation persists.

Note to Physician: Solvent presents aspiration hazard. Gastric lavage is indicated if material was taken internally. DDVP (Vapona®) is an organophosphate insecticide. If symptoms of cholinesterase inhibition are present, atropine sulfate by injection is antidotal. 2-PAM is also antidotal and may be administered in conjunction with atropine.

Storage and Disposal: Do not contaminate water, food or feed by storage or disposal.

Storage: Store in a cool place. Keep container tightly closed.

Pesticide Disposal: Wastes resulting from use of this product may be disposed of on site or at an approved waste disposal facility.

Container Disposal: Triple rinse (or equivalent). Then offer for recycling or reconditioning, or puncture and dispose of in a sanitary landfill, or incineration, or by burning if allowed by state and local authorities. If burned, stay out of smoke.

Warning(s): Keep out of reach of children.

Presentation: Pyrethrin Plus is packaged in a 5 gallon twin-pack containing two 2½ gallon plastic jugs. A case of four plastic 1 gallon jugs is also available.

Compendium Code No.: 14900001

SKUNK-OFF®

Thornell — **Deodorant Product**

Description: Does not contain enzymes, bacteria, nor oxidizers. Nontoxic, nonirritating, biodegradable, nonflammable.

Indications: To eliminate skunk odors from anything that has been sprayed by a skunk.

Works chemically through bonding, absorption and counteraction.

Dosage and Administration: For a fine spray, use short quick squeezes of the spray bottle. For a stream, use a sustained squeeze.

Wipe off any visible skunk oil and lightly coat the entire affected area with a fine spray. Saturate areas which have been directly hit, using a stream. Work in thoroughly if on hair or clothing. It is essential that SKUNK-OFF® gets into every place that the skunk spray has reached or at some later time a skunk odor may be detected. Clothing should be washed following treatment.

If pretreatment (tomato juice, shampoo, etc.) has occurred, dissolve one (1) full bottle of SKUNK-OFF® in two (2) quarts of warm water and completely saturate the animal or article. Repeat if any skunk odor remains.

Precaution(s): SKUNK-OFF® has an indefinite shelf life.

Caution(s): Although safe, as with all chemicals, it should be kept out of the reach of children. For external use only. Always spot test for color fastness before using on fabrics.

Presentation: 3.75 oz. squeeze spray bottle and 32 oz. professional size trigger spray bottle.

Compendium Code No.: 11210070

SKUNK-OFF® SHAMPOO

Thornell — **Deodorant Product**

Ingredient(s): SKUNK-OFF® is formulated with the ingredients of a mild (tearless/baby) shampoo plus the deodorizing components of the original Skunk-Off® liquid.

Indications: A mild shampoo expressly formulated to eliminate skunk odor.

Directions for Use: Wet coat thoroughly.

Shake bottle before using.

Work shampoo into coat.

Make certain that the shampoo has reached skin level and that all areas have been covered, including eye lids, between the toes and all other seemingly obscure areas. (There is no way to tell where the skunk spray has reached.) It is recommended that a minimum of 4 ounces (one half bottle) be used.

Thoroughly rinse then dry as usual.

If odor persists repeat procedure.

Caution(s): Care should be used to avoid direct contact with the eyes. Although SKUNK-OFF® shampoo is very mild (more so than many "tearless/baby" shampoos), in some cases it may cause minor eye irritation.

As with all chemicals keep out of reach of children.

Presentation: 8 fl oz (236 mL) and 1 gallon.

Compendium Code No.: 11210080

SKY-LYTES

Skylabs — **Electrolytes-Oral**

Active Ingredient(s):

Dextrose 56.6%
Citric acid 20.0%
Salt (NaCl) 10.0%
Potassium (K) 1.74%
Copper (Cu) 0.83%
Zinc (Zn) 1.18%

Ingredients: Dextrose, sodium chloride, citric acid, monopotassium phosphate, copper sulfate, zinc sulfate, red dye, artificial flavor.

Indications: A buffered electrolyte formula that provides essential elements needed by pigs that are dehydrated or show loss of body weight due to stress.

Dosage and Administration: Use in feed or water for five (5) to seven (7) days before, during, and after a stress situation occurs, or when one is anticipated.

Feed: Add one (1) bag (2.27 kg) to one (1) tonne of complete food, or 1,110 L of water.

Medicators: Make a stock solution by mixing 912 g of SKY-LYTES into 3.785 L. Meter at 29.5 mL per 3.785 L of drinking water.

Dispensers: Add 9 g per 3.785 L of drinking water.

Tank: Add 86.7 g per 37.85 L of drinking water, or 456 g per 227.0 L of drinking water.

Presentation: 1 lb and 30 lb.

Compendium Code No.: 10920021

SLEEPAWAY® Ⓒ

Fort Dodge — **Euthanasia Agent**

Sodium Pentobarbital-7.8% Isopropyl Alcohol-Euthanasia Solution

Active Ingredient(s): Composition: A non-sterile solution containing:

Sodium pentobarbital 26%
Isopropyl alcohol 7.8%
Propylene glycol 20.7%
Distilled water q.s.

Indications: For the humane euthanasia of cats and dogs.

Directions: Dogs and cats — 2 mL intravenously for the first 10 lb body weight; 1 mL for each additional 10 lb.

Precaution(s): Store at room temperature (approximately 25°C).

Caution(s): Federal law restricts this drug to use by or on the order of a licensed veterinarian. Do not use if material has precipitated.

Poison.

Warning(s): For euthanasia only. Must not be used for therapeutic purposes.

Carcasses of animals killed by euthanasia drugs should be disposed of in a manner that prevents their being consumed for food by people or animals due to the potential exposure to harmful drug residues. Keep out of reach of children.

Presentation: 100 mL bottles (NDC 0856-0471-01).

Compendium Code No.: 10031901 4713L

SLOW RELEASE CMPK BOLUS

PRN Pharmacal — **Calcium-Combination Therapy**

Active Ingredient(s): Each bolus contains:

Calcium .... 3.5 g
Magnesium .... 3.5 g
Phosphorus .... 2.0 g
Sodium .... 1.5 g
Potassium .... 800 mg
Vitamin D-3 .... 50,000 USP units
Vitamin E .... 300 I.U.

Indications: Nutritional Use: CMPK BOLUSES are a nutritional supplement for supplying additional nutrient intake in cattle. Where an additional intake of calcium, magnesium, and phosphorus are desired, CMPK BOLUS is the product of choice.

Dosage and Administration: Recommendations:

Cattle and Horses: 1 bolus per 250 lbs body weight per day. May be repeated as required.

Sheep and Swine: ½ bolus per 100 lbs body weight per day. May be repeated as required.

This bolus may be given orally with a balling gun or crushed and suspended in milk or water and given as a drench or sprinkled on the daily feed ration.

Precaution(s): Store in a cool, dry place. Avoid exposure to moisture.

Warning(s): For animal use only. Keep out of reach of children.

Presentation: 50 boluses.

Compendium Code No.: 10900180

SNAP® 3DX™ TEST KIT

Idexx Labs. — **Heartworm/Borrelia/Ehrlichia Test**

Canine Heartworm Antigen/Borrelia Burgdorferi/Ehrlichia Canis Antibody Test Kit

U.S. Vet. Lic. No.: 313

Components:

Item	Reagent	Volume 30 Test
1.	1 bottle Anti-HTWM/ *B. burgdorferi* / *E. canis* HRPO Conjugate	8.0 mL
2.	Test Devices	30
	Reagents contained in each device:	
3.	Substrate Solution	0.6 mL
4.	Wash Solution	0.4 mL

Other Components: Transfer pipets, sample tubes, reagent rack.

Indications: SNAP® Heartworm / Lyme / *E. canis*: SNAP® Heartworm Ag/*Borrelia burgdorferi* Ab/*Ehrlichia* canis Ab Test Kit is an enzyme immunoassay for the simultaneous detection of

S

Dirofilaria immitis (D. immitis) antigen, antibody to *Borrelia burgdorferi (B. burgdorferi)*, and antibody to *Ehrlichia canis (E. canis)* in canine whole blood, serum or plasma.

Test Principles: The SNAP® device is an assay technology developed by IDEXX Laboratories, Inc. In operation, the conjugate and the test sample are mixed and added to the SNAP® device which is then activated, releasing reagents stored within the device. Color development in the sample spot(s) is proportional to the concentration of heartworm antigen, *B. burgdorferi* antibody or *E. canis* antibody in the test sample. A Positive Control Spot develops color indicating assay reagents are active.

Test Procedure: Instructions for Use: Allow device, reagents and samples to come to room temperature — do not heat.

Important: Do not depress the activator until indicated.

Sample Information:

Samples must be at room temperature before the assay is run.

Serum or plasma, either fresh, previously frozen or stored at 2°-7°C (36°-45°F), may be used in this test. Serum or plasma may be stored for up to 7 days at 2°-7°C. For longer storage, sample should be frozen (-20°C or colder).

Previously frozen or older samples must be centrifuged before use.

Hemolyzed samples will not affect results.

EDTA or heparin in plasma will not affect results.

Whole blood may be used. Whole blood must be anticoagulated (e.g., EDTA, heparin) and may be used either fresh or after refrigeration 2°-7°C (36°- 45°F) for up to one week.

Test Procedure:

1. Gently mix the sample by inverting.
2. Using the pipet provided, dispense 2 drops of sample (whole blood, serum or plasma) into sample tube.
3. Holding bottle vertically, add 5 drops of Conjugate to the sample tube.
   Cap the sample tube and mix thoroughly by inverting tube 3-5 times.
4. Place the device on a flat surface. Add entire contents of sample tube to Sample Well.
   Sample will flow across Result Window, reaching Activate Circle in approximately 30 seconds to 2 minutes. Some sample may remain in Sample Well.
   Watch carefully for color in the Activate Circle.
   When color first appears in Activate Circle, push Activator firmly until it is flush with the device body.
   Note: Some samples may not flow to the Activate Circle within 2 minutes and, therefore, the circle may not turn color. In this case, press Activator after sample has flowed across the result window.
   Keep the device horizontal to ensure accurate results.

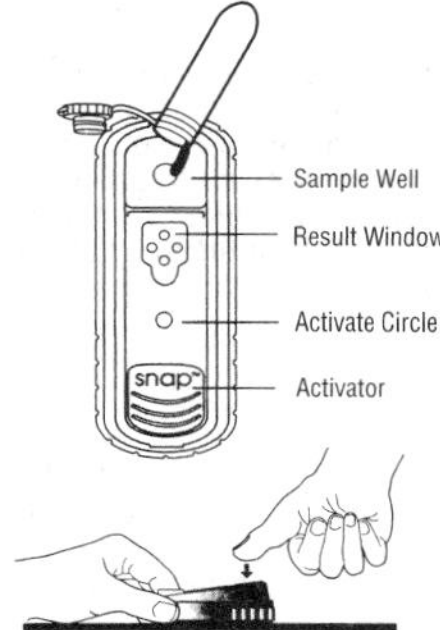

5. Wait eight minutes. Read result.

Interpretation of Results:

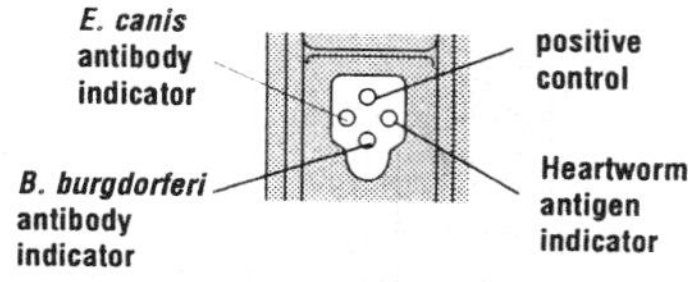

To determine the test result, read the reaction spots in the Result Window. Color development in the sample spots is proportional to the concentration of heartworm antigen, *B. burgdorferi* antibody or *E. canis* antibody in the sample. If no color develops in the positive control, repeat the test.

Negative Result: Only positive control develops color.

Positive Result:

1. Heartworm Ag: Positive control and Heartworm Ag sample spot develop color.
2. *E. canis* Ab and Heartworm Ag: Positive control, Heartworm Ag and *E. canis* Ab sample spots develop color.
3. *E. canis* Ab: Positive control and *E. canis* Ab sample spot develop color.
4. *B. burgdorferi* Ab: Positive control and *B. burgdorferi* Ab sample spot develop color.
5. *B. burgdorferi* Ab and *E. canis* Ab: Positive control, *B. burgdorferi* Ab and *E. canis* Ab sample spots develop color.
6. *B. burgdorferi* Ab and Heartworm Ag: Positive control, *B. burgdorferi* Ab and Heartworm Ag sample spots develop color.
7. *B. burgdorferi* Ab, *E. canis* Ab and Heartworm Ag: Positive control, Heartworm Ag, *B. burgdorferi* Ab and *E. canis* Ab sample spots develop color.

Invalid Results:

1. Background: If the sample is allowed to flow past the Activate Circle, background color may result. Some background color is normal. However, if colored background obscures test result, repeat the test.
2. No Color Development: If positive control does not develop color, repeat the test.

Storage: SNAP® devices and test reagents are stable until expiration date when stored at 2°- 7°C (36°-45°F).

Room temperature storage (optional): SNAP® devices and reagents may be stored at room temperature 15°-27°C (59°-80°F) for 90 days or until printed expiration date, whichever occurs first.

Once SNAP® devices and reagents are removed from 2°-7°C (36°-45°F) for more than 24 hours, the expiration date is 90 days or the printed expiration date, whichever occurs first.

If 90 day expiration date occurs prior to the printed expiration date, record the new date in the space provided on the kit label.

All components must be at room temperature before running the test - do not heat.

Caution(s): Use a separate sample tube and transfer pipet for each test.

During manufacturing, the bioactive spots are dyed for quality control purposes. This does not interfere with the test results or interpretation.

All wastes should be properly decontaminated prior to disposal.

Do not use components past expiration date.

Do not mix components from kits with different lot numbers.

The SNAP® device must be in a horizontal position on a flat surface while the test is performed.

Do not use a SNAP® device that has been activated prior to the addition of sample.

Do not expose device to extreme light after activation.

For veterinary use only.

Discussion: Heartworm disease is caused by the filarial nematode *D. immitis* and has worldwide distribution. The insect vector for *D. immitis* is the mosquito. Adult worms inhabit the blood and vascular tissue, especially in the heart and adjacent blood vessels. *D. immitis* often interferes with heart functions and blood circulation and may damage other vital organs.[1] The detection of heartworm antigen is diagnostic for infection by *D. immitis*.

The causative agent of Lyme Disease has been identified as the tick-borne spirochete *Borrelia burgdorferi*.[2] The organism is known to infect a wide variety of mammals and birds. In dogs, diagnosis of clinical Lyme Disease has been made following observation of typical clinical signs, and by demonstrating an elevated serological titer to *Borrelia burgdorferi*. Typical clinical signs, which vary during the course of the disease, can include skin lesions, fever, lethargy, anorexia, depression, generalized joint pain or arthritis and intermittent joint lameness. An assessment of exposure to *B. burgdorferi* can be made by measurement of canine antibody specific for *B. burgdorferi*.[3] The SNAP®) Lyme Antibody Test has been designed to demonstrate exposure to *B. burgdorferi*. Most Lyme-vaccinated dogs will be non-reactive on this test. However, in one study of 82 dog samples determined by Western blot to be from Lyme-vaccinated animals, 3 (3.6%) were reactive.

Canine ehrlichiosis is a tick-borne disease of dogs caused by the rickettsial parasite *E. canis*. Replication of the organism occurs within infected mononuclear cells and spreads to organs containing mononuclear phagocytes. Infection can result in thrombocytopenia, leukopenia and/or anemia. Clinical signs of infection include fever, dyspnea, weight loss, petechial hemorrhages and epistaxis.

Diagnosis of canine ehrlichiosis has been made by observation of typical clinical signs and by the measurement of a significant antibody titer to *E. canis*.[4]

A positive result in the SNAP® *E. canis* Antibody Test indicates a significant antibody titer to *E. canis*.

References: Available upon request.

Presentation: 30 test kits.

SNAP is either a registered trademark or trademark of IDEXX Laboratories, Inc. in the United States and/or other countries around the world.

U.S. Patent Nos. 5,726,010; 5,726,013; 5,780,333; 6,007,999; 6,025,338. Other patents pending.

Compendium Code No.: 11160512 06-04205-01

SNAP® CANINE HEARTWORM PF ANTIGEN TEST KIT

Idexx Labs. **Heartworm Test**

U.S. Vet. Lic. No.: 313

Description: SNAP® Canine Heartworm Antigen Test Kit is an enzyme immunoassay for the semi-quantitative detection of *Dirofilaria immitis (D. immitis)* antigen in canine and feline whole blood, serum or plasma.

Components:

Item	Reagent	Volume	
		15 Test	30 Test
1.	1 bottle Anti-HTWM: HRPO Conjugate	8.0 mL	8.0 mL
2.	Test Devices	15	30
	Reagents contained in each device:		
3.	Substrate Solution	0.6 mL	0.6 mL
4.	Wash Solution	0.4 mL	0.4 mL

Other Components: transfer pipets, sample tubes, reagent rack.

Test Principles: SNAP® is an enzyme immunoassay technology developed by Idexx Laboratories, Inc.[2] In operation, the conjugate and the test sample are mixed and added to the snap device which is then activated, releasing reagents stored within the device. Color development in high and low antigen indicators is proportional to *D. immitis* antigen concentration in the sample. A Positive Control Spot develops color indicating assay reagents are active. Color development in the Negative Control Spot indicates reactivity unrelated to the disease or an improperly performed test.

Test Procedure: Allow device, reagents and samples to come to room temperature - do not heat.

Important: Do not depress the activator until indicated.

Sample Information:

Samples must be at room temperature before running assay.

Serum or plasma, either fresh, previously frozen or stored at 2°-7°C (36°- 45°F), may be used in this test. Serum or plasma may be stored for up to 7 days at 2°-7°C. For longer storage, sample should be frozen (-20°C or colder).

Previously frozen or older samples must be centrifuged before use.

Hemolyzed samples will not affect results.

EDTA or heparin in plasma will not affect results.

Whole blood may be used. Whole blood must be anticoagulated (eg. EDTA, heparin) and may be used either fresh or after refrigeration 2°-7°C (36°-45°F) for up to one week.

Test Procedure:

1. Gently mix the sample by inverting.
2. Using the pipet provided, dispense 2 drops of sample (whole blood, serum or plasma) into sample tube.
3. Holding bottle vertically, add 5 drops of Conjugate to the sample tube.
   Cap the sample tube and mix thoroughly by inverting tube 3-5 times.
4. Place the device on a flat surface. Add entire contents of sample tube to Sample Well.
   Sample will flow across Result Window, reaching Activate Circle in approximately 30 seconds to 2 minutes. Some sample may remain in sample well.

Watch carefully for color in the Activate Circle.

When color first appears in Activate Circle, push Activator firmly until it is flush with the device body.

Note: Some samples may not flow to the Activate Circle within 2 minutes and, therefore, the circle may not turn color. In this case, press Activator after sample has flowed across the result window.

Keep the device horizontal to ensure accurate results.

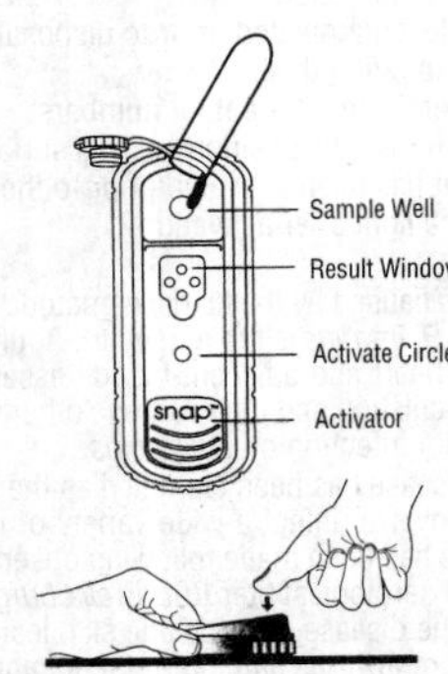

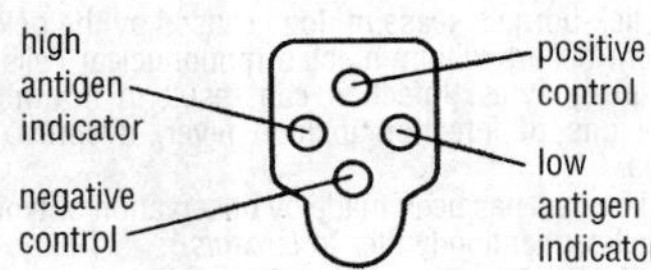

5. Wait six minutes. Read result.

Test Interpretation:

high antigen indicator
positive control
negative control
low antigen indicator

To determine the test result, read the reaction spots in the Result Window. Color development in antigen indicator spots is proportional to the heartworm antigen concentration in the sample indicating low or high antigen levels. If no color develops in the positive control, repeat the test.

Negative Result: Only positive control develops color.

Positive Result:

1. Low Antigen Level: Positive control and low antigen indicator develop color.

or

2. High Antigen Level: Positive control and both antigen indicators develop color.

Reaction with Negative Control: The negative control spot serves as a safeguard against false positives and helps indicate that the assay has been run properly.

1. Positive Result: If color in the high and/or low antigen indicator is darker than negative control, result is positive.

or

2. Invalid Result: If color in the negative control is equal to or darker than high and/or low antigen indicator, repeat the test.

Invalid Results:

1. Background: If the sample is allowed to flow past the activate circle, background color may result. Some background color is normal. However, if colored background obscures test result, repeat the test.
2. No Color Development: If positive control does not develop color, repeat the test.

Precaution(s): Snap devices and test reagents are stable until expiration date when stored at 2°-7°C (36°-45°F).

Room temperature storage (optional): Snap devices and reagents may be stored at room temperature 15°-27°C (59°-80°F) for 90 days or until printed expiration date, whichever occurs first.

Once snap devices and reagents are removed from 2°-7°C (36°-45°F) for more than 24 hours, the expiration date is 90 days or the printed expiration date, whichever occurs first.

If 90 day expiration date occurs prior to the printed expiration date, record the new date in the space provided on the kit label.

All components must be at room temperature before running the test—do not heat.

Caution(s): Use a separate sample tube and transfer pipet for each test.

During manufacturing the bioactive spots are dyed for quality control purposes. This does not interfere with the test results or interpretation.

All wastes should be properly decontaminated prior to disposal.

Do not use components past expiration date.

Do not mix components from kits with different lot numbers.

The snap device must be in a horizontal position on a flat surface while the test is performed.

Do not use a snap device that has been activated prior to the addition of sample.

Do not expose device to extreme light after activation.

For veterinary use only.

Discussion: Heartworm disease, caused by the filarial nematode, *D. immitis*, has a worldwide distribution. The insect vector for *D. immitis* is the mosquito. Adult worms inhabit the blood and vascular tissue, especially the heart and adjacent blood vessels. *D. immitis* often interferes with heart functions and blood circulation and may damage other vital organs.[1]

References:

1. Rawlings, C.A., et al. 1982. Four Types of Occult *Dirofilaria immitis* Infection in Dogs. JAVMA. 180: pp.1323-1326.
2. Patent Pending.

Presentation: 15 and 30 test kits.

Compendium Code No.: 11160461

SNAP® CANINE PARVOVIRUS ANTIGEN TEST KIT

Idexx Labs. **Parvovirus Test**

Canine Parvovirus Antigen Test Kit

U.S. Vet. Lic. No.: 313

Components:

Item	Component	Quantity
1.	1 bottle of extraction buffer	8.0 mL
2.	1 bottle of anti-parvovirus:HRPO conjugate	2.0 mL
3.	Snap® device Antibodies to CPV and control.	5
	Reagents contained in each device: 4. Wash Solution 5. Substrate Solution	0.4 mL 0.6 mL

Other Components: dacron swabs, test tubes, pipets, sample vials, reagent rack

Indications: SNAP® Canine Parvovirus Antigen Test Kit is an enzyme immunoassay for the detection of canine parvovirus (CPV) in feces.

Test Principles: SNAP® is an enzyme immunoassay technology developed by Idexx Laboratories, Inc. Upon mixing enzyme-conjugated antibody to CPV and the test sample, the antibody will bind to CPV antigen (if present). The sample/conjugate mixture is then added to the Snap® device and flows across the spotted matrix. The matrix-bound CPV antibody (sample spot) will capture the CPV-conjugated antibody complex. The device is then activated, releasing wash and substrate reagents stored within the device. Color development in the Sample Spot indicates the presence of CPV antigen in the sample. A Positive Control Spot should develop color to demonstrate that assay reagents are active. Color development in the Negative Control Spot indicates reactivity unrelated to the disease or an improperly performed test.

Test Procedure:

Sample Information: A large number of virus particles can be shed in feces and remain infectious for long periods.

Properly dispose of contaminated materials and disinfect work areas.

Canine fecal matter is required for this test. Swabs are provided for sampling.

Samples must be at room temperature before beginning test procedure.

Fecal samples may be stored at 2°-7°C (36°-45°F) for 24 hours. If longer storage is required, samples should be frozen.

Test Protocol:

1. Obtain a test tube, a swab, a pipet, a sample vial and a Snap® device for each sample to be tested. Fill the test tube to the line marked 1 (approx. 1 mL) with extraction buffer and place the tube in the rack provided. Using the swab, coat the swab lip with fecal material. Note: Only a thin coat of fecal material on the swab is required; do not coat the swab with excess feces. Immerse the swab in the extraction buffer and rotate the swab several times to release the sample into the buffer. Then, discard the swab and leave the test tube until the large particles in the sample have settled.
2. Using the pipet, dispense 4 drops of the fluid from the surface of the fecal extract into the sample vial.
3. Holding bottle vertical, add 4 drops of conjugate to the sample vial.
4. Cap the sample vial and mix thoroughly by inverting the vial 3-4 times.
5. Place the Snap® device or a horizontal surface. Add contents of the sample vial to sample well, being careful not to splash contents outside of the sample well. The sample will flow across the result window, reaching the activate circle in 30-60 seconds. Some sample may remain in the sample well.

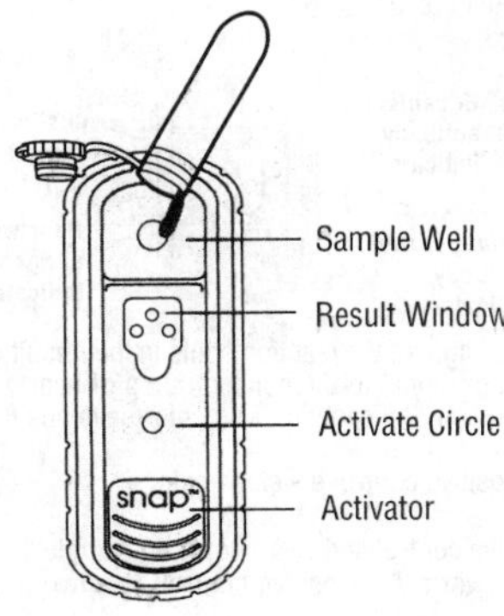

6. Watch carefully for sample or blue color in the activate circle. When color first appears in the activate circle, push activator firmly until it is flush with the device body. Keep the device horizontal to ensure accurate results. Note: Some samples may not flow to the activate circle within 1 minute and, therefore, the circle may not turn color. In this case, press the activator if the sample has flowed across the 3 spots of the result window.

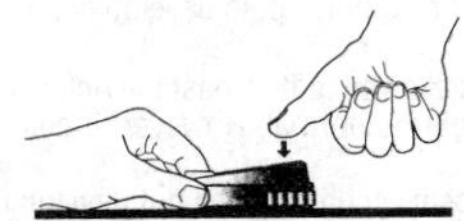

7. Wait 8 minutes. Read the result. Some positive samples will develop color prior to eight minutes.

Test Interpretation: To determine the test result, read the reaction spots in the result window and compare the color intensity of the sample spot to that of the negative control spot.

S

Color development in the positive control spot indicates that the test reagents are functional. If the positive control spot does not develop color, the result is invalid. Repeat the test.

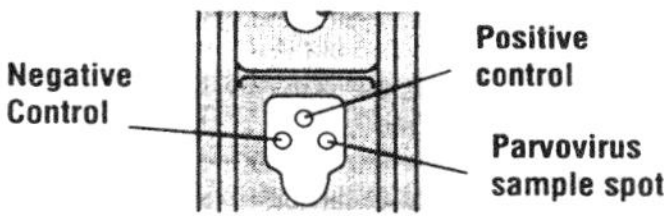

Negative Result: Only positive control spot develops color. Color does not develop in the sample spot or in the negative control spot.

Positive Result: Only positive control spot and sample spot develop color. Note: Color development in the sample spot is proportional to the level of CPV antigen in the sample. Less intense color development indicates a positive result with a low level of antigen in the sample.

Reaction with Negative Control: The negative control spot serves as a safeguard against false positives. If color in the sample spot is darker than the color in the negative control spot, the result is positive. If color in the negative control spot is equal to or darker than the color in the sample spot, the result is invalid and the sample should be retested.

Storage: Snap® devices and test reagents are stable until expiration date when stored at 2°-7°C (36°-45°F).

Room temperature storage (optional): Snap® devices and reagents may be stored at room temperature 15°-27°C (59°-80°F) for 90 days or until printed expiration date, whichever occurs first.

Once Snap® devices and reagents are removed from 2°-7°C (36°-45°F) for more than 24 hours, the expiration date is 90 days or the printed expiration date, whichever occurs first.

If the 90-day expiration date occurs prior to the printed expiration date, record the new date in the space provided on the kit label.

All components must be at room temperature before running the test - do not heat.

Caution(s): Use a separate swab, test tube, pipet and sample vial for each sample.

During manufacturing of the Snap® device, the bioactive spots are dyed for quality control purposes. This does not interfere with test results.

Do not use components past expiration date.

Do not mix components from different test kits.

The Snap® device must be in a horizontal position on a flat surface while the test is performed.

Do not use a Snap® device that has been activated prior to the addition of the sample.

Do not expose device to extreme light after activation.

Important: Do not depress the activator until step 6 of the test procedure.

For veterinary use only

Discussion: CPV infection is now recognized as one of the common causes of vomiting and diarrhea in dogs, particularly those younger than one year of age.[1] CPV is highly contagious and is transmitted principally by the fecal-oral route.[2] Rapid and accurate diagnosis of CPV infection allows the initiation of prompt treatment and quarantine of infected dogs.

References: Available upon request.

Presentation: 5 test kit.

SNAP® is a trademark of Idexx Laboratories, Inc. which is registered in the United States and other countries around the world.

Compendium Code No.: 11160472

SNAP® COMBO FeLV Ag/FIV Ab TEST KIT

Idexx Labs. **FeLV/FIV Test**

U.S. Vet. Lic. No.: 313

Description: SNAP® Combo FeLV Ag/FIV Ab Test Kit is an enzyme-linked immunosorbent assay (ELISA) for the simultaneous detection of feline leukemia virus (FeLV) antigen and antibody to feline immunodeficiency virus (FIV) in feline serum, plasma or whole blood.

Components:

Item	Reagent	Volume	
		15 Test	30 Test
1.	1 bottle Anti-FeLV/FIV Ag:HRPO Conjugate	3.5 mL	7 mL
2.	Snap® Device Monoclonal antibodies to p27, inactivated FIV antigen, and positive and negative controls	15	30
	Reagents contained in each device:		
3.	Wash Solution	0.4 mL	0.4 mL
4.	Substrate Solution	0.6 mL	0.6 mL

Other Components: Transfer pipets, sample tubes, reagent rack.

Indications: The detection of the FeLV group-specific viral antigen (p27) is diagnostic for FeLV infection. The measurement of specific antibody titer to FIV indicates that the animal has been exposed to the virus and is indicative of an active FIV infection.

Test Principles: The SNAP® Combo FeLV Ag/FIV Ab assay utilizes monoclonal antibodies to p27, inactivated FIV antigen, and positive and negative controls.

The conjugate mixture contains enzyme-conjugated antibody to p27 and enzyme-conjugated FIV antigen. Upon mixing the conjugate and the test sample, conjugated monoclonal antibody will bind p27 antigen (if present), and conjugated FIV antigen will bind to FIV antibody (if present). The sample/conjugate mixture is then added to the Snap® device and flows across the spotted matrix. The matrix-bound p27 antibody (FeLV spot) will capture the p27-conjugated antibody complex, while the matrix-bound FIV antigen (FIV spot) will capture the FIV antibody-conjugated antigen complex. The device is then activated, releasing wash and substrate reagents stored within the device.

Color development in the FeLV Ag sample spot indicates the presence of FeLV antigen, while color development in the FIV Ab sample spot indicates the presence of FIV antibody.

Test Procedure: Test device and all samples must be at room temperature - do not heat.

Important: Do not depress the activator until step 4.

Fresh serum, plasma or whole blood may be used in this test.

Whole blood must be anti-coagulated with heparin, EDTA or citrate.

Hemolyzed samples will not affect results.

Samples can either be fresh or refrigerated (2°-7°C) for up to 1 week. Thawed serum or plasma samples may be used.

1. Holding bottle vertical, add 4 drops of conjugate (blue cap) to the sample tube.
2. Using the pipet that is provided, transfer 3 drops (.15 mL) of sample (whole blood*, serum, or plasma) into sample tube.
   * .15 mL of whole blood is approximately 3 drops from a syringe with the needle removed.
3. Cap the sample tube and mix thoroughly by inverting tube 3-5 times.
4. Place the device on a flat surface. Add contents of sample tube to Sample Well, being careful not to splash contents outside of Sample Well.
   Sample will flow across Result Window, reaching Activate Circle in 30-60 seconds. Some samples may remain in sample well.
   Watch carefully for sample or blue color in the Activate Circle.
   When color first appears in Activate Circle push Activator firmly until it is flush with the device body.
   Note: Some samples may not flow to the activate circle within 60 seconds, and, therefore, the circle may not turn color. In this case, press the activator if sample has flowed across result window.
   Keep the device horizontal to ensure accurate results.

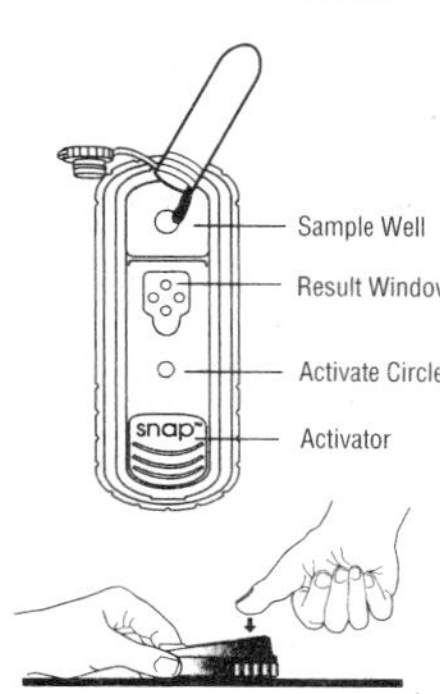

5. Read test result at 10 minutes
   Note: Positive control may develop sooner, but results are not complete until 10 minutes.

Test Interpretation: To determine test results, read the reaction spots in the Result Window. Color development in sample spot is proportional to the concentration of FeLV antigen or FIV antibody in the sample. If no color develops in the positive control spot, repeat the test.

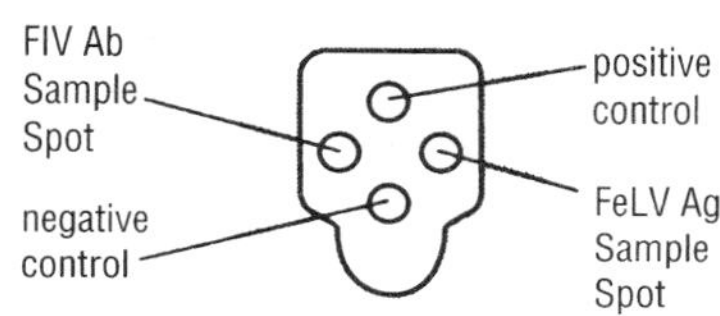

Negative Result: Only positive control spot develops color.

Positive Result:

FeLV Antigen: Positive control spot and FeLV Ag sample spot develop color.

FeLV Antigen and FIV Antibody: Positive control spot and both sample spots develop color.

FIV Antibody: Positive control spot and FIV Ab sample spot develop color.

Reaction with Negative Control: The negative control spot serves as a safeguard against false positives.

Positive Result: If color in the FIV Ab or FeLV Ag sample spot is darker than negative control spot, result is positive for that spot.

Invalid Result: If color in the negative control spot is equal to or darker than FIV Ab or FeLV Ag sample spot, the test is invalid for that sample spot.

Invalid Results:

1. Background: If the sample is allowed to flow past the activate circle, background color may result. Some background color is normal. However, if colored background obscures test result, repeat the test.
2. No Color Development: If positive control does not develop color, repeat the test.

Storage: Snap® devices and test reagents must be stored at 2°-7°C (36°-45°F).

Caution(s): Use a separate pipet for each sample.

During manufacturing the bioactive spots are dyed for quality control purposes. This does not interfere with the test results or interpretation.

FIV antigen used in the conjugate has been chemically inactivated. However, samples, sample tubes, pipets, conjugate and Snap® devices should be handled as though capable of transmitting FeLV and FIV. All waste should be properly decontaminated prior to disposal.

Do not use components past expiration date.

Do not mix components from kits with different lot numbers.

The Snap® device must be in a horizontal position on a flat surface while performing test.

Do not use a Snap® device that has been activated prior to the addition of sample.

Warning(s): For veterinary use only.

Presentation: 15 or 30 tests per kit.

Compendium Code No.: 11160481

SNAP* FELINE HEARTWORM ANTIGEN TEST

Idexx Labs. **Heartworm Test**

Feline Heartworm Antigen Test Kit

U.S. Vet. Lic. No.: 313

Components:

Item	Reagent	Amount	Amount
		5 Test	15 Test
1.	1 bottle Anti-HTWM: HRPO Conjugate	8.0 mL	8.0 mL
2.	Test Devices	5	15
	Reagents contained in each device:		
3.	Substrate Solution	0.6 mL	0.6 mL
4.	Wash Solution	0.4 mL	0.4 mL

Other Components: transfer pipets, sample tubes, reagent rack

Indications: SNAP* Feline Heartworm Antigen Test Kit is an enzyme immunoassay for the

S

semi-quantitative detection of *Dirofilaria immitis (D. immitis)* antigen in feline whole blood, serum or plasma.[1]

Test Procedure:

Sample Information: Samples must be at room temperature before beginning test procedure.

Serum or plasma, either fresh, previously frozen or stored at 2°-7°C (36°-45°F), may be used in this test. Serum or plasma may be stored for up to 7 days at 2°-7°C. For longer storage, sample should be frozen (-20°C or colder).

Previously frozen or older samples must be centrifuged before use.

Hemolyzed samples will not affect results.

EDTA or heparin in plasma will not affect results.

Whole blood may be used. Whole blood must be anticoagulated (e.g., EDTA, heparin) and may be used either fresh or after refrigeration 2°-7°C (36°-45°F) for up to one week.

Test Procedure:

1. Using the pipet provided, dispense 2 drops (.10 mL) of sample (whole blood, serum or plasma) into sample tube (blue cap).
2. Holding bottle vertically, add 5 drops of Conjugate to the sample tube (blue cap).
3. Cap the sample tube and mix thoroughly by inverting tube 3-5 times.
4. Place the device on a flat surface. Add entire contents of sample tube to Sample Well.
   Sample will flow across Result Window, reaching Activate Circle in approximately 30 seconds to 2 minutes. Some sample may remain in Sample Well.

Watch carefully for color in the Activate Circle.

- When color first appears in Activate Circle, push Activator firmly until it is flush with the device body.

Note: Some samples may not flow to the Activate Circle within 60 seconds and, therefore, the circle may not turn color. In this case, press Activator after sample has flowed across the Result Window.

Keep the device horizontal to ensure accurate results.

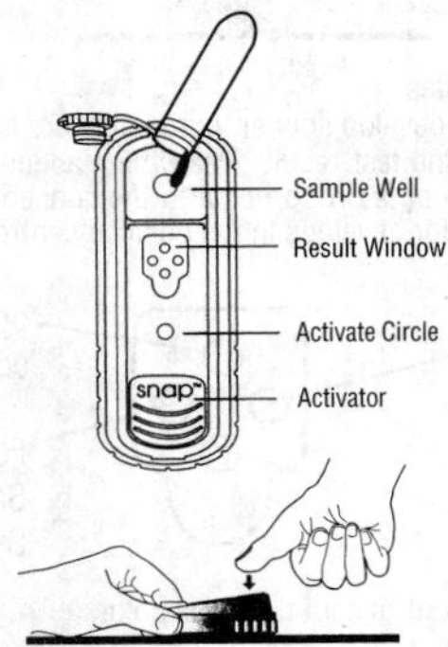

5. Read test results at ten minutes.
   Note: Positive control may develop sooner, but results are not complete until ten minutes.

Interpretation of Results: To determine the test result, read the reaction spots in the Result Window. Color development in antigen indicator spots is proportional to the heartworm antigen concentration in the sample indicating low or high antigen levels. If no color develops in the positive control, repeat the test.

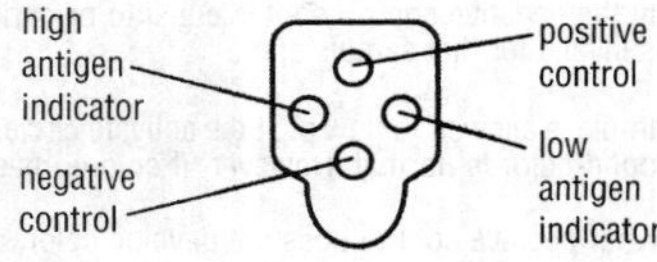

Negative Result: Only positive control develops color.

Positive Result

Low Antigen Level: Positive control and low antigen indicator develop color.

High Antigen Level: Positive control and both antigen indicators develop color.

Reaction with Negative Control: The negative control spot serves as a safeguard against false positives and helps indicate that the assay has been run properly.

Positive Result: If color in the high and/or low antigen indicator is darker than negative control, result is positive.

S

Invalid Result: If color in the negative control is equal to or darker than high and/or low antigen indicator, repeat the test.

Invalid Results

1. Background: If the sample is allowed to flow past the activate circle, background color may result. Some background color is normal. However, if colored background obscures test result, repeat the test.
2. No Color Development: If positive control does not develop color, repeat the test.

Storage: Snap devices and test reagents are stable until expiration date when stored at 2°-7°C (36°-45°F).

All components must be at room temperature before running the test. This may take up to 30 minutes, depending upon the temperature in your laboratory. Do not heat.

Caution(s): Use a separate sample tube and transfer pipet for each test.

During manufacturing the bioactive spots are dyed for quality control purposes. This does not interfere with the test results or interpretation.

Do not use components past expiration date.

Do not mix components from kits with different lot numbers.

The SNAP device must be in a horizontal position on a flat surface while the test is performed.

Do not use a SNAP device that has been activated prior to the addition of sample.

Discussion: Heartworm disease, caused by the filarial nematode, *D. immitis*, has a worldwide distribution. The insect vector for *D. immitis* is the mosquito. Adult worms inhabit the blood and vascular tissue, especially the heart and adjacent blood vessels. *D. immitis* often interferes with heart functions and blood circulation and may damage other vital organs.[2]

SNAP is an enzyme immunoassay technology developed by Idexx Laboratories, Inc. In operation, the conjugate and the test sample are mixed and added to the SNAP device which is then activated, releasing reagents stored within the device. Color development in high and low antigen indicators is proportional to *D. immitis* antigen concentration in the sample. A Positive Control Spot develops color indicating assay reagents are active. Color development in the Negative Control Spot indicates reactivity unrelated to the disease or an improperly performed test.

References: Available upon request.

Presentation: 5 or 15 tests per kit.

*SNAP is either a trademark or a registered trademark of Idexx Laboratories, Inc. in the United States and/or other countries.

Compendium Code No.: 11160620 06-04256-00

SNAP® FeLV ANTIGEN TEST KIT

Idexx Labs. **FeLV Test**

U.S. Vet. Lic. No.: 313

Description: SNAP® FeLV Antigen Test Kit is an enzyme-linked immunosorbent assay (ELISA) for the detection of feline leukemia virus (FeLV) antigen in feline serum, plasma or whole blood.

Components:

Item	Reagent	Volume	
		15 Test	30 Test
1.	1 bottle Anti-FeLV: HRPO Conjugate	3.5 mL	7 mL
2.	Snap® Device Monoclonal antibodies to p27, and positive and negative controls	15	30
	Reagents contained in each device:		
3.	Wash Solution	0.4 mL	0.4 mL
4.	Substrate Solution	0.6 mL	0.6 mL

Other Components: Transfer pipets, sample tubes, reagent rack.

Test Principles: The detection of the FeLV group-specific viral antigen (p27) is diagnostic for FeLV infection. The SNAP® FeLV Antigen assay utilizes monoclonal antibodies to p27, inactivated FIV antigen, and positive and negative controls.

The conjugate contains enzyme-conjugated antibody to p27. Upon mixing the conjugate and the test sample, conjugated monoclonal antibody will bind p27 antigen (if present). The sample/conjugate mixture is then added to the Snap® device and flows across the spotted matrix. The matrix-bound p27 antibody (FeLV spot) will capture the p27-conjugated antibody complex. The device is then activated, releasing wash and substrate reagents stored within the device.

Color development in the FeLV Ag sample spot indicates the presence of FeLV antigen.

Test Procedure: Test device and all samples must be at room temperature - do not heat.

Important: Do not depress the activator until step 4.

Fresh serum, plasma or whole blood may be used in this test.

Whole blood must be anti-coagulated with heparin, EDTA or citrate.

Hemolyzed samples will not affect results.

Samples can either be fresh or refrigerated (2°-7°C) for up to 1 week. Thawed serum or plasma samples may be used.

1. Holding bottle vertical, add 4 drops of conjugate to the sample tube.
2. Using the pipet that is provided, transfer 3 drops (.15 mL) of sample (whole blood*, serum, or plasma) into sample tube.
   * .15 mL of whole blood is approximately 3 drops from a syringe with the needle removed.
3. Cap the sample tube and mix thoroughly by inverting tube 3-5 times.
4. Place the device on a flat surface. Add contents of sample tube to Sample Well, being careful not to splash contents outside of Sample Well.
   Sample will flow across Result Window, reaching Activate Circle in 30-60 seconds. Some samples may remain in sample well.
   Watch carefully for sample or blue color in the Activate Circle.
   When color **first** appears in Activate Circle push Activator firmly until it is flush with the device body.
   Note: Some samples may not flow to the activate circle within 60 seconds, and, therefore, the circle may not turn color. In this case, press the activator if sample has flowed across result window.
   Keep the device horizontal to ensure accurate results.

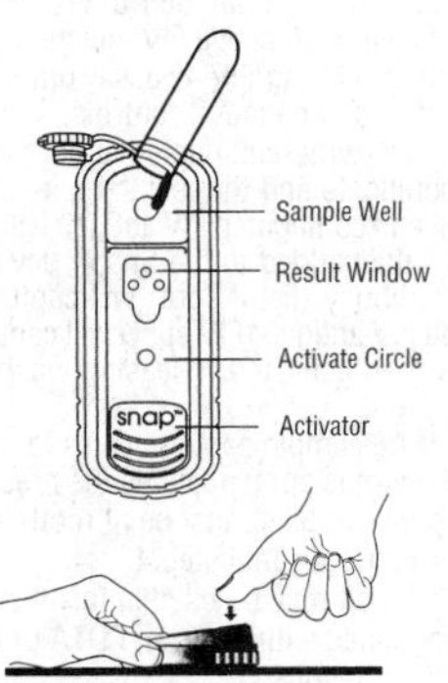

5. Read test result at 10 minutes
   Note: Positive control may develop sooner, but results are not complete until 10 minutes.

Test Interpretation: To determine test results, read the reaction spots in the Result Window. Color development in sample spot is proportional to the concentration of FeLV antigen in the sample. If no color develops in the positive control spot, repeat the test.

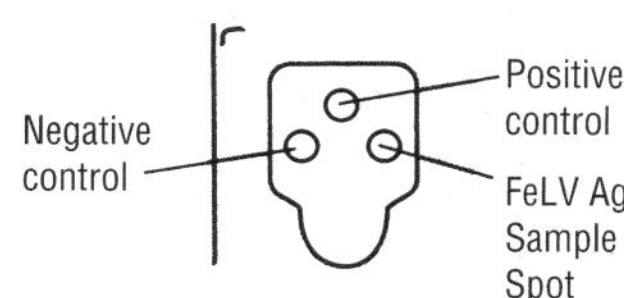

Negative Result: Only positive control spot develops color.
Positive Result: Positive control spot and FeLV Ag sample spot develop color.
Reaction with Negative Control: The negative control spot serves as a safeguard against false positives.

Positive Result: If color in the sample spot is darker than negative control spot, result is positive.

Invalid Result: If color in the negative control spot is equal to or darker than sample spot, the test is invalid.

Invalid Results:

1. Background: If the sample is allowed to flow past the activate circle, background color may result. Some background color is normal. However, if colored background obscures test result, repeat the test.
2. No Color Development: If positive control does not develop color, repeat the test.

Storage: Snap® devices and test reagents must be stored at 2°-7°C (36°-45°F).
Caution(s): Use a separate pipet for each sample.

During manufacturing the bioactive spots are dyed for quality control purposes. This does not interfere with the test results or interpretation.

Samples, sample tubes, pipets, conjugate and SNAP® should be handled as though capable of transmitting FeLV. All waste should be properly decontaminated prior to disposal.

Do not use components past expiration date.

Do not mix components from kits with different lot numbers.

The Snap® device must be in a horizontal position on a flat surface while performing test.

Do not use a Snap® device that has been activated prior to the addition of sample.

Warning(s): For veterinary use only.
Presentation: 15 or 30 tests per kit.
Compendium Code No.: 11160491

SNAP* FOAL IgG TEST KIT

Idexx Pharm. **IgG Test**

U.S. Vet. Lic. No.: 313
Components: Kit Components:

Item	Reagent	Volume
1.	Foal IgG SNAP* Devices	10
2.	10 bottles of Sample Diluent preserved with sodium azide	10 mL
3.	Anti-Equine IgG Alkaline Phosphate Conjugate preserved with sodium azide	5 mL
4.	1 bottle of Wash Solution preserved with gentamicin	100 mL
5.	1 bottle of Substrate Solution preserved with sodium azide	5 mL

Other Components: Membrane seating tool, micropipets.

Indications: SNAP* Foal IgG Test Kit is an enzyme-linked immunosorbent assay (ELISA) for the semi-quantitative measurement of IgG in equine serum, plasma or whole blood.

Equines are born with little or no circulating immunoglobulin. Neonatal immunity to infectious agents requires the uptake and absorption of maternal antibodies from colostrum. Failure of this passive transfer can occur as a result of premature lactation, deficient suckling, malabsorption or low levels of IgG in colostrum. Partial or complete failure of immune transfer occurs in 10-25% of all foals, and these animals are at a high risk of serious illness or death.[1,2]

Several studies have identified specific serum concentrations of IgG as indicators of the success of immune transfer.[2,3,4] Greater than 800 mg IgG per 100 mL serum is considered an adequate level of immunity. Levels of 400-800 mg/dL may be adequate, but foals at this level are possibly at risk. IgG levels between 200 and 400 mg/dL reflect a partial failure of immune transfer, while concentrations of less than 200 mg/dL suggest a total failure.

Rapid identification of low IgG levels is essential to the early initiation of treatment of immunodeficient foals. Furthermore, post-treatment testing allows a timely evaluation of the success of IgG supplementation.

Test Principles: SNAP* Foal IgG is an enzyme immunoassay designed to detect the presence of immunoglobulin G in serum, plasma or whole blood. In the SNAP* format, polyclonal antibodies to equine IgG, as well as calibration levels of equine IgG, have been spotted separately onto a fiber membrane on the device. Sample and reagents are applied onto the surface of the membrane and flow through the bioactive spots. Equine IgG, if present, is captured by the immobilized anti-IgG antibodies on the sample spot. Enzyme conjugated polyclonal antibodies are then added, and bind to the captured equine IgG forming an antibody-IgG-antibody sandwich. After washing away unbound material from the membrane, an enzyme substrate solution is added. Subsequent color development is proportional to the concentration of equine IgG captured.

Color will also develop in the IgG calibration spots. The spots contain equine IgG corresponding to serum sample IgG levels of 200 mg/dL, 400 mg/dL and 800 mg/dL. Since these spots are calibrated with specific levels of IgG, a comparison of color intensity between the sample and the controls allows an assessment of IgG level in the sample. In addition to their calibration function, these spots indicate that the assay reagents are active.

Test Procedure: Specimen Information: Serum, plasma or whole blood may be used in this test. Due to variation in hematocrit among foals, it is recommended that serum or plasma be used when maximum accuracy is desired. For serum or plasma, the sample can be either fresh or previously frozen. Whole blood must be anticoagulated with heparin, EDTA or citrate. Hemolyzed samples may be used without the risk of false positives.

Reagents must come to room temperature before starting the test procedure. Remove one SNAP* device, micropipet and bottle of sample diluent for each sample to be tested. Then, perform the steps below.

1. Dilute Sample:
   A. Serum or Plasma: When using serum or plasma 2 microliters of sample are required. Remove the cap and dropper tip from one bottle of Solution 2 Sample Diluent. Insert plunger in color coded end of microliter capillary pipet and push plunger down. Insert into sample; draw back exactly to the second line (2 microliters). Wipe excess sample from the outside of the pipet. Add the sample to the bottle of sample diluent by depressing the plunger. Draw sample diluent into pipet with plunger and then depress plunger to thoroughly rinse all sample from pipet into sample diluent bottle. Replace the tip and cap of the bottle and mix well.
   B. Whole Blood: Whole blood must be anticoagulated with heparin, EDTA or citrate. When using whole blood, 4 microliters are required. Remove the cap and dropper tip from one bottle of Solution 2 Sample Diluent. Insert plunger in color coded end of microliter capillary pipet and push plunger down. Insert into sample; draw back exactly to the fourth line (4 microliters). Wipe excess sample from the outside of the pipet. Add the sample to the bottle of sample diluent by depressing the plunger. Draw sample diluent into pipet with plunger and then depress plunger to thoroughly rinse all sample from pipet into sample diluent bottle. Replace the tip and cap of the bottle and mix well.
2. Wet Assay Device: Wet the assay device with Wash Solution by filling to the line on the inside of the device. Allow solution to be completely absorbed. To insure uniform flow through the bioactive membrane, press the sponge end of the seating tool firmly down on the membrane.
3. Add Diluted Sample: Mix the diluted sample thoroughly by gently shaking. Add 10 drops of diluted sample directly onto the center of the assay device. Wait 3 minutes.
4. Add Conjugate: Add 4 drops of Solution 3 (Phosphatase Conjugate) to the center of the assay device. Make sure that all four spots are covered with the blue conjugate. Wait 2 minutes.
5. Wash Assay Device: Add 5-10 drops of Wash Solution to assay device. Then, fill device with Wash Solution up to the line on the inside of the device. Allow Wash Solution to be absorbed. All blue color should be washed away.
5. Add Substrate: Add 4 drops of Solution 5 (Substrate Solution) being careful to cover all four spots. Wait 3 minutes for adequate color development.
6. Read Result: Determine the level of IgG in the sample by comparing sample spot to the calibration spots. (Optional: To preserve the result, add 10-15 drops of Wash Solution to assay device. Note: This may reduce color intensity of the reaction.)

Interpretation of Results: To determine the results of a test read the reaction spots on the SNAP* Foal IgG assay device. The spots are arranged as shown in the diagram.

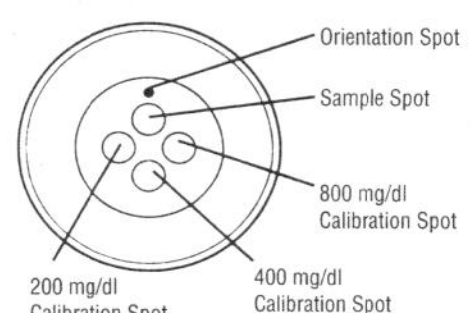

To determine the level of IgG in the test sample, compare the color of the sample spot to that of the three calibration spots. Possible test results and their interpretation are diagrammed below:

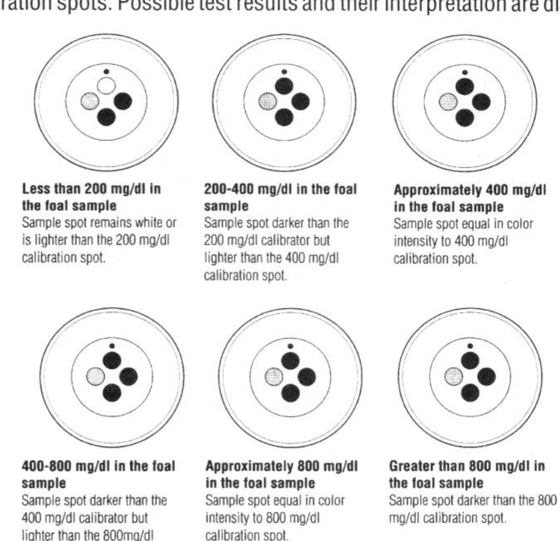

Less than 200 mg/dl in the foal sample
Sample spot remains white or is lighter than the 200 mg/dl calibration spot.
200-400 mg/dl in the foal sample
Sample spot darker than the 200 mg/dl calibrator but lighter than the 400 mg/dl calibration spot.
Approximately 400 mg/dl in the foal sample
Sample spot equal in color intensity to 400 mg/dl calibration spot.
400-800 mg/dl in the foal sample
Sample spot darker than the 400 mg/dl calibrator but lighter than the 800mg/dl calibration spot.
Approximately 800 mg/dl in the foal sample
Sample spot equal in color intensity to 800 mg/dl calibration spot.
Greater than 800 mg/dl in the foal sample
Sample spot darker than the 800 mg/dl calibration spot.

Storage: Store the kit containing reagents at 2°-7°C (36°-45°F). The SNAP* devices need not be refrigerated. After the bag seal is broken, bag should be tightly closed and stored at 2°-7°C (36°-45°F). All kit reagents and devices must be brought to room temperature prior to use and may be kept at room temperature throughout the day.

Caution(s): Drop reagents into the center of the SNAP* device, taking care to cover the four bioactive spots.

Do not use components past expiration date and do not intermix components from kits with different lot numbers.

Kit reagents (except wash solution) contain sodium azide as a preservative. Sink disposal requires flushing plumbing with large amounts of water to prevent formation of potentially explosive copper or lead azide complexes.

For veterinary use only.

References: Available upon request.
Presentation: 10 devices per kit.
*SNAP is either a registered trademark or a trademark of Idexx Laboratories, Inc. in the USA and/or other countries.
Compendium Code No.: 15070002 06-01415-02

SOA (SEX ODOR AEROSOL)

Intervet **Pheromone**

Active Ingredient(s): The active ingredient is Δ16-5α-androsten-3-ona (0.28 mg) with diluent and inert propellants. Contains no chlorofluorocarbons.

SOA contains a synthetic solution of the same pheromone which occurs naturally in the boar and is responsible for the "boar odor".

Indications: SOA can be used to determine if a gilt or sow is in "standing heat" and ready for artificial insemination.

SOA is a synthetic boar odor aerosol for heat detection in gilts and sows.

Dosage and Administration: Hold can about 20 inches from the head and spray directly at the nostrils of the gilt or sow. The spray should be applied for two seconds. If the gilt or sow is in estrus, the standing reflex will occur - ears pricked, tail cocked, rigid posture.

Applications: Each can contains approximately 30, two-second applications.
Precaution(s): Packed under pressure. Do not puncture, incinerate or expose to temperatures exceeding 122°F even when empty. Do not spray towards flame or hot objects. Inflammable.
Caution(s): For animal use only.
Presentation: 1.75 oz (55 g) aerosol can.
Holland Patent No. 69,11212
Compendium Code No.: 11061930

SOCUMB™-6 GR CII

Butler **Euthanasia Agent**
NADA No.: 045-737
Active Ingredient(s): Each mL of aqueous solution contains:
Pentobarbital sodium .... 6 grs. (389 mg)
Isopropyl alcohol 40.0%
Propylene glycol 2.5%
Edetate disodium 0.05%
Benzyl alcohol (preservative) 2.0%
Color added for identification.
Indications: For use as a euthanasia agent only in dogs and cats.
Dosage and Administration: Dogs and Cats: 1 mL per 10 pounds of body weight. Individual variation, particularly in cases of cardiac or circulatory deficiencies, may require higher doses in some animals. The intravenous route of injection is recommended. Intracardiac injection may be used when intravenous injection is impractical. The calculated dose should be injected rapidly. As with all pentobarbital euthanasia agents, terminal gasp may occur in the unconscious animal. Nervous or vicious animals may require tranquilization or sedation prior to injection for euthanasia.
Precaution(s): Store at a controlled room temperature between 15° and 30°C (59°-86°F).
Caution(s): Federal law restricts this drug to use by or on the order of a licensed veterinarian.
For veterinary use only. Keep out of the reach of children.
Warning(s): The product must not be used for anesthetic or therapeutic purposes.
Not for use in animals intended for food.
Presentation: 100 mL and 250 mL vials.
Compendium Code No.: 10821630

SODIUM ASCORBATE ℞

Neogen **Vitamin C**
Sterile Solution
Active Ingredient(s): Each mL of sterile aqueous solution contains:
Sodium Ascorbate .... 250 mg
Monothioglycerol .... 0.5% w/v
Edetate Disodium .... 0.1% w/v
Methylparaben (preservative) .... 0.18% w/v
Propylparaben (preservative) .... 0.02% w/v
Indications: For use as a nutritive supplement of Vitamin C in cattle, horses, sheep, swine, dogs and cats.
Dosage and Administration: Administer intramuscularly 1 to 10 mL, depending on condition, species, and body weight. Repeat daily or as indicated by desired response.
Precaution(s): Store at controlled room temperature between 15°-30°C (59°-86°F). Protect from light.
Since pressure may develop during long storage, precautions should be taken to release pressure before use. Storage under refrigeration is recommended to reduce possibility of pressure build-up.
Caution(s): Federal law restricts this drug to use by or on the order of a licensed veterinarian.
For animal use only.
Warning(s): Keep out of reach of children.
Presentation: 12 x 100 mL, amber glass vials per carton (NDC: 59051-9077-5).
Manufactured by: Sparhawk Laboratories, Lenexa, KS 66215.
Compendium Code No.: 14910112 0501

SODIUM ASCORBATE ℞

RXV **Vitamin C**
Injectable Solution (Equivalent to Vitamin C)
Active Ingredient(s): Each mL contains:
Sodium ascorbate .... 250 mg
Sodium bisulfite .... 0.2 mg
Sodium diversenate 0.025%
Phenol 0.5%
Water for injection .... q.s.
NaOH or HCl may be present to adjust pH.
Indications: For prevention and treatment of deficiencies of vitamin C.
Dosage and Administration: For intravenous or intramuscular use. 100-500 mg per 100 lbs of body weight daily.
Precaution(s): Since pressure may develop on long storage, precautions should be taken to wrap the container in a protective covering while it is being opened.
Caution(s): Federal law restricts this drug to use by or on the order of a licensed veterinarian.
Warning(s): For laboratory animal use only.
For animal use only.
Keep out of reach of children.
Presentation: 250 mL sterile multiple dose vials.
Compendium Code No.: 10910140

SODIUM ASCORBATE INJECTION ℞

Vedco **Vitamin C**
Active Ingredient(s): (Equivalent to Vitamin C): Each mL contains:
Sodium Ascorbate .... 250 mg
Sodium BiSulfite 0.2%
Disodium Edetate 0.025%
Phenol 0.5%
Water for Injection .... q.s.
NaOH or HCl may be present to adjust pH.
Sodium ascorbate is equivalent to vitamin C.
Indications: For prevention and treatment of deficiencies of Vitamin C in laboratory animals.
Dosage and Administration: For intramuscular or intravenous use.
Administer 100 mg to 500 mg per 100 lbs of body weight daily.
Precaution(s): Since pressure may develop in long storage, precautions should be taken to wrap the container in a protective covering while it is being opened.
Caution(s): Federal law restricts this drug to use by or on the order of a licensed veterinarian.
Warning(s): For laboratory animal use only.
Presentation: 100 mL and 250 mL vials.
Compendium Code No.: 10941850

SODIUM BICARBONATE ℞

Butler **Fluid Therapy**
Active Ingredient(s): Each 100 mL contains:
Sodium bicarbonate .... 8.4 g (100 mEq)
pH of 7.0 to 8.0.
The sterility of this product conforms to U.S.P. membrane testing methods.
Indications:
1. Respiratory acidosis caused by the retention of carbon dioxide.
2. Metabolic acidosis resulting from an accumulation of acid metabolites from metabolic disorders.
3. Renal acidosis caused by an inadequate excretion of hydrogen ions by the kidneys.

Dosage and Administration: If the carbon dioxide content of the plasma is unknown, an average dose would be 1 mL of undiluted sodium bicarbonate injection per pound of body weight administered in a liter of 5% dextrose, or isotonic saline, or other appropriate fluid therapy vehicle. The concentration of the bicarbonate solution and the route of administration is determined by the need of the patient. Undiluted sodium bicarbonate injection may be administered intravenously slowly and with caution, or following dilution to isotonicity (1.5%). For intravenous administration suitable concentrations range from isotonic (1.5%) to undiluted (8.4%), depending upon the clinical conditions and the requirements of the patient.
For subcutaneous injection, an isotonic solution (1.5%) of sodium bicarbonate injection can be prepared by diluting one (1) part of the product with five (5) to six (6) parts of sterile water.
A general average dose for all species may be 1 mL of sodium bicarbonate injection per pound of body weight administered intravenously, slowly with caution or diluted in an adequate quantity of intravenous fluid therapy solutions, e.g. sodium chloride injection (0.9%), or a 5% dextrose injection.
Contraindication(s): Alkalosis, especially respiratory alkalosis, convulsions or congestive heart failure.
Precaution(s): Store at temperatures between 59°-86°F (15°-30°C). Not for multiple dose use. Use only if the solution is clear. Any opened or unused portions should be discarded immediately. Sodium bicarbonate injection should not be boiled.
Caution(s): Federal (U.S.A.) law restricts this drug to use by or on the order of a licensed veterinarian.
The rapid injection of sodium bicarbonate may be extremely dangerous and may cause death by severe derangement of intra- or extra-cellular ionic concentrations. Hypertonic solutions must be employed with special care. In general, one or more liters of isotonic sodium bicarbonate may be administered to relieve acidosis. Because of the possibility of producing alkalosis by overcorrection of the bicarbonate deficit, repeated fractional doses should be used. Thus, the actual total amount of sodium bicarbonate given is governed by the successive clinical response in patients to each repeated fractional dose. Once the severe symptoms have been controlled, the size of each fractional dose and the frequency of administration should be decreased in order to gradually restore normal bicarbonate levels.
Caution should be exercised in patients with oliguria or anuria so that excessive retention of sodium will not occur. For veterinary use only. Keep out of the reach of children.
Overdose: Should alkalosis result from bicarbonate administration, the use of sodium bicarbonate should be stopped and the patient treated according to the degree of alkalosis. Sodium chloride injection (0.9%) intravenously is usually sufficient to restore plasma chloride levels. If alkalosis is severe, i.e. accompanied by hyperirritability or tetany, intravenous ammonium chloride (NH_4Cl) may be given as a ⅙ molar solution (167 mEq/L). Calcium gluconate may also be useful in controlling tetany.
Discussion: Acidosis is a result of an elevated concentration of hydrogen ions in the body fluids, which can result in the three conditions listed in the "Indications" section.
The administration of any sodium bicarbonate injection preparation directly increases the bicarbonate content of the plasma.
Presentation: 100 mL single dose vial.
Compendium Code No.: 10821641

SODIUM BICARBONATE 8.4% ℞

Neogen **Fluid Therapy**
Sterile Nonpyrogenic Solution
Active Ingredient(s): Description: SODIUM BICARBONATE 8.4% is a sterile nonpyrogenic preparation of sodium bicarbonate ($NaHCO_3$) in Water for Injection. Each 100 mL contains 8.4 grams of sodium bicarbonate (100 mEq/100 mL each of sodium and bicarbonate). This concentrated solution has an approximate pH of 7.8.
The total osmolar concentration of this product is approximately 2000 mOsm/L.
Indications: Sodium Bicarbonate is indicated in the treatment of metabolic acidosis which may be due to severe renal disease, uncontrolled diabetes, circulatory insufficiency due to shock or severe dehydration, cardiac arrest and severe primary lactic acidosis. Sodium Bicarbonate is also indicated in severe diarrhea which is often accompanied by a significant loss of bicarbonate. SODIUM BICARBONATE 8.4% is indicated in the treatment of metabolic acidosis in cattle, horses, sheep, swine and dogs depending upon causative factor.
Pharmacology: Actions: Sodium Bicarbonate is useful in the treatment of metabolic acidosis due to a wide variety of causes. Sodium Bicarbonate therapy increases plasma bicarbonate, buffers excess hydrogen ion concentration, raises blood pH and reverses the clinical manifestations of acidosis.
Dosage and Administration: SODIUM BICARBONATE 8.4% is injected intravenously. Caution should be taken in emergencies where very rapid infusion of large quantities of bicarbonate is indicated, such as in cardiac arrest. Sodium Bicarbonate solutions are hypertonic and may produce an undesirable rise in plasma sodium concentration during the process of correction of metabolic acidosis. During cardiac arrest, however, the risks from acidosis exceed those of hypernatremia. In cattle and horses, 200 to 300 mL of 8.4% solution may be given undiluted by rapid infusion using a needle and syringe.
SODIUM BICARBONATE 8.4% solution is often added to other intravenous fluids for the less urgent forms of metabolic acidosis. The amount of bicarbonate to be given over a 4 to 8 hour period is approximately 2 to 5 mEq per kg of body weight (1-2.5 mL/lb body weight) depending upon the severity of the acidosis as judged by the lowering of total CO_2 content, blood pH and clinical condition of the animal.

Bicarbonate therapy should always be planned in stepwise fashion since the degree of response from a given dose is not precisely predictable. Initially, an infusion of 2 to 5 mEq per kg of body weight over a period of 4 to 8 hours will produce a measurable improvement in the abnormal acid-base status of the blood. Completion of therapy is dependent upon the clinical response of the animal. If severe symptoms have abated, then frequency of administration and size of the dose should be reduced.

Contraindication(s): Sodium Bicarbonate is contraindicated in animals losing chloride by vomiting and in animals receiving diuretics known to produce a hypochloremic alkalosis.

Precaution(s): This is a sterile single dose vial. No preservatives have been added. Discard unused portion after use. Do not use if solution is hazy, cloudy, or contains a precipitate.

Store at room temperatures 15°C-30°C (59°F-86°F).

Caution(s): Federal law (U.S.A.) restricts this drug to use by or on the order of a licensed veterinarian.

Bicarbonate therapy is directed at producing a substantial correction of low total CO_2 content and blood pH, but risks of overdosage and alkalosis should be avoided. Repeated fractional doses and periodic monitoring by appropriate laboratory tests are therefore recommended to minimize the possibility of overdosage. Sodium Bicarbonate addition to parenteral solutions containing calcium should be avoided except where compatibility has been previously established. Precipitation or haze may result from sodium bicarbonate-calcium admixtures, and the resulting solution should not be administered. For animal use only.

Warning(s): Keep out of reach of children.

Overdosages: In case alkalosis occurs, the bicarbonate should be stopped and the animal managed according to the degree of alkalosis present. Sodium chloride injection (0.9%) may be given intravenously; potassium chloride also may be indicated if there is hypokalemia. Severe alkalosis may be accompanied by hyperirritability or tetany, and these symptoms may be controlled by calcium gluconate. An acidifying agent such as ammonium chloride may also be indicated in severe alkalosis.

Presentation: SODIUM BICARBONATE 8.4% is supplied in 100 mL single dose vials (NDC: 59051-9078-5).

Manufactured by: Omega Laboratories, Montreal, Quebec H3M 3E4.

Compendium Code No.: 14910122 L568-0201

SODIUM BICARBONATE 8.4% ℞

Phoenix Pharmaceutical **Fluid Therapy**

Sterile Nonpyrogenic Solution

Active Ingredient(s): Each mL contains:

Sodium Bicarbonate (equal to 1 mEq/mL) .... 84 mg
Water for injection .... q.s.

Indications: Sodium Bicarbonate is indicated in the treatment of metabolic acidosis which may be due to severe renal disease, uncontrolled diabetes, circulatory insufficiency due to shock or severe dehydration, cardiac arrest and severe primary lactic acidosis. Sodium Bicarbonate is also indicated in severe diarrhea which is often accompanied by a significant loss of bicarbonate. SODIUM BICARBONATE 8.4% is indicated in the treatment of metabolic acidosis in cattle, horses, sheep, swine and dogs depending upon causative factor.

Pharmacology: SODIUM BICARBONATE 8.4% is a sterile nonpyrogenic preparation of sodium bicarbonate ($NaHCO_3$) in water for injection.

This concentrated solution has an approximate pH of 7.8.

The total osmolar concentration of this product is approximately 2000 mOsm/L.

Actions: Sodium Bicarbonate is useful in the treatment of metabolic acidosis due to a wide variety of causes. Sodium Bicarbonate therapy increases plasma bicarbonate, buffers excess hydrogen ion concentration, raises blood pH and reverses the clinical manifestations of acidosis.

Dosage and Administration: SODIUM BICARBONATE 8.4% is injected intravenously. Caution should be taken in emergencies where very rapid infusion of large quantities of bicarbonate is indicated, such as in cardiac arrest. Sodium Bicarbonate solutions are hypertonic and may produce an undesirable rise in plasma sodium concentration during the process of correction of metabolic acidosis. During cardiac arrest, however, the risks from acidosis exceed those of hypernatremia. In cattle and horses, 200 to 300 mL of 8.4% solution may be given undiluted by rapid infusion using a needle and syringe.

SODIUM BICARBONATE 8.4% solution is often added to other intravenous fluids for the less urgent forms of metabolic acidosis. The amount of bicarbonate to be given over a 4 to 8 hour period is approximately 2 to 5 mEq per kg of body weight (1-2.5 mL/lb body weight) depending upon the severity of the acidosis as judged by the lowering of total CO_2 content, blood pH and clinical condition of the animal.

Bicarbonate therapy should always be planned in stepwise fashion since the degree of response from a given dose is not precisely predictable. Initially, an infusion of 2 to 5 mEq per kg of body weight over a period of 4 to 8 hours will produce a measurable improvement in the abnormal acid-base status of the blood. Completion of therapy is dependent upon the clinical response of the animal. If severe symptoms have abated, then frequency of administration and size of the dose should be reduced.

Contraindication(s): Sodium Bicarbonate is contraindicated in animals losing chloride by vomiting and in animals receiving diuretics known to produce a hypochloremic alkalosis.

Precaution(s): Store at room temperature 15°C-30°C (59°F-86°F).

The product is in a sterile single dose vial. No preservatives have been added. Discard unused portion after use. Do not use if solution is hazy, cloudy or contains a precipitate.

Caution(s): Federal law (U.S.A.) restricts this drug to use by or on the order of a licensed veterinarian.

Bicarbonate therapy is directed at producing a substantial correction of low total CO_2 content and blood pH, but risks of overdosage and alkalosis should be avoided. Repeated fractional doses and periodic monitoring by appropriate laboratory tests are therefore recommended to minimize the possibility of overdosage. Sodium Bicarbonate addition to parenteral solutions containing calcium should be avoided except where compatibility has been previously established. Precipitation or haze may result from sodium bicarbonate-calcium admixtures, and the resulting solution should not be administered. For veterinary use only. For animals use only.

Warning(s): Keep out of reach of children.

Overdose: In case alkalosis occurs, the bicarbonate should be stopped and the animal managed according to the degree of alkalosis present. Sodium chloride injection (0.9%) may be given intravenously; potassium chloride also may be indicated if there is hypokalemia. Severe alkalosis may be accompanied by hyperirritability or tetany, and these symptoms may be controlled by calcium gluconate. An acidifying agent such as ammonium chloride may also be indicated in severe alkalosis.

Presentation: SODIUM BICARBONATE 8.4% is supplied in 100 mL single dose vials (NDC 57319-357-05).

Compendium Code No.: 12560781 1099

SODIUM BICARBONATE 8.4% ℞

Vedco **Fluid Therapy**

Active Ingredient(s): Each mL contains:

Sodium bicarbonate (equal to 1 mEq/mL) .... 84 mg
Water for injection .... q.s.

The total osmolar concentration of the product is approximately 2,000 mOsm/L.

Indications: For the treatment of metabolic acidosis.

Dosage and Administration: Administer intravenously. Sodium bicarbonate is often given with other intravenous fluids for the less urgent forms of metabolic acidosis. The amount of bicarbonate to be given over a 4- to 8-hour period is approximately 2-5 mEq per kg of body weight, or 1-2.5 mL per lb., depending upon the severity of the acidosis.

Precaution(s): Store at a controlled room temperature between 15° and 30°C (59°-86°F).

SODIUM BICARBONATE 8.4% is in a sterile single dose vial. Preservatives have not been added. Discard the unused portion after use. Do not use if the solution is hazy, cloudy, or if it contains a precipitate.

Caution(s): Federal law restricts this drug to use by or on the order of a licensed veterinarian.

Warning(s): Keep out of reach of children.

Presentation: 100 mL bottle.

Compendium Code No.: 10941861

SODIUM IODIDE ℞

AgriLabs **Sodium Iodide**

Active Ingredient(s): Each 100 mL contains:

Sodium iodide........ 20 g
Water for injection .... q.s.

Indications: For use as an aid in the treatment of actinomycosis (lumpy jaw) of actinobacillosis (wooden tongue and necrotic stomatitis) in cattle.

Dosage and Administration: Administer intravenously slowly using aseptic procedures as follows: For actinomycosis or actinobacillosis in cattle, administer 15 mL per 100 lbs. of body weight. Repeat in 10 to 14 days. if necessary.

Contraindication(s): Do not use in pregnant animals or in animals exhibiting hyperthyroidism.

Precaution(s): Store at room temperature 59°-86°F (15°-30°C).

Caution(s): Federal law (U.S.A.) restricts this drug to use by or on the order of a licensed veterinarian. Not for human use. Keep out of the reach of children.

This is a sterile single dose vial. Preservatives have not been added. Discard any unused portion after use.

Warning(s): Animals vary in susceptibility to iodides. Administer cautiously until tolerance is determined. Discontinue treatment immediately if symptoms of iodinism appear. Not for intramuscular or subcutaneous use.

Not for use in lactating animals.

Presentation: 250 mL multiple dose vials.

Compendium Code No.: 10581700 Rev. 10-90

SODIUM IODIDE ℞

Vet Tek **Sodium Iodide**

20% Injection

Active Ingredient(s): Composition: Each 100 mL of sterile aqueous solution contains:

Sodium Iodide .... 20 grams
Water for Injection .... q.s.

Indications: For use as an aid in the treatment of actinomycosis (lumpy jaw) or actinobacillosis (wooden tongue) and necrotic stomatitis in cattle.

Dosage and Administration: Using aseptic procedures, administer slowly by intravenous injection. Inject carefully to avoid deposition outside of the vein. The usual dose is 30 mg per pound of body weight (15 mL/100 lb). May be repeated at weekly intervals, if necessary.

Contraindication(s): The use of SODIUM IODIDE is contraindicated in pregnancy and hyperthyroidism.

Precaution(s): Store between 15°C and 30°C (59°F-86°F).

Caution(s): Federal law restricts this drug to use by or on the order of a licensed veterinarian.

Animals vary in their susceptibility of iodides. Administer with caution until the animal's tolerance is determined. Discontinue treatment immediately if adverse reactions occur.

For animal use only.

Warning(s): Not for use in lactating dairy cows.

Keep out of the reach of children.

Presentation: 250 mL vials (NDC 60270-033-13).

Manufactured by: Phoenix Scientific, Inc., St. Joseph, MO 64506.

Compendium Code No.: 14200171 Iss. 3-94

SODIUM IODIDE 20% ℞

RXV **Sodium Iodide**

Injectable Solution-Sterile

Active Ingredient(s): Each 100 mL contains:

Sodium iodide........ 20 g
Water for injection .... q.s.

Indications: For use as an aid in the treatment of actinomycosis (lumpy jaw) or actinobacillosis (wooden tongue and necrotic stomatitis) in cattle.

Dosage and Administration: For intravenous injection only.

Cattle........ 15 mL/100 lbs body weight
(30 mg/lb of body weight)

Administer slowly, using aseptic procedures. Inject carefully to avoid deposition outside of the vein. May be repeated at once a week, if necessary.

Precaution(s): Store at controlled room temperature between 15°-30°C (59°-86°F).

Caution(s): Federal law restricts this drug to use by or on the order of a licensed veterinarian.

Animals vary in their susceptibility to iodides. Administer with caution until the animal's tolerance is determined. Discontinue treatment and consult a veterinarian if adverse reactions occur. No preservatives have been added. Discard any unused portion.

For animal use only.

Keep out of reach of children.

Warning(s): Not for use in pregnant animals, lactating dairy cows or animals exhibiting hyperthyroidism.

Presentation: 250 mL single dose vials.

Compendium Code No.: 10910150

SODIUM IODIDE 20% INJECTION ℞

Aspen **Sodium Iodide**

Active Ingredient(s): Each 100 mL of sterile aqueous solution contains:
Sodium iodide . . . . . 20 g
Water . . . . . q.s.

The product does not contain preservatives.

Indications: For use as an aid in the treatment of actinomycosis (lumpy jaw), actinobacillosis (wooden tongue) and necrotic stomatitis in cattle.

Dosage and Administration: Using aseptic procedures, administer slowly by intravenous injection. Inject carefully to avoid deposition outside of the vein. The usual dose is 30 mg per pound of body weight (15 mL/100 lb). May be repeated at weekly intervals, if necessary.

Contraindication(s): Hyperthyroidism and advanced pregnancy.

Precaution(s): Store between 15°C and 30°C (59°-86°F).

Caution(s): Federal law restricts this drug to use by or on the order of a licensed veterinarian. Animals vary in their susceptibility of iodides. Administer with caution until the animal's tolerance is determined. Discontinue treatment if adverse reactions occur.

The entire contents should be used upon entering.

Discard any unused solution.

Antidote(s): Epinephrine.

Warning(s): Do not administer to lactating dairy cattle. Keep out of the reach of children.

Presentation: 250 mL vials.

Compendium Code No.: 14750700

SODIUM IODIDE 20% INJECTION ℞

Phoenix Pharmaceutical **Sodium Iodide**

Active Ingredient(s): Composition: Each 100 mL of sterile aqueous solution contains:
Sodium Iodide . . . . . 20 g
Water for injection . . . . . q.s.

Indications: For use as an aid in the treatment of actinomycosis (lumpy jaw), actinobacillosis (wooden tongue) and necrotic stomatitis in cattle.

Dosage and Administration: Using aseptic procedures, administer slowly by intravenous injection. Inject carefully to avoid deposition outside of the vein. The usual dose is 30 mg per pound of body weight (15 mL/100 lb). May be repeated at weekly intervals, if necessary.

Contraindication(s): The use of sodium iodide is contraindicated in pregnancy and hyperthyroidism.

Precaution(s): Store between 15°C and 30°C (59°F-86°F).

Caution(s): Federal law restricts this drug to use by or on the order of a licensed veterinarian.

Animals vary in their susceptibility to iodides. Administer with caution until the animal's tolerance is determined. Discontinue treatment and consult veterinarian if adverse reactions occur.

For animal use only.

Warning(s): Not for use in lactating dairy cows.

Keep out of reach of children.

Presentation: 250 mL vials (NDC 57319-073-06).

Manufactured by: Phoenix Scientific, Inc., St. Joseph, MO 64503.

Compendium Code No.: 12560792 Rev. 5-02

SODIUM IODIDE 20% INJECTION ℞

Vedco **Sodium Iodide**

Active Ingredient(s): Each mL contains:
Sodium iodide . . . . . 200 mg
Propylene glycol . . . . . 10% v/v
Edetate disodium . . . . . 0.075% w/v
Benzyl alcohol . . . . . 0.25% v/v

Preservatives:
Methylparaben . . . . . 0.03% w/v
Propylparaben . . . . . 0.25% w/v

Indications: For use as an aid in the treatment of actinomycosis (lumpy jaw), actinobacillosis (wooden tongue) and necrotic stomatitis in cattle.

Dosage and Administration: Administer by slow intravenous injection, taking care to avoid perivascular deposition. The usual dose is 30 mg per pound of body weight (15 mL/100 lbs.). May be repeated once a week if necessary.

Contraindication(s): Animals vary in their susceptibility to iodides. Administer with caution until the animal's tolerance is determined. Discontinue treatment if signs of iodism or adverse reactions occur.

Precaution(s): Store at a controlled room temperature between 59-86°F (15-30°C).

Caution(s): Federal law restricts this drug to use by or on the order of a licensed veterinarian.

Keep out of the reach of children. Not for human use.

Warning(s): Not for use in lactating dairy cows.

Presentation: 250 mL containers.

Compendium Code No.: 10941870

SODIUM IODIDE SOLUTION 20% ℞

Butler **Sodium Iodide**

Active Ingredient(s): Each 100 mL of sterile aqueous solution contains:
Sodium iodide . . . . . 20 grams
Water for Injection . . . . . q.s.

Indications: For use as an aid in the treatment of actinomycosis (lumpy jaw) and actinobacillosis (wooden tongue) in cattle.

Dosage and Administration: Administer by slow intravenous injection, taking care to avoid perivascular deposition. The usual dose is 30 mg per pound of body weight (15 mL/100 lb). May be repeated at weekly intervals if necessary.

Contraindication(s): Do not give to animals in advanced pregnancy as it may result in abortion.

Precaution(s): Store between 15° and 30°C (59°-86°F).

Caution(s): Federal law restricts this drug to use by or on the order of a licensed veterinarian.

Animals vary in their susceptibility to iodides. Administer with caution until the animal's tolerance is determined. Discontinue treatment if signs of iodism or adverse reactions occur.

Warning(s): Not for use in lactating dairy animals.

For veterinary use only.

Keep out of the reach of children.

Presentation: 250 mL vials.

Compendium Code No.: 10821650

SODIUM PENTOBARBITAL INJECTION CII

Butler **General Anesthetic**

Active Ingredient(s): Composition: Each mL of sterile aqueous solution contains:
Sodium Pentobarbital . . . . . 1 gr (65 mg)
Ethyl Alcohol . . . . . 10% v/v
Propylene Glycol . . . . . 20% v/v
Benzyl Alcohol . . . . . 2% v/v

Indications: For use as a general anesthetic, primarily in dogs and cats, and for the symptomatic treatment of strychnine and other convulsant poisonings. Clinical experience and reports in the professional literature indicate that pentobarbital has been used in other domestic animal species (i.e., cattle, horses, swine, goats and sheep) as a sedative and general anesthetic, and in laboratory animals (i.e., rabbits, guinea pigs, gerbils, rats, mice, frogs, turtles and subhuman primates) as a general anesthetic. It is beyond the scope of this product information sheet to make a specific recommendations for the use of pentobarbital in these animals. Veterinarians who may wish to use pentobarbital in these species are advised to consult the published literature for specific information about dosage and proper usage.

Pharmacology: Description: SODIUM PENTOBARBITAL INJECTION is a barbituric acid derivative and is classified pharmacologically as a general anesthetic with a short duration of action.

Clinical Pharmacology: The major action of the barbiturates is to depress the central nervous system (CNS), including both the motor areas and sensory areas of the brain. Thus, barbiturates can be used to control convulsive seizures and to induce anesthesia. The level of CNS depression is dose related, varying in degree from mild sedation to deep anesthesia. Pentobarbital is metabolized principally by the hepatic microsomal enzyme system and excreted in the urine. Thus, the action of pentobarbital may be greatly prolonged in animals with liver or kidney disturbances. Substances that accelerate hepatic microsomal activity (e.g., phenytoin, chlorinated hydrocarbon pesticides) can significantly reduce the duration of pentobarbital anesthesia, while substances that suppress hepatic microsomal activity (e.g., chloramphenicol) can significantly prolong the duration of pentobarbital anesthesia. The effects of such substances may be detected for up to several weeks following administration or exposure and should be taken into consideration when using pentobarbital to induce anesthesia. In some animal species certain drugs (e.g., sulfonamides, aspirin) displace pentobarbital from plasma proteins, which leads to an increased blood level of unbound barbiturate for further depressant effect upon the CNS and prolongation of sleep time.

Dosage and Administration: Although various routes of administration (i.e., oral, intraperitoneal) have been used by some clinicians and for specific situations, only the intravenous route is recommended for induction of anesthesia. The intravenous dose is determined by the response desired and administered "to effect" as judged by the disappearance of normal reflexes. The usual anesthetic dose is 11 to 13 mg per pound of body weight (24-29 mg/kg), which is approximately 1 mL of SODIUM PENTOBARBITAL INJECTION per 5 pounds of body weight. Approximately one-half the anticipated dose should be injected at a moderately fast rate so that Stage II (the excitement stage) of anesthesia is bypassed. A pause for 1 to 5 minutes is recommended to allow the drug to exert its full effect. Thereafter, the remaining SODIUM PENTOBARBITAL INJECTION must be injected "to effect". Administer the remaining dose slowly in repeated small amounts over a period of several minutes with continuous monitoring of reflexes until the desired depth of surgical anesthesia is achieved. If preanesthetic agents are used (i.e., morphine, xylazine, tranquilizers) the dose of pentobarbital should be reduced by approximately one-half and given "to effect".

Contraindication(s): Do not use in animals suffering from severe respiratory depression, hepatic disturbances or renal disease.

Precaution(s): Store at controlled room temperature between 15°C and 30°C (59°F-86°F).

Do not use the solution if it has become cloudy or if a precipitate forms.

Caution(s): Federal law restricts this drug to use by or on the order of a licensed veterinarian.

When used to induce a state of deep surgical anesthesia, pentobarbital depresses the respiratory center. The use of an endotracheal catheter to maintain adequate airway and for administration of oxygen is recommended.

Barbiturates diffuse through the placenta into fetal tissue. The use of barbiturates in pregnant animals will depress the fetus and may result in an increased rate of fetal mortality.

Hypothermia may occur In animals that are anesthetized with barbiturates. Monitor body temperature and keep patient warm. Hypothermia may prolong recovery from pentobarbital anesthesia and may result in increase fatalities.

Extreme care should be taken in the presence of heart, liver or kidney diseases; patients with such conditions are poor anesthetic risks.

Individual variations in response to pentobarbital may occur due to age, sex, weight, nutritional status and prior or concurrent exposure to other drugs and chemical substances.

The anesthetic action of barbiturates can be potentiated by the administration of dextrose, fructose, lactate, pyruvate, and glutamate.

Emergence delirium in horses and emergence excitement in dogs may occur following barbiturate anesthesia.

Care should be taken to avoid inadvertent intraarterial injection, especially when performing intravenous injections in horses.

The accidental perivascular deposition of pentobarbital may result in severe inflammation with sloughing at the injection site.

Additional care should be employed when anesthetizing anemic or hypovolemic animals and animals with cardiac or respiratory problems. Liver pathology may delay detoxification. Elevated urea nitrogen or electrolyte imbalance may prolong anesthesia. Prolonged recovery may occur in hypothermia or in malnourished animals and following continuous use for a prolonged surgical procedure. For animal use only. Keep out of reach of children.

Warning(s): Not for use in animals intended for food.

Presentation: 100 mL vials x 12 per case (NDC 11695-0067-04).

Manufactured by: Veterinary Laboratories, Inc., Lenexa, Kansas 66215

Compendium Code No.: 10821660 S-0951-04 Rev: 1-97

SOFTGUARD™

Activon **Emollient**

Teat Dip Conditioning Additive

Available in Aqua Blue and Clear formulations

Ingredient(s): Aloe, Glycerin, Carbomer-940, Vitamin E, Allantoin, Methyl Paraben, Distilled Water, Triethanolamine, Methyl Gluceth 20. (Aqua Blue Additive also contains FD & C Blue #1 dye.)

Indications: Conditions, soothes, and protects udder and teats.

Designed for use with EfferCept® Vet teat dips.

Directions for Use: Shake well before using.

Mixing instructions:

1. Prepare EfferCept® Vet solution according to EfferCept® Vet label instructions.

2. Add Clear or Aqua Blue SoftGuard™ Additive at the rate of two ounces per gallon of finished EfferCept® Vet solution.
3. Stir or shake solution prior to every use.
4. When using as an udder pre-wash or pre-dip/spray, wipe the teat thoroughly before attaching milking equipment.
6. Aqua Blue SOFTGUARD™ is a strong colorant. Care should be given not to contaminate equipment/containers that contact or hold anything other then EfferCept® Vet solutions.

Container Yields:

32 Ounce Size: Conditions up to 16 gallons of teat dip/spray.

55 Ounce Size: Conditions up to 27.5 gallons of teat dip/spray.

Presentation: 32 ounce and 55 ounce sizes.

Compendium Code No.: 10600030

SOLE PACK™ HOOF DRESSING

Hawthorne **Hoof Product**

Active Ingredient(s): Pine tar, 4% iodine, potassium iodine and ichthammol.

Indications: For the relief of hard, dry, sore feet in horses of any breed. SOLE PACK™'s ingredients are quickly absorbed by all hoof horn in both wall and sole. Its rapid penetration and restoration of natural pliability of tough, dry, and hardened tissues of the foot permits expansion and contraction of the hoof. SOLE PACK™ keeps hooves growing and helps prevent cracking and chipping.

It is also recommended as an aid to prevent bacterial and fungal infections of the hoof and white line disease.

Directions: Clean and dry the hoof thoroughly before applying SOLE PACK™ Hoof Dressing. Apply SOLE PACK™ with a brush, working it well into the edge of the hair at the coronary band; brush vigorously into frog and sole. For best results, use 2 or 3 times each week.

For tough, dry and hardened hooves: Apply SOLE PACK™ daily until desired pliability is restored. Continue using SOLE PACK™ 2 or 3 times each week.

For bacterial and fungal infections on the hoof: Wash hoof thoroughly before each application. Each day, brush SOLE PACK™ Hoof Dressing vigorously into all affected areas, thoroughly saturating tissue. Continue treatment until all signs of infection are gone. For best results, use SOLE PACK™ in conjunction with Sole Pack™ "Dose Packs".

Caution(s): Keep out of reach of children.

Presentation: .473 liter (16 oz) brush/dauber applicator and .946 liter (32 oz) refill.

Compendium Code No.: 10670090

SOLE PACK™ HOOF PACKING

Hawthorne **Hoof Product**

Dose Packs

Active Ingredient(s): Pine tar, 4% iodine, potassium iodine and ichthammol.

Indications: A therapeutic hoof packing recommended for the relief of dry, hard, sore feet in horses and to maintain hoof pliability. SOLE PACK™ also combats bacterial and fungal infections and white line disease.

Directions: For use with leather or synthetic pads: Clean and trim the hoof. Use fingers to work SOLE PACK™ paste into cavities of food. Apply pad and shoe. For bandage applications: Clean the hoof and if necessary cut out abscess. Use your fingers to work SOLE PACK™ paste into hoof cavities. When necessary bandage foot normally or use polypropylene boot. For packing feet overnight, pack feet and cover with paper.

Presentation: 3.63 kg (8 lb) bulk and 56.7 gram (2 oz) dose pack-one dozen per box.

Compendium Code No.: 10670100

SOLO-JEC-7™

Aspen **Bacterin-Vaccine**

Canine Distemper-Hepatitis-Parainfluenza-Parvovirus Vaccine, Modified Live Virus-Leptospira Bacterin

U.S. Vet. Lic. No.: 124

Contents: A combination of antigenic, attenuated strains of canine distemper, canine parainfluenza, canine hepatitis and parvovirus propagated in cell line tissue cultures. The liquid diluent is Parvovirus Vaccine *Leptospira canicola-icterohaemorrhagiae* bacterin. The CD virus fraction has been proven safe and non-shedding when injected into susceptible dogs. The infectious canine hepatitis (CAV-1) fraction cross protects against respiratory disease caused by CAV-2. Contains gentamicin and a fungistat as preservatives.

Indications: For the vaccination of healthy susceptible dogs against disease caused by canine distemper, hepatitis (canine adenovirus type 1), canine adenovirus type 2, parainfluenza, parvovirus, *Leptospira canicola* and *Leptospira icterohaemorrhagiae.*

Dosage and Administration: The dry distemper-hepatitis-parainfluenza vaccine is rehydrated with 1 mL of liquid parvovirus vaccine-*Leptospira canicola-icterohaemorrhagiae* bacterin. Shake well and use entire contents when first opened.

Using aseptic technique, inject 1 mL intramuscularly or subcutaneously. Repeat dosage in 3 to 4 weeks. Annual revaccination with a single dose is recommended. Puppies vaccinated before 9 weeks of age should be revaccinated at 3 to 4 week intervals until 14 to 16 weeks of age. Regardless of age all dogs should receive 2 doses of vaccine in order to insure adequate levels of immunity against canine parainfluenza and parvovirus.

Contraindication(s): Do not vaccinate pregnant animals.

Precaution(s): Store out of direct sunlight at a temperature not over 45°F. Avoid freezing. Do not vaccinate pregnant animals. Burn containers and all unused contents.

Caution(s): Always use care when handling the dog and provide proper restraint when vaccinating.

Prepare the vaccine by injecting the liquid diluent into the vial containing the vaccine cake.

Shake well. Remove the entire contents back into the syringe. Push out air trapped in the syringe.

To give subcutaneously, inject under loose skin (back of neck or behind front leg) or to give IM, inject into the muscle of the hind limb.

Do not vaccinate into blood vessels. If blood enters the syringe freely or when the plunger is pulled back slightly, choose another injection site.

Under no circumstances is this product recommended for use in ferrets or mink. An occasional corneal opacity may occur following administration of the vaccine. This will disappear without untoward effect on the animal. Protective immunity may not be established in all puppies vaccinated at less than 16 weeks of age because of maternal antibody interference. Anaphylactoid reactions may occur.

Warning(s): For use in dogs only.

Presentation: Package contains one (1 dose) vial of dry vaccine, one (1 mL) vial of liquid diluent and one disposable syringe.

Compendium Code No.: 14750710

SOLO-JEC-7™

Boehringer Ingelheim **Bacterin-Vaccine**

Canine Distemper-Hepatitis-Parainfluenza-Parvovirus Vaccine, Modified Live Virus-Leptospira Bacterin

U.S. Vet. Lic. No.: 124

Description: SOLO-JEC-7™ vaccine is a combination of antigenic, attenuated strains of Canine Distemper, Canine Parainfluenza, Canine Hepatitis and Parvovirus propagated in cell line tissue cultures. The liquid diluent is Parvovirus Vaccine-*Leptospira canicola-icterohaemorrhagiae* Bacterin. The CD Virus fraction has been proven safe and non-shedding when injected into susceptible dogs. The infectious Canine Hepatitis (CAV-1) fraction cross protects against respiratory disease caused by CAV-2.

Preservatives: Gentamicin and a fungistat.

Indications: For the vaccination of healthy, susceptible dogs against disease caused by canine distemper, hepatitis (canine adenovirus type 1), canine adenovirus type 2, parainfluenza, parvovirus, *Leptospira canicola* and *L. icterohaemorrhagiae.*

For use in dogs only.

Directions: The dry Distemper-Hepatitis-Parainfluenza Vaccine is rehydrated with 1 mL of liquid Parvovirus Vaccine-*Leptospira canicola-icterohaemorrhagiae* Bacterin. Shake well and use entire contents when first opened.

Instructions: Read the carton information carefully.

Always use care when handling the dog and provide proper restraint when vaccinating.

Prepare the vaccine by injecting the liquid diluent into the vial containing the vaccine cake.

Shake well. Remove the entire contents back into the syringe. Push out air trapped in the syringe.

To give subcutaneously, inject under loose skin (back of neck or behind front leg) or to give IM, inject into the muscle of the hind limb.

Do not vaccinate into blood vessels. If blood enters the syringe freely or when the plunger is pulled back slightly, choose another injection site.

Dosage: Using aseptic technique, inject 1 mL intramuscularly or subcutaneously. Repeat the dosage in 3 to 4 weeks. Annual vaccination with a single dose is recommended. Puppies vaccinated before 9 weeks of age should be revaccinated at 3 to 4 week intervals until 14 to 16 weeks of age. Regardless of age, all dogs should receive 2 doses of vaccine in order to ensure adequate levels of immunity against canine parainfluenza and parvovirus.

Precaution(s): Store out of direct sunlight at a temperature between 35-45°F (2-7°C). Avoid freezing. Burn containers and all unused contents.

Caution(s): Do not vaccinate pregnant animals. Under no circumstances is this product recommended for use in ferrets or mink. An occasional transitory corneal opacity may occur following administration of the vaccine. This will disappear without untoward effect on the animal. Protective immunity may not be established in all puppies vaccinated at less than 16 weeks of age because of maternal antibody interference. Anaphylactoid reactions may occur.

Antidote(s): Epinephrine.

Presentation: 1 dose (1 mL) wth syringe and 25 x 1 dose (1 mL) without syringes.

Compendium Code No.: 10281011 BI 1223-3 6/99

SOLO-JEC-7™

Durvet **Bacterin-Vaccine**

Canine Distemper-Hepatitis-Parainfluenza-Parvovirus Vaccine, Modified Live Virus-Leptospira Bacterin

U.S. Vet. Lic. No.: 124

Contents: SOLO-JEC-7™ vaccine is a combination of antigenic, attenuated strains of canine distemper, canine parainfluenza, canine hepatitis and parvovirus propagated in cell line tissue cultures. The liquid diluent is Parvovirus Vaccine-Leptospira canicola-icterohaemorrhagiae Bacterin. The CD virus fraction has been proven safe and non-shedding when injected into susceptible dogs. The infectious canine hepatitis (CAV-1) fraction cross protects against respiratory disease caused by CAV-2.

Preservatives: Gentamicin and a fungistat.

Indications: For the vaccination of healthy, susceptible dogs against disease caused by canine distemper, hepatitis (canine adenovirus type 1), canine adenovirus type 2, parainfluenza, parvovirus, *Leptospira canicola* and *Leptospira icterohaemorrhagiae.*

Dosage and Administration: The dry Distemper-Hepatitis-Parainfluenza Vaccine is rehydrated with 1 mL of liquid Parvovirus Vaccine-Leptospira canicola-icterohaemorrhagiae bacterin. Shake well and use entire contents when first opened.

Using aseptic technique, inject 1 mL intramuscularly or subcutaneously. Repeat dosage in 3 to 4 weeks. Annual revaccination with a single dose is recommended. Puppies vaccinated before 9 weeks of age should be revaccinated at 3 to 4 week intervals until 14 to 16 weeks of age. Regardless of age all dogs should receive 2 doses of vaccine in order to insure adequate levels of immunity against canine parainfluenza and parvovirus.

Instructions: Read the carton information carefully.

Always use care when handling the dog and provide proper restraint when vaccinating.

Prepare the vaccine by injecting the liquid diluent into the vial containing the vaccine cake.

Shake well. Remove the entire contents back into the syringe. Push out air trapped in the syringe.

To give subcutaneously, inject under loose skin (back of neck or behind front leg) or to give IM, inject into the muscle of the hind limb.

Do not vaccinate into blood vessels. If blood enters the syringe freely or when the plunger is pulled back slightly, choose another injection site.

Contraindication(s): Do not vaccinate pregnant animals.

Precaution(s): Store out of direct sunlight at a temperature between 35-45°F (2-7°C). Avoid freezing. Burn containers and all unused contents.

Caution(s): Under no circumstances is this product recommended for use in ferrets or mink. An occasional transitory corneal opacity may occur following administration of the vaccine. This will disappear without untoward effect on the animal. Protective immunity may not be established in all puppies vaccinated at less than 16 weeks of age because of maternal antibody interference. Anaphylactoid reactions may occur.

Antidote(s): Epinephrine.

Warning(s): For use in dogs only.

Keep out of reach of children.

Presentation: Package contains one (1 dose) vial of dry vaccine, one (1 mL) vial of liquid diluent, and one disposable syringe.

Manufactured by: Boehringer Ingelheim Vetmedica, Inc.

Compendium Code No.: 10841480

SOLOXINE®

King Animal Health **Thyroid Therapy**

Active Ingredient(s): Each SOLOXINE® (levothyroxine sodium, U.S.P.) tablet provides synthetic crystalline levothyroxine sodium (L-thyroxine).

Dosage forms available: 0.1 mg, 0.2 mg, 0.3 mg, 0.4 mg, 0.5 mg, 0.6 mg, 0.7 mg, and 0.8 mg tablets.

Indications: Provides thyroid replacement therapy in all conditions of inadequate production of thyroid hormones. Hypothyroidism is the generalized metabolic disease resulting from deficiency of the thyroid hormones levothyroxine (T_4) and liothyronine (T_3). SOLOXINE® (levothyroxine sodium) will provide levothyroxine (T_4) as a substrate for the physiologic deiodination to liothyronine (T_3). Administration of levothyroxine sodium alone will result in complete physiologic thyroid replacement.

Pharmacology: Levothyroxine sodium acts, as does endogenous thyroxine, to stimulate metabolism, growth, development and differentiation of tissues. It increases the rate of energy exchange and increases the maturation rate of the epiphyses. Levothyroxine sodium is absorbed rapidly from the gastro-intestinal tract after oral administration. Following absorption, the compound becomes bound to the serum globulin fraction. For purposes of comparison, 0.1 mg of levothyroxine sodium elicits a clinical response approximately equal to that produced by one grain (65 mg) of desiccated thyroid.

Dosage and Administration: The initial recommended daily dose is 0.1 mg/10 lbs. (4.5 kg) of body weight. The dosage may then be adjusted according to the patient's response by monitoring T_4 blood levels at time intervals of four (4) weeks.

SOLOXINE® tablets may be administered orally or placed in the food.

Contraindication(s): Levothyroxine sodium therapy is contraindicated in thyrotoxicosis, acute myocardial infarction and uncorrected adrenal insufficiency. Use in pregnant bitches has not been evaluated.

Precaution(s): Store at a controlled room temperature of 15°C to 30°C (59°F to 86°F).

Caution(s): The effects of levothyroxine sodium therapy are slow in being manifested. Overdosage of any thyroid drug may produce the signs and symptoms of thyrotoxicosis including, but not limited to: Polydipsia, polyuria, polyphagia, reduced heat tolerance and hyperactivity or personality change. Administer with caution to animals with clinically significant heart disease, hypertension or other complications for which a sharply increased metabolic rate might prove hazardous.

Side Effects: There are no particular adverse reactions associated with levothyroxine sodium therapy at the recommended dosage levels. Overdosage will result in the signs of thyrotoxicosis listed above under Cautions.

Discussion: Canine hypothyroidism is usually primary, i.e., due to atrophy of the thyroid gland. In the majority of cases the atrophy is associated with lymphocytic thyroiditis and in the remainder it is non-inflammatory and yet of unknown etiology. Less than 10 percent of cases of hypothyroidism are secondary, i.e., due to deficiency of thyroid stimulating hormone (TSH). TSH deficiency may occur as a component of congenital hypopituitarism or as an acquired disorder in adult dogs, in which case it is invariably due to the growth of a pituitary tumor.

Hypothyroidism usually occurs in middle-aged and older dogs although the condition will sometimes be seen in younger dogs of the larger breeds. Neutered animals of either sex are also frequently affected, regardless of age. The following are clinical signs of hypothyroidism in dogs: Lethargy, lack of endurance, increased sleeping, reduced interest, alertness and excitability, slow heart rate, weak apex beat and pulse, low voltage on ECG, preference for warmth, low body temperature, cool skin, increased body weight, stiff and slow movements, dragging of front feet, head tilt, disturbed balance, unilateral facial paralysis, atrophy of epidermis, thickening of dermis, surface and follicular hyperkeratosis, pigmentation, puffy face, blepharoptosis, tragic expression, dry, coarse, sparse coat, slow regrowth after clipping, retarded turnover of hair (carpet coat of boxers), shortening or absence of estrus, lack of libido, dry feces, occasional diarrhea, hypercholesterolemia, normochromic, normocytic anemia, elevated serum creatinine phosphokinase.

Presentation: Bottles of 250 and 1,000 tablets.

Compendium Code No.: 11320051

SOLUBLE COLOSTRUM POWDER

Durvet **Large Animal Dietary Supplement**

Guaranteed Analysis: Minimum:

Vitamin A - Not Less Than .... 5500 I.U./tsp.
Vitamin D_3 - Not Less Than .... 2750 I.U./tsp.
Vitamin E - Not Less Than .... 2.75 I.U./tsp.

(Lactic acid producing microorganism 5 x 10^9/tsp.) (Equal number of each).

Ingredients: *Lactobacillus acidophilus* fermentation product dehydrated, *Lactobacillus casei* fermentation product dehydrated, *Bifido bacterium* fermentation product dehydrated, dried milk colostrum, vitamin A acetate (stability improved), (d-activated animal sterol) source of vitamin D_3, (d-alpha tocopherol acetate) source of vitamin E, calcium carbonate, rice mill by-product and dextrose.

S

Indications: A nutritional product for newborn calves, sheep and goats which contains a source of live (viable) naturally occurring microorganisms.

Directions for Use: (Feed 30 calves for 5 days.) Administer to newborn calves as soon as possible after birth: One teaspoonful in milk or milk replacer. Continue administration of product as long as calves are on milk replacer or milk.

Caution(s): For use in animals only.

Warning(s): Keep out of reach of children.

Presentation: 18 oz (NDC 30798-179-76).

Compendium Code No.: 10841491 2/98

SOLU-DELTA-CORTEF® ℞

Pharmacia & Upjohn **Corticosteroid Injection**

brand of prednisolone sodium succinate sterile powder-100 and 500 mg/10 mL*

NADA No.: 011-593

Active Ingredient(s): SOLU-DELTA-CORTEF® Sterile Powder contains prednisolone sodium succinate which is a salt of prednisolone that is particularly suitable for intravenous or intramuscular injection because it is highly water soluble, permitting administration of relatively large doses in a small volume of diluent. It is especially designed for intravenous use in situations requiring rapid and intense glucocorticoid and/or anti-inflammatory effect; however, it may be used by the intramuscular route in less acute conditions.

*Each mL (when mixed) of these preparations contains:

	100 mg	500 mg
Prednisolone sodium succinate equivalent to prednisolone	10 mg	50 mg
Monobasic sodium phosphate anhydrous	0.075 mg	0.075 mg
Dibasic sodium phosphate dried	0.81 mg	0.81 mg
Lactose hydrous	19.6 mg	19.6 mg
Tyloxapol	4.9 mg	4.9 mg
Chlorobutanol anhydrous (chloral deriv.) added as preservative	3.08 mg	3.08 mg

When necessary, pH was adjusted with sodium hydroxide and/or hydrochloric acid.

Indications: SOLU-DELTA-CORTEF® Sterile Powder is indicated for use in situations in which a rapid and intense adrenal glucocorticoid and/or anti-inflammatory effect is necessary. If the intravenous route is impracticable or the need is not so urgent, the intramuscular route may be used.

Inflammatory Conditions: As with the other adrenal steroids, SOLU-DELTA-CORTEF® has been found useful in alleviating lameness associated with acute localized and generalized arthritic conditions in horses, dogs, and cats. Treatment is usually required daily or on alternate days, depending on the severity or duration of the condition. Prednisolone sodium succinate has been used successfully to treat bursitis, carpitis, tendinitis, and myositis. Remission of the symptoms may be permanent, or symptoms may recur, depending on the cause and the extent of structural degeneration.

Generalized muscular soreness, stiffness, depression, and anorexia as a result of overtraining, shipping, unusual physical exertion, etc, respond promptly to prednisolone sodium succinate.

The intravenous administration is of particular value in treating acute laminitis (founder) in horses. It is important that the condition be detected early so that therapy may be instituted before there is irreparable damage to the laminae. It may be given at intervals of 12 to 24 hours, depending upon the response. Correction and/or treatment of the etiological factors is imperative and routine local antiphlogistic measures should be employed.

Allergic Reactions: SOLU-DELTA-CORTEF® is especially beneficial in treating acute hypersensitivity reactions resulting from treatment with a sensitizing drug or exposure to other allergenic agents. Usual manifestations are anaphylactoid reactions and urticaria. Less severe allergic manifestations, such as atopic and contact dermatitis, summer eczema, and conjunctivitis also may be treated. Response is usually rapid and complete, although in severe cases with extensive lesions, more prolonged adrenocorticoid therapy and other appropriate treatment may be indicated.

Overwhelming Infections with Severe Toxicity: In animals moribund from overwhelmingly severe infections for which specific antibacterial therapy is available (eg, critical pneumonia, peritonitis, endometritis, mastitis), intensive prednisolone sodium succinate therapy may aid in correcting the circulatory defect by counteracting the responsible inflammatory changes, thereby permitting the antibacterial agent to exert its full effect. As supportive therapy, this product combats the stress and improves the general attitude of the animal being treated. All necessary procedures for the establishment of a bacterial diagnosis should be carried out whenever possible before institution of therapy. In the presence of infection, prednisolone sodium succinate should be administered for the shortest possible time compatible with maintenance of an adequate clinical response, and antibacterial therapy should be continued for at least three days after the hormone has been withdrawn. Combined hormone and antibacterial therapy does not obviate the need for indicated surgical treatment.

Shock: For dogs, intravenous SOLU-DELTA-CORTEF® is indicated in the prevention and treatment of adrenal failure and shocklike states occurring in association with severe injury or other trauma, emergency surgery, anaphylactoid reactions and elective surgery in poor surgical risks. This hormone is recommended as an adjuvant to standard methods of combating shock, including use of plasma expanders. Because of interrelated physiologic activities, beneficial effects may not be exhibited until all such procedures have been employed. SOLU-DELTA-CORTEF® is an invaluable emergency kit drug.

Other Indications: SOLU-DELTA-CORTEF® has been found useful as supportive therapy in the treatment of stress-induced exhaustion, rattlesnake bite, toxemia, inflammatory ocular conditions and other stress conditions. Its employment in the treatment of these conditions is recommended as a measure supportive to standard procedures and time-honored treatments and will aid in recovery of the animal.

Pharmacology: Metabolic and Hormonal Effects: Prednisolone, a derivative of hydrocortisone, has greater glucocorticoid activity, greater anti-inflammatory activity, less sodium-retaining effect, and less potassium-losing effect than the parent compound.

The glucocorticoid activity of prednisolone is approximately 4 times that of hydrocortisone and 5 times that of cortisone as measured in experimental animals in terms of liver glycogen deposition, eosinopenic response, and thymic involution.

The anti-inflammatory activity of prednisolone is at least 4 times that of hydrocortisone. SOLU-DELTA CORTEF® exerts an inhibitory influence on the cellular, fibrous, and amorphous components of connective tissue and thereby suppresses the basic processes of inflammation. Vascular permeability is decreased, exudation diminished, and the migration of inflammatory cells markedly impaired.

Dosage and Administration: Directions for Using the Act-O-Vial® System:

1. Press down on plastic activator to force diluent into the lower compartment.
2. Gently agitate to effect solution.
3. Remove plastic tab covering center of stopper.
4. Sterilize top of stopper with a suitable germicide.
5. Insert 18 gauge or smaller needle squarely through center of plunger-stopper until tip is just visible. Invert vial and withdraw dose.

No additional diluent should be added, and the solution should be injected directly into the vein or muscle. If desired, the solution may be incorporated into the following infusion solutions: Dextrose 5% Injection, Dextrose 5% and Sodium Chloride Injection, Dextrose 10% Injection, Dextrose 10% and Sodium Chloride Injection, Ringer's Injection, Fructose 10%, and Lactated Potassic Saline Injection (Darrow's Solution) but must not be added to calcium infusion solutions. If the solution should become cloudy after reconstituting, it should not be used intravenously.

Horses: The dosage for horses is 50 to 100 mg as an initial dose. This may be given intravenously over a period of ½ to 1 minute, or intramuscularly, and may be repeated in inflammatory, allergic, or other stress conditions, at intervals of 12, 24, or 48 hours, depending upon the size of the animal, the severity of the condition, and the response to treatment. When steroid therapy is to be more prolonged, as in a chronic arthritic condition, Depo-Medrol® Sterile Aqueous Suspension containing methylprednisolone or Predef 2X® Sterile Aqueous Suspension containing isoflupredone acetate may be injected intramuscularly and continued daily, depending on the severity of the condition and response to treatment.

Dogs: The usual intravenous dose in shock and shocklike states ranges from 2.5 to 5 mg per lb of body weight as an initial dose, followed by equal maintenance doses at 1-, 3-, 6-, or 10-hour intervals as determined by the condition of the patient.

Dogs and Cats: The intramuscular dose in inflammatory, allergic, and less severe stress conditions, where immediate effect is not required, is usually 1 to 5 mg ranging upwards to 30 to 50 mg in large breeds of dogs. This may be repeated in 12 to 24 hours and continued for 3 to 5 days, if necessary. When steroid therapy is to be more prolonged, as in a chronic arthritic or dermal condition, DEPO-MEDROL Sterile Aqueous Suspension may be used. If permanent corticosteroid effect is required, oral therapy with prednisolone tablets may be substituted as soon as possible. When therapy is to be withdrawn after prolonged corticosteroid administration, the daily dose should be reduced gradually over a number of days, in stepwise fashion.

Choice of appropriate concentration of SOLU-DELTA-CORTEF® Sterile Powder will help minimize discard of unused drug. It is suggested that the 10 mg/mL formulation be used to treat cats and horses of any size as well as dogs weighing less than 40 pounds. For intravenous treatment of shock in dogs weighing over 40 pounds use the 50 mg/mL formulation. Do not use 50 mg/mL formulation in dogs and cats for intramuscular use.

All intravenous injections should be administered slowly.

Contraindication(s): Except when used for emergency therapy, prednisolone sodium succinate is contraindicated in animals with tuberculosis, Cushingoid syndrome, and peptic ulcer. Existence of congestive heart failure, diabetes, chronic nephritis, and osteoporosis are relative contraindications. In the presence of infection, appropriate antibacterial agents should also be administered and should be continued for at least 3 days after discontinuance of the hormone and disappearance of all signs of infection. Do not use in viral infections.

Precaution(s): Storage Conditions:

1. Store unreconstituted product at controlled room temperature 20° to 25°C (68° to 77°F) [see USP].
   Protect from light. Store in carton.
2. Do not store reconstituted product. Use immediately. Discard any unused reconstituted SOLU-DELTA-CORTEF® Sterile Powder.

Caution(s): Federal (USA) law restricts this drug to use by or on the order of a licensed veterinarian.

SOLU-DELTA-CORTEF® Sterile Powder may suppress systemic manifestations such as fever and also signs of toxemia. In some instances this alteration of the inflammatory reaction may be beneficial; however, it may also mask the signs of infection and tend to facilitate the spread of microorganisms. In infections characterized by overwhelming toxicity, prednisolone sodium succinate therapy in conjunction with indicated antibacterial therapy is effective in reducing mortality and morbidity. It is essential that the causative organism be known and an effective antibacterial agent be administered concurrently. The injudicious use of the adrenal hormones in animals with infections can be hazardous.

For intravenous or intramuscular use.

For use in animals only.

Warning(s): Clinical and experimental data have demonstrated that corticosteroids administered orally or parenterally to animals may induce the first stage of parturition when administered during the last trimester of pregnancy and may precipitate premature parturition followed by dystocia, fetal death, retained placenta and metritis.

Additionally, corticosteroids administered to dogs, rabbits, and rodents during pregnancy have resulted in cleft palate in offspring. Corticosteroids administered to dogs during pregnancy have also resulted in other congenital anomalies, including deformed forelegs, phocomelia, and anasarca.

Side Effects: The therapeutic use of SOLU-DELTA-CORTEF® Sterile Powder is unlikely to cause undesired accentuation of metabolic effects. However, if continued corticosteroid therapy is anticipated, a high protein intake should be provided to keep the animal in positive nitrogen balance. A retardant effect on wound healing has not been encountered, but such a possibility should also be considered when it is used in conjunction with surgery. Euphoria, or an improvement of attitude, and increased appetite are usual manifestations.

Undesirable effects of adrenocorticoid administration are sodium and water retention, potassium loss, glycosuria, hyperglycemia, and polyuria and polydipsia.

Presentation: SOLU-DELTA-CORTEF® Sterile Powder is available in 10 mL [100 mg/10 mL (NDC 0009-0623-02) or 500 mg/10 mL (NDC 0009-0996-02)] Act-O-Vial® Systems.

Compendium Code No.: 10490481 810 170 111

SOLUMINE

Durvet **Feed Additive**

Guaranteed Analysis: SOLUMINE Analysis:

Vitamin D_3: min. 1,892,700 IU/gallon, or 226,800 IU/lb in a liquid for all swine, poultry and cattle.

Ingredients: Propylene glycol, Chinese cinnamon, licorice extract, sodium bicarbonate, vitamin D_3 supplement liquid, xanthan gum.

Indications: Vitamin D_3 supplement aromatized from plant extract for all swine, poultry and cattle.

Directions: Shake well. Dilute before usage.

For Group Application:

Poultry and Swine:

Drinking water: Half a gallon of SOLUMINE in 256 gallons of drinking water. (Metric: 2 liters of SOLUMINE in 1,000 liters of drinking water).

Dilution: Mix a quarter gallon of SOLUMINE per gallon of stock solution with a proportioner set at 1:128. For best results use lukewarm water for stock solution. (Metric: 1 liter per 4 liters).

Swine:

Boar/sow/gilt: From 1 teaspoon (1 teaspoon = approx ⅙ ounce) to 1 tablespoon. (Metric: 5 mL to 20 mL).

Piglet: Half a teaspoon (Metric: 2.5 mL).

Beef Cattle:

Drinking water: 1 to 6 cups (1 cup = 8 ounces) of SOLUMINE per 256 gallons of drinking water (Metric: 250 mL to 1,450 mL of SOLUMINE per 1,000 liters drinking water).

Dilution: Mix half a cup to 3 cups per gallon of stock solution with a proportioner set at 1:128. For best results use lukewarm water for stock solution. (Metric: Mix 125 mL to 725 mL of SOLUMINE per 4 liters of stock solution with a proportioner set at 1:128).

Length of Supplementation: 7 to 15 days.

Note:

1. The final dilution can be obtained from the manufacturer.
2. When animals are facing high environmental temperature consumption of final product should be limited to quantity of normal water consumption.

Precaution(s): Protect from light. Store in cool, dry place.

Caution(s): Not for injection.

The viscosity of this product may vary inversely with the temperature at 74°F. 1.0 gram = 1 mL.

Presentation: 1 gallon and 5 gallons (18.9 L).

Manufactured by: Nutrapro Inc., 1905 Lamoureux, Suite 202, St. Hyacinthe, Québec, J2S 8B1, Canada.

Compendium Code No.: 10842090

SOLU/TET

Vedco **Water Medication**

Tetracycline Hydrochloride Soluble Powder-antibiotic

NADA No.: 140-578

Active Ingredient(s): Each pound contains: 25 g of tetracycline hydrochloride activity.

Indications: Antibiotic - For use in drinking water for swine, calves, and poultry for treatment and control of certain swine and calf diseases and control of specific diseases of poultry.

Dosage and Administration:

For Chickens and Turkeys: Chronic respiratory disease (air-sac infection), hexamitiasis, bluecomb (nonspecific enteritis), infectious sinusitis and synovitis.
As an aid in prevention: 100-200 mg/gallon.
For treatment: 200-400 mg/gallon.

For Swine: Bacterial enteritis.
As an aid in prevention: 100-200 mg/gallon
For treatment: 200-400 mg/gallon.

For Swine: Bacterial pneumonia:
As an aid in prevention: 200-400 mg/gallon.
For treatment: 400 mg/gallon.

For Calves: Bacterial diarrhea, bacterial pneumonia and shipping fever (hemorrhagic septicemia).
As an aid in prevention: 100-200 mg/gallon.
For treatment: 200-400 mg/gallon.

6.4 oz. will make:
100 gallons containing 100 mg of tetracycline hydrochloride per gallon.
50 gallons containing 200 mg of tetracycline hydrochloride per gallon.
25 gallons containing 400 mg of tetracycline hydrochloride per gallon.

Caution(s): For chickens and turkeys: Administer for not more than 21 days.

For calves: Administer for not more than five days. Prepare a fresh solution daily. Use as the sole source of tetracycline. Solutions are not stable for more than 24 hours. Do not supply unmedicated water or milk during treatment. Diagnosis should be reconsidered if improvement is not noticed within two to three days.

Livestock drug. Not for human use. Restricted drug, use only as directed.

Warning(s): Do not slaughter birds for food within four (4) days of treatment. Do not slaughter swine for food with four (4) days of treatment. Do not slaughter calves for food purposes within five (5) days of treatment. Not for use in chickens and turkeys producing eggs for human consumption. Keep out of reach of children.

Presentation: Packets containing 10 g, 62 per pail.

Compendium Code No.: 10941881

SOLU-TET® 324

Alpharma **Water Medication**

Tetracycline Hydrochloride Soluble Powder-Antibiotic

NADA No.: 140-578

Active Ingredient(s): Each packet contains: 202.5 grams of tetracycline hydrochloride activity.

Indications: Chickens: For control of chronic respiratory disease (CRD air sac infection) caused by *Mycoplasma gallisepticum* and *Escherichia coli;* infectious synovitis caused by *Mycoplasma synoviae* susceptible to tetracycline hydrochloride.

Dosage and Administration: Recommended Dosage Level:

CRD air sac disease: Use soluble powder in the drinking water at a drug level of 400-800 mg tetracycline hydrochloride per gallon per day.

Infectious synovitis: Use soluble powder in the drinking water at a drug level of 200-400 mg tetracycline hydrochloride per gallon per day.

Directions for Use: Administer for 7 to 14 days. Medicate at first clinical signs of disease or when experience indicates the disease may be a problem.

If improvement is not noted within 24 to 48 hours, consult a poultry veterinarian or poultry diagnostic laboratory.

General Cautions: Prepare fresh solutions at least once a day. Solutions are not stable for more than 24 hours. Use as a sole source of tetracycline.

Mixing Directions: To arrive at the recommended dosages, prepare stock solutions as follows:
200 mg/gallon — dissolve 1 packet (10 oz) in 30,280 mL warm water (8 gallons).
400 mg/gallon — dissolve 1 packet (10 oz) in 15,140 mL warm water (4 gallons).
800 mg/gallon — dissolve 1 packet (10 oz) in 7,570 mL warm water (2 gallon).

These stock solutions should then be metered into drinking water at approximately 1 ounce per gallon. At 200-800 mg/gallon this packet will medicate 253 to 1012 gallons of drinking water.

Note: The concentration of drug required in medicated water must be adequate to compensate for variations in the age and class of animals, feed consumption, and environmental temperature and humidity, each of which affects water consumption.

Caution(s): Do not use for more than 14 consecutive days.

Restricted drug (California). Use only as directed. For animal use only.

Warning(s): Do not slaughter birds for food within 4 days of treatment. Not for use in chickens producing eggs for human consumption.

Presentation: 10 oz (286 gram) packets.

Compendium Code No.: 10220570

SOMLETHOL CII

Webster **Euthanasia Agent**

(Pentobarbital Sodium) Euthanasia Injection

Active Ingredient(s): Composition: Each mL of aqueous solution contains:

Pentobarbital Sodium	8 gr (389 mg)
Isopropyl Alcohol	40.0% v/v
Propylene Glycol	2.3% v/v
Edetate Disodium	0.05% w/v
Benzyl Alcohol (preservative)	2.0% v/v

Color added for identification.

S

Manufactured by a non-sterilizing process.
Indications: For use only as a euthanasia agent in animals.
Dosage and Administration: Dogs and Cats- 1 mL per 10 pounds of body weight. Individual variation, particularly in cases of cardiac or circulatory deficiencies, may require higher dosage in some animals. The intravenous route of injection is recommended. Intracardiac injection may be used when intravenous injection is impractical. The calculated dose should be injected rapidly. As with all pentobarbital euthanasia agents, terminal gasp may occur in the unconscious animal. Nervous or vicious animals may require tranquilization or sedation prior to injection for euthanasia.
Precaution(s): Store at controlled room temperature between 15° and 30°C (59°-88°F).
Caution(s): Federal law restricts this drug to use by or on the order of a licensed veterinarian.
For animal use only.
Warning(s): This product must not be used for anesthetic or therapeutic purposes. Not for use in animals intended for food.
Keep out of reach of children. Poison.
Presentation: 250 mL (NDC 14043-0035-5).
Compendium Code No.: 11000010 Rev. 3-02

SOMNUMUNE®

AgriLabs **Bacterin**
Haemophilus somnus Bacterin
U.S. Vet. Lic. No.: 303
Active Ingredient(s): SOMNUMUNE® bacterin contains multiple inactivated whole cell cultures of *Haemophilus somnus* adjuvanted with aluminum hydroxide. Contains penicillin and streptomycin as preservatives.
Indications: For use in healthy cattle as an aid in the prevention and control of diseases caused by *Haemophilus somnus.*
Dosage and Administration: Shake well and administer 2 mL intramuscularly or subcutaneously to healthy calves three (3) months of age or older Repeat the dosage in two (2) to three (3) weeks. Revaccinate annually to maintain a high level of immunity.
Precaution(s): Store at 35-45°F (2-7°C). Do not freeze.
Caution(s): Use the entire contents when first opened. If anaphylactic reactions should occur, epinephrine should be administered immediately.
Warning(s): Do not vaccinate within 21 days before slaughter.
Presentation: 20 mL (10 dose) and 100 mL (50 dose) vials.
Compendium Code No.: 10580950

SOMNU SHIELD™

Novartis Animal Vaccines **Bacterin**
Haemophilus somnus Bacterin
U.S. Vet. Lic. No.: 303
Composition: The bacterin contains multiple inactivated whole cell cultures of *Haemophilus somnus* adjuvanted with aluminum hydroxide. Contains penicillin and streptomycin as preservatives.
Indications: For use in healthy cattle as an aid in the prevention and control of infections caused by *Haemophilus somnus.*
Dosage and Administration: Shake well before and during use. Administer a 2 mL dose intramuscularly or subcutaneously in healthy calves three (3) months of age or older. Repeat the dosage in two (2) to three (3) weeks. Revaccinate annually to maintain a high level of immunity.
Precaution(s): Store at 35°-45°F (2°-7°C). Do not freeze. Use the entire contents when first opened.
Caution(s): Anaphylactic reactions may occur following the use of the product. Symptomatic treatment: Epinephrine.
Warning(s): Do not vaccinate within 21 days prior to slaughter.
Discussion: *Haemophilus somnus* has long been recognized by veterinary researchers, diagnosticians, and practitioners as a major cause of death in feedlot calves due to encephalitis (brain infection). In the past five years, *H. somnus* has also been found to be a major cause of pneumonia, arthritis, and reproductive problems.
H. somnus infections occur most commonly in stress situations such as when cattle are grouped together in sale barns, feedlots, dairy herds, for shipping, etc., or when assembled for grazing fall and winter pasture.
The disease usually occurs one week to one month after cattle are grouped together. During an outbreak, some cattle will show signs of encephalitis, including blindness, staggering, and convulsions. Without prompt treatment with antibiotics, most of these animals will die. The brain damage caused by *H. somnus* is irreversible, so even if the animal is treated and survives it may have to be culled.
Concurrent with the encephalitis outbreak, other cattle will develop pneumonia. This pneumonia is indistinguishable from viral and Pasteurella shipping fever complex pneumonia, thus, *H. somnus* pneumonia can be easily misdiagnosed.
H. somnus infection is usually a systemic disease. The organism causes disease by blocking capillaries, thereby restricting the blood flow to vital organs. While the most common manifestations of *H. somnus* are encephalitis and pneumonia, all organs of the animal's body can be affected. Even if the animal is treated with antibiotics and recovers, damage due to the loss of blood supply to various body organs can cause chronic, debilitating disease problems. Common manifestations of this damage include arthritis, abortion, and sterility.
The damage caused by *H. somnus* to the joints of affected cattle makes them more susceptible to mycoplasma arthritis, thus turning a minor arthritis problem into a major one.
Disease and death losses from *H. somnus* infection can be greatly reduced or prevented by preconditioning cattle and calves before the stress of shipping and exposure with SOMNU SHIELD™.
Presentation: Available in 10 dose (20 mL) and 50 dose (100 mL) bottles.
Compendium Code No.: 11140482

SOMNU SHIELD™ XT

Novartis Animal Vaccines **Bacterin**
Haemophilus somnus Bacterin
U.S. Vet. Lic. No.: 303
Composition: The bacterin contains multiple inactivated whole cell cultures of *Haemophilus somnus* adjuvanted with Xtend III™. Contains penicillin and streptomycin as preservatives.
Indications: For use in healthy cattle as an aid in the prevention and control of infections caused by *Haemophilus somnus.*
Dosage and Administration: Shake well before using. Administer a 2 mL dose intramuscularly to healthy calves three (3) months of age or older. Repeat the dosage in four (4) to five (5) weeks. Vaccinate dairy cows during the drying-off period. Revaccinate annually to maintain a high level of immunity.
Precaution(s): Store at 35°-45°F (2°-7°C). Do not freeze. Use the entire contents when first opened.
Caution(s): Transient swelling may occur at the site of injection. Milk reduction and transient depression may be observed in lactating dairy cows for two to four days following vaccination. Anaphylactic reactions may occur following the use of the product. Symptomatic treatment: Epinephrine.
Warning(s): Do not vaccinate within 60 days prior to slaughter.
Presentation: Available in 50 dose (100 mL) bottles.
Compendium Code No.: 11140492

SOMUBAC®

Pfizer Animal Health **Bacterin**
Haemophilus Somnus Bacterin
U.S. Vet. Lic. No.: 189
Contents: SOMUBAC® consists of inactivated, standardized cultures of *Haemophilus somnus,* adjuvanted with aluminum hydroxide.
Indications: For vaccination of healthy cattle and calves as an aid in preventing disease caused by *Haemophilus somnus.*
Directions: Shake well before using. Administer a single 2-mL dose subcutaneously to healthy cattle 3 months of age or older, followed by a second dose 2-4 weeks later. In accordance with Beef Quality Assurance guidelines, this product should be administered subcutaneously (SC) under the skin. Annual revaccination with a single dose is recommended.
Precaution(s): Store at 2°-7°C. Do not freeze. Use entire contents when first opened. Sterilized syringes and needles should be used to administer this vaccine.
Caution(s): As with many vaccines, anaphylaxis may occur after use. Initial antidote of epinephrine is recommended and should be followed with appropriate supportive therapy.
Warning(s): Do not vaccinate within 21 days before slaughter.
For veterinary use only.
Presentation: 10 dose (20 mL) and 50 dose (100 mL) vials.
Compendium Code No.: 36900220 85-4255-05

SOOTHABLES™ COOL AID

A.A.H. **Topical Product**
Pet Health Aids-Hot Spot Spray
Ingredient(s): SOOTHABLES™ Cool Aid is specially formulated with Purified Water, SD Alcohol, Menthol, Clove Oil, Allantoin, Lanolin, Tea Tree Oil, Eucalyptus Oil, Peppermint Oil and Denatonium Benzoate.
Water soluble lanolin moisturizes without imparting a sticky, greasy feel to the skin or coat. Denatonium Benzoate (Bitrex) is a bittering agent which discourages licking and biting. Oils of Eucalyptus and Clove cool and soothe hot spot areas.
Indications: SOOTHABLES™ Cool Aid is designed to discourage chewing, licking and compulsive biting associated with allergic dermatitis, insect bites, rashes and dry itchy skin.
Non-sticky, non-greasy spray for dogs and cats.
Directions for Use: Hold spray 3-4 inches from affected areas. Part hair coat to allow spray to reach the skin. Safe for use on dogs and cats. May be used on dry or damp coat. Apply as often as needed.
Precaution(s): Store in a cool area.
Caution(s): This product is intended for topical use only. Avoid spraying into animal's eyes. If contact occurs, flush eyes with copious amounts of water. If skin becomes irritated or inflamed, discontinue use.
For animal use only.
Warning(s): Keep out of reach of children and pets.
Presentation: 8 fl oz (237 mL).
Compendium Code No.: 11180150

SOOTHABLES™ CRYSTAL-EAR

A.A.H. **Otic Cleanser**
Pet Health Aids-Gentle Ear Cleaner
Ingredient(s): SOOTHABLES™ Crystal-Ear is formulated with Purified Water, Polyethylene Glycol, Isopropyl Alcohol, Lactic Acid, Polyoxyethylene 20-Sorbitan Monolaurate, Tea Tree Oil and Aloe Vera.
Indications: The special blend of Tea Tree Oil and Aloe Vera in SOOTHABLES™ Crystal-Ear provides excellent cleaning and soothing properties without irritating the sensitive ear canal.
The build-up of waxy debris in the ear allows infection to persist underneath and can lead to otic health problems. A gentle ear flush, especially during the bath or grooming, is part of a standard preventive care program.
Directions for Use: Position the bottle close to but not touching the ear. Squeeze bottle gently, using the applicator top to apply 2 to 4 drops into the ear canal. Gently massage the base of the ear for several seconds. Allow animal to shake its head. Absorb any excess with cotton but do not swab the ear canal. To remove excessive dirt and waxy build-up apply 2 to 3 times daily for a period of several days. Then use once a week or as needed.
Precaution(s): Store in a cool area.
Caution(s): In case of increased irritation, discontinue use. Avoid contact with eyes. If contact occurs, flush the eyes with copious amount of water.
For animal use only.
Warning(s): Keep out of reach of children and pets.
Presentation: 8 fl oz (237 mL) bottle.
Compendium Code No.: 11180160

SOOTHABLES™ TENDER FOOT

A.A.H. **Topical Product**
Pet Health Aids-Foot Pad & Elbow Cream
Ingredient(s): Vitamin A, Vitamin D, Vitamin E, Riboflavin (Vit. B2), Panthenol (Vit. B5), Pyridoxine Hydrochloride (Vit. B6), d-Biotin (Vit. H), Niacinamide (Vit. B3), in a protective non-greasy moisturizing cream base.
Indications: Tender Foot is a specially compounded multi-vitamin cream. Use to protect, repair and restore lost resiliency to foot pads exposed to: Snow, ice and chemicals, hot sidewalks or black top, rough terrain, briars or nettles.
Also, use to soften and moisturize elbows calloused by lying on cement or other rough surfaces. Tender Foot cream is stabilized at the pH of normal animal skin.

Moisturizes and helps toughen dry, cracked, chapped foot pads. Moisturizes and softens calloused elbows.

For dogs and puppies.

Directions: Squeeze a ½" ribbon of Tender Foot on your finger or apply directly to the pad or elbow. Massage gently into your dog's foot pads and elbows. Use daily to moisturize and restore resiliency to dry, cracked, chapped or calloused skin and tissue.

Precaution(s): Store in a cool area.

Caution(s): For animal use only.

Warning(s): Keep out of reach of children and pets.

Presentation: 5 oz (141.7 g) tube.

Compendium Code No.: 11180180

SOW & GILT RESTART™ ONE-4

TechMix **Electrolytes-Oral**

Guaranteed Analysis:

Crude Protein	not less than 12.00%
Crude Fat	not less than 10.00%
Crude Fiber	not more than 0.50%
Salt (NaCl)	None Added
Vitamin A	not less than 20,000 I.Units/lb
Vitamin D	not less than 4,000 I.Units/lb
Vitamin E	not less than 25 I.Units/lb

Ingredients: Dried skim milk, dried whey, animal and vegetable fat (stabilized with BHA and lecithin), dextrose, fructose, sucrose, lactose, glycine, dibasic potassium phosphate, sodium bicarbonate, calcium lactate, magnesium gluconate, citric acid, potassium chloride, dried *Lactobacillus acidophilus* fermentation product, dried *Lactobacillus lactis* fermentation product, dried *Lactobacillus plantarum* fermentation product, dried *Bacillus subtilis* fermentation product, dried *Bacillus subtilis* fermentation extract, dried *Aspergillus oryzae* fermentation extract, dried *Trichoderma rescii* fermentation extract, dl-alpha tocopheryl acetate (source of vitamin E activity), choline bitartrate, vitamin A acetate, niacin supplement, d-activated animal sterol (source of vitamin D_3), ascorbic acid (vitamin C), d-calcium pantothenate, d-biotin, riboflavin supplement, vitamin B_{12} supplement, menadione dimenthylpyrimidinol bisulfite (source of vitamin K activity), thiamine hydrochloride, pyridoxine hydrochloride, folic acid, natural and artificial flavors added.

Indications: Combination of electrolytes, vitamins, microbial cultures and multiple sources of acidified energy intended to provide immediate essential nutrients to lactating sows and gilts that are off feed.

Dosage and Administration: For Sows and Gilts Still Eating Some Feed: Top dress two heaping scoops on the feed for one to four feedings.

For Sows and Gilts not Eating but Drinking Water or Fluids: Mix two heaping scoops in two quarts of drinking water for one to four feedings.

For Sows and Gilts not Eating or Drinking Substantial Amounts of Fluids: Mix two heaping scoops in one to two pints of lukewarm water and administer with a sow oral feeder. Administer for one to four feedings in six to eight hour intervals.

One heaping scoop equals approximately 2½ oz.

Caution(s): Sows and gilts with an elevated temperature or not consuming feed for a period of 36-48 hours should be treated and handled as designated by your veterinarian.

Presentation: 12x2 lb bags (24 lb pail) and 10 lb (4.5 kg) pail.

Compendium Code No.: 11440120

SOW BAC® CE II

Intervet **Bacterin-Toxoid**

Bordetella Bronchiseptica-Clostridium Perfringens Type C-Erysipelothrix Rhusiopathiae-Escherichia Coli-Pasteurella Multocida Bacterin-Toxoid

U.S. Vet. Lic. No.: 286

Contents: A chemically inactivated, adjuvanted product containing *Bordetella bronchiseptica, Clostridium perfringens* type C toxoid, *Erysipelothrix rhusiopathiae,* four major *Escherichia coli* antigens (K88, K99, F41, 987P) and *Pasteurella multocida* non-toxigenic type A and toxigenic type D.

Contains gentamicin, polymyxin B and thimerosal as preservatives.

Indications: For use in healthy pregnant swine as an aid in the prevention of colibacillosis, enterotoxemia, atrophic rhinitis and pneumonia in their nursing piglets and the prevention of erysipelas in healthy pregnant swine.

Dosage and Administration: When used alone, shake well and inject sow or gilt intramuscularly or subcutaneously with a 2 mL dose at 5 weeks and 2 weeks prefarrowing. Inject one 2 mL dose at 1-2 weeks before subsequent farrowings.

When packaged with ProSystem® Rota or ProSystem® TGE/Rota refer to insert for full directions.

Precaution(s): Store in the dark at not over 45°F (7°C). Do not freeze. Use entire contents when first opened; do not save partial contents.

Caution(s): Use only in healthy pregnant swine.

If allergic reaction occurs, treat with epinephrine.

For veterinary use only.

Warning(s): Do not vaccinate within 21 days of slaughter.

Presentation: 25 dose (50 mL) vials.

Compendium Code No.: 11061551 7112501

SOW BAC® E II

Intervet **Bacterin-Toxoid**

Bordetella Bronchiseptica-Erysipelothrix Rhusiopathiae-Escherichia Coli-Pasteurella Multocida Bacterin-Toxoid

U.S. Vet. Lic. No.: 286

Contents: This product contains the antigens listed above.

Contains thimerosal, gentamicin and polymyxin B as preservatives.

Indications: A chemically inactivated, adjuvanted product for use in healthy pregnant swine as an aid in the prevention of colibacillosis (caused by *E. coli* antigens K88, K99, F41, 987P), atrophic rhinitis and pneumonia (caused by *B. bronchiseptica* and *P. multocida* non-toxigenic type A and toxigenic types A and D) in their nursing piglets. This product is also used for the prevention of erysipelas in healthy pregnant swine caused by *E. rhusiopathiae.*

Dosage and Administration: Shake well, aseptically inject intramuscularly or subcutaneously with a 2 mL dose at 5 weeks and 2 weeks prefarrowing. Inject one 2 mL dose at 1-2 weeks before subsequent farrowing.

Precaution(s): Store in the dark at not over 45°F (7°C). Do not freeze. Do not save partial contents. Burn the container and all unused product.

Caution(s): Use only in healthy pregnant swine. If allergic reaction occurs, treat with epinephrine.

For veterinary use only.

Warning(s): Do not vaccinate within 21 days of slaughter.

Presentation: 25 doses (50 mL).

Compendium Code No.: 11062770 7872501

SOW BAC® TREC

Intervet **Bacterin-Toxoid-Vaccine**

Porcine Rotavirus-Transmissible Gastroenteritis Vaccine, Modified Live Virus-Bordetella Bronchiseptica-Clostridium Perfringens Type C-Erysipelothrix Rhusiopathiae-Escherichia Coli-Pasteurella Multocida Bacterin-Toxoid

U.S. Vet. Lic. No.: 286

Contents: The Rotavirus-TGE vaccine (ProSystem® TGE/Rota) contains two modified live G serotypes 5 and 4 of Serogroup A rotavirus, and a modified live TGE virus, in desiccated form. The bacterin-toxoid diluent (Sow Bac® CE II) is an adjuvanted liquid product containing *Bordetella bronchiseptica, Pasteurella multocida* non-toxigenic type A and toxigenic type D, *Erysipelothrix rhusiopathiae,* 4 major *E. coli* pilus antigens - K88, K99, F41 and 987P, and *C. perfringens* type C toxoid. Each serial of Sow Bac® CE II bacterin-toxoid is demonstrated to be compatible (non-viricidal) and therefore can be used as a diluent when packaged with the viral vaccine.

Contains gentamicin, polymyxin B and thimerosal as preservatives.

Indications: Porcine Rotavirus-Transmissible Gastroenteritis vaccine and *Bordetella bronchiseptica-Clostridium perfringens* Type C-*Erysipelothrix rhusiopathiae-Escherichia coli-Pasteurella multocida* bacterin-toxoid are used for the vaccination of healthy pregnant swine, to provide active protection against *Erysipelothrix rhusiopathiae*; and to provide sows and gilts with passive protection to their nursing pigs against 12 important pathogens:

1. Rotavirus (2 modified live G serotypes 5 and 4 of Serogroup A rotavirus).
2. TGE (transmissible gastroenteritis).
3. Atrophic rhinitis and pneumonia *(Bordetella bronchiseptica* and *Pasteurella multocida* non-toxigenic type A and toxigenic types A and D).
4. Colibacillosis *(Escherichia coli* pilus antigens K88, K99, F41 and 987P).
5. Enterotoxemia *(Clostridium perfringens* type C).

These etiologic agents are the most important causes of neonatal porcine diarrhea, atrophic rhinitis and pneumonia. They often occur in combination with each other causing increased morbidity and mortality losses. Furthermore, several of these diseases may produce similar clinical signs in baby pigs, therefore it is highly desirable to provide broad protection to nursing pigs. Laboratory confirmation of the cause of baby diarrhea is recommended since other viral, bacterial and coccidial agents also can cause similar disease signs.

Dosage and Administration: Dosage Guidelines: Follow directions carefully. Two vaccination programs may be used.

Intramuscular (Injection) vaccination method: To be used for sows and gilts having significant virulent TGE exposure within the prior 12 months.

1. Reconstitute ProSystem® TGE/Rota virus vaccine with Sow Bac® CE II bacterin-toxoid diluent, shake bacterin-toxoid well before and after addition to the virus vaccine.
2. Inject pregnant sow or gilt with 2.0 mL intramuscularly at 5 weeks and again at 2 weeks before each farrowing.

Oral and intramuscular (oral) vaccination method: To be used for sows and gilts not previously exposed to virulent TGE.

1. For initial use, each pregnant sow or gilt must receive at least 2 oral and 1 intramuscular dosings of ProSystem® TGE/Rota virus vaccine and 2 doses of Sow Bac® CE II bacterin-toxoid before farrowing. Refer to the five-step method for oral vaccination, as shown below, using desiccated viral vaccine.
   a. 5 weeks before farrowing - 1 oral dose ProSystem® TGE/Rota and 1 intramuscular dose of Sow Bac® CE II bacterin-toxoid.
   b. 3 weeks before farrowing - 1 oral dose ProSystem® TGE/Rota.
   c. 1 week before farrowing - 1 intramuscular dose of ProSystem® TGE/Rota rehydrated with Sow Bac® CE II bacterin-toxoid.
2. Subsequent farrowings - 2 weeks before farrowing, administer 1 oral dose of ProSystem® TGE/Rota and 1 intramuscular dose of ProSystem® TGE/Rota rehydrated with Sow Bac® CE II bacterin-toxoid.

For combination injection, reconstitute ProSystem® TGE/Rota dried vaccine with the accompanying Sow Bac® CE II bacterin-toxoid diluent. Shake well before use. If the bacterin-toxoid is given separately (e.g., at the time of oral vaccination with ProSystem® TGE/Rota), the 2.0 mL dose can be injected either intramuscularly or subcutaneously.

Recommended Methods for Oral Vaccination of Swine:

Step 1: Pour approximately 2 to 2½ gallons of cool water into a large plastic bucket. Add 5 - 10 cups of dry milk (any type of dry milk for human consumption is acceptable). Do not use hot water - it will destroy the vaccine.

Step 2: Stir milk mixture well. Drywall paddles attached to ½" drill make mixing easier.

Step 3: Remove metal ring and stopper. Reconstitute vaccine with milk mixture; add reconstituted vaccine to milk, and stir. (The bacterin-toxoid packaged in combination with viral vaccine must always be injected).

Step 4: Slowly add 40 lbs. of clean ground corn to the milk/vaccine mixture. Stir continuously, using an electric ½" drill and drywall paddle, until mixture thickens and drill pulls down. There should be no run-off seen. Mixing procedure takes approximately 3 minutes.

Step 5: Feed to pregnant sows and gilts in one of two ways:

1. Feed sows individually with approximately 4 lbs. of milk/vaccine/corn mixture.
2. Spread milk/vaccine/corn mixture in a row onto concrete, feeding 10 sows at a time.

For best TGE protection, sows and gilts which have never been exposed to virulent TGE virus should be vaccinated following the oral vaccination guidelines (above) and their baby pigs should be orally vaccinated with ProSystem® TGE (Transmissible Gastroenteritis vaccine).

Precaution(s): Store in the dark at not over 45°F (7°C). Do not freeze. Use vaccine immediately after reconstitution. Use entire contents when first opened. Burn the container and all unused contents.

Caution(s): Use in healthy pregnant swine only.

Conditions which interfere with lactation adversely affect immunity in baby pigs.

If allergic reaction follows use of this product, treat with epinephrine.

Although this product has been shown to be efficacious, some animals may be unable to develop or maintain an adequate immune response following vaccination if they are incubating any infectious disease, are malnourished or parasitized, or stressed due to shipment or adverse environmental conditions.

For highly TGE-susceptible (seronegative) sows and gilts, always use oral TGE vaccination program. For veterinary use only.

Warning(s): Do not vaccinate within 21 days of slaughter.
Trial Data: Safety and efficacy of the modified live rotaviruses and TGE have been demonstrated. The Rotavirus-TGE vaccine, rehydrated with the bacterin-toxoid, and the bacterin-toxoid alone have been evaluated for safety in pregnant swine as well as in laboratory animals. No adverse reactions were observed. Baby pigs are protected from enteritis, atrophic rhinitis, pneumonia, colibacillosis and enterotoxemia by receiving colostral and milk antibodies from vaccinated dams. Therefore it is mandatory that sows and gilts are lactating and baby pigs are nursing adequately.
Presentation: One 10 dose (20 mL) vial of each ProSystem® TGE/Rota and Sow Bac® CE II.
Compendium Code No.: 11061501 762711-01

SPECTAM® SCOUR-HALT™

AgriLabs **Spectinomycin**

NADA No.: 033-157
Active Ingredient(s): Each mL contains:
Spectinomycin .... 50 mg
Indications: Spectinomycin is specifically effective against *Escherichia coli*, the organism that causes 95% or more of the bacterial scour problems in baby pigs.
Dosage and Administration:
Pigs under 10 lbs.: One (1) pump (1 mL) twice a day.
Pigs over 10 lbs.: Two (2) pumps (2 mL) twice a day.
Each pump of the plunger delivers 1 mL of solution containing 50 mg of spectinomycin. Treatment may be continued twice a day for three (3) to five (5) days. If pigs do not improve within 48 hours, rediagnosis is suggested.
Caution(s): This product is intended for use only on pigs under four weeks of age or weighing less than 15 lbs.
Warning(s): Do not administer within 21 days of slaughter.
Presentation: 240 mL with pump, 500 mL and 1,000 mL without pump.
* ® SPECTAM is a registered trademark of Elf Sanofi
™ SCOUR-HALT is a trademark of Elf Sanofi
Compendium Code No.: 10580960

SPECTAM® SCOUR-HALT™

Durvet **Spectinomycin**

(Spectinomycin) Oral Solution
NADA No.: 033-157
Active Ingredient(s): Each mL contains:
Spectinomycin (from spectinomycin dihydrochloride pentahydrate) .... 50 mg
Indications: For use in baby pigs under four (4) weeks of age for the treatment and control of porcine enteric colibacillosis (scours) caused by *E. coli* susceptible to spectinomycin.
Dosage and Administration: Dose: Pigs under 10 lbs — 1 pump (1 mL) twice daily. Pigs over 10 lbs — 2 pumps (2 mL) twice daily.
Each pump of the plunger delivers 1 mL of solution containing 50 mg of spectinomycin. Treatment may be continued twice daily for 3 to 5 days. If pigs do not improve within 48 hours, rediagnosis is suggested.
Directions for Use: The 500 mL bottle of SPECTAM® SCOUR-HALT™ should be used only to refill the 240 mL container in the following manner:
1. Remove the cap and doser from the 240 mL bottle.
2. Unscrew the cap from the 500 mL bottle.
3. Pour (from the 500 mL bottle) the volume desired.
4. Re-insert the doser in the 240 mL bottle and screw the top on tightly.
5. Screw the top tightly on the 500 mL bottle.

Follow the detailed instructions for use shown on the carton containing the 240 mL bottle of SPECTAM® SCOUR-HALT™.
Caution(s): For animal use only. Not for human use.
Restricted Drug—Use only as directed (California).
Warning(s): This product is only intended for use in pigs under four weeks of age or weighing less than 15 lbs. Do not administer within 21 days of slaughter. Keep out of reach of children.
Presentation: 8 fl oz (240 mL) (NDC 30798-106-12) and 16.9 fl oz (500 mL) (NDC 30798-106-17) bottles.
® SPECTAM is a Registered Trademark of Elf Sanofi
™ SCOUR-HALT is a Trademark of Elf Sanofi
Compendium Code No.: 10841501 893

SPECTAM® WATER SOLUBLE

Bimeda **Spectinomycin**

(Spectinomycin) Water Soluble Antibiotic
NADA No.: 038-661
Active Ingredient(s): Each gram contains spectinomycin dihydrochloride pentahydrate equivalent to 0.5 g of spectinomycin activity. Highly water-soluble, it will not clog proportioners. High stability assures effectiveness over extended periods.
Indications: SPECTAM® Water Soluble antibiotic is indicated as an aid in the prevention or control of broiler losses due to chronic respiratory disease (CRD) associated with *Mycoplasma gallisepticum* (MG) and infectious synovitis associated with *Mycoplasma synoviae* (MS). It is also indicated as an effective means of increasing rate of weight gain and improving feed efficiency in floor-raised broilers.
Dosage and Administration: Mix in drinking water according to dosage directions. This mixture should be the only source of water for the first three (3) days of life, and for one (1) day following each vaccination.
For CRD associated with MG: Add contents to 250 gallons of water to provide 2 g of spectinomycin activity per gallon. For proportioners, dissolve contents of one-half (½) package in one (1) gallon of water. Meter at one (1) oz/gal.
For infectious synovitis associated with MS: Add contents to 500 gallons of water to provide 1 g of spectinomycin activity per gallon. For proportioners, dissolve contents of one-half (½) package in two (2) gallons of water. Meter at one (1) oz/gal.
For increased rate of weight gain and improved feed efficiency in floor-raised broiler chickens: Dissolve one-quarter (¼) bottle (50 g) in 50 gallons of water to provide 0.5 g of spectinomycin activity per gallon. For proportioners, dissolve contents of one-half (½) package in four (4) gallons of water. Meter at one (1) oz/gal.
Warning(s): Do not administer this drug within five (5) days of slaughter.
Do not administer to laying chickens.
Presentation: 1,000 g screw top, plastic jar (500 g activity per jar).
Compendium Code No.: 13990350

SPECTINOMYCIN HYDROCHLORIDE INJECTABLE

Durvet **Spectinomycin Injection**

Anti-Infective for Turkey Poults and Newly-Hatched Chicks
ANADA No.: 200-127
Active Ingredient(s): Contains per mL: spectinomycin dihydrochloride pentahydrate equivalent to 100 mg spectinomycin per mL; also benzyl alcohol, 9.45 mg, added as a preservative; and sterile water for injection.
Indications: SPECTINOMYCIN HYDROCHLORIDE INJECTABLE is for use in turkey poults and baby chicks as shown below:
Poults:
1. As an aid in the control of Chronic Respiratory Disease (CRD) associated with *Escherichia coli*.
2. As an aid in the control of airsacculitis associated with *Mycoplasma meleagridis* sensitive to spectinomycin.

Chicks: As an aid in the control of mortality and to lessen severity of infections caused by *Mycoplasma synoviae, Salmonella typhimurium, Salmonella infantis*, and *E. coli*.
Dosage and Administration: SPECTINOMYCIN HYDROCHLORIDE INJECTABLE is intended only for subcutaneous injection. The injection should be made under the loose skin on the top of the neck, halfway between the head and the base of the neck.
Thoroughly clean and sterilize syringes and needles before using (needles and syringes may be sterilized by boiling in water for 15 minutes).
Use all precautions to prevent contamination of contents of bottle.
Injection site should be disinfected with a suitable disinfectant such as 70% isopropyl alcohol just prior to injecting SPECTINOMYCIN HYDROCHLORIDE INJECTABLE.
Poults:
1. As an aid in the control of Chronic Respiratory Disease (CRD) associated with *E. coli*, inject newly-hatched turkey poults with SPECTINOMYCIN HYDROCHLORIDE INJECTABLE (5 mg spectinomycin) subcutaneously. See dilution table below for 5 mg concentration in saline solution.
2. As an aid in the control of airsacculitis associated with *M. meleagridis* sensitive to spectinomycin, inject newly-hatched turkey poults with 0.1 mL of SPECTINOMYCIN HYDROCHLORIDE INJECTABLE (10 mg spectinomycin) subcutaneously.

Chicks: As an aid in the control of mortality and to lessen severity of infections caused by *M. synoviae, S. typhimurium, S. infantis*, and *E. coli*, inject newly-hatched chicks subcutaneously with SPECTINOMYCIN HYDROCHLORIDE INJECTABLE diluted with sterile physiological saline solution to provide 2.5 to 5.0 mg of spectinomycin in a 0.2 mL dose. See dilution table below for 2.5 mg or 5.0 mg concentration in saline solution.

mL SPECTINOMYCIN HYDROCHLORIDE INJECTABLE	Dilution Table To administer SPECTINOMYCIN HYDROCHLORIDE INJECTABLE containing 100 mg spectinomycin/mL		Dose/chick mL
	mL sterile saline	Number of doses	
To provide 2.5 mg per 0.2 mL diluted dose:			
500 (1 bottle)	3,500	20,000	0.2
1,000 (2 bottles)	7,000	40,000	0.2
To provide 5.0 mg per 0.2 mL diluted dose:			
500 (1 bottle)	1,500	10,000	0.2
1,000 (2 bottles)	3,000	20,000	0.2

Precaution(s): Store at controlled room temperature, 20° to 25°C (68° to 77°F) [see USP]. Protect from freezing.
Caution(s): For large flock administration only, utilizing appropriate equipment with aseptic techniques. Discard any diluted solution remaining.
To assure sterility, there should be only one entry into the bottle.
Rarely, some individuals who handle spectinomycin develop serious reactions involving skin, nails, and eyes. Individuals who have experienced rash or other evidence of allergic reactions should avoid further contact with spectinomycin.
Warning(s): For use in 1 to 3-day old turkey poults and newly-hatched chicks.
Not for human use. Keep out of the reach of children.
Restricted Drug - Use only as directed (California).
For use in animals only.
For subcutaneous injection in turkey poults and newly-hatched chicks only.
Discussion: SPECTINOMYCIN HYDROCHLORIDE INJECTABLE is a clear, sterile solution of spectinomycin (from spectinomycin dihydrochloride pentahydrate) intended for subcutaneous injection in newly-hatched baby chicks and turkey poults. It is stable under normal conditions of storage and possesses excellent flow characteristics that make possible the use of a fine-gauge needle for injection.
Spectinomycin has an extremely low degree of toxicity. Subcutaneous injections of up to 50 mg per poult have caused no detectable ill effects. Doses of 90 mg per poult have produced transient ataxia and coma from which poults recovered in approximately four hours. Under post-mortem examination, no local tissue reaction has been observed following the injection of SPECTINOMYCIN HYDROCHLORIDE INJECTABLE.
Presentation: SPECTINOMYCIN HYDROCHLORIDE INJECTABLE, 100 mg/mL, is available in 500 mL (16.9 fl oz) rubber-stoppered glass bottles.
Manufactured by: Boehringer Ingelheim Animal Health, Inc.
Compendium Code No.: 10841510

SPECTRASOL™

KenVet **Disinfectant**

EPA Reg. No.: 1839-166-36208
Active Ingredient(s):
Octyl decyl dimethyl ammonium chloride 3.255%
Dioctyl dimethyl ammonium chloride 1.628%
Didecyl dimethyl ammonium chloride 1.628%
Alkyl (50% C_{14}, 40% C_{12}, 10% C_{16}) dimethyl benzyl ammonium chloride 4.339%
Inert Ingredients 89.150%
Total 100.000%
Indications: A disinfectant, detergent and cleaner for use on hard, non-porous surfaces.

S

Directions for Use: It is a violation of Federal law to use this product in a manner inconsistent with its labeling.

SPECTRASOL™ Disinfectant is a phosphate-free formulation designed to provide effective cleaning, deodorizing, and disinfection for hospitals and other institutions where housekeeping is of prime importance in controlling cross-contamination from treated surfaces.

This product, when used as directed, is formulated to disinfect hard non-porous inanimate environmental surfaces such as floors, walls, metal surfaces, stainless steel surfaces, porcelain, glazed ceramic tile, plastic surfaces and cabinets. For larger areas such as operating rooms and patient care facilities, this product is designed to provide both general cleaning and disinfecting.

This product deodorizes those areas which generally are hard to keep fresh smelling, such as garbage storage areas, empty garbage bins and cans and other areas which are prone to odors caused by microorganisms.

This product is formulated to a neutral pH and will not dull high-gloss floor finishes with repeated use.

Disinfection: To disinfect inanimate, hard non-porous surfaces, add 1 oz of this product per gallon of water. Apply solution with a mop, cloth, sponge, or hand-pump trigger sprayer so as to wet all surfaces thoroughly. Allow to remain wet for 10 minutes, then remove excess liquid. For heavily soiled areas, a pre-cleaning step is required. Prepare a fresh solution for each use.

Efficacy tests have demonstrated that this product is an effective bactericide and virucide in water up to 400 ppm hardness (as $CaCO_3$) in the presence of organic soil (5% blood serum).

Deodorization: To deodorize, apply this product as indicated under the heading Disinfection.

Bactericidal Activity: At the 1 oz per gallon dilution, this product demonstrates effective disinfectant activity against the organisms: *Pseudomonas aeruginosa, Salmonella choleraesuis, Staphylococcus aureus, Staphylococcus aureus* (clinical isolate), *Bordetella bronchiseptica, Corynebacterium ammoniagenes, Enterobacter aerogenes, Enterobacter cloacae, Enterobacter cloacae* (clinical isolate), *Enterococcus faecalis, Enterococcus faecalis* (clinical isolate), *Escherichia coli, Escherichia coli* (clinical isolate), *Fusobacterium necrophorum, Klebsiella pneumoniae* subsp. *pneumoniae, Lactobacillus casei* subsp. *rhamnosus, Listeria monocytogenes, Pasteurella multocida, Proteus vulgaris, Proteus mirabilis* ATCC 9921, *Proteus mirabilis* ATCC 25933, *Salmonella choleraesuis* subsp. *choleraesuis* serotype paratyphi B, *Salmonella choleraesuis* subsp. *choleraesuis* serotype typhi, *Salmonella choleraesuis* subsp. *choleraesuis* serotype typhimurium, *Salmonella choleraesuis* subsp. *choleraesuis* serotype pullorum, *Serratia marcescens, Shigella sonnei, Shigella flexneri* Type 2b, *Shigella dysenteriae, Staphylococcus aureus* subsp. *aureus, Staphylococcus epidermidis, Staphylococcus epidermidis* (clinical isolate), *Streptococcus pyogenes* (Clinical - Fresh Eating Strain BIRD M3), *Streptococcus pyogenes* Group A, *Xanthamonas maltophilia* (clinical isolate), Vancomycin resistant *Enterococcus faecalis*, and Methicillin resistant *Staphylococcus aureus.*

Fungicidal Activity: At the 1 oz per gallon dilution, this product demonstrates effective fungicidal activity against the pathogenic fungi *Trichophyton mentagrophytes, Canadida albicans*, and *Aspergillus niger.*

Virucidal Activity: This product when used on environmental inanimate hard non porous surfaces at 1 ounce per gallon of water exhibits effective virucidal activity against HIV-1, HIV-2, Herpes Simplex Type 1 (causative agent of fever blisters), Herpes Simplex Type 2 (genital disease), Influenza A_2/Hong Kong, Vaccinia, Pseudorabies, Bovine Rhinotracheitis, Feline Leukemia, Feline Picornavirus, and Canine Distemper.

Precautionary Statements: Hazards to Humans and Domestic Animals:

Danger: Keep out of reach of children.

Corrosive.

Causes eye and skin damage. Do not get in eyes, on skin, or on clothing. Wear goggles or face shield and rubber gloves when handing. Harmful or fatal if swallowed. Avoid contamination of food. Remove contaminated clothing and wash before reuse. Wash thoroughly with soap and water after handling.

Statement of Practical Treatment:

In case of contact, immediately flush eyes or skin with plenty of water for at least 15 minutes. For eyes, call a physician.

If swallowed, drink large quantities of water. Avoid alcohol. Call a physician immediately.

Note to Physician: Probable mucosal damage may contraindicate the use of gastric lavage.

Storage and Disposal: Do not contaminate water, food, or feed by storage or disposal.

Storage: Store in a dry place no lower in temperature than 50°F or higher than 120°F.

Container Disposal: Do not reuse empty container. Triple rinse empty container with water. Return metal drum then offer for reconditioning or puncture and dispose of in a sanitary landfill, or by other procedures approves by State and local authorities. Plastic containers may be disposed of in a sanitary landfill, incinerated, or if allowed by local authorities, by burning. If burned, stay out of smoke.

Pesticide Disposal: Pesticide wastes are acutely hazardous. Improper disposal of excess pesticide, spray mixture, or rinsate is a violation of Federal Law. If these wastes cannot be disposed of by use according to label instructions, contact your State Pesticide or Environmental Control Agency, or the Hazardous Waste representative at the nearest EPA Regional Office for guidance.

Disclaimer: Except as expressly provided herein, neither Loveland nor seller makes any warranties, guarantees, or representations of any kind, either by usage of trade, statutory or otherwise, with regard to the product sold, including, but not limited to merchantability, fitness for a particular purpose, use or eligibility of the product for any particular trade usage.

Unintended consequences may result because of, but not limited to, such factors as presence of other materials, or the manner of use or application, all of which are beyond the control of Loveland Industries, Inc. or seller. In no case shall seller be liable for consequential, special, or indirect damages resulting from the use or handling of this product. All such risks shall be assumed by the buyer or user.

Applicator's or grower's exclusive remedy against Loveland Industries, Inc. or seller for any cause of action relating to the product is a claim for damages, and in no event shall damages or any other recovery exceed the purchase price of the product in respect of which such claim is made.

Presentation: 1 US gallon (3.785 L).

Compendium Code No.: 11340040

SPECTRUM™

Westfalia•Surge **Udder Wash**

High Detergency Chlorhexidine Udder Wash plus Skin Conditioners

Active Ingredient(s): Contents:

chlorhexidine digluconate 0.6%

n-alkyl (60% C_{14}, 30% C_{16}, 5% C_{12}, 5% C_{18})
dimethyl benzyl ammonium chlorides 3.5%

n-alkyl (68% C_{12}, 32% C_{14}) dimethyl ethylbenzyl ammonium chlorides 3.5%

Inactive Ingredients: 92.4%*

*Contains skin conditioning agents.

Indications: SPECTRUM™ is a high detergency chlorhexidine udder wash plus skin conditioners.

Directions for Use: Prepare an udder wash solution by adding 1 oz. (30 mL) of SPECTRUM™ for each 4 gallons (15.1 L) of warm 100 - 110°F (38 - 43°C) water. Use a clean single service towel for each cow. Soak the towel in the udder wash solution and wash and massage the udder and teats. Never reuse towel or dip used towel back into solution. Thoroughly dry udder and teats with a second single service towel. Do not use as a teat dip.

Precaution(s): Storage Instructions: Store this product in a cool, dry area away from direct sunlight or heat to avoid deterioration. If frozen, separation may occur. Thaw completely and mix thoroughly before use. Keep containers closed to prevent contamination of this product.

Precautionary Statements: Danger. Contains materials which will cause severe eye irritation and possibly burn the eyes. May cause skin irritation. May be harmful or fatal if swallowed. Protect eyes and skin when handling. Do not take internally. Avoid breathing vapors. Do not mix with any other chemical products. Refer to Material Safety Data Sheet (MSDS).

First Aid:

If in Eyes: Flush with large volumes of water for at least 15 minutes. Call a physician immediately.

If Swallowed: Do not induce vomiting. Rinse mouth promptly, then give a large quantity of water. Avoid alcohol. Call a physician immediately. Do not give anything by mouth to an unconscious or convulsing person.

If on Skin: Flush with large volumes of water for at least 15 minutes while removing contaminated clothing and shoes. If irritation develops and persists, get medical attention.

Inhalation of Vapors: If breathing difficulty or irritation occurs, remove to fresh air. If symptoms persist, get medical attention.

For assistance with medical emergency, call 1-800-451-8346.

For farm, commercial and industrial use only.

Warning(s): Keep out of reach of children.

Presentation: Contact the company for container sizes available.

SPECTRUM is a Trademark of Westfalia•Surge, Inc.

Compendium Code No.: 10020260 Rev. 03-00

SPEC-TUSS™ ℞

Neogen **Expectorant**

Palatable Expectorant Powder

Active Ingredient(s): Contains:

Guaifenesin U.S.P. .... 7% (w/w)

Ammonium Chloride .... 75% (w/w)

Potassium Iodide U.S.P. .... 2% (w/w)

In a sweetened, flavored, palatable base.

Indications: A palatable powder used as an expectorant in horses.

Directions: Dissolve 1 lb in one gallon of water to make stock solution.

Dosage: Mix one pint of stock solution with 15 to 25 gallons of drinking water or ½ to 1 oz stock solution 3 times daily. ½-1 oz of SPEC-TUSS™ may be given in food or drinking water daily. For best results, animal should be kept on medicated food or water for 3-4 days.

One pound of SPEC-TUSS™ medicates 200-400 gallons of drinking water.

Caution(s): Federal law restricts this drug to use by or on the order of a licensed veterinarian.

For the horse only. For animal use only.

Warning(s): Keep out of reach of children.

Presentation: 1 lb (454 g) (NDC: 59051-8867-0).

Compendium Code No.: 14910401 L103-0701

SPF-LAC®

Pet-Ag **Milk Replacer**

Active Ingredient(s): Guaranteed Analysis:

Crude protein, min. 4.0%

Crude fat, min. 5.0%

Crude fiber .... None

Moisture, max. 85.0%

Ash, max. 1.0%

Ingredients: Skimmed milk, water, vegetable oils, casein, dextrose, glyceryl mono-stearate, tricalcium phosphate, sodium bicarbonate, carrageenan, choline chloride, iron sulfate, vitamin A supplement, vitamin E supplement, zinc sulfate, niacin supplement, calcium pantothenate, vitamin B_{12} supplement, copper sulfate, manganese sulfate, riboflavin, vitamin D_3 supplement, thiamine hydrochloride, menadione sodium bisulfite complex (source of vitamin K), pyridoxine hydrochloride, potassium iodide, and biotin.

Indications: A complete ready-to-feed, sterile formula for use as a replacement for the milk of sow's and other species having similar milk composition.

Dosage and Administration: SPF-LAC® Feeding Directions:

Laboratory Use: Originally developed for SPF pigs, SPF-LAC® is suitable for laboratory's conducting germ-free, specific pathogen free, or nutritional experiments requiring either sterile or conventional environments for newborn orphaned pigs and other animals. Feeding levels and frequency will vary with specific requirements of the animals and the experimental design.

Feeding Directions for Orphaned Pigs: It is always desirable for pigs or any animal to have access to colostrum milk. Special care and veterinary guidance may be necessary if colostrum milk is not available.

SPF-LAC® can be fed from a dish or pan. They will require auxiliary heat if less than one (1) week old. Maintain clean, dry quarters and wash all utensils.

First Week: Feed about one (1) can (12 oz.) per pig per day divided into three (3) meals. Offer a high milk prestarter on the fourth or fifth day. Make fresh water available when pigs start consuming dry feed.

Second and Third Weeks: Increase the amount of SPF-LAC® gradually to 18 oz. or 24 oz. per day divided into three (3) feedings. The quantity will depend upon the amount of prestarter consumed. SPF-LAC® can be decreased as prestarter consumption becomes significant. If necessary, mixing the prestarter with SPF-LAC® encourages consumption of dry-feed. SPF-LAC® can be discontinued during the third week.

Supplementing Nursing Pigs: SPF-LAC® is a supplement for use with nursing pigs particularly if there are large litters, runty pigs, or an inadequate milk supply from the sow.

A daily feeding of 4 oz. to 6 oz. is suggested. If nursing pigs do not readily drink SPF-LAC® from a dish or pan, bottle or tube feeding may be required.

A veterinarian should be consulted for advice about the care and feeding of pigs.

Precaution(s): Shake well. Refrigerate SPF-LAC® after opening. Discard after 72 hours. Do not freeze.

Presentation: 12.5 fl. oz. (355 mL) cans (12 per case).

Compendium Code No.: 10970251

SPRAVAC®

United **Vaccine**

Mink Distemper Vaccine, Modified Live Virus

U.S. Vet. Lic. No.: 245

Active Ingredient(s): The vaccine consists of two components: A freeze-dried distemper vaccine consisting of modified live canine distemper virus (SPRAVAC®) and a sterile diluent. The diluent is used to dissolve the SPRAVAC®.

Preservatives: Gentamicin and thimerosal.

Indications: SPRAVAC® is for use as an aid in the prevention of distemper in healthy, susceptible mink by spray administration.

Dosage and Administration: Mixing of the Vaccine:

1. Do not mix the vaccine until ready for use.
2. Mix only one pair of vials at a time, and use the entire contents within two (2) hours.
3. Disinfect rubber stoppers with alcohol.
4. Using a sterile transfer needle, transfer the diluent into the bottle of SPRAVAC®.
5. To do this, insert the short end of the double-pointed transfer needle into the diluent and turn the bottle upside down; then, insert the other end of the transfer needle into the SPRAVAC®. The diluent will be drawn into the SPRAVAC® bottle by vacuum.
6. After all the diluent has been transferred, shake gently to suspend evenly.

Dosage: Spray vaccinate mink of at least 10 weeks of age for 15 seconds, followed by an additional 3-minute contact. Up to six (6) mink per nest box may be vaccinated at one time.

Administration:

1. Use the atomizer distributed by United and the vaccine supplied in the package for spray distemper immunization of mink. The vaccine has been specially prepared for spray administration, and the atomizer has been calibrated to deliver the correct dose to each mink.
2. Before using the atomizer, make sure that the three (3) tiny capillary holes in the generator and the edges of the striking plate are clean of vaccine particles. (See #9).
3. Vaccinate on relatively calm days, preferably in the early morning or evening. Air drafts will tend to dissipate the vaccine spray and make it less effective.
4. Remove the tear away aluminum seal and stopper from the vaccine bottle and pour the vaccine into the reservoir of the sprayer, down through the chimney.
5. With the hose and connector supplied, attach the assembled atomizer to a source of compressed air regulated at 25 p.s.i (1.7 atmosphere, 1.76 kg/cm^2).
6. Enclose the mink to be vaccinated in nest boxes and holding the sprayer in an upright position, direct spray into the box for 15 seconds. Keep mink enclosed and in contact with the vapors for three (3) minutes. On extremely warm days, do not leave the mink enclosed for longer than three (3) minutes because of the danger of overheating.
7. Make sure that there is no interruption in spray coming from the nozzle. If the spray emits from the chimney instead of the nozzle, adjust the chimney up or down from the 5/8" (16 mm) height set at United until the spray comes out of the nozzle.
8. Discard the last 1 mL of vaccine remaining in the reservoir since the volume of spray is less consistent and the spray head will not deliver the vaccine uniformly enough to assure effective immunization.
9. Dismantle and clean the upper portions of the atomizer with soap and warm water before and after use. Rinse thoroughly with warm water and let air dry before reassembly. Do not disinfect with chemicals as they can leave residues that could kill the virus and destroy the vaccine.
10. Keep a record of brand name, quantity, serial number, expiration date, and place of purchase. Record the date of vaccination, the number, age and location of the mink.

Consult a veterinarian or United Vaccines Inc. for an alternate vaccinating schedule and before using the vaccine on a farm where disease exists or has occurred in the last 18 months.

Precaution(s): Store at 35-45°F (2-7°C).

Caution(s):

1. Burn the empty containers and any unused portion of the vaccine.
2. Incubating diseases (such as Aleutian disease), parasites, nutritional deficiencies (anemia), maternal antibodies and poor management practices (dehydration, adverse temperatures) will reduce the vaccine's effectiveness.
3. If shock occurs after vaccination, use atropine sulfate or epinephrine.
4. Should disease occur in an unvaccinated herd, the losses may be minimized by promptly vaccinating those animals which are not showing signs of the disease. The best procedure is to first vaccinate the mink located the farthest distance from those showing symptoms. Care should be taken to use a sterile needle for each animal and to disinfect handling gloves as often as is practical. Consult a veterinarian regarding the treatment and handling of sick animals.
5. Animals infected, yet not showing signs of disease at the time of vaccination, will not be protected by the vaccine. Symptoms of the disease may continue to develop for as long as two months after vaccination.

Presentation: 100 nest box doses.

Compendium Code No.: 11040110

S

SS PAC®

Schering-Plough **Bacterin**

Streptococcus suis Bacterin

U.S. Vet. Lic. No.: 301

Contents: *Streptococcus suis* serotype 2 bacterin, porcine isolates.

Contains gentamicin as preservative.

Indications: For vaccination of healthy pigs to aid in the prevention of meningitis, arthritis, pneumonia and septicemia caused by *Streptococcus suis* serotype 2.

Dosage and Administration: Read directions carefully before use. Shake occasionally during use. Administer a 1 mL dose intramuscularly to pigs at 10-12 days of age, followed by a 2 mL dose at approximately 3-5 weeks of age. This repeat dose is essential for maximum immune response. For best results, inject into the neck musculature behind the ear. Use sterile syringes and needles. Annual revaccination of breeding swine is recommended.

Precaution(s): Store at 2-7°C (35-45°F). Do not freeze.

Caution(s): Use entire contents when first opened. Transient local reactions may be observed at the injection site. If allergic reaction occurs, administer epinephrine.

Warning(s): Do not vaccinate within 60 days of slaughter.

Extreme caution should be used when injecting any oil emulsion vaccine to avoid injecting your finger or hand. Accidental injection can cause serious local reaction. Contact a physician immediately if accidental injection occurs. For veterinary use only.

Discussion: Disease caused by *Streptococcus suis* serotype 2 is usually introduced into a herd by healthy carrier pigs. Infection usually strikes young pigs - up to 130 pounds - causing sudden death, brain damage, pneumonia and arthritis, as well as slow growth. The *S. suis* bacterium is transmitted from pig to pig by nose-to-nose contact. Non-immune adults can also be affected. Infection is most prevalent in confined systems with high population density. Although outbreaks may be more frequent fall-to-spring or after sudden changes to colder weather, modern management conditions allow *S. suis* to occur year around. *S. suis* organisms harbor in nasal cavities and can persist in the tonsils of healthy carrier pigs even in the presence of antibodies and in pigs receiving penicillin-medicated feed for up to 512 days. In most cases clinical signs include a progression of anorexia, depression, reddening of skin, fever, incoordination, paralysis, paddling, opisthotonus, tremors and convulsions. In peracute cases, however, pigs may be found dead with no warning signs. The *S. suis* organism is commonly found in nearly all areas in which hogs are raised.

Presentation: 100 mL and 250 mL multiple dose vials.

Compendium Code No.: 10471851

STABILIZED-C

Alpharma **Water Additive**

Ingredient(s): Stabilized ascorbic acid.

Guaranteed Analysis: Per pack:

Ascorbic Acid . . . . 146 g

Indications: A stabilized vitamin concentrate for use in the drinking water of chickens, turkeys and swine.

Directions: Mix 1 pack (219 g) in 128 gallons of drinking water to produce 300 ppm ascorbic acid. Mix 1 pack (219 g) in 256 gallons of drinking water to produce 150 ppm ascorbic acid.

Precaution(s): Store in cool, dry place.

Caution(s): For oral animal use only. Not for human use. Keep out of reach of children

Presentation: 7.75 oz (219 g) packet.

Compendium Code No.: 10220581 AHF-026A 0005

STAFAC® 10

Phibro **Feed Medication**

Brand of Virginiamycin-Type A Medicated Article

NADA No.: 091-513

Active Ingredient(s):

Virginiamycin 2.2%

(Contains 10 g virginiamycin activity per lb)

Ingredients: Processed grain by-products, roughage products, calcium carbonate, carboxymethylcellulose

Indications: Improved feed efficiency. Increased rate of weight gain. Mix with swine and poultry feed.

Directions for Use: Important: Must be diluted in feed before use.

Mixing Directions: STAFAC® 10 Type A Medicated Article must be thoroughly mixed in the feed to assure even distribution. Determine the appropriate amount of STAFAC® 10 required from the table below. Dilute STAFAC® 10 with a portion of one of the feed ingredients (enough to make a quantity equal to 10 lb per ton) before final mixing.

Swine	Required level of virginiamycin activity per ton of Type C Medicated Feed (complete feed)	Required amount of STAFAC® 10 per ton of Type C Medicated Feed (complete feed)	Amount of virginiamycin activity provided to animal per lb body weight per day
Continuous Feed Programs From Weaning to Market Weight			
Weaning to 120 lb Increased rate of weight gain and improved feed efficiency	10 g	1.0 lb	
120 lb to market weight Increased rate of weight gain Improved feed efficiency	5-10 g 5 g	0.5-1.0 lb 0.5 lb	
Treatment of swine dysentery in nonbreeding swine weighing over 120 lb	100 g for 2 weeks	10.0 lb	2.27 mg
Treatment and control of swine dysentery in swine weighing up to 120 lb	100 g for 2 weeks followed by 50 g	10.0 lb 5.0 lb	2.27 mg 1.14 mg
Aid in control of swine dysentery in swine weighing up to 120 lb For use in animals or on premises with a history of swine dysentery but where symptoms have not yet occurred	25 g	2.5 lb	0.57 mg

Poultry	Required level of virginiamycin activity per ton of Type C Medicated Feed (complete feed)	Required amount of Stafac 10 per ton of Type C Medicated Feed (complete feed)
For use in broiler chickens Increased rate of weight gain Improved feed efficiency Prevention of necrotic enteritis caused by *Clostridium perfringens* susceptible to virginiamycin	5-15 g 5 g 20 g	0.5-1.5 lb 0.5 lb 2.0 lb
For use in growing turkeys Increased rate of weight gain and improved feed efficiency	10-20 g	1.0-2.0 lb

Feed continuously as sole ration.

Precaution(s): Store in cool, dry place. Close container after use.

Warning(s): Not for use in laying chickens.

Toxicology: STAFAC®-medicated feeds when used as directed can be safely administered to swine without fear of animal toxicity, residue problems, or environmental pollution. These aspects have been subjects of definitive laboratory studies. The safety and efficacy of virginiamycin have been demonstrated in numerous university and farm trials.

Presentation: 50 lb (22.7 kg) multiwall bag.
STAFAC is a registered trademark of Phibro Animal Health, for virginiamycin.
Active ingredient virginiamycin manufactured in Rixensart, Belgium, by Phibro Animal Health.
U.S. Patent Nos. 3,325,359 and 3,627,885; for use under U.S. Patent No. 3,017,272
Compendium Code No.: 36930141

STAFAC® 20

Phibro **Feed Medication**

Brand of Virginiamycin-Type A Medicated Article
NADA No.: 091-467
Active Ingredient(s):
Virginiamycin 4.4%
(Contains 20 g virginiamycin activity per lb)
Ingredients: Processed grain by-products, roughage products, calcium carbonate, carboxymethylcellulose
Indications: Improved feed efficiency. Increased rate of weight gain. Mix with swine and poultry feed.
Directions for Use: Important: Must be diluted in feed before use.
Mixing Directions: STAFAC® 20 Type A Medicated Article must be thoroughly mixed in the feed to assure even distribution. Determine the appropriate amount of STAFAC® 20 required from the table below. Dilute STAFAC® 20 with a portion of one of the feed ingredients (enough to make a quantity equal to 10 lb per ton) before final mixing.

Swine	Required level of virginiamycin activity per ton of Type C Medicated Feed (complete feed)	Required amount of Stafac 20 per ton of Type C Medicated Feed (complete feed)	Amount of virginiamycin activity provided to animal per lb body weight per day
Continuous Feed Programs From Weaning to Market Weight			
Weaning to 120 lb Increased rate of weight gain and improved feed efficiency	10 g	0.50 lb	
120 lb to market weight Increased rate of weight gain Improved feed efficiency	5-10 g 5 g	0.25-0.50 lb 0.25 lb	
Treatment of swine dysentery in nonbreeding swine weighing over 120 lb	100 g for 2 weeks	5.00 lb	2.27 mg
Treatment and control of swine dysentery in swine weighing up to 120 lb	100 g for 2 weeks followed by 50 g	5.00 lb 2.50 lb	2.27 mg 1.14 mg
Aid in control of swine dysentery in swine weighing up to 120 lb For use in animals or on premises with a history of swine dysentery but where symptoms have not yet occurred	25 g	1.25 lb	0.57 mg

Poultry	Required level of virginiamycin activity per ton of Type C Medicated Feed (complete feed)	Required amount of Stafac 20 per ton of Type C Medicated Feed (complete feed)
For use in broiler chickens Increased rate of weight gain Improved feed efficiency Prevention of necrotic enteritis caused by *Clostridium perfringens* susceptible to virginiamycin	 5-15 g 5 g 20 g	 0.25-0.75 lb 0.25 lb 1.00 lb
For use in growing turkeys Increased rate of weight gain and improved feed efficiency	10-20 g	0.50-1.00 lb

Feed continuously as sole ration.
Precaution(s): Store in cool, dry place. Close container after use.
Warning(s): Not for use in laying chickens.
Toxicology: STAFAC®-medicated feeds when used as directed can be safely administered to swine without fear of animal toxicity, residue problems, or environmental pollution. These aspects have been subjects of definitive laboratory studies. The safety and efficacy of virginiamycin have been demonstrated in numerous university and farm trials.
Presentation: 50 lb (22.7 kg) multiwall bag.
STAFAC is a registered trademark of Phibro Animal Health, for virginiamycin.
Active ingredient virginiamycin manufactured in Rixensart, Belgium, by Phibro Animal Health.
U.S. Patent Nos. 3,325,359 and 3,627,885; for use under U.S. Patent No. 3,017,272
Compendium Code No.: 36930151

STAFAC® 500

Phibro **Feed Medication**

(virginiamycin) Type A Medicated Article
NADA No.: 091-467
Active Ingredient(s):
Virginiamycin 50%
(Contains 227 g virginiamycin activity per lb)
Inert Ingredients: Calcium carbonate, carboxymethylcellulose, mineral oil
Indications: Mix with swine and poultry feed.
For use in swine and poultry feeds as specified below.
Directions for Use: Important: Must be diluted in feed before use.
Mixing Directions—Swine: STAFAC® 500 Type A Medicated Article must be thoroughly mixed in the feed to assure even distribution. Determine the appropriate amount of STAFAC® 500 required from the table below. Dilute STAFAC® 500 with a portion of one of the feed ingredients (enough to make a quantity equal to 10 lb per ton) before final mixing.

Swine	Required level of virginiamycin activity per ton of Type C Medicated Feed (complete feed)	Required amount of STAFAC® 500 per ton of Type C Medicated Feed (complete feed)	Amount of virginiamycin activity provided to animal per lb body weight per day
Continuous Feed Programs From Weaning to Market Weight			
Weaning to 120 lb Increased rate of weight gain and improved feed efficiency	10 g	20 g	
120 lb to market weight Increased rate of weight gain Improved feed efficiency	5-10 g 5 g	10-20 g 10 g	
Treatment of swine dysentery in nonbreeding swine weighing over 120 lb	100 g for 2 weeks	200 g	2.27 mg
Treatment and control of swine dysentery in swine weighing up to 120 lb	100 g for 2 weeks followed by 50 g	200 g 100 g	2.27 mg 1.14 mg
Aid in control of swine dysentery in swine weighing up to 120 lb For use in animals or on premises with a history of swine dysentery but where symptoms have not yet occurred	25 g	50 g	0.57 mg

Mixing Directions—Poultry: Mix 100 g STAFAC® 500 with enough of one of the feed ingredients to make 10 lb of an intermediate mix. Add 1 lb of the intermediate mix for each 5 g of virginiamycin needed to medicate a ton of feed.

Poultry	Required level of virginiamycin activity per ton of Type C Medicated Feed (complete feed)	Required amount of STAFAC® 500 per ton of Type C Medicated Feed (complete feed)
For use in broiler chickens Increased rate of weight gain Improved feed efficiency Prevention of necrotic enteritis caused by *Clostridium perfringens* susceptible to virginiamycin	 5-15 g 5 g 20 g	 10-30 g 10 g 40 g
For use in growing turkeys Increased rate of weight gain and improved feed efficiency	10-20 g	20-40 g

Feed continuously as sole ration.
Precaution(s): Store in dry place, below 25°C/77°F. Close container after use.
Warning(s): Not for use in laying chickens.
Presentation: 25 kg package.
U.S. Patent Nos. 3,325,359 and 3,627,885; for use under U.S. Patent No. 3,017,272.
Compendium Code No.: 36930330 301-8001-01

STAM-N-AID™ ℞

Neogen **Equine Dietary Supplement**

Guaranteed Analysis:

Nutrient	Per Lb	Per 3 oz Daily Supplement
Vitamin A	150 000 IU	28 000 IU
Vitamin D_3	21 000 USPU	3940 USPU
Vitamin E	5500 IU	1000 IU
Vitamin K	65 mg	12 mg
Thiamine (B_1)	225 mg	42 mg
Riboflavin (B_2)	250 mg	45 mg
d-Calcium Pantothenate	250 mg	55 mg
Niacin	1000 mg	180 mg
Pyridoxine (B_6)	850 mg	150 mg
Folic Acid	110 mg	20 mg
Vitamin B_{12}	2.5 mg	0.469 mg
Choline Chloride	4000 mg	750 mg
Biotin	5.5 mg	1.0 mg
Inositol	2200 mg	410 mg
Bioflavonoids	550 mg	100 mg
Rutin	550 mg	100 mg
Ascorbic Acid (Vitamin C)	1000 mg	180 mg
L-Lysine	6000 mg	1125 mg
Methionine	5400 mg	1000 mg
Magnesium	1500 mg	280 mg
Manganese*	1500 mg	280 mg
Iron*	1400 mg	260 mg
Copper*	375 mg	70 mg
Zinc*	2135 mg	400 mg
Iodine (organic)	20 mg	3 mg
Cobalt	55 mg	10 mg
Selenium	4.5 mg	0.9 mg
Potassium	8880 mg	1650 mg
Crude protein not less than	100 g (22.2%)	18880 mg

S

Nutrient	Per Lb	Per 3 oz Daily Supplement
Crude fat not less than	8 g (1.8%)	1.5 g
Crude fiber not less than	36 g (8.0%)	6.75 g

*Chelated Minerals

Ingredients: Feed supplement form of Vitamins A (acetate), DS (irradiated 7 dehydrocholesterol), E (dl-alpha tocopheryl acetate), K (MSBC), B_1, B_2, B_6, B_{12}, d-calcium pantothenate, niacin, folic acid, biotin, inositol, rutin, citrus bioflavonoids, choline chloride; l-lysine, methionine selenium; chelated manganese, iron, copper and zinc; apple flavor; ethoxyquin (antioxidant); processed grain by-products; dried fermented corn extratives; dried brewers yeast; dried extracted Streptomyces meal and fermentation solubles: dried extracted *Ashbya gossypfi* fermentation meal; dried *Aspergillus niger* fermentation solubles: dried *propionibacterium* fermentation solubles; dried *Bacillus subtillis* fermentation solubles; dried extracted *penicillium* meal, fermentation solubles and molasses.

In addition to the listed nutrients, the ingredients of STAM-N-AID™ supply, xanthophyll, and the following array of amino acids-arginine, cystine, glutamic acid, glycine, histidine, isoleucine, leucine, lysine, methionine, phenylalanine, threonine, tryptophan, tyrosine and valine.

Indications: A dietary supplement for the performance horse.

Dosage and Administration: 1 measure (3 oz) daily, mixed with the grain portion of the diet.

Caution(s): Federal law prohibits this drug to sale or use by or on the order of a licensed veterinarian. For animal use only.

Warning(s): Keep out of reach of children.

Presentation: 5 lb (NDC: 59051-8869-7) and 25 lb.

Compendium Code No.: 14910411 L110-1101 / L146-1101

STANISOL

Q.A. Laboratories **Topical Wound Dressing**

Active Ingredient(s): Each mL contains:

Salicylic acid .... 10.0 mg
Tannic acid .... 57.0 mg
Boric acid .... 26.0 mg

In an isopropanol, propylene glycol base.

Indications: For use as a topical application in the management of moist dermatitis in dogs and cats, and weeping skin wounds in large animals.

Dosage and Administration: Spray onto the affected areas. Repeat at 6- to 8-hour intervals until the lesion is dry. Continue using once a day until healing is complete. The solution may sting for a short time when initially applied.

Precaution(s): Store at a controlled room temperature, between 15-30°C (59-86°F).

Caution(s): Harmful if swallowed. Contact the nearest poison center immediately. Avoid contact with the eyes and mucous membranes.

Keep out of the reach of children. For external veterinary use only.

Presentation: 4 fl. oz. spray bottles.

Compendium Code No.: 13680060

STAPHAGE LYSATE (SPL)®

Delmont **Immunostimulant**

Staphylococcus Aureus Phage Lysate

U.S. Vet. Lic. No.: 339

Contents: Each milliliter contains: 120-180 million colony-forming unit equivalents of *S. aureus* and at least 100 million staphylococcus bacteriophage plaque-forming units.

Staphylococcus Aureus Phage Lysate — STAPHAGE LYSATE (SPL)® — is a bacteriologically sterile staphylococcal vaccine containing the components of *S. aureus*, a bacteriophage, and some culture medium ingredients (sodium chloride and ultrafiltered beef heart infusion broth) in solution.

SPL® is prepared by lysing cultures of *S. aureus*, Cowan Serologic Types I & III, with a polyvalent staphylococcus bacteriophage. Bacteriologic sterility is achieved by ultrafiltration. No chemical preservatives or inactivants are used in its preparation.

SPL® is standardized on the basis of bacterial cell count before phage lysis.

Indications: SPL® is indicated for the treatment of canine pyoderma and related staphylococcal hypersensitivity, or polymicrobial skin infections with a staphylococcal component.[2-9]

The use of SPL® has not been shown to affect adversely other treatment modalities, although the concomitant use of systemic corticosteroids is not advised. Abnormal thyroid conditions should be corrected before beginning therapy. The concomitant use of antibiotics may be beneficial.

Pharmacology: Clinical Pharmacology: Under experimental conditions, *S. aureus* or its cellular components induces cell-meditated immunity.[1]

In vitro, SPL® has been shown to stimulate lymphocyte responses in both T- and B-cell subpopulations in the blood of normal human subjects.

In canine pyoderma studies, SPL® has been used to treat and prevent recurrent skin infections.

These findings support the interpretation that SPL® in staphylococcal-sensitized subjects acts as an immunopotentiator of cell-meditated immunity.

Animal Pharmacology: An increased capability of macrophages to inactivate staphylococci has been demonstrated in laboratory animals following SPL® treatment.

SPL® also has been shown to act as an immunomodulator.

Dosage and Administration: SPL® is administered by subcutaneous injection. The severity of the infection and the response of the patient should be the guiding factors in adjusting the dosage regimen.

All highly allergic patients (or those predisposed to allergy) should first be skin-tested to assess their relative sensitivity to SPL®.

Although the chance of allergic reactions is very small, the patient should be observed for 45 minutes to 1 hour for immediate and for 48 hours for delayed reactions. Allergic reactions you might observe include weakness, vomiting, diarrhea, severe itching, and fast breathing.

For chronic, recurrent, refractory, or deep-seated infections, it may be necessary to increase cautiously the frequency and/or the dose to achieve the desired therapeutic response.

Following the initial injection, subsequent injections should avoid previous injection sites.

If an undue amount of local redness, itching, and/or swelling ensues, await a partial subsidence of the reactions, proceed with ½ the previous dose, and make incremental increases at longer intervals.

Staphylococcal infections or staphylococcal hypersensitivity:

Allergic Patients:

Skin Test — 0.05-0.1 mL intradermally.

Therapy — Initially, 0.2 mL subcutaneously, then incremental increases of 0.2 mL once a week to 1.0 mL (a total of 5 injections). When you reach 1.0 mL, continue weekly injections of 1.0 mL for approximately 10-12 weeks.

Nonallergic Patients[2]:

Skin Test — Not required for nonallergic patients.

Therapy — 0.5 mL subcutaneously 2 times a week for 10 to 12 weeks, then 0.5 to 1.0 mL every 1 or 2 weeks.

Concomitant antibiotic therapy is recommended for an initial 4- to 6-week period.

The maximum dose should be decreased in small dogs and can be increased cautiously, if necessary, in large dogs to 1.5 mL. This dose is continued until improvement is demonstrated, then the interval may be lengthened gradually to the longest interval that maintains adequate clinical control.

Contraindication(s): There are no known contraindications to the use of SPL® except that in highly allergic patients reduced desensitizing doses may be indicated.

Precaution(s): Store at 2-7°C (36-45°F). Do not freeze.

SPL® does not contain a preservative; therefore, it must be handled aseptically. Do not use if it becomes cloudy. (This would indicate contamination.) Use entire contents when first opened.

Caution(s): A separate, sterile syringe and needle should be used for each individual, and aseptic technique must be used in removing doses from either the 1 mL ampules or the 10 mL vials.

Caution should be exercised when administering SPL® to highly allergic patients (or those predisposed to allergy). See under Dosage and Administration.

In common with all antigens employed to stimulate the production of antibodies that are protective in the event of subsequent disease, SPL® presents the remote potential of host sensitization to staphylococcal or bovine protein. Although anaphylaxis-type reactions are rare, the clinician must bear this possibility in mind. Epinephrine and atropine are antidotes.

SPL® may cause vaccine-type or site-of-injection reactions (see under Adverse Reactions) and, if excessive, these reactions may be lessened by dose reduction.

Toxicology: Reproduction studies performed in rats and rabbits revealed no evidence of impaired fertility or harm to the fetus due to SPL®.

Adverse Reactions: SPL® may cause general vaccine-type reactions (i.e., malaise, fever, and/or chills). If excessive, these reactions may be lessened by dose reduction.

Transient reactions at the site of injection (i.e., redness, itching, and/or swelling) may occur in 2 to 3 hours and may last up to 3 days, steadily decreasing. If excessive, these reactions may be lessened by dose reduction.

References: Available upon request.

Presentation: SPL® (Serologic Types I & III) is supplied in: 1 mL ampules, boxes of 10, and 10 mL multidose vials.

Compendium Code No.: 11240002 V-106

STAPHYLOCOCCUS AUREUS BACTERIN-TOXOID

Hygieia **Bacterin-Toxoid**

Staphylococcus Aureus Bacterin-Toxoid

CA Vet. Biol. Lic. No.: 86

Contents: STAPHYLOCOCCUS AUREUS BACTERIN-TOXOID incorporates both cellular and toxoid antigens believed to be important in bovine mastitis. It utilizes a Freund's Incomplete type of oil adjuvant for maximum immune stimulation. In field trials, this vaccine has been shown to be safe for administration during lactation and pregnancy. The vaccine contains no antibiotics, so no milk withdrawal is required following vaccination of lactating animals.

Indications: This product is intended for use in otherwise healthy animals as an aid in the reduction of *Staphylococcus aureus* mastitis, in dairy cows and heifers.

Directions for Use: Administer 5 cc subcutaneously using a clean technique. Three doses spaced one month apart are recommended.

Precaution(s): Keep refrigerated at 35-47°F. Do not freeze. Shake well before using.

Entire contents of this bottle should be used when first opened.

Caution(s): This product contains an oil adjuvant. In the event of accidental self-injection, seek medical attention immediately.

Administration should be under the supervision of a licensed veterinarian. Occasionally anaphylactic or other adverse reactions may occur. If adverse reactions occur, appropriate therapy with epinephrine or other antianaphylactic drugs should be instituted immediately. Any adverse reactions following vaccination should be immediately reported to the manufacturer.

For sale in California only.

Warning(s): Do not vaccinate within 42 days of slaughter.

Discussion: Disease: *Staphylococcus aureus* is a gram-positive bacteria capable of causing severe mastitis and even death in susceptible dairy cows. Typically the bacteria colonize the udder and teat canal and generates a subclinical, chronic infection which responds, poorly to treatment. The reservoir of infection is the infected udder, and the organism is readily transmitted to uninfected herdmates at milking. In herds with subclinical mastitis due to *Staphylococcus aureus*, more than 30% of the animals may be infected. Most pathogenic strains produce toxins.

Vaccine: STAPHYLOCOCCUS AUREUS BACTERIN-TOXOID incorporates both cellular and toxoid antigens believed to be important in bovine mastitis. It utilizes a Freund's Incomplete type of oil adjuvant for maximum immune stimulation. In field trials, this vaccine has been shown to be safe for administration during lactation and pregnancy. The vaccine contains no antibiotics, so no milk withdrawal is required following vaccination of lactating animals.

Benefits: This vaccine has been shown to decrease shedding rates of *Staphylococcus aureus* bacteria when used according to label directions in infected animals. In controlled trials, vaccinates were significantly less likely to yield milk cultures positive for *Staphylococcus aureus* and showed significant improvement in milk quality by thirty days post-vaccination as shown by CMT scores. Unvaccinated control animals were four times more likely to be culled for mastitis than vaccinates.

Presentation: Available in 50 dose (250 cc) bottles.

Compendium Code No.: 15060030 Rev. 10/00

START TO FINISH® ENERGY PAK™ 100

Milk Specialties **Large Animal Dietary Supplement**

Nutritional Contents:

Crude Fat, not less than 99.0%
Free Fatty Acids, not more than 10%
Moisture, not more than 0.6%
Color .... white

Typical Fatty Acid Analysis (based on % of product):

C14:0 (myrisitic) 1.4%
C16:0 (palmitic) 28.0%
C16:1 (palmitoleic) 0.5%
C17:0 (heptadecanoic) 0.7%
C18:0 (stearic) 52.0%
C18:1 (oleic) 11.5%
C20:0 (eicsanoic) 1.5%
C20:1 (eicosenoic) 0.4%

S

Ingredients: ENERGY PAK™ 100 is manufactured by partially hydrogenating refined and deodorized animal fat. It is prilled to form a tiny spherical beadlet. The fat is stabilized to ensure maximum shelf life.

Indications: ENERGY PAK™ 100 is a dense source of calories for the performance horse.

Dosage and Administration: It should be added to the horse's grain mix at the rate of 2.5-5%.

Discussion: ENERGY PAK™ 100 contains 100% pure animal fat. It is white in color and is prilled to form a free flowing beadlet.

The white prilled ENERGY PAK™ 100 is non-dusty with a pleasant caramel aroma. It is ideal for pelleted feeds or for mixing with the horse's grain mix.

Presentation: Available in 50 lb bags.

Compendium Code No.: 10850110

START TO FINISH® MARE & FOAL PELLETS™

Milk Specialties — **Large Animal Dietary Supplement**

Nutritional Contents:

Crude Protein, not less than	30.0%
Crude Fat, not less than	10.0%
Crude Fiber, not more than	1.5%
Calcium, not less than	2.9%
Calcium, not more than	3.8%
Phosphorus, not less than	1.6%
Vitamin A, not less than	25,000 IU/lb
Vitamin D_3, not less than	2,600 IU/lb
Vitamin E, not less than	150 IU/lb
Trace Minerals:	
Magnesium	0.25%
Iron	380 ppm
Cobalt	11 ppm
Copper	120 ppm
Manganese	400 ppm
Zinc	400 ppm

Ingredients: Milk proteins, lactose, emulsified fats, minerals, vitamins and yeast culture.

Indications: A nutritional supplement for foals, mares and horses.

Dosage and Administration: Feeding Instructions:

Broodmares: Feed 1-1.5 lb of MARE & FOAL PELLETS™ along with enough grain to maintain a desirable body condition.

Orphan or Early Weaned Foals: At 2 months of age, should receive 1 lb of MARE & FOAL PELLETS™ per day along with Start To Finish® Mare Replacer™. Gradually build pellet intake so at 3 months of age the foal is consuming 2 lb of pellets/day.

Nursing Foals: At 2 weeks of age, should be offered small quantities of MARE & FOAL PELLETS™. Gradually build consumption until the foal consumes 2 lb of pellets per day.

Weanlings: 30 days before weaning, supply 2 lb of MARE & FOAL PELLETS™ with a small amount of grain. Slowly increase the grain level to support adequate growth and body condition.

Yearlings: Will need 1-1.5 lb MARE & FOAL PELLETS™ per day along with enough grain to obtain a desirable growth rate and body condition.

Long Yearlings/Two Year Olds: Should receive either 1 lb of MARE & FOAL PELLETS™ or 2 lb of Start To Finish Performance Pellets™ per day. The pellets should be fed along with 6-10 lb of grain per day.

All horses should be fed good quality hay or pasture and have access to free choice salt, and fresh clean water.

Presentation: Available in 25 lb and 50 lb bags.

Compendium Code No.: 10850120

START TO FINISH® MARE REPLACER™

Milk Specialties — **Milk Replacer**

Nutritional Contents:

Crude Protein, not less than	22.0%
Crude Fat, not less than	12.0%
Crude Fiber, not more than	0.15%
Calcium, not less than	0.75%
Calcium, not more than	1.25%
Phosphorus, not less than	0.65%
Copper, not less than	30 ppm
Zinc, not less than	120 ppm
Vitamin A, not less than	16,750 IU/lb
Vitamin D_3, not less than	1,675 IU/lb
Vitamin E, not less than	100 IU/lb

Ingredients: Whey protein sources, animal fats, vegetable oil, lecithin, lactose, vitamins, minerals and trace elements.

Indications: To be used as a milk replacer for foals.

Dosage and Administration: Mixing and Feeding Instructions:

Mixing: Mix ½ cup (¼ lb) of dry MARE REPLACER™ into one quart of warm water (100°F). For best mixing results, sprinkle the powder onto the water using a wire whisk to agitate the powder and water.

Feeding: Always ensure that the foal has received adequate colostrum intake during the first two days after birth.

First 24 hours on MARE REPLACER™: Feed 1 quart every 3 hours to achieve a total of 8 quarts in 8 feedings.

Second 24 hours: Alternate 1 quart then 1½ quarts every 3 hours for a total of 10 quarts in 8 feedings.

Third 24 hours: 1½ quarts every 3 hours for a total of 12 quarts in 8 feedings.

Fourth 24 hours to 3 months of age: 2 quarts every 4 hours for a total of 12 quarts in 6 feedings. Continue until the foal is weaned.

Discussion: Management Tips:

Thoroughly clean the mixing and feeding equipment after each feeding.

For best mixing results, sprinkle the MARE REPLACER™ powder into the water.

Feed the young foal in a shallow container so the young foal's nose can feel the bottom.

Once the foal drinks without submerging its nostrils, a deeper container can be used.

Presentation: 25 lb. pail and 25 lb. bag.

Compendium Code No.: 10850130

START TO FINISH® PERFORMANCE PELLETS™

Milk Specialties — **Large Animal Dietary Supplement**

Nutritional Contents: Specifications:

Crude Protein, not less than	20.0%
Crude Fat, not less than	10.0%
Crude Fiber, not more than	4.0%
Calcium, not less than	1.7%
Calcium, not more than	2.2%
Phosphorus, not less than	0.9%
Vitamin A, not less than	25,000 IU/lb
Vitamin D3, not less than	2,600 IU/lb
Vitamin E, not less than	250 IU/lb
Trace Minerals:	
Magnesium	0.23%
Iron	330 ppm
Cobalt	0.5 ppm
Copper	150 ppm
Manganese	400 ppm
Zinc	400 ppm

Ingredients: Cereal grains, saturated long chain triglycerides*, minerals, vitamins and a live yeast culture.

* From Start to Finish Energy Pak™ 100.

Indications: A high energy supplement to be administered to horses during exercise and work.

Dosage and Administration: Feeding Instructions:

Light Work: 1 lb of PERFORMANCE PELLETS™ per day fed along with 6-8 lbs of unfortified grain.

Medium Work: 1.5-2 lbs of PERFORMANCE PELLETS™ per day fed along with 8-10 lbs of unfortified grain.

Heavy Work: 2 lbs of PERFORMANCE PELLETS™ per day fed along with 10-14 lbs of unfortified grain.

All horses should receive at least 12 lbs of hay per day.

Presentation: Available in 20 lb pails and 50 lb bags.

Compendium Code No.: 10850140

START TO FINISH® SWEAT REPLACER™

Milk Specialties — **Electrolytes-Oral**

Ingredients:

Sodium, not less than	22.0%
Potassium, not less than	11.5%
Magnesium, not less than	0.5%
Chloride, not less than	40.0%

This product also contains trace elements.

Indications: A dietary electrolyte and trace element supplement for performance horses.

Dosage and Administration: Feeding Instructions:

Normal maintenance intake for performance horses at rest or being transported in hot weather is 1 ounce per day.

Horses at light to moderate work levels: 2 ounces per day.

Horses with intense work situations: 3-4 ounces per day.

All horses should have access to free choice salt and fresh, clean water.

Discussion: When performance horses sweat, they lose a significant amount of essential nutrients (including sodium, potassium and chloride) that are necessary for top performance. SWEAT REPLACER™ is formulated to quickly replace those nutrients lost in sweat by providing critical electrolytes and organic forms of trace elements. One ounce of SWEAT REPLACER™ will supply the amount of electrolytes and trace elements lost in about 2 liters of horse sweat.

Presentation: 20 lb and 50 lb pails with a measuring scoop.

Compendium Code No.: 10850151

STAT

PRN Pharmacal — **Dietary Supplement**

High Calorie Liquid Diet

Active Ingredient(s): Each ounce contains:

Fat (Polyunsaturated)	45%
Carbohydrate	33%
Protein	3.0%
Vitamin A	500 I.U.
Vitamin D_3	40 I.U.
Vitamin E	3 I.U.
Thiamine HCl (Vitamin B_1)	0.15 mg
Riboflavin 5'Phos Na (Vitamin B_2)	0.17 mg
Pyridoxine HCl (Vitamin B_6)	0.2 mg
Ascorbic Acid (Vitamin C)	6.0 mg
Nicotinamide	2.0 mg
Pantothenic Acid	1.0 mg
Folic Acid	0.04 mg
Sodium Benzoate	0.1%

Indications: A highly concentrated nutrient formula for animals.

STAT is designed to contain a maximum of nutritive value in a minimum of liquid volume.

As a supplement to other food STAT supplies added calories to help the patient gain weight.

Dosage and Administration: Shake well.

Calorie Content: 550 Kcal per 100 g of STAT.

2 Tablespoons T.I.D. (100 grams) will provide the caloric requirement of a 20 to 30 pound dog. This amount will supply more than the known daily vitamin requirements.

STAT may be fed "as is" to dogs unable to eat solid food. Mixed with water it may be used to combat dehydration and maintain nutritive balance.

Dog Dosage: 2 tbs T.I.D. per 20-30 lbs.

Adult Cat Dosage: 1 tbs (½) B.I.D.

Calf Dosage: 2 oz per calf T.I.D.

Baby Pig Dosage: 1 oz per pig T.I.D.

Precaution(s): Store in a cool, dry place.

Warning(s): Keep out of reach of children. For veterinary use only.

Presentation: 2 fl oz, 8 fl oz, 16 fl oz and 32 fl oz.

Compendium Code No.: 10900190

STAYBRED VL5™

Pfizer Animal Health **Bacterin**

Campylobacter Fetus-Leptospira Canicola-Grippotyphosa-Hardjo-Icterhaemorrhagiae-Pomona Bacterin

U.S. Vet. Lic. No.: 189

Description: STAYBRED VL5™ is a chemically inactivated, oil-adjuvanted suspension of Campylobacter fetus combined with chemically inactivated *Leptospira* cultures of *Leptospira canicola, L. grippotyphosa, L. hardjo, L. icterohaemorrhagiae,* and *L. pomona.*

Indications: STAYBRED VL5™ is for vaccination of healthy cows and heifers as an aid in preventing campylobacteriosis (vibriosis) caused by Campylobacter fetus; and leptospirosis caused by *Leptospira canicola, L. grippotyphosa, L. hardjo, L. icterohaemorrhagiae,* and *L. pomona.*

Directions:

1. General Directions: Vaccination of healthy cows and heifers is recommended. Shake well. Aseptically administer 2 mL intramuscularly. In accordance with Beef Quality Assurance guidelines, this product should be administered in the muscular region of the neck.
2. Primary Vaccination: Administer two 2-mL doses 2-4 weeks apart to all breeding-age cows and heifers 30-60 days before exposure or being added to the breeding herd.
3. Revaccination: Annual revaccination with a single dose is recommended.
4. Good animal husbandry and herd health management practices should be employed.

Precaution(s): Store at 2°-7°C. Prolonged exposure to higher temperatures may adversely affect potency. Do not freeze.

Use entire contents when first opened.

Sterilized syringes and needles should be used to administer this vaccine.

Caution(s): Occasional hypersensitivity reactions may occur up to 18 hours postvaccination. Owners should be advised to observe animals during this period. While this event appears to be rare overall, dairy cattle may be affected more frequently than other cattle. Animals affected may display excessive salivation, incoordination, and/or dyspnea. Animals displaying such signs should be treated immediately with epinephrine or equivalent. In nonresponsive animals, other modes of treatment should be considered.

As with many vaccines, anaphylaxis may occur after use. Initial antidote of epinephrine is recommended and should be followed with appropriate supportive therapy.

This product has been shown to be efficacious in healthy animals. A protective immune response may not be elicited if animals are incubating an infectious disease, are malnourished or parasitized, are stressed due to shipment or environmental conditions, are otherwise immunocompromised, or the vaccine is not administered in accordance with label directions.

Warning(s): Do not vaccinate within 21 days before slaughter.

For veterinary use only.

Discussion: Disease Description: Campylobacteriosis (vibriosis) is a venereal disease of cattle transmitted during breeding, either through coitus or artificial insemination with contaminated semen. Although the disease is often subclinical, in cows it causes temporary infertility, irregular estrus cycles, delayed conception, and occasionally, abortion.

Leptospirosis may be caused by several serovars of *Leptospira,* of which *L. canicola, L. grippotyphosa, L. hardjo, L. icterohaemorrhagiae,* and *L. pomona* are the most common that affect cattle. *Leptospira* localize in the kidneys, are shed in the urine, and cause anemia, bloody urine, fever, loss of appetite, and prostration in calves. Signs are usually subclinical in adult cattle. Infected pregnant cows, however, often abort, and dairy cows may exhibit a marked decrease in milk production. *Leptospira* spp. are known zoonotic pathogens.

Trial Data: Safety and Efficacy: Because the fractions of STAYBRED VL5™ are inactivated, they cannot replicate in vaccinated animals. Vaccine fractions stimulated satisfactory geometric mean antibody titers for protection. In safety studies of the STAYBRED VL5™ fractions, no adverse reactions to vaccination were reported.

Efficacy of each fraction of STAYBRED VL5™ was demonstrated in challenge-of-immunity tests. Cattle vaccinated with any fraction of STAYBRED VL5™, followed by challenge with a disease-causing strain of that fraction, showed no clinical signs or had significantly fewer signs than nonvaccinated control cattle. Serologic studies also demonstrated no immunologic interference among the fractions of STAYBRED VL5™.

Presentation: 10 dose and 50 dose vials.

Compendium Code No.: 36900701

75-4890-05

STERAMINE

Stearns **Disinfectant**

EPA Reg. No.: 3640-17

Active Ingredient(s):

n-Alkyl (10% C_{16}, 40% C_{12}, 50% C_{14}) dimethyl benzyl ammonium chloride	10.0%
Isopropanol	2.4%
Inert ingredients:	
Water	87.6%
Total	100.0%

Indications: For use in hospitals for the general disinfection of floors, walls, furniture, sinks, bath tubs, showers, toilets, etc.

For use in food processing plants, dairies, meat packers etc.

Used for bulk tank cleaning and for udder and teat washing.

A general deodorizer for garbage cans, drains, sewers, gratings, gutters, etc., utensils and other dairy equipment.

A sanitizer and deodorizer for pipeline milkers, milking machines and pipelines to remove milkstone, and thereby reduce the possibilities of a high bacteria count in milkstone formation.

STERAMINE is effective for the control of many forms of staphylococcus, streptococcus and coliform bacteria.

STERAMINE is effective for sanitizing applications in hard waters, and has been demonstrated by testing using the Chambers method, as outlined in Official Methods of Analysis of the Association of Official Agricultural Chemists (Ninth Ed., p. 70). It was found that 200 ppm (active) of the quaternary killed 99.999% of *E. coli* in 30 seconds in water of 50 ppm hardness.

Dosage and Administration:

1. Scrape and prewash all utensils and glassware.
2. Wash.
3. Rinse in clear water.
4. Sanitize in a solution of 1 oz. STERAMINE to four (4) gallons of water (200 ppm). Immerse all utensils for at least two (2) minutes, or for a contact time observed by the governing sanitation code.
5. Place sanitized utensils in a rack or drain board to air dry.

Hospitals: For the general disinfection of floors, walls, furniture, sinks, bath tubs, showers, toilets, etc., first wash with an effective detergent, then disinfect with a STERAMINE solution of 1 oz. per gallon (800 ppm). STERAMINE is effective at the above dilution for the control of many forms of staphylococcus, streptococcus and coliform bacteria. Apply thoroughly to porous and hard to clean surfaces.

Food processing plants, dairies, meat packers etc.: Clean the walls and floors with an effective detergent solution, then spray with STERAMINE at an 800 ppm dilution. For equipment, wash thoroughly in a suitable detergent, then dip in (or spray on) a STERAMINE solution of 1 oz. to four (4) gallons of water. Before re-use, rinse with potable water.

Bulk tank cleaning:

1. The pick-up tank truck driver should rinse out the tank at the time of pick-up with tepid water.
2. Make certain that the compressor is turned off.
3. Remove all detachable equipment and make a solution of a manual cleaner according to its label. Brush the interior, especially the bottom of the cover, and all equipment thoroughly.
4. Twice a week, clean with a milkstone remover for the control of milkstone.
5. Reassemble and thoroughly rinse with water at a temperature of 120°F and allow to drain.
6. Sanitize with a solution of STERAMINE at the rate of 1 oz. to four (4) gallons of water (200 ppm) at a temperature of 145°F or follow local health recommendations.
7. Before re-use, rinse with potable water.

Udder washing:

1. Udder and teats should be thoroughly washed with a solution of ½ oz. of STERAMINE to two (2) gallons of water and dried with a clean sponge or towel.
2. A new solution should be made for every eight (8) cows.

General deodorizing: When obnoxious odors appear about garbage cans, drains, sewers, gratings, gutters, etc., remove all refuse possible, then sprinkle or spray a solution of 4 oz. of STERAMINE per gallon of water over all surfaces.

Utensils and other dairy equipment:

1. Immediately following use, pre-rinse with tepid water.
2. Begin cleaning using a manual cleaner according to its label at a temperature as warm as the hand can stand.
3. Twice a week, follow the above with a milkstone remover for the control of milkstone.
4. Rinse thoroughly with water at 145°F.
5. Sanitize all utensils with STERAMINE at the rate of 1 oz. to four (4) gallons of water (200 ppm) at a temperature of 145°F or follow local health recommendations. Do not rinse.
6. Before re-use, rinse with potable water.

Pipeline milkers, milking machines and pipelines:

1. Immediately after milking, flush the entire system with warm water at 110°F until the water runs clear.
2. Circulate a concentration of pipeline cleaner according to label directions, opening and draining all valves at this time. Hand brush all parts not coming in contact with the solution.
3. Twice a week, circulate a solution of milkstone remover to remove milkstone, and thereby reduce the possibilities of a high bacteria count in milkstone formation.
4. Rinse with warm water at 110°F until the water runs out clear.
5. Sanitize with a solution of STERAMINE at the rate of 1 oz. to four (4) gallons of water (200 ppm) and circulate for 5-10 minutes, or follow local health recommendations.
6. Before re-use, rinse with potable water.

Caution(s): Danger. Corrosive. Keep out of the reach of children. Harmful if swallowed. Causes eye irritation. Do not get in the eyes or on skin.

In case of eye or skin contact, flush with plenty of water. For eyes, get medical attention. Dilute with water as directed.

Do not mix with soap. Where soap is used in cleaning instead of detergent, rinse with water before sanitizing.

Do not allow to come in contact with food.

Do not re-use the container. Destroy when empty.

Presentation: 1 gallon (3.79 L) containers.

Compendium Code No.: 10170040

STERILE PENICILLIN G BENZATHINE AND PENICILLIN G PROCAINE

Aspen **Penicillin Injection**

Active Ingredient(s): Each mL of suspension contains:

Penicillin G benzathine	150,000 units
Penicillin G procaine	150,000 units
Sodium formaldehyde sulfoxylate	1.75 mg
Lecithin	11.7 mg
Methylparaben (as preservative)	1.20 mg
Propylparaben (as preservative)	0.14 mg
Polysorbate 40	8.19 mg
Sorbitan monopalmitate	11.3 mg
Sodium citrate anhydrous	3.98 mg
Procaine hydrochloride	20.0 mg
Sodium carboxymethylcellulose	1.04 mg
Water for injection	q.s.

Indications: For the treatment of the following bacterial infections in beef cattle due to penicillin susceptible microorganisms that are susceptible to the serum levels common to this particular dosage form, such as:

1. Bacterial pneumonia (shipping fever complex) due to *Streptococcus spp., Corynebacterium pyogenes* and *Staphylococcus aureus.*
2. Upper respiratory infections such as rhinitis or pharyngitis due to *Corynebacterium pyogenes.*
3. Blackleg due to *Clostridium chauvoei.*

Pharmacology: Penicillin G is an antibiotic which shows a marked bactericidal effect against certain organisms during their growth phase. It is relatively specific in its action against gram-positive bacteria, but is usually ineffective against gram-negative organisms.

It is normally recommended that any bacterial infection be treated as early as possible and with a dosage that will give effective blood levels. Although the recommended dosage will give longer detectable penicillin blood levels than penicillin G procaine alone, it is recommended that a second dose be administered at 48 hours when treating a penicillin-susceptible bacterial infection.

Dosage and Administration: Warm to room temperature and shake well before using. A thoroughly cleaned, sterile needle and syringe should be used for each injection (needles and syringes may be sterilized by boiling in water for 15 minutes).

Before withdrawing the solution from the bottle, disinfect the rubber cap on the bottle with a suitable disinfectant, such as 70% alcohol. The injection site should be similarly cleaned with the disinfectant. Needles of 14 to 16 gauge and not more than one (1) inch long are adequate for injections.

A subcutaneous injection should be made by pinching up a fold of the skin between the thumb and forefinger. The mid-neck region is the preferred injection site. Insert the needle under the fold in a direction approximately parallel to the surface of the body. When the needle is inserted in this manner, the medication will be delivered underneath the skin between the skin and the muscles. Proper restraint, such as the use of a chute and nose lead is needed for proper administration of the product.

Beef cattle: 2 mL per 150 lbs of body weight given subcutaneously only (2,000 units penicillin G procaine and 2,000 units penicillin G benzathine per lb of body weight). The treatment should be repeated in 48 hours.

Important: Treatment in beef cattle should be limited to two (2) doses, given by subcutaneous injection only.

Precaution(s): Store under refrigeration between 2-8°C (36-46°F). Protect from freezing.

Caution(s): Penicillin G is a substance of low toxicity. However, side effects, or so-called allergic or anaphylactic reactions, sometimes fatal, have been know to occur in animals hypersensitive to penicillin and procaine. Such reactions can occur unpredictably with varying intensity. Animals administered penicillin G should be kept under close observation for at least one-half hour. Should allergic or anaphylactic reactions occur, discontinue the use of the product and immediately administer epinephrine following the manufacturer's recommendations. Call a veterinarian.

As with all antibiotic preparations, the use of the drug may result in the overgrowth of nonsusceptible organisms, including fungi. A lack of response by the treated animal, or the development of new signs or symptoms suggests that an overgrowth of nonsusceptible organisms has occurred. In such instances, consult a veterinarian.

Since bacterial drugs may interfere with the bacteriostatic action of tetracycline, it is advisable to avoid giving penicillin in conjunction with tetracyclines.

Warning(s): Beef cattle should be withheld from slaughter for food use for 30 days following last treatment. A withdrawal period has not been established for this product in pre-ruminating calves. Do not use in calves to be processed for veal.

Treatment in beef cattle must be limited to two (2) doses, by subcutaneous injection only. Do not inject intramuscularly.

Failure to use the subcutaneous route of administration may result in antibiotic residues in meat beyond the withdrawal time.

Restricted Drug (California).

Discussion: The use of antibiotics in the management of disease is based on an accurate diagnosis and an adequate course of treatment. When properly used in the treatment of diseases caused by penicillin-susceptible organisms, most animals treated show a noticeable improvement within 24 to 48 hours. If improvement does not occur within this period of time, the diagnosis and course of treatment should be re-evaluated. It is recommended that the diagnosis and treatment of animal diseases be carried out by a veterinarian. Since many diseases look alike but require different types of treatment, the use of professional veterinary and laboratory services can reduce treatment time, costs, and needless losses. Good housing, sanitation and nutrition are important in the maintenance of healthy animals and are essential in the treatment of disease.

Presentation: 100 mL and 250 mL vial.

Compendium Code No.: 14750740

STERILE PENICILLIN G BENZATHINE AND PENICILLIN G PROCAINE

G.C. Hanford **Penicillin Injection**

Active Ingredient(s): Each mL of suspension contains:

Penicillin G benzathine	150,000 units
Penicillin G procaine	150,000 units
Lecithin	11.7 mg
Sodium formaldehyde sulfoxylate	1.75 mg
Methylparaben (as preservative)	1.20 mg
Propylparaben (as preservative)	0.14 mg
Polysorbate 40	8.19 mg
Sorbitan monopalmitate	11.3 mg
Sodium citrate anhydrous	3.98 mg
Procaine hydrochloride	20.0 mg
Sodium carboxymethylcellulose	1.04 mg
Water for injection	q.s.

Indications: For the treatment of the following bacterial infections in beef cattle due to penicillin susceptible microorganisms that are susceptible to the serum levels common to this particular dosage form, such as:

1. Bacterial pneumonia (shipping fever complex) due to *Streptococcus spp., Corynebacterium pyogenes* and *Staphylococcus aureus.*
2. Upper respiratory infections such as rhinitis or pharyngitis due to *Corynebacterium pyogenes.*
3. Blackleg due to *Clostridium chauvoei.*

Pharmacology: Penicillin G is an antibiotic which shows a marked bactericidal effect against certain organisms during their growth phase. It is relatively specific in its action against gram-positive bacteria, but is usually ineffective against gram-negative organisms.

It is normally recommended that any bacterial infection be treated as early as possible and with a dosage that will give effective blood levels. Although the recommended dosage will give longer detectable penicillin blood levels than penicillin G procaine alone, it is recommended that a second dose be administered at 48 hours when treating a penicillin-susceptible bacterial infection.

Dosage and Administration: Warm to room temperature and shake well before using. A thoroughly cleaned, sterile needle and syringe should be used for each injection (needles and syringes may be sterilized by boiling in water for 15 minutes).

Before withdrawing the solution from the bottle, disinfect the rubber cap on the bottle with a suitable disinfectant, such as 70% alcohol. The injection site should be similarly cleaned with the disinfectant. Needles of 14 to 16 gauge and not more than one (1) inch long are adequate for injections.

A subcutaneous injection should be made by pinching up a fold of the skin between the thumb and forefinger. The mid-neck region is the preferred injection site. Insert the needle under the fold in a direction approximately parallel to the surface of the body. When the needle is inserted in this manner, the medication will be delivered underneath the skin between the skin and the muscles. Proper restraint, such as the use of a chute and nose lead is needed for proper administration of the product.

Beef cattle: 2 mL per 150 lb body weight given subcutaneously only (2,000 units penicillin G procaine and 2,000 units penicillin G benzathine per lb of body weight). The treatment should be repeated in 48 hours.

Important: Treatment in beef cattle should be limited to two (2) doses, given by subcutaneous injection only.

Precaution(s): Store under refrigeration between 2-8°C (36-46°F). Protect from freezing.

Caution(s): Penicillin G is a substance of low toxicity. However, side effects, or so-called allergic or anaphylactic reactions, sometimes fatal, have been know to occur in animals hypersensitive to penicillin and procaine. Such reactions can occur unpredictably with varying intensity. Animals administered penicillin G should be kept under close observation for at least one-half hour. Should allergic or anaphylactic reactions occur, discontinue the use of the product and immediately administer epinephrine following the manufacturer's recommendations. Call a veterinarian.

As with all antibiotic preparations, the use of the drug may result in the overgrowth of nonsusceptible organisms, including fungi. A lack of response by the treated animal, or the development of new signs or symptoms suggests that an overgrowth of nonsusceptible organisms has occurred. In such instances, consult a veterinarian.

Since bacterial drugs may interfere with the bacteriostatic action of tetracycline, it is advisable to avoid giving penicillin in conjunction with tetracyclines.

Warning(s): Beef cattle should be withheld from slaughter for food use for thirty (30) days following last treatment. A withdrawal period has not been established for this product in pre-ruminating calves. Do not use in calves to be processed for veal. Treatment in beef cattle must be limited to two (2) doses, by subcutaneous injection only. Do not inject intramuscularly.

Failure to use the subcutaneous route of administration may result in antibiotic residues in meat beyond the withdrawal time.

Restricted Drug (California) - Use only as directed.

Discussion: The use of antibiotics in the management of disease is based on an accurate diagnosis and an adequate course of treatment. When properly used in the treatment of diseases caused by penicillin-susceptible organisms, most animals treated show a noticeable improvement within 24 to 48 hours. If improvement does not occur within this period of time, the diagnosis and course of treatment should be re-evaluated. It is recommended that the diagnosis and treatment of animal diseases be carried out by a veterinarian. Since many diseases look alike but require different types of treatment, the use of professional veterinary and laboratory services can reduce treatment time, costs, and needless losses. Good housing, sanitation and nutrition are important in the maintenance of healthy animals and are essential in the treatment of disease.

Presentation: 24x100 mL, 12x250 mL and 12x500 mL vials.

Compendium Code No.: 10340031

STERILE PENICILLIN G PROCAINE

Aspen **Penicillin Injection**

Active Ingredient(s): Each mL contains:

Penicillin G procaine	300,000 units
Sodium citrate	10 mg
Povidone	5 mg
Lecithin	6 mg
Sodium carboxymethylcellulose	1 mg
Methylparaben	1.3 mg
Propylparaben	0.2 mg
Sodium formaldehyde sulfoxylate	0.2 mg
Procaine hydrochloride	20 mg
Water for injection	q.s.

Indications: For the treatment of cattle and sheep for bacterial pneumonia (shipping fever) caused by *Pasteurella multocida;* swine for erysipelas caused by *Erysipelothrix rhusiopathiae (insidiosa);* and horses for strangles caused by *Streptococcus equi.*

Dosage and Administration: STERILE PENICILLIN G PROCAINE Suspension should be injected deep within the fleshy muscles of the hip, rump, round or thigh. Do not inject subcutaneously, into a blood vessel or near a major nerve. The site of each injection should be changed. Use a 16 or 18 gauge needle, one and one-half (1½) inches long. The needle and syringe should be washed thoroughly before use and sterilized in boiling water for 15 to 20 minutes before use. The injection site should be washed with soap and water and painted with a disinfectant, such as 70% alcohol.

Warm the product to room temperature and shake well. Wipe the rubber stopper in the vial with 70% alcohol. Withdraw the suspension from the vial and inject deep into the muscle. Do not inject more than 10 mL into one site.

The dosage for cattle, sheep, swine and horses is 3,000 units per lb of body weight or 1 mL for each 100 lbs of body weight, once a day.

Continue the treatment for at least one (1) day after the symptoms disappear (usually 2 or 3 days).

Precaution(s): STERILE PENICILLIN G PROCAINE Suspension should be stored in a refrigerator at 36°-46°F (2°-8°C). Protect from freezing.

Caution(s): Exceeding the highest recommended daily dosage of 3,000 units per pound of body weight, administering at recommended levels for more than 4 consecutive days, and/or exceeding 10 mL intramuscularly per injection site may result in antibiotic residues beyond the withdrawal time.

Sensitivity reactions to penicillin or procaine such as hives or respiratory distress, sometimes fatal, have been known to occur in some animals. If signs of sensitivity do occur, stop using the medication and call a veterinarian. If respiratory distress is severe, the immediate injection of epinephrine may be helpful.

As with any antibiotic preparation, prolonged use may result in the overgrowth of nonsusceptible organisms, including fungi. If this condition is suspected, stop using the medication and consult a veterinarian.

Warning(s): Not for use in horses intended for food.

Milk that has been taken from animals during treatment and for 48 hours (4 milkings) after the last treatment with this drug must not be used for food.

Discontinue the use of this drug before treated animals are slaughtered for food 4 days in cattle, 8 days in sheep and 6 days in swine, and 7 days in non-ruminating calves.

Milk withholding time for the product is based on human safety standards. The milk plant may advise additional testing to ensure compliance with industry requirements. It is strongly recommended that the processor be consulted to avoid possible penalties.

Restricted Drug (under California law).

Presentation: 100 mL, 250 mL and 500 mL vials.

Compendium Code No.: 14750750

STERILE PENICILLIN G PROCAINE AQUEOUS SUSPENSION

Butler **Penicillin Injection**

Injectable Antibiotic

NADA No.: 065-505

Active Ingredient(s): Each mL contains: Penicillin G Procaine 300,000 units, sodium citrate 10 mg, povidone 5 mg, lecithin 6 mg, sodium carboxymethylcellulose 1 mg, methylparaben 1.3 mg, propylparaben 0.2 mg, sodium formaldehyde sulfoxylate 0.2 mg, procaine hydrochloride 20 mg, and Water for Injection q.s.

Indications: Penicillin G is an effective bactericide in the treatment of infections caused primarily by penicillin-sensitive organisms, such as *Streptococcus equi* and *Erysipelothrix insidiosa,* as well as the gram-negative organism *Pasteurella multocida.*

STERILE PENICILLIN G PROCAINE AQUEOUS SUSPENSION is indicated for the treatment of:

1. Cattle and Sheep: Bacterial pneumonia (shipping fever) caused by *Pasteurella multocida.*
2. Swine: Erysipelas caused by *Erysipelothrix insidiosa.*
3. Horses: Strangles caused by *Streptococcus equi.*

Dosage and Administration: The suspension should be administered by deep intramuscular injection within the fleshy muscles of the hip, rump, round or thigh, or into the neck, changing the site for each injection. Do not inject subcutaneously, into a blood vessel, or near a major nerve.

Use a 16- or 18-gauge needle, 1.5 inches long. The needle and syringe should be washed thoroughly before use. The needle and syringe should then be sterilized by placing them in boiling water for 15 to 20 minutes.

The injection site should be washed with soap and water and painted with a germicide such as tincture of iodine or 70% alcohol. The product should then be administered by using the following procedure:

1. Warm the vial to room temperature and shake thoroughly to ensure uniform suspension.
2. Wipe the rubber stopper in the top of the vial with a piece of absorbent cotton soaked in 70% alcohol.
3. Inject air into the vial for easier withdrawal.
4. After filling the syringe, make sure that the needle is empty by pulling back the plunger until a small air bubble appears. Then detach the needle from the syringe.
5. Insert the needle deeply into the muscle, attach the syringe and withdraw the plunger slightly. If blood appears, withdraw the needle and insert it in a different location.
6. Inject the dose slowly. Do not massage the site of injection.
7. Not more than 10 mL should be injected in one location.

Daily treatment should be continued for at least 48 hours after the temperature has returned to normal and other signs of infection have subsided. Animals treated with STERILE PENICILLIN G PROCAINE AQUEOUS SUSPENSION should show noticeable improvement within 36 to 48 hours.

The dosage for cattle, sheep, swine, and horses is 3,000 units per pound of body weight, or 1.0 mL for each 100 pounds of body weight once a day. The treatment should not exceed 7 days in non-lactating dairy and beef cattle, sheep, and swine, or 5 days in lactating dairy cattle. If improvement is not observed within 48 hours, consult a veterinarian.

Precaution(s): STERILE PENICILLIN G PROCAINE AQUEOUS SUSPENSION should be stored in a cold room at a temperature between 2° and 8°C (36°-46°F). Avoid freezing the product.

Caution(s): Sensitivity reactions to penicillin and procaine, such as hives or respiratory distress, may occur in some animals. If such signs of sensitivity occur, stop medication and call a veterinarian. In some instances, particularly if respiratory distress is severe, immediate injection of epinephrine or antihistamine may be necessary.

As with any antibiotic preparation, prolonged use may result in the overgrowth of nonsusceptible organisms, including fungi. If this condition is suspected, stop medication and consult a veterinarian.

Exceeding the highest recommended daily dosage of 3,000 units per pound of body weight, administering at recommended levels for more than 7 consecutive days, and/or exceeding 10 mL intramuscularly per injection site may result in antibiotic residues beyond the withdrawal time.

Livestock remedy - Not for human use.

Restricted drug (under California law); use only as directed.

For animal use only.

For intramuscular use only.

Warning(s):

1. Not for use in horses intended for food.
2. Milk that has been taken from animals during treatment and for 48 hours (4 milkings) after the last treatment must not be used for food. The daily treatment schedule should not exceed 7 days of treatment in non-lactating dairy and beef cattle, sheep and swine, or 5 days in lactating dairy cattle.
3. The drug should be discontinued for the following time periods before treated animals are slaughtered for food:

Cattle . . . 4 days
Sheep . . . 8 days
Swine . . . 6 days
Non-ruminating calves . . . 7 days

Presentation: STERILE PENICILLIN G PROCAINE AQUEOUS SUSPENSION is supplied in 100 mL and 250 mL multiple-dose vials.

Compendium Code No.: 10821670

STERILE SALINE SOLUTION ℞

Bimeda **Saline Solution**

Active Ingredient(s): Composition: Each 100 mL of sterile aqueous solution contains:

Sodium Chloride . . . 0.9 g

Millequivalents per liter:

Cations:

Sodium . . . 154 mEq/L

Anions:

Chloride . . . 154 mEq/L

Total osmolarity is 308 milliosmoles per liter.

This product contains no preservatives.

Indications: For use in the replacement therapy of sodium, chloride and water which may become depleted in many diseases. Because this solution is isotonic with body fluids, it may also be used as a solvent or diluent, for antibiotics and other pharmaceuticals and biologicals where compatible, and for washing mucous membranes and other tissue surfaces.

Dosage and Administration: Warm to body temperature and administer slowly by intravenous or subcutaneous injection. The amount and rate of administration must be judged by a veterinarian in relation to the condition being treated and the clinical response of the animal, being careful to avoid overhydration. When used as a solvent or diluent for pharmaceuticals and biologicals, follow the manufacturer's directions.

Precaution(s): Store between 15°C and 30°C (59°F-86°F). Use entire contents when first opened. Discard any unused solution.

Caution(s): Federal law restricts this drug to use by or on the order of a licensed veterinarian.

For animal use only.

Warning(s): Keep out of reach of children.

Presentation: 250 mL (NDC# 61133-2690-7), 500 mL (NDC# 61133-2690-8) and 1000 mL (NDC# 61133-2690-9) vials.

Manufactured by: Bimeda-MTC Animal Health Inc., Cambridge, Ontario, Canada N3C 2W4.

Compendium Code No.: 13990560 Iss. 2.00

STERILE SALINE SOLUTION ℞

RXV **Saline Solution**

Active Ingredient(s): Each 100 mL contains:

Sodium chloride . . . 0.9 g
Water for injection . . . q.s.

Indications: For the preparation of dilute solutions for injection, infusion or local application; for diluting water-based drugs and biological products used in the treatment of livestock.

Dosage and Administration: Use as required.

Precaution(s): Store at controlled room temperature between 15°-30°C (59°-86°F).

This product contains no preservatives. After a quantity has been withdrawn for use the remainder should be discarded. Solutions made from this product should be used promptly and with adequate precautions for maintaining sterility.

Caution(s): Federal law restricts this drug to use by or on the order of a licensed veterinarian.

Warning(s): For animal use only.

Keep out of reach of children.

Presentation: 100 mL, 250 mL, 500 mL and 1,000 mL vials.

Compendium Code No.: 10910160

STERILE WATER ℞

AgriLabs **Sterile Water**

For Injection, USP-Sterile-Nonpyrogenic

Active Ingredient(s): Contains:

Water For Injection, USP. . . . 100%

pH 5.0-7.0 (hypotonic).

Indications: This sterile water for injection is made by distillation and is suitable for use as a diluent for preparation of pharmaceutical solutions when made isotonic by addition of suitable solutes. This product contains no preservative; solutions made from this water should be used promptly or sterilized with adequate precautions for maintaining sterility.

Dosage and Administration: Use as required.

Precaution(s): Store between 15°C-30°C (59°F-86°F).

This is a single dose vial. After a quantity has been withdrawn for use the remainder should be discarded.

Do not use this product if seal is broken or solution is not clear. Contains no preservative. If entire contents are not used, discard unused portion.

Caution(s): Federal law restricts this drug to use by or on the order of a licensed veterinarian.

Additives may be incompatible. When introducing additives, use aseptic technique, mix thoroughly, and do not store.

For animal use only.

Warning(s): Keep out of reach children.

Presentation: 250 mL, 500 mL and 1000 mL sterile vials.

Compendium Code No.: 10581710 Iss. 5-99

STERILE WATER

G.C. Hanford **Sterile Water**

Sterile Water for Irrigation, USP

Active Ingredient(s): Sterile distilled water only. Does not contain antimicrobial or other ingredients.

Indications: Recommended for use in dogs, cats, cattle, swine and horses. This solution is indicated for use as a tracheal lavage, nasal irrigation solution or as an irrigation solution for flushing a body cavity.

Dosage and Administration: Use as required.

Contraindication(s): Do not use unless solution is clear and container intact.

Presentation: 100 mL (3.4 fl. oz.) single use container.

Compendium Code No.: 10340050 5/99

STERILE WATER ℞

Phoenix Pharmaceutical **Sterile Water**

Sterile-Nonpyrogenic

Active Ingredient(s): Contains:

Water for Injection, USP . . . 100%

This product contains no preservative.

pH 5.0 - 7.0 Hypotonic

Indications: This sterile water for injection is made by distillation and is suitable for use as a diluent for the preparation of pharmaceutical solutions when made isotonic by the addition of suitable solutes.

Dosage and Administration: Use as required.

Precaution(s): Store between 15°C and 30°C (59°F-86°F).

Do not use this product if seal is broken or if solution is not clear. If entire contents are not used, discard unused portion. Additives may be incompatible. When introducing additives, use aseptic technique, mix thoroughly, and do not store.

Solutions made from this water should be used promptly or sterilized with adequate precautions for maintaining sterility.

Caution(s): Federal law restricts this drug to use by or on the order of a licensed veterinarian.

For animal use only.

Warning(s): Keep out of reach of children.

Presentation: 100 mL (NDC 57319-078-05), 250 mL (NDC 57319-078-06), 500 mL (NDC 57319-078-07) and 1000 mL (NDC 57319-078-08) single dose vials.

Manufactured by: Phoenix Scientific, Inc., St. Joseph, MO 64503.

Compendium Code No.: 12560802 Rev. 3-02 / Rev. 4-02 / Rev. 3-01 / Rev. 12-01

STERILE WATER ℞

Vedco **Sterile Water**

Active Ingredient(s): Each 100 mL contains:

Sterile water for injection . . . . . 100 mL

Contains no preservative.

Indications: Water for injection as indicated for use as a sterile solvent or diluent for parenteral products such as sterile solids.

Dosage and Administration: For parenteral use only after the addition of suitable solutes to make an approximately isotonic solution. Approx. pH 5.8 (hypotonic).

Caution(s): Federal law restricts this drug to use by or on the order of a licensed veterinarian.

Keep out of the reach of children.

Do not use the product if the seal is broken or if the solution is not clear.

If the entire contents are not used, discard any unused portion. Solutions made from the water should be used promptly or sterilized with adequate precautions for maintaining sterility.

Presentation: 100 mL, 250 mL, 500 mL and 1,000 mL containers.

Compendium Code No.: 10941890

STERILE WATER FOR INJECTION

Butler **Sterile Water**

NDC No.: 11695-166-25/11695-166-00

Active Ingredient(s): Sterile water.

Indications: For use as a diluent for the preparation of pharmaceutical solutions.

Dosage and Administration: Use as required.

Precaution(s): Store at 35°-86°F (2°-30°F).

Caution(s): The product does not contain preservatives. Use the entire contents when first opened. Discard any unused solution. For veterinary use only.

Keep out of the reach of children. Restricted drug, use only as directed.

Presentation: 100 mL, 250 mL and 1,000 mL vials.

Compendium Code No.: 10821680

STERILE WATER FOR INJECTION

RXV **Sterile Water**

Active Ingredient(s): Contains:

Water for injection 100%

This product contains no preservatives.

Indications: For use as a diluent for the preparation of water-based solutions.

Dosage and Administration: Use as required.

Precaution(s): Store at controlled room temperature between 15°-30°C (59°-86°F).

Use entire contents when first opened. Discard any unused solution.

Caution(s): STERILE WATER FOR INJECTION is not suitable for intravascular injection without first having been made isotonic by the addition of a suitable solute.

Warning(s): For animal use only.

Keep out of reach of children.

Presentation: 100 mL, 250 mL, 500 mL and 1,000 mL vials.

Compendium Code No.: 10910170

STERILE WATER FOR INJECTION ℞

Vet Tek **Sterile Water**

Sterile-Nonpyrogenic

Active Ingredient(s): Contains:

Water For Injection USP 100%

pH 5.0 - 7.0 Hypotonic.

Indications: This sterile water for injection is made by distillation and is suitable for use as a diluent for preparation of pharmaceutical solutions when made isotonic by addition of suitable solutes. This product contains no preservative; solutions made from this water should be used promptly or sterilized with adequate precautions for maintaining sterility.

Dosage and Administration: Use as required.

Precaution(s): Store between 15°C-30°C (59°F-88°F).

Do not use this product if seal is broken or solution is not clear. Contains no preservative. If entire contents are not used, discard unused portion. Additives may be incompatible. When introducing additives, use aseptic technique, mix thoroughly, and do not store.

This is a single dose vial. After a quantity has been withdrawn for use the remainder should be discarded.

Caution(s): Federal law restricts this drug to use by or on the order of a licensed veterinarian.

For animal use only.

Keep out of reach of children.

Presentation: 250 mL, 500 mL and 1000 mL.

Compendium Code No.: 14200190 Iss. 3-98

STERILE WATER FOR INJECTION, USP

Aspen **Sterile Water**

Contents:

Water For Injection USP 100%

pH 5.0-7.0 (hypotonic).

Product is a single dose vial. After a quantity has been withdrawn for use the remainder should be discarded.

Sterile, non-pyrogenic.

Indications: This sterile water for injection is made by distillation and is suitable for use as a diluent for preparation of pharmaceutical solutions when made isotonic by addition of suitable solutes. This product contains no preservative; solutions made from this water should be used promptly or sterilized with adequate precautions for maintaining sterility.

Precaution(s): Store between 15°C-30°C (59°F-86°F).

Caution(s): Do not use this product if seal is broken or solution is not clear. Contains no preservative. If entire contents are not used, discard unused portion. Additives may be incompatible. When introducing additives, use aseptic technique, mix thoroughly, and do not store.

Warning(s): For animal use only.

Keep out of reach children.

Presentation: 250 mL, 500 mL and 1000 mL sterile vials.

Compendium Code No.: 14750760

STERILE WATER FOR INJECTION, USP ℞

Bimeda **Sterile Water**

Active Ingredient(s): Contains:

Water for injection U.S.P. 100%

This product is sterile and contains no preservatives.

Indications: STERILE WATER FOR INJECTION is suitable for use as a diluent for the preparation of pharmaceutical solutions when made isotonic by addition of suitable solutes.

Precaution(s): Store at controlled room temperature between 2° and 30°C (36°-86°F).

Handle under strict aseptic conditions. Solution made from sterile water should be used promptly or sterilized to maintain quality.

Unused portion remaining in bottle must be discarded.

Caution(s): Federal law restricts this drug to use by or on the order of a licensed veterinarian.

For animal use only.

Warning(s): Not for human use.

Keep out of reach of children.

Presentation: 250 mL (NDC# 61133-1297-7), 500 mL (NDC# 61133-1297-6) and 1,000 mL (NDC# 61133-1297-5) containers.

Manufactured by: Bimeda-MTC Animal Health Inc., Cambridge, Ontario, Canada N3C 2W4.

Compendium Code No.: 13990361

STOCK POWER

LeGear **Large Animal Dietary Supplement**

Active Ingredient(s): Roughage products, salt dicalcium phosphate, calcium carbonate, mineral oil, ferrous sulfate, natural and artificial flavors added, thiamine mononitrate, niacin supplement, d-calcium pantothenate, vitamin A acetate in gelatin, vitamin B_{12} supplement, riboflavin supplement, vitamin D_3 supplement, pyridoxine hydrochloride and potassium iodide.

Guaranteed analysis each pound contains not less than:

Calcium (Ca), min. 2.8%
Calcium (Ca), max. 3.30%
Phosphorus (P), min. 1.40%
Salt (NaCl), min. 9.0%
Salt (NaCl), max. 10.80%
Iron (Fe), min. 0.353%
Iodine (I), min. 0.0035%
Vitamin A, min. . . . . . 350,000 I.U./lb.
Vitamin D_3, min. . . . . . 35,000 I.U./lb.
Vitamin B_{12}, min. . . . . . 1 mg/lb.
Riboflavin, min. . . . . . 80 mg/lb.
d-Pantothenic acid, min. . . . . . 460 mg/lb.
Niacin, min. . . . . . 800 mg/lb.
Thiamine, min. . . . . . 71 mg/lb.
Vitamin B_6, min. . . . . . 65 mg/lb.

Indications: A vitamin and mineral supplement for horses, cattle, hogs, sheep, and goats.

Dosage and Administration:

Horses: Mix 1¼ lbs. of STOCK POWER with each 100 lbs. of concentrate or grain feed, or mix one (1) scoop per 4 lbs. of feed for each horse once a day.

Young colts and yearlings: Mix one and one-half (1½) scoops with the wet or dry feed for each young colt, or two (2) scoops for each yearling, regularly once a day.

Cattle: Mix 1½ lbs of STOCK POWER with each 100 lbs. of concentrate feed, or mix regularly once a day, one and one-quarter (1¼) scoops per 4 lbs. of feed.

Sheep and goats: Mix 2 lbs. with each 100 lbs. of grain and feed ration, or mix regularly once a day three (3) scoops with the grain feed for each six (6) lambs or kids weighing less than 50 lbs., or for each three (3) weighing from 50 to 100 lbs., or for each two (2) mature sheep or goats weighing over 100 lbs.

Hogs: Mix 1 lb. with each 100 lbs. of complete mixed feed ration or mix regularly once a day, two (2) scoops per 10 lbs. of feed.

Presentation: Available in 1 lb. canisters and 2 lb. canisters. Scoop included.

Compendium Code No.: 11530030

STOMADHEX™

Virbac **Dental Preparation**

Active Ingredient(s):

	C-100	C-300
	Cats and Small Dogs (up to 20 lbs)	Large Dogs (over 20 lbs)
Chlorhexidine	0.10 mg	0.33 mg
Nicotinamide	8.25 mg	25.7 mg
Excipient QS to	33.3 mg	111 mg

Indications: For clinical care period post dental procedure. To be used in dogs and cats.

Dosage and Administration: Directions for Use:

1. Dry the lip with absorbent paper - this is particularly necessary if the pet salivates freely.
2. Remove the patch from the blister pack by pushing through the foil. Place the patch on a dry index finger.
3. Position of the patch on the inside surface of the upper lip opposite the second premolar tooth.
4. Applying the patch -- Hold in place for three seconds.

Helpful Hints: Do not give food or water 5 minutes prior to applying the patch. The first patch should be applied immediately following the procedure. Your pet may drink 15 minutes after the patch is in position. STOMADHEX™ is used daily for 10 days after dental cleaning or as recommended by your veterinarian. The patch will remain attached unless there is excessive saliva when applied or the pet mechanically removes the patch.

Contraindication(s): No interaction has been reported with STOMADHEX™ and the use of antibiotics.

Safety: Chlorhexidine has long been used for its broad-spectrum pathogen kill. The safety of chlorhexidine is documented in many controlled studies conducted by various researchers in the 1950's and 1960's, including I.V. administration of 5 mg/kg daily for 15 days and 50-100 mg/kg administered via gavage daily for 9-16 months with no ill effects or lesions noted on the organs of the dogs upon microscopic examination. This work also demonstrates the lack of deleterious effect on normal flora.

Nicotinamide (Niacin) is an essential vitamin. The lack of this vitamin in the diet may cause oral lesions. The LD50 for Niacin was 5 grams per kilogram of body weight, making the active ingredients in STOMADHEX™ extremely safe.

Precaution(s): Store in a cool, dry place.
Discussion: Bioadhesive patch, using a new technology patented in Europe by ImmunoVet's parent company, Vétoquinol S.A. France, delivers a sustained release of Chlorhexidine and Nicotinamide (Niacin) for the critical care period which is 10 days post dental descaling or periodontal procedure. This is when good oral hygiene is of utmost importance. Heretofore, this need has been unfulfilled because prior options, including brushing, caused further damage to tissue or did not provide sufficient contact time for optimal benefit of the active ingredients.

STOMADHEX™ bio-adhesive delivery system is a breakthrough which aids in the control of dental plaque, tartar, and halitosis in dogs and cats. This sustained release system delivers active ingredients that disinfect the oral cavity. Disinfection reduces the pathogens that contribute to post-dental procedural complications.

A STOMADHEX™ patch is applied immediately after each dental procedure, then the additional nine patches are dispensed for the client's use on the pet.

STOMADHEX™ is safe, convenient and easily applied.

Trial Data:
Bacteriology

Pathogens: Reduction in cell count was dramatic after 7 days, and continued during the following week.

Anaerobes: The decrease in total Anaerobes was statistically significant ($p<0.01$)

Spirochetes: The trial showed a very significant reduction in the number of Spirochetes. ($p<0.001$). This coincided with a reduction of inflammation.

Clinical Efficacy

Halitosis: The breath was normal on all the dogs after 1 week. Statistically significant. ($p<0.02$)

Plaque: Moderate plaque found on only 4 dogs after 2 weeks. Statistically significant. ($p<0.001$)

Calculus: Little improvement was observed on the dogs having built-up calculus. Surgical scaling was required.

References: Available upon request.
Presentation: 20 blister pkgs of 10 patches per display carton for both C-100 and C-300.
Compendium Code No.: 10230560

STREP BAC® WITH IMUGEN® II

Intervet **Bacterin**
Streptococcus Suis Bacterin
U.S. Vet. Lic. No.: 286
Contents: This product contains the antigen listed above.

Contains gentamicin as a preservative.

Indications: For the vaccination of healthy swine as an aid in the prevention of meningitis and arthritis caused by *Streptococcus suis.*
Directions: Vaccinate swine with one 2 mL dose intramuscularly (IM). Give a second dose 2-3 weeks later. Pigs should be at least 3 weeks old at first vaccination. Revaccinate every six months.
Precaution(s): Shake well. Use entire contents when first opened. Store at 2° to 7°C (35°-45°F). Do not freeze.
Caution(s): In case of anaphylactoid reaction administer epinephrine.

For veterinary use only.

Warning(s): Do not vaccinate within 60 days before slaughter.
Presentation: 50 doses (100 mL).
Compendium Code No.: 11061990

STREPGUARD® WITH HAVLOGEN®*

Intervet **Bacterin**
Streptococcus Equi Bacterial Extract
U.S. Vet. Lic. No.: 286
Description: An adjuvanted, concentrated, enzyme extract of *Streptococcus equi.**+

Contains thimerosal as preservative.

Indications: Recommended for use in healthy horses as an aid in the prevention of strangles disease due to *Streptococcus equi* infection.
Dosage and Administration: Inject 1 mL intramuscularly using aseptic techniques. Repeat in 3-4 weeks. A 1 mL dose should be administered annually or prior to expected exposure.
Precaution(s): Store at 35° to 45°F (2° to 7°C). Shake well before using. Use entire contents when first opened.
Caution(s): Certain hypersensitive individuals may demonstrate local or generalized reactions, sometimes severe, following exposure to streptococcal proteins. To minimize reactions, free exercise is recommended after injection. Anaphylactoid reactions may occur.

For use in animals only.

Antidote(s): Epinephrine.
Warning(s): Do not vaccinate within 21 days before slaughter.
Presentation: 10 dose (10 x 1 mL) syringes with separate sterile needle and 10 doses (10 mL).
*Adjuvant—U.S. Patent Nos. 3,790,665 and 3,919,411.
+U.S. Patent No. 4,582,798.
Compendium Code No.: 11062000

S

STREPTOMYCIN ORAL SOLUTION

Contemporary Products **Water Medication**
25% Streptomycin Sulfate Oral Veterinary Solution
ANADA No.: 200-197
Active Ingredient(s): Each mL contains 250 mg streptomycin (as sulfate).

Preservatives: 0.5% Sodium Bisulfite and 0.25% phenol.

Indications: STREPTOMYCIN ORAL SOLUTION is indicated as an aid in the treatment of certain enteric diseases in which streptomycin-sensitive coliform bacteria (*Escherichia, Salmonella, Vibrio*, etc.) are implicated as either the cause or important complicating agents. STREPTOMYCIN ORAL SOLUTION is designed to be added to the drinking water.

Since it is already in solution, administration of STREPTOMYCIN ORAL SOLUTION is simple and rapid and can be used easily in standard automatic water proportioners.

Dosage and Administration: Dosage recommendations made below are based on normal water consumption.

Chickens = Normal water consumption = 100 chickens @ (2 lbs.) will consume 2 gallons of water per day.

Swine and Calves = Normal water consumption = 1 Swine @ (100 lbs.) will consume 1 gallon of water per day.

Normal water consumption = 1 Calf @ (100 lbs.) will consume 1 gallon of water per day.

Disease	Indications and Treatment — Action	Dosage
Chickens		
Non-specific Infectious Enteritis in Chickens	Treatment of non-specific infectious enteritis caused by organisms susceptible to streptomycin sulfate.	(Based on a 2 lb. Chicken) 1 tsp./2 gal. of drinking water = 10 mg streptomycin per pound of body weight. 1½ tsp./2 gal. of drinking water = 15 mg streptomycin per pound of body weight.
Swine and Calves		
Bacterial Enteritis of Swine and Calves	Treatment of bacterial enteritis caused by *Escherichia coli* and *Salmonella* spp. susceptible to streptomycin sulfate.	(Based on a 100 lb. Swine or 100 lb. Calf) 1½ tsp./2 gal. of drinking water = 10 mg streptomycin per pound of body weight. 2 tsp./2 gal. of drinking water = 15 mg streptomycin per pound of body weight.

Medicated water must be used within 24 hours.

Precaution(s): Store in a cool place.
Caution(s): Animals to be treated must actually be drinking enough water to provide the recommended level streptomycin (10-15 mg streptomycin per lb. body weight.

For oral veterinary use only.

The following word is required on this product to comply with the Agricultural Code of California: Hazardous.

Warning(s): Residue Warnings: Do not administer to chickens producing eggs for human consumption.

Do not administer to chickens within 4 days of slaughter.

Do not administer to calves within 2 days of slaughter.

Certain strains of bacteria may develop a tolerance for streptomycin. If favorable results are not obtained in 3 to 5 days, diagnosis should be re-determined.

Consult a veterinarian or poultry pathologist for diagnosis.

Keep out of reach of children.

Presentation: 1 gallon (3785 mL).
Compendium Code No.: 10620000

STREPVAX® II

Boehringer Ingelheim **Bacterin**
Streptococcus Equi Bacterial Extract (Strangles Vaccine)
U.S. Vet. Lic. No.: 124
Description: STREPVAX® II is a concentrated aluminum hydroxide-adsorbed suspension of purified antigens derived from *Streptococcus equi.* It contains the antigenic protein of this antigen but is essentially free of the toxic and irritant substances present in whole cell bacterins.
Indications: For use in healthy horses of all ages as an aid in the prevention of disease (strangles) due to *Streptococcus equi* infection.
Dosage and Administration: Shake well. Using aseptic technique, inject 1 mL intramuscularly preferably in the hind quarters. For primary vaccination give 3 doses at intervals of 3 weeks. Foals vaccinated when less than 3 months of age should receive an additional dose at 6 months. Revaccinate annually and prior to anticipated exposure, using a single 1 mL dose.
Precaution(s): Store out of direct sunlight at 35°-45°F (2°-70°C). Shake bottle well. Protect from freezing.
Caution(s): Anaphylactoid reactions may occur.

Field reports suggest that certain hypersensitive horses may demonstrate local or generalized reactions, sometimes severe, following exposure to streptococcal proteins. Studies indicate exercise following vaccination decreased incidence and duration of reactions.

Antidote(s): Epinephrine.
Warning(s): Do not vaccinate within 21 days before slaughter.

For veterinary use only.

Presentation: 1 dose (1 mL) and 10 dose (10 mL).
Compendium Code No.: 10281020

STRESS-DEX®

Neogen **Electrolytes-Oral**
Oral Electrolytes
Guaranteed Analysis:

Calcium (Ca)	
Min.	1.0%
Max.	1.4%
Phosphorus (P) Min.	0.8%
Salt (NaCl)	
Min.	6.0%
Max.	6.7%
Potassium (K) Min.	3.0%

Contains: Dextrose, Potassium Chloride, Sodium Chloride, Dicalcium Phosphate (Source of: Iron, Magnesium, Manganese, Copper, Cobalt, Zinc, Selenium), Sodium Saccharin, Artificial Coloring, Orange Flavor.

Indications: A balanced electrolyte-trace element powder to be used as a supplemental source of energy and of calcium, phosphorous, salt and potassium.
Dosage and Administration:

Horses: 1 to 2 oz. daily in one dose or divided into 2 doses, in feed or water.

Dogs: 50 to 100 lbs. one to 2 teaspoons daily in one dose or divided into 2 doses, in feed or water.

Caution(s): For veterinary use only.
Warning(s): Keep out of the reach of children.
Presentation: 20 oz (680 g) (NDC: 59051-9173-0), 4 lb (1.814 kg) (NDC: 59051-9174-6), 7 lb (3.175 kg) (NDC: 59051-9175-8), 12 lb (5.443 kg) (NDC: 59051-9176-0) and 20 lb (9.072 kg) (NDC: 59051-9177-0).
Compendium Code No.: 14910422 L424-0501

STRONGER IODINE TINCTURE 7%

Centaur **Topical Wound Dressing**

Topical Antiseptic

Active Ingredient(s):

Iodine . . . 7.0% w/v
Potassium Iodide . . . 5.0% w/v
Isopropyl Alcohol (99%) . . . 82.0% v/v
Inert Ingredients:
Water . . . q.s.

Indications: For use as an antiseptic for topical use, and as a counter-irritant in chronic inflammatory conditions. May be used as a pre- and post-operative dressing.

Directions: For superficial cuts, abrasions, insect bites or bruises, cleanse with soap and water. Apply lightly not more than once daily. If repeated, dilute with 3 volumes of water. Do not bandage.

Contraindication(s): Not for burns, deep wounds or body cavities.

Precaution(s): Danger. Flammable. Keep tightly closed when not in use. Store in a cool place.

Caution(s): If redness, irritation, or swelling persists or increases, discontinue use. Avoid contact with eyes and mucous membranes.

For animal use only.

Antidote(s): Thin starch or flour water paste. To vomit, take mustard and warm water. Call a physician at once.

Warning(s): Poison. Keep out of reach of children.

Presentation: 1 pint and 1 gallon (128 fl oz) 3.785 L containers.

Manufactured by: Unavet, North Kansas City, MO 64116.

Compendium Code No.: 14880280

STRONGHOLD™ TEAT SEALANT

WestAgro **Teat Preparation**

Active Ingredient(s): Contains: Tetrahydrofuran.

Indications: This product provides a physical barrier that aids in the prevention of mastitis in dry cows.

Directions for Use: Read and understand this label and the Material Safety Data Sheet (available from your dealer) before using this product.

Use in a well ventilated area. Do not pour unused product back into original container. Keep container tightly closed when not in use. Apply with a new disposable 3 oz. paper cup. Immediately discard applicator out of reach of children.

At Dry Off: At last milking prior to dry off, completely milk out cow. Infuse dry cow antibiotic into teat in accordance with label directions. If teat is wet or dirty, wipe with a dry towel. Dip entire length of each teat with STRONGHOLD™ Teat Sealant. For maximum protection, a second application may be applied after drying.

10 Days Prior to Calving: If teat is wet or dirty, wipe with a dry towel. dip entire length of each teat with STRONGHOLD™ Teat Sealant. dip should remain on teat for 3-7 days. Observe daily and re-dip if sealant is removed prior to calving. At calving, peel off any remaining sealant film prior to milking.

Precautionary Statements: Danger. Extremely flammable. Contains Tetrahydrofuran.

Contact with product can cause severe irritation to eyes. Wear safety glasses with side shields or goggles. Harmful if swallowed. Use in a well ventilated area. Avoid breathing fumes.

Caution: STRONGHOLD™ will damage Styrofoam™ and some plastic products.

First Aid:

Eye Contact: Immediately flush eyes with plenty of water for at least 15 minutes. Call a physician.

Skin Contact: Flush with water.

If Swallowed: Drink large quantities of water. Do not induce vomiting and get medical attention.

Chemtrec Emergency No.: 1-800-424-9300.

Storage and Disposal: Dispose of all measuring devices out of reach of children. Extremely flammable. Keep away from fire, sparks and heated surfaces. Keep container tightly closed when not in use. Avoid contamination of food or feed.

Warning(s): Keep out of reach of children.

Presentation: 1 quart.

U.S. Patent No. 5,192,536 and other Patent Pending.

Compendium Code No.: 10180060 0143-A0397

STRONGID® C

Pfizer Animal Health **Feed Medication**

(pyrantel tartrate) Equine Anthelmintic

Active Ingredient(s):

Pyrantel tartrate . . . 1.06% (4.8 g/lb)
Guaranteed Analysis:
Crude protein, not less than . . . 12.5%
Crude fat, not less than . . . 2.0%
Crude fiber, not less than . . . 22.0%

Ingredients: Dehydrated alfalfa meal, wheat middlings, ground corn, cane molasses, preserved with propionic acid.

Indications: For the prevention of *Strongylus vulgaris* larval infestation in horses.

For control of the following parasites in horses:

Large Strongyles (adults): *S. vulgaris, S. edentatus.*

Small Strongyles (adults and 4th-stage larvae): *Cyathostomum* spp., *Cylicocyclus* spp., *Cylicostephanus* spp., *Cylicodontophorus* spp. *Poteriostomum* spp., *Triodontophorus* spp.

Pinworms (adults and 4th-stage larvae): *Oxyuris equi.*

Ascarids (adults and 4th-stage larvae): *Parascaris equorum.*

Directions:

Mixing and Feeding Directions: STRONGID® C is to be administered on a continuous basis either as a top-dress or mixed in the horse's daily grain ration at the rate of 1.2 mg pyrantel tartrate per lb of body weight daily. To achieve this dose, administer 1 oz of STRONGID® C per 250 lb of body weight. (A STRONGID® C measuring cup is enclosed.) STRONGID® C should be administered for the entire period that the animal is at risk to internal parasites. Unprotected animals that have grazed may already have an established *S. vulgaris* larval infestation. Before administering STRONGID® C, these animals should be treated with a therapeutic dose of a larvicidal product.

Foals may be administered STRONGID® C as soon as consistent intake of grain mix is occurring. This is generally between 2-3 months of age.

STRONGID® C may be used in mares at any stage of pregnancy or lactation. Stallion fertility is not affected by the use of STRONGID® C.

Top-Dress Directions:

Body Weight (lb)	oz per Day of STRONGID® C
250	1
500	2
750	3
1000	4
1250	5

Medicated Grain Mix Directions:

lb of Medicated Grain Mix per 100 lb of Body Weight	lb of STRONGID® C	lb of Non-medicated Feed	Concentration (Grams/Ton)
2.0	25	1975	120
1.5	33	1967	160
1.0	50	1950	240
0.5	100	1900	480
0.2	250	1750	1200

Caution(s): Consult your veterinarian before using in severely debilitated animals and for assistance in the diagnosis, treatment, and control of parasitism. Do not mix in feeds containing bentonite.

Warning(s): Not for use in horses intended for food.

Presentation: 9 lb (30-day sample size) and 25 lb (11.3 kg) plastic pails.

Compendium Code No.: 36901391 03-4602-45-2, 03-4603-45-2

STRONGID® C 2X™

Pfizer Animal Health **Feed Medication**

(pyrantel tartrate) Equine Anthelmintic

Active Ingredient(s):

Pyrantel tartrate . . . 2.11% (9.6 g/lb)
Guaranteed Analysis:
Crude protein, not less than . . . 11.5%
Crude fat, not less than . . . 1.5%
Crude fiber, not more than . . . 22.0%

Ingredients: Dehydrated alfalfa meal, wheat middlings, cane molasses, preserved with propionic acid.

Indications: For the prevention of *Strongylus vulgaris* larval infestation in horses.

For the control of the following parasites in horses:

Large Strongyles (adults): *S. vulgaris, S. edentatus.*

Small Strongyles (adults and 4th-stage larvae): *Cyathostomum* spp., *Cylicocyclus* spp., *Cylicostephanus* spp., *Cylicodontophorus* spp., *Poteriostomum* spp., *Triodontophorus* spp.

Pinworms (adults and 4th-stage larvae): *Oxyuris equi.*

Ascarids (adults and 4th-stage larvae): *Parascaris equorum.*

Directions: Mixing and Feeding Directions: STRONGID® C 2X™ is to be administered on a continuous basis either as a top-dress or mixed in the horse's daily grain ration at the rate of 1.2 mg pyrantel tartrate per lb of body weight daily. To achieve this dose, administer 0.5 oz of STRONGID® C 2X™ per 250 lb of body weight. (A STRONGID® C 2X™ measuring cup is enclosed. Please note it is different in size and shape from the original Strongid® C measuring cup due to the higher concentration of STRONGID® C 2X™). STRONGID® C 2X™ should be administered for the entire period that the animal is at risk to internal parasites. Unprotected animals that have grazed may already have an established *S vulgaris* larval infestation. Before administering STRONGID® C 2X™, these animals should be treated with a therapeutic dose of a larvicidal product.

Foals may be administered STRONGID® C 2X™ as soon as consistent intake of grain mix is occurring. This is generally between 2-3 months of age.

STRONGID® C 2X™ may be used in mares at any stage of pregnancy or lactation. Stallion fertility is not affected by the use of STRONGID® C 2X™.

Top-Dress Directions:

Body Weight (lb)	oz per Day of STRONGID® C 2X™
250	0.5
500	1.0
750	1.5
1000	2.0
1250	2.5

Medicated Grain Mix Directions:

lb of Medicated Grain Mix per 100 lb of Body Weight	lb of STRONGID® C 2X™	lb of Non-medicated Feed	Concentration Grams/Ton
2.0	12.5	1987.5	120
1.5	16.5	1983.5	160
1.0	25.0	1975	240
0.5	50.0	1950	480
0.2	125.0	1875	1200

Caution(s): Consult your veterinarian before using in severely debilitated animals and for assistance in the diagnosis, treatment, and control of parasitism. Do not mix in feeds containing bentonite.

Warning(s): Not for use in horses intended for food.

Presentation: 10 lb (4.5 kg) pail and 50 lb (22.6 kg) bag.

Compendium Code No.: 36901402 01-5058-45-2 / 90-9648-45-1

STRONGID® C THIRTY

Pfizer Animal Health **Feed Medication**

(pyrantel tartrate) Equine Anthelmintic Medicated For Continuous Feeding

Active Ingredient(s):

Pyrantel tartrate .... 1.06% (4.8 g/lb)

Guaranteed Analysis:

Crude Protein, not less than 12.5%
Crude Fat, not less than 2.0%
Crude Fiber, not less than 22.0%

Ingredients: Dehydrated alfalfa meal, wheat middlings, ground corn, cane molasses, and preserved with propionic acid.

Indications: For the prevention of *Strongylus vulgaris* larval infestation in horses.

For control of the following parasites in horses:

Large Strongyles (adults) — *S. vulgaris, S. edentatus.*

Small Strongyles (adults and fourth-stage larvae) — *Cyathostomum* spp., *Cylicocyclus* spp., *Cylicostephanus* spp., *Cylicodontophorus* spp. *Poteriostomum* spp., *Triodontophorus* spp.

Pinworms (adults and fourth-stage larvae) — *Oxyuris equi.*

Ascarids (adults and fourth-stage larvae) — *Parascaris equorum.*

Directions: Mixing and Feeding Directions: STRONGID® C Thirty is to be administered on a continuous basis either as a top-dress or mixed in the horse's daily grain ration at the rate of 1.2 mg pyrantel tartrate per pound of body weight daily. To achieve this dose administer 1 oz of STRONGID® C Thirty per 250 lb of body weight. (A STRONGID® C Thirty measuring cup is enclosed.) STRONGID® C Thirty should be administered for the entire period that the animal is at risk to internal parasites. Unprotected animals that have grazed may already have an established *S. vulgaris* larval infestation. Before administering STRONGID® C Thirty, these animals should be treated with a therapeutic dose of a larvicidal product.

Foals may be administered STRONGID® C Thirty as soon as consistent intake of grain mix is occurring. This is generally between two to three months of age.

STRONGID® C Thirty may be used in mares at any stage of pregnancy or lactation. Stallion fertility is not affected by the use of STRONGID® C Thirty.

Top-Dress Directions:

Lb Body Weight	Ounces Per Day of STRONGID® C
250	1
500	2
750	3
1000	4
1250	5

(Measuring Cup Enclosed)

Medicated Grain Mix Directions:

Lb of Medicated Grain Mix Per 100 lb of Body Weight	Lb of STRONGID® C Thirty	Lb of Non-medicated Feed	Concentration Grams Per Ton
2.0	25	1975	120
1.5	33	1967	160
1.0	50	1950	240
0.5	100	1900	480
0.2	250	1750	1200

Caution(s): Consult your veterinarian before using in severely debilitated animals and for assistance in the diagnosis, treatment and control of parasitism. Do not mix in feeds containing bentonite.

Warning(s): Not for use in horses intended for food.

Presentation: 9 lb (4.08 kg).

Compendium Code No.: 36901411 03-9405-45-0

STRONGID® PASTE

Pfizer Animal Health **Parasiticide-Oral**

(pyrantel pamoate) Equine Anthelmintic

NADA No.: 129-831

Active Ingredient(s): STRONGID® Paste is a pale yellow to buff paste containing 43.9% w/w pyrantel pamoate in an inert vehicle. Each syringe contains 3.6 grams pyrantel base in 23.6 grams (20 mL) paste. Each milliliter contains 180 milligrams pyrantel base as pyrantel pamoate.

Indications: For the removal and control of mature infections of large strongyles *(Strongylus vulgaris, S. edentatus, S. equinus);* small strongyles: pinworms *(Oxyuris equi);* and large roundworms *(Parascaris equorum)* in horses and ponies.

Consult your veterinarian for assistance in the diagnosis, treatment, and control af parasitism.

Pharmacology: Composition: Pyrantel pamoate is a compound belonging to a family classified chemically as tetrahydropyrimidines. It is a yellow, water-insoluble crystalline salt of the tetrahydropyrimidine base and pamoic acid containing 34.7% base activity. The chemical structure and name are given below.

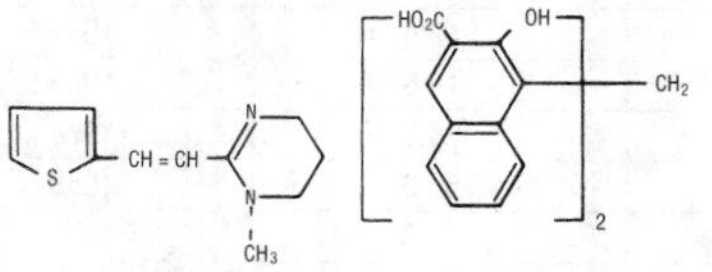

Chemical Name: (E)-1,4,5,6-tetrahydro-1-methyl-2-[2-(2-thienyl)-vinyl]-pyrimidine 4,4' methylenebis [3-hydroxy-2-naphtholate] (1:1).

Dosage and Administration:

Dosage and Treatment: STRONGID® Paste is to be administered as a single oral dose of 3 milligrams pyrantel base per pound of body weight. The syringe has four weight mark increments. Each weight mark indicates the recommended dose for 300 pounds of body weight.

Body Weight Range	Dosage	
	Volume	mg Pyrantel Base
Up to 300 lb	1/4 syringe (5 mL)	900 mg
301 to 600 lb	1/2 syringe (10 mL)	1800 mg
601 to 900 lb	3/4 syringe (15 mL)	2700 mg
901 to 1200 lb	1 full syringe (20 mL)	3600 mg

Note: Position screw-gauge over appropriate mark on plunger. Each milliliter contains 180 milligrams pyrantel base as pyrantel pamoate.

For maximum control of parasitism, it is recommended that foals (2-8 months of age) be dosed every 4 weeks. To minimize the potential source of infection that the mare may pose to the foal, the mare should be treated 1 month prior to anticipated foaling date followed by re-treatment 10 days to 2 weeks after birth of foal. Horses and ponies over 8 months of age should be routinely dosed every 6 weeks.

Administration: After removing the cap, the paste should be deposited on the dorsum of the tongue. Introduce the nozzle end of the syringe at the corner of the mouth. Direct the syringe backwards and depress the plunger to deposit the paste onto the tongue. Given in this manner, it is unlikely that rejection of the paste will occur. Raising the horse's head sometimes assists in the swallowing process. When only part of the paste has been used, replace the cap on the syringe nozzle.

Precaution(s): Recommended Storage: Store at room temperature, 59°-86°F (15°-30°C).

Caution(s): It is recommended that severely debilitated animals not be treated with this preparation.

Read entire brochure carefully before using this product.

Warning(s): Not for use in horses intended for food.

Keep out of reach of children.

Trial Data: Efficacy: Critical (worm count) studies in horses demonstrated that STRONGID® Paste (pyrantel pamoate) administered at the recommended dosage was efficacious against mature infections of *Strongylus vulgaris* (>90%), *S. edentatus* (69%), *S. equinus* (>90%), *Oxyuris equi* (81%), *Parascaris equorum* (>90%), and small strongyles (>90%).

Presentation: Available in 20 mL syringes.

Compendium Code No.: 36901420 23-4345-00-2

STRONGID® T ℞

Pfizer Animal Health **Parasiticide-Oral**

(pyrantel pamoate) Equine Anthelmintic Suspension

NADA No.: 091-739

Active Ingredient(s): STRONGID® T is a suspension of pyrantel pamoate in a palatable caramel-flavored vehicle. Each mL contains 50 mg of pyrantel base as pyrantel pamoate.

Indications: For the removal and control of mature infections of large strongyles *(Strongylus vulgaris, S. edentatus, S. equinus);* pinworms *(Oxyuris equi);* large roundworms *(Parascaris equorum);* and small strongyles in horses and ponies.

Pharmacology: Pyrantel pamoate is a compound belonging to a family classified chemically as tetrahydropyrimidines. It is a yellow, water-insoluble crystalline salt of the tetrahydropyrimidine base and pamoic acid containing 34.7% base activity. The chemical structure and name are given below:

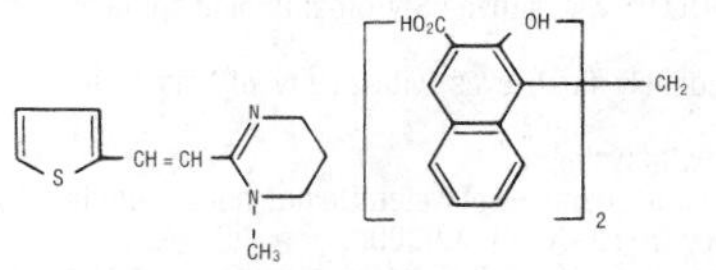

(E)-1,4,5,6-Tetrahydro-1-methyl-2-[2-(2-thienyl) vinyl] pyrimidine 4,4' methylenebis [3-hydroxy-2-naphthoate] (1:1)

Dosage and Administration: Dosage and Treatment: Administer 3 mg pyrantel base per lb of body weight (6 mL STRONGID® T per 100 lb of body weight). For maximum control of parasitism, it is recommended that foals (2-8 months of age) be dosed every 4 weeks. To minimize potential hazard that the mare may pose to the foal, she should be treated 1 month prior to anticipated foaling date followed by retreatment 10 days to 2 weeks after birth of foal. Horses over 8 months of age should be routinely dosed every 6 weeks.

Directions for Use: STRONGID® T may be administered by means of a stomach tube, dose syringe or by mixing into the feed.

Stomach Tube: Measure the appropriate dosage of STRONGID® T and mix in the desired quantity of water. Protect drench from direct sunlight and administer to the animal immediately following mixing. Do not attempt to store diluted suspension.

STRONGID® T is inactive against the common horse bot *(Gasterophilus* sp.). However, STRONGID® T may be administered concurrently with carbon disulfide observing the usual precautions with carbon disulfide.

Dose Syringe: Draw the appropriate dosage of STRONGID® T into a dose syringe and administer to the animal. Do not expose STRONGID® T to direct sunlight.

Feed: Mix the appropriate dosage of STRONGID® T in the normal grain ration. Fasting of animals prior to or following treatment is not required.

Precaution(s): Recommended Storage: Store below 30°C (86°F).

Caution(s): Federal law restricts this drug to use by or on the order of a licensed veterinarian.

It is recommended that severely debilitated animals not be treated with this preparation.

This product is a suspension and as such will separate. To insure uniform resuspension and to achieve proper dosage, it is extremely important that the product be shaken and stirred thoroughly before every use.

Keep out of the reach of children.

Warning(s): Not for horses or ponies intended for food.

Side Effects: Safety: STRONGID® T (pyrantel pamoate) is well tolerated by horses and ponies of all ages. Adverse drug response was not observed when dose rates up to 60 mg pyrantel base per lb of body weight were administered by stomach tube nor when 3 mg base per lb was given by intratracheal injection. The reproductive performance of pregnant mares and stud horses dosed with STRONGID® T has not been affected.

Trial Data: Efficacy: Critical (worm-count) studies in horses demonstrated that STRONGID® T administered at the recommended dosage was efficacious against mature infections of *Strongylus vulgaris* (>90%), *S. edentatus* (69%), *S. equinus* (>90%), *Oxyuris equi* (81%), *Parascaris equorum* (>90%), and small strongyles (>90%).

Presentation: 60 mL and 1 quart bottles.

Compendium Code No.: 36901431 75-7972-00

STRONG IODINE TINCTURE

Butler **Topical Antibacterial**

NDC No.: 11695-1719-1

Active Ingredient(s): Contains:

Iodine .... 7.0% w/v
Potassium iodide .... 5.0% w/v
Isopropyl alcohol (99%) .... 85.0% w/v
Water .... q.s.

Indications: An antiseptic and disinfectant for application to superficial cuts, abrasions, insect bites or minor bruises.

Dosage and Administration: Dilute one (1) part tincture iodine 7% with two (2) parts of propylene glycol. Cleanse the area with soap and water. Apply the dilution lightly not more than once a day.

Precaution(s): Store at 2°-30°C (36°-86°F).

Caution(s): Do not apply under a bandage. The product may irritate tender skin areas. In case of deep or puncture wounds or serious burns, consult a veterinarian. If redness, irritation, or swelling persists or increases, discontinue use of the product and consult a veterinarian. Avoid contact with the eyes and mucous membranes. Do not use on burns.

Not for use in deep cavity wounds or body cavities.

For animal use only.

Not for human use.

For external use only.

Keep out of the reach of children.

Flammable. Keep away from heat and open flame.

Keep the container closed.

May be fatal if swallowed.

Antidote(s): If swallowed, give starch paste, milk bread, egg white or activated charcoal. To vomit, take mustard and warm water. A 5% solution of sodium thiosulfate (photographic "hypo") may be administered orally at a rate of 10 mL per kilogram of body weight. Call a physician or poison control center.

Presentation: 1 gallon (3.785 L) containers.

Compendium Code No.: 10821690

STRONG IODINE TINCTURE 7%

Durvet **Topical Antibacterial**

Antiseptic/Disinfectant

Active Ingredient(s): Contains:

Iodine .... 7.0% w/v
Potassium Iodide .... 5.0% w/v
Isopropyl Alcohol (99%) .... 85.0% v/v
Water .... q.s.

Indications: For topical application on the skin of cattle, horses, sheep, swine and dogs to disinfect superficial wounds, cuts, abrasions, insect bites and minor bruises.

Directions for Use: If necessary, clip hair from area to be treated and cleanse with soap and water. Apply iodine with a swab.

Precaution(s): Flammable. Keep away from heat and open flame. Keep container closed when not in use. Protect from light. Store at 2°-30°C (36°-86°F).

Caution(s): May be fatal if swallowed. May cause burns. Call a physician or Poison Control Center.

Not for use in body cavities or deep wounds. Do not use on burns. Do not apply under bandage. Irritation may occur if used on tender skin areas. Avoid contact with eyes and mucous membranes. In case of deep or puncture wounds or serious burns consult a veterinarian. If redness, irritation, or swelling persists or increases, discontinue use and consult a veterinarian.

For animal use only.

Livestock drug.

Antidote(s): If swallowed give starch paste, milk, bread, egg whites or activated charcoal. Dilute by drinking 1 or 2 glasses of water. Call a physician or Poison Control Center immediately. Do not induce vomiting unless under the direct supervision of a physician. Do not give anything to an unconscious person. Avoid breathing vapors and contact with skin and eyes. For eyes, wash with water and contact Poison Control Center, physician or hospital emergency room immediately. Flush affected area with water for at least 15 minutes.

Warning(s): Keep out of reach of children.

Presentation: 16 oz (1 pt) (473 mL) (NDC 30798-495-31) and 1 gallon (3.785 L) (NDC 30798-495-35) containers.

Compendium Code No.: 10841521 Rev. 12-97 / Rev. 7-98

STYPT-STIX ℞

Vetus **Hemostatic**

Active Ingredient(s): Composed of a mixture of 75% silver nitrate and 25% potassium nitrate.

Indications: STYPT-STIX are useful for cauterization of skin or mucous membrane, and for removing warts and granulation tissue. They are ideal for stopping the bleeding of minor cuts, particularly those often encountered when clipping the nails of dogs or cats.

Dosage and Administration: Moisten the tip with distilled water and apply to the affected area. The strength of the action is controlled by dilution in water. One applicator is sufficient for one application.

Precaution(s): Store at room temperature in the closed package, in a dry place, protected from light, in the closed package. Silver nitrate is very sensitive to light and will turn black upon exposure to light. However, this does not affect its potency or utility. Silver nitrate will also turn tissue black, although the stain will gradually disappear.

Federal law prohibits dispensing this product without a prescription.

Caution(s): Federal law prohibits dispensing this product without a prescription.

Do not use in or near eyes.

Antidote(s): External - Immediately flush with copious amounts of water, then with a salt solution. Call a physician or local Poison Control Center.

Internal - Give copious amounts of salt water and follow with an emetic. Then administer a dose of Epsom salts and follow with milk. Call a physician.

Warning(s): Poison (see "Toxicology").

Toxicology: When ingested, silver nitrate is a violent poison which may be fatal. The symptoms include toxic gastroenteritis which may lead to coma, convulsions, paralysis, and profound alterations in respirations.

Discussion: Simple silver compounds such as this are commonly employed as caustics, antiseptics, and astringents. Since silver salts are completely precipitated by chlorides, the action of STYPT-STIX can be readily stopped by washing with a solution of common table salt.

Presentation: Available in a resealable foil pouch containing 100 six inch long applicator sticks.

Compendium Code No.: 14440820

SULFADIMETHOXINE INJECTION-40%

AgriPharm **Sulfadimethoxine**

Antibacterial

Sterile Multiple Dose Container

ANADA No.: 200-038

Active Ingredient(s): Each mL contains: 400 mg sulfadimethoxine compounded with 20% propylene glycol, 1% benzyl alcohol, 0.1 mg disodium edetate, 1 mg sodium formaldehyde sulfoxylate and pH adjusted with sodium hydroxide.

Indications: Cattle - For the treatment of bovine respiratory disease complex (shipping fever complex) and bacterial pneumonia associated with *Pasteurella* spp. sensitive to sulfadimethoxine; necrotic pododermatitis (foot rot) and calf diphtheria caused by *Fusobacterium necrophorum (Sphaerophorus necrophorus)*, sensitive to sulfadimethoxine.

Dosage and Administration: To be administered in amounts to provide 25 mg/lb (55 mg/kg) for initial dose, followed by 12.5 mg/lb (27.5 mg/kg) for maintenance doses every 24 hours.

During treatment period, make certain that animals maintain adequate water intake.

For intravenous use only in cattle.

Precaution(s): Store at 15°C-30°C (59°F-86°F).

Warning(s): Milk taken from animals during treatment and for 60 hours (5 milkings) after the latest treatment must not be used for food.

Do not administer within 5 days of slaughter. A withdrawal period has not been established for this product in pre-ruminating calves. Do not use in calves to be processed for veal.

For animal use only.

Restricted drug (California) - Use only as directed.

Not for human use.

Keep out of reach of children.

Presentation: 250 mL (8.5 fl oz) sterile multiple dose container.

Compendium Code No.: 14570930

SULFADIMETHOXINE INJECTION - 40%

Aspen **Sulfadimethoxine**

Antibacterial

ANADA No.: 200-038

Active Ingredient(s): Each mL contains 400 mg sulfadimethoxine compounded with 20% propylene glycol, 1% benzyl alcohol, 0.1 mg disodium edetate, 1 mg sodium formaldehyde sulfoxylate, and pH adjusted with sodium hydroxide.

Indications: SULFADIMETHOXINE INJECTION - 40% is indicated for the treatment of bovine respiratory disease complex (shipping fever complex) and bacterial pneumonia associated with *Pasteurella* spp. sensitive to sulfadimethoxine; necrotic pododermatitis (foot rot) and calf diphtheria caused by *Fuscobacterium necrophorum (Sphaerophorus necrophorus)* sensitive to sulfadimethoxine.

Pharmacology: Description: SULFADIMETHOXINE INJECTION - 40% is a low-dosage, rapidly absorbed, long-acting sulfonamide, effective for the treatment of shipping fever complex, bacterial pneumonia, calf diphtheria and foot rot in cattle. Sulfadimethoxine is a white, almost tasteless and odorless compound. Chemically, it is N' - (2,6-dimethoxy-4-pyrimidinyl) sulfanilamide. The structural formula is:

$H_2N-C_6H_4-SO_2-NH-C_4HN_2(OCH_3)_2$

Actions: Sulfadimethoxine has been demonstrated clinically or in the laboratory to be effective against a variety of organisms, such as streptococci, klebsiella, proteus, shigella, staphylococci, escherichia, and salmonella. The systemic sulfonamides which include sulfadimethoxine are bacteriostatic agents. Sulfonamides competitively inhibit bacterial synthesis of folic acid (pteroylglutamic acid) from para-aminobenzoic acid. Mammalian cells are capable of utilizing folic acid in the presence of sulfonamides.

The tissue distribution of sulfadimethoxine, as with all sulfonamides, is a function of plasma levels, degree of plasma protein binding, and subsequent distribution in the tissues of the lipid-soluble un-ionized form. The relative amounts are determined by both its pKa and by the pH of each tissue. Therefore, levels tend to be higher in less acid tissue and body fluids or those diseased tissues having high concentrations of leukocytes.

Slow renal excretion results from a high degree of tubular reabsorption, and plasma protein binding is very high, providing a blood reservoir of the drug. Thus, sulfadimethoxine maintains higher blood levels than most other long-acting sulfonamides. Single, comparatively low doses of sulfadimethoxine give rapid and sustained therapeutic blood levels.

To assure successful sulfonamide therapy (1) the drug must be given early in the course of the disease, and it must produce a high sulfonamide level in the body rapidly after administration, (2) therapeutically effective sulfonamide levels must be maintained in the body throughout the treatment period, (3) treatment should continue for a short period of time after the clinical signs have disappeared, and (4) the causative organisms must be sensitive to this class of drugs.

S

Dosage and Administration: SULFADIMETHOXINE INJECTION - 40% must be administered only by the intravenous route in cattle. Cattle should receive 1 mL of SULFADIMETHOXINE INJECTION - 40% per 16 pounds of body weight (55 mg/kg) as an initial dose, followed by 0.5 mL per 16 pounds of body weight (27.5 mg/kg) every 24 hours thereafter. Sulfadimethoxine boluses may be utilized for maintenance therapy in cattle. Representative weights and doses are indicated in the following table:

Each mL contains 400 mg sulfadimethoxine.

Animal Weight	Initial Dose 25 mg/lb (55 mg/kg)	Subsequent Daily Doses 12.5 mg/lb (27.5 mg/kg)
200 lb (113.6 kg)	15.6 mL	7.8 mL
500 lb (227.2 kg)	31.2 mL	15.6 mL
750 lb (340.9 kg)	46.9 mL	23.5 mL
1000 lb (454.5 kg)	62.5 mL	31.3 mL

Length of treatment depends on the clinical response. In most cases treatment for 3 to 5 days is adequate. Treatment should be continued until the animal is asymptomatic for 48 hours.

Contraindication(s): Limitations: Sulfadimethoxine is not effective in viral or rickettsial infections, and as with any anti-bacterial agent, occasional failures in therapy may occur due to resistant microorganisms. The usual precautions in sulfonamide therapy should be observed.

Precaution(s): Store at room temperature. Should crystallization occur at cold temperatures, crystals will dissolve either by storing at room temperature for several days or by heating the vial in warm water. Crystallization and redissolution do not impair the efficacy of the product.

Caution(s): During treatment period, make certain that animals maintain adequate water intake.

If animals show no improvement within 2 or 3 days, consult your veterinarian.

Tissue damage may result from perivascular infiltration.

Warning(s): Milk taken from animals during treatment and for 60 hours (5 milkings) after the latest treatment must not be used for food. Do not administer within 5 days of slaughter. A withdrawal period has not been established for this product in preruminating calves. Do not use in calves to be processed for veal.

Restricted Drug (California), use only as directed.

For animal use only - Not for human use - Keep out of reach of children.

Toxicology: Toxicity and Safety: Data regarding acute (LD_{50}) and chronic toxicities of sulfadimethoxine indicate the drug is very safe. The LD_{50} in mice is greater than 2 g/kg body weight when administered intraperitoneally and greater than 16 g/kg when administered orally. In dogs receiving massive single oral doses of 3.2 g/kg body weight, diarrhea was the only adverse effect observed. Dogs given 160 mg/kg body weight orally daily for 13 weeks showed no signs of toxicity.

In cattle, sulfadimethoxine has been shown to be safe through extensive clinical use with other dosage forms. In addition, studies with intravenous administration of SULFADIMETHOXINE INJECTION - 40% have demonstrated that hemolysis of erythrocytes does not occur by this route of administration. Sulfadimethoxine has a relatively high solubility at the pH normally occurring in the kidney, precluding the possibility of precipitation and crystalluria.

References: Available upon request.

Presentation: 250 mL sterile multiple dose containers.

Compendium Code No.: 14750771

SULFADIMETHOXINE INJECTION - 40%

Butler **Sulfadimethoxine**

Antibacterial

ANADA No.: 200-177

Active Ingredient(s): Composition: Each mL contains 400 mg sulfadimethoxine compounded with 20% propylene glycol, 1% benzyl alcohol (preservative), 0.1 mg disodium edetate, 1 mg sodium formaldehyde sulfoxylate, and pH adjusted with sodium hydroxide.

Indications: SULFADIMETHOXINE INJECTION - 40% (sulfadimethoxine) is indicated for the treatment of bovine respiratory disease complex (shipping fever complex) and bacterial pneumonia associated with *Pasteurella* spp sensitive to sulfadimethoxine; necrotic pododermatitis (foot rot) and calf diphtheria caused by *Fusobacterium necrophorum (Sphaerophorus necrophorus)*, sensitive to sulfadimethoxine.

Pharmacology: SULFADIMETHOXINE INJECTION - 40% (sulfadimethoxine) is a low-dosage, rapidly absorbed, long-acting sulfonamide, effective for the treatment of shipping fever complex, bacterial pneumonia, calf diphtheria and foot rot in cattle.

Sulfadimethoxine is a white, almost tasteless and odorless compound. Chemically, it is N^1-(2,6-dimethoxy-4-pyrimidinyl) sulfanilamide. The structural formula is:

OCH_3

H_2N– (benzene ring) –SO_2–NH– (pyrimidine ring, N, N)

OCH_3

Actions: Sulfadimethoxine has been demonstrated clinically or in the laboratory to be effective against a variety of organisms, such as streptococci, klebsiella, proteus, shigella, staphylococci, escherichia, and salmonella.[1,2]

The systemic sulfonamides which include sulfadimethoxine are bacteriostatic agents. Sulfonamides competitively inhibit bacterial synthesis of folic acid (pteroylglutamic acid) from para-aminobenzoic acid. Mammalian cells are capable of utilizing folic acid in the presence of sulfonamides.

The tissue distribution of sulfadimethoxine, as with all sulfonamides, is a function of plasma levels, degree of plasma protein binding, and subsequent passive distribution in the tissues of the lipid-soluble un-ionized form. The relative amounts are determined by both its pKa and by the pH of each tissue. Therefore, levels tend to be higher in less acid tissue and body fluids or those diseased tissues having high concentrations of leucocytes.[2]

Slow renal excretion results from a high degree of tubular reabsorption,[3] and plasma protein binding is very high, providing a blood reservoir of the drug. Thus, sulfadimethoxine maintains higher blood levels than most other long-acting sulfonamides. Single, comparatively low doses of sulfadimethoxine give rapid and sustained therapeutic blood levels.[1]

To assure successful sulfonamide therapy (1) the drug must be given early in the course of the disease, and it must produce a high sulfonamide level in the body rapidly after administration, (2) therapeutically effective sulfonamide levels must be maintained in the body throughout the treatment period, (3) treatment should continue for a short period of time after the clinical signs have disappeared, and (4) the causative organisms must be sensitive to this class of drugs.

Dosage and Administration: SULFADIMETHOXINE INJECTION - 40% (sulfadimethoxine) must be administered only by the intravenous route in cattle. Cattle should receive 1 mL of SULFADIMETHOXINE INJECTION - 40% (sulfadimethoxine) per 16 pounds of body weight (55 mg/kg) as an initial dose, followed by 0.5 mL per 16 pounds of body weight (27.5 mg/kg) every 24 hours thereafter. Sulfadimethoxine Boluses may be utilized for maintenance therapy in cattle. Representative weights and doses are indicated in the following table:

Animal Weight	Initial Dose 25 mg/lb (55 mg/kg)	Subsequent Daily Doses 12.5 mg/lb (27.5 mg/kg)
250 lb (113.6 kg)	15.6 mL	7.8 mL
500 lb (227.2 kg)	31.2 mL	15.6 mL
750 lb (340.9 kg)	46.9 mL	23.5 mL
1000 lb (454.5 kg)	62.5 mL	31.3 mL

Length of treatment depends on the clinical response. In most cases treatment for 3 to 5 days is adequate. Treatment should be continued until the animal is asymptomatic for 48 hours.

Directions for Intravenous Injection (Equipment needed):

1. A nose lead and/or halter sufficiently strong enough to effectively restrain or hold the animal's head steady so that the intravenous injection can be made with ease.
2. Hypodermic needles, 16 or 18 gauge and 2 inches long. Only new, sharp and sterile hypodermic needles should be used. Dull needles should be discarded. Extra needles should always be available in case the needles being used should become clogged.
3. Hypodermic syringes, 40 or 50 mL sterile disposable or reusable glass syringes should be available.
4. Alcohol (70%) or equally effective antiseptic for disinfecting the skin.

Preparation of the equipment: Glass syringes and regular hypodermic needles should be thoroughly cleaned and washed. Following this, the needles and syringes should be immersed in boiling water for 30 minutes prior to each injection. Regular hypodermic needles should not be used more than 3-4 times as repeated skin puncturing and boiling of the needles causes them to become quite dull. Disposable hypodermic needles and syringes should not be used more than once.

Restraint of animal: The cow should preferably be in a stanchion for maximum restraint. If this is not possible, the animal should be restrained in a manner to prevent excessive movement. A nose lead should be applied and the animal's head turned sidewise to stretch the skin and tense the muscles of the neck region.

Locating the jugular vein: When the animal has been restrained (as above), you will notice a long depression of the skin from below the angle of the jaw to just above the shoulder. This is known as the jugular furrow or jugular groove. The jugular vein is located just under the jugular groove.

Preparation of SULFADIMETHOXINE INJECTION - 40% (sulfadimethoxine) for injection: The rubber cap of the bottle should be thoroughly cleaned with 70% alcohol or another satisfactory antiseptic. The correct amount of SULFADIMETHOXINE INJECTION - 40% (sulfadimethoxine) for treatment should be calculated (see dosage directions) and that amount withdrawn into a syringe. One or two syringefuls of air should be injected into the bottle first to make withdrawing the drug easier. SULFADIMETHOXINE INJECTION - 40% (sulfadimethoxine) should preferably be at room temperature when filling syringes and when injecting intravenously.

Entering the vein: The skin of the injection area should be clean and free of dirt. Cotton saturated with 70% alcohol (or suitable antiseptic) should be used to wipe the injection site.

Apply pressure over the jugular vein close to the shoulder. This will reduce the flow of blood to the heart and cause the jugular vein to bulge or enlarge (See Figure 1) When the jugular vein has been "raised", insert the hypodermic needle at a 45 degree angle through the skin just underneath the jugular vein. The beveled edge of the hypodermic needles should be up.

After the skin has been punctured, the point of the needle should be directed toward the side of the vein and pushed into the center of the vein (See Figure 2). When the needle is in the center of the vein, there will be a free flow of blood back through the needle. Release external pressure when you are sure the needle is within the vein.

Injecting the SULFADIMETHOXINE INJECTION - 40% (sulfadimethoxine): After the needle has been accurately inserted into the jugular vein, firmly attach the syringe containing SULFADIMETHOXINE INJECTION - 40% (sulfadimethoxine) to the inserted hypodermic needle. Caution, be sure syringe is free of air. Exert firm pressure on the plunger of the syringe to inject the SULFADIMETHOXINE INJECTION - 40% (sulfadimethoxine) while the barrel is held firmly. The injection should be made moderately slow - never rapidly.

If the animal moves, causing resistance in pushing the plunger of the syringe, or if a bubble of the drug is noted under the skin, the needle is no longer within the vein. The needle should be repositioned.

When the injection is completed, quickly withdraw the syringe and needle with a quick pull and apply light pressure over the injection site with alcohol and cotton to minimize bleeding from the puncture site.

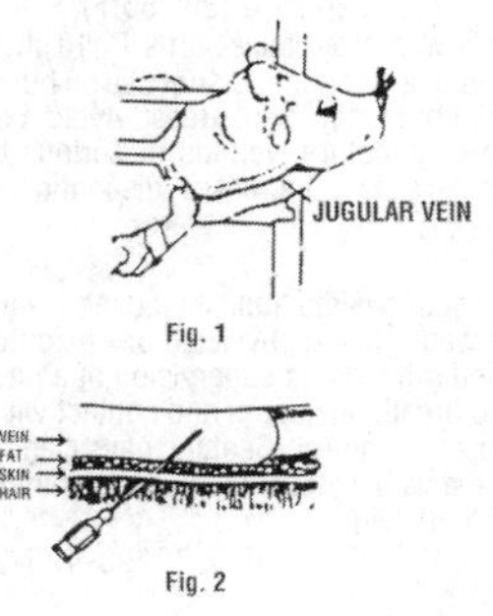

Fig. 1

Fig. 2

Precaution(s): Store at room temperature (15° and 30°C, 59° and 86°F). Should crystallization occur at cold temperatures, crystals will dissolve either by storing at room temperature for several days or by heating the vial in warm water. Crystallization and redissolution do not impair the efficacy of the product.

Caution(s): During treatment period, make certain that animals maintain adequate water intake.

If animals show no improvement within 2 or 3 days, consult your veterinarian.

Tissue damage may result from perivascular infiltration.

Sulfadimethoxine is not effective in viral or rickettsial infections, and as with any anti-bacterial agent, occasional failures in therapy may occur due to resistant microorganisms. The usual precautions in sulfonamide therapy should be observed.

For intravenous use only in cattle.

Restricted drug, Use only as directed - Not for human use (California).

For animal use only. Keep out of reach of children.

Warning(s): Milk taken from the animals during treatment and for 60 hours (5 milkings) after the latest treatment must not be used for food.

Do not administer within 5 days of slaughter.

Toxicology: Data regarding acute (LD_{50}) and chronic toxicities of sulfadimethoxine indicate the drug is safe. The LD_{50} in mice is greater than 2 g/kg body weight when administered intraperitoneally and greater than 16 g/kg when administered orally. In dogs receiving massive single oral doses of 3.2 g/kg body weight, diarrhea was the only adverse effect observed. Dogs given 160 mg/kg body weight orally daily for 13 weeks showed no signs of toxicity.

In cattle sulfadimethoxine has been shown to be safe through extensive clinical use with other dosage forms. In addition, studies with intravenous administration of sulfadimethoxine injection 40% have demonstrated that hemolysis of erythrocytes does not occur by this route of administration. Sulfadimethoxine has a relatively high solubility at the pH normally occurring in the kidney, precluding the possibility of precipitation and crystalluria.

References: Available upon request.

Presentation: 250 mL multiple dose vials (NDC 11695-3541-2).

Manufactured by: Phoenix Scientific, Inc., St. Joseph, MO 64506

Compendium Code No.: 10821700 Iss. 3-97

SULFADIMETHOXINE INJECTION-40%

Durvet **Sulfadimethoxine**

Antibacterial

ANADA No.: 200-177

Active Ingredient(s): Composition: Each mL contains 400 mg sulfadimethoxine compounded with 20% propylene glycol, 1% benzyl alcohol (preservative), 0.1 mg disodium edetate, 1 mg sodium formaldehyde sulfoxylate, and pH adjusted with sodium hydroxide.

Indications: SULFADIMETHOXINE INJECTION 40% is indicated for the treatment of bovine respiratory disease complex (shipping fever complex) and bacterial pneumonia associated with *Pasteurella* spp sensitive to sulfadimethoxine; necrotic pododermatitis (foot rot) and calf diphtheria caused by *Fusobacterium necrophorum (Sphaerophorus necrophorus),* sensitive to sulfadimethoxine.

Pharmacology: Description: SULFADIMETHOXINE INJECTION 40% is a low-dosage, rapidly absorbed, long-acting sulfonamide, effective for the treatment of shipping fever complex, bacterial pneumonia, calf diphtheria and foot rot in cattle.

Sulfadimethoxine is a white, almost tasteless and odorless compound. Chemically, it is N^1-(2,6-dimethoxy-4-pyrimidinyl) sulfanilamide. The structural formula is:

H_2N–(benzene ring)–SO_2•NH–(pyrimidine ring, N, N)–OCH_3, OCH_3

Actions: Sulfadimethoxine has been demonstrated clinically or in the laboratory to be effective against a variety of organisms, such as streptococci, klebsiella, proteus, shigella, staphylococci, escherichia, and salmonella.[1,2]

The systemic sulfonamides which include sulfadimethoxine are bacteriostatic agents. Sulfonamides competitively inhibit bacterial synthesis of folic acid (pteroylglutamic acid) from para-aminobenzoic acid. Mammalian cells are capable of utilizing folic acid in the presence of sulfonamides.

The tissue distribution of sulfadimethoxine, as with all sulfonamides, is a function of plasma levels, degree of plasma protein binding, and subsequent passive distribution in the tissues of the lipid-soluble un-ionized form. The relative amounts are determined by both its pKa and by the pH of each tissue. Therefore, levels tend to be higher in less acid tissue and body fluids or those diseased tissues having high concentrations of leucocytes.[2]

Slow renal excretion results from a high degree of tubular reabsorption,[3] and plasma protein binding is very high, providing a blood reservoir of the drug. Thus, sulfadimethoxine maintains higher blood levels than most other long-acting sulfonamides. Single, comparatively low doses of SULFADIMETHOXINE INJECTION 40% give rapid and sustained therapeutic blood levels.[1]

To assure successful sulfonamide therapy (1) the drug must be given early in the course of the disease, and it must produce a high sulfonamide level in the body rapidly after administration, (2) therapeutically effective sulfonamide levels must be maintained in the body throughout the treatment period, (3) treatment should continue for a short period of time after the clinical signs have disappeared, and (4) the causative organisms must be sensitive to this class of drugs.

Dosage and Administration: SULFADIMETHOXINE INJECTION 40% must be administered only by the intravenous route in cattle. Cattle should receive 1 mL of SULFADIMETHOXINE INJECTION 40% per 16 pounds of body weight (55 mg/kg) as an initial dose, followed by 0.5 mL per 16 pounds of body weight (27.5 mg/kg) every 24 hours thereafter. Sulfadimethoxine Boluses may be utilized for maintenance therapy in cattle. Representative weights and doses are indicated in the following table:

Animal Weight	Initial Dose 25 mg/lb. (55 mg/kg)	Subsequent Daily Doses 12.5 mg/lb. (27.5 mg/kg)
250 lb (113.6 kg)	15.6 mL	7.8 mL
500 lb (227.2 kg)	31.2 mL	15.6 mL
750 lb (340.9 kg)	46.9 mL	23.5 mL
1000 lb (454.5 kg)	62.5 mL	31.3 mL

Length of treatment depends on the clinical response. In most cases treatment for 3 to 5 days is adequate. Treatment should be continued until the animal is asymptomatic for 48 hours.

Directions for Intravenous Injection:

Equipment needed:

1. A nose lead and/or halter sufficiently strong enough to effectively restrain or hold the animal's head steady so that the intravenous injection can be made with ease.
2. Hypodermic needles, 16 or 18 gauge and 2 inches long. Only new, sharp and sterile hypodermic needles should be used. Dull needles should be discarded. Extra needles should always be available in case the needle being used should become clogged.
3. Hypodermic syringes, 40 or 50 mL sterile disposable or reusable glass syringes should be available.
4. Alcohol (70%) or equally effective antiseptic for disinfecting the skin.

Preparation of equipment: Glass syringes and regular hypodermic needles should be thoroughly cleaned and washed. Following this, the needles and syringes should be immersed in boiling water for 30 minutes prior to each injection. Regular hypodermic needles should not be used more than 3-4 times as repeated skin puncturing and boiling of the needles causes them to become quite dull. Disposable hypodermic needles and syringes should not be used more than once.

Restraint of animal: The cow should preferably be in a stanchion for maximum restraint. If this is not possible, the animal should be restrained in a manner to prevent excessive movement. A nose lead should be applied and the animal's head turned sidewise to stretch the skin and tense the muscles of the neck region.

Locating the jugular vein: When the animal has been restrained (as above), you will notice a long depression of the skin from below the angle of the jaw to just above the shoulder. This is known as the jugular furrow or jugular groove. The jugular vein is located just under the jugular groove.

Preparation of SULFADIMETHOXINE INJECTION 40% for injection: The rubber cap of the bottle should be thoroughly cleaned with 70% alcohol or other satisfactory antiseptic. The correct amount of SULFADIMETHOXINE INJECTION 40% for treatment should be calculated (see dosage directions) and that amount withdrawn into a syringe. One or two syringefuls of air should be injected into the bottle first to make withdrawing the drug easier. SULFADIMETHOXINE INJECTION 40% should preferably be at room temperature when filling syringes and when injecting intravenously.

Entering the vein: The skin of the injection area should be clean and free of dirt. Cotton saturated with 70% alcohol (or suitable antiseptic) should be used to wipe the injection site.

Apply pressure over the jugular vein close to the shoulder. This will reduce the flow of blood to the heart and cause the jugular vein to bulge or enlarge. (See Figure 1). When the jugular vein has been "raised", insert the hypodermic needle at a 45 degree angle through the skin just underneath the jugular vein. The beveled edge of the hypodermic needles should be up.

After the skin has been punctured, the point of the needle should be directed toward the side of the vein and pushed into the center of the vein (See Figure 2). When the needle is in the center of the vein, there will be a free flow of blood back through the needle. Release external pressure when you are sure the needle is within the vein.

Injecting the SULFADIMETHOXINE INJECTION 40%: After the needle has been accurately inserted into the jugular vein, firmly attach the syringe containing SULFADIMETHOXINE INJECTION 40% to the inserted hypodermic needle. Caution, be sure syringe is free of air. Exert firm pressure on the plunger of the syringe to inject the SULFADIMETHOXINE INJECTION 40% while the barrel is held firmly. The injection should be made moderately slow - never rapidly.

If the animal moves, causing resistance in pushing the plunger of the syringe, or if a bubble of the drug is noted under the skin, the needle is no longer within the vein. The needle should be repositioned.

When the injection is completed, quickly withdraw the syringe and needle with a quick pull and apply light pressure over the injection site with alcohol and cotton to minimize bleeding from the puncture site.

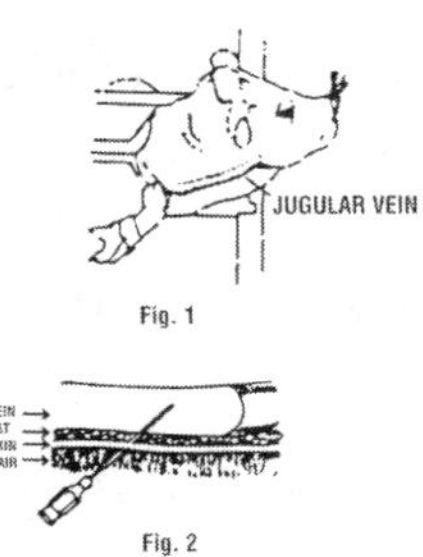

Fig. 1

Fig. 2

Precaution(s): Store at room temperature between 15° and 30°C (59° and 86°F). Should crystallization occur at cold temperatures, crystals will dissolve either by storing at room temperature for several days or by heating the vial in warm water. Crystallization and redissolution do not impair the efficacy of the product.

Caution(s): During treatment period, make certain that animals maintain adequate water intake.

If animals show no improvement within 2 or 3 days, consult a veterinarian.

Tissue damage may result from perivascular infiltration.

Limitations: Sulfadimethoxine is not effective in viral or rickettsial infections, and as with any anti-bacterial agent, occasional failures in therapy may occur due to resistant microorganisms. The usual precautions in sulfonamide therapy should be observed.

For intravenous use only in cattle.

For animal use only.

Restricted drug (California) - Use only as directed.

Not for human use.

Warning(s): Milk taken from animals during treatment and for 60 hours (5 milkings) after the latest treatment must not be used for food. Do not administer within 5 days of slaughter. A withdrawal period has not been established for this product in preruminating calves.

Do not use in calves to be processed for veal.

Keep out of reach of children.

Toxicology: Toxicity and Safety: Data regarding acute (LD_{50}) and chronic toxicities of sulfadimethoxine indicate the drug is safe. The LD_{50} in mice is greater than 2 g/kg body weight when administered intraperitoneally and greater than 16 g/kg when administered orally. In dogs receiving massive single oral doses of 3.2 g/kg body weight, diarrhea was the only adverse effect observed. Dogs given 160 mg/kg body weight orally daily for 13 weeks showed no signs of toxicity.

In cattle sulfadimethoxine has been shown to be safe through extensive clinical use with other dosage forms. In addition, studies with intravenous administration of SULFADIMETHOXINE INJECTION 40% have demonstrated that hemolysis of erythrocytes does not occur by this route of administration. Sulfadimethoxine has a relatively high solubility at the pH normally occurring in the kidney, precluding the possibility of precipitation and crystalluria.

References: Available upon request.

Presentation: 250 mL multiple dose vial (NDC 30798-588-13).

Manufactured by: Phoenix Scientific, Inc., St. Joseph, MO 64503.

Compendium Code No.: 10841531 Rev. 11-00

SULFADIMETHOXINE INJECTION-40%

Vedco **Sulfadimethoxine**

Antibacterial

ANADA No.: 200-038

Active Ingredient(s): Each mL contains: 400 mg sulfadimethoxine compounded with 20% propylene glycol, 1% benzyl alcohol, 0.1 mg disodium edetate, 1 mg sodium formaldehyde sulfoxylate and pH adjusted with sodium hydroxide.

Indications: Cattle: For the treatment of bovine respiratory disease complex (shipping fever complex) and bacterial pneumonia associated with *Pasteurella* spp sensitive to sulfadimethoxine; necrotic pododermatitis (foot rot) and calf diphtheria caused by *Fusobacterium necrophorum* sensitive to sulfadimethoxine.

Dosage and Administration: To be administered in amounts to provide 25 mg/lb (55 mg/kg) for initial dose, followed by 12.5 mg/lb (27.5 mg/kg) for maintenance doses every 24 hours.

During treatment period, make certain that animals maintain adequate water intake.

Warning(s): Milk taken from animals during treatment and for 60 hours (5 milkings) after the latest treatment must not be used for food.

Do not administer within 5 days of slaughter. A withdrawal period has not been established for this product in preruminating calves. Do not use in calves to be processed for veal.

For animal use only - Not for human use.

Keep out of reach of children.

Presentation: 250 mL (8.5 fl oz).

Compendium Code No.: 10491901

SULFADIMETHOXINE ORAL SOLUTION

AgriPharm **Water Medication**

Antibacterial

12.5% Concentrated Solution for Use in Drinking Water

ANADA No.: 200-192

Active Ingredient(s): Each fluid ounce contains 3.75 g sulfadimethoxine solubilized with sodium hydroxide.

Indications:

Broiler and Replacement Chickens: Use for the treatment of disease outbreaks of coccidiosis, fowl cholera, and infectious coryza.

Meat Producing Turkeys: Use for the treatment of disease outbreaks of coccidiosis and fowl cholera.

Dairy Calves, Dairy Heifers and Beef Cattle: Use in the treatment of shipping fever complex, bacterial pneumonia, calf diphtheria, and foot rot.

Dosage and Administration:

Chickens: For a 0.05% concentration, add 1 fl oz* to 2 gallons of drinking water or 25 fl oz to 50 gallons of drinking water.

Turkeys: For a 0.025% concentration, add 1 fl oz* to 4 gallons of drinking water or 25 fl oz to 100 gallons of drinking water.

Automatic Proportioners** Stock Solution - To make 2 gallons of stock solution use:

Chickens: 1 gal Sulfadimethoxine 12.5% Drinking Water Solution Concentrate plus 1 gal of water.

Turkeys: 2 qts Sulfadimethoxine 12.5% Drinking Water Solution Concentrate plus 6 qts of water.

Treatment Period: 6 consecutive days.

Sulfadimethoxine in Water:

Dairy Calves, Dairy Heifers and Beef Cattle: 25 mg/lb first day followed by 12.5 mg/lb/day for 4 days.

	Water Consumption	
	(Summer)	(Winter)
	1 gallon/† 100 lb b.w.	1 gallon/† 150 lb b.w.
First day add:		
1 pint (16 fl oz) to:	25 gallons	16 gallons
1 quart (32 fl oz) to:	50 gallons	33 gallons
1 gallon (128 fl oz) to:	200 gallons	127 gallons
Next 4 days add:		
1 pint (16 fl oz) to:	50 gallons	33 gallons
1 quart (32 fl oz) to:	100 gallons	66 gallons
1 gallon (128 fl oz) to:	400 gallons	266 gallons

†This dosage recommendation is based on a water consumption of 1 gallon per 100 lb of body weight per day, the expected water consumption rate for summer. Water consumption during cold months (winter) may drop markedly (30-40%). Accordingly, adjustments in drug concentration in drinking water must be made to insure proper drug intake.

For individual treatment of cattle, Sulfadimethoxine 12.5% Drinking Water Solution may be given as a drench. Administer using same mg/lb dose as outlined above. Four fluid ounces will medicate one-600 lb animal initially or two-600 lb animals on maintenance dose.

Treatment Period: 5 consecutive days.

*1 fl oz Sulfadimethoxine 12.5% Drinking Water Solution = 30 mL or 2 tablespoonfuls.

**Set proportioner to a feed rate of 1 fl oz of Sulfadimethoxine Stock Solution per gallon of water.

Precaution(s): Store at room temperature; if freezing occurs, thaw before using. Protect from light; direct sunlight may cause discoloration. Freezing or discoloration does not affect potency. Prepare a fresh stock solution daily.

Caution(s):

Chickens and Turkeys: If animals show no improvement within 5 days, discontinue treatment and re-evaluate diagnosis. Handle the recommended dilutions (chickens 0.05% and turkeys 0.025%) as regular drinking water. Administer as sole source of drinking water and sulfonamide medication.

Chickens and turkeys that have survived fowl cholera outbreaks should not be kept for replacements or breeders.

Cattle: During treatment period, make certain that animals maintain adequate water intake. If animals show no improvement within 2 or 3 days, re-evaluate diagnosis. Treatment should not be continued beyond 5 days.

Warning(s):

Chickens and Turkeys: Withdraw 5 days before slaughter. Do not administer to chickens over 16 weeks (112 days) of age or to turkeys over 24 weeks (168 days) of age.

Cattle: Withdraw 7 days before slaughter. For dairy calves, dairy heifers and beef cattle only. A withdrawal period has not been established for this product in pre-ruminating cattle. Do not use in calves to be processed for veal.

For use in animals only.

Restricted drug (California). Use only as directed.

Not for human use.

Keep out of reach of children.

Presentation: 3.785 L (1 gal) (128 fl oz).

Compendium Code No.: 14570940

SULFADIMETHOXINE ORAL SOLUTION

Aspen **Water Medication**

12.5% Concentrated Solution

ANADA No.: 200-030

Active Ingredient(s): Each fluid ounce contains 3.75 g of sulfadimethoxine solubilized with sodium hydroxide. This product is a 12.5% concentrated solution for use in drinking water.

Indications: For oral use in chickens, turkeys and cattle.

Broiler and Replacement Chickens: Use for the treatment of disease outbreaks of coccidiosis, fowl cholera, and infectious coryza.

Meat Producing Turkeys: Use for the treatment of disease outbreaks of coccidiosis and fowl cholera.

Dairy Calves, Dairy Heifers and Beef Cattle: Use in the treatment of shipping fever complex, bacterial pneumonia, calf diphtheria, and foot rot.

Dosage and Administration:

Chickens: For a 0.05% concentration, add 1 fl oz* to 2 gallons of drinking water, or 25 fl oz to 50 gallons of drinking water.

Turkeys: For a 0.025% concentration, add 1 fl oz* to 4 gallons of drinking water, or 25 fl oz to 100 gallons of drinking water.

Automatic proportioners** Stock Solution - To make 2 gallons of Stock Solution use:

Chickens: 1 gal SULFADIMETHOXINE 12.5% Drinking Water Solution Concentrate - plus - 1 gal of water.

Turkeys: 2 qts SULFADIMETHOXINE 12.5% Drinking Water Solution Concentrate - plus 6 qts of water.

Treatment Period: 6 consecutive days.

Dairy Calves, Dairy Heifers and Beef Cattle: 25 mg/lb first day followed by 12.5 mg/lb/day for 4 days.

	Sulfadimethoxine in Water Water Consumption	
	(Summer) 1 gallon/† 100 lb b.w.	(Winter) 1 gallon/† 150 lb b.w.
First day add:		
1 pint (16 fl oz) to:	25 gallons	16 gallons
1 quart (32 fl oz) to:	50 gallons	33 gallons
1 gallon (128 fl oz) to:	200 gallons	127 gallons
Next 4 days add:		
1 pint (16 fl oz) to:	50 gallons	33 gallons
1 quart (32 fl oz) to:	100 gallons	66 gallons
1 gallon (128 fl oz) to:	400 gallons	266 gallons

†This dosage recommendation is based on a water consumption of 1 gallon per 100 lb of body weight per day, the expected water consumption rate for summer. Water consumption during cold months (winter) may drop markedly (30-40%). Accordingly, adjustments in drug concentration in drinking water must be made to ensure proper drug intake.

For individual treatment of cattle, SULFADIMETHOXINE 12.5% Drinking Water Solution Concentrate may be given as a drench. Administer using the same mg/lb dosage as outlined above. Four fluid ounces will medicate one-600 lb animal initially, or two-600 lb animals on a maintenance dose.

Treatment Period: 5 consecutive days.

*1 fl oz SULFADIMETHOXINE 12.5% Drinking Water Solution Concentrate = 30 mL or 2 tablespoonfuls.

**Set the proportioner to a feed rate of 1 fl oz of SULFADIMETHOXINE stock solution per gallon of water.

Precaution(s): Store at room temperature. If freezing occurs, thaw before using. Protect from light, direct sunlight may cause discoloration. Freezing or discoloration does not affect potency. Prepare a fresh stock solution daily.

Caution(s): Chickens and Turkeys: If animals show no improvement within 5 days, discontinue treatment and re-evaluate diagnosis. Handle the recommended dilutions (chickens 0.05% and turkeys 0.025%) as regular drinking water. Administer as sole source of drinking water and sulfonamide medication.

Chickens and turkeys that have survived fowl cholera outbreaks should not be kept for replacements or breeders.

Cattle: During treatment period, make certain that animals maintain adequate water intake. If animals show no improvement within 2 or 3 days, re-evaluate diagnosis. Treatment should not be continued beyond 5 days.

Warning(s): Chickens and Turkeys: Withdraw 5 days before slaughter. Do not administer to chickens over 16 weeks (112 days) of age or to turkeys over 24 weeks (168 days) of age. Cattle: Withdraw 7 days before slaughter. For dairy calves, dairy heifers and beef cattle only. A withdrawal period has not been established for this product in preruminating calves. Do not use in calves to be processed for veal.

For animal use only.

Not for human use.

Keep out of reach of children.

Presentation: 1 gallon (3.875 L) containers.

Compendium Code No.: 14750780

SULFADIMETHOXINE ORAL SOLUTION

Butler **Water Medication**

Antibacterial

ANADA No.: 200-030

Active Ingredient(s): Each fluid ounce contains 3.75 g sulfadimethoxine solubilized with sodium hydroxide.

Indications:

Broiler and Replacement Chickens: For use in the treatment of disease outbreaks of coccidiosis, fowl cholera, and infectious coryza.

Meat Producing Turkeys: For use in the treatment of disease outbreaks of coccidiosis and fowl cholera.

Dairy Calves, Dairy Heifers and Beef Cattle: For use in the treatment of shipping fever complex, bacterial pneumonia, calf diphtheria and foot rot.

Dosage and Administration: For oral use in chickens, turkeys and cattle.

Chickens: Give a 0.05% concentration. Add 1 fl oz* to 2 gallons of drinking water, or 25 fl oz to 50 gallons of drinking water.

Turkeys: Give a 0.025% concentration. Add 1 fl oz* to 4 gallons of drinking water, or 25 fl oz to 100 gallons of drinking water.

Automatic Proportioners** Stock Solution: To Make 2 Gallons of Stock Solution Use:

Chickens: 1 gal of sulfadimethoxine 12.5% Drinking Water Solution Concentrate, plus 1 gal of water.

Turkeys: 2 qts of Sulfadimethoxine 12.5% Drinking Water Solution Concentrate, plus 6 qts of water.

Treatment Period: 6 consecutive days.

S

Sulfadimethoxine in Water:

Dairy calves, dairy heifers and beef cattle: Give a 25 mg/lb. dose the first day, followed by a 12.5 mg/lb./day dose for 4 days. See chart below:

	Water Consumption	
	(Summer)	(Winter)
	1 gallon/† 100 lb. body weight	1 gallon/† 150 lb. body weight
First day add:		
1 pint (16 fl oz) to:	25 gallons	16 gallons
1 quart (32 fl oz) to:	50 gallons	33 gallons
1 gallon (128 fl oz) to:	200 gallons	127 gallons
Next 4 days add:		
1 pint (16 fl oz) to:	50 gallons	33 gallons
1 quart (32 fl oz) to:	100 gallons	66 gallons
1 gallon (128 fl oz) to:	400 gallons	266 gallons

† The dosage recommendation is based on a water consumption of 1 gallon per 100 lbs. of body weight per day, the expected water consumption rate for summer. Water consumption during cold months (winter) may drop markedly (30-40%). Accordingly, adjustments in drug concentration in drinking water must be made to ensure proper drug intake.

For the individual treatment of cattle, Sulfadimethoxine 12.5% Drinking Water Solution may be given as a drench. Administer using the same mg/lb. dosage as outlined above. 4 fl oz will medicate 1-600 lb. animal initially, or 2-600 lb. animals on maintenance dose.

Treatment period: 5 consecutive days.

* 1 fl oz Sulfadimethoxine 12.5% Drinking Water Solution = 30 mL or 2 tablespoonfuls.

** Set the proportioner to a feed rate of 1 fl oz of sulfadimethoxine stock solution per gallon of water.

Prepare a fresh stock solution each day.

Precaution(s): Store at room temperature. If freezing occurs, thaw before using. Protect from light. Direct sunlight may cause discoloration. Freezing or discoloration does not affect potency.

Caution(s): Chickens and Turkeys: If the animals do not show improvement within 5 days, discontinue treatment and re-evaluate the diagnosis. Handle the recommended dilutions (chickens 0.05% and turkeys 0.025%) as regular drinking water. Administer as the sole source of drinking water and sulfonamide medication.

Chickens and turkeys that have survived fowl cholera outbreaks should not be kept for replacements or breeders.

Cattle: During the treatment period, make certain that the animals maintain adequate water intake. If the animals do not show improvement within two or three days, re-evaluate the diagnosis. The treatment should not be continued beyond five days.

Warning(s): Chickens and Turkeys: Withdraw 5 days before slaughter. Do not administer to chickens over 16 weeks (112 days) of age or to turkeys over 24 weeks (168 days) of age.

Cattle: Withdraw 7 days before slaughter. For dairy calves, dairy heifers and beef cattle only.

For animal use only.

Not for human use.

Keep out of the reach of children.

Presentation: 3.8 Liters (1 gallon).

Compendium Code No.: 10821710

SULFADIMETHOXINE ORAL SOLUTION

Durvet **Water Medication**

Antibacterial

ANADA No.: 200-192

Active Ingredient(s): Each fluid ounce contains 3.75 g of sulfadimethoxine solubilized with sodium hydroxide.

Indications:

Broiler and Replacement Chickens: Use for the treatment of disease outbreaks of coccidiosis, fowl cholera and infectious coryza.

Meat Producing Turkeys: Use for the treatment of disease outbreaks of coccidiosis and fowl cholera.

Dairy Calves, Dairy Heifers and Beef Cattle: Use for the treatment of shipping fever complex, bacterial pneumonia, calf diphtheria and foot rot.

Dosage and Administration:

Chickens: For a 0.05% concentrate, add 1 fl oz* to 2 gallons of drinking water, or 25 fl oz to 50 gallons of drinking water.

Turkeys: For a 0.025% concentrate, add 1 fl oz* to 4 gallons of drinking water, or 25 fl oz to 100 gallons of drinking water.

Automatic Proportioners** Stock Solution - To make 2 gallons of Stock Solution use:

Chickens: 1 gal of Sulfadimethoxine 12.5% Drinking Water Solution Concentrate, plus 1 gal of water.

Turkeys: 2 qts Sulfadimethoxine 12.5% Drinking Water Solution Concentrate, plus 6 qts of water.

Treatment Period—6 consecutive days.

Dairy Calves, Dairy Heifers and Beef Cattle: 25 mg/lb the first day, followed by 12.5 mg/lb/day for 4 days.

	Water Consumption	
	(Summer)	(Winter)
	1 gallon/† 100 lb. b.w.	1 gallon/† 150 lbs. b.w.
First Day Add:		
1 pint (16 fl oz) to:	25 gallons	16 gallons
1 quart (32 fl oz) to:	50 gallons	33 gallons
1 gallon (128 fl oz) to:	200 gallons	127 gallons
Next 4 Days Add:		
1 pint (16 fl oz) to:	50 gallons	33 gallons
1 quart (32 fl oz) to:	100 gallons	66 gallons
1 gallon (128 fl oz) to:	400 gallons	266 gallons

†This dosage recommendation is based on a water consumption of 1 gallon per 100 lb of body weight per day, the expected water consumption rate for summer. Water consumption during cold months (winter) may drop markedly (30-40%). Accordingly, adjustments in drug concentration in drinking water must be made to ensure proper drug intake.

For individual treatment of cattle, Sulfadimethoxine 12.5% Drinking Water Solution may be given as a drench. Administer using same mg/lb dosage as outlined above. Four fluid ounces will medicate one-600 lb animal initially, or two-600 lb animals on a maintenance dose.

Treatment Period—5 consecutive days.

* 1 fl oz Sulfadimethoxine 12.5% Drinking Water Solution = 30 mL or 2 tablespoonfuls.

** Set proportioner to a feed rate of 1 fl oz of Sulfadimethoxine Stock Solution per gallon of water.

Chickens and Turkeys: If animals do not show improvement within 5 days, discontinue treatment and re-evaluate diagnosis. Handle the recommended dilutions (chickens 0.05% and turkeys 0.025%) as regular drinking water. Administer as the sole source of drinking water and sulfonamide medication.

Chickens and turkeys that have survived fowl cholera outbreaks should not be kept for replacements or breeders.

Cattle: During treatment period, make certain that the animals maintain adequate water intake. If animals do not show improvement within 2 or 3 days, re-evaluate diagnosis. Treatment should not be continued beyond 5 days.

Precaution(s): Store at room temperature; if freezing occurs, thaw before using. Protect from light; direct sunlight may cause discoloration. Freezing or discoloration does not affect potency. Prepare a fresh stock solution daily.

Caution(s): For use in animals only.

Restricted Drug (California)-Use only as directed. Not for human use.

Warning(s): Chickens and Turkeys: Withdraw 5 days before slaughter.

Do not administer to chickens over 16 weeks (112 days) of age or to turkeys over 24 weeks (168 days) of age.

Cattle: Withdraw 7 days before slaughter. A withdrawal period has not been established for this product in pre-ruminating calves. Do not use in calves to be processed for veal.

Keep out of reach of children.

Presentation: 3.785 L (1 gal) (128 fl oz) (NDC 30798-587-37).

Compendium Code No.: 10841541 Iss. 6-97

SULFADIMETHOXINE ORAL SOLUTION

Vedco **Water Medication**

Antibacterial

12.5% Concentrate Solution for Use in Drinking Water

ANADA No.: 200-030

Active Ingredient(s): Each fluid ounce contains: 3.75 g sulfadimethoxine solubilized with sodium hydroxide.

Indications: For oral use in chickens, turkeys and cattle.

Broiler and Replacement Chickens: Use for the treatment of disease outbreaks of coccidiosis, fowl cholera and infectious coryza.

Meat Producing Trays: Use for the treatment of disease outbreaks of coccidiosis and fowl cholera.

Dairy Calves, Dairy Heifers and Beef Cattle: Use in the treatment of shipping fever complex, bacterial pneumonia, calf diphtheria and foot rot.

Dosage and Administration: Chickens: For a 0.05% concentration, add 1 fl oz* to 2 gallons of drinking water, or 25 fl oz to 50 gallons of drinking water.

Turkeys: For a 0.025% concentration, add 1 fl oz* to 4 gallons of drinking water, or 25 fl oz to 100 gallons of drinking water.

Automatic proportioners** Stock Solution - To make 2 gallons of Stock Solution use:

Chickens: 1 gal SULFADIMETHOXINE ORAL SOLUTION - plus - 1 gal of water.

Turkeys: 2 qts SULFADIMETHOXINE ORAL SOLUTION - plus 6 qts of water.

Treatment Period: 6 consecutive days.

Dairy Calves, Dairy Heifers and Beef Cattle: 25 mg/lb first day followed by 12.5 mg/lb/day for 4 days.

	Sulfadimethoxine in Water Water Consumption	
	(Summer) 1 gallon/† 100 lb b.w.	(Winter) 1 gallon/† 150 lb b.w.
First day add:		
1 pint (16 fl oz) to:	25 gallons	16 gallons
1 quart (32 fl oz) to:	50 gallons	33 gallons
1 gallon (128 fl oz) to:	200 gallons	127 gallons
Next 4 days add:		
1 pint (16 fl oz) to:	50 gallons	33 gallons
1 quart (32 fl oz) to:	100 gallons	66 gallons
1 gallon (128 fl oz) to:	400 gallons	266 gallons

†This dosage recommendation is based on a water consumption of 1 gallon per 100 lb of body weight per day, the expected water consumption rate for summer. Water consumption during cold months (winter) may drop markedly (30-40%). Accordingly, adjustments in drug concentration in drinking water must be made to ensure proper drug intake.

For individual treatment of cattle, SULFADIMETHOXINE ORAL SOLUTION may be given as a drench. Administer using the same mg/lb dosage as outlined above. Four fluid ounces will medicate one-600 lb animal initially, or two-600 lb animals on a maintenance dose.

Treatment Period: 5 consecutive days.

*1 fl oz SULFADIMETHOXINE ORAL SOLUTION = 30 mL or 2 tablespoonfuls.

**Set the proportioner to a feed rate of 1 fl oz of SULFADIMETHOXINE ORAL SOLUTION per gallon of water.

Chickens and Turkeys: If animals show no improvement within 5 days, discontinue treatment and re-evaluate diagnosis. Handle the recommended dilutions as regular drinking water. Administer as sole source of drinking water and sulfonamide medication.

**Chickens and turkeys that have survived fowl cholera outbreaks should not be kept for replacements or breeders.

Cattle: During treatment period, make certain that animals maintain adequate water intake. If animals show no improvement within 2 to 3 days, re-evaluate diagnosis. Treatment should not be continued beyond 5 days.

Precaution(s): Store at room temperature; if freezing occurs, thaw before using. Protect from light; direct sunlight may cause discoloration. Freezing or discoloration does not affect potency. Prepare a fresh stock solution daily.

Warning(s): Chickens and turkeys - withdraw 5 days before slaughter. Do not administer to chickens over 16 weeks of age or to turkeys over 24 weeks of age. Cattle - withdraw 7 days before slaughter. For dairy calves, dairy heifers and beef cattle only. A withdrawal period has not been established for this product in preruminating calves. Do not use in calves to be processed for veal.

For animal use only - Not for human use.

Keep out of reach of children.

Presentation: 1 gallon (3.785 L).

Compendium Code No.: 10941910

SULFADIMETHOXINE SOLUBLE POWDER

AgriPharm **Sulfadimethoxine**

Antibacterial

For Oral Use

ANADA No.: 200-031

Active Ingredient(s): Each packet contains 94.6 g (3.34 oz) of sulfadimethoxine in the form of the soluble sodium salt and disodium edetate.

Indications:

For Broiler and Replacement Chickens Only: Use for the treatment of disease outbreaks of coccidiosis, fowl cholera, and infectious coryza.

For Meat Producing Turkeys Only: Use for the treatment of disease outbreaks of coccidiosis and fowl cholera.

For Dairy Calves, Dairy Heifers and Beef Cattle: Use for the treatment of shipping fever complex, bacterial pneumonia, calf diphtheria, and foot rot.

Dosage and Administration:

Chickens: For a 0.05% concentration, add contents of packet to 50 gallons of water.

Turkeys: For a 0.025% concentration, add contents of packet to 100 gallons of water.

Automatic proportioners: To make stock solution, add contents of 5 packets to 2 gallons of water for chickens and to 4 gallons of water for turkeys. Set proportioner to feed at rate of 1 fl oz of stock solution per gallon of water.

Treatment Period: 6 consecutive days.

Sulfadimethoxine in Water:

Dairy Calves, Dairy Heifers and Beef Cattle: 25 mg/lb the first day followed by 12.5 mg/lb/day for 4 days.

Amount of Stock Solution for Cattle*	Water Consumption	
	(Summer)	(Winter)
	1 gallon/** 100 lb b.w.	1 gallon/** 150 lb b.w.
First day add:		
1 quart	10 gallons	7 gallons
2 quarts	20 gallons	14 gallons
1 gallon	40 gallons	28 gallons
Next 4 days add:		
1 quart	20 gallons	14 gallons
2 quarts	40 gallons	28 gallons
1 gallon	80 gallons	55 gallons

*Note: Make a cattle stock solution by adding 1 packet of SULFADIMETHOXINE SOLUBLE POWDER to 1 gallon of water.

**This dosage recommendation is based on a water consumption of 1 gallon per 100 lb of body weight per day, the expected water consumption rate for summer. Water consumption during cold months (winter) may drop markedly (30-40%). Accordingly, adjustments must be made in the dilution rates to compensate for this and insure proper drug intake.

For treatment of individual cattle, SULFADIMETHOXINE SOLUBLE POWDER stock solution for cattle may be given as a drench. Administer using same mg/lb dosage as outlined above.

Twenty fluid ounces of cattle stock solution will medicate one-600 lb animal initially or two-600 lb animals on maintenance dose. Contents of packet will medicate six-600 lb animals initially or twelve-600 lb animals on maintenance dose.

Treatment Period: 5 consecutive days.

Caution(s):

Chickens and Turkeys: If animals show no improvement within 5 days, discontinue treatment and re-evaluate diagnosis. Prepare a fresh stock solution daily. Handle the recommended dilutions (chickens 0.05% and turkeys 0.025%) as regular drinking water. Administer as sole source of drinking water and sulfonamide medication.

Chickens and turkeys that have survived fowl cholera outbreaks should not be kept for replacements or breeders.

Cattle: During treatment period, make certain that animals maintain adequate water intake. If animals show no improvement within 2 or 3 days, re-evaluate diagnosis. Treatment should not be continued beyond 5 days.

S

Warning(s):

Chickens and Turkeys: Withdraw 5 days before slaughter. Do not administer to chickens over 16 weeks (112 days) of age or to turkeys over 24 weeks (168 days) of age.

Cattle: Withdraw 7 days before slaughter. For dairy calves, dairy heifers and beef cattle only. A withdrawal period has not been established for this product in pre-ruminating calves. Do not use in calves to be processed for veal.

For animal use only.

Restricted drug (California) - Use only as directed.

Not for human use.

Keep out of reach of children.

Presentation: 25 packets, each containing 107 grams (3.77 oz).

Compendium Code No.: 14570950

SULFADIMETHOXINE SOLUBLE POWDER

Aspen **Sulfadimethoxine**

Antibacterial

ANADA No.: 200-258

Active Ingredient(s): Each packet contains 94.6 g (3.34 oz) sulfadimethoxine as sodium sulfadimethoxine.

Indications:

For Broiler and Replacement Chickens Only-Use for the treatment of disease outbreaks of coccidiosis, fowl cholera, and infectious coryza.

For Meat-producing Turkeys Only-Use for the treatment of disease outbreaks of coccidiosis and fowl cholera.

For Dairy Calves, Dairy Heifers, and Beef Cattle-Use for the treatment of shipping fever complex and bacterial pneumonia associated with *Pasteurella* spp. sensitive to sulfadimethoxine; and calf diphtheria and foot rot associated with *Sphaerophorus necrophorus* sensitive to sulfadimethoxine.

Dosage and Administration:

Species	Concentration	Use Direction
Chickens	0.05%	Contents of packet to 50 gal of water
Turkeys	0.025%	Contents of packet to 100 gal of water

Automatic Proportioners-To make stock solution, add contents of 5 packets to 2 gal of water for chickens and to 4 gal of water for turkeys. Set proportioner to feed at rate of 1 fl oz of stock solution per gal of water.

Treatment Period: 6 consecutive days.

Dairy Calves, Dairy Heifers, and Beef Cattle:

Dosage: 25 mg/lb the first day followed by 12.5 mg/lb/day for 4 days.

Sulfadimethoxine in Water:

	Amount of Stock Solution for Cattle*	Water Consumption	
		(Summer) 1 gal/100 lb body wt**	(Winter) 1 gal/150 lb body wt**
First Day Add	1 qt	10 gal	7 gal
	2 qt	20 gal	14 gal
	1 gal	40 gal	28 gal
Next 4 Days Add	1 qt	20 gal	14 gal
	2 qt	40 gal	28 gal
	1 gal	80 gal	56 gal

*Note: Make a cattle stock solution by adding 1 packet of SULFADIMETHOXINE SOLUBLE POWDER to 1 gal of water.

*Twenty fl oz of cattle stock solution will medicate 1-600 lb animal initially or 2-600 lb animals on maintenance dose. Contents of packet will medicate 6-600 lb animals initially or 12-600 lb animals on maintenance dose.

**This dosage recommendation is based on a water consumption of 1 gal per 100 lb of body weight per day, the expected water consumption rate for summer. Water consumption during cold months (winter) may drop markedly (30-40%). Accordingly, adjustments must be made in the dilution rates to compensate for this and insure proper drug intake.

For treatment of individual cattle, SULFADIMETHOXINE SOLUBLE POWDER stock solution for cattle may be given as a drench. Administer using same mg/lb dosage as outlined above.

Treatment Period: 5 consecutive days.

Caution(s):

Chickens and Turkeys-If animals show no improvement within 5 days, discontinue treatment and reevaluate diagnosis. Prepare a fresh stock solution daily. Handle the recommended dilutions (chickens 0.05% and turkeys 0.025%) as regular drinking water. Administer as sole source of drinking water and sulfonamide medication.

Chickens and turkeys that have survived fowl cholera outbreaks should not be kept for replacements or breeders.

Cattle-During treatment period, make certain that animals maintain adequate water intake. If animals show no improvement within 2 or 3 days, reevaluate diagnosis. Treatment should not be continued beyond 5 days.

Warning(s):

Chickens and Turkeys-Withdraw 5 days before slaughter. Do not administer to chickens over 16 weeks (112 days) of age or to turkeys over 24 weeks (168 days) of age.

Cattle: Withdraw 7 days before slaughter. For dairy calves, dairy heifers, and beef cattle only. A withdrawal period has not been established for this product in pre-ruminating calves. Do not use in calves to be processed for veal.

Restricted drug (California) - Use only as directed.

Not for human use.

Presentation: 25 x 107 g (3.77 oz) packets.

Manufactured by: Phoenix Scientific, Inc.

Compendium Code No.: 14750791

SULFADIMETHOXINE SOLUBLE POWDER

Durvet **Sulfadimethoxine**

Antibacterial

ANADA No.: 200-031

Active Ingredient(s): Each Packet Contains: 3.34 oz (94.6 g) Sulfadimethoxine in the form of the soluble sodium salt and disodium edetate.

Indications: For Broiler and Replacement Chickens Only: Use for the treatment of disease outbreaks of coccidiosis, fowl cholera and infectious coryza.

For Meat Producing Turkeys Only: Use for the treatment of disease outbreaks of coccidiosis and fowl cholera.

For Dairy Calves, Dairy Heifers and Beef Cattle: Use for the treatment of shipping fever complex, bacterial pneumonia, calf diphtheria and foot rot.

Dosage and Administration:

Chickens: For a 0.05% concentrate, add contents of 1 packet to 50 gallons of water.

Turkeys: For a 0.025% concentrate, add contents of 1 packet to 100 gallons of water.

Automatic proportioners: To make a stock solution, add the contents of 5 packets to 2 gallons of water for chickens, and to 4 gallons of water for turkeys. Set the proportioner to feed at a rate of 1 fl oz of stock solution per gallon of water.

Treatment Period—6 consecutive days.

Dairy Calves, Dairy Heifers and Beef Cattle: 25 mg/lb, followed by 12.5 mg/lb/day for 4 days.

Amount of Stock Solution for Cattle*	Sulfadimethoxine in Water Water Consumption	
	(Summer) 1 gallon/** 100 lb b.w.	(Winter) 1 gallon/** 150 lb b.w.
First Day Add:		
1 quart	10 gallons	7 gallons
2 quarts	20 gallons	14 gallons
1 gallon	40 gallons	28 gallons
Next 4 Days Add:		
1 quart	20 gallons	14 gallons
2 quarts	40 gallons	28 gallons
1 gallon	80 gallons	56 gallons

*Note: Make a cattle stock solution by adding 1 packet of SULFADIMETHOXINE SOLUBLE POWDER to 1 gallon of water.

**This dosage recommendation is based on a water consumption of 1 gallon per 100 lb of body weight per day, the expected water consumption rate for summer. Water consumption during cold months (winter) may drop markedly (30-40%). Accordingly, adjustments must be made in the dilution rates to compensate for this and ensure proper drug intake.

For treatment of individual cattle, SULFADIMETHOXINE SOLUTION POWDER stock solution for cattle may be given as a drench. Administer using mg/lb dosage as outlined above.

Twently fluid ounces of cattle stock solution will medicate one-600 lb animal initially, or two-600 lb animals on a maintenance dose. Contents of packet will medicate six-600 lb animals initially, or twelve-600 lb animals on a maintenance dose.

Treatment Period—5 consecutive days.

Chickens and Turkeys: If animals show no improvement within 5 days, discontinue treatment and re-evaluate the diagnosis. Prepare a fresh stock solution daily. Handle the recommended dilutions (chickens 0.05% and turkeys 0.025%) as regular drinking water. Administer as sole source of drinking water and sulfonamide medication.

Chickens and turkeys that have survived fowl cholera outbreaks should not be kept for replacements or breeders.

Cattle: During treatment period, ensure that animals maintain adequate water intake. If animals show no improvement within 2 or 3 days, re-evaluate diagnosis. Treatment should not be continued beyond 5 days.

Caution(s): For animal use only. Not for human use.

Warning(s): Chickens and Turkeys: Withdraw 5 days before slaughter. Do not administer to chickens over 16 weeks (112 days) of age or to turkeys over 24 weeks (168 days) of age.

Cattle: Withdraw 7 days before slaughter. For dairy calves, dairy heifers and beef cattle only. A withdrawal period has not been established for this product in pre-ruminating calves. Do not use in calves to be processed for veal. Keep out of reach of children.

Presentation: 25 x 107 g (3.77 oz) packets (NDC 30798-647-93).

Compendium Code No.: 10841551 6-99

SULFADIMETHOXINE SOLUBLE POWDER

Vedco **Sulfadimethoxine**

Antibacterial

ANADA No.: 200-031

Active Ingredient(s): Each packet contains 3.34 oz sulfadimethoxine in the form of the soluble sodium salt and disodium edate.

Indications: For oral use in chickens, turkeys and cattle.

For Broiler and Replacement Chickens Only: Use for the treatment of disease outbreaks of coccidiosis, fowl cholera, and infectious coryza.

For Meat Producing Turkeys Only: Use for the treatment of disease outbreaks of coccidiosis and fowl cholera.

Dairy Calves, Dairy Heifers and Beef Cattle: Use in the treatment of shipping fever complex, bacterial pneumonia, calf diphtheria, and foot rot.

Dosage and Administration: Chickens: For a 0.05% concentration, add contents of packet to 50 gallons of water.

Turkeys: For a 0.025% concentration, add contents of packet to 100 gallons of drinking water.

Automatic proportioners: To make stock solution, add contents of 5 packets to 2 gallons of water for chickens and to 4 gallons of water for turkeys. Set proportioner to feed at a rate of 1 fl oz of stock solution per gallon of water.

Treatment Period: 6 consecutive days.

Dairy Calves, Dairy Heifers and Beef Cattle: Dosage: 25 mg/lb first day followed by 12.5 mg/lb/day for 4 days.

Amount of Stock Solution for Cattle*	Sulfadimethoxine in Water Water Consumption	
	(Summer) 1 gallon/** 100 lb b.w.	(Winter) 1 gallon/** 150 lb b.w.
First Day Add:		
1 quart	10 gallons	7 gallons
2 quarts	20 gallons	14 gallons
1 gallon	40 gallons	28 gallons
Next 4 Days Add:		
1 quart	20 gallons	14 gallons
2 quarts	40 gallons	28 gallons
1 gallon	80 gallons	56 gallons

*Note: Make a cattle stock solution by adding 1 packet of SULFADIMETHOXINE SOLUBLE POWDER to 1 gallon of water.

**This dosage recommendation is based on a water consumption of 1 gallon per 100 lb of body weight per day, the expected water consumption rate for summer. Water consumption during cold months (winter) may drop markedly (30-40%). Accordingly, adjustments in drug concentration in drinking water must be made to ensure proper drug intake.

For treatment of individual cattle, SULFADIMETHOXINE SOLUBLE POWDER stock solution for cattle may be given as a drench. Administer using same mg/lb dosage as outlined above.

Twenty fluid ounces of cattle stock solution will medicate one-600 lb animal initially or two-600 lb animals on maintenance dose. Contents of packet will medicate six-600 lb animals initially or twelve-600 lb animals on maintenance dose.

Treatment Period: 5 consecutive days

Caution(s): Chickens and Turkeys: If animals show no improvement within 5 days, discontinue treatment and re-evaluate diagnosis. Prepare a fresh stock solution daily. Handle the recommended dilutions (chickens 0.05% and turkeys 0.025%) as regular drinking water. Administer as sole source of drinking water and sulfonamide medication.

Chickens and turkeys that have survived fowl cholera outbreaks should not be kept for replacements or breeders.

Cattle: During the treatment period, make certain that animals maintain adequate water intake.

If animals show no improvement within 2 or 3 days, re-evaluate diagnosis. Treatment should not be continued beyond 5 days.

For animal use only - Not for human use.

Warning(s): Chickens and Turkeys: Withdraw 5 days before slaughter. Do not administer to chickens over 16 weeks (112 days) of age or to turkeys over 24 weeks (168 days) of age.

Cattle: Withdraw 7 days before slaughter. For dairy calves, dairy heifers and beef cattle only. A withdrawal period has not been established for this product in preruminating calves. Do not use in calves to be processed for veal.

Keep out of reach of children.

Presentation: 3.77 oz (107 g) packets, 25 per pail.

Compendium Code No.: 10941921

SULFA-MAX® III CALF BOLUS

AgriLabs **Sulfamethazine**

Antibacterial-Sulfamethazine Sustained Release Calf Bolus

NADA No.: 120-615

Active Ingredient(s): Each Bolus Contains:

Sulfamethazine (formulated in a sustained release base) .... 123.8 gr. (8.02 g)

Indications: SULFA-MAX® III Calf Boluses (Sulfamethazine Sustained Release Boluses) are intended for oral administration to ruminating replacement calves (calves over one (1) month of age that are not on an all milk diet). SULFA-MAX® III Calf Boluses are indicated for the treatment of the following diseases when caused by one or more of the following pathogenic organisms sensitive to sulfamethazine: Bacterial Pneumonia *(Pasteurella* spp.), Colibacillosis (Bacterial Scours) *(E. coli),* and Calf Diphtheria *(Fusobacterium necrophorum).*

Dosage and Administration: SULFA-MAX® III Calf Boluses (Sulfamethazine Sustained Release Boluses) are designed to be administered orally to ruminating replacement calves (see Caution statment). SULFA-MAX® III Calf Bolus should be given according to the following dosage schedule:

Animal Body Wgt.	No. of Boluses
100 lbs.	2
150 lbs.	3
200 lbs.	4
250 lbs.	5
300 lbs.	6

The bolus may be divided for better approximation of correct dose; however, care should be taken not to crush the bolus. Care should also be taken to ensure the entire dose has been swallowed by the animal. Observe animals following administration to ensure the boluses are not regurgitated. Lubricate bolus before dosing animals.

SULFA-MAX® III Calf Bolus are designed to provide a therapeutic sulfamethazine level in approximately 6 hours and persist in providing this level for 72 hours (3 days). After 72 hours, all animals should be re-examined for persistence of observable disease signs. If signs are present, consult a veterinarian. It is strongly recommended that a second dose be given to provide an additional 72 hours of therapy, particularly in more severe cases. The above dosage schedule should be used at each 72-hour interval.

Caution(s): This drug, like all sulfonamides, may cause toxic reactions and irreparable injury unless administered with adequate and continuous supervision. Follow the recommended dosages carefully.

Fluid intake must be adequate at all times throughout the three-day therapy provided by the sustained release bolus.

This product has not been shown to be effective for non-ruminating calves.

For animal use only.

Not for human use.

Warning(s): Treated animals must not be slaughtered for food for at least 12 days after the last dose. Exceeding two (2) consecutive doses may cause violative tissue residues to remain beyond the withdrawal time. Do not use in calves under one (1) month of age or calves being fed an all-milk diet. Use in this class of calves may cause violative residues to remain beyond the withdrawal time. Do not use in female dairy cattle 20 months of age or older. Use of sulfamethazine in this class of cattle may cause milk residues.

Keep out of reach of children.

Presentation: Jars of 25 and 50 boluses.

® Registered Trademark of Agri Laboratories, Ltd.

Compendium Code No.: 10580981 8SUS021-401 / 8SUS036-401

SULFA-MAX® III CATTLE BOLUS

AgriLabs **Sulfamethazine**

Antibacterial Sulfamethazine Sustained Release Bolus

NADA No.: 120-615

Active Ingredient(s): Each Bolus Contains:

Sulfamethazine (formulated in a sustained release base) .... 495 gr. (32.1 g)

Indications: SULFA-MAX® III Boluses (Sulfamethazine Sustained Release Boluses) are intended for oral administration to beef cattle and non-lactating dairy cattle (see Warning). SULFA-MAX® III Boluses are indicated for the treatment of the following diseases when caused by one or more of the following pathogenic organisms sensitive to sulfamethazine: Bacterial Pneumonia and Bovine Respiratory Disease Complex (Shipping Fever Complex) *(Pasteurella* spp.), Colibacillosis (Bacterial Scours), *(E. coli),* Necrotic pododermatitis (Foot rot), Calf Diphtheria *(Fusobacterium necrophorum),* and Acute Metritis *(Streptococcus* spp.).

Dosage and Administration: SULFA-MAX® III Boluses (Sulfamethazine Sustained Release Boluses) are designed to be administered orally to beef cattle and non-lactating dairy cattle. SULFA-MAX® III boluses should be given according to the following dosage schedule:

Animal Body Wgt	No. of Boluses
200 lbs.	1
300 lbs.	1.5
400 lbs.	2
500 lbs.	2.5
600 lbs.	3
700 lbs.	3.5
800 lbs.	4
900 lbs.	4.5
1,000 lbs.	5

S

The bolus may be divided for better approximation of correct dose, however, care should be taken not to crush the bolus. Care should also be taken to ensure the entire dose has been swallowed by the animal. Observe animals following administration to ensure the boluses are not regurgitated. Lubricate SULFA-MAX® III Bolus before dosing animals.

SULFA-MAX® III Boluses are designed to provide a therapeutic sulfamethazine level in approximately 6 hours and persist in providing this level for 72 hours (3 days). After 72 hours, all animals should be re-examined for persistence of observable disease signs. If signs are present, consult a veterinarian. It is strongly recommended that a second dose be given to provide for an additional 72 hours of therapy, particularly in more severe cases. The above dosage schedule should be used at each 72-hour interval.

Caution(s): This drug, like all sulfonamides, may cause toxic reactions and irreparable injury unless administered with adequate and continuous supervision. Follow the recommended dosages carefully.

Fluid intake must be adequate at all times throughout the three-day therapy provided by the sustained release bolus.

For animal use only.

Not for human use.

Warning(s): Animals intended for human consumption should not be slaughtered for food for at least 12 days after the last dose. Exceeding two (2) consecutive doses may cause violative tissue residues to remain beyond the withdrawal time. Do not use in female dairy cattle 20 months of age or older. Use of sulfamethazine in this class of cattle may cause milk residues. Do not use in calves under one (1) month of age or calves being fed an all-milk diet. Use in this class of calves may cause violative residues to remain beyond the withdrawal time.

Keep out of reach of children.

Presentation: Boxes of 50 and 100 boluses.

® Registered Trademark of Agri Laboratories, Ltd.

Compendium Code No.: 10580971 8SUS039-401 / 8SUS040-401

SULFA-Q 20% CONCENTRATE

AgriPharm **Water Medication**

Active Ingredient(s): Each 100 mL contains:

Sulfaquinoxaline.......... 20 g

(dissolved in excess sodium hydroxide)

Indications: Poultry:

Coccidiosis: For use as an aid in the control of outbreaks in chickens *(Eimeria tenella, E. necatrix, E. acervulina, E. maxima* and *E. brunetti).*

For use as an aid in the control of outbreaks in turkeys *(Eimeria meleagrimitis* and *E. adenoeides).*

For use as an aid in the control of fowl cholera caused by *Pasteurella multocida,* sensitive to sulfaquinoxaline, and as an aid in the control of death losses and reduction of severity of disease in chickens and turkeys.

For use in the control of fowl typhoid caused by *Salmonella gallinarium* sensitive to sulfaquinoxaline, and as an aid in the control of death losses in chickens and turkeys.

Livestock:

Coccidiosis: For use as an aid in the control of outbreaks in cattle and calves *(Eimeria bovis* and *E. zurnii).*

Dosage and Administration: Poultry:

Coccidiosis: As an aid in the control of outbreaks in chickens *(Eimeria tenella, E. necatrix, E. acervulina, E. maxima* and *E. brunetti):* Give a dose of 12 fl. oz. (0.04%) per 50 gallon of water. Treat for two (2) to three (3) days, skip for three (3) days, then give a dose of 8 fl. oz. (0.025%) per 50 gallons of water and treat for two (2) more days. If bloody droppings appear, repeat the treatment at this level for two (2) more days. Do not change the litter unless absolutely necessary. Do not give flushing marshes.

As an aid in the control of outbreaks in turkeys *(Eimeria meleagrimitis* and *E. adenoeides):* Give a dose of 8 fl. oz. (0.025%) per 50 gallons of water. Treat for two (2) days, skip for three (3) days, treat for two (2) days, skip for three (3) days and treat for two (2) more days. Repeat if necessary. Do not change the litter unless absolutely necessary. Do not give flushing marshes.

Fowl cholera caused by *Pasteurella multocida,* sensitive to sulfaquinoxaline, as an aid in the control of death losses and reduction of severity of disease, fowl typhoid caused by *Salmonella gallinarium* sensitive to sulfaquinoxaline, and as an aid in the control of death losses in chickens and turkeys: Give a dose of 12 fl. oz. (0.04%) per 50 gallons of water. Use for two (2) to three (3) days. Move the birds to clean ground. If the disease recurs, repeat the treatment. If cholera has become established as the respiratory or chronic form, use feed medicated with SULFA-Q. Poultry which have survived typhoid outbreaks should not be kept for laying house replacements or breeders unless tests show they are not carriers.

Livestock:

Coccidiosis: As an aid in the control of outbreaks in cattle and calves *(Eimeria bovis* and *E. zurnii):* Give a dose of 5 fl. oz. (0.015%). Treat for three (3) to five (5) days.

For automatic drinking water proportioners: Dilute 32 fl. oz. of SULFA-Q 20% solution with water to make one (1) gallon of stock solution. When the stock solution is used in an automatic proportioner that meters 1 fl. oz. of stock solution per gallon of drinking water, this will provide 128 gallons of medicated water at the 0.04% dose. For a 0.025% dose, use 2 fl. oz. of SULFA-Q 20% solution.

Caution(s): Hazardous. Restricted drug. Use only as directed.

May cause toxic reactions unless the drug is evenly mixed in water at doses indicated and used according to directions.

Treated animals must actually consume enough medicated water to provide the recommended dose, which ranges from approximately 4 mg/lb. (0.15%) to 30 mg/lb. (0.1%), depending upon the treatment schedule.

Prolonged administration of SULFA-Q 20% at higher doses may result in depressed feed intake, deposition of sulfaquinoxaline crystals in the kidney and interference with normal blood clotting.

Causes skin and eye burns. Avoid contact with the eyes, skin or clothing. In case of contact, flush immediately with water for at least 15 minutes. For eyes, get medical attention.

Not for human use.

Keep out of the reach of children.

Warning(s): Do not give to dairy animals in production for food.

Do not treat chickens, turkeys or cattle within 10 days before slaughter for food.

Do not feed to laying chickens or laying turkeys in production for food.

Presentation: 1 gallon.

Compendium Code No.: 14570920

SULFASOL

Med-Pharmex **Water Medication**

Sulfadimethoxine Soluble Powder

ANADA No.: 200-238

Active Ingredient(s): Each packet contains 3.34 oz (94.6 g) sulfadimethoxine in the form of the soluble sodium salt and disodium edetate.

Indications:

For Broiler and Replacement Chickens Only - Use for the treatment of disease outbreaks of coccidiosis, fowl cholera, and infectious coryza.

For Meat-producing Turkeys Only - Use for the treatment of disease outbreaks of coccidiosis and fowl cholera.

For Dairy Calves, Dairy Heifers, and Beef Cattle - Use for the treatment of shipping fever complex and bacterial pneumonia associated with *Pasteurella* spp. sensitive to sulfadimethoxine; and calf diphtheria and foot rot associated with *Sphaerophorus necrophorus* sensitive to sulfadimethoxine.

Dosage and Administration:

Species	Concentration	Use Direction
Chickens	0.05%	Contents of packet to 50 gal of water
Turkeys	0.025%	Contents of packet to 100 gal of water

Automatic Proportioners - To make stock solution, add contents of 5 packets to 2 gal of water for chickens and to 4 gal of water for turkeys. Set proportioner to feed at rate of 1 fl oz stock solution per gal of water.

Treatment Period: 6 consecutive days.

Dairy Calves, Dairy Heifers, and Beef Cattle:

Dosage: 25 mg/lb first day followed by 12.5 mg/lb/day for 4 days.

	Amount of Stock Solution for Cattle*	Sulfadimethoxine in Water	
		Water Consumption	
		(Summer)* 1 gal/100 lb body weight**	(Winter)* 1 gal/150 lb body weight**
First Day Add	1 qt	10 gal	7 gal
	2 qt	20 gal	14 gal
	1 gal	40 gal	28 gal
Next 4 Days Add	1 qt	20 gal	14 gal
	2 qt	40 gal	28 gal
	1 gal	80 gal	56 gal

*Note: Make a cattle stock solution by adding 1 packet of Sulfadimethoxine Soluble Powder to 1 gal of water.

*Twenty fl oz of cattle stock solution will medicate 1 600 lb animal initially or 2 600 lb animals on maintenance dose. Contents of packet will medicate 6 600 lb animals initially or 12 600 lb animals on maintenance dose.

**This dosage recommendation is based on a water consumption of 1 gal per 100 lb of body weight per day, the expected water consumption rate for summer. Water consumption during cold months (winter) may drop markedly (30-40%). Accordingly, adjustments must be made in the dilution rates to compensate for this and insure proper drug intake.

For treatment of individual cattle, Sulfadimethoxine Solution Powder stock solution for cattle may be given as a drench.

Treatment Period: 5 consecutive days.

Chickens and Turkeys - If animals show no improvement within 5 days, discontinue treatment and reevaluate diagnosis. Prepare a fresh stock solution daily. Handle the recommended dilutions (chickens 0.05% and turkeys 0.025%) as regular drinking water. Administer as sole source of drinking water and sulfonamide medication.

Chickens and turkeys that have survived fowl cholera outbreaks should not be kept for replacements or breeders.

Cattle - During treatment period, make certain that animals maintain adequate water intake. If animals show no improvement within 2 or 3 days, reevaluate diagnosis. Treatment should not be continued beyond 5 days.

Warning(s):

Chickens and Turkeys - Withdraw 5 days before slaughter. Do not administer to chickens over 16 weeks (112 days) of age or to turkeys over 24 weeks (168 days) of age.

Cattle - Withdraw 7 days before slaughter. For dairy calves, dairy heifers, and beef cattle only. A withdrawal period has not been established for this product in pre-ruminating calves.

Do not use in calves to be processed for veal.

Restricted drug (California) - Use only as directed.

Not for human use.

Presentation: 3.77 oz (107 g) packet.

Compendium Code No.: 10270110

SULFASURE™ SR

Butler **Sulfamethazine**

Sulfamethazine Sustained Release Bolus Oral

NADA No.: 140-270

Active Ingredient(s): Each bolus contains:

Sulfamethazine.......... 30 grams

Indications: SULFASURE™ SR (sulfamethazine sustained release bolus) is indicated for the treatment of the following diseases in beef cattle and non-lactating dairy cattle: bovine respiratory disease complex (shipping fever complex) associated with *Pasteurella* spp.; bacterial pneumonia associated with *Pasteurella* spp.; necrotic pododermatitis (foot-rot) and calf diphtheria caused by *Fusobacterium necrophorum;* colibacillosis (bacterial scours) caused by *Escherichia coli;* coccidiosis caused by *Eimeria bovis* and *E. zurni;* acute mastitis caused by *Streptococcus* spp. (beef cattle only); acute metritis caused by *Streptococcus* spp.

Dosage and Administration: SULFASURE™ SR (sulfamethazine sustained release bolus) should be administered at the rate of 150 mg/lb body weight on the first day of treatment. Each bolus will treat 200 lbs of body weight. The bolus is scored to allow breaking for more accurate dosing, however, it must not be crushed. The bolus should be lubricated prior to administration and care taken to ensure the entire dose has been swallowed. Observe animal following dosing to ensure that regurgitation does not occur. If regurgitation occurs, clean regurgitated material and re-administer. If this is not practical, administer a new bolus.

Dosage Schedule:

Body Weight	No. Boluses
200 lbs	1
300 lbs	1.5
400 lbs	2
500 lbs	2.5
600 lbs	3
700 lbs	3.5
800 lbs	4
900 lbs	4.5
1000 lbs	5

Note: SULFASURE™ SR (sulfamethazine sustained release bolus) is designed to provide a therapeutic sulfamethazine level in approximately 6 hours, and persist in providing this level for 72 hours (3 days). After 72 hours, all animals should be re-examined for persistence of observable disease signs. If signs are present, consult a veterinarian. If signs of disease are significantly reduced, it is recommended that a second dose be given to provide for an additional 72 hours of therapy. No further doses should be administered.

Caution(s): This drug, like all sulfonamides, may cause toxic reactions and irreparable injury unless administered with adequate supervision. Follow recommended dosages carefully. Fluid intake must be adequate at all times throughout the three-day therapy provided by the sustained release bolus. If symptoms persist after using this preparation for 3 days, consult your veterinarian.

Warning(s): Do not use in female dairy cattle 20 months of age or older. Use of sulfamethazine in this class of cattle may cause milk residues. Do not use in calves under one (1) months of age or calves being fed an all milk diet. Use in these classes of calves may cause violative tissue residues to remain beyond the withdrawal time. Animals intended for human consumption must not be treated within 8 days of slaughtering.

For use in animals only.

Not for human use.

Keep out of the reach of children.

Presentation: 50 boluses.

SULFASURE™ is a Trademark of Fermenta Animal Health Company.

Compendium Code No.: 10821720

SULFASURE™ SR CALF BOLUS

Butler **Sulfamethazine**

Sulfamethazine Sustained Release Bolus Oral

NADA No.: 140-270

Active Ingredient(s): Each bolus contains:

Sulfamethazine.. 8.25 grams

Indications: SULFASURE™ sustained release calf bolus is intended for administration to ruminating beef and dairy calves only. These calves should be over one (1) month of age and no longer subsisting on an all milk diet.

SULFASURE™ sustained release calf bolus is indicated for the treatment of the following diseases: bacterial pneumonia associated with *Pasteurella* spp.; colibacillosis (bacterial scours) caused by *Escherichia coli;* calf diphtheria caused by *Fusobacterium necrophorum;* coccidiosis caused by *Eimeria bovis* and *E zurni.*

Dosage and Administration: SULFASURE™ SR Calf Boluses should be administered orally to ruminating beef and dairy calves at the rate of 165 mg/lb body weight on the first day of treatment. Each bolus will treat 50 lbs of body weight. The bolus is half-scored to allow breaking for more accurate dosing, however, it must not be crushed. The bolus should be lubricated prior to administration and care taken to ensure the entire dose has been swallowed. Observe animal following dosing to ensure regurgitation does not occur. If regurgitation occurs, clean regurgitated material and re-administer. If this is not practical, administer a new bolus.

Dosage Schedule:

Body Weight	No. Boluses
100 lbs	2
150 lbs	3
200 lbs	4
250 lbs	5
300 lbs	6

Note: Sulfamethazine sustained release calf boluses are designed to provide a therapeutic sulfamethazine level in approximately 6 hours, and persist in providing this level for 72 hours (3 days). After 72 hours, all animals should be re-examined for persistence of observable disease signs. If signs are present, consult a veterinarian. If signs of disease are significantly reduced, it is recommended that a second dose be given to provide for an additional 72 hours of therapy. No further doses should be administered.

Caution(s): This drug, like all sulfonamides, may cause toxic reactions and irreparable injury unless administered with adequate supervision. Follow recommended dosages carefully. Fluid intake must be adequate at all times throughout the three-day therapy provided by the sustained release bolus. If symptoms persist after using this preparation for 3 days, consult your veterinarian.

Warning(s): Do not use in female dairy cattle 20 months of age or older. Use of sulfamethazine in this class of cattle may cause milk residues. Do not use in calves under one (1) month of age or calves being fed an all milk diet. Use in these classes of calves may cause violative tissue residues to remain beyond the withdrawal time. Animals intended for human consumption must not be treated within 8 days of slaughtering.

For use in animals only.

Not for human use.

Keep out of reach of children.

Presentation: 50 boluses.

Compendium Code No.: 10821730

SULFASURE™ SR CALF BOLUS

Durvet **Sulfamethazine-Oral**

SMSR 6•80•8-Sulfamethazine Sustained Release Bolus-Oral Antibacterial

NADA No.: 140-270

Active Ingredient(s): Each calf bolus contains:

Sulfamethazine.. 8.25 grams

Indications: SULFASURE™ SR Calf Bolus is intended for administration to ruminating beef and dairy calves only. These calves should be over one (1) month of age and no longer subsisting on an all milk diet.

SULFASURE™ SR Calf Bolus is indicated for the treatment of the following diseases: bacterial pneumonia associated with *Pasteurella* spp.; colibacillosis (bacterial scours) caused by *Escherichia coli;* calf diphtheria caused by *Fusobacterium necrophorum;* coccidiosis caused by *Eimeria bovis* and *E. zurnii.*

Dosage and Administration: SULFASURE™ SR Calf Boluses should be administered orally to ruminating beef and dairy calves at the rate of 165 mg/lb body weight on the first day of treatment. Each bolus will treat 50 lbs of body weight. The bolus is scored to allow breaking for more accurate dosing, however, it must not be crushed. The bolus should be lubricated prior to administration and care taken to ensure the entire dose has been swallowed. Observe animal following dosing to ensure regurgitation does not occur. If regurgitation occurs, clean regurgitated material and readminister. If this is not practical, administer a new bolus.

Dosage Schedule:

Body Weight	No. Boluses
100 lbs	2
150 lbs	3
200 lbs	4
250 lbs	5
300 lbs	6

Note: SULFASURE™ SR Calf Boluses are designed to provide a therapeutic sulfamethazine level in approximately 6 hours, and persist in providing this level for 72 hours (3 days). After 72 hours, all animals should be re-examined for persistence of observable disease signs. If signs are present, consult a veterinarian. If signs of disease are significantly reduced, it is recommended that a second dose be given to provide for an additional 72 hours of therapy. No further doses should be administered.

Caution(s): This drug, like all sulfonamides, may cause toxic reactions and irreparable injury unless administered with adequate supervision. Follow recommended dosages carefully. Fluid intake must be adequate at all times throughout the three day therapy provided by the sustained release bolus. If symptoms persist after using this preparation for 3 days, consult your veterinarian.

For use in animals only.

Warning(s): Do not use in female dairy cattle 20 months of age or older. Use of sulfamethazine in this class of cattle may cause milk residues. Do not use in calves under one (1) month of age or calves being fed an all milk diet. Use in these classes of calves may cause violative tissue residues to remain beyond the withdrawal time. Animals intended for human consumption must not be treated within 8 days of slaughtering.

Keep out of reach of children.

Presentation: 25 (NDC 30798-739-66) and 50 (NDC 30798-739-69) boluses.

Compendium Code No.: 10841561 3/98

SULFASURE™ SR CATTLE BOLUS

Durvet **Sulfamethazine-Oral**

SMSR 6•80•8-Sulfamethazine Sustained Release Bolus

NADA No.: 140-270

Active Ingredient(s): Each bolus contains:

Sulfamethazine.. 30 grams

Indications: SULFASURE™ SR (Sulfamethazine Sustained Release Bolus) is indicated for the treatment of the following diseases in beef cattle and non-lactating dairy cattle: Bovine respiratory disease complex (shipping fever complex) associated with *Pasteurella* spp.; bacterial pneumonia associated with *Pasteurella* spp.; necrotic pododermatitis (foot-rot) and calf diphtheria caused by *Fusobacterium necrophorum;* colibacillosis (bacterial scours) caused by *Escherichia coli;* coccidiosis caused by *Eimeria bovis* and *E. zurnii;* acute mastitis caused by *Streptococcus* spp. (beef cattle only); acute metritis caused by *Streptococcus* spp.

Dosage and Administration: SULFASURE™ SR (Sulfamethazine Sustained Release Bolus) should be administered at the rate of 150 mg/lb body weight on the first day of treatment. Each bolus will treat 200 lbs of body weight. The bolus is scored to allow breaking for more accurate dosing, however, it must not be crushed. The bolus should be lubricated prior to administration and care taken to ensure the entire dose has been swallowed. Observe animal following dosing to ensure regurgitation does not occur. If regurgitation occurs, clean regurgitated material and readminister. If this is not practical, administer a new bolus.

Dosage Schedule:

Body Weight	No. Boluses
200 lbs	1
300 lbs	1.5
400 lbs	2
500 lbs	2.5
600 lbs	3
700 lbs	3.5
800 lbs	4
900 lbs	4.5
1000 lbs	5

Note: SULFASURE™ SR (Sulfamethazine Sustained Release Bolus) is designed to provide a therapeutic sulfamethazine level in approximately 6 hours, and persist in providing this level for 72 hours (3 days). After 72 hours, all animals should be re-examined for persistence of observable disease signs. If signs are present, consult a veterinarian. If signs of disease are significantly reduced, it is recommended that a second dose be given to provide for an additional 72 hours of therapy. No further doses should be administered.

Caution(s): This drug, like all sulfonamides, may cause toxic reactions and irreparable injury unless administered with adequate supervision. Follow recommended dosages carefully. Fluid intake must be adequate at all times throughout the three day therapy provided by the sustained release bolus. If symptoms persist after using this preparation for 3 days, consult your veterinarian.

For use in animals only.

Warning(s): Do not use in female dairy cattle 20 months of age or older. Use of sulfamethazine in this class of cattle may cause milk residues. Do not use in calves under one (1) month of age or calves being fed an all milk diet. Use in these classes of calves may cause violative tissue residues to remain beyond the withdrawal time. Animals intended for human consumption must not be treated within 8 days of slaughtering.

Keep out of reach of children.

Presentation: 50 (NDC 30798-738-69) and 100 (NDC 30798-738-70) boluses.

Compendium Code No.: 10841571 3/98

SULFODENE HC™ ANTI-ITCH LOTION FOR DOGS & CATS

Combe **Topical Corticosteroid**

Active Ingredient(s): 0.5% Hydrocortisone U.S.P.

Indications: Recommended as an aid to stop itching and for the treatment of hot spots.

Directions for Use: First clip hair from around affected area with blunt scissors, and gently wash the area with an anti-bacterial soap or shampoo. Then apply SULFODENE HC™ freely by squeezing product out of bottle's pinpoint applicator directly onto the affected area. If you prefer, apply SULFODENE HC™ freely with an applicator such as cotton-lipped swab or a soft, clean cloth or soft, disposable towel. Apply not more than 3 to 4 times daily for up to 7 consecutive days. SULFODENE HC™ is not harmful should your pet lick the problem skin area.

Caution(s): For external use only. Avoid contact with eyes. If condition worsens or if symptoms persist for more than seven days or clear up and occur again within a few days, stop use of this product and do not begin use of any hydrocortisone product unless you have consulted a veterinarian. If condition covers a large area of your pet's body, consult a veterinarian before using this product.

Warning(s): Keep out of reach of children. In case of accidental ingestion, seek professional assistance or contact a Poison Control Center immediately.

Presentation: 1.5 fl oz (44 mL).

Compendium Code No.: 10290090

SULFODENE® MEDICATED SHAMPOO & CONDITIONER FOR DOGS

Combe **Antidermatosis Shampoo**

Active Ingredient(s): Coal tar, sulfur, triclosan.

Other ingredients: Aloe vera.

Indications: For the temporary relief of itching, flaking and scaling.

Directions: Shake well before using. Moisten coat. Rub in shampoo to rich, conditioning lather. Rinse thoroughly. Dry and brush coat. Shampoo frequently for your dog's comfort and to keep the skin and coat clean, lustrous and odor free.

Contraindication(s): Not for use on cats.

Caution(s): For external use only. Avoid contact with eyes. If undue skin irritation develops or increases, discontinue use and consult veterinarian. Not recommended for use on puppies under six weeks of age.

Warning(s): Keep this and all medications out of reach of children. In case of accidental ingestion, seek professional assistance or contact a Poison Control Center immediately.

Presentation: 8 fl oz (236 mL) and 12 fl oz (354 mL) bottles.

7084015/7084515

Compendium Code No.: 10290102

SULFODENE® SKIN MEDICATION FOR DOGS

Combe **Topical Wound Dressing**

NADA No.: 005-236

Active Ingredient(s): 2-Mercaptobenzothiazole.

Also Contains: Isopropyl Alcohol 2.0%.

Indications: SULFODENE® medication is formulated to be effective as an aid in the treatment of certain common skin inflammations in dogs. It is recommended specifically as an aid for hot spots (moist dermatitis). Also, SULFODENE® is an effective first aid for scrapes and abrasions.

Directions for Use: Clip the hair from around the affected areas and apply SULFODENE® freely with an applicator such as cotton or soft, clean cloth twice a day. If the condition does not improve within 1 week, consult your veterinarian.

Precaution(s): Flammable. Keep away from heat or flame.

Caution(s): For external use only.

Warning(s): Rarely, minor allergic skin reactions occur in persons applying this product or in dogs following usage. Wash hands immediately after applying. Should this occur in dogs, discontinue use and wash the treated area with water. Keep away from the eyes. Keep this and all other medications away from children.

Discussion: Signs: These skin inflammations may be accompanied by itching so intense that the animal rubs, scratches and bites incessantly. Other signs associated with these skin inflammations include hair loss, redness, scaling and secondary infection.

Presentation: 4 fl oz (118 mL) and 8 fl oz (236 mL) containers.

Compendium Code No.: 10290112

SULFORAL

Med-Pharmex **Water Medication**

Sulfadimethoxine Concentrated Solution 12.5%

ANADA No.: 200-251

Active Ingredient(s): Each fluid ounce contains 3.75 g sulfadimethoxine solubilized with sodium hydroxide.

Indications: Antibacterial for use in drinking water.

For oral use in chickens, turkeys, and cattle.

Broiler and Replacement Chickens - Use for the treatment of disease outbreaks of coccidiosis, fowl cholera and infectious coryza.

Meat-Producing Turkeys - Use for the treatment of disease outbreaks of coccidiosis and fowl cholera.

Dairy Calves, Dairy Heifers and Beef Cattle - Use for the treatment of shipping fever complex, bacterial pneumonia, calf diphtheria and foot rot.

Dosage and Administration:

Species	Concentration	Use Directions
Chickens	0.05%	Add 1 fl oz* to 2 gallons of drinking water or 25 fl oz to 50 gallons of drinking water.
Turkeys	0.025%	Add 1 fl oz* to 4 gallons of drinking water or 25 fl oz to 100 gallons of drinking water.

Automatic Proportioners** Stock Solution: To make 2 gallons of stock solution use:

Chickens	1 gallon SULFORAL (sulfadimethoxine) 12.5% Drinking Water Solution Concentrate - plus - 1 gallon of water.
Turkeys	2 quarts SULFORAL (sulfadimethoxine) 12.5% Drinking Water Solution Concentrate - plus - 6 quarts of water.

Treatment Period - 6 consecutive days.

Dairy Calves, Dairy Heifers and Beef Cattle:

Dosage	SULFORAL (sulfadimethoxine) in Water		
25 mg/lb first day followed by 12.5 mg/lb/day for 4 days		Water Consumption	
		(Summer) 1 gallon/†100 lb b.w.	(Winter) 1 gallon/†100 lb b.w.
First Day	1 pint (16 fl oz) to:	25 gallons	16 gallons
	1 quart (32 fl oz) to:	50 gallons	33 gallons
	1 gallon (128 fl oz) to:	200 gallons	127 gallons
Next 4 Days Add	1 pint (16 fl oz) to:	50 gallons	33 gallons
	1 quart (32 fl oz) to:	100 gallons	66 gallons
	1 gallon (128 fl oz) to:	400 gallons	266 gallons

†This dosage recommendation is based on a water consumption of 1 gallon per 100 lb of body weight per day, the expected water consumption rate for summer. Water consumption during cold months (winter) may drop markedly (30-40%). Accordingly, adjustments in drug concentration in drinking water must be made to insure proper drug intake.

For individual treatment of cattle SULFORAL (sulfadimethoxine) 12.5% Drinking Water Solution may be given as a drench. Administer using same mg/lb dosage as outlined above. Four fluid ounces will medicate one-600 lb animal initially or two-600 lb animals on maintenance dose.

Treatment Period - 5 consecutive days.

*1 fl oz SULFORAL (sulfadimethoxine) 12.5% Drinking Water Solution = 30 mL or 2 tablespoonfuls.

**Set proportioner to a feed rate of 1 fl oz of SULFORAL (sulfadimethoxine) Stock Solution per gallon of water.

Precaution(s): Store at room temperature; if freezing occurs, thaw before using. Protect from light; direct sunlight may cause discoloration. Freezing or discoloration does not affect potency. Prepare a fresh solution daily.

Caution(s):

Chickens and Turkeys - If animals show no improvement within 5 days, discontinue treatment and re-evaluate diagnosis. Handle the recommended dilutions (chickens 0.05% and turkeys 0.025%) as regular drinking water. Administer as sole source of drinking water and sulfonamide medication.

Chickens and turkeys that have survived fowl cholera outbreaks should not be kept for replacements or breeders.

Cattle - During treatment period, make certain that animals maintain adequate water intake. If animals show no improvement within 2 or 3 days, re-evaluate diagnosis. Treatment should not be continued beyond 5 days.

Warning(s):

Chickens and Turkeys - Withdraw 5 days before slaughter. Do not administer to chickens over 16 weeks (112 days) of age or to turkeys over 24 weeks (168 days) of age.

Cattle - Withdraw 7 days before slaughter.

For dairy calves, dairy heifers and beef cattle only.

Restricted drug. Use only as directed - Not for human use.

Presentation: 1 gallon (128 fl oz).

Compendium Code No.: 10270120

SULF OXYDEX® SHAMPOO ℞

DVM **Antidermatosis Shampoo**

Antimicrobial Antiseborrheic Cleansing Moisturizing Formulation

Active Ingredient(s): Benzoyl peroxide 2.5% and micronized sulfur 2%.

Indications: For the relief of itching and scaling associated with seborrheic dermatitis, Schnauzer Comedo Syndrome, hyperkeratosis and follicular plugging in dogs and cats.

Product Description: SULF OXYDEX® Shampoo is a potent, antimicrobial, antiseborrheic, debriding formulation in a fragranced, soap-free, lathering shampoo base. This combination promotes follicular flushing and enhances keratolytic and keratoplastic activity.

Directions for Use: Shake well before use. Wet coat thoroughly. Begin by applying to affected areas, and then proceed to apply product over entire body. When the entire coat is treated, allow to stand 5-10 minutes. Rinse thoroughly with water. SULF OXYDEX® Shampoo may be used as often as necessary, or as directed by veterinarian. If condition worsens or does not improve after regular use of this product as directed, consult your veterinarian.

Precaution(s): Store at room temperature.

Caution(s): Federal law restricts this drug to use by, or on the order of a licensed veterinarian.

For external use only. Avoid contact with eyes. If contact occurs, rinse thoroughly with water. If irritation develops, discontinue and consult your veterinarian. May bleach colored fabrics.

Warning(s): Keep out of reach of children.

Presentation: 8 fl oz (237 mL) (NDC 47203-205-08), 12 fl oz (355 mL) (NDC 47203-205-12), and 1 gallon (3.78 L) (NDC 47203-205-28).

Compendium Code No.: 11420531 Rev 0399

SULFUR & TAR MEDICATED SHAMPOO

Davis **Antidermatosis Shampoo**

Active Ingredient(s): Contains refined coal tar solution U.S.P., sulfur, salicylic acid, zinc oxide, aloe and menthol.

Indications: Davis SULFUR & TAR MEDICATED SHAMPOO with aloe vera and menthol is a cleansing and grooming aid that may be used to relieve the itching, irritation and skin flaking associated with dandruff, seborrheic dermatitis, flea bites and nonspecific dermatoses. Eliminates odors, while grooming conditioners soften the horny layer of the skin and promote normalization of the coat and epidermal skin cells.

Dosage and Administration: Shake well before using.

Thoroughly wet the coat using warm water and enough Davis SULFUR & TAR MEDICATED SHAMPOO to work up a good lather. Massage the shampoo into the coat and the skin, then allow the pet to stand for 5-10 minutes. For the best results, rinse and repeat the procedure.

Some pets may be intolerant to full strength use. In such cases, dilute the shampoo in half with water and continue the treatment. If the condition does not improve, discontinue use and seek professional advice.

Caution(s): Keep out of the reach of children.

Do not use on cats. Do not use on cats, nursing bitches or puppies under four weeks of age. Do not use if the human or pet is allergic to the product.

Avoid contact with the eyes. In case of contact, flush thoroughly with water. Avoid prolonged contact with rectal and genital areas.

Presentation: 12 oz (355 mL) and 1 gallon (3.785 L) containers.

Compendium Code No.: 11410361

SULMET® DRINKING WATER SOLUTION 12.5%

Fort Dodge — **Water Medication**

Sulfamethazine Sodium

NADA No.: 006-084

Active Ingredient(s):

Sulfamethazine sodium 12.5%

Indications: For control and treatment of the following diseases when caused by one or more of the following pathogenic organisms susceptible to sulfamethazine.

For the treatment of:

Cattle: Bacterial pneumonia and bovine respiratory disease complex (shipping fever complex) *(Pasteurella* spp.); colibacillosis (bacterial scours) *(Escherichia coli);* necrotic pododermatitis (foot rot) *(Fusobacterium necrophorum);* calf diphtheria *(Fusobacterium necrophorum);* acute metritis *(Streptococcus* spp.).

Beef Cattle: Acute mastitis *(Streptococcus* spp.).

Swine: Porcine colibacillosis (bacterial scours) *(Escherichia coli);* bacterial pneumonia *(Pasteurella* spp.).

For the control of:

Chickens: Infectious coryza *(Haemophilus gallinarum);* coccidiosis *(Eimeria tenella, Eimeria necatrix);* acute fowl cholera *(Pasteurella multocida);* pullorum disease *(Salmonella pullorum).*

Turkeys: Coccidiosis *(Eimeria meleagrimitis, Eimeria adenoeides).*

For oral use in domestic animals and poultry. Not sterilized.

Dosage and Administration:

Dosage: Cattle, Calves and Swine:

1st Day: 6 tablespoons (3 fl oz) for each 100 lb body weight, providing approximately 112.5 mg/lb (247.5 mg/kg) body weight.

2nd, 3rd, and 4th Days: 3 tablespoons (1½ fl oz) for each 100 lb body weight, providing approximately 56.25 mg/lb (123.75 mg/kg) body weight.

Dosage: Poultry:

Add 2 tablespoons (1 fl oz) to each gallon of drinking water, or the contents of this container to 16 gallons. Following administration directions below, this will provide a recommended dose of approximately 61 to 89 mg/lb/day (134 to 196 mg/kg/day) body weight in chickens and 53 to 130 mg/lb/day (117 to 286 mg/kg/day) body weight in turkeys, depending upon the dosage, age and class of chickens or turkeys, ambient temperature, and other factors.

Administration: Cattle, Calves and Swine:

Add the required dose given above to that amount of water that will be consumed in 1 day; consumption should be carefully checked. Factors such as temperature, humidity and disease will cause variable fluid intake. As a generalization, the above animals will consume approximately 1 gallon per 100 lb body weight per day.

Administration: Chickens and Turkeys:

Add the required dose given above to that amount of water that will be consumed in 1 day. Water consumption should be carefully checked to insure adequate drug intake. As a generalization, 100 turkeys will drink 1 gallon of water per day for each week of age; chickens will consume one-half this amount.

Infectious Coryza (in chickens): Medicate for 2 consecutive days.

Acute fowl cholera and pullorum disease (in chickens): Medicate for 6 consecutive days.

Coccidiosis (in chickens and turkeys): Medicate as above for 2 days, then reduce amount of SULMET® Drinking Water Solution to one-half above for 4 additional days.

Precaution(s): Store at controlled room temperature 15° to 30°C (59° to 86°F).

Caution(s): For best advice in control and treatment of animal disease, consult a veterinarian.

Have only medicated water available during treatment, and check carefully to insure adequate SULMET® dosage and water intake. Cattle and calves not drinking or eating must be dosed by drench or with Sulmet® Oblets®. For best results, treat sick animals individually.

In poultry, consult a veterinarian or poultry pathologist for diagnosis. For control of outbreaks of disease, medication should be initiated as soon as the diagnosis is determined.

Medicated cattle, swine, chickens and turkeys must actually consume enough medicated water which provides the recommended dosages.

SULMET® works fast. If symptoms persist after using this preparation for 2 or 3 days, consult a veterinarian. Excessive dosage may cause toxic reactions; follow above dosage and administration instructions carefully. Hatchability of eggs laid during medication with sulfas and for short periods thereafter, may be adversely affected. Treatment of all diseases should be instituted early. Treatment should continue 24 to 48 hours beyond the remission of disease symptoms, but not to exceed a total of 5 consecutive days in cattle or swine.

Prepare fresh solutions daily.

Warning(s): Do not medicate chickens or turkeys producing eggs for human consumption. To avoid drug residues in edible flesh - withdraw medication from chickens and turkeys ten (10) days prior to slaughter for food.

Treated cattle must not be slaughtered for at least ten (10) days after the last dose. Exceeding five (5) consecutive days of treatment may cause violative tissue residue to remain beyond the withdrawal time.

Do not use in calves under one (1) month of age or calves being fed an all-milk diet. Use in these classes of calves may cause violative residues to remain beyond the withdrawal time.

Do not use in female dairy cattle 20 months of age or older. Use of sulfamethazine in this class of cattle may cause milk residues.

Withdraw medication from swine fifteen (15) days prior to slaughter for food.

Presentation: 12 x 16 oz. (NDC 0856-7972-65) and 4 x 1 gallon bottles (NDC 0856-7972-76).

Compendium Code No.: 10031911 — 6683B

SULMET® OBLETS®

Fort Dodge — **Sulfamethazine**

Antibacterial

NADA No.: 122-271

Active Ingredient(s): SULMET® OBLETS® 2.5 G contain 2.5 g sulfamethazine per tablet. SULMET® OBLETS® 5 G contain 5 g sulfamethazine per tablet.

Indications:

Calves: Bacterial pneumonia and bovine respiratory disease complex (shipping fever complex) *(Pasteurella* spp.); colibacillosis (bacterial scours) *(Escherichia coli);* calf diphtheria *(Fusobacterium necrophorum).*

Foals: Bacterial pneumonia (secondary infections associated with *Pasteurella* spp.); strangles *(Streptococcus equi);* bacterial enteritis *(Escherichia coli).*

Dosage and Administration: Once-A-Day Dosage By Mouth

SULMET® OBLETS® 2.5 G:

First Day: One OBLET® for each 25 lb body weight.

Following Days: One-half OBLET® for each 25 lb body weight.

The above dosage will provide approximately 100 mg/lb body weight the first day.

Weight of Animal	Dosage	
	1st Day	Following Days
25 lb	1 OBLET®	½ OBLET®
50 lb	2 OBLETS®	1 OBLET®
75 lb	3 OBLETS®	1½ OBLETS®
100 lb	4 OBLETS®	2 OBLETS®
125 lb	5 OBLETS®	2½ OBLETS®

SULMET® OBLETS® 5 G:

First Day: One OBLET® for each 50 lb body weight.

Following Days: One-half OBLET® for each 50 lb body weight.

The above dosage will provide approximately 100 mg/lb body weight the first day.

Weight of Animal	Dosage	
	1st Day No.	Following Days
50 lb	1 OBLET®	½ OBLET®
100 lb	2 OBLETS®	1 OBLET®
150 lb	3 OBLETS®	1½ OBLETS®
200 lb	4 OBLETS®	2 OBLETS®

Larger size OBLETS® are available and are easier to use with heavier animals. Give indicated dose once daily until animal's temperature and appearance are normal. Lubricate OBLETS® before dosing.

Caution(s): SULMET® sulfamethazine works fast. If symptoms persist after using this preparation for 2 or 3 days, consult a veterinarian. Excessive dosage may cause toxic reactions. Follow above dosages carefully. Fluid intake must be adequate while treating with SULMET®. For best advice in the control and treatment of disease, consult a veterinarian. Treatment of all diseases should be instituted early. Treatment should continue 24 to 48 hours beyond the remission of disease symptoms, but not to exceed 5 consecutive days.

For animal use only.

Warning(s): Treated cattle must not be slaughtered for at least 10 days after the last dose. Exceeding five (5) consecutive doses may cause violative tissue residue to remain beyond the withdrawal time. Do not use in calves under one (1) month of age or calves being fed an all-milk diet. Use in these classes of calves may cause violative residues to remain beyond the withdrawal time. Do not use in female dairy cattle 20 months of age or older. Use of sulfamethazine in this class of cattle may cause milk residues.

Not to be used in horses intended for food.

Presentation: OBLETS® 2.5 G - Bottles of 24 (NDC 0856-7974-91) or 100 (NDC 0856-7974-23).
OBLETS® 5 G - Bottles of 50 (NDC 0856-7981-18).

Manufactured by: PM Resources, Inc., Bridgeton, MO 63044

Compendium Code No.: 10031920 — 6932A (2.5 g); 6941A (5 g)

SULMET® SOLUBLE POWDER

Fort Dodge — **Water Medication**

Sodium Sulfamethazine

NADA No.: 122-272

Active Ingredient(s): Contents 100% sodium sulfamethazine.

Indications: For the control and treatment of the following diseases when caused by one or more of the following pathogenic organisms susceptible to sulfamethazine.

For the treatment of:

Cattle - Bacterial pneumonia and bovine respiratory disease complex (shipping fever complex) *(Pasteurella* spp.); colibacillosis (bacterial scours) *(Escherichia coli);* necrotic pododermatitis (foot rot) *(Fusobacterium necrophorum);* calf diphtheria *(Fusobacterium necrophorum);* acute metritis *(Streptococcus* spp.).

Beef Cattle - Acute mastitis *(Streptococcus* spp.).

Swine - Porcine colibacillosis (bacterial scours) *(Escherichia coli);* bacterial pneumonia *(Pasteurella* spp.).

For the control of:

Chickens - Infectious coryza *(Haemophilus gallinarum);* coccidiosis *(Eimeria tenella, Eimeria necatrix);* acute fowl cholera *(Pasteurella multocida);* pullorum disease *(Salmonella pullorum).*

Turkeys - Coccidiosis *(Eimeria meleagrimitis, Eimeria adenoeides).*

Dosage and Administration: Administration in Drinking Water: Prepare a 12.0% stock solution by adding the contents of this package to one gallon of water.

Dosage: Cattle, Calves and Swine:

1st Day: 6 tablespoons (3 fl oz) for each 100 lb body weight, providing approximately 108 mg/lb (237.6 mg/kg) body weight.

2nd, 3rd, 4th days: 3 tablespoons (1½ fl oz) for each 100 lb body weight, providing approximately 54 mg/lb. (118.8 mg/kg) body weight.

S

Dosage: Poultry:

Add 2 tablespoons (1 fl oz) to each gallon, or one gallon of stock solution to 128 gallons. Following administration directions, this will provide a recommended dose of approximately 58 to 85 mg/lb/day (128 to 187 mg/kg/day) body weight in chickens and 50 to 124 mg/lb/day (110 to 273 mg/kg/day) body weight in turkeys, depending upon the dosage, age, class of chickens or turkeys, ambient temperature and other factors.

Administration:

Cattle, Calves and Swine:

In drinking water: Add the required dose given above to that amount of water that will be consumed in one day; consumption should be carefully checked. Factors such as temperature, humidity and disease will cause variable fluid intake. As a generalization, the above animals will consume approximately 1 gallon per 100 lb body weight per day.

As a drench: Dilute the proper dose of stock solution, and drench or administer with dose syringe.

Cattle and calves not drinking must be dosed by drench or with Sulmet® Oblets®. For best results, pen-up animals to be treated, and treat sick animals individually.

Chickens and Turkeys:

Add the required dose to that amount of water that will be consumed in one day. Water consumption should be carefully checked to insure adequate drug intake. As a generalization, 100 turkeys will drink one gallon of water per day for each week of age; chickens will consume one-half this amount.

Infectious Coryza (in chickens): Medicate for 2 consecutive days.

Acute fowl cholera and pullorum disease (in chickens): Medicate for 6 consecutive days.

Coccidiosis (in chickens and turkeys): Medicate as above for 2 days, then reduce drug concentration to one-half above for 4 additional days.

Precaution(s): Store at controlled room temperature 15° to 30°C (59° to 86°F).

Caution(s): Prepare fresh solutions daily.

For best advice in control and treatment of animal disease, consult a veterinarian.

Have only medicated water available during treatment, and check carefully to insure adequate drug dosage and water intake. Cattle and calves not drinking or eating must be dosed by drench or with Sulmet® Oblets®. For best results, treat sick animals individually.

In poultry, consult a veterinarian or poultry pathologist for diagnosis. For control of outbreaks of disease, medication should be initiated as soon as the diagnosis is determined.

Medicated cattle, swine, chickens and turkeys must actually consume enough medicated water which provides the recommended dosages.

Sulmet® works fast. If symptoms persist after using this preparation for 2 or 3 days, consult a veterinarian. Excessive dosage may cause toxic reactions. Follow dosage and administration instructions carefully. Hatchability of eggs laid during medication with sulfas, and for short periods thereafter, may be adversely affected.

Treatment of all diseases should be instituted early. Treatment should continue 24 to 48 hours beyond the remission of disease symptoms, but not to exceed a total of 5 consecutive days in cattle or swine.

Warning(s): Do not medicate chickens or turkeys producing eggs for human consumption. To avoid drug residues in edible flesh withdraw medication from chickens and turkeys ten (10) days prior to slaughter for food.

Treated cattle must not be slaughtered for at least ten (10) days after the last dose. Exceeding five (5) consecutive days of treatment may cause violative tissue residue to remain beyond the withdrawal time.

Do not use in calves under one (1) month of age or calves being fed an all-milk diet. Use in these classes of calves may cause violative residues to remain beyond the withdrawal time.

Do not use in female dairy cattle 20 months of age or older. Use of sulfamethazine in this class of cattle may cause milk residues.

Withdraw medication from swine fifteen (15) days prior to slaughter for food.

Presentation: 1 lb (453.5 g) packets, 20 packets per pail (NDC 0856-7997-62).

Compendium Code No.: 10031931 6671B

SUNBUGGER CARPET DUST

Sungro **Parasiticide-Topical**

For Use on Carpets and Pets

EPA Reg. No.: 11474-89

Active Ingredient(s):

Pyrethrins	0.15%
Piperonyl Butoxide, Technical*	1.50%
Inert Ingredients:	98.35%
Total	100.00%

*Equivalent to 1.2% (butylcarbityl) (6-propyl-piperonyl) ether and 0.3% related compounds.

Indications: Kills fleas, ticks, lice, ants, roaches, and silverfish that live and breed in carpets.

For use in homes, vacation cabins, basements, pet sleeping quarters and storage areas, and on pets.

Directions for Use: It is a violation of Federal law to use this product in a manner inconsistent with its labeling.

Do not use in food serving areas while food is exposed.

Fleas and Other Insects in Carpets and Upholstery: Keep people and pets off treated carpet and upholstered furniture during treatment and until area is vacuumed.

Test hidden surface of carpet or upholstery before treating. If texture or color is affected, do not use.

Shake well before using. Punch plastic seal if present.

Carpet Treatment: Hold upside down and shake powder evenly across surface. Brush lightly with a broom to allow powder to penetrate carpet fibers. Wait 60 minutes, then vacuum. For severe problems or where ticks are known to be hiding, wait 2-3 hours before vacuuming. If powder adheres to a spot, brush it out and vacuum immediately. Apply to dry surfaces only. Do not allow powder to become wet. Clean carpet after using this product.

Upholstery Treatment: Remove all loose cushions. Sprinkle along creases, in corners. Brush gently, wait 60 minutes, vacuum. Sprinkle along underside of furniture. Do not use on exposed fabric; may cause staining. Remove bag from vacuum cleaner. Wrap securely in several layers of newspaper and discard in trash.

Fleas and Other Insects on and around Dogs, Cats and Premises:

To Control Fleas and Ticks on Dogs and Cats: Liberally apply powder to the animal, rubbing thoroughly to the skin. Begin with the neck and include the underbody, legs, feet and the base of the tail. Take care not to get the powder in animal's eyes, nose or mouth. Do not treat puppies or kittens less than four weeks of age. Do not apply directly to genitalia. Repeat as necessary.

Kennels: Surfaces of kennels should be dusted at the rate of (one) ounce per 50 square feet. Repeat as necessary.

Heavily infested basements, and crawl spaces: Should be dusted at the rate of (16) ounces per 1000 square feet. Repeat as necessary.

Precautionary Statements: Hazards to Humans and Domestic Animals:

Caution: Harmful if swallowed. Avoid breathing dust. Avoid contact with skin, eyes or clothing. Wash thoroughly with soap and water after handling. Do not contaminate feed, water or foodstuffs. Cover fish aquariums before use.

Statement of Practical Treatment:

If Swallowed: Call a physician or Poison Control Center immediately. Induce vomiting by giving victim 1 or 2 glasses of water and touching back of throat with finger. If person is unconscious, do not give anything by mouth and do not induce vomiting.

If in Eyes: Flush eyes with plenty of water. Get medical attention if irritation persists.

If on Skin: Wash with soap and warm water. Get medical attention if irritation persists.

If Inhaled: Remove victim to fresh air. If not breathing, give artificial respiration, preferably mouth-to-mouth. Get medical attention.

Environmental Hazards: Do not contaminate water by disposal of wastes. Apply this product only as specified on the label.

Storage and Disposal: Do not contaminate water, food, or feed by storage or disposal.

Storage: Store in original container in an area inaccessible to children and pets and away from heat and sunlight. Avoid exposure to moisture.

Disposal: Do not reuse empty container. Wrap container in several layers of newspaper before discarding in trash.

Warning(s): Keep out of reach of children.

Disclaimer: Buyer assumes all risks of use, storage or handling of this material not in strict accordance with directions given herewith.

Presentation: 16 ounces (0.45 kg), 12 per case. Treats four 10 x 10 carpets (400 sq. ft.).

Contains Pyrenone® - Registered Trademark of AgrEvo Environmental Health.

Compendium Code No.: 10100020

SUNBUGGER RESIDUAL ANT & ROACH SPRAY AQUEOUS

Sungro **Premise Insecticide**

EPA Reg. No.: 11474-34

Active Ingredient(s):	By weight
Diazinon (O,O-diethyl-O-(2-isopropyl-6-methyl-4-pyrimidinyl) phosphorothioate)	0.500%
Pyrethrins	0.052%
*Piperonyl Butoxide, Technical	0.260%
Inert Ingredients	99.188%

*Equivalent to 0.208% (butylcarbityl)(6-propyl piperonyl) ether and 0.052% related compounds.

Indications: A residual water base insecticide ready to use with flushing and quick knockdown characteristics kills brown dog ticks, fleas, roaches, ants.

Use in homes, institutions, non food areas of restaurants and food processing plants, warehouses, motels, hotels, garages.

For commercial/industrial use only.

This product authorized for use in USDA meat and poultry plants.

Directions for Use: It is a violation of federal law to use this product in a manner inconsistent with its labeling.

Indoor Use:

Use only in well ventilated areas. If clothing is sprayed during application, remove clothing immediately after spraying and launder before wearing again. Remove pets and cover fish bowls before spraying. Do not allow children to contact treated surfaces until surfaces are completely dry. Do not apply this pesticide when class rooms are in use. Do not apply this pesticide in the immediate area when occupants are present. Do not use in food areas or areas of food handling establishments, restaurants or other areas where food/feed is commercially prepared or processed. Do not use in serving areas while food is exposed or facility is in operation (serving areas include those where prepared foods are served such as dining rooms but exclude areas where food may be prepared or held). In the home, all food processing surfaces and utensils should be covered during treatment or thoroughly washed before reuse. Exposed food should be covered or removed.

Do not use this product in or on electrical equipment due to the possibility of shock hazard.

Non-food areas - includes garbage rooms, lavatories, floor drains (to sewers), entries and vestibules, offices, locker rooms, machine rooms, boiler rooms, garages, mop closets and storage (after canning or bottling).

Non-food Areas - Spot Treatment - As a spot treatment apply as a coarse low pressure fan spray to floor surface areas around water pipes, beneath cabinets, refrigerators, sinks, stoves, storage areas, dark corners of rooms and closets, cracks and crevices along baseboards and door stills and frames, and around garbage cans, plumbing and other utility installations, surfaces behind and beneath, lockers, tables, pallets and similar areas where cockroaches, ants, waterbugs, silverfish, spiders and cockroaches, ants, spiders, and silverfish hide. Pests driven out of hiding places should be sprayed directly. Spray ant trails, nests and points of entry. Repeat treatment as necessary. Do not use as a space spray.

To Kill Carpet Beetles: Spray edges of carpeting and under carpeting and rugs. Make localized applications to the floor and baseboards.

Spray directly into cracks, crevices, closets and infested areas of shelving. Repeat as necessary.

To Kill Fleas and Brown Dog Ticks: Clean premises thoroughly before treatment. Using a coarse cone or fan spray, treat the entire floor and carpet area. Special attention should be given to cracks, crevices and under carpet and rug edges. Also treat animal sleeping quarters, closets, upholstered furniture (with particular attention to seams), beds, under sofas and other furniture sleeping quarters, bedding should be cleaned or replaced with fresh bedding. Do not use this application in nurseries or any area where infants may sleep. Apply at the rate of approximately 1 gallon to 750 sq. ft. (17 fl. oz per 100 sq. ft.). To avoid reinfestation, pets must be treated simultaneously with an EPA approved insecticide labeled for use on animals. Application should be repeated as necessary. Humans and pets should avoid contact with treated surfaces (rugs, upholstered furniture, etc) for 4 hours after treatment.

Outdoor Use:

Precautions: When using outdoors, spray with the wind to your back. If clothing becomes wet from spraying during use, remove clothing after spraying. Wash affected body areas thoroughly with soap and water, and launder clothing before wearing again. Do not allow children or pets into a treated area until the treated area such as grass or soil has dried.

To Kill Flies, Mosquitoes, Wasps and Small Flying Moths: For use only as an aid in reducing annoyance from these pests. Spray the outside surfaces of screens, doors, window frames or wherever these insects may enter the room. Also treat surfaces around light fixtures on porches, in garages, and other places where these insects may alight or congregate.

To Kill Fleas, Chiggers, and Ants: For Treatment of localized infestation of these insects in outdoor areas, spray weeds and bushy non-crop areas around the home thoroughly. Avoid spraying desirable plants. For ants, thoroughly wet hills and runways. Repeat applications as infestations warrant and as reinfestation occurs.

Contraindication(s): Do not use on household pets or humans.

Precautionary Statements: Hazard to Humans and Domestic Animals: Causes substantial but temporary eye damage. Do not get into eyes or on clothing. Wear goggles or safety glasses. Harmful if swallowed. May be absorbed through skin. May cause skin sensitization following repeated contact with skin in susceptible individuals. Avoid repeated contact with skin. If sensitization reactions result, consult a physician. Avoid breathing of spray mist. Avoid contact with skin or clothing. Wash thoroughly after handling and before smoking or eating. Do not allow spray to contact food, feedstuffs or utensils. All food processing surfaces and utensils should be covered during treatment or thoroughly washed before reuse. Do not use on household pets or humans.

Statement of Practical Treatment:

If Swallowed: Contact a physician or Poison Control Center immediately. Drink one or two glasses of water and induce vomiting by touching back of throat with finger. Do not induce vomiting or give anything by mouth to an unconscious person.

If Inhaled: Remove victim to fresh air. Apply artificial respiration if indicated.

If on Skin: Remove contaminated clothing and wash affected areas with soap and water.

If in Eyes: Flush eyes with plenty of water. Call a physician. Note to Physician: Diazinone is an organophosphate insecticide. If symptoms of cholinesterase inhibition are present, atropine sulfate by injection is antidotal. 2-PAM is also antidotal and may be administered, but only in conjunction with atropine.

Environmental Hazards: This product is toxic to fish, birds, and wildlife including waterfowl. Birds and waterfowl feeding or drinking on treated areas may be killed. Keep out of lakes, streams, ponds, tidal marshes and estuaries. Shrimp and crab may be killed at application rates recommended on the label. Do not apply where fish, shrimp, crab and other aquatic life are important resources. Do not contaminate water by cleaning of equipment or disposal of equipment washwaters.

This pesticide is highly toxic to bees, exposed to direct treatment or residues on blooming plants where they feed. Do not apply this pesticide or allow it to drift to blooming plants if bees are visiting the treatment area. Do not apply this product or allow it to drift to food crops or any desirable vegetation at any time.

Storage and Disposal: Do not contaminate water food or feed by storage and disposal.

Containers Larger Than One Gallon:

Pesticide Storage and Procedure: Store upright at room temperature. Avoid exposure to extreme temperatures. In case of spill or leakage, soak up with an absorbent material such as sand, sawdust, earth, fuller's earth, etc. Dispose of with chemical wastes. Keep container closed. Protect from freezing. Do not transport or store under 32°F.

Pesticide Disposal: Waste resulting from the use of this product may be disposed of on site or at an approved waste disposal facility.

Container Disposal: Triple rinse (or equivalent). Then offer for recycling or reconditioning, or puncture and dispose of in a sanitary landfill, or by approved State and local procedures.

Containers of one gallon or Less:

Storage: Store in original container in a cool, dry place inaccessible to children and pets. Protect from freezing.

Disposal: Wrap container in several layers of newspaper and discard in trash.

Warning(s): Keep out of reach of children.

Disclaimer: Buyer assumes all risks of use, storage and handling of this material not in strict accordance with the directions given herewith.

Presentation: 1, 5, 15, 20, 30, 35 and 55 gallon containers.

Compendium Code No.: 10100031

SUN-DUST ROACH AWAY

Sungro **Premise Insecticide**

EPA Reg. No.: 11474-64

Active Ingredient(s):

	By Weight
Pyrethrins	1.0%
Piperonyl butoxide, technical*	10.0%
Amorphous silica gel	40.0%
Inert ingredients	49.0%
Total	100.0%

*Equivalent to 8.0% (butylcarbityl) (6-propylpiperonyl) ether and 2.0% related compounds.

Contains petroleum distillates.

Indications: A desiccant dust that provides quick control and kills for up to six months when left undisturbed.

Non-staining and relatively odorless. For use in residences, institutions, food plants, and on cats and dogs.

Dosage and Administration: It is a violation of federal law to use the product in a manner inconsistent with its labeling.

Fleas on dogs and cats: Liberally apply the powder to the animal, rubbing thoroughly to the skin. Begin with the neck and include the underbody, legs, feet and the base of the tail. Repeat as necessary, surfaces of kennels should be dusted at the rate of one (1) ounce per 50 square feet. Heavily infested lawns, basements and crawl spaces should be dusted at the rate of 16 ounces per 1,000 square feet. Repeat as necessary.

Applications within food areas: Food processing plants and warehouses, beverage plants, meat and poultry processing plants, hospitals and schools. Limit to crack and crevice treatment only. Using a bulbous duster apply a small amount of material directly into cracks and crevices such as expansion joints between different elements of construction or between equipment bases and the floor, wall voids, motor housing, junction boxes or switch boxes, conduits or hollow equipment legs where cockroaches, ants, silverfish, spiders, boxelder bugs and crickets hide. Care should be taken to avoid depositing the product onto exposed surfaces or introducing the material into the air. Avoid contamination of food or food processing surfaces.

Applications of the product in the food areas of food handling establishments, other than as a crack and crevice treatment, are not permitted.

Nonfood areas: Homes, institutions, hospitals, schools, truck trailers and railroad cars. To control crawling insects such as ants, cockroaches, silverfish, firebrats, spiders, boxelder bugs, ticks, lice, and fleas in animal quarters, distribute ROACH AWAY at the rate of two (2) ounces per 100 square feet of surface area. Apply a continuous visible film underneath and behind stairs, refrigerators and appliances. Treat on, around and behind moldings, shelving, baseboards, pipe openings, cracks, crevices, and other areas where insects hide. For severe infestations apply ROACH AWAY behind cabinets and walls, in crawl spaces and attics at a rate of 16 ounces per 1,000 square feet of surface area. Repeat the treatment as necessary.

Precaution(s):

Storage: Store in a cool, dry place. Keep the container closed.

Pesticide Disposal: Do not contaminate water, food, or feed by storage or disposal. Wastes resulting from the use of the product may be disposed of on-site or at an approved waste disposal facility.

Container Disposal: Triple rinse (or equivalent). Then offer for recycling or reconditioning, or puncture and dispose of in a sanitary landfill, or by incineration, or, if allowed by state and local authorities, by burning. If burned, stay out of smoke.

Buyer assumes all the risks of use, storage or handling of the product not in strict accordance with directions given herewith.

Caution(s): Keep out of the reach of children.

Precautionary Statement: Avoid inhalation. Containers larger than one pound may not be used or stored in food handling establishments.

Environmental Hazards: The product is toxic to fish. Do not apply in water. Do not apply where runoff is likely to occur. Do not apply when weather conditions favor drift from treated areas. Do not contaminate water by the cleaning of equipment or the disposal of wastes.

Statement of Practical Treatment:

If swallowed, do not induce vomiting unless directed by a physician. Contains petroleum solvent. Contact a physician or poison control center immediately.

If inhaled, remove victim to fresh air.

If on skin, wash contaminated skin with soap and water.

If on eyes, flush eyes with plenty of water for at least 15 minutes. Get medical attention immediately.

Presentation: 12x3 oz, 12x8 oz, 8x1 lb and 1x5 lb containers.

Compendium Code No.: 10100010

SUNGRO FLEA-ZY PET SHAMPOO

Sungro **Parasiticide Shampoo**

EPA Reg. No.: 11474-53

Active Ingredient(s):

Pyrethrins	0.05%
Piperonyl butoxide, technical*	0.50%
Inert ingredients	99.45%
Total	100.00%

*Equivalent to 0.4% of (butylcarbityl) (6-propylpiperonyl) ether and to 0.1% of related compounds.

Indications: A shampoo for use on cats and dogs which kills fleas and ticks and leaves a lustrous coat.

Directions for Use: It is a violation of federal law to use the product in a manner inconsistent with its labeling.

To shampoo and kill fleas and ticks, wet the pet's coat with warm water. Starting at the head, work the shampoo thoroughly into the hair. Allow the lather to penetrate the hair for five minutes before rinsing. Dry with a towel. The pet will have a clear, lustrous coat, free of fleas and ticks.

Precautionary Statements: Hazards to Humans and Domestic Animals: Do not swallow.

Storage and Disposal: Storage: Store only in the original container, tightly closed, in a secure area inaccessible to children.

Disposal: Do not re-use the container. Wrap the container in several layers of newspaper and discard it in the trash.

Warning(s): Keep out of reach of children.

Presentation: 1 and 5 gallon pails; 15, 20, 30, 35 and 55 gallon drums.

Compendium Code No.: 10100041

SUNGRO PERMITH

Sungro **Premise Insecticide**

EPA Reg. No.: 11474-67

Active Ingredient(s):

Permethrin [(3-phenoxyphenyl) methyl (cis/trans 3-(2,2-dichloroethenyl) 2,2-dimethylcyclopropanecarboxylate]*	0.50%
Inert ingredients	99.50%

*Cis/trans ratio: Min. 35% cis and Max. 65% trans.

Indications: A concentrated Permanone®, stable emulsion for use outdoors, and in homes, and nonfood areas of kennels, institutions, schools, and food/feed processing establishments.

For the control of fleas, brown dog ticks and lice on premises and on dogs. Apply with a conventional mechanical or compressed air equipment.

Directions for Use: It is a violation of federal law to use the product in a manner inconsistent with its labeling.

Shake well before use.

Indoor application: Do not use in the edible product areas of food/feed processing plants or other areas where food/feed is commercially prepared or processed. Do not use in areas while food is exposed.

Nonfood/feed areas include garbage rooms, lavatories, floor drains (to sewers), entries and vestibules, machine rooms, boiler rooms, garages, mop closets, etc.

Vacate the treated areas and ventilate before reoccupying. For maximum effectiveness, a combination of spot, surface treatment and fogging is recommended.

Surface spraying: To control fleas and ticks (adults and larvae): Thoroughly spray the infested areas, pet beds, resting quarters, nearby cracks and crevices, along and behind baseboards, mouldings, window and door frames, and entire areas of floor and floor coverings. Fresh bedding should be placed in animal quarters following treatment. Repeat the treatment as needed.

On livestock: To protect cattle (beef and dairy), goats, sheep, hogs and horses from horn flies, face flies, house flies, mosquitoes and gnats: Apply a light mist sufficient to wet the surface of the hair. For face flies, spray the face and head, but do not spray into the eyes.

To control stable flies, horse flies and deer flies: apply at a rate of 2 ounces per adult animal, sufficient to wet the hair thoroughly. Repeat the treatment once a day or at intervals necessary to give continued protection.

To control blood-sucking lice: Apply to the infested areas of the animal, using a stiff brush to get the spray to the base of the hair. Repeat every 3 weeks if required.

To control poultry lice: Spray roosts, walls and nests or cages thoroughly. This should be followed by spraying over the birds with a fine mist.

To control bedbugs and mites in poultry houses: Spray crevices of roost poles, cracks in walls, and cracks in nests where the bedbugs and mites hide.

On dogs: To control fleas, ticks and lice: Start spraying at the tail, moving the dispenser rapidly and making sure that the animal's entire body is covered, including the legs and underbody. While spraying, fluff the hair so that the spray will penetrate to the skin. Make sure that the spray wets thoroughly. Do not spray into the eyes or face. Avoid contact with genitalia. Repeat as necessary.

Note: Not recommended for use on puppies of less than four weeks of age.

Precautionary Statements: Hazards to Humans and Domestic Animals: Harmful if swallowed.

Avoid the contamination of feed and foodstuffs. Remove pets and birds, and cover fish aquaria before space spraying or surface applications.

Statement of Practical Treatment:

If swallowed, drink one to two glasses of water and induce vomiting by touching the back of the throat with a finger. Repeat until vomit fluid is clear. Call a physician immediately. Do not induce vomiting or give anything by mouth to an unconscious person.

If inhaled, remove the affected person to fresh air. Apply artificial respiration if indicated.

If on skin, remove contaminated clothing and wash the affected areas with soap and water.

If in eyes, flush eyes with plenty of water. Call a physician if irritation persists.

Environmental Hazards: The product is toxic to fish. Do not apply directly to lakes, ponds, streams, tidal marshes or estuaries. Do not contaminate water by the cleaning of equipment or the disposal of wastes.

Physical or Chemical Hazards: Wear a full-faced gas mask with the canister type recommended for general insecticide protection when applying indoors as a space spray or fog.

Storage and Disposal: Do not contaminate water, food or feed by storage or disposal.

Pesticide Storage and Spill Procedures: Store upright at room temperature. Do not expose to freezing temperatures. Avoid exposure to extreme temperatures. In case of spill or leakage, soak up with an absorbant material such as sand, sawdust, earth, fuller's earth, etc. Dispose of with chemical waste.

Pesticide Disposal: Pesticide, spray mixture or rinse water that cannot be used according to label instructions must be disposed of at or by an approved waste disposal facility.

Container Disposal: Triple rinse (or equivalent), then offer for recycling or reconditioning, or puncture and dispose of in a sanitary landfill, or by other approved state and local procedures.

Containers of one gallon and smaller: Do not transport or store below 32°F. Do not re-use the container. Wrap the container in several layers of newspaper and discard it in the trash.

Warning(s): Keep out of reach of children.

Disclaimer: The buyer assumes all risks of use, storage or handling of the product not in strict accordance with directions given herewith.

Presentation: 1 and 5 gallon pails; 15, 20, 30, 35 and 55 gallon drums.

Compendium Code No.: 10100051

SUNKLEEN 16

Sungro **Disinfectant**

Cleaner-Disinfectant-Fungicide-Detergent-Virucide-Mildewstat-Canine Parvocidal

EPA Reg. No.: 1839-101-11474

Active Ingredient(s):

n-Alkyl (60% C_{14}, 30% C_{16}, 5% C_{12}, 5% C_{18})
dimethyl benzyl ammonium chlorides 0.80%
n-Alkyl (68% C_{12}, 32% C_{14}) ethylbenzyl ammonium chlorides 0.80%
Inert Ingredients 98.40%
Total 100.00%

Indications: SUNKLEEN 16 is designed to provide effective cleaning, deodorizing and disinfection specifically for hospitals, nursing homes, schools, animal quarters, kennels, food processing plants, food service establishments, transportation terminals, office buildings, manufacturing facilities, lodging establishments, retail businesses and athletic/recreational facilities where housekeeping is of prime importance in controlling the hazard of cross contamination.

When used as directed, this product is formulated to disinfect hard, non-porous, inanimate environmental surfaces: floors, walls, metal surfaces, stainless steel surfaces, glazed porcelain, glazed ceramic tile, plastic surfaces, bathrooms, shower stalls, bathtubs, cabinets, tables, chairs (non-upholstered surfaces), and telephones. For larger areas: operating rooms, patient care facilities and restrooms, this product is designed to provide both general cleaning and disinfecting.

This product deodorizes those areas which generally are hard to keep fresh smelling, such as garbage storage areas, empty garbage bins and cans, toilet bowls, and other areas which are prone to odors caused by microorganisms.

Directions for Use: It is a violation of Federal Law to use this product in a manner inconsistent with its labeling.

Disinfection: To disinfect hard, inanimate, non-porous surfaces apply solution with a mop, cloth, sponge or hand pump trigger sprayer so as to wet all surfaces thoroughly. Allow to remain wet for 10 minutes and then let air dry.

General Disinfection: Add 4.5 ounces of this product per gallon of water.

Hospital Disinfection: Add 6 ounces of this product per gallon of water.

For heavily soiled areas, a pre-cleaning step is required. Prepare a fresh solution for each use.

To disinfect toilet bowls: Remove gross filth or soils from surfaces with bowl brush. Add 4.5 ounces of this product directly to the bowl water. Brush or swab the bowl completely using a scrub brush or toilet mop, making sure to get under the rim. Let stand for 10 minutes and flush.

To disinfect food processing premises: floors, walls, and storage areas, add 4.5 ounces of this product per gallon of water. For heavily soiled areas, a pre-cleaning step is required. Apply solution with a mop, cloth, sponge or hand pump trigger sprayer so as to wet all surfaces thoroughly. Allow to remain wet for 10 minutes, then remove excess liquid. Before using this product, food products and packaging materials must be removed from the area or carefully protected. After use, all surfaces in the area must be thoroughly rinsed with potable water.

S

To disinfect food service establishment food contact surfaces: countertops, appliances, tables, add 4.5 ounces of this product per gallon of water. For heavily soiled areas, a pre-cleaning step is required. Apply solution with a cloth, sponge or hand pump trigger sprayer so as to wet all surfaces thoroughly. Allow the surface to remain wet for 10 minutes, then remove excess liquid and rinse the surface with potable water. This product can not be used to clean the following food contact surfaces: utensils, glassware and dishes.

Disinfection of Poultry Equipment, Animal Quarters and Kennels: For disinfection of pre-cleaned poultry equipment (brooders, watering founts, feeding equipment), animal quarters and kennels, apply a solution of 6 ounces of this product per gallon of water. Remove all poultry, animals, and feed from premises, trucks, coops, and crates. Remove all litter and droppings from floors, walls and surfaces of facilities occupied or traversed by poultry or animals. Empty all troughs, racks, and other feeding and watering appliances. Thoroughly clean all surfaces with soap or detergent and rinse with water. Saturate the surfaces with the disinfecting solution for a period of 10 minutes. Ventilate building, coops, and other closed spaces. Do not house poultry or animals or employ equipment until treatment has been absorbed, set or dried. All treated equipment that will contact feed or drinking water must be rinsed with potable water before reuse.

Bactericidal Activity: When diluted at the rate of 4.5 ounces per gallon of water, this product exhibits disinfectant activity against the organisms: *Salmonella choleraesuis, Staphylococcus aureus*, and *Escherichia coli*. When diluted at the rate of 6 ounces per gallon of water, this product exhibits effective disinfectant activity against *Pseudomonas aeruginosa* in addition to the above microorganisms and meets all requirements for hospital use. *Virucidal Activity: This product, when used on environmental, inanimate, hard, non-porous surfaces at a dilution 18 ounces per gallon of water, exhibits effective virucidal activity against Canine Parvovirus.

For Disinfection Against Canine Parvovirus: Add 18 ounces of this product per gallon of water.

Mildewstat: To control mold and mildew (such as *Aspergillus niger* ATCC 6275) and the odors they cause on pre-cleaned, hard, non-porous surfaces add 4.5 ounces of this product per gallon of water. Apply solution with a cloth, mop or sponge making sure to wet all surfaces completely. Let air dry. Prepare a fresh solution for each use. Repeat application at weekly intervals or when mildew growth appears.

Fungicidal Activity: At the 4.5 ounces per gallon dilution, this product is also fungicidal against the pathogenic fungi, *Trichophyton mentagrophytes* (Athlete's Foot Fungus), when used as directed on hard surfaces found in bathrooms, shower stalls, locker rooms, exercise facilities or other clean, hard, non-porous, surfaces commonly contacted by bare feet.

Efficacy tests have demonstrated that this product is an effective bactericide and fungicide in the presence of organic soil (5% blood serum).

Contraindication(s): This product is not to be used as a terminal sterilant/high-level disinfectant on any surface or instrument that (1) is introduced directly into the human body either into or in contact with the bloodstream or normally sterile areas of the body, or (2) contacts intact mucous membranes but which does not ordinarily penetrate the blood barrier or otherwise enter normally sterile areas of the body.

Precautionary Statements: Hazards to Humans and Domestic Animals:

Danger: Keep out of reach of children. Corrosive. Causes irreversible eye damage and skin burns. Do not get in eyes, on skin, or on clothing. Wear goggles or face shield, rubber gloves and protective clothing. Harmful if swallowed. Remove contaminated clothing and wash before reuse. Wash thoroughly with soap and water after handling.

First Aid:

If in eyes: Hold eye open and rinse slowly and gently with water for 15-20 minutes. Remove contact lenses, if present, after the first 5 minutes, then continue rinsing eye. Call a poison control center or doctor for treatment advice.

If on skin or clothing: Take off contaminated clothing. Rinse skin with plenty of water for 15-20 minutes. Call poison control center or doctor for treatment advice.

If swallowed: Call poison control center or doctor immediately for treatment advice. Have person sip a glass of water if able to swallow. Do not induce vomiting unless told to do so by the poison control center or doctor. Do not give anything by mouth to an unconscious person.

If inhaled: Move person to fresh air. If person is not breathing, call 911 or an ambulance then give artificial respiration, preferably by mouth-to-mouth, if possible. Call a poison control center or doctor for further treatment advice.

Have the product container or label with you when calling a poison control center or doctor, or going for treatment.

Note to Physician: Probable mucosal damage may contraindicate the use of gastric lavage.

Environmental Hazards: This pesticide is toxic to fish. Do not discharge effluent containing this product into lakes, streams, ponds, estuaries, oceans or other waters unless in accordance with the requirements of a National Pollutant Discharge Elimination System (NPDES) permit and the permitting authority has been notified in writing prior to discharge. Do not discharge effluent containing this product to sewer systems without previously notifying the local sewage treatment plant authority. For guidance contact your State Water Board or Regional Office of the EPA.

Storage and Disposal: Do not contaminate water, food, or feed by storage or disposal.

Storage: Store in a dry place no lower in temperature than 50°F or higher than 120°F.

Container Disposal: Do not reuse empty container. Triple rinse empty container with water. Return metal drum or offer for reconditioning or puncture and dispose of in a sanitary landfill, or by other procedures approved by State and local authorities. Plastic containers may be disposed of in a sanitary landfill, incinerated, or if allowed by local authorities, by burning. If burned, stay out of smoke.

For containers 1 gallon or less: Do not reuse empty container. Rinse thoroughly before discarding in trash.

Pesticide Disposal: Pesticide wastes are acutely hazardous. Improper disposal of excess pesticide, spray mixture, or rinsate is a violation of Federal Law. If these wastes cannot be disposed of by use according to label instructions, contact your State Pesticide or Environmental Control Agency, or the Hazardous Waste representative at the nearest EPA Regional Office for guidance.

Warning(s): Keep out of reach of children.

Presentation: 1, 5, 6, 15, 20, 30, 35 and 55 gallon containers.

Compendium Code No.: 10100080

SUNKLEEN 45

Sungro **Disinfectant**

EPA Reg. No.: 1839-95-11474

Active Ingredient(s):

n-Alkyl (60% C14, 30% C16, 5% C12, 5% C18)
dimethyl benzyl ammonium chlorides 2.25%
n-Alkyl (68% C12, 32% C14) dimethyl ethylbenzyl ammonium chlorides 2.25%
Inert Ingredients 95.50%
Total 100.00%

Indications: SUNKLEEN 45 detergent/disinfectant has been designed specifically for hospitals, nursing homes, schools, food processing plants and other institutions where housekeeping is of prime importance.

SUNKLEEN 45 is a phosphate free concentrated detergent/disinfectant which provides effective cleaning, deodorizing, disinfection and sanitization, SUNKLEEN 45 detergent/disinfectant has been designed specifically for hospitals, nursing homes, schools, food processing plants and other institutions where housekeeping is of prime importance in controlling the hazard of cross contamination.

SUNKLEEN 45 when diluted at the rate of 2 ounces per gallon of water is an effective disinfectant against the organism *Psudomonas aeruginosa* and meets all requirements for hospital use. When used as directed SUNKLEEN 45 is formulated to disinfect inanimate hard surfaces such as walls, floors, sink tops, toilet bowls, tables, chairs, telephones and bed frames. For larger areas such as operating rooms, patient care facilities and restrooms, the product is designed to provide both general cleaning and disinfecting.

In addition, SUNKLEEN 45 deodorizes those areas which generally are hard to keep fresh smelling, such as garbage storage area, empty garbage bins and cans, toilet bowls and other areas which are prone to odors caused by microorganisms.

Disinfection - At 2 ounces per gallon dilution SUNKLEEN 45 exhibits effective disinfectant activity against the following:

Pseudomonas aeruginosa PRD-10, *Escherichia coli, Brevibacterium ammoniagenes, Klebsiella pneumoniae, Streptococcus faecallis, Salmonella schuttmuelleri, Shigella dysentariae, Salmonella chloeraesuis, Enterobacter aerogenes, Streptococcus salivarius, Staphylococcus aureus.*

At this level this product is also fungicidal against the Pathogenic fungi, *Trichophyton mentagrophytes.*

Virucidal Activity: The product when used on environmental inanimate hard surfaces at 2 ounces per gallon of water exhibits effective virucidal* activity against influenza A2-Asian (represntative of the common flu virus), Herpes simplex (representative agent of fever blisters and mononucleosis.), Adeno virus type 2 (causative agent of upper respiratory infections), and Vaccinia virus (representative of the pox virus group).

Efficacy tests have demonstrated that SUNKLEEN 45 is an effective bactericide, fungicide, and virucide* in the presence of organic soil (5% blood serum).

Mold and Mildewstat - SUNKLEEN 45 prevents and controls mold and mildew and the odors they cause on hard non-porous inanimate surfaces.

Sanitization - When used for sanitization of previously cleaned food equipment or food contact items limit active quaternaries to 200 ppm. At this level potable water rinse is required. SUNKLEEN 45 is an effective sanitizer when diluted in water up to 250 ppm hardness ($CaCO_3$).

Directions for Use: It is a violation of federal law to use this product in a manner inconsistent with its labeling.

Disinfection - To disinfect hard inanimate surfaces (such as walls, floors, tabletops), add 2 ounces SUNKLEEN 45 detergent/disinfectant per gallon of water. Apply solution with mop, cloth, or a sponge or mechanical sprayer so as to wet thoroughly. Allow to remain wet for 10 minutes and then let air dry.

To disinfect toilet bowls, add 2 ounces SUNKLEEN 45 detergent/disinfectant directly to bowl water. Swab the bowl completely using a scrub brush or toilet mop, making sure to get under the rim. Let stand for 10 minutes and flush.

For heavily soiled areas, a pre-cleaning step is required and recommended. Prepare a fresh solution for each use.

Mildewstat - To control mold and mildew on precleaned, hard non-porous surfaces (such as floors, walls, table tops) add 2 ounces SUNKLEEN 45 per gallon of water. Apply solution with a cloth, mop or sponge making sure to wet all surfaces completely. Let air dry. Prepare a fresh solution for each use. Repeat application at weekly intervals or when mildew growth reappears.

Sanitization - To sanitize previously cleaned and rinsed non-porous food contact surfaces, prepare 200 ppm active quaternary SUNKLEEN 45 solution by adding 2 ounces SUNKLEEN 45 to 3 ½ gallons of water.

To sanitize immobile items (such as tanks, chopping blocks, counter tops), flood the area with 200 ppm SUNKLEEN 45 solution or apply with a cloth or sponge, making sure to wet all surfaces completely for at least 60 seconds. Remove and rinse thoroughly with potable water. Prepare fresh solution for each use. To sanitize mobile items (such as drinking glasses, eating utensils), immerse in 200 ppm SUNKLEEN 45 solution for at least 60 seconds making sure to immerse completely. Remove and rinse thoroughly with potable water. Prepare a fresh solution daily or more frequently as soil is apparent.

Precautionary Statements: Hazard to Humans and Domestic Animals:

Danger: Keep out of reach of children. Causes eye and skin irritation. Do not get in eyes, skin or on clothing. Harmful if swallowed.

Statement of Practical Treatment: In case of contact, immediately flush eyes or skin with plenty of water for at least 15 minutes. For eyes, call a physician. Remove and wash contaminated clothing before reuse. If swallowed, drink milk, egg whites, gelatin solution or if these are not available, drink large quantities of water. Call a physician.

Note to Physician: Probable mucosal damage may contraindicate the use of gastric lavage. Measures against circulatory shock, respiratory depression and convulsions may be needed.

For sale to, use, and storage by service persons. Keep out of the reach of children.

Storage and Disposal: Do not contaminate water, food, or feed by storage and disposal.

Storage: Store in a dry place no lower in temperature than 50°F or higher than 120°F.

Container Disposal: Do not reuse empty container. Triple rinse empty container with water. Return metal drum then offer fro reconditioning or puncture and dispose of in a sanitary landfill, or by other procedures approved by state and local authorities. Plastic containers may be disposed of in a sanitary landfill, incinerated, or, if allowed by local authorities, by burning. If burned stay out of smoke.

Pesticide Disposal: Pesticide wastes are acutely hazardous. Improper disposal of excess pesticide, spray mixture or rinsate is a violation of Federal law. If these wastes cannot be disposed of by use according to label instructions, contact your State Pesticide or Environmental Control Agency, or the Hazardous Waste representative at the nearest EPA Regional Office for guidance.

Presentation: 1, 5, 6, 15, 20, 30, 35, and 55 gallon containers.

Compendium Code No.: 10100061

SUNKLEEN 90

Sungro **Disinfectant**

EPA Reg. No.: 1839-96-11474

Active Ingredient(s): By Wt.

n-Alkyl (60% C14, 30% C16, 5% C12, 5% C18) dimethyl benzyl ammonium chlorides	4.50%
n-Alkyl (68% C12, 32% C14) dimethyl ethylbenzyl ammonium chlorides	4.50%
Inert Ingredients	91.00%
Total	100.00%

Indications: SUNKLEEN 90 detergent/disinfectant has been designed specifically for hospitals, nursing homes, schools, food processing plants and other institutions where housekeeping is of prime importance.

SUNKLEEN 90 is a phosphate free concentrated detergent/disinfectant which provides effective cleaning, deodorizing, disinfection. SUNKLEEN 90 detergent/disinfectant has been designed specifically for hospitals, nursing homes, schools, food processing plants and other institutions where housekeeping is of prime importance in controlling the hazard of cross contamination.

SUNKLEEN 90 when diluted at the rate of 1 ounce per gallon of water is an effective disinfectant against the organism *Psudomonas aeruginosa* and meets all requirements for hospital use. When used as directed SUNKLEEN 90 is formulated to disinfect inanimate hard surfaces such as walls, floors, sink tops, toilet bowls, tables, chairs, telephones and bed frames. For larger areas such as operating rooms, patient care facilities and restrooms, the product is designed to provide both general cleaning and disinfecting.

In addition, SUNKLEEN 90 deodorizes those areas which generally are hard to keep fresh smelling, such as garbage storage area, empty garbage bins and cans, toilet bowls and other areas which are prone to odors caused by microorganisms.

Disinfection - At 1 ounce per gallon dilution SUNKLEEN 90 exhibits effective disinfectant activity against the following:

Pseudomonas aeruginosa PRD-10, *Salmonella typhi, Escherichia coli, Brevibacterium ammoniagenes, Klebsiella pneumoniae, Streptococcus faecallis, Salmonella schuttmuelleri, Shigella dysentariae, Salmonella chloeraesuis, Enterobacter aerogenes, Streptococcus salivarius, Staphylococcus aureus.*

At this level this product is also fungicidal against the Pathogenic fungi, *Trichophyton mentagrophytes.*

Virucidal Activity: The product when used on environmental inanimate hard surfaces at 1 ounce per gallon of water exhibits effective virucidal* activity against influenza A2-Asian (representative of the common flu virus), Herpes simplex (causative agent of fever blisters and mononucleosis), Adeno virus type 5 (causative agent of upper respiratory infections), and Vaccinia virus (representative of the pox virus group), and Influenza A/Brazil.

Efficacy tests have demonstrated that SUNKLEEN 90 is an effective bactericide, fungicide, and virucide* in the presence of organic soil (5% blood serum).

Mold and Mildewstat - SUNKLEEN 90 prevents and controls mold and mildew and the odors they cause on hard non-porous inanimate surfaces.

Directions for Use: It is a violation of federal law to use this product in a manner inconsistent with its labeling.

Disinfection - To disinfect hard inanimate surfaces (such as walls, floors, tabletops), add 1 ounce SUNKLEEN 90 detergent/disinfectant per gallon of water. Apply solution with mop, cloth, or a sponge or mechanical sprayer so as to wet thoroughly. Allow to remain wet for 10 minutes and then let air dry.

To disinfect toilet bowls, flush toilet add 1 ounce SUNKLEEN 90 detergent/disinfectant directly to bowl water. Swab the bowl completely using a scrub brush or toilet mop, making sure to get under the rim. Let stand for 10 minutes and flush.

For heavily soiled areas, a pre-cleaning step is required and recommended. Prepare a fresh solution for each use.

Mildewstat - To control mold and mildew on precleaned, hard non-porous surfaces (such as floors, walls, table tops) add 1 ounce SUNKLEEN 90 per gallon of water. Apply solution with a cloth, mop or sponge making sure to wet all surfaces completely. Let air dry. Prepare a fresh solution for each use. Repeat application at weekly intervals or when mildew growth reappears.

Precautionary Statements: Hazard to Humans and Domestic Animals:

Danger: Causes eye and skin damage. Do not get in eyes, skin or on clothing. Harmful or fatal if swallowed. Wear goggles or face shield and rubber gloves when handling. Avoid contamination of food.

Statement of Practical Treatment: In case of contact, immediately flush eyes or skin with plenty of water for at least 15 minutes. For eyes, call a physician. Remove and wash contaminated clothing before reuse.

If swallowed, drink promptly a large quantity of milk, egg whites, gelatin solution or if these are not available, drink large quantities of water. Avoid alcohol. Call a physician.

Note to Physician: Probable mucosal damage may contraindicate the use of gastric lavage. Measures against circulatory shock, respiratory depression and convulsions may be needed. If persistent, convulsions may be controlled by the catious intravenous injection of a shortacting barbiturate drug.

Storage and Disposal: Do not contaminate water, food, or feed by storage and disposal.

Storage: Store in a dry place no lower in temperature than 50°F or higher than 120°F.

Pesticide Disposal: Pesticide wastes are acutely hazardous. Improper disposal of excess pesticide, spray mixture or rinsate is a violation of Federal law. If these wastes cannot be disposed of by use according to label instructions, contact your State Pesticide or Environmental Control Agency, or the Hazardous Waste representative at the nearest EPA Regional Office for guidance.

Container Disposal: Do not reuse empty container. Triple rinse empty container with water. Return metal drum then offer fro reconditioning or puncture and dispose of in a sanitary landfill, or by other procedures approved by state and local authorities. Plastic containers may be disposed of in a sanitary landfill, incinerated, or, if allowed by local authorities, by burning. If burned stay out of smoke.

Warning(s): Keep out of reach of children.

Presentation: 1, 5, 6, 20, 30, 35, and 55 gallon containers.

Compendium Code No.: 10100071

SUPER II DAIRY & FARM SPRAY

Durvet **Topical Insecticide**

Ready-to-use Pyrethrin/Vapona

EPA Reg. No.: 47000-54-12281

Active Ingredient(s):

Pyrethrins	.05%
Piperonyl butoxide, technical*	.10%
N-octyl bicycloheptene dicarboximide**	.16%
Dichlorvos (2,2-dichlorovinyl, dimethyl phosphate)+	.465%
Related Compounds+	.035%
Other Ingredients:++	99.19%
Total	100.00%

*Consists of 0.08% (butylcarbityl) (6-propylpiperonyl) ether and 0.02% other related compounds.

**MGK 264

+Equivalent to .50%w of Vapona.

++Contains petroleum distillate.

Indications: For agricultural/commercial use only. Not for sale for any other uses.

Kills and repels horn flies, stable flies, mosquitoes and gnats.

For use in areas under general category of farm buildings, (farm yards); dairy and farm premises; feed lots, including around feed lots, stockyards, corrals, holding pens, fences, etc.; animal buildings, including barns, feeding areas, shelters and stables; dairy barns (including milk rooms, equipment and barnyards); and livestock feeding areas.

When properly applied, the repellent effect against above insects will last two days.

Directions for Use: It is a violation of Federal Law to use this product in a manner inconsistent with its labeling.

To protect livestock from attack by fleas, spray bedding and walls of pen, particularly cracks and crevices. Repeat treatment frequently until adequate control is obtained.

In a complete fly control program these sprays should be used in combination with residual insecticides and sanitary measures.

To develop a residual repellency to stable flies, mosquitoes and gnats on dairy cows, apply 1 to 2 ounces of SUPER II DAIRY & FARM SPRAY to each animal for a three day period. The spray should be applied with a good hydraulic-type hand sprayer so that the animal's entire body has been uniformly covered. Special care should be used in spraying the legs, belly and shoulders. Avoid areas around the nose, eyes and mouth. Avoid wetting the hide. Do not make direct application to livestock more frequently than once per day. Spray in the same manner again after two days have elapsed and every second day thereafter or when insects again disturb the animal. Be sure the teats and udder are washed with warm water prior to milking. Calves should be sprayed very lightly once a day instead of attempting to build up a residual repellency by spraying

S

more heavily. Brahman and Brahman cross cattle should not be treated as they may show hypersensitivity to organic phosphates.

For control of lice on livestock, spray the animals with 2 ounces of SUPER II DAIRY & FARM SPRAY. Immediately rub the spray into the hair, paying particular attention to infested areas. Repeat as necessary, but not more frequently than once every three weeks.

To kill flies, mosquitoes and gnats in the barn prior to milking, close all doors and windows and direct the spray toward the ceiling. The barn should remain closed for 10 to 20 minutes. Sweep up and destroy fallen insects. Repeat as necessary. Apply at the rate of one ounce spray per 1,000 cubic feet. Do not remain in the treated areas and ventilate the area after treatment is complete. Do not use this solution for fogging or misting in areas where animals have received direct application of dichlorvos or other organophosphate within 8 hours. Do not contaminate water, feed or foodstuffs, milk or milking utensils.

Precautionary Statements: Hazards to Humans and Domestic Animals: Harmful if swallowed, inhaled or absorbed through the skin. Avoid contact with skin. Wash thoroughly with soap and water after handling and before eating or smoking. Avoid prolonged breathing of spray mist.

Wear a pesticide respirator with an organic-vapor removing cartridge with a prefilter approved for pesticides (MSHA/NIOSH approval number prefix TX-23C), or a canister approved for pesticides (MSHA/NIOSH approval number prefix TC-14G), or a NIOSH approved respirator with an organic vapor (OV) cartridge or canister with any R, P or HE prefilter when applying indoor as a spray or fog.

If swallowed, consult a physician immediately. Avoid overspraying which will result in wetting the animals' hides. Avoid contamination of milk and milk handling equipment.

Statement of Practical Treatment:

If Swallowed: Do not induce vomiting. Contact a physician. Solvent poses an aspiration hazard.

If Inhaled: Remove to fresh air and apply artificial respiration if needed.

If On Skin: Wash with soap and water.

If In Eyes: Flush with water for 15 minutes. In all cases consult a physician.

Environmental Hazards: This product is toxic to fish and wildlife. Do not apply to any body of water. Do not contaminate water by disposal of equipment washwaters. Apply this product only as specified on this label.

Physical or Chemical Hazards: Do not use, pour, spill, or store near heat or open flame.

Storage and Disposal:

Prohibitions: Do not contaminate water, food, or feed by storage or disposal.

Pesticide Storage: Store in a cool, dry, secure area in original container.

Pesticide Disposal: Wastes resulting from the use of this product may be disposed of on site or at an approved waste disposal facility.

Container: (Plastic); Triple rinse (or equivalent). Then offer for recycling or reconditioning, or puncture and dispose of in a sanitary landfill, or incinerator, or, if allowed by state and local authorities, by burning. If burning, stay out of smoke.

Warning(s): Keep out of reach of children.

Disclaimer: Notice: Seller's guarantee shall be limited to the terms of the label and subject thereto the buyer assumes any risk to persons or property arising out of use or handling and accepts the product on these conditions.

Presentation: 1 gallon, 2.5 gallons and 5 gallons.

Compendium Code No.: 10841581 1/99

SUPER 14™

Farnam **Dietary Supplement**

14% Polyunsaturated Fatty Acids

Guaranteed Analysis: Each Pound Contains Not Less Than:

Crude Protein, min. 27%
Methionine, min. 0.7%
Crude Fat, min. 18%
Crude Fiber, max. 1.5%
Ash, max. 10%
Selenium, min. . . . . 0.7 ppm
Zinc, min. . . . . 1800 ppm
Vitamin A, min. . . . . 21,000 I.U.
Vitamin E, min. . . . . 150 I.U.
Vitamin B_6, min. . . . . 24 mg

Ingredients: Corn Oil, Soybean Oil, Soybean Flour, Dextrose, Vitamin A Acetate, Zinc Methionine, dl-alpha-Tocopheryl Acetate (source of Vitamin E), Pyridoxine Hydrochloride (source of Vitamin B_6), Calcium Silicate, Sodium Selenite, Mixed Tocopherols, Citric Acid, Ascorbic Acid (as preservatives), and Artificial Flavorings.

Indications: SUPER 14™ provides a specially formulated combination of polyunsaturated fatty acid nutrients useful in normal skin nutrition. Contains Corn Oil and Soybean Oil. High in Polyunsaturated Fatty Acids.

For all classes of horses, dogs and cats.

Directions: SUPER 14™ contains flavorizing agents which make the formula highly acceptable to all animals. Just feed morning and night on top of the grain.

Measuring Cup = 1 Tablespoon

For Horses: Feed 2-3 tablespoons of SUPER 14™ twice daily with the feed - once in the morning and once again in the evening. Sprinkle this amount over the feed or mix with the ration.

For Dogs and Cats: Sprinkle SUPER 14™ over the pet's ration once each day in the proper amount indicated below:

Weight of Pet	Amount per Day
Up to 15 lbs.	1/2 level Tablespoon
15 to 30 lbs.	1 level Tablespoon
30 to 60 lbs.	2 level Tablespoons
Over 60 lbs.	3 level Tablespoons

For horses and dogs with coats in particularly poor condition, feed twice the recommended level for the first two weeks and then reduce to the usual level.

Caution(s): If the condition persists, consult a veterinarian, since factors other than nutrition may be involved.

Warning(s): Not for human use.

Presentation: 1.36 kg (3 lb), 2.948 kg (6.5 lb) and 9.07 kg (20 lb).

Compendium Code No.: 10001010 9B9/9DD9 / 9B9/9AA9 / 9AA9

SUPER B COMPLEX ℞

Vedco **Vitamin B-Complex**

Active Ingredient(s): Composition: Each mL of sterile solution contains:

Thiamine Hydrochloride . . . . . 100 mg
Riboflavin 5 (Sodium Phosphate USP) . . . . . 5 mg
Pyridoxine Hydrochloride . . . . . 10 mg
Niacinamide . . . . . 100 mg
d-Panthenol . . . . . 10 mg
Cyanocobalamin . . . . . 100 mcg
Benzyl Alcohol (as preservative) . . . . . 1.5% v/v
Water for Injection . . . . . q.s.

Stabilized in citric acid buffer.

Indications: For use as a supplemental source of B complex vitamins for use in preventing or treating deficiencies in cattle, horses, swine, sheep, dogs and cats.

Dosage and Administration: Administer by intramuscular injection or subcutaneous injection. Dosage may be repeated once or twice weekly as needed.

Calves and Foals . . . . . 3 to 5 mL
Yearlings . . . . . 5 to 10 mL
Adult Cattle and Horses . . . . . 10 to 20 mL
Lambs and weaning pigs . . . . . 1 to 2 mL
Growing lambs and pigs . . . . . 2 to 3 mL
Adult sheep and swine . . . . . 3 to 5 mL
Dogs . . . . . 0.5 to 2 mL
Cats . . . . . 0.5 to 1 mL

May be repeated as indicated.

Precaution(s): Store at refrigerated temperature between 2-8°C (36-46°F).

Caution(s): Federal law restricts this drug to use by or on the order of a licensed veterinarian.

Not for intravenous use. Parenteral administration of thiamine has resulted in anaphylactic shock. Administer slowly and with caution in doses over 0.5 mL (50 mg thiamine).

For animal use only.

Warning(s): Keep out of reach of children.

Presentation: 100 mL, 250 mL and 500 mL.

Compendium Code No.: 10941931

SUPER B-PLEX

Neogen **Dietary Supplement**

With Electrolytes

Ingredients: Contains: Riboflavin (B_2), Sorbitol solution, Cobalt sulfate, Copper gluconate, Sodium benzoate, Ferric ammonium citrate, Sodium saccharin, Potassium chloride, Thiamine mononitrate, Pyridoxine HCl (B_6), Artificial flavor.

Indications: A water-dispersible blend of vitamins and electrolytes for horses and dogs.

Dosage and Administration:

Horses: 1 ounce daily in feed or water.

Dogs: 1 tablespoon (15 mL) daily in feed or water.

Precaution(s): Shake well before use.

Caution(s): For veterinary use only.

Warning(s): Keep out of reach of children.

Presentation: 128 fl oz (1 gallon) 3.785 L (NDC: 59051-9138-9).

Compendium Code No.: 14910431 L419-0501

SUPER CALCIUM DRENCH

Vedco **Calcium-Oral**

Guaranteed Analysis: (per 200 mL feeding): Calcium (ca), minimum: 11.5%, maximum 13.5%.

Ingredients: Water, calcium chloride, magnesium chloride, propylene glycol, potassium chloride, riboflavin supplement, vitamin B_{12} supplement, thiamin HCl, pyridoxine HCl and d-calcium pantothenate.

Indications: A ready to use blend of calcium, magnesium, potassium, b-complex vitamins and propylene glycol.

Dosage and Administration: Cows, provide 200 mL pre-calving and another 200 mL post-calving. Feed via drench gun or tube.

Caution(s): Not for human use. For livestock use only.

Warning(s): Keep out of reach of children.

Presentation: 3.8 liter (1 US gallon), provides 19 (200 mL) feedings.

Compendium Code No.: 10941940

SUPER CALCIUM GEL "62"

AgriPharm **Calcium-Oral**

Ingredient(s): Calcium chloride, water, magnesium chloride, cobalt sulfate, silicon dioxide, dextrose, sodium citrate.

Minimum contents of 300 mL dose:

Calcium . . . . . 54.0 g - 13.2% minimum
74.4 g - 18.2% maximum
Magnesium . . . . . 6.8 g
Cobalt . . . . . 0.6 g

Indications: For use as a high calcium nutritional supplement for dairy cattle during calving.

Dosage and Administration: Administer orally on back of tongue.

Prior to calving . . . . . 1 tube
After calving . . . . . 1 tube

Give one tube prior to calving and the second tube 12 to 24 hours after calving using the following directions:

1. Hold head of the cow in a slightly elevated position.
2. Place nozzle near rear of mouth. Use of hook nozzle recommended.
3. Discharge entire contents of the tube.
4. Hold up head of cow and allow animal time to swallow.

Not a drug. No withdrawal time.

Precaution(s): Do not freeze. Keep cool.

Warning(s): Keep out of the reach of children.

Presentation: 300 mL.

Compendium Code No.: 14570960

SUPERIOR-VITA-MIN BLEND™

Horses Prefer **Equine Dietary Supplement**

Guaranteed Analysis: (Minimum per lb):

Methionine	800 mg
Calcium (min)	1.00%
Calcium (max)	12.0%
Phosphorous (min)	4.0%
Salt (min)	0.8%
Salt (max)	1.6%
Manganese	0.4%
Iron	1%
Copper	.02%
Zinc	0.3%
Cobalt	.005%
Selenium	.00088%
Vitamin A	228,000 IU
Vitamin D_3	62,000 IU
Vitamin E	2,000 IU
Vitamin B_{12}	50 mg
Riboflavin	100 mg
d-Pantothenic Acid	20 mg
Niacin	60 mg
Choline	5,000 mg
Folic Acid	50 mg
Vitamin C	500 mg
Biotin	.02%

Ingredients: Corn Distillers Dried Solubles, Corn Distillers Dried Grains, Yeast Culture, Dried Molasses, Vitamin A Acetate (stability improved), D-Activated Animal Sterol (source of Vitamin D_3), DL-alpha-tocopheryl Acetate (source of Vitamin E), Vitamin B_{12} Supplement, Riboflavin Supplement, d-Calcium Pantothenate, Niacin Supplement, Choline Chloride, Folic Acid, Ascorbic Acid, DL-Methionine, Ferrous Sulfate, Copper Sulfate, Magnesium Oxide, Cobalt Carbonate, Potassium Chloride, Zinc Sulfate, Fermentation Products (Dried *Lactobacillus Acidophilus, Lactobacillus Lactis, Lactobacillus Plantarum, Streptococcus Cremoris, Lactobacillus Brevis, Pediococcus Acidilactici, Enterococcus Faecium* and *Pediococcus Pentacius),* Dicalcium Phosphate Calcium Carbonate, Salt, Pyridoxine Hydrochloride, Biotin, Sodium Selenite, Roughage Products, Oil and Flavor.

Indications: Complete daily nutrition with biotin and methionine.

Directions: Feeding Directions:

Recommended Dosage:

2-3 oz. per head/day for horses over 400 lbs.

1 oz. per head/day for horses under 400 lbs.

Note:

2 oz. per head per day supplies the recommended 15 mgs. of Biotin.

Do not feed more than 4 oz. per head/day.

Caution(s): Follow label directions. Feeding higher dosages will increase the intake of selenium above permitted levels.

Presentation: 5 lbs.

Compendium Code No.: 36950061

SUPER KETO DRENCH

Vedco **Acetonemia Preparations**

Guaranteed Analysis: (per 200 mL feeding):

Vitamin B_{12}	6000 mcg
Vitamin B_6	60 mg
Niacin	11,500 mg

Ingredients: Propylene glycol, niacin supplement, vitamin A acetate, de-activated animal sterol (source of vitamin D_3), cyanocobalamin (source of vitamin B_{12}), dl-alpha tocopherol acetate (source of vitamin E), riboflavin (source of vitamin B_6), choline bitartrate, and ascorbic acid.

Indications: Nutritional supplement for dairy cattle.

Dosage and Administration: Cows, provide 200 mL pre-calving and another 200 mL post-calving. Feed via drench gun or tube.

Caution(s): Not for human use. For livestock use only.

Warning(s): Keep out of reach of children.

Presentation: 3.8 liter (1 US gallon), provides 19 (200 mL) feedings.

Compendium Code No.: 10941950

SUPER POLY-BAC B® SOMNUS

Texas Vet Lab **Bacterin-Toxoid**

Haemophilus Somnus-Pasteurella Haemolytica-Multocida-Salmonella Typhimurium Bacterin-Toxoid

U.S. Vet. Lic. No.: 290

Contents: This product contains the antigens listed above.

Indications: For use in stocker and feeder calves as an aid in the prevention of respiratory disease associated with *Haemophilus somnus, Pasteurella haemolytica* A1, *Pasteurella haemolytica* A6 and *Pasteurella multocida* A3 and salmonellosis caused by *Salmonella typhimurium.*

Dosage and Administration: Instructions: Shake well and aseptically inject 2 mL subcutaneously in the side of the neck. Give a second dose 14 days after the first on the opposite side of the neck.

Precaution(s): Do not contaminate with dirt or chemicals. Use sterile equipment and adequately clean and disinfect bottle cap prior to each entry. Use entire contents when opened. Store at 2 to 7°C. Do not use if emulsion is broken as indicated by separation at the bottom of bottle.

Caution(s): May cause local swelling. Do not inject into muscle, may cause carcass trim. In case of anaphylactoid reaction, treat symptomatically. For veterinary use only.

Warning(s): Do not vaccinate within 60 days of slaughter.

Presentation: 50 dose (100 mL) and 100 dose (200 mL) bottles.

Compendium Code No.: 11080090

SUPER-TET® WITH HAVLOGEN®*

Intervet **Toxoid**

Tetanus Toxoid

U.S. Vet. Lic. No.: 286

Contents: Purified tetanus toxoid adsorbed with Havlogen®*.

Contains thimerosal as preservative.

Indications: Purified Tetanus Toxoid for vaccination of healthy horses, cattle, swine and sheep against Tetanus.

Dosage and Administration: For primary immunization, aseptically inject horses, cattle and swine with 1 mL or sheep with 0.5 mL intramuscularly and repeat the dose in 3 to 4 weeks. A dose should be administered annually.

Precaution(s): Store at 35° to 45°F (2° to 7°C). Shake well before using. Use entire contents when first opened.

Caution(s): Local reactions may occur if this product is given subcutaneously. Inject deep into the muscle only. Injury should be followed by a booster dose of a vaccine containing Tetanus Toxoid. Consult your veterinarian regarding indications and precautions for the use of tetanus antitoxin. Anaphylactoid reactions may occur.

For use in animals only.

Antidote(s): Epinephrine.

Warning(s): Do not vaccinate within 21 days before slaughter.

Presentation: 10 dose (10 x 1 mL) syringes and 10 dose (10 mL) vial.

*Adjuvant—U.S. Patent Nos. 3,790,665 and 3,919,411.

Compendium Code No.: 11062010

SUPER VITAMINS

Alpharma **Large Animal Dietary Supplement**

Ingredient(s): Sucrose, niacinamide, vitamin A supplement, menadione sodium bisulfite complex, sodium chloride, d-calcium pantothenic acid, vitamin D_3 supplement, riboflavin, vitamin E supplement, vitamin B_{12} supplement, pyridoxine HCl, thiamine HCl, folic acid.

Indications: A concentrated vitamin supplement for poultry and swine.

Directions: For use in drinking water or feed.

For Chickens:

For Starting, Growing and Laying Mashes: Mix 5 lbs with each ton of mash. For smaller batches, use 4 oz to each 100 lbs. If given in the drinking water, dissolve 2 level tablespoons in 5 gallons of water. This is equivalent to 1 lb per 100 gallons. For automatic medicators delivering 1 oz concentrate per gallon, add 1¼ bags per gallon as the concentrate.

For Breeder Mash: Mix 7½ lbs with each ton of mash. For smaller batches, use 6 oz to each 100 lbs. If given in the drinking water, dissolve 3 level tablespoons in 5 gallons of water. This is equivalent to 1½ lbs per 100 gallons.

For Swine:

For swine of all ages: Mix 4 oz with each 100 lbs of feed or 5 lbs per ton. When given in the drinking water, dissolve 4 tablespoons in each 10 gallons of water. This is equivalent to 1 lb per 100 gallons. For automatic medicator use, see directions for starting chickens. This product may be given to swine for as long as desired.

For Broilers and Turkeys:

For Starter and Grower Mashes: Mix 7½ lbs with each ton of mash. If given in the water, use at the rate of 1½ lbs (681 g) to each 100 gallons (378 liters) of water or 6 level tablespoons in each 10 gallons.

For Breeder Mash: Mix 10 lbs with each ton of mash. If given in the drinking water, use at the rate of 2 lbs to each 100 gallons. SUPER VITAMINS can be given to the birds either in the feed or in the water for as long as needed.

Precaution(s): Store in cool, dry place.

Caution(s): For oral animal use only.

Not for human use.

Keep out of reach of children.

Presentation: 16 oz (453.6 g).

Compendium Code No.: 10220591 AHF-035A 0003

SUPPRESSOR® ℞

RXV **Analgesic-Anti-inflammatory**

(Flunixin Meglumine Injection)

ANADA No.: 200-124

Active Ingredient(s): Each millimeter contains:

Flunixin Meglumine equivalent to Flunixin	50 mg
Edetate Disodium	0.1 mg
Sodium Formaldehyde Sulfoxylate	2.5 mg
Diethanolamine	4.0 mg
Propylene Glycol	207.2 mg
Phenol (as preservative)	5.0 mg
Water For Injection	q.s.

With hydrochloric acid to adjust pH.

Indications: SUPPRESSOR® (Flunixin Meglumine Injection) is recommended for the alleviation of inflammation and pain associated with musculoskeletal disorders in the horse. It is also recommended for the alleviation of visceral pain associated with colic in the horse.

Pharmacology: Flunixin meglumine is a potent, nonnarcotic, nonsteroidal, analgesic agent with anti-inflammatory and antipyretic activity. It is significantly more potent than pentazocine, meperidine and codeine as an analgesic in the rat yeast paw test. Flunixin is four times as potent on a mg per mg basis as phenylbutazone as measured by the reduction in lameness and swelling in the horse. Plasma half-life in horse serum is 1.6 hours following a single dose of 1.1 mg/kg. Measurable amounts are detectable in horse plasma at 8 hours post infection.

Dosage and Administration: The recommended dose for musculoskeletal disorders is 0.5 mg per pound (1 mL/100 lbs) of body weight once daily. Treatment may be given by intravenous or intramuscular injection and repeated for up to 5 days. Studies show onset of activity is within 2 hours. Peak response occurs between 12 and 16 hours and duration of activity is 24-36 hours.

The recommended dose for the alleviation of pain associated with equine colic is 0.5 mg per pound of body weight. Intravenous administration is recommended for prompt relief. Clinical studies show pain is alleviated in less than 15 minutes in many cases.

Treatment may be repeated when signs of colic recur. During clinical studies approximately 10% of the horses required one or two additional treatments.

The cause of colic should be determined and treated with concomitant therapy.

Compatibilities: The effect of SUPPRESSOR® (Flunixin Meglumine Injection) on pregnancy has not been determined. Studies to determine activity of SUPPRESSOR® (Flunixin Meglumine Injection) when administered concomitantly with other drugs have been conducted. Drug

compatibility should be monitored closely in patients requiring adjunctive therapy. Isolated reports of local reactions following intramuscular injection, particularly in the neck, have been received. These include localized swelling, sweating, induration, and stiffness.
Contraindication(s): There are no known contraindications to this drug when used as directed. Intra-arterial injection should be avoided. Horses inadvertently injected intra-arterially can show adverse reactions. Signs can be ataxia, incoordination, hyperventilation, hysteria, and muscle weakness. Signs are transient and disappear without antidotal medication within a few minutes. Do not use in horses showing hypersensitivity to flunixin meglumine.
Precaution(s): Store between 2° and 30°C (36° and 86°F).
Caution(s): Federal law restricts this drug to use by or on the order of a licensed veterinarian.
For animal use only.
Warning(s): Not for use in horses intended for food.
Keep out of reach of children.
Toxicology: Toxicity studies were conducted in horses. A threefold intramuscular dose of 1.5 mg per pound of body weight daily for 10 consecutive days was safe. No changes were observed in hematology, serum chemistry, or urinalysis values. Intravenous dosages of 0.5 mg/lb daily for 15 days; 1.5 mg/lb daily for 10 days; and 2.5 mg/lb daily for 5 days produced no changes in blood or urine parameters. No injection site irritation was observed following intramuscular injection of the 0.5 mg/lb recommended dose. Some irritation was observed following a 3-fold dose administered intramuscularly.
Side Effects: Isolated reports of local reactions following intramuscular injection, particularly in the neck have been received. These include localized swelling, sweating, induration, and stiffness. In rare instances, fatal or nonfatal clostridial infections or other infections have been reported in association with intramuscular use of flunixin meglumine. In addition, rare instances of anaphylactic-like reactions, some of which may have been fatal, have been reported primarily following intravenous use.
Presentation: 100 mL and 250 mL multidose vials.
Compendium Code No.: 10910180

SUPRASULFA III® CALF BOLUS

AgriPharm — **Sulfamethazine**
Sulfamethazine Sustained Release Bolus
NADA No.: 140-270
Active Ingredient(s): Each bolus contains:
Sulfamethazine.......... 8.25 grams
Indications: For administration to ruminating beef and dairy calves only. These calves should be over one (1) month of age and no longer subsisting on an all milk diet.

Indicated for the treatment of the following diseases: bacterial pneumonia associated with *Pasteurella* spp.; colibacillosis (bacterial scours) caused by *Escherichia coli;* calf diphtheria caused by *Fusobacterium necrophorum;* coccidiosis caused by *Eimeria bovis* and *E zurnii.*
Dosage and Administration: To administer orally to ruminating beef and dairy calves at the rate of 165 mg/lb body weight on the first day of treatment. Each bolus will treat 50 lbs of body weight. The bolus is scored to allow breaking for more accurate dosing, however, it must not be crushed. The bolus should be lubricated prior to administration and care taken to ensure the entire dose has been swallowed. Observe animal following dosing to ensure regurgitation does not occur. If regurgitation occurs, clean regurgitated material and readminister, if this is not practical, administer a new bolus.

Dosage Schedule:

Body Weight	No. Boluses
100 lbs	2
150 lbs	3
200 lbs	4
250 lbs	5
300 lbs	6

Caution(s): SUPRASULFA III® CALF BOLUS Boluses are designed to provide a therapeutic sulfamethazine level in approximately 6 hours, and persist in providing this level for 72 hours (3 days). After 72 hours, all animals should be re-examined for persistence of observable disease signs. If signs are present, consult a veterinarian. If signs of disease are significantly reduced, it is recommended that a second dose be given to provide an additional 72 hours of therapy. No further doses should be administered.

This drug, like all sulfonamides, may cause toxic reactions and irreparable injury unless administered with adequate and continuous supervision. Follow the recommended dosages carefully. Fluid intake must be adequate at all times throughout the three day therapy provided by the sustained release bolus. If symptoms persist after using this preparation for 3 days, consult your veterinarian.
Warning(s): Do not use in female dairy cattle 20 months of age or older. Use of sulfamethazine in this class of cattle may cause milk residues. Do not use in calves under one (1) month of age or calves being fed an all milk diet. Use in these classes of calves may cause violative tissue residues to remain beyond the withdrawal time. Animals intended for human consumption must not be treated within 8 days of slaughtering.
Restricted drug (California).
For animal use only. Keep out of the reach of children.
Presentation: 25 and 50 boluses.
Compendium Code No.: 14570970

SUPRASULFA III® CATTLE BOLUS

AgriPharm — **Sulfamethazine**
Sulfamethazine Sustained Release Bolus
NADA No.: 140-270
Active Ingredient(s): Each bolus contains:
Sulfamethazine.......... 30 grams
Indications: Indicated for the treatment of the following diseases in beef cattle and non-lactating dairy cattle: *Pasteurella* spp.; bacterial pneumonia associated with *Pasteurella* spp.; necrotic pododermatitis (foot-rot) and calf diphtheria caused by *Fusobacterium necrophorum;* coccidiosis (bacterial scours) caused by *Escherichia coli;* coccidiosis caused by *Eimeria bovis* and *E zurnii;* acute mastitis caused by *Streptococcus* spp. (beef cattle only); acute metritis caused by *Streptococcus* spp.
Dosage and Administration: SUPRASULFA III® (Sulfamethazine Sustained Release Bolus) should be administered at the rate of 150 mg/lb body weight on the first day of treatment. Each bolus will treat 200 lbs of body weight. The bolus is scored to allow breaking for more accurate dosing, however, it must not be crushed. The bolus should be lubricated prior to administration and care taken to ensure the entire dose has been swallowed. Observe animal following dosing to ensure regurgitation does not occur. If regurgitation occurs, clean regurgitated material and readminister, if this is not practical, administer a new bolus.

Dosage Schedule:

Body Weight	No. Boluses
200 lbs	1
300 lbs	1.5
400 lbs	2
500 lbs	2.5
600 lbs	3
700 lbs	3.5
800 lbs	4
900 lbs	4.5
1000 lbs	5

Caution(s): SUPRASULFA III® (Sulfamethazine Sustained Release Bolus) is designed to provide a therapeutic sulfamethazine level in approximately 6 hours, and persist in providing this level for 72 hours (3 days). After 72 hours, all animals should be re-examined for persistence of observable disease signs. If signs are present, consult a veterinarian. If signs of disease are significantly reduced, it is recommended that a second dose be given to provide an additional 72 hours of therapy. No further doses should be administered.

This drug, like all sulfonamides, may cause toxic reactions and irreparable injury unless administered with adequate and continuous supervision. Follow the recommended dosages carefully. Fluid intake must be adequate at all times throughout the three day therapy provided by the sustained release bolus. If symptoms persist after using this preparation for 3 days, consult your veterinarian.
Warning(s): Do not use in female dairy cattle 20 months of age or older. Use of sulfamethazine in this class of cattle may cause milk residues. Do not use in calves under one (1) month of age or calves being fed an all milk diet. Use in these classes of calves may cause violative tissue residues to remain beyond the withdrawal time. Animals intended for human consumption must not be treated within 8 days of slaughtering.

For animal use only. Restricted drug (California). Keep out of the reach of children.
Presentation: 50 and 100 boluses.
Compendium Code No.: 14570980

SURE-BLOCK™ TOPICAL PAIN RELIEVER

SureNutrition — **Analgesic-Topical**
Active Ingredient(s):
Capsaicin.......... .025%

Ingredients: Water, Carbomer, Capsicum Extract, Chamomile Extract, Germaben, Polysorbate 20, Triethanolomine, Propyl Gallate, Fragrance.
Indications: For the temporary relief of joint and tendon pain resulting from performance trauma and degenerative joint disease in horses.
Directions: Determine exact area of lameness. If necessary, consult your veterinarian for the necessary determination. Cover the affected area with a coating of SURE-BLOCK™ and rub in thoroughly. Apply to all sides of joints and tendons where possible. Apply to affected area not more than 4 times daily. Do not bandage. Wash hands with soap and water after application.
Precaution(s): Store at room temperature 15°-30°C (59°-86°F).
Caution(s): For external use only. Avoid contact with eyes and mucous membranes. Do not apply to open wounds or damaged, irritated, or broken skin. If rash or irritation occurs, discontinue use. Use only as directed. Discontinue use and consult your veterinarian if the condition worsens or fails to improve.
Warning(s): Keep this and all medications out of reach of children.

In case of ingestion, seek professional assistance or contact a poison control center immediately.
Presentation: 8 fl oz (236 mL).
Compendium Code No.: 12060040 — 0E1

SURE E&SE™

SureNutrition — **Vitamin E-Selenium**
Vitamin E & Selenium Supplement
Guaranteed Analysis: per lb:
Selenium, min.......... 71 ppm (32 mg)
Vitamin E, min.......... 20,000 IU

Ingredients: Wheat Middlings, Calcium Carbonate, dl-alphatocpheryl Acetate and Sodium Selenite.
Indications: SURE E&SE™ is a vitamin E and selenium supplement for horses.
Dosage and Administration: Feeding Directions:

Horses: Feed at the rate of 1 oz. per day. This will provide 2 mg of Selenium and 1,250 Int. Units of Vitamin E per day. 1 oz scoop enclosed.
Caution(s): Follow label directions. Higher levels of Selenium are not permitted.
For animal use only.
Warning(s): Keep out of reach of children.
Presentation: 5 lb (2.2 kg) and 20 lb (9 kg) pails.
Compendium Code No.: 12060050 — 0A1

SURELYTES™ PLUS CARBO LOAD

SureNutrition — **Electrolytes-Oral**
High Performance Equine Electrolytes-Glucose Polymers (Carbo Load)-Probiotic Enzymes (Lactobacillus Acidophilus)
Guaranteed Analysis:

	per lb:	per oz:
Crude Protein, min.	12.00%	3,400 mg
Calcium (Ca), min.	0.40%	110 mg
Calcium (Ca), max.	0.70%	190 mg
Salt (NaCl), min.	9.00%	2,550 mg
Salt (NaCl), max.	10.00%	2,835 mg
Phosphorus (P), min.	0.60%	170 mg
Magnesium (Mg), min.	0.40%	110 mg
Potassium (K)	5.90%	1,670 mg
Zinc (Zn), min.	0.04%	400 ppm
Carbo Load:	per lb:	per oz:
Glucose Polymers	50,000 mg	3,125 mg

Total Lactic Acid Producing Bacteria: 1.6×10^9 CFU/lb (1×10^8 CFU/oz)

S

Ingredients: Dextrose, Soy Protein Concentrate, Maltodextrin (Glucose Polymers), Potassium Chloride, Salt, Phosphorus Amino Acid Chelate, Magnesium Aspartate, Calcium Aspartate, Zinc Aspartate, Calcium Silicate (Anti-caking Agent) and Dried Fermentation Products of *Lactobacillus Acidophilus, Bifidobacterium Thermophilum, Bifidobacterium Longum* and *Enterococcus Faecium*.

Indications: High performance equine electrolytes with glucose polymers for horses in training and racing.

Dosage and Administration: Feeding Directions:

For maintenance levels of electrolytes: Mix one ounce per head per day into feed or water.

As a pre-race Carbo Load: Mix two ounces per head per day into feed or water for four days prior to race.

The enclosed scoop holds one ounce when rounded full.

Precaution(s): Store in a cool (60-80°F), dry place and keep container sealed.

Caution(s): For animal use only.

Warning(s): Keep out of reach of children.

Presentation: 5 lb (2.2 kg), 10 lb (4.4 kg) and 20 lb (8.8 kg) pails.

Compendium Code No.: 12060060 0BB1

SURE-START PLUS

AgriPharm **Large Animal Dietary Supplement**

Oral Paste

Guaranteed Analysis:

Vitamin A . . . 6,000,000 I.U./lb
Vitamin D . . . 750,000 I.U./lb
Niacin . . . 30,000 mg/lb
Zinc . . . 2,000 mg/lb

Total dried viable cultures of *Streptococcus faecium, Lactobacillus acidophilus*, and bifidobacteriums - 250 billion CFU/lb.

Ingredients: Colostrum whey, dried *Streptococcus faecium* fermentation product, *Lactobacillus acidophilus, Bifidobacterium thermophilum, Bifidobacterium longum*, corn oil, dextrose, niacin supplement, zinc oxide, silicon dioxide, vitamin A supplement, d-activated animal sterol (source of vitamin D), ddl-alpha tocopherol acetate (anti-oxidant), potassium sorbate (preservative), polysorbate 80, and FD&C blue color.

Indications: SURE-START PLUS contains a source of live, naturally occurring microorganisms, *Streptococcus faecium, Lactobacillus acidophilus, Bifidobacterium thermophilum* and *Bifidobacterium longum* for cattle and calves fortified with vitamins, minerals and colostrum.

Dosage and Administration: Administer orally on back of tongue.

Calves to long yearlings . . . 10 cc
(one full depression of handle)
Adult Cattle . . . 20 cc
(two full depressions of handle)

Repeat as necessary.

Precaution(s): Store in a cool place. Refrigeration recommended for extended storage periods.

Caution(s): For animal use only.

Keep out of reach of children.

Not intended for use as a source of antibody.

Presentation: 80 cc and 300 cc containers.

Compendium Code No.: 14570990

SURETIGHT™ PERFORMANCE LINIMENT

SureNutrition **Liniment**

Leg Tightener for Equine Athletes

Active Ingredient(s): Menthol 2%.

Water, Isopropanol, Menthol, Capsicum Extract, Chamomile Extract, Frankincense, Caprylates/C10-C30 Alkyl Acrylate Crosspolymer, Oil of Rosemary, Triethanolamine, Fragrance, Methyl Paraben, Diazolidinyl Urea, Propyl Paraben.

Contains: Menthol, capsaicin, boswellin and chamomile.

Indications: SURETIGHT™ Performance Liniment is recommended for use on the performance horse to reduce the symptoms of swelling, tenderness, and pain in ligaments and tendons caused by inflammation.

Directions: Shake well before using. Product is concentrated and does not need to be applied as generously as other liniments. Apply liniment directly to your hand and then massage thoroughly onto the horse's leg. Apply to all sides of injured ligaments or tendons. The importance of massage cannot be overemphasized as it improves circulation and reduces swelling and pain. Additional liniment can be used in more severe cases. The treated leg can be wrapped lightly with a thin cotton if desired. However, the effectiveness of this product is not dependent upon wrapping. Do not use plastic or wrap tightly. Apply to affected area not more than 4 times daily. Wash hands with soap and water after application.

Precaution(s): Store at room temperature 15°-30°C (59°-86°F).

Caution(s): For external use only. Avoid contact with eyes and mucous membranes. Do not apply to open wounds or damaged, irritated, or broken skin. If rash or irritation occurs, discontinue use. Use only as directed. Do not use with any other liniment. Discontinue use and consult your veterinarian if the condition worsens or fails to improve.

Warning(s): Keep this and all medications out of the reach of children.

In case of ingestion, seek professional assistance or contact a poison control center immediately.

Presentation: 16 fl oz (473 mL).

Compendium Code No.: 12060070 0E1

SURGICAL SCRUB AND HANDWASH

First Priority **Surgical Scrub**

Active Ingredient(s): 2% Chloroxylenol.

Ingredients: Purified Water, Sodium Laureth Sulfate, Propylene Glycol, Sodium Lauryl Sulfate, Polyquaternium-7, Hydroxyethylcellulose, Polysorbate-20, Fragrance, Sodium Hydroxymethylglycinate, FD and C Blue #1, FD and C Yellow #5.

Indications: SURGICAL SCRUB AND HANDWASH provides rapid bactericidal activity effective against a wide range of microorganisms including antibiotic-resistant bacteria. Its formula is uniquely kind to hands and is ideal for individuals that have a sensitivity to chlorhexidine or iodine scrubs. It contains emollients to prevent moisture loss and moisturizers to help maintain skin integrity even after frequent scrubbing.

Directions for Use: Remove jewelry. Wet hands and forearms with water and apply 5 mL (equivalent to the circumference of a golf ball) of scrub. Wash/scrub hands and forearms for 2 minutes paying particular attention to nails, cuticles, and interdigital spaces. Rinse thoroughly with water.

Health Care Personnel Handwash: Wet hands with water and apply 2 mL (equivalent to 2 pumps) of scrub. Wash in a vigorous manner. Rinse thoroughly and dry.

Preoperative Use on Patients: Apply Surgical Scrub generously (do not dilute). Spread using sterile gauze. Swab for 2 minutes. Wipe excess with sterile gauze.

Precaution(s): Storage: Store at controlled room temperature between 15°-30°C (59°-86°F).

Caution(s): For external use only. Avoid contact with eyes. Sold exclusively through veterinarians.

In case of accidental ingestion, seek professional assistance or contact the poison control center immediately.

For animal use only.

Warning(s): Keep out of reach of children.

Presentation: 1 gallon (3.785 L) (NDC# 58829-316-01).

Compendium Code No.: 11390810 Rev. 06-01

SURGICAL SCRUB & HANDWASH

Vet Solutions **Surgical Scrub**

2% Chloroxylenol-A Hydrating Broad Spectrum Antimicrobial Solution

Active Ingredient(s): 2% Chloroxylenol.

Ingredients: Deionized Water, Sodium Laureth Sulfate, Propylene Glycol, Sodium Lauryl Sulfate, Polyquaternium-7, Hydroxyethylcellulose, Polysorbate-20, Fragrance, Sodium Hydroxymethylglycinate, FD&C Blue No. 1, FD&C Yellow No. 5.

Indications: Vet Solutions SURGICAL SCRUB AND HANDWASH provides rapid bactericidal activity effective against a wide range of microorganisms including antibiotic-resistant bacteria. Its formula is uniquely kind to hands and is ideal for individuals that have a sensitivity to chlorhexidine or iodine scrubs. It contains emollients to prevent moisture loss and moisturizers to help maintain skin integrity even after frequent scrubbing.

Directions: Surgical Scrub:

1. Remove Jewelry.
2. Wet hands and forearms with water and apply 5 mL (equivalent to the circumference of a golf ball) of scrub.
3. Wash/scrub hands and forearms for 2 minutes paying particular attention to nails, cuticles, and interdigital spaces.
4. Rinse thoroughly with water.

Health Care Personnel Handwash:

1. Wet hands with water and apply 2 mL (equivalent to 2 pumps) of scrub.
2. Wash in a vigorous manner.
3. Rinse thoroughly and dry.

Preoperative use on Patients:

1. Apply Surgical Scrub generously (do not dilute).
2. Spread using sterile gauze.
3. Swab for 2 minutes.
4. Wipe excess with sterile gauze.

Precaution(s): Storage: Store at controlled room temperature.

Caution(s): For external use only. Avoid contact with eyes.

Sold exclusively through veterinarians.

Warning(s): Keep this and all drugs out of the reach of children. In case of accidental ingestion, seek professional assistance or contact the poison control center immediately.

Presentation: 12 fl. oz. (355 mL), 16 fl. oz., and 1 gallon.

Compendium Code No.: 10610170 990202

SURROUND™ 4

Biocor **Vaccine**

Bovine Rhinotracheitis-Virus Diarrhea-Parainfluenza 3-Respiratory Syncytial Virus Vaccine, Killed Virus

U.S. Vet. Lic. No.: 462

Contents: SURROUND™ 4 is an inactivated, multivalent immunogen containing the Cooper strain of IBR; New York and Singer strains of BVD; PI_3 and BRSV.

This product contains gentamicin and amphotericin B as preservatives and is adjuvanted with aluminum hydroxide and *Haemophilus somnus* cultures.

Indications: For use in the vaccination of healthy cattle against disease caused by the organisms represented.

Directions: Shake well. Administer 5 mL intramuscularly or subcutaneously. For initial vaccination, a second dose is required 2-4 weeks later. SURROUND™ 4 may be safely used in pregnant cows at any stage of gestation or very young calves nursing pregnant cows. Calves vaccinated before 6 months of age should be revaccinated at 6 months of age followed by a second dose 2-4 weeks later. Annual revaccination with a single 5 mL dose is recommended.

Precaution(s): Store at 35°F-45°F (2°C-7°C). Do not freeze. Use entire contents when first opened.

Caution(s): In case of anaphylactoid reactions, epinephrine should be administered immediately.

For veterinary use only.

Warning(s): Do not vaccinate within 21 days before slaughter.

Presentation: Code 68355 - 10 dose (50 mL) vials.
Code 68365 - 50 dose (250 mL) vials.

Compendium Code No.: 13940172 BAH1378-300 / BAH1379-300

SURROUND™ 4+HS

Biocor **Bacterin-Vaccine**

Bovine Rhinotracheitis-Virus Diarrhea-Parainfluenza 3-Respiratory Syncytial Virus Vaccine, Killed Virus-Haemophilus Somnus Bacterin

U.S. Vet. Lic. No.: 462

Contents: SURROUND™ 4+HS is an inactivated, multivalent immunogen containing the Cooper strain of IBR, New York and Singer strains of BVD; PI_3 and BRSV in combination with *Haemophilus somnus*.

This product contains gentamicin and amphotericin B as preservatives.

Indications: For use in the vaccination of healthy cattle against disease caused by the organisms represented.

Directions: Shake well. Administer 5 mL intramuscularly or subcutaneously. For initial vaccination, a second dose is required 2-4 weeks later. SURROUND™ 4+HS may be safely used in pregnant cows at any stage of gestation or very young calves nursing pregnant cows. Calves vaccinated before 6 months of age should be revaccinated at 6 months of age followed by a

second dose 2-4 weeks later. Annual revaccination with a with a single 5 mL dose is recommended.
Precaution(s): Store at 35°F-45°F (2°C-7°C). Do not freeze. Use entire contents when first opened.
Caution(s): In case of anaphylactoid reactions, epinephrine should be administered immediately.
For veterinary use only.
Warning(s): Do not vaccinate within 21 days before slaughter.
Presentation: Code 66955 - 10 dose (50 mL) vials.
Code 66965 - 50 dose (250 mL) vials.
Compendium Code No.: 13940182 BAH1398-300 / BAH1399-300

SURROUND™ 8

Biocor **Bacterin-Vaccine**

Bovine Rhinotracheitis-Virus Diarrhea-Parainfluenza 3 Vaccine, Killed Virus-Leptospira Canicola-Grippotyphosa-Hardjo-Icterohaemormagiae-Pomona Bacterin

U.S. Vet. Lic. No.: 462
Contents: SURROUND™ 8 is an inactivated, multivalent immunogen containing the Cooper strain of IBR; New York and Singer strains of BVD; and PI_3 in combination with the Leptospira serovars represented.
This product contains gentamicin and amphotericin B as preservatives and is adjuvanted with aluminum hydroxide and *Haemophilus somnus* cultures.
Indications: For use in the vaccination of healthy cattle against disease caused by the organisms represented.
Directions: Shake well. Administer 5 mL intramuscularly or subcutaneously. For initial vaccination, a second dose is required 2-4 weeks later. SURROUND™ 8 may be safely used in pregnant cows at any stage of gestation or very young calves nursing pregnant cows. Calves vaccinated before 6 months of age should be revaccinated at 6 months of age, followed by a second dose 2-4 weeks later. Annual revaccination with a single 5 mL dose is recommended.
Precaution(s): Store at 35°F-45°F (2°C-7°C). Do not freeze. Use entire contents when first opened.
Caution(s): In case of anaphylactoid reactions, epinephrine should be administered immediately.
For veterinary use only.
Warning(s): Do not vaccinate within 21 days before slaughter.
Presentation: Code 68255 - 10 dose (50 mL) vials.
Code 68265 - 50 dose (250 mL) vials.
Compendium Code No.: 13940192 BAH1358-300 / BAH1359-300

SURROUND™ 9

Biocor **Bacterin-Vaccine**

Bovine Rhinotracheitis-Virus Diarrhea-Parainfluenza 3-Respiratory Syncytial Virus Vaccine, Killed Virus-Leptospira Canicola-Grippotyphosa-Hardjo-Icterohaemorrhagiae-Pomona Bacterin

U.S. Vet. Lic. No.: 462
Contents: SURROUND™ 9 is an inactivated, multivalent immunogen containing the Cooper strain of IBR; New York and Singer strains of BVD; PI_3 and BRSV in combination with the Leptospira serovars represented.
This product contains gentamicin and amphotericin B as preservatives and is adjuvanted with aluminum hydroxide and *Haemophilus somnus* cultures.
Indications: For use in the vaccination of healthy cattle against disease caused by the organisms represented.
Directions: Shake well. Administer 5 mL intramuscularly or subcutaneously. For initial vaccination, a second dose is required 2-4 weeks later. SURROUND™ 9 may be safely used in pregnant cows at any stage of gestation or very young calves nursing pregnant cows. Calves vaccinated before 6 months of age should be revaccinated at 6 months of age, followed by a second dose 2-4 weeks later. Annual revaccination with a single 5 mL dose is recommended.
Precaution(s): Store at 35°F-45°F (2°C-7°C). Do not freeze. Use entire contents when first opened.
Caution(s): In case of anaphylactoid reactions, epinephrine should be administered immediately.
For veterinary use only.
Warning(s): Do not vaccinate within 21 days before slaughter.
Presentation: Code 68555 - 10 dose (50 mL) vials.
Code 68565 - 50 dose (250 mL) vials.
Compendium Code No.: 13940202 BAH1458-300 / BAH1459-300

SURROUND™ 9+HS

Biocor **Bacterin-Vaccine**

Bovine Rhinotracheitis-Virus Diarrhea-Parainfluenza 3-Respiratory Syncytial Virus Vaccine, Killed Virus, Haemophilus Somnus-Leptospira Canicola-Grippotyphosa-Hardjo-Icterohaemorrhagiae-Pomona Bacterin

S

U.S. Vet. Lic. No.: 462
Contents: SURROUND™ 9+HS is an inactivated, multivalent immunogen containing the Cooper stain of IBR; New York and Singer strains of BVD; PI_3 and BRSV in combination with *Haemophilus somnus* and the Leptospira serovars represented.
This product contains gentamicin and amphotericin B as preservatives.
Indications: For use in the vaccination of healthy cattle against disease caused by the organisms represented.
Directions: Shake well. Administer 5 mL intramuscularly or subcutaneously. For initial vaccination, a second dose is required 2-4 weeks later. SURROUND™ 9+HS may be safely used in pregnant cows at any stage of gestation or very young calves nursing pregnant cows. Calves vaccinated before 6 months of age should be revaccinated at 6 months of age, followed by a second dose 2-4 weeks later. Annual revaccination with a single 5 mL dose is recommended.
Precaution(s): Store at 35°F-45°F (2°C-7°C). Do not freeze. Use entire contents when first opened.
Caution(s): In case of anaphylactoid reactions, epinephrine should be administered immediately.
For veterinary use only.
Warning(s): Do not vaccinate within 21 days before slaughter.
Presentation: Code 68455 - 10 dose (50 mL) vials.
Code 68465 - 50 dose (250 mL) vials.
Compendium Code No.: 13940212 BAH1468-300 / BAH1469-300

SURROUND™ HS

Biocor **Bacterin**

Haemophilus Somnus Bacterin

U.S. Vet. Lic. No.: 462
Description: SURROUND™ HS is an inactivated bacterin of *Haemophilus somnus.*
Indications: Recommended for use in the vaccination of healthy cattle against disease caused by the *Haemophilus somnus* organisms.
Directions: Shake well. Administer 2 mL intramuscularly or subcutaneously. For initial vaccination, a second dose is required 2-4 weeks later. Ideally calves should be 4 months of age when vaccination procedure are instituted. Annual revaccination with a single 2 mL dose is recommended.
Precaution(s): Store at 35°F-45°F (2°C-7°C). Do not freeze. Use entire contents when first opened.
Caution(s): In case of anaphylactoid reactions, epinephrine should be administered immediately.
For veterinary use only.
Warning(s): Do not vaccinate within 21 days before slaughter.
Presentation: Code 69254 - 10 dose (20 mL) vials.
Code 69264 - 50 dose (100 mL) vials.
Compendium Code No.: 13940280 BAH468-700 / BAH469-700

SURROUND™ L5

Biocor **Bacterin**

Leptospira Canicola-Grippotyphosa-Hardjo-Icterohaemorrhagiae-Pomona Bacterin

U.S. Vet. Lic. No.: 462
Contents: SURROUND™ L5 contains inactivated cultures of *Leptospira canicola, L. grippotyphosa, L. hardjo, L. icterohaemorrhagiae,* and *L. pomona.*
Indications: Recommended for use in the vaccination of healthy cattle or swine against disease caused by the organisms represented.
Directions: Shake well. Administer 2 mL intramuscularly or subcutaneously in healthy cattle or swine. In swine a second vaccination in 2-4 weeks is required. Annual revaccination with a single 2 mL dose is recommended.
Precaution(s): Store at 35°F-45°F (2°C-7°C). Do not freeze. Use entire contents when first opened.
Caution(s): In case of anaphylactoid reactions, epinephrine should be administered immediately.
For veterinary use only.
Warning(s): Do not vaccinate within 21 days before slaughter.
Presentation: Code 65454 - 10 dose (20 mL) vials.
Code 65464 - 50 dose (100 mL) vials.
Compendium Code No.: 13940222 BAH478B-300 / BAH479B-300

SURROUND™ V-L5

Biocor **Bacterin**

Campylobacter Fetus-Leptospira Canicola-Grippotyphosa-Hardjo-Icterohaemorragiae-Pomona Bacterin

U.S. Vet. Lic. No.: 462
Contents: SURROUND™ V-L5 contains inactivated cultures of *Campylobacter fetus, Leptospira canicola, L. grippotyphosa, L. hardjo, L. icterohaemorrhagiae* and *L. pomona.*
Indications: Recommended for use in the vaccination of healthy cattle against disease caused by the organisms represented.
Directions: Shake well. Administer 5 mL intramuscularly or subcutaneously 2-6 weeks prior to breeding or adding to the breeding herd. In *Campylobacter fetus* infected herds or endemic areas, vaccinated cattle should be revaccinated at least 3 weeks later. Annual revaccination with a single 5 mL dose is recommended.
Precaution(s): Store at 35°F-45°F (2°C-7°C). Do not freeze. Use entire contents when first opened.
Caution(s): In case of anaphylactoid reactions, epinephrine should be administered immediately.
For veterinary use only.
Warning(s): Do not vaccinate within 21 days before slaughter.
Presentation: Code 69455 - 10 dose (50 mL) vials.
Code 69465 - 50 dose (250 mL) vials.
Compendium Code No.: 13940232 BAH488-300 / BAH489-300

SUSTAIN III®

Durvet **Sulfamethazine**

Antibacterial Sulfamethazine Sustained Release Bolus (72 Hours)

NADA No.: 120-615
Active Ingredient(s): Each Bolus Contains:
Sulfamethazine (formulated in a sustained release base) .... 495 grains (32.1 grams)
Indications: SUSTAIN III® boluses (Sulfamethazine Sustained Release Boluses) are intended for oral administration to beef cattle and non-lactating dairy cattle. (See Warning.) SUSTAIN III® boluses are indicated for the treatment of the following diseases when caused by one or more of the following pathogenic organisms sensitive to sulfamethazine: Bacterial Pneumonia and Bovine Respiratory Disease Complex (Shipping Fever Complex) *(Pasteurella* spp.), Colibacillosis (Bacterial Scours) *(E. coli)*, Necrotic pododermatitis (Foot rot), Calf Diphtheria *(Fusobacterium necrophorum)*, and Acute Metritis *(Streptococcus* spp.).
Dosage and Administration: SUSTAIN III® boluses (Sulfamethazine Sustained Release Boluses) are designed to be administered orally to beef cattle and non-lactating dairy cattle. (See Warning.) SUSTAIN III® boluses should be give according to the following dosage schedule:

Animal Body Weight	No. of Boluses
200 lbs.	1
300 lbs.	1.5
400 lbs.	2
500 lbs.	2.5
600 lbs.	3
700 lbs.	3.5
800 lbs.	4
900 lbs.	4.5
1,000 lbs.	5

The bolus may be divided for a better approximation of the correct dose; however, care should be taken not to crush the bolus. Care should also be taken to ensure that the entire dose has been swallowed by the animal. Observe the animals following administration to ensure that the boluses are not regurgitated. Lubricate SUSTAIN III® before dosing animals.

SUSTAIN III® boluses are designed to provide a therapeutic sulfamethazine level in approximately 6 hours and persist in providing this level for 72 hours (3 days). After 72 hours, all animals should be re-examined for the persistence of observable disease signs. If signs are present, consult a veterinarian. It is strongly recommended that a second dose be given to provide for an additional 72 hours of therapy, particularly in those more severe cases. The above dose schedule should be used at each 72-hour interval.

Caution(s): This drug, like all sulfonamides, may cause toxic reactions and irreparable injury unless administered with adequate and continuous supervision; follow the recommended dosages carefully.

Fluid intake must be adequate at all times throughout the three-day therapy provided by the sustained release bolus.

For animal use only.

Not for human use.

Warning(s): Animals intended for human consumption should not be slaughtered for food for at least 12 days after the last dose. Exceeding two consecutive doses may cause violative tissue residues to remain beyond the withdrawal time. Do not use in female dairy cattle 20 months of age or older. Use of sulfamethazine in this class of cattle may cause milk residues. Do not use in calves under one (1) months of age or calves being fed an all-milk diet. Use in these classes of calves may cause violative residues to remain beyond the withdrawal time.

Keep out of reach of children.

Presentation: Bottles of 10 (NDC 30798-109-65), 50 (NDC 30798-109-69) or 100 (NDC 30798-109-70) boluses.

SUSTAIN III® is registered trademark of Bimeda, Inc.

Compendium Code No.: 10841591 2/01 / 4/01 / 1/01

SUSTAIN® III CALF BOLUS

Bimeda **Sulfamethazine**

NADA No.: 120-615

Active Ingredient(s): Each bolus contains:

Sulfamethazine . . . . 8.02 g

Formulated in a sustained release base.

Indications: SUSTAIN® III Calf Boluses are intended for oral administration only to ruminating replacement calves (calves over one month of age that are not on a milk diet). SUSTAIN® III Calf Boluses are indicated for the treatment of the following diseases when caused by one or more of the following pathogenic organisms sensitive to sulfamethazine: Bacterial pneumonia *(Pasteurella* spp.), colibacillosis (bacterial scours) *(E. coli)*, and calf diphtheria *(Fusobacterium necrophorum)*.

Dosage and Administration: SUSTAIN® III Calf Boluses are to be given at a rate of two (2) boluses per 100 lbs. of body weight. This bolus may be divided for better approximation of correct dose, however, care should be taken not to crush the bolus. Care should be taken to ensure the entire dose has been swallowed by the animal. Observe animals following administration to ensure boluses are not regurgitated. Lubricate bolus before dosing animals. SUSTAIN® III Calf Boluses are designed to provide a therapeutic sulfamethazine level in approximately six (6) hours, and persist in providing this level for 72 hours (3 days). After 72 hours, all animals should be re-examined for persistence of observable disease signs. If signs are present, consult a veterinarian. It is strongly recommended that a second dose be given to provide for an additional 72 hours of therapy, particularly in those more severe cases. The above schedule should be used at each 72 hour interval.

Caution(s): This drug, like all sulfonamides, may cause toxic reactions and irreparable injury unless administered with adequate and continuous supervision. Follow recommended dosage carefully.

Fluid intake must be adequate at all times throughout the three-day therapy provided by the sustained release bolus. This product has not been shown to be effective for nonruminating calves.

Warning(s): Treated animals must not be slaughtered for food for at least 12 days after the last dose. Exceeding two consecutive doses may cause violative tissue residue to remain beyond the withdrawal time. Do not use in calves under one month of age or calves fed an all milk diet. Use in these classes of calves may cause violative tissue residue to remain beyond the withdrawal time. Do not use in female dairy cattle 20 months of age or older. Use of sulfamethazine in this class of cattle may cause milk residues.

Presentation: Bottles of 25 boluses and boxes of 50 boluses.

Compendium Code No.: 13990370

SUSTAIN III® CALF BOLUS

Durvet **Sulfamethazine**

Antibacterial Sulfamethazine Sustained Release Calf Bolus (72 Hours)

NADA No.: 120-615

Active Ingredient(s): Each Bolus Contains:

Sulfamethazine (formulated in a sustained release base) . . . . 123.8 grains (8.02 grams)

Indications: SUSTAIN III® Calf Boluses (Sulfamethazine Sustained Release Boluses) are intended for oral administration to ruminating replacement calves (calves over one (1) month old that are not on an all-milk diet). SUSTAIN III® Calf Boluses are indicated for the treatment of the following diseases when caused by one or more of the following pathogenic organisms sensitive to sulfamethazine: Bacterial Pneumonia *(Pasteurella* spp.), Colibacillosis (Bacterial Scours) *(E. coli)*, and Calf Diphtheria *(Fusobacterium necrophorum)*.

Dosage and Administration: SUSTAIN III® Calf Boluses (Sulfamethazine Sustained Release Boluses) are designed to be administered orally to ruminating replacement calves. (See Caution statement.) SUSTAIN III® Calf Boluses should be given according to the following dosage schedule:

Animal Body Wgt.	No. of Boluses
100 lbs.	2
150 lbs.	3
200 lbs.	4
250 lbs.	5
300 lbs.	6

The bolus may be divided for a better approximation of the correct dose; however, care should be taken not to crush the bolus. Care should also be taken to ensure that the entire dose has been swallowed by the animal. Observe animals following administration to ensure boluses are not regurgitated. Lubricate bolus before dosing animals.

SUSTAIN III® Calf Boluses are designed to provide a therapeutic sulfamethazine level in approximately 6 hours and persist in providing this level for 72 hours (3 days). After 72 hours, all animals should be re-examined for the persistence of observable disease signs. If signs are present, consult a veterinarian. It is strongly recommended that a second dose be given to provide for an additional 72 hours of therapy, particularly in those more severe cases. The above schedule should be used at each 72-hour interval.

Caution(s): This drug, like all sulfonamides, may cause toxic reactions and irreparable injury unless administered with adequate and continuous supervision; follow the recommended dosages carefully. Fluid intake must be adequate at all times throughout the three-day therapy provided by the sustained release bolus. The product has not been shown to be effective for non-ruminating calves.

For animal use only. Not for human use.

Warning(s): Treated animals must not be slaughtered for food for at least 12 days after the last dose. Exceeding two (2) consecutive doses may cause violative tissue residue to remain beyond the withdrawal time. Do not use in calves under one (1) month of age or calves being fed an all-milk diet. Use in these classes of calves may cause violative tissue residues to remain beyond the withdrawal time. Do not use in female dairy cattle 20 months of age or older. Use of sulfamethazine in this class may cause milk residues.

Keep out of reach of children.

Presentation: Bottles of 25 (NDC 30798-108-66) and 50 boluses (NDC 30798-108-69).

SUSTAIN III® is a trademark of Merial Limited.

Compendium Code No.: 10841601 5/98

SUSTAIN® III CATTLE BOLUS

Bimeda **Sulfamethazine**

Sulfamethazine Sustained-Release Bolus

NADA No.: 120-615

Active Ingredient(s): Each bolus contains:

Sulfamethazine . . . . 32.1 g (495 grains)

Formulated in a sustained release base.

Indications: SUSTAIN® III Boluses (sulfamethazine sustained-release boluses) are intended for oral administration to beef cattle and nonlactating dairy cattle. SUSTAIN® III Boluses are indicated for the treatment of the following diseases when caused by one or more of the following pathogenic organisms sensitive to sulfamethazine: Bacterial pneumonia and bovine respiratory disease complex (shipping fever complex) *(Pasteurella* spp.), colibacillosis (bacterial scours) *(E. coli)*, necrotic pododermatitis (foot rot), calf diphtheria *(Fusobacterium necrophorum)*, acute mastitis *(Streptococcus spp.)*, and acute metritis *(Streptococcus* spp.).

Dosage and Administration: SUSTAIN® III Boluses are designed to be administered orally to beef cattle and nonlactating dairy cattle. SUSTAIN® III Boluses should be given at a rate of one (1) bolus per 200 lbs. of body weight.

The bolus may be divided for better approximation of correct dose, however, care should be taken not to crush the bolus. Care should also be taken to ensure the entire dose has been swallowed by the animal. Observe animals following administration to ensure boluses are not regurgitated. Lubricate SUSTAIN® III before dosing animals.

SUSTAIN® III Boluses are designed to provide a therapeutic sulfamethazine level in approximately six (6) hours, and persist in providing this level for 72 hours (3 days). After 72 hours, all animals should be re-examined for persistence of observable disease signs. If signs are present, consult a veterinarian. It is strongly recommended that a second dose be given to provide for an additional 72 hours of therapy, particularly in those more severe cases. The above dose schedule should be used at each 72 hour interval.

Caution(s): This drug, like all sulfonamides, may cause toxic reactions and irreparable injury unless administered with adequate and continuous supervision. Follow recommended dosages carefully.

Fluid intake must be adequate at all times throughout the three-day therapy provided by the sustained release bolus.

Warning(s): Do not use in lactating dairy cattle. Animals intended for human consumption should not be slaughtered for food for at least 12 days after the last dose. Animals should not receive more than two doses of SUSTAIN® III Boluses because of the possibility of incurring residue violations. Do not use in calves under one month of age or in calves being fed an all-milk diet. Use in these classes of cattle may cause violative residues to remain beyond the withdrawal time. Do not use in female dairy cattle 20 months of age or older. Use of sulfamethazine in this class of cattle may cause milk residues.

Presentation: 50-count box and 100-count box.

Compendium Code No.: 13990381

SUVAXYN® AR/E/EC-4

Fort Dodge **Bacterin**

Bordetella Bronchiseptica-Erysipelothrix Rhusiopathiae-Escherichia Coli-Pasteurella Multocida Bacterin

U.S. Vet. Lic. No.: 112

Contents: This product contains the antigens listed above.

Contains gentamicin as a preservative.

Indications: For the vaccination of healthy swine as an aid in the prevention of clinical signs caused by *Bordetella bronchiseptica, Erysipelothrix rhusiopathiae, Escherichia coli* (K88, K99, 987P, and F41 types) and *Pasteurella multocida*.

Dosage and Administration: Aseptically inject 3 mL (3 cc) intramuscularly per animal. Sows and gilts: For primary vaccination, inject at 4 weeks and again at 2 weeks prior to farrowing. Revaccinate with a single dose between 4 and 2 weeks prior to subsequent farrowings.

Precaution(s): Store between 36° and 45°F (2° and 7°C). Avoid freezing. Shake well before using. Use entire contents when first opened.

Caution(s): Allergic reactions, although rare, may occur.

Transient local swelling may occur at site of injection.

For use in swine.

For veterinary use only.

Antidote(s): The antidote is epinephrine.

Warning(s): Do not vaccinate within 21 days before slaughter.

Presentation: 10 dose (30 mL) and 35 dose (105 mL) vials.

Compendium Code No.: 10031942 11294B

SUVAXYN® AR/T

Fort Dodge **Bacterin-Toxoid**

Bordetella Bronchiseptica-Pasteurella Multocida Bacterin-Toxoid

U.S. Vet. Lic. No.: 112

Contents: This product contains the antigens listed above.

Contains gentamicin as a preservative.

Indications: For the vaccination of healthy swine as an aid in the prevention of atrophic rhinitis caused by *Bordetella bronchiseptica* and *Pasteurella multocida* Serotype A and D toxin.

Dosage and Administration: Aseptically inject 2 mL (2 cc) intramuscularly or subcutaneously per animal.

Sows and gilts: For primary vaccination, inject at 4 weeks and again at 2 weeks prior to farrowing. Revaccinate 4 to 2 weeks prior to subsequent farrowings.

Pigs: Inject at 7 to 10 days of age or prior to weaning. Repeat with a second dose 2 to 3 weeks after first vaccination.

Breeding stock: Vaccinate with 2 doses given 2 weeks apart. Administer the first dose at 6 months of age or prior to introduction into a herd. Revaccinate boars with a single dose annually.

Precaution(s): Store between 36° and 45°F (2° and 7°C). Avoid freezing. Shake well before using. Use entire contents when first opened.

Caution(s): Allergic reactions, although rare, may occur.

For use in swine.

For veterinary use only.

Antidote(s): The antidote is epinephrine.

Warning(s): Do not vaccinate within 21 days before slaughter.

Presentation: 10 dose (20 mL) and 50 dose (100 mL) vials.

Compendium Code No.: 10031952 11547B

SUVAXYN® AR/T/E

Fort Dodge **Bacterin-Toxoid**

Bordetella Bronchiseptica-Erysipelothrix Rhusiopathiae-Pasteurella Multocida Bacterin-Toxoid

U.S. Vet. Lic. No.: 112

Contents: This product contains the antigens listed above.

Gentamicin is added as a preservative.

Indications: For the vaccination of healthy pigs as an aid in the prevention of atrophic rhinitis caused by *Bordetella bronchiseptica* by toxigenic strains of *Pasteurella multocida* serotypes A and D, and as an aid in the prevention of erysipelas caused by *Erysipelothrix rhusiopathiae*.

Dosage and Administration:

Sows and gilts: Administer a 2 mL dose intramuscularly, give two doses at least 2 weeks apart with a second dose administered 2 weeks prior to farrowing and revaccinate before each subsequent farrowing.

Piglets nursing non-immune dams: Vaccinate at 7 to 10 days of age or prior to weaning. Repeat with second dose 2 to 3 weeks later.

Piglets nursing immune dams: Vaccinate when maternal antibody levels will allow active immunization, usually after 6 weeks of age. Give a second dose 2 to 3 weeks later.

Breeding stock: Vaccinate all new breeding stock with two doses 2 to 3 weeks apart with the first dose at 6 months of age or prior to introduction into a herd.

Precaution(s): Please handle carefully and avoid accidental self-inoculation. Store in dark at 2° to 7°C (35° to 45°F). Avoid freezing. Use entire contents when first opened.

Caution(s): In case of anaphylactoid reaction, administer epinephrine.

For use in swine.

For veterinary use only.

Warning(s): Do not vaccinate within 21 days before slaughter.

Presentation: 10 dose (20 mL) and 50 dose (100 mL) vials.

Compendium Code No.: 10031962 11557B

SUVAXYN® E

Fort Dodge **Bacterin**

Erysipelothrix Rhusiopathiae Bacterin

U.S. Vet. Lic. No.: 112

Contents: This product contains the antigen listed above.

Indications: For the vaccination of healthy swine as an aid in the prevention of clinical signs caused by *Erysipelothrix rhusiopathiae*.

Dosage and Administration: Aseptically inject 2 mL (2 cc) intramuscularly or subcutaneously per animal. Pigs: Vaccinate at 7 to 10 days of age or prior to weaning. Repeat with second dose 2 to 3 weeks after the first vaccination. Breeding stock: Animals held for breeding should be vaccinated at the time of selection and 3 weeks later. All breeding stock should be vaccinated semiannually.

Precaution(s): Store between 2° and 7°C (36° and 45°F). Avoid freezing. Shake well before using. Use entire contents when first opened.

Caution(s): Allergic reactions, although rare, may occur.

For use in swine.

For veterinary use only.

Antidote(s): The antidote is epinephrine.

Warning(s): Do not vaccinate within 21 days before slaughter.

Presentation: 50 dose (100 mL) vials.

Compendium Code No.: 10031971 11315B

S

SUVAXYN® EC-4

Fort Dodge **Bacterin**

Escherichia Coli Bacterin

U.S. Vet. Lic. No.: 112

Contents: This product contains the antigen listed above.

Contains gentamicin as a preservative.

Indications: For the vaccination of healthy sows and gilts as an aid in the passive protection of nursing offspring against neonatal diarrhea due to *E. coli* K88, K99, 987P and F41.

Dosage and Administration: Sows and gilts, aseptically inject a 2 mL dose intramuscularly at four and two weeks prior to farrowing. Revaccinate with a single 2 mL dose between 4 and 2 weeks prior to subsequent farrowings.

Precaution(s): Store in dark at 2° to 7°C (36° to 45°F). Avoid freezing. Use entire contents when first opened.

Caution(s): In case of anaphylactoid reaction, administer epinephrine.

For use in swine.

For veterinary use only.

Warning(s): Do not vaccinate within 21 days before slaughter.

Presentation: 10 dose (20 mL) and 50 dose (100 mL) vials.

Compendium Code No.: 10031981 11275B

SUVAXYN® E-ORAL

Fort Dodge **Bacterial Vaccine**

Erysipelothrix Rhusiopathiae Vaccine, Avirulent Live Culture

U.S. Vet. Lic. No.: 112

Contents: This product contains the antigen listed above.

Indications: For use in healthy swine 6 weeks of age or older as an aid in the prevention of disease caused by *Erysipelothrix rhusiopathiae*.

Dosage and Administration: Dose: For oral use only. Resuspend the lyophilized cake with the supplied diluent. Dilute in an appropriate volume of skim milk or rehydrated non-medicated milk replacer and then administer at 1 ounce per gallon non-chlorinated drinking water using a proportional liquid dispenser. Vaccinate pigs at 6 weeks of age or older with 2 doses given 2 weeks apart.

Dosage is based on number of pigs not weight of pigs. Use at least one dose of vaccine per pig being vaccinated.

Directions:

Prepare the Pigs and the Water System:

1. Remove all disinfectants, medications, and sanitizers from feed and water system at least 72 hours prior to vaccination to assure antibacterial agents are removed. All materials used in administering this vaccine must be free of antibiotic or disinfectant residue to prevent inactivation of this vaccine. Do not administer this vaccine in chlorinated water.
2. Withhold drinking water at least 8 to 10 hours (overnight) prior to vaccination.
3. Flush water system (including medication proportioner) with clean skim milk or non-medicated milk replacer to remove all traces of antibacterial agents.

Prepare Proportioner Stock Solution:

4. The amount of stock solution needed for the proportioner is calculated based on how much the pigs will drink. Determine the total weight of pigs to be vaccinated. (No. Pigs X average weight per pig = total weight). Go to Table 1 to look up the amount of stock solution you'll need for pigs this size and number.
5. Add the amount of freshly prepared skim milk or non-medicated milk replacer from Table 1 to the stock solution container.

Mix the Vaccine into the Stock Solution:

6. Resuspend the dry vaccine in the accompanying diluent immediately before use. Use at least one dose of vaccine per pig.
7. Add the vaccine into the stock solution container and rinse the vial(s).
8. Mix vaccine thoroughly into the stock solution.

Vaccinate:

9. Insert proportioner hose into the stock solution, set proportioner to deliver 1 ounce per gallon, and start water flow. Continue until all of the vaccine stock solution has been administered (about 4-8 hours). Swirl vaccine solution each half hour or so during vaccination to ensure uniform dosing.

   Do not medicate or disinfect water system for 72 hours prior to and 72 hours following vaccination.

Table 1: Proportioner Stock Solution Amounts

Total weight of all pigs to be vaccinated	Estimated amount of water consumed in a 6 hour vaccinated period*	Stock Solution for Proportioner - ounces of stock solution needed to vaccinate pig
100 lb/45 kg	0.25 gallons/1 litre	0.25 ounces/7 grs
500 lb/223 kg	1.25 gallons/5 litres	1.25 ounces/35 grs
1,000 lb/453 kg	2.5 gallons/9.5 litres	2.5 ounces/71 grs
2,000 lb/907 kg	5.0 gallons/19 litres	5.0 ounces/140 grs
5,000 lb/2,300 kg	12.5 gallons/47 litres	12.5 ounces/350 grs
10,000 lb/4,500 kg	25 gallons/95 litres	25 ounces/700 grs
20,000 lb/9,000 kg	50 gallons/190 litres	50 ounces/1,420 kg
50,000 lb/23,000 kg	125 gallons/470 litres	125 ounces/3,540 kg
100,000 lb/45,300 kg	250 gallons/950 litres	250 ounces/7,100 kg

* Use this table to look up the amount of stock solution you'll need so all pigs drink enough during the vaccination period. Because pigs drink 8-12% of their body weight per day, the stock solution amount depends on the total number and total weight of the pigs. But the amount of vaccine you use is always one dose per pig, regardless of weight.

Precaution(s): Store in the dark at 35° to 45°F (2° to 7°C). Avoid freezing. Shake well before administration. Use entire contents when first opened. Chlorine or other antimicrobial agents, if present in the vaccine water, may inactivate the vaccine. Burn container and all unused contents.

Caution(s): Please follow administration instructions carefully to ensure proper efficacy of this live vaccine. Allergic reactions, although rare, may occur.

For use in swine.

For veterinary use only.

Antidote(s): The antidote is epinephrine.

Warning(s): Do not vaccinate within 21 days of slaughter.

Presentation: 100 doses (20 mL), 250 doses (50 mL) and 500 doses (100 mL) (1 vial vaccine, 1 vial diluent).

Patent Pending

Compendium Code No.: 10032703 2093E

SUVAXYN®-E (SWINE AND TURKEY)

Fort Dodge **Bacterin**

Erysipelothrix Rhusiopathiae Bacterin

U.S. Vet. Lic. No.: 112

Contents: This product contains the antigens listed above.

Indications: This inactivated and adjuvanted bacterin is for the vaccination of healthy swine and turkeys against clinical signs caused by *Erysipelothrix rhusiopathiae*.

Directions for Use:

Swine dosage: Aseptically inject 2 mL (2 cc) intramuscularly or subcutaneously per animal. Pigs: Vaccinate at 7 to 10 days of age or prior to weaning. Repeat with second dose 2 to 3 weeks after first vaccination. Breeding stock: Animals held for breeding should be vaccinated at the time of selection and 3 weeks later. All breeding stock should be vaccinated semiannually.

Turkey dosage: Aseptically inject 0.5 mL (0.5 cc) per bird of up to 10 lb. in weight and 1 mL (1 cc) above 10 lb. Vaccinate subcutaneously in the back of the neck at a point midway between the bird's head and the base of the neck. Insert the needle just under the skin in a direction away from the head and toward the base of the neck. Do not inject intradermally or into the muscle tissue of the neck or into the cervical vertebrae or at the base of the head. The usual recommended age for vaccination is 8 weeks. Repeat dose every 3 months.

Precaution(s): Store between 36° and 45°F (2° and 7°C). Avoid freezing. Shake well before using. Use entire contents when first opened.

This product is nonreturnable.

Caution(s): Allergic reactions, although rare, may occur.

This product should be stored, transported, and administered in accordance with the instructions and directions. The use of this product is subject to state laws, where applicable.

For veterinary use only.

Antidote(s): The antidote is epinephrine.

Warning(s): Do not vaccinate within 21 days before slaughter.

Presentation: Swine: 50 dose (100 mL) and 250 dose (500 mL) vials.
Turkey: 500 or 1,000 dose (500 mL) vials.

Compendium Code No.: 10032091 11317A

SUVAXYN® LE+B

Fort Dodge **Bacterin**

Erysipelothrix Rhusiopathiae-Leptospira Bratislava-Canicola-Grippotyphosa-Hardjo-Icterohaemorrhagiae-Pomona Bacterin

U.S. Vet. Lic. No.: 112

Contents: This product contains the antigens listed above.

Indications: This inactivated and adjuvanted product is for the vaccination of healthy swine against clinical signs caused by *Erysipelothrix rhusiopathiae* and the six Leptospira serovars indicated.

Dosage and Administration: Aseptically inject 2 mL (2 cc) intramuscularly per animal. Gilts: Since maternal antibodies will block vaccination response, administer first dose to gilts no sooner than 6 months of age and a second dose in 3 to 4 weeks. The second dose should be given no later than 2 weeks prior to breeding. Sows: For primary vaccination, inject one dose 6 weeks prior to breeding and again in 3 to 4 weeks. Revaccinate sows 8 to 2 weeks prior to subsequent breedings. Boars: Administer first dose no sooner than six months of age and a second dose in 3 to 4 weeks. Revaccinate every six months.

Precaution(s): Store between 36° and 45°F (2° and 7°C). Avoid freezing. Shake well before using. Use entire contents when first opened.

Caution(s): Allergic reactions, although rare, may occur. Do not mix with other vaccines or products, except as directed by manufacturer.

For use in swine.

For veterinary use only.

Antidote(s): The antidote is epinephrine.

Warning(s): Do not vaccinate within 21 days before slaughter.

Presentation: 50 doses (100 mL).

Compendium Code No.: 10031991 11427B

SUVAXYN® PLE

Fort Dodge **Bacterin-Vaccine**

Parvovirus Vaccine, Killed Virus-Erysipelothrix Rhusiopathiae-Leptospira Canicola-Grippotyphosa-Hardjo-Icterohaemorrhagiae-Pomona Bacterin

U.S. Vet. Lic. No.: 112

Contents: This product contains the antigens listed above.

Thimerosal and gentamicin added as preservative.

Indications: For the vaccination of healthy swine as an aid in the prevention of clinical signs caused by Porcine Parvovirus (PPV), *Erysipelothrix rhusiopathiae, Leptospira canicola, L. grippotyphosa, L. hardjo, L. icterohaemorrhagiae* and *L. pomona*.

Dosage and Administration: Vaccinate swine at six months of age or older with one 3 mL dose intramuscularly using aseptic technique. Revaccinate 3 to 4 weeks later. Gilts and sows should receive their second dose at least 2 weeks prior to breeding and should be revaccinated 8 to 2 weeks prior to each subsequent breeding. Revaccinate boars semiannually.

Precaution(s): Store in dark at 2° to 7°C (35° to 45°F). Avoid freezing. Use entire contents when first opened.

Caution(s): In case of anaphylactoid reaction, administer epinephrine.

For use in swine.

For veterinary use only.

Warning(s): Do not vaccinate within 21 days of slaughter.

Presentation: 10 dose (30 mL) and 35 dose (105 mL) vials.

Compendium Code No.: 10032002 11454D

SUVAXYN® PLE+B

Fort Dodge **Bacterin-Vaccine**

Parvovirus Vaccine, Killed Virus-Erysipelothrix Rhusiopathiae-Leptospira Bratislava-Canicola-Grippotyphosa-Hardjo-Icterohaemorrhagiae-Pomona Bacterin

U.S. Vet. Lic. No.: 112

Contents: This product contains the antigens listed above.

Contains gentamicin as a preservative.

Indications: For the vaccination of healthy swine as an aid in the prevention of clinical signs caused by Porcine Parvovirus, *Erysipelothrix rhusiopathiae, Leptospira bratislava, L. canicola, L. grippotyphosa, L. hardjo, L. icterohaemorrhagiae* and *L. pomona*.

Dosage and Administration: Aseptically inject 5 mL (5 cc) intramuscularly per animal.

Gilts: Since maternal antibodies will block vaccination response, administer first dose to gilts no sooner than 6 months of age and a second dose in 3 to 4 weeks. The second dose should be given no later than 2 weeks prior to breeding.

Sows: For primary vaccination, inject one dose 6 weeks prior to breeding and again in 3 to 4 weeks. Revaccinate sows 8 to 2 weeks prior to subsequent breedings.

Boars: Administer first dose no sooner than 6 months of age and a second dose in 3 to 4 weeks. Revaccinate every six months.

Precaution(s): Store between 35° and 45°F (2° and 7°C). Avoid freezing.

Shake well before using. Use entire contents when first opened.

Caution(s): Allergic reactions, although rare, may occur.

Do not mix with other vaccines or products, except as directed by manufacturer.

For use in swine.

For veterinary use only.

Antidote(s): The antidote is epinephrine.

Warning(s): Do not vaccinate within 21 days before slaughter.

Presentation: 10 dose (50 mL) and 50 dose (250 mL) vials.

Compendium Code No.: 10032012 11467C

SUVAXYN® PLE+B/PrV gpI⁻

Bacterin-Vaccine

Parvovirus-Pseudorabies Vaccine, Modified Live and Killed Virus, Erysipelothrix Rhusiopathiae-Leptospira Bratislava-Canicola-Grippotyphosa-Hardjo-Icterohaemorrhagiae-Pomona Bacterin

U.S. Vet. Lic. No.: 112

Contents: This product contains the antigens listed above.

Contains gentamicin as a preservative.

Indications: For the vaccination of healthy breeding swine as an aid in the prevention of clinical signs caused by Pseudorabies Virus (PRV), Porcine Parvovirus (PPV), *Erysipelothrix rhusiopathiae, Leptospira bratislava, L. canicola, L. grippotyphosa, L. hardjo, L. icterohaemorrhagiae*, and *L. pomona*.

Dosage and Administration: Dose: Aseptically rehydrate the vial of Pseudorabies Vaccine, Modified Live Virus, with one well-shaken vial of vaccine-bacterin diluent supplied. After rehydration, shake well. Aseptically inject 5 mL intramuscularly (neck region) per animal.

Sows: For primary vaccination, inject one dose 6 weeks prior to breeding. Vaccinate with a single dose of Suvaxyn® PLE+B three to four weeks later. Revaccinate sows with SUVAXYN® PLE+B/PrV gpI⁻ eight to two weeks prior to subsequent breedings.

Gilts: Since maternal antibodies will block vaccination response, administer first dose to gilts no sooner than 6 months of age. Vaccinate with Suvaxyn® PLE+B three to four weeks later, but no later than two weeks prior to breeding.

Boars: Administer one dose no sooner than 6 months of age. Vaccinate with a single dose of Suvaxyn® PLE+B three to four weeks later. Revaccinate with SUVAXYN® PLE+B/PrV gpI⁻ every six months.

Precaution(s): Store between 35° and 45°F (2° and 7°C). Avoid freezing.

Shake well before using. Use entire contents without delay after rehydration. Burn containers and all unused contents.

Do not mix with other vaccine or products.

Caution(s): Allergic reactions, although rare, may occur. Chemical disinfectants may destroy effectiveness of the vaccine and should not be used to sterilize equipment.

Note: Pigs previously vaccinated with PR-Vac® (SmithKline Beecham) or PrV/Marker Gold™ (SyntroVet) gpI⁻ deleted products will remain gpI⁻ seronegative (by Idexx HerdChek® and/or SmithKline Beecham ClinEase™ testing), after vaccination with the Fort Dodge Suvaxyn® PrV gpI⁻ product or SUVAXYN® PLE+B/PrV gpI⁻.

For use in swine only.

For veterinary use only.

Antidote(s): The antidote is epinephrine.

Warning(s): Do not vaccinate within 21 days before slaughter.

In the United States, distribution is limited to authorized recipients designated by proper State Officials and under such conditions as these officials may require.

Presentation: 10 dose (50 mL) vials.

Compendium Code No.: 10032022 11440B

SUVAXYN® PLE/PrV gpI⁻

Bacterin-Vaccine

Parvovirus-Pseudorabies Vaccine, Modified Live and Killed Virus-Erysipelothrix Rhusiopathiae-Leptospira Canicola-Grippotyphosa-Hardjo-Icterohaemorrhagiae-Pomona Bacterin

U.S. Vet. Lic. No.: 112

Contents: This product contains the antigens listed above.

Contains thimerosal and gentamicin as preservatives.

Indications: For the vaccination of healthy breeding swine as an aid in the prevention of clinical signs caused by Pseudorabies Virus (PRV), Porcine Parvovirus (PPV), *Erysipelothrix rhusiopathiae, Leptospira canicola, L. grippotyphosa, L. hardjo, L. icterohaemorrhagiae*, and *L. pomona*.

Dosage and Administration: Dose: Aseptically rehydrate with the accompanying diluent. Vaccinate swine at six months of age or older with one 3 mL dose intramuscularly using aseptic technique. Vaccinate 3 to 4 weeks later with 1 dose of Suvaxyn® PLE. Gilts and sows should receive the dose of Suvaxyn® PLE at least 2 weeks prior to breeding and should be revaccinated with Suvaxyn® PLE, 8 to 2 weeks prior to each subsequent breeding. Revaccinate boars semiannually.

Precaution(s): Store between 35° and 45°F (2° and 7°C). Avoid freezing. Shake well before/after rehydration. Use entire contents without delay after rehydration. Burn containers and all unused contents.

Do not mix with other vaccines or products.

Caution(s): Allergic reactions, although rare, may occur.

Note: Pigs previously vaccinated with PR-Vac® (SmithKline Beecham) or PrV/Marker Gold™ (SyntroVet) gpI⁻ deleted products will remain gpI⁻ seronegative (by Idexx HerdChek® and/or SmithKline Beecham ClinEase™ testing), after vaccination with the Fort Dodge Suvaxyn® PrV gpI⁻ product or SUVAXYN® PLE/PrV gpI⁻.

For use in swine only.

For veterinary use only.

Antidote(s): The antidote is epinephrine.

Warning(s): Do not vaccinate within 21 days before slaughter.

In the United States, distribution is limited to authorized recipients designated by proper State Officials and under such conditions as these officials may require.

Presentation: 1-10 dose bottle vaccine and 1-30 mL bottle vaccine-bacterin diluent.

Compendium Code No.: 10032031 15013C

SUVAXYN® PrV gpI⁻

Vaccine

Pseudorabies Vaccine, Modified Live Virus

U.S. Vet. Lic. No.: 112

Contents: This product contains the antigen listed above.

Contains gentamicin as a preservative.

Indications: SUVAXYN® PrV gpI⁻ is a modified live virus vaccine for the vaccination of healthy pigs as an aid in the prevention of pseudorabies (Aujeszky's disease) caused by pseudorabies virus (PRV).

Antibody produced solely by vaccination with this product can be differentiated from antibody produced by infection, using the Idexx HerdChek® Pseudorabies Virus gpI⁻ Antibody Test Kit.

Note: Pigs previously vaccinated with PR-Vac® (Pfizer) or PrV/Marker Gold™ (SyntroVet) gpI⁻ deleted products will remain gpI⁻ seronegative (by Idexx HerdChek® test), after vaccination with SUVAXYN® PrV gpI⁻ product.

Data shows the vaccine is safe and effective in pigs 3 days of age or older. This product will reduce death loss and challenge virus shedding. The vaccine may be safely used at any stage of gestation. Studies indicate the vaccine virus will not revert to virulence and that few, if any, adverse reactions in vaccinated pigs are to be expected. Additional studies have determined that shedding

of vaccine virus is minimal or nonexistent. SUVAXYN® PrV gpI⁻ shows no virulence for other domestic animals.
Dosage and Administration: For use in swine only. Aseptically rehydrate vaccine with sterile diluent supplied. Administer 2 mL intramuscularly at 3 days of age or older. Sterile syringes and needles should be used to administer this vaccine.

Pigs nursing non-immune dams may be vaccinated at any time after 3 days of age. Pigs nursing immune dams should be vaccinated when maternal antibody levels have declined, generally when pigs are three weeks to eight weeks of age. In an emergency situation where exposure is imminent, it may be desirable to immediately vaccinate all swine on the premises.

Semiannual revaccination is recommended for animals retained for breeding. Boars may be revaccinated at any time.
Precaution(s): Store between 2° to 7°C (35° to 45°F). Do not freeze. Use entire contents without delay after rehydration. Burn container and all unused contents.

Do not mix with other vaccines or products.
Caution(s): Allergic reactions, although rare, may occur.

For use in swine only.

For veterinary use only.
Antidote(s): The antidote is epinephrine.
Warning(s): Do not vaccinate within 21 days of slaughter.

Vaccination with SUVAXYN® PrV gpI⁻ may yield seropositive results in the official SN, ELISA, or latex agglutination tests. However, the Idexx HerdChek® Pseudorabies Virus gpI Antibody Test Kit differentiates SUVAXYN® PrV gpI⁻ vaccinates from infected animals based on gpI seroreactivity.

Although this product has been shown to be efficacious, some animals may be unable to develop or maintain an adequate immune response following vaccination if they are incubating any disease or are malnourished, parasitized or stressed due to shipment or adverse environmental conditions.

In the United States, distribution is limited to authorized recipients designated by proper State Officials and under such conditions as these officials may require.
Presentation: 10 dose and 25 dose vials.
Compendium Code No.: 10032042 11480D

SUVAXYN® RESPIFEND® APP

Fort Dodge **Bacterin**

Actinobacillus Pleuropneumoniae Bacterin
U.S. Vet. Lic. No.: 112
Contents: SUVAXYN® RESPIFEND® APP is an adjuvanted product containing chemically inactivated cultures of *Actinobacillus pleuropneumoniae* serotypes 1, 5 and 7.

Contains polymyxin B sulfate and gentamicin sulfate as preservatives.
Indications: For the vaccination of healthy swine as an aid in the prevention of pneumonia caused by *Actinobacillus pleuropneumoniae.*
Dosage and Administration: Aseptically inject 2 mL (2 cc) intramuscularly per animal.

Baby pigs: Inject at 4 weeks of age or older. Repeat with a second dose 3 to 4 weeks after the first vaccination.

Feeder pigs: Inject at time of arrival and repeat vaccination 3 to 4 weeks later.

Market hogs: Depending upon herd status, a third injection may be administered prior to high challenge periods.

Breeding stock: Vaccinate with two doses given 3 to 4 weeks apart. Administer the first dose at 6 months of age or prior to introduction into a herd. Revaccinate with a single dose semiannually.
Precaution(s): Store between 36° and 45°F (2° and 7°C). Avoid freezing. Shake well before using. Use entire contents when first opened.
Caution(s): Allergic reactions, although rare, may occur.

For use in swine.

For veterinary use only.
Antidote(s): The antidote is epinephrine.
Warning(s): Do not vaccinate within 60 days before slaughter.
Presentation: 50 dose (100 mL) vials.
Compendium Code No.: 10032051 11357C

SUVAXYN® RESPIFEND® HPS

Fort Dodge **Bacterin**

Haemophilus Parasuis Bacterin
U.S. Vet. Lic. No.: 112
Contents: This product contains the antigens listed above.
Indications: For the vaccination of healthy swine as an aid in the prevention of clinical signs, disease, and death due to Porcine Polyserositis and Arthritis Disease (Glässer's Disease) associated with *Haemophilus parasuis* serovars 4 and 5.
Dosage and Administration: Aseptically inject 2 mL (2 cc) intramuscularly per animal. Baby pigs: Inject 2 mL at 7 to 10 days of age or older. Repeat with second dose 2 to 3 weeks after first vaccination. Feeder pigs: Inject 2 mL at time of arrival and repeat vaccination 2 to 3 weeks later. Breeding stock: Vaccinate susceptible animals or breeding stock of unknown status with two doses given 2 to 3 weeks apart, prior to introduction into a herd.
Precaution(s): Store between 36° and 45°F (2° and 7°C). Avoid freezing. Shake well before using. Use entire contents when first opened.
Caution(s): Allergic reactions, although rare, may occur. Do not mix with other vaccines or products.

For use in swine.

For veterinary use only.
Antidote(s): The antidote is epinephrine.
Warning(s): Do not vaccinate within 21 days before slaughter.
Presentation: 50 doses (100 mL) and 125 doses (250 mL).
Compendium Code No.: 10032061 11507B

SUVAXYN® RESPIFEND® MH

Fort Dodge **Bacterin**

Mycoplasma Hyopneumoniae Bacterin
U.S. Vet. Lic. No.: 112
Contents: This product contains the antigen listed above.

Contains penicillin as a preservative.
Indications: This inactivated and adjuvanted bacterin is for the vaccination of healthy swine against clinical signs caused by *Mycoplasma hyopneumoniae.*
Dosage and Administration: Aseptically inject 2 mL (2 cc) intramuscularly. Baby pigs: Inject 2 mL at 7 to 10 days of age or prior to weaning. Repeat with second dose 2 to 3 weeks after first vaccination. Feeder pigs: Inject 2 mL at time of arrival and repeat vaccination 2 to 3 weeks later. Breeding stock: Vaccinate susceptible animals or breeding stock of unknown status with two doses given 2 to 3 weeks apart. The first dose should be given at 6 months of age or prior to introduction into a herd. Revaccinate with a single dose semiannually.
Precaution(s): Store between 36° and 45°F (2° and 7°C). Avoid freezing. Shake well before using. Use entire contents when first opened.
Caution(s): Allergic reactions, although rare, may occur.

For use in swine.

For veterinary use only.
Antidote(s): The antidote is epinephrine.
Warning(s): Do not vaccinate within 21 days before slaughter.
Presentation: 10 dose (20 mL), 50 dose (100 mL), 125 dose (250 mL), and 250 dose (500 mL) vials.
Compendium Code No.: 10032072 11528C

SUVAXYN® RESPIFEND® MH/HPS

Fort Dodge **Bacterin**

Haemophilus Parasuis-Mycoplasma Hyopneumoniae Bacterin
U.S. Vet. Lic. No.: 112
Contents: This product contains adjuvanted, inactivated cultures of strains representing *H. parasuis* serovars 4 and 5 and of *M. hyopneumoniae.*

Contains penicillin as a preservative.
Indications: For the vaccination of healthy swine as an aid in the prevention of clinical signs, disease, and death due to Porcine Polyserositis and Arthritis Disease (Glässer's Disease) associated with *Haemophilus parasuis* serovars 4 and 5, and as an aid in the prevention of respiratory disease associated with *Mycoplasma hyopneumoniae.*
Dosage and Administration: Aseptically inject 2 mL (2 cc) intramuscularly per animal. Baby pigs: Inject 2 mL at 7 to 10 days of age or older. Repeat with second dose 2 to 3 weeks after first vaccination. Feeder pigs: Inject 2 mL at time of arrival and repeat vaccination 2 to 3 weeks later. Breeding stock: Vaccinate susceptible animals or breeding stock of unknown status with two doses given 2 to 3 weeks apart, prior to introduction into a herd.
Precaution(s): Store between 36°F and 45°F (2° and 7°C). Avoid freezing. Shake well before using. Use entire contents when first opened.
Caution(s): Allergic reactions, although rare, may occur. Do not mix with other vaccines or products.

For use in swine.

For veterinary use only.
Antidote(s): The antidote is epinephrine.
Warning(s): Do not vaccinate within 21 days before slaughter.
Presentation: 50 doses (100 mL) and 125 doses (250 mL).
Compendium Code No.: 10032081 11517B

SWAT® FLY REPELLENT OINTMENT

Farnam **Topical Insecticide**

EPA Reg. No.: 270-103
Active Ingredient(s):
Piperonyl Butoxide, Technical* 0.5%
Pyrethrins I and II 0.2%
Di-n-propyl isocinchomeronate 1.0%
Inert Ingredients 98.3%

*Equivalent to 0.4% (butylcarbityl) (6-propylpiperonyl) ether and 0.1% related compounds.
Indications: For dogs, horses and ponies.

Fly repellent ointment for wounds and sores.
Dosage and Administration: It is a violation of federal law to use this product in a manner inconsistent with its labeling.

To treat superficial wounds, abrasions and scratches, apply enough ointment to cover the wound. Apply directly to the wound and use daily.
Precaution(s): Storage: Store in a cool, dry place.

Disposal: Do not reuse empty container. Wrap container and put it in trash collection.

This product is toxic to fish. Keep out of lakes, streams, or ponds. Do not apply where runoff is likely to occur. Do not contaminate water by cleaning of equipment or disposal of wastes.
Caution(s): Precautionary Statements: Not for human use. Wash hands after using.
Warning(s): Do not use on animals that are to be used for human consumption.

Keep out of reach of children.
Discussion: Repels house flies, stable flies, face flies, and horn flies from wounds and open sores. Also kills them on contact. Effective for hours.
Presentation: 6 oz. Also available: 6 oz. Clear Formula.
Compendium Code No.: 10000370

SWEETLIX® BLOAT GUARD® BLOCK MEDICATED

Sweetlix **Bloat Preparation**

NADA No.: 033-773
Active Ingredient(s):
Poloxalene* 6.6%

(Each lb contains 29.94 g/lb.)

*with 0.03% ethoxyquin and 0.095% BHT (both preservative)

Guaranteed Analysis:
Crude Protein, not less than 4.0%
Crude Fat, not less than 0.5%
Crude Fiber, not more than 12.5%
Salt (NaCl), not less than 19.5%
Salt (NaCl), not more than 23.0%
Iodine (I), not less than 0.0004%
Total Sugars (as invert), not less than 28.0%

Ingredients: Cane molasses, soybean hulls, salt, animal fat (preserved with BHA), manganous oxide, zinc oxide, ferrous carbonate, copper oxide, calcium iodate, cobalt carbonate.
Indications: For the control of legume (alfalfa, clover) bloat in dairy and beef cattle when consumed at the indicated rate.
Dosage and Administration:

1. To be fed at the rate of 0.8 oz of block per 100 lb of body weight per day. Example: 8 oz (0.5 lb) of block for a 1000 lb animal daily.

2. For adequate protection it is essential that each animal consume the total recommended dosage of SWEETLIX® BLOAT GUARD® Block daily.
3. Omit all salt from feed. Do not feed free choice sources of salt or mineral containing salt in any form. These blocks are an adequate source of salt.
4. Begin feeding blocks continuously. Feed blocks and full feed dry non-legume hay at least 48 hours prior to legume (alfalfa, clover) consumption. Repeat when block consumption is interrupted to maintain control.
5. Provide at least 1 block for each 5 head of cattle; add 1 additional block when each block has been half-consumed.
6. The location of the block is extremely important for adequate consumption. Place blocks where cattle congregate (watering, grazing and loafing areas) in order to limit the distance an animal must travel to have ready access to a block.
7. Controlled grazing practices (Strip Grazing) are recommended in order to limit the distance an animal must travel to have ready access to a block.
8. In some instances it may be necessary to confine cattle in a dry lot with additional SWEETLIX® BLOAT GUARD® Blocks for a period each day.

Caution(s): Access to, and intake of blocks may be limited during or directly after heavy rain or dew, and after frost or change of pasture. Variation in cattle routine may change their feeding and watering habits. Relocate blocks immediately as necessary. Special caution should be taken. Water high in salt and alkaline soils limit consumption and performance.

Presentation: 33.33 lb blocks.

BLOAT GUARD® is the registered trademark of SmithKline Beckman Corporation for its brand of poloxalene, U.S. Patent No. 3,465,083.

Compendium Code No.: 14920001

SWEETLIX® RABON® MINERAL/VITAMIN MOLASSES BLOCK

Sweetlix **Insecticide-Oral**

EPA Reg. No.: 40833-4

Active Ingredient(s):*

Tetrachlorvinphos: 2-Chloro-1-(2,4,5-trichlorophenyl) vinyl dimethyl phosphate	0.494%
Inert Ingredients**	99.506%
	100.000%

* Each lb contains 2.24 Rabon®

** Refers only to ingredients which are not larvicidal.

Guaranteed Analysis:

Calcium (Ca), not less than	4.5%
Calcium (Ca), not more than	5.5%
Phosphorus (P), not less than	4.0%
Salt (NaCl), not less than	15.0%
Salt (NaCl), not more than	18.0%
Potassium (K), not less than	2.0%
Magnesium (Mg), not less than	1.0%
Iodine (I), not less than	0.0069%
Selenium (Se), not less than	0.00216%
Vitamin A, min., IU/lb	100,000
Vitamin D_3, min., IU/lb	25,000
Vitamin E, min., IU/lb	25
Total Sugars (as invert), not less than	21.5%

Ingredients: Cane molasses, soybean hulls, dicalcium phosphate, salt, animal fat (preserved with BHA), potassium chloride, potassium sulfate, magnesium sulfate, magnesium oxide, vitamin A supplement, vitamin D_3 supplement, vitamin E supplement, riboflavin supplement, d-calcium pantothenate, thiamine mononitrate, niacin supplement, choline chloride, vitamin B_{12} supplement, folic acid, pyridoxine hydrochloride, biotin, menadione sodium bisulfite complex, ferrous carbonate, ferrous sulfate, zinc oxide, manganous oxide, manganese sulfate, copper oxide, copper sulfate, calcium iodate, ethylenediamine dihydriodide, cobalt carbonate, sodium selenite, yeast culture, ethoxyquin (a preservative).

Indications: For control of fecal flies in manure of treated cattle. Prevents development of face flies, horn flies, house flies and stable flies in the manure of treated cattle.

For control of fecal flies in manure of treated horses. Prevents development of house flies and stable flies in the manure of treated horses.

Directions for Use: It is a violation of Federal law to use this product in a manner inconsistent with its labeling.

1. Feed 1 block per 5 head of cattle or horses. This allows all animals equal access to blocks. Feed blocks at the rate of 0.5 oz per 100 lb of body weight. This intake will supply 6.87 g of larvicide per 100 lb of body weight.
2. Place blocks where animals congregate. Locate blocks throughout the pasture, placing them near water and loafing areas. Maintain adequate distance between blocks (10 ft minimum).
3. Do not allow animals to run out of blocks. When a block is half-consumed, place a new block near it. Place very small pieces in troughs or feed pans.
4. Cattle or horses will consume about 5 oz per head daily. When animals consume the block at the recommended rate, it will supply 3 mg of supplemental selenium.
5. Blocks can be fed to animals in confinement. Exact location of blocks to obtain desired consumption will vary between confinement feeding programs.
6. Feed as the only free choice source of salt, other minerals and vitamins.
7. SWEETLIX® RABON® Mineral/Vitamin Molasses Block prevents the development of fecal flies in the manure of treated cattle and horses, but it is not effective against existing adult flies. When starting a feeding program during the fly season, it may be necessary to use other control measures to reduce the population of existing adult flies. Supplemental fly control measures may be needed in and around buildings to control adult house flies and stable flies which can breed not only in animal manure but in other decaying matter on the premises. In order to achieve optimum fly control, SWEETLIX® RABON® Mineral/Vitamin Molasses Block should be used in conjunction with other good management and sanitation practices. Start feeding SWEETLIX® RABON® Mineral/Vitamin Molasses Block early in the spring before flies begin to appear and continue feeding throughout the summer and into the fall.

Precautionary Statements:

Hazards to Humans: Harmful if swallowed. Avoid contact with skin and eyes. Avoid breathing dust. Wash thoroughly with soap and water after handling and before eating or smoking. If in eyes, wash with plenty of water. If irritation persists, get medical attention. Wear long-sleeved shirt and pants; chemical resistant gloves; shoes and socks for protection when handling.

Environmental Hazards: This pesticide is toxic to fish. Do not contaminate water when disposing of equipment washwaters.

Storage and Disposal: Do not contaminate water, food, or feed by storage or disposal.

Storage: Store in a dry place in original container.

Container Disposal: Remove plastic wrap and place block in feeder. Dispose of plastic wrap in a sanitary landfill or by incineration, or, if allowed by State and local authorities, by burning. If burned, stay out of smoke.

Pesticide Disposal: Wastes resulting from the use of this product may be disposed of on-site or at an approved waste disposal facility.

Warning(s): SWEETLIX® RABON® Mineral/Vitamin Molasses Block may be fed to animals up to slaughter and to lactating cows without withholding the milk from market either during or after treatment.

Keep out of reach of children.

Presentation: 40 lb blocks (5 blocks weight 200 lb).

Compendium Code No.: 14920011

SWEETLIX® SAFE-GUARD® 20% NATURAL PROTEIN DEWORMING BLOCK FOR BEEF CATTLE

Sweetlix **Parasiticide-Oral**

(fenbendazole)

Active Ingredient(s):

Fenbendazole	750 mg/lb

Guaranteed Analysis:

Protein, not less than	20.00%
Fat, not less than	1.00%
Fiber, not more than	12.00%
Calcium (Ca), not more than	3.00%
Calcium (Ca), not less than	2.00%
Phosphorus (P), not less than	0.85%
Iodine (I), not less than	0.003%
Salt (NaCl), not more than	16.00%
Salt (NaCl), not less than	13.50%
Magnesium (Mg), not less than	0.60%
Manganese (Mn), not less than	0.01%
Cobalt (Co), not less than	0.004%
Copper (Cu), not less than	0.003%
Fluorine (F), not more than	0.01%
Ash, not more than	30.00%
Vitamin D_3, not less than	5,000 I.U. per pound
Vitamin A, not less than	20,000 I.U. per pound

Ingredients: Cottonseed meal, dehydrated alfalfa meal, salt, cane molasses, rice hulls, calcium carbonate, magnesium limestone, defluorinated phosphate, hemicellulose extract, bentonite, vitamin A supplement, potassium sulfate, magnesium sulfate, iron carbonate, cobalt carbonate, manganous oxide, iron oxide, mineral oil, dicalcium phosphate, monocalcium phosphate, magnesium oxide, d-activated animal sterol, calcium iodate, copper oxide, choline chloride, sodium bicarbonate, zinc sulfate, yeast culture, niacin, riboflavin supplement, meat and bone meal and cobalt sulfate.

Indications: For the removal and control of the following gastrointestinal parasites in beef cattle: lungworm *(Dictyocaulus viviparus)*, stomach worms: barberpole worm *(Haemonchus contortus)*, brown stomach worm *(Ostertagia ostertagi)*, small stomach worm *(Trichostrongylus axei)*, intestinal worms: hookworm *(Bunostomum phlebotomum)*, thread-necked intestinal worm *(Nematodirus helvetianus)*, small intestinal worms *(Cooperia punctata* and *C oncophora)*, bankrupt worm *(Trichostrongylus colubriformis)*, nodular worm *(Oesophagostomum radiatum)*.

Dosage and Administration: 1.67 mg fenbendazole per kg body weight per day for three (3) days. Total dose for the three (3) day period of 5 mg fenbendazole per kg of body weight (2.27 mg fenbendazole per pound).

Feeding Instructions: Adequate forage must be available at all times to cattle receiving supplemental block feeding.

SAFE-GUARD® (fenbendazole) 20% Natural Protein Deworming Block (Medicated) is designed for deworming pastured cattle by feeding these medicated blocks for three (3) days only as the sole source of salt.

It is essential to establish full cattle adaptation to supplemental block feeding prior to treating cattle with SAFE-GUARD® 20% Natural Protein Deworming Block (Medicated). Cattle behavior and per capita consumption must be established by feeding nonmedicated 20% Natural Protein Blocks prior to medicated block treatment. Adaptation to block feed intake for medicated treatment may take twelve (12) to nineteen (19) days of prior exposure to unmedicated feed blocks depending on consumption rates and environmental conditions. When cattle block consumption of 0.1 pound (1.6 ounces) per 100 pounds of body weight (or 1.0 pound for mature cattle) per day is attained for several days on the nonmedicated 20% Natural Protein Block, the three (3) day medicated treatment with SAFE-GUARD® 20% Protein Deworming Blocks (Medicated) may begin.

For effective treatment, the cattle must consume an average 0.1 pound of SAFE-GUARD® 20% Natural Protein Blocks (Medicated) per 100 pounds of body weight each day for the three (3) days of treatment. This is equivalent to an average of one (1) pound per head per day to mature cattle for the three days of treatment in order to provide a total dose of 2.27 mg fenbendazole per pound of body weight.

To commence deworming treatment, replace the nonmedicated blocks with SAFE-GUARD® 20% Natural Protein Deworming Blocks (Medicated). Place these medicated blocks at the same locations where cattle have demonstrated adequate per capita block intake (0.1 pound per 100 pounds of body weight per day).

Daily Treatment (to be continued for three (3) days):

Cattle Body Weight (Pounds)	Average Block Intake (lb/head/day)	Number of Head per Block*
500	½	16
750	¾	10
Mature Cattle	1	8

*Number of head fully treated by each block when consumed in three (3) days.

Following the three (3) day treatment any remaining SAFE-GUARD® 20% Natural Deworming Blocks (Medicated) should be removed from the pasture, and cattle may be returned to their normal supplemental feeding program. Remaining blocks, or portions of blocks, can be utilized for retreatment purposes if used prior to the expiration date.

It is essential that good block feeding husbandry practices be followed at all times. Block feeding techniques include, but are not limited to, a variety of practices. Blocks should be first located in those areas where cattle are seen to browse or loaf. It may be desirable to relocate unconsumed blocks to locations where obvious block consumption is identified. Increased consumption may often be obtained by moving feeding stations into shaded or loafing areas,

closer to water source, increasing the number of blocks available to the animals or combinations of these practices. Decreased consumption may often be obtained by the reverse of the above practices.
Caution(s): There are no known contraindications to the use of fenbendazole in cattle. Under conditions of continued exposure to parasites, retreatment may be needed after 6 to 8 weeks.

Consult your veterinarian for assistance in the diagnosis, treatment and control of parasitism.
Warning(s): Cattle must not be slaughtered within 16 days following last treatment.
Presentation: 25 lb blocks.
SWEETLIX® is the trademark of PM Ag Products Inc.
SAFE-GUARD® is the trademark of Hoechst Roussel Vet.
Compendium Code No.: 14920041

SWEETLIX® SAFE-GUARD* FREE-CHOICE MINERAL CATTLE DEWORMER

Sweetlix **Parasiticide-Oral**
(fenbendazole)
Active Ingredient(s):
Fenbendazole .... 1.90 grams/lb

Guaranteed Analysis:
Calcium, min. 13%
Calcium, max. 15%
Phosphorus, min. 6%
Salt, min. 35%
Salt, max. 37%

Feed Ingredients: Diacalcium phosphate, calcium carbonate, magnesium oxide, zinc sulfate, potassium iodide, dried cane molasses, sodium selenite, salt, mineral oil, rice hulls.
Indications: For the removal and control of the following parasites of cattle:

Lungworm: *(Dictyocaulus viviparus)*.

Stomach worms: Barberpole worm *(Haemonchus contortus)*, brown stomach worm *(Ostertagia ostertagi)*, small stomach worm *(Trichostrongylus axei)*.

Intestinal worms: Hookworm *(Bunostomum phlebotomum)*, thread-necked intestinal worm *(Nematodirus helvetianus)*, small intestinal worms *(Cooperia punctata, C oncophora)*, bankrupt worm *(Trichostrongylus colubriformis)*, nodular worm *(Oesophagostomum radiatum)*.
Dosage and Administration: This fenbendazole medicated free-choice mineral is to be fed to cattle for 3 to 6 days. The amount of this medicated free-choice feed given to a group of cattle is based on 1.91-ounce total consumption per 100 lbs body weight, to deliver a dosage of 2.27 mg fenbendazole per pound of body weight. The cattle must be allowed access to this medicated feed for sufficient time to receive this total dose. Under conditions of continued exposure to parasites, retreatment may be needed after 4-6 weeks. There are no known contraindications to the use of the drug in cattle.

This package treats 8,370 pounds of beef.

Weight of Cattle	Total oz Fed (over 3-5 days)	Head Treated per Package
400 lbs	7.65 oz	20.93
500 lbs	9.56 oz	16.74
600 lbs	11.47 oz	13.95
700 lbs	13.38 oz	11.96
1000 lbs	19.12 oz	8.37

Precaution(s): Store at room temperature.
Caution(s): Consult your veterinarian for assistance in the diagnosis, treatment, and control of parasitism.
Precaution(s): Store at room temperature.
Warning(s): Cattle must not be slaughtered within 13 days following last treatment. Because a withdrawal time has not been established, do not use in dairy cattle of breeding age.
*SAFE-GUARD is a trademark of Hoechst Roussel Vet.
Compendium Code No.: 14920031

SWIMMER'S EAR ASTRINGENT

Vet Solutions **Otic Cleanser**
Antiseptic Drying Gel and Deodorant
Ingredient(s): SD-Alcohol 40, Deionized Water, Butylene Glycol, Carbomer, Chloroxylenol, AMP, Fragrance, FD&C Blue No. 1.
Indications: Vet Solutions SWIMMER'S EAR ASTRINGENT is a unique drying gel and deodorant formulated to help maintain a moisture free environment for dogs and cats.
Directions: Clean ear canal prior to application. Apply a thin coating into ear canal. Massage base of the ear. To help maintain a moisture free environment, use once or twice weekly on a routine basis. Apply after swimming or bathing. May be used daily or as directed by veterinarian.
Precaution(s): Storage: Store this product at room temperature.
Caution(s): Do not apply to irritated or excoriated ears. Do not apply to ears with ruptured tympanic membranes. Avoid contact with eyes and mucous membranes. If contact occurs, immediately flush with water. If irritation or redness occurs, discontinue use and consult a veterinarian.

Sold exclusively through veterinarians.
Warning(s): Keep out of reach of children.
Presentation: 4 fl oz (120 mL).
Compendium Code No.: 10610210 010201

SWINE ACID-O-LITE®

TechMix **Electrolytes-Oral**
Guaranteed Analysis: Minimum:
Potassium (K) 10%
Sodium (NaCl) 10%
Phosphorus (P) 0.75%
Magnesium (Mg) 0.25%
Zinc (Zn) .... 1,500 ppm

Ingredients: Citric Acid, Potassium Chloride, Sodium Chloride, Dipotassium Phosphate, Magnesium Sulfate, Sodium Citrate, Zinc Methionine Complex, Manganese Sulfate, Copper Sulfate, Dextrose, Sodium Saccharin.
Indications: A water soluble acidified electrolyte for swine of any age.

SWINE ACID-O-LITE® is a palatable, water soluble acidified electrolyte specifically designed to treat or prevent shrink and dehydration in swine of all ages. The high level of electrolytes and acidification makes SWINE ACID-O-LITE® ideal and applicable as part of management programs for weaning and prior to shipment of both young and mature swine.
Directions for Use: Administer SWINE ACID-O-LITE® in the drinking water when pigs show signs of shrink or dehydration or 1 to 3 days prior to weaning, sorting or transporting pigs.

Administer at the following rates for 4 to 5 days:

Medicator Use: Mix one packet (8 oz or 227 grams) in water to make one gallon of stock solution. Set medicator at the rate of one ounce of stock solution per gallon of drinking water (1:128 ratio).

Stock Tanks: Mix one packet (8 oz or 227 grams) in 128 gallons of drinking water.

Feed Mixing: Add 1.5 lbs (3 8 oz packets) of SWINE ACID-O-LITE® to each ton of complete swine feed. Use SWINE ACID-O-LITE® in the feed for 7 days or until pigs no longer show signs of shrink or dehydration, or until feed intake has returned to normal.
Precaution(s): Store in a dry room at temperatures between 4°C and 30°C (40°F-86°F). Once bag is opened, seal with tape or binder and placed unused portion of SWINE ACID-O-LITE® in a dry air sealable container.
Caution(s): Pigs showing symptoms of coma, shock or too weak and dehydrated to eat normally should be treated by a veterinarian. This product is not nutritionally complete if administered by itself for long periods of time. It should not be administered beyond the recommended period without the addition of milk, milk replacers or prestarter pellets to young pigs or an appropriate ration for older pigs.
Discussion: Fluid-Electrolyte Balance: Water represents over 75 percent of the young piglet's body weight and over 50% of the body weight of mature pigs.

Electrolytes serve as the primary way in which the body balances its fluids in the three compartments of the body where fluid is stored. Through the electrolytes and their osmotic pressure, the body fluids are maintained at proper levels between the fluid inside the cell (intracellular), the fluid between cells (interstitial) and the fluid in the blood vascular system. Without adequate water and electrolytes, the body cannot maintain its proper fluid balance between the compartments resulting in tissue shrink or dehydration.

Dehydration of the cells and tissue leads to reduced growth, impaired maintenance and can result in death when the body looses between 7 to 15% of its normal body fluid. Young pigs, which have a high proportion of body fluid, are very subject to severe dehydration that contributes to the moderate to high mortality whenever they are exposed to stress and disease. Enteric infections caused by *E. coli*, TGE and rotavirus quickly dehydrate the body as fluids are lost from the loose, diarrhea conditions of the stools. This dehydration from the diarrhea makes the young piglet subject to shock and death in a matter of minutes or several hours.

Electrolyte Fortification: SWINE ACID-O-LITE® is a multiple electrolyte formula that provides five electrolytes to help maintain fluids in the cell as compared to many electrolyte formulas which only provide two or three electrolytes. SWINE ACID-O-LITE® provides three essential cations — potassium, magnesium and sodium and two anions — phosphate and chloride. These multiple sources of electrolytes help the fluids in the blood vessels, tissues and cells of the body because they are readily absorbed from the intestinal tract. SWINE ACID-O-LITE® was specially designed to assure rapid absorption of the electrolytes.

Water Acidification: The young pig has a limited ability to secrete acid in its digestive tract. *E. coli* are known to proliferate and grow in the digestive tract when the pig doesn't produce enough acid to maintain the proper pH. SWINE ACID-O-LITE® was specifically designed to promote gut acidification in a palatable and safe manner. The acidifier used in SWINE ACID-O-LITE® has been proven repeatedly to be highly palatable and effective for swine of any age.
Trial Data: Field Results: SWINE ACID-O-LITE® has been field tested in pigs at weaning and as an aid for improving consumption and absorption of commonly used water medications. SWINE ACID-O-LITE® can increase weight gain and reduce shrink of pigs following the stresses of weaning and transportation. Pigs will consume more water when SWINE ACID-O-LITE® is added to the water. Adequate water intake is necessary for optimum feed intake and efficient growth performance. Initial results show that finishing pigs given SWINE ACID-O-LITE® 24 hours before shipment had improvement in carcass yield and reduced shrink.
Presentation: 25-8 oz bags.
Compendium Code No.: 11440130

SWINE INFLUENZA VACCINE (H3N2 SUBTYPE)

SyntroVet **Vaccine**
Swine Influenza Vaccine, Killed Virus, H3N2 Subtype
U.S. Vet. Lic. No.: 314
Contents: This vaccine contains an inactivated swine influenza virus, Type A subtype H3N2 for the vaccination of healthy swine. The vaccine is adjuvanted to enhance immunity.

Contains gentamicin and thimerosal as preservatives.
Indications: For the vaccination of healthy swine 3 to 4 weeks of age or older against swine influenza caused by the H3N2 subtype.

Notice: This is a conditionally licensed vaccine. Efficacy and potency studies are in progress.
Dosage and Administration: For use in swine only. Shake well and administer 2 mL intramuscularly. For primary vaccination, administer a second dose in 2 to 3 weeks.
Precaution(s): Store at 35°-45°F (2°-7°C). Use entire contents when first opened.
Caution(s): Anaphylactoid reactions may occur.
Antidote(s): Epinephrine.
Warning(s): Do not vaccinate within 21 days of slaughter.
Presentation: 50 dose (100 mL) and 100 dose (200 mL) vials.
Compendium Code No.: 11170040

SWINE MASTER M PLUS™

AgriLabs **Bacterin**
Mycoplasma Hyopneumoniae Bacterin
U.S. Vet. Lic. No.: 165A
Contents: This product contains the antigen listed above.

Preservatives: Ampicillin, gentamicin, and thimerosal.
Indications: SWINE MASTER M PLUS™ is recommended for use as an aid in the prevention of pneumonia caused by *Mycoplasma hyopneumoniae* infection in swine.
Dosage and Administration: Using aseptic technique, inject 1 mL subcutaneously or intramuscularly at 7-10 days of age or older. Revaccinate with 1 mL 2 weeks after initial vaccination. Revaccinate with a single 1 mL dose annually.
Precaution(s): Store at 2°-7°C (35°-45°F). Do not freeze. Use entire contents when first opened.
Caution(s): Transient local reaction may occur at the injection site. If allergic response occurs, administer epinephrine.

Extreme caution should be used when injecting any oil emulsion vaccine to avoid injecting your finger or hand. Accidental injection can cause serious local reaction. Contact a physician immediately if accidental injection occurs.

For veterinary use only.

Warning(s): Do not vaccinate within 21 days of slaughter.

Presentation: 100 dose (100 mL) and 250 dose (250 mL) (NDC-0061-1166-09) vials.

Manufactured by: Schering-Plough Animal Health Corporation, Omaha, NE 68103.

Compendium Code No.: 10581021 P17911-11 / P17935-10

SYNANTHIC® BOVINE DEWORMER SUSPENSION, 9.06%

Fort Dodge **Parasiticide-Oral**

Oxfendazole

NADA No.: 140-854

Active Ingredient(s): Each mL contains 90.6 mg of oxfendazole.

Indications: SYNANTHIC® Bovine Dewormer Suspension, 9.06%, is a broad-spectrum anthelmintic effective for removal and control of the following parasites in cattle: lungworms, roundworms (including inhibited forms of *Ostertagia ostertagi)* and tapeworms, as indicated below:

Lungworms: *Dictyocaulus viviparus* (Adult, L_4)

Stomach Worms:

Barberpole Worms: *Haemonchus contortus* (Adult), *Haemonchus placei* (Adult)

Small Stomach Worms: *Trichostrongylus axei* (Adult)

Brown Stomach Worms: *Ostertagia ostertagi* (Adult, L_4, inhibited L_4)

Intestinal Worms:

Nodular Worms: *Oesophagostomum radiatum* (Adult)

Hookworms: *Bunostomum phlebotomum* (Adult)

Small Intestinal Worms: *Cooperia punctata* (Adult, L_4), *Cooperia oncophora* (Adult, L_4), *Cooperia mcmasteri* (Adult, L_4)

Tapeworms: *Moniezia benedeni* (Adult)

Directions: Determine the proper dose according to estimated body weight. Administer orally. The recommended dose of 2.05 mg/lb (4.5 mg/kg) is achieved when 2.5 mL of the suspension is given for each 110 lb (50 kg) of body weight.

Examples:

Cattle Weight	Dose
110 lb (50 kg)	2.5 mL
220 lb (100 kg)	5.0 mL
330 lb (150 kg)	7.5 mL
440 lb (200 kg)	10.0 mL
550 lb (250 kg)	12.5 mL
660 lb (300 kg)	15.0 mL
770 lb (350 kg)	17.5 mL
880 lb (400 kg)	20.0 mL
990 lb (450 kg)	22.5 mL
1100 lb (500 kg)	25.0 mL

Treatment may be repeated in 4-6 weeks.

Consult a veterinarian for assistance in the diagnosis, treatment and control of parasitism.

Contraindication(s): Safety: There are no contraindications for the use of SYNANTHIC® Bovine Dewormer Suspension, 9.06%, in cattle.

Precaution(s): Shake well before use. Avoid freezing. Protect from excessive heat. Store at temperatures not to exceed 104°F (40°C).

Caution(s): Use only as directed. Keep out of reach of children. Not for human use.

For animal use only.

Warning(s): Cattle must not be slaughtered until 7 days after treatment. Because a withdrawal time in milk has not been established, do not use in female dairy cattle of breeding age.

Presentation: 1000 mL (one liter) (NDC 0856-0875-75)
(treats 88 cattle weighing approximately 500 lbs each)
4000 mL (four liters) (NDC 0856-0875-76)
(treats 352 cattle weighing approximately 500 lbs each)

U.S. Patent No. 3,929,821; 4,080,461; and others.

Compendium Code No.: 10032120 0125B, 0124B

SYNANTHIC® BOVINE DEWORMER SUSPENSION, 22.5% ℞

Fort Dodge **Parasiticide-Oral**

Oxfendazole

NADA No.: 140-854

Active Ingredient(s): Each mL contains 225 mg of oxfendazole.

Manufactured by a non-sterilizing process.

Indications: SYNANTHIC® Bovine Dewormer Suspension, 22.5%, is a broad-spectrum anthelmintic effective for the removal and control of the following parasites in cattle: lungworms, roundworms (including inhibited forms of *Ostertagia ostertagi)* and tapeworms, as indicated below:

Lungworms: *Dictyocaulus viviparus* (adult, L_4)

Stomach Worms:

Barberpole Worms: *Haemonchus contortus* (Adult), *Haemonchus placei* (Adult)

Small Stomach Worms: *Trichostrongylus axei* (Adult)

Brown Stomach Worms: *Ostertagia ostertagi* (Adult, L_4, inhibited L_4)

Intestinal Worms:

Nodular Worms: *Oesophagostomum radiatum* (Adult)

Hookworms: *Bunostomum phlebotomum* (Adult)

Small Intestinal Worms: *Cooperia punctata* (Adult, L_4), *Cooperia oncophora* (Adult, L_4), *Cooperia mcmasteri* (Adult, L_4)

Tapeworms: *Moniezia benedeni* (Adult)

Dosage and Administration: The recommended dose for cattle is 2.05 mg/lb (4.5 mg/kg) of body weight. SYNANTHIC® Bovine Dewormer Suspension, 22.5%, may be administered either orally by accurate dose syringe or intraruminally with the Synanthic® Rumen Injector at the rate of 1 mL per 110 lb (50 kg) of body weight. This product should be shaken well immediately prior to use.

Before using the Synanthic® Rumen Injector, carefully read the instruction manual provided with the instrument for full information in regard to the proper care and use of the device.

When using the Synanthic® Rumen Injector, locate the correct target area on the left side of the animal (the triangle formed by the rear of the last rib, below the edge of the spine, and in front of the hip). Place the plastic shroud in the center of this area. Push the injector firmly into the animal's left side, at a right angle to the body surface, evenly depressing the plastic shroud. Pressing the injector firmly into the animal's side will activate the delivery system. Maintain pressure on the injector for 2-3 seconds to allow the full dose to be delivered. Withdraw the instrument.

The right side of the animal must not be used.

Appropriate cleanliness should always be observed. Always use a clean sharp needle; disinfect and replace as necessary. Use of the Synanthic® Rumen Injector on wet animals is not recommended. Clean the Synanthic® Rumen Injector before and after use.

Directions: Determine the proper dose according to estimated body weight. Administer orally or intraruminally. The recommended dose of 2.05 mg/lb (4.5 mg/kg) is achieved when 1 mL of the suspension is given for each 110 lb (50 kg) of body weight.

Examples:

Cattle Weight	Dose
110 lb (50 kg)	1.0 mL
220 lb (100 kg)	2.0 mL
330 lb (150 kg)	3.0 mL
440 lb (200 kg)	4.0 mL
550 lb (250 kg)	5.0 mL
660 lb (300 kg)	6.0 mL
770 lb (350 kg)	7.0 mL
880 lb (400 kg)	8.0 mL
990 lb (450 kg)	9.0 mL
1100 lb (500 kg)	10.0 mL

Treatment may be repeated in 4-6 weeks.

Consult a veterinarian for assistance in the diagnosis, treatment and control of parasitism.

Contraindication(s): Safety: There are no contraindications for the use of SYNANTHIC® Bovine Dewormer Suspension, 22.5%, in cattle.

Precaution(s): Shake well before use. Avoid freezing. Protect from excessive heat. Store at temperatures not to exceed 104°F (40°C).

Remove cap and protective seal and replace with blue cap prior to use. Do not squeeze sides of bottle.

Caution(s): Federal law restricts this drug to use by or on the order of a licensed veterinarian.

Use only as directed. Keep out of reach of children. Not for human use.

For animal use only.

Warning(s): Cattle must not be slaughtered until 7 days after treatment. Because a withdrawal time in milk has not been established, do not use in female dairy cattle of breeding age.

Presentation: 500 mL (NDC 0856-0881-80)
(treats 110 cattle weighing approximately 500 lbs each)
1000 mL (34 fl oz) (NDC 0856-0881-81)
(treats 220 cattle weighing approximately 500 lbs each)

U.S. Patent No. 3,929,821; 4,080,461; and others.

Compendium Code No.: 10032110 0134C

SYNERGIZED DELICE® POUR-ON INSECTICIDE

Schering-Plough **Premise and Topical Insecticide**

EPA No.: 773-72

Active Ingredient(s):

Permethrin: 3-(phenoxyphenyl)methyl (±)-cis, trans-3-(2,2-dichloroethenyl-2,2-dimethylcyclopropanecarboxylate* . . . 1.0%
Piperonyl Butoxide Technical** . . . 1.0%
Other Ingredients . . . 98.0%
Total 100.0%

*cis/trans ratio: Min. 35% (±) cis and max. 65% (±) trans

**Equivalent to Min. 0.8% (butylcarbityl)(6-propylpiperonyl) ether and 0.2% related compounds

Indications: For use on lactating and non-lactating dairy cattle, beef cattle and calves to control lice, horn flies, and face flies. It also aids in the control of horse flies, stable flies, house flies, mosquitoes and black flies.

For use on sheep to control sheep keds and lice.

For use in and around horse, beef, dairy, swine, sheep and poultry premises, animal hospital pens, kennels and "outside" meat processing premises to control house flies, stable flies, face flies, gnats, mosquitoes, black flies, fleas, and little house flies *(Fannia* spp.). It also aids in the control of cockroaches, ants, spiders, and crickets.

Directions for Use: It is a violation of Federal law to use this product in a manner inconsistent with its labeling.

Ready to Use—No dilution necessary.

Apply to lactating and non-lactating dairy cattle, beef cattle and calves for the control of lice, horn flies, face flies, aids in the control of horse flies, stable flies, mosquitoes, and black flies.

Application Instructions:

Dosage: Apply ½ fl oz (15 cc) per 100 lbs body wt of animal up to a maximum of 5 fl oz for any one animal.

Pour-On: Pour correct dose along back and down face.

Ready-To-Use Sprayer: Use undiluted in a mist sprayer to apply correct dose. Apply directly to neck, face, back, legs and ears.

Back Rubber Use: Mix one pint per gallon #2 diesel or mineral oil. Keep rubbing device charged. Results are improved by daily forced use.

Apply to sheep for the control of sheep keds and lice.

Application Instructions: Pour along the back. Apply ¼ fl oz (7.5 cc) per 50 lbs body wt of animal, up to a maximum of 3 fl oz for any one animal. For optimum control, all animals in the flock should be treated after shearing.

Premises: Apply in and around horse, beef, dairy, swine, sheep and poultry premises, animal hospital pens, kennels and "outside" meat processing premises to control house flies, stable flies, face flies, gnats, mosquitoes, black flies, fleas, little house flies *(Fannia* spp.), cockroaches, ants, spiders, and crickets.

Application Instructions: For use as a ready-to-use spot spray or premise spray, use undiluted in a mist sprayer. Apply directly to surface to leave a residual insecticidal coating, paying particular

S

attention to areas where insects crawl or alight. One gallon will treat approximately 7,300 square feet.

For cattle and sheep, repeat treatment as needed, but not more often than once every two weeks. For optimum lice control, two treatments at a 14-day interval are recommended.

Special Note: SYNERGIZED DELICE® Insecticide is not effective in controlling cattle grubs. SYNERGIZED DELICE® is an oil-based, ready-to-use product, that may leave an oily appearance on the hair coat of some animals. SYNERGIZED DELICE® should be used in an integrated pest management system which may involve repeated treatments and the use of other pest control practices.

Precautionary Statements: Hazards to Humans and Domestic Animals:

Caution: Harmful if absorbed through skin. Avoid contact with skin, eyes and clothing. Prolonged or frequently repeated skin contact may cause allergic reactions in some individuals. Wash thoroughly with soap and water after handling.

Statement of Practical Treatment:

If Swallowed: Call a physician immediately. Do not induce vomiting unless under medical attention.

If in Eyes: Immediately flush eyes with plenty of water. Get medical attention if discomfort persists.

If on Skin: Wash the skin with soap and water. Get medical attention.

Environmental Hazards: This product is extremely toxic to fish and other aquatic invertebrates. Do not add directly to water. Do not contaminate water when disposing of equipment washwaters. Apply this product only as specified on the label.

Physical or Chemical Hazards: Do not use or store near heat or open flame.

Storage and Disposal: Do not contaminate water, food or feed by storage or disposal.

Storage: Keep container sealed when not in use. Do not store near food or feed.

Pesticide Disposal: Wastes resulting from the use of this product may be disposed of on site or at an approved waste disposal facility.

Container Disposal: Triple rinse (or equivalent). Then offer for recycling or reconditioning, or puncture and dispose of in a sanitary landfill or by incineration, or, if allowed by State and local authorities, by burning. If burned, stay out of smoke.

Warning(s): Keep out of reach of children.

Disclaimer: Notice of Warranty: Schering-Plough Animal Health Corp. makes no warranty of merchantability, fitness for any particular purpose, or otherwise, expressed or implied concerning this product or its uses which extend beyond the use of the product under normal conditions in accord with the statements made on the label.

Presentation: 1 U.S. gallon (3.785 L) (NDC 0061-5074-06), 2.5 U.S. gallons (9.5 L) (NDC 0061-5074-02) and 55 U.S. gallons.

Compendium Code No.: 10471862

SYNERKYL® AQ WATER-BASED PET SPRAY

DVM **Parasiticide Spray**

EPA Reg. No.: 28293-116-41835

Active Ingredient(s):

Pyrethrins	0.112%
Permethrin [*(3-phenoxyphenyl) methyl (±) cis-trans-3-(2,2-dichloroethenyl)-2,2-dimethylcyclopropane-carboxylate]	0.101%
Related Compounds	0.009%
Inert Ingredients	99.778%
Total	100.000%

*cis-trans isomer ratio: Min. 35% (±) cis and Max. 65% (±) trans.

Indications: SYNERKYL® AQ Water-Based Pet Spray residually kills fleas on dogs and cats for up to 14 days, and will kill ticks for 4 days on dogs and 9 days on cats.

Directions for Use: It is a violation of Federal Law to use this product in a manner inconsistent with its labeling.

Read entire label before each use.

Use only on dogs and cats.

To Use: Use protective gloves or mitts to prevent contact with hands. Hold container upright. Shake well before using.

Spray the animal from a distance of 8-12 inches. Start spraying at the tail moving the dispenser rapidly and making sure that the animal's entire body is covered, including the legs and under the body. Fluff the hair while spraying so that the spray will penetrate to the skin. The spray should wet the ticks thoroughly. Do not spray in the face, eyes or on the genitalia. Reapply every 14 days for fleas on dogs and cats, every 4 days for ticks on dogs and every 9 days for ticks on cats. For cats, apply at the rate of 1 second per pound of body weight. For dogs, apply at the rate of 2 seconds per pound of body weight for thin or short haired dogs and up to 8 seconds per pound of body weight for heavy or long haired dogs.

Precautionary Statements: Hazards to Humans and Domestic Animals:

Caution: Harmful if swallowed. Avoid breathing vapors. Do not spray in eyes, face or on genitalia. Do not use on puppies and kittens under twelve (12) weeks. Consult a veterinarian before using this product on debilitated, aged, medicated, pregnant or nursing animals. Sensitivities may occur after using any pesticide product for pets. If signs occur, bathe your pet with mild soap and rinse with large amounts of water. If signs continue, consult a veterinarian immediately.

First Aid:

If Swallowed: Call a physician or Poison Control Center immediately.

If in Eyes: Flush with plenty of water. Get medical attention if irritation persists.

If on Skin: Wash with soap and warm water.

If Inhaled: Remove victim to fresh air and call a physician if effects occur.

Physical or Chemical Hazards: Do not use or store near heat or open flame.

Storage and Disposal: Store at room temperature and away from heat and open flame. Do not reuse empty container. Wrap original container in several layers of newspaper and discard in trash.

Warning(s): Keep out of reach of children.

Disclaimer: Warranty Statement: DVM's recommendations for use of this product are based upon tests believed to be reliable. The use of this product being beyond the control of the manufacturer, no guarantee, express or implied, is made as to the effects of such or the results to be obtained if not used in accordance with directions or established safe practice. The buyer must assume all responsibility, including injury or damage resulting from its misuse as such, or in combination with other materials.

Presentation: 16 fl oz (473 mL).

Compendium Code No.: 11420541 Rev 0998

SYNERKYL® PET DIP

DVM **Parasiticide Dip**

EPA Reg. No.: 28293-29-41835

Active Ingredient(s):

Pyrethrins	1.18%
Piperonyl Butoxide Technical*	11.84%
Inert Ingredients**	86.98%
Total	100.00%

*Equivalent to 9.47% (butylcarbityl) (6-propylpiperonyl) ether and 2.37% related compounds.

**Contains petroleum distillate.

Indications: Kills ticks, fleas and lice on cats and dogs.

Directions for Use: It is a violation of Federal law to use this product in a manner inconsistent with its labeling.

Read entire label before each use.

Use only on dogs and cats.

Dip or Sponge Bath: To control ticks, fleas and lice on cats and dogs, dilute the concentrate at the rate of 1 fluid ounce to 1 gallon of water and mix well to form a creamy emulsion dip. Dip or sponge the animal with the solution being careful to thoroughly wet the entire animal. Do not rinse. Allow solution to remain on animal. Reapply every two (2) weeks as needed.

Kennel: For control of insects in animal quarters and sleeping areas, dilute 1 ounce to 16 ounces of water and spray as a course spray. Spray cracks and crevices and other places insects can hide. Bedding should be removed and sprayed thoroughly. Remove pets before treating and ventilate area before allowing them to re-enter.

Precautionary Statements: Hazards to Humans and Domestic Animals:

Caution: Harmful if swallowed. Avoid breathing vapors. Avoid contact with eyes. In case of contact, immediately flush the eyes with plenty of water. Obtain medical attention if irritation persists. If swallowed, do not induce vomiting. Call a physician immediately. Avoid the contamination of feed and foodstuffs. Do not use on kittens or puppies under twelve (12) weeks of age. Consult a veterinarian before using this product on debilitated, medicated, aged, pregnant or nursing animals. Sensitivites may occur after using any pesticide product for pets. If signs of sensitivity occur, bathe your pet with mild soap and rinse with large amounts of water. If signs continue, consult a veterinarian immediately.

First Aid:

If Swallowed: Call a physician at once. Do not induce vomiting unless directed by a physician. Vomiting may cause aspiration pneumonia.

If on Skin: Wash with soap and water.

If in Eyes: Flush with plenty of water. Get medical attention if irritation persists.

Environmental Hazards: This product is toxic to fish. Do not apply directly to water. Do not contaminate water by cleaning equipment or disposal of waste.

Chemical and Physical Hazards: Do not use or store near heat or open flame.

Storage and Disposal:

Storage: Store in original container away from heat or open flame, in a locked storage area.

Disposal: Do not reuse bottle. Rinse thoroughly and wrap in newspaper before discarding in trash.

Warning(s): Keep out of reach of children.

Presentation: 64 fl oz (1.89 L).

Compendium Code No.: 11420561 Rev 0998

SYNOTIC® OTIC SOLUTION ℞

Fort Dodge **Otic Corticosteroid**

Fluocinolone Acetonide 0.01% And Dimethyl Sulfoxide 60%

NADA No.: 045-512

Active Ingredient(s): Formulation: Each mL of the solution contains 0.01% fluocinolone acetonide (6α,9α-difluoro-11β,16α,17,21-tetrahydroxypregna-1,4-diene-3,20-dione, cyclic 16,17-acetal with acetone) and 60% dimethyl sulfoxide in propylene glycol and citric acid.

Indications: SYNOTIC® Otic Solution Veterinary is indicated for the relief of pruritus and inflammation associated with acute and chronic otitis in the dog.

Pharmacology: General: Fluocinolone acetonide is an odorless crystalline powder essentially white in color. Other physical characteristics include:

Melting point	265°-277°C
Molecular weight	452.50

The structural formulation is:

Dimethyl sulfoxide (DMSO) an oxidation product of dimethyl sulfide, is the lowest member of the group of alkyl sulfoxides with a general formula of RSOR. Its structural formula is:

$$CH_3-\overset{\overset{\large O}{\|}}{S}-CH_3$$

It mixes freely with water with the evolution of heat and lowers the freezing point of aqueous solutions. It is soluble in many other compounds including ethanol, acetone, diethyl ether, glycerin, toluene, benzene and chloroform. DMSO is a solvent for many aromatic and unsaturated hydrocarbons as well as inorganic salts and nitrogen-containing compounds. DMSO has a high dielectric constant due to the polarity of the sulfur-oxygen bond. Its basicity is slightly greater than water due to enhanced electron density at the oxygen atom. It forms crystalline salts with strong protic acids and coordinates with Lewis acids. If modifies hydrogen bonding.

Propylene glycol is well established as being nonsensitizing, nontoxic and has antimicrobial activity. It has been selected for this formulation because of several useful properties: There is a low surface tension permitting great spreadability and penetration; its drying properties make it valuable in moist areas; the corticosteroid is highly soluble and stable in this vehicle; and a relatively slow rate of evaporation maintains the solution state for an adequate time to allow distribution and contact with all parts of the ear.

Fluocinolone acetonide is chemically related to prednisolone and possesses marked anti-inflammatory properties when applied topically. It has been shown to have over 100 times the anti-inflammatory activity of hydrocortisone. Fluocinolone acetonide decreases edema, inflammation, erythema, infiltration and pruritus with its associated scratching and excoriation. Following topical application of fluocinolone acetonide, especially at elevated dosage levels, systemic effects such as some adrenal suppression and weight loss have been observed. These effects, however, have been demonstrated to be reversible.

It has been demonstrated in the human, by both *in vivo* and *in vitro* methods, that DMSO enhances the percutaneous absorption of various compounds including steroids, vasoconstrictors, antiperspirants and dyes, as well as an anthelmintic (thiabendazole) and a skin antiseptic (hexachlorophene).[1,2,3,4,5] It was also shown in immature female rats that both estrogens and corticoids applied topically in DMSO exerted some of their usual biological effects.[6,7]

Dosage and Administration: The recommended dose of SYNOTIC® Otic Solution Veterinary is 4 to 6 drops (0.2 mL) per ear administered twice daily into the ear canal for a maximum period of 14 days. The total dosage used should not exceed 17 mL. It is recommended that the affected ear canal be cleansed by some appropriate method prior to the instillation of the solution. Following instillation, gentle external massage of the ear canal may aid in promoting an even distribution of the medication. Care should be taken to avoid contact of the medication with the dog's eyes. Contact of the bare hand with the medication should also be avoided.

Precaution(s): Very hygroscopic. Close vial tightly after use. Avoid freezing and excessive heat.

Caution(s): Federal law restricts this drug to use by or on the order of a licensed veterinarian.

There should be careful initial evaluation and follow-up of infected ears. Incomplete response or exacerbation of corticosteroid responsive lesions may be due to the presence of an infection which requires identification or antibiotic sensitivity testing, and the use of the appropriate antimicrobial agent. As with any corticosteroid, animals with a generalized infection should not be treated with this product without proper supportive antimicrobial therapy. Preparations with DMSO should not be used in pregnant animals since studies in chick embryos and guinea pigs have indicated it is teratogenic and embryotoxic.

SYNOTIC® (fluocinolone acetonide and dimethyl sulfoxide) Otic Solution Veterinary is recommended for topical application to the ear canal of the dog only.

Do not administer by any other route.

For animal use only.

Warning(s): Clinical and experimental data have demonstrated that corticosteroids administered orally or by injection to animals may induce the first stage of parturition if used during the last trimester of pregnancy and may precipitate premature parturition followed by dystocia, fetal death, retained placenta, and metritis.

Additionally, corticosteroids administered to dogs, rabbits, and rodents during pregnancy have resulted in cleft palate in offspring. Corticosteroids administered to dogs during pregnancy have also resulted in other congenital anomalies, including deformed forelegs, phocomelia and anasarca.

Toxicology:

Dimethyl Sulfoxide: Changes in the refractive index of the lens of the eye and nuclear cataracts have been observed in animals with the oral use of DMSO and appear to be related to high daily doses or a long duration of daily therapy. The lens changes were first observed in dogs receiving 5 g/kg of DMSO orally daily after 9 weeks of administration. Later studies revealed ocular effects at 4.5 mL/kg in 5-9 weeks and at 0.5-1 mL/kg for 19 weeks. These eye changes were slowly reversible but with a definite species difference, the dog being the slowest to exhibit improvement.

In a subsequent study conducted in dogs to determine the effects of a 90% dimethyl sulfoxide solution applied topically at a total daily dose of 20-60 mL for 21 consecutive days, no clinically meaningful ophthalmological effects were noted. No significant variations were observed in hematologic values or in other blood measurements including glucose, BUN, SGOT and plasma electrophoresis.

DMSO may facilitate the systemic absorption of other topically-applied drugs and may have a potentiating effect on drugs administered systemically. Medications containing DMSO as a vehicle should be used judiciously when administered in conjunction with other pharmaceutical preparations especially those affecting the cardiovascular and central nervous systems. Other medication should not be present at the site of its topical application. If other topical medications are indicated they should not be applied until after the medication containing DMSO is thoroughly dry.

DMSO is a potent solvent and may have a deleterious effect upon fabrics, plastics and other materials. Care should be taken to prevent physical contact with SYNOTIC® (fluocinolone acetonide and dimethyl sulfoxide) Otic Solution Veterinary when the drug is applied. Contact with the treated area should be avoided until drying of the treated ear canal has occurred.

Fluocinolone Acetonide: It is estimated that the maximum dosage dogs will tolerate, when fed fluocinolone acetonide daily for a period of 2 weeks, is less than 0.125 mg/kg. At this dose level animals lost weight and displayed diarrhea and intestinal inflammation. When dogs were fed fluocinolone acetonide daily for a period of three months the maximum daily dose tolerated is estimated to be between 0.05 and 0.125 mg/kg. At the lower dose the adrenal glands of treated dogs appeared somewhat smaller than the controls.

The intravenous lethal dose of fluocinolone acetonide in 50% aqueous propylene glycol is in excess of 50 mg/kg in mice and rabbits, in excess of 40 mg/kg in dogs, and in excess of 30 mg/kg in rats. The compound induced no pyrogenic response in rabbits nor sensitizing effects in guinea pigs. Gross or histologic effects were not encountered.

The lethal dose orally in dogs and cats exceeds 1 g/kg. There was lymphocytopenia in all animals and erythrocytosis in cats employed in this study.

Two g/kg of 0.05 to 0.2% fluocinolone acetonide applied daily 5 days per week for 3 weeks to the abraded skin of rabbits, resulted in neither local nor systemic toxicity.

Similar applications to intact skin for 13 weeks, including an additional group at 0.025%, resulted only in decreased body weight and adrenal size.

A small decrease in body weight was seen in dogs treated for 7 days with 0.5 mL (15 drops)/ear/day of SYNOTIC® (fluocinolone acetonide and dimethyl sulfoxide) Otic Solution Veterinary. In dogs which were treated for 21 days with 1.5 mL (45 drops)/ear/day of this formulation there was a slight loss of weight with changes in the adrenal glands consistent with corticosteroid treatment. This indicates absorption from the dogs' ears. This absorption, and concomitant effects, are probably enhanced by the action of DMSO.

In a subsequent study, dogs were treated with the recommended therapeutic dose of SYNOTIC® Otic Solution Veterinary at the rate of 12 drops (0.4 mL) per ear daily for 21 consecutive days. No significant changes were detected in clinical chemistry, urinalysis, or hematology. A reversible adrenal cortical atrophy with cortical cytoplasmic vacuolization was noted. An equivocal response was noted following ACTH administration on the day after SYNOTIC® Otic Solution Veterinary treatment was suspended, but after a one week recovery period, there was a definite eosinophile depression and recovery following ACTH administration, indicating normal adrenal function.

Side Effects: A transient, but mild, stinging sensation may be experienced by some animals when the solution is applied to denuded areas. The effect will disappear as healing progresses. A temporary increase in temperature of the area may also be noted.

Corticosteroid therapy will generally cause a remission of signs of allergic origin. However, until the causative agent is identified and removed from the animal's environment, the condition may recur when therapy is terminated.

Ordinarily, side effects are not encountered with topically applied corticosteroids; but as with all drugs, some animals may exhibit unfavorable local and/or systemic reactions. A local reaction may be due to sensitization to the corticosteroid or one of the other components of the solution.

It is known that DMSO enhances the percutaneous absorption of topically applied corticosteroids and the veterinarian should be aware of possible systemic reactions in this situation. Accordingly, this product is contraindicated wherever systemic corticosteroids would be dangerous. Adrenal suppression, weight loss and increased susceptibility to infections may be evidenced with the use of this drug, especially in overdosage. Therefore, care should be taken to assure that the recommended dosage is not exceeded.

In the presence of local and/or systemic side effects, the drug should be withdrawn. When a local reaction occurs other therapeutic measures should be instituted. Therapy can usually be resumed at a lower dose once systemic signs abate, without further recurrence of the problem.

Absorption of DMSO following topical application may result in an odorous breath described as oyster or garlic-like with an unpleasant taste. Some animals and clients may find this objectionable but these effects are transient and not considered to be of serious consequence.

References: Available upon request.

Presentation: SYNOTIC® (fluocinolone acetonide and dimethyl sulfoxide) Otic Solution Veterinary available in dropper vials of 8 mL (NDC 0856-0120-06) and 60 mL (NDC 0856-0120-14).

U.S. Pat. No. 3,126,375

Compendium Code No.: 10032131 0140B

SYNOVEX® C

Fort Dodge **Implant**

Calf Implants For Increased Rate of Weight Gain

NADA No.: 009-576

Active Ingredient(s): Each dosage consists of 4 pellets containing 100 mg progesterone and 10 mg estradiol benzoate per implantation. This product was manufactured by a non-sterilizing process.

SYNOVEX® C Calf Implants contain two pure steroid hormones, progesterone and estradiol benzoate. This formulation provides a complementary amount of each hormone for maximal growth stimulation.

Indications: SYNOVEX® C is recommended for use in suckling beef calves up to approximately 400 lbs of body weight. SYNOVEX® C is also recommended for improvement in rate of weight gain in steers weighing greater than 400 pounds and fed in confinement for slaughter when used as part of a re-implant program in which an initial SYNOVEX® C implant is followed at approximately 70 days by Synovex® S.

Dosage and Administration: Implant complete contents of one cartridge cell per calf at each implanting.

How to Implant with SYNOVEX® Pellets: Study the following instructions carefully, then proceed step by step, until the technique becomes routine. Many head can be implanted per hour by an experienced team, one member of which should be assigned to do nothing but the implantation. This person should maintain hand cleanliness and use sanitary instruments only.

Synovex® Gun:

Step 1 - Loading the Synovex® Gun: Load the Synovex® gun following the directions outlined in the instruction manual accompanying each Synovex® gun.

Step 2 - Restraint: Calves must be adequately restrained prior to implantation to minimize movement of the head. Heavier calves may be confined in a restraint mechanism (squeeze gate or head gate). The implant site on the back of the ear should be prepared by scrubbing with a generous-sized piece of cotton that has been soaked in a germicidal solution.

Step 3 - Implant Site: Divide the ear into three imaginary sections. The implanted pellets should be deposited in the center one-third of the ear. To accomplish this, the Synovex® gun needle should be inserted in the outer one-third of the ear. Implanting too close to the head may cause side effects. Care should be taken to avoid severing the major arteries of the ear.

Step 4 - Insert Needle: Grasp the ear with one hand. Holding the Synovex® gun firmly with the other hand, penetrate the skin. Thrust the needle under the skin taking care not to penetrate the cartilage. Ease the Synovex® gun forward (toward the base of the ear) until the full needle length is beneath the skin.

Step 5 - Pellet Implantation: When the needle is completely inserted, withdraw the needle approximately one-half inch. Then with continuous gentle pressure on the trigger, expel the pellets while continuing to slowly withdraw the needle. This technique allows the pellets to be deposited in a straight line in the path of the needle.

Step 6 - Inspection: Check the implant site. If properly administered, the implants should lie in a straight line under the skin.

Disinfect the Synovex® gun needle in a germicidal solution. You are now ready to implant the next animal.

Synovex® SX10® Gun*:

Step 1 - Loading the SX10® Gun: Load the SX10® gun following the directions outlined in the instruction manual accompanying each SX10® gun.

Step 2 - Restraint: The animal must be confined in a restraint mechanism (squeeze chute or head gate). The implant site on the back of the ear should be prepared by scrubbing with a generous-sized piece of cotton that has been soaked in a germicidal solution.

Note: If implanting horned cattle, greater safety is provided when the head is controlled by the use of a bull lead (nose tongs).

Step 3 - Implant Site: Divide the ear into three imaginary sections. The implanted pellets should be deposited in the center one-third of the ear. To accomplish this, the SX10® gun needle should be inserted in the outer one-third of the ear. Implanting too close to the head may cause abnormal sexual behavior. Care should be taken to avoid severing the major arteries of the ear.

Step 4 - Insert Needle: Just before grasping the ear with one hand, release the safety by striking the butt of the gun. Holding the SX10® gun firmly with the other hand, penetrate the skin. Thrust the needle under the skin taking care not to penetrate the cartilage. Ease the SX10® gun forward (toward the base of the ear) until the full needle length is beneath the skin.

Step 5 - Pellet Implantation: When the needle is completely inserted, activate the instrument by squeezing the trigger completely. Do not withdraw the needle, but allow the automatic needle retractor to release the pellets. This will allow the pellets to be deposited in a straight line in the path of the retracted needle.

Step 6 - Inspection: Check the implant site. If properly administered, the implants should lie in a straight line under the skin.

Disinfect the SX10® gun needle in a germicidal solution and recock the instrument by rotating the cocking grip left, pull back, rotate right, then push all the way forward. You are now ready to implant the next animal.

Note: Never sacrifice careful, clean technique for speed of implantation.

Precaution(s): Do not refrigerate — Store at controlled room temperature 15° to 30°C (59° to 86°F). Avoid excessive heat or humidity.
Caution(s): Bulling, rectal and vaginal prolapse, udder development, ventral edema and elevated tailheads have occasionally been reported in calves administered with SYNOVEX® C implants.
Restricted drug (California) — Use only as directed.
Warning(s): Implant pellets in the ear only. Any other location is in violation of federal law. Do not attempt salvage of implanted site for human or animal food.
Do not use in bull calves intended for reproduction, or in calves less than 45 days old.
Hazardous: Keep this and all drugs out of the reach of children.
For animal use only. For subcutaneous ear implantation only.
Presentation: 2 cartridges (20 doses) (NDC 0856-3903-02) and 10 cartridges (100 doses) (NDC 0856-3903-43). Each cartridge contains 10 rows of 4 pellets.
* U.S. Patent Nos. 4,223,674 and 4,474,572
Compendium Code No.: 10032140 6034A

SYNOVEX® H

Fort Dodge **Implant**
Heifer Implants
NADA No.: 011-427
Active Ingredient(s): Each dosage consists of 8 pellets containing 200 mg testosterone propionate and 20 mg estradiol benzoate per implantation. This product was manufactured by a non-sterilizing process.
Indications: SYNOVEX® H is recommended for use in heifers weighing 400 lbs or more.
When properly administered, SYNOVEX® H implants increase rate of weight gain and improve feed efficiency.
Dosage and Administration: Implant complete contents of one cartridge cell per heifer.
How to Implant with SYNOVEX® Pellets: Study the following instructions carefully, then proceed step by step, until the technique becomes routine. Many head can be implanted per hour by an experienced team, one member of which should be assigned to do nothing but the implantation. This person should maintain hand cleanliness and use sanitary instruments only.
Synovex® Gun:
Step 1 - Loading the Synovex® Gun: Load the Synovex® gun following the directions outlined in the instruction manual accompanying each Synovex® gun.
Step 2 - Restraint: The animal must be confined in a restraint mechanism (squeeze chute or head gate). The implant site on the back of the ear should be prepared by scrubbing with a generous-sized piece of cotton that has been soaked in a germicidal solution.
Note: If implanting horned cattle, greater safety is provided when the head is controlled by the use of a bull lead (nose tongs).
Step 3 - Implant Site: Divide the ear into three imaginary sections. The implanted pellets should be deposited in the center one-third of the ear. To accomplish this, the Synovex® gun needle should be inserted in the outer one-third of the ear. Implanting too close to the head may cause abnormal sexual behavior. Care should be taken to avoid severing the major arteries of the ear.
Step 4 - Insert Needle: Grasp the ear with one hand. Holding the Synovex® gun firmly with the other hand, penetrate the skin. Thrust the needle under the skin taking care not to penetrate the cartilage. Ease the Synovex® gun forward (toward the base of the ear) until the full needle length is beneath the skin.
Step 5 - Pellet Implantation: When the needle is completely inserted, withdraw the needle approximately one-half inch. Then with continuous gentle pressure on the trigger, expel the pellets while continuing to slowly withdraw the needle. This technique allows the pellets to be deposited in a straight line in the path of the needle.
Step 6 - Inspection: Check the implant site. If properly administered, the implants should lie in a straight line under the skin.
Disinfect the Synovex® gun needle in a germicidal solution. You are now ready to implant the next animal.
Synovex® SX10® Gun*:
Step 1 - Loading the SX10® Gun: Load the SX10® gun following the directions outlined in the instruction manual accompanying each SX10® gun.
Step 2 - Restraint: The animal must be confined in a restraint mechanism (squeeze chute or head gate). The implant site on the back of the ear should be prepared by scrubbing with a generous-sized piece of cotton that has been soaked in a germicidal solution.
Note: If implanting horned cattle, greater safety is provided when the head is controlled by the use of a bull lead (nose tongs).
Step 3 - Implant Site: Divide the ear into three imaginary sections. The implanted pellets should be deposited in the center one-third of the ear. To accomplish this, the SX10® gun needle should be inserted in the outer one-third of the ear. Implanting too close to the head may cause abnormal sexual behavior. Care should be taken to avoid severing the major arteries of the ear.
Step 4 - Insert Needle: Just before grasping the ear with one hand, release the safety by striking the butt of the gun. Holding the SX10® gun firmly with the other hand, penetrate the skin. Thrust the needle under the skin taking care not to penetrate the cartilage. Ease the SX10® gun forward (toward the base of the ear) until the full needle length is beneath the skin.
Step 5 - Pellet Implantation: When the needle is completely inserted, activate the instrument by squeezing the trigger completely. Do not withdraw the needle, but allow the automatic needle retractor to release the pellets. This will allow the pellets to be deposited in a straight line in the path of the retracted needle.
Step 6 - Inspection: Check the implant site. If properly administered, the implants should lie in a straight line under the skin.
Disinfect the SX10® gun needle in a germicidal solution and recock the instrument by rotating the cocking grip left, pull back, rotate right, then push all the way forward. You are now ready to implant the next animal.
Note: Never sacrifice careful, clean technique for speed of implantation.
Precaution(s): Do not refrigerate — Store at controlled room temperature 15° to 30°C (59° to 86°F). Avoid excessive heat or humidity.
Caution(s): Bulling, vaginal and rectal prolapse, udder development, ventral edema and elevated tailheads have occasionally been reported in heifers administered with SYNOVEX® H implants.
Restricted drug (California) — Use only as directed.
Warning(s): Not for dairy or beef replacement heifers. Implant pellets in the ear only. Any other location is in violation of federal law. Do not attempt salvage of implanted site for human or animal food.
Hazardous: Keep this and all drugs out of the reach of children.
For heifers only. For animal use only. For subcutaneous ear implantation only.
Presentation: 10 cartridges (100 doses) (NDC 0856-3901-40). Each cartridge contains 10 rows of 8 pellets.
* U.S. Patent Nos. 4,223,674 and 4,474,572
Compendium Code No.: 10032150 6042D

SYNOVEX® PLUS™

Fort Dodge **Implant**
(trenbolone acetate and estradiol benzoate) Implants for Steers and Heifers Fed in Confinement for Slaughter
NADA No.: 141-043
Active Ingredient(s): SYNOVEX® PLUS™ (trenbolone acetate and estradiol benzoate) is a growth promoting implant containing 200 mg of trenbolone acetate and 28 mg of estradiol benzoate. Each implant consists of 8 pellets.
Manufactured by a non-sterilizing process.
Indications: SYNOVEX® PLUS™ is recommended for increased rate of weight gain and improved feed efficiency in steers and for increased rate of weight gain in heifers fed in confinement for slaughter.
Dosage and Administration:
Directions: Implant complete contents of one cartridge cell per steer or heifer.
Dosage: One implant (eight pellets), containing 200 mg of trenbolone acetate and 28 mg of estradiol benzoate, is administered to each steer or heifer by subcutaneous implantation in the middle one-third of the ear.
The ten-dose cartridge of SYNOVEX® PLUS™ is designed to be used exclusively with a Synovex® implanting device.
How to Implant SYNOVEX® PLUS™ Pellets: For use with any Synovex® Gun: Study the following instructions carefully, then proceed step by step, until the technique becomes routine. Many head can be implanted per hour by an experienced team, one member of which should be assigned to do nothing but the implantation. Care should be taken to insure the hands of the person administering the implant are clean and only sanitary instruments are used.
Step 1 - Loading the SX10® Gun*: Load the SX10® gun following the directions outlined in the instruction manual accompanying each SX10® gun.
Step 2 - Restraint: The animal must be confined in a restraint mechanism (squeeze chute or head gate). The implant site on the back of the ear should be prepared by scrubbing with a generous-sized piece of cotton that has been soaked in a germicidal solution.
Note: If implanting horned cattle, greater safety is provided when the head is controlled by the use of a bull lead (nose tongs).
Step 3 - Implant Site: Divide the ear into three imaginary sections. The implanted pellets should be deposited in the center one-third of the ear. To accomplish this, the SX10® gun needle should be inserted in the outer one-third of the ear. Implanting too close to the head may cause abnormal sexual behavior. Care should be taken to avoid severing the major arteries of the ear.
Step 4 - Insert Needle: Just before grasping the ear with one hand, release the safety by striking the butt of the gun. Holding the SX10® gun firmly with the other hand, penetrate the skin. Thrust the needle under the skin taking care not to penetrate the cartilage. Ease the SX10® gun forward (toward the base of the ear) until the full needle length is beneath the skin.
Step 5 - Pellet Implantation: When the needle is completely inserted, activate the instrument by squeezing the trigger completely. Do not withdraw the needle, but allow the automatic needle retractor to release the pellets. This will allow the pellets to be deposited in a straight line in the path of the retracted needle.
Step 6 - Inspection: Check the implant site. If properly administered, the implants should lie in a straight line under the skin.
Disinfect the SX10® gun needle in a germicidal solution and recock the instrument by rotating the cocking grip left, pull back, rotate right, then push all the way forward. You are now ready to implant the next animal.
Note: Never sacrifice careful, clean technique for speed of implantation.
Precaution(s): Store unopened product at room temperature. Avoid excessive heat and humidity. Use product before the expiration date on the label.
Once the pouch is opened, unused product may be stored in the end-folded pouch (away from light) for up to six months under refrigerated conditions (2-8°C/36-47°F) or at room temperature (15-30°C/59-86°F) for up to one month.
Caution(s): Bulling, vaginal and rectal prolapse, udder development, ventral edema and elevated tailheads have occasionally been reported in heifers administered SYNOVEX® PLUS™ implants.
Restricted Drug (California) — Use only as directed.
Warning(s): Not for dairy or beef replacement heifers. Implant pellets in ear only. Any other location is a violation of Federal law. Do not attempt salvage of implanted site for human or animal food.
For animal use only.
Not for use in humans.
Keep this and all drugs out of the reach of children.
Trial Data: Studies have demonstrated that the administration of SYNOVEX® PLUS™ can result in decreased marbling scores when compared to non-implanted steers and heifers.
Presentation: One pouch contains ten 10-dose cartridges (100 implants) (NDC 0856-3904-10). Each cartridge contains 10 rows of 8 pellets.
* U.S. Patent Nos. 4,223,674 and 4,474,572
Compendium Code No.: 10032160 6053E

SYNOVEX® S

Fort Dodge **Implant**
Steer Implants For Increased Rate of Weight Gain and Improved Feed Efficiency
NADA No.: 009-576
Active Ingredient(s): Each dosage consists of 8 pellets containing 200 mg progesterone and 20 mg estradiol benzoate per implantation. This product was manufactured by a non-sterilizing process.
SYNOVEX® S Steer Implants contain two pure steroid hormones, progesterone and estradiol benzoate. This formulation provides a complementary amount of each hormone for maximal growth stimulation.
Indications: SYNOVEX® S is recommended for use in steers weighing 400 lbs or more.
When properly administered, SYNOVEX® S implants increase rate of weight gain and improve feed efficiency.
Dosage and Administration: Implant complete contents of one cartridge cell per steer.
How to Implant with SYNOVEX® Pellets: Study the following instructions carefully, then proceed step by step, until the technique becomes routine. Many head can be implanted per hour by an experienced team, one member of which should be assigned to do nothing but the implantation. This person should maintain hand cleanliness and use sanitary instruments only.
Synovex® Gun:
Step 1 - Loading the Synovex® Gun: Load the Synovex® gun following the directions outlined in the instruction manual accompanying each Synovex® gun.
Step 2 - Restraint: The animal must be confined in a restraint mechanism (squeeze chute or

head gate). The implant site on the back of the ear should be prepared by scrubbing with a generous-sized piece of cotton that has been soaked in a germicidal solution.

Note: If implanting horned cattle, greater safety is provided when the head is controlled by the use of a bull lead (nose tongs).

Step 3 - Implant Site: Divide the ear into three imaginary sections. The implanted pellets should be deposited in the center one-third of the ear. To accomplish this, the Synovex® gun needle should be inserted in the outer one-third of the ear. Implanting too close to the head may cause abnormal sexual behavior. Care should be taken to avoid severing the major arteries of the ear.

Step 4 - Insert Needle: Grasp the ear with one hand. Holding the Synovex® gun firmly with the other hand, penetrate the skin. Thrust the needle under the skin taking care not to penetrate the cartilage. Ease the Synovex® gun forward (toward the base of the ear) until the full needle length is beneath the skin.

Step 5 - Pellet Implantation: When the needle is completely inserted, withdraw the needle approximately one-half inch. Then with continuous gentle pressure on the trigger, expel the pellets while continuing to slowly withdraw the needle. This technique allows the pellets to be deposited in a straight line in the path of the needle.

Step 6 - Inspection: Check the implant site. If properly administered, the implants should lie in a straight line under the skin.

Disinfect the Synovex® gun needle in a germicidal solution. You are now ready to implant the next animal.

Synovex® SX10® Gun*:

Step 1 - Loading the SX10® Gun: Load the SX10® gun following the directions outlined in the instruction manual accompanying each SX10® gun.

Step 2 - Restraint: The animal must be confined in a restraint mechanism (squeeze chute or head gate). The implant site on the back of the ear should be prepared by scrubbing with a generous-sized piece of cotton that has been soaked in a germicidal solution.

Note: If implanting horned cattle, greater safety is provided when the head is controlled by the use of a bull lead (nose tongs).

Step 3 - Implant Site: Divide the ear into three imaginary sections. The implanted pellets should be deposited in the center one-third of the ear. To accomplish this, the SX10® gun needle should be inserted in the outer one-third of the ear. Implanting too close to the head may cause abnormal sexual behavior. Care should be taken to avoid severing the major arteries of the ear.

Step 4 - Insert Needle: Just before grasping the ear with one hand, release the safety by striking the butt of the gun. Holding the SX10® gun firmly with the other hand, penetrate the skin. Thrust the needle under the skin taking care not to penetrate the cartilage. Ease the SX10® gun forward (toward the base of the ear) until the full needle length is beneath the skin.

Step 5 - Pellet Implantation: When the needle is completely inserted, activate the instrument by squeezing the trigger completely. Do not withdraw the needle, but allow the automatic needle retractor to release the pellets. This will allow the pellets to be deposited in a straight line in the path of the retracted needle.

Step 6 - Inspection: Check the implant site. If properly administered, the implants should lie in a straight line under the skin.

Disinfect the SX10® gun needle in a germicidal solution and recock the instrument by rotating the cocking grip left, pull back, rotate right, then push all the way forward. You are now ready to implant the next animal.

For additional improvement in rate of weight gain in steers fed in confinement for slaughter, reimplant at approximately 70 days.

Note: Never sacrifice careful, clean technique for speed of implantation.

Precaution(s): Do not refrigerate — Store at controlled room temperature 15° to 30°C (59° to 86°F). Avoid excessive heat or humidity.

Caution(s): Bulling, rectal prolapse, ventral edema and elevated tailheads have occasionally been reported in steers administered with SYNOVEX® S implants.

Restricted drug (California) — Use only as directed.

Warning(s): Implant pellets in the ear only. Any other location is in violation of federal law. Do not attempt salvage of implanted site for human or animal food.

Hazardous: Keep this and all drugs out of the reach of children.

For steers only.

For animal use only.

For subcutaneous ear implantation only.

Trial Data: Studies have demonstrated that reimplantation of SYNOVEX® S can decrease marbling scores when compared to non-implanted controls.

Presentation: 10 cartridges (100 doses) (NDC 0856-3902-40). Each cartridge contains 10 rows of 8 pellets.

* U.S. Patent Nos. 4,223,674 and 4,474,572

Compendium Code No.: 10032170 6062D

SYNPHENOL-3™

V.P.L. **Disinfectant**

EPA Reg. No.: 11725-7-43591

Active Ingredient(s):

Ortho-phenylphenol	12.00%
Ortho-benzyl-para-chlorophenol	10.00%
Para-teritiary-amylphenol	4.00%
Inert ingredients	74.00%
Total	100.00%

Indications: SYNPHENOL-3™ is a synthetic detergent with a broad spectrum kill of gram-positive and gram-negative micro-organisms, provides effective cleaning and disinfecting in one operation, non-flammable and non-volatile in use dilutions, soluble, dilutes in hot, cold, soft, or hard water of up to 1,000 ppm water hardness.

The SYNPHENOL-3™ high foaming detergent system has been formulated to provide heavy-duty cleaning, wetting and penetration of soils and organic matter and easy rinsing of surfaces. The clinging foam is obtained at ½ oz. per gallon of water (1:256) to provide prolonged contact time.

SYNPHENOL-3™ at ½ oz. per gallon of water (1:256) provides residual control of odor-causing bacteria in the presence of moisture.

SYNPHENOL-3™ is recommended for use when used as directed on ceramic and glazed tile surfaces, stainless steel, aluminum, chrome, galvanized metal, glass and other nonporous surfaces such as treated wood, polyethylene, polypropylene, PVD (polyvinyl chloride), polystyrene, vinyl, fiberglass, viton, ethylene propylene, nitrite, acrylic and polyurethane.

SYNPHENOL-3™ at ½ oz. per gallon of water (1:256) is suited for disinfecting and cleaning in all animal care facilities and research centers, veterinary facilities, zoos, kennels, equine facilities including stables, stalls, breeding and foaling areas and transport vehicles.

Toxicity tests required by the U.S. Environment Protection Agency for SYNPHENOL-3™ disinfectant cleaner have been done, in conformity with the FDA and EPA Good Laboratory Practice Regulations.

Proven effective as a disinfectant by the following tests: A.O.A.C. (use dilution test method) in conformance with the 14th Edition 1984. All dilutions at (1:256). The following organisms tested at 1,000 ppm water hardness as calcium carbonate and 10% horse serum (as organic soil): *Staphylococcus aureus* (ATCC #6538), *Streptococcus pyogenes* (ATCC #9342), *Shigella sonnei* (ATCC #25931), *Klebsiella pneumoniae* (ATCC #4352), *Enterobacter aerogenes* (ATCC #13048), *Proteus vulgaris* (ATCC #13315), *Pseudomonas aeruginosa* (ATCC #15442), *Trichophyton mentagrophytes* (ATCC #9533 A.O.A.C. fungicidal test), *Pasteurella multocida* (ATCC #6529) (fowl cholera), *Pasteurella anapestifer, Beta streptococcus* (ATTC #19615), *Mycoplasma synoviae, Rhodococcus equi* (ATCC #6939), *Salmonella choleraesuis* Kunzendorf strain, *Taylorella equigenitalis* (C.E.M.), *Salmonella enteritidis* (ATCC #13076), *Aspergillus fumigatus* (ATTC #6285), *Salmonella choleraesuis* (ATCC #10708), *Salmonella schottmulleri* (ATTC #8749), *Salmonella pullorum* (ATTC #19945), *Salmonella gallinarum* (ATCC #9184), *Salmonella typhimurium* (ATCC #13311), *Salmonella arizonae* (#7:1,7,8), *Salmonella arizonae* PD 36, *Escherichia coli* (ATCC #11229), *Alcaligenes faecalis* strain #838, *Alcaligenes faecalis* Georgia strain, *Staphylococcus epidermidis*, Enterococci group D species, *Mycoplasma gallisepticum, Staphylococcus hyicus, Streptococcus equi* (ATCC #39506), *Streptococcus suis* (type II) and *Streptococcus pyogenes* (ATCC #19615).

*The following viruses tested in accordance with U.S. Environmental Protection Agency pesticide Assessment Guidelines on inanimate environmental surfaces. Tested at 1,000 ppm water hardness calcium carbonate and 10% serum (as organic soil): Herpes simplex type 1, Avian infections bronchitis virus, transmissible gastroenteritis virus (Purdue strains, ATCC #VR-763), canine parvovirus, strain CPV MLV (Cornell), parainfluenza virus type 1, Sendai strain ATCC #VR 105, avian rotavirus AVR-1, duck enteritis virus (D.V.E.), avian laryngotracheitis, Newcastle disease virus, avian influenza virus, pseudorabies virus (Aujeszky strain ATCC #VR-135), mouse hepatitis virus (strain MHV-A59 ATCC #VR-764), avian adenovirus, equine herpes virus ATCC #VR-700 (equine rhinopneumonitis), equine arteritis ATCC #VR-796 (equine viral arteritis) and influenza A-2/Hong Kong virus (ATCC #VR-544).

Hard surface mildewcidal test method: CSMA method 23 at 1,000 ppm water hardness as calcium carbonate and 10% serum (as organic soil): Aspergillus niger ATCC #6275 (black mold) and penicillium variable NRRL #3765 (green mold).

Directions for Use: It is a violation of federal law to use the product in a manner inconsistent with its labeling.

General use directions:

1. To clean, disinfect and deodorize walls, floors, tables, drinking fountains, sinks, refrigerators, stoves, restroom fixtures and garbage cans: Remove gross filth and heavy soil with a preliminary cleaning step prior to the application of SYNPHENOL-3™. Apply a solution of ½ oz. of SYNPHENOL-3™ per gallon of water (1:256) with a sponge, mop, mechanical spray device or a foaming apparatus making sure that all surfaces are wetted thoroughly. Allow the surface to remain wet for 10 minutes. Air dry.
2. To clean and disinfect such articles as combs, brushes, razors, scissors, instruments and rubber goods: All instruments and devices must be thoroughly cleaned to remove excess debris, rinsed and rough dried, including the hollows and lumens, before immersion in the solution. Soak for 10 minutes in a solution containing ½ oz. of SYNPHENOL-3™ per gallon of water (1:256).
3. To disinfect fabrics such as linens and uniforms: First rinse to remove gross filth or heavy soil, then soak for 10 minutes in a solution containing ½ oz. of SYNPHENOL-3™ per gallon of water (1:256).
4. To clean gross filth or heavy soil on surfaces prior to disinfection, use ½ oz. of SYNPHENOL-3™ per gallon of water (1:256).

Precautionary Statements:

Hazards to Humans and Domestic Animals: Danger. Corrosive. Causes eye and skin damage. Do not get in the eyes, on the skin, or on clothing. Wear goggles or a face shield and rubber gloves when handling. May be harmful or fatal if swallowed. Wash thoroughly with soap and water after handling and before eating, drinking or using tobacco. Remove contaminated clothing and wash before reuse.

Statement of Practical Treatment:

If on skin: Wash with plenty of soap and water. Get medical attention.

If in eyes: Hold the eyelids open and flush eyes with plenty of water. Get medical attention.

If swallowed: Call a physician immediately. Drink large quantities of water. Never give anything by mouth to an unconscious person. Avoid alcohol.

Note to Physician: Probable mucosal damage may contraindicate the use of gastric lavage. Measure against circulatory shock, respiratory depression and convulsion may be needed.

Storage and Disposal: Do not contaminate water food or feed by storage or disposal.

Pesticide Disposal: Pesticide wastes are acutely hazardous. Improper disposal of excess pesticide, spray mixture, or rinsate is a violation of federal law. If these wastes cannot be disposed of according to label instructions, contact a state pesticide or an environmental control agency, or the hazardous waste representative at the nearest EPA regional office for guidance.

Container Disposal (plastic): Triple rinse (or equivalent). Then offer for recycling or reconditioning, or puncture and dispose of in a sanitary landfill, or by incineration, or, if allowed by state and local authorities, by burning. If burned, stay out of smoke.

Warning(s): Keep out of the reach of children.

Presentation: 64 oz. containers.

Compendium Code No.: 11430310

SYN SHIELD™

Novartis Animal Vaccines **Vaccine**

Bovine Respiratory Syncytial Virus Vaccine, Killed Virus

U.S. Vet. Lic. No.: 303

Composition: The vaccine is prepared from a highly antigenic strain of BRSV propagated on an established bovine cell line. The vaccine is chemically inactivated and adjuvanted with Xtend III™ to provide long-lasting efficacy. Contains penicillin, streptomycin, amphotericin B, and thimerosal as preservatives.

Indications: For use in healthy cattle for the prevention of diseases caused by respiratory syncytial virus.

Dosage and Administration: Shake well before using. Administer a 2 mL dose intramuscularly to cattle. Repeat in four (4) to five (5) weeks. Calves vaccinated before weaning should be revaccinated after weaning. The vaccine may be administered to pregnant animals at any stage of gestation. Vaccinate dairy cows during the drying-off period. Revaccinate annually to maintain high levels of immunity.

Precaution(s): Store at 35°-45°F (2°-7°C). Do not freeze. Use the entire contents when first opened.

Caution(s): Transient swelling may occur at the site of injection. Milk reduction and transient

S

depression may be observed in lactating dairy cows two to four days following vaccination. Anaphylactic reactions may occur following the use of the vaccine. Symptomatic treatment: Epinephrine.

Warning(s): Do not vaccinate within 60 days before slaughter.

Discussion: Bovine respiratory syncytial virus (BRSV) was first isolated in the United States in 1974 and recently has been identified as a major contributing agent in the bovine respiratory disease (BRD) syndrome. It was named BRSV because it invades the cell lining of the air passages of the trachea and lungs and promotes the formation of large multinucleated cells called syncytial cells in the lung. BRSV appears to be widespread across the United States. In states where antibody prevalence testing has been done, 60% to 80% of the cattle tested are positive. Since research and information on BRSV are incomplete, we can only give a partial description of the disease syndrome produced by this virus.

An initial exposure to the virus usually produces: (1) a mild subclinical infection which occurs approximately five days after stress and exposure. Within 2-10 days after recovery from the primary infection some animals will exhibit (2) a severe clinical form of the disease, which if untreated will last 12-14 days and result in a high percentage of deaths. The course and severity of the disease can be aggravated by invasion of the weakened animal by other viral and bacterial pathogens.

1. The mild subclinical infection can affect animals of all ages. It is most commonly associated with other stressors such as inclement weather, overcrowding, nutritional and feed factors, fatigue, transport, etc. In most animals, the following symptoms occur but are usually not detected: anorexia, coughing, mild nasal and ocular discharge and fever ranging from 104-108°F. The animals tend to stand alone, head down, but appear to brighten up and run off when approached. During this phase, the virus is actively invading and replicating in the ciliated epithelial lining of the airways. This is the only stage of the disease in which the virus can be isolated from the animal and identified. The virus destroys the cilia, which are vital to the mechanism for clearing the air passages of the foreign particles. Dust is particularly aggravating and harmful to animals in this stage. Recovery usually follows this five- to seven-day infective phase, although the cough commonly persists.
2. In some animals a severe clinical form will occur 2-10 days after recovery from the milder form. These animals exhibit severe respiratory distress, a dry hacking cough, fever ranging from 105-109°F, nasal and ocular discharge, salivation and subcutaneous edema especially below the jaw and neck areas. The oxygen supply for many of these animals is so deficient that they will go completely off feed and water. Some will stand over the water trough unable to interrupt their breathing cycle long enough to drink. During this stage, BRS virus is not recoverable from the animal; however, the antibody titer does peak. Because of this many authors believe that the symptoms and lesions seen at this stage are a result of a hypersensitivity reaction in the animal. On the other hand, recent research demonstrates the virus present in large numbers in the cell lining of the infected lungs. Necropsy reveals firm, reddened, noncollapsed lungs characteristic of interstitial pneumonia. In addition, subpleural and interstitial air pockets and fluid accumulation are seen in all lobes of the lungs as well as at the base of the lungs.

The inflamed and weakened lungs resulting from either of these forms of BRSV are highly susceptible to invasion by bacterial pathogens such as *Pasteurella hemolytica* or *Haemophilus somnus*. In addition, viruses such as BVD, IBR or PI3 can and do contribute to the severity of BRSV disease or infect the animal weakened by it. Treatment is effective when it is instituted early, but it is very expensive both in terms of medical costs and production losses.

Trial Data: (Virus Re-isolation): BRSV was recovered from 75% of the controls (virus persisted for nine days), but from only 22% of the vaccinates (virus persisted for only two days). Re-isolation began the same day as challenge and was conducted over the 14-day period.

(Significance P = 0.02 level.)

	BRSV SN Titers*	
	Vaccinates	Controls
Prevaccination	1:4.5	1:3.0
6 weeks post 2nd vaccination or prechallenge	1:40	1:7
28 days post challenge	1:47	1:71

*Geometric mean SN titer.

Serum neutralization values demonstrated seroconversion in all 18 animals vaccinated with two doses of the vaccine. Six weeks post second vaccination, all BRSV vaccinated animals developed BRSV antibodies showing a 2-36 fold increase in antibody titer.

References: Available upon request.

Presentation: Available in 50 dose (100 mL) bottles.

Compendium Code No.: 11140503

T

T-4 POWDER ℞

Neogen **Thyroid Therapy**

Levothyroxine Sodium USP (0.22%)

Active Ingredient(s): Each pound (453.6 g) contains:

Levothyroxine Sodium USP . . . . . 0.22% (1.0 g)
One teaspoon contains. . . . . 12 mg of T-4
One tablespoon contains . . . . . 36 mg of T-4

Indications: For use in horses for correction of conditions associated with low circulating thyroid hormone (hypothyroidism).

Dosage and Administration:

Dosage: The suggested initial dose is 0.5 to 3.0 mg levothyroxine sodium (T-4) per 100 lbs of body weight (1 to 6 mg per 100 kg) once per day or in divided doses. Response to the administration of T-4 POWDER should be evaluated clinically until an adequate maintenance dose is established. In most horses, the total daily dose of T-4 is in the range of 6 to 36 mg. Serum T-3 and T-4 values can vary greatly among individual horses on thyroid supplementation. Dosages should be individualized and animals should be monitored daily for clinical signs of hyperthyroidism or hypersensitivity.

Administration: T-4 POWDER can be administered by mixing the daily dose in the concentrate or by top dressing on the grain, preferably rolled or ground. To facilitate the proper adhesion of T-4 POWDER to the ration, slightly moisten the grain with water or a liquid supplement.

Precaution(s): Store at controlled room temperature between 15°-30°C (59°-86°F) and protect from light. Avoid excessive heat (104°F).

Caution(s): Federal law restricts this drug to use by or on the order of a licensed veterinarian.

Administer with caution to animals with clinically significant heart disease, hypertension or other complications for which a sharply increased metabolic rate might prove hazardous. Use in pregnant mares has not been evaluated.

For animal use only.

Warning(s): Keep out of reach of children.

Presentation: 1 lb jars (12 per case) (NDC: 59051-9080-4) and 10 lb buckets (individually packaged) (NDC: 59051-9081-9).

Manufactured by: Sparhawk, Laboratories, Lenexa, KS 66215.

Compendium Code No.: 14910132 0501

T8 SOLUTION™ EAR RINSE

DVM **Otic Cleanser**

Active Ingredient(s): Purified Water USP, Benzyl Alcohol, Nonoxynol 12, PPG-12/PEG-50 Lanolin, Tromethamine Base, Tromethamine HCl and Tetrasodium Edetate.

Indications: For rinse of ears to aid in removal of wax and debris before use of medicated therapies.

Product Description: T8 SOLUTION™ is an alkaline (pH 8.5), water based formulation designed to gently cleanse and rinse ear canals in preparation for more extensive therapies.

A ready to use ear rinse and pretreatment solution for dogs and cats.

Directions for Use: Shake well before use. apply T8 SOLUTION™ liberally into ear canal. Gently massage base of ear to help break up and remove accumulated internal wax or crust. Use cotton or absorbent material to clean excess solution and debris from open area of ear. Repeat before introduction of medicated therapies or as directed by your veterinarian.

Precaution(s): Store at room temperature.

Caution(s): For external use on animals only.

Warning(s): Keep out of reach of children.

Presentation: 4 fl oz (118 mL) (NDC 47203-600-04) and 12 fl oz (355 mL) (NDC 47203-600-12). Patent Pending

Compendium Code No.: 11420640 Rev. 0102

TAKTIC® E.C.

Intervet **Premise and Topical Insecticide**

Emulsifiable Concentrate Miticide/Insecticide

EPA Reg. No.: 54382-3

Active Ingredient(s): Percent by Weight

Amitraz. 12.5
Inert Ingredients: 87.5
Total 100.0

This product contains Petroleum Distillate.

Indications: For the control of ticks, mange mites and lice on beef cattle, dairy cattle and swine.

Beef and Dairy Cattle:

Ticks and Lice: TAKTIC® E.C. will control the following ticks and lice on cattle: Lone Star Tick *(Amblyomma americanum),* Gulf Coast Tick *(A. maculatum),* Winter Tick *(Dermacentor albipictus),* Brown Dog Tick *(Rhipicephalus sanguineus),* American Dog Tick *(D. variabilis),* Rocky Mountain Wood Tick *(D. andersoni),* Spinose Ear Tick *(Otobius megnini),* Black-legged Tick *(Ixodes scapularis),* Tropical Bont Tick *(A. variegatum),* Cayenne Tick *(A. cajennense),* Cattle Tick *(Boophilus annulatus),* Southern Cattle Tick *(B. microplus),* Biting Louse *(Damalinia bovis),* Sucking Lice *(Haematopinus eurysternus, Linognathus vituli, Solenopotes capillatus).*

Mites: Scab and mange mites *(Chorioptes bovis, Psoroptes ovis* and *Sarcoptes scabiei* var. *bovis).*

Swine:

Mange Mite and Louse: *Sarcoptes scabiei* var. *suis* and *Haematopinus suis.*

Directions for Use: It is a violation of federal law to use this product in a manner inconsistent with its labeling.

Do not use on horses or dogs - can cause deaths.

Do not open container until ready to use.

Do not use on dogs or horses (May cause fatal colon impaction).

Use TAKTIC® E.C. with water only. Do not mix with oil or other solvents.

Beef and Dairy Cattle:

Spray: For control of ticks and lice, mix one can (760 mL) of TAKTIC® E.C. in 100 gallons of water; for control of mites, mix one can of TAKTIC® E.C. in 50 gallons of water. Use TAKTIC® E.C. solutions within 6 hours of mixing. Use up to 2 gallons of spray for a fully grown animal. It is important to wet the animal thoroughly and that the spray penetrates to the skin until run-off. For Lone Star ticks, cattle ticks, sucking lice and chewing lice, particular attention should be given to the legs, axilla and groin area, udder, tail regions and head, including the ears. For Gulf Coast ticks and ear ticks, treat the head, ears, shoulder area and neck with a low pressure spray. For control of lice, a second treatment 10-14 days later is recommended, to kill lice hatching from eggs.

Spray Dip Machine: For control of ticks and lice, mix one can (760 mL) of TAKTIC® E.C. in 100 gallons of water; for control of mites mix one can of TAKTIC® E.C. in 50 gallons of water. To control cattle scabies, applications should be made as instructed by USDA, APHIS, VS bulletins. Two treatments 7-10 days apart are required to control cattle scabies. Use TAKTIC® E.C. solutions within 6 hours of mixing. Use up to 2 gallons of spray for a fully grown animal. It is important to wet the animal thoroughly and that the spray penetrates to the skin until run-off.

Swine:

Important: Remove feed from pen and cover drinking bowls. Remove and destroy bedding. Hose out feces and excess feed. Use TAKTIC® E.C. solutions within 6 hours of mixing.

Spray: Mix one can (760 mL) TAKTIC® E.C. in 50 gallons of water (equivalent to ½ fl ounce per gallon of spray solution). A sprayer with a coarse nozzle delivering the solution at 70 to 150 psi is recommended. Spray the walls, floor and any fittings in the pen. Spray all animals (at the same time) whether visibly affected or not. Spray the animals until the mixture runs off, paying particular attention to treat the jowl, legs, inside the ears and underside of the body. It is important that the spray penetrates to the skin until runoff. A second treatment is recommended to break the parasites' life cycles. Make the application 7-10 days after the first treatment for mite control, and 10-14 days for lice control.

An alternate to spraying young pigs (piglets/weaners) is to dip them in a suitable-sized container. Dip 30 animals and then replace dip wash. Use dip wash to treat premises.

Do not treat animals more than 4 times per year.

Do not use TAKTIC® at the same time with any other amitraz containing product.

Contraindication(s): Do not use on dogs or horses (may cause fatal colon impaction).

Precautionary Statements: Hazards to Humans (and Domestic Animals):

Danger: Corrosive. Causes irreversible eye damage. Causes skin irritation. Harmful if swallowed or absorbed through skin or inhaled. Do not get in eyes, on skin or on clothing. Avoid breathing spray mist. Wear goggles of face shield. Prolonged or frequently repeated skin contact may cause allergic reaction in some individuals. Wash thoroughly with soap and water after handling. Remove contaminated clothing and wash before reuse.

Personal Protective Equipment (PPE):

Applicators and other handlers must wear:

- Chemical-resistant apron or coveralls over long-sleeved shirt and long pants.
- Chemical-resistant footwear plus socks.
- Chemical-resistant gloves.
- Chemical-resistant headgear for overhead exposure.
- Goggles or face shield, and chemical-resistant apron when cleaning equipment, mixing or loading.

Do not apply this product in a way that will contact workers or other persons, either directly or through drift. Only protected handlers may be in the area during application.

For livestock spray or dip applications in enclosed areas: Apply only in well-ventilated areas.

Follow manufacturer's instructions for cleaning/maintaining PPE. If no such instructions exist for washables, use detergent and hot water. Keep and wash PPE separately from other laundry.

User Safety Recommendations:

- Users should wash hands before eating, drinking, chewing gum, using tobacco, or using the toilet.
- Users should remove clothing immediately if pesticide gets inside. Then wash thoroughly and put on clean clothing.
- Users should remove PPE immediately after handling this product. Wash the outside of gloves before removing. As soon as possible, wash thoroughly and change into clean clothing.

Statement of Practical Treatment (First Aid):

If in Eyes: Hold eyelids open and flush with steady, gentle stream of water for 15 minutes. Get medical attention.

If on skin: Wash with plenty of soap and water. Get medical attention.

If Inhaled: Remove victim to fresh air. If not breathing, give artificial respiration, preferably mouth-to-mouth. Get medical attention.

If Swallowed: Call a physician or Poison Control Center. Do not induce vomiting. Drink promptly a large quantity of milk, egg whites, gelatin solution, or if these are not available, drink large quantities of water. Avoid alcohol.

Note to Physician: Amitraz, the active ingredient in this product, is not an organophosphorus compound. Do not use atropine as an antidote. Treat any overexposure symptomatically. Mucosal damage is probable which increases the risk of gastric lavage. The presence of petroleum distillate in this product may pose an aspiration pneumonia hazard.

Environmental Hazards: This pesticide is toxic to fish and aquatic invertebrates. Do not apply directly to water, or to areas where surface water is present or to intertidal areas below the mean water mark. Drift and runoff from treated areas may be hazardous to aquatic organisms in adjacent sites. Do not contaminate water when disposing of equipment washwaters or rinsate.

Physical or Chemical Hazards: Do not use or store near heat or open flame.

Storage and Disposal: Storage: Not for storage in and around the home environment. Store in original container in a locked dry place. Do not open the container until ready to use. Use entire contents of can when opened. Keep from freezing.

Pesticide Disposal: Do not contaminate water, food or feed by storage or disposal. Pesticide wastes are toxic. Improper disposal of excess pesticide, spray mixture or rinsate is a violation of federal law. If these wastes cannot be disposed of by use according to label instructions, contact your state pesticide or Environmental Control Agency, or the Hazardous Waste representative at the nearest EPA Regional Office for guidance.

Container Disposal: Triple rinse (or equivalent). Then offer for recycling or reconditioning, or puncture and dispose of in a sanitary landfill, or by other procedures approved by state and local authorities.

In case of spillage, cover with an absorbent such as soda ash, clay or sawdust. Sweep up and dispose of as directed under Storage and Disposal.

Do not reuse empty container.

Emergency Phone Nos.:

Human — 1-800-228-5635, Ext. 132

Animal — 1-800-345-4735, Ext. 104

Chemical (Spill, Leak, Fire or Exposure) — 1-800-424-9300

Warning(s): TAKTIC® E.C. can be used on lactating dairy animals, with no withholding period for milk following application. Also, there is no post-treatment slaughter interval on beef and dairy cattle.

Do not apply to swine within three days of slaughter.

Keep out of reach of children.

Disclaimer: Important Notice: Disclaimer: Read "Important Notice: Disclaimer" before buying or using. If terms are not acceptable, return at once unopened. Intervet warrants only that the product conforms to the chemical description on the label and is reasonably fit for the purpose stated on the label when used in accordance with the directions under normal conditions of use. This warranty does not extend to the use of this product contrary to label instructions or under abnormal conditions, or under conditions not reasonably foreseeable to Intervet, and user assumes the risk of any such use. Intervet makes no other warranty, express or implied, including any implied warranty of fitness for a particular purpose or of merchantability. In no case shall Intervet be liable for consequential, special, indirect or incidental damages resulting from the use or handling of this product. The foregoing conditions of sale and warranty can be varied only by an agreement in writing signed by a duly authorized representative of Intervet.

Presentation: 760 mL (25.7 fl oz) cans.

U.S. Patent Nos. 3,781,355 and 3,864,497

Compendium Code No.: 11062021 584300-B/584350-A

TAPE WORM TABS™ FOR CATS AND KITTENS

TradeWinds **Parasiticide-Oral**

Praziquantel Tapeworm Tablets

Active Ingredient(s): Each Tablet Contains 23 mg Praziquantel.

Indications: TAPE WORM TABS™ (praziquantel) Tapeworm Tablets will remove the common tapeworms, *Dipylidium caninum* and *Taenia taeniaeformis*, from cats and kittens.

Dosage and Administration: Administer to cats and kittens* only as follows:

4 pounds and under	½ tablet
5-11 pounds	1 tablet
Over 11 pounds	1½ tablets

*Not intended for use in kittens less than 6 weeks of age.

Fasting is neither necessary nor recommended.

Retreatment: Steps should be taken to control fleas and rodents on the premises in order to prevent reinfection; otherwise, retreatment will be necessary. This is especially true in cases of tapeworms transmitted by fleas *(Dipylidium caninum)* where reinfection is almost certain to occur if fleas are not removed from the animal and its environment. If reinfection occurs, tapeworm segments may be observed within one month of the initial treatment.

Description: TAPE WORM TABS™ (praziquantel) Tapeworm Tablets for Cats and Kittens are sized for easy oral administration to either adult cats or kittens. The tablets may be given directly in the mouth or crumbled and mixed with the food. If given with food, mix the tablet(s) with a small amount of the animal's usual ration. If all of the tablet(s) is/are not eaten, TAPE WORM TABS™ may not remove all tapeworms.

Warning(s): Consult your veterinarian before administering tablets to weak or debilitated animals.

Keep out of the reach of children. Not for human use.

Side Effects: Isolated incidents of either salivation or diarrhea have been reported following treatment, but were considered non-significant. If these signs are observed and they persist, consult your veterinarian.

Discussion: Tapeworm infection is one of the most common internal parasite problems actually observed by cat owners. The presence of tapeworms is indicated by the presence of tapeworm segments passed with the feces. Tapeworm segments are white, pinkish-white or yellow-white and similar in size and shape to flattened grains of rice. The segments are most frequently observed lying on the animal's droppings or, less often, moving across a freshly passed stool. Segments are also found on the hair around the anus of the animal, or occasionally on the animal's bedding. Cats become infected with tapeworms after eating fleas or small rodents (rats, mice) which are infected with tapeworm larvae. Consult your veterinarian for assistance in the diagnosis, treatment, and control of parasitism.

Presentation: 3 tablets.

Compendium Code No.: 12610030 TW70023

TAPE WORM TABS™ FOR DOGS AND PUPPIES

TradeWinds **Parasiticide-Oral**

Praziquantel Tapeworm Tablets

Active Ingredient(s): Each Tablet Contains 34 mg Praziquantel.

Indications: TAPE WORM TABS™ (praziquantel) Tapeworm Tablets will remove the common tapeworms, *Dipylidium caninum* and *Taenia pisiformis*, from dogs and puppies.

Dosage and Administration: Administer to dogs and puppies* only as follows:

5 pounds and under	½ tablet
6-10 pounds	1 tablet
11-15 pounds	1½ tablets
16-30 pounds	2 tablets
31-45 pounds	3 tablets
46-60 pounds	4 tablets
Over 60 pounds	5 tablets maximum

*Not intended for use in puppies less than 4 weeks of age.

Fasting is neither necessary nor recommended.

Retreatment: Steps should be taken to control fleas and small mammals on the premises in order to prevent reinfection; otherwise, retreatment will be necessary. This is especially true in cases of tapeworms transmitted by fleas *(Dipylidium caninum)* where reinfection is almost certain to occur if fleas are not removed from the animal and its environment. If reinfection occurs, tapeworm segments may be observed within one month of the initial treatment.

Description: TAPE WORM TABS™ (praziquantel) Tapeworm Tablets for Dogs and Puppies are sized for easy oral administration to either adult dogs or puppies. The tablets may be given directly in the mouth or crumbled and mixed with the food. If given with food, mix the tablet(s) with a small amount of the animal's usual ration. If all of the tablet(s) is/are not eaten, TAPE WORM TABS™ may not remove all tapeworms.

T

Warning(s): Consult your veterinarian before administering tablets to weak or debilitated animals.

Keep out of the reach of children. Not for human use.

Side Effects: Isolated incidents of either vomiting, diarrhea, poor appetite, or listlessness have been reported following treatment, but were considered non-significant. If these signs are observed and they persist, consult your veterinarian.

Discussion: Tapeworm infection is one of the most common internal parasite problems actually observed by dog owners. The presence of tapeworms is indicated by the presence of tapeworm segments passed with the feces. Tapeworm segments are white, pinkish-white or yellow-white and similar in size and shape to flattened grains of rice. The segments are most frequently observed lying on the animal's droppings or, less often, moving across a freshly passed stool. Segments are also found on the hair around the anus of the animal, or occasionally on the animal's bedding. Dogs become infected with tapeworms after eating fleas or small mammals (rabbits, hares) which are infected with tapeworm larvae. Consult your veterinarian for assistance in the diagnosis, treatment, and control of parasitism.

Presentation: 5 tablets.

Compendium Code No.: 12610040 TW70034

TARGET CANINE OVULATION KIT

BioMetallics **Ovulation Test**

Rapid Canine Progesterone Kit For Use in Veterinary Clinics

Components:

6 or 12 monoclonal antibody treated test cups.
6 or 12 sample applicators.
1 bottle of wash solution.
1 bottle of substrate buffer A.
1 bottle of substrate buffer B.
1 substrate mixing bottle.
1 bottle enzyme conjugate.
A color chart.

Indications: This kit will enable the user to determine the optimum time for fertilization.

Accurate timing is important for breeding success especially when the breeding is done with fresh chilled or frozen semen.

The main reason for unsuccessful breedings is improper timing.

Test Principles: The visible signs of heat and breeding time (such as vulval swelling, end of vaginal discharge, or flagging) are only an approximate indication of the time of ovulation. These signs can vary by more than a week.

Ovulation is triggered by the Luteinizing Hormone or LH which peaks two days before ovulation. Progesterone levels begin to rise at the same time as the LH surge. Ovulation occurs two days after the initial rise in progesterone. Predicting ovulation is accurately done by detecting the initial rise in progesterone.

After ovulation occurs, the ovacytes take 2-3 days to ripen, making the fertile period 5-6 days after the initial rise in progesterone.

With the TARGET CANINE OVULATION Timing kit, it is possible to detect the initial rise in progesterone. The progesterone level before ovulation is low (between 0 and 1.0 ng/mL). This corresponds to a bright blue test result. When the initial rise in progesterone occurs, the test result will be a light blue.

Test Procedure: Test Preparation (For Serum or Plasma): Allow all kit components and samples to come to room temperature. Collect the blood sample into an EDTA or heparin coated tube (purple top tube) or in a dry tube (red top tube). Immediately after sample collection, invert the tube several times to mix. Spin the blood down with a centrifuge or allow the blood to clot by staying at room temperature for ½ to 1 hr and pour the serum into a clean glass tube. If the sample is not run immediately, store the sample in the refrigerator. For long term storage the sample should be frozen. Label the sample with the name, sample day and cycle day. Do not use whole blood. Do not run test with cold kits.

Guideline for When to Test:

1. One serum sample should be run during the first five days of the proestrus cycle (characterized by the presence of blood and vulval swelling) in order to determine the baseline progesterone level. The baseline progesterone level varies between 0-1 ng/mL in individual dogs and gives a bright blue color result similar to the C1 color on the color chart.
2. Begin testing to determine the initial rise in progesterone about 11-13 days after observing the first day of vaginal bleeding and vulval swelling (the beginning of proestrus). If the first result is the baseline color, bright blue (C1), then the progesterone level is still very low.
3. Retest every two days until the test results are a light blue that is similar to the C2 color on the color chart. This first fading of the color from C1 to C2 represents the initial rise in the progesterone level; ovulation will occur 1-2 days later.
4. Retest every day until the test results are faint blue similar to the C3 color on the color chart. This means the egg is beginning to ripen and the fertile period begins 2-3 days later. After obtaining a C3 color, natural matings and inseminations with fresh semen should take place in 2 or 3 days and again in 2 days. If using frozen semen, inseminate in 2 or 3 days and every other day for a total of 3 times.
5. If a white result is obtained, mating or insemination should be done immediately.

Storage: Store the kit in the refrigerator when not in use. Do not freeze.

Always reseal the plastic bag after removing a test cup.

Caution(s): Timing during Step 2 (time of the enzyme) is important: one (1) minute.

Do not exchange test cups or reagents between different kits.

If you want to do a control, do steps 2-7, the result should be C1.

Discussion: Other Uses: The Target Canine Progesterone kit can also be used to accurately determine the right time for a Cesarean section. About 24 hours before normal whelping, progesterone levels drop back to low baseline levels (and the Target test result changes from white (C4) to bright blue (C1)). By daily testing just before the expected whelping date, the time for the C-section can be precisely determined and emergency surgery or premature puppies can be avoided. Progesterone levels can also be measured throughout pregnancy in order to confirm that the progesterone levels remain high (C4) and the bitch is maintaining a normal pregnancy.

Presentation: 6 and 12 test kits.

Compendium Code No.: 14850000

TARGET EQUINE PROGESTERONE KIT

BioMetallics **Progesterone Detection**

Components:

6, 12, or 20 monoclonal.
6, 12, or 20 sample applicators.
1 bottle of wash solution.
1 bottle of substrate buffer A.
1 bottle of substrate buffer B.
1 substrate mixing bottle.
1 bottle of enzyme conjugate.

Indications: For the determination of the mare's cycle.

Test Principles: Progesterone, a natural hormone that circulates in the mare's blood, is produced by the corpus luteum (CL) and fluctuates during a normal estrous cycle. Blood progesterone levels accurately reflect the different stages of the estrous cycle.

Test Procedure: Test Preparation (Serum, Plasma, or Whole Blood Sample):

For a whole blood sample, collect at least 6 drops of blood into a red or purple top tube. Run the test within 15 minutes after taking the blood sample. Invert the tube several times to mix before running the sample.

For a serum/plasma sample, collect blood into a labeled Red (serum) or a Purple (plasma) Top Tube. Allow the tube to stand for 20-30 min at room temperature or spin the sample down in a centrifuge. Pour the clear liquid into a clean glass tube.

For determining where the mare is in her cycle. A progesterone test is the most economical way to determine where the mare is in her reproductive cycle.

For determining whether there is a functional CL and thus, whether to use prostaglandin.

About 72 hours after a prostaglandin injection, or order to determine if the treatment was effective or if a second treatment is needed.

For monitoring the progesterone level during pregnancy.

For monitoring progesterone for embryo transfer.

Using TARGET with Prostaglandin: Prostaglandin is used when the mare has a functional corpus luteum (progesterone level is high) in order to induce heat (low level of progesterone).

In order for prostaglandin to be most effective, it is important to know where the mare is in her cycle at the time of injection in order to predict the result.

If a bright blue result is obtained on a first test, test again in 4 days to find out if your mare is approaching heat or is still in anestrus.

For an unbred mare, a white result indicates that the mare is in diestrus or may have a persistent corpus luteum. Prostaglandin may be used at the time of a white result to bring her into heat. About 72 hours after prostaglandin administration, a progesterone test will confirm heat (bright blue result). If the result is not bright blue, the CL has not fully regressed and could recover. Another treatment of prostaglandin is advisable in this case.

For a mare that has been bred, a white result 17-23 days after breeding can indicate pregnancy. Prostaglandin should not be used at this time, since it lowers progesterone and will cause an abortion of the pregnancy.

Using TARGET with Regu-Mater: TARGET is designed to recognize only the natural progesterone hormone. Regu-Mate® is a synthetic hormone and will not be detected by TARGET. When using TARGET to monitor pregnancy while Regu-Mate® is being given, a white result indicates the progesterone-deficient mare is producing enough progesterone to be taken off therapy.

Using TARGET to Monitor Pregnancy: Low levels of progesterone at any stage of pregnancy are a major cause of early embryo loss or late-term abortion. To determine if progesterone levels are adequate for pregnancy, test a sample 12-14 days after ovulation. Retest at various intervals during pregnancy to insure adequate progesterone levels are being maintained.

A white result indicates progesterone levels are adequate for pregnancy maintenance. The minimum safe level to maintain pregnancy is 4 ng/mL progesterone (a very faint blue result or white).

A bright blue or light blue result indicates a progesterone-deficient mare.

Using TARGET for Embryo Transfer: TARGET can be especially useful in embryo transfer programs where following the estrous cycles closely is essential in synchronizing the donor with a recipient mare.

Other Uses: TARGET can be used for pregnancy detection. A white result obtained 21-23 days after breeding indicates pregnancy. Note: TARGET indicates the presence of progesterone not specifically pregnancy. A positive indication of pregnancy should be confirmed by palpation or ultrasound.

Test Interpretation: No Cycling Occurs:

Winter Anestrus: No ovulation occurs during this time and therefore there is no progesterone. The test result is bright blue.

Transition Period: Developing follicles are detected by palpation. If ovulation has not occurred for the season, test result is bright blue.

Cycling Begins After the First Ovulation:

Estrus: The cycle begins. The normal cycle is 21-22 days. East heat (estrus) lasts 5-7 days. Progesterone levels are lowest during this time. The test result is bright blue.

After Ovulation (Day 0): The CL forms on the ovary and begins producing progesterone and the progesterone levels rise. The test result is light blue.

Diestrus: The progesterone concentration is very high during the 14-15 days of the diestrus period. The test result is white.

In the unbred mare, the CL regresses around day 16. The progesterone levels fall and the cycle is repeated.

In the pregnant mare, progesterone levels remain elevated beyond 17 days post breeding.

Storage: Store this kit in the refrigerator when not in use. Do not freeze.

Always reseal the plastic bag after removing a test cup.

Caution(s): Timing during Step 2 (time of the enzyme) is important: one (1) minute.

Do not exchange test cups or reagents between different kits.

Presentation: 6, 12, or 20 tests.

Compendium Code No.: 14850010

TARGET PROGESTERONE MILK TEST

BioMetallics **Progesterone Detection**

Rapid Test for Progesterone in Bovine Milk

Components:

20 monoclonal antibody treated test cups.
20 sample applicators.
1 bottle enzyme conjugate.
1 bottle wash solution.
1 bottle substrate buffer A.
1 bottle substrate buffer B.
1 substrate mixing bottle.

Indications: Recommended to confirm estrus, detect pregnancy, improve controlled breeding, define cycling, diagnose infertility disorders, and to monitor fertility treatment.

Test Procedure: Milk Sample Collection: Milk samples should be obtained preferably from the foremilk or milk jug and put into a clean container. Last milk can be used, but is less preferred. Initial strippings should not be used. Label samples with the cow number sampling date, and cycle day.

If a milk sample is not tested within 30 minutes it should be stored in the refrigerator. If the milk sample is to be tested more than 6 hours later, immediately after collection, add one drop of milk preservative (10% potassium dichromate) or ¼ milk preservative tablet to each 10 mLs of milk. Store milk in the refrigerator—do not freeze. It is not recommended to test samples more than 4-5 days after collection.

Test Kit Preparation: Allow samples and all kit reagents to come to room temperature before starting test (2-24 hrs). Use a timer while performing the test. Label each test cup to be used with the cow number and line up samples with respective cups.

When to Use TARGET:

1. Confirm estrus (heat): Take a milk sample on the day of suspected estrus. A bright blue test result indicates the cow is in estrus and ovulation is about to occur. The optimal time to inseminate is approximately 18 hours after obtaining a bright blue result.
2. Detect pregnancy or open cows: Take a milk sample 19 to 21 days after insemination. A bright blue test result indicates the cow is open and is in estrus. A white test result strongly indicates the cow is pregnant. An additional sample taken at 22 or 23 days increases the accuracy of a pregnancy determination—up to 95% accuracy if a white result is obtained on both tests.

   Pregnancy determination should be confirmed by a licensed veterinarian since high progesterone could indicate mid ovarian cycle because of inaccurately timed insemination, or development of a persistent corpus luteum. Furthermore, cows diagnosed with high progesterone on day 19-23 may return to estrus if fetal reabsorption occurs. A milk sample taken at the time of palpation can be used in conjunction with palpation results.
3. Improve prostaglandin controlled breeding: Take a milk sample prior to injection with prostaglandin. If the corpus luteum (CL) is functional (white result), continue with treatment. Prostaglandin injections after 50 days post-calving has been shown to reduce days open, reduce services per conception, and increase conception rate.
4. Define cycling: Take milk samples at 3 to 5 day intervals for a period of 3 weeks or more. A combination of low and high progesterone results (any shade of blue and white) indicates that ovarian activity has resumed (usually evident about 1 month post-calving).
5. Diagnose infertility disorders: After veterinarian confirmation of the presence of an ovarian cyst (by rectal palpation), TARGET is useful in determining the type of cyst. Take one milk sample at the day of palpation and 2 more samples at 7 day intervals for questionable cases.

   A bright blue test result (low progesterone) strongly indicates a follicular cyst or nonfunctional ovary.

   A white test result (high progesterone) strongly indicates the presence of a luteal cyst or cystic CL.
6. Monitor fertility treatment: Take a milk sample 10 days after treatment for a follicular cyst. If a white result (high progesterone) is obtained, the prescribed treatment was effective.

   Take a milk sample 2 to 4 days after treatment for a luteal cyst or cystic CL. If a bright blue result (low progesterone) is obtained, the prescribed therapy was effective.

Use of the Control: With TARGET, it is not necessary to use a control because of IPACT™ (Immuno Precision Color Technology)*, which is built into the kit during manufacturing.

*US Patent

If you want to do a control on the kit, do steps 2-5; the result should be bright blue.

Storage: Store entire kit in the refrigerator when not in use. Do not freeze.

Always reseal the ZipLoc bag after removing a test cup.

Caution(s): Timing during Step 2 (the time for the red bottle solution to be in contact with the test cup) is important: one (1) minute.

Never exchange reagents or test cups between different kits.

Discussion: The Importance of Testing for Progesterone: Progesterone, a hormone found in bovine milk, is produced by the corpus luteum (CL) during the estrous cycle and pregnancy. Milk progesterone levels accurately reflect the different stages of the estrous cycle and pregnancy status.

Normal lactating cows have heat cycles every 18-22 days and each heat cycle lasts 6-18 hours. Heat detection based on visual signs can be accurate.

Progesterone levels are lowest when the cow is in heat. After ovulation a CL forms on the ovary and begins producing progesterone, and progesterone levels are high from about Day 5 through Day 18.

If pregnant, progesterone levels continue at high level. If nonpregnant, around Day 18 the CL regresses and progesterone levels fall.

During the next estrous cycle, at Day 1 the cow is back in heat and progesterone levels are low.

Presentation: 20 tests.

Compendium Code No.: 14850020

TASTY PASTE® DOG & PUPPY WORMER

Farnam **Parasiticide-Oral**

(Piperazine Adipate)

Active Ingredient(s):

Piperazine (from adipate) . . . . 2.70 g (20.8%)

Indications: For control of roundworms (ascarids) *(Toxocara canis* and *Toxascaris leonina)* in puppies and adult dogs.

Dosage and Administration: For oral use in puppies and dogs. The contents will treat up to 90 lbs. of body weight.

Dosage: 30 mg piperazine per lb. of body weight.

Directions: Remove cap from nozzle. Push plunger just enough to fill nozzle. Turn the knurled wheel on the plunger so that the side nearest the barrel is at the weight mark corresponding to the weight of the dog. Add to the feed or insert the nozzle as far back in the dog's mouth as possible. Press the plunger down as far as it will go. For animals of up to 1 year of age administer every 2 or 3 months; for animals over 1 year old, administer periodically as necessary.

A repeat treatment should be given in 10 to 20 days to remove immature roundworms which may have entered the intestine from the lungs after the first dose. Laboratory fecal examinations should always be done to determine the need for treatment.

Consult your veterinarian for assistance in the diagnosis, treatment and control of parasitism.

Precaution(s): Store out of direct sunlight.

Caution(s): Although Piperazine is a drug with a wide margin of safety, occasionally an animal may show nausea, or muscular tremors. Such side effects are usually associated with overdosage. Therefore, recommended dosages should be followed carefully. Animals with known kidney pathology should be treated only by a veterinarian.

Do not use on sick or debilitated dogs.

Warning(s): Keep out of reach of children. Not for human use.

Presentation: 0.46 oz. (13 g) syringe (NDC 17135-232-12).

Compendium Code No.: 10000381 0E1/9DD8

TDC/TEAT DIP WITH CHLORHEXIDINE

Western Chemical **Teat Dip**

Active Ingredient(s):

Chlorhexidine gluconate 0.5%
Glycerin. 5.0%

Indications: Dairy farm teat dip as an aid in controlling organisms that cause mastitis.

Dosage and Administration: Use undiluted to dip teats.

Presentation: 15, 30 and 55 gallon drums.

Compendium Code No.: 10210020

T.D.N. MINI ROCKETS

DVM Formula **Large Animal Dietary Supplement**

Guaranteed Analysis: Per Capsule:

Vitamin A .... 87,500 IU
Vitamin B_{12} (Cyanocobalamin) .... 250 mcg
Vitamin C .... 125 mg
Vitamin D_3 .... 18,750 IU
Vitamin E .... 175 IU
Niacin .... 1,000 mg
Choline .... 50 mg
Lactic Acid Bacteria .... 750 million CFU

Ingredients: Vitamin A acetate, DL-alpha-tocopheryl acetate (vitamin E), d-activated animal sterol (vitamin D_3), niacinamide, cyanocobalamin (vitamin B_{12}), choline chloride, ascorbic acid (vitamin C), d-calcium pantothenate, riboflavin, cobalt carbonate, pyridoxine hydrochloride (vitamin B_6), iron sulfate, copper sulfate, zinc sulfate, chelated copper, chelated iron, zinc methionine, *Lactobacillus acidophilus* DDS-1, *Lactobacillus plantarum, Lactobacillus lactis, Lactobacillus casei, Enterococcus faecium,* dextrose, dry active yeast, *Lactobacillus fermentum,* bentonite, and silica.

Indications: A powerful capsule designed to stimulate appetite and combat stress associated with birth, weaning, antibiotic treatment, depressed appetite, or weather changes.

A concentrated source of yeast, direct fed microbials, antioxidant vitamins, and chelated minerals packed in a gelatin capsule designed for quick absorption.

All natural, no withholding.

Dosage and Administration: Up to two capsules per day depending on label directions.

Feeding Directions: Administer orally with approved balling gun.

Presentation: 6 capsule blister pack.

Compendium Code No.: 15030080

T.D.N. MINI ROCKETS™

Vets Plus **Large Animal Dietary Supplement**

Nutritional Gelatin Capsules

Guaranteed Analysis: (min. per capsule):

Vitamin A .... 87,500 IU
Vitamin D_3 .... 18,750 IU
Vitamin E .... 175 IU
Vitamin C .... 125 mg
Vitamin B_{12} .... 250 mcg
Niacin .... 1000 mg
Choline .... 50 mg
Lactic Acid Bacteria .... 750 Million CFU

(*Lactobacillus plantarum, Lactobacillus casei, Lactobacillus acidophilus, Lactobacillus fermentum,* and *Enterococcus faecium, Lactobacillus acidophilus* DDS-1)

Ingredients: Vitamin A acetate, DL-alpha-Tocopheryl Acetate (Vitamin E), D-Activated Animal Sterol (Vitamin D_3), Niacinamide, Cyanocobalamin (Vitamin B_{12}), Choline Chloride, Ascorbic Acid (Vitamin C), d-Calcium Pantothenate, Riboflavin, Cobalt Carbonate, Pyridoxine Hydrochloride (Vitamin B_6), Iron Sulfate, Copper Sulfate, Zinc Sulfate, Zinc Methionine, *Lactobacillus acidophilus* DDS-1, *Lactobacillus plantarum, Lactobacillus casei, Lactobacillus acidophilus, Lactobacillus fermentum, Enterococcus faecium,* Dextrose, Dry Active Yeast, Sodium bentonite, and Silica.

Indications: Administer to livestock during times of stress, such as: diet change, weaning, birth, depressed appetite, antibiotic treatment, shipping, or weather changes. T.D.N. MINI ROCKETS™ contain Lactic Acid Bacteria, including *Lactobacillus acidophilus* DDS-1, antioxidant vitamins, chelated minerals and yeast. This combination of essential elements strengthen the immune system and stimulate appetite and are packed in a fast-dissolving capsule for quick absorption.

Dosage and Administration:

	1st Day	2nd Day	3rd Day
Birth	2 capsules	2 capsules	1 capsule
Depressed appetite	2 capsules	1 capsule	as needed
Following Antibiotic Treatment	2 capsules	2 capsules	1 capsule
Disease conditions, Scours	2 capsules	2 capsules	2 capsules
Weather change	2 capsules	1 capsule	as needed

Feeding Directions: Place capsule into a balling gun. Hold the head of the animal in a slightly elevated position and place the balling gun into the back of the mouth. Deposit the capsule, insuring that the animal swallows the capsule. Do not give to animals that are unable to swallow. You may also break the capsule and top-dress the contents, if desired. If conditions do not improve, consult your veterinarian.

Precaution(s): Keep in a cool dry place.

Caution(s): Keep out of the reach of children.

Animal use only.

Presentation: 12x6-capsule blister packs per case and 18x50-capsule jars per case.

Compendium Code No.: 10730180

T.D.N. ROCKETS

DVM Formula **Large Animal Dietary Supplement**

Guaranteed Analysis: Per Capsule:

Vitamin A .... 350,000 IU
Vitamin B_{12} (Cyanocobalamin) .... 1,000 mcg
Vitamin C .... 500 mg
Vitamin D_3 .... 75,000 IU
Vitamin E .... 700 IU
Niacin .... 4,000 mg
Choline .... 200 mg
Lactic Acid Bacteria .... 3 billion CFU

Ingredients: Vitamin A acetate, DL-alpha-tocopheryl acetate (vitamin E), d-activated animal sterol (vitamin D_3), niacinamide, cyanocobalamin (vitamin B_{12}), choline chloride, ascorbic acid (vitamin C), d-calcium pantothenate, riboflavin, cobalt carbonate, pyridoxine hydrochloride (vitamin B_6), iron sulfate, copper sulfate, zinc sulfate, chelated copper, chelated iron, zinc methionine, *Lactobacillus acidophilus* DDS-1, *Lactobacillus plantarum, Lactobacillus lactis, Lactobacillus casei, Enterococcus faecium,* dextrose, dry active yeast, *Lactobacillus fermentum,* bentonite, and silica.

Indications: A powerful stress capsule designed to be used after calving or during sickness.

Stimulates appetite and promotes quick recovery after antibiotic treatment.

A concentrated source of yeast, direct fed microbials, antioxidant vitamins, and chelated minerals packed in a gelatin capsule designed for quick absorption.

All natural, no withholding.

Dosage and Administration: Up to two capsules per day depending on label directions.

Feeding Directions: Administer orally with approved balling gun.

Presentation: 4 capsule blister pack.

Compendium Code No.: 15030090

T.D.N. ROCKETS™

Vets Plus **Large Animal Dietary Supplement**

Nutritional Gelatin Capsules

Guaranteed Analysis: (min. per capsule):

Vitamin A .... 350,000 IU
Vitamin D_3 .... 75,000 IU
Vitamin E .... 700 IU
Vitamin C .... 500 mg
Vitamin B_{12} .... 1000 mcg
Niacin .... 4000 mg
Choline .... 200 mg
Lactic Acid Bacteria .... 3 Billion CFU

(*Lactobacillus plantarum, Lactobacillus casei, Lactobacillus acidophilus, Lactobacillus fermentum,* and *Enterococcus faecium, Lactobacillus acidophilus* DDS-1)

Ingredients: Vitamin A acetate, DL-alpha-Tocopheryl Acetate (Vitamin E), D-Activated Animal Sterol (Vitamin D_3), Niacinamide, Cyanocobalamin (Vitamin B_{12}), Choline Chloride, Ascorbic Acid (Vitamin C), d-Calcium Pantothenate, Riboflavin, Cobalt Carbonate, Pyridoxine Hydrochloride (Vitamin B_6), Iron Sulfate, Copper Sulfate, Zinc Sulfate, Zinc Methionine, *Lactobacillus plantarum, Lactobacillus casei, Lactobacillus acidophilus, Lactobacillus fermenium, Enterococcus faecium, Lactobacillus acidophilus* DDS-1, Dextrose, Dry Active Yeast, Sodium Bentonite, and Silica.

Indications: Administer to livestock during times of stress, such as: diet change, weaning, birth, depressed appetite, antibiotic treatment, shipping, or weather changes. T.D.N. ROCKETS™ contain Lactic Acid Bacteria, including *Lactobacillus acidophilus* DDS-1, antioxidant vitamins, chelated minerals and yeast. This combination of essential elements strengthen the immune system and stimulate appetite and are packed in a fast-dissolving capsule for quick absorption.

Dosage and Administration:

	1st Day	2nd Day	3rd Day
Freshening and cleaning	2 capsules	2 capsules	as needed
Depressed appetite	2 capsules	1 capsule	as needed
Following antibiotic treatment	2 capsules	2 capsules	1 capsule
Weather change	2 capsules	1 capsule	as needed

Feeding Directions: Place capsule into a balling gun. Hold the animal's head in a slightly elevated position and place the balling gun into the back of the mouth. Deposit the capsule, insuring that the animal swallows the capsule. Do not give to animals that are unable to swallow. You may also break open the capsule and top-dress the contents if desired. If conditions do not improve, consult your veterinarian.

Precaution(s): Keep in a cool dry place.

Caution(s): Keep out of the reach of children.

Animal use only.

Presentation: 12x4-capsule blister packs per case and 12x28-capsule jars per case.

Compendium Code No.: 10730190

TEARLESS FERRET SHAMPOO

Tomlyn **Grooming Shampoo**

Active Ingredient(s): Shampoo formula.

Indications: A deodorizing grooming shampoo for use on ferrets. It may also be used on other small mammals, rabbits, puppies and kittens.

Directions: Wet animal thoroughly with warm water. Apply shampoo along the back and work in well to produce a mild lather. Rinse thoroughly with warm water and towel dry.

Keep animal in a warm environment free from drafts until completely dry. Do not use on animals under 4 weeks of age.

To control odor in ferrets, bathe every 10 to 14 days.

Precaution(s): Store at room temperature.

Caution(s): For external animal use only.

Keep out of reach of children and pets.

Presentation: 12 x 8 fl oz (237 mL).

Compendium Code No.: 11220240 726-2

TEARLESS PUPPY SHAMPOO

Tomlyn **Grooming Shampoo**

Active Ingredient(s): Water (CAS 7732-18-5), PEG-80 sorbitan laurate (CAS 9005-64-5), Sodium trideceth sulfate (CAS 25446-78-0), PEG-150 distearate (CAS 9005-08-7), Cocamidopropyl hydroxysultaine (CAS 68139-30-0).

Indications: A mild grooming shampoo for use on puppies, kittens and ferrets.

Directions: Wet animal thoroughly with warm water. Apply TEARLESS PUPPY SHAMPOO along the back and work in well to produce a mild lather. Rinse thoroughly with warm water. Towel dry. Keep animal in a warm environment free from drafts until completely dry.

Do not use on kittens or ferrets under 4 weeks of age. To control odor in ferrets, bathe every 10 to 14 days.

Precaution(s): Store at room temperature.

Caution(s): For external animal use only.

Keep out of reach of children and pets.

Presentation: 12 x 12 fl oz (355 mL) and 4 x 1 gallon (128 fl oz - 3.79 L).

Compendium Code No.: 11220250 670-1, 671-2

TEARLESS SHAMPOO

Davis **Grooming Shampoo**

Ingredient(s): PEG-80 sorbitan laurate, sodium trideceth sulfate, PEG-150 distearate, cocamidopropyl hydroxysultaine, lauroamphocarboxyglycinate, sodium laureth-13 carboxylate, quaternium 15, fragrance.

Indications: For dogs, cats, puppies and kittens.

Extra mild formula that cleanses normal, dry or sensitive skin while leaving a clean fragrance. Ideal for texture building and frequent bathing.

Dosage and Administration: To use Davis TEARLESS PET SHAMPOO as a general grooming and cleansing shampoo, dilute 10 parts water (10:1) to 1 part shampoo. For extra dirty pets, dilute 3 parts water to 1 part shampoo (3:1).

Wet pet's coat thoroughly with warm water. Apply shampoo on head and ears, then lather. Repeat procedure with neck, chest, middle and hind quarter, finishing legs last. Rinse thoroughly.

Warning(s): For external use only.

Keep out of reach of children.

Discussion: Davis TEARLESS PET SHAMPOO is a special mild formula, non-irritating to the pet's eyes, that helps relieve skin irritation, adds body and texture, highlights color and prevents dryness while restoring skin's natural moisture. It is soap-free and excellent for dry, itchy, allergenic skin. Gentle enough for frequent use, even on puppies and kittens.

Davis TEARLESS PET SHAMPOO is pH balanced, easy on bather's hands and rinses residue free. Leaves coat with a clean fragrance and is designed for all colors. Safe for dogs, cats, puppies and kittens.

Presentation: 12 oz (355 mL) and 1 gallon (3.785 L).

Compendium Code No.: 11410371

TEAT DIP-LITE

Western Chemical **Teat Dip**

Active Ingredient(s):

Nonylphenoxypoly (ethyleneoxy) ethanol iodine complex 0.5%
Glycerin 2%

Indications: A dairy farm teat dip to be used undiluted as an aid in controlling organisms that cause mastitis.

Dosage and Administration: Use undiluted to dip teats.

Presentation: 15, 30 and 55 gallon drums.

Compendium Code No.: 10210040

TEAT DIP WITH GLYCERIN

Western Chemical **Teat Dip**

Active Ingredient(s):

Nonylphenoxypoly (ethyleneoxy) ethanol iodine complex 1.0%
Glycerin .... 5.0 or 10.0%

Indications: A dairy farm teat dip to be used undiluted as an aid in controlling organisms that cause mastitis.

Dosage and Administration: Use undiluted to dip teats.

Presentation: 15, 30 and 55 gallon drums.

Compendium Code No.: 10210030

TEAT ELITE

AgriPharm **Udder Product**

Active Ingredient(s): Contains: Vitamins A, D_3, E, B_2 (riboflavin), B_5 (panthenol), B_6 (pyridoxine), H (d-biotin), and B_3 (niacinamide) in a specially compounded base stabilized at pH of normal animal skin.

Indications: TEAT ELITE with multi-vitamins is for use as an aid in reducing dry, cracked and chapped udders in cattle. Contains humectants which assist in maintaining skin and tissue in natural moisture balance.

Milking machines, inclement weather and other factors strip natural moisture from the udders, leaving them dry and chapped.

The nonsticky, disappearing cream base discourages dirt and manure from sticking to udders.

Dosage and Administration: Apply once a day or as needed after milking to aid in reducing dryness, cracking and chapping associated with chapped udders in cattle.

Caution(s): For animal use only. Keep out of the reach of children.

If the animal shows signs of uncontrolled generalized infections, consult a veterinarian. Wash the teats and udder thoroughly before milking.

TEAT ELITE is not a substitute for balanced nutrition. Animals with signs of nutritional deficiency in the skin may require injections of therapeutic levels of vitamins. Consult a veterinarian for assistance in the diagnosis and treatment of nutritional deficiency.

Presentation: 1 lb. and 5 lb. containers.

Compendium Code No.: 14571000

TEAT GLO® SANITIZING TEAT DIP

Ecolab Food & Bev. Div. **Teat Dip**

Active Ingredient(s):

Iodine 1%
Specific gravity 1.055
Pounds per gallon 8.79

Contains nonylphenoxypolyethoxyethanol-iodine complex, providing 10,000 ppm titratable iodine.

(Contains a 10% emollient system).

Indications: For use as a teat dip in the prevention of mastitis.

Dosage and Administration: To Use: Directions For Teat Dipping

Post Milking: Immediately after milking, use TEAT GLO® at full strength. Submerge entire teat in TEAT GLO® solution. Allow to air dry. Do not wipe. Always use fresh, full strength TEAT GLO®. If product in dip cup becomes visibly dirty, discard contents and replenish with undiluted product. Do not reuse or return used product to the original container. Do not turn cows out in freezing weather until TEAT GLO® is completely dry.

Use proper procedures for udder washing or pre-milking teat dipping just prior to next milking to avoid contamination of milk.

Important: Do not mix TEAT GLO® with any other teat spray, dip or other products. If transferred from this container to any other, make sure that other container is thoroughly pre-cleaned and bears the proper container labeling for TEAT GLO®.

Caution(s): TEAT GLO® is not intended to cure or help the healing of chapped or irritated teats. In case of teat irritation or chapping, have the condition examined and, if necessary, treated by a veterinarian.

Warning(s): For cautionary and first aid information, consult the Material Safety Data Sheet (MSDS).

Presentation: Available in 55 gallon (208.2 L) drum.

Compendium Code No.: 14490141

TEAT GUARD™

Ecolab Food & Bev. Div. **Teat Dip**

Active Ingredient(s):

Nonylphenoxypolyethoxyethanol-iodine complex (providing 1% titratable iodine) 14.6%

Indications: For use as an aid in reducing the spread of organisms which may cause mastitis.

Dosage and Administration: Immediately after milking each cow, use TEAT GUARD™ at full strength. Submerge the entire teat in TEAT GUARD™ solution. Allow to air dry. Do not wipe.

Always use fresh, full strength TEAT GUARD™.

If product in dip cup becomes visibly dirty, discard contents and replenish with undiluted product. Do not reuse or return the used product to the original container.

Wash the entire udder and teats thoroughly just prior to the next milking with an appropriate udder wash product solution to avoid the contamination of milk. Use the proper procedures for udder washing. Apply daily for the first week of the dry period. Commence daily application one (1) week before calving.

Note: TEAT GUARD™ is not intended to cure or help the healing of chapped or irritated teats. In case of teat irritation or chapping, have the condition examined and if necessary, treated by a veterinarian.

M.S.D.S. available.

Precaution(s): Keep from freezing. If frozen, thaw completely and shake well before use.

Caution(s): Read label before using.

For food plant and other industrial use only.

Keep out of the reach of children.

Avoid contact with eyes. Prolonged use may cause irritation to eyes or skin. Wear rubber gloves, splash-proof glasses, goggles or a face shield.

First Aid:

Eyes: Flush immediately with plenty of cool running water. Remove contact lenses. Continue flushing for 15 minutes holding the eyelids apart to ensure rinsing of the entire eye.

Skin: Flush immediately with plenty of cool running water. Wash thoroughly with soap and water.

If swallowed: Do not induce vomiting. Rinse the mouth; then drink one or two large glasses of water. Never give anything by mouth to an unconscious person.

If irritation or discomfort persists, call a physician.

Presentation: 5 gallon, 15 gallon, and 55 gallon.

Compendium Code No.: 14490151

TEAT-KOTE®

Westfalia•Surge **Teat Dip**

Active Ingredient(s): Contains:

Nonylphenoxypoly (ethyleneoxy) ethanol iodine complex
(provides 1.75% titratable iodine) 11.5%

Contains lanolin and glycerin an a stable pH aqueous base.

Indications: This product has been tested under farm conditions of experimental exposure to known mastitis causing organisms and has been proven effective in reducing new infections of mastitis.

Dosage and Administration: Thoroughly cover at least the lower one-third (⅓) of each teat immediately after milking with TEAT-KOTE®. At the end of lactation, apply TEAT-KOTE® daily for one (1) week after last milking. In addition, begin application of TEAT-KOTE® about one (1) week prior to parturition.

If a common teat dip cup is used for application, a fresh solution should always be used at each milking. The teat dip cup should be emptied, cleaned and rinsed with potable water after each milking session or when cup becomes contaminated during milking. Do not pour remaining solution from dip cup back into the original container.

Precaution(s): Store TEAT-KOTE® in cool, dry place. Keep from freezing. If froze, thaw completely and mix well prior to use. Keep containers closed to prevent contamination of teat dip.

Caution(s): Danger - Keep out of the reach of children. Can cause eye damage. Protect eyes when handling. Do not get in eyes or on clothing. Harmful if swallowed. Avoid contamination of food.

First Aid:

Eyes: In case of contact with eyes, flush immediately with plenty of water for at least 15 minutes. Call a physician.

Internal: Do not take internally. If swallowed, promptly drink a large quantity of milk, egg whites, gelatin solution. If these are not available, drink large quantities of water. Avoid alcohol. Call a physician.

General Chemical Warnings: Always read label directions completely before using product. Always exercise caution when handling any chemicals. Avoid contact with eyes, skin and clothing. Never dispense any chemical product from its original container into another container for storage or resale. Never mix two or more products together. Mixing of products could result in release of toxic gases and/or render product ineffective for recommended use application.

Always use product in ventilated area. Avoid inhaling vapors or fumes. Always use product according to recommendations for particular application. Never exceed recommended usage without consulting trained personnel.

Presentation: Contact the company for container sizes available.

* TEAT-KOTE is a trademark of Westfalia•Surge, Inc.

Compendium Code No.: 10020141

TEAT KOTE 10/III™

Westfalia•Surge **Teat Dip**

Active Ingredient(s): Contains 10% triple emollient system.

Nonylphenoxypoly (ethyleneoxy) ethanol iodine complex 11.7%

Provides 1.0% of titratable iodine.

Indications: For use as a sanitizing teat dip for dairy cattle.

Dosage and Administration: Use at full strength. Do not dilute.

Thoroughly cover at least the lower one-third (⅓) of each teat immediately after milking with TEAT KOTE 10/III™. At the end of lactation, apply TEAT KOTE 10/III™ once a day for one (1) week after the last milking. In addition, begin application of TEAT KOTE 10/III™ about one (1) week prior to parturition.

If a common teat dip cup is used for application, a fresh solution should always be used at each milking. The teat dip cup should be emptied, cleaned and rinsed with potable water after each milking session or when the cup becomes contaminated during milking. Do not pour the remaining solution from the dip cup back into the original container.

Precaution(s): Store TEAT KOTE 10/III™ in a cool, dry place. Keep from freezing. If frozen, thaw completely and mix well prior to use. Keep containers closed to prevent contamination of the teat dip.

Caution(s): Danger. Keep out of the reach of children. Shake well before using. Can cause eye damage. Protect the eyes when handling. Do not get in the eyes or on clothing. Harmful if swallowed. Avoid contamination of food.

First Aid:

Eyes: In case of contact with the eyes, flush immediately with plenty of water for at least 15 minutes. Call a physician.

Internal: Do not take internally. If swallowed, promptly drink two to three glasses of milk (if unavailable, drink water). Avoid alcohol. Call a physician.

Handling Recommendations:

1. Always read the label directions completely before using the product.
2. Always exercise caution when handling any chemicals.
3. Avoid contact with the eyes, skin, and clothing.
4. Never dispense any chemical product from its original container into another container for storage or resale.
5. Never mix two or more products together. Mixing of products could result in the release of toxic gases and/or render the product ineffective for the recommended use application.
6. Always use the product in a ventilated area. Avoid inhaling vapors or fumes.
7. Always use the product according to the recommendations for a particular application.
8. Never exceed the recommended usage without consulting trained personnel.

Presentation: Contact the company for container sizes available.

Compendium Code No.: 10020131

TEK-TROL®

Bio-Tek **Disinfectant**

EPA No.: 11725-7

Active Ingredient(s):

ortho-Phenylphenol	12.0%
ortho-Benzyl-para-chlorophenol	10.0%
para-tertiary-Amylphenol	4.0%
Inert ingredients	74.0%
Total	100.0%

Indications: TEK-TROL® is a synthetic detergent which provides broad-spectrum kill of gram-positive and gram-negative micro-organisms, provides effective cleaning and disinfecting in one operation, nonflammable and nonvolatile in use dilutions, excellent solubility, dilutes in hot, cold, soft or hard water of up to 1,000 ppm water hardness.

The TEK-TROL® high foaming detergent system has been formulated to provide heavy duty cleaning, wetting and penetration of soils and organic matter and easy rinsing of surfaces. Clinging foam is obtained at ½ oz. per gallon of water (1:256) to provide prolonged contact time.

TEK-TROL® at ½ oz. per gallon of water (1:256) provides residual control of odor-causing bacteria in the presence of moisture.

TEK-TROL® is recommended for use when used as directed on ceramic and glazed tile surfaces, stainless steel, aluminum, chrome, galvanized metal, glass, and other nonporous surfaces such as treated wood, polyethylene, polypropylene, PVC (polyvinyl chloride), polystyrene, vinyl, fiberglass, viton, ethylene propylene, nitrile, acrylic, and polyurethane.

TEK-TROL® at ½ oz. per gallon of water (1:256) is suited for disinfecting and cleaning all areas of veterinary facilities, kennels and in poultry and turkey barns, breeder and laying operations.

Poultry house grow-out operations and hatcheries: Use in hatchers and setters, evaporative coolers, humidifying systems and ceiling fans, live haul equipment, chick busses, transfer trucks, trays, coop washing, polyethylene chick boxes, foot pans and feed bins.

Equine facilities: Use in stables, stalls, breeding and foaling areas and transport vehicles.

Directions for Use: It is a violation of federal law to use the product in a manner inconsistent with its labeling.

Hatching Egg Sanitizer: TEK-TROL® is recommended for use as a hatching egg sanitizer, with the best results being achieved in water temperatures ranging from 78°F to 110°F. The recommended dilution is ½ oz. per gallon of water (1:256), and may be applied through automatic washing systems, immersion tanks, foaming apparatus, low pressure sprayers, and fogging (wet misting) systems.

General Use Directions:

1. To clean, disinfect and deodorize walls, floors, tables, drinking fountains, sinks, refrigerators, stoves, restroom fixtures, and garbage cans: Remove gross filth and heavy soil with a preliminary cleaning step prior to the application of TEK-TROL®. Apply a solution of ½ oz. TEK-TROL® per gallon of water (1:256) with a sponge, mop, mechanical spray device, or foaming apparatus making sure that all surfaces are wetted thoroughly. Allow the surface to remain wet for 10 minutes. Air dry.
2. To clean and disinfect such articles as combs, brushes, razors, scissors, instruments and rubber goods: All instruments and devices must be thoroughly cleaned to remove excess debris, rinsed and rough dried, including hollows and lumens, before immersion in solutions. Soak for 10 minutes in a solution containing ½ oz. TEK-TROL® per gallon of water (1:256).
3. To disinfect fabrics such as sheets, linens, aprons and uniforms: First rinse to remove gross filth or heavy soil, then soak for 10 minutes in a solution containing ½ oz. of TEK-TROL® per gallon of water (1:256).
4. To clean gross filth or heavy soil on surfaces prior to disinfection, use ½ oz. of TEK-TROL® per gallon of water (1:256).

TEK-TROL® is an effective tuberculocide against *Mycobacterium bovis* in 10 minutes at 20°C when used on hard, nonporous inanimate surfaces. Follow the above directions, including removal of gross filth or heavy soil prior to the application of TEK-TROL®.

Directions for use in poultry houses, farm premises, swine-producing facilities, equine facilities, and veal barns: Do not use in milking stalls, milking parlors, or milk houses.

1. Remove all animals and feed from the premises.
2. Remove all trucks, coops, crates, water troughs and feed racks.
3. Remove all gross soil, litter, manure, droppings from animals and poultry from floors, walls and surfaces of barns, pens, stalls, chutes, and other facilities and fixtures occupied or traversed by animals and poultry.
4. Thoroughly clean and saturate all surfaces with a solution of ½ oz. TEK-TROL® per gallon of water (1:256). Use a high pressure sprayer or apply a layer of foam with a foaming apparatus.
5. Allow to remain in contact for at least 10 minutes.
6. Immerse halters, ropes and other types of equipment used in handling and restraining animals, forks, shovels, scrapers used for removing litter and manure, in a solution of TEK-TROL® at ½ oz. per gallon of water (1:256). Allow to remain in contact for 10 minutes.
7. Thoroughly scrub treated feed racks, troughs, automatic feeders, fountains, waterers, and mangers with a solution of TEK-TROL® at ½ oz. per gallon of water (1:256). Rinse with potable water before re-use.
8. Ventilate buildings, coops and other closed spaces. Do not house poultry or livestock or employ equipment until the treatment has been absorbed, set or dried.

TEK-TROL® is recommended for use in fogging (wet misting) operations as an adjunct either preceding or following regular cleaning and disinfecting procedures. Use at a dilution of ½ oz. per gallon of water (1:256). Check with a Bio-Tek representative to determine an effective fogging schedule for particular use sites. Leave the room when fogging. In well-ventilated areas, such as hatcheries, only 10 to 15 minutes is necessary before re-entering. If used in a poorly ventilated area, allow at least two (2) hours, or air thoroughly, before re-entry. Before fogging in a food processing area, all food and food packaging items must be removed or carefully protected. Treated food contact surfaces must be thoroughly scrubbed with TEK-TROL® at ½ oz. per gallon (1:256) and rinsed with potable water prior to re-use.

Precautionary Statements: Hazards to Humans and Domestic Animals: Danger. Corrosive. Causes eye and skin damage or skin irritation. Do not get in the eyes, on skin, or on clothing. Wear goggles or a face shield and rubber gloves when handling. Harmful or fatal if swallowed. Wash thoroughly with soap and water after handling and before eating, drinking or using tobacco. Remove contaminated clothing and wash before re-use.

Statement of Practical Treatment:

If on skin, wash with plenty of soap and water. Get medical attention.

If in eyes, hold eyelids open and flush eyes with plenty of water. Get medical attention.

If swallowed, call a physician immediately. Drink large quantities of water. Never give anything by mouth to an unconscious person. Avoid alcohol.

Note to Physician: Probable mucosal damage may contraindicate the use of gastric lavage. Measures against circulatory shock, respiratory depression and convulsion may be needed.

Storage and Disposal:

Pesticide Disposal: Pesticide wastes are acutely hazardous. Improper disposal of excess pesticide, spray mixture, or rinsate is a violation of federal law. If these wastes cannot be disposed of according to label instructions, contact a state pesticide or environmental control agency, or the hazardous waste representative at the nearest EPA regional office for guidance.

Do not contaminate water, food, or feed by storage or disposal.

Container Disposal: Triple rinse (or equivalent). Then offer for recycling or reconditioning, or puncture and dispose of in a sanitary landfill, or incineration, or if allowed by state and local authorities, by burning. If burned, stay out of smoke.

Warning(s): Keep out of the reach of children.

Discussion: Toxicity tests required by the U.S. Environmental Protection Agency for TEK-TROL® disinfectant cleaner have been done, in conformity with the FDA and EPA Good Laboratory Practice Regulations.

Proven effective as a disinfectant by the following tests: A.O.A.C. (use dilution test method) in conformance with the 14th Edition 1984. All dilutions at (1:256). The following organisms tested at 1,000 ppm water hardness as calcium carbonate and 10% horse serum (as organic soil): *Staphylococcus aureus* (ATCC #6538), *Streptococcus pyogenes* (ATCC #9342), *Shigella sonnei* (ATCC #25931), *Klebsiella pneumoniae* (ATCC #4352), *Enterobacter aerogenes* (ATCC #13048), *Proteus vulgaris* (ATCC #13315), *Pseudomonas aeruginosa* (ATCC #15442), *Mycobacterium bovis* (BCG) A.O.A.C. tuberculocidal test, *Trichophyton mentagrophytes* (ATCC #9533) A.O.A.C. fungicidal test, *Pasteurella multocida* (ATCC #6529); (fowl cholera), *P. anatipestifer*, Beta streptococcus (ATCC #19615), *Mycoplasma synoviae*, *Rhodococcus equi* (ATCC #6939), *Salmonella choleraesuis* (Kunzendorf strain), *Taylorella equigenitalis* (C.E.M. - Kentucky strain #3056, *Salmonella enteritidis* (ATCC #13076), *Aspergillus fumigatus* (ATCC #6285), *Salmonella choleraesius* (ATCC #10708), *S. schottmuelleri* (ATCC #8749), *S. pullorum* (ATCC #19945), *S. gallinarum* (ATCC #9184), *S. typhimurium* (ATCC #13311), *S. arizonae* (#7:1,7,8), *S. arizonae* (PD 36), *Escherichia coli* (ATCC #11229), *Alcaligenes faecalis* strain (#838), *A. faecalis* Georgia strain, *Staphylococcus epidermis*, enterococci group D species, *Mycoplasma gallisepticum*, *Staphylococcus hyicus*, *Streptococcus equi* (ATCC #39506), *Strept. suis* (type II), *Strept. pyogenes* (ATCC #19615), *Haemophilus parasuis* (ATCC #19417), and *Mycoplasma hyopneumoniae* (ATCC #25934).

The following viruses tested in accordance with U.S. Environmental Protection Agency Pesticide Assessment Guidelines on inanimate environmental surfaces. Tested at 1,000 ppm water hardness as calcium carbonate and 10% serum (as organic soil): Herpes simplex type 1; avian infectious bronchitis virus; transmissible gastro-enteritis virus Purdue strains (ATCC #VR-763); canine parvovirus, strain CPV MLV (Cornell); parainfluenza virus, type 1, Sendai strain (ATCC #VR-105); avian reovirus; porcine rotavirus (ATCC #VR-893); avian rotavirus (AVR-1); duck enteritis virus (D.V.E.); avian laryngotracheitis; Newcastle disease virus; avian influenza virus; pseudorabies virus, Aujeszky strain (ATCC #VR-135); mouse hepatitis virus, strain MHV-A59 (ATCC #VR-764); avian adenovirus; equine herpesvirus (ATCC #VR-700) (equine rhinopneumonitis); equine arteritis (ATCC #VR-796) (equine viral arteritis); influenza A-2/Hong Kong virus (ATCC #VR-544).

Hard surface mildewcidal test method: CSMA method 23 at 1,000 ppm water hardness as calcium carbonate and 10% serum (as organic soil): *Aspergillus niger* (ATCC #6275), black mold; Penicillium variable (NRRL #3765), green mold.

Presentation: Cases of 4 x 1 gallon jugs and 55 gallon drums.

Compendium Code No.: 13700040

TEK-TROL® HOG WASH

Bio-Tek **Grooming Shampoo**

Sow Shampoo

Indications: TEK-TROL® Brand Hog Wash Sow Shampoo with aloe is ideal for use prior to breeding, farrowing or transporting.

Directions for Use: Wash down sows with clear water to remove gross soils. Apply TEK-TROL® Brand Hog Wash at ½ oz per gallon dilutions, either by manual application or low pressure sprayer. Rinse again to remove further loosened soils. Repeat procedure. Bio-Tek recommends the use of the Tek-Trol® Applicator to insure accurate dilutions when applying TEK-TROL® Brand Hog Wash.

Precaution(s): Storage: Store in original packaging. Keep tightly sealed when not in use. Dispose of properly.

Warning(s): First Aid: Eye irritant. Avoid contact with eyes. If contact occurs, flush with liberal amounts of running water.

Presentation: 4 x 1 gallon (3.8 L) containers per case and 55 gallon drums.

Compendium Code No.: 13700080

TELAZOL® CIII

Fort Dodge **General Anesthetic**

Tiletamine HCl and Zolazepam HCl

NADA No.: 106-111

Active Ingredient(s): The product is supplied sterile in vials. The addition of 5 mL diluent produces a solution containing the equivalent of 50 mg tiletamine base, 50 mg zolazepam base and 57.7 mg mannitol per milliliter. This solution has a pH of 2 to 3.5 and is recommended for deep intramuscular injection.

Indications: TELAZOL® is indicated in cats for restraint or for anesthesia combined with muscle relaxation and in dogs for restraint and minor procedures of short duration (30 min. avg.) requiring mild to moderate analgesia. Minor surgery is considered to be laceration repair, draining of abscesses, castrations and other procedures requiring mild to moderate analgesia. (See Dogs under Administration and Dosage.)

Pharmacology: TELAZOL® (tiletamine HCl and zolazepam HCl) is a nonnarcotic, nonbarbiturate, injectable anesthetic agent for dogs and cats. Chemically, TELAZOL® is a combination of equal parts by weight of base of tiletamine hydrochloride (2-[ethylamino]-2-[2-thienyl]-cyclohexanone hydrochloride), an arylaminocycloalkanone dissociative anesthetic, and zolazepam hydrochloride (4-[o-fluorophenyl]-6, 8-dihydro-1,3, 8-trimethylpyrazolo [3, 4-e] [1, 4] diazepin-7 [1H]-1-hydrochloride), a nonphenothiazine diazepinone having minor tranquilizing properties.

Actions: TELAZOL® is a rapid-acting anesthetic combination of tiletamine hydrochloride and zolazepam hydrochloride. Tiletamine hydrochloride is a dissociative anesthetic agent whose pharmacologic action is characterized by profound analgesia, normal pharyngeal-laryngeal reflexes and cataleptoid anesthesia. The anesthetic state produced does not fit into the conventional classification of stages of anesthesia, but instead TELAZOL® produces a state of unconsciousness which has been termed "dissociative" anesthesia in that it appears to selectively interrupt association pathways to the brain before producing somesthetic sensory blockade. Cranial nerve and spinal reflexes remain active; however, these reflexes must not be confused with inadequate anesthesia. Analgesia results from apparent selective interruption of sensory inputs to the brain and usually persists after the anesthetic effect has subsided.

Protective reflexes, such as coughing and swallowing, are maintained under tiletamine anesthesia. Other reflexes, e.g., corneal, pedal, are maintained during tiletamine anesthesia, and should not be used as criteria for judging depth of anesthesia. The eyes normally remain open with the pupil dilated. It is suggested that a bland ophthalmic ointment be applied to the cornea if anesthesia is to be prolonged.

Used alone, tiletamine hydrochloride does not provide adequate muscle relaxation for abdominal surgical procedures. When combined with zolazepam hydrochloride, good muscle relaxation is generally attained during the phase of deep surgical anesthesia.

Following a single, deep intramuscular injection of TELAZOL® in cats and dogs, onset of anesthetic effect usually occurs within 5 to 12 minutes. Muscle relaxation is optimum for approximately the first 20 to 25 minutes after TELAZOL® is administered, and then diminishes. Recovery varies with the age and physical condition of the animal and the dose of TELAZOL® administered, but usually requires several hours. Recovery is extended with multiple injections, particularly in cats.

Repeated doses increase the duration of the effect of TELAZOL® but may not further diminish muscle tone. The quality of anesthesia with repeated doses varies because the ratio of the two components within the animal's body changes with each injection. This is due to the difference in the rates of metabolism and elimination of the two components. The quality of anesthesia will be improved and more predictable if the entire dose is given as a single injection rather than in several doses. The best method of evaluating the depth of TELAZOL® anesthesia is to monitor the patient for deliberate conscious response to nociceptive stimuli.

Copious salivation may occur during TELAZOL® anesthesia. Ptyalism may be controlled in dogs and cats by giving atropine sulfate, USP, 0.02 mg/lb (0.04 mg/kg) body weight, as concurrent medication. Exaggerated swallowing, reflex action and accumulation of saliva may give rise to vomiting and retching.

TELAZOL® has a wider margin of safety in cats than in dogs. Dogs have survived repeated dosage regimens of 13.6 mg/lb (30 mg/kg) (maximum safe dose) for eight successive days. This is approximately two times the maximum recommended therapeutic dose. Cats have survived dosage regimens of up to 32.7 mg/lb (72 mg/kg) (maximum safe dose) on alternate days for seven episodes. This is 4.6 times the maximum recommended therapeutic dose for cats. However, these reports should not obviate prudent anesthetic practices. Some degree of tolerance has been reported. This tolerance appears to be species-variable.

Cats: In cats, the duration of effect of zolazepam exceeds that of tiletamine so that as the animal recovers there is a greater degree of tranquilization than anesthetization. There is a slight lowering of blood pressure during the first hour after injection. Heart rate and electrocardiogram readings are unaffected by TELAZOL® (tiletamine HCl and zolazepam HCl). Arterial pO_2 levels are decreased three minutes after injection but usually return to normal within 15 to 35 minutes.

Dogs: In dogs, the duration of effect of tiletamine exceeds that of zolazepam so there is a lesser degree of tranquilization than anesthetization in this species. The total effect of TELAZOL® in dogs is of shorter duration than in cats.

Following administration of TELAZOL® in dogs, a marked, persistent tachycardia occurs within two minutes following either 4.5 or 9 mg/lb (10 or 20 mg/kg) TELAZOL® intramuscularly. Stroke volume decreases proportionately to the increased rate at the 4.5 mg/lb (10 mg/kg) dose, with little change in net cardiac output. There is an initial increase in systolic blood pressure, with a slight drop in pressure within five minutes. The systolic blood pressure remains at this decreased level throughout the duration of the anesthetic effect. Diastolic pressure increases throughout this same period. Following a 9 mg/lb (20 mg/kg) dose of TELAZOL® in dogs, the relationship between stroke volume and heart rate is disproportionate, with a resultant substantial decrease in cardiac output. Contractility and mean blood pressure are decreased, indicating direct myocardial depression. Ventricular function is adequate. During surgical manipulations, tachycardia and hypertension may be observed, and may be brought on by sympathetic reaction to painful stimuli. Epinephrine is markedly less arrhythmogenic in animals under TELAZOL® anesthesia than in those under halothane anesthesia.

During TELAZOL® anesthesia, the assurance of a patent airway is greatly enhanced by virtue of maintaining pharyngeal-laryngeal reflexes. During the first 15 minutes after intramuscular administration of 9 mg/lb (20 mg/kg) of TELAZOL®, the respiratory rate is doubled while the tidal volume is decreased to less than one-half of control values. Arterial pO_2 levels also decrease. This may be evidenced by hypoxemia and cyanosis. The pulmonary function usually returns to normal within 35 minutes after the administration of TELAZOL®.

Dosage and Administration: TELAZOL® is well tolerated by dogs and cats and should be administered by deep intramuscular injection in prescribed doses. At high doses, recovery is usually prolonged.

There may be pain on injection. This is especially prevalent in cats.

Fasting prior to induction of general anesthesia with TELAZOL® (tiletamine HCl and zolazepam HCl) is not essential; however, when preparing for elective surgery, it is advisable to withhold food for at least 12 hours prior to TELAZOL® administration.

As with other injectable anesthetic agents, the individual response to TELAZOL® is somewhat varied, depending upon the dose, general physical condition and age of the patient and duration of the surgical procedure. Therefore, recommendations for dosage regimens cannot be fixed absolutely.

Specific dosage requirements must be determined by evaluation of the health status and condition of the patient and of the procedure to be performed.

If adequate anesthesia is not produced by the recommended dosage regimen, supplemental anesthesia or another agent is indicated. This includes the use of barbiturates and volatile anesthetics. When used concurrently with TELAZOL® the dosage of these agents should be reduced.

Atropine sulfate, USP, 0.02 mg/lb (0.04 mg/kg), should be used as concurrent medication to control ptyalism.

Dogs: In healthy dogs, an initial intramuscular dosage of 3 to 4.5 mg/lb (6.6 to 9.9 mg/kg) TELAZOL® is recommended for diagnostic purposes; 4.5 to 6 mg/lb (9.9 to 13.2 mg/kg) for minor procedures of short duration, such as treatment of lacerations and wounds, castrations and other procedures requiring mild to moderate analgesia. When supplemental doses of TELAZOL® are required, such individual supplemental doses should be less than the initial dose, and the total dose given (initial dose plus supplemental dose or doses) should not exceed 12 mg/lb (26.4 mg/kg). The maximum safe dose is 13.6 mg/lb (29.92 mg/kg). (See Actions.) Results from TELAZOL® anesthesia in dogs will be more satisfactory if the procedures are completed within one hour and if the procedures can be completed following single dose administration. In order to maintain at least a 2X margin of safety in dogs, the use of this product is limited to procedures that call for low doses (see Indications). Studies show that there is variation in response to different dosages of TELAZOL® and that low doses do not give adequate levels of anesthesia, and in some instances do not give adequate analgesia, for extensive procedures.

Cats: In healthy cats, an initial TELAZOL® dosage of 4.4 to 5.4 mg/lb (9.7 to 11.9 mg/kg) is recommended for such procedures as dentistry, treatment of abscesses, foreign body removal and related types of surgery; 4.8 to 5.7 mg/lb (10.6 to 12.5 mg/kg) for minor procedures requiring mild to moderate analgesia, such as repair of lacerations, castrations and other procedures of short duration. Initial dosages of 6.5 to 7.2 mg/lb (14.3 to 15.8 mg/kg) are recommended for ovariohysterectomy and onychectomy. When supplemental doses of TELAZOL® are required, such individual supplemental doses should be given in increments that are less than the initial dose, and the total dose given (initial dose plus supplemental doses) should not exceed the maximum allowable safe dose of 32.7 mg/lb (72 mg/kg). (See Actions.)

Preparation of Solution: To each vial add 5 mL sterile water for injection, USP. Slight agitation will facilitate complete reconstitution. The resultant solution will contain 100 mg active ingredient per one milliliter.

Discard unused solution after 4 days when stored at room temperature or after 14 days when kept refrigerated. Only clear solutions should be administered.

Contraindication(s): The use of TELAZOL® is contraindicated in dogs and cats with pancreatic disease. TELAZOL® is excreted predominantly by the kidneys. Preexistent renal pathology or impairment of renal function may be expected to result in prolonged duration of anesthesia. TELAZOL® should not be used in dogs and cats with severe cardiac or pulmonary dysfunction. Because the teratogenic potential of TELAZOL® is unknown, it should not be used in pregnant bitches or queens at any stage of pregnancy. Also, a study has shown that TELAZOL® crosses the placental barrier and produces respiratory depression in the newborn; therefore, its use for Caesarean section is contraindicated.

Precaution(s): Store at controlled room temperature 15° to 30°C (59° to 86°F).

Caution(s): Federal law restricts this drug to use by or on the order of a licensed veterinarian.

The dosage of TELAZOL® should be reduced in geriatric dogs and cats, in animals in debilitated condition and in animals with impairment of renal function. Death has occurred in both cats and dogs following TELAZOL® administration. Preexisting pulmonary disease, renal disease (see Contraindications and Warnings) and shock were causally implicated at necropsy; however, death was drug attributable in at least one dog (of 1072) and one cat (of 1095). Cats and smaller dogs with small body masses in relation to large body surfaces should be protected from heat loss during TELAZOL® anesthesia. Body temperature should be monitored, and supplemental heat may be required to control hypothermia. As with other anesthetics, it is prudent to provide for hemostasis during any surgical procedure.

During TELAZOL® anesthesia, athetoid movement may occur. This athetosis should not be mistaken for lack of anesthesia nor is it indicative of lack of analgesia. Do not give additional anesthesia in an attempt to abolish the athetoid movement. Efforts to eliminate athetoid movement with additional doses of TELAZOL® can result in anesthetic overdosage. TELAZOL® does not abolish laryngeal, pharyngeal, pinnal, palpebral and pedal reflexes, and may not be adequate as the sole anesthetic for surgical procedures in these areas.

Endotracheal tubes are not well tolerated in connection with TELAZOL® anesthesia in the cat and their use may result in impaired respiration. After removal of the tube, normal respiration should resume.

The stimulation of surgical procedures aids in maintaining adequate ventilation. The anesthetized patient must be monitored throughout the procedure, and if cardiopulmonary problems do occur, measures must be taken to assure that alveolar ventilation and cardiovascular functions are maintained.

The eyes normally remain open with the pupils dilated. The use of a bland ophthalmic ointment is advisable to protect the corneas from desiccation. A study has indicated that the concurrent use of chloramphenicol will prolong the duration of anesthesia in cats.

Atropine (0.02 mg/lb) (0.04 mg/kg) should be used to control ptyalism.

Warning(s): For use in dogs and cats only. The principal route of excretion of both components in the cat is the urine; therefore, TELAZOL® is not recommended for use in cats suffering from renal insufficiency.

Balance studies in dogs indicated extensive biotransformation of both components with less than 4% of the dose excreted unchanged in the urine.

The safety of the use of TELAZOL® (tiletamine HCl and zolazepam HCl) in pregnant animals or on reproduction has not been established. TELAZOL® crosses the placental barrier and causes respiratory depression in the neonate. Phenothiazine-derivative drugs should not be used with TELAZOL® because the combination produces respiratory and myocardial depression, hypotension and hypothermia.

Pulmonary edema has been reported to occur in cats with the use of TELAZOL®. Signs and symptoms include dyspnea, lethargy, anorexia and abnormal behavior. Deaths have been reported occasionally in severely affected individuals. Cats should be observed closely for any signs and symptoms which may suggest pulmonary edema so that appropriate therapy may be instituted.

Adverse Reactions: Respiratory depression may occur following administration of high doses of TELAZOL®. If at any time respiration becomes excessively depressed and the animal becomes cyanotic, resuscitative measures should be instituted promptly. Adequate pulmonary ventilation using either oxygen or room air is recommended as a resuscitative measure.

Adverse reactions reported have included emesis during emergence, excessive salivation, transient apnea, vocalization, erratic recovery and prolonged recovery, excessive tracheal and bronchial secretions when atropine sulfate, USP, was not given before anesthesia, involuntary muscular twitching, hypertonicity, cyanosis, cardiac arrest, pulmonary edema and muscle rigidity during surgical procedures. Central nervous system stimulation and convulsions have also been reported. Tachycardia frequently occurs, particularly in the dog. This rise in heart rate usually last about 30 minutes. Either hypertension or hypotension may also occur. Insufficient anesthesia has been reported in dogs.

Death has been reported in dogs and cats following TELAZOL® administration.

Presentation: TELAZOL® (tiletamine HCl and zolazepam HCl) is available in individual vials of 5 mL solution when reconstituted (NDC 0856-9050-93).

Manufactured by: Wyeth-Lederle Parenterals, Inc., Carolina, Puerto Rico 00986

Compendium Code No.: 10032180 5080E

TEMARIL-P® TABLETS ℞

Pfizer Animal Health **Antitussive**

(trimeprazine with prednisolone) Antipruritic-Antitussive-Anti-inflammatory

NADA No.: 012-437

Active Ingredient(s): Composition: Each tablet contains trimeprazine tartrate (USP) 10-[3-(Dimethylamino)-2-methylpropyl] phenothiazine tartrate (2:1) equivalent to trimeprazine, 5 mg, and prednisolone, 2 mg.

Indications: Recommendations for use:

1. Antipruritic: TEMARIL-P® is recommended for the relief of itching regardless of cause. Its usefulness has been demonstrated for the relief of itching and the reduction of inflammation commonly associated with most skin disorders of dogs such as the eczema caused by internal disorders, otitis, and dermatitis (allergic, parasitic, pustular, and nonspecific). It often relieves pruritis which does not respond to other therapy. With any pruritus treatment, the cause should be determined and corrected; otherwise, signs are likely to recur following discontinuance of therapy.
2. Antitussive: TEMARIL-P® has been found to be effective therapy and adjunctive therapy in various cough conditions of dogs. Therefore, in addition to its antipruritic action, TEMARIL-P® is recommended for the treatment of "kennel cough" or tracheobronchitis, bronchitis including all allergic bronchitis and infections and coughs of nonspecific origin. (Coughs due to cardiac insufficiencies would not be expected to respond to TEMARIL-P® therapy.) As with any antitussive treatment, the etiology of the cough should be determined and eliminated if possible. Otherwise, symptoms are likely to recur following discontinuance of therapy.

Note: TEMARIL-P® may be administered to animals suffering from acute or chronic bacterial infections provided the infection is controlled by appropriate antibiotic or chemotherapeutic agents.

Pharmacology: Action: The exclusive TEMARIL-P® formula combines the antipruritic and antitussive action of trimeprazine with the anti-inflammatory action of prednisolone. A therapeutic effect is attained by administering the tablets twice daily.

Dosage and Administration: Recommended Dosage: The same dosage schedule may be followed for both antipruritic and antitussive therapy.

Weight of Dog	Initial Dosage
Up to 10 lb	½ tablet, twice daily
11-20 lb	1 tablet, twice daily
21-40 lb	2 tablets, twice daily
Over 40 lb	3 tablets, twice daily

After 4 days, reduce dosage to ½ of the initial dose or to an amount just sufficient to maintain remission of symptoms. Individual animal response will vary and dosage should be adjusted until proper response is obtained.

Precaution(s): Store in a dry, cool place at temperatures not above 25°C (77°F).

Caution(s): Federal law restricts this drug to use by or on the order of a licensed veterinarian.

All the cautions applicable to cortisone and to phenothiazine derivatives apply also to TEMARIL-P®.

Prolonged treatment with TEMARIL-P® must be withdrawn gradually. Use of corticosteroids, depending on dose, duration, and specific steroid, may result in inhibition of endogenous steroid production following drug withdrawal. In patients presently receiving or recently withdrawn from systemic steroid treatments, therapy with a rapidly acting corticosteroid should be considered in unusually stressful situations.

For use in dogs.

Warning(s): Clinical and experimental data have demonstrated that corticosteroids administered orally or by injection to animals may induce the first stage of parturition if used during the last trimester of pregnancy and may precipitate premature parturition followed by dystocia, fetal death, retained placenta, and metritis. Additionally, corticosteroids administered to dogs, rabbits, and rodents during pregnancy have resulted in cleft palate in offspring. Corticosteroids administered to dogs during pregnancy have also resulted in other congenital anomalies, including deformed forelegs, phocomelia, and anasarca. If a vasoconstrictor is needed, norepinephrine should be used in lieu of epinephrine. Phenothiazine derivatives may reverse the usual elevating action of epinephrine causing further lowering of blood pressure.

Side Effects: Possible side effects attributable to corticosteroids include sodium retention and potassium loss, negative nitrogen balance, suppressed adrenal cortical function, delayed wound healing, osteoporosis, elevated levels of SGPT and SAP, and vomiting and diarrhea (occasionally bloody). Cushings syndrome in dogs has been reported in association with prolonged or repeated steroid therapy. Possible increased susceptibility to bacterial invasion and/or the exacerbation of preexisting bacterial infection may occur in patients receiving corticosteroids. As noted above, however, this problem can be avoided by concomitant use of appropriate anti-infective agents. Possible side effects attributable to phenothiazine derivatives include sedation; protruding nictitating membrane; blood dyscrasias; intensification and prolongation of the action of analgesics, sedatives and general anesthetics; and potentiation of organophosphate toxicity and the activity of procaine hydrochloride.

It should be remembered that the premonitory signs of cortisone overdosage, such as sodium retention and edema, may not occur with prednisolone. Therefore, the veterinarians must be alert to detect less obvious side effects, such as blood dyscrasias, polydipsia and polyuria.

The appearance and severity of side effects are dose related and are minimal at the recommended dosage level. If troublesome side effects are encountered, the dosage of TEMARIL-P® should be reduced and discontinued unless the severity of the condition being treated makes its relief paramount.

References: Available upon request.

Presentation: Bottles of 100 and 1000.

U.S. Patent No. 2,837,518

Licensed under U.S. Patent No. 3,134,718

Compendium Code No.: 36901441 75-8548-09

TEMPO®

1% Dust Insecticide

Bayer

For Control of Crawling And Flying Insect Pests In Poultry And Livestock Facilities.

For Commercial Use Only

ACTIVE INGREDIENT:

Cyfluthrin, cyano(4-fluoro-3-phenoxyphenyl)methyl 3-(2,2-dichloroethenyl)-2,2-dimethylcyclopropanecarboxylate 1%

INERT INGREDIENTS: 99%

100%

STOP - Read The Label Before Use

KEEP OUT OF THE REACH OF CHILDREN

CAUTION

PRECAUCION AL USUARIO: Si usted no puede leer o entender inglés, no use este producto hasta que la etiqueta le haya sido explicada ampliamente.

(TO THE USER: If you cannot read or understand English, do not use this product until the label has been fully explained to you.)

PRECAUTIONARY STATEMENTS

HAZARDS TO HUMANS AND DOMESTIC ANIMALS

CAUTION: Causes moderate eye irritation. Harmful if swallowed, inhaled or absorbed through the skin. Do not get into eyes, on skin, or on clothing. Avoid breathing dust. If clothing becomes contaminated, remove and wash before reuse. Wash hands thoroughly with soap and warm water after handling. Keep out of reach of children.

Do not contaminate feed or food.

SYMPTOMS OF POISONING: In case of poisoning, call physician or Poison Control Center immediately. Have patient lie down and keep quiet.

STATEMENTS OF PRACTICAL TREATMENT

If in eyes: Hold eyelids open and flush with plenty of water. Call a physician if irritation persists. **If swallowed:** Call a physician or Poison Control Center. Administer water freely and induce vomiting by giving one dose (½ oz or 15 mL) of syrup of ipecac. If vomiting does not occur within 10 to 20 minutes, administer second dose. If syrup of ipecac is not available, induce vomiting by sticking finger down throat. Repeat until vomit fluid is clear. Never give anything by mouth to an unconscious person. Avoid alcohol. **If on skin:** Wash thoroughly with soap and water. Get medical attention if irritation occurs. **If inhaled:** Move victim to fresh air. If not breathing, give artificial respiration, preferably mouth-to-mouth. Get medical attention.

To Physician: No specific antidote is available. Treat the patient symptomatically.

ENVIRONMENTAL HAZARDS

This pesticide is toxic to fish. For terrestrial uses, do not apply directly to water, or to areas where surface water is present or to intertidal areas below the mean high water mark. Cover or remove any fish or aquatic organism tank within structures being treated. Disconnect any air supply sources to such tanks before applications are made and reconnect after any possibility of contamination has passed. Apply this product only as specified on the label.

DIRECTIONS FOR USE

It is a violation of Federal law to use this product in a manner inconsistent with its labeling.

IMPORTANT: Read these entire **Directions for Use** and **Conditions of Sale** before using TEMPO 1% Dust Insecticide.

CONDITIONS OF SALE: THE DIRECTIONS ON THIS LABEL WERE DETERMINED THROUGH RESEARCH TO BE APPROPRIATE FOR THE CORRECT USE OF THIS PRODUCT. THIS PRODUCT HAS BEEN TESTED UNDER DIFFERENT ENVIRONMENTAL CONDITIONS BOTH INDOORS AND OUTDOORS SIMILAR TO THOSE THAT ARE ORDINARY AND CUSTOMARY WHERE THE PRODUCT IS TO BE USED. INSUFFICIENT CONTROL OF PESTS OR PLANT INJURY MAY RESULT FROM THE OCCURRENCE OF EXTRAORDINARY OR UNUSUAL CONDITIONS, OR FROM FAILURE TO FOLLOW LABEL DIRECTIONS. IN ADDITION, FAILURE TO FOLLOW LABEL DIRECTIONS MAY CAUSE INJURY TO ANIMALS, MAN, AND DAMAGE TO THE ENVIRONMENT. BAYER OFFERS, AND THE BUYER ACCEPTS AND USES, THIS PRODUCT SUBJECT TO THE CONDITIONS THAT EXTRAORDINARY OR UNUSUAL ENVIRONMENTAL CONDITIONS, OR FAILURE TO FOLLOW LABEL DIRECTIONS ARE BEYOND THE CONTROL OF BAYER AND ARE, THEREFORE, THE RESPONSIBILITY OF THE BUYER.

Do not formulate this product into other end use products.

GENERAL INFORMATION

TEMPO 1% Dust Insecticide is a ready-to-use insecticide dust which provides effective knockdown and residual control of the pests listed on the label.

TEMPO 1% Dust Insecticide is for residual pest control in and around livestock and poultry housing facilities. Permitted areas of use include, **but are not limited to**, livestock housing structures, poultry houses, swine houses, cattle barns, horse stables and pet kennels.

Do not use in food/feed handling establishments, restaurants or other areas where food/feed is commercially prepared or processed.

INDOOR PESTS

Apply dust using hand or power dusters or other suitable equipment. Apply lightly and uniformly to infested areas. Pay particular attention to floors, walls and bedding, as well as, cracks and crevices; wall voids and around window and door frames. Apply 0.5 to 1 pound of TEMPO 1% Dust Insecticide per thousand square feet. Do not make application of TEMPO 1% Dust when animals are present in area of facility to be treated. Do not apply directly to animal feedstuffs or watering equipment. Repeat treatments as necessary to maintain adequate control.

OUTDOOR/PERIMETER PESTS

Make a residual treatment in voids, cracks and crevices in window and door frames, between elements of construction or void areas in door porches, eaves and in crawl spaces and other areas where pests hide.

Wasps and Bees: It is advisable to treat wasp and bee nests in the evening when insects are less active and have returned to the nest. Wear protective clothing if deemed necessary to avoid stings. Using hand-held or power duster or other suitable means, with extension tubes if necessary, thoroughly dust nest and entrance and surrounding areas where insects alight. To treat nests in wall voids, drill a hole in the area, dust entrance and surrounding areas. For best results check nests carefully one or two days after treatment to ensure complete kill, then remove and destroy nest to prevent emergence of newly-hatched insects. If removal is not feasible, retreat the nest, if necessary.

To help prevent invasion of structures by the listed outdoor pests, treat soil or other substrate adjacent to structure using TEMPO 1% Dust, TEMPO 20 WP or TEMPO 2 as per the registered label. Also treat the structure foundation where pests are active and may find entrance.

PESTS CONTROLLED BY TEMPO 1% DUST INSECTICIDE

I. INDOOR PREMISE PESTS

Ants (except Pharaoh), Bedbugs, Beetles (exposed adults & immature stages) (Cadelle, Centipedes, Cigarette, Cockroaches, Confused Flour, Darkling, Dermestid, Granary weevil, Hide, Larder, Leather, Lesser grain borer, Lesser mealworm, Merchant grain, Mealworm, Red flour, Rice weevil, Sawtoothed grain, Warehouse), Fire ants, Moths (Indian meal, Mediterranean flour), Spiders, Wasps, Yellow-jackets

II. OUTDOOR PESTS

Ants, Bees, Boxelder bugs, Centipedes, Cockroaches, Crickets, Fleas, Flies, Ground beetles, Hornets, Millipedes, Moths, Scorpions, Spiders, Ticks, Wasps, Yellow-jackets

STORAGE AND DISPOSAL

Do not contaminate water, food, or feed by storage or disposal.

Pesticide Disposal: Pesticide wastes are hazardous. Improper disposal of excess pesticide is a violation of Federal law. If these wastes cannot be disposed of by use according to label instructions, contact your State Pesticide or Environmental Control Agency, or the Hazardous Waste representative at the nearest EPA Regional Office for guidance.

Container Disposal: Do not use container in connection with food, feed, or drinking water. Completely empty container into application equipment. Offer for recycling or reconditioning, or puncture and dispose of in a sanitary landfill, or incineration, or if allowed by state and local authorities, by burning. If burned, stay out of smoke.

Storage: Store in a cool, dry place and in such a manner as to prevent cross contamination with other pesticides, fertilizers, food, and feed. Store in original containers and out of the reach of children, preferably in a locked storage area.

Handle and open container in a manner as to prevent spillage. If the container is leaking or material spilled for any reason or cause, carefully sweep material into a pile. Refer to Precautionary Statements on label for hazards associated with the handling of this material. Do not walk through spilled material. Dispose of pesticide as directed above. In spill or leak incidents, keep unauthorized people away. You may contact the Bayer Emergency Response Team for decontamination procedures or any other assistance that may be necessary. The Bayer Kansas City Emergency Response Telephone No. is 800-414-0244, or contact Chemtrec at 800-424-9300.

EPA Reg. No. 3125-485-11556
EPA Est. No. 34704-NB-001

SUPPLIED: Code 0375—4.50 kg (10 Pounds)

80003750, R.1
0375
905050
060796A

Manufactured For Bayer Corporation, Agriculture Division, Animal Health, Shawnee Mission, Kansas 66201 U.S.A.

Compendium Code No.: 10400350

TEMPO®

20 WP Insecticide

Bayer

For Commercial Use Only

For Broad-Spectrum Control Of Crawling, Flying, And Wood Infesting Insect Pests For Indoor And Outdoor Surfaces.

ACTIVE INGREDIENT:

Cyfluthrin, cyano(4-fluoro-3-phenoxyphenyl)methyl 3-(2,2-dichloroethenyl)-2,2-dimethylcyclopropanecarboxylate 20%
INERT INGREDIENTS 80%
100%

CAUTION

STOP - Read the label before use.

Keep out of reach of children.

PRECAUCION AL USUARIO: Si usted no puede leer o entender inglés, no use este producto hasta que la etiqueta le haya sido explicada ampliamente. (TO THE USER: If you cannot read or understand English, do not use this product until the label has been fully explained to you.)

PRECAUTIONARY STATEMENTS

HAZARDS TO HUMANS AND DOMESTIC ANIMALS

CAUTION: Causes moderate eye irritation. Harmful if swallowed, inhaled or absorbed through the skin. Do not get in eyes, on skin, or on clothing. Avoid breathing dust or spray mist.

Do not contaminate feed or food. Keep out of reach of children.

Wear safety glasses, goggles, or face shield when handling the undiluted material and wear a respirator when making general surface overhead treatments indoors.

Do not allow children or pets to enter treated areas until surfaces are dry. Wash thoroughly with soap and warm water after handling. Remove contaminated clothing and wash before reuse.

In case of poisoning: Call physician or Poison Control Center immediately. Have patient lie down and keep quiet.

STATEMENTS OF PRACTICAL TREATMENT

If in eyes, hold eyelids open and flush with plenty of water. Call a physician if irritation persists. **If swallowed,** call a physician or Poison Control Center. Administer water freely and induce vomiting by giving one dose (½ oz or 15mL) of syrup of ipecac. If vomiting does not occur within 10 to 20 minutes, administer second dose. If syrup of ipecac is not available, induce vomiting by sticking finger down throat. Repeat until vomit fluid is clear. Never give anything by mouth to an unconscious person. Avoid alcohol. **If on skin,** wash thoroughly with soap and water. Get medical attention if irritation occurs. **If inhaled,** remove victim to fresh air. If not breathing, give artificial respiration, preferably mouth to mouth. Get medical attention.

Note To Physician: No specific antidote is available. Treat the patient symptomatically.

ENVIRONMENTAL HAZARDS

This pesticide is toxic to fish. Remove from premises or tightly cover fish tanks and disconnect aerators when applying indoors where such containers are present. Do not apply directly to water, or to areas where surface water is present or to intertidal areas below the mean high water mark. Drift and runoff from treated areas may be hazardous to aquatic organisms in neighboring areas. Do not contaminate water when disposing of equipment washwaters.

Apply this product only as specified on this label.

This pesticide is highly toxic to bees exposed to direct treatment or residues on crops or weeds. Do not apply TEMPO 20 WP Insecticide or allow it to drift onto crops or weeds on which bees are actively foraging. Additional information may be obtained by consulting your Cooperative Extension Service.

DIRECTIONS FOR USE

It is a violation of Federal law to use this product in a manner inconsistent with its labeling.

IMPORTANT: Read these entire Directions for Use and Conditions of Sale before using TEMPO 20 WP Insecticide.

CONDITIONS OF SALE: THE DIRECTIONS ON THIS LABEL WERE DETERMINED THROUGH RESEARCH TO BE APPROPRIATE FOR THE CORRECT USE OF THIS PRODUCT. THIS PRODUCT HAS BEEN TESTED UNDER DIFFERENT ENVIRONMENTAL CONDITIONS BOTH INDOORS AND OUTDOORS SIMILAR TO THOSE THAT ARE ORDINARY AND CUSTOMARY WHERE THE PRODUCT IS TO BE USED. INSUFFICIENT CONTROL OF PESTS OR PLANT INJURY MAY RESULT FROM THE OCCURRENCE OF EXTRAORDINARY OR UNUSUAL CONDITIONS, OR FROM FAILURE TO FOLLOW LABEL DIRECTIONS. IN ADDITION, FAILURE TO FOLLOW LABEL DIRECTIONS MAY CAUSE INJURY TO ANIMALS, MAN, AND DAMAGE TO THE ENVIRONMENT. BAYER OFFERS, AND THE BUYER ACCEPTS AND USES, THIS PRODUCT SUBJECT TO THE CONDITIONS THAT EXTRAORDINARY OR UNUSUAL ENVIRONMENTAL CONDITIONS, OR FAILURE TO FOLLOW LABEL DIRECTIONS ARE BEYOND THE CONTROL OF BAYER AND ARE, THEREFORE, THE RESPONSIBILITY OF THE BUYER.

Do not formulate this product into other end-use products.

One level Tempo scoopful contains 5 grams of Tempo 20 WP. Do not use scoop for feed, food, or drinking water purposes.

GENERAL INFORMATION

TEMPO 20 WP Insecticide contains 20% active ingredient, which will provide effective knockdown and residual control of the pests listed in this label.

Tempo 20 WP is intended for use as a general surface, spot, or crack and crevice application in and around buildings and structures and their immediate surroundings and on various modes of transport. Permitted areas of use include, **but are not limited to**, grain mills, granaries, livestock housing structures, pet kennels, poultry houses, warehouses and similar structures as well as trucks, trailers and rail cars. Do not use in aircraft cabins.

Tempo 20 WP is intended to be mixed with water and applied with hand pressurized or power operated sprayers. Spray pressure should not exceed 50 PSI at the nozzle tip when used indoors. Add the appropriate amount of product when filling sprayer tank with water, shake or agitate as necessary to mix. Diluted spray mixture can be stored overnight and applied the following day; however, mixture should be agitated prior to application to prevent uneven distribution of product. Before leaving spray mixture unagitated for an extended period of time, release tank pressure and elevate nozzle and hose above tank outlet, activate trigger and drain all suspension from hose back into spray tank. Re-tighten spray tank lid and do not re-pressurize until starting spray again.

Tempo 20 WP will not stain or cause damage to any painted or varnished surface, plastic, fabric or other surface where water applied alone causes no damage.

TANK MIXING

The user, at his discretion, can tank mix pesticides currently registered for similar use patterns, unless the product labels specifically prohibit such use. It is always recommended that a small jar compatibility test using proper proportions of chemicals and water be run to check for physical compatibility prior to tank mixing.

GENERAL SURFACE APPLICATION

Use two level Tempo scoopsful of Tempo 20 WP per 1000 sq ft (see Note 1) in sufficient water to adequately cover the area being treated, but which will not allow dripping or run-off to occur (see Note 2). Use a low pressure system with a fan type nozzle to uniformly apply the suspension. Applications can be made to walls, floors, ceilings, between, behind and beneath equipment, around floor drains, window and door frames, and on the underside of shelves and in similar areas. Applications may be made to floor surfaces along walls and around air ducts, however, do not treat entire area of floor or floor coverings. Cover exposed food/feed or remove from area being treated. Re-application can be made at 10-day intervals, if necessary. Do not apply where electrical short circuits could occur. Use a dust or dry bait in these areas. It is recommended to wear safety glasses, goggles or face shield and a respirator when making a general surface treatment to overhead areas.

Note 1: Under conditions of severe pest infestation or when quicker knock-down and/or longer residual control is needed, use four level Tempo scoopsful of Tempo 20 WP per 1000 sq ft.

Note 2: Volume of Water Sprays Applied to A Vertical Surface to Attain Appropriate Coverage

Type of Surface	Quarts 1000 Sq Ft	Gallons 1000 Sq Ft
Ceramic tile (glazed)	0.75	0.2
Stainless steel	0.75	0.2
Latex painted plywood (semigloss)	4.0	1.0
Masonite (smooth)	6.3	1.5
Unpainted plywood	11.0	2.7
Unpainted particle board	11.7	3.0
Cement block (semigloss latex)	12.5	3.2
Cement block (unfinished)	145.5	36.3

SPOT, OR CRACK AND CREVICE APPLICATIONS TREATMENT

Mix two level Tempo scoopsful of Tempo 20 WP in one gallon of water to make a 0.05% active ingredient concentration (see Note 3). Use a low pressure system with a pin-point or variable pattern nozzle to apply the suspension in specific areas such as: cracks and crevices in floors, walls, expansion joints, areas around water and sewer pipes, wall voids, or voids in equipment where pests can hide as well as other similar areas. Spot treatments may also be made to areas **including but not limited to** storage areas, doors and windows, behind and under equipment and similar areas. Tempo 20 WP can be reapplied at 10-day intervals, if necessary. Do not apply where electrical short circuits could occur. Use a dust or dry bait in these areas.

Note 3: Under conditions of severe pest infestation or when quicker knock-down and/or longer residual control is needed, mix four level Tempo scoopsful of Tempo 20 WP in one gallon of water to make a 0.1% active ingredient concentration.

INDOOR PEST CONTROL

CRAWLING INSECT CONTROL

For **stored product pest control** of exposed adult and immature stages of insect pests, apply to cracks, crevices, and other surfaces where the pests have been seen or have harborage. Treat warehouses, production facilities, storage areas, rail cars, truck beds and other areas where products are stored before filling with the product. Tempo 20 WP may be used by pest control operators and grain producers to treat grain storage facilities and other areas noted above for stored product pest control. Cleaning of all areas prior to use of Tempo 20 WP will increase levels of control. Any foodstuffs infested with pests should be removed and destroyed.

For **use by pest control operators or livestock producers in livestock housing structures (including poultry houses) and pet kennels** to control crawling and flying insect pests. Apply as a general surface and/or a crack and crevice spray. Control will be enhanced when facilities

T

are cleaned and interior applications are supplemented with exterior perimeter treatments. Do not make interior applications of Tempo 20 WP in areas of facility where animals other than cattle or horses are present. Do not make applications to animal feedstuffs or watering equipment.

FLYING INSECT PEST CONTROL (General Surface Spray)

For control of flying insects indoors make application to surfaces as directed under Directions For Use, where the pests collect or rest. **Do not apply as a "space spray" application.**

OUTDOOR PEST CONTROL

For perimeter pest control, make a general surface application to outside surfaces of buildings, porches, patios, garages and other adjacent areas where pests have been seen or found. To help prevent infestations of buildings by occasional invaders, treat soil, turf or other substrates adjacent to buildings, the building foundation, walls, around doors and windows, soffit areas where these pests are active and may find entrance or harborage. Apply a minimum of 10 grams of Tempo 20 WP per 1000 sq ft in sufficient water to provide adequate coverage.

For control of the **imported red fire ant**, use a 0.1% suspension of Tempo 20 WP and thoroughly drench or inject the entire mound area. Treat all areas of the mound showing activity to provide contact control of the adult fire ants. Tempo 20 WP will provide contact activity and residual repellency in the active mound.

When using the injection treatment method for control of the imported red fire ant, it is essential that treatment be made to the bottom of the active mound. Apply suspension throughout the mound using a downward and upward motion of the injector tool. Multiple injection sites may be needed to ensure complete distribution of the suspension throughout the active mound.

Do not use Tempo 20 WP to treat fire ant mounds in any food crop production area, pasture or area where food crop production may occur.

PESTS CONTROLLED BY TEMPO *

I. INDOOR PREMISE PESTS

1. Crawling Pests

Ants (except Pharaoh), Bedbugs, Carpet beetle, Centipedes, Cockroaches (American, Asian, German, Oriental, brown-banded, smoky brown), Crickets, Darkling beetles, Earwigs, Firebrats, Millipedes, Pillbugs, Silverfish, Sowbugs, Spiders

2. Flying Pests

Clothes moths, Flies, Gnats, Midges, Mosquitoes, Moths, Yellow-jackets, Wasps

3. Stored Product Pests

Beetles (exposed adults & immature stages) (Cadelle, Cigarette, Confused flour, Dermestid, Drug-store, Granary weevil, Hide, Larder, Leather, Lesser grain borer, Lesser mealworm, Merchant grain, Mealworm, Red flour, Rice weevil, Sawtoothed grain, Warehouse), Moths (Indian meal, Mediterranean flour)

II. OUTDOOR/PERIMETER PESTS

Ants, Bees, Boxelder bugs, Carpenter ants, Cecidflies, Centipedes, Clusterflies, Cockroaches, Crickets, Elm leaf beetle, Fire ants, Firebrats, Flies, Fleas, Gnats, Ground beetles, Hornets, Imported red fire ants, Midges, Millipedes, Mosquitoes, Moths, Scorpions, Silverfish, Spiders, Ticks, Wasps, Yellow-jackets

*For **GENERAL SURFACE APPLICATION**, Use 10 grams of Tempo 20 WP per 1000 square feet in sufficient water to adequately cover the area being treated. Under conditions of severe pest infestation or when quicker knock-down and/or longer residual control is needed, use 20 grams of Tempo 20 WP per 1000 sq. ft.

*For **SPOT, OR CRACK AND CREVICE APPLICATIONS**, mix 10 grams of Tempo 20 WP in one gallon of water to make a 0.05% active ingredient concentration. Under conditions of severe pest infestation or when quicker knockdown and/or longer residual control is needed, mix 20 grams of Tempo 20 WP in one gallon of water to make a 0.1% active ingredient concentration.

STORAGE AND DISPOSAL

Do not contaminate water, food, or feed by storage or disposal.

Not For Storage In or Around the House

Pesticide Storage: Store in a cool, dry place and in such a manner as to prevent cross contamination with other pesticides, fertilizers, food, and feed. Store in original containers and out of the reach of children, preferably in a locked storage area.

Handle and open container in a manner as to prevent spillage. If the container is leaking or material spilled for any reason or cause, carefully sweep material into a pile. Refer to Precautionary Statements on label for hazards associated with the handling of this material. Do not walk through spilled material. Dispose of pesticide as directed below. In spill or leak incidents, keep unauthorized people away. You may contact the Bayer Emergency Response Team for decontamination procedures or any other assistance that may be necessary. The Bayer Kansas City Emergency Response Telephone Number is 800-414-0244, or contact Chemtrec at 800-424-9300.

Pesticide Disposal: Pesticide wastes are hazardous. Improper disposal of excess pesticide, spray mixture, or rinsate is a violation of Federal law. If these wastes cannot be disposed of by use according to label instructions, contact your State Pesticide or Environmental Control Agency, or the Hazardous Waste representative at the nearest EPA Regional Office for guidance.

Container Disposal: Do not use container in connection with food, feed, or drinking water. Completely empty container into application equipment. Triple rinse (or equivalent), and then offer for recycling or reconditioning, or puncture and dispose of in a sanitary landfill, or incineration, or if allowed by state and local authorities, by burning. If burned, stay out of smoke.

EPA Reg. No. 3125-380 EPA Est. No. 3125-MO-1

SUPPLIED: Code 0359—420 Grams 0359, R.4

909770 110299

Bayer Corporation, Garden and Professional Care, Box 4913, Kansas City, MO 64120-0013 U.S.A.

Compendium Code No.: 10400360

T

TEMPO®

SC Ultra Premise Spray

Bayer

For broad-spectrum control of crawling, flying, and wood-infesting insect pests in and around animal housing, warehouses, and processing and packing plants.

Shake well before using.

ACTIVE INGREDIENT:

Beta-cyfluthrin; Cyano(4-fluoro-3-phenoxyphenyl) methyl 3-(2,2-dichloroethenyl)-2,2-dimethylcyclopropanecarboxylate	11.8%
OTHER INGREDIENTS:	88.2%
	100.0%

Contains 1 lb cyano(4-fluoro-3-phenoxyphenyl) methyl 3-(2,2-dichloroethenyl)-2,2-dimethylcyclopropanecarboxylate per gallon.

STOP - Read the label before use. Keep out of reach of children.

CAUTION

PRECAUTIONARY STATEMENTS

HAZARDS TO HUMANS AND DOMESTIC ANIMALS

CAUTION: Harmful if swallowed, inhaled or absorbed through skin. Causes moderate eye irritation. Avoid contact with eyes, skin or clothing. Avoid breathing spray mist. Wash thoroughly with soap and water after handling and before eating, drinking or using tobacco. Remove contaminated clothing and wash before reuse.

FIRST AID

If swallowed: Call a poison control center or doctor immediately for treatment advice. Have person sip a glass of water if able to swallow. Do not induce vomiting unless told to do so by a poison control center or a doctor. Do not give anything by mouth to an unconscious person. **If on skin or clothing:** Take off contaminated clothing. Rinse skin immediately with plenty of water for 15-20 minutes. Call a poison control center or doctor for treatment advice. **If in eyes:** Hold eye open and rinse slowly and gently with water for 15-20 minutes. Remove contact lenses, if present, after the first 5 minutes, then continue rinsing eye. Call a poison control center for treatment advice. **If inhaled:** Move person to fresh air. If person is not breathing, call 911 or an ambulance, then give artificial respiration, preferably mouth-to-mouth if possible. Call a poison control center or doctor for further treatment advice. Have the product container with you when calling a poison control center or doctor, or going for treatment.

Note To Physician: No specific antidote is available. Treat the patient symptomatically.

ENVIRONMENTAL HAZARDS

This pesticide is extremely toxic to fish and aquatic invertebrates. Remove from premises or tightly cover fish tanks and disconnect aerators when applying indoors where such containers are present. Do not apply directly to water, to areas where surface water is present or to intertidal areas below the mean high water mark.

Do not apply when weather conditions favor drift from treated areas. Drift and runoff from treated areas may be hazardous to aquatic organisms in neighboring areas. Do not contaminate water when cleaning equipment or when disposing of equipment wash waters. Apply this product only as specified on this label.

This pesticide is highly toxic to bees exposed to direct treatment or residues on crops or weeds. Do not apply Tempo® SC Ultra insecticide or allow it to drift onto crops or weeds on which bees are actively foraging. Additional information may be obtained by consulting your Cooperative Extension Service.

DIRECTIONS FOR USE

It is a violation of Federal law to use this product in a manner inconsistent with its labeling.

IMPORTANT: Read these entire Directions for Use and Conditions of Sale before using Tempo® SC Ultra Insecticide.

CONDITIONS OF SALE: THE DIRECTIONS ON THIS LABEL WERE DETERMINED THROUGH RESEARCH TO BE APPROPRIATE FOR THE CORRECT USE OF THIS PRODUCT. THIS PRODUCT HAS BEEN TESTED UNDER DIFFERENT ENVIRONMENTAL CONDITIONS BOTH INDOORS AND OUTDOORS SIMILAR TO THOSE THAT ARE ORDINARY AND CUSTOMARY WHERE THE PRODUCT IS TO BE USED. INSUFFICIENT CONTROL OF PESTS OR PLANT INJURY MAY RESULT FROM THE OCCURRENCE OF EXTRAORDINARY OR UNUSUAL CONDITIONS, OR FROM FAILURE TO FOLLOW LABEL DIRECTIONS. IN ADDITION, FAILURE TO FOLLOW LABEL DIRECTIONS MAY CAUSE INJURY TO ANIMALS, MAN, AND DAMAGE TO THE ENVIRONMENT. BAYER OFFERS, AND THE BUYER ACCEPTS AND USES, THIS PRODUCT SUBJECT TO THE CONDITIONS THAT EXTRAORDINARY OR UNUSUAL ENVIRONMENTAL CONDITIONS, OR FAILURE TO FOLLOW LABEL DIRECTIONS ARE BEYOND THE CONTROL OF BAYER AND ARE, THEREFORE, THE RESPONSIBILITY OF THE BUYER.

GENERAL INFORMATION

FOR STRUCTURAL PEST CONTROL

Tempo® SC Ultra Insecticide is a liquid formulation containing 1 lb active ingredient per gallon, which will provide effective knockdown and residual control of the pests listed in this label.

Tempo® SC Ultra is intended for use as a general surface, spot, mist, or crack and crevice application in and around buildings and structures and their immediate surroundings. Permitted areas of use include, **but are not limited to**, dairies and dairy product processing plants, grain mills, granaries, greenhouses (structures only), industrial buildings, kitchens, laboratories, livestock housing structures, pet kennels, manufacturing establishments, poultry houses, meat, poultry and egg processing and packing plants, meat and produce canneries, stores, warehouses, and similar structures.

Tempo® SC Ultra is intended to be mixed with water and applied with hand pressurized, power operated sprayers or foam generating equipment. Spray pressure should not exceed 50 PSI at the nozzle tip when used indoors. Add the appropriate amount of product when filling sprayer tank with water, shake or agitate as necessary to mix. Diluted spray mixture can be stored overnight and applied the following day; however, mixture should be agitated prior to application to prevent uneven distribution of product. Before leaving spray mixture unagitated for an extended period of time, release tank pressure and elevate nozzle and hose above tank outlet, activate trigger and drain all dilution from hose back into spray tank. Retighten spray tank lid and do not repressurize until starting spray again.

Tempo® SC Ultra will not stain or cause damage to any painted or varnished household surface, plastic, fabric or other surface where water applied alone causes no damage.

TANK MIXING: The user, at his discretion, can tank mix pesticides currently registered for similar use patterns, unless the product labels specifically prohibit such use. See Extended Cockroach Control with Insect Growth Regulators, below. It is always recommended that a small jar compatibility test using proper proportions of chemicals and water be run to check for physical compatibility prior to tank mixing. Tempo® SC Ultra is not compatible with disinfectants and should not be tank mixed with them. Tempo® SC Ultra and disinfectants should be applied separately as per label directions.

GENERAL SURFACE APPLICATION

Use 8 milliliters of Tempo® SC Ultra per 1000 sq ft in sufficient water (under conditions of severe pest infestation or when quicker knock-down and/or residual control is needed, use 16 milliliters of Tempo® SC Ultra per 1000 sq ft) to adequately cover the area being treated, but which will not allow dripping or run-off to occur (see Note 1). Use a low pressure system with a fan type nozzle to uniformly apply the dilution. Applications can be made to walls, floors, ceilings, in and around cupboards, between, behind and beneath equipment, appliances, around floor drains, window and door frames, and on the underside of shelves, drawers and in similar areas. Applications may be made to floor surfaces along walls and around air ducts, however, do not treat entire area of floor or floor coverings. All food processing surfaces and utensils should be covered or thoroughly washed following treatment. Cover exposed foodstuffs or remove from area being treated. Re-application can be made at 10-day intervals, if necessary. Do not apply where electrical short circuits could occur. Use a dust or dry bait in these areas. It is recommended to wear safety glasses, goggles or face shield and a respirator when making a general surface treatment to overhead areas.

Note 1: Volume of Water Sprays Applied To A Vertical Surface to Attain Appropriate Coverage

Type of Surface	Quarts/1000 Sq Ft	Gallons/1000 Sq Ft
Ceramic tile (glazed)	0.75	0.2
Stainless steel	0.75	0.2
Latex painted plywood (semigloss)	4.0	1.0
Masonite (smooth)	6.3	1.5
Unpainted plywood	11.0	2.7
Unpainted particle board	11.7	3.0
Cement block (semigloss latex)	12.5	3.2
Cement block (unfinished)	145.5	36.3

SPOT, MIST OR CRACK AND CREVICE APPLICATIONS

Mix 8 milliliters of Tempo® SC Ultra in one gallon of water to make a dilution of 0.025% active ingredient concentration (under conditions of severe pest infestation or when quicker knock-down and/or longer residual control is needed use 16 milliliters of Tempo® SC Ultra in one gallon of water to make a dilution of 0.05% active ingredient concentration). Use a low pressure system with a pin-point or variable pattern nozzle or appropriate foam generating equipment to apply the suspension or sufficient volume of foam in specific areas such as: cracks and crevices in or behind baseboards, in floors, walls, expansion joints, areas around water and sewer pipes, wall voids, or voids in table legs and equipment where pests can hide as well as other similar areas. Spot treatments may also be made to areas **including but not limited to** storage areas, closets, around water pipes, doors and windows, behind and under refrigerators, cabinets, sinks, stoves and other equipment, the underside of shelves, drawers and similar areas. Tempo® SC Ultra can be reapplied at 10-day intervals, if necessary. Do not apply where electrical short circuits could occur. Use a dust or dry bait in these areas.

EXTENDED COCKROACH CONTROL WITH INSECT GROWTH REGULATORS

Use Tempo® SC Ultra in a tank mix combination with an Insect Growth Regulator (IGR) for extended control of American, Asian, German, oriental, brown-banded, smoky brown and other species of cockroaches. Use in food areas of food handling establishments only if all products in tank mix are registered for such use.

Make applications in accordance with those label instructions which are the same for each product. Prepare the tank mix using the recommended rate of Tempo® SC Ultra and the IGR of choice by adding the Tempo® SC Ultra first and making sure it's a well mixed dilution, then adding the correct amount of IGR according to it's label instructions. Follow all label instructions for use patterns and spray intervals from the IGR label to achieve maximum benefit.

Refer to the appropriate sections of the label for Tempo® SC Ultra and the label for the IGR of choice for additional precautions, restrictions, limitations, and application information.

FOOD/FEED HANDLING ESTABLISHMENT APPLICATIONS

Tempo® SC Ultra applications are permitted in both food/feed and non-food areas of food/feed handling establishments as a general surface, spot, or crack and crevice treatment. Food/feed handling establishments are defined as places other than private residences in which exposed food/feed is held, processed, prepared or served. Included also are areas for receiving, storing, packing (canning, bottling, wrapping, boxing), preparing, edible waste storage and enclosed processing systems (mills, dairies, edible oils, syrups) of food. Serving areas where food is exposed and the facility is in operation are also considered food areas.

General Surface Application: When the facility is in operation or foods are exposed do not apply as a general surface application in food handling areas. Do not apply directly to food products. Cover or remove all food processing and/or handling equipment during application. After application in food processing plants, bakeries, cafeterias and similar facilities, wash all equipment, benches, shelving and other surfaces which food will contact. Clean food handling or processing equipment and thoroughly rinse with clean, fresh water.

Spot, Crack and Crevice Application: Spot or crack and crevice applications may be made while the facility is in operation; however, food should be covered or removed from area being treated. Do not apply directly to food or food-handling surfaces.

INDOOR PEST CONTROL

CRAWLING INSECT PEST CONTROL

For **general household pests** and **occasional invaders** make applications in a manner as previously described under General Surface, Spot, or Crack and Crevice Application. Particular attention should be given to treating entry points and harborage areas.

For **pantry pest control** of exposed adult and immature stages of insects, make application to cupboards, shelving and storage areas. Particular attention should be given to treating cracks and crevices and other harborage areas. Remove all utensils, uncovered foodstuffs (or any with package opened), shelf paper and other objects before spraying. Allow treated surfaces to dry and cover shelves with clean paper before replacing any utensils, foodstuff or other items. Any foodstuff accidentally contaminated with spray dilution should be discarded.

For **stored product pest control** of exposed adult and immature stages of insect pests, apply to cracks, crevices, and other surfaces where the pests have been seen or have harborage. Treat warehouses, production facilities, storage areas, and other areas where products are stored before filling with the product. Tempo® SC Ultra may be used by pest control operators and grain producers to treat grain storage facilities and other areas noted above for stored product pest control. Cleaning of all areas prior to use of Tempo® SC Ultra will increase levels of control. Any foodstuffs infested with pests should be removed and destroyed.

For **use by pest control operators or livestock producers in livestock housing structures (including poultry houses) and pet kennels** to control crawling and flying insect pests. Apply as a general surface and/or a crack and crevice spray. Control will be enhanced when facilities are cleaned and interior applications are supplemented with exterior perimeter treatments. Do not make interior applications of Tempo® SC Ultra in areas of facility where animals are present. Do not make applications to animal feedstuffs or watering equipment.

FLYING INSECT PEST CONTROL (General Surface Spray)

For control of flying insects indoors make application to surfaces as directed under Directions For Use, where the pests collect or rest. **Do not apply as a "space spray" application.**

OUTDOOR PEST CONTROL

For control of flying insects outdoors use a 0.05% dilution and make applications to outside surfaces of buildings, porches, patios, garages and other areas where these pests have been seen or found. Use a 0.05% dilution and make pin stream applications directly to the nests of wasps, yellow-jackets and hornets. **For perimeter pest control**, make a general surface application to outside surfaces of buildings, porches, patios, garages and other adjacent areas where pests have been seen or found. To help prevent infestations of buildings by occasional invaders, treat soil, turf or other substrates adjacent to buildings, the building foundation, walls, around doors and windows, soffit areas where these pests are active and may find entrance or harborage. Apply a minimum of 8 milliliters of Tempo® SC Ultra per 1000 sq ft in sufficient water to provide adequate coverage.

For control of the **imported red fire ant**, use a 0.05% dilution of Tempo® SC Ultra and thoroughly drench or inject the entire mound area. Treat all areas of the mound showing activity to provide contact control of the adult fire ants. Tempo® SC Ultra will provide contact activity and residual repellency in the active mound.

When using the injection treatment method for control of the imported red fire ant, it is essential that treatment be made to the bottom of the active mound. Apply dilution or sufficient volume of foam throughout the mound using a downward and upward motion of the injector tool. Multiple injection sites may be needed to ensure complete distribution of the suspension throughout the active mound.

Do not use Tempo® SC Ultra to treat fire ant mounds in any food crop production area, pasture or area where food crop production may occur.

CONTROL OF WOOD INFESTING PESTS

For control of **wood infesting beetles** on structure surfaces, apply a 0.05% dilution of Tempo® SC Ultra. For treatment of small areas, apply by brushing or spraying the suspension evenly on wood surfaces. For large or overhead areas, apply as a coarse spray to thoroughly cover the area. Cover all surfaces below the area being sprayed with plastic sheeting or other material which can be disposed of by placing in trash if contamination from dripping occurs. Sprayed surfaces should be avoided until the treated area is completely dry.

For control of **above ground termites and wood-infesting beetles** in localized areas, apply a 0.05% dilution or sufficient volume of foam of Tempo® SC Ultra to voids and galleries in damaged wood, and in spaces between wooden structural members and between the sill plate and foundation where wood is vulnerable.

Such applications for termites are not a substitute for mechanical alteration, soil treatment or foundation treatment, but are merely a supplement. For active termite infestations, get a professional inspection.

PESTS CONTROLLED BY TEMPO® SC ULTRA*

I. INDOOR PREMISE PESTS

1. Crawling Pests

Ants (except Pharaoh), Bedbugs, Carpet beetles, Centipedes, Cockroaches (American, Asian, German, Oriental, brown-banded, smoky brown), Crickets, Darkling beetles, Earwigs, Firebrats, Millipedes, Pillbugs, Silverfish, Sowbugs, Spiders

2. Flying Pests

Clothes moths, Flies, Gnats, Midges, Mosquitoes, Moths, Wasps, Yellow-jackets

3. Pantry & Stored Product Pests

Beetles (exposed adults & immature stages) (Cadelle, Cigarette, Confused Flour, Dermestid, Drug-store, Granary weevil, Hide, Larder, Leather, Lesser grain borer, Lesser mealworm, Merchant grain, Mealworm, Red flour, Rice weevil, Sawtoothed grain, Warehouse), Moths (Indian meal, Mediterranean flour)

II. FOOD PROCESSING PESTS

(Same crawling & flying pests, pantry & stored product pests as for INDOOR PREMISE) and Fruitflies, Phoridflies and Sciaridflies

III. WOOD INFESTING PESTS

Beetles (Ambrosia, Deathwatch, False powderpost, Old house borer, Powderpost), Carpenter ants, Carpenter bees, Termites (Subterranean**, Formosan, Drywood)

IV. OUTDOOR/PERIMETER PESTS

Ants, Bees, Boxelder bugs, Carpenter ants, Cecidflies, Centipedes, Clusterflies, Cockroaches, Crickets, Elm leaf beetle, Fire ants, Firebrats, Flies, Fleas, Gnats, Ground beetles, Hornets, Imported red fire ants, Midges, Millipedes, Mosquitoes, Moths, Scorpions, Silverfish, Spiders, Ticks, Wasps, Yellow-jackets

* For **GENERAL SURFACE APPLICATION**, use 8 milliliters of Tempo® SC Ultra per 1000 square feet in sufficient water to adequately cover the area being treated.

* For **SPOT, CRACK AND CREVICE APPLICATIONS**, mix 8 milliliters Tempo® SC Ultra in one gallon of water to make a 0.025% active ingredient concentration.

**Only for control of above-ground, winged forms of subterranean termites.

STORAGE AND DISPOSAL

Do not contaminate water, food, or feed by storage or disposal.

Pesticide Storage: Store in a cool, dry place and in such a manner as to prevent cross contamination with other pesticides, fertilizers, food, and feed. Store in original containers and out of the reach of children, preferably in a locked storage area.

Handle and open container in a manner as to prevent spillage. If the container is leaking or material spilled for any reason or cause, carefully dam up spilled material to prevent runoff. Refer to Precautionary Statements on label for hazards associated with the handling of this material. Do not walk through spilled material. Absorb spilled material with absorbing type compounds and dispose of as directed for pesticides below. In spill or leak incidents, keep unauthorized people away. You may contact the Bayer Emergency Response Team for decontamination procedures or any other assistance that may be necessary. The Bayer Kansas City Emergency Response Telephone No. is 800-414-0244 or contact Chemtrec at 800-424-9300.

Pesticide Disposal: Pesticide wastes are hazardous. Improper disposal of excess pesticide, spray mixture, or rinsate is a violation of Federal law. If these wastes cannot be disposed of by use according to label instructions, contact your State Pesticide or Environmental Control Agency, or the Hazardous Waste representative at the nearest EPA Regional Office for guidance.

Container Disposal: Do not use container in connection with food, feed, or drinking water. Completely empty container into application equipment. Triple rinse (or equivalent). Then offer for recycling or reconditioning, or puncture and dispose of in a sanitary landfill, or incineration, or if allowed by state and local authorities, by burning. If burned, stay out of smoke.

EPA Reg. No. 11556-124 EPA Est. No. 432-TX-1

SUPPLIED:

Code 08711774-053499—240 mL 08714803-71005340, R.4

Code 08731643-066299—30.43 fl oz (900 mL) R.0

Mfg. for: Bayer Corporation, Agriculture Division, Animal Health, Shawnee Mission, Kansas 66201 U.S.A.

Compendium Code No.: 10400372

T

TENOSYNOVITIS VACCINE

Merial Select **Vaccine**

Tenosynovitis Vaccine, Modified Live Virus

U.S. Vet. Lic. No.: 279

Active Ingredient(s): The vaccine contains a live strain of tenosynovitis virus that has been modified by numerous passages through tissue cultures of chicken embryo origin.

Penicillin, streptomycin sulfate, and fungizone are added as bacteriostats and preservatives.

Notice: The vaccine meets the requirements of the U.S. Department of Agriculture in regards to safety, purity, potency and the capability to immunize normal, susceptible chickens.

Indications: The vaccine is recommended for subcutaneous injection into healthy one day old chickens. The virus has been shown to aid in the prevention of tenosynovitis (viral arthritis) in young chickens.

Chickens to be vaccinated must be healthy and free of all diseases. It is essential that the birds be maintained under good environmental conditions, and that the exposure to disease viruses be reduced as much as possible in the field.

Dosage and Administration: Frozen Vaccine:

Preparation of Vaccine for Use:

Important: Sterilize the vaccinating equipment by autoclaving for a minimum of 15 minutes at 121°C or by boiling in water for at least 20 minutes. Never allow chemical disinfectants to come into contact with the vaccinating equipment.

1. Add the contents of one (1) ampule to 1,600 mL of sterile diluent.
2. Remove only one (1) ampule of the vaccine at a time from the liquid nitrogen container and use immediately. Carefully observe all liquid nitrogen precautions, including wearing eye protection and gloves. Do not hold the ampule toward the face when removing it from a liquid nitrogen container. Never refreeze a vaccine ampule after thawing.
3. The contents of the ampule are thawed rapidly by immersing it in water at room temperature (15-25°C). Gently mix the ampule to disperse the contents. Break the ampule at its neck and quickly proceed as described below.
4. Remove the cover from the diluent container. Draw the contents of the ampule into a sterile 10 mL syringe fitted with an 18 or 20 gauge needle. Slowly add the contents of the vaccine ampule to the appropriate volume of diluent. Withdraw a small amount of the diluent, rinse the ampule once and add this to the vaccine-diluent mixture. Mix the contents of the bottle thoroughly by swirling and inverting the bottle. Do not shake.

Method of Vaccination: Give subcutaneously only.

1. Use a sterile automatic syringe with a 20-22 gauge, ⅜"-½" needle set to deliver 0.2 mL per dose. Check the accuracy of the delivery several times during the vaccination procedure.
2. Dilute the vaccine as directed, observing all precautions and warnings for handling.
3. Keep the bottle of diluted vaccine in an ice bath and agitate continuously.
4. Inject chickens under the loose skin at the back of the neck (subcutaneously). Hold the chicken by the back of the neck just below the head. The loose skin in this area is raised by gently pinching the thumb and forefinger. Insert the needle beneath the skin in a direction away from the head. Inject 0.2 mL per chicken. Avoid hitting the muscles and bones in the neck.
5. Use the entire contents of the container within one (1) hour after mixing.

Precaution(s):

Ampules: Store in a liquid nitrogen container.

Diluent: Store at room temperature.

Liquid nitrogen container: Store in a cool, well-ventilated area. Check the liquid nitrogen level once a day. Keep the container away from incubator intakes and chicken boxes.

Liquid Nitrogen Precautions: The liquid nitrogen containers and vaccine should be handled by properly trained personnel only. These persons should be familiar with the Union Carbide Publication, "Precautions and Safe Practices - Liquefied Atmospheric Gases", form #9888. Liquid nitrogen is extremely cold. Accidental contact with the skin or eyes can cause serious frostbite. Protect the eyes with goggles or a face shield, wear gloves and long sleeves when removing and handling frozen ampules, or when adding liquid nitrogen to the container. Storage and handling of liquid nitrogen containers should be in a well-ventilated area. Excessive amounts of nitrogen reduces the concentration of oxygen in the air of an unventilated space and can cause asphyxiation. If a person becomes drowsy or loses consciousness while working with liquid nitrogen, get the person to a well-ventilated area immediately. If breathing has stopped, apply artificial respiration and summon a physician immediately.

Caution(s): Use the entire contents when first opened.

Burn the container and all unused contents.

The ability of the vaccine to produce satisfactory results may depend on many factors, including, but not limited to, conditions of storage and handling by the user, administration of the vaccine, health and the responsiveness of individual chickens, and the degree of field exposure. Therefore, directions for use should be followed carefully.

The use of the vaccine is subject to applicable state and federal laws and regulations.

Warning(s): Do not vaccinate within 21 days before slaughter.

Presentation: 5 x 8,000 dose ampule of vaccine, with 1,600 mL of diluent.

Compendium Code No.: 11050431

TENO-VAXIN®

ASL **Vaccine**

Tenosynovitis Vaccine, Live Virus

U.S. Vet. Lic. No.: 226

Description: TENO-VAXIN® contains modified strain S-1133 of tenosynovitis virus, attenuated by serial chicken embryo passages.

Gentamicin is added as a bacteriostatic agent.

Indications: TENO-VAXIN® should be used on healthy susceptible chickens between 10 and 17 weeks of age intended for use a broiler-breeders replacements. Chickens to be vaccinated should be free of disease, in good health and maintained under good environmental conditions.

For vaccination of commercial broiler-breeder replacement chicken flocks against infectious tenosynovitis by drinking water method as directed below.

Dosage and Administration: Read full directions below carefully.

Rehydration of the Vaccine:

Do not open or mix vaccine until ready to begin vaccination. Use vaccine immediately after mixing.

1. Tear off the aluminum seal from the vial containing the dried vaccine.
2. Lift off the rubber stopper.
3. Carefully pour clean, cool, non-chlorinated water into the vaccine vial until the vial is approximately two-thirds full.
4. Put back the rubber stopper and shake vigorously until all material is dissolved.
5. The vaccine is now ready for drinking water use in accordance with the directions below. For best results be sure to follow directions carefully.

Drinking Water Administration: For chickens 10 to 17 weeks of age.

1. Remove all medications, sanitizers, and disinfectants from the drinking water, preferably 72 hours before vaccinating, and 24 hours following vaccination.
2. Scrub waterers thoroughly and rinse with fresh, clean water.
3. Withhold water for 2 hours before vaccinating to stimulate thirst.
4. Provide enough watering space so that at least two-thirds of the chickens can drink at one time.
5. Rehydrate the vaccine as directed above.
6. Add the 1,000 dose vial of rehydrated vaccine to 10 gallons of clean, cool, non-chlorinated water and mix thoroughly.
7. Do not use less than 1 dose per chicken.
8. Distribute the vaccine solution among the waterers provided for the chickens. Avoid placing waterers in direct sunlight.
9. Provide no other drinking water until all of the vaccine treated water has been consumed.

Precaution(s): Store vaccine in refrigerator under 45°F (7°C). Use entire contents of each vial when first opened. Burn containers and all unused contents.

Caution(s): Use only in states where permitted and in susceptible chickens 10 to 17 weeks of age. Do not use on premises where other susceptible chickens are maintained. Do not add vaccinates to premises with susceptible chickens.

Do not vaccinate chickens before 10 weeks or after 17 weeks of age.

Do not vaccinate chickens in production or use on premises with susceptible layers or young chickens.

Do not add vaccinated chickens to non-vaccinated susceptible flocks in production. The virus may spread from the vaccinates and decrease hatchability.

For drinking water use only.

Consult your poultry pathologist for further recommendations based on conditions existing in your area at any given time.

Care should be exercised to keep visitors away from vaccinated flocks.

Care should be taken to prevent contamination on hands, eyes or clothing with the vaccine.

Notice: All American Scientific Laboratories, Inc. vaccines released for sale meet the requirements of the licensing authority (U.S. Department of Agriculture) in regard to safety, purity, potency, and the capacity to immunize normal, susceptible chickens.

The capacity of this vaccine to produce satisfactory results depends on many factors, including, but not limited to, conditions of storage and handling by the user, administration of the vaccine, health and responsiveness of individual animals and degree of field exposure. Therefore, directions for use should be followed carefully.

The use of this vaccine is subject to applicable state and federal laws and regulations.

Warning(s): Do not vaccinate within 21 days before slaughter.

Discussion: Effective immunization helps to protect broiler-breeders against outbreaks of infectious tenosynovitis which can cause excessive mortality, poor growth rates and excessive trims at the processing plant.

Vaccination Programs: Many factors must be considered in determining the proper vaccination program for a particular farm or poultry operation. To be fully effective, the vaccine must be administered to healthy receptive chickens held in a proper environment under good management. In addition, the response may be modified by the age of the chickens and their immune status. Seldom does one vaccination under field conditions produce complete protection for all individuals in a given flock. The amount of protection required will vary with the type of operation and the degree of exposure that a flock is likely to encounter. For these reasons, a program of periodic revaccination may be required.

Presentation: Drinking water: 10 x 1,000 dose vials.

Compendium Code No.: 11020311 R0091R4

TENSYNVAC®

Intervet **Vaccine**

Tenosynovitis Vaccine, Modified Live Virus

U.S. Vet. Lic. No.: 286

Description: This product is a mild vaccine based on the temperature sensitive, highly attenuated 1133 strain of reovirus and is used for the prevention of Tenosynovitis (viral arthritis) in chickens and priming of breeder replacement stock. The immunizing capacity of this vaccine has been proven by the Master Seed Immunogenicity Test.

This vaccine contains gentamicin as a preservative.

Quality tested for purity, potency, and safety.

Indications: This vaccine is intended for subcutaneous administration at one day of age or older for prevention of Tenosynovitis (viral arthritis). The vaccine is also intended for the priming of breeder replacement stock.

Do not vaccinate with TENSYNVAC® if Marek's disease vaccine is administered, as interference phenomena may occur.

Dosage and Administration: Vaccination Programs: Many factors must be considered in determining a sound vaccination program for a particular farm or poultry complex. To be fully effective, the vaccine must be administered properly to healthy, receptive animals maintained in a proper environment under good management. In addition, the response may be influenced by the age of the animals and their immune status. Protection against reoviruses involves the maternal transfer of antibody through the yolk to progeny. To effect this transfer, an integrated program using both inactivated and modified live virus vaccine is recommended. In areas of high exposure, chicks can become susceptible during the first weeks of life. Therefore, early vaccination becomes mandatory in these areas. Revaccination should occur at 5 to 7 weeks of age and again at 9 to 11 weeks of age. In areas of lesser exposure, vaccination should occur at 5 to 6 weeks of age and again at 9 to 11 weeks of age. To complete the program for breeding birds, an inactivated reovirus vaccination is recommended between 16 to 22 weeks of age or 4 weeks prior to the onset of egg production.

Preparation of Vaccine:

For Subcutaneous Use: Sterilize vaccinating equipment by boiling it in water for 30 minutes or by autoclaving (20 minutes at 121°C). Do not use chemical disinfectants.

1. Use contents of 1,000 dose vial per 200 mL sterile diluent.
2. Remove the tear-off seal from vial containing the dried vaccine.
3. Remove center of aluminum seal of diluent bottle. Insert the syringe into the stopper and withdraw a small amount of diluent.
4. Add the diluent into the vial of vaccine and shake.
5. Withdraw the rehydrated vaccine into the syringe and add it to the rest of the diluent. Gently shake to mix. Withdraw a portion of the diluent with the syringe to flush the vial. Inject the liquid back into the diluent bottle. Remove the syringe.
6. Fill the previously sterilized automatic syringe according to the manufacturer's recommendations and set the dose for 0.2 mL.
7. The vaccine is now ready for use.

Subcutaneous Administration:

1. Dilute the vaccine as directed above, observing all precautions and warnings for handling.
2. Hold the chicken by the back of the neck just below the head. The loose skin in the area is raised by gently pinching with the thumb and forefinger. Insert the needle beneath the skin in a downward direction away from the head. Inject 0.2 mL per chicken. The bottle of vaccine should be kept in an ice bath and swirled frequently.
3. Avoid hitting the muscles and bones in the neck with the needle.
4. Entire contents of bottle must be used immediately after mixing or else discarded.

Records: Keep a record of vaccine, quantity, serial number, expiration date and place of purchase; the date and time of vaccination; the number, age, breed and locations of chickens; names of operators performing the vaccination and any observed reactions.

Precaution(s): Store vaccine between 2 and 7°C (35 and 45°F).
Do not spill or splash the vaccine.
Use entire contents when first opened.
Burn container and all unused contents.
This product is non-returnable.

Caution(s): Use of this vaccine at day of age can result in interference with Marek's disease vaccine causing problems with Marek's disease.

Vaccinate only healthy chickens. Although disease may not be evident, coccidiosis, mycoplasma infection, Marek's disease and other disease conditions may cause complications or reduce immunity.

All susceptible chickens on the same premises should be vaccinated at the same time.

Efforts should be taken to reduce stress conditions at the time of vaccination and during the post-vaccination period.

Do not dilute the vaccine or otherwise stretch the dosage.

Do not use TENSYNVAC® in combination with other vaccines.

For veterinary use only.

Notice: This vaccine has undergone rigid potency, safety and purity tests, and meets Intervet Inc. and USDA requirements. It is designed to stimulate effective immunity when used as directed. The user must be advised that the response to the vaccine depends upon many factors, including, but not limited to, conditions of storage and handling by the user, administration of the vaccine, health and responsiveness of individual chickens and the degree of field exposure. Therefore, directions should be followed carefully.

This product is not hazardous when used according to directions supplied. A material safety data sheet (MSDS) is available upon request. This and any other consumer information can be obtained by calling Intervet Customer Service at 1-800-441-8272 or 1-302-934-8051.

The use of this vaccine is subject to applicable federal and local laws and regulations.

Use only as directed.

Warning(s): Do not vaccinate within 21 days before slaughter or after 12 weeks of age.

Presentation: 10 x 1,000 doses for subcutaneous use with 10 x 200 mL bottles of sterile diluent per carton.

The vaccine is packaged in two separate units. One is a vial containing lyophilized virus and the other is a bottle of sterile diluent.

Compendium Code No.: 11062031 IAI 01609 AL 112

TERRAMYCIN® 10 (oxytetracycline) TM-10®

Phibro **Feed Medication**

Type A Medicated Article

NADA No.: 008-804

Active Ingredient(s):

Oxytetracycline (from oxytetracycline quaternary salt) equivalent to oxytetracycline hydrochloride (Terramycin®) . . . . 10 g/lb

Indications: A type A medicated article to be mixed in the feed of chickens; turkeys; swine; calves including pre-ruminating (veal) calves, beef cattle, and nonlactating dairy cattle; sheep and lobsters.

Recommended for increased rate of weight gain, improved feed efficiency, and for the control and treatment of ailments caused by microorganisms sensitive to oxytetracycline.

Directions:

Mixing and Use Directions: Thoroughly mix the amount of this premix according to the directions below with at least an equal amount by weight of feed formula ingredients prior to blending into a complete feed.

Indications for Use	Use Level of Terramycin	lb of TM-10®/ton
Chickens		
Increased rate of weight gain and improved feed efficiency	10-50 g/ton Use continuously	1-5
Control of infectious synovitis caused by *Mycoplasma synoviae;* control of fowl cholera caused by *Pasteurella multocida* susceptible to oxytetracycline	100-200 g/ton Feed continuously for 7-14 days	10-20
Control of chronic respiratory disease (CRD) and air sac infection caused by *Mycoplasma gallisepticum* and *Escherichia coli* susceptible to oxytetracycline	400 g/ton Feed continuously for 7-14 days	40
Reduction of mortality due to air sacculitis (air sac infection) caused by *Escherichia coli* susceptible to oxytetracycline	500 g/ton Feed for 5 days	50
Turkeys		
For growing turkeys for increased rate of weight gain and improved feed efficiency	10-50 g/ton Use continuously	1-5
Control of hexamitiasis caused by *Hexamita meleagrides* susceptible to oxytetracycline	100 g/ton Feed continuously for 7-14 days	10
Control of infectious synovitis caused by *Mycoplasma synoviae* susceptible to oxytetracycline	200 g/ton Feed continuously for 7-14 days	20
Control of complicating bacterial organisms associated with bluecomb (transmissible enteritis, coronaviral enteritis) susceptible to oxytetracycline	25 mg/lb of body weight daily Feed continuously for 7-14 days	83[1]
Swine		
Increased rate of weight gain and improved feed efficiency	10-50 g/ton Use continuously	1-5
Treatment of bacterial enteritis caused by *Escherichia coli* and *Salmonella choleraesuis* susceptible to oxytetracycline and treatment of bacterial pneumonia caused by *Pasteurella multocida* susceptible to oxytetracycline	10 mg/lb of body weight daily Feed continuously for 7-14 days	50[2]
For breeding swine for control and treatment of Leptospirosis (reducing the incidence of abortion and shedding of leptospirae) caused by *Leptospira pomona* susceptible to oxytetracycline	10 mg/lb of body weight daily Feed continuously for not more than 14 days	50[2]

Indications for Use	Use Level of Terramycin	lb of TM-10®/ton
Calves including pre-ruminating (veal) calves, beef cattle, and nonlactating dairy cattle		
For calves (up to 250 lb) for increased rate of weight gain and improved feed efficiency	0.05-0.1 mg/lb of body weight daily Use continuously	0.5-1.0[3]
For calves (250-400 lb) for increased rate of weight gain and improved feed efficiency	25 mg/head/day Use continuously	2.5[4]
For growing cattle (over 400 lb) for increased rate of weight gain, improved feed efficiency, and reduction of liver condemnation due to liver abscesses	75 mg/head/day Use continuously	7.5[4]
Prevention and treatment of the early stages of shipping fever complex (Feed 3-5 days before and after arrival in feedlots)	0.5-2.0 g/head/day	50-200[4]
Treatment of bacterial enteritis caused by *Escherichia coli* and bacterial pneumonia (shipping fever complex) caused by *Pasteurella multocida* susceptible to oxytetracycline	10 mg/lb of body weight daily Feed continuously for 7-14 days	500[5]
Sheep		
Increased rate of weight gain and improved feed efficiency	10-20 g/ton Use continuously	1-2
Treatment of bacterial enteritis caused by *Escherichia coli* and bacterial pneumonia caused by *Pasteurella multocida* susceptible to oxytetracycline	10 mg/lb of body weight daily Feed continuously for 7-14 days	120[6]
Lobsters		
Control of gaffkemia in lobsters caused by *Aerococcus viridans*	1 g/lb of medicated feed Feed for 5 days as the sole ration	200

[1] If bird weighs 10 lb, consuming 0.6 lb of complete feed per day.
[2] If pig weighs 100 lb, consuming 4 lb of complete feed per day.
[3] If calf weighs 100 lb, consuming 2 lb of complete starter feed per day.
[4] Include in feed supplements based on consumption of 2 lb of supplement per head per day.
[5] If cow weighs 500 lb, consuming 2 lb of supplement per head per day.
[6] If lamb weighs 60 lb, consuming 1 lb of supplement per head per day.

Precaution(s): Store in a dry, cool place.

Caution(s): For use in manufacturing medicated animal feeds only.

For use in dry feeds only. Not for use in liquid feed supplements.

Certain components of animal feeds, including medicated premixes, possess properties that may be a potential health hazard or a source of personal discomfort to certain individuals who are exposed to them. Human exposure should, therefore, be minimized by observing the general industry standards for occupational health and safety.

Precautions such as the following should be considered: dust masks or respirators and protective clothing should be worn; dust-arresting equipment and adequate ventilation should be utilized; personal hygiene should be observed; wash before eating or leaving a work site; be alert for signs of allergic reactions—seek prompt medical treatment if such reactions are suspected.

Warning(s):

Chickens:

At 400 g/ton use level, zero-day withdrawal period. In low calcium feeds withdraw 3 days before slaughter. Do not administer to chickens producing eggs for human consumption.

At 500 g/ton use level, 24-hour withdrawal period. In low calcium feeds withdraw 3 days before slaughter. Do not administer to chickens producing eggs for human consumption.

Turkeys: At 200 g/ton use level or higher, withdraw 5 days before slaughter. Zero-day withdrawal period for lower use levels. Do not administer to turkeys producing eggs for human consumption.

Swine: 5-day withdrawal at 10 mg/lb dosage.

Calves including pre-ruminating (veal) calves, beef cattle, and nonlactating dairy cattle: 5-day withdrawal at 10 mg/lb dosage. When used in milk replacers, the treatment claim (10 mg/lb) is limited to bacterial enteritis caused by *Escherichia coli* only.

Sheep: 5-day withdrawal at 10 mg/lb dosage.

Lobsters: Withdraw from feed 30 days before harvesting lobsters.

Presentation: 50 lb (22.6 kg) multi-wall paper bags.

Terramycin is a registered trademark of Pfizer Inc., licensed to Phibro Animal Health, for oxytetracycline.

Compendium Code No.: 36930160

TERRAMYCIN® 50

Phibro **Feed Medication**

(oxytetracycline) Type A Medicated Article

NADA No.: 095-143

Active Ingredient(s):

Oxytetracycline (from oxytetracycline dihydrate base) equivalent to oxytetracycline hydrochloride . . . . 50 g/lb

Indications: A type A medicated article to be mixed in the feed of chickens; turkeys; swine; calves including pre-ruminating (veal) calves, beef cattle, and nonlactating dairy cattle and sheep.

Recommended for increased rate of weight gain, improved feed efficiency, and for the control and treatment of ailments caused by microorganisms sensitive to oxytetracycline.

Directions: Mixing and Use Directions: Thoroughly mix the amount of this premix according to the directions below with at least an equal amount by weight of feed formula ingredients prior to blending into a complete feed.

Indications for Use	Oxytetracycline Amount	lb of TERRAMYCIN® 50/ton
Chickens		
Increased rate of weight gain and improved feed efficiency	10-50 g/ton Feed continuously	0.2-1.0
Control of infectious synovitis caused by *Mycoplasma synoviae;* control of fowl cholera caused by *Pasteurella multocida* susceptible to oxytetracycline	100-200 g/ton Feed continuously for 7-14 days	2-4

T

Indications for Use	Oxytetracycline Amount	lb of TERRAMYCIN® 50/ton
Control of chronic respiratory disease (CRD) and air sac infection caused by *Mycoplasma gallisepticum* and *Escherichia coli* susceptible to oxytetracycline	400 g/ton Feed continuously for 7-14 days	8
Reduction of mortality due to air sacculitis (air sac infection) caused by *Escherichia coli* susceptible to oxytetracycline	500 g/ton Feed continuously for 5 days	10
Turkeys		
For growing turkeys for increased rate of weight gain and improved feed efficiency	10-50 g/ton Feed continuously	0.2-1.0
Control of hexamitiasis caused by *Hexamita meleagrides* susceptible to oxytetracycline	100 g/ton Feed continuously for 7-14 days	2
Control of infectious synovitis caused by *Mycoplasma synoviae* susceptible to oxytetracycline	200 g/ton Feed continuously for 7-14 days	4
Control of complicating bacterial organisms associated with bluecomb (transmissible enteritis, coronaviral enteritis) susceptible to oxytetracycline	25 mg/lb of body weight daily Feed continuously for 7-14 days	16.7[1]
Swine		
Increased rate of weight gain and improved feed efficiency	10-50 g/ton Feed continuously	0.2-1.0
Treatment of bacterial enteritis caused by *Escherichia coli* and *Salmonella choleraesuis* susceptible to oxytetracycline and treatment of bacterial pneumonia caused by *Pasteurella multocida* susceptible to oxytetracycline	10 mg/lb of body weight daily Feed continuously for 7-14 days	10[2]
For breeding swine for control and treatment of Leptospirosis (reducing the incidence of abortion and shedding of leptospirae) caused by *Leptospira pomona* susceptible to oxytetracycline	10 mg/lb of body weight daily Feed continuously for not more than 14 days	10[2]
Calves including pre-ruminating (veal) calves, Beef Cattle, and Nonlactating Dairy Cattle		
For calves (up to 250 lb) for increased rate of weight gain and improved feed efficiency	0.05-0.1 mg/lb of body weight daily Feed continuously	0.1-0.2[3]
For calves (250-400 lb) for increased rate of weight gain and improved feed efficiency	25 mg/head/day Feed continuously	0.5[4]
For growing cattle (over 400 lb) for increased rate of weight gain, improved feed efficiency, and reduction of liver condemnation due to liver abscesses	75 mg/head/day Feed continuously	1.5[4]
Prevention and treatment of the early stages of shipping fever complex. (Feed 3-5 days before and after arrival in feedlots.)	0.5-2.0 g/head/day	10-40[4]
Treatment of bacterial enteritis caused by *Escherichia coli* and bacterial pneumonia (shipping fever complex) caused by *Pasteurella multocida* susceptible to oxytetracycline	10 mg/lb of body weight daily Feed continuously for 7-14 days	100[5]
Sheep		
Increased rate of weight gain and improved feed efficiency	10-20 g/ton Feed continuously	0.2-0.4
Treatment of bacterial enteritis caused by *Escherichia coli* and bacterial pneumonia caused by *Pasteurella multocida* susceptible to oxytetracycline	10 mg/lb of body weight daily Feed continuously for 7-14 days	24[6]

[1] If bird weighs 10 lb, consuming 0.6 lb of complete feed per day.
[2] If pig weighs 100 lb, consuming 4 lb of complete feed per day.
[3] If calf weighs 100 lb, consuming 2 lb of complete starter feed per day.
[4] Include in feed supplements based on consumption of 2 lb of supplement per head per day.
[5] If animal weighs 500 lb, consuming 2 lb of supplement per head per day.
[6] If lamb weighs 60 lb, consuming 1 lb of supplement per head per day.

Precaution(s): Store in a dry, cool place.

Caution(s): For use in manufacturing medicated animal feeds only.

For use in dry feeds only. Not for use in liquid feed supplements.

Warning(s): Chickens: At 500 g/ton use level withdraw 24 hours before slaughter. Zero day withdrawal period for lower use levels. In low calcium feeds withdraw 3 days before slaughter. Do not administer to chickens producing eggs for human consumption.

Turkeys: At 200 g/ton use level or higher, withdraw 5 days before slaughter. Zero-day withdrawal period for lower use levels. Do not administer to turkeys producing eggs for human consumption.

Calves including pre-ruminating (veal) calves, Beef Cattle, and Nonlactating Dairy Cattle: 5-day withdrawal before slaughter at 10 mg/lb dosage. When used in milk replacers, the treatment claim (10 mg/lb) is limited to bacterial enteritis caused by *Escherichia coli* only.

Sheep: 5-day withdrawal before slaughter at 10 mg/lb dosage.

Certain components of animal feeds, including medicated premixes, possess properties that may be a potential health hazard or a source of personal discomfort to certain individuals who are exposed to them. Human exposure should, therefore, be minimized by observing the general industry standards for occupational health and safety.

Precautions such as the following should be considered: dust masks or respirators and protective clothing should be worn; dust-arresting equipment and adequate ventilation should be utilized; personal hygiene should be observed; wash before eating or leaving a work site; be alert for signs of allergic reactions—seek prompt medical treatment if such reactions are suspected.

Presentation: 50 lb (22.6 kg) bags.

TERRAMYCIN is a registered trademark of Pfizer, Inc., licensed to Phibro Animal Health, for Oxytetracycline HCl.

Compendium Code No.: 36930111 101-9009-01

TERRAMYCIN® 100

Phibro **Feed Medication**

(oxytetracycline) Type A Medicated Article

NADA No.: 095-143

Active Ingredient(s):

Oxytetracycline (from oxytetracycline dihydrate base) equivalent to oxytetracycline hydrochloride . . . . 100 g/lb

Indications: A type A medicated article to be mixed in the feed of chickens; turkeys; swine; calves including pre-ruminating (veal) calves, beef cattle, and nonlactating dairy cattle and sheep.

Recommended for increased rate of weight gain, improved feed efficiency, and for the control and treatment of ailments caused by microorganisms sensitive to oxytetracycline.

Directions: Mixing and Use Directions: Thoroughly mix the amount of this premix according to the directions below with at least an equal amount by weight of feed formula ingredients prior to blending into a complete feed.

Indications for Use	Oxytetracycline Amount	lb of TERRAMYCIN® 100/ton
Chickens		
Increased rate of weight gain and improved feed efficiency	10-50 g/ton Feed continuously	0.1-0.5
Control of infectious synovitis caused by *Mycoplasma synoviae;* control of fowl cholera caused by *Pasteurella multocida* susceptible to oxytetracycline	100-200 g/ton Feed continuously for 7-14 days	1-2
Control of chronic respiratory disease (CRD) and air sac infection caused by *Mycoplasma gallisepticum* and *Escherichia coli* susceptible to oxytetracycline	400 g/ton Feed continuously for 7-14 days	4
Reduction of mortality due to air sacculitis (air sac infection) caused by *Escherichia coli* susceptible to oxytetracycline	500 g/ton Feed continuously for 5 days	5
Turkeys		
For growing turkeys for increased rate of weight gain and improved feed efficiency	10-50 g/ton Feed continuously	0.1-0.5
Control of hexamitiasis caused by *Hexamita meleagrides* susceptible to oxytetracycline	100 g/ton Feed continuously for 7-14 days	1
Control of infectious synovitis caused by *Mycoplasma synoviae* susceptible to oxytetracycline	200 g/ton Feed continuously for 7-14 days	2
Control of complicating bacterial organisms associated with bluecomb (transmissible enteritis, coronaviral enteritis) susceptible to oxytetracycline	25 mg/lb of body weight daily Feed continuously for 7-14 days	8.3[1]
Swine		
Increased rate of weight gain and improved feed efficiency	10-50 g/ton Feed continuously	0.1-0.5
Treatment of bacterial enteritis caused by *Escherichia coli* and *Salmonella choleraesuis* susceptible to oxytetracycline and treatment of bacterial pneumonia caused by *Pasteurella multocida* susceptible to oxytetracycline	10 mg/lb of body weight daily Feed continuously for 7-14 days	5[2]
For breeding swine for control and treatment of Leptospirosis (reducing the incidence of abortion and shedding of leptospirae) caused by *Leptospira pomona* susceptible to oxytetracycline	10 mg/lb of body weight daily Feed continuously for not more than 14 days	5[2]
Calves including pre-ruminating (veal) calves, Beef Cattle, and Nonlactating Dairy Cattle		
For calves (up to 250 lb) for increased rate of weight gain and improved feed efficiency	0.05-0.1 mg/lb of body weight daily Feed continuously	0.05-0.1[3]
For calves (250-400 lb) for increased rate of weight gain and improved feed efficiency	25 mg/head/day Feed continuously	0.25[4]
For growing cattle (over 400 lb) for increased rate of weight gain, improved feed efficiency, and reduction of liver condemnation due to liver abscesses	75 mg/head/day Feed continuously	0.75[4]
Prevention and treatment of the early stages of shipping fever complex. (Feed 3-5 days before and after arrival in feedlots.)	0.5-2.0 g/head/day	5-20[4]
Treatment of bacterial enteritis caused by *Escherichia coli* and bacterial pneumonia (shipping fever complex) caused by *Pasteurella multocida* susceptible to oxytetracycline	10 mg/lb of body weight daily Feed continuously for 7-14 days	50[5]
Sheep		
Increased rate of weight gain and improved feed efficiency	10-20 g/ton Feed continuously	0.1-0.2
Treatment of bacterial enteritis caused by *Escherichia coli* and bacterial pneumonia caused by *Pasteurella multocida* susceptible to oxytetracycline	10 mg/lb of body weight daily Feed continuously for 7-14 days	12[6]

[1] If bird weighs 10 lb, consuming 0.6 lb of complete feed per day.
[2] If pig weighs 100 lb, consuming 4 lb of complete feed per day.
[3] If calf weighs 100 lb, consuming 2 lb of complete starter feed per day.
[4] Include in feed supplement based on consumption of 2 lb of supplement per head per day.
[5] If animal weighs 500 lb, consuming 2 lb of supplement per head per day.
[6] If lamb weighs 60 lb, consuming 1 lb of supplement per head per day.

Precaution(s): Store in a dry, cool place.

Caution(s): For use in manufacturing medicated animal feeds only.

For use in dry feeds only. Not for use in liquid feed supplements.

Warning(s): Chickens: At 500 g/ton use level, withdraw 24 hours before slaughter. Zero-day withdrawal period for lower use levels. In low calcium feeds withdraw 3 days before slaughter. Do not administer to chickens producing eggs for human consumption.

Turkeys: At 200 g/ton use level or higher, withdraw 5 days before slaughter. Zero-day withdrawal period for lower use levels. Do not administer to turkeys producing eggs for human consumption.

Calves including pre-ruminating (veal) calves, Beef Cattle, and Nonlactating Dairy Cattle: 5-day withdrawal before slaughter at 10 mg/lb dosage. When used in milk replacers, the treatment claim (10 mg/lb) is limited to bacterial enteritis caused by *Escherichia coli* only.

Sheep: 5-day withdrawal before slaughter at 10 mg/lb dosage.

Certain components of animal feeds, including medicated premixes, possess properties that may be a potential health hazard or a source of personal discomfort to certain individuals who are exposed to them. Human exposure should, therefore, be minimized by observing the general industry standards for occupational health and safety.

Precautions such as the following should be considered: dust masks or respirators and protective clothing should be worn; dust-arresting equipment and adequate ventilation should be utilized; personal hygiene should be observed; wash before eating or leaving a work site; be alert for signs of allergic reactions—seek prompt medical treatment if such reactions are suspected.

Presentation: 50 lb (22.6 kg) bags.

TERRAMYCIN is a registered trademark of Pfizer, Inc., licensed to Phibro Animal Health, for Oxytetracycline HCl.

Compendium Code No.: 36930121 101-9008-01

TERRAMYCIN® 100 FOR FISH

Phibro **Feed Medication**

Type A Medicated Article

NADA No.: 038-439

Active Ingredient(s):

Oxytetracycline (from oxytetracycline quaternary salt) equivalent to oxytetracycline hydrochloride (TERRAMYCIN®) .... 100 g/lb

Indications: For Salmonids: For control of ulcer disease caused by *Hemophilus piscium*, furunculosis caused by *Aeromonas salmonicida*, bacterial hemorrhagic septicemia caused by *Aeromonas liquefaciens* and pseudomonas disease.

For Catfish: For control of bacterial hemorrhagic septicemia caused by *Aeromonas liquefaciens* and pseudomonas disease.

Directions: Feeding Directions—Salmonids and Catfish: Administer medicated feed daily for 10 days to provide a total dosage of 2.5-3.75 g of oxytetracycline per 100 lb of fish. If mortality is not reduced by the fifth day of treatment, the diagnosis should be reexamined.

Directions for Use: Thoroughly mix the amount of TERRAMYCIN® 100 for Fish indicated in the table below to make 1 ton of finished feed. Administer medicated feed daily for 10 days to provide a total dosage of 2.5-3.75 g of oxytetracycline per 100 lb of fish. If mortality is not reduced by the fifth day of treatment, the diagnosis should be reexamined.

Feeding Rate of Fish (% of Body Weight)	lb of TERRAMYCIN® 100 for Fish Per Ton of Feed	Level of TERRAMYCIN® in Finished Feed
0.5-0.75	100	5 g/lb
0.67-1.0	75	3.75 g/lb
1.0-1.5	50	2.5 g/lb
1.4-2.2	35	1.75 g/lb
2.0-3.0	25	1.25 g/lb
2.5-3.8	20	2000 g/ton
3.4-5.0	15	1500 g/ton
4.0-6.0	12.5	1250 g/ton
5.6-8.5	9	900 g/ton
7.1-9.3	7	700 g/ton
10.0-15.0	5	500 g/ton

Example: If feeding fish at a rate of 3% of body weight, add 20 lb of TERRAMYCIN® 100 for Fish to provide 2000 g/ton of finished feed.

If feeding fish at a rate of 5.5% of body weight, add 12.5 lb of TERRAMYCIN® 100 for Fish to provide 1250 g/ton of finished feed.

Table 1. Salmonid feeding rates, measured as percent of body weight:

Water Temp (°F)	Approximate Fish Length in Inches										
	<1	1-2	2-3	3-4	4-5	5-6	6-7	7-8	8-9	9-10	>10
49	9.4	7.8	6.3	4.7	3.5	2.8	2.4	2.0	1.8	1.5	1.4
50	9.9	8.1	6.5	4.9	3.7	2.9	2.5	2.1	1.9	1.6	1.5
51	10.3	8.5	6.8	5.1	3.8	3.1	2.6	2.2	1.9	1.7	1.5
52	10.7	8.9	7.1	5.3	4.0	3.2	2.7	2.3	2.0	1.8	1.6
53	11.2	9.3	7.5	5.6	4.2	3.4	2.8	2.4	2.1	1.9	1.7
54	11.6	9.7	7.8	5.8	4.4	3.5	2.9	2.5	2.2	1.9	1.8
55	12.2	10.1	8.2	6.1	4.6	3.7	3.0	2.6	2.3	2.0	1.8
56	12.7	10.5	8.5	6.4	4.8	3.8	3.2	2.7	2.4	2.1	1.9
57	13.4	11.0	8.9	6.7	5.0	4.0	3.3	2.8	2.5	2.2	2.0
58	14.0	11.5	9.3	6.9	5.2	4.2	3.5	3.0	2.6	2.3	2.1
59	14.5	12.0	9.7	7.2	5.4	4.4	3.6	3.1	2.7	2.4	2.2
60	15.1	12.6	10.1	7.6	5.7	4.6	3.8	3.2	2.8	2.5	2.3

The figures in this chart were obtained from U.S. Bureau of Sport Fisheries and Wildlife based upon "Feeding Tables for Trout," Deuel and Tunison, Feb 1944. Chart included for informational purposes only.

Table 2. Catfish feeding rates, measured as percent of body weight*:

Feeding Rates Based on Body Weight		Feeding Rates Based on Body Length	
Fish Weight	Feeding Rate	Fish Length	Feeding Rate
0-6 oz	3-5%	Hatching to 3"	3-5%
6 oz and up	3%	3" to market	3%

*Average fish feed consumption. These figures represent university, government, and industry recommended feeding levels and are not those of the manufacturer. Chart included for informational purposes only.

Precaution(s): Store in a dry, cool place.

Caution(s): For use in manufacturing medicated fish feeds only.

For use in dry feeds only. Not for use in liquid feed supplements.

Warning(s): Do not liberate or slaughter salmonids for food during treatment or for 21 days following last feeding of medicated feed. Do not use when water temperature is below 48.2°F (9°C).

Do not liberate or slaughter catfish for food during treatment or for 21 days following last feeding of medicated feed. Do not use when water temperature is below 62°F (16.7°C).

Certain components of animal feeds, including medicated premixes, possess properties that may be a potential health hazard or a source of personal discomfort to certain individuals who are exposed to them. Human exposure should, therefore, be minimized by observing the general industry standards for occupational health and safety.

Precautions such as the following should be considered: dust masks or respirators and protective clothing should be worn; dust-arresting equipment and adequate ventilation should be utilized; personal hygiene should be observed; wash before eating or leaving a work site; be alert for signs of allergic reactions—seek prompt medical treatment if such reactions are suspected.

Presentation: 50 lb (22.6 kg) bags.

TERRAMYCIN is a registered trademark of Pfizer, Inc., licensed to Phibro Animal Health, for Oxytetracycline.

Compendium Code No.: 36930222 101-9017-01

TERRAMYCIN® 200

Phibro **Feed Medication**

(oxytetracycline) Type A Medicated Article

NADA No.: 095-143

Active Ingredient(s):

Oxytetracycline (from oxytetracycline dihydrate base) equivalent to oxytetracycline hydrochloride .... 200 g/lb

Indications: A type A medicated article to be mixed in the feed of chickens; turkeys; swine; calves including pre-ruminating (veal) calves, beef cattle, and nonlactating dairy cattle and sheep.

Recommended for increased rate of weight gain, improved feed efficiency, and for the control and treatment of ailments caused by microorganisms sensitive to oxytetracycline.

Directions: Mixing and Use Directions: Thoroughly mix the amount of this premix according to the directions below with at least an equal amount by weight of feed formula ingredients prior to blending into a complete feed.

Indications for Use	Oxytetracycline Amount	lb of TERRAMYCIN® 200/ton
Chickens		
Increased rate of weight gain and improved feed efficiency	10-50 g/ton Feed continuously	0.05-0.25
Control of infectious synovitis caused by *Mycoplasma synoviae;* control of fowl cholera caused by *Pasteurella multocida* susceptible to oxytetracycline	100-200 g/ton Feed continuously for 7-14 days	0.5-1
Control of chronic respiratory disease (CRD) and air sac infection caused by *Mycoplasma gallisepticum* and *Escherichia coli* susceptible to oxytetracycline	400 g/ton Feed continuously for 7-14 days	2
Reduction of mortality due to air sacculitis (air sac infection) caused by *Escherichia coli* susceptible to oxytetracycline	500 g/ton Feed continuously for 5 days	2.5
Turkeys		
For growing turkeys for increased rate of weight gain and improved feed efficiency	10-50 g/ton Feed continuously	0.05-0.25
Control of hexamitiasis caused by *Hexamita meleagrides* susceptible to oxytetracycline	100 g/ton Feed continuously for 7-14 days	0.5
Control of infectious synovitis caused by *Mycoplasma synoviae* susceptible to oxytetracycline	200 g/ton Feed continuously for 7-14 days	1
Control of complicating bacterial organisms associated with bluecomb (transmissible enteritis, coronaviral enteritis) susceptible to oxytetracycline	25 mg/lb of body weight daily Feed continuously for 7-14 days	4.15[1]
Swine		
Increased rate of weight gain and improved feed efficiency	10-50 g/ton Feed continuously	0.05-0.25
Treatment of bacterial enteritis caused by *Escherichia coli* and *Salmonella choleraesuis* susceptible to oxytetracycline and treatment of bacterial pneumonia caused by *Pasteurella multocida* susceptible to oxytetracycline	10 mg/lb of body weight daily Feed continuously for 7-14 days	2.5[2]
For breeding swine for control and treatment of Leptospirosis (reducing the incidence of abortion and shedding of leptospirae) caused by *Leptospira pomona* susceptible to oxytetracycline	10 mg/lb of body weight daily Feed continuously for not more than 14 days	2.5[2]

Indications for Use	Oxytetracycline Amount	lb of TERRAMYCIN® 200/ton
Calves including pre-ruminating (veal) calves, Beef Cattle, and Nonlactating Dairy Cattle		
For calves (up to 250 lb) for increased rate of weight gain and improved feed efficiency	0.05-0.1 mg/lb of body weight daily Feed continuously	0.025-0.5[3]
For calves (250-400 lb) for increased rate of weight gain and improved feed efficiency	25 mg/head/day Feed continuously	0.125[4]
For growing cattle (over 400 lb) for increased rate of weight gain, improved feed efficiency, and reduction of liver condemnation due to liver abscesses	75 mg/head/day Feed continuously	0.375[4]
Prevention and treatment of the early stages of shipping fever complex. (Feed 3-5 days before and after arrival in feedlots.)	0.5-2.0 g/head/day	2.5-10[4]
Treatment of bacterial enteritis caused by *Escherichia coli* and bacterial pneumonia (shipping fever complex) caused by *Pasteurella multocida* susceptible to oxytetracycline	10 mg/lb of body weight daily Feed continuously for 7-14 days	25[5]
Sheep		
Increased rate of weight gain and improved feed efficiency	10-20 g/ton Feed continuously	0.05-0.1
Treatment of bacterial enteritis caused by *Escherichia coli* and bacterial pneumonia caused by *Pasteurella multocida* susceptible to oxytetracycline	10 mg/lb of body weight daily Feed continuously for 7-14 days	6[6]

1 If bird weighs 10 lb, consuming 0.6 lb of complete feed per day.
2 If pig weighs 100 lb, consuming 4 lb of complete feed per day.
3 If calf weighs 100 lb, consuming 2 lb of complete starter feed per day.
4 Include in feed supplement based on consumption of 2 lb of supplement per head per day.
5 If animal weighs 500 lb, consuming 2 lb of supplement per head per day.
6 If lamb weighs 60 lb, consuming 1 lb of supplement per head per day.

Precaution(s): Store in a dry, cool place.

Caution(s): For use in manufacturing medicated animal feeds only.

For use in dry feeds only. Not for use in liquid feed supplements.

Warning(s): Chickens: At 500 g/ton use level, withdraw 24 hours before slaughter. Zero-day withdrawal period for lower use levels. In low calcium feeds withdraw 3 days before slaughter. Do not administer to chickens producing eggs for human consumption.

Turkeys: At 200 g/ton use level or higher, withdraw 5 days before slaughter. Zero-day withdrawal period for lower use levels. Do not administer to turkeys producing eggs for human consumption.

Calves including pre-ruminating (veal) calves, Beef Cattle, and Nonlactating Dairy Cattle: 5-day withdrawal before slaughter at 10 mg/lb dosage. When used in milk replacers, the treatment claim (10 mg/lb) is limited to bacterial enteritis caused by *Escherichia coli* only.

Sheep: 5-day withdrawal before slaughter at 10 mg/lb dosage.

Certain components of animal feeds, including medicated premixes, possess properties that may be a potential health hazard or a source of personal discomfort to certain individuals who are exposed to them. Human exposure should, therefore, be minimized by observing the general industry standards for occupational health and safety.

Precautions such as the following should be considered: dust masks or respirators and protective clothing should be worn; dust-arresting equipment and adequate ventilation should be utilized; personal hygiene should be observed; wash before eating or leaving a work site; be alert for signs of allergic reactions—seek prompt medical treatment if such reactions are suspected.

Presentation: 50 lb (22.6 kg) bags.

TERRAMYCIN is a registered trademark of Pfizer, Inc., licensed to Phibro Animal Health, for Oxytetracycline HCl.

Compendium Code No.: 36930390 101-9010-01

TERRAMYCIN-343® SOLUBLE POWDER

Pfizer Animal Health **Water Medication**

(oxytetracycline HCl)-A broad-spectrum antibiotic

NADA No.: 008-622

Active Ingredient(s): The 4.78 oz (135.5 g) packet contains 102.4 grams of oxytetracycline HCl and will make:

512 gallons (1,938 L) containing 200 mg of oxytetracycline HCl per gallon.
256 gallons (969 L) containing 400 mg of oxytetracycline HCl per gallon.
128 gallons (484 L) containing 800 mg of oxytetracycline HCl per gallon.

The 9.55 oz (270.7 g) packet contains 204.8 grams of oxytetracycline HCl and will make:

1,024 gallons (3,876 L) containing 200 mg of oxytetracycline HCl per gallon.
512 gallons (1,938 L) containing 400 mg of oxytetracycline HCl per gallon.
256 gallons (969 L) containing 800 mg of oxytetracycline HCl per gallon.

The 4.5 lb (2041.2 g) tub contains 1543.5 grams of oxytetracycline HCl and will make:

7,718 gallons (29,215 L) containing 200 mg of oxytetracycline HCl per gallon.
3,859 gallons (14,608 L) containing 400 mg of oxytetracycline HCl per gallon.
1,930 gallons (7,306 L) containing 800 mg of oxytetracycline HCl per gallon.

Indications: For control and treatment of specific diseases in poultry, cattle, swine, sheep, and bees.

Chickens: Infectious synovitis caused by *Mycoplasma synoviae*.

Chronic respiratory disease (CRD) and air sac infection caused by *Mycoplasma gallisepticum* and *Escherichia coli*.

Fowl cholera caused by *Pasteurella multocida*.

Turkeys: Hexamitiasis caused by *Hexamita meleagridis*.

Infectious synovitis caused by *Mycoplasma synoviae*.

Growing Turkeys—Complicating bacterial organisms associated with bluecomb (transmissible enteritis, coronoviral enteritis).

Swine: Bacterial enteritis caused by *Escherichia coli* and *Salmonella choleraesuis*.

Bacterial pneumonia caused by *Pasteurella multocida*.

For Breeding Swine: Leptospirosis (reducing the incidence of abortions and shedding of leptospira) caused by *Leptospira pomona*.

Calves, Beef Cattle, Non-Lactating Dairy Cattle and Sheep: Bacterial enteritis caused by *Escherichia coli*.

Bacterial pneumonia (shipping fever complex) caused by *Pasteurella multocida*.

Honey Bees: For control of American Foulbrood caused by *Bacillus larvae*.

Directions for Use: For the control of the following poultry diseases caused by organisms susceptible to oxytetracycline: Add the following amount to 2 gallons of stock solution when proportioner is set to meter at the rate of 1 ounce per gallon (4.78 oz and 9.55 oz packets), or add 1 tub of soluble powder to the amounts of water listed below to make a stock solution for use in a proportioner set to meter at the rate of 1 ounce per gallon.

	Dosage	Packets/2 Gallons Stock Solution		Gal of Stock Solution per Tub
		4.78 oz packet	9.55 oz packet	
Chickens				
Infectious synovitis caused by *Mycoplasma synoviae*	200-400 mg/gal	½-1	¼-½	60-30
Chronic respiratory disease (CRD) and air sac infection caused by *Mycoplasma gallisepticum* and *Escherichia coli*	400-800 mg/gal	1-2	½-1	30-15
Fowl cholera caused by *Pasteurella multocida*	400-800 mg/gal	1-2	½-1	30-15
Turkeys				
Hexamitiasis caused by *Hexamita meleagridis*	200-400 mg/gal	½-1	¼-½	60-30
Infectious synovitis caused by *Mycoplasma synoviae*	400 mg/gal	1	½	30
Growing Turkeys—Complicating bacterial organisms associated with bluecomb (transmissible enteritis, coronaviral enteritis)	25 mg/lb body weight daily	Varies with age & water consumption (1 packet will treat 4,096 lb of turkeys)	Varies with age & water consumption (1 packet will treat 8,192 lb of turkeys)	Varies with age & water consumption (1 tub will treat 61,740 lb of turkeys)

Medicate continuously at the first clinical signs of disease and continue for 7-14 consecutive days. If improvement is not noted within 24-48 hours, consult a poultry diagnostic laboratory or poultry pathologist to determine diagnosis and advice on dosage.

For the control and treatment of the following diseases caused by organisms susceptible to oxytetracycline:

	Dosage
Swine	
Bacterial enteritis caused by *Escherichia coli* and *Salmonella choleraesuis* Bacterial pneumonia caused by *Pasteurella multocida* For Breeding Swine: Leptospirosis (reducing the incidence of abortions and shedding of leptospira) caused by *Leptospira pomona*	Administer in the drinking water at a level of 10 mg oxytetracycline HCl per lb of body weight daily. Administer up to 14 days.
Calves, Beef Cattle, Non-Lactating Dairy Cattle and Sheep	
Bacterial enteritis caused by *Escherichia coli* Bacterial pneumonia (shipping fever complex) caused by *Pasteurella multocida*	Administer in the drinking water at a level of 10 mg oxytetracycline HCl per lb of body weight daily. Administer up to 14 days.
The 4.78 oz packet will treat 10,240 lb of swine, cattle or sheep at 10 mg/lb. The 9.55 oz packet will treat 20,480 lb of swine, cattle or sheep at 10 mg/lb. The tub will treat 154,350 lb of swine, cattle or sheep at 10 mg/lb.	
Honey Bees	
For control of American Foulbrood caused by *Bacillus larvae*	200 mg/colony The drug is administered in 3 applications of sugar syrup or 3 dustings at 4- to 5-day intervals. The drug should be fed early in the spring or fall and consumed by the bees before main honey flow begins to avoid contamination of production honey.

Precaution(s): Recommended Storage: Store below 25°C (77°F).

Caution(s): Use as sole source of oxytetracycline. Prepare fresh solutions every 24 hours.

Special Note: The concentration of drug required in medicated water must be adequate to compensate for variation in the age of the animal, feed consumption rate, and the environmental temperature and humidity, each of which affects water consumption.

For use in drinking water only. Not for use in liquid feed supplements.

For oral use only.

For animal use only.

Restricted Drug(s) (California), not for human use, use only as directed.

Warning(s): Do not administer to turkeys, cattle or sheep within 5 days of slaughter. Zero-day slaughter withdrawal in swine. Do not administer to chickens or turkeys producing eggs for human consumption. Do not administer this product with milk or milk replacers. Administer 1 hour before or 2 hours after feeding milk or milk replacers.

Remove at least 6 weeks prior to main honey flow.

Keep out of reach of children.

Presentation: Packaged in 4.78 oz (135.5 g) packets (50 per pail), 9.55 oz (270.7 g) packets (25 per pail), and 4.5 lb (2041.2 g) tub.

Compendium Code No.: 36900271 01-4702-35-3 / 01-4536-35-4 / 05-9402-35-2

TERRAMYCIN® OPHTHALMIC OINTMENT

Pfizer Animal Health **Ophthalmic Antibiotic**

(oxytetracycline hydrochloride) Antibiotic with Polymyxin B Sulfate

NADA No.: 008-763

Active Ingredient(s): TERRAMYCIN® Ophthalmic Ointment with polymyxin B sulfate is a suspension of oxytetracycline hydrochloride and polymyxin B sulfate in a special petrolatum base. Each gram of ointment contains oxytetracycline HCl equivalent to 5 mg of oxytetracycline and 10,000 units of polymyxin B as the sulfate.

Indications: TERRAMYCIN® Ophthalmic Ointment with polymyxin B sulfate is indicated for the prophylaxis and local treatment of superficial ocular infections due to oxytetracycline- and polymyxin-sensitive organisms, including infections due to streptococci, rickettsiae, *E. coli,* and *A. aerogenes,* such as conjunctivitis, keratitis, pink eye, corneal ulcer, blepharitis in dogs, cats, cattle, sheep, and horses; ocular infections due to secondary bacterial complications of distemper in dogs, and bacterial inflammatory conditions which may occur secondary to other infectious diseases in the above species.

Pharmacology: TERRAMYCIN® (oxytetracycline HCl) is an antibiotic, bright yellow in color, possessing potent antimicrobial activity. It is one of the most versatile of the broad-spectrum antibiotics, and is effective in the treatment of infections due to gram-positive and gram-negative bacteria, both aerobic and anaerobic, spirochetes, rickettsiae, and certain of the larger viruses.

Polymyxin B sulfate is one of a group of related antibiotics derived from *Bacillus polymyxa.* The polymyxins are rapidly bactericidal, this action being exclusively against gram-negative bacteria.

The broad-spectrum effectiveness of TERRAMYCIN® against both gram-positive and gram-negative organisms is enhanced by the particular effectiveness of polymyxin B against infections associated with gram-negative organisms, especially those due to *Pseudomonas aeruginosa,* where polymyxin B is the antibiotic of choice. In addition, there is evidence to indicate that polymyxin B sulfate possesses some antifungal activity. The combined antibacterial effect of TERRAMYCIN® plus polymyxin is at least additive and, in many instances, an actual synergistic action is obtained.

Dosage and Administration: TERRAMYCIN® Ophthalmic Ointment with polymyxin B sulfate should be administered topically to the eye 2-4 times daily.

Precaution(s): Recommended storage: Store below 25°C (77°F).

Caution(s): Allergic reactions may occasionally occur. Treatment should be discontinued if reactions are severe.

Note: The use of oxytetracycline and other antibiotics may result in an overgrowth of resistant organisms such as Monilia, staphylococci, and other species of bacteria. If new infections due to nonsensitive bacteria or fungi appear during therapy, appropriate measures should be taken.

For animal use only.

Restricted Drug (California)—Use only as directed.

Not for human use.

Presentation: Available in ⅛ oz. tubes.

Compendium Code No.: 36901790 23-0223-50-4

TERRAMYCIN® SCOURS TABLETS

Pfizer Animal Health **Oxytetracycline-Oral**

(oxytetracycline HCl) A broad-spectrum antibiotic for use in beef and dairy calves

NADA No.: 011-060

Active Ingredient(s): Each tablet contains 250 mg of oxytetracycline HCl.

Indications: TERRAMYCIN® Scours Tablets are recommended for oral administration for the control and treatment of the following diseases in beef and dairy calves caused by organisms sensitive to oxytetracycline: bacterial enteritis caused by *Salmonella typhimurium* and *Escherichia coli* (colibacillosis) and bacterial pneumonia (shipping fever complex, pasteurellosis) caused by *Pasteurella multocida.*

Pharmacology: General Information: TERRAMYCIN® Scours Tablets is an oral formulation containing oxytetracycline, a versatile, broad-spectrum antibiotic that possesses potent antimicrobial activity, for use in beef and dairy calves.

Dosage and Administration: Dosage levels: For control of bacterial enteritis and bacterial pneumonia orally administer 1 tablet per 100 lb of body weight every 12 hours (5 mg/lb of body weight daily in divided doses) for up to 4 consecutive days.

For treatment of bacterial enteritis and bacterial pneumonia orally administer 2 tablets per 100 lb of body weight every 12 hours (10 mg/lb of body weight daily in divided doses) for up to 4 consecutive days.

Dosage should continue until the animal returns to normal and for 24-48 hours after symptoms have subsided. Treatment should not exceed 4 consecutive days.

Precaution(s): Recommended storage: Store below 25°C (77°F).

Caution(s): Exceeding the recommended dosage level of 2 tablets per 100 lb of body weight every 12 hours (10 mg/lb of body weight daily), or administering at this recommended level for more than 4 consecutive days, may result in antibiotic residues beyond the withdrawal time.

Organisms may vary in their degree of susceptibility to any chemotherapy. If no improvement is observed after recommended treatment, diagnosis and susceptibility should be reexamined.

Rarely do side reactions or allergic manifestations occur in calves treated with TERRAMYCIN®. If any unusual reactions are noted, discontinue use of the drug immediately and call a veterinarian.

Since bacteriostatic drugs may interfere with the bacterial action of penicillin, it is advisable to avoid giving TERRAMYCIN® in conjunction with penicillin.

Read entire package insert carefully before using this product.

For animal use only.

Restricted Drug (California)—Use only as directed.

Not for human use.

Warning(s): Discontinue treatment at least 7 days prior to slaughter. Not for use in lactating dairy cattle. A withdrawal period has not been established for this product in preruminating calves. Do not use in calves to be processed for veal.

Discussion: Care of sick animals: The use of antibiotics in the management of disease is based on an accurate diagnosis and an adequate course of treatment. When properly used in the treatment of diseases caused by oxytetracycline-susceptible organisms, most animals treated with TERRAMYCIN® Scours Tablets show a noticeable improvement within 24-48 hours. If improvement does not occur within this period of time, the diagnosis and course of treatment should be reevaluated. It is recommended that the diagnosis and treatment of animal diseases be carried out by a veterinarian. Since many diseases look alike but require different types of treatment, the use of professional veterinary and laboratory services can reduce treatment time, costs, and needless losses. Good housing, sanitation, and nutrition are important in the maintenance of healthy animals and are essential in the treatment of disease.

Presentation: Packaged in 24- and 100-tablet bottles.

Compendium Code No.: 36900280 75-7948-00

TERRAMYCIN® SOLUBLE POWDER

Pfizer Animal Health **Water Medication**

(oxytetracycline HCl) A Broad-Spectrum Antibiotic

NADA No.: 008-622

Active Ingredient(s): This packet contains 10 grams of oxytetracycline HCl.

Indications: For control and treatment of specific diseases in poultry, cattle, swine, sheep, and bees.

Chickens: Infectious synovitis caused by *Mycoplasma synoviae.*

Chronic respiratory disease (CRD) and air sac infection caused by *Mycoplasma gallisepticum* and *Escherichia coli.*

Fowl cholera caused by *Pasteurella multocida.*

Turkeys: Hexamitiasis caused by *Hexamita meleagridis.*

Infectious synovitis caused by *Mycoplasma synoviae.*

Growing turkeys—Complicating bacterial organisms associated with bluecomb (transmissible enteritis, coronoviral enteritis).

Swine: Bacterial enteritis caused by *Escherichia coli* and *Salmonella choleraesuis.*

Bacterial pneumonia caused by *Pasteurella multocida.*

For Breeding Swine: Leptospirosis (reducing the incidence of abortions and shedding of leptospira) caused by *Leptospira pomona.*

Calves, Beef Cattle, Non-Lactating Dairy Cattle and Sheep: Bacterial enteritis caused by *Escherichia coli.*

Bacterial pneumonia (shipping fever complex) caused by *Pasteurella multocida.*

Honey Bees: For control of American Foulbrood caused by *Bacillus larvae.*

Directions for Use: For the control of the following poultry diseases caused by organisms susceptible to oxytetracycline: Add the following amount to 2 gallons of stock solution when proportioner is set to meter at the rate of 1 ounce per gallon.

	Dosage	Packs/2 Gallons Stock Solution
Chickens		
Infectious synovitis caused by *Mycoplasma synoviae*	200-400 mg/gal	5-10
Chronic respiratory disease (CRD) and air sac infection caused by *Mycoplasma gallisepticum* and *Escherichia coli*	400-800 mg/gal	10-20
Fowl cholera caused by *Pasteurella multocida*	400-800 mg/gal	10-20
Turkeys		
Hexamitiasis caused by *Hexamita meleagridis*	200-400 mg/gal	5-10
Infectious synovitis caused by *Mycoplasma synoviae*	400 mg/gal	10
Growing Turkeys—Complicating bacterial organisms associated with bluecomb (transmissible enteritis, coronaviral enteritis)	25 mg/lb body weight daily	Varies with age & water consumption (1 packet will treat 400 lb of turkeys)

Medicate continuously at the first clinical signs of disease and continue for 7-14 consecutive days. If improvement is not noted within 24-48 hours, consult a poultry diagnostic laboratory or poultry pathologist to determine diagnosis and advice on dosage.

For the control and treatment of the following diseases caused by organisms susceptible to oxytetracycline:

	Dosage
Swine	
Bacterial enteritis caused by *Escherichia coli* and *Salmonella choleraesuis* Bacterial pneumonia caused by *Pasteurella multocida* For Breeding Swine: Leptospirosis (reducing the incidence of abortions and shedding of leptospira) caused by *Leptospira pomona*	Administer in the drinking water at a level of 10 mg oxytetracycline HCl per lb of body weight daily. Administer up to 14 days.
Calves, Beef Cattle, Non-Lactating Dairy Cattle and Sheep	
Bacterial enteritis caused by *Escherichia coli* Bacterial pneumonia (shipping fever complex) caused by *Pasteurella multocida*	Administer in the drinking water at a level of 10 mg oxytetracycline HCl per lb of body weight daily. Administer up to 14 days.
This packet will treat 1000 lb of swine, cattle or sheep at 10 mg/lb.	
Honey Bees	
For control of American Foulbrood caused by *Bacillus larvae*	200 mg/colony The drug is administered in 3 applications of sugar syrup or 3 dustings at 4- to 5-day intervals. The drug should be fed early in the spring or fall and consumed by the bees before main honey flow begins to avoid contamination of production honey.

Precaution(s): Recommended storage: Store below 25°C (77°F).

Caution(s): Use as sole source of oxytetracycline. Prepare fresh solutions every 24 hours.

Special Note: The concentration of drug required in medicated water must be adequate to compensate for variation in the age of the animal, feed consumption rate and the environmental temperature and humidity, each of which affects water consumption.

For use in drinking water only. Not for use in liquid feed supplements.

For animal use only.

Keep out of reach of children.

Restricted Drug(s) (California), Not for human use, Use only as directed.

For oral use only.

Warning(s): Do not administer to turkeys, cattle or sheep within 5 days of slaughter. Zero-day withdrawal in swine. Do not administer to chickens or turkeys producing eggs for human consumption. Do not administer this product with milk or milk replacers. Administer 1 hour before or 2 hours after feeding milk or milk replacers.

Remove at least 6 weeks prior to main honey flow.

Presentation: 6.4 oz (181.4 g) packet.

Compendium Code No.: 36900291 01-2358-35-4

TERRA-VET 100

Aspen **Oxytetracycline Injection**

(Oxytetracycline Hydrochloride)

ANADA No.: 200-068

Active Ingredient(s): Each mL contains:

Oxytetracycline HCl .... 100 mg
Water for injection .... 17.0% v/v
Magnesium chloride hexahydrate .... 5.76% w/v
Propylene glycol .... q.s.
Sodium formaldehyde sulfoxylate (as preservative) .... 1.3% w/v
With monoethanolamine for pH adjustment.

Indications: TERRA-VET 100 oxytetracycline hydrochloride injection is for the treatment of diseases in beef cattle, beef calves, nonlactating dairy cattle and dairy calves caused by pathogens sensitive to oxytetracycline HCl.

Pharmacology: Oxytetracycline is effective against a wide range of gram-negative and gram-positive organisms that are pathogenic for cattle. The antibiotic is primarily bacteriostatic in effect, and is believed to exert the antimicrobial action by the inhibition of microbial protein synthesis. The antibiotic activity of oxytetracycline is not appreciably diminished in the presence of body fluids, serum or exudates. Since the drugs in the tetracycline class have similar antimicrobial spectra, organisms can develop cross resistance among them. Oxytetracycline is concentrated by the liver in the bile and excreted in the urine and feces at high concentrations and in a biologically active form.

Dosage and Administration: 3-5 mg/lb of body weight per day for a maximum of four (4) consecutive days. For intravenous administration only.

A great many of the pathogens involved in cattle diseases are known to be susceptible to oxytetracycline hydrochloride therapy. Many strains or organisms, however, have shown resistance to oxytetracycline. In the case of certain colioforms, streptococci and staphylococci, it may be advisable to conduct culture and sensitivity testing to determine susceptibility of the infecting organism to oxytetracycline. In this manner, the likelihood of successful treatment with TERRA-VET 100 (Oxytetracycline Hydrochloride Injection) solution can be determined in advance.

Diseases for which TERRA-VET 100 (Oxytetracycline Hydrochloride Injection) is indicated in beef cattle, beef calves, non-lactating dairy cattle and dairy calves for treatment of the following disease conditions caused by one or more of the oxytetracycline sensitive pathogens listed as follows:

Disease	Causative Organism(s) Which Show Sensitivity to TERRA-VET 100 (Oxytetracycline Hydrochloride Injection)
Bacterial Pneumonia and Shipping Fever Complex Associated with *Pasteurella* spp.	*Pasteurella* spp.
Bacterial Enteritis (scours)	*Escherichia coli*
Necrotic Pododermatitis (Foot Rot)	*Fuscobacterium necrophorum*
Calf Diphtheria	*Fuscobacterium necrophorum*
Wooden Tongue	*Actinobacillus lignieresii*
Wound Infections; Acute Metritis; Traumatic Injury	Caused by oxytetracycline-susceptible strains of streptococcal and staphylococcal organisms.

Recommended Daily Dosages:

Treat at the first clinical signs of disease.

The intravenous injection of 3 to 5 mg of oxytetracycline hydrochloride per pound of body weight per day (3 to 5 mL per 100 lbs body weight) is the recommended dosage.

Severe foot-rot and the severe forms of the indicated diseases should be treated with 5 mg per pound of body weight. Surgical procedures may be indicated in some forms of foot-rot or other conditions.

In disease treatment, the daily dose of TERRA-VET 100 (Oxytetracycline Hydrochloride Injection) should be continued 24 to 48 hours following remission of disease symptoms; however, not to exceed a total of 4 consecutive days.

Dosage for Injection

Refer to the table below for proper dosage according to body weight of the animal.

Weight of the Animals, Lbs (Beef Cattle, Beef Calves, Non-Lactating Dairy Cattle, Dairy Calves)	Milligrams of Oxytetracycline Hydrochloride per 100 lbs of Body Weight Per Day	Daily Dosage of TERRA-VET 100 (Oxytetracycline Hydrochloride Injection) (mL)
50 lbs	300-500 mg	1.5-2.5 mL
100 lbs	300-500 mg	3-5 mL
200 lbs	300-500 mg	6-10 mL
300 lbs	300-500 mg	9-15 mL
400 lbs	300-500 mg	12-20 mL
500 lbs	300-500 mg	15-25 mL
600 lbs	300-500 mg	18-30 mL
800 lbs	300-500 mg	24-40 mL
1000 lbs	300-500 mg	30-50 mL
1200 lbs	300-500 mg	36-60 mL
1400 lbs	300-500 mg	42-70 mL

Precaution(s): Store at a temperature of 59°-86°F.

Note: The solution may darken on storage, but the potency remains unaffected.

Caution(s): Keep out of the reach of children.

If improvement does not occur within 24 to 48 hours, consult a veterinarian.

The improper or accidental injection of the drug outside the vein will cause local tissue irritation manifested by temporary swelling and discoloration at the injection site.

Shortly after injection, treated animals may have a transient hemoglobinuria (darkened urine).

Reactions of an allergic or anaphylactic nature, sometimes fatal, have been known to occur in hypersensitive animals following the injection of oxytetracycline solutions but such reactions are rare.

At the first sign of any adverse reaction or anaphylactic shock (noted by glassy eyes, increased salivation, grinding of the teeth, rapid breathing, muscular tremors, staggering, swelling of the eyelids or collapse), the product should be discontinued. Epinephrine solution at the recommended dosage levels should be administered and a veterinarian should be called immediately.

Because bacteriostatic drugs interfere with the bactericidal action of penicillin, do not give oxytetracycline hydrochloride in conjunction with penicillin.

As with other antibiotics, use of this drug may result in over-growth of nonsusceptible organisms. If any unusual symptoms occur in the absence of a favorable response following treatment, discontinue use immediately and call a veterinarian.

Warning(s): Discontinue treatment at least 22 days prior to slaughter.

Not for use in lactating dairy cattle.

A withdrawal period has not been established for this product in pre-ruminating calves. Do not use in calves to be processed for veal.

Do not use the drug for more than four (4) consecutive days. Use beyond four (4) days or a dosage higher than the maximum recommended dose may result in antibiotic residue in the tissues beyond the withdrawal time.

Restricted drug (California) - Use only as directed.

Discussion: The use of antibiotics, as with most medications used in the management of diseases, is based on accurate diagnosis and adequate treatment. When properly used in the treatment of diseases of oxytetracycline-susceptible organisms, animals usually show a noticeable improvement within 24 to 48 hours. If improvement does not occur within this period of time, the diagnosis and treatment of animal diseases should be carried out by a veterinarian. The use of professional veterinary and laboratory services can reduce treatment costs, time and needless losses. Good management, housing, sanitation and nutrition are essential in the care of animals and in the successful treatment of disease.

Presentation: 500 mL vials.

Compendium Code No.: 14750830

TERRA VET SOLUBLE POWDER

Aspen **Water Medication**

ANADA No.: 200-146

Active Ingredient(s): Each packet contains 10 grams of oxytetracycline HCl.

Indications: A broad spectrum antibiotic for control and treatment of specific diseases in poultry, cattle, sheep and swine.

Directions for Use:

For the control of the following poultry diseases caused by organisms susceptible to oxytetracycline: Add the following amount to two gallons of stock solution when proportioner is set to meter at the rate of one ounce per gallon.

	Dosage	Packets/2 Gallons Stock Solution
Chickens		
Infectious synovitis caused by *Mycoplasma synoviae*	200-400 mg/gal	5-10
Chronic respiratory disease (CRD) and air sac infection caused by *Mycoplasma gallisepticum* and *Escherichia coli*	400-800 mg/gal	10-20
Fowl cholera caused by *Pasteurella multocida*	400-800 mg/gal	10-20
Turkeys		
Hexamitiasis caused by *Hexamita meleagridis*	200-400 mg/gal	5-10
Infectious synovitis caused by *Mycoplasma synoviae*	400 mg/gal	10
Growing Turkeys—Complicating bacterial organisms associated with bluecomb (transmissible enteritis, coronaviral enteritis)	25 mg/lb body weight daily	varies with age & water consumption (1 packet will treat 400 pounds of turkeys.)

Medicate continuously at the first clinical signs of disease and continue for 7 to 14 consecutive days. If improvement is not noted within 24-48 hours, consult a poultry diagnostic laboratory or poultry pathologist to determine diagnosis and advice on dosage.

For the control and treatment of the following diseases caused by organisms susceptible to oxytetracycline:

	Dosage
Swine	
Bacterial enteritis caused by *Escherichia coli* and *Salmonella choleraesuis*	Administer in the drinking water at a level of 10 mg oxytetracycline HCl per pound of body weight daily. Administer up to 14 days.
Bacterial pneumonia caused by *Pasteurella multocida* For Breeding Swine: Leptospirosis (reducing the incidence of abortions and shedding of leptospira) caused by *Leptospira pomona.*	
Calves, Beef Cattle and Non-lactating Dairy Cattle	
Bacterial enteritis caused by *Escherichia coli*	Administer in the drinking water at a level of 10 mg oxytetracycline HCl per pound of body weight daily. Administer up to 14 days.
Bacterial pneumonia (shipping fever complex) caused by *Pasteurella multocida.*	
Sheep	
Bacterial enteritis caused by *Escherichia coli*	Administer in the drinking water at a level of 10 mg oxytetracycline HCl per pound of body weight daily. Administer up to 14 days.
Bacterial pneumonia (shipping fever complex) caused by *Pasteurella multocida.*	

Each packet will treat 1000 pounds of swine, cattle or sheep at 10 mg/pound.

Special Note: The concentration of drug required in medicated water must be adequate to compensate for variation in the age of the animal, feed consumption rate and the environmental temperature and humidity, each of which affects water consumption.

Precaution(s): Recommended Storage: Store below 77°F (25°C).

Caution(s): Use as sole source of oxytetracycline. Prepare fresh solutions every 24 hours.

For use in drinking water only.

Not for use in liquid feed supplements.

For animal use only.

Keep out of reach of children.

Restricted Drug(s) (California). Not for human use. Use only as directed.

Warning(s): Do not administer to turkeys, swine, cattle or sheep within 5 days of slaughter. Do

T

not administer to chickens or turkeys producing eggs for human consumption. Do not administer this product with milk or milk replacers. Administer 1 hour before or 2 hours after feeding milk or milk replacers.

A withdrawal period has not been established for this product in pre-ruminating calves. Do not use in calves to be processed for veal.

A milk discard period has not been established for this product in lactating dairy cattle. Do not use in female dairy cattle 20 months of age or older.

Presentation: 25 x 181.5 g (6.4 oz) packet.

Manufactured by: Phoenix Scientific, Inc., St. Joseph, MO 64503

Compendium Code No.: 14750820 800502

TERRA-VET SOLUBLE POWDER 343

Aspen **Water Medication**

(Oxytetracycline HCl)

ANADA No.: 200-247

Active Ingredient(s): Each packet contains 204.8 grams of oxytetracycline HCl. Each packet will make: 1,024 gallons (3,876 L) containing 200 mg oxytetracycline HCl per gallon; 512 gallons (1,938 L) containing 400 mg oxytetracycline HCl per gallon; 256 gallons (969 L) containing 800 mg oxytetracycline HCl per gallon.

Indications: A broad spectrum antibiotic for control and treatment of specific diseases in poultry, cattle, sheep and swine.

Directions for Use:

For the control of the following poultry diseases caused by organisms susceptible to oxytetracycline: Add the following amount to two gallons of stock solution when proportioner is set to meter at the rate of one ounce per gallon.

	Dosage	Packs/2 Gallons Stock Solution
Chickens		
Infectious synovitis caused by *Mycoplasma synoviae*	200-400 mg/gal	¼-½
Chronic respiratory disease (CRD) and air sac infection caused by *Mycoplasma gallisepticum* and *Escherichia coli*	400-800 mg/gal	½-1
Fowl cholera caused by *Pasteurella multocida*	400-800 mg/gal	½-1
Turkeys		
Hexamitiasis caused by *Hexamita meleagridis*	200-400 mg/gal	¼-½
Infectious synovitis caused by *Mycoplasma synoviae*	400 mg/gal	½
Growing Turkeys—Complicating bacterial organisms associated with bluecomb (transmissible enteritis, coronaviral enteritis)	25 mg/lb body weight daily	varies with age & water consumption (1 packet will treat 8192 pounds of turkeys.)

Medicate continuously at the first clinical signs of disease and continue for 7 to 14 consecutive days. If improvement is not noted within 24-48 hours, consult a poultry diagnostic laboratory or poultry pathologist to determine diagnosis and advice on dosage.

For the control and treatment of the following diseases caused by organisms susceptible to oxytetracycline.

	Dosage
Swine	
Bacterial enteritis caused by *Escherichia coli* and *Salmonella choleraesuis*	Administer in the drinking water at a level of 10 mg oxytetracycline HCl per pound of body weight daily. Administer up to 5 days.
Bacterial pneumonia caused by *Pasteurella multocida* For Breeding Swine: Leptospirosis (reducing the incidence of abortions and shedding of leptospira) caused by *Leptospira pomona.*	
Calves, Beef Cattle and Non-lactating Dairy Cattle	
Bacterial enteritis caused by *Escherichia coli*	Administer in the drinking water at a level of 10 mg oxytetracycline HCl per pound of body weight daily. Administer up to 5 days.
Bacterial pneumonia (shipping fever complex) caused by *Pasteurella multocida.*	
Sheep	
Bacterial enteritis caused by *Escherichia coli*	Administer in the drinking water at a level of 10 mg oxytetracycline HCl per pound of body weight daily. Administer up to 5 days.
Bacterial pneumonia (shipping fever complex) caused by *Pasteurella multocida.*	

Each packet will treat 20,480 pounds of swine, cattle or sheep at 10 mg/pound.

Special Note: The concentration of drug required in medicated water must be adequate to compensate for variation in the age of the animal, feed consumption rate and the environmental temperature and humidity, each of which affects water consumption.

Precaution(s): Recommended Storage: Store below 77°F (25°C).

Caution(s): Use as sole source of oxytetracycline. Not to be used for more than 14 consecutive days in chickens and turkeys or 5 consecutive days in cattle, swine or sheep. Prepare fresh solutions every 24 hours.

For use in drinking water only. Not for use in liquid feed supplements.

Restricted Drug(s) (California). Not for human use. Use only as directed.

For oral use only. For animal use only. Keep out of reach of children.

Warning(s): Do not administer to turkeys, swine, cattle or sheep within 5 days of slaughter. Do not administer to chickens or turkeys producing eggs for human consumption. Do not administer this product with milk or milk replacers. Administer 1 hour before or 2 hours after feeding milk or milk replacers. A withdrawal period has not been established for this product in preruminating calves. Do not use in calves to be processed for veal. A milk discard period has not been established for this product in lactating dairy cattle. Do not use in female dairy cattle 20 months of age or older.

Presentation: 25 x 272.2 g (9.6 oz) packet.

Manufactured by: Phoenix Scientific, Inc., St. Joseph, MO 64503

Compendium Code No.: 14750840 800507

TET 324™

Bimeda **Water Medication**

Tetracycline Hydrochloride Soluble Powder

NADA No.: 065-140

Active Ingredient(s): Contains:

Tetracycline hydrochloride activity . . . . 101.25 g

Indications:

Chickens: For the control of chronic respiratory disease (CRD air sac disease) caused by *Mycoplasma gallisepticum* and *Escherichia coli,* infectious synovitis caused by *Mycoplasma synoviae* sensitive to tetracycline hydrochloride.

Turkeys: For the control of infectious synovitis caused by *Mycoplasma synoviae,* bluecomb (transmissible enteritis) complicated by organisms sensitive to tetracycline hydrochloride.

Swine and Calves: For the control and treatment of bacterial enteritis (scours) caused by *Escherichia coli,* bacterial pneumonia associated with *Pasteurella* spp., *Hemophilus* spp., and *Klebsiella* spp., sensitive to tetracycline.

Dosage and Administration:

Chickens and Turkeys: Use the soluble powder in the drinking water at a drug level of tetracycline hydrochloride per gallon to provide 25 mg/lb. of body weight per day in divided doses.

Administer for three (3) to five (5) days. Medicate at the first clinical signs of disease or when experience indicates that the disease may be a problem.

Swine and Calves: Use the soluble powder in the drinking water at a drug level of tetracycline hydrochloride per gallon to provide 10 mg/lb. of body weight per day in divided doses. Administer for three (3) to five (5) days.

General cautions: Prepare fresh solutions at least once a day; solutions are not stable for more than 24 hours. Use as the sole source of tetracycline. Deliver the recommended dosage level in divided doses. The diagnosis should be reconsidered if improvement is not noticed within three (3) days.

Mixing directions: 5 oz. dissolved in 1,000 mL (approximately 34 fl. oz.) of warm water will provide a stock solution of 100 mg of tetracycline hydrochloride activity per mL. This stock solution, when metered at approximately 1 oz./gallon, will provide drinking water containing 2,957 mg of tetracycline hydrochloride activity per gallon.

The contents of the 5.0 oz. packet are sufficient to deliver the recommended daily dosage levels as follows:

At 25 mg/lb. of body weight, 4,050 total lbs. of chickens or turkeys to be medicated in divided doses.

At 10 mg/lb. of body weight, 10,125 total lbs. of calves or swine to be medicated in divided doses.

For individual calf treatment, 5 mL (1 measuring teaspoonful) twice a day for each 100 lbs. of body weight, administered as a drench or by dose syringe.

Special directions for baby calves and baby pigs: Administer the product one (1) hour before or two (2) hours after feeding milk or milk replacers. Provide clean (unmedicated) drinking water at all times.

Note: The product is to be administered twice a day in the drinking water of swine, calves and poultry. One-half (½) of the recommended daily dosage level of antibiotic is to be consumed during each administration period, thus providing the drug in divided doses.

Caution(s): Do not use for more than five consecutive days.

Warning(s): Do not slaughter birds for food within four (4) days of treatment.

Not for use in chickens and turkeys producing eggs for human consumption.

Do not slaughter animals for food purposes within four (4) days of treatment for swine, and within five (5) days of treatment for calves.

Presentation: 5 oz, 2 lb and 5 lb containers.

Compendium Code No.: 13990391

TET-324

Phoenix Pharmaceutical **Water Medication**

(Tetracycline Hydrochloride Soluble Powder 324) Antibiotic

ANADA No.: 200-136

Active Ingredient(s): Each pound contains 324 g of tetracycline hydrochloride.

Indications: For use in the control and treatment of the following conditions in swine, calves and poultry.

Swine: Bacterial enteritis (scours) caused by *Escherichia coli* and bacterial pneumonia associated with *Pasteurella* spp, *Hemophilus* spp and *Klebsiella* spp susceptible to tetracycline.

Calves: Bacterial enteritis (scours) caused by *Escherichia coli* and bacterial pneumonia (shipping fever complex) associated with *Pasteurella* spp, *Hemophilus* spp and *Klebsiella* spp susceptible to tetracycline.

Chickens: Control of chronic respiratory disease (CRD) and air sac infection caused by *Mycoplasma gallisepticum* and *Escherichia coli;* infectious synovitis caused by *Mycoplasma synoviae* susceptible to tetracycline.

Turkeys: Control of infectious synovitis caused by *Mycoplasma synoviae* and bluecomb (transmissible enteritis, coronaviral enteritis) caused by complicating bacterial organisms susceptible to tetracycline.

Dosage and Administration: Administer TET-324 (Tetracycline Hydrochloride Soluble Powder-324) in the drinking water of swine and calves at a drug level of tetracycline hydrochloride per gallon to provide approximately 10 mg/lb of body weight, daily, for 3 to 5 days.

Administer TET-324 (Tetracycline Hydrochloride Soluble Powder-324) in the drinking water of chickens and turkeys at a level of 25 mg/lb of body weight, daily, for 7 to 14 days.

Do not mix this product with milk or milk replacers. Administer one hour before or two hours after feeding milk or milk replacers. Drug use level must be adjusted to provide 10 mg/lb body weight daily in divided doses for swine and calves or, in the case of chickens and turkeys, 25 mg/lb.

Mixing Instructions: The enclosed 43 cc cup, when level full twice provides approximately 71.4 g (2.52 oz) of finished product which contains 51.0 g of tetracycline hydrochloride.

Swine: A stock solution of 71.4 g of product dissolved in 1500 mL (approximately 50 fl oz or 3 pints) of warm water provides about 34 mg of tetracycline hydrochloride activity per mL.

This stock solution metered at 1 oz/gallon will provide drinking water which contains approximately 1000 mg of tetracycline hydrochloride activity per gallon.

Calves: For individual dosing, prepare a solution of 71.4 g of product dissolved in 500 mL (approximately 16 fl oz or 1 pint) of warm water which provides about 100 mg of tetracycline hydrochloride activity per mL.

Administer 5 mL (1 measuring teaspoonful) of the stock solution (100 mg/mL) twice daily for each 100 lb of body weight as a drench or by dose syringe. This will provide the recommended dosage level of 10 mg/lb body weight daily in divided doses.

T

Chickens and Turkeys: A stock solution of 71.4 g of product dissolved in 1500 mL (approximately 50 fl oz or 3 pints) of warm water provides about 34 mg of tetracycline hydrochloride activity per mL.

This stock solution metered at 1 oz/gallon will provide drinking water which contains approximately 1000 mg of tetracycline hydrochloride activity per gallon.

Note: The concentration of the drug required in medicated water must be adequate to compensate for variation in the age of the animal, feed consumption and the environmental temperature and humidity, each of which affects water consumption.

The contents of the 2 lb container will provide sufficient drug to treat 64,800 total pounds of swine or calves for a single day at the recommended dosage level of 10 mg/lb of body weight in divided doses. The same container will treat 25,920 lb of poultry when supplied at 25 mg/lb.

The contents of the 5 lb container will provide sufficient drug to treat 162,000 total pounds of swine or calves for a single day at the recommended dosage level of 10 mg/lb of body weight in divided doses. The same container will treat 64,800 lb of poultry when supplied at 25 mg/lb.

Caution(s): Use as sole source of tetracycline. Not to be used in swine or calves for more than 5 days. Not to be used in chickens or turkeys for more than 14 consecutive days. When used in plastic or stainless steel waterers or automatic medicators, prepare fresh solution every 24 hours. When used in galvanized waterers, prepare fresh solution every 12 hours. If condition does not improve within 2 to 3 days, consult your veterinarian.

For animal use only.

Warning(s): Do not slaughter swine for food purposes within 4 days of treatment. Do not slaughter cattle for food purposes within 5 days of treatment. Do not slaughter poultry for food within 4 days of treatment. Not for use in poultry producing eggs for human consumption. A withdrawal period has not been established for this product in pre-ruminating calves. Do not use in calves to be processed for veal.

Keep out of reach of children.

Presentation: 2 lb (907.2 g) (NDC 57319-366-35) and 5 lb (2.26 kg) (NDC 57319-366-36).

Manufactured by: Phoenix Scientific, Inc., St. Joseph, MO 64503.

Compendium Code No.: 12560812 Rev. 1-02 / Rev. 10-00

TETANUS ANTITOXIN

Durvet **Antitoxin**

Tetanus Antitoxin, Equine Origin

U.S. Vet. Lic. No.: 303

Composition: This product is prepared from the blood of horses hyperimmunized with *Clostridium tetani* toxoid. Contains gentamicin and thimerosal as preservatives.

Indications: For use in cattle, horses, sheep, and swine as an aid in the prevention and treatment of tetanus caused by *Clostridium tetani.*

Dosage and Administration: Shake well before using. Administer the following doses intramuscularly or subcutaneously.

	Prevention	Treatment
Cattle and horses	1,500 units	10,000-25,000 units
Sheep and swine	500 units	5,000-12,500 units

The maximum volume recommended per injection site is 25 mL for cattle or horses and 10 mL for sheep or swine.

Precaution(s): Store in the dark at 35°-45°F (2°-7°C). Do not freeze. Use entire contents when first opened.

Caution(s): Horses-The preventative dose may cause infection site reactions. All Species-The treatment dose may cause severe injection site reactions and/or systemic reactions. Symptomatic treatment: Epinephrine.

Warning(s): Do not administer within 21 days prior to slaughter.

Presentation: 1,500 and 10,000 units.

Manufactured by: Advance Biologics, Inc., Freeman SD 57029.

Compendium Code No.: 10841901 3/01

TETANUS ANTITOXIN

Fort Dodge **Antitoxin**

Tetanus Antitoxin

U.S. Vet. Lic. No.: 112

Composition: This product is prepared from the blood of horses repeatedly injected with large doses of the toxin of *Clostridium tetani.*

Contains phenol and thimerosal as preservatives.

Indications: TETANUS ANTITOXIN is recommended for use in domestic animals for prevention and treatment of tetanus.

Dosage and Administration: 1500 units, minimum, if injected within 24 hours of exposure. Administer subcutaneously, intravenously or intraperitoneally. Increase dose relative to lapse of time following exposure to as much as 30,000 to 100,000 units in animals which are showing symptoms. Massive initial doses may succeed in effecting a cure where repeated smaller doses of the same aggregate volume may have no value.

It should always be remembered that good nursing and proper supportive treatment, in addition to administration of antitoxin, will improve the patient's chances for recovery.

Precaution(s): Store in dark at 2° to 7°C (35° to 45°F). Use all of this product at time container is first opened.

Caution(s): In case of anaphylactoid reaction, administer epinephrine.

It has been reported that biologicals of equine origin may in some manner be associated with the development of hepatitis (Theiler's Disease)[1,2] when injected into the equine species. The incidence of Theiler's Disease is rare and in affected animals may be manifested as hepatitis, icterus, anorexia, emaciation and death.

Warning(s): Do not administer to food-producing animals within 21 days before slaughter.

For veterinary use only.

References: Available upon request.

Presentation: 10,000 units and 10 x 1,500 units.

Compendium Code No.: 10032190 2780H

TETANUS ANTITOXIN, EQUINE ORIGIN

Colorado Serum **Antitoxin**

Tetanus Antitoxin, Equine Origin

U.S. Vet. Lic. No.: 188

Active Ingredient(s): TETANUS ANTITOXIN, EQUINE ORIGIN is prepared from the blood of healthy horses that have been hyperimmunized with repeated large doses of *Clostridium tetani* toxin. Each serial is tested for purity, safety, and antitoxin units in accordance with the applicable standard requirements issued by USDA.

Contains phenol and thimerosal as preservatives.

Indications: It is recommended for use in domestic animals as an aid in preventing and treating tetanus.

Dosage and Administration: TETANUS ANTITOXIN, EQUINE ORIGIN is recommended for use when a nonimmunized animal, or one whose immune status is unknown, suffers a deep penetrating wound that has or may become contaminated with soil. It provides quick, short-term protection. The antitoxin may also be administered to animals following castration, docking, and other operations performed on premises upon which tetanus infection has been a problem.

TETANUS ANTITOXIN, EQUINE ORIGIN confers immediate passive immunity lasting about 7-14 days. 1,500 units administered subcutaneously or intramuscularly is the recommended dose for prevention.

Large doses of TETANUS ANTITOXIN, EQUINE ORIGIN may provide a beneficial response in animals already infected with tetanus but the success of the treatment is not ensured. For treatment administer 10,000 to 50,000 units to horses and cattle and 3,000 to 15,000 units to sheep and swine. Animals that suffer slow healing puncture wounds or deep abrasions should be given a second dose of antitoxin in seven (7) days and additionally as considered necessary.

Precaution(s): Store in the dark at 2-7°C. Sterilize syringes and needles by boiling them in clean water. Use the entire contents when the bottle is first opened.

Caution(s): Anaphylaxis (shock) may occasionally follow the use of products of this nature. Epinephrine, or an equivalent drug, should be available for immediate use in these instances.

For veterinary use only.

Warning(s): Do not vaccinate within 21 days before slaughter.

Discussion: Tetanus is caused by a toxin (poison) produced by the growth of *Clostridium tetani,* an anaerobic (lives without air) micro-organism that may be carried into the wounds or sites of surgical operations.

Affected animals become stiff, have great difficulty swallowing and the pulse rate is increased. Breathing is labored. Spasmodic contractions of the muscle system occurs, extending muscles of the jaw. Thus, the term lockjaw is frequently applied. Legs are often spread, the tail is stiff with the abdominal muscles retracted. Tetanus stricken animals may be unusually sensitive to light and heat. The temperature of the animal generally remains normal, elevating only shortly before death.

Presentation: 1x1,500 unit, 10x1,500 unit and 1x15,000 unit vials.

Compendium Code No.: 11010321

TETANUS ANTITOXIN, EQUINE ORIGIN

Professional Biological **Antitoxin**

Tetanus Antitoxin, Equine Origin

U.S. Vet. Lic. No.: 188

Active Ingredient(s): TETANUS ANTITOXIN, EQUINE ORIGIN is prepared from the blood of healthy horses that have been hyperimmunized with repeated large doses of *Clostridium tetani* toxin. Each serial is tested for purity, safety, and antitoxin units in accordance with applicable standard requirements issued by USDA.

Contains phenol and thimerosal as a preservative.

Indications: It is recommended for use in domestic animals as an aid in preventing and treating tetanus.

Dosage and Administration: TETANUS ANTITOXIN, EQUINE ORIGIN is recommended for use when a nonimmunized animal, or one whose immune status is unknown, suffers a deep penetrating wound that has or may become contaminated with soil. It provides quick short-term protection. Antitoxin may also be administered to animals following castration, docking, and other operations performed on premises upon which tetanus infection has been a problem.

TETANUS ANTITOXIN, EQUINE ORIGIN confers immediate passive immunity lasting about 7-14 days. 1,500 units administered subcutaneously or intramuscularly is the recommended dose for prevention.

Large doses of TETANUS ANTITOXIN, EQUINE ORIGIN may provide beneficial response in animals already infected with tetanus but the success of treatment is not assured. For treatment administer 10,000 to 50,000 units to horses and cattle, 3,000 to 15,000 units to sheep and swine. Animals that suffer slow healing puncture wounds or deep abrasions should be given a second dose of antitoxin in seven (7) days and additionally as considered necessary.

Precaution(s): Store in the dark at 2° to 7°C. Sterilize syringes and needles by boiling in clean water. Use the entire contents when bottle is first opened.

Caution(s): Anaphylaxis (shock) may occasionally follow the use of products of this nature. Epinephrine, or equivalent, should be available for immediate use in these instances.

For veterinary use only.

Warning(s): Do not vaccinate within 21 days before slaughter.

Discussion: Tetanus is caused by a toxin (poison) produced by the growth of *Clostridium tetani,* an anaerobic (lives without air) micro-organism that may be carried into the wounds or sites of surgical operations.

Affected animals become stiff, have greater difficulty swallowing and the pulse rate is increased. Breathing is labored. Spasmodic contractions of the muscle system occurs, extending muscles of the jaw. Thus, the term lockjaw is frequently applied. Legs are often spread, tail stiff with abdominal muscles retracted. Tetanus stricken animals may be unusually sensitive to light and heat. The temperature of the animal generally remains normal, elevating only shortly before death.

Presentation: 1x1,500 unit, 10x1,500 unit and 1x15,000 unit vials.

Compendium Code No.: 14250031

TETANUS TOXOID

Fort Dodge **Toxoid**

Tetanus Toxoid

U.S. Vet. Lic. No.: 112

Contents: This product contains the antigen listed above.

The MetaStim™ adjuvant is added to enhance the immune response and to promote the proper rate of absorption following inoculation.

Formalin is used as an inactivating agent. Formalin, thimerosal, neomycin, polymyxin B and amphotericin B added as preservatives.

Indications: For vaccination of healthy horses, sheep and swine as an aid in the prevention of tetanus.

Dosage and Administration: Horses, inject one 1 mL dose intramuscularly using aseptic technique. Administer a second 1 mL dose 4 to 8 weeks after the first dose. Revaccinate annually using one 1 mL dose. For sheep, swine and smaller horses, administer a 0.5 mL dose according to the above schedule for horses.

Protective tetanus antibody titers usually occur two weeks after the second injection of the initial series. In the event of an injury during the course of the initial vaccination program, or if annual boosters have not been given, a prophylactic dose of at least 1500 units of tetanus antitoxin should be given.

Precaution(s): Store in dark at 2° to 7°C (35° to 45°F). Avoid freezing. Shake well.
Caution(s): Transitory local reactions at the injection site may occur. In case of anaphylactoid reaction, administer epinephrine.
For veterinary use only.
Warning(s): Do not vaccinate within 60 days before slaughter.
Presentation: 25 x 1 mL prefilled syringes with needles (25 doses), 10 mL (10 dose) vials, and 12 x 1 dose (syringe pouch packs).
Compendium Code No.: 10032201 2771E

TETANUS TOXOID-CONCENTRATED

Colorado Serum **Toxoid**
Tetanus Toxoid
U.S. Vet. Lic. No.: 188
Active Ingredient(s): Prepared by detoxifying tetanus toxin with a formaldehyde solution and moderate heat in such a manner that the antigenic properties remain intact.
The product is refined to remove most of the nonspecific components and concentrated to provide a low dose effective immunizing agent.
Each serial is tested for purity, safety, and potency in accordance with the applicable standard requirements issued by the United States Department of Agriculture.
Contains thimerosal as a preservative.
Indications: For the vaccination of cattle, horses, sheep, goats and swine against tetanus.
Dosage and Administration: The toxoid requires three (3) to four (4) weeks to establish an effective level of protection and should be used only in non-emergency instances. Booster injections should be made annually or at the time of injury regardless of interval.
Inject intramuscularly as follows:
For horses and cattle, at least two (2) doses of 1 mL each.
For sheep, goats and swine, two (2) doses of 0.5 mL each. The interval between doses should be approximately 30 days. Revaccinate all animals retained for breeding and those held beyond the normal marketing period annually. Use the full dose as recommended above.
Precaution(s): Shake well before using. Store in the dark at 2-7°C.
Sterilize syringes and needles by boiling in clean water.
Caution(s): Transitory local reaction may appear at the site of administration.
Anaphylaxis (shock) may sometimes follow the use of products of this nature. Epinephrine, or an equivalent drug, should be available for immediate use in these instances.
Use the entire contents when first opened. For veterinary use only.
Warning(s): Do not vaccinate within 21 days before slaughter.
Discussion: Tetanus is caused by a toxin (poison) produced by the growth of *Clostridium tetani*, an anaerobic (lives without air) micro-organism that may be carried into the wounds or sites of surgical operations.
Affected animals become stiff, have great difficulty swallowing and the pulse rate is increased. Breathing is labored. Spasmodic contractions of the muscle system occurs, extending muscles of the jaw. Thus, the term lockjaw is frequently applied. Legs are often spread, the tail is stiff with the abdominal muscles retracted. Tetanus stricken animals may be unusually sensitive to light and heat. The temperature of the animal generally remains normal, elevating only shortly before death.
Presentation: 10 x 1 dose (10 x 1 mL) and 10 dose (10 mL) vials.
Compendium Code No.: 11010330

TETANUS TOXOID-CONCENTRATED

Professional Biological **Toxoid**
Tetanus Toxoid, Concentrated
U.S. Vet. Lic. No.: 188
Active Ingredient(s): Prepared by detoxifying tetanus toxin with formaldehyde solution in such a manner as to allow the antigenic properties to remain intact. Product is purified and concentrated to provide a low dose effective immunizing agent. Each serial is tested for purity, safety and potency in accordance with applicable Standard Requirements issued by the United States Department of Agriculture.
Contains thimerosal as a preservative.
Indication(s): For the vaccination of healthy horses, cattle, sheep, goats and swine against tetanus.
Dosage and Administration: For primary immunization two doses should be administered subcutaneously or intramuscularly approximately 30 days apart. Use intramuscularly for horses as local reactions are more likely to occur if injected subcutaneously.
Horses or Cattle: 1 mL dose
Sheep, Goats, Swine: 0.5 mL dose
Annually, a single "Booster" vaccination is recommended.
Precaution(s): Shake well before using.
Use entire contents when first opened.
Store in the dark at 2 to 7°C.
Caution(s): A transitory local reaction may occur at injection site.
Anaphylactoid reaction sometimes follows administration of products of this nature. If noted, administer adrenalin or equivalent.
Warning(s): Do not vaccinate animals intended for food within 21 days before slaughter.
For veterinary use only.
Discussion: Tetanus is caused by a toxin (poison) produced by growth of *Clostridium tetani*, an anaerobic (lives without air) microorganism that may be carried into wounds or sites of surgical operations.
Affected animals become stiff, have great difficulty swallowing and the pulse rate is increased. Breathing is labored. Spasmodic contractions of the muscular system occur, extending muscles of the jaw. Thus the term "lockjaw" is frequently applied. Legs are often spread, tail stiff with abnormal muscles retracted. Tetanus stricken animals may be unusually sensitive to light and heat. Temperature of the animal generally remains normal, elevating only shortly before death.
Vaccination with tetanus toxoid is recommended for healthy domestic animals, not infected with tetanus, to establish an active immunity for prevention against tetanus. Protective antibody levels usually occur about two weeks after the second injection of the primary immunization series. In contrast, administration of Tetanus Antitoxin is recommended for immediate, emergency, passive treatment of exposed animals with an unknown vaccination history or with signs of tetanus infection. Refer to the product circular for Tetanus Antitoxin for full information.
Presentation: Available in single dose size packaged 10 vials to the carton and in 10 dose vials.
Compendium Code No.: 14250040

TETANUS TOXOID-UNCONCENTRATED

Colorado Serum **Toxoid**
Tetanus Toxoid, Unconcentrated
U.S. Vet. Lic. No.: 188
Contents: Prepared by detoxifying tetanus toxin with formaldehyde solution in such a manner as to allow the antigenic properties to remain intact. Each serial is tested for purity, safety and potency in accordance with applicable standard requirements issued by the United States Department of Agriculture.
Contains thimerosal as a preservative.
Indications: For the prevention of tetanus in horses, cattle, sheep, goats and swine.
Dosage and Administration: For primary immunization two doses should be administered subcutaneously or intramuscularly approximately 30 days apart. Use intramuscularly for horses as local reactions are more likely to occur if injected subcutaneously.
Horses or Cattle: 10 mL dose.
Sheep, Goats, Swine: 1 mL per 100 pounds.
Annually, a single "Booster" vaccination is recommended.
Precaution(s): Store in the dark at 2 to 7°C.
Shake well before using.
Use entire contents when first opened.
Caution(s): A transitory local reaction may occur at injection site.
Anaphylactoid reaction sometimes follows administration of products of this nature. If noted, administer adrenalin or equivalent.
Warning(s): Do not vaccinate meat animals within 21 days before slaughter.
Discussion: Tetanus is caused by a toxin (poison) produced by growth of *Clostridium tetani*, an anaerobic (lives without air) microorganism that may be carried into wounds or sites of surgical operations.
Affected animals become stiff, have great difficulty swallowing and the pulse rate is increased. Breathing is labored. Spasmodic contractions of the muscle system occurs, extending muscles of the jaw. Thus, the term "lockjaw" is frequently applied. Legs are often spread, tail stiff with abdominal muscles retracted. Tetanus stricken animals may be unusually sensitive to light and heat. Temperature of the animal generally remains normal, elevating only shortly before death.
Vaccination with tetanus toxoid is recommended for healthy domestic animals not infected with tetanus to establish an active immunity for prevention against tetanus. Protective antibody levels usually occur about two weeks after the second injection of the primary immunization series. In contrast, administration of Tetanus Antitoxin is recommended for immediate, emergency, passive treatment of exposed animals with an unknown vaccination history or with signs of tetanus infection.
Presentation: This product is packaged in 1 dose (10 mL) and 5 dose (50 mL) sizes.
Compendium Code No.: 11010341

TETGUARD™

Boehringer Ingelheim **Toxoid**
Tetanus Toxoid
U.S. Vet. Lic. No.: 124
Contents: TETGUARD™ is alum precipitated and purified.
Contains thimerosal as a preservative.
Indications: TETGUARD™ is recommended for vaccination of healthy horses, cattle, swine, and sheep to confer long-term, active immunity against tetanus.
Dosage and Administration: Shake well before use. Administer subcutaneously or intramuscularly, using aseptic technique.
Dosage: Horses, cattle and swine - 1 mL. Sheep - 0.5 mL. Repeat in 30 days. Revaccinate annually and prior to anticipated exposure.
Precaution(s): Store at 35-45°F (2-7°C). Protect from freezing. Use entire contents when first opened.
Caution(s): Anaphylactoid reactions may occur following use.
This product has been tested under laboratory conditions and shown to meet all Federal standards for safety and efficacy in normal healthy animals. This level of performance may be affected by conditions such as stress, weather, nutrition, disease, parasitism, other treatments, individual idiosyncrasies or impaired immunological competency. These factors should be considered by the user when evaluating product performance or freedom from reactions.
Antidote(s): Epinephrine.
Warning(s): Do not vaccinate within 21 days before slaughter.
Presentation: 1 mL (1 horse, cattle, swine dose; 2 sheep doses) and 20 mL (20 horse, cattle, swine doses; 40 sheep doses) vials.
Compendium Code No.: 10281060

TETNI-VAX®

AgriPharm **Bacterin-Toxoid**
Clostridium chauvoei-septicum-haemolyticum-novyi-tetani-perfringens Types C & D Bacterin-Toxoid
U.S. Vet. Lic. No.: 311
Active Ingredient(s): A formalin-inactivated, alum-precipitated bacterin-toxoid prepared from highly toxigenic cultures and culture filtrates of *Clostridium chauvoei, Cl. septicum, Cl. haemolyticum* (known elsewhere as *Cl. novyi* type D), *Cl. novyi, Cl. tetani*, and *Cl. perfringens* types C and D. TETNI-VAX® is an Electroferm® product produced by an electronically controlled deep culture process.
Indications: For the active immunization of healthy sheep and cattle against diseases caused by *Clostridium chauvoei, Cl. septicum, Cl. haemolyticum* (known elsewhere as *Cl. novyi* type D), *Cl. novyi, Cl. tetani*, and *Cl. perfringens* types C and D.
Although *Cl. perfringens* type B is not a significant problem in the U.S.A., immunity may be provided against the beta and epsilon toxins elaborated by *Cl. perfringens* type B. The immunity is derived from the combination of type C (beta) and type D (epsilon) fractions.
Dosage and Administration: Shake well. Using aseptic technique, inject 5 mL subcutaneously followed by a 2 mL dose in six (6) weeks. Revaccinate annually with 2 mL prior to periods of extreme risk, or parturition. For *Cl. novyi* and *Cl. haemolyticum*, revaccinate every five (5) to six (6) months. Vaccination should be scheduled so that pregnant ewes receive their second vaccination or annual booster two (2) to six (6) weeks before lambing commences in the flock. Lambs should be given their primary course beginning at 10 to 12 weeks of age.
Precaution(s): Store at 35°-45°F (2°-7°C). Protect from freezing.
Use the entire contents when first opened.

Caution(s): This product has been tested under laboratory conditions and has met all federal standards for safety and ability to immunize normal healthy animals. The level of performance may be affected by conditions of use such as stress, weather, nutrition, disease, parasitism, other treatments, individual idiosyncrasies or impaired immunological competency. These factors should be considered by the user when evaluating product performance or freedom from reactions.

Anaphylactic reactions may occur following use.

Antidote(s): Epinephrine.

Warning(s): Do not vaccinate within 21 days before slaughter.

Discussion: The specific toxoids and/or cellular antigens required for optimal disease protection are emphasized in the growth of Electroferm® cultures. These cultures are highly concentrated and, when divided for the blending of combination vaccines, make possible the production of the low volume dose. Exacting procedures are employed to ensure that each dose of combination vaccine contains an appropriate amount of each component.

All components of each serial of the final product are tested for potency using USDA-accepted laboratory and/or host animal tests.

Trial Data: The protective value of all components of TETNI-VAX® has been demonstrated through the most critical test procedures available. Vaccinated sheep withstood the challenge of massive doses of virulent live spores of *Cl. chauvoei, Cl. septicum, Cl. tetani, Cl. novyi* types B and D. *Cl. perfringens* types C and D, for which no host animal direct-challenge test exists, were evaluated by measuring the amount of antitoxin produced by cattle, sheep and laboratory animals.

Presentation: 10 dose (50 mL) and 50 dose (250 mL) vials.

TETNI-VAX is a registered trademark of Dealer Distribution of America.

Compendium Code No.: 14571310

TETNOGEN®

Fort Dodge — **Toxoid**

Tetanus Toxoid

U.S. Vet. Lic. No.: 112

Contents: This product contains the antigen listed above.

Indications: For the vaccination of healthy horses, cattle, sheep and swine against clostridium tetani.

Dosage and Administration: Shake well before using. Using aseptic technique, vaccinate healthy horses, cattle, swine with 1 mL; sheep with 0.5 mL, subcutaneously or intramuscularly. Administer a second dose 30 days later. Annual revaccination with a single dose is recommended.

Precaution(s): Do not freeze. Store between 2° and 7°C (35° and 45°F).

Caution(s): Use entire contents when first opened. In case of anaphylactic reactions, administer epinephrine.

Warning(s): Do not vaccinate within 21 days before slaughter.

For veterinary use only.

Presentation: Packages containing 10 dose vials and 12 x 1 dose (syringe pouch pack).

Compendium Code No.: 10032211 — 12173C, 12171A

TETNOGEN®-AT

Fort Dodge — **Antitoxin**

Tetanus Antitoxin, Equine origin

U.S. Vet. Lic. No.: 112

Contents: Tetanus antitoxin is prepared from the blood of healthy horses that have been hyperimmunized with repeated large doses of *Clostridium tetani* toxin. Each serial is tested for purity, safety, and antitoxin units in accordance with applicable Standard Requirements issued by USDA.

Tetanus Antitoxin contains phenol and thimerosal as preservatives.

Indications: TETNOGEN®-AT is recommended for use whenever a non-immunized animal, or one whose immune status is unknown, suffers a deep penetrating wound that has or may become contaminated with soil. It provides quick but short-term protection.

Antitoxin may also be administered to animals following castration, docking, and other operations performed on premises upon which tetanus infection has been a problem.

Dosage and Administration: Tetanus Antitoxin confers immediate passive immunity lasting about 7 to 14 days. 1500 units administered subcutaneously or intramuscularly is the recommended dose for prevention.

Large doses of Tetanus Antitoxin may provide beneficial response in animals already infected with tetanus, but success of treatment is not assured. For treatment, administer 10,000 to 50,000 units to horses and cattle, 3,000 to 15,000 units to sheep and swine. Animals that suffer slow healing puncture wounds or deep abrasions should be given a second dose of antitoxin in 7 days and additionally as considered necessary.

Precaution(s): Store in dark at 2° to 7°C (35° to 45°F). Sterilize needles and syringes by boiling in clean water. Use entire contents when first opened.

Caution(s): Anaphylaxis (shock) may occasionally follow the use of products of this nature. Epinephrine should be available for use in these instances.

Warning(s): Meat animals should not be vaccinated within 21 days before slaughter. If Tetanus Antitoxin must be used under emergency conditions, the animals so treated should be withheld from the market for 21 days after administration.

For veterinary use only.

Discussion: Tetanus is caused by a toxin (poison) produced by growth of *Clostridium tetani*, an anaerobic (lives without air) micro-organism that may be carried into the wounds or sites of surgical operations.

Affected animals become stiff, have great difficulty swallowing and the pulse rate is increased. Breathing is labored. Spasmodic contractions of the muscular system occurs, extending muscles of the jaw. Thus, the term "lockjaw" is frequently applied. Legs are often spread, tail stiff with abdominal muscles retracted. Tetanus stricken animals may be unusually sensitive to light and heat. Temperature of the animal generally remains normal, elevating only shortly before death.

Trial Data: A condition referred to as "serum hepatitis" infrequently occurs in horses. The literature associates this partially with the injection of biologics containing equine serum or tissue. This connection is based, at the present time, upon supposition and not upon scientific evidence, as efforts to experimentally reproduce such a condition in horses have not been successful. It seems prudent, however, in view of the published implication, to make the owners of horses aware of it. Some of the same publications that refer to "serum hepatitis" continue to recommend the use of Tetanus Antitoxin in horses that have suffered wounds that may have been contaminated with *Clostridium tetani* and the immunization status is unknown.

Presentation: Supplied in packages containing 10 x 1,500 unit vials and 1 x 10,000 unit vial.

Compendium Code No.: 10032221 — 12180A

TETRA BAC 324

AgriLabs — **Tetracycline-Oral**

Antibiotic

NADA No.: 065-496

Active Ingredient(s): Each pound contains 324 g of tetracycline hydrochloride.

Indications: For use in the control and treatment of the following conditions in swine, calves and poultry:

Swine: Bacterial enteritis (scours) caused by *Escherichia coli* and bacterial pneumonia associated with *Pasteurella* spp., *Hemophilus* spp., and *Klebsiella* spp. susceptible to tetracycline.

Calves: Bacterial enteritis (scours) caused by *Escherichia coli* and bacterial pneumonia (shipping fever complex) associated with *Pasteurella* spp., *Hemophilus* spp., and *Klebsiella* spp. susceptible to tetracycline.

Chickens: Control of chronic respiratory disease (CRD) and air sac infection caused by *Mycoplasma gallisepticum* and *Escherichia coli;* infectious synovitis caused by *Mycoplasma synoviae* susceptible to tetracycline.

Turkeys: Control of infectious synovitis caused by *Mycoplasma synoviae* and bluecomb (transmissible enteritis, coronaviral enteritis) caused by complicating bacterial organisms susceptible to tetracycline.

Dosage and Administration: Administer TETRA BAC 324 in the drinking water of swine and calves at a level of tetracycline hydrochloride per gallon to provide approximately 10 mg/lb. of body weight per day for three (3) to five (5) days.

Administer TETRA BAC 324 in the drinking water of chickens and turkeys at a level of 25 mg/lb. of body weight per day for 7-14 days.

Do not mix this product with milk or milk replacers. Administer one (1) hour before or two (2) hours after feeding milk or milk replacers. Drug use level must be adjusted to provide 10 mg/lb. of body weight per day in divided doses for swine and calves or, in the case of chickens and turkeys, 25 mg/lb.

Swine: A stock solution of 71.4 g dissolved in 1,500 mL (approximately 50 fl. oz. or 3 pt.) of warm water provides about 34 mg of tetracycline hydrochloride activity per mL.

Calves: For individual dosing, prepare a solution of 71.4 g dissolved in 500 mL (approximately 16 fl. oz. or 1 pt.) of warm water which provides about 100 mg of tetracycline hydrochloride activity per mL. Administer 5 mL (1 measuring teaspoonful) of the stock solution (100 mg/mL) twice a day for each 100 lb. of body weight as a drench or by a dose syringe. This will provide the recommended dosage level of 10 mg/lb. of body weight per day in divided doses.

Chickens and Turkeys: A stock solution of 71.4 g dissolved in 1,500 mL (approximately 50 fl. oz. or 3 pt.) of warm water provides about 34 mg of tetracycline hydrochloride activity per mL.

Enclosed cup will provide approximately 71.4 g when measured to the 3 oz. level.

This stock solution metered at 1 oz./gallon will provide drinking water which contains approximately 1,000 mg of tetracycline hydrochloride activity per gallon.

Note: The concentration of the drug required in medicated water must be adequate to compensate for variation in the age of the animal, feed consumption and the environmental temperature and humidity, each of which affects water consumption.

Caution(s): Use as the sole source of tetracycline. Not to be used in swine or calves for more than five consecutive days. Not to be used in chickens or turkeys for more than 14 consecutive days. When used in plastic or stainless steel waterers or automatic medicators, prepare fresh solution every 24 hours. When used in galvanized waterers, prepare fresh solutions every 12 hours. If the condition does not improve within two to three days, consult a veterinarian.

The contents of this container (5 lbs.) will provide sufficient drug to treat 162,000 total pounds of swine or calves for a single day at the recommended dosage level of 10 mg/lb. of body weight in divided doses. The same container will treat 64,800 lbs. of poultry when supplied at 25 mg/lb.

Warning(s): Do not slaughter swine for food purposes within four (4) days of treatment. Do not slaughter cattle for food purposes within five (5) days of treatment. Do not slaughter poultry for food within four (4) days of treatment. Not for use in poultry producing eggs for human consumption.

Keep out of reach of children.

Presentation: 5 oz. packets, and 2 lb. and 5 lb. bucket sizes.

Compendium Code No.: 10581031

TETRACYCLINE HYDROCHLORIDE SOLUBLE POWDER-324

Butler — **Tetracycline-Oral**

Antibiotic

NADA No.: 065-496

Active Ingredient(s): Each pound contains 324 g of tetracycline hydrochloride.

Indications: For use in the control and treatment of the following conditions in swine, calves and poultry.

Swine: Bacterial enteritis (scours) caused by *Escherichia coli* and bacterial pneumonia associated with *Pasteurella* spp., *Hemophilus* spp. and *Klebsiella* spp. susceptible to tetracycline.

Calves: Bacterial enteritis (scours) caused by *Escherichia coli* and bacterial pneumonia (shipping fever complex) associated with *Pasteurella* spp., *Hemophilus* spp., and *Klebsiella* spp. susceptible to tetracycline.

Chickens: Control of chronic respiratory disease (CRD) and air sac infection caused by *Mycoplasma gallisepticum* and *Escherichia coli;* infectious synovitis caused by *Mycoplasma synoviae* susceptible to tetracycline.

Turkeys: Control of infectious synovitis caused by *Mycoplasma synoviae* and bluecomb (transmissible enteritis, coronaviral enteritis) caused by complicating bacterial organisms susceptible to tetracycline.

Dosage and Administration: Administer TETRACYCLINE HYDROCHLORIDE SOLUBLE POWDER-324 in the drinking water of swine and calves at a drug level of tetracycline hydrochloride per gallon to provide approximately 10 mg/lb. of body weight per day for three (3) to five (5) days.

Administer TETRACYCLINE HYDROCHLORIDE SOLUBLE POWDER-324 in the drinking water of turkeys at a level of 25 mg/lb. of body weight per day for 7-14 days.

Do not mix the product with milk or milk replacers. Administer one (1) hour before or two (2) hours after feeding milk or milk replacers. The drug use level must be adjusted to provide 10 mg/lb. of body weight per day in divided doses for swine and calves or, in the case of chickens and turkeys, 25 mg/lb.

Swine: A stock solution of 71.4 g dissolved in 1,500 mL (approximately 50 fl. oz. or 3 pints) of warm water provides about 34 mg of tetracycline hydrochloride activity per mL. The enclosed cup will provide approximately 71.4 g when measured to the 3 oz. level.

Calves: For individual dosing, prepare a solution of 71.4 g dissolved in 500 mL (approximately 16 fl. oz. or 1 pint) of warm water which provides about 100 mg of tetracycline hydrochloride activity per mL. The enclosed cup will provide approximately 71.4 g when measured to the 3 oz. level.

Administer 5 mL (1 measuring teaspoonful) of the stock solution (100 mg/mL) twice a day for each 100 lb. of body weight as a drench or by a dose syringe. This will provide the recommended dosage level of 10 mg/lb. of body weight per day in divided doses.

Chickens and Turkeys: A stock solution of 71.4 g dissolved in 1,500 mL (approximately 50 fl. oz. or 3 pints) of warm water provides about 32 mg of tetracycline hydrochloride activity per mL. The enclosed cup will provide approximately 71.4 g when measured to the 3 oz. level.

This stock solution metered at 1 oz./gallon will provide drinking water which contains approximately 1,000 mg of tetracycline hydrochloride activity per gallon.

The contents of the container (2 lb.) will provide sufficient drug to treat 64,800 total pounds of swine or calves for a single day at the recommended dosage level of 10 mg/lb. of body weight in divided doses. The same container will treat 25,920 lbs. of poultry when supplied at 25 mg/lb.

Note: The concentration of the drug required in medicated water must be adequate to compensate for variation in the age of the animals, feed consumption and the environmental temperature and humidity, each of which affects water consumption.

Caution(s): Use as the sole source of tetracycline. Not to be used in swine or calves for more than five days. Not to be used in chickens or turkeys for more than 14 consecutive days. When used in plastic or stainless steel waterers or automatic medicators, prepare a fresh solution every 24 hours. When used in galvanized waterers, prepare a fresh solution every 12 hours. If the condition does not improve within two to three days, consult a veterinarian.

For veterinary use only.

Keep out of the reach of children.

Warning(s): Do not slaughter swine for food purposes within four (4) days of treatment.

Do not slaughter calves for food purposes within five (5) days of treatment.

Do not slaughter poultry for food within four (4) days of treatment.

Not for use in poultry producing eggs for human consumption.

Presentation: 2 lb. and 5 lb. containers.

Compendium Code No.: 10821750

TETRACYCLINE HYDROCHLORIDE SOLUBLE POWDER-324

Vedco **Tetracycline-Oral**

Antibiotic

NADA No.: 065-496

Active Ingredient(s): Each pound contains 324 g of tetracycline hydrochloride.

Indications: For use in the control and treatment of the following conditions in swine, calves and poultry.

Swine: Bacterial enteritis (scours) caused by *Escherichia coli* and bacterial pneumonia associated with *Pasteurella* spp., *Hemophilus* spp. and *Klebsiella* spp. susceptible to tetracycline.

Calves: Bacterial enteritis (scours) caused by *Escherichia coli* and bacterial pneumonia (shipping fever complex) associated with *Pasteurella* spp., *Hemophilus* spp., and *Klebsiella* spp. susceptible to tetracycline.

Chickens: Control of chronic respiratory disease (CRD) and air sac infection caused by *Mycoplasma gallisepticum* and *Escherichia coli;* infectious synovitis caused by *Mycoplasma synoviae* susceptible to tetracycline.

Turkeys: Control of infectious synovitis caused by *Mycoplasma synoviae* and bluecomb (transmissible enteritis, coronaviral enteritis) caused by complicating bacterial organisms susceptible to tetracycline.

Dosage and Administration: Administer TETRACYCLINE HYDROCHLORIDE SOLUBLE POWDER-324 in the drinking water of swine and calves at a drug level of tetracycline hydrochloride per gallon to provide approximately 10 mg/lb. of body weight per day, for three (3) to five (5) days.

Administer TETRACYCLINE HYDROCHLORIDE SOLUBLE POWDER-324 in the drinking water of chickens and turkeys at a level of 25 mg/lb. of body weight per day, for 7-14 days.

Do not mix the product with milk or milk replacers. Administer one (1) hour before or two (2) hours after feeding milk or milk replacers. The drug use level must be adjusted to provide 10 mg/lb. of body weight per day in divided doses for swine and calves or, in the case of chickens and turkeys, 25 mg/lb.

Mixing Instructions: The enclosed blue cup, when level full, provides approximately 71.4 g (2.52 oz.) of finished product which contains 51.0 g of tetracycline hydrochloride.

Swine: A stock solution of 71.4 g dissolved in 1,500 mL (approximately 50 fl. oz. or 3 pints) of warm water provides about 34 mg of tetracycline hydrochloride activity per mL.

The stock solution metered at 1 oz./gallon will provide drinking water which contains approximately 1,000 mg of tetracycline hydrochloride activity per gallon.

Calves: For individual dosing, prepare a solution of 71.4 g dissolved in 500 mL (approximately 16 fl. oz. or 1 pint) of warm water which provides about 100 mg of tetracycline hydrochloride activity per mL.

Administer 5 mL (1 measuring teaspoonful) of the stock solution (100 mg/mL) twice a day for each 100 lbs. of body weight as a drench or by a dose syringe. This will provide the recommended dosage level of 10 mg/lb. of body weight per day in divided doses.

Chickens and Turkeys: A stock solution of 71.4 g dissolved in 1,500 mL (approximately 50 fl. oz. or 3 pints) of warm water provides about 34 mg of tetracycline hydrochloride activity per mL.

The stock solution metered at 1 oz./gallon will provide drinking water which contains approximately 1,000 mg of tetracycline hydrochloride activity per gallon.

Note: The concentration of the drug required in medicated water must be adequate to compensate for variation in the age of the animals, feed consumption and the environmental temperature and humidity, each of which affects water consumption.

Caution(s): Use as the sole source of tetracycline. Not to be used in swine or calves for more than five days. Not to be used in chickens or turkeys for more than 14 consecutive days. When used in plastic or stainless steel waterers or automatic medicators, prepare a fresh solution every 24 hours. When used in galvanized waterers, prepare a fresh solution every 12 hours. If the condition does not improve within two to three days, consult a veterinarian.

For use in animals only.

Warning(s): Do not slaughter swine for food purposes within four (4) days of treatment.

Do not slaughter cattle for food purposes within five (5) days of treatment.

Do not slaughter poultry for food within four (4) days of treatment.

Not for use in poultry producing eggs for human consumption.

Keep out of the reach of children.

Presentation: 5 lb container.

Compendium Code No.: 10941961

TETRACYCLINE SOLUBLE POWDER 324

AgriPharm **Tetracycline-Oral**

Tetracycline Hydrochloride Soluble Powder

NADA No.: 065-496

Active Ingredient(s): Each pound contains:

Tetracycline hydrochloride .... 324 g

Indications: For use in the control and treatment of the following conditions in swine, calves and poultry:

Swine: Bacterial enteritis (scours) caused by *Escherichia coli* and bacterial pneumonia associated with *Pasteurella* spp., *Haemophilus* spp. and *Klebsiella* spp. susceptible to tetracycline.

Calves: Bacterial enteritis (scours) caused by *Escherichia coli* and bacterial pneumonia (shipping fever complex) associated with *Pasteurella* spp., *Haemophilus* spp. and *Klebsiella* spp. susceptible to tetracycline.

Chickens: For the control of chronic respiratory disease (CRD) and air sac infection caused by *Mycoplasma gallisepticum* and *Escherichia coli,* infectious synovitis caused by *Mycoplasma synoviae* susceptible to tetracycline.

Turkeys: For the control of infectious synovitis caused by *Mycoplasma synoviae* and bluecomb (transmissible enteritis, coronaviral enteritis) caused by complicating bacterial organisms susceptible to tetracycline.

Dosage and Administration: Administer TETRACYCLINE SOLUBLE POWDER 324 in the drinking water of swine and calves at a drug level of tetracycline hydrochloride per gallon to provide approximately 10 mg/lb. of body weight, each day, for three (3) to five (5) days.

Administer TETRACYCLINE SOLUBLE POWDER 324 in the drinking water of chickens and turkeys at a level of 25 mg/lb. of body weight, each day, for 7-14 days.

Do not mix the product with milk or milk replacers. Administer one (1) hour before or two (2) hours after feeding milk or milk replacers. The drug use level must be adjusted to provide 10 mg/lb. of body weight each day in divided doses for swine and calves, or in the case of chickens and turkeys, 25 mg/lb.

Mixing instructions: The enclosed blue cup, when level full, provides approximately 71.4 g (2.52 oz.) of finished product which contains 51 g of tetracycline hydrochloride.

Swine: A stock solution of 71.4 g dissolved in 1,500 mL (approximately 50 fl. oz. or 3 pt.) of warm water provides about 34 mg of tetracycline hydrochloride activity per mL.

This stock solution metered at 1 oz./gallon will provide drinking water which contains approximately 1,000 mg of tetracycline hydrochloride activity per gallon.

Calves: For individual dosing, prepare a solution of 71.4 g dissolved in 500 mL (approximately 16 fl. oz. or 1 pt.) of warm water which provides about 100 mg of tetracycline hydrochloride activity per mL.

Administer 5 mL (1 measuring teaspoonful) of the stock solution (100 mg/mL) twice a day for each 100 lbs. of body weight as a drench or by a dose syringe. This will provide the recommended dosage level of 10 mg/lb. of body weight each day in divided doses.

Chickens and Turkeys: A stock solution of 71.4 g dissolved in 1,500 mL (approximately 50 fl. oz. or 3 pt.) of warm water provides about 34 mg of tetracycline hydrochloride activity per mL.

This stock solution metered at 1 oz./gallon will provide drinking water which contains approximately 1,000 mg of tetracycline hydrochloride activity per gallon.

Note: The concentration of the drug required in medicated water must be adequate to compensate for the variation in the ages of the animals, feed consumption and the environmental temperature and humidity, each of which affects water consumption.

The contents of one (1) 2 lb. container will provide sufficient drug to treat 64,800 total pounds of swine or calves for a single day at the recommended dosage level of 10 mg/lb. of body weight in divided doses. The same container will treat 25,920 lbs. of poultry when supplied at 25 mg/lb.

The contents of one (1) 5 lb. container will provide sufficient drug to treat 162,000 total lbs. of swine or calves for a single day at the recommended dosage level of 10 mg/lb. of body weight in divided doses. The same container will treat 64,800 lbs. of poultry when supplied at 25 mg/lb.

Caution(s): For animal use only.

Restricted drug (California), use only as directed.

Keep out of the reach of children.

Use as the sole source of tetracycline. Not to be used in swine or calves for more than five days. Not to be used in chickens or turkeys for more than 14 consecutive days. When used in plastic or stainless steel waterers or automatic medicators, prepare a fresh solution every 24 hours. When used in galvanized waterers, prepare a fresh solution every 12 hours. If the condition does not improve within two or three days, consult a veterinarian.

Warning(s): Do not slaughter swine for food purposes within four (4) days of treatment.

Do not slaughter cattle for food purposes within five (5) days of treatment.

Do not slaughter poultry for food within four (4) days of treatment.

Not for use in poultry producing eggs for human consumption.

A withdrawal period has not been established for the product in preruminating calves. Do not use in calves to be processed for veal.

Presentation: 2 lb. and 5 lb. containers.

Compendium Code No.: 14571010

TETRASOL SOLUBLE POWDER

Med-Pharmex **Water Medication**

Tetracycline Hydrochloride Soluble Powder-Antibiotic

ANADA No.: 200-234

Active Ingredient(s): Each 5 oz packet contains 101.2 g of tetracycline hydrochloride.

Each pound contains 324 g of tetracycline hydrochloride.

Indications: For use in the control and treatment of the following conditions in swine, calves and poultry.

Swine and Calves: Control and treatment of bacterial enteritis (scours) caused by *Escherichia coli;* bacterial pneumonia associated with *Actinobacillus pleuropneumoniae, Pasteurella* spp. and *Klebsiella* spp. sensitive to tetracycline hydrochloride.

Chickens: Control of chronic respiratory disease (CRD) and air sac disease caused by *Mycoplasma gallisepticum* and *Escherichia coli;* infectious synovitis caused by *Mycoplasma synoviae* sensitive to tetracycline hydrochloride.

Turkeys: Control of infectious synovitis caused by a *Mycoplasma synoviae;* bluecomb (transmissible enteritis, coronaviral enteritis) complicated by organisms sensitive to tetracycline hydrochloride.

Dosage and Administration:

Swine and Calves: Use soluble powder in the drinking water at a drug level of tetracycline hydrochloride per gallon to provide 10 mg/lb of body weight per day in divided doses.

Caution: Do not use for more than 5 consecutive days.

T

Directions for Use: Administer for 3-5 days.

Chickens: CRD and air sac disease: Use soluble powder in the drinking water at a drug level of 400-800 mg tetracycline hydrochloride per gallon. Infectious synovitis: Use soluble powder in the drinking water at a drug level of 200-400 mg tetracycline hydrochloride per gallon.

Turkeys: Infectious synovitis: Use soluble powder in the drinking water at a drug level of 400 mg tetracycline hydrochloride per gallon. Bluecomb: Use soluble powder in the drinking water at a drug level of tetracycline hydrochloride per gallon to provide 25 mg/lb of body weight per day in divided doses.

Caution: Do not use for more than 14 consecutive days.

Chickens and Turkeys: Administer for 7-14 days. Medicate at first clinical signs of disease or when experience indicates the disease may be a problem.

Mixing Directions:

For Swine, Calves and Turkeys:

5 oz packet: 5 oz dissolved in 1,000 mL (approximately 34 fl oz) of warm water will provide a stock solution of 100 mg of tetracycline hydrochloride activity per mL. For Turkeys Only: This stock solution when metered at approximately 1 oz per gallon, will provide drinking water containing 2,957 mg of tetracycline hydrochloride activity per gallon.

2 lb and 5 lb: 2.52 oz (two scoops) dissolved in 500 mL (approximately 17 fl oz) of warm water will provide a stock solution of 100 mg of tetracycline hydrochloride activity per mL. For Turkeys Only: This stock solution when metered at approximately 1 oz per gallon, will provide drinking water containing 2,957 mg of tetracycline hydrochloride activity per gallon.

The contents of the 5 oz packet are sufficient to deliver the recommended daily dosage levels as follows:

At 25 mg/lb of body weight: 4,048 total lbs of turkeys to be medicated.

At 10 mg/lb of body weight: 10,120 total lbs of swine or calves to be medicated.

Individual calf treatment: 5 mL (1 measuring teaspoonful) twice daily for each 100 lbs of body weight administered as a drench or by dose syringe.

The contents of two scoops are sufficient to deliver the recommended daily dosage levels as follows:

At 25 mg/lb of body weight: 2,040 total lbs of turkeys to be medicated.

At 10 mg/lb of body weight: 5,100 total lbs of swine or calves to be medicated.

Individual calf treatment: 5 mL (1 measuring teaspoonful) twice daily for each 100 lbs of body weight administered as a drench or by dose syringe.

For Chickens and Turkeys:

To arrive at the recommended dosages, prepare stock solutions as follows:

200 mg/gallon - dissolve 1 packet (5 oz) in 15,140 mL warm water (4 gallons).

400 mg/gallon - dissolve 1 packet (5 oz) in 7,570 mL warm water (2 gallons).

800 mg/gallon - dissolve 1 packet (5 oz) in 3,785 mL warm water (1 gallon).

To arrive at the recommended dosages, use the enclosed contents of 2 scoops to prepare stock solutions as follows:

200 mg/gallon - dissolve 2 scoops (2.52 oz) in 7,570 mL warm water (2 gallons).

400 mg/gallon - dissolve 2 scoops (2.52 oz) in 3,785 mL warm water (1 gallon).

800 mg/gallon - dissolve 2 scoops (2.52 oz) in 1,892 mL warm water (0.5 gallon).

These stock solutions should then be metered into drinking water at approximately 1 oz per gallon.

At 200-800 mg/gallon the 5 oz packet will provide 126.5 to 506 gallons of medicated drinking water.

At 200-800 mg/gallon two scoops will provide 63.8 to 255 gallons of medicated drinking water.

Special Directions for Baby Calves and Baby Pigs: Administer this product one hour before or two hours after feeding milk or milk replacers. Provide clean (unmedicated) drinking water at all times.

Note: When using a watering trough, this product is to be administered twice a day in the drinking water of swine, calves and poultry. One-half of the recommended daily dosage level of antibiotic is to be consumed during each administration period, thus providing the drug in divided doses.

The contents of the 2 lb container will provide sufficient drug to treat 64,800 total pounds of swine or calves for a single day at the recommended dosage level of 10 mg/lb of body weight in divided doses. Or the contents of the container will treat 25,920 lbs of turkeys when supplied at 25 mg/lb or at 200-800 mg/gallon will provide 810 to 3,240 gallons of medicated drinking water for chickens or turkeys.

The contents of the 5 lb container will provide sufficient drug to treat 162,000 total pounds of swine or calves for a single day at the recommended dosage level of 10 mg/lb of body weight in divided doses. Or the contents of the container will treat 64,800 lbs of turkeys when supplied at 25 mg/lb or at 200-800 mg/gallon will provide 2,025 to 8,100 gallons of medicated drinking water for chickens or turkeys.

Caution(s): Prepare fresh solutions at least once a day. Solutions are not stable for more than 24 hours. Use as a sole source of tetracycline. Diagnosis should be reconsidered if improvement is not noticed within 3 days. The concentration of drug required in medicated water must be adequate to compensate for variations in the age and class of animals, feed consumption, and environmental temperature and humidity, each of which affects water consumption.

Warning(s):

Swine - Do not slaughter animals for food purposes within 4 days of treatment.

Calves - Do not slaughter animals for food purposes within 5 days of treatment.

A withdrawal period has not been established for this product in pre-ruminating calves.

Do not use in calves to be processed for veal.

Turkeys - Do not slaughter birds for food within 4 days of treatment.

Not for use in turkeys or chickens producing eggs for human consumption.

Restricted drug (California) - Use only as directed.

For use in animals only.

Keep out of reach of children.

Presentation: 5 oz (141.7 g) packets, 2 lb (907.2 g), and 5 lbs (2.27 kg).

Distributed by: Ellsworth Pharmaceuticals, Inc.

Compendium Code No.: 10270130

Active ingredients are cross-indexed with product names in the Green pages.

TETRAVET-CA™

Alpharma **Water Medication**

(Oxytetracycline HCl)-Antibiotic

NADA No.: 130-435

Active Ingredient(s): The packet contains 648 grams of oxytetracycline HCl and will treat 64,800 pounds of swine.

Indications: For the Control and Treatment of the Following Diseases in Swine: Bacterial enteritis caused by *Escherichia coli* and *Salmonella choleraesuis,* susceptible to oxytetracycline and Bacterial pneumonia caused by *Pasteurella multocida,* susceptible to oxytetracycline.

For Breeding Swine: Leptospirosis (reducing the incidence of abortions and shedding of leptospira) caused by *Leptospira pomona,* susceptible to oxytetracycline.

Directions for Use: Mixing Directions for Water Medication:

	Disease	Treatment Level
Swine	For the Control and Treatment of the Following Diseases in Swine — Bacterial enteritis caused by *Escherichia coli* and *Salmonella choleraesuis*, susceptible to oxytetracycline. Bacterial pneumonia caused by *Pasteurella multocida*, susceptible to oxytetracycline. For Breeding Swine: Leptospirosis (reducing the incidence of abortions and shedding of leptospira) caused by *Leptospira pomona*, susceptible to oxytetracycline.	10 mg/lb body weight

Mix fresh solutions daily. Use as sole source of drinking water. Do not mix this product directly with milk or milk replacers. Administer one hour before or two hours after feeding milk or milk replacers. Administer up to 5 days to swine.

Note: The concentration of drug required in medicated water must be adequate to compensate for variation in the age of the animal, feed consumption rate and the environmental temperatures and humidity, each of which affects water consumption.

Precaution(s): Recommended Packet Storage Conditions: Store below 77°F (25°C).

Caution(s): Use as sole source of oxytetracycline. Not to be used for more than 5 consecutive days in swine.

Livestock remedy. Not for human consumption. Hazardous remedy.

For use in drinking water only.

Not for use in liquid feed supplements.

Warning(s): Keep out of reach of children.

Presentation: 3.91 lb (1772 g) packets.

TETRAVET-CA is a trademark of Alpharma Inc.

Compendium Code No.: 10221320 AHL-467 0108

TETROXY®-100

Bimeda **Oxytetracycline Injection**

Active Ingredient(s): Contents:

Oxytetracycline hydrochloride .... 100 mg
Magnesium chloride hexahydrate .... 5.75% w/v
Water for injection 17.0%
Sodium formaldehyde sulfoxylate (as preservative) .... 1.3% w/v
Propylene glycol .... q.s.

Also contains 2-aminoethanol to adjust pH.

Indications: TETROXY®-100 is only for the treatment of diseases in beef cattle and nonlactating dairy cattle caused by pathogens susceptible to oxytetracycline HCl.

Dosage and Administration: For intravenous use only. Using aseptic conditions, slowly inject 3-5 mg/lb. of body weight per day for a maximum of four (4) consecutive days.

Warning(s): Discontinue treatment at least 19 days prior to slaughter. Not for use in lactating dairy cattle.

Presentation: 500 mL container.

Compendium Code No.: 13990401

TETROXY® HCA SOLUBLE POWDER

Bimeda **Water Medication**

(Oxytetracycline HCl) Antibiotic-Water Soluble Product

NADA No.: 200-144

Active Ingredient(s): Each 9.87 oz (280 g) packet contains 102.4 g of oxytetracycline HCl.

Each 19.74 oz (560 g) packet contains 204.8 g of oxytetracycline HCl.

Each 5 lb (2,270 g) container contains 830.2 g of oxytetracycline HCl.

Indications: Chickens: Control of infectious synovitis caused by *Mycoplasma synoviae,* chronic respiratory disease (CRD) and air sac infections caused by *Mycoplasma gallisepticum* and *Escherichia coli,* and fowl cholera caused by *Pasteurella multocida,* susceptible to oxytetracycline.

Turkeys: Control of hexamitiasis caused by *Hexamita meleagridis,* infectious synovitis caused by *Mycoplasma synoviae,* susceptible to oxytetracycline.

Growing Turkeys - Control of complicating bacterial organisms associated with bluecomb (transmissible enteritis, coronaviral enteritis), susceptible to oxytetracycline.

Swine:

For the Control and Treatment of the Following Diseases in Swine: Bacterial enteritis caused by *Escherichia coli* and *Salmonella choleraesuis,* bacterial pneumonia caused by *Pasteurella multocida,* susceptible to oxytetracycline.

For Breeding Swine: Leptospirosis (reducing the incidence of abortions and shedding of leptospira) caused by *Leptospira pomona,* susceptible to oxytetracycline.

Directions for Use: Mix fresh solutions daily. Use as sole source of drinking water. Do not mix this product directly with milk or milk replacers. Administer one hour before or two hours after feeding milk or milk replacers. If improvement is not noted within 24 to 48 hours, consult a poultry veterinarian or poultry pathologist laboratory - as a generalization, 200 chickens will drink one gallon of water per day for each week of age. Turkeys will consume twice that amount. Administer 7 to 14 days for chickens and turkeys and up to 5 days to swine.

Note: The concentration of drug required in medicated water must be adequate to compensate for variation in the age of the birds, feed consumption rate, and the environmental temperatures and humidity, each of which affects water consumption.

Mixing Instructions for Water Medication:

Each Packet Contains:		Chicken Dose		Turkey Dose			Swine Dose
Product Description	Grams of Activity	Treated Gallons	Mg per Treated Gallon	Treated Gallons	Mg per Treated Gallon	Lbs of Turkey Treated per Packet at 25 mg/lb	Lbs of Swine Treated per Packet at 10 mg/lb
TETROXY® HCA-280	102.4	512	200 mg	512	200 mg	4096	10,240
		256	400 mg	256	400 mg		
		128	800 mg				
TETROXY® HCA-560	204.8	1024	200 mg	1024	200 mg	8192	20,480
		512	400 mg	512	400 mg		
		256	800 mg				
TETROXY® HCA-2270	830.2	4151	200 mg	4151	200 mg	33,207	83,017
		2075	400 mg	2075	400 mg		
		1038	800 mg				

Dosage for Use in Water Proportioners: Add the following amount to one gallon of stock solution when proportioner is set to meter at the rate of one ounce per gallon.

Disease	Treatment Level	TETROXY® HCA-280	TETROXY® HCA-560	TETROXY® HCA-2270
Chickens				
Control of infectious synovitis caused by *Mycoplasma synoviae*, susceptible to oxytetracycline	200-400 mg	¼-½ pkt (70-140 g)	⅛-¼ pkt (70-140 g)	70-140 g
Control of chronic respiratory disease (CRD) and air sac infections caused by *Mycoplasma gallisepticum* and *Escherichia coli*, and fowl cholera caused by *Pasteurella multocida*, susceptible to oxytetracycline	400-800 mg	½-1 pkt (140-280 g)	¼-½ pkt (140-280 g)	140-280 g
Turkeys				
Control of hexamitiasis caused by *Hexamita meleagridis*, susceptible to oxytetracycline	200-400 mg	¼-½ pkt (70-140 g)	⅛-¼ pkt (70-140 g)	70-140 g
Control of infectious synovitis caused by *Mycoplasma synoviae*, susceptible to oxytetracycline	400 mg	½ pkt (140 g)	¼ pkt (140 g)	140 g
Growing Turkeys — Control of complicating bacterial organisms associated with bluecomb (transmissible enteritis, coronaviral enteritis), susceptible to oxytetracycline	25 mg/lb body weight	Varies with age & water consumption	Varies with age & water consumption	Varies with age & water consumption
Swine				
For the Control and Treatment of the Following Diseases in Swine: Bacterial enteritis caused by *Escherichia coli* and *Salmonella choleraesuis*, bacterial pneumonia caused by *Pasteurella multocida*, and leptospirosis in breeding swine (reducing the incidence of abortions and shedding of leptospira) caused by *Leptospira pomona*, susceptible to oxytetracycline	10 mg/lb body weight	Varies with age & water consumption	Varies with age & water consumption	Varies with age & water consumption

Precaution(s): Recommended Storage Conditions: Store below 77°F (25°C).

Caution(s): For use in drinking water only. Not for use in liquid feed supplements.

Use as sole source of oxytetracycline.

Not to be used for more than 14 consecutive days in chickens and turkeys or 5 consecutive days in swine.

Consult Material Safety Data Sheet prior to use.

Warning(s): Do not feed to birds producing eggs for human consumption.

Discontinue treatment of chickens, turkeys and swine 0 days prior to slaughter.

Livestock remedy - Not for human consumption - Hazardous remedy.

Keep out of reach of children.

Presentation: 40 x 9.87 oz (280 g) and 25 x 19.74 oz (560 g) packets and 5 lb (2.27 kg) (2,270 g) container.

TETROXY is a registered trademark of the Cross Vetpharm Group, DBA Bimeda, Inc.

Compendium Code No.: 13990610 8TET003-700 / 8TET005-700 / 8TET001-700

TETROXY® LA

Bimeda **Oxytetracycline Injection**

(Oxytetracycline Injection) Antibiotic

ANADA No.: 200-117

Active Ingredient(s): Each mL contains 200 mg of oxytetracycline base as amphoteric oxytetracycline and, on a w/v basis, 40.0% 2-pyrrolidone, 5.0% povidone, 1.8% magnesium oxide, 0.2% sodium formaldehyde sulfoxylate (as a preservative), monoethanolamine and/or hydrochloric acid as required to adjust pH.

Indications: TETROXY® LA is intended for use in the treatment of the following diseases in beef cattle, nonlactating dairy cattle and swine when due to oxytetracycline-susceptible organisms:

Cattle: In cattle, TETROXY® LA is indicated in the treatment of pneumonia and shipping fever complex associated with *Pasteurella* spp. and *Hemophilus* spp.; infectious bovine keratoconjunctivitis (pinkeye) caused by *Moraxella bovis;* foot-rot and diphtheria caused by *Fusobacterium necrophorum;* bacterial enteritis (scours) caused by *Escherichia coli;* wooden tongue caused by *Actinobacillus lignieresii,* leptospirosis caused by *Leptospira pomona;* and wound infections and acute metritis caused by strains of staphylococcal and streptococcal organisms sensitive to oxytetracycline.

Swine: In swine, TETROXY® LA is indicated in the treatment of bacterial enteritis (scours, colibacillosis) caused by *Escherichia coli;* pneumonia caused by *Pasteurella multocida;* and leptospirosis caused by *Leptospira pomona.*

In sows, TETROXY® LA is indicated as an aid in the control of infectious enteritis (baby pig scours, colibacillosis) in suckling pigs caused by *Escherichia coli.*

Pharmacology: TETROXY® LA (oxytetracycline injection 200 mg/mL) is a sterile, ready-to-use solution for the administration of the broad-spectrum antibiotic oxytetracycline by injection. Oxytetracycline is an antimicrobial agent that is effective in the treatment of a wide range of diseases caused by susceptible gram-positive and gram-negative bacteria.

Dosage and Administration: Read entire brochure carefully before using this product.

Cattle: TETROXY® LA is to be administered by intramuscular or intravenous injection to beef cattle and nonlactating dairy cattle.

A single dosage of 9 milligrams of TETROXY® LA per pound of body weight administered intramuscularly is recommended in the treatment of the following conditions: 1) bacterial pneumonia caused by *Pasteurella* spp. (shipping fever) in calves and yearlings, where re-treatment is impractical due to husbandry conditions, such as cattle on range, or where their repeated restraint is inadvisable; 2) infectious bovine keratoconjunctivitis (pinkeye) caused by *Moraxella bovis.*

TETROXY® LA can also be administered by intravenous or intramuscular injection at a level of 3 to 5 milligrams of oxytetracycline per pound of body weight per day. In the treatment of severe foot-rot and advanced cases of other indicated diseases, a dosage level of 5 milligrams per pound of body weight per day is recommended. Treatment should be continued 24 to 48 hours following remission of disease signs; however, not to exceed a total of four consecutive days. Consult your veterinarian if improvement is not noted within 24 to 48 hours of the beginning of treatment.

Swine: In swine, a single dosage of 9 milligrams of TETROXY® LA per pound of body weight administered intramuscularly is recommended in the treatment of bacterial pneumonia caused by *Pasteurella multocida* in swine, where re-treatment is impractical due to husbandry conditions or where repeated restraint is inadvisable.

TETROXY® LA can also be administered by intramuscular injection at a level of 3 to 5 milligrams of oxytetracycline per pound of body weight per day. Treatment should be continued 24 to 48 hours following remission of disease signs; however, not to exceed a total of four consecutive days. Consult your veterinarian if improvement is not noted within 24 to 48 hours of the beginning of treatment.

For sows, administer once intramuscularly 3 milligrams of oxytetracycline per pound of body weight approximately 8 hours before farrowing or immediately after completion of farrowing.

For swine weighing 25 lb of body weight and under, TETROXY® LA should be administered undiluted for treatment at 9 mg/lb but should be administered diluted for treatment at 3 or 5 mg/lb.

Body Weight	9 mg/lb Dosage	3 or 5 mg/lb Dosage		
	Volume of Undiluted TETROXY® LA	Volume of Diluted TETROXY® LA		
	9 mg/lb	3 mg/lb	Dilution*	5 mg/lb
5 lb	0.2 mL	0.6 mL	1:7	1.0 mL
10 lb	0.5 mL	0.9 mL	1:5	1.5 mL
25 lb	1.1 mL	1.5 mL	1:3	2.5 mL

*To prepare dilutions, add one part TETROXY® LA to three, five or seven parts of sterile water, or 5 percent dextrose solution as indicated; the diluted product should be used immediately.

Cattle Dosage Guide: At the first signs of pneumonia or pinkeye, administer a single dose of TETROXY® LA by deep intramuscular injection according to the following weight categories.*

Animal weight (lb)	Number of mL or cc
100	4.5
200	9.0
300	13.5
400	18.0
500	22.5
600	27.0
700	31.5
800	36.0
900	40.5
1000	45.0
1100	49.5
1200	54.0

*Do not administer more than 10 mL at any one injection site (1 to 2 mL per site in small calves). Discontinue treatment 28 days prior to slaughter.

Swine Dosage Guide: At the first signs of pneumonia, administer TETROXY® LA by deep intramuscular injection according to the following weight categories.*

Animal Weight (lb)	Number of mL or cc
10	0.5
25	1.1
50	2.3
75	3.4
100	4.5
125	5.6
150	6.8
175	7.9
200	9.0
225	10.1
250	11.3
275	12.4
300	13.5
325	14.6

*Do not administer more than 5 mL at any one injection site. Discontinue treatment 28 days prior to slaughter.

Directions for Use: TETROXY® LA is intended for use in the treatment of disease due to oxytetracycline-susceptible organisms in beef cattle, nonlactating dairy cattle and swine. A thoroughly cleaned, sterile needle and syringe should be used for each injection (needles and syringes may be sterilized by boiling in water for 15 minutes). In cold weather, TETROXY® LA should be warmed to room temperature before administration to animals. Before withdrawing the solution from the bottle, disinfect the rubber cap on the bottle with suitable disinfectant, such as 70 percent alcohol. The injection site should be similarly cleaned with the disinfectant. Needles of 16 to 18 gauge and 1 to 1½ inches long are adequate for intramuscular injections. Needles 2 to 3 inches are recommended for intravenous use.

Intramuscular Administration: Intramuscular injections should be made by directing the needle of suitable gauge and length into the fleshy part of a thick muscle such as in the rump, hip, or thigh regions; avoid blood vessels and major nerves. Before injecting the solution, pull back gently on the plunger. If blood appears in the syringe, a blood vessel has been entered; withdraw the needle and select a different site. No more than 10 mL should be injected intramuscularly at any one site in adult beef cattle and nonlactating dairy cattle, and not more than 5 mL per site in adult swine; rotate injection sites for each succeeding treatment. The volume administered per injection site should be reduced according to age and body size so that 1 to 2 mL per site is injected in small calves.

Intravenous Administration: TETROXY® LA may be administered intravenously to beef cattle and nonlactating dairy cattle. As with all highly concentrated materials, TETROXY® LA should be administered slowly by the intravenous route.

Preparation of the Animal for Injection:

1. Approximate location of vein. The jugular vein runs in the jugular groove on each side of the neck from the angle of the jaw to just above the brisket and slightly above and to the side of the windpipe. (See Fig. I.)
2. Restraint. A stanchion or chute is ideal for restraining the animal. With a halter, rope, or cattle leader (nose tongs), pull the animal's head around the side of the stanchion, cattle chute, or post in such a manner to form a bow in the neck (See Fig. II), then snub the head securely to prevent movement. By forming the bow in the neck, the outside curvature of the bow tends to expose the jugular vein and make it easily accessible. Caution: Avoid restraining the animal with a tight rope or halter around the throat or upper neck which might impede blood flow. Animals that are down present no problem so far as restraint is concerned.
3. Clip hair in area where injection is to be made (over the vein in the upper third of the neck). Clean and disinfect the skin with alcohol or other suitable antiseptic.

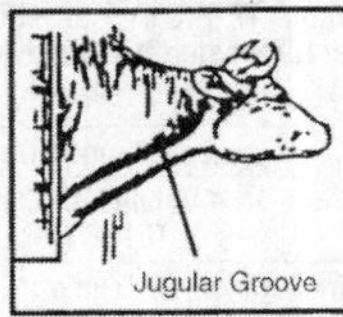

Figure I

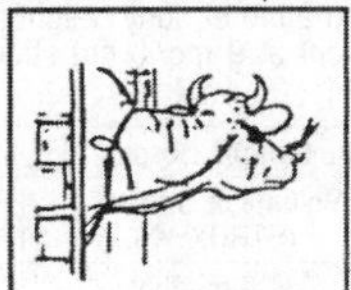
Figure II

Entering the Vein and Making the Injection:

1. Raise the vein. This is accomplished by tying the choke rope tightly around the neck close to the shoulder. The rope should be tied in such a way that it will not come loose and so that it can be untied quickly by pulling the loose end (See Fig. II). In thick-necked animals, a block of wood placed in the jugular groove between the rope and hide will help considerably in applying the desired pressure at the right point. The vein is a soft flexible tube through which blood flows back to the heart. Under ordinary conditions it cannot be seen or felt with the fingers. When the flow of blood is blocked at the base of the neck by the choke rope, the vein becomes enlarged and rigid because of the back pressure. If the choke rope is sufficiently tight, the vein stands out and can be easily seen and felt in thin-necked animals. As a further check in identifying the vein, tap it with the fingers in front of the choke rope. Pulsations that can be seen or felt with the fingers in front of the point being tapped will confirm the fact that the vein is properly distended. It is impossible to put the needle into the vein unless it is distended. Experienced operators are able to raise the vein simply by hand pressure, but the use of a choke rope is more certain.
2. Inserting the needle. This involves three distinct steps. First, insert the needle through the hide. Second, insert the needle into the vein. This may require two or three attempts before the vein is entered. The vein has a tendency to roll away from the point of the needle, especially if the needle is not sharp. The vein can be steadied with the thumb and finger of one hand. With the other hand, the needle point is placed directly over the vein, slanting it so that its direction is along the length of the vein, either toward the head or toward the heart. Properly positioned this way, a quick thrust of the needle will be followed by a spurt of blood through the needle, which indicates that the vein has been entered. Third, once in the vein, the needle should be inserted along the length of the vein all the way to the hub, exercising caution to see that the needle does not penetrate the opposite side of the vein. Continuous steady flow of blood through the needle indicates that the needle is still in the vein. If blood does not flow continuously, the needle is out of the vein (or clogged) and another attempt must be made. If difficulty is encountered, it may be advisable to use the vein on the other side of the neck.
3. While the needle is being placed in proper position in the vein, an assistant should get the medication ready so that the injection can be started without delay after the vein has been entered.
4. Making the injection. With the needle in position as indicated by continuous flow of blood, release the choke rope by a quick pull on the free end. This is essential—the medication cannot flow into the vein while it is blocked. Immediately connect the syringe containing TETROXY® LA to the needle and slowly depress the plunger. If there is resistance to depression of the plunger, this indicates that the needle has slipped out of the vein (or is clogged) and the procedure will have to be repeated. Watch for any swelling under the skin near the needle, which would indicate that the medication is not going into the vein. Should this occur, it is best to try the vein on the opposite side of the neck.
5. Removing the needle. When injection is complete, remove needle with straight pull. Then apply pressure over area of injection momentarily to control any bleeding through needle puncture, using cotton soaked in alcohol or other suitable antiseptic.

Precaution(s): Store at room temperature, 15°-30°C (59°-86°F). Keep from freezing.

TETROXY® LA does not require refrigeration; however, it is recommended that it be stored at room temperature, 15°-30°C (59°-86°F). The antibiotic activity of oxytetracycline is not appreciably diminished in the presence of body fluids, serum, or exudates.

Caution(s): Exceeding the highest recommended dosage level of drug per pound of body weight per day, administering more than the recommended number of treatments, and/or exceeding 10 mL intramuscularly per injection site in adult beef cattle and nonlactating dairy cattle, and 5 mL intramuscularly per injection site in adult swine, may result in antibiotic residues beyond the withdrawal period.

Reactions of an allergic or anaphylactic nature, sometimes fatal, have been known to occur in hypersensitive animals following the injection of oxytetracycline. Such adverse reactions can be characterized by signs such as restlessness, erection of hair, muscle trembling; swelling of eyelids, ears, muzzle, anus and vulva (or scrotum and sheath in males); labored breathing, defecation and urination, glassy-eyed appearance, eruption of skin plaques, frothing from the mouth and prostration. Pregnant animals that recover may subsequently abort. At the first sign of any adverse reaction, discontinue use of this product and administer epinephrine at the recommended dosage levels. Call a veterinarian immediately.

Shock may be observed following intravenous administration, especially where highly concentrated materials are involved. To minimize this occurrence, it is recommended that TETROXY® LA be administered slowly by this route.

Shortly after injection, treated animals may have transient hemoglobinuria resulting in darkened urine.

As with all antibiotic preparations, use of this drug may result in overgrowth of nonsusceptible organisms, including fungi. A lack of response by the treated animal, or the development of new signs, may suggest that an overgrowth of nonsusceptible organisms has occurred. If any of these conditions occur, consult your veterinarian.

Since bacteriostatic drugs may interfere with the bactericidal action of penicillin, it is advisable to avoid giving TETROXY® LA in conjunction with penicillin.

Care of Sick Animals: The use of antibiotics in the management of diseases is based on an accurate diagnosis and an adequate course of treatment. When properly used in the treatment of diseases caused by oxytetracycline-susceptible organisms, most animals that have been treated with oxytetracycline injection show a noticeable improvement within 24 to 48 hours. It is recommended that the diagnosis and treatment of animal diseases be carried out by a veterinarian. Since many diseases look alike but require different types of treatment, the use of professional veterinary and laboratory services can reduce treatment time, costs and needless losses. Good housing, sanitation and nutrition are important in the maintenance of healthy animals, and are essential in the treatment of diseased animals.

Warning(s): Discontinue treatment at least 28 days prior to slaughter of cattle and swine. Not for use in lactating dairy animals.

Livestock drug, not for human use.

Restricted drug, use only as directed.

Presentation: 250 mL (8.5 fl oz) and 500 mL (16.9 fl oz) vials.

Compendium Code No.: 13990301

TET-SOL 10

Alpharma **Water Medication**

Tetracycline Hydrochloride Soluble Powder-Antibiotic

NADA No.: 065-140

Active Ingredient(s): Each pound contains 25 g of tetracycline hydrochloride activity.

This packet contains 10 g of tetracycline hydrochloride activity.

Indications: For use in drinking water for swine, calves and poultry.

Swine: Control and treatment of bacterial enteritis (scours) caused by *Escherichia coli;* bacterial pneumonia associated with *Pasteurella* spp., *Actinobacillus pleuropneumoniae, Klebsiella* spp. sensitive to tetracycline hydrochloride.

Calves: Control and treatment of bacterial enteritis (scours) caused by *Escherichia coli;* bacterial pneumonia associated with *Pasteurella* spp., *Actinobacillus pleuropneumoniae, Klebsiella* spp. sensitive to tetracycline hydrochloride.

Chickens: Control of chronic respiratory disease (CRD air sac disease) caused by *Mycoplasma gallisepticum* and *Escherichia coli;* infectious synovitis caused by *Mycoplasma synoviae* sensitive to tetracycline hydrochloride.

Turkeys: Control of infectious synovitis caused by *Mycoplasma synoviae;* bluecomb (transmissible enteritis, corona viral enteritis) complicated by organisms sensitive to tetracycline hydrochloride.

Dosage and Administration: Recommended Dosage Level:

Swine: Use soluble powder in the drinking water at a drug level of tetracycline hydrochloride per gallon to provide 10 mg/lb of body weight per day in divided doses. (Administer for 3-5 days.)

Calves: Use soluble powder in the drinking water at a drug level of tetracycline hydrochloride per gallon to provide 10 mg/lb of body weight per day in divided doses. (Administer for 3-5 days.)

Special directions for baby calves and baby pigs: Administer this product one hour before or two hours after feeding milk or milk replacers. Provide clean (unmedicated) drinking water at all times. Note: This product is to be administered twice a day in the drinking water of swine, calves and poultry. One-half of the recommended daily dosage level of antibiotic is to be consumed during each administration period, thus providing the drug in divided doses.

Chickens:

CRD Air Sac Disease: Use soluble powder in the drinking water at a drug level of 400-800 mg tetracycline hydrochloride per gallon per day.

Infectious Synovitis: Use soluble powder in the drinking water at a drug level of 200-400 mg tetracycline hydrochloride per gallon per day. (Administer for 7-14 days.)

Turkeys:

Infectious Synovitis: Use soluble powder in the drinking water at a drug level of 400 mg tetracycline hydrochloride per gallon per day.

Bluecomb: Use soluble powder in the drinking water at a drug level of tetracycline hydrochloride per gallon to provide 25 mg/lb of body weight per day in divided doses. (Administer for 7-14 days.)

Directions for Use: Medicate at the first clinical signs of disease or when experience indicates that the disease may be a problem.

Mixing Instructions - 6.4 oz will make:

100 gal containing 100 mg of tetracycline hydrochloride/gal

50 gal containing 200 mg of tetracycline hydrochloride/gal

25 gal containing 400 mg of tetracycline hydrochloride/gal

12.5 gal containing 800 mg of tetracycline hydrochloride/gal

Precaution(s): Store below 77°F (25°C).

Caution(s): Prepare fresh solutions at least once a day; solutions are not stable for more than 24 hours. Use as a sole source of tetracycline. Deliver the recommended dosage level in divided doses. Diagnosis should be reconsidered if improvement is not noticed within 3 days. The concentration of drug required in medicated water must be adequate to compensate for variations in the age and class of animals, feed consumption, and environmental temperature and humidity, each of which affects water consumption.

For animal use only.

Restricted drug. Use only as directed (CA).

Warning(s): Do not slaughter birds/swine for food within 4 days of treatment.

Calves: Do not slaughter animals for food within 5 days of treatment. A withdrawal period has not been established for the product in pre-ruminating calves. Do not use in calves to be processed for veal.

Not for use in turkeys or chickens producing eggs for human consumption. Do not use for more than 14 consecutive days.

Do not use for more than 5 consecutive days in calves.

Presentation: 6.4 oz (181 g) packets.

Compendium Code No.: 10220600

TET-SOL™ 324

Alpharma **Water Medication**

Tetracycline Hydrochloride Soluble Powder-Antibiotic

NADA No.: 065-140

Active Ingredient(s): Each pound contains 324 g of tetracycline hydrochloride activity.

The packet contains 810 g of tetracycline hydrochloride activity.

Indications: For use in drinking water for swine, calves, and poultry.

Chickens: Control of chronic respiratory disease (CRD air sac disease) caused by *Mycoplasma gallisepticum* and *Escherichia coli;* infectious synovitis caused by *Mycoplasma synoviae* sensitive to tetracycline hydrochloride.

Turkeys: Control of infectious synovitis caused by *Mycoplasma synoviae;* bluecomb (transmissible enteritis, corona viral enteritis) complicated by organisms sensitive to tetracycline hydrochloride.

Swine and Calves: Control and treatment of bacterial enteritis (scours) caused by *Escherichia coli;* bacterial pneumonia associated with *Actinobacillus pleuropneumoniae, Pasteurella* spp., *Klebsiella* spp., sensitive to tetracycline hydrochloride.

Dosage and Administration: Recommended Dosage Level:

Chickens:

CRD air sac disease: Use soluble powder in the drinking water at a drug level of 400-800 mg tetracycline hydrochloride per gallon per day.

Infectious synovitis: Use soluble powder in the drinking water at a drug level of 200-400 mg tetracycline hydrochloride per gallon per day.

Turkeys:

Infectious synovitis: Use soluble powder in the drinking water at a drug level of 400 mg tetracycline hydrochloride per gallon per day.

Bluecomb: Use soluble powder in the drinking water at a drug level of tetracycline hydrochloride per gallon to provide 25 mg/pound of body weight per day in divided doses.

Directions for Use: Administer for 7-14 days. Medicate at first clinical signs of disease or when experience indicates the disease may be a problem.

Swine and Calves: Use soluble powder in the drinking water at a drug level of tetracycline hydrochloride per gallon to provide 10 mg/pound of body weight per day in divided doses.

Directions for Use: Administer for 3-5 days.

Mixing Directions:

Turkeys, Swine and Cattle: 40 oz dissolved in 8000 mL (approximately 2.1 gallons) of warm water will provide a stock solution of 100 mg of tetracycline hydrochloride activity per mL. This stock solution, when metered at approximately 1 ounce/gallon, will provide drinking water containing 2957 mg of tetracycline hydrochloride activity per gallon for turkeys.

The contents of this packet are sufficient to deliver the recommended daily dosage levels as follows:

At 25 mg/pound of body weight — 32,400 total pounds of turkeys to be medicated in divided doses.

At 10 mg/pound of body weight — 81,000 total pounds of calves or swine to be medicated in divided doses.

Individual calf treatment — 5 mL (1 measuring teaspoonful) twice daily for each 100 pounds body weight administered as a drench or by dose syringe.

Chickens and Turkeys: To arrive at the recommended dosages, prepare a stock solution as follows:

200 mg/gallon — dissolve 1 packet (40 oz) in 121,120 mL warm water (32 gallons).

400 mg/gallon — dissolve 1 packet (40 oz) in 60,560 mL warm water (16 gallons).

800 mg/gallon — dissolve 1 packet (40 oz) in 30,280 mL warm water (8 gallons).

These stock solutions should then be metered into drinking water at approximately 1 ounce per gallon. At 200-800 mg/gallon this packet will medicate 1012 to 4050 gallons of drinking water.

Special Directions for Baby Calves and Baby Pigs: Administer this product 1 hour before or 2 hours after feeding milk or milk replacers. Provide clean (unmedicated) drinking water at all times.

Note: This product is to be administered twice a day in the drinking water of swine, calves and poultry. One half of the recommended daily dosage level of antibiotic is to be consumed during each administration period, thus providing the drug in divided doses.

Precaution(s): Store below 77°F (25°C).

Caution(s): Prepare fresh solutions at least once a day. Solutions are not stable for more than 24 hours. Use as a sole source of tetracycline. Deliver the recommended dosage level in divided doses. Diagnosis should be reconsidered if improvement is not noticed within 3 days. The concentration of drug required in medicated water must be adequate to compensate for variations in the age and class of animals, feed consumption, and environmental temperature and humidity, each of which affects water consumption.

For animal use only.

Restricted drug. Use only as directed (CA).

Warning(s): Do not slaughter birds for food within 4 days of treatment.

Not for use in turkeys or chickens producing eggs for human consumption. Do not use for more than 14 consecutive days.

Swine - Do not slaughter animals for food purposes within 4 days of treatment.

Calves - Do not slaughter animals for food purposes within 5 days of treatment.

A withdrawal period has not been established for this product in pre-ruminating calves. Do not use in calves to be processed for veal.

Do not use for more than 5 consecutive days (swine and calves).

Presentation: 40 oz (1134 g) packets.

TET-SOL is a trademark of Alpharma Inc.

Compendium Code No.: 10220611 AHF-053-0112

TGE CELL™

Novartis Animal Vaccines **Vaccine**

Transmissible Gastroenteritis Vaccine, Modified Live Virus

U.S. Vet. Lic. No.: 303

Composition: TGE CELL™ is a modified live virus vaccine propagated on a stable cell line. Contains penicillin, streptomycin and amphotericin B as preservatives.

Indications: For use in healthy swine as an aid in the prevention and control of diseases caused by transmissible gastroenteritis virus.

Dosage and Administration: Aseptically rehydrate the vaccine with the accompanying diluent. Vaccinate sows and gilts twice with a 2 mL dose. The first dose may be administered orally or intramuscularly at six (6) weeks prior to farrowing. The second dose must be administered intramuscularly four (4) weeks later. For chronic diarrhea caused by TGE, vaccinate piglets with two (2) oral doses (2 mL per dose) at seven (7) days and at three (3) weeks of age. Do not return the piglets to the sow until 30 minutes after vaccinating.

Oral vaccination for sows and gilts: After withholding feed overnight, rehydrate the vaccine with the accompanying diluent and add each 2 mL dose to 1 qt. of cold milk. Mix each 1 qt. dose with ground corn until thickened and feed immediately.

Precaution(s): Store in the dark at 35°-45°F (2°-7°C). Do not freeze. Do not use chemical sterilization as traces of chemicals may inactivate the vaccine. Use the entire contents without delay after rehydration. Burn the container and any unused contents.

Caution(s): Anaphylactic reactions may occur following the use of biological products. Symptomatic treatment: Epinephrine.

For veterinary use only.

Warning(s): Do not administer within 21 days prior to slaughter.

Presentation: 10 dose (20 mL) bottles.

Compendium Code No.: 11140512

TGE SHIELD™

Novartis Animal Vaccines **Vaccine**

Transmissible Gastroenteritis Vaccine, Killed Virus

U.S. Vet. Lic. No.: 303

Composition: TGE SHIELD™ is prepared from a highly antigenic strain of TGE propagated on a stable cell line. The vaccine is chemically inactivated and adjuvanted with Xtend V™. Contains penicillin, streptomycin, amphotericin B, and thimerosal as preservatives.

Indications: For use in healthy swine as an aid in the prevention and control of disease caused by transmissible gastroenteritis virus.

Dosage and Administration: Shake well before using. Administer three (3) doses (2 mL/dose) intramuscularly to sows or gilts at 11, 6, and 2 weeks prior to farrowing and at six (6) and two (2) weeks prior to each subsequent farrowing.

Precaution(s): Store in the dark at 35°-45°F (2°-7°C). Do not freeze. Use the entire contents when first opened.

Caution(s): Anaphylactic reactions may occur following the use of the product. Symptomatic treatment: Epinephrine.

Warning(s): Do not vaccinate within 60 days prior to slaughter.

Discussion: Transmissible gastroenteritis (TGE) is a highly contagious, enteric disease of swine characterized by vomiting, severe diarrhea, and high mortality (often 100%) in piglets under two weeks of age. Although swine of all ages are susceptible to this viral infection, the mortality in swine over five weeks of age is very low. The disease is most frequently seen at farrowing time and commonly goes undiagnosed in growing, finishing or adult swine because of the mild clinical signs, which usually consist only of loss of appetite and diarrhea of a few days duration. However, lactating sows may become very sick demonstrating decreased appetite, fever, vomiting, diarrhea and a reduction of milk flow. Because suckling piglets passively acquire immunity from the sow's milk, any condition which arrests or reduces milk production will severely impair this protective immunity along with the general overall health of her piglets. Losses in the farrowing house can be devastating when baby pigs are affected. TGE can also be the cause of unresponsive bacterial scours in endemic herds, complicating existing *E. coli* scours in both baby and weaned pigs.

Trial Data: The efficacy of TGE SHIELD™ has been demonstrated by vaccination-challenge studies. Gilts were vaccinated with three doses (2 mL/dose) of vaccine administered intramuscularly. The three doses were given approximately four weeks apart and timed so that the last dose was administered at two weeks before farrowing. Results of the vaccination-challenge study are summarized in the following:

Test Group	% Mortality Post Challenge	SN Titer at Farrowing
Controls	34.0%	3.2
Vaccinates	5.5%	65.9

A six-fold increase in mortality from piglets born to nonvaccinated control gilts compared to piglets born to vaccinated gilts.

TGE SHIELD™ elicited a 20-fold increase in titer levels at farrowing compared to controls.

Presentation: Available in 50 dose (100 mL) bottles.

Compendium Code No.: 11140523

T

THERABLOAT® DRENCH CONCENTRATE

Pfizer Animal Health **Bloat Preparation**

poloxalene

NADA No.: 039-729

Active Ingredient(s): Each fl oz (approx. 30 mL) contains 25 grams of poloxalene.

Indications: THERABLOAT® Drench Concentrate will relieve legume bloat in cattle within minutes when used as directed. For best results administer at the earliest sign of bloat. If bloat has progressed in its severity to the degree that the animal is down, other means of treatment also are recommended (rumenotomy - rumen puncture). For oral use only—not for injection. May be used in lactating animals.

Dosage and Administration: For animals up to 500 lb, use 1 fl oz of Drench Concentrate. For animals over 500 lb, use 2 fl oz of Drench Concentrate.

Directions for Preparing Drench: Add the proper amount of concentrate to 1 pint of water. Mix well and administer using a drenching bottle. If a stomach tube is to be used, add concentrate to 1 gallon of water.

Precaution(s): Store at controlled room temperature 15°-30°C (59°-86°F).

Caution(s): Keep out of reach of children.

For animal use only. Restricted drug (California)—Use only as directed.

For veterinary use only. Not for human use.

Presentation: 2 fl oz (59.1 mL) plastic bottle.

Compendium Code No.: 36900751 85-8620-08

THERADERM® 2500

Westfalia•Surge **Teat Dip**

Active Ingredient(s): Nonylphenoxypoly (ethyleneoxy) ethanol iodine complex (provides 0.25% of titratable iodine). Contains 5% glycerin in a triple emollient system.

Indications: For use as a sanitizing teat dip for dairy cattle.

Dosage and Administration: Use at full strength. Do not dilute.

Pre dipping: Before milking, dip or spray each teat with THERADERM® 2500. After 15 to 30 seconds, dry each teat thoroughly with a single service paper towel. If the udder and teats are heavily soiled, wash with a sanitizing solution and dry before the application of THERADERM® 2500.

Post dipping: Immediately after milking, dip or spray each teat with THERADERM® 2500. Allow the teats to air dry.

If a common teat dip cup is used for application, a fresh solution should always be used at each milking. The teat dip cup should be emptied, cleaned and rinsed with potable water after each milking session or when the cup becomes contaminated during milking. Do not pour the remaining solution from the dip cup back into the original container.

Precaution(s): Store THERADERM® 2500 in a cool, dry place. Keep from freezing. If frozen, thaw completely and mix well prior to use. Keep containers closed to prevent contamination of the teat dip.

Caution(s): Danger. Keep out of the reach of children. Shake well before using. Can cause eye damage. Protect the eyes when handling. Do not get in the eyes or on clothing. Harmful if swallowed. Avoid contamination of food.

First Aid:

Eyes: In case of contact with the eyes, flush immediately with plenty of water for at least 15 minutes. Call a physician.

Internal: Do not take internally. If swallowed, promptly drink two to three glasses of milk (if unavailable, drink water). Avoid alcohol. Call a physician.

Handling Recommendations:

1. Always read the label directions completely before using the product.
2. Always exercise caution when handling any chemicals.
3. Avoid contact with the eyes, skin and clothing.
4. Never dispense any chemical product from its original container into another container for storage or resale.
5. Never mix two or more products together. Mixing of products could result in the release of toxic gases and/or render the product ineffective for the recommended use application.
6. Always use the product in a ventilated area. Avoid inhaling vapors or fumes.
7. Always use the product according to the recommendations for a particular application.
8. Never exceed the recommended usage without consulting trained personnel.

Presentation: Contact the company for container sizes available.

Compendium Code No.: 10020151

THERATEC™

Westfalia•Surge **Teat Dip**

Active Ingredient(s): Contains:

Nonylphenoxypoly (ethyleneoxy) ethanol iodine complex (provides 0.50% titratable iodine) 8.75%

Contains lanolin and glycerin in a stable pH aqueous base.

Indications: This product has been tested under farm conditions of experimental exposure to known mastitis causing organisms and has been proven effective in reducing new infections of mastitis.

Dosage and Administration:

Predipping: Before milking, dip or spray each teat with THERATEC™. After 15 to 30 seconds, dry each teat thoroughly with a single service paper towel. If the udder and teats are heavily soiled, wash with a sanitizing solution and dry before application of THERATEC™.

THERATEC™ has been tested under farm conditions and will not result in excess residues in milk when properly applied and dried prior to milking.

Postdipping: Immediately after milking, dip or spray each teat with THERATEC™. Allow teats to air dry.

Precaution(s): General Chemical Warnings:

Always read label directions completely before using product. Store THERATEC™ in cool, dry place. Keep from freezing. If frozen, thaw completely and mix well prior to use. Keep containers closed to prevent contamination of teat dip.

If a common teat dip cup is used for application, a fresh solution should always be used at each milking. The teat dip cut should be emptied, cleaned and rinsed with potable water after each milking session or when cup becomes contaminated during milking. Do not pour remaining solution from dip cup back into the original container.

Caution(s): Danger - Keep out of the reach of children. Can cause eye damage. Protect eyes when handling. Do not get in eyes or on clothing. Harmful if swallowed. Avoid contamination of food.

First Aid:

Eyes: In case of contact with eyes, flush immediately with plenty of water for at least 15 minutes. Call a physician.

Internal: Do not take internally. If swallowed, promptly drink a large quantity of milk, egg whites, gelatin solution. If these are not available, drink large quantities of water. Avoid alcohol. Call a physician.

Presentation: Contact the company for container sizes available.

* THERATEC is a trademark of Westfalia•Surge, Inc.

Compendium Code No.: 10020161

THERATEC® PLUS

Westfalia•Surge **Teat Dip**

Pre & Post Sanitizing Teat Dip with Added Emollient

Active Ingredient(s): Nonylphenoxypoly (ethyleneoxy) ethanol iodine complex (provides 0.5% of titratable iodine wt./wt.).

Contains 5% glycerin in a triple emollient system.

Indications: Pre and post sanitizing teat dip with added emollient.

Directions for Use:

Pre Dipping: Before milking, dip or spray each teat with THERATEC® Plus. After 15 to 30 seconds, dry each teat thoroughly with a single service paper towel. If the udder and teats are heavily soiled, wash with a sanitizing solution and dry before application of THERATEC® Plus.

Post Dipping: Immediately after milking, dip or spray each teat with THERATEC® Plus. Allow teats to air dry.

Precaution(s): Store this product in a cool, dry place. If frozen, thaw completely and mix well prior to use. Keep containers closed to prevent contamination of this product.

Warning(s): Danger: Keep out of reach of children.

Can cause eye damage.

Protect eyes when handling. Do not get in eyes or on clothing. Harmful if swallowed. Avoid contamination of food.

General Chemical Warnings:

Always read label directions completely before using product.

If a common teat dip cup is used for application, a fresh solution should always be used at each milking. The teat dip cup should be emptied, cleaned and rinsed with potable water after each milking session or when cup becomes contaminated during milking. Do not pour remaining solution from dip cup back into original container.

First Aid:

Eyes: In case of contact with eyes, flush immediately with plenty of water for at least 15 minutes. Call a physician.

Internal: If swallowed, promptly rinse mouth then give a large quantity of milk or water. Avoid alcohol. Contact a physician immediately. Never give anything by mouth to an unconscious person.

Refer to Material Safety Data Sheet.

Presentation: Contact the company for container sizes available.

THERATEC® is a Registered Trademark of Westfalia•Surge, Inc.

Compendium Code No.: 10020171

THERATRATE™

Westfalia•Surge **Teat Dip**

Iodine Teat Dip Concentrate

Active Ingredient(s):

Titratable Iodine 4.5%

Inert Ingredients*: 95.5%

*Includes glycerin as emollient.

Indications: Iodine teat dip concentrate.

Directions for Use:

Directions for Dilution: THERATRATE™ is formulated to be mixed with clean, potable water and when diluted correctly, will yield a 0.5% iodine teat dip product.

Dilution: 1 part THERATRATE™ with 9 parts water by volume.

Mixing Directions: Fill an empty, clean 55 gallon container with 40 gallons (334 lbs) of clean, potable water. Carefully weigh out 49 lbs of THERATRATE™ and pour into a 5 gallon container. Carefully pour the contents (49 lbs) of THERATRATE™ into the 55 gallon container. Now fill the empty container with 5 gallons of clear, potable water and swirl while filling. Pour that 5 gallons (42 lbs) of water/iodine concentrate mixture into the 55 gallon drum and mix thoroughly. The entire mixing process will net 50 gallons of ready-to-use product.

Note: If you are mixing product on a scale, measure the weight of the empty drum, then add water and concentrate according to weights listed above.

If frozen, thaw completely and mix well before using.

Caution(s): Do not use as is. This is a concentrate. Product must be diluted.

Warning(s): Danger: Keep out of reach of children. Can cause eye damage. May cause skin irritation. Vapors may be irritating to eyes. Protect eyes when handling. Do not get in eyes, on skin or on clothing. Harmful if swallowed. Avoid contamination of food.

General Chemical Warnings:

Always read label directions completely before using product.

Always exercise caution when handling any chemicals.

Avoid contact with eyes, skin and clothing.

Always use product in a ventilated area. Avoid inhaling vapors or fumes.

Never mix two or more products together. Mixing of products could result in release of toxic gases and/or render product ineffective for recommended use application.

Always use product according to recommendations for particular application.

Never exceed recommended usage without consulting trained personnel.

First Aid:

Eyes: In case of contact with eyes, flush immediately with plenty of water for at least 15 minutes. Call a physician.

External: Wash thoroughly. If irritation develops, contact a physician.

Internal: Do not take internally. If swallowed, rinse mouth then give promptly 2-3 glasses of milk (if unavailable, give water). Avoid alcohol. Call a physician. Never give anything by mouth to an unconscious person.

Refer to Material Safety Data Sheet.

Presentation: Contact the company for container sizes available.

Compendium Code No.: 10020181

THEREVAC®-SB

King Animal Health — Enema

Mini Enema-Stool Softener Evacuant

Active Ingredient(s): Each disposable gelatin ampule contains:

Docusate Sodium . . . . . 283 mg

Medicinal soft soap base of Polyethylene Glycol and Glycerine.

Indications: For relief of occasional constipation in dogs and cats. This product usually produces a bowel movement in 2 to 15 minutes.

Dosage and Administration: Administer rectally, as recommended by a veterinarian.

Non-irritating.

Precaution(s): Store at room temperature 15°-30°C (59°-86°F), below 50% relative humidity and avoid freezing.

Warning(s): Keep this and all drugs out of the reach of children. In case of accidental ingestion or overdose, seek professional assistance or contact a poison control center.

Presentation: Packs of five ampules.

Compendium Code No.: 11320061

THIA-DEX

Neogen — Thiamine

Thiamine B_1

Active Ingredient(s): Contains: Thiamine Hydrochloride (B_1), 500 mg per oz (approx. 83 mg per teaspoon), Dextrose, Flavor, Artificial Coloring and Sodium Saccharin.

Indications:

Horses: For the prevention and treatment of B_1 deficiencies in horses where horses are being fed poor-quality hay and grain.

Dogs: For the prevention and treatment of B_1 deficiencies in dogs where dogs are maintained on a diet deficient in B_1.

Dosage and Administration:

Horses: ½ to 1 ounce daily in feed.

Dogs: ½ to 2 teaspoons daily in feed or as directed by veterinarian.

Caution(s): For veterinary use only.

Warning(s): Keep out of the reach of children.

Presentation: 4 lb (1.814 kg) (NDC: 59051-9178-6) and 20 lb (9.072 kg) (NDC: 59051-9179-0).

Compendium Code No.: 14910441 — L431-0501 / L425-0301

THIAMINE HYDROCHLORIDE ℞

Vet Tek — Thiamine

200 mg/mL-Sterile Solution

Active Ingredient(s): Composition: Each mL of sterile aqueous solution contains:

Thiamine HCl . . . . . 200 mg
Disodium Edetate 0.01%
Benzyl Alcohol 1.5%
Water for Injection . . . . . q.s.

Indications: For the treatment of Vitamin B_1 deficiencies.

Dosage and Administration: To be determined by the veterinarian. For intramuscular use.

Precaution(s): Store between 15°C and 30°C (59°F-86°F). Do not expose to excessive heat.

Caution(s): Federal law restricts this drug to use by or on the order of a licensed veterinarian.

Anaphylactogenesis to parenteral Thiamine HCl has been reported. Administer slowly with caution in doses over 500 mg.

For animal use only.

Warning(s): Keep out of reach of children.

Presentation: 100 mL bottles (NDC 60270-043-10).

Manufactured by: Phoenix Scientific, Inc., St. Joseph, MO 64506.

Compendium Code No.: 14200201 — Iss. 7-95

THIAMINE HYDROCHLORIDE 200 MG ℞

Neogen — Thiamine

Sterile Solution

Active Ingredient(s): Each mL contains:

Thiamine Hydrochloride . . . . . 200 mg
Disodium Edetate . . . . . 0.01% w/v
Benzyl Alcohol (as preservative) . . . . . 1.5% v/v
Water for injection . . . . . q.s.

pH adjusted with Hydrochloric acid or Sodium Hydroxide.

Indications: For use as a supplemental source of thiamine in dogs, cats and horses.

Dosage and Administration: For intravenous or intramuscular use in dogs, cats and horses. Dosage may be repeated daily as needed.

Horses: 0.25 mL per 100 lbs body weight.

Dogs: 0.08 mL per 10 lbs up to 0.25 mL max.

Cats: 0.04 mL per 5 lbs up to 0.1 mL max.

Precaution(s): Store at controlled room temperature between 15°-30°C (59°-86°F).

Caution(s): Federal law restricts this drug to use by or on the order of a licensed veterinarian.

Anaphylactogenesis to parenteral thiamine has occurred. Administer slowly and with caution in doses over 0.25 mL (50 mg).

For animal use only.

Warning(s): Keep out of reach of children.

Presentation: 12 x 100 mL amber multi-dose vials per carton (NDC: 59051-9082-5).

Manufactured by: Omega Laboratories, Montreal, Quebec H2M 3E4.

Compendium Code No.: 14910142 — L569-0501

THIAMINE HYDROCHLORIDE 500 MG ℞

Neogen — Thiamine

Sterile Solution

Active Ingredient(s): Each mL contains:

Thiamine Hydrochloride . . . . . 500 mg
Disodium Edetate . . . . . 0.01% w/v
Benzyl Alcohol (as preservative) . . . . . 1.5% v/v
Water for Injection . . . . . q.s.

pH adjusted with Hydrochloric acid or Sodium Hydroxide.

Indications: For use as a supplemental source of thiamine in dogs, cats and horses.

Dosage and Administration: For intravenous or intramuscular use in horses, dogs and cats as determined by a veterinarian.

Precaution(s): Store at controlled room temperature between 15°-30°C (59°-86°F).

Caution(s): Federal law restricts this drug to use by or on the order of a licensed veterinarian.

Anaphylactogenesis to parenteral thiamine has occurred. Administer slowly and with caution in doses over 0.10 mL (50 mg).

For animal use only.

Warning(s): Keep out of reach of children.

Presentation: 12 x 100 mL amber multi-dose vials per carton (NDC: 59051-9083-5).

Manufactured by: Omega Laboratories, Montreal, Quebec H3M 3E4.

Compendium Code No.: 14910152 — 0201

THIAMINE HYDROCHLORIDE INJECTION ℞

Butler — Thiamine

Active Ingredient(s): Each mL contains:

Thiamine HCl . . . . . 500 mg
Disodium edetate 0.01%
Benzyl alcohol 1.5%
Water for injection . . . . . q.s.

Indications: For the treatment of vitamin B_1 deficiencies.

Dosage and Administration: To be determined by the veterinarian. For intramuscular use.

Precaution(s): Do not expose to excessive heat.

Caution(s): Federal law restricts this drug to use by or on the order of a licensed veterinarian.

For animal use only. For veterinary use only.

Anaphylactic reactions to parenteral thiamine HCl have been reported. Administer slowly and with caution in doses over 500 mg.

Presentation: 100 mL sterile multiple dose vials.

Compendium Code No.: 10821760

THIAMINE HYDROCHLORIDE INJECTION ℞

Phoenix Pharmaceutical — Thiamine

200 mg/mL

Active Ingredient(s): Composition: Each mL of sterile aqueous solution contains:

Thiamine HCl . . . . . 200 mg
Disodium Edetate 0.01%
Benzyl Alcohol 1.5%
Water for Injection . . . . . q.s.

Indications: For the treatment of Vitamin B_1 deficiencies.

Dosage and Administration: To be determined by a veterinarian. For intramuscular use.

Precaution(s): Store between 15°C and 30°C (59°F-86°F). Do not expose to excessive heat.

Caution(s): Federal law restricts this drug to use by or on the order of a licensed veterinarian.

Anaphylactogenesis to parenteral Thiamine HCl has been reported. Administer slowly with caution in doses over 500 mg.

For animal use only.

Warning(s): Keep out of reach of children.

Presentation: 100 mL sterile multiple dose vials (NDC 57319-095-05).

Manufactured by: Phoenix Scientific, Inc.

Compendium Code No.: 12560821 — Rev. 6-01

THIAMINE HYDROCHLORIDE INJECTION ℞

Vedco — Thiamine

Active Ingredient(s): Each mL contains:

Vitamin B_1, U.S.P. (thiamine HCl) . . . . . 200 mg or 500 mg
Monothioglycerol . . . . . 4 mg
Preservatives:
Methylparaben . . . . . 0.18% w/v
Proplyparaben . . . . . 0.02% w/v

Indications: For the treatment of vitamin B_1 deficiencies.

Dosage and Administration:

Dogs and Cats: 0.1 to 0.4 mL.

Cattle, Horses, Sheep and Swine: 0.4 to 1.0 mL per 100 lbs. of body weight intramuscularly. Repeat once a day as indicated.

Precaution(s): Store at 36-59°F (2-15°C).

Caution(s): Federal law restricts this drug to use by or on the order of a licensed veterinarian.

Keep out of the reach of children. Not for human use.

Sensitivity to parenterally administered thiamine hydrochloride has been reported. Administer slowly and with caution doses over 50 mg. Do not use if precipitated.

Presentation: Available in 100 mL multiple dose vials.

Compendium Code No.: 10941970

THIAMINE HYDROCHLORIDE SOLUTION ℞

Phoenix Pharmaceutical — Thiamine

500 mg/mL-Sterile Solution

Active Ingredient(s): Each mL contains:

Thiamine Hydrochloride . . . . . 500 mg
Disodium Edetate . . . . . 0.01% w/v
Benzyl Alcohol (as preservative) . . . . . 1.5% v/v
Water for Injection . . . . . q.s.

The pH is adjusted with Hydrochloric acid or Sodium Hydroxide.

Indications: For use as a supplemental source of thiamine in dogs, cats and horses.

Dosage and Administration: For intravenous or intramuscular use as determined by the veterinarian.

Precaution(s): Store at room temperature 15°-30°C (59°-86°F).

Caution(s): Federal law restricts this drug to use by or on the order of a licensed veterinarian.

Anaphylactogenesis to parenteral thiamine has occurred. Administer slowly and with caution in doses over 0.10 mL (50 mg).

For animal use only.

Warning(s): Keep out of reach of children.

Presentation: 100 mL bottles (NDC 57319-359-05).

Compendium Code No.: 12561110 — 1099

THRUSH TREATMENT

First Priority **Hoof Product**

Active Ingredient(s): Parachlorometaxylenol, propylene glycol and aloe vera in a specially prepared base.

Indications: Helps stop thrush before it starts. THRUSH TREATMENT is a unique blend of Aloe Vera and natural protein complexes which promote a healthy, conditioned hoof and is safe for every-day use. Easy to apply and will not stain or dry out hooves. Safe for use in all racing, shows and events.

Dosage and Administration: Clean hoof thoroughly, removing all debris. Apply a generous amount of THRUSH TREATMENT to the hoof daily. If thrush has already developed, use THRUSH TREATMENT for quick and effective relief.

Precaution(s): Store at controlled room temperature between 32°F and 90°F.

Caution(s): In case of prolonged contact with skin, flush with warm water. Avoid contact with eyes. If contact occurs, flush with warm water for 5 minutes and seek medical attention immediately.

Warning(s): Do not use on animals intended for food.

For animal use only. Keep out of reach of children.

Presentation: 16 fl oz (473 mL) with trigger sprayer.

Compendium Code No.: 11390711

THRUSH-XX™

Farnam **Hoof Product**

(Copper Naphthenate) Water-Resistant Protection Without Bandaging

Active Ingredient(s):

Copper naphthenate 37.5%
Inert Ingredients: 62.5%
Total 100.0%

Indications: As an aid in the treatment of thrush in horses and ponies due to organisms susceptible to copper naphthenate. Thrush is a disease of horses' hoofs characterized by a thick, black, foul-smelling discharge.

Dosage and Administration: Shake well before using.

Clean the hoof thoroughly by removing debris and necrotic material prior to application of THRUSH-XX™. A narrow paint brush (about 1" in diameter) may be used to assure thorough coverage. Apply THRUSH-XX™ daily.

Use THRUSH-XX™ as follows:

1. Remove cap.
2. With sharp instrument, punch a small hole in metal seal.
3. Replace with applicator cap; screw it down tightly.
4. Loosen nozzle a small amount.
5. Invert bottle and squeeze gently, using nozzle to regulate the flow of liquid.

Note: THRUSH-XX™ is easily removed from hands, clothing, and surfaces with a light grade fuel oil or any type of lighter fluid.

Precaution(s): Do not use, pour, spill, or store near heat or open flame.

Caution(s): For veterinary use only. Do not contaminate feed. Avoid contact around eyes. For use on horses and ponies only. Do not allow excess THRUSH-XX™ to run off and contact hair. Contact may result in hair loss.

Warning(s): This drug is not to be administered to horses that are to be slaughtered for use as food. Harmful if swallowed. For external use only.

Not for human use. Keep out of reach of children.

Presentation: 16 fl oz (473 mL).

Compendium Code No.: 10000390

THUJA-ZINC OXIDE

Butler **Topical Wound Dressing**

Active Ingredient(s): Contains:

Oil thuja 10.0%
Zinc oxide 10.0%

In a suitable base.

Indications: To be used for external application to superficial wounds and abrasions of horses.

Dosage and Administration: Cleanse the area and apply freely to the affected parts.

Precaution(s): Store at a controlled room temperature between 15° and 30°C (59°-86°F).

Caution(s): In the case of deep or puncture wounds or burns, consult a veterinarian. If redness, irritation, or swelling persists or increases, discontinue use of the product and consult a veterinarian.

For veterinary use only.

Keep out of the reach of children.

Warning(s): Not for use on animals intended for human consumption.

Presentation: 16 oz. (1 lb.) containers.

Compendium Code No.: 10821770

THUJA-ZINC OXIDE

Phoenix Pharmaceutical **Topical Wound Dressing**

Astringent-Antiseptic-Counterirritant-Topical Ointment

Active Ingredient(s): Composition:

Zinc Oxide .... 10% w/w

In a petrolatum and lanolin base containing oil of thuja and scarlet oil.

Indications: A protective astringent, antiseptic, counterirritant ointment for topical application to aid in the management of superficial wounds and abrasions of horses.

Dosage and Administration: Thoroughly cleanse and dry area of skin to be treated. Apply THUJA-ZINC OXIDE Ointment directly on the wound with a spatula or place on a piece of clean gauze.

Precaution(s): Store at a controlled room temperature, between 15° and 30°C (59°-86°F). Keep tightly closed when not in use.

Caution(s): Do not apply to irritated skin or if excessive irritation develops. Avoid getting into eyes or mucous membranes. In case of deep or puncture wounds or serious burns, consult a veterinarian. If redness, irritation, or swelling persists or increases, discontinue use and consult a veterinarian.

For animal use only.

Warning(s): Not for use on animals intended for food.

Keep out of reach of children.

Presentation: 16 oz. (1 lb) jars (NDC 57319-213-27).

Compendium Code No.: 12560831 Rev. 1-00

THUJA-ZINC OXIDE

Vedco **Topical Wound Dressing**

NDC No.: 50989-159-26

Active Ingredient(s):

Zinc oxide .... 10% w/w

In a petrolatum and lanolin ointment base containing oil of thuja and scarlet oil.

Indications: A protective astringent, antiseptic, counterirritant ointment for topical application to aid in the management of superficial wounds and abrasions of horses.

Dosage and Administration: Thoroughly cleanse and dry the area of the skin to be treated. Apply THUJA-ZINC OXIDE Ointment directly onto the wound with a spatula or place on a piece of gauze.

Precaution(s): Store at a controlled room temperature between 15° and 30°C (59°-86°F).

Keep the jar tightly closed when not in use.

Caution(s): Do not apply to irritated skin or if excessive irritation develops. Avoid getting into the eyes or on mucous membranes. In case of deep or puncture wounds or serious burns, consult a veterinarian. If redness, irritation, or swelling persists or increases, discontinue use and consult a veterinarian.

For animal use only.

Keep out of the reach of children.

Warning(s): Not for use on animals intended for food.

Presentation: 16 oz. (1 lb.) jars.

Compendium Code No.: 10941980

THYROID POWDER™

Eudaemonic **Thyroid Therapy**

Active Ingredient(s): THYROID POWDER™ is U.S.P. grade. It contains 15 grains of USP THYROID POWDER™ per 10.5 g (one large measure).

Eudaemonic thyroid has all of the naturally occurring thyroid hormones which include not less than 90% and not more than 110% of both levethyroxine (T4) and liothyronine (T3).

Indications: For use in horses as a supplemental source of thyroid.

Dosage and Administration: Horses: The usual starting dose is 10.5 g (1 large measure) a day in feed. The dose may need to be adjusted after 60 to 90 days depending upon the clinical response. When the clinical response is not sufficient, repeat the laboratory profile.

Presentation: 5 oz., 1 lb. (453.6 g), 2.31 lb. (1.05 kg) and 10 lb. (4.53 kg) containers.

Compendium Code No.: 14040020

THYRO-L® ℞

Vet-A-Mix **Thyroid Therapy**

Levothyroxine sodium powder supplement for horses

Active Ingredient(s): Each pound (453.6 g) contains:

Levothyroxine Sodium U.S.P. .... 0.22% (1.0 g)

One level teaspoonful contains approximately 12 mg of T-4.

One level tablespoonful contains approximately 36 mg of T-4.

Indications: For use in horses for correction of conditions associated with low circulating thyroid hormone (hypothyroidism).

Dosage and Administration: Dosage: The suggested initial dose is 0.5 to 3.0 mg levothyroxine sodium (T-4) per 100 pounds of body weight (1 to 6 mg per 100 kg) once per day or in divided doses. Response to the administration of THYRO-L® should be evaluated clinically until an adequate maintenance dose is established. In most horses, this is usually in the range of 6 to 36 mg total daily dose of T-4. Serum T-3 and T-4 values can vary greatly among individual horses on thyroid supplementation. Dosages should be individualized and animals should be monitored daily for clinical signs of hyperthyroidism or hypersensitivity.

Administration: THYRO-L® can be administered by mixing the daily dose in the concentrate or by top dressing on grain, preferably rolled or ground. To facilitate the proper adhesion of THYRO-L® to the ration, slightly moisten the grain with water or liquid supplement.

Precaution(s): Store at room temperature and protect from light. Avoid excessive heat (104°F).

Caution(s): Federal law restricts this drug to use by or on the order of a licensed veterinarian.

Administer with caution to animals with clinically significant heart disease, hypertension or other complications for which a sharply increased metabolic rate might prove hazardous. Use in pregnant mares has not been evaluated.

Warning(s): Keep out of the reach of children.

Presentation: 1 lb. (453.6 g) bottles and 10 lb. pails.

Compendium Code No.: 10500291 0800

THYROSYN TABLETS ℞

Vedco **Thyroid Therapy**

Active Ingredient(s): Each tablet contains:

Levothyroxine sodium .... 0.1 mg (yellow)
Levothyroxine sodium .... 0.2 mg (red)
Levothyroxine sodium .... 0.3 mg (green)
Levothyroxine sodium .... 0.4 mg (maroon)
Levothyroxine sodium .... 0.5 mg (white)
Levothyroxine sodium .... 0.6 mg (purple)
Levothyroxine sodium .... 0.7 mg (orange)
Levothyroxine sodium .... 0.8 mg (blue)

Indications: Provides thyroid replacement therapy in all conditions of inadequate production of thyroid hormone (hypothyroidism) in dogs.

Dosage and Administration: The initial recommended daily dose is 0.1 mg/10 lbs. of body weight. Dosage is then adjusted by monitoring the T-4 blood levels of the dog every four (4) weeks until an adequate maintenance dose is established.

Precaution(s): Protect from light and do not store above 104°F (40°C).

Caution(s): Federal (USA) law restricts this drug to use by or on the order of a licensed veterinarian.

Administer with caution to animals with primary hypertension, euthyroidsim and clinically diagnosed heart disease. Use in pregnant bitches has not been evaluated.

Warning(s): Keep out of reach of children.

Presentation: Bottles of 180 and 1,000 tablets.

Compendium Code No.: 10941991

THYRO-TABS® ℞

Vet-A-Mix **Thyroid Therapy**

(Levothyroxine sodium, USP)

Active Ingredient(s): THYRO-TABS® contain either 0.1 mg, 0.2 mg, 0.3 mg, 0.4 mg, 0.5 mg, 0.6 mg, 0.7 mg or 0.8 mg of levothyroxine sodium, USP per caplet.

Indications: For use in dogs for correction of conditions associated with low circulating thyroid hormone (hypothyroidism).

Pharmacology: Description: Each THYRO-TABS® Caplet contains synthetic crystalline levothyroxine sodium, USP.

The structural formula for levothyroxine sodium is:

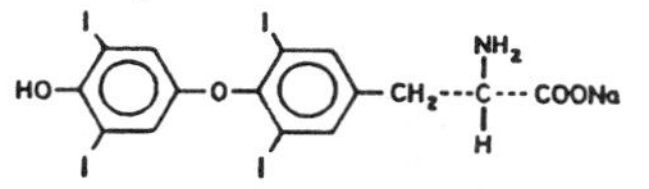

Mode of actions: Levothyroxine sodium provided by THYRO-TABS® Caplets cannot be distinguished from L-thyroxine endogenously secreted by the thyroid gland. L-thyroxine is a naturally circulating thyroid hormone released by the thyroid gland. The primary regulator of thyroid function is thyroid stimulating hormone (TSH) which is synthesized and secreted by the pars distalis of the adenohypophysis (anterior pituitary). The mediator from the hypothalamus which exerts a continuous influence over the pituitary release of TSH is thyrotropin-releasing hormone (TRH). Thyroid hormones influence virtually every body organ, either by their effect on growth and development or by the hormones' metabolic effects.

Dosage and Administration:

Dosages: The initial recommended daily dose is 0.1 to 0.2 mg/10 pounds (4.5 kg) body weight in single or divided doses. Dosage is then adjusted by monitoring the T-4 blood levels of the dog every four weeks until an adequate maintenance dose is established. The usual daily maintenance dose is 0.1 mg/10 lb (4.5 kg). A maximum of 0.8 to 1.0 mg total daily dose will be sufficient in most dogs over 80 pounds in body weight.

Administration: THYRO-TABS® Caplets may be administered orally or placed in the food.

Contraindication(s): Levothyroxine sodium therapy is contraindicated in thyrotoxicosis, acute myocardial infarction, and uncorrected adrenal insufficiency. Other conditions in which the use of L-thyroxine replacement therapy may be contraindicated or should be instituted with caution include primary hypertension, euthyroidism, and pregnancy.

Precaution(s): Storage: Store at controlled room temperature: 15°-30°C (59°-86°F) and protect from light.

Caution(s): Federal law restricts this drug to use by or on the order of a licensed veterinarian.

The clinical effects of levothyroxine sodium therapy are slow in being manifested. Overdosage of any thyroid drug may produce the signs and symptoms of thyrotoxicosis including, but not limited to: polydypsia, polyuria, polyphagia, reduced heat tolerance and hyperactivity or personality change. THYRO-TABS® 0.1 mg and 0.7 mg caplets contain FD&C Yellow #5 (tartrazine) which has been associated with allergic-type reactions (including bronchial asthma) in susceptible humans. It is unknown whether such a reaction could also occur in other animals.

Warning(s): The administration of levothyroxine sodium to dogs to be used for breeding purposes or in pregnant bitches has not been evaluated. There is evidence to suggest that administration to pregnant bitches may in some instances affect the normal development of the thyroid gland in the unborn pups.

Adverse Reactions: There are no specific adverse reactions associated with levothyroxine sodium administration at the recommended dosages. Overdosage will result in the signs of thyrotoxicosis listed above under cautions.

Discussion: Low serum circulating L-thyroxine (T-4) concentrations, coupled with clinical signs, are suggestive of hypothyroidism. Based on studies conducted by Vet-A-Mix and in cooperation with two commercial laboratories, the following parameters for T-4 concentrations in canine serum have been established:

Normal (euthyroid) - 18 to 32 ng/mL (1 .8 to 3.2 µg/dL)

Possible hypothyroid - 10 to 18 ng/mL (1 .0 to 1.8 µg/dL)

Hypothyroid - less than 10 ng/mL (< 1.0 µg/dL) The animal should be showing some clinical signs associated with hypothyroidism.

A resting serum T-4 concentration of 18 ng/mL or above signifies that hypothyroidism is unlikely in dogs. Normally, the greater the T-4 concentration exceeds this value, the less likely that a dog is hypothyroid. A dog with a T-4 value below 18 ng/mL that is exhibiting signs of hypothyroidism should be considered for levothyroxine replacement therapy.

T-4 measurements should be made at 30 day intervals to establish the proper maintenance dose during a therapeutic trial with THYRO-TABS® Caplets. A critical assessment of improvement in or resolution of clinical signs should be made after 12 weeks of levothyroxine sodium therapy. Further confirmation of the diagnosis could include withdrawal of the levothyroxine sodium therapy. A recurrence of clinical signs following cessation of therapy further supports the diagnosis. Correct diagnosis of hypothyroidism is important, since such a diagnosis normally commits an animal to life-long supplemental L-thyroxine replacement therapy. The principal objective of levothyroxine sodium administration is to achieve and maintain normal metabolism in the patient by providing an exogenous supply of synthetic L-thyroxine in amounts sufficient to maintain levels of the hormone within the animal's normal physiologic range. Animal adaptation may necessitate regular monitoring of serum T-4 concentrations during the first several months of treatment to establish proper maintenance doses.

The TSH Response Test may be used to provide a definitive diagnosis in dogs with borderline resting serum T-4 values. The TSH dose, post-dose sampling times, and interpretation of pre- and post-TSH injection responses depend somewhat on the reference laboratory used.

Occurrence of canine hypothyroidism: Hypothyroidism usually occurs in middle-aged and older dogs although the condition will sometimes be seen in younger dogs of the larger breeds. Neutered animals of either sex are also frequently affected, regardless of age. The condition is usually primary, failure of the thyroid gland, because of lymphocytic thyroiditis or other loss of follicular epithelium and resulting atrophy of the gland. Secondary hypothyroidism is relatively rare and usually due to a destructive pituitary tumor.

Clinical signs of canine hypothyroidism: Not all dogs with hypothyroidism will have classical clinical signs and laboratory findings. The following list of clinical signs and laboratory findings may vary in dogs with hypothyroidism depending upon the degree and length of time of the thyroid dysfunction:

Nerve and muscle function: lethargy, lack of endurance, increased sleeping, reduced alertness and interest, impaired cerebral function and dulled mental attitude, hypotonus, stiff and slow movements, dragging of forelimbs, head tilt, disturbed balance.

Metabolism: decreased oxygen consumption and lower metabolic rate, sensitivity and intolerance to cold, low body temperature, cool skin, preference for warmth, increased body weight, constipation, poor exercise tolerance, slow heart rate, weak pulse, weak apex heart beat, and low voltage on ECG.

Reproduction: reproductive failure, abortion, stillbirth, live birth of weak young, delayed puberty, reduced libido, impaired spermatogenesis, irregular estrus and anestrus, galactorrhea.

Skin and hair: myxedema of face, blepharoptosis, atrophy of epidermis, thickening of dermis, surface and follicular hyperkeratosis, hyperpigmentation, coarse and sparse coat, dry, dull and brittle hair, slow regrowth and retarded turnover of hair, bilateral alopecia.

Laboratory findings: low serum T-4 concentrations, hypercholesterolemia, hypertriglyceridemia, elevated serum creatine kinase, anemia (normochromic, normocytic).

References: Available upon request.

Presentation: THYRO-TABS® (levothyroxine sodium tablets, USP) is available as scored, color-coded caplets in 8 concentrations: 0.1 mg - yellow; 0.2 mg - pink; 0.3 mg green; 0.4 mg - maroon; 0.5 mg - white; 0.6 mg - purple; 0.7 mg - orange; 0.8 mg - blue; in bottles of 120 and 1000.

Compendium Code No.: 10500302

0898

THYROXINE-L POWDER ℞

Butler **Thyroid Therapy**

Levothyroxine sodium USP (.22%)

Active Ingredient(s): Each pound (453.6 g) contains:

Levothyroxine Sodium USP	0.22% (1.0 g)
One teaspoonful contains:	12 mg of T-4
One tablespoonful contains:	36 mg of T-4

Indications: For use in horses for correction of conditions associated with low circulating thyroid hormone (hypothyroidism).

Dosage and Administration: The suggested initial doses is 0.5 to 3.0 mg levothyroxine sodium (T-4) per 100 lbs of body weight (1 to 6 mg per 100 kg) once per day or in divided doses. Response to the administration of THYROXINE-L POWDER should be evaluated clinically until an adequate maintenance dose is established. In most horses, this is usually in the range of 6 to 36 mg total daily dose of levothyroxine sodium. Serum T-3 and T-4 values can vary greatly among individual horses on thyroid supplementation. Dosages should be individualized and animals should be monitored daily for clinical signs of hyperthyroidism or hypersensitivity.

THYROXINE-L POWDER can be administered by mixing the daily dose in the concentrate or by top dressing on the grain, preferably rolled or ground. To facilitate the proper adhesion of THYROXINE-L POWDER to the ration, slightly moisten the grain with water or a liquid supplement.

Precaution(s): Store at room temperature and protect from light. Avoid excessive heat (104°F).

Caution(s): Federal law restricts this drug to use by or on the order of a licensed veterinarian.

For animal use only.

Warning(s): Administer with caution to animals with clinically significant heart disease, hypertension or other complications for which a sharply increased metabolic rate might prove hazardous. Use in pregnant mares has not been evaluated.

Presentation: 1 lb jars and 10 lb buckets.

Manufactured by: Sparhawk Laboratories.

Compendium Code No.: 10821780

THYROXINE-L TABLETS ℞

Butler **Thyroid Therapy**

Active Ingredient(s): Each tablet contains either:

Levothyroxine sodium	0.1 mg
Levothyroxine sodium	0.2 mg
Levothyroxine sodium	0.3 mg
Levothyroxine sodium	0.4 mg
Levothyroxine sodium	0.5 mg
Levothyroxine sodium	0.6 mg
Levothyroxine sodium	0.7 mg
Levothyroxine sodium	0.8 mg

Indications: Provides thyroid replacement therapy in all conditions of inadequate production of thyroid hormones. Hypothyroidism is the generalized metabolic disease resulting from a deficiency of the thyroid hormones levothyroxine (T4) and liothyronine (T3). Levothyroxine sodium will provide levothyroxine (T4) as a substrate for the physiologic de-iodination to liothyronine (T3). Administration of levothyroxine sodium alone will result in complete physiologic thyroid replacement.

Pharmacology: Each levothyroxine sodium tablet provides synthetic crystalline levothyroxine sodium (L-thyroxine).

Levothyroxine sodium acts as does endogenous thyroxine, to stimulate metabolism, growth, development and differentiation on tissues. It increases the rate of energy exchange and increases the maturation rate of the epiphyses. Levothyroxine sodium is absorbed rapidly from the gastro-intestinal tract after oral administration. Following absorption, the compound becomes bound to the serum globulin fraction. For purposes of comparison 0.1 mg of levothyroxine sodium elicits a clinical response approximately equal to that produced by 1 grain (65 mg) of desiccated thyroid.

Dosage and Administration: The initial recommended dose is 0.1 mg per 10 lbs. of body weight. The dosage is then adjusted according to the patients' response by monitoring T4 blood levels at time intervals of four (4) weeks.

Thyroxine tablets may be administered orally or placed in the food.

Contraindication(s): Levothyroxine sodium therapy is contraindicated in thyrotoxicosis, acute myocardial infarction and incorrected adrenal insufficiency. Use in pregnant bitches has not been evaluated.

Precaution(s): Do not store at temperatures above 40°C (104°F) and protect from light.

Caution(s): Federal law restricts this drug to use by or on the order of a licensed veterinarian.

Keep this and all medications out of the reach of children.

The effects of levothyroxine sodium therapy are slow in being manifested. The overdose of any thyroid drug may produce the signs and symptoms of thyrotoxicosis including but not limited to polydipsia, polyuria, polyphagia, reduced heat tolerance and hyperactivity or personality change. Administer with caution to animals with clinically significant heart disease, hypertension or other complications for which a sharply increased metabolic rate might prove hazardous.

Side Effects: There are no particular adverse reactions connected with L-thyroxine therapy at the recommended dosage levels. An overdose will result in the signs of thyrotoxicosis listed above under cautions.

Discussion: Canine hypothyroidism is usually primary, i.e., due to atrophy of the thyroid gland. In the majority of cases the atrophy is associated with lymphocytic thyroiditis and in the remainder it is noninflammatory and as of yet unknown etiology. Less than 10% of cases of hypothyroidism are secondary, i.e., due to a deficiency of thyroid stimulating hormone (TSH). TSH deficiency may occur as a component of congenital hypopituitarism or as an acquired disorder in adult dogs, in which case it is invariably due to hypothyroidism in dogs:

Lethargy, lack of endurance, increased sleeping, reduced interest, alertness and excitability, slow heart rate, weak apex beat and pulse, low voltage on ECG, preference for warmth low body temperature, cool skin, increased body weight, stiff and slow movements, dragging of front feet, head tilt, disturbed balance, unilateral facial paralysis, atrophy of epidermis, thickening of dermis, surface and follicular hyperkeratosis, pigmentation, puffy face, blepharoptosis, tragic expression, dry, coarse, sparse coat, slow regrowth after clipping, retarded turnover of hair (carpet coat of boxers), shortening of absence of estrus, lack libido, dry feces, occasional diarrhea, hypercholesterolemia, normochromic, normocytic anemia and elevated serum creatinine phosphokinase.

Presentation: Bottles of 180 and 1,000 tablets.

Compendium Code No.: 10821790

THYROZINE ℞

RXV **Thyroid Therapy**

Active Ingredient(s): Each tablet contains either:

Levothyroxine sodium	0.1 mg
Levothyroxine sodium	0.2 mg
Levothyroxine sodium	0.3 mg
Levothyroxine sodium	0.4 mg
Levothyroxine sodium	0.5 mg
Levothyroxine sodium	0.6 mg
Levothyroxine sodium	0.7 mg
Levothyroxine sodium	0.8 mg

Indications: Provides thyroid replacement therapy in all conditions of inadequate production of thyroid hormones (hypothyroidism) in dogs.

Dosage and Administration: The initial recommended daily dose is 0.1 mg per 10 lbs. of body weight. The dose is then adjusted by monitoring the T-4 blood levels of the dog every four (4) weeks until an adequate maintenance dose is established.

Precaution(s): Protect from light and do not store above 104°F (40°C).

Caution(s): Federal law restricts this drug to use by or on the order of a licensed veterinarian.

Administer with caution to animals with primary hypertension, euthyroidism and clinically diagnosed heart disease.

Keep out of the reach of children.

Use in pregnant bitches has not been evaluated.

Presentation: 0.1 mg, 0.2 mg, 0.3 mg, 0.4 mg, 0.5 mg, 0.6 mg, 0.7 mg and 0.8 mg in bottles of 1,000 tablets.

Compendium Code No.: 10910190

THYROZINE POWDER ℞

Phoenix Pharmaceutical **Thyroid Therapy**

Active Ingredient(s): Composition: Each pound (453.6 g) contains:

Levothyroxine Sodium USP	0.22% (1.0 g)

One level teaspoonful contains 12 mg of T_4; one level tablespoonful contains 36 mg of T_4.

Indications: For use in horses and ponies for correction of conditions associated with low circulating thyroid hormone (hypothyroidism).

Dosage and Administration:

Dosage: Doses should be individualized and animals should be monitored daily for clinical signs of hyperthyroidism or hypersensitivity. Suggested initial doses are 1-10 mg levothyroxine sodium (T_4)/100 lb body weight (2-20 mg/100 kg) once per day or in divided doses. Response to the administration of THYROZINE POWDER should be evaluated clinically every week until an adequate maintenance dose is established. In most horses, this is usually in the range of 35 to 100 mg total daily dose of T_4 (1-3 level tablespoonfuls THYROZINE POWDER).

Administration: THYROZINE POWDER may be top dressed or mixed with the daily ration.

Precaution(s): Storage Conditions: Do not store above 30°C (86°F). Keep lid tightly closed and store in a dry location.

Caution(s): Federal law restricts this drug to use by or on the order of a licensed veterinarian.

Administer with caution to animals with clinically significant heart disease, hypertension or other complications for which a sharply increased metabolic rate might prove hazardous. Use in pregnant mares has not been evaluated.

Use only as directed.

Warning(s): Keep out of reach of children.

Presentation: 1 lb (453.6 g) and 10 lb (4.5 kg).

Manufactured by: First Priority.

Compendium Code No.: 12561120 Iss. 6-00

THYROZINE TABLETS ℞

Phoenix Pharmaceutical **Thyroid Therapy**

Levothyroxine Sodium Tablets, USP

Active Ingredient(s): Each tablet contains either:

Levothyroxine sodium USP	0.1 mg
Levothyroxine sodium USP	0.2 mg
Levothyroxine sodium USP	0.3 mg
Levothyroxine sodium USP	0.4 mg
Levothyroxine sodium USP	0.5 mg
Levothyroxine sodium USP	0.6 mg
Levothyroxine sodium USP	0.7 mg
Levothyroxine sodium USP	0.8 mg

Indications: Provides thyroid replacement therapy in all conditions of inadequate production of thyroid hormones. Hypothyroidism is the generalized metabolic disease resulting from deficiency of the thyroid hormones levothyroxine (T-4) and liothyronine (T-3). Levothyroxine sodium will provide levothyroxine (T-4) as a substrate for the physiologic deiodination to liothyronine (T-3). Administration of levothyroxine sodium alone will result in complete physiologic thyroid replacement.

Pharmacology: Each Levothyroxine Sodium Tablet provides synthetic crystalline levothyroxine sodium (L-thyroxine).

Action: Levothyroxine sodium acts as does endogenous thyroxine, to stimulate metabolism, growth, development and differentiation of tissues. It increases the rate of energy exchange and increases the maturation rate of the epiphyses. Levothyroxine sodium is absorbed rapidly from the gastro-intestinal tract after oral administration. Following absorption, the compound becomes bound to the serum alpha globulin fraction. For purposes of comparison, 0.1 mg of levothyroxine sodium elicits a clinical response approximately equal to that produced by one grain (65 mg) of desiccated thyroid.

Dosage and Administration: The initial recommended daily dose is 0.1 mg/10 lb body weight. Dosage is then adjusted according to the patient's response by monitoring T-4 blood levels at time intervals of four weeks.

Thyroxine tablets may be administered orally or placed in the food.

Contraindication(s): Levothyroxine sodium therapy is contraindicated in thyrotoxicosis, acute myocardial infraction and uncorrected adrenal insufficiency. Use in pregnant bitches has not been evaluated.

Precaution(s): Storage: Store at 15°-30°C (59°-86°F) and protect from light.

Tightly close the container after each use.

Caution(s): Federal law restricts this drug to use by or on the order of a licensed veterinarian.

The effects of levothyroxine sodium therapy are slow in being manifested. Overdosage of any thyroid drug may produce the signs and symptoms of thyrotoxicosis including, but not limited to, polydipsia, polyuria, polyphagia, reduced heat tolerance and hyperactivity or personality change. Administer with caution to animals with clinically significant heart disease, hypertension or other complications for which a sharply increased metabolic rate might prove hazardous.

For animal use only.

Warning(s): Keep out of reach of children.

Adverse Reactions: There are no particular adverse reactions connected with L-Thyroxine therapy at the recommended dosage levels. Overdose will result in the signs of thyrotoxicosis, listed above.

Discussion: Canine hypothyroidism is usually primary, i.e., due to atrophy of the thyroid gland. In the majority of cases, the atrophy is associated with lymphocytic thyroiditis and in the remainder it is noninflammatory, and as of yet, unknown etiology. Less than 10 percent of the cases of hypothyroidism are secondary, i.e., due to deficiency of the thyroid stimulating hormone (TSH). TSH deficiency may occur as a component of congenital hypopituitarism or as an acquired disorder in adult dogs, in which case it is invariably due to the growth of a pituitary tumor.

Hypothyroidism in the Dog: Hypothyroidism usually occurs in middle-aged and older dogs although the condition will sometimes be seen in younger dogs of the larger breeds. Neutered animals of either sex are also frequently affected, regardless of age. The following are clinical signs of hypothyroidism in dogs:

Lethargy, lack of endurance, increased sleeping, reduced interest, alertness and excitability, slow heart rate, weak apex beat and pulse, low voltage on ECG, preference for warmth, low body temperature, cool skin, increased body weight, stiff and slow movements, dragging of front feet, head tilt, disturbed balance, unilateral facial paralysis, atrophy of epidermis, thickening of dermis, surface and follicular hyperkeratosis, pigmentation, puffy face, blepharoptosis, tragic expression, dry, coarse, sparse coat, slow regrowth after clipping, retarded turnover of hair (carpet coat of boxers), shortening of absence of estrus, lack of libido, dry feces, occasional diarrhea, hypercholesterolemia, normochromic, normocytic anemia and elevated serum creatinine phosphokinase.

Presentation: 0.1 mg-light yellow (NDC 57319-331-31), 0.2 mg-pink (NDC 57319-332-31), 0.3 mg-light green (NDC 57319-333-31), 0.4 mg-light violet (NDC 57319-334-31), 0.5 mg-white (NDC 57319-335-31), 0.6 mg-violet (NDC 57319-336-31), 0.7 mg-light orange (NDC 57319-337-31), 0.8 mg-light blue (NDC 57319-338-31) in bottles of 180 and 1000 tablets.

Manufactured by: Lloyd, Inc.

Compendium Code No.: 12560841 Rev 06-01

TINCTURE IODINE 7%

Aspen **Topical Wound Dressing**

Active Ingredient(s):

Iodine	7.0% w/v
Potassium Iodide	5.0% w/v
Isopropyl Alcohol (99%)	85.0% v/v
Water	q.s.

Indications: An antiseptic and disinfectant for application to superficial cuts, abrasions, insect bites or minor bruises. Livestock remedy.

Dosage and Administration: Dilute 1 part tincture iodine 7% with 2 parts of propylene glycol. Cleanse area with soap and water. Apply dilution lightly not more than once daily.

Contraindication(s): Not for use in deep cavity wounds or body cavities.

Precaution(s): Flammable. Do not expose to heat, sparks, or open flame. Do not store above 120°F.

Keep container closed.

Caution(s): Do not apply under bandage. This product may irritate tender skin areas. In case of deep or puncture wounds or serious burns, consult veterinarian. If redness, irritation, or swelling persists or increases, discontinue use and consult veterinarian. Avoid contact with eyes and mucous membranes. Do not use on burns.

When used on or near the teats or udder of dairy animals the teats and udder should be thoroughly washed before next milking to prevent contamination of milk.

Antidote(s): If swallowed give starch paste, milk, bread, egg white or activated charcoal. To vomit, take mustard and warm water. A 5% solution of sodium thiosulfate (photographic "hypo") may be administered orally at a rate of 10 cc per kilogram of body weight. Call a physician or poison control center.

Warning(s): For animal use only. Not for human use. For external use only.

Presentation: 1 pint (4732 mL) and 1 gallon (3.785 L) containers.

Compendium Code No.: 14750850

TINCTURE IODINE 7%

Bimeda **Topical Wound Dressing**

Active Ingredient(s): Contains:

Iodine	7.0% w/v
Potassium iodide	5.0% w/v
Isopropyl alcohol (99%)	85.0% v/v
Water	q.s.

Indications: An antiseptic and disinfectant for application to superficial cuts, abrasions, insect bites or minor bruises.

Dosage and Administration: Dilute one (1) part TINCTURE IODINE 7% with two (2) parts of propylene glycol. Cleanse the area with soap and water. Apply the dilution lightly not more than once a day.

Warning(s): Keep out of the reach of children.

Presentation: 16 fl oz and 1 gallon containers.

Compendium Code No.: 13990411

TIP-TEST®: BLV

ImmuCell **Leukemia Test**

Bovine Leukemia Virus Antibody Test Kit

U.S. Vet. Lic. No.: 327

Contents: Materials Provided

10 Trays containing TIP-TEST®: BLV Tip and 4 reagent wells:
- #1) Sample well
- #2) Conjugate well
- #3) Wash solution well
- #4) Substrate well

20 Syringes
10 'Syringe-to-Tip' adapters
10 Wooden Stir Sticks
1 Vial Positive control serum

Materials Not Provided
1) Vacutainer™ anti-coagulant tube of clotting tube for blood collection.
2) Needle for blood collection.
3) 21 gauge needle or smaller for Positive Control Sampling.

Test Principles: TIP-TEST®: BLV is a reliable, easy-to-use method for the detection of antibodies to Bovine Leukemia Virus, the causative agent of bovine leukosis. The test relies upon the reaction of the antibodies with Bovine Leukemia Virus antigens attached to a small element inside a Tip that is connected to a 1 cc syringe. The Tip contains three elements, each designed to change color in response to a given condition. The three components are:
1) Test Element containing Bovine Leukemia Virus antigen
2) Negative Element, which establishes a baseline color to which all results are compared.
3) Positive Element, which turns purple color upon proper performance of the test and validates the integrity of the substrate.

A blood sample is obtained from a cow using an anti-coagulant tube or a clotting tube. A small amount whole blood, serum or plasma is transferred into the sample well of a disposable Tray which is provided with the test. This diluted sample is drawn into the Tip using a 1 cc syringe. Antibodies against Bovine Leukemia Virus bind to the test element. After a series of steps in which the reagents in subsequent wells contact the elements in the Tip, color development occurs. Reading this color development, visually, leads to the interpretation of the BLV status of the cow.

Sample Collection: Specimen Collection: Best results are obtained using fresh bovine blood taken in the proper manner. EDTA, citrate and heparin anticoagulants are compatible with the TIP-TEST®: BLV test kit. Whole blood, serum or plasma samples may be used.

Test Procedure: Bring test to room temperature. All Tip incubations are to be done in a horizontal position at room temperature.
1) Prepare Tip. Using wooden stir stick (provided), puncture cover of long well marked "Tip Inside" and remove Tip. Take care not to break stir stick. Attach an adapter (provided) to a 1 cc syringe (provided), and draw air into syringe to the 0.2 ml mark. Remove plug from Tip. Attach Tip to syringe/adapter. Set aside.
2) Prepare Sample. Obtain a 0.12 ml sample of bovine blood from anticoagulant tube (plasma or serum samples use 0.08 ml), using fresh 1 cc syringe (provided). Using wood stir stick, carefully puncture cover of well #1 and make a large hole, exposing diluent. Expel blood sample into well #1 and mix thoroughly with stir stick. Discard stick. Incubate for five minutes.
3) Draw Sample. (Well #1). Remove cap from Tip and expel storage buffer from Tip to waste. Immerse Tip into well #1 solution and slowly draw plunger up to the 0.2 ml mark. Fluid level should rise above top of elements. With Tip still fully immersed, slowly move sample fluid down just above the elements or to the 0.1 ml mark and draw up through elements to the 0.2 ml mark again and repeat. Keep fluid level above and below the elements for incubation. Incubate for five minutes. After incubation, slowly expel sample from Tip to waste. Wipe off any residual fluid from Tip.
4) Draw Conjugate. (Well #2). Carefully pierce and widen an opening in well #2 with Tip. At an angle, immerse Tip to the bottom of the well, and slowly draw plunger up allowing the fluid level to rise above top of elements or to approximately the 0.15 ml mark. Do not allow air to enter the bottom of the Tip. Move fluid in upward direction only (not up and down). Incubate for five minutes. After incubation, slowly expel conjugate from Tip to waste by fully depressing syringe plunger.
5) Wash Tip. (Well #3). Remove Tip from syringe/adapter, and expel any air and fluid from syringe. Pierce through well #3 with syringe/adapter (Tip not attached) and draw 0.6 ml of wash solution into the syringe. Re-attach Tip to syringe/adapter. With a steady drip, expel solution from syringe and Tip to waste. Remove Tip from syringe/adapter. Draw air into syringe. Re-attach Tip and slowly and completely expel air and remaining fluid from Tip. Wipe off any residual fluid from the end of the Tip.
6) Draw Substrate. (Well #4). Carefully pierce and widen an opening in well #4 with Tip. At an angle, immerse Tip to the bottom of the well, and slowly draw plunger up allowing the fluid level to rise above top of elements or to approximately the 0.15 ml mark. Do not allow air to enter the bottom of the Tip. Move fluid in upward direction only (not up and down). Incubate for five minutes. After incubation, slowly expel substrate from Tip to waste by full depressing the syringe plunger.
7) Wash Tip. (Well #3). Remove Tip from syringe/adapter, and expel any air and fluid from syringe. Immerse syringe/adapter into well #3 (Tip not attached) and draw 0.6 ml of wash solution into the syringe. Re-attach Tip to syringe/adapter. With a steady drip, expel solution from syringe and Tip to waste. Remove Tip from syringe/adapter. Draw air into syringe. Re-attach Tip and slowly and completely expel air and remaining fluid from Tip. Wipe off any residual fluid from the end of the Tip.
8) Read Results. Read result within 5 minutes, using Comparator Card provided for interpretation of results.

Interpretation of Results: Interpretation of Results and Limitations of the Procedure: Referring to the Comparator Card, choose the pattern of colors that most closely resemble the result you obtained.

BLV Negative: A result where the Test Element is the same white to slightly gray color as the Negative Element indicates that the animal is negative for BLV antibodies. While the Negative Element generally remains white, some samples that are negative for BLV antibodies can cause an overall graying of the Negative and Test Elements. When this occurs, carefully gauge the color on the Test Element. If the color of the Test Element is not clearly darker than the Negative Element, the result is negative for BLV antibodies.

BLV Positive: A Test Element that is darker than the Negative Element indicates that the animal is positive for BLV antibodies.

Invalid Results: Invalid results most commonly occur because of procedural errors, but can occasionally occur in relation to specific "problem" samples. The Positive and Negative Elements are procedural controls that help the user determine if the test has been run properly. The Positive Element generally turns dark purple, but occasionally can turn only moderately purple when the test is performed properly. If the Positive Element only becomes faintly purple or not purple at all, consider the test invalid. The Negative Element generally remains white to slightly gray when the test is performed properly. If the Negative Element changes color to purple (resembling the Positive Element), consider the test invalid. If the Negative Element displays a yellow color, consider the test invalid. Samples producing invalid results should be repeat tested; if the re-test is also invalid, contact ImmuCell Corporation for technical service. Test Elements that have irregular or "patchy" color development are valid results and should be scored based on the predominant color change in the Test Element.

As with any test, the reliability of a given result will increase if replicate testing is performed.

Storage: Store refrigerated at 2-7°C (35-45°F).

Caution(s):
1) Do not use beyond expiration date.
2) Do not peel back Tray cover. Cover helps prevent well-to-well cross contamination.
3) Read results within 5 minutes of completion of the test.
4) Bring test Tray to room temperature before use.
5) Positive Control serum included with each kit should be tested to verify conjugate integrity and proper performance by the user.
6) When sampling the Positive Control serum, use a 21 gauge needle or smaller.
7) While performing test, fluid movement in all steps should be slow and steady to ensure proper coverage of the elements and minimizing introduction of air into the Tip.
8) This product is intended for use by qualified professionals familiar with potential hazards. Avoid skin and eye contact and inhalation of reagents. Wash hands thoroughly after handling. In case of contact, immediately flush skin or eyes with copious amounts of water.
9) Wooden stir stick is breakable and may splinter under extreme pressure.
10) The reagent preservative contains sodium azide. If discarding waste into sink flush thoroughly with water.
11) For veterinary use only.

Discussion: TIP-TEST®: BLV is a test based on the 'ELISA' principle but requires no specialized equipment, and can be performed in about 25 minutes on-site using bovine blood, serum or plasma specimens. Using this test, the herd veterinarian can institute testing that can reduce the presence of BLV within herds, and limit the spread between herds.

Bovine Leukemia Virus (BLV) causes enzootic bovine leukosis in cattle characterized by a very short viremia and long latency period before onset of the disease[1]. The BLV seropositive rate is high for beef and dairy cattle at 10% and 44% respectively[2,3]. Once acquired, cattle can become a lifelong carrier of BLV[4]. Malignant lymphoma, a fatal clinical manifestation of the BLV infection, occur in 1-5% of BLV infected cattle in the U.S. Clinical cases of malignant lymphoma are most common in "enzootic leukosis herds" characterized by high antibody prevalence and significant mortality.[5] Clinical signs of malignant lymphoma become evident as the tumors invade different tissue and may include weight loss, decreased milk production, rear limb paralysis and persistent lymphocytosis, all of which contribute to significant economic losses. Other economic losses associated with BLV infections are due to restrictions on trade of infected animals and germplasm. BLV transmission occurs early in the life of a calf when virus is transmitted in the milk and horizontally through blood contaminated instruments used in animal husbandry. No vaccine or treatment is available to limit the spread of this disease. Therefore, the uses of biosecurity measures, herd management, routine testing and culling of animals are important aspects of controlling the spread of BLV infection.

Herd management practices that minimize spread and can lead to reduction of the prevalence of BLV include the following: a) instituting a testing program to determine the prevalence in a herd, b) prioritizing culling decisions based, in part, on the BLV status of individual cows, c) testing purchased animals prior to introduction into the herd, d) avoiding feeding colostrum from BLV positive individuals, e) separating calves from BLV positive dams and f) use sanitized instruments in routine animal husbandry practices. Unfortunately these practices are hampered by the high costs, slow turn-around-time for laboratory testing (several days for ELISA results) and the inconvenience of sending specimens. The fastest method of testing is the ELISA method, wherein serum samples from suspected animals are tested for the presence of antibodies specific to BLV antigens incorporated into the test. The ELISA method is specific (99.4%) and sensitive, but requires specialized equipment. Thus, there is a need for a test that rapid, sensitive and can be done on-site, or in the herd veterinarian's office or clinic.

Trial Data: Sensitivity and Specificity: In a blinded, multi-center study, TIP-TEST®: BLV was used to test 100 specimens from adult dairy cows whose serological status for Bovine Leukemia Virus was determined by AGID and ELISA testing. Fifty positive samples were selected based on positive results from AGID and ELISA test assay. Fifty negative samples were selected from an isolated farm where all animals repeat test negative on AGID and ELISA semi-annually.

The overall average sensitivity was 100%, i.e. TIP-TEST®: BLV detected 100% of the AGID seropositive cows.

The overall average specificity was 98.7% (range of 96-100%); i.e. 98.7% of the animals negative by AGID serological testing also tested negative by TIP-TEST®: BLV.

References: Available upon request.

Presentation: 10 tests per kit.

Vacutainer™ is a trademark of Becton Dickinson & Co.

Compendium Code No.: 11200070 Revision 4/2001

TIP-TEST®: JOHNE'S

ImmuCell **Johne's Disease Test**

Mycobacterium paratuberculosis Antibody Test Kit

U.S. Vet. Lic. No.: 327

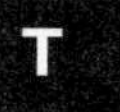

Contents: Materials Provided: Trays containing the TIP-TEST®: JOHNE'S tip and 4 reagent wells:
1) Sample well, containing an *M. phlei* antigen to absorb cross-reacting (non-specific) antibodies in the sample

#2) Conjugate well
#3) Wash solution well
#4) Substrate well

Syringes and 'syringe-to-tip' adapter
Wooden Stir Stick
Positive control serum

Materials Not Provided
1) Vacutainer™ anti-coagulant tube or clotting tube for blood collection
2) Needle for blood collection

Indications: For use by veterinarians, to help limit the spread of Johne's disease within and between herds.

Test Principles: TIP-TEST®: JOHNE'S is a reliable, easy-to-use method for the detection of antibodies to *Mycobacterium paratuberculosis*, the causative agent of Johne's disease. The test relies upon the reaction of the antibodies with *M. paratuberculosis* antigens attached to a small element inside a tip that is connected to a 1 cc syringe. The tip contains three elements, each designed to change color in response to a given condition. The three components are:

1) Test Element containing *M. paratuberculosis* antigen,
2) Negative Element which establishes a baseline color to which all results are compared, and
3) Positive Element which turns purple in color upon proper performance of the test.

A blood sample is obtained from a cow using an anti-coagulant tube or a clotting tube. A small amount of whole blood, serum or plasma is transferred into the sample well of a disposable tray which is provided with the test. Non-specific antibodies are absorbed in the sample well by binding to *M. phlei* antigens in the diluent. This diluted sample is drawn into the tip using a 1 cc syringe. Antibodies against *M. paratuberculosis* bind to the test element. After a series of steps in which the reagents in subsequent wells contact the elements in the tip, color development occurs. Reading this color development, visually leads to the interpretation of the Johne's status of the cow.

Sensitivity and Specificity: In a blinded, multi-center study TIP-TEST®: JOHNE'S was used to test 100 specimens from adult dairy cows whose Johne's fecal culture and clinical status was followed through to slaughter. The overall average sensitivity was 76.1% (range 70-81.2%), i.e. the test detected 76.1% of the culture-positive cows in varying clinical stages of Johne's Disease. In animals with clinical signs of the disease and positive fecal cultures, the test was 88-92.8% sensitive. In animals that were subclinical, but shed *M. paratuberculosis* the test was 42.8-66.7% sensitive.

The overall average specificity was 91.1% (range of 80-100%), i.e. 91.1% of the animals negative by fecal culture also tested negative by this test.

Sample Collection: Best results are obtained using fresh bovine blood taken in the proper manner. Serum or plasma may also be used.

Test Procedure: Bring test to room temperature.

1) Prepare Tip. Using wooden stir stick provided, puncture cover of long well marked 'Tip Inside' and remove Tip. Take care not to break stir stick. Remove plug from Tip. Attach an adapter (provided) to a 1 cc syringe, and draw air into syringe to the 0.2 mL mark. Attach Tip to syringe/adapter Set aside.
2) Prepare Sample. Obtain a 0.075 mL sample of bovine blood from anticoagulant tube (plasma or serum samples use 0.05 mL), using fresh 1 cc syringe (provided). Using wooden stir stick, carefully puncture cover of well #1 and make a large hole, exposing diluent. Expel blood sample into well #1 and mix thoroughly with stir stick. Discard stick. Incubate for five minutes.
3) Draw Sample (Well #1). Remove cap from Tip and expel storage buffer from Tip to waste. Immerse Tip into well #1 solution and slowly draw plunger up to the 0.2 mL mark. Fluid level should rise above top of element. With Tip still fully immersed, slowly move sample fluid down and up through element twice, always keeping fluid level above the top of the element. Incubate for five minutes in horizontal position. After incubation, slowly expel sample from Tip to waste. Wipe off any residual fluid from Tip.
4) Draw Conjugate (Well #2). Carefully pierce well #2 with Tip, immerse Tip fully and slowly draw plunger up to approx. the 0.2 mL mark. Fluid level should rise above top of elements, but air should not enter the bottom of the Tip. Move fluid in upward direction only (not up and down). Incubate for five minutes in horizontal position. After incubation, slowly expel conjugate from Tip to waste.
5) Wash Tip (Well #3). Remove Tip from syringe/adapter, and expel any air and fluid from syringe by fully depressing plunger. Pierce through well #3 with syringe/adapter (Tip not attached) and draw plunger to 0.8 mL mark, bringing the wash solution to approximately the 0.6 mL mark. Re-attach Tip to syringe/adapter. Slowly expel solution from syringe and Tip to waste. Remove Tip from syringe/adapter. Draw 0.2 mL of air into syringe. Re-attach Tip and slowly expel air and residual fluid from Tip. Wipe off any residual fluid from the end of the Tip.
6) Draw Substrate (Well #4). Carefully pierce well #4 with Tip, immerse Tip fully and slowly draw plunger up to approx. the 0.2 mL mark. Fluid level should rise above top of elements, but air should not enter the bottom of the Tip. Incubate for five minutes in horizontal position. After incubation, slowly expel substrate from Tip to waste.
7) Wash Tip (Well #3). Remove Tip from syringe/adapter, and expel any air and fluid from syringe by fully depressing plunger. Immerse syringe/adapter into well #3 (Tip not attached) and draw plunger to 0.8 mL mark, bringing the wash solution to approximately the 0.6 mL mark. Re-attach Tip to syringe/adapter Slowly expel solution from syringe and Tip to waste. Remove Tip from syringe/adapter. Draw 0.2 mL of air into syringe. Re-attach Tip and slowly expel air and residual fluid from Tip. Wipe off any residual fluid from the end of the Tip.
8) Read Results. Read result within 5 minutes, using comparator card provided for interpretation of results.

Interpretation of Results: Interpretation of Results and Limitations of the Procedure: Referring to the Comparator Card, choose the pattern of colors which most closely resembles the result you obtained.

Johne's Negative: A result where the Test Element is the same white to slightly gray color as the Negative Element indicates that the animal is negative for Johne's antibodies. While the Negative Element generally remains white, some samples that are negative for Johne's antibodies can cause an overall graying of the Negative and Test Elements. When this occurs, carefully gauge the color on the Test Element. If the color of the Test Element is not clearly darker than the Negative Element, the result is negative for Johne's antibodies.

Johne's Positive: A Test Element that is clearly darker than the Negative Element indicates that the animal is positive for Johne's antibodies. A result where the Test Element is slightly darker than the Negative Element indicates that the animal is 'Johne's suspect', and should be retested in 3-6 months. A re-test where the Test Element remains slightly darker than the Negative Element ('Johne's suspect') may have Johne's disease, or may indicate a true 'false positive' due to the presence of cross reacting antibodies. If the Test Element is dramatically darker than the Negative Element, this animal should be considered Johne's positive. While there is generally a direct relationship between increasing levels of Johne's antibodies and disease progression, some animals have clinical or microbiological Johne's disease without development of a strong antibody response, and some animals in very late stage clinical Johne's disease may not have detectable antibodies at all[6]. It may be prudent to test an animal that is positive for Johne's antibodies by another method such as culture, AGID test, or other laboratory assay to confirm a diagnosis of Johne's disease.

While this test provides an absorbing antigen to reduce false positive reactions due to environmental *Mycobacteria*, it does not eliminate the possibility that a false positive result might occur.

Invalid Results: Invalid results most commonly occur because of procedural errors, but can occasionally occur in relation to specific 'problem' samples. The Positive and Negative Elements are procedural controls, and help the user determine if the test has been run properly, or if a specific sample contains interfering substances. The Positive Element generally turns dark purple, but occasionally can turn only moderately purple when the test is properly run. If the Positive Element only becomes faintly purple or not purple at all, consider the test invalid. The Negative Element generally remains white to slightly gray when the test is properly run. If the Negative Element changes color to purple (resembling the Positive Element), consider the test invalid. If the Negative Element displays a yellow color, consider the test invalid. Samples producing invalid results should be repeat tested; if the re-test is also invalid, contact ImmuCell Corporation technical service. Test Elements that have irregular or 'patchy' color development are valid results and should be scored based on the predominant color change in the Test Element.

User-to-user Interpretation Differences: In blinded clinical trials, user-to-user differences were noted in the interpretation of TIP-TEST®: JOHNE'S results (see Sensitivity and Specificity). An inverse relationship was noted between user's interpretations and sensitivity/specificity. Among users who scored more specimens positive, sensitivity was highest (81.2% overall), but specificity was lowest (80% overall). Among users who scored fewer specimens positive, sensitivity was lowest (70% overall), but specificity was highest (100%). Therefore, 'over interpretation' leads to somewhat higher sensitivity and lower specificity, while 'under interpretation' leads to somewhat lower sensitivity and higher specificity. Keep this in mind when making management decisions within a given herd.

Storage: Store refrigerated at 2-7°C (35-45°F).

Caution(s):

1) Do not use beyond expiration date.
2) Do not peel back tray cover. Cover helps prevent well-to-well cross contamination.
3) Read results within 5 minutes of completion of the test.
4) Bring test tray to room temperature before use.
5) Positive Control serum included with each kit should be tested to verify kit validity.
6) While performing test, fluid movement in all steps should be slow and steady to ensure proper coverage of the elements in fluid and to minimize the introduction of air into the tip.
7) This product is intended for use by qualified professionals familiar with potential hazards. Avoid skin and eye contact and inhalation of reagents. Wash hands thoroughly after handling. In case of contact, immediately flush skin or eyes with copious amounts of water.
8) Wooden stir stick is breakable and may splinter under extreme pressure.
9) For veterinary use only.

Discussion: TIP-TEST®: JOHNE'S is a test based on the 'ELISA' principle but requires no specialized equipment, and can be performed in about 25 minutes on-site using bovine blood, serum or plasma specimens. Using this test, the herd veterinarian can institute testing that, when used with other testing methods, can reduce the presence of Johne's disease within herds, and limit the spread between herds.

Johne's disease, first described in 1895 by Johne & Frothingham, is a slow-developing, often chronic "wasting" disease of ruminant animals which is caused by the bacterium *Mycobacterium paratuberculosis*[1]. Economic losses are seen in lower milk production (2-19% loss), lower carcass weight at time of slaughter, restrictions in sale of stock, and early culling of infected animals[2,3]. Commonly, the disease persists on farm by fecal contamination from animals that are either chronically ill or asymptomatic shedders (*M. paratuberculosis* organisms are highly resistant to environmental degradation and can remain viable in manure and stagnant water for more than a year[4]). The purchase of infected cattle with no overt clinical signs[5] contributes to the persistence on farm and to establishment in uninfected herds. Identification of animals with clinical or subclinical Johne's disease is therefore an important aspect of controlling the spread of infection.

Herd management practices that minimize spread and can lead to reduction of the prevalence of Johne's disease include the following: a) instituting a testing program to determine the prevalence in a herd, b) prioritizing culling decisions based, in part, on the Johne's status of individual cows, c) testing purchased animals prior to introduction into the herd, d) avoiding feeding or pooling colostrum from Johne's positive individuals, and e) separating calves from Johne's positive dams. Unfortunately these practices are hampered by the high costs and slow turn-around-time for laboratory testing (several days for ELISA results, and 4-16 weeks for culture), the inconvenience of sending specimens, and the fear that results will not be held in confidence. The fastest method of testing for Johne's disease, and the method recommended as part of proposed certification programs is the ELISA method, wherein serum samples from suspected animals are tested for the presence of antibodies specific to *M. paratuberculosis* antigens incorporated into the test[6,7]. The ELISA method is specific and relatively sensitive (approx. 45%[8]), but requires specialized equipment and must be performed in a certified laboratory. Thus, there is a need for a test that is rapid, sensitive and can be done on-site, or in the herd veterinarian's office or clinic.

References: Available upon request.

Presentation: 25 tests per kit.

Compendium Code No.: 11200031

TISSUE-BOND™

Vedco **Topical Wound Dressing**

(Formulated Cyanoacrylate)

Active Ingredient(s): Description: TISSUE-BOND™ contains purified n-butyl cyanoacrylate monomer, stabilizer, and a certified D&C dye which permits differentiation from body fluids.

Indications: TISSUE-BOND™ is indicated for veterinary use only. This liquid form is indicated for wound management in a variety of situations including: lacerations and abrasions, cat declaws, cuts, tail docking.

Pharmacology: Actions: TISSUE-BOND™ is a monomeric formulation which, upon contact with an alkaline pH environment, polymerizes to form a thin, flexible waterproof bandage.

TISSUE-BOND™ polymerizes in about one second after contact with moist wound surfaces. Dry surfaces slow the polymerization process.

TISSUE-BOND™ can seal off capillary ends, acting as a hemostatic agent. It also seals off exposed nerve endings.

Dosage and Administration: Administration: Proper administration of the wound site is critical for using TISSUE-BOND™ successfully.

If antiseptic treatment is desired for the wound site, wash the area with a povidone solution.

After preparing the wound site, use sterile gauze to remove any accumulation of blood or moisture from the wound.

Do not apply TISSUE-BOND™ over a pool of blood or fluid. This causes improper polymerization of the bandage and results in premature sloughing of the bandage.

Directions for Use: When using the 2 mL bottle, insert the applicator tip snugly into the tip of the bottle. The 1 mL bottle is tapered for direct application.

Hold the tip of the bottle, or applicator tip, directly over the wound.

Squeeze the bottle to release the TISSUE-BOND™ drops one-at-a-time until the wound is completely covered.

Do not over apply. A light, thin coat is better than a thick, heavy coat. Too much TISSUE-BOND™ will lose flexibility and could develop microscopic cracks.

Use of the Applicator Tip (2 mL): The applicator tip fits snugly into the tip of the 2 mL TISSUE-BOND™ bottle. This allows better control of the size and placement of the drops.

The tips may be bent to provide easier access to tight places.

Each 2 mL bottle package contains several applicator tips that can be reused, or disposed of, if contaminated.

The applicator tip may be left in place over a prolonged period of time. However, upon removal of the tip, remember to wipe the tip of the bottle before replacing the cap.

Removal of TISSUE-BOND™: TISSUE-BOND™ can be removed from skin or other surfaces with dimethylsulfoxide or acetone (finger-nail polish remover).

Contraindication(s): TISSUE-BOND™ is contraindicated for management of infected and deep puncture wounds.

Precaution(s): Storage Conditions: TISSUE-BOND™ may be stored at room temperature. Avoid prolonged exposure to temperatures above 32°C, (90°F). The product should not be used beyond the expiration date.

Caution(s): Avoid contact with skin and eyes.

Avoid contact with clothing, stains are permanent.

Avoid contact with metal instruments.

Presentation: 2 x 1 mL tapered bottles and 1 x 2 mL dropper bottle with applicator tips.

Compendium Code No.: 10942320

TISSUMEND™

V.P.L. **Surgical Glue**

Synthetic Absorbable Liquid Tissue Adhesive (a methoxypropyl cyanoacrylate composition)

Active Ingredient(s): TISSUMEND™ Bioabsorbable Liquid Tissue Adhesive is a patented, unique absorbable biopolymer consisting of a methoxypropyl cyanoacrylate monomer, polymeric modifiers, and D&C Violet #2 FDA approved dye.

Indications: TISSUMEND™ Liquid is indicated for the closure of surgical wounds, declaws, tail dockings, incision sites, debrided trauma wounds and hemostasis.

Directions: Application: Wounds should be properly prepared before using TISSUMEND™. The tissue may be cleaned prior to applying TISSUMEND™ but residual saline or medications should be removed prior to application as these may interfere with appropriate polymerization and adhesion. It is recommended to remove excess blood or fluid before application as copious amounts of fluid may interfere with polymerization.

To apply, simply coat the intended tissue area with TISSUMEND™ until tissue is completely covered with the polymer. Close the tissue together and hold for 30 seconds to one minute allowing for secure polymerization.

For multiple applications, portions of the pipette tip may be aseptically trimmed. Do not over-apply TISSUMEND™ Liquid. A light thin coat is better than a thick, heavy coat.

Contraindication(s): TISSUMEND™ Liquid is contraindicated in the management of infected wounds or situations where tissue closure would be detrimental to the patient. This product is not intended for intravenous administration or other routes of administration other than topical application.

Precaution(s): Storage: TISSUMEND™ Liquid may be stored at room temperature. Avoid prolonged exposure of TISSUMEND™ Liquid to temperatures above 32°C (90°F). The product should not be used beyond the indicated expiration date.

Caution(s): To be used by or under the supervision of a licensed veterinarian and is not intended for human application.

Avoid contact with skin and eyes. Avoid contact with clothing since the stain may be permanent. Avoid contact with metal instruments.

Accidental Application: TISSUMEND™ may be removed from surfaces with chloroform, dimethylsulfoxide or acetone. These removal agents should not be used in situations that may cause injury or harm to the patient.

Veterinary use only.

Discussion: Description and Function: TISSUMEND™ represents the most advanced tissue adhesive and is designed to better suit the needs of the veterinary surgeon that routinely uses tissue adhesives.

TISSUMEND™ has the following advantages over current cyanoacrylate adhesives:

- Unlike octyl and butyl cyanoacrylates, TISSUMEND™ is broken down by hydrolysis and eventually absorbed.
- Reduced exothermic properties upon polymerizing resulting in reduced cytotoxicity and enhanced tissue acceptance.
- Forms an exceptional adhesive joint that is favorably compliant with tissue.

TISSUMEND™ Liquid polymerizes to form a strong bond between moist tissue surfaces within 30 seconds after application. TISSUMEND™ provides the surgeon hemostatic properties in combination with superior adhesive qualities.

Presentation: TISSUMEND™ Liquid Biopolymer Bioabsorbable Tissue Adhesive is supplied in individual prefilled pipettes (0.2 mL). Each package contains 36 prefilled pipettes.

TISSUMEND™ Tissue Adhesive is a trademark of Veterinary Products Laboratories.

Compendium Code No.: 11430480 01-1676

TISSUVAX® 6 VACCINE

Schering-Plough **Bacterin-Vaccine**

Canine Distemper-Hepatitis-Parainfluenza-Parvovirus Vaccine, Modified Live Virus, Leptospira Bacterin

U.S. Vet. Lic. No.: 298

Active Ingredient(s): TISSUVAX® 6 is a combination of a lyophilized suspension of canine distemper, hepatitis, and parainfluenza modified live viruses and a liquid diluent composed of a parvovirus (feline isolate) and Leptospira bacterin. The lyophilized suspension of canine distemper, hepatitis, and parainfluenza modified live viruses is propagated in a stable cell line of canine origin and backfilled with an inert gas. The liquid modified live parvovirus is propagated in a stable cell line of feline origin, and combined with inactivated cultures of *Leptospira canicola* and *L. icterohaemorrhagiae,* which have been processed to be non-viricidal when used as a diluent to rehydrate the canine distemper-hepatitis-parainfluenza vaccine.

Production of the viral components by the stable cell line process ensures maximum uniformity with regard to safety and immunogenicity. The immunogenicity and safety of the product have been demonstrated by vaccination and challenge tests in healthy susceptible dogs. Data indicates that the development of corneal opacity is not associated with the use of the product. Contains neomycin, polymyxin B, and a fungistat as preservatives.

Indications: For the immunization of healthy unexposed puppies and dogs against canine distemper, canine hepatitis, canine parvovirus-induced disease, respiratory disease induced by canine adenovirus type 2, and canine parainfluenza, as well as leptospirosis caused by *L. canicola* and *L. icterohaemorrhagiae.*

Dosage and Administration: Aseptically rehydrate the vaccine with the accompanying diluent. Using aseptic technique, inject 1 mL either subcutaneously or intramuscularly. Two (2) doses of the vaccine are required for initial immunization in order to develop a higher level of immunity against canine parainfluenza and parvovirus. Susceptible puppies and dogs should receive two (2) doses two (2) to four (4) weeks apart.

The age at which maternal antibody no longer interferes with the development of active immunity varies according to the bitch's titer and the quantity of colostral antibodies absorbed by the puppy. In some instances, interference may last for as long as four (4) months. Therefore, dogs vaccinated at younger than 16 weeks of age should receive one (1) dose every two (2) to four (4) weeks until reaching this age. An annual booster dose is recommended for all dogs.

Precaution(s): Store at 35°-45°F (2°-7°C).

Caution(s): Use the entire contents when first opened. Do not use chemicals to sterilize syringes and needles. Burn the container and all unused contents. In case of an anaphylactic reaction, administer epinephrine. It is generally recommended to avoid the vaccination of pregnant dogs. Central nervous system reactions have been temporally associated with the administration of modified live canine distemper vaccines. Clinical experience indicates that the incidence of such reactions is extremely low.

The product is tested before release for sale and meets all tests required by the United States government, as well as the laboratories of Pitman-Moore, Inc.

For veterinary use only.

Presentation: 25 x 1 dose vials.

* ® Registered trademark of Schering-Plough Animal Health Corporation.

Compendium Code No.: 10471870

TITANIUM™ 3

AgriLabs **Vaccine**

Bovine Rhinotracheitis-Virus Diarrhea Vaccine, Modified Live Virus (IBR-BVD)

U.S. Vet. Lic. No.: 213

Contents: This product contains the antigens listed above.

Contains neomycin as a preservative

Indications: For the vaccination of healthy cattle as an aid in the prevention of disease caused by bovine rhinotracheitis virus and bovine virus diarrhea virus, Type I and Type II.

Dosage and Administration: Rehydrate the desiccated vial with accompanying diluent and shake well. Inject 2 mL intramuscularly or subcutaneously using aseptic techniques. Annual revaccination is recommended. Calves vaccinated before weaning should be revaccinated 30 days after weaning when the possible influence of maternal antibodies is decreased.

Contraindication(s): Do not use in pregnant animals or in calves nursing pregnant animals. Abortions may result.

Precaution(s): Store at 35° to 45°F (2° to 7°C). Do not freeze. Use entire contents when first rehydrated. Burn container and all unused contents.

Caution(s): Allergic reactions may follow the use of vaccine.

Antidote(s): Epinephrine.

Warning(s): Do not vaccinate within 21 days before slaughter.

For use in animals only.

Presentation: 10 dose (20 mL) and 50 dose (100 mL) vials.

Manufactured by: Diamond Animal Health, Inc.

Compendium Code No.: 10581050

TITANIUM® 3

Intervet **Vaccine**

Bovine Rhinotracheitis-Virus Diarrhea Vaccine, Modified Live Virus

U.S. Vet. Lic. No.: 213

Contents: This product contains the antigens listed above.

Indications: For the vaccination of healthy cattle as an aid in the prevention of disease caused by bovine rhinotracheitis virus (IBR) and bovine virus diarrhea virus, Type I and Type II (BVD).

Dosage and Administration: Rehydrate the desiccated vial with accompanying diluent and shake well. Inject 2 mL subcutaneously or intramuscularly using aseptic technique. Annual revaccination is recommended. Calves vaccinated before weaning should be revaccinated 30 days after weaning when the possible influence of maternal antibodies is decreased.

Contraindication(s): Do not use in pregnant cows or in calves nursing pregnant cows, abortions may result.

Precaution(s): Store at 35° to 45°F (2° to 7°C). Do not freeze. Use entire contents when first opened. Burn container and all unused contents.

Caution(s): Allergic reactions may follow the use of vaccines.

For use in animals only.

Antidote(s): Epinephrine.

Warning(s): Do not vaccinate within 21 days before slaughter.

Presentation: 50 doses (100 mL).

TITANIUM® is a registerd trademark of Agri Laboratories, Ltd.

Manufactured by: Diamond Animal Health, Inc., Des Moines, IA 50327.

Compendium Code No.: 11062661 03313

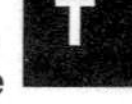

TITANIUM® 3+BRSV

Intervet **Vaccine**

Bovine Rhinotracheitis-Virus Diarrhea-Respiratory Syncytial Virus Vaccine, Modified Live Virus

U.S. Vet. Lic. No.: 213

Contents: This product contains the antigens listed above.

Indications: For the vaccination of healthy cattle as an aid in the prevention of disease caused by bovine rhinotracheitis virus (IBR), bovine virus diarrhea virus, Type I and Type II (BVD), bovine respiratory syncytial virus (BRSV).

Dosage and Administration: Rehydrate the desiccated vial with the accompanying diluent and shake well. Inject 2 mL subcutaneously or intramuscularly, using aseptic technique, followed by a second dose of monovalent bovine respiratory syncytial virus vaccine (Titanium® BRSV) to be given 14 to 28 days after the first dose. Annual revaccination is recommended. Calves vaccinated before weaning should be revaccinated 30 days after weaning when the possible influence of maternal antibodies is decreased.

Contraindication(s): Do not use in pregnant cows or in calves nursing pregnant cows, abortions may result.

Precaution(s): Store at 35° to 45°F (2° to 7°C). Do not freeze. Use entire contents when first opened. Burn container and all unused contents.
Caution(s): Allergic reactions may follow the use of vaccines.
For use in animals only.
Antidote(s): Epinephrine.
Warning(s): Do not vaccinate within 21 days before slaughter.
Presentation: 10 doses (20 mL) and 50 doses (100 mL).
TITANIUM® is a registered trademark of Agri Laboratories, Ltd.
Manufactured by: Diamond Animal Health, Inc., Des Moines, IA 50327.
Compendium Code No.: 11062670 01830-2

TITANIUM™ 3+BRSV LP

AgriLabs **Bacterin-Vaccine**
Bovine Rhinotracheitis-Virus Diarrhea-Respiratory Syncytial Virus Vaccine, Modified Live Virus-Leptospira pomona Bacterin (IBR-BVD-BRSV-Lepto P)
U.S. Vet. Lic. No.: 213
Contents: This product contains the antigens listed above.
Contains neomycin as a preservative.
Indications: For the vaccination of healthy cattle as an aid in the prevention of disease caused by bovine rhinotracheitis virus (IBR), bovine virus diarrhea virus, Type I and Type II (BVD), bovine respiratory syncytial virus (BRSV) and a bacterin (diluent) to be used as an aid in the prevention of disease caused by *Leptospira pomona.*
Dosage and Administration: Aseptically add the accompanying bottle of Lepto P bacterin (diluent) to the bottle of desiccated Titanium™ 3+BRSV. Agitate until dissolved and use entire contents immediately. Inject 2 mL intramuscularly or subcutaneously for cattle using aseptic techniques. Immunization against bovine respiratory syncytial virus requires a second dose of bovine respiratory syncytial virus (Titanium™ BRSV) vaccine given 14 to 28 days after the first dose. Annual revaccination is recommended. Calves vaccinated before weaning should be revaccinated 30 days after weaning when the possible influence of maternal antibodies is decreased.
Contraindication(s): Do not use in pregnant animals or in calves nursing pregnant animals. Abortions may follow use of this vaccine in pregnant animals.
Precaution(s): Store at 35° to 45°F (2° to 7°C). Do not freeze. Use entire contents when first rehydrated. Burn container and all unused contents.
Caution(s): Allergic reactions may follow the use of vaccine. For use in animals only.
Antidote(s): Epinephrine.
Warning(s): Do not vaccinate within 21 days before slaughter.
Presentation: 50 dose (100 mL) vial.
Manufactured by: Diamond Animal Health, Inc.
Compendium Code No.: 10581061

TITANIUM® 3+BRSV LP

Intervet **Bacterin-Vaccine**
Bovine Rhinotracheitis-Virus Diarrhea-Respiratory Syncytial Virus Vaccine, Modified Live Virus-Leptospira Pomona Bacterin
U.S. Vet. Lic. No.: 213
Contents: This product contains the antigens listed above.
Indications: For the vaccination of healthy cattle as an aid in the prevention of disease caused by bovine rhinotracheitis virus (IBR), bovine virus diarrhea virus, Type I and Type II (BVD), bovine respiratory syncytial virus (BRSV) and *Leptospira pomona.*
Dosage and Administration: Rehydrate the desiccated vial with the accompanying diluent and shake well. Inject 2 mL subcutaneously or intramuscularly using aseptic technique, followed by a second dose of monovalent bovine respiratory syncytial virus vaccine (Titanium® BRSV) to be given 14 to 28 days after the first dose. Annual revaccination is recommended. Calves vaccinated before weaning should be revaccinated 30 days after weaning when the possible influence of maternal antibodies is decreased.
Contraindication(s): Do not use in pregnant cows or in calves nursing pregnant cows, abortions may result.
Precaution(s): Store at 35° to 45°F (2° to 7°C). Do not freeze. Use entire contents when first opened. Burn container and all unused contents.
Caution(s): Allergic reactions may follow the use of vaccines. For use in animals only.
Antidote(s): Epinephrine.
Warning(s): Do not vaccinate within 21 days before slaughter.
Presentation: 10 doses (20 mL) and 50 doses (100 mL).
TITANIUM® is a registered trademark of Agri Laboratories, Ltd.
Manufactured by: Diamond Animal Health, Inc., Des Moines, IA 50327.
Compendium Code No.: 11062681 03289-2 / 03290-2

TITANIUM™ 4

AgriLabs **Vaccine**
Bovine Rhinotracheitis-Virus Diarrhea-Parainfluenza$_3$ Vaccine, Modified Live Virus (IBR-BVD-PI$_3$)
U.S. Vet. Lic. No.: 213
Contents: This product contains the antigens listed above.
Contains neomycin as a preservative.
Indications: For the vaccination of healthy cattle as an aid in the prevention of disease caused by bovine rhinotracheitis virus, bovine virus diarrhea virus, Type I and Type II and bovine parainfluenza$_3$ virus.
Dosage and Administration: Rehydrate the desiccated vial with accompanying diluent and shake well. Inject 2 mL intramuscularly or subcutaneously using aseptic techniques. Annual revaccination is recommended. Calves vaccinated before weaning should be revaccinated 30 days after weaning when the possible influence of maternal antibodies is decreased.
Contraindication(s): Do not use in pregnant animals or in calves nursing pregnant animals. Abortions may result.
Precaution(s): Store at 35° to 45°F (2° to 7°C). Do not freeze. Use entire contents when first rehydrated. Burn container and all unused contents.
Caution(s): Allergic reactions may follow the use of vaccine. For use in animals only.
Antidote(s): Epinephrine.
Warning(s): Do not vaccinate within 21 days before slaughter.
Presentation: 50 dose (100 mL) vial.
Manufactured by: Diamond Animal Health, Inc.
Compendium Code No.: 10581071

TITANIUM™ 4 L5

AgriLabs **Bacterin-Vaccine**
Bovine Rhinotracheitis-Virus Diarrhea-Parainfluenza$_3$ Vaccine, Modified Live Virus-Leptospira canicola-grippotyphosa-hardjo-icterohaemorrhagiae-pomona Bacterin (IBR-BVD-PI$_3$-Lepto 5)
U.S. Vet. Lic. No.: 213
Contents: This product contains the antigens listed above.
Contains neomycin as a preservative.
Indications: For the vaccination of healthy cattle as an aid in the prevention of disease caused by bovine rhinotracheitis (IBR), bovine virus diarrhea, Type I and Type II (BVD), and bovine parainfluenza$_3$ viruses (PI$_3$) and a bacterin (diluent) to be used as an aid in the prevention of disease caused by *Leptospira canicola-grippotyphosa-hardjo-icterohaemorrhagiae* and *Leptospira pomona* (Lepto 5).
Dosage and Administration: Rehydrate the desiccated vial with accompanying diluent and shake well. Inject 2 mL intramuscularly or subcutaneously using aseptic techniques. Annual revaccination is recommended. Calves vaccinated before weaning should be revaccinated 30 days after weaning when the possible influence of maternal antibodies is decreased.
Contraindication(s): Do not use in pregnant animals or in calves nursing pregnant animals. Abortions may result.
Precaution(s): Store at 35° to 45°F (2° to 7°C). Do not freeze. Use entire contents when first rehydrated. Burn container and all unused contents.
Caution(s): Allergic reactions may follow the use of vaccine. For use in animals only.
Antidote(s): Epinephrine.
Warning(s): Do not vaccinate within 21 days before slaughter.
Presentation: 10 dose (20 mL) vial.
Manufactured by: Diamond Animal Health, Inc.
Compendium Code No.: 10581081

TITANIUM™ 5

AgriLabs **Vaccine**
Bovine Rhinotracheitis-Virus Diarrhea-Parainfluenza$_3$-Respiratory Syncytial Virus Vaccine, Modified Live Virus (IBR-BVD-PI$_3$-BRSV)
U.S. Vet. Lic. No.: 213
Contents: This product contains the antigens listed above.
Contains neomycin as a preservative
Indications: For the vaccination of healthy cattle as an aid in the prevention of disease caused by bovine rhinotracheitis virus (IBR), bovine virus diarrhea virus, Type I and Type II (BVD), parainfluenza$_3$ virus (PI$_3$) and respiratory syncytial virus (BRSV).
Dosage and Administration: Rehydrate the desiccated vial with accompanying diluent and shake well. Inject 2 mL intramuscularly or subcutaneously using aseptic techniques. Immunization against bovine respiratory syncytial virus requires a second dose of bovine respiratory syncytial virus (Titanium™ BRSV) vaccine to be given 14 to 28 days after the first dose. Annual revaccination is recommended. Calves vaccinated before weaning should be revaccinated 30 days after weaning when the possible influence of maternal antibodies is decreased.
Contraindication(s): Do not use in pregnant animals or in calves nursing pregnant animals. Abortions may result.
Precaution(s): Store at 35° to 45°F (2° to 7°C). Do not freeze. Use entire contents when first rehydrated. Burn container and all unused contents.
Caution(s): Allergic reactions may follow the use of vaccine.
Antidote(s): Epinephrine.
Warning(s): Do not vaccinate within 21 days before slaughter. For use in animals only.
Presentation: 10 dose (20 mL) and 50 dose (100 mL) vials.
Manufactured by: Diamond Animal Health, Inc.
Compendium Code No.: 10581090

TITANIUM® 5

Intervet **Vaccine**
Bovine Rhinotracheitis-Virus Diarrhea-Parainfluenza$_3$-Respiratory Syncytial Virus Vaccine, Modified Live Virus
U.S. Vet. Lic. No.: 213
Contents: This product contains the antigens listed above.
Indications: For the vaccination of healthy cattle as an aid in the prevention of disease caused by bovine rhinotracheitis virus (IBR), bovine virus diarrhea virus, Type I and II (BVD), bovine parainfluenza$_3$ virus (PI$_3$) and bovine respiratory syncytial virus (BRSV).
Dosage and Administration: Rehydrate the desiccated vial with accompanying diluent and shake well. Inject 2 mL subcutaneously or intramuscularly using aseptic technique, followed by a second dose of monovalent bovine respiratory syncytial virus vaccine (Titanium® BRSV) to be given 14 to 28 days after the first dose. Annual revaccination is recommended. Calves vaccinated before weaning should be revaccinated 30 days after weaning when the possible influence of maternal antibodies is decreased.
Contraindication(s): Do not use in pregnant cows or in calves nursing pregnant cows, abortions may result.
Precaution(s): Store at 35° to 45°F (2° to 7°C). Do not freeze. Use entire contents when first opened. Burn container and all unused contents.
Caution(s): Allergic reactions may follow the use of vaccines. For use in animals only.
Antidote(s): Epinephrine.
Warning(s): Do not vaccinate within 21 days before slaughter.
Presentation: 10 doses (20 mL) and 50 doses (100 mL).
TITANIUM® is a registered trademark of Agri Laboratories, Ltd.
Manufactured by: Diamond Animal Health, Inc., Des Moines, IA 50327.
Compendium Code No.: 11062691 03283-2 / 03284-2

TITANIUM™ 5 L5

AgriLabs **Bacterin-Vaccine**
Bovine Rhinotracheitis-Virus Diarrhea-Parainfluenza$_3$-Respiratory Syncytial Virus Vaccine, Modified Live Virus-Leptospira canicola-grippotyphosa-hardjo-icterohaemorrhagiae-pomona Bacterin (IBR-BVD-PI$_3$-BRSV-Lepto 5)
U.S. Vet. Lic. No.: 213
Contents: This product contains the antigens listed above.
Contains neomycin as a preservative.
Indications: For the vaccination of healthy cattle as an aid in the prevention of disease caused by bovine rhinotracheitis (IBR), bovine virus diarrhea virus, Type I and Type II (BVD), bovine

parainfluenza$_3$ viruses (PI$_3$) and bovine respiratory syncytial virus (BRSV) and a bacterin (diluent) to be used as an aid in the prevention of disease caused by *Leptospira canicola-grippotyphosa-hardjo-icterohaemorrhagiae* and *Leptospira pomona* (Lepto 5).
Dosage and Administration: Rehydrate the desiccated vial with accompanying diluent and shake well. Inject 2 mL intramuscularly or subcutaneously using aseptic techniques, followed by a second dose of monovalent Titanium™ BRSV in 14 to 28 days. Annual revaccination is recommended. Calves vaccinated before weaning should be revaccinated 30 days after weaning when the possible influence of maternal antibodies is decreased.
Contraindication(s): Do not use in pregnant animals or in calves nursing pregnant animals. Abortions may result.
Precaution(s): Store at 35° to 45°F (2° to 7°C). Do not freeze. Use entire contents when first rehydrated. Burn container and all unused contents.
Caution(s): Allergic reactions may follow the use of vaccine.
For use in animals only.
Antidote(s): Epinephrine.
Warning(s): Do not vaccinate within 21 days before slaughter.
Presentation: 5 dose (10 mL), 10 dose (20 mL) and 50 dose (100 mL) vials.
Manufactured by: Diamond Animal Health, Inc.
Compendium Code No.: 10581101

TITANIUM® 5 L5

Intervet **Bacterin-Vaccine**

Bovine Rhinotracheitis-Virus Diarrhea-Parainfluenza$_3$-Respiratory Syncytial Virus Vaccine, Modified Live Virus-Leptospira Canicola-Grippotyphosa-Hardjo-Icterohaemorrhagiae-Pomona Bacterin
U.S. Vet. Lic. No.: 213
Contents: This product contains the antigens listed above.
Indications: For the vaccination of healthy cattle as an aid in the prevention of disease caused by bovine rhinotracheitis virus (IBR), bovine virus diarrhea virus, Type I and Type II (BVD), bovine parainfluenza$_3$ virus (PI$_3$) and bovine respiratory syncytial virus (BRSV) and *Leptospira canicola, L. grippotyphosa, L. hardjo, L. icterohaemorrhagiae* and *L. pomona.*
Dosage and Administration: Rehydrate the desiccated vial with accompanying diluent and shake well. Inject 2 mL subcutaneously or intramuscularly using aseptic technique, followed by a second dose of monovalent bovine respiratory syncytial virus vaccine (Titanium® BRSV) to be given 14 to 28 days after the first dose. Annual revaccination is recommended. Calves vaccinated before weaning should be revaccinated 30 days after weaning when the possible influence of maternal antibodies is decreased.
Contraindication(s): Do not use in pregnant cows or in calves nursing pregnant cows, abortions may result.
Precaution(s): Store at 35° to 45°F (2° to 7°C). Do not freeze. Use entire contents when first opened. Burn container and all unused contents.
Caution(s): Allergic reactions may follow the use of vaccines. For use in animals only.
Antidote(s): Epinephrine.
Warning(s): Do not vaccinate within 21 days before slaughter.
Presentation: 10 doses (20 mL) and 50 doses (100 mL).
TITANIUM® is a registered trademark of Agri Laboratories, Ltd.
Manufactured by: Diamond Animal Health, Inc., Des Moines, IA 50327.
Compendium Code No.: 11062701 03287-2 / 03288-2

TITANIUM® 5+P.H.M. BAC®-1

AgriLabs **Vaccine**

Bovine Rhinotracheitis-Virus Diarrhea-Parainfluenza$_3$-Respiratory Syncytial Virus Vaccine, Modified Live Virus-Pasteurella Haemolytica-Multocida Vaccine, Avirulent Live Culture
U.S. Vet. Lic. No.: 213
Contents: This product contains the antigens listed above.
From the Signature cell line® IBR-BVD-PI$_3$-BRSV-P.h.-P.m.
Contains streptomycin as a preservative.
Indications: For the vaccination of healthy cattle as an aid in the prevention of disease caused by infectious bovine rhinotracheitis virus (IBR), bovine virus diarrhea virus, Type I and Type II (BVD), bovine parainfluenza$_3$ viruses (PI$_3$) and bovine respiratory syncytial virus (BRSV) and disease caused by *Pasteurella haemolytica* and *Pasteurella multocida.*
Directions: Asepticaly rehydrate P.H.M. BAC®-1 (bacterial component) with the accompanying diluent, agitate until dissolved, then use the mixture to rehydrate TITANIUM®5 (viral component), shake well. Inject 2 mL intramuscularly using aseptic technique. Immunization against BRSV requires a second dose of bovine respiratory syncytial virus vaccine (Titanium® BRSV) to be given 14 to 28 days after the first dose. Annual revaccination is recommended. Calves vaccinated before weaning should be revaccinated 30 days after weaning when the possible influence of maternal antibodies is decreased.
Contraindication(s): Do not use in pregnant cows or in calves nursing pregnant cows. Abortions may result.
Precaution(s): Store in the dark at 35° to 45°F (2° to 7°C). Do not freeze.
Use entire contents when first opened. Care should be taken to avoid chemical or microbial contamination of the product. Burn container and all unused contents.
Caution(s): Allergic reactions may follow the use of vaccines.
Antidote(s): Epinephrine.
Warning(s): Do not vaccinate within 21 days before slaughter.
For use in animals only.
Presentation: 10 dose (20 mL) and 50 dose (100 mL) vials.
Manufactured by: Diamond Animal Health, Inc., Des Moines, Iowa 50317 U.S.A.
Compendium Code No.: 10581040

TITANIUM® 5+P.H.M. BAC®-1

Intervet **Vaccine**

Bovine Rhinotracheitis-Virus Diarrhea-Parainfluenza$_3$-Respiratory Syncytial Virus-Pasteurella Haemolytica-Multocida Vaccine, Modified Live Virus and Avirulent Live Culture
U.S. Vet. Lic. No.: 286
Contents: TITANIUM® 5+P.H.M. BAC®-1 is a multi-antigenic modified and avirulent live vaccine.
The five viral antigens and two bacterial antigens (as listed above) are combined in the proper ratio, stabilized, and desiccated respectively.
Contains streptomycin as a preservative.
Indications: For the vaccination of healthy cattle as an aid in the prevention of disease caused by Infectious Bovine Rhinotracheitis (IBR), Bovine Virus Diarrhea (BVD) Type I and Type II, Parainfluenza$_3$ (PI$_3$), Bovine Respiratory Syncytial Virus (BRSV) and respiratory disease caused by *Pasteurella haemolytica* and *Pasteurella multocida.*
Dosage and Administration: Directions: Aseptically add the accompanying bottle of diluent to Once PMH® (bacterial component). Agitate until dissolved and aseptically add this rehydrated Once PMH® to the Titanium® 5 (IBR BVD-PI$_3$-BRSV viral component) vial. Shake well and use entire contents immediately.
Dosage: Inject 2 mL intramuscularly for cattle of all ages, using aseptic technique. Immunization against Bovine Respiratory Syncytial Virus requires a second dose of monovalent modified live Bovine Respiratory Syncytial Virus vaccine (Titanium® BRSV) to be given 14 to 28 days after the first dose. Annual revaccination is recommended. Calves vaccinated before weaning should be revaccinated 30 days after weaning when the possible influence of maternal antibodies is decreased.
Contraindication(s): Do not use in pregnant animals or in calves nursing pregnant animals. Abortion may follow use of this vaccine.
Precaution(s): Store in the dark at 35°-45°F (2°C-7°C). Do not freeze. Use entire contents when first rehydrated. Burn the containers and all unused contents.
Caution(s): Allergic reactions may follow the use of product of this nature.
Scientific evidence demonstrates the inability of some animals of an occasional herd to develop antibodies to Bovine Viral Diarrhea virus after vaccination. This affected animal may exhibit symptoms similar to mucosal disease.
Administer only to healthy animals. Animals infected by disease agents may suffer adverse reaction after vaccination. For veterinary use only.
Antidote(s): Epinephrine.
Warning(s): Do not vaccinate within 21 days before slaughter.
Trial Data: Safety of the combined vaccine was demonstrated under field conditions.
Vaccine antigenicity and lack of antigenic interference were determined by measuring antibody response of serologically negative calves to vaccination for IBR-BVD-PI$_3$-BRSV. Lack of interference between the viral and bacterial antigens was determined by *in vitro* and *in vivo* studies.
Vaccine efficacy was demonstrated by resistance of vaccinated calves to challenge with virulent IBR, PI$_3$, BRSV, *P. haemolytica* or *P. multocida* in comparison to non-vaccinated controls and by measuring antibody levels to the viruses before and after vaccination.
Discussion: Serologic surveys indicate the five viruses and two strains of *Pasteurella* are widespread in the cattle population. The viruses and bacteria are considered contributors to the respiratory disease complex of cattle. Multiple virus infections do occur, and *Pasteurella* infection may exacerbate the disease signs. *Pasteurella* may also play a primary role in respiratory diseases.
Signs of IBR may include high fever, hyperpnea, dyspnea, and severe inflammation of the nasal mucosa with formation of mucoid plaques. BVD manifests itself in many ways making diagnosis difficult. Since diarrhea may be one of the lesser signs seen, it is unfortunate the word diarrhea is associated with the name of the disease. A transient diarrhea may be unnoticed until more severe signs are observed in the herd. Respiratory signs, rough hair coat, laminitis, and decreased weight gains are also seen. Generally, morbidity is high and mortality is low; however, complications with other conditions are common and will increase the severity and mortality.
BVD is often obscured or confused with other conditions of the respiratory disease complex. BVD in pregnant animals may cause abortions or malformed and weak calves at birth. Chronic disease with erosions in the alimentary tract is referred to as "Mucosal Disease" and is usually fatal.
Disease signs caused by PI$_3$ virus generally appear within 14 days after shipment and arrival of calves at their destination. Signs are weakness, depression, watery to mucopurulent nasal discharge, fever, coughing, and weight loss.
BRSV infections generally affect weaned calves although susceptible cattle of any age may become infected. BRSV signs follow an incubation of 5 to 7 days and may include fever, cough, nasal discharge, ocular discharge, anorexia, hyperpnea, pulmonary edema and emphysema, and denuding of the ciliated epithelium, leading to secondary bacterial pneumonia and associated sequela. BRSV signs vary in severity but may rapidly progress to a crisis phase.
Pasteurella haemolytica and *Pasteurella multocida* are associated with many diseases and are major causative pathogens for bovine respiratory diseases. They may be a primary agent but more frequently they are secondary invaders when resistance of animals is reduced by primary infections by viruses or other organisms, or by various stresses. The major disease associated with *P. haemolytica* and *P. multocida* is pneumonia of cattle.
Presentation: 10 doses (20 mL) and 50 doses (100 mL).
TITANIUM® is a registered trademark of Agri Laboratories, Ltd.
Distributed by: Agri Laboratories, Ltd., St. Joseph, MO 64505.
Compendium Code No.: 11062710 Rev. 97801

TITANIUM™ BRSV

AgriLabs **Vaccine**

Bovine Respiratory Syncytial Virus Vaccine, Modified Live Virus
U.S. Vet. Lic. No.: 213
Contents: This product contains the antigens listed above.
Indications: For the vaccination of healthy cattle as an aid in the prevention of disease caused by bovine respiratory syncytial virus (BRSV).
Directions: Rehydrate with accompanying diluent and shake well. Inject 2 mL intramuscularly or subcutaneously using aseptic techniques. Repeat the dose in 14 to 28 days. Annual revaccination is recommended. Calves vaccinated before weaning should be revaccinated 30 days after weaning when the possible influence of maternal antibodies is decreased.
Precaution(s): Store at 35° to 45°F (2° to 7°C). Do not freeze. Use entire contents when first opened. Burn container and all unused contents.
Caution(s): Allergic reactions may follow the use of vaccines.
Antidote(s): Epinephrine.
Warning(s): Do not vaccinate within 21 days before slaughter. For use in animals only.
Presentation: 10 dose (20 mL) and 50 dose (100 mL) vials.
Manufactured by: Diamond Animal Health, Inc., Des Moines, Iowa 50317 U.S.A.
Compendium Code No.: 10581111 01627-1

TITANIUM® BRSV

Intervet **Vaccine**

Bovine Respiratory Syncytial Virus Vaccine, Modified Live Virus
U.S. Vet. Lic. No.: 213
Contents: This product contains the antigens listed above.
Indications: For the vaccination of healthy cattle as an aid in the prevention of disease caused by bovine respiratory syncytial virus (BRSV).
Directions: Rehydrate with accompanying diluent and shake well. Inject 2 mL subcutaneously

or intramuscularly using aseptic technique, followed by a second dose of monovalent bovine respiratory syncytial virus vaccine to be give 14 to 28 days after the first dose. Annual revaccination is recommended. Calves vaccinated before weaning should be revaccinated 30 days after weaning when the possible influence of maternal antibodies is decreased.
Precaution(s): Store at 35° to 45°F (2° to 7°C). Do not freeze. Use entire contents when first opened. Burn container and all unused contents.
Caution(s): Allergic reactions may follow the use of vaccines. For use in animals only.
Antidote(s): Epinephrine.
Warning(s): Do not vaccinate within 21 days before slaughter.
Presentation: 50 doses (100 mL).
TITANIUM® is a registered trademark of Agri Laboratories, Ltd.
Manufactured by: Diamond Animal Health, Inc., Des Moines, IA 50327.
Compendium Code No.: 11062720 03293-2

TITANIUM™ BRSV 3

AgriLabs **Vaccine**

Bovine Rhinotracheitis-Parainfluenza$_3$-Respiratory Syncytial Virus Vaccine, Modified Live Virus (IBR-PI$_3$-BRSV)
U.S. Vet. Lic. No.: 213
Contents: This product contains the antigens listed above.
Contains neomycin as a preservative.
Indications: For the vaccination of healthy cattle as an aid in the prevention of disease caused by bovine rhinotracheitis virus (IBR), parainfluenza$_3$ viruses (PI$_3$) and respiratory syncytial virus (BRSV).
Dosage and Administration: Rehydrate with accompanying diluent and shake well. Aseptically inject 2 mL intramuscularly or subcutaneously followed by a second dose of monovalent Titanium™ BRSV in 14 to 28 days. Annual revaccination is recommended. Calves vaccinated before weaning should be revaccinated 30 days after weaning when the possible influence of maternal antibodies is decreased.
Contraindication(s): Do not use in pregnant animals or in calves nursing pregnant animals. Abortions may result.
Precaution(s): Store at 35° to 45°F (2° to 7°C). Do not freeze. Use entire contents when first rehydrated. Burn container and all unused contents.
Caution(s): Allergic reactions may follow the use of vaccine.
For use in animals only.
Antidote(s): Epinephrine.
Warning(s): Do not vaccinate within 21 days before slaughter.
Presentation: 50 dose (100 mL) vial.
Manufactured by: Diamond Animal Health, Inc.
Compendium Code No.: 10581121

TITANIUM® BRSV 3

Intervet **Vaccine**

Bovine Rhinotracheitis-Parainfluenza$_3$-Respiratory Syncytial Virus Vaccine, Modified Live Virus
U.S. Vet. Lic. No.: 213
Contents: This product contains the antigens listed above.
Indications: For the vaccination of healthy cattle as an aid in the prevention of disease caused by bovine rhinotracheitis virus (IBR), bovine parainfluenza$_3$ virus (PI$_3$) and bovine respiratory syncytial virus (BRSV).
Dosage and Administration: Rehydrate the desiccated vial with the accompanying diluent and shake well. Inject 2 mL subcutaneously or intramuscularly, using aseptic technique, followed by a second dose of monovalent bovine respiratory syncytial virus vaccine (Titanium® BRSV) to be given 14 to 28 days after the first dose. Annual revaccination is recommended. Calves vaccinated before weaning should be revaccinated 30 days after weaning when the possible influence of maternal antibodies is decreased.
Contraindication(s): Do not use in pregnant cows or in calves nursing pregnant cows, abortions may result.
Precaution(s): Store at 35° to 45°F (2° to 7°C). Do not freeze. Use entire contents when first opened. Burn container and all unused contents.
Caution(s): Allergic reactions may follow the use of vaccines.
For use in animals only.
Antidote(s): Epinephrine.
Warning(s): Do not vaccinate within 21 days before slaughter.
Presentation: 10 doses (20 mL) and 50 doses (100 mL).
TITANIUM® is a registered trademark of Agri Laboratories, Ltd.
Manufactured by: Diamond Animal Health, Inc., Des Moines, IA 50327.
Compendium Code No.: 11062731 03285-2 / 03286-2

TITANIUM™ IBR

AgriLabs **Vaccine**

Bovine Rhinotracheitis Vaccine, Modified Live Virus (IBR)
U.S. Vet. Lic. No.: 213
Contents: This product contains the antigens listed above.
Contains neomycin as a preservative
Indications: For the vaccination of healthy cattle as an aid in the prevention of disease caused by bovine rhinotracheitis virus (IBR).
Dosage and Administration: Rehydrate with desiccated vial with accompanying diluent and shake well. Inject 2 mL subcutaneously or intramuscularly using aseptic techniques. Annual revaccination is recommended. Calves vaccinated before weaning should be revaccinated 30 days after weaning when the possible influence of maternal antibodies is decreased.
Contraindication(s): Do not use in pregnant animals or in calves nursing pregnant animals. Abortions may result.
Precaution(s): Store at 35° to 45°F (2° to 7°C). Do not freeze. Use entire contents when first rehydrated. Burn container and all unused contents.
Caution(s): Allergic reactions may follow the use of vaccine.
Antidote(s): Epinephrine.
Warning(s): Do not vaccinate within 21 days before slaughter.
For use in animals only.
Presentation: 10 dose (20 mL) and 50 dose (100 mL) vials.
Manufactured by: Diamond Animal Health, Inc.
Compendium Code No.: 10581130

TITANIUM® IBR

Intervet **Vaccine**

Bovine Rhinotracheitis Vaccine, Modified Live Virus
U.S. Vet. Lic. No.: 213
Contents: This product contains the antigens listed above.
Indications: For the vaccination of healthy cattle as an aid in the prevention of disease caused by bovine rhinotracheitis virus (IBR).
Dosage and Administration: Rehydrate the desiccated vial with the accompanying diluent and shake well. Inject 2 mL subcutaneously or intramuscularly using aseptic technique. Annual revaccination is recommended. Calves vaccinated before weaning should be revaccinated 30 days after weaning when the possible influence of maternal antibodies is decreased.
Contraindication(s): Do not use in pregnant cows or in calves nursing pregnant cows, abortions may result.
Precaution(s): Store at 35° to 45°F (2° to 7°C). Do not freeze. Use entire contents when first opened. Burn container and all unused contents.
Caution(s): Allergic reactions may follow the use of vaccine.
For use in animals only.
Antidote(s): Epinephrine.
Warning(s): Do not vaccinate within 21 days before slaughter.
Presentation: 50 doses (100 mL).
TITANIUM® is a registered trademark of Agri Laboratories. Ltd.
Manufactured by: Diamond Animal Health, Inc., Des Moines, IA 50327.
Compendium Code No.: 11062740 03298-2

TITANIUM™ IBR-LP

AgriLabs **Bacterin-Vaccine**

Bovine Rhinotracheitis Vaccine, Modified Live Virus-Leptospira pomona Bacterin (IBR-Lepto P)
U.S. Vet. Lic. No.: 213
Contents: This product contains the antigens listed above.
Contains neomycin as a preservative.
Indications: For the vaccination of healthy cattle as an aid in the prevention of disease caused by bovine rhinotracheitis virus (IBR) and a bacterin (diluent) to be used as an aid in the prevention of disease caused by *Leptospira pomona* (Lepto P).
Dosage and Administration: Aseptically add the accompanying bottle of Leptospira Pomona Bacterin (diluent) to the bottle of desiccated vaccine. Agitate until dissolved and use entire contents immediately. Inject 2 mL intramuscularly or subcutaneously using aseptic techniques. Annual revaccination is recommended. Calves vaccinated before weaning should be revaccinated 30 days after weaning when the possible influence of maternal antibodies is decreased.
Contraindication(s): Do not use in pregnant animals or in calves nursing pregnant animals. Abortions may result.
Precaution(s): Store at 35° to 45°F (2° to 7°C). Do not freeze. Use entire contents when first rehydrated. Burn container and all unused contents.
Caution(s): Allergic reactions may follow the use of vaccine.
For use in animals only.
Antidote(s): Epinephrine.
Warning(s): Do not vaccinate within 21 days before slaughter.
Presentation: 50 dose (100 mL) vial.
Manufactured by: Diamond Animal Health, Inc.
Compendium Code No.: 10581141

TITERCHEK™ CDV/CPV

Synbiotics **Distemper-Parvovirus Test**

Canine Distemper-Parvovirus Antibody Test Kit
U.S. Vet. Lic. No.: 312
Test Description: TITERCHEK™ CDV/CPV is an ELISA based assay used for the determination of antibody levels to Canine Distemper Virus (CDV) and Canine Parvovirus (CPV) in canine serum or plasma samples.
Contents: Contents of Kit: The following items are packaged in each kit:

	16 test	24 test	48 test
CDV Antigen Coated Wells	2 x 8	3 x 8	6 x 8
CPV Antigen Coated Wells	2 x 8	3 x 8	6 x 8
Bottle A - Positive Control (Red Cap)	1.0 mL	2.0 mL	3.0 mL
Bottle B - Negative Control/Sample Diluent (Gray Cap)	3.0 mL	5.0 mL	7.0 mL
Bottle C - Conjugate (Blue Cap)	2.0 mL	3.0 mL	5.0 mL
Bottle D - Chromogenic Substrate (Green Cap)	3.0 mL	5.0 mL	7.0 mL
Bottle E - 10X Wash Solution (Orange Cap)	100 mL	100 mL	100 mL
Direction Insert	1	1	1
Disposable Sample Loops	50	50	100
Well Holder	1	1	1

Additional material required but not provided: Deionized or distilled water; squirt bottles (2); timer.
Indications: For the determination of Canine Distemper Virus and Canine Parvovirus antibody levels.
Test Principles: Color coded plastic wells are coated with either purified canine distemper virus (CDV) antigen or canine parvovirus (CPV) antigen. Serum or plasma samples are incubated in the coated wells followed by incubation with polyclonal rabbit anti-dog IgG conjugated to Hrp. Antibodies to CDV and/or CPV, if present in the canine samples, are bound to the specific antigen coated wells and, in turn, bind the anti-dog IgG conjugate. The free, unbound enzyme-linked conjugate is washed away and a chromogenic substrate is added. For CDV, a positive test result is intended to indicate a serum neutralization titer of 1:16 or greater, and a negative test result should indicate a serum neutralization titer of less than 1:16. For CPV, a positive test result is intended to indicate a hemagglutination titer of 1:80 or greater; and a negative test result should indicate a hemagglutination titer of less than 1:80.

TITERCHEK™ CDV/CPV is highly specific, sensitive and simple to perform. Test results can be obtained in 15 minutes. The diagnostic kit contains a positive control and a negative control which must be included each time the assay is performed. Visual comparison of the color of samples to the positive control for each assay will allow accurate detection of the presence of CDV and/or CPV antibody in the sample.

Sample Collection: Sample Information: One microliter (1 µL) of serum or plasma is required. Use only canine samples for test specimens. Samples may be stored at 2°-7°C (36°-45°F) up to seven days. If longer storage is desired, samples may be stored at -20°C or below. Severely hemolyzed or lipemic serum may produce background color. When in doubt, obtain a better quality sample.

Test Procedure: Preparation of Wash Solution: Allow wash concentrate to come to room temperature. Mix gently by inversion. Dilute wash concentrate 10-fold with distilled or deionized water (1 part concentrate to 9 parts dH_2O) in a squirt bottle. Reconstituted wash solution may be stored at 2°-7°C (36°-45°F).

A. Set Up and Sample Incubation:

1. Remove and place CDV wells (white rim) in top half of holder, one well for Positive Control (Bottle A - Red Cap), one well for Negative Control (Bottle B - Gray Cap), and one well for each sample to be tested. Place CPV wells (red rim) in bottle half of holder; one well for Positive Control, one well for Negative Control and one well for each sample to be tested. Leave the required number of wells attached to each other.
2. Add 1 drop of Positive Control (Bottle A - Red Cap) into the first CDV well and first CPV well.
3. Place 1 drop of Negative Control/Sample Diluent (Bottle B - Gray Cap) into the second CDV well and to each CDV test sample well. Place 1 drop of Negative Control/Sample Diluent to the second CPV well and to each CPV test sample well.
4. Using a separate sample loop for each sample, add 1 loopful (1 µL) of each sample to each of the CDV and CPV sample wells. Mix sample in diluent thoroughly by twisting the handle of the loop between the thumb and forefinger. Be careful not to splash from well to well. Incubate for 5 minutes at room temperature (21°-25°C; 70°-78°F).
If several samples are run simultaneously, only one set of CDV and CPV controls are needed.

B. Blot and Wash:

5. Discard the fluid from wells into sink or appropriate container. Wash wells once by vigorously filling the wells to overflowing the diluted wash solution (see Preparation of Wash Solution for preparation).
Discard excess fluid into sink or appropriate container. Invert holder and blot firmly onto a paper towel to remove final drops.

C. Conjugate:

6. Add 1 drop of Conjugate (Bottle C - Blue Cap) into each well. Gently tap the holder for 10-15 seconds and incubate for 5 minutes at room temperature (21°-25°C; 70°-78°F).

D. Blot and Wash:

7. Discard the fluid from wells into sink or appropriate container. Wash by vigorously filling the wells to overflowing with diluted wash solution. Discard the fluid from the wells and blot after each wash. Repeat the washing procedure three (3) times. Wash two more times with distilled or deionized water to remove bubbles.
Discard excess fluid into sink or appropriate container. Invert holder and blot firmly onto a paper towel to remove final drops.

E. Develop:

8. Place 2 drops of Chromogenic Substrate (Bottle D - Green Cap) into each well. Mix by gently tapping the holder several times. Incubate 5 minutes.
After incubating, gently tap holder for 5 seconds and read results immediately. See Interpretation of Results section.

Test Interpretation:

F. Interpretation of Results:

9. Compare each CDV sample well with the CDV positive and negative control wells. Compare each CPV sample well with the CPV positive and negative control wells.
Development of a blue color in the sample well that is of equal or greater intensity than the color of the Positive Control well is considered to be positive (CDV SN titer ≥ 1:16 or CPV HI titer ≥ 1:80.
No blue color in the sample well or color that is of less intensity than the color of the Positive Control Well is considered to be negative (CDV SN titer <1:16 or CPV HI titer <1:80).
For the test to be valid, the fluid in the positive control well must be distinctly blue, while that in the negative control well must show no color change from initial substrate color. Results should be interpreted immediately after the 5 minute incubation period in Step 7. Wells can be detached and compared alongside the positive control well using a white background for easier visual inspection.

Storage: Storage and Stability: Store the test kit and unused diluted wash solution at 2°-7°C (36°-45°F). Do not freeze. Reagents should be stable until expiration date provided they have been stored properly.

Caution(s):

1. Allow kit to come to room temperature (21°-25°C; 70°-78°F) prior to use.
2. Use separate sample loop for each sample.
3. Do not expose kit to direct sunlight.
4. Do not use expired reagents or mix from different kit lots.
5. Follow instructions exactly. Improper washing or contamination of reagents may produce non-specific color development.
6. For veterinary use only.

Good Techniques = Accurate Results

Serum or plasma must be used as a sample.

Hemolyzed and lipemic serum samples may be used, however, severely hemolyzed and lipemic samples may produce a background color. When in doubt, obtain a better quality sample.

Washing is the most important step. Wells cannot be overwashed. Underwashing will result in color development in the negative control and negative sample wells.

Prolonged incubation for more than 5 minutes in step 8 may result in non-specific color development. If no color is seen after 5 minutes, the sample is negative.

Always compare results to the positive control. The kit negative control is used to verify good washing technique. It should not be used to differentiate positive from negative results.

Do not use the test kit past the expiration date and do not intermix components from different serial numbers.

Trial Data: Research Results: In order to evaluate the sensitivity and specificity of TITERCHEK™, the veterinary diagnostic laboratories of Kansas State University (KSU), University of Georgia (UGA), University of Wisconsin (UW) and Synbiotics Corporation each tested samples for which CDV serum neutralization or CPV hemagglutination titers had been determined in the respective laboratories. Results of these studies are summarized below.

CDV Sensitivity:

	Samples	Correct	Identified
UGA	53	41	77%
KSU	62	56	90%
UW	54	46	85%
Synbiotics	99	97	98%

CDV Specificity:

	Samples	Correct	Identified
UGA	8	7	88%
KSU	2	2	100%
UW	11	11	100%
Synbiotics	57	53	93%

CPV Sensitivity:

	Samples	Correct	Identified
UGA	60	55	92%
KSU	64	61	95%
UW	51	38	75%
Synbiotics	103	91	88%

CPV Specificity:

	Samples	Correct	Identified
UGA	1	1	100%
KSU	56	55	98%
UW	69	68	99%
Synbiotics	44	42	95%

References: Available upon request.
Presentation: 5-14 test kit.
Compendium Code No.: 11150540 03-1300-0302

TITERVAC™ 5

Aspen **Vaccine**

Bovine Rhinotracheitis-Virus Diarrhea-Parainfluenza$_3$-Respiratory Syncytial Virus Vaccine, Modified Live Virus

U.S. Vet. Lic. No.: 124

Contents: This product contains the antigens listed above.
Preservative: Neomycin.

Indications: Recommended for the vaccination of healthy, susceptible cattle as an aid in the reduction of diseases caused by Bovine Rhinotracheitis (IBR), Bovine Virus Diarrhea (BVD) Types 1 and 2, Parainfluenza$_3$ (PI$_3$), and Bovine Respiratory Syncytial virus (BRSV).

Directions: Rehydrate the vaccine by aseptically adding the accompanying liquid diluent to the vaccine vial.

Dosage: Using aseptic technique, inject 2 mL intramuscularly. Repeat in 14 to 28 days and once annually. Calves vaccinated before 6 months of age should be revaccinated at 6 months. A 2 mL booster dose is recommended prior to time of stress or exposure.

Contraindication(s): It is possible that healthy appearing cattle can be persistently infected with or incubating virulent BVD virus at time of vaccination. In view of these findings and suggested causes, BVD vaccine is contraindicated in persistently infected cattle and use should be limited only to healthy, immunocompetent, unstressed, non-pregnant cattle.

Precaution(s): Store out of direct sunlight at a temperature between 35-45°F (2-7°C). Avoid freezing. Shake well before using. Use entire contents when first opened.

Caution(s): Stressed cattle should not be vaccinated. Do not use in pregnant cows or in calves nursing pregnant cows. Burn containers and all unused contents. Injection site swelling may occur. Anaphylactoid reactions may occur.

Antidote(s): Epinephrine.

Warning(s): Do not vaccinate within 21 days of slaughter.

Animal inoculation only. Accidental injection to humans can cause serious local reactions. Contact a physician immediately if accidental injection occurs.

Presentation: 10 dose vial of MLV vaccine (20 mL vial sterile water diluent) and 50 dose vial of MLV vaccine (100 mL vial sterile water diluent).

Manufactured by: Boehringer Ingelheim Vetmedica, Inc., St. Joseph, Missouri 64506 U.S.A.

Compendium Code No.: 14750880 26313-00

TITERVAC™ 5-HS

Aspen **Vaccine**

Bovine Rhinotracheitis-Virus Diarrhea-Parainfluenza$_3$-Respiratory Syncytial Virus Vaccine, Modified Live Virus-Haemophilus Somnus Bacterin

U.S. Vet. Lic. No.: 124

Contents: This product contains the antigens listed above.
Preservative: Neomycin.

Indications: Recommended for the vaccination of healthy, susceptible cattle as an aid in the reduction of diseases caused by Bovine Rhinotracheitis (IBR) virus, Bovine Virus Diarrhea (BVD) Types 1 and 2, Parainfluenza$_3$ (PI$_3$), Bovine Respiratory Syncytial virus (BRSV), and *Haemophilus somnus.*

Directions: Rehydrate the modified live virus vaccine by aseptically adding the accompanying bottle of liquid bacterin.

Dosage: Using aseptic technique, inject 2 mL intramuscularly. Repeat in 14 to 28 days and once annually. Calves vaccinated before 6 months of age should be revaccinated at 6 months. A 2 mL booster dose is recommended prior to time of stress or exposure.

Contraindication(s): It is possible that healthy appearing cattle can be persistently infected with or incubating virulent BVD virus at time of vaccination. In view of these findings and suggested causes, BVD vaccine is contraindicated in persistently infected cattle and use should be limited only to healthy, immunocompetent, unstressed, non-pregnant cattle.

Precaution(s): Store out of direct sunlight at a temperature between 35-45°F (2-7°C). Avoid freezing. Shake well before using. Use entire contents when first opened.

Caution(s): Stressed cattle should not be vaccinated. Do not use in pregnant cows or in calves

nursing pregnant cows. Burn containers and all unused contents. Injection site swelling may occur. Anaphylactoid reactions may occur.
Antidote(s): Epinephrine.
Warning(s): Do not vaccinate within 21 days of slaughter.
Animal inoculation only. Accidental injection to humans can cause serious local reactions. Contact a physician immediately if accidental injection occurs.
Presentation: 10 dose vial of MLV vaccine (20 mL vial of liquid bacterin diluent) and 50 dose vial of MLV vaccine (100 mL vial of liquid bacterin diluent).
Manufactured by: Boehringer Ingelheim Vetmedica, Inc., St. Joseph, Missouri 64506 U.S.A.
Compendium Code No.: 14750890 26407-00

TITERVAC™ 10

Aspen **Bacterin-Vaccine**

Bovine Rhinotracheitis-Virus Diarrhea-Parainfluenza$_3$-Respiratory Syncytial Virus Vaccine, Modified Live Virus-Leptospira Canicola-Grippotyphosa-Hardjo-Icterohaemorrhagiae-Pomona Bacterin
U.S. Vet. Lic. No.: 124
Contents: This product contains the antigens listed above.
Preservative: Neomycin.
Indications: Recommended for the vaccination of healthy, susceptible cattle as an aid in the reduction of diseases caused by Bovine Rhinotracheitis (IBR) virus, Bovine Virus Diarrhea (BVD) Types 1 and 2, Parainfluenza$_3$ (PI$_3$) virus, Bovine Respiratory Syncytial virus (BRSV), *Leptospira canicola, L. grippotyphosa, L. hardjo, L. icterohaemorrhagiae*, and *L. pomona.*
Directions: Rehydrate the modified live virus vaccine by aseptically adding the accompanying bottle of liquid bacterin.
Dosage: Using aseptic technique, inject 2 mL intramuscularly. Repeat in 14 to 28 days and once annually. Calves vaccinated before 6 months of age should be revaccinated at 6 months. A 2 mL booster dose is recommended prior to time of stress or exposure.
Contraindication(s): It is possible that healthy appearing cattle can be persistently infected with or incubating virulent BVD virus at time of vaccination. In view of these findings and suggested causes, BVD vaccine is contraindicated in persistently infected cattle and use should be limited only to healthy, immunocompetent, unstressed, non-pregnant cattle.
Precaution(s): Store out of direct sunlight at a temperature between 35-45°F (2-7°C). Avoid freezing. Shake well before using. Use entire contents when first opened. Burn containers and all unused contents.
Caution(s): Stressed cattle should not be vaccinated. Do not use in pregnant cows or in calves nursing pregnant cows. Injection site swelling may occur. Anaphylactoid reactions may occur.
Antidote(s): Epinephrine.
Warning(s): Do not vaccinate within 21 days of slaughter.
Animal inoculation only. Accidental injection to humans can cause serious local reactions. Contact a physician immediately if accidental injection occurs.
Presentation: 10 dose vial of MLV vaccine (20 mL vial of liquid bacterin diluent) and 50 dose vial of MLV vaccine (100 mL vial of liquid bacterin diluent).
Manufactured by: Boehringer Ingelheim Vetmedica, Inc., St. Joseph, Missouri 64506 U.S.A.
Compendium Code No.: 14750860 27406-00

TITERVAC™ 10-HS

Aspen **Bacterin-Vaccine**

Bovine Rhinotracheitis-Virus Diarrhea-Parainfluenza$_3$-Respiratory Syncytial Virus Vaccine, Modified Live Virus-Haemophilus Somnus-Leptospira Canicola-Grippotyphosa-Hardjo-Icterohaemorrhagiae-Pomona Bacterin
U.S. Vet. Lic. No.: 124
Contents: This product contains the antigens listed above.
Preservative: Neomycin.
Indications: Recommended for the vaccination of healthy, susceptible cattle as an aid in the reduction of diseases caused by Bovine Rhinotracheitis (IBR) virus, Bovine Virus Diarrhea (BVD) Types 1 and 2, Parainfluenza$_3$ (PI$_3$) virus, Bovine Respiratory Syncytial virus (BRSV), *Haemophilus somnus, Leptospira canicola, L. grippotyphosa, L. hardjo, L. icterohaemorrhagiae*, and *L. pomona.*
Directions: Rehydrate the modified live virus vaccine by aseptically adding the accompanying bottle of liquid bacterin.
Dosage: Using aseptic technique, inject 2 mL intramuscularly. Repeat in 14 to 28 days and once annually. Calves vaccinated before 6 months of age should be revaccinated at 6 months. A 2 mL booster dose is recommended prior to time of stress or exposure.
Contraindication(s): It is possible that healthy appearing cattle can be persistently infected with or incubating virulent BVD virus at time of vaccination. In view of these findings and suggested causes, BVD vaccine is contraindicated in persistently infected cattle and use should be limited only to healthy, immunocompetent, unstressed, non-pregnant cattle.
Precaution(s): Store out of direct sunlight at a temperature between 35-45°F (2-7°C). Avoid freezing. Shake well before using. Use entire contents when first opened. Burn containers and all unused contents.
Caution(s): Stressed cattle should not be vaccinated. Do not use in pregnant cows or in calves nursing pregnant cows. Injection site swelling may occur. Anaphylactoid reactions may occur.
Antidote(s): Epinephrine.
Warning(s): Do not vaccinate within 21 days of slaughter.
Animal inoculation only. Accidental injection to humans can cause serious local reactions. Contact a physician immediately if accidental injection occurs.
Presentation: 10 dose vial of MLV vaccine (20 mL vial of liquid bacterin diluent) and 50 dose vial of MLV vaccine (100 mL vial of liquid bacterin diluent).
Manufactured by: Boehringer Ingelheim Vetmedica, Inc., St. Joseph, Missouri 64506 U.S.A.
Compendium Code No.: 14750870 27507-00

T-LUX® SHAMPOO

Virbac **Antidermatosis Shampoo**

NDC No.: 51311-029-08
Active Ingredient(s): Contains solubilized tar equivalent to 4% coal tar, sulfur 2% and salicylic acid 2% in a golden clear shampoo base.
Indications: T-LUX® Shampoo is an antiseptic cleansing agent for the control of dandruff, seborrhea, and eczema in dogs. The formula provides therapeutic benefits while leaving the hair coat clean and lustrous.
Dosage and Administration: Using warm water, wet the coat thoroughly. Massage T-LUX® into the wet hair coat. Lather freely. Rinse and repeat. Allow the lather to remain on the hair and skin for 5-10 minutes, then rinse well. May be used once a day, or as directed by a veterinarian.
Caution(s): For topical use only. Not for use on cats. Avoid contact with the eyes.
Keep out of the reach of children.
Presentation: 8 oz. (237 mL), 16 oz. (473 mL), and 1 gallon (3.79 L) containers.
Compendium Code No.: 10230570

TM-50®

Phibro **Feed Medication**

Type A Medicated Article-Contains Terramycin®
NADA No.: 008-804
Active Ingredient(s):
Oxytetracycline (from oxytetracycline quaternary salt) equivalent to oxytetracycline hydrochloride (Terramycin®) .... 50 g/lb
Indications: A type A medicated article to be mixed in the feed of chickens; turkeys; swine; calves including pre-ruminating (veal) calves, beef cattle, and nonlactating dairy cattle; sheep and lobsters.
Recommended for increased rate of weight gain, improved feed efficiency, and for the control and treatment of ailments caused by microorganisms sensitive to oxytetracycline.
Directions: Mixing and Use Directions: Thoroughly mix the amount of this premix according to the directions below with at least an equal amount by weight of feed formula ingredients prior to blending into a complete feed.

Indications for Use	Oxytetracycline Amount	lb of TM-50®/ton
Chickens		
Increased rate of weight gain and improved feed efficiency	10-50 g/ton Feed continuously	0.2-1.0
Control of infectious synovitis caused by *Mycoplasma synoviae;* control of fowl cholera caused by *Pasteurella multocida* susceptible to oxytetracycline	100-200 g/ton Feed continuously for 7-14 days	2-4
Control of chronic respiratory disease (CRD) and air sac infection caused by *Mycoplasma gallisepticum* and *Escherichia coli* susceptible to oxytetracycline	400 g/ton Feed continuously for 7-14 days	8
Reduction of mortality due to air sacculitis (air sac infection) caused by *Escherichia coli* susceptible to oxytetracycline	500 g/ton Feed continuously for 5 days	10
Turkeys		
For growing turkeys for increased rate of weight gain and improved feed efficiency	10-50 g/ton Feed continuously	0.2-1.0
Control of hexamitiasis caused by *Hexamita meleagrides* susceptible to oxytetracycline	100 g/ton Feed continuously for 7-14 days	2
Control of infectious synovitis caused by *Mycoplasma synoviae* susceptible to oxytetracycline	200 g/ton Feed continuously for 7-14 days	4
Control of complicating bacterial organisms associated with bluecomb (transmissible enteritis, coronaviral enteritis) susceptible to oxytetracycline	25 mg/lb of body weight daily Feed continuously for 7-14 days	16.7[1]
Swine		
Increased rate of weight gain and improved feed efficiency	10-50 g/ton Feed continuously	0.2-1.0
Treatment of bacterial enteritis caused by *Escherichia coli* and *Salmonella choleraesuis* susceptible to oxytetracycline and treatment of bacterial pneumonia caused by *Pasteurella multocida* susceptible to oxytetracycline	10 mg/lb of body weight daily Feed continuously for 7-14 days	10[2]
For breeding swine for control and treatment of Leptospirosis (reducing the incidence of abortion and shedding of leptospirae) caused by *Leptospira pomona* susceptible to oxytetracycline	10 mg/lb of body weight daily Feed continuously for not more than 14 days	10[2]
Calves including pre-ruminating (veal) calves, Beef Cattle, and Nonlactating Dairy Cattle		
For calves (up to 250 lb) for increased rate of weight gain and improved feed efficiency	0.05-0.1 mg/lb of body weight daily Feed continuously	0.1-0.2[3]
For calves (250-400 lb) for increased rate of weight gain and improved feed efficiency	25 mg/head/day Feed continuously	0.5[4]
For growing cattle (over 400 lb) for increased rate of weight gain, improved feed efficiency, and reduction of liver condemnation due to liver abscesses	75 mg/head/day Feed continuously	1.5[4]
Prevention and treatment of the early stages of shipping fever complex (Feed 3-5 days before and after arrival in feedlots)	0.5-2.0 g/head/day	10-40[4]
Treatment of bacterial enteritis caused by *Escherichia coli* and bacterial pneumonia (shipping fever complex) caused by *Pasteurella multocida* susceptible to oxytetracycline	10 mg/lb of body weight daily Feed continuously for 7-14 days	100[5]
Sheep		
Increased rate of weight gain and improved feed efficiency	10-20 g/ton Feed continuously	0.2-0.4
Treatment of bacterial enteritis caused by *Escherichia coli* and bacterial pneumonia caused by *Pasteurella multocida* susceptible to oxytetracycline	10 mg/lb of body weight daily Feed continuously for 7-14 days	24[6]
Lobsters		
Control of gaffkemia in lobsters caused by *Aerococcus viridans*	1 g/lb of medicated feed Feed for 5 days as the sole ration	40

[1] If bird weighs 10 lb, consuming 0.6 lb of complete feed per day.
[2] If pig weighs 100 lb, consuming 4 lb of complete feed per day.
[3] If calf weighs 100 lb, consuming 2 lb of complete starter feed per day.
[4] Include in feed supplement based on consumption of 2 lb of supplement per head per day.
[5] If animal weighs 500 lb, consuming 2 lb of supplement per head per day.
[6] If lamb weighs 60 lb, consuming 1 lb of supplement per head per day.

Precaution(s): Store in a dry, cool place.

Caution(s): For use in manufacturing medicated animal feeds only.

For use in dry feeds only. Not for use in liquid feed supplements.

Warning(s): Chickens: At 500 g/ton use level, withdraw 24 hours before slaughter. Zero-day withdrawal period for lower use levels. In low calcium feeds withdraw 3 days before slaughter. Do not administer to chickens producing eggs for human consumption.

Turkeys: At 200 g/ton use level or higher, withdraw 5 days before slaughter. Zero-day withdrawal period for lower use levels. Do not administer to turkeys producing eggs for human consumption.

Calves including pre-ruminating (veal) calves, Beef Cattle, and Nonlactating Dairy Cattle: 5-day withdrawal before slaughter at 10 mg/lb dosage. When used in milk replacers, the treatment claim (10 mg/lb) is limited to bacterial enteritis caused by *Escherichia coli* only.

Sheep: 5-day withdrawal before slaughter at 10 mg/lb dosage.

Lobsters: Withdraw from feed 30 days before harvesting lobsters.

Certain components of animal feeds, including medicated premixes, possess properties that may be a potential health hazard or a source of personal discomfort to certain individuals who are exposed to them. Human exposure should, therefore, be minimized by observing the general industry standards for occupational health and safety.

Precautions such as the following should be considered: dust masks or respirators and protective clothing should be worn; dust-arresting equipment and adequate ventilation should be utilized; personal hygiene should be observed; wash before eating or leaving a work site; be alert for signs of allergic reactions—seek prompt medical treatment if such reactions are suspected.

Presentation: 50 lb (22.6 kg) bags.

TM-50 is a Phibro Animal Health registered trademark for Oxytetracycline HCl.
Terramycin is a registered trademark of Pfizer Inc., licensed to Phibro Animal Health, for Oxytetracycline HCl.

Compendium Code No.: 36930171 101-9001-101

TM-50®D

Phibro **Feed Medication**

Type A Medicated Article-Contains Terramycin®

NADA No.: 008-804

Active Ingredient(s):

Oxytetracycline (from oxytetracycline quaternary salt) equivalent to oxytetracycline hydrochloride (Terramycin®) . . . . . 50 g/lb

Indications: A type A medicated article to be mixed in the feed of chickens; turkeys; swine; calves including pre-ruminating (veal) calves, beef cattle, and nonlactating dairy cattle; sheep; honey bees and lobsters.

Recommended for increased rate of weight gain, improved feed efficiency, and for the control and treatment of ailments caused by microorganisms sensitive to oxytetracycline.

Directions: Mixing and Use Directions: Thoroughly mix the amount of this premix according to the directions below with at least an equal amount by weight of feed formula ingredients prior to blending into a complete feed.

Indications for Use	Oxytetracycline Amount	lb of TM-50®D/ton
Chickens		
Increased rate of weight gain and improved feed efficiency	10-50 g/ton Feed continuously	0.2-1.0
Control of infectious synovitis caused by *Mycoplasma synoviae;* control of fowl cholera caused by *Pasteurella multocida* susceptible to oxytetracycline	100-200 g/ton Feed continuously for 7-14 days	2-4
Control of chronic respiratory disease (CRD) and air sac infection caused by *Mycoplasma gallisepticum* and *Escherichia coli* susceptible to oxytetracycline	400 g/ton Feed continuously for 7-14 days	8
Reduction of mortality due to air sacculitis (air sac infection) caused by *Escherichia coli* susceptible to oxytetracycline	500 g/ton Feed continuously for 5 days	10
Turkeys		
For growing turkeys for increased rate of weight gain and improved feed efficiency	10-50 g/ton Feed continuously	0.2-1.0
Control of hexamitiasis caused by *Hexamita meleagrides* susceptible to oxytetracycline	100 g/ton Feed continuously for 7-14 days	2
Control of infectious synovitis caused by *Mycoplasma synoviae* susceptible to oxytetracycline	200 g/ton Feed continuously for 7-14 days	4
Control of complicating bacterial organisms associated with bluecomb (transmissible enteritis, coronaviral enteritis) susceptible to oxytetracycline	25 mg/lb of body weight daily Feed continuously for 7-14 days	16.7[1]
Swine		
Increased rate of weight gain and improved feed efficiency	10-50 g/ton Feed continuously	0.2-1.0
Treatment of bacterial enteritis caused by *Escherichia coli* and *Salmonella choleraesuis* susceptible to oxytetracycline and treatment of bacterial pneumonia caused by *Pasteurella multocida* susceptible to oxytetracycline	10 mg/lb of body weight daily Feed continuously for 7-14 days	10[2]
For breeding swine for control and treatment of Leptospirosis (reducing the incidence of abortion and shedding of leptospirae) caused by *Leptospira pomona* susceptible to oxytetracycline	10 mg/lb of body weight daily Feed continuously for not more than 14 days	10[2]
Calves including pre-ruminating (veal) calves, Beef Cattle, and Nonlactating Dairy Cattle		
For calves (up to 250 lb) for increased rate of weight gain and improved feed efficiency	0.05-0.1 mg/lb of body weight daily Feed continuously	0.1-0.2[3]
For calves (250-400 lb) for increased rate of weight gain and improved feed efficiency	25 mg/head/day Feed continuously	0.5[4]
For growing cattle (over 400 lb) for increased rate of weight gain, improved feed efficiency, and reduction of liver condemnation due to liver abscesses	75 mg/head/day Feed continuously	1.5[4]
Prevention and treatment of the early stages of shipping fever complex (Feed 3-5 days before and after arrival in feedlots)	0.5-2.0 g/head/day	10-40[4]
Treatment of bacterial enteritis caused by *Escherichia coli* and bacterial pneumonia (shipping fever complex) caused by *Pasteurella multocida* susceptible to oxytetracycline	10 mg/lb of body weight daily Feed continuously for 7-14 days	100[5]
Sheep		
Increased rate of weight gain and improved feed efficiency	10-20 g/ton Feed continuously	0.2-0.4
Treatment of bacterial enteritis caused by *Escherichia coli* and bacterial pneumonia caused by *Pasteurella multocida* susceptible to oxytetracycline	10 mg/lb of body weight daily Feed continuously for 7-14 days	24[6]
Honey Bees		
Control of American Foulbrood caused by *Bacillus larvae*, and European Foulbrood caused by *Streptococcus pluton* susceptible to oxytetracycline	200 mg/colony	See Mixing Directions below
Lobsters		
Control of gaffkemia in lobsters caused by *Aerococcus viridans*	1 g/lb of medicated feed Feed for 5 days as the sole ration	40

[1] If bird weighs 10 lb, consuming 0.6 lb of complete feed per day.
[2] If pig weighs 100 lb, consuming 4 lb of complete feed per day.
[3] If calf weighs 100 lb, consuming 2 lb of complete starter feed per day.
[4] Include in feed supplement based on consumption of 2 lb of supplement per head per day.
[5] If animal weighs 500 lb, consuming 2 lb of supplement per head per day.
[6] If lamb weighs 60 lb, consuming 1 lb of supplement per head per day.

Mixing and Use Directions for Honey Bees: Due to the high drug concentration of this product, an intermediate mixture must be prepared for use with bees. To prepare this intermediate mixture add 7 lb of TM-50®D to 100 lb of powdered sugar and mix well. This mixture contains approximately 200 mg of oxytetracycline hydrochloride activity per oz.

Dusting Directions: Apply 1 oz (200 mg oxytetracycline) of this mixture per colony. Apply the dust on the outer parts or ends of the frames.

Syrup Directions: Use 1 oz (200 mg oxytetracycline) of this mixture per 5 lb jar containing 1:1 sugar syrup (equal parts sugar and water w/w) per colony. Dissolve in a small quantity of water before adding to syrup. Bulk feed the syrup using feeder pails or division board feeders or by filling the combs.

Administer in 3 applications of sugar syrup or 3 dustings at 4- to 5-day intervals. The drug should be fed in the spring or fall and consumed by the bees before main honey flow begins to avoid contamination of production honey.

Extender Patty Directions: Use 4 oz (800 mg oxytetracycline) of this mixture mixed with 165 g of vegetable shortening (Crisco® or equivalent) and 330 g of sugar. The patties are placed on the top bars of the brood nest frames.

Precaution(s): Store in a dry, cool place.

Caution(s): For use in manufacturing medicated animal feeds only.

For use in dry feeds only. Not for use in liquid feed supplements.

Warning(s): Chickens: At 500 g/ton use level, withdraw 24 hours before slaughter. Zero-day withdrawal period for use in lower levels. In low calcium feeds withdraw 3 days before slaughter. Do not administer to chickens producing eggs for human consumption.

Turkeys: At 200 g/ton use level or higher, withdraw 5 days before slaughter. Zero-day withdrawal period for lower use levels. Do not administer to turkeys producing eggs for human consumption.

Calves including pre-ruminating (veal) calves, Beef Cattle, and Nonlactating Dairy Cattle: 5-day withdrawal before slaughter at 10 mg/lb dosage. When used in milk replacers, the treatment claim (10 mg/lb) is limited to bacterial enteritis caused by *Escherichia coli* only.

Sheep: 5-day withdrawal before slaughter at 10 mg/lb dosage.

Honey Bees: Remove at least 6 weeks prior to main honey flow.

This mixture should be fed in the spring or fall and consumed by the bees before main honey flow begins to avoid contamination of production honey. Honey stored during medication periods in combs for surplus honey should be removed following final medication of the bee colony and must not be used for human food. Honey from bee colonies likely to be infected with foulbrood should not be used for preparation of medicated syrup supplements since it may be contaminated with spores of foulbrood and may result in spreading the disease. Remove at least 6 weeks before main honey flow. Do not use in a manner contrary to state apiary laws and regulations. Each state has specific regulations relative to disease control and medications. Contact the appropriate official or state departments of agriculture for specific inter- and intrastate laws and regulations.

Lobsters: Withdraw from feed 30 days before harvesting lobsters.

Certain components of animal feeds, including medicated premixes, possess properties that may be a potential health hazard or a source of personal discomfort to certain individuals who are exposed to them. Human exposure should, therefore, be minimized by observing the general industry standards for occupational health and safety.

Precautions such as the following should be considered: dust masks or respirators and protective clothing should be worn; dust-arresting equipment and adequate ventilation should be utilized; personal hygiene should be observed; wash before eating or leaving a work site; be

alert for signs of allergic reactions—seek prompt medical treatment if such reactions are suspected.
Presentation: 50 lb (22.6 kg) bags.
TM-50 is a Phibro Animal Health registered trademark for Oxytetracycline HCl.
Terramycin is a registered trademark of Pfizer Inc., licensed to Phibro Animal Health, for Oxytetracycline HCl.
Crisco® is a trademark of Proctor & Gamble, Cincinnati, OH 45202.
Compendium Code No.: 36930181 101-9003-01

TM-100®

Phibro **Feed Medication**

Type A Medicated Article-Contains Terramycin®
NADA No.: 008-804
Active Ingredient(s):
Oxytetracycline (from oxytetracycline quaternary salt) equivalent to oxytetracycline hydrochloride (Terramycin®) .... 100 g/lb
Indications: A type A medicated article to be mixed in the feed of chickens; turkeys; swine; calves including pre-ruminating (veal) calves, beef cattle, and nonlactating dairy cattle; sheep and lobsters.

Recommended for increased rate of weight gain, improved feed efficiency, and for the control and treatment of ailments caused by microorganisms sensitive to oxytetracycline.
Directions: Mixing and Use Directions: Thoroughly mix the amount of this premix according to the directions below with at least an equal amount by weight of feed formula ingredients prior to blending into a complete feed.

Indications for Use	Oxytetracycline Amount	lb of TM-100®/ton
Chickens		
Increased rate of weight gain and improved feed efficiency	10-50 g/ton Feed continuously	0.1-0.5
Control of infectious synovitis caused by *Mycoplasma synoviae;* control of fowl cholera caused by *Pasteurella multocida* susceptible to oxytetracycline	100-200 g/ton Feed continuously for 7-14 days	1-2
Control of chronic respiratory disease (CRD) and air sac infection caused by *Mycoplasma gallisepticum* and *Escherichia coli* susceptible to oxytetracycline	400 g/ton Feed continuously for 7-14 days	4
Reduction of mortality due to air sacculitis (air sac infection) caused by *Escherichia coli* susceptible to oxytetracycline	500 g/ton Feed continuously for 5 days	5
Turkeys		
For growing turkeys for increased rate of weight gain and improved feed efficiency	10-50 g/ton Feed continuously	0.1-0.5
Control of hexamitiasis caused by *Hexamita meleagrides* susceptible to oxytetracycline	100 g/ton Feed continuously for 7-14 days	1
Control of infectious synovitis caused by *Mycoplasma synoviae* susceptible to oxytetracycline	200 g/ton Feed continuously for 7-14 days	2
Control of complicating bacterial organisms associated with bluecomb (transmissible enteritis, coronaviral enteritis) susceptible to oxytetracycline	25 mg/lb of body weight daily Feed continuously for 7-14 days	8.3[1]
Swine		
Increased rate of weight gain and improved feed efficiency	10-50 g/ton Feed continuously	0.1-0.5
Treatment of bacterial enteritis caused by *Escherichia coli* and *Salmonella choleraesuis* susceptible to oxytetracycline and treatment of bacterial pneumonia caused by *Pasteurella multocida* susceptible to oxytetracycline	10 mg/lb of body weight daily Feed continuously for 7-14 days	5[2]
For breeding swine for control and treatment of Leptospirosis (reducing the incidence of abortion and shedding of leptospirae) caused by *Leptospira pomona* susceptible to oxytetracycline	10 mg/lb of body weight daily Feed continuously for not more than 14 days	5[2]
Calves including pre-ruminating (veal) calves, Beef Cattle, and Nonlactating Dairy Cattle		
For calves (up to 250 lb) for increased rate of weight gain and improved feed efficiency	0.05-0.1 mg/lb of body weight daily Feed continuously	0.05-0.1[3]
For calves (250-400 lb) for increased rate of weight gain and improved feed efficiency	25 mg/head/day Feed continuously	0.25[4]
For growing cattle (over 400 lb) for increased rate of weight gain, improved feed efficiency, and reduction of liver condemnation due to liver abscesses	75 mg/head/day Feed continuously	0.75[4]
Prevention and treatment of the early stages of shipping fever complex (Feed 3-5 days before and after arrival in feedlots)	0.5-2.0 g/head/day	5-20[4]
Treatment of bacterial enteritis caused by *Escherichia coli* and bacterial pneumonia (shipping fever complex) caused by *Pasteurella multocida* susceptible to oxytetracycline	10 mg/lb of body weight daily Feed continuously for 7-14 days	50[5]
Sheep		
Increased rate of weight gain and improved feed efficiency	10-20 g/ton Feed continuously	0.1-0.2
Treatment of bacterial enteritis caused by *Escherichia coli* and bacterial pneumonia caused by *Pasteurella multocida* susceptible to oxytetracycline	10 mg/lb of body weight daily Feed continuously for 7-14 days	12[6]
Lobsters		
Control of gaffkemia in lobsters caused by *Aerococcus viridans*	1 g/lb of medicated feed Feed for 5 days as the sole ration	20

1 If bird weighs 10 lb, consuming 0.6 lb of complete feed per day.
2 If pig weighs 100 lb, consuming 4 lb of complete feed per day.
3 If calf weighs 100 lb, consuming 2 lb of complete starter feed per day.
4 Include in feed supplement based on consumption of 2 lb of supplement per head per day.
5 If animal weighs 500 lb, consuming 2 lb of supplement per head per day.
6 If lamb weighs 60 lb, consuming 1 lb of supplement per head per day.

Precaution(s): Store in a dry, cool place.
Caution(s): For use in manufacturing medicated animal feeds only.
For use in dry feeds only. Not for use in liquid feed supplements.
Warning(s): Chickens: At 500 g/ton use level, withdraw 24 hours before slaughter. Zero-day withdrawal period in lower use levels. In low calcium feeds withdraw 3 days before slaughter. Do not administer to chickens producing eggs for human consumption.

Turkeys: At 200 g/ton use level or higher, withdraw 5 days before slaughter. Zero-day withdrawal period for lower use levels. Do not administer to turkeys producing eggs for human consumption.

Calves including pre-ruminating (veal) calves, Beef Cattle, and Nonlactating Dairy Cattle: 5-day withdrawal before slaughter at 10 mg/lb dosage. When used in milk replacers, the treatment claim (10 mg/lb) is limited to bacterial enteritis caused by *Escherichia coli* only.

Sheep: 5-day withdrawal before slaughter at 10 mg/lb dosage.

Lobsters: Withdraw from feed 30 days before harvesting lobsters.

Certain components of animal feeds, including medicated premixes, possess properties that may be a potential health hazard or a source of personal discomfort to certain individuals who are exposed to them. Human exposure should, therefore, be minimized by observing the general industry standards for occupational health and safety.

Precautions such as the following should be considered: dust masks or respirators and protective clothing should be worn; dust-arresting equipment and adequate ventilation should be utilized; personal hygiene should be observed; wash before eating or leaving a work site; be alert for signs of allergic reactions—seek prompt medical treatment if such reactions are suspected.
Presentation: 50 lb (22.6 kg) bags.
TM-100 is a Phibro Animal Health registered trademark for Oxytetracycline HCl.
Terramycin is a registered trademark of Pfizer Inc., licensed to Phibro Animal Health, for Oxytetracycline HCl.
Compendium Code No.: 36930191 101-9002-01

TM-100®D

Phibro **Feed Medication**

Type A Medicated Article-Contains Terramycin®
NADA No.: 008-804
Active Ingredient(s):
Oxytetracycline (from oxytetracycline quaternary salt) equivalent to oxytetracycline hydrochloride (Terramycin®).... 100 g/lb
Indications: A type A medicated article to be mixed in the feed of chickens; turkeys; swine; calves including pre-ruminating (veal) calves, beef cattle, and nonlactating dairy cattle; sheep; honey bees and lobsters.

Recommended for increased rate of weight gain, improved feed efficiency, and for the control and treatment of ailments caused by microorganisms sensitive to oxytetracycline.
Directions: Mixing and Use Directions: Thoroughly mix the amount of this premix according to the directions below with at least an equal amount by weight of feed formula ingredients prior to blending into a complete feed.

Indications for Use	Oxytetracycline Amount	lb of TM-100®D/ton
Chickens		
Increased rate of weight gain and improved feed efficiency	10-50 g/ton Feed continuously	0.1-0.5
Control of infectious synovitis caused by *Mycoplasma synoviae;* control of fowl cholera caused by *Pasteurella multocida* susceptible to oxytetracycline	100-200 g/ton Feed continuously for 7-14 days	1-2
Control of chronic respiratory disease (CRD) and air sac infection caused by *Mycoplasma gallisepticum* and *Escherichia coli* susceptible to oxytetracycline	400 g/ton Feed continuously for 7-14 days	4
Reduction of mortality due to air sacculitis (air sac infection) caused by *Escherichia coli* susceptible to oxytetracycline	500 g/ton Feed continuously for 5 days	5
Turkeys		
For growing turkeys for increased rate of weight gain and improved feed efficiency	10-50 g/ton Feed continuously	0.1-0.5
Control of hexamitiasis caused by *Hexamita meleagrides* susceptible to oxytetracycline	100 g/ton Feed continuously for 7-14 days	1
Control of infectious synovitis caused by *Mycoplasma synoviae* susceptible to oxytetracycline	200 g/ton Feed continuously for 7-14 days	2
Control of complicating bacterial organisms associated with bluecomb (transmissible enteritis, coronaviral enteritis) susceptible to oxytetracycline	25 mg/lb of body weight daily Feed continuously for 7-14 days	8.3[1]
Swine		
Increased rate of weight gain and improved feed efficiency	10-50 g/ton Feed continuously	0.1-0.5
Treatment of bacterial enteritis caused by *Escherichia coli* and *Salmonella choleraesuis* susceptible to oxytetracycline and treatment of bacterial pneumonia caused by *Pasteurella multocida* susceptible to oxytetracycline	10 mg/lb of body weight daily Feed continuously for 7-14 days	5[2]
For breeding swine for control and treatment of Leptospirosis (reducing the incidence of abortion and shedding of leptospirae) caused by *Leptospira pomona* susceptible to oxytetracycline	10 mg/lb of body weight daily Feed continuously for not more than 14 days	5[2]

T

Indications for Use	Oxytetracycline Amount	lb of TM-100®D/ton
Calves including pre-ruminating (veal) calves, Beef Cattle, and Nonlactating Dairy Cattle		
For calves (up to 250 lb) for increased rate of weight gain and improved feed efficiency	0.05-0.1 mg/lb of body weight daily Feed continuously	0.05-0.1[3]
For calves (250-400 lb) for increased rate of weight gain and improved feed efficiency	25 mg/head/day Feed continuously	0.25[4]
For growing cattle (over 400 lb) for increased rate of weight gain, improved feed efficiency, and reduction of liver condemnation due to liver abscesses	75 mg/head/day Feed continuously	0.75[4]
Prevention and treatment of the early stages of shipping fever complex (Feed 3-5 days before and after arrival in feedlots)	0.5-2.0 g/head/day	5-20[4]
Treatment of bacterial enteritis caused by *Escherichia coli* and bacterial pneumonia (shipping fever complex) caused by *Pasteurella multocida* susceptible to oxytetracycline	10 mg/lb of body weight daily Feed continuously for 7-14 days	50[5]
Sheep		
Increased rate of weight gain and improved feed efficiency	10-20 g/ton Feed continuously	0.1-0.2
Treatment of bacterial enteritis caused by *Escherichia coli* and bacterial pneumonia caused by *Pasteurella multocida* susceptible to oxytetracycline	10 mg/lb of body weight daily Feed continuously for 7-14 days	12[6]
Honey Bees		
Control of American Foulbrood caused by *Bacillus larvae*, and European Foulbrood caused by *Streptococcus pluton* susceptible to oxytetracycline	200 mg/colony	See Mixing Directions below
Lobsters		
Control of gaffkemia in lobsters caused by *Aerococcus viridans*	1 g/lb of medicated feed Feed for 5 days as the sole ration	20

[1] If bird weighs 10 lb, consuming 0.6 lb of complete feed per day.

[2] If pig weighs 100 lb, consuming 4 lb of complete feed per day.

[3] If calf weighs 100 lb, consuming 2 lb of complete starter feed per day.

[4] Include in feed supplement based on consumption of 2 lb of supplement per head per day.

[5] If animal weighs 500 lb, consuming 2 lb of supplement per head per day.

[6] If lamb weighs 60 lb, consuming 1 lb of supplement per head per day.

Mixing and Use Directions for Honey Bees: Due to the high drug concentration of this product, an intermediate mixture must be prepared for use with bees. To prepare this intermediate mixture add 7 lb of TM-100®D to 200 lb of powdered sugar and mix well. This mixture contains approximately 200 mg of oxytetracycline hydrochloride activity per oz.

Dusting Directions: Apply 1 oz (200 mg oxytetracycline) of this mixture per colony. Apply the dust on the outer parts or ends of the frames.

Syrup Directions: Use 1 oz (200 mg oxytetracycline) of this mixture per 5 lb jar containing 1:1 sugar syrup (equal parts sugar and water w/w) per colony. Dissolve in a small quantity of water before adding to syrup. Bulk feed the syrup using feeder pails or division board feeders or by filling the combs.

Administer in 3 applications of sugar syrup or 3 dustings at 4- to 5-day intervals. The drug should be fed in the spring or fall and consumed by the bees before main honey flow begins to avoid contamination of production honey.

Extender Patty Directions: Use 4 oz (800 mg oxytetracycline) of this mixture mixed with 165 g of vegetable shortening (Crisco® or equivalent) and 330 g of sugar. The patties are placed on the top bars of the brood nest frames.

Precaution(s): Store in a dry, cool place.

Caution(s): For use in manufacturing medicated animal feeds only.

For use in dry feeds only. Not for use in liquid feed supplements.

Warning(s): Chickens: At 500 g/ton use level, withdraw 24 hours before slaughter. Zero-day withdrawal period for lower use levels. In low calcium feeds withdraw 3 days before slaughter. Do not administer to chickens producing eggs for human consumption.

Turkeys: At 200 g/ton use level or higher, withdraw 5 days before slaughter. Zero-day withdrawal period for lower use levels. Do not administer to turkeys producing eggs for human consumption.

Calves including pre-ruminating (veal) calves, Beef Cattle, and Nonlactating Dairy Cattle: 5-day withdrawal before slaughter at 10 mg/lb dosage. When used in milk replacers, the treatment claim (10 mg/lb) is limited to bacterial enteritis caused by *Escherichia coli* only.

Sheep: 5-day withdrawal before slaughter at 10 mg/lb dosage.

Honey Bees: Remove at least 6 weeks prior to main honey flow.

This mixture should be fed in the spring or fall and consumed by the bees before main honey flow begins to avoid contamination of production honey. Honey stored during medication periods in combs for surplus honey should be removed following final medication of the bee colony and must not be used for human food. Honey from bee colonies likely to be infected with foulbrood should not be used for preparation of medicated syrup supplements since it may be contaminated with spores of foulbrood and may result in spreading the disease. Remove at least 6 weeks before main honey flow. Do not use in a manner contrary to state apiary laws and regulations. Each state has specific regulations relative to disease control and medications. Contact the appropriate official or state departments of agriculture for specific inter- and intrastate laws and regulations.

Lobsters: Withdraw from feed 30 days before harvesting lobsters.

Certain components of animal feeds, including medicated premixes, possess properties that may be a potential health hazard or a source of personal discomfort to certain individuals who are exposed to them. Human exposure should, therefore, be minimized by observing the general industry standards for occupational health and safety.

Precautions such as the following should be considered: dust masks or respirators and protective clothing should be worn; dust-arresting equipment and adequate ventilation should be utilized; personal hygiene should be observed; wash before eating or leaving a work site; be alert for signs of allergic reactions—seek prompt medical treatment if such reactions are suspected.

Presentation: 50 lb (22.6 kg) bags.

TM-100 is a Phibro Animal Health registered trademark for Oxytetracycline HCl.

Terramycin is a registered trademark of Pfizer Inc., licensed to Phibro Animal Health, for Oxytetracycline HCl.

Crisco® is a trademark of Proctor & Gamble, Cincinnati, OH 45202.

Compendium Code No.: 36930201 101-9004-01

ToDAY®

Fort Dodge **Mastitis Therapy**

Cephapirin Sodium

NADA No.: 097-222

Active Ingredient(s): Each 10 mL disposable syringe contains 200 mg of cephapirin activity in a stable peanut oil gel. This product was manufactured by a non-sterilizing process.

Indications: For lactating cows only.

For the Treatment of Bovine Mastitis: ToDAY® (cephapirin sodium) for Intramammary Infusion should be used at the first signs of inflammation or at the first indication of any alteration in the milk. Treatment is indicated immediately upon determining, by C.M.T. or other tests, that the leucocyte count is elevated, or that a susceptible pathogen has been cultured from the milk.

ToDAY® for Intramammary Infusion has been shown to be efficacious in the treatment of mastitis in lactating cows caused by susceptible strains of *Streptococcus agalactiae* and *Staphylococcus aureus* including strains resistant to penicillin.

Pharmacology: ToDAY® (cephapirin sodium) is a cephalosporin which possesses a wide range of antimicrobial activity against gram-positive and gram-negative organisms. It is derived biosynthetically from 7-aminocephalosporanic acid.

Action: Cephapirin is bactericidal to susceptible organisms; it is known to be highly active against *Streptococcus agalactiae* and *Staphylococcus aureus* including strains resistant to penicillin.

To determine the susceptibility of bacteria to cephapirin in the laboratory, the class disc, Cephalothin Susceptibility Test Discs, 30 mcg, should be used.

Dosage and Administration: Infuse the entire contents of one syringe (10 mL) into each infected quarter immediately after the quarter has been completely milked out. Repeat once only in 12 hours. If definite improvement is not noted within 48 hours after treatment, the causal organism should be further investigated. Consult your veterinarian.

Milk out udder completely. Wash the udder and teats thoroughly with warm water containing a suitable dairy antiseptic and dry, preferably using individual paper towels. Carefully scrub the teat end and orifice with 70% alcohol, using a separate swab for each teat. Allow to dry.

ToDAY® (cephapirin sodium) is packaged with the Opti-Sert® Protective Cap.

For partial insertion: Twist off upper portion of the Opti-Sert® Protective Cap to expose 3-4 mm of the syringe tip.

For full insertion: Remove protective cap to expose the full length of the syringe tip.

Insert syringe tip into the teat canal and expel the entire contents of one syringe into each infected quarter. Withdraw the syringe and gently massage the quarter to distribute the suspension into the milk cistern. Do not milk out for 12 hours.

Do not infuse contents of the mastitis syringe into the teat canal if the Opti-Sert® Protective Cap is broken or damaged.

Re-infection — The use of antibiotics, however effective, for the treatment of mastitis will not significantly reduce the incidence of this disease in the herd unless their use is fortified by good herd management, and sanitary and mechanical safety measures are practiced to prevent reinfection.

Precaution(s): Store at controlled room temperature 15° to 30°C (59° to 86°F); avoid excessive heat.

Caution(s): ToDAY® should be administered with caution to subjects which have demonstrated some form of allergy, particularly to penicillin. Such reactions are rare; however, should they occur, consult your veterinarian.

Warning(s):

1. Milk that has been taken from animals during treatment and for 96 hours after the last treatment must not be used for food.
2. Treated animals must not be slaughtered for food until 4 days after the last treatment.
3. Administration of more than the prescribed dose may lead to residue of antibiotic in milk longer than 96 hours.

Presentation: Carton containing 12 x 10 mL syringes (NDC 0856-02727-1).

Opti-Sert® Protective Cap — U.S. Patent No. 4,850,970

Compendium Code No.: 10032230 4940B

TOLAZINE™ INJECTION ℞

Lloyd **Alpha-Adrenergic Antagonist**

Tolazoline HCl, USP 100 mg/mL Sterile Solution-Xylazine Reversing Agent and Antagonist

NADA No.: 140-994

Active Ingredient(s): Each mL contains: tolazoline hydrochloride equivalent to 100 mg base activity, chlorobutanol 5.0 mg, tartaric acid 7.8 mg, sodium citrate dihydrate 7.8 mg and water for injection. The pH is adjusted with hydrochloric acid and sodium citrate.

Indications: TOLAZINE™ should be used in horses when it is desirable to reverse the effects of sedation and analgesia caused by xylazine.

Pharmacology: TOLAZINE™ contains tolazoline hydrochloride with the chemical name 1H-Imidazole,4,5-dihydro-2-(phenylmethyl)-monohydrochloride. Tolazoline hydrochloride has a molecular weight of 196.68 and the molecular formula is $C_{10}H_{12}N_2 \bullet HCl$. The structural formula is:

$C_6H_5-CH_2-$(imidazoline ring: N, N–H) · HCl

Clinical Pharmacology: Tolazoline belongs to the synthetic group of alpha-adrenergic blocking agents known as the imidazoline derivatives. It is a mixed alpha-1 and alpha-2 adrenergic receptor antagonist that competitively inhibits alpha-adrenoceptors. Tolazoline is also a direct peripheral vasodilator that decreases the peripheral resistance and increases venous capacitance.

Xylazine is an alpha-2 adrenergic agonist with sedative and analgesic properties related to central nervous system depression. Administration of TOLAZINE™ reverses xylazine's central nervous system depressant effects resulting in rapid recovery from sedation. The competitive

T

blocking of the alpha-2 adrenergic receptor by TOLAZINE™ displaces xylazine from these sites and thereby rapidly cancels the effect of the xylazine.

Onset of arousal is usually apparent within 5 minutes of TOLAZINE™ administration, depending on the depth and duration of xylazine-induced sedation.

Dosage and Administration: The TOLAZINE™ dose is 4.0 mg/kg body weight or 1.8 mg/lb (4 mL/100 kg or 4 mL/220 lb) to reverse the sedative effects of xylazine. The carefully calculated dose of TOLAZINE™ should be given slowly by intravenous injection. Administration rate should approximate 1 mL/second.

The table demonstrates the correct injection volume based on body weight:

Body Weight (kg)	Body Weight (lb)	TOLAZINE™ injection Volume
250 kg	550 lb	10 mL
500 kg	1100 lb	20 mL

Precaution(s): Protect from light. Store at controlled room temperature 15° to 30°C (59° to 86°F).

Caution(s): Federal law restricts this drug to use by or on the order of a licensed veterinarian.

The safety of TOLAZINE™ has not been evaluated in horses with metabolically unstable conditions. TOLAZINE™ should not be administered to animals exhibiting signs of stress, debilitation, cardiac disease, sympathetic blockage, hypovolemia or shock.

The safety of TOLAZINE™ has not been evaluated for reversing xylazine used as a preanesthetic to a general anesthetic

The safety of TOLAZINE™ has not been established in pregnant mares, lactating mares, horses intended for breeding, or foals.

TOLAZINE™ should be administered carefully and at a slow rate to allow venous dilution to occur prior to the drug reaching the brain and heart. An administration rate of 1 mL/second was shown to be safe at the recommended dose.

TOLAZINE™ reverses the analgesic effects of xylazine as well as the sedative effects. If the animal was given xylazine for its analgesic properties, reversal may result in return of normal pain perception.

Warning(s): Keep out of reach of children. Not for human use.

This drug is for use in horses only and not for use in food-producing animals.

Avoid contact with eyes, skin and mucous membranes. In case of eye contact flush with plenty of water. Exposed skin should be washed with soap and water. In case of accidental oral exposure or injection, seek emergency medical attention.

Users with cardiovascular disease (for example, hypertension or ischemic heart disease) should take special precautions to avoid accidental exposure to this product.

To report adverse reactions in users or to obtain a copy of the material safety data sheet for this product, call 1-800-831-0004.

Note to Physician: This product contains an alpha-2 adrenoreceptor antagonist. Epinephrine should not be used to treat hypotension in humans resulting from exposure to this product since tolazoline may cause "epinephrine reversal" (further reduction in blood pressure, followed by an exaggerated rebound).

Toxicology: Safety: The safety of TOLAZINE™ alone without prior xylazine administration was evaluated in healthy horses. TOLAZINE™ was administered at 1, 3, and 5 times the recommended dose of 4 mg/kg, every 6 hours for 3 doses. When administered alone, TOLAZINE™ caused gastrointestinal hypermotility as horses defecated or attempted to defecate with flatulence within minutes after injection. Some horses exhibited abdominal discomfort (mild colic) and displayed transient diarrhea. Gastrointestinal disturbances were seen in all dose groups.

The safety of TOLAZINE™ was evaluated following administration of xylazine in healthy horses. The frequency of gastrointestinal disturbances was decreased in the presence of xylazine. Most horses experienced xylazine-induced hypomotility. A return to normal intestinal motility occurred within 5 minutes after TOLAZINE™ administration. A single incidence of mild colic was observed at three times the recommended TOLAZINE™ dose, and one instance of transient diarrhea was exhibited at three times the recommended TOLAZINE™ dose.

The heart rate may briefly increase immediately after TOLAZINE™ injection at the recommended dose with return to pretreatment rates within 5-10 minutes. The degree and duration of tachycardia increased with higher doses, although the increased rate usually lasted less than 60 minutes.

When TOLAZINE™ was administered at higher than the recommended dose in healthy horses, intraventricular conduction was slowed, as demonstrated by a prolongation of the QRS complex of the ECG. This effect was not observed at the 1X dose, only a mild prolongation occurred in a single horse at the 2X dose, and it was seen in most horses that received the 3X and 5X doses. Abnormalities of intraventricular conduction can predispose to ventricular arrhythmias and possibly death.

Overdoses of TOLAZINE™ at 5 times the recommended dose have been associated with fatalities in horses.

TOLAZINE™ reverses blood pressure reduction induced by xylazine in healthy horses, and may result in mild hypertension in some animals at the recommended dose.

TOLAZINE™ at doses less than or equal to 5 times the recommended dose did not affect any hematologic, serum biochemical, or urinalysis measurements.

Side Effects: Temporary side effects of TOLAZINE™ may be mild increases in blood pressure; tachycardia; peripheral vasodilatation, evidenced by injected mucous membranes of the gingiva and conjunctiva; and sweating. A few horses may show hyperalgesia of the lips, evidenced by licking or flipping of the lips. Some horses may exhibit piloerection soon after dosing. Clear lacrimal and nasal discharges may be noted. Muscle fasciculations may be observed. Some horses may show signs of temporary apprehensiveness. All clinical side effects should dissipate within 60-120 minutes.

The potential for side effects increases when higher than recommended doses are given or when TOLAZINE™ is given without prior administration of xylazine.

Presentation: 100 mL multiple-dose vial.

Compendium Code No.: 11350020

ToMORROW®

Fort Dodge **Mastitis Therapy**

Cephapirin Benzathine

NADA No.: 108-114

Active Ingredient(s): Each 10 mL disposable syringe contains 300 mg of cephapirin activity in a stable peanut oil gel. This product was manufactured by a non-sterilizing process.

Indications: For the treatment of mastitis in dairy cows during the dry period.

ToMORROW® has been shown by extensive clinical studies to be efficacious in the treatment of mastitis in dry cows, when caused by *Streptococcus agalactiae* and *Staphylococcus aureus* including penicillin-resistant strains.

Treatment of the dry cow with ToMORROW® is indicated in any cow known to harbor any of these organisms in the udder at drying off.

Pharmacology: ToMORROW® (cephapirin benzathine) for Intramammary Infusion into the Dry Cow is a product which provides a wide range of bactericidal activity against gram-positive and gram-negative organisms. It is derived biosynthetically from 7-aminocephalosporanic acid.

Action: In the non-lactating mammary gland, ToMORROW® (cephapirin benzathine) provides bactericidal levels of the active antibiotic, cephapirin, for a prolonged period of time. This prolonged activity is due to the low solubility of the cephapirin benzathine and to the slow release gel base.

Cephapirin is bactericidal to susceptible organisms; it is known to be highly active against *Streptococcus agalactiae* and *Staphylococcus aureus* including strains resistant to penicillin.

To determine the susceptibility of bacteria to cephapirin in the laboratory, the class disc, Cephalothin Susceptibility Test Discs, 30 mcg, should be used.

Dosage and Administration: ToMORROW® (cephapirin benzathine) is for use in dry cows only. Infuse each quarter at the time of drying off with a single 10 mL syringe. Use no later than 30 days prior to calving.

Completely milk out all four quarters. The udder and teats should be thoroughly washed with warm water containing a suitable dairy antiseptic and dried, preferably using individual paper towels. Carefully scrub the teat end and orifice with 70% alcohol, using a separate swab for each teat. Allow to dry.

ToMORROW® is packaged with the Opti-Sert® Protective Cap.

For partial insertion: Twist off upper portion of the Opti-Sert® Protective Cap to expose 3-4 mm of the syringe tip.

For full insertion: Remove protective cap to expose the full length of the syringe tip.

Insert syringe tip into the teat canal and expel the entire contents of syringe into the quarter. Withdraw the syringe and gently massage the quarter to distribute the medication.

Do not infuse contents of the mastitis syringe into the teat canal if the Opti-Sert® Protective Cap is broken or damaged.

Precaution(s): Store at controlled room temperature 15° to 30°C (59° to 86°F); avoid excessive heat.

Caution(s): ToMORROW® should be administered with caution to subjects which have demonstrated some form of allergy, particularly to penicillin. Such reactions are rare; however, should they occur, consult your veterinarian.

Warning(s):

1. For use in dry cows only.
2. Not to be used within 30 days of calving.
3. Milk from treated cows must not be used for food during the first 72 hours after calving.
4. Any animal infused with this product must not be slaughtered for food until 42 days after the latest infusion.

Presentation: Carton containing 12 x 10 mL syringes (NDC 0856-02731-1).

Opti-Sert® Protective Cap — U.S. Patent No. 4,850,970

Compendium Code No.: 10032241 4980B

TOPICAL FUNGICIDE

Durvet **Topical Antifungal**

Active Ingredient(s):

Benzalkonium chloride 0.15%

Other ingredients: Allantoin

Indications: For use on cattle, sheep, horses, dogs and cats as an aid in the control of summer itch, girth itch, foot rot, ringworm and other fungal problems.

Dosage and Administration: Soak affected area liberally with TOPICAL FUNGICIDE solution. Apply daily until hair begins to grow. Leave treated areas uncovered. Rinse treated areas with clear water before reapplying. Results should be apparent in a matter of days. If no improvement is noted within seven days, consult veterinarian.

Note: Efficiency is neutralized by soap or detergent residues.

Warning(s): In case of contact with eyes or mucous membranes, flush immediately with water. Obtain medical attention for eye inflammation.

For external veterinary use only.

Not for human use.

Presentation: 16 fl. oz. and 32 fl. oz.

Compendium Code No.: 10841610

TOPICAL FUNGICIDE

First Priority **Topical Antifungal**

Active Ingredient(s):

Benzalkonium Chloride 0.15%

Other Ingredients: Allantoin.

Indications: For use on horses, dogs and cats as an aid in the control of summer itch, girth itch, ringworm and other fungal problems.

Directions for Use: Soak affected area liberally with TOPICAL FUNGICIDE solution. Apply daily until hair begins to grow. Leave treated areas uncovered. Rinse treated areas with clear water before reapplying. Results should be apparent in a matter of days. If improvement is not noted within seven days, consult veterinarian.

Note: Efficiency is neutralized by soap or detergent residues.

Caution(s): In case of contact with the eyes or mucous membranes, flush immediately with water. Obtain medical attention for eye inflammation.

For external veterinary use only.

Warning(s): Not for use on animals intended for food.

Not for human use. Keep out of reach of children.

Presentation: 16 fl oz (473 mL) (NDC# 58829-195-16) and 32 fl oz (960 mL) (NDC# 58829-195-32) with trigger sprayers.

Compendium Code No.: 11390723 Rev. 06-01 / Iss. 2-98

TOPICAL FUNGICIDE

Vedco **Topical Antifungal**

Active Ingredient(s): Contains:

Benzalkonium chloride 0.15%

Other ingredients: Carbamide, allantoin.

Indications: For use on horses, dogs and cats as an aid in the control of summer itch, girth itch, ringworm and other fungal problems.

Dosage and Administration: Soak the affected area liberally with TOPICAL FUNGICIDE solution. Apply once a day until the hair begins to grow. Leave the treated areas uncovered. Rinse the treated areas with clear water before re-applying. Results should be apparent in a matter of days. If improvement is not noted within seven (7) days, consult a veterinarian.

Note: Efficiency is neutralized by soap or detergent residues.

Caution(s): Keep out of the reach of children. Not for human use.

In case of contact with eyes or mucous membranes, flush immediately with water. Obtain medical attention for eye inflammation.

Warning(s): Not for use on animals intended for food.

Presentation: 16 fl. oz. containers.

Compendium Code No.: 10942000

TOP LINE™

AgriLabs **Parasiticide-Topical**

(ivermectin) Pour-On for Cattle

Active Ingredient(s): Contains 5 mg ivermectin/mL.

Indications: TOP LINE™ Pour-On applied at the recommended dose level of 500 mcg/kg is indicated for the effective control of these parasites.

Gastrointestinal Roundworms: *Ostertagia ostertagi* (including inhibited stage) (adults and L_4), *Haemonchus placei* (adults and L_4), *Trichostrongylus axei* (adults and L_4), *T. colubriformis* (adults and L_4), *Cooperia* spp (adults and L_4), *Strongyloides papillosus* (adults), *Oesophagostomum radiatum* (adults and L_4), *Trichuris* spp (adults).

Lungworms: *Dictyocaulus viviparus* (adults and L_4).

Cattle Grubs (parasitic stages): *Hypoderma bovis, H. lineatum.*

Mites: *Sarcoptes scabiei* var. *bovis.*

Lice: *Linognathus vituli, Haematopinus eurysternus, Damalinia bovis, Solenopotes capillatus.*

Horn Flies: *Haematobia irritans.*

Pharmacology: Mode of Action: Ivermectin as a member of the avermectin family kills certain parasitic roundworms and ectoparasites, such as mites, lice, horn flies and other insects. Its action is unique to the avermectin class of antiparasitic agents. This action involves a chemical that serves as a signal from one nerve cell to another, or from a nerve cell to a muscle cell. This chemical, a neurotransmitter, is called gamma-aminobutyric acid or GABA.

In roundworms, ivermectin stimulates the release of GABA from nerve endings and enhances binding of GABA to special receptors at nerve junctions, thus interrupting nerve impulses — thereby paralyzing and killing the parasite.

The enhancement of the GABA effect in arthropods such as mites, lice, and horn flies resembles that in roundworms except that nerve impulses are interrupted between the nerve ending and the muscle cell. Again, this leads to paralysis and death.

Ivermectin has no measurable effect against flukes or tapeworms, presumably because they do not have GABA as a nerve impulse transmitter.

The principal peripheral neurotransmitter in mammals, acetylcholine, is unaffected by ivermectin. Ivermectin does not readily penetrate the central nervous system of mammals where GABA functions as a neurotransmitter.

Dosage and Administration:

Treatment of Cattle for Horn Flies: TOP LINE™ Pour-On controls horn flies *(Haematobia irritans)* for up to 28 days after dosing. For best results TOP LINE™ Pour-On should be part of a parasite control program for both internal and external parasites based on the epidemiology of these parasites. Consult your veterinarian or an entomologist for the most effective timing of applications.

The dose rate is 1 mL for each 22 lb of body weight. The formulation should be applied along the topline in a narrow strip extending from the withers to the tailhead.

When to Treat Cattle with Grubs: TOP LINE™ Pour-On effectively controls all stages of cattle grubs. However, proper timing of treatment is important. For the most effective results, cattle should be treated as soon as possible after the end of the heel fly (warble fly) season. While this is not peculiar to ivermectin, destruction of *Hypoderma* larvae (cattle grubs) at the period when these grubs are in vital areas may cause undesirable host-parasite reactions. Killing *Hypoderma lineatum* when it is in the esophageal tissues may cause bloat; killing *H bovis* when it is in the vertebral canal may cause staggering or paralysis. Cattle should be treated either before or after these stages of grub development.

Cattle treated with TOP LINE™ Pour-On at the end of the fly season may be re-treated with TOP LINE™ during the winter without danger of grub-related reactions. For further information and advice on a planned parasite control program, consult your veterinarian.

Squeeze-Measure-Pour System (8.5 fl oz/250 mL Bottle with 25 mL Metering Cup): Attach the metering cup to the bottle.

Set the dose by turning the top section of the cup to align the correct body weight with the pointer on the knurled cap. When body weight is between markings, use the higher setting.

Hold the bottle upright and squeeze it to deliver a slight excess of the required dose as indicated by the calibration lines.

By releasing the pressure, the dose automatically adjusts to the correct level. Tilt the bottle to deliver the dose. The off (Stop) position will close the system between dosing.

Squeeze-Measure-Pour System (33.8 fl oz/1 Liter Bottle with 50 mL Metering Cup): Attach the metering cup to the bottle.

Set the dose by turning the top section of the cup to align the correct body weight with the pointer on the knurled cap. When body weight is between markings, use the higher setting.

Hold the bottle upright and squeeze it to deliver a slight excess of the required dose as indicated by the calibration lines.

By releasing the pressure, the dose automatically adjusts to the correct level. Tilt the bottle to deliver the dose. When 220 lb (10 mL) or 330 lb (15 mL) dose is required, turn the pointer to "Stop" before delivering the dose. The off (Stop) position will close the system between dosing.

Collapsible Pack (84.5 fl oz/2.5 L Pack and 169 fl oz/5 L Pack): Connect the applicator gun to the collapsible pack as follows:

Attach the open end of the draw-off tubing to the dosing equipment. (Because of the solvents used in the formulation, only the Protector Drench Gun from Instrument Supplies Limited, or equivalent, is recommended. Other applicators may exhibit compatibility problems, resulting in locking, incorrect dosage or leakage.)

Replace the shipping cap with the draw-off cap and tighten down. Attach draw-off tubing to the draw-off cap.

Gently prime the applicator gun, checking for leaks.

Follow the manufacturer's directions for adjusting the dose.

When the interval between uses of the applicator gun is expected to exceed 12 hours, disconnect the gun and draw-off tubing from the product container and empty the product from the gun and tubing back into the product container. To prevent removal of special lubricants from the Protector Drench Gun, the gun and tubing must not be washed.

Contraindication(s): This product is for application to skin surface only. Do not give orally or parenterally.

Ivermectin has been associated with adverse reactions in sensitive dogs; therefore, TOP LINE™ Pour-On is not recommended for use in species other than cattle.

Precaution(s): This product is flammable.

Keep away from heat, sparks, open flame, and other sources of ignition.

Store away from excessive heat (104°F/40°C) and protect from light.

Cloudiness in the formulation may occur when TOP LINE™ Pour-On is stored at temperatures below 32°F. Allowing to warm at room temperature will restore the normal appearance without affecting efficacy.

Environmental Safety: Studies indicate that when ivermectin comes in contact with the soil, it readily and tightly binds to the soil and becomes inactive over time. Free ivermectin may adversely affect fish or certain water-borne organisms on which they feed. Do not permit cattle to enter lakes, streams or ponds for at least six hours after treatment. Do not contaminate water by direct application or by the improper disposal of drug containers. Dispose of containers in an approved landfill or by incineration.

Caution(s): Consult your veterinarian for assistance in the diagnosis, treatment and control of parasitism.

Use only in well-ventilated areas or outdoors.

Close container tightly when not in use.

Cattle should not be treated when the hair or hide is wet since reduced efficacy may be experienced.

Do not use when rain is expected to wet cattle within six hours after treatment.

Antiparasitic activity of ivermectin will be impaired if the formulation is applied to areas of the skin with mange scabs or lesions, or with dermatoses or adherent materials, e.g., caked mud or manure.

Warning(s): Cattle must not be treated within 48 days of slaughter for human consumption. Because a withdrawal time in milk has not been established, do not use on female dairy cattle of breeding age.

Not for use in humans.

This product should not be applied to self or others because it may be irritating to human skin and eyes and absorbed through the skin. To minimize accidental skin contact, the user should wear a long-sleeved shirt and rubber gloves. If accidental skin contact occurs, wash immediately with soap and water. If accidental eye exposure occurs, flush eyes immediately with water and seek medical attention.

Keep this and all drugs out of the reach of children.

Safety: Studies conducted in the U.S.A. have demonstrated the safety margin for ivermectin. Based on plasma levels, the topically applied formulation is expected to be at least as well tolerated by breeding animals as is the subcutaneous formulation which had no effect on breeding performance.

Presentation: TOP LINE™ Pour-On is available in an 8.5 fl oz/250 mL bottle with a squeeze-measure-pour system, a 33.8 fl oz/1 L bottle with a squeeze-measure-pour system, or in an 84.5 fl oz/2.5 L collapsible pack and a 169 fl oz/5 L collapsible pack intended for use with appropriate automatic dosing equipment.

U.S. Pat 4,199,569

Compendium Code No.: 10581150

TORBUGESIC® CIV

Fort Dodge **Analgesic**

Butorphanol Tartrate Injection

NADA No.: 135-780

Active Ingredient(s): Each mL of TORBUGESIC® contains:

Butorphanol base (as butorphanol tartrate, USP)	10 mg
Citric acid, USP	3.3 mg
Sodium citrate, USP	6.4 mg
Sodium chloride, USP	4.7 mg
Benzethonium chloride, USP	0.1 mg
Water for injection, USP	q.s.

Indications: TORBUGESIC® (butorphanol tartrate) is indicated for the relief of pain associated with colic in adult horses and yearlings. Clinical studies in the horse have shown that TORBUGESIC® alleviates abdominal pain associated with torsion, impaction, intussusception, spasmodic and tympanic colic and postpartum pain.

Pharmacology:

Description: TORBUGESIC® (butorphanol tartrate) is a totally synthetic, centrally acting, narcotic agonist-antagonist analgesic with potent antitussive activity. It is a member of the phenanthrene series. The chemical name is Morphinan-3, 14-diol, 17-(cyclobutylmethyl)-,(-)-, (S-(R*,R*))-2,3-dihydroxybutanedioate (1:1) (salt). It is a white, crystalline, water soluble substance having a molecular weight of 477.55; its molecular formula is $C_{21}H_{29}NO_2 \bullet C_4H_6O_6$.

Chemical Structure:

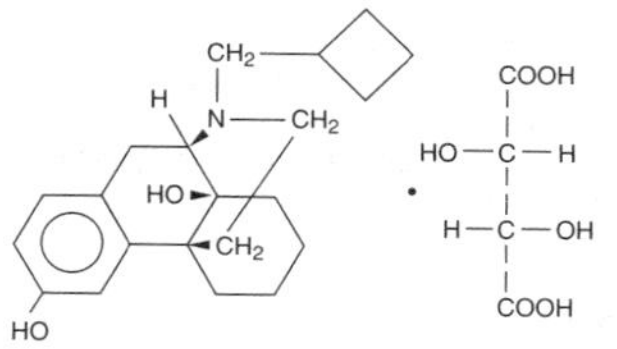

Clinical Pharmacology:

Comparative Pharmacology: In animals, butorphanol has been demonstrated to be 4 to 30 times more potent than morphine and pentazocine (Talwin®-V) respectively.[1] In humans, butorphanol has been shown to have 5 to 7 times the analgesic activity of morphine and 20 times that of pentazocine.[2,3] Butorphanol has 15 to 20 times the oral antitussive activity of codeine or dextromethorphan in dogs and guinea pigs.[4]

As an antagonist, butorphanol is approximately equivalent to nalorphine and 30 times more potent than pentazocine.[1]

Cardiopulmonary depressant effects are minimal after treatment with butorphanol as demonstrated in dogs[5], humans[6,7] and horses.[8] Unlike classical narcotic agonist analgesics which are associated with decreases in blood pressure, reduction in heart rate and concomitant release of histamine, butorphanol does not cause histamine release.[1] Furthermore, the cardiopulmonary effects of butorphanol are not distinctly dosage-related but rather reach a ceiling effect beyond which further dosage increases result in relatively lesser effects.

Reproduction: Studies performed in mice and rabbits revealed no evidence of impaired fertility or harm to the fetus due to butorphanol tartrate. In the female rat, parenteral administration was associated with increased nervousness and decreased care for the newborn, resulting in a decreased survival rate of the newborn. This nervousness was seen only in the rat species.

Equine Pharmacology: Following intravenous injection in horses, butorphanol is largely eliminated from the blood within 3 to 4 hours. The drug is extensively metabolized in the liver and excreted in the urine.

In ponies, butorphanol given intramuscularly at a dosage of 0.22 mg/kg, was shown to alleviate experimentally induced visceral pain for about four hours.[9]

In horses, intravenous dosages of butorphanol ranging from 0.05 to 0.4 mg/kg were shown to be effective in alleviating visceral and superficial pain for at least 4 hours, as illustrated in the following figure:

Analgesic Effects of Butorphanol Given at Various Dosages in Horses with Abdominal Pain

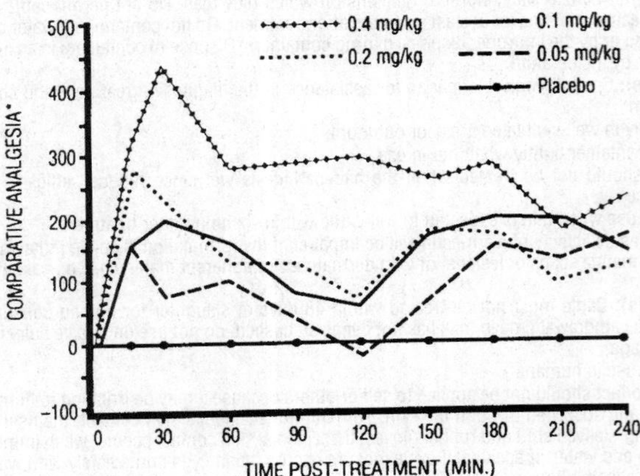

*Pain threshold in butorphanol-treated colicky horses relative to placebo controls.

A definite dosage-response relationship was detected in that butorphanol dosage of 0.1 mg/kg was more effective than 0.05 mg/kg but not different from 0.2 mg/kg in alleviating deep abdominal pain.

Dosage and Administration: The recommended dosage in the horse is 0.1 mg of butorphanol per kilogram of body weight (0.05 mg/lb) by intravenous injection. This is equivalent to 5 mL of TORBUGESIC® for each 1,000 lbs body weight. The dose may be repeated within 3 to 4 hours but treatment should not exceed 48 hours. Pre-clinical model studies and clinical field trials in horses demonstrate that the analgesic effects of TORBUGESIC® are seen within 15 minutes following injection and persist for about 4 hours.

Precaution(s): Store at controlled room temperature 15° to 30°C (59° to 86°F).

Caution(s): Federal law restricts this drug to use by or on the order of a licensed veterinarian.

TORBUGESIC®, a potent analgesic, should be used with caution with other sedative or analgesic drugs as these are likely to produce additive effects.

There are no well-controlled studies using butorphanol in breeding horses, weanlings and foals. Therefore, the drug should not be used in these groups.

Warning(s): Not for use in horses intended for food. Not for human use.

Toxicology:

Acute Equine Studies: Rapid intravenous administration of butorphanol at a dosage of 2 mg/kg (20 times the recommended dosage) to a previously unmedicated horse resulted in a brief episode of inability to stand, muscle fasciculation, a convulsive seizure of 6 seconds duration and recovery within three minutes. The same dosage administered after 10 successive daily 1 mg/kg dosages of butorphanol resulted only in transient sedative effects. During the 10-day course of administration at 1 mg/kg (10 times the recommended use level) in two horses, the only detectable drug effects were transient behavioral changes typical of narcotic agonist activity. These included muscle fasciculation about the head and neck, dysphoria, lateral nystagmus, ataxia and salivation. Repeated administration of butorphanol at 1 mg/kg (10 times the recommended dose) every four hours for 48 hours caused constipation in one of two horses.

Subacute Equine Studies: Horses were found to tolerate butorphanol given intravenously at dosages of 0.1, 0.3 and 0.5 mg/kg every 4 hours for 48 hours followed by once daily injections for a total of 21 days. The only detectable drug effects were slight transient ataxia observed occasionally in the high dosage group. No clinical, laboratory, or gross or histopathologic evidence of any butorphanol-related toxicity was encountered in the horses.

Adverse Reactions: In clinical trials in horses, the most commonly observed side effect was slight ataxia which lasted 3 to 10 minutes. Marked ataxia was reported in 1.5% of the 327 horses treated. Mild sedation was reported in 9% of the horses.

References: Available upon request.

Presentation: TORBUGESIC® (butorphanol tartrate) is supplied in 10 mL (NDC 0856-2033-10) and 50 mL (NDC 0856-2033-20) vials.

Compendium Code No.: 10032260 4540G

TORBUGESIC®-SA Ⓒ

Fort Dodge **Analgesic**

Butorphanol Tartrate, USP Injection

NADA No.: 141-047

Active Ingredient(s): Each mL of TORBUGESIC®-SA contains 2 mg butorphanol base (as butorphanol tartrate, USP); 3.3 mg citric acid, USP; 6.4 mg sodium citrate, USP; 4.7 mg sodium chloride, USP; and 0.1 mg benzethonium chloride, USP; q.s. with water for injection, USP.

Indications: TORBUGESIC®-SA (butorphanol tartrate, USP) is indicated for the relief of pain in cats caused by major or minor trauma, or pain associated with surgical procedures.

Pharmacology:

Description: Butorphanol tartrate, USP is a synthetic, centrally acting, narcotic agonist-antagonist analgesic with potent antitussive activity. The results from laboratory and clinical studies suggest the existence of several distinct types of receptors that are responsible for the activity of opioid and opioid-like drugs. When activated, the μ(mu)-receptors are involved in analgesia, respiratory depression, miosis, physical dependence and feelings of well-being (euphoria). When activated, the κ(kappa)-receptors are involved in analgesia, as well as less intense (as compared to μ-receptors) miosis and respiratory depression. Butorphanol is considered to be a weak antagonist at the μ-receptor, but a strong agonist at the κ-receptor. Thus, butorphanol provides analgesia with a lower incidence and/or intensity of adverse reactions (e.g., miosis and respiratory depression) than traditional opioids.

Butorphanol tartrate is a member of the phenanthrene series. The chemical name is Morphinan-3, 14-diol, 17-(cyclobutylmethyl)-, (-)-, (S- (R*, R*))-2,3-dihydroxybutanedioate (1:1) (salt). It is a white, crystalline, water soluble substance having a molecular weight of 477.55; its molecular formula is $C_{21}H_{29}NO_2 \bullet C_4H_6O_6$.

Chemical Structure:

Clinical Pharmacology:

Feline Pharmacology: The magnitude and duration of analgesic activity of butorphanol were studied in cats under controlled laboratory conditions using both a visceral pain model and a somatic pain model.[1,2] Subcutaneous butorphanol dosages of 0.4 mg/kg produced analgesia significantly ($p<0.05$) greater than the placebo for up to two hours in the somatic pain model. At the label dose (0.4 mg/kg), cardiopulmonary depressant effects were minimal after treatment with butorphanol as demonstrated in cats.[1,2]

Clinical studies confirmed the analgesic effect of butorphanol administered subcutaneously in the cat. In field trials the overall analgesic effect was rated as satisfactory in approximately 75% of butorphanol treated cats. The duration of activity in cats responding to butorphanol ranged from 15 minutes to 8 hours. However, in 70% of responding cats the duration of activity was 3 to 6 hours following subcutaneous administration.

Safety Studies in Cats: Daily subcutaneous injections of butorphanol in cats, beginning at a dosage of 2 mg/kg the first week and doubling each week to a final dosage of 16 mg/kg on the fourth week, resulted in no deaths. No evidence of toxicity was observed during the first three weeks of the experiment, other than pain on injection. During the fourth week, transient incoordination, salivation, or mild seizures were observed within the first hour in the cats following the 16 mg/kg dosage (40 times the recommended clinical dosage). No other clinical, serum chemistry, or gross necropsy evidence of drug toxicity was encountered in any of the cats.

In subacute safety studies, butorphanol was injected subcutaneously to each of six cats at dosages of 0 (saline), 0.4, 1.2 or 2.0 mg/kg, every six hours for six days and continued once daily for a total of 21 days. The only adverse clinical effect observed was pain on injection. Histopathologic changes indicative of minimal to slight irritation were noted at the injection sites in 3 of 6 cats in the low dose group, 4 of 6 cats in the middle dose group and 6 of 6 cats in the high dose group. Histopathologic changes of focal renal tubular dilation were noted in half of the cats in the high dose group.

Dosage and Administration: The recommended dosage in cats is 0.4 mg of butorphanol per kilogram body weight (0.2 mg/lb) given by subcutaneous injection. This is equivalent to 1.0 mL of TORBUGESIC®-SA per 10 lbs of body weight.

Pre-clinical model studies and clinical field trials in cats demonstrated that the analgesic effects of TORBUGESIC®-SA are seen within 20 minutes and persist in the majority of responding cats for 3 to 6 hours following subcutaneous injection (see Feline Pharmacology). The dose may be repeated up to 4 times per day for up to 2 days.

Precaution(s): Store at controlled room temperature 15° to 30°C (59° to 86°F).

Caution(s): Federal law restricts this drug to use by or on the order of a licensed veterinarian.

TORBUGESIC®-SA, a potent analgesic, should be used with caution with other sedative or analgesic drugs as these are likely to produce additive effects.

Safety for use in pregnant female cats, breeding male cats or kittens less than 4 months of age has not been determined. Use of TORBUGESIC®-SA can therefore not be recommended in these groups.

Warning(s): Not for human use.

Adverse Reactions: In clinical trials in cats, pain on injection, mydriasis, disorientation, swallowing/licking and sedation were reported.

References: Available upon request.

Presentation: 10 mL vials TORBUGESIC®-SA (butorphanol tartrate, USP) Veterinary Injection, 2 mg base activity per mL.

NDC 0856-4531-01 — 10 mL — vials

Compendium Code No.: 10032251 4530C

TORBUTROL® Ⓒ

Fort Dodge **Antitussive**

Butorphanol Tartrate-Injection and Tablets

NADA No.: 102-990 (Injection)/103-390 (Tablets)

Active Ingredient(s): Each mL of injectable solution contains:

Butorphanol tartrate . . . . 0.5 mg base activity

Each tablet contains either:

Butorphanol tartrate . . . . 1 mg, 5 mg, or 10 mg base activity

Indications: TORBUTROL® is indicated for the relief of chronic non-productive cough associated with tracheobronchitis, tracheitis, tonsillitis, laryngitis and pharyngitis originating from inflammatory conditions of the upper respiratory tract.

Pharmacology:

Description: TORBUTROL® (butorphanol tartrate) is a narcotic agonist-antagonist analgesic with potent antitussive activity. It is a member of the phenanthrene series. The chemical name is levo-N-cyclobutylmethyl-6, 10 α, β-dihydroxy-1,2,3,9,10,10a-hexahydro-(4H)-10, 4a- iminoethanophenanthrene tartrate (1:1). It is a white crystalline water soluble substance having a molecular weight of 477.56, and its molecular formula is $C_{21}H_{29}NO_2 \bullet C_4H_6O_6$.

Chemical Structure:

Clinical Pharmacology: In dogs, the antitussive properties of butorphanol given s.c. were four times more potent than morphine, 10 times more potent than pentazocine (Talwin®-V), and 100 times more potent than codeine. Orally butorphanol is approximately 15 to 20 times more active than either codeine or dextromethorphan.[1]

Butorphanol given intravenously in large doses (3 mg/kg) to dogs temporarily reduced aortic blood pressure. Aortic pressure returned to baseline control values within 15 to 30 minutes. Changes in cardiac contractile force and cardiac rate were of the same magnitude as the changes in aortic pressure. No appreciable effect on expired carbon dioxide was seen.[2] Studies in anesthetized dogs at equianalgetic doses indicate that butorphanol has less potential than morphine for causing airway constriction, hypotension and histamine release.[3] In conscious dogs butorphanol produced minimal cardiovascular and respiratory effects.[4]

The specific site of action of butorphanol is not known. Butorphanol probably exerts analgesic and antitussive effects via the central nervous system (subcortical, possibly the hypothalamus).

Reproduction studies, performed in mice and rabbits, revealed no evidence of impaired fertility or harm to the fetus due to butorphanol tartrate. In the rat species the female, on parenteral administration, showed increased nervousness and decreased care for the newborn, resulting in a decreased survival rate of the newborn. This nervousness was seen only in the rat species. There are no well-controlled studies in pregnant bitches but, although there is no well-defined risk, the use of TORBUTROL® in pregnant bitches is not recommended.

Dosage and Administration: The usual parenteral dose of TORBUTROL® is 0.025 mg of butorphanol base activity per lb of body weight. This is the equivalent of ½ mL (0.5 mL) for each 10 lbs of body weight. It should be administered by subcutaneous injection, and repeated at intervals of 6 to 12 hours as required. If necessary, the dose may be increased to a maximum of 0.05 mg/lb or 1 mL/10 lbs body weight. Treatment should not normally be required for longer than seven days.

The usual oral dose of TORBUTROL® is 0.25 mg of butorphanol base activity per lb of body weight. This is the equivalent of one 5 mg tablet per 20 lbs of body weight. The dose should be repeated at intervals of 6 to 12 hours as required. If necessary, the dose may be increased to a maximum of one 5 mg tablet for each 10 lbs of body weight. Treatment should not normally be required for longer than seven days.

Contraindication(s):

1. The safety of TORBUTROL® has not been determined in dogs afflicted with heartworm disease *(Dirofilaria immitis)*.
2. TORBUTROL® should not be used in dogs with a history of liver disease.
3. Since TORBUTROL® can be effective in totally suppressing cough, it should not be used in conditions of the lower respiratory tract associated with copious mucus production.

Precaution(s): Store at controlled room temperature 15° to 30°C (59° to 86°F).

Caution(s): Federal law restricts this drug to use by or on the order of a licensed veterinarian.

TORBUTROL® has been shown to have potent analgesic activity in rodents; it is undesirable to administer other sedative or analgesic drugs during treatment with TORBUTROL® (butorphanol tartrate) as these are likely to produce an additive effect.

Cough suppression may be accompanied by mild sedation; the degree of sedation is dose related. If sedation is considered undesirable or unnecessary, the dose should be reduced.

Warning(s): For use in dogs only.

Toxicology: Toxicity studies indicate that the LD_{50} in dogs by oral administration is greater than 50 mg/kg. In studies of 4.5 and 13 weeks duration, the following effects were noted in some but not all dogs at 4.6 times the recommended therapeutic dose level BID given parenterally: Decreased activity, weight loss, salivation, elevated SGPT and/or SAP and mild proliferative changes of the bile duct epithelium.

Adverse Reactions: The most frequent adverse reaction reported in 264 dogs treated with oral TORBUTROL® was slight sedation in 6 dogs (2.3%). Other less frequent adverse reactions which have been reported include anorexia/nausea and diarrhea (reported incidence less than 1%).

Following the marketing of TORBUTROL® Veterinary Injection transient sedation and ataxia have been reported rarely as side effects in dogs.

References: Available upon request.

Presentation: Injectable solution is available in 10 mL vials (NDC 0856-2030-19).

Tablets are available in bottles of 100 at 1 mg (NDC 0856-2025-60), 5 mg (NDC 0856-2026-60) and 10 mg (NDC 0856-2027-60) strengths.

Compendium Code No.: 10032271 4520H

TORPEX™ ℞

Boehringer Ingelheim **Bronchodilator**

Aerosol Albuterol Sulfate, HFA

NADA No.: 141-180

Active Ingredient(s): The active ingredient of TORPEX™ is albuterol sulfate, USP racemic α^1 - [*(tert*-butylamino) methyl]-4-hydroxy-*m*-xylene-α, α^1-diol sulfate (2.1)(salt), a relatively selective $beta_2$-adrenergic bronchodilator.

Each drug canister contains a microcrystalline suspension of albuterol sulfate in propellant HFA-134a (1,1,1, 2-tetrafluoroethane), ethanol, and oleic acid.

This product does not contain chlorofluorocarbon (CPC) propellant.

Indications: For the immediate relief of bronchospasm and bronchoconstriction associated with reversible airway obstruction in horses. In most bronchoconstricted horses, the effect of a single dose (3-6 actuations) of drug lasts for at least one hour although some individual animals may exhibit clinically significant bronchodilation for up to seven (7) hours. Treatment of hoses with small airway disease should include comprehensive reduction of dust and airborne allergens, irritants, or toxins.

Dosage and Administration: Administration: Prior to each use:

1. Shake or invert the product two or three times. When the canister is empty, the spray from the device will decrease sharply. This will be obvious to the drug administrator.
2. Inspect the delivery device and bulb to ensure that they are dry and free of debris.
3. Make sure the bulb is properly attached to the device.
4. The device must be primed before the first use, and when it has not been used for more than two weeks. To prime, hold the device in the upright position and "test fire" two actuations (puffs) away from the horse, and your face.

Insert the bulb into the horse's left nostril avoiding the false nostril. Determine the breathing pattern by observing the air flow-direction vane on the device. To deliver a puff, actuate the device with sharp, crisp finger pressure on the trigger during inspiration. Administer the appropriate number of puffs during sequential inspirations. Remove the device from the nostril. Remove the bulb from the device and clean according to the instructions below.

Dosage: Each actuation (puff) of the device delivers 120 mcg of albuterol sulfate. One dose is three (3) puffs, totaling 360 mcg. Administer one dose. If the desired clinical effect is not achieved, one dose may be repeated immediately for a total of six (6) puffs.

Do not administer more frequently than every six (6) hours. Do not administer more than 4 treatments within 24 hours. Do not use for more than five (5) consecutive days.

In most bronchoconstricted horses, the minimum duration of effect from a single treatment (3-6 puffs) of drug is one hour, but effects may persist for up to seven (7) hours.

Device Cleaning:

Bulb: Remove the bulb and immerse it in warm water with mild soap or detergent. Agitate the bulb a few times and manually remove any foreign material. Rinse thoroughly in clean potable water. Shake out excess water. Allow the interior surface of the bulb to air dry or dry with a non-tinting absorbent cloth prior to use. Thorough cleansing is recommended if the bulb will be used for multiple horses.

Equine inhaler: Inspect the device for debris. Remove debris with a cotton swab.

Precaution(s): Storage: Store at room temperature between 15°C and 25°C (59°F and 77°F). For best results, use at room temperature. Occasional excursions outside storage temperature range will not affect drug delivery. Avoid exposing product to extreme heat and cold for prolonged periods.

Contents under pressure. Do not puncture. Do not store near heat or flame. Exposure to temperatures above 120°F may cause bursting. Never throw container into fire or incinerator.

Caution(s): Federal (U.S.A.) law restricts this drug to use by or on the order of a licensed veterinarian.

The safety of TORPEX™ in horses used for breeding purposes, pregnant or lactating mares has not been evaluated.

Warning(s): Not for use in horses intended for human consumption.

Human Warning: Avoid spraying into eyes. Keep out of reach of children. Avoid human inhalation. People with heart disorders, hypersensitivity to aerosol albuterol, and pregnant or nursing women should contact their physician prior to use of this product. Although uncommon, adverse effects of albuterol in humans after therapeutic inhalation may include increased heart rate, irregular heart rhythm, and tremors. Consult a physician immediately if any of these symptoms develop after accidental human inhalation.

Adverse Reactions: Sweating, muscle tremors, or excitement have been shown to occur as an adverse reaction to $beta_2$-agonists in horses. During clinical trials in which 459 treatments of up to 6 actuations were administered, sweating was reported in 10.7% of horses prior to treatment, in 11.1% after drug treatment, and in 3.5% after placebo treatment. Mild trembling was reported in <1% of observations prior to treatment, after drug treatment, or after placebo treatment. Mild excitement was reported in 5.0% of horses prior to treatment, 4.8% after drug treatment, and 1.3% after placebo treatment. In most cases, signs dissipated within 30 minutes.

For a copy of the Material Safety Data Sheet (MSDS) or to report a suspected adverse reaction, call 1-800-821-7467.

Discussion: TORPEX™ is a pressurized metered dose aerosol drug unit for inhalation that is contained in a hand-held, manually-actuated dispensing device for drug administration to the lungs of horses.

Presentation: TORPEX™ is supplied in a pressurized aluminum canister within an actuator system equipped with a detachable nasal delivery bulb. Each valve actuation delivers 120 mcg of albuterol sulfate. In addition to priming doses, net weight of 6.7 grams of formulated product provides adequate drug to deliver 200 puffs to the horse.

U.S. Patent Nos. 5,225,183; 5,666,948; 5,062,423

TORPEX™ a registered trademark of Boehringer Ingelheim Vetmedica, Inc., St Joseph, MO 64506.

Jointly developed for Equine Health by 3M and Boehringer Ingelheim Vetmedica, Inc.

Manufactured by: 3M Animal Care Products.

Compendium Code No.: 10281341 BI 4333-5 5/02, 433303L-03-0111

TOTALON® POUR-ON DEWORMER

Schering-Plough **Parasiticide-Topical**

(Levamisole) Topical Anthelmintic

NADA No.: 139-877

Active Ingredient(s): Each mL contains:

Levamisole . . . . 200 mg

Indications: TOTALON® (levamisole) is a broad-spectrum anthelmintic and is effective against the following nematode infections in cattle.

Stomach Worms: *Haemonchus, Trichostrongylus, Ostertagia.*

Intestinal Worms: *Trichostrongylus, Cooperia, Nematodirus, Bunostomum, Oesophagostomum, Chabertia.*

Lungworms: *Dictyocaulus.*

Dosage and Administration: The recommended dose of TOTALON® (levamisole) is 2.5 mL per 110 lbs. (50 kg) of body weight. Apply topically to the back of the animal. For example:

Body Weight (lbs.)	Dose
200-300	5 mL
300-400	7.5 mL
400-500	10 mL
500-600	12.5 mL
600-700	15 mL
700-80	17.50 mL
800-900	20 mL

Use of the Applicator Gun: Remove the cap and inner seal from the bottle. Firmly seal the tube adaptor supplied with the applicator gun. Carefully estimate the cattle weight and select the desired mL setting. Squeeze the handle completely while directing the fluid along the backline of the animal.

Use of the Dosing Device: Remove the cap and inner seal from the calibrated dosing chamber of the bottle. Carefully estimate the cattle weight and calculate the dose. Squeeze the bottle to fill the calibrated cylinder to the desired graduation mark. Pour evenly along the backline of the animal. Do not squeeze the bottle during the application of the dose.

Do not treat animals immediately before dipping or prior to exposure to heavy rain. Cattle maintained under conditions of constant helminth exposure may require retreatment within two (2) to four (4) weeks after the first treatment.

Precaution(s): Store at room temperature: 15-30°C (59-86°F). For the storage of unused material, remove the delivery tube system and replace the original cap. Dispose of empty containers and wastes resulting from the cleanup of spills in approved landfills in accordance with federal, state and local regulations.

Warning(s): Cattle must not be slaughtered within nine (9) days following the last treatment with this drug. Because a withdrawal time in milk has not been established, do not use on female dairy cattle of breeding age.

Human Warning: The product is absorbed through intact skin.

Rubber gloves should be used to protect the hands of the operator. Use only in well ventilated areas. In case of skin contact, immediately flush with water while removing contaminated clothing and wash with soap and water.

If in eyes, flush with water for 15 minutes. Get medical attention if irritation persists.

If inhaled, remove victim to fresh air. Apply artificial respiration, if indicated.

If swallowed, induce vomiting. Never give anything by mouth to an unconscious person.

Keep out of the reach of children.

Side Effects: In clinical trials, an accumulation of desquamated epidermal flakes was noted at the application site in 8% of the animals 7-10 days after treatment. The skin flaking was not clinically significant and disappeared spontaneously within 30 days after TOTALON® (levamisole) administration without a residual effect. Two types of skin reactions have been observed on cattle treated with TOTALON® (levamisole). An accumulation of desquamated epidermal flakes has been noted at the application site 7-10 days after treatment. This skin flaking was not clinically significant and disappeared spontaneously within 30 days without residual effect. A local sensitivity type reaction has also been observed after the use of the product. While the reaction is infrequent, affected cattle may develop localized inflammation at the area of application. Drying and peeling of the skin can occur. Resolution takes place within a few weeks. If adverse skin reactions are severe, consult a veterinarian.

Muzzle foam may be observed within a few hours. If this condition persists, a veterinarian should be consulted.

Consult a veterinarian for assistance in the diagnosis, treatment and control of parasitism and before using in severely debilitated animals.

Presentation: 500 mL and 2 L plastic containers.

* ® Registered trademark of Janssen Pharmaceutica N.V.

Compendium Code No.: 10471881

TOXIBAN™

Vet-A-Mix **Adsorbent**

Active Ingredient(s): TOXIBAN™ Granules contain 47.5% MedChar™, 10% Kaolin and 42.5% wetting and dispersing agents, including sorbitol, and is free-flowing and wettable for rapid reconstitution in water. It may also be mixed in the dry form with food.

TOXIBAN™ Suspension contains 10.4% charcoal and 6.25% kaolin in an aqueous base. It is a stable suspension which is intended for use as a convenient emergency treatment of small animals or small numbers of large animals.

TOXIBAN™ Suspension with Sorbitol is a convenient, ready-to-use, activated charcoal suspension containing 10% MedChar™, 10% sorbitol and 6.25% kaolin in an aqueous base with special suspending agents and preservatives intended for use as an emergency treatment of small animals.

MedChar™, (a medicinal grade of activated charcoal), contained in all three products, is a small particle size type of vegetable charcoal that possesses a relatively high activity as an adsorbent of organic chemicals. It has been processed by Vet-A-Mix to enhance its adsorptive power and reduce dustiness. Its adsorptive activity exceeds the USP standard for activated charcoal.

Indications: TOXIBAN™ Granules, TOXIBAN™ Suspension and TOXIBAN™ Suspension with Sorbitol are intended for use as adsorbents of orally ingested toxicants.

Indications And Usage: TOXIBAN™ Granules, TOXIBAN™ Suspension and TOXIBAN™ Suspension with Sorbitol are most effective when administered as soon as ingestion of a toxicant is suspected. They can also be used in some toxic emergencies when absorption of the toxicant is nearly complete or the exposure was via a parenteral route. This application usually involves repetitive or multiple dose activated charcoal use. Multiple doses of charcoal may be useful in adsorbing toxins which undergo enterohepatic circulation. Drugs such as digitoxin which are subject to biliary secretion are constantly secreted into the gastrointestinal tract and are reabsorbed resulting in prolonged toxicity. Frequent doses of activated charcoal can adsorb those toxins, interrupt the enterohepatic circulation, thereby preventing their reabsorption, and enhance toxicant elimination from the body into the gastrointestinal tract. Treatment with TOXIBAN™ should be designed to inactivate at least 80% of an ingested toxicant. Normal body detoxification mechanisms combined with specific or symptomatic antidotal therapy are used to inactivate or counteract the toxicant that is not adsorbed by TOXIBAN™.

Adsorption of a toxin can occur anywhere along the gastrointestinal tract. However, to be most effective, TOXIBAN™ should be administered as soon as ingestion of a toxicant is suspected or at the onset of signs of toxicosis. If an oral emetic, such as syrup of ipecac, hydrogen peroxide, or apomorphine is used, TOXIBAN™ should not be used until after emesis. There should be a delay of thirty to sixty minutes between the conclusion of emesis and the administration of TOXIBAN™ Granules, TOXIBAN™ Suspension or TOXIBAN™ Suspension with Sorbitol to avoid regurgitation of the treatment.

When gastric lavage is used to facilitate stomach evacuation, a single dose of TOXIBAN™ may be administered in the early stages of this procedure. The primary advantage of using TOXIBAN™ with gastric lavage is that early administration of activated charcoal permits prompt adsorption of the toxicant. The only disadvantage is that the lavage returns will be black, thus making it difficult to visually evaluate the ingesta. Only TOXIBAN™ Suspension or Granules should be used with this technique. After completion of the lavage procedure, TOXIBAN™ Suspension with Sorbitol may be administered via the lavage tube before its removal.

Multiple dose activated charcoal is also used in what is termed gastrointestinal dialysis in which the toxin passively diffuses along a concentration gradient between blood perfusing the gastrointestinal tract and the luminal fluids. Multiple treatment doses adsorb the toxin preventing its reabsorption which further maximizes the concentration gradient which permits diffusion of even more toxin into the GI tract. While not all toxins respond to this treatment, lipophilic, uncharged and not extensively protein bound compounds are effectively eliminated in this way. Phenobarbital and theophylline are examples of toxins which can be eliminated more rapidly using this concept.

TOXIBAN™ Suspension with Sorbitol should not be used in each dose of the multiple dose activated charcoal regimen unless it is necessary to achieve catharsis. Since TOXIBAN™ Suspension with Sorbitol contains sorbitol, it may produce excessive catharsis and resultant fluid and electrolyte problems if used at each dosage interval (see cautions). TOXIBAN™ Suspension should be used at the dosage intervals when TOXIBAN™ Suspension with Sorbitol is not being used.

Catharsis should only be used intermittently during multiple dose activated charcoal use.

There are no specific recommendations established for when to stop multiple dose charcoal therapy. Clinical judgment should be used in conjunction with consideration of which agents were ingested, serum concentration, clinical status of the animal, and any pertinent considerations specific to the animal being treated.

If catharsis of activated charcoal does not occur within eight hours following the use of TOXIBAN™ Suspension with Sorbitol, an additional dose of sorbitol at 1.5 mg per kilogram may be administered. Or if desired, a saline cathartic such as magnesium citrate or sodium or magnesium sulfate may be used at a dosage of 1 gram/kilogram if the patient's renal function is not compromised.

In most herds with accidental acute poisonings, the dosages of the toxicant are obviously unknown and the decision relative to which animals to treat and the dosage levels of TOXIBAN™ Granules are judgmental. In instances involving valuable or prized animals or small herds it is probably prudent to treat all animals which were possibly exposed. In large herds, treatment with TOXIBAN™ maybe delayed until signs of toxicosis are elicited. In any case, overdosing with TOXIBAN™ will cause no untoward effects.

TOXIBAN™ Granules will be used to treat acute toxicosis in most cases, but it may be administered daily or mixed in feed in subacute or chronic toxicosis, to enhance the body clearance and excretion of certain already absorbed drugs or toxicants. An example of the latter is the hastening of excretion of chlorinated hydrocarbon insecticides from body fat of food-producing animals. When TOXIBAN™ is administered repeatedly on a daily basis, TOXIBAN™ will also depress the action of oral antibacterials, such as sulfonamides and antibiotics, when used concurrently with such drugs.

Chlorinated Hydrocarbon Insecticides: Chemicals in this group include aldrin, chlordane, DDT, dieldrin, endrin, heptachlor, lindane, mirex, methoxychlor, perthane, DDS, and toxaphene. Clinical signs of poisoning from these compounds usually occur within 24 hours after ingestion or dermal application and are predominantly neuromuscular, characterized by hyperexcitability and tonoclonic convulsions. TOXIBAN™ should be administered whenever signs are noted. It may be necessary to control convulsions, before or after administering TOXIBAN™, by use of light anesthesia with pentobarbital or chloral hydrate or by tranquilizing. The animal should be cooled if body temperature increases exceedingly. If toxicosis is from dermal applications the pesticide should be removed by bathing with water and soap. TOXIBAN™ administration should be repeated every 6 to 8 hours until signs subside.

Organophosphate Insecticides: Chemicals in this large group include Abate, azinphos methyl, azodrin, bidrin, carbophenothion, Ciodrin, chlorfenvinphos, coumaphos, dasanit, demeton, fensulfothion, dichlofenthion, dichlorvos, dimethoate, dioxathion, disulfoton, dursban, dyfonate, EPN, ethion, famphur, fenthion, Imidan, malathion, methyl parathion, methyl trithion, mevinphos, mocap, parathion, naled, phorate, phosdrin, phosphamidon, rabon, ronnel, Ruelene, tepp, and trichlorfon.

Carbamate Insecticides: These chemicals include baygon, BUX, carbaryl, carbofuran, and landrin. The organophosphate (O-P) and carbamate insecticides have largely replaced the chlorinated hydrocarbons for agricultural use. Both of these types of chemicals are acetylcholinesterase inhibitors, and acute toxicosis is due to over stimulation of the parasympathetic nervous system. Signs generally include salivation, gastrointestinal hypermotility, dyspnea, miosis, twitching and stiffness of skeletal muscles. Small animals may exhibit excess CNS stimulation. Signs of poisoning by carbamates and O-P pesticides are usually evident within minutes to hours after ingestion, but may be delayed for several days in the case of the systemic O-P compounds, such as coumaphos and ruelene.

Atropine sulfate is the preferred pharmacologic antidote for carbamates and O-P insecticides. The recommended dosage is 0.5 mg/kg body weight in all animals. The average horse may receive 65 mg; the average dog may receive 2 mg. Initially, approximately ¼ of the dose should be injected intravenously, and the rest given intramuscularly or subcutaneously.

If animals are known or thought to have ingested any of these toxicants, TOXIBAN™ should be given first followed by atropine when signs first appear. Atropinization usually lasts 2 to 4 hours, and if signs persist, atropine injections should be repeated every 2 to 4 hours. Two or three doses of atropine injections may be necessary. TOXIBAN™ administration should be repeated every 6 to 8 hours until signs subside.

Oximes, such as 2-PAM (protopam chloride, TMB-4, pralidoxime) are useful treatments for O-P toxicosis, but not for carbamate poisoning. Intravenous dosages of 20 mg/kg body weight are recommended and can be given with atropine and TOXIBAN™. The opiates, succinylcholine and phenothiazine tranquilizers are contraindicated for treatment of carbamate and O-P poisonings.

Alkaloids: Strychnine, nicotine (cigarettes) and many poisonous principles in weeds are alkaloids. TOXIBAN™ is effective in inactivating alkaloids, but the animal must be treated to alleviate the signs due to the absorbed alkaloids.

Animals poisoned with strychnine should be anesthetized with intravenous injections of pentobarbital sodium or by other suitable methods and then given TOXIBAN™ by oral infusion. The prognosis is poor in animals poisoned by nicotine, but TOXIBAN™ should be given by oral infusion followed by artificial respiration and administration of oxygen. Animals known or thought to have ingested a toxic alkaloid should be given prophylactic doses of TOXIBAN™.

Synthetic Herbicides and Fungicides: Generally speaking the organic herbicides and fungicides are not toxic at their normal application rates. Animals may be poisoned by voluntary ingestion of the pure chemical or by careless incorporation into rations during farm feed mixing.

Ethylene Glycol: TOXIBAN™ is effective and increases survival rate if used early in the treatment of cases of ethylene glycol (antifreeze) poisoning. To be effective, TOXIBAN™ must be administered within 4 hours after ingestion of the antifreeze occurs. Any history of ethylene glycol ingestion should be handled as a medical emergency and the animal treated immediately unless advanced clinical signs have occurred. Tests for ethylene glycol must be conducted before TOXIBAN™ is administered to prevent false positive reactions.

Miscellaneous Use for TOXIBAN™: TOXIBAN™ is indicated whenever synthetic organic drugs have been administered accidentally or mistakenly in overdoses. Included in this list are the barbiturates, tranquilizers, narcotics, salicylates (aspirin), pyrazolon drugs (phenylbutazone), stimulants, and diuretics.

TOXIBAN™ can be used in cases of toxic bacterial enteritis and in ruminants with toxic overload as an adsorbent of putrefactive toxins, as well as the catecholamines and bacterial endotoxins. It should be used as an adjunct with other treatments, such as rumenotomies, fluid therapy, and restoration of acid-base balance by adding sodium bicarbonate at about 2 mg per kg mixed in the slurry with the TOXIBAN™. Charcoal has been reported to adsorb mercuric salts, but is not considered a generally satisfactory antidote for heavy metal poisoning.

TOXIBAN™ is indicated in "garbage poisoning" of dogs.

Pharmacology: Clinical Pharmacology: Activated charcoal is the most valuable single emergency antidote, since it acts by inactivating many organic toxicants by adsorption, a surface-active phenomenon. It is considered a universal antidote. Charcoal, with a small particle size, is most effective; plant charcoal is more effective than animal charcoal. Most organic ring compounds are adsorbed by charcoal in a more-or-less nondiscriminatory manner. Nevertheless, adsorption sites are somewhat selective and larger heterocyclic molecules may be adsorbed competitively in place of smaller molecules. Therefore, the dose of charcoal needed to inactivate a given dose of toxicant depends on the following factors: (1) the intrinsic activity of the charcoal type; (2) the dose of toxicant; (3) the types and amounts of other competitive compounds in the gastrointestinal ingesta.

It has been reported that 1 gram of activated charcoal would adsorb the following substances in the amounts (in mg) indicated in parentheses: mercuric chloride (1800), sulfanilamide (1000), strychnine nitrate (950), morphine hydrochloride (800), atropine sulfate (700), nicotine (700), salicylic acid (550), phenol (400), phenobarbital (350), and alcohol (300). These data were derived from *in vitro* aqueous solutions, however, and do not reflect the true situation in the gastrointestinal compartments. In *in vivo* systems, natural substances in ingesta adsorb or absorb low levels of most toxicants. Conversely, normal non-toxic compounds present in ingesta compete for binding sites on orally administered charcoal.

It has been determined that charcoal inactivation of a toxicant in gastrointestinal contents, appears to be approximately stoichiometric and dose related in a linear fashion up to 70% to 85% . Above these levels increased levels of charcoal are needed to improve the percent of inactivation. This has been shown to occur with strychnine in canine gastric contents and phorate and carbofuran in bovine rumen fluids. See Graph.

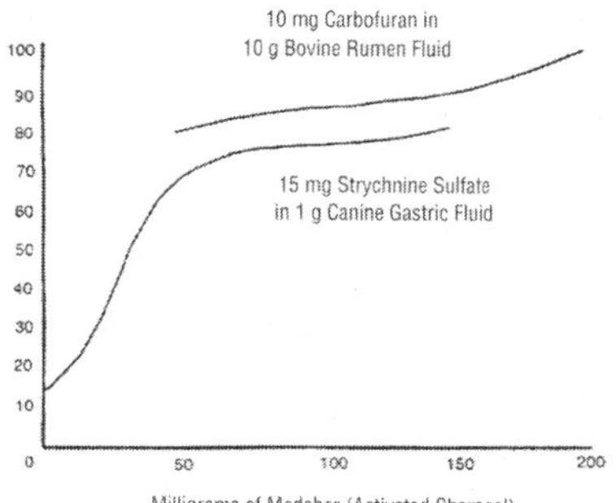

In Vitro Adsorption for Rumen Contents Spiked with Carbofuran and for Canine Gastric Contents Spiked with Strychnine Sulfate

As a general rule it is safe to assume that 1 gram of MedChar activated charcoal will adsorb 70 mg to 90 mg of an ingested organic toxicant.

Sorbitol is a hexahydric sugar alcohol which primarily serves as an osmotic cathartic. It is poorly absorbed during its transit through the gastrointestinal tract. Sorbitol that is absorbed is metabolized by the liver and slowly converted to fructose. Insulin is not necessary for intracellular transport of sorbitol. Therefore, customary cathartic doses can be safely used by animals with diabetes mellitus.

As a hyperosmotic cathartic, sorbitol produces a hygroscopic action resulting in increased water in the large intestine and increased intraluminal pressure which stimulates catharsis. Sorbitol does not compromise the adsorptive capacity of activated charcoal.

Activated charcoal given alone becomes stationary in the gastrointestinal tract, releasing its adsorbed toxin which may subsequently be absorbed by the intestinal mucosa to again produce toxicoses. Sorbitol is an effective cathartic for use with activated charcoal in monogastric animals. It promotes passage of the activated charcoal and adsorbed toxin via the feces.

Kaolin is a naturally occurring hydrated aluminum silicate which is powdered and refined for pharmaceutical use. It is not absorbed from the gut after oral administration. Colloidal kaolin is an intestinal protectant for inflamed GI mucosa. Its well-known adsorptive properties in removing bacteria and endotoxins from gastrointestinal contents aid in preventing absorption of these and other GI toxins.

Dosage and Administration: Administration: Give TOXIBAN™ Suspension or TOXIBAN™ Suspension with Sorbitol orally by causing the animal to drink the calculated dose either as is or mixed with a small amount of cold water. To reduce viscosity and improve flow, shake the container thoroughly. The container has headroom which allows for the addition of water to reduce viscosity and improve flow. Rinse the liquid receptacle with cold water and administer the rinsing. Consult a veterinarian should administration by stomach tube be needed.

Directions for Professional Use Only: TOXIBAN™ Suspension or TOXIBAN™ Suspension with Sorbitol can be poured through a funnel attached to a stomach tube in most animals. Alternate methods are use of a stomach pump or syringe to inject the suspension through a stomach tube.

Dilute suspensions of TOXIBAN™ Granules should be stirred or agitated frequently during administration to keep the liquid uniform and prevent equipment clogging. A stomach tube or rumen tube is preferred for administration in all animals, but an oral drench may be used in an emergency.

An effective method for administering activated charcoal slurries to large animals is to use a plastic enema bag or a calf milk feeding bag. These containers allow manipulation of the slurry to keep it agitated as it is introduced into the stomach tube. Administration equipment should be flushed with a dose of cold water before removing the stomach tube. Equipment used to administer TOXIBAN™ cleans easily with water and detergent or water alone.

Stomach tubes can be passed nasogastrically or orogastrically. First measure from tip of nose to the last rib to predetermine the length of tube needed to be inserted. The position of the tube can be checked by injecting one mL of sterile saline. Coughing will normally occur if the trachea has been intubated. For a detailed description of oral administration of liquids refer to pages 536 - 540 of the 5th edition of Handbook of Veterinary Procedures and Emergency Treatment by Kirk et al.

Poisoned animals should be watched closely after treatment, since specific or systemic treatment may need be repeated. Repeated doses of activated charcoal given every 4 to 6 hours for 24 to 48 hours may interrupt the hepatoenteric circulation of the toxicant in cases of acute toxicosis.

Dosage:

TOXIBAN™ Granules: To make a thin suspension mix one volume measure with 5 to 7 parts of cold water (Ex: one level cup TOXIBAN™ Granules to 6 cupfuls water) and shake or stir vigorously for 10-30 seconds until good suspension is obtained.

Large Animals - The recommended dosage is 0.75 to 2.0 grams per kilogram (0.35 to 0.9 grams per pound) body weight. One pound (453.6 grams) will normally treat an animal weighing 225 to 600 kilograms (500 to 1300 pounds).

Small Animals - 2 to 4 grams per kg (1 to 2 grams per pound) body weight.

TOXIBAN™ Granules				
Measure	Equivalent Measure	MedChar	Kaolin	Sorbitol
1 level teaspoonful	2.0 g	1.0 g	0.2 g	0.6 g
1 level tablespoonful	5.0 g	2.4 g	0.5 g	1.4 g
1 level cupful	120.0 g	57.0 g	12.0 g	33.0 g
One pound	453.6 g	215.5 g	45.4 g	124.7 g
One kilogram	1,000 g	475.0 g	100.0 g	275.0 g

TOXIBAN™ Suspension or TOXIBAN™ Suspension with Sorbitol:

Small Animals - 10 to 20 mL per kg (5 to 10 mL per pound) body weight.

Large Animals - 4 to 12 mL per kg (2 to 6 mL per pound) body weight.

TOXIBAN™ Suspension and TOXIBAN™ Suspension with Sorbitol*				
Measure	Equivalent Measure	MedChar	Kaolin	Sorbitol
1 level teaspoonful	5 mL	0.5 g	0.3 g	0.5 g
1 level tablespoonful	15 mL	1.5 g	0.9 g	1.5 g
1 level cupful	240 mL	25.0 g	15.0 g	25.0 g
One liter	1,000 mL	104.0 g	62.5 g	104.0 g

*TOXIBAN™ Suspension does not contain therapeutic amounts of sorbitol 2 grams TOXIBAN™ Granules is equivalent to the charcoal activity of 9 mL TOXIBAN™ Suspension.

Contraindication(s): There are no known absolute contraindications to the use of activated charcoal. However, it is not equally effective as an adsorbent for all toxins. Chemicals that are not effectively adsorbed by activated charcoal include caustic materials (bleach, lye), ethanol and methanol, fertilizer, fluoride, heavy metal salts, iodides, nitrate and nitrite, sodium chloride and chlorate. It should be used with caution, if at all, in animals that have ingested corrosive agents since the activated charcoal may not be advised if the animal has significant fluid and/or electrolyte abnormalities. It should not be given simultaneously or shortly before the oral administration of other therapeutic agents such as antibiotics, vitamins, or amino acids. Antibiotic therapy should be administered parenterally when TOXIBAN™ is used.

Caution(s): All three TOXIBAN™ products are adjuncts in the management of poisoning emergencies. Prior to their use, proper basic life support measures must be implemented as well as the appropriate gastric emptying technique if indicated. Since more than an hour may pass before activated charcoal can be administered without regurgitation after an emetic has been given, it may be more effective to give TOXIBAN™ immediately because adsorption of a toxicant may be a more effective removal than vomition.

When TOXIBAN™ therapy is used, it should be noted the products will produce black stools. These stools may have a diarrhea consistency and may persist for several hours. Since a profound cathartic effect may occur following the use of TOXIBAN™ Suspension with Sorbitol, proper attention should be provided to the animal's fluid and electrolyte needs.

TOXIBAN™ Suspension with Sorbitol should be used cautiously in animals receiving multiple dose activated charcoal therapy. If TOXIBAN™ Suspension with Sorbitol is used at each dosage interval, profound catharsis may develop resulting in dehydration and even hypotension.

Presentation: TOXIBAN™ Granules, 12 x 454 g (1 lb) per carton and 5 kg (11 lb) pails.
TOXIBAN™ Suspension, 12 x 240 mL per carton.
TOXIBAN™ Suspension with Sorbitol, 12 x 240 mL per carton.

Compendium Code No.: 10500312 0101

TOXIVAC® AD+E

Boehringer Ingelheim **Bacterin-Toxoid**

Bordetella bronchiseptica-Erysipelothrix rhusiopathiae-Pasteurella multocida Bacterin-Toxoid

U.S. Vet. Lic. No.: 319

Contents: The bacterin-toxoid is adjuvanted and contains cell free and nontoxic antigens of *Pasteurella multocida* as well as inactivated cultures of *Bordetella bronchiseptica* and *Erysipelothrix rhusiopathiae.* Gentamicin is added as a preservative.

Indications: For use as an aid in the prevention of disease due to infection by *Bordetella bronchiseptica, Erysipelothrix rhusiopathiae* and toxigenic strains of *Pasteurella multocida* types A and D.

Dosage and Administration: Shake well.

Sows or Gilts: Vaccinate intramuscularly with two (2) doses (2 mL each) at five (5) weeks and two (2) weeks prior to initial farrowing. Vaccinate with one (1) dose (2 mL) at three (3) weeks prior to subsequent farrowings. Vaccinate all new replacement breeding stock with two (2) doses (2 mL each) spaced a minimum of two (2) to three (3) weeks apart prior to entry into the breeding herd.

Boars: Initially vaccinate intramuscularly with two (2) doses (2 mL each) spaced a minimum of two (2) to three (3) weeks apart. Revaccinate annually.

Pigs: Vaccinate intramuscularly with one (1) dose (2 mL) at three (3) to four (4) weeks of age.

Precaution(s): Store in the dark under refrigeration not over 45°F or 7°C.

Caution(s): Use the entire contents when first opened. In case of an anaphylactic reaction, epinephrine is symptomatic treatment.

Warning(s): Do not vaccinate within 21 days of slaughter.

Presentation: 100 mL (50 dose) vials.

Compendium Code No.: 10281070

TOXIVAC® PLUS PARASUIS

Boehringer Ingelheim **Bacterin-Toxoid**

Bordetella bronchiseptica-Erysipelothrix rhusiopathiae-Haemophilus parasuis-Pasteurella multocida Bacterin-Toxoid

U.S. Vet. Lic. No.: 319

Contents: The bacterin-toxoid is adjuvanted and contains cell free and nontoxic antigens of *Pasteurella multocida* as well as inactivated cultures of *Bordetella bronchiseptica, Erysipelothrix rhusiopathiae,* and *Haemophilus parasuis.* Gentamicin is added as a preservative.

Indications: TOXIVAC® Plus Parasuis is intended to aid in the prevention of disease in swine due to infection caused by *Bordetella bronchiseptica, Erysipelothrix rhusiopathiae, Haemophilus parasuis* and *Pasteurella multocida* associated with atrophic rhinitis.

Dosage and Administration: Shake well.

Sows or Gilts: Vaccinate intramuscularly with two (2) doses (2 mL each) at five (5) weeks and two (2) weeks prior to farrowing and with one (1) dose (2 mL) at three (3) weeks prior to subsequent farrowings.

New breeding stock should be vaccinated with two (2) doses (2 mL each) spaced three (3) weeks apart prior to entry into the breeding herd.

Boars should initially be vaccinated with two (2) doses (2 mL) each spaced three (3) weeks apart and revaccinated annually with one (1) 2 mL dose.

Pigs should be vaccinated with one (1) dose (2 mL) at 3-4 weeks of age. *Haemophilus parasuis* requires a second dose given 2-4 weeks after the first.

Precaution(s): Store in the dark under refrigeration at not over 45°F or 7°C.

Caution(s): Use the entire contents when first opened. In case of an anaphylactic reaction, epinephrine is symptomatic treatment.

Warning(s): Do not vaccinate within 21 days of slaughter.

Discussion: Atrophic rhinitis continues to be one of the most complex disease syndromes that swine practitioners and producers face today. Management factors that affect the environment, nutrition and husbandry have a significant impact on the severity of the disease. The two bacterial pathogens most associated with this complex are *Bordetella bronchiseptica* and toxigenic *Pasteurella multocida*, types A and D.

Erysipelothrix rhusiopathiae is a gram-positive rod that causes the disease erysipelas. The two major serotypes are serotypes 1 and 2. Erysipelas in swine may be manifested as an acute, subacute (signs and lesions less severe), or chronic (arthritis, endocarditis) syndrome. Abortion in later stages of pregnancy is sometimes seen. Acute septicemic erysipelas occurs suddenly with death in one or more animals. Very high fevers (107°F), leg stiffness and cutaneous lesions may be seen in some. Subacute and chronic cases may be observed in the same herd. Erysipelas can kill swine of any age.

Glasser's disease is associated with *Haemophilus parasuis* worldwide. *H. parasuis* is best known as the etiologic agent of Glasser's disease, which is characterized by polyserositis and arthritis. Pigs of about five to eight weeks of age are the most commonly affected, however the range can be highly variable, especially in minimal disease operations or where nonimmune swine are comingled with more conventionally raised animals which commonly carry the organism as part of their normal respiratory flora. Morbidity and mortality reports are also variable with a wide spectrum of clinical signs possible. Peracute or acute death may occur or any combination of high fever (105°-107°F), malaise, anorexia, respiratory distress, edema, cyanosis, lameness, reluctance to move or CNS signs are possible. Cross postmortem lesions of fibrinous pleuritis, pericarditis, arthritis and meningitis with or without pneumonia are commonly observed. Diagnosis is based upon history, clinical signs, findings at necropsy and isolation of the small gram-negative highly pleomorphic rod. *H. parasuis* is an extremely diverse organism in nature and varies greatly in pathogenic properties. The most commonly identified U.S. serotypes are 2, 4 and 5. Other common serotypes have recently been identified. Autogenous and other *H. parasuis*-containing biologicals have been used to help control the disease in naive herds. It was suggested recently that strains may differ antigenically and that if homologous and heterologous protection are desired, vaccine isolates need to be selected carefully.

Trial Data: A recent trial* at Boehringer demonstrated the cross-protective properties of TOXIVAC® Plus Parasuis. Fifteen pigs were vaccinated at three to four weeks of age and again three weeks later. Five comparable nonvaccinated control animals were also included. Pigs were challenged with a serotype not in the vaccine. They were monitored daily for fever and clinical signs of Glasser's disease. All five controls became febrile (range = 106.4° to 107.7°F) on Day 1 and remained so until death which occurred between Days 3 and 5 postchallenge. Clinically, the following were observed in controls before death: Depression, labored breathing, severe lameness and CNS (staggering) signs. All vaccinates remained clinically normal.

*Data on file Boehringer Ingelheim.

Presentation: 100 mL (50 dose) vials.

Compendium Code No.: 10281090

TRACHIVAX®

Schering-Plough **Vaccine**

Fowl Laryngotracheitis Vaccine, Modified Live Virus

U.S. Vet. Lic. No.: 165A

Active Ingredient(s): TRACHIVAX® is a live fowl laryngotracheitis vaccine containing a carefully selected virus strain that has been modified by passage in chicken embryos. The vaccine contains gentamicin as a preservative.

Indications: For the vaccination of healthy chickens four weeks of age or older, as an aid in the prevention of laryngotracheitis through immunization by the eye drop method.

Dosage and Administration:

When to Vaccinate: Vaccinate initially at four (4) weeks of age.

Replacement chickens vaccinated initially at four (4) weeks of age should be revaccinated at 10 weeks of age or older.

Vaccination Program: The development of a durable, strong protection depends upon the use of an effective vaccination program as well as many other circumstances such as administration techniques, environment and flock health at the time of vaccination. Also, the immune response to one (1) vaccination under field conditions is seldom complete for all animals within a given flock. Even when vaccination is successful, the protection stimulated in individual animals against different diseases may not be life-long.

If necessary, the vaccine may be used to aid in limiting the spread of an outbreak; however, only birds not yet infected with the virulent outbreak virus can be protected.

Examination of birds for vaccination takes is unnecessary and so-called takes are not to be expected. As with all live virus vaccines, a mild transitory reaction may occur. This is generally limited to a mild, localized eye reaction of short duration.

Preparation of the Vaccine:

1. Do not open and mix the vaccine until ready for use.
2. Mix only one (1) vial at a time and use the entire contents within two (2) hours.
3. Remove the tear-off aluminum seal and stopper from the vial containing the dried vaccine.
4. Remove the tear-off aluminum seal and stopper from the bottle containing the diluent.
5. Hold the diluent bottle firmly in an upright position and insert the vaccine vial on the adapter of the diluent bottle. The neck of the vaccine vial should snap into position and should be seated securely on the adapter on the diluent bottle.
6. Invert the two (2) containers so that the vaccine vial is on the bottom and allow the diluent to flow into the vaccine vial. If the diluent does not flow freely, squeeze the bottle gently and the diluent will flow into the vaccine vial. The vaccine vial should be completely filled with diluent to prevent excess foaming.
7. Hold the joined containers by the ends and shake vigorously until the vaccine plug is completely dissolved.
8. Return the joined containers to their original position (diluent bottle on the bottom). Allow the rehydrated vaccine to flow into the diluent bottle. If the vaccine does not flow into the diluent bottle, tap or squeeze the diluent bottle gently and release to draw the vaccine into the diluent bottle. Be sure that all of the product is removed from the vaccine vial.
9. Remove the vaccine vial and adapter from the neck of the diluent bottle and insert the dropper applicator into the plastic diluent bottle.
10. The vaccine is now ready for eye drop use.

How to Vaccinate: Vaccination for laryngotracheitis by the eye drop method is conducted by allowing one (1) full drop of rehydrated vaccine to fall into the open eye of the bird and holding until the bird swallows. Hold the dropper bottle in a vertical position throughout the vaccination to avoid wasting the vaccine.

Records: Keep a record of the vaccine type, quantity, serial number, expiration date, and place of purchase; the date and time of vaccination; the number, age, and location of the birds; the names of operators performing the vaccination and any observed reactions.

Precaution(s): The vaccine must be stored refrigerated between 35° to 45°F (2° to 7°C).

Caution(s): For veterinary use only.

1. Vaccinate healthy birds only. Although disease may not be evident, coccidiosis, chronic respiratory disease, mycoplasma infection, lymphoid leukosis, infectious bursal disease, Marek's disease, or other disease conditions may cause serious complications or reduce protection.
2. Increased eye reactions may be noticed if the birds ar incubating coryza or other infectious organisms, or if there is an excess amount of ammonia or dust in the air of the housing facilities.
3. All birds within a house should be vaccinated on the same day. Isolate other susceptible birds on the premises from the birds being vaccinated.
4. In outbreak situations, vaccinate healthy birds first, progressing toward outbreak areas in order to vaccinate diseased birds last.
5. Do not spill or spatter the vaccine. Use the entire contents of the vial when first opened. Burn the empty bottles, caps and all unused vaccine and accessories.
6. Wash hands thoroughly after using the vaccine.
7. Do not dilute the vaccine or otherwise stretch the dosage.

Warning(s): Do not vaccinate within 21 days before slaughter.

Presentation: Supplied in 10 x 1,000 dose combo pak units with diluent.

Compendium Code No.: 10471890

TRANQUIVED INJECTABLE (Dogs and Cats) ℞

Vedco **Analgesic-Sedative**

(Xylazine Sterile Solution) 20 mg/mL Injection

NADA No.: 139-236

Active Ingredient(s): TRANQUIVED is supplied as a sterile solution. Each mL contains:

Xylazine hydrochloride equivalent to base activity	20 mg
Methylparaben	0.9 mg
Propylparaben	0.1 mg

Water for injection. pH adjusted with citric acid and sodium citrate.

Indications: Xylazine should be used in dogs and dogs when it is desirable to produce a state of sedation accompanied by a shorter period of analgesia. Xylazine has been used successfully as follows:

1. Diagnostic procedures - examination of mouth and ears, abdominal palpation, rectal palpation, vaginal examination, catheterization of the bladder and radiographic examinations of head and extremities.
2. Orthopedic procedures, such as application of casting materials and splints.
3. Dental procedures.
4. Minor surgical procedures of short duration such as debridement, removal of cutaneous neoplasms and suturing of lacerations.
5. To calm and facilitate restraint of fractious animals.
6. Major surgical procedures:
   a. When used as a preanesthetic to general anesthesia.
   b. When used in conjunction with local anesthetics.

Pharmacology: Xylazine, a nonnarcotic compound, is a sedative and analgesic as well as a muscle relaxant. Its sedative and analgesic activity is related to central nervous system depression. Its muscle relaxant effect is based on inhibition of the intraneural transmission of impulses in the central nervous system. The principal pharmacological activities develop within 10 to 15 minutes after intramuscular or subcutaneous injection, and within 3 to 5 minutes following intravenous administration.

A sleeplike state, the depth of which is dose-dependent, is usually maintained for 1 to 2 hours, while analgesia lasts from 15 to 30 minutes. The centrally-acting muscle relaxant effect causes relaxation of the skeletal musculature complementing sedation and analgesia.

In animals under the influence of xylazine, the respiratory rate is reduced as in natural sleep. Following treatment with xylazine, the heart rate is decreased and a transient change in the conductivity of the cardiac muscle may occur as evidenced by a partial atrioventricular block. This resembles the atrioventricular block often observed in apparently normal animals. Intravenous administration of xylazine causes a transient rise in blood pressure, followed by a slight decrease.

Xylazine has no effect on blood clotting time or other hematological parameters.

Dosage and Administration:

1. Dosage:

   Intravenous - 0.5 mL/20 lb body weight (0.5 mg/lb or 1.1 mg/kg).

   Intramuscular or subcutaneous - 1.0 mL/20 lb body weight (1.0 mg/lb or 2.2 mg/kg).

   In large dogs (over 50 lbs), a dosage of 0.5 mg/lb administered intramuscularly may provide sufficient sedation and/or analgesia for most procedures.

   Since vomiting may occur (see Side Effects), fasting for 6-24 hours prior to the use of xylazine may reduce the incidence; the I.V. route results in the least vomiting.

   Following the injection of xylazine, the animal should be allowed to rest quietly until the full effect has been reached.

   These dosages produce sedation which is usually maintained for one (1) to two (2) hours, and analgesia which lasts for 15 to 30 minutes.
2. Preanesthetic to Local Anesthesia: Xylazine at the recommended dosages can be used in conjunction with local anesthetics, such as procaine or lidocaine.
3. Preanesthetic to General Anesthesia: Xylazine at the recommended dosage rates produces an additive effect to central nervous system depressants such as pentobarbital sodium, thiopental sodium and thiamylal sodium. Therefore, the dosage of such compounds should be reduced and administered to the desired effect. In general, ⅓ to ½ of the calculated dosage of the barbiturates will be needed to produce a surgical plane of anesthesia. Postanesthetic or emergence excitement has not been observed in animals preanesthetized with xylazine.

   Xylazine has been used successfully as a preanesthetic agent for pentobarbital sodium, thiopental sodium, thiamylal sodium, nitrous oxide, ether, halothane and methoxyflurane anesthesia.

Precaution(s): Protect from heat. Do not store over 30°C (86°F).

Caution(s): Federal law restricts this drug to use by or on the order of a licensed veterinarian.

Clinical results with xylazine have not revealed any detrimental effects when compound is administered to pregnant dogs. However, until more definitive studies are completed, xylazine is not recommended for use in these animals. Careful consideration should be given before administering to dogs or cats with significantly depressed respiration, severe pathologic heart disease, advanced liver or kidney disease, severe endotoxic or traumatic shock and stress conditions such as extreme heat, cold or fatigue. Analgesic effect is variable, and depth should be carefully assayed prior to surgical/clinical procedures. In spite of sedation, the practitioner and handlers should proceed with caution since defense reactions may not be diminished. Do not use xylazine in conjunction with tranquilizers. Since an additive effect results from the use of xylazine and the barbiturate compounds, it should be used with caution with these central nervous system depressants. Products known to produce respiratory depression or apnea, such as thiamylal sodium, should be given at a reduced dosage and, when injected intravenously, should be administered slowly.

When intravenous administration is desired, avoid perivascular injection in order to achieve the desired effect. Studies have shown negligible evidence of tissue irritation, however, following perivascular injection of xylazine. Bradycardia and an arrhythmia in the form of incomplete atrioventricular block have been reported following xylazine administration. Although clinically the importance of this effect is questioned, a standard dose of atropine given prior to or following xylazine injection will greatly decrease the incidence. While sedation usually lasts from 1 to 2 hours, recovery periods in excess of 4 to 5 hours have been reported in dogs and cats.

Warning(s): This drug is for use in dogs and cats only.

Safety: Xylazine has been tested in dogs at 4 times the recommended dose. Doses of this magnitude produced muscle tremors, emesis and long periods of sedation.

Side Effects: Emesis occurs occasionally in dogs, and frequently in cats, soon after the administration of xylazine, but before clinical sedation is evident. When observed, emesis usually occurs only a single time, after which there is no further emetic effect. The use of antiemetics may delay this phenomenon. The occurrence of emesis may be considered a desirable effect when xylazine is administered as a preanesthetic to general anesthesia. Xylazine used at recommended dosage levels may occasionally cause slight muscle tremors, bradycardia with partial A-V heart block and a reduced respiratory rate. Should excessive respiratory depression occur following the use of TRANQUIVED (xylazine), administer yohimbine to rapidly reverse the xylazine-induced effects. Gaseous extension of the stomach may occur in dogs treated with xylazine making radiographic interpretation more difficult. Movement in response to sharp auditory stimuli may be observed. Increased urination may occur in cats following the use of xylazine.

Presentation: 20 mL multiple-dose vials.

Compendium Code No.: 10942010

TRANQUIVED INJECTABLE (Horses) ℞

Vedco **Analgesic-Sedative**

(Xylazine Sterile Solution) 100 mg/mL Injection

NADA No.: 140-442

NDC No.: 50989-234-11

Active Ingredient(s): Each mL contains:

Xylazine hydrochloride equivalent to base activity	100 mg
Methylparaben	0.9 mg
Propylparaben	0.1 mg
Sodium citrate dihydrate	0.5 mg

Water for injection. The pH is adjusted with citric acid and sodium citrate.

Indications: Xylazine should be used in horses when it is desirable to produce a state of sedation accompanied by a shorter period of analgesia. Xylazine has been used successfully as follows:

1. Diagnostic procedures, such as oral and ophthalmic examinations, abdominal palpation, rectal palpation, vaginal examination, catheterization of the bladder and radiographic examinations.
2. Orthopedic procedures, such as the application of casting materials and splints.
3. Dental procedures.
4. Minor surgical procedures of short duration, such as debridement, removal of cutaneous neoplasms and suturing of lacerations.
5. To calm and facilitate the handling of fractious animals.
6. Major surgical procedures:
   a. When used as a pre-anesthetic to general anesthesia.
   b. When used in conjunction with local anesthetics.

Pharmacology: Xylazine, a non-narcotic compound, is a sedative and analgesic as well as a muscle relaxant. Its sedative and analgesic activity is related to central nervous system depression. Its muscle-relaxant effect is based upon inhibition of the intraneural transmission of impulses in the central nervous system. The principal pharmacological activities develop within 10 to 15 minutes after intramuscular injection, and within three to five minutes following intravenous administration.

A sleeplike state, the depth of which is dose-dependent, is usually maintained for one to two hours, while analgesia lasts from 15 to 30 minutes. The muscle-relaxant effect causes relaxation of the skeletal musculature complementing sedation and analgesia.

In animals under the influence of xylazine, the respiratory rate is reduced as in natural sleep. Following treatment with xylazine, the heart rate is decreased and a transient change in the conductivity of the cardiac muscle may occur, as evidenced by a partial atrioventricular block. This resembles the atrioventricular block often observed in normal horses.[1,2,3,4] Although a partial A-V block may occasionally occur following the intramuscular injection of xylazine, the incidence is less than when it is administered intravenously. Intravenous administration of xylazine causes a transient rise in blood pressure, followed by a slight decrease.

Xylazine does not have an effect on blood clotting time or on other hematologic parameters.

Dosage and Administration:

1. Dosage:
   Intravenous - 0.5 mL/100 lbs. of body weight (0.5 mg/lb., or 1.1 mg/kg).
   Intramuscular - 1.0 mL/100 lbs. of body weight (1 mg/lb., or 2.2 mg/kg).
   Following the injection of xylazine, the animal should be allowed to rest quietly until the full effect has been reached.
   These dosages produce sedation which is usually maintained for one (1) to two (2) hours, and analgesia which lasts for 15 to 30 minutes.
2. Pre-anesthetic to local anesthesia: Xylazine at the recommended dosages can be used in conjunction with local anesthetics, such as procaine or lidocaine.
3. Pre-anesthetic to general anesthesia: Xylazine, at the recommended dosage rates, produces an additive effect to central nervous system depressants such as pentobarbital sodium, thiopental sodium and thiamylal sodium. Therefore, the dosage of such compounds should be reduced and administered to the desired effect. In general, only one-third (⅓) to one-half (½) of the calculated dosage of the barbiturates will be needed to produce a surgical plane of anesthesia. Postanesthetic or emergence excitement has not been observed in animals pre-anesthetized with xylazine.
   Xylazine has been used successfully as a pre-anesthetic agent for pentobarbital sodium, thiopental sodium, thiamylal sodium, nitrous oxide, ether, halothane, glyceryl guaiacolate and methoxyflurane anesthesia.

Precaution(s): Protect from heat. Do not store at temperatures over 30°C (86°F).

Caution(s): Federal law restricts this drug to use by or on the order of a licensed veterinarian.

Careful consideration should be given before administering to horses with significantly depressed respiration, severe pathologic heart disease, advanced liver or kidney disease, severe endotoxic or traumatic shock and stress conditions such as extreme heat, cold, high altitude or fatigue.

Do not use xylazine in conjunction with tranquilizers.

Since an additive effect results from the use of xylazine with the barbiturate compounds, it should be used with caution with these central nervous system depressants. Products known to produce respiratory depression or apnea, such as thiamylal sodium, should be given at a reduced dosage and, when injected intravenously, should be administered slowly. When intravenous administration is desired, avoid perivascular injection in order to achieve the desired effect. Studies have shown negligible evidence of tissue irritation following perivascular injection of xylazine.

Intracarotid arterial injection should be avoided. As with many compounds, including tranquilizers, immediate violent seizures followed by collapse may result from inadvertent administration into the carotid artery. Although the reaction with xylazine is usually transient and recovery may be rapid and complete, special care should be taken to assure that the needle is in the jugular vein rather than the carotid artery.

Bradycardia and an arrhythmia in the form of incomplete atrioventricular block have been reported following xylazine administration. Although clinically the importance of this effect is questioned,[1,2,3,4] a standard dose of atropine given prior to or following xylazine injection will greatly decrease the incidence.

The analgesic effect is variable, and depth should be carefully assayed prior to surgical/clinical procedures. Variability of analgesia occurs most frequently at the distal extremities of the horse. In spite of sedation, the practitioner and handlers should proceed with caution since defense reactions may not be diminished.

Sedation for transport is most successful if actual transportation is begun after the full effect of the drug has been reached and the animal's stability is maintained while standing. In addition, it should be noted that animals under the influence of xylazine can be aroused by noise or other stimuli and this may increase the risk of injury.

Warning(s): Not for human use. The drug is for use in horses only and should not be administered to food-producing animals.

Toxicology: Xylazine has been tested in horses at five times the recommended dose. Doses of this magnitude may produce convulsions and long periods of sedation.

Side Effects: Xylazine used at the recommended dosage levels may occasionally cause slight muscle tremors, bradycardia with partial A-V heart block and a reduced respiratory rate. Movement in response to sharp auditory stimuli may be observed. Sweating, rarely profuse, has been reported following administration.

References: Available upon request.

Presentation: 50 mL vials.

Compendium Code No.: 10942020

TREMBLEX™

L.A.H.I. (New Jersey) **Vaccine**

Avian Encephalomyelitis Vaccine, Live Virus

U.S. Vet. Lic. No.: 196

Active Ingredient(s): Description: This product is a live virus avian encephalomyelitis vaccine of chicken embryo origin manufactured from SPF (Specific Pathogen Free) eggs.

Contains neomycin as a preservative.

This vaccine was carefully produced and passed all tests in accordance with the U.S. Government requirements.

Indications: For administration to chickens for the prevention of avian encephalomyelitis. For drinking water or aerosol use.

When administered to susceptible birds, a mild infection results which stimulates immunity.

This product should be administered either by the drinking water or aerosol method to growing chickens which are intended for use as breeder replacements or commercial layers in areas where avian encephalomyelitis is known to exist.

This product should be administered between ten weeks of age and four weeks before egg production begins.

Dosage and Administration: Preparation of Vaccine for Drinking Water Use: Open the bottle of vaccine by removing the aluminum tear seal and rubber stopper. Fill the bottle about ¾ full of clean non-sanitized water. Replace the stopper, shake well and pour all the contents into a pint jar ¾ full of non-sanitized water. Shake well and mix with approximately 10 U.S. or 8.3 Imperial gallons of non-sanitized water.

If the water in your area is extremely hard or contains excessive minerals, add a commercial powdered milk to the drinking water at the rate of 1 tablespoonful to each gallon of water as a stabilizer.

Method of Vaccination: Keep all medication and disinfectants from the drinking water 24 hours before and 24 hours after vaccination. Rinse waterers with clean non-sanitized water. Water starve birds for at least two hours prior to vaccination. Provide adequate space so that at least two-thirds of the birds can drink at one time.

Divide mixed vaccine into the waterers. Provide no other drinking water until all vaccine has been consumed.

Preparation of Vaccine for Aerosol Use: Remove the aluminum overseal and stopper from the vaccine bottle. Fill the bottle about ¾ full of clean non-sanitized water. Pour the entire contents into the reservoir of a sprayer containing 70 mL of deionized water or 5 mL of glycerine and 65 mL of deionized water. Before the vaccination the sprayer should be calibrated so that 100 mL will be delivered in 3 minutes.

Method of Vaccination: Confine the birds to a corner of the house with fences and direct the stream from the sprayer over the heads of the birds. Extreme caution should be taken to prevent birds from smothering during this operation.

Contraindication(s): Birds to be vaccinated should be free of all diseases, including the latent form of diseases such as chronic respiratory disease (CRD), coccidiosis, blackhead, parasitic disease, etc. If there are susceptible birds on the premises, the virus may spread from the vaccinated to the susceptible birds and affect egg production or cause disease in chicks under six weeks of age.

Precaution(s): Keep vaccine in the dark, between 2-7°C (35-45°F).

Use entire contents when first opened. Burn this container and all unused contents.

Caution(s): It is imperative that the user of this product comply with the indications for use, contraindications, and method of vaccination stated on the direction sheet. The vaccine must be prepared and administered as directed to obtain best results.

Warning(s): Do not vaccinate within 21 days before slaughter.

Care should be taken to avoid contaminating hands, eyes and clothing with the vaccine.

For veterinary use only.

Presentation: 1,000 and 10,000 dose vials.

Compendium Code No.: 10080382

TREMOR BLEN® D

Merial Select **Vaccine**

Avian Encephalomyelitis Vaccine, Live Virus

U.S. Vet. Lic. No.: 279

Contents: This vaccine contains live avian encephalomyelitis virus.

Contains gentamicin as a bacteriostatic agent.

Notice: Merial Select's vaccines have met the requirements of the USDA in regard to safety, purity, potency, and the capability to protect susceptible chickens. This vaccine has been tested by the Master Seed immunogenicity test for efficacy.

Indications: For the vaccination of healthy chickens between ten weeks of age and four weeks before production by wing web stab or drinking water as an aid in the prevention of avian encephalomyelitis.

This vaccine is recommended for the protection of healthy chickens. It is essential that the chickens be maintained under good environmental conditions and that exposure to disease viruses be reduced as much as possible.

Dosage and Administration:

Wing Web Method:

1. Pull up on the plastic tear-flip-up top to remove the aluminum seal from the bottle containing the vaccine. Carefully pry up one edge of the rubber stopper to permit air to replace the vacuum in the bottle, then remove the stopper.
2. Remove the aluminum seal from the bottle containing the diluent, and transfer the entire contents to the bottle containing the vaccine. Replace the stopper and shake the contents vigorously until the vaccine is evenly suspended.
3. To apply the vaccine, dip the two-pronged applicator supplied in the package into the vaccine and stab into the webbed portion of the wing from the underside. Avoid stabbing through feathers which may wipe off the vaccine.
4. The applicator is designed to carry the proper amount of vaccine in the grooves of the needles. The needles should be touched briefly to the inner lip of the bottle before withdrawing to avoid wasting vaccine which may drop from the needles. Dip the applicator before each application.

Drinking Water Vaccination Using Pouring Application: Drinking water vaccination is recommended for healthy chickens between ten weeks of age and four weeks before production.

1. Remove all medications, sanitizers and disinfectants from the drinking water 72 hours (three days) prior to vaccination.
2. Provide sufficient waterers so that all the chickens can drink at one time. Shut off water supply and allow chickens to consume all the water in the lines.
3. Raise water lines above the chickens' heads. Clean and rinse the waterers thoroughly.
4. Withhold all water from the chickens for a minimum of two hours in warm weather to four hours in cool weather prior to vaccination to stimulate thirst. Withdrawal time should be reduced if half-house brooding is in process.
5. Do not open or mix vaccine until ready to vaccinate.
6. Drinking water for vaccine delivery should contain one ounce (29 gm) of non-fat dry milk per gallon (3.8 liters) of non-chlorinated water, or should contain milk product based stabilizer prepared according to the manufacturer's instructions.
7. Reconstitute the vaccine in 3 gallons (11 liters) of milk-water during cool weather or 4 gallons (15 liters) of milk-water during warm weather for each 1,000 doses.
8. Distribute vaccine solution among waterers. Avoid direct sunlight.
9. Lower waterers and allow the chickens to drink freely. Add the remaining vaccine solution to the water lines as the chickens drink.
10. Do not provide additional drinking water until all the vaccine is consumed.

Drinking Water Vaccination Using Proportioner Application: Drinking water vaccination is recommended for healthy chickens between ten weeks of age and four weeks before production. Several types of medicator/proportioners are commercially available. Set proportioner to deliver one ounce (30 mL) of vaccine concentrate per one gallon (3.8 liters) of water.

1. Remove all medications, sanitizers and disinfectants from the drinking water 72 hours (three days) prior to vaccination.
2. Clean all containers, hoses and waterers prior to vaccination.
3. Withhold all water from the chickens for a minimum of two hours in warm weather to four hours in cool weather prior to vaccination to stimulate thirst. Withdrawal time should be reduced if half-house brooding is in process.
4. Do not open or mix vaccine until ready to vaccinate.
5. Calculate to supply vaccine solution at a rate of 3 gallons (11 liters) per 1,000 chickens in cool weather and 4 gallons (15 liters) per 1,000 chickens in warm weather. The age of the chickens should be considered when calculating water supply. Always use non-chlorinated water when vaccinating chickens.
   Example:
   1,000 chickens in cool weather x 3 gallons (11 liters) = 3 gallons (11 liters).
   1,000 chickens in warm weather x 4 gallons (15 liters) = 4 gallons (15 liters).
6. Prepare vaccine stock solution as follows:
   a. Determine the quantity of vaccine concentrate required by multiplying one ounce (30 mL) x gallons of water needed for vaccine/drinking water.
   Example:
   For 1,000 chickens: 3 gallons x 1 ounce (30 mL) = 3 ounces (90 mL).
   b. Add 3 ounces (85 gm) of non-fat dry milk per 16 ounces (480 mL) of cool water, or use a commercial milk product based stabilizer according to the manufacturer's instructions. For 1,000 chickens add 0.5 ounces (16 gm) non-fat dry milk to the 3 ounces (90 mL) of water.
   c. Reconstitute the dried vaccine with the milk solution. Rinse the vaccine vial to remove all the vaccine.
7. Insert proportioner hose into the vaccine stock solution and start water flow. Continue until all solution has been consumed before changing water supply to direct flow.
8. Do not medicate or use disinfectants for 24 hours after vaccination.

Precaution(s): To preserve its potency during storage, the vaccine should be kept in a refrigerator at 35 to 45°F (2 to 7°C). Do not freeze. Improper storage or handling may result in a loss of potency. Do not remove from refrigeration until ready for use.

Mix only the amount of vaccine to be used immediately and use promptly. Use all at one time and do not stretch the dosage.

Burn all vaccine containers, applicators, and unused vaccine when the vaccination is completed.

Caution(s): This vaccine is not recommended for layer or breeder replacement birds that are sick or debilitated, under stress, or under ten weeks of age. It should not be used on birds that are within four weeks of egg production.

Vaccinate only healthy birds.

Do not use for vaccination except under conditions previously outlined.

To ensure that the progeny is protected, eggs for hatching should not be taken from the flock until four weeks following vaccination.

Birds vaccinated during production may suffer a 5 to 15 percent drop in egg production for a period of two to three weeks and will pass virus through the egg to any progeny hatched from eggs produced during this period.

Vaccinated pullets should not be added to non-vaccinated flocks in production.

Do not expose chicks under four weeks of age.

This vaccine is prepared for the vaccination of healthy birds. Improper handling or administration may result in variable responses.

Do not vaccinate diseased chickens.

Vaccinate all chickens on the premises at one time. Administer a minimum of one dose per chicken.

Avoid stress conditions during and following vaccination.

Do not place chickens in contaminated facilities.

Exposure to disease must be minimized as much as possible.

The capability of this vaccine to produce satisfactory results depends upon many factors, including, but not limited to, conditions of storage and handling by the user, administration of the vaccine, health and responsiveness of individual chickens, and degree of field exposure. Therefore, directions for use should be followed carefully. The use of this vaccine is subject to applicable state and federal laws and regulations.

For veterinary use only.

Warning(s): Do not vaccinate within 21 days of slaughter.

Presentation: 25 x 1,000 dose size without diluent for water administration only.

Compendium Code No.: 11050442 0699

TREMORMUNE™ AE

Biomune **Vaccine**

Avian Encephalomyelitis Vaccine, Live Virus

U.S. Vet. Lic. No.: 368

Contents: TREMORMUNE™ AE contains live avian encephalomyelitis virus vaccine for the vaccination of chickens as an aid in the prevention of avian encephalomyelitis.

Contains gentamicin and amphotericin B as preservatives.

Indications: Administer by wing web to healthy, susceptible chickens at least eight weeks of age but at least four weeks prior to the start of egg production as an aid in the prevention of avian encephalomyelitis due to avian encephalomyelitis virus.

Dosage and Administration: Remove seal and stopper from vaccine vial and diluent vial. Pour entire contents of diluent vial into vaccine vial, insert stopper, and shake well. The vaccine is ready for use and should be used within one hour. Hold each individual bird and spread the wing with the underside facing up. Dip the applicator into the vaccine so that the grooves fill with liquid and deliver 0.01 mL per bird. Insert the double-pronged applicator into the web portion of the wing avoiding blood vessels, muscle, and bone.

Precaution(s): Federal regulations prohibit repackaging or sale of the contents of this package in fractional units. Do not accept if seal is broken.

Store vaccine at 35-45°F (2-7°C).

Use entire contents immediately after rehydrating. Burn containers and all unused contents.

Caution(s): All birds on a farm should be vaccinated at one time.

Warning(s): Do not vaccinate within 21 days of slaughter.

Presentation: 10 x 1000 doses.

Compendium Code No.: 11290430 665

TREMVAC®

Intervet **Vaccine**

Avian Encephalomyelitis Vaccine, Live Virus

U.S. Vet. Lic. No.: 286

Description: TREMVAC®, a live virus vaccine, is prepared from the tested and proven Calnek strain of Avian Encephalomyelitis Virus which was backpassaged through SPF (Specific Pathogen Free) chickens to assure its full potential. The vaccine virus has been propagated in fertile eggs from SPF flocks. The immunizing capability of this vaccine has also been proved by the Master Seed Immunogenicity Test.

This vaccine contains gentamicin as a preservative.

Quality tested for purity, potency, and safety.

Indications: TREMVAC® is indicated for the immunization of commercial layers, commercial layer breeders, and broiler breeders against Avian Encephalomyelitis. This vaccine is recommended for use via drinking water in chickens 8-17 weeks of age.

Dosage and Administration: Preparation of Vaccine:

For Drinking Water Use: Do not open and mix the vaccine until ready to begin vaccination. Use vaccine immediately after mixing.

1. Remove the tear-off aluminum seal and stopper from vial containing the vaccine.
2. Carefully pour clean, cool water (non-chlorinated) into the vial until the vial is approximately two-thirds full.
3. Insert the rubber stopper and shake vigorously until all material is dissolved.
4. The vaccine is now ready for drinking water use in accordance with directions below. For best results, be sure to follow directions carefully!

Drinking Water Administration:

For Chickens 8-17 Weeks of Age:

1. Do not use any disinfectants in the drinking water for 48 hours before vaccination and for 24 hours after vaccination.
2. Withhold drinking water from the birds until they are thirsty. Withholding periods will vary from 2 to 8 hours according to age of birds and climatic conditions. Be careful in hot weather.
3. Scrub and rinse waterers thoroughly with fresh, clean water. Do not use disinfectants for cleaning the waterers.
4. Rehydrate the vaccine as directed above.
5. Mix the rehydrated vaccine with clean, cool, non-chlorinated water in accordance with the following chart:

Birds	Water Per 1,000 Doses Vaccine
Chickens 8-17 weeks of age	13 gal. (49.2 liters)

   As an aid in preserving the virus, 3.2 ounces of non-fat powdered milk may be added with each 10 gallons of water used for mixing the vaccine. Add the dried milk first and mix until dissolved. Then add the rehydrated vaccine from the vial and mix thoroughly.
6. Distribute the vaccine solution, as prepared above, among the waterers provided for the birds. Avoid placing the waterers in direct sunlight.

7. Do not provide any other drinking water until all the vaccine-water solution has been consumed. Elapsed time should not exceed 3 hours.

Records: Keep a record of vaccine, quantity, serial number, expiration date, and place of purchase; the date and time of vaccination; the number, age, breed and locations of birds; names of operators performing the vaccination and any observed reactions.

Precaution(s): Store vaccine between 2 and 7°C (35 and 45°F).

Do not spill or splash the vaccine.

Use entire contents when first opened.

Burn containers and all unused contents.

This product is non-returnable.

Caution(s): Vaccinate only healthy birds. Although disease may not be evident, concurrent disease conditions may cause complications or reduce immunity.

All susceptible birds on the same premises should be vaccinated at the same time.

Do not use less than 1 dose per bird.

For veterinary use only.

Notice: This vaccine has undergone rigid potency, safety and purity tests, and meets Intervet Inc. and USDA requirements. It is designed to stimulate effective immunity when used as directed, but the user must be advised that the response to the product depends upon many factors, including, but not limited to, conditions of storage and handling by the user, administration of the vaccine, health and responsiveness of individual birds, and the degree of field exposure. Therefore, directions should be followed carefully.

This product is not hazardous when used according to directions supplied. A material safety data sheet (MSDS) is available upon request. This and any other consumer information can be obtained by calling Intervet Customer Service at 1-800-441-8272 or 1-302-934-8051.

Use only as directed.

Warning(s): Do not vaccinate within 21 days before slaughter or 35 days prior to onset or during egg production.

Presentation: 10 x 1,000 doses and 10 x 10,000 doses for drinking water use.

Compendium Code No.: 11062081 01407 AL100

TREMVAC-FP®

Intervet **Vaccine**

Avian Encephalomyelitis-Fowl Pox Vaccine, Live Virus

U.S. Vet. Lic. No.: 286

Description: The Avian Encephalomyelitis portion of this vaccine is prepared from the tested and proven Calnek strain of Avian Encephalomyelitis Virus which was back passaged through SPF (Specific Pathogen Free) chickens to assure its full potential. The Fowl Pox portion of this vaccine is prepared from a proven strain of Fowl Pox virus which was back passaged through Specific Pathogen Free (SPF) chickens to assure its full potential. The immunizing capability of this vaccine has been proven by the Master Seed Immunogenicity Test.

This vaccine contains gentamicin as a preservative.

Quality tested for purity, potency, and safety.

Indications: This combination vaccine is indicated for the immunization of commercial layers, commercial layer breeders, broiler breeders and turkey breeder replacements against Avian Encephalomyelitis and Fowl Pox. This combination vaccine is indicated for immunization of chickens 8-17 weeks of age and turkeys 10-22 weeks of age against Avian Encephalomyelitis and Fowl Pox via wing-web stick method.

Dosage and Administration: Preparation of Vaccine: Do not open and mix the vaccine until ready to begin vaccination. Use vaccine immediately after mixing.

1. Remove the tear-off seal and stopper from the vaccine vial.
2. Remove the seal and stopper from the vial of 10 mL diluent.
3. Pour one-half of diluent from diluent vial into vial of vaccine. Insert the rubber stopper and shake until resuspended.
4. Pour resuspended vaccine into diluent vial. Add rubber stopper and shake well. Vaccine is now ready for use.

Wing-Web Administration:

For Chickens From 8-17 Weeks of Age and for Turkeys 10-22 Weeks of Age:

1. Vaccine is applied to the web of the wing. Use the enclosed two-pronged applicator.
2. Vaccinate by dipping the applicator in the vaccine mixture and stabbing the webbed portion of the wing from beneath. Avoid feathered areas of the web.
3. At about 7 to 10 days after vaccination, a few birds should be examined for takes. A good take reaction, indicating that a satisfactory vaccination job was done, shows swelling of the skin at the point of vaccination with scab formation. The scabs will fall off about 2 to 3 weeks following vaccination. Good immunity is established 2 to 3 weeks after vaccination.

Records: Keep a record of vaccine, quantity, serial number, expiration date, and place of purchase; the date and time of vaccination; the number, age, breed and locations of chickens; names of operators performing the vaccination and any observed reactions.

Precaution(s): Store vaccine between 2 and 7°C (35 and 45°F).

Do not spill or splash the vaccine.

Use entire contents when first opened.

Burn containers and all unused contents.

This product is non-returnable.

Caution(s): Vaccinate only healthy chickens. Although disease may not be evident, concurrent disease conditions may cause complications or reduce immunity.

All susceptible birds on the same premises should be vaccinated at the same time.

Efforts should be taken to reduce stress conditions at the time of vaccination.

Do not use less than 1 dose per bird.

For veterinary use only.

Notice: This vaccine has undergone rigid potency, safety and purity tests, and meets Intervet Inc. and USDA requirements. It is designed to stimulate effective immunity when used as directed, but the user must be advised that the response to the product depends upon many factors, including, but not limited to, conditions of storage and handling by the user, administration of the vaccine, health and responsiveness of the individual chickens, and the degree of field exposure. Therefore, directions should be followed carefully.

This product is not hazardous when used according to directions supplied. A material safety data sheet (MSDS) is available upon request. This and any other consumer information can be obtained by calling Intervet Customer Service at 1-800-441-8272 or 1-302-934-8051.

The use of this vaccine is subject to applicable federal and local laws and regulations.

Use only as directed.

Warning(s): Do not vaccinate within 21 days of slaughter or 35 days prior to onset and during egg production.

Presentation: 10 x 1,000 doses with 10 x 10 mL sterile diluent for wing-web administration.

Compendium Code No.: 11062071 01706 AL101

TREMVAC-FP-CAV™

Intervet **Vaccine**

Avian Encephalomyelitis-Chicken Anemia Virus-Fowl Pox Vaccine, Live and Modified Live Virus

U.S. Vet. Lic. No.: 286

Description: TREMVAC-FP-CAV™ is a live virus vaccine containing Avian Encephalomyelitis Virus prepared from the Calnek strain, a modified Fowl Pox Virus, and Chicken Anemia Virus prepared from a modified U.S. field isolate. The vaccine is packaged in two separate units. One is a vial containing freeze-dried Avian Encephalomyelitis Virus and Fowl Pox Virus (Tremvac-FP®). The second is a vial containing Chicken Anemia Virus suspension (CAV-Vac®) to be used as the wing web diluent.

This vaccine contains gentamicin and amphotericin B as preservatives.

Quality tested for purity, potency, and safety.

Indications: This combination vaccine is indicated for the immunization of breeder chickens for prevention of disease due to Avian Encephalomyelitis Virus and Fowl Pox Virus. The Chicken Anemia Virus portion prevents disease due to chicken infectious anemia in progeny of vaccinated breeders. Properly vaccinated chickens are protected throughout the laying cycle. The vaccine should be administered one time to breeder chickens via the wing web stick method from 10 to 12 weeks of age.

Dosage and Administration: Preparation of Vaccine: Do not open the vaccine until ready to begin vaccination. Use vaccine immediately after opening.

1. Remove the tear-off seal and stopper from the vial containing the freeze-dried Tremvac-FP®.
2. Remove the seal and stopper from the CAV-Vac® vial.
3. Pour one-half of the CAV-Vac® from the vial into Tremvac-FP® vial. Insert the rubber stopper and shake until dissolved.
4. Pour the dissolved Tremvac-FP® into the CAV-Vac® vial. Re-insert the rubber stopper and shake well. The vaccine is now ready for use.

Wing-Web Administration:

For Chickens from 10 to 12 Weeks of Age:

1. Vaccine is applied to the web of the wing. Use the enclosed two-pronged applicator.
2. Vaccinate by dipping the applicator in the vaccine mixture and stabbing the webbed portion of the wing from beneath. Avoid feathered areas of the web.
3. Periodically during use, re-insert stopper and shake vaccine well.
4. At about 7 to 10 days after vaccination, a few birds should be examined for takes. A good take reaction, indicating that a satisfactory vaccination job was done, shows swelling of the skin at the point of vaccination with scab formation. The scabs will fall off in about 2 to 3 weeks following vaccination.

Records: Keep a record of vaccine, quantity, serial number, expiration date, and place of purchase; the date and time of vaccination; the number, age, breed and locations of chickens; names of operators performing the vaccination and any observed reactions.

Precaution(s): Store vaccine in refrigerator between 2° and 7°C (35° and 45°F).

Do not spill or splash the vaccine.

Use entire contents when first opened.

Burn containers and all unused contents.

This product is non-returnable.

Caution(s): Use of this product in chickens younger than three weeks of age may cause clinical signs of chicken anemia. Do not vaccinate breeder chickens in lay.

Vaccinate only healthy chickens. Although disease may not be evident, concurrent disease conditions may cause complications or reduce immunity.

All susceptible chickens on the same premises should be vaccinated at the same time.

Efforts should be taken to reduce stress conditions at the time of vaccination.

Do not use less than one dose per bird.

Following vaccination, virus may be shed in the feces. Thus, care should be taken to avoid spread of the vaccine virus to young chickens or to unexposed chickens in lay.

For veterinary use only.

Notice: This vaccine has undergone rigid potency, safety and purity tests, and meets Intervet Inc. and USDA requirements. It is designed to stimulate effective immunity when used as directed, but the user must be advised that the response to the product depends upon many factors, including, but not limited to, conditions of storage and handling by the user, administration of the vaccine, health and responsiveness of the individual chickens, and the degree of field exposure. Therefore, directions should be followed carefully.

This product is not hazardous when used according to directions supplied. A material safety data sheet (MSDS) is available upon request. This and any other consumer information can be obtained by calling Intervet Inc. Customer Service at 1-800-441-8272 or 1-302-934-8051.

The use of this vaccine is subject to applicable local and federal laws and regulations.

Use only as directed.

Warning(s): Do not vaccinate within 21 days of slaughter or 6 weeks prior to onset of or during lay.

Presentation: 10 x 1,000 dose vial Tremvac-FP® with 10 x 1,000 doses (10 mL/vial) CAV-Vac® as diluent.

U.S. Patent No. 5,686,077

Compendium Code No.: 11062850 Rev. 24501 AL192

TREPONEMA BACTERIN

Novartis Animal Vaccines **Bacterin**

U.S. Vet. Lic. No.: 303

Contents: Contains chemically inactivated culture of *Treponema* sp. and SuprImm® adjuvant.

Indications: For the vaccination of healthy cattle six months of age or older as an aid in the reduction of clinical signs of digital dermatitis caused by *Treponema* sp.

Dosage and Administration: Three 4 mL doses at three week intervals administered subcutaneously. Bi-annual boosters are recommended.

Precaution(s): Store at 2-7°C. Shake thoroughly before use. Use entire contents when first opened.

Caution(s): In case of anaphylactoid reaction, administer epinephrine. This product is conditionally licensed. Potency and efficacy studies are in progress.

For veterinary use only.

Warning(s): Do not vaccinate within 60 days of slaughter.

Presentation: 25 dose (100 mL) and 50 dose (200 mL) bottles.

Compendium Code No.: 11140720

TRESADERM® ℞

Merial **Topical Antimicrobial-Antifungal-Corticosteroid (thiabendazole, dexamethasone, neomycin sulfate solution) Dermatologic Solution**

NADA No.: 042-633

Active Ingredient(s): Description: Dermatologic Solution TRESADERM® (thiabendazole, dexamethasone, neomycin sulfate solution) contains the following active ingredients per mL: 40 mg thiabendazole, 1 mg dexamethasone, 3.2 mg neomycin (from neomycin sulfate). Inactive ingredients: glycerin, propylene glycol, purified water, hypophosphorous acid, calcium hypophosphite; about 8.5% ethyl alcohol and about 0.5% benzyl alcohol.

Indications: Dermatologic Solution TRESADERM® is indicated as an aid in the treatment of certain bacterial, mycotic, and inflammatory dermatoses and otitis externa in dogs and cats. Both acute and chronic forms of these skin disorders respond to treatment with TRESADERM®. Many forms of dermatoses are caused by bacteria (chiefly *Staphylococcus aureus, Proteus vulgaris* and *Pseudomonas aeruginosa).* Moreover, these organisms often act as opportunistic or concurrent pathogens that may complicate already established mycotic skin disorders, or otoacariasis caused by *Otodectes cynotis.* The principle etiologic agents of dermatomycoses in dogs and cats are species of the genera *Microsporum* and *Trichophyton.*

The efficacy of neomycin as an antibacterial agent with activity against both gram-negative and gram-positive pathogens, is well documented. Detailed studies in various laboratories have verified the significant activity thiabendazole displays against the important dermatophytes. Dexamethasone, a synthetic adrenocorticoid steroid, inhibits the reaction of connective tissue to injury and suppresses the classic inflammatory manifestations of skin disease. The formulation for TRESADERM® combines these several activities in a complementary form for control of the discomfort and direct treatment of dermatisis and otitis externa produced by the above mentioned infectious agents.

Dosage and Administration: Prior to the administration of Dermatologic Solution TRESADERM®, remove the ceruminous, purulent or foreign material from the ear canal, as well as the crust which may be associated with dermatoses affecting other parts of the body. The design of the container nozzle safely allows partial insertion into the ear canal for ease of administration. The amount to apply and the frequency of treatment are dependent upon the severity and extent of the lesions. Five to 15 drops should be instilled into the ear twice daily. In treating dermatoses affecting other than the ear, the surface of the lesions should be well moistened (2 to 4 drops per square inch) with Dermatologic Solution TRESADERM® twice daily. The volume required will be dependent upon the size of the lesion.

Application of TRESADERM® should be limited to a period of not longer than one week.

Precaution(s): Store in a refrigerator 36-46°F (2-8°C).

Caution(s): Federal (U.S.A.) law restricts this drug to use by or on the order of a licensed veterinarian.

On rare occasions dogs may be sensitive to neomycin. In these animals, application of the drug will result in erythema of the treated area, which may last for 24 to 48 hours. Also, evidence of transient discomfort has been noted in some dogs when the drug was applied to fissured or denuded areas. The expression of pain may last 2 to 5 minutes. Application of Dermatologic Solution TRESADERM® should be limited to periods not longer than one week.

While systemic side effects are not likely with topically applied corticosteroids, such a possibility should be considered if use of the solution is extensive and prolonged. If signs of salt and water retention or potassium excretion are noticed (increased thirst, weakness, lethargy, oliguria, gastrointestinal disturbances or tachycardia), treatment should be discontinued and appropriate measures taken to correct the electrolyte and fluid imbalance.

For topical use in dogs and cats.

Avoid contact with eyes.

Warning(s): Keep this and all drugs out of the reach of children.

The Material Safety Data Sheet (MSDS) contains more detailed occupational safety information. To report adverse effects in users, to obtain an MSDS, or for assistance call 1-800-672-6372.

Presentation: Dermatologic Solution TRESADERM® Veterinary is supplied in 7.5 mL and 15 mL dropper bottles, each in 12 bottle boxes.

TRESADERM is a registered trademark of Merial.

(Merial Limited: Registered in England and Wales [Reg. No. 3332751] with registered offices at 27 Knightsbridge, London, SW1X 7QT, England and domesticated in Delaware, USA as Merial LLC).

Compendium Code No.: 11110792 7612105

TREXONIL™ ℞

Wildlife **Carfentanil Antagonist**

(Naltrexone Hydrochloride) Sterile Injection

NADA No.: 141-074

Active Ingredient(s): Each mL contains: 50 mg naltrexone hydrochloride; 8.6 mg sodium chloride; USP; 1.8 mg of methylparaben and 0.2 mg of propylparaben, NF; water for injection, USP.

Indications: For use as an antagonist to carfentanil citrate immobilization in free-ranging or confined elk and moose *(Cervidae).*

Pharmacology: TREXONIL™ is a sterile injectable solution which contains naltrexone hydrochloride as the active ingredient.

The pH is adjusted with hydrochloric acid or sodium hydroxide. Naltrexone hydrochloride is 17-(cyclopropylmethyl)-4, 5-epoxy-3, 14 dihydroxy-morphinan-6-one hydrochloride. It has a chemical formula of $C_{20}H_{23}NO_4HCl$ and a molecular weight of 377.9.

Naltrexone Structural Formula:

Naltrexone hydrochloride is a cyclopropyl derivative of oxymorphone. It is structurally similar to naloxone and nalorphine and is metabolized by the liver. Studies in rats and mice have indicated that naltrexone has undetectable or minimal narcotic agonist effects. Its relative opiate antagonistic potency is 40 times that of nalorphine and 2-3 times that of naloxone.

Dosage and Administration: 100 mg of TREXONIL™ (naltrexone hydrochloride) should be used for each mg of carfentanil citrate previously administered. Administer one-quarter of the calculated dose intravenously and three-quarters of the calculated dose subcutaneously.

Contraindication(s): Available data are inadequate to recommend the use of naltrexone in pregnant animals. Avoid using during breeding season.

Precaution(s): Protect from light. Store at controlled room temperature 15-30°C (59-86°F).

Caution(s): Federal law restricts this drug to use by or on the order of a licensed veterinarian.

Intrathoracic, intra-abdominal or intramuscular injection should be avoided. The user of TREXONIL™ must be proficient in appropriate procedures necessary to handle problems resulting from animals being in lateral or sternal recumbency for extended periods of time. Users must also have necessary equipment, supplies and experienced personnel to handle such situations that may occur during or following immobilization and reversal procedures to minimize possible injury to the animal or personnel.

Reversal of the effects of carfentanil citrate immobilization in elk and moose is usually accomplished within 3 to 10 minutes of administration of TREXONIL™. However, in clinical trials, animals may have required as little as 2 minutes or a period of greater than 10 minutes to reverse from the effects of carfentanil citrate. Doses lower than the proposed dose resulted in signs of renarcotization, including open-mouth breathing, hypermetria, ataxia and subtle changes in behavior and responsiveness.

After administering naltrexone hydrochloride to an animal that has been immobilized with carfentanil citrate, it may rise quickly and be fully conscious in as little as 2 minutes. All necessary procedures should have been accomplished and personnel advised that the reversal agent has been administered.

Side effects associated with carfentanil administration, such as muscle tremors or heavy panting, may not immediately abate upon administration of the reversal agent.

Animals should, if possible, be monitored until any side effects associated with carfentanil administration subside.

Warning(s): Keep out of the reach of children. Do not use in domestic food-producing animals. Do not use 45 days before or during the hunting season.

Adverse Reactions: Doses of up to 500 mg (5X) naltrexone per mg carfentanil citrate administered were given with no adverse reactions.

References: Available upon request.

Presentation: TREXONIL™ is supplied in 20 mL multiple use vials.

Compendium Code No.: 10520030

TRIAMCINOLONE ACETONIDE TABLETS ℞

Boehringer Ingelheim **Steroidal Anti-inflammatory**

NADA No.: 137-694

Active Ingredient(s): Each tablet contains 0.5 mg or 1.5 mg of triamcinolone acetonide.

Indications: Triamcinolone acetonide is a highly potent glucocorticoid effective in the treatment of inflammation and related disorders in dogs and cats. It is indicated in the management and treatment of acute arthritis and allergic and dermatologic disorders.

Pharmacology: Triamcinolone acetonide is a highly potent synthetic glucocorticoid and anti-inflammatory agent.[1] Its advantage over the older corticoids lies in its ability to achieve equal anti-inflammatory effect with a lower dose.[2,3,4] Triamcinolone has very weak sodium-retaining effects and is probably the least electrolyte-retaining compound of the corticosteroid group.[2,4] Triamcinolone has a plasma half-life of approximately 300 minutes and is classified as an intermediate acting glucocorticoid, whereas the acetonide salt has a longer duration of action and a higher lipid-water distribution co-efficient.[1,2,3,4]

Glucocorticoids exert a regulatory influence of lymphocytes, erythrocytes and eosinophils of the blood and on the structure and function of lymphoid tissues.[1,4,5] A primary feature of the glucocorticoids is their anti-inflammatory activity with minimum sodium and water retention, which is often associated with the mineralocorticoids.[1,2,3,4,5,6] Glucocorticoids not only inhibit the early phases of the inflammatory process (edema, fibrin deposition, capillary dilatation, migration of leukocytes into the inflamed area and phagocytic activity) but also the later manifestations (capillary proliferation, fibroblast proliferation and deposition of collagen).[3,4,6] The exact mechanism is not known, but the glucocorticoids obviously suppress the normal tissue response to injury and alleviate symptoms from many conditions.2

As with other adrenal steroids, triamcinolone acetonide has been found useful in alleviating the pain and lameness associated with acute localized arthritic conditions and generalized arthritic conditions. Glucocorticoids have been used successfully to treat traumatic arthritis, osteoarthritis and generalized arthritic conditions in dogs. Remission of musculoskeletal conditions may be permanent, or the symptoms may recur, depending upon the cause and extent of structural degeneration.[1,2,3,4,5] Glucocorticoids also relieve pruritus and inflammation of allergic dermatitis, acute moist dermatitis, dry eczema, urticaria, bronchial asthma, pollen sensitivities and otitis externa in dogs and allergic dermatitis and moist and dry eczema in cats. The symptoms may be expected to recur if the cause of the allergic reaction is still present, in which case retreatment may be indicated. In treating acute hypersensitivity reactions, such as anaphylactic shock, appropriate treatment such as intravenous prednisolone sodium succinate should be used.[1,2,3,4,5]

In dogs and cats moribund from overwhelmingly severe infections for which antibacterial therapy is available (e.g., critical pneumonia, pyometritis), a glucocorticoid may be lifesaving, acting to inhibit the inflammatory reaction, which itself may be lethal; preventing vascular collapse and preserving the integrity of the blood vessels; modifying the animal's reaction to drugs; and preventing or reducing the exudative reaction which often complicates certain infections. As supportive therapy, it improves the general attitude of the animal being treated. All necessary procedures for the establishment of a bacterial diagnosis should be carried out whenever possible before the institution of therapy. Corticosteroid therapy in the presence of infection should be administered for the shortest possible time compatible with the maintenance of an adequate response, and antibacterial therapy should be continued for at least three days after the hormone has been withdrawn. Combined hormone and antibacterial therapy does not obviate the need for indicated surgical treatment.[1,2,3,4,5,6]

Dosage and Administration: The keystone of satisfactory therapeutic management with triamcinolone acetonide, as with other steroids, is the individualization of dosage in reference to the severity of the disease, the anticipated duration of steroid therapy and the animal's threshold or tolerance for steroid excess. The prime objective of steroid therapy should be to achieve a satisfactory degree of control with a minimum effective dose.

The initial suppressive dose level of 0.5-1.0 mg per 10 lbs. of body weight per day should be administered until a satisfactory clinical response is obtained, a period not to exceed 14 days. If a satisfactory response is not obtained in 14 days, a re-evaluation of the case to confirm the original diagnosis should be made. As soon as a satisfactory clinical response is obtained, the daily dose should be reduced gradually, either to termination of treatment in the case of acute conditions (e.g., seasonal asthma, dermatitis, acute ocular inflammations) or to the minimal effective maintenance dose level in the case of chronic conditions (e.g., rheumatoid arthritis). Symptoms of adrenal insufficiency following withdrawal may persist for several days, weeks or years. Some cases have resulted in death. To minimize the adverse effects from withdrawal or a reduction in dosage, cautiously decrease the dosage in a gradual manner. In dogs, dosing in the morning may also be beneficial in minimizing effects because nocturnal pituitary/adrenal activity will be less inhibited. In chronic conditions, and in rheumatoid arthritis especially, it is important that the reduction in dosage from initial maintenance dose levels be accomplished slowly. The maintenance dose level should be adjusted from time to time as required by a fluctuation in the activity of the disease and the animal's general status. Maintenance dosage levels of 0.125-0.25 mg per 10 lbs. of body weight per day are recommended. Accumulated experience has shown that the long-term benefits to be gained from continued steroid maintenance are probably greater the lower the maintenance dose level. In rheumatoid arthritis in particular, maintenance steroid therapy should be at the lowest possible level.

Important: In the therapeutic management of animals with chronic diseases, such as rheumatoid arthritis, triamcinolone should be regarded as a highly valuable adjunct, to be used in conjunction with but not as a replacement for standard therapeutic measures.

Recommended Dosage Schedule:

Body Weight	Initial Daily Dosage	Maintenance Daily Dosage
5 lbs.	0.25-0.5 mg	0.0625-0.125 mg
10 lbs.	0.5-1.0 mg	0.125-0.25 mg
20 lbs.	1.0-2.0 mg	0.25-0.5 mg
30 lbs.	1.5-3.0 mg	0.375-0.75 mg
60 lbs.	3.0-6.0 mg	0.75-1.5 mg

Contraindication(s): Do not use in viral infections. Except for emergency therapy, do not use in animals with tuberculosis, chronic nephritis, Cushingoid syndrome and peptic ulcers. Existence of congestive heart failure, diabetes and osteoporosis are relative contraindications.

Precaution(s): Because of its inhibitory effect on fibroplasia, triamcinolone may mask the signs of infection and enhance the dissemination of the infecting organism. Hence, all animals receiving triamcinolone should be watched for any evidence of intercurrent infection. Should infection occur, it must be brought under control by the use of appropriate antibacterial measures or administration of triamcinolone should be discontinued.

The usual early sign of cortisone or hydrocortisone overdosage (i.e., increase in body weight due to fluid retention) is not a reliable index of overdosage because this anti-inflammatory steroid manifests little sodium-retaining activity. Hence, the recommended dosage levels should not be exceeded, and all animals receiving triamcinolone acetonide should be under close medical supervision.

The use of corticosteroids may result in the inhibition of endogenous steroid production which sometimes persists for weeks following drug withdrawal. In patients presently receiving or recently withdrawn from corticosteroid treatments, the administration of a rapid acting, corticosteroid before, during and after an unusually stressful situation is recommended.

Caution(s): Federal law restricts this drug to use by or on the order of a licensed veterinarian.

For oral use in dogs and cats only.

Warning(s): Not for human use. Clinical and experimental data have demonstrated that corticosteroids administered orally or parenterally to animals may induce the first stage of parturition when administered during the last trimester of pregnancy and may precipitate premature parturition followed by dystocia, fetal death, retained placenta and metritis.

Additionally, corticosteroids administered to dogs, rabbits and rodents during pregnancy have produced cleft palate in offspring. Other congenital anomalies including deformed forelegs, phocomelia and anasarca have been reported in the offspring of dogs which received corticosteroids during pregnancy.

Side Effects: As with the use of any corticosteroid, side effects and metabolic alterations can be anticipated when the treatment is intensive or prolonged in animals with diabetes mellitus, the use of triamcinolone acetonide may be associated with an increase in the insulin requirement. Negative nitrogen balance may occur, particularly in animals that require protracted maintenance therapy.[3,4,5]

Polydipsia or polyuria may occur with high dosage or with frequent administration. The likelihood of their occurrence may be minimized by giving as brief a course of corticosteroid therapy as possible, and by waiting for the re-appearance of symptoms before repeating therapy. If polydipsia or polyuria should occur, therapy should then be resumed at a lower dosage level.

Other adverse reactions that have occurred with the use of corticosteroids are SAP and SGPT enzyme elevations, weight loss, anorexia, vomiting and diarrhea (occasionally bloody). Anaphylactic reactions have occasionally been seen following administration.

Cushing's syndrome in dogs has been reported in association with prolonged or repeated steroid therapy.

References: Available upon request.

Presentation: TRIAMCINOLONE ACETONIDE TABLETS, 0.5 mg: Bottles of 1,000 tablets.
TRIAMCINOLONE ACETONIDE TABLETS, 1.5 mg: Bottles of 500 tablets.

Compendium Code No.: 10281100

TRIAMTABS ℞

Vetus **Steroidal-Anti-inflammatory**

Triamcinolone Acetonide Tablets

NADA No.: 137-694

Active Ingredient(s): Each tablet contains 0.5 mg or 1.5 mg of triamcinolone acetonide.

Indications: For oral use in dogs and cats only. Triamcinolone acetonide is a highly potent glucocorticoid effective in the treatment of inflammation and related disorders in dogs and cats. It is indicated in the management and treatment of acute arthritis and allergic and dermatologic disorders.

Dosage and Administration: The keystone of satisfactory therapeutic management with triamcinolone acetonide, as with other steroids, is individualization of dosage in reference to the severity of the disease, the anticipated duration of steroid therapy and the animal's threshold or tolerance for steroid excess. The prime objective of steroid therapy should be to achieve satisfactory degree of control with a minimum effective dose.

The initial suppressive dose level of 0.5-1.0 mg per 10 pounds of body weight daily should be administered until a satisfactory clinical response is obtained, a period not to exceed 14 days. If a satisfactory response is not obtained in 14 days, re-evaluation of the case to confirm the original diagnosis should be made. As soon as a satisfactory clinical response is obtained, the daily dose should be reduced gradually, either to termination of treatment in the case of acute conditions (e.g. seasonal asthma, dermatitis, acute ocular inflammations) or to the minimal effective maintenance dose level in the case of chronic conditions (e.g. rheumatoid arthritis).

Symptoms of adrenal insufficiency following withdrawal may persist for several days, weeks or years. Some cases have resulted in death. To minimize the adverse effects from withdrawal or reduction in dosage, cautiously decrease dosage in a gradual manner. In dogs, dosing in the morning may also be beneficial in minimizing effects because nocturnal pituitary/adrenal activity will be less inhibited. In chronic conditions, and in rheumatoid arthritis especially, it is important that the reduction in dosage from initial to maintenance dose levels be accomplished slowly. The maintenance dose level should be adjusted from time to time as required by fluctuation in the activity of the disease and the animal's general status. Maintenance dosage levels of 0.125-0.25 mg per 10 pounds of body weight daily are recommended. Accumulated experience has shown that the long-term benefits to be gained from continued steroid maintenance are probably greater the lower the maintenance dose level. In rheumatoid arthritis in particular, maintenance steroid therapy should be at the lowest possible level.

Important: In the therapeutic management of animals with chronic diseases, such as rheumatoid arthritis, triamcinolone should be regarded as a highly valuable adjunct, to be used in conjunction with but not a replacement for standard therapeutic measures.

Recommended Dosage Schedule:

Body Weight	Initial Daily Dosage	Maintenance Daily Dosage
5 lbs	0.25 to 0.5 mg	0.0625 to 0.125 mg
10 lbs	0.5 to 1.0 mg	0.125 to 0.25 mg
20 lbs	1.0 to 2.0 mg	0.25 to 0.50 mg
30 lbs	1.5 to 3.0 mg	0.375 to 0.75 mg
60 lbs	3.0 to 6.0 mg	0.75 to 1.50 mg

Contraindication(s): Do not use in viral infections. Except for emergency therapy do not use in animals with tuberculosis, chronic nephritis cushingoid syndrome and peptic ulcers. Existence of congestive heart failure, diabetes and osteoporosis are relative contraindications.

Caution(s): Federal law restricts this drug to use by or on the order of a licensed veterinarian.

Because of its inhibitory effect on fibroplasia, triamcinolone may mask the signs of infection and enhance dissemination of the infecting organism. Hence, all animals receiving triamcinolone should be watched for evidence of intercurrent infection. Should infection occur, it must be brought under control by use of appropriate antibacterial measures or administration of triamcinolone should be discontinued.

Because this anti-inflammatory steroid manifests little sodium-retaining activity, the usual sign of cortisone or hydrocortisone overdosage (i.e., increase in body weight due to fluid retention) is not a reliable index of overdosage. Hence, recommended dosage levels should not be exceeded, and all animals receiving triamcinolone acetonide should be under close medical supervision.

Use of corticosteroids may result in the inhibition of endogenous steroid production which sometimes persist for weeks following drug withdrawal. In patients presently receiving or recently withdrawn from corticosteroid treatments, administration of a rapid acting corticosteroid before, during and after an unusually stressful situation is recommended.

Single or multiple doses of 1 mg/kg of a corticosteroid induced hepatopathy in the dog and rabbit in a study by Rogers and Ruebner in 1977. The condition was determined in the dog by a biopsy of the liver and was accompanied by elevated serum glutamic-pyruvic transaminase, SAP and SGGT (in some dogs) and increased bromsulphalein retention.

Warning(s): Not for human use. Clinical and experimental data have demonstrated that corticosteroids administered orally or parenterally to animals may induce the first stage of parturition when administered during the last trimester of pregnancy and may precipitate premature parturition followed by dystocia, fetal death, retained placenta and metritis.

Additionally, corticosteroids administered to dogs, rabbits and rodents during pregnancy have produced cleft palate. Other congenital anomalies including deformed forelegs, phocomelia and anasarca have been reported in the offspring of dogs which received corticosteroids during pregnancy.

Side Effects: Adverse Reactions: As with the use of any corticosteroid, side effects and metabolic alterations can be anticipated when treatment is intensive or prolonged. In animals with diabetes mellitus, use of triamcinolone acetonide may be associated with an increase in the insulin requirement. Negative nitrogen balance may occur, particularly in animals that require protracted maintenance therapy.

Polydipsia or polyuria may occur with high dosage or frequent administration. The likelihood of their occurrence may be minimized by giving as brief a course of corticosteroid therapy as possible, and by waiting for the reappearance of symptoms before repeating therapy. If polydipsia or polyuria should occur, therapy should then be resumed as a lower dosage level. Other adverse reactions that have occurred with the use of corticosteroids are SAP and SGPT enzyme elevations, weight loss, anorexia, vomiting and diarrhea (occasionally bloody). Anaphylactic reactions have occasionally been seen following administrations.

Cushings Syndrome in dogs has been reported in association with prolonged or repeated steroid therapy.

Discussion: Triamcinolone acetonide is a highly potent synthetic glucocorticoid and anti-inflammatory agent. Its advantage over the older corticoids lies in its ability to achieve equal anti-inflammatory effect with a lower dose. Triamcinolone has very weak sodium-retaining effects and is probably the least electrolyte-retaining compound of the corticosteroid group. Triamcinolone has a plasma half-life of approximately 300 minutes and is classified as an intermediate acting glucocorticoid, whereas the acetonide salt has a longer duration of action and a higher lipid-water distribution coefficient.

Actions: Glucocorticoids exert a regulatory influence on lymphocytes, erythrocytes and eosinophils of the blood and on the structure and function of lymphoid tissues. A primary feature of the glucocorticoids is their anti-inflammatory activity with minimum sodium and water retention, which is often associated with the mineralocorticoids.

Glucocorticoids not only inhibit the early phases of the inflammatory process (edema, fibrin deposition, capillary dilation, migration of leukocytes into the inflamed area and phagocytic activity) but also the later manifestations (capillary proliferation, fibroblast proliferation and deposition of collagen). The exact mechanism is not known, but the glucocorticoids obviously suppress normal tissue response to injury and alleviate symptoms from many conditions.

As with other adrenal steroids, triamcinolone acetonide has been found useful in alleviating the pain and lameness associated with acute localized arthritic conditions and generalized arthritic conditions. Glucocorticoids have been used successfully to treat traumatic arthritis, osteoarthritis and generalized arthritic conditions in dogs. Remission of musculoskeletal conditions may be permanent, or symptoms may recur, depending on the cause and extent of structural degeneration. Glucocorticoids also relieve pruritis and inflammation of allergic dermatitis, acute moist dermatitis, dry eczema, uticaria, bronchial asthma, pollen sensitivities and otitis externa in dogs and allergic dermatitis and moist and dry eczema in cats. Symptoms may be expected to recur if the cause of the allergic reaction is still present, in which case retreatment may be indicated. In treating acute hypersensitivity reactions, such as anaphylactic shock, appropriate treatment such as intravenous prednisolone sodium succinate should be used.

In dogs and cats moribund from overwhelmingly severe infections for which antibacterial therapy is available (e.g. critical pneumonia, pyometritis) a glucocorticoid may be lifesaving, acting to inhibit the inflammatory reaction which itself may be lethal; preventing vascular collapse and preserving the integrity of the blood vessels; modifying the animal's reaction to drugs; and preventing or reducing the exudative reaction which often complicates certain infections. As supportive therapy, it improves the general attitude of the animal being treated. All necessary procedures for the establishment of a bacterial diagnosis should be carried out whenever possible before institution of therapy. Corticosteroid therapy in the presence of infection should be administered for the shortest possible time compatible with maintenance of an adequate response, and antibacterial therapy should be continued for at least three days after the hormone has been withdrawn. Combined hormone and antibacterial therapy does not obviate the need for indicated surgical treatment.

References: Available upon request.

Presentation: 0.5 mg bottles of 1000 tablets; 1.5 mg bottles of 500 tablets.

Compendium Code No.: 14440830

TRIANGLE® 1 + TYPE II BVD

Fort Dodge **Vaccine**

Bovine Virus Diarrhea Vaccine, Killed Virus

U.S. Vet. Lic. No.: 112

Contents: This product contains the antigens listed above.

Thimerosal, neomycin, and polymyxin B added as preservatives.

Indications: For vaccination of healthy cattle as an aid in the prevention of disease caused by bovine virus diarrhea (BVD) types I and II.

Dosage and Administration: Cattle, inject one 2 mL dose intramuscularly or subcutaneously using aseptic technique. Repeat in 14 to 28 days. A 2 mL booster dose is recommended annually or prior to time of stress or exposure. Calves vaccinated under six months of age should be revaccinated at six months of age. May be administered to pregnant animals at any stage of gestation. Protect animals from exposure for at least 14 days after the last dose of vaccine.

Precaution(s): Store in dark at 2° to 7°C (35° to 45°F). Avoid freezing. Shake well. Use entire contents when first opened.

Caution(s): In case of anaphylactoid reaction, administer epinephrine.

Warning(s): Do not vaccinate within 21 days before slaughter.

For veterinary use only.

Presentation: 10 doses (20 mL)and 50 doses (100 mL).

Compendium Code No.: 10032300 0855B

TRIANGLE® 3 + TYPE II BVD

Fort Dodge **Vaccine**

Bovine Rhinotracheitis-Virus Diarrhea-Parainfluenza-3 Vaccine, Killed Virus

U.S. Vet. Lic. No.: 112

Contents: This product contains the antigens listed above.

Thimerosal, neomycin, and polymyxin B added as preservatives.

Indications: For vaccination of healthy cattle as an aid in the prevention of disease caused by infectious bovine rhinotracheitis (IBR), bovine viral diarrhea (BVD types I and II) and parainfluenza-3 (PI-3).

Dosage and Administration: Cattle, inject one 2 mL dose intramuscularly or subcutaneously using aseptic technique. Repeat in 14 to 28 days. A 2 mL booster dose is recommended annually or prior to time of stress or exposure. Calves vaccinated under six months of age should be revaccinated at six months of age. May be administered to pregnant animals at any stage of gestation. Protect animals from exposure for at least 14 days after the last dose of vaccine.

Precaution(s): Store in dark at 2° to 7°C (35° to 45°F). Avoid freezing. Shake well. Use entire contents when first opened.

Caution(s): Transient swelling may occur at the injection site. In case of anaphylactoid reaction, administer epinephrine.

Warning(s): Do not vaccinate within 21 days before slaughter.

For veterinary use only.

Presentation: 10 doses (20 mL) and 50 doses (100 mL).

Compendium Code No.: 10032310 1835B

TRIANGLE® 3 V5L

Fort Dodge **Bacterin-Vaccine**

Bovine Rhinotracheitis-Virus Diarrhea-Parainfluenza-3 Vaccine, Killed Virus-Campylobacter Fetus-Leptospira Canicola-Grippotyphosa-Hardjo-Icterohaemorrhagiae-Pomona Bacterin

U.S. Vet. Lic. No.: 112

Contents: This product contains the antigens listed above.

The vaccine contains a dual adjuvant system plus an oil adjuvant to stimulate immunity. The vaccine uses the Immune-Guard™ inactivant and process to kill viral components.

Neomycin and polymyxin B added as preservatives.

Indications: For vaccination of healthy cattle to protect against disease caused by bovine rhinotracheitis (IBR), bovine virus diarrhea (BVD), parainfluenza-3 (PI-3), *Campylobacter fetus, Leptospira pomona, hardjo, grippotyphosa, canicola* and *icterohaemorrhagiae*.

Dosage and Administration: Cattle, inject one 10 mL dose subcutaneously using aseptic technique in the neck or behind the shoulder. In noninfected herds and susceptible animals a second dose should be administered 2 to 4 weeks later. The last injection should precede the breeding season by 4 to 8 weeks. Protect animals from exposure for at least 14 days after the last dose of vaccine. Revaccinate annually. Safety data in pregnant animals has not been accumulated.

Precaution(s): Store in dark at 2° to 7°C (35° to 45°F). Avoid freezing. Shake well. Use entire contents when first opened.

Caution(s): Transitory injection site swelling, fever, malaise and temporarily lowered milk production may occur following use of this product. In case of anaphylactoid reaction, administer epinephrine.

Warning(s): Do not vaccinate within 60 days before slaughter.

For veterinary use only.

Presentation: 10 doses (100 mL) and 50 doses (500 mL).

Compendium Code No.: 10032320 1978I

TRIANGLE® 4+HS

Fort Dodge **Bacterin-Vaccine**

Bovine Rhinotracheitis-Virus Diarrhea-Parainfluenza-3-Respiratory Syncytial Virus Vaccine, Killed Virus-Haemophilus Somnus Bacterin

U.S. Vet. Lic. No.: 112

Contents: This product contains the antigens listed above.

The vaccine contains the Enhance™ dual adjuvant system. The vaccine uses the Immune-Guard® inactivant and process to kill viral components. The *Haemophilus somnus* fraction is an extracted bacterial antigen.

Formalin, thimerosal, neomycin and polymyxin B added as preservatives.

Indications: For vaccination of healthy cattle as an aid in the prevention of disease caused by infectious bovine rhinotracheitis (IBR), bovine virus diarrhea (BVD), parainfluenza-3 (PI-3), bovine respiratory syncytial virus (BRSV) and *Haemophilus somnus.*

Dosage and Administration: Cattle, inject one 5 mL dose intramuscularly or subcutaneously using aseptic technique. Repeat in 14 to 28 days. A 5 mL booster dose is recommended annually or prior to time of stress or exposure. Calves vaccinated under 6 months of age should be revaccinated at 6 months of age. Protect animals from exposure for at least 14 days after the last dose of vaccine.

Precaution(s): Store in dark at 2° to 7°C (35° to 45°F). Avoid freezing. Shake well. Use entire contents when first opened.

Caution(s): Transient swelling and soreness may occur at injection site. In case of anaphylactoid reaction, administer epinephrine.

Warning(s): Do not vaccinate within 21 days before slaughter.

For veterinary use only.

Presentation: 10 doses (50 mL) and 50 doses (250 mL).

Compendium Code No.: 10032340 1757E

TRIANGLE® 4+PH/HS

Fort Dodge **Bacterin-Vaccine**

Bovine Rhinotracheitis-Virus Diarrhea-Parainfluenza-3-Respiratory Syncytial Virus Vaccine, Killed Virus-Haemophilus Somnus-Pasteurella Haemolytica Bacterin

U.S. Vet. Lic. No.: 112

Contents: This product contains the antigens listed above.

The vaccine contains the Enhance™ dual adjuvant system. The vaccine uses the Immune-Guard® inactivant and process to kill the viral components.

Thimerosal, neomycin and polymyxin B added as preservatives.

Indications: For vaccination of healthy cattle as an aid in the prevention of disease caused by infectious bovine rhinotracheitis (IBR), bovine viral diarrhea (BVD), parainfluenza-3 (PI-3), bovine respiratory syncytial virus (BRSV), *Haemophilus somnus* and *Pasteurella haemolytica.*

Dosage and Administration: Cattle, inject one 5 mL dose intramuscularly or subcutaneously using aseptic technique. Repeat in 14 to 28 days. A 5 mL booster dose is recommended annually or prior to time of stress or exposure. Calves vaccinated under 6 months of age should be revaccinated at 6 months of age. Protect animals from exposure for at least 14 days after the last dose of vaccine. Transient swelling and soreness may occur at the injection site. Safety data in pregnant animals has not been accumulated.

Precaution(s): Store in dark at 2° to 7°C (35° to 45°F). Avoid freezing. Shake well. Use entire contents when first opened.

Caution(s): In case of anaphylactoid reaction, administer epinephrine.

Warning(s): Do not vaccinate within 21 days before slaughter.

For veterinary use only.

Presentation: 10 doses (50 mL) and 50 doses (250 mL).

Compendium Code No.: 10032360 2115E

TRIANGLE® 4+PH-K

Fort Dodge **Bacterin-Vaccine**

Bovine Rhinotracheitis-Virus Diarrhea-Parainfluenza-3-Respiratory Syncytial Virus Vaccine, Killed Virus-Pasteurella Haemolytica Bacterin

U.S. Vet. Lic. No.: 112

Contents: The vaccine contains the Enhance™ dual adjuvant system. The vaccine uses the Immune-Guard® inactivant and process to kill viral components. The *Pasteurella haemolytica* fraction is an extracted bacterial antigen.

Thimerosal, neomycin and polymyxin B added as preservatives.

Indications: For vaccination of healthy cattle as an aid in the prevention of disease caused by infectious bovine rhinotracheitis (IBR), bovine virus diarrhea (BVD), parainfluenza-3 (PI-3), bovine respiratory syncytial virus (BRSV) and *Pasteurella haemolytica.*

Dosage and Administration: Cattle, inject one 5 mL intramuscularly or subcutaneously using aseptic technique. Repeat in 14 to 28 days. A 5 mL booster dose is recommended annually or prior to time of stress or exposure. Calves vaccinated under 6 months of age should be revaccinated at 6 months of age. Protect animals from exposure for at least 14 days after the last dose of vaccine.

Precaution(s): Store in dark at 2° to 7°C (35° to 45°F). Avoid freezing. Shake well. Use entire contents when first opened.

Caution(s): In case of anaphylactoid reaction, administer epinephrine. Transient swelling and soreness may occur at the injection site.

Warning(s): Do not vaccinate within 21 days before slaughter.

For veterinary use only.

Presentation: 10 dose (50 mL) and 50 dose (250 mL) vials.

Compendium Code No.: 10032350 1745G

TRIANGLE® 4 + TYPE II BVD

Fort Dodge **Vaccine**

Bovine Rhinotracheitis-Virus Diarrhea-Parainfluenza-3-Respiratory Syncytial Virus Vaccine, Killed Virus

U.S. Vet. Lic. No.: 112

Contents: This product contains the antigens listed above.

Thimerosal, neomycin, and polymyxin B added as preservatives.

Indications: For vaccination of healthy cattle as an aid in the prevention of diseases caused by infectious bovine rhinotracheitis (IBR), bovine virus diarrhea (BVD types I and II), parainfluenza-3 (PI-3) and bovine respiratory syncytial (BRSV) viruses.

Dosage and Administration: Cattle, inject one 2 mL dose intramuscularly or subcutaneously using aseptic technique. Repeat in 14 to 28 days. A 2 mL booster dose is recommended annually or prior to time of stress or exposure. Calves vaccinated under six months of age should be revaccinated at six months of age. May be administered to pregnant animals at any stage of gestation. Protect animals from exposure for at least 14 days after the last dose of vaccine.

Precaution(s): Store in dark at 2° to 7°C (35° to 45°F). Avoid freezing. Shake well. Use entire contents when first opened.

Caution(s): Transient swelling may occur at the injection site. In case of anaphylactoid reaction, administer epinephrine.

Warning(s): Do not vaccinate within 21 days before slaughter.

For veterinary use only.

Presentation: 10 doses (20 mL) and 50 doses (100 mL).

Compendium Code No.: 10032330 1785B, 1787B

TRIANGLE® 8 + TYPE II BVD

Fort Dodge **Bacterin-Vaccine**

Bovine Rhinotracheitis-Virus Diarrhea-Parainfluenza-3 Vaccine, Killed Virus-Leptospira Canicola-Grippotyphosa-Hardjo-Icterohaemorrhagiae-Pomona bacterin

U.S. Vet. Lic. No.: 112

Contents: This product contains the antigens listed above.

Thimerosal, neomycin, and polymyxin B added as preservatives.

Indications: For vaccination of healthy cattle as an aid in the prevention of disease caused by infectious bovine rhinotracheitis (IBR), bovine viral diarrhea (BVD types I and II), parainfluenza-3 (PI-3) viruses and *Leptospira pomona, L. hardjo, L. grippotyphosa, L. canicola* and *L. icterohaemorrhagiae.*

Dosage and Administration: Cattle, inject one 5 mL dose intramuscularly or subcutaneously using aseptic technique. Repeat in 14 to 28 days. A 5 mL booster dose is recommended annually or prior to time of stress or exposure. Calves vaccinated under six months of age should be revaccinated at six months of age. May be administered to pregnant animals at any stage of gestation. Protect animals from exposure for at least 14 days after the last dose of vaccine.

Precaution(s): Store in dark at 2° to 7°C (35° to 45°F). Avoid freezing. Shake well. Use entire contents when first opened.

Caution(s): In case of anaphylactoid reaction, administer epinephrine.

Warning(s): Do not vaccinate within 21 days before slaughter. For veterinary use only.

Presentation: 10 doses (50 mL) and 50 doses (250 mL).

Compendium Code No.: 10032370 1866B

TRIANGLE® 9+HS

Fort Dodge **Bacterin-Vaccine**

Bovine Rhinotracheitis-Virus Diarrhea-Parainfluenza-3-Respiratory Syncytial Virus Vaccine, Killed Virus-Haemophilus Somnus-Leptospira Canicola-Grippotyphosa-Hardjo-Icterohaemorrhagiae-Pomona Bacterin

U.S. Vet. Lic. No.: 112

Contents: This product contains the antigens listed above.

The vaccine contains a dual adjuvant system to stimulate immunity. The vaccine uses the Immune-Guard™ inactivation process for the viral components.

Thimerosal, neomycin and polymyxin B added as preservatives.

Indications: For vaccination of healthy cattle as an aid in the prevention of disease caused by infectious bovine rhinotracheitis (IBR), bovine virus diarrhea (BVD), parainfluenza-3 (PI-3), bovine respiratory syncytial virus (BRSV), *Haemophilus somnus, Leptospira pomona, hardjo, grippotyphosa, canicola* and *icterohaemorrhagiae.*

Dosage and Administration: Cattle, inject one 5 mL dose intramuscularly using aseptic technique. Repeat in 14 to 28 days. A 5 mL booster dose is recommended annually or prior to time of stress or exposure. Calves vaccinated under 6 months of age should be revaccinated at 6 months of age. May be administered to pregnant animals at any stage of gestation. Protect animals from exposure for at least 14 days after the last dose of the vaccine.

Precaution(s): Store in dark at 2° to 7°C (35° to 45°F). Avoid freezing. Shake well. Use entire contents when first opened.

Caution(s): In case of anaphylactoid reaction, administer epinephrine.

Warning(s): Do not vaccinate within 21 days before slaughter. For veterinary use only.

Presentation: 10 dose (50 mL) and 50 dose (250 mL).

Compendium Code No.: 10032390 1855D

TRIANGLE® 9+PH-K

Fort Dodge **Bacterin-Vaccine**

Bovine Rhinotracheitis-Virus Diarrhea-Parainfluenza-3-Respiratory Syncytial Virus Vaccine, Killed Virus-Leptospira Canicola-Grippotyphosa-Hardjo-Icterohaemorrhagiae-Pomona-Pasteurella Haemolytica Bacterin

U.S. Vet. Lic. No.: 112

Contents: This product contains the antigens listed above.

The vaccine contains the Enhance™ dual adjuvant system to stimulate immunity. The vaccine uses the Immune-Guard™ inactivant and process to kill viral components. The *Pasteurella haemolytica* fraction is an extracted outer membrane antigen.

Thimerosal, neomycin and polymyxin B added as preservatives.

Indications: For vaccination of healthy cattle as an aid in prevention of disease caused by infectious bovine rhinotracheitis (IBR), bovine virus diarrhea (BVD), parainfluenza-3 (PI-3), bovine respiratory syncytial virus (BRSV), *Pasteurella haemolytica, Leptospira pomona, hardjo, grippotyphosa, canicola* and *icterohaemorrhagiae.*

Dosage and Administration: Cattle, inject one 5 mL dose intramuscularly using aseptic technique. Repeat in 14 to 28 days. A 5 mL booster dose is recommended annually or prior to time of stress or exposure. Calves vaccinated under 6 months of age should be revaccinated at 6 months of age. May be administered to pregnant animals at any stage of gestation. Protect animals from exposure for at least 14 days after the last dose of vaccine.

Precaution(s): Store in dark at 2° to 7°C (35° to 45°F). Avoid freezing. Shake well. Use entire contents when first opened.

Caution(s): In case of anaphylactoid reaction, administer epinephrine.

Warning(s): Do not vaccinate within 21 days before slaughter. For veterinary use only.

Presentation: 10 dose (50 mL) and 50 dose (250 mL) vials.

Compendium Code No.: 10032400 1777D

TRIANGLE® 9 + TYPE II BVD

Fort Dodge **Bacterin-Vaccine**

Bovine Rhinotracheitis-Virus Diarrhea-Parainfluenza-3-Respiratory Syncytial Virus Vaccine, Killed Virus-Leptospira Canicola-Grippotyphosa-Hardjo-Icterohaemorrhagiae-Pomona Bacterin

U.S. Vet. Lic. No.: 112

Contents: This product contains the antigens listed above.

Thimerosal, neomycin, and polymyxin B added as preservatives.

Indications: For vaccination of healthy cattle as an aid in the prevention of disease caused by infectious bovine rhinotracheitis (IBR), bovine viral diarrhea (BVD types I and II), parainfluenza-3 (PI-3), bovine respiratory syncytial (BRSV) viruses, *Leptospira pomona, L. hardjo, L. grippotyphosa, L. canicola* and *L. icterohaemorrhagiae.*

Dosage and Administration: Cattle, inject one 5 mL dose intramuscularly or subcutaneously using aseptic technique. Repeat in 14 to 28 days. A 5 mL booster dose is recommended annually or prior to time of stress or exposure. Calves vaccinated under six months of age should be revaccinated at six months of age. May be administered to pregnant animals at any stage of gestation. Protect animals from exposure for at least 14 days after the last dose of vaccine.

Precaution(s): Store in dark at 2° to 7°C (35° to 45°F). Avoid freezing. Shake well. Use entire contents when first opened.

Caution(s): In case of anaphylactoid reaction, administer epinephrine.

Warning(s): Do not vaccinate within 21 days before slaughter. For veterinary use only.

Presentation: 10 doses (50 mL) and 50 doses (250 mL).

Compendium Code No.: 10032380 1886B

TRIBRISSEN® 48% INJECTION ℞

Schering-Plough **Trimethoprim-Sulfadiazine**

Sterile Injection

NADA No.: 106-965

Active Ingredient(s): TRIBRISSEN® 48% Injection is a sterile aqueous suspension of trimethoprim* in a solution of the sodium salt of sulfadiazine for intravenous administration. Each mL contains: trimethoprim 80 mg and sulfadiazine 400 mg.

Vehicle contains the inactive ingredients: diethanolamine 6 mg, sodium hydroxide 55 mg (additional may be added to adjust pH), polysorbate 80 0.2 mg, sodium metabisulfite 1 mg (at time of manufacture) and water for injection, q.s.

Indications: TRIBRISSEN® therapy is indicated in horses where potent systemic antibacterial action against sensitive organisms is required. TRIBRISSEN® 48% Injection is indicated where control of bacterial infections is required during treatment of: Acute strangles, acute urogenital infections, respiratory tract infections, wound infections and abscesses. TRIBRISSEN® is well tolerated by foals.

Pharmacology: TRIBRISSEN® is a combination of trimethoprim and sulfadiazine in the ratio of 1 part to 5 parts by weight, which provides effective antibacterial activity against a wide range of bacterial infections in animals.

Trimethoprim is 2,4 diamino-5-(3,4,5-trimethoxybenzyl) pyrimidine.

Actions:

Microbiology: Trimethoprim blocks bacterial production of tetrahydrofolic acid from dihydrofolic acid by binding to and reversibly inhibiting the enzyme dihydrofolate reductase.

Sulfadiazine, in common with other sulfonamides, inhibits bacterial synthesis of dihydrofolic acid by competing with para-aminobenzoic acid.

TRIBRISSEN® thus imposes a sequential double blockade on bacterial metabolism. This deprives bacteria of nucleic acids and proteins essential for survival and multiplication and produces a high level of antibacterial activity which is usually bactericidal.

Although both sulfadiazine and trimethoprim are antifolate, neither affects the folate metabolism of animals. The reasons are: animals do not synthesize folic acid and cannot, therefore, be directly affected by sulfadiazine; and although animals must reduce their dietary folic acid to tetrahydrofolic acid, trimethoprim does not affect this reduction because its affinity for dihydrofolate reductase of mammals is significantly less than for the corresponding bacterial enzyme.

TRIBRISSEN® is active against a wide spectrum of bacterial pathogens, both gram-negative and gram-positive. The following *in vitro* data are available, but their clinical significance is unknown. In general, species of the following genera are sensitive to TRIBRISSEN®:

Very Sensitive: Escherichia, Streptococcus, Proteus, Salmonella, Pasteurella, Shigella and Haemophilus.

Sensitive: Staphylococcus, Neisseria, Klebsiella, Fusiformis, Corynebacterium, Clostridium and Bordetella.

Moderately Sensitive: Moraxella, Nocardia and Brucella.

Not Sensitive: Mycobacterium, Leptospira, Pseudomonas and Erysipelothrix.

As a result of the sequential double blockade of the metabolism of susceptible organisms by trimethoprim and sulfadiazine, the minimum inhibitory concentration (MIC) of TRIBRISSEN® is markedly less than that of either of the components used separately. Many strains of bacteria that are not susceptible to one of the components are susceptible to TRIBRISSEN®. A synergistic effect between trimethoprim and sulfadiazine in combination has been shown experimentally both *in vitro* and *in vivo* (in dogs).

TRIBRISSEN® is bactericidal against susceptible strains and is often effective against sulfonamide-resistant organisms. *In vitro* sulfadiazine is usually only bacteriostatic.

The following table shows MICs, using the above ratio, of bacteria which were susceptible to both trimethoprim (TMP) and sulfadiazine (SDZ). The organisms are those most commonly involved in conditions for which TRIBRISSEN® is indicated.

Average Minimum Inhibitory Concentration (MIC-mcg/mL):

Bacteria	TMP Alone	SDZ Alone	TMP/SDZ	
			TMP	SDZ
Escherichia coli	0.31	26.5	0.07	1.31
Proteus species	1.3	24.5	0.15	2.85
Staphylococcus aureus	0.6	17.6	0.13	2.47
Pasteurella species	0.06	20.1	0.03	0.56
Salmonella species	0.15	61.0	0.05	0.95
β *Streptococcus*	0.5	24.5	0.15	2.85

The following table demonstrates the marked effect of the trimethoprim and sulfadiazine combination against sulfadiazine-resistant strains of normally susceptible organisms.

Average Minimum Inhibitory Concentration of Sulfadiazine-Resistant Strains (MIC-mcg/mL):

Bacteria	TMP Alone	SDZ Alone	TMP/SDZ	
			TMP	SDZ
Escherichia coli	0.32	>245	0.27	5.0
Proteus species	0.66	>245	0.32	6.2

The precise *in vitro* MIC of the combination varies with the ratio of the drugs present, but action of TRIBRISSEN® occurs over a wide range of ratios with an increase in the concentration of one of its components compensating for a decrease in the other. It is usual, however, to determine MIC's using a constant ratio of one part trimethoprim in twenty parts of the combination.

Susceptibility Testing: In testing susceptibility to TRIBRISSEN®, it is essential that the medium used does not contain significant amounts of interfering substances which can bypass the metabolic blocking action, e.g. thymidine or thymine.

The standard SxT disc is appropriate for testing by the disc diffusion method.

Following parenteral administration, TRIBRISSEN® is rapidly absorbed and widely distributed throughout body tissues. Concentrations of trimethoprim are usually higher in tissues than in blood. The levels of trimethoprim are high in lung, kidney and liver, as would be expected from its physical properties.

Serum concentration in horses following intravenous administration indicate rapid dissolution of trimethoprim particles and a steady rate of elimination of both components, with half lives of about three hours and clearance within 24 hours.

Usually, the concentration of an antibacterial in the blood and the *in vitro* MIC of the infecting organism indicate an appropriate period between doses of a drug. This does not hold entirely for TRIBRISSEN® because trimethoprim, in contrast to sulfadiazine, localizes in the tissues and therefore, its concentration and ratio to sulfadiazine are higher there than in blood. Serum levels following dosing give an indication, however, of the probable duration of effectiveness of a single dose.

The following table shows the average serum concentrations of trimethoprim and sulfadiazine in 11 adult horses following administration of a single IV dose of 22 mg/kg.

Average Serum Concentration (mcg/mL):

Trimethoprim (3.6 mg/kg)					Sulfadiazine (18 mg/kg)				
1 h	3 h	6h	8h	24h	1 h	3 h	6h	8h	24h
1.15	0.64	0.17	0.07	<0.02	27.2	16.4	7.5	4.5	0.09

Excretion of TRIBRISSEN® is chiefly by the kidneys, by both glomerular filtration and tubular secretion. Urine concentrations of both trimethoprim and sulfadiazine are severalfold higher than blood concentrations. Neither trimethoprim nor sulfadiazine interferes with the excretion pattern of the other.

Dosage and Administration: The recommended dose is 2 mL TRIBRISSEN® 48% Injection per 100 lbs (45 kg) body weight per day. Shake well before using. Administer by intravenous injection. The usual course of treatment is a single, daily dose for 5 to 7 days. The daily dose may be halved and given morning and evening.

Continue acute infection therapy for two to three days after clinical signs have subsided.

A convenient dosage guide is:

250 lb body weight-5 mL daily
500 lb body weight-10 mL daily
750 lb body weight-15 mL daily
1000 lb body weight-20 mL daily
1250 lb body weight-25 mL daily

If no improvement of acute infections is seen in three to five days, re-evaluate diagnosis.

TRIBRISSEN® 48% Injection may be used alone or in conjunction with oral dosing. Following an initial injection, therapy can be maintained using Tribrissen® 400 Oral Paste.

A complete blood count should be done periodically in patients receiving TRIBRISSEN® for prolonged periods. If significant reduction in the count of any formed blood element should be noted, treatment with TRIBRISSEN® should be discontinued.

Contraindication(s): TRIBRISSEN® should not be used in horses showing marked liver parenchymal damage, blood dyscrasias, or in those with a history of sulfonamide sensitivity.

Precaution(s): Water should be readily available to horses receiving sulfonamide therapy.

Caution(s): Federal law restricts this drug to use by or on the order of a licensed veterinarian.

Rapid IV injection or excessive dosage may result in acute toxicity.

Following administration intramuscularly, subcutaneously or by accidental perivascular infiltration, swelling, pain and minor tissue damage have occasionally be observed.

Serious, sometimes fatal, shock-like reactions accompanied by convulsions and collapse occurring within seconds to minutes following injection have been reported.

Individual animal hypersensitivity may result in local or generalized reactions, sometimes fatal. Anaphylactoid reactions, although rare, may also occur.

Antidote(s): Epinephrine.

Warning(s): Not for use in horses intended for food.

Keep out of the reach of children.

Toxicology: Toxicity is low. The acute toxicity (LD_{50}) of TRIBRISSEN® is more than 5 g/kg orally in rats and mice. No significant changes were recorded in rats given doses of 600 mg/kg per day for 90 days.

Horses have tolerated up to five times the recommended daily dose for seven days or the recommended daily dose for 21 consecutive days without clinical effects or histopathological changes.

Lengthening of clotting time was seen in some of the horses on high or prolonged doses in one of two trials. The effect, which may have been related to a resolving infection, was not seen in a second similar trial.

Slight to moderate reductions in hematopoietic activity following high, prolonged dosage in several species have been recorded. This is usually reversible by folinic acid (leucovorin) administration or by stopping the drug. During long-term treatment of horses, periodic platelet counts and white and red blood cell counts are advisable.

Research has shown that TRIBRISSEN® produces minimal to no effect on the composition of fecal flora. However, any antibacterial compound has the potential to produce an adverse effect on the alimentary tract of the horse. In rare instances, horses have developed diarrhea during TRIBRISSEN® treatment. If fecal consistency changes during TRIBRISSEN® therapy, discontinue treatment immediately and institute appropriate symptomatic measures.

Teratology: The effects of TRIBRISSEN® 48% Injection on pregnancy has not been determined. Studies to date show there is no detrimental effect on stallion spermatogenesis with or following the recommended dose of TRIBRISSEN® 48% Injection.

Adverse Reactions: Transient pruritis has been reported following the first dose in a small number of horses. This resolved spontaneously within 24 hours and did not recur after subsequent doses.

Presentation: TRIBRISSEN® 48% Injection is available in 100 mL multiple dose vials.

*Mfd. under Pat. 3,956,327.

Compendium Code No.: 10471990

TRIBRISSEN® 400 ORAL PASTE ℞

Schering-Plough **Potentiated Sulfa**

(Trimethoprim and sulfadiazine)

NADA No.: 131-918

Active Ingredient(s): TRIBRISSEN® 400 Oral Paste contains 67 mg trimethoprim* and 333 mg sulfadiazine per gram.

Manufactured under patent 3,956,327.

Indications: TRIBRISSEN® therapy is indicated in horses where potent systemic antibacterial action against sensitive organisms is required. TRIBRISSEN® 400 Oral Paste is indicated where the control of bacterial infections is required during treatment of acute strangles, respiratory tract infections, acute urogenital infections, and wound infections and abscesses.

TRIBRISSEN® is well tolerated by foals.

Pharmacology: TRIBRISSEN® is a combination of trimethoprim and sulfadiazine in the ratio of one part to five parts by weight, which provides effective antibacterial activity against a wide range of bacterial infections in animals.

Trimethoprim is 2,4 diamino-5-(3,4,5-trimethoxybenzyl) pyrimidine.

Trimethoprim blocks bacterial production of tetrahydrofolic acid from dihydrofolic acid by binding to and reversibly inhibiting the enzyme dihydrofolate reductase.

Sulfadiazine, in common with other sulfonamides, inhibits bacterial synthesis of dihydrofolic acid by competing with para-aminobenzoic acid.

TRIBRISSEN® thus imposes a sequential double blockade on bacterial metabolism. This deprives bacteria of nucleic acids and proteins essential for survival and multiplication and produces a high level of antibacterial activity which is usually bactericidal.

Although both sulfadiazine and trimethoprim are antifolate, neither affects the folate metabolism of animals. The reasons are: animals do not synthesize folic acid and cannot, therefore, be directly affected by sulfadiazine; and although animals must reduce their dietary folic acid to tetrahydrofolic acid, trimethoprim does not affect this reduction because its affinity for dihydrofolate reductase of mammals is significantly less than that for the corresponding bacterial enzyme.

TRIBRISSEN® is active against a wide spectrum of bacterial pathogens, both gram-positive and gram-negative. The following *in vitro* data are available, but their clinical significance is unknown. In general, species of the following genera are sensitive to TRIBRISSEN®:

Very sensitive: Escherichia, Streptococcus, Proteus, Salmonella, Pasteurella, Shigella, Haemophilus.

Sensitive: Staphylococcus, Neisseria, Klebsiella, Fusiformis, Corynebacterium, Clostridium, Bordetella.

Moderately sensitive: Moraxella, Nocardia, Brucella.

Not sensitive: Mycobacterium, Leptospira, Pseudomonas, Erysipelothrix.

As a result of the sequential double blockade of the metabolism of susceptible organisms by trimethoprim and sulfadiazine, the minimum inhibitory concentration (MIC) of TRIBRISSEN® is markedly less than that of either of the components used separately. Many strains of bacteria that are not susceptible to one of the components are susceptible to TRIBRISSEN®. A synergistic effect between trimethoprim and sulfadiazine in combination has been shown experimentally both *in vitro* and *in vivo* (in dogs).

TRIBRISSEN® is bactericidal against susceptible strains and is often effective against sulfonamide-resistant organisms. *In vitro* sulfadiazine is usually only bacteriostatic.

The precise *in vitro* MIC of the combination varies with the ratio of the drugs present, but the action of TRIBRISSEN® occurs over a wide range of ratios with an increase in the concentration of one of its components compensating for a decrease in the other. It is usual, however, to determine MICs using a constant ratio of one part trimethoprim in twenty parts of the combination.

The following table shows MICs, using the above ratio of bacteria which were susceptible to both trimethoprim (TMP) and sulfadiazine (SDZ). The organisms are those most commonly involved in conditions for which TRIBRISSEN® is indicated.

Average minimum inhibitory concentration (MIC - mcg/mL):

Bacteria	TMP Alone	SDZ Alone	TPM/SDZ
Escherichia coli	0.31	26.5	0.07/1.31
Proteus species	1.30	24.5	0.15/2.85
Staphylococcus aureus	0.60	17.6	0.13/2.47
Pasteurella species	0.06	20.1	0.03/0.56
Salmonella species	0.15	61.0	0.05/0.95
β Streptococcus	0.50	24.5	0.15/2.85

The following table demonstrates the marked effect of the trimethoprim and sulfadiazine combination against sulfadiazine-resistant strains of normally susceptible organisms.

Average minimum inhibitory concentration of sulfadiazine-resistant strains (MIC - mcg/mL):

Bacteria	TMP Alone	SDZ Alone	TMP/SDZ
Escherichia coli	0.32	>245	0.27/5.0
Proteus species	0.66	>245	0.32/6.2

Susceptibility Testing: In testing susceptibility to TRIBRISSEN®, it is essential that the medium used does not contain significant amounts of interfering substances which can bypass the metabolic blocking action; e.g., thymidine or thymine.

The standard SxT disc is appropriate for testing by the disc diffusion method.

Following oral administration, TRIBRISSEN® is rapidly absorbed and widely distributed throughout body tissues. Concentrations of trimethoprim are usually higher in tissues than in the blood. The levels of trimethoprim are high in the lung, kidney and liver, as would be expected from its physical properties.

Serum trimethoprim concentrations in horses following oral administration indicate rapid absorption of the drug; peak concentrations occur in two to three hours. The mean serum elimination half-life is two to three hours. Sulfadiazine absorption is slower, requiring three to six hours to reach peak concentration. The mean serum elimination half-life for sulfadiazine is about seven hours.

Usually, the concentration of an antibacterial in the blood and the *in vitro* MIC of the infecting organism indicate an appropriate period between doses of a drug. This does not hold entirely for TRIBRISSEN® because trimethoprim, in contrast to sulfadiazine, localizes in the tissues and, therefore, its concentration and ratio to sulfadiazine are higher there than in blood.

The following shows the average serum concentrations of trimethoprim and sulfadiazine in eleven adult horses observed on day 3 of three consecutive daily doses of TRIBRISSEN® 400 Oral Paste.

Average serum concentration (mcg/mL):

Trimethoprim (5 mg/kg): 1 hr. - 0.71; 3 hrs. - 0.95; 6 hrs. - 0.37; 10 hrs. - 0.04; 24 hrs. - <0.04.

T

Sulfadiazine (25 mg/kg): 1 hr. - 8.0; 3 hrs. - 15.8; 6 hrs. - 9.9; 10 hrs. - 5.6; 24 hrs. - 0.6.

Excretion of TRIBRISSEN® is chiefly by the kidneys, by both glomerular filtration, and tubular secretion. Urine concentrations of both trimethoprim and sulfadiazine are severalfold higher than blood concentrations. Neither trimethoprim nor sulfadiazine interferes with the excretion pattern of the other.

Dosage and Administration: The recommended dose is 3.75 g TRIBRISSEN® 400 Oral Paste per 110 lbs. (50 kg) of body weight per day. Administer orally once a day by means of the Dial-A-Dose® syringe. Each marking on the syringe doses 110 lbs. of body weight. When administering TRIBRISSEN® 400 Oral Paste, the oral cavity should be empty. Deposit the paste on the back of the tongue by depressing the plunger that has been previously set to deliver the correct dose.

The usual course of treatment is once a day for five (5) to seven (7) days.

Continue acute infection therapy for two (2) to three (3) days after the clinical signs have subsided.

If improvement of acute infections is not seen in three (3) to five (5) days, re-evaluate the diagnosis.

A complete blood count should be done periodically in patients receiving TRIBRISSEN® for prolonged periods. If a significant reduction in the count of any formed blood element is noted, treatment with TRIBRISSEN® should be discontinued.

Contraindication(s): TRIBRISSEN® should not be used in horses showing marked liver parenchymal damage, blood dyscrasias, or in those with a history of sulfonamide sensitivity.

Precaution(s): Water should be readily available to horses receiving sulfonamide therapy.

Caution(s): Federal (USA) law restricts the drug to use by or on the order of a licensed veterinarian.

Keep out of the reach of children.

Individual animal hypersensitivity may result in local or generalized reactions. Anaphylactic reactions, although rare, may also occur.

Antidote(s): Epinephrine.

Warning(s): Not for use in horses intended for food.

Toxicology: Toxicity is low. The acute toxicity (LD_{50}) of TRIBRISSEN® is more than 50 g/kg orally in rats and mice.

Significant changes were not recorded in rats given doses of 600 mg/kg per day for 90 days.

The effect of TRIBRISSEN® 400 Oral Paste on pregnancy has not been determined. Studies to date show that there is not any detrimental effect on stallion spermatogenesis with or following the recommended dose of TRIBRISSEN® 400 Oral Paste.

Side Effects: Adverse reactions of consequence have not been noted following not administration of TRIBRISSEN® 400 Oral Paste. During clinical trials, one case of anorexia and one case of loose feces following treatment with the drug were reported.

Lengthening of clotting time was seen in some of the horses on high or prolonged dosing in one of two trials. The effect, which may have been related to a resolving infection, was not seen in a second similar trial.

Slight to moderate reductions in hematopoietic activity following high, prolonged dosage in several species have been recorded. This is usually reversible by folinic acid (leucovorin) administration or by stopping use of the drug. During the long-term treatment of horses, periodic platelet counts and white and red blood cell counts are advisable.

In rare instances, horse have developed diarrhea during TRIBRISSEN® treatment. If fecal consistency changes during TRIBRISSEN® therapy, discontinue treatment immediately and institute appropriate symptomatic measures.

Presentation: 37.5 g Dial-A-Dose® syringes.

TRIBRISSEN is a registered trademark of Schering-Plough Animal Health Corporation.
Dial-A-Dose is a registered trademark of Plas-Pak Industries, Inc.

Compendium Code No.: 10471980

TRIBRISSEN® TABLETS ℞

Schering-Plough **Potentiated Sulfa**

NADA No.: 095-614

Active Ingredient(s):

TRIBRISSEN® 30 mg: Each white sugar-coated unscored tablet contains 5 mg trimethoprim and 25 mg sulfadiazine.

TRIBRISSEN® 120 mg: Each white sugar-coated unscored tablet contains 20 mg trimethoprim and 100 mg sulfadiazine.

TRIBRISSEN® 480 mg: Each white scored tablet contains 80 mg trimethoprim and 400 mg sulfadiazine.

TRIBRISSEN® 960 mg: Each white unscored tablet contains 160 mg trimethoprim and 800 mg sulfadiazine.

Indications: TRIBRISSEN® therapy is indicated for use in dogs where potent systemic antibacterial action against sensitive organisms is required, either alone or as an adjunct to surgery or debridement with associated infection.

TRIBRISSEN® Tablets are indicated where the control of bacterial infections is required during treatment of acute urinary tract infections, acute bacterial complications of canine distemper, acute respiratory tract infections, acute alimentary tract infections, wound infections and abscesses.

Pharmacology: Description: TRIBRISSEN® is a combination of trimethoprim and sulfadiazine in the ratio of 1 part to 5 parts by weight, which provides effective antibacterial activity against a wide range of bacterial infections in animals.

Trimethoprim is 2,4 diamino-5-(3,4,5-trimethoxybenzyl) pyrimidine.

N NH₂ N CH₂ NH₂ CH₃O OCH₃ OCH₃

Actions:

Microbiology: Trimethoprim blocks bacterial production of tetrahydrofolic acid by binding to and reversibly inhibiting the enzyme dihydrofolate reductase.

Sulfadiazine, in common with other sulfonamides, inhibits bacterial synthesis of dihydrofolic acid by competing with para-aminobenzoic acid.

TRIBRISSEN® thus imposes a sequential double blockade on bacterial metabolism. This deprives bacteria of nucleic acids and proteins essential for survival and multiplication and produces a high level of antibacterial activity which is usually bactericidal.

Although both sulfadiazine and trimethoprim are antifolate, neither affects the folate metabolism of animals. The reasons are: animals do not synthesize folic acid and cannot, therefore, be directly affected by sulfadiazine; and although animals must reduce their dietary folic acid to tetrahydrofolic acid, trimethoprim does not affect this reduction because its affinity for dihydrofolate reductase of mammals is significantly less than that for the corresponding bacterial enzyme.

TRIBRISSEN® is active against a wide spectrum of bacterial pathogens, both gram-negative and gram-positive. The following *in vitro* data are available, but their clinical significance is unknown. In general, species of the following genera are sensitive to TRIBRISSEN®:

Very Sensitive: Escherichia, Streptococcus, Proteus, Salmonella, Pasteurella, Shigella, Haemophilus.

Sensitive: Staphylococcus, Neisseria, Klebsiella, Fusiformis, Corynebacterium, Clostridium, Bordetella.

Moderately Sensitive: Moraxella, Nocardia, Brucella.

Not Sensitive: Mycobacterium, Leptospira, Pseudomonas, Erysipelothrix.

As a result of the sequential double blockade of the metabolism of susceptible organisms by trimethoprim and sulfadiazine, the minimum inhibitory concentration (MIC) of TRIBRISSEN® Tablets is markedly less than that of either of the components used separately. Many strains of bacteria that are not susceptible to one of the components are susceptible to TRIBRISSEN®. A synergistic effect between trimethoprim and sulfadiazine in combination has been shown experimentally both *in vitro* and *in vivo* (in dogs).

TRIBRISSEN® is bactericidal against susceptible strains and is often effective against sulfonamide-resistant organisms. *In vitro* sulfadiazine is usually only bacteriostatic.

The precise *in vitro* MIC of the combination varies with the ratio of the drugs present, but the action of TRIBRISSEN® Tablets occurs over a wide range of ratios with an increase in the concentration of one of its components compensating for a decrease in the other. It is usual, however, to determine MICs using a constant ratio of one part trimethoprim in twenty parts of the combination.

The following table shows MICs, using the above ratio of bacteria which were susceptible to both trimethoprim (TMP) and sulfadiazine (SDZ). The organisms are those most commonly involved in conditions for which TRIBRISSEN® is indicated.

Average Minimum Inhibitory Concentration (MIC - mcg/mL):

Bacteria	TMP Alone	SDZ Alone	TMP/SDZ
Escherichia coli	0.31	26.5	0.07/1.31
Proteus species	1.3	24.5	0.15/2.85
Staphylococcus aureus	0.6	17.6	0.13/2.47
Pasteurella species	0.06	20.1	0.03/0.56
Salmonella species	0.15	61.0	0.05/0.95
β Streptococcus	0.5	24.5	0.15/2.85

The following table demonstrates the marked effect of the trimethoprim and sulfadiazine combination against sulfadiazine-resistant strains of normally susceptible organisms.

Average Minimum Inhibitory Concentration of Sulfadiazine-Resistant Strains (MIC - mcg/mL):

Bacteria	TMP Alone	SDZ Alone	TMP/SDZ
Escherichia coli	0.32	>245	0.27/5.0
Proteus species	0.66	>245	0.32/6.2

Susceptibility Testing: In testing susceptibility to TRIBRISSEN®, it is essential that the medium used does not contain significant amounts of interfering substances which can bypass the metabolic blocking action; e.g., thymidine or thymine.

The standard SxT disc is appropriate for testing by the disc diffusion method.

Following oral administration, TRIBRISSEN® is rapidly absorbed and widely distributed throughout the body tissues. Concentrations of trimethoprim are usually higher in tissues than in blood. The levels of trimethoprim are high in the lung, kidney and liver, as would be expected from its physical properties.

Studies with labeled trimethoprim in dogs have shown that about two-thirds of the dose is excreted in the urine in 24 hours.

Therapeutic serum levels are detected one to three hours after dosing. In dogs, peak blood levels occur three to four hours after oral administration.

Usually the concentration of an antibacterial in the blood and the *in vitro* MIC of the infecting organism indicate an appropriate period between doses of a drug. This does not hold entirely for TRIBRISSEN® because trimethoprim, in contrast to sulfadiazine, localizes in the tissues and, therefore, its concentration and ratio to sulfadiazine are higher there than in blood. Serum levels following dosing give an indication, however, of the probable duration of effectiveness of a single dose.

The following table shows the average serum concentrations of trimethoprim and sulfadiazine in six adult dogs following administration of a single oral dose of 30 mg/kg on two separate occasions.

Average Serum Concentration (mcg/mL):

Trimethoprim (5 mg/kg)				Sulfadiazine (25 mg/kg)			
1 hr.	3 hr.	6 hr.	24 hr.	1 hr.	3 hr.	6 hr.	24 hr.
1.36	1.52	0.51	<0.047	21.6	30.1	27.3	9.8

Excretion of TRIBRISSEN® is chiefly by the kidneys, by both glomerular filtration, and tubular secretion. Urine concentrations of TRIBRISSEN® are severalfold higher than blood concentrations. Neither trimethoprim nor sulfadiazine interferes with the excretion pattern of the other.

Dosage and Administration: The schedule below provides for a dose of 30 mg/2.5 lb per day (approximately 30 mg/kg per day).

Weight of Dog	TRIBRISSEN® Tablet
2.5 lb	1 x 30 mg tablet
10.0 lb	1 x 120 mg tablet
40.0 lb	1 x 480 mg tablet
80 lb	1 x 960 mg tablet

The recommended dose may be given once daily or one-half the daily dose may be administered every 12 hours.

Administer for two to three days after symptoms have subsided.

If no improvement of acute infections is seen in 3 to 5 days, re-evaluate the diagnosis.

TRIBRISSEN® Tablets may be used alone or in conjunction with Tribrissen® 24% Injection.

Therapy with TRIBRISSEN® Tablets is not recommended for more than 14 days. A complete blood count should be done periodically in patients receiving TRIBRISSEN® for prolonged

T

periods. If a significant reduction in the count of any formed blood element is noted, treatment with TRIBRISSEN® should be discontinued.

Contraindication(s): TRIBRISSEN® should not be used in dogs showing marked liver parenchymal damage, blood dyscrasias, or in those with a history of sulfonamide sensitivity.

Precaution(s): Storage: Store at 15°-30°C (59°-86°F) in a dry place.

Caution(s): Federal (U.S.A.) law restricts this drug to use by or on the order of a licensed veterinarian.

Water should be readily available to dogs receiving sulfonamide therapy.

Individual animal hypersensitivity may result in local or generalized reactions, sometimes fatal. Anaphylactic reactions, although rare, may also occur.

Antidote(s): Epinephrine.

Warning(s): Keep out of reach of children. Not for human use.

Toxicology: Toxicity and Side Effects: Toxicity is low. The acute toxicity (LD_{50}) of TRIBRISSEN® is more than 5 g/kg orally in rats and mice.

No significant changes were recorded in rats given doses of 600 mg/kg per day for 90 days.

Dogs can tolerate up to ten times the recommended therapeutic dose without exhibiting ill effect. Dogs dosed at 300 mg/kg per day for a period of 20 days revealed only slight changes in hematologic values.

Slight to moderate reductions in hematopoietic activity following high, prolonged dosage in several species have been recorded. This is usually reversible by folinic acid (leucovorin) administration or by stopping use of the drug. During the long-term treatment of dogs, periodic platelet counts and white and red blood cell counts are advisable.

Teratology: Dogs given therapeutic doses (30 mg/kg per day) of TRIBRISSEN® continuously and at interrupted intervals throughout pregnancy gave birth to normal progeny. From these studies, it appears that TRIBRISSEN® can safely be given to dogs during gestation.

Adverse Reactions: Conditions reported following use of trimethoprim/sulfadiazine include polyarthritis, urticaria, facial swelling, fever, hemolytic anemia, polydypsia/polyuria, vomiting, anorexia, diarrhea and seizures. Keratitis sicca possibly due to the prolonged use of trimethoprim/sulfadiazine has been reported. The condition has also been associated with the prolonged use of other sulfonamide-containing products.

Hepatitis possibly due to sulfonamide hypersensitivity has been diagnosed following trimethoprim/sulfadiazine therapy.

Presentation: TRIBRISSEN® 30 mg Tablets are available in bottles of 100 (NDC 0061-5078-01). TRIBRISSEN® 120 mg Tablets are available in bottles of 100 (NDC 0061-5079-01) and 1000 (NDC 0061-5079-02).
TRIBRISSEN® 480 mg Tablets are available in bottles of 100 (NDC 0061-5070-01) and 250 (NDC 0061-5070-02).
TRIBRISSEN® 960 mg Tablets are available in bottles of 100 (NDC 0061-5081-01).

Compendium Code No.: 10472001 Rev. 12/97

TRICAINE-S

Western Chemical **Anesthetic-Aquaculture**

Tricaine Methanesulfonate

ANADA No.: 200-226

Active Ingredient(s): Tricaine methanesulfonate.

Indications: TRICAINE-S is intended for the anesthesia, tranquilization and temporary immobilization of fish, amphibians, and other aquatic, cold-blooded animals. It has long been recognized as a valuable tool for the proper handling of these animals during manual spawning (fish stripping), weighing, measuring, marking, surgical operations, transport, photography, and research.

Chemistry: TRICAINE-S is the methanesulfonate of meta-amino benzoic acid ethylester, or simply ethyl *m*-amino benzoate. It is thus an isomer of benzocaine having the formula $C_9H_{11}O_2N + CH_3SO_3H$ and the following structure:

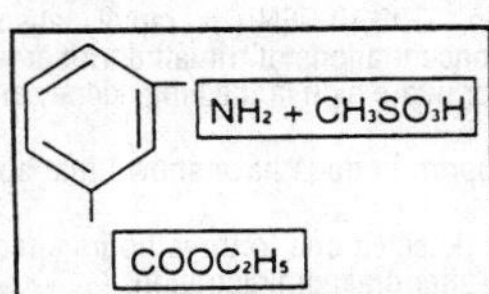

TRICAINE-S is a fine white crystalline powder. Its molecular weight is 261.3. Soluble to 11%, it forms clear, colorless, acid solutions in water.

Dosage and Administration:

I. Guidelines for Use on Fish:

TRICAINE-S is effective and safe for the anesthesia of fish when used as directed. Its use is governed by, and can be tailored to, the needs of individual fishery personnel. Sedation and various rates of anesthetization are controlled by the concentration. The versatility of TRICAINE-S is demonstrated by the fact that it has been used in fisheries at levels ranging from 10 to 1,000 mg/liter[3]. The action of the anesthetic is slowed at cooler temperatures, in extremely soft water (approximately 10 mg/liter of $CACO_3$, or less), and in larger fish[4]. Also, efficacy may vary with species[4]. Thus, it is imperative that preliminary tests of anesthetic solutions be made against small numbers of fish to determine the desired rates of anesthesia and exposure times for the specific lots of fish under prevailing conditions.

The following tables may be used as guidelines in selecting concentrations of TRICAINE-S for the anesthetization of various fishes:

Table 1 - Concentrations Required for Rapid Anesthesia (Induction time less than 2-5 minutes; used in spawning, marking, measuring, and some surgical operations):

Fish	Temperature	Concentration (mg/liter)	Max. tolerated exposure time* (min.)	Recovery time in fresh water (min.)
Salmonidae[4]	7-17°C (45-63°F)	80-135	4-12	3-19
(Pacific and Atlantic salmon; trout; chars; etc.)				
Esocidae[5]	8-12°C (46-54°F)	150	8-28	8-31
(Northern Pike; muskellunge)				
Cyprinidae[3]	16°C (61°F)	150-200		
(Carp; goldfish)				
Ictaluridae[2]	7-27°C (45-81°F)	140-270	4-11	3-24
(Channel catfish)				
Centrarchidae[4]	10-27°C (50-81°F)	260-330	3-5	7-11
(Bluegill; largemouth bass)				
Percidae[3]	10-16°C (50-61°F)	100-120	7-18	5-40
(Walleye)				
Pet and Tropical[1]				
Live-bearers	24-27°C (75-81°F)	85	12 hrs.	
Egg layers	24-27°C (75-81°F)	75	12 hrs.	

* Maximum tolerated exposure time (in minutes) of fish to TRICAINE-S solution.

Table 2 - Concentrations Required for Moderately Rapid Anesthesia (Induction time less than 15-20 minutes; used in surgical operations and in spawning and marking where longer exposures are more important than rapid immobilization):

Fish	Temperature	Concentration (mg/liter)	Maximum tolerated exposure time* (min.)	Recovery time in fresh water (min.)
Salmonidae[4]	7-17°C (45-63°F)	50-60	30 or >	2-20
(Pacific and Atlantic salmon; trout; chars; etc.)				
Ictaluridae[2]	7-27°C (45-81°F)	70	30 or >	1-10
(Channel catfish)				

* Maximum tolerated exposure time (in minutes) of fish to TRICAINE-S solution.

Table 3 - Concentrations Required for Sedation (Induction within 15 minutes; used in fish transport):

Fish	Temperature	Concentration (mg/liter)	Maintenance of sedation (hr.)
Salmonidae[4]	7-17°C (45-63°F)	15-30	6
(Pacific and Atlantic salmon; trout; chars; etc.)			
Esocidae[5]		40	
(Chain pickerel)			
Ictaluridae[2]	7-27°C (45-81°F)	20-40	6
(Channel catfish)			
Centrarchidae[8]		25	8-13
(Bluegills)			
Pet and Tropical[1]			
[Bettas, Piranhas, etc. (uncrowded)	24-27°C (75-81°F)	66	48
Goldfish]	24-27°C (75-81°F)	37	48

Important: Since, in many cases, relatively rapid rates of anesthesia can be achieved only by exceeding the lethal concentration of TRICAINE-S, it is necessary to return anesthetized fish to fresh water before they are overexposed. Excessive exposures are avoided by observing the following sensory and motor responses of the fish which characterize progressively deeper levels of anesthesia:

Sedation - Decreased reactivity to visual and vibrational stimuli; opercular activity reduced.

Total loss of equilibrium - Fish turns over; locomotion ceases; fish swims or extends fins in response to pressure on caudal fin or peduncle.

Total loss of reflex - No response to pressure on caudal fin or peduncle; opercular rate slow and erratic.

Medullary collapse - Opercular activity ceases.

Laboratory and field investigations[3,9] have shown that the action of TRICAINE-S is readily reversed when the fish are transferred to fresh water before opercular activity ceases. Additional exposure following medullary collapse may result in mortality. A rough estimate of the safe total exposure can be made by multiplying the time required for anesthesia by a factor of 2 or 3.

Water: Since TRICAINE-S is very soluble (1:9) in water, it dissolves with equal readiness in spring water, tap water, or sea-water. Do not use distilled or deionized water, or water containing chlorine, heavy metals (copper, zinc, etc.), or other toxic contaminants. The anesthetic solution should be well oxygenated, and its temperature should be similar to that of the water from which the fish are taken. In the field, many water quality problems are eliminated by using natural water to which the fish are acclimated, provided the water does not possess high chemical or biologic oxygen demand.

Methods of Application:

1. General anesthesia: For most situations where rapid or moderately rapid anesthesia is required, TRICAINE-S may be applied in a bath, i.e., the fish are immersed in the anesthetic solution. Containers may be of glass, plastic, steel, aluminum, or other suitable material. However, do not use galvanized or brass containers unless treated or sealed to prevent dissolution of zinc. Size of container is determined by individual needs, but the fish should not be overcrowded. Discard anesthetic solutions when a loss in potency is noted, or when the solutions become fouled with mucus or excrement.
2. For surgery and certain physiologic studies, the fish may be anesthetized to loss of reflex, removed from the anesthetic, and then positioned so that the gills are bathed in a sedating concentration of TRICAINE-S. Some investigators have developed flowing, re-circulating systems for bathing the gills with anesthetic during surgery.

   Large fishes such as sharks and rays are anesthetized within minutes by spraying the gills with a 1 g/liter solution of TRICAINE-S.[10] The application is made by means of water pistol, bulb syringe, hand pump, etc.
3. Transport - TRICAINE-S been used to sedate fish during transport. It is more successful in cold than in warm water, and it is instrumental in reducing injuries because of hyperactivity. Fish are usually transported by means of distribution units (tank trucks), or by air in plastic bags.[11,12] In either case, the fish should be fasted before-hand to reduce metabolic wastes. Also, some workers suggest pretransport sedation for several hours to lower metabolism. With distribution units, the fish may be fasted and sedated prior to loading. The anesthetic solution is prepared in the distribution unit and oxygenated. Then, the fish are added and temperature acclimated.

   In air shipments, the anesthetic solution is placed in a suitable plastic bag, the sedated fish are added, the bag inflated with oxygen, tied securely, and placed in a second bag. This bag is also tied, and then placed on ice in an insulated container[13]. A modification of this method involves complete anesthesia of the fish, and placing them in water bags which contain no anesthetic. In any case, upon arrival, the fish should be acclimated slowly to new environmental temperatures.

Preparation of TRICAINE-S Solutions: Prior to use, TRICAINE-S may be weighed out into amounts which are convenient for the volume of water to be used. A handy unit is 2 g since this quantity in 5 gallons of water yields a concentration of about 100 mg/liter. For rough approximations, one level teaspoonful contains 2.0 to 2.5 g. Thus, a level teaspoonful of anesthetic in 5 gallons gives a concentration of about 120 mg/liter.

To convert mg/liter into g/gal.: multiply number of mg by 0.00378.

e.g. 80 mg/liter = 80 x 0.00378 = 0.302 g/gal.

To convert mg/liter into a ratio of TRICAINE-S to water: divide 1,000,000 by the number of mg.

e.g. 80 mg/liter = 1,000,000 ÷ 80 = 1:12,500

Limitations in Use: Since TRICAINE-S is taken up into the blood of fish, residues of the drug may occur in edible tissues. However, the residues dissipate rapidly after the fish are placed in fresh water[14]. Thus, treated fish which may be used for food must be held in fresh water above 10°C (50°F) for a period of 21 days.

Withdrawal in fresh water is unnecessary for non-food fishes such as goldfish, bait fish, and ornamentals. Also, withdrawal is unnecessary for sublegal sizes of the following species of fish because they are not used as food immediately following anesthesia (Table 4).

Table 4 - Sublegal Sizes of Fish Species Not Used as Food Immediately after Anesthesia[15]:

Species	Size (in.)
Pink salmon	6
Chum salmon	6
Coho salmon	6
Sockeye salmon	6
Chinook salmon	6
Cutthroat trout	6
Steelhead trout	8
Rainbow trout	6
Atlantic salmon	10
Brown trout	6
Brook trout	6
Lake trout	5
Splake trout	6
Grayling	6
Northern pike	12
Muskellunge	12
Channel catfish	6
Flathead catfish	6
Bluegill	3
Redear sunfish	3
Smallmouth bass	5
Largemouth bass	5
Walleye	6

II. Guidelines for Use on Amphibians:

Table 5 - Effects of Varying Concentrations of TRICAINE-S on Salamanders

Salamander	Concentration*	Duration of Anesthesia*	Remarks
Embryos	1:10,000 (3b)	2 days	No adverse effects.
Ambystoma opacum	1:3,000 (3c)	to 30 min.	
Larvae	1:10,000 (3b)	2 days	No adverse effects.
	1:12,000 (3f)	10-15 min.	
	1:20,000 (3f)	10-15 min.	
Ambystoma opacum	1:3,000 (3c)	to 30 min.	No adverse effects.
	1:1,000 (3b)	few min.	No adverse effects.
Adults	1:3,000 (3b)	3 days	
Newts	1:1,000 (3b)	few min.	No adverse effects.
	1:10,000 (3b)	2 days	
Triturus sp.	1:1,000 (3k)	20 min.	No adverse effects.
Triturus uridescens	1:3,000 (3g)	1 hour	No adverse effects.
Mole salamanders			
Ambystoma opacum	1:3,000 (3c)	to 30 min.	No adverse effects.
Ambystoma tigrinum	1:2,000 (3j)	15-30 min.	No adverse effects.
Ambystoma punctatum	1:2,000 (3j)	15-30 min.	No adverse effects.
Mud-puppy			
Necturus maculosus	1:1,500 (3i)	to 6 hours	See below.**

* When an individual of any of the species listed is exposed at the designated concentration, the data available suggests that the animal may be safely maintained under anesthesia for the time noted. Prolonging exposure to the anesthetic beyond the time indicated may cause deaths. See Cautions.

**Remarks: Maintenance dose, 0.1 of induction concentration. At exposure to induction concentration for more than 20-30 minutes, renal circulation becomes sluggish or stops.

Table 6 - Effects of Varying Concentrations of TRICAINE-S on Frogs:

Frog	Concentration*	Duration of Anesthesia*	Remarks
Embryos	1:1,000 (3b)	few min.	No adverse effects.
	1:10,000 (3b)	2 days	
	1:15,000 (3h)	3 days	
Tadpoles	1:1,000 (3j)	30 min.	No adverse effects.
	1:3,000 (3f)	10-15 min.	
	1:10,000 (3b)	2 days	
	1:15,000 (3h)	3 days	
Rana sp.	1:5,000 (3k)	5 hours	No adverse effects.
	1:1,000 (3j)	15-30 min.	
	1:3,333 (3a)	2 min.	
Rana pipiens	variable (3d)	1 hour	
Adults	1:1,000 (3e)	30 min.	No adverse effects.
Leopard frog			
Rana pipiens	1:3,000 (3c)	to 30 min.	No adverse effects.
Eastern wood frog			
Rana sylvatica	1:8,000 (3l)	5-10 min.	Only slightly under anesthesia.

* When an individual of any of the species listed is exposed at the designated concentration, the data available suggests that the animal may be safely maintained under anesthesia for the time noted.

Prolonging exposure to the anesthetic beyond the time indicated, may cause deaths. See Cautions.

Precaution(s): Store at room temperature (approximately 25°C). Keep tightly closed.

Caution(s):

1. Avoid inhaling TRICAINE-S or getting it into the eyes.
2. Always conduct preliminary tests with TRICAINE-S to determine desired rates of anesthesia and optimal length of exposure.
3. Do not overexpose fish to lethal levels of TRICAINE-S.
4. Do not anesthetize more fish than can be handled effectively.
5. Do not contaminate eggs or sperm with TRICAINE-S when stripping fish.
6. Do not use water containing chlorine, or other toxic agents.
7. Insure adequate oxygen in anesthetic solution.
8. Discard anesthetic solutions when fouled with mucus or metabolic wastes.
9. Do not discard TRICAINE-S solutions into water supplies or natural waters.
10. Store TRICAINE-S solutions in a cool place away from light.*
11. Discard stock solutions of TRICAINE-S after several days.*
12. Treated fish destined for food must be held in fresh water above 10°C (50°F) for 21 days before use.

* The color of TRICAINE-S solutions may change rapidly to yellow or brown when exposed to light. This does not affect activity in any significant way. However, for best results, use freshly prepared solutions. A 10 percent solution stored at room temperature shows no significant loss of potency after three days, but after 10 days, a brownish color and an activity decrease of 5 percent is observed.

Warning(s): Do not use within 21 days of harvesting fish for food.

When used in food fish, use should be restricted to Ictaluridae, Salmonidae, Esocidae, and Percidae and water temperature should exceed 10°C (50°F).

In other fish and other cold-blooded animals (poikilotherms), TRICAINE-S should be limited to hatchery or laboratory use.

Keep out of reach of children.

Toxicology: Comparative toxicologic studies carried out on fish and frogs gave the following results:

Fish Toxicity Studies - The toxicity of TRICAINE-S was measured by standard methods in laboratory bioassays with rainbow trout, brown trout, brook trout, lake trout, northern pike, channel catfish, bluegill, largemouth bass, and walleye. The 24, 48 and 96 hour LC_{50} (lethal concentration for 50 percent of the animals) values for trout ranged from 52 to 31 mg/liter; for northern pike, from 56 to 48 mg/liter; for catfish, from 66 to 50 mg/liter, for bluegill and largemouth bass, from 61 to 39 mg/liter; and for walleye, the values were 49 to 46 mg/liter.

Safety index: The safety indices for TRICAINE-S refer to the margin between concentrations which cause anesthesia and mortality. They are expressed by the quotient of the lethal concentration for 50 percent of the fish (LC_{50}) and the effective concentration for 50 percent of the fish (EC_{50}).

Safety Indices for Rainbow Trout and Channel Catfish at 12°C (54°F).

Species	Exposure (min.)	LC_{50} (mg/liter)	EC_{50} (mg/liter)	Index
Rainbow trout[1]	15	65	32	2.0
"	30	57	32	1.8
"	60	56	29	1.9
Channel catfish[2]	15	139	47	3.0
"	30	118	45	2.6
"	60	110	46	2.4

Frog Toxicity Studies[3] - Frogs were put into various concentrations of TRICAINE-S for 30 minutes and then transferred to tap water in order to determine the LC_{50}. The LC_{50} was 6.2 percent TRICAINE-S. Therefore, the anesthetic must be used in very high concentration before it is fatal to frogs.

References: Available upon request.

Presentation: Bottles of 3.5 oz (100 grams) and 2.2 lb (1 kilogram).

Sold under licensing agreement between Western Chemical Inc. and R. & L. Secor, Trustees.

Compendium Code No.: 10210050

TRICHGUARD®

Fort Dodge **Vaccine**

Tritrichomonas Foetus Vaccine, Killed Protozoa

U.S. Vet. Lic. No.: 112

Contents: This product contains the antigen listed above.

Neomycin and polymyxin B are added as preservatives.

Indications: For vaccination of healthy cattle as an aid in the prevention of disease caused by *Tritrichomonas foetus.*

Dosage and Administration: Cattle, inject one 2 mL dose subcutaneously under aseptic conditions. A second dose should be administered 2 to 4 weeks later. The last injection should precede the breeding season by 4 weeks. Revaccinate annually.

Precaution(s): Store in dark at 2° to 7°C (35° to 45°F). Avoid freezing. Shake well. Use entire contents when first opened.

Caution(s): In case of anaphylactoid reaction, administer epinephrine.

Warning(s): Do not vaccinate within 60 days before slaughter.

For veterinary use only.

Presentation: 10 dose (20 mL) and 50 dose (100 mL) vials.

U.S. Patent Nos. 5,223,253 and 5,679,353

Compendium Code No.: 10032411 1796H

T

TRICHGUARD® V5L

Fort Dodge **Bacterin-Vaccine**

Tritrichomonas Foetus Vaccine, Killed Protozoa-Campylobacter Fetus-Leptospira Canicola-Grippotyphosa-Hardjo-Icterohaemorrhagiae-Pomona Bacterin

U.S. Vet. Lic. No.: 112

Contents: Killed, concentrated cultures of *Tritrichomonas foetus, Campylobacter fetus* var. *venerealis* and *Leptospira canicola, grippotyphosa, hardjo, icterohaemorrhagiae* and *pomona* organisms suspended in special oil adjuvant.

Neomycin and polymyxin B added as preservatives.

Indications: For vaccination of healthy cattle as an aid in the prevention of disease caused by *Tritrichomonas foetus, Campylobacter fetus, Leptospira canicola, L. grippotyphosa, L. hardjo, L. icterohaemorrhagiae* and *L. pomona.*

Dosage and Administration: Cattle, inject one 5 mL dose subcutaneously under aseptic conditions in the neck or behind the shoulder. A second dose should be administered 2 to 4 weeks later. The last injection should precede the breeding season by 4 weeks. Revaccinate annually.

Precaution(s): Store in dark at 2° to 7°C (35° to 45°F). Avoid freezing. Shake well. Use entire contents when first opened.

Caution(s): Transient swelling may occur at injection site. In case of anaphylactoid reaction, administer epinephrine.

Warning(s): Do not vaccinate within 60 days before slaughter. For veterinary use only.

Presentation: 10 dose (50 mL) and 50 dose (250 mL) vials.

U.S. Patent No. 5,223,253 and 5,679,353

Compendium Code No.: 10032421 1075E

TRICLOSAN DEODORIZING SHAMPOO

Davis **Grooming Shampoo**

Active Ingredient(s): Triclosan.

Indications: A deodorizing formula with coat conditioners for dogs, cats, puppies and kittens.

Directions for Use: To use Davis TRICLOSAN DEODORIZING SHAMPOO as a general grooming and cleansing shampoo, dilute 10 parts water to 1 part shampoo (10:1). For extra deodorizing, dilute 4 parts water to 1 part shampoo (4:1) or apply shampoo undiluted.

Wet pet's coat thoroughly with warm water. Do not get shampoo into eyes. Apply shampoo to head and ears, then lather. Repeat procedure with neck, chest, middle and hind quarter, finishing legs last. Allow pet to stand for 5 to 10 minutes. Rinse pet thoroughly. For best results, repeat procedure.

Warning(s): For external use only. Keep out of reach of children.

Presentation: 12 fl oz (355 mL) and one gallon (3.785 L).

Compendium Code No.: 11410380

TRICLOSAN HAND SOAP

Davis **Hand Soap**

Active Ingredient(s): Contains .05% triclosan in a moisturizing solution.

Indications: Davis TRICLOSAN HAND SOAP is a hand soap formulated for professionals in the animal health industry. Especially formulated for routine and frequent washings.

Directions for Use: Apply enough Davis TRICLOSAN HAND SOAP to create a good lather and rinse thoroughly.

Warning(s): For external veterinary use only. Keep out of reach of children.

Presentation: 12 fl oz (355 mL) and 1 gallon (3.785 L).

Compendium Code No.: 11410391

TRIENAMINE™ ℞

Phoenix Pharmaceutical **Antihistamine**

Tripelennamine Hydrochloride Injection 20 mg/mL

ANADA No.: 200-162

Active Ingredient(s): Composition: Each mL of sterile aqueous solution contains:

Tripelennamine Hydrochloride USP .... 20 mg

Indications: For use in cattle and horses in conditions in which antihistaminic therapy may be expected to lead to alleviation of some signs of disease.

Pharmacology: Tripelennamine hydrochloride is a white, crystalline material which is stable, nonhygroscopic, and readily soluble in water.

Action: Tripelennamine hydrochloride is characterized by its capacity to antagonize many of the pharmacologic effects of histamine.

Dosage and Administration: Warm the solution to near body temperature.

Using aseptic precautions, administer intravenously or intramuscularly as specified below. Intramuscular injections should be made into the heavy musculature of the hind leg or cervical area.

The doses specified below may be repeated in 6 to 12 hours if necessary.

Cattle: Administer intravenously or intramuscularly at a dose of 0.5 mg per lb of body weight (2.5 mL for each 100 lbs of body weight). For a more rapid onset of action, the intravenous route of administration is recommended.

Horses: Administer intramuscularly only at a dose of 0.5 mg per lb of body weight (2.5 mL for each 100 lbs of body weight).

Precaution(s): Storage: Protect from light. Store between 15°C and 30°C (59°F-86°F). Avoid excessive heat (104°F).

Caution(s): Federal law restricts this drug to use by or on the order of a licensed veterinarian.

Central nervous system stimulation in the form of hyperexcitability, nervousness, and muscle tremors lasting up to 20 minutes have been noted in horses, particularly following intravenous administration; therefore, only the intramuscular route of administration should be used in horses.

Overdosage of tripelennamine hydrochloride may give rise to excitement, ataxia, and convulsions.

Depression of the central nervous system and incoordination may occur when the drug is used at therapeutic dose levels.

Disturbances in gastrointestinal function may occur in some instances.

While poisonous snake bites have been treated with antihistaminic drugs, other conjunctive therapy is required because of toxic reactions associated with the protein complex of venom.

For parental use.

For animal use only.

Warning(s): Do not use in horses intended for food purposes.

Milk that has been taken during treatment and for 24 hours (two milkings) after the last treatment must not be used for food.

Treated cattle must not be slaughtered for food during treatment and for four days following the last treatment.

A withdrawal period has not been established for this product in pre-ruminating calves. Do not use in calves to be processed for veal. Keep out of reach of children.

Presentation: TRIENAMINE™ (Tripelennamine Hydrochloride Injection) is supplied in 250 mL (NDC 57319-353-06) and 500 mL (NDC 57319-353-07) multiple dose vials, containing 20 mg Tripelennamine Hydrochloride USP per mL.

Manufactured by: Phoenix Scientific, Inc., St. Joseph, MO 64503.

Compendium Code No.: 12560852 Rev. 5-01 / Rev. 5-01

TRIFECTANT™

Evsco **Disinfectant**

Broad Spectrum Disinfectant

EPA Reg. No.: 62432-1-74510

Active Ingredient(s):

Potassium peroxymonosulfate 20.4%
Sodium Chloride 1.5%
Other Ingredients 78.1%
Total 100.0%

Equivalent to 9.75% available chlorine.

Indications: Broad Spectrum Disinfectant: TRIFECTANT™ is effective against numerous microorganisms affecting animals: viruses, gram positive and gram negative bacteria, fungi (molds and yeasts), and mycoplasma. Efficacy was determined in the presence of hard water and organic material. TRIFECTANT™ passes the AOAC germicidal and detergent sanitizer test at a concentration of 0.5% (1:200) in the presence of 200 ppm hard water.

Effective Against:

Poultry:

Bacteria: *Streptococcus pyogenes, Campylobacter pyloridis, Klebsiella pneumoniae, Escherichia coli, Salmonella typhimurium, Salmonella choleraesuis, Pseudomonas aeruginosa, Staphylococcus aureus, Staphylococcus epidermidis, Mycoplasma gallisepticum, Clostridium perfringens, Bordetella avium.*

Viruses: Newcastle Disease, Infectious Bronchitis, Infectious Bursal Disease, Avian Laryngotracheitis, Avian Influenza, Marek's Disease, Egg Drop Syndrome Adenovirus, Turkey Herpes Virus, Duck Viral Enteritis.

Fungi: *Aspergillus flavus, Aspergillus fumigatus, Candida albicans.*

Swine:

Bacteria: *Pasteurella multocida, Bordetella bronchiseptica, Actinobacillus pleuropneumonia, Treponema hyodysenteriae, Clostridium perfringens.*

Viruses: Hog Cholera, Swine Influenza, Porcine Parvovirus, Rotaviral Diarrhea, Vesicular stomatitis, Pseudorabies, Porcine Reproductive and Respiratory Syndrome (PRRS), African Swine Fever, Foot and Mouth Disease.

Fungi: *Fusarium moniliforme.*

Bovine:

Bacteria: *Moraxella bovis, Mycobacterium bovis, Haemophilus somnus.*

Viruses: Calf rotavirus, Infective Bovine Rhinotracheitis, Bovine Adenovirus Type 4, Pseudorabies, Foot and Mouth Disease.

Fungi: *Fusarium moniliforme.*

Equine:

Bacteria: *Clostridium perfringens,* Fistulous Withers (Poll Evil), *Taylorella equigenitalis, Streptococcus equi* (Strangles), *Pseudomonas mallei* (Glanders), *Bordetella bronchiseptica.*

Viruses: African Horse Sickness, Equine Viral Arteritis (Pink Eye), Critical Exantherma, Myeloencephalopathy, Rhinopneumonitis, Equine Infectious Anemia (Swamp Fever), Equine Papilomatosis, Equine Contagious Abortion, Adenovirus Pneumonia, Equine Influenza (The Cough).

Fungi: *Trichophyton* spp. (Ringworm), *Trichophyton* spp. (Mud Fever), *Fusarium moniliforme.*

Companion Animals:

Bacteria: *Staphylococcus aureus, Streptococcus pyogenes, Klebsiella pneumoniae, Pseudomonas aeruginosa.*

Viruses: Canine Parvovirus, Distemper, *Leptospira canicola,* Feline Parvovirus, Feline herpes, Feline calicivirus.

Fungi: *Microsporum canis.*

Emergency Disease Control: Controls Foot and Mouth Disease virus (see Directions for Use).

Directions for Use: It is a violation of Federal law to use this product in a manner inconsistent with its labeling.

This powder is easily diluted for use in manual or machine operations.

TRIFECTANT™ Dilution Chart: Fill container with desired amount of water and add TRIFECTANT™ powder to achieve recommended solution concentration.

Quantity of Water	1% Solution	2% Solution
1 quart	0.3 oz	0.7 oz
1 gallon	1.3 oz	2.7 oz
10 gallons	13.4 oz	26.7 oz
50 gallons	66.8 oz	133.5 oz

1.3 oz measuring scoop is provided.

General Instructions - Poultry and Farm Premises:

1. Remove all poultry or other animals and feeds from premises, trucks or other vehicles, coops, crates or other enclosures.
2. Remove all litter droppings and manure from floors, walls and surfaces of barns pens, stalls, chutes and other facilities and fixtures occupied or traversed by poultry or other animals.
3. Empty all troughs, racks, and other feeding and watering appliances.
4. Heavily soiled surfaces should be cleaned with a heavy-duty soap or detergent, like Antec's Biosolve, and rinsed with water.
5. Saturate surfaces with the recommended disinfecting solution for a period of 10 minutes.
6. Immerse all halters, ropes, and other types of equipment used in handling and restraining animals, as well as forks, shovels, and scrapers used for removing litter and manure.
7. Ventilate buildings, cars, boats, coops, and other closed spaces. Do not house poultry or livestock or employ equipment until treatment has been absorbed, set, or dried.
8. Thoroughly scrub treated feed racks, mangers, troughs, automatic feeders, fountains, and waterers with soap or detergent, and rinse with potable water before reuse.

Add 1.3 oz (1 scoop) of TRIFECTANT™ to one gallon of warm water. Solutions are stable for 7 days. Do not soak metal objects in TRIFECTANT™ for long periods-10 minutes is the maximum necessary contact time. One gallon of solution is sufficient to treat 135 square feet.

Poultry Production/Ratite Production:

Hatcheries: TRIFECTANT™ at 1% solution can be used for cleaning and disinfecting hatchers, setters, evaporative coolers, humidifying systems, ceiling fans, chicken houses, transfer trucks, trays, and plastic chick boxes (use 2% solution for *Mycoplasma, Aspergillus flavus* and *Aspergillus fumigatus)*. TRIFECTANT™ at 1-2% solution is recommended for use in fogging (wet misting) operations as a supplemental measure, either before or after regular cleaning and disinfecting procedures. Fog (wet mist) until the area is moist, using automatic foggers according to manufacturer's use directions.

Broiler/Breeder Houses: Follow General Instructions above to remove birds and preclean area to be treated. Spray floors and walls with TRIFECTANT™ at 1% solution. Thoroughly wash waterers and feeders with a 1% solution of TRIFECTANT™ (use 2% solution for *Mycoplasma, Aspergillus flavus* and *Aspergillus fumigatus)*. After contact for 10 minutes, rinse with water.

Do not house poultry or use equipment until treatment has dried.

For Air Sanitizing: Use TRIFECTANT™ at 1-2% solution and fog until surfaces are moist. Allow at least 2 hours before entering treated area. Rinse foggers and sprayers with water following use.

Processing Plants: Spray TRIFECTANT™ at 1% solution to disinfect and clean walls, ceilings and floors.

Swine Production: Follow General Instructions above to remove swine and preclean area to be treated. TRIFECTANT™ at 1% solution is recommended for cleaning and disinfecting farrowing units, nurseries, finisher houses and processing plants (use 2% solution for *Mycoplasma, Aspergillus flavus* and *Aspergillus fumigatus)* and agricultural production equipment such as trucks, waterproof footwear (such as rubber boots), and associated livestock equipment and instruments.

TRIFECTANT™ at 1-2% solution is recommended for use in fogging (wet misting) operations or as a supplemental measure either before or after regular cleaning and disinfecting procedures. Fog (wet mist) until the area is moist, using automatic foggers according to manufacturer's use directions. Rinse foggers and sprayers with water following use.

Bovine Production: A 1% solution of TRIFECTANT™ is recommended to clean and disinfect areas associated with bovine housing, hospital pens and feedlot facilities and agricultural production equipment such as trucks, waterproof footwear (such as rubber boots), and associated livestock equipment and instruments.

Equine Production:

Broad Spectrum Equine Disinfectant/Detergent/Wash:

For Cleaning and Disinfecting Stables, Equipment and Aerial Disinfection:

Applications: For cleaning and disinfecting all surfaces, equipment, utensils and instruments in stables.

Uses:

Stables, Stalls, Tack, Equipment and Feed Rooms: Thoroughly clean and dry surfaces, then wash the area manually or with a pressure washer with a 1% TRIFECTANT™ solution. Rinse with clean water.

Blankets and Saddle Pads: Shampoo by hand or spray lightly with a hand sprayer and leave to dry. Shake or vacuum to remove residue.

Aerial Spraying to control airborne diseases: Use a hand held sprayer with fine setting or an automatic spraying system. Spray a 1% solution for 2-3 minutes twice daily. Rinse sprayers with water after use.

Companion Animals:

Applications: A 1% solution of TRIFECTANT™ is recommended as a "one step" cleaning and disinfection procedure for all surfaces, equipment, instruments, utensils and cages within grooming and boarding facilities, kennels, catteries and animal transportation vehicles.

Emergency Disease Control:

Controls: Foot and Mouth Disease virus: A 1% solution of TRIFECTANT™ is recommended to clean and disinfect agricultural facilities and equipment, military facilities and equipment, airport facilities and equipment, port facilities and equipment, rail facilities and equipment, quarantine facilities and equipment, slaughter facilities and equipment, and other shipping facilities and equipment where animals or soils suspected of harboring foot and mouth disease virus might have been previously present.

Within these facilities, treated objects include, but are not limited to, vehicles, farm equipment (including tractors, ploughing shares, cars and trucks, farm engines, harvesters, loaders, mowers, tillers and slaughter machinery), military equipment (including tank and troop carriers), and shipping equipment (pallets, bins and containers).

Spray TRIFECTANT™ at 1% solution to disinfect and clean walls, ceilings, floors, decks, container surfaces, vehicles, wheels, waterproof footwear (such as rubber boots), livestock equipment, utensils and instruments.

Precautionary Statements: Hazards to Humans and Domestic Animals:

Danger: Powder is corrosive. Causes skin burns and irreversible eye damage. Harmful if swallowed, absorbed through skin, or inhaled. Do not get in eyes, on skin, or on clothing. Wear protective clothing and rubber gloves. Avoid breathing dust. Wear goggles, face shield, or safety glasses. Wash thoroughly with soap and water after handling. Remove contaminated clothing and wash before reuse. Corrosive statement refers to powder only, not in use solution.

First Aid:

If in Eyes: Hold eyelids open and flush with a steady, gentle stream of water for 15 minutes. Get prompt medical attention.

If on Skin: Wash with plenty of soap and water. Get medical attention if irritation persists.

If Inhaled: If symptoms of coughing, choking, or wheezing are troublesome, remove to fresh air and seek medical attention.

If Swallowed: Drink promptly a large quantity of water. Avoid alcohol. Get immediate medical attention.

Notice to Physician: Probable mucosal damage may contraindicate the use of gastric lavage.

Storage and Disposal: Storage: Store in a cool, dry place in tightly closed container away from children. Always replace lid after use.

Disposal: Wash empty container thoroughly and dispose in trash. Do not mix this product with other chemicals.

Warning(s): Keep out of reach of children.

Presentation: 10 lb (4.54 kg).

TRIFECTANT is a registered trademark of Antec International Limited.

U.S. Patent No. 4,822,512

Manufactured by: Antec International Limited.

Distributed by: Vétoquinol N.-A., Inc., 2000, Chemin Georges, Lavaltrie, Québec, J0K 1H0 Canada.

Compendium Code No.: 10050340 10LB/trifect/vetoq/12.01

TRI-HIST® GRANULES ℞

Neogen **Antihistamine**

Antihistamine-Decongestant

Active Ingredient(s): Each ounce contains:

Pyrilamine Maleate U.S.P. .... 600 mg

Pseudoephedrine HCl U.S.P. .... 600 mg

in a palatable corn meal base.

Indications: Recommended for use as an antihistamine and decongestant in horses.

Dosage and Administration: ½ ounce (1 level tablespoon) per 1,000 lbs body weight or as recommended by a veterinarian. Can be mixed with feed and repeated at 12 hour intervals if needed.

Caution(s): Federal law restricts this drug to use by or on the order of a licensed veterinarian.

Do not use at least 72 hours prior to sporting events.

For equine use only.

For animal use only.

Warning(s): Keep out of reach of children.

Presentation: 20 oz (567 g) (NDC: 59051-8874-6) and 5 lb (2.268 kg) (NDC: 59051-8874-7).

Compendium Code No.: 14910451 L100-0997 Rev 0701, L308-0299 Rev 1101

TRIOPTIC-P™ ℞

Pfizer Animal Health **Ophthalmic Antibiotic**

(bacitracin-neomycin-polymyxin) Sterile Veterinary Ophthalmic Ointment-Antibacterial

NADA No.: 065-016

Active Ingredient(s): Each gram contains bacitracin zinc 400 units, neomycin sulfate 5 mg (equivalent to 3.5 mg of neomycin base), polymyxin B sulfate 10,000 units, in a base of white petrolatum and mineral oil.

Indications: In the treatment of superficial bacterial infections of the eyelid and conjunctiva in dogs and cats when due to organisms susceptible to the antibiotics contained in the ointment. Laboratory tests should be conducted including *in vitro* culturing and susceptibility tests on samples collected prior to treatment.

Pharmacology: The 3 antibiotics present in TRIOPTIC-P™ Veterinary Ophthalmic Ointment provide a broad spectrum of activity against the gram-positive and gram-negative bacteria commonly involved in superficial infections of the eyelid and conjunctiva. Bacitracin is effective against gram-positive bacteria including hemolytic and non-hemolytic Streptococci and Staphylococci. Resistant strains rarely develop. Neomycin is effective against both gram-positive and gram-negative bacteria including Staphylococci, *Escherichia coli, Haemophilus influenzae,* and many strains of Proteus and Pseudomonas. Polymyxin B is bactericidal to gram-negative bacteria especially Pseudomonas. No resistant strains have been found to develop *in vivo.*

Dosage and Administration: Apply a thin film over the cornea 3 or 4 times daily in dogs and cats. The area should be properly cleansed prior to use. Foreign bodies, crusted exudates, and debris should be carefully removed.

Precaution(s): Store at room temperature.

Caution(s): Federal law restricts this drug to use by or on the order of a licensed veterinarian.

Sensitivity to TRIOPTIC-P™ Veterinary Ophthalmic Ointment is rare; however, if a reaction occurs, discontinue use of the preparation. As with any antibiotic preparation, prolonged use may result in the overgrowth of nonsusceptible organisms including fungi. Appropriate measures should be taken if this occurs. If infection does not respond to treatment in 2 or 3 days, the diagnosis and therapy should be reevaluated.

Care should be taken not to contaminate the applicator tip of the tube during application of the preparation. Do not allow the applicator tip to come in contact with any tissue.

Adverse Reactions: Do not use this product as a presurgical ocular lubricant. Adverse reactions of ocular irritation and corneal ulcerations have been reported in association with such use.

Itching, burning or inflammation may occur in animals sensitive to the product. Discontinue use in such cases.

Presentation: 3.5-gram (⅛-oz), sterile, tamper-proof tubes.

Manufactured by: Altana Inc., Melville, NY 11747, USA

Compendium Code No.: 36901450 75-8276-03

TRIOPTIC-S® ℞

Pfizer Animal Health **Ophthalmic Antimicrobial-Corticosteroid**

(bacitracin-neomycin-polymyxin-hydrocortisone acetate 1%) Sterile Veterinary Ophthalmic Ointment-Antibacterial

NADA No.: 065-015

Active Ingredient(s): Each gram contains bacitracin zinc USP 400 units, neomycin sulfate 0.5% (equivalent to 3.5 mg neomycin base), polymyxin B sulfate USP 10,000 units, hydrocortisone acetate USP 1.0% in a base of white petrolatum and mineral oil.

Indications: TRIOPTIC-S® may be used in acute or chronic conjunctivitis, when caused by organisms susceptible to the antibiotics contained in this ointment. Laboratory tests should be conducted including in vitro culturing and susceptibility tests on samples collected prior to treatment.

Pharmacology: The overlapping spectra of these 3 antibiotics provide effective bactericidal action against most commonly occurring gram-positive and gram-negative bacteria associated with infections of the eyes. The range of bactericidal activity encompasses many bacteria which are, or have become, resistant to other antibiotics, notably Pseudomonas and Staphylococcus. In susceptible organisms, resistance rarely develops, even on repeated or prolonged usage. Hydrocortisone acetate exerts a marked anti-inflammatory action at the tissue level and effectively suppresses inflammation in many disorders of the anterior segment of the eye. Local application to the eye often gives rapid relief of pain and photophobia, particularly in lesions of the cornea.

The combined anti-inflammatory and antimicrobial activity of bacitracin, neomycin, polymyxin, hydrocortisone acetate 1% veterinary ophthalmic ointment permits effective management of many disorders of the anterior segment of the eye in which combined activity is needed.

Dosage and Administration: Apply a thin film over the cornea 3 or 4 times daily. The area to be treated should be properly cleansed prior to use. Foreign bodies, crusted exudates, and debris should be carefully removed. Insert the tip of the tube beneath the lower lid and express a small quantity of the ointment into the conjunctival sac in dogs and cats.

Contraindication(s): Ophthalmic preparations containing corticosteroids are contraindicated in the treatment of deep, ulcerative lesions of the cornea where the inner layer (endothelium) is involved, in fungal infections, and in the presence of viral infections.

Precaution(s): Store at room temperature. Keep container tightly closed.

Caution(s): Federal law restricts this drug to use by or on the order of a licensed veterinarian.

Sensitivity to this ophthalmic ointment is rare; however, if a reaction occurs, discontinue use of the preparation.

The prolonged use of antibiotic-containing preparations may result in overgrowth of nonsusceptible organisms including fungi. Appropriate measures should be taken if this occurs. If infection does not respond to treatment in 2 or 3 days, the diagnosis and therapy should be reevaluated. Animals under treatment with this product should be observed for usual signs of corticosteroid overdose which include polydipsia, polyuria and occasionally, an increase in weight.

Use of corticosteroids, depending on dose, duration, and specific steroid, may result in inhibition of endogenous steroid production following drug withdrawal. In patients presently receiving or recently withdrawn from systemic corticosteroid treatments, therapy with a rapidly acting corticosteroid should be considered in unusually stressful situations.

Care should be taken not to contaminate the applicator tip during administration of the preparation.

All topical ophthalmic preparations containing corticosteroids, with or without an antimicrobial agent, are contraindicated in the initial treatment of corneal ulcers. They should not be used until the infection is under control and corneal regeneration is well under way.

Adverse Reactions: Itching, burning or inflammation may occur in animals sensitive to the product. Discontinue use in such cases.

SAP and SGPT (ALT) enzyme elevations, polydipsia, and polyuria have occurred following parenteral or systemic use of synthetic corticosteroids in dogs. Vomiting and diarrhea (occasionally bloody) have been observed in dogs.

Cushings syndrome in dogs has been reported in association with prolonged or repeated steroid therapy.

Trial Data: Clinical and experimental data have demonstrated that corticosteroids administered orally or by injection to animals may induce the first stage of parturition if used during the last trimester of pregnancy and may precipitate premature parturition followed by dystocia, fetal death, retained placenta, and metritis.

Additionally, corticosteroids administered to dogs, rabbits, and rodents during pregnancy have resulted in cleft palate in offspring. Corticosteroids administered to dogs during pregnancy have also resulted in other congenital anomalies, including deformed forelegs, phocomelia, and anasarca.

Presentation: 3.5-gram (1/8-oz), sterile, tamper-proof tube.

Manufactured by: Altana Inc., Melville, NY 11747, USA

Compendium Code No.: 36901460 75-8274-02

TRI-OTIC® ℞

Med-Pharmex **Otic Antimicrobial-Corticosteroid**

Gentamicin Sulfate USP, Betamethasone Valerate, USP and Clotrimazole, USP Ointment

ANADA No.: 200-229

Active Ingredient(s): Each gram of gentamicin-betamethasone-clotrimazole ointment contains gentamicin sulfate USP equivalent to 3 mg gentamicin base; betamethasone valerate, USP equivalent to 1 mg betamethasone; and 10 mg clotrimazole, USP in a mineral oil-based system containing a plasticized hydrocarbon gel.

Indications: Gentamicin-betamethasone-clotrimazole ointment is indicated for the treatment of canine acute and chronic otitis externa associated with yeast *(Malassezia pachydermatis*, formerly *Pityrosporum canis)* and/or bacteria susceptible to gentamicin.

Pharmacology:

Gentamicin: Gentamicin sulfate is an aminoglycoside antibiotic active against a wide variety of pathogenic gram-negative and gram-positive bacteria. *In vitro* tests have determined that gentamicin is bactericidal and acts by inhibiting normal protein synthesis in susceptible microorganisms. Specifically, gentamicin is active against the following organisms commonly isolated from canine ears: *Staphylococcus aureus*, other *Staphylococcus* spp., *Pseudomonas aeruginosa*, *Proteus* spp., and *Escherichia coli*.

Betamethasone: Betamethasone valerate is a synthetic adrenocorticoid for dermatologic use. Betamethasone, an analog of prednisolone, has a high degree of corticosteroid activity and a slight degree of mineralocorticosteroid activity. Betamethasone valerate, the 17-valerate ester of betamethasone, has been shown to provide anti-inflammatory and anti-pruritic activity in the topical management of corticosteroid-responsive otitis externa. Topical corticosteroids can be absorbed from normal, intact skin. Inflammation can increase percutaneous absorption. Once absorbed through the skin, topical corticosteroids are handled through pharmacokinetic pathways similar to systemically administered corticosteroids.

Clotrimazole: Clotrimazole is a broad-spectrum antifungal agent that is used for the treatment of dermal infections caused by various species of pathogenic dermatophytes and yeasts. The primary action of clotrimazole is against dividing and growing organisms.

In vitro, clotrimazole exhibits fungistatic and fungicidal activity against isolates of *Trichophyton rubrum, Trichophyton mentagrophytes, Epidermophyton floccosum, Microsporum canis, Candida* spp. and *Malassezia pachydermatis (Pityrosporum canis)*. Resistance to clotrimazole is very rare among the fungi that cause superficial mycoses.

In an induced otitis externa infected with *Malassezia pachydermatis*, 1% clotrimazole in the gentamicin-betamethasone-clotrimazole ointment vehicle was effective both microbiologically and clinically in terms of reduction of exudate odor and swelling.

In studies of the mechanism of action, the minimum fungicidal concentration of clotrimazole caused leakage of intracellular phosphorus compounds into the ambient medium with concomitant breakdown of cellular nucleic acids and accelerated potassium efflux. These events began rapidly and extensively after addition of the drug. Clotrimazole is very poorly absorbed following dermal application.

Gentamicin-Betamethasone-Clotrimazole: By virtue of its three active ingredients, gentamicin-betamethasone-clotrimazole ointment has antibacterial, anti-inflammatory, and antifungal activity.

In component efficacy studies, the compatibility and additive effect of each of the components were demonstrated. In clinical field trials, gentamicin-betamethasone-clotrimazole was effective in the treatment of otitis externa associated with bacteria and *Malassezia pachydermatis*. Gentamicin sulfate USP, betamethasone valerate, USP and clotrimazole, USP ointment reduced discomfort, redness, swelling, exudate, and odor, and exerted a strong antimicrobial effect.

Dosage and Administration: The external ear should be thoroughly cleaned and dried before treatment. Remove foreign material, debris, crusted exudates, etc., with suitable non-irritating solutions. Excessive hair should be clipped from the treatment area. After verifying that the eardrum is intact, instill 4 drops (2 drops from the 215 g bottle) of gentamicin-betamethasone-clotrimazole ointment twice daily into the ear canal of dogs weighing less than 30 lbs. Instill 8 drops (4 drops from the 215 g bottle) twice daily into the ear canal of dogs weighing 30 lbs or more. Therapy should continue for 7 consecutive days.

Contraindication(s): If hypersensitivity to any of the components occurs, treatment should be discontinued and appropriate therapy instituted. Concomitant use of drugs known to induce ototoxicity should be avoided. Do not use in dogs with known perforation of eardrums.

Precaution(s): Store between 2° and 25°C (36° and 77°F).

Shake well before use when using the 215 gram bottle.

Caution(s): Federal law restricts this drug to use by or on the order of a licensed veterinarian.

The use of gentamicin-betamethasone-clotrimazole ointment has been associated with deafness or partial hearing loss in a small number of sensitive dogs (eg. geriatric). The hearing deficit is usually temporary. If hearing or vestibular dysfunction is noted during the course of treatment, discontinue use of gentamicin-betamethasone-clotrimazole ointment immediately and flush the ear canal thoroughly with a non-ototoxic solution. Corticosteroids administered to dogs, rabbits, and rodents during pregnancy have resulted in cleft palate in offspring. Other congenital anomalies including deformed forelegs, phocomelia, and anasarca have been reported in offspring of dogs which received corticosteroids during pregnancy.

Clinical and experimental data have demonstrated that corticosteroids administered orally or parenterally to animals may induce the first stage of parturition if used during the last trimester of pregnancy and may precipitate premature parturition followed by dystocia, fetal death, retained placenta and metritis.

Identification of infecting organisms should be made either by microscopic roll smear evaluation or by culture as appropriate. Antibiotic susceptibility of the pathogenic organism(s) should be determined prior to use of this preparation.

If overgrowth of nonsusceptible bacteria, fungi or yeasts occur, or if hypersensitivity develops, treatment should be discontinued and appropriate therapy instituted.

Administration of recommended doses of gentamicin-betamethasone-clotrimazole ointment beyond 7 days may result in delayed wound healing.

Avoid ingestion. Adverse systemic reactions have been observed following the oral ingestion of some topical corticosteroid preparations. Patients should be closely observed for the usual signs of adrenocorticoid overdosage which include sodium retention, potassium loss, fluid retention, weight gain, polydipsia and/or polyuria. Prolonged use or overdosage may produce adverse immunosuppressive effects.

Use of corticosteroids, depending on dose, duration, and specific steroid, may result in endogenous steroid production inhibition following drug withdrawal. In patients presently receiving or recently withdrawn from corticosteroid treatments, therapy with a rapidly acting corticosteroid should be considered in especially stressful situations.

Before instilling any medication into the ear, examine the external ear canal thoroughly to be certain the tympanic membrane is not ruptured in order to avoid the possibility of transmitting infection to the middle ear as well as damaging the cochlea or vestibular apparatus from prolonged contact.

Warning(s): For otic use in dogs only.

Keep this and all drugs out of the reach of children.

Toxicology: Clinical and safety studies with gentamicin sulfate USP, betamethasone valerate, USP and clotrimazole, USP ointment have shown a wide safety margin at the recommended dose level in dogs (see Cautions/Side Effects).

Side Effects:

Gentamicin: While aminoglycosides are absorbed poorly from skin, intoxication may occur when aminoglycosides are applied topically for prolonged periods of time to large wounds, burns, or any denuded skin, particularly if there is renal insufficiency. All aminoglycosides have the potential to produce reversible and irreversible vestibular, cochlear and renal toxicity.

Betamethasone: Side effects such as SAP and SGPT enzyme elevations, weight loss, anorexia, polydipsia, and polyuria have occurred following the use of parenteral or systemic synthetic corticosteroids in dogs. Vomiting and diarrhea (occasionally bloody) have been observed in dogs and cats.

Cushing's syndrome in dogs has been reported in association with prolonged or repeated steroid therapy.

Clotrimazole: The following have been reported occasionally in humans in connection with the use of clotrimazole: erythema, stinging, blistering, peeling, edema, pruritus, urticaria, and general irritation of the skin not present before therapy.

Presentation: Gentamicin-betamethasone-clotrimazole ointment is available in 7.5 gram and 15 gram tubes as well as in 10 gram, 25 gram and 215 gram plastic bottles.

Compendium Code No.: 10270141

TRIPELENNAMINE HYDROCHLORIDE ℞

AgriLabs **Antihistamine**

Injection 20 mg/mL

ANADA No.: 200-162

Active Ingredient(s): Each mL of sterile aqueous solution contains:

Tripelennamine Hydrochloride USP .... 20 mg

Indications: For use in cattle and horses in conditions in which antihistaminic therapy may be expected to lead to alleviation of some signs of disease.

Pharmacology: Tripelennamine hydrochloride is a white, crystalline material which is stable, nonhygroscopic, and readily soluble in water.

Tripelennamine hydrochloride is characterized by its capacity to antagonize many of the pharmacologic effects of histamine.

Dosage and Administration: This product is for parenteral use.

Warm the solution to near body temperature.

Using aseptic precautions, administer intravenously or intramuscularly as specified below. Intramuscular injections should be made into the heavy musculature of the hind leg or cervical area.

The doses specified below may be repeated in 6 to 12 hours if necessary.

Cattle-Administer intravenously or intramuscularly at a dose of 0.5 mg per lb of body weight (2.5 mL for each 100 lbs of body weight). For a more rapid onset of action, the intravenous route of administration is recommended.

Horses-Administer intramuscularly only at a dose of 0.5 mg per lb of body weight (2.5 mL for each 100 lbs of body weight).

Precaution(s): Protect from light. Store between 15°C and 30°C (59°F-86°F). Avoid excessive heat (104°F).

Caution(s): Federal law restricts this drug to use by or on the order of a licensed veterinarian.

Central nervous system stimulation in the form of hyperexcitability, nervousness, and muscle tremors lasting up to 20 minutes have been noted in horses, particularly following intravenous administration; therefore, only the intramuscular route of administration should be used in horses.

Overdosage of tripelennamine hydrochloride may give rise to excitement, ataxia, and convulsions.

Depression of the central nervous system and incoordination may occur when the drug is used at therapeutic dose levels.

Disturbances in gastrointestinal function may occur in some instances.

While poisonous snake bites have been treated with antihistaminic drugs, other conjunctive therapy is required because of toxic reactions associated with the protein complex of venom.

For animal use only.

Warning(s): Do not use in horses intended for food purposes.

Milk that has been taken during treatment and for 24 hours (two milkings) after the last treatment must not be used for food.

Treated cattle must not be slaughtered for food during treatment and for four days following the last treatment.

A withdrawal period has not been established for this product in pre-ruminating calves. Do not use in calves to be processed for veal. Keep out of reach of children.

Presentation: Tripelennamine Hydrochloride Injection is supplied in 500 mL multiple dose vials.

Manufactured by: Phoenix Scientific, Inc., St. Joseph, MO 64506

Compendium Code No.: 10581720 Rev. 4-96

TRIPELENNAMINE HYDROCHLORIDE ℞

Aspen **Antihistamine**

Injection 20 mg/mL

ANADA No.: 200-162

Active Ingredient(s): Each mL of sterile aqueous solution contains:

Tripelennamine Hydrochloride USP . . . . 20 mg

Indications: For use in cattle and horses in conditions in which antihistaminic therapy may be expected to lead to alleviation of some signs of disease.

Pharmacology: Tripelennamine hydrochloride is a white, crystalline material which is stable, nonhygroscopic, and readily soluble in water.

Tripelennamine hydrochloride is characterized by its capacity to antagonize many of the pharmacologic effects of histamine.

Dosage and Administration: Warm the solution to near body temperature.

Using aseptic precautions, administer intravenously or intramuscularly as specified below. Intramuscular injections should be made into the heavy musculature of the hind leg or cervical area.

The doses specified below may be repeated in 6 to 12 hours if necessary.

Cattle: Administer intravenously or intramuscularly at a dose of 0.5 mg per lb of body weight (2.5 mL for each 100 lbs of body weight). For a more rapid onset of action, the intravenous route of administration is recommended.

Horses: Administer intramuscularly only at a dose of 0.5 mg per lb of body weight (2.5 mL for each 100 lbs of body weight).

Precaution(s): Protect from light. Store between 15°C and 30°C (59°F-86°F). Avoid excessive heat (104°F).

Caution(s): Federal law restricts this drug to use by or on the order of a licensed veterinarian.

Central nervous system stimulation in the form of hyperexcitability, nervousness, and muscle tremors lasting up to 20 minutes have been noted in horses, particularly following intravenous administration; therefore, only the intramuscular route of administration should be used in horses.

While poisonous snake bites have been treated with antihistaminic drugs, other conjunctive therapy is required because of toxic reactions associated with the protein complex of venom.

Warning(s): Do not use in horses intended for food purposes.

Milk that has been taken during treatment and for 24 hours (two milkings) after the last treatment must not be used for food.

Treated cattle must not be slaughtered for food during treatment and for four days following the last treatment.

A withdrawal period has not been established for this product in pre-ruminating calves. Do not use in calves to be processed for veal. For animal use only. Keep out of reach of children.

Overdose: Overdosage of tripelennamine hydrochloride may give rise to excitement, ataxia, and convulsions.

Side Effects: Depression of the central nervous system and incoordination may occur when the drug is used at therapeutic dose levels.

Disturbances in gastrointestinal function may occur in some instances.

Presentation: Tripelennamine Hydrochloride Injection is supplied in 500 mL multiple dose vials, containing 20 mg Tripelennamine Hydrochloride USP per mL.

Compendium Code No.: 14750900

TRIPELENNAMINE HYDROCHLORIDE ℞

Butler **Antihistamine**

Injection 20 mg per mL

ANADA No.: 200-162

Active Ingredient(s): Composition: Each mL of sterile aqueous solution contains:

Tripelennamine Hydrochloride USP . . . . 20 mg

Indications: For use in cattle and horses in conditions in which antihistaminic therapy may be expected to lead to alleviation of some signs of disease.

Pharmacology: Tripelennamine hydrochloride is a white, crystalline material which is stable, nonhygroscopic, and readily soluble in water.

Action: Tripelennamine hydrochloride is characterized by its capacity to antagonize many of the pharmacologic effects of histamine.

Dosage and Administration: Warm the solution to near body temperature.

Using aseptic precautions, administer intravenously or intramuscularly as specified below. Intramuscular injections should be made into the heavy musculature of the hind leg or cervical area.

The doses specified below may be repeated in 6 to 12 hours if necessary.

Cattle—Administer intravenously or intramuscularly at a dose of 0.5 mg per lb of body weight (2.5 mL for each 100 lbs of body weight). For a more rapid onset of action, the intravenous route of administration is recommended.

Horses—Administer intramuscularly only at a dose of 0.5 mg per lb of body weight (2.5 mL for each 100 lbs of body weight).

Precaution(s): Protect from light. Store between 15°C and 30°C (59°F-86°F). Avoid excessive heat (104°F). @P1 = **Caution(s):** Federal law restricts this drug to use by or on the order of a licensed veterinarian.

Central nervous system stimulation in the form of hyperexcitability, nervousness, and muscle tremors lasting up to 20 minutes have been noted in horses, particularly following intravenous administration; therefore, only the intramuscular route of administration should be used in horses.

Overdosage of tripelennamine hydrochloride may give rise to excitement, ataxia, and convulsions.

Depression of the central nervous system and incoordination may occur when the drug is used at therapeutic dose levels.

Disturbances in gastrointestinal function may occur in some instances.

While poisonous snake bites have been treated with antihistaminic drugs, other conjunctive therapy is required because of toxic reactions associated with the protein complex of venom.

For animal use only. Keep out of reach of children.

Warning(s): Do not use in horses intended for food purposes.

Milk that has been taken during treatment and for 24 hours (two milkings) after the last treatment must not be used for food.

Treated cattle must not be slaughtered for food during treatment and for four days following the last treatment.

A withdrawal period has not been established for this product in pre-ruminating calves. Do not use in calves to be processed for veal.

Presentation: 100 mL and 250 mL multiple dose vials.

Manufactured by: Phoenix Scientific, Inc., St. Joseph, MO 64506

Compendium Code No.: 10821800 Rev. 4-96

TRIPELENNAMINE HYDROCHLORIDE ℞

Vet Tek **Antihistamine**

Injection 20 mg/mL

ANADA No.: 200-162

Active Ingredient(s): Composition: Each mL of sterile aqueous solution contains:

Tripelennamine Hydrochloride USP . . . . 20 mg

Indications: For use in cattle and horses in conditions in which antihistaminic therapy may be expected to lead to alleviation of some signs of disease.

Pharmacology: Description: Tripelennamine hydrochloride is a white, crystalline material which is stable, nonhygroscopic, and readily soluble in water.

Action: Tripelennamine hydrochloride is characterized by its capacity to antagonize many of the pharmacologic effects of histamine.

Dosage and Administration: Warm the solution to near body temperature.

Using aseptic precautions, administer intravenously or intramuscularly as specified below. Intramuscular injections should be made into the heavy musculature of the hind leg or cervical area.

The doses specified below may be repeated in 6 to 12 hours if necessary.

Cattle: Administer intravenously or intramuscularly at a dose of 0.5 mg per lb of body weight (2.5 mL for each 100 lbs of body weight). For a more rapid onset of action, the intravenous route of administration is recommended.

Horses: Administer intramuscularly only at a dose of 0.5 mg per lb of body weight (2.5 mL for each 100 lbs of body weight).

Precaution(s): Storage: Protect from light. Store between 15°C and 30°C (59°F-86°F). Avoid excessive heat (104°F).

Caution(s): Federal law restricts this drug to use by or on the order of a licensed veterinarian.

Central nervous system stimulation in the form of hyperexcitability, nervousness, and muscle tremors lasting up to 20 minutes have been noted in horses, particularly following intravenous administration; therefore, only the intramuscular route of administration should be used in horses.

Overdosage of tripelennamine hydrochloride may give rise to excitement, ataxia, and convulsions.

Depression of the central nervous system and incoordination may occur when the drug is used at therapeutic dose levels.

Disturbances in gastrointestinal function may occur in some instances.

While poisonous snake bites have been treated with antihistaminic drugs, other conjunctive therapy is required because of toxic reactions associated with the protein complex of venom.

For use in cattle and horses.

For animal use only.

For parenteral use.

Warning(s): Do not use in horses intended for food purposes.

Milk that has been taken during treatment and for 24 hours (two milkings) after the last treatment must not be used for food.

Treated cattle must not be slaughtered for food during treatment and for four days following the last treatment.

A withdrawal period has not been established for this product in pre-ruminating calves. Do not use in calves to be processed for veal. Keep out of reach of children.

Presentation: 250 mL (NDC 60270-578-13) and 500 mL (NDC 60270-578-17) multiple dose vials.

Manufactured by: Phoenix Scientific, Inc., St. Joseph, MO 64506.

Compendium Code No.: 14200211 Iss. 2-96

TRIPLE CAST™

Neogen **Medicated Bandage**

Ingredient(s): Package Contains: Gauze impregnated with zinc oxide, acacia, glycerine, castor oil, white petrolatum and calamine.

Indications: TRIPLE CAST™ is a premium poultice bandage. It is effective supportive care for tenderness and helps in reducing inflammation associated with such equine ailments as bowed tendons, edema (stocking up), suspensory ligament damage, wind puffs and minor bone conditions (sesamoiditis, splints, etc.) It is also an effective light support after intra-articular injections.

Directions for Use: As per veterinarian.

Precaution(s): Store at room temperature between 15°-30°C (59°-86°F).

Caution(s): If skin sensitivity or irritation develops, discontinue use and consult a veterinarian.

Warning(s): Keep out of reach of children.

Presentation: 1 medicated roll 4" x 10 yds (10 cm x 9 m) (NDC: 59051-8880-0).

Compendium Code No.: 14910461 L507-0501

TRIPLE-E®

Fort Dodge **Vaccine**

Encephalomyelitis Vaccine, Eastern, Western and Venezuelan, Killed Virus

U.S. Vet. Lic. No.: 112

Contents: This product contains the antigens listed above.

Contains gentamicin as a preservative.

Indications: For the vaccination of healthy horses against Eastern, Western and Venezuelan equine encephalomyelitis.

Dosage and Administration: Using aseptic technique, vaccinate healthy horses with a 1 mL dose intramuscularly followed by a second 1 mL dose 2 to 4 weeks later. A booster is recommended annually, or in the event of a threatened epizootic. Horses subject to repeated exposure to field virus may benefit from revaccination with a single dose every three months.

Precaution(s): Shake well before using. Use entire contents when first opened.

Store between 2°C and 7°C (35°F and 45°F). Do not freeze. Use new, non-chemically sterilized needles and syringes.

Caution(s): Do not mix with other vaccines. Local reactions are rare. To minimize such reactions, ensure that injections are administered in deep muscle tissue. The use of a biological may produce anaphylaxis and/or other inflammatory immune-mediated hypersensitivity reactions.

Antidote(s): Epinephrine, corticosteroids and antihistamines may all be indicated depending on the nature and severity of the reaction.*

Warning(s): Do not vaccinate within 21 days of slaughter. For veterinary use only.

References: Available upon request.*

Presentation: Packages containing 12 x 1 dose (syringe pouch pack) and 1 x 10 mL tank vial (10 doses).

Compendium Code No.: 10032430 12241A

TRIPLE-E® T INNOVATOR

Fort Dodge **Toxoid-Vaccine**

Encephalomyelitis Vaccine-Tetanus Toxoid, Eastern, Western & Venezuelan, Killed Virus

U.S. Vet. Lic. No.: 112

Contents: This product contains the antigens listed above.

Thimerosal, neomycin and polymyxin B added as preservatives.

Indications: For vaccination of healthy horses as an aid in the prevention of equine encephalomyelitis due to Eastern, Western and Venezuelan viruses and tetanus.

Dosage and Administration: Inject one 1 mL dose intramuscularly using aseptic technique. Administer a second 1 mL dose 3 to 4 weeks after the first dose. Revaccinate annually using a one 1 mL dose.

Precaution(s): Store in the dark at 2° to 7°C (35° to 45°F). Avoid freezing. Shake well. Use entire contents when first opened.

Caution(s): In some instances, transient local reactions may occur at the injection site.

In case of anaphylactoid reaction, administer epinephrine. For veterinary use only.

Warning(s): Do not vaccinate within 21 days before slaughter.

Presentation: 1 dose (1 mL) vial.

Compendium Code No.: 10032810 16391A

TRIPLE HISTAMINE ℞

RXV **Antihistamine**

(Tripelennamine Hydrochloride Injection)

ANADA No.: 200-162

Active Ingredient(s): Each mL contains:

Tripelennamine hydrochloride USP .... 20 mg

Indications: For use in cattle and horses in conditions in which antihistaminic therapy may be expected to lead to alleviation of some signs of disease.

Pharmacology: Tripelennamine hydrochloride is a white, crystalline material which is stable, nonhygroscopic, and readily soluble in water.

Tripelennamine hydrochloride is characterized by its capacity to antagonize many of the pharmacologic effects of histamine.

Dosage and Administration: Warm the solution to near body temperature.

Using aseptic precautions, administer intravenously or intramuscularly as specified below. Intramuscular injections should be made into the heavy musculature of the hind leg or cervical area.

The doses specified below may be repeated in 6 to 12 hours if necessary.

Cattle: Administer intravenously or intramuscularly at a dose of 0.5 mg per lb of body weight (2.5 mL for each 100 lbs of body weight). For a more rapid onset of action, the intravenous route of administration is recommended.

Horses: Administer intramuscularly only at a dose of 0.5 mg per lb of body weight (2.5 mL for each 100 lbs of body weight).

Precaution(s): Protect from light. Store between 15°C and 30°C (59°F-86°F). Avoid excessive heat (104°F).

Caution(s): Federal law restricts this drug to use by or on the order of a licensed veterinarian.

Central nervous system stimulation in the form of hyperexcitability, nervousness, and muscle tremors lasting up to 20 minutes have been noted in horses, particularly following intravenous administration; therefore, only the intramuscular route of administration should be used in horses.

Overdosage of tripelennamine hydrochloride may give rise to excitement, ataxia, and convulsions.

Depression of the central nervous system and incoordination may occur when the drug is used at therapeutic dose levels.

Disturbances in gastrointestinal function may occur in some instances.

While poisonous snake bites have been treated with antihistaminic drugs, other conjunctive therapy is required because of toxic reactions associated with the protein complex of venom.

Warning(s): A withdrawal period has not been established for this product in pre-ruminating calves. Do not use in calves to be processed for veal.

Do not use in horses intended for food purposes.

Milk that has been taken during treatment and for 24 hours (two milkings) after the last treatment must not be used for food.

Treated cattle must not be slaughtered for food during treatment and for four days following the last treatment.

Presentation: Supplied in 250 mL and 500 mL multiple dose vials.

Compendium Code No.: 10910200

TRIPLE-NO-CHEW

Q.A. Laboratories **Topical Product**

Active Ingredient(s):

2 oz. container: Deionized water, isopropyl alcohol, oleoresin capsicum, carbomer, sucrose octyl acetate, polysorbate 60, orange peel bitter, propylene glycol, sodium hydroxide, FD&C red #40.

4 oz. container: Isopropyl alcohol, deionized water, oleoresin capsicum, sucrose octyl acetate, orange peel bitter, propylene glycol, polysorbate 60, FD&C red #40.

Indications: TRIPLE-NO-CHEW contains three active bittering agents from tabasco pepper, orange peel and denatured alcohol to discourage licking, biting and chewing.

Dosage and Administration: Shake well before using. Apply to bandages, casts, hair, or household furniture twice a day or as directed by a veterinarian.

Caution(s): Avoid contact with broken skin, eyes or mucous membranes. If in contact, wash with copious amounts of cool water immediately. If redness or irritation occurs or if accidently swallowed, call a physician or poison control center.

Before applying to extensive areas of furniture, test the effect of the product on a small, inconspicuous area.

Flammable. Keep away from heat or open flame.

Sold only through veterinarians.

Keep out of the reach of children.

Presentation: 2 oz. container and 4 oz. container with sprayer.

Compendium Code No.: 13680070

TRIPLE PYRETHRINS FLEA & TICK SHAMPOO

Davis **Parasiticide Shampoo**

EPA Reg. No.: 50591

Active Ingredient(s):

Pyrethrins	0.15%
Piperonyl butoxide, technical*	1.00%
N-octyl bicycloheptene dicarboximide	0.50%
Di-n-propyl isocinchomeronate	0.50%
Inert ingredients	97.85%
Total	100.00%

*Equivalent to 0.80% of (butylcarbityl) (6-propyl-piperonyl) ether and 0.20% of related compounds.

Indications: A concentrated, lathering shampoo enriched with coconut extract, lanolin and aloe. Removes loose dandruff, dirt and scales. Leaves the coat soft and shining. Kills fleas, lice and ticks on dogs, cats, puppies and kittens (avoid treatment of nursing puppies and kittens under six weeks of age). Repels gnats, flies, and mosquitoes for two or three days.

Dosage and Administration: It is a violation of federal law to use the product in a manner inconsistent with its labeling.

The product may be used full strength or diluted with two (2) parts of water. Thoroughly soak the animal with warm water taking two (2) to three (3) minutes to wet the hair. Do not apply the shampoo around the eyes. Apply the shampoo on the head and ears, then lather; repeat the procedure with the neck, chest, middle and hindquarters, finishing with the legs last. Let the animal stand two (2) to five (5) minutes, then rinse the animal thoroughly. In extremely dirty, or scaly animals, the above procedure may be repeated. May be used every 7-10 days.

Precaution(s): Store in a cool area. Do not re-use the container. Wrap it and put it in the trash.

Caution(s): Keep out of the reach of children.

Precautionary Statement: Hazards to Humans and Domestic Animals:

Humans: Causes eye and skin irritation. Do not get in the eyes or on skin or on clothing. Harmful if swallowed. Wash thoroughly with soap and water after handling. Remove contaminated clothing and wash before reuse.

Environmental Hazards: The product is toxic to fish. Keep out of lakes, streams, ponds, tidal marshes and estuaries. Do not wash the animal where runoff is likely to occur.

Statement of Practical Treatment:

If in eyes: Flush with plenty of water. Get medical attention.

If swallowed: Promptly drink a large quantity of milk, egg whites, gelatin solution, or if these are not available, drink large quantities of water. Avoid alcohol.

If on skin: Wash with plenty of soap and water. Get medical attention if irritation persists.

Presentation: 12 oz (355 mL) and 1 gallon (3.785 L) containers.

Compendium Code No.: 11410401

TRIPLEVAC®

Intervet **Vaccine**

Newcastle-Bronchitis Vaccine, B_1 Type, B_1 Strain, Mass. and Conn. Types, Live Virus

U.S. Vet. Lic. No.: 286

Description: This vaccine is prepared from the proven B_1 strain of Newcastle disease virus and the mild Massachusetts and Connecticut types of infectious bronchitis virus. The viruses have been propagated using SPF substrates.

This vaccine contains gentamicin as a preservative.

Quality tested for purity, potency, and safety.

Indications: Drinking Water: Vaccination of healthy chickens two weeks of age or older for protection against Newcastle disease and Massachusetts and Connecticut types bronchitis.

Beak-O-Vac or Coarse Spray: Vaccination of healthy chickens one day of age or older (spray) for protection against Newcastle disease and Massachusetts and Connecticut types bronchitis. If chickens are vaccinated earlier than two weeks of age, revaccination is recommended for optimum protection.

Dosage and Administration: Vaccination Programs: Many factors must be considered in determining a sound vaccination program for a particular farm or poultry complex. To be fully effective, the vaccine must be administered properly to healthy, receptive birds maintained in a proper environment under good management. In addition, the response may be influenced by the age of the birds and their immune status. Seldom does one live virus vaccination under field conditions produce lifetime protection for all individuals in a given flock. The level of immunity required will vary with operational practices and the degree of exposure. Therefore, a program of periodic revaccinations may be necessary.

Preparation of Vaccine:

For Beak-O-Vac Use: Do not open and mix the vaccine until ready to begin vaccination. Use vaccine immediately after mixing.

1. Remove the tear-off seal and stopper from the bottle of vaccine.
2. Remove the seal and stopper from the bottle of diluent.
3. Pour a small amount of diluent into the vial of vaccine.
4. Insert the rubber stopper and shake the vial.
5. Pour the rehydrated vaccine back into the bottle containing the rest of the diluent. Replace the stopper and shake.
6. Place the vaccine into an appropriate container.

The vaccine is now ready for use by the following method. For best results, be sure to follow directions carefully!

Beak-O-Vac Administration - For Chickens One Day of Age:

1. Attach the container holding the vaccine to the Beak-O-Vac machine and adjust for delivery of 33-35 doses per mL.
2. Hold the chicken in such a manner that the chicken's beak is opened in the direction of the nozzle so that the vaccine is deposited on the roof of the mouth as the beak is turned.

Preparation of Vaccine:

For Drinking Water or Coarse Spray Use: Do not open and mix the vaccine until ready to begin vaccination. Use vaccine immediately after mixing.

1. Remove the tear-off seal and stopper from the vial containing the dried vaccine.
2. Carefully pour clean, cool non-chlorinated tap water into the vaccine vial until the vial is approximately two-thirds full.
3. Insert the rubber stopper and shake vigorously until all material is dissolved.
4. The vaccine is now ready for drinking water or coarse spray use in accordance with the directions below. For best results, be sure to follow directions carefully!

Drinking Water Administration - For Chickens Two Weeks of Age or Older:

1. Do not use any disinfectants in the drinking water for 48 hours before vaccinating and 24 hours after vaccination.
2. Withhold the water from the chickens until they are thirsty. Withholding periods will vary from 2 to 8 hours according to age of chickens and weather conditions.
3. Scrub waterers and rinse thoroughly with fresh, clean water. Do not use disinfectants for cleaning waterers.
4. Mix rehydrated vaccine with clean, cool, non-chlorinated tap water in accordance with chart below.

Age of Chickens	Water Per 1,000 Doses Vaccine
2-4 weeks	6 gal. (23 liters)
4-8 weeks	10 gal. (38 liters)
8 weeks or older	16 gal. (60 liters)

As an aid in preserving the virus, 3.2 ounces (100 g) of non-fat powdered milk may be added to each 10 gallons (38 liters) of water used for mixing vaccine. Add the dried milk first and agitate until dissolved. Then add the rehydrated vaccine from the vial and mix thoroughly.

5. Distribute the vaccine solution, as prepared above, in the waterers provided for the chickens. Avoid placing waterers in direct sunlight.
6. Provide no other drinking water until all the vaccine-water solution has been consumed.

Coarse Spray Administration - For Chickens One Day of Age:

1. Use rehydrated vaccine as indicated for a specific coarse spray vaccination machine. For example, a machine which dispenses 20 mL to a box of 100 chickens; - total volume for 2,000 doses is 400 mL, and 10,000 doses is 2,000 mL of deionized water. Mix thoroughly.
2. Add the vaccine solution to the reservoir on the machine.
3. Prime and adjust machine as instructed in manual accompanying the specific machine.
4. Place boxes holding 100 chickens each on the conveyor belt or in machine. Activate spray head.

Coarse Spray Administration - For Chickens Two Days of Age or Older:

1. Initial spray vaccination should be coarse spray, i.e. Hardi®.
2. Do not use any disinfectants or skim milk in sprayer.
3. Use sprayer only for administration of vaccines.
4. Shut off all fans while spray vaccinating. Turn on fan immediately after spraying. Be careful in hot weather.
5. Spray chickens by walking slowly through the house.
6. Follow the manufacturer's directions regarding water volume.
7. Use only clean, cool, deionized water.
8. Individual(s) spraying chickens should wear face mask and goggles.

Records: Keep a record of vaccine, quantity, serial number, expiration date, and place of purchase; the date and time of vaccination; the number, age, breed, and locations of chickens; name of operators performing the vaccination and any observed reactions.

Precaution(s): Store vaccine between 2 and 7°C (35 and 45°F).

Do not spill or splash the vaccine.

Use entire contents when first opened.

Burn containers and all unused contents.

This product is non-returnable.

Caution(s): Vaccinate only healthy chickens. Although disease may not be evident, coccidiosis, Mycoplasma infection, infectious bursal disease, Marek's disease, reovirus infection and other disease conditions may cause complications or reduce immunity.

All susceptible chickens on the same premises should be vaccinated at the same time.

The revaccination of laying hens with live Newcastle/Bronchitis vaccine may be detrimental to the flock and cannot be generally recommended. Consult your Intervet representative for more information.

Efforts should be taken to reduce stress conditions at the time of vaccination and during the reaction period.

Do not dilute the vaccine or otherwise stretch the dosage.

For veterinary use only.

Notice: This vaccine has undergone rigid potency, safety and purity tests, and meets Intervet Inc. and USDA requirements and is designed to stimulate effective immunity when used as directed. The user must be advised that the response to the vaccine depends on many factors, including, but not limited to, conditions of storage and handling by the user, administration of the vaccine, health and responsiveness of the individual chickens, and the degree of field exposure. Therefore, directions should be followed carefully!

This product is not hazardous when used according to directions supplied. A material safety data sheet (MSDS) is available upon request. This and any other consumer information can be obtained by calling Intervet Customer Service at 1-800-441-8272 or 1-302-934-8051.

The use of this vaccine is subject to applicable federal and local laws and regulations.

Use only as directed.

Warning(s): Do not vaccinate within 21 days before slaughter.

Newcastle virus occasionally causes conjunctivitis in humans. Avoid any contact of vaccine with eyes.

Presentation: 10 x 2,000 doses for drinking water or coarse spray use. 10 x 2,000 doses with diluent for Beak-O-Vac use.

10 x 10,000 doses for drinking water or coarse spray use. 10 x 10,000 doses with diluent for Beak-O-Vac use.

10 x 25,000 doses for drinking water or coarse spray use.

Compendium Code No.: 11062091 20108 AL 89-2.0

TRI-REO®

Fort Dodge **Vaccine**

Avian Reovirus Vaccine, Killed Virus

U.S. Vet. Lic. No.: 112

Contents: This product contains the antigen listed above.

Gentamicin and amphotericin B added as preservatives.

Indications: For the subcutaneous or intramuscular revaccination of healthy chickens 10 weeks of age as an aid in the prevention of signs and lesions associated with avian reovirus infections which cause malabsorption syndrome. Progeny of vaccinates are aided in the prevention of signs of malabsorption associated with reovirus disease via maternal antibodies. It is essential for best protection to prime birds at least once with live virus vaccine for tenosynovitis.

Dosage and Administration: Inject 0.5 mL (0.5 cc) intramuscularly or subcutaneously (in the lower neck region) using aseptic technique. Vaccinate only healthy birds.

Precaution(s): Store in the dark at 36° to 45°F (2° to 7°C). Do not freeze. Warm to 72°F (22°C) and shake well before using. Use entire contents when first opened.

Caution(s): If birds are vaccinated during lay, a drop in egg production may occur.

Warning(s): Do not vaccinate within 42 days before slaughter.

In case of accidental human injection seek immediate medical attention, stating the vaccine is an oil emulsion type.

For veterinary use only.

Presentation: 1,000 dose (500 mL) vials.

Compendium Code No.: 10032291 10331C

TRISOL™

KenVet **Hand Soap**

Active Ingredient(s):

Triclosan 0.5%

Indications: An antimicrobial hand lotion soap effective against gram positive and gram negative bacteria, fungi, and yeasts @P1 = **Directions for Use:** Wet hands and apply a small amount of TRISOL™. Lather and wash 10-15 seconds and rinse. Use before and after each patient.

Caution(s): For external use only.

Avoid contact with eyes.

In rare instances of local sensitivity, discontinue use.

Presentation: 1 gallon (3.78 litres).

Compendium Code No.: 11340050

TRI-TEC 14™ FLY REPELLENT

Farnam **Insect Repellent**

EPA Reg. No.: 270-251

Active Ingredient(s):

Cypermethrin [(±) -alpha-cyano-(3-phenoxyphenyl) methyl-(±)-cis, trans 3-(2,2-dichloroethenyl)-2, 2- dimethylcyclopropanecarboxylate] 0.150%
Pyrethrins 0.200%
Piperonyl Butoxide Technical* 1.600%
Butoxylpolypropylene Glycol 5.000%
Inert Ingredients 93.05%

*Equivalent to 1.28% (butylcarbityl) (6-propylpiperonyl) ether and 0.32% of related compounds.

Indications: Gentle, water base formula for horses and ponies. Up to 14 days fly control. Ready-to-use TRI-TEC 14™ Fly Repellent's insecticide/repellent/sunscreen formula provides repellency, quick knock-down and long-lasting protection from flies, gnats, and mosquitoes. The special sun-screening agent in TRI-TEC 14™ protects against both forms of the sun's harmful ultra-violet rays.

Directions for Use: It is a violation of Federal law to use this product in a manner inconsistent with its labeling.

Wash hands with soap and water after use. Shake well before using. To protect horses from horse flies, house flies, stable flies, face flies, horn flies, deer flies, gnats, mosquitoes, lice and deer ticks that may transmit Lyme Disease: Thoroughly brush the horse's coat prior to application to remove loose dirt and debris. For dirty horses, shampoo and rinse thoroughly.

Wait until coat is completely dry before applying TRI-TEC 14™ Fly Repellent.

TRI-TEC may be applied either as a spray or as a wipe. For horse's face, always apply as a wipe using a piece of clean absorbent cloth, toweling (Turkish) or sponge. Wear rubber glove or mitt when applying as a wipe. Spray or wipe horse's entire body while brushing against the lay of the coat to ensure adequate coverage. Avoid getting spray into horse's eyes, nose or mouth. Application should be liberal for best residual results. Reapply every 5 to 7 days under normal conditions for initial applications. As protection builds, reapply every 10 to 14 days as needed. Also, reapply each time animal is washed or is exposed to heavy rain.

Precautionary Statements: Hazards to Humans and Domestic Animals: Caution:

Humans: For animal use only. Not for use on humans. Harmful if swallowed. Avoid contact with eyes, skin or clothing. Avoid breathing spray mist. Avoid contamination of food. Wash hands with soap and water after use.

Horses: Avoid contact with eyes or mucous membranes. Harmful if swallowed. Avoid breathing spray mist. Avoid contamination of food.

Statement of Practical Treatment:

If Swallowed: Contact a physician or Poison Control Center immediately. Drink 1 or 2 glasses of water and induce vomiting by touching back of throat with finger or by administering syrup of ipecac. Do not induce vomiting or give anything by mouth to an unconscious person.

If Inhaled: Remove victim to fresh air. Apply artificial respiration and/or seek medical attention if indicated.

If on Skin: Remove contaminated clothing and wash skin thoroughly with soap and water.

If in Eyes: Immediately flush eyes with plenty of water. Get medical attention if irritation persists.

Environmental Hazards: This product is toxic to fish. Keep out of lakes, streams and ponds. Do not contaminate water by cleaning of equipment or disposal of wastes. Do not apply to any body of water. Do not contaminate water when disposing of equipment washwaters.

Storage and Disposal:

Storage: Store in a cool, dry place.

Pesticide Disposal: Securely wrap empty original container in several layers of newspaper and discard in trash.

Container Disposal: Do not reuse empty container. Wrap container and put in trash.

Warning(s): Not for use on horses intended for human consumption.

Keep out of reach of children.

Disclaimer: Limited Warranty and Disclaimer: Buyer assumes all risk of use, storage or handling of this material not in strict accordance with directions and usage. In no event shall seller's liability exceed the purchase price of this product.

Presentation: 32 fl oz (0.946 L) with sprayer and 128 fl oz (3.785 L).

Compendium Code No.: 10000401

TRITOP® ℞

Pharmacia & Upjohn **Topical Antimicrobial-Corticosteroid**

Neomycin sulfate, isoflupredone acetate, tetracaine hydrochloride topical ointment

NADA No.: 030-025

Active Ingredient(s): TRITOP® Topical Ointment (neomycin sulfate, isoflupredone acetate, tetracaine hydrochloride ointment) contains in each gram the potent anti-inflammatory agent isoflupredone acetate 1 mg (0.1%); the antibiotic neomycin sulfate, 5 mg (0.5%) (equivalent to 3.5 mg neomycin); and the topical anesthetic tetracaine hydrochloride, 5 mg (0.5%).

Indications: TRITOP® Topical Ointment is indicated as treatment or adjunctive therapy of certain ear and skin conditions in dogs, cats and horses caused by or associated with neomycin susceptible organisms and/or allergy. In addition, it is indicated as superficial dressing applied to minor cuts, wounds, lacerations, abrasions, and for post surgical application where reduction of pain and inflammatory response is deemed desirable.

TRITOP® Topical Ointment is useful in treating such conditions as acute otitis externa in dogs and to a lesser degree, chronic otitis externa in dogs. It also is effective in treating anal gland infections and moist dermatitis in the dog and is a useful dressing for minor cuts, lacerations, abrasions, and post surgical therapy in the horse, cat, and dog.

TRITOP® Topical Ointment may also be used following amputation of dewclaws, tails and claws, following ear trimming and castrating operations.

This combination is well suited for the treatment or adjunctive therapy of many ear and skin conditions, as well as a dressing for superficial wounds occurring in dogs, cats and horses. Its action is specific as to anti-inflammatory, bactericidal, and anesthetic properties.

Pharmacology:

Isoflupredone Acetate: It has been reported by research workers that isoflupredone acetate is 14 times as potent as hydrocortisone as an anti-inflammatory steroid as measured by the cotton pellet implantation assay.

Isoflupredone acetate markedly inhibits inflammatory reaction through its controlling influence on connective tissue and vascular components. Topically applied isoflupredone acetate is rapidly effective. In otitis externa, wounds of the concha, ulcerations of the ear flaps, and irritated lesions of the skin, the inflammatory response may also be effectively inhibited by isoflupredone acetate. Chronic conditions respond more slowly and relapses are more frequent.

Neomycin: Neomycin is an antibiotic substance derived from cultures of the soil organism *Streptomyces fradiae*. Its antimicrobial range includes both gram-positive and gram-negative organisms commonly responsible for or associated with otic infections, such as staphylococci, streptococci, *Escherichia coli, Aerobacter aerogenes*, and many strains of Proteus and Pseudomonas organisms. It is not active against fungi. Neomycin is unusually nontoxic for epithelial cells in tissue culture and is nonirritating in therapeutic concentrations. The presence of neomycin in TRITOP® Topical Ointment affords control of infections caused by neomycin susceptible organisms.

Tetracaine: Tetracaine hydrochloride is a topical anesthetic agent that is more potent than either procaine or cocaine in comparable concentrations and has greater ability than procaine to penetrate mucous membranes. The duration of anesthetic action of tetracaine exceeds that produced by either butacaine or phenacaine.

Many investigators have demonstrated that local anesthesia plays a significant part in the promotion of healing, especially where pain is a prominent factor. It is believed that trauma stimulates local pain receptors, which results in reflex vasodilation, edema, tenderness, and muscular spasm.

If the reflex is abolished through use of a local anesthetic such as tetracaine, amelioration of these tissue changes that interfere with healing is favored. The local anesthetic action of tetracaine has proved to be of great value in alleviating the pain reflex in painful skin and ear conditions.

Dosage and Administration: In treatment of otitis externa and other inflammatory conditions of the external ear canal, a quantity of ointment sufficient to fill the external ear canal may be applied one to three times daily. When used on the skin or mucous membranes, cleanse the affected area, apply a small amount of the ointment and spread or rub in gently. The involved area may be treated one to three times a day and these daily applications continued in accordance with the clinical response. Limit treatment to the period when local anesthesia is essential to control self-inflicted trauma.

Precaution(s): Store at controlled room temperature 20° to 25°C (68° to 77°F) [see USP].

Incomplete response or exacerbation of corticosteroid responsive lesions may be due to the presence of non-susceptible organisms or to prolonged use of antibiotic-containing preparations resulting in over-growth of non-susceptible organisms, particularly Monilia. Thus, if improvement is not noted within two or three days, or if redness, irritation, or swelling persists or increases, the diagnosis should be redetermined and appropriate therapeutic measures initiated.

Tetracaine and neomycin have the potential to sensitize. Care should be taken to observe animals being treated for evidence of hypersensitivity or allergy to TRITOP® Topical Ointment (neomycin sulfate, isoflupredone acetate, tetracaine hydrochloride ointment). If such signs are noted, therapy with TRITOP® Topical Ointment should be stopped.

Caution(s): Federal (USA) law restricts this drug to use by or on the order of a licensed veterinarian.

Before instilling any medication into the ear, examine the external ear canal thoroughly to be certain the tympanic membrane is not ruptured in order to avoid the possibility of transmitting infection to the middle ear as well as damaging the cochlea or vestibular apparatus from prolonged contact. If hearing or vestibular dysfunction is noted during the course of treatment discontinue use of TRITOP® Topical Ointment.

For use in animals only.

Warning(s): Not for human use.

Presentation: TRITOP® Topical Ointment is available in 10 gram tubes with a special applicator tip.

Compendium Code No.: 10490490

TRI-TUSSIN™ POWDER ℞

Creative Science **Expectorant**

Active Ingredient(s): Contents:

Guaifenesin U.S.P.	7% (w/w)
Ammonium Chloride	75% (w/w)
Potassium Iodide U.S.P.	2% (w/w)

In a sweetened, flavored, palatable base.

Indications: A palatable powder used in water as an expectorant in large animals.

Directions: Dissolve one pound of product in 1 gallon of water to make stock solution.

Dosage: Swine and Poultry: Mix one pint of stock solution with 25 to 50 gallons of drinking water. Cattle, Horse and Sheep: Mix 1 pint of stock solution with 15 to 25 gallons of drinking water or ½ to 1 oz stock solution 3 times daily.

For horses and cattle, ½-1 oz of TRI-TUSSIN™ may be given in feed or drinking water daily.

For best results, animals should be kept on medication feed or water for 3-4 days.

Allow no other sources of drinking water during treatment.

One pound of powder medicates 200-400 gal. of drinking water.

Precaution(s): Store in a cool dry place.

Caution(s): Federal law restricts this drug to use by or on the order of a licensed veterinarian.

For animal use only.

Keep out of reach of children.

Presentation: 1 lb (454 g) jar and 25 lb pail.

Compendium Code No.: 13760040

TRIVAC-ARK®

Intervet **Vaccine**

Newcastle-Bronchitis Vaccine, B_1 Type, B_1 Strain, Mass. and Ark. Types, Live Virus

U.S. Vet. Lic. No.: 286

Description: This vaccine is prepared from a B_1 strain of Newcastle disease virus and the mild Massachusetts and mild Arkansas types of infectious bronchitis virus. The viruses have been propagated using SPF substrates.

This vaccine contains gentamicin as a preservative.

Quality tested for purity, potency, and safety.

Indications: Coarse Spray: Vaccination of healthy chickens 1 day of age or older for protection against Newcastle disease and Massachusetts and Arkansas types bronchitis. If chickens are vaccinated earlier than 2 weeks of age, revaccination is recommended for optimum protection.

Dosage and Administration: Vaccination Programs: Many factors must be considered in determining a sound vaccination program for a particular farm or poultry complex. To be fully effective, the vaccine must be administered properly to healthy, receptive birds maintained in a proper environment under good management. In addition, the response may be influenced by the age of the birds and their immune status. Seldom does one live virus vaccination under field conditions produce lifetime protection for all individuals in a given flock. The level of immunity required will vary with operational practices and the degree of exposure. Therefore a program of periodic revaccinations may be necessary.

Preparation of Vaccine:

For Coarse Spray Use: Do not open and mix the vaccine until ready to begin vaccination. Use vaccine immediately after mixing.

1. Remove the tear-off seal and stopper from vial containing the dried vaccine.
2. Carefully pour clean, cool, deionized water into the vaccine vial until the vial is approximately two-thirds full.
3. Insert the rubber stopper and shake vigorously until all material is dissolved.
4. The vaccine is now ready for coarse spray use in accordance with directions below. For best results, be sure to follow directions carefully!

Coarse Spray Administration:

For Chickens One Day of Age:

1. Use rehydrated vaccine as indicated for specific coarse spray vaccination machine. For example, a machine which dispenses 20 mL to a box of 100 chickens; total volume for 2,000 doses is 400 mL, and 10,000 doses is 2,000 mL of deionized water. Mix thoroughly.
2. Add the vaccine solution to reservoir on the machine.
3. Prime and adjust machine as instructed in manual accompanying the specific machine.
4. Place boxes holding 100 chickens each on the conveyor belt or in machine. Activate spray head.

Coarse Spray Administration:

For Chickens Two Days of Age or Older:

1. Initial spray vaccination should be coarse spray, i.e. Hardi® spray nozzle number 10 with grey swirls.
2. Do not use any disinfectants or skim milk in sprayer.
3. Use sprayer only for administration of vaccine.
4. Shut off all fans while spray vaccinating. Turn on fan immediately after spraying. Be careful in hot weather.
5. Spray chickens by walking slowly through the house.
6. Follow the manufacturer's directions regarding water volume.
7. Use only clean, cool, deionized water.
8. Individual(s) spraying chickens should wear face mask and goggles.

Records: Keep a record of vaccine, quantity, serial number, expiration date and place of purchase; the date and time of vaccination, the number, age, breed and location of chickens; names of operators performing the vaccination and any observed reactions.

Precaution(s): Store vaccine between 2 and 7°C (35 and 45°F).

Do not spill or splash the vaccine.

Use entire contents when first opened.

Burn containers and all unused contents.

This product is non-returnable.

Caution(s): Vaccinate only healthy chickens. Although disease may not be evident, coccidiosis, Mycoplasma infection, infectious bursal disease, Chicken Infectious Anemia, Marek's disease, reovirus infection and other disease conditions may cause complications or reduce immunity.

All susceptible chickens on the same premises should be vaccinated at the same time.

The revaccination of laying hens with live Newcastle/Bronchitis vaccine may be detrimental to the flock and cannot be generally recommended. Consult your Intervet representative for more information.

Efforts should be taken to reduce stress conditions at the time of vaccination and during the reaction period.

Do not dilute the vaccine or otherwise stretch the dosage.

For veterinary use only.

Notice: This vaccine has undergone rigid potency, safety and purity tests, and meets Intervet Inc. and USDA requirements and is designed to stimulate effective immunity when used as directed. The user must be advised that the response to the vaccine depends on many factors, including, but not limited to, conditions of storage and handling by the user, administration of the vaccine, health and responsiveness of the individual chickens, and the degree of field exposure. Therefore, directions should be followed carefully!

This product is not hazardous when used according to directions supplied. A material safety data sheet (MSDS) is available upon request. This and any other consumer information can be obtained by calling Intervet Customer Service at 1-800-441-8272 or 1-302-934-8051.

The use of this vaccine is subject to applicable federal and local laws and regulations.

Use only as directed.

Warning(s): Do not vaccinate within 21 days before slaughter.

Newcastle virus occasionally causes conjunctivitis in humans. Avoid any contact of vaccine with eyes.

Presentation: 10 x 10,000 doses and 10 x 25,000 doses for coarse spray use.

Compendium Code No.: 11062101 20902 AL 173

TRIVIB 5L®

Fort Dodge **Bacterin**

Campylobacter Fetus-Leptospira Canicola-Grippotyphosa-Hardjo-Icterohaemorrhagiae-Pomona Bacterin

U.S. Vet. Lic. No.: 112

Contents: Killed, concentrated cultures of *Campylobacter fetus* var. *venerealis* and *Leptospira pomona, hardjo, grippotyphosa, canicola* and *icterohaemorrhagiae* organisms suspended in a special oil adjuvant.

Indications: For vaccination of healthy cattle to protect against *Campylobacter fetus, Leptospira pomona, hardjo, grippotyphosa, canicola* and *icterohaemorrhagiae* infections.

Dosage and Administration: Cattle, inject one 5 mL dose subcutaneously using aseptic technique in the neck or behind the shoulder. In non-infected herds and susceptible animals a second dose should be administered 2 to 4 weeks later. The last injection should precede the breeding season by 4 to 8 weeks. Revaccinate annually.

Precaution(s): Store in dark at 2° to 7°C (35° to 45°F). Avoid freezing. Shake well. Use entire contents when first opened.

Caution(s): In case of anaphylactoid reaction, administer epinephrine.

Warning(s): Do not vaccinate within 60 days before slaughter.

For veterinary use only.

Presentation: 10 doses (50 mL) and 50 doses (250 mL).

Compendium Code No.: 10032471 1067G

TROVAC®-AIV H5

Merial Select **Vaccine**

Avian Influenza-Fowl Pox Vaccine, Live Fowl Pox Vector, H5 Subtype

U.S. Vet. Lic. No.: 279

Contents: This vaccine contains a live strain of fowl pox vectored virus that has been shown to aid in the prevention of avian influenza subtype H5 and fowl pox.

Penicillin and streptomycin sulfate are added as bacteriostatic agents.

Contains amphotericin B as a fungistatic agent.

Notice: This vaccine meets the requirements of the U.S. Department of Agriculture in regard to safety, purity, potency and the ability to protect susceptible chickens.

Indications: This vaccine is recommended for initial use in healthy one-day-old chickens. Chickens vaccinated any time after one day of age should not have received a prior fowl pox vaccination. Vaccinates have been proven to remain immune to fowl pox for ten weeks and immune to avian influenza subtype H5 for 20 weeks after the initial vaccination. This vaccine may be combined with Select Laboratories' Marek's Disease Vaccines, Serotypes 2&3, Live Virus, product codes MHSF-3115 and MHSF-3175. It is essential that the chickens be maintained under good environmental conditions, and that exposure to disease viruses be reduced as much as possible.

Dosage and Administration:

Preparation of Vaccine for Subcutaneous Injection:

Important: Sterilize vaccinating equipment by autoclaving 15 minutes at 121°C or by boiling in water for 20 minutes. Never allow any chemical disinfectant to come in contact with vaccinating equipment.

1. For each 1,000 doses of vaccine, use 200 mL of sterile diluent.
2. Do not open and rehydrate the vaccine until ready to start vaccinating.
3. Tear off the aluminum seal from a bottle of diluent and remove the stopper.
4. Using a sterile syringe, remove 2 mL of diluent and add to the dried vaccine.
5. Allow the vaccine to dissolve, and transfer the dissolved vaccine back into the bottle of diluent.
6. Rinse the vaccine vial to be sure of removing all the vaccine.
7. Replace the stopper and thoroughly mix the vaccine and diluent by swirling and inverting.
8. Use the vaccine-diluent mixture immediately as described below.

Subcutaneous Injection Method:

1. Use a sterile automatic syringe with a 20-22 gauge, ⅜-½ inch needle that is set to accurately deliver 0.2 mL. Check the accuracy of delivery several times during the vaccination procedure.
2. Dilute the vaccine only as directed, observing all precautions and warnings for handling.
3. Keep the bottle of diluted vaccine in an ice bath and agitate continuously.
4. Hold the chicken by the back of the neck, just below the head. The loose skin in this area is raised by gently pinching with the thumb and forefinger. Insert the needle beneath the skin in a direction away from the head. Inject 0.2 mL per chicken. Avoid hitting the muscles and bones in the neck.
5. Use entire contents of bottle within one hour after mixing.

Directions for Addition of Blue Dye to Sterile Diluent: Blue dye may be aseptically added to sterile diluent using the following procedures:

1. 0.5 mL blue dye may be added to each 200 mL diluent.
2. Swab top of rubber stoppers on dye vial and diluent container with alcohol; let dry.
3. Using a sterile syringe and needle, withdraw 0.5 mL dye.
4. Inject dye into diluent container and mix well.
5. Add vaccine according to the manufacturer's recommendations.
6. Properly dispose of the dye container and any unused contents at the end of the day.

Precaution(s): Store at 35-45°F (2-7°C). Do not freeze.

Use entire contents when first opened.

Burn this container and all unused contents.

Caution(s): This product may only be distributed and used as part of an official USDA animal disease control program.

Do not vaccinate diseased birds.

Vaccinate all birds on the premises at one time.

Administer a minimum of one dose for each bird.

Avoid stress conditions during and following vaccination.

Do not place chickens in contaminated facilities.

Exposure to disease must be minimized as much as possible.

For veterinary use only.

The ability of this vaccine to produce satisfactory results may depend on many factors, including - but not limited to - conditions of storage and handling by the user, administration of the vaccine, health and responsiveness of individual chickens and degree of field exposure. Therefore, directions for use should be followed carefully. The use of this vaccine is subject to applicable local and federal laws and regulations.

Warning(s): Do not vaccinate within 21 days before slaughter.

Presentation: 50 x 1,000 doses.

Compendium Code No.: 11050451

TRUSTGARD™ 5L

Vedco **Bacterin**

Leptospira Canicola-Grippotyphosa-Hardjo-Icterohaemorrhagiae-Pomona Bacterin

U.S. Vet. Lic. No.: 124

Composition: This product consists of chemically inactivated aluminum hydroxide adsorbed, highly antigenic whole cultures of the organisms listed. Contains gentamicin and a fungistat as preservatives.

Indications: Recommended for the vaccination of healthy, susceptible cattle and swine as an aid in the reduction of diseases caused by *Leptospira canicola, L. grippotyphosa, L. hardjo, L. icterohaemorrhagiae* and *L. pomona*.

Dosage and Administration: Using aseptic technique, inject 2 mL intramuscularly. A second dose is recommended 3 to 6 weeks later. Cattle and swine vaccinated at an early age should be revaccinated after weaning. Repeat with a single 2 mL booster dose annually or prior to each breeding.

Precaution(s): Store out of direct sunlight at a temperature between 35-45°F (2-7°C). Avoid freezing. Shake well before using. Use entire contents when first opened.

Caution(s): Anaphylactoid reactions may occur.

Antidote(s): Epinephrine.

Warning(s): Do not vaccinate within 21 days before slaughter.

Presentation: 10 doses (20 mL) and 50 doses (100 mL).

Manufactured by: Boehringer Ingelheim Vedmedica, Inc., St. Joseph, MO 64506.

Compendium Code No.: 10942331 18413-00

TRUSTGARD™ 7

Vedco **Bacterin-Toxoid**

Clostridium Chauvoei-Septicum-Novyi-Sordellii-Perfringens Types C & D Bacterin-Toxoid

U.S. Vet. Lic. No.: 124

Composition: Prepared from cultures of the organisms listed. Alum precipitated.

Indications: Recommended for the vaccination of healthy, susceptible cattle and sheep as an aid in the reduction of diseases caused by *Clostridium chauvoei, Cl. septicum, Cl. novyi, Cl. sordellii* and *Cl. perfringens* Types C and D. Although *Clostridium perfringens* Type B is not a significant problem in the U.S.A., immunity may be provided against the beta and epsilon toxins elaborated by *Clostridium perfringens* Type B. This immunity is derived from the combination of Type C (beta) and Type D (epsilon) fractions.

Dosage and Administration: Cattle: Using aseptic technique, inject 5 mL subcutaneously. Repeat in 21 to 28 days and once annually.

Sheep: Using aseptic technique, inject 2.5 mL subcutaneously. Repeat in 21 to 28 days and once annually.

Precaution(s): Store out of direct sunlight at a temperature between 35-45°F (2-7°). Avoid freezing. Shake well before using. Use entire contents when first opened.

Caution(s): Anaphylactoid reactions may occur.

Antidote(s): Epinephrine.

Warning(s): Do not vaccinate within 21 days before slaughter.

Presentation: 10 cattle doses or 20 sheep doses (50 mL), 50 cattle doses or 100 sheep doses (250 mL), and 200 cattle doses or 400 sheep doses (1000 mL).

Manufactured by: Boehringer Ingelheim Vedmedica, Inc., St. Joseph, MO 64506.

Compendium Code No.: 10942341 13316-00 / 13317-00 / 13318-00

TRUSTGARD™ 7/HS

Vedco **Bacterin-Toxoid**

Clostridium Chauvoei-Septicum-Novyi-Sordellii-Perfringens Types C & D-Haemophilus Somnus Bacterin-Toxoid

U.S. Vet. Lic. No.: 124

Composition: Prepared from cultures of the organisms listed. Alum precipitated.

Indications: Recommended for the vaccination of healthy, susceptible cattle as an aid in the reduction of diseases caused by *Clostridium chauvoei, Cl. septicum, Cl. novyi, Cl. sordellii, Cl. perfringens* Types C and D and *Haemophilus somnus*. Although *Clostridium perfringens* Type B is not a significant problem in the U.S.A., immunity may be provided against the beta and epsilon toxins elaborated by *Clostridium perfringens* Type B. This immunity is derived from the combination of Type C (beta) and Type D (epsilon) fractions.

Dosage and Administration: Using aseptic technique, inject 5 mL subcutaneously. Repeat in 21 to 28 days and once annually.

Precaution(s): Store out of direct sunlight at a temperature between 35-45°F (2-7°). Avoid freezing. Shake well before using. Use entire contents when first opened.

Caution(s): Transient swelling at the injection site may occur. Anaphylactoid reactions may occur.

Antidote(s): Epinephrine.

Warning(s): Do not vaccinate within 21 days before slaughter.

Presentation: 10 doses (50 mL), 50 doses (250 mL), and 200 doses (1,000 mL).

Manufactured by: Boehringer Ingelheim Vedmedica, Inc., St. Joseph, MO 64506.

Compendium Code No.: 10942351 18719-00 / 18720-00

TRUSTGARD™ 8

Vedco **Bacterin-Toxoid**

Clostridium Chauvoei-Septicum-Haemolyticum-Novyi-Sordellii-Perfringens Types C & D Bacterin-Toxoid

U.S. Vet. Lic. No.: 124

Composition: Prepared from cultures of the organisms listed. Alum precipitated.

Indications: Recommended for the vaccination of healthy, susceptible cattle and sheep as an aid in the reduction of diseases caused by *Clostridium chauvoei, Cl. septicum, Cl. haemolyticum, Cl. novyi, Cl. sordellii* and *Cl. perfringens* Types C and D. Although *Clostridium perfringens* Type B is not a significant problem in the U.S.A., immunity may be provided against the beta and epsilon toxins elaborated by *Clostridium perfringens* Type B. This immunity is derived from the combination of Type C (beta) and Type D (epsilon) fractions.

Dosage and Administration: Cattle: Using aseptic technique, inject 5 mL subcutaneously. Repeat in 21 to 28 days and once annually.

Sheep: Using aseptic technique, inject 2.5 mL subcutaneously. Repeat in 21 to 28 days and once annually.

Precaution(s): Store out of direct sunlight at a temperature between 35-45°F (2-7°C). Avoid freezing. Shake well before using. Use entire contents when first opened.

Caution(s): Anaphylactoid reactions may occur.

Antidote(s): Epinephrine.

Warning(s): Do not vaccinate within 21 days before slaughter.

Presentation: 10 cattle doses or 20 sheep doses (50 mL) and 50 cattle doses or 100 sheep doses (250 mL).

Manufactured by: Boehringer Ingelheim Vedmedica, Inc., St. Joseph, MO 64506.

Compendium Code No.: 10942361 24211-00 / 24212-00

TRUSTGARD™ CD

Vedco **Toxoid**

Clostridium Perfringens Types C & D Toxoid

U.S. Vet. Lic. No.: 124

Composition: Prepared from cultures of *Clostridium perfringens* Types C and D. Alum precipitated.

Indications: Recommended for the vaccination of healthy, susceptible sheep and cattle as an aid in the reduction of enterotoxemia caused by the toxins of *Clostridium perfringens* Types C and D. Although *Cl. perfringens* Type B is not a significant problem in the U.S.A., immunity may be provided against the beta and epsilon toxins elaborated by *Cl. perfringens* Type B. This immunity is derived from the combination of Type C (beta) and Type D (epsilon) fractions.

Dosage and Administration: Sheep: Using aseptic technique, inject 2 mL subcutaneously. Repeat in 21 to 28 days and once annually.

Cattle: Using aseptic technique, inject 5 mL subcutaneously. Repeat in 21 to 28 days and once annually.

Precaution(s): Store out of direct sunlight at a temperature between 35-45°F (2-7°C). Avoid freezing. Shake well before using. Use entire contents when first opened.

Caution(s): Anaphylactoid reactions may occur.

Antidote(s): Epinephrine.

Warning(s): Do not vaccinate within 21 days before slaughter.

Presentation: 10 cattle doses or 25 sheep doses (50 mL) and 50 cattle doses or 125 sheep doses (250 mL).

Manufactured by: Boehringer Ingelheim Vedmedica, Inc., St. Joseph, MO 64506.

Compendium Code No.: 10942371 10907-00 / 10908-00

TRUSTGARD™ CD/T

Vedco **Toxoid**

Clostridium Perfringens Types C & D-Tetanus Toxoid

U.S. Vet. Lic. No.: 124

Composition: Prepared from cultures of the organisms listed. Alum precipitated.

Indications: Recommended for the vaccination of healthy, susceptible sheep, goats and cattle as an aid in the reduction of enterotoxemia and tetanus caused by the toxins of *Clostridium perfringens* Types C and D and *Clostridium tetani*. Although *Cl. perfringens* Type B is not a significant problem in the U.S.A., immunity may be provided against the beta and epsilon toxins elaborated by *Cl. perfringens* Type B. This immunity is derived from the combination of Type C (beta) and Type D (epsilon) fractions.

Dosage and Administration: Cattle: Using aseptic technique, inject 5 mL subcutaneously. Repeat in 21 to 28 days and once annually.

Sheep and Goats: Using aseptic technique, inject 2 mL subcutaneously. Repeat in 21 to 28 days and once annually.

Precaution(s): Store out of direct sunlight at 35-45°F (2-7°C). Avoid freezing. Shake well before using. Use entire contents when first opened.

Caution(s): Anaphylactoid reactions may occur.

Antidote(s): Epinephrine.

Warning(s): Do not vaccinate within 21 days before slaughter.

Presentation: 10 cattle doses or 25 sheep/goat doses (50 mL) and 50 cattle doses or 125 sheep/goat doses (250 mL).

Manufactured by: Boehringer Ingelheim Vedmedica, Inc., St. Joseph, MO 64506.

Compendium Code No.: 10942381 20305-00 / 20306-00

TRUSTGARD™ HS

Vedco **Bacterin**

Haemophilus Somnus Bacterin

U.S. Vet. Lic. No.: 124

Composition: Contains inactivated cultures of *Haemophilus somnus*.

Preservative: Neomycin.

Indications: Recommended for the vaccination of healthy, susceptible cattle 4 months of age or older as an aid in the reduction of diseases caused by *Haemophilus somnus*.

Dosage and Administration: Using aseptic technique, inject 2 mL intramuscularly in healthy calves 4 months of age or older. Repeat in 21 days and once annually.

Precaution(s): Store out of direct sunlight at a temperature between 35-45°F (2-7°C). Avoid freezing. Shake well before using. Use entire contents when first opened.

Caution(s): Analyphylactoid reactions may occur.

Antidote(s): Epinephrine.

Warning(s): Do not vaccinate within 21 days before slaughter.

Presentation: 10 doses (20 mL) and 50 doses (100 mL).

Manufactured by: Boehringer Ingelheim Vedmedica, Inc., St. Joseph, MO 64506.

Compendium Code No.: 10942391 15016-00 / 15017-00

TRUSTGARD™ MB

Vedco **Bacterin**

Moraxella Bovis Bacterin

U.S. Vet. Lic. No.: 124

Composition: This vaccine contains inactivated isolates of *Moraxella bovis*.

Indications: For use in prevention and control of pinkeye (infectious bovine keratoconjunctivitis) in healthy cattle caused by *Moraxella bovis*.

Dosage and Administration: Shake well. Administer a 2 mL dose subcutaneously to cattle 2 months of age or older. Repeat vaccination in 21 days.

Precaution(s): Store out of direct sunlight at a temperature between 35-45°F (2-7°C). Do not freeze. Shake well before and during use. Use entire contents when first opened.

Caution(s): Anaphylactoid reactions may occur.

Antidote(s): Epinephrine.

Warning(s): Do not vaccinate within 21 days before slaughter.

Presentation: 10 doses (20 mL) and 50 doses (100 mL).

Manufactured by: Boehringer Ingelheim Vetmedica, Inc., St. Joseph MO 64506.

Compendium Code No.: 10942401 05205-00 / 05206-00

TRUSTGARD™ VIBRIO/5L

Vedco **Bacterin**

Campylobacter Fetus-Leptospira Canicola-Grippotyphosa-Hardjo-Icterohaemorrhagiae-Pomona Bacterin

U.S. Vet. Lic. No.: 124

Composition: Chemically inactivated aluminum hydroxide adsorbed whole cultures of the organisms listed. Contains gentamicin and Amphotericin B as preservatives.

Indications: Recommended for the vaccination of healthy, susceptible cattle as an aid in the reduction of infertility, delayed conception or abortion caused by *Campylobacter fetus* and leptospirosis caused by *Leptospira canicola, L. grippotyphosa, L. hardjo, L. icterohaemorrhagiae* and *L. pomona*.

Dosage and Administration: Using aseptic technique, inject 5 mL intramuscularly in healthy cattle of any age. Repeat in 14 to 21 days. Administer a single 5 mL booster dose annually.

Precaution(s): Store out of direct sunlight at a temperature between 35-45°F (2-7°C). Avoid freezing. Shake well before using. Use entire contents when first opened.

Caution(s): Anaphylactoid reactions may occur.

Antidote(s): Epinephrine.

Warning(s): Do not vaccinate within 21 days before slaughter.

Presentation: 10 doses (50 mL) and 50 doses (250 mL).

Manufactured by: Boehringer Ingelheim Vetmedica, Inc., St. Joseph MO 64506.

Compendium Code No.: 10942411 17605-00 / 17606-00

TRYAD®

Loveland **Disinfectant**

EPA Reg. No.: 134-67

Active Ingredient(s):

N-alkyl (50% C_{14}, 40% C_{12}, 10% C_{16}) dimethyl benzyl ammonium chloride	5.00%
Inert ingredients	95.00%
Total	100.00%

The product contains sodium hydroxide and compatible detergents.

Indications: TRYAD® is a multiple-use cleanser, disinfectant and deodorant for hatcheries and livestock buildings.

Fungicidal against *Trichophyton interdigitale, Aspergillus niger* and *Candida albicans*.

Dosage and Administration: It is a violation of federal law to use the product in a manner inconsistent with its labeling.

TRYAD® has been tested and shown to be bactericidal and fungicidal by official methods. At a use dilution of one (1) part TRYAD® to 500 parts water, the test pathogenic fungi, *Trichophyton interdigitale, Aspergillus niger* and *Candida albicans* were killed on inanimate surfaces when subjected to the A.O.A.C. fungicidal test. Use dilutions of one (1) part TRYAD® to 250 parts water (½ oz./gallon) are generally recommended.

Hatchery: TRYAD® can be used for cleaning, disinfecting and deodorizing floors, walls and equipment throughout the hatchery. Add one (1) part TRYAD® to 250 parts of water or approximately ½ oz. to each gallon of water. Hot or cold water may be used. Use 1 oz. per gallon on surfaces which are difficult to clean or disinfect.

Incubators and hatchers: Remove loose waste material and scrub all surfaces with TRYAD® solution by brushing. Use a fresh solution for each piece of equipment.

Seller and hatcher trays: Soak the trays if possible and then scrub to properly clean and disinfect. TRYAD® may be used in automatic tray washing equipment.

Racks and other hatchery equipment: Brush with the TRYAD® solution. Scrape away any adhering dirt and repeat the disinfectant applications.

Floors and walls: Sweep or vacuum and remove all loose dirt accumulation. Using 1 oz. of TRYAD® to each two (2) gallons of water, scrub or mop all accessible surfaces. Following this, prepare a fresh solution of the same strength and spray all surfaces until they are thoroughly wet.

Poultry and livestock buildings: Use as a disinfecting spray in properly cleaned and prepared buildings. Follow this procedure:

1. Remove all animals, poultry and feed from premises, coops and crates.
2. Remove all litter and manure from floors, walls and surfaces of pens, stalls, chutes and other facilities and fixtures occupied or traversed by animals.
3. Empty all troughs, racks and other feeding and watering equipment.
4. Saturate all surfaces with the TRYAD® solution using 1 oz. TRYAD® per gallon of water.
5. Immerse all halters, ropes and other types of equipment used in handling and restraining animals. Treat forks, shovels and scrapers the same way.
6. Ventilate buildings, coops and other closed spaces. Do not house poultry, livestock or employ equipment until the treatment has been absorbed, set or dried.

7. All treated feed racks, mangers, troughs, automatic feeders, fountains and waterers must be thoroughly scrubbed with detergents and rinsed with potable water prior to reuse.

Other applications: Use for cleaning, disinfecting and deodorizing cages, kennels, feeding pans, trucks and other equipment. One-half (½) ounce of TRYAD® to each gallon of water is recommended. Use 1 oz. per gallon of water where previous disease conditions have existed.

For washing hatching eggs: Use ½ oz. TRYAD® per gallon of water in non-recirculating egg washing equipment. Do not reuse the egg wash water.

Precaution(s): Keep from freezing.

Do not contaminate water, food or feed by storage or disposal. Open dumping is prohibited. Do not reuse the empty container.

Store in the original container only. Keep the container tightly closed when not in use. Do not store under excessive temperatures or other conditions that might adversely affect the container.

Pesticide Disposal: Pesticide wastes are acutely hazardous. Improper disposal of excess pesticide, spray mixture, or rinsate is a violation of federal law. If these wastes cannot be disposed of according to label instructions, contact the state pesticide or environmental control agency, or the hazardous waste representative at the nearest EPA regional office for guidance.

Container Disposal: Triple rinse (or equivalent). Then offer for recycling or reconditioning, or puncture and dispose of in a sanitary landfill, or by incineration, or if allowed by state and local authorities, by burning. If burned, stay out of smoke.

Caution(s): Precautionary Statements:

Hazards to Humans: Keep out of the reach of children. The undiluted product is corrosive and causes eye damage and skin irritation. Do not get in the eyes, on the skin or on clothing. Wear goggles or a face shield and rubber gloves when handling. Harmful or fatal if swallowed. Avoid contamination of food.

First Aid:

In case of contact, immediately flush the eyes or the skin with plenty of water for at least 15 minutes. For the eyes, call a physician. Remove and wash the contaminated clothing before reuse.

If swallowed, promptly drink a large quantity of milk, egg whites, gelatin solution or if these are not available, drink large quantities of water. Avoid alcohol. Call a physician immediately.

Note to Physician: Probable mucosal damage may contraindicate the use of gastric lavage.

Statement of Practical Treatment:

If swallowed: Call a physician or poison control center immediately. Do not induce vomiting.

If inhaled: Remove the victim to fresh air. Apply artificial respiration if indicated.

If on the skin: Remove contaminated clothing and wash the affected areas with soap and water.

If in the eyes: Flush the eyes with plenty of water. Call a physician immediately.

Presentation: 1 gallon (3.785 L) containers.

Compendium Code No.: 10860360

TRYPTOPHAN PLUS GEL™

Horses Prefer — **Equine Dietary Supplement**

Guaranteed Analysis: (Minimum per tube):

Protein	99 mg
L-Tryptophan	2 mg
Dextrose	19 mg
Calcium Chloride	57 mg
Sodium Chloride	880 mg
Potassium Chloride	70 mg
Magnesium Sulfate	70 mg
Niacinamide	592 mg
Pyridoxine Hydrochloride	35 mg
Thiamine Hydrochloride	35 mg
Riboflavin	16 mg

Ingredients: Dextrose, Cane Molasses, L-Tryptophan, Propylene Glycol, Niacinamide, Beef Peptone, Calcium Chloride, Magnesium Sulfate, Potassium Chloride, Thiamine Hydrochloride, Pyridoxine Hydrochloride, Riboflavin Supplement, Lactic Acid, Apple Flavor and Ethoxyquin as a Preservative.

Indications: Suggested Use: TRYPTOPHAN PLUS GEL™ is formulated to provide horses with vitamins, minerals and aminoacid L-Tryptophan during times of need like exercise, and trailering.

Directions: Administer orally 1½ to 2 hours prior to competition, strenuous exercise, racing or shipping.

Dosage:

Adults Horses	16 cc - 32 cc

Precaution(s): Store in a cool, dry place. Do not freeze.

Caution(s): For animal use only.

Warning(s): Keep out of reach of children.

Presentation: 32 cc tube.

Compendium Code No.: 36950071

TRYPZYME®-V AEROSOL SPRAY

V.P.L. — **Topical Wound Dressing**

NADA No.: 031-555

Active Ingredient(s): Each gram delivered to the wound site contains:

Trypsin, crystalline, N.F.	0.12 mg
Balsam Peru, N.F.	87.00 mg
Castor oil, U.S.P.	788.00 mg

With an emulsifier and propellants (water dispersible).

Inert propellant 25% of total content.

Indications: TRYPZYME®-V is for use as an aid in the treatment of external wounds and assists healing by facilitating the removal of necrotic tissue, exudate and organic debris.

For use on dogs, cats, horses and cattle.

Dosage and Administration: Shake well before each use.

Hold the can upright approximately 12 inches from the area to be treated. Press the valve and coat rapidly. The wound may be left unbandaged or apply a wet dressing. Apply twice a day or as often as necessary. To remove, wash gently with warm water.

Caution(s): Flammable. The contents under pressure.

Warning(s): Do not use near fire or an open flame. Do not use on fresh arterial clots. Do not puncture or incinerate. Do not expose to temperature above 120°F.

Presentation: 4 oz. (113.4 g) containers.

Compendium Code No.: 11430320

TRYPZYME®-V LIQUID

V.P.L. — **Topical Wound Dressing**

NADA No.: 031-555

Active Ingredient(s): Each gram delivered to the wound site contains:

Trypsin, crystalline, N.F.	0.12 mg
Balsam Peru, N.F.	87.00 mg
Castor oil, U.S.P.	788.00 mg

With an emulsifier and propellants (water dispersible).

Indications: TRYPZYME®-V is for use as an aid in the treatment of external wounds and assists healing by facilitating the removal of necrotic tissue, exudate and organic debris.

For use on dogs, cats, horses and cattle.

Dosage and Administration: Apply twice a day or as often as necessary. When applied to a sensitive area, a temporary stinging sensation may be noted.

Warning(s): Do not apply in the eyes. Do not use on fresh arterial clots. Keep out of the reach of children.

Presentation: 1 fl. oz. containers.

Compendium Code No.: 11430330

TSV-2®

Pfizer Animal Health — **Vaccine**

Bovine Rhinotracheitis-Parainfluenza$_3$ Vaccine, Modified Live Virus

U.S. Vet. Lic. No.: 189

Description: The vaccine is prepared by growing attenuated virus strains on a bovine cell line. The virus fractions are combined and stabilized by freeze-drying. A sterile diluent is supplied for rehydration.

Contains gentamicin as preservative.

Indications: TSV-2® is for vaccination of healthy cattle, including pregnant cows, as an aid in preventing infectious bovine rhinotracheitis caused by infectious bovine rhinotracheitis (IBR) virus and disease caused by parainfluenza$_3$ (PI$_3$) virus.

Directions:

1. General Directions: Vaccination of healthy cattle, including pregnant cows, is recommended. Aseptically rehydrate the freeze-dried vaccine with the sterile diluent provided, shake well, and administer 2 mL intranasally using a cannula or a syringe with the needle removed. Place half the dose (1 mL) in each nostril.
2. Primary Vaccination: Administer a single 2-mL dose to healthy cattle. Calves vaccinated before the age of 6 months should be revaccinated after 6 months of age to avoid possible maternal antibody interference with immunization.
3. Revaccination: Annual revaccination with a single dose is recommended.
4. Good animal husbandry and herd health management practices should be employed.

Precaution(s): Store at 2°-7°C. Prolonged exposure to higher temperatures and/or direct sunlight may adversely affect potency. Do not freeze.

Use entire contents when first opened.

Sterilized syringes and needles should be used to administer this vaccine. Do not sterilize with chemicals because traces of disinfectant may inactivate the vaccine.

Burn containers and all unused contents.

Caution(s): As with many vaccines, anaphylaxis may occur after use. Initial antidote of epinephrine is recommended and should be followed with appropriate supportive therapy.

This product has been shown to be efficacious in healthy animals. A protective immune response may not be elicited if animals are incubating an infectious disease, are malnourished or parasitized, are stressed due to shipment or environmental conditions, are otherwise immunocompromised, or the vaccine is not administered in accordance with label directions.

Warning(s): Do not vaccinate within 21 days before slaughter.

For veterinary use only.

Discussion: TSV-2® is unique in that the virus strains it contains are temperature-specific. Tests have shown that they will not grow *in vivo* at or above 39°C,[1] the normal bovine body temperature. This restricts viral replication to the nasal mucosa, which is constantly ventilated and maintained at temperatures less than 39°C, even in the febrile animal. At this localized site, the temperature-specific viruses replicate and stimulate local and systemic immunity.[2] Because the temperature-specific strains cannot grow in the internal body organs or developing fetus, pregnant cows may be safely vaccinated. Stimulation of a localized immune response also results in a rapid onset of protection.[3,4]

Disease Description: IBR is a prevalent viral respiratory disease characterized by fever, nasal discharge, conjunctivitis, a hyperemic muzzle ("red nose"), coughing, and increased respiration. In pregnant cows, IBR virus can also cause abortions.

PI$_3$ is a common viral respiratory infection, sometimes mild or inapparent, but often associated with bovine respiratory disease complex.

Trial Data: Safety and Efficacy: Safety of the temperature-specific IBR strain was demonstrated in a test where it was administered to 1,019 pregnant cows in 12 herds.[5] No abortions attributed to IBR were observed. In a controlled challenge-of-immunity test, 5 of 5 susceptible vaccinates were protected from a virulent IBR challenge that clinically affected all 5 nonvaccinated control calves. In a second challenge-of-immunity test, all 25 vaccinated calves were protected from a virulent PI$_3$ challenge that produced clinical signs or temperature increase in 6 of 7 nonvaccinated control calves. In an onset-of-protection study, 2 pairs of susceptible calves remained clinically normal when subjected to contact challenge 72 and 48 hours after vaccination with virulent IBR virus. One calf challenged 24 hours postvaccination remained normal, another exhibited mild clinical signs. All control calves and calves used for contact challenge were clinically affected.[4]

References: Available upon request.

Presentation: 1 dose, 10 dose and 25 dose vials.

Compendium Code No.: 36900410 — 75-4904-06

TUBERCULIN OT ℞

Synbiotics — **Tuberculosis Test**

U.S. Vet. Lic. No.: 107

Composition: Tuberculin, mammalian, human isolates, intradermic is prepared from culture filtrates of *Mycobacterium tuberculosis* (strain Pn, C, and Dt) which are heat-inactivated and concentrated to 40% of their original volume by evaporation.

The cultures are grown on a synthetic media and tested in accordance with U.S.D.A. requirements.[1]

Indications: For intradermal testing of cattle, goats, swine and nonhuman primates for mammalian tuberculosis.

Test Procedure: Equipment: Intradermic tuberculin syringes graduated in hundredths of a mL and is equipped with a 26 gauge needle, ⅜ inch in length. The needle should be cleaned with alcohol and dried before each use.

T

Intradermic test: For cattle and goats, inject 0.1 mL between the superficial layers of the caudal fold skin; cattle (2½ inches), goats (1 inch) distal to the base of the tail. For swine, inject 0.1 mL into the skin on the upper surface of the ear. Care should be exercised to ensure that the point of the needle does not penetrate through the skin.

For nonhuman primates, follow the procedure recommended in the current "Laboratory Animal Management: Nonhuman Primates" - National Academy Press, or equivalent.

If the skin is clean, it is not necessary to disinfect or otherwise clean the surface. Soiled skin should be cleaned with cotton, either dry or moistened with 50% alcohol. Strong disinfectants must not be applied near the injection site. Care must be taken to ensure that all traces of alcohol are removed from both the injection site and needle prior to each injection. This is necessary to avoid any inflammation from the disinfectant which might be mistaken for a reaction.

A positive reaction is indicated by an induration (swelling) of the skin at the site of injection. The test should be interpreted at 72 ± 6 hours by palpation and observation (additional observations may be made at 48, 96 and 120 hours).

Precaution(s): Store in the dark at 35°-45°F (2°-7°C). Protect from freezing.

Caution(s): The test should not be repeated at less than 60-day intervals.

Veterinarians interested in the use of the product should contact regulatory officials within their state or country for specific directions and legal requirements pertaining to its use.

The product has been tested under laboratory conditions and shown to meet all federal standards for safety and use in normal healthy animals. The level of performance may be affected by conditions of use such as stress, weather, nutrition, disease, parasitism, other treatments, individual idiosyncrasies or impaired immunologic competency. These factors should be considered by the user when evaluating product performance or freedom from reaction.

Restricted to use by or under the direction of a veterinarian.

References: United States Code of Federal Regulations, Title 9, Part 113, 200.

Presentation: 1 x 10 mL vials (100 tests per vial).

Compendium Code No.: 11150391

TUBERCULIN PPD ℞

Synbiotics **Tuberculosis Test**

U.S. Vet. Lic. No.: 107

Active Ingredient(s): TUBERCULIN PPD bovis, intradermic contains 1.0 + 0.1 mg per mL of tuberculoprotein derived from cultures of *Mycobacterium bovis* concentrated by ultrafiltration and purified by ammonium sulfate precipitation and dialysis.

Each serial lot is produced and tested in accordance with current USDA regulations and must meet the requirements set forth for purity, safety, potency and special chemical characteristics prior to release for marketing.

Indications: For intradermal testing of cattle for bovine tuberculosis.

Test Procedure: Equipment: Intradermic tuberculin syringes graduated in hundredths of a mL and is equipped with a 26 gauge needle, ⅜-inch in length. The needle should be cleaned with alcohol and dried before each use.

Intradermic test: Inject 0.1 mL of TUBERCULIN PPD bovis, intradermic between the superficial layers of the caudal fold skin approximately 2½-inches distal to the base of the tail. Care should be exercised to ensure that the point of the needle does not penetrate through the skin.

If the skin is clean, it is not necessary to disinfect or otherwise clean the surface. Soiled skin should be cleaned with cotton, either dry or moistened with 50% alcohol. Strong disinfectants must not be applied near the injection site. Care must be taken to ensure that all traces of alcohol are removed from both the injection site and needle prior to each injection. This is necessary to avoid any inflammation from the disinfectant which might be mistaken for a reaction.

A positive reaction is indicated by an induration (swelling) of the skin at the site of injection. The test should be interpreted at 72 ± 6 hours by palpation and observation.

Precaution(s): Store in the dark at 35°-45°F (2°-7°C). Protect from freezing.

Caution(s): The test should not be repeated at less than 60-day intervals.

Veterinarians interested in the use of the product should contact regulatory officials within their state or country for specific directions and legal requirements pertaining to its use.

The product has been tested under laboratory conditions and shown to meet all federal standards for safety and use in normal healthy animals. The level of performance may be affected by conditions of use such as stress, weather, nutrition, disease, parasitism, other treatments, individual idiosyncrasies or impaired immunologic competency. These factors should be considered by the user when evaluating product performance or freedom from reaction.

This PPD reagent must be used in accordance with the uniform methods and rules adopted by the United States Animal Health Association and approved by USDA. Under this agreement, accredited veterinarians are restricted to the use of the single caudal fold test procedure for official testing. Other procedures concerning retesting of suspected animals by comparative cervical test (C-C test) or for cleanup testing of infected herds in the United States (0.2 mL intradermal dose, caudal fold or cervical site) can only be conducted as approved by State or Federal Regulatory Veterinarians.

Restricted to use by or under the direction of a veterinarian.

Discussion: TUBERCULIN PPD bovis, intradermic was developed by the United States Department of Agriculture (USDA) and is to be used for the official Tuberculin test in cattle. The purified protein derivative (PPD) of *Mycobacterium bovis* strain AN-5 is considered more specific than the mammalian O.T. for bovine tuberculosis and has been adopted for official use under the Cooperative United States, Federal and State Bovine Tuberculosis Eradication Program.

References:

1. Konyha, L.D., "Replacement of Mammalian Tuberculin with an *M. bovis* PPD Tuberculin for Field Testing for Tuberculosis." Proceedings 19th Annual Meeting. American Association of Veterinary Laboratory Diagnosticians. (1976). 345-350.
2. United States Code of Federal Regulations, Title 9, Part 113, 203.

Presentation: 1 x 10 mL vials (100 tests per vial).

Compendium Code No.: 11150400

TUCOPRIM® POWDER ℞

Pharmacia & Upjohn **Potentiated Sulfa**

trimethoprim and sulfadiazine

ANADA No.: 200-244

Active Ingredient(s): TUCOPRIM® Powder contains 67 mg trimethoprim and 333 mg sulfadiazine per gram.

Indications: Trimethoprim/sulfadiazine is indicated in horses where potent systemic antibacterial action against sensitive organisms is required. Trimethoprim/sulfadiazine is indicated where control of bacterial infections is required during treatment of: Acute strangles, acute urogenital infections, respiratory tract infections, wound infections and abscesses.

Trimethoprim/sulfadiazine is well tolerated by foals.

Pharmacology: TUCOPRIM® Powder is a combination of trimethoprim and sulfadiazine in the ratio of 1 part to 5 parts by weight, which provides effective antibacterial activity against a wide range of bacterial infections in animals.

The chemical structure of trimethoprim is

The chemical name of trimethoprim is 2,4 diamino-5-(3,4,5-trimethoxybenzyl) pyrimidine.

Actions:

Microbiology: Trimethoprim blocks bacterial production of tetrahydrofolic acid from dihydrofolic acid by binding to and reversibly inhibiting the enzyme dihydrofolate reductase.

Trimethoprim/sulfadiazine thus imposes a sequential double blockade on bacterial metabolism. This deprives bacteria of nucleic acids and proteins essential for survival and multiplication and produces a high level of antibacterial activity which is usually bactericidal.

Although both sulfadiazine and trimethoprim are antifolate, neither affects the folate metabolism of animals. The reasons are: animals do not synthesize folic acid and cannot, therefore, be directly affected by sulfadiazine; and although animals must reduce their dietary folic acid to tetrahydrofolic acid, trimethoprim does not affect this reduction because its affinity for dihydrofolate reductase of mammals is significantly less than for the corresponding bacterial enzyme.

Trimethoprim/sulfadiazine is active against a wide spectrum of bacterial pathogens, both gram-negative and gram-positive. The following *in vitro* data are available, but their clinical significance is unknown. In general, species of the following genera are sensitive to trimethoprim/sulfadiazine:

Very Sensitive: Escherichia, Streptococcus, Proteus, Salmonella, Pasteurella, Shigella, Haemophilus.

Sensitive: Staphylococcus, Neisseria, Klebsiella, Fusiformis, Corynebacterium, Clostridium, Bordetella.

Moderately Sensitive: Moraxella, Nocardia, Brucella.

Not Sensitive: Mycobacterium, Leptospira, Pseudomonas, Erysipelothrix.

As a result of the sequential double blockade of the metabolism of susceptible organisms by trimethoprim and sulfadiazine, the minimum inhibitory concentration (MIC) of trimethoprim/sulfadiazine is markedly less than that of either of the components used separately. Many strains of bacteria that are not susceptible to one of the components are susceptible to the combination. A synergistic effect between trimethoprim and sulfadiazine in combination has been shown experimentally both *in vitro* and *in vivo* (in dogs).

Trimethoprim/sulfadiazine is bactericidal against susceptible strains and is often effective against sulfonamide-resistant organisms. *In vitro* sulfadiazine is usually only bacteriostatic.

The precise *in vitro* MIC of the combination varies with the ratio of the drugs present, but action of trimethoprim/sulfadiazine occurs over a wide range of ratios with an increase in the concentration of one of its components compensating for a decrease in the other. It is unusual, however, to determine MICs using a constant ratio of one part trimethoprim in twenty parts of the combination.

The following table shows MICs, using the above ratio, of bacteria which were susceptible to both trimethoprim (TMP) and sulfadiazine (SDZ). The organisms are those most commonly involved in conditions for which trimethoprim/sulfadiazine is indicated.

Average Minimum Inhibitory Concentration (MIC-mcg/mL):

Bacteria	TMP	SDZ	TMP/SDZ	
			TMP	SDZ
Escherichia coli	0.31	26.5	0.07	1.31
Proteus species	1.3	24.5	0.15	2.85
Staphylococcus aureus	0.6	17.6	0.13	2.47
Pasteurella species	0.06	20.1	0.03	0.56
Salmonella species	0.15	61.0	0.05	0.95
β *Streptococcus*	0.5	24.5	0.15	2.85

The following table demonstrates the marked effect of the trimethoprim and sulfadiazine combination against sulfadiazine-resistant strains of normally susceptible organisms:

Average Minimum Inhibitory Concentration of Sulfadiazine-Resistant Strains (MIC-mcg/mL):

Bacteria	TMP Alone	SDZ Alone	TMP/SDZ	
			TMP	SDZ
Escherichia coli	0.32	>245	0.27	5.0
Proteus species	0.66	>245	0.32	6.2

Susceptibility Testing: In testing susceptibility to trimethoprim/sulfadiazine, it is essential that the medium used does not contain significant amounts of interfering substances which can bypass the metabolic blocking action, e.g., thymidine or thymine.

The standard SxT disc is appropriate for testing by the disc diffusion method.

Following oral administration, trimethoprim/sulfadiazine is rapidly absorbed and widely distributed throughout body tissues. Concentrations of trimethoprim are usually higher in tissues than in blood. The levels of trimethoprim are high in lung, kidney and liver, as would be expected from its physical properties.

Serum trimethoprim concentrations in horses following oral administration indicate rapid absorption of the drug; peak concentrations occur in 1.5 hours. The mean serum elimination half-life is 2 to 2.5 hours. Sulfadiazine absorption is slower requiring 2.5 to 6 hours to reach peak concentrations. The mean serum elimination half-life for sulfadiazine is about 4 to 5.5 hours.

Usually, the concentration of an antibacterial in the blood and the *in vitro* MIC of the infecting organism indicate an appropriate period between doses of a drug. This does not hold entirely for trimethoprim/sulfadiazine because trimethoprim, in contrast to sulfadiazine, localizes in tissues and therefore, its concentration and ratio to sulfadiazine are higher there than in blood.

The following table shows the average concentration of trimethoprim and sulfadiazine, as measured in either serum or plasma, in 24 adult horses observed after a single dose of TUCOPRIM® Powder:

Average Plasma Concentration (mcg/mL):

Trimethoprim (5 mg/kg)					Sulfadiazine (25 mg/kg)				
1 hr	3 hr	6 hr	10 hr	24 hr	1 hr	3 hr	6 hr	10 hr	24 hr
0.82	0.69	0.36	0.12	<0.25	9.9	18.8	17.3	9.0	1.6

Excretion of trimethoprim/sulfadiazine is chiefly by the kidneys, by both glomerular filtration and tubular secretion. Urine concentrations of both trimethoprim and sulfadiazine are severalfold higher than blood concentrations. Neither trimethoprim nor sulfadiazine interferes with the excretion pattern of the other.

Dosage and Administration: The recommended dose is 3.75 g TUCOPRIM® Powder per 50 kg (110 lbs) body weight per day. Each level, loose-filled scoop contains 15 grams which is sufficient to treat 200 kg (440 lbs) of body weight. Since product contents may settle, gentle agitation during scooping is recommended. Administer orally once a day in a small amount of palatable feed.

The usual course of treatment is a single, daily dose for five to seven days. Continue acute infection therapy for two or three days after clinical signs have subsided. If no improvement of acute infections is seen in three to five days, re-evaluate diagnosis.

Trimethoprim/sulfadiazine may be used alone or in conjunction with intravenous dosing. Following treatment with trimethoprim/sulfadiazine 48% injection, therapy can be maintained using oral powder.

A complete blood count should be done periodically in patients receiving trimethoprim/sulfadiazine for prolonged periods. If significant reduction in the count of any formed blood element is noted, treatment with trimethoprim/sulfadiazine should be discontinued.

Contraindication(s): Trimethoprim/sulfadiazine should not be used in horses showing marked liver parenchymal damage, blood dyscrasias or in those with a history of sulfonamide sensitivity.

Precaution(s): Storage Conditions: Store at or below 30°C.

Caution(s): Federal (USA) law restricts this drug to use by or on the order of a licensed veterinarian.

Water should be readily available to horses receiving sulfonamide therapy.

Antidote(s): Epinephrine.

Warning(s): Not for human use. Keep out of reach of children.

Not for use in horses intended for food.

Toxicology: Toxicity and Side Effects: Toxicity is low. The acute toxicity (LD_{50}) of trimethoprim/sulfadiazine is more than 5 g/kg orally in rats and mice. No significant changes were recorded in rats given doses of 600 mg/kg per day for 90 days.

Horses treated intravenously with trimethoprim/sulfadiazine 48% injection have tolerated up to five times the recommended daily dose for seven days or on the recommended daily dose for 21 consecutive days without clinical effects or histopathological changes.

Lengthening of clotting time was seen in some of the horses on high or prolonged dosing in one of two trials. The effect, which may have been related to a resolving infection, was not seen in a second similar trial.

Slight to moderate reductions in hematopoietic activity following high, prolonged dosage in several species have been recorded. This is usually reversible by folinic acid (leucovorin) administration or by stopping the drug. During long-term treatment of horses, periodic platelet counts and white and red blood cell counts are advisable.

In rare instances, horses have developed diarrhea during trimethoprim/sulfadiazine treatment. If fecal consistency changes during trimethoprim/sulfadiazine therapy, discontinue treatment immediately and institute appropriate symptomatic measures.

Teratology: The effect of trimethoprim/sulfadiazine on pregnancy has not been determined. Studies to date show that there is no detrimental effect on stallion spermatogenesis with or following the recommended dose of trimethoprim/sulfadiazine.

Adverse Reactions: No adverse reactions of consequence have been noted following administration of trimethoprim/sulfadiazine. During clinical trials, one case of anorexia and one case of loose feces following treatment with the drug were reported.

Individual animal hypersensitivity may result in local or generalized reactions, sometimes fatal. Anaphylactoid reactions, although rare, may also occur.

Presentation: TUCOPRIM® Powder is available in the following package sizes:
200 gram bottle (NDC 0009-7703-01).
2000 gram pails (NDC 0009-7703-02).

Manufactured by: Pharmacia & Upjohn Animal Health Limited, Corby, Northants, NN17 4DS, England

Compendium Code No.: 10490501 802 610 002 / 802 034 002

TUMIL-K® ℞

King Animal Health **Mineral Supplement**

Active Ingredient(s): Each 0.65 g (¼ level teaspoonful) of powder contains: Potassium gluconate 2 mEq (468 mg) in a palatable protein base.

Each tablet contains:

Potassium gluconate . . . . . . 2 mEq (468 mg)

Indications: For use as a supplement in potassium deficient states in cats and dogs.

Dosage and Administration:

Powder: The suggested dose of TUMIL-K® for adult cats and dogs is 0.65 g (¼ level teaspoonful) per 10 lbs. (4.5 kg) of body weight twice a day with food. The dosage may be adjusted to satisfy the patient's need. For use in kittens and puppies, consult a veterinarian.

Tablets: The suggested dose of TUMIL-K® for adult cats and dogs is one (1) tablet per 10 lbs. (4.5 kg) of body weight twice a day. The dosage may be adjusted to satisfy the patient's need.

Precaution(s): Store at a controlled room temperature of 59°-86°F (15°-30°C).

Caution(s): Federal law restricts this drug to use by or on the order of a licensed veterinarian.

Use with caution in the presence of cardiac disease, particularly in digitalized patients or in the presence of renal disease.

Do not administer in diseases where high potassium levels may be encountered, such as severe renal insufficiency or adrenal insufficiency.

Warning(s): Keep this and all medications out of the reach of children.

Presentation: 4 oz. powder.
Bottles of 100 tablets.

Compendium Code No.: 11320071

TUMIL-K® GEL ℞

King Animal Health **Mineral Supplement**

Active Ingredient(s): Each 2.34 g (½ teaspoon) contains 2 mEq (468 mg) of potassium gluconate in a palatable base.

Indications: For use as a supplement in potassium deficient states in cats and dogs.

Dosage and Administration: The suggested dose of TUMIL-K® for adult cats and dogs is 2.34 g (½ teaspoon) per 10 lbs. (4.5 kg) of body weight twice a day. The dosage may be adjusted to satisfy the patient's need.

TUMIL-K® is highly palatable. To initiate interest in taste, place a small amount on the animal's nose or on the roof of its mouth. The gel may be placed on the paw after initial interest has been established.

Precaution(s): Store at a controlled room temperature of 59°-86°F (15°-30°C).

Caution(s): Federal law restricts this drug to use by or on the order of a licensed veterinarian.

Use with caution in the presence of cardiac disease, particularly in digitalized patients or in the presence of renal disease.

Do not administer in diseases where high potassium levels may be encountered, such as severe renal insufficiency or adrenal insufficiency.

Warning(s): Keep this and all medications out of the reach of children.

Presentation: 5 oz. (142 g) container (NDC No. 0689-0134-01).

Compendium Code No.: 11320081

TUNAVITE™

Vedco **Small Animal Dietary Supplement**

Tuna Flavored Vitamins & Minerals

Ingredient(s): Malt Syrup, Corn Syrup, Soybean Oil, Calcium Phosphate, Cod Liver Oil, Cane Molasses, Methylcellulose, Poultry By-Products, Fish By-Products, Taurine, Water, Choline Bitartrate, Magnesium Sulfate, Nicotinamide, dl-Alpha Tocopheryl Acetate (Vitamin E), Sodium Benzoate (Preservative), Iron Proteinate, Calcium Pantothenate (Source of Calcium and Pantothenic Acid), Riboflavin 5' Phosphate Sodium (Source of Vitamin B_2 and Phosphorus), Salt, Thiamine HCl, Pyridoxine HCl, Vitamin A Supplement, Vitamin D_3 Supplement, Zinc Sulfate, Menadione Sodium Bisulfate Complex, Manganese Sulfate, Potassium Iodide (source of Iodine and Potassium), Cobalt Sulfate, Copper Sulfate, Folic Acid, Tuna Oil and Cyanocobalamin (Vitamin B_{12}).

Indications: A tuna flavored vitamin and mineral supplement for cats.

Directions for Use: To supplement your adult cat's diet give one level teaspoon (approx. 6 grams) daily. For kittens over 4 weeks: Give one-half level teaspoon (approx. 3 grams) daily.

Its highly palatable flavor aids in easy administration. To acquaint pet to the flavor put a small amount on your cat's paw or nose.

Presentation: 3 oz (85.0 g) tube (NDC 50989-608-20).

Compendium Code No.: 10942420

TWIN-PEN™

AgriLabs **Penicillin Injection**

Sterile Penicillin G Benzathine and Penicillin G Procaine

NADA No.: 065-500

Active Ingredient(s): Each mL of suspension contains:

Penicillin G benzathine	150,000 units
Penicillin G procaine	150,000 units
Lecithin	11.7 mg
Sodium formaldehyde sulfoxylate	1.75 mg
Methylparaben (as preservative)	1.20 mg
Propylparaben (as preservative)	0.14 mg
Polysorbate 40	8.19 mg
Sorbitan monopalmitate	11.3 mg
Sodium citrate anhydrous	3.98 mg
Procaine hydrochloride	20.0 mg
Sodium carboxymethylcellulose	1.04 mg
Water for injection	q.s.

Indications: Sterile penicillin G benzathine and penicillin G procaine in aqueous suspension is indicated for treatment of the following bacterial infections in beef cattle due to penicillin susceptible microorganisms that are susceptible to the serum levels common to the particular dosage form, such as:

1. Bacterial pneumonia (shipping fever complex) *(Streptococcus* spp., *Corynebacterium pyogenes, Staphylococcus aureus).*
2. Upper respiratory infections such as rhinitis or pharyngitis *(Corynebacterium pyogenes).*
3. Blackleg *(Clostridium chauvoei).*

Dosage and Administration:

Beef Cattle: 2 mL per 150 lbs. of body weight given subcutaneously only (2,000 units penicillin G procaine and 2,000 units penicillin G benzathine per lb. of body weight). Treatment should be repeated in 48 hours.

Important: Treatment in beef cattle must be limited to two (2) doses given by subcutaneous injection only.

The recommended dosage for beef cattle should be administered by subcutaneous injection only. Failure to use the subcutaneous route of administration may result in antibiotic residues in meat beyond the withdrawal time.

A thoroughly cleaned, sterile needle and syringe should be used for each injection (needles and syringes may be sterilized by boiling in water for 15 minutes).

Before withdrawing the solution from the bottle, disinfect the rubber cap on the bottle with a suitable disinfectant, such as 70 percent alcohol. The injection site should be similarly cleaned with the disinfectant. Needles of 14 to 16 gauge and not more than one (1) inch long are adequate for injections.

A subcutaneous injection should be made by pinching up a fold of the skin between the thumb and forefinger. The mid-neck region is the preferred injection site. Insert the needle under the fold in a direction approximately parallel to the surface of the body. When the needle is inserted in this manner, the medication will be delivered underneath the skin between the skin and the muscles. Proper restraint, such as the use of a chute and nose lead is needed for proper administration of the product.

Precaution(s): Sterile penicillin G benzathine and penicillin G procaine in aqueous suspension should be stored under refrigeration below 59°F (15°C). Avoid freezing. Warm to room temperature, and shake well before using.

Caution(s): Exceeding the recommended doses and dosage levels may result in antibiotic residues beyond the withdrawal time. Do not inject the material intramuscularly.

Penicillin G is a substance of low toxicity. However, side effects, or so-called allergic or anaphylactic reactions, sometimes fatal, have been known to occur in animals hypersensitive to penicillin and procaine. Such reactions can occur unpredictably with varying intensity. Animals administered penicillin G should be kept under close observation for at least one-half hour. Should allergic or anaphylactic reactions occur, discontinue use of the product and immediately administer epinephrine following the manufacturer's recommendations. Call a veterinarian.

As with all antibiotic preparations, use of the drug may result in the overgrowth of nonsusceptible organisms, including fungi. A lack of response by the treated animal, or the development of new signs or symptoms suggests that an overgrowth of nonsusceptible organisms has occurred. In such instances, consult a veterinarian.

Since bacterial drugs may interfere with the bacteriostatic action of tetracyclines, it is advisable to avoid giving penicillin in conjunction with tetracyclines.

For veterinary use only.

Restricted drug (California). Use only as directed.

Warning(s): Beef cattle should be withheld from slaughter for food use for 30 days following last treatment.

Discussion: Penicillin G is an antibiotic which shows a marked bactericidal effect against certain organisms during their growth phase. It is relatively specific in its action against gram-positive bacteria but is usually ineffective against gram-negative organisms.

It is normally recommended that any bacterial infection be treated as early as possible and with a dosage that will give effective blood levels. Although the recommended dosage will give longer detectable penicillin blood levels than penicillin G procaine alone, it is recommended that a second dose be administered at 48 hours when treating a penicillin-susceptible bacterial infection.

The use of antibiotics in the management of disease is based on an accurate diagnosis and an adequate course of treatment. When properly used in the treatment of diseases caused by penicillin-susceptible organisms, most animals treated show a noticeable improvement within 24 to 48 hours. If improvement does not occur within this period of time, the diagnosis and course of treatment should be re-evaluated. It is recommended that the diagnosis and treatment of animal diseases be carried out by a veterinarian. Since many diseases look alike but require different types of treatment, the use of professional veterinary and laboratory services can reduce treatment time, costs, and needless losses. Good housing, sanitation and nutrition are important in the maintenance of healthy animals and are essential in the treatment of disease.

Presentation: Available in 100 mL and 250 mL vials.

Compendium Code No.: 10581160

TWINVAX®-99

Schering-Plough **Vaccine**

Newcastle-Bronchitis Vaccine, B_1 Type, B_1 Strain-Mass. & Ark. Types Live Virus

U.S. Vet. Lic. No.: 165A

Active Ingredient(s): TWINVAX®-99 is a combination live virus vaccine prepared from mild reaction, modified infectious bronchitis viruses (Massachusetts and Arkansas types) and the B_1 strain Newcastle virus. The vaccine contains gentamicin as a preservative.

Indications: For the vaccination of healthy chickens two weeks of age or older as an aid in preventing Newcastle disease and Massachusetts and Arkansas types of bronchitis.

Dosage and Administration:

When to Vaccinate:

Initial Vaccination: Two (2) weeks of age or older via the water method.

Revaccination: Birds vaccinated initially before four (4) weeks of age should be revaccinated by water or spray methods at four (4) weeks of age or older with the appropriate vaccine.

Vaccination Program: The development of a durable, strong protection to both diseases depends upon the use of an effective vaccination program as well as many circumstances such as administration techniques, environment and flock health at the time of vaccination. Also, the immune response to one (1) vaccination under field conditions is seldom complete for all animals within a given flock. Even when vaccination is successful, the protection stimulated in individual animals against different diseases may not be life-long. Therefore, a program of periodic revaccination may be necessary.

Preparation of the Vaccine:

1. Assemble the equipment needed to vaccinate the entire flock at one time.
2. Do not open and mix the vaccine until ready for use.
3. Remove the tear-off aluminum seal from the vaccine vial without disturbing the rubber stopper.
4. Use cool, clean, nonchlorinated tap water to which powdered milk has been added as directed under How to Vaccinate.
5. Hold the vial submerged in a pail of water or under a running stream of water. Lift the lip of the rubber stopper so that the water (milk added) is sucked into the vial.
6. Reseat the stopper and shake to thoroughly dissolve the vaccine.

How to Vaccinate:

1. Drinking Water Method: Do not mix the vaccine into the drinking water until ready for use. Drinking water for vaccination should be mixed with powdered milk to prevent inactivation from chlorine or other water additives and also to stabilize the vaccine virus. The powdered milk should be added to the water at the rate of one (1) heaped teaspoon per three (3) U.S. gallons or 2.5 imperial gallons (3 g per 11 L); or one (1) heaped cupful per 80 U.S. gallons or 66 imperial gallons (90 g per 300 L).

   Withhold water from the birds for several hours before vaccinating so that the birds are thirsty. Thoroughly clean and rinse all watering containers so that no residual disinfectants remain. Dilute the vaccine immediately before use with cool, clean, nonchlorinated water (milk added). Pour the dissolved vaccine material into the following amounts of water and mix thoroughly.

Each 5,000 Birds	U.S. Gallons	Imperial Gallons	Metric Liters
2 to 4 weeks	12.5	10	50
4 to 8 weeks	25.0	20	100
Over 8 weeks	50.0	40	200

   Distribute the diluted vaccine so that all of the birds are able to drink within a 1-hour period and do not add any more water until the vaccine is consumed. Avoid placing water in direct sunlight.
2. Spray Method: Use this method for revaccination only. Proper spray application of the vaccine is only accomplished through the use of a clean sprayer emitting a very a fine aerosol (mist) which floats and disseminates easily through the air. Only use the spray method in houses that can be closed during vaccination and for at least 15 minutes thereafter. Cross winds, drafts, or operating ventilation fans prevent effective application.

   Rehydrate the vaccine according to the above instructions. Further dilute each 5,000 doses of vaccine to 500 mL using distilled water. Place the vaccine in the sprayer container and set at the lowest output. Spray droplets of 17 to 20 microns average size and the application of about 700 doses of vaccine per minute are desirable.

   Apply the vaccine over all of the birds at the rate of one (1) dose per square foot, or one (1) dose per bird, whichever is greater.

   Use protective goggles during vaccination to avoid eye contact with Newcastle vaccine.

Records: Keep a record of the vaccine type, quantity, serial number, expiration date, and place of purchase; the date and time of vaccination; the number, age, breed, and location of the birds; the names of operators performing the vaccination; and any observed reactions.

Contraindication(s): As will all bronchitis vaccines, the initial vaccination of layer or breeder replacement stock should be conducted before 16 weeks of age to avoid possible damage to reproductive organs. For the same reason, at least one revaccination with a bronchitis vaccine should be conducted before 16 weeks of age.

Precaution(s): Store at 35° to 45° F (2° to 7°C).

Caution(s): For veterinary use only.

1. Vaccinate healthy birds only. Although disease may not be evident, coccidiosis, chronic respiratory disease, mycoplasma infection, or other disease conditions may cause serious complications or reduce protection.
2. All birds within a house should be vaccinated on the same day. Isolate other susceptible birds on the premises from the birds being vaccinated.
3. In outbreak situations, vaccinate healthy birds first, progressing toward outbreak areas in order to vaccinate diseased birds last.
4. Do not spill or spatter the vaccine. Use the entire contents of the vial when first opened. Burn the empty bottles, caps, and all unused vaccine and accessories.
5. Wash hands thoroughly after using the vaccine.
6. Do not dilute the vaccine or otherwise stretch the dosage.
7. Newcastle virus occasionally causes inflammation of the eyelids in humans, lasting two or three days. Avoid contact of the eyes with the vaccine.

The use of the vaccine is subject to state laws wherever applicable.

Warning(s): Do not vaccinate within 21 days before slaughter.

Presentation: Supplied in 10 x 5,000 dose units.

Compendium Code No.: 10472010

TWINVAX®-MR

Schering-Plough **Vaccine**

Newcastle-Bronchitis Vaccine, B_1 Type, B_1 Strain-Mass. & Conn. Types Live Virus

U.S. Vet. Lic. No.: 165A

Active Ingredient(s): TWINVAX®-MR is a combination live virus vaccine prepared from selected mild reaction infectious bronchitis virus strains (B_1 strain, Connaught Massachusetts and Connecticut types) and the B_1 strain Newcastle virus. The vaccine contains gentamicin as a preservative.

Indications: For vaccinating healthy chickens as an aid in preventing infectious bronchitis and Newcastle disease.

Dosage and Administration:

When to Vaccinate: Initial Vaccination:

Beak-O-Vac Method: One (1) day of age.

Water Method: Two (2) weeks to 16 weeks of age.

Revaccination: Birds vaccinated initially before four (4) weeks of age should be revaccinated by water or spray methods at four (4) weeks of age or older with the appropriate vaccine.

Vaccination Program: The development of a durable, strong protection to disease depends upon the use of an effective vaccination program as well as many circumstances such as administration techniques, environment and flock health at the time of vaccination. Also, the immune response to one (1) vaccination under field conditions is seldom complete for all animals within a given flock. Even when vaccination is successful, the protection stimulated in individual animals against different diseases may not be life-long. Therefore, a program of periodic revaccination may be necessary.

Preparation of the Vaccine:

For Beak-O-Vac Use:

1. Do not open and mix the vaccine until ready for use.
2. Mix only one (1) vial at a time and use the entire contents within two (2) hours.
3. Remove the tear-off aluminum seal and stopper from the vial containing the dried vaccine.
4. Remove the tear-off aluminum seal and stopper from the bottle containing the diluent. Insert the long end of the adapter into the diluent bottle.
5. Hold the diluent bottle firmly in an upright position and insert the vaccine vial on the adapter of the diluent bottle. The neck of the vaccine vial should snap into position and should be seated securely on the adapter on the diluent bottle.
6. Invert the two (2) containers so that the vaccine vial is on the bottom and allow the diluent to flow into the vaccine vial. If the diluent does not flow freely, squeeze the bottle gently and the diluent will flow into the vaccine vial. The vaccine vial should be completely filled with diluent to prevent excess foaming.
7. Hold the joined containers by the ends and shake vigorously until the vaccine plug is completely dissolved.
8. Return the joined containers to their original position (diluent bottle on the bottom). Allow the rehydrated vaccine to flow into the diluent bottle. If the vaccine does not flow into the diluent bottle, tap or squeeze the diluent bottle gently and release to draw the vaccine into the diluent bottle. Be sure that all of the product is removed from the vaccine vial.
9. Remove the vaccine vial and adapter from the neck of the diluent bottle.
10. The vaccine is now ready for beak-o-vac use.

For Water Use:

1. Assemble the vaccine and equipment needed to vaccinate the entire flock at one time.
2. Do not open and mix the vaccine until ready for use.
3. Remove the tear-off aluminum seal from the vaccine vial without disturbing the rubber stopper.
4. Use cool, clean, nonchlorinated tap water to which powdered milk has been added as directed under How to Vaccinate.
5. Holding the vial submerged in a pail of water or under a running stream of water, lift the lip of the rubber stopper so that the water (milk added) is sucked into the vial.
6. Reseat the stopper and shake to thoroughly dissolve the vaccine.

How to Vaccinate:

1. Drinking Water Method: Do not mix the vaccine into the drinking water until ready for use. Drinking water for vaccination should be mixed with powdered milk to prevent inactivation from chlorine or other water additives and also to stabilize the vaccine virus. The powdered milk should be added to the water at the rate of one (1) heaped teaspoon per three (3) U.S. gallons or 2.5 imperial gallons (3 g per 11 L); or one (1) heaped cupful per 80 U.S. gallons or 66 imperial gallons (90 g per 300 L).

   Withhold water from the birds for several hours before vaccinating so that the birds are thirsty. Thoroughly clean and rinse all watering containers so that no residual disinfectants remain. Dilute the vaccine immediately before use with cool, clean, nonchlorinated water (milk added). Pour the dissolved vaccine material into the following amounts of water and mix thoroughly.

Each 100 Birds	U.S. Gallons	Imperial Gallons	Metric Liters
2 to 4 weeks	2.5	2	10
4 to 8 weeks	5.0	4	20
Over 8 weeks	10.0	8	40

   Distribute the diluted vaccine so that all of the birds are able to drink within a 1-hour period and do not add any more water until the vaccine is consumed. Avoid placing water in direct sunlight.
2. Spray Method: For revaccination only. Proper spray application of the vaccine is

accomplished through the use of a clean sprayer only. The droplet size of the spray is important: a fine mist (spray droplets of 5-20 microns) will produce a stronger immune response, but may also elicit strong reactions. A coarse spray (spray droplets of 30-50 microns) will produce less respiratory reactions, but will also reduce immunity. Environmental conditions, bird strain and bird health will determine which droplet size is appropriate for an operation. Only use the spray method in houses that can be closed during vaccination and for 15 minutes thereafter. Cross winds, drafts or operating ventilation fans will prevent effective application.

Rehydrate the vaccine according to the above instructions "Preparation of the Vaccine for Beak-O-Vac Use".

Further dilute each 2,500 doses (75 mL) of vaccine to 250 mL, each 5,000 doses (150 mL) of vaccine to 500 mL, or each 10,000 doses (300 mL) of vaccine to 1,000 mL using distilled water. Place the rehydrated vaccine in the sprayer container. Apply the vaccine at the rate of one (1) dose per square foot or one (1) dose per bird, whichever is greater. The vaccine should be applied at the rate of 700 doses of vaccine per minute. See the manufacturer's directions for the spray applicator to choose for more specific application directions.

Use protective goggles during vaccination to avoid eye contact with Newcastle vaccine.

3. Beak-O-Vac Method: Only use this method for the vaccination of day-old chicks in the hatchery. Proper beak-o-vac application of the vaccine is only accomplished through the use of a clean disinfectant-free beak-o-vac machine (or equivalent automatic debeaking vaccinating machine) adjusted to deliver 33 to 34 doses per mL of the final rehydrated vaccine.

   Using an appropriate clean sterile disinfectant-free tubing, hook up the final mixed vaccine to the beak-o-vac machine. Make sure that all of the air bubbles are removed from the delivery tubing and that the proper dosage is delivered consistently with each debeaking action of the machine.

   Hold the chicks so that the mouth of the bird is open and across the spray bar at the vaccine delivery point to ensure that the vaccine is sprayed directly into the entire oral cavity of the bird; thus, exposing the upper respiratory tissues to the vaccine virus.

   Beak-o-vac machine operators should use protective goggles during vaccination to avoid eye contact with Newcastle vaccine.

Records: Keep a record of the vaccine type, quantity, serial number, expiration date, and place of purchase; the date and time of vaccination; the number, age, breed, and location of the birds; the names of operators performing the vaccination; and any observed reactions.

Contraindication(s): As will all bronchitis vaccines, the initial vaccination of layer or breeder replacement stock should be conducted before 16 weeks of age to avoid possible damage to reproductive organs. For the same reason, at least one revaccination with a bronchitis vaccine should be conducted before 16 weeks of age.

Precaution(s): Store at 35° to 45° F (2° to 7°C).

Caution(s): For veterinary use only.

1. Vaccinate healthy birds only. Although disease may not be evident, coccidiosis, chronic respiratory disease, mycoplasma infection, lymphoid leukosis, infectious bursal disease, Marek's disease, or other disease conditions may cause serious complications or reduce protection.
2. All birds within a house should be vaccinated on the same day. Isolate other susceptible birds on the premises from the birds being vaccinated.
3. In outbreak situations, vaccinate healthy birds first, progressing toward outbreak areas in order to vaccinate diseased birds last.
4. Do not spill or spatter the vaccine. Use the entire contents of the vial when first opened. Burn the empty bottles, caps, and all unused vaccine and accessories.
5. Wash hands thoroughly after using the vaccine.
6. Do not dilute the vaccine or otherwise stretch the dosage.
7. Newcastle virus occasionally causes inflammation of the eyelids in humans, lasting two or three days. Avoid contact of the eyes with the vaccine.

Warning(s): Do not vaccinate within 21 days before slaughter.

Presentation: Supplied in 10 x 2,500, 10 x 10,000, and 10 x 20,000 dose units. Diluent can be purchased separately.

Compendium Code No.: 10472020

TYLAN® 40

Elanco **Feed Medication**

Tylosin Phosphate-Type A Medicated Article

NADA No.: 012-491

Active Ingredient(s):

Tylosin (as tylosin phosphate) .... 40 g per lb

Ingredients: Roughage products, calcium carbonate and mineral oil.

Indications:

Swine: For increased rate of weight gain and improved feed efficiency.

For prevention and/or control of porcine proliferative enteropathies (ileitis) associated with *Lawsonia intracellularis.*

For prevention of swine dysentery (bloody scours) caused by *Serpulina hyodysenteriae.*

For maintaining weight gains and feed efficiency in the presence of atrophic rhinitis.

For treatment and control of swine dysentery (bloody scours) caused by *Serpulina hyodysenteriae* following initial medication with TYLAN® Soluble in drinking water.

Beef Cattle: For reduction of incidence of liver abscesses caused by *Fusobacterium necrophorum* and *Actinomyces pyogenes.*

Chickens: For increased rate of weight gain and improved feed efficiency.

Laying Chickens: For improving feed efficiency.

Broiler and Replacement Chickens: To aid in the control of chronic respiratory disease caused by *Mycoplasma gallisepticum.*

Dosage and Administration:

Mixing and Feeding Directions for Swine Feeds:

For increased rate of weight gain and improved feed efficiency:

Feed	TYLAN® 40 Per Ton of Type C Feed	Tylosin Per Ton of Type C Feed
Pre-Starter or Starter	0.5 to 2.5 lbs	20 to 100 g
Grower	0.5 to 1 lb	20 to 40 g
Finisher	0.25 to 0.5 lbs	10 to 20 g
Feed continuously as the only ration.		

For prevention and/or control of porcine proliferative enteropathies: Feed 100 g of tylosin per ton (2.5 pounds of TYLAN® 40 per ton) of complete feed as the sole ration for 21 days.

For prevention of swine dysentery (bloody scours): Feed 100 g of tylosin per ton (2.5 pounds of TYLAN® 40 per ton) of complete feed for at least three weeks. Follow with 40 g of tylosin per ton (1 pound of TYLAN® 40 per ton) of complete feed until pigs reach market weight.

For maintaining weight gains and feed efficiency in the presence of atrophic rhinitis: Feed 100 g of tylosin per ton (2.5 pounds of TYLAN® 40 per ton) of complete feed. Feed continuously as the only ration.

For the treatment and control of swine dysentery (bloody scours): Treat with TYLAN® Soluble (250 mg tylosin per gallon) in drinking water for 3 to 10 days and follow with 40 to 100 g of tylosin per ton (1 to 2.5 pounds of TYLAN® 40) of complete feed for two to six weeks.

Mixing and Feeding Directions for Beef Cattle Feeds:

For reduction of the incidence of liver abscesses in beef cattle caused by *Fusobacterium necrophorum* and *Actinomyces pyogenes:*

TYLAN® 40 Per Ton of Type C Feed	Tylosin Per Ton of Type C Feed
0.2 to 0.25 lbs	8 to 10 g
To be fed so that each animal receives not more than 90 mg per head per day and not less than 60 mg per head per day. Feed continuously as the only ration.	

Mixing and Feeding Directions for Chicken Feeds:

For increased rate of weight gain and improved feed efficiency:

TYLAN® 40 Per Ton of Type C Feed	Tylosin Per Ton of Type C Feed
0.1 to 1.25 lbs	4 to 50 g
Feed continuously as the only ration.	

Mixing and Feeding Directions for Broiler and Replacement Chicken Feeds:

To aid in the control of chronic respiratory disease caused by *Mycoplasma gallisepticum:*

	TYLAN® 40 Per Ton of Type C Feed	Tylosin Per Ton of Type C Feed
Broilers	20 to 25 lbs	800 to 1000 g
Replacement Chickens	25 lbs	1000 g

For Broiler and Replacement Chickens: Administer in the feed to chickens 0 to 5 days of age, follow with second administration in feed for 24 to 48 hours at 3 to 5 weeks of age.

Mixing and Feeding Directions for Laying Chicken Feeds:

For improving feed efficiency:

	TYLAN® 40 Per Ton of Type C Feed	Tylosin Per Ton of Type C Feed
Laying Chickens	0.5 to 1.25 lbs	20 to 50 g

Precaution(s): Not to be used after the date printed on the bottom of the bag.

Caution(s): For use in swine, beef cattle and chicken feeds only.

Do not feed undiluted.

Must be thoroughly mixed in feeds before use.

To insure adequate mixing, an intermediate blending step should be used prior to manufacturing a complete feed. Do not use in any finished feed (supplement, concentrate or complete feed) containing in excess of 2% bentonite.

TYLAN® 40 may be irritating to unprotected skin and eyes. When mixing and handling TYLAN® 40 use protective clothing and impervious gloves. In case of accidental eye exposure, flush eyes with plenty of water. Exposed skin should be washed with plenty of soap and water. Remove and wash contaminated clothing. Seek medical attention if irritation becomes severe or persists. The material safety data sheet (MSDS) contains more detailed occupational safety information. To report adverse effects in users or obtain a copy of the MSDS, call 1-800-428-4441.

Diagnosis should be confirmed by a veterinarian when results are not satisfactory.

Notice: Organisms vary in their degree of susceptibility to any chemotherapeutic. If no improvement is observed after recommended treatment, diagnosis and susceptibility should be reconfirmed.

Warning(s): Withdraw 5 days before slaughter when fed to chickens at 800 to 1000 grams per ton.

Presentation: 50-lb. multiwall, flat bottom bag.

TYLAN® is a Trademark of Eli Lilly and Company.

Compendium Code No.: 103101411 BG 0516 AMB

TYLAN®40 SULFA-G™

Elanco **Feed Medication**

Tylosin Phosphate and Sulfamethazine Elliptical Pellets-Type A Medicated Article

NADA No.: 041-275

Active Ingredient(s):

Tylosin (as tylosin phosphate) .... 40 g per lb

Sulfamethazine .... 8.8% (40 g per lb)

Ingredients: Roughage products, calcium carbonate, and mineral oil.

Indications: For maintaining weight gains and feed efficiency in the presence of atrophic rhinitis; lowering the incidence and severity of *Bordetella bronchiseptica* rhinitis; prevention of swine dysentery (bloody scours) caused by *Serpulina hyodysenteriae;* control of swine pneumonias caused by bacterial pathogens *(Pasteurella multocida* and/or *Actinomyces pyogenes).*

Directions: Important: Must be thoroughly mixed in feeds before use.

Do not feed undiluted.

Do not use in any finished feed (supplement, concentrate or complete feed) containing in excess of 2% bentonite.

Mixing and Feeding Directions: Thoroughly mix 2.5 pounds TYLAN® 40 SULFA-G™ in one ton of Type C Feed to provide 100 grams of tylosin and 100 grams of sulfamethazine per ton.

Precaution(s): Not to be used after the date printed on bag.

TYLAN® 40 SULFA-G™ may be irritating to unprotected skin and eyes. When mixing and handling TYLAN® 40 SULFA-G™ use protective clothing and impervious gloves. In case of accidental eye exposure, flush eyes with plenty of water. Exposed skin should be washed with plenty of soap and water. Remove and wash contaminated clothing. Seek medical attention if irritation becomes severe or persists. The material safety data sheet (MSDS) contains more detailed occupational safety information. To report adverse effects in users or obtain a copy of the MSDS, call 1-800-428-4441.

Caution(s): For use in swine feeds only.

Warning(s): Feeds containing TYLAN® 40 SULFA-G™ must be withdrawn 15 days before swine are slaughtered.

Presentation: 50 lb (22.68 kg) bags.

TYLAN® 40 SULFA-G™ is a trademark of Eli Lilly and Company.

Compendium Code No.: 10310151 BG 1305 AMB (L-I-Mar-01)

TYLAN® 50 INJECTION

Elanco **Tylosin**

Tylosin-50 mg per mL

NADA No.: 012-965

Active Ingredient(s): TYLAN® 50 Injection is a sterile solution of tylosin base in 50% propylene glycol with 4% benzyl alcohol and water for injection. Each mL contains 50 mg of tylosin activity (as tylosin base).

Indications: In beef cattle and nonlactating dairy cattle, TYLAN® 50 Injection is indicated for use in the treatment of bovine respiratory complex (shipping fever, pneumonia) usually associated with *Pasteurella multocida* and *Actinomyces pyogenes;* foot rot (necrotic pododermatitis) and diphtheria caused by *Fusobacterium necorphorum* and metritis caused by *Actinomyces pyogenes.*

In swine, TYLAN® 50 Injection is indicated for use in the treatment of swine arthritis caused by *Mycoplasma hyosynoviae;* swine pneumonia caused by *Pasteurella* spp. swine erysipelas caused by *Erysipelothrix rhusiopathiae;* acute swine dysentery associated with *Treponema hyodysenteriae* when followed by appropriate medication in the drinking water and/or feed.

Pharmacology: TYLAN® has an antibacterial spectrum that is essentially gram-positive, but it is also active against certain spirochetes, large viruses, and certain gram-negative organisms (not including coliforms). It has also been found to be active against certain *Mycoplasma* species.

Dosage and Administration: TYLAN® 50 Injection is administered intramuscularly.

Beef Cattle and Nonlactating Dairy Cattle—Inject intramuscularly 8 mg per pound of body weight one time daily (1 mL per 6.25 pounds). Treatment should be continued for 24 hours following the remission of disease signs, not to exceed 5 days. Do not inject more than 10 mL per site. This formulation is recommended for use in calves weighing less than 200 pounds.

Swine—Inject intramuscularly 4 mg per pound of body weight (1 mL per 12.5 pounds) twice daily. Treatment should be continued for 24 hours following remission of disease signs, not to exceed 3 days. Do not inject more than 5 mL per site.

Precaution(s): Adverse reactions, including shock and death may result from overdosage in baby pigs.

Do not attempt injection into pigs weighing less than 6.25 pounds (0.5 mL), unless the syringe is capable of accurately delivering 0.1 mL.

If tylosin medicated drinking water is used as a followup treatment for swine dysentery the animal should thereafter receive feed containing 40 to 100 g of tylosin per ton for 2 weeks to assure depletion of tissue residues.

Store at 72°F (22°C) or below.

Caution(s): Do not mix TYLAN® 50 Injection with other injectable solutions as this may cause a precipitation of the active ingredients. Do not administer to horses or other equines. Injection of tylosin in equines has been fatal.

Warning(s): Discontinue use in cattle 21 days before slaughter. Discontinue use in swine 14 days before slaughter. Do not use in lactating dairy cattle.

A withdrawal period has not been established for this product in pre-ruminating calves. Do not use in calves to be processed for veal.

Side Effects: Side effects consisting of an edema of the rectal mucosa, anal protrusion, diarrhea, erythema, and pruritus have been observed in some hogs following the use of tylosin. Discontinuation of treatment effected an uneventful recovery from the reaction.

Presentation: TYLAN® 50 Injection is supplied in 100 mL vials with aluminum sealed rubber stoppers.

Compendium Code No.: 10310161 PI 3294 AMP

TYLAN® 100

Elanco **Feed Medication**

Tylosin Phosphate-Type A Medicated Article

NADA No.: 015-166

Active Ingredient(s):

Tylosin (as tylosin phosphate) .... 100 g per lb

Ingredients: Roughage products, calcium carbonate and mineral oil.

Indications:

Swine:

For increased rate of weight gain and improved feed efficiency.

For prevention and/or control of porcine proliferative enteropathies (ileitis) associated with *Lawsonia intracellularis.*

For prevention of swine dysentery (bloody scours) caused by *Serpulina hyodysenteriae.*

For maintaining weight gains and feed efficiency in the presence of atrophic rhinitis.

For treatment and control of swine dysentery (bloody scours) caused by *Serpulina hyodyenteriae* following initial medication of Tylan® Soluble in drinking water.

Beef Cattle:

For reduction of incidence of liver abscesses caused by *Fusobacterium necrophorum* and *Actinomyces pyogenes.*

Chickens:

For increased rate of weight gain and improved feed efficiency.

Laying Chickens:

For improving feed efficiency.

Broiler and Replacement Chickens:

To aid in the control of Chronic Respiratory Disease caused by *Mycoplasma gallisepticum.*

Directions:

Mixing and Feeding Directions for Swine Feeds:

For increased rate of weight gain and improved feed efficiency:

Feed	TYLAN® 100 Per Ton of Type C Feed	Tylosin Per Ton of Type C Feed
Pre-Starter or Starter	0.2 to 1.0 lbs	20 to 100 g
Grower	0.2 to 0.4 lbs	20 to 40 g
Finisher	0.1 to 0.2 lbs	10 to 20 g
Feed continuously as the only ration.		

For prevention and/or control of porcine proliferative enteropathies: Feed 100 g of tylosin per ton (1.0 pounds of TYLAN® 100 per ton) of complete feed as the sole ration for 21 days.

Caution: Diagnosis should be confirmed by a veterinarian when results are not satisfactory.

For prevention of swine dysentery (bloody scours): Feed 100 g of tylosin per ton (1.0 pounds of TYLAN® 100 per ton) of complete feed for at least three weeks. Follow with 40 grams of tylosin per ton (0.4 pounds of TYLAN® 100 per ton) of complete feed until pigs reach market weight.

For maintaining weight gains and feed efficiency in the presence of atrophic rhinitis: Feed 100 g of tylosin per ton (1.0 pounds of TYLAN® 100 per ton) of complete feed. Feed continuously as the only ration.

For the treatment and control of swine dysentery (bloody scours): Treat with TYLAN® Soluble (250 mg tylosin per gallon) in drinking water for 3 to 10 days and follow with 40 to 100 g of tylosin per ton (0.4 to 1.0 pounds of TYLAN® 100) of complete feed for two to six weeks.

Mixing and Feeding Directions for Beef Cattle Feeds:

For reduction of incidence of liver abscesses in beef cattle caused by *Fusobacterium necrophorum* and *Actinomyces pyogenes:*

TYLAN® 100 Per Ton of Type C Feed	Tylosin Per Ton of Type C Feed
0.08 to 0.10 lbs	8 to 10 g
To be fed so that each animal receives not more than 90 mg per head and not less than 60 mg per head per day. Feed continuously as the only ration.	

Mixing and Feeding Directions for Chicken Feeds:

For increased rate of weight gain and improved feed efficiency:

TYLAN® 100 Per Ton of Type C Feed	Tylosin Per Ton of Type C Feed
0.04 to 0.5 lbs	4 to 50 g
Feed continuously as the only ration.	

Mixing and Feeding Directions for Broiler and Replacement Chicken Feeds:

To aid in the control of chronic respiratory disease caused by *Mycoplasma gallisepticum:*

	TYLAN® 100 Per Ton of Type C Feed	Tylosin Per Ton of Type C Feed
Broilers	8 to 10 lbs	800 to 1000 g
Replacement Chickens	10 lbs	1000 g

For Broiler and Replacement Chickens: Administer in the feed to chickens 0 to 5 days of age, follow with second administration in feed for 24 to 48 hours at 3 to 5 weeks of age.

Mixing and Feeding Directions for Laying Chicken Feeds:

Improving feed efficiency:

	TYLAN® 100 Per Ton of Type C Feed	Tylosin Per Ton of Type C Feed
Laying Chickens	0.2 to 0.5 lbs	20 to 50 g

Precaution(s): Not to be used after the date printed on the bottom of the bag.

Caution(s): For use in swine, beef cattle and chicken feeds only.

Do not feed undiluted.

Must be thoroughly mixed in feeds before use.

To insure adequate mixing, an intermediate blending step should be used prior to manufacturing a complete feed. Do not use in any finished feed (supplement, concentrate or complete feed) containing in excess of 2% bentonite.

Notice: Organisms vary in their degree of susceptibility to any chemotherapeutic. If no improvement is observed after recommended treatment, diagnosis and susceptibility should be reconfirmed.

Warning(s): Withdraw 5 days before slaughter when fed to chickens at 800 to 1000 grams per ton.

TYLAN® 100 may be irritating to unprotected skin and eyes. When mixing and handling TYLAN® 100 use protective clothing and impervious gloves. In case of accidental eye exposure, flush eyes with plenty of water. Exposed skin should be washed with plenty of soap and water. Remove and wash contaminated clothing. Seek medical attention if irritation becomes severe or persists. The material safety data sheet (MSDS) contains more detailed occupational safety information. To report adverse effects in users or obtain a copy of the MSDS, call 1-800-428-4441.

Presentation: 50 lb (22.68 kg) multiwall, flat bottom bag.

TYLAN® is a trademark of Eli Lilly and Company.

Compendium Code No.: 10310121 BG 0505 AMB

TYLAN® 100 CAL

Elanco **Feed Medication**

Tylosin Phosphate-Type A Medicated Article

NADA No.: 012-491

Active Ingredient(s):

Tylosin (as tylosin phosphate) .... 100 g per lb

Ingredients: Calcium carbonate and mineral oil.

Indications:

Swine:

For increased rate of weight gain and improved feed efficiency.

For prevention and/or control of porcine proliferative enteropathies (ileitis) associated with *Lawsonia intracellularis.*

For prevention of swine dysentery (bloody scours) caused by *Serpulina hyodysenteriae.*

For maintaining weight gain and feed efficiency in the presence of atrophic rhinitis.

For treatment and control of swine dysentery (bloody scours) caused by *Serpulina hyodysenteriae* following initial medication with TYLAN® Soluble in drinking water.

Beef Cattle:

For reduction of incidence of liver abscesses caused by *Fusobacterium necrophorum* and *Actinomyces pyogenes.*

Chickens:

For increased rate of weight gain and improved feed efficiency.

Broilers and Replacement Chickens:

To aid in the control of Chronic Respiratory Disease caused by *Mycoplasma gallisepticum.*

Laying Chickens:

For improved feed efficiency.

Directions: Do not feed undiluted.

Important: Must be thoroughly mixed in feeds before use.

To insure adequate mixing, an intermediate blending step should be used prior to manufacturing a complete feed.

Do not use in any finished feed (supplement, concentrate or complete feed) containing in excess of 2% bentonite.

Mixing and Feeding Directions for Swine Feeds:
For increased rate of weight gain and improved feed efficiency.

Feed	TYLAN® 100 CAL Per Ton of Type C Feed	Tylosin Per Ton of Type C Feed
Pre-Starter or Starter	0.2 to 1.0 lbs	20 to 100 g
Grower	0.2 to 0.4 lbs	20 to 40 g
Finisher	0.1 to 0.2 lbs	10 to 20 g
Feed continuously as the only ration.		

For prevention and/or control of porcine proliferative enteropathies: Feed 100 g of tylosin per ton (1.0 pound TYLAN® 100 CAL per ton) of complete feed as the sole ration for 21 days. Caution: Diagnosis should be confirmed by a veterinarian when results are not satisfactory.

For prevention of swine dysentery (bloody scours): Feed 100 g of tylosin per ton (1.0 pound TYLAN® 100 CAL per ton) of complete feed for at least three weeks. Follow with 40 g tylosin per ton (0.4 pounds TYLAN® 100 CAL per ton) of complete feed until pigs reach market weight.

For maintaining weight gains and feed efficiency in the presence of atrophic rhinitis: Feed 100 g of tylosin per ton (1.0 pound TYLAN® 100 CAL per ton) of complete feed. Feed continuously as the only ration.

For the treatment and control of swine dysentery (bloody scours): Treat with TYLAN® Soluble (250 mg tylosin per gallon) in drinking water for 3 to 10 days and follow with 40 to 100 g tylosin per ton (0.4 to 1.0 pound TYLAN® 100 CAL) of complete feed for two to six weeks.

Notice: Organisms vary in their degree of susceptibility to any chemotherapeutic. If no improvement is observed after recommended treatment, diagnosis and susceptibility should be reconfirmed.

Mixing and Feeding Directions for Beef Cattle Feeds:
For reduction of incidence of liver abscesses in beef cattle caused by *Fusobacterium necrophorum* and *Actinomyces pyogenes*.

TYLAN® 100 CAL Per Ton of Type C Feed	Tylosin Per Ton of Type C Feed
0.08 to 0.10 lbs	8 to 10 g
To be fed so that each animal receives not more than 90 mg per head per day and not less than 60 mg per head per day. Feed continuously as the only ration.	

Mixing and Feeding Directions for Chicken Feeds:
For increased rate of weight gain and improved feed efficiency.

TYLAN® 100 CAL Per Ton of Type C Feed	Tylosin Per Ton of Type C Feed
0.04 to 0.5 lb	4 to 50 g
Feed continuously as the only ration.	

Mixing and Feeding Directions for Broilers and Replacement Chicken Feeds:
To aid in the control of chronic respiratory disease caused by *Mycoplasma gallisepticum*.

	TYLAN® 100 CAL Per Ton of Type C Feed	Tylosin Per Ton of Type C Feed
Broilers	8 to 10 lbs	800 to 1000 g
Replacement Chickens	10 lbs	1000 g

For Broiler and Replacement Chickens: Administer in the feed to chickens 0 to 5 days of age, follow with second administration in feed for 24 to 48 hours at 3 to 5 weeks of age.

Mixing and Feeding Directions for Laying Chicken Feeds:
Improving feed efficiency.

	TYLAN® 100 CAL Per Ton of Type C Feed	Tylosin Per Ton of Type C Feed
Laying Chickens	0.2 to 0.5 lbs	20 to 50 g

Precaution(s): Not to be used after the date printed on the bottom of the bag.

TYLAN® 100 CAL may be irritating to unprotected skin and eyes. When mixing and handling TYLAN® 100 CAL use protective clothing and impervious gloves. In case of accidental eye exposure, flush eyes with plenty of water. Exposed skin should be washed with plenty of soap and water. Remove and wash contaminated clothing. Seek medical attention if irritation becomes severe or persists. The material safety data sheet (MSDS) contains more detailed occupational safety information. To report adverse effects in users or obtain a copy of the MSDS, call 1-800-428-4441.

Caution(s): For use in swine, beef cattle, and chicken feeds only.

Warning(s): Withdraw 5 days before slaughter when fed to chickens at 800 to 1000 grams per ton.

Presentation: 50 lb (22.68 kg) bag.

TYLAN® is a trademark of Eli Lilly and Company.

Compendium Code No.: 10310180 BG 0614 AMB

TYLAN® 200 INJECTION

Elanco **Tylosin**

Tylosin-200 mg per mL

NADA No.: 012-965

Active Ingredient(s): TYLAN® 200 Injection is a sterile solution of tylosin base in 50% propylene glycol with 4% benzyl alcohol and water for injection. Each mL contains 200 mg of tylosin activity (as tylosin base).

Indications: In beef cattle and nonlactating dairy cattle, TYLAN® 200 Injection is indicated for use in the treatment of bovine respiratory complex (shipping fever, pneumonia) usually associated with *Pasteurella multocida* and *Actinomyces pyogenes;* foot rot (necrotic pododermatitis) and diphtheria caused by *Fusobacterium necorphorum* and metritis caused by *Actinomyces pyogenes.*

In swine, TYLAN® 200 Injection is indicated for use in the treatment of swine arthritis caused by *Mycoplasma hyosynoviae;* swine pneumonia caused by *Pasteurella* spp. swine erysipelas caused by *Erysipelothrix rhusiopathiae;* acute swine dysentery associated with *Treponema hyodysenteriae* when followed by appropriate medication in the drinking water and/or feed.

Pharmacology: TYLAN® has an antibacterial spectrum that is essentially gram-positive, but it is also active against certain spirochetes, large viruses, and certain gram-negative organisms (not including coliforms). It has also been found to be active against certain *Mycoplasma* species.

Dosage and Administration: TYLAN® 200 Injection is administered intramuscularly.

Beef Cattle and Nonlactating Dairy Cattle—Inject intramuscularly 8 mg per pound of body weight one time daily (1 mL per 25 pounds). Treatment should be continued for 24 hours following remission of disease signs, not to exceed 5 days. Do not inject more than 10 mL per site.

Swine—Inject intramuscularly 4 mg per pound of body weight (1 mL per 50 pounds) twice daily. Treatment should be continued for 24 hours following the remission of disease signs, not to exceed 3 days. Do not inject more than 5 mL per site.

Precaution(s): Adverse reactions, including shock and death may result from overdosage in baby pigs.

Do not attempt injection into pigs weighing less than 25 pounds (0.5 mL), with the common syringe. It is recommended that TYLAN® 50 Injection be used in pigs weighing less than 25 pounds.

Store at 72°F (22°C) or below.

Caution(s): Do not mix TYLAN® 200 Injection with other injectable solutions as this may cause a precipitation of the active ingredients. Do not administer to horses or other equines. Injection of tylosin in equines has been fatal.

If tylosin medicated drinking water is used as a followup treatment for swine dysentery the animal should thereafter receive feed containing 40 to 100 grams of tylosin per ton for 2 weeks to assure depletion of tissue residues.

Warning(s): Discontinue use in cattle 21 days before slaughter. Discontinue use in swine 14 days before slaughter. Do not use in lactating dairy cattle.

A withdrawal period has not been established for this product in pre-ruminating calves. Do not use in calves to be processed for veal.

Side Effects: Side effects consisting of an edema of the rectal mucosa, anal protrusion, diarrhea, erythema, and pruritus have been observed in some hogs following the use of tylosin. Discontinuation of treatment effected an uneventful recovery from the reaction.

Presentation: TYLAN® 200 Injection is supplied in 100 mL, 250 mL, and 500 mL vials with aluminum sealed rubber stoppers.

Compendium Code No.: 10310131 PI 3314 AMP

TYLAN® SOLUBLE

Elanco **Water Medication**

Tylosin Tartrate

NADA No.: 013-076

Active Ingredient(s):

Tylosin, as the tartrate. . . . . 100 g

Indications:

Chickens: As an aid in the treatment of chronic respiratory disease (CRD) caused by *Mycoplasma gallisepticum* sensitive to tylosin in broiler and replacement chickens. For the control of chronic respiratory disease (CRD) caused by *Mycoplasma gallisepticum* sensitive to tylosin at time of vaccination or other stress in chickens. For the control of chronic respiratory disease (CRD) caused by *Mycoplasma synoviae* sensitive to tylosin in broiler chickens.

Turkeys: For maintaining weight gains and feed efficiency in the presence of infectious sinusitis caused by *Mycoplasma gallisepticum* sensitive to tylosin.

Swine: For the treatment and control of swine dysentery caused by *Serpulina hyodysenteriae* or other pathogens sensitive to tylosin.

Dosage and Administration:

Mixing Directions:

Chickens and Turkeys: To assure thorough dissolution, place the TYLAN® (contents of the jar) in a mixing container and add one gallon of water (3790 mL) to the material. Mix this concentrated solution with water to make 50 gallons (189 liters) of treated drinking water.

Swine: To assure thorough dissolution, place the TYLAN® (contents of the jar) in a mixing container and add one gallon of water (3790 mL) to the material. Mix this concentrated solution with water to make 400 gallons of treated drinking water resulting in 250 mg/gallon.

Always add the water to the powder. Do not pour the powder into the water. Prepare a fresh TYLAN® solution every three days. When mixing and handling tylosin, use protective clothing and impervious gloves.

Directions for Use:

Chickens should be treated for three days; however, treatment may be administered for one to five days depending upon severity of infection. Treated chickens must consume enough medicated water to provide 50 mg per pound of body weight per day. Only medicated water should be available to the birds.

Turkeys should be treated for three days; however, treatment may be administered for two to five days depending upon severity of infection. Treated turkeys must consume enough medicated water to provide 60 mg per pound of body weight per day. Only medicated water should be available to the birds.

Swine should be treated for three to ten days, depending upon severity of infection. Treated swine must consume enough medicated water to provide a therapeutic dose. Only medicated water (250 mg/gal) should be available

Notice: Organisms vary in their degree of susceptibility to any chemotherapeutic. If no improvement is observed after recommended treatment, diagnosis and susceptibility should be reconfirmed.

Precaution(s): Store in a cool, dry place.

Warning(s): Chickens must not be slaughtered for food within 24 hours after treatment. Turkeys must not be slaughtered for food within five days after treatment. Swine must not be slaughtered for food within 48 hours after treatment. Do not use in layers producing eggs for human consumption.

Avoid contact with human skin. Exposure to tylosin may cause a rash.

Presentation: 100 g in cases of 10.

TYLAN® is a trademark of Eli Lilly and Co.

Compendium Code No.: 10310170

TYLOSIN INJECTION

AgriLabs **Tylosin**

Tylosin Injection 200 mg/mL

NADA No.: 138-955

Active Ingredient(s): Each mL contains 200 mg of tylosin activity (as tylosin base) in 50% propylene glycol, 4% benzyl alcohol and water for injection, q.s.

Indications: TYLOSIN INJECTION is indicated for use in the treatment of bovine respiratory complex (shipping fever, pneumonia) associated with *Pasteurella multocida* and *Actinomyces pyogenes;* foot rot (necrotic pododermatitis) and calf diphtheria caused by *Fusobacterium necrophorum* and metritis caused by *Actinomyces pyogenes* in beef cattle and nonlactating dairy cattle.

In swine, TYLOSIN INJECTION is indicated for use in the treatment of swine arthritis caused by *Mycoplasma hyosynoviae;* pneumonia caused by *Pasteurella* spp.,; erysipelas caused by

Erysipelothrix rhusiopathiae; and acute swine dysentery associated with *Treponema hyodysenteriae* when followed by appropriate medication in the drinking water and/or feed.

Dosage and Administration: For intramuscular injection only.

Beef Cattle and Nonlactating Dairy Cattle — Inject 8 mg per pound of body weight (1 mL per 25 pounds) once daily. Treatment should be continued 24 hours after symptoms of the disease have stopped, not to exceed 5 days. Do not inject more than 10 mL per injection site.

Swine — Inject 4 mg per pound of body weight (1 mL per 50 pounds) twice daily. Treatment should be continued 24 hours after symptoms of the disease have stopped, not to exceed 3 days. Do not inject more than 5 mL per injection site.

Precaution(s): Store at 72°F (22°C) or below.

Caution(s): Do not mix TYLOSIN INJECTION with other injectable solutions as this may cause precipitation of the active ingredients. Do not administer to horses or other equine species. Injection of tylosin in equines has been fatal.

Adverse reactions, including shock and death may result from overdosage in baby pigs. Do not attempt injection into pigs weighing less than 25 pounds (0.5 mL). It is recommended that TYLOSIN INJECTION 50 mg/mL be used in pigs weighing less than 25 pounds.

Warning(s): Discontinue use in cattle 21 days before slaughter. Discontinue use in swine 14 days before slaughter. Do not use in lactating dairy cattle.

A withdrawal period has not been established for this product in pre-ruminating calves. Do not use in calves to be processed for veal.

If tylosin medicated drinking water is used as a follow-up treatment for swine dysentery, the animal should thereafter receive feed containing 40 to 100 grams of tylosin per ton for 2 weeks to assure depletion of tissue residues.

Presentation: 250 mL and 500 mL vials.

Compendium Code No.: 10581171

TYLOSIN INJECTION

Aspen — **Tylosin**

Antibiotic Sterile

NADA No.: 138-955

Active Ingredient(s): Each mL contains:

Tylosin activity (as tylosin base)........ 200 mg
Propylene glycol........ 50%
Benzyl alcohol........ 4%
Water for injection........ q.s.

Indications: TYLOSIN INJECTION is indicated for use in the treatment of bovine respiratory complex (shipping fever and pneumonia) associated with *Pasteurella multocida* and *Corynebacterium pyogenes*, foot rot (necrotic pododermatitis) and calf diphtheria caused by *Fusobacterium necrophorum* and metritis caused by *Corynebacterium pyogenes* in beef cattle and nonlactating dairy cattle.

In swine, TYLOSIN INJECTION is indicated for use in the treatment of swine arthritis caused by *Mycoplasma hyosynoviae,* pneumonia caused by *Pasteurella* spp., erysipelas caused by *Erysipelothrix rhusiopathiae,* and acute swine dysentery associated with *Treponema hyodysenteriae* when followed by the appropriate medication in the drinking water and/or feed.

Dosage and Administration: For intramuscular injection only. Use automatic syringe equipment only.

Beef Cattle and Nonlactating Dairy Cattle: Inject 8 mg per lb of body weight (1 mL of the 50 mg product per 6.25 lbs and 1 mL of the 200 mg product per 25 lbs) once a day. The treatment should be continued for 24 hours after the symptoms of the disease have stopped, not to exceed five (5) days. Do not inject more than 10 mL per injection site.

Tylosin Injection 50 mg/mL is recommended for use in calves weighing less than 200 lbs.

Swine: Inject 4 mg per lb of body weight (1 mL per 12.5 lbs) twice a day. The treatment should be continued for 24 hours after the symptoms of the disease have stopped, not to exceed three (3) days. Do not inject more than 5 mL per injection site.

Precaution(s): Store at 72°F (22°C) or below.

Caution(s): Keep out of the reach of children.

Do not mix Tylosin Injection 50 mg/mL with other injectable solutions, as this may cause precipitation of the active ingredients.

Do not administer to horses or other equine species. Injection of tylosin in equines has been fatal.

Do not attempt injection into pigs weighing less than 25 lb (0.5 mL). It is recommended that Tylosin Injection 50 mg/mL be used in pigs weighing less than 25 pounds.

If tylosin-medicated drinking water is used as a follow-up treatment for swine dysentery, the animal should thereafter receive feed containing 40-100 g of tylosin per ton for two weeks to ensure depletion of tissue residues.

Warning(s): Discontinue use in cattle 21 days before slaughter. Discontinue use in swine 14 days before slaughter. Do not use in lactating dairy cattle.

A withdrawal period has not been established for this product in pre-ruminating calves. Do not use in calves to be processed for veal.

Presentation: 250 mL and 500 mL sterile multiple dose vials.

Compendium Code No.: 14750910

TYLOSIN INJECTION

Boehringer Ingelheim — **Tylosin**

Antibiotic - Sterile

NADA No.: 138-955

Active Ingredient(s): TYLOSIN INJECTION is available in two concentrations containing either 50 mg/mL or 200 mg/mL tylosin base.

Each mL contains:

	50 mg/mL	200 mg/mL
Tylosin base	50.0 mg	200.0 mg
Propylene glycol	50% v/v	50% v/v
Benzyl alcohol	4% v/v	4% v/v
Water for injection	q.s.	q.s.

Indications: TYLOSIN INJECTION is indicated for use in the treatment of bovine respiratory complex (shipping fever, pneumonia) usually associated with *Pasteurella multocida* and *Corynebacterium pyogenes;* foot rot (necrotic pododermatitis) and calf diphtheria caused by *Fusobacterium necrophorum,* and metritis caused by *Corynebacterium pyogenes* in beef cattle and nonlactating dairy cattle.

In swine, TYLOSIN INJECTION is indicated for use in the treatment of swine arthritis caused by *Mycoplasma hyosynoviae*; swine pneumonia caused by *Pasteurella* spp.; swine erysipelas caused by *Erysipelothrix rhusiopathiae;* acute swine dysentery associated with *Treponema hyodysenteriae* when followed by appropriate medication in the drinking water and/or feed.

Dosage and Administration: The product is recommended for intramuscular injection only in beef cattle, nonlactating dairy cattle and swine.

Beef Cattle and Nonlactating Dairy Cattle: Inject intramuscularly 8 mg per pound of body weight once a day (1 mL of the 50 mg product per 6.25 pounds or 1 mL of the 200 mg product per 25 pounds). The treatment should be continued for 24 hours after symptoms of the disease have stopped, not to exceed five (5) days. Do not inject more than 10 mL per site. The 50 mg formulation is recommended for use in calves weighing less than 200 pounds.

Swine: Inject intramuscularly 4 mg per pound of body weight (1 mL of the 50 mg product per 12.5 pounds or 1 mL of the 200 mg product per 50 pounds) twice a day. The treatment should be continued for 24 hours after symptoms of the disease have stopped, not to exceed three (3) days. Do not inject more than 5 mL per site.

Precaution(s): Store at 72°F (22°C) or below.

Caution(s): Keep out of the reach of children.

Do not mix TYLOSIN INJECTION with other injectable solutions as it may cause precipitation of the active ingredients. Do not administer to horses or other equines. Injection of tylosin in equines has been fatal.

Do not attempt injection of the 50 mg product into pigs weighing less than 6.25 pounds (0.5 mL) unless the syringe is capable of accurately delivering 0.1 mL. Do not attempt injection of the 200 mg product into pigs weighing less than 25 pounds (0.5 mL). It is recommended that the 50 mg formulation be used in pigs weighing less than 25 pounds.

If tylosin-medicated drinking water is used as follow-up treatment for swine dysentery, the animal should thereafter receive feed containing 40 to 100 g of tylosin per ton for two weeks to ensure depletion of tissue residues.

Warning(s): Discontinue use in cattle 21 days before slaughter. Discontinue use in swine 14 days before slaughter. Do not use in lactating dairy cattle.

Overdose: Adverse reactions including shock and death may result from overdosage in baby pigs.

Side Effects: Side effects consisting of edema of the rectal mucosa, anal protrusion, diarrhea, erythema and pruritus have been observed in some hogs following the use of tylosin. Discontinuation of treatment effected an uneventful recovery.

Presentation: TYLOSIN INJECTION, 50 mg/mL is available in 100 mL vials.

TYLOSIN INJECTION, 200 mg/mL is available in 100 mL, 250 mL and 500 mL vials. The 500 mL size is for use via automatic syringe only.

Compendium Code No.: 10281110

TYLOVED INJECTION

Vedco — **Tylosin**

Tylosin Base

NADA No.: 138-955

Active Ingredient(s): Each mL contains:

Tylosin Base........ 200.0 mg
Propylene Glycol........ 50% v/v
Benzyl Alcohol........ 4% v/v
Water for Injection........ q.s.

Indications: TYLOVED INJECTION is indicated for use in the treatment of bovine respiratory complex (shipping fever, pneumonia) usually associated with *Pasteurella multocida* and *Actinomyces pyogenes;* foot-rot (necrotic pododermatitis) and calf diphtheria caused by *Fusobacterium necrophorum* and metritis caused by *Actinomyces pyogenes* in beef cattle and nonlactating dairy cattle.

In swine, TYLOVED INJECTION is indicated for use in the treatment of swine arthritis caused by *Mycoplasma hyosynoviae;* swine pneumonia caused by *Pasteurella* spp.; swine erysipelas caused by *Erysipelothrix rhusiopathiae;* acute swine dysentery associated with *Serpulina hyodysenteriae* when followed by appropriate medication in the drinking water and/or feed.

Dosage and Administration: For intramuscular injection only in beef cattle, nonlactating dairy cattle, and swine.

Beef Cattle and Nonlactating Dairy Cattle - Inject intramuscularly 8 mg per pound of body weight once daily (1 mL of the product per 25 pounds). Treatment should be continued 24 hours after symptoms of the disease have stopped, not to exceed 5 days. Do not inject more than 10 mL per site.

Swine - Inject intramuscularly 4 mg per pound of body weight (1 mL of the product per 50 pounds) twice daily. Treatment should be continued 24 hours after symptoms of the disease have stopped, not to exceed 3 days. Do not inject more than 5 mL per site.

If tylosin medicated drinking water is used as a follow-up treatment for swine dysentery, the animal should thereafter receive feed containing 40 to 100 grams of tylosin per ton for 2 weeks to assure depletion of tissue residues.

Contraindication(s): Do not administer to horses or other equines. Injection of tylosin in equines has been fatal.

Adverse reactions, including shock and death may result from overdosage in baby pigs.

Do not attempt injection of the 200 mg product into pigs weighing less than 25 pounds (0.5 mL).

Precaution(s): Store at 72°F (22°C) or below.

Do not mix TYLOVED INJECTION with other injectable solutions as this may cause precipitation of the active ingredients.

Warning(s): Discontinue use in cattle 21 days before slaughter. Discontinue use in swine 14 days before slaughter. Do not use in lactating dairy cattle.

A withdrawal period has not been established for this product in pre-ruminating calves. Do not use in calves to be processed for veal.

Keep out of reach of children.

Side Effects: Side effects consisting of edema of the rectal mucosa, anal protrusion, diarrhea, erythema and pruritus have been observed in some hogs following the use of tylosin. Discontinuation of treatment effected an uneventful recovery.

Presentation: TYLOVED INJECTION, 200 mg/mL is available in 250 mL and 500 mL vials. The 500 mL size is for use via automatic syringe only.

Compendium Code No.: 10942031

TYPHIMUNE®

Biomune — **Bacterin**

Salmonella typhimurium Bacterin, Containing a Patented Immune Enhancer

U.S. Vet. Lic. No.: 368

Contents: TYPHIMUNE® bacterin is an inactivated bacterial vaccine adjuvanted with aluminum hydroxide. It also contains a patented biological adjuvant which acts as an immune enhancer to ensure the level of response to vaccination and provide long-lasting immunity. The bacterin contains three antigenic strains of *Salmonella typhimurium*, the most common species of Salmonella identified in cases of paratyphoid (salmonellosis) in columbiformes, specifically pigeons and doves.

The bacterin has been carefully produced and has undergone purity, sterility, safety, efficacy and potency tests to meet Biomune, Inc. requirements and USDA regulations.

Indications: TYPHIMUNE® bacterin is indicated for use as an aid in the prevention of Salmonella (paratyphoid) infection in birds of the columbiforme species. Young birds may be vaccinated at weaning age. Initially, two vaccinations are recommended two (2) to four (4) weeks apart. Thereafter, boosters are recommended semi-annually to annually depending on the risk of infection.

Dosage and Administration: The product should be shaken well before use and periodically during use. Vaccination is accomplished by using a syringe and small gauge needle to inject 0.5 mL of bacterin either intramuscularly in the pectoral muscle or subcutaneously at the base of the neck and midline at the level of the shoulders in the direction away from the head and toward the base of the neck. Withdraw slightly on the syringe plunger prior to injection to ensure that delivery of the bacterin is not into a blood vessel. Caution should be taken to administer the subcutaneous venous plexus present in pigeons and doves. Aseptic technique should be followed using alcohol to clean the injection site and a new sterile syringe and needle between each bird.

See the package insert for complete information.

Precaution(s): Store in the dark at 35°-45°F.

Use the entire contents when first opened.

Caution(s): Vaccinate only healthy birds.

For veterinary use only.

Warning(s): Vaccinations should be completed at least two (2) to three (3) weeks prior to racing, exhibition or the onset of egg production. Do not vaccinate within 21 days of slaughter.

Discussion: Paratyphoid is a highly infectious and fatal disease commonly occurring in these birds. Clinical expression of the disease varies from a septicemic form displaying diarrhea, depression and nervous disorders to an articular form characterized by the swelling of joints, drooping of wings or lameness.

Presentation: 100 doses (10 x 5 mL).

Compendium Code No.: 11290341

Disclaimer

Every effort has been made to ensure the accuracy of the information published. However, it remains the responsibility of the readers to familiarize themselves with the product information contained on the product label or package insert.

Inclusion or omission of products does not imply endorsement or criticism by the Publisher or anyone involved in the publication. Inclusion does not imply product availability and/or product registration. The Publisher, Editorial Team and all those involved in the production of this book cannot be held responsible for publication errors or any consequence that could result from the use of published information.

UAA (UNIVERSAL ANIMAL ANTIDOTE) GEL

Vedco **Antidote**

Ingredient(s): Contains: Activated hardwood charcoal and thermally activated attapulgite clay in an aqueous gel suspension.

Indications: For use as emergency first aid for combating poisoning caused by the accidental ingestion of insecticides, herbicides, organic chemicals, and intestinal toxins from bacteria. UAA GEL is also indicated for food poisoning (garbage intoxication) in dogs and cats, and grain overload in ruminants.

Dosage and Administration: Recommended Oral Dosage:

Dogs and Cats: 1 to 3 mL per kilogram (2.2 lb) of body weight. The use of a stomach tube is recommended with this syringe.

Large Animals: 1 to 3 mL per kilogram (2.2 lb) of body weight. A dose syringe may be used. However, the use of a stomach tube is recommended for comatose or severely debilitated animals. For cattle and horses, it is recommended that the entire contents of one tube (300 mL) of UAA be given.

Proper supportive therapies such as parenteral fluids and injectable antidotes (to counteract the physiological effects of the poison) are recommended as a part of the treatment. If indicated or necessary repeat the dosage of UAA GEL after 1 to 4 hours, or until the symptoms subside.

Precaution(s): Shake well before use. Protect from freezing.

Caution(s): UAA GEL may not be very effective in the treatment of heavy metal poisoning from lead, arsenic, or mercury.

For veterinary use only.

Warning(s): Keep out of reach of children.

Presentation: 8 fl oz bottle, 60 mL tube and 300 mL tube with easy dose syringe.

Compendium Code No.: 10942040

UDDER BALM

Aspen **Udder Product**

Frost Protection and Sun Screen

Ingredient(s): Water, mineral oil, glycerol stearate, stearic acid, propylene glycol, glycerin, sorbitol, lanolin, vitamin E, vitamins A and D, aloe vera, methylparaben, sodium hydroxide, propylparaben, fragrance, FD&C yellow #5, cetearyl alcohol, ethyl dihydroxypropyl PABA.

Indications: UDDER BALM aids in the protection against the effects of extremes in weather, low humidity, warm and cold temperatures. Daily application of UDDER BALM aids in soothing and softening chapped and irritated skin.

UDDER BALM is recommended for use on teats, udders, hands and other skin areas that are exposed to frequent washing and temperature changes.

Directions for Use: Thoroughly dry udder and each teat before application of UDDER BALM. Apply UDDER BALM liberally to entire teat and udder area after each milking. Be sure to coat teat orifice.

Caution(s): Before milking, thoroughly wash the entire udder and teat area to avoid contamination of milk.

Warning(s): For animal use only.

Keep out of reach of children.

Presentation: 4 oz (113.3 g) and 1 lb (16 oz).

Compendium Code No.: 14750920

UDDER BALM

First Priority **Udder Product**

Frost Protection-Sunscreen

Ingredient(s): Water, mineral oil, stearic acid, glyceryl stearate, petrolatum, glycerin, cetyl alcohol, propylene glycol, lanolin, triethanolamine, lemon fragrance, methylparaben, aloe vera, vitamin A, vitamin E, propylparaben, PABA, vitamin D, artificial color.

Indications: UDDER BALM aids in the protection against the effects of extremes in weather, low humidity, warm and cold temperatures. Daily application of UDDER BALM aids in soothing and softening chapped and irritated skin.

UDDER BALM is recommended for use on teats, udders, hands and other skin areas that are exposed to frequent washing and temperature changes.

Directions for Use: Thoroughly dry udder and each teat before application of UDDER BALM. Apply UDDER BALM liberally to entire teat and udder area after each milking. Be sure to coat teat orifice.

Precaution(s): Storage: Store at controlled room temperature between 15°-30°C (59°-86°F). Keep container tightly closed when not in use.

Caution(s): Before milking, thoroughly wash the entire udder and teat area to avoid contamination of milk.

Warning(s): Keep out of reach of children.

Presentation: 4 oz (113.3 g) tube (NDC# 58829-210-04), 1 lb (16 oz, 453.6 g) (NDC# 58829-210-16) and 4 lb (1.8 kg) (NDC# 58829-210-18).

Sold to veterinarians only.

Compendium Code No.: 11390733 Rev. 05-98 / Rev. 07-01 / Iss. 3-97

UDDER BALM

Vedco **Udder Product**

Active Ingredient(s): Contains:

Chloroxylenol . . . . 1% w/w

Vitamins A, D_3 and E in a water-miscible emollient base.

Preservatives:

Methylparaben . . . . 0.15% w/w

Propylparaben . . . . 0.02% w/w

Artificial color and fragrance added.

Indications: A soothing water-miscible creme for topical application to aid in the management of superficial wounds, cuts, abrasions and irritations such as chapped teats and udders.

Dosage and Administration: Thoroughly wash the affected areas with soap and warm water. Dry with a clean cloth. Apply the creme night and morning, gently massaging. Repeat as indicated.

Contraindication(s): Do not use on cats.

Precaution(s): Store at a controlled room temperature between 59-86°F (15-30°C).

Caution(s): Keep out of the reach of children.

Avoid contact with the eyes and mucous membranes. Do not apply to large areas of broken skin. In case of deep or puncture wounds or serious burns consult a veterinarian. If redness, irritation, or swelling persists or increases, discontinue use and consult a veterinarian. Keep tightly closed when not in use.

To avoid contamination of milk, thoroughly wash udder and teats before milking.

Presentation: 16 oz. (1 lb.) containers.

Compendium Code No.: 10942050

UDDER CLEANITIZER®

Westfalia•Surge **Udder Wash**

High Detergency Udder Wash/Sprinkler Pen Solution

Active Ingredient(s): Contents:

n-alkyl (60% C_{14}, 30% C_{16}, 5% C_{12}, 5% C_{18})

dimethyl benzyl ammonium chlorides 9%

n-alkyl (68% C_{12}, 32% C_{14}) dimethyl ethylbenzyl ammonium chlorides 9%

Inactive Ingredients: 82%

Indications: UDDER CLEANITIZER® is a high detergency udder wash and sprinkler pen solution.

Directions for Use: Prepare an udder wash solution by adding 1 oz. (30 mL) of UDDER CLEANITIZER® for each 12 gallons (45.4 L) of warm 100 - 110°F (38 - 43°C) water. Use a clean single service towel for each cow. Soak the towel in the udder wash solution and wash and massage the udder and teats. Never reuse towel or dip used towel back into solution. Thoroughly dry udder and teats with a second single service towel.

Automatic metering devices used to inject udder wash directly into water should be checked with a test kit to ensure proper proportioning. Solution strength should be a minimum of 125 ppm active quaternary. Do not use as a teat dip.

Precaution(s): Storage Instructions: Store this product in a cool, dry area away from direct sunlight or heat to avoid deterioration. If frozen, separation may occur. Thaw completely and mix thoroughly before use. Keep containers closed to prevent contamination of this product.

Precautionary Statements: Danger. Contains materials which will cause severe eye irritation and possibly burn the eyes. May cause skin irritation. May be harmful or fatal if swallowed. Protect eyes and skin when handling. Do not take internally. Avoid breathing vapors. Do not mix with any other chemical products. Refer to Material Safety Data Sheet (MSDS).

First Aid:

If in Eyes: Flush with large volumes of water for at least 15 minutes. Call a physician immediately.

If Swallowed: Do not induce vomiting. Rinse mouth promptly, then give a large quantity of water. Avoid alcohol. Call a physician immediately. Do not give anything by mouth to an unconscious or convulsing person.

If on Skin: Flush with large volumes of water for at least 15 minutes while removing contaminated clothing and shoes. If irritation develops and persists, get medical attention.

Inhalation of Vapors: If breathing difficulty or irritation occurs, remove to fresh air. If symptoms persist, get medical attention.

For assistance with medical emergency, call 1-800-451-8346.

For farm, commercial and industrial use only.

Warning(s): Keep out of reach of children.

Presentation: Contact the company for container sizes available.

UDDER CLEANITIZER is a Trademark of Westfalia•Surge, Inc.

Compendium Code No.: 10020270 Rev. 03-00

UDDER COMFORT CREAM

Phoenix Pharmaceutical **Udder Product**

Ingredient(s): Water, Mineral Oil, Stearic Acid, Glyceryl Stearate, Petrolatum, Glycerin, Cetyl Alcohol, Propylene Glycol, Lanolin, Triethanolamine, Lemon Fragrance, Methylparaben, Aloe Vera, Vitamin A, Vitamin E, Propylparaben, PABA, Vitamin D, Artificial Color.

Indications: UDDER COMFORT CREAM aids in the protection against the effects of extremes in weather, low humidity, warm and cold temperatures. Daily application of UDDER COMFORT CREAM aids in soothing and softening chapped and irritated skin.

UDDER COMFORT CREAM is recommended for use on teats, udders, hands and other skin areas that are exposed to frequent washing and temperature changes.

Directions: Thoroughly dry udder and each teat before application of UDDER COMFORT CREAM. Apply UDDER COMFORT CREAM liberally to entire teat and udder area after each milking. Be sure to coat teat orifice.

Caution(s): Before milking, thoroughly wash entire udder and teat area to avoid contamination of milk.

For animal use only.

Warning(s): Keep out of reach of children.

Presentation: 1 lb (NDC 57319-296-27).

Manufactured by: First Priority, Inc., Elgin, IL 60123.

Compendium Code No.: 12560862 Rev. 10-01

UDDERGOLD® GERMICIDAL BARRIER TEAT DIP (ACTIVATOR)

Alcide **Teat Dip**

Active Ingredient(s): 2.64% Lactic Acid.

Contains: Isopropyl alcohol, thickening agents, FD&C yellow no. 5 and sodium benzoate as a preservative.

Indications: UDDERGOLD® Germicidal Barrier Teat Dip is used as an aid in reducing the spread of organisms which may cause mastitis. The gel formulation provides a protective barrier over the teat end until the next milking.

For use only with UdderGold® Base.

Directions for Use: Add equal volumes of UDDERGOLD® base and activator to a clean container and mix until the color is uniform throughout. Only enough product should be mixed for one milking of the herd. The average amount of product used is less than ¼ ounce per cow per milking. Discard any unused teat dip. Rinse dip cups and equipment with tap water after each milking.

Application: Immediately after milking, dip teats ⅔ to all their length in UDDERGOLD® Germicidal Teat Dip. Allow to air dry. Do not wipe. Always use freshly mixed, full strength UDDERGOLD® Germicidal Teat Dip. If product in dip cup becomes visibly dirty, discard contents and refill with fresh UDDERGOLD® teat dip. Do not turn cows out in freezing weather until teat dip is completely dry. Prior to the next milking, pre-dip or wash teats thoroughly with a compatible pre-dip or udder wash using proper procedures.

When a cow is being dried off, dip the teats once a day for several days after last milking. Under normal conditions UDDERGOLD® Germicidal Teat Dip will remain on teats for at least 24 hours.

Approximately 10 days prior to calving, dip teats twice daily with UDDERGOLD® teat dip.

Note 1: If teat irritation occurs, discontinue use until irritation subsides. Consult your veterinarian and milking equipment service personnel if irritation persists.

Note 2: The gold color in the mixed product fades with time. At higher temperatures the fading is more rapid. However, this will not affect the efficacy of the product.

Caution(s): For external use only. Not for use in sanitizing dairy equipment. Do not mix with any other teat dip or other product. Avoid contact with food. Avoid contact with eyes. If contact occurs, flush eyes with large quantities of water. See a physician if irritation develops.

Storage and Disposal: Store at room temperature. Protect from heat and freezing. Always store away from continuous artificial light or direct sunlight.

Disposal: Unused teat dip may be diluted with water and flushed down drain. Do not reuse containers. Empty containers should be thoroughly rinsed with water and taken to a recycling center.

Avoid freezing: If product is exposed to freezing temperatures, components must be mixed thoroughly prior to use.

Warning(s): Keep out of the reach of children.

Disclaimer: Distributor's and Alcide's liability on any claim, whether in negligence or any other tort or in contract or otherwise, with respect to products delivered hereunder, shall not exceed the purchase price of the products sold or, if Distributor and Alcide shall so elect, buyer shall be entitled only to replacement of product. In no event shall Distributor and Alcide be liable for buyer's incidental or consequential damages.

Presentation: Available in 1, 5, 15 and 55 gallon sizes.

U.S. Patent No. 4,891,216
Mexico Patents 155,546 and 171,177
Foreign Patents Issued and Pending
UDDERGOLD® is a registered trademark of Alcide Corporation.

Compendium Code No.: 14760080 L1611A Rev. 01 4-99

UDDERGOLD® GERMICIDAL BARRIER TEAT DIP (BASE)

Alcide **Teat Dip**

Active Ingredient(s): 0.64% Sodium Chlorite in a gel formulation.

Contains: Thickening agents and emollients.

Indications: UDDERGOLD® Germicidal Barrier Teat Dip is used as an aid in reducing the spread of organisms which may cause mastitis. The gel formulation provides a protective barrier over the teat end until the next milking.

For use only with UdderGold® Activator.

Directions for Use: Add equal volumes of UDDERGOLD® base and activator to a clean container and mix until the color is uniform throughout. Only enough product should be mixed for one milking of the herd. The average amount of product used is less than ¼ ounce per cow per milking. Discard any unused teat dip. Rinse dip cups and equipment with tap water after each milking.

Application: Immediately after milking, dip teats ⅔ to all their length in UDDERGOLD® Germicidal Teat Dip. Allow to air dry. Do not wipe. Always use freshly mixed, full strength UDDERGOLD® Germicidal Teat Dip. If product in dip cup becomes visibly dirty, discard contents and refill with fresh UDDERGOLD® teat dip. Do not turn cows out in freezing weather until teat dip is completely dry. Prior to the next milking, pre-dip or wash teats thoroughly with a compatible pre-dip or udder wash using proper procedures.

When a cow is being dried off, dip the teats once a day for several days after last milking. Under normal conditions UDDERGOLD® Germicidal Teat Dip will remain on teats for at least 24 hours.

Approximately 10 days prior to calving, dip teats twice daily with UDDERGOLD® teat dip.

Note 1: If teat irritation occurs, discontinue use until irritation subsides. Consult your veterinarian and milking equipment service personnel if irritation persists.

Note 2: The gold color in the mixed product fades with time. At higher temperatures the fading is more rapid. However, this will not affect the efficacy of the product.

Caution(s): For external use only. Not for use in sanitizing dairy equipment. Do not mix with any other teat dip or other product. Avoid contact with food. Avoid contact with eyes. If contact occurs, flush eyes with large quantities of water. See a physician if irritation develops.

Storage and Disposal: Store at room temperature. Protect from heat and freezing. Always store away from continuous artificial light or direct sunlight.

Disposal: Unused teat dip may be diluted with water and flushed down drain. Do not reuse containers. Empty containers should be thoroughly rinsed with water and taken to a recycling center.

Avoid freezing: If product is exposed to freezing temperatures, components must be mixed thoroughly prior to use.

Warning(s): Keep out of the reach of children.

Disclaimer: Distributor's and Alcide's liability on any claim, whether in negligence or any other tort or in contract or otherwise, with respect to products delivered hereunder, shall not exceed the purchase price of the products sold or, if Distributor and Alcide shall so elect, buyer shall be entitled only to replacement of product. In no event shall Distributor and Alcide be liable for buyer's incidental or consequential damages.

Presentation: Available in 1, 5, 15 and 55 gallon sizes.

U.S. Patent No. 4,891,216
Mexico Patents 155,546 and 171,177
Foreign Patents Issued and Pending
UDDERGOLD® is a registered trademark of Alcide Corporation.

Compendium Code No.: 14760090 L1611B Rev. 01 4-99

UDDERGOLD® PLUS GERMICIDAL BARRIER TEAT DIP (ACTIVATOR)

Alcide **Teat Dip**

Sanitizer

Active Ingredient(s): 3.0% Mandelic Acid.

Contains: 5% glycerin, isopropyl alcohol, thickening agents, FD&C yellow no. 5 and sodium benzoate as a preservative.

Indications: UDDERGOLD® Plus Germicidal Barrier Teat Dip is used as an aid in reducing the spread of organisms which may cause mastitis. The gel formulation provides a protective barrier over the teat end until the next milking.

For use only with UdderGold® Plus Base.

Directions for Use: Add equal volumes of UDDERGOLD® Plus base and activator to a clean container and mix until the color is uniform throughout. Only enough product should be mixed for one milking of the herd. The average amount of product used is less than ¼ ounce per cow per milking. Discard any unused teat dip. Rinse dip cups and equipment with tap water after each milking.

Application: Immediately after milking, dip teats ⅔ to all their length in UDDERGOLD® Plus Germicidal Barrier Teat Dip. Allow to air dry. Do not wipe. Always use freshly mixed, full strength UDDERGOLD® Plus Germicidal Teat Dip. If product in dip cup becomes visibly dirty, discard contents and refill with fresh UDDERGOLD® Plus teat dip. Do not turn cows out in freezing weather until teat dip is completely dry. Prior to the next milking, pre-dip or wash teats thoroughly with a compatible pre-dip or udder wash using proper procedures. When a cow is being dried off, dip the teats once a day for several days after last milking. Under normal conditions UDDERGOLD® Plus Germicidal Teat Dip will remain on teats for at least 24 hours.

Approximately 10 days prior to calving, dip teats twice daily with UDDERGOLD® teat dip.

Note 1: If teat irritation occurs, discontinue use until irritation subsides. Consult your veterinarian and milking equipment service personnel if irritation persists.

Note 2: The gold color in the mixed product fades with time. At higher temperatures the fading is more rapid. However, this will not affect the efficacy of the product.

Caution(s): For external use only. Not for use in sanitizing dairy equipment. Do not mix with any other teat dip or other product. Avoid contact with food. Avoid contact with eyes. If contact occurs, flush eyes with large quantities of water. See a physician if irritation develops.

Storage and Disposal: Store at room temperature. Protect from heat and freezing. Always store away from continuous artificial light or direct sunlight.

Disposal: Unused teat dip may be diluted with water and flushed down drain. Do not reuse containers. Empty containers should be thoroughly rinsed with water and taken to a recycling center.

Avoid freezing: If product is exposed to freezing temperatures, components must be mixed thoroughly prior to use.

Warning(s): Keep out of the reach of children.

Disclaimer: UMS's and Alcide's liability on any claim, whether in negligence or any other tort or in contract or otherwise, with respect to products delivered hereunder, shall not exceed the purchase price of the products sold or, if UMS and Alcide shall so elect, buyer shall be entitled only to replacement of product. In no event shall UMS and Alcide be liable for buyer's incidental or consequential damages.

Presentation: Available in 1, 5, 15 and 55 gallon sizes.

U.S. Patents 4,891,216, 4,986,990 and 5,185,161
Mexico Patents 161,768 and 171,177
European Patents 287,074 and 176,558
Foreign Patents Issued and Pending
UDDERGOLD® Plus is a registered trademark of Alcide Corporation.

Distributed by: Universal Marketing Services, 5545 Avenida de los Robles, Visalia, CA 93291.

Compendium Code No.: 14760100 L8009A Rev. 01 1-99

UDDERGOLD® PLUS GERMICIDAL BARRIER TEAT DIP (BASE)

Alcide **Teat Dip**

Sanitizer

Active Ingredient(s): 0.64% Sodium Chlorite in a gel formulation.

Contains: Thickening agents and emollients.

Indications: UDDERGOLD® Plus Germicidal Barrier Teat Dip is used as an aid in reducing the spread of organisms which may cause mastitis. The gel formulation provides a protective barrier over the teat end until the next milking.

For use only with UdderGold® Plus Activator.

Directions for Use: Add equal volumes of UDDERGOLD® Plus base and activator to a clean container and mix until the color is uniform throughout. Only enough product should be mixed for one milking of the herd. The average amount of product used is less than ¼ ounce per cow per milking. Discard any unused teat dip. Rinse dip cups and equipment with tap water after each milking.

Application: Immediately after milking, dip teats ⅔ to all their length in UDDERGOLD® Plus Germicidal Barrier Teat Dip. Allow to air dry. Do not wipe. Always use freshly mixed, full strength UDDERGOLD® Plus Germicidal Teat Dip. If product in dip cup becomes visibly dirty, discard contents and refill with fresh UDDERGOLD® Plus teat dip. Do not turn cows out in freezing weather until teat dip is completely dry. Prior to the next milking, pre-dip or wash teats thoroughly with a compatible pre-dip or udder wash using proper procedures. When a cow is being dried off, dip the teats once a day for several days after last milking. Under normal conditions UDDERGOLD® Plus Germicidal Teat Dip will remain on teats for at least 24 hours.

Approximately 10 days prior to calving, dip teats twice daily with UDDERGOLD® teat dip.

Note 1: If teat irritation occurs, discontinue use until irritation subsides. Consult your veterinarian and milking equipment service personnel if irritation persists.

Note 2: The gold color in the mixed product fades with time. At higher temperatures the fading is more rapid. However, this will not affect the efficacy of the product.

Caution(s): For external use only. Not for use in sanitizing dairy equipment. Do not mix with any other teat dip or other product. Avoid contact with food. Avoid contact with eyes. If contact occurs, flush eyes with large quantities of water. See a physician if irritation develops.

Storage and Disposal: Store at room temperature. Protect from heat and freezing. Always store away from continuous artificial light or direct sunlight.

Disposal: Unused teat dip may be diluted with water and flushed down drain. Do not reuse containers. Empty containers should be thoroughly rinsed with water and taken to a recycling center.

Avoid freezing: If product is exposed to freezing temperatures, components must be mixed thoroughly prior to use.

Warning(s): Keep out of the reach of children.

Disclaimer: UMS's and Alcide's liability on any claim, whether in negligence or any other tort or in contract or otherwise, with respect to products delivered hereunder, shall not exceed the purchase price of the products sold or, if UMS and Alcide shall so elect, buyer shall be entitled only to replacement of product. In no event shall UMS and Alcide be liable for buyer's incidental or consequential damages.

Presentation: Available in 1, 5, 15 and 55 gallon sizes.

U.S. Patents 4,891,216, 4,986,990 and 5,185,161
Mexico Patents 161,768 and 171,177
European Patents 287,074 and 176,558
Foreign Patents Issued and Pending
UDDERGOLD® Plus is a registered trademark of Alcide Corporation.

Distributed by: Universal Marketing Services, 5545 Avenida de los Robles, Visalia, CA 93291.

Compendium Code No.: 14760110 L8009B Rev. 01 1-99

UDDER MOIST

A.A.H. **Udder Cream**

Udder Moisturizer Cream

Ingredient(s): Contains: Vitamins A, D, E, Riboflavin, Panthenol, Pyridoxine Hydrochloride, Biotin and Niacinamide in a specially compounded base stabilized at pH of normal animal skin.

Indications: Vitamin enriched UDDER MOIST can be used as an aid in reducing dry, cracked and chapped udders in cattle. Contains humectants which assist in maintaining the natural moisture balance of skin and tissue.

The non-sticky, disappearing cream base discourages dirt and manure from sticking to udders.

Directions: Apply daily or as needed after milking to aid in reducing dryness, cracking and chapping associated with chapped udders in cattle.

Caution(s): UDDER MOIST is not a substitute for balanced nutrition. Animals with signs of nutritional deficiency in the skin may require injections of therapeutic levels of vitamins. Wash the teats and udder thoroughly before milking. Consult your veterinarian for assistance in the diagnosis and treatment of nutritional deficiency.

If animal shows signs of uncontrolled generalized infections, consult your veterinarian.

For use in animals only.

Warning(s): Keep out of reach of children.

Discussion: Milking machines, inclement weather and other factors strip natural moisture from the udders, leaving them dry and chapped.

UDDER MOIST is a unique blend of 8 vitamins which are naturally present in healthy skin. Helps promote natural moisture balance essential in treating and preventing chapped udders in cattle.

Presentation: 12 x 16 oz (454 g) jars per case.

Compendium Code No.: 11180260 1001

UDDER OINTMENT™

LeGear **Udder Product**

Active Ingredient(s): Lanolin, petrolatum, benzethonium chloride, cetyl alcohol, vitamins A, D_3, and E.

Indications: Combines lanolin, antiseptics, vitamin A, vitamin D_3, and vitamin E to soften, soothe and promote the healing of scratched, chapped and abraded skin.

Dosage and Administration:

Chapped Teats, Scratches and Bruises: Apply generously after every milking, Rub in well.

Galls, Fetter Burns, Cracked Heels and Saddle Sores: Rub in well, then apply a light coating after rubbing.

To soothe and soften chapped and rough skin, massage a liberal amount of the ointment into the affected areas several times each day.

Caution(s): Wash the teats and udder of treated animals prior to milking.

Presentation: Available in 14 oz. jars and 4 lb. pails.

Compendium Code No.: 11530040

ULTRABAC® 7

Pfizer Animal Health **Bacterin-Toxoid**

Clostridium Chauvoei-Septicum-Novyi-Sordellii-Perfringens Types C & D Bacterin-Toxoid

U.S. Vet. Lic. No.: 189

Description: ULTRABAC® 7 consists of killed, standardized cultures of *Cl. chauvoei, Cl. septicum, Cl. novyi, Cl. sordellii,* and *Cl. perfringens* types C and D, with an adjuvant.

Indications: For use in healthy cattle and sheep as an aid in preventing blackleg caused by *Clostridium chauvoei,* malignant edema caused by *Cl. septicum,* black disease caused by *Cl. novyi,* gas-gangrene caused by *Cl. sordellii,* and enterotoxemia and enteritis caused by *Cl. perfringens* types B, C, and D. Although *Cl. perfringens* type B is not a significant problem in North America, immunity is provided by the beta toxoid of type C and the epsilon toxoid of type D.

Directions: Shake well.

Cattle: Aseptically administer 5 mL subcutaneously, followed by a second dose 4-6 weeks later. In accordance with Beef Quality Assurance guidelines, this product should be administered subcutaneously (SC) under the skin.

Sheep: Aseptically administer 2½ mL subcutaneously, followed by a second dose 4-6 weeks later. Annual revaccination with a single dose is recommended.

Precaution(s): Store at 2°-7°C. Do not freeze. Use entire contents when first opened.

Caution(s): As with many vaccines, anaphylaxis may occur after use. Initial antidote of epinephrine is recommended and should be followed with appropriate supportive therapy.

Warning(s): Do not vaccinate within 21 days before slaughter. For veterinary use only.

Presentation: 10 dose, 50 dose, and 200 dose plastic vials. Color coded labels.

Compendium Code No.: 36900230 85-4381-04

ULTRABAC® 7/SOMUBAC®

Pfizer Animal Health **Bacterin-Toxoid**

Clostridium Chauvoei-Septicum-Novyi-Sordellii-Perfringens Types C & D-Haemophilus Somnus Bacterin-Toxoid

U.S. Vet. Lic. No.: 189

Description: ULTRABAC® 7 consists of killed, standardized cultures of *Cl. chauvoei, Cl. septicum, Cl. novyi, Cl. sordellii, Cl. perfringens* types C and D, and *H. somnus,* with an adjuvant.

Indications: For use in healthy cattle and calves 3 months of age or older as an aid in preventing blackleg caused by *Clostridium chauvoei,* malignant edema caused by *Cl. septicum,* black disease caused by *Cl. novyi,* gas-gangrene caused by *Cl. sordellii,* enterotoxemia and enteritis caused by *Cl. perfringens* types B, C, and D, and disease caused by *Haemophilus somnus.* Although *Cl. perfringens* type B is not a significant problem in North America, immunity is provided by the beta toxoid of type C and the epsilon toxoid of type D.

Directions: Shake well. Aseptically administer 5 mL subcutaneously, followed by a second dose 4-6 weeks later. In accordance with Beef Quality Assurance guidelines, this product should be administered subcutaneously (SC) under the skin. Annual revaccination with a single dose is recommended.

Precaution(s): Store at 2°-7°C. Do not freeze.

Use entire contents when first opened.

Caution(s): As with many vaccines, anaphylaxis may occur after use. Initial antidote of epinephrine is recommended and should be followed with appropriate supportive therapy.

Warning(s): Do not vaccinate within 21 days before slaughter. For veterinary use only.

Presentation: 10 dose, 50 dose, and 200 dose plastic vials. Color coded labels.

Compendium Code No.: 36900240 85-4384-05

ULTRABAC® 8

Pfizer Animal Health **Bacterin-Toxoid**

Clostridium Chauvoei-Septicum-Haemolyticum-Novyi-Sordellii-Perfringens Types C & D Bacterin-Toxoid

U.S. Vet. Lic. No.: 189

Description: ULTRABAC® 8 consists of killed, standardized cultures of *Cl. chauvoei, Cl. septicum, Cl. haemolyticum, Cl. novyi, Cl. sordellii,* and *Cl. perfringens* types C and D, with an adjuvant.

Indications: For use in healthy cattle and sheep as an aid in preventing blackleg caused by *Clostridium chauvoei,* malignant edema caused by *Cl. septicum,* bacillary hemoglobinuria caused by *Cl. haemolyticum,* black disease caused by *Cl. novyi,* gas-gangrene caused by *Cl. sordellii,* and enterotoxemia and enteritis caused by *Cl. perfringens* types B, C, and D. Although *Cl. perfringens* type B is not a significant problem in North America, immunity is provided by the beta toxoid of type C and the epsilon toxoid of type D.

Directions: Shake well.

Cattle: Aseptically administer 5 mL subcutaneously, followed by a second dose 4-6 weeks later. In accordance with Beef Quality Assurance guidelines, this product should be administered subcutaneously (SC) under the skin.

Sheep: Aseptically administer 2½ mL subcutaneously, followed by a second dose 4-6 weeks later. For *Cl. haemolyticum,* repeat the dose every 5-6 months in animals subject to reexposure. Annual revaccination with a single dose is recommended.

Precaution(s): Store at 2°-7°C. Do not freeze.

Use entire contents when first opened.

Caution(s): As with many vaccines, anaphylaxis may occur after use. Initial antidote of epinephrine is recommended and should be followed with appropriate supportive therapy.

Warning(s): Do not vaccinate within 21 days before slaughter.

For veterinary use only.

Presentation: 10 dose, 50 dose, and 200 dose plastic vials. Color coded labels.

Compendium Code No.: 36900250 85-4387-04

ULTRABAC® CD

Pfizer Animal Health **Bacterin-Toxoid**

Clostridium Perfringens Types C & D Bacterin-Toxoid

U.S. Vet. Lic. No.: 189

Description: ULTRABAC® CD consists of killed, standardized cultures of *Cl. perfringens* types C and D, with an adjuvant.

Indications: For use in healthy cattle and sheep as an aid in preventing enterotoxemia and enteritis caused by *Cl. perfringens* types B, C, and D. Although *Cl. perfringens* type B is not a significant problem in North America, immunity is provided by the beta toxoid of type C and the epsilon toxoid of type D.

Directions: Shake well.

Cattle: Aseptically administer 5 mL subcutaneously, followed by a second dose 4-6 weeks later. In accordance with Beef Quality Assurance guidelines, this product should be administered subcutaneously (SC) under the skin.

Sheep: Aseptically administer 1 mL subcutaneously, followed by a second dose 4-6 weeks later. Annual revaccination with a single dose is recommended.

Precaution(s): Store at 2°-7°C. Do not freeze.

Use entire contents when first opened.

Caution(s): As with many vaccines, anaphylaxis may occur after use. Initial antidote of epinephrine is recommended and should be followed with appropriate supportive therapy.

Warning(s): Do not vaccinate within 21 days before slaughter.

For veterinary use only.

Presentation: 10 dose and 50 dose plastic vials. Color coded labels.

Compendium Code No.: 36900260 85-4388-04

ULTRA BOSS® POUR-ON INSECTICIDE

Schering-Plough **Topical Insecticide**

EPA No.: 773-84

Active Ingredient(s):

Permethrin: (3-phenoxyphenyl)methyl (±)-cis, trans-3-(2,2-dichloroethenyl-2,2-dimethylcyclopropanecarboxylate* 5.00%
Piperonyl Butoxide Technical** 5.00%
Inert Ingredients*** 90.00%
Total 100.00%

*cis/trans ratio Min 35% (±) cis and Max 65% (±) trans

**Equivalent to 4.5% (butylcarbityl) (6-propylpiperonyl) ether and 0.5% related compounds

***contains petroleum distillates

Indications: Pour-on insecticide for cattle and sheep.

For lactating and non-lactating dairy cattle and beef cattle and calves.

Controls lice and flies on cattle - controls keds and lice on sheep.

Directions for Use: It is a violation of Federal law to use this product in a manner inconsistent with its labeling.

Ready to Use - No dilution necessary.

Apply to	Target Species	Dosage
Lactating and non-lactating dairy cattle and beef cattle and calves	Lice, Horn flies, Face flies Aids in control of Horse flies, Stable flies, Mosquitoes, Black flies and Ticks	Apply 3 mL per 100 lbs. body weight of animal up to a maximum of 30 mL for any one animal. Pour along back and down face. Back Rubber Use: Mix 100 mL per gallon of #2 diesel oil or mineral oil. Keep rubbing device charged. Results improved by daily forced use.
Sheep	Sheep keds, Lice	Pour along back. Apply 1.5 mL per 50 lbs. of body weight of animal up to a maximum of 18 mL for any one animal.

For cattle and sheep, repeat treatment as needed but not more than once every two weeks. For optimum lice control, two treatments at 14-day intervals are recommended.

Special Note: ULTRAS BOSS® Pour-On Insecticide is not effective against cattle grubs.

Precautionary Statements: Hazards to Humans and Domestic Animals:

Caution - Harmful if swallowed or absorbed through the skin. Avoid contact with skin, eyes or clothing. Wash thoroughly with soap and water after handling. Prolonged or frequently repeated skin contact may cause allergic reactions in some individuals.

Statement of Practical Treatment:

If Swallowed: Call a physician immediately. Do not induce vomiting unless under medical attention.

Note to Physician: Solvent represents aspiration hazard. Gastric lavage is indicated if material was taken internally.

If in Eyes: Immediately flush eyes with plenty of water. Get medical attention if irritation persists.

If on Skin: Wash skin with plenty of soap and water. Get medical attention if irritation persists.

Environmental Hazards: This product is extremely toxic to fish and other aquatic invertebrates. Do not add directly to water. Do not contaminate water by cleaning of equipment or disposal of wastes. Apply this product only as specified on label.

Storage and Disposal: Do not contaminate water, food or feed by storage or disposal.

Storage: Keep container sealed when not in use. Do not store near food or feed.

Pesticide disposal: Wastes resulting from the use of this product may be disposed of on-site or at an approved waste-disposal facility.

Container disposal: Triple rinse (or equivalent). Then offer for recycling or reconditioning, or puncture and dispose of in a sanitary landfill or incineration, or, if allowed by state and local authorities, by burning. If burned, stay out of smoke.

Warning(s): Keep out of reach of children.

Disclaimer: Notice of Warranty: Schering-Plough Animal Health Corporation makes no warranty of merchantability, fitness for any particular purpose, or otherwise expressed or implied concerning this product or its uses which extend beyond the use of this product under normal conditions and in accord with the statement on the label.

Presentation: 1 U.S. quart (0.946 L) in a Squeeze 'N' Measure™ bottle (NDC 0061-5260-02) and 1 U.S. gallon (3.785 L) (NDC 0061-5260-01).

Compendium Code No.: 10472031 Rev. 8/99

ULTRACHOICE™ 7

Pfizer Animal Health **Bacterin-Toxoid**

Clostridium Chauvoei-Septicum-Novyi-Sordellii-Perfringens Types C & D Bacterin-Toxoid

U.S. Vet. Lic. No.: 189

Description: This product consists of killed, standardized cultures of *Clostridium chauvoei, Cl. septicum, Cl. novyi, Cl. sordellii,* and *Cl. perfringens* types C and D, with a special, water-soluble adjuvant (Stimugen™).

Contains formalin as preservative.

Indications: For use in healthy cattle and sheep as an aid in preventing blackleg caused by *Cl. chauvoei;* malignant edema caused by *Cl. septicum;* black disease caused by *Cl. novyi;* gas-gangrene caused by *Cl. sordellii;* and enterotoxemia and enteritis caused by *Cl. perfringens* types B, C, and D. Although *Cl. perfringens* type B is not a significant problem in North America, immunity is provided by the beta toxoid of type C and the epsilon toxoid of type D.

Directions: Shake well. Cattle: Aseptically administer 2 mL. In accordance with Beef Quality Assurance guidelines, this product should be administered subcutaneously (SC) under the skin. Healthy cattle should receive 2 doses administered 4-6 weeks apart. Sheep: Aseptically administer 1 mL subcutaneously in the neck, followed by a second dose 4-6 weeks later. Annual revaccination with a single dose is recommended.

Precaution(s): Store at 2°-7°C. Do not freeze. Use entire contents when first opened.

Caution(s): Temporary local swelling at injection site may occur after administration. As with many vaccines, anaphylaxis may occur after use. Initial antidote of epinephrine is recommended and should be followed with appropriate supportive therapy.

Warning(s): Do not vaccinate within 21 days before slaughter.

For veterinary use only.

Presentation: 10 doses, 50 doses and 250 doses.

Compendium Code No.: 36900760 85-5064-01

ULTRACHOICE™ 8

Pfizer Animal Health **Bacterin-Toxoid**

Clostridium Chauvoei-Septicum-Novyi-Sordellii-Perfringens Types C & D Bacterin-Toxoid

U.S. Vet. Lic. No.: 189

Description: This product consists of killed, standardized cultures of *Clostridium chauvoei, Cl. septicum, Cl. haemolyticum, Cl. novyi, Cl. sordellii,* and *Cl. perfringens* types C and D, with a special, water-soluble adjuvant (Stimugen™).

Contains formalin as preservative.

Indications: For use in healthy cattle and sheep as an aid in preventing blackleg caused by *Cl. chauvoei;* malignant edema caused by *Cl. septicum;* bacillary hemoglobinuria caused by *Cl. haemolyticum;* black disease caused by *Cl. novyi;* gas-gangrene caused by *Cl. sordellii;* and enterotoxemia and enteritis caused by *Cl. perfringens* types B, C, and D. Although *Cl. perfringens* type B is not a significant problem in North America, immunity is provided by the beta toxoid of type C and the epsilon toxoid of type D.

Directions: Shake well. Cattle: Aseptically administer 2 mL. In accordance with Beef Quality Assurance guidelines, this product should be administered subcutaneously (SC) under the skin. Healthy cattle should receive 2 doses administered 4-6 weeks apart. Sheep: Aseptically administer 1 mL subcutaneously in the neck, followed by a second dose 4-6 weeks later. For *Cl. haemolyticum* repeat the dose every 6 months in animals subject to reexposure. Annual revaccination with a single dose is recommended.

Precaution(s): Store at 2°-7°C. Do not freeze. Use entire contents when first opened.

Caution(s): Temporary local swelling at injection site may occur after administration. As with many vaccines, anaphylaxis may occur after use. Initial antidote of epinephrine is recommended and should be followed with appropriate supportive therapy.

Warning(s): Do not vaccinate within 21 days before slaughter.

For veterinary use only.

Presentation: 10 doses, 50 doses and 250 doses.

Compendium Code No.: 36900770 85-5067-01

ULTRACHOICE™ CD

Pfizer Animal Health **Bacterin-Toxoid**

Clostridium Perfringens Types C & D Bacterin-Toxoid

U.S. Vet. Lic. No.: 189

Description: This product consists of killed, standardized cultures of *Clostridium perfringens* types C and D, with a special, water-soluble adjuvant (Stimugen™).

Contains formalin as preservative.

Indications: For use in healthy cattle and sheep as an aid in preventing enterotoxemia and enteritis caused *by Cl. perfringens* types B, C, and D. Although *Cl. perfringens* type B is not a significant problem in North America, immunity is provided by the beta toxoid of type C and the epsilon toxoid of type D.

Directions: Shake well. Cattle: Aseptically administer 2 mL. In accordance with Beef Quality Assurance guidelines, this product should be administered subcutaneously (SC) under the skin. Healthy cattle should receive 2 doses administered 4-6 weeks apart. Sheep: Aseptically administer 1 mL subcutaneously in the neck, followed by a second dose 4-6 weeks later. Annual revaccination with a single dose is recommended.

Precaution(s): Store at 2°-7°C. Do not freeze. Use entire contents when first opened.

Caution(s): Temporary local swelling at injection site may occur after administration. As with many vaccines, anaphylaxis may occur after use. Initial antidote of epinephrine is recommended and should be followed with appropriate supportive therapy.

Warning(s): Do not vaccinate within 21 days before slaughter.

For veterinary use only.

Presentation: 10 doses and 50 doses.

Compendium Code No.: 36900780 85-5061-01

ULTRA-DYNE™

Westfalia•Surge **Udder Wash**

3.5% Iodine Detergent Udder Wash

Active Ingredient(s):

Titratable iodine 3.5%

Indications: 3.5% iodine detergent udder wash.

Directions for Use:

For Udder Washing: Prepare a fresh solution of 25 p.p.m. iodine. Wash teats with solution using a separate towel for each cow. (Do not reuse the towel.) Dry teats with separate towel for each cow and examine each quarter with strip cup. After milking, use an approved teat dip. Submerge entire teat and allow to dry. Do not wipe.

Use Dilution: 1 oz ULTRA-DYNE™ in 13 gallons of water gives 25 p.p.m. titratable iodine. 1 oz ULTRA-DYNE™ in 6½ gallons of water gives 50 p.p.m. titratable iodine.

Always use fresh solution. Change solution when the solution becomes visually dirty.

If frozen, thaw completely and mix well before using.

Contraindication(s): Do not use as a teat dip.

Precautionary Statements:

Danger: Corrosive. Contains phosphoric acid. Causes severe burns to eyes. May cause skin burns. May be harmful or fatal if swallowed. Protect eyes and skin when handling. Do not take internally. Avoid breathing vapors. Avoid contamination of food. Refer to Material Safety Data Sheet (MSDS).

First Aid:

If in Eyes: Flush immediately with large volumes of water for at least 15 minutes. Call a physician immediately.

If Swallowed: Do not induce vomiting. Rinse mouth promptly then give a small amount/glass of water. Call a physician immediately. Do not give anything by mouth to an unconscious or convulsing person.

If on Skin: Flush immediately with large volumes of water for at least 15 minutes while removing contaminated clothing and shoes. If irritation persists, get medical attention.

Inhalation of Vapors: If breathing difficulty or irritation occurs, remove to fresh air. If symptoms persist, get medical attention.

Warning(s): Keep out of reach of children.

Presentation: Contact the company for container sizes available.

Compendium Code No.: 10020191

ULTRA™ EAR MITICIDE

Bimeda **Otic Parasiticide**

Active Ingredient(s): Contains:

Rotenone 0.12%
Cube resins 0.16%
Inert ingredients 99.72%

Indications: Kills ear mites on dogs, cats and rabbits. Dislodges and dissolves blockages due to ear wax.

Directions for Use: It is a violation of federal law to use the product in a manner inconsistent with its labeling.

While holding the pet firmly, fill each ear canal half full of EAR MITICIDE and massage the base of the ear to ensure that the insecticide action penetrates the ear wax. Repeat the treatment every other day until the condition is relieved. Improvement is usually noted after two (2) applications.

Precautionary Statements: Hazardous to Humans and Domestic Animals: Harmful if swallowed. Avoid inhaling vapors. Avoid contact with skin.

Environmental Hazards: This product is toxic to fish, birds, and other wildlife. Do not apply directly to water. Do not contaminate water by the cleaning of equipment or the disposal of wastes.

Warning(s): Keep out of the reach of children.

Presentation: 2 oz. dropper bottle with applicator tip.

Compendium Code No.: 13990430

ULTRAGROOM™ SHAMPOO

Virbac **Grooming Shampoo**

Ingredient(s): Contains: Chitosanide, urea and glycerin are present in encapsulated (Spherulites®) and free forms. Peach fragrance is present in free form. Purified water, sodium lauryl sulfate, lauramide DEA, sodium chloride, citric acid, sodium hydroxide, DMDM hydantoin in free form. Also contains FD&C color.

Indications: ULTRAGROOM™ is a routine grooming shampoo for dogs and cats of any age.

Directions for Use: Shake well before use. Wet the coat with warm water and apply sufficient shampoo to create a rich lather. Massage ULTRAGROOM™ into wet coat, lather freely. Rinse and repeat as necessary.

Caution(s): For topical use only. Avoid contact with eyes. In case of contact, flush eyes with water and seek medical attention if irritation persists.

Available through licensed veterinarians only.

Warning(s): Keep out of reach of children.

Discussion: ULTRAGROOM™ contains Spherulites®, an exclusive and patented encapsulation system developed by Virbac to provide slow release of ingredients long after the shampoo is rinsed off.

Presentation: 1 gallon (3.79 L).

Compendium Code No.: 10230580

ULTRAMECTRIN™ INJECTION

RXV **Parasiticide Injection**

(ivermectin) Injection 1% Sterile Solution

NADA No.: 128-409

Active Ingredient(s): ULTRAMECTRIN™ Injection is a clear, ready-to-use, sterile solution containing 1% ivermectin, 40% glycerol formal, and propylene glycol, q.s. ad 100%. ULTRAMECTRIN™ Injection is formulated to deliver the recommended dose level of 200 mcg ivermectin/kilogram of body weight in cattle when given subcutaneously at the rate of 1 mL/110 lb (50 kg). In swine, ULTRAMECTRIN™ Injection is formulated to deliver the recommended dose level of 300 mcg ivermectin/kilogram of body weight when given subcutaneously in the neck at the rate of 1 mL per 75 lb (33 kg).

Indications: A parasiticide for the treatment and control of internal and external parasites in cattle and swine.

Cattle: ULTRAMECTRIN™ Injection is indicated for the effective treatment and control of the following harmful species of gastrointestinal roundworms, lungworms, grubs, sucking lice, and mange mites in cattle:

Gastrointestinal Roundworms (adults and fourth-stage larvae): *Ostertagia ostertagi* (including inhibited *O. ostertagi), O. lyrata, Haemonchus placei, Trichostrongylus axei, T. colubriformis, Cooperia oncophora, C. punctata, C. pectinata, Oesophagostomum radiatum, Bunostomum phlebotomum, Nematodirus helvetianus* (adults only), *N. spathiger* (adults only).

Lungworms (adults and fourth-stage larvae): *Dictyocaulus viviparus.*

Cattle Grubs (parasitic stages): *Hypoderma bovis, H. lineatum.*

Sucking Lice: *Linognathus vituli, Haematopinus eurysternus, Solenopotes capillatus.*

Mites (scabies): *Psoroptes ovis* (syn. *P. communis* var. *bovis), Sarcoptes scabiei* var. *bovis.*

Further studies have shown that ULTRAMECTRIN™ Injection given at the recommended dosage controls infections of *Dictyocaulus viviparus* and *Ostertagia ostertagi* for 21 days after treatment; *Oesophagostomum radiatum, Haemonchus placei, Trichostrongylus axei, Cooperia punctata* and *Cooperia oncophora* for 14 days after treatment.

Swine: ULTRAMECTRIN™ Injection is indicated for the effective treatment and control of the following harmful species of gastrointestinal roundworms, lungworms, lice, and mange mites in swine:

Gastrointestinal Roundworms:

Large roundworm: *Ascaris suum* (adults and fourth-stage larvae).

Red stomach worm: *Hyostrongylus rubidus* (adults and fourth-stage larvae).

Nodular worm: *Oesophagostomum* spp (adults and fourth-stage larvae).

Threadworm: *Strongyloides ransomi* (adults).

Somatic Roundworm Larvae:

Threadworm: *Strongyloides ransomi* (somatic larvae).

Sows must be treated at least seven days before farrowing to prevent infection in piglets.

Lungworms:

Metastrongylus spp (adults).

Lice:

Haematopinus suis.

Mange Mites:

Sarcoptes scabiei var. *suis.*

Reindeer: For the treatment and control of warbles *(Oedemagena tarandi)* in reindeer.

Pharmacology: Product Description: Ivermectin is derived from the avermectins, a family of potent, broad-spectrum antiparasitic agents isolated from fermentation of *Streptomyces avermitilis.*

Mode of Action: Ivermectin is a member of the macrocyclic lactone class of endectocides which have a unique mode of action. Compounds of the class bind selectively and with high affinity to glutamate-gated chloride ion channels which occur in invertebrate nerve and muscle cells. This leads to an increase in the permeability of the cell membrane to chloride ions with hyperpolarization of the nerve or muscle cell, resulting in paralysis and death of the parasite. Compounds of this class may also interact with other ligand-gated chloride channels, such as those gated by the neurotransmitter gamma-aminobutyric acid (GABA).

The wide margin of safety is attributable to the fact that mammals do not have glutamate-gated chloride channels, the macrocyclic lactones have a low affinity for other mammalian ligand-gated chloride channels and they do not readily cross the blood-brain barrier.

Dosage and Administration: Dosage:

Cattle: ULTRAMECTRIN™ Injection should be given only by subcutaneous injection under the loose skin in front of or behind the shoulder at the recommended dose level of 200 mcg of ivermectin per kilogram of body weight. Each mL of ULTRAMECTRIN™ contains 10 mg of ivermectin, sufficient to treat 110 lb (50 kg) of body weight (maximum 10 mL per injection site).

Body Weight (lb)	Dose Volume (mL)
220	2
330	3
440	4
550	5
660	6
770	7
990	9
1100	10

Swine: ULTRAMECTRIN™ Injection should be given only by subcutaneous injection in the neck of swine at the recommended dose level of 300 mcg of ivermectin per kilogram (2.2 lb) of body weight. Each mL of ULTRAMECTRIN™ contains 10 mg of ivermectin, sufficient to treat 75 lb of body weight.

	Body Weight (lb)	Dose Volume (mL)
Growing Pigs	19	¼
	38	½
	75	1
	150	2
Breeding Animals (Sows, Gilts, and Boars)	225	3
	300	4
	375	5
	450	6

Administration:

Cattle: ULTRAMECTRIN™ Injection is to be given subcutaneously only, to reduce risk of potentially fatal clostridial infection of the injection site. Animals should be appropriately restrained to achieve the proper route of administration. Use of a 16-gauge ½ to ¾" needle is suggested. Inject under the loose skin in front of or behind the shoulder (see illustration).

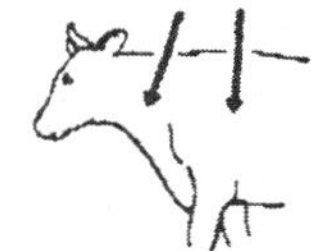

When using the 200 mL or 500 mL pack size, use only automatic syringe equipment.

Use sterile equipment and sanitize the injection site by applying a suitable disinfectant. Clean, properly disinfected needles should be used to reduce the potential for injection site infection. No special handling or protective clothing is necessary.

Swine: ULTRAMECTRIN™ Injection is to be given subcutaneously in the neck. Animals should be appropriately restrained to achieve the proper route of administration. Use of a 16- or 18-gauge needle is suggested for sows and boars, while an 18- or 20-gauge needle may be appropriate for young animals. Inject under the skin, immediately behind the ear (see illustration).

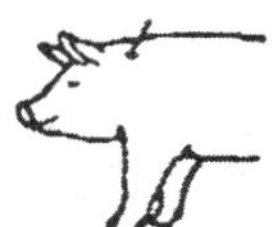

When using the 200 mL or 500 mL pack size, use only automatic syringe equipment. As with any injection, sterile equipment should be used. The injection site should be cleaned and disinfected with alcohol before injection. The rubber stopper should also be disinfected with alcohol to prevent contamination of the contents. Mild and transient pain reactions may be seen in some swine following subcutaneous administration.

Recommended Treatment Program:

Swine: At the time of initiating any parasite control program, it is important to treat all breeding animals in the herd. After the initial treatment, use ULTRAMECTRIN™ Injection regularly as follows:

Breeding Animals:

Sows: Treat prior to farrowing, preferably 7-14 days before, to minimize infection of piglets.

Gilts: Treat 7-14 days prior to breeding. Treat 7-14 days prior to farrowing.

Boars: Frequently and need for treatments are dependent upon exposure.

Treat at least two times a year.

Feeder Pigs (Weaners/Growers/Finishers): All weaner/feeder pigs should be treated before placement in clean quarters.

Pigs exposed to contaminated soil or pasture may need retreatment if reinfection occurs.

Note:

1. ULTRAMECTRIN™ Injection has a persistent drug level sufficient to control mite infestations throughout the egg to adult life cycle. However, since the ivermectin effect is not immediate, care must be taken to prevent reinfestation from exposure to untreated animals or contaminated facilities. Generally, pigs should not be moved to clean quarters or exposed to uninfested pigs for approximately one week after treatment. Sows should be treated at least one week before farrowing to minimize transfer of mites to newborn baby pigs.
2. Louse eggs are unaffected by ULTRAMECTRIN™ Injection and may require up to three weeks to hatch. Louse infestations developing from hatching eggs may require retreatment.
3. Consult a veterinarian for aid in the diagnosis and control of internal and external parasites of swine.

Special Minor Use:

Reindeer: For the treatment and control of warbles *(Oedemagena tarandi)* in reindeer, inject 200 micrograms ivermectin per kilogram of body weight, subcutaneously. Follow use directions for cattle as described under Administration.

Consult your veterinarian for assistance in the diagnosis, treatment and control of parasitism.

Contraindication(s): ULTRAMECTRIN™ Injection for Cattle and Swine has been developed specifically for use in cattle, swine, and reindeer only. This product should not be used in other animal species as severe adverse reactions, including fatalities in dogs, may result.

Precaution(s): Protect product from light.

Environmental Safety: Studies indicate that when ivermectin comes in contact with the soil, it readily and tightly binds to the soil and becomes inactive over time. Free ivermectin may adversely affect fish and certain water-borne organisms on which they feed. Do not permit water runoff from feedlots or production sites to enter lakes, streams, or ponds. Do not contaminate water by direct application or by the improper disposal of drug containers. Dispose of containers in an approved landfill or by incineration.

Caution(s): Transitory discomfort has been observed in some cattle following subcutaneous administration. A low incidence of soft tissue swelling at the injection site has been observed. These reactions have disappeared without treatment. For cattle, divide doses greater than 10 mL between two injection sites to reduce occasional discomfort or site reaction.

Use sterile equipment and sanitize the injection site by applying a suitable disinfectant. Clean, properly disinfected needles should be used to reduce the potential for injection site infections.

Observe cattle for injection site reactions. Reactions may be due to clostridial infection and should be aggressively treated with appropriate antibiotics. If injection site infections are suspected, consult your veterinarian.

ULTRAMECTRIN™ effectively controls all stages of cattle grubs. However, proper timing of treatment is important. For most effective results, cattle should be treated as soon as possible after the end of the heel fly (warble fly) season.

Destruction of *Hypoderma* larvae (cattle grubs) at the period when these grubs are in vital areas may cause undesirable host-parasite reactions including the possibility of fatalities. Killing *Hypoderma lineatum* when it is in the tissue surrounding the esophagus (gullet) may cause salivation and bloat; killing *H. bovis* when it is in the vertebral canal may cause staggering or paralysis. These reactions are not specific to treatment with ULTRAMECTRIN™, but can occur with any successful treatment of grubs. Cattle should be treated either before or after these stages of grub development. Consult your veterinarian concerning the proper time for treatment.

Cattle treated with ULTRAMECTRIN™ after the end of the heel fly season may be retreated with ULTRAMECTRIN™ during the winter for internal parasites, mange mites, or sucking lice without danger of grub-related reactions. A planned parasite control program is recommended.

This product is not for intravenous or intramuscular use.

Warning(s): Do not treat cattle within 35 days of slaughter. Because a withdrawal time in milk has not been established, do not use in female dairy cattle of breeding age.

Do not treat swine within 18 days of slaughter.

Do not treat reindeer within 8 weeks (56 days) of slaughter.

Keep this and all drugs out of the reach of children.

Presentation: ULTRAMECTRIN™ Injection for Cattle and Swine is available in three ready-to-use pack sizes:

The 50 mL pack is a multiple-dose, rubber-capped bottle. Each bottle contains sufficient solution to treat 10 head of 550 lb (250 kg) cattle or 100 head of 38 lb (17.3 kg) swine.

The 200 mL pack is a soft, collapsible pack designed for use with automatic syringe equipment. Each pack contains sufficient solution to treat 40 head of 550 lb (250 kg) cattle or 400 head of 38 lb (17.3 kg) swine.

The 500 mL pack is a soft, collapsible pack designed for use with automatic syringe equipment. Each pack contains sufficient solution to treat 100 head of 550 lb (250 kg) cattle or 1000 head of 38 lb (17.3 kg) swine.

Compendium Code No.: 10910210

ULTRAMECTRIN™ POUR-ON

RXV **Parasiticide-Topical**

(ivermectin) Pour-On 5 mg per mL

NADA No.: 140-841

Active Ingredient(s): ULTRAMECTRIN™ Pour-On is an 0.5% w/v blue-colored solution of ivermectin.

Indications: ULTRAMECTRIN™ Pour-On applied at the recommended dose level of 500 mcg/kg is indicated for the effective control of these parasites.

Gastrointestinal Roundworms: *Ostertagia ostertagi* (including inhibited stage) (adults and L_4), *Haemonchus placei* (adults and L_4), *Trichostrongylus axei* (adults and L_4), *T. colubriformis* (adults and L_4), *Cooperia* spp. (adults and L_4), *Strongyloides papillosus* (adults), *Oesophagostomum radiatum* (adults and L_4), *Trichuris* spp. (adults).

Lungworms: *Dictyocaulus viviparus* (adults and L_4).

Cattle Grubs (parasitic stages): *Hypoderma bovis, H. lineatum.*

Mites: *Sarcoptes scabiei* var. *bovis.*

Lice: *Linognathus vituli, Haematopinus eurysternus, Damalinia bovis, Solenopotes capillatus.*

Horn Flies: *Haematobia irritans.*

Pharmacology: Mode of Action: Ivermectin as a member of the avermectin family kills certain parasitic roundworms and ectoparasites, such as mites, lice, horn flies and other insects. Its action is unique to the avermectin class of antiparasitic agents. This action involves a chemical that serves as a signal from one nerve cell to another, or from a nerve cell to a muscle cell. This chemical, a neurotransmitter, is called gamma-amino-butyric acid or GABA.

In roundworms, ivermectin stimulates the release of GABA from nerve endings and enhances binding of GABA to special receptors at nerve junctions, thus interrupting nerve impulses — thereby paralyzing and killing the parasite.

The enhancement of the GABA effect in arthropods such as mites, lice, and horn flies resembles that in roundworms except that nerve impulses are interrupted between the nerve ending and the muscle cell. Again, this leads to paralysis and death.

Ivermectin has no measurable effect against flukes or tapeworms, presumably because they do not have GABA as a nerve impulse transmitter.

The principal peripheral neurotransmitter in mammals, acetylcholine, is unaffected by ivermectin. Ivermectin does not readily penetrate the central nervous system of mammals where GABA functions as a neurotransmitter.

Dosage and Administration:

Treatment of Cattle for Horn Flies: ULTRAMECTRIN™ Pour-On controls horn flies *(Haematobia irritans)* for up to 28 days after dosing. For best results, ULTRAMECTRIN™ Pour-On should be part of a parasite control program for both internal and external parasites based on the epidemiology of these parasites. Consult your veterinarian or an entomologist for the most effective timing of applications.

Dosage: The dose rate is 1 mL for each 22 lb of body weight. The formulation should be applied along the topline in a narrow strip extending from the withers to the tailhead.

Administration:

Squeeze-Measure-Pour System (33.8 fl oz/1 Liter Bottles with 50 mL Metering Cup: Attach the metering cap to the bottle.

Set the dose by turning the top section of the cup to align the correct body weight with the pointer on the knurled cap. When body weight is between markings, use the higher setting.

Hold the bottle upright and squeeze it to deliver a slight excess of the required dose as indicated by the calibration lines.

By releasing the pressure, the dose automatically adjusts to the correct level. Tilt the bottle to deliver the dose. When 220 lb (10 mL) or 330 lb (15 mL) dose is required, turn the pointer to "Stop" before delivering the dose. The off (Stop) position will close the system between dosing.

Collapsible Pack (84.5 fl oz/2.5 L Pack and 169 fl oz/5 L Pack): Connect the applicator gun to the collapsible pack as follows:

Attach the open end of the draw-off tubing to the dosing equipment. (Because of the solvents used in the formulation, only the Protector Drench Gun from Instrument Supplies Limited, or equivalent, is recommended. Other applicators may exhibit compatibility problems resulting in locking, incorrect dosage or leakage.) Replace the shipping cap with the draw-off cap and tighten down. Attach draw-off tubing to the draw-off cap.

Gently prime the applicator gun, checking for leaks.

Follow the manufacturer's directions for adjusting the dose.

When the interval between uses of the applicator gun is expected to exceed 12 hours, disconnect the gun and draw-off tubing from the product container and empty the product from the gun and tubing back into the product container. To prevent removal of special lubricants from the Protector Drench Gun, the gun and tubing must not be washed.

When to Treat Cattle with Grubs: ULTRAMECTRIN™ Pour-On effectively controls all stages of cattle grubs. However, proper timing of treatment is important. For the most effective results, cattle should be treated as soon as possible after the end of the heel fly (warble fly) season. While this is not peculiar to ivermectin, destruction of *Hypoderma* larvae (cattle grubs) at the period when these grubs are in vital areas may cause undesirable host-parasite reactions. Killing *Hypoderma lineatum* when it is in the esophageal tissues may cause bloat; killing *H. bovis* when it is in the vertebral canal may cause staggering or paralysis. Cattle should be treated either before or after these stages of grub development.

Cattle treated with ULTRAMECTRIN™ Pour-On at the end of the fly season may be re-treated with ULTRAMECTRIN™ during the winter without danger of grub-related reactions. For further information and advice on a planned parasite control program, consult your veterinarian.

Safety: Studies conducted in the U.S.A. have demonstrated the safety margin for ivermectin. Based on plasma levels, the topically applied formulation is expected to be at least as well tolerated by breeding animals as is the subcutaneous formulation which had no effect on breeding performance.

Consult your veterinarian for assistance in the diagnosis, treatment and control of parasitism.

Precaution(s): Flammable!

Keep away from heat, sparks, open flame, and other sources of ignition.

Store away from excessive heat (104°F/40°C) and protect from light.

Use only in well-ventilated areas or outdoors.

Close container tightly when not in use.

Cloudiness in the formulation may occur when ULTRAMECTRIN™ (ivermectin) Pour-On is stored at temperatures below 32°F. Allowing to warm at room temperature will restore the normal appearance without affecting efficacy.

Environmental Safety: Studies indicate that when ivermectin comes in contact with the soil, it readily and tightly binds to the soil and becomes inactive over time. Free ivermectin may adversely affect fish or certain water-borne organisms on which they feed. Do not permit cattle to enter lakes, streams, or ponds for at least six hours after treatment. Do not contaminate water by direct application or by the improper disposal of drug containers. Dispose of containers in an approved landfill or by incineration.

Caution(s): Cattle should not be treated when hair or hide is wet since reduced efficacy may be experienced.

Do not use when rain is expected to wet cattle within six hours after treatment.

This product is for application to skin surface only. Do not give orally or parenterally.

Antiparasitic activity of ivermectin will be impaired if the formulation is applied to areas of the skin with mange scabs or lesions, or with dermatoses or adherent materials, e.g., caked mud or manure.

Ivermectin has been associated with adverse reaction in sensitive dogs; therefore, ULTRAMECTRIN™ Pour-On is not recommended for use in species other than cattle.

Warning(s): Cattle must not be treated within 48 days of slaughter for human consumption. Because a withdrawal time in milk has not been established, do not use on female dairy cattle of breeding age.

Not for use in humans.

This product should not be applied to self or others because it may be irritating to human skin and eyes and absorbed through the skin. To minimize accidental skin contact, the user should wear a long-sleeved shirt and rubber gloves. If accidental skin contact occurs, wash immediately with soap and water. If accidental eye exposure occurs, flush eyes immediately with water and seek medical attention.

Keep this and all drugs out of the reach of children.

Presentation: ULTRAMECTRIN™ Pour-On is available in a 33.8 fl oz/1 L bottle with a squeeze-measure-pour system, or in an 84.5 fl oz/2.5 L collapsible pack and a 169 fl oz/5 L collapsible pack intended for use with appropriate automatic correct dosing equipment.

U.S. Pat. 4,199,569

Compendium Code No.: 10910220

ULTRASPOT™ BY ABSORBINE®

W.F. Young **Parasiticide-Topical**

EPA Reg. No.: 68688-56-1543

Active Ingredient(s):

Permethrin*: [CAS #52645-53-1]	45.00%
Other Ingredient	55.00%
Total	100.00% [w/w]

* Cis/trans ratio: max 55% (±) cis and min 45% (±) trans

Indications: For biting fly protection. Kills and repels horse flies, deer flies, gnats, mosquitoes, black flies, horn flies, face flies, stable flies and house flies for up to two weeks. Kills and repels members of the *Culicoidae* and *Simuliidae,* vectors that may cause Sweet Itch, for up to two weeks.

Sweat and water resistant. Field tested. Protects up to 14 days.

For use on horses only.

Directions for Use: It is a violation of Federal law to use this product in a manner inconsistent with its labeling.

Read all directions before using this product.

Do not use on horses intended for slaughter.

Not for use on foals under three (3) months of age.

Ready to use, no dilution necessary.

Hold tube in upright position pointing away from the user's face and body, and twist off cap. Break off tip or cut with scissors. Using the cc guide marks on the tube apply ULTRASPOT™ as follows:

1. Streak 1 cc on top of the croup.
2. Streak 1 cc on the forehead under the forelock; taking care to avoid the eyes and mucous membranes.
3. Spot 1 cc over the dorsum of the carpus (from of the knee) on each of the front legs (2 cc total).
4. Spot 1 cc over the plantar surface of the tarsus (behind the hock) on each of the hind legs (2 cc in total).

Place empty applicator in trash. Do not reapply for 14 days.

May be used with Absorbine® UltraShield® Brand Residual Insecticide and Repellent.

Precautionary Statements: Hazards to Humans and Domestic Animals:

Caution: Harmful if swallowed or absorbed through skin. Causes moderate eye irritation. Avoid contact with skin, eyes or clothing. Wash thoroughly with soap and water after handling.

Sensitivities can occur after using any pesticide product for animals. If signs of sensitivity occur, wash area with mild soap and rinse with large amounts of water. If signs continue, consult a veterinarian immediately.

First Aid:

If Swallowed: Call a poison control center or doctor immediately for treatment advice. Have person sip a glass of water, if able to swallow. Do not induce vomiting unless told to do so by a poison control center or doctor.

If on Skin or Clothing: Take off contaminated clothing. Rinse skin immediately with plenty of water for 15 to 20 minutes. Call a poison control center or doctor for treatment advice.

If in Eyes: Hold eye open and rinse slowly and gently with water for 15 to 20 minutes. Remove contact lenses, if present, after first 5 minutes, then continue rinsing eyes. Call a poison control center for treatment advice.

Hot Line Number: Have the product container or label with you when calling a poison control center or doctor, or going for treatment. You may also contact 1-800-628-9653 for emergency medical treatment information.

Environmental Hazards: This product is extremely toxic to fish. Do not apply directly to water, or areas where surface water is present, or to intertidal areas below the mean high water mark. Do not contaminate water when cleaning equipment or disposing of equipment washwaters.

Chemical Hazards: Combustible. Do not use or store near heat or open flame.

Storage and Disposal: Do not contaminate water, food or feed by storage or disposal.

Pesticide Storage: Store in cool, dry place. Protect from freezing.

Pesticide Disposal: Call your local solid waste agency or [1-800-CLEANUP or equivalent organization] for disposal instructions. Unless otherwise instructed, place in trash. Never pour unused product down the drain or on the ground.

Container Disposal: Do not reuse empty container. Place in trash.

Warning(s): Do not use on horses intended for slaughter.

Keep out of reach of children.

Disclaimer: Warranty: W.F. Young, Inc., warrants that this product conforms to the chemical description on the label. W.F. Young, Inc., neither makes nor authorizes any agent or representative to make, any other warranty of fitness or of merchantability, guarantee or representation, express or implied, concerning this material. W.F. Young, Inc's maximum liability for breach of this warranty shall not exceed the purchase price of this product. Buyer and user acknowledge and assume all risks and liabilities resulting from the handling, storage and use of this material which extend beyond the use of the product under normal conditions in accord with statements made on the label.

Presentation: 2 x 6 cc and 8 x 6 cc applicators.

Compendium Code No.: 10990270 RM315950 / RM315854

UNIPET NUTRITABS®

Pharmacia & Upjohn **Small Animal Dietary Supplement**

Active Ingredient(s): Each tablet supplies: Vitamins: vitamin A, 1100 I.U.; vitamin D, 110 I.U.; vitamin E, 2.5 I.U.; thiamine (B_1), 0.2 mg; riboflavin (B_2), 0.5 mg; pantothenic acid, 2 mg; niacin, 2.25 mg; pyridoxine (B_6), 0.22 mg; folic acid, 0.04 mg; vitamin B_{12}, 4 mcg. Minerals: *calcium, 160 mg; *phosphorus, 100 mg; iron, 6.75 mg; zinc, 2.5 mg. *Supplied by bone meal and calcium phosphate.

Indications: A vitamin-mineral supplement for puppies and dogs.

Dosage and Administration: Suggested daily dosage:

Puppies: ½ to 1 tablet.

Dogs: 1 to 4 tablets.

Precaution(s): Keep container tightly closed.

Store at room temperature.

Warning(s): Not for human use. Keep out of reach of children.

Presentation: Available in bottles of 50, 150 and 300 tablets.

Manufactured by: Global Pharm Inc.

Compendium Code No.: 10490510

UNIPRIM® POWDER ℞

Macleod **Potentiated Sulfa**

ANADA No.: 200-033

Active Ingredient(s): UNIPRIM® Powder contains 67 mg trimethoprim and 333 mg sulfadiazine per gram.

Indications: Trimethoprim/sulfadiazine is indicated in horses where potent systemic antibacterial action against sensitive organisms is required. Trimethoprim/sulfadiazine is indicated where control of bacterial infections is required during treatment of: Acute strangles, acute urogenital infections, respiratory tract infections, wound infections and abscesses.

Trimethoprim/sulfadiazine is well-tolerated by foals.

Pharmacology: UNIPRIM® Powder is a combination of trimethoprim and sulfadiazine in the ratio of 1 part to 5 parts by weight, which provides effective antibacterial activity against a wide range of bacterial infections in animals.

Trimethoprim is 2, 4 diamino-5-(3,4,5- trimethoxybenzyl) pyrimidine.

Actions:

Microbiology: Trimethoprim blocks bacterial production of tetrahydrofolic acid from dihydrofolic acid by binding to and reversibly inhibiting the enzyme dihydrofolate reductase.

Sulfadiazine, in common with other sulfonamides, inhibits bacterial synthesis of dihydrofolic acid by competing with *para*-aminobenzoic acid.

Trimethoprim/sulfadiazine thus imposes a sequential double blockade of bacterial metabolism. This deprives bacteria of nucleic acids and proteins essential for survival and multiplication, and produces a high level of antibacterial activity which is usually bactericidal.

Although both sulfadiazine and trimethoprim are antifolate, neither affects the folate metabolism of animals. The reasons are: animals do not synthesize folic acid and cannot, therefore, be directly affected by sulfadiazine; and although animals must reduce their dietary folic acid to tetrahydrofolic acid, trimethoprim does not affect this reduction because its affinity for dihydrofolate reductase of mammals is significantly less than for the corresponding bacterial enzyme.

Trimethoprim/sulfadiazine is active against a wide spectrum of bacterial pathogens, both gram-negative and gram-positive. The following *in vitro* data are available, but their clinical significance is unknown. In general, species of the following genera are sensitive to trimethoprim/sulfadiazine:

Very Sensitive: Escherichia, Streptococcus, Proteus, Salmonella, Pasteurella, Shigella, Haemophilus.

Sensitive: Staphylococcus, Neisseria, Klebsiella, Fusiformis, Corynebacterium, Clostridium, Bordetella.

Moderately Sensitive: Moraxella, Nocardia, Brucella.

Not Sensitive: Mycobacterium, Leptospira, Pseudomonas, Erysipelothrix.

As a result of the sequential double blockade of the metabolism of susceptible organisms by trimethoprim and sulfadiazine, the minimum inhibitory concentration (MIC) of trimethoprim/sulfadiazine is markedly less than that of either of the components used separately. Many strains of bacteria that are not susceptible to one of the components are susceptible to trimethoprim/sulfadiazine. A synergistic effect between trimethoprim and sulfadiazine in combination has been shown experimentally both *in vitro* and *in vivo* (in dogs).

Trimethoprim/sulfadiazine is bactericidal against susceptible strains and is often effective against sulfonamide-resistant organisms. *In vitro* sulfadiazine is usually only bacteriostatic.

The precise *in vitro* MIC of the combination varies with the ratio of the drugs present, but action of trimethoprim/sulfadiazine occurs over a wide range of ratios with an increase in the concentration of one of its components compensating for a decrease in the other. It is unusual, however, to determine MIC's using a constant ratio of one part trimethoprim in twenty parts of the combination.

The following table shows MIC's, using the above ratio, of bacteria which were susceptible to both trimethoprim (TMP) and sulfadiazine (SDZ). The organisms are those most commonly involved in conditions for which trimethoprim/sulfadiazine is indicated:

Average Minimum Inhibitory Concentration (MIC-mcg/mL):

Bacteria	TMP Alone	SDZ Alone	TMP/SDZ	
			TMP	SDZ
Escherichia coli	0.31	26.5	0.07	1.31
Proteus species	1.30	24.5	0.15	2.85
Staphylococcus aureus	0.60	17.6	0.13	2.47
Pasteurella species	0.06	20.1	0.03	0.56
Salmonella species	0.15	61.0	0.05	0.95
β *Streptococcus*	0.50	24.5	0.15	2.85

The following table demonstrates the marked effect of the trimethoprim and sulfadiazine combination against sulfadiazine resistant strains of normally susceptible organisms:

Average Minimum Inhibitory Concentration of Sulfadiazine-Resistant Strains (MIC-mcg/mL):

Bacteria	TMP Alone	SDZ Alone	TMP/SDZ	
			TMP	SDZ
Escherichia coli	0.32	>245	0.27	5.0
Proteus species	0.66	>245	0.32	6.2

Susceptibility Testing: In testing susceptibility to trimethoprim/sulfadiazine, it is essential that the medium used does not contain significant amounts of interfering substances which can bypass the metabolic blocking action, e.g., thymidine or thymine.

The standard SxT disc is appropriate for testing by the disc diffusion method.

Following oral administration, trimethoprim/sulfadiazine is rapidly absorbed and widely distributed throughout the body tissues. Concentrations of trimethoprim are usually higher in tissues than in blood. The levels of trimethoprim are high in lung, kidney and liver, as would be expected from its physical properties.

Serum trimethoprim concentrations in horses following oral administration indicate rapid absorption of the drug; peak concentrations occur in 1.5 hours. The mean serum elimination half-life is 2 to 2.5 hours. Sulfadiazine absorption is slower requiring 2.5 to 6 hours to reach peak concentrations. The mean serum elimination half-life for sulfadiazine is about 4 to 5.5 hours.

Usually, the concentration of an antibacterial in the blood and the *in vitro* MIC of the infecting organism indicate an appropriate period between doses of a drug. This does not hold entirely for trimethoprim/sulfadiazine because trimethoprim, in contrast to sulfadiazine, localizes in tissues and therefore, its concentration and ratio to sulfadiazine are higher there than in blood.

The following table shows the average concentration of trimethoprim and sulfadiazine, as measured in either serum or plasma, in twenty-four adult horses observed after a single dose of UNIPRIM® Powder:

Average Serum/Plasma Concentration (mcg/mL):

Trimethoprim (5 mg/kg)					Sulfadiazine (25 mg/kg)				
1h	3h	6h	10h	24h	1h	3h	6h	10h	24h
0.82	0.69	0.36	0.12	<.025	9.9	18.8	17.3	9.0	1.6

Excretion of trimethoprim/sulfadiazine is chiefly by the kidneys, by both glomerular filtration and tubular secretion. Urine concentrations of both trimethoprim and sulfadiazine are severalfold higher than blood concentrations. Neither trimethoprim nor sulfadiazine interferes with the excretion pattern of the other.

Dosage and Administration: The recommended dose is 3.75 g trimethoprim/sulfadiazine per 110 lbs (50 kg) body weight per day. Administer trimethoprim/sulfadiazine powder orally once a day in a small amount of palatable feed.

The usual course of treatment is a single, daily dose for five to seven days.

Continue acute infection therapy for two or three days after clinical signs have subsided.

If no improvement of acute infections is seen in three to five days, re-evaluate diagnosis.

Trimethoprim/sulfadiazine may be used alone or in conjunction with intravenous dosing. Following treatment with trimethoprim/sulfadiazine 48% injection, therapy can be maintained using oral powder.

A complete blood count should be done periodically in patients receiving trimethoprim/sulfadiazine for prolonged periods. If significant reduction in the count of any formed blood element is noted, treatment with trimethoprim/sulfadiazine should be discontinued.

Contraindication(s): Trimethoprim/sulfadiazine should not be used in horses showing marked liver parenchymal damage, blood dyscrasias or in those with a history of sulfonamide sensitivity.

Precaution(s): Store at or below 30°C (86°F).

Caution(s): Federal (U.S.A.) law restricts this drug to use by or on the order of a licensed veterinarian.

Water should be readily available to horses receiving sulfonamide therapy.

Individual animal hypersensitivity may result in local or generalized reactions, sometimes fatal. Anaphylactoid reactions, although rare, may also occur.

Antidote(s): Epinephrine.

Warning(s): Not for use in horses intended for food.

Toxicology: Toxicity is low. The acute toxicity of trimethoprim/sulfadiazine is more than 5 g/kg orally in rats and mice. No significant changes were recorded in rats given doses of 600 mg/kg per day for 90 days.

Horses treated intravenously with trimethoprim/sulfadiazine 48% injection have tolerated up to five times the recommended daily dose for 21 consecutive days without clinical effects or histopathological changes.

Teratology: The effect of trimethoprim/sulfadiazine on pregnancy has not been determined. Studies to date show that there is no detrimental effect on stallion spermatogenesis with or following the recommended dose of trimethoprim/sulfadiazine.

Adverse Reactions: No adverse reactions of consequence have been noted following administration of trimethoprim/sulfadiazine. During clinical trials, one case of anorexia and one case of loose feces following treatment with the drug were reported.

Other Side Effects: Lengthening of clotting time was seen in some of the horses on high or prolonged dosing in one of two trials. The effect, which may have been related to a resolving infection, was not seen in a second similar trial.

Slight to moderate reductions in hematopoietic activity following high, prolonged dosage in several species have been recorded. This is usually reversible by folinic acid (leucovorin) administration or by stopping the drug. During the long-term treatment of horses, periodic platelet counts and white and red blood cell counts are advisable.

Presentation: UNIPRIM® Powder is available in 37.5 g and 1,125 g packets.

Compendium Code No.: 14160000

UNIVAC 5

TradeWinds **Vaccine**

Canine Distemper-Adenovirus Type 2-Parainfluenza-Parvovirus Vaccine, Modified Live and Killed Virus

U.S. Vet. Lic. No.: 462

Contents: This product contains the antigens listed above.

The Adenovirus fraction is inactivated. The remaining virus fractions are live, and attenuated to assure safety.

This product contains gentamicin and amphotericin B as preservatives.

Indications: UNIVAC 5 is recommended for use in the vaccination of healthy dogs against disease caused by Canine Distemper, Infectious Canine Hepatitis, Canine Parvovirus and respiratory disease caused by Canine Adenovirus Type 2 and Parainfluenza.

Directions: Aseptically rehydrate vial of desiccated antigens by injecting the liquid product into the vial containing the vaccine cake. Shake well. Remove the entire contents back into the syringe. Push out air trapped in the syringe. Administer entire contents (1 mL) intramuscularly or subcutaneously. To give subcutaneously, vaccinate under loose skin (back of neck). To give intramuscularly, vaccinate in large muscle of hind limb. Do not vaccinate into blood vessels. If blood enters the syringe, choose another injection site.

Persistence of maternal origin antibody in puppies should receive consideration in determining vaccination programs. Ideally, puppies should be vaccinated at 9 weeks of age with revaccination every 2-4 weeks until at least 18 weeks of age. Dogs vaccinated after 18 weeks of age should receive a 1 mL dose followed by a second dose 2-4 weeks later. Annual revaccination with a single 1 mL dose is recommended.

Precaution(s): Store at 35°F-45°F (2°C-7°C). Do not freeze. Use entire contents when first rehydrated. Burn these containers, including syringe and needle.

Caution(s): Do not vaccinate pregnant bitches. In case of anaphylactoid reactions, epinephrine should be administered immediately.

For veterinary use only.

Presentation: 1 dose (1 mL).

Manufactured by: Biocor Animal Health Inc., Omaha, NE 68134 U.S.A.

Compendium Code No.: 12610050 TW11901-1200

UNIVAC 7

TradeWinds **Bacterin-Vaccine**

Canine Distemper-Adenovirus Type 2-Parainfluenza-Parvovirus Vaccine, Modified Live and Killed Virus-Leptospira Bacterin

U.S. Vet. Lic. No.: 462

Contents: This product contains the antigens listed above.

The Adenovirus and Leptospira fractions are inactivated. The remaining virus fractions are live, and attenuated to assure safety.

This product contains gentamicin and amphotericin B as preservatives.

Indications: UNIVAC 7 is recommended for use in the vaccination of healthy dogs against disease caused by Canine Distemper, Infectious Canine Hepatitis, Canine Parvovirus, *Leptospira canicola* and *L. icterohaemorrhagiae* and respiratory disease caused by Canine Adenovirus Type 2 and Parainfluenza.

Directions: Aseptically rehydrate vial of desiccated antigens by injecting the liquid product into the vial containing the vaccine cake. Shake well. Remove the entire contents back into the syringe. Push out air trapped in the syringe. Administer entire contents (1 mL) intramuscularly or subcutaneously. To give subcutaneously, vaccinate under loose skin (back of neck). To give intramuscularly, vaccinate in large muscle of hind limb. Do not vaccinate into blood vessels. If blood enters the syringe, choose another injection site.

Persistence of maternal origin antibody in puppies should receive consideration in determining vaccination programs. Ideally, puppies should be vaccinated at 9 weeks of age with revaccination every 2-4 weeks until at least 18 weeks of age. Dogs vaccinated after 18 weeks of age should receive a 1 mL dose followed by a second dose 2-4 weeks later. Annual revaccination with a single 1 mL dose is recommended.

Precaution(s): Store at 35°F-45°F (2°C-7°C). Do not freeze. Use entire contents when first rehydrated. Burn these containers, including syringe and needle.

Caution(s): Do not vaccinate pregnant bitches. In case of anaphylactoid reactions, epinephrine should be administered immediately.

For veterinary use only.

Presentation: 1 dose (1 mL).

Manufactured by: Biocor Animal Health Inc., Omaha, NE 68134 U.S.A.

Compendium Code No.: 12610060 TW9501-801

UNIVAC PARVO

TradeWinds **Vaccine**

Parvovirus Vaccine, Modified Live Virus

U.S. Vet. Lic. No.: 462

Contents: This product contains the antigen listed above.

This product contains gentamicin, amphotericin B and thimerosal as preservatives.

Indications: Recommended for use in the vaccination of healthy dogs against disease caused by Canine Parvovirus.

Directions: Shake well. Aseptically remove entire contents into the syringe. Push out any air trapped in the syringe. Administer entire contents (1 mL) subcutaneously or intramuscularly. To give subcutaneously, vaccinate under loose skin (back of neck). To give intramuscularly, vaccinate in large muscle of hind limb. Do not vaccinate into blood vessels. If blood enters the syringe, choose another injection site.

Persistence of maternal origin antibody in puppies should receive consideration in determining vaccination programs. Ideally, puppies should be vaccinated at 9 weeks of age with revaccination every 2-4 weeks until at least 18 weeks of age. Dogs vaccinated after 18 weeks of age should receive a 1 mL dose followed by a second dose 2-4 weeks later. Annual revaccination with a single 1 mL dose is recommended.

Precaution(s): Store at 35°F-45°F (2°C-7°C). Do not freeze. Use entire contents when first rehydrated. Burn this container, including syringe and needle.

Caution(s): Do not vaccinate pregnant bitches. In case of anaphylactoid reactions, epinephrine should be administered immediately.

For veterinary use only.

Presentation: 1 dose (1 mL).

Manufactured by: Biocor Animal Health Inc., Omaha, NE 68134 U.S.A.

Compendium Code No.: 12610070 TW11301-200

UNIVAX-BD®

Schering-Plough **Vaccine**

Bursal Disease Vaccine, Live Virus

U.S. Vet. Lic. No.: 165A

Active Ingredient(s): UNIVAX-BD® is a live virus vaccine of tissue culture origin containing a carefully selected mild strain of bursal disease virus grown in tissue culture and combined with stabilizing agents. The product is supplied as a lyophilized vaccine contained in vials sealed under vacuum. The vaccine contains gentamicin as a preservative.

Indications: For the vaccination of healthy chickens two weeks of age or older as an aid in preventing infectious bursal disease.

Dosage and Administration:

When to Vaccinate: Vaccinate at two (2) weeks of age or older. Good management practices should be followed to reduce exposure of the birds to the virulent infectious bursal disease virus during the first several weeks of life.

Vaccination Program: The development of a durable, strong protection depends upon the use of an effective vaccination program as well as many other circumstances such as administration techniques, environment and flock health at the time of vaccination. Also, the immune response to one (1) vaccination under field conditions is seldom complete for all animals within a given flock. Even when vaccination is successful, the protection stimulated in individual animals against different diseases may not be life-long. Therefore, under certain circumstances revaccination may be necessary.

Preparation of the Vaccine:

1. Assemble the vaccine and equipment needed to vaccinate the entire flock at one time.
2. Do not open and mix the vaccine until ready for use.
3. Remove the tear-off aluminum seal from the vaccine vial without disturbing the rubber stopper.
4. Use cool, clean, nonchlorinated drinking water.
5. Holding the vial submerged in a pail of water or under a running stream of water, lift the lip of the rubber stopper so that the water is sucked into the vial.
6. Reseat the stopper and shake the vial to thoroughly dissolve the vaccine.

How to Vaccinate: Withhold water from the birds for several hours before vaccinating so the birds are thirsty. Thoroughly clean and rinse all watering containers so that no residual disinfectants remain. Dilute the vaccine immediately before use with cool, clean, nonchlorinated water. Pour the dissolved vaccine material into the following amounts of water and mix thoroughly:

Each 1,000 Birds	U.S. Gallons	Imperial Gallons	Metric Liters
2 to 4 weeks	2½	2	10
4 to 8 weeks	5	4	20
Over 8 weeks	10	8	40

Distribute the diluted vaccine so that all of the birds are able to drink within a 1-hour period and do not add any more water until the vaccine is consumed. Avoid placing water in direct sunlight.

Records: Keep a record of the vaccine type, quantity, serial number, expiration date, and place of purchase; the date and time of vaccination; the number, age, breed, and location of the birds; the names of operators performing the vaccination and any observed reactions.

Precaution(s): Store at 35° to 45°F (2° to 7°C).

Caution(s): For veterinary use only.

1. Vaccinate healthy birds only. Although disease may not be evident, coccidiosis, chronic respiratory disease, mycoplasma infection, lymphoid leukosis, infectious bursal disease, Marek's disease, or other disease conditions may cause serious complications or reduce protection.
2. All birds within a house should be vaccinated on the same day. Isolate other susceptible birds on the premises from the birds being vaccinated.
3. In outbreak situations, vaccinate healthy birds first, progressing toward outbreak areas in order to vaccinate diseased birds last.
4. Do not spill or spatter the vaccine. Use the entire contents of the vial when first opened. Burn the empty bottles, caps, and all unused vaccine and accessories.
5. Wash hands thoroughly after using the vaccine.
6. Do not dilute the vaccine or otherwise stretch the dosage.
7. Use only in states where permitted and on premises with a history of bursal disease.

The use of the vaccine is subject to state laws wherever applicable.

Warning(s): Do not vaccinate within 21 days before slaughter.

Presentation: Supplied in 10 x 1,000 dose units, 10 x 5,000 dose units, and 10 x 20,000 dose units.

Compendium Code No.: 10472040

UNIVAX™ PLUS

Schering-Plough **Vaccine**

Bursal Disease Vaccine, Live Virus

U.S. Vet. Lic. No.: 165A

Contents: UNIVAX™ Plus is a live virus vaccine containing two live bursal disease viruses. The vaccine viruses have been demonstrated in controlled studies to provide protection against standard and variant bursal disease viruses.

The vaccine viruses are grown in chicken embryos and cell culture, and are combined with stabilizing agents. The product is supplied as a lyophilized vaccine contained in vials sealed under vacuum.

This vaccine contains gentamicin as a preservative.

Indications: For use in chickens at 1 day of age by subcutaneous route of administration of by drinking water at 2 weeks or older as an aid in preventing bursal disease associated with infection by standard and variant bursal disease viruses.

Dosage and Administration:

When to Vaccinate: Vaccinate subcutaneously at 1 day of age or by drinking water at 2 weeks or older. Good management practices should be followed to reduce exposure of birds to virulent infectious bursal disease virus during the first several weeks of life.

Vaccination Program: The development of a durable, strong protection depends upon the use of an effective vaccination program as well as many circumstances such as administration techniques, environment and flock health at time of vaccination. Also, the immune response to one vaccination under field conditions is seldom complete for all birds within a given flock. Even when vaccination is successful, the protection stimulated in individual birds against different diseases may not be life long. Therefore, under certain circumstances revaccination may be necessary.

Preparation of the Vaccine:

Subcutaneous Route of Administration:

1. Do not open and mix the vaccine until ready for use.
2. Mix only one vial at a time and use entire contents within 2 hours.
3. Lift up top of seal on vaccine vial to expose rubber stopper. Using sterile needle and 5 or 10 mL syringe, remove a small amount (5 mL) of diluent and transfer this to the vaccine vial. Vacuum in the vaccine vial will readily pull in the diluent. Release the vacuum remaining in the vial.
4. Vigorously shake vaccine vial with transferred diluent to rehydrate the vaccine.
5. Using the same sterile needle and syringe, completely transfer the rehydrated vaccine to remaining diluent. Rinse syringe and vaccine vial by withdrawing additional diluent and repeating the process.
6. Vigorously shake final rehydrated vaccine for 20-30 seconds to mix thoroughly.
7. The vaccine is now ready for use.

Drinking Water Method:

1. Assemble the vaccine and equipment needed to vaccinate the entire flock at one time.
2. Do not open and mix the vaccine until ready for use.
3. Remove the tear-off aluminum seal from the vaccine vial without disturbing the rubber stopper.
4. Use cool, clean, non-chlorinated tap water to which powdered milk has been added as directed under "How to Vaccinate".
5. Holding vial submerged in a pail of water or under a running stream of water, lift the lip of the rubber stopper so that the water (milk added) is sucked into the vial.
6. Reseat the stopper and shake the vial to thoroughly dissolve the vaccine.

How to Vaccinate:

By Subcutaneous Route of Administration: Insert a filling tube (large, sharpened transfer tube) into the bottle of vaccine. Connect the filling tube by means of rubber or plastic tubing to an automatic vaccinator fitted with a 22 gauge ½ inch needle. The automatic vaccinator should be calibrated accurately ahead of time to deliver 0.2 mL.

By Drinking Water Method: Do not mix the vaccine into the drinking water until ready for use. Drinking water for vaccination should be mixed with powdered milk to prevent inactivation from chlorine or other water additives and also to stabilize the vaccine virus. The powdered milk should be added to the water at the rate of 3 grams per 11 liters (one heaped teaspoon per 3 U.S. gallons or 2.5 Imp. gallons); or 90 grams per 300 liters (one heaped cupful per 80 U.S. gallons or 66 Imp. gallons).

The following schedule is a general guideline for the amount of water to use with the vaccine. These amounts will vary depending upon the individual management conditions, climate, age and sex of the birds.

Withhold water for several hours before vaccinating so birds are thirsty. Thoroughly clean and rinse all watering containers so that no residual disinfectants remain. Dilute the vaccine immediately before use with cool, clean, non-chlorinated water (milk added). Pour the dissolved vaccine material into the following amounts of water and mix thoroughly.

Each 1 000 Birds	U.S. Gallons	Imperial Gallons	Metric Liters
2 to 4 Weeks	2-½	2	10
4 to 8 Weeks	5	4	20
Over 8 Weeks	10	8	40

Distribute diluted vaccine so that all birds are able to drink within a 1 hour period and do not add any more water until the vaccine is consumed. Avoid placing water in direct sunlight.

Records: Keep a record of vaccine type, quantity, serial number, expiration date, and place of purchase; the date and time of vaccination; the number, age, breed, and location of the birds; names of operators performing the vaccination and any observed reactions.

Precaution(s): Store at 2° to 7°C (35° to 45°F).

Do not dilute the vaccine or otherwise stretch the dosage.

Do not spill or spatter the vaccine. Use entire contents of vial when first opened. Burn empty bottles, caps and all unused vaccine and accessories.

Caution(s): For subcutaneous use only in day old birds. For use by drinking water in birds 2 weeks or older.

All birds within a house should be vaccinated on the same day. Isolate other susceptible birds on the premises from birds being vaccinated.

Vaccinate only healthy birds. Although disease may not be evident, coccidiosis, chronic respiratory disease, mycoplasma infection, lymphoid leukosis, Marek's disease, or other disease conditions may cause serious complications or reduce protection.

In outbreak situations, vaccinate healthy birds first progressing toward outbreak areas in order to vaccinate diseased birds last.

Warning(s): Do not vaccinate within 21 days before slaughter.

Use only in states where permitted and on premises with a history of bursal disease.

The use of this vaccine is subject to state laws wherever applicable.

Wash hands thoroughly after using the vaccine.

For veterinary use only.

Compendium Code No.: 10472050

UNIVERSAL MEDICATED SHAMPOO

Vet Solutions — **Antidermatosis Shampoo**

Active Ingredient(s): 2% Chloroxylenol, 2% Salicylic Acid, 2% Sodium Thiosulfate (source of soluble sulfur).

Ingredients: Deionized Water, Sodium C14-16 Olefin Sulfonate, Propylene Glycol, Cocamide DEA, Polyquaternium-10, Fragrance, Citric Acid, Methylchloroisothiazolinone, Methylisothiazolinone, FD&C Blue No. 1.

Indications: Vet Solutions UNIVERSAL MEDICATED SHAMPOO may be used as adjunctive therapy for the most common dermatological conditions. For dogs and cats.

Deep cleansing action, removes scales and crusts, antibacterial, antifungal, deodorizing, gentle for routine use.

Directions: Shake well. With tepid water, thoroughly wet animal's coat. Massage small amounts of shampoo into the coat while continuously adding water to get better dispersion. Continue until a generous lather is generated. Rinse well and repeat procedure. Shampoo may be used weekly or as often as recommended by your veterinarian.

Precaution(s): Storage: Store at controlled room temperature.

Caution(s): Keep out of reach of children. For topical use only. Avoid contact with eyes. If eye contact occurs, immediately flush with water.

Sold exclusively through veterinarians.

Presentation: 16 fl. oz. (473 mL) and 1 gallon.

Compendium Code No.: 10610180 990804

UPJOHN J-5 BACTERIN™

Pharmacia & Upjohn — **Bacterin**

Escherichia Coli Bacterin

U.S. Vet. Lic. No.: 357

Contents: This product contains the antigen listed above.

Indications: *Escherichia Coli* Bacterin is recommended for use in healthy dairy cattle as an aid in the prevention of clinical mastitis caused by *E coli.* For effective mastitis control, this product should be used in conjunction with acceptable good management practices.

Directions: Shake well. Three doses are required. Administer each 5 mL dose subcutaneously, one hand-width cranial to the shoulder. Vaccinate cows or heifers at 7 and 8 months of gestation followed by the third dose within two weeks postpartum.

Precaution(s): Store at 35°F to 45°F (2°C to 7°C).

Do not freeze. Use entire contents when first opened.

Caution(s): Local swelling occasionally occurs and may persist at the injection site. In case of anaphylactoid reactions, epinephrine should be administered immediately.

Warning(s): Do not vaccinate within 60 days before slaughter.

Presentation: 20 dose (100 mL) (NDC 0009-3637-05) and 50 dose (250 mL) (NDC 0009-3637-06) vials.

Manufactured by: Poultry Health Laboratories, Davis, CA 95616.

Compendium Code No.: 10490192 801 349 001 / 801 350 001

UREA WOUND POWDER

First Priority — **Topical Wound Dressing**

Antiseptic Dusting Powder

Active Ingredient(s):

Urea 83%

Indications: Urea creates a chemical action to debride the wound and remove dead tissue through proeolytic action. An antiseptic dusting powder for surface wounds.

Dosage and Administration: Thoroughly cleanse entire area to be treated. Sprinkle compound evenly on surface wounds several times daily.

Precaution(s): Store at controlled room temperature between 15° and 30°C (59°F-86°F).

Keep tightly closed when not in use.

Caution(s): In case of deep or puncture wounds or serious burns consult a veterinarian. If redness, irritation or swelling persists or increases, discontinue use and consult a veterinarian. Avoid contact with the eyes and mucous membranes. Do not apply to large areas of broken skin.

Warning(s): Do not use on animals intended for food.

Keep out of reach of children.

Presentation: 6 oz (170 g).

Compendium Code No.: 11390741

UROEZE® ℞

King Animal Health — **Urinary Acidifier**

Active Ingredient(s): Each one-quarter level teaspoon (650 mg) contains: Ammonium chloride 400 mg in a palatable amino acid protein base.

Indications: For use as a urinary acidifier in cats and dogs.

Dosage and Administration: The suggested dose of UROEZE® Powder for adult cats and dogs is one-quarter (¼) level teaspoonful per 10 lbs. (4.5 kg) of body weight twice a day with food. The suggested dose of UROEZE® Tablets for adult cats and dogs is one (1) tablet per 10 lbs. (4.5 kg) of body weight twice a day with food.

The dosage may then be adjusted to accomplish the desired urine pH (approximately 6).

Contraindication(s): Not intended for use in kittens.

Precaution(s): Store at a controlled room temperature of 15°-30°C (59°-86°F).

Caution(s): Federal law restricts this drug to use by or on the order of a licensed veterinarian.

May cause gastric mucosal irritation.

Do not administer to animals with severe liver or kidney damage, or to animals exhibiting acidosis.

Warning(s): Keep this and all medication out of the reach of children.

Presentation: 4 oz. and 16 oz. powder.

Compendium Code No.: 11320091

UROEZE® 200 ℞

King Animal Health — **Urinary Acidifier**

Active Ingredient(s): Each one-quarter level teaspoonful (0.65 g) powder contains: 200 mg ammonium chloride in a palatable protein base.

Each scored tablet contains 200 mg ammonium chloride.

Indications: For use as a urinary acidifier in cats and dogs.

Dosage and Administration: The suggested dose of UROEZE® 200 Powder for adult cats and dogs is 0.65 g (¼ level teaspoonful) per 10 lbs. (4.5 kg) of body weight twice a day with food. The suggested dose of UROEZE® 200 Tablets for adult cats and dogs is one (1) tablet per 10 lbs. (4.5 kg) of body weight twice a day with food. The daily dose may vary with different diets depending on the alkalinity of the diet. The dosage should be adjusted to maintain the urine pH consistently below 6.6.

Contraindication(s): Not intended for use in kittens.

Precaution(s): Store at a controlled room temperature of 15°-30°C (59°-86°F).

Caution(s): Federal law restricts this drug to use by or on the order of a licensed veterinarian.

May cause gastric mucosal irritation.

Do not administer to animals with severe liver or kidney damage or to animals exhibiting acidosis.

Presentation: Powder: 4 oz. bottles.

Tablets: Bottles of 100 and 500 tablets.

Compendium Code No.: 11320101

UTERINE BOLUS

Butler **Uterine Bolus**

NDC No.: 11695-4115-3

Active Ingredient(s): Each bolus contains:

Urea . . . . 13.4 g

Indications: For use as an antiseptic and proteolytic aid in beef and dairy cattle and sheep.

Dosage and Administration: For intra-uterine or topical use only. Insert the boluses into the uterus or dissolve in one (1) pint warm water to make a flush.

Cattle . . . . 2-4 boluses

Sheep . . . . ½-1 bolus

For topical application, dissolve four (4) boluses into one (1) pint of warm water and thoroughly flush the wound.

Repeat the treatment in 24 to 48 hours, if necessary.

Precaution(s): Store in a cool, dry place.

Caution(s): Strict cleanliness must be observed in order to prevent the introduction of further infection. Thoroughly cleanse the hands and arms of the operator and the external genital parts of the animal with soap and water before inserting the boluses or flush.

Do not administer orally.

Do not use in deep or puncture wounds or for serious burns.

For animal use only.

Keep out of the reach of children.

Keep the container tightly closed when not in use.

Presentation: Jars of 50 boluses.

Compendium Code No.: 10821810

UTERINE BOLUS

Durvet **Uterine Bolus**

NDC No.: 30798-017-69

Active Ingredient(s): Each bolus contains:

Urea . . . . 13.4 g

Indications: For use as an antiseptic and proteolytic aid in beef and dairy cattle, and sheep.

Dosage and Administration: For intrauterine or topical use only. Insert the boluses into the uterus or dissolve it in one (1) pint of warm water to make a flush.

Cattle: Give two (2) to four (4) boluses.

Sheep: Give one-half (½) to one (1) bolus.

For topical application, dissolve four (4) boluses in one (1) pint of warm water and thoroughly flush the wound.

Repeat the treatment in 24 to 48 hours if necessary.

Precaution(s): Store in a cool, dry place. Keep the container tightly closed when not in use.

Caution(s): Do not administer orally.

Strict cleanliness must be observed to prevent the introduction of further infections. Thoroughly cleanse the hands and the arms of the operator and the external genital parts of the animal with soap and water before inserting the boluses or flush.

Do not use in deep or puncture wounds or for serious burns.

Keep out of the reach of children.

For animal use only.

Presentation: 50 boluses

Compendium Code No.: 10841620

UTERINE BOLUS

First Priority **Uterine Bolus**

Antiseptic and Proteolytic Bolus

Active Ingredient(s): Each bolus contains:

Urea . . . . 13.4 g

Indications: For use as an antiseptic and proteolytic aid in beef, dairy cattle and sheep.

Dosage and Administration: For intrauterine or topical use only. Insert boluses into uterus or dissolve in one pint warm water to make a flush.

Cattle: 2-4 boluses

Sheep: ½-1 boluses

For topical application, dissolve 4 boluses in one pint of warm water and thoroughly flush wound.

Repeat treatment in 24 to 48 hours if necessary.

Contraindication(s): Do not administer orally.

Do not use in deep or puncture wounds or for serious burns.

Precaution(s): Store in a cool, dry place.

Keep container tightly closed when not in use.

Caution(s): Strict cleanliness must be observed to prevent introduction of further infections. Thoroughly cleanse hands and arms of operator and external genital parts of the animal with soap and water before inserting boluses or flush.

Warning(s): For use in animals only.

Keep out of reach of children.

Presentation: 50 boluses.

Compendium Code No.: 11390750

UTERINE BOLUS

Phoenix Pharmaceutical **Uterine Bolus**

Antiseptic and Proteolytic Bolus

Active Ingredient(s): Composition: Each bolus contains:

Urea . . . . 13.4 g

Indications: For use as an antiseptic and proteolytic aid in beef and dairy cattle and sheep.

Dosage and Administration: For intra-uterine or topical use only. Insert boluses into uterus, or dissolve one pint of warm water to make a flush.

Cattle: 2-4 boluses.

Sheep: ½-1 bolus.

For topical application, dissolve 4 boluses in one pint of warm water and thoroughly flush wound.

Repeat treatment in 24 to 48 hours, if necessary.

Precaution(s): Store in a cool, dry place. Keep container tightly closed when not in use.

Caution(s): Do not administer orally.

Strict cleanliness must be observed to prevent the introduction of further infection. Thoroughly cleanse hands and arms of operator and external genital parts of the animal with soap and water before inserting boluses or flush.

Do not use in deep or puncture wounds or for serious burns.

For animal use only.

Warning(s): Keep out of reach of children.

Presentation: Jars of 50 boluses (NDC 57319-391-12).

Manufactured by: Phoenix Scientific, Inc., St. Joseph, MO 64503.

Compendium Code No.: 12560872 Rev. 2-02

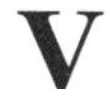

V

VACCINE STABILIZER

Alpharma **Pasteurella Stabilizer**

Active Ingredient(s): The product contains nonfat milk, maltodextrin, sodium caseinate, isolated soy protein, whey, lactose, calcium caseinate, artificial flavor, carrageenan, lecithin, sugar and salt.

Indications: A stabilizing agent compatible with live fowl cholera vaccines.

Dosage and Administration: Consult the vaccine label or the package insert for instructions on dilution.

Caution(s): For oral animal use only.

Not for human consumption.

Keep out of the reach of children.

Presentation: 16 oz. (453.6 g).

Compendium Code No.: 10220620

V.A. CHICKVAC™

Fort Dodge **Vaccine**

Tenosynovitis Vaccine, Modified Live Virus

U.S. Vet. Lic. No.: 112

Contents: This product contains the antigen listed above.

Contains gentamicin and amphotericin B as preservatives.

Indications: V.A. CHICKVAC™ is recommended for subcutaneous administration to healthy chickens 1 to 10 days of age as an aid in the prevention of tenosynovitis (viral arthritis).

Directions: Read in full, follow directions carefully.

1. Use Fort Dodge Animal Health, Inc., diluent only. Store diluent at not over 80°F (27°C).
2. Rehydrate only 1 vial of vaccine with 1 bottle of Fort Dodge Animal Health, Inc. diluent.
3. Remove the central tab of the aluminum seal of the vaccine vial, leaving the outer ring intact. Sanitize the rubber stopper with alcohol. Also, sanitize with alcohol the rubber stopper of the container of diluent.
4. Using a sterile syringe and needle, penetrate the stopper of the diluent container and withdraw 3 mL (3 cc) diluent. Then, insert needle through stopper of vaccine vial and discharge syringe contents.
5. Remove syringe and needle. Pull back on syringe plunger to admit 2 or 3 mL of air. This is very important.
6. Reinsert needle into vaccine vial. Barely penetrate the stopper. Expel the air into the vial (to break vacuum).
7. With syringe and needle still in place, invert the vial and pull back plunger so that all of the contents (the rehydrated vaccine) are drawn from vial into syringe.
8. Insert the needle into diluent container (through the stopper) and expel syringe contents into diluent. Rotate container gently so that mixture is uniform. The vaccine is ready for use.
9. An automatic syringe with 22- to 20-gauge needles, 3/8 inch to 1/2 inch in length, is recommended. Make certain that all equipment is sterilized. Change needles frequently.
10. Inject each bird subcutaneously in the back of the neck with 0.2 mL of the vaccine.
11. Use all vaccine from 1 vial (1,000 doses) within 1 hour after rehydrating. Avoid placing the vaccine near heat. Do not expose to direct sunlight.

Records: Keep a record of vaccine serial number and expiration date; date of receipt and date of vaccination; where vaccination took place; and any reactions observed.

Precaution(s): Store this vaccine at not over 45°F (7°C).

Use entire contents of vial when first opened.

Burn vaccine container and all unused contents.

This product should be stored, transported, and administered in accordance with the directions.

This product is nonreturnable.

Caution(s): This product may reduce the efficacy of Marek's Disease Vaccines when administered at one day of age. Use only in states where permitted.

The use of the vaccine is subject to applicable state laws.

Warning(s): Do not vaccinate within 21 days before slaughter.

Do not vaccinate birds in egg production.

For veterinary use only.

Presentation: 10 x 1,000 doses.

Compendium Code No.: 10032481 10970A

VALBAZEN® CATTLE DEWORMER PASTE

Pfizer Animal Health **Parasiticide-Oral**

(albendazole)

NADA No.: 128-070

Active Ingredient(s):

Albendazole 30%

Indications: VALBAZEN® is a broad-spectrum anthelmintic effective in the removal and control of the following internal parasites of cattle:

Adult Liver Flukes: *(Fasciola hepatica).*

Heads and Segments of Tapeworms: *(Moniezia benedeni, M. expansa).*

Adult and 4th Stage Larvae of Stomach Worms: Brown Stomach Worms, including 4th stage inhibited larvae *(Ostertagia ostertagi),* Barberpole Worm *(Haemonchus contortus, H. placei),* Small Stomach Worm *(Trichostrongylus axei).*

Adult and 4th Stage Larvae of Intestinal Worms: Thread-necked Intestinal Worm *(Nematodirus spathiger, N. helvetianus),* Small Intestinal Worm *(Cooperia punctata* and *C. oncophora)*

Adult Stages of Intestinal Worms: Hookworm *(Bunostomum phlebotomum),* Bankrupt Worm *(Trichostrongylus colubriformis),* Nodular Worm *(Oesophagostomum radiatum)*

Adult and 4th Stage Larvae of Lungworms: *(Dictyocaulus viviparus).*

Dosage and Administration: VALBAZEN® Cattle Dewormer Paste should be administered to cattle at the recommended rate of 10 mg/kg (4.54 mg/lb) of body weight. The following table indicates recommended dosing schedule.

Wt. of Animal	Cattle (4.54 mg/lb) Gun Setting No.	Depress Trigger
65-200 lb	1	Once
201-340 lb	2	Once
341-475 lb	3	Once
476-600 lb	4	Once
601-915 lb	3	Twice
916-1050 lb	4	Twice

One paste cartridge contains enough VALBAZEN® to treat twenty-four 500-lb animals.

Important: Accurate estimates of the weight of the cattle to be treated are essential for most effective results with this product. Animals constantly exposed to internal parasites should be retreated as necessary.

Directions for Use: This cartridge is intended for use only with the dosing gun designed for this product.

To prepare dosing gun for administration of VALBAZEN® Cattle Dewormer Paste, follow these steps:

1. Depress elongated lever at rear of gun and retract plunger rod fully. Be sure to leave trigger free while retracting rod.
2. Insert large end of cartridge into the gun handle and turn the cartridge clockwise until tight.
3. Remove small cap from nozzle end of cartridge.
4. Loosen thumbscrew, select proper dose setting on the dial for the body weight of the animal to be treated, then tighten thumbscrew.
5. Depress trigger repeatedly until paste begins to extrude from nozzle. Discard ejected paste. This will ensure a full initial dose.
6. Place nozzle well back in the mouth of the animal.
7. Depress trigger 1 or 2 times as indicated to deliver a full dose for the weight range selected.
8. Remove cartridge by turning counterclockwise. Replace cap on nozzle if contents not fully used.

Precaution(s): Store at controlled room temperature 15°-30°C (59°-86°F). Protect from freezing.

Caution(s): Do not administer to female cattle during first 45 days of pregnancy or for 45 days after removal of bulls. Consult your veterinarian for assistance in the diagnosis, treatment, and control of parasitism.

Keep this and all medication out of reach of children.

For use in animals only.

Warning(s): Cattle must not be slaughtered within 27 days following last treatment. Because a withdrawal time in milk has not been established, do not use in female dairy cattle of breeding age.

Presentation: 205 g (7.2 oz)

U.S. Patent Nos. 3,915,986 and 3,956,499

Compendium Code No.: 36900310 90-8786-06

VALBAZEN® SUSPENSION

Pfizer Animal Health **Parasiticide-Oral**

(albendazole) Broad-Spectrum Dewormer

NADA No.: 110-048

Active Ingredient(s):

Albendazole. 11.36%

(Equivalent to 113.6 mg/mL)

Indications: For removal and control of: Liver flukes, tapeworms, stomach worms, intestinal worms, lungworms.

VALBAZEN® is a broad-spectrum anthelmintic effective in the removal and control of the following internal parasites in cattle and sheep:

Parasite	Cattle	Sheep
Adult Liver Flukes	*Fasciola hepatica*	*Fasciola hepatica, Fascioloides magna*
Heads and Segments of Tapeworms	*Moniezia benedeni, M. expansa*	Common Tapeworms *(Moniezia expansa),* Fringed Tapeworms *(Thysanosoma actinioides)*
Adult and 4th Stage Larvae of Stomach Worms	Brown Stomach Worms, including 4th stage inhibited larvae *(Ostertagia ostertagi),* Barberpole Worm *(Haemonchus contortus, H. placei),* Small Stomach Worm *(Trichostrongylus axei)*	Brown Stomach Worms *(Ostertagia circumcincta, Marshallagia marshalli),* Barberpole Worm *(Haemonchus contortus),* Small Stomach Worm *(Trichostrongylus axei)*
Adult and 4th Stage Larvae of Intestinal Worms	Thread-necked Intestinal Worm *(Nematodirus spathiger, N. helvetianus),* Small Intestinal Worm *(Cooperia punctata, C. oncophora)*	Thread-necked Intestinal Worm *(Nematodirus spathiger, N. fificollis),* Cooper's Worms *(Cooperia oncophora),* Bankrupt Worm *(Trichostrongylus colubriformis),* Nodular Worm *(Oesophagostomum columbianum),* Large-mouth Bowel Worm *(Chabertia ovina)*
Adult Stages of Intestinal Worms	Hookworm *(Bunostomum phlebotomum),* Bankrupt Worm *(Trichostrongylus colubriformis),* Nodular Worm *(Oesophagostomum radiatum)*	
Adult and 4th Stage Larvae of Lungworms	*Dictyocaulus viviparus*	Adult and Larval Stages of Lungworms

Dosage and Administration: VALBAZEN® Suspension should be administered to cattle at the recommended rate of 4 mL/100 lb of body weight (equivalent to 4.54 mg of albendazole/lb, 10 mg/kg) and to sheep at the recommended rate of 0.75 mL/25 lb of body weight (equivalent to 3.4 mg of albendazole/lb, 7.5 mg/kg). The following table indicates recommended dosing schedules.

Cattle		Sheep	
Body Weight	Dosage	Body Weight	Dosage
250 lb	10 mL	25 lb	0.75 mL
500 lb	20 mL	50 lb	1.5 mL
750 lb	30 mL	75 lb	2.25 mL
1000 lb	40 mL	100 lb	3.0 mL
1250 lb	50 mL	200 lb	6.0 mL
1500 lb	60 mL	300 lb	9.0 mL

Cattle: 1 liter of VALBAZEN® 11.36% Suspension will treat 50 animals weighing 500 lb.

Sheep: 1 liter of VALBAZEN® 11.36% Suspension will treat 664 animals weighing 50 lb.

VALBAZEN® 11.36% Suspension should be given orally using any type of standard dosing gun or dose syringe.

Important: Accurate estimates of the weight of the cattle and sheep to be treated are essential for most effective results with this product. Animals constantly exposed to internal parasites should be retreated as necessary.

Precaution(s): Shake well before using.

Store at controlled room temperature of 15°-30°C (59°-86°F).

Protect from freezing.

Caution(s): Do not administer to female cattle during first 45 days of pregnancy or for 45 days after removal of bulls. Do not administer to ewes during the first 30 days of pregnancy or for 30 days after removal of rams. Consult your veterinarian for assistance in the diagnosis, treatment, and control of parasitism.

Keep this and all medication out of reach of children.

For use in animals only.

Warning(s): Cattle must not be slaughtered within 27 days following last treatment. Sheep must not be slaughtered within 7 days following last treatment. Because a withdrawal time in milk has not been established, do not use in female dairy cattle of breeding age.

Presentation: 500 mL, 1 liter, 5 liter.

U.S. Patent Nos. 3,915,986 and 3,956,499

Compendium Code No.: 36900300 80-8784-05

V.A.L.® SYRUP

Fort Dodge **Vitamin B-Complex**

Active Ingredient(s): Product Analysis: Per fluid ounce:

Thiamine hydrochloride . . . . . 2 mg
Riboflavin . . . . . 2 mg
Calcium pantothenate . . . . . 12 mg
Nicotinamide . . . . . 15 mg
Pyridoxine hydrochloride . . . . . 2 mg
Protein hydrolysates (as source of amino acids) . . . . . 3.5 g
Liver fraction 1 . . . . . 1.5 g

Additional Ingredients: Niacinamide, sodium benzoate, cane sugar, glycerin, vanillin, ethyl vanillin, ethyl alcohol, purified water (q.s.).

Alcohol 4.75% by volume.

Indications: Highly palatable source of B-vitamins, amino acids and liver fraction 1. Use in animals as a dietary B-complex vitamin supplement.

Dosage and Administration:

Horses and Cattle . . . . . 1 to 2 Tbsp. twice per day

Dogs and Cats weighing:

under 12 lbs . . . . . 1 tsp. per day
12 to 30 lbs. . . . . . 2 tsp. per day
30 to 50 lbs. . . . . . 3 tsp. per day
over 50 lbs . . . . . 4 tsp. per day

For growing puppies and kittens double the dosage.

Warning(s): Keep out of reach of children.

Presentation: 8 fl oz (236 mL) and 1 gallon containers.

Compendium Code No.: 10032491 9203F

VANGUARD® 5

Pfizer Animal Health **Vaccine**

Canine Distemper-Adenovirus Type 2-Parainfluenza-Parvovirus Vaccine, Modified Live Virus

U.S. Vet. Lic. No.: 189

Description: VANGUARD® 5 contains attenuated strains of CD virus, CAV-2, CPI virus, and CPV propagated on an established canine cell line. The CPV fraction was attenuated by low passage on the canine cell line and at that passage level has immunogenic properties capable of overriding maternal antibodies. Some puppies in the field may have higher levels of maternal antibodies than those evaluated in our pivotal efficacy study. VANGUARD® 5 is packaged in freeze-dried form with inert gas in place of vacuum.

Contains penicillin and streptomycin as preservatives.

Indications: VANGUARD® 5 is for vaccination of healthy dogs as an aid in preventing canine distemper caused by canine distemper (CD) virus, infectious canine hepatitis (ICH) caused by canine adenovirus type 1 (CAV-1), respiratory disease caused by canine adenovirus type 2 (CAV-2), canine parainfluenza caused by canine parainfluenza (CPI) virus, and canine parvoviral enteritis caused by canine parvovirus (CPV).

Directions:

1. General Directions: Vaccination of healthy dogs is recommended. Aseptically rehydrate the freeze-dried vaccine with the sterile diluent provided, shake well, and administer 1 mL subcutaneously or intramuscularly.
2. Primary Vaccination: Healthy dogs should receive 2 doses administered 3-4 weeks apart. If dogs are vaccinated before the age of 4 months, they should be revaccinated with a single dose upon reaching 4 months of age. (Maternal antibodies may interfere with development of an adequate immune response in puppies less than 4 months old.)
3. Revaccination: Annual revaccination with a single dose is recommended.

Precaution(s): Store at 2°-7°C. Prolonged exposure to higher temperatures and/or direct sunlight may adversely affect potency. Do not freeze.

Use entire contents when first opened.

Sterilized syringes and needles should be used to administer this vaccine. Do not sterilize with chemicals because traces of disinfectant may inactivate the vaccine.

Burn containers and all unused contents.

Caution(s): Vaccination of pregnant bitches should be avoided.

As with many vaccines, anaphylaxis may occur after use. Initial antidote of epinephrine is recommended and should be followed with appropriate supportive therapy.

This product has been shown to be efficacious in healthy animals. A protective immune response may not be elicited if animals are incubating an infectious disease, are malnourished or parasitized, are stressed due to shipment or environmental conditions, are otherwise immunocompromised, or the vaccine is not administered in accordance with label directions.

Warning(s): For use in dogs only.

For veterinary use only.

Discussion: Disease Description: CD is a universal, high-mortality viral disease with variable manifestations. Approximately 50% of nonvaccinated, nonimmune dogs infected with CD virus develop clinical signs, and approximately 90% of those dogs die.[1] ICH, caused by CAV-1, is a universal, sometimes fatal, viral disease of dogs characterized by hepatic and generalized endothelial lesions. CAV-2 causes respiratory disease which in severe cases may include pneumonia and bronchopneumonia. CPI is a common viral upper respiratory disease. Uncomplicated CPI may be mild or subclinical, with signs becoming more severe if concurrent infection with other respiratory pathogens exists. CPV infection results in enteric disease characterized by sudden onset of vomiting and diarrhea, often hemorrhagic. Leukopenia commonly accompanies clinical signs. Susceptible dogs of any age can be affected, but mortality is greatest in puppies. In puppies 4-12 weeks of age CPV may occasionally cause myocarditis that can result in acute heart failure after a brief and inconspicuous illness. Following infection many dogs are refractory to the disease for a year or more. Similarly, seropositive bitches may transfer to their puppies CPV antibodies which can interfere with active immunization of the puppies through 16 weeks of age.

Trial Data: Safety and Efficacy: Laboratory evaluation demonstrated that VANGUARD® 5 aided in preventing disease caused by CD, ICH, CAV-2 respiratory disease, CPI, and CPV, and that no immunologic interference existed among the vaccine fractions.

It has been demonstrated that CAV-2 vaccine cross-protects against ICH caused by CAV-1. The CAV-2 fraction in Vanguard® vaccines is used as a replacement for CAV-1 because it has significant advantages. Some CAV-1 vaccines may produce undesirable reactions, including persistent kidney infections, uveitis, and corneal opacity ("blue eye"), which have not been reported after vaccination with CAV-2.[2] In addition, the CAV-2 strain used in Vanguard® vaccines has been specially selected for freedom from oncogenic properties characteristic of adenoviruses.

Studies demonstrated that the CAV-2 fraction in VANGUARD® 5 not only protects against ICH, but against CAV-2 respiratory disease as well.[3] Although conventional CAV-1 (ICH) vaccines cross-protect against CAV-2, they may not prevent subclinical infection and spread of the CAV-2 agent. Canine adenovirus type 2 challenge virus was not recovered from CAV-2-vaccinated dogs.

The CPV fraction in VANGUARD® 5 was subjected to comprehensive safety and efficacy testing. It was shown safe and reaction-free in laboratory tests and in clinical trials under field conditions. Product safety was demonstrated by oral administration of multiple doses of the vaccine strain to susceptible dogs, which remained normal. The CPV virus in VANGUARD® 5 shares a characteristic with other live CPV vaccine strains in that the vaccinal virus may be present in the feces following administration. Although this CPV vaccinal virus was found occasionally and in low titers in the feces of vaccinated dogs, testing demonstrated that the vaccine strain did not revert to virulence following 6 consecutive backpassages in susceptible dogs.

Susceptible test dogs all developed CPV antibody titers after vaccination and were protected following oral administration of virulent CPV. Conversely, after challenge exposure, nonvaccinated control dogs all developed clinical signs of CPV infection, including vomiting and diarrhea with blood and mucus in the feces. Challenge virus was isolated from the feces of 5/5 control dogs, but only 1/20 vaccinates, and all controls developed marked lymphopenia, while no lymphopenia was demonstrated in vaccinates.

Further research demonstrated a stronger correlation of CPV immunogenicity to number of attenuating virus passages than to antigenic mass; immunogenicity of the vaccinal strain was shown to decline as the number of passages increased. The low-passage vaccinal virus in VANGUARD® 5 is therefore highly immunogenic and capable of stimulating active immunity in the presence of maternal antibodies at the levels shown in Table 1. Studies demonstrating that capability involved forty-one 6- to 8-week-old puppies (32 vaccinates and 9 controls) with the range of maternal antibody titers shown in Table 2. By 14 days after vaccination, 91% of vaccinates' titers were well above the protective threshold. By 21 days, all dogs, including the dog with the initial SN titer of 1:64 seroconverted, giving a group seroconversion rate of 100%. In contrast, seropositive sentinel littermate dogs' CPV antibody titers declined, demonstrating that initial antibody titers were indeed of maternal origin and no adventitious exposure occurred during the study.

Table 1. Pre- and Postvaccination Serum Neutralization (SN) Titers

Number of Dogs	Prevaccination	Postvaccination		
		7 Days	14 Days	21 Days
5	2	39.2	768.0	1433.6
2	4	3.0	36.0	192.0
11	8	45.1	457.5	488.7
9	16	33.8	263.1	739.6
4	32	40.0	450.0	640.0
1	64	32.0	32.0	128.0
Average	13.8	37.3	410.8	696.0

Table 2. Initial Serum Neutralization (SN) Titers of Vaccinates and Controls.

SN Titers	# Vaccinates Included	# Controls Included
1:2	5	0
1:4	2	1
1:8	11	2
1:16	9	4
1:32	4	2
1:64	1	0

References: Available upon request.

Presentation: Cartons of 25 x 1 dose vials.

U.S. Patent No. 3,616,203

Compendium Code No.: 36901470 75-4982-04

VANGUARD® 5/B

Pfizer Animal Health **Bacterin-Vaccine**

Canine Distemper-Adenovirus Type 2-Parainfluenza-Parvovirus Vaccine, Modified Live Virus-Bordetella Bronchiseptica Bacterin

U.S. Vet. Lic. No.: 189

Description: The vaccine component of VANGUARD® 5/B contains attenuated strains of CD virus, CAV-2, CPI virus, and CPV propagated on an established canine cell line. The CPV fraction was attenuated by low passage on the canine cell line and at that passage level has immunogenic properties capable of overriding maternal antibodies. Some puppies in the field may have higher levels of maternal antibodies than those evaluated in our pivotal efficacy study. The vaccine is packaged in freeze-dried form with inert gas in place of vacuum. The bacterin component, containing inactivated whole cultures of *B. bronchiseptica,* is supplied as diluent.

Contains penicillin and streptomycin as preservatives.

Indications: VANGUARD® 5/B is for vaccination of healthy dogs as an aid in the prevention and control of canine distemper caused by canine distemper (CD) virus, infectious canine hepatitis (ICH) caused by canine adenovirus type 1 (CAV-1), respiratory disease caused by canine adenovirus type 2 (CAV-2), canine parainfluenza caused by canine parainfluenza (CPI) virus, canine parvoviral enteritis caused by canine parvovirus (CPV), and infectious tracheobronchitis ("kennel cough") caused by *Bordetella bronchiseptica.*

Directions:

1. General Directions: Vaccination of healthy dogs is recommended. Aseptically rehydrate the freeze-dried vaccine (Vanguard® 5) with the liquid bacterin provided (CoughGuard® B), shake well, and administer 1 mL subcutaneously or intramuscularly.
2. Primary Vaccination: Healthy dogs should receive 2 doses administered 2-4 weeks apart. If dogs are vaccinated before the age of 4 months, they should be revaccinated with a single dose upon reaching 4 months of age. (Maternal antibodies may interfere with development of an adequate immune response in puppies less than 4 months old.) Where *B. bronchiseptica* and canine virus exposure is likely, such as breeding, boarding, and showing situations, an additional booster may be indicated or annual revaccination should be timed 2-4 weeks prior to these events.
3. Revaccination: Annual revaccination with a single dose is recommended.

Precaution(s): Store at 2°-7°C. Prolonged exposure to higher temperatures and/or direct sunlight may adversely affect potency. Do not freeze.

Use entire contents when first opened.

Sterilized syringes and needles should be used to administer this vaccine. Do not sterilize with chemicals because traces of disinfectant may inactivate the vaccine.

Burn containers and all unused contents.

Caution(s): Vaccination of pregnant bitches should be avoided.

Although the *Bordetella* fraction of VANGUARD® 5/B has been specifically designed to be nontoxic, a small, nonirritating, sterile nodule may appear in some puppies after subcutaneous inoculation. For puppies, therefore, intramuscular vaccination may be advisable. Stinging has been reported in up to 10% of dogs vaccinated intramuscularly.

As with many vaccines, anaphylaxis may occur after use. Initial antidote of epinephrine is recommended and should be followed with appropriate supportive therapy.

This product has been shown to be efficacious in healthy animals. A protective immune response may not be elicited if animals are incubating an infectious disease, are malnourished or parasitized, are stressed due to shipment or environmental conditions, are otherwise immunocompromised, or the vaccine is not administered in accordance with label directions.

Warning(s): For use in dogs only.

For veterinary use only.

Discussion: Disease Description: CD is a universal, high-mortality viral disease with variable manifestations. Approximately 50% of nonvaccinated, nonimmune dogs infected with CD virus develop clinical signs, and approximately 90% of those dogs die.[1] ICH, caused by CAV-1, is a universal, sometimes fatal, viral disease of dogs characterized by hepatic and generalized endothelial lesions. CAV-2 causes respiratory disease which in severe cases may include pneumonia and bronchopneumonia. CPI is a common viral upper respiratory disease. Uncomplicated CPI may be mild or subclinical, with signs becoming more severe if concurrent infection with other respiratory pathogens exists. CPV infection results in enteric disease characterized by sudden onset of vomiting and diarrhea, often hemorrhagic. Leukopenia commonly accompanies clinical signs. Susceptible dogs of any age can be affected, but mortality is greatest in puppies. In puppies 4-12 weeks of age CPV may occasionally cause myocarditis that can result in acute heart failure after a brief and inconspicuous illness. Following infection many dogs are refractory to the disease for a year or more. Similarly, seropositive bitches may transfer to their puppies CPV antibodies which can interfere with active immunization of the puppies through 16 weeks of age. Although there is no single cause for kennel cough, *B. bronchiseptica* is a primary etiological agent in the kennel cough complex.[4,5] The outstanding sign of *B. bronchiseptica* infection is a harsh, dry cough which is aggravated by activity or excitement. The coughing occurs in paroxysms, followed by retching or gagging in attempts to clear small amounts of mucus from the throat. Body temperature may be elevated as secondary bacterial invasion takes place. Antibiotics are generally recognized as poor agents to treat the primary disease. In contrast, immunoprophylaxis for *B. bronchiseptica* provides an effective means to aid in the control of the disease.[6]

Trial Data: Safety and Efficacy: Laboratory evaluation demonstrated that VANGUARD® 5/B aided in preventing disease caused by CD, ICH, CAV-2 respiratory disease, CPI, CPV, and *B. bronchiseptica,* and that no immunologic interference existed among the vaccine fractions.

It has been demonstrated that CAV-2 vaccine cross-protects against ICH caused by CAV-1. The CAV-2 fraction in Vanguard® vaccines is used as a replacement for CAV-1 because it has significant advantages. Some CAV-1 vaccines may produce undesirable reactions, including persistent kidney infections, uveitis, and corneal opacity ("blue eye"), which have not been reported after vaccination with CAV-2.[2] In addition, the CAV-2 strain used in Vanguard® vaccines has been specially selected for freedom from oncogenic properties characteristic of adenoviruses.

Studies demonstrated that the CAV-2 fraction in VANGUARD® 5/B not only aids in preventing ICH, but against CAV-2 respiratory disease as well.[3] Although conventional CAV-1 (ICH) vaccines cross-protect against CAV-2, they may not prevent subclinical infection and spread of the CAV-2 agent. Canine adenovirus type 2 challenge virus was not recovered from CAV-2-vaccinated dogs.

The CPV fraction in VANGUARD® 5/B was subjected to comprehensive safety and efficacy testing. It was shown safe and reaction-free in laboratory tests and in clinical trials under field conditions. Product safety was demonstrated by oral administration of multiple doses of the vaccine strain to susceptible dogs, which remained normal. The CPV virus in VANGUARD® 5/B shares a characteristic with other live CPV vaccine strains in that the vaccinal virus may be present in the feces following administration. Although this CPV vaccinal virus was found occasionally and in low titers in the feces of vaccinated dogs, testing demonstrated that the vaccine strain did not revert to virulence following 6 consecutive backpassages in susceptible dogs.

Susceptible test dogs all developed CPV antibody titers after vaccination and were protected following oral administration of virulent CPV. Conversely, after challenge exposure, nonvaccinated control dogs all developed clinical signs of CPV enteritis, including vomiting and diarrhea with blood and mucus in the feces. Challenge virus was isolated from the feces of 5/5 control dogs, but only 1/20 vaccinates, and all controls developed marked lymphopenia, while no lymphopenia was demonstrated in vaccinates.

Further research demonstrated a stronger correlation of CPV immunogenicity to number of attenuating virus passages than to antigenic mass; immunogenicity of the vaccinal strain was shown to decline as the number of passages increased. The low-passage vaccinal virus in VANGUARD® 5/B is therefore highly immunogenic and capable of stimulating active immunity in the presence of maternal antibodies at the levels shown in Table 1. Studies demonstrating that capability involved forty-one 6- to 8-week-old puppies (32 vaccinates and 9 controls) with the range of maternal antibody titers shown in Table 2. By 14 days after vaccination, 91% of vaccinates' titers were well above the protective threshold. By 21 days, all dogs, including the dog with the initial SN titer of 1:64 seroconverted, giving a group seroconversion rate of 100%. In contrast, seropositive sentinel littermate dogs' CPV antibody titers declined, demonstrating that initial antibody titers were indeed of maternal origin and no adventitious exposure occurred during the study.

The *B. bronchiseptica* fraction in VANGUARD® 5/B is prepared from a highly antigenic strain which has been inactivated and processed to be nontoxic when administered to dogs. Historically, *Bordetella* bacterins have had a tendency toward toxic reactions characterized by lethargy, anorexia, and vomiting 1-6 hours after administration; however, the *B. bronchiseptica* fraction is safe and effective. In an extensive field trial in which over 3,268 doses of the *B. bronchiseptica* fraction were administered, no reports of these reactions were received.

When VANGUARD® 5/B was administered subcutaneously to adult dogs, serious reactions to the *B. bronchiseptica* fraction were not noted. In puppies, however, petite nodules developed. These were nonirritating, sterile, and transitory in nature. This mild reaction was not observed in puppies when VANGUARD® 5/B was administered by the intramuscular route. A postvaccinal sting has been reported in less than 10% of dogs vaccinated intramuscularly.

In tests conducted with normal, susceptible dogs under controlled conditions, experimental infection with the virulent BC strain of *B. bronchiseptica* resulted in coughing and other respiratory signs typical of kennel cough. In the usual research model, palpation of the throat is necessary to produce coughing. Due to the severity of the challenge in the test, coughing was spontaneous for extended periods beginning 2-5 days after challenge. (Data on file, Pfizer Animal Health.)

Clinical signs of coughing were significantly ($p = 0.05$) reduced when vaccinates were experimentally exposed to the virulent BC strain of *B. bronchiseptica* (Table 3).

Table 1. Pre- and Postvaccination Serum Neutralization (SN) Titers

Number of Dogs	Prevaccination	Postvaccination		
		7 Days	14 Days	21 Days
5	2	39.2	768.0	1433.6
2	4	3.0	36.0	192.0
11	8	45.1	457.5	488.7
9	16	33.8	263.1	739.6
4	32	40.0	450.0	640.0
1	64	32.0	32.0	128.0
Average	13.8	37.3	410.8	696.0

Table 2. Initial Serum Neutralization (SN) Titers of Vaccinates and Controls.

SN Titers	# Vaccinates Included	# Controls Included
1:2	5	0
1:4	2	1
1:8	11	2
1:16	9	4
1:32	4	2
1:64	1	0

Table 3. Reduction in coughing associated with experimental challenge exposure of dogs with the virulent BC strain of *B. bronchiseptica*

Treatment	Total No. of Dogs	Mean Percent (%) Cough Reduction*
Vaccinated	548	77±12**
Nonvaccinated control	233	-

*Results of 89 efficacy tests ranged from 50% (minimum) to 96% (maximum) cough reduction in vaccinates.

**Standard deviation.

References: Available upon request.

Presentation: Cartons of 25 x 1 dose vials.

U.S. Patent No. 3,616,203

Compendium Code No.: 36901480 75-4970-05

VANGUARD® 5/CV

Pfizer Animal Health **Vaccine**

Canine Distemper-Adenovirus Type 2-Coronavirus-Parainfluenza-Parvovirus Vaccine, Modified Live and Killed Virus

U.S. Vet. Lic. No.: 189

Description: The freeze-dried component of VANGUARD® 5/CV contains attenuated strains of CD virus, CAV-2, CPI virus, and CPV propagated on an established canine cell line. The CPV fraction was attenuated by low passage on the canine cell line and at that passage level has immunogenic properties capable of overriding maternal antibodies. Some puppies in the field may have higher levels of maternal antibodies than those evaluated in our pivotal efficacy study. The liquid component, containing a preparation of inactivated CCV propagated on an established canine cell line with an adjuvant, is used to rehydrate the freeze-dried component, which is packaged with inert gas in place of vacuum.

Contains penicillin and streptomycin as preservatives.

Indications: VANGUARD® 5/CV is for vaccination of healthy dogs as an aid in preventing canine distemper caused by canine distemper (CD) virus, infectious canine hepatitis (ICH) caused by canine adenovirus type 1 (CAV-1), respiratory disease caused by canine adenovirus type 2 (CAV-2), canine parainfluenza caused by canine parainfluenza (CPI) virus, and disease caused by canine parvovirus (CPV) and canine coronavirus (CCV).

V

Directions:

1. General Directions: Vaccination of healthy dogs is recommended. Aseptically rehydrate the freeze-dried vaccine (Vanguard® 5) with the accompanying vial of liquid vaccine (FirstDose® CV), shake well, and administer 1 mL subcutaneously or intramuscularly.
2. Primary Vaccination: Healthy dogs should receive 2 doses administered 3-4 weeks apart. If dogs are vaccinated before the age of 4 months, they should be revaccinated with a single dose upon reaching 4 months of age. (Maternal antibodies may interfere with development of an adequate immune response in puppies less than 4 months old.)
3. Revaccination: Annual revaccination with a single dose is recommended.

Precaution(s): Store at 2°-7°C. Prolonged exposure to higher temperatures and/or direct sunlight may adversely affect potency. Do not freeze.

Use entire contents when first opened.

Sterilized syringes and needles should be used to administer this vaccine. Do not sterilize with chemicals because traces of disinfectant may inactivate the vaccine.

Burn containers and all unused contents.

Caution(s): Vaccination of pregnant bitches should be avoided.

As with many vaccines, anaphylaxis may occur after use. Initial antidote of epinephrine is recommended and should be followed with appropriate supportive therapy.

This product has been shown to be efficacious in healthy animals. A protective immune response may not be elicited if animals are incubating an infectious disease, are malnourished or parasitized, are stressed due to shipment or environmental conditions, are otherwise immunocompromised, or the vaccine is not administered in accordance with label directions.

Warning(s): For use in dogs only.

For veterinary use only.

Discussion: Disease Description: CD is a universal, high-mortality viral disease with variable manifestations. Approximately 50% of nonvaccinated, nonimmune dogs infected with CD virus develop clinical signs, and approximately 90% of those dogs die.[1] ICH, caused by CAV-1, is a universal, sometimes fatal, viral disease of dogs characterized by hepatic and generalized endothelial lesions. CAV-2 causes respiratory disease which in severe cases may include pneumonia and bronchopneumonia. CPI is a common viral upper respiratory disease. Uncomplicated CPI may be mild or subclinical, with signs becoming more severe if concurrent infection with other respiratory pathogens exists. CPV infection results in enteric disease characterized by sudden onset of vomiting and diarrhea, often hemorrhagic. Leukopenia commonly accompanies clinical signs. Susceptible dogs of any age can be affected, but mortality is greatest in puppies. CCV also causes enteric disease. Characteristics include depression, anorexia, fever, vomiting, and diarrhea. Particularly in puppies, potentially life-threatening dehydration may result from severe diarrhea.

Laboratory procedures are frequently employed to differentiate CPV and CCV infections due to their clinical similarities. Laboratory diagnosis based solely on hemagglutination (HA) tests, however, may not distinguish between the 2 agents because HA tests can yield positive results when either CPV or CCV is present, particularly at low levels of HA activity. The result may be a false positive diagnosis for either virus when in fact the other is the agent of disease. Comprehensive protection thus requires vaccination for both CPV and CCV.

Trial Data: Safety and Efficacy: VANGUARD® 5/CV was subjected to comprehensive safety testing. It was shown safe in laboratory tests and in clinical trials under field conditions. Laboratory evaluation demonstrated that VANGUARD® 5/CV aided in preventing disease caused by CD, ICH, CAV-2 respiratory disease, CPI, CPV, and CCV, and that no immunologic interference existed among the vaccine fractions.

It has been demonstrated that CAV-2 vaccine cross-protects against ICH caused by CAV-1. The CAV-2 fraction in Vanguard® vaccines is used as a replacement for CAV-1 because it has significant advantages. Some CAV-1 vaccines may produce undesirable reactions, including persistent kidney infections, uveitis, and corneal opacity ("blue eye"), which have not been reported after vaccination with CAV-2.[2] In addition, the CAV-2 strain used in Vanguard® vaccines has been specially selected for freedom from oncogenic properties characteristic of adenoviruses.

Studies demonstrated that the CAV-2 fraction in VANGUARD® 5/CV not only protects against ICH, but against CAV-2 respiratory disease as well.[3] Although conventional CAV-1 (ICH) vaccines cross-protect against CAV-2, they may not prevent subclinical infection and spread of the CAV-2 agent. Canine adenovirus type 2 challenge virus was not recovered from CAV-2-vaccinated dogs.

Safety of the CPV fraction in VANGUARD® 5/CV was demonstrated by oral administration of multiple doses of the vaccine strain to susceptible dogs, which remained normal. The CPV virus in VANGUARD® 5/CV shares a characteristic with other live CPV vaccine strains in that the vaccinal virus may be present in the feces following administration. Although this CPV vaccinal virus was found occasionally and in low titers in the feces of vaccinated dogs, testing demonstrated that the vaccine strain did not revert to virulence following 6 consecutive backpassages in susceptible dogs.

Safety of the CCV fraction in VANGUARD® 5/CV was assessed in a field trial in which 5,999 doses were administered. Postvaccinal reactions occurred in 0.78% of vaccinates. Stinging and pain were observed in 0.08% of vaccinates, transient lameness or swelling were observed in 0.28% of vaccinates, anaphylaxis was observed in 0.12% of vaccinates, and gastroenteritis was observed in 0.30% of vaccinates.

Efficacy of the CPV fraction in VANGUARD® 5/CV was demonstrated in challenge-of-immunity studies. Susceptible test dogs all developed CPV antibody titers after vaccination and were protected following oral administration of virulent CPV. Conversely, after challenge exposure, nonvaccinated control dogs all developed clinical signs of CPV enteritis, including vomiting and diarrhea with blood and mucus in the feces. Challenge virus was isolated from the feces of 5/5 control dogs, but only 1/20 vaccinates, and all controls developed marked lymphopenia, while no lymphopenia was demonstrated in vaccinates.

V

Further research demonstrated a stronger correlation of CPV immunogenicity to number of attenuating virus passages than to antigenic mass; immunogenicity of the vaccinal strain was shown to decline as the number of passages increased. The low-passage vaccinal virus in VANGUARD® 5/CV is therefore highly immunogenic and capable of stimulating active immunity in the presence of maternal antibodies at the levels shown in Table 1. Studies demonstrating that capability involved forty-one 6- to 8-week-old puppies (32 vaccinates and 9 controls) with the range of maternal antibody titers shown in Table 2. By 14 days after vaccination, 91% of vaccinates' titers were well above the protective threshold. By 21 days, all dogs, including the dog with the initial SN titer of 1:64 seroconverted, giving a group seroconversion rate of 100%. In contrast, seropositive sentinel littermate dogs' CPV antibody titers declined, demonstrating that initial antibody titers were indeed of maternal origin and no adventitious exposure occurred during the study.

Table 1. Pre- and Postvaccination Serum Neutralization (SN) Titers

Number of Dogs	Prevaccination	Postvaccination		
		7 Days	14 Days	21 Days
5	2	39.2	768.0	1433.6
2	4	3.0	36.0	192.0
11	8	45.1	457.5	488.7
9	16	33.8	263.1	739.6
4	32	40.0	450.0	640.0
1	64	32.0	32.0	128.0
Average	13.8	37.3	410.8	696.0

Table 2. Initial Serum Neutralization (SN) Titers of Vaccinates and Controls

SN Titers	# Vaccinates Included	# Controls Included
1:2	5	0
1:4	2	1
1:8	11	2
1:16	9	4
1:32	4	2
1:64	1	0

Efficacy of the CCV fraction was demonstrated in a challenge-of-immunity study involving 20 vaccinated puppies and 10 controls. Twenty 6- to 7-week-old puppies received 1 dose of vaccine given by the subcutaneous route, followed by a second subcutaneous dose 21 days later. Vaccinates and controls were challenged with virulent CCV 21 days postvaccination. Puppies vaccinated with CCV demonstrated significant differences in reduction of clinical signs, virus shed, and reduction of diarrhea postchallenge when compared to the control group. There was a significant reduction of IFA detectable CCV antigen detected in the intestine at 19 days postchallenge in vaccinates compared to the control group. Serological responses of vaccinates were equal to or higher than the control group.

References: Available upon request.

Presentation: Cartons of 25 x 1 dose vials.

U.S. Patent Nos. 4,567,042; 4,567,043; and 4,824,785

Compendium Code No.: 36901490 75-4972-06

VANGUARD® 5/CV-L

Pfizer Animal Health **Bacterin-Vaccine**

Canine Distemper-Adenovirus Type 2-Coronavirus-Parainfluenza-Parvovirus Vaccine, Modified Live and Killed Virus-Leptospira Bacterin

U.S. Vet. Lic. No.: 189

Description: VANGUARD® 5/CV-L is a freeze-dried preparation of attenuated strains of CD virus, CAV-2, CPI virus, CPV, and inactivated whole cltures of *L. canicola* and *L. icterohaemorrhagiae* plus a liquid preparation of inactivated CCV with an adjuvant. All viruses were propagated on established cell lines. The CPV fraction was attenuated by low passage on the canine cell line and at that passage level has immunogenic properties capable of overriding maternal antibodies. Some puppies in the field may have higher levels of maternal antibodies than those evaluated in our pivotal efficacy study. The liquid component is used to rehydrate the freeze-dried component, which is packaged with inert gas in place of vacuum.

Contains penicillin and streptomycin as preservatives.

Indications: VANGUARD® 5/CV-L is for vaccination of healthy dogs as an aid in preventing canine distemper caused by canine distemper (CD) virus, infectious canine hepatitis (ICH) caused by canine adenovirus type 1 (CAV-1), respiratory disease caused by canine adenovirus type 2 (CAV-2), canine parainfluenza caused by canine parainfluenza (CPI) virus, disease caused by canine parvovirus (CPV) and canine coronavirus (CCV), and leptospirosis caused by *Leptospira canicola* and *L. icterohaemorrhagiae.*

Directions:

1. General Directions: Vaccination of healthy dogs is recommended. Aseptically rehydrate the freeze-dried vaccine (Vanguard® 5/L) with the accompanying vial of liquid vaccine (FirstDose® CV), shake well, and administer 1 mL subcutaneously or intramuscularly immediately after rehydration.
2. Primary Vaccination: Healthy dogs should receive 2 doses administered 3-4 weeks apart. If dogs are vaccinated before the age of 4 months, they should be revaccinated with a single dose upon reaching 4 months of age. (Maternal antibodies may interfere with development of an adequate immune response in puppies less than 4 months old.)
3. Revaccination: Annual revaccination with a single dose is recommended.

Precaution(s): Store at 2°-7°C. Prolonged exposure to higher temperatures and/or direct sunlight may adversely affect potency. Do not freeze.

Use entire contents when first opened.

Sterilized syringes and needles should be used to administer this vaccine. Do not sterilize with chemicals because traces of disinfectant may inactivate the vaccine.

Burn containers and all unused contents.

Caution(s): Vaccination of pregnant bitches should be avoided.

As with many vaccines, anaphylaxis may occur after use. Initial antidote of epinephrine is recommended and should be followed with appropriate supportive therapy.

This product has been shown to be efficacious in healthy animals. A protective immune response may not be elicited if animals are incubating an infectious disease, are malnourished or parasitized, are stressed due to shipment or environmental conditions, are otherwise immunocompromised, or the vaccine is not administered in accordance with label directions.

Warning(s): For use in dogs only.

For veterinary use only.

Discussion: Disease Description: CD is a universal, high-mortality viral disease with variable manifestations. Approximately 50% of nonvaccinated, nonimmune dogs infected with CD virus develop clinical signs, and approximately 90% of those dogs die.[1] ICH, caused by CAV-1, is a universal, sometimes fatal, viral disease of dogs characterized by hepatic and generalized endothelial lesions. CAV-2 causes respiratory disease which in severe cases may include pneumonia and bronchopneumonia. CPI is a common viral upper respiratory disease. Uncomplicated CPI may be mild or subclinical, with signs becoming more severe if concurrent infection with other respiratory pathogens exists. CPV infection results in enteric disease characterized by sudden onset of vomiting and diarrhea, often hemorrhagic. Leukopenia commonly accompanies clinical signs. Susceptible dogs of any age can be affected, but mortality is greatest in puppies. CCV also causes enteric disease. Characteristics include depression, anorexia, fever, vomiting, and diarrhea. Particularly in puppies, potentially life-threatening dehydration may result from severe diarrhea. Leptospirosis occurs in dogs of all ages, with a wide range of clinical signs and chronic nephritis generally following acute infection. Infection with *L. canicola* and *L. icterohaemorrhagiae* cannot be differentiated clinically.

Laboratory procedures are frequently employed to differentiate CPV and CCV infections due to their clinical similarities. Laboratory diagnosis based solely on hemagglutination (HA) tests, however, may not distinguish between the 2 agents because HA tests can yield positive results when either CPV or CCV is present, particularly at low levels of HA activity. The result may be a false positive diagnosis for either virus when in fact the other is the agent of disease. Comprehensive protection thus requires vaccination for both CPV and CCV.

Trial Data: Safety and Efficacy: VANGUARD® 5/CV-L was subjected to comprehensive safety tests. It was shown safe in laboratory tests and in clinical trials under field conditions. Laboratory evaluation demonstrated that VANGUARD® 5/CV-L aided in preventing disease caused by CD, ICH, CAV-2 respiratory disease, CPI, CPV, CCV, and leptospirosis caused by *L. canicola* and *L. icterohaemorrhagiae*, and that no immunologic interference existed among the vaccine fractions.

It has been demonstrated that CAV-2 vaccine cross-protects against ICH caused by CAV-1. The CAV-2 fraction in Vanguard® vaccines is used as a replacement for CAV-1 because it has significant advantages. Some CAV-1 vaccines may produce undesirable reactions, including persistent kidney infections, uveitis, and corneal opacity ("blue eye"), which have not been reported after vaccination with CAV-2.[2] In addition, the CAV-2 strain used in Vanguard® vaccines has been specially selected for freedom from oncogenic properties characteristic of adenoviruses.

Studies demonstrated that the CAV-2 fraction in VANGUARD® 5/CV-L not only protects against ICH, but against CAV-2 respiratory disease as well.[3] Although conventional CAV-1 (ICH) vaccines cross-protect against CAV-2, they may not prevent subclinical infection and spread of the CAV-2 agent. Canine adenovirus type 2 challenge virus was not recovered from CAV-2-vaccinated dogs.

Safety of the CPV fraction in VANGUARD® 5/CV-L was demonstrated by oral administration of multiple doses of the vaccine strain to susceptible dogs, which remained normal. The CPV virus in VANGUARD® 5/CV-L shares a characteristic with other live CPV vaccine strains in that the vaccinal virus may be present in the feces following administration. Although this CPV vaccinal virus was found occasionally and in low titers in the feces of vaccinated dogs, testing demonstrated that the vaccine strain did not revert to virulence following 6 consecutive backpassages in susceptible dogs.

Safety of the CCV fraction in VANGUARD® 5/CV-L was assessed in a field trial in which 5,999 doses were administered. Postvaccinal reactions occurred in 0.78% of vaccinates. Stinging and pain were observed in 0.08% of vaccinates, transient lameness or swelling were observed in 0.28% of vaccinates, anaphylaxis was observed in 0.12% of vaccinates, and gastroenteritis was observed in 0.30% of vaccinates.

Efficacy of the CPV fraction in VANGUARD® 5/CV-L was demonstrated in challenge-of-immunity studies. Susceptible test dogs all developed CPV antibody titers after vaccination and were protected following oral administration of virulent CPV. Conversely, after challenge exposure, nonvaccinated control dogs all developed clinical signs of CPV enteritis, including vomiting and diarrhea with blood and mucus in the feces. Challenge virus was isolated from the feces of 5/5 control dogs, but only 1/20 vaccinates, and all controls developed marked lymphopenia, while no lymphopenia was demonstrated in vaccinates.

Further research demonstrated a stronger correlation of CPV immunogenicity to number of attenuating virus passages than to antigenic mass; immunogenicity of the vaccinal strain was shown to decline as the number of passages increased. The low-passage vaccinal virus in VANGUARD® 5/CV-L is therefore highly immunogenic and capable of stimulating active immunity in the presence of maternal antibodies at the levels shown in Table 1. Studies demonstrating that capability involved forty-one 6- to 8-week-old puppies (32 vaccinates and 9 controls) with the range of maternal antibody titers shown in Table 2. By 14 days after vaccination, 91% of vaccinates' titers were well above the protective threshold. By 21 days, all dogs, including the dog with the initial SN titer of 1:64 seroconverted, giving a group seroconversion rate of 100%. In contrast, seropositive sentinel littermate dogs' CPV antibody titers declined, demonstrating that initial antibody titers were indeed of maternal origin and no adventitious exposure occurred during the study.

Table 1. Pre- and Postvaccination Serum Neutralization (SN) Titers

Number of Dogs	Prevaccination	Postvaccination		
		7 Days	14 Days	21 Days
5	2	39.2	768.0	1433.6
2	4	3.0	36.0	192.0
11	8	45.1	457.5	488.7
9	16	33.8	263.1	739.6
4	32	40.0	450.0	640.0
1	64	32.0	32.0	128.0
Average	13.8	37.3	410.8	696.0

Table 2. Initial Serum Neutralization (SN) Titers of Vaccinates and Controls

SN Titers	# Vaccinates Included	# Controls Included
1:2	5	0
1:4	2	1
1:8	11	2
1:16	9	4
1:32	4	2
1:64	1	0

Efficacy of the CCV fraction was demonstrated in a challenge-of-immunity study involving 20 vaccinated puppies and 10 controls. Twenty 6- to 7-week-old puppies received 1 dose of vaccine given by the subcutaneous route, followed by a second subcutaneous dose 21 days later. Vaccinates and controls were challenged with virulent CCV 21 days postvaccination. Puppies vaccinated with CCV demonstrated significant differences in reduction of clinical signs, virus shed, and reduction of diarrhea postchallenge when compared to the control group. There was a significant reduction of IFA detectable CCV antigen detected in the intestine at 19 days postchallenge in vaccinates compared to the control group. Serological responses of vaccinates were equal to or higher than the control group.

References: Available upon request.

Presentation: Cartons of 25 x 1 dose vials.

U.S. Patent Nos. 4,567,042; 4,567,043; and 4,824,785

Compendium Code No.: 36901500 75-4973-05

VANGUARD® 5/L

Pfizer Animal Health **Bacterin-Vaccine**

Canine Distemper-Adenovirus Type 2-Parainfluenza-Parvovirus Vaccine, Modified Live Virus-Leptospira Bacterin

U.S. Vet. Lic. No.: 189

Description: The vaccine component of VANGUARD® 5/L contains attenuated strains of CD virus, CAV-2, CPI virus, and CPV propagated on an established canine cell line. The CPV fraction was attenuated by low passage on the canine cell line and at that passage level has immunogenic properties capable of overriding maternal antibodies. Some puppies in the field may have higher levels of maternal antibodies than those evaluated in our pivotal efficacy study. The vaccine is packaged in freeze-dried form with inert gas in place of vacuum. The bacterin component, containing inactivated whole cultures of *L. canicola* and *L. icterohaemorrhagiae*, is supplied as diluent.

Contains penicillin and streptomycin as preservatives.

Indications: VANGUARD® 5/L is for vaccination of healthy dogs as an aid in preventing canine distemper caused by canine distemper (CD) virus, infectious canine hepatitis (ICH) caused by canine adenovirus type 1 (CAV-1), respiratory disease caused by canine adenovirus type 2 (CAV-2), canine parainfluenza caused by canine parainfluenza (CPI) virus, canine parvoviral enteritis caused by canine parvovirus (CPV), and leptospirosis caused by *Leptospira canicola* and *L. icterohaemorrhagiae*.

Directions:

1. General Directions: Vaccination of healthy dogs is recommended. Aseptically rehydrate the freeze-dried vaccine (Vanguard® 5) with the liquid bacterin provided (Leptoferm C-I®), shake well, and administer 1 mL subcutaneously or intramuscularly.
2. Primary Vaccination: Healthy dogs should receive 2 doses administered 3-4 weeks apart. If dogs are vaccinated before the age of 4 months, they should be revaccinated with a single dose upon reaching 4 months of age. (Maternal antibodies may interfere with development of an adequate immune response in puppies less than 4 months old.)
3. Revaccination: Annual revaccination with a single dose is recommended.

Precaution(s): Store at 2°-7°C. Prolonged exposure to higher temperatures and/or direct sunlight may adversely affect potency. Do not freeze.

Use entire contents when first opened.

Sterilized syringes and needles should be used to administer this vaccine. Do not sterilize with chemicals because traces of disinfectant may inactivate the vaccine.

Burn containers and all unused contents.

Caution(s): Vaccination of pregnant bitches should be avoided.

As with many vaccines, anaphylaxis may occur after use. Initial antidote of epinephrine is recommended and should be followed with appropriate supportive therapy.

This product has been shown to be efficacious in healthy animals. A protective immune response may not be elicited if animals are incubating an infectious disease, are malnourished or parasitized, are stressed due to shipment or environmental conditions, are otherwise immunocompromised, or the vaccine is not administered in accordance with label directions.

Warning(s): For use in dogs only.

For veterinary use only.

Discussion: Disease Description: CD is a universal, high-mortality viral disease with variable manifestations. Approximately 50% of nonvaccinated, nonimmune dogs infected with CD virus develop clinical signs, and approximately 90% of those dogs die.[1] ICH, caused by CAV-1, is a universal, sometimes fatal, viral disease of dogs characterized by hepatic and generalized endothelial lesions. CAV-2 causes respiratory disease which in severe cases may include pneumonia and bronchopneumonia. CPI is a common viral upper respiratory disease. Uncomplicated CPI may be mild or subclinical, with signs becoming more severe if concurrent infection with other respiratory pathogens exists. CPV infection results in enteric disease characterized by sudden onset of vomiting and diarrhea, often hemorrhagic. Leukopenia commonly accompanies clinical signs. Susceptible dogs of any age can be affected, but mortality is greatest in puppies. In puppies 4-12 weeks of age CPV may occasionally cause myocarditis that can result in acute heart failure after a brief and inconspicuous illness. Following infection many dogs are refractory to the disease for a year or more. Similarly, seropositive bitches may transfer to their puppies CPV antibodies which can interfere with active immunization of the puppies through 16 weeks of age. Leptospirosis occurs in dogs of all ages, with a wide range of clinical signs and chronic nephritis generally following acute infection. Infection with *L. canicola* and *L. icterohaemorrhagiae* cannot be differentiated clinically.

Trial Data: Safety and Efficacy: Laboratory evaluation demonstrated that VANGUARD® 5/L aided in preventing disease caused by CD, ICH, CAV-2 respiratory disease, CPI, CPV, and leptospirosis caused by *L. canicola* and *L. icterohaemorrhagiae*, and that no immunologic interference existed among the vaccine fractions.

It has been demonstrated that CAV-2 vaccine cross-protects against ICH caused by CAV-1. The CAV-2 fraction in Vanguard® vaccines is used as a replacement for CAV-1 because it has significant advantages. Some CAV-1 vaccines may produce undesirable reactions, including persistent kidney infections, uveitis, and corneal opacity ("blue eye"), which have not been reported after vaccination with CAV-2.[2] In addition, the CAV-2 strain used in Vanguard® vaccines has been specially selected for freedom from oncogenic properties characteristic of adenoviruses.

Studies demonstrated that the CAV-2 fraction in VANGUARD® 5/L not only protects against ICH, but against CAV-2 respiratory disease as well.[3] Although conventional CAV-1 (ICH) vaccines cross-protect against CAV-2, they may not prevent subclinical infection and spread of the CAV-2 agent. Canine adenovirus type 2 challenge virus was not recovered from CAV-2-vaccinated dogs.

The CPV fraction in VANGUARD® 5/L was subjected to comprehensive safety and efficacy testing. It was shown safe and reaction-free in laboratory tests and in clinical trials under field conditions. Product safety was demonstrated by oral administration of multiple doses of the vaccine strain to susceptible dogs, which remained normal. The CPV virus in VANGUARD® 5/L shares a characteristic with other live CPV vaccine strains in that the vaccinal virus may be present in the feces following administration. Although this CPV vaccinal virus was found occasionally and in low titers in the feces of vaccinated dogs, testing demonstrated that the vaccine strain did not revert to virulence following 6 consecutive backpassages in susceptible dogs.

Susceptible test dogs all developed CPV antibody titers after vaccination and were protected following oral administration of virulent CPV. Conversely, after challenge exposure, nonvaccinated control dogs all developed clinical signs of CPV enteritis, including vomiting and diarrhea with blood and mucus in the feces. Challenge virus was isolated from the feces of 5/5 control dogs, but only 1/20 vaccinates, and all controls developed marked lymphopenia, while no lymphopenia was demonstrated in vaccinates.

Further research demonstrated a stronger correlation of CPV immunogenicity to number of attenuating virus passages than to antigenic mass; immunogenicity of the vaccinal strain was shown to decline as the number of passages increased. The low-passage vaccinal virus in VANGUARD® 5/L is therefore highly immunogenic and capable of stimulating active immunity in the presence of maternal antibodies at the levels shown in Table 1. Studies demonstrating that capability involved forty-one 6- to 8-week-old puppies (32 vaccinates and 9 controls) with the range of maternal antibody titers shown in Table 2. By 14 days after vaccination, 91% of vaccinates' titers were well above the protective threshold. By 21 days, all dogs, including the dog with the initial SN titer of 1:64 seroconverted, giving a group seroconversion rate of 100%. In contrast, seropositive sentinel littermate dogs' CPV antibody titers declined, demonstrating that initial antibody titers were indeed of maternal origin and no adventitious exposure occurred during the study.

Table 1. Pre- and Postvaccination Serum Neutralization (SN) Titers

Number of Dogs	Prevaccination	Postvaccination		
		7 Days	14 Days	21 Days
5	2	39.2	768.0	1433.6
2	4	3.0	36.0	192.0
11	8	45.1	457.5	488.7
9	16	33.8	263.1	739.6
4	32	40.0	450.0	640.0
1	64	32.0	32.0	128.0
Average	13.8	37.3	410.8	696.0

Table 2. Initial Serum Neutralization (SN) Titers of Vaccinates and Controls

SN Titers	# Vaccinates Included	# Controls Included
1:2	5	0
1:4	2	1
1:8	11	2
1:16	9	4
1:32	4	2
1:64	1	0

References: Available upon request.
Presentation: Cartons of 25 x 1 dose vials.
U.S. Patent No. 3,616,203
Compendium Code No.: 36901510 75-4983-04

VANGUARD® CPV (killed)

Pfizer Animal Health **Vaccine**

Canine Parvovirus Vaccine, Killed Virus

U.S. Vet. Lic. No.: 189

Description: VANGUARD® CPV (killed) contains a strain of CPV propagated on an established canine cell line and is chemically inactivated.

Contains penicillin and streptomycin as preservatives.

Indications: VANGUARD® CPV (killed) is for vaccination of healthy dogs as an aid in preventing canine parvoviral enteritis caused by canine parvovirus (CPV).

Directions:

1. General Directions: Vaccination of healthy dogs is recommended. Shake well. Aseptically administer 1 mL subcutaneously or intramuscularly.
2. Primary Vaccination: Healthy dogs should receive 2 doses administered 3-4 weeks apart. If dogs are vaccinated before the age of 4 months, they should be revaccinated with 2 doses 3-4 weeks apart after reaching the age of 4 months. (Maternal antibodies may interfere with development of an adequate immune response in puppies less than 4 months old.)
3. Revaccination: Annual revaccination with a single dose is recommended.

Precaution(s): Store at 2°-7°C. Prolonged exposure to higher temperatures may adversely affect potency. Do not freeze.

Use entire contents when first opened.

Caution(s): As with any vaccine, anaphylaxis may occur after use. Initial antidote of epinephrine is recommended and should be followed with appropriate supportive therapy.

This product has been shown to be efficacious in healthy animals. A protective immune response may not be elicited if animals are incubating an infectious disease, are malnourished or parasitized, are stressed due to shipment or environmental conditions, are otherwise immunocompromised, or the vaccine is not administered in accordance with label directions.

Warning(s): For use in dogs only.

For veterinary use only.

Discussion: Disease Description: CPV is generally transmitted through direct contact with infectious feces. The virus also can be carried on dogs' hair and feet or other contaminated objects, and can remain infective for more than 6 months at room temperature.[1] Incubation period of CPV infection ranges from 4-14 days.[2,3] Vomiting usually is the first clinical sign, with diarrhea following within 24 hours. Dogs mildly affected may recover spontaneously without additional clinical manifestations. In more severe cases, depression, anorexia, vomiting (consisting chiefly of gastric juices), bloody diarrhea, and fever may be observed.[3] Leukopenia commonly accompanies clinical signs.[2] Course of CPV disease may be aggravated by concurrent parasitism or infection with other enteric pathogens.[1,3] Following infection many dogs are refractory to the disease for a year or more. Similarly, seropositive bitches may transfer to their puppies CPV antibodies which can interfere with active immunization of the puppies through 16 weeks of age.

Trial Data: Safety and Efficacy: Safety of VANGUARD® CPV (killed) was confirmed in field tests involving 600 dogs. No postvaccination reactions were reported. Because it is chemically inactivated, VANGUARD® CPV (killed) poses no danger of viral shed or reversion to virulence.

Efficacy of VANGUARD® CPV (killed) was demonstrated in challenge-of-immunity studies. All dogs vaccinated with 2 doses resisted rigorous challenge with virulent CPV. After challenge some vaccinates experienced a single incidence of vomiting or slightly loose stool. White blood cell counts of all vaccinates remained essentially unchanged. In contrast, all nonvaccinated control dogs developed severe clinical signs of CPV disease after challenge. Among controls, anorexia, depression, vomiting, diarrhea, and mucoid feces were observed. Marked leukopenia occurred in 80% of these dogs.

References: Available upon request.
Presentation: 10 dose vials.
Compendium Code No.: 36901520 75-4962-06

VANGUARD® DA$_2$MP

Pfizer Animal Health **Vaccine**

Canine Distemper-Adenovirus Type 2-Measles-Parainfluenza Vaccine, Modified Live Virus

U.S. Vet. Lic. No.: 189

Description: VANGUARD® DA$_2$MP contains highly attenuated strains of CD virus, measles virus, CAV-2, and CPI virus propagated on an established canine cell line and freeze-dried to preserve stability.

Contains penicillin and streptomycin as preservatives.

Indications: VANGUARD® DA$_2$MP is for vaccination of healthy dogs 6-12 weeks of age as an aid in preventing canine distemper caused by canine distemper (CD) virus, infectious canine hepatitis (ICH) caused by canine adenovirus type 1 (CAV-1), respiratory disease caused by canine adenovirus type 2 (CAV-2), and canine parainfluenza caused by canine parainfluenza (CPI) virus.

Directions:

1. General Directions: Vaccination of healthy dogs 6-12 weeks of age is recommended. Aseptically rehydrate the freeze-dried vaccine with the sterile diluent provided, shake well, and administer 1 mL intramuscularly.
2. Primary Vaccination: Administer a single 1-mL dose to healthy dogs between 6 and 12 weeks of age.
3. Revaccination: Dogs should be revaccinated at 14-16 weeks of age with a canine distemper, canine adenovirus type 2, and canine parainfluenza vaccine. In most cases, a complete immunization program will also include vaccination for canine parvovirus, *Leptospira canicola,* and *L. icterohaemorrhagiae.* At the discretion of the veterinarian, annual revaccination with a single dose against any or all of these pathogens is recommended.

Precaution(s): Store at 2°-7°C. Prolonged exposure to higher temperatures and/or direct sunlight may adversely affect potency. Do not freeze.

Use entire contents when first opened.

Sterilized syringes and needles should be used to administer this vaccine. Do not sterilize with chemicals because traces of disinfectant may inactivate the vaccine.

Burn containers and all unused contents.

Caution(s): Vaccination of pregnant bitches should be avoided.

As with many vaccines, anaphylaxis may occur after use. Initial antidote of epinephrine is recommended and should be followed with appropriate supportive therapy.

This product has been shown to be efficacious in healthy animals. A protective immune response may not be elicited if animals are incubating an infectious disease, are malnourished or parasitized, are stressed due to shipment or environmental conditions, are otherwise immunocompromised, or the vaccine is not administered in accordance with label directions.

Warning(s): For use in dogs only.

For veterinary use only.

Discussion: Disease Description: CD is a universal, high-mortality viral disease with variable manifestations. ICH, caused by CAV-1, is a universal, sometimes fatal, viral disease of dogs characterized by hepatic and generalized endothelial lesions. CAV-2 respiratory infection is commonly associated with infectious tracheobronchitis ("kennel cough") in dogs of all ages. CPI is a common viral upper respiratory disease. Uncomplicated CPI may be mild or subclinical, with signs becoming more severe if concurrent infection with other respiratory pathogens exists.

Trial Data: Safety and Efficacy: Laboratory evaluation demonstrated that VANGUARD® DA$_2$MP immunized dogs against CD, ICH, CAV-2 respiratory disease, and CPI, and that no significant immunologic interference existed among the vaccine fractions. No adverse reactions to vaccination were observed in any of the test dogs. The viral fractions of the vaccine all have an extensive clinical history of safe and effective use in other Pfizer Animal Health vaccines.

Protection against CD is desirable at the earliest possible age. However, successful vaccination may not be possible in puppies with maternal antibodies against CD. By 12 weeks of age, maternal CD antibodies decline in almost all dogs to levels that do not neutralize attenuated vaccine virus. Measles virus stimulates heterotypic protection against CD in puppies regardless of circulating CD antibody levels. The resistance provided by measles virus, however, does not appear to be as effective in very young puppies as in those 6 weeks of age or older. Thus, a combined CD and measles virus vaccine increases the probability of protecting puppies against CD during the period when they commonly carry maternal antibodies. For example, studies showed that 45/76 experimental dogs at 6 weeks of age had maternal antibody levels sufficient to interfere with active immunization. When vaccinated with a combination distemper-measles vaccine at 6 weeks of age, 63/67 puppies (94%) were protected, 42 of them by the measles virus fraction.[1] Figure 1 shows the proportion of puppies at various ages protected by measles and CD virus fractions, and overall percentages of protection in puppies inoculated with a combination distemper-measles vaccine.

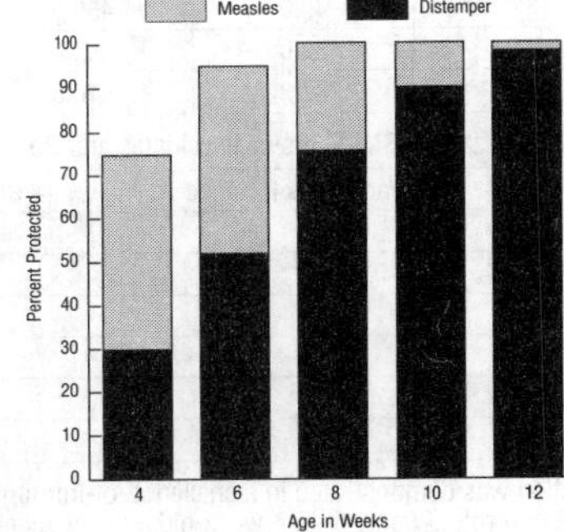

Figure 1. Protection Against Canine Distemper Challenge Afforded by Distemper-Measles Virus Fractions in a Combined Vaccine

Use of measles vaccine in adult bitches may produce high levels of measles antibodies that can interfere with successful protection of puppies in the next generation. Thus, VANGUARD® DA$_2$MP is recommended for use in puppies 6-12 weeks of age. Heterotypic immunity should not be relied on for protection after 16 weeks of age.

It has been demonstrated that CAV-2 vaccine cross-protects against ICH caused by CAV-1. The CAV-2 fraction in Vanguard® vaccines is used as a replacement for CAV-1 because it has significant advantages. Some CAV-1 vaccines may produce undesirable reactions, including persistent kidney infections, uveitis, and corneal opacity ("blue eye"), which have not been reported after vaccination with CAV-2.[2] In addition, the CAV-2 strain used in Vanguard® vaccines has been specially selected for freedom from oncogenic properties characteristic of adenoviruses.

Studies demonstrated that the CAV-2 fraction in VANGUARD® DA$_2$MP not only protects against ICH, but against CAV-2 respiratory disease as well.[3] Although conventional CAV-1 (ICH) vaccines cross-protect against CAV-2, they may not prevent subclinical infection and spread of the CAV-2 agent. Canine adenovirus type 2 challenge virus was not recovered from CAV-2-vaccinated dogs.

A test of the CPI immunizing agent showed that hemorrhagic lung lesions characteristic of infection were absent or greatly diminished in vaccinated dogs necropsied after challenge. Nonvaccinated control dogs all had characteristic lung lesions, in some cases distributed in all lobes.[4]

References: Available upon request.

Presentation: Cartons of 25 x 1 dose vials.

Compendium Code No.: 36901530 75-4952-06

VANGUARD® DA$_2$P

Pfizer Animal Health **Vaccine**

Canine Distemper-Adenovirus Type 2-Parainfluenza Vaccine, Modified Live Virus

U.S. Vet. Lic. No.: 189

Description: VANGUARD® DA$_2$P contains attenuated strains of CD virus, CAV-2, and CPI virus propagated on an established canine cell line and freeze-dried to preserve stability.

Contains penicillin and streptomycin as preservatives.

Indications: VANGUARD® DA$_2$P is for vaccination of healthy dogs as an aid in preventing canine distemper caused by canine distemper (CD) virus, infectious canine hepatitis (ICH) caused by canine adenovirus type 1 (CAV-1), respiratory disease caused by canine adenovirus type 2 (CAV-2), and canine parainfluenza caused by canine parainfluenza (CPI) virus.

Directions:

1. General Directions: Vaccination of healthy dogs is recommended. Aseptically rehydrate the freeze-dried vaccine with the sterile diluent provided, shake well, and administer 1 mL subcutaneously or intramuscularly.
2. Primary Vaccination: Healthy dogs should receive 2 doses administered 3-4 weeks apart. If dogs are vaccinated before the age of 4 months, they should be revaccinated upon reaching 4 months of age. (Maternal antibodies may interfere with development of an adequate immune response in puppies less than 4 months old.)
3. Revaccination: Annual revaccination with a single dose is recommended.

Precaution(s): Store at 2°-7°C. Prolonged exposure to higher temperatures and/or direct sunlight may adversely affect potency. Do not freeze.

Use entire contents when first opened.

Sterilized syringes and needles should be used to administer this vaccine. Do not sterilize with chemicals because traces of disinfectant may inactivate the vaccine.

Burn containers and all unused contents.

Caution(s): Vaccination of pregnant bitches should be avoided.

As with many vaccines, anaphylaxis may occur after use. Initial antidote of epinephrine is recommended and should be followed with appropriate supportive therapy.

This product has been shown to be efficacious in healthy animals. A protective immune response may not be elicited if animals are incubating an infectious disease, are malnourished or parasitized, are stressed due to shipment or environmental conditions, are otherwise immunocompromised, or the vaccine is not administered in accordance with label directions.

Warning(s): For use in dogs only.

For veterinary use only.

Discussion: Disease Description: CD is a universal, high-mortality viral disease with variable manifestations. Approximately 50% of nonvaccinated, nonimmune dogs infected with CD virus develop clinical signs, and approximately 90% of those dogs die.[1] The disease is considered airborne and is highly contagious. It more frequently and acutely affects puppies under 3 months of age. Early clinical signs of CD include anorexia, diarrhea, and dehydration. As the disease progresses, fever, depression, vomiting, and bloody diarrhea may be observed and accompanied by signs of respiratory distress. Coughing, labored breathing, inflammation of tissues around the eyes and nose, and mucopurulent oculonasal discharge may occur. Neurological complications manifested by muscle tremors, incoordination, convulsive seizures, and paralysis of the rear quarters are typical signs of the terminal stage of CD.

ICH, caused by CAV-1, is transmitted principally in urine, and can affect dogs of all ages. ICH is characterized by fever, leukopenia, enlarged tonsils, hepatitis, nephritis, and occasionally, uveitis with corneal opacity ("blue eye"). Additional clinical signs of ICH are similar to those of CD: depression, anorexia, vomiting, and oculonasal inflammation and discharge. While oral lesions may accompany ICH and help distinguish the disease from CD, dual ICH-CD infections also may occur. Clinical signs of this syndrome may be particularly severe.

CAV-2 infections are primarily respiratory, clinically evidenced by pneumonia, bronchitis, tonsillitis, and pharyngitis. Depression, anorexia, fever, labored breathing, and coughing may be associated with these conditions. Infection with CAV-2 may predispose the respiratory tract to secondary bacterial infections. CAV-2 has not been associated with corneal opacity, uveitis or virus localization in the kidneys, which may accompany CAV-1 infections.[2]

CPI is a highly contagious respiratory virus which contributes to upper respiratory disease and infectious tracheobronchitis. A characteristic clinical sign of CPI infection is coughing that may be intensified by activity or excitement. Environmental factors such as drafts, cold, and high humidity may enhance susceptibility to the disease. Typically, CPI is self-limiting, with a course of 5-10 days duration. However, secondary bacterial infections of the respiratory tract are not uncommon, and may complicate the clinical syndrome.

Trial Data: Safety and Efficacy: Safety of VANGUARD® DA$_2$P was confirmed in laboratory and field tests.[3] In more than 15,000 vaccinated dogs, no significant postvaccination reactions attributable to the vaccine were reported. These findings are particularly important since adverse side effects sometimes follow vaccination with modified live ICH vaccine. After vaccination with ICH vaccine, persistent kidney infections may occur, causing virus shedding in urine. Uveitis and corneal opacity also are occasionally observed 1-2 weeks after vaccination.[2] Vaccination with the CAV-2 fraction in VANGUARD® DA$_2$P, however, produced no such lesions. Challenge virus was not recovered from vaccinated dogs, and was not isolated from tissues taken at necropsy. Ocular lesions were not observed in any of 172 dogs inoculated intravenously with multiple doses of CAV-2 vaccine virus, while intravenous inoculation of 32 dogs with ICH vaccine produced ocular lesions in 22%. Additionally, the strain of CAV-2 in this product has been shown free of oncogenic properties characteristic of canine adenovirus.

Efficacy of VANGUARD® DA$_2$P was demonstrated in challenge-of-immunity studies.[3] Dogs vaccinated with the CAV-2 vaccine were completely protected against challenge with virulent ICH virus that produced clinical disease in 100% of nonvaccinated control dogs. Vaccinates were also protected against challenge with virulent CAV-2 that caused severe respiratory syndromes in susceptible controls. After challenge with virulent CD virus, 95% of dogs vaccinated with the CD vaccine remained healthy. In contrast, all nonvaccinated control dogs developed clinical signs of CD, and 80% died. After challenge with virulent CPI virus, no clinical signs of disease were observed among dogs vaccinated with CPI vaccine, while all nonvaccinated controls revealed clinical signs and severe lung lesions typical of CPI.

References: Available upon request.

Presentation: Cartons of 25 x 1 dose vials.

U.S. Patent No. 3,616,203

Compendium Code No.: 36901800 75-4945-08

VANGUARD® DA$_2$PL

Pfizer Animal Health **Bacterin-Vaccine**

Canine Distemper-Adenovirus Type 2-Parainfluenza Vaccine, Modified Live Virus-Leptospira Bacterin

U.S. Vet. Lic. No.: 189

Description: The vaccine component of VANGUARD® DA$_2$PL contains attenuated strains of CD virus, CAV-2, and CPI virus propagated on an established canine cell line and freeze-dried to preserve stability. The bacterin component, containing inactivated whole cultures of *L. canicola* and *L. icterohaemorrhagiae,* is supplied as diluent.

Contains penicillin and streptomycin as preservatives.

Indications: VANGUARD® DA$_2$PL is for vaccination of healthy dogs as an aid in preventing canine distemper caused by canine distemper (CD) virus, infectious canine hepatitis (ICH) caused by canine adenovirus type 1 (CAV-1), respiratory disease caused by canine adenovirus type 2 (CAV-2), canine parainfluenza caused by canine parainfluenza (CPI) virus, and leptospirosis caused by *Leptospira canicola* and *L. icterohaemorrhagiae.*

Directions:

1. General Directions: Vaccination of healthy dogs is recommended. Aseptically rehydrate the freeze-dried vaccine (Vanguard® DA$_2$P) with the liquid bacterin provided (Leptoferm C-I®), shake well, and administer 1 mL subcutaneously or intramuscularly.
2. Primary Vaccination: Healthy dogs should receive 2 doses administered 3-4 weeks apart. If dogs are vaccinated before the age of 4 months, they should be revaccinated with a single dose upon reaching 4 months of age. (Maternal antibodies may interfere with development of an adequate immune response in puppies less than 4 months old.)
3. Revaccination: Annual revaccination with a single dose is recommended.

Precaution(s): Store at 2°-7°C. Prolonged exposure to higher temperatures and/or direct sunlight may adversely affect potency. Do not freeze.

Use entire contents when first opened.

Sterilized syringes and needles should be used to administer this vaccine. Do not sterilize with chemicals because traces of disinfectant may inactivate the vaccine.

Burn containers and all unused contents.

Caution(s): Vaccination of pregnant bitches should be avoided.

As with many vaccines, anaphylaxis may occur after use. Initial antidote of epinephrine is recommended and should be followed with appropriate supportive therapy.

This product has been shown to be efficacious in healthy animals. A protective immune response may not be elicited if animals are incubating an infectious disease, are malnourished or parasitized, are stressed due to shipment or environmental conditions, are otherwise immunocompromised, or the vaccine is not administered in accordance with label directions.

Warning(s): For use in dogs only.

For veterinary use only.

Discussion: Disease Description: CD is a universal, high-mortality viral disease with variable manifestations. Approximately 50% of nonvaccinated, nonimmune dogs infected with CD virus develop clinical signs, and approximately 90% of those dogs die.[1] The disease is considered airborne and is highly contagious. It more frequently and acutely affects puppies under 3 months of age. Early clinical signs of CD include anorexia, diarrhea, and dehydration. As the disease progresses, fever, depression, vomiting, and bloody diarrhea may be observed and accompanied by signs of respiratory distress. Coughing, labored breathing, inflammation of tissues around the eyes and nose, and mucopurulent oculonasal discharge may occur. Neurological complications manifested by muscle tremors, incoordination, convulsive seizures, and paralysis of the rear quarters are typical signs of the terminal stage of CD.

ICH, caused by CAV-1, is transmitted principally in urine, and can affect dogs of all ages. ICH is characterized by fever, leukopenia, enlarged tonsils, hepatitis, nephritis, and occasionally, uveitis with corneal opacity ("blue eye"). Additional clinical signs of ICH are similar to those of CD: depression, anorexia, vomiting, and oculonasal inflammation and discharge. While oral lesions may accompany ICH and help distinguish the disease from CD, dual ICH-CD infections also may occur. Clinical signs of this syndrome may be particularly severe.

CAV-2 infections are primarily respiratory, clinically evidenced by pneumonia, bronchitis, tonsillitis, and pharyngitis. Depression, anorexia, fever, labored breathing, and coughing may be associated with these conditions. Infection with CAV-2 may predispose the respiratory tract to secondary bacterial infections. CAV-2 has not been associated with corneal opacity, uveitis or virus localization in the kidneys, which may accompany CAV-1 infections.[2]

CPI is a highly contagious respiratory virus which contributes to upper respiratory disease and infectious tracheobronchitis. A characteristic clinical sign of CPI infection is coughing that may be intensified by activity or excitement. Environmental factors such as drafts, cold, and high humidity may enhance susceptibility to the disease. Typically, CPI is self-limiting, with a course of 5-10 days duration. However, secondary bacterial infections of the respiratory tract are not uncommon, and may complicate the clinical syndrome.

Infection with *Leptospira* bacteria occurs chiefly through exposure to contaminated water. Leptospires commonly localize in the kidneys, and may be shed in urine for months or years. Sudden onset of depression, anorexia, vomiting, and diarrhea is characteristic of acute leptospirosis; jaundice, fever, and generalized weakness also may occur. Subsequently, body temperature may drop to below normal, and weakness may advance to muscular pain, stiffness, and tremors. Labored breathing, coughing, and intense thirst typically accompany these signs. In severe cases, blood may be observed in the vomitus, stool, and urine.

Trial Data: Safety and Efficacy: Safety of VANGUARD® DA_2PL was confirmed in laboratory and field tests.[3] In more than 16,000 vaccinated dogs, no significant postvaccination reactions attributable to the vaccine were reported. These findings are particularly important since adverse side effects sometimes follow vaccination with modified live ICH vaccine. After vaccination with ICH vaccine, persistent kidney infections may occur, causing virus shedding in urine. Uveitis and corneal opacity also are occasionally observed 1-2 weeks after vaccination.[2] Vaccination with the CAV-2 fraction in VANGUARD® DA_2PL, however, produced no such lesions. Challenge virus was not recovered from vaccinated dogs, and was not isolated from tissues taken at necropsy. Ocular lesions were not observed in any of 172 dogs inoculated intravenously with multiple doses of CAV-2 vaccine virus, while intravenous inoculation of 32 dogs with ICH vaccine produced ocular lesions in 22%. Additionally, the strain of CAV-2 in this product has been shown free of oncogenic properties characteristic of canine adenovirus.

Efficacy of VANGUARD® DA_2PL was demonstrated in challenge-of-immunity studies.[3] Dogs vaccinated with the CAV-2 vaccine were completely protected against challenge with virulent ICH virus that produced clinical disease in 100% of nonvaccinated control dogs. Vaccinates were also protected against challenge with virulent CAV-2 that caused severe respiratory syndromes in susceptible controls. After challenge with virulent CD virus, 95% of dogs vaccinated with the CD vaccine remained healthy. In contrast, all nonvaccinated control dogs developed clinical signs of CD, and 80% died. After challenge with virulent CPI virus, no clinical signs of disease were observed among dogs vaccinated with CPI vaccine, while all nonvaccinated controls revealed clinical signs and severe lung lesions typical of CPI. Comparable results were obtained after challenge with virulent *Leptospira.* Ninety percent of dogs vaccinated with the *Leptospira* bacterin were protected, while 100% of nonvaccinated control dogs became infected when challenged with *L. canicola.* Similarly, challenge with *L. icterohaemorrhagiae* produced disease in all controls, but had no clinical effect on vaccinates.

References: Available upon request.

Presentation: Cartons of 25 x 1 dose vials.

U.S. Patent No. 3,616,203

Compendium Code No.: 36901540 75-4947-07

VANGUARD® DM

Pfizer Animal Health **Vaccine**

Canine Distemper-Measles Vaccine, Modified Live Virus

U.S. Vet. Lic. No.: 189

Description: VANGUARD® DM contains highly attenuated strains of CD virus and measles virus propagated on an established canine cell line and freeze-dried to preserve stability.

Contains penicillin and streptomycin as preservatives.

Indications: VANGUARD® DM is for initial vaccination of healthy dogs 6-12 weeks of age as an aid in preventing canine distemper caused by canine distemper (CD) virus.

Directions:

1. General Directions: VANGUARD® DM is specifically designed for the temporary protection of puppies against canine distemper. Vaccination of healthy dogs 6-12 weeks of age is recommended. Aseptically rehydrate the freeze-dried vaccine with the sterile diluent provided, shake well, and administer 1 mL intramuscularly within 1 hour after rehydration.
2. Primary Vaccination: Administer a single 1-mL dose to healthy dogs between 6 and 12 weeks of age, followed by 1 dose of a vaccine containing canine distemper virus at 14-16 weeks of age.
3. Revaccination: Annual revaccination with a single dose of a vaccine containing canine distemper virus is recommended.

Precaution(s): Store at 2°-7°C. Prolonged exposure to higher temperatures and/or direct sunlight may adversely affect potency. Do not freeze.

Use entire contents when first opened.

Sterilized syringes and needles should be used to administer this vaccine. Do not sterilize with chemicals because traces of disinfectant may inactivate the vaccine.

Burn containers and all unused contents.

Caution(s): Vaccination of pregnant bitches should be avoided.

As with many vaccines, anaphylaxis may occur after use. Initial antidote of epinephrine is recommended and should be followed with appropriate supportive therapy.

This product has been shown to be efficacious in healthy animals. A protective immune response may not be elicited if animals are incubating an infectious disease, are malnourished or parasitized, are stressed due to shipment or environmental conditions, are otherwise immunocompromised, or the vaccine is not administered in accordance with label directions.

Warning(s): For use in dogs only.

For veterinary use only.

Discussion: Disease Description: CD is a universal, high-mortality viral disease with variable manifestations. Approximately 50% of nonvaccinated, nonimmune dogs infected with CD virus develop clinical signs, and approximately 90% of those dogs die.[1] The disease is considered airborne and is highly contagious. It more frequently and acutely affects puppies under 3 months of age. Early clinical signs of CD include anorexia, diarrhea, and dehydration. As the disease progresses, fever, depression, vomiting, and bloody diarrhea may be observed and accompanied by signs of respiratory distress. Coughing, labored breathing, inflammation of tissues around the eyes and nose, and mucopurulent oculonasal discharge may occur. Neurological complications manifested by muscle tremors, incoordination, convulsive seizures, and paralysis of the rear quarters are typical signs of the terminal stage of CD.

Trial Data: Safety and Efficacy: Protection against CD is desirable at the earliest possible age. Puppies may be successfully immunized by modified live virus CD vaccine providing they do not have circulating antibodies against CD. When passive antibodies are present, whether acquired maternally or from inoculation of CD antiserum, vaccination will be unsuccessful until the antibodies decline to a level which will not interfere with vaccine virus.

Measles virus (MV) stimulates immunity to CD in puppies in the presence of circulating CD antibodies.[3] Thus, because the immune status of a puppy is often unknown, combination distemper-measles vaccination is a practical alternative to CD vaccination alone. Immunity provided by MV generally is most effective in puppies 6 weeks of age or older;[2] younger puppies may not be immunologically competent to respond to vaccination.

Controlled experiments to determine effectiveness of VANGUARD® DM in puppies of various ages showed that the vaccine protected 63/67 puppies (94%) against CD at 6 weeks of age. Of these puppies, 45 had levels of maternal antibodies sufficient to interfere with active immunization by CD virus. Forty-two of these 45 puppies (93%) were protected by the measles virus fraction. Figure 1 compares the protection of VANGUARD® DM with the protection of either modified live CD virus vaccine or modified live MV vaccine in puppies 4-12 weeks old.

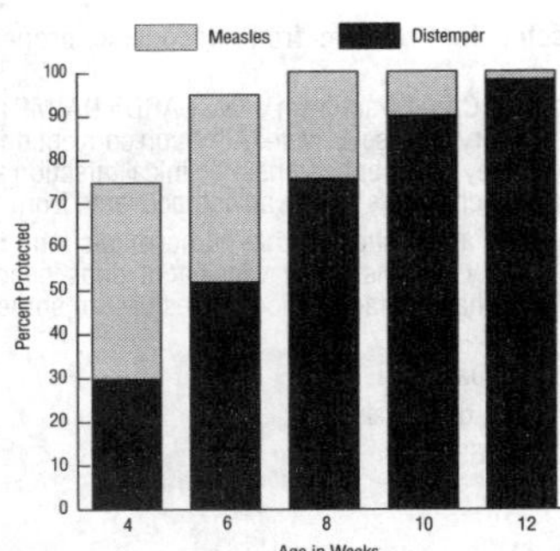

Figure 1. Relationship Between Canine Distemper Virus and Measles Virus in Protection of Puppies with VANGUARD® DM

Immunity stimulated by MV does not interfere with subsequent active immunization by CD virus. It may actually stimulate a more rapid serological response and, in many cases, a higher level of antibodies. Because repeated use of this vaccine may produce high levels of MV antibodies, which can interfere with MV immunization of puppies in the next generation, it should not be used on female puppies over 12 weeks of age, or older bitches. Use of vaccines containing the MV antigen is not indicated in dogs more than 16 weeks old.[2]

Throughout developmental testing, and in field studies conducted by private practitioners, no significant postvaccination reactions attributable to use of VANGUARD® DM were reported.

References: Available upon request.

Presentation: Cartons of 25 x 1 dose vials.

U.S. Patent No. 3,616,203

Compendium Code No.: 36901550 75-4942-05

VANGUARD® LCI

Pfizer Animal Health **Bacterin**

Leptospira Canicola-Icterohaemorrhagiae Bacterin

U.S. Vet. Lic. No.: 189

Contents: This product contains the antigens listed above.

Contains penicillin and streptomycin as preservatives.

Indications: For vaccination of healthy dogs as an aid in preventing leptospirosis caused by *Leptospira canicola* and *L. icterohaemorrhagiae.*

Directions: Shake well. Aseptically administer 1 mL subcutaneously or intramuscularly. Healthy dogs should receive 2 doses administered 3-4 weeks apart. If dogs are vaccinated before the age of 4 months, they should be revaccinated with a single dose upon reaching 4 months of age. (Maternal antibodies may interfere with development of an adequate immune response in puppies less than 4 months old.) Annual revaccination with a single dose is recommended.

Precaution(s): Store at 2°-7°C. Prolonged exposure to higher temperatures may adversely affect potency. Do not freeze. Use entire contents when first opened. Sterilized syringes and needles should be used to administer this vaccine.

Caution(s): Recommended for use by veterinary professionals in the context of a veterinarian-client-patient relationship that includes knowledge of the animal's health status and history.

Vaccination of pregnant bitches should be avoided. As with many vaccines, anaphylaxis may occur after use. Initial antidote of epinephrine is recommended and should be followed with appropriate supportive therapy. This product has been shown to be efficacious in healthy animals. A protective immune response may not be elicited if animals are incubating an infectious disease, are malnourished or parasitized, are stressed due to shipment or environmental conditions, are otherwise immunocompromised, or the vaccine is not administered in accordance with label directions.

For use in dogs only.

Presentation: 50 x 1 mL vials of liquid bacterin.

Compendium Code No.: 36901920 21-5308-00

VANGUARD® PLUS 4

Pfizer Animal Health **Vaccine**

Canine Distemper-Adenovirus Type 2-Parvovirus Vaccine, Modified Live Virus

U.S. Vet. Lic. No.: 189

Description: The vaccine component of VANGUARD® Plus 4 contains attenuated strains of CD virus, CAV-2, and CPV propagated on an established canine cell line. The CPV fraction is high titer (>107.0 $TCID_{50}$/dose) and was attenuated by low passage (35 passes from the canine isolate with a maximum of 2 additional passes allowed for production) on the canine cell line which gives it the immunogenic properties capable of overriding maternal antibody interference at the levels indicated in Table 2. Some puppies in the field may have higher levels of maternal antibodies than those evaluated in our pivotal efficacy study. The vaccine is packaged in freeze-dried form with inert gas in place of vacuum.

Contains penicillin and streptomycin as preservatives.

Indications: VANGUARD® Plus 4 is for vaccination of healthy dogs 6 weeks of age or older as an aid in preventing canine distemper caused by canine distemper (CD) virus, infectious canine hepatitis (ICH) caused by canine adenovirus type 1 (CAV-1), respiratory disease caused by canine adenovirus type 2 (CAV-2), and canine parvoviral enteritis caused by canine parvovirus (CPV).

Directions:

1. General Directions: Vaccination of healthy dogs is recommended. Aseptically rehydrate the freeze-dried vaccine (VANGUARD® Plus 4) with the sterile diluent provided, shake well, and administer 1 mL subcutaneously or intramuscularly.
2. Primary Vaccination: Healthy dogs 6 weeks of age or older should receive 3 doses, each administered 3 weeks apart.
3. Revaccination: Annual revaccination with a single dose is recommended.

Precaution(s): Store at 2°-7°C. Prolonged exposure to higher temperatures and/or direct sunlight may adversely affect potency. Do not freeze.

Use entire contents when first opened.

Sterilized syringes and needles should be used to administer this vaccine. Do not sterilize with chemicals because traces of disinfectant may inactivate the vaccine.

Burn containers and all unused contents.

Caution(s): Vaccination of pregnant bitches should be avoided.

As with many vaccines, anaphylaxis may occur after use. Initial antidote of epinephrine is recommended and should be followed with appropriate supportive therapy.

This product has been shown to be efficacious in healthy animals. A protective immune response may not be elicited if animals are incubating an infectious disease, are malnourished or parasitized, are stressed due to shipment or environmental conditions, are otherwise immunocompromised, or the vaccine is not administered in accordance with label directions.

For veterinary use only.

Discussion: Disease Description: CD is a universal, high-mortality viral disease with variable manifestations. Approximately 50% of nonvaccinated, nonimmune dogs infected with CD virus develop clinical signs, and approximately 90% of those dogs die.[1] ICH, caused by CAV-1, is a universal, sometimes fatal, viral disease of dogs characterized by hepatic and generalized endothelial lesions. CAV-2 causes respiratory disease, which in severe cases may include pneumonia and bronchopneumonia. CPV infection results in enteric disease characterized by sudden onset of vomiting and diarrhea, often hemorrhagic. Leukopenia commonly accompanies clinical signs. Susceptible dogs of any age can be affected, but mortality is greatest in puppies. In puppies 4-12 weeks of age CPV may occasionally cause myocarditis that can result in acute heart failure after a brief and inconspicuous illness. Following infection many dogs are refractory to the disease for a year or more. Similarly, seropositive bitches may transfer to their puppies CPV antibodies which can interfere with active immunization of the puppies through 16 weeks of age.

Trial Data: Safety and Efficacy: Laboratory evaluation demonstrated that VANGUARD® Plus 4 aided in preventing disease caused by CD, ICH, CAV-2 and CPV, and that no immunologic interference existed among the vaccine fractions. Extensive field safety trials conducted by Pfizer Animal Health showed it to be safe and reaction-free in dogs as young as 6 weeks of age under normal usage conditions.

It has been demonstrated that CAV-2 vaccine cross-protects against ICH caused by CAV-1. The CAV-2 fraction in Vanguard® vaccines is used as a replacement for CAV-1 because it has significant advantages. Some CAV-1 vaccines may produce undesirable reactions, including persistent kidney infections, uveitis, and corneal opacity ("blue eye"), which have not been reported after vaccination with CAV-2.[2] In addition, the CAV-2 strain used in Vanguard® vaccines has been specially selected for freedom from oncogenic properties characteristic of adenoviruses.

Studies conducted at Pfizer demonstrated that CAV-2 not only protects against ICH, but against CAV-2 respiratory disease as well.[3] Although conventional CAV-1 (ICH) vaccines cross-protect against CAV-2, they may not prevent subclinical infection and spread of the CAV-2 agent. Canine adenovirus type 2 challenge virus was not recovered from CAV-2-vaccinated dogs in tests conducted at Pfizer.

The CPV fraction in VANGUARD® Plus 4 was subjected to comprehensive safety and efficacy testing at Pfizer. It was shown safe and reaction-free in laboratory tests and in clinical trials under field conditions. Product safety was further demonstrated by a backpassage study, which included oral administration of multiple doses of the vaccine strain to susceptible dogs, all of whom remained normal. The CPV virus in VANGUARD® Plus 4 shares a characteristic with other live CPV vaccine strains in that the vaccine virus may be present in the feces following administration. Although this CPV vaccine virus was found occasionally and in low titers in the feces of vaccinated dogs, testing demonstrated that the vaccine master seed did not revert to virulence following 6 consecutive backpassages in susceptible dogs.

Research at Pfizer demonstrated that 3 doses of the vaccine with increased CPV virus titer can overcome serum neutralization (SN) titers associated with maternal antibody. Serum neutralization titers as low as 1:4 have been shown by others to interfere with active immunization using conventional modified live vaccines.[4,5] A clinical trial was conducted with fifty 6-week-old puppies [25 vaccinates (SN titer range <2-256) and 25 nonvaccinated controls (SN titer range 4-1024)] (Table 1). The group of vaccinates received 3 doses, with vaccinations administered 3 weeks apart beginning at 6 weeks of age.

Table 1. Initial Serum Neutralization (SN) Titers of Vaccinates and Controls:

SN Titers	# Vaccinates Included	# Controls Included
<1:2	3	0
1:4	4	3
1:8	1	3
1:16	4	1
1:32	2	5
1:64	3	1
1:128	6	3
1:256	2	3
1:512	0	5
1:1024	0	1

After 1 vaccination, 13/25 puppies exhibited a 4-fold or greater increase in CPV SN titer (seroconversion) (Table 2). Twelve of these 13 puppies had maternal SN titers ≥1:16 at the time of the first vaccination with the remaining puppy having an SN titer of 1:64. Another 9 puppies with initial SN titers between 1:16 and 1:256 seroconverted after the second vaccination. Their maternal antibody SN titers had declined to ≥1:64 at the time of the second vaccination. Similarly, the last 3 vaccinates, with initial SN titers of 1:128, seroconverted after the third vaccination, after their maternal antibody CPV titer dropped ≥1:64. Therefore, in this study, when 3 doses of vaccine were given beginning at 6 weeks of age, all 25 vaccinates, even those with the highest maternal antibody levels, became actively immunized (GM = 1:1176; range of SN titers 128-4096). All 50 dogs were challenged 3 weeks after the third vaccination with a heterologous CPV challenge virus. Fourteen of 25 nonvaccinated control dogs died or showed illness severe enough to warrant euthanasia, while all 25 vaccinates remained essentially healthy.

Table 2. Postvaccination Serum Neutralization (SN) Titers Geometric Mean (Range)[a]:

Groups	N	Prevaccination	Postvaccination 1	Postvaccination 2	Postvaccination 3[b]
All Vaccinated Dogs	25	1:24 (<2-256)	1:108 (8-1024)	1:605 (8-4096)	1:1176 (128->4096)
Responders Post 1st Vaccination	13	1:6 (<2-64)	1:460 (64-1024)	1:1745 (256-4096)	1:1410 (256-4096)
Responders Post 2nd Vaccination	9	1:87 (16-256)	1:20 (8-64)	1:376 (256-1024)	1:1625 (256-4096)
Responders Post 3rd Vaccination	3	1:128 (128)	1:32 (16-64)	1:25 (8-64)	1:203 (128-256)
Nonvaccinated Control Dogs	25	1:64 (4-1024)	1:9 (<2-64)	1:3 (<2-64)	<1:2 (<2-4)

[a] Dogs were vaccinated at 6, 9, and 12 weeks of age.

[b] Pre-challenge SN titers

The high-titer, low-passage vaccine virus in VANGUARD® Plus 4 is therefore highly immunogenic and capable of stimulating active immunity in the presence of maternal antibodies.

References: Available upon request.

Presentation: 25 x 1 dose vials.

U.S. Patent No. 3,616,203

Compendium Code No.: 36901861 75-5309-01

VANGUARD® PLUS 4/LCI

Pfizer Animal Health **Bacterin-Vaccine**

Canine Distemper-Adenovirus Type 2-Parvovirus Vaccine, Modified Live Virus-Leptospira Bacterin

U.S. Vet. Lic. No.: 189

Description: The vaccine component of VANGUARD® Plus 4/Lci contains attenuated strains of CD virus, CAV-2, and CPV propagated on an established canine cell line. The CPV fraction is high titer (>$10^{7.0}$ $TCID_{50}$/dose) and was attenuated by low passage (35 passes from the canine isolate with a maximum of 2 additional passes allowed for production) on the canine cell line which gives it the immunogenic properties capable of overriding maternal antibody interference at the levels indicated in Table 2. Some puppies in the field may have higher levels of maternal antibodies than those evaluated in our pivotal efficacy study. The vaccine is packaged in freeze-dried form with inert gas in place of vacuum. The bacterin component, containing inactivated whole cultures of *Leptospira canicola* and *L. icterohaemorrhagiae*, is supplied as diluent.

Contains penicillin and streptomycin as preservatives.

Indications: VANGUARD® Plus 4/Lci is for vaccination of healthy dogs 6 weeks of age or older as an aid in preventing canine distemper caused by canine distemper (CD) virus, infectious canine hepatitis (ICH) caused by canine adenovirus type 1 (CAV-1), respiratory disease caused by canine adenovirus type 2 (CAV-2), canine parvoviral enteritis caused by canine parvovirus (CPV), and leptospirosis caused by *L. canicola* and *L. icterohaemorrhagiae.*

Directions:

1. General Directions: Vaccination of healthy dogs is recommended. Aseptically rehydrate the freeze-dried vaccine (Vanguard® Plus 4) with the liquid bacterin provided (Vanguard® Lci), shake well, and administer 1 mL subcutaneously or intramuscularly.
2. Primary Vaccination: Healthy dogs 6 weeks of age or older should receive 3 doses, each administered 3 weeks apart.
3. Revaccination: Annual revaccination with a single dose is recommended.

Precaution(s): Store at 2°-7°C. Prolonged exposure to higher temperatures and/or direct sunlight may adversely affect potency. Do not freeze.

Use entire contents when first opened.

Sterilized syringes and needles should be used to administer this vaccine. Do not sterilize with chemicals because traces of disinfectant may inactivate the vaccine.

Burn containers and all unused contents.

Caution(s): Vaccination of pregnant bitches should be avoided.

As with many vaccines, anaphylaxis may occur after use. Initial antidote of epinephrine is recommended and should be followed with appropriate supportive therapy.

This product has been shown to be efficacious in healthy animals. A protective immune response may not be elicited if animals are incubating an infectious disease, are malnourished or parasitized, are stressed due to shipment or environmental conditions, are otherwise immunocompromised, or the vaccine is not administered in accordance with label directions.

For use in dogs only.

For veterinary use only.

Discussion: Disease Description: CD is a universal, high-mortality viral disease with variable manifestations. Approximately 50% of nonvaccinated, nonimmune dogs infected with CD virus develop clinical signs, and approximately 90% of those dogs die.[1] ICH, caused by CAV-1, is a universal, sometimes fatal, viral disease of dogs characterized by hepatic and generalized endothelial lesions. CAV-2 causes respiratory disease, which in severe cases may include pneumonia and bronchopneumonia. CPV infection results in enteric disease characterized by sudden onset of vomiting and diarrhea, often hemorrhagic.

Leukopenia commonly accompanies clinical signs. Susceptible dogs of any age can be affected, but mortality is greatest in puppies. In puppies 4-12 weeks of age CPV may occasionally cause myocarditis that can result in acute heart failure after a brief and inconspicuous illness. Following infection many dogs are refractory to the disease for a year or more. Similarly, seropositive bitches may transfer to their puppies CPV antibodies, which can interfere with active immunization of the puppies through 16 weeks of age. Leptospirosis occurs in dogs of all ages, with a wide range of clinical signs and chronic nephritis generally following acute infection. Infection with *L. canicola* and *L. icterohaemorrhagiae* cannot be differentiated clinically.

Trial Data: Safety and Efficacy: Laboratory evaluation demonstrated that VANGUARD® Plus 4/Lci aided in preventing disease caused by CD, ICH, CAV-2, CPV, *L. canicola* and *L. icterohaemorrhagiae,* and that no immunologic interference existed among the vaccine fractions. Extensive field safety trials conducted by Pfizer Animal Health showed it to be safe and reaction-free in dogs as young as 6 weeks of age under normal usage conditions.

It has been demonstrated that CAV-2 vaccine cross-protects against ICH caused by CAV-1. The CAV-2 fraction in Vanguard® vaccines is used as a replacement for CAV-1 because it has significant advantages. Some CAV-1 vaccines may produce undesirable reactions, including persistent kidney infections, uveitis, and corneal opacity ("blue eye"), which have not been reported after vaccination with CAV-2.[2] In addition, the CAV-2 strain used in Vanguard® vaccines has been specially selected for freedom from oncogenic properties characteristic of adenoviruses.

Studies conducted at Pfizer demonstrated that CAV-2 not only protects against ICH, but against CAV-2 respiratory disease as well.[3] Although conventional CAV-1 (ICH) vaccines cross-protect against CAV-2, they may not prevent subclinical infection and spread of the CAV-2 agent. Canine adenovirus type 2 challenge virus was not recovered from CAV-2-vaccinated dogs in tests conducted at Pfizer.

The CPV fraction in VANGUARD® Plus 4/Lci was subjected to comprehensive safety and efficacy testing at Pfizer. It was shown safe and reaction-free in laboratory tests and in clinical trials under field conditions. Product safety was further demonstrated by a backpassage study, which included oral administration of multiple doses of the vaccine strain to susceptible dogs, all of whom remained normal. The CPV virus in VANGUARD® Plus 4/Lci shares a characteristic with other live CPV vaccine strains in that the vaccine virus may be present in the feces following administration. Although this CPV vaccine virus was found occasionally and in low titers in the feces of vaccinated dogs, testing demonstrated that the vaccine master seed did not revert to virulence following 6 consecutive backpassages in susceptible dogs.

Research at Pfizer demonstrated that 3 doses of the vaccine with increased CPV virus titer can overcome serum neutralization (SN) titers associated with maternal antibody. Serum neutralization titers as low as 1:4 have been shown by others to interfere with active immunization using conventional modified live vaccines.[4,5] A clinical trial was conducted with fifty 6-week-old puppies [25 vaccinates (SN titer range <2-256) and 25 nonvaccinated controls (SN titer range 4-1024)] (Table 1).

Table 1. Initial Serum Neutralization (SN) Titers of Vaccinates and Controls:

SN Titers	# Vaccinates Included	# Controls Included
<1:2	3	0
1:4	4	3
1:8	1	3
1:16	4	1
1:32	2	5
1:64	3	1
1:128	6	3
1:256	2	3
1:512	0	5
1:1024	0	1

The group of vaccinates received 3 doses, with vaccinations administered 3 weeks apart beginning at 6 weeks of age. After 1 vaccination, 13/25 puppies exhibited a 4-fold or greater increase in CPV SN titer (seroconversion) (Table 2).

Table 2. Postvaccination Serum Neutralization (SN) Titers Geometric Mean (Range)[a]:

Groups	N	Prevaccination	Postvaccination		
			1	2	3[b]
All Vaccinated Dogs	25	1:24 (<2-256)	1:108 (8-1024)	1:605 (8-4096)	1:1176 (128->4096)
Responders Post 1st Vaccination	13	1:6 (<2-64)	1:460 (64-1024)	1:1745 (256-4096)	1:1410 (256-4096)
Responders Post 2nd Vaccination	9	1:87 (16-256)	1:20 (8-64)	1:376 (256-1024)	1:1625 (256-4096)
Responders Post 3rd Vaccination	3	1:128 (128)	1:32 (16-64)	1:25 (8-64)	1:203 (128-256)
Nonvaccinated Control Dogs	25	1:64 (4-1024)	1:9 (<2-64)	1:3 (<2-64)	<1:2 (<2-4)

[a] Dogs were vaccinated at 6, 9, and 12 weeks of age.
[b] Pre-challenge SN titers

Twelve of these 13 puppies had maternal SN titers ≤1:16 at the time of the first vaccination with the remaining puppy having an SN titer of 1:64. Another 9 puppies with initial SN titers between 1:16 and 1:256 seroconverted after the second vaccination. Their maternal antibody SN titers had declined to ≤1:64 at the time of the second vaccination. Similarly, the last 3 vaccinates, with initial SN titers of 1:128, seroconverted after the third vaccination, after their maternal antibody CPV titer dropped ≤1:64. Therefore, in this study, when 3 doses of vaccine were given beginning at 6 weeks of age, all 25 vaccinates, even those with the highest maternal antibody levels, became actively immunized (GM = 1:1176; range of SN titers 128-4096). All 50 dogs were challenged 3 weeks after the third vaccination with a heterologous CPV challenge virus. Fourteen of 25 nonvaccinated control dogs died or showed illness severe enough to warrant euthanasia, while all 25 vaccinates remained essentially healthy. The high-titer, low-passage vaccine virus in VANGUARD® Plus 4/Lci is therefore highly immunogenic and capable of stimulating active immunity in the presence of maternal antibodies.

References: Available upon request.

Presentation: 25 x 1 dose vials.

U.S. Patent No. 3,616,203

Compendium Code No.: 36901930 75-5307-00

VANGUARD® PLUS 5

Pfizer Animal Health **Vaccine**

Canine Distemper-Adenovirus Type 2-Parainfluenza-Parvovirus Vaccine, Modified Live Virus

U.S. Vet. Lic. No.: 189

Description: VANGUARD® Plus 5 contains attenuated strains of CD virus, CAV-2, CPI virus, and CPV propagated on an established canine cell line. The CPV fraction is high titer ($10^{7.0}$ $TCID_{50}$/dose) and was attenuated by low passage (35 passes from the canine isolate with a maximum of 2 additional passes allowed for production) on the canine cell line which gives it the immunogenic properties capable of overriding maternal antibody interference at the levels indicated in Table 2. Some puppies in the field may have higher levels of maternal antibodies than those evaluated in our pivotal efficacy study. VANGUARD® Plus 5 is packaged in freeze-dried form with inert gas in place of vacuum.

Contains penicillin and streptomycin as preservatives.

Indications: VANGUARD® Plus 5 is for vaccination of healthy dogs 6 weeks of age or older as an aid in preventing canine distemper caused by canine distemper (CD) virus, infectious canine hepatitis (ICH) caused by canine adenovirus type 1 (CAV-1), respiratory disease caused by canine adenovirus type 2 (CAV-2), canine parainfluenza caused by canine parainfluenza (CPI) virus, and canine parvoviral enteritis caused by canine parvovirus (CPV).

Directions:

1. General Directions: Vaccination of healthy dogs is recommended. Aseptically rehydrate the freeze-dried vaccine with the sterile diluent provided, shake well, and administer 1 mL subcutaneously or intramuscularly.
2. Primary Vaccination: Healthy dogs 6 weeks of age or older should receive 3 doses, each administered 3 weeks apart.
3. Revaccination: Annual revaccination with a single dose is recommended.

Precaution(s): Store at 2°-7°C. Prolonged exposure to higher temperatures and/or direct sunlight may adversely affect potency. Do not freeze.

Use entire contents when first opened.

Sterilized syringes and needles should be used to administer this vaccine. Do not sterilize with chemicals because traces of disinfectant may inactivate the vaccine.

Burn containers and all unused contents.

Caution(s): Vaccination of pregnant bitches should be avoided.

As with many vaccines, anaphylaxis may occur after use. Initial antidote of epinephrine is recommended and should be followed with appropriate supportive therapy.

This product has been shown to be efficacious in healthy animals. A protective immune response may not be elicited if animals are incubating an infectious disease, are malnourished or parasitized, are stressed due to shipment or environmental conditions, are otherwise immunocompromised, or the vaccine is not administered in accordance with label directions.

For use in dogs only.

Warning(s): For veterinary use only.

Discussion: Disease Description: CD is a universal, high-mortality viral disease with variable manifestations. Approximately 50% of nonvaccinated, nonimmune dogs infected with CD virus develop clinical signs, and approximately 90% of those dogs die.[1] ICH, caused by CAV-1, is a universal, sometimes fatal, viral disease of dogs characterized by hepatic and generalized endothelial lesions. CAV-2 causes respiratory disease which in severe cases may include pneumonia and bronchopneumonia. CPI is a common viral upper respiratory disease. Uncomplicated CPI may be mild or subclinical, with signs becoming more severe if concurrent infection with other respiratory pathogens exists. CPV infection results in enteric disease characterized by sudden onset of vomiting and diarrhea, often hemorrhagic. Leukopenia commonly accompanies clinical signs. Susceptible dogs of any age can be affected, but mortality is greatest in puppies. In puppies 4-12 weeks of age CPV may occasionally cause myocarditis that can result in acute heart failure after a brief and inconspicuous illness. Following infection many dogs are refractory to the disease for a year or more. Similarly, seropositive bitches may transfer to their puppies CPV antibodies which can interfere with active immunization of the puppies through 16 weeks of age.

Trial Data: Safety and Efficacy: Laboratory evaluation demonstrated that VANGUARD® Plus 5 immunized dogs against CD, ICH, CAV-2 respiratory disease, CPI, and CPV, and that no immunologic interference existed among the vaccine fractions. Extensive field safety trials conducted by Pfizer Animal Health showed it to be safe and reaction-free in dogs as young as 6 weeks of age under normal usage conditions.

It has been demonstrated that CAV-2 vaccine cross-protects against ICH caused by CAV-1. The CAV-2 fraction in Vanguard vaccines is used as a replacement for CAV-1 because it has significant advantages. Some CAV-1 vaccines may produce undesirable reactions, including persistent kidney infections, uveitis, and corneal opacity ("blue eye"), which have not been reported after vaccination with CAV-2.[2] In addition, the CAV-2 strain used in Vanguard® vaccines has been specially selected for freedom from oncogenic properties characteristic of adenoviruses.

Studies conducted at Pfizer demonstrated that CAV-2 not only protects against ICH, but against CAV-2 respiratory disease as well.[3] Although conventional CAV-1 (ICH) vaccines cross-protect against CAV-2, they may not prevent subclinical infection and spread of the CAV-2 agent. Canine adenovirus type 2 challenge virus was not recovered from CAV-2-vaccinated dogs in tests conducted at Pfizer.

The CPV fraction in VANGUARD® Plus 5 was subjected to comprehensive safety and efficacy testing at Pfizer. It was shown safe and reaction-free in laboratory tests and in clinical trials under field conditions. Product safety was further demonstrated by a backpassage study which included oral administration of multiple doses of the vaccine strain to susceptible dogs, all of whom remained normal. The CPV virus in VANGUARD® Plus 5 shares a characteristic with other live CPV vaccine strains in that the vaccine virus may be present in the feces following administration. Although this CPV vaccine virus was found occasionally and in low titers in the feces of vaccinated dogs, testing demonstrated that the vaccine master seed did not revert to virulence following 6 consecutive backpassages in susceptible dogs.

Table 1. Initial Serum Neutralization (SN) Titers of Vaccinates and Controls

SN Titers	# Vaccinates Included	# Controls Included
<1:2	3	0
1:4	4	3
1:8	1	3
1:16	4	1
1:32	2	5
1:64	3	1
1:128	6	3
1:256	2	3
1:512	0	5
1:1024	0	1

Table 2. Postvaccination Serum Neutralization (SN) Titers Geometric Mean (Range)[a]

Groups	N	Pre-vaccination	Postvaccination		
			1	2	3[b]
All Vaccinated Dogs	25	1:24 (<2-256)	1:108 (8-1024)	1:605 (8-4096)	1:1176 (128->4096)
Responders Post 1st Vac.	13	1:6 (<2-64)	1:460 (64-1024)	1:1745 (256-4096)	1:1410 (256-4096)
Responders Post 2nd Vac.	9	1:87 (16-256)	1:20 (8-64)	1:376 (256-1024)	1:1625 (256-4096)
Responders Post 3rd Vac.	3	1:128 (128)	1:32 (16-64)	1:25 (8-64)	1:203 (128-256)
Nonvaccinated Control Dogs	25	1:64 (4-1024)	1:9 (<2-64)	1:3 (<2-64)	<1:2 (<2-4)

[a] Dogs were vaccinated at 6, 9, and 12 weeks of age.
[b] Pre-challenge SN titers

Research at Pfizer demonstrated that 3 doses of the vaccine with increased CPV virus titer can overcome serum neutralization (SN) titers associated with maternal antibody. Serum neutralization titers as low as 1:4 have been shown by others to interfere with active immunization using conventional modified live vaccines.[4,5] A clinical trial was conducted with fifty 6-week-old puppies [25 vaccinates (SN titer range -256) and 25 nonvaccinated controls (SN titer range 4-1024)] (Table 1). The group of vaccinates received 3 doses, with vaccinations administered 3 weeks apart beginning at 6 weeks of age. After 1 vaccination, 13/25 puppies exhibited a 4-fold or greater increase in CPV SN titer (seroconversion) (Table 2). Twelve of these 13 puppies had maternal SN titers ≤1:16 at the time of the first vaccination with the remaining puppy having an SN titer of 1:64. Another 9 puppies with initial SN titers between 1:16 and 1:256 seroconverted after the second vaccination. Their maternal antibody SN titers had declined to ≤1:64 at the time of the second vaccination. Similarly, the last 3 vaccinates, with initial SN titers of 1:128, seroconverted after the third vaccination, after their maternal antibody CPV titer dropped ≤1:64.

Therefore, in this study, when 3 doses of vaccine were given beginning at 6 weeks of age, all 25 vaccinates, even those with the highest maternal antibody levels, became actively immunized (GM = 1:1176; range of SN titers 128-4096). All 50 dogs were challenged 3 weeks after the third vaccination with a heterologous CPV challenge virus. Fourteen of 25 nonvaccinated control dogs died or showed illness severe enough to warrant euthanasia, while all 25 vaccinates remained essentially healthy. The high-titer, low-passage vaccine virus in VANGUARD® Plus 5 is therefore highly immunogenic and capable of stimulating active immunity in the presence of maternal antibodies.

References: Available upon request.

Presentation: 1 dose.

U.S. Patent No. 3,616,203

Compendium Code No.: 36901560 75-5303-00

VANGUARD® PLUS 5/CV

Pfizer Animal Health **Vaccine**

Canine Distemper-Adenovirus Type 2-Coronavirus-Parainfluenza-Parvovirus Vaccine, Modified Live and Killed Virus

U.S. Vet. Lic. No.: 189

Description: VANGUARD® Plus 5/CV is a freeze-dried preparation of attenuated strains of CD virus, CAV-2, CPI virus, and CPV, plus a liquid preparation of inactivated CCV with an adjuvant. The CPV fraction is high titer (>$10^{7.0}$ $TCID_{50}$/dose) and was attenuated by low passage (35 passes from the canine isolate with a maximum of 2 additional passes allowed for production) on the canine cell line which gives it the immunogenic properties capable of overriding maternal antibody interference at the levels indicated in Table 2. Some puppies in the field may have higher levels of maternal antibodies than those evaluated in our pivotal efficacy study. All viruses were propagated on established cell lines. The liquid component is used to rehydrate the freeze-dried component, which is packaged with inert gas in place of vacuum.

Contains penicillin and streptomycin as preservatives.

Indications: VANGUARD® Plus 5/CV is for vaccination of healthy dogs 6 weeks of age or older as an aid in preventing canine distemper caused by canine distemper (CD) virus, infectious canine hepatitis (ICH) caused by canine adenovirus type 1 (CAV-1), respiratory disease caused by canine adenovirus type 2 (CAV-2), canine parainfluenza caused by canine parainfluenza (CPI) virus, and enteritis caused by canine coronavirus (CCV) and canine parvovirus (CPV).

Directions:

1. General Directions: Vaccination of healthy dogs is recommended. Aseptically rehydrate the freeze-dried vaccine (Vanguard® Plus 5) with the accompanying vial of liquid vaccine (FirstDose® CV), shake well, and administer 1 mL subcutaneously or intramuscularly.
2. Primary Vaccination: Healthy dogs 6 weeks of age or older should receive 3 doses, each administered 3 weeks apart.
3. Revaccination: Annual revaccination with a single dose is recommended.

Precaution(s): Store at 2°-7°C. Prolonged exposure to higher temperatures and/or direct sunlight may adversely affect potency. Do not freeze.

Use entire contents when first opened.

Sterilized syringes and needles should be used to administer this vaccine. Do not sterilize with chemicals because traces of disinfectant may inactivate the vaccine.

Burn containers and all unused contents.

Caution(s): Vaccination of pregnant bitches should be avoided.

As with many vaccines, anaphylaxis may occur after use. Initial antidote of epinephrine is recommended and should be followed with appropriate supportive therapy.

This product has been shown to be efficacious in healthy animals. A protective immune response may not be elicited if animals are incubating an infectious disease, are malnourished or parasitized, are stressed due to shipment or environmental conditions, are otherwise immunocompromised, or the vaccine is not administered in accordance with label directions.

Warning(s): For use in dogs only.

For veterinary use only.

Discussion: Disease Description: CD is a universal, high-mortality viral disease with variable manifestations. Approximately 50% of nonvaccinated, nonimmune dogs infected with CD virus develop clinical signs, and approximately 90% of those dogs die.[1] ICH, caused by CAV-1, is a universal, sometimes fatal, viral disease of dogs characterized by hepatic and generalized endothelial lesions. CAV-2 causes respiratory disease which in severe cases may include pneumonia and bronchopneumonia. CPI is a common viral upper respiratory disease. Uncomplicated CPI may be mild or subclinical, with signs becoming more severe if concurrent infection with other respiratory pathogens exists. CPV infection results in enteric disease characterized by sudden onset of vomiting and diarrhea, often hemorrhagic. Leukopenia commonly accompanies clinical signs. Susceptible dogs of any age can be affected, but mortality is greatest in puppies. In puppies 4-12 weeks of age CPV may occasionally cause myocarditis that can result in acute heart failure after a brief and inconspicuous illness. Following infection many dogs are refractory to the disease for a year or more. Similarly, seropositive bitches may transfer to their puppies CPV antibodies which can interfere with active immunization of the puppies through 16 weeks of age. CCV also causes enteric disease in susceptible dogs of all ages worldwide.[2] Highly contagious, the virus is transmitted primarily through direct contact with infectious feces, and may cause clinical enteritis within 1-4 days after exposure. Severity of disease may be exacerbated by concurrent infection with other agents.[3] Primary signs of CCV infection include anorexia, vomiting, and diarrhea. Frequency of vomiting usually diminishes within a day or 2 after onset of diarrhea, but diarrhea may linger through the course of infection, and stools occasionally may contain streaks of blood. With CCV infection most dogs remain afebrile and leukopenia is not observed in uncomplicated cases.[2-4]

Trial Data: Safety and Efficacy: Laboratory evaluation demonstrated that VANGUARD® Plus 5/CV immunized dogs against CD, ICH, CAV-2 and CPI respiratory disease, and enteritis caused by CCV and CPV infection, and that no immunologic interference existed among the vaccine fractions. Extensive field safety trials conducted by Pfizer Animal Health showed it to be safe and essentially reaction-free in dogs as young as 6 weeks of age under normal usage conditions.

It has been demonstrated that CAV-2 vaccine cross-protects against ICH caused by CAV-1. The CAV-2 fraction in Vanguard® vaccines is used as a replacement for CAV-1 because it has significant advantages. Some CAV-1 vaccines may produce undesirable reactions, including persistent kidney infections, uveitis, and corneal opacity ("blue eye"), which have not been reported after vaccination with CAV-2.[5] In addition, the CAV-2 strain used in Vanguard® vaccines has been specially selected for freedom from oncogenic properties characteristic of adenoviruses.

Studies conducted at Pfizer demonstrated that CAV-2 not only protects against ICH, but against CAV-2 respiratory disease as well.[6] Although conventional CAV-1 (ICH) vaccines cross-protect against CAV-2, they may not prevent subclinical infection and spread of the CAV-2 agent. Canine adenovirus type 2 challenge virus was not recovered from CAV-2-vaccinated dogs in tests conducted at Pfizer.

The CPV fraction in VANGUARD® Plus 5/CV was subjected to comprehensive safety and efficacy testing at Pfizer. It was shown safe and essentially reaction-free in laboratory tests and in clinical trials under field conditions. Product safety was further demonstrated by a backpassage study which included oral administration of multiple doses of the vaccine strain to susceptible dogs, all of whom remained normal. The CPV virus in VANGUARD® Plus 5/CV shares a characteristic with other live CPV vaccine strains in that the vaccine virus may be present in the feces following administration. Although this CPV vaccine virus was found occasionally and in low titers in the feces of vaccinated dogs, testing demonstrated that the vaccine master seed did not revert to virulence following 6 consecutive backpassages in susceptible dogs.

Research at Pfizer demonstrated that 3 doses of the vaccine with increased CPV virus titer can overcome serum neutralization (SN) titers associated with maternal antibody. Serum neutralization titers as low as 1:4 have been shown by others to interfere with active immunization using conventional modified live vaccines.[7,8] A clinical trial was conducted with fifty 6-week-old puppies [25 vaccinates (SN titer range <2-256) and 25 nonvaccinated controls (SN titer range 4-1024)] (Table 1). The group of vaccinates received 3 doses, with vaccinations administered 3 weeks apart beginning at 6 weeks of age. After 1 vaccination, 13/25 puppies exhibited a 4-fold or greater increase in CPV SN titer (seroconversion) (Table 2). Twelve of these 13 puppies had maternal SN titers ≤1:16 at the time of the first vaccination with the remaining puppy having an SN titer of 1:64. Another 9 puppies with initial SN titers between 1:16 and 1:256 seroconverted after the second vaccination. Their maternal antibody SN titers had declined to ≤1:64 at the time of the second vaccination. Similarly, the last 3 vaccinates, with initial SN titers of 1:128, seroconverted after the third vaccination, after their maternal antibody CPV titer dropped ≤1:64. Therefore, in this study, when 3 doses of vaccine were given beginning at 6 weeks of age, all 25 vaccinates, even those with the highest maternal antibody levels, became actively immunized (GM = 1:1176; range of SN titers 128-4096). All 50 dogs were challenged 3 weeks after the third vaccination with a heterologous CPV challenge virus. Fourteen of 25 nonvaccinated control dogs died or showed illness severe enough to warrant euthanasia, while all 25 vaccinates remained essentially healthy. The high-titer, low-passage vaccine virus in VANGUARD® Plus 5/CV is therefore highly immunogenic and capable of stimulating active immunity in the presence of maternal antibodies.

Table 1. Initial Serum Neutralization (SN) Titers of Vaccinates and Controls

SN Titers	# Vaccinates Included	# Controls Included
<1:2	3	0
1:4	4	3
1:8	1	3
1:16	4	1
1:32	2	5
1:64	3	1
1:128	6	3
1:256	2	3
1:512	0	5
1:1024	0	1

Table 2. Postvaccination Serum Neutralization (SN) Titers Geometric Mean (Range)[a]

Groups	N	Prevaccination	Postvaccination		
			1	2	3[b]
All Vaccinated Dogs	25	1:24 (<2-256)	1:108 (8-1024)	1:605 (8-4096)	1:1176 (128->4096)
Responders Post 1st Vaccination	13	1:6 (<2-64)	1:460 (64-1024)	1:1745 (256-4096)	1:1410 (256-4096)
Responders Post 2nd Vaccination	9	1:87 (16-256)	1:20 (8-64)	1:376 (256-1024)	1:1625 (256-4096)
Responders Post 3rd Vaccination	3	1:128 (128)	1:32 (16-64)	1:25 (8-64)	1:203 (128-256)
Nonvaccinated Control Dogs	25	1:64 (4-1024)	1:9 (<2-64)	1:3 (<2-64)	<1:2 (<2-4)

[a]Dogs were vaccinated at 6, 9, and 12 weeks of age.

[b]Pre-challenge SN titers

The efficacy of the CCV fraction of VANGUARD® Plus 5/CV was demonstrated in an extensive vaccination challenge study. Sixteen 7- to 8-week-old puppies were vaccinated with Vanguard® Plus 5/CV-L (vaccinates) and 17 with Vanguard® Plus 5 (controls). All puppies received three 1-mL doses at 3-week intervals. Three weeks following the third vaccination, puppies were challenged with a virulent strain of CCV (CV-6). Clinical observations, temperatures, weights, and blood parameters were monitored for 21 days following infection. CCV vaccinates demonstrated a reduction in the occurrence of diarrhea and amount of virulent CCV shed when compared to controls. At 21 days postchallenge, fluorescent antibody staining for virulent CCV of small intestinal sections demonstrated a significant reduction ($P<0.05$) in detectable CCV antigen between CCV vaccinates and controls (Table 3).

Table 3. Fluorescent Antibody Staining of Small Intestinal Sections 21 Days Following Challenge

	Gut Section	% Dogs Fluorescent Antibody Positive	
		Vaccinates	Controls
Duodenum	1	0	89
	2	0	100
	3	0	100
Jejunum	4	0	89
	5	0	100
Ileum	6	12.5	56
	7	0	78
	8	12.5	78
	9	0	67
	10	12.5	56

References: Available upon request.

Presentation: 25 x 1 dose vials with accompanying bacterin diluent.

U.S. Patent Nos. 3,616,203; 4,567,042; 4,567,043; and 4,824,785

Compendium Code No.: 36901570 75-5305-00

VANGUARD® PLUS 5/CV-L

Pfizer Animal Health **Bacterin-Vaccine**

Canine Distemper-Adenovirus Type 2-Coronavirus-Parainfluenza-Parvovirus Vaccine, Modified Live and Killed Virus-Leptospira Bacterin

U.S. Vet. Lic. No.: 189

Description: VANGUARD® Plus 5/CV-L is a freeze-dried preparation of attenuated strains of CD virus, CAV-2, CPI virus, CPV, and inactivated whole cultures of *L. canicola* and *L. icterohaemorrhagiae,* plus a liquid preparation of inactivated CCV with an adjuvant. The CPV fraction is high titer ($10^{7.0}$ $TCID_{50}$/ dose) and was attenuated by low passage (35 passes from the canine isolate with a maximum of 2 additional passes allowed for production) on the canine cell line which gives it the immunogenic properties capable of overriding maternal antibody interference at the levels indicated in Table 2. Some puppies in the field may have higher levels of maternal antibodies than those evaluated in our pivotal efficacy study. All viruses were propagated on established cell lines. The liquid component is used to rehydrate the freeze-dried component, which is packaged with inert gas in place of vacuum.

Contains penicillin and streptomycin as preservatives.

Indications: VANGUARD® Plus 5/CV-L is for vaccination of healthy dogs 6 weeks of age or older as an aid in preventing canine distemper caused by canine distemper (CD) virus, infectious canine hepatitis (ICH) caused by canine adenovirus type 1 (CAV-1), respiratory disease caused by canine adenovirus type 2 (CAV-2), canine parainfluenza caused by canine parainfluenza (CPI) virus, enteritis caused by canine coronavirus (CCV) and canine parvovirus (CPV), and leptospirosis caused by *Leptospira canicola* and *L. icterohaemorrhagiae.*

Directions:

1. General Directions: Vaccination of healthy dogs is recommended. Aseptically rehydrate the freeze-dried vaccine (VANGUARD® Plus 5/L) with the accompanying vial of liquid vaccine (FirstDose® CV), shake well, and administer 1 mL subcutaneously or intramuscularly.
2. Primary Vaccination: Healthy dogs 6 weeks of age or older should receive 3 doses, each administered 3 weeks apart.
3. Revaccination: Annual revaccination with a single dose is recommended.

Precaution(s): Store at 2°-7°C. Prolonged exposure to higher temperatures and/or direct sunlight may adversely affect potency. Do not freeze.

Use entire contents when first opened.

Sterilized syringes and needles should be used to administer this vaccine. Do not sterilize with chemicals because traces of disinfectant may inactivate the vaccine.

Burn containers and all unused contents.

Caution(s): Vaccination of pregnant bitches should be avoided.

As with many vaccines, anaphylaxis may occur after use. Initial antidote of epinephrine is recommended and should be followed with appropriate supportive therapy.

This product has been shown to be efficacious in healthy animals. A protective immune response may not be elicited if animals are incubating an infectious disease, are malnourished or parasitized, are stressed due to shipment or environmental conditions, are otherwise immunocompromised, or the vaccine is not administered in accordance with label directions.

For use in dogs only.

Warning(s): For veterinary use only.

Discussion: Disease Description: CD is a universal, high-mortality viral disease with variable manifestations. Approximately 50% of nonvaccinated, nonimmune dogs infected with CD virus develop clinical signs, and approximately 90% of those dogs die.[1] ICH, caused by CAV-1, is a universal, sometimes fatal, viral disease of dogs characterized by hepatic and generalized endothelial lesions. CAV-2 causes respiratory disease which in severe cases may include pneumonia and bronchopneumonia. CPI is a common viral upper respiratory disease. Uncomplicated CPI may be mild or subclinical, with signs becoming more severe if concurrent infection with other respiratory pathogens exists. CPV infection results in enteric disease characterized by sudden onset of vomiting and diarrhea, often hemorrhagic. Leukopenia commonly accompanies clinical signs. Susceptible dogs of any age can be affected, but mortality is greatest in puppies. In puppies 4-12 weeks of age CPV may occasionally cause myocarditis that can result in acute heart failure after a brief and inconspicuous illness. Following infection many dogs are refractory to the disease for a year or more. Similarly, seropositive bitches may transfer to their puppies CPV antibodies which can interfere with active immunization of the puppies through 16 weeks of age. CCV also causes enteric disease in susceptible dogs of all ages worldwide.[2] Highly contagious, the virus is transmitted primarily through direct contact with infectious feces, and may cause clinical enteritis within 1-4 days after exposure. Severity of disease may be exacerbated by concurrent infection with other agents.[3] Primary signs of CCV infection include anorexia, vomiting, and diarrhea. Frequency of vomiting usually diminishes within a day or 2 after onset of diarrhea, but diarrhea may linger through the course of infection, and stools occasionally may contain streaks of blood. With CCV infection most dogs remain afebrile and leukopenia is not observed in uncomplicated cases.[2-4] Leptospirosis occurs in dogs of all ages, with a wide range of clinical signs and chronic nephritis generally following acute infection. Infection with *L. canicola* and *L. icterohaemorrhagiae* cannot be differentiated clinically.

Trial Data: Safety and Efficacy: Laboratory evaluation demonstrated that VANGUARD® Plus 5/CV-L immunized dogs against CD, ICH, CAV-2 and CPI respiratory disease, enteritis caused by CCV and CPV, and leptospirosis caused by *L. canicola* and *L. icterohaemorrhagiae,* and that no immunologic interference existed among the vaccine fractions. Extensive field safety trials conducted by Pfizer Animal Health showed it to be safe and essentially reaction-free in dogs as young as 6 weeks of age under normal usage conditions.

It has been demonstrated that CAV-2 vaccine cross-protects against ICH caused by CAV-1. The CAV-2 fraction in Vanguard® vaccines is used as a replacement for CAV-1 because it has significant advantages. Some CAV-1 vaccines may produce undesirable reactions, including persistent kidney infections, uveitis, and corneal opacity ("blue eye"), which have not been reported after vaccination with CAV-2.[5] In addition, the CAV-2 strain used in Vanguard® vaccines has been specially selected for freedom from oncogenic properties characteristic of adenoviruses.

Studies conducted at Pfizer demonstrated that CAV-2 not only protects against ICH, but against CAV-2 respiratory disease as well.[6] Although conventional CAV-1 (ICH) vaccines cross-protect against CAV-2, they may not prevent subclinical infection and spread of the CAV-2 agent. Canine adenovirus type 2 challenge virus was not recovered from CAV-2-vaccinated dogs in tests conducted at Pfizer.

The CPV fraction in VANGUARD® Plus 5/CV-L was subjected to comprehensive safety and efficacy testing at Pfizer. It was shown safe and essentially reaction-free in laboratory tests and in clinical trials under field conditions. Product safety was further demonstrated by a backpassage study which included oral administration of multiple doses of the vaccine strain to susceptible dogs, all of whom remained normal. The CPV virus in VANGUARD® Plus 5/CV-L shares a characteristic with other live CPV vaccine strains in that the vaccine virus may be present in the feces following administration. Although this CPV vaccine virus was found occasionally and in low titers in the feces of vaccinated dogs, testing demonstrated that the vaccine master seed did not revert to virulence following 6 consecutive backpassages in susceptible dogs.

Research at Pfizer demonstrated that 3 doses of the vaccine with increased CPV virus titer can overcome serum neutralization (SN) titers associated with maternal antibody. Serum neutralization titers as low as 1:4 have been shown by others to interfere with active immunization using conventional modified live vaccines.[7,8] A clinical trial was conducted with fifty 6-week-old puppies [25 vaccinates (SN titer range -256) and 25 nonvaccinated controls (SN titer range 4-1024)] (Table 1). The group of vaccinates received 3 doses, with vaccinations administered 3 weeks apart beginning at 6 weeks of age. After 1 vaccination, 13/25 puppies exhibited a 4-fold or greater increase in CPV SN titer (seroconversion) (Table 2). Twelve of these 13 puppies had maternal SN titers ≤1:16 at the time of the first vaccination with the remaining puppy having an SN titer of 1:64. Another 9 puppies with initial SN titers between 1:16 and 1:256 seroconverted after the second vaccination. Their maternal antibody SN titers had declined to ≤1:64 at the time of the second vaccination. Similarly, the last 3 vaccinates, with initial SN titers of 1:128, seroconverted after the third vaccination, after their maternal antibody CPV titer dropped ≤1:64. Therefore, in this study, when 3 doses of vaccine were given beginning at 6 weeks of age, all 25 vaccinates, even those with the highest maternal antibody levels, became actively immunized (GM = 1:1176; range of SN titers 128-4096). All 50 dogs were challenged 3 weeks after the third vaccination with a heterologous CPV challenge virus. Fourteen of 25 nonvaccinated control dogs died or showed illness severe enough to warrant euthanasia, while all 25 vaccinates remained essentially healthy. The high-titer, low-passage vaccine virus in VANGUARD® Plus 5/CV-L is therefore highly immunogenic and capable of stimulating active immunity in the presence of maternal antibodies.

The efficacy of the CCV fraction of VANGUARD® Plus 5/CV-L was demonstrated in an extensive vaccination challenge study. Sixteen 7- to 8-week-old puppies were vaccinated with VANGUARD® Plus 5/CV-L (vaccinates) and 17 with Vanguard® Plus 5/L (controls). All puppies received three 1-mL doses at 3-week intervals. Three weeks following the third vaccination, puppies were challenged with a virulent strain of CCV (CV-6). Clinical observations, temperatures, weights, and blood parameters were monitored for 21 days following infection. CCV vaccinates demonstrated a reduction in the occurrence of diarrhea and amount of virulent CCV shed when compared to controls. At 21 days postchallenge, fluorescent antibody staining for virulent CCV of small intestinal sections demonstrated a significant reduction (P) in detectable CCV antigen between CCV vaccinates and controls (Table 3).

Table 1. Initial Serum Neutralization (SN) Titers of Vaccinates and Controls

SN Titers	# Vaccinates Included	# Controls Included
<1:2	3	0
1:4	4	3
1:8	1	3
1:16	4	1
1:32	2	5
1:64	3	1
1:128	6	3
1:256	2	3
1:512	0	5
1:1024	0	1

Table 2. Postvaccination Serum Neutralization (SN) Titers Geometric Mean (Range)[a]

Groups	N	Prevaccination	Postvaccination		
			1	2	3[b]
All Vaccinated Dogs	25	1:24 (<2-256)	1:108 (8-1024)	1:605 (8-4096)	1:1176 (128->4096)
Responders Post 1st Vaccination	13	1:6 (<2-64)	1:460 (64-1024)	1:1745 (256-4096)	1:1410 (256-4096)
Responders Post 2nd Vaccination	9	1:87 (16-256)	1:20 (8-64)	1:376 (256-1024)	1:1625 (256-4096)
Responders Post 3rd Vaccination	3	1:128 (128)	1:32 (16-64)	1:25 (8-64)	1:203 (128-256)
Nonvaccinated Control Dogs	25	1:64 (4-1024)	1:9 (<2-64)	1:3 (<2-64)	<1:2 (<2-4)

[a]Dogs were vaccinated at 6, 9, and 12 weeks of age.
[b]Pre-challenge SN titers

Table 3. Fluorescent Antibody Staining of Small Intestinal Sections 21 Days Following Challenge

	Gut Section	% Dogs Fluorescent Antibody Positive	
		Vaccinates	Controls
Duodenum	1	0	89
	2	0	100
	3	0	100
Jejunum	4	0	89
	5	0	100
	6	12.5	56
	7	0	78
	8	12.5	78
Ileum	9	0	67
	10	12.5	56

References: Available upon request.

Presentation: 1 dose vial with accompanying bacterin diluent.

U.S. Patent Nos. 3,616,203; 4,567,042; 4,567,043; and 4,824,785

Compendium Code No.: 36901580

75-5306-00

VANGUARD® PLUS 5/L

Pfizer Animal Health **Bacterin-Vaccine**

Canine Distemper-Adenovirus Type 2-Parainfluenza-Parvovirus Vaccine, Modified Live Virus-Leptospira Bacterin

U.S. Vet. Lic. No.: 189

Description: The vaccine component of VANGUARD® Plus 5/L contains attenuated strains of CD virus, CAV-2, CPI virus, and CPV propagated on an established canine cell line. The CPV fraction is high titer ($10^{7.0}$ $TCID_{50}$/dose) and was attenuated by low passage (35 passes from the canine isolate with a maximum of 2 additional passes allowed for production) on the canine cell line which gives it the immunogenic properties capable of overriding maternal antibody interference at the levels indicated in Table 2. Some puppies in the field may have higher levels of maternal antibodies than those evaluated in our pivotal efficacy study. The vaccine is packaged in freeze-dried form with inert gas in place of vacuum. The bacterin component, containing inactivated whole cultures of *L. canicola* and *L. icterohaemorrhagiae,* is supplied as diluent.

Contains penicillin and streptomycin as preservatives.

Indications: VANGUARD® Plus 5/L is for vaccination of healthy dogs 6 weeks of age or older as an aid in preventing canine distemper caused by canine distemper (CD) virus, infectious canine hepatitis (ICH) caused by canine adenovirus type 1 (CAV-1), respiratory disease caused by canine adenovirus type 2 (CAV-2), canine parainfluenza caused by canine parainfluenza (CPI) virus, canine parvoviral enteritis caused by canine parvovirus (CPV), and leptospirosis caused by *Leptospira canicola* and *L. icterohaemorrhagiae.*

Directions:

1. General Directions: Vaccination of healthy dogs is recommended. Aseptically rehydrate the freeze-dried vaccine (VANGUARD® Plus 5) with the liquid bacterin provided (Leptoferm C-I®), shake well, and administer 1 mL subcutaneously or intramuscularly.
2. Primary Vaccination: Healthy dogs 6 weeks of age or older should receive 3 doses, each administered 3 weeks apart.
3. Revaccination: Annual revaccination with a single dose is recommended.

Precaution(s): Store at 2°-7°C. Prolonged exposure to higher temperatures and/or direct sunlight may adversely affect potency. Do not freeze.

Use entire contents when first opened.

Sterilized syringes and needles should be used to administer this vaccine. Do not sterilize with chemicals because traces of disinfectant may inactivate the vaccine.

Burn containers and all unused contents.

Caution(s): Vaccination of pregnant bitches should be avoided.

As with many vaccines, anaphylaxis may occur after use. Initial antidote of epinephrine is recommended and should be followed with appropriate supportive therapy.

This product has been shown to be efficacious in healthy animals. A protective immune response may not be elicited if animals are incubating an infectious disease, are malnourished or parasitized, are stressed due to shipment or environmental conditions, are otherwise immunocompromised, or the vaccine is not administered in accordance with label directions.

For use in dogs only.

Warning(s): For veterinary use only.

Discussion: Disease Description: CD is a universal, high-mortality viral disease with variable manifestations. Approximately 50% of nonvaccinated, nonimmune dogs infected with CD virus develop clinical signs, and approximately 90% of those dogs die.[1] ICH, caused by CAV-1, is a universal, sometimes fatal, viral disease of dogs characterized by hepatic and generalized endothelial lesions. CAV-2 causes respiratory disease which in severe cases may include pneumonia and bronchopneumonia. CPI is a common viral upper respiratory disease. Uncomplicated CPI may be mild or subclinical, with signs becoming more severe if concurrent infection with other respiratory pathogens exists. CPV infection results in enteric disease characterized by sudden onset of vomiting and diarrhea, often hemorrhagic. Leukopenia commonly accompanies clinical signs. Susceptible dogs of any age can be affected, but mortality is greatest in puppies. In puppies 4-12 weeks of age CPV may occasionally cause myocarditis that can result in acute heart failure after a brief and inconspicuous illness. Following infection many dogs are refractory to the disease for a year or more. Similarly, seropositive bitches may transfer to their puppies CPV antibodies which can interfere with active immunization of the puppies through 16 weeks of age. Leptospirosis occurs in dogs of all ages, with a wide range of clinical signs and chronic nephritis generally following acute infection. Infection with *L. canicola* and *L. icterohaemorrhagiae* cannot be differentiated clinically.

Trial Data: Safety and Efficacy: Laboratory evaluation demonstrated that VANGUARD® Plus 5/L immunized dogs against CD, ICH, CAV-2 respiratory disease, CPI, CPV, and leptospirosis caused by *L. canicola* and *L. icterohaemorrhagiae,* and that no immunologic interference existed among the vaccine fractions. Extensive field safety trials conducted by Pfizer Animal Health showed it to be safe and reaction-free in dogs as young as 6 weeks of age under normal usage conditions.

It has been demonstrated that CAV-2 vaccine cross-protects against ICH caused by CAV-1. The CAV-2 fraction in Vanguard® vaccines is used as a replacement for CAV-1 because it has significant advantages. Some CAV-1 vaccines may produce undesirable reactions, including persistent kidney infections, uveitis, and corneal opacity ("blue eye"), which have not been reported after vaccination with CAV-2.[2] In addition, the CAV-2 strain used in Vanguard® vaccines has been specially selected for freedom from oncogenic properties characteristic of adenoviruses.

Studies conducted at Pfizer demonstrated that CAV-2 not only protects against ICH, but against CAV-2 respiratory disease as well.[3] Although conventional CAV-1 (ICH) vaccines cross-protect against CAV-2, they may not prevent subclinical infection and spread of the CAV-2 agent. Canine adenovirus type 2 challenge virus was not recovered from CAV-2-vaccinated dogs in tests conducted at Pfizer.

Table 1. Initial Serum Neutralization (SN) Titers of Vaccinates and Controls

SN Titers	# Vaccinates Included	# Controls Included
<1:2	3	0
1:4	4	3
1:8	1	3
1:16	4	1
1:32	2	5
1:64	3	1
1:128	6	3
1:256	2	3
1:512	0	5
1:1024	0	1

The CPV fraction in VANGUARD® Plus 5/L was subjected to comprehensive safety and efficacy testing at Pfizer. It was shown safe and reaction-free in laboratory tests and in clinical trials under field conditions. Product safety was further demonstrated by a backpassage study which included oral administration of multiple doses of the vaccine strain to susceptible dogs, all of whom remained normal. The CPV virus in VANGUARD® Plus 5/L shares a characteristic with other live CPV vaccine strains in that the vaccine virus may be present in the feces following administration. Although this CPV vaccine virus was found occasionally and in low titers in the feces of vaccinated dogs, testing demonstrated that the vaccine master seed did not revert to virulence following 6 consecutive backpassages in susceptible dogs.

Table 2. Postvaccination Serum Neutralization (SN) Titers Geometric Mean (Range)[a]

Groups	N	Pre-vaccination	Postvaccination 1	2	3[b]
All Vaccinated Dogs	25	1:24 (<2-256)	1:108 (8-1024)	1:605 (8-4096)	1:1176 (128->4096)
Responders Post 1st Vac.	13	1:6 (<2-64)	1:460 (64-1024)	1:1745 (256-4096)	1:1410 (256-4096)
Responders Post 2nd Vac.	9	1:87 (16-256)	1:20 (8-64)	1:376 (256-1024)	1:1625 (256-4096)
Responders Post 3rd Vac.	3	1:128 (128)	1:32 (16-64)	1:25 (8-64)	1:203 (128-256)
Nonvaccinated Control Dogs	25	1:64 (4-1024)	1:9 (<2-64)	1:3 (<2-64)	<1:2 (<2-4)

[a] Dogs were vaccinated at 6, 9, and 12 weeks of age.

[b] Pre-challenge SN titers

Research at Pfizer demonstrated that 3 doses of the vaccine with increased CPV virus titer can overcome serum neutralization (SN) titers associated with maternal antibody. Serum neutralization titers as low as 1:4 have been shown by others to interfere with active immunization using conventional modified live vaccines.[4,5] A clinical trial was conducted with fifty 6-week-old puppies [25 vaccinates (SN titer range -256) and 25 nonvaccinated controls (SN titer range 4-1024)] (Table 1). The group of vaccinates received 3 doses, with vaccinations administered 3 weeks apart beginning at 6 weeks of age. After 1 vaccination, 13/25 puppies exhibited a 4-fold or greater increase in CPV SN titer (seroconversion) (Table 2). Twelve of these 13 puppies had maternal SN titers ≤1:16 at the time of the first vaccination with the remaining puppy having an SN titer of 1:64. Another 9 puppies with initial SN titers between 1:16 and 1:256 seroconverted after the second vaccination. Their maternal antibody SN titers had declined to ≤1:64 at the time of the second vaccination. Similarly, the last 3 vaccinates, with initial SN titers of 1:128, seroconverted after the third vaccination, after their maternal antibody CPV titer dropped ≤1:64. Therefore, in this study, when 3 doses of vaccine were given beginning at 6 weeks of age, all 25 vaccinates, even those with the highest maternal antibody levels, became actively immunized (GM = 1:1176; range of SN titers 128-4096). All 50 dogs were challenged 3 weeks after the third vaccination with a heterologous CPV challenge virus. Fourteen of 25 nonvaccinated control dogs died or showed illness severe enough to warrant euthanasia, while all 25 vaccinates remained essentially healthy. The high-titer, low-passage vaccine virus in VANGUARD® Plus 5/L is therefore highly immunogenic and capable of stimulating active immunity in the presence of maternal antibodies.

References: Available upon request.

Presentation: 1 dose.

U.S. Patent No. 3,616,203

Compendium Code No.: 36901590 75-5304-00

VANGUARD® PLUS CPV

Pfizer Animal Health **Vaccine**

Parvovirus Vaccine, Modified Live Virus

U.S. Vet. Lic. No.: 189

Description: VANGUARD® Plus CPV contains a strain of CPV attenuated by low passage on an established canine cell line. The vaccine is high titer ($10^{7.0}$ $TCID_{50}$/dose) and was attenuated by low passage (35 passes from the canine isolate with a maximum of 2 additional passes allowed for production) on the canine cell line which gives it the immunogenic properties capable of overriding maternal antibody interference at the levels indicated in Table 2. Some puppies in the field may have higher levels of maternal antibodies than those evaluated in our pivotal efficacy study. Vanguard Plus CPV is packaged in liquid form.

Contains penicillin, streptomycin, and amphotericin B as preservatives.

Indications: VANGUARD® Plus CPV is for vaccination of healthy dogs 6 weeks of age or older for the prevention of canine parvoviral enteritis caused by canine parvovirus (CPV).

Directions:

1. General Directions: Vaccination of healthy dogs is recommended. Shake well. Aseptically administer 1 mL subcutaneously or intramuscularly.
2. Primary Vaccination: Healthy dogs 6 weeks of age or older should receive 3 doses, each administered 3 weeks apart.
3. Revaccination: Annual revaccination with a single dose is recommended.

Precaution(s): Store at 2°-7°C. Prolonged exposure to higher temperatures and/or direct sunlight may adversely affect potency. Do not freeze.

Use entire contents when first opened.

Sterilized syringes and needles should be used to administer this vaccine. Do not sterilize with chemicals because traces of disinfectant may inactivate the vaccine.

Burn containers and all unused contents.

Caution(s): Vaccination of pregnant bitches should be avoided.

As with many vaccines, anaphylaxis may occur after use. Initial antidote of epinephrine is recommended and should be followed with appropriate supportive therapy.

This product has been shown to be efficacious in healthy animals. A protective immune response may not be elicited if animals are incubating an infectious disease, are malnourished or parasitized, are stressed due to shipment or environmental conditions, are otherwise immunocompromised, or the vaccine is not administered in accordance with label directions.

For use in dogs only.

Warning(s): For veterinary use only.

Discussion: Disease Description: CPV is generally transmitted through direct contact with infectious feces. The virus also can be carried on dogs' hair and feet or other contaminated objects and can remain infective for more than 6 months at room temperature.[1] With an incubation period of 4-14 days, CPV infection results in enteric disease characterized by sudden onset of vomiting and diarrhea, often hemorrhagic.[2,3] Leukopenia commonly accompanies clinical signs.[2] Course of CPV disease may be aggravated by concurrent parasitism or infection with other enteric pathogens.[1,3] Susceptible dogs of any age can be affected, but mortality is greatest in puppies. In puppies 4-12 weeks of age CPV may occasionally cause myocarditis that can result in acute heart failure after a brief and inconspicuous illness. Following infection many dogs are refractory to the disease for a year or more. Similarly, seropositive bitches may transfer to their puppies CPV antibodies which can interfere with active immunization of the puppies through 16 weeks of age.

Trial Data: Safety and Efficacy: VANGUARD® Plus CPV was subjected to comprehensive safety and efficacy testing at Pfizer Animal Health. Extensive field safety trials conducted by Pfizer showed it to be safe and reaction-free in dogs as young as 6 weeks of age under normal usage conditions.

Product safety was further demonstrated by a backpassage study which included oral administration of multiple doses of the vaccine strain to susceptible dogs, all of whom remained normal. VANGUARD® Plus CPV vaccine virus shares a characteristic with other live CPV vaccine strains in that the vaccine virus may be present in the feces following administration. Although this CPV vaccine virus was found occasionally and in low titers in the feces of vaccinated dogs, testing demonstrated that the vaccine master seed did not revert to virulence following 6 consecutive backpassages in susceptible dogs.

Table 1. Initial Serum Neutralization (SN) Titers of Vaccinates and Controls

SN Titers	# Vaccinates Included	# Controls Included
<1:2	3	0
1:4	4	3
1:8	1	3
1:16	4	1
1:32	2	5
1:64	3	1
1:128	6	3
1:256	2	3
1:512	0	5
1:1024	0	1

Research at Pfizer demonstrated that 3 doses of the vaccine with increased CPV virus titer can overcome serum neutralization (SN) titers associated with maternal antibody. Serum neutralization titers as low as 1:4 have been shown by others to interfere with active immunization using conventional modified live vaccines.[4,5] A clinical trial was conducted with fifty 6-week-old puppies [25 vaccinates (SN titer range -256) and 25 nonvaccinated controls (SN titer range 4-1024)] (Table 1). The group of vaccinates received 3 doses, with vaccinations administered 3 weeks apart beginning at 6 weeks of age. After 1 vaccination, 13/25 puppies exhibited a 4-fold or greater increase in CPV SN titer (seroconversion) (Table 2). Twelve of these 13 puppies had maternal SN titers ≤1:16 at the time of the first vaccination with the remaining puppy having an SN titer of 1:64. Another 9 puppies with initial SN titers between 1:16 and 1:256 seroconverted after the second vaccination. Their maternal antibody SN titers had declined to ≤1:64 at the time of the second vaccination. Similarly, the last 3 vaccinates, with initial SN titers of 1:128, seroconverted after the third vaccination, after their maternal antibody CPV titer dropped ≤1:64. Therefore, in this study, when 3 doses of vaccine were given beginning at 6 weeks of age, all 25 vaccinates, even those with the highest maternal antibody levels, became actively immunized (GM = 1:1176; range of SN titers 128-4096). All 50 dogs were challenged 3 weeks after the third vaccination with a heterologous CPV challenge virus. Fourteen of 25 nonvaccinated control dogs died or showed illness severe enough to warrant euthanasia, while all 25 vaccinates remained essentially healthy. The high-titer, low-passage vaccine virus in Vanguard Plus CPV is therefore highly immunogenic and capable of stimulating active immunity in the presence of maternal antibodies.

Table 2. Postvaccination Serum Neutralization (SN) Titers Geometric Mean (Range)[a]

Groups	N	Prevaccination	Postvaccination		
			1	2	3[b]
All Vaccinated Dogs	25	1:24 (<2-256)	1:108 (8-1024)	1:605 (8-4096)	1:1176 (128->4096)
Responders Post 1st Vaccination	13	1:6 (<2-64)	1:460 (64-1024)	1:1745 (256-4096)	1:1410 (256-4096)
Responders Post 2nd Vaccination	9	1:87 (16-256)	1:20 (8-64)	1:376 (256-1024)	1:1625 (256-4096)
Responders Post 3rd Vaccination	3	1:128 (128)	1:32 (16-64)	1:25 (8-64)	1:203 (128-256)
Nonvaccinated Control Dogs	25	1:64 (4-1024)	1:9 (<2-64)	1:3 (<2-64)	<1:2 (<2-4)

[a] Dogs were vaccinated at 6, 9, and 12 weeks of age.

[b] Pre-challenge SN titers

References: Available upon request.

Available upon request.

Presentation: 1 dose.

Compendium Code No.: 36901600 75-5301-00

VANGUARD® PLUS CPV/CV

Pfizer Animal Health **Vaccine**

Canine Coronavirus-Parvovirus Vaccine, Modified Live and Killed Virus

U.S. Vet. Lic. No.: 189

Description: VANGUARD® Plus CPV/CV is a liquid preparation of attenuated strains of CPV and inactivated CCV with an adjuvant. The CPV fraction is high titer ($>10^{7.0}$ $TCID_{50}$/dose) and was attenuated by low passage (35 passes from the canine isolate with a maximum of 2 additional passes allowed for production) on the canine cell line which gives it the immunogenic properties capable of overriding maternal antibody interference at the levels indicated in Table 2. Some puppies in the field may have higher levels of maternal antibodies than those evaluated in our pivotal efficacy study. Both viruses were propagated on established cell lines.

Contains penicillin and streptomycin as preservatives.

Indications: VANGUARD® Plus CPV/CV is for vaccination of healthy dogs 6 weeks of age or older as an aid in preventing enteritis caused by canine coronavirus (CCV) and canine parvovirus (CPV).

Directions:

1. General Directions: Vaccination of healthy dogs is recommended. Shake well. Aseptically administer 1 mL subcutaneously or intramuscularly.
2. Primary Vaccination: Healthy dogs 6 weeks of age or older should receive 3 doses, each administered 3 weeks apart.
3. Revaccination: Annual revaccination with a single dose is recommended.

Precaution(s): Store at 2°-7°C. Prolonged exposure to higher temperatures and/or direct sunlight may adversely affect potency. Do not freeze.

Use entire contents when first opened.

Sterilized syringes and needles should be used to administer this vaccine. Do not sterilize with chemicals because traces of disinfectant may inactivate the vaccine.

Burn containers and all unused contents.

Caution(s): Vaccination of pregnant bitches should be avoided.

As with many vaccines, anaphylaxis may occur after use. Initial antidote of epinephrine is recommended and should be followed with appropriate supportive therapy.

This product has been shown to be efficacious in healthy animals. A protective immune response may not be elicited if animals are incubating an infectious disease, are malnourished or parasitized, are stressed due to shipment or environmental conditions, are otherwise immunocompromised, or the vaccine is not administered in accordance with label directions.

Warning(s): For use in dogs only.

For veterinary use only.

Discussion: Disease Description: CPV infection results in enteric disease characterized by sudden onset of vomiting and diarrhea, often hemorrhagic. Leukopenia commonly accompanies clinical signs. Susceptible dogs of any age can be affected, but mortality is greatest in puppies. In puppies 4-12 weeks of age CPV may occasionally cause myocarditis that can result in acute heart failure after a brief and inconspicuous illness. Following infection many dogs are refractory to the disease for a year or more. Similarly, seropositive bitches may transfer to their puppies CPV antibodies which can interfere with active immunization of the puppies through 16 weeks of age. CCV also causes enteric disease in susceptible dogs of all ages worldwide.[1] Highly contagious, the virus is transmitted primarily through direct contact with infectious feces, and may cause clinical enteritis within 1-4 days after exposure. Severity of disease may be exacerbated by concurrent infection with other agents.[2] Primary signs of CCV infection include anorexia, vomiting, and diarrhea. Frequency of vomiting usually diminishes within a day or 2 after onset of diarrhea, but diarrhea may linger through the course of infection, and stools occasionally may contain streaks of blood. With CCV infection most dogs remain afebrile and leukopenia is not observed in uncomplicated cases.[1-3]

Trial Data: Safety and Efficacy: Laboratory evaluation demonstrated that VANGUARD® Plus CPV/CV immunized dogs against enteritis caused by CCV and CPV infection, and that no immunologic interference existed between the vaccine fractions. Extensive field safety trials conducted by Pfizer Animal Health have shown the 2 fractions to be safe and essentially reaction-free in dogs as young as 6 weeks of age under normal usage conditions.

Safety of the CPV fraction was further demonstrated by a backpassage study which included oral administration of multiple doses of the vaccine strain to susceptible dogs, all of whom remained normal. The CPV virus in VANGUARD® Plus CPV/CV shares a characteristic with other live CPV vaccine strains in that the vaccine virus may be present in the feces following administration. Although this CPV vaccine virus was found occasionally and in low titers in the feces of vaccinated dogs, testing demonstrated that the vaccine master seed did not revert to virulence following 6 consecutive backpassages in susceptible dogs.

Research at Pfizer demonstrated that 3 doses of a vaccine with increased CPV virus titer can overcome serum neutralization (SN) titers associated with maternal antibody. Serum neutralization titers as low as 1:4 have been shown by others to interfere with active immunization using conventional modified live vaccines.[4,5] A clinical trial was conducted with fifty 6-week-old puppies [25 vaccinates (SN titer range <2-256) and 25 nonvaccinated controls (SN titer range 4-1024)] (Table 1). The group of vaccinates received 3 doses, with vaccinations administered 3 weeks apart beginning at 6 weeks of age. After 1 vaccination, 13/25 puppies exhibited a 4-fold or greater increase in CPV SN titer (seroconversion) (Table 2). Twelve of these 13 puppies had maternal SN titers ≤1:16 at the time of the first vaccination with the remaining puppy having an SN titer of 1:64. Another 9 puppies with initial SN titers between 1:16 and 1:256 seroconverted after the second vaccination. Their maternal antibody SN titers had declined to ≤1:64 at the time of the second vaccination. Similarly, the last 3 vaccinates, with initial SN titers of 1:128, seroconverted after the third vaccination, after their maternal antibody CPV titer dropped ≤1:64. Therefore, in this study, when 3 doses of vaccine were given beginning at 6 weeks of age, all 25 vaccinates, even those with the highest maternal antibody levels, became actively immunized (GM = 1:1176; range of SN titers 128-4096). All 50 dogs were challenged 3 weeks after the third vaccination with a heterologous CPV challenge virus. Fourteen of 25 nonvaccinated control dogs died or showed illness severe enough to warrant euthanasia, while all 25 vaccinates remained essentially healthy. The high-titer, low-passage vaccine virus in VANGUARD® Plus CPV/CV is therefore highly immunogenic and capable of stimulating active immunity in the presence of maternal antibodies.

Table 1. Initial Serum Neutralization (SN) Titers of Vaccinates and Controls

SN Titers	# Vaccinates Included	# Controls Included
<1:2	3	0
1:4	4	3
1:8	1	3
1:16	4	1
1:32	2	5
1:64	3	1
1:128	6	3
1:256	2	3
1:512	0	5
1:1024	0	1

Table 2. Postvaccination Serum Neutralization (SN) Titers Geometric Mean (Range)[a]

Groups	N	Prevaccination	Postvaccination		
			1	2	3[b]
All Vaccinated Dogs	25	1:24 (<2-256)	1:108 (8-1024)	1:605 (8-4096)	1:1176 (128->4096)
Responders Post 1st Vaccination	13	1:6 (<2-64)	1:460 (64-1024)	1:1745 (256-4096)	1:1410 (256-4096)
Responders Post 2nd Vaccination	9	1:87 (16-256)	1:20 (8-64)	1:376 (256-1024)	1:1625 (256-4096)
Responders Post 3rd Vaccination	3	1:128 (128)	1:32 (16-64)	1:25 (8-64)	1:203 (128-256)
Nonvaccinated Control Dogs	25	1:64 (4-1024)	1:9 (<2-64)	1:3 (<2-64)	<1:2 (<2-4)

[a]Dogs were vaccinated at 6, 9, and 12 weeks of age.

[b]Pre-challenge SN titers

The efficacy of the CCV fraction of VANGUARD® Plus CPV/CV was demonstrated in an extensive vaccination challenge study. Sixteen 7- to 8-week-old puppies were vaccinated with Vanguard® Plus 5/CV-L (vaccinates) and 17 with Vanguard® Plus 5/L (controls). All puppies received three 1-mL doses at 3-week intervals. Three weeks following the third vaccination, puppies were challenged with a virulent strain of CCV (CV-6). Clinical observations, temperatures, weights, and blood parameters were monitored for 21 days following infection. CCV vaccinates demonstrated a reduction in the occurrence of diarrhea and amount of virulent CCV shed when compared to controls. At 21 days postchallenge, fluorescent antibody staining for virulent CCV of small intestinal sections demonstrated a significant reduction ($P<0.05$) in detectable CCV antigen between CCV vaccinates and controls (Table 3).

V

Table 3. Fluorescent Antibody Staining of Small Intestinal Sections 21 Days Following Challenge

	Gut Section	% Dogs Fluorescent Antibody Positive	
		Vaccinates	Controls
Duodenum	1	0	89
	2	0	100
	3	0	100
Jejunum	4	0	89
	5	0	100
	6	12.5	56
	7	0	78
Ileum	8	12.5	78
	9	0	67
	10	12.5	56

References: Available upon request.

Presentation: 1 dose.

U.S. Patent Nos. 4,567,042; 4,567,043; and 4,824,785

Compendium Code No.: 36901610 75-5302-00

VAPONA® CONCENTRATE INSECTICIDE

Boehringer Ingelheim **Premise Insecticide**

EPA Reg. No.: 4691-130

Active Ingredient(s): By Weight

Dichlorvos (CAS# 62-73-7)* 40.2%

Related Compounds* 3.0%

Other Ingredients** 56.8%

Total 100.0%

This product contains 3.88 lbs. of Dichlorvos per gallon.

*Equivalent to 43.2% w/w Vapona® Insecticide.

**Contains petroleum hydrocarbons.

Indications: Use as a beef cattle, lactating dairy cattle spray; indoor application for dairy barns, poultry houses, swine confinement facilities, or other animal buildings; outdoor application for feedlots, holding pens, corrals and other livestock holding facilities.

Controls flies, gnats and mosquitoes on cattle and around livestock and poultry premises.

Directions for Use: It is a violation of Federal law to use this product in a manner inconsistent with its labeling.

For agricultural/commericial use only. Not for sale for any other uses.

This product must be mixed with water or diesel oil, depending on use, prior to using. It is suitable for use in conventional power or low pressure knapsack sprayers, mist blowers or non-thermal foggers. Select the specific site, method of use and insect problem, then dilute as directed. Follow the remarks for the safe use and best results in using this product. Do not store diluted product. Prior to use, read the Precautionary Statements.

Livestock Use Directions - Dilute in water only.

For direct application to beef and dairy cattle (including lactating). Do not make direct application to livestock more frequently than once per day.

Must be diluted prior to application.

Use	Insects Controlled	Dilution VAPONA® in Water	Remarks
Dairy Cattle (including lactating), Beef Cattle	Horn Flies, Face Flies, Stable Flies, House Flies, Mosquitoes	1 gal. in 50 gal. or 5 oz. in 2 gal. (1% Dilution)	Apply 1 to 2 fl. oz. of diluted solution (do not exceed 2 oz.) per animal daily as a fine mist spray. Be sure to cover all parts of animal for best results. Do not apply in combination with other dermal organophosphate pesticides (e.g. trichlorfon). Brahman and Brahman cross cattle should not be treated as they may show hypersensitivity to organophosphates. Do not wet the hide. Do not apply to calves under 6 months of age. One day withdrawal is required on beef cattle.

Indoor Premise/Area Use Directions - Dilute in water only.

For indoor application to livestock facilities.

Use	Insects Controlled	Dilution VAPONA® in Water	Remarks
Dairy Barns, Poultry Houses, Swine Barns, Other Animal Buildings	Flies, Gnats, Mosquitoes, Roaches, Sowbugs, Ants	1 gal. in 100 gal. or 2 oz. in 1.5 gal. (0.5% Dilution)	Apply as a space spray mist to open air space at the rate of 1 quart (32 oz.) of diluted solution per 8,000 cubic feet or as a coarse wet spray to indoor surfaces at the rate of 1 quart of diluted solution per 1,000 sq. ft. Before applying reduce air movement as much as possible by closing doors, windows, and other openings. Do not use this solution in areas where animals have received a direct organophosphate pesticide application within eight hours. If animals are present, ventilate treated area immediately following spray application. Do not contaminate water, feed, or foodstuffs, milk or milking utensils.
		1 gal. in 50 gal. or 5 oz. in 2 gal. (1.0% Dilution)	Apply as above at the rate of 1 pint (16 oz.) per 8,000 cubic feet or 1 pint (16 oz.) per 1,000 sq. ft. when a reduced quantity of water is desired and equipment can adequately provide coverage of area to be treated.
Manure Piles	Fly Maggots	1 gal. in 100 gal. or 2 oz. in 1.5 gal. (0.5% Dilution)	Apply as above at the rate of 1 to 2 qts. of solution per 100 sq. ft. of manure once a week.

Outdoor Area Use Directions - Dilute in water (misting) or diesel oil (fogger).

For outdoor area treatment of livestock holding facilities.

Use	Insects Controlled	Dilution VAPONA® in Diluent	Remarks
Cattle Feedlots, Stockyards, Holding Pens, Corrals	Flies, Gnats, Mosquitoes	1 gal. in 100 gal. or 1 qt. in 25 gal. (0.5% Dilution)	Apply at an overall application rate of approximately 5 gallons of diluted solution per acre. Fog or mist during the time insects are most active, usually late afternoon and when there is little wind. Particular attention should be given or to areas where flies congregate such as around feed bunks, fences, and walls buildings. Avoid direct application to exposed feed and water. Animals may be present during treatment.

Precautionary Statements: Hazards to Humans and Domestic Animals: Danger. Poisonous if swallowed, inhaled or absorbed through the skin and eyes. Rapidly absorbed through skin. Repeated inhalation or skin contact may without symptoms, progressively increase susceptibility to dichlorvos (DDVP) poisoning. Do not swallow or get in eyes, on skin or on clothing. Do not breathe vapor. Do not contaminate food or feed products.

Personal Protective Equipment (PPE): Some materials that are chemical-resistant to this product are listed below. If you want more options follow the instructions of category "C" on an EPA chemical-resistance category selection chart in the Worker Protection Standard.

Applicators and other Handlers Must Wear: Coveralls over long-sleeved shirt and long pants, chemical-resistant gloves such as Barrier Laminate, Butyl Rubber, Nitrile Rubber, Neoprene Rubber, Polyvinyl Chloride or Viton, chemical-resistant footwear plus socks, protective eyewear, chemical-resistant headgear for overhead exposure, chemical-resistant apron required for mixing/loading and cleaning equipment, respirator with either an organic vapor removing ON cartridge with a prefilter approved for pesticides (MSHA/NIOSH approval number prefix TX-23C) or a canister approved for pesticides (MSHA/NIOSH approval number TC-14G).

Discard clothing and other absorbent materials that have been drenched or heavily contaminated with this product's concentrate. Do not reuse them. Follow manufacturer's instructions for cleaning/maintaining PPE. If no such instructions for washables, use detergent and hot water. Keep and wash PPE separately from other laundry.

Statement of Practical Treatment:

If Swallowed: Call a physician or Poison Control Center immediately. Induce vomiting by giving victim 1 or 2 glasses of water and by touching back of throat with finger. Never induce vomiting or give anything by mouth to an unconscious or convulsing person.

If Inhaled: Remove victim to fresh air immediately. Apply artificial respiration if indicated. Get medical attention.

If in Eyes: Hold eyelids open and flush with a steady gentle stream of water for 15 minutes. Get medical attention.

If on Skin: Remove contaminated clothing immediately and wash affected area with soap and water. Call a physician immediately. Wash clothing before reuse.

Note to Physician - Poisoning Symptoms: Symptoms include weakness, headache, tightness in chest, blurred vision, non-reactive pinpoint pupils, salivation, sweating, nausea, vomiting, diarrhea, and abdominal cramps.

Treatment: Atropine is the specific therapeutic antagonist of choice against parasympathetic nervous stimulation. If there are signs of parasympathetic stimulation, Atropine Sulfate should be injected at 10 minute intervals in doses of 1 to 2 milligrams until complete atropinization has occurred. Pralidoxime chloride (2-PAM) may also be used as an effective antidote in addition to and while maintaining full atropinization. In adults, an initial dose of 1 gram of 2-PAM should be injected preferably as an infusion in 250 cc of saline over a 15 to 30 minute period. If this is not practical, 2-PAM may be administered slowly by intravenous injection as a 5 percent solution in water over not less than two minutes. After about an hour, a second dose of 1 gram of 2-PAM will be indicated if muscle weakness has not been relieved. For infants and children the dose of 2-PAM is 0.25 gram. Morphine is an improper treatment. Clear chest by postural drainage. Oxygen administration may be necessary. Observe patient continuously for 48 hours. Repeated exposure to cholinesterase inhibitors may without warning cause prolonged susceptibility to very small doses of any cholinesterase inhibitor. Allow no further exposure until cholinesterase regeneration has been attained as determined by blood test.

Environmental Hazards: This pesticide is highly toxic to fish, birds and other wildlife. Do not apply to water, or to areas where surface water is present or to intertidal areas below the mean high water mark. Do not apply where runoff is likely to occur or when weather conditions favor drift from areas treated. Drift and runoff from treated areas may be hazardous to aquatic organisms in treated areas. Do not contaminate water when disposing of equipment washwaters.

Physical or Chemical Hazards: Do not use or store near heat or open flame. Do not use with thermal foggers or heat-generating devices.

Storage and Disposal: Not for use or storage in or around the home.

Do not contaminate water, food or feed by storage or disposal.

Storage: Store in original container only. Store in a safe place where children or animals cannot reach the product or its diluted emulsion. Protect from freezing.

Container Disposal: Triple-rinse (or equivalent). Then puncture and dispose of in a sanitary landfill, or by other procedures approved by State and local authorities.

Pesticide Disposal: Pesticide wastes are acutely hazardous. Improper disposal of excess pesticide, spray mixture, or rinsate is a violation of Federal law. If these wastes cannot be disposed of by use according to label instructions, contact the State Pesticide or Environmental Control Agency, or the Hazardous Waste representative at the nearest EPA Regional Office for guidance.

Warning(s): This product can be used on lactating dairy cattle and requires only 1-day withdrawal period when used on beef cattle.

Danger. Poison.

Keep out of reach of children.

Disclaimer: Warranty and Limitations of Damages: Seller warrants that this material conforms to its chemical description and is reasonably fit for the purposes stated on the label when used in accordance with directions under normal conditions of use and Buyer assumes the risk of any use contrary to such directions. Seller makes no other express or implied warranty of Fitness or of Merchantability, and no agent of Seller is authorized to do so except in writing and with specific reference to this warranty. In no event shall Seller's liability for any breach of warranty exceed the purchase price of the material as to which a claim is made.

Presentation: 2.5 gallons (9.5 L).

Compendium Code No.: 10281122 BI 6576-1 10/00

VARIANT VAX-BD™

Schering-Plough **Vaccine**

Bursal Disease Vaccine, Live Virus

U.S. Vet. Lic. No.: 165A

Contents: A live virus vaccine containing a bursal disease virus derived from a field strain. The vaccine was attenuated by serial passage in cell culture and has been demonstrated in controlled studies to provide protection against standard and variant bursal disease viruses.

The vaccine virus is grown in chicken embryos and combined with stabilizing agents. The product is supplied as a lyophilized vaccine contained in vials sealed under vacuum. Contains gentamicin as a preservative.

Indications: For use in chickens at 1 day of age by subcutaneous route of administration or by drinking water at 2 weeks or older as an aid in preventing bursal disease associated with infection by standard and variant bursal disease viruses.

Dosage and Administration: When to Vaccinate: Vaccinate subcutaneously at 1 day of age or by drinking water at 2 weeks or older. Good management practices should be followed to reduce exposure of birds to virulent infectious bursal disease virus during the first several weeks of life.

Preparation of the Vaccine:

Subcutaneous Route of Administration:

Do not open and mix the vaccine until ready for use.

Mix only one vial at a time and use entire contents within 2 hours.

Lift up top of seal on vaccine vial to expose rubber stopper. Using sterile needle and 5 or 10 mL syringe, remove a small amount (5 mL) of diluent from the diluent bottle and transfer this to the vaccine vial. Vacuum in the vaccine vial will readily pull in the diluent. Release the vacuum remaining in the vial.

Vigorously shake vaccine vial with transferred diluent to rehydrate the vaccine.

Using the same sterile needle and syringe, completely transfer the rehydrated vaccine to remaining diluent in the diluent bottle. Rinse syringe and vaccine vial by withdrawing additional diluent in diluent bottle. Rinse syringe and vaccine vial by withdrawing additional diluent and repeating the process.

Vigorously shake the final rehydrated vaccine for 20-30 seconds to mix thoroughly.

The vaccine is now ready for use.

Drinking Water Method:

Assemble the vaccine and equipment needed to vaccinate the entire flock at one time.

Do not open and mix the vaccine until ready for use.

Remove the tear-off aluminum seal from the vaccine vial without disturbing the rubber stopper.

Use cool, clean, non-chlorinated tap water to which powdered milk has been added as directed under How to Vaccinate.

Holding vial submerged in a pail of water or under a running stream of water, lift the top of the rubber stopper so that the water (milk added) is sucked into the vial.

Reseat the stopper and shake the vial to thoroughly dissolve the vaccine.

How to Vaccinate:

By Subcutaneous Route of Administration: Insert a filling tube (large, sharpened transfer tube) into the bottle of vaccine. Connect the filling tube by means of rubber or plastic tubing to an automatic vaccinator fitted with a 22 gauge ½ inch needle. The automatic vaccinator should be calibrated accurately ahead of time to deliver 0.2 mL.

By Drinking Water Method: Do not mix the vaccine into the drinking water until ready for use. Drinking water for vaccination should be mixed with powdered milk to prevent inactivation from chlorine or other water additives and also to stabilize the vaccine virus. The powdered milk should be added to the water at a rate of 3 grams per 11 liters (one heaped teaspoon per 3 U.S. gallons or 2.5 Imp. gallons); or 90 grams per 300 liters (one heaped cupful per 80 gallons or 66 Imp. gallons).

Withhold water for several hours before vaccinating so birds are thirsty. Thoroughly clean and rinse all watering containers so that no residual disinfectants remain. Dilute the vaccine immediately before use with cool, clan, non-chlorinated water (milk added). Pour the dissolved vaccine material into the following amounts of water and mix thoroughly.

Each 1000 Birds	U.S. Gallons	Imperial Gallons	Metric Liters
2 to 4 Weeks	2½	2	10
4 to 8 Weeks	5	4	20
Over 8 Weeks	10	8	40

Distribute diluted vaccine so that all birds are able to drink within a 1 hour period and do not add any more water until the vaccine is consumed. Avoid placing water in direct sunlight.

Records: Keep a record of vaccine type, quantity, serial number, expiration date, and place of purchase; the date and time of vaccination; the number, age, breed, and location of the birds; names of operators performing the vaccination and any observed reactions.

Precaution(s): Store at 2° to 7°C (35° to 45°F).

Do not dilute the vaccine or otherwise stretch the dosage.

Do not spill or splatter the vaccine. Use entire contents of vial when first opened. Burn empty bottles, caps and all unused vaccine and accessories.

Caution(s): Use only in states where permitted and on premises with a history of bursal disease.

For subcutaneous use only in day old birds. For use by drinking water in birds 2 weeks or older.

All birds within a house should be vaccinated on the same day. Isolate other susceptible birds on the premises from birds being vaccinated.

Vaccinate only healthy birds. Although disease may not be evident, coccidiosis, chronic respiratory disease, mycoplasma infection, lymphoid leukosis, Marek's disease, or other disease conditions may cause serious complications or reduce protection.

In outbreak situations, vaccinate healthy birds first, progressing toward outbreak areas in order to vaccinate diseased birds last.

Warning(s): Do not vaccinate within 21 days of slaughter. Wash hands thoroughly after using the vaccine.

The use of this vaccine is subject to state laws wherever applicable.

For veterinary use only.

Discussion: Vaccination Program: The development of a durable, strong protection against this disease depends upon the use of an effective vaccination program as well as many circumstances such as administration techniques, environment and flock health at time of vaccination. Also, the immune response to one vaccination under field conditions is seldom compete for all birds within a given flock. Even when vaccination is successful, the protection stimulated in individual animals against different diseases may not be life long. Therefore, a program of periodic revaccination may be necessary.

Presentation: 5000 dose vials.

Compendium Code No.: 10472061

VECTORMUNE® FP-LT

Biomune **Vaccine**

Fowl Pox-Laryngotracheitis Vaccine, Live Fowl Pox Vector

U.S. Vet. Lic. No.: 368

Description: VECTORMUNE® FP-LT contains a genetically engineered, live virus vaccine for the vaccination of chickens as an aid in the prevention of fowl pox and laryngotracheitis. The fowl pox vaccine has been genetically engineered to contain and express key protective laryngotracheitis virus antigens.

Contains gentamicin and amphotericin B as preservatives.

Indications: Administer by wing web to healthy, susceptible chickens at least eight weeks old but at least four weeks prior to the start of egg product. Chickens receiving this vaccine must not have been previously vaccinated with a fowl pox vaccine.

Dosage and Administration: Remove seal and stopper from vaccine vial and diluent vial. Pour entire contents of diluent vial into vaccine vial. Insert stopper and shake well. The vaccine is ready for use and should be used within one hour. Hold each individual bird and spread the wing with the underside facing up. Dip the two-pronged wing web applicator into the vaccine so that grooves fill with liquid and deliver 0.01 mL per bird. Insert the double-pronged applicator into the web portion of the wing avoiding blood vessels, muscle and bone. Seven to ten days after vaccination, observe several chickens for evidence of "takes" that include swelling and/or scab formation at the site of injection.

Precaution(s): Store vaccine at 35-45°F (2-7°C).

Use entire contents immediately after rehydrating. Burn containers and all unused contents.

Caution(s): All birds on a farm should be vaccinated at one time.

Warning(s): Do not vaccinate within 21 days of slaughter.

Presentation: 10 x 1,000 doses with sterile diluent and wing-web applicators packaged separately.

Compendium Code No.: 11290480 April 11, 2002

VECTORMUNE® FP-LT+AE

Biomune **Vaccine**

Avian Encephalomyelitis-Fowl Pox-Laryngotracheitis Vaccine, Live Virus, Live Fowl Pox Vector

U.S. Vet. Lic. No.: 368

Description: VECTORMUNE® FP-LT+AE contains a genetically engineered, live virus vaccine for the vaccination of chickens as an aid in the prevention of fowl pox and laryngotracheitis. The vaccine also contains a conventional live virus for vaccination as an aid in the prevention of avian encephalomyelitis. The fowl pox vaccine has been genetically engineered to contain and express key protective laryngotracheitis virus antigens.

Contains gentamicin and amphotericin B as preservatives.

Indications: Administer by wing web to healthy, susceptible chickens at least eight weeks old but at least four weeks prior to the start of egg product. Chickens receiving this vaccine must not have been previously vaccinated with a fowl pox vaccine.

Dosage and Administration: Remove seal and stopper from vaccine vial and diluent vial. Pour entire contents of diluent vial into vaccine vial. Insert stopper and shake well. The vaccine is ready for use and should be used within one hour. Hold each individual bird and spread the wing with the underside facing up. Dip the two-pronged wing web applicator into the vaccine so that the grooves fill with liquid and deliver 0.01 mL per bird. Insert the double-pronged applicator into the web portion of the wing avoiding blood vessels, muscle and bone. Seven to ten days after vaccination, observe several chickens for evidence of "takes" that include swelling and/or scab formation at the site of injection.

Precaution(s): Store vaccine at 35-45°F (2-7°C).

Use entire contents immediately after rehydrating. Burn containers and all unused contents.

Caution(s): All birds on a farm should be vaccinated at one time.

Warning(s): Do not vaccinate within 21 days of slaughter.

Presentation: 10 x 1,000 doses with sterile diluent and wing-web applicators packaged separately.

Compendium Code No.: 11290490 June 7, 2001

VECTORMUNE® FP-N

Biomune **Vaccine**

Newcastle Disease-Fowl Pox Vaccine, Live Fowl Pox Vector

U.S. Vet. Lic. No.: 368

Description: VECTORMUNE® FP-N is a genetically engineered, live virus vaccine for the vaccination of chickens as an aid in the prevention of Newcastle disease and fowl pox. The fox pox vector used in this vaccine has been genetically modified to contain and express genes for the key protective Newcastle disease virus (NDV) antigens, as well as the full complement of protective fowl pox virus (FPV) antigens.

Contains gentamicin and amphotericin B as preservatives.

Indications: For the vaccination of healthy chickens as an aid in the prevention of Newcastle disease and fowl pox. The vaccine may be used subcutaneously in NDV maternal antibody negative chickens at one day of age or older or by wing web in FPV susceptible chickens at nine weeks of age or older. NDV susceptible or primed chickens ay be vaccinated by the wing web route. Chickens receiving this vaccine must not have been previously vaccinated with a fowl pox product.

Dosage and Administration: Subcutaneous: Aseptically transfer 5 to 10 mL of sterile diluent from the 100 mL diluent bottle to the vaccine vial and mix until the lyophilized material is rehydrated. Transfer the rehydrated vaccine back to the diluent bottle and mix. Administer 0.2 mL per bird subcutaneously in the loose skin on the back of the neck, just below the head.

Wing Web: Aseptically transfer the entire 5 mL of sterile diluent to the vaccine vial and mix until the lyophilized material is rehydrated. Administer one dose per bird using a two-pronged wing web applicator designed to deliver 0.01 mL per bird. Stab the underside of the webbed portion of the wing, avoiding blood vessels, bones, wing muscles and feathered areas.

Precaution(s): Store vaccine at 35-45°F (2-7°C).

Use entire contents immediately after rehydrating. Burn containers and all unused contents.

Warning(s): Do not vaccinate within 21 days of slaughter.

Presentation: 10 x 500 doses and 10 x 1,000 doses with sterile diluent and wing web applicators packaged separately.

Patent Number 6,123,949

Compendium Code No.: 11290500 Feb. 26, 2001

VEDADINE BOLUS

Vedco — **Topical Wound Dressing**

PVP Iodine-pH Balanced

Active Ingredient(s): Each bolus contains: 250 mg. Available iodine as polyvinylpyrrolidone iodine complex in a urea base.
Indications: Uses: To prepare a solution of iodine for flushing wounds, or for topical disinfection.
Dosage and Administration: Dissolve one bolus in 50 to 100 mL of water. Apply as a soak or cleanse area with solution on gauze.
Caution(s): For topical use only.
Not for human use.
For veterinary use only.
Warning(s): Keep out of reach of children.
Presentation: 50 boluses (NDC 50989-247-49).
Compendium Code No.: 10942430

VEDA-K_1 CAPSULES

Vedco — **Vitamin K_1-Oral**

Active Ingredient(s): Each capsule contains:

Phytonadione	25 mg

Indications: Vitamin K_1 capsules are indicated in dogs and cats to counter hypoprothrombinemia induced by ingestion of coumarin-based compounds, common ingredients in commercial rodenticides, and other drug induced hypoprothrombinemia where it is definitely shown that the result is due to interference with vitamin K metabolism, e.g. salicylates.
Dosage and Administration: Dogs and Cats: Acute hypoprothrombinemia (with hemorrhage) - Administer orally at the rate of 2.5-5 mg/kg of body weight (1 capsule per each 11 pounds of body weight for higher dosage) once a day as conditions require for up to three (3) weeks. The frequency and amount of oral administration should be guided by regular determination of prothrombin time.

Note: Regular determinations of prothrombin time response should be performed to guide in the initial and subsequent administration of Vitamin K_1 oral capsules. The dosage should be adjusted accordingly.
Precaution(s): Protect from light at all times.
Caution(s): Keep out of the reach of children.

Temporarily resistance to prothrombin-depressing anticoagulants may result, especially when larger doses of phytonadione are used.

It is recommended that Vitamin K_1 capsules be used in follow-up therapy only after an administration of Vitamin K_1 injection and hospitalization is no longer required. An immediate coagulant effect should not be expected after the administration of phytonadione when administered orally. Phytonadione will not counteract the anticoagulant action of heparin.

Repeated large doses of Vitamin K_1 are not warranted in hepatic disease if the response to the initial therapy is unsatisfactory. Failure to respond to Vitamin K_1 may indicate that the condition being treated is inherently unresponsive to Vitamin K_1.
Presentation: 50 capsule, 25 mg containers.
Compendium Code No.: 10942060

VEDA-K_1 INJECTION

Vedco — **Vitamin K_1-Injection**

Active Ingredient(s): Each mL contains:

Phytonadione	10 mg
Polyoxyethylated fatty acid derivative	70 mg
Dextrose	37.5 mg
Water	q.s.
Benzyl alcohol (added as a preservative)	0.9%

Indications: Vitamin K_1 injection is indicated in cattle, calves, horses, swine, sheep, goats, dogs and cats to counter hypoprothrombinemia induced by ingestion of courmarin based compounds, common ingredients in commercial rodenticides. Vitamin K_1 injection is also indicated to counter hypoprothrombinemia caused by consumption of bishydroxycoumarin found in spoiled and moldy sweet clover.
Dosage and Administration:
Cattle, Calves, Horses, Swine, Sheep and Goats:

Acute hypoprothrombinemia (with hemorrhage): 0.5-2.5 mg/kg of body weight, intravenously, at a rate not to exceed 10 mg/minute in mature animals and 5 mg/minute in newborn and very young animals.

Nonacute hypoprothrombinemia: 0.5-2.5 mg/kg of body weight, intramuscularly or subcutaneously.
Dogs and Cats:

Acute hypoprothrombinemia (with hemorrhage): 0.25-2.5 mg/kg of body weight, intravenously, at a rate not to exceed 5 mg/minute.

Nonacute hypoprothrombinemia: 0.25-2.5 mg/kg of body weight, intramuscularly or subcutaneously.
Precaution(s): Protect from light. Store in a dark place.
Caution(s): For animal use only. Not for human use. Keep out of the reach of children.

Intravenous use: Severe reactions, including fatalities, have occurred during and immediately after intravenous injections of phytonadione, even when precautions have been taken to dilute the Vitamin K_1 and to avoid rapid infusion. Typically, these severe reactions have resembled hypersensitivity or anaphylaxis, including shock and cardiac and or respiratory arrest. Some animals have exhibited these severe reactions on receiving vitamin K_1 injection for the first time. Therefore, the intravenous route should be restricted to those situations where other routes are not feasible and the serious risk involved is considered justified.

Pain, swelling, and tenderness at the injection site may occur. The possibility of allergic sensitivity, including an anaphylactic reaction, should be kept in mind.
Presentation: 30 mL and 100 mL vials.
Compendium Code No.: 10942070

VEDALAX™ AND VEDALAX™ TUNA

Vedco — **Laxative**

Hairball Preparation

Ingredients:

VEDALAX™: Malt syrup, corn syrup, petrolatum, cane molasses, soybean oil, mineral oil, water, hydrolyzed gelatin by-products, sorbic acid, potassium sorbate.

VEDALAX™ Tuna: Malt syrup, corn syrup, petrolatum, cane molasses, soybean oil, mineral oil, water, hydrolyzed gelatin by-products, sorbic acid, potassium sorbate, artificial tuna flavor.
Indications: A gentle preparation which can aid in the elimination and prevention of hairballs.

Hairballs accumulate in the digestive tract and can interfere with regular digestion and elimination.
Directions for Use: The highly palatable flavor of VEDALAX™ aids in easy administration.

To acquaint pet to the flavor of VEDALAX™, place a small amount on nose or paw.

For Hair Balls: Feed adult cats ½-1 teaspoonful for 2-3 days then ¼-½ teaspoonful for 2-3 times a week. For kittens under 4 weeks old: Administer half doses.

Feed adult dogs ½-1 teaspoonful 2-3 times a week.
Presentation: VEDALAX™: 3 oz (85 g) tube (NDC 50989-609-20).
VEDALAX™ Tuna: 3 oz (85 g) tube (NDC 50989-594-20).
Compendium Code No.: 10942440

VEDALYTE 8X POWDER

Vedco — **Electrolytes-Oral**

Active Ingredient(s): Contains:

Calcium lactate trihydrate	1.28%
Magnesium citrate soluble purified	0.65%
Potassium chloride	1.27%
Sodium chloride	9.68%
Sodium citrate dihydrate	7.36%
Dextrose monohydrate	79.76%

Indications: A powdered electrolyte concentrate for use in preparing a balanced electrolyte solution with 5% dextrose.
Dosage and Administration: Dissolve one (1) package (16 oz.) in 40 gallons of drinking water.
Precaution(s): Do not store above 30°C (86°F). Store in a cool, dry place.
Caution(s): The product contains citrate salts which in some cases may be incompatible with tetracycline antibiotics.
For animal use only.
Warning(s): Keep out of reach of children.
Presentation: 16 oz (1 lb) packages, 25 per pail (NDC 50989-243-26).
Compendium Code No.: 10942101

VEDA-SORB BOLUS

Vedco — **Adsorbent**

Active Ingredient(s): Each bolus contains: Activated attapulgite, carob powder, citrus pectin, magnesium trisilicate, and colloidal aluminum silicate.
Indications: For the relief of simple diarrhea of cattle and horses.
Dosage and Administration: Horses and Cattle: Two (2) to three (3) boluses. Repeat at 4-hour intervals if necessary. Discontinue after three (3) days.
Caution(s): Keep out of the reach of children. For veterinary use only.

If symptoms appear indicating dryness of throat such as difficulty in swallowing, etc., discontinue the use of the product. If symptoms persist after using the preparation for two to three days, consult a veterinarian.
Presentation: 50 bolus containers.
Compendium Code No.: 10942080

VEDA-SORB JR BOLUS

Vedco — **Adsorbent**

NDC No.: 50989-362-49
Active Ingredient(s): Each bolus contains: Activated attapulgite, carob flour, pectin, and magnesium trisilicate, in a suitable base.
Indications: For use as an aid in the relief of simple noninfectious diarrhea of colts and calves.
Dosage and Administration: Administer orally. Give two (2) boluses to calves and foals.

Repeat the treatment at 4- to 6-hour intervals as needed. Discontinue use of the product after three (3) days. If symptoms persist after using the preparation for three (3) days, consult a veterinarian.
Precaution(s): Store at a controlled room temperature between 15°-30°C (59°-86°F).
Caution(s): For animal use only.
Keep out of the reach of children.
Presentation: 50 boluses.
Compendium Code No.: 10942090

VELENIUM™ ℞

Fort Dodge — **Vitamin E-Selenium**

(Selenium, Vitamin E) Injection

ANADA No.: 200-109
Active Ingredient(s): Each mL contains: 10.95 mg sodium selenite (equivalent to 5 mg selenium), 50 mg (68 USP units) vitamin E (as *d*-alpha tocopheryl acetate), 250 mg polysorbate 80, 2% benzyl alcohol (preservative), water for injection q.s. Sodium hydroxide and/or hydrochloric acid may be added to adjust pH.
Indications: VELENIUM™ (selenium, vitamin E) is recommended for the prevention and treatment of STD syndrome in weanling calves and breeding beef cattle. Clinical signs are: stiffness and lameness; chronic, persistent diarrhea; unthriftiness; abortions and/or weak premature calves.
Pharmacology:

Description: VELENIUM™ (selenium, vitamin E) is an emulsion of selenium-tocopherol for the prevention and treatment of Selenium-Tocopherol Deficiency (STD) syndrome in weanling calves and breeding beef cattle.

Actions: It has been demonstrated that selenium and tocopherol exert physiological effects and that these effects are intertwined with sulfur metabolism. Additionally, tocopherol appears to have a significant role in the oxidation process, thus suggesting an interrelationship between selenium and tocopherol in overcoming sulfur-induced depletion and restoring normal metabolism. Although oral ingestion of adequate amounts of selenium and tocopherol would seemingly restore normal metabolism, it is apparent that the presence of sulfur and, perhaps, other factors interfere during the digestive process with proper utilization of selenium and tocopherol. When selenium and tocopherol are injected, they bypass the digestive process and exert their full metabolic effects promptly on cell metabolism. Anti-inflammatory action has been demonstrated by selenium-tocopherol in the Selye Pouch Technique and experimentally induced polyarthritis study in rats.
Dosage and Administration: Inject subcutaneously or intramuscularly. Weanling calves: 1 mL per 200 pounds of body weight. Breeding beef cows: 1 mL per 200 pounds of body weight during the middle third of pregnancy, and 30 days before calving.

Contraindication(s): Do not use in adult dairy cattle. Premature births and abortions have been reported in dairy cattle injected with this product during the third trimester of pregnancy.

Storage: Store between 2° and 30°C (36° and 86°F). Protect from freezing.

Caution(s): Federal law restricts this drug to use by or on the order of a licensed veterinarian.

Anaphylactoid reactions, some of which have been fatal, have been reported in cattle administered the VELENIUM™ product. Signs include excitement, sweating, trembling, ataxia, respiratory distress, and cardiac dysfunction.

Warning(s): Use only as directed in weanling calves and breeding beef cows. Discontinue use 30 days before the treated cattle are slaughtered for human consumption.

For veterinary use only.

Toxicology: Selenium is toxic if administered in excess. A fixed dose schedule is therefore important (read package insert for each selenium-tocopherol product carefully before using).

Discussion: Selenium-Tocopherol Deficiency (STD) syndrome produces a variety and complexity of symptoms often interfering with a proper diagnosis. Even in selenium deficient areas there are other disease conditions which produce similar clinical signs. It is imperative that all these conditions be carefully considered prior to treatment of STD syndrome. Serum selenium levels, elevated SGOT, and creatine levels may serve as aids in arriving at a diagnosis of STD, when associated with other indices.

Important: Use only the selenium-tocopherol product recommended for each species. Each formulation is designed for the species indicated to produce the maximum efficacy and safety.

Presentation: 100 mL sterile, multiple dose vial (NDC 0856-4602-01).

Compendium Code No.: 10032501 4600B

VENTIPULMIN® SYRUP ℞

Boehringer Ingelheim **Bronchodilator**

Clenbuterol HCl (72.5 mcg/mL)

NADA No.: 140-973

Active Ingredient(s): Each mL contains clenbuterol HCL 72.5 mcg.

Indications: VENTIPULMIN® Syrup (clenbuterol hydrochloride) is indicated for the management of horses affected with airway obstruction, such as occurs in chronic obstructive pulmonary disease (COPD).

Pharmacology: Clenbuterol (4-amino-alpha-[(tert-butylamino) methyl]-3, 5-dichlorobenzyl alcohol hydrochloride) is a beta-2-adrenergic agonist which provides bronchodilating properties as well as other effects, with minimum effect on the cardiovascular system. It is provided as a colorless, palatable syrup. VENTIPULMIN® Syrup (clenbuterol hydrochloride) is antagonized by beta-adrenergic blocking agents.

Dosage and Administration: Administer orally twice a day (b.i.d.)

Initial dose is 0.5 mL/100 lbs body weight (0.8 mcg/kg) twice daily.

Dosage Schedule:

Initial dosage: administer 0.5 mL/100 lbs (0.8 mcg/kg) for 3 days (6 treatments);

If no improvement, administer 1.0 mL/100 lbs (1.6 mcg/kg) for 3 days (6 treatments);

If no improvement, administer 1.5 mL/100 lbs (2.4 mcg/kg) for 3 days (6 treatments);

If no improvement, administer 2.0 mL/100 lbs (3.2 mcg/kg) for 3 days (6 treatments);

If no improvement, horse is non-responder to clenbuterol and treatment should be discontinued.

Recommended duration of treatment at effective dose is 30 days. At the end of this 30-day treatment period, drug should be withdrawn to determine recurrence of signs. If signs return, the 30-day treatment regimen may be repeated. If repeating treatment, the step-wise dosage schedule should be repeated.

Dosage Calculation Chart:

Lbs Body Weight	mL/treatment at 0.5 mL/100# (0.8 mcg/kg)	mL/treatment at 1.0 mL/100# (1.6 mcg/kg)	mL/treatment at 1.5 mL/100# (2.4 mcg/kg)	mL/treatment at 2.0 mL/100# (3.2 mcg/kg)
500	2.5	5.0	7.5	10.0
600	3.0	6.0	9.0	12.0
700	3.5	7.0	10.5	14.0
800	4.0	8.0	12.0	16.0
900	4.5	9.0	13.5	18.0
1000	5.0	10.0	15.0	20.0
1100	5.5	11.0	16.5	22.0
1200	6.0	12.0	18.0	24.0
1300	6.5	13.0	19.5	26.0
1400	7.0	14.0	21.0	28.0
1500	7.5	15.0	22.5	30.0
1600	8.0	16.0	24.0	32.0
1700	8.5	17.0	25.5	34.0
1800	9.0	18.0	27.0	36.0

Administer two treatments per day.

Directions for Administration: Remove safety cap and seal; replace with enclosed plastic dispensing cap. Remove cover from dispensing tip and connect syringe (without needle). Draw out appropriate volume of VENTIPULMIN® Syrup. Administer orally to the horse. Replace cover on dispensing tip to prevent leakage.

Contraindication(s): VENTIPULMIN® Syrup antagonizes the effects of prostaglandin F_2 alpha and oxytocin. VENTIPULMIN® Syrup should not be used in pregnant mares near term. Because tachycardia may occur, VENTIPULMIN® Syrup should not be used in horses suspected of having cardiovascular impairment.

Precaution(s): Store at controlled room temperature (15-30°C) (59-86°F). Avoid freezing.

The safety cap should be placed on the bottle when not in use.

Caution(s): Federal (U.S.A.) law restricts this drug to use by or on the order of a licensed veterinarian.

Warning(s): Federal (U.S.A.) law prohibits the extralabel use of this drug in food animals.

For use in horses not intended for food.

The effect on reproduction in breeding stallions and brood mares has not been determined. Treatment starting with dosages higher than the initial dose is not recommended.

Human Warnings: This product is not for human use or for use in animals intended for food. Keep out of the reach of children. In case of accidental ingestion, contact a physician immediately. Ingestion of VENTIPULMIN® Syrup may cause undesirable reactions. Clenbuterol, like other beta adrenergic agonists, can produce significant cardiovascular effects in some people as evidenced by elevated pulse rate, blood pressure changes and/or ECG changes.

Adverse Reactions: Mild sweating, muscle tremor, restlessness, urticaria and tachycardia may be observed in some horses during the first few days of treatment. May cause elevated creatine kinase (CK) serum levels. Ataxia was observed in 3 out of 239 horses (1.3%) in clinical studies.

Presentation: VENTIPULMIN® Syrup is available in 100 mL and 330 mL plastic bottles.

Compendium Code No.: 10281130

VETADINE

Centaur **Topical Antibacterial**

Povidone-Iodine Topical Solution USP-Antiseptic-Microbicide

Active Ingredient(s): 10% Polyvinyl Pyrrolidone-Iodine Complex (Titratable Iodine 1.0%).

Indications: Povidone-iodine topical solution U.S.P. Antiseptic-microbicide. Virtually non-irritating, film-forming, non-staining to skin, fur and natural fibers.

Directions for Use: For minor wounds and infections, apply directly to affected area full strength. May be covered with gauze or adhesive bandage.

Precaution(s): Avoid storage in excessive heat.

Caution(s): In case of deep or puncture wounds or serious burns, consult veterinarian. If redness, irritation, swelling or pain persists or increases, or if infection occurs, discontinue use and consult a veterinarian.

Avoid contact with eyes.

For animal use only.

Warning(s): Keep out of reach of children.

Presentation: 1 pint (16 fl oz) 473 mL and 1 gallon (128 fl oz) 3.785 L containers.

Manufactured by: Unavet, North Kansas City, MO 64116.

Compendium Code No.: 14880290

VETADINE SCRUB

Vedco **Surgical Scrub**

Active Ingredient(s):

Povidone-iodine (0.75% titratable) 7.5%

Indications: Surgical scrub.

Dosage and Administration: A germicidal cleanser for pre-operative and post-operative skin washing and a shampoo for bacterial and fungal skin infections in animals. Used routinely it also helps to prevent infections in cuts, scratches, abrasions, and burns. Nonstaining to skin, hair and natural fabrics. Avoid storing at excessive heat.

Caution(s): Keep out of the reach of children.

In case of deep or puncture wounds or serious burns, consult a veterinarian. If irritation or infection persists, discontinue use and consult a veterinarian.

Presentation: 1 gallon containers.

Compendium Code No.: 10942110

VETADINE SOLUTION

Vedco **Topical Antibacterial**

Active Ingredient(s):

Povidone-iodine (1.0% titratable) 10%

Indications: Kills gram-negative and gram-positive bacteria, fungi, viruses, protozoa, and yeasts. Film-forming, virtually nonirritating and nonstaining to skin, hair and natural fabrics.

Dosage and Administration: Apply full-strength as often as needed. Wet the area thoroughly to ensure complete coverage and penetration but avoid "pooling". May be covered with bandage if necessary.

Precaution(s): Avoid storing at excessive heat.

Caution(s): Keep out of the reach of children. For veterinary use only.

Avoid contact with the eyes. May be harmful if swallowed. If infection or irritation persists, discontinue use and consult a veterinarian.

Presentation: 1 gallon containers.

Compendium Code No.: 10942120

VETA-K_1® CAPSULES ℞

Bimeda **Vitamin K_1-Oral**

Active Ingredient(s): Each capsule contains 25 mg of phytonadione with excipients in an artificially colored soft gelatin shell.

Indications: VETA-K_1® Capsules are indicated in dogs and cats to counter hypoprothrombinemia induced by ingestion of coumarin-based compounds, common ingredients of commercial rodenticides, and other drug induced hypoprothrombinemia where it is definitely shown that the result is due to interference with vitamin K metabolism, e.g. salicylates.

Pharmacology: Actions: VETA-K_1® Capsules for oral administration possesses the same type and degree of activity as does naturally occurring vitamin K. The primary function of vitamin K is to stimulate the production via the liver of active prothrombin from a precursor protein. The mechanism by which vitamin K promotes the formation of prothrombin at the molecular level has not been established.

Dosage and Administration: Dogs and Cats:

Hypoprothrombinemia (with hemorrhage) — Administer orally at the rate of 2.5-5 mg/kg body weight (1 capsule for each 22 pounds of body weight for lower dosage or 1 capsule for each 11 pounds body weight for higher dosage) daily as conditions require up to 3 weeks.

Frequency and amount of oral administration should be guided by regular determination of prothrombin time.

The smallest effective dose should be sought to minimize the risk of adverse reaction.

Note: Regular determinations of prothrombin time response should be performed to guide in the initial and subsequent administration of VETA-K_1® oral capsules. The dosage should be adjusted accordingly.

Contraindication(s): Hypersensitivity to any component of this medication.

Precaution(s): Protect from light at all times.

Caution(s): Federal law restricts this drug to use by or on the order of a licensed veterinarian.

Temporary resistance to prothrombin-depressing anticoagulants may result, especially when larger doses of phytonadione are used.

For animal use only.

Not for human use.

Warning(s): It is recommended that VETA-K_1® oral capsules be used in follow-up therapy only after administration of a phytonadione injection and hospitalization is no longer required. An immediate coagulant effect should not be expected after administration of phytonadione when administered orally.

Phytonadione will not counteract the anticoagulant action of heparin.

Repeated large doses of vitamin K_1 are not warranted in hepatic disease if the response to the initial therapy is unsatisfactory. Failure to respond to vitamin K_1 may indicate that the condition being treated is inherently unresponsive to vitamin K_1.

Keep out of reach of children.

Presentation: VETA-K_1® oral capsules are available in bottles of 50 capsules each.

Manufactured by: Banner Gelatin Production Corp., Chatsworth, California 91311-0230

Compendium Code No.: 13990441 8VET001-800

VETA-K_1® INJECTION ℞

Bimeda **Vitamin K_1-Injection**

(Phytonadione) Aqueous Colloidal Solution-10 mg/mL

Active Ingredient(s): Each mL Contains: Phytonadione 10 mg; Polyoxyethylated fatty acid derivative 65 mg; Dextrose monohydrate 37.5 mg; Butylated hydroxyanisole 1 mg; Butylated hydroxytoluene 1 mg; Citric acid 8.4 mg; Sodium phosphate 17.2 mg with Benzyl Alcohol 0.9% w/v added as a preservative.

Indications: VETA-K_1® Injection is indicated in coagulation disorders which are due to faulty formation of factors II, VII, IX and X when caused by vitamin K deficiency or interference with vitamin K activity.

VETA-K_1® Injection is indicated in cattle, calves, horses, swine, sheep, goats, dogs, and cats to counter hypoprothrombinemia induced by ingestion of anticoagulant rodenticides.

VETA-K_1® Injection is also indicated to counter hypoprothrombinemia caused by consumption of bishydroxycoumarin found in spoiled and moldy sweet clover.

Pharmacology: Description: Phytonadione is a vitamin, which is a clear, yellow to amber, viscous, odorless or nearly odorless liquid. It is insoluble in water, soluble in chloroform and slightly soluble in ethanol. It has a molecular weight of 450.70.

Phytonadione is 2-methyl-3-phytyl-1,4-naphthoquinone. Its empirical formula is $C_{31}H_{46}O_2$.

VETA-K_1® Injection is a yellow, sterile, aqueous colloidal solution of Vitamin K_1, with a pH of 5.0 to 7.0, available for injection by intravenous, intramuscular, and subcutaneous routes.

Clinical Pharmacology: VETA-K_1® Injection aqueous colloidal solution of vitamin K_1 for parenteral injection, possesses the same type and degree of activity as does naturally-occurring vitamin K, which is necessary for the production via the liver of active prothrombin (factor II), proconvertin (factor VII), plasma thromboplastin component (factor IX), and Stuart factor (factor X). The prothrombin test is sensitive to the levels of three of these four factors -- II, VII and X. Vitamin K is an essential cofactor for a microsomal enzyme that catalyzes the post-translational carboxylation of multiple, specific, peptide-bound glutamic acid residues in inactive hepatic precursors of factors II, VII, IX and X. The resulting gamma-carboxyglutamic acid residues convert the precursors into active coagulation factors that are subsequently secreted by liver cells into the blood.

Phytonadione is readily absorbed following intramuscular administration. After absorption, phytonadione is initially concentrated in the liver, but the concentration declines rapidly. Very little vitamin K accumulates in tissues. Little is known about the metabolic fate of vitamin K. Almost no free unmetabolized vitamin K appears in bile or urine.

In normal animals, phytonadione is virtually devoid of pharmacodynamic activity. However, in animals deficient in vitamin K, the pharmacological action of vitamin K is related to its normal physiological function, that is, to promote the hepatic biosynthesis of vitamin K dependent clotting factors.

The action of the aqueous colloidal solution, when administered intravenously, is generally detectable within an hour or two and hemorrhage is usually controlled within 3 to 6 hours. A normal prothrombin level may often be obtained in 12 to 14 hours.

Dosage and Administration: Cattle, Calves, Horses, Swine, Sheep, and Goats:

Acute hypoprothrombinemia (with hemorrhage) and Non-acute hypoprothrombinemia: 0.5-2.5 mg/kg subcutaneously or intramuscularly.

Dogs and Cats:

Acute hypoprothrombinemia (with hemorrhage) and Non-acute hypoprothrombinemia: 0.25-5.0 mg/kg subcutaneously or intramuscularly. Use higher end of dose for second generation rodenticides.

Whenever possible, VETA-K_1® Injection should be given by the subcutaneous or intramuscular route. When intravenous administration is considered unavoidable, the drug should be diluted and injected very slowly, not exceeding 1 mg per minute.

Directions for Dilution: VETA-K_1® Injection may be diluted with 0.9% Sodium Chloride Injection, 5% Dextrose, Injection, or 5% Dextrose and Sodium Chloride Injection. Other diluents should not be used. When dilutions are indicated, administration should be started immediately after mixture with the diluent, and unused portions of the dilution should be discarded.

Whole blood or component therapy may be indicated if bleeding is excessive. This therapy, however, does not correct the underlying disorder and VETA-K_1® Injection should be given concurrently. In the event of shock or excessive blood loss, the use of whole blood or component therapy is indicated.

Drug Interactions: Temporary resistance to prothrombin-depressing anticoagulants may result, especially when larger doses of phytonadione are used. If relatively large doses have been employed, it may be necessary when reinstituting anticoagulant therapy to use somewhat larger doses of prothrombin-depressing anticoagulant, or to use one which acts on a different principle, such as heparin sodium.

Contraindication(s): Hypersensitivity to any component of this medication.

Precaution(s): Storage: Protect from light at all times. Store in a dark place at controlled room temperature between 15° and 30°C (59°-86°F).

Caution(s): Federal (U.S.A.) law restricts this drug to use by or on the order of a licensed veterinarian.

Laboratory tests: Prothrombin time should be checked regularly as clinical conditions indicate.

Parenteral drug products should be inspected visually for particulate matter and discoloration prior to administration, whenever solution and container permit.

*Intravenous Use: Severe reactions, including fatalities, have occurred during and immediately after intravenous injection of phytonadione, even when precautions have been taken to dilute the phytonadione and to avoid rapid infusion. Typically these severe reactions have resembled hypersensitivity or anaphylaxis, including shock and cardiac and/or respiratory arrest. Some animals have exhibited these severe reactions on receiving phytonadione for the first time. Therefore the intravenous route should be restricted to those situations where other routes are not feasible and the serious risk involved is considered justified.

An immediate coagulant effect should not be expected after administration of phytonadione. A minimum of 1 to 2 hours is required for measurable improvement in the prothrombin time. Whole blood or component therapy may be necessary if the bleeding is severe. Phytonadione will not counteract the anticoagulant action of heparin. When vitamin K_1 is used to correct excessive anticoagulant-induced hypoprothrombinemia, anticoagulant therapy still being indicated, the patient is again faced with the clotting hazards existing prior to starting the anticoagulant therapy. Phytonadione is not a clotting agent, but overzealous therapy with vitamin K_1 may restore conditions which originally permitted thromboembolic phenomena. Dosage should be kept as low as possible, and prothrombin time should be checked regularly as clinical conditions indicate.

Repeated large doses of vitamin K are not warranted in liver disease if the response to initial use of the vitamin is unsatisfactory. Failure to respond to vitamin K may indicate that the condition being treated is inherently unresponsive to vitamin K.

For animal use only.

Warning(s): Keep out of reach of children.

Adverse Reactions: Deaths have occurred following intravenous injection. (See Caution*). Pain, swelling and tenderness at the injection site may occur. Intramuscular injection may result in hematomas. The possibility of allergic sensitivity, including an anaphylactoid reaction, should be kept in mind.

Presentation: 100 mL multiple dose vial (NDC # 61133-6003-1).

VETA-K_1® is a Registered Trademark of Bimeda, Inc.

Manufactured by: Bimeda-MTC Animal Health Inc., Cambridge, ON, Canada N3C 2W4.

Compendium Code No.: 13990491 8VIT064A

VETAKET® INJECTION CIII

Lloyd **General Anesthetic**

Ketamine Hydrochloride Injection, USP

ANADA No.: 200-055

Active Ingredient(s): Each 10 mL vial contains the equivalent of 100 mg ketamine base per milliliter and contains not more than 0.1 mg/mL benzethonium chloride as a preservative.

Indications: VETAKET® (ketamine hydrochloride injection, USP) may be used in cats for restraint or as the sole anesthetic agent for diagnostic or minor, brief, surgical procedures that do not require skeletal muscle relaxation. It may be used in subhuman primates for restraint.

Pharmacology: Ketamine hydrochloride is a rapid-acting, nonnarcotic, nonbarbiturate agent for anesthetic use in cats and for restraint in subhuman primates. It is chemically designated *dl* 2-(o-chlorophenyl)-2-(methylamino) cyclohexanone hydrochloride and is supplied as a slightly acid (pH 3.0 to 5.0) solution for intramuscular injection.

Action: Ketamine hydrochloride is a rapid-acting agent whose pharmacological action is characterized by profound analgesia, normal pharyngeal-laryngeal reflexes, mild cardiac stimulation and respiratory depression. Skeletal muscle tone is variable and may be normal, enhanced or diminished. The anesthetic state produced does not fit into the conventional classification of stages of anesthesia, but instead ketamine hydrochloride produces a state of unconsciousness which has been termed "dissociative" anesthesia in that it appears to selectively interrupt association pathways to the brain before producing somesthetic sensory blockade.

In contrast to other anesthetics, protective reflexes, such as coughing and swallowing, are maintained under ketamine hydrochloride anesthesia. The degree of muscle tone is dependent upon level of dose; therefore, variations in body temperature may occur. At low dosage levels there may be an increase in muscle tone and a concomitant slight increase in body temperature. However, at high dosage levels there is some diminution in muscle tone and a resultant decrease in body temperature, to the point where supplemental heat may be advisable.

In cats, there is usually some transient cardiovascular stimulation, increased cardiac output with slight increase in mean systolic pressure with little or no change in total peripheral resistance. At higher doses respiratory rate is usually decreased.

The assurance of a patent airway is greatly enhanced by virtue of maintained pharyngeal-laryngeal reflexes. Although some salivation is occasionally noted, the persistence of the swallowing reflex aids in minimizing the hazards associated with ptyalism. Salivation may be effectively controlled with atropine sulfate in dosages of 0.04 mg/kg (0.02 mg/lb) in cats and 0.01 to 0.05 mg/kg (0.005 to 0.025 mg/lb) in subhuman primates.

Other reflexes, e.g., corneal, pedal, etc., are maintained during ketamine hydrochloride anesthesia, and should not be used as criteria for judging depth of anesthesia. The eyes normally remain open with the pupils dilated. It is suggested that a bland ophthalmic ointment be applied to the cornea if anesthesia is to be prolonged.

Following administration of recommended doses, cats become ataxic in about 5 minutes with anesthesia usually lasting from 30 to 45 minutes at higher doses. At the lower doses, complete recovery usually occurs in 4 to 5 hours but with higher doses recovery time is more prolonged and may be as long as 24 hours.

In studies involving 14 species of subhuman primates represented by at least 10 anesthetic episodes for each species, the median time to restraint ranged from 1.5 [*Aotus trivirgatus* (night monkey) and *Cebus capucinus* (white-throated capuchin)] to 5.3 minutes [*Macaca nemestrina* (pig-tailed macaque)]. The median duration of restraint ranged between 20 and 55 minutes in all but five of the species studied. Total time from injection to end of restraint ranged from 43 [*Saimiri sciureus* (squirrel monkey)] to 183 minutes [*Macaca nemestrina* (pig-tailed macaque)] after injection. Recovery is generally smooth and uneventful. The duration is dose related.

By single intramuscular injection, ketamine hydrochloride usually has a wide margin of safety in cats and subhuman primates. In cats, cases of prolonged recovery and death have been reported.

Dosage and Administration: Ketamine hydrochloride is well tolerated by cats and subhuman primates when administered by intramuscular injection.

Fasting prior to the induction of anesthesia or restraint with ketamine hydrochloride is not essential; however, when preparing for elective surgery, it is advisable to withhold food for at least six hours prior to the administration of ketamine hydrochloride.

Anesthesia may be of shorter duration in immature cats. Restraint in subhuman primate neonates (less than 24 hours of age) is difficult to achieve.

As with other anesthetic agents, the individual response to ketamine hydrochloride is somewhat varied depending upon the dose, general condition, and age of the subject so that dosage recommendations cannot be absolutely fixed.

Dosage:

Cats: A dose of 11 mg/kg (5 mg/lb) is recommended to produce restraint. Dosages from 22 to 33 mg/kg (10 to 15 mg/lb) produce anesthesia that is suitable for diagnostic or minor surgical procedures that do not require skeletal muscle relaxation.

Subhuman primates: The recommended restraint dosages of ketamine hydrochloride injection for the following species are: *Cercocebus torquatus* (white-collared mangabey), *Papio cynocephalus* (yellow baboon), *Pan troglodytus verus* (chimpanzee), *Papio anubis* (olive baboon), *Pongo pygmaeus* (orangutan), *Macaca nemestrina* (pig-tailed macaque) 5 to 7.5 mg/kg: *Presbytis entellus* (entellus langur) 3 to 5 mg/kg: *Gorilla gorilla gorilla* (gorilla) 7 to 10 mg/kg: *Aotus trivirgatus* (night monkey) 10 to 12 mg/kg: *Macaca mulatta* (rhesus monkey) 5 to 10 mg/kg: *Cebus capucinus* (white-throated capuchin) 13 to 15 mg/kg; and *Macaca fascicularis* (crab-eating macaque), *Macaca radiata* (bonnet macaque) and *Saimiri sciureus* (squirrel monkey) 12 to 15 mg/kg.

A single intramuscular injection produces restraint suitable for TB testing, radiography, physical examination, or blood collection.

Contraindication(s): Ketamine hydrochloride is contraindicated in cats and subhuman primates suffering from renal or hepatic insufficiency.

Ketamine hydrochloride is detoxified by the liver and excreted by the kidneys; therefore, any preexistent hepatic or renal pathology or impairment of function can be expected to result in prolonged anesthesia; related fatalities have been reported.

Caution(s): Federal law restricts this drug to use by or on the order of a licensed veterinarian.

In cats, doses in excess of 50 mg/kg during any single procedure should not be used. The maximum recommended dose in subhuman primates is 40 mg/kg.

To reduce the incidence of emergence reactions, animals should not be stimulated by sound or handling during the recovery period. However, this does not preclude the monitoring of vital signs.

Apnea, respiratory arrest, cardiac arrest, and death have occasionally been reported with ketamine used alone, and more frequently when used in conjunction with sedatives or other anesthetics. Close monitoring of patients is strongly advised during induction, maintenance, and recovery from anesthesia.

For intramuscular use in cats and subhuman primates only.

Adverse Reactions: Respiratory depression may occur following administration of high doses of ketamine hydrochloride. If at any time respiration becomes excessively depressed and the animal becomes cyanotic, resuscitative measures should be instituted promptly. Adequate pulmonary ventilation using either oxygen or room air is recommended as a resuscitative measure.

Adverse reactions reported have included emesis, salivation, vocalization, erratic recovery and prolonged recovery, spastic jerking movements, convulsions, muscular tremors, hypertonicity, opisthotonos, dyspnea, and cardiac arrest. In the cat, myoclonic jerking and/or mild tonic convulsions can be controlled by ultrashort-acting barbiturates which should be given to effect. The barbiturates should be administered intravenously at a dose level of one-sixth to one-fourth the usual dose for the product being used. Acepromazine may also be used. However, recent information indicates that some phenothiazine derivatives may potentiate the toxic effects of organic phosphate compounds such as found in flea collars and certain anthelmintics. A study has indicated that ketamine hydrochloride alone does not potentiate the toxic effects of organic phosphate compounds.

Trial Data: Clinical Studies: Ketamine hydrochloride has been clinically studied in subhuman primates in addition to those species listed under Dosage and Administration. Dosages for restraint in these additional species, based on limited clinical data, are: *Cercopithecus aethiops* (grivet), *Papio papio* (guinea baboon) 10 to 12 mg/kg; *Erythrocebus patas patas* (patas monkey) 3 to 5 mg/kg; *Hylobates lar* (white-handed gibbon) 5 to 10 mg/kg; *Lemur catta* (ringtailed lemur) 7.5 to 10 mg/kg; *Macaca fuscata* (Japanese macaque) 5 mg/kg; *Macaca speciosa* (stumptailed macaque) and *Miopithecus talapoin* (mangrove monkey) 5 to 7.5 mg/kg; and *Symphalangus syndactylus* (siamangs) 5 to 7 mg/kg.

Presentation: 10 mL vial (NDC 061311-487-10).

Manufactured by: Taylor Pharmaceuticals, Decatur, IL 62525.

Compendium Code No.: 11350030 0799

VETA-LAC® CANINE

Vet-A-Mix **Milk Replacer**

Powdered milk replacer for puppies and food supplement for dogs

Guaranteed Analysis:

Crude Protein, minimum 25.0%
Crude Fat, minimum 35.0%
Crude Fiber, maximum 1.0%
Moisture, maximum 5.0%
Ash, maximum 8.0%

Per 400 grams: (All values are minimum quantities unless otherwise stated.)

Protein: DL-methionine 1000 mg; Minerals: Calcium, minimum 0.7%; Calcium, maximum 0.9%; Phosphorus 0.6%; Potassium 1,650 mg, 0.4%; Sodium 2,200 mg, 0.55%; Chloride 3,200 mg, 0.8%, Magnesium 650 mg, 0.16%; Iron 48 mg; Copper 6 mg; Manganese 3 mg; Zinc 2 mg; Iodine 2 mg; Vitamins and others: Vitamin A 8,800 IU; Vitamin D 1,300 IU; Vitamin E 18 IU; Thiamine 3 mg; Riboflavin 8 mg; Pantothenic acid 8 mg; Niacin 40 mg; Pyridoxine 3 mg; Folic acid 1 mg; Vitamin B_{12} 88 mcg; Choline 440 mg; *Ascorbic acid 1 mg, *Inositol 4 mg; *Cobalt 1 mg.

*Not recognized as essential nutrients by AAFCO Dog Nutrient Profiles.

Ingredients: Dried milk protein, animal fat, magnesium sulfate, sodium citrate, sodium phosphate, dicalcium phosphate, DL-methionine, choline bitartrate, lecithin, vitamin B_{12} supplement, vegetable oil, polyoxyethylene sorbitan, polyethylene glycol monoleate, ferrous sulfate, niacin, vitamin E supplement, copper sulfate, vitamin A supplement, pantothenic acid, manganese sulfate, riboflavin, saccharin sodium, folic acid supplement, inositol, vitamin D_3 supplement, pyridoxine hydrochloride, thiamine mononitrate, cobalt sulfate, zinc oxide, ethylenediamine dihydriodide, ascorbic acid, artificial flavorings and ethoxyquin, a preservative.

Indications: A powdered milk replacer for puppies and food supplement for dogs.

Directions: Directions for Mixing VETA-LAC® Canine: Add three level measures of VETA-LAC® Canine powder to 8 fluid ounces (½ pint or 1 cup) of very warm water and shake or stir vigorously. The mixture may be stored in a covered container under refrigeration for several days. Emulsification of fats is improved by refrigeration and only brief mixing is needed just before feeding. If a smaller amount of reconstituted liquid is required, mix one measure of medium to firmly packed VETA-LAC® Canine powder with three measures of very warm water as described above.

This product is intended for intermittent or supplemental feeding only.

Feeding Orphan Puppies: A veterinarian should be consulted for advice about the care and feeding of puppies. Feed young puppies whenever they are hungry, but avoid overfeeding. Feed from a dropper or small nipple bottle. Experience will soon tell you how much and how often to feed. VETA-LAC® Canine may be fed either at body temperature or refrigerator temperature, but avoid sudden changes or wide variations in temperature.

Strong newborn puppies should normally be fed six times during each 24 hours (weak or very small animals should be fed every two hours) for the first few days. The number of feedings may be reduced to four times every 24 hours during the second week.

By the third or fourth week, feeding three times per day is usually sufficient. Puppies should be eating from a bowl and a small amount of dry meal can be added to the liquid to make a gruel-like mixture.

Gradually decrease the amount of liquid being fed and increase the amount of regular ration. This change from all liquid feeding to the regular ration should be made in not less than two (2) to three (3) weeks. For the best results, continue to feed small or supplemental amounts of reconstituted liquid after weaning.

Reconstituted VETA-LAC® Canine Feeding Guide:

Weight of Puppy	Measures reconstituted liquid to feed daily*
4 oz.	1
8 oz.	2
1 lb	3
2 lb	6
3 lb	10

*1 measure = 1 fluid ounce = approximately 2 tablespoonfuls.

Feeding Pregnant and Lactating Bitches: Mix VETA-LAC® Canine powder into the daily ration at the rate of one (1) level measure (approximately 15 g) per 5 lb (2.2 kg) body weight until two weeks after giving birth.

Presentation: 400 g bottles and 5 kg (11 lb) pails.

Compendium Code No.: 10500341 1200

VETA-LAC® FELINE

Vet-A-Mix **Milk Replacer**

Powdered milk replacer for kittens and food supplement for cats

Guaranteed Analysis:

Crude Protein, minimum 35.0%
Crude Fat, minimum 20.0%
Crude Fiber, maximum 1.0%
Moisture, maximum 5.0%
Ash, maximum 8.0%

Per 200 grams: Vitamin A 4,400 IU; Vitamin D 650 IU; Vitamin E 9 IU; Vitamin B_{12} 44 mcg; Ascorbic acid 500 mcg; Thiamine 1.5 mg; Riboflavin 4 mg; Niacin 20 mg; Folic acid 0.5 mg; Pyridoxine 1.5 mg; Pentothenic acid 4 mg; Choline 220 mg; Taurine 220 mg; DL-Methionine 500 mg; Inositol 2 mg; Calcium, minimum 1.0%; Calcium, maximum 1.2%; Phosphorus, minimum 0.8%; Magnesium 350 mg; Iron 24 mg; Copper 3 mg; Cobalt 0.5 mg; Manganese 1.5 mg; Zinc 1 mg; Iodine 1 mg; Potassium 1,430 mg; Sodium 980 mg; Chloride 2,850 mg.

Ingredients: Milk protein (from dried skim milk and/or milk protein concentrates), edible animal fats, magnesium sulfate, sodium citrate, sodium phosphate, dicalcium phosphate, DL-methionine, choline bitartrate, lecithin, vitamin B_{12} supplement, taurine, vegetable oil, polyoxyethylene sorbitan, polyethylene glycol monoleate, ferrous sulfate, niacin, vitamin E supplement, copper sulfate, vitamin A supplement, pantothenic acid, manganese sulfate, riboflavin, saccharin sodium, folic acid supplement, inositol, vitamin D_3 supplement, pyridoxine hydrochloride, thiamine mononitrate, cobalt sulfate, zinc oxide, ethylenediamine dihydriodide, ascorbic acid, artificial flavorings and ethoxyquin, a preservative.

Indications: A powdered milk replacer for kittens and food supplement for cats.

Directions: Directions for Mixing VETA-LAC® Feline: Add three level measures of VETA-LAC® Feline powder to 4 fluid ounces (½ cup) of very warm water and shake or stir vigorously. This mixture may be stored in a covered container under refrigeration for several days. Emulsification of fats is improved by refrigeration and only brief mixing is needed just before feeding. If a smaller amount of reconstituted liquid is required, mix one measure of medium to firmly packed VETA-LAC® Feline powder with three measures of very warm water as described above.

Feeding VETA-LAC® Feline to Orphan Kittens: A veterinarian should be consulted for advice about the care and feeding of kittens. Feed young kittens whenever they are hungry but avoid overfeeding. Feed from a dropper or small nipple bottle. Experience will soon tell you how much and how often to feed. VETA-LAC® Feline may be fed either at body temperature or refrigerator temperature, but avoid sudden changes or wide variations in temperature.

Strong newborn kittens should normally be fed six times during each 24 hours (weak or very small animals should be fed every two hours) for the first few days. The number of feedings may be reduced to four times every 24 hours during the second week.

By the third or fourth week, feeding three times per day is usually sufficient. Kittens should be eating from a bowl and a small amount of dry meal can be added to the liquid to make a gruel-like mixture.

Gradually decrease the amount of liquid being fed and increase the regular amount of ration. This change from all liquid feeding to the regular ration should be made in not less than two to three weeks. For the best results, continue to feed small or supplemental amounts of reconstituted liquid after weaning.

Reconstituted VETA-LAC® Feline Feeding Guide:

Weight of Kitten	Measures reconstituted liquid to feed daily*
2 oz	1
4 oz	2
8 oz	4
1 lb	6
2 lb	12

*1 measure = approximately 1 tablespoonful.

Feeding VETA-LAC® Feline to Pregnant and Lactating Queens: Mix VETA-LAC® Feline powder into the daily ration at the rate of 2 level measures (approximately 15 g) per 5 lb (2.2 kg) body weight until two weeks after giving birth.

Presentation: 200 g bottles.

Compendium Code No.: 10500351 0998

VETALAR® CIII

Fort Dodge **General Anesthetic**

Ketamine Hydrochloride Injection, USP

NADA No.: 045-290

Active Ingredient(s): VETALAR® (ketamine hydrochloride) is supplied as a slightly acid (pH 3.5 to 5.5) solution for intramuscular injection in a concentration containing the equivalent of 100 mg ketamine base per milliliter and contains not more than 0.1 mg/mL of benzethonium chloride as a preservative.

Indications: VETALAR® may be used in cats for restraint or as the sole anesthetic agent for diagnostic or minor, brief, surgical procedures that do not require skeletal muscle relaxation. It may be used in subhuman primates for restraint.

Pharmacology:

Description: VETALAR® (ketamine hydrochloride injection, USP) is a rapid-acting, nonnarcotic, nonbarbiturate agent for anesthetic use in cats and for restraint in subhuman primates. It is chemically designated *dl*-2-(o-chlorophenyl)-2-(methylamino) cyclohexanone hydrochloride.

Action: VETALAR® is a rapid-acting agent whose pharmacological action is characterized by profound analgesia, normal pharyngeal-laryngeal reflexes, mild cardiac stimulation and respiratory depression. Skeletal muscle tone is variable and may be normal, enhanced or diminished. The anesthetic state produced does not fit into the conventional classification of stages of anesthesia, but instead VETALAR® produces a state of unconsciousness which has been termed "dissociative" anesthesia in that it appears to selectively interrupt association pathways to the brain before producing somesthetic sensory blockade.

In contrast to other anesthetics, protective reflexes, such as coughing and swallowing are maintained under VETALAR® anesthesia. The degree of muscle tone is dependent upon level of dose; therefore, variations in body temperature may occur. At low dosage levels there may be an increase in muscle tone and a concomitant slight increase in body temperature. However, at high dosage levels there is some diminution in muscle tone and a resultant decrease in body temperature, to the point where supplemental heat may be advisable.

In cats, there is usually some transient cardiovascular stimulation, increased cardiac output with slight increase in mean systolic pressure with little or no change in total peripheral resistance. At higher doses the respiratory rate is usually decreased.

The assurance of a patent airway is greatly enhanced by virtue of maintained pharyngeal-laryngeal reflexes. Although some salivation is occasionally noted, the persistence of the swallowing reflex aids in minimizing the hazards associated with ptyalism. Salivation may be effectively controlled with atropine sulfate in dosages of 0.04 mg/kg (0.02 mg/lb) in cats and 0.01 to 0.05 mg/kg (0.005 to 0.025 mg/lb) in subhuman primates.

Other reflexes, e.g., corneal, pedal, etc., are maintained during VETALAR® (ketamine hydrochloride injection, USP) anesthesia, and should not be used as criteria for judging depth of anesthesia. The eyes normally remain open with the pupils dilated. It is suggested that a bland ophthalmic ointment be applied to the cornea if anesthesia is to be prolonged.

Following administration of recommended doses, cats become ataxic in about 5 minutes with anesthesia usually lasting from 30 to 45 minutes at higher doses. At the lower doses, complete recovery usually occurs in 4 to 5 hours but with higher doses recovery time is more prolonged and may be as long as 24 hours.

In studies involving 14 species of subhuman primates represented by at least 10 anesthetic episodes for each species, the median time to restraint ranged from 1.5 [*Aotus trivirgatus* (night monkey) and *Cebus capucinus* (white-throated capuchin)] to 5.3 minutes [*Macaca nemestrina* (pig-tailed macaque)]. The median duration of restraint ranged between 20 and 55 minutes in all but five of the species studied. Total time from injection to end of restraint ranged from 43 [*Saimiri sciureus* (squirrel monkey)] to 183 minutes [*Macaca nemestrina* (pig-tailed macaque)] after injection. Recovery is generally smooth and uneventful. The duration is dose related.

By single intramuscular injection, VETALAR® usually has a wide margin of safety in cats and subhuman primates. In cats, cases of prolonged recovery and death have been reported.

Dosage and Administration: VETALAR® is well tolerated by cats and subhuman primates when administered by intramuscular injection.

Fasting prior to induction of anesthesia or restraint with VETALAR® is not essential; however, when preparing for elective surgery, it is advisable to withhold food for at least six hours prior to administration of VETALAR®.

Anesthesia may be of shorter duration in immature cats. Restraint in subhuman primate neonates (less than 24 hours of age) is difficult to achieve.

As with other anesthetic agents, the individual response to VETALAR® is somewhat varied depending upon the dose, general condition and age of the subject so that dosage recommendations cannot be absolutely fixed.

Dosage:

Cats: A dose of 11 mg/kg (5 mg/lb) is recommended to produce restraint. Dosages from 22 to 33 mg/kg (10 to 15 mg/lb) produce anesthesia that is suitable for diagnostic or minor surgical procedures that do not require skeletal muscle relaxation.

Subhuman primates: The recommended restraint dosages of VETALAR® (ketamine hydrochloride injection, USP) for the following species are: *Cercocebus torquatus* (white-collared mangabey), *Papio cynocephalus* (yellow baboon), *Pan troglodytes verus* (chimpanzee), *Papio anubis* (olive baboon), *Pongo pygmaeus* (orangutan), *Macaca nemestrina* (pig-tailed macaque) 5 to 7.5 mg/kg; *Presbytis entellus* (entellus langur) 3 to 5 mg/kg; *Gorilla gorilla gorilla* (gorilla) 7 to 10 mg/kg; *Aotus trivirgatus* (night monkey) 10 to 12 mg/kg; *Macaca mulatta* (rhesus monkey) 5 to 10 mg/kg; *Cebus capucinus* (white-throated capuchin) 13 to 15 mg/kg; and *Macaca fascicularis* (crab-eating macaque), *Macaca radiata* (bonnet macaque) and *Saimiri sciureus* (squirrel monkey) 12 to 15 mg/kg.

A single intramuscular injection produces restraint suitable for TB testing; radiography, physical examination or blood collection.

Contraindication(s): VETALAR® is contraindicated in cats and subhuman primates suffering from renal or hepatic insufficiency.

VETALAR® is detoxified by the liver and excreted by the kidneys; therefore, any preexistent hepatic or renal pathology or impairment of function can be expected to result in prolonged anesthesia; related fatalities have been reported.

Caution(s): Federal law restricts this drug to use by or on the order of a licensed veterinarian.

In cats, doses in excess of 50 mg/kg during any single procedure should not be used. The maximum recommended dose in subhuman primates is 40 mg/kg.

To reduce the incidence of emergence reactions, animals should not be stimulated by sound or handling during the recovery period. However, this does not preclude the monitoring of vital signs.

Apnea, respiratory arrest, cardiac arrest and death have occasionally been reported with ketamine used alone, and more frequently when used in conjunction with sedatives or other anesthetics. Close monitoring of patients is strongly advised during induction, maintenance and recovery from anesthesia.

Warning(s): For intramuscular use in cats and subhuman primates only.

Adverse Reactions: Respiratory depression may occur following administration of high doses of VETALAR® (ketamine hydrochloride injection, USP). If at any time respiration becomes excessively depressed and the animal becomes cyanotic, resuscitative measures should be instituted promptly. Adequate pulmonary ventilation using either oxygen or room air is recommended as a resuscitative measure.

Adverse reactions reported have included emesis, salivation, vocalization, erratic recovery and prolonged recovery, spastic jerking movements, convulsions, muscular tremors, hypertonicity, opisthotonos, dyspnea and cardiac arrest. In the cat, myoclonic jerking and/or mild tonic convulsions can be controlled by ultrashort-acting barbiturates which should be given to effect. The barbiturates should be administered intravenously at a dose level of one-sixth to one-fourth the usual dose for the product being used. Acepromazine may also be used. However, recent information indicates that some phenothiazine derivatives may potentiate the toxic effects of organic phosphate compounds such as found in flea collars and certain anthelmintics. A study has indicated that ketamine hydrochloride alone does not potentiate the toxic effects of organic phosphate compounds.

Trial Data:

Clinical studies: VETALAR® has been clinically studied in subhuman primates in addition to those species listed under Dosage and Administration. Dosages for restraint in these additional species, based on limited clinical data, are: *Cercopithecus aethiops* (grivet), *Papio papio* (guinea baboon) 10 to 12 mg/kg; *Erythrocebus patas patas* (patas monkey) 3 to 5 mg/kg; *Hylobates lar* (white-handed gibbon) 5 to 10 mg/kg; *Lemur catta* (ringtailed lemur) 7.5 to 10 mg/kg; *Macaca fuscata* (Japanese macaque) 5 mg/kg; *Macaca speciosa* (stumptailed macaque) and *Miopithecus talapoin* (mangrove monkey) 5 to 7.5 mg/kg; and *Symphalangus syndactylus* (siamangs) 5 to 7 mg/kg.

Presentation: Each 10 mL vial contains 100 mg/mL (NDC 0856-2012-01).

Compendium Code No.: 10032510 4550G

VETALOG® PARENTERAL ℞

Fort Dodge **Corticosteroid Injection**

Sterile Triamcinolone Acetonide Suspension USP

NADA No.: 012-198

Active Ingredient(s): Description: VETALOG® Parenteral (sterile triamcinolone acetonide suspension USP) is available for veterinary use as a sterile suspension in vials providing 2 mg or 6 mg triamcinolone acetonide per mL with 0.9% (w/v) benzyl alcohol as a preservative, sodium chloride for isotonicity, 0.75% carboxymethylcellulose sodium and 0.04% polysorbate 80. Sodium hydroxide or hydrochloric acid may have been added to adjust the pH. At the time of manufacture, the air in the container is replaced by nitrogen.

Indications: VETALOG® Parenteral is indicated for the treatment of inflammation and related disorders in dogs, cats and horses. It is also indicated for use in dogs and cats for the management and treatment of acute arthritis, allergic and dermatologic disorders.

Rationale for Use:

Inflammation and Related Disorders:

Dogs, Cats and Horses: Injection of VETALOG® Parenteral provides rapid relief from pain and reduces inflammation and swelling.

Depending on the nature of the condition, VETALOG® Parenteral may be injected intramuscularly, intra-articularly or intrasynovially. The usual pattern of response is improvement of motion and decrease of pain within 24 hours, followed by diminution of swelling.

The extent of return to normal is limited by the degree of irreversible pathologic change present. Triamcinolone acetonide will not reverse permanent pathologic changes.

Allergic and Dermatologic Disorders:

Dogs and Cats: Intramuscular or subcutaneous administration of VETALOG® Parenteral (sterile triamcinolone acetonide suspension USP) has been found to provide prompt and prolonged relief in the management of allergic symptoms such as conjunctivitis or reactions to insect bites and in various dermatoses. Inflammation, edema and pruritus are suppressed and discomfort is eased, usually within 24 hours. Since scratching is reduced or eliminated, lesions are permitted to heal more rapidly. In many cases a single injection is sufficient to terminate symptomatology. If necessary, repeat treatments can be administered.

Intralesional administration of VETALOG® Parenteral is effective for treatment of dermatological disorders such as moist eczema, frictional acanthosis, and other dermatitides in dogs and cats. Inflammation and pruritus are often abated within one to three days. A single intralesional injection is often sufficient to effect remission or elimination of the lesion within a period of one to two weeks.

Pharmacology: Actions: Triamcinolone acetonide is a highly potent synthetic glucocorticoid which is primarily effective because of its anti-inflammatory activity. The apparent analgesic effect is a result of the anti-inflammatory properties of the drug.

Dosage and Administration:

Intramuscular or Subcutaneous:

Dogs and Cats: The dose is a single injection of 0.05 mg to 0.1 mg triamcinolone acetonide per pound of body weight in inflammatory or allergic disorders and 0.1 mg per pound of body weight in dermatologic disorders. Remission of symptoms, if not permanent, usually lasts 7 to 15 days. After this time, if symptoms recur, the dose may be repeated or oral corticosteroid therapy may be instituted.

Horses: The dose is 0.01 mg to 0.02 mg triamcinolone acetonide per pound of body weight as a single injection; the usual range is 12 mg to 20 mg.

Intralesional:

Dogs and Cats: The usual intralesional dosage is 1.2 mg to 1.8 mg triamcinolone acetonide. Injections should be circumscribed around the lesion in various sites to insure adequate distribution of the dose. Injections should be spaced 0.5 cm to 2.5 cm apart, depending on the size of the lesion. The spacing of the dose also reduces pain and/or pressure necrosis.

The dose injected at any one site should not exceed 0.6 mg to minimize local tissue intolerance and atrophy, and should be made well into the cutis to prevent subsequent rupture of the epidermis. When treating dogs and cats with multiple lesions, do not exceed a total dose of 6 mg. Repeat courses of treatment may be administered if necessary.

It is preferable to employ a tuberculin syringe with a small bore needle (23-25 gauge) for accuracy of dose measurement and ease of administration.

Intra-articular and Intrasynovial:

Dogs, Cats and Horses: The dose for intra-articular or intrasynovial administration is dependent on the size of the joint to be treated and on the severity of symptoms. A single injection of 1 mg to 3 mg triamcinolone acetonide for cats and dogs and 6 mg to 18 mg for horses is recommended. After three or four days, injections may be repeated, depending on the severity of symptoms and the clinical response. If initial results are inadequate or too transient, dosage may be increased but the recommended dose should not be exceeded.

Routine aseptic preparation of the area should be made prior to all intra-articular injections. A thorough understanding of the pertinent anatomic relationships is essential. The inadvertent administration of the corticosteroid into the soft tissues surrounding a joint is not harmful, but is the most common cause of failure to achieve the desired local results.

Following intra-articular administration, pain and other local symptoms may continue for a short time before effective relief is obtained, but an increase in joint discomfort is rare. A marked increase in pain accompanied by local swelling, further restriction of joint motion, fever and malaise are suggestive of a septic arthritis. If these complications should occur and the diagnosis of sepsis is confirmed, antimicrobial therapy should be instituted immediately and continued until all evidence of infection has disappeared.

Contraindication(s): Do not use in viral infections. Except for emergency therapy, do not use in animals with tuberculosis, chronic nephritis, or cushingoid syndrome. Existence of congestive heart failure, diabetes, and osteoporosis are relative contraindications.

Precaution(s): Storage: Store at room temperature; avoid freezing.

Caution(s): Federal law restricts this drug to use by or on the order of a licensed veterinarian.

VETALOG® Parenteral (sterile triamcinolone acetonide suspension USP) should not be used to alleviate pain or reduce inflammation arising from infectious states unless concomitant antimicrobial therapy is given.

Because of the anti-inflammatory action of corticosteroids, signs of infection may be hidden and it may be necessary to stop treatment until diagnosis is made.

Overdosage of some glucocorticoids may result in sodium retention, fluid retention, potassium loss and weight gains.

Corticosteroids have been used in the treatment of laminitis; VETALOG® Parenteral (sterile triamcinolone acetonide suspension USP) is not recommended for that use. Cases of laminitis have been reported following the administration of VETALOG® Parenteral (sterile triamcinolone acetonide suspension USP); the mechanism of that response has not been fully elucidated. Care is necessary when using any corticosteroid in the equine species.

Use of corticosteroids, depending on dose, duration and specific steroid, may result in inhibition of endogenous steroid production following drug withdrawal. In patients presently receiving or recently withdrawn from systemic corticosteroid treatments, therapy with a rapidly acting corticosteroid should be considered in unusually stressful situations.

Usage in Pregnancy: The safety of most corticosteroid drugs for use during all stages of pregnancy has not been adequately established. However, clinical and experimental data have demonstrated that corticosteroids administered orally or by injection to animals may induce the first stage of parturition if used during the last trimester of pregnancy and may precipitate premature parturition followed by dystocia, fetal death, retained placenta and metritis. Additionally, corticosteroids administered to dogs, rabbits and rodents during pregnancy have resulted in cleft palate in offspring. Corticosteroids administered to dogs during pregnancy have also resulted in other congenital anomalies including deformed forelegs, phocomelia and anasarca. Therefore, before use of corticosteroids in pregnant animals, the possible benefits to the pregnant animal should be weighed against potential hazards to its developing embryo or fetus.

Warning(s): Not for use in horses intended for food.

Adverse Reactions: As with any corticosteroid, polydipsia or polyuria may occur with high dosage or frequent administration of triamcinolone acetonide. The likelihood of their occurrence may be minimized by giving as brief a course of corticosteroid therapy as possible, and by waiting for the reappearance of symptoms before repeating therapy. If polydipsia or polyuria should occur, therapy should be discontinued until these unwanted effects have disappeared; therapy should then be resumed at a lower dosage level.

Other adverse reactions that have occurred with the use of corticosteroids are weight loss, anorexia and diarrhea (occasionally bloody). Anaphylactic reactions have occasionally been seen following administration.

Intra-articular injection in leg injuries of the horse may produce osseous metaplasia.

Side effects such as serum alkaline phosphatase (SAP) and serum glutamic pyruvic transaminase (SGPT) enzyme elevations have occurred following use of synthetic corticosteroids in dogs.

Cushing's Syndrome in dogs has been reported in association with prolonged or repeated steroid therapy.

Presentation: VETALOG® Parenteral (sterile triamcinolone acetonide suspension USP) is supplied for veterinary use in two concentrations and various vial sizes:

NDC 53501-973-50 — 2 mg/mL — 100 mL vial (For Horses Only)*
NDC 53501-973-30 — 2 mg/mL — 25 mL vial
NDC 53501-976-31 — 6 mg/mL — 25 mL vial (For Horses Only)*
NDC 53501-976-20 — 6 mg/mL — 5 mL vial
NDC 53501-976-30 — 6 mg/mL — 3 mL vial (For Horses Only)

*To limit the number of entries through the stopper, these two vials are for use in horses only.

Manufactured by: Bristol Myers Squibb S.p.A., Contrada Fontana del Ceraso, 03012 Anagni (Fr), Italy.

Compendium Code No.: 10032532 12800B

VETALYTE PLUS I.V. SOLUTION ℞

RXV **Electrolyte Injection**

Active Ingredient(s): Each 100 mL contains:

Dextrose monohydrate	5 g
Sodium chloride	536 mg
Sodium gluconate	510 mg
Sodium acetate	271 mg
Potassium chloride	37 mg
Magnesium chloride • $6H_2O$	42 mg
Milliequivalents per 1000 mL:	
Sodium	148 mEq
Potassium	5 mEq
Magnesium	4 mEq
Total cations	157 mEq
Chloride	101 mEq
Gluconate	23 mEq
Acetate	33 mEq
Total anions	157 mEq

This product contains no preservative.

Indications: As a fluid and electrolyte replenisher in the treatment of dehydration and electrolyte depletion in cattle.

Dosage and Administration: Administer intravenously.

Cattle .... 2 to 5 mL/lb of body weight

One to three times daily or as needed.

Precaution(s): Store at controlled room temperature between 15°-30°C (59°-86°F).

Entire contents should be used upon entering. Discard any unused portion.

Caution(s): Federal law restricts this drug to use by or on the order of a licensed veterinarian.

Solution should be warmed to room temperature and administered slowly.

Warning(s): For animal use only.

Keep out of reach of children.

Presentation: 1000 mL vials.

Compendium Code No.: 10910240

VETASYL™ FIBER TABLETS FOR CATS

Virbac **Laxative**

Active Ingredient(s): VETASYL™ contains psyllium husks, barley malt extract powder, acacia and thiamine HCl (vitamin B_1).

Guaranteed analysis: 5% minimum non-crude fiber.

Indications: A natural dietary fiber supplement for cats.

Dosage and Administration: For cats weighing over 7 lbs., sprinkle one (1) capsule per day on the food. For cats and kittens under 7 lbs., use one-half (½) capsule (250 mg) per day. A veterinarian may give specific directions. Follow professional advice closely.

Note: For the best results, cats should have an ample supply of water available.

Precaution(s): Store at room temperature.

Caution(s): Keep out of the reach of children.

Presentation: Bottles of 60-500 mg, 60-1000 mg and 180-1000 mg tablets.

Compendium Code No.: 10230590

VET BIOSIST™

Cook **Topical Wound Dressing**

Tissue Repair Sheet

Composition: VET BIOSIST™ tissue repair sheets are composed of a biocompatible matrix. The single layered lyophilized sheets are not synthetic, but are a naturally-occurring derivative of the submucosal layer of the porcine small intestine which has been disinfected to remove bacterial and viral components. This "natural" material contains collagen (Types I, III and V), fibronectin, decorin, hyaluronic acid, chondroitin sulphate A, heparan sulphate, and growth factors (TGFβ, FGF-2, and VEGF).

Indications: VET BIOSIST™ is for use as a surgical patch for soft tissue repair or reinforcement. It promotes wound healing and tissue remodeling by providing a biocompatible, absorbable scaffold for tissue ingrowth. It is suitable for dermal tissue repair applications where the skin cannot be sutured together or when subdermal tissues are damaged. Other potential applications of this surgical patch include repairs of internal organs, cleft palate, periodontal tissue, and corneal ulcers. VET BIOSIST™ has also been used in surgery as an anti-adhesion barrier, a suture reinforcement sheet, and a hemostatic plug.

Dosage and Administration: Suggested Instructions for Use: Always handle VET BIOSIST™ using sterile technique. Prepare wound area using standard methods to insure wound is free of debris and necrotic tissue. Debride the wound to insure the wound edges contain viable tissue. When necessary, it is recommended that VET BIOSIST™ is not applied until excessive exudate, bleeding, acute swelling and infection are controlled.

To apply, cut the dry sheet with sterile scissors into a patch slightly larger than the outline of the wound area. Rehydrate the patch by placing it in a bowl of sterile saline or other isotonic solution for at least one (1) minute before placing the patch over the wound surface. In dermal applications, place the edge of the patch under the edge of the intact tissue to encourage tissue overgrowth during wound healing. Secure the patch to the wound edges using sutures or small surgical clips.

In large area wounds, multiple sheets may need to be used and several evenly spaced sutures may be placed through the patch and into the wound bed to enhance overall contact between the tissue and the patch. If excess exudate collects under the patch, small openings can be cut in the patch to allow the exudate to drain.

Use an appropriate dressing to maintain a moist wound environment. The optimum dressing is determined by wound location, size, depth, and surgeon preference. For external wounds, it is recommended that the VET BIOSIST™ patch be covered with an aqueous gel and a non-adhesive dressing. Cover this dressing with a dry exterior dressing that will protect the wound and maintain internal moisture. Leave the moist interior dressing undisturbed for at least three (3) days or until the VET BIOSIST™ patch begins to be absorbed into the underlying tissue. The VET BIOSIST™ patch should not be removed.

Caution(s): VET BIOSIST™ is not for use in humans or *in vitro* diagnostics.

Initial application of this product may produce mild, localized inflammation. If this condition worsens or persists beyond five (5) days. the product should be removed. If noticeable wound infection occurs, appropriate oral antibiotic therapy should be administered. If infection persists, the product should be removed and the wound should be surgically debrided. When used in high pressure applications, sheets may need to be placed in multiple layers to provide adequate strength. This product is derived from a porcine source. Animals with known sensitivity to porcine material should not be exposed to this product.

Storage: VET BIOSIST™ sheets are stable for 12 months when kept dry and stored in the original, unopened packaging at room temperature.

Sterility: Supplied sterile in easy open packages, for one-time use. Re-sterilization of this product will result in product degradation.

Presentation: Available:

Multilaminate Sheet: Multilaminate sheets are packaged in double peel-pouches. The surface characteristics of both sides of the multilaminate sheet are the same. Each single layer sheet is available as 70 mm x 100 mm or (2) 70 mm x 200 mm and a multilayer sheet 70 mm x 100 mm is used for internal hernia repairs. Supplied sterile in easy open packages, for one time use.

Ocular Disc: Ocular discs are packaged in double peel-pouches with the rough side indicated by a notch. Experiments have shown that cell ingrowth increases if the rough side is placed against the wound. Each disc is 10 mm in diameter. Four individual discs are supplied sterile in sealed sections of easy open packages, for one time use.

Compendium Code No.: 12850000 V-BSRS1099

VETERINARY LINIMENT

First Priority **Counterirritant**

Ingredient(s): Composition: Witch Hazel, Aloe Vera, Parachlorometaxylenol, Menthol, Wormwood, Thymol, Potassium Iodide, Iodine in an Isopropyl Alcohol base.

Indications: Use as a warm-up prior to exercise and as an effective, soothing body wash or brace after workouts. VETERINARY LINIMENT is specially formulated to quickly stimulate blood flow to legs and muscles. As a stimulating brace, or for temporary relief of sprains, strains, and general soreness, VETERINARY LINIMENT is an effective treatment that will not blister or stain. Safe for use in all racing, shows and events.

Dosage and Administration: As a warm-up prior to exercise: Apply a moderate amount of VETERINARY LINIMENT and gently massage into the skin. Then lightly apply a second application to wet the skin.

For relief of muscle soreness or stiffness: Apply as above, then wrap with a bandage or standing wrap if desired. May be used for legs, shoulders, hips, backs or stifles to minimize muscle, tendon, and ligament soreness after workouts.

As a body wash or refreshing brace: Mix 1 part VETERINARY LINIMENT with 8 parts water. Use after workouts to refresh and cool.

Precaution(s): Store at controlled room temperature between 32°F and 90°F.

Caution(s): Not for use on deep or puncture wounds. If redness, irritation or swelling persists or increases, discontinue use and consult a veterinarian.

For animal use only.

Warning(s): Keep out of reach of children.

Presentation: 16 fl oz (473 mL) and 1 gallon (3.785 L) (NDC# 58829-282-01).

Compendium Code No.: 11390762 Iss. 12-98

VETERINARY SURFACTANT

Vedco **Enema-Cerumenolytic**

Active Ingredient(s): Contains water, propylene glycol, dioctyl sodium sulfosuccinate, 5%.

Indications:

Horses: For use an enema and a laxative.

Dogs and Cats: For use as an enema and a cerumenolytic agent.

Dosage and Administration:

Horses: For use as an enema, administer 4-6 ounces in one (1) gallon water. For use as a laxative, administer orally eight (8) ounces in one (1) gallon water or mineral oil.

Dogs and Cats: For use as an enema, administer 2-3 ounces of a mixture of 5 mL VETERINARY SURFACTANT per ounce of water. For use as a cerumenolytic agent, administer two (2) to three (3) drops in each ear.

Note: Cooler temperatures cause the product to become cloudy. Place in warm water or bring to room temperature (68-74°F).

Caution(s): Not for human use. Keep out of the reach of children. For veterinary use only.

Presentation: 1 gallon containers.

Compendium Code No.: 10492130

VETERINARY SURFACTANT (D.S.S.) ℞

First Priority **Laxative**

Laxative-Stool Softener-Lubricant

Active Ingredient(s): Water miscible solution of Dioctyl Sodium Sulfosuccinate 5%.

Ingredients: Water, Propylene Glycol, Dioctyl Sodium Sulfosuccinate.

Indications: To be used as an aid in the relief of constipation and impactions caused by hard fecal masses in horses, dogs and cats.

Directions for Use:

Horses: For use as an enema, administer 4-6 ounces in 1 gallon water. For use as a laxative, administer orally with the aid of a stomach tube 8 ounces in 1 gallon water or mineral oil.

Dogs and Cats: For use as an enema, administer 2-3 ounces of a mixture of 5 mL VETERINARY SURFACTANT (D.S.S.) per ounce of water.

Precaution(s): Storage: Store at controlled room temperature between 15°-30°C (59°-86°F). Keep container tightly closed when not in use.

Caution(s): Federal law restricts this drug to use by or on the order of a licensed veterinarian.

For animal use only.

Warning(s): Keep out of reach of children.

Presentation: 1 gallon (3.785 L) (NDC# 58829-220-01).

Compendium Code No.: 11390772 Rev. 08-01

VETISULID®

Fort Dodge **Sulfachlorpyridazine**

Sodium Sulfachlorpyridazine Powder and Sulfachlorpyridazine Boluses

NADA No.: 033-373 (Powder)/033-127 (Bolus)

Active Ingredient(s): Description: Bottles of VETISULID® Powder (Sodium Sulfachlorpyridazine Powder) for oral use contain 54 g sodium sulfachlorpyridazine powder (equivalent to 50 g sulfachlorpyridazine).

VETISULID® Boluses (Sulfachlorpyridazine Boluses) for oral administration contain 2 g sulfachlorpyridazine per bolus.

Indications: VETISULID® Powder and VETISULID® Boluses are especially indicated for the treatment of diarrhea caused or complicated by *E. coli* (colibacillosis) in calves under 1 month of age; VETISULID® Powder is also indicated for the treatment of colibacillosis in swine.

Pharmacology: Actions: Sulfachlorpyridazine is a broad spectrum antibacterial compound which is effective in the treatment of infections caused by gram-positive and gram-negative organisms that are commonly susceptible to sulfonamide therapy and which has been proven by laboratory and field experiments to be highly effective against diseases caused by *Escherichia coli.*

Sulfachlorpyridazine has a rapid onset of action in several species of animals following both oral and parenteral administration. In comparison with other sulfonamides, the administration of comparatively effective oral doses of sulfachlorpyridazine to dogs produces blood concentrations that reach maximum levels in 1 to 3 hours. The blood level declines to 1 to 2 mg-percent after 12 hours and the drug is completely excreted in the urine within 48 hours. In experimental studies in which cattle are given the recommended dosage of sulfachlorpyridazine intravenously, the blood level rises to above 12 mg-percent within 1 hour and 6 hours later it falls to 3 to 4 mg-percent; after 18 hours no sulfonamide can be detected. In swine given the recommended dosage of sulfachlorpyridazine either intramuscularly or orally, the blood level reaches 5.5 mg-percent after 1.5 hours. The blood level declines to 1 to 2 mg-percent within 6 hours; after 12 hours practically no sulfonamide can be detected. Laboratory studies with other species of animals have demonstrated similar responses in blood and urine following oral or parenteral administration of sulfachlorpyridazine.

Sulfachlorpyridazine is readily soluble at normal urinary pH making it unlikely that crystallization of the free and acetylated forms will occur.

Studies with laboratory animals indicate that sulfachlorpyridazine attains a high concentration in the bile; the concentrations in the liver and kidneys approximately parallel that of the blood, thus demonstrating excellent penetration of tissues.

Dosage and Administration:

Calves: The recommended daily dose is 30 to 45 mg of sulfachlorpyridazine per lb of body weight administered in 2 divided doses for 1 to 5 days, as follows:

It is suggested that therapy be initiated by administering VETISULID® Injection (see package information accompanying that product for complete information) intravenously and continuing therapy with the oral administration of either VETISULID® Boluses or VETISULID® Powder.

VETISULID® Boluses (Sulfachlorpyridazine Boluses)—Administer 1 bolus orally for each 100 lb of body weight twice daily.

VETISULID® Powder (Sodium Sulfachlorpyridazine Powder)—To prepare a solution for treatment, mix the contents of a 54 g bottle of VETISULID® Powder (equivalent to 50 g sulfachlorpyridazine) with sufficient milk or milk substitute to treat a number of calves totaling 2200 to 3300 lb of body weight (e.g., 20 calves from 110 to 165 lb each). Use immediately. Administer fresh solution twice daily.

Example administration for a single calf: Each level teaspoon of VETISULID® Powder contains approximately 2800 mg of sulfachlorpyridazine. The daily dose of VETISULID® Powder is 30-45 mg per pound body weight divided into two equal treatments.

To treat a single 130 pound calf, mix ¾ teaspoon to 1 level teaspoon of VETISULID® Powder with sufficient milk, or milk substitute, to be consumed at one feeding. Repeat every 12 hours for up to 5 days duration. Mix VETISULID® Powder with milk just prior to each treatment.

Swine:

VETISULID® Powder—The recommended daily oral dose is 20 to 35 mg of sulfachlorpyridazine per lb of body weight administered in 2 divided doses for 1 to 5 days. The dose may be administered either individually or by herd treatment. Prepare fresh solution at time of use.

Individual Pig Treatment—To prepare a solution for treatment, add the contents of a 54 g bottle of VETISULID® Powder to 5 cups (40 ounces) of water. Draw the prepared solution into a syringe graduated in milliliters and administer it to each pig orally using the following dosage schedule:

Pig Weight in Pounds	Dose per Pig
5.0	2 mL twice daily
10.0	4 mL twice daily

Important: When treating the pigs individually, make certain the entire recommended dose is swallowed by each pig.

Herd Treatment—To prepare a solution for treatment, add the contents of a 54 g bottle of VETISULID® Powder to 15 gallons of water. Since the daily water consumption of pigs varies tremendously, that quantity of VETISULID® Powder medicated drinking water will treat the following numbers of pigs according to their body weight. Prepare fresh solution at time of use.

Pig Weight in Pounds	Number of Pigs Treated
12.5	220-400
25.0	110-200
50.0	60-100
100.0	30-50

If the recommended quantity of medicated drinking water is consumed, replace it with normal or unmedicated water until it is time for the next dose to be administered.

Precaution(s): Storage: Store at room temperature; avoid excessive heat (104°F).

Caution(s): The diagnosis should be reconfirmed if symptoms persist for 2 to 3 days.

To insure adequate urine flow and to prevent crystalluria, water should be readily available to animals receiving sulfachlorpyridazine therapy.

Warning(s): Treated, ruminating calves must not be slaughtered for food during treatment and for 7 days after the last oral treatment. Treated swine must not be slaughtered for food during treatment and for 4 days after the last treatment.

A withdrawal period has not been established for these products in pre-ruminating calves. Do not use in calves to be processed for veal.

Trial Data: Veterinary laboratories have confirmed the exceptional activity of sulfachlorpyridazine against *E. coli* by both *in vitro* and *in vivo* tests. In one study, 64 out of 70 *E. coli* strains that were isolated from clinical cases of colibacillosis in calves were sensitive to sulfachlorpyridazine. Another sensitivity study involving calves revealed 225 isolates of *E. coli* that were sensitive to sulfachlorpyridazine out of a total of 226 isolates examined. Pretreatment and post-treatment identifications of various serotypes of *E. coli* were made in this study. In all serotypes, except one, the number of isolates cultured from the feces of treated calves was reduced following treatment with sulfachlorpyridazine. Results from a study in swine revealed that 110 out of 118 strains of *E. coli* isolated from swine enteritis were sensitive to sulfachlorpyridazine. Clinical studies confirm its efficacy in treating *E. coli* infections.

Presentation: VETISULID® Boluses (Sulfachlorpyridazine Boluses), bottles of 50 (NDC 53501-221-30) and 100 (NDC 53501-221-45) boluses.

VETISULID® Powder (Sodium Sulfachlorpyridazine Powder), bottles of 1.9 oz (54 grams) of powder (53501-235-10).

Compendium Code No.: 10032551 12750D

VETISULID® INJECTION

Fort Dodge **Sulfachlorpyridazine**

Sodium Sulfachlorpyridazine Injection

NADA No.: 033-318

Active Ingredient(s): Description: VETISULID® Injection (Sodium Sulfachlorpyridazine Injection) is a sterile, aqueous solution for intravenous use. Each mL provides 215 mg (21.5%) sodium sulfachlorpyridazine (equivalent to 200 mg sulfachlorpyridazine), 16 mg benzyl alcohol and sodium hydroxide to adjust the pH.

Indications: VETISULID® Injection (Sodium Sulfachlorpyridazine Injection), is especially indicated for the treatment of diarrhea caused or complicated by *E. coli* (colibacillosis) in calves under 1 month of age.

Pharmacology: Actions: Sulfachlorpyridazine is a broad spectrum antibacterial compound which is effective in the treatment of infections caused by gram-positive and gram-negative organisms that are commonly susceptible to sulfonamide therapy and which has been proven by laboratory and field experiments to be highly effective against diseases caused by *Escherichia coli.*

Sulfachlorpyridazine has a rapid onset of action in several species of animals following both oral and parenteral administration. In comparison with other sulfonamides, the administration of comparatively effective oral doses of sulfachlorpyridazine to dogs produces blood concentrations that reach maximum levels in 1 to 3 hours. The blood level declines to 1 to 2 mg-percent after 12 hours and the drug is completely excreted in the urine within 48 hours. In experimental studies in which cattle are given the recommended dosage of sulfachlorpyridazine intravenously, the blood level rises to above 12 mg-percent within 1 hour and 6 hours later it falls to 3 to 4 mg-percent; after 18 hours no sulfonamide can be detected. In swine given the recommended dosage of sulfachlorpyridazine either intramuscularly or orally, the blood level reaches 5.5 mg-percent after 1.5 hours. The blood level declines to 1 to 2 mg-percent within 6 hours; after 12 hours practically no sulfonamide can be detected. Laboratory studies with other species of animals have demonstrated similar responses in blood and urine following oral or parenteral administration of sulfachlorpyridazine.

Sulfachlorpyridazine is readily soluble at normal urinary pH making it unlikely that crystallization of the free and acetylated forms will occur.

Studies with laboratory animals indicate that sulfachlorpyridazine attains a high concentration in the bile; the concentrations in the liver and kidneys approximately parallel that of the blood, thus demonstrating excellent penetration of tissues.

Dosage and Administration:

Calves: The recommended daily dose is 30 to 45 mg of sulfachlorpyridazine per lb of body weight administered in 2 divided doses for 1 to 5 days, as follows:

VETISULID® Injection (Sodium Sulfachlorpyridazine Injection) — Administer intravenously 1 mL per 10 lb of body weight morning and night.

It is suggested that therapy be initiated by administering VETISULID® Injection intravenously and continuing therapy with the oral administration of either Vetisulid® Boluses or Vetisulid® Powder.

Precaution(s): Storage: VETISULID® Injection: Protect from light. Store at room temperature; avoid freezing.

Caution(s): The diagnosis should be reconfirmed if symptoms persist for 2 to 3 days.

To insure adequate urine flow and to prevent crystalluria, water should be readily available to animals receiving sulfachlorpyridazine therapy.

Sodium sulfachlorpyridazine injection for use in calves only.

Warning(s): Treated, ruminating calves must not be slaughtered for food during treatment and for 5 days after the last intravenous treatment. A withdrawal period has not been established for these products in pre-ruminating calves. Do not use in calves to be processed for veal.

Trial Data: Veterinary laboratories have confirmed the exceptional activity of sulfachlorpyridazine against *E. coli* by both *in vitro* and *in vivo* tests. In one study, 64 out of 70 *E. coli* strains that were isolated from clinical cases of colibacillosis in calves were sensitive to sulfachlorpyridazine. Another sensitivity study involving calves revealed 225 isolates of *E. coli* that were sensitive to sulfachlorpyridazine out of a total of 226 isolates examined. Pretreatment and post-treatment identifications of various serotypes of *E. coli* were made in this study. In all serotypes, except one, the number of isolates cultured from the feces of treated calves was reduced following treatment with sulfachlorpyridazine. Results from a study in swine revealed that 110 out of 118 strains of *E. coli* isolated from swine enteritis were sensitive to sulfachlorpyridazine. Clinical studies confirm its efficacy in treating *E. coli* infections.

Presentation: VETISULID® Injection (Sodium Sulfachlorpyridazine Injection) is supplied in 250 mL multiple dose vials.

Manufactured by: Phoenix Scientific, Inc., St. Joseph, MO 64506

Compendium Code No.: 10032641 12759A

VET-KEM® BREAKAWAY® FLEA & TICK COLLAR FOR CATS

Wellmark **Parasiticide Collar**

EPA Reg. No.: 2724-275

Active Ingredient(s):

Propoxur (CAS #114-26-1) 10.0%
Other Ingredients: 90.0%
Total 100.0%

Indications: Kills fleas and ticks up to 5 months. Controls Lyme disease-carrying ticks. For cats of all sizes.

Directions for Use: It is a violation of Federal Law to use this product in a manner inconsistent with its labeling.

Read entire label before each use.

1. Buckle collar around cat's neck. Thread flat end of the collar through buckle hole and tighten as necessary, so that at least 2 ridges are covered by the buckle. Since the plastic buckle is molded into the collar, the possibility of neck irritation and buckle failure is reduced. Fit collar snug enough to prevent placement of the cat's leg or lower jaw through the collar, yet loose enough to be rotated about the neck.
2. Leave 1 to 2 extra inches on the collar for adjustment; cut off excess length and dispose of in trash.
3. Check periodically and adjust fit it necessary, especially when kittens are rapidly growing.
4. May be used in addition to regular collar. Replace collar when effectiveness diminishes. To release the collar, squeeze buckle between thumb and finger and pull sharply.

Precautionary Statements: Hazards to Humans and Domestic Animals — Caution: Do not get dust or collar in mouth, harmful if swallowed. Do not get dust in eyes, will cause temporary pupillary constriction.* The dust released by this collar is a cholinesterase inhibitor.

Humans: Do not open package until ready to use. Do not allow children to play with this collar. Dust will form on this collar during storage. Wash hands thoroughly with soap and water after handling collar.

Animals: Consult a veterinarian before using this product on debilitated, aged, medicated, pregnant or nursing cats. Do not use on kittens under 12 weeks of age. Do not use this product on cats simultaneously or within 30 days before or after treatment with or exposure to cholinesterase-inhibiting drugs, pesticides, or chemicals. However, flea and tick collars may be immediately replaced. When collar is first worn, observe neck area every few days for irritation. Remove collar at the first sign of irritation or adverse reaction. Sensitivities may occur after using any pesticide product for pets. If signs of sensitivity occur, remove collar and bathe your pet with mild soap and rinse with large amounts of water.

First Aid:

If swallowed, call physician, veterinarian, or Poison Control Center. Drink 1 or 2 glasses of water and induce vomiting by touching back of throat with finger. If person is unconscious, do not give anything by mouth and do not induce vomiting. If in eyes, flush eyes with plenty of water. Get medical attention if irritation persists.

Note to Physician/Veterinarian: *Atropine and *homatropine are antidotal only if symptoms of cholinesterase inhibition are present.

In case of emergency or for product use information, call 1-800-766-7661.

Storage and Disposal: Store in original unopened container away from children. Do not reuse container or reuse collar. Wrap and put in trash.

Warning(s): Do not allow children to play with this collar.

Use only on cats.

Disclaimer: Seller makes no warranty, expressed or implied, concerning the use of this product other than indicated on the label. Buyer assumes all risk of use and handling of this material when such use and handling are contrary to label instructions.

Discussion: Unique Feature: This collar is designed to stretch under the weight of an average size adult cat. It helps the cat to free itself ("breakaway") if the collar gets snagged on a fixed object. If the collar is fitted improperly, so that it is loose enough for a cat to work the collar over its leg or jaw, this release feature may not stretch adequately to allow the extra room necessary for the cat to free itself.

What to Expect:

For Fleas:

1. This BREAKAWAY® collar is designed to kill adult fleas.
2. This collar starts killing fleas as soon as it is placed around the cat's neck.
3. Protection against fleas will be achieved within a few days, providing continuous protection for 5 months.
4. Replace collar every 5 months to help control flea infestations on your pet.

For Ticks:

1. Ticks are tougher to kill than fleas and are killed more slowly.
2. Full projection against adult and immature ticks will be achieved within a few days, providing continuous protection for 5 months.
3. Adult ticks will be killed over the entire pet. Dead ticks will fall off or may be easily removed.
4. Replace collar every 5 months for continuous protection from ticks.

Presentation: 0.37 oz (10.5 g) collar.

BREAKAWAY® and VET-KEM® are registered trademarks of Wellmark International.

Compendium Code No.: 10930050 43905E

VET-KEM® BREAKAWAY® PLUS FLEA & TICK COLLAR FOR CATS

Wellmark **Parasiticide Collar**

EPA Reg. No.: 2724-491

Active Ingredient(s):

Propoxur (CAS #114-26-1) 10.0%
(S)-Methoprene (CAS #65733-16-6) 2.1%
Other Ingredients: 87.9%
Total: 100.0%

Indications: Kills immature fleas, adult fleas and flea eggs up to 8 months. Kills ticks up to 6 months including those carrying Lyme disease. For cats of all sizes - works from head to tail. Plus Precor® - Kills flea eggs.

Directions for Use: It is a violation of Federal Law to use this product in a manner inconsistent with its labeling.

Read entire label before each use. Use only on cats and kittens 12 weeks of age and older.

1. Buckle collar around cat's neck. Thread flat end of the collar through buckle hole and tighten as necessary, so that at least 2 ridges are covered by the buckle. Since the plastic buckle is molded into the collar, the possibility of neck irritation and buckle failure is reduced. Collar should fit snug enough to prevent placement of the cat's leg or lower jaw through the collar, yet loose enough to be rotated about the neck.
2. Leave 1-2 extra inches on the length of the collar for adjustment, cut off excess, and dispose of in trash.
3. Check periodically and adjust fit if necessary, especially when kittens are rapidly growing.
4. Replace in 8 months for continuous protection from adult fleas and flea egg hatch. Replace in 6 months for continuous protection from ticks. To release the collar, squeeze buckle between thumb and finger and pull sharply. Collar does not need replacement if cat becomes wet.

Contraindication(s): Do not use on kittens under 12 weeks of age.

Precautionary Statements: Hazards to Humans and Domestic Animals - Caution: Do not get dust or collar in mouth. Harmful if swallowed or absorbed through skin. Do not get dust in eyes, will cause temporary constriction of the pupils*. The dust released by this collar is a cholinesterase inhibitor. Avoid contact with skin, eyes or clothing.

Humans: Do not open package until ready to use. Do not allow children to play with this collar. Pesticidal dust will form on this collar during storage. Wash hands thoroughly with soap and water after handling collar.

Animals: Consult a veterinarian before using this product on debilitated, aged, medicated, pregnant, or nursing cats. Do not use on kittens under 12 weeks of age. Do not use this product on cats simultaneously or within 30 days before or after treatment with or exposure to cholinesterase inhibiting drugs or pesticides (e.g. carbaryl or propoxur, etc.). However, flea and tick collars may be immediately replaced. When collar is first worn, observe neck area every few days for irritation. Remove collar at the first sign of irritation or adverse reaction. Sensitivities may occur after using any pesticide product for pets. If signs of sensitivity occur, remove collar and bathe your cat with mild soap and rinse with large amounts of water.

First Aid:

If swallowed: Call poison control center or doctor immediately for treatment advice. Have person sip a glass of water if able to swallow. Do not induce vomiting unless told to do so by the poison control center or doctor. Do not give anything by mouth to an unconscious person.

If on skin or clothing: Take off contaminated clothing. Rinse skin immediately with plenty of water for 15-20 minutes. Call a poison control center or doctor for treatment advice.

If in eyes: Hold eye open and rinse slowly and gently with water for 15-20 minutes. Remove contact lenses, if present, after the first 5 minutes, then continue rinsing eye. Call a poison control center or doctor for treatment advice.

Note to Physician/Veterinarian: *Atropine is antidotal only if symptoms of cholinesterase inhibition are present.

In case of emergency, call 1-800-766-7661 or a Poison Control Center. Have the product container or label with you when calling a poison control center or doctor or going for treatment.

Storage and Disposal: Store in original unopened package away from children. Wrap used collar and put in trash. Collar should be left in place once fitted on cat. If collar is temporarily removed, do not set it on wood or other surfaces.

Warning(s): Do not allow children to play with this collar.

Disclaimer: Seller makes no warranty, expressed or implied, concerning the use of this product other than indicated on the label. Buyer assumes all risk of use and handling of this material when such use and handling are contrary to label instructions.

Discussion: Unique Feature: This collar is designed to stretch under the weight of an average sized adult cat. It helps the cat to free itself ("breakaway") if the collar gets snagged on a fixed object. If the collar is fitted improperly, so that it is loose enough for a cat to work the collar over its leg or jaw, this release feature may not stretch adequately to allow the extra room necessary for the cat to free itself.

To minimize flea infestation, use appropriate products to:

1. Treat the pet.
2. Treat the indoor environment, especially where pets spend time resting.
3. Treat the outdoor environment when necessary.

What to Expect:

For Fleas:

1. This BREAKAWAY® Plus collar is designed to kill adult fleas and flea eggs.
2. This collar begins working to kill fleas and flea eggs as soon as it is placed around the cat's neck.
3. Protection against fleas and flea eggs will be achieved within 48 hours, providing continuous protection for 8 months.
4. Replace collar every 8 months to help control adult flea infestations on your pet.

For Ticks:

1. Ticks are tougher to kill than fleas and are killed more slowly.
2. Full protection against adult and immature ticks will be achieved within a few days, providing continuous protection for 6 months.
3. Adult ticks will be killed over the entire pet. Dead ticks will fall off or may be easily removed.
4. Replace collar every 6 months for continuous protection from ticks.

Presentation: 0.37 oz (10.5 g) collar.

Precor® and VET-KEM® BREAKAWAY® Plus Flea & Tick Collar for Cats are registered trademarks of Wellmark International.

Compendium Code No.: 10930150 43967

VET-KEM® OVITROL® PLUS FLEA & TICK SHAMPOO FOR DOGS & CATS

Wellmark **Parasiticide Shampoo**

EPA Reg. No.: 2724-485

Active Ingredient(s):

(S)-Methoprene (CAS #65733-16-6)	1.10%
Pyrethrins (CAS #8003-34-7)	0.15%
Piperonyl Butoxide (CAS #51-03-6)	1.05%
Other Ingredients	98.25%
Total	100.00%

Contains Precor® Insect Growth Regulator plus Pyrethrins, an adulticide.

Indications: OVITROL® Plus Flea Tick Shampoo is a concentrated lathering shampoo enriched with oatmeal, coconut extract, lanolin, and aloe. It soothes sensitive skin and leaves the coat soft, shining, and manageable. The shampoo removes loose dandruff, dirt, and scales. Precor® Insect Growth Regulator provides 28 days of control of pre-adult fleas before they become biting adults.

Directions for Use: It is a violation of Federal Law to use this product in a manner inconsistent with its labeling. For topical use only. Do not ingest.

Read entire label before each use. Use only on dogs, cats, puppies or kittens.

OVITROL® Plus Flea & Tick Shampoo may be used full strength or diluted with 2 parts water. Thoroughly wet animal with warm water. Do not apply shampoo around eyes. Apply shampoo on head and ears, then lather; repeat procedure with neck, chest, middle and hind quarters, finishing legs last. Continue to work lather in for 3 to 5 minutes (this is an important part of the grooming procedure), then rinse animal thoroughly. For extremely dirty or scaly animals, the above procedure may be repeated. Repeat every 7 to 10 days, if necessary, for adult flea relief. Flea egg hatch inhibition will last far 28 days. Do not use on puppies or kittens under 12 weeks old.

Precautionary Statements: Caution - Hazards to Humans and Domestic Animals:

Humans: Causes moderate eye irritation. Harmful if absorbed through skin. Avoid contact with eyes, skin or clothing. Wash thoroughly with soap and water after handling.

Animals: Do not use on pets less than 12 weeks old. Consult a veterinarian before using this product on debilitated, aged, animals on medication, or pregnant or nursing animals. Sensitivities may occur after using ANY pesticide product for pets. If signs of sensitivity occur, bathe your pet with mild soap and rinse with large amounts of water. If signs continue, consult a veterinarian immediately.

First Aid in Humans/Animals:

If in Eyes: Flush eyes with plenty of water. Call a physician/veterinarian if irritation persists.

If on Skin: Wash with plenty of soap and water. Get medical attention if irritation persists.

In case of emergency or for product use information call 1-800-766-7661

Storage and Disposal:

Storage - Store in a cool area.

Disposal - Do not reuse empty container. Wrap and put in trash.

Warning(s): Keep out of reach of children.

Disclaimer: Seller makes no warranty, expressed or implied, concerning the use of this product other than indicated on the label. Buyer assumes all risk of use and handling of this material when such use and handling are contrary to label instructions.

Presentation: 12 fl oz (355 mL).

OVITROL®, Precor® Insect Growth Regulator and VET-KEM® are registered trademarks of Wellmark International.

Compendium Code No.: 10930060 06653A

VET-KEM® OVITROL® PLUS FLEA, TICK & BOT SPRAY

Wellmark **Flea Control & Topical Parasiticide**

EPA Reg. No.: 2724-404

Active Ingredient(s):

(S)-Methoprene (CAS #65733-16-6)	0.27%
Pyrethrins (CAS #8003-34-7)	0.20%
Piperonyl Butoxide (CAS #51-03-6)	0.37%
N-octyl Bicycloheptene Dicarboximide (CAS #113-48-4)	0.62%
Other Ingredients:	98.54%
Total	100.00%

Contains Precor® Insect Growth Regulator plus Pyrethrins, an adulticide.

Indications: OVITROL® Plus controls fleas, flea larvae, ticks, lice, mosquitoes, gnats, house flies, stable flies, horn flies, face flies, and horse bots. Botfly eggs and flea eggs sprayed with OVITROL® Plus will not hatch into adults.

Directions for Use: It is a violation of Federal Law to use this product in a manner inconsistent with its labeling.

Read entire label before each use.

Use only on dogs, puppies, cats, kittens, horses and ponies.

Shake well before using.

For Dogs and Cats:

For Fleas: A light even coverage of the hair coat will provide effective flea control. For best results, ruffle the coat while spraying against the natural lay of the hair. Cover animal's eyes with hand. With a firm fast stroke, spray head, ears, and, chest. With cloth, rub into face around mouth, nose, and eyes. Then spray the neck, middle and hind quarters, finishing with legs and tail last. Avoid spraying rectum and genitals. Apply at the rate of 1 or 2 squeezes of the trigger sprayer [0.10 fluid ounce] per pound of body weight. For larger dogs, spray until damp, not saturated. Do not allow animals, cats in particular, to become' chilled. Repeat every 2 months, if necessary.

For Ticks: Make sure spray thoroughly wets individual ticks.

For Puppies and Kittens:

For Fleas: Leaving the eyes, nose, and mouth exposed, treat puppies and kittens weighing less than 3 pounds by wrapping the animal in a towel that has been lightly sprayed with OVITROL® Plus, for 5 to 10 minutes. Or lightly spray a brush or cotton ball and work thoroughly into the hair coat. Fleas may then be removed from the coat by picking or combing. Puppies and kittens over 3 pounds may be treated the same as dogs and cats as described above. Repeat every 2 months, if necessary. Do not allow animal to become chilled. Do not use on puppies and kittens under 12 weeks of age.

For Horses and Ponies:

For Flies: Remove excess dirt and dust by brushing coat. Apply spray directly to horse's coat, giving particular attention to legs, shoulders, flanks, neck, and topline. To treat face, dampen a cloth with spray and rub on face and head, being careful to avoid eyes. Repeat every 2 months, if necessary.

For Prevention of Hatch of Horse Botfly Eggs: Spray any infested areas directly at the first sign of visible eggs, paying particular attention to legs, shoulders, flanks, neck, and topline. Spray to the point of dampness but not to the point of runoff of the spray. For a high degree of botfly egg control, spray animals every 3-5 days during the botfly season.

Consult a veterinarian before using this product on debilitated, aged, pregnant, nursing, or animals on medication.

Precautionary Statements: Hazards to Humans — Caution: Harmful if swallowed or absorbed through skin. Avoid contact with skin, eyes, or clothing. May cause dermal sensitization (skin allergy).

First Aid in Humans:

If in eyes, flush with plenty of water. Get medical attention if irritation persists. If on skin, remove contaminated clothing and wash affected areas with soap and water. Get medical attention if irritation persists. If swallowed, call Vet-Kem at 1-800-766-7661 or physician or Poison Control Center. Drink 1 or 2 glasses of water and induce vomiting by touching the back of tine throat with finger. Do not induce vomiting or give anything by mouth to an unconscious person.

Hazards to Animals — Caution: Sensitivities may occur after using any pesticide product for pets. If signs of sensitivity occur, bathe your pet with mild soap and rinse with large amounts of water. If signs continue, consult a veterinarian immediately. Some cats may be sensitive to products containing pyrethrins. Excessive salivation and ear and paw flicking may occur; however, these effects are temporary and not harmful. May cause dermal sensitization (skin allergy).

First Aid in Animals: Consult Vet-Kem at 1-800-766-7661 or a veterinarian or an animal poison control center.

Physical Hazards: Combustible. Do not use or store near heat or open flame.

For more information, or in case of emergency, call 1-800-766-7661.

Storage and Disposal: Do not contaminate water, food, or feed by storage or disposal.

Storage: Do not store near heat or open frame. Store away from children and animals.

Disposal: Do not reuse empty container. Wrap and put in trash.

Warning(s): Do not treat horses destined for food.

Keep out of reach of children.

Disclaimer: Seller makes no warranty, expressed or implied, concerning the use and handling of this product other than indicated on the label. Buyer assumes all risks of use and handling of this material when such use and handling are contrary to label instructions.

Discussion: OVITROL® Plus combines the adult flea killing power of natural pyrethrins with the long-lasting egg-killing power of Precor® Insect Growth Regulator. This highly effective combination of ingredients provides quick relief from biting fleas and continuous killing of flea eggs laid on the animal, breaking the flea life cycle. The elimination of both adult fleas and flea eggs is important because adult fleas live on your pet, causing discomfort and skin irritation, while the vast number of eggs that they lay fall off and develop in your house. If fleas are already developing in your house, then use a Siphotrol® premise product. Effective flea control requires treatment of your pets, house, and yard.

OVITROL® Plus contains Precor® Insect Growth Regulator, which effectively kills botfly eggs that have been glued to the hairs on the forelegs, shoulders, and faces of horses, by adult botflies (*Gasterophilus* spp.). If left untreated, botfly larvae emerge from these eggs and are taken into the mouth of the horse. After botfly larvae are swallowed, they attach to the stomach and small intestinal linings in tremendous numbers, where they can remain for months before passing out in the feces. Adult botflies emerge from pupae in the soil to begin the cycle all over again. Botflies have been implicated as a cause of some stomach and intestinal conditions in horses.

Presentation: 1 pt (16 fl oz) (2 month protection).

OVITROL®, Precor® Insect Growth Regulator, and VET-KEM® are registered trademarks of Wellmark International.

Compendium Code No.: 10930071 68403A/68405A

VET-KEM® OVITROL PLUS® SPOT ON® FLEA & TICK CONTROL FOR DOGS AND PUPPIES (UNDER 30 LBS.)

Wellmark **Flea Control & Topical Parasiticide**

EPA Reg. No.: 40849-72-2724

Active Ingredient(s):

Permethrin (CAS #57645-53-1)	45.0%
(S)-Methoprene (CAS #65733-16-6)	3.0%
Other Ingredients	52.0%
Total	100.0%

Contains Precor® Insect Growth Regulator (IGR).

Indications: OVITROL PLUS® prevents eggs from developing into adult fleas for up to 3 months. OVITROL PLUS® also kills and repels fleas, ticks and mosquitoes for up to 30 days.

Directions for Use: It is a violation of Federal Law to use this product in a manner inconsistent with its labeling.

Read entire label before each use. Use only on dogs and puppies.

1. Bend at perforation and tear off first month's applicator.
2. Hold applicator upright and snap tip back, away from face and body.
3. Position the tip of the applicator on the dog's back between the shoulder blades. Apply half of the contents of the applicator.
4. Invert the applicator to an upright position and move to the dog's hind quarters. Position the tip of the applicator at the base of the tail and apply the remaining contents of the applicator.
5. Do not reapply product for 30 days.

Although OVITROL PLUS® is applied only between the shoulder blades and at the base of the tail, the dog's skin and hair oils carry the product aver the entire body for protection against fleas, ticks, and flea eggs. Do not bathe the dog for 5 days before or 5 days after treatment. OVITROL PLUS® is most effective when used as part of a total flea and tick management program. Use other Vet-Kem products registered for residential area control of these pests in conjunction with this treatment.

Contraindication(s): Intended for use on dogs or puppies 6 months of age or older. Do not use on cats.

Precautionary Statements: Hazards to Humans and Domestic Animals — Caution:

Humans: Avoid contact with skin or clothing. Wash thoroughly with soap and water after handling.

Domestic Animals: Do not use on cats. Cats which actively groom or engage in close physical contact with recently treated dogs may be at risk of toxic exposure. Do not use on puppies less than 6 months of age. Consult a veterinarian before using this product on debilitated, aged, medicated, pregnant or nursing animals. Sensitivities may occur after using any pesticide product for pets. If signs of sensitivity occur, bathe your pet with a mild soap and rinse with large amounts of water. If signs continue, consult a veterinarian immediately. In the event of an emergency, contact the National Animal Poison Control Center at (800) 345-4735.

First Aid: If on skin, wash with plenty of soap and water. Get medical attention if irritation persists.

Environmental Hazards: This product is toxic to fish.

Physical or Chemical Hazards: Combustible. Do not use or store near heat or open flame.

In case of emergency, or for product use information call 1-800-766-7661.

Warning(s): Keep out of reach of children.

Storage and Disposal:

Storage: Store in a cool dry area in a location out of reach of children and pets.

Disposal: Do not reuse empty applicator, wrap and discard in trash.

Presentation: Three 1 cc applicators (3 month supply).

OVITROL PLUS®, Precor® Insect Growth Regulator, SPOT ON® and VET-KEM® are registered trademarks of Wellmark International.

Compendium Code No.: 10930080 77617

VET-KEM® OVITROL PLUS® SPOT ON® FLEA & TICK CONTROL FOR DOGS AND PUPPIES (OVER 30 LBS.)

Wellmark **Flea Control & Topical Parasiticide**

EPA Reg. No.: 40849-72-2724

Active Ingredient(s):

Permethrin (CAS #52645-53-1)	45.0%
(S)-Methoprene (CAS #65733-16-6)	3.0%
Other Ingredients:	52.0%
Total	100.0%

Contains Precor® Insect Growth Regulator (IGR).

Indications: OVITROL PLUS® prevents eggs from developing into adult fleas for up to 3 months.

OVITROL PLUS® also kills and repels fleas, ticks and mosquitoes for up to 30 days.

Directions for Use: It is a violation of Federal Law to use this product in a manner inconsistent with it labeling.

Read entire label before each use. Use only on dogs and puppies.

1. Bend at perforation and tear off first month's applicator.
2. Hold applicator upright and snap tip back, away from face and body.
3. Position the tip of the applicator on the dog's back between the shoulder blades. Apply half of the contents of the applicator.
4. Invert the applicator to an upright position and move to the dog's hind quarters. Position the tip of the applicator at the base of the tail and apply the remaining contents of the applicator.
5. Do not reapply product for 30 days.

Although OVITROL PLUS® is applied only between the shoulder blades and at the base of the tail, the dog's skin and hair oils carry the product over the entire body for protection against fleas, ticks, and flea eggs. Do not bathe the dog for 5 days before or 5 days after treatment. OVITROL PLUS® is most effective when used as part of a total flea and tick management program. Use other Vet-Kem products registered for residential area control of these pests in conjunction with this treatment.

Contraindication(s): Intended for use on dogs or puppies 6 months of age or older. Do not use on cats.

Precautionary Statements: Hazards to Humans and Domestic Animals — Caution:

Humans: Avoid contact with skin or clothing. Wash thoroughly with soap and water after handling

Domestic Animals: Do not use on cats. Cats which actively groom or engage in close physical contact with recently treated dogs may be at risk of toxic exposure. Do not use on puppies less than 6 months of age. Consult a veterinarian before using this product on debilitated, aged, medicated, pregnant or nursing animals. Sensitivities may occur after using any pesticide product for pets. If signs of sensitivity occur, bathe your pet with a mild soap and rinse with large amounts of water. If signs continue, consult a veterinarian immediately. In the event of an emergency, contact the National Animal Poison Control Center at (800) 345-4735.

First Aid: If on skin, wash with plenty of soap and water. Get medical attention if imitation persists.

Environmental Hazards: This product is toxic to fish.

Physical or Chemical Hazards: Combustible. Do not use or store near heat or open flame.

In case of emergency, or for product use information call 1-800-766-7661.

Storage and Disposal:

Storage: Store in a cool dry area in a location out of reach of children and pets.

Disposal: Do not reuse empty applicator; wrap and discard in trash.

Warning(s): Keep out of reach of children.

Presentation: Three 2 cc applicators (3 month supply).

OVITROL PLUS®, Precor® Insect Growth Regulator, SPOT ON® and VET-KEM® are registered trademarks of Wellmark International.

Compendium Code No.: 10930090 77607

VET-KEM® OVITROL® SPOT ON® FLEA CONTROL FOR CATS

Wellmark **Flea Control**

EPA Reg. No.: 2724-488

Active Ingredient(s):

(S)-Methoprene (CAS #65733-16-6)	3.6%
Other Ingredients:	96.4%
Total	100.0%

Contains Precor® Insect Growth Regulator (IGR).

Indications: Kills and prevents flea eggs from hatching for up to 1 month on cats and kittens.

Directions for Use: It is a violation of Federal Law to use this product in a manner inconsistent with its labeling.

Read entire label before each use.

Use only on cats or kittens over 12 weeks of age.

1. Bend at perforation and tear off 1st month's applicator.
2. Hold applicator upright and snap tip back, away from face and body.
3. Prior to application of the product, gently lift the cat's haircoat on the back between the shoulder blades, position the tip of the applicator on the cat's exposed skin and squeeze out the entire contents of the applicator onto the cat's skin.
4. Repeat every month.

Precautionary Statements: Hazards to Humans — Caution: Causes moderate eye irritation. Harmful it swallowed or absorbed through skin. Avoid contact with eyes, skin, or clothing. Wash thoroughly with soap and water after handling.

Hazards to Domestic Animals — Caution: Do not use on kittens less than 12 weeks old. Consult a veterinarian before using this product on debilitated, aged, medicated, pregnant or nursing animals. Sensitivity may occur after using any pesticide product for pets. If signs of sensitivity occur, bathe your pet with mild soap and rinse with large amounts of water. It signs continue. consult a veterinarian immediately.

First Aid:

If in eyes, flush eyes with plenty of water. Call a physician if irritation persists.

If swallowed, call a physician or Poison Control Center. Drink 1 or 2 glasses of water and induce vomiting by touching back of throat with finger. If person is unconscious, do not give anything by mouth and do not induce vomiting.

If on skin, wash with plenty of soap and water. Get medical attention. Be sure to read full directions and precautions on the label. In case of emergency or for product use information, call 1-800-766-7661.

Storage and Disposal: Do not contaminate water, food, or teed by storage or disposal. Store in a cool dry place. Do not reuse empty applicator. Wrap and discard in trash.

Warning(s): Keep out of reach of children.

Discussion: OVITROL® SPOT ON® Flea Control contains a topically applied long-lasting insect growth regulator specifically formulated for cats and killers, which prevents flea eggs from maturing into adults. A single application of OVITROL® will last for up to 1 month. OVITROL® provides relief from flea infestations for 1 month by controlling and preventing flea eggs on your cat/kitten. Normal insecticides will not kill the flea eggs, but OVITROL® kills flea eggs, thereby breaking the flea life cycle. After application, through its natural movement, your cat's skin and hair oils carry OVITROL® over the pet's body for protection against flea eggs. Once fleas are evident on your pet, there is already an infestation of their preadult stages in your home. To kill existing adult flea populations, you may need to treat the home, pet's bed, and yard with traditional flea products approved for use on pets, around the home, or in your yard. As with all flea products, OVITROL® is most effective when used as part of a total program aimed at reducing fleas in the cat's environment. Be sure to treat the animal's bedding and surroundings with Vet-Kem flea products registered for these uses.

Presentation: Three 1 cc applicators (3 month supply).

OVITROL®, Precor® Insect Growth Regulator, SPOT ON® and VET-KEM® are registered trademarks of Wellmark International.

Compendium Code No.: 10930100 54607

VET-KEM® PARAMITE® SPONGE-ON FOR DOGS

Wellmark **Parasiticide Lotion**

EPA Reg. No.: 2724-169

Active Ingredient(s):

Phosmet (CAS# 732-11-6)	11.75%
Other Ingredients*	88.25%
Total	100.00%

*Contains aromatic petroleum solvent.

Indications: For the control of fleas, ticks and sarcoptic mange. Gives 16 days of residual control of fleas and Brown Dog ticks. Use only on dogs.

Directions for Use: It is a violation of Federal Law to use this product in a manner inconsistent with its labeling.

Read entire label before each use.

Fleas and ticks: Mix 1 oz (2 Tbsp) PARAMITE® with 1 gallon water. Sponge on solution until skin is wet. For maximum residual control, allow to dry on animal. Allow animal to dry before handling.

Sarcoptic mange on dogs is characterized by loss of hair, thickened skin, and intense itching caused by the *Sarcoptes* mite. Mix 1 oz (2 Tbsp) PARAMITE® with 1 gallon water. Sponge on dog until skin is wet and allow to shake dry. Do not rinse. If no improvement is seen within 14 days, consult your veterinarian. If mange mites reinfest your dog, retreatment may be necessary.

Do not reapply product for 7 days. Do not use on dogs under 12 weeks.

Food utensils such as tablespoons or measuring cups should not be used for food purposes after use with insecticides. Assure containers are disposed of properly or thoroughly closed following use.

Contraindication(s): Use only on dogs. Do not use on cats or other animals.

Precautionary Statements:

Hazards To Humans: Danger: Corrosive. Causes irreversible eye damage. May be fatal if swallowed. Harmful if absorbed through skin. Avoid contact with eyes, skin, or clothing. Avoid breathing vapor. Use only in well ventilated areas. Applicators must wear safety glasses, long-sleeved shirt, long pants, elbow-length waterproof gloves, waterproof apron, and unlined waterproof boots. Wash all contaminated clothing with soap and hot water before reuse. Wash thoroughly with soap and water before eating, drinking, or using tobacco. Not intended for human use.

Hazards to Domestic Animals: Danger: Corrosive. Causes irreversible eye damage. May be fatal if swallowed. Do not use this product on animals simultaneously or within 30 days before or after treatment with or exposure to cholinesterase inhibiting drugs, pesticides, or chemicals. However, flea and tick collars may be immediately replaced. Consult a veterinarian before using this product on debilitated, aged, pregnant, nursing, or medicated animals. Sensitivities may occur after using any pesticide product for pets. If signs of sensitivity occur, bathe your pet with mild soap and rinse with large amounts of water. If signs continue, consult a veterinarian immediately. Improper dilution of this product could cause serious injury to dogs. Do not use on cats or other animals.

First Aid:

If in eyes, hold eyelids open and flush with a steady gentle stream of water for 15 minutes. Get medical attention.

If swallowed, call a physician/veterinarian or Poison Control Center immediately. Do not induce vomiting. Do not give anything by mouth to an unconscious person. Avoid alcohol.

If on skin, wash promptly with soap and water. Remove contaminated clothing. Get medical attention if irritation persists.

If inhaled, remove victim to fresh air. If not breathing, give artificial respiration, preferably mouth to mouth. Get medical attention.

Note to Physician/Veterinarian: PARAMITE® is an organophosphorous insecticide and cholinesterase inhibitor. Atropine is antidotal. 2-PAM is also antidotal and may be administered with atropine. If ingested do not induce vomiting. May present aspiration hazard. Usual symptoms of poisoning in animals include salivation, labored breathing, gastrointestinal disturbance, tremors, staggering, and pin-point pupils.

Physical or Chemical Hazards: Do not use or store near heat or open flame. Protect from temperatures below 20°F.

For more information and in case of emergency call 1-800-766-7661.

Storage and Disposal: Do not contaminate water, food, or feed by storage or disposal.

Storage: Store in original container away from children. Disposal: Do not reuse container. Rinse thoroughly before discarding in trash.

Warning(s): Keep out of reach of children.

Disclaimer: Seller makes no warranty, expressed or implied, concerning the use of this product other than indicated on the label. Buyer assumes all risk of use and handling of this material when such use and handling are contrary to label instructions.

Presentation: 128 fl oz (1 gal) 3.8 L.

PARAMITE® and VET-KEM® are registered trademarks of Wellmark International.

Compendium Code No.: 10930110 61813C/61815F

VET-KEM® SIPHOTROL® PLUS II PREMISE SPRAY

Wellmark **Flea Control & Premise Insecticide**

with Precor® Insect Growth Regulator (IGR)

EPA Reg. No.: 2724-490

Active Ingredient(s):

(S)-Methoprene (CAS #65733-16-6)	0.085%
Permethrin (CAS #52645-53-1)	0.350%
Phenothrin (CAS #26002-80-2)	0.300%
N-octyl bicycloheptene dicarboximide (CAS #113-48-4)	2.000%
Piperonyl butoxide (CAS #51-03-6)	1.400%
Other Ingredients*:	95.865%
Total	100.000%

* contains petroleum distillates

SIPHOTROL® II contains Precor® Insect Growth Regulator.

Indications: SIPHOTROL® Plus II Premise Spray (SIPHOTROL® Plus II) kills adult fleas, hatching flea eggs, and ticks. Precor®, the unique ingredient in SIPHOTROL® Plus II provides 30 weeks' protection by preventing eggs from ever developing into biting fleas. For best results, use SIPHOTROL® Plus II with VET-KEM® on-animal products for complete control of fleas and ticks.

100% knock down for adult fleas in 10 minutes. Kills both adult and immature fleas and ticks. Treats 2000 square feet. Leaves no lingering odor, no stains, no sticky mess. Prevents reinfestation and flea build-up for 30 weeks. Easy to apply water-based aerosol.

Directions for Use: It is a violation of Federal Law to use this product in a manner inconsistent with its labeling.

Read entire label before use.

Shake well before using.

For Use in the Home/Garage/Kennel:

1. Identify treatment areas, especially those where pets frequent, such as in and around pet's sleeping and resting areas. These are the primary areas where fleas, their eggs, and ticks are found. Before treatment, a test application should be made to upholstery, drapery, light-colored, delicate fabrics, or wood surfaces in an inconspicuous place.
2. Prepare treatment areas. All food processing surfaces and utensils should be covered during treatment or thoroughly washed after product use. Exposed food should be covered or removed. Remove pets and cover and unplug aquariums before spraying. Remove motor vehicles before using in garages. For best results with Surface/Carpet treatments, vacuum thoroughly before spraying and discard vacuum bag in outside trash. This product may also be used for infested surfaces inside motor vehicles.
3. Apply treatment. For flea/tick infestations, a single can treats 2000 square feet. Hold container upside down 2-3 feet from surface, point actuator towards the surface, and push button. Using a sweeping motion, apply a light uniform spray to all surfaces of furniture, rugs, carpets, drapes, and around all pet resting areas. Avoid thoroughly wetting surfaces. Mist treated areas only until "slightly damp". Do not over-treat. Reapply in 14 days, if necessary.

   Important: Only complete and proper application to carpets, upholstery, drapes, and other fabrics will provide thorough flea/tick elimination. Keep children and pets out of areas during treatment. Vacate room after treatment and before reoccupying, ventilate until surfaces are dry.
4. For best results, eliminate fleas/ticks on your pet with appropriate VET-KEM® on-animal products.

Contraindication(s): Not for use on humans or pets.

Precautionary Statements: Hazards to Humans and Domestic Animals - Caution: Avoid contact with skin or clothing. Wash thoroughly with soap and water after handling. Prolonged or frequently repeated skin contact may cause allergic reactions in some individuals.

First Aid:

If on Skin or Clothing: Take off contaminated clothing. Rinse skin immediately with plenty of water for 15-20 minutes. Call a poison control center or doctor for treatment advice.

If Swallowed: Call a poison control center or doctor immediately for treatment advice. Do not induce vomiting unless told to do so by a poison control center or doctor. Do not give any liquid to the person. Do not give anything by mouth to an unconscious person.

Note to Physician/Veterinarian: Contains petroleum distillates - vomiting may cause aspiration pneumonia.

In case of emergency, call 1-800-766-7661 or a poison control center. Have the product container or label with you when calling a poison control center or doctor or going for treatment.

Physical or Chemical Hazards: Contents under pressure. Do not use or store near heat or open flame. Do not puncture or incinerate container. Exposure to temperatures above 130°F may cause bursting.

Storage and Disposal:

Storage: Store in a cool dry area. Do not transport or store below 32°F.

Disposal: Place container in trash. Do not incinerate or puncture.

Warning(s): Keep out of reach of children.

Disclaimer: Seller makes no warranty, expressed or implied, concerning the use of this product other than indicated on the label. Buyer assumes all risk of use and handling of this material when such use and handling are contrary to label instructions.

Presentation: 16 oz (454 mL) can.

Precor® Insect Growth Regulator and VET-KEM® SIPHOTROL® Plus II Premise Spray are registered trademarks of Wellmark International.

Compendium Code No.: 10930170 60852

VET-KEM® SIPHOTROL® PLUS AREA TREATMENT FOR HOMES

Wellmark **Flea Control & Premise Insecticide**

EPA Reg. No.: 2724-483

Active Ingredient(s):

(S)-Methoprene (CAS #65733-16-6)	0.09%
Permethrin (CAS #52645-53-1)	0.50%
Other Ingredients:	99.41%
Total	100.00%

Contains Precor® Insect Growth Regulator (IGR) plus Permethrin, an adulticide.

Contains no CFC or other ozone-depleting substances. Federal regulations prohibit CFC propellants in aerosols.

Indications: Kills both adult and pre-adult fleas. Kills adult ticks. Stops flea eggs and larvae from developing for 30 weeks.

Directions for Use: It is a violation of Federal Law to use this product in a manner inconsistent with its labeling.

In the home, all food processing surfaces and utensils should be covered during treatment or thoroughly washed before use. Exposed food should be covered or removed.

Shake well before using.

A single can (16 oz) treats 2000 square feet.

Remove protective cap, hold container upside down and spray from a distance of 2 to 3 feet. Remove birds and cover and unplug aquariums before spraying.

Fleas (Adults and Larvae) and Ticks (Adults):

For Use in Home: For best results, pay special attention to areas your pets frequent.

Avoid thoroughly wetting the area that needs treating.

To kill adult fleas, flea larvae, and adult ticks in your home, hold container upside down 2 to 3 feet from surface, point actuator towards the surface, and push button.

For Surface/Carpet Spray: Vacuum thoroughly before spraying.

A test application should be made to upholstery or drapery fabrics in an inconspicuous place before use. Apply uniformly with a sweeping motion to rugs, carpets, drapes, and all surfaces of upholstered furniture. Treat surfaces uniformly from one end to the other. Only complete coverage of carpets, upholstery, drapes, and other fabrics will provide thorough flea/tick elimination.

For Use in Pet Areas: Pay special attention to areas where pets frequent, such as in and around sleeping and resting areas. Treat pet bedding and other pet resting areas as these are primary hiding areas for fleas/ticks. For best results, pets should be treated before they return to the treated areas.

Precautionary Statements: Hazards to Humans and Domestic Animals — Caution: Harmful if swallowed. May be absorbed through skin. Avoid inhalation of spray mist. Avoid contact with skin, eyes, or clothing. Wash thoroughly after handling and before smoking or eating. Avoid contamination of feed and foodstuffs. Remove pets and birds and cover and unplug aquariums before space spraying or surface applications. This product is not for use on humans. Vacate room after treatment and ventilate before reoccupying. Do not allow children or pets to contact treated areas until surfaces are dry.

First Aid:

If inhaled, remove affected person to fresh air. Apply artificial respiration if indicated.

If in eyes, flush with plenty of water. Contact a physician if irritation persists.

If on skin, wash affected area immediately with soap and water Get medical attention if irritation persists.

Physical or Chemical Hazards: Contents under pressure. Do not use or store near heat or open flame. Do not puncture or incinerate container. Exposure to temperatures above 130°F may cause bursting.

For information or in an emergency call 1-800-766-7661

Storage and Disposal: Store in a cool dry area. Do not transport or store below 32°F. Wrap container in several layers of newspaper and dispose of in trash. Do not incinerate or puncture.

Warning(s): Keep out of reach of children.

Disclaimer: Seller makes no warranty, expressed or implied, concerning the use of this product other than indicated on the label. Buyer assumes all risk of use and handling of this material when such use and handling are contrary to label instructions.

Presentation: 16 oz (454 g) can.

Precor® Insect Growth Regulator, SIPHOTROL® and VET-KEM® are registered trademarks of Wellmark International.

Compendium Code No.: 10930120 60802E

VET-KEM® SIPHOTROL® PLUS AREA TREATMENT PUMP SPRAY FOR HOMES

Wellmark **Flea Control & Premise Insecticide**

EPA Reg. No.: 2724-401

Active Ingredient(s):

(S)-Methoprene (CAS #65733-16-6)	0.01%
Permethrin (CAS #52645-53-1)	0.28%
Other Ingredients:	99.71%
Total	100.00%

Contains Precor® Insect Growth Regulator plus Permethrin, an adulticide.

Indications: SIPHOTROL® Plus Area Treatment Pump Spray for Homes contains a unique combination of ingredients that kills preadult fleas before they grow up to bite. It reaches fleas hidden in carpets, rugs, upholstery, and pet bedding; protects your home from flea build-up; pets and family from bites. One treatment gives continuous protection against pre-adult fleas for 7 months. Kills fleas, ticks, roaches, silverfish, earwigs, and ants. Leaves no bad smell, no sticky mess, no stains.

Directions for Use: It is a violation of Federal Law to use this product in a manner inconsistent with its labeling. Read entire label before each use. Shake well before using.

Fleas: For maximum effectiveness, treat entire carpeted area. Adjust spray nozzle to create a fine spray. Treat carpets, rugs, drapes, and all surfaces of upholstered furniture. Old pet bedding should be removed and replaced with clean fresh bedding after treatment of pet area. Retreat as necessary. Use in homes, garages, attics, apartments, and hotels. One bottle will treat a surface area equivalent to approximately three 10' x 10' rooms. Avoid wetting furniture and carpeting. A fine spray applied uniformly is all that is necessary to kill fleas. To kill ticks, roaches, silverfish, earwigs, and ants in the environment, apply directly to pests.

Contraindication(s): Do not spray on pets or humans.

Precautionary Statements: Hazards to Humans and Domestic Animals — Caution: Harmful if absorbed through the skin. Causes eye irritation. Avoid contact with skin, eyes, or clothing. Wash thoroughly after handling. Leave treated areas and do not return for at least 1 hour. Do not spray on pets or humans. Avoid contamination of food and foodstuffs. Do not use in edible product areas of food processing plants, restaurants, or other areas where food is commercially prepared, processed, or stored. Do not use in serving areas while food is exposed. Remove birds and cover aquariums before spraying.

First Aid:

If on skin, remove contaminated clothing and wash affected areas with soap and water. Get medical attention if irritation persists.

If in eyes, flush eyes with plenty of water. Get medical attention if irritation persists.

Physical or Chemical Hazards: Do not use or store near heat or open flame.

In case of emergency or for product use information, call 1-800-766-7661.

Storage and Disposal:

Storage: Store in original container away from children. Protect from freezing or high temperatures.

Disposal: Do not reuse empty container. Wrap and put in trash.

Warning(s): Keep out of reach of children.

Disclaimer: Seller makes no warranty, expressed or implied, concerning the use of this product other than indicated on the label. Buyer assumes all risk of use and handling of this material when such use and handling are contrary to label instructions.

Discussion: SIPHOTROL® Plus Area Treatment Pump Spray is designed for use on all fabrics and carpeting; however, some natural fibers (such as wool) and synthetics may be adversely affected by any liquid product. Always test a hidden area prior to use. Lighter colored carpets may show some soiling after treatment. To help avoid soiling carpets, allow product to dry completely before walking on treated areas. To protect pets against fleas outdoors, use a Vet-Kem flea and tick collar, pet spray, pet sponge-on, pet spot on, or pet shampoo.

Presentation: 24 fl oz (710 mL) (7 month protection).

Precor® Insect Growth Regulator, SIPHOTROL® Plus, and VET-KEM® are registered trademarks of Wellmark International.

Compendium Code No.: 10930130 63253/63255

VET-KEM® SIPHOTROL PLUS® FOGGER

Wellmark **Flea Control & Premise Insecticide**

EPA Reg. No.: 2724-454

Active Ingredient(s):

(S)-Methoprene (CAS #65733-16-6)	0.09%
Permethrin (52645-53-1	0.15%
Other Ingredients	99.33%
Total	100.00%

Indications: SIPHOTROL PLUS® Fogger kills adult fleas, hatching flea eggs, and ticks. Precor®, the ingredient in the SIPHOTROL PLUS® Fogger, provides 30 weeks protection by preventing eggs from ever developing into biting fleas. This product enables you to fill an entire room with insect-killing fog while you are away. For best results, use SIPHOTROL PLUS® Fogger together with other Vet-Kem® products for complete control of fleas and ticks.

Kills adult fleas and ticks. Stops hatching eggs and larvae from developing into adult fleas for 30 weeks. Prevents flea infestation and flea build-up for 30 weeks. Treats 6,000 cubic feet.

Directions for Use: It is a violation of Federal Law to use this product in a manner inconsistent with its labeling.

In the home, all food processing surfaces and utensils should be covered during treatment, or thoroughly washed before use. Exposed food should be covered or removed. Shake well before using.

1. Vacuum thoroughly before fogging. To ensure unobstructed flow of fogger mist, open inside doors and cabinets. Remove or cover exposed food, dishes, utensils, food preparation equipment, and surfaces. Remove pets and birds and remove or cover (and turn off) aquariums. Close outside doors and windows. Turn off all ignition sources such as pilot lights (shut off gas valves), other open flames, or running electrical appliances that cycle off and on (i.e., refrigerators, thermostats, etc.). Call your gas, utility or management company if you need assistance with your pilot lights.
2. Use one container for each 6000 cubic feet of area (a room 30' X 25' with an 8' ceiling). Do not use more than 1 fogger per room. Do not use in small enclosed spaces such as closets, cabinets, or under counters or tables. Do not use in a room 5' x 5' or smaller; instead, allow fog to enter from other rooms.
3. Remove all motor vehicles before fogging garage.
4. Elevate fogger by placing on stand or table covered by newspaper in center of room to be fogged. Newspapers should be spread on the floor for several feet around area of release.
5. Before activating, tilt can away from face (container sprays straight up). Press down firmly on edge of actuator tab until it locks into place.
6. After activating fogger, leave room or house at once. Keep treated area closed for at least 2 hours, then open all doors and windows and allow treated area to air for 1 hour before returning.
7. For best results, spot treat with a Vet-Kem® premise product under beds, furniture, or obstructed areas where fogger mist may not penetrate.

Precautionary Statements: Hazards to Humans and Domestic Animals:

Caution: Use only when area to be treated is vacated by humans and pets. Harmful if inhaled, swallowed, or absorbed through the skin. Avoid breathing vapors or spray mist. May cause eye irritation. Avoid contact with eyes, skin, and clothing. Wash thoroughly with soap and water after using. In case of contact, immediately flush eyes or skin with plenty of water. Obtain medical attention if irritation persists. Avoid contamination of food, foodstuffs, and food preparation areas. Leave room or house at once after activating fogger. If pet is exposed to wet surface, wash fur with soap and water.

First Aid:

If Swallowed: Call a physician/veterinarian or Poison Control Center immediately. Do not induce vomiting.

Note to Physician/Veterinarian: May present aspiration hazard.

If Inhaled: Remove individual to fresh air. If not breathing, give artificial respiration, preferably mouth to mouth. Get medical attention.

If on Skin: Remove contaminated clothing and wash affected areas with soap and water. Get medical attention if irritation persists.

If in Eyes: Flush eyes with plenty of water. Obtain medical attention if irritation persists. Contact veterinarian if pets are exposed during application.

Physical or Chemical Hazards: Extremely Flammable. Contents under pressure. Keep away from heat, sparks, and open flame. Do not puncture or incinerate container. Exposure to temperatures above 130°F may cause bursting. This product contains a highly flammable ingredient. It may cause a fire or explosion if not used properly. Follow the "Directions for Use" on this label very carefully.

Storage and Disposal: Storage: Store in a cool, dry area away from heat or open flame.

V

Disposal: Do Not Puncture or Incinerate! If empty: Place in trash or offer for recycling if available. If partly filled: Call your local solid waste agency or 1-800-CLEANUP for disposal instructions.

Warning(s): Keep out of reach of children.

Disclaimer: Seller makes no warranty, expressed or implied, concerning the use of this product other than indicated on the label. Buyer assumes all risk of use and handling of this material when such use and handling are contrary to label instructions.

Presentation: 6 oz aerosol spray.

Precor® Insect Growth Regulator and VET-KEM® SIPHOTROL PLUS® Fogger are registered trademarks of Wellmark International.

Compendium Code No.: 10930180 April, 2002

VET-KEM® TICKAWAY™ TICK COLLAR FOR DOGS

Wellmark **Parasiticide Collar**

EPA Reg. No.: 2724-254

Active Ingredient(s):

Propoxur (CAS #114-26-1)	10%
Other Ingredients:	90%
Total	100%

Indications: Kills tick up to 5 months. Kills Lyme disease and Rocky Mountain Spotted Fever carrying ticks. Kills fleas up to 5 months. One size fits all.

Directions for Use: It is a violation of Federal Law to use this product in a manner inconsistent with its labeling.

Read entire label before each use.

Use only on dogs.

1. Buckle collar around dog's neck. Fit collar snug enough to prevent placement of the dog's leg or lower jaw through the collar, yet loose enough to be rotated about the neck. Generally, 2 or 3 fingers should fit between the collar and dog's neck.
2. Leave 2 to 3 extra inches on the collar for adjustment; cut off excess length and dispose of in trash.
3. Check periodically and adjust fit if necessary, especially when puppies are rapidly growing.
4. May be used in addition to regular collar. Replace collar when effectiveness diminishes.

Contraindication(s): Do not use on puppies under 12 weeks of age.

Precautionary Statements: Hazards to Humans and Domestic Animals - Caution: Do not get dust or collar in mouth, harmful if swallowed. Do not get dust in eyes, will cause temporary pupillary constriction.* The dust released by this collar is a cholinesterase inhibitor.

Humans: Do not open package until ready to use. Do not allow children to handle this collar. Dust will form on this collar during storage. Wash hands thoroughly with soap and water after handling collar.

Animals: Consult a veterinarian before using this product on debilitated, aged, medicated, pregnant, or nursing dogs. Do not use on puppies under 12 weeks of age. Do not use this product on dogs simultaneously or within 30 days before or after treatment with or exposure to cholinesterase inhibiting drugs, pesticides, or chemicals. However, flea and tick collars may be immediately replaced. When collar is first worn, observe neck area every few days for irritation. Remove collar at the first sign of irritation or adverse reaction. Sensitivities may occur after using any pesticide product for pets. If signs of sensitivity occur, remove collar and bathe your pet with mild soap and rinse with large amounts of water.

First Aid:

If Swallowed, call physician, veterinarian, or Poison Control Center. Drink 1 or 2 glasses of water and induce vomiting by touching back of throat with finger. If person is unconscious, do not give anything by mouth and do not induce vomiting.

If in Eyes, flush eyes with plenty of water. Get medical attention if irritation persists.

Note to Physician/Veterinarian: *Atropine and *homatropine are antidotal only if symptoms of cholinesterase inhibition are present.

In case of emergency or for product use information, call 1-800-766-7661.

Storage and Disposal: Store in original unopened container away from children. Do not reuse container or reuse collar. Wrap and put in trash.

Warning(s): Do not allow children to play with this collar.

Disclaimer: Seller makes no warranty, expressed or implied, concerning the use of this product other than indicated on the label. Buyer assumes all risk of use and handling of this material when such use and handling are contrary to label instructions.

Discussion: What to Expect:

For Ticks:

1. Ticks are tougher to kill than fleas and are killed more slowly.
2. Full protection against adult and immature ticks will be achieved within a few days, providing continuous protection for up to 5 months.
3. Adult ticks will be killed over the entire pet. Dead ticks will fall off or may be easily removed.
4. Replace collar every 5 months for continuous protection from ticks. If your dog goes swimming or is out in the rain, it is not necessary to remove the collar. The continuous action collar will rapidly replace any tick and flea killing material removed.

For Fleas:

1. This VET-KEM® collar is designed to kill adult fleas.
2. This collar starts killing fleas as soon as it is placed around dog's neck.
3. Protection against fleas will be achieved within a few days, providing continuous protection for up to 5 months.
4. Replace collar every 5 months to help control flea infestations on your pet.

Presentation: 1.2 oz (34 g) collar.

VET-KEM® and TICKAWAY™ are trademarks of Wellmark International.

Compendium Code No.: 10930160 46557

VET-KEM® TRIPLE ACTION FLEA & TICK SHAMPOO FOR DOGS, CATS, & HORSES

Wellmark **Parasiticide Shampoo**

EPA Est. No.: 68688-32-2724

Active Ingredient(s):

Pyrethrins	0.15%
Piperonyl Butoxide, Technical*	1.00%
N-octyl bicycloheptene dicarboximide	0.50%
Di-n-propyl isocinchomeronate	0.50%
Other Ingredients	97.85%
Total	100.00%

*Equivalent to 0.80% of (butylcarbityl)(6-propylpiperonyl) ether and 0.20% related compounds.

Contains aloe, coconut extract, and lanolin.

Indications: A concentrated lathering shampoo enriched with aloe, coconut extract, and lanolin. Removes loose dandruff, dirt, and scales. Leaves coat soft and shining.

Kills fleas, ticks and lice.

Repels gnats, flies and mosquitoes for 2 to 3 days.

Controls stable flies, horse flies, deer flies, face flies, gnats and mosquitoes on horses and foals.

Directions for Use: It is a violation of Federal Law to use this product in a manner inconsistent with its labeling.

Read entire label before each use. Use only on dogs, puppies, cats, kittens, horses and foals.

May be used full strength or diluted with 2 parts water. Thoroughly soak animal with warm water taking 2 to 3 minutes to wet hair. Do not apply shampoo around eyes. Apply shampoo on head and ears, then lather. Repeat procedure with neck, chest, middle and hind quarters, finishing legs last. Let animal stand 3 to 5 minutes (this is an important part of the grooming procedure), then rinse animal thoroughly, In extremely dirty or scaly animals, the above procedure may be repeated. May be used every 7 to 10 days. Do not use on puppies or kittens under 12 weeks old.

Horses and Foals (Horses and foals not for slaughter): Follow above procedure. Repeat treatment as necessary.

Consult a veterinarian before using this product on debilitated, aged, pregnant or nursing animals, or animals on medication.

Contraindication(s): Do not use on puppies or kittens under 12 weeks old.

Precautionary Statements: Hazards to Humans and Domestic Animals — Warning:

Humans: Causes eye and skin irritation. Do not get in eyes or on skin or on clothing. Harmful if swallowed. Wash thoroughly with soap and water after handling. Remove contaminated clothing and wash before reuse.

Animals: Do not use on pets and foals less than 12 weeks old. Sensitivities may occur after using any pesticide product for pets. If signs occur, bathe your pet with mild soap and rinse with large amounts of water. If signs continue, consult a veterinarian immediately.

First Aid:

If in eyes, hold eyelids open and flush with a steady, gentle stream of water for 15 minutes. Get medical attention.

If swallowed, drink promptly a large quantity of milk, egg whites, gelatin solution, or if these are not available, drink large quantities of water. Avoid alcohol.

If on skin, wash with plenty of soap and water. Get medical attention if irritation persists.

Environmental Hazards: This product is toxic to fish. Keep out of lakes, streams, ponds, tidal marshes, and estuaries Do not wash animals where runoff is likely to occur.

In case of emergency or for product use information, call 1-800-766-7861.

Storage and Disposal:

Storage - Store in a cool area.

Disposal - Do not reuse container. Wrap and put in trash.

Warning(s): Not for use on horses and foals intended for slaughter.

Keep out of reach of children.

Disclaimer: Seller makes no warranty, expressed or implied, concerning the use of this product other than indicated on the label. Buyer assumes all risk of use and handling of this material when such use and handling are contrary to label instructions.

Presentation: 12 fl oz (355 mL) and 1 gallon.

VET-KEM® is a registered trademark of Wellmark International.

Compendium Code No.: 10930141 05453G

VET LUBE

Phoenix Pharmaceutical **Lubricant**

All Purpose Non-Spermicidal Lubricating Jelly

Ingredient(s): Purified Water, Propylene Glycol, Sodium Carboxymethylcellulose, Methyl and Propyl Parahydroxybenzoate.

Indications: A virtually non-toxic formula which minimizes irritation to the skin of the operator and the delicate mucous membranes of the animal.

Directions: For coating hands, arms, instruments and subject areas in performing gynecological procedures and rectal examinations. Apply liberally immediately before use.

Precaution(s): Storage: Store at controlled room temperature between 15°-30°C (59°-86°F). Keep container tightly closed when not in use.

Caution(s): For animal use only.

Warning(s): Keep out of reach of children.

Presentation: 1 gallon (3.785 L) containers (NDC 57319-454-09).

Manufactured by: First Priority, Inc., Elgin, IL 60123.

Compendium Code No.: 12560882 Rev. 01-02

VETRACHLORACIN® OPHTHALMIC OINTMENT ℞

Pharmaderm **Ophthalmic Antibiotic**

Chloramphenicol 1%

NADA No.: 065-460

Active Ingredient(s): Each gram contains chloramphenicol 10 mg, in a light mineral oil, white petrolatum, polyoxyethylene sorbitan monostearate base.

Indications: Chloramphenicol Veterinary Ophthalmic Ointment 1% is appropriate for use in dogs and cats for the topical treatment of bacterial conjunctivitis caused by pathogens susceptible to chloramphenicol.

Pharmacology: Actions: Chloramphenicol is a broad-spectrum antibiotic providing rapid clinical response and having therapeutic activity against susceptible strains of a number of gram-positive and gram-negative organisms including *Escherichia coli, Staphylococcus aureus* and *Streptococcus hemolyticus.*

Dosage and Administration: Application of the ointment should be preceded by cleansing to remove discharge and crusts. The ointment is applied every three hours around the clock for 48 hours, after which night instillations may be omitted. A small amount of ointment should be placed in the lower conjunctival sac. Treatment should be continued for two days after the eye appears normal. Therapy for cats should not exceed 7 days.

Contraindication(s): Chloramphenicol products must not be used in meat, egg or milk-producing animals. The length of time that residues persist in milk or tissues has not been determined.

Precaution(s): Store at room temperature.

Caution(s): Federal law restricts this drug to use by or on the order of a licensed veterinarian.

Most susceptible bacteria will respond to chloramphenicol therapy in a few days. If improvement is not noted in this period of time, a change of therapy should be considered.

When infection is suspected as the cause of a disease process, especially in purulent or catarrhal conjunctivitis, attempts should be made to determine through susceptibility testing, which antibiotics will be effective prior to applying ophthalmic preparations.

Warning(s): Not for use in animals which are raised for food production. Prolonged use in cats may produce blood dyscrasias.

For veterinary use only.

Presentation: 3.5 g (⅛ oz) sterile tamper proof tubes.

Compendium Code No.: 10880040

VetRED® CANINE HEARTWORM ANTIGEN TEST KIT

Synbiotics **Heartworm Test**

U.S. Vet. Lic. No.: 312

Description: Rapid whole blood assay for the routine detection of canine heartworm antigen.

Components: Each kit contains:

A two well agglutination slides with detachable blood sample well	25
B card slide holders	3
C pipette tips	25
D dropper bottle negative control reagent (green cap)	1 vial 1.1 mL
E dropper bottle test reagent (black cap)	1 vial 0.9 mL
F dropper bottle positive control reagent (red cap)	1 vial 0.7 mL
G stirrers	25

Additional VetRED® equipment required and supplied separately:

H 10 microliter (uL) fixed volume micropipette

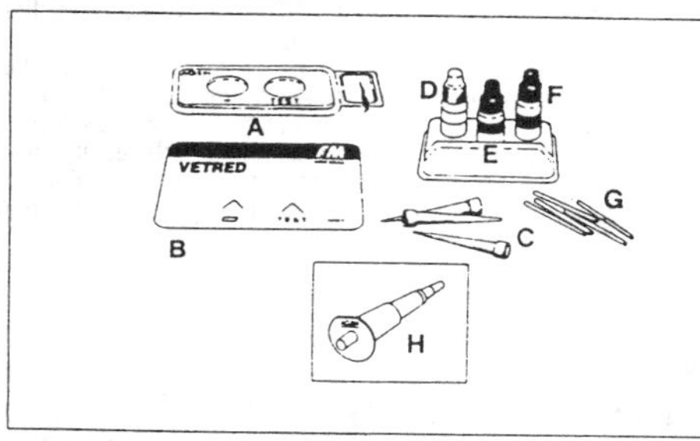

Indications: VetRED® Canine Heartworm Antigen Test is recommended for the routine diagnostic screening of dogs for heartworm infection status (positive or negative) or to positively confirm a diagnosis when clinical history and/or clinical signs suggest heartworm disease. The performance of the VetRED® Canine Heartworm Antigen Test is independent of circulating microfilariae and can be used to detect amicrofilaraemic infections. This test can also be used to monitor treatment response to adulticide therapy.

Test Principles: VetRED® Canine Heartworm Antigen Test is a canine red blood cell agglutination test that is both rapid and simple to perform. The test reagent is made by chemically combining two different monoclonal antibodies to make a single bifunctional antibody. When this reagent is mixed with dog whole blood, part of the bifunctional antibody binds to dog red blood cells and the other part is free to bind to soluble adult *Dirofilaria immitis* antigen. If a diagnostic level of adult *D immitis* antigen is present in the blood sample, the red blood cells will agglutinate in a clearly visible manner.

Test Procedure: Specimen Information: The test should be performed on fresh whole blood without anticoagulant. If any delay between sample collection and testing is necessary, either heparin or EDTA anticoagulant may be used. Anticoagulated whole blood samples should be stored at 2°-7°C (35°-45°F). Samples should be tested as soon as possible and within 48 hours of collection. Blood stored for more than 48 hours or hemolyzed whole blood samples should not be used.

1. Blood Collection: Collect blood sample with a sterile needle and syringe. If performing test immediately, tear off blood collection well from two well agglutination slide and dispense blood into the well. If test is to be delayed, dispense blood into a heparin or EDTA collection tube and store at 2°-7°C (35°-45°F).
2. Dispensing Blood: Place the clean agglutination slide in card slide holder. Put a clean pipette tip firmly onto the micropipette and dispense one pipette full (10 uL) of blood into both wells of the agglutination slides. Stored blood should be mixed well before dispensing.
3. Dispensing Negative Control: Take the Green Capped bottle of negative control, remove the cap, wipe tip dry with a clean tissue, hold the bottle vertically and dispense one drop of reagent into the (—) well. Immediately replace the Green Cap.
4. Dispensing Test Reagent: Take the Black Capped bottle of test reagent, remove cap, wipe tip dry with a clean tissue, hold the bottle vertically and dispense one drop of reagent into the Test well and immediately replace the Black Cap.
5. Mixing Reagents: Take a clean stirrer, stir and spread the contents thoroughly over the entire surface of the (—) well for 4-5 seconds. Using the same stirrer repeat the procedure for the Test well. Always stir the (—) well first.
6. Developing Test: Immediately commence rocking the slide continuously for 2 minutes ensuring a swirling motion occurs to the contents of both wells. Do not splash or mix contents from one well to another.
7. Reading Test: At 2 minutes, stop rocking the slide and check for any agglutination by comparing the Test well with the (—) well. Do not mix or read test beyond 2 minutes.
8. Positive Control Test Validation: If no agglutination is observed in the Test well, take the Red Capped bottle of positive control, remove cap, wipe tip dry with a clean tissue, hold the bottle vertically and dispense one drop of reagent into the Test well only. Immediately replace the Red Cap and recommence rocking slide. Agglutination will occur within 30 seconds, validating kit components and correct test procedure.

Interpretation of Results: The presence of heartworm antigen from adult worms is indicated when the Test well shows any agglutination when compared to the negative control well (-well).

The Test well agglutination reaction depends on the amount of heartworm antigen present in the blood. A test result should be interpreted in the context of all available clinical information and history for the particular dog being tested.

In any heartworm area, some dogs may be infected with very low numbers of worms. In cases where infection consists of immature worms or 1-2 adult worms, the amount of antigen in the blood may be undetectable. Low worm number infections can have high microfilarial counts but undetectable levels of heartworm antigen in the blood.

Note: Correct assay procedure and satisfactory performance of the kit components are indicated by agglutination of the Test well after the addition of the positive control reagent. Occasionally a second drop of positive control reagent may have to be added to cause agglutination of the Test well. Agglutination of the (—) well invalidates the test result.

Storage: Store test kit reagents at 2°-7°C (35°-45°F). Do not freeze.

Do not use the kit after the expiration date which is stated on the package label.

Contraindications: The test cannot be used on feline whole blood samples.

Caution(s):

1. VetRED® should only be used with canine whole blood samples. Hemolyzed blood or blood stored for more than 48 hours should not be used.
2. The micropipette is reusable and should be retained for subsequent VetRED® Kits. All other kit components are disposable and should not be reused.
3. Use a separate sterile disposable syringe and needle for each blood collection prior to testing.
4. Allow stored blood and test reagents to come to room temperature and ensure the stored blood is thoroughly mixed prior to use.
5. Do not touch the wells with the fingers or contaminate them with other materials.
6. Prior to use, dropper bottle tips must be wiped dry with a separate, clean tissue and dropper bottles must be held vertically to dispense reagent volumes accurately. Do not shake dropper bottles or touch dropper tips to the contents of any well.
7. Immediately replace color coded caps on their respective color coded bottles after use. Do not mix color coded caps on bottles.
8. Do not use expired kits.
9. For veterinary use only.

Discussion: Life Cycle: Heartworm disease in dogs has a worldwide distribution and is caused by the filarial nematode *D immitis.* Adult *D immitis* worms are found in the right ventricle and pulmonary arteries of infected dogs. The adult female worm produces first stage larvae (microfilariae) which can circulate in the peripheral blood. When ingested by a suitable mosquito vector while taking a blood meal, these microfilariae undergo development to become infective third stage larvae. When these larvae are transferred to other dogs during feeding by these infected mosquitoes, they undergo further development for approximately 70-80 days. After this time immature adults begin to migrate to the distal pulmonary arteries and eventually grow to occupy the main pulmonary artery. Some 6-8 months after infection by the third stage larvae, the parasites will have matured. Secreted adult heartworm antigen, as well as microfilariae, may then be found in the peripheral blood.

Presentation: One kit (to process 25 samples).

VetRED® is a registered trademark of Agen Biomedical Limited.

USA Pat. No. 5,086,002

Compendium Code No.: 11150420

VETRIN™ CANINE PAIN RELIEF TABLETS

Farnam **Non-Steroidal Anti-Inflammatory**

Canine Aspirin Arthritis Pain Relief

Active Ingredient(s): Each tablet contains either:

Aspirin . . . . 100 mg

Aspirin . . . . 325 mg

Ingredients: Aspirin, Natural Roast Beef and Liver Flavors, Stearic Acid and Magnesium Stearate. Contains no artificial flavors or colors.

VETRIN™ is manufactured in compliance with the Food and Drug Administration's Current Good Manufacturing Procedures.

Indications: For use in relief of pain, fever and inflammation, particularly as associated with arthritis and joint problems.

VETRIN™ is a chewable tablet with a highly palatable flavor base used in the care of arthritic dogs. Aids in temporary relief of pain, fever and inflammation.

Dosage and Administration: Recommended Dosage: 8-12 mg per 1 pound of body weight every 12 hours.

100 mg: Approximately 1 tablet per 8-12 lbs of body weight every 12 hours.

325 mg: Approximately 1 tablet per 30-40 lbs of body weight every 12 hours.

Contraindication(s): Not for use in cats.

Precaution(s): Store at room temperature.

Caution(s): If vomiting or diarrhea occur, stop administration and consult your veterinarian. If symptoms persist more than three days, discontinue use and contact your veterinarian. In case of accidental overdose, contact a health professional immediately.

For use in dogs only.

Warning(s): Keep out of reach of children and pets.

Presentation: 100 mg: Bottles of 100 Snap 'N Chew Tablets (Toy and Small Breeds) (NDC 61731-726-01).
325 mg: Bottles of 100 Snap 'N Chew Tablets (Large and Giant Breeds) (NDC 61731-724-01).

Compendium Code No.: 10000970 0AA0

VETRO-BIOTIC® OINTMENT ℞

Pharmaderm **Topical Antibiotic**

(Neomycin and Polymyxin B Sulfate and Bacitracin Zinc Ointment USP)-Topical First Aid Antibiotic for Cats and Dogs

Active Ingredient(s): Each gram contains: neomycin sulfate 5 mg equivalent to 3.5 mg of neomycin base, polymyxin B sulfate equal to 5,000 polymyxin B units, and bacitracin zinc equal to 400 bacitracin units in a base of white petrolatum.

Indications: First aid to prevent infection in minor cuts, scrapes and burns in cats and dogs.

Directions: Clean the affected area. Apply a small amount of this product (an amount equal to the surface area of the tip of a finger) on the area 1 to 3 times daily.

Precaution(s): Store at room temperature.

Caution(s): Federal law restricts this drug to use by or on the order of a licensed veterinarian.

Warning(s): For external use only. Do not use in the eyes or apply over large areas of the body. In case of deep or puncture wounds, animal bites, or serious burns, consult your veterinarian. Stop use and consult your veterinarian if the condition persists or gets worse, or if a rash or other allergic reaction develops. Do not use longer than one week unless directed by your veterinarian. Keep this and all drugs out of the reach of children. In case of accidental ingestion, seek professional assistance or contact a Poison control Center immediately.

Presentation: 1 oz or 30 gram tubes.

Compendium Code No.: 10880050 R3/00

VETRO-CORT® LOTION ℞

Pharmaderm **Topical Corticosteroid**

1% Hydrocortisone Lotion-Anti-inflammatory/Antipruritic

Active Ingredient(s): Each mL contains 10 mg of hydrocortisone in a vehicle consisting of carbomer 940, propylene glycol, polysorbate 40, propylene glycol stearate, cholesterol and related sterols, isopropyl myristate, sorbitan palmitate, cetyl alcohol, triethanolamine, sorbic acid, simethicone and purified water.

Indications: For the temporary relief of itching associated with minor skin irritations, inflammation and rashes due to eczema, insect bites, *tick bites, poison ivy, poison oak, or poison sumac, soaps, detergents, seborrheic dermatitis, psoriasis.

Directions: Shake well before using. Apply to affected area not more than 3 to 4 times daily.

Precaution(s): Store at room temperature.

Caution(s): Federal law restricts this drug to use by or on the order of a licensed veterinarian.

*Rashes associated with tick bites can be an indicator of Lyme disease or other tick-transmitted diseases. If rash appears, consult a veterinarian.

For external use only. Do not use in the eyes or nose. Not for prolonged use. Do not apply to large areas of the body. Do not use where infection (pus) is present, since the drug may allow infection to be spread. If redness, irritation, or swelling persists or increases, discontinue use and consult your veterinarian.

In case of accidental ingestion, seek professional assistance or contact a Poison Control Center immediately.

Warning(s): For animal use only.

Not for use on animals intended as food.

Keep this and all drugs out of the reach of children.

Presentation: 118 mL (4 fl oz).

Compendium Code No.: 10880060

VETROLIN® BATH

Equicare **Grooming Shampoo**

Ingredient(s): Shampoo formula, conditioners, PABA sunscreen, fragrance.

Indications: Concentrated conditioning shampoo for horses. It may also be used on dogs.

Directions for Use: Mix 2-4 oz of VETROLIN® Bath in a pail of water. Wet horse's coat thoroughly and lather entire body. Let stand for 3 minutes. Rinse.

For sheen, follow with Vetrolin® Shine.

Warning(s): Keep away from eyes.

Presentation: 946 mL (32 fl oz) and 64 fl oz.

Compendium Code No.: 14470191

VETROLIN® LINIMENT

Equicare **Counterirritant**

Active Ingredient(s): Alcohol (64%), green soap, camphor, methyl salicylate, oils of cedarwood, sassafras, spike, thyme and rosemary.

Indications: VETROLIN® is an aromatic camphor and soap analgesic concentrate to be used as a counter-irritant aid in the temporary relief of minor stiff and sore muscles caused by overexertion.

Dosage and Administration: Recommended Dilutions:

1. Body Wash: Dilute one (1) ounce with one (1) quart of warm water.
2. Brace: Dilute four (4) ounces with one (1) quart of warm water. Apply freely and rub briskly.

May be used full strength.

Precaution(s): Cap tightly between uses.

Caution(s): Do not apply to irritated skin or if excessive irritation develops. Avoid contact with the eyes or mucous membranes.

For external use only.

Flammable liquid.

Warning(s): Not to be used on horses intended for food.

Keep out of the reach of children.

Presentation: 32 oz and 1 gallon (128 fl oz/3.785 L).

Compendium Code No.: 14470201

VETROLIN® SHINE

Equicare **Grooming Spray**

Ingredient(s): Conditioners, vitamins, PABA sunscreen, fragrance.

Indications: Sheen and conditioner for horses.

Directions for Use: After shampooing, remove excess water. Spray a fine mist over entire horse. Brush in direction of hair growth.

For best results, bathe your horse with Vetrolin® Bath conditioning shampoo before applying VETROLIN® Shine.

Warning(s): Keep away from eyes.

Presentation: 32 fl oz with sprayer and 64 fl oz (1.89 L).

Compendium Code No.: 14470211

VETROPOLYCIN® HC OPHTHALMIC OINTMENT ℞

Pharmaderm **Ophthalmic Antimicrobial-Corticosteroid**

Bacitracin-Neomycin-Polymyxin with Hydrocortisone Acetate 1% Veterinary Ophthalmic Ointment

NADA No.: 065-015

Active Ingredient(s): Each gram contains bacitracin zinc 400 units, neomycin sulfate 5 mg (equivalent to 3.5 mg of neomycin base), polymyxin B sulfate 10,000 units, hydrocortisone acetate 10 mg (1%), in a base of white petrolatum and mineral oil.

Indications: It may be used in acute or chronic conjunctivitis, when caused by organisms susceptible to the antibiotics contained in this ointment. Laboratory tests should be conducted including *in vitro* culturing and susceptibility tests on samples collected prior to treatment.

Pharmacology: Actions: The overlapping spectra of these three antibiotics provide effective bactericidal action against most commonly occurring gram-positive and gram-negative bacteria associated with infections of the eyes. The range of bactericidal activity encompasses many bacteria which are, or have become, resistant to other antibiotics, notably Pseudomonas and Staphylococcus. In susceptible organisms, resistance rarely develops, even on repeated or prolonged usage. Hydrocortisone acetate exerts a marked anti-inflammatory action at the tissue level and effectively suppresses inflammation in many disorders of the anterior segment of the eye. Local application to the eye often gives rapid relief of pain and photophobia, particularly in lesions of the cornea.

The combined anti-inflammatory and antimicrobial activity of VETROPOLYCIN® HC (Bacitracin-Neomycin-Polymyxin-Hydrocortisone Acetate 1%) Veterinary Ophthalmic Ointment permits effective management of many disorders of the anterior segment of the eye in which combined activity is needed.

Dosage and Administration: Apply a thin film over the cornea three or four times daily. The area to be treated should be properly cleansed prior to use. Foreign bodies, crusted exudates and debris should be carefully removed. Insert the tip of the tube beneath the lower lid and express a small quantity of the ointment into the conjunctival sac in dogs and cats.

Contraindication(s): Ophthalmic preparations containing corticosteroids are contraindicated in the treatment of those deep, ulcerative lesions of the cornea where the inner layer (endothelium) is involved, in fungal infections and in the presence of viral infections.

Precaution(s): Store at room temperature.

Caution(s): Federal law restricts this drug to use by or on the order of a licensed veterinarian.

Sensitivity to this ophthalmic ointment is rare, however, if a reaction occurs, discontinue use of the preparation.

The prolonged use of antibiotic-containing preparations may result in overgrowth of nonsusceptible organisms including fungi. Appropriate measures should be taken if this occurs. If infection does not respond to treatment in two or three days, the diagnosis and therapy should be reevaluated. Animals under treatment with this product should be observed for usual signs of corticosteroid overdose which include polydipsia, polyuria and occasionally an increase in weight.

Use of corticosteroids, depending on dose, duration, and specific steroid, may result in inhibition of endogenous steroid production following drug withdrawal. In patients presently receiving or recently withdrawn from systemic corticosteroid treatments, therapy with a rapidly acting corticosteroid should be considered in unusually stressful situations. Care should be taken not to contaminate the applicator tip during administration of the preparation.

Warning(s): All topical ophthalmic preparations containing corticosteroids with or without an antimicrobial agent, are contraindicated in the initial treatment of corneal ulcers. They should not be used until the infection is under control and corneal regeneration is well under way. Clinical and experimental data have demonstrated that corticosteroids administered orally or by injection to animals may induce the first stage of parturition if used during the last trimester of pregnancy and may precipitate premature parturition followed by dystocia, fetal death, retained placenta, and metritis.

Additionally corticosteroids administered to dogs, rabbits, and rodents during pregnancy have resulted in cleft palate in offspring. Corticosteroids administered to dogs during pregnancy have also resulted in other congenital anomalies, including deformed forelegs, phocomelia, and anasarca.

Adverse Reactions: Itching, burning or inflammation may occur in animals sensitive to the product. Discontinue use in such cases.

SAP and SGPT (ALT) enzyme elevations, polydypsia and polyuria have occurred following parenteral or systemic use of synthetic corticosteroids in dogs. Vomiting and diarrhea (occasionally bloody) have been observed in dogs.

Cushings syndrome in dogs has been reported in association with prolonged or repeated steroid therapy.

Presentation: 3.5 g (⅛ oz) sterile tamper proof tubes.

Compendium Code No.: 10880070

VETROPOLYCIN® OPHTHALMIC OINTMENT ℞

Pharmaderm **Ophthalmic Antibiotic**

Bacitracin-Neomycin-Polymyxin Veterinary Ophthalmic Ointment

NADA No.: 065-016

Active Ingredient(s): Each gram contains bacitracin zinc 400 units, neomycin sulfate 5 mg (equivalent to 3.5 mg of neomycin base), polymyxin B sulfate 10,000 units, in a base of white petrolatum and mineral oil.

Indications: In the treatment of superficial bacterial infections of the eyelid and conjunctiva in dogs and cats when due to organisms susceptible to the antibiotics contained in the ointment. Laboratory tests should be conducted including *in vitro* culturing and susceptibility tests on samples collected prior to treatment.

Pharmacology: Actions: The three antibiotics present in VETROPOLYCIN® (Bacitracin-Neomycin-Polymyxin) Veterinary Ophthalmic Ointment provide a broad spectrum of activity against the gram-positive and gram-negative bacteria commonly involved in superficial infections of the eyelid and conjunctiva. Bacitracin is effective against gram-positive bacteria including hemolytic and non-hemolytic Streptococci and Staphylococci. Resistant strains rarely develop. Neomycin is effective against both gram-positive and gram-negative bacteria including Staphylococci, *Escherichia coli* and *Haemophilus influenza* and many strains of Proteus and Pseudomonas. Polymyxin B is bactericidal to gram-negative bacteria especially Pseudomonas. No resistant strains have been found to develop *in vivo*.

Dosage and Administration: Apply a thin film over the cornea three or four times daily in dogs and cats. The area should be properly cleansed prior to the use of VETROPOLYCIN® (Bacitracin-Neomycin-Polymyxin) Veterinary Ophthalmic Ointment. Foreign bodies, crusted exudates, and debris should be carefully removed.

Precaution(s): Store at room temperature.

Caution(s): Federal law restricts this drug to use by or on the order of a licensed veterinarian.

Sensitivity to VETROPOLYCIN® (Bacitracin-Neomycin-Polymyxin) Veterinary Ophthalmic Ointment is rare; however, if a reaction occurs, discontinue use of the preparation. As with any antibiotic preparation, prolonged use may result in the overgrowth of nonsusceptible organisms including fungi. Appropriate measures should be taken if this occurs. If infection does not respond to treatment in two or three days, the diagnosis and therapy should be re-evaluated.

Care should be taken not to contaminate the applicator tip of the tube during application of the preparation. Do not allow the applicator tip to come in contact with any tissue.

Do not use this product as a pre-surgical ocular lubricant. Adverse reactions of ocular irritation and corneal ulceration have been reported in association with such use.

Adverse Reactions: Itching, burning or inflammation may occur in animals sensitive to the product. Discontinue use in such cases.

Presentation: 3.5 g (⅛ oz) sterile tamper proof tubes.

Compendium Code No.: 10880080

VETR$_x$™ CAGED BIRD REMEDY

Goodwinol **Respiratory Product**

Active Ingredient(s): Made with 3.3% (v-v) alcohol U.S.P. The mixture contains Canada balsam, camphor, oil origanum, oil rosemary, blended in a corn oil base.

Indications: For use as an aid in the treatment of respiratory problems of caged birds and for the gentle treatment of scaly-face and scaly-leg mite problems.

Recommended for canaries, parakeets (budgies), love birds, parrots, cockatiels, finches, macaws.

For internal and external applications.

Dosage and Administration:

Treatment of Respiratory Problems: Respiratory conditions in birds are of a complicated nature, and no one product can prove effective in all instances.

Make certain that the cage is clean, warm and dry.

Before use, VETR$_x$™ should be warmed. To warm, loosen the cap, place the bottle in a pan of warm water. When all of the ingredients are dispersed, shake well.

Mix one (1) teaspoonful of warm VETR$_x$™ into one-half (½) cup of warm water. VETR$_x$™ mixes with warm water, and floats on top of cold water.

With an eye dropper drip two (2) drops of diluted solution into the nostrils. Do this twice a day for four (4) days. If this is difficult to perform, then, in its place, using the fingers, rub two (2) drops full strength under the wings. Do this twice a day for four (4) days. The body heat of the bird will vaporize VETR$_x$™, and the bird will inhale the vapors.

Put three (3) drops of the solution down the throat of the bird at night. Continue for four (4) days.

Add two (2) drops (full strength from bottle) into clean drinking water once a day for five (5) days. Globules may rise to the top, they contain medication, and birds will often pick at it.

Preventive Therapy: Keeping a bird healthy before sickness strikes is the owner's responsibility. Keep birds away from drafts and excessive cold or heat. Sudden drops in temperature can be a source of danger. All varieties of caged birds have sensitive respiratory systems. What begins as a minor cold or sniffles can evolve into a life threatening condition. Never position the cage close to windows, doors, heating ducts, fans, or air conditions.

Make certain that the cage is clean and dry at all times, with clean litter on the floor. Try to change the drinking water often, and keep it at a moderate temperature.

VETR$_x$™ can help prevent sickness. Sprinkle a few drops of warm VETR$_x$™ in the litter every five (5) days.

Mix three (3) drops of warm VETR$_x$™ in the drinking water each time it is changed.

Once a week, rub two (2) to three (3) drops of warm VETR$_x$™ under the bird's wing. Body heat will cause the aromatic oils in VETR$_x$™ to vaporize into a medicinal vapor that will help keep nasal passages clear.

VETR$_x$™ does not stain, and will not harm feathers or wings.

Treatment:

Scaly-legs and feet : Use VETR$_x$™, at room temperature, directly from the bottle. Using a cotton swab, apply to scaly areas. Rub in well with a swab or fingers. Do this every day, once a day, for one (1) week. After the fifth or sixth day, scales should come off by themselves or with gentle hand rubbing. Thereafter, apply to the bird's feed and legs three (3) times a month. Avoid soaking the feathers.

The moderate use of VETR$_x$™ will not harm feathers.

Scaly-face: Apply VETR$_x$™, at room temperature, directly from the bottle. Using a cotton swab, apply two (2) times a day to the scaly area. Do this for five (5) days, an improvement should be noted. Use sparingly, and apply a thin film. Keep VETR$_x$™ out of the bird's eyes. When the eyelids are involved, work carefully and slowly.

The combination of pure lard and strong essential oils in VETR$_x$™ will help to penetrate effectively to where the mites burrow into the skin. To discourage the presence of mites, rub perches with warm VETR$_x$™ (full strength from bottle) two (2) times each month.

Caution(s): Avoid contact with the eyes. If respiratory conditions persist, it is important to contact a veterinarian.

For animal use only. Not for human consumption. Use only as directed. Keep all medication out of the reach of children.

Discussion:

Respiratory Problems: Stress conditions can often lead to respiratory ailments in birds. These involve the transporting of birds away from their usual setting, extreme changes in weather conditions or house heating, and crowding of birds into a cage that is too small.

Symptoms to look for: Changes in the bird's appearance or posture that indicate signs of stress. Wet, watery eyes, and eyes closing in a sleeping posture. Tail-bobbing. In severe respiratory involvement, tail-bobbing will often be noted while a bird is at rest.

Signs of effortful breathing. An unhealthy bird will continue to breathe quickly, not smoothly.

Huddling and ruffling of feathers.

Unusual respiratory sounds, such as hissing or whistling, clicking sounds in the neck and head, intermittent cough or sneeze, change or loss of voice or song.

Sitting low on the perch, and crouching over its feet.

Loss of appetite, often accompanied by increased drinking of water.

Scaly-face and Scaly-leg Mite Problems:

Canaries, lovebirds and budgerigars are the most commonly affected by mites. Parakeets, parrots, cockatiels and finches are also susceptible.

Microscopic mites (or bugs) burrow into the skin and feather follicles.

Birds seem to get the mites from their parents when they are babies in the nests. Contact with infected birds also appears to be a cause. They cause white, scaly deposits. The most common areas affected are eyelids, beak corners, legs and toes. On parakeets, the disease usually begins on the face and feet. Scales are crusty, thick, white or off-white in color. Small holes, where the mite has burrowed, can be detected. The mite can damage the beak's growth plate and cause a crooked beak that will have to be trimmed so that the bird can eat. On canaries, the crusty scale often begins on the undersurface of the feet, and then spreads to form scabs over the toes. If the condition is severe and unyielding, microscopic examination by a veterinarian can confirm the presence of the scale mites.

Important: As canaries grow older, there is an increase in the thickness of the scales of the feet. This is normal, and should not be confused with scaly-leg disease.

Presentation: 2 fl. oz. (59 mL) and 1 quart containers.

Compendium Code No.: 14380020

VETR$_x$™ EQUINE FORMULA

Goodwinol **Respiratory Product**

Active Ingredient(s): Made with 3.3% (v-v) alcohol U.S.P. The mixture contains Canada balsam, camphor, oil origanum, oil rosemary, blended in a corn oil base.

Indications: For use as an aid in the treatment of respiratory problems in horses.

Dosage and Administration: VETR$_x$™ may be used for acute respiratory infection or in conjunction with antibiotics. In addition, it may be used pre-race for non-specific respiratory problems.

Route of Administration:

1. 1 oz. orally two (2) to three (3) times per day for sick or coughing animals or 1 oz. before a race for non-specific respiratory ailments.
2. 10 mL intranasally via a syringe or plastic catheter.
3. Aerosol spraying of stables and bedding. Light sprayers are very effective for the misting of VETR$_x$™ in the living area.

Note: Make certain that the sprayer is free of any residue. Use only clean bottles to spray.

If symptoms persist consult a veterinarian.

Presentation: 1 quart container.

Compendium Code No.: 14380031

VETR$_x$™ FOR CATS AND KITTENS

Goodwinol **Respiratory Product**

Active Ingredient(s): Made with 3.3% (v-v) alcohol U.S.P. The mixture contains Canada balsam, camphor, oil origanum, oil rosemary, blended in a corn oil base.

Indications: For treating all breeds of cats and kittens. For use as an aid in the treatment of upper respiratory ailments produced by congestion or allergy. When a cat looses its sense of smell due to congestion, it also loses its appetite, further weakening the pet.

Symptoms to look for: Sniffling, sneezing, nasal discharge and noisy breathing.

Dosage and Administration:

Dosages and Preparing Suggestions: For the best results, use VETR$_x$™ warm. Put the bottle in a container of warm water and let it stand for a few minutes or warm quickly over medium heat will the spout in an open (upright) position. Always test the temperature of the product before applying.

Apply two (2) drops directly into each nostril for adult cats, one (1) drop for kittens. Repeat in five (5) minutes. Repeat the application three (3) to four (4) times a day. If possible, isolate the pet and treat with VETR$_x$™ in a warm water vaporizer, following the manufacturer's directions.

If upper respiratory symptoms persist, consult a veterinarian.

Presentation: 2 fl. oz. (59 mL) and 1 quart.

Compendium Code No.: 14380040

VETR$_x$™ FOR DOGS AND PUPPIES

Goodwinol **Respiratory Product**

Active Ingredient(s): Made with 3.3% (v-v) alcohol U.S.P. The mixture contains Canada balsam, camphor, oil origanum, oil rosemary, blended in a corn oil base.

Indications: For use as an aid in the treatment of all breeds of dogs and puppies. Effective for the relief of upper respiratory ailments produced by congestion or allergy. When a dog loses its sense of smell due to congestion, it also loses its appetite, further weakening the pet.

Symptoms to look for: Sniffling, sneezing, nasal discharge and noisy breathing.

Dosage and Administration:

Dosages and Preparing Suggestions: For the best results, use VETR$_x$™ warm. Put the bottle in a container of warm water and let it stand for a few minutes or warm quickly over medium heat will the spout in an open (upright) position. Always test the temperature of the product before applying.

Apply two (2) drops directly into each nostril for adult dogs, one (1) drop for puppies. Repeat in five (5) minutes. Repeat the application three (3) to four (4) times a day. If possible, isolate the pet and treat with VETR$_x$™ in a warm water vaporizer, following the manufacturer's directions.

If upper respiratory symptoms persist, consult a veterinarian.

Presentation: 2 fl. oz. (59 mL) and 1 quart.

Compendium Code No.: 14380050

VETR$_x$™ GOAT & SHEEP REMEDY

Goodwinol **Respiratory Product**

Active Ingredient(s): Made with 3.3% (v-v) alcohol U.S.P. The mixture contains Canada balsam, camphor, oil origanum, oil rosemary, blended in a corn oil base.

Indications: To aid in the treatment of respiratory infections and ear mites in goats and sheep.

For internal and external applications.

Dosage and Administration:

Respiratory Problems:

Symptoms: Coughing, sneezing, rattling sounds, possible loss of appetite.

Treatment: Three (3) drops in each nostril four (4) times a day for three (3) days for adult animals.

Two (2) drops in each nostril three (3) times a day for three (3) days for kids and lambs.

Can be safely used in conjunction with any prescribed veterinary medication.

Caution(s): For animal use only. Not for human consumption. Use only as directed.

Keep away from children.

If upper respiratory symptoms persist for 48 hours, consult a licensed veterinarian.

Presentation: 2 fl. oz. (59 mL) and 1 quart container.

Compendium Code No.: 14380060

VETR$_x$™ PIGEON REMEDY

Goodwinol **Respiratory Product**

Active Ingredient(s): Made with 3.3% (v-v) alcohol U.S.P. The mixture contains Canada balsam, camphor, oil origanum, oil rosemary, blended in a corn oil base.

Indications: For use as an aid in the tratment of respiratory disease (CRD) in racing and show pigeons.

Colds, sneezing, pneumonia, roup and throat canker.

For internal and external application.

Dosage and Administration: Always use VETR$_x$™ warm.

Treatments: Place the spout in an open (upright) position. Put the bottle in a small pan of water. Heat at medium temperature. Always test the temperature of the product before applying internally or externally.

Prepare Solution: Into one-half (½) a cup of very warm water, mix one (1) teaspoon of VETR$_x$™ Pigeon Remedy. Use the solution for the following treatments.

Nostrils and Throat: Using a medicine dropper, treat both nostrils with two (2) drops in each. Continue the treatment twice a day for seven (7) days. During the 7-day treatment, one (1) drop may also be put down the bird's throat each time the nostrils are treated. This will help to keep the throat passages clean.

Eye Pack: If the eyes are badly swollen, make a pack about one-inch square from hospital cotton. Dip the pack into the solution and place over the infected eye. Then, with another piece of cotton, gently drip the warm solution over the eye pack. Continue for about five (5) minutes each day for several days, until improvement is noted.

Under Wings: Put a drop of VETR$_x$™ full strength (warm) from the bottle under the wings of each bird to be treated. When the bird puts its head under either wing while resting, the vapors will help to relieve cold symptoms.

Vaporizer: If deciding to use a vaporizer, make certain it is a hot water model. Follow the manufacturer's directions. Fill the cup with VETR$_x$™ and operate the vaporizer for at least one (1) hour while birds are roosting, not more than twice a week.

Caution(s): For animal use only. Not for human consumption. Use only as directed. Keep all medication out of the reach of children.

Discussion:

General Precautions - Preventing Sickness: While treating birds, follow the usual precautions, because respiratory problems are contagious. Isolate infected birds as soon as possible. Clean out all lofts in which sick birds have roosted. Keep the birds as clean and dry as possible, and free from drafts. Recovered birds can be carriers of disease. Once respiratory problems have infected a loft, watch carefully for signs of a fresh outbreak among a new crop of young birds. If a bird is losing weight and not eating or drinking, hand feeding is recommended. Some breeders soak a small piece of bread in milk, and place it down the bird's throat. Do this regularly to keep up body weight during stress periods. Once the disease is under control, six (6) drops of VETR$_x$™ per gallon of clean drinking water can be effective. Watch for evidences of disease in birds coming home from races or shows. Diseases are often contracted in baskets. Many pigeon fanciers spray VETR$_x$™ solution routinely in the lofts and place a few drops in the litter every time they change it. Other owners, as a preventive measure, routinely treat nostrils and throats, and place VETR$_x$™ under the wings of birds returning from races or shows. They do the same for young birds, or any birds even suspected of catching colds.

If symptoms persist consult a veterinarian.

Presentation: 2 fl. oz. (59 mL) and 1 quart.

Compendium Code No.: 14380070

VETR$_x$™ POULTRY REMEDY

Goodwinol **Respiratory Product**

Active Ingredient(s): Made with 3.3% (v-v) alcohol U.S.P. The mixture contains Canada balsam, camphor, oil origanum, oil rosemary, blended in a corn oil base.

Indications: For use as an aid in the treatment of respiratory problems in all varieties of poultry, including bantams, ducks, turkeys, geese, and game birds.

Effective reliefs for colds, roup, scaly legs, and eye worm and as a conditioner for show preparations. For internal and external application.

Dosage and Administration:

Dosages and Preparing Solution: The directions below apply to bantams and mature poultry of similar size, unless otherwise noted. For larger or smaller birds, change the dosage in proportion to the size of the bird.

Use VETR$_x$™ warm, unless otherwise specified. To warm, place the spout in an open position. Put the bottle in a small pan of water. Heat at medium temperature. Always test the temperature of the product before applying internally or externally.

To prepare the solution, add one (1) teaspoonful of warm VETR$_x$™ to one (1) cup of very warm water. VETR$_x$™ mixes with hot water, but floats on top of cold water.

Colds and Roup: Symptoms of colds are watery eyes, droopy appearance, and an unusual tendency to shake or turn the head.

To treat colds, drip VETR$_x$™ solution into the bird's nostrils. Place a few drops of warm VETR$_x$™, straight from the bottle, down the throat of the infected bird at night. Also, rub some warm VETR$_x$™ from the bottle over the head of birds and under wings. If a cold develops into more severe roup, change to a stronger solution of one (1) teaspoonful of VETR$_x$™ in one-half (½) cup of hot water. Treat the same as for colds. Also, swab the throat and wash the head and eyes with the stronger solution four (4) or five (5) times a day. Keep the nostrils, eyes, and throat as clean as possible.

Flock Care: If colds infect many in a flock, spray warm VETR$_x$™ solution over as many birds as possible. Use any small sprayer, and keep the sprayer in a pan of hot water before using. For birds in a flock which look droopy, rub warm VETR$_x$™, full strength, over their heads, eyes, and under their wings. Also, provide plenty of clean, cool drinking water for the flock. Add a few drops of VETR$_x$™ to the drinking water each time it is changed. It will float on the water and get on the beaks and nostrils of the birds each time they drink.

Vaporizer: If deciding to use a vaporizer, make certain that it is a hot water model. Follow the manufacturer's directions. Fill the cup with VETR$_x$™ full strength and operate the vaporizer for at least one (1) hour while birds are roosting.

Preventing Colds and Roup: To help prevent colds, sprinkle a few drops of VETR$_x$™ in the litter every four (4) or five (5) days. Add a few drips to the drinking water every time it is changed. Rub one (1) or two (2) drops of warm, full-strength VETR$_x$™ under the wings.

For Show Birds: To protect birds from colds while traveling to and from shows, place a few drops of warm VETR$_x$™ under one (1) wing. It does not stain, or harm feathers, wing, or color. Rubbing VETR$_x$™ on the legs brings out the true color and helps to protect them from mites and lice. When the birds return from shows, keep them separated from the flock for one (1) week. Wash their feet and heads with a warm solution, and rub warm VETR$_x$™ from the bottle on the heads and under wings.

Scaly Legs: When shanks of the bird appear dry, rub them with a small amount of cold VETR$_x$™ from the bottle. In cases of heavy scale, apply cold VETR$_x$™ and rub in thoroughly all over the shanks and toes. Repeat every three (3) days until the legs are completely free of scale.

"Eye Worm": The tiny worm works its way under the third eyelid and causes a pus pocket to form. The bird will blink excessively and rub its eye at the base of the wing feather. To treat, hold the bird under one (1) arm so that both hands are free. Open the bird's mouth while turning its head to the side and tilting down to the cleft in the roof of the mouth can be seen. Dip a small cotton swab into warm VETR$_x$™. Press the swab right into the cleft. Do this slowly. Watch for VETR$_x$™ to come from each side of the bird's beak and pus coming from the corner of each eye. Remove the pus and rest the bird for awhile. The treatment may have to be repeated two (2) or three (3) times before results are seen.

Tonic Feeder for Breeding: To keep breeding birds healthy for maximum production of breeding eggs.

Keep three (3) quarts of laying mash indoors for a few hours until it reaches room temperature. Warm a bottle of VETR$_x$™. Pour the entire bottle onto the mash and mix well by rubbing the mash between the hands. Let it stand in a warm room over night. Next day, put the treated mash in a container with a tight lid and let it stand for about two (2) weeks. Mix one (1) tablespoon of treated mash, once a day, in feed for every 20 birds. If feeding 10 birds or less, one (1) teaspoon is enough. Be sure to stir the treated mash thoroughly into feed.

General Precautions: While treating poultry and other birds, follow the usual precautions. Isolate infected birds as soon as possible. Clean out all coops lofts in which sick birds have been. Keep the birds as clean and dry as possible, and free from drafts. Watch for evidences of disease in birds coming home from shows. Diseases are often contracted in baskets.

If symptoms persist consult a veterinarian.

Caution(s): For animal use only. Not for human consumption. Use only as directed. Keep all medication out of the reach of children.

Presentation: 2 fl. oz. (59 mL) and 1 quart.

Compendium Code No.: 14380080

VETR$_x$™ RABBIT REMEDY

Goodwinol **Respiratory Product**

Active Ingredient(s): Made with 3.3% (v-v) alcohol U.S.P. The mixture contains Canada balsam, camphor, oil origanum, oil rosemary, blended in a corn oil base.

Indications: For use as an aid in the treatment of all standard breeds of rabbits raised commercially, as a hobby, or for showing.

Effective relief for snuffles, pneumonia, ear mites, or ear canker.

Dosage and Administration:

Snuffles and Pneumonia:

Symptoms: Snuffles or colds produce sneezing, watery eyes, and a pus-filled nasal discharge. Watch for rabbits rubbing their noses with their front feet. Check inside the front paws of the animals suspected of having snuffles. Matted fur here can indicate snuffles. Rabbits with advanced snuffles will often have badly matted fur around the nostrils.

Frequently snuffles can develop into pneumonia. Signs of pneumonia are difficult breathing and gasping.

Treatment: Use VETR$_x$™ Rabbit Remedy warm. To warm, place the spout in an open position. Put the bottle in a small pan of water. Heat at medium temperature. Always test the temperature of the product before applying. Place two (2) drops of warm VETR$_x$™ on each side of the nostrils, and to any scabbed area. Repeat two (2) or three (3) times a day until symptoms disappear. Eight (8) drops per gallon in clean drinking water can help respiratory ailments.

Ear Mites or Ear Canker:

Symptoms: The rabbit will shake its head a great deal and scratch at its ears. Brown, scaly scabs appear inside the ears. Symptoms are caused by tiny mites which burrow into the skin of the ear and cause tissue damage. Check rabbits' ears routinely for symptoms.

Treatment: Use VETR$_x$™ warm. Shake the bottle well to mix the contents.

Apply by the drop or with a cotton swab . Be sure to dampen the entire affected area. Do not dig off the scabs. The scab should eventually be shaken off by the rabbit. After 24 hours, dampen the entire affected area for the second time. Repeat again after 36 hours. Wait three (3) more days and add two (2) drops into the ears. This should result in clean mite-free ears. If, at this time, scabs have not been shaken off by the rabbit, use a damp cotton swab and gently remove the remaining scales and crusts from the ear.

Note: VETR$_x$™ will leave an oily film on the skin and fur. This will not burn the skin or remove hair. It is helpful in destroying any mites or mite ova which may be present.

General Precautions: While treating infected animals, follow the usual precautions. Isolate infected animals as soon as possible. Clean all hutches and nest boxes which sick rabbits have occupied. Keep rabbits as clean and as dry as possible. In case of snuffles, keep the animals away from drafts. Cold symptoms in rabbits tend to subside and then recur. So, if rabbits have a tendency to catch a cold, watch them carefully for early symptoms. When a rabbit has been to a show, it is wise to isolate it from the others for several days. Treat the ears and nose as described above.

Caution(s): For animal use only. Not for human consumption. Use only as directed.

Keep all medication out of the reach of children.

If symptoms persist consult a veterinarian.

Presentation: 2 fl. oz. (59 mL) and 1 quart.

Compendium Code No.: 14380090

VETR$_x$™ SMALL FUR ANIMAL REMEDY

Goodwinol **Respiratory Product**

For commercially raised, domestic pets, and laboratory research animals.

Active Ingredient(s): 3.3% (v/v) alcohol U.S.P., Canada balsam, camphor, oil of origanum, oil of rosemary, corn oil.

Indications: As an aid in treating hamsters, guinea pigs, gerbils, mice, rats, ferrets, chinchillas, lemmings, mink.

Effective relief from respiratory infections, colds, wheezing, snuffles. This product can help alleviate many respiratory problems common to small animals. For conditions that do not respond, the advice of a veterinarian should be sought.

For internal and external applications.

Dosage and Administration:

Symptoms: These conditions (colds, snuffles, pneumonia) are characterized by a change in respiration, often reflected in rate, depth, noisiness and distress. Coughing, sneezing, snorting and wheezing may also occur. Occasional symptoms are watery eyes and a pus-filled nasal discharge. Animals whose lung tissue is affected have a reduced oxygen exchange level and show "air hunger", exaggerated breathing effort, with difficulty in drawing or expelling air.

Frequently, colds can develop into pneumonia, since it is believed the same bacteria which result in colds can move down the respiratory passages into the lungs. Signs of pneumonia are loud gasping noises and increased difficulty in breathing.

Treatment: Use VETR$_x$™ Remedy warm. To warm, open cap and put bottle in small pan of heated water. Shake well. Always test temperature of product before applying.

Depending upon size of animal, place one or two drops of warm VETR$_x$™ on each side of nostril. Apply one drop, by hand, to any scabbed area. Repeat twice daily, until symptoms disappear.

To clean, fresh water (changed daily) add eight drops per gallon. Globules may rise to the top. These contain some medication that can be helpful if consumed internally.

Note: VETR$_x$™ will leave an oily film on skin and fur. This will not burn skin or remove hair. It will, in fact, help destroy any mites or mite ova which may be present.

General Precautions: Respiratory infections are often contagious and can affect nearby animals.

Isolate infected animals as soon as possible. Clean all cages and hutches which sick animals have occupied. Keep animals as clean and dry as possible. Keep animals away from drafts. Change litter daily. When putting down fresh litter, you can add two drops of warm VETR$_x$™ to floor of cage.

Caution(s): For animal use only. Not for human consumption. Use only as directed. Keep this and all medication out of the reach of children. If symptoms persist for more than 48 hours consult a licensed veterinarian.

Discussion:

General Information on Temperature Conditions: As a general rule, mice, rats, hamsters, lemmings and gerbils require some extra heat in cold weather. It is recommended that they be kept indoors or in a heated shed, with the nest temperature approximately 70°F.

Guinea pigs, chinchilla, mink and ferrets are well suited to outdoor cages and pens, as long as these quarters are weatherproofed.

General Information on Feeding: Many owners and breeders feed their animals some table scraps, and find that animals thrive. There are, however, some recommended guide lines for nutrition.

Mice and Rats: Cubed diets and pellets obtained from animal foodstuff compounders are a complete diet.

For the remainder of the small rodents, the basic ration can be mouse and rat pellets, supplemented with green vegetables, and possibly sunflower seeds. Lemmings and gerbils will probably satisfy their water need from the fresh vegetables. Hamsters should not be fed oats or similar grains which might damage the mucous membrane of their cheek pouches.

Basic diet of guinea pigs and chinchillas can consist of commercially available pellets. Guinea pig diets must be supplemented with greens or other sources of vitamin C. Roughage in the form of good quality hay is also necessary for these three species.

Ferrets and mink are carnivores, and their staple diet is usually fresh meat or fish. When feeding raw meat, care must be taken to insure the diet includes vitamins and minerals, particularly calcium.

Feeding utensils for all animals must be cleaned regularly.

This product is based on a formula in use since 1874.

Presentation: 2 fl oz and 1 quart.

Compendium Code No.: 14380100

VIBRALONE™-L5

Intervet **Bacterin**

Campylobacter Fetus-Leptospira Canicola-Grippotyphosa-Hardjo-Icterohaemorrhagiae-Pomona Bacterin

U.S. Vet. Lic. No.: 286

Contents: A chemically inactivated suspension of the organisms listed.

Contains formaldehyde as preservative.

Indications: For use in healthy cattle as an aid in preventing Vibriosis and Leptospirosis.

Dosage and Administration: 5 mL. Inject intramuscularly. Initial vaccination requires two doses 2 to 4 weeks apart. Annual revaccination is recommended. In either case, vaccination should be completed 30-60 days prior to breeding.

Precaution(s): Shake well before using. Store at 35° to 45°F (2° to 7°C). Use entire contents when first opened.

Caution(s): Anaphylactoid reactions may occur.

For use in animals only.

Antidote(s): Epinephrine.

Warning(s): Do not vaccinate within 21 days before slaughter.

Presentation: 10 doses (50 mL) and 50 doses (250 mL).

Compendium Code No.: 11062780 9811001 / 9815001

VIBRIN®

Pfizer Animal Health **Bacterin**

Campylobacter Fetus Bacterin

U.S. Vet. Lic. No.: 189

Description: VIBRIN® is prepared from an inactivated, concentrated suspension of *Campylobacter fetus,* bovine isolate, in a patented repository base.[1]

Indications: VIBRIN® is for vaccination of healthy cows and heifers as an aid in preventing campylobacteriosis (vibriosis) caused by *Campylobacter fetus.*

Directions:

1. General Directions: Vaccination of healthy cows and heifers is recommended. Shake well. Aseptically administer 2 mL subcutaneously in the upper part of the neck. In accordance with Beef Quality Assurance guidelines, this product should be administered subcutaneously (SC) under the skin.
2. Primary Vaccination: Administer a single 2-mL dose to all breeding cows and heifers between 30 days and 7 months before breeding. Pregnant animals can be safely vaccinated.[2,4]
3. Revaccination: Annual revaccination with a single dose is recommended between 30 days and 7 months before breeding.
4. Good animal husbandry and herd health management practices should be employed.

Precaution(s): Store at 2°-7°C. Prolonged exposure to higher temperatures may adversely affect potency. Do not freeze.

Use entire contents when first opened.

Sterilized syringes and needles should be used to administer this vaccine.

Caution(s): As with many vaccines, anaphylaxis may occur after use. Initial antidote of epinephrine is recommended and should be followed with appropriate supportive therapy.

This product has been shown to be efficacious in healthy animals. A protective immune response may not be elicited if animals are incubating an infectious disease, are malnourished or parasitized, are stressed due to shipment or environmental conditions, are otherwise immunocompromised, or the vaccine is not administered in accordance with label directions.

Warning(s): To avoid vaccination site trim-out, do not vaccinate within 60 days before slaughter.

For veterinary use only.

Discussion: Disease Description: Campylobacteriosis is a venereal disease of cattle transmitted during breeding, either through coitus or artificial insemination with contaminated semen. Although the disease is often subclinical, in cows it causes temporary infertility, irregular estrus cycles, delayed conception, and occasionally, abortion.

Trial Data: Safety and Efficacy: Chemical inactivation renders VIBRIN® incapable of causing or spreading infectious disease. The special adjuvant base enhances and prolongs antigenic stimulation and may produce a localized vaccine granuloma. These are noninflammatory, however, and usually disappear in several weeks. Field use and extensive, controlled tests in breeding cattle under experimental conditions demonstrated that the serotype of *Campylobacter fetus* used in VIBRIN® was effective in prevention of campylobacteriosis.[2,3] Pregnancy rates in vaccinated heifers were up to 44% higher than in nonvaccinated control heifers. All research conducted on VIBRIN® indicated a single dose is effective and there is no advantage in using 2 injections.[2,4,5]

References: Available upon request.

Presentation: 10 dose and 50 dose vials.

U.S. Patent Nos. 3,329,573 and 3,435,112

Compendium Code No.: 36900850 75-4935-08

V

VIBRIO-LEPTO 5

AgriLabs **Bacterin**

Campylobacter fetus-Leptospira canicola-grippotyphosa-hardjo-icterohaemorrhagiae-pomona Bacterin

U.S. Vet. Lic. No.: 272

Contents: This bacterin contains inactivated cultures of *Campylobacter fetus, Leptospira canicola, L grippotyphosa, L hardjo, L icterohaemorrhagiae,* and *L pomona.*

Indications: Recommended for the vaccination of healthy cattle against diseases caused by these organisms represented.

Dosage and Administration: Shake well. Administer 5 mL IM or SC 2 to 6 weeks prior to breeding or adding to the breeding herd. In Campylobacter infected herds or endemic areas, vaccinated animals should be revaccinated at least 3 weeks later. Annual revaccination with a single 5 mL dose is recommended.

Precaution(s): Store at 35°F-45°F (2°C-7°C). Use entire contents when first opened.

Caution(s): In case of anaphylactoid reactions, epinephrine should be administered immediately.

Warning(s): Do not vaccinate within 21 days before slaughter. For veterinary use only.

Presentation: 10 dose (50 mL) and 50 dose (250 mL) vials.

Compendium Code No.: 10581180

VIBRIO-LEPTO-5™

Boehringer Ingelheim **Bacterin**

Campylobacter Fetus-Leptospira Canicola-Grippotyphosa-Hardjo-Icterohaemorrhagiae-Pomona Bacterin

U.S. Vet. Lic. No.: 124

Composition: Chemically inactivated aluminum hydroxide adsorbed whole cultures of the organisms listed. Contains gentamicin and Amphotericin B as preservatives.

Indications: Recommended for the vaccination of healthy, susceptible cattle against infertility, delayed conception or abortion caused by *Campylobacter fetus* and leptospirosis caused by *Leptospira canicola, L. grippotyphosa, L. hardjo, L. icterohaemorrhagiae* and *L. pomona.*

Dosage and Administration: Using aseptic technique, inject 5 mL intramuscularly in healthy cattle of any age. Repeat in 14 to 21 days. Administer a single 5 mL booster dose annually.

Precaution(s): Store out of direct sunlight at a temperature between 35-45°F (2-7°C). Avoid freezing. Shake well before using. Use entire contents when first opened.

Caution(s): Anaphylactoid reactions may occur.

Antidote(s): Administer epinephrine.

Warning(s): Do not vaccinate within 21 days before slaughter.

Presentation: 50 mL (10 dose) and 250 mL (50 dose) vials.

Compendium Code No.: 10281150

VIBRIO-LEPTO 5

Durvet **Bacterin**

Campylobacter Fetus-Leptospira Canicola-Grippotyphosa-Hardjo-Icterohaemorrhagiae-Pomona Bacterin

U.S. Vet. Lic. No.: 272

Contents: This product contains the antigens listed above.

Indications: For the vaccination of healthy cattle against diseases caused by *C. fetus* and the Leptospira serovars represented.

Directions: Shake well. Administer 5 mL intramuscularly or subcutaneously 2-6 weeks prior to breeding or when adding to the breeding herd. In *Campylobacter fetus* infected herds or endemic areas, vaccinated animals should be revaccinated at least 3 weeks later. Annual revaccination with a single dose is recommended.

Precaution(s): Store at 35°F-45°F (2°C-7°C). Use entire contents when first opened.

Caution(s): In case of an anaphylactoid reactions, administer epinephrine immediately.

For veterinary use only.

Warning(s): Do not vaccinate within 21 days before slaughter.

Presentation: 10 doses (50 mL) and 50 doses (250 mL).

Manufactured by: BioCor, Inc., Omaha, NE 68134.

Compendium Code No.: 10841631 3/93

VIBRIO-LEPTO 5

Premier Farmtech **Bacterin**

Campylobacter fetus-Leptospira canicola-grippotyphosa-hardjo-icterohaemorrhagiae-pomona Bacterin, Aluminum Hydroxide Adsorbed

U.S. Vet. Lic. No.: 272

Contents: Inactivated cultures of *Campylobacter fetus, Leptospira canicola, L grippotyphosa, L hardjo, L icterohaemorrhagiae* and *L pomona,* aluminum hydroxide adsorbed.

Indications: For the immunization of healthy cattle against these infections.

Dosage and Administration: Shake well. Inject 5 mL IM or SC 2 to 6 weeks prior to breeding or being added to the breeding herd. Revaccinate once annually to maintain a high level of immunity. In vibrio infected herds or endemic areas, 2 doses, at least 3 weeks apart, are recommended for primary immunization.

Precaution(s): Store at 35°F - 45°F (2°C - 7°C). Use entire contents when first opened.

Caution(s): In case of anaphylactoid reactions, epinephrine should be administered immediately.

Antidote(s): Epinephrine.

Warning(s): Do not vaccinate within 21 days before slaughter.

For veterinary use only.

Presentation: 10 dose (50 mL) and 50 dose (250 mL) vials.

Compendium Code No.: 10320030

VIBRIO LEPTO 5 (OIL BASE)

Aspen **Bacterin**

Campylobacter Fetus-Leptospira Canicola-Grippotyphosa-Hardjo-Icterohaemorrhagiae-Pomona Bacterin

U.S. Vet. Lic. No.: 303

Composition: This bacterin contains inactivated cultures of *Campylobacter fetus, Leptospira canicola, grippotyphosa, hardjo, icterohaemorrhagiae,* and *pomona* adjuvanted with oil. Contains penicillin, streptomycin, and thimerosal as preservatives.

Indications: For use in healthy cattle as an aid in the prevention and control of disease caused by *Campylobacter fetus, Leptospira canicola, grippotyphosa, hardjo, icterohaemorrhagiae,* and *pomona.*

Dosage and Administration: Shake well before using. Administer 2 mL intramuscularly 2-4 weeks prior to breeding.

Precaution(s): Store in the dark at 35°-45°F (2°-7°C). Do not freeze. Use entire contents when first opened.

Caution(s): Transient swelling may occur at the site of injection. Milk reduction and transient depression may be observed in lactating dairy cows for 3-6 days following vaccination. Anaphylactic reactions may occur following the use of this biological. Symptomatic treatment: Epinephrine.

Warning(s): Do not vaccinate within 60 days prior to slaughter.

Presentation: 10 dose (20 mL) and 50 dose (100 mL) vials.

Compendium Code No.: 14750930

VIBRIO-LEPTO 5 VACCINE

Aspen **Bacterin**

Campylobacter fetus-Leptospira canicola-grippotyphosa-hardjo-icterohaemorrhagiae-pomona Bacterin

U.S. Vet. Lic. No.: 272

Active Ingredient(s): Contains inactivated cultures of *Campylobacter fetus, Leptospira canicola, L. grippotyphosa, L. hardjo, L. icterohaemorrhagiae* and *L. pomona.*

Indications: For the immunization of healthy cattle against infections caused by *Campylobacter fetus, Leptospira canicola, L. grippotyphosa, L. hardjo, L. icterohaemorrhagiae* and *L. pomona.*

Dosage and Administration: Shake well. Inject 5 mL intramuscularly or subcutaneously two (2) to six (6) weeks prior to breeding, or being added to the breeding herd. Revaccinate once annually to maintain a high level of immunity.

Precaution(s): Store at 35°-45°F (2°-7°C). Do not freeze.

Caution(s): Use the entire contents when first opened.

If an allergic response occurs, epinephrine should be administered immediately.

Antidote(s): Epinephrine.

Warning(s): Do not vaccinate within 21 days before slaughter. For veterinary use only.

Presentation: 10 dose (50 mL) and 50 dose (250 mL) vials.

Compendium Code No.: 14750940

VIBRIO/LEPTOFERM-5™

Pfizer Animal Health **Bacterin**

Campylobacter Fetus-Leptospira Canicola-Grippotyphosa-Hardjo-Icterohaemorrhagiae-Pomona Bacterin

U.S. Vet. Lic. No.: 189

Contents: This product contains the antigens listed above.

Indications: For vaccination of healthy cows and heifers as an aid in preventing disease caused by *Campylobacter fetus, Leptospira canicola, L. grippotyphosa, L. hardjo, L. icterohaemorrhagiae,* and *L. pomona.*

Directions: Shake well. Aseptically administer 2 mL intramuscularly. In accordance with Beef Quality Assurance guidelines, this product should be administered in the muscular region of the neck. Administer two 2-mL doses 2-4 weeks apart to all breeding-age cows and heifers 30-60 days before exposure or being added to the breeding herd. Annual revaccination with a single dose is recommended.

Precaution(s): Store at 2°-7°C. Do not freeze. Use entire contents when first opened. Occasional hypersensitivity reactions may occur up to 18 hours postvaccination. While this event appears to be rare overall, dairy cattle may be affected more frequently than other cattle.

Warning(s): Do not vaccinate within 21 days before slaughter.

For veterinary use only.

Presentation: 10 dose (20 mL) and 50 dose (100 mL) vials.

Compendium Code No.: 36900011 85-4918-05

VIBROGEN

Novartis (Aqua Health) **Bacterin**

Vibrio Anguillarum-Ordalii Bacterin

U.S. Vet. Lic. No.: 335

Contents: VIBROGEN has been shown to be safe and effective for use with 2 grams or larger salmonids. This bacterin contains formalin inactivated cultures of *Vibrio anguillarum* and *Vibrio ordalii.* No other preservative is added.

Indications: For the immunization of healthy salmonids against vibriosis caused by *Vibrio anguillarum* and *Vibrio ordalii.*

Dosage and Administration: Vaccination Program: Vaccination should precede exposure of vaccinates to the disease agent by 14 days if holding water temperatures are 10°-12°C. A longer period of time should be allowed if temperatures are below 10°C.

Methods:

For immersion and spray delivery, dilute entire contents of this vial with 9 liters of clean hatchery water.

Immersion Delivery: Measure diluted bacterin in a suitable plastic container. Add fish to attain a density of 500 g per liter of diluted bacterin. Expose fish for 30 seconds, then drain bacterin from fish. Return fish to holding facility. Repeat until a total of 20 groups have been vaccinated.

Spray Delivery: Pressurize spray unit to 2.1 kg/cm² (30 psi) with compressed gas (O_2, N_2 or air) to deliver 10 liters of diluted bacterin in 12-14 minutes. Adjust nozzle of unit so that 5 seconds contact time is achieved. Dewater fish from holding facility and place in unit. Expose fish to spray for 5 seconds then return to holding facility. Ten liters of diluted bacterin will vaccinate approximately 250 kg, depending on fish size.

Precaution(s): Shake well before using. Store between 2-7°C (35-45°F). Do not freeze. Use entire contents when first opened. Vaccinal solution and hatchery water ambient temperature should be within 2°C.

Caution(s): Vaccinate healthy fish only.

Revaccination can be done if immunity is required for longer than 300 days.

For veterinary use only.

Warning(s): Do not vaccinate within 21 days of slaughter.

Presentation: 1000 mL bottle.

Distributed by: Mr. J. Zinn, Buhl, Idaho 83316

Compendium Code No.: 14970082 L-23-0

VIBROGEN-2™

Novartis (Aqua Health) **Bacterin**

Vibrio Anguillarum-Ordalii Bacterin

U.S. Vet. Lic. No.: 335

Contents: VIBROGEN-2™ has been shown to be safe and effective for use with 2 grams or larger salmonids. This bacterin contains formalin inactivated cultures of *Vibrio anguillarum* and *Vibrio ordalii.* No other preservative is added.

Indications: For the immunization of healthy salmonids against vibriosis caused by *Vibrio anguillarum* and *Vibrio ordalii.*
Dosage and Administration: Vaccination Program: Vaccination should precede exposure of vaccinates to the disease agent by 14 days if holding water temperatures are 10°-12°C. A longer period of time should be allowed if temperatures are below 10°C.
Methods:
For immersion and spray delivery, dilute entire contents of this vial with 9 liters of clean hatchery water.
Immersion Delivery: Measure diluted bacterin in a suitable plastic container. Add fish to attain a density of 500 grams per liter of diluted bacterin. Expose fish for 30 seconds, then drain bacterin from fish. Return fish to holding facility. Repeat until a total of 20 groups have been vaccinated.
Spray Delivery: Pressurize spray unit to 2.1 kg/cm^2 (30 psi) with compressed gas (O_2, N_2 or air) to deliver 10 liters of diluted bacterin in 12-14 minutes. Adjust nozzle of unit so that 5 seconds contact time is achieved. Dewater fish from holding facility and place in unit. Expose fish to spray for 5 seconds then return to holding facility. Ten liters of diluted bacterin will vaccinate approximately 250 kg, depending on fish size.
Precaution(s): Shake well before using. Store between 2-7°C (35-45°F). Do not freeze. Use entire contents when first opened. Vaccinal solution and hatchery water ambient temperature should be within 2°C.
Caution(s): Vaccinate healthy fish only.
Revaccination can be done if immunity is required for longer than 300 days.
For veterinary use only.
Warning(s): Do not vaccinate within 21 days of slaughter.
Presentation: 1000 mL bottle.
Distributed by: Mr. J. Zinn, Buhl, Idaho 83316
Compendium Code No.: 14970092 L-22-0

VIB SHIELD®

Novartis Animal Vaccines **Bacterin**
Campylobacter fetus Bacterin
U.S. Vet. Lic. No.: 303
Composition: The bacterin contains inactivated whole cultures of *Campylobacter fetus* subspecies *venerealis* which are adsorbed onto aluminum hydroxide.
Indications: For use in healthy cattle as an aid in the prevention and control of bovine vibriosis.
Dosage and Administration: Administer a single, 2 mL dose to cattle, subcutaneously or intramuscularly, two (2) to four (4) weeks prior to breeding. Revaccinate annually to maintain high levels of immunity.
Precaution(s): Store at 35°-45°F (2°-7°C). Do not freeze. Use the entire contents when first opened.
Caution(s): Anaphylactic reactions may occur with the use of any bacterin. Symptomatic treatment: Epinephrine.
Warning(s): Do not vaccinate within 21 days of slaughter.
Discussion: Bovine genital campylobacteriosis, previously known as vibriosis, is a venereal disease of cattle caused by *Campylobacter fetus* subsp. *venerealis.* The bacterium is a gram-negative curved rod with a polar flagellum. The disease is spread from bull to cow and cow to bull during breeding. It can also be spread through artificial insemination if the semen or pipettes are contaminated.
Infection with *Campylobacter* is subclinical and remains restricted to the vaginal and uterine mucosa of the cow and the mucous membranes of the prepuce and penis of the bull. The uterine infection at the time of conception usually destroys the embryo at its earliest stages. However, in some instances, the embryo survives, becomes infected and is usually aborted in the second trimester of gestation. The presence of the disease is suspected when conception rates for a newly infected herd drops dramatically to 40-50% or lower. Definite diagnoses can be made by identifying the organism in the cervico-vaginal mucus of the cow or preputial fluid from the suspected bull.
In herds where artificial insemination (A.I.) can be instituted, the disease can be eliminated from the herd if proper procedures are followed. In herds where A.I. is not feasible then vaccination is the only effective means of eliminating the disease from the herd.
Presentation: Available in 50 dose (100 mL) bottles.
Compendium Code No.: 11140532

VIB SHIELD® L5

Novartis Animal Vaccines **Bacterin**
Campylobacter fetus-Leptospira canicola-grippotyphosa-hardjo-icterohaemorrhagiae-pomona Bacterin
U.S. Vet. Lic. No.: 303
Composition: The bacterin contains inactivated antigenic cultures of *Campylobacter fetus, Leptospira canicola, grippotyphosa, hardjo, icterohaemorrhagiae,* and *pomona* adjuvanted with aluminum hydroxide. Contains penicillin and streptomycin as preservatives.
Indications: For use in healthy cattle as an aid in the prevention and control of diseases caused by *Campylobacter fetus, Leptospira canicola, grippotyphosa, hardjo, icterohaemorrhagiae,* and *pomona.*
Dosage and Administration: Shake well before using. Administer 2 mL subcutaneously or intramuscularly to cows two (2) to four (4) weeks prior to breeding. Revaccinate prior to each breeding to maintain high levels of immunity.
Precaution(s): Store at 35°-45°F (2°-7°C). Do not freeze. Use the entire contents when first opened.
Caution(s): Anaphylactic reactions may occur with the use of the bacterin. Symptomatic treatment: Epinephrine.
Warning(s): Do not vaccinate within 21 days of slaughter.
Discussion: Bovine genital campylobacteriosis, previously known as vibriosis, is a venereal disease of cattle caused by *Campylobacter fetus.* The disease is spread from bull to cow and cow to bull during breeding. It can also be spread through artificial insemination if the pipette or semen is contaminated.
Infection with Campylobacter is subclinical and remains restricted to the vaginal and uterine mucosa of the cow and the mucous membrane of the penis and sheath of the bull. The uterine infection usually destroys the embryo at its earliest stages. However, in some instances, the embryo survives, becomes infected and is aborted in the second trimester of pregnancy. The presence of the disease should be suspected when conception rates for a newly infected herd drop below 90%.
Definite diagnosis can be made by identifying the organism in the cervical or vaginal mucus of the cow or in preputial fluid from the infected bull.
The disease has been present in cattle herds for many years and has come to be known as the "repeat breeder syndrome".
Vaccination of the heifers, cows, and bulls prior to breeding is the only practical way to eliminate this insidious, costly disease.
Leptospirosis: Although leptospirosis is not the threat to the livestock industry that it once was, the organism should not be forgotten. Leptospirosis is prevalent in all domestic animals, as well as wildlife populations such as skunks, opossums, and raccoons.
The organism will not survive by itself in the environment. Animals that recover from leptospirosis may become carriers, and the organism may be shed in the urine for various periods of time.
The susceptible animal ingests the organism, usually through feed or in water contaminated by animals shedding the organism in their urine.
Clinical signs in infected cattle are, for the most part, not observed. A particularly observant herdsman may notice a day or two of lowered feed consumption, and in the case of milk cows, lowered milk production. The most frequent clinical sign of leptospirosis is abortion in the last trimester of gestation. Red colored urine due to hemoglobinuria may be seen also.
Trial Data: In a severe prebreeding challenge (controls = 21 cows and vaccinates = 20 cows), nearly twice as many cows became pregnant in the vaccinated group. These animals were challenged with two different strains of *Campylobacter (Vibrio) fetus.* This demonstrates protection against the heterologous challenges most likely to occur in a herd.

Group	% Conception Rate
Controls	43%
Vaccinates	80%

References: Available upon request.
Presentation: Available in 10 dose (20 mL) and 50 dose (100 mL) bottles.
Compendium Code No.: 11140542

VIB SHIELD® L5 HARDJO BOVIS

Novartis Animal Vaccines **Bacterin**
Campylobacter Fetus-Leptospira Canicola-Grippotyphosa-Hardjo-Icterohaemorrhagiae-Pomona Bacterin
U.S. Vet. Lic. No.: 303
Composition: This bacterin contains inactivated cultures of *Campylobacter fetus, Leptospira canicola, grippotyphosa, hardjo-bovis, icterohaemorrhagiae,* and *pomona* adjuvanted with aluminum hydroxide. Contains thimerosal as a preservative.
Indications: For use in healthy cattle as an aid in the prevention and control of disease caused by *Campylobacter fetus, Leptospira canicola, grippotyphosa, hardjo, icterohaemorrhagiae,* and *pomona.*
Dosage and Administration: Shake well before using. Administer 2 mL intramuscularly 2-4 weeks prior to breeding.
Precaution(s): Store in the dark at 35°-45°F (2°-7°C). Do not freeze. Use entire contents when first opened.
Caution(s): Anaphylactic reactions may occur following the use of this biological. Symptomatic treatment: Epinephrine.
For veterinary use only.
Warning(s): Do not vaccinate within 21 days prior to slaughter.
Presentation: 10 dose (20 mL) and 50 dose (100 mL) bottles.
Compendium Code No.: 11140770 F278 / F279

VIB SHIELD® PLUS

Novartis Animal Vaccines **Bacterin**
Campylobacter fetus Bacterin
U.S. Vet. Lic. No.: 303
Composition: The bacterin contains inactivated whole cultures of *Campylobacter fetus* subspecies *venerealis* adjuvanted with Xtend III™ for maximum and long lasting immunity. Contains penicillin and streptomycin as preservatives.
Indications: For use in healthy cattle as an aid in the prevention and control of bovine vibriosis.
Dosage and Administration: Shake well before and during use. Administer a single 2 mL dose of bacterin deep intramuscularly to breeding stock. Vaccinate dairy cows during the drying-off period. Vaccinate beef cows anytime within 12 months of breeding. Revaccinate annually.
Precaution(s): Store at 35°-45°F (2°-7°C). Do not freeze. Use the entire contents when first opened.
Caution(s): Anaphylactic reactions may occur with any bacterin. Symptomatic treatment: Epinephrine.
Warning(s): The product causes persistent swellings at the site of injection. Do not vaccinate within 60 days of slaughter.
Discussion: Bovine genital campylobacteriosis, previously known as vibriosis, is a venereal disease of cattle caused by *Campylobacter fetus* subsp. *venerealis.* The bacterium is a gram negative curved rod with a polar flagellum. The disease is spread from bull to cow and cow to bull during breeding. It can also be spread through artificial insemination if the semen or pipettes are contaminated.
Infection with Campylobacter is subclinical and remains restricted to the vaginal and uterine mucosa of the cow and the mucous membranes of the prepuce and penis of the bull. The uterine infection at the time of conception usually destroys the embryo at its earliest stages, however, in some instances the embryo survives, becomes infected and is usually aborted in the second trimester of gestation. The presence of the disease is suspected when conception rates for a newly infected herd drop dramatically to 40-50% or lower. Definite diagnoses can be made by identifying the organism in the cervico-vaginal mucous of the cow or preputial fluid from the suspected bull.
In herds where artificial insemination (A.I.) can be instituted, the disease can be eliminated from the herd if proper procedures are followed. In herds where A.I. is not feasible then vaccination is the only effective means of eliminating the disease from the herd.
Trial Data: In a severe prebreeding challenge (controls = 15 cows and vaccinates = 17 cows), nearly twice as many cows became pregnant in the vaccinated group. These animals were challenged with two different strains of *Campylobacter (Vibrio) fetus.* This demonstrates protection against the heterologous challenges most likely to occur in a herd.

Group	% Conception Rate
Controls	66.6%
Vaccinates	100%

References: Available upon request.
Presentation: Available in 10 dose (20 mL) and 50 dose (100 mL) bottles.
Compendium Code No.: 11140552

VIB SHIELD® PLUS L5

Novartis Animal Vaccines **Bacterin**

Campylobacter fetus-Leptospira canicola-grippotyphosa-hardjo-icterohaemorrhagiae-pomona Bacterin

U.S. Vet. Lic. No.: 303

Composition: This bacterin contains inactivated antigenic cultures of *Campylobacter fetus, Leptospira canicola, L. grippotyphosa, L. hardjo, L. icterohaemorrhagiae* and *L. pomona* adjuvanted with Xtend III®.

Contains thimerosal, penicillin and streptomycin as preservatives.

Indications: For use in healthy cattle as an aid in the prevention and control of diseases caused by *Campylobacter fetus, Leptospira canicola, L. grippotyphosa, L. hardjo, L. icterohaemorrhagiae* and *L. pomona.*

Dosage and Administration: Shake well before using. Administer a 2 mL dose intramuscularly to cows 2-4 weeks prior to breeding. Revaccinate prior to each breeding to maintain high levels of immunity.

Precaution(s): Store at 35°-45°F (2°-7°C). Do not freeze. Use the entire contents when first opened.

Caution(s): Transient swelling may occur at the site of injection. Milk reduction and transient depression may be observed in lactating dairy cows for 3-6 days following vaccination. Anaphylactic reactions may occur following the use of the product. Symptomatic treatment: Epinephrine.

For veterinary use only.

Warning(s): Do not vaccinate within 60 days of slaughter.

Presentation: Available in 10 dose (20 mL) and 50 dose (100 mL) bottles.

Compendium Code No.: 11140562

VI BURSA C.E.™

L.A.H.I. (New Jersey) **Vaccine**

Bursal Disease Vaccine, Live Virus

U.S. Vet. Lic. No.: 196

Active Ingredient(s): This product is a live virus vaccine containing a chicken embryo propagated Bursal Disease Virus for protection against Infectious Bursal (Gumboro) Disease.

Contains neomycin as a preservative.

This vaccine was carefully produced and passed all tests in accordance with the U.S. Government requirements.

Indications: When administered to susceptible birds, the vaccine stimulates immunity.

Effective use of this vaccine is an aid in protecting young and older chickens against outbreaks of Infectious Bursal Disease, which can cause excessive mortality, immunosuppression and poor growth rates.

Dosage and Administration: In chicks with no detectable maternal antibodies one vaccination at 10 days of age is recommended.

In chicks with maternal antibodies 2 vaccinations are recommended, one at 10-14 days of age and the second at 2-3 weeks after the first vaccination.

Preparation of Vaccine for Drinking Water Use: Remove the aluminum overseal and stopper and add clean non-sanitized water. Replace the stopper and shake well. Pour the contents into a quart jar ¾ full of non-sanitized water. Shake well and dilute the vaccine as the case may be as outlined in the charts below. A dried skim milk powder should be used as a vaccine stabilizer at the rate of 8.0 grams per gallon of water. The powdered milk is added prior to the reconstitution of the vaccine.

Method of Vaccination: Withhold all medication and disinfectants from the drinking water 24 hours before and 24 hours after vaccinating. Rinse waterers with clean non-sanitized water and remove all water from chicks for at least two hours prior to vaccination. Provide adequate space so that at least two-thirds of the birds can drink at one time.

Add mixture to water as per following charts:

1000 Dose:

Age of Birds	Heavy per 1000 birds	Leghorn per 1000 birds
3 Weeks	3 Gals. of Water	3 Gals. of Water
4 Weeks-8 Weeks	8 Gals. of Water	5 Gals. of Water

2500 Dose:

Age of Birds	Heavy per 2500 birds	Leghorn per 2500 birds
3 Weeks	7 Gals. of Water	7 Gals. of Water
4 Weeks-8 Weeks	20 Gals. of Water	12 Gals. of Water

10,000 Dose:

Age of Birds	Heavy per 10,000 birds	Leghorn per 10,000 birds
3 Weeks	30 Gals. of Water	30 Gals. of Water
4 Weeks-8 Weeks	80 Gals. of Water	50 Gals. of Water

15,000 Dose:

Age of Birds	Heavy per 15,000 birds	Leghorn per 15,000 birds
3 Weeks	45 Gals. of Water	45 Gals. of Water
4 Weeks-8 Weeks	120 Gals. of Water	80 Gals. of Water

Divide the mixed vaccine into the waterers. Provide no other drinking water until all vaccine has been consumed.

Contraindication(s): Vaccinate healthy chickens only. Check with your poultry pathologist before vaccinating birds suspected of having been recently exposed to infectious Bursal Disease.

Precaution(s): Keep vaccine in the dark between 2-7°C (35-45°F).

Use entire contents when first opened. Burn this container and all unused contents.

Caution(s): This vaccine is not effective when birds are derived from strongly immune parent stock. Therefore, the immune status of the flock to be vaccinated should be determined prior to using this vaccine. Use this vaccine when parental antibody to Bursal Disease Virus (Gumboro Disease) is at its minimum.

While immunity begins to develop immediately, it generally requires 10 days to two weeks for birds to establish immunity to Gumboro disease following vaccination, during which time they should not be placed in contaminated premises or otherwise exposed to Gumboro disease.

Distribution in each state shall be limited to authorized recipients designated by proper state officials under such additional conditions as these authorities may require.

Recommended use shall be restricted to premises having a history of the disease.

All susceptible birds on any farm should be vaccinated at the same time. If this is not possible, individual lots may be vaccinated if strict isolation and separate caretakers are provided for the vaccinated and unvaccinated lots of birds.

It is imperative that the user of this product comply with the indications for use, contraindication, cautions and methods of vaccination stated on the direction sheet packed with the product. The vaccine must be prepared and administered as directed to obtain best results.

Warning(s): Do not vaccinate within 21 days before slaughter.

Care should be taken to avoid contaminating your hands, eyes and clothing with the vaccine.

For veterinary use only.

Presentation: 1000, 2500, 10,000, and 15,000 dose vials.

Compendium Code No.: 10080392

VI BURSA-G™

L.A.H.I. (New Jersey) **Vaccine**

Bursal Disease Vaccine, Live Virus

U.S. Vet. Lic. No.: 196

Active Ingredient(s): Description: This product is a live virus vaccine containing a chicken tissue culture propagated bursal disease virus for protection against infectious bursal (Gumboro) disease.

Gentamicin and a amphotericin B added as preservatives.

This vaccine was carefully produced and passed all tests in accordance with the U.S. Government requirements.

Indications: In chicks with no detectable maternal antibodies one vaccination at 10 days of age is recommended. For drinking water use.

In chicks with maternal antibodies 2 vaccinations are recommended, one at 10-14 days of age and the second at 2-3 weeks after the first vaccination.

Dosage and Administration: Preparation of Vaccine for Drinking Water Use: Remove the aluminum overseal and stopper and add clean, non-sanitized water. Replace the stopper and shake well. Pour the contents into a quart jar ¾ full of non-sanitized water. Shake well and dilute the vaccine for 1,000, 2,500 and 10,000 doses as the case may be as outlined in the chart below. A dried skim milk powder should be used as a vaccine stabilizer at the rate of 8.0 grams per gallon of water. The powdered milk is added prior to the reconstitution of the vaccine.

Method of Vaccination: Withhold all medication and disinfectants from the drinking water 24 hours before and 24 hours after vaccinating. Rinse waterers with clean, non-sanitized water and remove all water from chicks for at least two hours prior to vaccination. Provide adequate space so that at least two-thirds of the birds can drink at one time.

Add mixture to water as per following chart:

Age of Birds	Heavy			Leghorn		
	per 1,000 birds	per 2,500 birds	per 10,000 birds	per 1,000 birds	per 2,500 birds	per 10,000 birds
3 Weeks	3 Gals. of Water	7 Gals. of Water	30 Gals. of Water	3 Gals. of Water	7 Gals. of Water	30 Gals. of Water
4 Weeks-8 Weeks	8 Gals. of Water	20 Gals. of Water	50 Gals. of Water	5 Gals. of Water	12 Gals. of Water	50 Gals. of Water

Contraindication(s): Vaccinate healthy chickens only. Check with your poultry pathologist before vaccinating birds suspected of having been recently exposed to infectious Bursal Disease.

Precaution(s): Keep vaccine in the dark between 2-7°C (35-45°F).

Use entire contents when first opened. Burn this container and all unused contents.

Caution(s): When administered to susceptible birds, a mild form of the disease results which stimulates immunity.

Effective use of this vaccine is an aid in protecting young chickens against outbreaks of infectious bursal disease, which can cause excessive mortality, immunosuppression and poor growth rates.

The immune status of the flock to be vaccinated should be determined prior to the use of this vaccine. The vaccine can be used in the presence of maternal antibodies. However, even in the presence of low levels of maternal antibodies may interfere with complete protection. Thus, in order to obtain satisfactory protection it is recommended that revaccination be conducted 2-3 weeks after the first vaccination.

While immunity begins to develop immediately, it generally requires 10 days to two weeks for birds to establish immunity to Gumboro disease following vaccination, during which time they should not be placed in contaminated premises or otherwise exposed to Gumboro disease.

Distribution in each state shall be limited to authorized recipients designated by proper state officials under such additional conditions as these authorities may require.

Recommended use shall be restricted to premises having a history of the disease.

All susceptible birds on any farm should be vaccinated at the same time. If this is not possible, individual lots may be vaccinated if strict isolation and separate caretakers are provided for the vaccinated and unvaccinated lots of birds.

It is imperative that the user of this product comply with the indications for use, contraindications, and method of vaccination stated on the direction sheet. The vaccine must be prepared and administered as directed to obtain the best results.

Warning(s): Do not vaccinate within 21 days before slaughter.

Care should be taken to avoid contaminating your hands, eyes and clothing with the vaccine.

For veterinary use only.

Presentation: 1,000, 2,500 and 10,000 doses.

Compendium Code No.: 10080402

VI BURSA-K™

L.A.H.I. (New Jersey) **Vaccine**

Bursal Disease Vaccine, Killed Virus

U.S. Vet. Lic. No.: 196

Active Ingredient(s): This product is a betapropiolactone (BPL) inactivated oil base emulsion of an antigenic strain of infectious bursal disease virus.

The vaccine is manufactured in accordance with a detailed production outline, which has been filed with the Veterinary Services of the USDA. Only specific pathogen free (SPF) eggs are used for production purposes. Seed virus is derived from a master seed virus lot which has been fully tested for purity, safety and immunogenicity. The fill volume for this product is 500 mL in a 625 mL plastic bottle. The bottles are sealed with a rubber stopper and an aluminum overseal.

Quality Control: The flocks producing SPF eggs are under constant observation by experienced personnel and routinely sampled and tested serologically to confirm absence of exposure to a large variety of avian pathogens. Shipments from the supplier are accompanied by regular reports on test results for each flock from which eggs were obtained.

The product is fully tested for purity, safety and potency according to the standard requirements for bursal disease vaccine, killed virus, published as part 113, in particular, 113.120 and 113.132

of title 9 of the federal regulations by the Animal and Plant Health Inspection Service of the U.S. Department of Agriculture. Each serial is tested for: Bacteria and fungi; safety and potency tests in chickens.

Samples and complete test reports on each serial are submitted to the Veterinary Services of the USDA and no merchandise is released for shipment until this government agency has given its release agreement.

Indications: This product is recommended for subcutaneous or intramuscular vaccination in chickens three weeks of age or older for the prevention of infectious bursal disease.

Dosage and Administration: Immediately prior to use, shake the vaccine vigorously for 30 seconds to one (1) minute. Remove the aluminum overseal and the vaccine is ready to use.

Method of Vaccination: The vaccine should be administered subcutaneously in the neck or intramuscularly in the leg. No other route is suggested or implied. Subcutaneous inoculation should be given in the mid-portion of the neck. Each bird should receive 0.5 mL of vaccine. Intramuscular injection in a dose of 0.5 mL should be given in the back of leg into the thigh muscle.

Precaution(s): The vaccine shall be stored in the dark in a refrigerator between 35-45°F (2-7°C).

Expiration date: 24 months.

Caution(s): It is imperative that the user of this product comply with the indications for use, contraindications, cautions and method of vaccination stated on the direction sheet packed with the product. The vaccine must be prepared and administered as directed to obtain the best results. For veterinary use only.

Warning(s): Do not market birds for at least six (6) weeks after vaccinating so that there is no swelling at the site of vaccine administration.

Presentation: 1,000 doses.

Compendium Code No.: 10080422

VI BURSA-K+V

L.A.H.I. (New Jersey) **Vaccine**

Bursal Disease Vaccine, Killed Virus, Standard and Variant

U.S. Vet. Lic. No.: 196

Active Ingredient(s): This product is a suspension of killed infectious bursal disease viruses of chicken tissue culture, chicken embryo and bursal tissue origin emulsified in an oil base.

The vaccine is manufactured in accordance with a detailed production outline, which has been filed with the Veterinary Services of the USDA. Seed virus is derived from a master seed virus lot, which has been fully tested for purity, safety and immunogenicity. Only specific pathogen free (SPF) eggs and chickens are used for production purposes.

Quality Control: The flocks producing SPF eggs are under constant observation by experienced personnel and routinely sampled and tested serologically to confirm absence of exposure to a large variety of avian pathogens. Shipments from the supplier are accompanied by regular reports on test results for each flock from which eggs were obtained.

The product is fully tested for purity, safety and potency according to the standard requirements for bursal disease vaccine, killed virus, chicken tissue culture origin, published as part 113, in particular, 113.166 of title 9 of the federal regulations by the Animal and Plant Health Inspection Service of the USDA.

Each serial is tested for: Bacteria and fungi; safety and potency tests in chickens according to 9 CFR 113.132 (challenge against standard and variant IBD viruses).

Indications: This product is recommended for initial vaccination and revaccination of broiler breeders for the passive protection of progeny broilers against standard and variant infectious bursal disease. The initial vaccination is administered to pullets three weeks of age or older. Revaccination is recommended between 16-20 weeks of age.

Dosage and Administration: Immediately prior to use, shake bottle vigorously for 30 seconds to one (1) minute. Remove aluminum overseal. Should greater than four (4) hours elapse between the first and last use it is recommended that the bottle be shaken again before continuing with vaccinations.

Method of Vaccination: Inject each bird with a 0.5 mL dose either for initial vaccination or revaccination. The vaccine should be administered subcutaneously in the neck or intramuscularly in the leg.

Precaution(s): The vaccine shall be stored in the dark in a refrigerator between 35-45°F (2-7°C).

Expiration date: 24 months.

Caution(s): It is imperative that the user of this product comply with indications for use, contraindications, cautions and method of vaccination stated on the label. The vaccine must be prepared and administered as directed to obtain best results. For veterinary use only.

Warning(s): Do not market birds for at least six (6) weeks after vaccinating so that there is no swelling at the site of vaccine administration.

Presentation: The product is distributed in 625 mL sterile plastic bottles filled with 500 mL of finished product (1,000 doses). Full directions for use are given on the label of each bottle.

Compendium Code No.: 10080412

VI BURSA-L™

L.A.H.I. (New Jersey) **Vaccine**

Bursal Disease Vaccine, Live Virus

U.S. Vet. Lic. No.: 196

Active Ingredient(s): This product is a live virus vaccine containing a chicken tissue culture propagated bursal disease virus for protection against infectious bursal (Gumboro) disease.

Gentamicin and a fungistat are added as preservatives.

This vaccine was carefully produced and passed all tests in accordance with the U.S. Government requirements.

Indications: This vaccine should be administered to birds three weeks of age or older. For drinking water use.

Dosage and Administration: Preparation of Vaccine for Drinking Water Use: Remove the aluminum overseal and stopper and add clean, non-sanitized water. Replace the stopper and shake well. Pour the contents into a quart jar ¾ full of non-sanitized water. Shake well and dilute as outlined in the chart below. A dried skim milk powder should be used as a vaccine stabilizer at the rate of 8.0 grams per gallon of water. The powdered milk is added prior to the reconstitution of the vaccine.

Method of Vaccination: Withhold all medication and disinfectants from the drinking water 24 hours before and 24 hours after vaccinating. Rinse waterers with clean, non-sanitized water and remove all water from chicks for at least two hours prior to vaccination. Provide adequate space so that at least two-thirds of the birds can drink at one time.

Add mixture to water as per following chart:

Age of Birds	Heavy		Leghorn	
	per 1,000 birds	per 10,000 birds	per 1,000 birds	per 10,000 birds
3 Weeks	3 Gals. of Water	30 Gals. of Water	3 Gals. of Water	30 Gals. of Water
4 Weeks-8 Weeks	8 Gals. of Water	50 Gals. of Water	8 Gals. of Water	50 Gals. of Water

Contraindication(s): Chickens to be vaccinated should be free of all diseases, including the latent form of diseases such as chronic respiratory disease (CRD), coccidiosis, parasitic disease, etc. Check with your poultry pathologist before vaccinating birds suspected of having been recently exposed to infectious Bursal Disease.

Precaution(s): Keep vaccine in the dark between 2-7°C (35-45°F).

Use entire contents when first opened. Burn this container and all unused contents.

Caution(s): When administered to susceptible birds, a mild form of the disease results which stimulates immunity.

Effective use of this vaccine is an aid in protecting young chickens against outbreaks of infectious bursal disease, which can cause excessive mortality, immunosuppression and poor growth rates.

This vaccine is not effective when birds are derived from strongly immune parent stock. Therefore, the immune status of the flock to be vaccinated should be determined prior to using this vaccine. Use this vaccine when parental antibody to Bursal Disease Virus (Gumboro Disease) is at its minimum.

While immunity begins to develop immediately, it generally requires 10 days to two weeks for birds to establish immunity to Gumboro disease following vaccination, during which time they should not be placed in contaminated premises or otherwise exposed to Gumboro disease.

Distribution in each state shall be limited to authorized recipients designated by proper state officials - under such additional conditions as these authorities may require.

Recommended use shall be restricted to premises having a history of the disease.

All susceptible birds on any farm should be vaccinated at the same time. If this is not possible, individual lots may be vaccinated if strict isolation and separate caretakers are provided for the vaccinated and unvaccinated lots of birds.

It is imperative that the user of this product comply with the indications for use, contraindications, and method of vaccination stated on the direction sheet. The vaccine must be prepared and administered as directed to obtain the best results.

Warning(s): Do not vaccinate within 21 days before slaughter.

Care should be taken to avoid contaminating your hands, eyes and clothing with the vaccine. For veterinary use only.

Presentation: 1,000, 2,500 and 10,000 doses.

Compendium Code No.: 10080432

VICETON® ℞

Bimeda **Chloramphenicol**

Chloramphenicol Tablets

NADA No.: 055-059

Active Ingredient(s): Each tablet contains:

Chloramphenicol . . . . . 100 mg
Chloramphenicol . . . . . 250 mg
Chloramphenicol . . . . . 500 mg
Chloramphenicol . . . . . 1 g

Indications: Chloramphenicol Tablets are recommended for oral treatment of the following conditions in dogs:

- Bacterial pulmonary infections caused by susceptible microorganisms such as: *Staphylococcus aureus, Streptococcus pyogenes* and *Brucella bronchiseptica.*
- Infections of the urinary tract caused by susceptible microorganisms such as: *Escherichia coli, Proteus vulgaris, Corynebacterium renale, Streptococcus* spp. and hemolytic *Staphylococcus.*
- Enteritis caused by susceptible microorganisms such as: *E. coli, Proteus* spp., *Salmonella* spp., and *Pseudomonas* spp.
- Infections associated with canine distemper caused by susceptible microorganisms such as: *Brucella bronchiseptica, E. coli, P. aeruginosa, Proteus* spp., *Shigella* spp. and *Neisseria catarrhalis.*

Additional adjunctive therapy should be used when indicated. Most susceptible infectious disease organisms will respond to chloramphenicol therapy in three to five days when the recommended dosage regime is followed. If no response to chloramphenicol therapy is obtained in three to five days, discontinue its use and review the diagnosis. Also, a change of therapy should be considered.

Laboratory tests should be conducted including *in vitro* culturing and susceptibility tests on samples collected prior to treatment.

Pharmacology: Chloramphenicol is a broad-spectrum antibiotic shown to have specific therapeutic activity against a wide variety of organisms. Its activity was first demonstrated in culture filtrates from a species of soil organism collected in Venezuela, later designated as *Streptomyces venezuelae.* The antibiotic was subsequently isolated from culture filtrates, identified chemically, and later synthesized.

Aqueous solutions of chloramphenicol are neutral in pH. Chloramphenicol is stable for several years at room temperature and forms colorless to yellowish-white crystals in the shape of elongated plates or fine needles. It is only slightly soluble in water, but soluble in alcohol and propylene glycol.

Chloramphenicol is exceptionally stable in the presence of high pH, although it is destroyed at pH's in excess of 10. Dissolved in distilled water, it can withstand boiling for five hours.

Actions: At low concentrations, chloramphenicol exerts a bacteriostatic effect on a wide range of pathogenic organisms, including many gram-positive and gram-negative bacteria, spirochetes, several rickettsiae and certain large viruses and Mycoplasma (PPLO). At high concentrations, it inhibits growth of animal and plant cells.

Chloramphenicol exerts its bacteriostatic action by inhibiting protein synthesis in susceptible organisms. Complete suppression of the assimilation of ammonia and of the incorporation of amino acids, particularly glutamic acid, together with an increased formation of ribonucleic acid (RNA), lead to an inhibition of bacterial growth.

Chloramphenicol antagonizes the actions of such antibiotics as penicillin and streptomycin, which act only on growing cells, but is synergistic to tetracycline, which also acts by inhibiting protein synthesis. It is possible the chloramphenicol would produce similar synergism with other antibiotics which act by inhibiting protein synthesis.

In this respect, the experimentally demonstrated synergistic action between chloramphenicol and gamma-globulin should be mentioned. Clinical observations in man and corresponding investigations in laboratory animals experimentally infected with various pathogenic bacteria have shown that a combination of chloramphenicol with gamma-globulin or specific antisera has a greater therapeutic effect than would be expected from a mere addition of the individual effects.

Many experiments have revealed that the development of resistance to chloramphenicol is rare compared with that occurring with other important antibiotics. Bacterial resistance may develop some strains against chloramphenicol but has been encountered only infrequently in clinical usage.

Chloramphenicol achieves maximum serum levels very rapidly following oral, intravenous and intraperitoneal administration. Intramuscular injection with chloramphenicol, except certain soluble forms, results in a somewhat delayed absorption and lower serum levels than when given by the oral, intravenous, or intraperitoneal route.

Chloramphenicol diffuses readily into all body tissues, but at different concentrations. Highest concentrations are found in the liver and kidney of dogs indicating that these organs are the main route of inactivation and excretion for the metabolites. The lungs, spleen, heart and skeletal muscles contain concentrations similar to that of the blood.

Chloramphenicol reaches significant concentration in the aqueous and vitreous humors of the eye from the blood.

A significant difference from other antibiotics is its marked ability to diffuse into the cerebrospinal fluid. Within three to four hours after administration, the concentration in the cerebrospinal fluid has reached, on the average, 50% of the concentration in the serum. If the meninges are inflamed, the percentage may be even higher.

Chloramphenicol diffuses readily into milk, pleural and ascitic fluids and crosses the placenta attaining concentrations of about 75% of that of the maternal blood.

Chloramphenicol is rather rapidly metabolized, mainly in the liver, by conjugation with glucuronic acid.

Dosage and Administration: Dogs — 25 mg/lb body weight every 6 hours for oral administration.

Contraindication(s): Because of potential antagonism, chloramphenicol should not be administered simultaneously with penicillin or streptomycin.

Precaution(s): Store at or below 25°C (77°F) in a dry place.

Caution(s): Federal law restricts this drug to use by or on the order of a licensed veterinarian.

1. This antibiotic contains a chemical structure (nitrobenzene group) that is characteristic of a group of drugs long known to depress hematopoietic activity of the bone marrow.
2. *In vitro*-tissue culture studies using canine bone marrow cells have demonstrated that extremely high concentrations of chloramphenicol inhibit both uptake of iron by the nucleated red cells and incorporation of iron into heme.
3. Chloramphenicol products should not be administered in conjunction with or two hours prior to the induction of general anesthesia with pentobarbital because of prolonged recovery time.
4. Chloramphenicol products should not be administered to dogs maintained for breeding purposes. Some experiments indicate that chloramphenicol causes, in experimental animals, particularly females, significant disorders in morphology as well as in function of the gonads.

Warning(s): Not for use in animals which are raised for food production. Chloramphenicol products should not be administered in conjunction with or 2 hours prior to the induction of general anesthesia with pentobarbital because of prolonged recovery.

Chloramphenicol products should not be administered to dogs maintained for breeding purposes. Some experiments indicate that chloramphenicol causes in experimental animals, particularly in females, significant disorders in morphology as well as in function of the gonads.

Keep out of reach of children.

Toxicology: Approximately 55% of a single daily dose can be recovered from the urine of a treated dog. A small fraction of this is in the form of unchanged chloramphenicol.

A single intravenous dose of 150 mg/kg (approximately 68 mg/lb) in propylene glycol is the maximum dose tolerated by the dog. No toxic effect was observed when dogs were administered orally, 200 mg/kg (approximately 91 mg/lb) daily for over four months. In the mouse, the LD-50 is 150-250 mg/kg (68 to 114 mg/lb) body weight by intravenous injection and 1,500 mg/kg (approximately 681 mg/lb) by the oral administration.

Adverse Reactions: Certain individual dogs may exhibit transient vomiting or diarrhea after an oral dose of 25 mg/lb body weight.

References: Available upon request.

Presentation: 100 mg: Bottles of 500's.
250 mg: Bottles of 500's, 1,000's.
500 mg: Bottles of 500's.
1 gram: Bottles of 100's.

Compendium Code No.: 13990450

VI CLEMCOL-C™

L.A.H.I. (New Jersey) **Vaccine**

Pasteurella multocida Vaccine, Avirulent Live Culture, Avian Isolate

U.S. Vet. Lic. No.: 196

Active Ingredient(s): *Pasteurella multocida* vaccine is a freeze dried avirulent live culture of a turkey isolate.

This vaccine was carefully produced and passed all tests in accordance with the U.S. Government requirements.

Indications: For prevention of fowl cholera in chickens.

When administered by the wing-web application in chickens, antibodies are produced which provide immunity against infection caused by *Pasteurella multocida* type 1 strain. The level and duration of immunity is dependant on many factors including the health of the birds, nutrition, stress factors, concurrent disease and climatic conditions.

This vaccine is administered initially to chickens 6 to 12 weeks of age and repeated once at about 18 to 20 weeks of age prior to initiation of lay. For wing-web application.

Dosage and Administration: Preparation of Vaccine: The active agent of the vaccine is supplied in a dried form in the bottle labelled "Vaccine". Open the bottle by removing the aluminum tear seal and rubber stopper. Open the diluent and pour a small quantity of diluent into the bottle of vaccine, replace the stopper and shake well. Pour the mixture back into the bottle containing the remainder of the diluent and shake mixture vigorously. Do not open or mix the vaccine until ready to use.

Method of Vaccination: Vaccination is accomplished by double dipping the needle applicator in the mixed vaccine and piercing the "web of the wing" from the underside. Do not apply through feathers, muscle or bone. The applicator must be redipped between each application.

Examination for Takes: Normally no clinical reaction is observed. At 5 to 10 days following vaccination, a swelling of the skin (subcutaneous granuloma) will develop in the wing web at the point of inoculation. The absence of this local reaction may mean that the birds were immune before vaccination or that improper vaccination methods were used. Examination for these takes may be used to assure that proper vaccination has been conducted. Immunity will normally develop within 14 days after vaccination.

Contraindication(s): Initial vaccination in chickens over 12 weeks of age may be undesirable because larger granulomas may develop at the site of inoculation and this may result in downgrading of carcasses at slaughter.

Precaution(s): Keep vaccine in the dark between 2-7°C (35-45°F).

Use entire contents when first opened. Burn this container and all unused contents.

Caution(s): It is imperative that the user of this product comply with the indications for use, contraindication, and method of vaccination stated on the direction sheet. The vaccine must be prepared and administered as directed to obtain best results.

Chickens to be vaccinated should be free of all diseases including the latent form of diseases such as chronic respiratory disease (CRD), coccidiosis, black-head, parasitic diseases, mycoplasma infection, infectious bursal disease, Marek's disease, etc.

All susceptible birds on any farm should be vaccinated at the same time. If this is not possible, individual lots may be vaccinated if strict isolation and separate caretakers are provided for the vaccinated and unvaccinated lots of birds.

Withhold all antibiotics and sulfas from feed and water for 3 days before and 5 days following vaccination.

Warning(s): Do not vaccinate within 21 days before slaughter.

Care should be taken to avoid contaminating hands, eyes and clothing with the vaccine.

For veterinary use only.

Presentation: 500 doses - rehydrate to 5 mL.

Compendium Code No.: 10080442

VICTOR GALL REMEDY

Fiebing **Topical Wound Dressing**

Active Ingredient(s):

Methylene blue U.S.P.	0.34%
Isopropyl alcohol	35.2%

Indications: For dressing sore shoulders, saddle galls and wire cuts on horses and cattle.

Dosage and Administration: Apply freely to the affected area. The application may be repeated several times a day until the wound is healed.

Caution(s): For external use only.

Flammable. Keep away from heat or flame.

Not for human use.

Keep out of the reach of children.

Presentation: 7 oz. and 1 gallon plastic bottles.

Compendium Code No.: 10590021

VIGILQUAT

Alex C. Fergusson **Disinfectant**

EPA Reg. No.: 833-71

Active Ingredient(s):

Alkyl (C_{14}, 50%; C_{12}, 40%; C_{16}, 10%) dimethyl benzyl ammonium chloride	4.00%
Octyl decyl dimethyl ammonium chloride	3.00%
Didecyl dimethyl ammonium chloride	1.5%
Dioctyl dimethyl ammonium chloride	1.5%
Inert ingredients	90.00%
Total	100.00%

Indications: Disinfectant, sanitizer, fungicide, deodorizer with organic soil tolerance for hospitals, institutions, industries, schools, dairies and other farm uses.

Dosage and Administration: It is a violation of federal law to use the product in a manner inconsistent with its labeling.

Apply VIGILQUAT with a cloth, mop or mechanical spray device. When applied with a mechanical spray device, surfaces must be sprayed until thoroughly wetted. Treated surfaces must remain wet for 10 minutes. A fresh solution should be prepared once a day or when the used solution becomes visibly dirty.

Disinfection of poultry equipment, animal quarters, and kennels: Poultry brooders, watering founts, feeding equipment and other animal quarters (such as stalls and kennel areas) can be disinfected after a thorough cleaning by applying a solution of 1.75 oz. VIGILQUAT in five (5) gallons of water. Small utensils should be immersed in the solution.

Prior to disinfection, all poultry, other animals and their feeds must be removed from the premises. This includes emptying all troughs, racks, and other feeding and watering appliances. Remove all litter and droppings from floors, walls, and other surfaces occupied or traversed by poultry or other animals.

After disinfection, ventilate buildings, coops, and other closed spaces. Do not house poultry, or other animals or employ equipment until the treatment has been absorbed, set or dried.

All treated equipment that will contact feed or drinking water must be rinsed with potable water before re-use.

Disinfection in hospitals, nursing homes and other health care institutions: For disinfecting floors, walls, countertops, bathing areas, lavatories, bedframes, tables, chairs, garbage pails and other nonporous surfaces.

Add 3.0 oz. VIGILQUAT to five (5) gallons of water. Apply to previously cleaned hard surfaces. At this use-level, VIGILQUAT is effective against *Pseudomonas aeruginosa*, *Staphylococcus aureus* and *salmonella choleraesuis* in the presence of 5% blood serum when evaluated by AOAC use-dilution test.

Disinfection in institutions, industry and schools: Add 1.75 oz. of VIGILQUAT to five (5) gallons of water. At 0.5 oz. to 3.0 gallons of water use level, the fungicidal effectiveness of VIGILQUAT in the presence of 5% blood serum against *Trichophyton mentagrophytes* has been shown utilizing the AOAC fungicidal test.

Egg shell sanitizing: Thoroughly clean all eggs. Thoroughly mix 1 oz. of the product with five (5) gallons of warm water to produce 150 ppm VIGILQUAT. The sanitizer temperature should not exceed 130°F. Spray the warm sanitizer so that the eggs are thoroughly wetted. Allow the eggs to thoroughly dry before casing or breaking. Do not apply a potable water rinse. The solution should not be re-used to sanitize eggs.

Sanitizing of food processing equipment and other hard surfaces in food contact locations: For sanitizing food processing equipment, dairy equipment, food utensils, dishes, silverware, glasses, sink tops, countertops, refrigerated storage and display equipment and other hard nonporous surfaces. No potable water rinse is required.

Wash and rinse all articles thoroughly, then apply a solution of 1 oz. VIGILQUAT in five (5) gallons of water (150 ppm active). Surfaces should remain wet for at least one (1) minute followed by adequate draining and air drying. A fresh solution should be prepared once a day or when the used solution becomes visibly dirty. For mechanical application, the use solution may not be re-used for sanitizing applications.

Apply to sink tops, countertops, refrigerated storage and display equipment and other stationary hard surfaces with a cloth or brush or mechanical spray device. No potable water rinse is required.

Dishes, silverware, glasses, cooking utensils and other similar size food processing equipment can be sanitized by immersion in a 1 oz. per five (5) gallon dilution of VIGILQUAT.

No potable water rinse is required.

At 1 oz. per five (5) gallons, VIGILQUAT fulfills the criteria of Appendix F of the Grade A Pasteurized Milk Ordinances 1978 recommendations of the U.S. Public Health Services in waters up to 800 ppm of hardness calculated as $CaCO_3$, when evaluated by the AOAC Germicidal and Detergent Sanitizer Method against *Escherichia coli* and *Staphylococcus auerus*.

The udders, flanks, and teats of dairy cows can be sanitized by washing with a solution of 1 oz. VIGILQUAT in five (5) gallons of warm water. No potable water rinse is required. Use a fresh towel for each cow. Avoid contamination of the sanitizing solution by dirt and soil. Do not dip the used towel back into the sanitizing solution. When the solution becomes visibly dirty, discard and provide a fresh solution.

Precaution(s):

Storage: Keep the container closed when not in use. Store indoors.

Disposal: Do not contaminate water, food or feed by storage or disposal, or by the cleaning of equipment. In the case of a spill, flood the area with a large quantity of water washing to a sewer or a collection vessel.

Wastes resulting from the use of the product may be disposed of on-site or at an approved waste disposal facility.

Do not re-use the empty container. Triple rinse, puncture and dispose of the container in a sanitary landfill or by incineration.

Caution(s): Precautionary Statements:

Hazards to Humans and Domestic Animals: Danger. Keep out of the reach of children. Corrosive. Causes eye damage and skin irritation. Do not get in eyes, on skin, or on clothing. Wear goggles or a face shield and rubber gloves when handling the product. Harmful if swallowed. Do not inhale spray mist. Avoid the contamination of food.

Statement of Practical Treatment:

In case of contact, immediately flush eyes or skin with plenty of water for at least 15 minutes. For eyes, call a physician. Remove and wash contaminated clothing before re-use.

If swallowed, promptly drink a large quantity of egg whites, gelatin solution; or if these are not available, drink large quantities of water. Avoid alcohol. Call a physician immediately.

Note to Physician: Probable mucosal damage may contraindicate the use of gastric lavage. Measures against circulatory shock, respiratory depression, and convulsion may be needed.

Presentation: 1 gallon containers (4 to a case) or 55 gallon drums.

Compendium Code No.: 10150020

VI MARK® BURSAL DISEASE-MAREK'S DISEASE VACCINE (Live Virus, Chicken and Turkey Herpesvirus)

L.A.H.I. (New Jersey) **Vaccine**

Bursal Disease-Marek's Disease Vaccine, Live Virus, Live Chicken and Turkey Herpesvirus, Cell Associated

U.S. Vet. Lic. No.: 196

Active Ingredient(s): Description: This product is of chicken tissue culture origin using SPF (Specific Pathogen Free) eggs. The product contains the SB_1 strain of chicken herpesvirus, the FC-126 strain of turkey herpesvirus and bursal disease virus. The product is packaged in two separate units. One is an ampule containing frozen live chicken and turkey herpesvirus and frozen live bursal disease virus and the other is a bottle of sterile diluent. The ampules are in canisters containing liquid nitrogen.

Gentamicin and amphotericin B are added as preservatives to the vaccine suspension in the ampule.

All vaccines released for sale meet the requirements of the licensing authority (U.S. Department of Agriculture) in regard to safety, purity, potency and the capacity to immunize normal susceptible birds.

Indications: This product is used for the prevention of bursal disease and very virulent Marek's disease in chickens. Give subcutaneously only.

This vaccine is recommended for use in healthy one-day-old chicks. The virus will infect chicks even though they may be carrying maternal precipitating antibodies to Marek's disease herpesvirus (MDHV).

Good management practices are recommended to reduce exposure for at least two weeks following vaccination.

Dosage and Administration: Preparation of Vaccine: Read warning advice on handling vaccine ampule.

Sterilize vaccinating equipment by boiling in water for 20 minutes or by autoclaving (15 minutes at 120°C). Do not use chemical disinfectants.

1. Before withdrawing vaccine from liquid-nitrogen refrigerator, protect hands with gloves. Wear long sleeves and use a face mask or goggles. It is possible an accident could occur with either the liquid nitrogen or the vials of vaccine. When removing a vial from the cane, hold palm of gloved hand away from body and face.
2. When withdrawing package of vials from canister in liquid-nitrogen refrigerator, expose only the vial at a time. After removing the vial, the cane holding the remaining vials should be replaced immediately in the canister of the liquid-nitrogen refrigerator.
3. The contents of the ampule are thawed rapidly by immersing in water at room temperature. Shake ampule to disperse contents. Then break ampule at the neck and immediately proceed as below. Caution: Ampules have been known to explode on sudden temperature change. Do not thaw in hot or ice cold water.
4. Draw contents of the ampule into a 10 cc sterile syringe.
5. Dilute immediately by filling the syringe slowly from a portion of the contents of the diluent bottle, after removing the center of the aluminum seal.
6. The contents of the syringe are then added to the remaining diluent. It is important that this be done slowly. Insert the syringe needle through the center of the rubber stopper of the diluent bottle. Slowly empty the syringe, allowing the vaccine to run down the side of the bottle. Gently shake the bottle as the vaccine is being mixed. Withdraw a portion of the diluent with the syringe to flush ampule. Inject the washing back into the diluent bottle. Remove the syringe.
7. Fill the automatic syringe according to the manufacturer's recommendations and set the dosage for 0.20 mL.
8. The vaccine and vaccinating syringe are now ready for use.

Method of Vaccination: Subcutaneous Administration:

1. Dilute the vaccine as directed above observing all precautions and warnings for handling.
2. Hold the chick by the back of the neck just below the head. The loose skin in the area is raised by gently pinching with the thumb and forefinger. Insert the needle beneath the skin in a downward direction away from the head. Inject 0.2 mL per chick. The bottle of vaccine should be kept in an ice bath and swirled frequently.
3. Avoid hitting the muscles and bones in the neck.
4. Entire contents of bottle must be used within 2 hours after mixing or discarded.

Contraindication(s): Birds to be vaccinated should be maintained under good environmental conditions to prevent unnecessary exposure to Marek's disease virus.

Precaution(s): Important: Storage Conditions:

Ampule - Store in liquid nitrogen refrigerator.

Diluent - Diluent may be stored at room temperature until a few hours prior to use. The diluent at the time of use should have the same temperature as the thawed vaccine.

Container - Store liquid nitrogen container securely in upright position in a dry, well-ventilated area.

Burn containers and all unused contents.

Keep vaccine ampule frozen in liquid nitrogen until ready to vaccinate.

Do not refreeze vaccine.

The entire contents should be used immediately upon thawing.

Do not mix Marek's vaccine with other vaccines or antibiotics.

Keep liquid nitrogen containers away from incubator intakes and chick boxes.

Caution(s): The capacity of this vaccine to produce satisfactory results depends on many factors, including but not limited to conditions of storage and handling by the user, administration of the vaccine, health and responsiveness of individual animals and degree of field exposure. Therefore, directions for use should be followed carefully.

The use of this vaccine is subject to applicable state and federal laws and regulations.

Warning(s): Do not vaccinate within 21 days of slaughter.

Liquid nitrogen container and vaccine should be handled only by properly trained personnel who are thoroughly conversant with the Union Carbide publication and instruction booklet regarding the use of, precautions and safe procedures for liquefied atmospheric gases (particularly liquid nitrogen).

When removing ampule cane, handling frozen ampules, or adding liquid nitrogen, wear long sleeves, a plastic face shield and gloves to protect the skin from contact with the liquid nitrogen. All storage and handling of the liquid nitrogen container must be in a dry, well-ventilated area. Do not inhale liquid nitrogen vapors. If drowsiness occurs, get fresh air quickly; then, ventilate entire area. If breathing difficulty occurs, apply artificial respiration. If any of these difficulties persist or there is a loss of consciousness, summon a physician immediately.

Care should be exercised to prevent contaminating hands, eyes and clothing with the vaccine.

For veterinary use only.

Presentation: 1000 doses with a 200 mL diluent.

Compendium Code No.: 10080462

VI MARK® BURSAL DISEASE-MAREK'S DISEASE VACCINE (Modified Live Virus, Turkey Herpesvirus)

L.A.H.I. (New Jersey) **Vaccine**

Bursal Disease-Marek's Disease Vaccine, Modified Live Virus, Live Turkey Herpesvirus, Cell Associated

U.S. Vet. Lic. No.: 196

Active Ingredient(s): Description: This product is of chicken tissue culture origin using SPF (Specific Pathogen Free) eggs. The product contains the FC-126 strain of turkey herpesvirus, and bursal disease virus and is used for the prevention of Marek's disease and Bursal disease in chickens. The product is packaged in two separate units. One is an ampule containing frozen live turkey herpesvirus and frozen live bursal disease virus and the other is a bottle of sterile diluent. The ampules are in canisters containing liquid nitrogen.

Gentamicin and amphotericin B are added as preservatives to the vaccine suspension in the ampule.

All vaccines released for sale meet the requirements of the licensing authority (U.S. Department of Agriculture) in regard to safety, purity, potency and the capacity to immunize normal susceptible birds.

Indications: This vaccine is recommended for use in healthy one-day-old chicks. The virus will infect chicks even though they may be carrying maternal precipitating antibodies to Marek's disease herpesvirus (MDHV). For subcutaneous vaccination.

Good management practices are recommended to reduce exposure for at least two weeks following vaccination.

Dosage and Administration: Preparation of Vaccine: Read warning advice on handling vaccine ampule.

Sterilize vaccinating equipment by boiling in water for 20 minutes or by autoclaving (15 minutes at 120°C). Do not use chemical disinfectants.

1. Before withdrawing vaccine from liquid-nitrogen refrigerator, protect hands with gloves. Wear long sleeves and use a face mask or goggles. It is possible an accident could occur with either the liquid nitrogen or the vials of vaccine. When removing a vial from the cane, hold palm of gloved hand away from body and face.
2. When withdrawing package of vials from canister in liquid-nitrogen refrigerator, expose only the vial at a time. After removing the vial, the cane holding the remaining vials should be replaced immediately in the canister of the liquid-nitrogen refrigerator.
3. The contents of the ampule are thawed rapidly by immersing in water at room temperature. Shake ampule to disperse contents. Then break ampule at the neck and immediately proceed as below. Caution: Ampules have been known to explode on sudden temperature change. Do not thaw in hot or ice cold water.
4. Draw contents of the ampule into a 10 cc sterile syringe.
5. Dilute immediately by filling the syringe slowly from a portion of the contents of the diluent bottle, after removing the center of the aluminum seal.
6. The contents of the syringe are then added to the remaining diluent. It is important that this be done slowly. Insert the syringe needle through the center of the rubber stopper of the diluent bottle. Slowly empty the syringe, allowing the vaccine to run down the side of the bottle. Gently shake the bottle as the vaccine is being mixed. Withdraw a portion of the diluent with the syringe to flush ampule. Inject the washing back into the diluent bottle. Remove the syringe.
7. Fill the automatic syringe according to the manufacturer's recommendations and set the dosage for 0.20 mL.
8. The vaccine and vaccinating syringe are now ready for use.

Method of Vaccination: Subcutaneous Administration:

1. Dilute the vaccine as directed above observing all precautions and warnings for handling.
2. Hold the chick by the back of the neck just below the head. The loose skin in the area is raised by gently pinching with the thumb and forefinger. Insert the needle beneath the skin

in a downward direction away from the head. Inject 0.2 mL per chick. The bottle of vaccine should be kept in an ice bath and swirled frequently.
3. Avoid hitting the muscles and bones in the neck.
4. Entire contents of bottle must be used within 2 hours after mixing or discarded.

Contraindication(s): Birds to be vaccinated should be healthy and free from all diseases. It is essential that the birds be maintained under good environmental conditions to prevent unnecessary exposure to Marek's disease virus.

Precaution(s): Important: Storage Conditions:

Ampule - Store in liquid nitrogen refrigerator.

Diluent - Diluent may be stored at room temperature until a few hours prior to use. The diluent at the time of use should have the same temperature as the thawed vaccine.

Container - Store liquid nitrogen container securely in upright position in a dry, well-ventilated area.

Burn containers and all unused contents.

Keep vaccine ampule frozen in liquid nitrogen until ready to vaccinate.

Do not refreeze vaccine.

Do not use vaccine that has been thawed other than immediately before use.

Keep liquid nitrogen containers away from incubator intakes and chick boxes.

Caution(s): The capacity of this vaccine to produce satisfactory results depends on many factors, including but not limited to conditions of storage and handling by the user, administration of the vaccine, health and responsiveness of individual animals and degree of field exposure. Therefore, directions for use should be followed carefully.

The use of this vaccine is subject to applicable state and federal laws and regulations.

Warning(s): Do not vaccinate within 21 days of slaughter.

Liquid nitrogen container and vaccine should be handled only by properly trained personnel who are thoroughly conversant with the Union Carbide publication and instruction booklet regarding the use of, precautions and safe procedures for liquefied atmospheric gases (particularly liquid nitrogen).

When removing ampule cane, handling frozen ampules, or adding liquid nitrogen, wear long sleeves, a plastic face shield and gloves to protect the skin from contact with the liquid nitrogen. All storage and handling of the liquid nitrogen container must be in a dry, well-ventilated area. Do not inhale liquid nitrogen vapors. If drowsiness occurs, get fresh air quickly; then, ventilate entire area. If breathing difficulty occurs, apply artificial respiration. If any of these difficulties persist or there is a loss of consciousness, summon a physician immediately.

Care should be exercised to prevent contaminating your hands, eyes and clothing with the vaccine.

For veterinary use only.

Presentation: 1,000 dose virus ampule, 200 mL diluent.

Compendium Code No.: 10080472

VI MARK® MAREK'S DISEASE VACCINE (Live Chicken and Turkey Herpesvirus)

L.A.H.I. (New Jersey) **Vaccine**

Marek's Disease Vaccine, Live Chicken and Turkey Herpesvirus, Cell Associated

U.S. Vet. Lic. No.: 196

Active Ingredient(s): Description: The product is of chicken tissue culture origin using SPF (Specific Pathogen Free) eggs. The product contains the SB-1 strain of chicken herpesvirus and the FC-126 strain of turkey herpesvirus, and is used for the prevention of Marek's disease in chickens.

The product is packaged in two separate units. One is an ampule containing frozen live chicken and turkey herpesvirus of chicken tissue culture origin and the other is a bottle of sterile diluent. The ampules are inserted on metal canes. The canes are in canisters containing liquid nitrogen.

Gentamicin and amphotericin B are added as preservatives to the virus suspension in the ampule.

All vaccines released for sale meet the requirements of the licensing authority (U.S. Department of Agriculture) in regard to safety, purity, potency and the capacity to immunize normal susceptible birds.

Indications: The vaccine is recommended for use in healthy one-day-old chicks for the prevention of Marek's disease. The virus will infect chicks even though they may be carrying maternal antibodies to Marek's disease herpesvirus (MDHV). For subcutaneous vaccination.

Good management practices are recommended to reduce exposure for at least two weeks following vaccination.

Dosage and Administration: Preparation of Vaccine: Caution: Read the warning advice on handling the vaccine ampule.

Sterilize the vaccinating equipment by boiling in water for 20 minutes or by autoclaving (15 minutes at 120°C). Do not use chemical disinfectants.

1. Before withdrawing vaccine from liquid-nitrogen refrigerator, protect hands with gloves. Wear long sleeves and use a face mask or goggles. It is possible an accident could occur with either the liquid nitrogen or the vials of vaccine. When removing a vial from the cane, hold palm of the gloved hand away from body and face.
2. When withdrawing the package of vials from canister in liquid-nitrogen refrigerator, expose only the vial to be used immediately. The manufacturer recommends handling only one vial at a time. After removing the vial, the cane holding the remaining vials should be replaced immediately in the canister of the liquid-nitrogen refrigerator.
3. The contents of the ampule are thawed rapidly by immersing in water at room temperature. Shake ampule to disperse contents. Then break ampule at the neck and immediately proceed as below. Caution: Ampules have been known to explode on sudden temperature change. Do not thaw in hot or ice cold water.
4. Draw contents of the ampule into a 10 cc sterile syringe.
5. Dilute immediately by filling the syringe slowly from a portion of the contents of the diluent bottle, after removing the center of the aluminum seal.
6. The contents of the filled syringe are then added to the remaining diluent. It is important that this be done slowly. Insert the syringe needle through the center of the rubber stopper of the diluent bottle. Slowly empty the syringe, allowing the vaccine to run down the side of the bottle. Gently shake the bottle as the vaccine is being mixed. Withdraw a portion of the diluent with the syringe to flush the ampule. Inject the washing back into the diluent bottle. Remove the syringe.
7. Fill the automatic syringe according to the manufacturer's recommendations and set the dosage for 0.20 mL.
8. The vaccine and vaccinating syringe are now ready for use.

Method of Vaccination: Subcutaneous Administration:

1. Dilute the vaccine as directed above observing all precautions and warnings for handling.
2. Hold the chick by the back of the neck just below the head. The loose skin in the area is raised by gently pinching with the thumb and forefinger. Insert the needle beneath the skin in a downward direction away from the head. Inject 0.2 mL per chick. The bottle of vaccine should be kept in an ice bath and swirled frequently.
3. Avoid hitting the muscles and bones in the neck.
4. Entire contents of the bottle must be used within 2 hours after mixing or discarded.

Contraindication(s): Birds to be vaccinated should be healthy and free from all diseases. It is essential that the birds be maintained under good environmental conditions to prevent unnecessary exposure to Marek's disease virus.

Precaution(s): Important: Storage Conditions:

Ampule - Store in a liquid nitrogen refrigerator.

Diluent - The diluent may be stored at room temperature until a few hours prior to use. The diluent at the time of use should have the same temperature as the thawed vaccine.

Container - Store the liquid nitrogen container securely in an upright position in a dry, well-ventilated area.

Burn containers and all unused contents.

Keep vaccine ampule frozen in liquid nitrogen until ready to vaccinate.

Do not refreeze vaccine.

Do not use vaccine that has been thawed other than immediately before use.

Do not mix Marek's disease vaccine with other vaccines or antibiotics unless authorized by your veterinarian.

Keep liquid nitrogen containers away from incubator intakes and chick boxes.

Caution(s): The capacity of this vaccine to produce satisfactory results depends on many factors, including, but not limited to, conditions of storage and handling by the user, administration of the vaccine, health and responsiveness of individual animals and the degree of field exposure. Therefore, the directions for use should be followed carefully.

The use of this vaccine is subject to applicable state and federal laws and regulations.

Warning(s): Do not vaccinate within 21 days before slaughter.

Liquid nitrogen container and vaccine should be handled only by properly trained personnel who are thoroughly conversant with the Union Carbide publication and instruction booklet regarding the use of, precautions and safe practices for liquefied atmospheric gases (particularly liquid nitrogen).

When removing the ampule cane, handling frozen ampules, or adding liquid nitrogen, wear long sleeves, a plastic face shield and gloves to protect the skin from contact with the liquid nitrogen. All storage and handling of the liquid nitrogen container must be in a dry, well-ventilated area. Do not inhale liquid nitrogen vapors. If drowsiness occurs, get fresh air quickly, then ventilate the entire area. If breathing difficulty occurs, apply artificial respiration. If any of these difficulties persist or there is a loss of consciousness, summon a physician immediately.

Care should be exercised to prevent contaminating the hands, eyes and clothing with the vaccine.

For veterinary use only.

Presentation: 1,000 doses.

Compendium Code No.: 10080492

VI MARK® MAREK'S DISEASE VACCINE (Live Chicken Herpesvirus)

L.A.H.I. (New Jersey) **Vaccine**

Marek's Disease Vaccine, Live Chicken Herpesvirus, Cell Associated

U.S. Vet. Lic. No.: 196

Active Ingredient(s): Description: This product is of chicken tissue culture origin using SPF (Specific Pathogen Free) eggs. The product contains the SB_1 strain of chicken herpesvirus and is used for the prevention of very virulent Marek's disease in chickens. The product is packaged in two separate units. One is an ampule containing frozen live chicken herpesvirus of chicken culture origin and the other is a bottle of sterile diluent. The ampules are inserted on metal canes. The canes are in canisters containing liquid nitrogen.

Gentamicin and amphotericin B are added as preservatives to the vaccine suspension in the ampule.

All vaccines released for sale meet the requirements of the licensing authority (U.S. Department of Agriculture) in regard to safety, purity, potency and the capacity to immunize normal susceptible birds.

Indications: This vaccine is recommended for use in healthy one-day-old chicks. The virus will infect chicks even though they may be carrying maternal precipitating antibodies to Marek's disease herpesvirus (MDHV).

Good management practices are recommended to reduce exposure for at least two weeks following vaccination.

Dosage and Administration: Preparation of Vaccine: Read warning advice on handling vaccine ampule.

Sterilize vaccinating equipment by boiling in water for 20 minutes or by autoclaving (15 minutes at 120°C). Do not use chemical disinfectants.

1. Before withdrawing vaccine from liquid-nitrogen refrigerator, protect hands with gloves. Wear long sleeves and use a face mask or goggles. It is possible an accident could occur with either the liquid nitrogen or the vials of vaccine. When removing a vial from the cane, hold palm of gloved hand away from body and face.
2. When withdrawing package of vials from canister in liquid-nitrogen refrigerator, expose only the vial to be used immediately. The manufacturer recommends handling only one vial at a time. After removing the vial, the cane holding the remaining vials should be replaced immediately in the canister of the liquid-nitrogen refrigerator.
3. The contents of the ampule are thawed rapidly by immersing in water at room temperature. Shake ampule to disperse contents. Then break ampule at the neck and immediately proceed as below. Caution: Ampules have been known to explode on sudden temperature change. Do not thaw in hot or ice cold water.
4. Draw contents of the ampule into a 10 cc sterile syringe.
5. Dilute immediately by filling the syringe slowly from a portion of the contents of the diluent bottle, after removing the center of the aluminum seal.
6. The contents of the filled syringe are then added to the remaining diluent. It is important that this be done slowly. Insert the syringe needle through the center of the rubber stopper of the diluent bottle. Slowly empty the syringe, allowing the vaccine to run down the side of the bottle. Gently shake the bottle as the vaccine is being mixed. Withdraw a portion of the diluent with the syringe to flush ampule. Inject the washing back into the diluent bottle. Remove the syringe.
7. Fill the automatic syringe according to the manufacturer's recommendations and set the dosage for 0.20 mL.
8. The vaccine and vaccinating syringe are now ready for use.

Method of Vaccination: Subcutaneous Administration:

1. Dilute the vaccine as directed above observing all precautions and warnings for handling.
2. Hold the chick by the back of the neck just below the head. The loose skin in the area is

V

raised by gently pinching with the thumb and forefinger. Insert the needle beneath the skin in a downward direction away from the head. Inject 0.2 mL per chick. The bottle of vaccine should be kept in an ice bath and swirled frequently.
3. Avoid hitting the muscles and bones in the neck.
4. Entire contents of bottle must be used within 1 hour after mixing or discarded.

Contraindication(s): Birds to be vaccinated should be healthy and free from all diseases. It is essential that the birds be maintained under good environmental conditions to prevent unnecessary exposure to Marek's disease virus.

Precaution(s): Important: Storage Conditions:

Ampule - Store in liquid nitrogen refrigerator.

Diluent - Diluent may be stored at room temperature until a few hours prior to use. The diluent at the time of use should have the same temperature as the thawed vaccine.

Container - Store liquid nitrogen container securely in upright position in a dry, well-ventilated area.

Burn containers and all unused contents.

Keep vaccine ampule frozen in liquid nitrogen until ready to vaccinate.

Do not refreeze vaccine.

Do not use vaccine that has been thawed other than immediately before use.

Keep liquid nitrogen containers away from incubator intakes and chick boxes.

Caution(s): The capacity of this vaccine to produce satisfactory results depends on many factors, including but not limited to conditions of storage and handling by the user, administration of the vaccine, health and responsiveness of individual animals and degree of field exposure. Therefore, directions for use should be followed carefully.

The use of this vaccine is subject to applicable state and federal laws and regulations.

Warning(s): Do not vaccinate within 21 days before slaughter.

Liquid nitrogen container and vaccine should be handled only by properly trained personnel who are thoroughly conversant with the Union Carbide publication and instruction booklet regarding the use of, precautions and safe procedures for liquefied atmospheric gases (particularly liquid nitrogen).

When removing ampule cane, handling frozen ampules, or adding liquid nitrogen, wear long sleeves, a plastic face shield and gloves to protect the skin from contact with the liquid nitrogen. All storage and handling of the liquid nitrogen container must be in a dry, well-ventilated area. Do not inhale liquid nitrogen vapors. If drowsiness occurs, get fresh air quickly; then, ventilate entire area. If breathing difficulty occurs, apply artificial respiration. If any of these difficulties persist or there is a loss of consciousness, summon a physician immediately.

Care should be exercised to prevent contaminating hands, eyes and clothing with the vaccine.

For veterinary use only.

Presentation: 1,000 dose virus ampule with a 200 mL diluent.

Compendium Code No.: 10080502

VI MARK® MAREK'S DISEASE VACCINE (Live Turkey Herpesvirus)

L.A.H.I. (New Jersey) **Vaccine**

Marek's Disease Vaccine, Live Turkey Herpesvirus, Cell Associated

U.S. Vet. Lic. No.: 196

Active Ingredient(s): Description: This product is of chicken tissue culture origin using SPF (Specific Pathogen Free) eggs. The product contains the FC-126 strain of turkey herpesvirus and is used for the prevention of Marek's disease in chickens. The product is packaged in two separate units. One is an ampule containing frozen live turkey herpesvirus of chicken culture origin and the other is a bottle of sterile diluent. The ampules are inserted on metal canes. The canes are in canisters containing liquid nitrogen.

Gentamicin and amphotericin B are added as preservatives to the vaccine suspension in the ampule.

All vaccines released for sale meet the requirements of the licensing authority (U.S. Department of Agriculture) in regard to safety, purity, potency and the capacity to immunize normal susceptible birds.

Indications: This vaccine is recommended for use in healthy one-day-old chicks. The virus will infect chicks even though they may be carrying maternal precipitating antibodies to Marek's disease herpesvirus (MDHV). For subcutaneous vaccination.

Good management practices are recommended to reduce exposure for at least two weeks following vaccination.

Dosage and Administration: Preparation of Vaccine: Read warning advice on handling vaccine ampule.

Sterilize vaccinating equipment by boiling in water for 20 minutes or by autoclaving (15 minutes at 120°C). Do not use chemical disinfectants.

1. Be sure to select proper size virus ampule for mixing with diluent. The diluent must be chilled before use.
2. Before withdrawing vaccine from liquid-nitrogen refrigerator, protect hands with gloves. Wear long sleeves and use a face mask or goggles. It is possible an accident could occur with either the liquid nitrogen or the vials of vaccine. When removing a vial from the cane, hold palm of gloved hand away from body and face.
3. When withdrawing package of vials from canister in liquid-nitrogen refrigerator, expose only the vial to be used immediately. The manufacturer recommends handling only one vial at a time. After removing the vial, the cane holding the remaining vials should be replaced immediately in the canister of the liquid-nitrogen refrigerator.
4. The contents of the ampule are thawed rapidly by immersing in water at room temperature. Shake ampule to disperse contents. Then break ampule at the neck and immediately proceed as below. Caution: Ampules have been known to explode on sudden temperature change. Do not thaw in hot or ice cold water.
5. Draw contents of the ampule into a 10 cc sterile syringe.
6. Dilute immediately by filling the syringe slowly from a portion of the contents of the diluent bottle, after removing the center of the aluminum seal.
7. The contents of the filled syringe are then added to the remaining diluent. It is important that this be done slowly. Insert the syringe needle through the center of the rubber stopper of the diluent bottle. Slowly empty the syringe, allowing the vaccine to run down the side of the bottle. Gently shake the bottle as the vaccine is being mixed. Withdraw a portion of the diluent with the syringe to flush ampule. Inject the washing back into the diluent bottle. Remove the syringe.
8. Fill the automatic syringe according to the manufacturer's recommendations and set the dosage for 0.20 mL.
9. The vaccine and vaccinating syringe are now ready for use.

Method of Vaccination: Subcutaneous Administration:

1. Dilute the vaccine as directed above observing all precautions and warnings for handling.
2. Hold the chick by the back of the neck just below the head. The loose skin in the area is raised by gently pinching with the thumb and forefinger. Insert the needle beneath the skin in a downward direction away from the head. Inject 0.2 mL per chick. The bottle of vaccine should be kept in an ice bath and swirled frequently.
3. Avoid hitting the muscles and bones in the neck.
4. Entire contents of bottle must be used within 2 hours after mixing or discarded.

Contraindication(s): Birds to be vaccinated should be healthy and free from all diseases. It is essential that the birds be maintained under good environmental conditions to prevent unnecessary exposure to Marek's disease virus.

Precaution(s): Important: Storage Conditions:

Ampule - Store in liquid nitrogen refrigerator.

Diluent - Diluent may be stored at room temperature until a few hours prior to use. The diluent at the time of use should have the same temperature as the thawed vaccine.

Container - Store liquid nitrogen container securely in upright position in a dry, well-ventilated area.

Burn containers and all unused contents.

Keep vaccine ampule frozen in liquid nitrogen until ready to vaccinate.

Do not refreeze vaccine.

Do not use vaccine that has been thawed other than immediately before use.

Keep liquid nitrogen containers away from incubator intakes and chick boxes.

Caution(s): The capacity of this vaccine to produce satisfactory results depends on many factors, including but not limited to conditions of storage and handling by the user, administration of the vaccine, health and responsiveness of individual animals and degree of field exposure. Therefore, directions for use should be followed carefully.

The use of this vaccine is subject to applicable state and federal laws and regulations.

Warning(s): Do not vaccinate within 21 days before slaughter.

Liquid nitrogen container and vaccine should be handled only by properly trained personnel who are thoroughly conversant with the Union Carbide publication and instruction booklet regarding the use of, precautions and safe procedures for liquefied atmospheric gases (particularly liquid nitrogen).

When removing ampule cane, handling frozen ampules, or adding liquid nitrogen, wear long sleeves, a plastic face shield and gloves to protect the skin from contact with the liquid nitrogen. All storage and handling of the liquid nitrogen container must be in a dry, well-ventilated area. Do not inhale liquid nitrogen vapors. If drowsiness occurs, get fresh air quickly; then, ventilate entire area. If breathing difficulty occurs, apply artificial respiration. If any of these difficulties persist or there is a loss of consciousness, summon a physician immediately.

Care should be exercised to prevent contaminating hands, eyes and clothing with the vaccine.

For veterinary use only.

Presentation: 1,000 doses.

Compendium Code No.: 10080512

VI NU CHICK VAC-K™

L.A.H.I. (New Jersey) **Vaccine**

Newcastle Disease Vaccine, Killed Virus

U.S. Vet. Lic. No.: 196

Active Ingredient(s): This product consists of one inactivated virus strain capable of preventing Newcastle disease in chickens. The virus used in this product is a highly antigenic strain.

The vaccine is manufactured in accordance with a detailed production outline, which has been filed with the Veterinary Services of the USDA. Only specific pathogen free (SPF) eggs are used for production purposes. Seed virus is derived from a master seed virus lot which has been fully tested for purity, safety and immunogenicity. The fill volume for these products is 500 mL in a 625 mL plastic bottle. The bottles are sealed with a rubber stopper and an aluminum overseal.

The flocks producing SPF eggs are under constant observation by experienced personnel and routinely sampled and tested serologically to confirm absence of exposure to a large variety of avian pathogens. Shipments from the supplier are accompanied by regular reports on test results for each flock from which eggs were obtained.

These products are fully tested for purity, safety and potency according to the standard requirements for Newcastle disease and infectious bronchitis vaccines published as part 113, in particular, section 113.125 of title 9 of the federal regulations by the Animal and Plant Health Inspection Service of the USDA, and according to the production outline submitted to the U.S. Department of Agriculture.

Each serial is tested for: Bacteria, fungi, and salmonella.

Potency is tested according to the outline approved by the USDA.

Indications: This product is used for vaccination of one day old chicks for the prevention of Newcastle disease. In chicks having varying levels of antibodies to Newcastle disease, vaccination can also be done using the live Newcastle disease B_1 vaccines simultaneously.

Dosage and Administration: Immediately prior to use, shake the bottle vigorously for 30 seconds to one (1) minute. Remove the aluminum overseal and the product is ready for use.

Method of Vaccination: The vaccine should be administered subcutaneously in the mid-portion of the neck or intramuscularly in the leg. Inject each chick with 0.1 mL dose. For simultaneous live and killed Newcastle disease vaccination, use additionally the live Newcastle disease B_1 vaccine as per recommendations for that vaccine.

Precaution(s): The vaccine shall be stored in the dark in a refrigerator between 2-7°C (35-45°F).

Expiration date: 18 months.

Caution(s): It is imperative that the user of this product comply with the indications for use, contraindications, cautions and method of vaccination stated on the directions sheet packed with the product. The vaccine must be prepared and administered as directed to obtain the best results.

For veterinary use only.

Warning(s): Do not market birds for at least six (6) weeks after vaccinating so that there is no swelling at the site of vaccine administration.

Presentation: 5,000 doses.

Compendium Code No.: 10080532

VIODINE™ MEDICATED SHAMPOO

Equicare **Antidermatosis Shampoo**

Active Ingredient(s): Povidone-iodine 5%.

Indications: An aid in the treatment and prevention of bacterial and fungal skin infections common to animals.

For use on horses, cattle, swine, dogs and cats.

Directions for Use: Shake gently. Wet animal with water and apply a sufficient amount of shampoo to work into a rich lather. For maximum effectiveness allow lather to remain for 3 minutes. Rinse thoroughly. Repeat daily or as needed.

Precaution(s): Avoid storing at excessive heat.

Caution(s): For external use only. Avoid contact with eyes. If infection or irritation persists, discontinue use and consult a veterinarian.

Do not use in conjunction with other medications or pesticides.

For veterinary use.

Warning(s): Keep out of reach of children. May be harmful if swallowed.

Presentation: 473 mL (16 fl oz).

Compendium Code No.: 14470220

VIOKASE®-V ℞

Fort Dodge **Enzyme Preparation**

Whole Pancreas-Not an Extract-Not Enteric Coated

Active Ingredient(s): Description: VIOKASE®-V is activated whole raw pancreas; a pancreatic enzyme concentrate of porcine origin containing standardized amylase, protease and lipase activities plus esterases, peptidases, nucleases and elastase.

Each 425 mg tablet contains:

Lipase . . . 9,000 USP units
Protease . . . 57,000 USP units
Amylase . . . 64,000 USP units

Each 2.8 grams (1 teaspoonful) of powder contains:

Lipase . . . 71,400 USP units
Protease . . . 388,000 USP units
Amylase . . . 460,000 USP units

Indications: As a digestive aid; replacement therapy where digestion of protein, carbohydrate and fat is inadequate due to exocrine pancreatic insufficiency.

Dosage and Administration: The VIOKASE®-V tablets are administered before each meal. VIOKASE®-V powder is added to moistened dog food (canned or dry). Thorough mixing is necessary to bring the enzymes into close contact with the food particles. Incubation at room temperature for 15-20 minutes before feeding appears to enhance the digestive process. Frequent feeding, at least 3 times daily, is important.

Usual Dosage:

Dogs: 2-3 tablets or ¾-1 teaspoonful (2.8 g/teaspoonful) with each meal.

Cats: ½-1 tablet or ¼-¾ teaspoonful (2.8 g/teaspoonful) with each meal.

Note: No one regimen will be successful for every patient. The above dosage should be adjusted according to the severity of the pancreatic exocrine deficiency and weight of the animal. In cases of chronic insufficiency, the dosage should be increased until desired results are obtained.

Each tablet contains sufficient pancreatic enzymes to digest *(in vitro):* 33 g fat; 57 g protein; 64 g starch.

Each 2.8 grams (1 teaspoonful) contains sufficient pancreatic enzymes to digest *(in vitro):* 260 g fat; 388 g protein; 460 g starch.

Treatment in Acute and Chronic Pancreatitis: The most important aspect of the treatment of acute pancreatitis is initiation of vigorous therapy aimed at combating pain and shock, restoring blood volume, blood pressure and renal function, with reducing pancreatic secretions and combating secondary infection of necrotic tissue. Animals surviving an acute attack should be placed on a bland and easily digested diet (such as Prescription Diet®, i/d) and supplemented with VIOKASE®-V.

In chronic pancreatitis, replacement therapy must be given for the duration of the animal's life. Three daily feedings of a bland and easily digested diet containing sufficient quantities of good quality proteins and carbohydrates and low levels of fat are recommended (i.e., Prescription Diet®, i/d). VIOKASE®-V is given with each meal at a dosage level sufficient to keep the feces normal.

Precaution(s): Store in tightly closed container in a dry place at a temperature not exceeding 25°C (77°F).

Caution(s): Federal law restricts this drug to use by or on the order of a licensed veterinarian.

Discontinue use in animals with symptoms of sensitivity.

Discussion: Background Information: A review of the literature over the past 20 years, together with clinical experience, prompts the conclusion that pancreatitis is an important disease in the dog. Evidence of the disease was observed in approximately 3% of a series of dogs necropsied at the Angell Memorial Animal Hospital. Others have classified disease of the pancreas into 4 distinctive categories: acute necrotic pancreatitis; subacute or chronic pancreatitis; pancreatic fibrosis; and collapse or atrophy of the acinar pancreatic tissue. Only acute and chronic pancreatitis is readily recognized clinically.

Dogs that acquire acute pancreatitis usually recover, but are subject to exacerbations of the chronic inflammatory process that may persist. Complete healing of the acute lesion may not occur, and progressive destruction of the gland may take place over a period of months, even in the absence of clinical signs.

Chronic pancreatitis is characterized by acute exacerbations of pancreatic inflammation that occur after the remission of acute pancreatitis. Signs of the disease are similar to those of acute pancreatitis but are usually less severe.

Steatorrhea, diarrhea, weight loss and increased appetite characterize the digestive impairment caused by failure of pancreatic exocrine secretion. Secretion ceases when the acinar tissue is destroyed in the course of chronic pancreatitis. This sequela does not become evident until virtually total destruction of the acinar pancreas has occurred, because as little as 12 to 20 percent of the exocrine pancreas can secrete enough pancreatic juice to sustain digestion. Thus, digestive impairment is a relatively late event in the pathogenesis of chronic pancreatitis. Transient episodes of fetid diarrhea may occur at the time of an acute exacerbation, and may be caused by a temporary reduction of pancreatic exocrine secretion. However, food engorgement or the ingestion of fatty food often precipitates an exacerbation of chronic pancreatitis and the character of the food, rather than the absence of pancreatic enzymes, may cause the diarrhea.

The veterinarian should not be too concerned about whether the pancreatic lesion is acute or chronic. Their primary concern should be to recognize pancreatic inflammatory disease and begin treatment. The differentiation of acute and chronic pancreatitis is then made on the basis of history, and is of importance in advancing a prognosis.

VIOKASE®-V will replace pancreatic enzymes' secretions after total pancreatectomy.

Presentation: VIOKASE®-V Tablets—425 mg each in bottles of 100 (NDC 0856-9301-63) and 500 (NDC 0856-9301-70).

VIOKASE®-V Powder—Bottles of 4 ounce (NDC 0856-9303-12), 8 ounce (NDC 0856-9303-25) and 12 ounce (NDC 0856-9303-22).

Compendium Code No.: 10032581 5300E

VIONATE® VITAMIN MINERAL POWDER

ARC **Dietary Supplement**

Guaranteed Analysis: (guarantees are minimum, unless otherwise stated):

Vitamin A . . . 220,000 I.U. per kg
Vitamin D_3 . . . 22,000 I.U. per kg
Vitamin B_1 (Thiamine Mononitrate) . . . 39.6 mg per kg
Vitamin B_2 (Riboflavin) . . . 79.2 mg per kg
Vitamin B_6 (Pyridoxine Hydrochloride) . . . 9.98 mg per kg
Vitamin B_{12} . . . 0.15 mg per kg
Calcium pantothenate . . . 110 mg per kg
Niacin . . . 275 mg per kg
Folic acid . . . 2.2 mg per kg
Calcium Chloride . . . 6,720 mg per kg
Ascorbic acid . . . 2,494.8 mg per kg
Vitamin E . . . 119.9 I.U. per kg
94,802.4 mg per kg
Calcium (Ca) . . . (min) 9.5% 113,762 mg per kg
(max) 11.4% 47,828 mg per kg
Phosphorus (P) . . . 4.79% 4,994 mg per kg
Sodium (NaCl) . . . (min) 0.5% 14,982 mg per kg
(max) 1.5% 22 mg per kg
Iodine (I) . . . 0.0022% 550 mg per kg
Iron (Fe) . . . 0.055% 5.5 mg per kg
Cobalt (Co) . . . 0.00055% 55 mg per kg
Copper (Cu) . . . 0.0055% 423.06 mg per kg
Magnesium (Mg) . . . 0.0424% 75.68 mg per kg
Manganese (Mn)

Ingredients: Degermed corn meal; dibasic calcium phosphate, calcium carbonate; salt (sodium chloride); ferrous carbonate; magnesium oxide; niacin; calcium pantothenate; riboflavin; BHT (butylated hydroxytoluene) as a preservative; dl-atocopheryl acetate; vitamin A palmitate; thiamine mononitrate; manganous oxide; cupric sulfate; calcium iodate; pyridoxine hydrochloride; cobalt carbonate; folic acid; d-activated animal sterol (source of vitamin D_3); cyanocobalamin (a source of vitamin B_{12}).

Indications: Vitamin mineral powder for pets including dogs, cats, birds, horses, rabbits and hamsters.

Dosage and Administration: Suggested Daily Dosage Table:

Sprinkle on food and mix well. Do not dip wet utensils into powder. Keep dry.

	Daily Amount per Animal	Daily Amount for Several Animals
Dogs	1 teaspoon per 15 lbs body weight	1 tablespoon per 45 lbs body weight
	1 tablespoon per 45 lbs body weight	¼ cup per 180 lbs body weight
Puppies	⅔ teaspoon per 5 lbs body weight	1 tablespoon per 20 lbs body weight
	1 teaspoon per 7 lbs body weight	¼cup per 80 lbs body weight
Bitches in Whelp or Lactating	1 tablespoon per 22 lbs body weight	¼ cup per 100 lbs body weight
Cats	¾ teaspoon	2½ tablespoons/10 cats
Kittens	½ teaspoon	1 tablespoon/4-6 kittens
Rabbits	¾ teaspoon	2½ tablespoons/10 rabbits
Hamsters, Gerbils, Mice	⅛ teaspoon	1 teaspoon/8 animals
Mink and Chinchilla (Lactating Females)	½ teaspoon	4 tablespoons/16 animals 1 cup/96 animals
(Other Adults and Kits)	⅓ teaspoon	1 tablespoon/9 animals 1 cup/144 animals
Fox Cub	¾ teaspoon	4 tablespoons/16 animals 1 cup/64 animals
Fox Adult	½ teaspoon	4 tablespoons/24 animals 1 cup/96 animals
Monkeys (Small)	⅓-½ teaspoon	1-2 tablespoons/12 animals ¼-½ cup/48 animals
(Large)	1-2 teaspoons	¼-½ cup/12 animals 1-2 cups/48 animals

To mix with large amounts of feed, add at a level of 1% of the ration: e.g. 1 oz per 6 lbs of feed, or 1 lb per 100 lbs of feed. To mix with pelleted foods add a few drops of cooking oil, add VIONATE® and mix well.

Birds Suggested Daily Dosage Table

(for other animals see other panel)

Mix with food daily. Keep dry.

	Daily Amount per Animal	Daily Amount for Several Animals
Small Birds (Parakeets, Finches, Canaries, etc.)	⅛ teaspoon	1 teaspoon for 8-10 birds 1 tablespoon for 25 birds ¼ cup for 100 birds
Medium Birds (Cockatiels, Small Parrots, Lovebirds, Mynahs, etc.)	⅛-¼ teaspoon	1-2 teaspoons for 8-10 birds 1-2 tablespoons for 25 birds ¼-½ cup for 100 birds
Large Birds (Large Parrots, Cockatoos, Macaws, etc.)	¼-½ teaspoon	2-4 teaspoons for 8-10 birds
Very Large Birds (Pheasants, Geese, Swans, Ostriches, Peacocks, Emues, etc.)	½-1 teaspoon	1-2 tablespoons for 6 birds ⅛-¼ cup for 12 birds ¼-½ cup for 25 birds

To mix with bird seed or pelleted food, add a small amount of cooking oil, honey or syrup and then stir in the VIONATE® Powder.

Precaution(s): Keep tightly closed. Store at room temperature; avoid excessive heat (104°F) (40°C).

Caution(s): For oral use in animals only.

Presentation: 8 oz. (227 g), 2 lb. and 10 lb. containers.

Compendium Code No.: 10960101

V

V.I.P.-20™ IODINE SHAMPOO

Equicare **Antidermatosis Shampoo**

Active Ingredient(s): Povidone-iodine.

Indications: A medicated shampoo for use on horses and dogs.

Directions for Use: Wet animal thoroughly with water. Add 1 to 2 ounces of V.I.P.-20™ Shampoo to a large pail, spray water into pail to create an abundance of suds. Apply sudsy solution to animal's body, rub briskly and work into a rich lather. Rinse thoroughly with clean water. Scrape or wipe off excess water. If irritation occurs, discontinue use and consult a veterinarian.

Precaution(s): Product may discolor if exposed to direct sunlight. Store at room temperature.

Caution(s): Do not use in conjunction with other medications or insecticides.

Avoid contamination of feed or foodstuffs.

Warning(s): Harmful or fatal if swallowed. If ingested seek medical attention.

For external animal use only. Avoid contact with eyes or mucous membranes. Keep out of reach of children. If irritation occurs, seek medical attention. For animal use only.

Presentation: 32 oz and 3.785 L (1 gallon).

Compendium Code No.: 14470181

VIP® FLEA CONTROL SHAMPOO

V.P.L. **Parasiticide Shampoo**

EPA Reg. No.: 4758-141

Active Ingredient(s):

d-Limonene	5.0%
Inert Ingredients	95.0%
Total	100.0%

Indications: Kills fleas and conditions and deodorizes the coats of dogs and cats, puppies and kittens.

Directions for Use: It is a violation of Federal law to use the product in a manner inconsistent with its labeling.

Wet the dog or cat with warm water and apply a small amount of shampoo along the back of the animal. Work well into the coat, starting at the head and working backwards. Include the legs and feet. When the lather is of desired consistency, continue to work into the coat for 10 minutes to kill fleas. Rinse thoroughly with warm water and dry. When washing cats, kittens or puppies, dry with a cloth immediately after rinsing to prevent chilling.

Zone control: To effectively control fleas, treatment may be required in three (3) insect zones where fleas live. These zones are the pet, the home, and the yard. VIP® Flea Control Shampoo treats the pet insect zone. Ask a veterinarian how to control fleas for the comfort and well-being of the pet and family.

Precautionary Statements: Hazards to Humans and Domestic Animals:

Warning: Causes eye irritation. Do not get into the eyes. Harmful if swallowed. While washing pets, avoid getting shampoo into the animal's eyes. Do not use on kittens or puppies under six weeks of age.

May be used in conjunction with organophosphates and carbamate based insecticides. Does not inhibit acetylcholinesterase activity.

Statement of Practical Treatment:

If Swallowed: Call a physician or poison control center. Give a glass or two of water and induce vomiting by touching the back of the throat with a finger, or, if available, by administration of syrup of ipecac. Never give anything by mouth or induce vomiting in an unconscious person.

If in Eyes: Flush eyes with plenty of water. Get medical attention.

Storage and Disposal: Disposal: Do not re-use the container. Wrap the container and discard it with the trash.

Warning(s): Keep out of the reach of children.

Presentation: 12 fl oz (355 mL) and 1 gallon (3.785 L) containers.

Compendium Code No.: 11430341

VIP® FLEA DIP

V.P.L. **Parasiticide Dip**

EPA Reg. No.: 4758-144

Active Ingredient(s):

d-Limonene	78.20%
Inert ingredients	21.80%
Total	100.00%

Indications: Kills fleas and conditions and deodorizes the coats on dogs and cats, puppies and kittens.

Dosage and Administration: It is a violation of federal law to use the product in a manner inconsistent with its labeling.

Important: For guaranteed effectiveness, keep the diluted mixture out of sunlight. Do not use full strength. Mix only the amount needed in an 8-hour period. To kill fleas, dilute with water as directed.

Degree of Flea Infestation:

Dilution rate:

Light - 1.5 oz./gallon (1.5 oz. = 3 tbsp.).

Medium - 2.0 oz./gallon (2.0 oz. = 4 tbsp.).

Heavy - 2.5 oz./gallon (2.5 oz. = 5 tbsp.).

Be sure that the concentrate is well mixed with water. Wet the animal with water first. Sponge or pour the mixture on the pet until the coat is thoroughly wet. Rub well into fur, on ears, legs and paws. Avoid eye, scrotal or anal area. For the best results do not rinse, but allow to dry naturally. Towel all young animals dry immediately after dipping to prevent chilling. Wash hands with soap and water after using.

Zone control: To effectively control fleas, treatment may be required in three (3) insect zones where fleas live. These zones are the pet, the home, and the yard. VIP® Flea Dip treats the pet insect zone. Ask a veterinarian for specific recommendations on how to control fleas for the comfort and well being of the pet and family.

Precaution(s):

Storage: Do not use or store near heat or open flames. Keep out of sunlight. Store in a cool, dark area. Product effectiveness cannot be guaranteed after prolonged exposure to light.

Disposal: Do not re-use the container. Rinse thoroughly before discarding in the trash. Securely wrap the original container in several layers of newspaper and discard it in the trash.

Caution(s): Keep out of the reach of children.

Precautionary Statements:

Hazards to Humans and Domestic Animals: May cause eye injury. Do not get in eyes or on clothing. Wear eye protection when mixing concentrate with water. Harmful if swallowed. Wash thoroughly with soap and water after handling. Use with caution on nursing animals. Do not use on puppies or kittens under six weeks of age. Some individuals and pets may be sensitive to the product. If irritation develops, discontinue use.

May be used in conjunction with organophosphates and carbamate based insecticides. Does not inhibit acetylcholinesterase activity.

Statement of Practical Treatment:

If the concentrate is swallowed: Call a physician or poison control center. Give milk or water, but do not induce vomiting except under medical supervision because of an aspiration hazard. Do not give anything by mouth to an unconscious person.

If on skin: Wash off with soap and water. Get medical attention if irritation develops.

If in eyes: Flush eyes with plenty of water. Get medical attention.

Presentation: 8 fl. oz. (237 mL) and 1 gallon (3.785 L) containers.

Compendium Code No.: 11430350

VIP® FLY REPELLENT OINTMENT

V.P.L. **Topical Insecticide**

EPA Reg. No.: 4758-11

Active Ingredient(s):

Butoxypolypropylene glycol	10.00%
Piperonyl butoxide, technical*	1.00%
Pyrethrins	0.15%
Inert ingredients	88.85%
Total	100.00%

*Equivalent to 0.80% (butylcarbityl) (6-propylpiperonyl) ether and 0.20% of related compounds.

Indications: Repels biting flies on dogs and cats. Kills ticks on ears and between toes.

Dosage and Administration: It is a violation of federal law to use the product in a manner inconsistent with its labeling.

Spread lightly on the tips and edges of the ears to aid in repelling biting flies, houseflies and mosquitoes from these areas of the animal's body.

To kill ticks, spread a light film on the ears and between toes. Make sure that the ointment makes contact with ticks.

Precaution(s): Do not re-use the empty container. Wrap the container and put it in the trash collection.

Caution(s): Keep out of the reach of children.

Toxicology: Acute oral LD_{50}:

Piperonyl butoxide	7,500 mg/kg
Pyrethrins	1,500 mg/kg

Presentation: 2 oz. (57 g) jars.

Compendium Code No.: 11430360

ViraCHEK®/CV

Synbiotics **FIP Test**

Feline Infectious Peritonitis Antibody Test Kit

U.S. Vet. Lic. No.: 312

Contents: The following items are packaged in each kit:

	24 test	48 test	96 test
Antigen coated wells	2x12 wells	4x12 wells	8x12 wells
Vial A—Positive Control Serum	1.0 mL	1.0 mL	1.5 mL
Vial B—Negative Control/Sample Diluent	3.0 mL	3.0 mL	7.0 mL
Vial C—Protein A Hrp Conjugate	3.0 mL	3.0 mL	5.0 mL
Vial D—TMB Chromogen	3.0 mL	3.0 mL	7.0 mL
Vial E—Substrate buffer	3.0 mL	3.0 mL	7.0 mL
Vial F—10X Wash Concentrate	100.0 mL	100.0 mL	100.0 mL

Additional material provided: Disposable Sample Loops, Holder for microwells, Direction insert with instructions for conducting the test.

Additional material required: Deionized or distilled water, Squirt bottles (2), Timer.

Indications: For the detection of antibodies to feline coronavirus.

Test Principles: The plastic wells are coated with purified coronavirus antigen. Protein A derived from *Staphylococcus aureus* is conjugated to HRP. The serum or plasma sample is incubated in the coated wells followed by incubation with the Protein A conjugate. Antibodies to FCoV, if present in the feline sample, are bound to the well and in turn bind the Protein A conjugate. The free enzyme-linked Protein A is washed away and a chromogenic substrate is added. The development of a distinctly blue color indicates the presence of antibody to FCoV. In the absence at FCoV antibody, no color change will be observed.

ViraCHEK®/CV is highly specific, sensitive and simple to perform. Test results can be obtained in 30 minutes. The diagnostic kit contains a positive control and a negative control which should be included each time the assay is performed. Visual comparison of the color of samples to the negative control will allow accurate detection of the presence of FCoV antibody in the sample.

Sample Collection: One microliter (1 µL) of serum or plasma is required. Use only feline samples for test specimens. Samples may be stored at 2°-7°C up to seven days. If longer storage is desired, samples may be stored at -20°C. Severely hemolyzed or lipemic serum may produce background color. When in doubt, obtain a better quality sample.

Test Procedure: Preparation of Wash Solution: Allow wash concentrate to come to room temperature. Mix gently by inversion. Dilute wash concentrate 10-fold using distilled or deionized water (1 part concentrate to 9 parts dH_2O) in a squirt bottle. Diluted wash solution may be stored at 2°-7°C.

For use with serum or plasma only. (No whole blood.)

Note: Prior to use, allow kit components to come to room temperature (21°-25°C; 70°-78°F).

A. Set Up and Sample Incubation

1. Remove and place in holder one well for Positive (+) Control, one well for Negative (-) Control/Sample Diluent, and one well for each sample. Leave the wells attached to each other.
2. Add 1 drop of Positive Control (Bottle A — Red Cap) into the first well.
3. Add 1 drop of Negative Control/Sample Diluent (Bottle B — Gray Cap) into the second well and to each test sample well.
4. Using a separate sample loop for each sample, add 1 loopful (1 µL) of each Sample to appropriate wells (well 3, 4, etc.) and swirl. Gently tap the holder for 10-15 seconds being careful not to splash from well to well.

   Incubate for 10 minutes at room temperature (21°-25°C; 70°-78°F). If several specimens are run simultaneously, only one set of controls is needed.

B. Blot and Wash

5. Discard the fluid from the wells by inverting and blotting onto a paper towel. Wash wells once by vigorously filling the wells to overflowing with diluted wash solution. (See Preparation of Wash Solution section.) Discard the fluid from the wells, and blot after wash.

C. Conjugate

6. Add 1 drop of Protein A conjugate (Bottle C — Blue Cap) into each well. Gently tap the holder for 10-15 seconds and incubate 10 minutes at room temperature (21°-25°C; 70°-78°F).

D. Blot and Wash

7. Discard the fluid from the wells by inverting and blotting onto a paper towel. Wash by vigorously filling the wells to overflowing with diluted wash solution. Discard the fluid from the wells, and blot after each wash. Repeat the washing procedure three (3) times. Wash two more times with distilled or deionized water to remove bubbles.
Blot dry on a paper towel.

E. Develop

8. Place 1 drop of Chromogen (Bottle D — Green Cap) into each well followed by 1 drop of Substrate Buffer (Bottle E — White Cap). Mix by gently tapping the holder several times. Incubate 5 minutes. After incubating, gently tap holder for 5 seconds and read results immediately. See Interpretation of Results section.

Good Techniques = Accurate Results

Serum or plasma may be used as a sample.

Hemolyzed and lipemic serum samples may be used however, severely hemolyzed and lipemic samples may produce background color. When in doubt, obtain a better quality sample.

Washing is the most important step. Wells cannot be overwashed. Underwashing will result in color development in the negative control and negative sample wells.

Prolonged incubation for more than 5 minutes in step 8 may result in non-specific color development. If no color is seen after 5 minutes, the sample is negative.

Always compare results to the negative control. The kit positive is engineered to be a moderate antibody level and is used to verify proper addition of reagents and good washing technique. It should not be used to differentiate positive from negative results.

Do not use the test kit past the expiration date and do not intermix components from different serial numbers.

Store kit at 2°-7°C (36°-45°F). Allow kit to come to room temperature before use.

Interpretation of Results:

1. For the test to be valid, the fluid in the positive control well must be distinctly blue, while that in the negative control well should remain clear.
2. A color change in the test sample well of greater intensity than the negative control well indicates the animal has previously been exposed to, or currently has an active infection with FCoV and may be capable of transmitting virus by shedding of coronavirus in fecal material. It is important that a positive diagnosis of FIP be supported by other clinical data and findings.
3. No color development in the test sample well strongly suggests a lack of clinical disease due to FIP.

A Positive result (antibody to feline coronavirus is present) is indicated by any degree of blue color in the sample well when read immediately after the 5 minute incubation period.

A Negative result (antibody to feline coronavirus is absent) is indicated by no blue color development in the sample well. A Negative test result indicates that the animal is free of the virus or has not yet sero-converted after exposure. Cats may sero-convert in as little as 4 weeks or as long as twelve weeks after becoming infecting with Feline Coronavirus. Care must be taken when interpreting positive test results it cats under six months of age as maternal FCoV antibodies may be present.

For the test to be valid, the fluid in the Positive Control well must be distinctly blue, while that in the Negative Control well must be clear.

Results should be interpreted immediately after the five minute incubation period. Prolonged incubation may result in non-specific color development. Wells can be detached and compared alongside the negative control well against a white background for easier visual inspection.

Caution(s):

1. Allow kit to come to room temperature (21°-25°C; 70°-78°F) prior to use.
2. Use separate sample loop for each sample.
3. Do not expose kit to direct sunlight.
4. Do not use expired reagents or mix from different kit lots.
5. Follow instructions exactly. Improper washing or contamination of reagents may produce nonspecific color development.
6. For veterinary use only.

Storage: Store the test kit and unused diluted wash solution at 2°-7°C (36°-45°F. Do not freeze. Reagents should be stable until expiration date provided they have been stored properly.

Discussion: Feline infectious peritonitis (FIP) a currently the leading infectious cause of death among young cats 3 months to 3 years of age and also in cats older than 10 years, especially those originating from purebred catteries and other large multi-cat households. Feline enteric coronavirus (FeCV) is a highly infectious virus and is endemic in multiple-cat households. FeCV poses a considerable health risk to cats as it is generally thought to be the precursor of FIP. The ultimate control of FIP in catteries is linked to the control and prevention of FeCV infection. FeCV is included in the broad classification of Feline Coronavirus (FCoV). The presence of antibodies to FCoV indicates the possibility of FeCV and/or FIP infection. A positive titer does not necessarily mean that the cat has FeCV and/or FIP; however, a positive FCoV serology should be considered in conjunction with other clinical findings and symptomology to support a diagnosis of FeCV and/or FIP. A negative antibody titer strongly suggests lack of clinical disease due to FeCV and/or FIP.

References: Available upon request.

Presentation: 32-94 test kits.

Compendium Code No.: 11150431

03-1200-1098

ViraCHEK®/EIA

Synbiotics **EIA Test**

Equine Infectious Anemia Virus Antibody Test Kit

U.S. Vet. Lic. No.: 312

Contents: Each kit contains:

	48 Test	96 Test
EIA Antigen Coated Wells	4 X 12	8 X 12
Bottle A - EIA antigen - HRP conjugate (Blue Cap)	2.5 mL	5.0 mL
Bottle B - EIA Positive Control (Red Cap)	1.0 mL	1.6 mL
Bottle C - EIA Negative Control (Grey Cap)	1.0 mL	1.6 mL
EIA Antigen Coated Wells	4 X 12	8 X 12
Bottle D - Chromogen (Green Cap)	2.5 mL	7.5 mL
Bottle E - Substrate Buffer (White Cap)	2.5 mL	7.5 mL
Bottle F - 10X Wash Concentrate	100 mL	100 mL
Microwell holder		

Additional material required but not provided:
50 µl pipet; disposable pipet tips
Deionized or distilled water
Squirt Bottles (2); Timer
Optional: Microwell plate reader

Indications: For the detection of antibodies to equine infectious anemia virus.

Test Principles: The plastic wells are coated with EIA recombinant antigen. The same EIA recombinant is labeled with the enzyme Horseradish peroxidase (HRP). The serum sample is incubated simultaneously with the coated wells and enzyme-labeled EIA antigen. Antibodies to EIA, if present in the equine sample, are bound to the well and enzyme-labeled EIA antigen at the same time. The free enzyme-labeled EIA antigen is washed away and a chromogenic substrate is added. The development of a dark blue color indicates the presence of antibody to EIA. In the absence of EIA antibody, little or no color change will be observed.

ViraCHEK®/EIA is highly specific, sensitive and simple to perform. Test results can be obtained in 20 minutes. The diagnostic kit contained a Positive Control and a Negative Control which must be included each time the assay is performed. Visual comparison of the color of the sample to the Positive Control will allow accurate detection of the presence of EIA antibody in the sample. If desired, test results may be determined by use of a microwell plate reader.

Test Procedure:

Sample Information: 50 µl of serum is required. Use only equine samples for test specimens. Samples may be stored at 2°-7°C for up to seven days. If longer storage is desired, samples may be stored at -20°C. Severely hemolyzed or lipemic serum may produce background color. When in doubt, obtain a better quality sample.

Preparation of Wash Solution: Allow 10X Wash Concentrate to come to room temperature. Mix gently by inversion. Dilute wash concentrate 10-fold (1 part concentrate to 9 parts distilled water) in a wash bottle.

Only use Serum samples to perform test.

Prior to use, allow kit components to come to room temperature (70°-78°F; 21°-25°C).

A. Preparation:

1. Calculate required number of wells:
   - 1 well for positive control
   - 1 well for negative control
   - 1 well for each sample

   Note: When testing a high number of samples in an assay, Synbiotics strongly recommends including one Negative Control well and one Positive Control well for every 22 samples tested within a run.

   Remove required number of wells.
   Leave wells attached to each other.
   Place in well holder.
   Note: If a microwell plate reader will be used to read the results, leave the appropriate space empty so that the plate reader will blank on air.

B. Conjugate:

2. Add 1 drop Bottle A - Conjugate (Blue Cap) into each well.

C. Sample Addition:

3. Controls
   Add 1 drop Bottle B - Positive Control (Red Cap) into the first well.
   Add 1 drop Bottle C - Negative Control (Grey Cap) into the second well.
   Samples
   Pipette 50 µL of sample into the next well following the controls.
   Repeat for each additional sample into subsequent wells. Use a separate pipette tip for each sample.
   Wait 10 minutes. (Tap side of well holder for the first 15 seconds of the 10 minute incubation period. Be careful not to splash reagents.)

D. Blot and Wash:

4. Discard fluid from wells into sink or appropriate container.
   Invert holder and blot firmly onto a paper towel to remove final drops.
5. Flush wells vigorously:
   - Wash by vigorously filling the wells to overflowing with diluted wash solution (See section Preparation of Wash Solution for preparation).
   - Direct a forceful stream into each well. (Oversplashing will not contaminate adjacent wells).
   - Shake out excess wash solution.
   - Repeat wash cycle 5 times.

   Wash wells 2 more times with distilled or deionized water to remove bubbles.
   Blot against a paper towel to dry wells.

E. Develop:

6. Add 1 drop of Bottle D (Green Cap) to each well.
   Add 1 drop of Bottle E (White Cap) to each well.
   Wait 10 minutes. (Tap side of well holder for the first 15 seconds of the 10 minute incubation period. Be careful not to splash reagents.)
   Tap side of well holder again for the last 15 seconds of the 10 minute incubation period. Be careful not to splash reagents.
   Read results at exactly 10 minutes.

Good Procedure Techniques:

Only serum may be used as a sample.

Hemolyzed and lipemic samples may be used however, severely hemolyzed and lipemic samples may produce background color. When in doubt, obtain a better quality sample.

Washing is the most important step.

Microwells cannot be overwashed.

Underwashing may result in nonspecific blue color development in the negative control and sample wells.

Prolonged incubation for more than 10 minutes in step 6 may result in non-specific color development.

Always compare results to the Positive Control. Wells can be detached and compared alongside the Positive Control well against a white background for easier visual inspection.

Test Interpretation:

A. Controls - For a valid test, the Positive Control must produce a distinct blue color and the Negative Control must produce no color. If color does not develop in the Positive Control or if there is any color development in the Negative Control well, results are invalid and the test should be repeated.

B. Evaluation of Test Wells -

1. Samples producing color of equal or greater intensity than the Positive Control are Positive for antibodies to EIA.
2. Samples producing color of less intensity than the Positive Control are Negative for antibodies to EIA.
3. After the test is completed, the Positive Control well can be detached and held next to the test well for easier comparison of color intensity.
4. If desired, results may be read on a microwell plate reader using an air blank. For single wavelength readers, set the wavelength of the plate reader at 630 nm. For plate readers with dual wavelength capability, set the test wavelength at 630 nm and reference wavelength at 490 nm. Samples producing an Optical Density (O.D.) equal to or greater than the O.D. of the Positive Control are Positive for EIA antibodies. Any sample with an O.D. less than the Positive Control is negative.
5. Any questionable sample should be sent to the National Veterinary Services Laboratory (NVSL) for verification. Positive test results should be verified using the Agar Gal Immunodiffusion (AGID) test.

Storage: Store the test kit and unused diluted wash solution at 2°-7°C (36°-45°F). Do not freeze. Reagents are stable until expiration date provided they have been stored properly.

Caution(s):

1. Allow kit to come to room temperature (21°-25°C; 70°-78°F) prior to use.
2. Use separate pipet tip for each sample.
3. Do not expose kit to direct sunlight.
4. Do not use expired reagents or mix from different kit lots.
5. Follow instructions exactly. Improper washing or contamination of reagents may produce nonspecific color development.
6. For veterinary use only.
7. Sale and use restricted to laboratories approved by State and Federal (U.S.D.A.) animal health officials.

Presentation: 16-46 or 32-94 test kits.

ViraCHEK®/EIA is a registered trademark of Synbiotics Corporation.

Compendium Code No.: 11150441

ViraCHEK®/FeLV

Synbiotics **FeLV Test**

U.S. Vet. Lic. No.: 312

Contents:

	Test Kit	Lab Pack
Anti-FeLV coated wells	4 x 12 wells	12 x 12 wells
Bottle A - HRP monoclonal antibody conjugate (blue cap)	1 vial (2.5 mL)	1 vial (7.5 mL)
Bottle B - FeLV positive control (red cap)	1 vial (1.0 mL)	1 vial (3.0 mL)
Bottle C - FeLV negative control (gray cap)	1 vial (1.0 mL)	1 vial (3.0 mL)
Bottle D - chromogen (green cap)	1 vial (2.5 mL)	1 vial (7.5 mL)
Bottle E - substrate buffer (white cap)	1 vial (2.5 mL)	1 vial (7.5 mL)

Materials required, but not provided: Marking pen, timer, wash bottle, deionized/distilled water or normal saline, and precision pipettes.

Indications: For use in the detection of feline leukemia virus.

Test Principle: The plastic wells contain antibodies directed against the FeLV group specific antigen, p27. A monoclonal antibody, directed against the p27 is labelled with horseradish peroxidase (HRP). The specimen (either whole blood, plasma or serum) is incubated simultaneously with the solid phase and enzyme-labelled antibodies. The virus and free group-specific antigen are bound to the well and the enzyme-linked antibody at the same time. The free enzyme-linked antibody is washed away and a chromogenic substrate is added. The development of a distinctly blue color indicates the presence of FeLV. In the absence of FeLV, a color change will not be observed.

Test Procedure:

Specimen: 50 microliters (0.05 mL) of either whole blood (anticoagulated with EDTA, heparin, etc.), plasma or serum is required. Use feline samples only for test specimens. The specimens may be stored at 2°-8°C for up to seven (7) days. If longer storage is required, store at -20°C. Hemolysis does not significantly interfere with the test if adequate washing is performed.

Test procedure:

Set up and conjugate:

1. Place one (1) well in the holder for the positive control, one (1) well for the negative control and one (1) well for each specimen. Leave the wells attached to each other.
2. Place one (1) drop of positive control (bottle B - red cap), negative control (bottle C - grey cap) or 50 mcg of the specimen into the appropriate wells.

   If several specimens are run simultaneously, only one (1) set of controls is needed.

   If a device is not available to accurately pipet 50 mcg of the specimen, four (4) drops from a 20-gauge needle or six (6) drops from a 22-gauge needle may be used. Be sure to hold the needle in a vertical position to deliver the sample drops.
3. Place one (1) drop of the HRP monoclonal antibody conjugate (bottle A - blue cap) into each well. Mix gently by tapping the holder several times (10-15 seconds). Incubate for five (5) minutes at room temperature(70°-78°F, 21°-25°C).

Blot and wash:

4. Discard the fluid from the wells by inverting and blotting onto a paper towel.
5. Rinse by filling the wells to overflowing with normal (isotonic) saline solution when using whole blood, or with distilled or deionized water when using serum or plasma. Discard the fluid from the wells, and blot after each wash. Repeat washing five (5) times and blot dry on a paper towel after the final rinse.

Develop:

6. Place one (1) drop of chromogen (bottle D - green cap) into each well, followed by one (1) drop of substrate buffer (bottle E - white cap). Mix by gently tapping the holder several times. Incubate for five (5) minutes. After incubating, gently tap the holder for five (5) seconds.

Interpretation of results:

7. For the test to be valid, the fluid in the positive control well must be distinctly blue, while that in the negative control well must not show any color change from the initial substrate color.

   A color change in the test sample of greater intensity than the negative control indicates active FeLV infection. Because infection is transient in cats that develop immunity, p27 antigen positive animals should be isolated and retested in three (3) or four (4) weeks. A positive second test would indicate persistent infection while a negative second sample would indicate immune clearance of FeLV. Persistent FeLV infection is accompanied by a high risk that the cat will develop lymphosarcoma or one (1) of the other FeLV associated diseases. An infected cat will shed FeLV and is a potential source of infection. A negative test indicates that the cat has little likelihood of having active FeLV infection at the time of testing.

Precaution(s):

1. Store the test kit at 2°-8°C.
2. Allow the components to come to room temperature (70°-78°F, 21°-25°C) prior to use. The color intensity will vary with temperature.
3. Follow the instructions exactly. Improper washing or contamination of the reagents may produce nonspecific color development. Immediate intense color development usually indicates inadequate washing.
4. Do not store below 2°C as a precaution against freezing.
5. Properly stored reagents are stable until the expiration date.

Caution(s):

1. Use a separate pasteur pipet for each specimen.
2. Include positive and negative controls (provided in the test kit) each time a test is performed.
3. Handle all of the samples as if capable of transmitting FeLV. Burn all the unused biological components.
4. Do not mix reagents from different kit lots.
5. For veterinary use only.

Discussion: Feline leukemia virus (FeLV) is a contagious oncogenic RNA virus that causes both neoplastic and non-neoplastic disease in pet cats.[1] The most prevalent diseases caused by FeLV include lymphosarcoma, myelogenous leukemia, thymic atrophy, nonregenerative anemia and panleukopenia-like disease. Because FeLV is immunosuppressive, it predisposes infected cats to a variety of secondary diseases.[2]

Since FeLV can be transmitted horizontally, it is important that FeLV-infected cats be identified and separated from noninfected cats. The group specific antigen, p27, is found in high levels in infected cats and its presence is diagnostically significant for FeLV infection. VIRACHEK®/FeLV is an immunoenzymetric assay using antibodies that specifically recognize p27 in cat blood. The assay provides for the rapid and accurate diagnosis and identification of FeLV infected cats.

References: Available upon request.

Presentation: Available in 2 sizes: Regular (16-46 tests) and Lab Pack (48-140 tests).

Compendium Code No.: 11150451

VIRA SHIELD® 2

Novartis Animal Vaccines **Vaccine**

Bovine Virus Diarrhea Vaccine, Killed Virus

U.S. Vet. Lic. No.: 303

Composition: The vaccine is prepared from two highly antigenic Type I and Type II cytopathic and noncytopathic strains of virus propagated on an established bovine cell line. The vaccine is chemically inactivated and adjuvanted with Xtend III™ to provide maximum efficacy. Contains penicillin, streptomycin and amphotericin B as preservatives.

Indications: For use in healthy cattle for the prevention of diseases caused by bovine virus diarrhea.

Dosage and Administration: Shake well before using. Administer a 2 mL dose intramuscularly to cattle. Repeat in four (4) to five (5) weeks. Calves vaccinated before weaning should be revaccinated after weaning. The vaccine may be administered to pregnant animals at any stage of gestation. Vaccinate dairy cows during the drying-off period. Revaccinate annually to maintain high levels of immunity.

In a herd where it is suspected that animals are persistently infected carriers, vaccinate all brood stock over six (6) months of age with two (2) doses of VIRA SHIELD® 2, four (4) to five (5) weeks apart. Three (3) weeks following the second vaccination take blood serum samples from each animal and have each tested for BVD antibodies. Any vaccinated animals with a titer below 1:16 should be suspected to be persistently infected carriers and serum samples from these animals submitted for BVD virus isolation. Animals which are identified as persistently infected carriers should be culled from the herd and any of their calves should be isolated as suspect until they are old enough to test.

Precaution(s): Store at 35°-45°F (2°-7°C). Do not freeze. Use the entire contents when first opened.

Caution(s): Transient swelling may occur at the site of injection. Milk reduction and transient depression may be observed in lactating dairy cows for two to four days following vaccination. Anaphylactic reactions may occur following the use of the vaccine. Symptomatic treatment: Epinephrine.

Warning(s): Do not vaccinate within 60 days before slaughter.

Discussion: Bovine viral diarrhea virus is one of the most important bovine viral pathogens in the world. The complexity of the virus and its involvement in multiple bovine disease processes are only now beginning to be understood. Neutralizing antibodies for this virus have been detected in 50% to 90% of the clinically normal cattle tested in the United States. The virus is associated with (a) severe bovine respiratory disease; (b) reproductive disorders, including infertility, abortion, and neonatal defects and (c) enteric disorders including bovine viral diarrhea, acute mucosal disease and chronic mucosal disease.

a) Bovine respiratory disease: If a normal susceptible herd is exposed to the BVD virus at the same time it undergoes environmental stress such as dust, inclement weather, overcrowding, transport, interruption of usual nutritional cycles, etc., the stage is set for an outbreak of bovine respiratory disease. The BVD virus causes immunosuppression and the environmental stressors cause irritation and reduced resistance which allows other viral and bacterial pathogens to rapidly multiply in each animal causing the symptoms of severe bovine respiratory disease. Viruses involved include IBR, PI_3, and BRSV; bacteria include *Pasteurella haemolytica, Pasteurella multocida* and *Haemophilus somnus.*

b) Reproductive disorders: If infection of a susceptible cow with the BVD virus occurs:
1. At breeding it can interfere with fertilization;
2. Between 42 and 100 days of gestation it can cause fetal death followed by abortion or mummification;
3. Between 100 and 150 days the virus can cause congenital defects primarily associated with neurological defects such as incomplete development of the cerebellum, cataracts or small, incomplete development of brains;
4. Between 42 and 114 days with a noncytopathic strain the calf may become immunotolerant to the BVD virus. These calves may be born smaller, weak, and show a slow growth rate or may appear quite healthy and develop normally. These calves are persistently infected with the noncytopathic BVD virus and are a source of infection for the herd as well as their own fetuses. In addition, it is these persistently infected animals which are susceptible to mucosal disease.

c) Enteric disorders: These can be divided into two categories depending upon the immunological status of the animal at the time of infection.
1. Bovine viral diarrhea: If susceptible cattle are infected with BVD virus, the infection is usually subclinical: however some show symptoms which include mild depression, inappetence, acute nasal discharge, diarrhea and a drop in milk production. The morbidity is high in susceptible herds, but mortality is usually zero.
2. Mucosal disease: When an animal which is persistently infected by and immunotolerant to noncytopathic BVD virus is infected with a cytopathic BVD strain, it will become superinfected with acute mucosal disease. The animal so infected will show severe erosive lesions of the mouth, esophagus, gastrointestinal tract, nasal cavity, genital areas, and digital areas. Symptoms include severe diarrhea, mucopurulent nasal discharge (thick pus filled), depression, lameness, high fever, anorexia, and dehydration. Death may occur early but usually within 3-10 days from onset of symptoms. This is now classified as acute mucosal disease. A few of the animals do not die in this acute phase but survive only to steadily waste away with a continuation of the above symptoms and lesions. Animals with the chronic mucosal disease ultimately die, although some may survive for up to 18 months.

Herd vaccination, testing, and the elimination of persistently infected animals are essential to control the disease. Since sheep, goats and wild ruminants like deer and elk serve as host reservoirs for this virus, a continual vaccination program is essential.

Presentation: Available in 10 dose (20 mL) and 50 dose (100 mL) bottles.

Compendium Code No.: 11140572

VIRA SHIELD® 2+BRSV

Novartis Animal Vaccines **Vaccine**

Bovine Virus Diarrhea-Respiratory Syncytial Virus Vaccine, Killed Virus

U.S. Vet. Lic. No.: 303

Composition: The vaccine is prepared from highly antigenic Type I and Type II strains of bovine virus diarrhea (cytopathic and noncytopathic) and bovine respiratory syncytial viruses propagated on an established bovine cell line. The vaccine is chemically inactivated and adjuvanted with Xtend III®. Contains penicillin, streptomycin, amphotericin B, and thimerosal as preservatives.

Indications: For use in healthy cattle as an aid in the prevention of diseases caused by bovine virus diarrhea and respiratory syncytial viruses.

Dosage and Administration: Shake well before using. Administer a 5 mL dose intramuscularly to cattle. Repeat in four (4) to five (5) weeks. Calves vaccinated before weaning should be revaccinated after weaning. The vaccine may be administered to pregnant animals at any stage of gestation. Vaccinate dairy cows during the drying-off period. Revaccinate annually to maintain high levels of immunity.

Precaution(s): Store at 35°-45°F (2°-7°C). Do not freeze. Use the entire contents when first opened.

Caution(s): Transient swelling may occur at the site of injection. Milk reduction and transient depression may be observed in lactating dairy cows for three to six days following vaccination. Anaphylactic reactions may occur following the use of the vaccine. Symptomatic treatment: Epinephrine.

For veterinary use only.

Warning(s): Do not vaccinate within 60 days before slaughter.

Discussion: Bovine Viral Diarrhea Virus: Neutralizing antibodies for bovine viral diarrhea virus have been detected in 50% to 90% of the clinically normal cattle tested in the United States. The virus is associated with (A) severe bovine respiratory disease; (B) reproductive disorders, and (C) enteric disorders.

A) Bovine Respiratory Disease: If a susceptible herd is exposed to the BVD virus when it undergoes environmental stress such as inclement weather, transport, etc., the stage is set for bovine respiratory disease. The BVD virus causes immunosuppression and the environmental stressors cause irritation and reduced resistance which allow other pathogens to produce severe bovine respiratory disease. Viruses involved include IBR, PI_3, and BRSV; bacteria include *Pasteurella haemolytica, Pasteurella multocida* and *Haemophilus somnus.*

B) Reproductive Disorders: If infection of a susceptible cow with the BVD virus occurs:
1. At breeding it can interfere with fertilization;
2. Between 42 and 100 days of gestation it can cause fetal death or;
3. Between 100 and 150 days the virus can cause congenital defects such as incomplete development of the cerebellum, cataracts or incomplete development of the brain;
4. Between 42 and 114 days with a noncytopathic strain the calf may become immunotolerant to the BVD virus. These calves may be born weak and show a slow growth rate or may appear quite healthy and develop normally. They are persistently infected with the noncytopathic BVD virus and are a source of infection for the herd and their own fetuses. These persistently infected animals are susceptible to mucosal disease.

V

C) Enteric Disorders: These can be divided into two categories.
1. Bovine Viral Diarrhea: If susceptible cattle are infected with BVD virus, the infection is usually subclinical: however, some show symptoms which include mild depression, inappetence, acute nasal discharge, diarrhea and a drop in milk production. The morbidity is high in susceptible herds, but mortality is usually low.
2. Mucosal Disease: When an animal which is persistently infected by noncytopathic BVD virus is infected with a cytopathic BVD strain, it will become superinfected with acute mucosal disease. It will show severe erosive lesions of the digestive tract, nasal cavity, genital areas, and hooves. Symptoms include severe diarrhea, pus-filled nasal discharge, depression, lameness, high fever, anorexia, and dehydration. Death usually occurs within 3-10 days from the onset of symptoms. A few of these animals survive only to steadily waste away. Animals with this chronic mucosal disease ultimately die, although some may survive for up to 18 months.

Herd vaccination, testing, and the elimination of persistently infected animals are essential to control the disease. Since sheep, goats and wild ruminants like deer and elk serve as host reservoirs for this virus, a continual vaccination program is essential.

Bovine Respiratory Syncytial Virus (BRSV): BRSV was first isolated in the United States in 1974 and is a major contributing agent in the bovine respiratory disease (BRD) syndrome. BRSV is widespread across the United States; 60% to 80% of the cattle tested are positive. Since information on BRSV is incomplete, we can only give a partial description of the disease syndrome produced.

An initial exposure to the virus usually produces: (1) a mild subclinical infection which occurs approximately five days after stress and exposure. Within 2-10 days after recovery from the primary infection some animals will exhibit (2) a severe clinical form of the disease, which can last 12-14 days and result in a high percentage of deaths.
1. The mild subclinical infection can affect animals of all ages. It is most commonly associated with other stressors such as inclement weather, transport, etc. The following symptoms occur but are usually not detected: anorexia, coughing, mild nasal and ocular discharge and fever ranging from 104°-108°F. The animals tend to stand alone, head down, but appear to brighten up and run off when approached. The virus destroys the cilia, which are vital for clearing the air passages of the foreign particles. Dust is particularly aggravating and harmful. Recovery usually follows this infective phase, although the cough commonly persists.
2. In some animals a severe clinical form will occur 2-10 days after recovery from the milder form. These animals exhibit severe respiratory distress, a dry hacking cough, fever ranging from 105°-109°F, nasal and ocular discharge, salivation and subcutaneous edema especially below the jaw and neck areas. The oxygen supply for many of these animals is so deficient that they will go completely off feed and water. Necropsy reveals firm, reddened, noncollapsed lungs characteristic of interstitial pneumonia. In addition, subpleural and interstitial air pockets and fluid accumulation are seen.

BRSV affected animals are highly susceptible to bacterial pathogens such as *Pasteurella hemolytica* or *Haemophilus somnus.* In addition, viruses such as BVD, IBR or PI3 sometimes contribute to the severity of BRSV disease. Treatment is sometimes effective when it is instituted early, but it is very expensive both in terms of medical costs and production losses.

Trial Data: Host Animal Immunogenicity Study - Vira Shield® 2 (Killed Virus):

Group	Pre Vac. Titer*	2 Week Post 2nd Vac. Titer*
Vaccinates (20)	<1:2	1:428
Controls (11)	<1:2	<1:2

*Geometric mean titers.

Vaccinated intramuscularly 28 days apart. All animals bled two weeks post second vaccination.

Virus Re-isolation: BRSV was recovered from 75% of the controls (virus persisted for nine days), but from only 22% of the vaccinates (virus persisted for only two days). Re-isolation began the same day as challenge and was conducted over the 14-day period.

	BRSV SN Titers*	
	Vaccinates	Controls
Prevaccination	1:4.5	1:3.0
6 weeks post 2nd vaccination or prechallenge	1:40	1:7
28 days post challenge	1:47	1:71

*Geometric mean SN titer.

Serum neutralization values demonstrated seroconversion in all 18 animals vaccinated with two doses of the vaccine. Six weeks post second vaccination, all BRSV vaccinated animals developed BRSV antibodies showing a 2-36 fold increase in antibody titer.

Presentation: Available in 50 dose (250 mL) bottles.

Compendium Code No.: 11140582

VIRA SHIELD® 3

Novartis Animal Vaccines **Vaccine**

Bovine Rhinotracheitis-Virus Diarrhea Vaccine, Killed Virus.

U.S. Vet. Lic. No.: 303

Active Ingredient(s): This vaccine is prepared from highly antigenic strains of IBR and BVD (cytopathic Type 1 and noncytopathic Type 2) viruses propagated on an established bovine cell line. The vaccine is chemically inactivated and adjuvanted with Xtend III®. Contains amphotericin B, penicillin, and thimerosal as preservatives.

Indications: For use in healthy cattle as an aid in the prevention of disease caused by infectious bovine rhinotracheitis and bovine virus diarrhea viruses.

Dosage and Administration: Shake well before using. Administer 5 mL intramuscularly. Revaccinate in 4-5 weeks. Calves vaccinated before weaning should be revaccinated after weaning. This vaccine may be administered to pregnant animals at any stage of gestation. Vaccinate dairy cows during the dry off period. Revaccinate annually to maintain high levels of immunity.

Precaution(s): Store in the dark at 35°-45°F (2°-7°C). Do not freeze. Use entire contents when first opened.

Caution(s): Transient swelling may occur at the site of injection. Milk reduction and transient depression may be observed in lactating dairy cows for 3-6 days following vaccination. Anaphylactic reactions may occur following the use of this biological. Symptomatic treatment: Epinephrine.

For veterinary use only.

Warning(s): Do not vaccinate within 60 days prior to slaughter.

Discussion: Infectious Bovine Rhinotracheitis is caused by Bovine Herpes Virus 1, which is also responsible for the disease syndrome known as infectious pustular vulvovaginitis and balanoposthitis (IPV-IPB). It appears that the latter (IPV) was the primary form of the disease until the animals were concentrated into high population units such as beef feedlots and large dairy herds. The virus is associated with A) upper respiratory tract infections (IBR) and bovine respiratory disease, B) conjunctivitis and C) reproductive disorders including IPB, abortion and neonatal death.

Clinical signs: Conjunctival, nasal, and tracheal discharges, IPB, and IPV.

Bovine Viral Diarrhea Virus is one of the most important bovine viral pathogens in the world. The complexity of the virus and its involvement in multiple bovine disease processes are only now beginning to be understood. Neutralizing antibodies for this Pestivirus have been detected in 50% to 90% of the clinically normal cattle tested in the United States. The virus is associated with A) Bovine Respiratory Disease; B) reproductive disorders including infertility, abortion, and neonatal defects and C) enteric disorders including Bovine Viral Diarrhea, Acute Mucosal Disease and Chronic Mucosal Disease. In addition, the newly recognized Type 2 strains of BVD have been implicated in severe disease outbreaks where the animals often show hemorrhagic symptoms and death losses approach 100% of affected animals.

Clinical signs: Hemorrhagic syndrome, neurological defects in calves, nasal discharge, oral ulcers, GI ulcers, infertility, abortion, genital ulcers, erosions of the coronary band and interdigital cleft, and immunosuppression.

Trial Data: South Dakota State University Research: A portion of the study was designed to prove protection against a BVD Type 2 challenge (Strain 890). In June of 1994, six 500- to 700- lb calves received two vaccinations, four weeks apart, with Vira Shield® 5 which has IBR and BVD fractions identical to those found in the Vira Shield® 3 and Vira Shield® 3+VL5. The controls were three seronegative, unvaccinated calves (400 lbs) from the same herd. Eleven months after vaccination, the calves were challenged intranasally with NVSL BVD challenge strain 890. Clinical scores on each animal were recorded daily from three days prechallenge to 14 days post challenge.[1]

Graph 1: Vaccinated vs. Non-Vaccinated Cattle
Respiratory Study

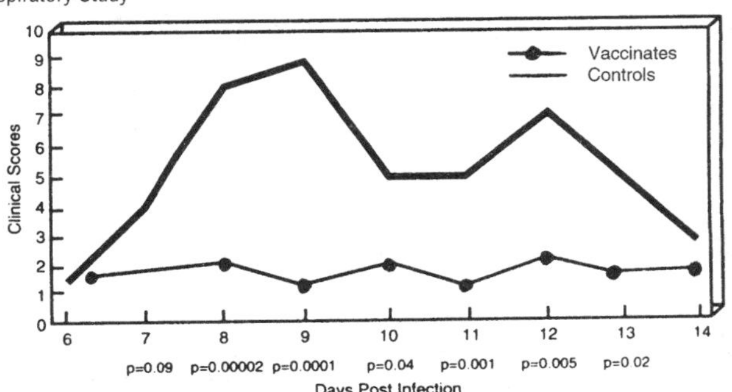

Clinical parameters included in Graph 1 are: temperature; dyspnea; depression; nasal discharge; lacrimation; conjunctivitis; and inflammation of the nasal mucosa. The clinical scores from days 8 through 13 were statistically significant at the values indicated.

Graph 2: Vaccinated vs. Non-Vaccinated Cattle
Diarrhea Study

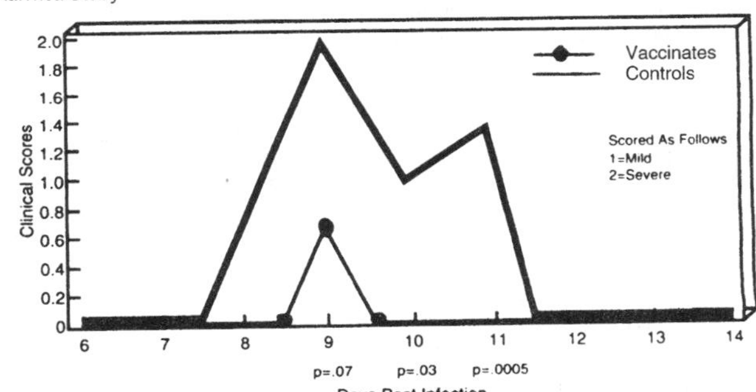

The clinical scores determining severity of diarrhea are presented in Graph 2. Note the statistically significant difference between vaccinates and controls for days 8 through 11.[1] This study demonstrates that for up to 11 months post vaccination, Vira Shield® significantly protected against type 2 BVDV 890.

Tests for cell-mediated immunity against BVDV, IBRV and BRSV were included in this study. The results show that Vira Shield® demonstrated a unique cell mediated activation, lasting for 11 months, against all these viruses.[1] This confirms previous research with IBR and BRSV vaccines that cell-mediated immunity is produced by Vira Shield®.[2]

References: [1]Chase, C., Hurley, D. (AABP 1995). [2]Ellis, J.A., et al., JAVMA, 1995; 206, 3:354-361.

Presentation: Available in 50 dose (250 mL) bottles.

Compendium Code No.: 11140592

VIRA SHIELD® 3+VL5

Novartis Animal Vaccines **Bacterin-Vaccine**

Bovine Rhinotracheitis-Virus Diarrhea Vaccine, Killed Virus-Campylobacter Fetus-Leptospira Canicola-Grippotyphosa-Hardjo-Icterohaemorrhagiae-Pomona Bacterin

U.S. Vet. Lic. No.: 303

Composition: This product contains an IBR virus, a cytopathic Type 1 BVD virus, and a noncytopathic Type 2 BVD virus propagated on an established bovine cell line and cultures of *Campylobacter fetus, Leptospira canicola, grippotyphosa, hardjo, icterohaemorrhagiae,* and *pomona.* The product is chemically inactivated and adjuvanted with Xtend III®. Contains amphotericin B, penicillin, streptomycin, and thimerosal as preservatives.

Indications: For use in healthy heifers and cows as an aid in the prevention of disease caused by infectious bovine rhinotracheitis and bovine virus diarrhea viruses, and *Campylobacter fetus, Leptospira canicola, grippotyphosa, hardjo, icterohaemorrhagiae,* and *pomona.*

Dosage and Administration: Shake well before using. Administer 5 mL intramuscularly 2-4 weeks prior to breeding. Revaccinate with Vira Shield® 3 (Bovine Rhinotracheitis-Virus Diarrhea Vaccine) in 4-5 weeks. Revaccinate annually.

Precaution(s): Store in the dark at 35°-45°F (2°-7°C). Do not freeze. Use entire contents when first opened.

Caution(s): Transient swelling may occur at the site of injection. Milk reduction and transient depression may be observed in lactating dairy cows for 3-6 days following vaccination. Anaphylactic reactions may occur following the use of this biological. Symptomatic treatment: Epinephrine.

For veterinary use only.

Warning(s): Do not vaccinate within 60 days prior to slaughter.

Discussion: Infectious Bovine Rhinotracheitis is caused by Bovine Herpes Virus 1, which is also responsible for the disease syndrome known as infectious pustular vulvovaginitis and balanoposthitis (IPV-IPB). It appears that the latter (IPV) was the primary form of the disease until the animals were concentrated into high population units such as beef feedlots and large dairy herds. The virus is associated with A) upper respiratory tract infections (IBR) and bovine respiratory disease, B) conjunctivitis and C) reproductive disorders including IPB, abortion and neonatal death.

Clinical signs: Conjunctival, nasal, and tracheal discharges, IPB, and IPV.

Bovine Viral Diarrhea Virus is one of the most important bovine viral pathogens in the world. The complexity of the virus and its involvement in multiple bovine disease processes are only now beginning to be understood. Neutralizing antibodies for this Pestivirus have been detected in 50% to 90% of the clinically normal cattle tested in the United States. The virus is associated with A) Bovine Respiratory Disease; B) reproductive disorders including infertility, abortion, and neonatal defects and C) enteric disorders including Bovine Viral Diarrhea, Acute Mucosal Disease and Chronic Mucosal Disease. In addition, the newly recognized Type 2 strains of BVD have been implicated in severe disease outbreaks where the animals often show hemorrhagic symptoms and death losses approach 100% of affected animals.

Clinical signs: Hemorrhagic syndrome, neurological defects in calves, nasal discharge, oral ulcers, GI ulcers, infertility, abortion, genital ulcers, erosions of the coronary band and interdigital cleft, and immunosuppression.

Bovine genital Campylobacteriosis, previously known as Vibriosis, is a venereal disease of cattle caused by *Campylobacter fetus.* This disease is spread from bull to cow and cow to bull during breeding. It can also be spread through artificial insemination if the pipette or semen is contaminated.

Infection with *Campylobacter* is subclinical and remains restricted to the vaginal and uterine mucosa of the cow and the mucous membrane of the penis and sheath of the bull. The uterine infection usually destroys the embryo at its earliest stages. However, in some instances, the embryo survives, becomes infected and is aborted in the second trimester of pregnancy. The presence of the disease should be suspected when conception rates for a newly infected herd drop below 90%.

Definite diagnosis can be made by identifying the organism in the cervical or vaginal mucus of the cow or in preputial fluid from the infected bull.

This disease has been present in our cattle herds for many years and has come to be known as the "repeat breeder syndrome".

Vaccination of the heifers, cows, and bulls prior to breeding is the only practical way to eliminate this insidious, costly disease.

Leptospirosis is a contagious disease of both man and animals and has been estimated to cause losses in excess of 100 million dollars per year to the livestock industry, according to the USDA. This loss is due primarily to abortions and stillbirths in breeding stock, lowered milk production, and by sickness and death in young animals. Abortion rates can be 30% or higher in affected cattle herds before the disease can be stopped.

The causative organisms belong to a group of pathogens called *Leptospira interrogans*, with five major serovars incriminated: *L grippotyphosa, L hardjo, L pomona, L canicola,* and *L icterohaemorrhagiae.*

This disease is spread to our domestic livestock by the shedding of the organisms in the urine, which contaminates feed or water. These organisms survive well in surface waters. The organism may be found in the udder and be secreted in the milk to suckling calves, thus infecting them.

Many wildlife species may be infected with these organisms, with some of the more common ones being rats, raccoons, skunks, foxes, and opossums. Dogs are also often infected.

The incubation period varies from 1 to 4 days and is followed by a leptospiremia (bacteria in the blood) which lasts for 1-5 days. With the appearance of antibody in the animal's blood, the leptospiremic phase is terminated. The organisms may remain in the kidney and multiply in this location, then are shed in the urine for months or years, infecting other farm animals.

Young animals that are actually ill with leptospirosis may show a transient fever, loss of appetite, and difficulty in breathing, with death losses approaching 15% due to severe anemia. Lactating cows exhibit a loss of milk production with a milk secretion that is yellow, clotted, and often blood-tinged. Severely affected animals develop anemia, jaundice, hemoglobinuria and pneumonia.

Treatment of this disease using antibiotics is sometimes effective, but costly. Good husbandry and a solid immunization program using a Novartis Animal Vaccines, Inc. Federally approved vaccine, such as VIRA SHIELD® 3+VL5, is the economical route in preventing this disease in cattle.

Trial Data: South Dakota State University Research: A portion of the study was designed to prove protection against a BVD Type 2 challenge (Strain 890). In June of 1994, six 500- to 700- lb calves received two vaccinations, four weeks apart, with Vira Shield® 5 which has IBR and BVD fractions identical to those found in the Vira Shield® 3 and VIRA SHIELD® 3+VL5. The controls were three seronegative, unvaccinated calves (400 lbs) from the same herd. Eleven months after vaccination, the calves were challenged intranasally with NVSL BVD challenge strain 890. Clinical scores on each animal were recorded daily from three days prechallenge to 14 days post challenge.[1]

Graph 1: Vaccinated vs. Non-Vaccinated Cattle
Respiratory Study

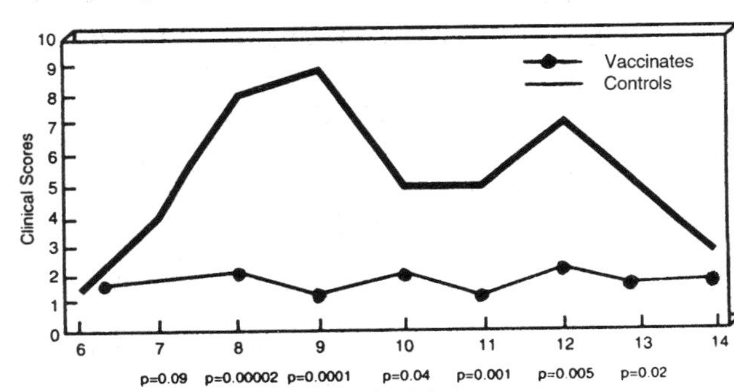

Clinical parameters included in Graph 1 are: temperature; dyspnea; depression; nasal discharge; lacrimation; conjunctivitis; and inflammation of the nasal mucosa. The clinical scores from days 8 through 13 were statistically significant at the values indicated.

V

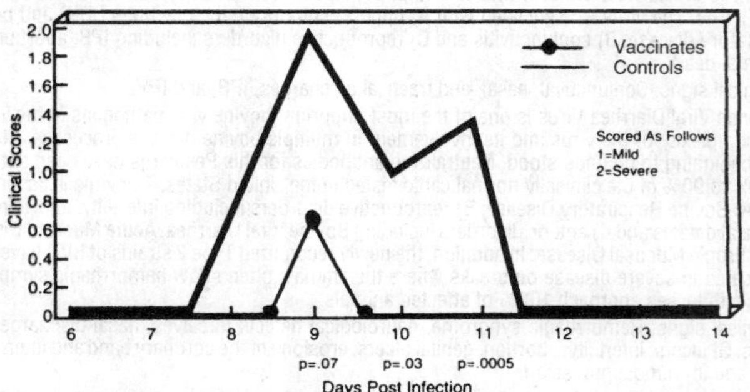

The clinical scores determining severity of diarrhea are presented in Graph 2. Note the statistically significant difference between vaccinates and controls for days 8 through 11.[1] This study demonstrates that for up to 11 months post vaccination, Vira Shield® significantly protected against type 2 BVDV 890.

Tests for cell-mediated immunity against BVDV, IBRV and BRSV were included in this study. The results show that Vira Shield® demonstrated a unique cell mediated activation, lasting for 11 months, against all these viruses.[1] This confirms previous research with IBR and BRSV vaccines that cell-mediated immunity is produced by Vira Shield®.[2]

References: Available upon request.

Presentation: Available in 10 dose (50 mL) and 50 dose (250 mL) bottles.

Compendium Code No.: 11140603

VIRA SHIELD® 4

Novartis Animal Vaccines **Vaccine**

Bovine Rhinotracheitis-Virus Diarrhea-Parainfluenza 3 Vaccine, Killed Virus

U.S. Vet. Lic. No.: 303

Contents: This product contains an IBR virus, a cytopathic Type 1 BVD virus, a noncytopathic Type 2 BVD virus, and a PI_3 virus propagated on an established bovine cell line. The vaccine is chemically inactivated and adjuvanted with Xtend III®. Contains amphotericin B, penicillin, streptomycin, and thimerosal as preservatives.

Indications: For use in healthy cattle as an aid in the prevention of diseases caused by infectious bovine rhinotracheitis, bovine virus diarrhea, and parainfluenza Type 3 viruses.

Dosage and Administration: Shake well before using. Administer 5 mL intramuscularly or subcutaneously. Revaccinate in 4 to 5 weeks. This vaccine may be administered to pregnant animals at any stage of gestation. Vaccinate dairy cows during the dry-off period. Revaccinate annually.

Precaution(s): Store in the dark at 35°-45°F (2°-7°C). Do not freeze. Use entire contents when first opened.

Caution(s): Transient swelling may occur at the site of injection. Anaphylactic reactions may occur following the use of this biological. Symptomatic treatment: Epinephrine.

Warning(s): Do not vaccinate within 60 days prior to slaughter.

Discussion: Infectious bovine rhinotracheitis (IBR) is caused by bovine herpes virus 1, which is also responsible for the disease syndrome known as infectious pustular vulvovaginitis and balanoposthitis (IPV-IPB). It appears the latter (IPV) was the primary form of the disease until the animals were concentrated into high population units such as beef feedlots and large dairy herds. The virus is associated with A) upper respiratory tract infections (IBR) and bovine respiratory disease; B) conjunctivitis; and C) reproductive disorders including IPV, abortion, and neonatal disease.

Bovine viral diarrhea (BVD) virus is one of the most important bovine viral pathogens in the world. The complexity of the virus and its involvement in multiple bovine disease processes are only now beginning to be understood. Neutralizing antibodies for this pestivirus have been detected in 50% to 90% of the clinically normal cattle tested in the United States. The virus is associated with A) bovine respiratory disease; B) reproductive disorders including infertility, abortion, and neonatal defects; and C) enteric disorders including bovine viral diarrhea, acute mucosal disease, and chronic mucosal disease. In addition, the newly recognized Type 2 strains of BVD have been implicated in severe disease outbreaks where the animals often show hemorrhagic symptoms and death losses approach 100% of affected animals.

Parainfluenza 3 (PI_3) is a paramyxovirus belonging to the same family as BRSV. PI_3 virus has been isolated, identified, and studied in relation to bovine respiratory disease (BRD) syndrome. PI_3 virus is commonly isolated from animals suffering from BRD, although it appears to be more of a contributing agent rather than a primary pathogen. By itself, PI_3 virus produces a rather benign infection of the lung. PI_3 antibodies have been detected in approximately 90% of the cattle tested in the United States. It most commonly invades the lungs, causing a fibrinous pleuritis and pneumonia.

Trial Data: Product Comparisons of Antibody to Cytopathic Type 1 BVD Virus Over 12 Months:

Group	Days After First Vaccination							
	0	34	89	146	205	256	314	366
Control	<2	<2	<2	<2	<2	<2	<2	<2
VIRA SHIELD® 4	<2	10	94	94	59	51	64	87
Vaccine B	<2	3	11	7	4	3	2	3
Vaccine C	<2	3	13	9	5	5	5	6
Vaccine D	<2	<2	3	2	2	2	3	2

Product Comparison of Antibody to IBR Virus Over 12 Months:

Group	Days After First Vaccination							
	0	34	89	146	205	256	314	366
Control	<2	<2	<2	<2	<2	<2	<2	<2
VIRA SHIELD® 4	<2	<2	12	6	7	7	9	6
Vaccine B	<2	<2	2	<2	<2	<2	<2	<2
Vaccine C	<2	<2	3	<2	<2	<2	<2	<2
Vaccine D	<2	<2	2	<2	<2	<2	<2	<2

Product Comparisons of Antibody to Noncytopathic Type 2 BVD Virus Over 12 Months:

Group	Days After First Vaccination							
	0	34	89	146	205	256	314	366
Control	<2	<2	<2	<2	<2	<2	<2	<2
VIRA SHIELD® 4	<2	10	64	81	44	32	20	17
Vaccine B	<2	<2	2	<2	<2	<2	<2	2
Vaccine C	<2	<2	2	2	2	<2	<2	<2
Vaccine D	<2	<2	3	3	2	2	2	2

Study conducted at the University of Nebraska by Merwin L. Frey, D.V.M., Ph.D.

Geometric mean antibody titers to indicated virus at indicated levels in non-vaccinated control calves (n=7) and in four groups of calves (n=8 or 9) given respectively, 1 of 4 different killed vaccines (all received 2 doses, at 0 and 34 days).

Conclusions: Because of their safety, the use of inactivated vaccines will almost certainly continue to increase. Four federally licensed, inactivated BVDV-IBRV vaccines were compared in this trial. Only one of the four was effective in eliciting high SN titers that persisted over a one-year period.

Presentation: Available in 10 dose (50 mL), 20 dose (100 mL) and 50 dose (250 mL) bottles.

Compendium Code No.: 11140612

VIRA SHIELD® 4+L5

Novartis Animal Vaccines **Bacterin-Vaccine**

Bovine Rhinotracheitis-Virus Diarrhea-Parainfluenza 3 Vaccine, (Killed Virus)-Leptospira Canicola-Grippotyphosa-Hardjo-Icterohaemorrhagiae-Pomona Bacterin

U.S. Vet. Lic. No.: 303

Contents: This product contains an IBR virus, a cytopathic Type 1 BVD virus, a noncytopathic Type 2 BVD virus, and a PI_3 virus propagated on an established bovine cell line, and cultures of *Leptospira canicola, grippotyphosa, hardjo, icterohaemorrhagiae,* and *pomona.* The product is chemically inactivated and adjuvanted with Xtend III®. Contains amphotericin B, penicillin, streptomycin, and thimerosal as preservatives.

Indications: For use in healthy cattle as an aid in the prevention of diseases caused by infectious bovine rhinotracheitis, bovine virus diarrhea, parainfluenza type 3 viruses and *Leptospira canicola, grippotyphosa, hardjo, icterohaemorrhagiae,* and *pomona.*

Dosage and Administration: Shake well before using. Administer a 5 mL dose intramuscularly. Revaccinate with Vira Shield® 4 (Bovine Rhinotracheitis-Virus Diarrhea-Parainfluenza 3 Vaccine) in 4-5 weeks. Vaccinate dairy cows during the dry-off period. Revaccinate annually.

Precaution(s): Store at 35°-45°F (2°-7°C). Do not freeze. Use entire contents when first opened.

Caution(s): Transient swelling may occur at the site of injection. Anaphylactic reactions may occur following the use of this biological. Symptomatic treatment: Epinephrine.

Warning(s): Do not vaccinate within 60 days prior to slaughter.

Discussion: Infectious bovine rhinotracheitis (IBR) is caused by bovine herpes virus 1, which is also responsible for the disease syndrome known as infectious pustular vulvovaginitis and balanoposthitis (IPV-IPB). It appears the latter (IPV) was the primary form of the disease until the animals were concentrated into high population units such as beef feedlots and large dairy herds. The virus is associated with A) upper respiratory tract infections (IBR) and bovine respiratory disease; B) conjunctivitis; and C) reproductive disorders including IPV, abortion, and neonatal disease.

Bovine viral diarrhea (BVD) virus is one of the most important bovine viral pathogens in the world. The complexity of the virus and its involvement in multiple bovine disease processes are only now beginning to be understood. Neutralizing antibodies for this pestivirus have been detected in 50% to 90% of the clinically normal cattle tested in the United States. The virus is associated with A) bovine respiratory disease; B) reproductive disorders including infertility, abortion, and neonatal defects; and C) enteric disorders including bovine viral diarrhea, acute mucosal disease, and chronic mucosal disease. In addition, the newly recognized Type 2 strains of BVD have been implicated in severe disease outbreaks where the animals often show hemorrhagic symptoms and death losses approach 100% of affected animals.

Parainfluenza 3 (PI_3) is a paramyxovirus belonging to the same family as BRSV. PI_3 virus has been isolated, identified, and studied in relation to bovine respiratory disease (BRD) syndrome. PI_3 virus is commonly isolated from animals suffering from BRD, although it appears to be more of a contributing agent rather than a primary pathogen. By itself, PI_3 virus produces a rather benign infection of the lung. PI_3 antibodies have been detected in approximately 90% of the cattle tested in the United States. It most commonly invades the lungs, causing a fibrinous pleuritis and pneumonia.

Leptospirosis is a contagious disease of man and animals that is caused by the bacteria *Leptospira interrogans;* five major serovars are implicated in cattle: *L. hardjo, L. grippotyphosa, L. pomona, L. canicola,* and *L. icterohaemorrhagiae.* The disease is spread by bacteria shedding in urine, contaminating feed and water consumed by other animals. Suckling animals may also be infected through the milk. Many wildlife species can carry leptospirosis and potentially infect domestic animals. Clinical signs include abortions, stillbirths, and lowered milk production in adult animals, and sickness and death in young animals.

Trial Data: Product Comparisons of Antibody to Cytopathic Type 1 BVD Virus Over 12 Months:

Group	Days After First Vaccination							
	0	34	89	146	205	256	314	366
Control	<2	<2	<2	<2	<2	<2	<2	<2
Vira Shield® 4	<2	10	94	94	59	51	64	87
Vaccine B	<2	3	11	7	4	3	2	3
Vaccine C	<2	3	13	9	5	5	5	6
Vaccine D	<2	<2	3	2	2	2	3	2

Product Comparison of Antibody to IBR Virus Over 12 Months:

Group	Days After First Vaccination							
	0	34	89	146	205	256	314	366
Control	<2	<2	<2	<2	<2	<2	<2	<2
Vira Shield® 4	<2	<2	12	6	7	7	9	6
Vaccine B	<2	<2	2	<2	<2	<2	<2	<2
Vaccine C	<2	<2	3	<2	<2	<2	<2	<2
Vaccine D	<2	<2	2	<2	<2	<2	<2	<2

V

Product Comparisons of Antibody to Noncytopathic Type 2 BVD Virus Over 12 Months:

Group	Days After First Vaccination							
	0	34	89	146	205	256	314	366
Control	<2	<2	<2	<2	<2	<2	<2	<2
Vira Shield® 4	<2	10	64	81	44	32	20	17
Vaccine B	<2	<2	2	<2	<2	<2	<2	2
Vaccine C	<2	<2	2	2	2	<2	<2	<2
Vaccine D	<2	<2	3	3	2	2	2	2

Study conducted at the University of Nebraska by Merwin L. Frey, D.V.M., Ph.D.

Geometric mean antibody titers to indicated virus at indicated levels in non-vaccinated control calves (n=7) and in four groups of calves (n=8 or 9) given respectively, 1 of 4 different killed vaccines (all received 2 doses, at 0 and 34 days).

Conclusions: Because of their safety, the use of inactivated vaccines will almost certainly continue to increase. Four federally licensed, inactivated BVDV-IBRV vaccines were compared in this trial. Only one of the four was effective in eliciting high SN titers that persisted over a one-year period.

Presentation: Available in 10 dose (50 mL), 20 dose (100 mL) and 50 dose (250 mL) bottles.

Compendium Code No.: 11140622

VIRA SHIELD® 5

Novartis Animal Vaccines **Vaccine**

Bovine Rhinotracheitis-Virus Diarrhea-Parainfluenza 3-Respiratory Syncytial Virus Vaccine, Killed Virus

U.S. Vet. Lic. No.: 303

Composition: This vaccine contains an IBR virus, a cytopathic Type 1 BVD virus, a noncytopathic Type 2 BVD virus, a PI_3 virus, and a BRS virus propagated on an established bovine cell line. The vaccine is chemically inactivated and adjuvanted with Xtend III®. Contains amphotericin B, gentamicin and thimerosal as preservatives.

Indications: For use in healthy cattle as an aid in the prevention of diseases caused by infectious bovine rhinotracheitis, bovine virus diarrhea Type 1, bovine virus diarrhea Type 2, parainfluenza Type 3, and bovine respiratory syncytial viruses.

Dosage and Administration: Shake well before using. Administer 5 mL intramuscularly or subcutaneously. Revaccinate in 4-5 weeks. This vaccine may be administered to pregnant animals at any stage of gestation. Vaccinate dairy cows during the dry off period. Revaccinate annually.

Precaution(s): Store in the dark at 35°-45°F (2°-7°C). Do not freeze. Use entire contents when first opened.

Caution(s): Transient swelling may occur at the site of injection. Anaphylactic reactions may occur following the use of this biological. Symptomatic treatment: Epinephrine.

Warning(s): Do not vaccinate within 60 days prior to slaughter.

Discussion: Technical Disease Information:

Infectious Bovine Rhinotracheitis (IBR): Infectious Bovine Rhinotracheitis is caused by Bovine Herpes Virus 1, which is also responsible for the disease syndrome known as infectious pustular vulvovaginitis and balanoposthitis (IPV-IPB). It appears that the latter (IPV) was the primary form of the disease until the animals were concentrated into high population units such as beef feedlots and large dairy herds. The virus is associated with A) upper respiratory tract infections (IBR) and bovine respiratory disease, B) conjunctivitis and C) reproductive disorders including IPV, abortion and neonatal death.

Bovine Virus Diarrhea (BVD): Bovine Viral Diarrhea virus is one of the most important bovine viral pathogens in the world. The complexity of the virus and its involvement in multiple bovine disease processes are only now beginning to be understood. Neutralizing antibodies for this Pestivirus have been detected in 50% to 90% of the clinically normal cattle tested in the United States. The virus is associated with A) Bovine Respiratory Disease; B) reproductive disorders including infertility, abortion, and neonatal defects and C) enteric disorders including Bovine Viral Diarrhea, Acute Mucosal Disease and Chronic Mucosal Disease. In addition, the Type 2 strains of BVD have been implicated in severe disease outbreaks where the animals often show hemorrhagic symptoms and death losses approach 100% of affected animals.

Parainfluenza 3 (PI_3): Parainfluenza-3 is a Paramyxovirus belonging to the same family as BRSV. PI_3 virus has been isolated, identified and studied in relation to Bovine Respiratory Disease (BRD) syndrome. The PI_3 virus is commonly isolated from animals suffering from BRD, although it appears to be more of a contributing agent rather than a primary pathogen. By itself PI_3 virus produces a rather benign infection of the lung. PI_3 antibodies have been detected in approximately 90% of the cattle tested in the United States. It most commonly invades the lungs causing a fibrinous pleuritis and pneumonia.

Bovine Respiratory Syncytial Virus (BRSV): Bovine Respiratory Syncytial Virus was first isolated in the United States in 1974 and recently has been identified as a major contributing agent in the Bovine Respiratory Disease (BRD) syndrome. It was named BRSV because this Pneumovirus invades the cell lining of the trachea and lungs and because it promotes the formation of large multinucleated cells called syncytial cells in the epithelium and interstitial spaces of the lung. BRSV appears to be widespread across the United States. In states where antibody prevalence testing has been done, 60% to 80% of the cattle tested are positive.

An initial exposure to the virus usually produces: 1) a Mild Subclinical Infection which occurs approximately 5 days after stress and exposure. Within 2-10 days after recovery from this primary infection some animals will exhibit 2) a Severe Clinical Form of this disease, which if untreated will last 12-14 days and result in a high percentage of deaths. At any of these stages the course and severity of the disease can be aggravated by invasion of the weakened animal by other viral and bacterial pathogens.

Trial Data: South Dakota State University Research: A portion of the study was designed to prove protection against a BVD Type 2 challenge (Strain 890). In June of 1994, six 500- to 700- lb calves received two vaccinations, four weeks apart, with VIRA SHIELD® 5. The controls were three seronegative, unvaccinated calves (400 lbs) from the same herd. Eleven months after vaccination, the calves were challenged intranasally with NVSL BVD challenge strain 890. Clinical scores on each animal were recorded daily from three days prechallenge to 14 days post challenge.[1]

Graph 1: Vaccinated vs. Non-Vaccinated Cattle
Respiratory Study

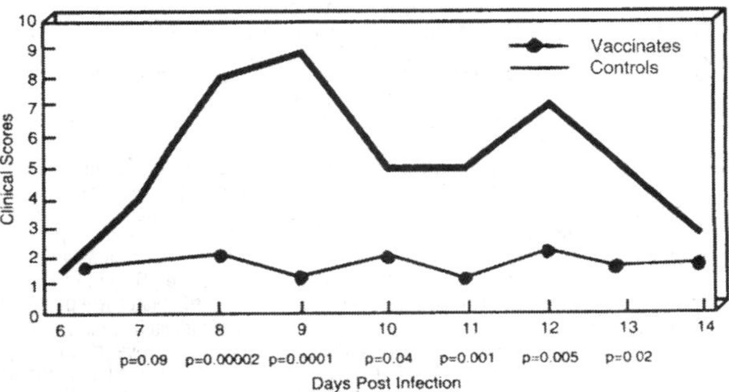

Clinical parameters included in Graph 1 are: temperature; dyspnea; depression; nasal discharge; lacrimation; conjunctivitis; and inflammation of the nasal mucosa. The clinical scores from days 8 through 13 were statistically significant at the values indicated.

Graph 2: Vaccinated vs. Non-Vaccinated Cattle
Diarrhea Study

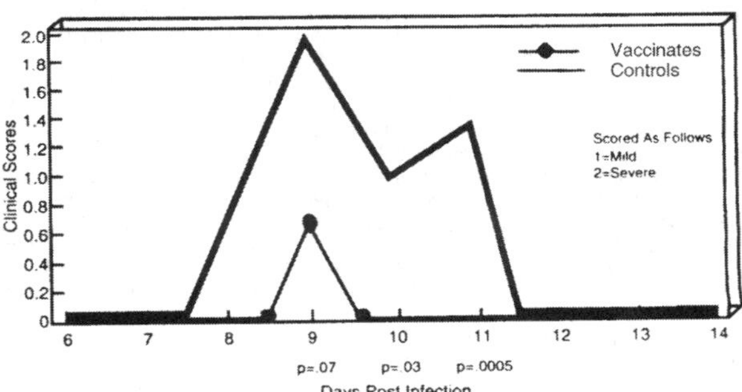

The clinical scores determining severity of diarrhea are presented in Graph 2. Note the statistically significant difference between vaccinates and controls for days 8 through 11.[1] This study demonstrates that for up to 11 months post vaccination, Vira Shield® significantly protected against type 2 BVDV 890.

Tests for cell-mediated immunity against BVDV, IBRV and BRSV were included in this study. The results show that VIRA SHIELD® 5 demonstrated a unique cell-mediated activation, lasting for 11 months, against all these viruses.[1] This confirms previous research with IBR and BRSV vaccines that cell-mediated immunity is produced by VIRA SHIELD® 5.[2]

References: Available upon request.

Presentation: Available in 10 dose (50 mL), 20 dose (100 mL) and 50 dose (250 mL) bottles.

Compendium Code No.: 11140633 MP-F197-NOV01

VIRA SHIELD® 5+L5

Novartis Animal Vaccines **Bacterin-Vaccine**

Bovine Rhinotracheitis-Virus Diarrhea-Parainfluenza 3-Respiratory Syncytial Virus Vaccine, Killed Virus-Leptospira Canicola-Grippotyphosa-Hardjo-Icterohaemorrhagiae-Pomona Bacterin

U.S. Vet. Lic. No.: 303

Composition: This product contains an IBR virus, a cytopathic Type 1 BVD virus, a noncytopathic Type 2 BVD virus, a PI_3 virus and a BRS virus propagated on an established bovine cell line and cultures of *Leptospira canicola, grippotyphosa, hardjo, icterohaemorrhagiae,* and *pomona.* The product is chemically inactivated and adjuvanted with Xtend III®. Contains amphotericin B, gentamicin and thimerosal as preservatives.

Indications: For use in healthy cattle as an aid in the prevention of disease caused by infectious bovine rhinotracheitis, bovine virus diarrhea Type 1, bovine virus diarrhea Type 2, parainfluenza Type 3, bovine respiratory syncytial viruses and *Leptospira canicola, grippotyphosa, hardjo, icterohaemorrhagiae,* and *pomona.*

Dosage and Administration: Shake well before using. Administer 5 mL intramuscularly. Revaccinate with Vira Shield® 5 (Bovine Rhinotracheitis-Virus Diarrhea-Parainfluenza 3-Respiratory Syncytial Virus Vaccine) in 4-5 weeks. Vaccinate dairy cows during the dry off period. Revaccinate annually.

Precaution(s): Store in the dark at 35°-45°F (2°-7°C). Do not freeze. Use entire contents when first opened.

Caution(s): Transient swelling may occur at the site of injection. Anaphylactic reactions may occur following the use of this biological. Symptomatic treatment: Epinephrine.

Warning(s): Do not vaccinate within 60 days prior to slaughter.

Discussion: Technical Disease Information:

Infectious Bovine Rhinotracheitis (IBR): Infectious Bovine Rhinotracheitis is caused by Bovine Herpes Virus 1, which is also responsible for the disease syndrome known as infectious pustular vulvovaginitis and balanoposthitis (IPV-IPB). It appears that the latter (IPV) was the primary form of the disease until the animals were concentrated into high population units such as beef feedlots and large dairy herds. The virus is associated with A) upper respiratory tract infections (IBR) and bovine respiratory disease, B) conjunctivitis and C) reproductive disorders including IPB, abortion and neonatal death.

Bovine Virus Diarrhea (BVD): Bovine Viral Diarrhea Virus is one of the most important bovine viral pathogens in the world. The complexity of the virus and its involvement in multiple bovine disease processes are only now beginning to be understood. Neutralizing antibodies for this Pestivirus have been detected in 50% to 90% of the clinically normal cattle tested in the United States. The virus is associated with A) Bovine Respiratory Disease; B) reproductive disorders including infertility, abortion , and neonatal defects and C) enteric disorders including Bovine Viral Diarrhea, Acute Mucosal Disease and Chronic Mucosal Disease. In addition, the Type 2 strains of BVD have been implicated in severe disease outbreaks where the animals often show hemorrhagic symptoms and death losses approach 100% of affected animals.

Parainfluenza 3 (PI_3): Parainfluenza-3 is a Paramyxovirus belonging to the same family as BRSV. PI_3 virus has been isolated, identified and studied in relation to Bovine Respiratory Disease (BRD) syndrome. PI_3 virus is commonly isolated from animals suffering from BRD, although it appears to be more of a contributing agent rather than a primary pathogen. By itself PI_3 virus produces a rather benign infection of the lung. PI_3 antibodies have been detected in approximately 90% of the cattle tested in the United States. It most commonly invades the lungs causing a fibrinous pleuritis and pneumonia.

Bovine Respiratory Syncytial Virus (BRSV): Bovine Respiratory Syncytial Virus (BRSV) was first isolated in the United States in 1974 and recently has been identified as a major contributing agent in the Bovine Respiratory Disease (BRD) syndrome. It was named BRSV because this Pneumovirus invades the cell lining of the trachea and lungs and because it promotes the formation of large multinucleated cells called syncytial cells in the epithelium and interstitial spaces of the lung. BRSV appears to be widespread across the United States. In states where antibody prevalence testing has been done, 60% to 80% of the cattle tested are positive.

An initial exposure to the virus usually produces: 1) a Mild Subclinical Infection which occurs approximately 5 days after stress and exposure. Within 2-10 days after recovery from this primary infection some animals exhibit 2) a Severe Clinical Form of this disease, which, if untreated will last 12-14 days and result in a high percentage of deaths. At any of these stages the course and severity of the disease can be aggravated by invasion of the weakened animal by other viral and bacterial pathogens.

Leptospirosis: Although leptospirosis is not the threat to our livestock industry that it once was, we can't forget about this organism. Leptospirosis is prevalent in all domestic animals, as well as wildlife populations such as skunks, opossums and raccoons.

This organism will not survive by itself in the environment. Animals that recover from leptospirosis may become carriers, and the organism may be shed in the urine for various periods of time. The susceptible animal ingests this organism, usually through feed or in water contaminated by animals shedding the organism in their urine.

Clinical signs in infected cattle are, for the most part, not observed. A particularly observant herdsman may notice a day or two of lowered feed consumption, and in the case of milk cows, lowered milk production. The most frequent clinical sign of leptospirosis is an abortion in the last trimester of gestation. Red colored urine due to hemoglobinuria may be seen also.

Trial Data: South Dakota State University Research: A portion of the study was designed to prove protection against a BVD Type 2 challenge (Strain 890). In June of 1994, six 500- to 700- lb. calves received two vaccinations, four weeks apart, with Vira Shield® 5. The controls were three seronegative, unvaccinated calves (400 lbs.) from the same herd. Eleven months after vaccination, the calves were challenged intranasally with NVSL BVD challenge strain 890. Clinical scores on each animal were recorded daily from three days prechallenge to 14 days post challenge.[1]

Graph 1: Vaccinated vs. Non-Vaccinated Cattle
Respiratory Study

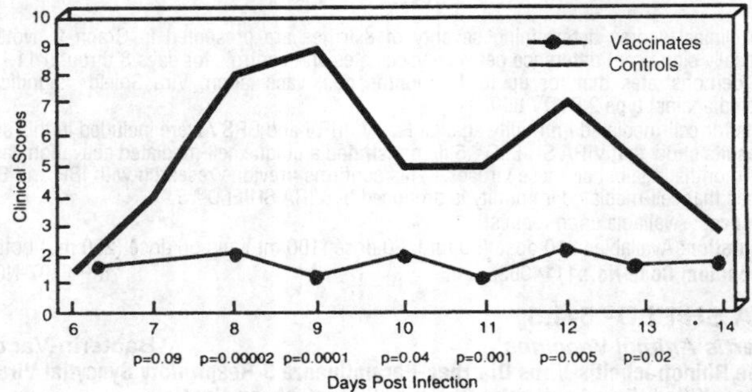

Clinical parameters included in Graph 1 are: temperature; dyspnea; depression; nasal discharge; lacrimation; conjunctivitis; and inflammation of the nasal mucosa. The clinical scores from days 8 through 13 were statistically significant at the values indicated.

Graph 2: Vaccinated vs. Non-Vaccinated Cattle
Diarrhea Study

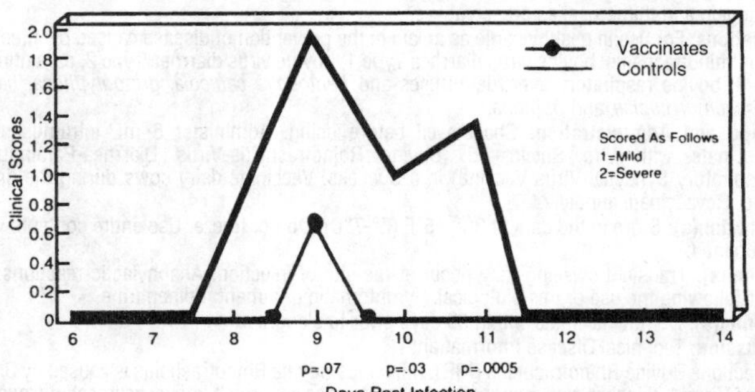

The clinical scores determining severity of diarrhea are presented in Graph 2. Note the statistically significant difference between vaccinates and controls for days 8 through 11.[1] This study demonstrates that for up to 11 months post vaccination, Vira Shield® significantly protected against Type 2 BVDV 890.

Tests for cell-mediated immunity against BVDV, IBRV and BRSV were included in this study. The results show that Vira Shield® 5 demonstrated a unique cell mediated activation, lasting for 11 months, against all these viruses.[1] This confirms previous research with IBR and BRSV vaccines that cell-mediated immunity is produced by Vira Shield® 5.[2]

References: Available upon request.

Presentation: Available in 10 dose (50 mL) and 50 dose (250 mL) bottles.

Compendium Code No.: 11140643 MP-F197-NOV01

VIRA SHIELD® 5+L5 SOMNUS

Novartis Animal Vaccines **Bacterin-Vaccine**

Bovine Rhinotracheitis-Virus Diarrhea-Parainfluenza 3-Respiratory Syncytial Virus Vaccine, Killed Virus-Haemophilus Somnus-Leptospira Canicola-Grippotyphosa-Hardjo-Icterohaemorrhagiae-Pomona Bacterin

U.S. Vet. Lic. No.: 303

Composition: This product contains an IBR virus, a cytopathic Type 1 BVD virus, a noncytopathic Type 2 BVD virus, a PI_3 virus and a BRS virus propagated on an established bovine cell line and cultures of *Haemophilus somnus, Leptospira canicola, grippotyphosa, hardjo, icterohaemorrhagiae,* and *pomona.* The product is chemically inactivated and adjuvanted with Xtend III®. Contains amphotericin B, gentamicin and thimerosal as preservatives.

Indications: For use in healthy breeding cattle as an aid in the prevention of disease caused by infectious bovine rhinotracheitis, bovine virus diarrhea Type 1, bovine virus diarrhea Type 2, parainfluenza Type 3, bovine respiratory syncytial viruses, *Haemophilus somnus* and *Leptospira canicola, grippotyphosa, hardjo, icterohaemorrhagiae,* and *pomona.*

Dosage and Administration: Shake well before using. Administer 5 mL intramuscularly. Revaccinate with Vira Shield® 5 + Somnus (Bovine Rhinotracheitis-Virus Diarrhea-Parainfluenza 3-Respiratory Syncytial Virus Vaccine, Killed Virus-*Haemophilus somnus* Bacterin) in 4-5 weeks. Vaccinate dairy cows during the dry off period. Revaccinate annually.

Precaution(s): Store in the dark at 35°-45°F (2°-7°C). Do not freeze. Use entire contents when first opened.

Caution(s): Transient swelling may occur at the site of injection. Anaphylactic reactions may occur following the use of this biological. Symptomatic treatment: Epinephrine.

For veterinary use only.

Warning(s): Do not vaccinate within 60 days prior to slaughter.

Discussion: Technical Disease Information:

Infectious Bovine Rhinotracheitis (IBR): Infectious Bovine Rhinotracheitis is caused by Bovine Herpes Virus 1, which is also responsible for the disease syndrome known as infectious pustular vulvovaginitis and balanoposthitis (IPV-IPB). It appears that the latter (IPV) was the primary form of the disease until the animals were concentrated into high population units such as beef feedlots and large dairy herds. The virus is associated with A) upper respiratory tract infections (IBR) and bovine respiratory disease, B) conjunctivitis and C) reproductive disorders including IPB, abortion and neonatal death.

Bovine Virus Diarrhea (BVD): Bovine Viral Diarrhea Virus is one of the most important bovine viral pathogens in the world. The complexity of the virus and its involvement in multiple bovine disease processes are only now beginning to be understood. Neutralizing antibodies for this Pestivirus have been detected in 50% to 90% of the clinically normal cattle tested in the United States. The virus is associated with A) Bovine Respiratory Disease; B) reproductive disorders including infertility, abortion , and neonatal defects and C) enteric disorders including Bovine Viral Diarrhea, Acute Mucosal Disease and Chronic Mucosal Disease. In addition, the Type 2 strains of BVD have been implicated in severe disease outbreaks where the animals often show hemorrhagic symptoms and death losses approach 100% of affected animals.

Parainfluenza 3 (PI_3): Parainfluenza-3 is a Paramyxovirus belonging to the same family as BRSV. PI_3 virus has been isolated, identified and studied in relation to Bovine Respiratory Disease (BRD) syndrome. PI_3 virus is commonly isolated from animals suffering from BRD, although it appears to be more of a contributing agent rather than a primary pathogen. By itself PI_3 virus produces a rather benign infection of the lung. PI_3 antibodies have been detected in approximately 90% of the cattle tested in the United States. It most commonly invades the lungs causing a fibrinous pleuritis and pneumonia.

Bovine Respiratory Syncytial Virus (BRSV): Bovine Respiratory Syncytial Virus (BRSV) was first isolated in the United States in 1974 and recently has been identified as a major contributing agent in the Bovine Respiratory Disease (BRD) syndrome. It was named BRSV because this Pneumovirus invades the cell lining of the trachea and lungs and because it promotes the formation of large multinucleated cells called syncytial cells in the epithelium and interstitial spaces of the lung. BRSV appears to be widespread across the United States. In states where antibody prevalence testing has been done, 60% to 80% of the cattle tested are positive.

An initial exposure to the virus usually produces: 1) a Mild Subclinical Infection which occurs approximately 5 days after stress and exposure. Within 2-10 days after recovery from this primary infection some animals exhibit 2) a Severe Clinical Form of this disease, which, if untreated will last 12-14 days and result in a high percentage of deaths. At any of these stages the course and severity of the disease can be aggravated by invasion of the weakened animal by other viral and bacterial pathogens.

Leptospirosis: Although leptospirosis is not the threat to our livestock industry that it once was, we can't forget about this organism. Leptospirosis is prevalent in all domestic animals, as well as wildlife populations such as skunks, opossums and raccoons.

This organism will not survive by itself in the environment. Animals that recover from leptospirosis may become carriers, and the organism may be shed in the urine for various periods of time. The susceptible animal ingests this organism, usually through feed or in water contaminated by animals shedding the organism in their urine.

Clinical signs in infected cattle are, for the most part, not observed. A particularly observant herdsman may notice a day or two of lowered feed consumption, and in the case of milk cows, lowered milk production. The most frequent clinical sign of leptospirosis is an abortion in the last trimester of gestation. Red colored urine due to hemoglobinuria may be seen also.

Haemophilus somnus: *Haemophilus somnus* has long been recognized by veterinary researchers, diagnosticians, and practitioners as a major cause of death in feedlot calves due to encephalitis (brain infection). Recently, *H. somnus* has also been found to be a major cause of pneumonia, arthritis, myocarditis, and reproductive problems.

H. somnus infections occur most commonly in stress situations such as when cattle are grouped together in sale barns, feedlots, dairy herds, for shipping, etc. or when assembled for grazing fall and winter pasture.

The disease usually occurs one week to one month after cattle are grouped together. During an outbreak, some cattle will show signs of encephalitis, including blindness, staggering, and convulsions. Without prompt treatment with antibiotics, most of these animals will die. The brain damage caused by *H. somnus* is irreversible, so even if the animal is treated and survives it may have to be culled.

Concurrent with the encephalitis outbreak, other cattle will develop pneumonia. This pneumonia is indistinguishable from viral and *Pasteurella* shipping fever complex pneumonia, thus *H. somnus* pneumonia can be easily misdiagnosed.

H. somnus infection is usually a systemic disease. The organism causes disease by blocking capillaries, thereby restricting the blood flow to vital organs. While the most common manifestations of *H. somnus* are encephalitis and pneumonia, all organs of the animal's body can be affected. Even if the animal is treated with antibiotics and recovers, damage due to the loss of blood supply to various body organs can cause chronic, debilitating disease problems. Common manifestations of this damage include arthritis, myocarditis, abortion, and sterility.

Trial Data: South Dakota State University Research: A portion of the study was designed to prove protection against a BVD Type 2 challenge (Strain 890). In June of 1994, six 500- to 700- lb. calves received two vaccinations, four weeks apart, with Vira Shield® 5. The controls were three seronegative, unvaccinated calves (400 lbs.) from the same herd. Eleven months after vaccination, the calves were challenged intranasally with NVSL BVD challenge strain 890. Clinical scores on each animal were recorded daily from three days prechallenge to 14 days post challenge.[1]

Graph 1: Vaccinated vs. Non-Vaccinated Cattle
Respiratory Study

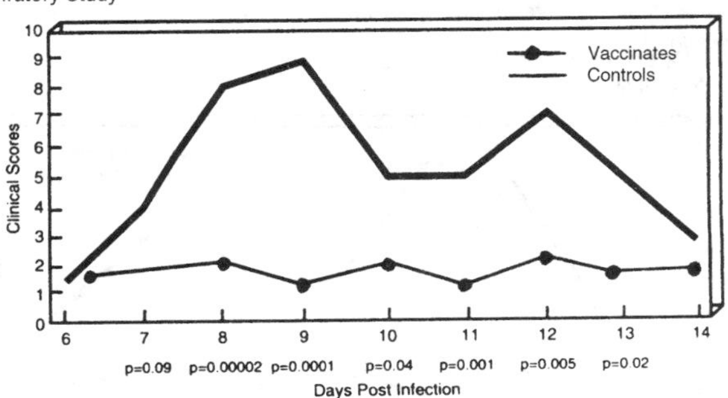

Clinical parameters included in Graph 1 are: temperature; dyspnea; depression; nasal discharge; lacrimation; conjunctivitis; and inflammation of the nasal mucosa. The clinical scores from days 8 through 13 were statistically significant at the values indicated.

Graph 2: Vaccinated vs. Non-Vaccinated Cattle
Diarrhea Study

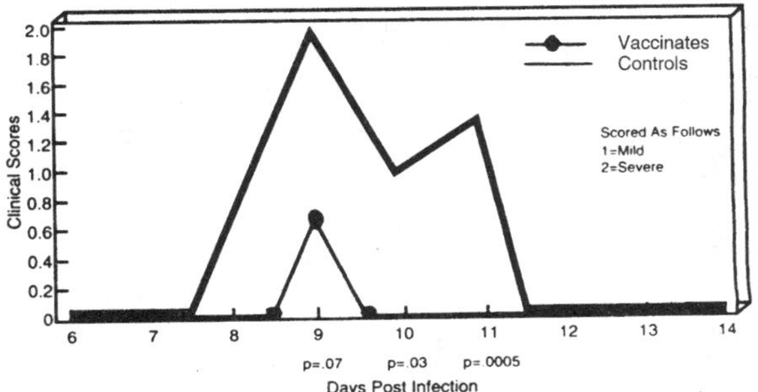

The clinical scores determining severity of diarrhea are presented in Graph 2. Note the statistically significant difference between vaccinates and controls for days 8 through 11.[1] This study demonstrates that for up to 11 months post vaccination, Vira Shield® significantly protected against Type 2 BVDV 890.

Tests for cell-mediated immunity against BVDV, IBRV and BRSV were included in this study. The results show that Vira Shield® 5 demonstrated a unique cell mediated activation, lasting for 11 months, against all these viruses.[1] This confirms previous research with IBR and BRSV vaccines that cell-mediated immunity is produced by Vira Shield® 5.[2]

References: Available upon request.

Presentation: Available in 10 dose (50 mL) and 50 dose (250 mL) bottles.

Compendium Code No.: 11140692 MP-F197-NOV01

VIRA SHIELD® 5+SOMNUS

Novartis Animal Vaccines **Bacterin-Vaccine**

Bovine Rhinotracheitis-Virus Diarrhea-Parainfluenza 3-Respiratory Syncytial Virus Vaccine, Killed Virus-Haemophilus Somnus Bacterin

U.S. Vet. Lic. No.: 303

Composition: This product contains an IBR virus, a cytopathic Type 1 BVD virus, a noncytopathic Type 2 BVD virus, a PI_3 virus, and a BRS virus propagated on an established bovine cell line and cultures of *Haemophilus somnus.* The product is chemically inactivated and adjuvanted with Xtend III®. Contains amphotericin B, gentamicin and thimerosal as preservatives.

Indications: For use in healthy cattle as an aid in the prevention of diseases caused by infectious bovine rhinotracheitis, bovine virus diarrhea Type 1, bovine virus diarrhea Type 2, parainfluenza Type 3, bovine respiratory syncytial viruses and *Haemophilus somnus.*

Dosage and Administration: Shake well before using. Administer 5 mL intramuscularly at 3 months of age or older. Repeat in 4-5 weeks. This vaccine may be administered to pregnant animals at any stage of gestation. Vaccinate dairy cows during the dry off period. Revaccinate annually.

Precaution(s): Store in the dark at 35°-45°F (2°-7°C). Do not freeze. Use entire contents when first opened.

Caution(s): Transient swelling may occur at the site of injection. Anaphylactic reactions may occur following the use of this biological. Symptomatic treatment: Epinephrine.

Warning(s): Do not vaccinate within 60 days prior to slaughter.

Discussion: Technical Disease Information:

Infectious Bovine Rhinotracheitis (IBR): Infectious Bovine Rhinotracheitis is caused by Bovine Herpes Virus 1, which is also responsible for the disease syndrome known as infectious pustular vulvovaginitis and balanoposthitis (IPV-IPB). It appears that the latter (IPV) was the primary form of the disease until the animals were concentrated into high population units such as beef feedlots and large dairy herds. The virus is associated with A) upper respiratory tract infections (IBR) and bovine respiratory disease, B) conjunctivitis and C) reproductive disorders including IPV, abortion and neonatal death.

Bovine Virus Diarrhea (BVD): Bovine Viral Diarrhea Virus is one of the most important bovine viral pathogens in the world. The complexity of the virus and its involvement in multiple bovine disease processes are only now beginning to be understood. Neutralizing antibodies for this Pestivirus have been detected in 50% to 90% of the clinically normal cattle tested in the United States. The virus is associated with A) Bovine Respiratory Disease; B) reproductive disorders including infertility, abortion, and neonatal defects and C) enteric disorders including Bovine Viral Diarrhea, Acute Mucosal Disease and Chronic Mucosal Disease. In addition, the Type 2 strains of BVD have been implicated in severe disease outbreaks where the animals often show hemorrhagic symptoms and death losses approach 100% of affected animals.

Parainfluenza 3 (PI_3): Parainfluenza-3 is a Paramyxovirus belonging to the same family as BRSV. PI_3 virus has been isolated, identified and studied in relation to Bovine Respiratory Disease (BRD) syndrome. PI_3 virus is commonly isolated from animals suffering from BRD, although it appears to be more of a contributing agent rather than a primary pathogen. By itself PI_3 virus produces a rather benign infection of the lung. PI_3 antibodies have been detected in approximately 90% of the cattle tested in the United States. It most commonly invades the lungs causing a fibrinous pleuritis and pneumonia.

Bovine Respiratory Syncytial Virus (BRSV): Bovine Respiratory Syncytial Virus (BRSV) was first isolated in the United States in 1974 and recently has been identified as a major contributing agent in the Bovine Respiratory Disease (BRD) syndrome. It was named BRSV because this Pneumovirus invades the cell lining of the trachea and lungs and because it promotes the formation of large multinucleated cells called syncytial cells in the epithelium and interstitial spaces of the lung. BRSV appears to be widespread across the United States. In states where antibody prevalence testing has been done, 60% to 80% of the cattle tested are positive. Since research and information on BRSV are incomplete, we can give only a partial description of the disease syndrome produced by this virus.

An initial exposure to the virus usually produces: 1) a Mild Subclinical Infection which occurs approximately 5 days after stress and exposure. Within 2-10 days after recovery from this primary infection some animals will exhibit 2) a Severe Clinical Form of this disease, which if untreated will last 12-14 days and result in a high percentage of deaths. At any of these stages the course and severity of the disease can be aggravated by invasion of the weakened animal by other viral and bacterial pathogens.

Haemophilus somnus: *Haemophilus somnus* has long been recognized by veterinary researchers, diagnosticians, and practitioners as a major cause of death in feedlot calves due to encephalitis (brain infection). Recently, *H. somnus* has also been found to be a major cause of pneumonia, arthritis, myocarditis, and reproductive problems.

H. somnus infections occur most commonly in stress situations such as when cattle are grouped together in sale barns, feedlots, dairy herds, for shipping, etc. or when assembled for grazing fall and winter pasture.

The disease usually occurs one week to one month after cattle are grouped together. During an outbreak, some cattle will show signs of encephalitis, including blindness, staggering, and convulsions. Without prompt treatment with antibiotics, most of these animals will die. The brain damage caused by *H. somnus* is irreversible, so even if the animal is treated and survives it may have to be culled.

Concurrent with the encephalitis outbreak, other cattle will develop pneumonia. This pneumonia is indistinguishable from viral and *Pasteurella* shipping fever complex pneumonia, thus *H. somnus* pneumonia can be easily misdiagnosed.

H. somnus infection is usually a systemic disease. The organism causes disease by blocking capillaries, thereby restricting the blood flow to vital organs. While the most common manifestations of *H. somnus* are encephalitis and pneumonia, all organs of the animal's body can be affected. Even if the animal is treated with antibiotics and recovers, damage due to the loss of blood supply to various body organs can cause chronic, debilitating disease problems. Common manifestations of this damage include arthritis, myocarditis, abortion, and sterility.

Trial Data: South Dakota State University Research: A portion of the study was designed to prove protection against a BVD Type 2 challenge (Strain 890). In June of 1994, six 500- to 700- lb. calves received two vaccinations, four weeks apart, with Vira Shield® 5. The controls were three seronegative, unvaccinated calves (400 lbs.) from the same herd. Eleven months after vaccination, the calves were challenged intranasally with NVSL BVD challenge strain 890. Clinical scores on each animal were recorded daily from three days prechallenge to 14 days post challenge.[1]

Graph 1: Vaccinated vs. Non-Vaccinated Cattle
Respiratory Study

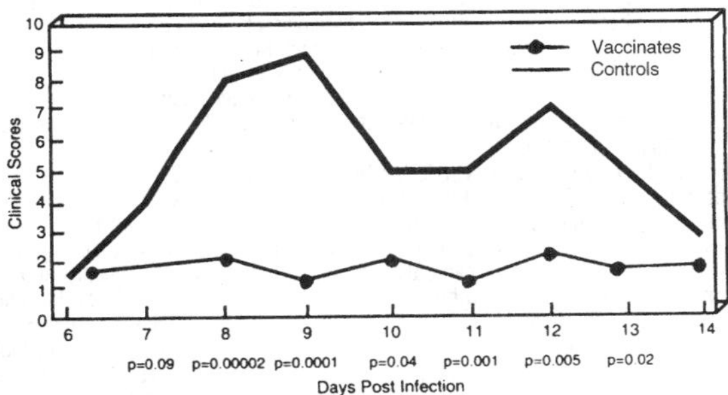

Clinical parameters included in Graph 1 are: temperature; dyspnea; depression; nasal discharge; lacrimation; conjunctivitis; and inflammation of the nasal mucosa. The clinical scores from days 8 through 13 were statistically significant at the values indicated.

Graph 2: Vaccinated vs. Non-Vaccinated Cattle
Diarrhea Study

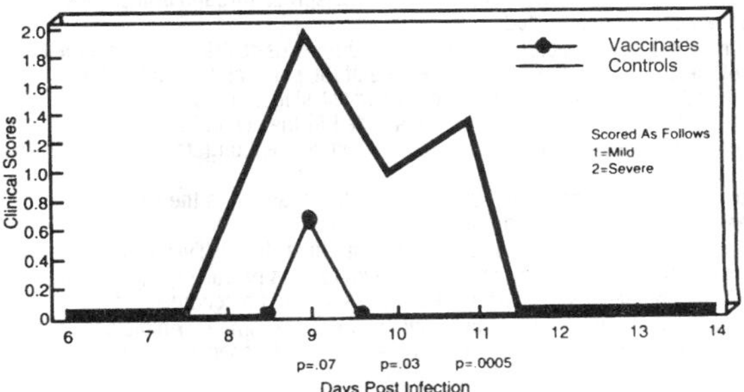

The clinical scores determining severity of diarrhea are presented in Graph 2. Note the statistically significant difference between vaccinates and controls for days 8 through 11.[1] This

V

The active ingredient in this collar, Nylar® will not kill adult parasites. Therefore, if the dog or its environment is heavily infested with fleas when the collar is first applied, the collar's flea and flea egg sterilizing benefit will not be apparent for several weeks until all pre-existing environmental flea life cycle stages have developed and either found a host or died. In these circumstances it is necessary to use other means (e.g., insecticide treatments, applied to both the pet and its environment) to kill existing flea stages on the pet and in its environment. Tick infestation must always be controlled by products labelled for ticks. The collar and its active ingredient in the dog's haircoat are not affected by normal wetting or bathing. Replace collar as needed.

Presentation: 1 collar (42 g).

Nylar®, is a registered trademark of McLaughlin, Gormley, King Co.

Compendium Code No.: 10230630

VIRBAC KNOCKOUT® IGR HOUSEHOLD PUMP SPRAY

Virbac **Premise Insecticide**

EPA Reg. No.: 2382-158

Active Ingredient(s):

Pyriproxyfen	0.005%
Permethrin[1]	0.500%
Piperonyl butoxide[2]	1.000%
Inert Ingredients	98.495%

[1]cis-trans isomer ration: min. 35% (±), max. 65% (±) trans.

[2]Equivalent to 0.8% of (butylcarbityl) (6-propylpiperonyl) ether and 0.2% of related compounds.

With Nylar® Insect Growth Regulator

Indications: To kill fleas, ticks and other pests for up to 3 weeks.

To break the flea life cycle and reinfestation for more than 12 months.

Directions for Use: It is a violation of Federal law to use this product in a manner inconsistent with its labeling.

VIRBAC KNOCKOUT® Household Pump Spray contains a unique combination of ingredients that kills both adult and pre-adult fleas (before they grow up to bite). A single application immediately kills adult insects in your home and in the pet's environment and continues to kill these pests for up to 3 weeks. This provides an initial period of protection against preexisting insects, especially adult fleas and ticks, while the Nylar® (pyriproxyfen) Insect Growth Regulator goes to work to prevent development and kill immature stages of fleas that are already in the pet's environment. A single treatment with this product continues, for at least 12 months, to prevent all new fleas from developing in treated areas since pyriproxyfen kills all new flea eggs and immature fleas before they can become adult fleas. Protects your home from reinfestation and flea buildup and your pets and family from flea bites. Leaves no odor or moss and, used as directed, does not stain furnishings or fabrics. Treat by spraying surfaces, at the rate of approximately five trigger squeezes (10 mL) for each four square feet. Spray all areas frequented by the pet, where most flea eggs accumulate and where flea larvae develop to provide a source of new fleas to reinfest your pet. Pay special attention to areas and surfaces where the pet spends most of its time and sleeps, including pet beds and bedding, areas of carpet, rugs and flooring, cracks and joints in wood flooring, and surfaces and crevasses of furniture. Also treat inside kennels, upholstery and carpets of vehicles and boats used to transport pets. Use a registered Virbac flea and tick control product on your pets, in conjunction with this environment treatment, to achieve an integrated parasite control program.

Contraindication(s): Do not apply directly to pets.

Precautionary Statements: Hazards to Humans and Domestic Animals - Caution: Avoid contamination of food or feedstuffs. Do not apply directly to pets. Keep children and pets off treated surfaces until dry.

Storage and Disposal: Storage: Store in a cool area. Disposal: Do not reuse empty container. Wrap in several layers of newspaper and discard in trash.

Warning(s): Keep out of reach of children.

Presentation: 16 fl oz (473 mL).

Nylar® Registered Trademark of McLaughlin, Gormley King Co.

Compendium Code No.: 10230640

VIRBAC KNOCKOUT® ROOM AND AREA FOGGER

Virbac **Household Insecticide**

EPA Reg. No.: 11715-313-2382

Active Ingredient(s):

2-[1-Methyl-2- [4-phenoxyphenoxy] ethoxy] pyridine*	0.100%
Pyrethrins	0.050%
N-Octyl bicycloheptene dicarboximide®	0.400%
Permethrin [**(3-Phenoxyphenyl) methyl (+ or -) cis-trans-3-(2,2-dichloroethenyl) 2,2-dimethylcyclopropate-carboxylate]	0.400%
Related compounds	0.035%
Inert Ingredients	99.015%

*MGK® 264, Insecticide Synergist

**Cis-trans isomers ratio: Max. 55% (+ or -) cis and Min. 45% (+ or -) trans.

Indications: Kills adult and pre-adult fleas, including flea eggs for 7 months (30 weeks).

Also kills cockroaches, spiders, ants, and ticks, including deer ticks and other toxoid species that may carry and transmit Lyme Disease.

Directions for Use: It is a violation of Federal law to use this product in a manner inconsistent with its labeling.

Read all directions and cautions completely before use.

For use only when building has been vacated by human beings and pets. Ventilate area for 30 minutes before reentry.

For best results, treat all infested areas. Use one fogger for each 6,000 cubic feet (approximately 27 ft. x 8 ft. ceiling) of unobstructed area. Use additional units for remote rooms or where the free flow of fog is not assured.

Note: Do not use more than one unit per average size room. Do not use this unit in a cabinet or under a counter or table. Do not use this unit in an area less than 100 cubic feet.

Preparation: Remove or cover exposed food, dishes, utensils, surfaces and food-handling equipment. Shut off fans and air conditioners. Put out all flames and pilot lights. Close outside doors and windows. Remove pets and birds, but leave pets' bedding as this is a primary hiding place for fleas and must be treated for best results. No need to discard pet bedding after treatment. Cover or remove fish tanks and bowls.

Leave rugs, draperies, and upholstered furniture in place. This product will not harm furniture when used as directed. Open interior closet doors and cabinets or areas to be treated. [Cover waxed wood floors and waxed furniture in the immediate areas surrounding the fogger.] [Newspapers may be used.] For more effective control of storage pests and cockroaches, open all cupboard doors and drawers for better penetration of fog. Remove all infested foodstuffs and dispose of in outdoor trash. For flea and tick control, thoroughly vacuum all carpeting, upholstered furniture, along baseboards, under furniture and in closets. Put vacuum bag into a sack and dispose of in outside trash. Mop all hard floor surfaces.

Read all directions and cautions completely before use.

To Start Fogging: Shake fogger well before using. Hold can at arm's length with top of can pointing away from face and eyes. Push down on finger pad until it locks. This will start fogging action. Set canister in an upright position on a table, stand, etc. (up to 30 inches in height in the center of the area) and place several thicknesses of newspaper under the canister to prevent marring of the surface. Treat the whole dwelling, using multiple units in homes with more than one level and numerous rooms. Leave the building at once.

Do not re-enter building for two hours. After two hours, open all outside doors and windows, turn on air conditioners and/or fans and let treated area air for 30 minutes before reoccupying. If additional units are used for remote rooms or where free flow of fog is not assured, increase airing-out time accordingly.

Precautionary Statements:

Hazards to Humans and Domestic Animals: Harmful if swallowed. Avoid breathing vapors or spray mist. Avoid contact with skin or eyes. In case of contact, flush with plenty of water. Wash with soap and water after use. Obtain medical attention if irritation persists. Avoid contamination of food or feedstuffs. Do not use in serving areas while food is exposed or facility is in operation. Serving areas are areas where foods are served such as dining rooms, but excluding ares where foods may be prepared or held. Do not use in food areas or food handling establishments, restaurants or other areas where food is commercially prepared or processed. In the home, all food processing surfaces and utensils should be covered during treatment or thoroughly washed before use. Exposed food should be covered or removed. Non-food areas are areas such as garbage rooms, lavatories, floor drains (to sewers), entries and vestibules, offices, locker rooms, machine rooms, garages, mop closets and storage (after canning or bottling). Not for use in USDA meat and poultry plants. Remove pets, birds, and cover fish aquariums before spraying.

Sold only to veterinarians.

Statement of Practical Treatment:

If swallowed: Call a physician or Poison Control Center immediately. If in eyes: Flush with plenty of water. Get medical attention if irritation persists. If on skin or clothing: Remove contaminated clothing and wash before reuse. Wash skin with soap and warm water. Get medical attention if irritation persists. If inhaled: Remove victim to fresh air if effects occur, and call a physician.

Physical or Chemical Hazards: Contents under pressure. Keep away from heat, sparks, and open flame. Do not puncture or incinerate container. Exposure to temperatures above 130°F may cause bursting. Extremely flammable.

Storage and Disposal:

Storage: Store in a cool, dry area away from heat or open flame.

Disposal: Replace cap and discard container in trash.

Warning(s): Keep out of reach of children.

Presentation: 6 oz (170 g).

One unit treats up to 6,000 cubic feet of unobstructed space (27 x 27 x 8).

Nylar® is a registered trademark of McLaughlin Gormley King Co.

Compendium Code No.: 10230650

VIRBAC® LONG ACTING KNOCKOUT™

Virbac **Topical Insecticide**

EPA Reg. No.: 2382-124

Active Ingredient(s):

Pyriproxyfen: 2-[1-methyl-2-(phenoxyphenoxy) ethoxy] pyridine	0.05%
Permethrin: (3*-Phenoxyphenyl) methyl (±)cis-trans-3-(2,2-dichloroethenyl) 2,2-dimethylcyclopropate-carboxylate]	2.00%
Inert Ingredients	97.95%
	100.00%

*cis-trans isomer ratio: min. 35% (±) max. 65% (±) trans.

Indications: Kills fleas for 2 months and ticks (including Lyme vectors) for 1 month. Pyrlproxyfen IGR sterilizes fleas for up to 3 months.

Directions for Use: It is a violation of Federal law to use this product in a manner inconsistent with its labeling. To prevent harm to you and your pet, read entire label before use. Spray over entire haircoat making sure the coat is thoroughly wetted to the skin. Spray against the lay of the hair, ruffling the coat on long-haired dogs. Weight of dog, length of hair and density of coat will determine amount of spray to be applied to wet the skin (average dose approximately 7.5 g/kg). This 16 oz bottle should be sufficient for four applications at a two month interval to an average 30-35 lb dog. Lighter applications will reduce period effectiveness and require more frequent treatments. Allow dog to air dry or blow dry. Do not towel dry.

Precautionary Statements: Hazards to Humans and Domestic Animals:

Hazards to Humans: Causes moderate eye irritation. Avoid contact with eyes or clothing. Avoid breathing spray mist. Use only in a well ventilated area. Avoid contamination of food. Wash exposed skin with soap and water after using. Remove contaminated clothing and wash before reuse.

Hazards to Animals: Do not use on cats. For use only on adult dogs. Consult a veterinarian before treating pregnant, nursing, sick, old or debilitated dogs or dogs undergoing drug or other pesticide treatment. Do not spray in eyes, face or on genitalia. Until dry, do not confine treated dog in area without adequate cross ventilation. In event of adverse reaction, shampoo dog with a non-pesticidal shampoo to remove pesticide residue and immediately seek veterinary advice.

Statement of Practical Treatment:

If in Eyes: Flush with plenty of water. Call a physician if irritation persists.

Physical or Chemical Hazards: Do not use or store near heat or open flame.

Storage and Disposal:

Storage: Store in cool area away from heat and open flame.

Disposal: Do not reuse empty container. Wrap in several layers of newspaper and discard in trash.

Warning(s): Keep out of reach of children.

Sold only to veterinarians.

Presentation: 16 oz (473 mL).

Nylar® is a registered trademark of McLaughlin Gormley King Co.

Compendium Code No.: 10230660

VIRBAC PYRETHRIN DIP™

Virbac **Topical Insecticide**

EPA Reg. No.: 2382-89

Active Ingredient(s):

Pyrethrins 1.00%
Piperonyl butoxide, technical* 4.00%
N-octyl bicycloheptene dicarboximide 6.00%
Di-n-propyl isocinchomeronate 4.00%
Inert ingredients........ 85.00%
Total 100.00%

*Equivalent to 3.20% of (butylcarbityl) (6-propylpiperonyl) ether and 0.80% of related compounds.

Indications: For cats, kittens, dogs and puppies. Pyrethrin formula-fly repellent kills and repels fleas, ticks, lice, gnats, mosquitoes and flies.

Directions for Use: It is a violation of Federal Law to use this product in a manner inconsistent with its labeling. Shake well before using.

For Cats, Kittens, Dogs and Puppies: Dilution: To kill fleas, ticks and lice thoroughly mix ½ oz (1 tablespoon) of Dip with 1 gal. warm water. For use under more severe reinfestation pressure, dilute at the rate of 1 fl oz (2 tablespoons) per gallon. Do not dilute more dip than will be used in a 24 hr. period.

Application: Dip should be applied to dry or damp (not wet) coat. Sponge, dip or spray animal with diluted VIRBAC PYRETHRIN DIP™ making sure all areas are soaked to the skin. Let animal drip dry. Do not rinse off. Use VIRBAC PYRETHRIN DIP™ as directed by your veterinarian and as often as necessary without interval restrictions on frequency of dipping.

Precautionary Statements: Hazards to Humans and Domestic Animals: Wash thoroughly with soap and water after handling. Do not use on kittens or puppies less than 6 weeks of age unless prescribed by a veterinarian.

Storage and Disposal: Storage: Protect from freezing. If frozen, allow to warm to room temperature and shake well before using. Keep tightly sealed in original container. Disposal: Do not reuse empty container. Wrap container and put in trash.

Warning(s): Keep out of reach of children.

Presentation: 4 fl oz (118 mL) and 1 gallon (3.79 L).

Compendium Code No.: 10230481

VIRBAC® YARD SPRAY CONCENTRATE

Virbac **Household Insecticide**

Insecticidal

EPA Reg. No.: 2382-122

Active Ingredient(s):

Esfenvalerate: (S) -cyano (3-phenoxyphenyl) methyl-(S)-
4 chloro-alpha-(1-methylethyl) benzeneacetate........ 0.44%
Inert Ingredients........ 99.56%
100.00%

Indications: Residual action insecticide concentrate for use outdoors on residential lawns and around residential premises only to kill fleas and ticks. Kills deer ticks and other Ixodid species that carry and transmit Lyme disease.

Directions for Use: It is a violation of Federal Law to use this product in a manner inconsistent with its labeling. To kill fleas and ticks harboring in lawns, backyards, dog kennels and runs, apply Yard Spray Concentrate through the hose end sprayer provided with this product or by compressed air sprayer or watering can. For best results, lawn should be mowed a day or two before spraying.

For use with Hose End Spray Applicator: The hose end applicator cap is calibrated to deliver the correct dilution rate, and when attached to this bottle will treat 6000 square feet. To treat smaller areas, stop spraying when the appropriate amount of concentrate has been used (e.g., half the concentrate should be used for a 3000 square foot yard), reclose bottle with original cap and store bottle for next application. Separate mixing of the concentrate or other application equipment is not required. First ensure the hose faucet is turned off. Then screw end of hose into the black end of the sprayer cap. Remove bottle cap (save for closing after use). Secure sprayer cap to bottle by turning bottle counter-clockwise. Turn on faucet. Spray using a slow, even sweeping motion, being sure to cover the entire lawn surface where pets frequent. Spray under ornamentals and trees but avoid soaking young or flowering plants. Flea populations are greatest where the pet spends the most time. Therefore be sure to thoroughly soak these areas (e.g., shaded areas such as underbrushes, trees, porches, inside pet kennel and wherever your pet frequents). Repeat treatment may be necessary at 7 to 14 day intervals.

For Compressed Air Sprayer or Watering Can Application: Mix two (2) fluid ounces of the concentrate per one (1) gallon of water and apply at the rate of one (1) gallon of diluted spray per 1000 square feet to surfaces of kennels, exercise runs, patios, on and under porches, crawl spaces and other outdoor areas pets frequent.

Precautionary Statements: Hazards to Humans and Domestic Animals:

Caution: Harmful if swallowed, absorbed through skin or inhaled, causes moderate eye irritation. Avoid breathing vapors or spray mist and contact with skin, eyes or clothing. In case of contact, flush with plenty of water. Avoid contamination of food or foodstuffs. Do not spray plants used for food or feed. Keep pets and children out of treated area until after spray has dried. Do not spray on animals.

Statement of Practical Treatment:

If Swallowed: Call a physician or Poison Control Center immediately. Do not induce vomiting because of aspiration pneumonia hazard.

If in Eyes: Flush with plenty of water. Get immediate medical attention.

If Inhaled: Remove victim to fresh air or, if not breathing, give artificial respiration, preferably mouth-to-mouth. Get medical attention.

If on Skin: Wash skin with soap and warm water after use. Get medical attention if irritation persists.

If on Clothing: Remove contaminated clothing and wash before re-use.

Environmental Hazards: This pesticide is highly toxic to fish and aquatic invertebrates. Do not apply directly to water. Drift from treated areas may be hazardous to organisms in adjacent aquatic sites. Do not contaminate water when disposing of equipment washwaters.

Storage and Disposal:

Storage: Store in closed container in a cool, dry place.

Disposal: Do not reuse empty container. Wrap container in newspaper and discard in trash.

Warning(s): Keep out of the reach of children.

Sold only by veterinarians.

Presentation: 16 fl oz (473 mL).

Compendium Code No.: 10230670

VIRKON®-S

Farnam, Livestock Div. **Disinfectant**

Broad Spectrum Disinfectant

EPA Reg. No.: 62432-1-270

Active Ingredient(s):

Potassium peroxymonosulfate 20.4%
Sodium Chloride........ 1.5%
Inert Ingredients........ 78.1%
Total 100.0%

Equivalent to 9.75% available chlorine.

Indications: For use in cleaning and disinfecting industrial, animal and agricultural facilities.

VIRKON®-S is effective against numerous microorganisms affecting animals: viruses, gram positive and gram negative bacteria, fungi (molds and yeasts) and mycoplasma. Efficacy was determined under AOAC guidelines in the presence of hard water and organic material.

Effective Against:

Viruses: Avian influenza virus, Avian laryngotracheitis virus, Avian infectious bronchitis virus, Bovine adenovirus type 4, Calf rotavirus, Canine parvovirus, Equine arteritis virus, Feline calicivirus, Infectious bronchitis virus, Infectious bursal disease (gumboro) virus, Infectious bovine rhinotracheitis virus, Newcastle disease virus, Parainfluenza virus, Porcine Reproductive and Respiratory Syndrome (PRRS), Porcine parvovirus, Pseudorabies virus, Turkey herpes virus.

Bacteria: *Actinobacillus pleuropneumoniae, Bordetella avium (alcaligenes faecalis), Bordetella bronchiseptica, Brucella abortus* (fistulous withers), *Campylobacter pyloridis, Clostridium perfringens, Eschericia coli, Haemophilus somnus, Klebsiella pneumoniae, Moraxella bovis, Mycoplasma gallisepticum, Pasteurella multocida, Pseudomonas aeruginosa, Salmonella choleraesuis, Salmonella typhimurium, Serpulina (treponema) hyodysenteriae, Staphylococcus aureus, Staphylococcus epidermidis, Streptococcus equi* (strangles), *Streptococcus pyogenes, Taylorella equigenitalis.*

Fungi: *Aspergillus fumigatus, Candida albicans, Fusarium moniliforme.*

Directions for Use: Federal law prohibits the use of this product in a manner inconsistent with its labeling.

This powder is easily diluted for use in manual or machine operations.

Solutions are stable for 7 days. Do not soak metal objects for longer than 10 minutes. One gallon of solution treats 135 sq. ft.

Dilution Chart: Fill container with desired amount of warm water and mix in appropriate amount of VIRKON®-S powder.

Quantity of Water	Amount of Powder for 1% Solution	Amount of Powder for 2% Solution
1 gal	1.3 oz	2.7 oz
10 gals	13.4 oz	26.7 oz
50 gals	66.8 oz	133.5 oz

1.3 oz measuring scoop provided.

Poultry and Rattite Production:

Controls: The above listed viruses, bacteria and fungi.

Hatcheries: VIRKON®-S at 1% solution can be used to clean and disinfect hatchers, setters, evaporative coolers, humidifying systems, ceiling fans, chicken houses, transfer trucks, trays, and plastic chick boxes (use 2% solution for *Mycoplasma* and *Aspergillus fumigatus).* VIRKON®-S at 1-2% solution is recommended for use in fogging (wet misting) operations, either before or after regular cleaning and disinfecting procedures. Fog (wet mist) until the area is moist, using automatic foggers according to manufacturer's use directions.

Broiler/Breeder Houses: Remove chickens, feed, and water troughs, then remove manure and litter. Spray dry floors and walls with VIRKON®-S at 1% solution. Thoroughly wash waterers and feeders with a 1% solution of VIRKON®-S (use 2% solution for *Mycoplasma* and *Aspergillus fumigatus).* After 10 minutes, rinse with potable water and let dry.

Do not house poultry or equipment in treated areas until treatment has dried.

For Air Sanitizing: Use VIRKON®-S at 1-2% solution and fog until surfaces are moist. Allow at least 2 hours before entering treated area. Rinse foggers and sprayers with water following use.

VIRKON®-S passes the AOAC germicidal and detergent sanitizer test at a concentration of 0.5% (1:200) in the presence of 200 ppm hard water.

Processing Plants: Spray VIRKON®-S at 1% solution to disinfect and clean walls, ceilings and floors.

Swine Production:

Controls: The above listed viruses, bacteria and fungi.

Applications: VIRKON®-S at 1% solution is recommended for cleaning and disinfecting farrowing units, nurseries, finisher houses and processing plants (use 2% solution for *Mycoplasma* and *Aspergillus fumigatus).*

VIRKON®-S at 1-2% solution is recommended for use in fogging (wet misting) operations, either preceding or following regular cleaning and disinfectant procedures. Fog (wet mist) until the area is moist, using automatic foggers according to manufacture's use directions. Rinse foggers and sprayers with water following use.

Bovine Production:

Controls: The above listed viruses, bacteria and fungi.

Applications: VIRKON®-S at 1% solution is recommended to clean and disinfect areas associated with bovine housing, hospital pens and feedlot facilities.

Equine Production, Broad Spectrum Equine Disinfectant/Detergant/Wash for Cleaning and Disinfecting Stables, Equipment and Aerial Disinfection:

Controls: The above listed viruses, bacteria and fungi.

Applications: For cleaning and disinfection of all surfaces, equipment, utensils and instruments.

Uses:

On Animal: Shampoo infected area with VIRKON®-S using a clean sponge. Rinse with clean water. Apply three times a day. Repeat as necessary.

Stable, Stalls, Tack, Equipment and Feed Rooms: Thoroughly clean and dry surfaces, then wash the area manually or with a pressure washer with a 1% solution of VIRKON®-S. Rinse with clean water.

Blankets and Saddle Pads: Shampoo by hand or spray lightly with a hand sprayer and leave to dry. Shake or vacuum to remove residue.

Aerial Spraying: To control airborne diseases; use a hand held sprayer with a fine setting or an automatic spraying system. Spray a 1% solution for 2-3 minutes twice daily. Rinse sprayers with water after use.

Companion Animals:

Controls: The above listed viruses, bacteria and fungi.

Applications: A 1% solution of VIRKON®-S is recommended as a "one step" cleaning and disinfection procedure for all surfaces, equipment, instrument utensils and cages in grooming and boarding facilities, kennels, catteries animal transport vehicles.

Precautionary Statements: Hazards to Humans and Domestic Animals:

Danger. Powder is corrosive. May cause skin burns and irreversible eye damage. Harmful if swallowed, absorbed through skin, or inhaled. Do not get in eyes, on skin, or on clothing. Wear protective clothing and rubber gloves. Avoid breathing dust. Wear goggles, face shield, or safety glasses. Wash thoroughly with soap and water after handling. Remove contaminated clothing and wash before reuse. Corrosive statement refers to powder only, not in-use solution.

Statement of Practical Treatment:

If in Eyes: Hold eyelids open and flush with a steady, gentle stream of water for 15 minutes. Get prompt medical attention.

If on Skin: Wash with plenty of soap and water. Get medical attention if irritation persists.

If Inhaled: If symptoms of coughing, choking, or wheezing are troublesome, remove to fresh air and seek medical attention.

If Swallowed: Drink promptly a large quantity of water. Avoid alcohol. Get immediate medical attention.

Notice to Physician: Probable mucosal damage may contraindicate the use of gastric lavage.

Storage and Disposal:

Storage: Store in a cool, dry place in a tightly closed container away from children. Always reseal bag after use.

Disposal: Wash empty container thoroughly and dispose in trash. Do not mix this product with other chemicals.

Warning(s): Keep out of reach of children.

Presentation: 10 lbs (4.54 kg) and 20 lbs (9.07 kg).

VIRKON-S is a registered trademark of Antec International Limited.

Manufactured by: Antec International Limited.

U.S. Patent No. 4,822,512

Compendium Code No.: 14990010 9DD7

VIROCID®

Merial Select **Disinfectant**

Concentrated Broad Spectrum Disinfectant

EPA Reg. No.: 71355-1

Active Ingredient(s):

Alkyl* Dimethyl Benzyl Ammonium Chloride *(50% C_{14}; 40% C_{12}; 10% C_{16})	17.060% (by wt)
Didecyl Dimethyl Ammonium Chloride	7.800%
Glutaraldehyde	10.725%
Inert ingredients	64.415%
	100.000%

Indications: VIROCID® is effective against:

Bacteria: *Salmonella Choleraesuis* (ATCC 10708), *Staphylococcus aureus* (ATCC 6538), *Pseudomonas aeruginosa* (ATCC 15442).

Fungus: *Tricophyton mentagrophytes* (ATCC 9533) on environmental surfaces.

Virus: Infectious Bursal Disease of Chickens (SPAFAS Strain 2512) on environmental surfaces.

Application:

Disinfection of non-food surfaces, farm, animal, and poultry housing facilities and equipment:

1. Farm Equipment and animal housing buildings (poultry & turkey grow-out houses, laying houses, swine production and housing, barns and large animal buildings)
2. Hatchers, Setters, and chick processing facilities.
3. Food processing plants (slaughterhouses).
4. Trays, racks, carts, chick boxes, cages and other hard surfaces.
5. Veterinary hospitals.

Directions for Use: It is a violation of federal law to use this product in a manner inconsistent with its labelling.

1. Farm equipment and animal housing buildings (poultry & turkey grow-out houses, laying houses, swine production and housing, barns and large animal buildings):
   For disinfection of hard, non-porous surfaces: stainless, galvanised and painted steel, copper, aluminum, finished wood, vinyl, plastics, glazed tiles, brick walls, sandwich panels and feeding/drinking equipment:
   A. Remove all animals and feed from premises, vehicles and enclosures. Remove all litter and manure from floors, walls and surfaces of barns, pens, stalls, chutes, and other facilities and fixtures occupied or traversed by animals. Empty all troughs, racks, and other feeding and watering appliances.
   B. Thoroughly clean all surfaces with soap or detergent and rinse with water. Saturate all surfaces with 1:400 disinfecting solution by using a course spray, mop, or sponge. Surfaces must remain wet for 10 minutes.
   C. Ventilate buildings and other closed spaces. Do not house animals or employ equipment until treatment has been absorbed or dried.
   D. Thoroughly scrub treated feed racks, troughs, and other feeding and water appliances with soap or detergent and rinse with potable water before reuse.
   E. Disinfection of equipment: Immerse all halters, ropes, and other types of restraining equipment used in handling and restraining animals, as well as forks, shovels, and scrapers used for removing litter and manure in a 1:400 dilution for 10 minutes. Allow to air dry.
   F. Fresh disinfecting solution should be made daily.
2. Hatcheries: Remove all animals from the area. Thoroughly clean all surfaces (hatchers, setters, trays, racks, carts, sexing tables, chick boxes, cages) with soap or detergent, then rinse with water. Saturate all surfaces with 1:400 disinfecting solution by using a course spray, mop, or sponge. Surfaces must remain wet for 10 minutes. Do not house animals or employ equipment until surfaces have been absorbed or dried. Fresh disinfection solution should be made daily or if visibly soiled.
3. Food processing plants (including Chicken Processing Facilities): Before using this product, all food products and packaging materials must be removed from the room or carefully protected. Thoroughly clean all surfaces with soap or detergent, then rinse with water. Disinfect hard, non-porous surfaces by applying 1:400 solution with a course spray, mop, or sponge. All surfaces must remain thoroughly wet for 10 minutes. Allow to air dry. A potable water rinse is required for all surfaces that come into contact with food.
4. Trucks and other vehicles: Clean all vehicles including mats, crates, cabs, and wheels with high pressure water. Use 1:400 disinfecting solution to treat all vehicles. Leave all treated surfaces exposed to disinfectant solution wet for 10 minutes. Allow to air dry.
5. Veterinary hospitals: For disinfection of the following hard non-porous surfaces: floors, walls, ceilings, counters, cages, feeding/drinking equipment, and handling/restraining equipment. Remove animals and feed from the premises. Thoroughly clean all surfaces with soap or detergent, then rinse with water. Saturate surfaces with 1:400 disinfecting solution by using a course spray, mop, or sponge. Surfaces must remain wet for 10 minutes. Do not house livestock or employ equipment until surfaces have been absorbed or dried. Thoroughly scrub treated feeding and watering equipment with soap or detergent and rinse with potable water before reuse. Fresh disinfection solution should be made daily or if visibly soiled.

Precautionary Statements: Hazard to Humans and Domestic Animals: Danger. Corrosive. Causes irreversible eye damage and skin burns. May be fatal if absorbed through the skin. Do not get in eyes, on skin, or on clothing. Wear protective eyewear, protective clothing, and rubber gloves. Harmful if inhaled. Avoid breathing vapor. Harmful if swallowed. Prolonged or frequently repeated skin contact may cause allergic reaction in some individuals.

Wash thoroughly with soap and water after handling and before eating, drinking, or using tobacco. Remove contaminated clothing and wash before reuse.

First Aid Statements:

If in Eyes: Hold eyelids open and flush with a steady, gentle stream of water for 15-20 minutes. Remove contact lenses, if present, after the first 5 minutes, then continue rinsing eyes. Call a poison control center or doctor for treatment advice.

If on Skin: Remove contaminated clothing. Rinse skin immediately with plenty of water for 15-20 minutes. Call a poison control center or doctor for treatment advice.

If Swallowed: Call a poison control center or doctor for treatment advice. Have individual sip a glass of water if able to swallow. Do not induce vomiting unless told to do so by the poison control center or doctor. Do not give anything by mouth to an unconscious person.

If Inhaled: Move person to fresh air. If person is not breathing, call 911 or an ambulance, then give artificial respiration, preferably mouth-to-mouth, if possible. Call a poison control center or doctor for further treatment advice.

Note to Physician: Probable mucosal damage may contraindicate the use of gastric lavage.

Environmental Hazards: This pesticide is toxic to fish. Do not discharge effluent containing this product into lakes, streams, ponds, estuaries, oceans or other waters unless in accordance with the requirements of a National Pollutant Discharge Elimination System (NPDES) permit and the permitting authority has been notified in writing prior to discharge. Do not discharge effluent containing this product into sewer systems without previously notifying the local sewage treatment plant authority. For guidance contact your State Water Board or Regional Office of the EPA.

Storage and Disposal: Do not contaminate water, food, or feed by storage and disposal.

Storage: Store in a cool, dry place in tightly closed container away from children. Avoid temperatures below 23°F and above 113°F.

Disposal of pesticide: Pesticide wastes are acutely hazardous. Improper disposal of excess pesticide, spray mixture or rinsate is a violation of Federal Law. If these wastes cannot be disposed of by use according to label instructions, contact your State Pesticide or Environmental Control Agency, or the Hazardous Waste representatives at the nearest EPA Regional Office for guidance.

Disposal of container: Triple rinse. Then offer for recycling or puncture and dispose in a sanitary landfill. Disposal by incineration, or if allowed by state and local authorities, by burning. If burned, stay out of smoke.

Warning(s): Keep out of reach of children.

Disclaimer: Limited Warranty and Disclaimer: The manufacturer warrants (a) that this product conforms to the chemical description on the label; (b) that this product is a reasonable fit for the purposes set forth in the directions for use when it is used in accordance with such directions; and (c) that the directions, warnings and other statements on the label are based upon responsible expert's evaluation of reasonable tests of effectiveness and of toxicity to laboratory animals. Tests have not been made on all varieties or in all states or under all conditions. The manufacturer neither makes nor intends, nor does it authorize any agent or representative to make, any other warranties, expressed or implied, and it expressly excludes and disclaims all implied warranties or merchantability and fitness for particular purpose. This warranty does not extend to, and the buyer shall be solely responsible for, any and all loss or damage which results from the use of this product in any manner which is inconsistent with the label directions, warnings or cautions. Buyer's exclusive remedy and manufacturer's or seller's exclusive liability for any and all claims, losses, damages, or injuries resulting from the use or handling of this product, whether or not such liability is based in the contract, negligence, strict liability in tort of otherwise, shall be limited, at the manufacturer's option, to replacement of, or the repayment of the purchase price for, the quantity of product with respect to which damages are claimed. In no event shall manufacturer or seller be liable for special, indirect or consequential damages resulting from the use or handling of this product.

Presentation: 4 x 5 L.

Compendium Code No.: 11050461 CL-043

VISION® 7 SOMNUS WITH SPUR®*

Intervet **Bacterin-Toxoid**

Clostridium Chauvoei-Septicum-Novyi-Sordellii-Perfringens Types C&D-Haemophilus Somnus Bacterin-Toxoid

U.S. Vet. Lic. No.: 286

Contents: This product contains the antigens listed above.

Contains formaldehyde as preservative.

Indications: For use in healthy cattle as an aid in preventing diseases caused by *Clostridium chauvoei* (Blackleg), *septicum* (Malignant edema), *novyi* (Black disease), *sordellii, perfringens* Types C and D (Enterotoxemia), and *Haemophilus somnus*.

Dosage and Administration: Cattle: 2 mL. Inject subcutaneously. Repeat in 3 to 4 weeks.

Precaution(s): Shake well before using. Store at 35° to 45°F (2° to 7°C). Use entire contents when first opened.

Caution(s): Anaphylactoid reactions may occur. For use in animals only.

Antidote(s): Epinephrine.

Warning(s): Do not vaccinate within 21 days before slaughter.

Presentation: 10 doses (20 mL), 50 doses (100 mL) and 250 doses (500 mL).

*Adjuvant—U.S. Patent Nos. 3,790,665 and 3,919,411.

Compendium Code No.: 11062150

VISION® 7 WITH SPUR®*

Intervet **Bacterin-Toxoid**

Clostridium Chauvoei-Septicum-Novyi-Sordellii-Perfringens Types C & D Bacterin-Toxoid

U.S. Vet. Lic. No.: 286

Contents: This product contains the antigens listed above.

Contains formaldehyde as preservative.

Indications: For use in healthy cattle and sheep as an aid in preventing diseases caused by *Clostridium chauvoei* (Blackleg), *septicum* (Malignant edema), *novyi* (Black disease), *sordellii* and *perfringens* Types C and D (Enterotoxemia).

Dosage and Administration: Cattle: 2 mL, Sheep: 2 mL. Inject subcutaneously. Repeat in 3 to 4 weeks. Annual revaccination is recommended.

Precaution(s): Shake well before using. Store at 35° to 45°F (2° to 7°C). Use entire contents when first opened.
Caution(s): Anaphylactoid reactions may occur. For use in animals only.
Antidote(s): Epinephrine.
Warning(s): Do not vaccinate within 21 days before slaughter.
Presentation: 10 doses (20 mL), 50 doses (100 mL), and 250 doses (500 mL).
*Adjuvant—U.S. Patent Nos. 3,790,665 and 3,919,411.
Compendium Code No.: 11062160

VISION® 8 SOMNUS WITH SPUR®*

Intervet **Bacterin-Toxoid**
Clostridium Chauvoei-Septicum-Haemolyticum-Novyi-Sordellii-Perfringens Types C&D-Haemophilus Somnus Bacterin-Toxoid
U.S. Vet. Lic. No.: 286
Contents: This product contains the antigens listed above.
Contains formaldehyde as preservative.
Indications: For use in healthy cattle as an aid in preventing diseases caused by *Clostridium chauvoei* (Blackleg), *septicum* (Malignant edema), *haemolyticum* (Bacillary hemoglobinuria), *novyi* (Black disease), *sordellii, perfringens* Types C and D (Enterotoxemia), and *Haemophilus somnus.*
Dosage and Administration: Cattle: 2mL. Inject subcutaneously. Repeat in 3 to 4 weeks. In animals subject to reexposure to *Cl. haemolyticum* revaccinate every 5 to 6 months.
Precaution(s): Shake well before using. Store at 35° to 45°F (2° to 7°C). Use entire contents when first opened.
Caution(s): Anaphylactoid reactions may occur. For use in animals only.
Antidote(s): Epinephrine.
Warning(s): Do not vaccinate within 21 days before slaughter.
Presentation: 50 doses (100 mL).
*Adjuvant—Intervet's Proprietary Technology
Compendium Code No.: 11062170

VISION® 8 WITH SPUR®*

Intervet **Bacterin-Toxoid**
Clostridium Chauvoei-Septicum-Haemolyticum-Novyi-Sordellii-Perfringens Types C & D Bacterin-Toxoid
U.S. Vet. Lic. No.: 286
Contents: This product contains the antigens listed above.
Contains formaldehyde as preservative.
Indications: For use in healthy cattle and sheep as an aid in preventing disease caused by *Clostridium chauvoei* (Blackleg), *septicum* (Malignant edema), *haemolyticum* (Bacillary Hemoglobinuria/Red Water), *novyi* (Black disease), *sordellii* and *perfringens* Types C and D (Enterotoxemia).
Dosage and Administration: Cattle: 2 mL, Sheep: 2 mL. Inject subcutaneously. Repeat in 3 to 4 weeks. In animals subject to reexposure to *Cl. haemolyticum* revaccinate every 5 to 6 months. Annual revaccination is recommended.
Precaution(s): Shake well before using. Store at 35° to 45°F (2° to 7°C). Use entire contents when first opened.
Caution(s): Anaphylactoid reactions may occur. For use in animals only.
Antidote(s): Epinephrine.
Warning(s): Do not vaccinate within 21 days before slaughter.
Presentation: 10 doses (20 mL), 50 doses (100 mL), and 250 doses (500 mL).
*Adjuvant—U.S. Patent Nos. 3,790,665 and 3,919,411.
Compendium Code No.: 11062180

VISION® CD•T WITH SPUR®*

Intervet **Bacterin-Toxoid**
Clostridium Perfringens Types C & D-Tetani Bacterin-Toxoid
U.S. Vet. Lic. No.: 286
Contents: This product contains the antigens listed above.
Contains formaldehyde as a preservative.
Indications: For use in healthy cattle, sheep and goats as an aid in preventing disease caused by *Clostridium perfringens* Types C and D (Enterotoxemia) and *Clostridium tetani* (Tetanus).
Dosage and Administration: 2 mL: Cattle, sheep and goats. Inject subcutaneously. Repeat the dose in 3 to 4 weeks. Annual revaccination is recommended.
Precaution(s): Shake well before using. Store at 35° to 45°F (2° to 7°C). Use entire contents when first opened.
Caution(s): Anaphylactoid reactions may occur. For use in animals only.
Antidote(s): Epinephrine.
Warning(s): Do not vaccinate within 21 days before slaughter.
Presentation: 50 doses (100 mL).
*Adjuvant—U.S. Patent Nos. 3,790,665 and 3,919,411.
Compendium Code No.: 11062200

VISION® CD WITH SPUR®*

Intervet **Bacterin-Toxoid**
Clostridium Perfringens Types C & D Bacterin-Toxoid
U.S. Vet. Lic. No.: 286
Contents: This product contains the antigens listed above.
Contains formaldehyde as a preservative.
Indications: For use in healthy cattle, sheep and goats as an aid in the prevention of Enterotoxemia caused by *Clostridium perfringens* Types C and D.
Dosage and Administration: 2 mL: Cattle, sheep and goats. Inject subcutaneously. Repeat the dose in 3 to 4 weeks. Annual vaccination is recommended.
Precaution(s): Shake well before using. Store at 35° to 45°F (2° to 7°C). Use entire contents when first opened.
Caution(s): Anaphylactoid reactions may occur. For use in animals only.
Antidote(s): Epinephrine.
Warning(s): Do not vaccinate within 21 days before slaughter.
Presentation: 10 doses (20 mL), 50 doses (100 mL), and 250 doses (500 mL).
*Adjuvant—U.S. Patent Nos. 3,790,665 and 3,919,411.
Compendium Code No.: 11062190

VI SO BRONC®

L.A.H.I. (New Jersey) **Vaccine**
Newcastle Bronchitis Vaccine, B_1 Type, LaSota Strain, Mass. Type, Live Virus
U.S. Vet. Lic. No.: 196
Description: This product is manufactured from SPF (Specific Pathogen Free) eggs and is a combination live virus vaccine of chicken embryo origin for the prevention of Newcastle Disease and Massachusetts Type Infectious Bronchitis.

The strains of viruses in this product were carefully selected to protect against field challenges yet provide minimum reaction when used as directed.

This vaccine was carefully produced and passed all tests in accordance with the U.S. Government requirements.

Contains neomycin as a preservative.

Indications: This product is recommended for initial vaccination and revaccination of chickens for the prevention of Newcastle Disease and Massachusetts Type Infectious Bronchitis. Initial vaccination is administered to birds at 2 weeks of age by the intranasal or intraocular routes, and at 5 weeks of age by the drinking water route. Aerosol spray application of the vaccine is recommended for revaccination only. This product is also used in replacement birds before 16 weeks of age that were previously vaccinated.

This vaccine will stimulate protective antibodies in susceptible birds. However, the duration of immunity resulting from the use of this vaccine is not permanent, therefore, revaccinations are necessary.

Consult your poultry pathologist for recommendations on revaccination based on conditions existing in your area at any given time.

Dosage and Administration: Read instructions before use.

1,000 Doses - Rehydrate to 30 mL:

Preparation of Vaccine for Intranasal and Intraocular Use: Remove the aluminum tear seal and rubber stopper from the vaccine bottle. Pour some of the diluent into the bottle. Replace the rubber stopper and shake vigorously. Pour the mixed vaccine back into the bottle containing the remaining diluent and attach the dropper tip. The vaccine is now ready for use.

Method of Vaccination: The vaccine may be administered by way of the nostril, (intranasally) or the eye, (intraocularly). When the vaccine is administered by way of the nostril, the beak is held shut, a finger is placed over one nostril and a drop of vaccine, from the applicator, is dropped into the other nostril.

When used intraocularly, birds are held on their side and one drop of the mixed vaccine allowed to fall into the open eye. Hold the birds until the drop of vaccine disappears. Take care to prevent injury to the cornea of the eye with the dropper tip.

Preparation of Vaccine for Aerosol Use: Remove the aluminum overseal and stopper from the vaccine bottle and pour part of the diluent into the bottle. Shake well and pour the vaccine back into the remaining diluent. Pour the entire contents into the reservoir of a sprayer containing 70 mL of deionized water or 5 mL of glycerine and 65 mL of deionized water. Before the vaccination, the sprayer should be calibrated so that 100 mL will be delivered in 3 minutes.

Method of Vaccination: Confine the birds to a corner of the house with fences and direct the stream from the sprayer over the heads of the birds. Extreme caution should be taken to prevent birds from smothering during this operation.

1,000 Doses and 2,500 Doses:

Preparation of Vaccine for Drinking Water Use: Remove the aluminum overseal and stopper and add clean non-sanitized water. Replace the stopper and shake well. Pour the contents into a quart jar ¾ full of non-sanitized water. Shake well and dilute the vaccine for 1000 doses or 2500 doses as the case may be as outlined in the chart below. A dried skim milk powder should be used as a vaccine stabilizer at the rate of 8.0 grams per gallon of water. The powdered milk is added prior to the reconstitution of the vaccine.

Method of Vaccination: Withhold all medication and disinfectants from the drinking water 24 hours before and 24 hours after vaccinating. Rinse waterers with clean non-sanitized water and remove all water from chicks for at least two hours prior to vaccination. Provide adequate space so that at least two-thirds of the birds can drink at one time.

Add mixture to water as per following chart:

1,000 Doses:

Age of Birds	Heavy per 1,000 birds	Leghorn per 1,000 birds
5 to 8 weeks	8 Gals. of Water	5 Gals. of Water
9 to 15 weeks	10 Gals. of Water	8 Gals. of Water
16 to 20 weeks	13 Gals. of Water	10 Gals. of Water

2,500 Doses:

Age of Birds	Heavy per 2,500 birds	Leghorn per 2,500 birds
5 to 8 weeks	20 Gals. of Water	12 Gals. of Water
9 to 15 weeks	25 Gals. of Water	20 Gals. of Water
16 to 20 weeks	30 Gals. of Water	25 Gals. of Water

Divide the mixed vaccine into the waterers.

Provide no other drinking water until all vaccine has been consumed.

Contraindication(s): Vaccinate healthy chickens only.

If there are susceptible laying birds on the premises there is the possibility that the virus might spread from the vaccinated to the susceptible birds and affect egg production.

Precaution(s): Keep vaccine in the dark - between 2-7°C (35-45°F).

Use entire contents when first opened. Burn this container and all unused contents.

Caution(s): It is imperative that the user of this product comply with the "Indications", "Contraindications" and "Method of Vaccination" stated in the direction sheet. The vaccine must be prepared and administered as directed to obtain best results.

Warning(s): Do not vaccinate within 21 days before slaughter.

Care should be taken to avoid contaminating hands, eyes and clothing with the vaccine. Newcastle Disease virus can cause a mild inflammation of the conjunctiva lasting for 3 to 5 days.

For veterinary use only.

Presentation: 1,000 and 2,500 doses.

Compendium Code No.: 10080543 41995

VI SO BRONC® (Drinking Water Use)

L.A.H.I. (New Jersey) **Vaccine**

Newcastle Bronchitis Vaccine, B_1 Type, LaSota Strain, Mass. Type, Live Virus

U.S. Vet. Lic. No.: 196

Description: This product is manufactured from SPF (Specific Pathogen Free) eggs and is a combination live virus vaccine of chicken embryo origin for the prevention of Newcastle Disease and Massachusetts Type Infectious Bronchitis.

The strains of viruses in this product were carefully selected to protect against field challenges yet provide minimum reaction when used as directed.

This vaccine was carefully produced and passed all tests in accordance with the U.S. Government requirements.

Contains neomycin as a preservative.

Indications: This product is recommended for initial vaccination and revaccination of chickens for the prevention of Newcastle Disease and Massachusetts Type Infectious Bronchitis. Initial vaccination is administered to birds at 5 weeks of age. This product is also used in replacement birds before 16 weeks of age that were previously vaccinated.

This vaccine will stimulate protective antibodies in susceptible birds. However, the duration of immunity resulting from the use of this vaccine is not permanent, therefore, revaccinations are necessary.

Consult your poultry pathologist for recommendations on revaccination based conditions existing in your area at any given time.

For drinking water use.

Dosage and Administration: Read instructions before use.

10,000 Doses:

Preparation of Vaccine: Remove the aluminum overseal and stopper and add clean non-sanitized water. Replace the stopper and shake well. Pour the contents into a quart jar ¾ full of non-sanitized water. Shake well and dilute as outlined in the chart below.

Method of Vaccination: Keep all medication and disinfectants from the drinking water 24 hours before and 24 hours after vaccination. Rinse waterers with clean non-sanitized water. Water starve the birds for at least two hours prior to vaccination. Provide adequate space so that at least two-thirds of the birds can drink at one time.

Add mixture to water as per following chart:

Age of Birds	Heavy	Leghorn
5-8 Weeks	80 Gals. of Water	50 Gals. of Water
9-15 Weeks	100 Gals. of Water	80 Gals. of Water
16-20 Weeks	130 Gals. of Water	100 Gals. of Water

Divide mixed vaccine into the waterers.

Provide no other drinking water until all vaccine has been consumed.

Contraindication(s): Vaccinate healthy chickens only that are free of PPLO and without previous history of a respiratory disease.

If there are susceptible laying birds on the premises there is the possibility that the virus might spread from the vaccinated to the susceptible birds and affect egg production.

Precaution(s): Keep vaccine in the dark - between 2-7°C (35-45°F).

Use entire contents when first opened. Burn this container and all unused contents.

Caution(s): It is imperative that the user of this product comply with the "Indications", "Contraindications", and "Method of Vaccination" stated on the direction sheet. The vaccine must be prepared and administered as directed to obtain best results.

If chicks are to be vaccinated at a very young age, the vaccination must be done at the point of destination to avoid violation of the Postal Laws and Regulations.

Warning(s): Do not vaccinate within 21 days before slaughter.

Care should be taken to avoid contaminating your hands, eyes and clothing with the vaccine since the Newcastle Disease virus can cause a mild inflammation of the conjunctiva lasting for 3 to 5 days.

For veterinary use only.

Presentation: 10,000 dose vial.

Compendium Code No.: 10080671 117158

VI SO HOL™

L.A.H.I. (New Jersey) **Vaccine**

Newcastle Bronchitis Vaccine, B_1 Type, LaSota Strain, Mass. Type, Live Virus

U.S. Vet. Lic. No.: 196

Description: This product is manufactured from SPF (Specific Pathogen Free) eggs and is a combination live virus vaccine of chicken embryo origin for the prevention of Newcastle Disease and Massachusetts Type Infectious Bronchitis in chickens.

The virus strains in this product are the Massachusetts Type, Holland Strain - high egg passages of bronchitis virus and the B_1 type, LaSota Strain of Newcastle Disease virus.

These viruses were carefully selected to protect against field challenges yet provide minimum reaction when used as directed.

This vaccine was carefully produced and passes all tests in accordance with the U.S. Government requirements.

Contains neomycin as a preservative.

Indications: This product is recommended for initial intranasal or intraocular vaccination of chickens at two weeks of age; initial aerosol vaccination of chickens at six weeks of age and initial water vaccination of chickens at five weeks of age.

Parental immunity and immunological incompetence are major factors in preventing young birds from developing immunity. The duration of immunity resulting from vaccination is also directly related to the age of the birds and their susceptibility.

Consult your poultry pathologist for recommendations on revaccination based on conditions existing in your area at any given time.

Dosage and Administration: Read instructions before use.

1,000 Doses - Rehydrate to 30 mL:

Preparation of Vaccine for Intranasal and Intraocular Use: Remove the aluminum tear seal and rubber stopper from the vaccine bottle. Pour some of the diluent into the bottle. Replace the rubber stopper and shake vigorously. Pour the mixed vaccine back into the bottle containing the remaining diluent and attach the dropper tip. The vaccine is now ready for use.

Method of Vaccination: The vaccine may be administered by way of the nostril (intranasally) or the eye (intraocularly). When the vaccine is administered by way of the nostril, the beak is held shut, a finger is placed over one nostril and a drop of vaccine, from the applicator, is dropped into the other nostril.

When used intraocularly, birds are held on their side and one drop of the mixed vaccine allowed to fall into the open eye. Hold the bird until the drop of vaccine disappears. Take care to prevent injury to the cornea of the eye with the dropper tip.

Preparation of Vaccine for Aerosol Use: Remove the aluminum overseal and stopper from the vaccine bottle and pour part of the diluent into the bottle. Shake well and pour the vaccine back into the remaining diluent. Pour the entire contents into the reservoir of a sprayer containing 70 mL of deionized water or 5 mL of glycerine and 65 mL of deionized water. Before the vaccination the sprayer should be calibrated so that 100 mL will be delivered in 3 minutes.

Method of Vaccination: Confine the birds to a corner of the house with fences and direct the stream from the sprayer over the heads of the birds. Extreme caution should be taken to prevent birds from smothering during this operation.

1,000 and 2,500 Doses:

Preparation of Vaccine for Drinking Water Use: Remove the aluminum overseal and stopper and add clean non-sanitized water. Replace the stopper and shake well. Pour the contents into a quart jar ¾ full of non-sanitized water. Shake well and dilute the vaccine for 1000 or 2500 doses as the case may be as outlined in the chart below. A dried skim milk powder should be used as a vaccine stabilizer at the rate of 8.0 grams per gallon of water. The powdered milk is added prior to the reconstitution of the vaccine.

Method of Vaccination: Withhold all medication and disinfectants from the drinking water 24 hours before and 24 hours after vaccination. Rinse waterers with clean non-sanitized water and remove all water from chicks for at least two hours prior to vaccination. Provide adequate space so that at least two-thirds of the birds can drink at one time.

Add mixture to water as per following chart:

1,000 Doses:

Age of Birds	Heavy per 1,000 birds	Leghorn per 1,000 birds
5-8 Weeks	8 Gals of Water	5 Gals of Water
9-15 Weeks	10 Gals of Water	8 Gals of Water

2,500 Doses:

Age of Birds	Heavy per 2,500 birds	Leghorn per 2,500 birds
5-8 Weeks	20 Gals of Water	12 Gals of Water
9-15 Weeks	25 Gals of Water	20 Gals of Water

Divide the mixed vaccine into the waterers.

Provide no other drinking water until all vaccine has been consumed.

Contraindication(s): Vaccinate healthy chickens only.

If there are susceptible laying birds on the premises there is the possibility that the virus might spread from the vaccinated to the susceptible birds and affect egg production.

Precaution(s): Keep vaccine in the dark - between 2-7°C (35-45°F).

Use entire contents when first opened. Burn this container and all unused contents.

Caution(s): It is imperative that the user of this product comply with the "Indications", "Contraindications", and "Method of Vaccination" stated on the direction sheet. The vaccine must be prepared and administered as directed to obtain best results.

Warning(s): Do not vaccinate within 21 days before slaughter.

Care should be taken to avoid contaminating hands, eyes and clothing with the vaccine. Newcastle Disease virus can cause inflammation of the eyelids in humans.

For veterinary use only.

Presentation: 1,000 and 2,500 doses.

Compendium Code No.: 10080553 95A

VI SO HOL™ (Drinking Water Use)

L.A.H.I. (New Jersey) **Vaccine**

Newcastle Bronchitis Vaccine, B_1 Type, LaSota Strain, Mass. Type, Live Virus

U.S. Vet. Lic. No.: 196

Description: This product is manufactured from SPF (Specific Pathogen Free) eggs and is a combination live virus vaccine of chicken embryo origin for the prevention of Newcastle Disease and Massachusetts Type Infectious Bronchitis.

The strains of viruses in this product were carefully selected to protect against field challenges yet provide minimum reaction when used as directed.

This vaccine was carefully produced and passed all tests in accordance with the U.S. Government requirements.

Contains neomycin as a preservative.

Indications: This product is recommended for initial vaccination and revaccination of chickens for the prevention of Newcastle Disease and Massachusetts Type Infectious Bronchitis. Initial vaccination is administered to birds at 5 weeks of age. This product is also used in replacement birds before 16 weeks of age that were previously vaccinated.

This vaccine will stimulate protective antibodies in susceptible birds. However, the duration of immunity resulting from the use of this vaccine is not permanent, therefore, revaccinations are necessary.

Consult your poultry pathologist for recommendations on revaccination based conditions existing in your area at any given time.

For drinking water use.

Dosage and Administration: Read instructions before use.

10,000 Doses:

Preparation of Vaccine: Remove the aluminum overseal and stopper and add clean non-sanitized water. Replace the stopper and shake well. Pour the contents into a quart jar ¾ full of non-sanitized water. Shake well and dilute as outlined in the chart below.

Method of Vaccination: Keep all medication and disinfectants from the drinking water 24 hours before and 24 hours after vaccinating. Rinse waterers with clean non-sanitized water. Water starve the birds for at least two hours prior to vaccination. Provide adequate space so that at least two-thirds of the birds can drink at one time.

Add mixture to water as per following chart:

Age of birds	Heavy	Leghorn
5-8 Weeks	80 Gals. of Water	50 Gals. of Water
9-15 Weeks	100 Gals. of Water	80 Gals. of Water
16-20 Weeks	130 Gals. of Water	100 Gals. of Water

Divide mixed vaccine into the waterers.

Provide no other drinking water until all vaccine has been consumed.

Contraindication(s): Vaccinate healthy chickens only that are free of PPLO and without previous history of a respiratory disease.

If there are susceptible laying birds on the premises there is the possibility that the virus might spread from the vaccinated to the susceptible birds and affect egg production.

Precaution(s): Keep vaccine in the dark - between 2-7°C (35-45°F).

Use entire contents when first opened. Burn this container and all unused contents.

Caution(s): It is imperative that the user of this product comply with the "Indications", "Contraindications", and "Method of Vaccination" stated on the direction sheet. The vaccine must be prepared and administered as directed to obtain best results.

If chicks are to be vaccinated at a very young age, the vaccination must be done at the point of destination to avoid violation of the Postal Laws and Regulations.

Warning(s): Do not vaccinate within 21 days before slaughter.

Care should be taken to avoid contaminating hands, eyes and clothing with the vaccine. Newcastle Disease virus can cause a mild inflammation of the conjunctiva lasting for 3 to 5 days.

For veterinary use only.

Presentation: 10,000 dose vial.

Compendium Code No.: 10080681 117158

VI-SORBIN®

Pfizer Animal Health **Dietary Supplement**

Vitamin-Iron Preparation with Sorbitol

Guaranteed Analysis: Per Teaspoon (5 mL): (All values are minimum quantities unless otherwise stated.)

Minerals

Calcium

Minimum 0.0%

Maximum 0.5%

Phosphorus 0.0%

Salt

Minimum 0.0%

Maximum 0.5%

Iron .... 10.0 mg

Vitamins and Others:

Pyridoxine .... 1.5 mg

Folic Acid .... 0.4 mg

Vitamin B_{12} .... 8.3 mcg

Ingredients: Sorbitol, Water, Ferric Pyrophosphate, Sodium Citrate Dihydrate, Citric Acid, Cherry Flavor, Methylparaben, Pyridoxine Hydrochloride, Polyparaben, Folic Acid, FD&C Green #3, Cyanocobalamin.

Indications: A palatable, nutritional, vitamin and iron supplement. Useful for both young and very old animals and for horses on the racing circuit.

Directions: Administer directly or mix with food when possible.

Dogs: 1-3 teaspoons daily, depending upon size. Cats: ½ teaspoon daily (mix in milk if desired). Puppies and kittens: ¼ teaspoon daily. Calves, and foals up to yearlings: ½ fl oz daily. Yearlings and adult horses: 1 fl oz daily.

Precaution(s): Important: Protect from light. Dispense only in amber bottles. Do not refrigerate.

Caution(s): For veterinary use only.

Presentation: 1 gallon (3.785 L) containers.

Licensed under U.S. Pat. No. 2,850,429

Compendium Code No.: 36901620 85-8850-09

VI-SORBITS®

Pfizer Animal Health **Small Animal Dietary Supplement**

Guaranteed Analysis: per tablet: (All values are minimum quantities)

Minerals:

Calcium

Minimum 4.5%

Maximum 5.5%

Phosphorus 4.0%

Potassium 0.55%

Salt

Minimum 0.20%

Maximum 0.70%

Chloride 0.20%

Magnesium 0.25%

Iron .... 9.0 mg

Copper .... 0.45 mg

Vitamins:

Vitamin A .... 1,250 IU

Vitamin D .... 125 IU

Vitamin E .... 2.0 IU

Thiamine .... 1.0 mg

Riboflavin (B_2) .... 1.0 mg

Pantothenic Acid .... 0.5 mg

Niacin .... 10.0 mg

Pyridoxine (B_6) .... 1.0 mg

Folic Acid .... 0.2 mg

Vitamin B_{12} .... 8.0 mcg

Ingredients: Wheat germ, calcium phosphate, pork liver powder, corn syrup, sorbitol, linoleic acid, ferrous fumarate, gelatin, poultry fat, magnesium sulfate, niacinamide, cyanocobalamin, thiamine mononitrate, vitamin E supplement, vitamin A palmitate, vitamin D supplement, cupric acetate, pyridoxine hydrochloride, riboflavin, d-calcium pantothenate, folic acid, ethoxyquin.

Indications: VI-SORBITS® are a source of supplemental vitamins and iron when used as recommended. VI-SORBITS® have special flavor appeal for dogs. Regularly scheduled examinations by your veterinarian help assure a healthy, happy dog.

Dosage and Administration: Suggested daily dosage: One tablet per day, or as directed by your veterinarian, given whole or crumbled on food. Available only from your veterinarian.

Precaution(s): Store at controlled room temperature 15°-30°C (59°-86°F).

Caution(s): Keep out of reach of children.

Presentation: Plastic bottles of 50 and 200 tablets.

Compendium Code No.: 36901630 85-8866-12

VITA-15™ INJECTION ℞

Neogen **Vitamin-Mineral Injection**

Active Ingredient(s): Each mL formulated to contain:

Pyridoxine HCl .... 10 mg

Riboflavin 5'PO4-Na .... 10 mg

d-Panthenol .... 15 mg

Niacinamide .... 100 mg

Inositol .... 10 mg

Choline chloride .... 10 mg

Biotin .... 10 mcg

L-Lysine HCl .... 20 mg

Glycine .... 20 mg

Cobalt Gluconate .... 2 mg

Benzyl Alcohol 2.0%

Water for injection .... q.s.

Indications: A source of nutritional factors for use in horses.

Dosage and Administration: Intramuscular or intravenous. Horse: 1 mL per 100 lbs body weight. Repeat once or twice weekly or as indicated.

Precaution(s): Avoid exposure to light. Store at controlled room temperature between 15°C-30°C (59°F-86°F).

Caution(s): Federal Law restricts this drug to use by or on the order of a licensed veterinarian.

Sold to licensed veterinarians only.

For animal use only.

Warning(s): Keep out of reach of children.

Presentation: 100 mL sterile multiple dose vials (NDC: 59051-8882-5).

Manufactured by: Omega Laboratories, Montreal, QC.

Compendium Code No.: 14910471 L112-0501

VITA•B-1 CRUMBLES

Horse Health **Thiamine**

Feed Supplement

Guaranteed Analysis: Each pound contains not less than:

Crude Protein, min. 11%

Crude Fat, min. 4%

Crude Fiber, max. 16%

Calcium, min. 8%

Calcium, max. 9%

Thiamine (Vitamin B1), min. .... 8,000 mg

Ingredients: Dehydrated Alfalfa Meal, Wheat Middlings, Ground Limestone, Oat Hulls, Vegetable Oil, Thiamine Hydrochloride, Cane Molasses, Propionic and Acetic Acids (Preservatives).

Indications: A quality feed supplement for all classes of horses.

Dosage and Administration: Feeding Instructions: Feed ½ oz. to 1 oz. in daily grain ration (1 ounce measuring scoop enclosed).

Caution(s): For animal use only.

Warning(s): Keep out of reach of children.

Presentation: 1.13 kg (2.5 lb), 6.8 kg (15 lb) and 9.09 kg (20 lb).

Compendium Code No.: 15000070 0D1 / 9BB9

VITA•B-1 POWDER

Horse Health **Thiamine**

Feed Supplement

Guaranteed Analysis: Each pound contains not less than:

Calcium, min. 8%

Calcium, max. 9%

Thiamine (Vitamin B1) min. .... 8,000 mg

Ingredients: Processed Grain Products, Calcium Carbonate, Cane Molasses, Thiamine Hydrochloride, Propionic and Acetic Acids (Preservatives).

Indications: A quality feed supplement for all classes of horses.

Dosage and Administration: Feeding Instructions: Feed ½ oz. to 1 oz. in daily grain ration (1 ounce measuring scoop enclosed).

Caution(s): For animal use only.

Warning(s): Keep out of reach of children.

Presentation: 6.8 kg (15 lb) pail.

Compendium Code No.: 15000110 9BB9

VITA•BIOTIN™ CRUMBLES

Horse Health **Biotin**

Feed Supplement

Guaranteed Analysis:

Crude Protein, min. 10.5%

Crude Fat, min. 3.0%

Crude Fiber, max. 17.5%

Calcium (Ca), min. 8.0%

Calcium (Ca), max. 9.0%

Biotin, min. .... 100 mg/lb

Ingredients: Dehydrated Alfalfa Meal, Ground Limestone, Wheat Middlings, Oat Hulls, Biotin, Vegetable Oil, Cane Molasses, Natural and Artificial Flavorings, Propionic and Acetic Acids (preservatives).

Indications: A quality feed supplement for all classes of horses.

Dosage and Administration: Feeding Instructions: Feed ½ oz. to 1 ounce in daily grain ration (1 ounce measuring scoop enclosed).

Caution(s): For animal use only.

Warning(s): Keep out of reach of children.

Presentation: 1.13 kg (2.5 lb) and 9.07 kg (20 lb).

Compendium Code No.: 15000080 0D1

VITA BOOST PASTE™

AgriLabs **Large Animal Dietary Supplement**

Guaranteed Analysis:

	(per 15 cc)	(per pound)
Methionine, min	100 mg	3026.66 mg
Vitamin A, min	200,000 IU	6,053,333.3 IU
Vitamin E, min	400 IU	12,106.6 IU
Vitamin D, min	50,000 IU	1,513,333.3 IU
Vitamin B_{12}, min	500 mcg	15,133.33 mg
Niacin	200 mg	6,053.33 mg
Choline, min	100 mg	3,026.66 mg
Yeast cells, min	10 billion CFU	302.66 billion CFU
L. acid bacteria, min	5 billion	151.33 billion
Bacillus, min	10 billion	302.66 billion
Protease, min	2500 PC	75,666.6 PC
Amylase	1500 RAU	45,400 RAU

Ingredients: Vitamin A acetate, D-activated animal sterol (source of vitamin D_3), cyanocobalamin (source of vitamin B_{12}), dl-tocopheral acetate (source of vitamin E), riboflavin, *Aspergillus oryzae* fermentation product, d-Pantothenic acid, niacin, folic acid, pyridoxine hydrochloride, choline bitartrate, zinc proteinate, manganese proteinate, dried *Bacillus coagulans* fermentation product, dried *Bacillus licheniformis* fermentation product, dried *Bacillus subtilis* fermentation product, dried *Lactobacillus casei* fermentation product, dried *Lactobacillus fermentum* fermentation product, dried *Lactobacillus plantarum,* DL methionine, *Sacchromyces cerevisiae,* dextrose, vegetable oil, ethoxyquin, and beef peptone.

Note: VITA BOOST PASTE™ contains no iron or copper and may be used in veal calves and sheep.

Indications: A source of live (viable) naturally occurring micro-organisms, amino acids, enzymes, yeast, and vitamins.

Directions for Use: Use at calving, birth, weaning, shipping, weather or ration changes and post antibiotic treatment. Administer on back of tongue. Each click administers 5 mL.

Recommended Usage:

Beef and Dairy Calves, birth to 350 lbs. . . . . 10 mL (2 clicks)
Beef and Dairy Cattle, over 350 lbs. . . . . 15 mL (3 clicks)
Veal Calves . . . . . 10 mL (2 clicks)
Sheep/Goats/Swine - Growing . . . . . 5 mL (1 click)
Mature Animal . . . . . 10 mL (2 clicks)
Horses . . . . . 15 mL (3 clicks)
Foals, to 6 month of age . . . . . 10 mL (2 clicks)

Precaution(s): Do not freeze. Store in cool dry place. Protect from direct sunlight.

Caution(s): No withdrawal time. For livestock use only. Keep out of reach of children.

Presentation: 10 ounces (300 mL).

Compendium Code No.: 10581190

VITA CHARGE® 28 DISPERSIBLE POWDER

BioZyme **Large Animal Dietary Supplement**

with the Amaferm® advantage

Active Ingredient(s): **Aspergillus oryzae* fermentation extract.

Guaranteed Analysis: Per Pound:

Copper . . . . . 4.0 mg Min.
Zinc . . . . . 11.4 mg Min.
Manganese . . . . . 6.4 mg Min.
Cobalt . . . . . 0.80 mg Min.
Vitamin A . . . . . 1,000,000 IU Min.
Vitamin D_3 . . . . . 786,000 IU Min.
Vitamin E . . . . . 16,000 IU Min.
Vitamin B_{12} . . . . . 13,200 mcg Min.
Ascorbic Acid . . . . . 640 mg Min.
Riboflavin . . . . . 320 mg Min.
d-Pantothenic Acid . . . . . 1,280 mg Min.
Niacin . . . . . 3,840 mg Min.
Folic Acid . . . . . 96 mg Min.
Pyridoxine . . . . . 160 mg Min.
Choline . . . . . 3,200 mg Min.
Bacillus subtilis, minimum . . . . . 10 billion CFU Min.

Ingredients: Vitamin A supplement, d-activated animal sterol (a source of vitamin D_3), cyanocobalamin (source of vitamin B_{12}), dl-alpha-tocopherol acetate (source of vitamin E), riboflavin supplement, calcium pantothenate, niacin supplement, folic acid, pyridoxine hydrochloride, choline bitartrate, zinc methionine, manganese methionine, copper lysine, cobalt glucoheptonate, dried *Bacillus subtilis* fermentation product, dextrose, dried *Aspergillus oryzae* fermentation extract*, artificial flavor.

Indications: A digestive enhancer fortified with vitamins and minerals. Supplement for beef and dairy calves and cattle.

Dosage and Administration:

Calves: ⅓ oz per calf, daily, in milk or milk replacer or top dress on food.

Cattle: ⅔ top dress on feed daily.

Caution(s): Due to the copper level, do not feed to sheep. Follow label directions.

Presentation: 2 lb jar, 5 lb and 25 lb pail.

*Amaferm® is a product of a patented process, U.S. Patent #3043748

Compendium Code No.: 14960030

VITA CHARGE® CALF BOLUS

BioZyme **Large Animal Dietary Supplement**

with the Amaferm® advantage

Active Ingredient(s): **Aspergillus oryzae* fermentation extract.

Guaranteed Analysis:

Ash . . . . . 19.5% Max.
Calcium
Min. 0.6%
Max. 0.8%
Phosphorus . . . . . 0.4% Min.
Salt
Min. 1.0%
Max. 2.0%
Magnesium . . . . . 0.1% Min.
Potassium . . . . . 5.0% Min.
Zinc . . . . . 4100.0 ppm Min.
Cobalt . . . . . 1590.0 ppm Min.
Selenium . . . . . 32.0 ppm Min.
Vitamin A . . . . . 2,185,000 IU/lb Min.
Vitamin D . . . . . 832,000 IU/lb Min.
Vitamin E . . . . . 2,590 IU/lb Min.
Choline . . . . . 1,050 mg/lb Min.
Niacin . . . . . 32,300 mg/lb Min.
d-Pantothenic Acid . . . . . 78.0 mg/lb Min.
Riboflavin . . . . . 52.0 mg/lb Min.
Thiamine . . . . . 11.0 mg/lb Min.
Vitamin B_{12} . . . . . 130 mcg/lb Min.

Ingredients: Dried whey, cellulose, dried *Aspergillus oryzae* fermentation extract, vitamin A supplement, d-activated animal sterol (a source of vitamin D_3), dl-alpha-tocopherol acetate (source of vitamin E), choline chloride, niacin, calcium pantothenate, riboflavin, vitamin B_{12} supplement, thiamine hydrochloride, potassium chloride, yeast culture, dicalcium phosphate, zinc sulfate, ferrous sulfate, copper sulfate, manganese sulfate, calcium iodate, cobalt sulfate, sodium selenite, dextrose corn sugar.

Indications: A digestive enhancer fortified with vitamins and minerals. Supplement for beef/dairy calves.

Dosage and Administration: Two (2) 6-gram boluses per calf, daily, for calves under 350 lbs.

Caution(s): Due to the copper level, do not feed to sheep. Follow label directions.

Presentation: 50 bolus jar and 200 bolus jar.

*Amaferm® is a product of a patented process, U.S. Patent #3043748

Compendium Code No.: 14960040

VITA CHARGE® EQUINE

BioZyme **Equine Dietary Supplement**

with the Amaferm® advantage

Guaranteed Analysis:

		App. per 2 oz
Crude Protein	11.0% Min.	6.2 g
Crude Fat	3.0% Min.	1.7 g
Crude Fiber	4.0% Max.	2.2 g
Calcium (Ca)	4.0% Min./5.0% Max.	2.8 g
Phosphorus (P)	4.0% Min.	1.9 g
Salt (NaCl)	3.5% Min./4.5% Max.	2.2 g
Magnesium (Mg)	2.0% Min.	1.1 g
Potassium (K)	2.0% Min.	1.1 g
Cobalt (Co)	90.0 ppm Min.	50.0 mg
Copper (Cu)	2,000.0 ppm Min.	110.0 mg
Iodine	150.0 ppm Min.	8.5 mg
Iron (Fe)	5,000.0 ppm Min.	280.0 mg
Manganese (Mn)	6,000.0 ppm Min.	340.0 mg
Selenium (Se)	50.0 ppm Min.	2.5 mg
Zinc (Zn)	7,400.0 ppm Min.	470.0 mg
Vitamin A	500,000 IU/lb Min.	62,500 IU
Vitamin D_3	48,000 IU/lb Min.	6,000 IU
Vitamin E	3,000 IU/lb Min.	375 IU
Vitamin B_{12}	1.20 mg/lb Min.	150.0 mcg
Menadione (Vitamin K)	20.0 mg/lb Min.	2.5 mg
Riboflavin	400.0 mg/lb Min.	50.0 mg
d-Pantothenic Acid	800.0 mg/lb Min.	100.0 mg
Thiamine	480.0 mg/lb Min.	60.0 mg
Pyridoxine Hydrochloride	120.0 mg/lb Min.	15.0 mg
Niacin	1,900.0 mg/lb Min.	240.0 mg
Folic Acid	40.0 mg/lb Min.	5.0 mg
Choline	1,500.0 mg/lb Min.	187.0 mg
Biotin	24.0 mg/lb Min.	3.0 mg

Ingredients: Yeast culture, dicalcium phosphate, monocalcium phosphate, corn distillers dried grains with solubles, heat processed soybean meal, zinc sulfate, ferrous sulfate, copper sulfate, manganese sulfate, calcium iodate, cobalt sulfate, sodium selenite, monocalcium phosphate, vitamin A supplement, d-activated animal sterol (source of vitamin D_3), dl-alpha-tocopherol acetate (source of vitamin E), choline chloride, niacin, calcium pantothenate, riboflavin, vitamin B_{12} supplement, thiamine hydrochloride, ascorbic acid, biotin, salt, dried *Aspergillus oryzae* fermentation extract, magnesium oxide, potassium chloride, calcium carbonate, mineral oil, dimethylprimidinol bisulfate (source of vitamin K), natural flavors.

Indications: Amaferm® blended in a highly palatable meal with vitamins, trace minerals and yeast culture for all horses; work, show, pleasure, breeding and racing.

Dosage and Administration: Feeding Directions: Should be top-dressed or mixed in grain rations.

Mature horses: 2 oz per head, daily.

Foals to 6 months of age: 1 oz per head, daily.

Precaution(s): Store in a cool, dry place. Protect from sunlight.

Caution(s): For oral use in horses only. Due to the copper level, do not feed to sheep. Follow label directions. The addition of higher levels of selenium is not permitted.

Warning(s): Not for human consumption. Keep out of reach of children.

Presentation: 7 lb and 20 lb pail.

Compendium Code No.: 14960061

05/00

VITA CHARGE® GEL CAP

BioZyme **Large Animal Dietary Supplement**

with the Amaferm® advantage

Active Ingredient(s): **Aspergillus oryzae* fermentation extract.

Guaranteed Analysis:

Crude Protein . . . 2.0% Min.
Calcium (Ca) . . . 0.3% Min. - 0.4% Max.
Phosphorus (P) . . . 0.2% Min.
Magnesium (Mg) . . . 0.15% Min.
Potassium (K) . . . 7.0% Min.
Cobalt (Co) . . . 2000 ppm Min.
Copper (Cu) . . . 1500.0 ppm Min.
Iodine . . . 120 ppm Min.
Manganese (Mn) . . . 4500 ppm Min.
Selenium (Se) . . . 40 ppm Min.
Zinc (Zn) . . . 5600 ppm Min.
Vitamin A . . . 2,800,000 IU/lb Min.
Vitamin D_3 . . . 1,000,000 IU/lb Min.
Vitamin E . . . 3500 IU/lb Min.
Vitamin B_{12} (Cyanocobalamin) . . . 180 mcg/lb or 0.180 mg/lb Min.
Riboflavin . . . 70 mg/lb Min.
d-Pantothenic Acid . . . 100 mg/lb Min.
Thiamine . . . 12 mg/lb Min.
Niacin . . . 44,000 mg/lb Min.
Choline . . . 1200 mg/lb Min.

Ingredients: Monocalcium phosphate, dicalcium phosphate, dextrose corn sugar, dried *Aspergillus oryzae* fermentation extract, vitamin A supplement, d-activated animal sterol (source of vitamin D_3), dl-alpha-tocopherol acetate (source of vitamin E), choline chloride, niacin, calcium pantothenate, riboflavin, vitamin B_{12} supplement, thiamine hydrochloride, potassium chloride, yeast culture, zinc sulfate, ferrous sulfate, copper sulfate, manganese sulfate, calcium iodate, cobalt sulfate, sodium selenite, cobalt carbonate.

Indications: A digestive enhancer fortified with vitamins and minerals. Supplement for beef and dairy cattle.

Dosage and Administration: One (1) 21-gram gel cap per head, daily, for cattle over 350 lbs.

Administer with proper procedure according to animal's ability to accommodate gel cap bolus size.

Caution(s): Due to the copper level, do not feed to sheep. Follow label directions.

Presentation: Box of 50 gel caps and pail of 200 gel caps.

*Amaferm® is a product of a patented process, U.S. Patent #3043748

Compendium Code No.: 14960070

VITA CHARGE® PASTE

BioZyme **Large Animal Dietary Supplement**

with the Amaferm® advantage

Active Ingredient(s): **Aspergillus oryzae* fermentation extract.

Guaranteed Analysis: Per 15 mL (gram):

Calcium
Min. . . . 0.00026%
Max. . . . 0.00032%
Phosphorus . . . 0.0% Min.
Salt
Min. . . . 0.17%
Max. . . . 0.22%
Sodium . . . 73.19 mg Min.
Magnesium . . . 0.0% Min.
Potassium . . . 1.71% Min.
Zinc . . . 0.068% Min.
Vitamin A . . . 200,000 IU Min.
Vitamin D_3 . . . 50,000 IU Min.
Vitamin E . . . 400 IU Min.
Vitamin B_{12} . . . 500 mcg Min.
Bacillus subtilis . . . 200 million CFU Min.

Ingredients: Vegetable oil, silicon dioxide, dried *Aspergillus oryzae* fermentation extract, wheat bran, wheat middlings, potassium chloride, dextrose, sodium bicarbonate, niacin, whey protein concentrate, sodium chloride, zinc sulfate, manganese proteinate, zinc proteinate, manganese sulfate, choline chloride, d-biotin, sodium selenite, calcium pantothenate, pyridoxine hydrochloride, folic acid, cobalt carbonate, calcium iodate, vitamin E supplement, vitamin A supplement, polysorbate 80, d-activated animal sterol (source of vitamin D_3), vitamin B_{12} supplement, dried *Bacillus subtilis* fermentation product, dried whey sodium sulfate, corn starch lecithin, artificial flavoring and coloring.

Indications: A highly palatable digestive enhancer fortified with vitamins and minerals. Supplement for horses, beef/dairy cattle, swine, sheep and goats.

Dosage and Administration:

Beef and Dairy Cattle birth to 350 lbs: 10 mL
Beef and Dairy Cattle over 350 lbs: 15 mL
Sheep/Goats/Swine - Growing Animal: 5 mL
Mature Animal: 10 mL
Horses: 15 mL
Foals to 6 months of age: 10 mL

Administer VITA CHARGE® Paste orally on back of tongue. Consistency of paste prevents the animal from spitting it out. Each click delivers 5 mL; three clicks (trigger fully depressed), 15 mL. For best results, leave capped when not in use.

Presentation: 80 mL and 300 mL tube.

*Amaferm® is a product of a patented process, U.S. Patent #3043748

Compendium Code No.: 14960090

V

VITA CHARGE® POWER DRENCH

BioZyme **Electrolytes-Oral**

with the Amaferm® advantage

Guaranteed Analysis:

Calcium (Ca) . . . 8.2% Min./9.8% Max.
Salt (NaCl) . . . 3.2% Min./4.2% Max.
Magnesium (Mg) . . . 5.0% Min.
Potassium (K) . . . 10.0% Min.
Zinc (Zn) . . . 225.0 ppm Min.
Vitamin A . . . 500,000 IU/lb Min.
Vitamin D_3 . . . 6,000 IU/lb Min.
Vitamin E . . . 500 IU/lb Min.
Vitamin B_{12} . . . 0.015 mg/lb or 15.0 mcg/lb
Niacin . . . 3,000.0 mg/lb
Choline . . . 200.0 mg/lb

Ingredients: Ground Limestone, Calcium Propionate, Potassium Chloride, Yeast Culture, Dextrose, Magnesium Oxide, Salt, Dried Whey, Niacin, Dried *Aspergillus oryzae* Fermentation Extract, dl-alpha-Tocopheryl Acetate (Source of Vitamin E), Zinc Methionine Complex, Betaine Monohydrate, Vitamin A Supplement, D-Activated Animal Sterol (Source of Vitamin D_3).

Indications: A source of vitamins, electrolytes, energy, yeast and dried *Aspergillus oryzae* fermentation extract designed to hydrate animals with essential electrolytes when they experience stressful situations such as heat, sickness, calving and shipping. Use on dairy cows, beef cows, calves, feedlot cattle, sick and convalescing animals.

Dosage and Administration: Administer by drenching with fluid feeder or mix thoroughly into 5 gallons drinking water. Also may be top-dressed onto grain or TMR mix.

During stress, administer at rate of 1 pound per 1 to 2 gallons warm water to cattle over 1,000 pounds, and ½ pound per 2 to 4 quarts water to cattle less than 1,000 pounds. Administer immediately on first day of calving or shipping/receiving. Administer to sick cattle for up to 3 days.

Note: Two 8 oz scoops = 1 lb.

Precaution(s): Seal after using to keep product integrity (freshness).

Presentation: 25 lb (11.34 kg) pail.

Compendium Code No.: 14960141 10/01

VITA•E & SELENIUM POWDER

Horse Health **Vitamin E-Selenium**

Feed Supplement

Guaranteed Analysis: Per Pound:

Crude Protein, min. . . . 5.5%
Crude Fat, min. . . . 2.5%
Crude Fiber, max. . . . 2.5%
Calcium, min. . . . 7.5%
Calcium, max. . . . 8.5%
Selenium, min. . . . 70 ppm
Vitamin E, min. . . . 20,000 IU

Ingredients: Corn, ground limestone, Vitamin E Supplement, Sodium Selenite, Cane Molasses, Propionic and Acetic Acid (as preservatives).

Indications: A quality feed supplement for all classes of horses.

Dosage and Administration: Feeding Directions:

Horses: Feed ¼ to ½ ounce daily (½ ounce provides 1 mg Selenium) (1 ounce measuring scoop enclosed).

Precaution(s): Store in area inaccessible to children and animals.

Caution(s): Follow label directions. The addition to feed of higher levels of this premix containing selenium is not permitted. Excessive amounts of Selenium may be toxic.

For animal use only.

Warning(s): Keep out of reach of children.

Presentation: 1.81 kg (2.5 lb) and 11.34 kg (25 lb).

Compendium Code No.: 15000100 9BB9

VITA E 300

AgriPharm **Vitamin E**

Injectable d-Alpha-Tocopherol

Active Ingredient(s): Each mL contains: 300 IU's of vitamin E (as d-alpha-tocopherol, a natural source of vitamin E) compounded with 2% benzyl alcohol (preservative) in a water emulsifiable base.

Indications: VITA E 300 Injectable Tocopherol (natural-source vitamin E) is a clear, sterile, non-aqueous solution of d-alpha-tocopherol for use as an aid in the prevention of vitamin E deficiencies in swine, cattle, and sheep.

This product is intended as a supplemental source of natural vitamin E.

Dosage and Administration: Intramuscular or subcutaneous use only. If dose is greater than 5 mL, equally divide the dose and inject at two different sites.

Suggested Dosage:	mL	International Units (I.U.)
Swine		
Sows and Gilts 2 wks pre-partum 2 wks pre-breeding	 4-6 4-6	 1200-1800 1200-1800
Pigs At birth Weaning	 1-2 2-3	 300-600 600-900
Cattle (Dairy and Beef)		
Cows and heifers 2 to 3 wks pre-partum At calving	 8-10 8-10	 2400-3000 2400-3000
Calves At birth Weaning	 4-6 4-6	 1200-1800 1200-1800
Yearlings	5-6	1500-1800
Sheep		
Ewes 2-3 wks pre-partum At lambing	 4-5 4-5	 1200-1500 1200-1500
Lambs At birth Weaning	 2-3 2-3	 600-900 600-900
Finishing Lambs	3-4	900-1200

Precaution(s): Store between 2° and 30°C (36° and 86°F) in a dark place.

Caution(s): Do not add water to the solution.

Do not exceed the recommended dosage. Occasionally, reactions of an anaphylactic or allergic nature may occur. Should such reactions occur, treat immediately with injection of epinephrine.

Warning(s): Intramuscular or subcutaneous use only.
Not for human use.
Keep out of the reach of children.
Discussion: Natural tocopherols in feedstuffs can be destroyed through processing, ensiling and storage. A reduced vitamin E intake can result in marginal deficiencies that may not be visible. Intramuscular or subcutaneous injections offer an efficient and rapid method to increase vitamin E status of animals.
Presentation: 250 mL vials.
Compendium Code No.: 14571020

VITA E-AD

AgriPharm **Vitamins A-D-E**

Injectable d-Alpha-Tocopherol with AD

Active Ingredient(s): Each mL contains: 300 IU's of vitamin E (as d-alpha-tocopherol, a natural source of vitamin E); 100,000 IU's vitamin A propionate; 10,000 IU's vitamin D_3; compounded with 2% benzyl alcohol (preservative) in a water emulsifiable base.
Indications: VITA E-AD Injectable d-alpha-tocopherol with AD is a clear, sterile, non-aqueous solution of vitamin A, vitamin D_3, and vitamin E. The product is intended as a supplemental source of vitamin A, D, and E in cattle.
Dosage and Administration: Intramuscular or subcutaneous administration only. If dose is greater than 5 mL, equally divide the dose and inject at two different sites.
Suggested Dosage:
Cattle (Dairy and Beef):
Cows and Heifers:
2-3 wks pre-partum . . . 8-10 mL
At calving . . . 8-10 mL
End of lactation . . . 8-10 mL
Calves:
At birth . . . 4-6 mL
At weaning . . . 4-6 mL
Yearlings . . . 5-6 mL
Precaution(s): Store between 2° and 30°C (36° and 86°F) in a dark place.
Caution(s): Do not add water to the solution.
Do not exceed recommended dosage. Occasionally, reactions of an anaphylactic or allergic nature may occur. Should such reactions occur, treat immediately with injection of epinephrine.
Warning(s): Intramuscular or subcutaneous administration only.
Not for human use.
Keep out of reach of children.
Discussion: Natural vitamin A (carotenes), and tocopherols can be destroyed in feedstuffs through processing, ensiling and storage. Due to these losses, reduced intakes of fat-soluble vitamins can occur in animals maintained in continual confinement compared to animals allowed to graze lush pasture. Intramuscular or subcutaneous injections offer an efficient and rapid method to increase vitamin A, vitamin D and vitamin E status of animals.
Presentation: 250 mL vials.
Compendium Code No.: 14571030

VITA•E & SELENIUM CRUMBLES™

Horse Health **Vitamin E-Selenium**

Vitamin E & Selenium Supplement

Guaranteed Analysis:
Crude Protein, min. . . . 10.0%
Crude Fat, min. . . . 3.5%
Crude Fiber, max. . . . 15.0%
Calcium, min. . . . 8.5%
Calcium, max. . . . 9.5%
Selenium, min. . . . 70 ppm
Vitamin E, min. . . . 20,000 IU/lb
Ingredients: Dehydrated Alfalfa Meal, Wheat Middlings, Ground Limestone, Sodium Selenite, Vitamin E Supplement, Vegetable Oil, Cane Molasses, Propionic and Acetic Acids (preservatives).
Indications: A vitamin E and selenium supplement for all classes of horses.
Directions: Top dress daily grain ration with ¼ to ½ scoop (1 ounce measuring scoop enclosed).
Each ½ ounce contains 1 mg Selenium.
Precaution(s): Store in area inaccessible to children and animals.
Caution(s): Follow label directions. The addition to feed of higher levels of this premix with Selenium is not permitted. Excessive amounts of Selenium may be toxic.
For animal use only.
Warning(s): Keep out of reach of children.
Presentation: 1.13 kg (2.5 lb) and 9.09 kg (20 lb).
Compendium Code No.: 15000090 0D1

VITA FERM® BREEDER BOOSTER+MAG

BioZyme **Large Animal Dietary Supplement**

with the Amaferm® advantage

Guaranteed Analysis:
Crude Protein . . . 7.0% Min.
Crude Fat . . . 1.0% Min.
Crude Fiber . . . 3.0% Max.
Calcium . . . 8.0% Min./9.0% Max.
Phosphorus (P) . . . 6.0% Min.
Salt (NaCl) . . . 9.2% Min./10.2% Max.
Magnesium (Mg) . . . 10.0% Min.
Potassium (K) . . . 2.0% Min.
Cobalt (Co) . . . 40.0 ppm Min.
Copper (Cu) . . . 2,500.0 ppm Min.
Iodine . . . 120.0 ppm Min.
Manganese (Mn) . . . 3,000.0 ppm Min.
Selenium (Se) . . . 26.0 ppm Min.
Zinc (Zn) . . . 5,000.0 ppm Min.
Vitamin A . . . 300,000 IU/lb. Min.
Vitamin D_3 . . . 40,000 IU/lb. Min.
Vitamin E . . . 400 IU/lb. Min.
Vitamin B_{12} . . . 0.013 mg or 13.0 mcg/lb. Min.
Riboflavin . . . 5.5 mg/lb. Min.
d-Pantothenic Acid . . . 8.5 mg/lb. Min.
Thiamine . . . 1.0 mg/lb. Min.
Niacin . . . 50.0 mg/lb. Min.
Choline . . . 500.0 mg/lb. Min.
Ingredients: Monocalcium Phosphate, Dicalcium Phosphate, Corn Distillers Dried Grains with Solubles, Magnesium Oxide, Salt, Calcium Carbonate, Zinc Sulfate, Ferrous Sulfate, Copper Sulfate, Manganese Sulfate, Calcium Iodate, Cobalt Sulfate, Sodium Selenite, Potassium Chloride, Dried *Aspergillus Oryzae* Fermentation Extract, Copper Amino Acid Complex, Cottonseed Meal, Heat Processed Soybean Meal, Vitamin A Supplement, D-Activated Animal Sterol (Source of Vitamin D_3), dl-alpha-tocopheryl Acetate (Source of Vitamin E), Choline Chloride, Niacin, Calcium Pantothenate, Riboflavin, Vitamin B_{12} Supplement, Thiamine Hydrochloride, Mineral Oil.
Indications: Amaferm® blended with vitamins, macro and trace minerals, some protein meals (for palatability). Formulated with key nutrients to optimize cycling and conception, plus high magnesium to help prevent grass tetany.
Dosage and Administration: Feeding Directions: Feed to beef or dairy cattle free-choice at the rate of 4 oz per head, daily. Regulate consumption with salt or protein meals.
Caution(s): Due to the copper level, do not feed to sheep. Follow label directions. The addition of higher levels of selenium is not permitted.
Presentation: 50 lb bags.
Compendium Code No.: 14960150 02/01

VITA FERM® CATTLEMAN'S BEEFMAKER

BioZyme **Large Animal Dietary Supplement**

with the Amaferm® advantage

Guaranteed Analysis:
Crude Protein . . . 9.5% Min.
Crude Fat . . . 1.0% Min.
Crude Fiber . . . 3.5% Max.
Calcium . . . 11.0% Min./12.0% Max.
Phosphorus (P) . . . 4.0% Min.
Salt (NaCl) . . . 13.5% Min./15.5% Max.
Magnesium (Mg) . . . 2.0% Min.
Potassium (K) . . . 1.0% Min.
Cobalt (Co) . . . 25.0 ppm Min.
Copper (Cu) . . . 640.0 ppm Min.
Iodine . . . 50.0 ppm Min.
Manganese (Mn) . . . 1,900.0 ppm Min.
Selenium (Se) . . . 16.0 ppm Min.
Zinc (Zn) . . . 2,350.0 ppm Min.
Vitamin A . . . 190,000 IU/lb. Min.
Vitamin D_3 . . . 10,000 IU/lb. Min.
Vitamin E . . . 100 IU/lb. Min.
Ingredients: Corn Distillers Dried Grains with Solubles, Calcium Carbonate, Monocalcium Phosphate, Dicalcium Phosphate, Salt, Magnesium Oxide, Zinc Sulfate, Ferrous Sulfate, Copper Sulfate, Manganese Sulfate, Calcium Iodate, Cobalt Sulfate, Sodium Selenite, Dried *Aspergillus Oryzae* Fermentation Extract, Potassium Chloride, Mineral Oil, Vitamin A Supplement, D-Activated Animal Sterol (Source of Vitamin D_3), dl-alpha-tocopheryl Acetate (Source of Vitamin E).
Indications: An Amaferm®-based, vitamin and mineral mix designed to fill basic nutrient needs of cattle on fair to good-quality forage. Ideally suited for background and yearling cattle on grass, but can be used for cows as well.
Dosage and Administration: Feeding Directions: Feed to beef cattle at the rate of 4 oz per head, daily. Use salt or protein meals to regulate consumption.
Caution(s): Due to the copper level, do not feed to sheep. Follow label directions. The addition of higher levels of selenium is not permitted.
Presentation: 50 lb bags.
Compendium Code No.: 14960160 05/00

VITA FERM® CATTLEMAN'S BEEFMAKER+MAG

BioZyme **Large Animal Dietary Supplement**

with the Amaferm® advantage

Guaranteed Analysis:
Crude Protein . . . 9.5% Min.
Crude Fat . . . 1.0% Min.
Crude Fiber . . . 3.5% Max.
Calcium . . . 7.5% Min./8.5% Max.
Phosphorus (P) . . . 4.0% Min.
Salt (NaCl) . . . 8.0% Min./9.0% Max.
Magnesium (Mg) . . . 11.5% Min.
Cobalt (Co) . . . 25.0 ppm Min.
Copper (Cu) . . . 640.0 ppm Min.
Iodine . . . 50.0 ppm Min.
Manganese (Mn) . . . 1,900.0 ppm Min.
Selenium (Se) . . . 16.0 ppm Min.
Zinc (Zn) . . . 2,300.0 ppm Min.
Vitamin A . . . 200,000 IU/lb. Min.
Vitamin D_3 . . . 10,000 IU/lb. Min.
Vitamin E . . . 100 IU/lb. Min.
Ingredients: Corn Distillers Dried Grains with Solubles, Magnesium Oxide, Monocalcium Phosphate, Dicalcium Phosphate, Calcium Carbonate, Salt, Zinc Sulfate, Ferrous Sulfate, Copper Sulfate, Manganese Sulfate, Calcium Iodate, Cobalt Sulfate, Sodium Selenite, Dried *Aspergillus Oryzae* Fermentation Extract, Mineral Oil, Vitamin A Supplement, D-Activated Animal Sterol (Source of Vitamin D_3), dl-alpha-tocopheryl Acetate (Source of Vitamin E), Choline Chloride, Niacin, Calcium Pantothenate, Riboflavin, Vitamin B_{12} Supplement, Thiamine Hydrochloride.
Indications: An Amaferm®-based, vitamin and mineral mix designed to fill basic nutrient needs of cattle grazing lush pastures or small grain forages. Ideally suited for background and yearling cattle, but can be used for cows as well.
Dosage and Administration: Feeding Directions: Feed to beef cattle at the rate of 4 oz per head, daily. Use salt or protein meals to regulate consumption.
Caution(s): Due to the copper level, do not feed to sheep. Follow label directions. The addition of higher levels of selenium is not permitted.
Presentation: 50 lb bags.
Compendium Code No.: 14960170 05/00

VITA FERM® CONCEPT-AID

BioZyme **Large Animal Dietary Supplement**
with the Amaferm® advantage
Guaranteed Analysis:

Crude Protein	9.0% Min.
Crude Fat	2.0% Min.
Crude Fiber	2.0% Max.
Calcium	10.0% Min.
Phosphorus (P)	10.0% Min.
Magnesium (Mg)	2.5% Min.
Potassium (K)	4.0% Min.
Cobalt (Co)	40.0 ppm Min.
Copper (Cu)	1,290.0 ppm Min.
Iodine	80.0 ppm Min.
Manganese (Mn)	3,750.0 ppm Min.
Selenium (Se)	27.0 ppm Min.
Zinc (Zn)	4,650.0 ppm Min.
Vitamin A	400,000 IU/lb. Min.
Vitamin D_3	40,000 IU/lb. Min.
Vitamin E	400 IU/lb. Min.
Vitamin B_{12}	0.019 mg Min.
Riboflavin	7.0 mg/lb. Min.
d-Pantothenic Acid	10.0 mg/lb. Min.
Niacin	65.0 mg/lb. Min.
Choline	575.0 mg/lb. Min.

Ingredients: Monocalcium Phosphate, Dicalcium Phosphate, Heat Processed Soybean Meal, Corn Distillers Dried Grains with Solubles, Potassium Chloride, Calcium Carbonate, Magnesium Oxide, Zinc Sulfate, Ferrous Sulfate, Copper Sulfate, Manganese Sulfate, Calcium Iodate, Cobalt Sulfate, Sodium Selenite, Cottonseed Meal, Yeast Culture, Dried *Aspergillus Oryzae* Fermentation Extract, Potassium Sulfate, Zinc Proteinate, Manganese Proteinate, Copper Proteinate, Vitamin A Supplement, D-Activated Animal Sterol (Source of Vitamin D_3), dl-alpha-tocopheryl Acetate (Source of Vitamin E), Choline Chloride, Niacin, Calcium Pantothenate, Riboflavin, Vitamin B_{12} Supplement, Thiamine Hydrochloride.

Indications: Amaferm® blended with a highly fortified, complete vitamin, mineral, proteinated trace mineral formulas specifically designed to target cycling, egg production and conception. A premier breeding mineral for all breeding age cows, heifers and bulls; especially beneficial in intensive A.I. and E.T. breeding environments.

Dosage and Administration: Feeding Directions: Feed at the recommended rate of 4 oz per head, daily. If fed free-choice, regulate consumption with salt or protein meals.

Caution(s): Due to the copper level, do not feed to sheep. Follow label directions. The addition of higher levels of selenium is not permitted.

Presentation: 50 lb bags.

Compendium Code No.: 14960180 05/00

VITA FERM® CONCEPT-AID+MAG

BioZyme **Large Animal Dietary Supplement**
with the Amaferm® advantage
Guaranteed Analysis:

Crude Protein	9.0% Min.
Crude Fat	3.5% Min.
Crude Fiber	2.5% Max.
Calcium	8.5% Min.
Phosphorus (P)	10.0% Min.
Magnesium (Mg)	8.0% Min.
Potassium (K)	4.0% Min.
Cobalt (Co)	40.0 ppm Min.
Copper (Cu)	1,300 ppm Min.
Iodine	80.0 ppm Min.
Manganese (Mn)	3,650.0 ppm Min.
Selenium (Se)	26.0 ppm Min.
Zinc (Zn)	4,650.0 ppm Min.
Vitamin A	400,000 IU/lb. Min.
Vitamin D_3	40,000 IU/lb. Min.
Vitamin E	400 IU/lb. Min.
Vitamin B_{12}	0.014 mg/lb. Min.
Riboflavin	5.0 mg/lb. Min.
d-Pantothenic Acid	9.50 mg/lb. Min.
Niacin	50.0 mg/lb. Min.
Choline	500.0 mg/lb. Min.

Ingredients: Monocalcium Phosphate, Dicalcium Phosphate, Heat Processed Soybean Meal, Corn Distillers Dried Grains with Solubles, Potassium Chloride, Calcium Carbonate, Magnesium Oxide, Zinc Sulfate, Ferrous Sulfate, Copper Sulfate, Manganese Sulfate, Calcium Iodate, Cobalt Sulfate, Sodium Selenite, Cottonseed Meal, Yeast Culture, Dried *Aspergillus Oryzae* Fermentation Extract, Potassium Sulfate, Zinc Proteinate, Manganese Proteinate, Copper Proteinate, Vitamin A Supplement, D-Activated Animal Sterol (Source of Vitamin D_3), dl-alpha-tocopheryl Acetate (Source of Vitamin E), Choline Chloride, Niacin, Calcium Pantothenate, Riboflavin, Vitamin B_{12} Supplement, Thiamine Hydrochloride.

Indications: Amaferm® blended with a highly fortified, complete vitamin, mineral, proteinated trace mineral formulas specifically designed to target cycling, egg production and conception. A premier breeding mineral for all breeding age cows, heifers and bulls; especially beneficial in intensive A.I. and E.T. breeding environments.

Dosage and Administration: Feeding Directions: Feed at the recommended rate of 4 oz per head, daily. If fed free-choice, regulate consumption with salt or protein meals.

Caution(s): Due to the copper level, do not feed to sheep. Follow label directions. The addition of higher levels of selenium is not permitted.

Presentation: 50 lb bags.

Compendium Code No.: 14960190 05/00

VITA FERM® CONCEPT-AID A•P

BioZyme **Large Animal Dietary Supplement**
with the Amaferm® advantage
Guaranteed Analysis:

Crude Protein	9.0% Min.
Crude Fat	2.0% Min.
Crude Fiber	4.0% Max.
Magnesium (Mg)	4.0% Min.
Potassium (K)	5.0% Min.
Cobalt (Co)	88.0 ppm Min.
Copper (Cu)	2,600.0 ppm Min.
Iodine	160.0 ppm Min.
Manganese (Mn)	7,800.0 ppm Min.
Selenium (Se)	20.0 ppm Min.
Zinc (Zn)	9,750.0 ppm Min.
Vitamin A	1,000,000 IU/lb Min.
Vitamin D_3	200,000 IU/lb Min.
Vitamin E	1,600 IU/lb Min.
Vitamin B_{12}	0.070 mg/lb or 70.0 mcg/lb Min.
Riboflavin	20.0 mg/lb Min.
d-Pantothenic Acid	40.0 mg/lb Min.
Niacin	200.0 mg/lb Min.
Choline	1,200.0 mg/lb Min.

Ingredients: Potassium sulfate, yeast culture, corn distillers dried grains with solubles, wheat midds, dried *Aspergillus oryzae* fermentation extract, monocalcium phosphate, dicalcium phosphate, calcium carbonate, zinc sulfate, ferrous sulfate, copper sulfate, manganese sulfate, calcium iodate, cobalt sulfate, sodium selenite, zinc proteinate, manganese proteinate, copper proteinate, vitamin A supplement, d-activated animal sterol (source of vitamin D_3), dl-alpha-tocopherol acetate (source of vitamin E), choline chloride, niacin, calcium pantothenate, riboflavin, vitamin B_{12} supplement, thiamine hydrochloride, magnesium oxide, mineral oil, potassium chloride, active dry yeast, cobalt carbonate.

Indications: Amaferm® blended with highly fortified, proteinated trace minerals and vitamins specifically designed to target cycling, egg production and conception. Also excellent for use in high-stress situations such as weaning and pre-conditioning.

Dosage and Administration: Feeding Directions: Feed 1 ounce per head per day if fed without other Vita Ferm® products; ½ ounce hd/day if fed with other Vita Ferm® products.

Caution(s): Due to the copper level, do not feed to sheep. Follow label directions. The addition of higher levels of selenium is not permitted.

Presentation: 50 lb bags.

Compendium Code No.: 14960052 05/00

VITA FERM® COW CALF 5

BioZyme **Large Animal Dietary Supplement**
with the Amaferm® advantage
Guaranteed Analysis:

Crude Protein	12.0% Min.
Crude Fat	1.4% Min.
Crude Fiber	5.0% Max.
Calcium	5.5% Min./6.5% Max.
Phosphorus (P)	5.0% Min.
Salt (NaCl)	18.5% Min./22.0% Max.
Magnesium (Mg)	2.0% Min.
Potassium (K)	2.0% Min.
Cobalt (Co)	40.0 ppm Min.
Copper (Cu)	1,000.0 ppm Min.
Iodine	80.0 ppm Min.
Manganese (Mn)	3,000.0 ppm Min.
Selenium (Se)	25.0 ppm Min.
Zinc (Zn)	3,500.0 ppm Min.
Vitamin A	400,000 IU/lb. Min.
Vitamin D_3	40,000 IU/lb. Min.
Vitamin E	200 IU/lb. Min.
Vitamin B_{12}	0.018 mg or 18.0 mcg/lb. Min.
Riboflavin	7.0 mg/lb. Min.
d-Pantothenic Acid	12.0 mg/lb. Min.
Thiamine	1.5 mg/lb. Min.
Niacin	64.0 mg/lb. Min.
Choline	740.0 mg/lb. Min.

Ingredients: Corn Distillers Dried Grains with Solubles, Monocalcium Phosphate, Dicalcium Phosphate, Salt, Zinc Sulfate, Ferrous Sulfate, Copper Sulfate, Manganese Sulfate, Calcium Iodate, Cobalt Sulfate, Sodium Selenite, Calcium Carbonate, Heat Processed Soybean Meal, Magnesium Oxide, Potassium Chloride, Dried *Aspergillus Oryzae* Fermentation Extract, Potassium Sulfate, Vitamin A Supplement, D-Activated Animal Sterol (Source of Vitamin D_3), dl-alpha-tocopheryl Acetate (Source of Vitamin E), Choline Chloride, Niacin, Calcium Pantothenate, Riboflavin, Vitamin B_{12} Supplement, Thiamine Hydrochloride.

Indications: Amaferm® blended with vitamins, macro and trace minerals, protein meals (for palatability) and salt added for free-choice use. A highly versatile and highly palatable, all-purpose, free-choice mineral for cattle of all ages.

Dosage and Administration: Feeding Directions: Feed to beef or dairy cattle at the rate of 4 oz per head, daily. Regulate consumption with salt or protein meals.

Caution(s): Due to the copper level, do not feed to sheep. Follow label directions. The addition of higher levels of selenium is not permitted.

Presentation: 50 lb bags.

Compendium Code No.: 14960200 10/01

VITA FERM® DAIRY BASEMIX 12:16

BioZyme **Large Animal Dietary Supplement**
with the Amaferm® advantage
Guaranteed Analysis:

Calcium	11.5% Min./13.8% Max.
Phosphorus (P)	16.0% Min.
Magnesium (Mg)	3.0% Min.
Potassium (K)	3.0% Min.
Copper (Cu)	1,000.0 ppm Min.
Manganese (Mn)	3,500.0 ppm Min.
Selenium (Se)	27.0 ppm Min.
Zinc (Zn)	4,000.0 ppm Min.
Vitamin A	460,000 IU/lb. Min.
Vitamin D_3	60,000 IU/lb. Min.
Vitamin E	1,200 IU/lb. Min.
Vitamin B_{12}	0.020 mg or 20.0 mcg/lb. Min.
Riboflavin	8.0 mg/lb. Min.

V

d-Pantothenic Acid . . . . . 10.0 mg/lb. Min.
Thiamine . . . . . 1.5 mg/lb. Min.
Niacin . . . . . 75.0 mg/lb. Min.
Choline . . . . . 375.0 mg/lb. Min.

Ingredients: Monocalcium Phosphate, Dicalcium Phosphate, Monosodium Phosphate, Heat Processed Soybean Meal, Potassium Chloride, Magnesium Oxide, Zinc Sulfate, Ferrous Sulfate, Copper Sulfate, Manganese Sulfate, Calcium Iodate, Cobalt Sulfate, Sodium Selenite, Dried *Aspergillus Oryzae* Fermentation Extract, Vitamin A Supplement, D-Activated Animal Sterol (Source of Vitamin D_3), dl-alpha-tocopheryl Acetate (Source of Vitamin E), Choline Chloride, Niacin, Calcium Pantothenate, Riboflavin, Vitamin B_{12} Supplement, Thiamine Hydrochloride, Potassium Sulfate, Magnesium Sulfate, Mineral Oil.

Indications: Amaferm® blended with a complete vitamin/mineral basemix for on-farm ration mixing. One of three Vita Ferm® basemixes available; formulated with varying calcium to phosphorus ratios to balance a variety of grass, legume and grain combinations. For lactating dairy cows.

Dosage and Administration: Feeding Directions: Basemix 12:16 is designed to be used in lactating dairy cow rations that contain forages from legume and grain silage sources. Rations containing a legume to grain silage forage ratio (dry matter basis) of from 2:1 to 1:2 are acceptable for the use of 12:16. Provide 7 oz per adult animal, daily, in the grain mix or complete ration.

Caution(s): Due to the copper level, do not feed to sheep. Follow label directions. The addition of higher levels of selenium is not permitted.

Presentation: 50 lb bags.

Compendium Code No.: 14960210 05/00

VITA FERM® DAIRY BASEMIX 18:6

BioZyme **Large Animal Dietary Supplement**

with the Amaferm® advantage

Guaranteed Analysis:

Calcium . . . . . 17.0% Min./20.0% Max.
Phosphorus (P) . . . . . 6.0% Min.
Salt (NaCl) . . . . . 9.2% Min./11.0% Max.
Magnesium (Mg) . . . . . 4.2% Min.
Potassium (K) . . . . . 4.2% Min.
Cobalt (Co) . . . . . 25.0 ppm Min.
Copper (Cu) . . . . . 650.0 ppm Min.
Manganese (Mn) . . . . . 2,000.0 ppm Min.
Selenium (Se) . . . . . 16.5 ppm Min.
Zinc (Zn) . . . . . 2,500.0 ppm Min.
Vitamin A . . . . . 270,000 IU/lb. Min.
Vitamin D_3 . . . . . 30,000 IU/lb. Min.
Vitamin E . . . . . 680 IU/lb. Min.
Vitamin B_{12} . . . . . 0.010 mg or 10.0 mcg/lb. Min.
Riboflavin . . . . . 4.5 mg/lb. Min.
d-Pantothenic Acid . . . . . 7.5 mg/lb. Min.
Thiamine . . . . . 1.0 mg/lb. Min.
Niacin . . . . . 80.0 mg/lb. Min.
Choline . . . . . 200.0 mg/lb. Min.

Ingredients: Calcium Carbonate, Monocalcium Phosphate, Dicalcium Phosphate, Salt, Heat Processed Soybean Meal, Potassium Chloride, Magnesium Oxide, Zinc Sulfate, Ferrous Sulfate, Copper Sulfate, Manganese Sulfate, Calcium Iodate, Cobalt Sulfate, Sodium Selenite, Dried *Aspergillus Oryzae* Fermentation Extract, Vitamin A Supplement, D-Activated Animal Sterol (Source of Vitamin D_3), dl-alpha-tocopheryl Acetate (Source of Vitamin E), Choline Chloride, Niacin, Calcium Pantothenate, Riboflavin, Vitamin B_{12} Supplement, Thiamine Hydrochloride, Potassium Sulfate, Magnesium Sulfate, Mineral Oil.

Indications: Amaferm® blended with a complete vitamin/mineral basemix for on-farm ration mixing. One of three Vita Ferm® basemixes available; formulated with varying calcium to phosphorus ratios to balance a variety of grass, legume and grain combinations. For lactating dairy cows.

Dosage and Administration: Feeding Directions: Basemix 18:6 is designed for use in lactating dairy cow rations which consist of forages primarily from grain silage sources. Rations containing a legume to grain silage ratio of 1:3 (dry matter basis) or less are recommended for the use of 18:6. Provide 12 oz per adult animal, daily, in the grain mix or complete ration.

Caution(s): Due to the copper level, do not feed to sheep. Follow label directions. The addition of higher levels of selenium is not permitted.

Presentation: 50 lb bags.

Compendium Code No.: 14960220 05/00

VITA FERM® DAIRY BASEMIX 18:12

BioZyme **Large Animal Dietary Supplement**

with the Amaferm® advantage

Guaranteed Analysis:

Calcium . . . . . 16.5% Min./19.8% Max.
Phosphorus (P) . . . . . 12.0% Min.
Magnesium (Mg) . . . . . 1.5% Min.
Potassium (K) . . . . . 1.8% Min.
Cobalt (Co) . . . . . 40.0 ppm Min.
Copper (Cu) . . . . . 1,000.0 ppm Min.
Manganese (Mn) . . . . . 3,500.0 ppm Min.
Selenium (Se) . . . . . 27.0 ppm Min.
Sulfur (S) . . . . . 6,000.0 ppm Min.
Zinc (Zn) . . . . . 4,000.0 ppm Min.
Vitamin A . . . . . 460,000 IU/lb. Min.
Vitamin D_3 . . . . . 60,000 IU/lb. Min.
Vitamin E . . . . . 1,200 IU/lb. Min.
Vitamin B_{12} . . . . . 0.020 mg or 20.0 mcg/lb. Min.
Riboflavin . . . . . 8.0 mg/lb. Min.
d-Pantothenic Acid . . . . . 10.0 mg/lb. Min.
Thiamine . . . . . 1.5 mg/lb. Min.
Niacin . . . . . 75.0 mg/lb. Min.
Choline . . . . . 375.0 mg/lb. Min.

Ingredients: Monocalcium Phosphate, Dicalcium Phosphate, Calcium Carbonate, Heat Processed Soybean Meal, Zinc Sulfate, Ferrous Sulfate, Copper Sulfate, Manganese Sulfate, Calcium Iodate, Cobalt Sulfate, Sodium Selenite, Potassium Sulfate, Magnesium Sulfate, Potassium Chloride, Magnesium Oxide, Dried *Aspergillus Oryzae* Fermentation Extract, Mineral Oil, Vitamin A Supplement, D-Activated Animal Sterol (Source of Vitamin D_3), dl-alpha-tocopheryl Acetate (Source of Vitamin E), Choline Chloride, Niacin, Calcium Pantothenate, Riboflavin, Vitamin B_{12} Supplement, Thiamine Hydrochloride.

Indications: Amaferm® blended with a complete vitamin/mineral basemix for on-farm ration mixing. One of three Vita Ferm® basemixes available; formulated with varying calcium to phosphorus ratios to balance a variety of grass, legume and grain combinations. For lactating dairy cows.

Dosage and Administration: Feeding Directions: Feed to dairy cattle at the rate of 7 oz per head, daily. Free-choice salt should be provided as Basemix 18:12 contains no salt.

Caution(s): Due to the copper level, do not feed to sheep. Follow label directions. The addition of higher levels of selenium is not permitted.

Presentation: 50 lb bags.

Compendium Code No.: 14960230 05/00

VITA FERM® EQUINE

BioZyme **Equine Dietary Supplement**

with the Amaferm® advantage

Guaranteed Analysis:

		App. per 4 oz
Crude Protein	14.0% Min.	18.1 g
Crude Fat	1.5% Min.	1.7 g
Crude Fiber	5.5% Max.	6.0 g
Calcium (Ca)	5.0% Min./6.0% Max.	6.4 g
Phosphorus (P)	4.5% Min.	5.1 g
Salt (NaCl)	12.0% Min./14.0% Max.	14.8 g
Magnesium (Mg)	1.0% Min.	1.1 g
Potassium (K)	2.0% Min.	2.3 g
Cobalt (Co)	40.0 ppm Min.	4.5 mg
Copper (Cu)	1,000.0 ppm Min.	112.0 mg
Iodine	39.0 ppm Min.	4.5 mg
Iron (Fe)	2,300.0 ppm Min.	261.0 mg
Manganese (Mn)	3,000 ppm Min.	350.0 mg
Selenium (Se)	26.0 ppm Min.	2.5 mg
Zinc (Zn)	3,700.0 ppm Min.	400.0 mg
Vitamin A	250,000 IU/lb. Min.	62,500 IU
Vitamin D_3	20,000 IU/lb. Min.	5,000 IU
Vitamin E	1,500 IU/lb. Min.	375 IU
Vitamin B_{12}	600 mcg/lb. Min.	150.0 mcg
Menadione (Vitamin K)	10.0 mg/lb. Min.	2.5 mg
Riboflavin	200.0 mg/lb. Min.	50.0 mg
d-Pantothenic Acid	400.0 mg/lb. Min.	100.0 mg
Thiamine	250.0 mg/lb. Min.	60.0 mg
Pyridoxine Hydrochloride	60.0 mg/lb. Min.	15.0 mg
Niacin	970.0 mg/lb. Min.	240.0 mg
Folic Acid	20.0 mg/lb. Min.	5.0 mg
Choline	1,000.0 mg/lb. Min.	250.0 mg
Biotin	12.0 mg/lb. Min.	3.0 mg

Ingredients: Monocalcium Phosphate, Dicalcium Phosphate, Corn Distillers Dried Grains with Solubles, Cottonseed Meal, Wheat Midds, Salt, Heat Processed Soybean Meal, Zinc Sulfate, Ferrous Sulfate, Copper Sulfate, Manganese Sulfate, Calcium Iodate, Cobalt Sulfate, Sodium Selenite, Potassium Chloride, Calcium Carbonate, Vitamin A Supplement, D-Activated Animal Sterol (Source of Vitamin D_3), dl-alpha-Tocopheryl Acetate (Source of Vitamin E), Choline Chloride, Niacin, Calcium Pantothenate, Riboflavin, Vitamin B_{12} Supplement, Thiamine Hydrochloride, Folic Acid, Menadione Dimethylprimidinol Bisulfate (source of Vitamin K), Pyridoxine Hydrochloride, Ascorbic Acid, Biotin, Dried *Aspergillus Oryzae* Fermentation Extract, Magnesium Oxide, Yeast Culture.

Indications: Amaferm® blended with vitamins, macro and trace minerals and some protein meals (for palatability). Designed for all horses: work, show, pleasure, breeding and racing. Formulated to meet the nutrition needs of the active horse.

Dosage and Administration: Feeding Directions: Feed as a top-dress on grains or as free-choice in pasture. Feed at the rate of 4 oz per adult horse, daily.

Note: May overconsume if fed free-choice; use salt to control consumption.

Caution(s): Due to the copper level, do not feed to sheep. Follow label directions. The addition of higher levels of selenium is not permitted.

Presentation: 50 lb bags.

Compendium Code No.: 14960240 05/00

VITA FERM® EWE AND LAMB

BioZyme **Dietary Supplement**

with the Amaferm® advantage

Guaranteed Analysis:

Crude Protein . . . . . 13.5% Min.
Crude Fat . . . . . 2.0% Min.
Crude Fiber . . . . . 6.0% Max.
Calcium (Ca) . . . . . 5.0% Min./6.0% Max.
Phosphorus (P) . . . . . 5.0% Min.
Salt (NaCl) . . . . . 12.5% Min./15.0% Max.
Magnesium (Mg) . . . . . 2.0% Min.
Potassium (K) . . . . . 2.5% Min.
Cobalt (Co) . . . . . 15.0 ppm Min.
Iodine . . . . . 33.0 ppm Min.
Manganese (Mn) . . . . . 140.0 ppm Min.
Selenium (Se) . . . . . 8.0 ppm Min.
Zinc (Zn) . . . . . 1,000.0 ppm Min.
Vitamin A . . . . . 300,000 IU/lb. Min.

Vitamin D_3	38,000 IU/lb. Min.
Vitamin E	800 IU/lb. Min.
Riboflavin	7.0 mg/lb. Min.
d-Pantothenic Acid	13.0 mg/lb. Min.
Thiamine	2.0 mg/lb. Min.
Niacin	64.0 mg/lb. Min.
Choline	650.0 mg/lb. Min.

Ingredients: Monocalcium Phosphate, Dicalcium Phosphate, Wheat Midds, Cottonseed Meal, Corn Distillers Dried Grains with Solubles, Salt, Heat Processed Soybean Meal, Calcium Carbonate, Potassium Chloride, Magnesium Oxide, Yeast Culture, Potassium Sulfate, Dried *Aspergillus Oryzae* Fermentation Extract, Zinc Sulfate, Ferrous Sulfate, Manganese Sulfate, Cobalt Sulfate, Calcium Iodate, Sodium Selenite, Vitamin A Supplement, D-Activated Animal Sterol (Source of Vitamin D_3), dl-alpha-Tocopheryl Acetate (Source of Vitamin E), Choline Chloride, Niacin, Calcium Pantothenate, Riboflavin, Vitamin B_{12} Supplement, Thiamine Hydrochloride.

Indications: Amaferm® blended with vitamins, macro and trace minerals, and protein meals formulated to meet the nutrition needs of sheep consuming primarily forages. Designed for sheep of all ages and production levels.

Dosage and Administration: Feeding Directions: Feed to sheep at the rate of 1 to 1.5 oz per adult animal, daily. Can be fed free-choice on pasture or top-dressed on grain. Use salt to control free-choice consumption.

Caution(s): Follow label directions. The addition of higher levels of selenium is not permitted.

Presentation: 50 lb bags.

Compendium Code No.: 14960250 05/00

VITA FERM® FAR OUT DRY COW

BioZyme **Large Animal Dietary Supplement**

with the Amaferm® advantage

Guaranteed Analysis:

Crude Protein	12.5% Min.
Crude Fat	3.0% Min.
Crude Fiber	4.0% Max.
Calcium	7.2% Min./8.6% Max.
Phosphorus (P)	7.0% Min.
Magnesium (Mg)	1.4% Min.
Potassium (K)	2.0% Min.
Copper (Cu)	700.0 ppm Min.
Iodine	16.0 ppm Min.
Manganese (Mn)	3,000.0 ppm Min.
Selenium (Se)	20.0 ppm Min.
Zinc (Zn)	2,900.0 ppm Min.
Vitamin A	300,000 IU/lb. Min.
Vitamin D_3	80,000 IU/lb. Min.
Vitamin E	1,500 IU/lb. Min.

Ingredients: Monocalcium Phosphate, Dicalcium Phosphate, Corn Distillers Dried Grains with Solubles, Heat Processed Soybean Meal, Potassium Sulfate, Wheat Midds, Calcium Carbonate, Sodium Selenite, Yeast Culture, Manganese Sulfate, Dried *Aspergillus Oryzae* Fermentation Extract, Zinc Sulfate, dl-Alpha-Tocopheryl Acetate (Source of Vitamin E), D-Activated Animal Sterol (Source of Vitamin D_3), Vitamin A Supplement, Choline Chloride, Niacin, Calcium Pantothenate, Riboflavin, Vitamin B_{12} Supplement, Thiamine Hydrochloride, Ferrous Sulfate, Copper Sulfate, Calcium Iodate, Cobalt Sulfate, Mineral Oil.

Indications: Amaferm® blended with high levels of quality vitamins and trace minerals. Formulated to supply the correct nutrient balance for dairy cows receiving a recommended, grass haylage diet. Designed for dry dairy cows up until 30 days prior to freshening.

Dosage and Administration: Feeding Directions: Feed to dairy cows at a rate of 0.5 lb per head, daily, up until 30 days prior to freshening.

Caution(s): Due to the copper level, do not feed to sheep. Follow label directions. The addition of higher levels of selenium is not permitted.

Presentation: 50 lb bags.

Compendium Code No.: 14960260 05/00

VITA FERM® FEEDLOT FORMULA

BioZyme **Large Animal Dietary Supplement**

with the Amaferm® advantage

Guaranteed Analysis:

Calcium	18.0% Min./21.6% Max.
Phosphorus (P)	4.0% Min.
Magnesium (Mg)	1.0% Min.
Potassium (K)	1.8% Min.
Cobalt (Co)	4.0 ppm Min.
Copper (Cu)	200.0 ppm Min.
Iodine	80.0 ppm Min.
Manganese (Mn)	2,200.0 ppm Min.
Selenium (Se)	15.5 ppm Min.
Vitamin A	60,000 IU/lb. Min.
Vitamin D_3	8,000 IU/lb. Min.
Vitamin E	200 IU/lb. Min.

Ingredients: Calcium Carbonate, Sodium Sesquicarbonate, Monocalcium Phosphate, Dicalcium Phosphate, Potassium Sulfate, Dried *Aspergillus Oryzae* Fermentation Extract, Potassium Chloride, Sodium Selenite, Mineral Oil, Zinc Sulfate, Ferrous Sulfate, Copper Sulfate, Manganese Sulfate, Calcium Iodate, Cobalt Sulfate, D-Activated Animal Sterol (Source of Vitamin D_3), dl-alpha-tocopheryl Acetate (Source of Vitamin E), Vitamin A Supplement, Vitamin B_{12} Supplement, Choline Chloride, Niacin, Calcium Pantothenate, Riboflavin, Thiamine Hydrochloride.

Indications: An Amaferm®-based, vitamin and mineral mix designed to balance the nutrient requirements of diets for fattening cattle.

Dosage and Administration: Feeding Directions: Feed to beef cattle at the rate of 4 oz per head, daily, incorporated in a prepared feed.

Caution(s): Due to the copper level, do not feed to sheep. Follow label directions. The addition of higher levels of selenium is not permitted.

Presentation: 50 lb bags.

Compendium Code No.: 14960270 11/01

VITA FERM® FESCUE FIBER BUSTER

BioZyme **Large Animal Dietary Supplement**

with the Amaferm® advantage

Guaranteed Analysis:

Crude Protein	7.0% Min.
Crude Fat	0.5% Min.
Crude Fiber	3.0% Max.
Calcium	12.0% Min./13.0% Max.
Phosphorus (P)	6.0% Min.
Salt (NaCl)	9.0% Min./10.0% Max.
Magnesium (Mg)	2.0% Min.
Potassium (K)	3.0% Min.
Cobalt (Co)	40.0 ppm Min.
Copper (Cu)	2,500.0 ppm Min.
Iodine	120.0 ppm Min.
Manganese (Mn)	3,000.0 ppm Min.
Selenium (Se)	27.0 ppm Min.
Zinc (Zn)	5,000.0 ppm Min.
Vitamin A	450,000 IU/lb. Min.
Vitamin D_3	40,000 IU/lb. Min.
Vitamin E	400 IU/lb. Min.
Vitamin B_{12}	0.017 mg or 17.0 mcg/lb. Min.
Riboflavin	7.0 mg/lb. Min.
d-Pantothenic Acid	11.0 mg/lb. Min.
Thiamine	1.5 mg/lb. Min.
Niacin	64.0 mg/lb. Min.
Choline	550.0 mg/lb. Min.

Ingredients: Monocalcium Phosphate, Dicalcium Phosphate, Corn Distillers Dried Grains with Solubles, Calcium Carbonate, Salt, Potassium Chloride, Magnesium Oxide, Zinc Sulfate, Ferrous Sulfate, Copper Sulfate, Manganese Sulfate, Calcium Iodate, Cobalt Sulfate, Sodium Selenite, Dried *Aspergillus Oryzae* Fermentation Extract, Copper Amino Acid Complex, Cottonseed Meal, Vitamin A Supplement, D-Activated Animal Sterol (Source of Vitamin D_3), dl-alpha-tocopheryl Acetate (Source of Vitamin E), Choline Chloride, Niacin, Calcium Pantothenate, Riboflavin, Vitamin B_{12} Supplement, Thiamine Hydrochloride, Heat Processed Soybean Meal.

Indications: Amaferm® blended with vitamins, macro and trace minerals, some protein meals (for palatability). Formulated to provide nutrients lacking in fescue forages and to help offset the effects of high endophyte fescue, pasture and hay.

Dosage and Administration: Feeding Directions: Feed to beef or dairy cattle free-choice at the rate of 4 oz per head, daily. Regulate consumption with salt or protein meals.

Caution(s): Due to the copper level, do not feed to sheep. Follow label directions. The addition of higher levels of selenium is not permitted.

Presentation: 50 lb bags.

Compendium Code No.: 14960280 11/01

VITA FERM® FESCUE POWER KEG

BioZyme **Large Animal Dietary Supplement**

with the Amaferm® advantage

Guaranteed Analysis:

Crude Protein	20.0% Min.
Crude Fat	2.5% Min.
Crude Fiber	3.0% Max.
Calcium	3.5% Min./4.5% Max.
Phosphorus (P)	3.0% Min.
Salt (NaCl)	6.0% Min./7.0% Max.
Magnesium (Mg)	4.5% Min.
Potassium (K)	1.5% Min.
Cobalt (Co)	8.0 ppm Min.
Copper (Cu)	630.0 ppm Min.
Iodine	38.0 ppm Min.
Manganese (Mn)	760.0 ppm Min.
Selenium (Se)	5.1 ppm Min.
Zinc (Zn)	2,400.0 ppm Min.
Vitamin A	100,000 IU/lb. Min.
Vitamin D_3	20,000 IU/lb. Min.
Vitamin E	120 IU/lb. Min.
Vitamin B_{12}	0.0030 mg or 3.0 mcg/lb. Min.
Riboflavin	2.5 mg/lb. Min.
d-Pantothenic Acid	4.7 mg/lb. Min.
Thiamine	0.80 mg/lb. Min.
Niacin	26.0 mg/lb. Min.
Choline	745.0 mg/lb. Min.

Ingredients: Condensed Fermented Corn Extractives, Corn Distillers Dried Grains with Solubles, Soybean Meal, Monocalcium Phosphate, Dicalcium Phosphate, Heat Processed Soybean Meal, Magnesium Oxide, Calcium Sulfate, Salt, Cottonseed Meal, Potassium Chloride, Zinc Sulfate, Ferrous Sulfate, Copper Sulfate, Manganese Sulfate, Calcium Iodate, Cobalt Sulfate Sodium Selenite, Calcium Carbonate, Dried *Aspergillus Oryzae* Fermentation Extract, Vitamin A Supplement, D-Activated Animal Sterol (Source of Vitamin D_3), dl-alpha-tocopheryl Acetate (Source of Vitamin E), Choline Chloride, Niacin, Calcium Pantothenate, Riboflavin, Vitamin B_{12} Supplement, Thiamine Hydrochloride, Copper Proteinate.

Indications: Amaferm® blended with vitamins, macro and trace minerals, salt, condensed corn extractives, dried grains with solubles, soybean meal, heat processed soybean meal and cottonseed meal. Formulated for cattle on fescue grass and hay and where additional protein and energy intake are desired.

Dosage and Administration: Feeding Directions:

1. Provide 1 Power Keg for each 25-30 adult, beef cattle.
2. Provide plenty of good quality forage at all times.
3. Free-choice salt should be provided.
4. Provide a fresh, clean water supply at all times.
5. Make Power Kegs available in more than 1 location in large pastures or where more than 1 water source is available.
6. Consumption should be approximately .75-1.25 lbs./hd/day. Consumption can vary with weather and feed conditions.

7. The above feeding directions are guidelines. Use good management practices adapted to varying weather conditions.
8. If over consumed, move keg farther from water or loafing area and/or offer additional free-choice salt.

Caution(s): Due to the copper level, do not feed to sheep. Follow label directions. The addition of higher levels of selenium is not permitted.

Presentation: 200 lb kegs.

Compendium Code No.: 14960290 05/00

VITA FERM® FORMULA

BioZyme **Large Animal Dietary Supplement**

with the Amaferm® advantage

Guaranteed Analysis:

Crude Protein	20.0% Min.
Crude Fat	2.0% Min.
Crude Fiber	8.0% Max.
Calcium (Ca)	2.25% Min./2.75% Max.
Phosphorus (P)	1.3% Min.
Salt (NaCl)	1.75% Min./2.25% Max.
Magnesium (Mg)	2.0% Min.
Potassium (K)	4.7% Min.
Cobalt (Co)	65.0 ppm Min.
Copper (Cu)	1,700.0 ppm Min.
Iodine	130.0 ppm Min.
Manganese (Mn)	5,000 ppm Min.
Selenium (Se)	40.0 ppm Min.
Zinc (Zn)	6,200.0 ppm Min.
Vitamin A	900,000 IU/lb. Min.
Vitamin D_3	100,000 IU/lb. Min.
Vitamin E	1,000 IU/lb. Min.
Vitamin B_{12}	0.045 mg or 45.0 mcg/lb. Min.
Riboflavin	19.0 mg/lb. Min.
d-Pantothenic Acid	30.0 mg/lb. Min.
Thiamine	4.0 mg/lb. Min.
Niacin	150.0 mg/lb. Min.
Choline	1,500.0 mg/lb. Min.

Ingredients: Corn Distillers Dried Grains with Solubles, Cottonseed Meal, Wheat Midds, Heat Processed Soybean Meal, Potassium Chloride, Zinc Sulfate, Ferrous Sulfate, Copper Sulfate, Manganese Sulfate, Calcium Iodate, Cobalt Sulfate, Sodium Selenite, Monocalcium Phosphate, Dicalcium Phosphate, Calcium Carbonate, Potassium Sulfate, Dried *Aspergillus Oryzae* Fermentation Extract, Magnesium Oxide, Yeast Culture, Salt, Vitamin A Supplement, D-Activated Animal Sterol (Source of Vitamin D_3), dl-alpha-Tocopheryl Acetate (Source of Vitamin E), Choline Chloride, Niacin, Calcium Pantothenate, Riboflavin, Vitamin B_{12} Supplement, Thiamine Hydrochloride.

Indications: Amaferm® blended with high levels of quality vitamins and trace minerals. A vitamin/trace mineral premix. Designed to complement any existing beef feeding programs.

Dosage and Administration: Feeding Directions: Feed 2.5 oz per head, daily to adult beef cattle.

Caution(s): Due to the copper level, do not feed to sheep. Follow label directions. The addition of higher levels of selenium is not permitted.

Presentation: 50 lb bags.

Compendium Code No.: 14960300 05/00

VITA FERM® GRASS ENHANCER

BioZyme **Large Animal Dietary Supplement**

with the Amaferm® advantage

Guaranteed Analysis:

Crude Protein	6.5% Min.
Crude Fat	0.5% Min.
Crude Fiber	3.0% Max.
Calcium	11.5% Min./12.5% Max.
Phosphorus (P)	7.0% Min.
Salt (NaCl)	9.5% Min./10.5% Max.
Magnesium (Mg)	2.6% Min.
Potassium (K)	3.5% Min.
Cobalt (Co)	40.0 ppm Min.
Copper (Cu)	2,500.0 ppm Min.
Iodine	120.0 ppm Min.
Manganese (Mn)	3,000.0 ppm Min.
Selenium (Se)	27.0 ppm Min.
Zinc (Zn)	5,000.0 ppm Min.
Vitamin A	400,000 IU/lb. Min.
Vitamin D_3	40,000 IU/lb. Min.
Vitamin E	300 IU/lb. Min.
Vitamin B_{12}	0.017 mg or 17.0 mcg/lb. Min.
Riboflavin	7.0 mg/lb. Min.
Thiamine	1.5 mg/lb. Min.
d-Pantothenic Acid	11.0 mg/lb. Min.
Niacin	70.0 mg/lb. Min.
Choline	550.0 mg/lb. Min.

Ingredients: Monocalcium Phosphate, Dicalcium Phosphate, Corn Distillers Dried Grains with Solubles, Calcium Carbonate, Salt, Potassium Chloride, Magnesium Oxide, Zinc Sulfate, Ferrous Sulfate, Copper Sulfate, Manganese Sulfate, Calcium Iodate, Cobalt Sulfate, Sodium Selenite, Dried *Aspergillus Oryzae* Fermentation Extract, Copper Amino Acid Complex, Cottonseed Meal, Vitamin A Supplement, D-Activated Animal Sterol (Source of Vitamin D_3), dl-alpha-tocopheryl Acetate (Source of Vitamin E), Choline Chloride, Niacin, Calcium Pantothenate, Riboflavin, Vitamin B_{12} Supplement, Thiamine Hydrochloride, Heat Processed Soybean Meal.

Indications: Amaferm® blended with vitamins, macro and trace minerals, some protein meals (for palatability). Formulated to provide nutrients lacking in most grasses and mature forages. Best suited for beef cattle on summer and early fall pastures.

Dosage and Administration: Feeding Directions: Feed free-choice to beef or dairy cattle at the rate of 4 oz per adult animal, daily. Regulate consumption with salt or protein meals.

Caution(s): Due to the copper level, do not feed to sheep. Follow label directions. The addition of higher levels of selenium is not permitted.

Presentation: 50 lb bags.

Compendium Code No.: 14960310 04/01

VITA FERM® HIGH MAG

BioZyme **Large Animal Dietary Supplement**

with the Amaferm® advantage

Guaranteed Analysis:

Crude Protein	11.0% Min.
Crude Fat	1.0% Min.
Crude Fiber	5.0% Max.
Calcium	3.5% Min./4.5% Max.
Phosphorus (P)	3.8% Min.
Salt (NaCl)	16.7% Min./20.0% Max.
Magnesium (Mg)	10.0% Min.
Copper (Cu)	1,000.0 ppm Min.
Iodine	80.0 ppm Min.
Manganese (Mn)	3,000.0 ppm Min.
Selenium (Se)	25.0 ppm Min.
Zinc (Zn)	3,700.0 ppm Min.
Vitamin A	400,000 IU/lb. Min.
Vitamin D_3	40,000 IU/lb. Min.
Vitamin E	200 IU/lb. Min.
Vitamin B_{12}	0.018 mg or 18.0 mcg/lb. Min.
Riboflavin	7.0 mg/lb. Min.
d-Pantothenic Acid	12.0 mg/lb. Min.
Thiamine	2.5 mg/lb. Min.
Niacin	70.0 mg/lb. Min.
Choline	650.0 mg/lb. Min.

Ingredients: Corn Distillers Dried Grains with Solubles, Magnesium Oxide, Salt, Monocalcium Phosphate, Dicalcium Phosphate, Corn Distillers Dried Grains with Solubles, Cottonseed Meal, Zinc Sulfate, Ferrous Sulfate, Copper Sulfate, Manganese Sulfate, Calcium Iodate, Cobalt Sulfate, Sodium Selenite, Heat Processed Soybean Meal, Dried *Aspergillus Oryzae* Fermentation Extract, Calcium Carbonate, Yeast Culture, Potassium Sulfate, Vitamin A Supplement, D-Activated Animal Sterol (Source of Vitamin D_3), dl-alpha-tocopheryl Acetate (Source of Vitamin E), Choline Chloride, Niacin, Calcium Pantothenate, Riboflavin, Vitamin B_{12} Supplement, Thiamine Hydrochloride, Mineral Oil.

Indications: Amaferm® blended with vitamins, macro and trace minerals, protein meals (for palatability) and salt added for free-choice use. Helps ensure against grass tetany.

Dosage and Administration: Feeding Directions: Feed to beef cattle at the rate of 4 oz per head, daily. Regulate consumption with salt or protein meals. Free-choice salt should be provided.

Caution(s): Due to the copper level, do not feed to sheep. Follow label directions. The addition of higher levels of selenium is not permitted.

Presentation: 50 lb bags.

Compendium Code No.: 14960320 10/01

VITA FERM® MILK-N-MORE MEDICATED MILK REPLACER WITH DECOQUINATE

BioZyme **Milk Replacer**

with the Amaferm® advantage

Active Ingredient(s):

Decoquinate	45.42 g/ton (22.71 mg/lb.)

Guaranteed Analysis:

Crude Protein (not less than)	20.00%
Crude Fat (not less than)	20.00%
Crude Fiber (not more than)	0.15%
Calcium (not less than)	0.70%
Calcium (not more than)	1.20%
Phosphorus (not less than)	0.60%
Vitamin A (not less than)	50,000 IU/lb.
Vitamin D_3 (not less than)	10,000 IU/lb.
Vitamin E (not less than)	150 IU/lb.
Zinc (not less than)	115.00 ppm
Iron (not less than)	65.00 ppm
Manganese (not less than)	90.00 ppm
Copper (not less than)	10.00 ppm
Selenium (not less than)	0.30 ppm

Ingredients: Dried skimmed milk, Animal fat (preserved with BHA and citric acid), Dried whey, Dried whey protein concentrate, Dried buttermilk, Limestone, Sodium phosphate, Lecithin, Vitamin A supplement, D-activated animal sterol (source of Vitamin D_3), Alpha-tocopheryl acetate (source of Vitamin E), Riboflavin supplement, d-Calcium pantothenate, Niacin supplement, *Aspergillus oryzae* fermentation extract, Vitamin B_{12} supplement, Menadione sodium bisulfite complex (source of Vitamin K), Folic acid, Thiamin hydrochloride, Pyridoxine hydrochloride, Ascorbic acid (source of Vitamin C), Sodium bicarbonate, Manganese sulfate, Manganese proteinate, Zinc sulfate, Zinc proteinate, Ferrous sulfate, Copper sulfate, Copper proteinate, Sodium selenite, Cobalt sulfate, Ethylenediamine dihydriodide, and Artificial flavor.

Indications: For the prevention of coccidiosis in ruminating and non-ruminating calves and cattle caused by *E. bovis* and *E. zuernii*.

A milk replacer to be fed to herd replacement calves.

Directions: Important: Feed high quality colostrum for the first three days of life. It is important for the calf to receive colostrum as soon after birth as possible to insure establishment of immunity. Feed 3-4 lbs within one hour of birth and another 3-4 lbs six hours later. A third feeding the first day is recommended. Force feed with an esophageal tube if necessary. Do not allow the calf to nurse. Colostrum should be fed at the rate of 8% to 12% of body weight per day for the first three days. (One quart of colostrum weighs approximately 2.2 lbs).

After the third day start feeding milk replacer according to the guidelines below. Again, calves should be fed at the rate of 8% to 12% of body weight (1 qt reconstituted milk replacer weighs approximately 2.0 lbs) daily.

Mixing and Feeding Directions: Mix 4 dry oz (one cup provided in bag) per qt of warm water (110-120°F).

Feed reconstituted milk replacer at 104°F in divided feedings. Use only clean, sanitized feeding and mixing equipment (pails, bottles, nipples, etc.).

VITA FERM® MILK-N-MORE MEDICATED MILK REPLACER WITH NEO/OTC

Each gallon of milk replacer will provide 22.71 mg Decoquinate and 1 g of Amaferm® per day. Feed at a rate to provide 22.71 mg Decoquinate per 100 lbs body weight per day.

Weight, lbs.	Quarts Reconstituted Milk Replacer
50	2.0
60	2.4
70	2.8
80	3.2
90	3.6
100	4.0
110	4.4
120	4.8
130	5.2
140	5.6
150	6.0

The above feeding schedule is on a per head per day basis. These quantities should be divided into at least two feedings per day. Calves should not be weaned until they are consuming at least 2 pounds of dry feed daily for three consecutive days.

Calves should have access to fresh, clean water at all times.

Keep a good quality non-medicated calf starter ration in front of the calves starting day 3-5. Keep starter fresh and mold free by removing old and replacing with fresh daily. Switch to an appropriate medicated calf starter after weaning.

Warning(s): Do not feed to cattle producing milk for food.

Presentation: 50 lb (22.7 kg) bags.

Compendium Code No.: 14960330

VITA FERM® MILK-N-MORE MEDICATED MILK REPLACER WITH NEO/OTC

BioZyme **Milk Replacer**

with the Amaferm® advantage

Active Ingredient(s):

Neomycin base. . . . . 200 g/ton
Oxytetracycline. . . . . 100 g/ton

Guaranteed Analysis:

Crude Protein (not less than) 20.00%
Crude Fat (not less than) 20.00%
Crude Fiber (not more than). 0.15%
Calcium (not less than) 0.70%
Calcium (not more than) 1.20%
Phosphorus (not less than) 0.60%
Vitamin A (not less than) . . . . . 50,000 IU/lb.
Vitamin D_3 (not less than) . . . . . 10,000 IU/lb.
Vitamin E (not less than) . . . . . 150 IU/lb.
Zinc (not less than) . . . . . 115.00 ppm
Iron (not less than) . . . . . 65.00 ppm
Manganese (not less than). . . . . 90.00 ppm
Copper (not less than) . . . . . 10.00 ppm
Selenium (not less than) . . . . . 0.30 ppm

Ingredients: Dried skimmed milk, Animal fat (preserved with BHA and citric acid), Dried whey, Dried whey protein concentrate, Dried buttermilk, Limestone, Sodium phosphate, Lecithin, Vitamin A supplement, D-activated animal sterol (source of Vitamin D_3), Alpha-tocopheryl acetate (source of Vitamin E), Riboflavin supplement, d-Calcium pantothenate, Niacin supplement, *Aspergillus oryzae* fermentation extract, Vitamin B_{12} supplement, Menadione sodium bisulfite complex (source of Vitamin K), Folic acid, Thiamin hydrochloride, Pyridoxine hydrochloride, Ascorbic acid (source of Vitamin C), Sodium bicarbonate, Manganese sulfate, Manganese proteinate, Zinc sulfate, Zinc proteinate, Ferrous sulfate, Copper sulfate, Copper proteinate, Sodium selenite, Cobalt sulfate, Ethylenediamine dihydriodide, and Artificial flavor.

Indications: A milk replacer to be fed to herd replacement calves. Aid in the prevention of bacterial enteritis (Scours).

Directions: Important: Feed high quality colostrum for the first three days of life. It is important for the calf to receive colostrum as soon as possible after birth as possible to insure establishment of immunity. Feed 3-4 lbs within one hour of birth and another 3-4 lbs six hours later. A third feeding the first day is recommended. Force feed with an esophageal tube if necessary. Do not allow the calf to nurse. Colostrum should be fed at the rate of 8% to 12% of body weight per day for the first three days. (One qt of colostrum weighs approximately 2.2 lbs).

After the third day start feeding milk replacer according to the guidelines below. Again, calves should be fed at the rate of 8% to 12% of body weight (1 qt reconstituted milk replacer weighs approximately 2.0 lbs) daily.

Mixing and Feeding Directions: Mix 4 dry oz (one cup provided in bag) per qt of warm water (110-120°F).

Feed reconstituted milk replacer at 104°F in divided feedings. Use only clean, sanitized feeding and mixing equipment (pails, bottles, nipples, etc.).

Each gallon of reconstituted milk replacer will supply 100 mg of Neomycin base and 50 mg of Oxytetracycline and 1 g of Amaferm® per day. Feeding at the following rates will provide 50-150 mg of Neomycin base and 25-75 mg of Oxytetracycline per day.

Weight, lbs	Quarts Reconstituted Milk Replacer
50	2.0
60	2.4
70	2.8
80	3.2
90	3.6
100	4.0
110	4.4
120	4.8
130	5.2
140	5.6
150	6.0

The above feeding schedule is on a per head per day basis. These quantities should be divided into at least two feedings per day. Calves should not be weaned until they are consuming at least 2 lbs of dry feed daily for three consecutive days.

Calves should have access to fresh, clean water at all times.

Keep a good quality non-medicated calf starter ration in front of the calves starting day 3-5. Keep starter fresh and mold free by removing old and replacing with fresh daily. Switch to an appropriate medicated calf starter after weaning.

Warning(s): All use levels in milk replacer require a 30 day withdrawal before slaughter. A withdrawal period has not been established for pre-ruminant calves. Do not use in calves to be processed for veal.

Presentation: 50 lb (22.7 kg) bags.

Compendium Code No.: 14960340

VITA FERM® MILK-N-MORE NON-MEDICATED MILK REPLACER

BioZyme **Milk Replacer**

with the Amaferm® advantage

Guaranteed Analysis:

Crude Protein (not less than) 20.00%
Crude Fat (not less than). 20.00%
Crude Fiber (not more than) 0.15%
Calcium (not less than). 0.70%
Calcium (not more than). 1.20%
Phosphorus (not less than). 0.60%
Vitamin A (not less than). . . . . 50,000 IU/lb.
Vitamin D_3 (not less than). . . . . 10,000 IU/lb.
Vitamin E (not less than). . . . . 150 IU/lb.
Zinc (not less than). . . . . 115.00 ppm
Iron (not less than) . . . . . 65.00 ppm
Manganese (not less than) . . . . . 90.00 ppm
Copper (not less than) . . . . . 10.00 ppm
Selenium (not less than). . . . . 0.30 ppm

Ingredients: Dried skimmed milk, Animal fat (preserved with BHA and citric acid), Dried whey, Dried whey protein concentrate, Dried buttermilk, Limestone, Sodium phosphate, Lecithin, Vitamin A supplement, D-activated animal sterol (source of Vitamin D_3), Alpha-tocopheryl acetate (source of Vitamin E), Riboflavin supplement, d-Calcium pantothenate, Niacin supplement, *Aspergillus oryzae* fermentation extract, Vitamin B_{12} supplement, Menadione sodium bisulfite complex (source of Vitamin K), Folic acid, Thiamin hydrochloride, Pyridoxine hydrochloride, Ascorbic acid (source of Vitamin C), Sodium bicarbonate, Manganese sulfate, Manganese proteinate, Zinc sulfate, Zinc proteinate, Ferrous sulfate, Copper sulfate, Copper proteinate, Sodium selenite, Cobalt sulfate, Ethylenediamine dihydriodide, and Artificial flavor.

Indications: A milk replacer to be fed to herd replacement calves.

Directions: Important: Feed high quality colostrum for the first three days of life. It is important for the calf to receive colostrum as soon as possible after birth as possible to insure establishment of immunity. Feed 3-4 lbs within one hour of birth and another 3-4 lbs six hours later. A third feeding the first day is recommended. Force feed with an esophageal tube if necessary. Do not allow the calf to nurse. Colostrum should be fed at the rate of 8% to 12% of body weight per day for the first three days. (One qt of colostrum weighs approximately 2.2 lbs).

After the third day start feeding milk replacer according to the guidelines below. Again, calves should be fed at the rate of 8% to 12% of body weight (1 qt reconstituted milk replacer weighs approximately 2.0 lbs) daily.

Mixing and Feeding Directions: Mix 4 dry oz (one cup provided in bag) per qt of warm water (110-120°F).

Feed reconstituted milk replacer at 104°F in divided feedings. Use only clean, sanitized feeding and mixing equipment (pails, bottles, nipples, etc.).

Feeding according to the following schedule, each gallon will provide at least 1 g of Amaferm® per head per day:

Weight	45-60	60-80	over 80 lb
Age, Days	Quarts	Quarts	Quarts
1-3 days	colostrum	colostrum	colostrum
4-7	2.0	3.0	3.5
8-14	2.5	3.5	4.0
15-42	3.0	4.0	4.0
42-56	2.0	3.0	3.0

The above feeding schedule is on a per head per day basis. These quantities should be divided into at least two feedings per day. Calves should not be weaned until they are consuming at least 2 lbs of dry feed daily for three consecutive days.

Calves should have access to fresh, clean water at all times.

Keep a good quality calf starter ration in front of the calves starting day 3-5. Keep starter fresh and mold free by removing old and replacing with fresh daily.

Presentation: 25 lb (11.34 kg) and 50 lb (22.7 kg).

Compendium Code No.: 14960350

VITA FERM® NATURAL PROTEIN PASTURE FORMULA (NPPF)

BioZyme **Large Animal Dietary Supplement**

with the Amaferm® advantage

Guaranteed Analysis:

Crude Protein . . . . . 24.0% Min.
Crude Fat . . . . . 1.5% Min.
Crude Fiber . . . . . 7.5% Max.
Calcium. . . . . 3.4% Min./4.4% Max.
Phosphorus (P) . . . . . 5.0% Min
Magnesium (Mg) . . . . . 5.5% Min.
Potassium (K). . . . . 1.5% Min.
Copper (Cu) . . . . . 400.0 ppm Min.
Iodine . . . . . 30.0 ppm Min.
Manganese (Mn). . . . . 1,200.0 ppm Min.
Selenium (Se). . . . . 10.0 ppm Min.
Zinc (Zn). . . . . 1,500.0 ppm Min.
Vitamin A . . . . . 160,000 IU/lb. Min.
Vitamin D_3. . . . . 16,000 IU/lb. Min.

Vitamin E .... 80 IU/lb. Min.
Vitamin B_{12}.......... 0.008 mg or 8.0 mcg/lb. Min.
Riboflavin.......... 3.7 mg/lb. Min.
d-Pantothenic Acid.......... 7.0 mg/lb. Min.
Niacin.......... 50.0 mg/lb. Min.
Choline.......... 800.0 mg/lb. Min.

Ingredients: Cottonseed Meal, Monocalcium Phosphate, Dicalcium Phosphate, Magnesium Oxide, Corn Distillers Dried Grains with Solubles, Heat Processed Soybean Meal, Wheat Midds, Potassium Chloride, Zinc Sulfate, Ferrous Sulfate, Copper Sulfate, Manganese Sulfate, Calcium Iodate, Cobalt Sulfate, Sodium Selenite, Yeast Culture, Dried *Aspergillus Oryzae* Fermentation Extract, Vitamin A Supplement, D-Activated Animal Sterol (Source of Vitamin D_3), dl-alpha-tocopheryl Acetate (Source of Vitamin E), Choline Chloride, Niacin, Calcium Pantothenate, Riboflavin, Vitamin B_{12} Supplement, Thiamine Hydrochloride.

Indications: Amaferm® blended with vitamins, macro and trace minerals and all-natural protein meals to supplement more of the nutrition needs of calves and cows on poor quality forages. Ideal for replacement and first-calf heifers.

Dosage and Administration: Feeding Directions: Feed to adult beef or dairy cattle at the rate of 10 oz per head, daily. Regulate consumption with salt or protein meals. Free-choice salt should be provided.

Caution(s): Due to the copper level, do not feed to sheep. Follow label directions. The addition of higher levels of selenium is not permitted.

Presentation: 50 lb bags.

Compendium Code No.: 14960360 05/00

VITA FERM® PASTURE FORMULA

BioZyme **Large Animal Dietary Supplement**

with the Amaferm® advantage

Guaranteed Analysis:

Calcium (Ca) .... 10.0% Min./12.0% Max.
Phosphorus (P) .... 10.0% Min.
Magnesium (Mg) .... 3.2% Min.
Potassium (K) .... 5.8% Min.
Cobalt (Co).......... 40.0 ppm Min.
Copper (Cu) .... 1,000.0 ppm Min.
Iodine.......... 80.0 ppm Min.
Manganese (Mn) .... 3,000.0 ppm Min.
Selenium (Se) .... 25.0 ppm Min.
Zinc (Zn) .... 3,500.0 ppm Min.
Vitamin A.......... 400,000 IU/lb. Min.
Vitamin D_3 .... 40,000 IU/lb. Min.
Vitamin E .... 200 IU/lb. Min.
Vitamin B_{12}.......... 0.020 mg or 20.0 mcg/lb. Min.
Riboflavin.......... 7.0 mg/lb. Min.
d-Pantothenic Acid.......... 11.0 mg/lb. Min.
Thiamine .... 1.4 mg/lb. Min.
Niacin.......... 60.0 mg/lb. Min.
Choline.......... 500.0 mg/lb. Min.

Ingredients: Monocalcium Phosphate, Dicalcium Phosphate, Potassium Chloride, Cottonseed Meal, Corn Distillers Dried Grains with Solubles, Calcium Carbonate, Magnesium Oxide, Wheat Midds, Zinc Sulfate, Ferrous Sulfate, Copper Sulfate, Manganese Sulfate, Calcium Iodate, Cobalt Sulfate, Sodium Selenite, Dried *Aspergillus Oryzae* Fermentation Extract, Potassium Sulfate, Vitamin A Supplement, D-Activated Animal Sterol (Source of Vitamin D_3), dl-alpha-tocopheryl Acetate (Source of Vitamin E), Choline Chloride, Niacin, Calcium Pantothenate, Riboflavin, Vitamin B_{12} Supplement, Thiamine Hydrochloride.

Indications: Amaferm® blended with vitamins, macro and trace minerals, with a low level of protein meal. No salt added. Being lower in palatability than other Vita Ferm® formulations, this product is generally used when poorer pasture conditions exist.

Dosage and Administration: Feeding Directions: Feed to beef or dairy cattle at the rate of 4 oz per head, daily. Regulate consumption with salt or protein meals. Free-choice salt should be provided.

Caution(s): Due to the copper level, do not feed to sheep. Follow label directions. The addition of higher levels of selenium is not permitted.

Presentation: 50 lb bags.

Compendium Code No.: 14960370 05/00

VITA FERM® POWER KEG

BioZyme **Large Animal Dietary Supplement**

with the Amaferm® advantage

Guaranteed Analysis:

Crude Protein.......... 20.0% Min.
Crude Fat .... 3.0% Min.
Crude Fiber.......... 4.0% Max.
Calcium .... 3.5% Min./4.5% Max.
Phosphorus (P) .... 3.0% Min.
Salt (NaCl) .... 6.0% Min./7.0% Max.
Magnesium (Mg) .... 3.0% Min.
Potassium (K) .... 1.5% Min.
Cobalt (Co).......... 8.0 ppm Min.
Copper (Cu) .... 330.0 ppm Min.
Iodine.......... 38.0 ppm Min.
Manganese (Mn) .... 750.0 ppm Min.
Selenium (Se) .... 4.3 ppm Min.
Zinc (Zn) .... 860.0 ppm Min.
Vitamin A.......... 100,000 IU/lb. Min.
Vitamin D_3 .... 20,000 IU/lb. Min.
Vitamin E .... 125 IU/lb. Min.
Vitamin B_{12}.......... 0.0030 mg or 3.0 mcg/lb. Min.
Riboflavin.......... 3.0 mg/lb. Min.
d-Pantothenic Acid.......... 5.0 mg/lb. Min.
Thiamine .... 1.0 mg/lb. Min.
Niacin.......... 30.0 mg/lb. Min.
Choline.......... 850.0 mg/lb. Min.

Ingredients: Condensed Fermented Corn Extractives, Corn Distillers Dried Grains with Solubles, Monocalcium Phosphate, Dicalcium Phosphate, Soybean Meal, Heat Processed Soybean Meal, Calcium Sulfate, Salt, Magnesium Oxide, Cottonseed Meal, Potassium Chloride, Zinc Sulfate, Ferrous Sulfate, Copper Sulfate, Manganese Sulfate, Calcium Iodate, Cobalt Sulfate, Sodium Selenite, Calcium Carbonate, Dried *Aspergillus Oryzae* Fermentation Extract, Vitamin A Supplement, D-Activated Animal Sterol (Source of Vitamin D_3), dl-alpha-tocopheryl Acetate (Source of Vitamin E), Choline Chloride, Niacin, Calcium Pantothenate, Riboflavin, Vitamin B_{12} Supplement, Thiamine Hydrochloride, Copper Proteinate.

Indications: Amaferm® blended with vitamins, macro and trace minerals, salt, condensed corn extractives, dried grains with solubles, soybean meal, heat processed soybean meal and cottonseed meal. Formulated for use on all cattle where additional protein and energy intake are desired.

Dosage and Administration: Feeding Directions:

1. Provide 1 Power Keg for each 25-30 adult, beef cattle.
2. Provide plenty of good quality forage at all times.
3. Free-choice salt should be provided.
4. Provide a fresh, clean water supply at all times.
5. Make Power Kegs available in more than 1 location in large pastures or where more than 1 water source is available.
6. Consumption should be approximately .75-1.5 lbs/hd/day. Consumption can vary with weather and feed conditions.
7. The above feeding directions are guidelines. Use good management practices adapted to varying weather conditions.
8. If over consumed, move keg farther from water or loafing area and/or offer additional free-choice salt.

Caution(s): Due to the copper level, do not feed to sheep. Follow label directions. The addition of higher levels of selenium is not permitted.

Presentation: 200 lb kegs.

Compendium Code No.: 14960380 05/00

VITA FERM® PRO-GEST

BioZyme **Large Animal Dietary Supplement**

with the Amaferm® advantage

Guaranteed Analysis:

Crude Protein .... 11.0% Min.
Crude Fat .... 3.0% Min.
Crude Fiber.......... 7.0% Max.

Ingredients: Yeast culture, wheat middlings, dried *Aspergillus oryzae* fermentation extract.

Indications: Amaferm® blended with yeast in a wheat bran carrier. Use in any livestock feeding situation to stimulate feed intake and increase the digestion efficiency of all rations, including calf weaning and starting rations. Ideal for use in "all-natural-beef" feeding programs.

Dosage and Administration: Feeding Directions: Can be top dressed or mixed in rations.

Lactating Dairy: 1.5 oz./day
Beef Cattle: 1 oz./day
Calves: 0.5 oz./day
Horses: 1 oz./day
Sheep: 0.5 oz./day
Poultry: 40 lbs./ton of complete feed
Swine:
Weaning and starter diet: 40 lbs./ton of complete feed
Grower finisher diet: 14 lbs./ton of complete feed
Lactating sows and last 30 days of gestation: 5 lbs./ton of complete feed

Presentation: 50 lb bags.

Compendium Code No.: 14960102 05/00

VITA FERM® PRO-GEST 30

BioZyme **Feed Additive**

with the Amaferm® advantage

Guaranteed Analysis:

Crude Protein .... 21.0% Min.
Crude Fat .... 2.0% Min.
Crude Fiber.......... 9.3% Max.

Ingredients: Corn Distillers Dried Grains with Solubles, Wheat Middlings, Dried *Aspergillus oryzae* Fermentation Extract.

Indications: Amaferm® blended in a wheat bran carrier. Use in any livestock feeding situation to stimulate feed intake and increase digestion efficiency of lactating dairy rations, calf weaning and starting rations.

Dosage and Administration: Feeding Directions: Can be top-dressed or mixed in rations.

Lactating Dairy: 1.5 oz./day
Beef Cattle: 1 oz./day
Calves: 0.5 oz./day
Horses: 1 oz./day
Sheep: 0.5 oz./day
Poultry: 40 lbs./ton of complete feed
Swine:
Weaning and starter diet: 40 lbs./ton of complete feed
Grower finisher diet: 14 lbs./ton of complete feed
Lactating sows and last 30 days of gestation: 5 lbs./ton of complete feed

Presentation: 50 lb. bags.

Compendium Code No.: 14960112 05/00

VITA FERM® ROUGHAGE FORTIFIER

BioZyme **Large Animal Dietary Supplement**

with the Amaferm® advantage

Guaranteed Analysis:

Crude Protein .... 7.0% Min.
Crude Fat .... .5% Min.
Crude Fiber.......... 3.0% Max.
Calcium.......... 12.0% Min./14.4% Max.
Phosphorus (P) .... 8.0% Min.
Salt (NaCl).......... 7.7% Min./9.2% Max.
Magnesium (Mg) .... 3.0% Min.
Potassium (K).......... 3.5% Min.
Cobalt (Co) .... 40.0 ppm Min.
Copper (Cu) .... 2,500.0 ppm Min.
Iodine .... 120.0 ppm Min.

Manganese (Mn) .... 3,000.0 ppm Min.
Selenium (Se) .... 26.0 ppm Min.
Zinc (Zn) .... 5,000.0 ppm Min.
Vitamin A .... 400,000 IU/lb. Min.
Vitamin D_3 .... 40,000 IU/lb. Min.
Vitamin E .... 400 IU/lb. Min.
Vitamin B_{12} .... 0.012 mg or 12.0 mcg/lb. Min.
d-Pantothenic Acid .... 8.5 mg/lb. Min.
Thiamine .... 1.2 mg/lb. Min.
Niacin .... 50.0 mg/lb. Min.
Choline .... 450.0 mg/lb. Min.

Ingredients: Monocalcium Phosphate, Dicalcium Phosphate, Calcium Carbonate, Corn Distillers Dried Grains with Solubles, Salt, Cottonseed Meal, Potassium Chloride, Magnesium Oxide, Zinc Sulfate, Ferrous Sulfate, Copper Sulfate, Manganese Sulfate, Calcium Iodate, Cobalt Sulfate, Sodium Selenite, Heat Processed Soybean Meal, Dried *Aspergillus Oryzae* Fermentation Extract, Copper Amino Acid Complex, Vitamin A Supplement, D-Activated Animal Sterol (Source of Vitamin D_3), dl-alpha-tocopheryl Acetate (Source of Vitamin E), Choline Chloride, Niacin, Calcium Pantothenate, Riboflavin, Vitamin B_{12} Supplement, Thiamine Hydrochloride, Mineral Oil.

Indications: Amaferm® blended with vitamins, macro and trace minerals, some protein meals (for palatability). Formulated to provide nutrients lacking in high fiber and poor quality roughages. Ideally suited for beef cattle on winter pasture or hay, but can be used year round.

Dosage and Administration: Feeding Directions: Feed to cattle at the rate of 4 oz per adult animal, daily. Regulate consumption with salt or protein meals. Feed with free-choice salt.

Caution(s): Due to the copper level, do not feed to sheep. Follow label directions. The addition of higher levels of selenium is not permitted.

Presentation: 50 lb bags.

Compendium Code No.: 14960390 03/02

VITA FERM® SHEEP & GOAT KEG

BioZyme **Dietary Supplement**

with the Amaferm® advantage

Guaranteed Analysis:

Crude Protein .... 20.0% Min.
Crude Fat .... 3.0% Min.
Crude Fiber .... 4.0% Max.
Calcium .... 2.5% Min./3.5% Max.
Phosphorus (P) .... 3.0% Min.
Salt (NaCl) .... 8.0% Min./9.0% Max.
Magnesium (Mg) .... 1.2% Min.
Potassium (K) .... 1.5% Min.
Cobalt (Co) .... 3.5 ppm Min.
Iodine .... 30.0 ppm Min.
Manganese (Mn) .... 48.0 ppm Min.
Selenium (Se) .... 3.0 ppm Min.
Zinc (Zn) .... 325.0 ppm Min.
Vitamin A .... 80,000 IU/lb. Min.
Vitamin D_3 .... 10,000 IU/lb. Min.
Vitamin E .... 330 IU/lb. Min.
Vitamin B_{12} .... 0.0040 mg or 4.0 mcg/lb. Min.
Riboflavin .... 4.0 mg/lb. Min.
d-Pantothenic Acid .... 6.0 mg/lb. Min.
Thiamine .... 1.0 mg/lb. Min.
Niacin .... 37.0 mg/lb. Min.
Choline .... 1,000.0 mg/lb. Min.

Ingredients: Condensed Fermented Corn Extractives, Corn Distillers Dried Grains with Solubles, Monocalcium Phosphate, Dicalcium Phosphate, Salt, Heat Processed Soybean Meal, Cottonseed Meal, Magnesium Oxide, Calcium Carbonate, Potassium Chloride, Dried *Aspergillus Oryzae* Fermentation Extract, Zinc Sulfate, Ferrous Sulfate, Copper Sulfate, Manganese Sulfate, Calcium Iodate, Cobalt Sulfate Sodium Selenite, Vitamin A Supplement, D-Activated Animal Sterol (Source of Vitamin D_3), dl-alpha-tocopheryl Acetate (Source of Vitamin E), Choline Chloride, Niacin, Calcium Pantothenate, Riboflavin, Vitamin B_{12} Supplement, Thiamine Hydrochloride, Calcium Iodate.

Indications: Amaferm® blended with vitamins, macro and trace minerals, salt, condensed corn extractives, dried grains with solubles, soybean meal, heat processed soybean meal and cottonseed meal. Formulated for adult sheep and goats on pasture.

Dosage and Administration: Feeding Directions:

1. Provide 1 Sheep and Goat Keg per 60 adult sheep or 75 adult goats.
2. Provide plenty of good quality forage at all times.
3. Free-choice salt should be provided.
4. Provide a fresh, clean water supply at all times.
5. Make Sheep and Goat Kegs available in more than 1 location in large pastures or where more than 1 water source is available.
6. Consumption should be approximately 4 oz per head/day. Consumption can vary with weather and feed conditions.
7. The above feeding directions are guidelines. Use good management practices adapted to varying weather conditions.
8. If over consumed, move keg farther from water or loafing area and/or offer additional free-choice salt.

Caution(s): VITA FERM® Sheep & Goat Keg has been formulated with no added copper; however, natural levels of copper are contained in the ingredients utilized to formulate VITA FERM® Sheep & Goat Keg. Protein meals and some mineral constituents contain acceptable levels of copper. When utilizing VITA FERM® Sheep & Goat Keg as a vitamin supplement, all food sources should be tested for both copper and molybdenum. The total copper intake and the copper to molybdenum ratio should be calculated prior to feeding a supplement or feed to sheep. The ideal copper to molybdenum ratio should be between 6 to 10 parts copper to 1 part molybdenum. Do not utilize VITA FERM® Sheep & Goat Keg vitamin/mineral supplement until these calculations are performed and evaluated by a livestock nutritionist or veterinarian.

Note: Some breeds of sheep and some individuals within a breed of sheep are extremely sensitive to any level of copper in feed, pasture or supplements. Certain breeds of goats may require additional copper supplementation.

Presentation: 200 lb kegs.

Compendium Code No.: 14960400 05/00

VITA FERM® SURE CHAMP AND VITA START PELLETS

BioZyme **Large Animal Dietary Supplement**

with the Amaferm® advantage

Guaranteed Analysis:

Crude Protein .... 25.0% Min.
Crude Fat .... 2.5% Min.
Crude Fiber .... 9.0% Max.
Calcium (Ca) .... 2.3% Min./2.7% Max.
Phosphorus (P) .... 1.0% Min.
Magnesium (Mg) .... 0.5% Min.
Potassium (K) .... 2.0% Min.
Copper (Cu) .... 350.0 ppm Min.
Iodine .... 25.0 ppm Min.
Manganese (Mn) .... 550.0 ppm Min.
Selenium (Se) .... 6.7 ppm Min.
Zinc (Zn) .... 1,150.0 ppm Min.
Vitamin A .... 70,000 IU/lb. Min.
Vitamin D_3 .... 7,000 IU/lb. Min.
Vitamin E .... 80 IU/lb. Min.
Vitamin B_{12} .... 0.005 mg or 5.0 mcg/lb. Min.
Riboflavin .... 3.0 mg/lb. Min.
Niacin .... 2,500.0 mg/lb. Min.
Choline .... 1,000.0 mg/lb. Min.

Ingredients: Corn Distillers Dried Grains with Solubles, Cottonseed Meal, Heat Processed Soybean Meal, Calcium Carbonate, Dried Molasses, Potassium Sulfate, Monocalcium Phosphate, Dicalcium Phosphate, Vitamin A Supplement, D-Activated Animal Sterol (Source of Vitamin D_3), dl-alpha-Tocopheryl Acetate (Source of Vitamin E), Choline Chloride, Niacin, Calcium Pantothenate, Riboflavin, Vitamin B_{12} Supplement, Thiamine Hydrochloride, Potassium Chloride, Zinc Sulfate, Ferrous Sulfate, Copper Sulfate, Manganese Sulfate, Calcium Iodate, Cobalt Sulfate, Sodium Selenite, Dried *Aspergillus Oryzae* Fermentation Extract, Zinc Proteinate, Manganese Proteinate, Copper Proteinate, Ethoxyquin Preservative.

Indications: Pelletized 25%, all-natural protein derived from highly-digestible sources, Amaferm® blended with high levels of vitamins and minerals. Contains no urea, screenings or fillers. Ideal for starting calf and show calf rations.

Dosage and Administration: Feeding Directions: Feed to beef cattle at the rate of 1 lb per head, daily, top-dressed over ration or mixed in complete ration. Cattle starting on feed should receive 3-5 lbs long stem hay per day.

Caution(s): Due to the copper level, do not feed to sheep. Follow label directions. The addition of higher levels of selenium is not permitted.

Presentation: 50 lbs bags.

Compendium Code No.: 14960410 12/01

VITA FERM® SURE START 2

BioZyme **Large Animal Dietary Supplement**

with the Amaferm® advantage

Guaranteed Analysis:

Crude Protein .... 24.0% Min.
Crude Fat .... 3.0% Min.
Crude Fiber .... 7.0% Max.
Calcium (Ca) .... 2.5% Min./3.5% Max.
Phosphorus (P) .... 0.8% Min.
Salt (NaCl) .... 1.2% Min./1.7% Max.
Potassium (K) .... 2.0% Min.
Cobalt (Co) .... 16.0 ppm Min.
Copper (Cu) .... 175.0 ppm Min.
Manganese (Mn) .... 280.0 ppm Min.
Selenium (Se) .... 3.0 ppm Min.
Zinc (Zn) .... 700.0 ppm Min.
Vitamin A .... 75,000 IU/lb. Min.
Vitamin D_3 .... 7,500 IU/lb. Min.
Vitamin E .... 200 IU/lb. Min.
Vitamin B_{12} .... 0.011 mg/lb. or 11.0 mcg/lb. Min.
Thiamin .... 35.0 mg/lb. Min.
Niacin .... 750.0 mg/lb. Min.
Choline .... 1,100.0 mg/lb. Min.

Ingredients: Corn Distillers Dried Grains with Solubles, Heat Processed Soybean Meal, Calcium Carbonate, Yeast Culture, Soybean Meal, Cottonseed Meal, Potassium Chloride, Dried Molasses, Salt, Zinc Amino Acid Complex, Manganese Amino Acid Complex, Copper Amino Acid Complex, Cobalt Glucoheptonate, Monocalcium Phosphate, Dicalcium Phosphate, Wheat Midds, Magnesium Oxide, Dried *Aspergillus Oryzae* Fermentation Extract, Sodium Selenite, Niacin, Vitamin A Supplement, D-Activated Animal Sterol (Source of Vitamin D_3), dl-alpha-Tocopheryl Acetate (source of Vitamin E), Choline Chloride, Calcium Pantothenate, Riboflavin, Vitamin B_{12} Supplement, Thiamin Hydrochloride, Zinc Sulfate, Manganese Sulfate, Calcium Iodate.

Indications: Amaferm® blended with vitamins, trace minerals, and natural protein at levels to meet the needs of non-preconditioned, stressed calves.

Dosage and Administration: Feeding Directions: Feed to newly weaned or received beef calves at the rate of 2 lbs per head per day.

Presentation: 50 lb bags.

Compendium Code No.: 14960420 07/01

VITA FERM® SURE START PAC

BioZyme **Large Animal Dietary Supplement**

with the Amaferm® advantage

Guaranteed Analysis:

Crude Protein .... 16.0% Min.
Crude Fat .... 2.5% Min.
Crude Fiber .... 5.0% Max.
Calcium (Ca) .... 7.8% Min./9.3% Max.
Phosphorus (P) .... 2.0% Min.
Salt (NaCl) .... 5.0% Min./6.0% Max.
Potassium (K) .... 4.0% Min.
Cobalt (Co) .... 64.0 ppm Min.
Copper (Cu) .... 785.0 ppm Min.
Manganese (Mn) .... 1,515.0 ppm Min.
Selenium (Se) .... 12.0 ppm Min.

Zinc (Zn) .... 2,600.0 ppm Min.
Vitamin A .... 300,000 IU/lb. Min.
Vitamin D_3 .... 30,000 IU/lb. Min.
Vitamin E .... 800 IU/lb. Min.
Vitamin B_{12} .... 0.012 mg/lb. or 12.0 mcg/lb. Min.
Thiamine .... 105.0 mg/lb. Min.
Niacin .... 3,000.0 mg/lb. Min.
Choline .... 825.0 mg/lb. Min.

Ingredients: Corn Distillers Dried Grains with Solubles, Calcium Carbonate, Heat Processed Soybean Meal, Monocalcium Phosphate, Dicalcium Phosphate, Potassium Chloride, Salt, Soybean Meal, Cottonseed Meal, Zinc Amino Acid Complex, Manganese Amino Acid Complex, Copper Amino Acid Complex, Cobalt Glucoheptonate, Wheat Midds, Dried Molasses, Dried *Aspergillus Oryzae* Fermentation Extract, Zinc Sulfate, Ferrous Sulfate, Copper Sulfate, Manganese Sulfate, Calcium Iodate, Cobalt Sulfate, Sodium Selenite, Niacin, Vitamin A supplement, D-Activated Animal Sterol (Source of Vitamin D_3), dl-alpha-tocopheryl Acetate (Source of Vitamin E), Choline chloride, Calcium Pantothenate, Riboflavin, Vitamin B_{12} Supplement, Thiamine Hydrochloride, Magnesium Oxide.

Indications: Amaferm® blended with key vitamins, minerals, trace minerals at levels to meet the needs of non-preconditioned, stressed calves. Use where adequate protein is available.

Dosage and Administration: Feeding Directions: Feed to newly weaned or received beef calves at the rate of ½ lb per head per day.

Presentation: 50 lb bags.

Compendium Code No.: 14960430 07/01

VITA FERM® UP CLOSE DRY COW

BioZyme **Large Animal Dietary Supplement**

with the Amaferm® advantage

Guaranteed Analysis:

Crude Protein .... 16.0% Min.
Crude Fat .... 4.0% Min.
Crude Fiber .... 5.0% Max.
Calcium .... 5.0% Min./7.0% Max.
Phosphorus (P) .... 3.0% Min.
Magnesium (Mg) .... 6.0% Min.
Potassium (K) .... 0.5% Min.
Cobalt (Co) .... 27.0 ppm Min.
Copper (Cu) .... 500.0 ppm Min.
Iodine .... 18.0 ppm Min.
Manganese (Mn) .... 2,000.0 ppm Min.
Selenium (Se) .... 12.0 ppm Min.
Zinc (Zn) .... 2,000.0 ppm Min.
Vitamin A .... 300,000 IU/lb. Min.
Vitamin D_3 .... 80,000 IU/lb. Min.
Vitamin E .... 2,000 IU/lb. Min.
Niacin .... 15,000.0 mg/lb. Min.

Ingredients: Corn Distillers Dried Grains with Solubles, Heat Processed Soybean Meal, Calcium Carbonate, Magnesium Oxide, Wheat Midds, Monocalcium Phosphate, Dicalcium Phosphate, Monosodium Phosphate, Niacin, Zinc Sulfate, Ferrous Sulfate, Copper Sulfate, Manganese Sulfate, Calcium Iodate, Cobalt Sulfate, Sodium Selenite, Potassium Chloride, Yeast Culture, Dried *Aspergillus Oryzae* Fermentation Extract, Vitamin A Supplement, D-Activated Animal Sterol (Source of Vitamin D_3), dl-Alpha-Tocopheryl Acetate (Source of Vitamin E), Choline Chloride, Calcium Pantothenate, Riboflavin, Vitamin B_{12} Supplement, Cobalt Carbonate.

Indications: Amaferm® blended with high levels of quality vitamins and trace minerals. Designed to supply the correct nutrient balance for dairy or beef cows during the last 30 days of pregnancy.

Dosage and Administration: Feeding Directions: Feed to dairy or beef cows at the rate of 0.5 lb per head, daily, during the last 30 days of gestation.

Caution(s): Due to the copper level, do not feed to sheep. Follow label directions. The addition of higher levels of selenium is not permitted.

Presentation: 50 lb bags.

Compendium Code No.: 14960440 05/00

VITA FERM® VITA GROW 32 NATURAL

BioZyme **Large Animal Dietary Supplement**

with the Amaferm® advantage

Guaranteed Analysis:

Crude Protein .... 32.0% Min.
Crude Fat .... 2.0% Min.
Crude Fiber .... 12.0% Max.
Calcium (Ca) .... 3.0% Min./4.0% Max.
Phosphorus (P) .... 0.9% Min.
Salt (NaCl) .... 5.0% Min./6.0% Max.
Potassium (K) .... 1.0% Min.
Copper (Cu) .... 175.0 ppm Min.
Iodine .... 16.0 ppm Min.
Manganese (Mn) .... 250 ppm Min.
Selenium (Se) .... 4.0 ppm Min.
Zinc (Zn) .... 590.0 ppm Min.
Vitamin A .... 34,000 IU/lb. Min.
Vitamin D_3 .... 3,400 IU/lb. Min.
Vitamin E .... 40 IU/lb. Min.
Riboflavin .... 2.0 mg/lb. Min.
d-Pantothenic Acid .... 4.0 mg/lb. Min.
Thiamine .... 3.0 mg/lb. Min.
Niacin .... 35.0 mg/lb. Min.
Choline .... 1,000.0 mg/lb. Min.

Ingredients: Cottonseed Meal, Calcium Carbonate, Heat Processed Soybean Meal, Corn Distillers Dried Grains with Solubles, Salt, Dried Molasses, Monocalcium Phosphate, Dicalcium Phosphate, Zinc Sulfate, Ferrous Sulfate, Copper Sulfate, Manganese Sulfate, Calcium Iodate, Cobalt Sulfate, Sodium Selenite, Potassium Chloride, Magnesium Oxide, Dried *Aspergillus Oryzae* Fermentation Extract, Ethoxyquin Preservative, Vitamin A Supplement, D-Activated Animal Sterol (Source of Vitamin D_3), dl-alpha-Tocopheryl Acetate (Source of Vitamin E), Choline Chloride, Niacin, Calcium Pantothenate, Riboflavin, Vitamin B_{12} Supplement, Thiamine Hydrochloride, Cobalt Carbonate.

Indications: A pelletized 32%, all-natural protein supplement blended with Amaferm® and adequate levels of vitamins and minerals that, when mixed with grain, provides ample nutrition for growing and finishing beef or dairy cattle.

Dosage and Administration: Feeding Directions: Feed to cattle at the rate of 1.5 lbs per head, daily.

Caution(s): Due to the copper level, do not feed to sheep. Follow label directions. The addition of higher levels of selenium is not permitted.

Presentation: 50 lb bags.

Compendium Code No.: 14960450 05/00

VITA-HOOF®

Equicare **Hoof Product**

Ingredient(s): Petrolatum, lanolin, soybean oil, povidone-iodine, urea, wheat germ oil, cod liver oil.

Indications: Hoof conditioner and dressing for use on horses.

Directions for Use: Apply daily to complete hoof, deep into heel, and to coronary band. For maximum effectiveness also apply to the pastern area and massage into the skin. To improve absorption during cold weather, VITA-HOOF® should be warmed prior to application.

Presentation: 1 quart (0.95 L) and 1 gallon.

U.S. Patent 4,604,283

Compendium Code No.: 14470241

VITA-JEC® A & D "500"

AgriPharm **Vitamins A-D**

Active Ingredient(s): Each mL contains:

Vitamin A propionate .... 500,000 I.U.
Vitamin D_3 .... 75,000 I.U.
Vitamin E (antioxidant) .... 5 I.U.
Benzyl alcohol .... 2% v/v
Ethyl alcohol .... 8% v/v

0.75% B.H.A. and 0.75% B.H.T. as preservatives.

Indications: A water emulsifiable solution to be used as a supplemental source of vitamins A and D_3 in cattle.

Dosage and Administration: Administer by deep intramuscular injection. Dosage may be repeated after 60 days, if needed.

Calves .... ½ to 1 mL
Yearlings/Feedlot .... 1 to 3 mL
Adult Cattle .... 3 to 6 mL

Precaution(s): Store at controlled temperature between 2°-30°C (36°-86°F). Protect from light. Refrigerate unused portion.

Caution(s): Do not exceed recommended dosage. If intended dose is greater than 4 mL in cattle, divide dose equally and give in 2 different sites.

Not for human use.

Keep out of reach of children.

Warning(s): Do not administer to food producing animals within 60 days of slaughter.

Presentation: 100 mL, 250 mL and 500 mL vials.

Compendium Code No.: 14571040

VITA-JEC® B-COMPLEX

AgriPharm **Vitamin B-Complex**

Active Ingredient(s): Each mL contains:

Thiamine HCl .... 12.5 mg
Riboflavin (as 5' phosphate sodium) .... 2 mg
Niacinamide .... 100 mg
d-Panthenol .... 10 mg
Pyridoxine HCl .... 5 mg
Cyanocobalamin (cryst.) .... 5 mcg
Benzyl alcohol (preservative) .... 1.5% v/v
Water for injection .... q.s.

Stabilized in a buffered base.

Indications: A sterile aqueous solution of B-complex vitamins for use in preventing or treating deficiencies of these vitamins in cattle, horses, sheep, and swine.

Dosage and Administration: Administer intramuscularly or subcutaneously. The dosage may be repeated once or twice a week as needed.

Lambs and Weanling pigs .... 1-2 mL
Growing Lambs and Pigs .... 2-3 mL
Adult Sheep and Swine .... 3-5 mL
Calves and Foals .... 3-5 mL
Yearlings .... 5-10 mL
Adult Cattle and Horses .... 10-20 mL

Precaution(s): Store at a temperature between 36°-46°F (2°-8°C).

Caution(s): For animal use only.

Keep out of the reach of children.

Not for intravenous use. Anaphylactic reactions to parenteral thiamine HCl have been reported. Administer slowly and with caution in doses over 4 mL (50 mg thiamine).

Presentation: 250 mL and 500 mL vials.

Compendium Code No.: 14571060

VITA-JEC® B COMPLEX FORTIFIED

AgriPharm **Vitamin B-Complex**

Active Ingredient(s): Each mL contains:

Thiamine HCl .... 100 mg
Riboflavin 5' sodium phosphate U.S.P. .... 5 mg
Niacinamide .... 100 mg
d-Panthenol .... 10 mg
Pyridoxine HCl .... 10 mg
Cyanocobalamin (vitamin B_{12}) .... 100 mcg
Benzyl alcohol (preservative) .... 1.5% v/v
Water for injection .... q.s.

Stabilized in a citric acid buffer.

Indications: For use as a supplemental source of B complex vitamins for cattle, sheep, and swine.

Dosage and Administration: Administer intramuscularly or subcutaneously. Dosage may be repeated once or twice weekly as needed.

Calves . . . 3 to 5 mL
Yearlings . . . 5 to 10 mL
Adult Cattle. . . . 10 to 20 mL
Lambs and Weanling Pigs . . . 1 to 2 mL
Growing Lambs and Pigs. . . . 2 to 3 mL
Adult Sheep and Swine . . . 3 to 5 mL
Precaution(s): Store at refrigerated temperatures between 2°-8°C (36°-46°F). Protect from light. Refrigerate unused portion.
Caution(s): Not for intravenous use. Parenteral administration of thiamine has resulted in anaphylactic shock. Administer slowly and with caution in doses over 0.5 mL (50 mg thiamine).
Warning(s): For animal use only. Keep out of reach of children.
Presentation: 100 mL, 250 mL and 500 mL vials.
Compendium Code No.: 14571050

VITA-JEC® B-COMPLEX WITH CYANO PLUS

AgriPharm **Vitamin B-Complex Injection**

Active Ingredient(s): Each mL of sterile aqueous solution contains:
Thiamine Hydrochloride (B_1) . . . 12.5 mg
Niacinamide . . . 12.5 mg
Pyridoxine Hydrochloride (B_6) . . . 5.0 mg
d-Panthenol . . . 5.0 mg
Riboflavin (B_2) (as Riboflavin 5' phosphate sodium) . . . 2.0 mg
Cyanocobalamin (B_{12}) . . . 1000 mcg
with benzyl alcohol 1.5% v/v as preservative, ammonium sulfate 0.1%.
Indications: For use as a supplemental source of B complex vitamins in cattle, swine and sheep.
Dosage and Administration: Subcutaneous or intramuscular injection is recommended. May be administered intravenously at the discretion of a veterinarian. The following are suggested dosages, depending on the condition of the animal and the desired response.
Adult Cattle: 1 to 2 mL per 500 pounds of body weight.
Calves, Swine and Sheep: 1 to 2 mL. May be repeated once or twice weekly.
Precaution(s): Store at controlled room temperature between 15° to 30°C (59°-86°F).
Protect from light.
Caution(s): Hypersensitivity reactions to the parenteral administration of products containing thiamine have been reported. Administer with caution and keep treated animals under close observation.
Warning(s): For animal use only. Keep out of reach of children.
Presentation: 250 mL (8.5 fl oz).
Compendium Code No.: 14571071

VITA-JEC® THIAMINE HCL ℞

RXV **Thiamine**

Active Ingredient(s): Each mL contains:
Thiamine hydrochloride . . . 200 mg
Disodium edetate . . . 0.01% w/v
Benzyl alcohol (as preservative) . . . 1.5% w/v
Water for injection . . . q.s.
pH adjusted with hydrochloric acid or sodium hydroxide.
Indications: For use as a supplemental source of thiamine in dogs, cats and horses.
Dosage and Administration: For intravenous or intramuscular use in horses, dogs and cats.
Horses . . . 0.25 mL/100 lbs bw
Dogs . . . 0.08 mL/10 lbs bw to 0.25 mL maximum
Cats . . . 0.04 mL/5 lbs bw to 0.1 mL maximum
Precaution(s): Store at controlled room temperature between 15°-30°C (59°-86°F).
Caution(s): Federal law restricts this drug to use by or on the order of a licensed veterinarian.
Anaphylactogenesis reactions to parenteral thiamine has occurred. Administer slowly and with caution in doses over 0.25 mL (50 mg).
Warning(s): For animal use only.
Keep out of reach of children.
Presentation: 100 mL and 250 mL vials.
Compendium Code No.: 10910250

VITA-JEC® VITAMIN B_{12} (Cyano 1,000 mcg/mL) ℞

RXV **Vitamin B_{12}**

Active Ingredient(s): Each mL contains:
Cyanocobalamin. . . . 1000 mcg
Benzyl alcohol (as preservative) . . . 1.5% v/v
Sodium chloride . . . 0.8% w/v
Water for injection . . . q.s.
pH buffered with acetic acid.
Indications: For use in vitamin B_{12} deficiency associated with cobalt deficiency in cattle and sheep, and for vitamin B_{12} deficiency associated with inadequate vitamin B_{12} intake or intestinal malabsorption in swine.
Dosage and Administration: For intramuscular or subcutaneous use.
Cattle and Sheep . . . 1 to 2 mL
Swine . . . 0.1 to 2.0 mL
Dosage may be repeated at weekly intervals if necessary.
Precaution(s): Store at temperature between 2°-30°C (36°-86°F).
Caution(s): Federal law restricts this drug to use by or on the order of a licensed veterinarian.
Warning(s): For animal use only. Keep out of reach of children.
Presentation: 100 mL, 250 mL and 500 mL vials.
Compendium Code No.: 10910270

V

VITA-JEC® VITAMIN B_{12} (Cyano 3,000 mcg/mL) ℞

RXV **Vitamin B_{12}**

Active Ingredient(s): Each mL contains:
Cyanocobalamin. . . . 3000 mcg
Benzyl alcohol (as preservative) . . . 1.5% v/v
Sodium chloride . . . 0.8% w/v
Water for injection . . . q.s.
pH buffered with acetic acid.
Indications: For use in vitamin B_{12} deficiency associated with cobalt deficiency in cattle and sheep and for vitamin B_{12} deficiency associated with inadequate vitamin B_{12} intake or intestinal malabsorption in swine.
Dosage and Administration: Administer intramuscularly or subcutaneously.
Cattle and Sheep . . . ⅓ to ⅔ mL
Swine . . . 1/10 to ⅔ mL
Dosage may be repeated at weekly intervals, if necessary.
Precaution(s): Store at temperature between 2°-30°C (36°-86°F).
Caution(s): Federal law restricts this drug to use by or on the order of a licensed veterinarian.
Warning(s): For animal use only. Keep out of reach of children.
Presentation: 100 mL and 250 mL vials.
Compendium Code No.: 10910280

VITA-JEC® VITAMIN K1 INJECTABLE ℞

RXV **Vitamin K_1-Injection**

Active Ingredient(s): Each mL contains:
Phytonadione . . . 10 mg
Polyoxyethylated fatty acid derivative . . . 70 mg
Dextrose . . . 37.5 mg
Water . . . q.s.
with benzyl alcohol 0.9% added as a preservative.
Indications: For the control of acute hypoprothrombinemia (with hemorrhage) and non-acute hypoprothrombinemia in cattle, calves, horses, swine, sheep, goats, dogs and cats.
Dosage and Administration:
Cattle, Calves, Horses, Swine, Sheep and Goats:
Acute Hypoprothrombinemia (with Hemorrhage):
Mature Animals: 0.5-2.5 mg/kg body weight injected intravenously at a rate not to exceed 10 mg/minute.
Newborn and Very Young Animals: 0.5-2.5 mg/kg body weight injected intravenously at a rate not to exceed 5 mg/minute.
Non-Acute Hypoprothrombinemia:
All Ages: 0.5-2.5 mg/kg body weight injected intramuscularly or subcutaneously.
Dogs and Cats:
Acute Hypoprothrombinemia (with Hemorrhage):
All Ages: 0.25-2.5 mg/kg body weight injected intravenously at a rate not to exceed 5 mg/minute.
Non-Acute Hypoprothrombinemia:
All Ages: 0.25-2.5 mg/kg body weight injected intramuscularly or subcutaneously.
Precaution(s): Protect from light. Store in a dark place. Store in a cool place between 2°-8°C (36°-46°F).
Caution(s): Federal law restricts this drug to use by or on the order of a licensed veterinarian.
Warning(s): Not for human use.
Keep out of reach of children.
Presentation: 100 mL vials.
Compendium Code No.: 10910290

VITA-KEY® ANTIOXIDANT CONCENTRATE

Vita-Key **Equine Dietary Supplement**

Guaranteed Analysis:

	Per Ounce	Per Pound
Crude Protein, minimum	2.4 g	8.50%
Methionine, minimum	550 mg	1.94%
Lysine, minimum	326 mg	1.15%
Fat, minimum	425 mg	1.50%
Fiber, maximum	3.1 g	11.00%
Cobalt, minimum from cobalt glucoheptonate complex	10 mg	353 ppm
Copper, minimum from copper lysine complex	60 mg	2,114 ppm
Iodine, minimum from ethylenediamine dihydroiodide	1 mg	35 ppm
Manganese, minimum from manganese methionine complex	100 mg	3,524 ppm
Zinc, minimum from zinc methionine complex	150 mg	5,286 ppm
Selenium, minimum	1 mg	35.2 ppm
Vitamin A, minimum	20,000 I.U.	320,000 I.U.
Vitamin D_3, minimum	5,000 I.U.	80,000 I.U.
Vitamin E, minimum	2,000 I.U.	32,000 I.U.
Vitamin B_{12}, minimum	0.4 mg	6.4 mg
Menadione, minimum	4 mg	64 mg
Riboflavin, minimum	40 mg	640 mg
d-Pantothenic Acid, minimum	65 mg	1,040 mg
Thiamine, minimum	125 mg	2,000 mg
Niacin, minimum	125 mg	2,000 mg
Vitamin B_6, minimum	25 mg	400 mg
Folic Acid, minimum	25 mg	400 mg
Biotin, minimum	0.3 mg	4.8 mg
Ascorbic Acid, minimum	1,500 mg	24,000 mg
Beta-Carotene, minimum	2 mg	32 mg

Ingredients: *Saccharomyces cerevisiae* yeast and the media on which it was grown, vitamin E supplement, ascorbic acid, beta-carotene, zinc methionine complex, cobalt glucoheptonate complex, copper lysine complex, manganese methionine complex, ethylenediamine dihydroiodide, vitamin A supplement, vitamin D supplement, vitamin B_{12} supplement, riboflavin supplement, niacin supplement, calcium pantothenate, menadione sodium bisulfite complex, pyridoxine hydrochloride, folic acid, thiamine mononitrate, sodium selenite, d-biotin, and diatomaceous earth.
Indications: A nutritional vitamin, yeast and trace mineral supplement for older, stressed horses, and performance horses.
Directions: Feeding Directions: Apply to horses daily grain ration (with 2 oz of corn oil for best results) and mix thoroughly, using the following basic guidelines. Feed the higher recommended levels (as listed below) during periods of reduced feed intake, stress, adaptation to diets, or to nutritionally support horses for optimum performance. Divide VITA-KEY® Antioxidant Concentrate amounts equally by number of feedings per day.

*Note: The acclimation period varies for each individual horse.
Older Horses: 1-2 oz daily.
Stressed Horses: 1-2 oz daily.
Weight Gain: 1-2 oz daily.
Performance Horses: 1-2 oz daily.
Breeding Stock: 1-2 oz daily.
Weanlings: ½-1 oz daily.
The enclosed measuring cup, level full, is one ounce.

*Note: Because of VITA-KEY®'s high vitamin and mineral content, the smell and taste may be offensive to some animals. Mixing with 2 oz of corn oil will help. If problems still persist, feed 25% of recommended feeding level for 5 days, 50% of recommended feeding level for the next 5 days, and then the full 100% of the recommended feeding level.

Contraindication(s): Do not feed to sheep or any other livestock sensitive to copper.

Precaution(s): Store in a cool, dry and clean place, keeping container tightly closed.

Caution(s): Do not feed wet, moldy, or insect-infested feed.

VITA-KEY® Antioxidant Concentrate is only part of a well balanced diet and should be fed with a properly balanced ration (proteins, fat, fiber, minerals, quantity consumed, etc.).

VITA-KEY® Antioxidant Concentrate is a nutritional feed additive. It contains no drugs or hormones and does not replace antibiotics. No withdrawal.

Vitamins degrade over time and with exposure to air, sunlight, temperature, and moisture. Use this product as directed by your veterinarian, and in a timely manner.

VITA-KEY, L.C. makes no warranties, either expressed or implied as to the use of this product, other than the actual guaranteed analysis on the label when the product is stored as recommended and analyzed in a timely manner.

Presentation: 5 lbs (2.27 kg) and 20 lbs.

VITA-KEY® contains Zinpro, Cuplex, Manpro, and Copro, which are registered trademarks of Zinpro Corporation.

Compendium Code No.: 14770001

VITA-KEY® BIOTIN ZM-80

Vita-Key **Equine Dietary Supplement**

A biotin, zinc methionine and dl-methionine supplement designed to improve and maintain healthy hooves, fortified with Diamond V Yeast Culture

Guaranteed Analysis:

	Per oz	Per lb
Biotin	15 mg	240 mg
Zinc from Zinc Methionine Complex	200 mg	0.0325%
Methionine	3,000 mg	10.57%

Ingredients: Dried *Saccharomyces cerevisiae* fermentation product, d-biotin, zinc methionine complex®, dl-methionine.

Indications: Preventive supplementation of the formula described above may be beneficial for horses subject to: Moist stalling conditions; rough terrain; Extreme moisture variations which cause frequent expansion and contraction of the hoof wall; nutritional deficiencies.

Dosage and Administration: A 5 pound container is a 80 day supply for one horse. VITA-KEY® Biotin ZM-80 should be supplemented at the rate of 1 ounce per day.

Clinical Trials: For supplementation to be effective it must be given daily over a considerable period of time. Research reported by Hoffmann-LaRoche Laboratories indicates the following times are required for a hoof to grow enough to replace itself; Lippizzaners - 11 months, Shires - 15 months, Ponies - 20 months.

In a clinical study involving 70 horses with a history of hoof problems, 60% were judged by veterinarians to have a complete recovery after supplementing biotin for 12 months. The remaining showed marked and significant improvement.

Discussion: The following conditions may indicate significant deficiencies: Splitting or cracking hooves; poor hoof white-line health; hoof abscesses; poor frog health or thrush; brittle; dry mane and tail; dry, flaky skin.

Presentation: 5 lb and 20 lb.

Compendium Code No.: 14770012

VITA-KEY® BROOD MARE SUPPLEMENT

Vita-Key **Large Animal Dietary Supplement**

Guaranteed Analysis:

	Per oz	Per lb
Zinc, from zinc methionine complex	100 mg	0.352%
Manganese, from manganese methionine complex	100 mg	0.352%
Copper, from copper lysine complex	60 mg	0.211%
Iron, from iron methionine	32 mg	0.112%
Cobalt, from cobalt glucoheptonate complex	5 mg	0.0176%
Selenium	1 mg	0.00352%
Vitamin A, minimum	25,000 IU	400,000 IU
Vitamin D_3, minimum	4,000 IU	64,000 IU
Vitamin E, minimum	500 IU	8,000 IU
Vitamin B_{12}, minimum	0.15 mg	2.4 mg
Menadione, minimum	1.5 mg	24 mg
Riboflavin, minimum	25 mg	400 mg
d-Pantothenic Acid, minimum	40 mg	640 mg
Thiamine, minimum	40 mg	640 mg
Niacin, minimum	100 mg	1,600 mg
Vitamin B_6, minimum	8 mg	128 mg
Folic Acid, minimum	10 mg	160 mg
Biotin, minimum	1.25 mg	20 mg
Ascorbic Acid, minimum	500 mg	8,000 mg
Bera-Carotene, minimum	250 mg	4,000 mg
Methionine, minimum	539 mg	1.90%
Lysine, minimum	255 mg	0.90%

Ingredients: Dried *Saccharomyces cerevisiae* fermentation product, Zinc Methionine Complex®, Cobalt Glucoheptonate Complex®, Copper Lysine Complex®, Manganese Methionine Complex®, Ferric Methionine Complex®, sodium selenite, beta-carotene, vitamin E supplement, ascorbic acid, vitamin A supplement, vitamin D supplement, vitamin B_{12} supplement, riboflavin supplement, niacin supplement, calcium pantothenate, menadione sodium bisulfite complex, folic acid, pyridoxine hydrochloride, thiamine mononitrate, d-biotin.

Indications: A concentrated source of bioavailable trace minerals and vitamins, including high levels of Beta-carotene, for the brood mare.

VITA-KEY® Brood Mare Supplement is recommended for use 30 days prior to parturition (foaling) and until pregnancy is confirmed.

Dosage and Administration: Use 1 to 2 oz daily for 30 days prior to parturition and until pregnancy is confirmed.

Presentation: 5#, a 40 day supply at the 2 oz dose.

Compendium Code No.: 14770021

VITA-KEY® EQUINE SUPPLEMENT

Vita-Key **Equine Dietary Supplement**

Guaranteed Analysis:

	Per Ounce	Per Pound
Crude Protein, minimum	2.5 g	9.00%
Lysine, minimum	320 mg	1.12%
Methionine, minimum	567 mg	2.00%
Crude Fat, minimum	0.5 g	1.76%
Crude Fiber, maximum	3.1 g	11.00%
Cobalt, minimum from cobalt glucoheptonate complex	9 mg	317 ppm
Copper, minimum from copper lysine complex	60 mg	2,114 ppm
Iodine, minimum from ethylenediamine dihydroiodide	1 mg	35 ppm
Iron, minimum from iron methionine complex	25 mg	882 ppm
Manganese, minimum from manganese methionine complex	100 mg	3,524 ppm
Zinc, minimum from zinc methionine complex	125 mg	4,409 ppm
Selenium, minimum	0.5 mg	17.62 ppm
Vitamin A, minimum	20,000 I.U.	320,000 I.U.
Vitamin D_3, minimum	5,000 I.U.	80,000 I.U.
Vitamin E, minimum	600 I.U.	9,600 I.U.
Vitamin B_{12}, minimum	0.2 mg	3.2 mg
Menadione, minimum	2 mg	32 mg
Riboflavin, minimum	30 mg	480 mg
d-Pantothenic Acid, minimum	50 mg	800 mg
Thiamine, minimum	100 mg	1,600 mg
Niacin, minimum	125 mg	2,000 mg
Vitamin B_6, minimum	15 mg	240 mg
Folic Acid, minimum	12 mg	192 mg
Biotin, minimum	1.5 mg	24 mg
Ascorbic Acid, minimum	600 mg	9,600 mg

Ingredients: *Saccharomyces cerevisiae* yeast and the media on which it was grown, zinc methionine complex, cobalt glucoheptonate complex, copper lysine complex, manganese methionine complex, ferric methionine complex, sodium selenite, ethylenediamine dihydroiodide, vitamin E supplement, ascorbic acid, vitamin A supplement, vitamin D supplement, vitamin B_{12} supplement, riboflavin supplement, niacin supplement, calcium pantothenate, d-pantothenic acid, menadione sodium bisulfite complex, folic acid, pyridoxine hydrochloride, thiamine mononitrate, d-biotin and diatomaceous earth.

Indications: A vitamin, yeast culture and trace mineral supplement for performance horses.

Directions: Feeding Directions: Apply to horse's daily grain ration (with 2 oz of corn oil for best results) and mix thoroughly, using the following basic guidelines. Feed the higher recommended feeding levels (as listed below), during periods of reduced feed intake, stress, adaptation to diets, to horses on poorly, fortified diets, or to nutritionally support horses for optimum performance. Divide supplemented amounts equally by number of feedings per day.

*Note: The acclimation period varies for each individual horse.
Racing and Training Horses: 2 oz daily.
Performance Horses: 2 oz daily.
Mares in Foal: 2 oz daily.
Breeding Stock: 1 to 2 oz daily.
Weanlings: 1 oz daily.
Yearlings: 1 to 2 oz daily.
Pleasure Horses: Normal use - 2 oz daily, Light use 1 oz daily.
Horses in Poor Condition: 2 oz daily.
The enclosed measuring cup, level full, is approximately one ounce.

*Note: Because of VITA-KEY®'s high vitamin and mineral content, the smell and taste may be offensive to some animals. In this case mix with 2 oz of corn oil. If problems still persist, feed 25% of recommended feeding level for 5 days, 50% of recommended feeding level for the next 5 days, and then the full 100% of the recommended feeding level.

Contraindication(s): Do not feed to sheep or any other livestock sensitive to copper.

Precaution(s): Store in a cool, dry and clean place, in shaded area, keeping container tightly closed.

Caution(s): Do not feed wet, moldy, or insect-infested feed.

VITA-KEY® Equine Supplement is only part of a well balanced diet and should be fed with a properly balanced ration (proteins, fat, fiber, minerals, quantity consumed, etc.).

VITA-KEY® Equine Supplement is a nutritional feed additive. It contains no drugs or hormones and does not replace antibiotics. No withdrawal.

Vitamins degrade over time and with exposure to air, sunlight, temperature, and moisture. Use this product as directed, and in a timely manner.

VITA-KEY, L.C. makes no warranties, either expressed or implied as to the use of this product, other than the actual guaranteed analysis on the label when the product is stored as recommended and analyzed in a timely manner.

Presentation: 5 lbs (2.27 kg) and 20 lbs.

VITA-KEY® Equine Supplement contains Zinpro, Cuplex, Meth-Iron, Manpro, and Copro, which are registered trademarks of Zinpro Corporation.

Compendium Code No.: 14770031

VITA-KEY® MARE & FOAL SUPPLEMENT

Vita-Key **Equine Dietary Supplement**

Guaranteed Analysis:

	Per Ounce	Per Pound
Crude Protein, minimum	2.268 g	8.00%
Lysine, minimum	2,000 mg	7.05%
Methionine, minimum	680 mg	2.40%
Crude Fat, minimum	354 mg	1.25%
Crude Fiber, maximum	2.835 g	10.00%
Cobalt, minimum from cobalt glucoheptonate complex	14 mg	494 ppm
Copper, minimum from copper lysine complex	70 mg	2,469 ppm
Iodine, minimum from ethylenediamine dihydroiodide	1 mg	35 ppm
Manganese, minimum from manganese methionine complex	110 mg	3,880 ppm
Zinc, minimum from zinc methionine complex	200 mg	7,055 ppm
Selenium, minimum	0.5 mg	17.62 ppm
Vitamin A, minimum	20,000 I.U.	320,000 I.U.
Vitamin D_3, minimum	5,000 I.U.	80,000 I.U.
Vitamin E, minimum	600 I.U.	9,600 I.U.
Vitamin B_{12}, minimum	0.2 mg	3.2 mg
Menadione, minimum	2 mg	32 mg
Riboflavin, minimum	30 mg	480 mg
d-Pantothenic Acid, minimum	50 mg	800 mg
Thiamine, minimum	100 mg	1,600 mg
Niacin, minimum	125 mg	2,000 mg
Vitamin B_6, minimum	15 mg	240 mg
Folic Acid, minimum	12 mg	192 mg
Biotin, minimum	1.5 mg	24 mg
Ascorbic Acid, minimum	2,250 mg	36,000 mg

Ingredients: *Saccharomyces cerevisiae* yeast and the media on which it was grown, zinc methionine complex, cobalt glucoheptonate complex, copper lysine complex, manganese methionine complex, sodium selenite, ethylenediamine dihydroiodide, vitamin E supplement, ascorbic acid, vitamin A supplement, vitamin D supplement, vitamin B_{12} supplement, riboflavin supplement, niacin supplement, calcium pantothenate, d-pantothenic acid, menadione sodium bisulfite complex, folic acid, pyridoxine hydrochloride, thiamine mononitrate, d-biotin and diatomaceous earth.

Indications: A vitamin, yeast culture and trace mineral supplement for pregnant and lactating mares, and for weanling and yearling foals. Recommended as an aid to meet foals' nutritional needs from fetus through yearling.

Directions: Feeding Directions: Apply to horse's daily grain ration (with 2 oz of corn oil for best results) and mix thoroughly, using the following basic guidelines. Feed the higher recommended feeding levels (as listed below), during periods of reduced feed intake, stress, adaptation to diets, to horses on poorly, fortified diets, or to nutritionally support horses for optimum performance.

Divide supplemented amounts equally by number of feedings per day.

*Note: The acclimation period varies for each individual horse.

Pregnant Mares: 2-4 oz daily.
Lactating Mares: 2-4 oz daily.
Brood Mares: 2-4 oz daily.
Weanlings: 1-2 oz daily.
Yearlings: 2-3 oz daily.
Horses in Poor Condition: 2-4 oz daily.
The enclosed measuring cup, level full, is one ounce.

*Note: Because of VITA-KEY®'s high vitamin and mineral content, the smell and taste may be offensive to some animals. In this case mix with 2 oz of corn oil. If problems still persist, feed 25% of recommended feeding level for 5 days, 50% of recommended feeding level for the next 5 days, and then the full 100% of the recommended feeding level.

Contraindication(s): Do not feed to sheep or any other livestock sensitive to copper.

Precaution(s): Store in a cool, dry and clean place, in shaded area, keeping container tightly closed.

Caution(s): Do not feed wet, moldy, or insect-infested feed.

VITA-KEY® Mare and Foal Supplement is only part of a well balanced diet and should be fed with a properly balanced ration (proteins, fat, fiber, minerals, quantity consumed, etc.).

VITA-KEY® Mare and Foal Supplement is a nutritional feed additive. It contains no drugs or hormones and does not replace antibiotics. No withdrawal.

Vitamins degrade over time and with exposure to air, sunlight, temperature, and moisture. Use this product as directed, and in a timely manner.

VITA-KEY, L.C. makes no warranties, either expressed or implied as to the use of this product, other than the actual guaranteed analysis on the label when the product is stored as recommended and analyzed in a timely manner.

Presentation: 5 lbs (2.27 kg) and 20 lbs.

VITA-KEY® Mare & Foal Supplement contains Zinpro, Cuplex, Manpro, and Copro, which are registered trademarks of Zinpro Corporation.

Compendium Code No.: 14770041

VITA-KEY® SHOW CATTLE CONCENTRATE, PHASE II

Vita-Key **Large Animal Dietary Supplement**

Guaranteed Analysis:

	Per Pound
Crude Protein, minimum	10.0%
Methionine, minimum	4.0%
Lysine, minimum	2.0%
Crude Fat, minimum	1.4%
Crude Fiber, maximum	9.0%
Zinc, minimum from zinc methionine complex	1.268%
Cobalt, minimum from cobalt glucoheptonate complex	880 ppm
Copper, minimum from copper lysine complex	4,220 ppm
Manganese, minimum from manganese methionine complex	7,000 ppm
Iodine, minimum from ethylenediamine dihydroiodide	105 ppm
Selenium, minimum	53 ppm
Vitamin A, minimum	800,000 I.U.
Vitamin D_3, minimum	150,000 I.U.
Vitamin E, minimum	6,000 I.U.
Thiamine, minimum	2,880 mg
Niacin, minimum	9,600 mg
Total Bacteria*, minimum colony forming units	8 billion

(**Streptococcus faecium, Lactobacillus acidophilus, Lactobacillus casei, Lactobacillus lactis, Bifidobacterium bifidum, Streptococcus diacetilactis.*)

Ingredients: *Saccharomyces cerevisiae* yeast and the media on which it was grown, dried *Saccharomyces cerevisiae* fermentation product, zinc methionine complex, cobalt glucoheptonate complex, copper lysine complex, manganese methionine complex, vitamin E supplement, vitamin A supplement, vitamin D supplement, niacin supplement, thiamine mononitrate, sodium selenite, ethylenediamine dihydroiodide, dried *Streptococcus faecium* fermentation product, dried *Lactobacillus acidophilus* fermentation product, dried *Lactobacillus casei* fermentation product, dried *Lactobacillus lactis* fermentation product, dried *Bifidobacterium bifidum* fermentation product, dried *Streptococcus diacetilactis* fermentation product, protease, amylase, lipase, and diatomaceous earth.

Indications: A nutritional supplement for cattle with vitamins, specific amino acid complexed trace minerals, live direct-fed microbials, enzymes, and yeast culture.

Directions: Feeding Directions: Apply to cattle's daily grain ration and mix thoroughly, using the following basic guidelines. Feed the higher recommended levels (as listed below) during periods of reduced feed intake, stress, adaptation of cattle to feedlot diets, or to nutritionally support cattle for optimum performance. Divide supplemented amounts equally by number of feedings per day.

*Note: The acclimation period varies for each individual animal.

Show Cattle Weighing:

110 to 200 pounds: ½ oz daily.
200 to 300 pounds: 1 oz daily.
300 pounds and up: 1 oz to 2 oz daily.

Beef Cows and Bulls: 1 oz to 2 oz daily.
Donor Cows (21 days before flushing): 2 oz daily.
A.I. and Recipient Cows (21 days before breeding): 2 oz daily.
The enclosed measuring cup, level full, is one ounce.

*Note: Because of VITA-KEY®'s high vitamin and mineral content, the smell and taste may be offensive to some animals. If problems occur, feed 25% of recommended feeding level for 5 days, 50% of recommended feeding level for the next 5 days, and then the full 100% of the recommended feeding level.

Contraindication(s): Do not feed to sheep or any other livestock sensitive to copper.

Precaution(s): Store in a cool (not to exceed 78 degrees Fahrenheit), dry and clean place, keeping container tightly closed. Refrigerate for longer shelf life.

Caution(s): Do not feed wet, moldy, or insect-infested feed.

VITA-KEY® Show Cattle Concentrate is only part of a well balanced diet and should be fed with a properly balanced ration (proteins, fat, fiber, minerals, quantity consumed, etc.).

VITA-KEY® Show Cattle Concentrate is a nutritional feed additive. It contains no drugs or hormones and does not replace antibiotics. No withdrawal.

Vitamins and microbes degrade over time and with exposure to air, sunlight, temperature, and moisture. Use this product as directed, and in a timely manner.

VITA-KEY, L.C. makes no warranties, either expressed or implied as to the use of this product, other than the actual guaranteed analysis on the label when the product is stored as recommended and analyzed in a timely manner.

Presentation: 5 lb and 20 lb.

VITA-KEY® Show Cattle Concentrate contains Zinpro, Cuplex, Manpro, and Copro, which are registered trademarks of Zinpro Corporation.

Compendium Code No.: 14770050

VITA-KEY® SHOW CATTLE SUPPLEMENT, PHASE I

Vita-Key **Large Animal Dietary Supplement**

Guaranteed Analysis:

	Per Pound
Crude Protein, minimum	7.0%
Crude Fat, minimum	25.0%
Crude Fiber, minimum	7.0%
Cobalt, min. from cobalt glucoheptonate complex	0.044%
Copper, min. from copper lysine complex	0.211%
Manganese, min. from manganese methionine complex	0.352%
Zinc, min. from zinc methionine complex	0.634%
Iodine, min. from ethylenediamine dihydriodide	0.00528%
Selenium, minimum	0.00264%
Vitamin A, minimum	400,000 I.U.
Vitamin D_3, minimum	75,000 I.U.
Vitamin E, minimum	3,000 I.U.
Thiamine, minimum	1,440 mg
Niacin, minimum	4,800 mg
Methionine, minimum	2.14%
Lysine, minimum	0.82%

Ingredients: Dried *Saccharomyces cerevisae* fermentation product, animal digest, animal fat, Zinc Methionine Complex®, Cobalt Glucoheptonate Complex®, Copper Lysine Complex®, Manganese Methionine Complex®, dried *Lactobacillus acidophilus* ferm. prod., dried *Lactobacillus casei* ferm. prod., dried *Lactobacillus lactis* ferm. prod., dried *Bifidobacterium bifidum* ferm. prod., dried *Streptococcus diacetilactis* ferm. prod., vitamin E supplement, vitamin D supplement, niacin supplement, thiamine mononitrate, dried whey, sodium selenite.

Indications: A vitamin, trace mineral and microbial culture product to supplement the diet of cattle.

Feeding Directions: Apply to cattle's daily grain ration and mix thoroughly, using the following basic guidelines. Feed the higher recommended levels as listed below, during periods of reduced feed intake, stress, adaptation of cattle to feedlot diets, or to nutritionally challenge optimum performance. Divide supplement amounts equally by number of feedings per day.

*Note: the acclimation period varies for each animal.

As a Supplement to:

Show Cattle Weighing;
100-200 lbs . . . . . 1 oz daily
200-300 lbs . . . . . 2 oz daily
300 lbs and up . . . . . 2 oz to 4 oz daily
Cows and Bulls: . . . . . 2 oz to 4 oz daily
Donor Cows (21 days before flushing) . . . . . 4 oz daily
AI Recipient Cows (21 days pre-breeding) . . . . . 4 oz daily

Presentation: 5#, an 80 day supply.
20#, a 320 day supply.

Compendium Code No.: 14770060

VITA-KEY® SWINE SUPPLEMENT

Vita-Key **Large Animal Dietary Supplement**

Guaranteed Analysis:

	Per Ounce	Per Pound
Crude Protein, minimum	2.75 g	10.00%
Lysine, minimum	1,418 mg	5.00%
Methionine, minimum	212 mg	0.75%
Crude Fat, not less than	0.50 g	2.00%
Crude Fiber, not more than	2.75 g	9.00%
Chromium, minimum	0.38 mg	13.3 ppm
Cobalt, minimum from cobalt glucoheptonate complex	10 mg	350 ppm
Copper, minimum from copper lysine complex	62 mg	2180 ppm
Iodine, minimum from ethylenediamine dihydroiodide	0.88 mg	31 ppm
Iron, minimum from iron methionine	32 mg	1120 ppm
Manganese, minimum from manganese methionine complex	19 mg	660 ppm
Zinc, minimum from zinc methionine and zinc lysine complex	62 mg	2180 ppm
Selenium, minimum	0.5 mg	17.6 ppm
Vitamin A, minimum	20,000 I.U.	320,000 I.U.
Vitamin D_3, minimum	3,500 I.U.	56,000 I.U.
Vitamin E, minimum	150 I.U.	2,400 I.U.
Vitamin B_{12}, minimum	0.08 mg	1.28 mg
Menadione, minimum	3.3 mg	52.8 mg
Riboflavin, minimum	16 mg	256 mg
d-Pantothenic Acid, minimum	50 mg	800 mg
Thiamine, minimum	5 mg	80 mg
Niacin, minimum	80 mg	1,280 mg
Vitamin B_6, minimum	10 mg	160 mg
Folic Acid, minimum	8 mg	128 mg
Biotin, minimum	.24 mg	3.84 mg
Total Bacteria*, minimum colony forming units	250 million	4 billion

(**Streptococcus faecium, Lactobacillus acidophilus, Lactobacillus casei, Lactobacillus lactis, Bifidobacterium bifidum, Streptococcus diacetilactis*)

Ingredients: *Saccharomyces cerevisiae* yeast and the media on which it was grown, dried *Saccharomyces cerevisiae* fermentation product, zinc lysine complex, zinc methionine complex, copper lysine complex, ferric methionine complex, cobalt glucoheptonate complex, manganese methionine complex, chromium tripicolinate, sodium selenite, ethylenediamine dihydroiodide, vitamin E supplement, vitamin A supplement, vitamin D supplement, vitamin B_{12} supplement, riboflavin supplement, niacin supplement, calcium pantothenate, menadione sodium bisulfite complex, folic acid, pyridoxine hydrochloride, thiamine mononitrate, d-biotin, dried *Streptococcus faecium* fermentation product, dried *Lactobacillus acidophilus* fermentation product, dried *Lactobacillus casei* fermentation product, dried *Lactobacillus lactis* fermentation product, dried *Bifidobacterium bifidum* fermentation product, dried *Streptococcus diacetilactis* fermentation product, protease, amylase, lipase, and diatomaceous earth.

Indications: A vitamin and trace mineral supplement for swine with chromium, live direct fed microbials, enzymes, and yeast culture.

Directions: Feeding Directions: Apply to the daily grain ration and mix thoroughly, using the following basic guidelines. Feed the higher recommended levels as listed below, during periods of reduced feed intake, stress, adaptation to diets, to swine on poorly fortified diets, or to nutritionally support swine for optimum performance. The lower recommended feeding levels as listed below are designed for swine on premium quality commercially fortified diets. Divide supplemented amounts equally by number of feedings per day.

*Note: The acclimation period varies for each individual animal.

Swine Weighing Between:
22 to 44 pounds: .25 to .5 oz daily.
44 to 110 pounds: .5 to .75 oz daily.
110 to 220 pounds: .5 to 1.0 oz daily.
Over 220 pounds: 1.0 oz daily.
Bred Gilts: 1.0 oz daily.
Sows: 1.0 oz daily.
Boars: 1.0 oz daily.
Lactating Sows: 2.0 to 3.0 oz daily.

The enclosed measuring cup, level full, is approximately one ounce.

*Note: Because of VITA-KEY® Swine Supplement's high vitamin and mineral content, the smell and taste may be offensive to some animals. If problems still persist, feed 25% of recommended feeding level for 5 days, 50% of recommended feeding level for the next 5 days, and then the full 100% of the recommended feeding level.

Contraindication(s): Do not feed to sheep or any other livestock sensitive to copper.

Precaution(s): Store in a cool, dry and clean place, in shaded area, keeping container tightly closed.

Caution(s): Do not feed wet, moldy, or insect-infested feed.

VITA-KEY® Swine Supplement is only part of a well balanced diet and should be fed with a properly balanced ration (proteins, fat, fiber, minerals, quantity consumed, etc.).

VITA-KEY® Swine Supplement is a nutritional feed additive. It contains no drugs or hormones and does not replace antibiotics. No withdrawal.

Vitamins and microbials degrade over time and with exposure to air, sunlight, temperature, and moisture. Use this product as directed, and in a timely manner.

VITA-KEY, L.C. makes no warranties, either expressed or implied as to the use of this product, other than the actual guaranteed analysis on the label when the product is stored as recommended and analyzed in a timely manner.

Presentation: 5 lbs (2.27 kg) and 20 lbs.

VITA-KEY® Swine Supplement contains Zinpro, Cuplex, Meth-Iron, Manpro, and Copro, which are registered trademarks of Zinpro Corporation.

Compendium Code No.: 14770071

VI-TAL

Loveland **Large Animal Dietary Supplement**

Active Ingredient(s): Each packet of VI-TAL contains:

Vitamin A . . . . . 2,600,000 I.U.
Vitamin D_3 . . . . . 600,000 I.C.U.
Vitamin E . . . . . 800 I.U.
Riboflavin . . . . . 250 mg
d-Pantothenic acid . . . . . 1,500 mg
Niacin . . . . . 2,000 mg
Vitamin B_{12} . . . . . 2,500 mcg
Menadione sodium bisulfite complex (source of vitamin K) . . . . . 1,040 mg
Thiamine mononitrate . . . . . 125 mg
Folic acid . . . . . 75 mg
Pyridoxine hydrochloride . . . . . 250 mg

Also contains electrolytes and trace minerals from potassium chloride, sodium chloride, magnesium sulfate, calcium gluconate, sodium bicarbonate, manganese sulfate, zinc sulfate, copper sulfate, ethylene diamine dihydriodide and cobalt sulfate.

Indications: VI-TAL is a concentrated water-dispersible supplement of essential vitamins, electrolytes and trace minerals to aid in growth, productivity and to stimulate water consumption and maintain the balance of body fluids in livestock and poultry.

When receiving and placing poultry and livestock: For use as an aid in alleviating stress due to scours, vaccination, castration, dehorning and debeaking, during temperature extremes, to stimulate appetite through improved nutrition, as an aid in nutritional buildup when feed intake is below normal.

Dosage and Administration: Mixing Directions:

For a high level supplementation, mix one (1) packet per 128 gallons of water.

For a moderate level supplementation, mix one (1) packet per 256 gallons of water.

For a low level supplementation, mix one (1) packet per 384 gallons of water.

Note: For water proportioners delivering 1 oz. of the stock solution per gallon of drinking water, the high, moderate and low levels outlined above are for one (1) packet per one (1) gallon, two (2) gallons and three (3) gallons of the stock solution, respectively. Prepare fresh solutions each day.

Water Supplementation:

Offer for 3-5 days: When receiving and placing poultry and livestock, to aid in alleviating stress due to scours, vaccination, castration, dehorning and debeaking, during temperature extremes, to stimulate appetite through improved nutrition, use the high or moderate level as outlined in the mixing directions.

Offer for 1-2 days: Before and after transportation, use the high level as outlined in the mixing directions.

Supplementation for 10 days or more: For aid in nutritional buildup when feed intake is below normal, use the low level as outlined in the mixing directions.

Feed Supplementation: Thoroughly mix two (2) packets per ton of complete feed. Use for five (5) or more days.

Consumption Guide: A 6 oz. packet per 128 gallons of water will treat the following poultry and livestock each day:

Chickens (Age):
1 week 28,500
3 weeks 8,500
5 weeks 5,300
8 weeks 3,100

Replacement Pullets:
9 weeks 3,000
12 weeks 2,300
Non-laying hens 2,500
Laying hens 1,800
Laying hens (summer) 1,400

Ducks (Age):
1-3 weeks 2,500

Turkeys:
1 week 10,600
3 weeks 5,120
6 weeks 2,130
10 weeks 1,250
15 weeks 750-800

Hogs:
25 lbs 300
50 lbs 200
100 lbs 125

Calves:
300 lbs 40
500 lbs 25
Lambs (feedlot) 125-250

Beef cattle:
700 lbs 20
1,200 lbs 10
Dairy cattle 5-10

In hot weather with a higher water consumption, divide the above numbers in half.

Presentation: 6 oz. packets.

Compendium Code No.: 10860370

VITAL E®-300

Schering-Plough **Vitamin E**

Injectable Tocopherol

Active Ingredient(s): Each mL contains 300 I.U. of vitamin E (as d-alpha-tocopherol, a natural-source of vitamin E) compounded with 20% ethyl alcohol and 1% benzyl alcohol (preservative) in an emulsifiable base.

Indications: VITAL E®-300 (natural-source of vitamin E) is a clear, sterile, non-aqueous solution of d-alpha-tocopherol for use as a supplemental source of natural vitamin E in swine, cattle and sheep.

Dosage and Administration: Injection by intramuscular or subcutaneous administration only. May be repeated. If the dosage is greater than 5 mL, equally divide the dosage and inject at two different sites.

Swine:

Sows and Gilts:

2 wks pre-partum .... 4-6 mL (1200-1800 I.U.)
2 wks pre-breeding .... 4-6 mL (1200-1800 I.U.)

Pigs:

At Birth .... 1-2 mL (300-600 I.U.)
Weaning .... 2-3 mL (600-900 I.U.)

Cattle (Dairy and Beef):

Cows and Heifers:

2-3 wks pre-partum .... 8-10 mL (2400-3000 I.U.)
At calving .... 8-10 mL (2400-3000 I.U.)

Calves:

At birth .... 4-6 mL (1200-1800 I.U.)
Weaning .... 4-6 mL (1200-1800 I.U.)
Yearlings .... 5-6 mL (1500-1800 I.U.)

Sheep:

Ewes:

2-3 wks pre-partum .... 4-5 mL (1200-1500 I.U.)
At lambing .... 4-5 mL (1200-1500 I.U.)

Lambs:

At birth .... 2-3 mL (600-900 I.U.)
Weaning .... 2-3 mL (600-900 I.U.)
Finishing Lambs .... 3-4 mL (900-1200 I.U.)

Precaution(s): Store between 2° and 30°C (36° and 86°F) in a dark place. Store partially used vials under refrigeration (36°-55°F).

Caution(s): Do not add water to solution.

Anaphylactoid or allergic reactions, which have resulted in deaths, abortions, and/or premature births, have been reported in individual animals as well as entire herds. Should such reactions or hypersensitivity occur, treat immediately with injection of epinephrine and/or antihistamines.

Do not exceed recommended dosage.

Warning(s): Not for human use. Keep out of reach of children.

Discussion: Natural tocopherols in feedstuffs can be destroyed through processing, ensiling, and storage. A reduced vitamin E intake can result in marginal deficiencies that may not be visible. Intramuscular or subcutaneous injections offer an efficient and rapid method to increase vitamin E status of animals.

Presentation: 8.5 fl oz (250 mL) multi-dose amber glass vials (NDC 0061-1017-01).

Compendium Code No.: 10472091 Rev. 11/99

VITAL E®+A ℞

Schering-Plough **Vitamins A-E**

(Injectable A-Tocopherol) (Vitamins A and E)

Active Ingredient(s): Each mL contains 200,000 I.U. vitamin A and 300 I.U. vitamin E (as d-alpha-tocopherol, a natural source of vitamin E). Also contains 20% ethyl alcohol, 1% benzyl alcohol (preservative) in an emulsifiable base.

Vitamin A activity is provided as retinyl palmitate, the biological storage form of vitamin A; and vitamin E activity is provided as d-alpha-tocopherol, the natural and biologically active form of vitamin E.

Indications: Injectable A-Tocopherol is a clear, sterile, non-aqueous solution of vitamin A and vitamin E. The product is intended as a supplemental source of vitamins A and E.

Dosage and Administration: Administer by intramuscular or subcutaneous injection only. May be repeated as needed. If the dosage is greater than 5 mL, equally divide the dosage and inject at two different sites.

Suggested Dosage:

Swine:

Sows and Gilts .... 4-6 mL
Weaning Pigs .... 1-2 mL
Newborn Pigs .... ½-1 mL

Cattle (Dairy and Beef):

Cows and Heifers .... 8-10 mL
Yearlings .... 5-6 mL
Calves .... 4-6 mL

Precaution(s): Store between 2° and 30°C (36° and 86°F) in a dark place. Store partially used vials under refrigeration (36°-55°F).

Caution(s): Federal (USA) law restricts this drug to use by or on the order of a licensed veterinarian.

Do not add water to solution.

Anaphylactoid or allergic reactions, which have resulted in deaths, abortions, and/or premature births, have been reported in individual animals as well as entire herds. Should such reactions or hypersensitiivty occur, treat immediately with injection of epinephrine and/or antihistamines.

Do not exceed recommended dosage.

Warning(s): Not for human use. Keep out of reach of children.

Discussion: Natural vitamin A (carotenes), and tocopherols can be destroyed in feedstuffs through processing, ensiling and storage. Due to these losses, reduced intakes of fat-soluble vitamins can occur in animals maintained in continual confinement compared to animals allowed to graze lush pasture. Intramuscular or subcutaneous injections offer an efficient and rapid method to increase vitamin A and vitamin E status of animals.

Presentation: 8.5 fl oz (250 mL) (NDC 0061-1024-01).

Compendium Code No.: 10472081 Rev. 11/99

VITAL E®-A+D

Schering-Plough **Vitamins A-D-E**

Injectable A+D Tocopherol (Vitamins A, D_3, and E)

Active Ingredient(s): Each mL contains 100,000 I.U. of vitamin A, 10,000 I.U. of vitamin D_3 and 300 I.U. of vitamin E (as d-alpha-tocopherol, a natural source of vitamin E). Also contains 20% ethyl alcohol and 1% benzyl alcohol (preservative) in an emulsifiable base.

Indications: Injectable A+D-Tocopherol is a clear, sterile, non-aqueous solution of vitamin A, vitamin D_3 and vitamin E. VITAL E®-A+D is intended as a supplemental source of natural vitamins A, D and E.

Dosage and Administration: Injection by intramuscular or subcutaneous administration only. May be repeated. If the dosage is greater than 5 mL, equally divide the dosage and inject at two different sites.

Suggested Dosage:

Cattle (Dairy and Beef):

Cows and Heifers:

2-3 wks pre-partum .... 8-10 mL
At calving .... 8-10 mL
End of lactation .... 8-10 mL

Calves:

At birth .... 4-6 mL
Weaning .... 4-6 mL
Yearlings .... 5-6 mL

Precaution(s): Store between 2° and 30°C (36° and 86°F) in a dark place. Store partially used vials under refrigeration (36°-55°F).

Caution(s): Anaphylactoid or allergic reactions, which have resulted in deaths, abortions, and/or premature births, have been reported in individual animals as well as entire herds. Should such reactions or hypersensitivity occur, treat immediately with injection of epinephrine and/or antihistamines.

Do not exceed recommended dosage.

Do not add water to solution.

Warning(s): Not for human use. Keep out of reach of children.

Discussion: Natural vitamin A (carotenes) and tocopherols can be destroyed in feedstuffs through processing, ensiling, and storage. Due to these losses, reduced intakes of fat-soluble vitamins can occur in animals maintained in continual confinement compared to animals allowed to graze lush pasture. Intramuscular or subcutaneous injections offer an efficient and rapid method to increase vitamin A, vitamin D, and vitamin E status of animals.

Vitamin A activity is provided as retinyl palmitate, the biological storage-form of vitamin A, and vitamin E activity is provided as d-alpha-tocopherol, the natural and biologically active form of vitamin E.

Presentation: 8.5 fl oz (250 mL) multi-dose amber glass vials (NDC 0061-1041-01).

Compendium Code No.: 10472101 Rev. 11/99

VITA-LYTE ℞

Phoenix Pharmaceutical **Large Animal Dietary Supplement**

Guaranteed Analysis:

Vitamin E, minimum .... 122 I.U./lb.
Sodium (Na), maximum 6.00%
Sodium (Na), minimum 5.50%
Potassium (K), minimum 1.40%
Magnesium (Mg), minimum 0.15%

Lactic acid bacteria, minimum (*Lactobacillus acidophilus, L. casei, L. fermentum, L. plantarum, Streptococcus faecium*)

Total .... 907,200,000 CFU/lb.

Ingredients: Glucose, guar gum, sodium chloride, sodium bicarbonate, potassium chloride, lecithin, citric acid, magnesium sulfate, glycine, dried *Lactobacillus acidophilus* fermentation product, dried *Lactobacillus casei* fermentation product, *Lactobacillus fermentum* fermentation product, *Lactobacillus plantarum* fermentation product, dried *Streptococcus faecium* fermentation product, sodium sulfate, sodium silico aluminate, monocalcium phosphate, corn syrup solids, active yeast *(saccharomyces cerevisiae)*, vitamin A acetate, d-activated animal sterol (source of vitamin D_3), vitamin E supplement, vitamin B_{12} supplement, riboflavin supplement, niacin supplement, calcium pantothenate, menadione dimethylpyrimidinol bisulphite, folic acid, pyridoxine hydrochloride, thiamine hydrochloride, d-biotin, fumaric acid, dried citrus pulp, ascorbic acid, zinc proteinate, cobalt proteinate, ferrous proteinate, copper proteinate, buttermilk, cellulose gum and manganese proteinate.

Contains a source of live (viable) naturally occurring microorganisms.

Indications: A blend of ingredients as a source of electrolytes, nutrients and sugars for energy in young calves, veal, foals and lambs.

Dosage and Administration:

Mixing: Mix ⅔ cup (100 g) into 2 quarts warm water or milk replacer and shake or mix thoroughly.

Calves, Veal and Foals: Feed above mixture per calf twice a day for 2 days. Receiving calves should be given 2 feedings prior to the regular milk program.

Lambs: Feed above mixture at the rate of 4 fluid ounces per 5 lbs. body weight, 3 times a day for 2 days.

Caution(s): Federal law restricts this drug to use by or on the order of a licensed veterinarian.

For animal use only.

Warning(s): Keep out of reach of children.

Presentation: 100 grams (NDC 57319-273-32).

Manufactured by: Advantech, Ltd., Fort Dodge, IA 50501.

Compendium Code No.: 12560891 Rev. 06-01

VITAMIN AD₃

AgriLabs **Vitamins A-D**

Active Ingredient(s): Each mL contains:

Vitamin A propionate .... 500,000 I.U.
Vitamin D_3 .... 75,000 I.U.
Vitamin E (antioxidant) .... 5 I.U.
Ethyl alcohol .... 8% v/v
Benzyl alcohol .... 2% v/v
B.H.A. (as preservative) .... 0.75% w/v
B.H.T. (as preservative) .... 0.75% w/v

In an emulsifiable base.

V

Indications: A water emulsifiable solution to be used as a supplemental source of vitamins A and D in cattle.
Dosage and Administration: Administer by deep intramuscular injection. The dosage may be repeated after 60 days if needed.
Cattle:
Calves . . . ½ to 1 mL
Yearling/Feedlot . . . 1 to 3 mL
Adult cattle . . . 3 to 6 mL
Precaution(s): Store at temperatures between 2°-30° (36°-86°F). Refrigerate unused portion. Protect from light.
Caution(s): For intramuscular use only. Do not exceed the recommended dosage. If the intended dose is greater than 4 mL in cattle, divide the dose equally and give in two different sites.
Keep out of the reach of children.
For veterinary use only.
Warning(s): Do not administer to food producing animals within 60 days of slaughter.
Presentation: 100 mL, 250 mL and 500 mL containers.
Compendium Code No.: 10581200

VITAMIN AD

Butler **Vitamins A-D**

Active Ingredient(s): Each mL contains:
Vitamin A . . . 500,000 I.U.
Vitamin D_3 . . . 75,000 I.U.
Benzyl alcohol . . . 2% v/v
Ethyl alcohol . . . 8%
Vitamin E (antioxidant) 5 I.U., B.H.A. 0.75%, and B.H.T. 0.75% as preservatives in an emulsifiable base.
Indications: A water emulsifiable solution to be used as a supplemental source of vitamins A and D in cattle, sheep and swine.
Dosage and Administration: For intramuscular use.
The dosage may be repeated in two (2) or three (3) months, as needed.
Calves . . . 0.5 to 1 mL
Yearlings . . . 1 to 2 mL
Adult cattle . . . 2 to 4 mL
Lambs . . . 0.25 to 0.5 mL
Growing lambs . . . 0.5 to 1 mL
Adult sheep . . . 1 to 2 mL
Weaning pigs . . . 0.25 to 0.5 mL
Growing pigs . . . 0.5 to 1 mL
Adult swine . . . 1 to 2 mL
Precaution(s): Store in a dark, cool place, not above 10°C (50°F). Keep from freezing.
Caution(s): Not for human use. Keep out of the reach of children.
Warning(s): Do not inject into meat animals within 60 days of marketing.
Presentation: 100 mL and 250 mL vials.
Compendium Code No.: 10821830

VITAMIN A & D ℞

Vedco **Vitamins A-D**

Active Ingredient(s): Each mL contains:
Vitamin A . . . 500,000 I.U.
Vitamin D . . . 75,000 I.U.
Benzyl alcohol . . . 2% v/v
Ethyl alcohol . . . 8%
Vitamin E (antioxidant) . . . 5 I.U.
B.H.A. and B.H.T. (as preservatives in a base) . . . 0.75% each
Indications: A water emulsifiable solution to be used as a supplemental source of vitamins A and D in cattle, sheep and swine.
Dosage and Administration: For intramuscular use. May be repeated in two (2) or three (3) months, as needed.
Calves . . . 0.5 to 1 mL
Yearlings . . . 1 to 2 mL
Adult Cattle . . . 2 to 4 mL
Lambs . . . 0.25 to 0.5 mL
Growing Lambs . . . 0.5 to 1 mL
Adult Sheep . . . 1 to 2 mL
Weaning Pigs . . . 0.25 to 0.5 mL
Growing Pigs . . . 0.5 to 1 mL
Adult Swine . . . 1 to 2 mL
Precaution(s): Store in a dark, cool place, not above 50°F (10°C). Keep from freezing.
Caution(s): Federal law restricts this drug to use by or on the order of a licensed veterinarian.
Warning(s): Keep out of reach of children.
Presentation: 100 mL, 250 mL and 500 mL vials.
Compendium Code No.: 10942141

VITAMIN A & D "500"

AgriPharm **Vitamins A-D**

Active Ingredient(s): Each mL contains:
Vitamin A propionate . . . 500,000 I.U.
Vitamin D_3 . . . 75,000 I.U.
Vitamin E (antioxidant) . . . 5 I.U.
Benzyl alcohol . . . 2% v/v
Ethyl alcohol . . . 8% v/v
Preservatives:
BHT . . . 0.75%
BHA . . . 0.75%
Indications: A water emulsifiable solution to be used as a supplemental source of vitamin A and D_3 in cattle.
Dosage and Administration: Administer by deep intramuscular injection. The dosage may be repeated after 60 days, if needed.
Calves . . . ½ to 1 mL
Yearlings and feedlot cattle . . . 1 to 3 mL
Adult cattle . . . 3 to 6 mL
Precaution(s): Store at a controlled temperature between 59°-86°F (15°-30°C).
Protect form light.
Refrigerate the unused potion.
Caution(s): For animal use only.
Keep out of the reach of children.
Do not exceed the recommended dosage. If the intended dose is greater then 4 mL in cattle, divide the dose equally and give in 2 different sites.
Warning(s): Do not administer to food producing animals within 60 days of slaughter.
Presentation: 100 mL, 250 mL and 500 mL containers.
Compendium Code No.: 14571080

VITAMIN A D B_{12} INJECTION ℞

Vedco **Vitamins A-B_{12}-D**

Active Ingredient(s): Each mL contains:
Vitamin A . . . 500,000 I.U.
Vitamin D_3 . . . 75,000 I.U.
Cyanocobalamin (B_{12}) . . . 500 mcg
In a emulsifiable base.
Vitamin E (antioxidant) . . . 5 I.U. per mL
Benzyl alcohol . . . 2% v/v
Ethyl alcohol . . . 15%
B.H.A. and B.H.T. (as preservatives in a base) . . . 0.75% each
Indications: For use as a supplemental source of vitamins A, D and B_{12} in cattle, sheep and swine.
Dosage and Administration: For intramuscular use.
Calves . . . 0.5 to 1 mL
Yearling Cattle . . . 1 to 2 mL
Adult Cattle . . . 2 to 4 mL
Lambs . . . 0.25 to 0.5 mL
Fattening Lambs . . . 0.5 to 1 mL
Adult Sheep . . . 1 to 2 mL
Weaning Pigs . . . 0.25 to 0.5 mL
Growing Pigs . . . 0.5 to 1 mL
Adult Swine . . . 1 to 2 mL
These suggested dosages may be repeated after 60 days, if necessary.
Precaution(s): Store at a controlled room temperature, between 59-86°F (15-30°C). Protect from light and excessive heat. Keep partially used vials under refrigeration.
Caution(s): Federal law restricts this drug to use by or on the order of a licensed veterinarian.
Keep out of the reach of children.
Warning(s): Do not inject into meat animals within 60 days of marketing.
Presentation: 100 mL and 250 mL containers.
Compendium Code No.: 10942150

VITAMIN AD INJECTION

Aspen **Vitamins A-D**

Active Ingredient(s): Each mL of sterile solution contains:
Vitamin A . . . 500,000 I.U.
Vitamin D_3 . . . 75,000 I.U.
Vitamin E (antioxidant) . . . 5 I.U.
Ethyl alcohol . . . 8%
Benzyl alcohol . . . 2% v/v
B.H.A. (as a preservative in an emulsifiable base) . . . 0.75%
B.H.T. (as a preservative in an emulsifiable base) . . . 0.75%
Indications: For use as a supplemental source of vitamins A and D in cattle, sheep and swine.
Dosage and Administration: Inject intramuscularly, using a sterile 14 to 18 gauge needle, 1-2 inches long. Injection should be made into a heavily muscled area, preferably high on the rump, using aseptic technique.
Calves . . . 0.5 to 1 mL
Yearling Cattle . . . 1 to 2 mL
Adult Cattle . . . 2 to 4 mL
Lambs . . . 0.25 to 0.5 mL
Fattening Lambs . . . 0.5 to 1 mL
Adult Sheep . . . 1 to 2 mL
Weanling Pigs . . . 0.25 to 0.5 mL
Growing Pigs . . . 0.5 to 1 mL
Adult Swine . . . 1 to 2 mL
These suggested dosages may be repeated in two to three months, as needed.
Precaution(s): Store at a controlled room temperature, between 59° and 86°F (15°-30°C). Keep partially used vials under refrigeration. Keep from freezing.
Caution(s): Keep out of the reach of children.
Presentation: 250 mL and 500 mL vials.
Compendium Code No.: 14750950

VITAMIN AD$_3$ INJECTION

Bimeda **Vitamins A-D**

Active Ingredient(s): Each mL contains:
Vitamin A (as vitamin A propionate) . . . 500,000 I.U.
Vitamin D_3 . . . 75,000 I.U.
Vitamin E . . . 5 I.U.
Ethyl alcohol . . . 8%
Benzyl alcohol (preservative) . . . 2%
BHT . . . 0.75%
BHA . . . 0.75%
Emulsifiable base, q.s. . . . 1.0 mL
Indications: An emulsifiable solution of vitamins A and D_3 for use in cattle.
Dosage and Administration: For intramuscular administration.
Calves . . . ¼ to 1 mL
Yearlings and feedlot cattle . . . 1 to 2 mL
Beef and dairy cows . . . 1 to 2 mL
Breeding cattle . . . 1 to 2 mL
For breeding animals, the dosage may be repeated in two (2) or three (3) months as needed.
Caution(s): For animal use only. Not for human use. Keep out of the reach of children.
Warning(s): For market animals, administer at least 60 days before marketing.
Presentation: 100 mL, 250 mL and 500 mL containers.
Compendium Code No.: 13990460

VITAMIN AD INJECTION ℞

Phoenix Pharmaceutical **Vitamins A-D**

Active Ingredient(s): Composition: Each mL of sterile solution contains:

Vitamin A .... 500,000 IU
Vitamin D_3 .... 75,000 IU

In an emulsifiable base with vitamin E (antioxidant), N-methylpyrrolidone, polyoxyethylated (30) castor oil, propylene glycol dicaprylate, polyoxyethylene (20) sorbitan monooleate and benzyl alcohol 2%.

Indications: For use as a supplemental nutritive source of vitamins A and D in cattle, sheep and swine.

Dosage and Administration: Inject intramuscularly or subcutaneously preferably in the neck area using aseptic technique.

Calves: ½ to 1 mL.
Adult Cattle: 2 to 4 mL.
Lambs: ¼ to ½ mL.
Adult Sheep: 1 to 2 mL.
Weaning Pigs: ¼ to ½ mL.
Adult Swine: 1 to 2 mL.
These suggested dosages may be repeated after 60 days, if necessary.

Precaution(s): Store at controlled room temperature between 15° and 30°C (59-86°F).
Protect from light and excessive heat.

Caution(s): Federal law restricts this drug to use by or on the order of a licensed veterinarian.
For animal use only.

Warning(s): Do not inject into meat animals within 60 days of marketing.
Keep out of reach of children.

Presentation: 100 mL (NDC 57319-454-05) and 250 mL (NDC 57319-424-06) vials.

Manufactured by: Veterinary Laboratories, Inc., Lenexa, KS 66215.

Compendium Code No.: 12560902 Rev. 11-00

VITAMIN B-COMPLEX

AgriLabs **Vitamin B-Complex**

Active Ingredient(s): Each mL contains:

Thiamine hydrochloride .... 12.5 mg
Riboflavin 5' sodium phosphate U.S.P. .... 2 mg
Pyridoxine hydrochloride .... 5 mg
Niacinamide .... 100 mg
d-Panthenol .... 10 mg
Cyanocobalamin (vitamin B_{12}) .... 5 mcg
Benzyl alcohol (as preservative) .... 1.5% v/v
Stabilized in a buffered base
Water for injection .... q.s.

Indications: For use as a supplemental source of B-complex vitamins in cattle, sheep, and swine.

Dosage and Administration: Administer by intramuscular or subcutaneous injection. The dosage may be repeated once or twice a week as needed.

Calves .... 3 to 5 mL
Yearlings .... 5 to 10 mL
Adult Cattle .... 10 to 20 mL
Lambs and Weanling Pigs .... 1 to 2 mL
Growing Lambs and Pigs .... 2 to 3 mL
Adult Sheep and Swine .... 3 to 5 mL

Precaution(s): Store at refrigerated temperature between 2°-8°C (36°-46°F).

Caution(s): Not for intravenous use. Parenteral administration of thiamine has resulted in anaphylactic shock. Administer slowly and with caution in doses over 4.0 mL (50 mg thiamine).
For veterinary use only.

Warning(s): Keep out of reach of children.

Presentation: 100 mL and 250 mL bottles.

Compendium Code No.: 10581211

VITAMIN B COMPLEX

AgriPharm **Vitamin B-Complex**

Active Ingredient(s): Each mL contains:

Thiamine HCl .... 12.5 mg
Riboflavin 5' Phosphate Sodium .... 2 mg
Niacinamide .... 12.5 mg
d-Panthenol .... 5 mg
Pyridoxine HCl .... 5 mg
Cobalt (As Cyanocobalamin) .... 0.2 ppm
Benzyl Alcohol (Preservative) 1.5%
Water for injection .... q.s.

Indications: An aqueous solution of B-vitamins to provide a supplemental nutritional supply of these vitamins and complexed cobalt to cattle, sheep and swine.

Dosage and Administration: Administer intramuscularly. Sheep and Swine: 5 to 10 mL. Cattle: 10 to 20 mL. Repeat daily as indicated.

Precaution(s): Store between 15°C and 30°C (59°F-86°F). Keep from freezing.

Caution(s): Not for intravenous use. Anaphylactogenesis to parenteral thiamine HCl has been reported. Administer slowly and with caution in doses over 50 mg.

Warning(s): For animal use only.
Keep out of reach of children.

Presentation: 100 mL.

Compendium Code No.: 14571090

V

VITAMIN B COMPLEX

Aspen **Vitamin B-Complex**

Active Ingredient(s): Each mL contains:

Thiamine HCl .... 12.5 mg
Riboflavin (as 5' phosphate sodium) .... 2 mg
Niacinamide .... 12.5 mg
d-Panthenol .... 5 mg
Pyridoxine HCl .... 5 mg
Cobalt (as Cyanocobalamin) .... 0.2 ppm
Benzyl alcohol (preservative) 1.5%
Water .... q.s.

Indications: An aqueous solution of B-vitamins to provide a supplemental supply of these vitamins and complexed cobalt to cattle, sheep, and swine.

Dosage and Administration: Administer intramuscularly.

Sheep and Swine .... 5-10 mL
Cattle .... 10-20 mL
Repeat once a day, as indicated.

Precaution(s): Store at a controlled room temperature, 59°-86°F (15°-30°C). Keep from freezing.

Caution(s): For animal use only.
Keep out of the reach of children.
Anaphylactic reactions to parenteral thiamine HCl has been reported. Administer slowly and with caution in doses over 50 mg.

Presentation: 250 mL and 500 mL vials.

Compendium Code No.: 14750960

VITAMIN B COMPLEX ℞

Butler **Vitamin B-Complex**

Sterile Solution

Active Ingredient(s): Each mL contains:

Thiamine Hydrochloride .... 50 mg
Riboflavin 5' Phosphate Sodium .... 2 mg
Pyridoxine Hydrochloride .... 2 mg
Niacinamide .... 100 mg
d-Panthenol .... 10 mg
Cobalt (as Cyanocobalamin) .... 0.4 ppm
Benzyl Alcohol (as preservative) .... 1.5% v/v
Water for Injection .... q.s.
Stabilized in a buffered base.

Indications: As a supplemental source of B complex vitamins and complexed cobalt for use in preventing or treating deficiencies in cattle, horses, sheep, swine, dogs and cats.

Dosage and Administration: Administer by intramuscular or subcutaneous injection. Dosage may be repeated once or twice weekly as needed.

Calves and Foals .... 3 to 5 mL
Yearlings .... 5 to 10 mL
Adult Cattle and Horses .... 10 to 20 mL
Lambs and Weaning Pigs .... 1 to 2 mL
Growing Lambs and Pigs .... 2 to 3 mL
Adult Sheep and Swine .... 3 to 5 mL
Dogs .... 0.5 to 2 mL
Cats .... 0.5 to 1 mL

Precaution(s): Store between 15°C-30°C (59°F-86°F).

Caution(s): Federal law restricts this drug to use by or on the order of a licensed veterinarian.
Not for intravenous use. Parenteral administration of thiamine has resulted in anaphylactic shock. Administer slowly and with caution in doses over 1.0 mL (50 mg thiamine).
For animal use only.

Warning(s): Keep out of reach of children.

Presentation: 100 mL vials (NDC 11695-3560-1).

Manufactured by: Phoenix Scientific, Inc., St. Joseph, MO 64508.

Compendium Code No.: 10821841 Iss. 6-94

VITAMIN-B COMPLEX

Durvet **Vitamin B-Complex**

Injectable

Active Ingredient(s): Each mL Contains:

Thiamine Hydrochloride .... 12.5 mg
Riboflavin 5' Sodium Phosphate .... 2 mg
Pyridoxine Hydrochloride .... 5 mg
Niacinamide .... 12.5 mg
d-Panthenol .... 5 mg
Cobalt (as Cyanocobalamin) .... 2 ppm
Benzyl Alcohol (as preservative) 1.5%
Water for Injection .... q.s.

Indications: A sterile aqueous solution of B vitamins to provide a supplemental nutritional supply of these vitamins and complexed cobalt to cattle, sheep and swine.

Dosage and Administration: Administer intramuscularly.

Sheep and Swine: 5 to 10 mL
Adult Cattle: 10 to 20 mL
Repeat daily as indicated.

Precaution(s): Store between 15°C-30°C (59°F-86°F). Keep from freezing.

Caution(s): Anaphylactogenesis to parenteral Thiamine HCl has been reported. Administer slowly and with caution in doses over 50 mg.
For animal use only.

Warning(s): Keep out of reach of children.

Presentation: 100 mL (NDC 30798-038-10), 250 mL (NDC 30798-038-13) and 500 mL (NDC 30798-038-17) vials.

Compendium Code No.: 10841661 Rev. 10-95

VITAMIN B COMPLEX

Phoenix Pharmaceutical **Vitamin B-Complex**

Active Ingredient(s): Each mL contains:

Thiamine HCl .... 12.5 mg
Riboflavin 5' Phosphate Sodium .... 2 mg
Niacinamide .... 12.5 mg
d-Panthenol .... 5 mg
Pyridoxine HCl .... 5 mg
Cobalt (as Cyanocobalamin) .... 0.2 ppm
Benzyl Alcohol (Preservative) 1.5%
Water .... q.s.

Indications: An aqueous solution of B-Vitamins to provide a supplemental nutritional supply of these vitamins and Complexed Cobalt to cattle, sheep, and swine.

Dosage and Administration: Administer intramuscularly.

Sheep and Swine: 5 to 10 mL.
Cattle: 10 to 20 mL.
Repeat daily as indicated.

Precaution(s): Store between 15°C and 30°C (59°F-86°F). Keep from freezing.
Caution(s): Anaphylactogenesis to parenteral Thiamine HCl has been reported. Administer slowly and with caution in doses over 50 mg. For animal use only.
Warning(s): Keep out of reach of children.
Presentation: 100 mL (NDC 57319-089-05) and 250 mL (NDC 57319-089-06) vials.
Manufactured by: Phoenix Scientific, Inc., St. Joseph, MO 64503.
Compendium Code No.: 12560912 Rev. 6-01 / Rev. 7-01

VITAMIN B COMPLEX ℞

Vedco **Vitamin B-Complex**

Active Ingredient(s): Each mL contains:
Thiamine hydrochloride (B_1) .... 12.5 mg
Riboflavin (B_2) (as riboflavin 5' phosphate sodium) .... 2.0 mg
Niacinamide .... 12.5 mg
Pyridoxine hydrochloride (B_6) .... 5.0 mg
d-panthenol .... 5.0 mg
Cyanocobalamin (B_{12}) .... 5.0 mcg
Citric acid .... 0.5% w/v
Benzyl alcohol (preservative) .... 1.5% v/v
Indications: For use as a supplement of B-complex vitamins.
Dosage and Administration: Administer intramuscularly.
Dogs and Cats: 0.5 to 2 mL depending upon size.
Calves, Sheep, Foals and Swine: 5 mL per 100 pounds of body weight.
Adult Cattle and Horses: 1 to 2 mL per 100 pounds of body weight.
May be repeated once a day, as indicated.
Precaution(s): Store at a controlled room temperature, between 36-49°F (2-8°C).
Caution(s): Federal law restricts this drug to use by or on the order of a licensed veterinarian.
Not for human use.
Hypersensitivity reactions to the parenteral administration of thiamine have been reported. Administer with caution and keep treated animals under close observation.
Warning(s): Keep out of reach of children.
Presentation: 100 mL, 250 mL and 500 mL containers.
Compendium Code No.: 10942161

VITAMIN B COMPLEX FORTE INJECTION

Bimeda **Vitamin B-Complex**

(Sterile Aqueous Solution)
Active Ingredient(s): Each mL contains:
Thiamine hydrochloride .... 100 mg
Riboflavin 5' sodium phosphate .... 5 mg
Pyridoxine hydrochloride .... 10 mg
Niacinamide .... 100 mg
d-Panthenol .... 10 mg
Cyanocobalamin (Vitamin B_{12}) .... 100 mcg
Benzyl alcohol (as preservative) .... 1.5% w/v
Water for injection .... q.s.
Indications: An aqueous solution of B complex vitamins to provide a supplemental nutritional source of these vitamins to cattle, horses, sheep, swine, dogs and cats.
Dosage and Administration: Administer by subcutaneous or intramuscular injection.
Calves and Foals .... 3-5 mL
Yearlings .... 5-10 mL
Adult Cattle and Horses .... 10-20 mL
Lambs .... 1-2 mL
Growing Lambs .... 2-3 mL
Adult Sheep .... 3-5 mL
Weanling Pigs .... 1-2 mL
Growing Pigs .... 2-3 mL
Adult Pigs .... 3-5 mL
Dogs .... 0.5-2 mL
Cats .... 0.5-1 mL
Repeat once or twice weekly, or as indicated.
Precaution(s): Storage: Avoid exposure to direct sunlight. Store below 86°F. Avoid freezing.
Caution(s): Not for intravenous use. Parenteral administration of thiamine has resulted in anaphylactic shock. Administer slowly and with caution in doses over 0.5 mL (50 mg thiamine).
For veterinary use only. For animal use only.
Warning(s): Keep out of reach of children.
Presentation: 100 mL (NDC# 61133-204-06) and 250 mL (NDC# 61133-2040-4) bottles.
Compendium Code No.: 13990471 71VIT0081 / Rev. 4.00

VITAMIN B COMPLEX FORTIFIED

Aspen **Vitamin B-Complex**

Active Ingredient(s): Each mL contains:
Thiamine HCl .... 100 mg
Riboflavin 5' Phosphate Sodium .... 5 mg
Niacinamide .... 100 mg
d-Panthenol .... 10 mg
Pyridoxine HCl .... 10 mg
Cobalt (As Cyanocobalamin) .... 4.0 ppm
Benzyl Alcohol (Preservative) 1.5%
Citric Acid .... 5 mg
Water For Injection .... q.s.
Indications: An aqueous solution of B complex vitamins to provide a supplemental nutritional supply of these vitamins and complexed cobalt to cattle, sheep and swine.
Dosage and Administration: Administer intramuscularly or subcutaneously. Sheep and Swine: 5 to 10 mL. Cattle: 10 to 20 mL. Repeat daily as indicated.
Precaution(s): Store between 15°C and 30°C (59°F-86°F).
Keep from freezing.
Caution(s): Anaphylactogenesis to parenteral Thiamine HCl has been reported. Administer slowly and with caution in doses over 50 mg.
Warning(s): For animal use only. Keep out of reach of children.
Presentation: 250 mL and 500 mL vials.
Compendium Code No.: 14750970

VITAMIN B COMPLEX FORTIFIED

Phoenix Pharmaceutical **Vitamin B-Complex**

Active Ingredient(s): Each mL contains:
Thiamine HCl .... 100 mg
Riboflavin 5' Phosphate Sodium .... 5 mg
Niacinamide .... 100 mg
d-Panthenol .... 10 mg
Pyridoxine HCl .... 10 mg
Cobalt (as Cyanocobalamin) .... 4.0 ppm
Benzyl Alcohol (Preservative) 1.5%
Citric Acid .... 5 mg
Water .... q.s.
Indications: An aqueous solution of B Complex vitamins to provide a supplemental nutritional supply of these vitamins and Complexed Cobalt to cattle, sheep, and swine.
Dosage and Administration: Administer intramuscularly or subcutaneously.
Sheep and Swine: 5 to 10 mL.
Cattle: 10 to 20 mL.
Repeat daily as indicated.
Precaution(s): Store between 15°C and 30°C (59°F-86°F). Keep from freezing.
Caution(s): Anaphylactogenesis to parenteral Thiamine HCl has been reported. Administer slowly and with caution in doses over 50 mg.
For animal use only.
Warning(s): Keep out of reach of children.
Presentation: 100 mL (NDC 57319-090-05) and 250 mL (NDC 57319-090-06) vials.
Manufactured by: Phoenix Scientific, Inc., St. Joseph, MO 64503.
Compendium Code No.: 12560922 Rev. 5-02 / Rev. 8-01

VITAMIN B COMPLEX WITH CYANO PLUS

AgriPharm **Vitamin B-Complex**

Vitamin B-Complex Injection
Active Ingredient(s): Each mL of sterile aqueous solution contains:
Thiamine Hydrochloride (B_1) .... 12.5 mg
Niacinamide .... 12.5 mg
Pyridoxine Hydrochloride (B_6) .... 5.0 mg
d-Panthenol .... 5.0 mg
Riboflavin (B_2) (as Riboflavin 5' phosphate sodium) .... 2.0 mg
Cyanocobalamin (B_{12}) .... 1000 mcg
with benzyl alcohol 1.5% v/v as preservative, ammonium sulfate 0.1%.
Indications: For use as a supplemental source of B complex vitamins in cattle, swine and sheep.
Dosage and Administration: Subcutaneous or intramuscular injection is recommended. May be administered intravenously at the discretion of a veterinarian. The following are suggested dosages, depending on the condition of the animal and the desired response.
Adult Cattle: 1 to 2 mL per 500 pounds of body weight.
Calves, Swine and Sheep: 1 to 2 mL. May be repeated once or twice weekly.
Precaution(s): Store at controlled room temperature between 15° to 30°C (59°-86°F). Protect from light.
Caution(s): Hypersensitivity reactions to the parenteral administration of products containing thiamine have been reported. Administer with caution and keep treated animals under close observation.
Warning(s): For animal use only. Keep out of reach of children.
Presentation: 100 mL and 250 mL (8.5 fl oz).
Compendium Code No.: 14571101

VITAMIN B-1 POWDER

AHC **Thiamine**

Ingredient(s): Thiamine hydrochloride, dextrose, FD & C red #40, natural and artificial flavorings.
Analysis, each ounce contains not less than:
Vitamin B-1 .... 500 mg
Indications: Thiamine hydrochloride feed supplement.
Directions for Use: VITAMIN B-1 is 100% water soluble and may be administered in feed or drinking water.
Each teaspoon contains 82 mg's of Thiamine Hydrochloride.
Horses: Supplement regular ration as needed with ½ teaspoonful twice daily.
Dogs: Supplement regular ration with ¼ to ½ teaspoonful daily.
Other Small Animals: Supplement regular ration as needed with ⅛ to ¼ teaspoonful daily.
Reseal after each use.
Caution(s): For veterinary use only.
For animal use only.
Keep out of reach of children.
Presentation: 1½ pounds.
Compendium Code No.: 10770061

VITAMIN B12 ℞

Butler **Vitamin B_{12}**

Active Ingredient(s): Each mL contains:

	1,000 mcg	3,000 mcg	5,000 mcg
Cyanocobalamin	1,000 mcg	3,000 mcg	5,000 mcg
Benzyl alcohol (as preservative)	1.5% v/v	1.5% v/v	1.5% v/v
Sodium chloride	0.8% w/v	0.8% w/v	0.8% w/v

pH adjusted with acetic acid.
Water for injection .... q.s.
Indications: For use in vitamin B_{12} deficiency associated with cobalt deficiency in cattle and sheep, and for vitamin B_{12} deficiency associated with inadequate vitamin B_{12} intake or intestinal malabsorption in swine.
Dosage and Administration: Inject intramuscularly or subcutaneously. The dosage may be repeated once a week, if necessary.

	1,000 mcg	3,000 mcg	5,000 mcg
Cattle and Sheep	1.0-2 mL	0.35-0.66 mL	0.2-0.4 mL
Swine	0.5-2 mL	0.20-0.66 mL	0.1-0.4 mL

Precaution(s): Store at a temperature between 36°-86°F (2°-30°C).
Caution(s): Federal law (U.S.A.) restricts this drug to use by or on the order of a licensed veterinarian.
For veterinary use only.
Keep out of the reach of children.
Presentation: 100 mL vials.
Compendium Code No.: 10821850

VITAMIN B_{12} ℞

Vedco **Vitamin B_{12}**

Active Ingredient(s): Each mL contains:

	1,000 mcg	3,000 mcg	5,000 mcg
Cyanocobalamin (B_{12})	1,000 mcg	3,000 mcg	5,000 mcg
Sodium chloride	0.22% w/v	0.9% w/v	0.22% w/v
Ammonium sulfate	0.1% w/v	0.1% w/v	0.1% w/v
Citric acid	0.01% w/v	0.01% w/v	0.01% w/v
Sodium citrate	0.008% w/v	0.008% w/v	0.008% w/v
Benzyl alcohol (preservative)	1.0% v/v	1.5% v/v	1.0% v/v

Indications: For use as an aid in the management of vitamin B_{12} deficiencies in horses, dogs and cats.
Dosage and Administration: Inject subcutaneously or intramuscularly.
Horses . . . 1 to 2 mL
Dogs and Cats . . . 0.25 to 0.5 mL
May be repeated once or twice a week, as indicated by the condition and response of the animal.
Precaution(s): Store at a controlled room temperature, between 59-86°F (15-30°C). Avoid exposure to light.
Caution(s): Federal law restricts this drug to use by or on the order of a licensed veterinarian.
Keep out of the reach of children. Not for use by humans.
Presentation: 1,000 mcg: 100 mL and 500 mL vials.
3,000 mcg: 100 mL vials.
5,000 mcg: 100 mL vials.
Compendium Code No.: 10942170

VITAMIN B_{12} 1000 mcg ℞

Phoenix Pharmaceutical **Vitamin B_{12}**

(Cyanocobalamin) Injection

Active Ingredient(s): Composition: Each mL of sterile aqueous solution contains:
Cyanocobalamin (B_{12}) . . . 1000 mcg
Sodium Chloride . . . 0.8% w/v
Benzyl Alcohol (preservative) . . . 1.5% v/v
Indications: For use as an aid in the management of vitamin B_{12} deficiencies in cattle, horses, dogs and cats.
Dosage and Administration: Inject subcutaneously or intramuscularly.
Cattle and Horses: 1 to 2 mL
Dogs and Cats: 0.25 to 0.50 mL
May be repeated once or twice weekly, as indicated by condition and response.
Precaution(s): Store between 15°C and 30°C (59°F-86°F). Avoid exposure to light.
Caution(s): Federal law restricts this drug to use by or on the order of a licensed veterinarian.
For animal use only.
Warning(s): Keep out of reach of children.
Presentation: 100 mL (NDC 57319-091-05) and 250 mL (NDC 57319-091-06) vials.
Manufactured by: Phoenix Scientific, Inc., St. Joseph, MO 64503.
Compendium Code No.: 12560932 Rev. 8-01 / Iss. 3-99

VITAMIN B_{12} 1000 mcg ℞

Vet Tek **Vitamin B_{12}**

Cyanocobalamin Injection

Active Ingredient(s): Composition: Each mL of sterile aqueous solution contains:
Cyanocobalamin (B_{12}) . . . 1000 mcg
Sodium Chloride . . . 0.8% w/v
Benzyl Alcohol (preservative) . . . 1.5% v/v
Indications: For use as supplemental nutritive source of Vitamin B_{12} in cattle, horses, dogs and cats.
Dosage and Administration: Inject subcutaneously or intramuscularly.
Cattle and Horses—1 to 2 mL
Dogs and Cats—0.25 to 0.5 mL
May be repeated once or twice weekly, as indicated by condition and response.
Precaution(s): Store between 15°C and 30°C (59°F-86°F). Avoid exposure to light.
Caution(s): Federal law restricts this drug to use by or on the order of a licensed veterinarian.
For animal use only.
Warning(s): Keep out of reach of children.
Presentation: 100 mL (NDC 60270-039-10), 250 mL (NDC 60270-039-13) and 500 mL (NDC 60270-039-17) bottles.
Manufactured by: Phoenix Scientific, Inc., St. Joseph, MO 64506.
Compendium Code No.: 14200221 Rev. 12-98 / Rev. 6-96 / Rev. 10-99

VITAMIN B_{12} 1000 MCG INJECTION ℞

Aspen **Vitamin B_{12}**

Active Ingredient(s): Each mL contains:
Cyanocobalamin (B_{12}) . . . 1000 mcg
Benzyl alcohol (as preservative) . . . 1.5% v/v
Sodium chloride . . . 0.8% w/v
Water for injection . . . q.s.
Indications: For use as an aid in the management of vitamin B_{12} deficiencies in cattle, horses, dogs and cats.
Dosage and Administration: Inject intramuscularly or subcutaneously.
Cattle and Horses . . . 1 to 2 mL
Dogs and Cats . . . 0.25 to 0.5 mL
May be repeated once or twice weekly, as indicated by condition and response.
Precaution(s): Store at temperatures between 36°-86°F (2°-30°C).
Avoid exposure to light.
Caution(s): Federal law (U.S.A.) restricts this drug to use by or on the order of a licensed veterinarian. Keep out of the reach of children.
Presentation: 250 mL and 500 mL vials.
Compendium Code No.: 14750981

VITAMIN B_{12} 3000 MCG ℞

Neogen **Vitamin B_{12}**

Cyanocobalamin 3000 mcg-Sterile Solution

Active Ingredient(s): Each mL contains:
Cyanocobalamin . . . 3000 mcg
Benzyl Alcohol (as preservative) . . . 1.5% v/v
Sodium Chloride . . . 0.8% w/v
Water for injection . . . q.s.
pH buffered with Acetic Acid.
Indications: For use in vitamin B_{12} deficiency associated with cobalt deficiency in cattle and sheep and for vitamin B_{12} deficiency associated with inadequate vitamin B_{12} intake or intestinal malabsorption in swine and horses.
Dosage and Administration: Inject intravenously, intramuscularly or subcutaneously. Dosage may be repeated in weekly intervals if necessary.
Cattle and Sheep . . . ⅓ to ⅔ mL
Swine . . . ⅒ to ⅔ mL
Horse . . . ⅓ to ⅔ mL
Precaution(s): Store at temperature between 2°-30°C (36°-86°F).
Caution(s): Federal law restricts this drug to use by or on the order of a licensed veterinarian.
For animal use only.
Warning(s): Keep out of reach of children.
Presentation: 12 x 100 mL amber glass multi-dose vials per carton (NDC: 59051-9087-5).
Manufactured by: Omega Laboratories, Montreal, Quebec H3M 3F4.
Compendium Code No.: 14910162 L570-0201

VITAMIN B_{12} 3000 mcg ℞

Phoenix Pharmaceutical **Vitamin B_{12}**

(Cyanocobalamin) Injection

Active Ingredient(s): Composition: Each mL of sterile aqueous solution contains:
Cyanocobalamin (B_{12}) . . . 3000 mcg
Sodium Chloride . . . 0.8% w/v
Benzyl Alcohol (preservative) . . . 1.5% v/v
Indications: For use as a supplemental nutritive source of vitamin B_{12} in cattle, horses, sheep, swine, dogs and cats.
Dosage and Administration: Inject subcutaneously or intramuscularly.
Cattle, Horses, Sheep and Swine: 1 to 2 mL
Dogs and Cats: 0.25 to 0.5 mL
Suggested dosage may be repeated at 1 to 2 week intervals, as indicated by condition and response.
Precaution(s): Store between 15°C and 30°C (59°F-86°F). Avoid exposure to light.
Caution(s): Federal law restricts this drug to use by or on the order of a licensed veterinarian.
For animal use only.
Warning(s): Keep out of reach of children.
Presentation: 100 mL vials (NDC 57319-103-05).
Manufactured by: Phoenix Scientific, Inc., St. Joseph, MO 64503.
Compendium Code No.: 12560942 Rev. 8-01

VITAMIN B_{12} 3000 mcg ℞

Vet Tek **Vitamin B_{12}**

Cyanocobalamin Injection

Active Ingredient(s): Composition: Each mL of sterile aqueous solution contains:
Cyanocobalamin (B_{12}) . . . 3000 mcg
Sodium Chloride . . . 0.8% w/v
Benzyl Alcohol (preservative) . . . 1.5% v/v
Indications: For use as supplemental nutritive source of Vitamin B_{12} in cattle, horses, sheep, swine, dogs and cats.
Dosage and Administration: Inject subcutaneously or intramuscularly.
Cattle, Horses, Sheep and Swine—1 to 2 mL
Dogs and Cats—0.25 to 0.5 mL
Suggested dosage may be repeated at 1 to 2 week intervals, as indicated by condition and response.
Precaution(s): Store between 15°C and 30°C (59°F-86°F). Avoid exposure to light.
Caution(s): Federal law restricts this drug to use by or on the order of a licensed veterinarian.
For animal use only.
Warning(s): Keep out of reach of children.
Presentation: 100 mL bottles (NDC 60270-040-10).
Manufactured by: Phoenix Scientific, Inc., St. Joseph, MO 64503.
Compendium Code No.: 14200231 Rev. 8-96

VITAMIN B_{12} 5000 MCG ℞

Neogen **Vitamin B_{12}**

Cyanocobalamin 5000-Sterile Solution

Active Ingredient(s): Each mL contains:
Cyanocobalamin . . . 5000 mcg
Benzyl Alcohol (as preservative) . . . 1.5% v/v
Sodium Chloride . . . 0.8% w/v
pH buffered with Acetic Acid
Water for injection . . . q.s.
Indications: For use in vitamin B_{12} deficiency associated with cobalt deficiency in cattle and sheep and for vitamin B_{12} deficiency associated with inadequate vitamin B_{12} intake or intestinal malabsorption in swine and horses.

Dosage and Administration: Inject intravenously, intramuscularly or subcutaneously. Dosage may be repeated in weekly intervals if necessary.
Cattle and Sheep .... 0.2 to 0.4 mL
Swine .... 0.1 to 0.4 mL
Horse .... 0.2 to 0.4 mL
Precaution(s): Store at temperatures between 2°-30°C (36°-86°F).
Caution(s): Federal law restricts this drug to use by or on the order of a licensed veterinarian.
For animal use only.
Warning(s): Keep out of reach of children.
Presentation: 12 x 100 mL amber glass multi-dose vials per carton (NDC: 59051-9088-5).
Manufactured by: Omega Laboratories, Montreal, QC H3M 3E4.
Compendium Code No.: 14910172 L571-0501

VITAMIN B_{12} 5000 mcg ℞

Phoenix Pharmaceutical **Vitamin B_{12}**

(Cyanocobalamin) Injection

Active Ingredient(s): Each mL of sterile aqueous solution contains:
Cyanocobalamin .... 5000 mcg
Benzyl Alcohol (as preservative) .... 1.5% w/v
Sodium Chloride .... 0.8% w/v
Water for Injection .... q.s.
Indications: For use in Vitamin B_{12} deficiency associated with cobalt deficiency in cattle and sheep and for Vitamin B_{12} deficiency associated with inadequate Vitamin B_{12} intake or intestinal malabsorption in swine.
Dosage and Administration: Inject intramuscularly or subcutaneously. Dosage may be repeated at weekly intervals if necessary.
Cattle and Sheep: 0.2 to 0.4 mL
Swine: 0.1 to 0.4 mL
Precaution(s): Store between 15°C and 30°C (59°F-86°F). Avoid exposure to light.
Caution(s): Federal law restricts this drug to use by or on the order of a licensed veterinarian.
For animal use only.
Warning(s): Keep out of reach of children.
Presentation: 100 mL vials (NDC 57319-111-05).
Manufactured by: Phoenix Scientific, Inc., St. Joseph, MO 64503.
Compendium Code No.: 12560953 Rev. 7-01

VITAMIN B_{12} INJECTION 1000 MCG ℞

Bimeda **Vitamin B_{12}**

Cyanocobalamin 1000 Injection

Active Ingredient(s): Composition: Each mL contains:
Cyanocobalamin (B_{12}) .... 1000 mcg
Sodium Chloride .... 0.8% w/v
Sodium phosphate monobasic .... 0.20% w/v
Benzyl alcohol .... 1.5% w/v
Water for injection .... q.s.
Indications: For use as a supplemental source of Vitamin B_{12} or for prevention and treatment of Vitamin B_{12} deficiency.
Dosage and Administration: Cattle and Sheep: 1 or 2 mL weekly by intramuscular injection. Administer slowly utilizing aseptic technique.
Precaution(s): Storage: 15°C-30°C (59°F-86°F).
Caution(s): Federal law restricts this drug to use by or on the order of a licensed veterinarian.
For animal use only.
Warning(s): Not for human use.
Keep out of reach of children.
Presentation: 250 mL bottles.
Manufactured by: Bimeda-MTC Animal Health Inc., Cambridge, Ontario, Canada N3C 2W4.
Compendium Code No.: 13990481 Iss. 3.99

VITAMIN B_{12} INJECTION (1,000 mcg/mL) ℞

AgriLabs **Vitamin B_{12}**

Active Ingredient(s): Each mL of sterile aqueous solution contains:
Cyanocobalamin (B_{12}) .... 1,000 mcg
Sodium chloride .... 0.8% w/v
Benzyl alcohol (preservative) .... 1.5% v/v
Buffered with acetic acid.
Indications: For use as a supplemental source of vitamin B_{12} in cattle, horses, sheep, swine, dogs and cats.
Dosage and Administration: Inject subcutaneously or intramuscularly.
Cattle, Horses, Sheep and Swine .... 1 to 2 mL
Dogs and Cats .... 0.25 to 0.5 mL
The suggested dosage may be repeated at 1- to 2-week intervals, as indicated by condition and response.
Precaution(s): Store at a temperature between 2° and 30°C (36°-86°F). Avoid exposure to light.
Caution(s): Federal law restricts this drug to use by or on the order of a licensed veterinarian.
Not for human use.
Keep out of the reach of children.
Presentation: 100 mL, 250 mL and 250 mL bottles.
Compendium Code No.: 10581730 Iss. 2-91

VITAMIN B_{12} INJECTION 3000 MCG ℞

Bimeda **Vitamin B_{12}**

Cyanocobalamin 3000 Injection

Active Ingredient(s): Composition: Each mL of sterile aqueous solution contains:
Cyanocobalamin (B_{12}) .... 3000 mcg
Sodium Chloride .... 0.6% w/v
Sodium Acetate Trihydrate .... 0.73% w/v
Benzyl Alcohol (preservative) .... 1.5% v/v
Indications: For use as a supplemental source of vitamin B_{12} in cattle, horses, sheep, swine, dogs and cats.
Dosage and Administration: Inject subcutaneously or intramuscularly.
Cattle, Horses, Sheep and Swine: .... 1 to 2 mL
Dogs and Cats .... 0.25 to 0.5 mL
Suggested dosage may be repeated at 1 to 2 week intervals as indicated by condition and response.
Precaution(s): Store between 15°C and 30°C (59°F-86°F). Avoid exposure to light.
Caution(s): Federal law restricts this drug to use by or on the order of a licensed veterinarian.
For animal use only.
Warning(s): Keep out of reach of children.
Presentation: 100 mL and 250 mL sterile multiple dose vials.
Manufactured by: Bimeda-MTC Animal Health Inc., Cambridge, ON, Canada N3C 2W4.
Compendium Code No.: 13990570 Rev.05.02

VITAMIN B_{12} INJECTION (3,000 mcg/mL) ℞

AgriLabs **Vitamin B_{12}**

Active Ingredient(s): Each mL of sterile aqueous solution contains:
Cyanocobalamin (B_{12}) .... 3,000 mcg
Benzyl alcohol (as preservative) .... 1.5% w/v
Sodium chloride .... 0.8% w/v
Water for injection .... q.s.
Buffered with acetic acid.
Indications: For use in vitamins B_{12} deficiency associated with cobalt deficiency in cattle and sheep and for vitamins B_{12} deficiency associated with inadequate vitamin B_{12} intake or intestinal malabsorption in swine.
Dosage and Administration: Inject subcutaneously or intramuscularly. The dosage may be repeated once a week if necessary.
Cattle and Sheep .... ⅓ to ⅔ mL
Swine .... ⅒ to ⅔ mL
Precaution(s): Store at a temperature between 2° and 30°C (36°-86°F). Avoid exposure to light.
Caution(s): Federal law restricts this drug to use by or on the order of a licensed veterinarian.
Not for human use.
Warning(s): Keep out of reach of children.
Presentation: 250 mL bottles.
Compendium Code No.: 10581740 Iss. 12-88

VITAMIN B_{12} INJECTION 5000 MCG ℞

Bimeda **Vitamin B_{12}**

Cyanocobalamin 5000 Injection

Active Ingredient(s): Composition: Each mL of sterile aqueous solution contains:
Cyanocobalamin .... 5000 mcg
Sodium chloride .... 0.6% w/v
Sodium acetate trihydrate .... 0.73% w/v
Benzyl alcohol (preservative) .... 1.5% w/v
Indications: For use in Vitamin B_{12} deficiency associated with cobalt deficiency in cattle and sheep and for Vitamin B_{12} deficiency associated with inadequate Vitamin B_{12} intake or intestinal malabsorption in swine.
Dosage and Administration: Inject subcutaneously or intramuscularly. Dosage may be repeated in weekly intervals if necessary.
Cattle and Sheep: 0.2 to 0.4 mL
Swine: 0.1 to 0.4 mL
Precaution(s): Store between 15°C and 30°C (59°F-86°F). Avoid exposure to light.
Caution(s): Federal law restricts this drug to use by or on the order of a licensed veterinarian.
For animal use only.
Warning(s): Keep out of reach of children.
Presentation: 100 mL sterile-multiple dose vials (NDC# 61133-0218-9).
Manufactured by: Bimeda-MTC Animal Health Inc., Cambridge, Ontario, Canada N3C 2W4.
Compendium Code No.: 13990580 Iss. 4.00

VITAMIN B_{12}-IRON GEL™

Horses Prefer **Iron-Oral**

Guaranteed Analysis: (Minimum per tube):
Iron 1.4%
Vitamin B_{12} .... 4,000 mcg
Ingredients: Iron Proteinate, Vitamin B_{12} Supplement, Liver Powder, Beef Peptone, Propylene Glycol, Methyl Paraben, Propylparaben, Ethoxyquin as a Preservative, and Apple Flavor.
Indications: Suggested Use: VITAMIN B_{12}-IRON GEL™ is formulated to provide horses with supplemental Iron and Vitamin B_{12} which may be lacking in horse's regular diet.
Directions: Administer single dose tube onto back of horse's tongue. For more information consult your veterinarian.
Precaution(s): Store below 85°F.
Caution(s): For animal use only.
Warning(s): Keep out of reach of children.
Presentation: 32 cc tube.
Compendium Code No.: 36950081

VITA-MIN BIOTIN

Farnam **Biotin**

Nutritional Crumbles-Equine Feed Supplement

Guaranteed Analysis: Per Pound:
Calcium, min. 8%
Calcium, max. 9%
Biotin, min. .... 100 mg
Ingredients: Dehydrated Alfalfa Meal, Ground Limestone, Wheat Middlings, Oat Hulls, Biotin, Vegetable Oil, Cane Molasses and Propionic and Acetic Acids (as preservatives).
Indications: VITA-MIN BIOTIN is a quality blend equine feed supplement for all classes of horses.
Dosage and Administration: Feeding Instructions: Feed ½ scoop to 1 ounce in daily feed ration (1 ounce measuring scoop enclosed).
Caution(s): For animal use only.
Warning(s): Keep out of reach of children.
Presentation: 1.13 kg (2.5 lb) and 9.07 kg (20 lb).
Compendium Code No.: 10000980 0D1

VITAMIN C ℞

AgriLabs **Vitamin C**

Injectable Solution

Active Ingredient(s): Composition: Each mL of sterile aqueous solution contains:
Sodium Ascorbate . . . . . 250 mg
Benzyl Alcohol (preservative) . . . . . 1.5% v/v
Sodium Metabisulfite . . . . . 0.2% w/v

Indications: For use as a nutritive supplement of vitamin C in guinea pigs and primates.

Dosage and Administration: Administer intramuscularly 1 to 10 mL, depending on condition, species, and body weight. Repeat daily or as indicated by desired response.

Precaution(s): Store between 15° and 30°C (59°-86°F). Protect from light.

Since pressure may develop on long storage, precautions should be taken to release pressure before use. Storage under refrigeration will reduce possibility of pressure build-up.

Caution(s): Federal law restricts this drug to use by or on the order of a licensed veterinarian.

For animal use only.

Warning(s): Keep out of reach of children.

Presentation: 250 mL vial.

Compendium Code No.: 10581750 Iss. 1-97

VITAMIN C ℞

Butler **Vitamin C**

Active Ingredient(s): Each mL of sterile aqueous solution contains:
Sodium ascorbate . . . . . 250 mg
Benzyl alcohol (preservative) . . . . . 1.5% v/v
Sodium metabisulfite . . . . . 0.2% w/v

Indications: For use as a supplement of vitamin C in cattle, horses, sheep, swine, dogs and cats.

Dosage and Administration: Administer intramuscularly 1 to 10 mL depending upon the condition, species, and body weight. Repeat each day or as indicated by the response.

Precaution(s): Since pressure may develop upon long storage, precautions should be taken to release the pressure before use. Storage under refrigeration will reduce the possibility of pressure build-up.

Store at a controlled room temperature between 59°-86°F (15°-30°C). Protect from light.

Caution(s): Federal law restricts this drug to use by or on the order of a licensed veterinarian.

For animal use only. Keep out of the reach of children.

Presentation: 100 mL containers.

Compendium Code No.: 10821860

VITAMIN C ℞

Phoenix Pharmaceutical **Vitamin C**

Injectable Solution

Active Ingredient(s): Composition: Each mL of sterile aqueous solution contains:
Sodium Ascorbate . . . . . 250 mg
Benzyl Alcohol (preservative) . . . . . 1.5% v/v
Sodium Metabisulfite . . . . . 0.2% w/v

Indications: For use as a nutritive supplement of vitamin C in guinea pigs and primates.

Dosage and Administration: Administer intramuscularly 1 to 10 mL, depending on condition, species, and body weight. Repeat daily or as indicated by desired response.

Precaution(s): Store between 15°C and 30°C (59°F-86°F). Protect from light.

Since pressure may develop on long storage, precautions should be taken to release the pressure before use. Storage under refrigeration will reduce the possibility of pressure build-up.

Caution(s): Federal law restricts this drug to use by or on the order of a licensed veterinarian.

For animal use only.

Warning(s): Keep out of reach of children.

Presentation: 100 mL (NDC 57319-068-05) and 250 mL (NDC 57319-068-06) vials.

Manufactured by: Phoenix Scientific, Inc., St. Joseph, MO 64503.

Compendium Code No.: 12560962 Rev. 4-02

VITAMIN C ℞

Vet Tek **Vitamin C**

NDC No.: 60270-582-13

Active Ingredient(s): Each mL of injectable sterile aqueous solution contains:
Sodium ascorbate . . . . . 250 mg
Benzyl alcohol (preservative) . . . . . 1.5% v/v
Sodium metabisulfite . . . . . 0.2% w/v

Indications: For use as a nutritive supplement of vitamin C in guinea pigs and primates.

Dosage and Administration: Administer intramuscularly 1 to 10 mL depending on condition, species, and body weight. Repeat daily or as indicated by response.

Precaution(s): Protect from light. Store between 15°C-30°C (59°F-86°F). Keep from freezing.

Since pressure may develop upon long storage, precautions should be taken to release pressure before use. Storage under refrigeration will reduce possibility of pressure buildup.

Caution(s): Federal law restricts this drug to use by or on the order of a licensed veterinarian.

For animal use only.

Keep out of reach of children.

Presentation: 250 mL.

Compendium Code No.: 14200240

VITAMIN E-300

AgriLabs **Vitamin E**

Injectable Tocopherol (300 I.U. Vitamins E per mL)

Active Ingredient(s): Each mL contains: 300 International Units of vitamin E (as d-alpha-tocopherol, a natural source of vitamin E), compounded with 20% ethyl alcohol and 1% benzyl alcohol (preservative) in an emulsifiable base.

Indications: VITAMIN E-300 is for use as a supplemental source of natural vitamin E in swine, cattle, and sheep.

Dosage and Administration: Intramuscular or subcutaneous administration only. May be repeated. If dose is greater than 5 mL, equally divide the dose and inject at two different sites.

Suggested Dosage:
Swine:
Sows and Gilts:
2 wks pre-partum . . . . . 4-6 mL (1200-1800 I.U.)
2 wks pre-breeding . . . . . 4-6 mL (1200-1800 I.U.)
Pigs:
At birth . . . . . 1-2 mL (300-600 I.U.)
Weaning . . . . . 2-3 mL (600-900 I.U.)
Cattle (Dairy and Beef):
Cows and Heifers:
2-3 wks pre-partum . . . . . 8-10 mL (2400-3000 I.U.)
At calving . . . . . 8-10 mL (2400-3000 I.U.)
Calves:
At birth . . . . . 4-6 mL (1200-1800 I.U.)
Weaning . . . . . 4-6 mL (1200-1800 I.U.)
Yearlings . . . . . 5-6 mL (1500-1800 I.U.)
Sheep:
Ewes:
2-3 wks pre-partum . . . . . 4-5 mL (1200-1500 I.U.)
At lambing . . . . . 4-5 mL (1200-1500 I.U.)
Lambs:
At birth . . . . . 2-3 mL (600-900 I.U.)
Weaning . . . . . 2-3 mL (600-900 I.U.)
Finishing lambs . . . . . 3-4 mL (900-1200 I.U.)

Precaution(s): Store between 2° and 30°C (36° and 86°F) in a dark place. Store partially used vials under refrigeration (36°-55°F).

Caution(s): Anaphylactoid or allergic reactions, which have resulted in deaths, abortions, and/or premature births, have been reported in individual animals as well as entire herds. Should such reactions or hypersensitivity occur, treat immediately with injection of epinephrine and/or antihistamines.

Do not exceed recommended dosage. Do not add water to the solution.

Restricted drug (California)—use only as directed.

Warning(s): Not for human use.

Keep out of the reach of children.

Discussion: VITAMIN E-300 (natural-source of vitamin E is a clear, sterile, non-aqueous solution of d-alpha-tocopherol.

Natural tocopherols in feedstuffs can be destroyed through processing, ensiling, and storage. A reduced vitamin E intake can result in marginal deficiencies that may not be visible. Intramuscular or subcutaneous injections offer an efficient and rapid method to increase vitamin E status of animals.

Presentation: 8.5 fl oz (250 mL) vials.

Compendium Code No.: 10581220

VITAMIN E 300

Durvet **Vitamin E**

Injectable Tocopherol

Active Ingredient(s): Each mL contains 300 IU's of vitamin E (as d-alpha-tocopherol, a natural source of vitamin E) compounded with 2% benzyl alcohol (preservative) in a water emulsifiable base.

Indications: Injectable tocopherol (natural-source vitamin E) is a clear, sterile, non-aqueous solution of d-alpha-tocopherol for use as an aid in the prevention of vitamin E deficiencies in swine, cattle, and sheep.

This product is intended as a supplemental source of natural vitamin E.

Dosage and Administration: Intramuscular or subcutaneous use only. If dose is greater than 5 mL, equally divide the dose and inject at two different sites.

Suggested Dosage:	mL	International Units (I.U.)
Swine		
Sows and Gilts		
2 wks pre-partum	4-6	1200-1800
2 wks pre-breeding	4-6	1200-1800
Pigs		
At birth	1-2	300-600
Weaning	2-3	600-900
Cattle (Dairy and Beef)		
Cows and Heifers		
2 to 3 wks pre-partum	8-10	2400-3000
At calving	8-10	2400-3000
Calves		
At birth	4-6	1200-1800
Weaning	4-6	1200-1800
Yearlings	5-6	1500-1800
Sheep		
Ewes		
2-3 wks pre-partum	4-5	1200-1500
At lambing	4-5	1200-1500
Lambs		
At birth	2-3	600-900
Weaning	2-3	600-900
Finishing Lambs	3-4	900-1200

Precaution(s): Store at temperature between 2°-30°C (36°-86°F) in a dark place.

Caution(s): Do not add water to solution.

Do not exceed recommended dosage. Occasionally, reactions of an anaphylactic or allergic nature may occur. Should such reactions occur, treat immediately with injection of epinephrine.

Warning(s): Intramuscular or subcutaneous use only.

For animal use only.

Keep out of reach of children.

Discussion: Natural tocopherols in feedstuffs can be destroyed through processing, ensiling and storage. A reduced vitamin E intake can result in marginal deficiencies that may not be visible. Intramuscular or subcutaneous injections offer an efficient and rapid method to increase vitamin E status of animals.

Presentation: 250 mL vials.

Compendium Code No.: 10841640

VITAMIN E+AD

Durvet **Vitamins A-D-E**

NDC No.: 30798-156-13

Active Ingredient(s): Each mL contains:

Vitamin E (as d-alpha-tocopherol, (a natural source of vitamin E) .... 300 I.U.
Vitamin A propionate .... 100,000 I.U.
Vitamin D_3 .... 10,000 I.U.
Benzyl alcohol (preservative) 2%

In a water emulsifiable base.

Indications: Injectable VITAMIN E+AD is a clear, sterile, nonaqueous solution of vitamin A, vitamin D_3 and vitamin E. The product is intended as a supplemental source of vitamin A, D, and E in cattle.

Dosage and Administration: For intramuscular or subcutaneous administration only. If the dose is greater than 5 mL, divide the dose equally and inject it at two (2) different sites.

Cattle (dairy and beef):

Cows and heifers (2 to 3 weeks pre-partum, at calving and at the end of lactation): Give an 8-10 mL dose.

Calves (at birth and at weaning): Give a 4-6 mL dose.

Yearlings: Give a 5-6 mL dose.

Precaution(s): Store between 36° and 86°F (2° and 30°C) in a dark place.

Caution(s): Natural vitamin A (carotenes) and tocopherols in feedstuffs can be destroyed through processing, ensiling and storage. Due to these losses, reduced intakes of fat-soluble vitamins can occur in animals maintained in continual confinement compared to animals allowed to graze the pasture.

Do not exceed the recommended dose. Occasionally an anaphylactic reaction or an allergic response may occur. If such reactions occur, treat immediately with an injection of epinephrine.

Do not add water to the solution.

Keep out of the reach of children.

Not for human use.

For veterinary use only.

Presentation: 250 mL vials.

Compendium Code No.: 10841650

VITAMIN E-AD 300

AgriLabs **Vitamins A-D-E**

Injectable A+D Tocopherol (Vitamins A, D_3, and E)

Active Ingredient(s): Each mL contains: 100,000 I.U. vitamin A, 10,000 I.U. vitamin D_3, and 300 I.U. vitamin E (as d-alpha-tocopherol, a natural source of vitamin E). Also contains 20% ethyl alcohol, 1% benzyl alcohol (preservative) in an emulsifiable base.

Indications: The product is intended as a supplemental source of vitamin A, D, and E.

Dosage and Administration: Intramuscular or subcutaneous administration only. May be repeated as needed. If dose is greater than 5 mL, equally divide the dose and inject at two different sites.

Suggested Dosage:

Cattle (Dairy and Beef):

Cows and Heifers:
2-3 wks pre-partum .... 8-10 mL
At calving .... 8-10 mL
End of lactation .... 8-10 mL

Calves:
At birth .... 4-6 mL
At weaning .... 4-6 mL

Yearlings .... 5-6 mL

Precaution(s): Store between 2° and 30°C (36° and 86°F) in a dark place. Store partially used vials under refrigeration (36°-55°F).

Caution(s): Anaphylactoid or allergic reactions, which have resulted in deaths, abortions, and/or premature births, have been reported in individual animals as well as entire herds. Should such reactions or hypersensitivity occur, treat immediately with injection of epinephrine and/or antihistamines.

Do not exceed recommended dosage. Do not add water to solution.

Restricted drug (California)—use only as directed.

Warning(s): Not for human use.

Keep out of reach of children.

Intramuscular or subcutaneous injection only.

Discussion: Injectable A+D Tocopherol is a clear, sterile, non-aqueous solution of vitamin A, vitamin D_3, and vitamin E.

Natural vitamin A (carotenes) and tocopherols can be destroyed in feedstuffs through processing, ensiling, and storage. Due to these losses, reduced intakes of fat-soluble vitamins can occur in animals maintained in continual confinement compared to animals allowed to graze lush pasture. Intramuscular or subcutaneous injections offer an efficient and rapid method to increase vitamin A, vitamin D, and vitamin E status of animals.

Vitamin A activity is provided as retinyl palmitate, the biological storage-form of vitamin A; and vitamin E activity is provided as d-alpha-tocopherol, the natural and biologically active form of vitamin E.

Presentation: 8.5 fl oz (250 mL).

Compendium Code No.: 10581230

VITA-MIN E & SELENIUM

Farnam **Vitamin E-Selenium**

Nutritional Crumbles-Equine Feed Supplement

Guaranteed Analysis: Per Pound:

Crude Protein, min. 10.0%
Crude Fat, min. 3.5%
Crude Fiber, max. 15.0%
Calcium, min. 8.5%
Calcium, max. 9.5%
Selenium (Se) .... 70 ppm
Vitamin E, min. .... 20,000 IU

Ingredients: Dehydrated Alfalfa Meal, Ground Limestone, Wheat Middlings, Sodium Selenite, Vitamin E Supplement, Vegetable Oil, Cane Molasses and Propionic and Acetic Acids (as preservatives).

Indications: VITA-MIN & SELENIUM is a quality blend equine feed supplement for all classes of horses.

Dosage and Administration: Feeding Instructions: Top dress daily grain ration with ¼ to ½ scoop. (1 ounce measuring scoop enclosed).

Each ½ oz contains 1 mg Selenium.

Precaution(s): Store in area inaccessible to children and animals.

Caution(s): Follow label directions. The addition to feed of higher levels of this premix containing Selenium is not permitted. Excessive amounts of Selenium may be toxic.

For animal use only.

Warning(s): Keep out of reach of children.

Presentation: 1.13 kg (2.5 lb) and 9.07 kg (20 lb).

Compendium Code No.: 10000990 0E1 / 0D1

VITAMIN E & SELENIUM POWDER

AHC **Equine Dietary Supplement**

Feed Supplement

Guaranteed Analysis: Each pound contains not less than:

Vitamin E .... 20,000 IU
Selenium .... 45.4 mg (0.01%) (100 ppm)

(A ½ ounce provides approximately 625 IU Vitamin E and 1.5 mg Selenium.)

Ingredients: rice hulls, calcium carbonate, d-alpha tocopheryl acetate, mineral oil, sodium selenite and magnesium-mica.

Indications: A Vitamin E and Selenium feed supplement for horses, formulated to supply supplemental Vitamin E and selenium that may be lacking or in insufficient quantities in the horse's regular feed.

Dosage and Administration: Recommended Dosage: Feed ½ ounce (3 teaspoons) daily for 1000 lb of body weight with regular feed.

Note: The addition to feed of higher levels of this supplement containing selenium is not permitted.

Precaution(s): Reseal after each use.

Caution(s): For animal use only.

Keep out of reach of children

Presentation: 2.5 lb jar and 5 lb pail.

Compendium Code No.: 10770070

VITAMIN E DISPERSIBLE LIQUID

Alpharma **Water Additive**

Ingredient(s): Vitamin E (as dl-alpha-tocopheryl acetate), polysorbate 80, and n-propyl alcohol; may also contain potassium sorbate or polyethylene glycol 400 monooleate.

Guaranteed to contain: 400 IU of vitamin E (as dl-alpha-tocopheryl acetate) per gram.

Indications: A nutritional supplement for use in healthy or sick or convalescing poults.

Directions: Water dispersible vitamin E for use in poultry drinking water. Use 3 oz per gallon of stock solution. One gallon of stock solution medicates 128 gallons of water. Contents of this bottle will provide at least 266 IU of vitamin E for 1,364 gallons of drinking water.

Precaution(s): Store in cool, dry place.

Caution(s): For oral animal use only.

Keep out of reach of children.

Presentation: 32 oz bottles.

Compendium Code No.: 10220641 AHL-270 0005

VITAMIN K_1 ℞

Vet Tek **Vitamin K Injection**

(Phytonadione Injection) 10 mg/mL-Aqueous Colloidal Solution

Active Ingredient(s): Each mL contains:

Phytonadione .... 10 mg

Inactive ingredients:

Polyoxyethylated fatty acid derivative .... 70 mg
Dextrose .... 37.5 mg
Water for Injection, q.s. .... 1 mL

Added as preservative:

Benzyl alcohol 0.9%

Indications: VITAMIN K_1 Injection is indicated in coagulation disorders which are due to faulty formation of factors II, VII, IX and X when caused by vitamin K deficiency or interference with vitamin K activity.

VITAMIN K_1 Injection is indicated in cattle, calves, horses, swine, sheep, goats, dogs, and cats to counter hypoprothrombinemia induced by ingestion of anticoagulant rodenticides.

VITAMIN K_1 Injection is also indicated to counter hypoprothrombinemia caused by consumption of bishydroxycoumarin found in spoiled and moldy sweet clover.

Pharmacology: Description: Phytonadione is a vitamin, which is a clear, yellow to amber, viscous, odorless or nearly odorless liquid. It is insoluble in water, soluble in chloroform and slightly soluble in ethanol. It has a molecular weight of 450.70.

Phytonadione is 2-methyl-3-phytyl-1,4-naphthoquinone. Its empirical formula is $C_{31}H_{46}O_2$.

VITAMIN K_1 Injection is a yellow, sterile, aqueous colloidal solution of vitamin K_1, with a pH of 5.0 to 7.0, available for injection by the intravenous, intramuscular, and subcutaneous routes.

Clinical Pharmacology: VITAMIN K_1 Injection aqueous colloidal solution of vitamin K_1 for parenteral injection, possesses the same type and degree of activity as does naturally-occurring vitamin K, which is necessary for the production via the liver of active prothrombin (factor II), proconvertin (factor VII), plasma thromboplastin component (factor IX), and Stuart factor (factor X). The prothrombin test is sensitive to the levels of three of these four factors - II, VII, and X. Vitamin K is an essential cofactor for a microsomal enzyme that catalyzes the post-translational carboxylation of multiple, specific, peptide-bound glutamic acid residues in inactive hepatic precursors of factors II, VII, IX, and X. The resulting gamma-carboxyglutamic acid residues convert the precursors into active coagulation factors that are subsequently secreted by liver cells into the blood.

Phytonadione is readily absorbed following intramuscular administration. After absorption, phytonadione is initially concentrated in the liver, but the concentration declines rapidly. Very little vitamin K accumulates in tissues. Little is known about the metabolic fate of vitamin K. Almost no free unmetabolized vitamin K appears in bile or urine.

In normal animals, phytonadione is virtually devoid of pharmacodynamic activity. However, in animals deficient in vitamin K, the pharmacological action of vitamin K is related to its normal physiological function, that is, to promote the hepatic biosynthesis of vitamin K dependent clotting factors.

The action of the aqueous colloidal solution, when administered intravenously, is generally detectable within an hour or two and hemorrhage is usually controlled within 3 to 6 hours. A normal prothrombin level may often be obtained in 12 to 14 hours.

Dosage and Administration:

Cattle, Calves, Horses, Swine, Sheep, and Goats: Acute hypoprothrombinemia (with hemorrhage) and Non-acute hypoprothrombinemia — 0.5-2.5 mg/kg subcutaneously or intramuscularly.

Dogs and Cats: Acute hypoprothrombinemia (with hemorrhage) and Non-acute hypoprothrombinemia — 0.25-5 mg/kg subcutaneously or intramuscularly. Use higher end of dose for second generation rodenticides.

Whenever possible, VITAMIN K_1 Injection should be given by subcutaneous or intramuscular route. When intravenous administration is considered unavoidable, the drug should be diluted and injected very slowly, not exceeding 1 mg per minute.

Directions for Dilution: VITAMIN K_1 Injection may be diluted with 0.9% Sodium Chloride Injection, 5% Dextrose Injection, or 5% Dextrose and Sodium Chloride Injection. Other diluents should not be used. When dilutions are indicated, administration should be started immediately after mixture with the diluent, and unused portions of the dilution should be discarded.

Whole blood or component therapy may be indicated if bleeding is excessive. This therapy, however, does not correct the underlying disorder and VITAMIN K_1 Injection should be given concurrently. In the event of shock or excessive blood loss, the use of whole blood or component therapy is indicated.

Drug Interactions: Temporary resistance to prothrombin-depressing anticoagulants may result, especially when larger doses of phytonadione are used. If relatively large doses have been employed, it may be necessary when reinstituting anticoagulant therapy to use somewhat larger doses of the prothrombin-depressing anticoagulant, or to use one which acts on a different principle, such as heparin sodium.

Contraindication(s): Hypersensitivity to any component of this medication.

Precaution(s): Storage: Protect from light at all times. Store in a dark place. Store at controlled room temperature 15°-30°C (59°-86°F).

Caution(s): Federal law restricts this drug to use by or on the order of a licensed veterinarian.

Intravenous Use: Severe reactions, including fatalities, have occurred during and immediately after intravenous injection of phytonadione, even when precautions have been taken to dilute the phytonadione and to avoid rapid infusion. Typically these severe reactions have resembled hypersensitivity or anaphylaxis, including shock and cardiac and/or respiratory arrest. Some patients have exhibited these severe reactions on receiving phytonadione for the first time. Therefore the intravenous route should be restricted to those situations where other routes are not feasible and the serious risk involved is considered justified.

An immediate coagulant effect should not be expected after administration of phytonadione. It takes a minimum of 1 to 2 hours for measurable improvement in the prothrombin time. Whole blood or component therapy may also be necessary if bleeding is severe.

Phytonadione will not counteract the anticoagulant action of heparin.

When vitamin K_1 is used to correct excessive anticoagulant-induced hypoprothrombinemia, anticoagulant therapy still being indicated, the patient is again faced with the clotting hazards existing prior to starting the anticoagulant therapy. Phytonadione is not a clotting agent, but overzealous therapy with vitamin K_1 may restore conditions which originally permitted thromboembolic phenomena. Dosage should be kept as low as possible, and prothrombin time should be checked regularly as clinical conditions indicate.

Repeated large doses of vitamin K are not warranted in liver disease if the response to initial use of the vitamin is unsatisfactory. Failure to respond to vitamin K may indicate that the condition being treated is inherently unresponsive to vitamin K.

Laboratory Tests: Prothrombin time should he checked regularly as clinical conditions indicate.

Parenteral drug products should be inspected visually for particulate matter and discoloration prior to administration, whenever solution and container permit.

For animal use only.

Warning(s): Keep out of reach of children.

Adverse Reactions: Deaths have occurred after intravenous administration (see Caution).

Pain, swelling, and tenderness at the injection site may occur. Intramuscular injection may result in hematomas.

The possibility of allergic sensitivity, including an anaphylactoid reaction, should be kept in mind.

Presentation: VITAMIN K_1 Injection is supplied in 100 mL bottles.

Manufactured by: Phoenix Scientific Inc., St. Joseph, MO 64503.

Compendium Code No.: 14200251 Rev. 03-01

VITAMIN K_1 INJECTION ℞

Butler **Vitamin K_1-Injection**

Active Ingredient(s): VITAMIN K_1 INJECTION is a yellow, sterile aqueous colloidal solution of vitamin K_1 (phytonadione), available for injection by the intravenous, intramuscular and subcutaneous routes. Each mL contains:

Phytonadione .... 10 mg

Inactive ingredients:

Polyoxyethylated fatty acid derivative .... 70 mg

Dextrose .... 37.5 mg

Water for injection .... q.s.

Added as a preservative:

Benzyl alcohol 0.9%

Indications: VITAMIN K_1 INJECTION is indicated in cattle, calves, horses, swine, sheep, goats, dogs and cats to counter hypoprothrombinemia induced by ingestion of coumarin-based compounds, common ingredients in commercial rodenticides. VITAMIN K_1 INJECTION is also indicated to counter hypoprothrombinemia caused by consumption of bishydroxycoumarin found in spoiled and moldy sweet clover.

Pharmacology: VITAMIN K_1 INJECTION, an aqueous colloidal solution of vitamin K_1 for parenteral injection, possesses the same type and degree of activity as does naturally occurring vitamin K. The primary function of vitamin K is to stimulate the production via the liver of active prothrombin from a precursor protein. The mechanism by which vitamin K promotes formation of prothrombin at the molecular level has not been established.

The action of the aqueous colloidal solution, when administered intravenously, is generally detectable within an hour or two and hemorrhage is usually controlled within three to six hours. A normal prothrombin level may often be obtained in 12 to 14 hours.

Dosage and Administration: Cattle, Calves, Horses, Swine, Sheep and Goats:

Acute hypoprothrombinemia (with hemorrhage): Intravenously, 0.5-2.5 mg/kg of body weight, at a rate not to exceed 10 mg per minute in mature animals and 5 mg per minute in newborn and very young animals.

Nonacute hypoprothrombinemia: Intramuscularly or subcutaneously, 0.5-2.5 mg/kg of body weight.

Dogs and Cats:

Acute hypoprothrombinemia (with hemorrhage): Intravenously, 0.25-2.5 mg/kg of body weight, at a rate not to exceed 5 mg per minute.

Nonacute hypoprothrombinemia: Intramuscularly or subcutaneously, 0.25-2.5 mg/kg of body weight.

Whenever possible, VITAMIN K_1 INJECTION should be given by the intramuscular or subcutaneous routes. When intravenous injection is considered unavoidable, the drug should be given very slowly, at the rate indicated above. Monitor prothrombin time and adjust dosage accordingly.

Regular determinations of prothrombin time response should be performed to guide in the initial and subsequent administration of VITAMIN K_1 INJECTION. The dosage should be adjusted accordingly.

The frequency and amount of subsequent doses should be guided by regular determination of prothrombin time response and clinical condition. If in six (6) to eight (8) hours after parenteral administration the prothrombin time has not been shortened satisfactorily, the dose should be repeated.

In the event of shock or excessive blood loss, the use of whole blood or component therapy is indicated. The smallest effective dose should be sought to minimize the risk of adverse reaction.

VITAMIN K_1 INJECTION may be diluted with 0.9% sodium chloride injection, 5% dextrose injection, or 5% dextrose with sodium chloride injection. Other diluents should not be used. When dilutions are indicated, administration should be started immediately after mixture with the diluent, and unused portions of the dilution should be discarded.

Contraindication(s): Hypersensitivity to any component of this medication.

Precaution(s): Store in a cool, dark place between 2° and 8°C (36°-48°F). Protect from light at all times. Temporary resistance to prothrombin-depressing anticoagulants may result, especially when larger doses of phytonadione are used.

Caution(s): Federal (U.S.A.) law restricts this drug to use by or on the order of a licensed veterinarian.

Not for human use. Keep out of the reach of children.

Warning(s): Intravenous use: Severe reactions, including fatalities, have occurred during and immediately after intravenous injection of phytonadione, even when precautions have been taken to dilute the vitamin K_1 and to avoid rapid infusion. Typically, these severe reactions have resembled hypersensitivity or anaphylaxis, including shock and cardiac and/or respiratory arrest. Some animals have exhibited these severe reactions on receiving VITAMIN K_1 INJECTION for the first time. Therefore, the intravenous route should be restricted to those situations where other routes are not feasible and the serious risk involved is considered justified.

An immediate coagulant effect should not be expected after administration of phytonadione. A minimum of one (1) to two (2) hours is required for measurable improvement in the prothrombin time. Whole blood or component therapy may be necessary if the bleeding is severe.

Phytonadione will not counteract the anticoagulant action of heparin.

Repeated large doses of vitamin K are not warranted in hepatic disease if the response to the initial therapy is unsatisfactory. Failure to respond to vitamin K may indicate that the condition being treated is inherently unresponsive to vitamin K.

Side Effects: Deaths have occurred following intravenous injection (see warning for intravenous use).

Pain, swelling, and tenderness at the injection site may occur. The possibility of allergic sensitivity, including an anaphylactic reaction, should be kept in mind.

Presentation: 100 mL multiple dose vials.

Compendium Code No.: 10821870

VITAMIN K_1 INJECTION ℞

Neogen **Vitamin K_1-Injection**

(Phytonadione) 10 mg/mL-Aqueous Colloidal Sterile Solution

Active Ingredient(s): Each milliliter contains:

Phytonadione .... 10 mg

Inactive ingredients:

Polyoxyethylated fatty acid derivative .... 70 mg

Dextrose .... 37.5 mg

Water for Injection, q.s .... 1 mL

Added as preservative:

Benzyl alcohol .... 1.5% v/v

Indications: VITAMIN K_1 INJECTION is indicated in coagulation disorders which are due to faulty formation of factors II, VII, IX and X when caused by vitamin K deficiency or interference with vitamin K activity.

VITAMIN K_1 INJECTION is indicated in cattle, calves, horses, swine, sheep, goats, dogs, and cats to counter hypoprothrombinemia induced by ingestion of anticoagulant rodenticides.

VITAMIN K_1 INJECTION is also indicated to counter hypoprothrombinemia caused by consumption of bishydroxycoumarin found in spoiled and moldy sweet clover.

Pharmacology: Description: Phytonadione is a vitamin, which is a clear, yellow to amber, viscous, odorless or nearly odorless liquid. It is insoluble in water, soluble in chloroform and slightly soluble in ethanol. It has a molecular weight of 450.70.

Phytonadione is 2-methyl-3-phytyl-1, 4-naphthoquinone. Its empirical formula is $C_{31}H_{46}O_2$.

VITAMIN K_1 INJECTION is a yellow, sterile, aqueous colloidal solution of vitamin K1, with a pH of 5.0 to 7.0, available for injection by the intravenous, intramuscular, and subcutaneous routes.

Clinical Pharmacology: VITAMIN K_1 INJECTION aqueous colloidal solution of vitamin K1 for parenteral injection, possesses the same type and degree of activity as does naturally-occurring vitamin K, which is necessary for the production via the liver of active prothrombin (factor II), proconvertin (factor VII), plasma thromboplastin component (factor IX), and Stuart factor (factor X). The prothrombin test is sensitive to the levels of three of these four factors—II, VII, and X. Vitamin K is an essential cofactor for a microsomal enzyme that catalyzes the posttranslational carboxylation of multiple, specific, peptide-bound glutamic acid residues in inactive hepatic precursors of factors II, VII, IX, and X. The resulting gamma-carboxyglutamic acid residues convert the precursors into active coagulation factors that are subsequently secreted by liver cells into the blood.

Phytonadione is readily absorbed following intramuscular administration. After absorption, phytonadione is initially concentrated in the liver, but the concentration declines rapidly. Very little vitamin K accumulates in tissues. Little is known about the metabolic fate of vitamin K. Almost no free unmetabolized vitamin K appears in bile or urine.

In normal animals, phytonadione is virtually devoid of pharmacodynamic activity. However, in animals deficient in vitamin K, the pharmacological action of vitamin K is related to its normal physiological function, that is, to promote the hepatic biosynthesis of vitamin K dependent clotting factors.

The action of the aqueous colloidal solution, when administered intravenously, is generally detectable within an hour or two and hemorrhage is usually controlled within 3 to 6 hours. A normal prothrombin level may often be obtained in 12 to 14 hours.

Dosage and Administration:

Cattle, Calves, Horses, Swine, Sheep, and Goats: Acute hypoprothrombinemia (with hemorrhage) and Non-acute hypoprothrombinemia — 0.5-2.5 mg/kg subcutaneously or intramuscularly.

Dogs and Cats: Acute hypoprothrombinemia (with hemorrhage) and Non-acute hypoprothrombinemia — 0.25-5 mg/kg subcutaneously or intramuscularly. Use higher end of dose for second generation rodenticides.

Whenever possible, VITAMIN K_1 INJECTION should be given by the subcutaneous or intramuscular route. When intravenous administration is considered unavoidable, the drug should be diluted and injected very slowly, not exceeding 1 mg per minute.

Direction For Dilution: VITAMIN K_1 INJECTION may be diluted with 0.9% Sodium Chloride Injection, 5% Dextrose Injection, or 5% Dextrose and Sodium Chloride Injection. Other diluents should not be used. When dilutions are indicated, administration should be started immediately after mixture with diluent, and unused portions of the dilution should be discarded.

Whole blood or component therapy may be indicated if bleeding is excessive. This therapy, however, does not correct the underlying disorder and VITAMIN K_1 INJECTION should be given concurrently. In the event of shock or excessive blood loss, the use of whole blood or component therapy is indicated.

Drug Interactions: Temporary resistance to prothrombin-depressing anticoagulants may result, especially when larger doses of phytonadione are used. If relatively large doses have been employed, it may be necessary when reinstituting anticoagulant therapy to use somewhat larger doses of the prothrombin-depressing anticoagulant, or to use one which acts on a different principle, such as heparin sodium.

Contraindication(s): Hypersensitivity to any component of this medication.

Precaution(s): Storage: Protect from light at all times. Store in dark place. Store at controlled room temperature 15°-30°C (59°-86°F).

Caution(s): Federal law restricts this drug to use by or on the order of a licensed veterinarian.

Laboratory Tests: Prothrombin time should be checked regularly as clinical conditions indicate.

Parenteral drug products should be inspected visually for particulate matter and discoloration prior to administration, whenever solution and container permit.

Intravenous Use: Severe reactions, including fatalities, have occurred during and immediately after intravenous injection of phytonadione, even when precautions have been taken to dilute the phytonadione and to avoid rapid infusion. Typically these severe reactions have resembled hypersensitivity or anaphylaxis, including shock and cardiac and/or respiratory arrest. Some patients have exhibited these severe reactions on receiving phytonadione for the first time. Therefore the intravenous route should be restricted to those situations where other routes are not feasible and the serious risk involved is considered justified.

An immediate coagulant effect should not be expected after administration of phytonadione. It takes a minimum of 1 to 2 hours for measurable improvement in the prothrombin time. Whole blood or component therapy may also be necessary if bleeding is severe.

Phytonadione will not counteract the anticoagulant action of heparin.

When vitamin K1 is used to correct excessive anticoagulant-induced hypoprothrombinemia, anticoagulant therapy still being indicated, the patient is again faced with the clotting hazards existing prior to starting the anticoagulant therapy. Phytonadione is not a clotting agent, but overzealous therapy with vitamin K1 may restore conditions which originally permitted thromboembolic phenomena. Dosage should be kept as low as possible, and prothrombin time should be checked regularly as clinical conditions indicate.

Repeated large doses of vitamin K are not warranted in liver disease if the response to initial use of the vitamin is unsatisfactory. Failure to respond to vitamin K may indicate that the condition being treated is inherently unresponsive to vitamin K.

For animal use only.

Warning(s): Keep out of reach of children.

Adverse Reactions: Deaths have occurred after intravenous administration. (See Cautions.)

Pain, swelling, and tenderness at the injection site may occur. Intramuscular injection may result in hematomas.

The possibility of allergic sensitivity, including an anaphylactoid reaction, should be kept in mind.

Presentation: 100 mL multiple dose vial.

Manufactured by: Omega Laboratories, Montreal, Quebec, H3M 3E4.

Compendium Code No.: 14910182 L527-0801

VITAMIN K_1 INJECTION ℞

Phoenix Pharmaceutical **Vitamin K**

(phytonadione injection) 10 mg/mL Aqueous Colloidal Solution

Active Ingredient(s): Each mL contains:

Phytonadione . . . . 10 mg

Inactive ingredients:

Polyoxyethylated fatty acid derivative . . . . 70 mg

Dextrose . . . . 37.5 mg

Water for Injection, q.s. . . . . 1 mL

Added as preservative:

Benzyl alcohol 0.9%

Indications: VITAMIN K_1 INJECTION is indicated in coagulation disorders which are due to faulty formation of factors II, VII, IX and X when caused by vitamin K deficiency or interference with vitamin K activity.

VITAMIN K_1 INJECTION is indicated in cattle, calves, horses, swine, sheep, goats, dogs, and cats to counter hypoprothrombinemia induced by ingestion of anticoagulant rodenticides.

VITAMIN K_1 INJECTION is also indicated to counter hypoprothrombinemia caused by consumption of bishydroxycoamarin found in spoiled and moldy sweet clover.

Pharmacology: Description: Phytonadione is a vitamin, which is a clear, yellow to amber, viscous, odorless or nearly odorless liquid. It is insoluble in water, soluble in chloroform and slightly soluble in ethanol. It has a molecular weight of 450.70.

Phytonadione is 2-methyl-3-phytyl-1,4-naphthoquinone. Its empirical formula is $C_{31}H_{46}O_2$.

VITAMIN K_1 INJECTION is a yellow, sterile, aqueous colloidal solution of vitamin K_1, with a pH of 5.0 to 7.0, available for injection by the intravenous, intramuscular, and subcutaneous routes.

Clinical Pharmacology: VITAMIN K_1 INJECTION aqueous colloidal solution of vitamin K_1 for parenteral injection, possesses the same type and degree of activity as does naturally-occurring vitamin K, which is necessary for the production via the liver of active prothrombin (factor II), proconvertin (factor VII), plasma thromboplastin component (factor IX), and Stuart factor (factor X). The prothrombin test is sensitive to the levels of three of these four factors - II, VII, and X. Vitamin K is an essential cofactor for a microsomal enzyme that catalyzes the post-translational carboxylation of multiple, specific, peptide-bound glutamic acid residues in inactive hepatic precursors of factors II, VII, IX, and X. The resulting gamma-carboxyglutamic acid residues convert the precursors into active coagulation factors that are subsequently secreted by liver cells into the blood.

Phytonadione is readily absorbed following intramuscular administration. After absorption, phytonadione is initially concentrated in the liver, but the concentration declines rapidly. Very little vitamin K accumulates in tissues. Little is known about the metabolic fate of vitamin K. Almost no free unmetabolized vitamin K appears in bile or urine.

In normal animals, phytonadione is virtually devoid of pharmacodynamic activity. However, in animals deficient in vitamin K, the pharmacological action of vitamin K is related to its normal physiological function, that is, to promote the hepatic biosynthesis of vitamin K dependent clotting factors.

The action of the aqueous colloidal solution, when administered intravenously, is generally detectable within an hour or two and hemorrhage is usually controlled within 3 to 6 hours. A normal prothrombin level may often be obtained in 12 to 14 hours.

Dosage and Administration: Cattle, Calves, Horses, Swine, Sheep, and Goats: Acute hypoprothrombinemia (with hemorrhage) and Non-acute hypoprothrombinemia—0.5-2.5 mg/kg subcutaneously or intramuscularly.

Dogs and Cats: Acute hypoprothrombinemia (with hemorrhage) and Non-acute hypoprothrombinemia—0.25-5 mg/kg subcutaneously or intramuscularly. Use higher end of dose for second generation rodenticides.

Whenever possible, VITAMIN K_1 INJECTION should be given by subcutaneous or intramuscular route. When intravenous administration is considered unavoidable, the drug should be diluted and injected very slowly, not exceeding 1 mg per minute.

Directions For Dilution: VITAMIN K_1 INJECTION may be diluted with 0.9% Sodium Chloride Injection, 5% Dextrose Injection, or 5% Dextrose and Sodium Chloride Injection. Other diluents should not be used. When dilutions are indicated, administration should be started immediately after mixture with the diluent, and unused portions of the dilution should be discarded.

Whole blood or component therapy may be indicated if bleeding is excessive. This therapy, however, does not correct the underlying disorder and VITAMIN K_1 INJECTION should be given concurrently. In the event of shock or excessive blood loss, the use of whole blood or component therapy is indicated.

Drug Interactions: Temporary resistance to prothrombin-depressing anticoagulants may result, especially when larger doses of phytonadione are used. If relatively large doses have been employed, it may be necessary when reinstituting anticoagulant therapy to use somewhat larger doses of the prothrombin-depressing anticoagulant, or to use one which acts on a different principle, such as heparin sodium.

Contraindication(s): Hypersensitivity to any component of this medication.

Precaution(s): Storage: Protect from light at all times. Store in a dark place. Store at controlled room temperature 15°30°C (59°-86°F).

Caution(s): Federal law restricts this drug to use by or on the order of a licensed veterinarian.

Intravenous Use-Severe reactions, including fatalities, have occurred during and immediately after Intravenous injection of phytonadione, even when precautions have been taken to dilute the phytonadione and to avoid rapid infusion. Typically these severe reactions have resembled hypersensitivity or anaphylaxis, including shock and cardiac and/or respiratory arrest. Some patients have exhibited these severe reactions on receiving phytonadione for the first time. Therefore the intravenous route should be restricted to those situations where other routes are not feasible and the serious risk involved is considered justified.

An immediate coagulant effect should not be expected after administration of phytonadione. It takes a minimum of 1 to 2 hours for measurable improvement in the prothrombin time. Whole blood or component therapy may also be necessary if bleeding is severe.

Phytonadione will not counteract the anticoagulant action of heparin.

When vitamin K_1 is used to correct excessive anticoagulant-induced hypoprothrombinemia, anticoagulant therapy still being indicated, the patient is again faced with the clotting hazards existing prior to starting the anticoagulant therapy. Phytonadione is not a clotting agent, but overzealous therapy with vitamin K_1 may restore conditions which originally permitted thrombuembolic phenomena. Dosage should he kept as low as possible, and prothrombin time should be checked regularly as clinical conditions indicate.

Repeated large doses of vitamin K are not warranted in liver disease if the response to initial use of the vitamin is unsatisfactory. Failure to respond to vitamin K may indicate that the condition being treated is inherently unresponsive to vitamin K.

For animal use only.

Adverse Reactions: Deaths have occurred after intravenous administration (see Caution). Pain, swelling, and tenderness at the injection site my occur. Intramuscular injection may result in hematomas. The possibility of allergic sensitivity, including an anaphylactoid reaction, should be kept in mind.

Trial Data: Laboratory Tests: Prothrombin time should be checked regularly as clinical conditions indicate. Parenteral drug products should be inspected visually for particulate matter and discoloration prior to administration, whenever solution and container permit.

Presentation: VITAMIN K_1 INJECTION is supplied in 100 mL bottles (NDC 57319-258-05).

Manufactured by: Phoenix Scientific Inc.

Compendium Code No.: 12560981 Rev. 7-01

VITAMIN K_1 ORAL CAPSULES ℞

Butler **Vitamin K_1-Oral**

Active Ingredient(s): Each capsule contains:

Phytonadione . . . . 25 mg

With excipients in an artificially colored soft gelatin shell.

Indications: VITAMIN K_1 CAPSULES are indicated in dogs and cats to counter hypoprothrombinemia induced by ingestion of coumarin-based compounds, common ingredients of commercial rodenticides, and other drug induced hypoprothrombinemia where it has been definitely shown that the result is due to interference with vitamin K metabolism, e.g. salicylates.

Pharmacology: VITAMIN K_1 CAPSULES for oral administration possesses the same type and degree of activity as naturally occurring vitamin K. The primary function of vitamin K is to stimulate the production via the liver of active prothrombin from a precursor protein. The mechanism by which vitamin K promotes formation of prothrombin at the molecular level has not been established.

Dosage and Administration:

Dogs and Cats: Acute hypoprothrombinemia (with hemorrhage) - Administer orally at the rate of 2.5-5 mg/kg of body weight (1 capsule per each 22 lbs. of body weight for lower dosage, or 1 capsule per each 11 lbs. of body weight for higher dosage) once a day as conditions require up to three (3) weeks.

The frequency and amount of oral administration should be guided by the regular determination of prothrombin time.

The smallest effective dose should be sought to minimize the risk of adverse reactions.

Note: Regular determinations of prothrombin time response should be performed to guide in the initial and subsequent administration of VITAMIN K_1 ORAL CAPSULES. The dosage should be adjusted accordingly.
Contraindication(s): Hypersensitivity to any component of this medication.
Precaution(s): Protect from light at all times.
Caution(s): Federal law restricts this drug to use by or on the order of a licensed veterinarian.
It is recommended that VITAMIN K_1 ORAL CAPSULES be used in follow-up therapy only after the administration of phytonadione injection and hospitalization is no longer required. An immediate coagulant effect should not be expected after administration of phytonadione when administered orally.
Phytonadione will not counteract the anticoagulant action of heparin.
Repeated large doses of vitamin K_1 are not warranted in hepatic disease if the response to the initial therapy is unsatisfactory. Failure to respond to vitamin K_1 may indicate that the condition being treated is inherently unresponsive to vitamin K_1.
Temporary resistance to prothrombin-depressing anticoagulants may result, especially when larger doses of phytonadione are used.
For animal use only. Not for human use.
For veterinary use only.
Keep out of reach of children.
Presentation: VITAMIN K_1 ORAL CAPSULES are available in bottles of 50 capsules each (NDC 11695-2461-1).
Compendium Code No.: 10821880

VITAMIN K_1 ORAL CAPSULES ℞

Phoenix Pharmaceutical **Vitamin K_1-Oral**
25 mg Phytonadioine
Active Ingredient(s): Each capsule contains:
Phytonadione .... 25 mg
With excipients in an artificially colored soft gelatin shell.
Indications: VITAMIN K_1 CAPSULES are indicated in dogs and cats to counter hypoprothrombinemia induced by ingestion of coumarin-based compounds, common ingredients of commercial rodenticides, and other drug induced hypoprothrombinemia where it has been definitely shown that the result is due to interference with Vitamin K metabolism, e.g. salicylates.
Pharmacology: Actions: VITAMIN K_1 CAPSULES for oral administration possess the same type and degree of activity as naturally occurring Vitamin K. The primary function of Vitamin K is to stimulate the production via the liver of active prothrombin from a precursor protein. The mechanism by which Vitamin K promotes formation of prothrombin at the molecular level has not been established.
Dosage and Administration: Dogs and Cats: Hypoprothrombinemia (with hemorrhage)—Administer orally at the rate of 2.5-5 mg/kg of body weight (1 capsule per each 22 pounds of body weight for lower dosage, or 1 capsule per each 11 pounds of body weight for higher dosage) daily as conditions require up to 3 weeks.
Frequency and amount of oral administration should be guided by the regular determination of prothrombin time.
The smallest effective dose should be sought to minimize the risk of adverse reactions.
Note: Regular determinations of prothrombin time response should be performed to guide in the initial and subsequent administration of VITAMIN K_1 ORAL CAPSULES. The dosage should be adjusted accordingly.
Contraindication(s): Hypersensitivity to any component of this medication.
Precaution(s): Protect from light at all times.
Caution(s): Federal law restricts this drug to use by or on the order of a licensed veterinarian.
It is recommended that VITAMIN K_1 ORAL CAPSULES be used in follow-up therapy only after administration of phytonadione injection and hospitalization is no longer required. An immediate coagulant effect should not be expected after administration of phytonadione when administered orally.
Phytonadione will not counteract the anticoagulant action of heparin.
Repeated large doses of Vitamin K_1 are not warranted in hepatic disease if the response to the initial therapy is unsatisfactory. Failure to respond to Vitamin K_1 may indicate that the condition being treated is inherently unresponsive to Vitamin K_1.
Temporary resistance to prothrombin-depressing anticoagulants may result, especially when larger doses of phytonadione are used.
For animal use only.
Warning(s): Keep out of reach of children.
Presentation: VITAMIN K_1 ORAL CAPSULES are available in bottles of 50 capsules [NDC 57319-287-12 (Banner Gelatin)] [NDC 57319-395-12 (Jice)] each.
Manufactured by: Banner Gelatin Production Corp., Chatsworth, CA 91311-0230 and Jice Pharmaceuticals, Lowell, MI 49331.
Compendium Code No.: 12560972 Rev. 11-01 / Rev. 06-01

VITAMIN K-1 ORAL CAPSULES ℞

RXV **Vitamin K_1-Oral**
Active Ingredient(s): Each capsule contains 25 mg of Phytonadione.
Description: VITAMIN K-1 CAPSULES contain phytonadione with excipients in an artificially colored soft gelatin shell.
Indications: VITAMIN K-1 CAPSULES are indicated in dogs and cats to counter hypoprothrombinemia induced by ingestion of coumarin-based compounds, common ingredients of commercial rodenticides, and other drug induced hypoprothrombinemia where it has been definitely shown that the result is due to interference with vitamin K metabolism, e.g. salicylates.
Pharmacology: Actions: VITAMIN K-1 CAPSULES for oral administration possesses the same type and degree of activity as naturally occurring vitamin K. The primary function of vitamin K is to stimulate the production via the liver of active prothrombin from a precursor protein. The mechanism by which vitamin K promotes formation of prothrombin at the molecular level has not been established.
Dosage and Administration: Dogs and Cats:
Hypoprothrombinemia (with hemorrhage) - Administer orally at the rate of 2.5-5 mg/kg body weight (1 capsule per each 22 pounds of body weight for lower dosage or 1 capsule per each 11 pounds of body weight for higher dosage) daily as conditions require up to 3 weeks. Frequency and amount of oral administration should be guided by regular determination of prothrombin time.
The smallest effective dose should be sought to minimize the risk of adverse reactions.
Note: Regular determinations of prothrombin time response should be performed to guide in the initial and subsequent administration of VITAMIN K-1 ORAL CAPSULES. The dosage should be adjusted accordingly.
Contraindication(s): Hypersensitivity to any component of this medication.
Precaution(s): Protect from light at all times.
Caution(s): VITAMIN K-1 ORAL CAPSULES are sold only to licensed veterinarians.
It is recommended that VITAMIN K-1 ORAL CAPSULES be used in follow-up therapy only after the administration of Vitamin K-1 Injection and hospitalization are no longer required. An immediate coagulant effect should not be expected after administration of phytonadione when administered orally.
Phytonadione will not counteract the anticoagulant action of heparin.
Repeated large doses of VITAMIN K-1 are not warranted in hepatic disease if the response to the initial therapy is unsatisfactory. Failure to respond to VITAMIN K-1 may indicate that the condition being treated is inherently unresponsive to VITAMIN K-1.
Temporary resistance to prothrombin-depressing anticoagulants may result, especially when larger doses of phytonadione are used.
For animal use only.
Not for human use.
Warning(s): Keep out of reach of children.
Presentation: VITAMIN K-1 ORAL CAPSULES are available in bottles of 50 capsules each.
Compendium Code No.: 10910370 Iss. 01-01

VITAMINS AD$_3$E DISPERSIBLE LIQUID

Alpharma **Water Additive**
Active Ingredient(s):
400,000 IU vitamin A per gram
100,000 IU vitamin D_3 per gram
200 IU vitamin E per gram
Ingredients: Polysorbate 80, Vitamin E (dl-alpha-tocopheryl acetate), Vitamin D_3 (D-Activated animal sterol), Vitamin A (Retinyl Proprionate), Water, BHT, Potassium Sorbate.
Indications: A supplementary nutrition for hogs, chickens, turkeys, calves, and beef cattle.
Directions: Water dispersible vitamin A, D_3 and E for use in drinking water during periods of reduced feed intake. Use 1 oz to 128 gallons of drinking water. This will supply 88,593 IU A, 22,148 IU D_3 and 44.3 IU vitamin E in each gallon of drinking water.
Mix fresh solutions daily.
Precaution(s): Store in cool, dry place.
Caution(s): For oral animal use only.
Not for human use.
Keep out of reach of children.
Presentation: 16 oz.
Compendium Code No.: 10220651 AHL-271 0008

VITAMINS AND ELECTROLYTES

Durvet **Large Animal Dietary Supplement**
Water Soluble Powder
Guaranteed Analysis:

	Per 8 oz.	Per lb.
Vitamin A	2,500,000 IU	5,000,000 IU
Vitamin D_3	1,000,000 IU	2,000,000 IU
Vitamin E	1,000 IU	2,000 IU
Riboflavin	750 mg	1,500 mg
d-Pantothenic Acid	1,250 mg	2,500 mg
Niacin	2,500 mg	5,000 mg
Vitamin B_{12}	2.5 mg	5.0 mg
Menadione Sodium Bisulfite	1,000 mg	2,000 mg
Folic Acid	65 mg	130 mg
Thiamine Mononitrate	250 mg	500 mg
Pyridoxine Hydrochloride	250 mg	500 mg
Ascorbic Acid	3,750 mg	7,500 mg

Ingredients: Vitamin A supplement, d-activated animal sterol (source of vitamin D_3), alpha tocopheryl acetate (source of vitamin E), riboflavin supplement, d-calcium pantothenate, niacin supplement, vitamin B_{12} supplement, menadione sodium bisulfite (source of vitamin K), folic acid, thiamine mononitrate, pyridoxine hydrochloride, ascorbic acid, sodium chloride, calcium chloride, magnesium sulfate, ferric ammonium citrate, potassium chloride and dextrose.
Indications: A water soluble premix of vitamins and electrolytes formulated to be a nutrient supplement applicable for use in poultry, swine, ruminants and horses.
Directions for Use:
As a Water Additive:
For Automatic Proportioners delivering 1 oz. of the stock solution per gallon of drinking water: Dissolve 8 oz. per gallon of the stock solution.
For Drinking Water: Dissolve 4 oz. in 55 gallons or 8 oz. in 110 gallons.
Always mix fresh solutions daily.
As a Feed Additive: Thoroughly mix 8 oz. per ton of the complete ration containing the regular levels of fortification.
Presentation: 8 oz and 25 lbs (NDC 30798-487-47).
Compendium Code No.: 10841671 2/99

VITAMINS AND ELECTROLYTES CONCENTRATE

Alpharma **Dietary Supplement**
Ingredient(s): Sodium chloride, potassium chloride, niacinamide, vitamin A supplement, d-calcium pantothenic acid, ascorbic acid, vitamin E supplement, vitamin D_3 supplement, biotin supplement, sodium bicarbonate, sodium citrate, riboflavin, menadione sodium bisulfite complex, vitamin B_{12} supplement, thiamine HCl, magnesium sulfate, pyridoxine HCl, folic acid, ferrous sulfate, copper sulfate, zinc sulfate, manganese sulfate, cobalt sulfate, calcium lactate, potassium sulfate, magnesium carbonate, ethylenediamine dihydriodide.
Guaranteed analysis per pound:
Vitamin A .... 16,000,000 I.U.
Vitamin D_3 .... 6,400,000 I.U.
Vitamin E .... 10,000 I.U.
Vitamin B_{12} .... 20 mg
Riboflavin .... 6,600 mg

V

Niacinamide . . . . 66,000 mg
d-Pantothenic acid . . . . 28,000 mg
Menadione SBC . . . . 6,000 mg
Folic acid . . . . 840 mg
Thiamine HCl . . . . 4,050 mg
Pyridoxine HCl . . . . 2,000 mg
Ascorbic acid . . . . 20,000 mg
Biotin . . . . 100 mg

Indications: A vitamin and electrolyte concentrate used to ensure adequate intake of essential vitamins and electrolytes.

Directions: Use VITAMINS AND ELECTROLYTES CONCENTRATE in 256 gallons (968 L) water to assure adequate intake of essential vitamins and electrolytes.

Precaution(s): Store in cool, dry place.

Caution(s): For oral animal use only.

Not for human use.

Keep out of reach of children.

Presentation: 4 oz. (113.5 g).

Compendium Code No.: 10220661 AHF-047 0005

VITAMINS AND ELECTROLYTES CONCENTRATE

Durvet **Large Animal Dietary Supplement**

Guaranteed Analysis: Per 4 oz:

Vitamin A . . . . 2,500,000 I.U.
Vitamin D_3 . . . . 1,000,000 ICU
Vitamin E . . . . 1,000 I.U.
Riboflavin . . . . 750 mg
d-Pantothenic acid . . . . 1,250 mg
Niacin . . . . 2,500 mg
Vitamin B_{12} . . . . 2.5 mg
Menadione sodium bisulfite . . . . 1,000 mg
Folic acid . . . . 65 mg
Thiamine mononitrate . . . . 250 mg
Pyridoxine hydrochloride . . . . 250 mg
Ascorbic acid . . . . 3,750 mg

Ingredients: Vitamin A supplement, d-activated animal sterol (source of vitamin D_3), alpha tocopheryl acetate (source of vitamin E), riboflavin supplement, d-calcium pantothenate, niacin supplement, vitamin B_{12} supplement, menadione sodium bisulfite (source of vitamin K), folic acid, thiamine mononitrate, pyridoxine hydrochloride, ascorbic acid, sodium chloride, calcium chloride, magnesium sulfate, ferric ammonium citrate, potassium chloride and dextrose.

Indications: A water soluble premix of vitamins and electrolytes formulated as a supplement for use in poultry, swine, ruminants and horses when normal feed intakes are reduced.

Dosage and Administration:

As a water additive:

For automatic proportioners delivering 1 oz. of the stock solution per gallon of drinking water: Dissolve 4 oz. per gallon of the stock solution.

For drinking water: Dissolve 2 oz. in 55 gallons or 4 oz. in 110 gallons.

Mix fresh solutions each day.

As a feed additive: Thoroughly mix 4 oz. per ton of the complete ration containing the regular levels of fortification.

Discontinue use in water and feed when poultry and animals return to normal feed intakes.

Presentation: 4 oz.

Compendium Code No.: 10841681

VITAMINS & ELECTROLYTES CONCENTRATE

Fort Dodge **Dietary Supplement**

Active Ingredient(s):

Guaranteed Analysis	Per Pound	Per Kilo
Potassium, (K) %	0.75	0.75
Vitamin A, I.U.	16,000,000	35,273,600
Vitamin D_3, I.C.U.	2,400,000	5,291,040
Vitamin E, I.U.	12,000	26,455
Vitamin B_{12}, mg	3.5	7.7
Riboflavin, mg	2,000	4,409
Niacin, mg	32,000	70,547
d-Pantothenic Acid, mg	1,000	2,205
(Calcium d-Pantothenate, mg)	(1,087)	(2,396)
d-Biotin, mg	100	220

Ingredients: Citric acid, sodium bicarbonate, vitamin A supplement, D-activated animal sterol (source of vitamin D_3), vitamin E supplement, vitamin B_{12} supplement, riboflavin supplement, niacin supplement, calcium pantothenate, folic acid, d-biotin, ascorbic acid, salt, potassium chloride.

Indications: VITAMINS AND ELECTROLYTES CONCENTRATE is a balanced formula for use in the feed or drinking water. A supplementary nutritional product, VITAMINS AND ELECTROLYTES CONCENTRATE is indicated for both healthy birds and sick or convalescent birds eating less than normal.

Directions:

For drinking-water use: Mix the contents of this pouch in 256 gallons (973 liters) or 1 oz. VITAMINS AND ELECTROLYTES CONCENTRATE (28.4 grams) in 64 gallons (243 liters) of drinking water of poultry and give for 3 to 5 days. This dosage may be repeated whenever needed.

For use in automatic proportioners: Mix the contents of this pouch in water sufficient to make 2 gallons (7.6 liters) of stock solution. Set the proportioner to deliver 1 fluid ounce (30 mL) per gallon (3.8 liters) of drinking water. Prepare fresh stock solutions daily.

For feed use: Mix pouch contents in 1,000 pounds (454.5 kg) of complete feed. Give for 3 to 5 days. This dosage may be repeated whenever needed.

Precaution(s): Do not store above 100°F (38°C).

Caution(s): Keep out of reach of children.

For oral use only in poultry.

Not for human use.

Presentation: 4 ounce (113.5 gram) pouches (NDC 53501-016-81).

Compendium Code No.: 10032611 12541A

VITAMINS & ELECTROLYTES "PLUS"

AgriLabs **Electrolytes-Oral**

Water Soluble Powder-Vitamins-Electrolytes-Microbes and Acidifiers

Active Ingredient(s):

Specifications:	per 4 oz.	per lb.
Vitamin A (IU)	2,500,000	10,000,000
Vitamin D_3 (IU)	1,000,000	4,000,000
Vitamin E (IU)	2,000	8,000
Riboflavin (mg)	750	3,000
d-pantothenic Acid (mg)	2,000	8,000
Folic Acid (mg)	125	500
Thiamine Mononitrate (mg)	375	1,500
Niacinamide (mg)	5,000	20,000
Pyridoxine HCl (mg)	300	1,200
Ascorbic Acid (mg)	3,750	15,000
Vitamin B_{12} (mg)	2.5	10
Vitamin K (mg)	1,000	4,000
Lactobacillus Acidophilus (CFU)	4 billion	16 billion
Streptococcus Facium (CFU)	4 billion	16 billion

Ingredients: Vitamin A Supplement, Vitamin D Supplement, Vitamin E Supplement, Menadione Sodium Bisulfite Complex (source of Vitamin K), Niacin Supplement, Riboflavin Supplement, Calcium Pantothenate, Pyridoxine Hydrochloride, Folic Acid, Thiamine Mononitrate, Vitamin B_{12} Supplement, Citric Acid, Ascorbic Acid, Magnesium Sulfate, Calcium Chloride, Potassium Chloride, Sodium Chloride, Iron Sulfate Monohydrate, *Lactobacillus Acidophilus, Streptococcus Facium,* Dextrose.

Indications: A water soluble nutritional premix containing vitamins, electrolytes, organic acidifiers and naturally occurring microorganisms for use in cattle, swine, sheep, horses, ruminants, poultry, and turkeys during periods of stress or reduced feed intake.

Directions: Use Directions:

Drinking Water: Mix contents of the pouch (4 oz.) in 128 gallons of water.

For Automatic Proportions: Mix contents of the pouch (4 oz.) in one gallon of water to prepare a stock solution. Set the proportioner to deliver one (1) fluid ounce of stock solution per gallon of drinking water. Prepare fresh stock solution daily.

Feed Use: Mix contents of the pouch (4 oz.) per 500 lbs. of complete feed.

Provide for 3-5 days. Dosage may be repeated whenever needed.

Caution(s): For animal and poultry use only.

Warning(s): Keep out of reach of children.

Presentation: 40 x 4 oz packets per bucket.

Compendium Code No.: 10581241 Iss: 933

VITAMINS & ELECTROLYTES (SOLUBLE)

Fort Dodge **Dietary Supplement**

Nutritional Supplement

Active Ingredient(s):

Guaranteed Minimum Analysis	Per Pound	Per Kilo
Salt (Min.) %	0.60	0.60
Salt (Max.) %	0.90	0.90
Potassium, (K) %	1.000	1.000
Vitamin A, I.U.	5,000,000	11,023,000
Vitamin D_3, I.C.U.	750,000	1,653,450
Vitamin E, I.U.	2,500	5,512
Riboflavin, mg	500	1,102
d-Pantothenic Acid, mg	4,000	8,818
(Calcium d-Pantothenate, mg)	(4,348)	(9,586)

Ingredients: Dextrose, vitamin A supplement, D-activated animal sterol (source of vitamin D_3), vitamin E supplement, riboflavin supplement, calcium pantothenate, folic acid, menadione sodium bisulfite complex, thiamine mononitrate, potassium chloride, salt.

Indications: VITAMINS & ELECTROLYTES SOLUBLE For Poultry is a balanced formula for use in the feed or drinking water. A supplementary nutritional product, VITAMINS & ELECTROLYTES is indicated for both healthy birds and sick or convalescent birds eating less feed than normal.

Directions:

For drinking-water use: Mix 1 pouch of VITAMINS & ELECTROLYTES in 128 gallons (486 liters), or 1 ounce (28.4 grams) in 16 gallons (61 liters) of drinking water of poultry and give for 3 to 5 days. This dosage may be repeated whenever needed.

For use in automatic proportioners: To make a stock solution, mix the contents of 1 pouch of VITAMINS & ELECTROLYTES in 1 U.S. gallon (3.8 liters) of water. Set the proportioner to deliver 1 fluid ounce (30 mL) per gallon (3.8 liters) of drinking water. Prepare fresh solutions daily.

For feed use: Mix the contents of 1 pouch in 500 pounds (227 kg) of complete feed. Give for 3 to 5 days. This dosage may be repeated whenever needed.

Caution(s): Keep out of reach of children.

For oral use only.

Not for human use.

Presentation: 8 oz (227 g) pouches (NDC 53501-015-06).

Compendium Code No.: 10032601 12513C

VITAMINS E-K-A PLUS D_3

Alpharma **Water Additive**

Ingredient(s): Vitamin E supplement, sodium chloride, potassium chloride, vitamin A supplement, sodium citrate, menadione sodium bisulfite complex, vitamin D_3 supplement.

Guaranteed analysis per pound:

Vitamin A . . . . 16,400,000 IU
Vitamin D_3 . . . . 2,048,000 IU
Vitamin E . . . . 68,000 IU
Vitamin K Activity (As menadione sodium bisulfite complex) . . . . 6,060 mg

Indications: For use as a supplement for vitamins E, K, A, and D_3 in chickens, turkeys, swine, and other livestock.

Dosage and Administration: Mix 4 oz (one packet) in 256 gallons, or mix 8 oz. (one packet) in

512 gallons of drinking water for routine use. This product may be used at higher concentrations if conditions warrant. Administer this product for 1 to 3 days.
Precaution(s): Store in cool, dry place.
Caution(s): For oral animal use only.
Not for human use.
Keep out of reach of children.
Presentation: 4 oz. (113.4 g), 8 oz (226.8 g) packages.
Compendium Code No.: 10220671 AHF-022A 0003, AHF-032A 0003

VITA OIL

Hawthorne **Liniment**

Veterinary Liniment

Active Ingredient(s): Mineral oil, turpentine, peppers, mustard flour and other spices.
Indications: For the temporary relief of muscular soreness, minor sprains, stiffness caused by overexertion.

VITA OIL has no alcohol or other quickly evaporative substances that can dry skin, but instead is a combination of natural oils and spices that remains moist and active for hours.
Directions: For temporary relief of sore, stiff muscles: Thoroughly rub in all the VITA OIL the skin will absorb. For best results: Apply hot compress, either moist or dry, or sponge with hot water to open pores. Towel dry, then rub in VITA OIL. Repeat as necessary.

As a sweat: Apply full strength VITA OIL to affected area. Wrap with plastic wrap and cover with blanket or bandage.

As a leg brace: Dilute two ounces of VITA OIL with one pint of witch hazel and one pint of rubbing alcohol. Shake thoroughly.

As a body wash: Add two ounces of VITA OIL to one quart of rubbing alcohol, witch hazel or water.
Precaution(s): Keep lid fastened securely when not in use.
Caution(s): Keep away from eyes and mucous membranes. If excessive irritation develops or affected area does not respond to treatment, consult a veterinarian.
Warning(s): Keep out of children's reach.
Presentation: 16 fl oz (1 pt) and 32 fl oz (1 qt).
Trade Mark Reg. U.S. Pat Off.
Compendium Code No.: 10670120

VITA PAK

Alpharma **Water Additive**

Ingredient(s): Sodium bicarbonate, citric acid, sodium chloride, niacinamide, vitamin A supplement, d-calcium pantothenic acid, ascorbic acid, vitamin E supplement, potassium chloride, vitamin D_3 supplement, riboflavin, menadione sodium bisulfite complex, biotin supplement, vitamin B_{12} supplement, thiamine HCl, pyridoxine HCl, folic acid, magnesium sulfate.

Guaranteed analysis per pound:
Vitamin A .... 12,800,000 IU
Vitamin D_3 .... 5,120,000 IU
Vitamin E .... 8,000 IU
Vitamin B_{12} .... 16 mg
Riboflavin .... 5,280 mg
Niacinamide .... 52,800 mg
d-Pantothenic Acid .... 22,400 mg
MSBC .... 4,800 mg
Folic Acid .... 672 mg
Thiamine HCl .... 3,264 mg
Pyridoxine HCl .... 1,600 mg
Ascorbic Acid .... 16,000 mg
Biotin .... 80 mg
Contains the electrolytes of sodium, potassium, magnesium and bicarbonate.
Indications: Effervescent vitamin concentrate for use in poultry drinking water.
Directions: Use VITA PAK effervescent vitamin concentrate in 256 gallons (968 L) of drinking water to assure adequate intake of essential vitamins and electrolytes.

Note: Do not mix in closed containers of any kind.
Precaution(s): Store in cool, dry place.
Caution(s): For oral animal use only.
Keep out of reach of children.
Presentation: 5 oz (141.7 g) packet.
Compendium Code No.: 10220631 AHF-041 0006

VITA PLUS®

Farnam **Equine Dietary Supplement**

Guaranteed Analysis: Each pound contains not less than:

	Per Ounce	Per Pound
Crude Protein, min	10.00%	10.00%
Lysine	0.50%	0.50%
Methionine	0.20%	0.20%
Crude Fat, min	8.00%	8.00%
Crude Fiber, max	12.00%	12.00%
Calcium, min	638 mg	2.25%
Calcium, max	780 mg	2.75%
Phosphorous, min	425 mg	1.50%
Salt, min	567 mg	2.00%
Salt, max	709 mg	2.50%
Potassium, min	241 mg	0.850%
Magnesium, min	12.5 mg	0.044%
Iodine, min	1 mg	35 ppm
Zinc, min	20 mg	705 ppm
Iron, min	100 mg	3,527 ppm
Cobalt, min	0.05 mg	18 ppm
Copper, min	4.0 mg	141 ppm
Manganese, min	10 mg	300 ppm
Selenium, min	10 mcg	0.4 ppm
Vitamin A, min	25,000 I.U.	400,000 I.U.
Vitamin D_3, min	2,500 I.U.	40,000 I.U.
Vitamin E, min	25 I.U.	400 I.U.
Vitamin B_{12}, min	200 mcg	3,200 mcg
Riboflavin, min	25 mg	400 mg
d-Pantothenic Acid	62.5 mg	1,000 mg
Thiamine	12.5 mg	200 mg
Niacin, min	125 mg	2,000 mg
Vitamin B_6, min	5 mg	80 mg
Choline, min	106 mg	1,186 mg

Ingredients: Dehydrated Alfalfa Meal, Wheat Middlings, Ground Corn, Dicalcium Phosphate, Soybean Oil, Potassium Chloride, Dried Whey, Ferrous Sulfate, Salt, Ground Limestone, Choline Chloride, Magnesium Sulfate, Manganese Sulfate, Wheat Germ Meal, Sodium Selenite, L-Lysine, DL Methionine, Wheat Germ Oil, Vitamin A Acetate, Cholecalciferol (Source of Vitamin D_3), alpha-Tocopherol Acetate (Source of Vitamin E), Riboflavin, Cyanocobalamin (Source of Vitamin B_{12}), Lecithin, Niacinamide, d-Calcium Pantothenate, Potassium Iodide, Thiamine Mononitrate, Pyridoxine Hydrochloride (Vitamin B_6), Zinc Sulfate, Copper Sulfate, Ethylene Diamine Dihydriodide, Cobalt Sulfate, propionic and acetic acids (as preservatives).
Indications: Nutritional feed supplement for all classes of horses.
Directions: Divide the daily dosage of VITA PLUS® into two feedings - one in the morning and one again in the evening. Sprinkle the proper amount over the feed or mix with the ration.
One Scoop = 1 oz.
Adult Horses: 2 ounces per day
Foals, Weanlings and Ponies: 1 ounce per day
Broodmares: 4 ounces per day
Precaution(s): Store in area inaccessible to children and animals.
Caution(s): Follow label directions. The addition to feed of higher levels of this premix containing selenium is not permitted.
Excessive amounts of selenium may be toxic.
Warning(s): Keep out of reach of children.
Presentation: 3 lbs, 7 lbs (3.18 kg), 20 lbs and 100 lbs.
VITA PLUS® Registered Trademark No. 821,234
Compendium Code No.: 10000411

VITA-PLUS® WITH EQUITROL®

Farnam **Larvicide**

EPA Reg. No.: 270-165
Active Ingredient(s):
Tetrachlorvinphos: 2-Chloro-1-(2,4,5-trichlorophenyl) vinyl dimethyl phosphate 1.234%*
Inert Ingredients 98.766%**

* Contains 5.597 gms. Rabon® per pound. ** Refers only to ingredients which are not larvicidal.

Guaranteed Analysis: Contains Not Less Than:

	Per Ounce:	Per Pound:
Lysine		0.05%
Methionine		0.05%
Calcium (Min.)	766 mg	2.75%
Calcium (Max.)	836 mg	3.75%
Phosphorus (Min.)	326 mg	1.15%
Salt (Min.)	255 mg	0.9%
Salt (Max.)	397 mg	1.4%
Potassium (K)	241 mg	0.85%
Magnesium (Mg)	12.5%	0.044%
Copper (Cu)	4.0 mg	141 ppm
Selenium (Se)	120 mcg	4 ppm
Zinc (Zn)	20.0 mg	705 ppm
Iodine (I)	1.0 mg	35 ppm
Iron (Fe)	100.0 mg	3,527 ppm
Cobalt (Co)	0.05 mg	18 ppm
Manganese (Mn)	10.0 mg	353 ppm
Vitamin A	25,000 IU	400,000 IU
Vitamin D3	2,500 IU	40,000 IU
Vitamin E	25 IU	400 IU
Vitamin B12	200 mcg	3,200 mcg
Riboflavin (B2)	25 mg	400 mg
d-Pantothenic Acid	62.5 mg	1,000 mg
Thiamine (B1)	12.5 mg	200 mg
Niacin	125.0 mg	2,000 mg
Vitamin B6	5.0 mg	80 mg
Choline	106.0 mg	1,696 mg
Polyunsaturated Fatty Acids (as glycerides)		2.75%

Feed Ingredients: Wheat Middlings, Dehydrated Alfalfa Meal, Wheat Germ Meal, Molasses, Corn, Dicalcium Phosphate, Salt, Dried Whey, Vitamin A Supplement, Vitamin D_3 Supplement, Vitamin E Supplement, Vitamin B_{12} Supplement, Riboflavin Supplement, Niacin, Calcium Pantothenate, Choline Chloride, Thiamine Mononitrate, Pyridoxine Hydrochloride (Vitamin B_6), Sodium Selenite, L Lysine Hydrochloride, dL-Methionine, Zinc Amino Acid Chelate, Manganese Amino Acid Chelate, Iron Amino Acid Chelate, Copper Amino Acid Chelate, Iodine Amino Acid Chelate, and Cobalt Amino Acid Chelate, Magnesium Sulfate, Potassium Chloride, propionic acid and acetic acid (preservatives).
Indications: VITA-PLUS® WITH EQUITROL® is a nutritional feed supplement with the additional benefit of Equitrol® Feed-Thru Fly Control. Fed as directed, VITA-PLUS® WITH EQUITROL® will prevent the development of House and Stable Flies in manure, while providing a healthy balance of vitamins, trace minerals, amino acids, selenium, balanced electrolytes and polyunsaturates.
Directions for Use: It is a violation of Federal law to use this product in a manner inconsistent with its labeling.

Feed the recommended dosage to each horse separately to make certain he receives his full portion. This product should be fed topdressed or mixed with the horse's total ration to provide 70 mg of Rabon® per 100 lbs. of body weight. For an occasional finicky eater who does not accept new feeds readily, mix VITA-PLUS® WITH EQUITROL® with sweet feed or grain ration.

Begin feeding VITA-PLUS® WITH EQUITROL® early in the spring before flies appear and continue feeding throughout the summer and into the fall until cold weather restricts fly activity.

VITA-PLUS® WITH EQUITROL® prevents the development of house flies and stable flies in the manure of treated horses but is not effective against existing adult flies.

In some cases, supplemental fly control measures may be needed in and around paddocks and buildings to control adult house flies and stable flies which can breed not only in manure but in other decaying vegetable matter or silage on the premises.

In order to achieve optimum fly control VITA-PLUS® WITH EQUITROL® should be used in conjunction with other good management and sanitation practices.

Daily Dosage:

300-500 lb. Horse	Feed 4⁄5 oz. (One VITA-PLUS® WITH EQUITROL® measuring cup filled to the blue line) per horse per day.
500-700 lb. Horse	Feed 1 1⁄5 oz. (One VITA-PLUS® WITH EQUITROL® measuring cup filled to the red line) per horse per day.
700-900 lb. Horse	Feed 1 3⁄5 oz. (One VITA-PLUS® WITH EQUITROL® measuring cup filled to the green line) per horse per day.
900-1100 lb. horse	Feed 2 oz. (One VITA-PLUS® WITH EQUITROL® measuring cup filled to the black line) per horse per day.
For larger horses over 1100 lbs. of body weight feed 1⁄2 oz for each 250 lbs. of body weight.	

(VITA-PLUS® WITH EQUITROL® measuring cup is marked in orange at the 1⁄2 oz. level)

Precautionary Statements: Hazards to Humans:

Caution: Keep out of reach of children. Harmful if swallowed. Avoid contact with skin and eyes. Avoid breathing dust. Wash thoroughly with soap and water after handling and before eating or smoking. If in eyes, wash with plenty of water for 15 minutes. If irritation persists, see a physician. Wear long-sleeved shirt and pants; chemical resistant gloves; shoes and socks for protection when handling.

Environmental Hazards: This product is toxic to fish. Do not apply directly to water. Do not contaminate water when disposing of equipment washwaters or rinsate.

Caution: Follow label directions. The addition to feed or higher levels of this premix containing Selenium is not permitted.

Storage and Disposal: Do not contaminate water, food or feed by storage or disposal.

Storage: Store tightly closed in cool dry place, inaccessible to children and pets.

Pesticide Disposal: Pesticide that cannot be used according to label instructions must be disposed of according to Federal, State or local procedures under the Resource Conservation and Recovery Act.

Disposal: Completely empty container. Then dispose of empty container in a sanitary landfill or by incineration or, if allowed by State and local authorities, by burning. If burned, stay out of smoke. Wastes resulting from the use of this product may be disposed of on site or at an approved waste disposal facility.

Warning(s): Do not use on horses intended for slaughter.

Presentation: 7.5 lbs (3.40 kg) and 25 lbs.

®Rabon is a registered trademark of E.I. Du Pont de Vemours and Company, Wilmington, DE

Compendium Code No.: 10000421

VIT-E-LYTE "PLUS"

Bimeda **Electrolytes-Oral**

Soluble Powder-Vitamins-Electrolytes-Microbes and Acidifiers

Active Ingredient(s):

Specifications	Minimum per 4 oz	Minimum per lb
Vitamin A (IU)	2,500,000	10,000,000
Vitamin D_3 (IU)	1,000,000	4,000,000
Vitamin E (IU)	2,000	8,000
Riboflavin (mg)	750	3,000
d-pantothenic Acid (mg)	2,000	8,000
Folic Acid (mg)	125	500
Thiamine (mg)	375	1,500
Niacin (mg)	5,000	20,000
Pyridoxine (mg)	300	1,200
Ascorbic Acid (mg)	3,750	15,000
Vitamin B_{12} (mg)	2.5	10

Total colony forming units not less than 32 billion per pound (8 billion per 4 oz) *(Streptococcus faecium, Lactobacillus acidophilus)*.

Ingredients: Vitamin A acetate, Vitamin D_3 Supplement, Vitamin E Supplement, Menadione Sodium Bisulfite Complex (source of Vitamin K), Niacinamide, Riboflavin, Calcium Pantothenate, Pyridoxine Hydrochloride, Folic Acid, Thiamine Hydrochloride, Vitamin B_{12} Supplement, Citric Acid, Ascorbic Acid, Magnesium Sulfate, Calcium Chloride, Potassium Chloride, Sodium Chloride, Ferrous Sulfate, Dried *Streptococcus faecium* fermentation product, Dried *Lactobacillus acidophilus* fermentation product, Dextrose.

Indications: A soluble supplement which contains vitamins, electrolytes, organic acidifiers and a source of live (viable) occurring micro-organisms. For use in water or feed for swine, horses, ruminants and poultry during periods leading to reduced feed intake.

Directions: Use Directions:

Drinking Water: Mix contents of the pouch (4 oz) in 128 gallons of water.

For Automatic Proportions: Mix contents of the pouch (4 oz) in one gallon of water to prepare a stock solution. Set the proportioner to deliver one (1) fluid ounce of stock solution per gallon of drinking water. Prepare fresh stock solution daily.

Feed Use: Mix contents of the pouch (4 oz) per 500 lbs of complete feed.

Provide for 3-5 days. Dosage may be repeated as needed.

Caution(s): For animal and poultry use only.

Warning(s): Keep out of reach of children.

Presentation: 4 oz (113.5 g) pouch.

Compendium Code No.: 13990620

VI-TREMPOX™

L.A.H.I. (New Jersey) **Vaccine**

Avian Encephalomyelitis-Fowl Pox Vaccine, Live Virus

U.S. Vet. Lic. No.: 196

Active Ingredient(s): Avian encephalomyelitis and fowlpox live virus vaccine.

This product is a live virus vaccine of chicken embryo origin manufactured from SPF (Specific Pathogen Free) eggs for the prevention of fowl pox and avian encephalomyelitis in chickens.

This vaccine was carefully produced and passed all tests in accordance with the U.S. Government requirements.

Contains neomycin as a preservative.

Indications: This vaccine is for wing-web application to chickens 12 weeks of age and older.

It is used in breeder replacements and commercial layers in areas where avian encephalomyelitis and fowl pox are known to exist.

Dosage and Administration: Preparation of Vaccine: The active agent of the vaccine is supplied in a dried form in the bottle labeled 'Vaccine'. Open the bottle by removing the aluminum tear seal and rubber stopper. Open the diluent and pour a small quantity into the bottle of vaccine, replace the rubber stopper, and shake well. Pour the mixture back into the bottle of diluent and shake mixture vigorously. Do not open or mix the vaccine until ready for use.

Method of Vaccination: Vaccination is accomplished by dipping the double needle in the mixed vaccine and piercing the "web of the wing" from the underside. Do not apply through feathers, muscle or bone. The applicator must be redipped between each application.

Birds from the flock should be examined for evidence of a "take" to insure that the vaccine was applied properly.

The evidence of a successful vaccination will appear at the point of vaccination in from 7 to 10 days after vaccination. Brownish, black scabs will be found on both the under and upper surfaces of the web of the wing through which the needle vaccinator was thrust.

Contraindication(s): Birds to be vaccinated should be free of all diseases, including the latent form of diseases such as chronic respiratory disease (CRD), coccidiosis, blackhead, parasitic disease, etc.

Precaution(s): Keep vaccine in the dark, between 2-7°C (35-45°F).

Use entire contents when first opened. Burn this container and all unused contents.

Caution(s): When administered to susceptible birds, a mild infection results which stimulates immunity. No vaccine confers immediate protection. While immunity begins to develop immediately, it takes 2 to 3 weeks for birds to establish maximum immunity to fowl pox and avian encephalomyelitis following vaccination, during which time they should not be placed in contaminated premises.

All susceptible birds on any farm should be vaccinated at the same time. If this is not possible individual lots may be vaccinated if strict isolation and separate caretakers are provided for the vaccinated and unvaccinated lots of birds.

It is imperative that the user of this product comply with the indications for use, contraindications, and method of vaccination stated on the direction sheet. The vaccine must be prepared and administered as directed to obtain best results.

Warning(s): Do not vaccinate within 21 days before slaughter.

Care should be taken to avoid contaminating hands, eyes, and clothing with the vaccine.

For veterinary use only.

Presentation: 500 and 1,000 doses.

Compendium Code No.: 10080572

VIVOMUNE®

Biomune **Vaccine**

Bursal Disease Vaccine, Live Virus, Mild-Intermediate Strain

U.S. Vet. Lic. No.: 280

Contents: This vaccine contains a live mild-intermediate strain of infectious bursal disease virus.

Contains gentamicin and amphotericin B as preservatives.

This vaccine is thoroughly tested before sale and meets the requirements of the U.S. Department of Agriculture.

Indications: For drinking water use.

This vaccine is recommended for the vaccination of healthy chickens at two weeks of age. Careful consideration and determination of the immune status of the flock to be vaccinated is recommended. Vaccinate when passive resistance (parental antibody) to infectious bursal disease subsides.

Dosage and Administration:

1. Discontinue water medication 48 hours before vaccination. Do not resume any medication in the water for 24 hours after all vaccine water has been consumed. The waterers should be thoroughly cleaned before use. Do not use disinfecting solutions during cleaning as the disinfectant residue may destroy the vaccine virus. Drinking containers must be free from all disinfecting solutions and medications for 48 hours prior to vaccination and for 24 hours after vaccination.
2. Deprive the birds of water for two hours prior to vaccination.
3. Tear off the aluminum seal from the vial containing the dried vaccine and remove the stopper.
4. Use clean, cold, nonchlorinated water for rehydration of the dried vaccine. Mix a 1,000 dose vial of vaccine with 2 gallons (7.5 L) of water, a 10,000 dose vial of vaccine with 20 gallons (75 L) of water, or a 25,000 dose vial of vaccine with 50 gallons (187.5 L) of water.
5. A dried milk powder may be beneficial as a stabilizer. It is used in the water at the rate of 7.5 grams per gallon (3.75 L), 15 grams per 2 gallons (7.5 L), 150 grams per 20 gallons (75 L), or 375 grams per 50 gallons (187.5 L). Add the milk powder before the vaccine is added.
6. Provide enough waterers so that all birds may have an opportunity to drink the vaccine-treated water.
7. Avoid exposure of the waterers to direct sunlight.
8. Do not resume watering until water containing vaccine has been consumed. Then continue watering with untreated water for 24 hours before resuming the normal watering practice.
9. Vaccinating with less than one dose per bird may fail to protect satisfactorily.

Precaution(s): Use entire contents of vial immediately after mixing.

Do not over dilute or otherwise extend the dosage.

Store the vaccine at 35°-45°F (2°-7°C).

Do not spill or splatter the vaccine. Burn empty bottles and unused vaccine.

Warning(s): Do not vaccinate within 21 days of slaughter.

Presentation: 10 x 1,000, 10 x 2,000, 10 x 5,000, 10 x 10,000, and 10 x 25,000 dose vials.

Compendium Code No.: 11290352

VL5-1X

Durvet **Bacterin**

Campylobacter Fetus-Leptospira Canicola-Grippotyphosa-Hardjo-Icterohaemorrhagiae-Pomona Bacterin

U.S. Vet. Lic. No.: 303

Composition: This bacterin contains inactivated cultures of *Campylobacter fetus, Leptospira canicola, grippotyphosa, hardjo, icterohaemorrhagiae,* and *pomona* adjuvanted with aluminum hydroxide. Contains penicillin, streptomycin, and thimerosal as preservatives.

Indications: For use in healthy cattle as an aid in the prevention and control of disease caused by *Campylobacter fetus, Leptospira canicola, grippotyphosa, hardjo, icterohaemorrhagiae,* and *pomona.*

Dosage and Administration: Shake well before using. Administer 2 mL intramuscularly 2-4 weeks prior to breeding.

Precaution(s): Store in the dark at 35°-45°F (2°-7°C). Do not freeze. Use entire contents when first opened.

Caution(s): Anaphylactic reactions may occur following the use of this biological. Symptomatic treatment: Epinephrine.

Warning(s): Do not vaccinate within 21 days prior to slaughter.

Presentation: 10 dose (20 mL) and 50 dose (100 mL) vials.

Manufactured by: Advance Biologics, Inc.

Compendium Code No.: 10841690

VL5-1X PLUS™

Durvet **Bacterin**

Campylobacter Fetus-Leptospira Canicola-Grippotyphosa-Hardjo-Icterohaemorrhagiae-Pomona Bacterin

U.S. Vet. Lic. No.: 303

Composition: This bacterin contains inactivated cultures of *Campylobacter fetus, Leptospira canicola grippotyphosa, hardjo, icterohaemorrhagiae,* and *pomona* adjuvanted with oil. Contains penicillin, streptomycin, and thimerosal as preservatives.

Indications: For use in healthy cattle as an aid in the prevention and control of disease caused by *Campylobacter fetus, Leptospira canicola, grippotyphosa, hardjo, icterohaemorrhagiae,* and *pomona.*

Dosage and Administration: Shake well before using. Administer 2 mL intramuscularly 2-4 weeks prior to breeding.

Precaution(s): Store in the dark at 35°-45°F (2°-7°C). Do not freeze. Use entire contents when first opened.

Caution(s): Transient swelling may occur at the site of injection. Milk reduction and transient depression may be observed in lactating dairy cows for 3-6 days following vaccination. Anaphylactic reactions may occur following the use of this biological. Symptomatic treatment: Epinephrine.

Warning(s): Do not vaccinate within 60 days prior to slaughter.

Presentation: 10 doses (20 mL) and 50 doses (100 mL).

Manufactured by: Advance Biologics, Inc., Freeman, SD 57029.

Compendium Code No.: 10841701

3/01

V-MAX™ M

Phibro **Feed Medication**

(virginiamycin) Type A Medicated Article

NADA No.: 140-998

Active Ingredient(s):

Virginiamycin 30%

(Contains 136.2 g virginiamycin activity per lb)

Inert Ingredients: Processed grain by-products, silicon dioxide, mineral oil.

Indications: For use in complete feeds (Type C) for cattle fed in confinement for slaughter to improve feed efficiency, reduce the incidence of liver abscesses and increase rate of weight gain.

Directions:

Cattle fed in confinement for slaughter	Virginiamycin required mg/hd/day	Virginiamycin (g/tons) of complete feed (90% dry matter basis)
Improved feed efficiency	70-240	1.0-16.0
Reduction of incidence of liver abscesses	85-240	13.5-1.60
Increased rate of weight gain	100-340	16.0-22.5

Mixing Directions:

Type C Medicated Feeds for cattle fed in confinement for slaughter—V-MAX™ M Type A Medicated Article must be diluted to a Type C Medicated Feed before being fed. Thoroughly mix the V-MAX™ M Type A Medicated Article, using recommended equipment, to make 1 ton of Type C Medicated Feed to provide 11.0-22.5 g of virginiamycin per ton of complete feed on a 90% dry matter basis.

The Table below shows the amount of V-MAX™ M needed to medicate a ton of feed containing the approved levels of virginiamycin.

lb of V-MAX™ M Type A Medicated Article per ton of Type C Medicated Feed (complete feed 90% dry matter basis)	grams virginiamycin per ton of Type C Medicated Feed (complete feed 90% dry matter basis)
.08	11.0
.10	13.5
.12	16.0
.13	18.0
.15	20.0
.17	22.5

Recommended Equipment: A micro-ingredient weighing and delivery system capable of weighing and delivering 0.5 to 1000 gram of drug per batch of feed should be used. The weighing pan and delivery system should be cleaned daily when in continuous production or following each use to prevent drug build-up and/or carryover.

Feed continuously as sole ration.

Precaution(s): Store in a cool, dry place.

Close container after use.

Caution(s): Not for use in animals intended for breeding.

Must be diluted in feed before use.

Presentation: 50 lb (22.7 kg) bags.

V-MAX is a trademark of Phibro Animal Health, for virginiamycin.

U.S. Patent Nos. 3,325,359 and 3,627,885; for use under U.S. Patent No. 3,017,272

Compendium Code No.: 36930231

VOLAR®

Intervet **Bacterin**

Fusobacterium Necrophorum Bacterin-Footrot Bacterin

U.S. Vet. Lic. No.: 286

Contents: An inactivated and adjuvanted bivalent culture of *Fusobacterium necrophorum.* Contains gentamicin and thimerosal as preservatives.

Indications: For vaccination of beef and dairy cattle as an aid in the prevention of Acute Footrot caused by *Fusobacterium necrophorum* and as an aid in the prevention and treatment of Chronic Footrot in sheep.*

Dosage and Administration: Directions and Recommendations for Use:

Cattle: For vaccination of healthy cattle, two doses are required. Aseptically inject a 5 mL dose intramuscularly or subcutaneously in the neck. Repeat in 3 to 4 weeks. A booster dose should be given annually or at any time endemic conditions exist or exposure is imminent. VOLAR® has been shown to be effective against acute Footrot in beef and dairy cattle but not against chronic foot conditions.

Sheep: For vaccination of healthy sheep, two doses are required. Aseptically inject a 3 mL dose intramuscularly or subcutaneously in the neck area. Repeat in 3 to 4 weeks. A booster dose should be given annually or at any time endemic conditions exist or exposure is imminent. For best results, sheep should be receiving a free choice mineral supplement providing 40 to 80 mg of zinc as zinc methionine per head per day.

Precaution(s): Shake well before using. Store at 35° to 45°F (2° to 7°C). Use entire contents when first opened.

Caution(s): Anaphylactoid reactions may occur.

Antidote(s): Epinephrine.

Warning(s): Do not vaccinate within 21 days before slaughter.

Discussion: Disease: Acute Footrot in cattle is an infection caused by *Fusobacterium necrophorum* initially characterized by necrosis of the interdigital skin with subsequent extension into deeper subcutaneous tissues. Clinical manifestations including swelling and acute lameness.†

Chronic Footrot in sheep is a synergistic infection caused by two gram negative bacteria, *Fusobacterium necrophorum* and *Bacteroides noduses.*†† The disease begins as an interdigital dermatitis which can extend into the adjacent hard horn. Sequential necrosis and regeneration of tissue result in eventual overgrowth and separation of horny tissues.

Trial Data: Safety: VOLAR® has been shown to be safe in beef and dairy cattle, including pregnant cows, when used in accordance with label recommendations. Studies involving over 800 pregnant cows shows no difference in calving rates between controls and animals vaccinated twice, in either early or late pregnancy.

VOLAR® has been shown to be safe in sheep, including pregnant ewes, when used in accordance with label recommendations. A study involving over 530 pregnant ewes shows no difference in lambing rates between controls and animals vaccinated twice in either early or late pregnancy.

References: Available upon request.

Presentation: 10 cattle doses/16 sheep doses (50 mL) and 50 cattle doses/83 sheep doses (250 mL).

*Patent Pending

Compendium Code No.: 11062210

VPL FLY REPELLENT OINTMENT

V.P.L. **External Parasiticide**

EPA Reg. No.: 270-103-43591

Active Ingredient(s):

Piperonyl butoxide technical* 0.5%

Pyrethrins I and II 0.2%

Di-n-propyl isocinchomeronate 1.0%

Inert ingredients 98.3%

Total 100.0%

*Equivalent to 0.4% (butylcarbityl) (6-propylpiperonyl) ether and 0.1% of related compounds.

Indications: Repels houseflies, stable flies, face flies and horn flies from wounds and open sores. Also kills them on contact. For dogs, ponies and horses.

Dosage and Administration: It is a violation of federal law to use the product in a manner inconsistent with its labeling.

Use for the treatment of superficial wounds, abrasions, sores and scratches. Apply enough ointment to cover the wound. Apply directly to the wound and use once a day.

Precaution(s):

Storage: Store tightly closed in a cool, dry place away from heat and sunlight.

Disposal: Do not re-use the empty jar. Wrap the jar and put it in the trash.

Caution(s): Keep out of the reach of children. Not for human use. Wash hands after using.

The product is toxic to fish. Keep out of lakes, streams or ponds. Do not apply where run-off is likely to occur. Do not contaminate water by the cleaning of equipment, or the disposal of wastes.

Warning(s): Do not use on horses that are to be used for human consumption.

Presentation: 2 oz. and 6 oz. jars.

Compendium Code No.: 11430380

V.T.D.

Interchem **Disinfectant**

EPA Reg. No.: 1839-100-33431

Active Ingredient(s):

N-alkyl (60% C_{14}, 30% C_{16}, 5% C_{12}, 5% C_{18}) dimethyl benzyl ammonium chloride 4.50%

N-alkyl (68% C_{12}, 32% C_{14}) dimethyl ethylbenzyl ammonium chloride 4.50%

Inert ingredients 91.00%

Total 100.000%

Indications: V.T.D. (Veterinary Type Disinfectant) is an effective bactericide, fungicide (against pathogenic fungi) and virucide in the presence of organic soil (5% blood serum).

Bactericidal activity: When used as directed. V.T.D. demonstrates effective disinfectant activity against *Pseudomonas aeruginosa, Escherichia coli, Klebsiella pneumoniae, Salmonella*

V

schuttmuelleria, Salmonella choleraesuis, Streptococcus faecallis, Shigella dysenteriae, Enterobacter aerogenes and *Staphylococcus aureus.* When used as directed, this formulation is an effective disinfectant against *Pseudomonas aeruginosa* in animal hospitals and laboratories.

Virucidal activity: When used at the 1 oz. to one (1) gallon dilution rate, V.T.D. exhibits effective virucidal activity on inanimate hard surfaces against canine distemper, canine parvovirus, pseudorabies virus, vaccine virus, influenza A_2, herpes complex and adenovirus type 2.

Dosage and Administration: It is a violation of federal law to use the product in a manner inconsistent with its labeling.

V.T.D. is designed specifically for use in animal hospitals, animal laboratories, kennels, pet shops, zoos and pet animal quarters. When used as directed, the formulation is designed to disinfect, deodorize and clean inanimate hard surfaces such as walls, floors, sink-tops, furniture, operating tables, kennel runs, cages, and feeding and watering equipment.

In addition, V.T.D. will deodorize those areas which generally are hard to keep fresh smelling such as garbage storage areas, empty garbage bins and cans, and any other areas which are prone to odors caused by micro-organisms.

Disinfection: For disinfecting, add 1 oz. of V.T.D. to one (1) gallon of water and apply the solution with a mop, cloth, sponge or mechanical sprayer so as to wet all surfaces thoroughly. Allow to remain wet for 10 minutes and then let air dry.

For feeding and watering equipment, rinse with potable water after disinfecting.

For heavily soiled or contaminated areas, a precleaning step is required. Prepare a fresh solution for each use.

Mildewstat: To control mold and mildew on precleaned hard nonporous surfaces, add 1 oz. to one (1) gallon of water. Apply the solution with a cloth, mop or sponge making sure to wet all surfaces completely. Let air dry. Prepare a fresh solution for each use. Repeat the application at weekly intervals or when mildew growth re-appears.

Precaution(s): Do not contaminate water, food, or feed by storage and disposal.

Storage: Store in a dry place no lower in temperature than 50°F or higher than 120°F.

Container Disposal: Do not re-use the empty container. Triple rinse the empty container with water. Rinse the metal drum, then offer for reconditioning or puncture and dispose of in a sanitary landfill site, or by other procedures approved by state and local authorities. Plastic containers may be disposed of in a sanitary landfill site, incinerated or if allowed by local authorities by burning. If burned, stay out of smoke.

Pesticide Disposal: Pesticide wastes are acutely hazardous. Improper disposal of excess pesticide, spray mixture, or rinsate is a violation of federal law. If these wastes cannot be disposed of according to label instructions, contact the State Pesticide or Environmental Control Agency, or the Hazardous Waste representative at the nearest EPA regional office for guidance.

Caution(s): Precautionary Statements:

Hazard to Humans and Domestic Animals:

Danger - Keep out of the reach of children. Causes severe eye and skin damage. Do not get in eyes, on skin or on clothing. Wear goggles or a face shield and rubber gloves when handling. Harmful or fatal if swallowed. Avoid the contamination of food.

Statement of Practical Treatment: In case of contact, immediately flush eyes or skin with plenty of water for at least 15 minutes. For eyes, call a physician. Remove and wash all contaminated clothing before re-use.

If swallowed, promptly drink a large quantity of milk, egg whites, gelatin solution or if these are not available, drink large quantities of water. Call a physician immediately.

Note to Physician: Probable muscosal damage may contraindicate the use of gastric lavage. Measures against circulatory shock as well as oxygen and measures to support breathing manually or mechanically may be needed. If persistent, convulsions may be controlled by the cautious intravenous injection of a short acting barbituate drug.

Presentation: 1 gallon, 5 gallon, 30 gallon, and 55 gallon containers.

Compendium Code No.: 10200010

V-TERGENT®

Veterinary Specialties — **Detergent**

Detergent-Deodorant

Active Ingredient(s): Contains:

Benzethonium chloride 1.6%
Isopropyl alcohol 13.5%

Indications: Recommended to clean and deodorize pets, kennels, litter boxes, carpets, floors, cages, hands and arms.

Directions for Use:

Undiluted: As a deodorant shampoo on pets sprayed by skunks or whose coats are soiled by grease or oils. Wet the hair of the animal before applying and rinse thoroughly after completing the shampoo.

Diluted: 1-3 teaspoons per gallon of water (hard or soft) as a cleanser and deodorizer for kennels, catteries, litter boxes, cages, utensils, walls, floors and carpets.

Other uses: Soaking and deodorizing mops. Cleaning and deodorizing garbage cans.

Not germicidal in these applications. Do not use with common laundry detergents or soaps.

Caution(s): Keep out of reach of children.

Warning(s): Avoid getting the concentrate in eyes. In case of eye contact, wash thoroughly with water. If irritation persists (human), get medical attention.

Presentation: One dozen bottles containing 8 ounces (237 mL) each.

Compendium Code No.: 10950020

VVMD-VAC®

Fort Dodge — **Vaccine**

Marek's Disease Vaccine, Serotypes 2 & 3, Live Virus

U.S. Vet. Lic. No.: 112

Contents: This product contains the antigens listed above.

Contains gentamicin as a preservative.

Indications: This product is recommended for the subcutaneous vaccination of healthy one-day-old chicks or the *in ovo* vaccination of 18 to 19 day old embryonated chicken eggs, to aid in the prevention of the signs and lesions of Marek's disease. Use only the Fort Dodge Animal Health sterile diluent included.

Directions: Read in full, follow directions carefully.

Directions for Subcutaneous Administration:

1. Vaccinate healthy one-day-old chicks only.
2. Avoid early exposure of chicks to Marek's disease, to allow for development of protection.
3. The exact amount of diluent is provided for each shipment of vaccine. Use Fort Dodge Animal Health diluent only. Store diluent at not over 80°F (27°C).
4. Wear protective clothing when withdrawing vaccine from liquid-nitrogen refrigerator; protect hands with gloves, wear long sleeves, and use a face mask or goggles.
5. Before opening liquid-nitrogen refrigerator, prepare a clean, wide-mouthed container with a capacity of 1 to 5 gallons (3.8-19 liters). Half-fill this container with water 80°F (27°C).
6. When withdrawing a cane of vials from the liquid-nitrogen refrigerator, expose only the vial to be used immediately. When removing a vial from the cane, hold palm of gloved hand away from face and body. Dilute only 1 vial at a time. Immediately replace cane with remaining vials into the canister in the liquid-nitrogen refrigerator.
7. Place the vial into prepared container half-filled with water 80°F (27°C). The frozen material thaws rapidly. When thawed, towel-dry vial.
8. The vials are pre-scored below the gold band. Before snapping off the top portion, wrap vial with a cloth, holding the top part away from face and body.
9. For subcutaneous route of vaccination, use 200 mLs of diluent per 1,000 doses of vaccine. For example: 1,000 doses of vaccine-200 mLs of diluent; 3,000 doses of vaccine-600 mLs of diluent.
10. Using a sterile mixing syringe with a 1½-inch (3.8 cm) 18-gauge needle, draw up a small volume of diluent. Then draw the contents from the vaccine vial into the syringe and swirl gently. Insert needle into diluent bottle and slowly expel contents of syringe. Mix well by gently swirling the bottle. Withdraw a small amount of the reconstituted vaccine and use to rinse each vial injecting the rinses back into reconstituted vaccine. The vaccine is ready for use.
11. While vaccinating, maintain the diluted vaccine (in the diluent bottle) at 70° to 80°F (21° to 27°C). If the temperature cannot be held as low as 80°F (27°C), place the diluent bottle containing the diluted vaccine in an ice bath.
12. For vaccination, an automatic syringe with 22- to 20-gauge needles, ⅜- to ½-inch (0.95 to 1.27 cm) long, is recommended. Make certain that all equipment is sterilized and change needles frequently.
13. Inject each chick subcutaneously with 0.2 mL of the vaccine.
14. After diluting, use the vaccine within 2 hours. Do not save any vaccine that has been diluted. Burn vaccine containers and all unused contents.

Directions for use with Embrex Inovoject® Egg Injection System:

1. Vaccinate using the *in ovo* route of vaccination in 18 to 19 day-old healthy embryonated chicken eggs only.
2. The exact amount of diluent is provided for each shipment of vaccine. Use Fort Dodge Animal Health diluent only. Store diluent at not over 80°F (27°C).
3. Sanitize the Inovoject® Egg Injection System in accordance with the procedures described in the Inovoject® operator's manual.
4. Wear protective clothing when withdrawing vaccine from liquid-nitrogen refrigerator; protect hands with gloves, wear long sleeves, and use a face mask or goggles.
5. Before opening liquid-nitrogen refrigerator, prepare a clean, wide-mouthed container with a capacity of 1 to 5 gallons (3.8-19 liters). Half-fill this container with water at 80°F (27°C).
6. When withdrawing a cane of vials from the liquid-nitrogen refrigerator, expose only the vials to be used immediately. When removing a vial from the cane, hold palm of gloved hand away from face and body. Dilute only 4 vials at a time. Immediately replace the cane with remaining vials into the canister in the liquid-nitrogen refrigerator.
7. Place the vials into a prepared container half-filled with water 80°F (27°C). The frozen material thaws rapidly. When thawed, towel-dry vial.
8. The vials are pre-scored below the gold band. Before snapping off the top portion, wrap the vial with a cloth, holding the top part away from face and body.
9. For *in ovo* route of vaccination, use 50 mLs diluent per 1,000 doses of vaccine. For example: 4,000 doses of vaccine - 200 mL diluent.
10. Using 4 sterile mixing syringes with a 1½-inch (3.8 cm) 18-gauge needle, draw up a small amount of diluent into each syringe. Then draw the contents from one vaccine vial into the syringe and swirl gently. Repeat this step with the other 3 syringes. Insert needle into diluent container and slowly expel contents of syringe. Repeat this step with the other 3 syringes. Mix well by gently swirling the container. Withdraw a small amount of the reconstituted vaccine and use to rinse each vial injecting the rinses back into reconstituted vaccine. The vaccine is ready for use.
11. While vaccinating, maintain the diluted vaccine (in the diluent container) at 70° to 80°F (21° to 27°C). If the temperature cannot be held as low as 80°F (27°C), place the diluent container containing the diluted vaccine in an ice bath.
12. Carefully read and follow the Inovoject® operator's manual before initiating vaccination. Failure to follow instructions for Inovoject® operation may result in personal injury and/or embryonic morbidity and mortality.
13. The Inovoject® Egg Injection machine is equipped with an automatic injection system which utilizes a 20-gauge needle and deposits the vaccine about 1-inch deep into the egg.
14. Inject each egg *in ovo* with 0.05 mL of the vaccine solution.
15. After diluting, use the vaccine solution within 2 hours. Do not save any vaccine that has been diluted. Burn all unused material.

Records: Keep a record of vaccine serial number and expiration date; date of receipt and date of vaccination; where vaccination takes place; and any reactions observed.

Precaution(s): Store in liquid nitrogen. Dilute before using. Use entire contents when first opened. Burn vaccine container and all unused contents.

This product is nonreturnable.

Caution(s): This product should be stored, transported, and administered in accordance with the instructions and directions.

The use of this vaccine is subject to state laws, wherever applicable.

Combining this product with other biological products is not recommended.

Warning(s): Do not vaccinate within 21 days before slaughter.

Take all precautionary measures, including the use of gloves and face shield or goggles, to avoid potential hazards of handling liquid nitrogen and the possibility of explosion of glass vials as they are taken from the liquid-nitrogen refrigerator or canister or holding cane, or as they are placed in the thawing container. When removing the vial from the cane, hold palm of the gloved hand away from face and body.

Only vaccines, diluents etc., that have been approved by Embrex and are labeled appropriately for *in ovo* use can be used in the Inovoject® Egg Injection System.

Before using this vaccine, be certain to read directions.

For veterinary use only.

Disclaimer: Having cautioned the user concerning the handling of liquid nitrogen and the possibility of explosion of glass ampules as they are removed from the nitrogen or holding cane, or when placed in the thawing container, and having no control over the safety measures taken other than cautioning against possible dangers, Fort Dodge Animal Health shall not be responsible for personal injury and/or property damage resulting from said handling and/or the possibility of explosion.

Presentation: 5 x 1,000 doses.
Inovoject is a registered trademark of Embrex, Inc.
U.S. Patent No. 3,642,574 (turkey herpesvirus/MD-Vac); Patent Pending (chicken herpesvirus)
Compendium Code No.: 10032621 10745A

vWF ZYMTEC™

DMS Laboratories **ELISA Test**

Reagents and Materials Provided: All reagents, including the microtiter wells, are stable through the expiration date printed on each label when stored at 2-7°C.

Standards: Five vials, each containing 1.5 mL of plasma with a known concentration of vWF:Ag stated in terms of % of normal for the species to be tested in ELISA Dilution Buffer (EDB) with preservatives including 0.02% Thimerosal. Ready to use. See Master Matrix Data Form for exact values.

Controls: Two vials, each containing 0.2 mL of plasma with a specified level of vWF:Ag stated in terms of % of normal for the species to be tested. See Master Matrix Data Form for exact values.

Coated Microtiter Wells: Eight strips, each containing 12 wells coated with a rabbit anti-vWF antibody.

Sandwich Antibody: One vial containing 0.5 mL of concentrated goat anti-vWF antibody, stabilized in a buffer with preservatives including 0.02% Thimerosal.

Wash Buffer Concentrate (10X): One bottle containing 125 mL of PBS-Tween Solution. Preservatives include 0.02% Thimerosal.

Secondary Antibody Conjugate: One vial containing 0.5 mL of concentrated swine anti-goat antibody conjugated with horseradish peroxidase (HRP), stabilized in a protein solution with preservatives including 0.02% Thimerosal.

Conjugate Dilution Buffer (CDB): One vial containing 10 mL of buffered saline solution with detergents and 0.02% Thimerosal as preservative. Mix gently before use. Avoid foaming. Do not dilute.

ELISA Dilution Buffer (EDB): Two bottles, each containing 60 mL of buffered saline solution with protein stabilizers and 0.02% Thimerosal as preservative. Mix gently before use. Avoid foaming. Do not dilute.

Substrate Buffer: One bottle containing 25 mL of citrate phosphate buffer pH 5.6 with hydrogen peroxide. Preservatives include 0.02% Thimerosal. Mix gently before use. Do not dilute.

Stop Solution: One bottle containing 10 mL of 4.5N H_2SO_4. Ready to use.

Warning: Avoid contact, can cause severe burns.

Chromogen: Four hermetically-sealed packages, each containing a 5 mg tablet of O-Phenylenediamine Dihydrochloride (OPD).

Warning: Harmful if swallowed, inhaled or absorbed through the skin. May induce contact hypersensitivity.

Microtiter Well Holder: One reusable microtiter well holder with a capacity to hold 96 wells.

Humidified Incubation Chamber: Black, plastic box with sponge to provide a humidified environment.

Master Matrix Data Form: This sheet is provided as a worksheet when setting up your ELISA plate. It also provides the actual values for the Standards and Controls supplied with this kit. Make copies before use.

Materials Required But Not Provided:
- Micropipettes for dispensing 10-100 µL
- Test tubes
- ELISA plate reader
- Assorted glassware for the preparation of reagents and buffer solutions
- Timer
- Vortex Mixer
- Absorbent paper (paper towel)

Indications: An ELISA Assay for the *in vitro* determination of von Willebrand Factor (vWF) in plasma.

Intended Use: vWF zymtec™ can be used with other tests to identify those patients likely to be afflicted with von Willebrand's disease (vWD) and to identify asymptomatic carriers of the vWD trait[1,2]. vWF zymtec™ provides a quantitative measure of vWF:Ag (von Willebrand Factor Antigen) based on the protein's antigenic properties. This sensitive assay can measure extremely low levels of vWF, such as those seen with homozygous type III von Willebrand's disease[3,4]. The vWF zymtec™ Assay can be used to evaluate many mammalian plasma samples[3,13,14] simultaneously and is well-suited for screening programs[2].

Test Principles: The assay principle is represented in Figure 1. The vWF:Ag in the patient's plasma binds to the capture antibody, rabbit anti-vWF, which has been adsorbed to the surface of polystyrene microtiter wells. After the removal of unbound plasma, the goat anti-vWF sandwich antibody is added to each microtiter well where it binds to vWF:Ag. The unbound sandwich is washed out of the wells and swine anti-goat antibody (Secondary Antibody Conjugate) labeled with horseradish peroxidase (HRP) is added. After incubation, the microtiter wells are washed, followed by the addition of chromogenic substrate (hydrogen peroxide and OPD). The reaction is stopped by the addition of dilute sulfuric acid. When the absorbance at 490nm is plotted against % vWF:Ag, the resultant standard curve is used to determine the sample vWF:Ag concentrations.

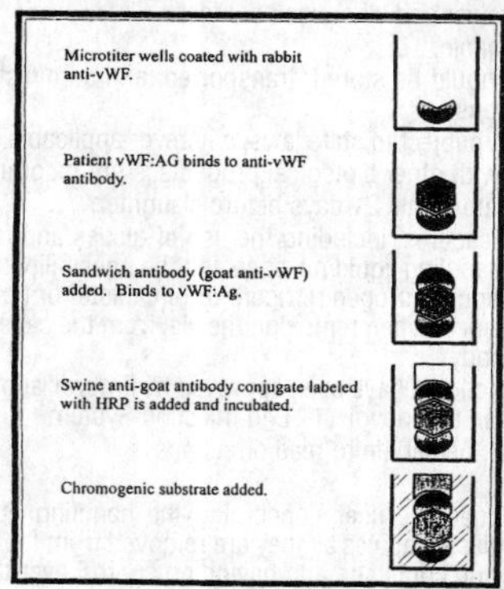

Microtiter wells coated with rabbit anti-vWF.
Patient vWF:AG binds to anti-vWF antibody.
Sandwich antibody (goat anti-vWF) added. Binds to vWF:Ag.
Swine anti-goat antibody conjugate labeled with HRP is added and incubated.
Chromogenic substrate added.

Figure 1
Modified Double-Sandwich ELISA for vWF:Ag Measurements

V

Test Procedure: Reagent Preparation: Bring all reagents to room temperature (20-25°C) before use. Mix all reagents and sample thoroughly before dilution.

1. Wash Solution: Add 100 mL of Wash Buffer Concentrate to 900 mL of distilled or deionized water to make a total of 1.0 liter of the working solution. The working solution is stable for one week from the date of preparation when stored at room temperature (20-25°C) or for one month at 2-7°C.
   Note: Crystal formation in the concentrate is common when storage temperatures are low. Redissolve crystals by warming the concentrate to 30-35°C before dilution.
2. Sandwich Antibody: Dilute 1:51 in EDB. After dilution, the Sandwich Antibody is stable for one day when stored at 2-7°C. Example: Diluting 60.0 µL of antibody in 3.0 mL of EDB will provide working solution sufficient for as many as 30 wells.
3. Secondary Antibody Conjugate: Dilute 1:101 in CDB for about 60 minutes before application. After dilution, the Secondary Antibody Conjugate is stable for one day when stored at 2-7°C. Example: Diluting 30.0 µL of Conjugate in 3.0 mL of CDB will provide working conjugate solution sufficient for as many as 30 wells.
4. Chromogen Substrate Solution: OPD is highly hydroscopic and will react with moisture in the air. Open only one package at a time and use immediately. To prepare the working chromogen substrate, add one 5 mg OPD tablet to 5.0 mL of Substrate Buffer. One tablet is sufficient for up to 50 wells. Prepare just prior to use. The chromogen substrate is stable for one hour when kept from excessive heat and light. Chromogen Substrate Solution is very unstable and remaining quantities should be discarded.

Specimen Collection and Handling: Blood should be collected by clean venipuncture through sodium citrate anticoagulant or into a blue-top Vacutainer® tube. Only 3.8% sodium citrate anticoagulant should be used in a 1:10 final dilution (1 part citrate to 9 parts blood). Inspect the specimen for clots. If any clots are present, discard the sample. If the sample is free of clots and significant hemolysis, centrifuge as soon as possible. Transfer the plasma into a labeled specimen vial. Store at 2-7°C if testing is to take place within one week after collection. If testing is to take place more than one week after collection, specimens should be stored at -20°C. Avoid repeated freezing and thawing.

Warning: Handle all specimens as if capable of transmitting disease.

Calibration and Quality Control: Standards are provided with each kit for the purpose of calibration. Five levels of plasma vWF are provided and must be run to establish a proper standard curve for the assay. (See Calculation of Results section.) The Standards and Controls must be run with each assay of patient samples.

Do not use the standard curve shown in this package insert for calculation purposes.

Two levels of Control plasma have been provided as a quality control check. The Control supplies are in both the normal and abnormal ranges. The values may vary from lot to lot and are stated on the vial labels.

In accordance with good laboratory practice, each laboratory should use quality control routines to establish inter- and intra-assay precision and performance characteristics.

Loading the Microtiter Plate: The microtiter well holder supplied is labeled 1-12 for columns and A-H for rows. Figure 2 illustrates a format to test four patients in duplicate.

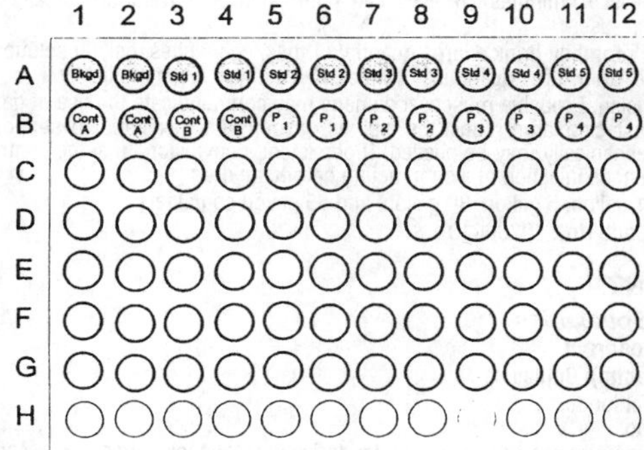

Figure 2

1. Make several copies of the ELISA Matrix Worksheet before beginning. Using one of the copies as your worksheet, record the position and assay function of each microtiter well as illustrated in Figure 2. For future information and reference, record the lot number of each of the kit reagents.
2. Beginning at the top of the plate, insert one strip of 12 wells in Row A and a second 12-well strip in Row B.

Procedure: Bring all reagents to room temperature (20-25°C) before use.

1. Refer to the daily Job List for samples to be evaluated. Using the appropriate Matrix sheet, assign Plate location for wells that will be used to evaluate each specimen. Insert required wells into well holder.
2. Dilute each plasma and Control sample 1:201 in ELISA Diluent Buffer (EDB). Add 10 µL of sample to 2.0 mL EDB, and mix by vortexing.
3. Add 100 µL of EDB to each of the wells that will be used to evaluate the background absorbance associated with the coated wells.
4. Add 100 µL of each Standard to the assigned wells (duplicate).
5. Pipette 100 µL of each diluted plasma Sample and diluted Control into the assigned wells.
6. Place the microtiter plate in the Humidified Incubation Chamber. Incubate at 20-25°C (room temperature) for 1.0 hour. Keep plate level during incubation.
7. Remove the plate from the Humidified Incubation Chamber and aspirate the contents of the wells.
8. Fill each well with appropriately diluted Wash Solution and aspirate. Repeat three times, for a total of four washes. Finally, invert the plate on absorbent paper (paper towel) and blot the excess fluid from the wells.
9. Pipette 100 µL of appropriately EDB-diluted (1:51) Sandwich Antibody to each well. Return the plate to the Humidified Incubation Chamber and incubate at 20-25°C (room temperature) for 1.0 hour.
10. Wash and blot the wells as described in Step 8.
11. Pipette 100 µL of appropriately CDB-diluted (1:101) Secondary Antibody to each well. Return the plate to the Humidified Incubation Chamber and incubate at 20-25°C (room temperature) for 30 minutes.
12. Wash and blot the wells as described in Step 8.

13. Immediately prepare Chromogen Substrate Solution by adding one OPD tablet to 5 mL of Substrate Solution. Allow tablet to dissolve completely and mix well. See Reagent Preparation Section, Step 4.
14. Add 100 µL of Chromogen Substrate Solution to each well.
15. Use the black plastic box provided, or cover the plate with a black cloth, or place the plate in a drawer to avoid light. Incubate at 20-25°C (room temperature) for precisely 20 minutes.
16. After 20 minutes, add 100 µL of Stop Solution to each well.
17. Determine the absorbance at 490 nm of the contents of each well.

    Note: Stability of the Chromophoric Reaction - The absorbance of the final reaction can be measured up to one hour after the addition of the Stop Solution if the microtiter plates are stored in a darkened, humidified chamber. However, good laboratory practice dictates that the measurements be made as soon as possible.

Interpretation of Results: Test Results: Results are reported as % vWF:Ag compared to an established pooled plasma standard from normal, healthy animals.

Calculation of Results: A conventional data reduction software program with the ability to handle log/log data transformation with the application of quadratic curve fitting techniques is a useful tool to calculate the results. However, if your laboratory is not equipped to conveniently handle such data analysis, you will find, on page 13 of the Assay Manual, semi-logarithmic one cycle x 100 divisions cross-sectional sheet. Use this sheet to plot and draw the required standard curves.

Before use, make an adequate number of copies.

Typical data points are shown in Figure 3 and a standard curve is shown in Figure 4.

Note: Do not use this example standard curve to interpret your assay data.

Figure 3 - Typical vWF Data:

Microtiter Well Position	Standard Value Percentage (%)	Absorbance Reading at 490 nm	Average Absorbance	% vWF from Curve
A 01	blank 0.001	0.001		
A 02	blank 0.001	0.003	0.002	
A 03	100	0.864		
A 04	100	0.787	0.826	
A 05	75	0.729		
A 06	75	0.716	0.723	
A 07	50	0.510		
A 08	50	0.543	0.527	
A 09	25	0.308		
A 10	25	0.312	0.310	
A 11	12.5	0.153		
A 12	12.5	0.155	0.154	
B 01	Control A	0.683		
B 02	Control A	0.677	0.680	67.05%
B 03	Control B	0.076		
B 04	Control B	0.072	0.074	0%
B 05	Patient 1	0.907		
B 06	Patient 1	0.893	0.900	112.50%
B 07	Patient 2	0.555		
B 08	Patient 2	0.545	0.550	51.56%

Sample Calculations, Manual Technique:

1. Using the absorbance reading from the plate reader, calculate the average value for each of the Standards, Controls, Blanks and Patient Samples, i.e., $\frac{A1 + A2}{2}$ = Average Absorbance Value.
2. Using the average absorbance values calculated in Step 1, subtract the Average Blank Value from each of the Standards, Controls and Patient Absorbance Values.
3. Make a copy of page 13 of the Assay Manual and use it to plot the data points calculated in Step 2.
4. Plot the average absorbance reading for each of the five Standards. Draw the best fit smooth curve through these data points.
5. Using the standard curve, determine the values of Controls A and B. The % vWF from the curve must be within ± 10% of the expected values. If not, the test is invalid. The expected values are provided with each kit.
6. Using the sta ... it.

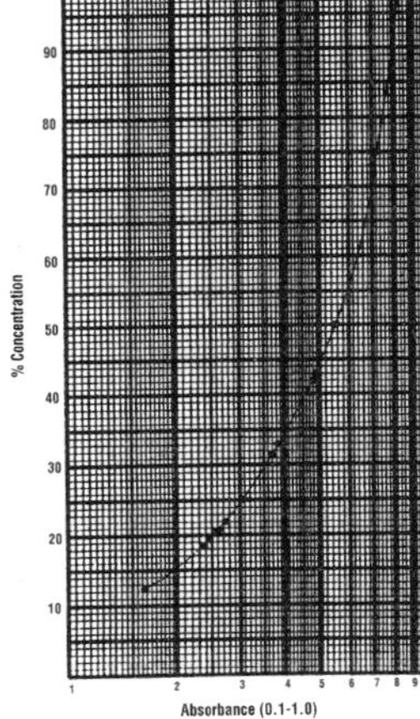

Figure 4 Typical Standard Curve

Table 1 - Interpretation of Test Results: Diagnosis of von Willebrand's Disease

Bleeding Time **	von Willebrand Factor Antigen (%)+	Interpretation
Normal	70 or greater	Normal range is 70-180%
Normal	70-79	Lower end of normal; caution advised for breeding stock. Mates should have higher levels and offspring should be tested.
Normal	50-69	Borderline normal (equivocal results) or heterozygous carrier of vWD gene. Recommend retesting and/or breeding only to higher-testing mates. Offspring should be tested.
Normal	less than 50	Type I vWD. This is the most common form of vWD. Heterozygous carrier of vWD*. Recommend breeding only to higher-testing mates. Offspring should be tested.
Elevated	less than 50	Type I vWD. Has exhibited some bleeding problem (e.g. hematuria, epistaxis, melaena, post-surgical bleeding).* Clinically affected animals should not be used for breeding.
Normal or Elevated	less than 50	Type II vWD. Clinically affected animals exhibit severe bleeding symptoms. Multimeric analysis of vWF reveals absence of high molecular weight multimers. These animals should not be used for breeding.
Elevated	less than 0.01	Type III vWD. Exhibits bleeding symptoms and homozygous for vWD. This animal is the product of two asymptomatic, heterozygous carrier parents and should not be used for breeding.
Normal	greater than 180	Probably reflects stress, improper sample collection, or activation from disease. Recommend retesting. Test invalid for prediction of genetic status for vWD trait.

+ Formerly called factor VIII-related antigen; measured by ELISA methodology. When measured by Clotting or RIA methods, normal ranges may vary slightly.

* Development of concomitant thyroid dysfunction may aggravate existing vWD or increase the risk of bleeding in some previously asymptomatic carriers.

** Abnormal bleeding time is not specific for vWD; homeostatic disorders including thrombocytopenia and platelet dysfunction will also cause variable prolongation of bleeding time test.

Interpretation of Test Results: Patients testing in the normal range (See Table 1) are at low risk of transmitting the vWD trait. Patients that are free of the vWD trait, when bred to a normal-testing mate, should only produce offspring of normal genotype with vWF:Ag levels of 70% or greater.

Patients testing in the borderline range (50-69% vWF:Ag) cannot be accurately classified as free of the vWD trait or as carriers on the basis of this single measurement. It is recommended that patients testing in this range be bred only to mates testing well within the normal range. Their offspring should be tested to identify normal individuals and to further clarify the vWD status of the parents.

Healthy patients testing in the abnormal range (0-49% vWF:Ag) are considered to be carriers of the vWD trait and can transmit the defect to some of their offspring[5-9].

When using the vWF:Ag test as a genetic predictor of vWD status, certain caveats apply before one considers test results falling within the normal range to be valid. Plasma from patients that are or have been ill or vaccinated within 10-14 days or from females tested during estrus, pregnancy or lactation may be transiently higher or lower than the true baseline and, therefore, can result in misclassification. Patients with endocrine disease, especially thyroid dysfunction, can also have fluctuating levels of vWF[8-11].

Limitations, Precautions and General Comments:

1. Strict adherence to the exact procedures described in this package insert and careful techniques must be exercised to obtain reliable results with this test kit. Numerous conditions which are unrelated to vWD may cause abnormal plasma vWF levels.
2. Poor sample collection techniques must be avoided. Hemolysis or clots in samples will cause gross inaccuracies in test results.
3. Standards are provided as a set of 5. Do not mix standards from a different set without matching lot numbers.
4. A standard curve must be established for every run.
5. Chromogen substrate solution is light sensitive and should be protected from direct light.
6. Sodium azide is known to interfere with horseradish peroxidase activity.
7. Reagents should not be used after the expiration date shown on each label.

Performance Characteristics: This patented technology, which Iatric Corporation is licensed to use, employs a modified double-antibody sandwich ELISA for measuring vWF:Ag. It provides parallel accuracy to the Laurell Method but is more sensitive. It provides accurate results below 1% vWF:Ag, compared to the lower limit of detection of 7% by Laurell. The performance characteristics of the ELISA on which vWF zymtec™ is based have been previously reported by the developers in numerous journals[3,4,12,13,14]. Over 600 randomly chosen, individual canine plasma samples were analyzed in these studies, as well as feline, equine and other mammalian plasma samples. The reproducibility of this assay is ± 8% (intra-and inter-assay variation) with a coefficient of variation of less than 9%[3,12].

The results obtained with vWF zymtec™ are comparable to those reported by the developers of the ELISA-based methodology used in vWF zymtec™[3,4]. The values used by the developers to categorize patient results are shown in Table 1.

Discussion: Summary and Explanation of Assay: vWF zymtec™ is a multispecies enzyme-linked immunosorbent assay (ELISA) which was developed[3,4] and adapted for vWF:Ag measurements[3]. The assay measures the chromophoric products of the enzyme-catalyzed oxidation of the substrate O-Phenylenediamine Dihydrochloride (OPD). The amount of enzyme activity is proportional to the amount of vWF antigen present. After prescribed incubation periods, the reaction is stopped and the endpoint absorbance is measured at 490nm using a microplate reader. A standard curve is constructed by plotting optical density against sample concentration on semi-log paper to obtain results expressed as percent vWF:Ag. Standard quadratic curve fitting techniques may be employed.

References: Available upon request.

vWF ZYMTEC™

Presentation: This kit contains sufficient materials to test up to 40 patients. It is designed to test 16 patients when tested in batches of 4, when each patient is of the same species.

vWF zymtec is a trademark of DMS Laboratories, Inc.

vWF zymtec is manufactured under a license agreement with Health Research, Inc., Albany NY, 12209, to U.S. Patents 5,196,311 and 5,202,264 and foreign patents corresponding to PCT/US90/06194.

Manufactured by: Vetazyme Corporation, 1706 West Fourth Street, Tempe, Arizona 85281.

Compendium Code No.: 14810060 PN30300001, 10/30/96

V

W

WARBEX® FAMPHUR POUR-ON FOR CATTLE

Schering-Plough **Topical Insecticide**

NADA No.: 034-697

Active Ingredient(s):

0,0-dimethyl 0-[p-(dimethylsulfamoyl) phenyl] phosphorothioate* 13.2%
Inert ingredients. 86.8%

*Famphur (1 gallon contains 1.04 pounds of famphur).

Indications: WARBEX® Pour-On is for the control of cattle grubs and the reduction of lice infestations.

Dosage and Administration: Apply WARBEX® using a graduated dipper or calibrated applicator at the rate of 1 ounce per 200 pounds body weight from the shoulder to the tail head. Do not exceed a maximum of 4 ounces on any animal. Follow the suggested schedule below:

Average Cattle Weight	Dosage	One Gallon Treats
200 lb	1 oz	128 head
400 lb	2 oz	64 head
600 lb	3 oz	42 head
800 lb	4 oz (maximum)	32 head

One treatment of WARBEX® will effectively control cattle grubs and reduce cattle lice infestations.

Use in a well ventilated area.

For Grub Control:

Apply as soon as possible after heel fly activity ceases. It is important to treat before the grub larvae reach the gullet or spinal area as the rapid killing of large numbers of larvae may possibly cause a host-parasite reaction. Appropriate timing of treatment of cattle should be judged by their origin; as a general guide, the treatment should be applied to cattle in or from the following areas as shown below:

Southwestern states. . . . . April/May
Southern states . . . . June/July
Central states . . . . August/September
Northern states . . . . October/November

Consult a veterinarian, extension entomologist or county agent to confirm the best time for application in your area.

Treatment within 6-8 weeks of grub emergence will be less effective and carcass damage may result from dead grubs.

Treatment is less effective on wet animals or animals exposed to rain after treatment.

For Lice Control:

Initial treatment (lice) must be made at the times recommended for grub control. If lice re-infestation occurs, animals may be retreated 40 days after the last treatment.

Contraindication(s): Do not treat Brahman bulls.

Precaution(s): Disposal of Containers: Drain container completely. Add one-half gallon water, one-quarter cup of detergent and one-quarter pound of lye. Tighten the closure. Rotate to wet all surfaces and let stand for at least 15 minutes. Drain completely and rinse several times with water. Bury the rinse solution at least 18 inches deep in an isolated area away from water supplies. Dispose of container according to applicable Federal, state and local laws.

Environmental Hazards: This product is toxic to fish, birds and other wildlife. Birds feeding on treated animals may be killed. Birds killed by famphur may pose a hazard to birds of prey (e.g., hawks, eagles, vultures, owls). Do not apply directly to water. Do not apply directly to areas where run-off occurs, do not contaminate wells, wetlands or any body of water by cleaning of equipment or disposal of wastes. Apply this product only as specified on the label. Use of this product in a manner inconsistent with its labeling is a violation of Federal law.

Caution(s): Flammable: Keep away from heat, sparks and open flame including hot branding irons and cautery dehorning equipment.

Keep out of the reach of children. Harmful or fatal if swallowed or absorbed through the skin. Avoid contact with the skin, eyes, and clothing. Wash thoroughly after handling. Do not contaminate food or feed products.

First Aid: If poisoning should occur, call a physician.

Note to Physicians: The product may cause cholinesterase inhibition. Atropine is antidotal. Pralidoxime chloride (2-P.A.M.; PROTOPAM chloride) may be effective as an adjunct to atropine. Use according to label directions.

Do not use on calves of less than three months of age; animals stressed from castration, overexcitement or dehorning; sick or convalescent animals. Animals may become dehydrated and under stress following shipment. Do not treat until they are in good condition. On occasion, cattle treated with WARBEX® may show signs of organophosphate poisoning such as excessive salivation, stiffness of limbs and bloat. Atropine is antidotal. A veterinarian should be consulted. Brahman and Brahman crossbreds are less tolerant of cholinesterase-inhibiting insecticides than other breeds.

Note: Do not treat Brahman bulls.

WARBEX® is a cholinesterase inhibitor. Do not use any drug, pesticide, insecticide, or chemicals having cholinesterase-inhibiting activity either simultaneously or within a few days before or after treatment with WARBEX®. Keep swine away from areas where run-off occurs.

The use of WARBEX may pose a hazard to the following Federally designated endangered/threatened species known to be found in certain areas within the named locations.

Bald Eagle: Arizona, California [within 10 miles of the lower Colorado River from Blythe (CA) to Yuma (AZ)], New Mexico, Oklahoma [west of the 100th meridian] and Texas [west of the 100th meridian].

Yellow Shouldered Blackbird: Southern coastal areas of Puerto Rico from Cabo Rojo to Guayama.

Mississippi Sandhill Crane: Mississippi [within ½ mile of all known nesting, foraging and roosting areas].

This product may not be used in areas where adverse impact on the Federally designated endangered/threatened species noted above is likely. If the user is in doubt whether or not the above named endangered/threatened species may be affected, he should contact either the U.S. Fish and Wildlife Service Office [Endangered Species Specialist] or personnel of the State and Fish and Game office.

To further reduce the impact of WARBEX® use on the bald eagle, and to eliminate or reduce the impact on wildlife, all cattle and any birds associated with the cattle found dead within 35 days of treatment with WARBEX® must be disposed of immediately to prevent the carcasses posing a threat to raptors and scavengers.

Notice: It is a Federal offense to use any pesticide product in a manner that results in the death of an endangered species.

Emergency Numbers:

1-800-228-5635: 24-Hour emergency medical assistance.

1-800-424-9300: 24-Hour chemical emergency [spill, leak, fire, exposure or accident].

1-800-548-2423: 24-Hour emergency animal poison control center.

1-800-541-7459: Customer service number to obtain product information, including copies of MSDS and to report incidents of WARBEX® poisonings of fish or wildlife.

Antidote(s): Atropine.

Warning(s): Do not slaughter within 35 days after treatment. Do not treat lactating dairy cows or dry cows within 21 days of refreshing.

Precautionary Statements:

Persons handling WARBEX® Pour-On must wear long-sleeved shirt and long pants, socks and shoes and chemical resistant (such as nitrile or butyl) gloves.

User Safety Recommendations:

Users should: Wash hands before eating, drinking, chewing gum, using tobacco or using the toilet. Remove clothing immediately if pesticide gets inside. Then wash thoroughly and put on clean clothing. Wash outside of gloves before removing. As soon as possible, wash thoroughly and change into clean clothing.

Disclaimer: Schering-Plough Animal Health Corporation warrants that the material contained herein conforms to the chemical description on the label and is fit for the use therein described when used in accordance with the directions on the label. Any damages arising from a breach of this warranty shall be limited to direct damages, and shall not include consequential commercial damages such as loss of profits or values, etc. Buyer assumes the risk of any use contrary to label instructions.

Presentation: 1 gallon (4 per case) metal containers.

* ® Registered trademark of Schering-Plough Animal Health Corporation.

Compendium Code No.: 10472111

WAR PAINT™ INSECTICIDAL PASTE

Loveland **Topical Insecticide**

EPA Reg. No.: 58864-2-36208

Active Ingredient(s):

Permethrin: (*(3-phenoxyphenyl) methyl (±) cis, trans-3-
(2,2-dichloroethyenyl)-2,2-dimethylcyclopropanecarboxylate 7.0%
Related Reaction Products 0.6%
**Piperonyl Butoxide, Technical. 14.0%
N-octyl bicycloheptene dicarboximide. 21.0%
Inert Ingredients 57.4%
Total 100.0%

*cis-trans isomer ratio: Min. 35% (±) cis and Max. 65% (±) trans

**Equivalent to Min. 11.2% (butylcarbityl) (6-propylpiperonyl) ether and Max. 2.0% related compounds.

Indications: Kills and repels face flies, horn lies, stable flies, house flies, black flies and bot flies on horses and foals.

Directions for Use: It is a violation of Federal law to use this product in manner inconsistent with its labeling. Do not apply to a wet animal since the product will not adhere to moist surfaces.

Full Body Fly Control: Adult horses: For the treatment of pastured horses, and those that are not going to be ridden for a period of weeks, it is recommended that a full dose, 12 grams, of WAR PAINT™ be applied as a single treatment. This should provide adequate fly control for approximately one week on pastured horses.

Apply one (1) gram under each eye, two (2) grams on back and two (2) grams on each leg below the hock or knee — grams total as a single treatment. Do not repeat treatment for seven (7) days. See application techniques.

Local Fly Control: For horses that are to be ridden and handled frequently, lesser amounts of WAR PAINT™ applied more frequently are a better choice. Lesser amounts of WAR PAINT™ applied discreetly and prudently to the horse can provide effective local fly control for several days to a week. If this technique is used, remember not to apply more than 12 grams of WAR PAINT™ to a horse in any 7-day period. See application technique.

How to Apply WAR PAINT™:

Full Body Control: Apply 12 grams: One (1) gram under each eye, two (2) grams on back and two (2) grams on each leg.

Bot Fly Control: Apply over eggs instead of on front of legs.

Stable Fly Control: Apply to the front of each leg: A one inch wide by four inch long stripe just below the knee and hock. These stripes will apply two grams to each leg.

Face Fly Control: Apply under each eye: A one inch stripe along the lower eyelid. (This will apply one (1) gram to each eye.)

Application Techniques:

Face Flies: Apply one (1) gram under each eye. Maximum control is achieved if WAR PAINT™ is applied under the eye, close to the eyelid. WAR PAINT™ should not be applied directly into the eye. Treatment may be repeated when flies again reach bothersome levels. Invert tube while squeezing and apply a narrow ribbon of paste under each eye, from corner to corner along the lower lid. Smooth out with dome top on applicator tube to a one inch wide stripe under the eye. A one inch wide stripe under the eye will apply approximately one (1) gram of WAR PAINT™ to each eye.

Horn Flies, Black Flies and House Flies: Apply two (2) grams to the back. To apply WAR PAINT™ to the back of the horse utilizing the squeeze tube applicator, invert the container and touch the tip of the applicator to a spot on the midline of the back just behind the withers. Squeeze the container and move the applicator tip to apply paste in a four inch long ribbon. Smooth out ribbon with dome top on tube to a one inch wide stripe. A four inch long by one inch wide stripe will apply approximately two (2) grams of WAR PAINT™ to the back of the horse.

Stable Flies and Bot Flies: Apply two (2) grams to each leg. When applying WAR PAINT™ to the legs of a horse, utilizing the squeeze tube applicator, it is easiest to apply the material to the front of the horse's leg. Start at a place on the front of the leg four inches below the knee or the hock. Invert the container and touch the tip of the applicator to the spot to be treated. While squeezing the container, move the applicator tip up the horse's leg four inches toward the knee or hock, then stop and smooth out with dome top on tube to a one inch wide stripe.

Bot Flies: To kill and repel bot flies during the egg laying season, WAR PAINT™ should be applied over the bot eggs already on the horse. A four inch by one inch wide strip should be painted over the area where the bot eggs exist. This should be done instead of applying WAR PAINT™ to the front of the leg since this application will also control stable flies.

Foals: The same technique for applying WAR PAINT™ can be used on foals, except only ½ of the adult amount should be used.

12 grams will treat two foals. Since the foals' eyes are smaller than adult horses, a one inch wide stripe under each eye of a foal will apply only ½ gram of WAR PAINT™ under each eye. When applying WAR PAINT™ to a foal's back and legs, make the stripe only two inches long instead of the four inch long stripe used on adult horses. This will insure that a foal will receive one-half of the adult horse dose. Remember, 12 grams should treat two foals.

Precautions for Use: Do not apply to the hair of a wet animal since the product will not adhere to moist surfaces. WAR PAINT™, once applied to the hair of the horse, cannot be wiped off. Therefore, it should not be applied within two or three weeks of an anticipated show or event in which the presence of small amounts of WAR PAINT™ on the horse's hair would have an adverse effect on the horse's appearance. WAR PAINT™ will stain clothing and once it is on clothing, it is difficult to remove. Therefore, care should be taken in applying WAR PAINT™ to the horse to avoid getting it on clothing. If WAR PAINT™ does get on clothing, nail polish remover is helpful in removing it, but it often takes frequent applications of nail polish remover with frequent washing to remove the material from clothing. Do not use nail polish remover to remove WAR PAINT™ from a horse's hair. As with any product, certain horses may be sensitive to one of the ingredients in WAR PAINT™ and develop some local irritation. If irritation occurs, discontinue use. If irritation persists, consult your veterinarian.

Precautionary Statements: Hazards to Humans and Domestic Animals:

Caution: Harmful if swallowed or absorbed through the skin. Avoid contact with skin, eyes or clothing. Do not contaminate food or foodstuff. Wash thoroughly with soap after handling.

Statement of Practical Treatment: If Swallowed: Contact a physician or poison control center immediately. If on Skin: Immediately remove contaminated clothing, wipe material from skin and wash affected area with plenty of soap and water. Contact a physician if irritation persists. Wash clothing prior to reuse. If in Eyes: Flush eyes with plenty of water. Contact a physician of irritation persists.

Environmental Hazards: This product is toxic to fish and other aquatic animals. Do not contaminate any body of water with this product by cleaning of equipment or disposal of wastes.

Storage and Disposal: For squeeze tube containers: Do not contaminate water, food or feed by storage or disposal. Storage: Tightly close cap and store in a dry place (preferably locked). Avoid extreme temperatures. Pesticide Disposal: Wastes resulting from the use of this product may be disposed of on site or at an approved waste disposal facility. Container Disposal: Dispose of empty tube in a sanitary landfill or by incineration, or, if allowed by state and local authorities, by burning. If burned, stay out of smoke.

Warning(s): Do not use this product on horses intended for human food.

Keep out of reach of children.

Disclaimer: Except as expressly provided herein, neither Loveland nor seller makes any warranties, guarantees, or representations of any kind, either by usage of trade, statutory or otherwise, with regard to the product sold, including, but not limited to merchantability, fitness for a particular purpose, use or eligibility of the product for any particular trade usage.

Unintended consequences may result because of, but not limited to, such factors as presence of other materials, or the manner of use or application, all of which are beyond the control of Loveland Industries, Inc. or seller. In no case shall seller be liable for consequential, special, or indirect damages resulting from the use or handling of this product. All such risks shall be assumed by the buyer or user.

Applicator's or grower's exclusive remedy against Loveland Industries, Inc. or seller for any cause of action relating to the product is a claim for damages, and in no event shall damages or any other recovery exceed the purchase price of the product in respect of which such claim is made.

Presentation: 96 gram tube.

Compendium Code No.: 10860380

WART SHIELD™

Novartis Animal Vaccines — **Vaccine**

Wart Vaccine, Killed Virus

U.S. Vet. Lic. No.: 303

Composition: A formalin inactivated vaccine which contains virus-laden tissue extracts derived from bovine papillomas.

Contains amphotericin B, gentamicin, and thimerosal as preservatives.

Indications: For prophylactic use only as an aid in the control of viral papillomas (warts) in cattle. Each serial is tested for purity and safety in accordance with U.S.D.A. regulations.

Dosage and Administration: Shake well before using. Inject subcutaneously. If more than 10 mL is administered, choose two (2) or more locations to deliver the total dose.

Mature cattle .... 10-50 mL
Calves .... 10-35 mL

Repeat the dose in three (3) to five (5) weeks.

WART SHIELD™ can be used in cattle of all sizes and ages, with the dosage variable depending upon the size and degree of involvement of the animals. Since the papilloma virus is so hardy, it is recommended that a vaccination program be continued for at least one (1) year after the last warts have been noticed in a herd.

Precaution(s): Store in the dark at 35°-45°F (2°-7°C). Do not freeze. Use the entire contents when first opened.

Caution(s): Anaphylactic reactions may occur following the use of the product. Symptomatic treatment: Epinephrine.

For veterinary use only.

Warning(s): Do not vaccinate within 21 days of slaughter.

Discussion: Papillomas (warts) in cattle are caused by the bovine papilloma virus. They are a form of benign, self-limiting epithelial tumor that usually occurs in young animals (less than one year of age). Warts can appear as cauliflower-like growths or as small, scattered elevations on the skin. While they can occur anywhere on the body, including the mucous membranes of the reproductive tract, they are usually limited to the skin of the head, neck and shoulders. The incubation period is about 30 days, and the duration varies considerably, from one to twelve months.

The papilloma virus replicates within the wart tissue; therefore, the surface of the wart contains infective virus. If affected animals rub against objects such as fences or stanchions, the virus can be transferred to these objects, where it is very resistant to destruction. If other animals receive skin abrasions from these objects, the virus is easily transferred. Other objects, such as tattoo pliers, needles, and surgical instruments, have also been implicated in spreading the virus among animals.

Different remedies for warts have been suggested, including various chemical treatments, with limited results. Surgical removal has also been tried, but it has the disadvantage that, if it is done too early in the course of the wart development, it may actually stimulate regrowth and spread of the warts.

References: Available upon request.

Presentation: Available in 100 mL bottles.

Compendium Code No.: 11140672

WARTSOFF™

Creative Science — **Topical Product**

Wart Ointment

Active Ingredient(s): Contains: Castor oil, 43% (w/w), Salicylic acid, 18% (w/w), Inert ingredients, 39% (w/w).

Indications: For use in removal of external warts from cattle, horses, goats and dogs.

Directions: Apply directly on the wart twice daily. Rub in well leaving wart completely covered with WARTSOFF™. Apply to teats and udders of dairy cows after milking. If no benefit is apparent after two weeks of treatment, or for warts that grow rapidly, consult a veterinarian.

Caution(s): Wash treated teats and udders before each milking. Avoid contact with eyes.

For animal use only.

Warning(s): Wash hands thoroughly with soap and warm water after applying the product to animals.

Not for human use.

Keep out of reach of children.

Presentation: 4 oz (113 g) container.

Compendium Code No.: 13760031

WART-VAC

Durvet — **Vaccine**

Wart Vaccine, Killed Virus

U.S. Vet. Lic. No.: 303

Composition: This vaccine contains inactivated virus-laden tissue extracts derived from bovine papillomas. Contains amphotericin B, gentamicin, and thimerosal as preservatives.

Indications: For prophylactic use only in cattle as an aid in the control of viral papillomas (warts).

Dosage and Administration: Shake well before using. Administer subcutaneously.

Mature cattle: 10-50 mL

Calves: 10-35 mL

If greater than 10 mL is administered, choose 2 or more locations to deliver total dose. Revaccinate in 3-5 weeks.

Precaution(s): Store in the dark at 35°-45°F (2°-7°C). Do not freeze. Use entire contents when first opened.

Caution(s): Anaphylactic reactions may occur following the use of this biological. Symptomatic treatment: Epinephrine.

Warning(s): Do not vaccinate within 21 days prior to slaughter.

Presentation: 100 mL vials.

Manufactured by: Advance Biologics, Inc.

Compendium Code No.: 10841710

WART VACCINE

AgriLabs — **Vaccine**

Wart Vaccine, Killed Virus

U.S. Vet. Lic. No.: 303

Active Ingredient(s): The formalin inactivated vaccine contains virus-laden tissue extracts derived from bovine papillomas. Contains amphotericin B, gentamicin, and thimerosal as preservatives.

Each serial is tested for purity and safety in accordance with U.S.D.A. regulations.

Indications: For prophylactic use only as an aid in the control of viral papillomas (warts) in cattle.

Dosage and Administration: Shake well before using. Inject subcutaneously. If greater than 10 mL is administered, choose two (2) or more locations to deliver the total dose.

Mature Cattle .... 10-50 mL
Calves .... 10-35 mL

Repeat in 3-5 weeks.

Precaution(s): Store in the dark at 35°-45°F (2°-7°C). Do not freeze.

Caution(s): Use the entire contents when first opened. Anaphylactic reactions may occur following the use of the biological. Symptomatic treatment: Epinephrine. For veterinary use only.

Warning(s): Do not vaccinate within 21 days before slaughter.

Presentation: 100 mL vials.

Compendium Code No.: 10581250

WART VACCINE

Colorado Serum — **Vaccine**

Wart Vaccine, Killed Virus

U.S. Vet. Lic. No.: 188

Active Ingredient(s): Wart vaccine, killed virus.

Indications: For use as an aid in the prophylactic treatment of viral warts (papillomas) in cattle only.

Dosage and Administration: The dose for calves is 10 mL injected subcutaneously preferably at two (2) sites along the side of the neck. For older cattle, the dose should be increased to 15 mL. In each instance a repeat dose should be administered in three (3) to five (5) weeks.

Precaution(s): Shake well before using. Store in the dark at 2-7°C.

Caution(s): Anaphylactic reactions sometimes follow administration of products of this nature. If noted, administer adrenaline or an equivalent drug. Use the entire contents when first opened.

For veterinary use only.

Warning(s): Do not vaccinate within 21 days before slaughter.

Presentation: 50 mL vials.

Compendium Code No.: 11010350

WATERLESS ANTIBACTERIAL HAND CLEANER

Davis — **Hand Cleanser**

Ingredient(s): Contains: 62% ethyl alcohol, water, thickening agent, emollients, skin moisturizers, aloe vera gel and fragrance.

Indications: Davis ANTIBACTERIAL HAND CLEANER is safe and effective for use before and after handling animals with skin conditions associated with bacteria, fungi or other microorganisms.
Directions for Use: Squeeze a small amount of the gel directly onto hands. Apply evenly over hands with a washing motion. Hands should feel dry in 15 seconds. Repeat application if desired.
No water or hand towels are needed. Evaporates quickly, leaving no sticky residue.
Caution(s): Keep away from open flame.
If eye contact occurs, flush with water for 15 minutes and seek medical attention. Not tested for use on animals.
Warning(s): Keep out of reach of children.
For external use only.
Presentation: 8 fl oz (236 mL).
Compendium Code No.: 11410410

WATERLESS SPRAY-ON SHAMPOO

Davis **Grooming Shampoo**

Ingredient(s): Cleaning formula, chamomile and sunflower oil.
Indications: A grooming shampoo for dogs, cats, puppies and kittens to be used in-between baths for touch-ups, after surgery or any situation when there is insufficient time for a full bath.
Directions for Use: Spray coat thoroughly with Davis WATERLESS SHAMPOO, beginning at the head and working towards the hindquarter, finishing legs last. Massage into the coat until a silky lather appears. No water is needed. Gently towel off, brush and dry the coat.
Warning(s): Do not get into eyes.
For external use only.
Keep out of reach of children.
Presentation: 32 oz and 1 gallon (3.785 L).
Compendium Code No.: 11410421

WAX-O-SOL™ 25%

Life Science **Otic Cleanser**

NDC No.: 49759-602-05
Active Ingredient(s): Contains 25% hexamethyltetracosane in mineral oil.
Indications: WAX-O-SOL™ is intended as a cleansing agent for the removal of ear wax in dogs and cats.
Dosage and Administration: To help soften and loosen ear wax accumulation, fill the ear canal with WAX-O-SOL™ 25% and gently massage for several minutes. The excess may be removed with cotton or paper towel.
Caution(s): For animal use only.
For external use only.
Keep out of reach of children.
Presentation: 1 fl oz (30 mL) bottle with dropper, 12 per box, and 16 oz (pint).
Compendium Code No.: 10870170

WAZINE® 17

Fleming **Water Medication**

Turkey, Chicken and Swine Wormer
NADA No.: 010-005
Active Ingredient(s): Each 100 mL contains 17 grams piperazine base (present as sulfate).
Inert Ingredients: Water, color, flavoring, preservatives and stabilizer.
Indications: For use in drinking water for the removal of large roundworms (*Ascaridia* spp.) from turkeys, chickens and large roundworms *(Ascaris suum)* and nodular worms (*Oesophagostomum* spp.) from swine.
Directions: One pint (16 fluid ounces) of provides 1 treatment for:
800 turkeys up to 12 weeks of age
400 turkeys over 12 weeks of age
1600 chickens 4-6 weeks of age
800 over 6 weeks of age
64 25-lb. (11.4 kg) pigs
32 50-lb. (22.7 kg) pigs
16 100-lb. (45.5 kg) pigs
8 200-lb. (90.9 kg) pigs
For best results, remove water in the evening (except during hot weather). Then, early the next morning, begin water medicated with WAZINE® 17. Provide medicated water only, distributed in waterers sufficient in number so that all birds or animals have access to water. The medicated water should be consumed in 1 day or less. Worming every 30 days is necessary to break the large roundworm life cycle.
Turkeys - Under 12 weeks of age: for each 100 birds, use 2 fluid ounces (60 mL) of WAZINE® 17 in 2 U.S. gallons (7.6 liters) of drinking water.
Over 12 weeks of age: for each 100 birds, use 4 fluid ounces (120 mL) of WAZINE® 17 in 4 U.S. gallons (15 liters) of drinking water.
Worm turkeys at 4-6 weeks of age and thereafter at 30 days, or as needed.
Chickens - 4 to 6 weeks of age: for each 100 birds, use 1 fluid ounce (30 mL) of WAZINE® 17 in 1 U.S. gallon (3.8 liters) of drinking water.
Over 6 weeks of age: for each 100 birds, use 2 fluid ounces (60 mL) of WAZINE® 17 in 2 U.S. gallons (7.6 liters) of drinking water.
Treat broilers at 4 weeks of age and thereafter at 30 days, or as needed. Treat replacement pullets at 8, 12, and 16 weeks of age.
Swine - For each 100 pounds (45.5 kilograms) of herd weight: give 1 fluid ounce (30 mL) of WAZINE® 17 per U.S. gallon (3.8 liters) of drinking water. Treat sows and gilts breeding and up to 2 weeks before farrowing, treat boars at any time, and treat pigs 1 week after weaning and every 30 days thereafter.
Precaution(s): Store above 32°F (0°C).
Caution(s): Keep out of reach of children. For animal use only. Do not give to sick, feverish, underweight or physically weak birds or animals. Consult your veterinarian for assistance in the diagnosis, treatment and control of parasitism.
Warning(s): Do not medicate prior to slaughter within 14 days for turkeys and chickens and 21 days for swine. Do not use in chickens producing eggs for human consumption.
Presentation: 8 fl. oz., 16 fl. oz. (1 U.S. pt.) and 1 gallon.
Compendium Code No.: 10120020

WAZINE® 34

Fleming **Water Medication**

Wormer
NADA No.: 010-005
Active Ingredient(s): Each 100 mL contains 34 grams piperazine base (present as sulfate).
Inert Ingredients: Water, color, flavoring, preservatives and stabilizer.
Indications: For use in drinking water for the removal of large roundworms (*Ascaridia* spp.) from turkeys, chickens and large roundworms *(Ascaris suum)* and nodular worms (*Oesophagostomum* spp.) from swine.
Directions: For best results, remove water in the evening (except during hot weather). Then, early the next morning, give WAZINE® 34 in the drinking water. Provide medicated water only, distributed in waterers sufficient in number so that all birds or animals have access to water. The medicated water should be consumed in 1 day or less. Worming every 30 days helps break the large roundworm life cycle.
Turkeys:
Under 12 weeks of age: for each 1000 birds, use 10 fluid oz. (300 mL) of WAZINE® 34 in 20 U.S. gallons (76 liters) of drinking water.
Over 12 weeks of age: for each 1000 birds, use 20 fluid oz. (600 mL) of WAZINE® 34 in 40 U.S. gallons (150 liters) of drinking water.
Worm turkeys at 4-6 weeks of age and thereafter at 30 days or as needed.
Chickens:
4 to 6 weeks of age: for each 1000 birds, use 5 fluid oz. (150 mL) of WAZINE® 34 in 10 U.S. gallons (38 liters) of drinking water.
Over 6 weeks of age: for each 1000 birds, use 10 fluid oz. (300 mL) of WAZINE® 34 in 20 U.S. gallons (76 liters) of drinking water.
Treat replacement pullets at 8, 12, and 16 weeks of age. Treat broilers at 4 weeks of age or as needed.
Swine:
For each 100 lb. (45.5 kg) of herd weight: give ½ fluid ounce (15 mL) of WAZINE® 34 per U.S. gallon (3.8 liters) of drinking water. Treat sows and gilts before breeding and up to 2 weeks before farrowing, treat boars at any time, and treat pigs 1 week after weaning and every 30 days thereafter.
For use in automatic water proportioners: Mix 1 part WAZINE® 34 with 1 part water and set proportioner to deliver 1 fluid ounce (30 mL) per gallon of drinking water and give for 1 day.
One gallon (3.8 liters) of WAZINE® 34 provides a treatment for:
Turkeys: 12,800 up to 12 weeks of age, 6,400 over 12 weeks of age, or
Chickens: 25,600 4 to 6 weeks of age, 12,800 over 6 weeks of age, or
Swine: 1,024 25-lb. (11.4 kg) pigs, or 512 50-lb. (22.7 kg) pigs, or 256 100-lb. (45.5 kg) pigs, or 128 200-lb. (90.9 kg) pigs.
Precaution(s): Store above 32°F (0°C).
Caution(s): Keep out of reach of children. For animal use only.
Do not give to sick, feverish, underweight or physically weak birds or animals. Consult your veterinarian for assistance in the diagnosis, treatment and control of parasitism.
Warning(s): Do not medicate prior to slaughter as follows:
Turkeys - 14 days Chickens - 14 days Swine - 21 days
Do not use in chickens producing eggs for human consumption.
Presentation: 1 U.S. gallon (3.785 L), 5 gallon and 55 gallon.
Compendium Code No.: 10120030

WAZINE® SOLUBLE

Fleming **Water Medication**

Piperazine Wormer
NADA No.: 010-005
Active Ingredient(s): Piperazine dihydrochloride (piperazine base equivalent to 230 grams).
Indications: For removing large roundworms from turkeys, chickens (*Ascaridia* spp.), and swine *(Ascaris suum)*, and nodular worms *(Oesophagostomum* spp.) from swine.
Directions: WAZINE® Soluble may be given in either the drinking water or feed according to the dosages below. Starting in the morning, give the required quantity of medicated water or feed as the sole source of water/feed until consumed, which should require 1 day or less. Withdraw non-medicated water or feed the evening before giving medicated water/feed. Do not withhold water during hot weather.
Provide sufficient watering or feeding space so that all birds/pigs have access to medicated water/feed. It is recommended that the entire contents of this package be used at one time. Worming ever 30 days helps break the large roundworm life cycle.
Turkeys: One package of WAZINE® Soluble will treat turkeys as follows:

Age	Turkeys	Water	Feed	Piperazine Base/Bird
Under 12 wks	2300	50 gal	200 lb.	100 mg
Over 12 wks	1150	50 gal	200 lb.	200 mg

Worm turkeys at 4-6 weeks of age and thereafter at 30 days or as needed.
Chickens: One package of WAZINE® Soluble will treat chickens as follows:

Age	Chickens	Water	Feed	Piperazine Base/Bird
Under 6 wks	4600	50 gal	200 lb.	50 mg
Over 6 wks	2300	50 gal	200 lb.	100 mg

Worm replacement pullets at 8, 12, and 16 weeks of age, and broilers at 4 weeks of age or as needed.
Swine: One package of WAZINE® Soluble will treat 4600 lbs. live weight providing 50 mg piperazine base per pound of body weight. (Examples: 92 50-lb. pigs or 30 150-lb. pigs, etc.). Mix each package with 50 gallons of water or 200 lbs. of feed.
In general, worm swine every 30 days. Worm sows and gilts before breeding and up to 2 weeks before farrowing; boars at any time; and pigs one week after weaning and every 30 days thereafter.
For use in automatic water proportioners: Dissolve each package in 50 fl. oz. (1½ qts) of water to make a stock solution. Set proportioner to deliver 1 fl. oz. (30 mL) per gallon of drinking water, so that each package of WAZINE® Soluble medicates 50 gallons of water.
Caution(s): Don't give product to sick, feverish, underweight or physically weak birds or pigs.
Consult your veterinarian for assistance in the diagnosis, treatment and control of parasitism.
Keep out of reach of children. For animal use only.
Warning(s): Withdraw medication prior to slaughter as follows:
Chickens - 14 days Turkeys - 14 days Swine - 21 days.
Do not use in chickens producing eggs for human consumption.
Presentation: 16 oz (454 g) bag and 50 kg.
Compendium Code No.: 10120040

WEIGHT BUILDER™

Farnam **Large Animal Dietary Supplement**

Premium Concentrated High Calorie Supplement

Guaranteed Analysis:

Crude protein, minimum	14%
Crude fat, minimum	40%
Crude fiber, maximum	11%
Calcium, minimum	0.8%
Calcium, maximum	1.2%
Phosphorus, minimum	0.5%

Ingredients: Vegetable fat, distillers' dried grains with solubles, heat stabilized flax meal, calcium carbonate, propionic acid, BHT/BHA (as a preservative).

Indications: To enhance skin and coat condition. To increase calorie intake for weight gain.

Dosage and Administration: Feeding Instructions: Includes 2 oz scoop.

To improve skin and coat condition, feed one scoop (2 oz) daily with regular grain ration.

For weight gain, feed 2 scoops (4 oz) daily with regular grain ration.

Depending on a horse's activity level and condition, more WEIGHT BUILDER™ may be fed with no adverse effects.

Precaution(s): Store in cool, dry place in the sealed bucket.

Warning(s): For animal use only.

Keep out of reach of children.

Presentation: 8 lb (3.632 kg) (32-day supply) and 28 lb (12.7 kg) (112-day supply).

Compendium Code No.: 10000430

WELADOL® ANTISEPTIC SHAMPOO

Veterinary Specialties **Antidermatosis Shampoo**

Antibacterial-Antiseptic

Active Ingredient(s): Contains: Polyalkyleneglycol-iodine complex in a shampoo base. Available iodine - 1%.

Indications: WELADOL® Antiseptic Shampoo is indicated as an aid in the control of bacterial skin infections in dogs and cats.

Directions for Use: Shake well before using.

Apply liquid petrolatum to eyes before shampooing. Avoid contact with eyes.

Wet the hair coat with warm water. Apply WELADOL® Antiseptic Shampoo over the entire body using additional warm water to aid in application. Rinse the hair coat thoroughly and repeat procedure. Use as indicated.

Note: This product tends to discolor metal. Do not allow it to come in contact with jewelry.

Warning(s): For external use only.

Keep out of reach of children.

Presentation: A one gallon bottle. Also available as one dozen bottles containing 8 ounces (237 mL) each.

Compendium Code No.: 10950030

WEST NILE VIRUS VACCINE

Fort Dodge **Vaccine**

West Nile Virus Vaccine, Killed Virus

U.S. Vet. Lic. No.: 112

Contents: This product contains the antigen listed above.

Thimerosal, neomycin and polymyxin B added as preservatives.

Indications: For the vaccination of healthy horses as an aid in the prevention of disease caused by West Nile Virus.

Dosage and Administration: Dose: Inject one 1 mL dose intramuscularly using aseptic technique.

Administer a second 1 mL dose 3 to 6 weeks after the first dose.

Revaccinate annually using one 1 mL dose.

Precaution(s): Store in the dark at 2° to 7°C (35° to 45°F). Avoid freezing. Shake well. Use entire contents when first opened.

Caution(s): In some instances, transient local reactions may occur at the injection site. In case of anaphylactoid reaction, administer epinephrine.

Warning(s): Do not vaccinate within 21 days before slaughter.

For veterinary use only.

Discussion: This product license is conditional.

Efficacy and potency test studies are in progress.

Owners should be advised that vaccinated horses may develop IgG and/or IgM antibody to West Nile Virus, which may affect their ability to export the animal.

Presentation: 10 doses (10 mL).

Patent Pending

Compendium Code No.: 10032721 16663C

WEST-VET® PREMISE® DISINFECTANT

WestAgro **Disinfectant**

EPA Reg. No.: 4959-15-AA

Active Ingredient(s):

Alpha-(p-nonylphenyl)-omega-hydroxypoly (oxyethylene)-iodine complex	18.05%
Phosphoric acid	16.00%
Inert ingredients	65.95%
Total	100.00%

(Providing 1.75% titratable iodine.)

Indications: For cleaning, disinfecting, and sanitizing animal housing and equipment; for sanitizing poultry drinking water; for use as a shoe bath prior to entering barns and poultry houses; for use as a deodorant, for sanitizing food-processing equipment.

PREMISE® Disinfectant is tuberculocidal at a dilution of 3 oz. to 5 gallons of water.

PREMISE® Disinfectant is not adversely affected by water hardness or low-temperature water.

PREMISE® Disinfectant has its own built-in indicator of germicidal activity. When the amber color disappears, a fresh solution should be prepared.

Also effective against canine parvovirus and *E. coli*.

Dosage and Administration: It is a violation of federal law to use the product in a manner inconsistent with its labeling.

Sanitizing buildings and equipment on the farm:

To sanitize surfaces of buildings, equipment, or utensils which have previously been thoroughly cleaned, use 1 oz. of PREMISE® Disinfectant in 5 gallons of water. Spray or swab the solution onto surfaces to be sanitized. Allow to drain dry without rinsing.

Sanitizing poultry drinking water: Add 1 oz. of PREMISE® Disinfectant to every 10 gallons of drinking water. Regular use in the drinking water also helps to keep the waterers free of slime and mineral deposits.

Food plant sanitization: Use 1 oz. of PREMISE® Disinfectant in each 5 gallons of water as the final sanitizing rinse on previously cleaned food-processing equipment and utensils. Drain, but do not rinse. When used at this dilution (1:640), PREMISE® Disinfectant does not require a final potable water-rinse, as prescribed in Federal Food Additive Regulation 178.1010.

Shoe bath: To help prevent tracking disease organisms into poultry houses, farrowing houses, and hog barns, place a shoe bath inside the doorway, containing 3 oz. of PREMISE® Disinfectant per gallon of water. After scraping shoes outside the doorway, stand in the shoe bath for 30 seconds prior to entering building interior. Change the shoe bath once a day.

Deodorant: PREMISE® Disinfectant destroys many odors as it sanitizes and disinfects. For general deodorant applications (garbage pails, refuse containers, etc.), swab or spray on a solution of 1 oz. of disinfectant per gallon of water.

Cleaning and disinfecting building and equipment on the farm: Before proceeding as indicated below, remove all animals and feeds from premises, cars, boats, trucks, and other equipment. Remove all litter and manure from floors, walls, and surfaces of barns, pens, stalls, chutes, and other facilities and fixtures occupied or traversed by animals. Empty all troughs, racks, and other feeding and watering appliances, saturating all surfaces with PREMISE® Disinfectant solution. Immerse all halters, ropes, and other types of equipment used in handling and restraining animals; as well as forks, shovels, and scrapers. Ventilate buildings, cars, boats, and other closed spaces. Do not house livestock or employ equipment until the treatment has been absorbed, set, or dried. All treated feed racks, mangers, troughs, automatic feeders, fountains, and waterers must be thoroughly rinsed with potable water prior to re-use.

Then, clean and disinfect in one step with PREMISE® Disinfectant. Use ½ oz. of PREMISE® Disinfectant per gallon of water. Scrub the surfaces to be cleaned and disinfected with a good brush or with a power sprayer. Start at the highest point of the building or equipment being cleaned, and work downwards. Let the solution drain dry without rinsing.

Precaution(s):

Storage: Keep the container closed when not in use. Do not store below 25°F or above 100°F for extended periods.

Disposal: Do not contaminate water, food, or feed by storage or disposal, or the cleaning of equipment. In case of a spill, flood the area with a large quantity of water, washing to the sewer or collection vessel.

Wastes resulting from the use of the product may be disposed of on site or at an approved waste disposal facility. Do not re-use the empty container. Triple rinse, puncture, and dispose of the container in a sanitary landfill or by incineration.

Caution(s): Keep out of the reach of children.

Precautionary Statements:

Hazards to Humans and Domestic Animals: Corrosive. Causes eye damage and skin irritation. Do not get in the eyes, on skin, or on clothing. Protect eyes and skin when handling. Harmful if swallowed. Avoid contamination of food.

First Aid:

In case of contact, immediately flush eyes or skin with plenty of water for at least 15 minutes. For eyes, call a physician. Remove and wash contaminated clothing before re-use.

If swallowed, promptly drink a large quantity of milk, egg whites, gelatin solution, or if these are not available, drink large quantities of water. Call a physician immediately.

Note to Physician: Probable mucosal damage may contraindicate the use of gastric lavage. Measures against circulatory shock, respiratory depression, and convulsions may be needed.

Presentation: 1 U.S. gallon (3.78 L) containers.

Compendium Code No.: 10180020

WEST-VET® PREPODYNE® SCRUB

WestAgro **Surgical Scrub**

NDC No.: 33392-039-11

Active Ingredient(s): PREPODYNE® Scrub contains a poloxamer-iodine complex.

Titratable iodine (in a lathering base) 0.75%

Indications: PREPODYNE® Scrub is an antibacterial, antifungal, antiseptic germicidal cleanser. It can be used for general handwashing and as a pre-operative and a post-operative scrub.

PREPODYNE® Scrub also destroys a broad range of micro-organisms including *Salmonella typhosa, Salmonella choleraesuis, Escherichia coli, Shigella sonnei, Proteus vulgaris, Serratia marcescens, Streptococcus pyogenes, Pseudomonas aeruginosa, Staphylococcus aureus, Staphylococcus albus* and Staphylococcus 80/81 (antibiotic resistant).

Dosage and Administration:

For general use: Wet hands with water. Pour approximately 5 mL of PREPODYNE® Scrub into the palm of the hand and spread over both hands, rubbing thoroughly. Add enough water to make a lather. Rinse thoroughly under running water.

For pre-operative use: Place approximately 5 mL of PREPODYNE® Scrub in the palm of the hand. Lather with water. Scrub with a brush around nails, under nails, and in nail and cuticle areas. Scrub the entire hand and arm up to the elbow and into the elbow creases for five (5) minutes. Rinse and repeat.

Caution(s): Keep out of the reach of children. For professional veterinary use only.

Presentation: Available as a ready-to-use 0.75% aqueous iodine solution in 1 gallon plastic containers.

* PREPODYNE is a licensed trademark of Alfa Laval, AB.

Compendium Code No.: 10180030

WEST-VET® PREPODYNE® SOLUTION

WestAgro **Surgical Preparation**

NDC No.: 33392-040-11

Active Ingredient(s): PREPODYNE® Solution contains a poloxamer-iodine complex.

Titratable iodine 1%

Contains patented, Advanced Conditioning Technology™ (ACT).

Indications: An antiseptic, PREPODYNE® Solution can be used for both pre-and post-surgical application as well as for general skin application. It can also be used for preparing the skin prior to injections, aspirations, lavages, or emergency treatment of lacerations and abrasions.

The iodine complex releases its iodine at a pre-determined rate, resulting in a topical antiseptic solution with prolonged germ-killing action. The solution is effective against gram-negative and gram-positive bacteria as well as against fungi and other disease-causing organisms.

PREPODYNE® Solution also destroys a broad range of micro-organisms including *Staphylococcus aureus, Staphylococcus aureus* (antibiotic resistant), *Staphylococcus epidermidis, Streptococcus pyogenes, Corynebacterium diphtheriae, Serratia marcescens,*

Escherichia coli, Salmonella typhosa, Salmonella choleraesuis, Proteus vulgaris, Pseudomonas aeruginosa, Shigella sonnei and *Candida albicans.*

Dosage and Administration: PREPODYNE® Solution retains its germicidal activity in up to 10% blood. Application, by swab or spray, should be confined to the prepared skin area of the operative site; the solution should not be allowed to pool. Bandages or tape can be applied to the treated area without their adhesiveness being affected by the solution.

Caution(s): Keep out of the reach of children. For professional veterinary use only.

Presentation: Available as a ready-to-use 1% aqueous iodine solution in 1 gallon plastic containers.

* PREPODYNE is licensed trademark of Alfa Laval, AB.

Compendium Code No.: 10180040

WEST-VET® ULTRADINE®

WestAgro **Teat Dip**

Active Ingredient(s): Contains 1.0% iodine and glycerin.

Indications: A teat dip concentrate effective for both pre-dipping and post-dipping procedures.

Dosage and Administration: Before starting or continuing to use ULTRADINE® teat dip, consult a veterinarian if a cow's teats are sore or chapped.

Pre-dipping:

1. Make sure that the udder is clean and dry.
2. Clean the teats and forestrip. If water is used, use a minimal amount. Thoroughly dry with a clean, single service paper towel.
3. Dip or spray the cow's teats with ULTRADINE® teat dip solution.
4. Allow a 15 to 30 second contact time.
5. Attach the milker unit.

Post-dipping:

1. Immediately after removing the inflations, dip or spray each teat with ULTRADINE® teat dip solution.
2. If the outside temperature is below freezing, allow the dip to air-dry on the teats before turning the cow out of the milking parlor.

Dilution Directions to Prepare ULTRADINE® 0.25% Iodine Teat Dip Solution: One (1) quart (32 fl. oz.) of ULTRADINE® teat dip concentrate should be reconstituted to one (1) gallon of 0.25% (V/V) iodine teat dip solution. Pour the entire contents into a clean one (1) gallon container and add 3 qt. of clean, potable water to make one (1) gallon of the teat dip solution. Shake or swirl the entire contents to ensure thorough mixing.

Precaution(s): If the product has frozen, thaw in a warm room and shake well before using. Keep the container closed when not in use. Do not re-use the empty container. Dispose of it in a safe manner.

The dip solution should be changed if it becomes visible dirty or if sediment is introduced.

Caution(s): Dilute with the proper amount of water before use as a teat dip. Do not use the concentrate as a teat dip. Follow the dilution directions.

Warning(s): Keep out of the reach of children. Do not take internally, avoid contact with the eyes.

First Aid: If swallowed, drink large quantities of water and seek medical advice. If in eyes, flush with water for at least 15 minutes and get prompt medical attention.

Trial Data: Efficacy of ULTRADINE® Teat Dip Solution in controlling new infections caused by major mastitis pathogens:

Treatment	Number of New Infections
Control (no dip used)	33
ULTRADINE® Teat Dip Solution	8
Percent reduction	75.8%

The study was conducted at Cornell University in accordance with Protocol B procedures as described by the National Mastitis Council. The challenge organisms included *Staphylococcus aureus* and *Streptococcus agalactia.*

Presentation: 32 fl oz (1 qt) (12 per case) (NDC 33392-171-13) and 5 gallon containers.

Compendium Code No.: 10180051

WGS

Durvet **Water Additive**

Guaranteed Analysis:

Crude Protein (Min %)	14%
Glycine (Min %)	10%
Sodium (Min %)	4.0%
(Max %)	7.5%
Potassium (Max %)	5.2%
Vitamin A Supplement (Min %)	68,040 IU/lb
Vitamin D_3 Supplement (Min %)	13,607 IU/lb
Vitamin E Supplement (Min %)	3,765 IU/lb

Ingredients: Dextrose, glycine, sodium chloride, potassium chloride, egg product, horse radish, kaolin, montmorillonite clay, soybean lecithin, psyllium powder, sodium bicarbonate, calcium gluconate, citric acid, citrus peels (citrus pomace DEH), apple pomace dried, vitamin C (ascorbic acid), vitamin E (A tocopherol), locust bean gum, betaine HCl, Chinese cinnamon, sodium aluminosilicate, vitamin A supplement, vitamin B_1 (thiamin HCl), vitamin B_{12} supplement, vitamin B_2 (riboflavin), vitamin B_3 (niacin), vitamin B_5 (D-calcium pantothenate), vitamin B_6 (pyridoxine HCl), vitamin B_9 (folic acid), vitamin D_3 supplement, vitamin H (biotin), menadione sodium bisulfite complex (source of vitamin K_3 activity), *Yucca schidigera,* zinc methionine, inositol, iodine ethylenediamine dihydriodide, vanillin, xanthan gum, sodium saccharin, sodium benzonate, silicon dioxide, propylene glycol, allspice, ethoxyquin as preservative, copper sulfate, cobalt sulfate, benzyl acetate, amyl butyrate, gamma undecalactone, ethyl butyrate.

Indications: Vitamin, mineral and protein supplement aromatized with plant extracts for all swine and calves.

Directions: Shake well. Dilute before usage.

Swine:

Direction 1: Top dress: 1 teaspoon (⅛ ounce) of WGS per piglet birth to 30 lbs. 2 teaspoons (¼ ounce) of WGS per piglet 30-66 lbs. 1 ounce (30 g) of WGS per piglet 66 lbs +, or

Direction 2: Mix 2 ounces (2 mini-cups) of WGS in 2 ounces of lukewarm water, and feed 1 cc per piglet 11 lb (5 kg) twice a day as long as needed. Half a teaspoon (2 grams) of WGS per 11 lb (5 kg) of life weight.

Calf:

Direction 1: 2 ounces per day (120 lbs or 55 kg) (2 mini-cup), or

Direction 2: Mix 1 ounce (1 mini-cup) of WGS with milk or half gallon of lukewarm water per meal twice a day as long as needed. Feed half an ounce (15 grams) of WGS per day as long as needed.

Length of Supplementation: 7 to 15 days.

Note: Feeding Vitamins other than Vitamins A, D, E to ruminants older than three months of age may not have a beneficial effect.

Precaution(s): Protect from light. Store in cool, dry place.

Caution(s): Not for injection.

Always follow directions.

Presentation: 2 oz, 4.4 lb, 11 lb (5 kg), 22 lb (10 kg) and 44 lb (20 kg).

Manufactured by: Nutrapro Inc., 1905 Lamoureux, Suite 202, St. Hyacinthe, Québec, J2S 8B1, Canada.

Compendium Code No.: 10842101

WHITE LINIMENT

Butler **Liniment**

Counterirritant-Rubefacient

Active Ingredient(s): Composition:

Turpentine	6.0% v/v
Stronger Ammonia Water	4.0% w/v
Ammonium Chloride	1.5% w/v
Camphor	1.0% w/v

Indications: For use as an aid in the temporary relief of minor stiffness and soreness of muscles and joints in horses caused by overexertion.

Directions for Use: Apply topically to horses only. Apply 2 or 3 times daily to affected areas. Massage gently to stimulate local circulation. Do not bandage treated areas.

Precaution(s): Store at controlled room temperature between 15° and 30°C (59°-86°F).

Protect from freezing.

Keep tightly closed when not in use.

Shake well before use.

Caution(s): Do not apply to irritated skin or if excessive irritation develops. Avoid getting into eyes or on mucous membranes.

Restricted drug - Use only as directed.

Warning(s): Not for use on horses intended for food.

For veterinary use only.

Keep out of the reach of children.

Presentation: 1 gallon (3.8 L) containers (NDC 11695-086-07).

Compendium Code No.: 10821891 Rev. 7-86

WHITE LINIMENT

Durvet **Liniment**

Active Ingredient(s): Turpentine, stronger ammonia water, ammonium chloride, and camphor formulated in an aqueous base with emollients, surfactants and stabilizers.

Indications: For use as an aid in the temporary relief of minor stiffness and soreness of muscles and joints caused by overexertion in horses.

Dosage and Administration: Shake well before using.

Apply topically to horses only. Apply two (2) or three (3) times a day to the affected area. Massage gently to stimulate local circulation. Do not bandage the treated areas.

Precaution(s): Store at a controlled room temperature between 59°-86°F (15° and 30°C). Protect from freezing. Keep tightly closed when not in use.

Caution(s): Do not apply to irritated skin or if excessive irritation develops.

Avoid getting into the eyes or on mucous membranes.

For topical use only.

For animal use only.

Warning(s): Not for use on horses intended for food.

Keep out of reach of children.

Presentation: 1 gallon (3.785 L) (NDC 30798-015-35).

Compendium Code No.: 10841721

WHOLE BLOOD CALF IgG MIDLAND QUICK TEST KIT™

Midland BioProducts **IgG Test**

Description: A qualitative test of immunity levels to determine the health and value of your calf.

Contents: Each kit contains: cassette, 0.2 mL pipette, dilution vial, and instructions.

Indications: The WHOLE BLOOD CALF IgG MIDLAND QUICK TEST KIT™ is designed to detect immunoglobulin G (IgG) in newborn calves, in a rapid test format, without the use of elaborate laboratory equipment.

Test Principles: The WHOLE BLOOD CALF IgG MIDLAND QUICK TEST KIT™ consists of a 4 mm strip enclosed in a plastic cassette, incorporating both complexing and detection reagents. Using the pipette provided, sample is transferred to the dilution vial and mixed.

A portion of the diluted sample is then transferred to the sample well of the cassette. If bovine IgG is greater than 10 mg/mL, it complexes with a complexing agent in the cassette. The complex then migrates through the test strip and bypasses the immobilized detection line (position "T") but reacts with the immobilized control line (position "C") causing a single red colored line to develop. However, if the bovine IgG is less than 10 mg/mL, it will not complex with complexing agent. The free complexing reagent will migrate through the test strip and react with both the immobilized "T" and "C" lines causing the development of two red lines. Excess sample will be absorbed in an upper filter.

As noted above, regardless of the concentration of the IgG sample, a line should develop at the "C" position. This has been incorporated into the cassette as a control mechanism. If no line is observed at the "C" position, then the test should be considered invalid and should be repeated with a new, unused kit. If the same results are obtained in the repeated test, contact Midland BioProducts at 1.800.370.6367.

Whole Blood Sample Information: The WHOLE BLOOD CALF IgG MIDLAND QUICK TEST KIT™ is based upon an average of hematocrits from normal, healthy calves. Due to variations in hematocrits among calves, it is recommended that the Plasma Calf IgG Midland Quick Test Kit™ be used when testing sick calves, or when maximum accuracy is desired.

Test Procedure:

Step 1: Sample Collection: Contact your veterinarian for proper collection technique. Collection supplies are not included in the kit.

You will need: collection tubes containing anticoagulant, blood collection needle, and marking pen.

1. Label the collection tube with calf number, date, time of collection, etc.
2. Collect approximately 2 mL of whole blood using a collection tube and needle.
3. Gently mix the sample blood with the anticoagulant.
4. Remaining sample may be stored refrigerated, in the collection tube, for 4-7 days. Do not freeze the whole blood.

Step 2: Procedure

1. Obtain sample (see Sample Collection).
2. Remove the cassette from the foil pouch by tearing at the notched end.
3. Discard the foil pouch and desiccant.
4. Label or otherwise identify each cassette so that it can be associated with the collected sample.
5. Gently mix the sample. Using a clean pipette from the pouch provided with the kit, completely depress the bulb and submerge the pipette into the sample. Gently release the bulb, which will allow the sample to be drawn into the pipette.
   The pipette will not be completely full.
   Quickly releasing the bulb increases the likelihood that air will be drawn into the pipette which may affect the accuracy of the test.
6. Remove the cap from the dilution vial and transfer the sample into it. Rinse the pipette by repeatedly drawing up and expressing its contents into the dilution vial.
7. Recap the dilution vial and invert several times to thoroughly mix the sample. Avoid shaking. Shaking will harm the sample and possibly affect the accuracy of the cassette.
8. Once the sample is thoroughly mixed, remove the cap from the dilution vial. Using the empty pipette from step 6, completely depress the bulb and submerge the pipette into the dilution vial. Gently release the bulb, which will allow the diluted sample to be drawn into the pipette.
9. Express two to four drops of the diluted sample into the sample well of the cassette, making sure that it is on a level surface.
10. Allow the test to proceed for 20 minutes, then read the results. For accuracy, do not read results after 40 minutes.

Test Interpretation:

Step 3: Interpretation of Results

A. IgG levels <10 mg/mL Indicated by Two lines; One at the "T" position and One at the "C" position. Even a faint line at the "T" position indicates <10 mg/mL IgG.

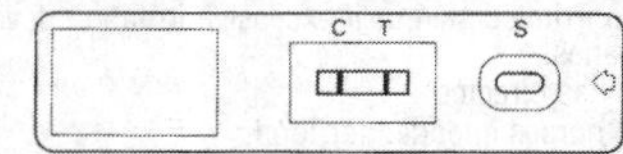

Low to Marginal IgG

B. IgG levels >10 mg/mL Indicated by One line at the "C" position.

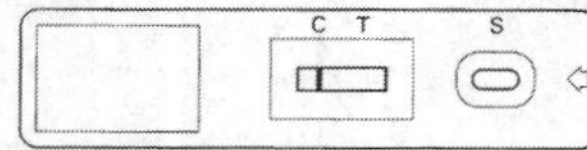

Satisfactory to High IgG Results

Storage: Avoid temperature and humidity extremes.

Do not freeze the dilution vial.

Do not remove the cassette from the foil pouch until ready for use. Even though the foil pouch includes a desiccant packet, exposure to high humidity conditions should be minimized.

Caution(s): Do not use components past expiration date and do not mix components from kits with different lot numbers.

The dilution vial in this kit contains sodium azide. Sodium azide may react with lead or copper plumbing to form highly explosive metal azides. On disposal, flush with a large volume of water to prevent azide build-up. For further information, refer to the manual issued by the Centers for Disease Control.

Do not ingest desiccant.

Dispose of all kit components in an appropriate manner.

Discussion: Failure of Passive Transfer (FPT): Calves are born virtually devoid of any detectable level of immunoglobulin G (IgG). The neonatal calf's immunity to infectious agents relies on the ingestion and absorption of maternal IgG from colostrum in mother's milk. This process, termed passive transfer, is a critical determinant of calf health.[6] Failure of passive transfer (FPT) may occur as a result of inadequate suckling, poor absorption of IgG, low levels of IgG in colostrum, or environmental stress. Despite a number of studies that have shown an increased risk of morbidity and mortality in FPT calves,[1,2,3,4] its prevalence in the field remains high. In fact, it is not uncommon to find herds with 40% of calves in this classification.[5]

The calf's ability to absorb IgG is optimal at birth and progressively declines in absorptive efficiency. The highest rate of absorption occurs during the first 4 hours followed by a gradual slowing until 12 hours. From 12 to 24 hours there is a substantial decline in absorption. Estimated closure time for IgG is approximately 24 hours.[8]

A number of studies have identified the specific concentrations of IgG that indicate adequate passive transfer.[5,6,7] Serum IgG concentrations of less than 10 mg/mL are considered to show FPT, while serum IgG concentrations above 10 mg/mL are considered to have an adequate level of immunity.

The rapid identification of calves with adequate IgG levels can be used to assess management and husbandry practices. In addition, if low IgG levels are detected, intervention strategies may be developed in conjunction with your health professional to optimize calf health and farm productivity.

References: Available upon request.

Presentation: Kits are packaged and sold in the following sizes: Packages of 6, 12, and 24.

Patent Pending

Compendium Code No.: 15010022 9007 rev. 4

WHOLE BLOOD FOAL IgG MIDLAND QUICK TEST KIT™

Midland BioProducts **IgG Test**

Description: A qualitative test of immunity levels to determine the health and value of newborn foals.

Contents: Contents for 4 mg/mL (400 mg/dL) kit and the 8 mg/mL (800 mg/dL) kit:

Each kit contains: cassette, 0.2 mL pipette, dilution vial, and instructions.

Indications: The WHOLE BLOOD FOAL IgG MIDLAND QUICK TEST KIT™ is designed to detect immunoglobulin G (IgG) concentrations from 0 to 7 day old foals, in a rapid test format without elaborate laboratory equipment.

Test Procedure:

Step 1: Sample Collection: Collection supplies are not included with the kit. Contact a veterinarian for proper collection technique.

1. Label the collection tube with foal no., date, age, etc.
2. Collect approximately 2 mL of whole blood in a collection tube using a collection needle and holder. Alternately, whole blood may be collected with a syringe and needle, then gently expelled into the collection tube.
3. If using an anticoagulant tube (i.e., a purple top tube), gently mix the sample blood with the anticoagulant in the tube.
4. Sample may be stored refrigerated in the anticoagulant collection tube for 7 to 14 days. Do not freeze whole blood. If sample is from a syringe, use immediately.

Step 2: Procedure

1. Obtain the foal whole blood sample (see "Sample Collection").
2. Next, in the foil pouch, remove the Cassette from the foil pouch by tearing at the notched end on the side of the pouch. Discard the Cassette foil pouch and the desiccant inside the pouch.
3. Label or otherwise identify the Cassette so that each foal whole blood sample can be associated with its Cassette.
4. In the kit, take the dilution vial and remove the seal and septum (cap) from the dilution vial.
5. Using a clean pipette provided with the kit, completely depress the bulb, and put the pipette in the foal whole blood sample. Release the bulb, which will allow the sample to be drawn into the pipette. Note: The pipette will not be completely full. Quickly releasing the bulb increases the likelihood that air will be drawn into the pipette which may effect the accuracy of the test.
6. Transfer the foal whole blood sample in the pipette to the dilution vial. Rinse the pipette by repeatedly drawing up and expressing its contents back into the dilution vial.
7. Put the septum (cap) on the dilution vial and invert several times to thoroughly mix the sample. Avoid shaking.
8. Once the sample is thoroughly mixed, remove the septum from the dilution vial. Using the pipette from step 5 and 6, completely depress the bulb and submerge the pipette into the diluted sample in the dilution vial. Gently release the bulb, which will allow the diluted sample to be drawn into the pipette.
9. Express 2 to 4 drops of the diluted sample into the sample well of the Cassette (marked "S"), making sure that the Cassette is on a level surface. Allow the test to proceed for 20 minutes, then read the results. For accuracy, do not read the results before 20 minutes or after 40 minutes.

Test Interpretation:

Step 3: Interpretation of Test Results

Example of WHOLE BLOOD FOAL IgG MIDLAND QUICK TEST KIT™ cassette results (Control = "C", Test = "T" and Sample = "S"):

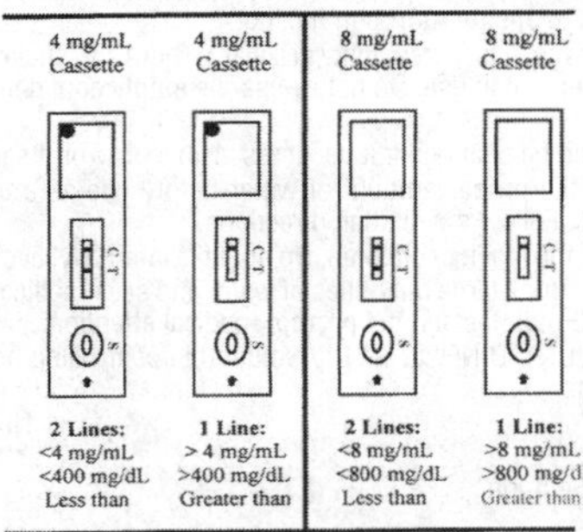

Storage: Avoid prolonged temperature and humidity extremes.

Do not remove the cassette from the foil pouch until ready for use.

Even though the foil pouch includes a desiccant packet, exposure to high humidity conditions should be minimized.

If the buffer in the dilution vial freezes, thaw before using.

Caution(s): Do not use components past expiration date and do not mix components from kits from different lot numbers.

The dilution vial in this kit contains sodium azide. Sodium azide may react with lead or copper plumbing to form highly explosive metal azides. On disposal, flush with a large volume of water to prevent azide build-up. For further information, refer to the manual issued by the Centers for Disease Control.

Do not ingest the desiccant or the buffer solution.

Dispose of all kit components in an appropriate manner.

Discussion: Failure of Passive Transfer (FPT): Foals are born devoid of any detectable level of immunoglobulin G (IgG). The neonatal foal's immunity to infectious agents relies on the ingestion and absorption of maternal IgG from colostrum in mother's milk. This process, termed passive transfer, is a critical determinant of foal health. Failure of passive transfer (FPT) may occur as a result of inadequate suckling, poor absorption of IgG, low levels of IgG in colostrum, or environmental stress.[2] FPT in foals ranges as high as 24%.[3] As a result, the foal is at a greater risk of developing severe respiratory illness, diarrhea and other septicemic illnesses.[3,4,5,6]

The foal's ability to absorb IgG is optimal at birth and progressively declines in absorptive efficiency. The highest rate of absorption occurs during the first 12 hours. From 12 to 24 hours there is a substantial decline in absorption. Estimated closure time for IgG is approximately 24 hours.[3,7]

Studies have identified the specific concentrations of IgG that indicate adequate passive transfer.[6,7,8] Serum IgG concentration: less than 4 mg/mL (400 mg/dL) are considered to show FPT. While serum IgG concentrations between 4 mg/mL (400 mg/dL) and 8 mg/mL (800 mg/dL) may have an adequate level of immunity, they are considered to have partial failure of passive transfer (PFPT). Serum IgG concentrations above 8 mg/mL (800 mg/dL) are considered to have an adequate level of immunity.

The rapid identification of foals with adequate IgG levels can be used to assess management and husbandry practices. In addition, if low IgG levels are detected, intervention strategies may be developed in conjunction with your health professional to optimize foal health and farm productivity.

References: Available upon request.

Presentation: Kits are packaged and sold in the following sizes:
4 mg/mL (400 mg/dL): Packages of 6, 12 and 24 tests.
8 mg/mL (800 mg/dL): Packages of 6, 12 and 24 tests.

Patent Pending

Compendium Code No.: 15010032 9047 rev. 0

WILDNIL™ Ⓒ

Wildlife **Tranquilizer**

Carfentanil Citrate Sterile Injection

NADA No.: 139-633

Active Ingredient(s): Carfentanil citrate is methyl 4-(1-oxopropyl) phenylaminol-1-(2 phenylethyl)-4-piperidinecarboxylate-2 hydroxy-1, 2, 3-propanetricarboxylate (1:1).

Each mL contains:

Carfentanil citrate (equivalent to 3 mg carfentanil) . . . . 4.46 mg
Sodium chloride . . . . 8 mg
Methylparaben . . . . 1.8 mg
Propylparaben . . . . 0.2 mg

In water for injection.

Indications: Carfentanil citrate is for the immobilization of free ranging or confined members of the family cervidae (deer, elk, moose).

Pharmacology: Carfentanil citrate is a synthetic opiate with a clinical potency 10,000 times that of morphine.[1] Carfentanil citrate is a Schedule II Controlled drug substance.

Structural Formula:

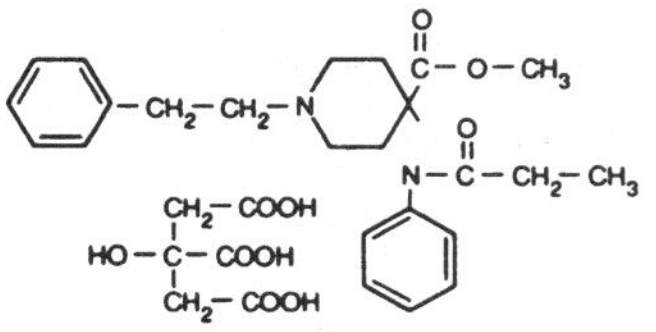

Carfentanil citrate has a morphine-like analgesic mode of action and produces rapid immobilization following intramuscular injection.

Dosage and Administration:

a. Recommended Dose Range for Cervidae:

Species	Dose (mg/kg)
Moose *(Alces americana)*	.006 - .014
Elk *(Cervus elaphus)*	.005 - .020
Axis deer *(Axis axis)*	.005 - .010
Sitka deer *(Odocoileus hemionus sitkensis)*	.005 - .011

For members of the family Cervidae, a dose range of .005-.020 mg/kg has been found to be safe and effective. Immobilization is usually achieved 2 to 10 minutes following administration. The lower end of the dose range is suggested for those animals of quiet temperament, under confinement, that have not been pursued prior to administration of the drug, or in poor physical condition. The upper dose range is suggested for animals of excitable temperament following extensive pursuit or in instances where an extremely short time to effect is desirable.

Some exotic species of deer (Elks, Pampas, Muntjac, and Indian hog deer) may require a higher dose for immobilization. The highest dose required for immobilization in clinical trials was 0.064 mg/kg in Muntjac deer.

The most effective dose rate will vary due to conditions of use. The upper end of the dose range may also be appropriate for animals being pursued by vehicle or aircraft when an extremely quick knockdown time is desired or when individuals are known to be highly excitable. In all instances, all factors including nutritional, reproductive and health status of an animal as well as environmental conditions (temperature, cover and terrain) must be evaluated by the user and best professional judgement used.

b. Administration:

Inject dose deep into a large muscle mass of the neck, shoulder, back or hindquarter. Intrathoracic, intra-abdominal or subcutaneous injection is to be avoided. To ensure proper dosage for animals weighing less than 50 kg, remove required calculated dose of carfentanil citrate with a tuberculin syringe. Dilute to appropriate volume with sterile water for injection prior to administration.

For administration to free-range animals or captive animals, request information on Dan-Inject equipment.

Contraindication(s): Do not use carfentanil citrate in animals that display clinical signs of severe cardiovascular or respiratory disease or impairment. Available data are inadequate to recommend use of carfentanil citrate in pregnant animals. Avoid using during breeding season. Never use carfentanil citrate unless the antidote or antagonist is on hand.

Precaution(s): Store at controlled room temperature (59-86°F) in a facility consistent with appropriate Drug Enforcement Agency regulations regarding Schedule II Class drugs. Protect from prolonged exposure to excessive heat.

Caution(s): Federal law restricts this drug to use by or on the order of a licensed veterinarian.

The licensed veterinarian shall be engaged in zoo and exotic animal practice, wildlife management programs or research.

Veterinarians using carfentanil citrate should be familiar with clinical procedures such as measurement of pulse and respiration, prevention of aspiration, relief of bloat, obstetrics, control of shock and hemorrhage, recognition of hyperventilation and heat exhaustion, the immobilization of fractures, etc. In cases of severe excitement during induction or delayed recovery, continued observation is necessary to correct any of the above and to ensure the animal does not injure itself.

Adequate ventilation - especially in cages or crates - is mandatory; keep head and neck in position to ensure patent air passage and to prevent aspiration of stomach contents.

In animals that are recumbent for a considerable length of time, care should be taken to avoid eye damage; shading to prevent retinal burning is advisable and a bland opthalmic ointment is beneficial. Predatory birds such as magpies have been known to peck at the eyes of recumbent animals. Following carfentanil citrate administration, a brief period of visual adjustment occurs and it may be necessary to direct animals away from hazards such as water, ravines, trees, etc.

Care should be used not to dart animals in the abdomen (intraperitoneally) or against bone. The ideal locations are the heavy muscles of the shoulder or rump. Use a heavy initial dose and avoid subsequent fractional doses. Injection into fat depots results in slow absorption; use needles of adequate length.

As with any anesthetic or immobilization procedure in wild or exotic species, extreme care must be exercised when the drug is used during high environmental temperatures or following extended pursuit or any other activity that may result in elevated body temperatures. Supplies and equipment to shade the animal and control hyperthermia should be available when using carfentanil citrate during periods of hot weather. High ambient temperatures increase risk when using carfentanil citrate. Spraying and/or shading animals is useful to lower body temperature. Never use when the temperature is over 100°F and restrict use to days when temperature is less than 85°F. High humidity and/or extreme altitude cause stress.

Lateral recumbency is hazardous in all ruminants. When using carfentanil citrate, one must be prepared to employ proper procedures to handle problems resulting from lateral or sternal recumbency. Lateral recumbency may call for immediate position correction and injection of the antidote diprenorphine. Animals in or near water may require immediate assistance to prevent drowning or aspiration.

Prolonged periods of lateral recumbency in heavy animals have caused radial paralysis. Adequate padding may be helpful and diprenorphine should be administered as soon as feasible.

Animals that exhibit hyperexcitability, anxiety and hyperventilation should either: Be given one additional dose of carfentanil citrate to quiet them to prevent excessive hyperventilation and alkalosis or administered diprenorphine as an antidote.

The transportation of animals given carfentanil citrate requires careful surveillance to prevent excessive struggling, injury or death. Do not transport more than one animal in a sling, stall or crate.

Antidote(s): Naltrexone HCl is antidotal and rapidly reverses the effect of carfentanil citrate. Administer 100 mg of naltrexone HCl for each milligram of carfentanil citrate. The calculated dose of antagonist may be administered ¼ intravenously and ¾ subcutaneously. Intramuscular administration may be employed if a slower recovery is desired. Reversal of the effects of carfentanil citrate are usually observed in 2 to 10 minutes.

Warning(s): Carfentanil is an extremely potent drug and must be handled with extreme care to avoid risk to users. Avoid accidental administration to humans. Please read human warning section carefully.

Do not administer 45 days before or during hunting season. Do not use in domestic animals intended for food.

Carfentanil citrate must never be used unless adequate amounts of the reversal agent, naltrexone HCl, are immediately available.

Human Warnings:

Treatment of Accidental Human Exposure: Carfentanil citrate is an extremely potent drug and is to be used only by individuals experienced in handling potent immobilizing agents in zoos, exotic animal and wildlife practices, wildlife management procedures and biological research.

As with all potent drugs capable of producing rapid immobilization in wild animals, carfentanil citrate must be treated with extreme respect and caution. Human safety is critical.

Since carfentanil citrate may be employed in locations distant from emergency medical facilities, users must always observe the following precautions:

1. User should seek professional medical attention immediately if the drug is accidentally ingested or injected.
2. At least two people in the field team should be able to recognize signs of toxicity if accidental exposure should occur. They should be familiar with emergency, cardiopulmonary resuscitation procedures plus have first aid kits containing resuscitation aids available.
3. Work in pairs when loading syringes or darts with carfentanil citrate. Wear rubber gloves when loading syringes to avoid accidental spills on hands.
4. Do not spray, squirt or spill the drug when filling syringes.
5. Wash at once with large volumes of water if WILDNIL™ (carfentanil citrate) comes in contact with skin or mucous membranes.
6. Practice good medical techniques. Do not become careless. Do not hold used needles in mouth. Always ensure that darts and syringes contain proper dose.
7. All reasonable efforts should be made to locate and retrieve any loaded darts that missed the target animal.
8. Respect all dart guns, darts and power delivery syringes as though they were cocked and loaded.

Information for Physicians: Carfentanil citrate is a powerful synthetic opiate. Accidental human exposure may produce severe central nervous system depression resulting in respiratory depression or failure followed by coma. Depending on route of administration, effects may be noted within 2 to 30 minutes. Treatment should start immediately by administering an appropriate opiate antagonist providing airway support, plus cardiopulmonary resuscitation techniques.

Side Effects: Seven drug related fatalities were reported during clinical trials that involved the immobilization of 509 members of the family Cervidae (deer, elk, moose). Mortalities were attributed to hyperthermia, acute myopathy and/or narcotic recycling in 3.8% (6/158) of moose and less than 1% (1/295) of elk immobilized in clinical trials.

Other reported adverse reactions were as follows: tachycardia, tachypnea, excitement during induction, respiratory depression, erratic breathing, thrashing, struggling, hiccuping, padding, torticollis, penile prolapse, excessive salivation, regurgitation of rumen contents and delayed renarcotization. Signs of acute toxicity may include extreme respiratory or cardiovascular depression. Antagonist or antidote should be administered immediately to effect.

References: Available upon request.

Presentation: Carfentanil citrate is supplied in a 10 mL multiple use vial.

™ Registered trademark of Janssen Pharmaceutica, Beerse, Belgium.

Compendium Code No.: 10520040

WIND-AID®

Hawthorne **Antitussive**

Breathing Aid

Active Ingredient(s):

	Each 1 U.S. fl oz contains:	Each 32 U.S. fl oz contains:
Potassium iodide	1.9 g	30.6 g

Eucalyptus oil, peppermint oil, glycerine in aqueous base.

Indications: For use as an aid for the relief of equine bronchial congestion, minor throat irritation and minor wind problems.

Dosage and Administration: Shake well.

For minor wind problems, administer two ounces orally with dose syringe two hours prior to exercise or racing.

For equine bronchial congestion with minor wind problems, give two ounces orally two or three times daily.

Caution(s): Keep away from children. For veterinary use only.

Presentation: 1 U.S. fl oz syringe and 32 U.S. fl oz.

Compendium Code No.: 10670110

WINSTROL®-V STERILE SUSPENSION Ⓒⅲ

Pharmacia & Upjohn **Anabolic Agent**

Stanozolol

NADA No.: 030-844

Active Ingredient(s): WINSTROL®-V Sterile Suspension contains 50 mg stanozolol per mL.

Indications: Anabolic therapy with WINSTROL®-V Sterile Suspension is indicated whenever excessive tissue breakdown or extensive repair processes are proceeding. Such processes usually diminish protein reserves in the tissues, thus leading to negative nitrogen balance. WINSTROL®-V is indicated to reverse tissue-depleting processes and restore constructive metabolism. Anabolic therapy is intended primarily as an adjunct to other specific and supportive therapy, including nutrition therapy. Optimal results can be expected only when dietary intake is adequate and well balanced.

Dogs and Cats: WINSTROL®-V Sterile Suspension is indicated when the therapeutic objective is to improve appetite, promote weight gain, and increase strength and vitality. For these reasons WINSTROL®-V is recommended for anorexia, unthriftiness, weight loss, debility, cachexia, inanition and poor hair coat when these accompany disease, trauma, or old age. Since certain skin conditions occurring in older dogs (alopecia and some types of eczema, for example) are caused by metabolic disorders based on negative nitrogen balance, WINSTROL®-V may help to control such conditions.

Horses: WINSTROL®-V Sterile Suspension is recommended as an aid for treating debilitated horses when the therapeutic objective is to improve appetite, promote weight gain, improve general physical conditions, and accelerate recovery. Clinical conditions most amenable to treatment are debilitated states resulting from illness, surgery, traumatic injuries, or plain overwork. In clinical investigations, the administration of WINSTROL®-V frequently had a marked effect on horses exhibiting diminished vitality and vigor due to overexertion.

Pharmacology: WINSTROL®-V Sterile Suspension contains stanozolol which is 17-methyl-2'*H*-5α-androst-2-eno[3,2-c] pyrazol-17β-ol. It is a member of a unique series of heterocyclic steroids synthesized at the Sterling-Winthrop Research Institute. The unique endocrinologic activity of this compound was produced by the fusion of a pyrazole ring to a steroid nucleus. When administered to animals, WINSTROL®-V was found to have an unusual pattern of biologic activity in that its anabolic (tissue-building) effect far outweighed its weak androgenic (masculinizing) influence.

Clinical Pharmacology: WINSTROL®-V Sterile Suspension is classified as "anabolic steroid" because of the pronounced stimulatory effects on constructive metabolism. Stanozolol increases the retention of nitrogen and minerals, reverses tissue-depleting processes, and promotes better utilization of dietary protein. Its anabolic effects lead to improvement in appetite, increased vigor, and notable gains in weight. In this respect, it differs greatly from other steroids, such as the androgens, estrogens, and corticosteroids. Methyltestosterone also possesses anabolic action, but its predominant androgenic activity makes it unsuitable for long-term anabolic therapy. Although the frequently undesirable virilizing effects of the male sex hormones may be overcome by androgen-estrogen combinations, this does not improve their anabolic function. The corticosteroids (cortisone, prednisone, prednisolone, dexamethasone) comprise an entirely different group of steroids, which are well known for their anti-inflammatory and antirheumatic activities. As a rule, prolonged use of the corticosteroids results in a catabolic (tissue-wasting) effect which may be relieved by anabolic therapy.

In a wide variety of tests in animals, WINSTROL®-V was shown to possess high anabolic potency, whereas its androgenic effect was very low. Extensive clinical investigations by veterinary practitioners have confirmed its anabolic action and therapeutic usefulness in dogs, cats, and horses.

Dosage and Administration: Whenever indicated, anabolic therapy should be prescribed in conjunction with or as a follow-up to other therapeutic measures.

Dogs and Cats: Because WINSTROL®-V Sterile Suspension is absorbed slowly, injections may be given at weekly intervals. The suspension is best administered by deep intramuscular injection into the thigh. The recommended dose for cats and small breeds of dogs is 0.5 mL (25 mg) and for larger dogs, 1 mL (50 mg). If desired, Winstrol®-V Tablets and WINSTROL®-V Sterile Suspension can be combined in a regimen of therapy. Many investigating clinicians gave an initial dose of the injectable form and then dispensed tablets for daily administration at home.

Horses: Only WINSTROL®-V Sterile Suspension is recommended for administration to horses. The recommended dose is 25 mg per 100 pounds of body weight intramuscularly, equivalent to 5 mL (250 mg) for a 1,000 pound animal. Deep intramuscular injection in the gluteal region is recommended. Medication may be repeated at weekly intervals up to and including four weeks. In clinical trials, many animals required no more than one or two doses to achieve desirable therapeutic results.

Contraindication(s): Because the data regarding use during pregnancy are insufficient, WINSTROL®-V Sterile Suspension should not be administered to pregnant dogs and cats. In the absence of data on the effects of WINSTROL®-V Sterile Suspension on stallions and pregnant mares or the teratogenicity on offspring, WINSTROL®-V should not be used in these animals.

Precaution(s): Store at controlled room temperature 20° to 25°C (68° to 77°F) [USP].

Caution(s): Federal (USA) law restricts this drug to use by or on the order of a licensed veterinarian.

When receiving anabolic therapy, animals with impaired cardiac and renal function should be watched closely for the possibility of sodium and water retention. Special caution should be exercised in aged dogs suffering from chronic interstitial nephritis. In such cases, the progress of the disorder should be checked by means of laboratory tests and treatment discontinued if the drug appears to aggravate the disease.

Warning(s): Not for use in horses intended for food. Not for human use. Keep out of reach of children.

Side Effects: Mild androgenic effects may be noted after prolonged therapy with excessively high doses.

Presentation: WINSTROL®-V Sterile Suspension is available in 10 mL and 30 mL multiple-dose vials.

Manufactured by: Abbott Laboratories.

Compendium Code No.: 10490520

WINSTROL®-V TABLETS Ⓒⅲ

Pharmacia & Upjohn **Anabolic Agent**

Stanozolol

NADA No.: 015-506

Active Ingredient(s): Each scored tablet contains 2 mg stanozolol.

Indications: Anabolic therapy with WINSTROL®-V Tablets is indicated whenever excessive tissue breakdown or extensive repair processes are proceeding. Such processes usually diminish protein reserves in the tissues, thus leading to negative nitrogen balance. WINSTROL®-V is indicated to reverse tissue-depleting processes and restore constructive metabolism. Anabolic therapy is intended primarily as an adjunct to other specific and supportive therapy, including nutrition therapy. Optimal results can be expected only when dietary intake is adequate and well balanced.

Dogs and Cats: WINSTROL®-V Tablets are indicated when the therapeutic objective is to improve appetite, promote weight gain, and increase strength and vitality. For these reasons WINSTROL®-V is recommended for anorexia, unthriftiness, weight loss, debility, cachexia, inanition and poor hair coat when these accompany disease, trauma, or old age. Since certain skin conditions occurring in older dogs (alopecia and some types of eczema, for example) are caused by metabolic disorders based on negative nitrogen balance, WINSTROL®-V may help to control such conditions.

Pharmacology: WINSTROL®-V Tablets contain stanozolol which is 17-methyl-2'*H* 5α-androst-2-eno[3,2-c] pyrazol-17β-ol. It is a member of a unique series of heterocyclic steroids synthesized at the Sterling-Winthrop Research Institute. The unique endocrinologic activity of this compound was produced by the fusion of a pyrazole ring to a steroid nucleus. When administered to animals, WINSTROL®-V was found to have an unusual pattern of biologic activity in that its anabolic (tissue-building) effect far outweighed its weak androgenic (masculinizing) influence.

Clinical Pharmacology: WINSTROL®-V Tablets are classified as "anabolic steroids" because of their pronounced stimulatory effects on constructive metabolism. Stanozolol increases the retention of nitrogen and minerals, reverses tissue-depleting processes, and promotes better utilization of dietary protein. Its anabolic effects lead to improvement in appetite, increased vigor, and notable gains in weight. In this respect, it differs greatly from other steroids, such as the androgens, estrogens, and corticosteroids. Methyltestosterone also possesses anabolic action, but its predominant androgenic activity makes it unsuitable for long-term anabolic therapy. Although the frequently undesirable virilizing effects of the male sex hormones may be overcome by androgen-estrogen combinations, this does not improve their anabolic function. The corticosteroids (cortisone, prednisone, prednisolone, dexamethasone) comprise an entirely different group of steroids, which are well known for their anti-inflammatory and antirheumatic activities. As a rule, prolonged use of the corticosteroids results in a catabolic (tissue-wasting) effect which may be relieved by anabolic therapy.

In a wide variety of tests in animals, WINSTROL®-V was shown to possess high anabolic potency, whereas its androgenic effect was very low. Extensive clinical investigations by veterinary practitioners have confirmed its anabolic action and therapeutic usefulness in dogs and cats.

Dosage and Administration: Whenever indicated, anabolic therapy should be prescribed in conjunction with or as a follow-up to other therapeutic measures.

Dogs and Cats: The suggested oral dose for cats and small breeds of dogs is ½ to 1 tablet twice daily and for large breeds of dogs, 1 to 2 tablets twice daily, depending on body weight. If preferred, the WINSTROL®-V Tablets can be crushed and administered in feed. Treatment should be continued for at least several weeks, depending on the condition and response of the animal. In certain chronic conditions, especially in aged dogs, treatment can be continued for several months without untoward reactions.

If desired, WINSTROL®-V Tablets and Winstrol®-V Sterile Suspension can be combined in a regimen of therapy. Many investigating clinicians gave an initial dose of the injectable form and then dispensed tablets for daily administration at home.

Contraindication(s): Because the data regarding use during pregnancy are insufficient, WINSTROL®-V should not be administered to pregnant dogs and cats.

Precaution(s): Store at controlled room temperature 20° to 25°C (68° to 77°F) [see USP].

Caution(s): Federal (USA) law restricts this drug to use by or on the order of a licensed veterinarian.

When receiving anabolic therapy, animals with impaired cardiac and renal function should be watched closely for the possibility of sodium and water retention. Special caution should be exercised in aged dogs suffering from chronic interstitial nephritis. In such cases, the progress of the disorder should be checked by means of laboratory tests and treatment discontinued if the drug appears to aggravate the disease.

Warning(s): Not for human use. Keep out of reach of children.

Adverse Reactions: Mild androgenic effects may be noted after prolonged therapy with excessively high doses.

Presentation: WINSTROL®-V Tablets are available in bottles of 500 tablets.

Manufactured by: Searle, Ltd. Puerto Rico, Inc.

Compendium Code No.: 10490530

WIPE® FLY PROTECTANT

Farnam **Parasiticide-Topical**

EPA Reg. No.: 270-37

Active Ingredient(s):

Pyrethrins	0.20%
*Piperonyl Butoxide, Technical	0.50%
Di-n-propyl isocinchomeronate	1.00%
Butoxypolypropylene Glycol	20.00%
Inert Ingredients	78.30%
Total	100.00%

*Equivalent to 0.4% (butylcarbityl) (6-propylpiperonyl) ether and 0.1% of related compounds.

Indications: WIPE® Fly Protectant provides effective, long-lasting fly protection for horses and ponies. Repels horse flies, house flies, stable flies, deer flies, gnats, and mosquitoes. Also kills them on contact. Actually helps remove dirt and dandruff, imparts a high sheen to the hair when brushed out. Has a light, bright, pleasing fragrance.

Directions for Use: It is a violation of Federal law to use this product in a manner inconsistent with its labeling.

Shake well before using.

Before applying WIPE® to your horse, brush him down thoroughly to remove loose dust and dirt.

Moisten, but do not soak, a folded piece of Turkish toweling (approximately 12" x 15") or an Applicator Mitt with WIPE®. Rub briskly against the growth direction of the hair. Give special attention to the shanks, legs, shoulders, neck and facial areas of the horse where flies tend to cause the greatest problems. Add more WIPE® to the applicator as needed, applying approximately one to two ounces for the total application on a daily basis (the variance will depend on the size of the horse). Groom with a brush. To killed attached ticks, dab WIPE® directly on the tick with a saturated cloth.

(After long-standing non-use, mix contents by inverting several times.)

A Few Important Points to Remember:

- To keep applicator moist, keep in an airtight container between uses.
- Daily applications of WIPE® may build up repellency allowing a reduction in amount used in subsequent applications.
- Apply in early morning for maximum efficacy.
- The amount of WIPE® needed depends on temperature, humidity, and cleanliness of the horse's coat. Experiment with the amount applied to determine how much your horse needs.

Use only Turkish toweling or Wipe® Applicator Mitt (not a substitute material) to apply WIPE®. Avoid excessive amounts of WIPE® on your horse. Do not soak the skin.

Precautionary Statements: Hazards to Humans and Domestic Animals:

Caution: Harmful if swallowed. Keep out of reach of children. Wash hands thoroughly after using.

Environmental Hazards: This product is toxic to fish. Do not apply directly to water. Keep out of lakes, ponds, or streams. Do not contaminate water by cleaning of equipment or disposal of wastes.

Storage and Disposal:

Storage: Store in a cool, dry place.

Pesticide Disposal: Securely wrap original container in several layers of newspaper and discard in trash.

Container Disposal: Do not reuse empty container. Wrap container and put in trash.

Warning(s): Do not apply to horses to be used for food.

Presentation: 16 fl oz (473 mL) 32 fl oz and 1 gallon.

Compendium Code No.: 10000441

WIPE® II BRAND FLY SPRAY WITH CITRONELLA

Farnam **Parasiticide-Topical**

EPA Reg. No.: 270-263

Active Ingredient(s):

Pyrethrins 0.1%
Piperonyl Butoxide Technical* 1.0%
Butoxypolypropylene Glycol 7.5%
Inert Ingredients** 91.4%
Total 100.00%

*Equivalent to 0.8% (butylcarbityl) (6-propylpiperonyl) ether and 0.2% of related compounds.

**Contains Petroleum Distillate

Indications: Kills and repels six fly species, gnats, mosquitoes on horses.

Directions for Use: It is a violation of Federal law to use this product in a manner inconsistent with its labeling.

WIPE® II Brand Fly Spray with Citronella has been especially developed for use on horses. It provides a protective hair coating against flies while imparting a high sheen to the hair when brushed out. 1-2 ounces per head per day gives adequate to protection. Apply by either soft cloth or fine mist spray.

Use to Wipe On: First, brush animal to remove excess dirt and dust. Moisten (but do not wet to the point of dripping) a soft cloth and rub over the hair. It is best to apply by rubbing against the hair growth. Give special attention to the legs, shoulders shanks, neck and facial areas where flies most often are seen.

Only a light application is required. Avoid using an excessive amount on your horses. Do not wet skin.

After application, brush out thoroughly to bring out bright sheen on coat.

Repeat daily or as required.

Use As a Spray: WIPE® II Brand Fly Spray with Citronella may be applied as a fine mist spray to stable area and over and around stabled horses for fast paralysis and kill of flies. Do not wet horse's skin or exceed two ounces per application.

Precautionary Statements: Hazards to Humans and Domestic Animals:

Caution: Harmful if swallowed. Remove or cover exposed foods before spraying. Do not apply to dairy animals.

Statement of Practical Treatment:

If Swallowed: Do not induce vomiting unless directed by a physician. Petroleum distillate may cause aspiration. Contact a physician immediately.

If in Eyes: Flush with plenty of water. Contact a physician if irritation persists.

If Inhaled: Remove victim to fresh air. Apply artificial respiration if indicated.

If on Skin: Remove contaminated clothing and wash affected areas with plenty of soap and water.

Environmental Hazards: This product is toxic to fish. Do not apply directly to water. Do not apply where run-off is likely to occur. Do not contaminate water by cleaning of equipment or disposal of wastes. Apply this product only as specified on the label.

Physical or Chemical Hazards: Do not use or store near heat or open flame.

Storage and Disposal: Do not contaminate water, food or feed by storage or disposal.

Pesticide Storage and Spill Procedure: Store upright at room temperature. In case of spill or leakage, soak up with an absorbent material such as sand, sawdust, earth, fuller's earth, etc. Dispose of with chemical waste.

Pesticide Disposal: Pesticide, spray mixture or rinse water that cannot be used according to label instructions must be disposed of at or by an approved waste disposal facility.

Storage: Store in original container inaccessible to children and pets.

Disposal: Do not reuse container. Wrap container in several layers of newspaper and discard in trash.

Disclaimer: Buyer assumes all risk of use, storage or handling of this product not in strict accordance with directions given herein.

Presentation: 32 fl oz (946.4 mL) refill and sprayer.

Compendium Code No.: 10000451

WIPE OUT® DAIRY WIPES

ImmuCell **Udder Product**

Active Ingredient(s): Nisin 50 µg/mL.

Indications: Proven against the leading organisms that cause mastitis.

Directions for Use:

1. Cut along dotted line.
2. Place refill roll in bucket.
3. Take wipe from center of roll.
4. Pull first wipe through lid opening.
5. Close lid and pull wipe through.

Use one pre-treated WIPE OUT® Dairy Wipe per cow to clean, sanitize and dry the entire teat area, especially at the teat opening. WIPE OUT® Dairy Wipes will leave the teat dry and ready to milk. Use of a paper towel for drying is not required.

Warning(s): The bag is not a toy. Dispose of bag properly to avoid possible suffocation.

Keep this and all medicines out of children's reach,

Presentation: Available in 500-count buckets (4 in a case), or 500-count replacement bags (4 in a case).

WIPE OUT® is a registered trademark of ImmuCell Corporation.

Compendium Code No.: 11200041

WITNESS® CPV

Synbiotics **Parvovirus Test**

Canine Parvovirus Antigen Test Kit

U.S. Vet. Lic. No.: 312A

Kit Contents: 10 pouches, each containing 1 test device.

10 tubes containing 1.0 mL of sample extraction buffer.
10 sampling swabs.
10 transfer pipettes.
Instructions for use.

Indications: For the detection of canine parvovirus antigen.

Test Principles: The WITNESS® CPV test is a simple test, based on rapid immunomigration (RIM) technology, which detects the presence of canine parvovirus antigen in canine feces. Sensitized particles bound to the CPV antigen present within the sample (fecal extract) migrate along a membrane. The complex is then captured on a sensitized reaction zone where its accumulation causes the formation of a clearly visible purple band. A purple band in the control window ensures that the test was performed correctly.

Test Procedure:

1. Sample extraction:

For each sample to be tested, you will need one sampling swab and one tube of pre-dispensed sample extraction buffer. Remove the stopper from the tube. Coat the swab with a thin layer of feces.

Immerse the feces coated swab into the sample extraction buffer in the tube. Swirl the swab in the buffer. Remove as much fecal material from the swab as possible by swirling vigorously and pressing the swab against the side of the tube.

When removing the swab from the test tube, press the swab against the side of the tube repeatedly until no more liquid comes from the swab.

Completely remove the swab from the tube and discard appropriately.

2. Sample application:

For each sample to be tested, you will need one device, one pipette and the tube of extracted sample.

Prepare the device by tearing open the pouch and placing the test device on a flat horizontal surface for the duration of the test.

Squeeze the pipette near the sealed end. Immerse the open end of the pipette into the extracted fecal solution. Release the pressure slightly to draw up a small amount of sample into the pipette.

Holding the pipette vertically, transfer three drops of sample to the sample well, Window #1. Allow sample drops to fall onto membrane at Window #1. Do not touch pipette tip directly to the membrane.

If migration does not pass Window #2 by one minute, add one additional drop of sample.

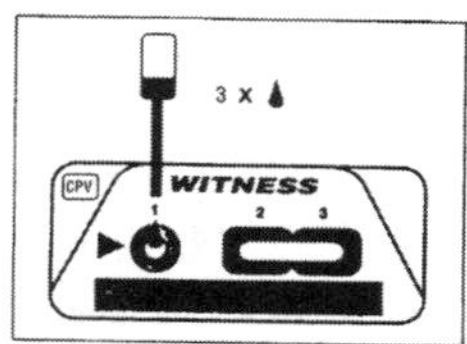

3. Reading test:

Wait five minutes, observe the presence or absence of pink/purple bands in Windows #2 and #3.

Sample results are read in Window #2. The control band is read in Window #3.

Notes: The test is complete and may be read before 5 minutes if pink/purple bands are visible in both Windows #2 and #3. The presence of a pink/purple band only in Window #3 does not mean that the test is complete as a band in Window #2 may develop slower than the time control band in Window #3. Wait a full 5 minutes before declaring a result as negative.

Interpretation of Results: Results:

Validation: Test is validated if a pink/purple band is present in Window #3.

Negative for canine parvovirus (CPV) antigen: No band in Window #2, with one pink/purple band in Window #3.

Positive for CPV antigen: One pink/purple band in Window #2, with one pink/purple band in Window #3.

Invalid test: No pink/purple band in Window #3.

Note: A test result should always be interpreted in the context of all available clinical information and history for the dog.

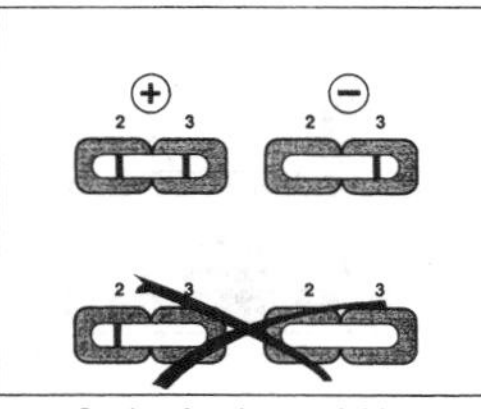

Sample Information and Storage: Canine fecal material is required for this test. Stool samples may be stored at 2°C7°C (35°F45°F) for 48 hours. If longer storage is required, the samples may he frozen.

Caution(s):

Do not use components after expiration date.

Refrigeration is not required. Store the test kit at 2°C25°C (35°F77°F). Do not freeze.

Use the test within 10 minutes after opening the sealed pouch.

Avoid touching or damaging the membrane at Windows #1, #2 or #3.

The WITNESS® CPV device should be placed on a flat horizontal surface while performing the test.

Use a separate extraction pipette for each sample.

Hold extraction pipette vertically when dispensing sample.

For veterinary use only.

Note: Samples from healthy vaccinated animals may falsely produce a positive result when tested 4 to 10 days after canine parvovirus vaccination.

Discussion: Canine Parvovirus (CPV) is a member of the feline parvovirus subgroup. It is closely related to feline panleukopenia virus and mink enteritis virus, and is considered endemic to nearly all populations of domesticated and wild canines.

CPV causes two forms of disease: myocarditis and enteritis. Due to maternal antibody protection, the myocardial form is rare. The enteric form, however, is prevalent and can be fatal to puppies and geriatric dogs. CPV enteritis causes severe, often bloody diarrhea, vomiting, leukopenia and dehydration.

Transmission is fecal-oral and most infections occur from exposure to contaminated feces. CPV is highly contagious and stable under a variety of environmental conditions. Rapid diagnosis of CPV allows for quarantine and prompt treatment of infected dogs. Diagnosis may be difficult in milder cases. WITNESS® CPV detects all strains of canine parvovirus shed in the feces. Positive results with WITNESS® CPV indicate the presence of canine parvovirus.

Presentation: 5 and 10 test kits.

Manufactured by: Agen Biomedical Limited, Australia.

Compendium Code No.: 11150463

WITNESS® FeLV

Synbiotics **FeLV Test**

Feline Leukemia Virus Antigen Test Kit

U.S. Vet. Lic. No.: 312A

Contents: 10 pouches, each containing 1 test device.

10 disposable pipettes.

1 buffer dropper bottle (2.2 mL).

Instructions for use.

Indications: WITNESS® FeLV is indicated for use when history and/or clinical signs may suggest infection by FeLV or as a screening test prior to an FeLV vaccination. Cats should also be tested prior to entry into FeLV negative households or catteries.

Test Principles: WITNESS® FeLV is a simple test, based on rapid immunomigration (RIM) technology, which detects the presence of the FeLV antigen p27 in cats' blood. Sensitized particles bound to p27 antigen present within the sample (whole blood, serum, or plasma) migrate along a nitrocellulose strip. The complex is then captured on a sensitized reaction line where its accumulation causes the formation of a clearly visible pink/purple band. A pink/purple band in the control window ensures that the test was performed correctly.

Test Procedure: Sample Information:

The test can be performed on whole blood, serum, or plasma.

Whole blood samples must be anticoagulated with EDTA or heparin.

Samples should be collected with a sterile needle and syringe.

Hemolysis does not significantly interfere with the test, but strongly hemolyzed samples may partly obscure a weak positive band.

Sample Storage: It is recommended to test samples immediately after collection. If samples are kept at room temperature, they should be tested within 4 hours. If testing is further delayed, samples should be refrigerated at 2-7°C (35-45°F) for up to 2 days. For prolonged storage, samples (serum and plasma only) should be kept frozen at -20°C (-4°F).

Important: Allow sample and buffer drops to fall onto membrane at window #1. Do not touch pipette tip, sample or buffer drops, or buffer bottle tip directly to the membrane.

1. Sample application:

   Tear open the pouch provided and place the test device on a flat horizontal surface for the duration of the test.

   Squeeze the provided pipette near the sealed end. Insert the open end of the pipette into an anticoagulated whole blood, serum, or plasma sample. Release the pressure slightly to draw up a small amount of sample into the pipette.

   Holding the pipette vertically, transfer one drop of sample to the sample well, window #1.

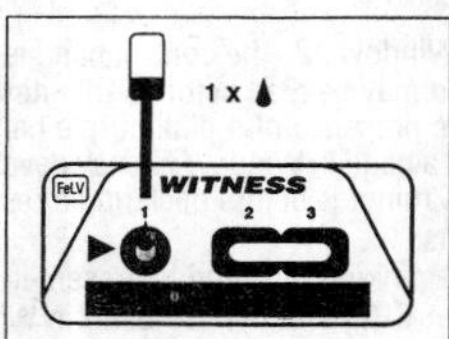

2. Buffer dispensing:

   Remove the cap from the buffer bottle, hold it vertically and add two drops of buffer to the sample well window #1.

   If migration does not pass window #2 by one minute, add one additional drop of buffer.

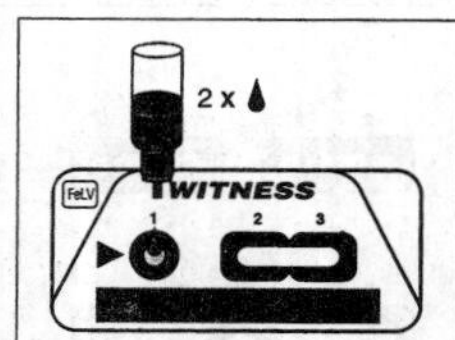

3. Reading test:

   Wait five minutes, observe the presence or absence of pink/purple bands in reading windows #2 and #3.

   Sample results are read in window #2. The control band is read in window #3

Notes:

The test is complete and may be read before 5 minutes if pink/purple bands are visible in both windows #2 and #3.

The presence of a pink/purple band only in window #3 before 5 minutes does not mean that the test is complete. A pink/purple band in window #2 may develop slower than the control pink/purple band in window #3.

Test Interpretation:

Validation:

Valid test: Test is validated if a pink/purple band is present in the reading window #3.

Interpretation:

Negative for FeLV antigen: No band in reading window #2, with one pink/purple band in window #3.

Positive for FeLV antigen: One pink/purple band in reading window #2, with one pink/purple band in window #3.

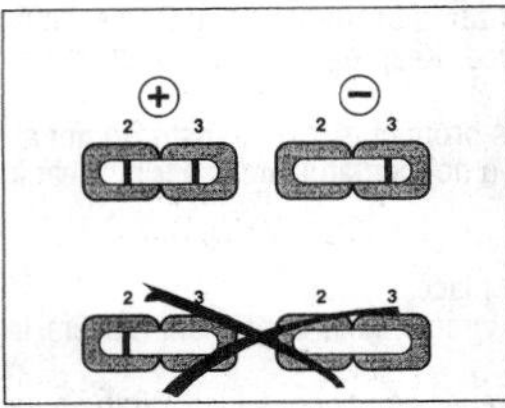

Invalid Test:

Invalid test: No pink/purple band in control window #3.

Note: A test result should always be interpreted in the context of all available clinical information and history for the cat being tested.

Caution(s): Do not use components after expiration date.

Refrigeration not required. Store the test kit at 2-25°C (35-77°F). Do not freeze.

Use the test within 10 minutes after opening the sealed pouch.

Avoid touching or damaging membrane at windows #1, #2, #3.

The WITNESS® device should be placed on a flat, horizontal surface while performing the test.

Use a separate pipette for each sample.

Hold pipette and buffer bottle vertically when dispensing sample and buffer.

Handle all samples as if capable of transmitting FeLV.

For veterinary use only.

Note: Prior to use, test and control bands appear yellow. The bands are dyed yellow for quality control purposes. The dye does not interfere with the test results and will wash away while the test is developing.

Discussion: Feline Leukemia Virus (FeLV) is a contagious retrovirus which is endemic particularly among high density or close contact cat populations in many areas of the world. Transmission occurs essentially by contact, mainly through saliva or nasal secretions and by biting or licking. One major source of the virus is persistently viremic, mostly clinically healthy, carrier rats. Vertical (congenital) transmission is also described. A variety of outcomes are possible after cats are exposed to FeLV. Infected cats can become persistently viremic, and many of these cats will die from non-neoplastic diseases. Exposed cats may also develop immunity through the production of virus neutralizing antibodies. Some cats develop an atypical infection where viral replication incompletely contained with intermittent antigenemia and occasional shedding of virus. Diagnosis of FeLV infection is usually by detection of the viral antigen, p27, which is in high quantities in the blood of viremic cats.

Presentation: 10 test kits.

Manufactured by: AGEN Biomedical Limited, Brisbane, Australia 4110

Compendium Code No.: 11150471

WITNESS® FHW

Synbiotics **Heartworm Test**

Feline Heartworm Antibody Test Kit

U.S. Vet. Lic. No.: 312A

Kit Contents: 5 or 25 pouches, each containing 1 test device; 5 or 25 disposable pipettes; 1 buffer dropper bottle (2.2 mL); Instructions for use.

Indications: A large percentage of naturally infected cats test antigen negative due to low worm burdens and low levels of detectable circulating antigen. Clinical signs and serology must be considered in the event of a negative antigen assay. Antibody can develop in response to precardiac heartworm larvae that never complete their development. When used in conjunction with other tests and the evaluation of clinical signs, the antibody test aids in the correct diagnosis of infection. In contrast, a negative antibody test provides strong evidence that a cat is not currently infected.

Test Principles: WITNESS® FHW is a simple test, based on rapid immunomigration (RIM) technology, using highly specific recombinant antigen to quickly identify antibodies in heartworn infected cats. Sensitized colloidal gold particles bound to anti-FHW antibodies present within the sample (whole blood, serum, or plasma) migrate along a nitrocellulose strip. The complex is then captured on a sensitized reaction line where its accumulation causes the formation of a clearly visible pink/purple band. A pink/purple band in the control window ensures that the test was performed correctly.

Test Procedure: Sample Information:

The test can be performed on whole blood, serum, or plasma.

Whole blood samples must be anticoagulated with EDTA or heparin.

Samples should be collected with a sterile needle and syringe.

Hemolysis does not significantly interfere with the test, but strongly hemolyzed samples may partly obscure a weak positive band.

Important: Allow sample and buffer drops to fall onto membrane at window #1. Do not touch pipette tip, sample or buffer drops, or buffer bottle tip directly to the membrane.

1. Sample application

   Tear open the pouch provided and place the test device on a flat horizontal surface for the duration of the test.

   Squeeze the provided pipette near the sealed end. Insert the open end of the pipette into an anticoagulated whole blood, serum, or plasma sample. Release the pressure slightly to draw up a small amount of sample into the pipette.

   Holding the pipette vertically, transfer one drop of sample to the sample well, window #1.

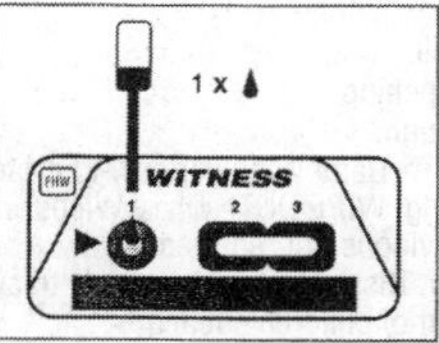

2. Buffer dispensing

   Remove the cap from the buffer bottle, hold it vertically and add two drops of buffer to the sample well window #1.

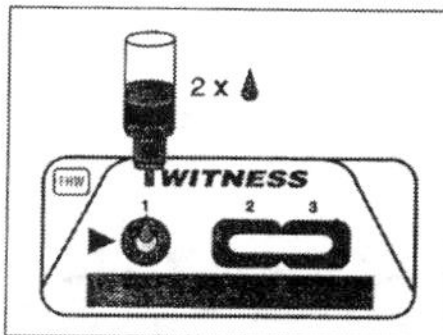

3. Reading test

Wait five minutes, observe the presence or absence of pink/purple bands in reading windows #2 and #3.

Sample results are read in window #2. The control band is read in window #3.

Notes: The test is complete and may be read before 5 minutes if pink/purple bands are visible in both windows #2 and #3.

The presence of a pink/purple band only in window #3 before 5 minutes does not mean that the test is complete. A pink/purple band in window #2 may develop slower than the control pink/purple band in window #3.

Interpretation of Results: Validation:

Valid test: Test is validated if a pink/purple band is present in the reading window #3.

Interpretation:

Negative for *D. immitis* antibodies: No band in reading window #2, with one pink/purple band in window #3.

Positive for *D. immitis* antibodies: One pink/purple band in reading window #2, with one pink/purple band in window #3.

Invalid Test

Invalid test: No pink/purple band in control window #3.

Note: A test result should always be interpreted in the context of all available clinical information and history for the cat being tested.

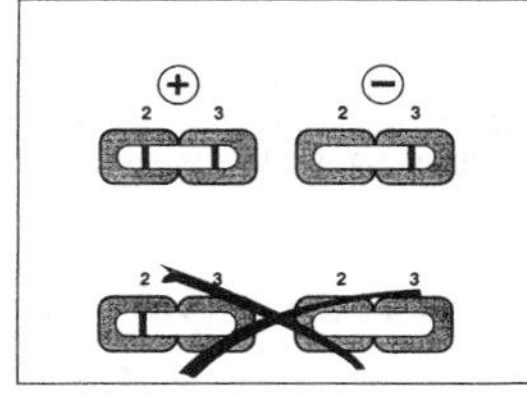

Storage: Sample Storage: It is recommended to test samples immediately after collection. If samples are kept at room temperature, they should be tested within 4 hours. If testing is further delayed, samples should be refrigerated at 2-7°C (35-45°F) for up to 7 days. For prolonged storage, samples (serum and plasma only) should be kept frozen at -20°C (-4°F).

Disposal of Samples and Test Devices: Handle all samples as if capable of transmitting disease. Dispose of samples and used devices appropriately.

Refrigeration not required. Store the test kit at 2-25°C (35-77°F). Do not freeze.

Caution(s): Do not use components after expiration date.

Use the test within 10 minutes after opening the sealed pouch.

Avoid touching or damaging membrane at windows #1, #2, #3.

The WITNESS® device should be placed on a flat, horizontal surface while performing the test.

Use a separate pipette for each sample.

Hold pipette and buffer bottle vertically when dispensing sample and buffer.

Handle all samples as if capable of transmitting disease.

For veterinary use only.

Note: Prior to use, test and control bands appear yellow. The bands are dyed yellow for quality control purposes. The dye does not interfere with the test results and will wash away while the test is developing.

Discussion: General Information: Feline heartworm (FHW) disease has reached worldwide distribution and is caused by the filarial nematode *Dirofilaria immitis*. More cats presenting with coughing, intermittent vomiting, abnormal heart and lung sounds are being diagnosed with FHW. Heartworm infection is more difficult to detect in cats due to fewer worms present and lower incidence of circulating microfilaria.

The effect that heartworm has in cats is often more significant than in dogs being due mainly to the cats intense response to the parasite and their smaller body size. A true prevalence of heartworm in cats may be understated due to their greater tendency to either spontaneously eliminate the parasite or die from the infection. The life span of the parasite is typically shorter in cats and infections may be self limiting after 2 or 3 years although heartworms are capable of causing severe disease.

Presentation: 5 or 25 test kits.

Manufactured by: AGEN Biomedical Limited, Brisbane, Australia 4110.

Compendium Code No.: 11150491 RM 1027-A, Rev. 03/00

WITNESS® HW

Synbiotics **Heartworm Test**

Canine Heartworm Antigen Test Kit

U.S. Vet. Lic. No.: 312A

Test Description: Canine heartworm antigen test kit.

Contents: 10 or 25 pouches, each containing 1 test device; 10 or 25 disposable pipettes; 1 buffer dropper bottle (2.2 mL); Instructions for use.

Indications: An early and accurate heartworm diagnosis in an infected dog will allow treatment before the appearance of serious cardiovascular symptoms. The WITNESS® HW test for the detection of the soluble *D. immitis* antigen is recommended for use when clinical history and/or clinical signs suggest heartworm disease. The performance of the WITNESS® HW test is independent of circulating microfilariae and can be used to detect amicrofilaraemic or "occult" infections, or for rapid screening for heartworm infection.

Test Principles: The WITNESS® HW test is a simple test, based on rapid immunomigration (RIM) technology, which detects the presence of adult *D. immitis* antigen in dogs' blood. Sensitized particles bound to the heartworm antigen present within the sample (whole blood, serum or plasma) migrate along a nitrocellulose strip. The complex is then captured on a sensitized reaction zone where its accumulation causes the formation of a clearly visible pink/purple band. A pink/purple band in the control window ensures that the test was performed correctly.

Test Procedure: Sample Information:

The test can be performed on whole blood, serum, or plasma.

Whole blood samples must be anticoagulated with EDTA or heparin.

Samples should be collected with a sterile needle and syringe.

Hemolysis does not significantly interfere with the test, but strongly hemolyzed samples may partly obscure a weak positive band.

Important: Allow sample and buffer drops to fall onto membrane at window #1. Do not touch pipette tip, sample or buffer drops, or buffer bottle tip directly to the membrane.

1. Sample application

Tear open the pouch provided and place the test device on a flat horizontal surface for the duration of the test.

Squeeze the provided pipette near the sealed end. Insert the open end of the pipette into an anticoagulated whole blood, serum, or plasma sample. Release the pressure slightly to draw up a small amount of sample into the pipette.

Holding the pipette vertically, transfer one drop of sample to the sample well, window #1.

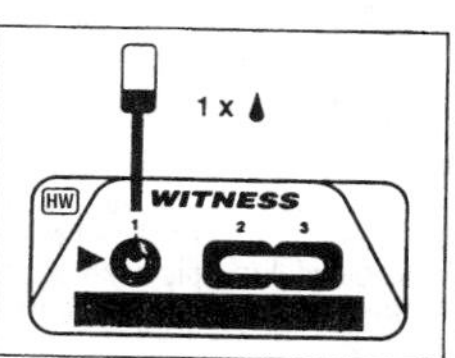

2. Buffer dispensing

Remove the cap from the buffer bottle, hold it vertically and add two drops of buffer to the sample well window #1.

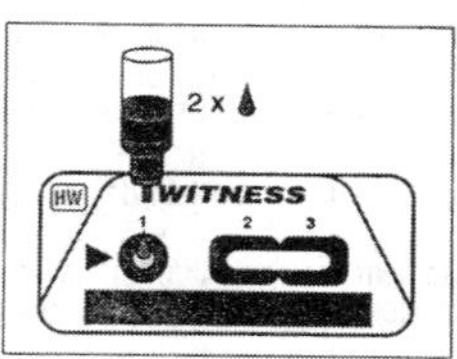

3. Reading test

Wait ten minutes, observe the presence or absence of pink/purple bands in reading windows #2 and #3.

Sample results are read in window #2. The control band is read in window #3.

Notes: The test is complete and may be read before 10 minutes if pink/purple bands are visible in both windows #2 and #3.

The presence of a pink/purple band only in window #3 before 10 minutes does not mean that the test is complete. A pink/purple band in window #2 may develop slower than the control pink/purple band in window #3.

Test Interpretation: Results:

Validation:

Valid test: Test is validated if a pink/purple band is present in the reading window #3.

Interpretation:

Negative for HW antigen: No band in reading window #2, with one pink/purple band in window #3.

Positive for HW antigen: One pink/purple band in reading window #2, with one pink/purple band in window #3.

Invalid Test:

Invalid test: No pink/purple band in control window #3.

Note: A test result should always be interpreted in the context of all available clinical information and history for the dog.

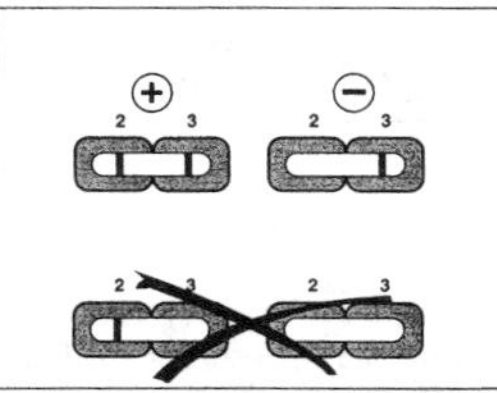

Storage: Refrigeration not required. Store the test kit at 2-25°C (35-77°F). Do not freeze.

Sample Storage: It is recommended to test samples immediately after collection. If samples are kept at room temperature, they should be tested within 4 hours. If testing is further delayed, samples should be refrigerated at 2-7°C (35-45°F) and may be held for up to 24 hours.

Caution(s): Do not use components after expiration date.

Use the test within 10 minutes after opening the sealed pouch. Avoid touching or damaging membrane at windows #1, #2, #3.

The WITNESS® device should be placed on a flat, horizontal surface while performing the test.

Use a separate pipette for each sample.

Hold pipette and buffer bottle vertically when dispensing sample and buffer.

Note: Prior to use, test and control bands appear yellow. The bands are dyed yellow for quality control purposes. The dye does not interfere with the test results and will wash away while the test is developing.

For veterinary use only.

Discussion: General Information: Heartworm disease in dogs has a worldwide distribution and is caused by the filarial nematode *Dirofilaria immitis*. Adult *D. immitis* worms are found in the right ventricle and pulmonary arteries of infected dogs. The adult female worm produces first stage larvae (microfilariae) which can circulate in the peripheral blood. When ingested by a suitable mosquito vector while taking a blood meal, these microfilariae undergo development to become infective third stage larvae. When these larvae are transferred to other dogs during feeding by these infected mosquitoes, they undergo further development for approximately 70-80 days. After this time, immature adults begin to migrate to the distal pulmonary arteries and eventually grow to occupy the heart and the main pulmonary artery. Some 6-8 months after infection by the third stage larvae, the parasites will have matured. Secreted adult heartworm antigen may then be found in the peripheral blood.

Presentation: 10 or 25 test kits.

Manufactured by: AGEN Biomedical Limited, Brisbane, Australia 4110.

Licensed under U.S. Patent No. 4,839,275.

Compendium Code No.: 11150482 RM 789-C Rev. 7/99

WITNESS® RELAXIN

Synbiotics **Pregnancy Test**

Canine Pregnancy Test Kit

Test Description: Canine pregnancy test kit.

Contents: 5 pouches, each containing 1 test device and desiccant; 1 Buffer dropper bottle (2 mL); Instructions for use; 5 pipettes.

Indications: The WITNESS® Relaxin tests offers an early, inexpensive and reliable means of determining the success or failure of a planned mating or unwanted exposure. A sudden decrease of serum relaxin level may indicate that abortion has occurred.

Test Principles: WITNESS® Relaxin is a simple test, based on Rapid Immuno-Migration (RIM) technology, using the combination of anti-canine relaxin antibodies to quickly identify this hormone in biological samples (serum or plasma) from the bitch. Sensitized colloidal gold particles bind to relaxin molecules present in the sample. The complexes migrate along a nitrocellulose strip and are then captured on a sensitized reaction line where its accumulation causes the formation of a clearly visible pink/purple band. A control band, located at the end of the reading window, ensures that the test was performed correctly.

Sample Collection: Sample Information:

The test can be performed on serum or plasma (anticoagulated with EDTA, sodium citrate or heparin). Do not use whole blood.

Samples should always be collected with a sterile needle and syringe.

Hemolysis does not significantly interfere with the test, but strongly hemolyzed samples may partly obscure a weak positive line (due to hemoglobin background).

Test Procedure: Important: Allow sample and buffer drops to fall onto membrane at window #1. Do not touch pipette tip, sample or buffer drops, or buffer bottle tip directly to the membrane.

1. Sample application:

   Tear open the pouch provided and place the test device on a flat horizontal surface for the duration of the test.

   Squeeze the provided pipette near the sealed end. Insert the open end of the pipette into a serum or plasma sample. Release the pressure slightly to draw up a small amount of sample into the pipette.

   Holding the pipette vertically, transfer two drops of sample to the sample well, window #1.

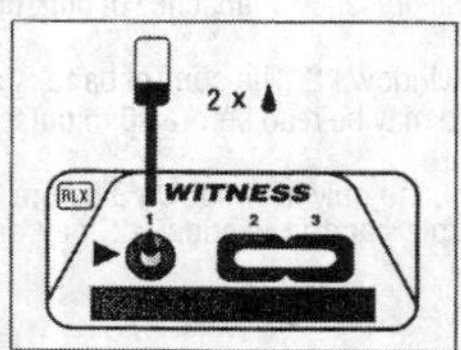

2. Buffer dispensing:

   Remove the cap from the buffer bottle, hold it vertically and add two drops of buffer to the sample well window #1.

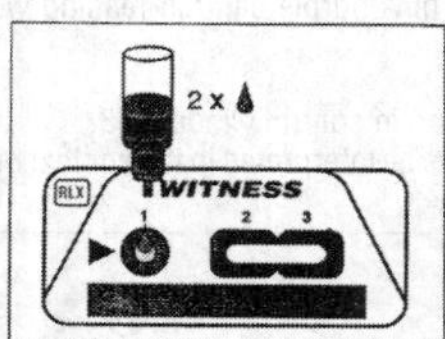

3. Reading test:

   Wait ten minutes, observe the presence or absence of pink/purple bands in reading windows #2 and #3.

   Sample results are read in window #2. The control band is read in window #3.

   Notes: The test is complete and may be read before 10 minutes if pink/purple bands are visible in both windows #2 and #3.

   The presence of a pink/purple band only in window #3 before 10 minutes does not mean that the test is complete. A pink/purple band in window #2 may develop slower than the control pink/purple band in window #3.

Interpretation of Results: Validation:

Valid test: Test is validated if a pink/purple band is present in the reading window #3.

Interpretation:

Negative for relaxin: No band in reading window #2, with one pink/purple band in window #3.

Positive for relaxin: One pink/purple band in reading window #2, with one pink/purple band in window #3.

Note: For more information, consult General Information section (see Discussion).

Negative Samples: Any negative result is considered indicative of non-pregnancy; however, two negative results one week apart may be required for confirmation of this status, especially when date of mating is unknown.

Positive Samples: A positive result is considered indicative of pregnancy. A weak positive result may be observed at the beginning of the pregnancy. It is recommended to repeat the test on a fresh sample one week later to confirm pregnancy.

Invalid Test:

Invalid test: No pink/purple band in control window #3.

Note: A test result should always be interpreted in the context of all available clinical information and history of the dog.

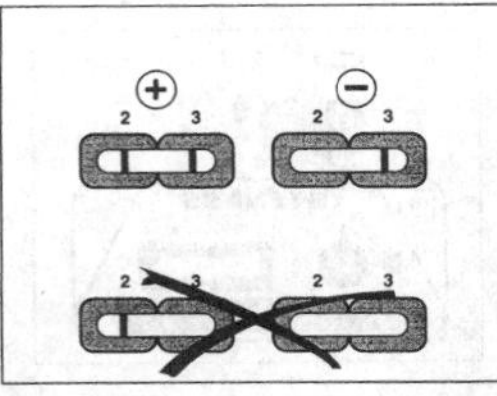

Storage: Refrigeration not required. Store the test kit at 2-25°C (35-77°F). Do not freeze.

Sample Storage: It is recommended to test samples immediately after collection. If samples are kept at room temperature, they should be tested within 4 hours. If testing is further delayed, samples should be refrigerated at 2-7°C (35-45°F) and may be held for up to 48 hours.

Caution(s): Do not use components after expiration date.

Use the test within 10 minutes after opening the sealed pouch.

Avoid touching or damaging membrane at windows #1, #2, #3.

The WITNESS® device should be placed on a flat, horizontal surface while performing the test.

Use a separate pipette for each sample.

Hold pipette and buffer bottle vertically when dispensing.

For veterinary use only.

Note: Prior to use, test and control bands appear yellow. The hands are dyed yellow for quality control purposes. The dye does not interfere with the test results and will wash away while the test is developing.

Discussion: General Information: The WITNESS® Relaxin kit is intended to determine pregnancy in the bitch, by measuring relaxin levels in plasma and serum samples. The presence of significant amounts of this hormone is a reliable indicator of pregnancy. A sudden decrease in relaxin may indicate that abortion has occurred. The WITNESS® Relaxin kit detects relaxin produced by the developing placenta(s) as early as day 20 after the luteinizing hormone (LH) surge. It is suspected that factors such as breed, size of the bitch and litter size may have some influences on the level of serum relaxin. Although approximately 80% of pregnant bitches are detected between 20 and 28 days post-LH surge, some may not be detected as positive until day 31. Since canine serum have a fertile intrauterine lifespan of 6 to 7 days after breeding (Concannon et al. 1983), initial detection post-breeding may vary. For example, a bitch detected positive for relaxin 22 days post-LH, will be claimed positive 24 days post-breeding if bred 2 days before the LH surge and 16 days post-breeding if the breeding occurred 6 days after.

Presentation: 5 test kits.

Compendium Code No.: 11150512 03-0087-1101

WONDER DUST™ WOUND POWDER

Farnam **Topical Wound Dressing**

Active Ingredient(s):

Iodoform	2.0%
Potassium alum	5.0%
Flowers of sulfur	2.0%
Tannic acid	2.0%
Activated charcoal	5.0%
Copper sulfate	13.0%
Hydrated lime	71.0%

Indications: WONDER DUST™ is a dressing powder and blood coagulant for use on certain types of wounds, cuts and abrasions. Formulated for use on horses and show stock. A caustic and drying agent for slow-healing lesions and excessive granulated tissue (proud flesh). Also for use on other livestock as a blood-stop powder after castrating, docking or dehorning. It contains a deodorant to remove objectionable odors from foul or infected wounds.

Dosage and Administration: Shake well before using. Open the nozzle by turning the tip up. Hold the nozzle two (2) inches to four (4) inches from the wound. Squeeze the container firmly, puffing the powder freely over the entire surface of the wound. Use WONDER DUST™ with or without bandages. Repeat the application as often as necessary.

Caution(s): Keep out of the reach of children.

Keep out of the eyes.

Not for human use. For veterinary use only.

Presentation: 4 oz. (113 g).

Compendium Code No.: 10000460

WONDER WORMER™ FOR HORSES

Farnam **Parasiticide-Oral**

Active Ingredient(s):

Piperazine phosphate monohydrate 100%

Equivalent to 42% piperazine base.

Indications: For control of four major internal parasites: Large strongyles or bloodworms *(Strongylus vulgaris)*, large roundworms or Ascarids *(Parascaris equorum)*, small strongyles and pinworms *(Oxyuris equi)*. Recommended for the treatment of all horses and ponies. Excellent for horses in heavy training and valuable race and show horses.

Dosage and Administration: The prescribed dosage for horses is 50 mg of piperazine base (119 mg of WONDER WORMER™) per pound of body weight. Each foil pack contains 3.75 oz. by weight - enough to treat one (1) adult horse weighing 900 lbs.

Table of Recommended Dosages		
Yearlings	Approx. 600 lbs.	2.50 oz.
Adults	Approx. 900 lbs.	3.75 oz.

For horses over 900 lbs. in weight, increase dosage proportionately according to the above table.

Dose each horse individually. Carefully determine the weight of the animal to be treated and determine the correct dosage. Mix WONDER WORMER™ thoroughly with the amount of grain the horse will consume in a single feeding. Horses must be individually confined during treatment so that consumption of medicated feed can be observed and accurately measured. Do not give the horse additional feed that day until the treated feed is fully consumed. Most horses will take the medicated feed readily and should be given plenty of good hay when all of the grain is consumed.

For finicky eaters mix WONDER WORMER™ into molasses and water (50/50) and add the mixture to the amount of grain the horse will consume in a single feeding. For the horse that refuses to eat medicated feed, consult a veterinarian.

Note: Horses are constantly subject to reinfestation, particularly through grazing in confined pastures. Therefore, periodic worming and good stable sanitation are essential. For the most effective control of internal parasites, treat horses with WONDER WORMER™ every eight to ten weeks.

Precaution(s): Store out of direct sunlight.

Caution(s): Although piperazine is a drug with a wide margin of safety, occasionally an animal may show nausea, vomiting, or muscular tremors. Such side effects are usually associated with overdosage. Therefore, the recommended dosages should be followed carefully. Animals with known kidney pathology should be treated only by a veterinarian.

Consult your veterinarian for assistance in the diagnosis, treatment and control of parasitism.

Do not treat heavily parasitized animals with this drug.

If heavy parasitism is suspected due to poor physical condition, consult a veterinarian before treating these horses.

Warning(s): This drug is not to be administered to horses that are to be slaughtered for use in food.

Keep out of the reach of children.

Not for human use.

Presentation: 3.75 oz. (106 g).

Compendium Code No.: 10000470

WOUND-KOTE GENTIAN VIOLET

Farnam **Topical Wound Dressing**

Active Ingredient(s):

Propylene glycol	19.37%
Glycerin	6.31%
Urea	1.80%
Sodium propionate	1.40%
Methyl violet	0.51%
Acriflavine	0.03%

Indications: A quick-drying, penetrating antiseptic dressing and gall lotion for horses and cattle.

Spray on surface wounds, minor cuts and skin abrasions, harness galls, cowpox sores.

WOUND-KOTE dries up cowpox lesions and controls secondary infections.

Dosage and Administration: Shake well:

Remove the protective cap. Point the nozzle opening towards the wound or the area to be treated. Spray from a distance of two (2) to four (4) inches. Release the spray by pressing the valve stem down for just an instant. The slightest amount of spray you can quickly release over the area to be treated will provide an adequate dosage. The application may be repeated once a day or more often until healing takes place. Whenever possible, clean and dry the affected area before applying. Do not use on exceedingly large areas or in deep wounds.

Precaution(s): Contents are under pressure. Do not place in hot water or near radiators, stoves or other sources of heat. Do not puncture or incinerate container, even when empty, or store at temperatures above 120°F.

Container may explode if heated.

Caution(s): In case of deep or puncture wounds or serious burns, consult veterinarian. If redness, irritation, or swelling persists or increases, discontinue use of the product, consult a veterinarian.

Keep out of the reach of children.

Livestock remedy: Not for human use. Avoid contact with the eyes and mucous membranes. Do not apply to large areas of the body. Do not apply at all to cats. Note that the spray will stain clothing.

For veterinary use only.

Presentation: 5 oz. (142 g).

Compendium Code No.: 10000480

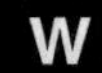

Disclaimer

Every effort has been made to ensure the accuracy of the information published. However, it remains the responsibility of the readers to familiarize themselves with the product information contained on the product label or package insert.

Inclusion or omission of products does not imply endorsement or criticism by the Publisher or anyone involved in the publication. Inclusion does not imply product availability and/or product registration. The Publisher, Editorial Team and all those involved in the production of this book cannot be held responsible for publication errors or any consequence that could result from the use of published information.

X-Y-Z

XENODINE®

V.P.L. **Antiseptic**

Active Ingredient(s): Iodine - 1%.

Indications: Topical antiseptic/disinfectant for use on horses, dogs and farm animals.

To aid in wound healing and in prevention of topical bacterial and fungal infections. These include wounds, cuts, abrasions, ears, hooves, udders, declaws, ear cropping, naval dipping, tail docking, castrations, and surgical site preparations.

Dosage and Administration: Cleanse affected areas thoroughly and apply XENODINE® two or three times daily, or as needed. Apply a sufficient amount of XENODINE® to cover the affected area. For more rapid release of the active ingredient, XENODINE® must be applied to a moist surface. The wound site may be covered or bandaged after application.

In case of deep or puncture wounds or serious burns, additional or alternative therapy may be warranted. If redness, irritation or swelling persists or increases, discontinue use and consult your veterinarian.

Contraindication(s): This product should not be used on cats or kittens.

Precaution(s): Store at room temperature; avoid excessive heat 104°F (40°C).

Caution(s): For external use only. Do not allow animals to consume product or lick at site of product application.

Note: When used on or near the teats or udders of dairy animals, the teats and udders should be thoroughly washed before the next milking to prevent contamination of milk.

Warning(s): For veterinary use only.

Keep out of reach of children.

Presentation: 12 x 1 fl oz (30 mL) and 8 fl oz (240 mL).

Xenodine and Polyhydroxydine are trademarks of Xenovet, a division of eMDee Corporation.

Compendium Code No.: 11430391

XENODINE® SPRAY

V.P.L. **Antiseptic**

Active Ingredient(s): Iodine - 1%.

Indications: Topical antiseptic/disinfectant for use on horses, dogs and farm animals.

To aid in wound healing and in prevention of topical bacterial and fungal infections. These include wounds, cuts, abrasions, ears, hooves, udders, declaws, ear cropping, naval dipping, tail docking, castrations, and surgical site preparations.

Dosage and Administration: Cleanse affected areas thoroughly and apply XENODINE® two or three times daily, or as needed. Apply a sufficient amount to cover the affected area. For more rapid release of the active ingredient, XENODINE® must be applied to a moist surface. The wound site may be covered or bandaged after application. When using the pump spray, adjust the nozzle by turning counter clockwise approximately ¼ turn or until the desired spray pattern is obtained. Hold the container 10 to 12 inches (25 to 30 cm) from the skin.

In case of deep or puncture wounds or serious burns, additional or alternative therapy may be warranted. If redness, irritation or swelling persists or increases, discontinue use and consult your veterinarian.

Contraindication(s): This product should not be used on cats or kittens.

Precaution(s): Store at room temperature; avoid excessive heat 104°F (40°C).

Cold temperatures below 40°F (4°C) may make XENODINE® Solution difficult to spray. Place the bottle in warm water or hold at room temperature until the solution flows freely.

Caution(s): For external use only. Do not allow animals to consume product or lick at site of product application.

Note: When used on or near the teats or udders of dairy animals, the teats and udders should be thoroughly washed before the next milking to prevent contamination of milk.

Warning(s): For veterinary use only.

Keep out of reach of children.

Presentation: 12 fl oz (360 mL).

Compendium Code No.: 11430401

X-JECT E ℞

Vetus **Analgesic-Sedative**

Xylazine 100 mg/mL

ANADA No.: 200-139

Active Ingredient(s): Each mL contains 100 mg xylazine, (base equivalent), 0.9 mg methylparaben, 0.1 mg propylparaben, water for injection; citric acid and sodium citrate for pH adjustment to 5.5 ± 0.3.

Xylazine Hydrochloride (Equivalent to 10% base)	11.4%
Inert Ingredients	88.6%
	100%

Indications: X-JECT E (xylazine) should be used in horses and *Cervidae* (Fallow Deer, Mule Deer, Sika Deer, White-Tailed Deer and Elk) when it is desirable to produce a state of sedation accompanied by a shorter period of analgesia.

Horses: X-JECT E (xylazine) has been used successfully as follows:

1. Diagnostic procedures-oral and ophthalmic examinations, abdominal palpation, rectal palpation, vaginal examination, catheterization of the bladder and radiographic examinations.
2. Orthopedic procedures, such as application of casting materials and splints.
3. Dental procedures.
4. Minor surgical procedures of short duration such as debridement, removal of cutaneous neoplasms and suturing of lacerations.
5. To calm and facilitate handling of fractious animals.
6. Therapeutic medication for sedation and relief of pain following injury or surgery.
7. Major surgical procedures:
   a. When used as a preanesthetic to general anesthesia.
   b. When used in conjunction with local anesthetics.

Cervidae: X-JECT E (xylazine) may be used for the following:

1. To calm and facilitate handling of fractious animals.
2. Diagnostic procedures.
3. Minor surgical procedures.
4. Therapeutic medication for sedation and relief of pain following injury or surgery.
5. As a preanesthetic to local anesthesia. X-JECT E (xylazine) at the recommended dosages can be used in conjunction with local anesthetics, such as procaine or lidocaine.

Pharmacology: X-JECT E (xylazine), a non-narcotic compound, is a sedative and analgesic as well as a muscle relaxant. Its sedative and analgesic activity is related to central nervous system depression. Its muscle relaxant effect is based on inhibition of the intraneural transmission of impulses in the central nervous system. The principal pharmacological activities develop within 10 to 15 minutes after intramuscular injection in horses and *Cervidae*, and within 3 to 5 minutes following intravenous administration in horses.

A sleeplike state, the depth of which is dose-dependent, is usually maintained for 1 to 2 hours, while analgesia lasts from 15 to 30 minutes. The centrally acting muscle relaxant effect causes relaxation of the skeletal musculature, complementing sedation and analgesia.

In horses and *Cervidae* under the influence of X-JECT E (xylazine), the respiratory rate is reduced as in natural sleep. Following treatment with X-JECT E (xylazine), the heart rate is decreased and a transient change in the conductivity of the cardiac muscle may occur, as evidenced by a partial atrioventricular block. This resembles the atrioventricular block often observed in normal horses.[1,2,3,4] Partial A-V block may occasionally occur following intramuscular injection of X-JECT E (xylazine). When given intravenously in horses, the incidence of partial A-V block is higher. Intravenous administration causes a transient rise in blood pressure in horses, followed by a slight decrease.

Dosage and Administration:

Horses:

1. Dosage:
   Intravenously-0.5 mL/100 lbs body weight (0.5 mg/lb).
   Intramuscularly-1.0 mL/100 lbs body weight (1.0 mg/lb).
   Following injection of X-JECT E (xylazine) the animal should be allowed to rest quietly until the full effect has been reached. These dosages produce sedation which is usually maintained for 1 to 2 hours, and analgesia which lasts for 15 to 30 minutes.
2. Preanesthetic to Local Anesthesia:
   X-JECT E (xylazine) at the recommended dosages can be used in conjunction with local anesthetics, such as procaine or lidocaine.
3. Preanesthetic to General Anesthesia:
   X-JECT E (xylazine) at the recommended dosage rates produces an additive effect to central nervous system depressants such as pentobarbital sodium, thiopental sodium and thiamyl sodium.
   Therefore, the dosage of such compounds should be reduced and administered to the desired effect. In general, only ⅓ to ½ of the calculated dosage of the barbiturates will be needed to produce a surgical plane of anesthesia. Post-anesthetic or emergence excitement has not been observed in animals preanesthetized with X-JECT E (xylazine).
   X-JECT E (xylazine) has been used successfully as a preanesthetic agent for pentobarbital sodium, thiopental sodium, thiamylal sodium, nitrous oxide, ether, halothane, glyceryl guaiacolate and methoxyflurane anesthesia.

Cervidae:

Administer intramuscularly, either by hand syringe or syringe dart, in the heavy muscles of the croup or shoulder.

Dosage Range:

Fallow Deer *(Dama dama)*-2.0 to 4.0 mL/100 lbs body weight (2.0 to 4.0 mg/lb).

Mule Deer *(Odocoileus hemionus)*-1.0 to 2.0 mL/100 lbs body weight (1.0 to 2.0 mg/lb).

Sika Deer *(Cervus nippon)*-1.0 to 2.0 mL/100 lbs body weight (1.0 to 2.0 mg/lb).

White-Tailed Deer *(Odocoileus virginianus)*-1.0 to 2.0 mL/100 lbs body weight (1.0 to 2.0 mg/lb).

Elk *(Cervus canadensis)*-0.25 to 0.5 mL/100 lbs body weight (0.25 to 0.5 mg/lb).

Following injection of X-JECT E (xylazine) the animal should be allowed to rest quietly until the full effect has been reached. These dosages produce sedation which is usually maintained for 1 to 2 hours and analgesia which lasts for 15 to 30 minutes.

Precaution(s): Store at controlled room temperature (15° to 30°C or 59° to 86°F).

Caution(s): Federal law restricts this drug to use by or on the order of a licensed veterinarian.

Careful consideration should be given before administering to horses and *Cervidae* with significantly depressed respiration, severe pathologic heart disease, advanced liver or kidney disease, severe endotoxic or traumatic shock and stress conditions such as extreme heat, cold, high altitude or fatigue.

Do not use X-JECT E (xylazine) in conjunction with tranquilizers.

Analgesic effect is variable, and depth should be carefully assayed prior to surgical/clinical procedures. Variability of analgesia occurs most frequently at the distal extremities of horses and *Cervidae*. In spite of sedation, the practitioner and handlers should proceed with caution since defense reactions may not be diminished.

Horses: Since an additive effect results from the use of X-JECT E (xylazine) and the barbiturate compounds, it should be used with caution with these central nervous system depressants. Products known to produce respiratory depression or apnea, such as thiamylal sodium should be given at a reduced dosage and, when injected intravenously, should be administered slowly. When intravenous administration of X-JECT E (xylazine) is desired, avoid perivascular injection in order to achieve the desired effect. Studies have shown negligible evidence of tissue irritation, however, following perivascular injection of xylazine.

Intracarotid Arterial Injection Should be Avoided. As with many compounds, including tranquilizers, immediate violent seizures followed by collapse may result from inadvertent administration into the carotid artery. Although the reaction with X-JECT E (xylazine) is usually transient and recovery may be rapid and complete, special care should be taken to assure that the needle is in the jugular vein rather than the carotid artery.

Bradycardia and arrhythmia in the form of incomplete atrioventricular block have been reported following xylazine administration. Although clinically the importance of this effect is questioned,[1,2,3,4] a standard dose of atropine given prior to or following xylazine will greatly decrease the incidence.

Sedation for transport is most successful if actual transportation is begun after the full effect of the drug has been reached and the animal's stability is maintained while standing. In addition, it should be noted that animals under the influence of xylazine can be aroused by noise or other stimuli and this may increase the risk of injury.

Cervidae: As in all ruminants, it is preferable to administer X-JECT E (xylazine) to fasted *Cervidae* as a safeguard against aspiration of food material into the lungs and/or bloat during deep sedation.

Care should be taken to administer X-JECT E (xylazine) in the heavy muscles of the croup or shoulder. Injections given subcutaneously, intraperitoneally or into fat deposits will give unpredictable results.

Intra-arterial injection should be avoided, as with many compounds, including tranquilizers, immediate violent seizures followed by collapse may result from inadvertent administration into an artery.

The animal should not be disturbed during induction or until the full effect of the drug has been reached which is usually 10 to 15 minutes following injection.

The usual time to initial effect of the drug is 2 to 5 minutes. The administrator of the drug should be fully cognizant of this interval prior to administration of drug to free-ranging deer or elk, especially at night or in heavily wooded areas.

If the animal has been underdosed (faulty injection or miscalculation on weight) it is advisable to wait one hour before administering a second dose.

Adequate ventilation-especially in cages or crates-is mandatory; keep head and neck in position to insure patient air passage and to prevent aspiration of stomach contents.

During sedation, animals should be prevented from assuming lateral recumbency. A sternal recumbent position is desirable.

While under the effects of X-JECT E (xylazine) the animal should be protected from extreme hot or cold environments.

Efforts should be made to prevent patient from rising until almost complete recovery is attained.

The transportation of *Cervidae* given X-JECT E (xylazine) should be carefully monitored to prevent excessive struggling, injury or death.

Hyperthermic reactions may occur, especially if the subject is in a highly excited state when the drug is administered. Hosing the head and entire body with cold water has usually proven to be an effective deterrent.

The safety of X-JECT E (xylazine) has not been demonstrated in pregnant *Cervidae*. Avoid use during the breeding season.

Cervidae should be observed closely until all of the sedative effects of X-JECT E (xylazine) are gone.

Care should be taken at all times when administering X-JECT E (xylazine) to *Cervidae*. This is due to the method of administration (usually darting), the difficulty in estimating body weights and the accepted theory that wild animals are more unpredictable in their response to sedatives and analgesics than the domesticated species.

Warning(s): Do not use in *Cervidae* less than 15 days before or during the hunting season.

This drug should not be administered to domestic food-producing animals. Not for use in horses intended for food.

Avoid accidental administration to humans. Should such exposure occur, notify a physician immediately. Artificial respiration may be indicated.

In *Cervidae*, occasional capture-associated deaths occur. Clinical trials reveal a mortality rate of approximately 3.5% attendant with the administration of xylazine.

Side Effects: X-JECT E (xylazine) in horses and *Cervidae*, used at recommended dosage levels may occasionally cause slight muscle tremors, bradycardia with partial A-V heart block and a reduced respiratory rate. Movement in response to sharp auditory stimuli may be observed.

In horses, sweating, rarely profuse, has been reported following administration. In *Cervidae*, salivation, various vocalizations (bellowing, bleating, groaning, grunting, snoring) on expiration, audible grinding of molar teeth, protruding tongue and elevated temperatures have also been noted in some cases.

Trial Data: Safety: X-JECT E (xylazine) is tolerated at 10 times the recommended dose in horses and at doses above the recommended range in *Cervidae*. However, some elevated doses produced muscle tremors and long periods of sedation.

References: Available upon request.

Presentation: X-JECT E (xylazine 100 mg/mL for intravenous or intramuscular use) is available in 50 mL multiple dose vials.

Compendium Code No.: 14440870

X-JECT SA ℞

Vetus **Analgesic-Sedative**

Xylazine 20 mg/mL

ANADA No.: 200-184

Active Ingredient(s): Each mL contains 20 mg xylazine (base equivalent), 0.9 mg methylparaben, 0.1 mg propylparaben, water for injection; citric acid and sodium citrate for pH adjustment to 5.5 ± 0.3.

Xylazine Hydrochloride (Equivalent to 2% base)	2.3%
Inert Ingredients	97.7%
	100%

Indications: X-JECT SA (xylazine) should be used in dogs and cats when it is desirable to produce a state of sedation accompanied by a shorter period of analgesia. X-JECT SA (xylazine) has been used successfully as follows:

1. Diagnostic procedures - examination of mouth and ears, abdominal palpation, rectal palpation, vaginal examination, catheterization of the bladder and radiographic examinations.
2. Orthopedic procedures, such as application of casting materials and splints.
3. Dental procedures.
4. Minor surgical procedures of short duration such as debridement, removal of cutaneous neoplasms and suturing of lacerations.
5. To calm and facilitate restraint of fractious animals.
6. Therapeutic medication for sedation and relief of pain following injury or surgery.
7. Major surgical procedures:
   a. When used as a preanesthetic to general anesthesia.
   b. When used in conjunction with local anesthetics.

Pharmacology: X-JECT SA (xylazine), a non-narcotic compound, is a sedative and analgesic as well as muscle relaxant. Its sedative and analgesic activity is related to central nervous system depression. Its muscle-relaxant effect is based upon inhibition of the intraneural transmission of impulses in the central nervous system. The principal pharmacological activities develop within 10 to 15 minutes after intramuscular or subcutaneous injection, and within 3 to 5 minutes following intravenous administration.

A sleeplike state, the depth of which is dose-dependent, is usually maintained for 1 to 2 hours, while analgesia lasts from 15 to 30 minutes. The centrally-acting muscle relaxant effect causes relaxation of the skeletal musculature complementing sedation and analgesia.

In animals under the influence of X-JECT SA (xylazine), the respiratory rate is reduced as in natural sleep. Following treatment with X-JECT SA (xylazine), the heart rate is decreased and a transient change in the conductivity of the cardiac muscle may occur as evidenced by a partial atrioventricular block. This resembles the atrioventricular block often observed in apparently normal animals.[1] Intravenous administration of X-JECT SA (xylazine) causes a transient rise in blood pressure, followed by a slight decrease.

Dosage and Administration:

1. Dosage:

   Intravenously - 0.5 mL/20 lbs body weight (0.5 mg/lb).

   Intramuscularly or Subcutaneously - 1 mL/20 lbs body weight (1 mg/lb).

   In large dogs (over 50 lbs), a dosage of 0.5 mg/lb administered intramuscularly may provide sufficient sedation and/or analgesia for most procedures.

   Since vomiting may occur (see Side Effects), fasting for 6-24 hours prior to the use of X-JECT SA (xylazine) may reduce the incidence; the I.V. route results in the least vomiting.

   Following injection of X-JECT SA (xylazine), the animal should be allowed to rest quietly until the full effect has been reached.

   These dosages produce sedation which is usually maintained for 1 to 2 hours and analgesia which lasts for 15 to 30 minutes.

2. Preanesthetic to Local Anesthesia:

   X-JECT SA (xylazine) at the recommended dosages can be used in conjunction with local anesthetics, such as procaine or lidocaine.

3. Preanesthetic to General Anesthesia:

   X-JECT SA (xylazine), at the recommended dosage rates, produces an additive effect to central nervous system depressants such as pentobarbital sodium, thiopental sodium and thiamylal sodium. Therefore, the dosage of such compounds should be reduced and administered to the desired effect. In general, ⅓ to ½ of the calculated dosage of the barbiturates will be needed to produce a surgical plane of anesthesia. Post-anesthetic or emergence excitement has not been observed in animals preanesthetized with X-JECT SA (xylazine).

   X-JECT SA (xylazine) has been used successfully as a pre-anesthetic agent for pentobarbital sodium, thiopental sodium, thiamylal sodium, nitrous oxide, ether, halothane and methoxyflurane anesthesia.

Caution(s): Federal law restricts this drug to use by or on the order of a licensed veterinarian.

Clinical results with xylazine have not revealed any detrimental effects when the compound is administered to pregnant dogs or cats. However, until more definitive studies are completed, X-JECT SA (xylazine) is not recommended for use in these animals.

Careful consideration should be given before administering to dogs or cats with significantly depressed respiration, severe pathologic heart disease, advanced liver or kidney disease, severe endotoxic or traumatic shock and stress conditions such as extreme heat, cold or fatigue.

Analgesic effect is variable, and depth should be carefully assayed prior to surgical/clinical procedures. In spite of sedation, the practitioner and handlers should proceed with caution since defense reactions may not be diminished.

Do not use X-JECT SA (xylazine) in conjunction with tranquilizers.

Since an additive effect results from the use of X-JECT SA (xylazine) and the barbiturate compounds, it should be used with caution with these central nervous system depressants. Products known to produce respiratory depression or apnea, such as thiamylal sodium, should be given at a reduced dosage and, when injected intravenously, should be administered slowly.

When intravenous administration is desired, avoid perivascular injection in order to achieve the desired effect. Studies have shown negligible evidence of tissue irritation, however, following perivascular injection of xylazine.

Bradycardia and an arrhythmia in the form of incomplete atrioventricular block have been reported following xylazine administration. Although clinically the importance of this effect is questioned, a standard dose of atropine given prior to or following X-JECT SA (xylazine) will greatly decrease the incidence.

While sedation usually lasts from 1 to 2 hours, recovery periods in excess of 4 to 5 hours have been reported in both dogs and cats.

Warning(s): The drug is for use in dogs and cats only.

Side Effects: Emesis occurs occasionally in dogs, and frequently in cats, soon after the administration of X-JECT SA (xylazine), but before clinical sedation is evident. When observed, emesis usually occurs only a single time, after which there is no further emetic effect. The use of antiemetics may delay this phenomenon. The occurrence of emesis may be considered a desirable effect when X-JECT SA (xylazine) is administered as a preanesthetic to general anesthesia.

X-JECT SA (xylazine) used at the recommended dosage levels may occasionally cause slight muscle tremors, bradycardia with partial A-V heart block and a reduced respiratory rate. Should excessive respiratory depression occur following the use of X-JECT SA (xylazine), administer respiratory stimulants and provide artificial respiration.

Movement in response to sharp auditory stimuli may be observed.

Increased urination may occur in cats following the use of X-JECT SA (xylazine).

Trial Data: X-JECT SA (xylazine) is tolerated in dogs and cats at 10 times the recommended dose. However, doses of this magnitude produce muscle tremors, emesis and long periods of sedation.

References: Available upon request.

Presentation: X-JECT SA (xylazine) is available in 20 mL multiple dose vials.

Compendium Code No.: 14440880

XYLA-JECT® 20 mg/mL INJECTABLE ℞

Phoenix Pharmaceutical **Analgesic-Sedative**

(xylazine) Sedative and Analgesic

ANADA No.: 200-184

Active Ingredient(s): Each mL contains 20 mg XYLA-JECT® (xylazine, base equivalent present as the hydrochloride), 0.9 mg methylparaben, 0.1 mg propylparaben, water for injection, citric acid and sodium citrate for pH adjustment to 5.5 ± 0.3.

Xylazine hydrochloride (equivalent to 2% base)	2.3%
Inert ingredients	97.7%
Total	100.0%

Indications: XYLA-JECT® (xylazine) should be used in dogs and cats when it is desirable to produce a state of sedation accompanied by a shorter period of analgesia. XYLA-JECT® (xylazine) has been used successfully as follows:

1. Diagnostic procedures: Examination of mouth and ears, abdominal palpation, rectal palpation, vaginal examination, catheterization of the bladder and radiographic examinations.
2. Orthopedic procedures, such as the application of casting materials and splints.
3. Dental procedures.
4. Minor surgical procedures of short duration such as debridement, removal of cutaneous neoplasms and suturing of lacerations.
5. To calm and facilitate the restraint of fractious animals.
6. Therapeutic medication for sedation and the relief of pain following injury or surgery.
7. Major surgical procedures:
   a. When used as a pre-anesthetic to general anesthesia.
   b. When used in conjunction with local anesthetics.

Pharmacology: XYLA-JECT® (xylazine), a non-narcotic compound, is a sedative and analgesic as well as a muscle relaxant. Its sedative and analgesic activity is related to central nervous system depression. Its muscle-relaxant effect is based upon inhibition of the intraneural transmission of impulses in the central nervous system. The principal pharmacological activities develop within 10 to 15 minutes after intramuscular or subcutaneous injection, and within 3 to 5 minutes following intravenous administration.

A sleeplike state, the depth of which is dose-dependent, is usually maintained for 1 to 2 hours, while analgesia lasts from 15 to 30 minutes. The centrally-acting muscle relaxant effect causes relaxation of the skeletal musculature complementing sedation and analgesia.

In animals under the influence of XYLA-JECT® (xylazine), the respiratory rate is reduced as in natural sleep. Following treatment with XYLA-JECT® (xylazine), the heart rate is decreased and a transient change in the conductivity of the cardiac muscle may occur, as evidenced by a partial atrioventricular block. This resembles the atrioventricular block often observed in apparently normal animals.[1] Intravenous administration of XYLA-JECT® (xylazine) causes a transient rise in blood pressure, followed by a slight decrease.

XYLA-JECT® (xylazine) has no effect on blood clotting time or other hematologic parameters.

Dosage and Administration:

1. Dosage:

   Intravenously: 0.5 mL/20 lbs of body weight (0.5 mg/lb).

   Intramuscularly or Subcutaneously: 1 mL/20 lbs of body weight (1 mg/lb).

   In large dogs (over 50 lbs), a dosage of 0.5 mg/lb administered intramuscularly may provide sufficient sedation and/or analgesia for most procedures.

   Since vomiting may occur (see Side Effects), fasting for 6-24 hours prior to the use of XYLA-JECT® (xylazine) may reduce the incidence; the I.V. route results in the least vomiting.

   Following the injection of XYLA-JECT® (xylazine), the animal should be allowed to rest quietly until the full effect has been reached.

   These dosages produce sedation which is usually maintained for 1 to 2 hours, and analgesia which lasts for 15 to 30 minutes.

2. Pre-anesthetic to Local Anesthesia: XYLA-JECT® (xylazine) at the recommended dosages can be used in conjunction with local anesthetics, such as procaine or lidocaine.
3. Pre-anesthetic to General Anesthesia: XYLA-JECT® (xylazine) at the recommended dosage rates, produces an additive effect to central nervous system depressants such as pentobarbital sodium, thiopental sodium and thiamylal sodium. Therefore, the dosage of such compounds should be reduced and administered to the desired effect. In general, ⅓ to ½ of the calculated dosage of the barbiturates will be needed to produce a surgical plane of anesthesia. Post-anesthetic or emergence excitement has not been observed in animals pre-anesthetized with XYLA-JECT® (xylazine).

   XYLA-JECT® (xylazine) has been used successfully as a pre-anesthetic agent for pentobarbital sodium, thiopental sodium, thiamylal sodium, nitrous oxide, ether, halothane and methoxyflurane anesthesia.

Precaution(s): Store between 15°C and 30°C (59°F and 86°F).

Caution(s): Federal law restricts this drug to use by or on the order of a licensed veterinarian.

Clinical results with xylazine have not revealed any detrimental effects when the compound is administered to pregnant dogs or cats. However, until more definitive studies are completed, XYLA-JECT® (xylazine) is not recommended for use in these animals.

Careful consideration should be given before administering to dogs or cats with significantly depressed respiration, severe pathologic heart disease, advanced liver or kidney disease, severe endotoxic or traumatic shock and stress conditions such as extreme heat, cold, or fatigue.

Analgesic effect is variable, and the depth should be carefully assayed prior to surgical/clinical procedures. In spite of sedation, the practitioner and handlers should proceed with caution since defense reactions may not be diminished.

Do not use XYLA-JECT® (xylazine) in conjunction with tranquilizers.

Since an additive effect results from the use of XYLA-JECT® (xylazine) and the barbiturate compounds, it should be used with caution with these central nervous system depressants. Products known to produce respiratory depression or apnea, such as thiamylal sodium, should be given at a reduced dosage and, when injected intravenously, should be administered slowly.

When intravenous administration is desired, avoid perivascular injection in order to achieve the desired effect. Studies have shown negligible evidence of tissue irritation following the perivascular injection of xylazine.

Bradycardia and an arrhythmia in the form of incomplete atrioventricular block have been reported following xylazine administration. Although clinically the importance of this effect is questioned,[1] a standard dose of atropine given prior to or following XYLA-JECT® (xylazine) will greatly decrease the incidence.

While sedation usually lasts from 1 to 2 hours, recovery periods in excess of 4 to 5 hours have been reported in both dogs and cats.

For use in dogs and cats only.

Warning(s): Not for human use.

Keep out of reach of children.

Toxicology: Safety: XYLA-JECT® (xylazine) is tolerated in dogs and cats at 10 times the recommended dose. However, doses of this magnitude produced muscle tremors, emesis and long periods of sedation.

Side Effects: Emesis occurs occasionally in dogs, and frequently in cats, soon after the administration of XYLA-JECT® (xylazine), but before clinical sedation is evident. When observed, emesis usually occurs only a single time, after which there is no further emetic effect. The use of anti-emetics may delay this phenomenon. The occurrence of emesis may be considered a desirable effect when XYLA-JECT® (xylazine) is administered as a pre-anesthetic to general anesthesia.

XYLA-JECT® (xylazine) used at the recommended dosage levels may occasionally cause slight muscle tremors, bradycardia with partial A-V heart block and a reduced respiratory rate. Should excessive respiratory depression occur following the use of XYLA-JECT® (xylazine), administer respiratory stimulants and provide artificial respiration.

Movement in response to sharp auditory stimuli may be observed.

Increased urination may occur in cats following the use of XYLA-JECT® (xylazine).

References: Available upon request.

Presentation: Supplied in 20 mL multiple dose vials as a sterile solution (NDC 57319-362-26).

Manufactured by: Phoenix Scientific, Inc., St. Joseph, MO 64503.

Compendium Code No.: 12561012 Rev. 8-01

XYLA-JECT® 100 mg/mL INJECTABLE ℞

Phoenix Pharmaceutical **Analgesic-Sedative**

(Xylazine) Sedative and Analgesic

ANADA No.: 200-139

Active Ingredient(s): Each mL contains 100 mg XYLA-JECT® (xylazine, base equivalent), 0.9 mg methylparaben, 0.1 mg propylparaben, water for injection; citric acid and sodium citrate for pH adjustment to 5.5 ± 0.3.

Xylazine hydrochloride (equivalent to 10% base)	11.4%
Inert Ingredients	88.6%
Total	100.0%

Indications: XYLA-JECT® (xylazine) should be used in horses and *Cervidae* (Fallow Deer, Mule Deer, Sika Deer, White-Tailed Deer and Elk) when it is desirable to produce a state of sedation accompanied by a shorter period of analgesia.

Horses: XYLA-JECT® (xylazine) has been used successfully as follows:

1. Diagnostic procedures-oral and opthalmic examinations, abdominal palpation, rectal palpation, vaginal examination, catheterization of the bladder and radiographic examinations.
2. Orthopedic procedures, such as application of casting materials and splints.
3. Dental procedures.
4. Minor surgical procedures of short duration such as debridement, removal of cutaneous neoplasms and suturing of lacerations.
5. To calm and facilitate handling of fractious animals.
6. Therapeutic medication for sedation and relief-of pain following injury or surgery.
7. Major surgical procedures:
   a. When used as a preanesthetic to general anesthesia.
   b. When used in conjunction with local anesthetics.

Cervidae: XYLA-JECT® (xylazine) may be used for the following:

1. To calm and facilitate handling of fractious animals.
2. Diagnostic procedures.
3. Minor surgical procedures.
4. Therapeutic medication for sedation and relief of pain following injury or surgery.
5. As a preanesthetic to local anesthesia. XYLA-JECT® (xylazine) at the recommended dosages can be used in conjunction with local anesthetics, such as procaine or lidocaine.

Pharmacology: XYLA-JECT® (xylazine), a non-narcotic compound, is a sedative and analgesic as well as muscle relaxant. Its sedative and analgesic activity is related to central nervous system depression. Its muscle relaxant effect is based on inhibition of the intraneural transmission of impulses in the central nervous system. The principal pharmacological activities develop within 10 to 15 minutes after intramuscular injection in horses and *Cervidae,* and within 3 to 5 minutes following intravenous administration in horses.

A sleeplike state, the depth of which is dose-dependent, is usually maintained for 1 to 2 hours, while analgesia lasts from 15 to 30 minutes. The centrally-acting muscle relaxant effect causes relaxation of the skeletal musculature, complementing sedation and analgesia.

In horses and *Cervidae* under the influence of XYLA-JECT® (xylazine), the respiratory rate is reduced as in natural sleep. Following treatment with XYLA-JECT® (xylazine), the heart rate is decreased and a transient change in the conductivity of the cardiac muscle may occur, as evidenced by a partial atrioventricular block. This resembles the atrioventricular block often observed in normal horses.[1,2,3,4] Partial A-V block may occasionally occur following intramuscular injection of XYLA-JECT® (xylazine). When given intravenously in horses, the incidence of partial A-V block is higher. Intravenous administration causes a transient rise in blood pressure in horses, followed by a slight decrease.

XYLA-JECT® (xylazine) has no effect on blood clotting time or other hematologic parameters.

Dosage and Administration:

Horses:

1. Dosage:
   Intravenously: 0.5 mL/100 lbs body weight (0.5 mg/lb)
   Intramuscularly: 1.0 mL/100 lbs body weight (1.0 mg/lb)
   Following injection of XYLA-JECT® (xylazine), the animal should be allowed to rest quietly until the full effect has been reached. These dosages produce sedation which is usually maintained for 1 to 2 hours, and analgesia which lasts for 15 to 30 minutes.
2. Preanesthetic to Local Anesthesia: XYLA-JECT® (xylazine) at the recommended dosages can be used in conjunction with local anesthetics, such as procaine or lidocaine.
3. Preanesthetic to General Anesthesia: XYLA-JECT® (xylazine) at the recommended dosage rates produces an additive effect to central nervous system depressants such as pentobarbital sodium, thiopental sodium and thiamylal sodium. Therefore, the dosage of such compounds should be reduced and administered to the desired effect. In general, only ⅓ to ½ of the calculated dosage of the barbiturates will be needed to produce a surgical plane of anesthesia. Post-anesthetic or emergence excitement has not been observed in animals preanesthetized with XYLA-JECT® (xylazine).

XYLA-JECT® (xylazine) has been used successfully as a preanesthetic agent for pentobarbital sodium, thiopental sodium, thiamylal sodium, nitrous oxide, ether, halothane, glyceryl guaiacolate and methoxyflurane anesthesia.

Cervidae: Administer intramuscularly, either by hand syringe or syringe dart, in the heavy muscles of the croup or shoulder.

Dosage Range:

Fallow Deer *(Dama dama):* 2.0 to 4.0 mL/100 lbs body weight (2.0 to 4.0 mg/lb)

Mule Deer *(Odocoileus hemionus),* Sika Deer *(Cervus nippon)* and White-Tailed Deer *(Odocoileus virginianus):* 1.0 to 2.0 mL/100 lbs body weight (1.0 to 2.0 mg/lb)

Elk *(Cervus canadensis):* 0.25 to 0.5 mL/100 lbs body weight (0.25 to 0.5 mg/lb)

Following injection of XYLA-JECT® (xylazine), the animal should be allowed to rest quietly until the full effect has been reached. These dosages produce sedation which is usually maintained for 1 to 2 hours and analgesia which lasts for 15 to 30 minutes.

Precaution(s): Store at controlled room temperature (15° to 30°C or 59° to 86°F).

Caution(s): Federal law restricts this drug to use by or on the order of a licensed veterinarian.

Careful consideration should be given before administering to horses and *Cervidae* with significantly depressed respiration, severe pathologic heart disease, advanced liver or kidney disease, severe endotoxic or traumatic shock and stress conditions such as extreme heat, cold, high altitude or fatigue.

Do not use XYLA-JECT® (xylazine) in conjunction with tranquilizers.

Analgesic effect is variable, and depth should be carefully assayed prior to surgical/clinical procedures. Variability of analgesia occurs most frequently at the distal extremities of horses and *Cervidae.* In spite of sedation, the practitioner and handlers should proceed with caution since defense reactions may not be diminished.

Horses: Since an additive effect results from the use of XYLA-JECT® (xylazine) and the barbiturate compounds, it should be used with caution with these central nervous system depressants. Products known to produce respiratory depression or apnea, such as thiamylal sodium, should be given at a reduced dosage and, when injected intravenously, should be administered slowly. When intravenous administration of XYLA-JECT® (xylazine) is desired, avoid perivascular injection in order to achieve the desired effect. Studies have shown negligible evidence of tissue irritation, however, following perivascular injection of xylazine.

Intracarotid arterial injection should be avoided. As with many compounds, including tranquilizers, immediate violent seizures followed by collapse may result from inadvertent administration into the carotid artery. Although the reaction with XYLA-JECT® (xylazine) is usually transient and recovery may be rapid and complete, special care should be taken to assure that the needle is in the jugular vein rather than the carotid artery.

Bradycardia and arrhythmia in the form of incomplete atrioventricular block have been reported following xylazine administration. Although clinically the importance of this effect is questioned,[1,2,3,4] a standard dose of atropine given prior to or following xylazine will greatly decrease the incidence.

Sedation for transport is most successful if actual transportation is begun after the full effect of the drug has been reached and the animal's stability is maintained while standing. In addition, it should be noted that animals under the influence of xylazine can be aroused by noise or other stimuli and this may increase the risk of injury.

Cervidae: As in all ruminants, it is preferable to administer XYLA-JECT® (xylazine) to fasted *Cervidae* as a safeguard against aspiration of food material into the lungs and/or bloat during deep sedation.

Care should be taken to administer XYLA-JECT® (xylazine) in the heavy muscles of the croup or shoulder. Injections given subcutaneously, intraperitoneally or into fat deposits will give unpredictable results.

Intra-arterial injection should be avoided, as with many compounds, including tranquilizers, immediate violent seizures followed by collapse may result from inadvertent administration into an artery.

The animal should not be disturbed during induction or until the full effect of the drug has been reached which is usually 10 to 15 minutes following injection.

The usual time to initial effect of the drug is 2 to 5 minutes. The administrator of the drug should be fully cognizant of this interval prior to administration of drug to free-ranging deer or elk, especially at night or in heavily wooded areas.

If the animal has been underdosed (faulty injection or miscalculation on weight) it is advisable to wait one hour before administering a second dose.

Adequate ventilation, especially in cages or crates, is mandatory; keep head and neck in position to insure patent air passage and to prevent aspiration of stomach contents.

During sedation, animals should be prevented from assuming lateral recumbency. A sternal recumbent position is desirable.

While under the effects of XYLA-JECT® (xylazine), the animal should be protected from extreme hot or cold environments.

Efforts should be made to prevent patient from rising until almost complete recovery is attained.

The transportation of *Cervidae* given XYLA-JECT® (xylazine) should be carefully monitored to prevent excessive struggling, injury or death.

Hyperthermic reactions may occur, especially if the subject is in a highly excited state when the drug is administered. Hosing the head and entire body with cold water has usually proven to be an effective deterrent.

The safety of XYLA-JECT® (xylazine) has not been demonstrated in pregnant *Cervidae.* Avoid use during the breeding season.

Cervidae should be observed closely until all of the sedative effects of XYLA-JECT® (xylazine) are gone.

Care should be taken at all times when administering XYLA-JECT® (xylazine) to *Cervidae.* This is due to the method of administration (usually darting), the difficulty in estimating body weights and the accepted theory that wild animals are more unpredictable in their response to sedatives and analgesics than the domesticated species.

Warning(s): This drug should not be administered to domestic food-producing animals. Not for use in horses intended for food.

Do not use in *Cervidae* less than 15 days before or during the hunting season.

Avoid accidental administration to humans. Should such exposure occur, notify a physician immediately. Artificial respiration may be indicated. In *Cervidae,* occasional capture-associated deaths occur. Clinical trials reveal a mortality rate of approximately 3.5% attendant with the administration of xylazine.

Not for human use.

Keep out of reach of children.

Toxicology: Safety: XYLA-JECT® (xylazine) is tolerated at 10 times the recommended dose in horses and at doses above the recommended range in *Cervidae.* However, some elevated doses produced muscle tremors and long periods of sedation.

Side Effects: XYLA-JECT® (xylazine), in horses and *Cervidae,* used at recommended dosage levels may occasionally cause slight muscle tremors, bradycardia with partial A-V heart block and a reduced respiratory rate. Movement in response to sharp auditory stimuli may be observed.

In horses, sweating, rarely profuse, has been reported following administration. In *Cervidae,* salivation, various vocalizations (bellowing, bleating, groaning, grunting, snoring) on expiration, audible grinding of molar teeth, protruding tongue and elevated temperatures have also been noted in some cases.

References: Available upon request.

Presentation: XYLA-JECT® is supplied in 50 mL multiple dose vials (NDC 57319-314-04).

Manufactured by: Phoenix Scientific, Inc., St. Joseph, MO 64503.

Compendium Code No.: 12561002 Rev. 8-00

XYLAZINE-20 INJECTION ℞

Butler **Analgesic-Sedative**

Xylazine Sterile Solution 20 mg per mL

NADA No.: 139-236

Active Ingredient(s): XYLAZINE-20 INJECTION is supplied as a sterile solution. Each mL contains xylazine hydrochloride equivalent to 20 mg of base activity, methylparaben 0.9 mg, propylparaben 0.1 mg, and water for injection. The pH is adjusted with citric acid and sodium citrate.

Indications: Xylazine should be used in dogs when it is desirable to produce a state of sedation accompanied by a shorter period of analgesia. Xylazine has been used successfully as follows:

1. Diagnostic procedures, such as examination of mouth and ears, abdominal palpation, rectal palpation, vaginal examination, catheterization of the bladder and radiographic examinations of the head and extremities.
2. Orthopedic procedures, such as the application of casting materials and splints.
3. Dental procedures.
4. Minor surgical procedures of short duration, such as debridement, removal of cutaneous neoplasms and suturing of lacerations.
5. To calm and facilitate the handling of fractious animals.
6. Major surgical procedures:
   a. When used as a pre-anesthetic to general anesthesia.
   b. When used in conjunction with local anesthetics.

Pharmacology: Xylazine, a non-narcotic compound, is a sedative and analgesic as well as a muscle relaxant.[1] Its sedative and analgesic activity is related to central nervous system depression. Its muscle relaxant effect is based on inhibition of the intraneural transmission of impulses in the central nervous system. The principal pharmacological activities develop within 10 to 15 minutes after intramuscular or subcutaneous injection, and within three to five minutes following intravenous administration.

A sleeplike state, the depth of which is dose-dependent, is usually maintained for one to two hours, while analgesia lasts from 15 to 30 minutes. The muscle relaxant effect causes relaxation of the skeletal musculature complementing sedation and analgesia.

In animals under the influence of xylazine, the respiratory rate is reduced as in natural sleep. Following treatment with xylazine, the heart rate is decreased and a transient change in the conductivity of the cardiac muscle may occur as evidenced by a partial atrioventricular block. This resembles the atrioventricular block often observed in apparently normal animals.[2] Intravenous administration of xylazine causes a transient rise in blood pressure, followed by a slight decrease.

Xylazine does not have an effect on blood clotting time or on other hematological parameters.

Dosage and Administration:

1. Dosage:

   Intravenous - 0.5 mL/20 lbs. of body weight (0.5 mg/lb., or 1.1 mg/kg).

   Intramuscular or subcutaneous - 1.0 mL/20 lbs. of body weight (1.0 mg/lb., or 2.2 mg/kg).

   In large dogs (over 50 lbs.), a dosage of 0.5 mg/lb. administered intramuscularly may provide sufficient sedation and/or analgesia for most procedures.

   Since vomiting may occur (see Side Effects), fasting for 6-24 hours prior to the use of xylazine may reduce the incidence; the I.V. route results in the least vomiting.

   Following the injection of xylazine, the animal should be allowed to rest quietly until the full effect has been reached.

   These dosages produce sedation which is usually maintained for one (1) to two (2) hours and analgesia which lasts for 15 to 30 minutes.
2. Pre-anesthetic to local anesthesia: Xylazine at the recommended dosages can be used in conjunction with local anesthetics, such as procaine or lidocaine.
3. Pre-anesthetic to general anesthesia: Xylazine at the recommended dosage rates produces an additive effect to central nervous system depressants such as pentobarbital sodium, thiopental sodium and thiamylal sodium. Therefore, the dosage of such compounds should be reduced and administered to the desired effect. In general, one-third (⅓) to one-half (½) of the calculated dosage of the barbiturates will be needed to produce a surgical plane of anesthesia. Postanesthetic or emergence excitement has not been observed in animals pre-anesthetized with xylazine.

   Xylazine has been used successfully as a pre-anesthetic agent for pentobarbital sodium, thiopental sodium, thiamylal sodium, nitrous oxide, ether, halothane and methoxyflurane anesthesia.

Precaution(s): Protect from heat. Do not store at temperatures over 86°F (30°C).

Caution(s): Federal law restricts this drug to use by or on the order of a licensed veterinarian.

Clinical results with xylazine have not revealed any detrimental effects when the compound is administered to pregnant dogs. However, until more definitive studies are completed, xylazine is not recommended for use in these animals.

Careful consideration should be given before administering to dogs with significantly depressed respiration, severe pathologic heart disease, advanced liver or kidney disease, severe endotoxic or traumatic shock and stress conditions such as extreme heat, cold, or fatigue.

The analgesic effect is variable, and depth should be carefully assayed prior to surgical/clinical procedures. In spite of sedation, the practitioner and handlers should proceed with caution since defense reactions may not be diminished.

Do not use xylazine in conjunction with tranquilizers.

Since an additive effect results from the use of xylazine and the barbiturate compounds, it should be used with caution with these central nervous system depressants. Products known to produce respiratory depression or apnea, such as thiamylal sodium, should be given at a reduced dosage and, when injected intravenously, should be administered slowly.

When intravenous administration is desired, avoid perivascular injection in order to achieve the desired effect. Studies have shown negligible evidence of tissue irritation following perivascular injection of xylazine.

Bradycardia and an arrhythmia in the form of incomplete atrioventricular block have been reported following xylazine administration. Although clinically the importance of this effect is questioned,[2] a standard dose of atropine given prior to or following xylazine injection will greatly decrease the incidence.

While sedation usually lasts from one to two hours, recovery periods in excess of four to five hours have been reported in dogs.

Warning(s): The drug is for use in dogs only.

Not for human use. The drug should not be adminstered to food-producing animals.

Toxicology: Xylazine has been tested in dogs at four times the recommended dose. Doses of this magnitude produced muscle tremors, emesis and long periods of sedation.

Side Effects: Emesis occurs occasionally in dogs soon after the administration of xylazine, but before clinical sedation is evident. When observed, emesis usually occurs only a single time, after which there is no further emetic effect. The use of anti-emetics may delay this phenomenon. The occurrence of emesis may be considered a desirable effect when xylazine is administered as a pre-anesthetic to general anesthesia.

Xylazine used at the recommended dosage levels may occasionally cause slight muscle tremors, bradycardia with partial A-V heart block and a reduced respiratory rate. Should excessive respiratory depression occur following the use of xylazine, administer respiratory stimulants and provide artificial respiration.

Gaseous extension of the stomach may occur in dogs treated with xylazine making radiographic interpretation more difficult.[3]

Movement in response to sharp auditory stimuli may be observed.

References: Available upon request.

Presentation: 20 mL multiple-dose vials.

Compendium Code No.: 10821910

XYLAZINE-100 INJECTION ℞

Butler **Analgesic-Sedative**

Xylazine Sterile Solution 100 mg per mL

NADA No.: 140-442

Active Ingredient(s): XYLAZINE-100 INJECTION is supplied as a sterile solution. Each mL contains xylazine hydrochloride equivalent to 100 mg of base activity, methylparaben 0.9 mg, propylparaben 0.1 mg, and water for injection. The pH is adjusted with citric acid and sodium citrate.

Indications: Xylazine should be used in horses when it is desirable to produce a state of sedation accompanied by a shorter period of analgesia. Xylazine has been used successfully as follows:

1. Diagnostic procedures, such as oral and ophthalmic examinations, abdominal palpation, rectal palpation, vaginal examination, catheterization of the bladder and radiographic examinations.
2. Orthopedic procedures, such as the application of casting materials and splints.
3. Dental procedures.
4. Minor surgical procedures of short duration, such as debridement, removal of cutaneous neoplasms and suturing of lacerations.
5. To calm and facilitate handling of fractious animals.
6. Major surgical procedures:
   a. When used as a pre-anesthetic to general anesthesia.
   b. When used in conjunction with local anesthetics.

Pharmacology: Xylazine, a non-narcotic compound, is a sedative and analgesic as well as a muscle relaxant. Its sedative and analgesic activity is related to central nervous system depression. Its muscle-relaxant effect is based on inhibition of the intraneural transmission of impulses in the central nervous system. The principal pharmacological activities develop within 10 to 15 minutes after intramuscular injection, and within three to five minutes following intravenous administration.

A sleeplike state, the depth of which is dose-dependent, is usually maintained for one to two hours, while analgesia lasts from 15 to 30 minutes. The muscle-relaxant effect causes relaxation of the skeletal musculature complementing sedation and analgesia.

In animals under the influence of xylazine, the respiratory rate is reduced as in natural sleep. Following treatment with xylazine, the heart rate is decreased and a transient change in the conductivity of the cardiac muscle may occur, as evidenced by a partial atrioventricular block. This resembles the atrioventricular block often observed in normal horses.[1,2,3,4] Although a partial A-V block may occasionally occur following intramuscular injection of xylazine, the incidence is less than when it is administered intravenously. Intravenous administration of xylazine causes a transient rise in blood pressure, followed by a slight decrease.

Xylazine does not have an effect on blood clotting time or on other hematologic parameters.

Dosage and Administration:

1. Dosage:
   Intravenous - 0.5 mL/100 lbs. of body weight (0.5 mg/lb., or 1.1 mg/kg).
   Intramuscular - 1.0 mL/100 lbs. of body weight (1 mg/lb., or 2.2 mg/kg).
   Following the injection of xylazine, the animal should be allowed to rest quietly until the full effect has been reached.
   These dosages produce sedation which is usually maintained for one (1) to two (2) hours, and analgesia which lasts for 15 to 30 minutes.
2. Pre-anesthetic to local anesthesia: Xylazine at the recommended dosages can be used in conjunction with local anesthetics, such as procaine or lidocaine.
3. Pre-anesthetic to general anesthesia: Xylazine, at the recommended dosage rates, produces an additive effect to central nervous system depressants such as pentobarbital sodium, thiopental sodium and thiamylal sodium. Therefore, the dosage of such compounds should be reduced and administered to the desired effect. In general, only one-third (⅓) to one-half (½) of the calculated dosage of the barbiturates will be needed to produce a surgical plane of anesthesia. Postanesthetic or emergence excitement has not been observed in animals pre-anesthetized with xylazine.
   Xylazine has been used successfully as a pre-anesthetic agent for pentobarbital sodium, thiopental sodium, thiamylal sodium, nitrous oxide, ether, halothane, glyceryl guaiacolate and methoxyflurane anesthesia.

Precaution(s): Protect from heat. Do not store at temperatures over 86°F (30°C).

Caution(s): Federal law restricts this drug to use by or on the order of a licensed veterinarian.

Careful consideration should be given before administering to horses with significantly depressed respiration, severe pathologic heart disease, advanced liver or kidney disease, severe endotoxic or traumatic shock and stress conditions such as extreme heat, cold, high altitude or fatigue.

Do not use xylazine in conjunction with tranquilizers.

Since an additive effect results from the use of xylazine with the barbiturate compounds, it should be used with caution with these central nervous system depressants. Products known to produce respiratory depression or apnea, such as thiamylal sodium, should be given at a reduced dosage and, when injected intravenously, should be administered slowly. When intravenous administration is desired, avoid perivascular injection in order to achieve the desired effect. Studies have shown negligible evidence of tissue irritation following perivascular injection of xylazine.

Intracarotid arterial injection should be avoided. As with many compounds, including tranquilizers, immediate violent seizures followed by collapse may result from inadvertent administration into the carotid artery. Although the reaction with xylazine is usually transient and recovery may be rapid and complete, special care should be taken to assure that the needle is in the jugular vein rather than the carotid artery.

Bradycardia and an arrhythmia in the form of incomplete atrioventricular block have been reported following xylazine administration. Although clinically the importance of this effect is questioned,[1,2,3,4] a standard dose of atropine given prior to or following xylazine injection will greatly decrease the incidence.

The analgesic effect is variable, and depth should be carefully assayed prior to surgical/clinical procedures. Variability of analgesia occurs most frequently at the distal extremities of the horse. In spite of sedation, the practitioner and handlers should proceed with caution since defense reactions may not be diminished.

Sedation for transport is most successful if actual transportation is begun after the full effect of the drug has been reached and the animal's stability is maintained while standing. In addition, it should be noted that animals under the influence of xylazine can be aroused by noise or other stimuli and this may increase the risk of injury.

Warning(s): Not for human use. The drug is for use in horses only and should not be administered to food-producing animals.

Toxicology: Xylazine has been tested in horses at five times the recommended dose. Doses of this magnitude may produce convulsions and long periods of sedation.

Side Effects: Xylazine used at the recommended dosage levels may occasionally cause slight muscle tremors, bradycardia with partial A-V heart block and a reduced respiratory rate. Movement in response to sharp auditory stimuli may be observed. Sweating, rarely profuse, has been reported following administration.

References: Available upon request.

Presentation: 50 mL multiple-dose vials.

Compendium Code No.: 10821900

XYLAZINE HCL INJECTION ℞

Boehringer Ingelheim **Analgesic-Sedative**

100 mg/mL Xylazine Base Sedative

NADA No.: 140-442

Active Ingredient(s): Each mL contains: Xylazine HCl equivalent to 100 mg xylazine base; 0.9 mg methylparaben and 0.1 mg propylparaben as preservatives; 6.12 mg sodium citrate dihydrate; water for injection, qs.

Hydrochloric acid and/or sodium citrate dihydrate may also be used, as necessary, for pH adjustment.

Indications: XYLAZINE HCL INJECTION should be used in horses when it is desirable to produce a state of sedation. It has been successfully used when conducting various diagnostic, orthopedic and dental procedures and for minor surgical procedures of short duration. It may also be used as a pre-anesthetic to local or general anesthesia.

Pharmacology: Xylazine is pharmacologically classified as a non-narcotic sedative.[1,2,3,4] The drug causes sedation by acting upon α-adrenergic receptors in the brain to prevent the release of norepinephrine.[5] Xylazine also produces muscle relaxation by inhibiting the intraneural transmission of impulses in the central nervous system.[1,4]

Deep sedation develops in the horse within 10 to 15 minutes after intramuscular injection, and within three to five minutes following intravenous administration.[1,2,4,6,7] Deep sedation lasts 15 to 20 minutes, while a sleep-like state, the depth of which is dose-dependent, is usually maintained for one to two hours following intramuscular administration of the drug at the recommended dosage.[1,2,4,6,7] Recovery is complete within 30-40 minutes following intravenous injection.[1,2,6,7]

In animals under the influence of xylazine, the respiratory and pulse rates are reduced as in a natural sleep.[1,3,4,5] The intramuscular injection of xylazine produces only negligible effects on the cardiovascular and respiratory systems. However, intravenous administration in the horse may cause transient changes in the conductivity of the cardiac muscle, evidenced by partial atrioventricular (AV) blocks, bradycardia, decreased cardiac output and a rise in arterial blood pressure.[1,3,4,5,6,7] These actions are transient and can be counteracted to a large degree by the administration of atropine prior to or following xylazine injection.[1,3,4,5] Xylazine does not have an effect on blood clotting time or other hematologic parameters.[4]

Although not devoid of undesirable attributes, xylazine seems to possess certain properties which make it a better sedative for horses than any other compound currently in use.[6,7] It is more dependable, results in less respiratory depression and greater cardiovascular stability and has resulted in a higher percentage of quiet recoveries from surgical anesthesia in the horse than when promazine hydrochloride or acepromazine maleate is used for pre-anesthetic medication.[1,7]

Dosage and Administration: For intravenous or intramuscular administration in horses.

The recommended dosage for intravenous administration is 0.5 mL/100 lbs. of body weight (0.5 mg/lb). The recommended dosage for intramuscular administration is 1.0 mL/100 lbs. of body weight (1.0 mg/lb). Following administration of XYLAZINE HCL INJECTION, the animal should be allowed to rest quietly until the full effect has been reached. These dosages produce a state of sedation which is usually maintained for one (1) to two (2) hours.

Pre-anesthetic to Local Anesthesia: At the recommended dosage rates, XYLAZINE HCL INJECTION may be used in conjunction with local anesthetics, such as procaine and lidocaine.

Pre-anesthetic to General Anesthesia: At the recommended dosage rates, XYLAZINE HCL INJECTION produces an additive effect to central nervous system depressants, such as sodium pentobarbital, sodium thiopental and sodium thiamylal. Accordingly, the dosage of such compounds should be reduced and administered to the desired effect. Generally, one-third (⅓) to one-half (½) of the calculated dosage of the barbiturates will be needed to produce a surgical plane of anesthesia. Postanesthetic or emergence excitement has not been observed in animals pre-anesthetized with XYLAZINE HCL INJECTION.

XYLAZINE HCL INJECTION has been successfully used as a pre-anesthetic agent for sodium pentobarbital, sodium thiopental, sodium thiamylal, nitrous oxide, ether, halothane, glyceryl guaiacolate and methoxyflurane anesthesia.

Contraindication(s): Xylazine should not be used in conjunction with neuroleptics or tranquilizers.[1,4,5]

Precaution(s): Debilitated animals with depressed respiration, cardiac disease, renal and liver impairment, shock or any other stress conditions should be carefully monitored whenever xylazine is administered.[1]

Because xylazine produces an additive effect to central nervous system depressants, caution should be taken when administering barbiturate compounds in conjunction with xylazine. These drugs should be given at a reduced dosage to the desired effect, and when injected intravenously, should be given slowly.

Arrythmias, resulting in partial AV blocks, and bradycardia are transient changes which may occur, but that can be counteracted to a large degree by the administration of atropine prior to or following xylazine injection.[1,3,4,5]

The analgesic effect is variable, and sedative depth should be carefully determined prior to surgical/clinical procedures. The variability of analgesia occurs most frequently at the distal extremities of the horse. In spite of sedation, the practitioner should proceed with caution, since defense reactions may not be diminished. Sedation for transport is most successful if the actual transportation is initiated after the full effect of the drug has been obtained and the animal's stability maintained in the standing position. It should be noted that animals under the influence of xylazine are particularly sensitive to noise and care should be taken accordingly, to avoid risk of injury.

Caution(s): Federal law restricts this drug to use by or on the order of a licensed veterinarian.

Keep out of the reach of children.

Warning(s): Intracarotid arterial injection should be avoided. As with many drugs, including tranquilizers, immediate and violent seizure followed by collapse may result from inadvertent administration into the carotid artery. Although the reaction with xylazine is usually transient and the recovery rapid and complete, special care should be taken to ensure that the needle is in the jugular vein rather than the carotid artery.

Do not use in horses intended for food.

Toxicology: Xylazine is tolerated in horses at 10 times the recommended dosage, however, doses of this magnitude produce muscle tremors and long periods of sedation.[4]

Side Effects: The deep sedation produced by xylazine is characterized by lowering of the head, drooping of the eyelids and lower lip and a marked reluctance to move.[1,6] Most horses given xylazine sweat around the ears and poll region, and may seem particularly sensitive to sharp auditory stimuli during the recovery period.[1,4,6,7] The respiratory and pulse rate are reduced as in natural sleep.[1,3,4,5] Transient changes in the conductivity of the cardiac muscle (resulting in partial AV blocks), bradycardia, decreased cardiac output and a rise in arterial blood pressure may occur following intravenous administration.[1,3,4,5,6,7]

References: Available upon request.

Presentation: 50 mL multiple-dose vials.

Compendium Code No.: 10281170

XYLAZINE HCL INJECTION ℞

RXV **Analgesic-Sedative**

(Xylazine) 100 mg/mL-Sedative and Analgesic

ANADA No.: 200-139

Active Ingredient(s):

Xylazine hydrochloride (equivalent to 10% base) 11.4%
Inert Ingredients: 88.6%
Total 100.0%

Description: Each mL contains 100 mg xylazine, (base equivalent), 0.9 mg methylparaben, 0.1 mg propylparaben, water for injection; citric acid and sodium citrate for pH adjustment to 5.5 ± 0.3.

Indications: XYLAZINE HCL INJECTION (xylazine) should be used in horses and *Cervidae* (Fallow Deer, Mule Deer, Sika Deer, White-Tailed Deer and Elk) when it is desirable to produce a state of sedation accompanied by a shorter period of analgesia.

Horses: XYLAZINE HCL INJECTION (xylazine) has been used successfully as follows:

1. Diagnostic procedures - oral and ophthalmic examinations, abdominal palpation, rectal palpation, vaginal examination, catheterization of the bladder and radiographic examinations.
2. Orthopedic procedures, such as application of casting materials and splints.
3. Dental procedures.
4. Minor surgical procedures of short duration such as debridement, removal of cutaneous neoplasms and suturing of lacerations.
5. To calm and facilitate handling of fractious animals.
6. Therapeutic medication for sedation and relief of pain following injury or surgery.
7. Major surgical procedures:
   a. When used as a preanesthetic to general anesthesia.
   b. When used in conjunction with local anesthetics.

Cervidae: XYLAZINE HCL INJECTION (xylazine) may be used for the following:

1. To calm and facilitate handling of fractious animals.
2. Diagnostic procedures.
3. Minor surgical procedures.
4. Therapeutic medication for sedation and relief of pain following injury or surgery.
5. As a preanesthetic to local anesthesia. XYLAZINE HCL INJECTION (xylazine) at the recommended dosages can be used in conjunction with local anesthetics, such as procaine or lidocaine.

Pharmacology: XYLAZINE HCL INJECTION (xylazine), a non-narcotic compound, is a sedative and analgesic as well as muscle relaxant. Its sedative and analgesic activity is related to central nervous system depression. Its muscle relaxant effect is based on inhibition of the intraneural transmission of impulses in the central nervous system. The principal pharmacological activities develop within 10 to 15 minutes after intramuscular injection in horses and *Cervidae*, and within 3 to 5 minutes following intravenous administration in horses.

A sleeplike state, the depth of which is dose-dependent, is usually maintained for 1 to 2 hours, while analgesia lasts from 15 to 30 minutes. The centrally-acting muscle relaxant effect causes relaxation of the skeletal musculature, complementing sedation and analgesia.

In horses and *Cervidae* under the influence of XYLAZINE HCL INJECTION (xylazine), the respiratory rate is reduced as in natural sleep. Following treatment with XYLAZINE HCL INJECTION (xylazine), the heart rate is decreased and a transient change in the conductivity of the cardiac muscle may occur, as evidenced by a partial atrioventricular block. This resembles the atrioventricular block often observed in normal horses.[1,2,3,4] Partial A-V block may occasionally occur following intramuscular injection of XYLAZINE HCL INJECTION (xylazine). When given intravenously in horses, the incidence of partial A-V block is higher. Intravenous administration causes a transient rise in blood pressure in horses, followed by a slight decrease.

XYLAZINE HCL INJECTION (xylazine) has no effect on blood clotting time or other hematologic parameters.

Dosage and Administration:

Horses:

1. Dosage:
   Intravenously - 0.5 mL/100 lbs body weight (0.5 mg/lb).
   Intramuscularly - 1.0 mL/100 lbs body weight (1.0 mg/lb).
   Following injection of XYLAZINE HCL INJECTION (xylazine) the animal should be allowed to rest quietly until the full effect has been reached.
   These dosages produce sedation which is usually maintained for 1 to 2 hours, and analgesia which lasts for 15 to 30 minutes.
2. Preanesthetic to Local Anesthesia: XYLAZINE HCL INJECTION (xylazine) at the recommended dosages can be used in conjunction with local anesthetics, such as procaine or lidocaine.
3. Preanesthetic to General Anesthesia: XYLAZINE HCL INJECTION (xylazine) at the recommended dosage rates produces an additive effect to central nervous system depressants such as pentobarbital sodium, thiopental sodium and thiamyl sodium. Therefore, the dosage of such compounds should be reduced and administered to the desired effect. In general, only ⅓ to ½ of the calculated dosage of the barbiturates will be needed to produce a surgical plane of anesthesia. Post-anesthetic or emergence excitement has not been observed in animals preanesthetized with XYLAZINE HCL INJECTION (xylazine).

XYLAZINE HCL INJECTION (xylazine) has been used successfully as a preanesthetic agent for pentobarbital sodium, thiopental sodium, thiamylal sodium, nitrous oxide, ether, halothane, glyceryl guaiacolate and methoxyflurane anesthesia.

Cervidae: Administer intramuscularly, either by hand syringe or syringe dart, in the heavy muscles of the croup or shoulder.

Dosage Range:

Fallow Deer *(Dama dama)* - 2.0 to 4.0 mL/100 lbs body weight (2.0 to 4.0 mg/lb).

Mule Deer *(Odocoileus hemionus)* - 1.0 to 2.0 mL/100 lbs body weight (1.0 to 2.0 mg/lb).

Sika Deer *(Cervus nippon)* - 1.0 to 2.0 mL/100 lbs body weight (1.0 to 2.0 mg/lb).

White-Tailed Deer *(Odocoileus virginianus)* - 1.0 to 2.0 mL/100 lbs body weight (1.0 to 2.0 mg/lb).

Elk *(Cervus canadensis)* - 0.25 to 0.5 mL/100 lbs body weight (0.25 to 0.5 mg/lb).

Following injection of XYLAZINE HCL INJECTION (xylazine) the animal should be allowed to rest quietly until the full effect has been reached. These dosages produce sedation which is usually maintained for 1 to 2 hours and analgesia which lasts for 15 to 30 minutes.

Precaution(s): Store at controlled room temperature (15° to 30°C or 59° to 86°F).

Caution(s): Federal law restricts this drug to use by or on the order of a licensed veterinarian.

Careful consideration should be given before administering to horses and *Cervidae* with significantly depressed respiration, severe pathologic heart disease, advanced liver or kidney disease, severe endotoxic or traumatic shock and stress conditions such as extreme heat, cold, high altitude or fatigue.

Do not use XYLAZINE HCL INJECTION (xylazine) in conjunction with tranquilizers.

Analgesic effect is variable, and depth should be carefully assayed prior to surgical/clinical procedures. Variability of analgesia occurs most frequently at the distal extremities of horses and *Cervidae*. In spite of sedation, the practitioner and handlers should proceed with caution since defense reactions may not be diminished.

Horses: Since an additive effect results from the use of XYLAZINE HCL INJECTION (xylazine) and the barbiturate compounds, it should be used with caution with these central nervous system depressants. Products known to produce respiratory depression or apnea, such as thiamylal sodium should be given at a reduced dosage and, when injected intravenously, should be administered slowly. When intravenous administration of XYLAZINE HCL INJECTION (xylazine) is desired, avoid perivascular injection in order to achieve the desired effect. Studies have shown negligible evidence of tissue irritation, however, following perivascular injection of xylazine.

Intracarotid arterial injection should be avoided. As with many compounds, including tranquilizers, immediate violent seizures followed by collapse may result from inadvertent administration into the carotid artery. Although the reaction with XYLAZINE HCL INJECTION (xylazine) is usually transient and recovery may be rapid and complete, special care should be taken to assure that the needle is in the jugular vein rather than the carotid artery.

Bradycardia and arrhythmia in the form of incomplete atrioventricular block have been reported following xylazine administration. Although clinically the importance of this effect is questioned,[1,2,3,4] a standard dose of atropine given prior to or following xylazine will greatly decrease the incidence.

Sedation for transport is most successful if actual transportation is begun after the full effect of the drug has been reached and the animal's stability is maintained while standing. In addition, it should be noted that animals under the influence of xylazine can be aroused by noise or other stimuli and this may increase the risk of injury.

Cervidae: As in all ruminants, it is preferable to administer XYLAZINE HCL INJECTION (xylazine) to fasted *Cervidae* as a safeguard against aspiration of food material into the lungs and/or bloat during deep sedation.

Care should be taken to administer XYLAZINE HCL INJECTION (xylazine) in the heavy muscles of the croup or shoulder. Injections given subcutaneously, intraperitoneally or into fat deposits will give unpredictable results.

Intra-arterial injection should be avoided, as with many compounds, including tranquilizers, immediate violent seizures followed by collapse may result from inadvertent administration into an artery.

The animal should not be disturbed during induction or until the full effect of the drug has been reached which is usually 10 to 15 minutes following injection.

The usual time to initial effect of the drug is 2 to 5 minutes. The administrator of the drug should be fully cognizant of this interval prior to administration of drug to free-ranging deer or elk, especially at night or in heavily wooded areas.

If the animal has been underdosed (faulty injection or miscalculation on weight) it is advisable to wait one hour before administering a second dose.

Adequate ventilation, especially in cages or crates, is mandatory; keep head and neck in position to insure patient air passage and to prevent aspiration of stomach contents.

During sedation, animals should be prevented from assuming lateral recumbency. A sternal recumbent position is desirable.

While under the effects of XYLAZINE HCL INJECTION (xylazine) the animal should be protected from extreme hot or cold environments.

Efforts should be made to prevent patient from rising until almost complete recovery is attained.

The transportation of *Cervidae* given XYLAZINE HCL INJECTION (xylazine) should be carefully monitored to prevent excessive struggling, injury or death.

Hyperthermic reactions may occur, especially if the subject is in a highly excited state when the drug is administered. Hosing the head and entire body with cold water has usually proven to be an effective deterrent.

The safety of XYLAZINE HCL INJECTION (xylazine) has not been demonstrated in pregnant *Cervidae*. Avoid use during the breeding season.

Cervidae should be observed closely until all of the sedative effects of XYLAZINE HCL INJECTION (xylazine) are gone.

Care should be taken at all times when administering XYLAZINE HCL INJECTION (xylazine) to *Cervidae*. This is due to the method of administration (usually darting), the difficulty in estimating body weights and the accepted theory that wild animals are more unpredictable in their response to sedatives and analgesics than the domesticated species.

Warning(s): This drug should not be administered to domestic food-producing animals. Not for use in horses intended for food.

Avoid accidental administration to humans. Should such exposure occur, notify a physician immediately. Artificial respiration may be indicated.

In *Cervidae*, occasional capture-associated deaths occur. Clinical trials reveal a mortality rate of approximately 3.5% attendant with the administration of xylazine.

Keep out of reach of children.

Side Effects: XYLAZINE HCL INJECTION (xylazine) in horses and *Cervidae*, used at recommended dosage levels may occasionally cause slight muscle tremors, bradycardia with partial A-V heart block and a reduced respiratory rate. Movement in response to sharp auditory stimuli may be observed.

In horses, sweating, rarely profuse, has been reported following administration. In *Cervidae*, salivation, various vocalizations (bellowing, bleating, groaning, grunting, snoring) on expiration, audible grinding of molar teeth, protruding tongue and elevated temperatures have also been noted in some cases.

Trial Data: Safety: XYLAZINE HCL INJECTION (xylazine) is tolerated at 10 times the recommended dose in horses and at doses above the recommended range in *Cervidae*. However, some elevated doses produced muscle tremors and long periods of sedation.

References: Available upon request.

Presentation: XYLAZINE HCL INJECTION (xylazine) is available in 50 mL multiple dose vials.

Manufactured by: Phoenix Scientific, Inc., St. Joseph, MO 64503.

Compendium Code No.: 10910311 Rev. 4-00

XYLAZINE HCL INJECTION ℞

Vet Tek **Analgesic-Sedative**

(Xylazine) 100 mg/mL-Sedative and Analgesic

ANADA No.: 200-139

Active Ingredient(s):

Xylazine hydrochloride (Equivalent to 10% base) 11.4%
Inert Ingredients: 88.6%
Total 100.0%

Each mL contains 100 mg xylazine, (base equivalent), 0.9 mg methylparaben, 0.1 mg propylparaben, water for injection; citric acid and sodium citrate for pH adjustment to 5.5 ± 0.3.

Indications: XYLAZINE HCL INJECTION (xylazine) should be used in horses and *Cervidae* (Fallow Deer, Mule Deer, Sika Deer, White-Tailed Deer and Elk) when it is desirable to produce a state of sedation accompanied by a shorter period of analgesia.

Horses: XYLAZINE HCL INJECTION (xylazine) has been used successfully as follows:

1. Diagnostic procedures - oral and ophthalmic examinations, abdominal palpation, rectal palpation, vaginal examination, catheterization of the bladder and radiographic examinations.
2. Orthopedic procedures, such as application of casting materials and splints.
3. Dental procedures.
4. Minor surgical procedures of short duration such as debridement, removal of cutaneous neoplasms and suturing of lacerations.
5. To calm and facilitate handling of fractious animals.
6. Therapeutic medication for sedation and relief of pain following injury or surgery.
7. Major surgical procedures:
   a. When used as a preanesthetic to general anesthesia.
   b. When used in conjunction with local anesthetics.

Cervidae: XYLAZINE HCL INJECTION (xylazine) may be used for the following:

1. To calm and facilitate handling of fractious animals.
2. Diagnostic procedures.
3. Minor surgical procedures.
4. Therapeutic medication for sedation and relief of pain following injury or surgery.
5. As a preanesthetic to local anesthesia. XYLAZINE HCL INJECTION (xylazine) at the recommended dosages can be used in conjunction with local anesthetics, such as procaine or lidocaine.

Pharmacology: XYLAZINE HCL INJECTION (xylazine), a non-narcotic compound, is a sedative and analgesic as well as a muscle relaxant. Its sedative and analgesic activity is related to central nervous system depression. Its muscle relaxant effect is based on inhibition of the intraneural transmission of impulses in the central nervous system. The principal pharmacological activities develop within 10 to 15 minutes after intramuscular injection in horses and *Cervidae*, and within 3 to 5 minutes following intravenous administration in horses.

A sleeplike state, the depth of which is dose-dependent, is usually maintained for 1 to 2 hours, while analgesia lasts from 15 to 30 minutes. The centrally-acting muscle relaxant effect causes relaxation of the skeletal musculature, complementing sedation and analgesia.

In horses and *Cervidae* under the influence of XYLAZINE HCL INJECTION (xylazine), the respiratory rate is reduced as in natural sleep. Following treatment with XYLAZINE HCL INJECTION (xylazine), the heart rate is decreased and a transient change in the conductivity of the cardiac muscle may occur, as evidenced by a partial atrioventricular block. This resembles the atrioventricular block often observed in normal horses.[1,2,3,4] Partial A-V block may occasionally occur following intramuscular injection of XYLAZINE HCL INJECTION (xylazine). When given intravenously in horses, the incidence of partial A-V block is higher. Intravenous administration causes a transient rise in blood pressure in horses, followed by a slight decrease.

XYLAZINE HCL INJECTION (xylazine) has no effect on blood clotting time or other hematologic parameters.

Dosage and Administration:

Horses:

1. Dosage:
   Intravenously - 0.5 mL/100 lbs body weight (0.5 mg/lb).
   Intramuscularly - 1.0 mL/100 lbs body weight (1.0 mg/lb).
   Following injection of XYLAZINE HCL INJECTION (xylazine) the animal should be allowed to rest quietly until the full effect has been reached.
   These dosages produce sedation which is usually maintained for 1 to 2 hours, and analgesia which lasts for 15 to 30 minutes.
2. Preanesthetic to Local Anesthesia:
   XYLAZINE HCL INJECTION (xylazine) at the recommended dosages can be used in conjunction with local anesthetics, such as procaine or lidocaine.
3. Preanesthetic to General Anesthesia:
   XYLAZINE HCL INJECTION (xylazine) at the recommended dosage rates produces an additive effect to central nervous system depressants such as pentobarbital sodium, thiopental sodium and thiamyl sodium. Therefore, the dosage of such compounds should be reduced and administered to the desired effect. In general, only ⅓ to ½ of the calculated dosage of the barbiturates will be needed to produce a surgical plane of anesthesia. Post-anesthetic or emergence excitement has not been observed in animals preanesthetized with XYLAZINE HCL INJECTION (xylazine).
   XYLAZINE HCL INJECTION (xylazine) has been used successfully as a preanesthetic agent for pentobarbital sodium, thiopental sodium, thiamylal sodium, nitrous oxide, ether, halothane, glyceryl guaiacolate and methoxyflurane anesthesia.

Cervidae:

Administer intramuscularly, either by hand syringe or syringe dart, in the heavy muscles of the croup or shoulder.

Dosage Range:

Fallow Deer *(Dama dama)* - 2.0 to 4.0 mL/100 lbs body weight (2.0 to 4.0 mg/lb).

Mule Deer *(Odocoileus hemionus)* - 1.0 to 2.0 mL/100 lbs body weight (1.0 to 2.0 mg/lb).

Sika Deer *(Cervus nippon)* - 1.0 to 2.0 mL/100 lbs body weight (1.0 to 2.0 mg/lb).

White-Tailed Deer *(Odocoileus virginianus)* - 1.0 to 2.0 mL/100 lbs body weight (1.0 to 2.0 mg/lb).

Elk *(Cervus canadensis)* - 0.25 to 0.5 mL/100 lbs body weight (0.25 to 0.5 mg/lb).

Following injection of XYLAZINE HCL INJECTION (xylazine) the animal should be allowed to rest quietly until the full effect has been reached. These dosages produce sedation which is usually maintained for 1 to 2 hours and analgesia which lasts for 15 to 30 minutes.

Precaution(s): Store at controlled room temperature (15° to 30°C or 59° to 86°F).

Caution(s): Federal law restricts this drug to use by or on the order of a licensed veterinarian.

Careful consideration should be given before administering to horses and *Cervidae* with significantly depressed respiration, severe pathologic heart disease, advanced liver or kidney disease, severe endotoxic or traumatic shock and stress conditions such as extreme heat, cold, high altitude or fatigue.

Do not use XYLAZINE HCL INJECTION (xylazine) in conjunction with tranquilizers.

Analgesic effect is variable, and depth should be carefully assayed prior to surgical/clinical procedures. Variability of analgesia occurs most frequently at the distal extremities of horses and *Cervidae*. In spite of sedation, the practitioner and handlers should proceed with caution since defense reactions may not be diminished.

Horses: Since an additive effect results from the use of XYLAZINE HCL INJECTION (xylazine) and the barbiturate compounds, it should be used with caution with these central nervous system depressants. Products known to produce respiratory depression or apnea, such as thiamylal sodium should be given at a reduced dosage and, when injected intravenously, should be administered slowly. When intravenous administration of XYLAZINE HCL INJECTION (xylazine) is desired, avoid perivascular injection in order to achieve the desired effect. Studies have shown negligible evidence of tissue irritation, however, following perivascular injection of xylazine.

Intracarotid Arterial Injection Should be Avoided. As with many compounds, including tranquilizers, immediate violent seizures followed by collapse may result from inadvertent administration into the carotid artery. Although the reaction with XYLAZINE HCL INJECTION (xylazine) is usually transient and recovery may be rapid and complete, special care should be taken to assure that the needle is in the jugular vein rather than the carotid artery.

Bradycardia and arrhythmia in the form of incomplete atrioventricular block have been reported following xylazine administration. Although clinically the importance of this effect is questioned,[1,2,3,4] a standard dose of atropine given prior to or following xylazine will greatly decrease the incidence.

Sedation for transport is most successful if actual transportation is begun after the full effect of the drug has been reached and the animal's stability is maintained while standing. In addition, it should be noted that animals under the influence of xylazine can be aroused by noise or other stimuli and this may increase the risk of injury.

Cervidae: As in all ruminants, it is preferable to administer XYLAZINE HCL INJECTION (xylazine) to fasted *Cervidae* as a safeguard against aspiration of food material into the lungs and/or bloat during deep sedation.

Care should be taken to administer XYLAZINE HCL INJECTION (xylazine) in the heavy muscles of the croup or shoulder. Injections given subcutaneously, intraperitoneally or into fat deposits will give unpredictable results.

Intra-arterial injection should be avoided, as with many compounds, including tranquilizers, immediate violent seizures followed by collapse may result from inadvertent administration into an artery.

The animal should not be disturbed during induction or until the full effect of the drug has been reached which is usually 10 to 15 minutes following injection.

The usual time to initial effect of the drug is 2 to 5 minutes. The administrator of the drug should be fully cognizant of this interval prior to administration of drug to free-ranging deer or elk, especially at night or in heavily wooded areas.

If the animal has been underdosed (faulty injection or miscalculation on weight) it is advisable to wait one hour before administering a second dose.

Adequate ventilation-especially in cages or crates-is mandatory; keep head and neck in position to insure patient air passage and to prevent aspiration of stomach contents.

During sedation, animals should be prevented from assuming lateral recumbency. A sternal recumbent position is desirable.

While under the effects of XYLAZINE HCL INJECTION (xylazine) the animal should be protected from extreme hot or cold environments.

Efforts should be made to prevent patient from rising until almost complete recovery is attained.

The transportation of *Cervidae* given XYLAZINE HCL INJECTION (xylazine) should be carefully monitored to prevent excessive struggling, injury or death.

Hyperthermic reactions may occur, especially if the subject is in a highly excited state when the drug is administered. Hosing the head and entire body with cold water has usually proven to be an effective deterrent.

The safety of XYLAZINE HCL INJECTION (xylazine) has not been demonstrated in pregnant *Cervidae*. Avoid use during the breeding season.

Cervidae should be observed closely until all of the sedative effects of XYLAZINE HCL INJECTION (xylazine) are gone.

Care should be taken at all times when administering XYLAZINE HCL INJECTION (xylazine) to *Cervidae*. This is due to the method of administration (usually darting), the difficulty in estimating body weights and the accepted theory that wild animals are more unpredictable in their response to sedatives and analgesics than the domesticated species.

Warning(s): This drug should not be administered to food-producing animals. Not for use in horses intended for food.

Avoid accidental administration to humans. Should such exposure occur, notify a physician immediately. Artificial respiration may be indicated.

In *Cervidae*, occasional capture-associated deaths occur. Clinical trials reveal a mortality rate of approximately 3.5% attendant with the administration of xylazine.

Do not use in *Cervidae* less than 15 days before or during the hunting season.

Not for human use.

Keep out of reach of children.

Side Effects: XYLAZINE HCL INJECTION (xylazine) in horses and *Cervidae*, used at recommended dosage levels may occasionally cause slight muscle tremors, bradycardia with partial A-V heart block and a reduced respiratory rate. Movement in response to sharp auditory stimuli may be observed.

In horses, sweating, rarely profuse, has been reported following administration. In *Cervidae*, salivation, various vocalizations (bellowing, bleating, groaning, grunting, snoring) on expiration, audible grinding of molar teeth, protruding tongue and elevated temperatures have also been noted in some cases.

Trial Data: Safety: XYLAZINE HCL INJECTION (xylazine) is tolerated at 10 times the recommended dose in horses and at doses above the recommended range in *Cervidae*. However, some elevated doses produced muscle tremors and long periods of sedation.

References: Available upon request.

Presentation: XYLAZINE HCL INJECTION (xylazine) is available in 50 mL multiple dose vials (NDC 60270-581-05).

Manufactured by: Phoenix Scientific Inc., St. Joseph, MO 64503.

Compendium Code No.: 14200261 Rev. 7-96/Rev. 4-00

XYLAZINE HCL INJECTION 100 MG ℞

AgriLabs **Analgesic-Sedative**

(Xylazine)

ANADA No.: 200-139

Active Ingredient(s): Each mL contains 100 mg xylazine, (base equivalent), 0.9 mg methylparaben, 0.1 mg propylparaben, water for injection; citric acid and sodium citrate for pH adjustment to 5.5 ± 0.3.

Xylazine hydrochloride (equivalent to 10% base)	11.4%
Inert ingredients	88.6%
	100.0%

Indications: XYLAZINE HCL INJECTION (xylazine) should be used in horses and *Cervidae* (Fallow Deer, Mule Deer, Sika Deer, White-Tailed Deer and Elk) when it is desirable to produce a state of sedation accompanied by a shorter period of analgesia.

Horses: XYLAZINE HCL INJECTION (xylazine) has been used successfully as follows:

1. Diagnostic procedures - oral and ophthalmic examinations, abdominal palpation, rectal palpation, vaginal examination, catheterization of the bladder and radiographic examinations.
2. Orthopedic procedures, such as application of casting materials and splints.
3. Dental procedures.
4. Minor surgical procedures of short duration such as debridement, removal of cutaneous neoplasms and suturing of lacerations.
5. To calm and facilitate handling of fractious animals.
6. Therapeutic medication for sedation and relief of pain following injury or surgery.
7. Major surgical procedures:
   a. When used as a preanesthetic to general anesthesia.
   b. When used in conjunction with local anesthetics.

Cervidae: XYLAZINE HCL INJECTION (xylazine) may be used for the following:

1. To calm and facilitate handling of fractious animals.
2. Diagnostic procedures.
3. Minor surgical procedures.
4. Therapeutic medication for sedation and relief of pain following injury or surgery.
5. As a preanesthetic to local anesthesia. XYLAZINE HCL INJECTION (xylazine) at the recommended dosages can be used in conjunction with local anesthetics, such as procaine or lidocaine.

Pharmacology: XYLAZINE HCL INJECTION (xylazine), a non-narcotic compound, is a sedative and analgesic as well as muscle relaxant. Its sedative and analgesic activity is related to central nervous system depression. Its muscle relaxant effect is based on inhibition of the intraneural transmission of impulses in the central nervous system. The principal pharmacological activities develop within 10 to 15 minutes after intramuscular injection in horses and *Cervidae*, and within 3 to 5 minutes following intravenous administration in horses.

A sleeplike state, the depth of which is dose-dependent, is usually maintained for 1 to 2 hours, while analgesia lasts from 15 to 30 minutes. The centrally-acting muscle relaxant effect causes relaxation of the skeletal musculature, complementing sedation and analgesia.

In horses and *Cervidae* under the influence of XYLAZINE HCL INJECTION (xylazine), the respiratory rate is reduced as in natural sleep. Following treatment with XYLAZINE HCL INJECTION (xylazine), the heart rate is decreased and a transient change in the conductivity of the cardiac muscle may occur, as evidenced by a partial atrioventricular block. This resembles the atrioventricular block often observed in normal horses.[1,2,3,4] Partial A-V block may occasionally occur following intramuscular injection of XYLAZINE HCL INJECTION (xylazine). When given intravenously in horses, the incidence of partial A-V block is higher. Intravenous administration causes a transient rise in blood pressure in horses, followed by a slight decrease.

XYLAZINE HCL INJECTION (xylazine) has no effect on blood clotting time or other hematologic parameters.

Dosage and Administration:

Horses:

1. Dosage:
   Intravenously - 0.5 mL/100 lbs body weight (0.5 mg/lb).
   Intramuscularly - 1.0 mL/100 lbs body weight (1.0 mg/lb).
   Following injection of XYLAZINE HCL INJECTION (xylazine) the animal should be allowed to rest quietly until the full effect has been reached.
   These dosages produce sedation which is usually maintained for 1 to 2 hours, and analgesia which lasts for 15 to 30 minutes.
2. Preanesthetic to Local Anesthesia: XYLAZINE HCL INJECTION (xylazine) at the recommended dosages can be used in conjunction with local anesthetics, such as procaine or lidocaine.
3. Preanesthetic to General Anesthesia: XYLAZINE HCL INJECTION (xylazine) at the recommended dosage rates produces an additive effect to central nervous system depressants such as pentobarbital sodium, thiopental sodium and thiamyl sodium. Therefore, the dosage of such compounds should be reduced and administered to the desired effect. In general, only ⅓ to ½ of the calculated dosage of the barbiturates will be needed to produce a surgical plane of anesthesia. Post-anesthetic or emergence excitement has not been observed in animals preanesthetized with XYLAZINE HCL INJECTION (xylazine).
   XYLAZINE HCL INJECTION (xylazine) has been used successfully as a preanesthetic agent for pentobarbital sodium, thiopental sodium, thiamylal sodium, nitrous oxide, ether, halothane, glyceryl guaiacolate and methoxyflurane anesthesia.

Cervidae: Administer intramuscularly, either by hand syringe or syringe dart, in the heavy muscles of the croup or shoulder.

Dosage Range:

Fallow Deer *(Dama dama)* - 2.0 to 4.0 mL/100 lbs body weight (2.0 to 4.0 mg/lb).

Mule Deer *(Odocoileus hemionus)* - 1.0 to 2.0 mL/100 lbs body weight (1.0 to 2.0 mg/lb).

Sika Deer *(Cervus nippon)* - 1.0 to 2.0 mL/100 lbs body weight (1.0 to 2.0 mg/lb).

White-Tailed Deer *(Odocoileus virginianus)* - 1.0 to 2.0 mL/100 lbs body weight (1.0 to 2.0 mg/lb).

Elk *(Cervus canadensis)* - 0.25 to 0.5 mL/100 lbs body weight (0.25 to 0.5 mg/lb).

Following injection of XYLAZINE HCL INJECTION (xylazine) the animal should be allowed to rest quietly until the full effect has been reached. These dosages produce sedation which is usually maintained for 1 to 2 hours and analgesia which lasts for 15 to 30 minutes.

Precaution(s): Store at controlled room temperature (15° to 30°C or 59° to 86°F).

Caution(s): Federal law restricts this drug to use by or on the order of a licensed veterinarian.

Careful consideration should be given before administering to horses and *Cervidae* with significantly depressed respiration, severe pathologic heart disease, advanced liver or kidney disease, severe endotoxic or traumatic shock and stress conditions such as extreme heat, cold, high altitude or fatigue.

Do not use XYLAZINE HCL INJECTION (xylazine) in conjunction with tranquilizers.

Analgesic effect is variable, and depth should be carefully assayed prior to surgical/clinical procedures. Variability of analgesia occurs most frequently at the distal extremities of horses and *Cervidae*. In spite of sedation, the practitioner and handlers should proceed with caution since defense reactions may not be diminished.

Horses: Since an additive effect results from the use of XYLAZINE HCL INJECTION (xylazine) and the barbiturate compounds, it should be used with caution with these central nervous system depressants. Products known to produce respiratory depression or apnea, such as thiamylal sodium should be given at a reduced dosage and, when injected intravenously, should be administered slowly. When intravenous administration of XYLAZINE HCL INJECTION (xylazine) is desired, avoid perivascular injection in order to achieve the desired effect. Studies have shown negligible evidence of tissue irritation, however, following perivascular injection of xylazine.

Intracarotid Arterial Injection Should be Avoided. As with many compounds, including tranquilizers, immediate violent seizures followed by collapse may result from inadvertent administration into the carotid artery. Although the reaction with XYLAZINE HCL INJECTION (xylazine) is usually transient and recovery may be rapid and complete, special care should be taken to assure that the needle is in the jugular vein rather than the carotid artery.

Bradycardia and arrhythmia in the form of incomplete atrioventricular block have been reported following xylazine administration. Although clinically the importance of this effect is questioned,[1,2,3,4] a standard dose of atropine given prior to or following xylazine will greatly decrease the incidence.

Sedation for transport is most successful if actual transportation is begun after the full effect of the drug has been reached and the animal's stability is maintained while standing. In addition, it should be noted that animals under the influence of xylazine can be aroused by noise or other stimuli and this may increase the risk of injury.

Cervidae: As in all ruminants, it is preferable to administer XYLAZINE HCL INJECTION (xylazine) to fasted *Cervidae* as a safeguard against aspiration of food material into the lungs and/or bloat during deep sedation.

Care should be taken to administer XYLAZINE HCL INJECTION (xylazine) in the heavy muscles of the croup or shoulder. Injections given subcutaneously, intraperitoneally or into fat deposits will give unpredictable results.

Intra-arterial injection should be avoided, as with many compounds, including tranquilizers, immediate violent seizures followed by collapse may result from inadvertent administration into an artery.

The animal should not be disturbed during induction or until the full effect of the drug has been reached which is usually 10 to 15 minutes following injection.

The usual time to initial effect of the drug is 2 to 5 minutes. The administrator of the drug should be fully cognizant of this interval prior to administration of drug to free-ranging deer or elk, especially at night or in heavily wooded areas.

If the animal has been underdosed (faulty injection or miscalculation on weight) it is advisable to wait one hour before administering a second dose.

Adequate ventilation- especially in cages or crates- is mandatory; keep head and neck in position to insure patient air passage and to prevent aspiration of stomach contents.

During sedation, animals should be prevented from assuming lateral recumbency. A sternal recumbent position is desirable.

While under the effects of XYLAZINE HCL INJECTION (xylazine) the animal should be protected from extreme hot or cold environments.

Efforts should be made to prevent patient from rising until almost complete recovery is attained.

The transportation of *Cervidae* given XYLAZINE HCL INJECTION (xylazine) should be carefully monitored to prevent excessive struggling, injury or death.

Hyperthermic reactions may occur, especially if the subject is in a highly excited state when the drug is administered. Hosing the head and entire body with cold water has usually proven to be an effective deterrent.

The safety of XYLAZINE HCL INJECTION (xylazine) has not been demonstrated in pregnant *Cervidae*. Avoid use during the breeding season.

Cervidae should be observed closely until all of the sedative effects of XYLAZINE HCL INJECTION (xylazine) are gone.

Care should be taken at all times when administering XYLAZINE HCL INJECTION (xylazine) to *Cervidae*. This is due to the method of administration (usually darting), the difficulty in estimating body weights and the accepted theory that wild animals are more unpredictable in their response to sedatives and analgesics than the domesticated species.

Keep out of reach of children.

Warning(s): Do not use in *Cervidae* less than 15 days before or during the hunting season.

This drug should not be administered to domestic food-producing animals. Not for use in horses intended for food.

Avoid accidental administration to humans. Should such exposure occur, notify a physician immediately. Artificial respiration may be indicated.

In *Cervidae*, occasional capture-associated deaths occur. Clinical trials reveal a mortality rate of approximately 3.5% attendant with the administration of xylazine.

Side Effects: XYLAZINE HCL INJECTION (xylazine) in horses and *Cervidae*, used at recommended dosage levels may occasionally cause slight muscle tremors, bradycardia with partial A-V heart block and a reduced respiratory rate. Movement in response to sharp auditory stimuli may be observed.

In horses, sweating, rarely profuse, has been reported following administration. In *Cervidae*, salivation, various vocalizations (bellowing, bleating, groaning, grunting, snoring) on expiration, audible grinding of molar teeth, protruding tongue and elevated temperatures have also been noted in some cases.

Trial Data: Safety: XYLAZINE HCL INJECTION (xylazine) is tolerated at 10 times the recommended dose in horses and at doses above the recommended range in *Cervidae*. However, some elevated doses produced muscle tremors and long periods of sedation.

References: Available upon request.

Presentation: XYLAZINE HCL INJECTION (xylazine) is available in 50 mL multiple dose vials.

Compendium Code No.: 10581760 Iss. 3-00

YELLOW LITE

AgriPharm **Large Animal Dietary Supplement**

Soluble Granules

Guaranteed Analysis: Each 1 lb contains:

Zinc (Zn) minimum . . . . 0.14% (1,400 ppm)
Vitamin E minimum . . . . 1,000 I.U.
Lactic acid bacteria *(L. acidophilus, L. casei, L. fermentum, L. plantarum, S. faecium)* min . . . . 3,870,000,000 CFU
Sodium (Na) max. 2.50%
Sodium (Na) min 2.00%
Potassium (K) min 1.50%

Ingredients: Citric acid, glucose, potassium chloride, salt, dl-alpha tocopherol acetate (source of vitamin E), silicon dioxide, zinc sulfate, dried *Lactobacillus acidophilus* fermentation product, dried *Lactobacillus casei* fermentation product, dried *Lactobacillus fermentum* fermentation product, dried *Lactobacillus plantarum* fermentation product, dried *Streptococcus faecium* fermentation product, copper sulfate, fumaric acid, active yeast *(Saccharomyces cerevisiae),* vitamin A acetate, d-activated animal sterol (source of vitamin D_3), vitamin B_{12} supplement, riboflavin, niacin, d-calcium pantothenate, menadione dimethylpyrimidinol bisulfite (source of vitamin K_3), folic acid, pyridoxine HCl, thiamine, d-biotin, ascorbic acid, magnesium sulfate, FD&C yellow No. 5, ethylene diamine dihydriodide, sodium bicarbonate, iron sulfate, manganous sulfate, natural and artificial flavorings.

Indications: A buffered electrolyte water acidifier with vitamins.

Contains a source of live (viable) naturally occurring microorganisms.

Dosage and Administration: When using proportioners, use warm water.

All Weaned Pigs: Use at the rate of one package (16 ounces) to 128 gallons of drinking water for one (1) week prior and two (2) weeks after weaning.

All Feeder Pigs: Use same rate as weaned pigs, administer from arrival for two (2) weeks.

All Young Pigs: For pigs who have been on heavy medication. Use same rate as above for two weeks after medication is discontinued.

Incoming Cattle: Use at the rate of one package (16 ounces) to 64 gallons of drinking water.

Calves, Lambs, Rabbits: Use at the rate of one package (16 ounces) to 128 gallons of drinking water, (or mix one (1) teaspoon per one (1) gallon of water).

Dogs, Foxes, Mink: Use at the rate of one package (16 ounces) to 128 gallons of drinking water, (or mix one (1) teaspoon per one (1) gallon of water).

Dairy/Veal calves: Add ½ tsp. per gallon of milk replacer. Use twice a day and continue until weaning.

Precaution(s): Store in a dark, cool, dry place.

Caution(s): For animal use only. Keep out of reach of children.

Presentation: 1 lb and 3 lb containers.

Compendium Code No.: 14571110

YOBINE® INJECTION ℞

Lloyd **Narcotic Antagonist**

Yohimbine Sterile Solution 2 mg/mL-Xylazine Reversing Agent and Antidote

NADA No.: 140-866

Active Ingredient(s): Each mL contains:

Yohimbine (as the hydrochloride) . . . . 2.0 mg
Methylparaben . . . . 0.9 mg
Propylparaben . . . . 0.1 mg
Citric acid . . . . 3.34 mg
Water for injection . . . . q.s.

The pH is adjusted with sodium hydroxide.

Indications: YOBINE® should be used in dogs when it is desirable to reverse the effects of xylazine. YOBINE® has been used successfully to reverse the sedative effects of xylazine and to reverse the cardiac effects of xylazine such as arrythmia and bradycardia when xylazine is administered alone.

Pharmacology: Yohimbine as an indolealkylamine alkaloid that acts primarily by blocking central alpha-2 adrenoreceptors that are stimulated by xylazine. Yohimbine is an alpha-2 adrenergic receptor antagonist that easily penetrates the blood-brain barrier.[1] It competitively blocks and antagonizes central nervous system depression or sedation and the bradycardia and respiratory depression caused by xylazine.[2]

Xylazine, an alpha-2 adrenergic agonist with potent sedative, analgesic and muscle relaxant properties, has been used extensively as an analgesic-sedative restraining agent. It has also been used as a pre-anesthetic agent for many general anesthetics. The central nervous system depressant effect, as well as other pharmacologic effects of xylazine, is dose-dependent.

Yohimbine is useful to counteract sedation after standard doses of xylazine. The competitive selective blocking of the alpha-2 adrenergic receptor by yohimbine displaces xylazine from these sites and thereby rapidly cancels the effect of the xylazine.

Yohimbine, when used at the prescribed dose, will reverse the effects of xylazine used alone in dogs.[3] Yohimbine abbreviates the anesthesia and chemical restraint of the xylazine.

The reversal of the sedative effects of xylazine by I.V. injection of yohimbine is rapid, usually occurring within one to three minutes, regardless of the route of administration of xylazine.[4]

Dosage and Administration: For intravenous injection, the usual dose is 0.5 mL per 20 lbs. of body weight (0.05 mg/lb. or 0.11 mg/kg) to reverse the sedative effects of xylazine. The carefully calculated dose of YOBINE® should be given by slow intravenous injection.

Contraindication(s): Doses in excess of those recommended should not be given. While YOBINE® is tolerated in dogs at 0.25 mg/lb. of body weight, doses of this magnitude may occasionally produce seizures and muscle tremors of short duration.

Precaution(s): Protect from heat and light. Do not store over 30°C (86°F).

The safety of YOBINE® in pregnant dogs or in dogs intended for breeding has not been established.

Careful consideration should be given before administering to dogs known to be epileptic or seizure prone. The drug reverses the analgesic effects of xylazine as well as the sedative effects. If the animal was given xylazine for its analgesic properties, reversal may result in the return of normal pain perception.

Caution(s): Federal law restricts this drug to use by or on the order of a licensed veterinarian.

Warning(s): Not for human use. This drug should not be administered to food-producing animals.

Side Effects: Occasionally a dog that has been injected with yohimbine will show signs of apprehensiveness but this state quickly subsides.

References: Available upon request.

Presentation: 20 mL multiple-dose vials.

Compendium Code No.: 11350040

ZENIQUIN® ℞

Pfizer Animal Health **Marbofloxacin**

(marbofloxacin) Tablets

NADA No.: 141-151

Active Ingredient(s): Each scored, coated tablet contains either:

Marbofloxacin . . . . 25 mg, 50 mg, 100 mg, or 200 mg

Indications: ZENIQUIN® (marbofloxacin) tablets are indicated for the treatment of infections in dogs and cats associated with bacteria susceptible to marbofloxacin.

Pharmacology: Description: Marbofloxacin is a synthetic broad-spectrum antibacterial agent from the fluoroquinolone class of chemotherapeutic agents. Marbofloxacin is the non-proprietary designation for 9-fluoro-2,3-dihydro-3-methyl-10-(4-methyl-1-piperazinyl)-7-oxo-7H-pyrido[3,2,1-ij][4,1,2] benzoxadiazine-6-carboxylic acid. The empirical formula is $C_{17}H_{19}FN_4O_4$ and the molecular weight is 362.36. The compound is soluble in water; however, solubility decreases in alkaline conditions. The N-octanol/water partition coefficient (Kow) is 0.835 measured at pH 7 and 25°C.

Figure 1: Chemical structure of marbofloxacin.

Clinical Pharmacology: Marbofloxacin is rapidly and almost completely absorbed from the gastrointestinal tract following oral administration to fasted animals. Divalent cations are generally known to diminish the absorption of fluoroquinolones. The effects of concomitant feeding on the absorption of marbofloxacin have not been determined. (See Drug Interactions.) In the dog, approximately 40% of an oral dose of marbofloxacin is excreted unchanged in the urine.[1] Excretion in the feces, also as unchanged drug, is the other major route of elimination in dogs. Ten to 15% of marbofloxacin is metabolized by the liver in dogs. *In vitro* plasma protein binding of marbofloxacin in dogs was 9.1% and in cats was 7.3%. In the cat, approximately 70% of an oral dose is excreted in the urine as marbofloxacin and metabolites with approximately 85% of the excreted material as unchanged drug. Pharmacokinetic parameters related to intravenous dosing were estimated in a study of 6 healthy adult beagle dogs, and are summarized in Table 1. The absolute bioavailability following dosing of oral tablets to the same animals was 94%.

Marbofloxacin plasma concentrations were determined over time in healthy adult beagle dogs (6 dogs per dosage group) following single oral doses of 1.25 mg/lb or 2.5 mg/lb. Absorption of orally administered marbofloxacin increases proportionally over the dose range of 1.25 to 2.5 mg/lb. Marbofloxacin plasma concentrations were determined over time in 7 healthy adult male cats following a single oral dose of 2.5 mg/lb. Plasma pharmacokinetic parameters following oral dosing of dogs and cats are summarized in Figure 2 and 3 and in Table 2. Based on the terminal elimination half-life and the dosing interval, steady-state levels are reached after the third dose and are expected to be approximately 25% greater in dogs and 35% greater in cats than those achieved after a single dose. Marbofloxacin is widely distributed in canine tissues. Tissue concentrations of marbofloxacin were determined in healthy male beagle dogs (4 dogs per time period) at 2, 18 and 24 hours after a single oral dose (1.25 or 2.5 mg/lb) and are summarized in Tables 3a and 3b.

Table 1: Mean pharmacokinetic parameters following intravenous administration of marbofloxacin to 6 adult beagle dogs at a dosage of 2.5 mg/lb.

Parameter	Estimate ± SD* n=6
Total body clearance, (mL/h•kg)	94 ± 8
Volume of distribution at steady state, V_{SS}, (L/kg)	1.19 ± 0.08
$AUC_{0\text{-}inf}$ (µg•h/mL)	59 ± 5
Terminal plasma elimination half-life, $t_{½}$(h)	9.5 ± 0.7

* SD = standard deviation

Table 2: Mean pharmacokinetic parameters following oral administration of marbofloxacin tablets to adult beagle dogs at a nominal dosage of 1.25 mg/lb or 2.5 mg/lb and to cats at 2.5 mg/lb.†

Parameter	Dog Estimate ± SD* (1.25 mg/lb) n=6	Dog Estimate ± SD* (2.5 mg/lb) n=6	Cat Estimate ± SD* (2.5 mg/lb) n=7
Time of maximum concentration, T_{max}(h)	1.5 ± 0.3	1.8 ± 0.3	1.2 ± 0.6
Maximum concentration, C_{max} (µg/mL)	2.0 ± 0.2	4.2 ± 0.5	4.8 ± 0.7
$AUC_{0\text{-}inf}$ (µg•h/mL)	31.2 ± 1.6	64 ± 8	70 ± 6
Terminal plasma elimination half-life, $t_{½}$(h)	10.7 ± 1.6	10.9 ± 0.6	12.7 ± 1.1

† mean actual dosages administered to dogs were 1.22 mg/lb and 2.56 mg/lb, respectively, and the mean actual dosage administered to cats was 2.82 mg/lb.

* SD = standard deviation

Figure 2: Mean plasma concentrations (µg/mL) following single oral administration of marbofloxacin to adult beagle dogs at dosages of 1.25 mg/lb or 2.5 mg/lb.

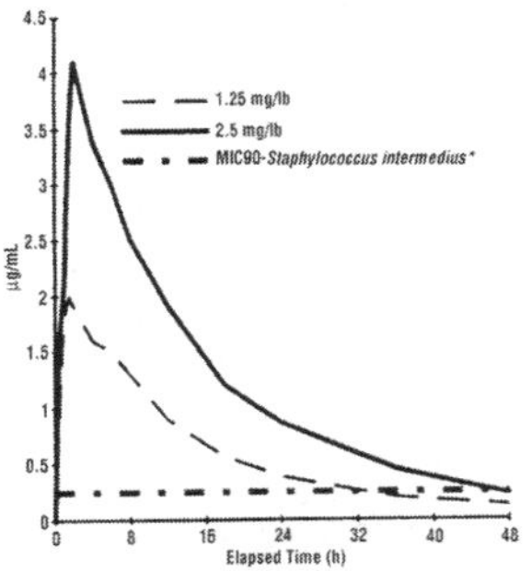

* See Table 4 in Microbiology section for MIC data.

X-Z

Figure 3: Mean plasma concentrations (µg/mL) following single oral administration of marbofloxacin to adult cats at a dosage of 2.5 mg/lb.

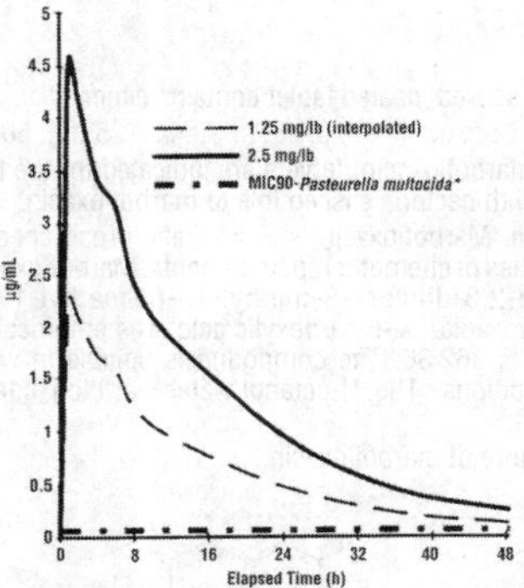

* See Table 5 in Microbiology section for MIC data.

Table 3a: Tissue distribution following a single oral administration of marbofloxacin tablets to adult beagle dogs at a dosage of 1.25 mg/lb*.

Tissue	Marbofloxacin Concentrations (µg/g ± SD)		
	2 hours n=4	18 hours n=4	24 hours n=4
bladder	4.8 ± 1.1	2.6 ± 1.5	1.11 ± 0.19
bone marrow	3.1 ± 0.5	1.5 ± 1.5	0.7 ± 0.2
feces	15 ± 9	48 ± 40	26 ± 11
jejunum	3.6 ± 0.5	1.3 ± 1.0	0.7 ± 0.3
kidney	7.1 ± 1.7	1.4 ± 0.5	0.9 ± 0.3
lung	3.0 ± 0.5	0.8 ± 0.2	0.57 ± 0.19
lymph node	5.5 ± 1.1	1.3 ± 0.3	1.0 ± 0.3
muscle	4.1 ± 0.3	1.0 ± 0.3	0.7 ± 0.2
prostate	5.6 ± 1.4	1.8 ± 0.6	1.1 ± 0.4
skin	1.9 ± 0.6	0.41 ± 0.13	0.32 ± 0.08

* SD = standard deviation

Table 3b: Tissue distribution following a single oral administration of marbofloxacin tablets to adult beagle dogs at a dosage of 2.5 mg/lb.

Tissue	Marbofloxacin Concentrations (µg/g ± SD*)		
	2 hours n=4	18 hours n=4	24 hours n=4
bladder	12 ± 4	6 ± 7	1.8 ± 0.4
bone marrow	4.6 ± 1.5	1.28 ± 0.13	0.9 ± 0.3
feces	18 ± 3	52 ± 17	47 ± 28
jejunum	7.8 ± 1.1	2.0 ± 0.3	1.1 ± 0.3
kidney	12.7 ± 1.7	2.7 ± 0.3	1.6 ± 0.2
lung	5.48 ± 0.17	1.45 ± 0.19	1.0 ± 0.2
lymph node	8.3 ± 0.7	2.3 ± 0.5	2.03 ± 0.06
muscle	7.5 ± 0.5	1.8 ± 0.3	1.20 ± 0.12
prostate	11 ± 3	2.7 ± 1.0	2.0 ± 0.5
skin	3.20 ± 0.33	0.705 ± 0.013	0.46 ± 0.09

* SD = standard deviation

Microbiology: The primary action of fluoroquinolones is to inhibit the bacterial enzyme, DNA gyrase. In susceptible organisms, fluoroquinolones are rapidly bactericidal at relatively low concentrations. Marbofloxacin is bactericidal against a broad range of gram-negative and gram-positive organisms. The minimum inhibitory concentrations (MICs) of pathogens isolated in clinical field studies performed in the United States were determined using National Committee for Clinical Laboratory Standards (NCCLS) standards, and are shown in Tables 4 and 5.

Table 4: MIC Values* (µg/mL) of marbofloxacin against pathogens isolated from skin, soft tissue and urinary tract infections in dogs enrolled in clinical studies conducted during 1994-1996.

Organism	No. of Isolates	MIC_{50}	MIC_{90}	MIC Range
Staphylococcus intermedius	135	0.25	0.25	0.125-2
Escherichia coli	61	0.03	0.06	0.015-2
Proteus mirabilis	35	0.06	0.125	0.03-0.25
Beta-hemolytic *Streptococcus*, (not Group A or Group B)	25	1	2	0.5-16
Streptococcus, Group D enterococcus	16	1	4	0.008-4
Pasteurella multocida	13	0.015	0.06	≤0.008-0.5
Staphylococcus aureus	12	0.25	0.25	0.25-0.5
Enterococcus faecalis	11	2	2	1-4
Klebsiella pneumoniae	11	0.06	0.06	0.01-0.06
Pseudomonas spp.	9	**	**	0.06-1
Pseudomonas aeruginosa	7	**	**	0.25-1

*The correlation between *in vitro* susceptibility data (MIC) and clinical response has not been determined.

**MIC_{50} and MIC_{90} not calculated due to insufficient number at isolates.

Table 5: MIC Values* (µg/mL) of marbofloxacin against pathogens isolated from skin and soft tissue infections in cats enrolled in clinical studies conducted in 1995 and 1998.

Organism	No. of Isolates	MIC_{50}	MIC_{90}	MIC Range
Pasteurella multocida	135	0.03	0.06	≤0.008-0.25
Beta-hemolytic *Streptococcus*	22	1	1	0.06-1
Staphylococcus aureus	21	0.25	0.5	0.125-1
Corynebacterium spp.	14	0.5	1	0.25-2
Staphylococcus intermedius	11	0.25	0.5	0.03-0.5
Enterococcus faecalis	10	2.0	2.0	1.0-2.0
Escherichia coli	10	0.03	0.03	0.015-0.03
Bacillus spp.	10	0.25	0.25	0.125-0.25

* The correlation between *in vitro* susceptibility data (MIC) and clinical response has not been determined.

Dosage and Administration: The recommended dosage for oral administration to dogs and cats is 1.25 mg marbofloxacin per lb of body weight once daily, but the dosage may be safely increased to 2.5 mg/lb.

For the treatment of skin and soft tissue infections, ZENIQUIN® tablets should be given for 2-3 days beyond the cessation of clinical signs for a maximum of 30 days. For the treatment of urinary tract infections, ZENIQUIN® tablets should be administered for at least 10 days. If no improvement is noted within 5 days, the diagnosis should be reevaluated and a different course of therapy considered.

Drug Interactions: Compounds (e.g., sucralfate, antacids, and mineral supplements) containing divalent and trivalent cations (e.g., iron, aluminum, calcium, magnesium, and zinc) can interfere with the absorption of quinolones which may result in a decrease in product bioavailability. Therefore, the concomitant oral administration of quinolones with foods, supplements, or other preparations containing these compounds should be avoided.

Contraindication(s): Marbofloxacin and other quinolones have been shown to cause arthropathy in immature animals of most species tested, the dog being particularly sensitive to this side effect. Marbofloxacin is contraindicated in immature dogs during the rapid growth phase (small and medium breeds up to 8 months of age, large breeds up to 12 months of age and giant breeds up to 18 months of age). Marbofloxacin is contraindicated in cats under 12 months of age. Marbofloxacin is contraindicated in dogs and cats known to be hypersensitive to quinolones.

Precaution(s): Store below 30°C (86°F).

Caution(s): Federal law restricts this drug to use by or on the order of a licensed veterinarian.

Federal law prohibits the extralabel use of this drug in food-producing animals.

Quinolones should be used with caution in animals with known or suspected central nervous system (CNS) disorders. In such animals, quinolones have, in rare instances, been associated with CNS stimulation which may lead to convulsive seizures. Quinolones have been shown to produce erosions of cartilage of weight-bearing joints and other signs of arthropathy in immature animals of various species. The use of fluoroquinolones in cats has been reported to adversely affect the retina. Such products should be used with caution in cats. The safety of marbofloxacin in animals used for breeding purposes, pregnant, or lactating has not been demonstrated.

To report suspected adverse effects, and/or obtain a copy of the MSDS, call 1-800-366-5280.

Warning(s): Human Warning: For use in animals only. Keep out of reach of children. Avoid contact with eyes. In case of contact, immediately flush eyes with copious amounts of water for 15 minutes. In case of dermal contact, wash skin with soap and water. Consult a physician if irritation persists following ocular or dermal exposure. Individuals with a history of hypersensitivity to fluoroquinolones should avoid this product. In humans, there is a risk of user photosensitization within a few hours after excessive exposure to quinolones. If excessive accidental exposure occurs, avoid direct sunlight.

For oral use in dogs and cats only.

Adverse Reactions: The following clinical signs were reported during the course of clinical field studies in dogs receiving marbofloxacin at dosages up to 2.5 mg/lb daily: decreased or loss of appetite (5.4%), decreased activity (4.4%), and vomiting (2.9%). The following signs were reported in less than 1% of cases in dogs: increased thirst, soft stool/diarrhea, behavioral changes, shivering/shaking/tremors, and ataxia. One dog which had a seizure the day before study enrollment experienced a seizure while on marbofloxacin therapy.

The following clinical signs were reported during clinical field studies in cats receiving 1.25 mg/lb/day: diarrhea (2.1%) and soft stool (1.4%). Vomiting was reported in less than 1% of cases in cats.

Trial Data: Effectiveness Confirmation: Clinical effectiveness was confirmed in bacterial skin and soft tissue infections in dogs and cats and urinary tract infections (cystitis) in dogs associated with bacteria susceptible to marbofloxacin. Bacterial pathogens isolated in clinical field studies are provided in the Microbiology section.

Target Animal Safety:

Dogs: The toxicity of marbofloxacin was assessed in 12- to 14-month-old beagle dogs administered marbofloxacin at 2.5, 7.5 and 12.5 mg/lb/day for 42 days. Vomiting, reddened skin (usually involving the ears) and reddened mucous membranes were occasionally observed in all groups, including controls, but were noted most frequently in the 12.5 mg/lb group. Decreased food consumption and weight loss were significant in the 7.5 mg/lb and 12.5 mg/lb groups. No clinical lameness was noted in any of the treated animals. Minimal to slight lesions in the articular cartilage were observed in 1/8 placebo-treated animals and in 3/8 animals given 12.5 mg marbofloxacin/lb. Macroscopically, these lesions were vesicles, raised areas, or depressed, light-colored areas. Microscopically, these lesions were characterized by the presence of one or more of the following: fissuring, erosion, chondrocyte proliferation, fibrillation, or vertical splitting of the articular cartilage. These cartilage lesions in treated dogs were similar to those in control dogs, and were not typical of those produced by fluoroquinolones. In addition to the above pathologic alterations, red areas of articular cartilage were noted macroscopically in 0/8 placebo-treated dogs and in 2/8 dogs from each of the three marbofloxacin-treated groups. These areas usually correlated microscopically with areas of vascularity of the articular surface, but could not be confirmed microscopically in all animals. They consisted of large blood vessels in mature fibrous connective tissue, with no indication of active vascularization due to drug-induced damage. They were considered most likely to be developmental anomalies or normal variations of the joint surface and were not considered to be related to drug treatment.

Marbofloxacin was administered to 12- to 14-month-old beagle dogs at a dosage of 25 mg/lb/day for 12 days. Decreased food consumption, vomiting, dehydration, excessive salivation, tremors, reddened skin, facial swelling, decreased activity and weight loss were seen in treated dogs. No clinical lameness was noted. As in the 42 day study, grossly visible, focal, red areas of articular cartilage were seen. These findings were noted in 2/6 placebo-treated dogs and in 4/6 marbofloxacin-treated dogs. The foci were areas of fibrocartilage with prominent vascularization or increased vascularization of subchondral bone. Due to the appearance microscopically and macroscopically, these red foci were described as likely to be developmental anomalies or normal variations in articular cartilage.

Marbofloxacin administered to 3- to 4-month-old large breed, purpose-bred mongrel dogs at a dosage of 5 mg/lb/day for 14 days resulted in marked lameness in all dogs due to articular cartilage lesions. Lameness was accompanied by decreased appetite and activity.

Cats: Marbofloxacin was administered for 42 consecutive days to 24 cats approximately 8 months old (8 cats per treatment group) at the dosages of 2.5, 7.5 and 12.5 mg/lb/day (5.5, 16.5 and 27.5 mg/kg/day). Treatment with marbofloxacin did not produce adverse effects on body weights, food consumption, serum chemistry, urinalysis or organ weight parameters. Decreased segmented neutrophil counts were observed in some cats in all treatment groups, including the placebo group, but mean counts were significantly lower in the marbofloxacin-treated groups. In some cats, absolute neutrophil counts were below normal reference values (as low as 615 neutrophils/μL in a marbofloxacin-treated cat and as low as 882 neutrophils/μL in a placebo-treated cat). Other hematological observations were not adversely affected. Clinical signs were occasionally noted in cats in the highest dosage group: excessive salivation in 4/8 cats and redness of ear pinnae in 2/8 cats. Macroscopic changes in the articular cartilage of femurs were seen in one cat receiving 7.5 mg/lb and in 3 cats receiving 12.5 mg/lb. Microscopically, these gross lesions were related to a focal or multifocal chondropathy. Microscopic chondropathy not associated with macroscopic observations was also present in one cat treated with 2.5 mg/lb daily (1X the upper end of the dose range) and one additional cat treated with 7.5 mg/lb daily. There was no evidence of lameness during the course of the study. A perivascular to diffuse dermatitis was seen microscopically in one mid-dose cat and 4 high-dose cats. Funduscopic exam by a board-certified ophthalmologist and histologic examination of retina and optic nerve by ocular pathologists revealed no lesions in any of the treatment groups.

Marbofloxacin was also administered orally to 6 cats approximately 8 months of age for 14 consecutive days at a dosage of 25 mg/lb/day (55 mg/kg/day). Clinical signs associated with drug intolerance were excessive salivation in 5/6 cats and redness of ear pinnae in all cats after 8 days of treatment. Emesis was noted occasionally in several cats and diminished activity was noted in one cat. Decreased food intake was noted in some animals, primarily males, when compared to controls. Perivascular to diffuse dermatitis was seen microscopically in the pinnae of all treated animals and in the standard skin samples of several animals. There was focal or multifocal articular chondropathy in 2/6 treated animals. One treated cat had a duodenal mucosal erosion and one treated cat had a pyloric ulcer. There were no observations of lameness and no adverse effects on hematology, clinical chemistry, urinalysis, or organ weight parameters. Funduscopic examination by a board-certified ophthalmologist and histologic examination of retina and optic nerve by ocular pathologists revealed no lesions.

A study was conducted to investigate the effect of marbofloxacin on articular cartilage of skeletally mature cats 12-14 months of age. Forty cats were randomly assigned to 4 groups of 10 cats each. Groups received placebo or marbofloxacin at dosages of 1.25, 3.75 or 7.5 mg/lb/day (2.75, 8.25 or 16.5 mg/kg/day) for 42 consecutive days. There were no treatment-related pathological changes in the joints or other tissues. Emesis and soft stools was noted in all treatment groups, including placebo, and increased in frequency with increasing dose and duration of treatment. Emesis was more apparent in the high-dose males.

References: Available upon request.

Presentation: Marbofloxacin is supplied in 25-mg, 50-mg, 100-mg, and 200-mg scored, coated tablets.

25 mg - 100 and 250 tablets
50 mg - 100 and 250 tablets
100 mg - 50 tablets
200 mg - 50 tablets

Compendium Code No.: 36901641 75-8485-04

ZEV

Dominion **Antitussive**

Active Ingredient(s): Active ingredients include: Ammonium carbonate, camphor and menthol. Other ingredients include: Canada balsam, carrageenan, licorice fluid extract, pine needle oil and sorbitol.

Indications: Horses with coughs, bronchial irritation or nasal congestion are often impossible to work or exercise in a normal fashion. This cough remedy and conditioner will help cure these irritations and allow horses to return to work sooner.

As a digestive aid, this product helps horses get the most from their feeds, assisting in overall appearance, health and performance.

Dosage and Administration: This liquid formulation can be added to feeds, or it can be administered orally.

For coughs of colds, bronchial irritation or stable cough, add 3 or 4 tablespoons to the horse's feed, two or three times per day.

Or, mix 3 or 4 tablespoons with equal parts of honey, molasses or corn syrup. This mixture is then placed well back in the horses mouth. This should be repeated two to three times per day. Treatment should continue for one week.

For nasal congestion, add 4 tablespoons to a half pail of hot water, then place in stall or where horse can breathe vapors freely.

As a conditioner, add two or three tablespoons to feed, twice daily, for two weeks. After the first two weeks, feed twice weekly.

Warning(s): For veterinary use only.

Presentation: 2 L and 4 L plastic containers.

Compendium Code No.: 15080081

ZIMECTERIN® PASTE 1.87%

Farnam **Parasiticide-Oral**

(Ivermectin) Anthelmintic and Boticide

NADA No.: 134-314

Active Ingredient(s):

Ivermectin 1.87%

Indications: Consult your veterinarian for assistance in the diagnosis, treatment, and control of parasitism. ZIMECTERIN® (ivermectin) Paste provides effective control of the following parasites in horses: Large strongyles (adults) — *Strongylus vulgaris* (also early forms in blood vessels), *S edentalus* (also tissue stages), *S equinus, Triodontophorus* spp; Small strongyles including those resistant to some benzimidazole class compounds (adults and fourth-stage larvae) — *Cyathostomum* spp, *Cylicocyclus* spp, *Cylicostephanus* spp, *Cylicodontophorus* spp; Pinworms (adults and fourth-stage larvae) — *Oxyuris equi*; Ascarids (adults and third- and fourth-stage larvae) — *Parascaris equorum;* Hairworms (adults) — *Trichostrogylus axei;* Large-mouth Stomach Worms (adults) — *Habronema muscae;* Bots (oral and gastric stages) — *Gasterophilus* spp; Lungworms (adults and forth-stage larvae) — *Dictyocaulus arnfieldi;* Intestinal Threadworms (adults) — *Strongyloides westeri;* Summer Sores caused by *Habronema* and *Draschia* spp cutaneous third-stage larvae; Dermatitis caused by neck threadworm microfilarie, *Onchocerca* sp.

Dosage and Administration: The syringe contains sufficient paste to treat one 1250 lb horse at the recommended dose rate of 91 mcg ivermectin per lb (200 mcg/kg) body weight. Each weight marking on the syringe plunger delivers enough paste to treat 250 lb body weight.

(1) While holding plunger, turn the knurled ring on the plunger ¼ turn to the left and slide it so the side nearest the barrel is at the prescribed weight marking. (2) Lock the ring in place by making a ¼ turn to the right. (3) Make sure that the horse's mouth contains no feed. (4) Remove the cover from the tip of the syringe. (5) Insert the syringe tip into the horse's mouth at the space between the teeth. (6) Depress the plunger as far as it will go, depositing paste on the back of the tongue. (7) Immediately raise the horse's head for a few seconds after dosing.

Precaution(s): Ivermectin and excreted ivermectin residues may adversely affect aquatic organisms. Do not contaminate ground or surface water. Dispose of the ZIMECTERIN® (ivermectin) Paste syringe in an approved landfill or by incineration.

Caution(s): ZIMECTERIN® (ivermectin) Paste has been formulated specifically for use in horses only. This product should not be used in other animal species as severe reactions, including fatalities in dogs, may result.

Note to User: Swelling and itching reactions after treatment with ZIMECTERIN® Paste have occurred in horses carrying heavy infections of neck threadworm *(Onchocerca* sp) microfiliariae. These reactions were most likely the result of microfiliarae dying in large numbers. Symptomatic treatment may be advisable. Consult your veterinarian should any such reactions occur. Healing of summer sores involving extensive tissue changes may require other appropriate therapy in conjunction with treatment with ZIMECTERIN® (ivermectin) Paste. Reinfection, and measures for its prevention, should also be considered. Consult your veterinarian if the condition does not improve.

Warning(s): Do not use on horses intended for food purposes.

Refrain from smoking and eating when handling. Wash hands after use. Avoid contact with eyes. Keep this and all drugs out of the reach of children.

Side Effects: Safety — ZIMECTERIN® (ivermectin) Paste may be used in horses of all ages, including mares at any stage of pregnancy. Stallions may be treated without adversely affecting their fertility.

Discussion:

Parasite Control Program: All horses should be included in a regular parasite control program with particular attention being paid to mares, foals and yearlings. Foals should be treated initially at 6 to 8 weeks of age, and routine treatment repeated as appropriate. Consult your veterinarian for a control program to meet your specific needs. ZIMECTERIN® (ivermectin) Paste effectively controls gastrointestinal nematodes and bots of horses. Regular treatment will reduce the chances of verminous arteritis caused by *S vulgaris.*

Product Advantages: Broad-spectrum control, ZIMECTERIN® Paste kills important internal parasites, including bots and the arterial stages of *Strongyles vulgaris,* with a single dose. ZIMECTERIN® Paste is a potent anti-parasitic agent that is neither a benzimidazole nor an organophosphate.

Presentation: 0.21 oz (6.08 g).
Contents will treat up to 1250 lb body weight.

ZIMECTERIN Reg TM Farnam Companies, Inc.

Compendium Code No.: 10000491

ZIMECTERIN® PASTE 1.87%

Merial **Parasiticide-Oral**

(ivermectin) Anthelmintic and Boticide

NADA No.: 134-314

Active Ingredient(s): Each syringe contains:

Ivermectin 1.87%

Indications: ZIMECTERIN® (ivermectin) Paste provides effective control of the following parasites in horses:

Large Strongyles (adults) — *Strongylus vulgaris* (also early forms in blood vessels), *S. edentalus* (also tissue stages), *S. equinus, Triodontophorus* spp.

Small Strongyles including those resistant to some benzimidazole class compounds (adults and fourth-stage larvae) — *Cyathostomum* spp, *Cylicocyclus* spp, *Cylicostephanus* spp, *Cylicodontophorus* spp.

Pinworms (adults and fourth-stage larvae) — *Oxyuris equi.*

Ascarids (adults and third- and fourth-stage larvae) — *Parascaris equorum.*

Hairworms (adults) — *Trichostrogylus axei.*

Large-mouth Stomach Worms (adults) — *Habronema muscae.*

Bots (oral and gastric stages) — *Gastrophilus* spp.

Lungworms (adults and forth-stage larvae) — *Dictyocaulus arnfieldi.*

Intestinal Threadworms (adults) — *Strongyloides westeri.*

Summer Sores caused by *Habronema* and *Draschia* spp cutaneous third-stage larvae.

Dermatitis caused by neck threadworm microfilariae, *Onchocerca* sp.

Dosage and Administration: The syringe contains sufficient paste to treat one 1,250 lb horse at the recommended dose rate of 91 mcg ivermectin per lb (200 mcg/kg) body weight. Each weight marking on the syringe plunger delivers enough paste to treat 250 lb body weight.

(1) While holding plunger, turn the knurled ring on the plunger ¼ turn to the left and slide it so the side nearest the barrel is at the prescribed weight marking. (2) Lock the ring in place by making a ¼ turn to the right. (3) Make sure that the horse's mouth contains no feed. (4) Remove the cover from the tip of the syringe. (5) Insert the syringe tip into the horse's mouth at the space between the teeth. (6) Depress the plunger as far as it will go, depositing paste on the back of the tongue. (7) Immediately raise the horse's head for a few seconds after dosing.

Parasite Control Program: All horses should be included in a regular parasite control program with particular attention being paid to mares, foals and yearlings. Foals should be treated initially at 6 to 8 weeks of age, and routine treatment repeated as appropriate. Consult your veterinarian for a control program to meet your specific needs. ZIMECTERIN® (ivermectin) Paste effectively controls gastrointestinal nematodes and bots of horses. Regular treatment will reduce the chances of verminous arteritis caused by *Strongylus vulgaris.*

Consult your veterinarian for assistance in the diagnosis, treatment, and control of parasitism.

Precaution(s): Environmental Safety: Ivermectin and excreted ivermectin residues may adversely affect aquatic organisms. Do not contaminate ground or surface water. Dispose of the syringe in an approved landfill or by incineration.

Caution(s): ZIMECTERIN® (ivermectin) Paste has been formulated specifically for use in horses only. This product should not be used in other animal species as severe reactions, including fatalities in dogs, may result.

Note to User: Swelling and itching reactions after treatment with ZIMECTERIN® (ivermectin) Paste have occurred in horses carrying heavy infections of neck threadworm *(Onchocerca* sp) microfilariae. These reactions were most likely the result of microfilariae dying in large numbers. Symptomatic treatment may be advisable. Consult your veterinarian should any such reactions occur. Healing of summer sores involving extensive tissue changes may require other appropriate therapy in conjunction with treatment with ZIMECTERIN® Paste. Reinfection, and measures for its prevention, should also be considered. Consult your veterinarian if the condition does not improve.

For oral use in horses only.

Warning(s): Do not use on horses intended for food purposes.

Not for use in humans. Keep this and all drugs out of the reach of children.

Refrain from smoking and eating when handling. Wash hands after use. Avoid contact with eyes.

The Material Safety Data Sheet (MSDS) contains more detailed occupational safety information. To report adverse reactions in users, to obtain more information, or to obtain an MSDS, contact Merial at 1-888-637-4251.

Discussion: Product Advantages: Broad-spectrum Control — ZIMECTERIN® Paste kills important internal parasites, including bots and the arterial stages of *S. vulgaris,* with a single dose. ZIMECTERIN® Paste is a potent anti-parasitic agent that is neither a benzimidazole nor an organophosphate.

Trial Data: Animal Safety: ZIMECTERIN® (ivermectin) Paste may be used in horses of all ages, including mares at any stage of pregnancy. Stallions may be treated without adversely affecting their fertility.

Presentation: 0.21 oz (6.08 g) syringe.

ZIMECTERIN is a registered trademark of Merial.
Merial Limited: Registered in England and Wales [Reg. No. 3332751] with registered offices at 27 Knightsbridge, London SW1X 7QT, England and domesticated in Delaware, USA as Merial LLC.
U.S. Patent No. 4,199,569

Compendium Code No.: 11110920 09265800/9355500

ZINC OXIDE 20% OINTMENT

AgriPharm **Antiseptic**

Astringent-Antiseptic Topical Ointment

Active Ingredient(s): Contains zinc oxide 20% in a petrolatum, mineral oil and lanolin ointment base.

Indications: A protective astringent and antiseptic ointment for topical application to aid in the management of superficial wounds and abrasions of horses, cattle, sheep and swine.

Dosage and Administration: Thoroughly cleanse and dry area of skin to be treated. Apply ointment directly to wound with spatula or first place on piece of gauze. Protect treated area to prevent licking.

Precaution(s): Store at controlled room temperature between 15° and 30°C (59°-86°F).

Keep tightly closed when not in use.

Caution(s): Avoid getting into eyes or on mucous membranes. In case of deep of puncture wounds or serious burns consult veterinarian. If redness, irritation, or swelling persists or increases, discontinue use and consult veterinarian.

Warning(s): For animal use only.

Keep out of reach of children.

Presentation: 18 lb.

Compendium Code No.: 14571121

ZINC PLUS™ TABLETS

Butler **Small Animal Dietary Supplement**

Oral nutrient supplement

Active Ingredient(s): Each tablet contains:

Zinc	30 mg
as Zinc-Amino Acid complex	
Manganese	3 mg
Copper	1.8 mg
Cobalt	.4 mg
as metal complexes	
Vitamin E	40 I.U.
Vitamin C	150 mg
Vitamin B_1	7 mg
Vitamin B_2	7 mg
Niacin	30 mg
Vitamin B_6	5 mg
Vitamin B_{12}	20 mcg
Biotin	5 mcg
d-Calcium Pantothenate	20 mg
Choline Bitartrate	10 mg

in a flavored base containing liver, animal proteins, lecithin, yeast, and dextrose.

Indications: Recommended for use as an oral nutritional supplement to supply essential trace minerals, B complex vitamins, and Vitamins E and C. Certain dermatological conditions respond well to oral supplementation of the diet with trace minerals and vitamins used in conjunction with anti-inflammatory or antihistamine treatments.

Dosage and Administration: Recommended Dosages:

Dogs	1 to 4 tablets daily
Puppies	½ to 1 tablet daily
Cats	½ to 1 tablet daily

Feed free choice or crumble and mix with food.

Contraindication(s): None known.

Caution(s): Keep out of the reach of children.

Presentation: Bottle of 120 chewable tabs, 12 per box.

Compendium Code No.: 10821920

ZINPRO+3

Zinpro **Feed Additive**

Typical Analysis:

Zinc	2.53%
Manganese	1.40%
Copper	0.88%
Cobalt	0.09%
Total Amino Acids	10.12%
Aspartic Acid	0.33%
Threonine	0.24%
Serine	0.59%
Glutamic Acid	0.60%
Proline	0.50%
Glycine	0.45%
Alanine	0.26%
Cystine	0.24%
Valine	0.37%
Methionine	5.04%
Isoleucine	0.24%
Leucine	0.40%
Tyrosine	0.14%
Phenylalanine	0.24%
Histidine	0.06%
Lysine	0.10%
Arginine	0.33%

Indications: A nutritional feed additive for livestock. It combines zinc, manganese and copper amino acid complexes plus cobalt glucoheptonate.

Physical Description: A light-to-medium brown granular powder. ZINPRO+3 weighs approximately 38 lbs/cu ft.

Dosage and Administration:

Beef and Dairy Cattle: Feed at the rate of ½ ounce (14 grams) per head daily, or 1 lb per 32 head daily.

Each ½ ounce of ZINPRO+3 will supply 360 mg zinc from zinc methionine; 200 mg manganese from manganese amino acid complex; 125 mg copper from copper amino acid complex, and 12 mg cobalt from cobalt glucoheptonate.

Contraindication(s): Do not feed to sheep or related species.

Toxicology: When correctly used, there is no toxicity hazard in the use of ZINPRO+3.

Presentation: ZINPRO+3 is packaged in 50 lb multiwall bags.

Compendium Code No.: 11300210

ZINPRO 40

Zinpro **Feed Additive**

Zinc Methionine

Typical Analysis:

Zinc	4.0%
Methionine	8.0%
Protein	5.4%
Fat	0.0%
Fiber	13.9%
Ash	51.5%
Calcium	8.5%
Salt	2.8%

Indications: A nutritional feed additive for livestock and poultry. When used as a commercial feed ingredient it must be declared as zinc methionine.

Physical Description: A light brown granular powder with characteristic methionine-like odor. ZINPRO 40 weighs approximately 32 lbs/cu ft.

Feeding Instructions:

*Swine: Add 2 lbs (908 grams) per ton of complete ration.

Laying Hens, Broilers and Turkeys: Add 2 lbs (908 grams) per ton of complete ration.

Dairy Cattle: Feed 9 grams per head daily, or 2 lbs per 100 head daily.

Beef Cattle: Feed 9 grams per head daily, or 2 lbs per 100 head daily.

*Sheep: Feed 1 gram per head daily, or 1 lb per 454 head daily.

Horses: Feed 4.5 grams per head daily.

*Double recommended levels during periods of reduced feed intake.

Toxicology: When correctly used, there is no toxicity hazard in the use of ZINPRO 40.

Presentation: ZINPRO 40 is packaged in 50 lb multiwall bags.

Compendium Code No.: 11300200

ZINPRO 100

Zinpro **Feed Additive**

Zinc Methionine

Typical Analysis:

Zinc	10.0%
Methionine	20.0%
Protein	11.8%
Fat	0.0%
Fiber	15.0%
Ash	20.0%
Salt	1.2%

Indications: A nutritional feed additive for livestock and poultry. When used as a commercial feed ingredient it must be declared as zinc methionine.

Physical Description: A light brown granular powder with characteristic methionine-like odor. ZINPRO 100 weighs approximately 35 lbs/cu ft.

Feeding Instructions:

*Swine: Add 0.8 lb (360 grams) per ton of complete ration.

Laying Hens, Broilers and Turkeys: Add 0.8 lb (360 grams) per ton of complete ration.

Dairy Cattle: Feed 3.6 grams per head daily, or 1 lb per 125 head daily.
Beef Cattle: Feed 3.6 grams per head daily, or 1 lb per 125 head daily.
*Sheep: Feed 0.4 grams per head daily, or 1 lb per 1,250 head daily.
Horses: Feed 2.0 grams per head daily.
*Double recommended levels during periods of reduced feed intake.
Toxicology: When correctly used, there is no toxicity hazard in the use of ZINPRO 100.
Presentation: ZINPRO 100 is packaged in 25 lb and 50 lb multiwall bags.
Compendium Code No.: 11300181

ZINPRO 180

Zinpro **Feed Additive**
Zinc Methionine
Typical Analysis:
Zinc 18.0%
Methionine 36.0%
Protein 19.5%
Fat 0.0%
Fiber 0.0%
Ash 35.8%
Salt 1.7%
Indications: A nutritional feed additive for livestock and poultry. When used as a commercial feed ingredient it must be declared as zinc methionine.
Physical Description: Water soluble tan powder with characteristic methionine-like odor. ZINPRO 180 weighs approximately 28 lbs/cu ft.
Solubility: One part ZINPRO 180 will dissolve in two parts hot water. One percent solution has pH of 4.5-5.0.
Feeding Instructions:
*Swine: Add 0.44 lb (200 grams) per ton of complete ration.
Laying Hens, Broilers and Turkeys: Add 0.44 lb (200 grams) per ton of complete ration.
Dairy Cattle: Feed 2.0 grams per head daily, or 1 lb per 225 head daily.
Beef Cattle: Feed 2.0 grams per head daily, or 1 lb per 225 head daily.
*Sheep: Add 1.0 gram to the daily ration of 5 head, or 1 ounce to the daily ration of 140 head.
Horses: Feed 1 gram per head daily.
*Double recommended levels during periods of reduced feed intake.
Toxicology: When correctly used, there is no toxicity hazard in the use of ZINPRO 180.
Presentation: ZINPRO 180 is packaged in 6.67 oz foil pak (50 packets/pail) and 50 lb multiwall bags with 2 mil inserted polyethylene liners.
Compendium Code No.: 11300191

ZINPRO SULFATE & DL-METHIONINE LIQUID

Alpharma **Water Medication**
Oral Supplement
Active Ingredient(s): Ingredients: Water, zinc sulfate, hydrochloric acid, dl-methionine.
Indications: An oral supplement for poultry.
Directions: Shake well before use.
Mix 16 oz into 128 gallons of water to produce a supplemented poultry drinking water.
Caution(s): For animal use only. Not for human use.
Presentation: 1 gallon (3785 mL).
Compendium Code No.: 10221330 AHL-300 0109

ZOAMIX®

Alpharma **Feed Medication**
Coccidiostat-Type A Medicated Article
NADA No.: 011-116
Active Ingredient(s):
Zoalene (3,5-dinitro-o-toluamide) 25%
Inactive ingredients:
Roughage product, ground limestone, mineral oil 75%
Indications: Zoalene is to be fed continuously as an aid for the prevention and control of cecal and intestinal coccidiosis in chickens and intestinal coccidiosis in turkeys.
Directions: It is suggested that a mixture of ZOAMIX® and some feed ingredient be prepared prior to mixing in with the finished ration. This will insure thorough and even distribution in the feed.
For chickens grown for meat purposes: Use 1 lb (454 g) of ZOAMIX® per 2,000 lb (909 kg) of finished product to produce a feed containing 0.0125% zoalene. ZOAMIX® should be thoroughly blended into the finished feed. Feed containing zoalene should be fed continuously as the only ration from the time chicks are placed in floor pens until they are slaughtered for meat.
For replacement chickens: Feed containing zoalene can be used in a program to raise replacement birds. When used under conditions of exposure to coccidiosis, it will allow immunity to develop adequate to protect against losses due to the disease when the birds are placed on nonmedicated feed for egg laying purposes. The following chart outlines the type of feeding program to follow where complete formulated feed is the sole ration:

Growing conditions	Starter ration			Grower ration*		
	% Zoalene per ton	ZOAMIX® to be added per ton of feed (lb)	ZOAMIX® to be added per ton of feed (g)	% Zoalene in feed	ZOAMIX® to be added per ton of feed (lb)	ZOAMIX® to be added per ton of feed (g)
Severe exposure to coccidiosis expected	0.0125	1	454	0.0083 to 0.0125	⅔ to 1	303 to 454
Light to moderate exposure to coccidiosis expected	0.0083 to 0.0125	⅔ to 1	303 to 454	0.004 to 0.0083	⅓ to ⅔	151 to 303

* Grower ration not to be fed to birds over 14 weeks of age.

For turkeys grown for meat purposes only: When turkey poults are reared in confinement and severe exposure to coccidiosis is usually a problem, use 1½ lb (681 g) of ZOAMIX® per ton (2,000 lb) of feed to produce a finished feed containing 0.0187% zoalene. Under the usual conditions of rearing turkey poults, or when turkey poults are on range, use 1 lb (454 g) of ZOAMIX® per 2,000 lb (909 kg) of feed to produce a finished feed containing 0.0125% zoalene. The feed containing zoalene should be fed continuously until the birds are 14 to 16 weeks of age.
Caution(s): For use in preparation of feeds for chickens and turkeys only.
Livestock remedy - not for human use.
Combinations with other drugs: Use only in accordance with the current New Animal Drug Regulation for zoalene, Section 558.680 of the Regulations promulgated under the Federal Food, Drug and Cosmetic Act.
Consult a veterinarian or poultry pathologist if losses exceed 0.5% in a two-day period.
Avoid inhaling dust.
Avoid contact with eyes.
Warning(s): Not to be fed to laying birds.
Presentation: 50 lb (22.67 kg) bag.
Compendium Code No.: 10220681 AHG-009 0002

ZOOLOGIC® BENE-BAC™ LARGE MAMMAL

Pet-Ag **Large Animal Dietary Supplement**
Guaranteed Analysis: Total Viable Lactic Acid Producing Bacteria provides 20 million CFU per gram. *(Lactobacillus acidophilus, Lactobacillus plantarum, Streptococcus faecium, Lactobacillus casei)*
Ingredients: Dried *Lactobacillus acidophilus* fermentation product, dried *Lactobacillus plantarum* fermentation product, dried *Streptococcus faecium* fermentation product, dried *Lactobacillus casei* fermentation product, vegetable oil, sugar, silicon dioxide, artificial color, Polysorbate 80, preserved with tertiary butyl hydroquinone and ethoxyquin.
Indications: Contains a source of live (viable) naturally occurring beneficial intestinal microorganisms for mammals.
Directions for Use: Administer orally on back of tongue.
Usage Amounts: 1 gram up to 10 lbs body weight. Additional 1 gram for each 10 lbs body weight up to 90 lbs. 10 grams for 100 lbs body weight and over.
Times of Administration:
Newborns: At 12 to 24 hours of age and days 4 and 7.
Post Anthelmintic/Post Antibiotic Therapy: 1, 3, and 7 days post therapy.
Transportation: On days 3 and 1 prior to transportation and first day following transportation.
Precaution(s): Storage: Avoid extreme heat. Store at normal room temperature.
Presentation: 1.06 oz (30 g) (12 per case).
Compendium Code No.: 10970261

ZOOLOGIC® BENE-BAC™ POWDER

Pet-Ag **Dietary Supplement**
Beneficial Bacteria
Ingredient(s): Guaranteed total live (viable) Lactic Acid Product Bacteria: 10 million Colony Forming Units (CFU) per gram *(Lactobacillus fermentum, Enterococcus faecium, Lactobacillus plantarum, Lactobacillus acidophilus)*.
Sucrose, maltodextrin, silicon dioxide, dried *Lactobacillus fermentum,* dried *enterococcus faecium,* dried *L. plantarum,* and dried *L. acidophilus* fermentation products.
Indications: For domestic, exotic and wildlife mammals.
A source of live naturally-occurring microorganisms.
Recommended as part of the management program for all mammals subjected to changing environmental or nutritional conditions or after antibiotic therapy.
Help for animals under adverse conditions such as: simple intestinal stress, antibiotic therapy, post surgery, birth, weaning, worming, traveling.
Directions for Use: Initial Treatment: Provide one dosage from table below on days 1, 3, 5 and 7, and then one dosage per week until weaned.

Body Weight	Amount of BBP
< ½ lb (227 g)	¼ level teaspoon
½ - 1 lb	½ level teaspoon
1 lb - 5 lbs	1 level teaspoon
5 lbs - 20 lbs	2 level teaspoons
20 lbs+	3 level teaspoons

For Maintenance: Use above recommended daily dosage once weekly. Treat animals by top dressing BENE-BAC™ Powder on moistened or oiled dry food or fresh fruits or vegetables. Discard uneaten food after no more than 8 hours and thoroughly wash dishes.
Regular use of BBP for normal maintenance is recommended.
General Information: If several animals are maintained in a common cage, use the approximate total weight of all animals to determine feeding level. Mix with feed so that all animals receive appropriate dose.
One level teaspoon equals approximately 2.7 grams of BENE-BAC™ Powder.
Wash all feeding dishes, water bottles or water dishes, thoroughly with hot, soapy water and rinse well after each use.
Be sure to contact your veterinarian for any illness.
Precaution(s): Store in cool, dry conditions.
Presentation: 16 oz (454 g).
Compendium Code No.: 10970361

ZOOLOGIC® MILK MATRIX 20/14

Pet-Ag **Milk Replacer**
Active Ingredient(s): Guaranteed Analysis:
Crude protein, min. 20.0%
Crude fat, min. 14.0%
Crude fiber 0.1%
Moisture, max. 6.0%
Ash, max. 8.5%
Copper, max. 0.003%
Ingredients: Dried whey, dried skimmed milk, animal and vegetable fat (preserved with BHA), dried whey protein concentrate, malto dextrins, dried corn syrup, dried milk protein, lecithin, calcium carbonate, dicalcium phosphate, natural and artificial flavors added, vitamin E supplement, magnesium sulfate, ferrous sulfate, dried *Lactobacillus casei* fermentation product, dried *Lactobacillus fermentum* fermentation product, dried *Streptococcus faecium* fermentation product, dried *Lactobacillus plantarum* fermentation product, manganese sulfate, vitamin A supplement, vitamin D_3 supplement, copper sulfate, zinc sulfate, vitamin B_{12} supplement, calcium pantothenate, niacin supplement, riboflavin supplement, thiamine mononitrate, folic acid, pyridoxine hydrochloride, menadione sodium bisulfite complex, ethylenediamine dihydroiodide, biotin, and sodium selenite.
Indications: A milk replacer and nutritional supplement containing a medium level of lactose. Part of an integrated system designed to virtually match any mammal's milk.

Dosage and Administration:

Mixing Directions: Reconstituting milk replacers with water is most accurately accomplished by weighing the individual components. If weighing is not possible, use the following volume measurements to reconstitute Milk Matrix 20/14 powder to the indicated concentrations:

Powder	Water	% Solids	% Protein	% Fat	% Carbohydrate
3 vols.	4 vols.	27.1	5.4	4.3	13.8
1 vol.	2 vols.	19.8	4.0	3.2	10.1
2 vols.	5 vols.	16.6	3.3	2.6	8.5
1 vol.	3 vols.	14.2	2.8	2.3	7.2

A volume is a measurement such as a teaspoon, tablespoon, cup, etc. The table below indicates the approximate weight-volume relationship of Milk Matrix 20/14 and water.

	Milk Matrix 20/14*	Water
Enclosed scoop	6.8 g	14.0 g
Standard measuring tablespoon	7.8 g	15.0 g
¼ standard measuring cup	31.7 g	60.0 g
⅓ standard measuring cup	42.3 g	80.0 g
1 cup	127.0 g	240.0 g

*Weights determined by scooping powder from the container and leveling. These values are only guidelines and can vary 5-10% due to variation in production.

Milk Replacer: Milk Matrix 20/14 may be used alone or blended with other products in the Matrix family to formulate a milk replacer with nutrient levels that closely match a species' natural milk.

As a general rule, liquid or reconstituted milk replacer should be fed at a rate of 10% to 20% of the body weight per day or as tolerated and required for steady growth and proper stool condition. Divide the total daily amount into 6-12 feedings per day, depending upon age, condition, species and staffing.

Reconstituted milk replacers should be refrigerated and used within 24 hours. Feed at room or body temperature depending upon the size and condition of the animal.

Weaning Food Supplement: Because of its highly digestible milk nutrients, the formula used during suckling is an excellent supplement during weaning as a transition from milk to solid food. Add to the diet at the rate of one (1) teaspoon of powder per 10 lbs. of body weight.

Precaution(s):

Unblended Product: After opening, refrigeration is recommended but not necessary. Discard if unused after three months.

Blended Powder: Refrigerate for up to one month.

Note: To extend the storage life of opened or blended powder, freeze in a sealed container and discard after six months. Unopened product may be frozen to extend shelf life for six months beyond the expiration date.

Warning(s): Contains a high level of copper. Do not feed to sheep or related species.

Presentation: 24 oz. can (4 per case) and 25 lb. pail (1 each).

Compendium Code No.: 10970270

ZOOLOGIC® MILK MATRIX 20/20

Pet-Ag **Milk Replacer**

Active Ingredient(s): Guaranteed Analysis:

Crude protein, min. 20.0%
Crude fat, min. 20.0%
Crude fiber, max. 0.15%
Moisture, max. 6.0%
Ash, max. 8.0%

Ingredients: Dried whey, dried whey protein concentrate, dried whey product, dried skimmed milk, animal and vegetable fat (preserved with BHA and BHT), lecithin, dried milk protein, vitamin A supplement, vitamin D_3 supplement, vitamin E supplement, vitamin B_{12} supplement, folic acid, choline chloride, riboflavin supplement, niacin supplement, calcium carbonate, calcium pantothenate, thiamine mononitrate, ferrous sulfate, copper sulfate, cobalt sulfate, zinc sulfate, ethylenediamine dihydroiodide, sodium selenite, manganese sulfate, magnesium oxide, silicon dioxide, polyoxyethylene glycol (400) mono and dioleates, and artificial flavor.

Indications: A milk replacer and nutritional supplement containing a low level of lactose. Part of an integrated system designed to virtually match any mammal's milk.

Dosage and Administration:

Mixing Directions: Reconstituting milk replacers with water is most accurately accomplished by weighing the individual components. If weighing is not possible, use the following volume measurements to reconstitute Milk Matrix 20/20 powder to the indicated concentrations:

Powder	Water	% Solids	% Protein	% Fat	% Carbohydrate
3 vols.	4 vols.	28.6	5.7	5.7	13.4
1 vol.	2 vols.	21.1	4.2	4.2	9.9
2 vols.	5 vols.	17.6	3.5	3.5	8.3
1 vol.	3 vols.	15.1	3.0	3.0	7.1

A volume is a measurement such as a teaspoon, tablespoon, cup, etc. The table below indicates the approximate weight-volume relationship of Milk Matrix 20/20 and water.

	Milk Matrix 20/20*	Water
Enclosed scoop	8.0 g	14.0 g
Standard measuring tablespoon	8.2 g	15.0 g
¼ standard measuring cup	32.5 g	60.0 g
⅓ standard measuring cup	43.3 g	80.0 g
1 cup	130.0 g	240.0 g

*Weights determined by scooping powder from the container and leveling. These values are only guidelines and can vary 5-10% due to variation in production.

Milk Replacer: Milk Matrix 20/20 may be used alone or blended with other products in the Matrix family to formulate a milk replacer with nutrient levels that closely match a species' natural milk.

As a general rule, liquid or reconstituted milk replacer should be fed at a rate of 10% to 20% of the body weight per day or as tolerated and required for steady growth and proper stool condition. Divide the total daily amount into 6-12 feedings per day, depending upon age, condition, species and staffing.

Reconstituted milk replacers should be refrigerated and used within 24 hours. Feed at room or body temperature depending upon the size and condition of the animal.

Weaning Food Supplement: Because of its highly digestible milk nutrients, the formula used during suckling is an excellent supplement during weaning as a transition from milk to solid food. Add to the diet at the rate of one (1) teaspoon of powder per 10 lbs. of body weight.

Precaution(s):

Unblended Product: After opening, refrigeration is recommended but not necessary. Discard if unused after three months.

Blended Powder: Refrigerate for up to one month.

Note: To extend the storage life of opened or blended powder, freeze in a sealed container and discard after six months. Unopened product may be frozen to extend shelf life for six months beyond the expiration date.

Presentation: 24 oz. can (4 per case) and 25 lb. pail (1 each).

Compendium Code No.: 10970280

ZOOLOGIC® MILK MATRIX 23/30

Pet-Ag **Milk Replacer**

Active Ingredient(s): Guaranteed Analysis:

Crude protein, min. 23.0%
Crude fat, min. 30.0%
Crude fiber, max. 0.2%
Moisture, max. 5.0%
Ash, max. 8.0%

Ingredients: Dried whey protein concentrate, dried whey, vegetable and animal fat (preserved with BHA), dried whey product, lecithin, dl methionine, l lysine, vitamin A acetate, vitamin D_3 supplement, vitamin E supplement, vitamin B_{12} supplement, folic acid, choline chloride, riboflavin supplement, niacin supplement, calcium pantothenate, thiamine mononitrate, sodium propionate, citric acid, potassium sorbate, calcium propionate (preservatives), ferrous sulfate, cobalt sulfate, zinc sulfate, manganese sulfate, magnesium oxide, ethylenediamine dihydroiodide, silicon dioxide, sodium selenite, and artificial flavor.

Indications: A milk replacer and nutritional supplement containing a medium level of lactose. Part of an integrated system designed to virtually match any mammal's milk.

Dosage and Administration:

Mixing Directions: Reconstituting milk replacers with water is most accurately accomplished by weighing the individual components. If weighing is not possible, use the following volume measurements to reconstitute Milk Matrix 23/30 powder to the indicated concentrations:

Powder	Water	% Solids	% Protein	% Fat	% Carbohydrate
3 vols.	4 vols.	26.0	6.0	7.8	9.1
1 vol.	2 vols.	19.0	4.4	5.7	6.6
2 vols.	5 vols.	15.8	3.6	4.7	5.5
1 vol.	3 vols.	13.5	3.1	4.1	4.7

A volume is a measurement such as a teaspoon, tablespoon, cup, etc. The table below indicates the approximate weight-volume relationship of Milk Matrix 23/30 and water.

	Milk Matrix 23/30*	Water
Enclosed scoop	6.5 g	14.0 g
Standard measuring tablespoon	7.2 g	15.0 g
¼ standard measuring cup	30.0 g	60.0 g
⅓ standard measuring cup	40.0 g	80.0 g
1 cup	120.0 g	240.0 g

*Weights determined by scooping powder from the container and leveling. These values are only guidelines and can vary 5-10% due to variation in production.

Milk Replacer: Milk Matrix 23/30 may be used alone or blended with other products in the Matrix family to formulate a milk replacer with nutrient levels that closely match a species' natural milk.

As a general rule, liquid or reconstituted milk replacer should be fed at a rate of 10% to 20% of the body weight per day or as tolerated and required for steady growth and proper stool condition. Divide the total daily amount into 6-12 feedings per day, depending upon age, condition, species and staffing.

Reconstituted milk replacers should be refrigerated and used within 24 hours. Feed at room or body temperature depending upon the size and condition of the animal.

Weaning Food Supplement: Because of its highly digestible milk nutrients, the formula used during suckling is an excellent supplement during weaning as a transition from milk to solid food. Add to the diet at the rate of one (1) teaspoon of powder per 10 lbs. of body weight.

Precaution(s):

Unblended Product: After opening, refrigeration is recommended but not necessary. Discard if unused after three months.

Blended Powder: Refrigerate for up to one month.

Note: To extend the storage life of opened or blended powder, freeze in a sealed container and discard after six months. Unopened product may be frozen to extend shelf life for six months beyond the expiration date.

Presentation: 24 oz. can (4 per case) and 25 lb. pail (1 each).

Compendium Code No.: 10970290

ZOOLOGIC® MILK MATRIX 25/13

Pet-Ag **Milk Replacer**

Active Ingredient(s): Guaranteed Analysis:

Crude protein, min. 25.0%
Crude fat, min. 13.0%
Crude fiber, max. 0.15%
Moisture, max. 6.0%
Ash, max. 8.0%

Ingredients: Dried whey, dried whey protein concentrate, dried skimmed milk, vegetable and animal fat (preserved with BHA), lecithin, vitamin A supplement, vitamin D_3 supplement, vitamin E supplement, vitamin B_{12} supplement, folic acid, choline chloride, riboflavin supplement, niacin supplement, calcium pantothenate, thiamine mononitrate, menadione sodium bisulfite complex, citric acid and potassium sorbate (preservatives), ferric ammonium citrate, copper sulfate, cobalt sulfate, zinc sulfate, manganese sulfate, magnesium oxide, ethylenediamine dihydroiodide, silicon dioxide, polyoxyethylene glycol (400) mono and dioleates, sodium selenite, ascorbic acid, and artificial flavor.

Indications: A milk replacer and nutritional supplement containing a low level of lactose. Part of an integrated system designed to virtually match any mammal's milk.

Dosage and Administration:

Mixing Directions: Reconstituting milk replacers with water is most accurately accomplished by weighing the individual components. If weighing is not possible, use the following volume measurements to reconstitute Milk Matrix 25/13 powder to the indicated concentrations:

Powder	Water	% Solids	% Protein	% Fat	% Carbohydrate
3 vols.	4 vols.	27.7	6.9	4.0	13.3
1 vol.	2 vols.	20.3	5.1	2.9	9.7
2 vols.	5 vols.	16.9	4.2	2.4	8.1
1 vol.	3 vols.	14.5	3.6	2.1	7.0

A volume is a measurement such as a teaspoon, tablespoon, cup, etc. The table below indicates the approximate weight-volume relationship of Milk Matrix 25/13 and water.

	Milk Matrix 25/13*	Water
Enclosed scoop	7.5 g	14.0 g
Standard measuring tablespoon	7.8 g	15.0 g
¼ standard measuring cup	30.5 g	60.0 g
⅓ standard measuring cup	40.6 g	80.0 g
1 cup	122.0 g	240.0 g

*Weights determined by scooping powder from the container and leveling. These values are only guidelines and can vary 5-10% due to variation in production.

Milk Replacer: Milk Matrix 25/13 may be used alone or blended with other products in the Matrix family to formulate a milk replacer with nutrient levels that closely match a species' natural milk.

As a general rule, liquid or reconstituted milk replacer should be fed at a rate of 10% to 20% of the body weight per day or as tolerated and required for steady growth and proper stool condition. Divide the total daily amount into 6-12 feedings per day, depending upon age, condition, species and staffing.

Reconstituted milk replacers should be refrigerated and used within 24 hours. Feed at room or body temperature depending upon the size and condition of the animal.

Weaning Food Supplement: Because of its highly digestible milk nutrients, the formula used during suckling is an excellent supplement during weaning as a transition from milk to solid food. Add to the diet at the rate of one (1) teaspoon of powder per 10 lbs. of body weight.

Precaution(s):

Unblended Product: After opening, refrigeration is recommended but not necessary. Discard if unused after three months.

Blended Powder: Refrigerate for up to one month.

Note: To extend the storage life of opened or blended powder, freeze in a sealed container and discard after six months. Unopened product may be frozen to extend shelf life for six months beyond the expiration date.

Presentation: 24 oz. can (4 per case) and 25 lb. pail (1 each).

Compendium Code No.: 10970300

ZOOLOGIC® MILK MATRIX 30/55

Pet-Ag **Milk Replacer**

Guaranteed Analysis:

Crude protein, min. 30.0%
Crude fat, min. 55.0%
Crude fiber, max. 0.25%
Moisture, max. 5.0%
Ash, max. 8.0%

Ingredients: Animal fat (preserved with BHA and citric acid), casein, dicalcium phosphate, calcium carbonate, lecithin, potassium chloride, choline chloride, magnesium sulfate, vitamin E supplement, vitamin A supplement, zinc methionine, ferrous sulfate, calcium pantothenate, vitamin B_{12} supplement, niacin supplement, manganese sulfate, copper sulfate, vitamin D_3 supplement, riboflavin supplement, thiamine mononitrate, pyridoxine hydrochloride, menadione sodium bisulfite complex, folic acid, calcium iodate, biotin, sodium selenite, mono and diglycerides.

Indications: A milk replacer and nutritional supplement containing a low level of lactose. Part of an integrated system designed to virtually match any mammal's milk.

Dosage and Administration: Mixing Directions: Reconstituting milk replacers with water is most accurately accomplished by weighing the individual components. If weighing is not possible, use the following volume measurements to reconstitute Milk Matrix 30/55 powder to the indicated concentrations:

Powder	Water	% Solids	% Protein	% Fat	% Carbohydrate
1 vol.	1 vol.	26.8	8.3	14.7	0
3 vols.	4 vols.	21.3	6.6	11.7	0
2 vols.	5 vols.	12.4	3.8	6.8	0
1 vol.	3 vols.	10.8	3.3	5.9	0

A volume is a measurement such as a teaspoon, tablespoon, cup, etc. The table below indicates the approximate weight-volume relationship of Milk Matrix 30/55 and water.

	Milk Matrix 30/55*	Water
Enclosed scoop	5.5 g	14.0 g
Standard measuring tablespoon	5.5 g	15.0 g
¼ standard measuring cup	25.0 g	60.0 g
⅓ standard measuring cup	33.3 g	80.0 g
1 cup	100.0 g	240.0 g

*Weights determined by scooping powder from the container and leveling. These values are only guidelines and can vary 5-10% due to variation in production.

Milk Replacer: Milk Matrix 30/55 may be used alone or blended with other products in the Matrix family to formulate a milk replacer with nutrient levels that closely match a species' natural milk.

As a general rule, liquid or reconstituted milk replacer should be fed at a rate of 10% to 20% of the body weight per day or as tolerated and required for steady growth and proper stool condition. Divide the total daily amount into 6-12 feedings per day, depending upon age, condition, species and staffing.

Reconstituted milk replacers should be refrigerated and used within 24 hours. Feed at room or body temperature depending upon the size and condition of the animal.

Weaning Food Supplement: Because of its highly digestible milk nutrients, the formula used during suckling is an excellent supplement during weaning as a transition from milk to solid food. Add to the diet at the rate of one (1) teaspoon of powder per 10 lbs. of body weight.

Precaution(s): Unblended Product: After opening, refrigeration is recommended but not necessary. Discard if unused after three months.

Blended Powder: Refrigerate for up to one month.

Note: To extend the storage life of opened or blended powder, freeze in a sealed container and discard after six months. Unopened product may be frozen to extend shelf life for six months beyond the expiration date.

Presentation: 24 oz can (4 per case), 6 lb pail (4 per case), and 20 lb pail (1 each).

Compendium Code No.: 10970311

ZOOLOGIC® MILK MATRIX 33/40

Pet-Ag **Milk Replacer**

Guaranteed Analysis:

Crude protein, min. 33.0%
Crude fat, min. 40.0%
Crude fiber . . . . . None
Moisture, max. 5.0%
Ash, max. 6.0%

Ingredients: Vegetable oil (preserved with BHA, BHT, propyl gallate and citric acid), casein, dried skimmed milk, egg yolk, l arginine, dl methionine, calcium carbonate precipitated, potassium phosphate monobasic, dried corn syrup, calcium hydroxide, salt, lecithin, monocalcium phosphate, sodium hydroxide, choline chloride, potassium chloride, magnesium carbonate, magnesium sulfate, vitamin A supplement, zinc sulfate, vitamin E supplement, iron sulfate, niacin supplement, copper sulfate, calcium pantothenate, vitamin B_{12} supplement, manganese sulfate, vitamin D_3 supplement, folic acid, riboflavin, thiamine hydrochloride, calcium iodate, and pyridoxine hydrochloride.

Indications: A milk replacer and nutritional supplement containing a low level of lactose. Part of an integrated system designed to virtually match any mammal's milk.

Dosage and Administration:

Mixing Directions: Reconstituting milk replacers with water is most accurately accomplished by weighing the individual components. If weighing is not possible, use the following volume measurements to reconstitute Milk Matrix 33/40 powder to the indicated concentrations:

Powder	Water	% Solids	% Protein	% Fat	% Carbohydrate
1 vol.	1 vol.	27.0	9.1	11.5	3.8
3 vols.	4 vols.	21.7	7.4	9.1	3.0
1 vol.	2 vols.	15.6	5.3	6.6	2.2
1 vol.	3 vols.	11.0	3.7	4.6	1.5

A volume is a measurement such as a teaspoon, tablespoon, cup, etc. The table below indicates the approximate weight-volume relationship of Milk Matrix 33/40 and water.

	Milk Matrix 33/40*	Water
Enclosed scoop	5.4 g	14.0 g
Standard measuring tablespoon	5.8 g	15.0 g
¼ standard measuring cup	21.5 g	60.0 g
⅓ standard measuring cup	28.6 g	80.0 g
1 cup	86.0 g	240.0 g

*Weights determined by scooping powder from the container and leveling. These values are only guidelines and can vary 5-10% due to variation in production.

Milk Replacer: Milk Matrix 33/40 may be used alone or blended with other products in the Matrix family to formulate a milk replacer with nutrient levels that closely match a species' natural milk.

As a general rule, liquid or reconstituted milk replacer should be fed at a rate of 10% to 20% of the body weight per day or as tolerated and required for steady growth and proper stool condition. Divide the total daily amount into 6-12 feedings per day, depending upon age, condition, species and staffing.

Reconstituted milk replacers should be refrigerated and used within 24 hours. Feed at room or body temperature depending upon the size and condition of the animal.

Weaning Food Supplement: Because of its highly digestible milk nutrients, the formula used during suckling is an excellent supplement during weaning as a transition from milk to solid food. Add to the diet at the rate of one (1) teaspoon of powder per 10 lbs. of body weight.

Precaution(s):

Unblended Product: Refrigerate after opening. Discard if unused after one months.

Blended Powder: Refrigerate for up to one month.

Note: To extend the storage life of opened or blended powder, freeze in a sealed container and discard after six months. Unopened product may be frozen to extend shelf life for six months beyond the expiration date.

Presentation: 24 oz. can (4 per case) and 5 lb. pail (4 per case).

Compendium Code No.: 10970322

ZOOLOGIC® MILK MATRIX 42/25

Pet-Ag **Milk Replacer**

Guaranteed Analysis:

Crude protein, min. 42.0%
Crude fat, min. 25.0%
Crude fiber . . . . . None
Moisture, max. 5.0%
Ash, max. 7.0%

Ingredients: Vegetable oil (preserved with BHA, BHT, propyl gallate and citric acid), casein, dried skimmed milk, egg yolk, calcium carbonate precipitated, potassium phosphate monobasic, l arginine, dried corn syrup, calcium hydroxide, salt, lecithin, monocalcium phosphate, sodium hydroxide, choline chloride, potassium chloride, magnesium carbonate, taurine, magnesium sulfate, vitamin A supplement, zinc sulfate, vitamin E supplement, iron sulfate, niacin supplement, copper sulfate, calcium pantothenate, vitamin B_{12} supplement, manganese sulfate, vitamin D_3 supplement, folic acid, riboflavin, thiamine hydrochloride, calcium iodate, and pyridoxine hydrochloride.

ZOOLOGIC® MILK MATRIX 42/25

Indications: A milk replacer and nutritional supplement containing a medium level of lactose. Part of an integrated system designed to virtually match any mammal's milk.

Dosage and Administration:

Mixing Directions: Reconstituting milk replacers with water is most accurately accomplished by weighing the individual components. If weighing is not possible, use the following volume measurements to reconstitute Milk Matrix 42/25 powder to the indicated concentrations:

Powder	Water	% Solids	% Protein	% Fat	% Carbohydrate
1 vol.	1 vol.	28.8	12.4	8.3	5.2
3 vols.	4 vols.	23.3	10.0	6.7	4.2
1 vol.	2 vols.	16.9	7.3	4.9	3.0
2 vols.	5 vols.	14.0	6.0	4.1	2.5

A volume is a measurement such as a teaspoon, tablespoon, cup, etc. The table below indicates the approximate weight-volume relationship of Milk Matrix 42/25 and water.

	Milk Matrix 42/25*	Water
Enclosed scoop	5.7 g	14.0 g
Standard measuring tablespoon	6.4 g	15.0 g
¼ standard measuring cup	25.5 g	60.0 g
⅓ standard measuring cup	34.0 g	80.0 g
1 cup	102.0 g	240.0 g

*Weights determined by scooping powder from the container and leveling. These values are only guidelines and can vary 5-10% due to variation in production.

Milk Replacer: Milk Matrix 42/25 may be used alone or blended with other products in the Matrix family to formulate a milk replacer with nutrient levels that closely match a species' natural milk.

As a general rule, liquid or reconstituted milk replacer should be fed at a rate of 10% to 20% of the body weight per day or as tolerated and required for steady growth and proper stool condition. Divide the total daily amount into 6-12 feedings per day, depending upon age, condition, species and staffing.

Reconstituted milk replacers should be refrigerated and used within 24 hours. Feed at room or body temperature depending upon the size and condition of the animal.

Weaning Food Supplement: Because of its highly digestible milk nutrients, the formula used during suckling is an excellent supplement during weaning as a transition from milk to solid food. Add to the diet at the rate of one (1) teaspoon of powder per 10 lbs. of body weight.

Precaution(s):

Unblended Product: Refrigerate after opening. Discard if unused after one months.

Blended Powder: Refrige.rate for up to one month.

Note: To extend the storage life of opened or blended powder, freeze in a sealed container and discard after six months. Unopened product may be frozen to extend shelf life for six months beyond the expiration date.

Presentation: 24 oz. can (4 per case) and 5 lb. pail (4 per case).

Compendium Code No.: 10970332

Product Index

Products are listed alphabetically by trade name; page numbers indicate the location of the product monograph.

The information presented has been supplied by the manufacturers and distributors. Inclusion or omission of products does not imply endorsement or otherwise, by the publisher or anyone involved in the publication. It must be pointed out that the information is presented as a reference, and it remains the responsibility of the readers to familiarize themselves with the information contained on the label or package insert accompanying each product. Reference to names is not intended as a violation of any trademarks or patents. The Publisher, Editorial Team and all those involved in the production of the book are not responsible for any errors or consequences that could result from the use of published information.